To John,

the always cheerful supplier of paperclips and wisdom

Beccles, September 1995

Christine Reuter
Peter Reuter

Thieme Leximed
Reuter/Reuter
Medical Dictionary
English-German

**Thieme Leximed
Medical Dictionary**
in 2 Volumes

Volume 1: English-German
Volume 2: Deutsch-Englisch

Thieme Leximed

Medical Dictionary
English-German

Peter Reuter
Christine Reuter

1995
Georg Thieme Verlag Stuttgart · New York

Dr. med. Peter Reuter
Christine Reuter, Übersetzerin
The Pines
2 Upper Grange Road
Beccles
Suffolk
UK

Library of Congreß Cataloging-in-Publication Data

Reuter, Peter:
Thieme Leximed: medical dictionary; English-German/
Christine Reuter. – Stuttgart; New York: Thieme 1995
NE: Reuter, Christine; Leximed; HST

Any reference to or mention of manufactures or specific brand names should not be interpreted as an endorsement or advertisement for any company or product.
Some of the product names, patents and registered designs referred to in this book are in fact registered trademarks or proprietary names even though specific reference to this fact is not always made in the text. therefore, the appearance of a neme without designnation as proprietary is not to be construed as a representation by the publisher that it is in the public domain.
This book, including all parts therof, is legally protected by copyright. any use, exploitation orcommercialization outside the narrow limits set by copyright legislation, without the publisher`s consent, is illegal and liable to prosecution. This applies in particular to photostat reproduction copying, mimeographingor duplication of any kind, translating, prepartion of microfims, and electronic data processing and storage.

© 1995, Georg Thieme Verlag, Rüdigerstraße 14, D-70469 Stuttgart, Germany
Data preparation by BiLex Dr. Peter Reuter Christine Reuter, Beccles, UK
Typesetting by Langenscheidt KG, Berlin, Germany
Printed in Finnland by Werner Söderström Osakeyhtiö, SF 06100 Porvoo
ISBN 3-13 -100471

Für unsere Töchter
Kim, Ann und Lauren

Preface

During our studies, and what is more, through the daily dealing with the language in theory and praxis whilst working in an English-speaking country, we most certainly developed an intuitive understanding of the standards a bilingual medical dictionary is obliged to comply with.Thus, when we first started to work out a draft for the present dictionary, some five years ago, it was our intention to create a reference that would represent a source of information heretofore unprecedented in scope and accuracy. Building upon our medical and linguistic training and experience, it was our ambition to achieve a harmonious and unique synthesis of medical and English-German dictionaries, for users in both medical and linguistic fields.

To meet those requirements, we had to go far beyond the simple translation of words. In its entirety, this book – page after page, entry by entry – has been designed and compiled to satisfy the demands of a broad spectrum of demanding users. A specialised type of software, tailored for data gathering and processing for wordbooks, made it possible not only to include additional features, such as syllabification and pronounciation, but also greatly aided in achieving high quality and topicality.

Over the last years, building on this groundwork, medical books from all corners of clinical and preclinical medicine, not to mention articles in international medical journals, have been scanned. The vocabulary selected has been revised time and again in order to cover all medical and linguistic aspects. Whenever necessary, we actively sought advice and help from physicians and other medical personnel as well as linguists.

The rather unusual approach to simultaneously emphasize both, theory and praxis, research and clinical routine, the study of the medical literature and of the layman's language, has enabled us to compile a unique collection of contemporary Anglo-American medical words. We are convinced that this dictionary will come up to the highest standards of both quality and quantity. Nevertheless, if only due to the limitation of the space available, no book will ever be a fully comprehensive dictionary.

From the very beginning, we have been aware of the importance and necessity of a rather unusually strong support through a publisher. Hence our delight at the acceptance of our idea through the Board under the direction of Dr. G. Hauff. Above all, the collaboration with Mr. A. Menge and Mr. P. Hemming set a very high standard indeed, and inspired us during the planning stage as well as during the actual work on the dictionary.

For most of the time whenever the going got rough Mr. F. Hübner, Langenscheidt KG, Munich, undoubtedly was our main source of help and advice in the hour of need. His ever present calmness of mind together with his untiring readiness to help secured us safe passage through troubled waters.

Beccles, Suffolk
Great Britain,
September 1994

Vorwort

Während des Studiums und, natürlich erst Recht, durch die Auseinandersetzung mit der Sprache in Theorie und Praxis während der Arbeit in einem englischsprachigen Land kann man ein Gefühl dafür entwickeln, welche Anforderungen ein zweisprachiges medizinisches Wörterbuch erfüllen muß. Als wir vor fünf Jahren damit begannen, ein erstes Rahmenkonzept für dieses Buch zu erarbeiten, war es deshalb unser Ziel ein Werk zu konzipieren, das sowohl Benutzern aus dem medizinischen als auch dem sprachlichen Bereich ein Maximum an Information bietet. Auf der Grundlage unserer Erfahrung in beiden Bereichen, strebten wir eine harmonische Synthese aus einem medizinischen und einem englisch-deutschen Wörterbuch an.

Um diesem Anspruch gerecht werden zu können, haben wir bewußt den engen Rahmen einfacher Wortgleichungen weit hinter uns gelassen. Das gesamte Werk – Seite für Seite, Eintrag für Eintrag – wurde so bearbeitet und gestaltet, daß es einem breiten Benutzerspektrum angepaßt ist. Durch Datenerfassung und Datenverwaltung auf einer speziellen Wörterbuchsoftware konnten nicht nur besondere Serviceleistungen, wie z.B. Silbentrennpunkte, Aussprache etc. eingeplant werden, sondern es war auch eine Qualitätssteigerung und Aktualisierung im inhaltlichen Bereich erzielbar.

Auf dieser Basis wurden in den letzten Jahren Werke aus allen Bereichen der vorklinischen und klinischen Medizin ausgewertet. Hinzu kam das Studium von Beiträgen in internationalen Fachzeitschriften. Alle ausgewählten Begriffe wurden mehrfach unter medizinischen und sprachlichen Aspekten bearbeitet. Wo immer nötig, ergänzte die Diskussion mit und Beratung durch Mediziner und Linguisten das erworbene Material.

Die ungewöhnliche simultane Schwerpunktsetzung auf Theorie und Praxis Forschung und klinischen Alltag, Literaturstudium und Laiensprache hat eine einzigartige Sammlung aktueller anglo-amerikanischer Medizinvokabeln ermöglicht. Zweifellos erfüllt dieses Buch, sowohl unter qualitativen als auch quantitativen Aspekten, höchste Ansprüche. Trotzdem darf man aber nicht vergessen, daß es, schon auf Grund des Umfangs, kein allumfassendes Wörterbuch sein kann.

Von Anfang an waren wir uns der Notwendigkeit einer außergewöhnlich guten Unterstützung durch einen Verleger bewußt. Über die Akzeptanz unserer Ideen durch die Verlagsleitung des Thieme Verlags unter Führung von Herrn Dr. G. Hauff haben wir uns daher ganz besonders gefreut. Vor allem die Zusammenarbeit mit Herrn A. Menge und Herrn P. Hemming hat wesentliche Impulse bei der Planung des Werkes und während der Bearbeitungszeit gegeben, ohne die die Umsetzung der Vision in ein konkretes Projekt kaum möglich gewesen wäre.

Die für uns aber in vielen Phasen und unter wichtigen Aspekten herausragende Quelle von Rat und Tat in Not und Pein war Herr F. Hübner von der Langenscheidt KG, München. Seine Ruhe im Sturm und unermüdliche Hilfsbereitschaft halfen uns, manche Krise zu meistern.

Peter Reuter / Christine Reuter

Contents	page/Seite	Inhaltsverzeichnis
A Guide to the Dictionary	X	**Hinweise zur Benutzung des Wörterbuches**
I. Organisation of Entries	X	I. Anordnung der Einträge
1. Alphabetization of Main Entries	X	1. Alphabetische Einordnung der
	XI	Hauptstichwörter
2. Alphabetization and Abbreviation of Subentries	XI	2. Alphabetisierung und Abkürzung von Untereinträgen
3. Alphabetization of Eponyms	XII	3. Alphabetische Einordnung von Eponymen
4. Spelling	XII	4. Orthographie
	XII	
II. General Structure of Entries	XII	II. Allgemeiner Stichwortaufbau
1. Typeface	XII	1. Schriftbild
2. Subdivision of Entries	XIII	2. Unterteilung der Stichwörter
3. Syllabification	XIII	3. Silbentrennung
4. Homographs	XIII	4. Homonyme
5. Parts Of Speech	XIII	5. Wortarten
6. Irregular Forms	XIII	6. Unregelmäßige Formen
7. Tilde	XIII	7. Tilde
8. Phrasal Verbs		8. Phrasal Verbs
9. Restrictive Labels	XIII	9. Bestimmende Zusätze
III. Cross-References	XV	III. Verweise
A Guide to Pronounciation	XV	**Hinweise zur Verwendung der Lautschrift**
Phonetic Symbols	XV	Lautschriftsymbole
1. Vowels and Diphthongs	XVI	1. Vokale und Diphthonge
2. Consonants	XVI	2. Konsonanten
3. Additional Symbols used for non-English Entries	XVI	3. Zusätzliche Symbole für nicht-englische Stichwörter
4. Stress Marks	XVII	4. Betonungsakzente
Abbreviations Used in this Dictionary	XVII	**Verzeichnis der verwandten Abkürzungen**
Medical Dictionary	1–838	**Medizinisches Wörterbuch**
English-German		**Englisch-Deutsch**
Appendix	A 1	**Anhang**
Contents Appendix	A 1	Inhaltsverzeichnis Anhang
Weights and Measures	A 2–A 6	Maße und Gewichte
Conversions Tables for Temperatures	A 7	Umrechnungstabellen für Temperaturen
Anatomical Plates	A 8–A 65	Anatomische Tafeln

A Guide to the Dictionary

I. Organization of Entries

1. Alphabetization of Main Entries

Main entries are alphabetized using a letter-for-letter system. When a main entry consists of more than one word, i.e. compound entries, such main entry is alphabetized as though all one word on the sequence of letters, regardless of spaces or hyphens that may occur between them [for rules governing eponyms see below]. Thus the following sequence could be found:

    heart ...
    heart attack ...
    heartbeat ...
    heart disease ...
    heart-disease cell ...

Main entries are printed in the singular form. If the use of the plural form is more common or mandatory, this plural form is given. A cross-reference might be found to lead the user from the singular form entry to the appropriate entry under which the translation can be found. If necessary, irregular forms and variant spellings are listed in the proper alphabetical order. There again is a cross-reference to the relevant main entry.

    vis·cus *sing* → viscera.

Capitalized entries commonly precede lower case entries.

    Ba·cil·lus [bəˈsɪləs] *n* ...
    ba·cil·lus [bəˈsɪləs] *n* ...

Umlauts are ignored in alphabetization and ä, ö, ü will be treated as a, o, u, respectively.

    mud fever ...
    Mueller-Hinton: M.-H. agar ...
    mulberry cell ...
    Müller: arteries of M. ...
    müllerian: m. capsule ...

In the alphabetization of chemical, biochemical and pharmacological terms italic prefixes (e.g. *o-*, *p-*, *m-*) numbers (e.g. 3,5-diiodothyronine), Greek letters (e.g. α-dextrinase) and the prefixes L-, D-, l-, d- are ignored. In the case of terms in which the prefix is spelled out and closed up, the entry will be alphabetized according to the rules given above. Under these rules ⟨epsilon-aminocaproic acid⟩ is found under e, whereas ⟨ε-aminocaproic acid⟩ is found under a.

    epsilon-aminocaproic acid ... under ... e
    ε-aminocaproic acid ... under ... a

Abbreviations, contractions and acronyms are alphabetized as written on a letter-for-letter basis.

    fly¹ [flaɪ] (*v:* **flew, flown**) **I** *n* Fliegen *nt*, ...
    fly² [flaɪ] *n bio.* Fliege *f.*
    fly agaric *bio.* Fliegenpilz *m*, Amanita...
    Fm *abbr.* → fermium.
    FMN *abbr.* → flavin mononucleotide.
    FMN adenylyltransferase FMN- ...
    FNTC *abbr.* → fine-needle ...
    F₀ *abbr.* → oligomycin-sensitivity-...
    foam [fəʊm] **I** *n* Schaum *m.* **II** *vt, vi...*

Multiple-word terms like ⟨**lateral nasal branches of anterior ethmoidal nerve**⟩ are ordinarily given as subentries under a logical main entry. Thus the term mentioned before is to be found as a subentry of the main entry ⟨**nasal branch**⟩.

    nasal branch ...
        lateral n.es of anterior ethmoidal nerve ...

Although this system may at first be confusing to the user accustomed to language dictionaries, it offers the chance to compile related terms.

Hinweise zur Benutzung des Wörterbuches

I. Anordnung der Einträge

1. Alphabetische Einordnung der Hauptstichwörter

Hauptstichwörter werden streng alphabetisch auf der Grundlage eines Buchstaben--für-Buchstaben-Systems eingeordnet. Bestehen sie aus mehreren Wörtern (Komposita), werden sie unabhängig von Leerräumen oder Bindestrichen als natürliche Einheit betrachtet und ebenfalls nach ihrer Buchstabenfolge eingeordnet [die Einordnung von Eponymen wird weiter unten besprochen]. Auf dieser Grundlage ergibt sich folgendes Beispiel:

Hauptstichwörter erscheinen in ihrer Singularform. Ist die Pluralform die geläufigere oder die vorgeschriebene Form, wird sie als Haupteintrag angegeben. Die Singularform wird in der Regel ebenfalls aufgenommen und mit einem Verweis auf das Stichwort, unter dem die Übersetzung erfolgt, versehen. Unregelmäßige Formen und abweichende Schreibweisen werden gemäß ihrer alphabetischen Reihenfolge eingeordnet. Auch hier erfolgt ein Verweis auf den relevanten Haupteintrag.

Großgeschriebene Einträge werden gewöhnlich vor kleingeschriebenen Varianten eingeordnet.

Umlaute werden bei der Alphabetisierung nicht besonders berücksichtigt, d.h. ä, ö, ü werden als a, o bzw. u eingeordnet.

Bei der alphabetischen Einordnung von Einträgen aus der Chemie, der Biochemie und der Pharmakologie werden kursiv geschriebene Vorsilben (z.B. *o-*, *p-*, *m-*) numerische Präfixe (z.B. 3,5-diiodothyronine), griechische Buchstaben (z.B. α-dextrinase) und die Präfixe L-, D-, l-, d- nicht beachtet. Wird das Präfix ausgeschrieben und mit dem folgenden Substantiv verbunden, erfolgt die Einordnung nach den oben beschriebenen Regeln. Der Eintrag ⟨epsilon-aminocaproic acid⟩ ist deshalb unter e zu finden, während der Eintrag ⟨ε-aminocaproic acid⟩ unter a eingeordnet ist.

Abkürzungen, Kurzwörter und Akronyme werden ebenfalls alphabetisch aufgeführt.

Mehrworteinträge, also komplexe Komposita, wie z.B. ⟨**lateral nasal branches of anterior ethmoidal nerve**⟩ erscheinen in der Regel als Untereinträge zu einem logischen Überbegriff. Das vorgenannte Beispiel wird deshalb als Untereintrag zu dem Hauptstichwort ⟨**nasal branch**⟩ eingeordnet.

Auch wenn dieses System dem an allgemeinsprachlichen Wörterbüchern orientierten Benutzer zunächst verwirrend erscheinen mag, so bietet es doch die Möglichkeit, inhaltlich verwandte Begriffe sinnvoll zusammenzufassen.

2. Alphabetization and Abbreviation of Subentries

In subentries the main entry word is represented by its initial letter only.

Subentries are alphabetized letter by letter just like the main entries. The abbreviation for the main entry, or the plural form of that abbreviation, or the spelled-out plural is always completely disregarded in alphabetizing subentries. The same applies to prepositions, conjunctions and articles as well as the apostrophe-s denoting the possessive in eponymic terms.

In the case of a main entry consisting of more than one word, the first letter of the first word represents the main entry.

Subentries may be either singular or plural. Regular English plural forms are represented by the addition of an ⟨s⟩ to the initial letter.

Irregular English plural forms are sometimes spelled out, or the last letter or last syllable of the plural form is added to the initial letter.
Latin and Greek plurals are treated the same way.

3. Alphabetization of Eponyms

Unfortunately, the use of apostrophe-s for eponymic terms is becoming progressively less common, leading to an inconsistent mixture of forms in the medical literature and in medical dictionaries. Users of this dictionary should therefore be aware that the variation in forms seen in this dictionary is only a reflection of the forms found in the literature and not a guide to the usage of apostrophe-s.

This dictionary follows the most frequently used spelling of names. Alphabetization is determined precisely by that spelling. This procedure has also been followed for the prefixes ⟨Mac⟩ and ⟨Mc⟩. If you cannot find an entry, please check under the alternative spelling.

To make alphabetization simpler, eponymic terms, regardless of whether they are made up of one or several names of persons, are listed as subentries of the name or names comprising the eponym. Thus the following sequence is found:

As subentries, compound eponymic terms are alphabetized on the usual letter-for-letter basis. The apostrophe-s, if one occurs, does not count for alphabetization. Thus, under the main entry ⟨Duchenne⟩, the following subentries appear in this order:

As subentries eponymic terms consisting of more than one name and which are hyphenated are represented by the initial letter of each name with hyphen(s) between them.

---

ax·is ['æksɪs] *n, pl* **ax·es** ...
  a. of contraction Kontraktionsrichtung *f*, -achse.
  a. of heart Herzachse.

nu·cle·us ['n(j)u:klɪəs] *n* ...
  n. of abducens nerve ...
  n. of accessory nerve ...
  n.i of acoustic nerve ...
  n. of ansa lenticularis ...
  n. of Burdach's column/tract ...
  n. of caudal colliculus ...
  n.i of cerebellum ...

bone cyst ...
  aneurysmal b.

lymph node ...
  abdominal l.s ...
  anorectal l.s → pararectal l.s.
  aortic l.s, lateral ...
  apical l.s ...

gan·gli·on *n, pl* **-gli·ons, -gli·a** ...
  g.lia of autonomic plexuses ...
  g.lia of sympathetic plexuses ...
  g.lia of sympathetic trunk ...

Erb: E.'s atrophy ...
  E.'s disease ...
Erb-Charcot: E.-C. disease ...
Erb-Duchenne: E.-D. paralysis ...
Erb-Goldflam: E.-G. disease ...

Duchenne: D. atrophy ...
  D.'s disease ...
  D. gait ...
  D.'s muscular dystrophy ...
  D.'s paralysis ...
  D.'s sign ...
  D.'s syndrome ...
  D.'s type ...

Chédiak-Higashi: C.-H. anomaly ...
  C.-H. disease ...
  C.-H. syndrome ...

---

2. Alphabetisierung und Abkürzung von Untereinträgen

In Unterstichworten wird das Hauptstichwort durch den Anfangsbuchstaben ersetzt.

Untereinträge werden genauso wie Hauptstichwörter alphabetisch eingeordnet. Die Abkürzung für das Hauptstichwort, die Pluralform der Abkürzung oder die ausgeschriebene Pluralform werden bei der Einordnung nicht berücksichtigt. Das gleiche gilt für Präpositionen, Konjunktionen und Artikel als auch für das Apostroph-s bei Eponymen.

Handelt es sich bei dem Haupteintrag um ein Kompositum, so wird es im Untereintrag durch den ersten Buchstaben des ersten Wortes repräsentiert.

Untereinträge können im Singular oder im Plural stehen. Regelmäßige englische Pluralformen werden durch Anhängung von ⟨s⟩ an den Anfangsbuchstaben gebildet.

Unregelmäßige englische Pluralformen werden zum Teil ausgeschrieben, zum Teil wird der letzte Buchstabe oder die letzte Silbe der Pluralform an den Anfangsbuchstaben angehängt.
Lateinische und griechische Pluralformen werden nach denselben Regeln behandelt.

3. Alphabetische Einordnung von Eponymen

Leider wird immer mehr auf eine Apostrophierung von Eponymen verzichtet, was zum Vorhandensein einer unausgewogenen Mischung in der medizinischen Literatur und in medizinischen Wörterbüchern führt. Die Benutzer dieses Wörterbuches sollten sich vergegenwärtigen, daß die angegebenen Formen aus der Literatur übernommen wurden und auf keinen Fall als Richtlinien für die Verwendung von Apostroph-s zu sehen sind.

Das Wörterbuch enthält Eponyme in ihrer allgemein gebräuchlichen Schreibweise, durch die auch die alphabetische Einordnung bestimmt ist. Das gilt ebenfalls für die Vorsilben ⟨Mac⟩ und ⟨Mc⟩. Im Zweifelsfall ist es ratsam, alternative Schreibweisen nachzuschlagen, wenn ein Eintrag nicht sofort gefunden werden kann.

Zur Vereinfachung der Einordnung werden Eponyme als Untereinträge unter dem/den Namen der betreffenden Person(en) verzeichnet. Es ergibt sich daher folgende Reihenfolge:

Als Untereinträge werden Eponyme aufgrund ihrer Buchstabenfolge eingeordnet. Apostroph-s wird nicht für die Alphabetisierung berücksichtigt. Deshalb erscheinen die folgenden Termini als Untereinträge des Hauptstichwortes ⟨Duchenne⟩ in der folgenden Reihenfolge:

Eponyme, die mehr als einen Namen enthalten und die mit Bindestrich(en) verbunden sind, werden als Untereinträge durch den Anfangsbuchstaben jedes Namens verbunden durch Bindestrich(e) dargestellt.

XII

For names beginning with prefixes such as ⟨van⟩, ⟨von⟩, ⟨de⟩ etc. and which may be used either with or without the prefix, the spelling is based on the most common usage. In many cases such names have been entered in this dictionary with and without the prefix. In such a case cross-references are inserted, but a double-check should always be made.

Eponyme, die mit einem Namenszusatz wie z.B. ⟨van⟩, ⟨von⟩, ⟨de⟩ etc. beginnen und die wahlweise mit oder ohne Namenszusatz geschrieben werden können, werden in ihrer allgemein gebräuchlichen Form in das Wörterbuch aufgenommen. In vielen Fällen werden beide Schreibweisen geführt. Auch wenn dann in der Regel mit Verweisen gearbeitet wird, so ist es doch ratsam, alternative Schreibweisen zu überprüfen.

4. Spelling

Because of the dominance of American spelling in the international medical literature, this dictionary is based on American English as far as spelling, and pronunciation are concerned.
Occasionally, it is necessary to include the British spelling, which is then marked accordingly.

tumour *n Brit.* → tumor 1.

4. Orthographie

Die Dominanz des amerikanischen Englisch in der internationalen medizinischen Literatur hat dazu geführt, daß dieses Wörterbuch sich in puncto Rechtschreibung und Aussprache auf amerikanisches Englisch stützt.
Gelegentlich ist es nötig, britische Schreibweisen aufzunehmen, die dann entsprechend gekennzeichnet werden.

II. General Structure of Entries

1. Typeface

Four different styles of type are used for the following categories of information.

boldface type for the main entry

lightface type for subentries, illustrative phrases and idiomatic expressions

plainface type for the translation

italic type for all explanations, definitions, and restrictive labels.

II. Allgemeiner Stichwortaufbau

1. Schriftbild

Vier verschiedene Schriftarten werden zur Gliederung der Einträge eingesetzt:

Halbfett für den Haupteintrag

Auszeichnungsschrift für Untereinträge, Anwendungsbeispiele und Redewendungen

Grundschrift für die Übersetzung

Kursiv für alle erklärenden Zusätze, Definitionen und bestimmende Zusätze.

2. Subdivision of Entries

The main entry appears in large boldface type flush left to the margin of the column.

If the entry word is used in more than one grammatical form, Roman numerals are used to distinguish the various parts of speech (i.e. noun, adjective, adverb, transitive verb, intransitive verb etc.).

bleach [bli:tʃ] **I** *n* ... **II** *vt* ... **III** *vi* ...

Arabic numerals are used to distinguish the various meanings of the entry. This consecutive numbering is used regardless of the Roman numerals mentioned above.

cool [ku:l] **I** *n* Kühle *f*, Frische *f*. **II** *adj* **1.** kühl ... **2.** fieberfrei. **3.** *fig.* kühl, ... **III** *vt* **4.** (ab-)kühlen ... **5.** abkühlen ... **IV** *vi* kühl

2. Unterteilung der Stichwortartikel

Das Hauptstichwort erscheint in halbfetter Schrift nach links ausgerückt.

Hat das Stichwort mehrere grammatische Bedeutungen, werden die einzelnen Wortarten (d.h. Substantiv, Adjektiv, Adverb, transitives Verb, intransitives Verb etc.) durch römische Ziffern unterschieden.

Arabische Ziffern werden zur Unterscheidung der verschiedenen Bedeutungsfacetten eingesetzt. Ihre fortlaufende Numerierung ist unabhängig von den obengenannten römischen Ziffern.

3. Syllabification

For single-word entries of more than one syllable, syllabification is shown by boldfaced centered dots in between the syllables.

er·go·cal·cif·e·rol ...

For combining forms, eponyms, abbreviations, and compound entries (with or without hyphen), no syllable dividers are given.

adren(o)- *pref.* Nebennieren-, Adren(o)-.
left-handed *adj* **1.** linkshändig. **2.** *phys.* linksdrehend, lävorotatorisch.
paraperitoneal hernia Hernia paraperitonealis.

The syllable division for the spelled entry and the syllable division for the pronunciation can differ, as they are determined by entirely different sets of rules.

If there are alternative pronunciations for the main entry, the syllabification given is according to the first pronunciation.

pha·ryn·ge·al [fə'rɪndʒ(ɪ)əl, færɪn'dʒi:əl] *adj* ...

3. Silbentrennung

Bei mehrsilbigen Stichwörtern wird die Silbentrennung durch halbfett auf Mitte stehende Punkte zwischen den Silben angezeigt.

Für Wortbildungselemente, Eponyme, Abkürzungen und Komposita (mit oder ohne Bindestrich) werden keine Silbentrennpunkte angegeben.

Die Silbentrennung des geschriebenen Eintrags kann sich von der Silbentrennung der Aussprache unterscheiden, da sie nach unterschiedlichen Regeln vorgenommen werden.

Wenn mehrere alternative Aussprachen angegeben werden, beruht die Silbentrennung auf der ersten angegebenen Möglichkeit.

XIII

4. Homographs

Main entries that are spelled identically but are of different derivation are marked with superior numbers.

os¹ [ɑs] *n, pl* **o·ra** ['ɔ:rə, 'ɔʊrə] *anat.* (Körper-)Öffnung *f*, ...
os² [ɑs] *n, pl* **os·sa** ['ɑsə] *anat.* Knochen *m*,

4. Homonyme

Hauptstichwörter gleicher Schreibung aber unterschiedlicher Herkunft werden durch Exponenten gekennzeichnet.

5. Parts of Speech

Main entries that consist of a single word or a hyphenated compound entry are given a part-of-speech label, i.e. an italicized abbreviation preceding the translation(s) for that part of speech. [see also 'Abbreviations used in this Dictionary', page XIV]

ha·lo·pro·gin [-'prɑdʒɪn] *n pharm.* Haloprogin *nt*.

5. Wortarten

Haupteinträge, die aus einem Wort oder einem mit Bindestrich geschriebenen Kompositum bestehen, erhalten eine Wortartangabe, d.h. eine kursive Abkürzung, die vor der/den Übersetzung(en) der betreffenden Wortart steht. [siehe auch 'Verzeichnis der verwandten Abkürzungen']

If the entry word is used in more than one grammatical form, the appropriate italicized part-of-speech label is given immediately after every Roman numeral.

sam·ple ['sæmpəl, 'sɑ:m-] I *n* 1. Probe *f*. 2. ... 3. *stat.* ... II *adj* Muster- ... III *vt* 5. eine Stichprobe machen ... 6. ...

Gehört ein Haupteintrag mehreren grammatikalischen Kategorien an, steht die entsprechende kursive Wortartbezeichnung unmittelbar hinter jeder römischen Ziffer.

6. Irregular Forms

Irregular English and Latin plural forms are generally given. Regular English plural forms are only given to avoid possible confusion amongst users whose mother tongue is not English.

hal·lux ['hæləks] *n, pl* **hal·lu·ces** ['hæljəsi:z] Großzehe *f*, ...
stri·a ['straɪə] *n, pl* **stri·ae** ['straɪ,i:] 1. *anat.* Streifen *m*, ...
life [laɪf] *n, pl* **lives** 1. Leben *nt*. ...

6. Unregelmäßige Formen

Unregelmäßige englische und lateinische Pluralformen werden in der Regel angegeben. Regelmäßige Pluralformen englischer Einträge werden nur dann angegeben, wenn die Angabe Benutzern, deren Muttersprache nicht englisch ist, weiterhilft.

For irregular verbs the past tense and past participle are given.

break [breɪk] (*v:* broke; broken) I *n* 1. (Ab-, Zer-, Durch-, Entzwei-)Brechen ... II *vt* 5. ab-, auf-, durchbrechen ... III *vi* 11. brechen ...

Bei unregelmäßigen Verben werden Präteritum und Partizip Perfekt angegeben.

7. Tilde

In phraseological examples, idioms etc. the main entry is replaced by a **lightfaced** ⟨~⟩.

bite ... II *vt* 6. beißen. **to ~ one's nails** an den Nägeln kauen. ...

7. Tilde

In Anwendungsbeispielen, Redewendungen etc. wird das Stichwort durch eine **halbfette** ~ ersetzt.

8. Phrasal Verbs

Phrasal verbs are covered in subentries following the translation(s) of the main entry.

let [let] (**let; let**) *vt* lassen; jdm. erlauben. **to ~ sb./sth. alone** jdn./etw. in Ruhe lassen...
let down *vt* jdn. im Stich lassen ...
let in I *vt* (her-, hin-)einlassen; ...
let out *vt* heraus-, hinauslassen (*of* ...
let through *vt* durchlassen.

8. Phrasal Verbs

Phrasal verbs werden als Untereinträge im Anschluß an die Übersetzung(en) des Haupteintrags behandelt.

9. Restrictive Labels

Restrictive labels (e.g. subject labels, usage labels etc.) are used to mark entries that are limited (in whole or in part) to a particular region, time, subject, or level of usage etc. Sometimes more than one label is given.

Phy·co·my·ce·tes *pl bio., micro.* niedere Pilze *pl*, Algenpilze *pl* ...

9. Bestimmende Zusätze

Bestimmende Zusätze ⟨restrictive labels⟩ (z.B. Sachgebietsangaben, Stilangaben etc.) werden dazu verwendet, Einträge zu kennzeichnen, die in ihrer Gesamtheit oder in Teilbedeutungen Einschränkungen unterliegen. Wenn nötig, können mehrere Labels verwendet werden.

If the label applies to the entire entry it appears before the first part-of-speech label, or after it if there is only one part of speech.

ga·lac·ta·gogue *pharm.* I *n* Galaktagogum *nt*, Laktagogum *nt*. II *adj* ...

Wenn der Zusatz für die gesamte Übersetzung gilt, steht er vor der ersten Wortartangabe oder direkt hinter ihr, wenn es nur eine gibt.

If the label applies to a certain part of speech only, it follows the part-of-speech label and precedes the subsequent translation(s).

spi·nal I *n inf.* → spinal anesthesia 1. II *adj* ... Wirbel-.

Gilt die Einschränkung nur für eine Wortart, steht sie unmittelbar hinter der Wortartangabe aber vor der Übersetzung.

If the restriction applies to a certain meaning only, it follows the Arabic numeral and precedes the translation(s).

si·nus 1. Höhle *f* ... 2. *anat.* Knochenhöhle *f* ... 3. *patho.* Fistelgang *m* ...

Wenn das Label nur für eine Bedeutung gilt, erscheint die entsprechende Abkürzung direkt hinter einer arabischen Ziffer aber vor der betreffenden Übersetzung.

III. Cross-References

Cross-references which are mainly used to assist in finding the less-commonly used entries quickly and easily, as well as to save room, are indicated by arrows. They are used in the following cases:

Cross-reference from main entry to main entry.

Cross-reference from a main entry to a subentry or a part of speech or a specific meaning of another main entry.

Cross-reference from a subentry or a part of speech or a specific meaning of one main entry to another main entry.

Cross-reference from a subentry to a subentry of the same main entry.

Cross-reference from a subentry of a main entry to a subentry of another main entry.

ga·lac·ta·gogue *pharm*. **I** *n* Galaktagogum *nt*, Laktagogum *nt*. **II** *adj* ...

adenomatous polyposis coli → adenomatosis of the colon.
neu·tro·cyte *n* → neutrophil 1.
neu·tro·phil·ic *adj* → neutrophil II.

limiting membrane Grenzmembran *f*, -schicht *f*.
  anterior l. → Bowman's membrane.
e·ryth·ro·phil [ɪˈrɪθrəfɪl] **I** *n* erythrophile Zelle *f od*. Substanz *f*. **II** *adj* → erythrophilic.
mac·u·la 1. Fleck *m* ... **2.** Macula *f*... **3.** → macula lutea.

muscular atrophy:
  Duchenne-Aran m. → Aran-Duchenne m.
  familial spinal m. → Hoffmann's m.

hypersensitivity reaction Überempfindlichkeitsreaktion *f*.
  delayed h. → hypersensitivity, type IV.
  immediate h. → hypersensitivity, type I.

III. Verweise

Verweise, die primär dabei helfen sollen, weniger gebräuchliche Einträge schnell und leicht zu finden, als auch Platz zu sparen, werden durch Pfeile gekennzeichnet. Sie kommen in den folgenden Fällen zur Anwendung:

Verweis von einem Hauptstichwort zu einem anderen Hauptstichwort.

Verweis von einem Haupteintrag zu einem Untereintrag oder einer Wortart oder einer einzelnen Bedeutung eines anderen Hauptstichwortes.

Verweis von einem Untereintrag oder einer Wortart oder einer speziellen Bedeutung eines Haupteintrages zu einem anderen Haupteintrag.

Verweis von einem Untereintrag zu einem anderen Untereintrag desselben Stichwortes.

Verweis von einem Untereintrag auf einen Untereintrag eines anderen Haupteintrages.

A Guide to Pronunciation

The pronunciation of this dictionary is indicated by the alphabet of the ⟨International Phonetic Association⟩ (IPA) and is based on ⟨A Pronouncing Dictionary of American English⟩ by John S. Kenyon and Thomas A. Knott, Merriam-Webster 1953.

The first pronunciation shown is generally the one considered to be in most frequent use, although there may be very little difference in usage between any consecutive pronunciations.

For every single-word main entry listed in this dictionary the pronunciation is shown in parenthesis immediately following the entry word.

mon·o·some ['mɑnəsoʊm] *n* ...
mon·o·so·mia [ˌ-'soʊmɪə] *n* ...
mon·o·so·mic [ˌ-'soʊmɪk] *adj* ...

No pronunciation is given for compound entries, whether hyphenated or written as two or more separate words. For their pronunciation the user must consult the respective simple entries.

Entries that follow a word which they are derived from, often have only stress marks and part of the pronunciation given.

hy·po ['haɪpoʊ] *n* ....
hy·po·a·cid·i·ty [ˌ-ə'sɪdətɪ] *n*...
hy·po·ac·tive [ˌ-'æktɪv] ...
hy·po·ac·tiv·i·ty [ˌ-æk'tɪvətɪ] *n* ...
hy·po·a·cu·sis [ˌ-ə'k(j)uːsɪs] *n* ...

If the pronunciation changes for different parts of speech, the variant pronunciations are given immediately after the entry preceding the first part of speech.

re·cord [*n*, *adj* 'rekərd; *v* rɪ'kɔːrd] **I** *n* .... **II** *adj* ....

Hinweise zur Verwendung der Lautschrift

Die in diesem Wörterbuch angebenen Aussprachen benutzen die Zeichen der ⟨International Phonetic Association⟩ (IPA) und basieren auf dem Werk ⟨A Pronouncing Dictionary of American English⟩ von John S. Kenyon and Thomas A. Knott, Merriam-Webster 1953.

Die erste angegebene Aussprache wird als die allgemein übliche angesehen, auch wenn es kaum Unterschiede in der Häufigkeit der Verwendung zu folgenden Formen geben mag.

Für jedes einfache Hauptstichwort dieses Wörterbuches wird die Aussprache in eckigen Klammern unmittelbar hinter dem Stichwort angegeben.

Für Komposita wird keine Aussprache angegeben, unabhängig davon, ob die einzelnen Worte durch Bindestriche verbunden sind oder nicht. Ihre Aussprache muß bei den jeweiligen Gliedern des Terminus nachgeschlagen werden.

Hauptstichwörter, die auf einen Eintrag folgen, vom dem sie abgeleitet sind, erhalten häufig nur Betonungsakzente und Teilumschrift.

Gibt es für verschiedene Wortarten eines Stichwortes unterschiedliche Aussprachen, so werden die verschiedenen Aussprachen unmittelbar hinter dem Stichwort vor der ersten Wortartangabe aufgeführt.

Phonetic Symbols
1. Vowels and Diphthongs

[æ]	hat	[hæt]
[e]	red	[red]
[eɪ]	rain	[reɪn]
[ɑ]	got	[gɑt]
[ɑː]	car	[kɑːr]
[eə]	chair	[tʃeər]
[iː]	key	[kiː]
[ɪ]	in	[ɪn]
[ɪə]	fear	[fɪər]
[aɪ]	eye	[aɪ]
[f]	fast	[fæst]

Lautschriftsymbole
1. Vokale und Diphthonge

[ɔː]	raw	[rɔː]
[ʊ]	sugar	['ʃʊgər]
[uː]	super	['suːpər]
[ʊə]	crural	['krʊərəl]
[ʌ]	cut	[kʌt]
[aʊ]	out	[aʊt]
[ɜ]	hurt	[hɜrt]
[oʊ]	focus	['foʊkəs]
[ɔɪ]	soil	[sɔɪl]
[ə]	hammer	['hæmər]
[ɔ̃ː]	chaiselongue	[ʃeɪz'lɔ̃ːŋg]

[ː] This symbol indicates the long pronunciation of a vowel.

[ː] Dieses Symbol gibt die lange Betonung eines Vokals an.

2. Consonants

[r]	**arm**	[ɑːrm]
[s]	salt	[sɔːlt]
[v]	vein	[veɪn]
[w]	wave	[weɪv]
[z]	zoom	[zuːm]
[tʃ]	chief	[tʃiːf]
[j]	yoke	[joʊk]

2. Konsonanten

[dʒ]	bridge	[brɪdʒ]
[ŋ]	pink	[pɪŋk]
[ʃ]	shin	[ʃɪn]
[ʒ]	vision	['vɪʒn]
[θ]	throat	[θroʊt]
[ð]	there	[ðeər]
[x]	loch	[lɑx]

[b] [d] [g] [h] [k] [l] [m] [n] [p] [t]
The use of these consonants in English and German pronunciation ist the same.

[b] [d] [g] [h] [k] [l] [m] [n] [p] [t]
Die Verwendung dieser Konsonanten ist im Deutschen und Englischen gleich.

3. Additional Symbols used for non-English Entries 3. Zusätzliche Symbole für nicht-englische Stichwörter

[a]	natif	[naˈtɪf]	Backe	[bakə]
[ã]	emploi	[ãˈplwa]		
[ɛ̃]	pain	[pɛ̃]		
[ɛ]	lettre	[ˈlɛtrə]	Bett	[bɛt]
[i]	iris	[iˈris]	Titan	[tiˈtaːn]
[o]	dos	[do]	Hotel	[hoˈtel]
[y]	durée	[dyˈre]	mürbe	[ˈmyrbə]
[ɔ]	note	[nɔt]	toll	[tɔl]
[u]	nourrir	[nuˈriːr]	mutieren	[muˈtiːrən]
[õ]	bon	[bõn]		
[œ]	neuf	[nœf]	Mörser	[ˈmœrzər]
[ɥ]	cuisse	[kɥis]		
[ø]	feu	[fø]	Ödem	[øˈdeːm]
[ɲ]	baigner	[bɛˈɲe]		
[œ̃]	lundi	[lœ̃di]		
[œj]	feuille	[fœj]		
[ɑːj]	tenailles	[təˈnɑːj]		
[ij]	cochenille	[koʃˈnij]		
[ɛj]	sommeil	[sɔˈmɛj]		
[aj]	maille	[maj]		
[ç]			Becher	[ˈbɛçər]

4. Stress Marks

[ˈ] indicates primary stress. The syllable following it is pronounced with greater prominence than other syllables in the word.

[ˌ] indicates secondary stress. Syllables marked for secondary stress are pronounced with greater prominence than those bearing no stress mark at all but with less prominence than those marked for primary stress.

4. Betonungsakzente

[ˈ] steht für den Hauptakzent. Die auf das Zeichen folgende Silbe wird stärker betont als die anderen Silben des Wortes.

[ˌ] steht für den Nebenakzent. Silben, die mit diesem Symbol gekennzeichnet sind, werden stärker betont als nicht markierte Silben aber schwächer als mit einem Hauptakzent markierte Silben.

Abbreviations Used in this Dictionary — Verzeichnis der verwandten Abkürzungen

English	Abbr.	German
arteria, arteriae	A., Aa.	Arteria, Arteriae
also	a.	auch
abbreviation, acronym, contraction	abbr.	Abkürzung, Akronym, Kontraktion
adjective	jdj	Adjektiv
adverb	adv	Adverb
general	allg.	allgemein
anatomy	anat.	Anatomie
andrology	andro.	Andrologie
anesthesiology	anes.	Anästhesiologie
articulatio, articulationes	Artic., Articc.	Articulatio, Articulationes
Bacterium	Bact.	Bacterium
bacteriology	bact.	Bakteriologie
relating to (in German)	betr.	betreffend
biology	bio.	Biologie
biochemistry	biochem.	Biochemie
botany	bot.	Botanik
British	Brit.	britisch
respectively, or (in German)	bzw.	beziehungsweise
carcinoma	Ca.	Carcinoma
cardiology	card.	Kardiologie
chemistry	chem.	Chemie
(general) surgery	chir.	(Allgemein-)Chirurgie
clinical medicine	clin.	Klinische Medizin
cytology	cyto.	Zytologie
dentistry, odontology	dent.	Zahnheilkunde, Odontologie
dermatology and venereology	derm.	Dermatologie und Venerologie
electricity	electr.	Elektrizitätslehre
embryology	embryo.	Embryologie
emergency medicine	emerg.	Notfallmedizin
endocrinology	endo.	Endokrinologie
epidemiology	epidem.	Epidemiologie
et cetera	etc.	et cetera
something (in German)	etw.	etwas
feminine	f	Femininum; weiblich
figurative(ly)	fig.	figurativ, übertragen
foramen, foramina	For., Forr.	Foramen, Foramina
forensic medicine	forens.	Rechtsmedizin, forensische Medizin
French	French	Französisch
gastroenterology	GE	Gastroenterologie
genetics	genet.	Genetik
geriatrics	geriat.	Geriatrie
ganglion, ganglia	Ggl., Ggll.	Ganglion, Ganglia
glandula, glandulae	Gl., Gll.	Glandula, Glandulae
general practice, general medicine	GP	Allgemeinmedizin
gynecology and obstetrics	gyn.	Gynäkologie und Geburtshilfe
physiotherapy	heilgymn.	Heil-, Krankengymnastik
hematology	hema.	Hämatologie
histology	histol.	Histologie
historical	histor.	geschichtlich, historisch
ear, nose and throat (ENT)	HNO	Hals-Nasen-Ohrenheilkunde

Abbreviations Used in this Dictionary		Verzeichnis der verwandten Abkürzungen
heart, thorax and vascular surgery	HTG	Herz-, Thorax- und Gefäßchirurgie
hygiene	hyg.	Hygiene
intensive care medicine	IC	Intensivmedizin, -pflege
immunology, allergology	immun.	Immunologie, Allergologie
incisura, incisurae	Inc., Incc.	Incisura, Incisurae
informal	inf.	umgangssprachlich
someone, to someone, someone, of someone (in German)	jd., jdm., jdn., jds.	jemand, jemandem, jemanden, jemandes
chemical/clinical pathology, clinical biochemistry	lab.	Labormedizin, Klinische Chemie
ligamentum, ligamenta	Lig., Ligg.	Ligamentum, Ligamenta
musculus, musculi	M., Mm.	Musculus, Musculi
masculine	m	Masculinum; männlich
mathematics	mathe.	Mathematik
internal medicine	med.	Innere Medizin
microbiology	micro.	Mikrobiologie
nervus, nervi	N., Nn.	Nervus, Nervi
noun	n	Substantiv, Hauptwort
nucleus, nuclei	Nc., Ncc.	Nucleus, Nuclei
neonatology	neonat.	Neonatologie
nephrology	nephro.	Nephrologie
neurology	neuro.	Neurologie
neurosurgery	neurochir.	Neurochirurgie
neuter	nt	Neutrum; sächlich
obstetrics	obst.	Geburtshilfe
occupational medicine	occup.	Arbeitsmedizin
or (in German)	od.	oder
old, obsolete	old	veraltet, obsolet
oncology	oncol.	Onkologie
ophthalmology	ophthal.	Augenheilkunde, Ophthalmologie
optics	opt.	Optik
orthopedic surgery, traumatology	ortho.	Orthopädie, Unfallchirurgie, Traumatologie
oneself	o.s.	sich (in englisch)
parasitology	parasit.	Parasitologie
pathology	patho.	Pathologie
pediatrics	ped.	Kinderheilkunde, Pädiatrie
perinatology	perinat.	Perinatologie
pharmacology and toxicology	pharm.	Pharmakologie und Toxikologie
photography	photo.	Photographie
physics	phys.	Physik
physiology	physiol.	Physiologie
plural	pl	Plural, Mehrzahl
plastic surgery, cosmetic surgery	plastchir.	plastische/kosmetische Chirurgie
prefix	pref.	Vorsilbe, Präfix
preposition	prep	Präposition
processus, processus	Proc., Procc.	Processus, Processus
psychiatry	psychia.	Psychiatrie
psychology	psycho.	Psychologie
pulmonology, pneumology	pulmo.	Pulmo(no)logie, Pneumo(no)logie
radiology, nuclear medicine, radiotherapy	radiol.	Radiologie, Nuklearmedizin, Strahlentherapie

XIX

Abbreviations Used in this Dictionary		Verzeichnis der verwandten Abkürzungen
recessus, recessus	Rec., Recc.	Recessus, Recessus
rehabilitation	rehab.	Rehabilitation
rheumatology	rheumat.	Rheumatologie
oneself (in German)	s.	sich
somebody	sb.	jemand (in englisch)
singular	sing	Singular, Einzahl
slang	sl.	Slang
someone	s.o.	jemand (in englisch)
sociology	socio.	Soziologie
sports medicine	sport.	Sportmedizin
statistics	stat.	Statistik
something	sth.	etwas (in englisch)
suffix	suf.	Nachsilbe, Suffix
technology	techn.	Technik
tropical medicine	tropic.	Tropenmedizin
and (in German)	u.	und
urology	urol.	Urologie
(US) American	US	(US-)amerikanisch
vena, venae	V., Vv.	Vena, Venae
verb	v	Verb
intransitive verb	vi	intransitives Verb
virology	virol.	Virologie
reflexive verb	vr	reflexives Verb
transitive verb	vt	transitives Verb
zoology	zoo.	Zoologie

A

A *abbr.* **1.** → absorbance. **2.** → acute 1. **3.** → adenine. **4.** → adenosine. **5.** → admittance. **6.** → ampere. **7.** → Angström unit. **8.** → anterior 1. **9.** → artery 1. **10.** → mass number.
Å *abbr.* → Angström unit.
A *abbr.* → alpha.
a *abbr.* **1.** → atto-. **2.** → absorption coefficient, specific. **3.** → ampere.
å *abbr.* → Angtröm unit.
α *abbr.* **1.** → alpha. **2.** → Bunsen coefficient.
AA *abbr.* → amino acid.
AA amyloidosis reaktiv-sekundäre Amyloidose *f.*
AAC *abbr.* **1.** → antibiotic-associated colitis. **2.** → antigen-antibody complex.
A antigen Antigen A *nt.*
AA protein AA-Protein *nt,* Amyloidprotein-A *nt.*
Aaron ['eərən, 'ɑːr-]: **A.'s sign** (von) Aaron-Zeichen *nt,* -Symptom *nt.*
Aarskog ['ɑːrskɑg]: **A.'s syndrome** Aarskog-Syndrom *nt.*
Aarskog-Scott [skɑt]: **A.-S. syndrome** → Aarskog's syndrome.
AAS *abbr.* → anthrax antiserum.
Aase [ɑːz]: **A. syndrome** Aase-Syndrom *nt.*
AAV *abbr.* → adeno-associated virus.
Ab *abbr.* → antibody.
a·bac·te·ri·al [ˌeɪbæk'tɪərɪəl] *adj* frei von Bakterien, bakterienfrei, abakteriell.
Abadie [æbə'diː]: **A.'s sign 1.** Abadie'-Zeichen *nt.* **2.** *ortho.* Abadie-Rocher-Zeichen *nt.*
A band *histol.* A-Band *nt,* A-Streifen *m,* A-Zone *f,* anisotrope Bande *f.*
a·ban·don [ə'bændən] *vt (Hoffnung)* aufgeben; verzichten auf; jdn. verlassen *od.* im Stich lassen.
a·bar·og·no·sis [ˌæbærəg'nəʊsɪs] *n* Abarognosis *f,* Baragnosis *f.*
ab·ar·tic·u·lar gout [æbɑːr'tɪkjələr] extraartikuläre/viszerale Gicht *f.*
a·ba·sia [ə'beɪzɪə, ʒ(ɪ)ə] *n* Gehunfähigkeit *f,* Abasie *f.*
a·ba·sic [ə'beɪzɪk] *adj* Abasie betr., gehunfähig, abatisch.
a·bate [ə'beɪt] **I** *vt* vermindern, verringern, *(Schmerzen)* lindern, dämpfen; *(Temperatur)* senken. **II** *vi* abnehmen, nachlassen, s. legen, s. vermindern, abflauen, zurückgehen, abklingen.
a·bate·ment [ə'beɪtmənt] *n* Abnehmen *nt,* Nachlassen *nt,* Abflauen *nt,* Abklingen *nt*; Senkung *f,* Verminderung *f,* Linderung *f.*
a·bat·ic [ə'bætɪk] *adj* → abasic.
ab·bau ['apbaʊ] *n chem., biochem.* **1.** Abbau *m.* **2.** Abbauprodukt *nt.*
Abbé ['æbiː, 'ɑbə]: **A.'s flap** Abbé'-Hautlappen *m.*
A.'s image formation theory Abbe'-Bildentstehungstheorie *f.*
A.'s operation *ortho.* Abbé-Operation *f.*
A.'s rings *chir.* Abbe-Ringe *pl.*

Abbé-Zeiss [zaɪs]: **A.-Z. apparatus** (Thoma-)Zeiss-Zählkammer *f.*
A.-Z. counting cell → A.-Z. apparatus.
A.-Z. counting chamber → A.-Z. apparatus.
Abbott ['æbət]: **A.'s method** *ortho.* Skliosebehandlung *f* nach Abbott.
Abbott-Miller ['mɪlər]: **A.-M. tube** Miller--Abbott-Sonde *f.*
Abbott-Rawson ['rɔːsən]: **A.-R. tube** Abbott-Rawson-Sonde *f.*
ABC *abbr.* **1.** → antigen-binding capacity. **2.** → aspiration biopsy cytology.
ab·do·men ['æbdəmən, æb'dəʊ-] *n* Bauch *m,* Unterleib *m,* Abdomen *nt.*
abdomin- *pref.* → abdomino.
ab·dom·i·nal [æb'dɑmɪnl] *adj* Abdomen *od.* Bauch(höhle) betr., abdominal, abdominell, Bauch-, Abdominal-.
abdominal actinomycosis abdominale/intestinale Aktinomykose *f.*
abdominal aneurysm Aneurysma *nt* der Bauchschlagader, Abdominalaneursma *nt.*
abdominal angina Morbus Ortner *m,* Ortner-Syndrom II *nt,* Angina abdominalis/intestinalis, Claudicatio intermittens abdominalis.
abdominal aorta Bauchschlagader *f,* Abdominalaorta *f,* Aorta abdominalis, Pars abdominalis aortae.
abdominal aponeurosis Bauchdeckenaponeurose *f.*
abdominal apoplexy intraabdominale Spontanblutung *f.*
abdominal apron *patho., chir.* Fettschürze *f.*
abdominal ballottement *gyn.* Ballottement *nt* des kindlichen Kopfes.
abdominal bleeding abdominelle Blutung *f.*
abdominal brain Plexus c(o)eliacus.
abdominal breathing Bauchatmung *f.*
abdominal canal Leistenkanal *m,* Canalis inguinalis.
abdominal cavity Bauchraum *m,* -höhle *f,* Cavitas abdominalis.
abdominal cramps Bauchkrämpfe *pl.*
abdominal distension abdominelles Spannungsgefühl *nt.*
abdominal drain 1. Bauchhöhlendrainage *f.* **2.** Bauchhöhlendrain *m.*
abdominal dropsy Bauchwassersucht *f,* Aszites *m,* Ascites *m.*
abdominal epilepsy abdominale Epilepsie *f.*
abdominal esophagus → abdominal part of esophagus.
abdominal examination abdominelle Untersuchung *f.*
abdominal exploration *chir.* Exploration *f* des Bauchraums, abdominelle Exploration *f.*
abdominal fascia, internal Fascia transversalis.
abdominal fibromatosis abdominale Fibromatose *f.*

abdominal film → abdominal radiograph.
abdominal fissure *embryo.* Bauchwandspalte *f.*
abdominal fistula (äußere) Bauchfistel *f.*
ab·dom·i·nal·gia [æbˌdɑmɪ'nældʒ(ɪ)ə] *n* Abdominal-, Bauch-, Leibschmerzen *pl,* Abdominalgie *f.*
abdominal girth Bauchumfang *m.*
abdominal guarding abdominelle Abwehrspannung *f.*
abdominal hemorrhage abdominelle Blutung *f.*
abdominal hernia Bauch(wand)hernie *f,* Laparozele *f,* Hernia abdominalis/ventralis.
abdominal hysterectomy → abdominohysterectomy.
abdominal hysteropexy *gyn.* transabdominelle Hysteropexie *f,* Laparohysteropexie *f.*
abdominal hysterotomy → abdominohysterotomy.
abdominal incision Bauchschnitt *m.*
abdominal influenza Darmgrippe *f.*
abdominal injury → abdominal trauma.
abdominal membrane Bauchfell *nt,* Peritoneum *nt.*
abdominal muscle, straight Rektus *m* abdominis, M. rectus abdominis.
abdominal muscle deficiency syndrome ventrales Defektsyndrom *nt,* Bauchdeckenaplasie *f,* Pflaumenbauchsyndrom *nt,* prune-belly syndrome *(nt).*
abdominal myomectomy *gyn.* transabdominelle Myomektomie *f,* Laparomyomektomie *f.*
abdominal nephrectomy vordere/transabdominelle Nephrektomie *f.*
abdominal opening of uterine tube abdominelle Tubenöffnung *f,* Ostium abdominale tubae uterinae.
abdominal organ Abdominal-, Bauchhöhlenorgan *nt.*
abdominal orifice of uterine tube → abdominal opening of uterine tube.
abdominal pad *chir.* Bauchtuch *nt.*
abdominal pain Bauch-, Leib, Abdominalschmerzen *pl,* Schmerzen *pl* im Abdomen, Abdominalgie *f.*
lower a. Unterbauch-, Unterleibsschmerzen, Schmerzen im Unterbauch/Unterleib.
upper a. Oberbauchschmerzen, Schmerzen im Oberbauch.
abdominal palpation Palpation *f* des Abdomens/der Bauchdecke.
abdominal part: a. of aorta Bauchschlagader *f,* Abdominalaorta *f,* Aorta abdominalis, Pars abdominalis aortae.
a. of autonomic nervous system Bauchabschnitt *m* des vegetativen Nervensystems, Pars abdominalis systematis autonomici, Pars abdominalis autonomica.
a. of esophagus Bauchabschnitt *m* der Speiseröhre, Pars abdominalis (o)esophagi.
a. of thoracic duct Bauchabschnitt *m* des

abdominal perfusion

Ductus thoracicus, Pars abdominalis ductus thoracici.
a. of ureter Bauchabschnitt *m* des Harnleiters, Pars abdominalis ureteris.
abdominal perfusion abdominelle Durchblutung/Perfusion *f*.
abdominal peritoneum Peritoneum *nt* der Bauchwand, parietales Peritoneum *nt*, Peritoneum parietale.
abdominal pregnancy Bauchhöhlenschwangerschaft *f*, Abdominalschwangerschaft *f*, -gravidität *f*, abdominale Schwangerschaft *f*, Graviditas abdominalis.
abdominal pulse Puls *m* über der Aorta abdominalis, Pulsus abdominalis.
abdominal radiograph Röntgenaufnahme *f* des Abdomens, Abdomenaufnahme *f*.
plain a. Abdomenleeraufnahme, Abdomenübersicht(saufnahme) *f*.
abdominal raphe Linea alba.
abdominal reflex Bauchdeckenreflex *m* *abbr.* BDR, Bauchhautreflex *m* *abbr.* BHR.
abdominal region 1. → abdominal cavity. **2. ~s** *pl anat.* Bauchwandfelder *pl*, -regionen *pl*, Regiones abdominales.
abdominal respiration Bauchatmung *f*.
abdominal retractor *chir.* **1.** Bauchdeckenhaken *m*. **2.** Bauchdeckenhalter *m*.
abdominal ribs falsche Rippen *pl*, Costae spuriae.
abdominal rigidity *patho., chir.* bretthartes Abdomen *nt*.
abdominal ring: deep a. innerer Leistenring *m*, A(n)nulus inguinalis profundus.
external a. äußerer Leistenring *m*, A(n)nulus inguinalis superficialis.
internal a. → deep a.
superficial a. → external a.
abdominal roentgenogram → abdominal radiograph.
abdominal sac *embryo.* Abdominalsack *m*.
abdominal salpingectomy *gyn.* transabdominelle Salpingektomie *f*, Zölio-, Laparosalpingektomie *f*.
abdominal salpingotomy *gyn.* transabdominelle Salpingotomie *f*, Zölio-, Laparosalpingotomie *f*.
abdominal section *chir.* **1.** operative Eröffnung *f* der Bauchhöhle, Zölio-, Laparotomie *f*. **2.** Bauch(decken)schnitt *m*.
abdominal sonogram Bauchsonogramm *nt*.
abdominal surgery Abdominal-, Bauchchirurgie *f*.
abdominal testis Bauch-, Abdominalhoden *m*.
abdominal trauma Bauch-, Abdominalverletzung *f*, -trauma *nt*.
blunt a. stumpfes Bauchtrauma.
penetrating a. perforierendes/penetrierendes Bauchtrauma.
abdominal typhoid Bauchtyphus *m*, Typhus (abdominalis) *m*, Febris typhoides.
abdominal veins, subcutaneous subkutane Bauchdeckenvenen *pl*, Vv. subcutaneae abdominis.
abdominal version *gyn.* äußere Wendung *f*.
abdominal vertebrae Lenden-, Lumbalwirbel *pl*, Vertebrae lumbales.
abdominal viscera Baucheingeweide *pl*, abdominelle Viszera *pl*.
abdominal wall fold *embryo.* Bauchwandfalte *f*.
abdominal x-ray → abdominal radiograph.
abdominal zones → abdominal region 2.

abdomino- *pref.* Bauch(höhlen)-, abdomino-, Abdominal-, Abdomino-.
ab·dom·i·no·car·di·ac reflex [æb,dɑmɪnəʊˈkɑːrdɪæk] abdominokardialer Reflex *m*.
ab·dom·i·no·cen·te·sis [ˌ-senˈtiːsɪs] *n* Bauchpunktion *f*, Abdominozentese *f*.
ab·dom·i·no·cys·tic [ˌ-ˈsɪstɪk] *adj* Abdomen u. Gallenblase betr. *od.* verbindend.
ab·dom·i·no·gen·i·tal [ˌ-ˈdʒɛnɪtl] *adj* Abdomen u. Genitalien betr., abdominogenital.
ab·dom·i·no·hys·ter·ec·to·my [ˌ-hɪstəˈrɛktəmɪ] *n gyn.* transabdominelle Hysterektomie *f*, Laparohysterektomie *f*, Hysterectomia abdominalis.
ab·dom·i·no·hys·te·rot·o·my [ˌ-hɪstəˈrɑtəmɪ] *n gyn.* transabdominelle Hysterotomie *f*, Abdomino-, Laparo-, Zöliohysterotomie *f*.
ab·dom·i·no·jug·u·lar reflux [ˌ-dʒʌgjələr, -ˈdʒʊːɡjə-] hepatojugulärer Reflux *m*.
ab·dom·i·no·pel·vic [ˌ-ˈpɛlvɪk] *adj* Bauch- u. Beckenhöhle betr., abdominopelvin.
abdominopelvic cavity Bauch- u. Beckenhöhle *f*.
ab·dom·i·no·per·i·ne·al [ˌ-pɛrɪˈniːəl] *adj* Abdomen u. Perineum betr. *od.* verbindend, abdominoperineal.
abdominoperineal excision of the rectum *chir.* Miles-Operation *f*, abdominoperineale Rektumamputation *f*.
abdominoperineal resection *chir.* abdominoperineale Rektumamputation *f*, Miles-Operation *f*.
ab·dom·i·no·sac·ro·per·i·ne·al [ˌ-ˌsækrəʊpɛrɪˈniːəl] *adj* abdominosakroperineal.
abdominosacroperineal approach *chir.* abdominosakroperinealer Zugang *m*.
ab·dom·i·nos·co·py [æbˌdɑmɪˈnɑskəpɪ] *n* **1.** Untersuchung *f* od. Exploration *f* des Bauchraums. **2.** Bauchspiegelung *f*, Laparoskopie *f*.
ab·dom·i·no·scro·tal [æbˌdɑmɪnəʊˈskrəʊtl] *adj* Abdomen u. Scrotum betr. *od.* verbindend.
ab·dom·i·no·tho·rac·ic [ˌ-θɔːˈræsɪk, -θə-] *adj* Abdomen u. Thorax betr. *od.* verbindend, abdominothorakal, thorakoabdominal.
ab·dom·i·no·u·te·rot·o·my [ˌ-juːtəˈrɑtəmɪ] *n* → abdominohysterotomy.
ab·dom·i·no·vag·i·nal [ˌ-ˈvædʒənl, -vəˈdʒaɪnl] *adj* Abdomen u. Vagina betr. *od.* verbindend, abdominovaginal.
ab·dom·i·no·ves·i·cal [ˌ-ˈvɛsɪkl] *adj* Abdomen u. Harnblase betr. *od.* verbindend, abdominovesikal, vesikoabdominal.
ab·du·cens [æbˈd(j)uːsənz] *n* → abducent nerve.
abducens nucleus Abduzenskern *m*, Nc. abducens, Nc. n. abducentis.
abducens paralysis Abduzensparese *f*.
ab·du·cent [æbˈd(j)uːsənt] *adj* abduzierend, von der Längsachse wegbewegend.
abducent nerve Abduzens *m*, Abducens *m*, VI. Hirnnerv *m*, N. abducens [VI].
ab·duct [æbˈdʌkt] *vt* **1.** von der Längsachse wegbewegen, abduzieren. **2.** entführen, gewaltsam mitnehmen.
ab·duc·tion [æbˈdʌkʃn] *n* **1.** Wegbewegung *f* von der Längsachse, Abduktion *f*. **2.** Entführung *f*.
abduction contracture Abduktionskontraktur *f*.
ab·duc·tor [æbˈdʌktər] *n* → abductor muscle.
abductor digiti minimi manus (muscle) Abduktor *m* digiti minimi manus, M. abductor digiti minimi manus.
abductor digiti minimi pedis (muscle) Abduktor *m* digiti minimi pedis, M. abductor digiti minimi pedis.
abductor hallucis (muscle) Abduktor *m* hallucis, M. abductor hallucis.
abductor indicis (muscle) Abduktor *m* indicis, M. interosseus dorsalis manus I.
abductor muscle Abduktionsmuskel *m*, Abduktor *m*, M. abductor.
a. of great toe → abductor hallucis (muscle).
a. of little finger → abductor digiti minimi manus (muscle).
a. of little toe → abductor digiti minimi pedis (muscle).
long a. of thumb → abductor pollicis longus (muscle).
short a. of thumb → abductor pollicis brevis (muscle).
abductor pollicis brevis (muscle) Abduktor *m* pollicis brevis, M. abductor pollicis brevis.
abductor pollicis longus (muscle) Abduktor *m* pollicis longus, M. abductor pollicis longus.
abductor pollicis (muscle) Abduktor *m* pollicis, M. abductor pollicis.
Abel [ˈeɪbəl] **A.'s bacillus** Ozäna-Bakterium *nt*, Klebsiella (pneumoniae) ozaenae, Bact. ozaenae.
ab·em·bry·on·ic pole [æbˌɛmbrɪˈɑnɪk] *embryo.* abembryonaler Pol *m*.
ab·ep·i·thy·mia [æbˌɛpəˈθiːmɪə] *n neuro.* Paralyse *f* des Plexus solaris.
Abercrombie [ˈæbərkrʌmbɪ] **A.'s degeneration/syndrome** amyloide Degeneration *f*; Amyloidose *f*.
Abernethy [ˈæbərniːθɪ, -nɛθ-] **A.'s fascia** Fascia iliaca.
ab·er·rant [əˈbɛrənt, ˈæbər-] *adj* **1.** an atypischer Stelle liegend, atypisch gebildet, aberrant. **2.** anomal, von der Norm abweichend.
aberrant complex (*EKG*) aberrierende Überleitung *f*.
aberrant duct aberrierender Kanal/Gang *m*.
aberrant ductules aberrante *od.* blinde Ductus efferentes u. epididymidis, Ductuli aberrantes.
aberrant fibers of Déjérine Déjérine-Fasern *pl*, Fibrae aberrantes.
aberrant goiter Struma aberrans.
aberrant pancreas heterotopes/ektopes Pankreas(gewebe *nt*) *nt*, Pankreasektopie *f*, -heteropie *f*.
ab·er·ra·tio [ˌæbəˈreɪʃɪəʊ] *n* → aberration.
ab·er·ra·tion [ˌæbəˈreɪʃn] *n* **1.** *phys., bio.* Abweichung *f*, Aberration *f*. **2.** *patho.* Aberration *f*. **3.** Abirrung *f*, Abweichung *f*. **4.** *psycho.* (geistige) Verwirrung *f*, Umnachtung *f*, (Geistes)Gestörtheit *f*.
ab·er·rom·e·ter [æbəˈrɑmɪtər] *n* Aberrationsmesser *m*.
a·be·ta·lip·o·pro·tein·e·mia [eɪˌbeɪtəˌlɪpəˌprəʊtiːˈniːmɪə] *n* Abetalipoproteinämie *f*, A-Beta-Lipoproteinämie *f*, Bassen-Kornzweig-Syndrom *nt*.
ABG *abbr.* → arterial blood gases.
a·bi·at·ro·phy [ˌeɪbaɪˈætrəfɪ, ˌæbɪ-] *n* vorzeitiger *od.* endogener Vitalitätsverlust *m*.
A bile A-Galle *f*, Choledochusgalle *f*.
a·bil·i·ty test [əˈbɪlətɪ] Eignungstest *m*.
a·bi·o·gen·e·sis [ˌeɪbaɪəʊˈdʒɛnəsɪs, ˌæbɪ-] *n* Abiogenese *f*.
a·bi·o·ge·net·ic [ˌ-dʒəˈnɛtɪk] *adj* Abiogenese betr., von Abiogenese gekennzeichnet, abiogenetisch.
a·bi·og·e·nous [ˌeɪbaɪˈɑdʒənəs, ˌæbɪ-] *adj* → abiogenetic.
abi·on·er·gy [ˌ-ˈɑnərdʒɪ] *n* → abiosis 2.
a·bi·o·sis [ˌ-ˈəʊsɪs] *n* **1.** Abwesenheit *f* von

Leben, Abiose *f.* 2. Abiotrophie *f*, Vitalitätsverlust *m*.
a·bi·ot·ic [ˌ-'atɪk] *adj* abiotisch.
a·bi·o·tro·phia [ˌ-ə'trəʊfɪə] *n* → abiosis 2.
a·bi·o·troph·ic [ˌ-ə'trafɪk, -'trəʊf-] *adj* abiotroph, abiotrophisch.
a·bi·ot·ro·phy [ˌ-'ɑtrəfɪ] *n* → abiosis 2.
a·bil·i·ty [ə'bɪlətɪ] *n, pl* **-ties** 1. Fähigkeit *f*, Vermögen *nt*, Können *nt*. 2. **~ties** *pl* Anlagen *pl*, Talente *pl*, Begabungen *pl*. 3. *techn.* Leistungsfähigkeit *f*. 4. *psycho.* Ability *f*. 5. Geschicklichkeit *f*.
a. to absorb Absorptionsvermögen.
a. to hear Hörfähigkeit.
ability test Eignungstest *m*.
ab·ir·ri·tant [æb'ɪrɪtənt] **I** *n* reizlinderndes Mittel *nt*. **II** *adj* reizlindernd.
ab·ir·ri·ta·tion [æbˌɪrɪ'teɪʃn] *n* 1. *patho.* verminderte Reizbarkeit *f*. 2. Schwäche *f*, Schlaffheit *f*, Erschlaffung *f*, Tonusmangel *m*, Atonie *f*.
ab·ir·ri·ta·tive [æb'ɪrɪtetɪv] *adj* → abirritant II.
ab·lac·tate [æb'læktet] *vt* abstillen.
ab·lac·ta·tion [ˌæblæk'teɪʃn] *n* Abstillen *nt*, Ablaktation *f*, Ablactatio *f*.
ab·late [æb'leɪt] *vt chir.* entfernen, abtragen; amputieren.
ab·la·tio [æb'leɪʃɪəʊ] *n* → ablation 2.
ab·la·tion [æb'leɪʃn] *n* 1. *patho.* Ablösung *f*, Abtrennung *f*, Abhebung *f*, Ablation *f*, Ablatio *f*. 2. *chir.* (operative) Entfernung *f*, Abtragung *f*, Amputation *f*, Ablatio *f*.
ab·la·tive [æb'leɪtɪv] *adj* entfernend, amputierend, ablativ.
ablative surgery amputierende/ablative Chirurgie *f*, Amputation *f*.
a·bleph·a·ria [ˌeɪblef'eərɪə] *n embryo., patho.* Alepharie *f*.
a·bleph·a·ron [eɪ'blefərən] *n* → ablepharia.
a·bleph·a·ry [eɪ'blefərɪ] *n* → ablepharia.
a·blep·sia [eɪ'blepsɪə] *n* Verlust *m* od. Verminderung *f* des Sehvermögens; Blindheit *f*, Erblindung *f*, Amaurose *f*.
a·blep·sy [eɪ'blepsɪ] *n* → ablepsia.
ab·lu·ent ['æblʊənt] **I** *n* Reinigungs-, Waschmittel *nt*, Detergens *nt*. **II** *adj* reinigend.
ab·lu·mi·nal [ab'luːmɪnl] *adj* vom Lumen weg gerichtet.
ab·lu·tion [ə'bluːʃn] *n* (Ab-)Waschen *nt*, Reinigen *nt*; (Ab-)Waschung *f*, Reinigung *f*.
ab·lu·to·ma·ni·a [abˌluːtə'meɪnɪə, -jə] *n* Waschzwang *m*, Ablutomanie *f*.
ab·nor·mal [æb'nɔːrml] *adj* 1. abnorm(al), von der Norm abweichend, anormal, ungewöhnlich. 2. ungewöhnlich hoch *od.* groß, abnorm(al).
abnormal cessation of menses *gyn.* Amenorrhoe *f*, Amenorrhoea *f*.
ab·nor·mal·cy [æb'nɔːrmlsɪ] *n, pl* **-cies** → abnormality.
ab·nor·mal·i·ty [ˌæbnɔː'rmælətɪ] *n, pl* **-ties** 1. Abnormalität *f*. 2. Anomalie *f*.
ab·nor·mi·ty [æb'nɔːrmətɪ] *n, pl* **-ties** 1. → abnormality. 2. Fehlbildung *f*.
ABO antigen ABO-Antigen *nt*.
ABO compatibility *hema.* ABO-Verträglichkeit *f*, ABO-Kompatibilität *f*.
ABO cross-match *hema.* ABO-Kreuzprobe *f*.
ABO cross-matching → ABO cross-match.
ABO incompatibility *hema.* ABO-Unverträglichkeit *f*, ABO-Inkompatibilität *f*.
a·bol·ish [ə'bɑlɪʃ] *vt* abschaffen, aufheben.
a·bol·ish·ment [ə'bɑlɪʃmənt] *n* → abolition.
ab·o·li·tion [ˌæbə'lɪʃn] *n* Abschaffung *f*, Aufhebung *f*.

ab·o·rad [æb'əʊræd] *adj* vom Mund weg (führend), aborad.
ab·o·ral [æb'ɔːrəl, -'əʊr-] *adj* vom Mund weg (führend), mundfern, aboral.
a·bort [ə'bɔːrt] **I** *n* → abortion 1, 2. **II** *vt* 1. eine Fehlgeburt herbeiführen, abtreiben. 2. (*Krankheit*) im Anfangsstadium unterdrücken. **III** *vi* 3. abortieren, eine Fehlgeburt haben. 4. (*Organ*) verkümmern.
a·bort·ed [ə'bɔːrtɪd] *adj* zu früh geboren; verkümmert, zurückgeblieben, abortiv.
a·bor·ti·cide [ə'bɔːrtɪsaɪd] *n* 1. → abortifacient 1. 2. Abtötung *f* der Leibesfrucht.
a·bor·ti·fa·cient [əˌbɔːrtə'feɪʃnt] **I** *n* Abortivmittel *nt*, Abortivum *nt*, Abortifaciens *nt, inf.* Abtreibemittel *nt*. **II** *adj* eine Fehlgeburt verursachend, abortiv.
a·bor·tion [ə'bɔːrʃn] *n* 1. Fehlgeburt *f*, Abgang *m*, Abort(us) *m*. 2. Schwangerschaftsunterbrechung *f*, -abbruch *m*, Abtreibung *f*. **to have an ~** eine Abtreibung vornehmen lassen, abtreiben (lassen). **to procure an ~** eine Abtreibung vornehmen lassen (*on* bei). 3. (*a. fig.*) Mißgeburt *f*, -gestalt *f*. 4. (*Entwicklung*) vorzeitiger Abbruch *m*; (*Organ*) Verkümmerung *f*, Fehlbildung *f*.
a·bor·tion·ist [ə'bɔːrʃnɪst] *n* 1. Abtreiber(in *f*) *m*. 2. Abtreibungsbefürworter(in *f*) *m*.
a·bor·tive [ə'bɔːrtɪv] **I** *n* → abortifacient I. **II** *adj* 1. → abortifacient II. 2. unfertig, unvollständig entwickelt, verkümmert, zurückgeblieben, abortiv. 3. abgekürzt (verlaufend), vorzeitig, verfrüht, gemildert, abortiv.
abortive poliomyelitis abortive Verlaufsform *f* der Poliomyelitis.
a·bor·tus [ə'bɔːrtəs] *n* → abortion 1.
abortus bacillus Bang'-Bazillus *m*, Brucella abortus, Bact. abortus Bang.
abortus-Bang-ring test Abortus-Bang-Ringprobe *f*, ABR-Probe *f*.
ABO system ABO-System *nt*.
a·bou·lia [ə'buːlɪə] *n* → abulia.
a·bove [ə'bʌv] **I** *adv* oben, darüber, oberhalb; vor-, oben-. **II** *prep* über, oberhalb.
above-average *adj* überdurchschnittlich, über dem Durchschnitt.
above-elbow *adj abbr.* **AE** oberhalb des Ellenbogens (liegend), Oberarm-.
above-elbow amputation Oberarmamputation *f*.
above-elbow cast Oberarmgips(verband *m*) *m*.
above-knee *adj abbr.* **AK** oberhalb des Kniegelenks (liegend), Oberschenkel-, Bein-.
above-knee amputation Oberschenkelamputation *f*, Amputation *f* durch den Oberschenkel.
above-knee prosthesis Oberschenkelprothese *f*.
above-knee stump Oberschenkelstumpf *m*.
ABP *abbr.* 1. → androgen binding protein. 2. → arterial blood pressure.
a·bra·chia [eɪ'breɪkɪə] *n embryo.* Abrachie *f*.
a·bra·chi·a·tism [eɪ'breɪkɪətɪzəm] *n* → abrachia.
a·bra·chi·o·ce·pha·lia [eɪˌbreɪkɪəʊsɪ'feɪlɪə] *n embryo.* Abrachiocephalie *f*, -cephalus *m*.
a·bra·chi·o·ceph·a·lus [ˌ-'sefələs] *n embryo.* Abrachiocephalus *m*, Abrachius acephalus.
a·bra·chi·us [eɪ'breɪkɪəs] *n embryo.* Abrachius *m*.
a·brad·ant [ə'breɪdnt] *n, adj* → abrasive.
a·brade [ə'breɪd] **I** *vt* 1. abschaben, abreiben. 2. *chir.* (*Haut*) abschürfen, aufscheuern. **II** *vi s.* abreiben; verschleißen.

Abrahams ['eɪbrəhəm]: **A.' sign** Abrahams-Zeichen *nt*.
Abrami [ə'brɑːmɪ]: **A.'s disease** hämolytische Anämie *f*.
Abrams ['eɪbrəmz]: **A.'s reflex** Abrams'--Lungenreflex *m*.
A.'s heart reflex Abrams'-Herzreflex *m*.
a·brase [ə'breɪz] *vt, vi* → abrade.
a·bra·sio [ə'breɪsɪəʊ] *n* → abrasion.
a·bra·sion [ə'breɪʒn] *n* 1. Abschürfen *nt*, Abschaben *nt*, Abreiben *nt*. 2. (Haut-)Abschürfung *f*, Ablederung *f*.
a·bra·sive [ə'breɪsɪv] **I** *n* Schleif-, Poliermittel *nt*, Schmirgel *m*. **II** *adj* abreibend, abschleifend, schmirgelartig, Schleif-.
ab·re·act [ˌæbrɪ'ækt] *vt psycho.* abreagieren.
ab·re·ac·tion [ˌæbrɪ'ækʃn] *n psycho.* Abreaktion *f*.
Abrikosov [æbrɪ'kɒsəf]: **A.'s tumor** Myoblastenmyom *nt*, Myoblastom *nt*, Abrikossoff-Geschwulst *f*, -Tumor *m*, Granularzelltumor *m*.
Abrikossoff → Abrikosov.
a·brin ['eɪbrən, eɪ'brɪn, 'æb-] *n* Abrin *nt*.
a·bro·sia [ə'brəʊzɪə] *n* Nahrungsmangel *m*.
ABR test → abortus-Bang-ring test.
ab·rupt [ə'brʌpt] *adj* 1. abrupt, plötzlich, jäh. 2. schroff.
ab·scess ['æbses] *n* Abszeß *m*.
abscess cavity Abszeßhöhle *f*.
abscess fistula Abszeßfistel *f*.
abscess formation Abszeßbildung *f*, -formation *f*, Abszedierung *f*.
abscess-forming *adj* abszessbildend, abszedierend.
abscess-forming pneumonia abszedierende Pneumonie *f*.
abscess-forming pyelonephritis abszedierende Pyelonephritis *f*.
abscess membrane Abszeßmembran *f*.
ab·sces·sus [əb'sesəs] *n* → abscess.
ab·scise ['æbsaɪz] *vt* ab-, wegschneiden, abtrennen, entfernen.
ab·scis·sa [æb'sɪsə] *n, pl* **-sas, -sae** [-siː] *mathe.* Abszisse *f*.
ab·scis·sion [æb'sɪʒn, -'sɪʃ-] *n chir.* Abschneiden *nt*, Abtrennung *f*, Wegschneiden *nt*, Entfernung *f*.
ab·sence ['æbsəns] *n* 1. Abwesenheit *f*, Fehlen *nt*, Nichtvorhandensein *nt*; Mangel *m* (*of* an); Fernbleiben *nt* (*from* von). 2. *psychia.* Absence *f*. 3. *neuro.* Petit-mal(-Epilepsie *f*) *nt abbr.* **PM**.
a. of menses *gyn.* Amenorrhoe *f*, Amenorrhoea *f*.
absence seizure *neuro.* Petit-mal(-Epilepsie *f*) *nt abbr.* **PM**.
ab·sent [æb'sənt] *adj* abwesend, fehlend, nicht vorhanden. **to be ~ from** ausbleiben, ausfallen, fehlen.
absent development of speech (motorische) Hörstummheit *f*, Audimutitas *f*, fehlende *od.* verzögerte Sprachentwicklung *f*.
absent pulse *card.* fehlender Puls(schlag *m*) *m*.
Ab·sid·ia [ən'sɪdɪə] *n micro.* Absidia *f*.
ab·so·lute ['æbsəluːt] *adj* 1. absolut, uneingeschränkt, unumschränkt. 2. *chem.* rein, unvermischt, absolut. 3. *phys.* absolut unabhängig, nicht relativ.
absolute accommodation *ophthal.* absolute Akkommodation *f*.
absolute agraphia völlige/totale/ataktische Agraphie *f*.
absolute alcohol absoluter Alkohol *m*, Alcoholus absolutus.
absolute configuration *chem.* absolute Konfiguration *f*.
absolute glaucoma absolutes Glaukom *nt*, Glaucoma absolutum.

absolute hemianopia/hemianopsia *ophthal.* absolute Hemianop(s)ie *f.*
absolute humidity *phys.* absolute Feuchtigkeit *f.*
absolute hyperopia *ophthal.* absolute Weitsichtigkeit/Hyperopie *f.*
absolute leukocytosis absolute Leukozytose *f.*
absolute refractoriness *physiol.* absolute Refraktärität *f.*
absolute scale Kelvin-Skala *f.*
absolute scotoma *ophthal.* absolutes Skotom *nt.*
absolute sterility *gyn.* absolute Sterilität *f.*
absolute temperature *abbr.* **T** *phys.* absolute Temperatur *f abbr.* T.
absolute temperature scale Kelvin-Skala *f.*
absolute threshold Absolutschwelle *f,* Reizschwelle *f,* Reizlimen *nt abbr.* RL.
absolute unit absolute Einheit *f.*
absolute viscosity absolute/dynamische Zähigkeit/Viskosität *f abbr.* η.
ab·sorb [æb'sɔːrb] *vt* ab-, resorbieren, ein-, aufsaugen, in s. aufnehmen.
ab·sor·ba·ble [æb'sɔːrbəbl] *adj* ab-, resorbierbar.
absorbable suture *chir.* ab-/resorbierbares Nahtmaterial *nt,* ab-/resorbierbare Naht *f.*
ab·sorb·ance [æb'sɔːrbəns] *n abbr.* **A** *phys.* Extinktion *f abbr.* E.
ab·sorb·ate [æb'sɔːrbənt] *n* absorbierte Substanz *f,* Absorbent *nt.*
ab·sor·be·fa·cient [æb,sɔːrbə'feɪʃnt] **I** *n* absorptionsförderndes/absorbierendes Mittel *nt.* **II** *adj* Absorption fördernd, re-, absorbierend.
ab·sorb·en·cy [æb'sɔːrbənsɪ] *n* → absorbance.
absorbancy index Extinktionskoeffizient *m.*
ab·sorbed dose [æb'sɔːrbd] *radiol.* Energiedosis *f.*
ab·sorb·ent [æb'sɔːrbənt] **I** *n* saugfähiger Stoff *m,* absorbierende Struktur/Substanz *f,* Absorber *m,* Absorbens *nt.* **II** *adj* saugfähig, ein-, aufsaugend, absorbierend, resorbierend.
absorbent cotton (Verbands-)Watte *f,* Tupfer *m.*
absorbent gland *old* → lymph node.
absorbent system lymphatisches System *nt,* Lymphsystem *nt,* Systema lymphaticum.
ab·sorb·ing [æb'sɔːrbɪŋ] *adj* ab-, resorbierend, Absorptions-, Aufnahme-.
absorbing epithelium resorbierendes Epithel *nt,* Saumzellen *pl,* Enterozyten *pl.*
ab·sorp·tion [æb'sɔːrpʃn] *n* **1.** Absorption *f,* Resorption *f,* Aufnahme *f;* Einverleibung *f.* **2.** *phys.* Absorption *f.* **3.** *fig.* Versunkensein *nt,* Vertieftsein *nt.*
absorption atelectasis (*Lunge*) Absorptions-, Resorptions-, Obstruktionsatelektase *f.*
absorption band *phys.* Absorptionsbande *f,* -streifen *m.*
absorption coefficient Extinktionskoeffizient *f.*
molar a. *abbr.* **E** molarer Extinktionskoeffizient *abbr.* E.
specific a. *abbr.* **a** spezifischer Extinktionskoeffizient *abbr.* a.
absorption constant → absorption coefficient.
absorption lacunae Howship'-Lakunen *pl.*
absorption lines *phys.* Absorptionslinien *pl.*
absorption maximum *phys.* Absorptionsmaximum *nt.*

absorption spectrophotometer Absorptionsspektrophotometer *nt.*
absorption spectrum *phys.* Absorptionsspektrum *nt.*
ab·sorp·tive [æb'sɔːrptɪv] *adj* Absorption betr., ab-, adsorptiv, absorbierend, Absorptions-.
ab·sorp·tiv·i·ty [,æbsɔːrp'tɪvətɪ] *n phys.* Extinktionskoeffizient *m.*
abst. *abbr.* → abstract I.
ab·stain [æb'steɪn] *vi* s. enthalten (*from*).
ab·stain·er [æb'steɪnər] *n* Abstinenzler(in *f*) *m.*
ab·sten·tion [æb'stenʃn] *n* Enthaltung *f* (*from* von).
ab·ster·gent [æb'stɜːrdʒənt] **I** *n* **1.** Abführmittel *nt.* **2.** Reinigungsmittel *nt.* **II** *adj* **3.** abführend. **4.** reinigend.
ab·sti·nence ['æbstɪnəns] *n* Enthaltung *f,* Enthaltsamkeit *f,* Abstinenz *f* (*from* von).
abstinence symptoms Entzugssymptome *pl,* -symptomatik *f.*
abstinence syndrome Entzugssyndrom *nt.*
ab·sti·nent ['æbstɪnənt] *adj* enthaltsam (*from* von), mäßig, abstinent.
abstr. *abbr.* → abstract I.
ab·stract [*n* 'æbstrækt; *adj* æb'strækt] **I** *n abbr.* **abst., abstr.** Auszug *m,* Abriß *m,* Inhaltsangabe *f,* Übersicht *f.* **II** *adj* abstrakt; rein begrifflich, theoretisch.
a·bu·lia [ə'b(j)uːlɪə] *n psycho., psychia.* krankhafte Willenlosig-, Entschlußlosigkeit *f,* Abulie *f.*
a·bu·lic [ə'b(j)uːlɪk] *adj* Abulie betr., von Abulie betroffen.
Abuna [ə'buːnə]: **A. splint** *ortho.* Fingerschiene *f* nach Abuna.
a·bun·dance [ə'bʌndəns] *n* Überfluß *m,* Reichtum *m* (*of* an), Fülle *f* (*of* von).
a·bun·dant [ə'bʌndənt] *adj* reich(lich), üppig; reich (*in, with* an).
a·buse [*n* ə'bjuːs; *v* ə'bjuːz] **I** *n* **1.** Mißbrauch *m,* mißbräuchliche Anwendung *f,* Abusus *m.* **2.** Mißhandlung *f;* (*sexueller*) Mißbrauch *m.* **II** *vt* **3.** mißbrauchen; übermäßig beanspruchen; (*Gesundheit*) Raubbau treiben mit. **4.** mißhandeln; (sexuell) mißbrauchen, s. vergehen an.
a·bu·sive [ə'bjuːsɪv] *adj* **1.** Mißbrauch treibend. **2.** mißbräuchlich. **3.** beleidigend, ausfallend.
AC *abbr.* **1.** → acromioclavicular. **2.** → adenylate cyclase. **3.** → air conduction. **4.** → alternating current. **5.** → anodal closure.
A.C. *abbr.* **1.** → acromioclavicular. **2.** → air conduction. **3.** → alternating current.
Ac *abbr.* → actinium.
ac *abbr.* [ante cibum] *pharm.* vor dem Essen, ante cibum.
a·ca·cia [ə'keɪʃə] *n* Gummi arabicum.
a·cal·cer·o·sis [eɪ,kælsə'rəʊsɪs] *n patho.* systemischer Kalziummangel *m.*
a·cal·cu·lia [,eɪkæl'kjuːlɪə] *n neuro.* Akalkulie *f.*
a·cal·cu·lous cholecystitis [eɪ'kælkjələs] nicht-steinbedingte Gallenblasenentzündung/Cholezystitis *f.*
acanth- *pref.* → acantho-.
a·can·tha [ə'kænθə] *n* **1.** *anat.* Wirbelsäule *f;* Dornfortsatz *m.* **2.** *bio.* Stachel *m,* Dorn *m.*
ac·an·tha·ceous [ækən'θeɪʃəs] *adj* stachelig, dornig.
a·can·tha·me·bi·a·sis [ə,kænθəmɪ'baɪəsɪs] *n* Acanthamoeba-Infektion *f.*
A·can·tha·moe·ba [ə,kænθə'miːbə] *n micro.* Akanthamöbe *f,* Acanthamoeba *f.*
a·can·thes·the·sia [ə,kænθes'θiːʒ(ɪ)ə] *n neuro.* Akanthästhesie *f.*
A·can·thi·a lec·tu·la·ria [ə'kænθɪə ,lektjʊ-

'leərɪə] *n micro.* Bettwanze *f,* Cimex lectularius, Acanthia lectularia.
acantho- *pref.* Dorn(en)-, Akanth(o)-, Acanth(o)-.
A·can·tho·ceph·a·la [ə,kænθə'sefələ] *pl, sing* **-lus** [-ləs] *micro.* Kratzer *pl,* Kratzwürmer *pl,* Acanthocephala *f.*
a·can·tho·ceph·a·lans [,-'sefələns] *pl* → Acanthocephala.
a·can·tho·ceph·a·li·a·sis [,-,sefə'laɪəsɪs] *n* Akanthozephaliasis *f.*
A·can·tho·ceph·a·lus *sing* → Acanthocephala.
A·can·tho·chei·lo·ne·ma [,-keɪləʊ'niːmə] *micro.* Acanthocheilonema *f.*
a·can·tho·chei·lo·ne·mi·a·sis [,-keɪləʊnə-'maɪəsɪs] *n* Mansonellainfektion *f,* Mansonelliasis *f,* Mansonellose *f.*
a·can·tho·cyte [ə'kænθəsaɪt] *n* stechapfelförmiger Erythrozyt *m,* Akanthozyt *m.*
a·can·tho·cy·to·sis [ə,kænθəsaɪ'təʊsɪs] *n* Akanthozytose *f.*
a·can·thoid [ə'kænθɔɪd] *adj* stachelförmig, spitz, dornartig.
ac·an·thol·y·sis [æ,kæn'θɑləsɪs] *n* Akantholyse *f.*
a·can·tho·lyt·ic [ə,kænθə'lɪtɪk] *adj* Akantholyse betr., akantholytisch.
ac·an·tho·ma [ækən'θəʊmə] *n, pl* **-ma·ta** [-mətə], **-mas** Akanthom *nt,* Acanthoma *nt.*
a·can·tho·pel·vis [ə,kænθə'pelvɪs] *n* Akanthopelvis *f.*
a·can·tho·pel·yx [,-'pelɪks] *n* → acanthopelvis.
ac·an·tho·sis [ækən'θəʊsɪs] *n, pl* **-ses** [-siːz] Akanthose *f,* Acanthosis *f.*
ac·an·thot·ic [,-'θɑtɪk] *adj* von Akanthose gekennzeichnet, akanthotisch.
a·can·thro·cyte [ə'kænθrəsaɪt] *n* → acanthocyte.
a·can·thro·cy·to·sis [ə,kænθrəsaɪ'təʊsɪs] *n* → acanthocytosis.
a·cap·nia [ə'kæpnɪə] *n* Akapnie *f;* Hypokapnie *f.*
a·cap·ni·al [ə'kæpnɪəl] *adj* → acapnic.
a·cap·nic [ə'kæpnɪk] *adj* Akapnie betr., akapnoisch.
acar- *pref.* → acaro-.
a·car·bi·a [ə'kɑːrbɪə] *n* Akarbie *f.*
a·car·di·a [eɪ'kɑːrdɪə] *n embryo.* Akardie *f.*
a·car·di·ac [eɪ'kɑːrdɪæk] *adj* von Akardie betroffen, akardial.
a·car·di·a·cus [,eɪkɑːr'daɪəkəs] *n* → acardius.
a·car·di·us [eɪ'kɑːrdɪəs] *n embryo.* Akardier *m,* Akardi(k)us *m,* Acardi(c)us *m.*
a·car·i·an [ə'kærɪən] *adj* Milben betr. Zecken betr., zecken-, milbenartig, Milben-, Zecken-.
ac·a·ri·a·sis [ækə'raɪəsɪs] *n, pl* **-ses** [-siːz] Akarinose *f,* Akariosis *f,* Acariasis *f,* Acarinosis *f,* Acaridosis *f.*
a·car·i·cide [ə'kærəsaɪd] **I** *n* Akarizid *nt.* **II** *adj* milben(ab)tötend, akarizid.
ac·a·rid ['ækərɪd] *n* Milbe *f* od. Zecke *f* der Ordnung Acarina.
A·car·i·dae [ə'kærɪdiː] *pl micro.* Acaridae *pl.*
ac·a·ri·dan [ə'kærɪdən] *n* → acarid.
ac·a·ri·di·a·sis [ə,kærə'daɪəsɪs] *n* → acariasis.
Ac·a·ri·na [ækə'raɪnə, -riːnə] *pl* Acarina *pl.*
ac·a·rine ['ækəraɪn, -riːn] *n* Acarine *f.*
ac·a·ri·no·sis [,ækərɪ'nəʊsɪs] *n* → acariasis.
ac·a·ri·o·sis [,-'əʊsɪs] *n* → acariasis.
acaro- *pref.* Milben-, Acar(o)-.
ac·a·ro·der·ma·ti·tis [,ækərəʊ,dɜːrmə'taɪtɪs] *n* Milbendermatitis *f,* Acarodermatitis *f,* Skabies *f.*
ac·a·roid ['ækərɔɪd] *adj* milbenähnlich, zeckenartig.

ac·a·ro·tox·ic [ˌækərəʊˈtɑksɪk] *adj* milben(ab)tötend.
Ac·a·rus [ˈækərəs] *n micro.* Acarus *m.*
A. scabiei Krätzmilbe *f*, Acarus scabiei, Sarcoptes scabiei.
ac·a·rus [ˈækərəs] *n, pl* **-ri** [-raɪ, -riː] *micro.* Acarus *m.*
a·car·y·ote [əˈkærɪəʊt eɪ-] *n* kernlose Zelle *f.*
a·cat·a·la·se·mia [eɪˌkætləˈsiːmɪə] *n* → acatalasia.
a·cat·a·la·sia [eɪˌkætəˈleɪʒ(ɪ)ə, -zɪə] *n* Akatalasämie *f*, Akatalasie *f*, Takahara-Krankheit *f.*
a·cat·a·lep·sia [ˌ-ˈlepsɪə] *n* Unsicherheit *f* von Diagnose *od.* Prognose, Akatalepsie *f.*
a·cat·a·lep·sy [eɪˈkætəlepsɪ] *n* → acatalepsia.
a·cat·a·ma·the·sia [eɪˌkætəməˈθiːʒ(ɪ)ə] *n* Akatamathesie *f.*
a·cat·a·pha·sia [ˌ-ˈfeɪʒ(ɪ)ə, -zɪə] *n psychia.* Akataphasie *f.*
ac·a·tas·ta·sia [ˌækətæsˈteɪʒ(ɪ)ə, -zɪə] *n* Unregelmäßigkeit *f*, Normabweichung *f.*
ac·a·tas·tat·ic [ˌ-ˈtætɪk] *adj* unregelmäßig, von der Norm abweichend.
ac·a·this·ia [ˌækəˈθiːʒ(ɪ)ə, -zɪə] *n* → akathisia.
a·cau·dal [eɪˈkɔːdl] *adj* → acaudate.
a·cau·date [eɪˈkɔːdeɪt] *adj bio.* schwanzlos.
ACC *abbr.* → anodal closure contraction.
Acc *abbr.* → accommodation 1.
ac·cel·er·ant [ækˈselərənt] **I** *n* → accelerator 1. **II** *adj* beschleunigend, akzelerierend.
ac·cel·er·ate [ækˈseləreɪt] **I** *vt* beschleunigen, akzelerieren; *(Entwicklung)* fördern, beschleunigen. **II** *vi* schneller werden, Geschwindigkeit erhöhen, s. beschleunigen, akzelerieren.
ac·cel·er·at·ed reaction [ækˈseləreɪtɪd] *chem.* beschleunigte Reaktion *f.*
accelerated rejection *chir. (Transplantation)* beschleunigte Abstoßung(sreaktion) *f.*
accelerated respiration beschleunigte Atmung *f.*
ac·cel·er·a·tion [ækˌseləˈreɪʃn] *n* **1.** Beschleunigung *f*, Geschwindigkeitsänderung *f*, Akzeleration *f.* **2.** Beschleunigen *nt.* **3.** *bio.* Akzeleration *f*, Entwicklungsbeschleunigung *f.*
a. of the pulse Pulserhöhung *f.*
acceleration period Beschleunigungsphase *f.*
acceleration phase → acceleration period.
acceleration sensor Beschleunigungssensor *m.*
acceleration work Beschleunigungsarbeit *f.*
ac·cel·er·a·tor [ækˈseləreɪtər] *n* **1.** *phys., chem., techn.* Beschleuniger *m*, Akzelerator *m.* **2.** *chem.* Katalysator *m.* **3.** *old* → sympathetic nervous system.
accelerator factor Proakzelerin *nt*, Proaccelerin *nt*, Acceleratorglobulin *nt*, labiler Faktor *m*, Faktor V *m abbr.* F V.
accelerator globulin *abbr.* **AcG** → accelerator factor.
ac·cel·er·in [ækˈselərɪn] *n* Akzelerin *nt*, Accelerin *nt*, Faktor VI *m abbr.* F VI.
ac·cel·er·om·e·ter [ækˌseləˈrɑmɪtər] *n* Beschleunigungsmesser *m.*
ac·cen·tu·ate [ækˈsentʃuːeɪt] *vt* akzentuieren, betonen; hervorheben; *(Frequenz)* anheben.
ac·cen·tu·a·tion [ækˌsentʃuːˈeɪʃn] *n* Betonung *f*; *(Frequenz)* Anhebung *f.*
ac·cept [ækˈsept] *vt* **1.** *(Patient)* (zur Behandlung) annehmen, akzeptieren. **2.** *(Hypothese)* akzeptieren, gelten lassen. **3.** *(Notwendigkeit, Dringlichkeit)* einsehen, anerkennen.
ac·cept·a·bil·i·ty [ækˌseptəˈbɪlətɪ] *n* Annehmbarkeit *f*, Akzeptierbarkeit *f*; Erträglichkeit *f*; Zulässigkeit *f.*
ac·cept·a·ble [ækˈseptəbl] *adj* akzeptabel, annehmbar *(to* für); *(Medikament)* zulässig.
ac·cept·ance [ækˈseptəns] *n* Akzeptierung *f*, Akzeptanz *f*, Annahme *f*; Anerkennung *f*, Zustimmung *f.*
ac·cept·ed [ækˈseptɪd] *adj* (allgemein) anerkannt, akzeptiert.
ac·cep·tor [ækˈseptər] *n chem.* Akzeptor *m*, Acceptor *m.*
acceptor control *biochem.* Akzeptorkontrolle *f.*
acceptor control index/ratio Akzeptorkontrollindex *m*, -ratio *f.*
acceptor molecule Akzeptormolekül *nt.*
ac·cess [ˈækses] *n* **1.** Zutritt *m*, Zugang *m (to* zu). **to be easy of ~** *fig. (Person)* zugänglich sein. **to have/gain ~ to** Zutritt haben/erhalten zu. **2.** *chir.* operativer Zugang *m*; *(Gefäß)* Zugang *m*, (liegender) Katheter *m.* **3.** Anfall *m*, Ausbruch *m (einer Krankheit).*
a. of fever Fieberanfall *m.*
ac·ces·si·bil·i·ty [ækˌsesəˈbɪlətɪ] *n (a. fig.)* Zugänglichkeit *f*, Erreichbarkeit *f.*
ac·ces·si·ble [ækˈsesɪbl] *adj* (leicht) zugänglich *od.* erreichbar *(to* für); *(Person)* zugänglich.
ac·ces·so·ry [ækˈsesərɪ, ɪk-, ək-] **I** *n (a. techn.)* Zubehör(teile *pl) nt*; Zusatz *m.* **II** *adj* **1.** akzessorisch, zusätzlich, begleitend, ergänzend, Neben-, Bei-, Hilfs-, Zusatz-. **2.** untergeordnet, nebensächlich, Neben-.
accessory bones akzessorische Knochen *pl*, Ossa accessoria.
accessory breasts → accessory mammae.
accessory cartilages of nose akzessorische Nasenknorpel *pl*, Cartilagines nasales accessoriae.
accessory chromosome überzähliges Chromosom *nt.*
accessory cramp Schiefhals/Torticollis *m* bei Akzessoriuslähmung.
accessory diaphragm Urogenitaldiaphragma *nt*, Diaphragma urogenitale.
accessory floccule/flocculus Paraflocculus *m.*
accessory ganglia Ggll. intermedia.
accessory ligament akzessorisches Ligament *nt*, Lig. accessorium.
a. of humerus Lig. coracohumerale.
plantar a.s Ligg. accessoria plantaria.
volar a.s Ligg. accessoria volaria.
accessory mammae zusätzliche/akzessorische Brustdrüsen *pl*, Mammae aberrantes/accessoriae/erraticae.
accessory nerve Akzessorius *m*, XI. Hirnerv *m*, N. accessorius [XI].
spinal a. → accessory nerve.
vagal a. Ramus internus n. accessorii.
accessory nipples *embryo.* akzessorische Brustwarzen *pl*; Polythelie *f.*
accessory nucleus Edinger-Westphal-Kern, Nc. oculomotorius accessorius.
a. of ventral column of spinal chord Akzessoriuskern, Nc. n. accessorii, Nc. accessorius.
accessory olive Nebenolive *f.*
accessory organs of eye Hilfsorgane *pl* des Auges, Adnexa oculi, Organa oculi accessoria.
accessory pancreas Nebenbauchspeicheldrüse *f*, Nebenpankreas *nt*, Pancreas accessorium.

accommodation phosphene

accessory placenta akzessorische Plazenta *f*, Placenta accessoria.
accessory process Proc. accessorius.
accessory recess of elbow Rec. sacciformis artic. cubiti.
accessory sign Begleit-, Nebensymptom *nt.*
accessory sinuses of nose (Nasen-)Nebenhöhlen *pl*, Sinus paranasales.
accessory spleen Nebenmilz *f*, Lien accessorius.
accessory symptom Begleit-, Nebensymptom *nt.*
accessory thyroid akzessorische Schilddrüse *f*, Gl. thyroidea accessoria.
ac·ci·dent [ˈæksɪdənt] *n* **1.** Unfall *m*, Unglück(sfall *m) nt.* **to have an ~** verunglücken, einen Unfall haben. **2.** Zufall *m*, zufälliges Ereignis *nt.* **by ~** zufällig; versehentlich. **~ at work** Betriebs-, Arbeitsunfall *m.*
ac·ci·den·tal [ˌæksɪˈdentl] *adj* **1.** Unfall betr., durch Unfall, Unfall-. **2.** zufällig (hinzukommend *od.* eintretend), versehentlich, akzident(i)ell, Zufalls-.
accidental abortion akzidentaler/traumatischer Abort *m.*
accidental afterimage *ophthal.* negatives Nachbild *nt.*
accidental albuminuria akzidentelle Albuminurie/Proteinurie *f.*
accidental death Unfalltod *m.*
accidental hemorrhage *gyn. Brit.* Plazentalösung *f*, Abruptio placentae.
accidental host *micro.* Fehlwirt *m.*
accidental image *ophthal., psycho.* Nachbild *nt.*
accidental injury Unfallverletzung *f.*
accidental involution akzidentelle Involution *f.*
accidental membrane Pseudomembran *f.*
accidental murmur akzidentelles (Herz-)Geräusch *nt.*
accidental parasite *micro.* Zufallsparasit *m.*
accidental proteinuria → accidental albuminuria.
accident and emergency (department) (allgemeine) Notaufnahme *f.*
accident-prone *adj* unfallgefährdet.
ACCI *abbr.* → anodal closure clonus.
ac·cli·ma·ta·tion [əˈklaɪməˈteɪʃn] *n* → acclimation.
ac·cli·mate [ˈækləmeɪt, əˈklaɪmɪt] *vt, vi* → acclimatize.
ac·cli·ma·tion [ækləˈmeɪʃn, ˌæklə-] *n* Eingewöhnung *f*, Anpassung *f*, Akklimatisation *f*, Akklimatisierung *f.*
a. to high altitude Höhenanpassung, -akklimatisation *f.*
ac·cli·ma·ti·za·tion [əˌklaɪmətəˈzeɪʃn, -taɪ-] *n* → acclimation.
ac·cli·ma·tize [əˈklaɪmətaɪz] **I** *vt (a. fig.)* akklimatisieren *od.* gewöhnen *(to* an), eingewöhnen *(to* in). **II** *vi (a. fig.)* s. akklimatisieren *od.* gewöhnen *(to* an), s. eingewöhnen *(to* in).
ac·com·mo·date [əˈkɑmədeɪt] **I** *vt* **1.** anpassen, angleichen, akkommodieren *(to* an). **2.** jdn. versorgen *(with* mit). **3.** unterbringen, aufnehmen können. **II** *vi* s. anpassen *(to* an); s. einstellen *(to* auf); *ophthal.* s. akkommodieren.
ac·com·mo·da·tion [əˌkɑməˈdeɪʃn] *n* **1.** *abbr.* **Acc** *(a. ophthal.)* Einstellung *f*, Angleichung *f*, Anpassung *f*, Akkommodation *f (to* an) *abbr.* **A.** **2.** Versorgung *f (with* mit). **3.** Unterbringung *f*, -kunft *f.*
accommodation apparatus *physiol.* Akkommodationsapparat *m.*
accommodation phosphene *patho., neuro.* Akkommodationsphosphen *nt.*

accommodation reflex *physiol.* Naheinstellungsreaktion *f*, -reflex *m*, Akkommodationsreflex *m*.
accommodation spasm *ophthal.* Akkommodationskrampf *m*.
accommodation system *physiol.* Akkommodationssystem *nt*.
ac·com·mo·da·tive [əˈkɑmədeɪtɪv] *adj* akkommodativ.
accommodative asthenopia *ophthal.* akkommodative Asthenopie *f*.
accommodative capacity Akkommodationsfähigkeit *f*.
accommodative strabismus *ophthal.* Strabismus accommodativus.
ac·com·mo·dom·e·ter [ə͵kɑməˈdɑmɪtər] *n* Akkommodometer *nt*.
ac·com·pa·ny·ing [əˈkʌmpəniːɪŋ] *adj* begleitend, Begleit-.
accompanying artery Begleitarterie *f*, A. comitans.
  a. of ischiatic nerve Begleitarterie des N. ischiadicus, A. comitans n. ischiadici/sciatici.
  a. of median nerve Begleitarterie des N. medianus, A. comitans n. mediani.
accompanying vein Begleitvene *f*, V. comitans.
  a. of hypoglossal nerve Begleitvene des N. hypoglossus, V. comitans n. hypoglossi.
ac·com·plish [əˈkʌmplɪʃ] *vt* schaffen, vollbringen, ausführen, etw. zustande bringen.
ac·cord [əˈkɔːrd] **I** *n* Übereinstimmung *f*, Einigkeit *f*. **II** *vi* s./einander entsprechen, übereinstimmen (*with* mit).
ac·cor·di·on graft [əˈkɔːrdjən, -dɪən] Mesh-Graft *f*/*nt*, Mesh-Transplantat *nt*, Maschen-, Gittertransplantat *nt*.
ac·couche·ment [əˈkuːʃmənt, -mɑ̃ːŋ] *n gyn.* Geburt *f*, Entbindung *f*, Partus *m*.
ac·cou·cheur [͵ækuːˈʃɜr] *n* Geburtshelfer *m*.
accoucheur's hand Geburtshelferhand *f*.
ac·cou·cheuse [͵ækuːˈʃɜz] *n* Hebamme *f*.
ac·count [əˈkaʊnt] **I** *n* Bericht *m*, Darstellung *f*. **to give an ~ of** Bericht erstatten über. **II** *vi* erklären (*for*). **to ~ (to s.o.) for** jdm. Rechenschaft ablegen über, s. (jdm. gegenüber) verantworten für.
ac·cre·tio [əˈkriːʃɪəʊ] *n* → accretion 1.
ac·cre·tion [əˈkriːʃn] *n* **1.** pathologische Verwachsung *f*, Verklebung *f*. **2.** Anwachsen *nt*, Wachstum *nt*, Zuwachs *m*, Zunahme *f*. **3.** → accumulation.
accretion lines *dent.* Retzius'-Streifung *f*.
ac·cu·mu·late [əˈkjuːmjəleɪt] **I** *vt* ansammeln, auf-, anhäufen, akkumulieren; (*a. techn.*) (auf-)speichern, (*a. psycho.*) (auf-)stauen. **II** *vi* anwachsen, s. auf- od. anhäufen, s. ansammeln *od.* akkumulieren; (*a. psycho.*) s. (auf-)stauen.
ac·cu·mu·la·tion [ə͵kjuːmjəˈleɪʃn] *n* Ansammlung *f*, Auf-, Anhäufung *f*, Akkumulation *f*; (Auf-)Speicherung *f*; (*a. psycho.*) (Auf-)Stauung *f*.
accumulation disease Speicherkrankheit *f*, Thesaurismose *f*.
ac·cu·mu·la·tive [əˈkjuːmjəleɪtɪv, -lətɪv] *adj* (an-)wachsend, an-, aufhäufend, akkumulierend, Häufungs-.
ac·cu·ra·cy [ˈækjərəsɪ] *n* Genauigkeit *f*, Präzision *f*; Richtigkeit *f*, Exaktheit *f*.
ac·cu·rate [ˈækjərɪt] *adj* genau, exakt, richtig, akurat; (*Person*) sorgfältig; (*Test, Diagnose*) präzise, exakt.
ACD blood [acid citrate dextrose] Frischblut *nt* mit ACD-Stabilisator.
ACD solution [acid citrate dextrose] ACD-Lösung *f*, ACD-Stabilisator *m*.
ACE *abbr.* → angiotensin converting enzyme.

a·ce·bu·to·lol [æsɪˈbjuːtəɔl, -əʊl] *n pharm.* Acebutolol *nt*.
ACE inhibitor Angiotensin-Converting-Enzym-Hemmer *m*, ACE-Hemmer *m*.
A cells 1. (*Pankreas*) A-Zellen *pl*, α-Zellen *pl*. **2.** (*Adenohypophyse*) azidophile Zellen, α-Zellen *pl*. **3.** amakrine Zellen *pl*.
A cell tumor (*Pankreas*) Glukagonom *nt*, Glucagonom *nt*, A-Zell(en)-Tumor *m*.
a·cel·lu·lar [eɪˈseljələr] *adj* zellfrei, nicht aus Zellen bestehend, azellulär.
a·ce·no·cou·ma·rin [ə͵siːnəʊˈkuːmərɪn] *n* → acenocoumarol.
a·ce·no·cou·ma·rol [͵-ˈkuːmərɔl, -əʊl] *n pharm.* Acenocoumarol *nt*.
a·cen·tric [eɪˈsentrɪk] **I** *n* → acentric chromosome. **II** *adj* nicht im Zentrum (liegend), nichtzentral, azentrisch.
acentric chromosome azentrisches Chromosom *nt*.
a·ce·pha·lia [͵eɪsɪˈfeɪlɪə] *n embryo.* Azephalie *f*, Acephalie *f*.
a·ceph·a·lism [eɪˈsefəlɪzəm] *n* → acephalia.
a·ceph·a·lo·bra·chia [eɪ͵sefələʊˈbreɪkɪə] *n embryo.* Azephalobrachie *f*.
a·ceph·a·lo·bra·chi·us [͵-ˈbreɪkɪəs] *n embryo.* Azephalobrachius *m*.
a·ceph·a·lo·car·dia [͵-ˈkɑːrdɪə] *n embryo.* Azephalokardie *f*.
a·ceph·a·lo·car·di·us [͵-ˈkɑːrdɪəs] *n embryo.* Azephalokardius *m*.
a·ceph·a·lo·chi·ria [͵-ˈkaɪrɪə] *n embryo.* Azephalochirie *f*.
a·ceph·a·lo·chi·rus [͵-ˈkaɪrəs] *n embryo.* Azephalochirus *m*.
a·ceph·a·lo·gas·ter [͵-ˈgæstər] *n embryo.* Azephalogaster *m*.
a·ceph·a·lo·gas·tria [͵-ˈgæstrɪə] *n embryo.* Azephalogastrie *f*.
a·ceph·a·lo·po·dia [͵-ˈpəʊdɪə] *n embryo.* Azephalopodie *f*.
a·ceph·a·lo·po·di·us [͵-ˈpəʊdɪəs] *n embryo.* Azephalopodius *m*.
a·ceph·a·lo·rha·chia [͵-ˈreɪkɪə] *n embryo.* Azephalorrhachie *f*.
a·ceph·a·lo·sto·mia [͵-ˈstəʊmɪə] *n embryo.* Azephalostomie *f*.
a·ceph·a·lo·sto·mus [eɪ͵sefəˈlɑstəməs] *n embryo.* Azephalostomus *m*.
a·ceph·a·lo·tho·ra·cia [eɪ͵sefələʊθəːˈreɪsɪə] *n* Azephalothoracie *f*.
a·ceph·a·lo·tho·rus [͵-ˈθɔːrəs] *n embryo.* Azephalothorus *m*.
a·ceph·a·lous [eɪˈsefələs] *adj embryo.* ohne Kopf, kopflos, azephal.
a·ceph·a·lus [eɪˈsefələs] *n*, *pl* **-li** [-laɪ, -liː] *embryo.* kopflose Mißgeburt *f*, Azephaler *m*, Acephalus *m*, Acephalus *m*.
a·ceph·a·ly [eɪˈsefəlɪ] *n* → acephalia.
a·cer·vu·lus [əˈsɜrvjələs] *n*, *pl* **-li** [-laɪ] Hirnsand *m*, Acervulus *m* (cerebri).
a·ces·cent [əˈsesənt] *adj* säuerlich, leicht sauer.
a·ces·o·dyne [əˈsesədaɪn] *adj* schmerzlindernd, -stillend.
ac·e·tab·u·lar [͵æsɪˈtæbjələr] *adj* Azetabulum *nt* betr., azetabular, azetabulär, Hüftpfannen-, Acetabulum-.
acetabular angle Pfannendachwinkel *m*.
acetabular artery 1. Azetabulumast *m* der A. circumflexa femoris medialis, Ramus acetabularis a. circumflexae femoris medialis. **2.** Hüftkopfarterie *f*, *old* A. acetabuli, Ramus acetabularis a. obturatoriae.
acetabular bone *old* → acetabulum.
acetabular branch: a. of medial circumflex femoral artery → acetabular artery 1.
  a. of obturator artery → acetabular artery 2.
acetabular cavity → acetabulum.
acetabular dysplasia (Hüft-)Pfannendysplasie *f*, Acetabulumdysplasie *f*.

acetabular edge Pfannen-, Azetabulumrand *m*, Limbus acetabuli, Margo acetabulaːːː.
acetabular fossa Fossa acetabuli/acetabularis.
acetabular fracture Hüftpfannenbruch *m*, -fraktur *f*, Acetabulumfraktur *f*.
acetabular index *ortho.* Pfannendachwinkel *m*.
acetabular labrum Pfannenlippe *f*, Labrum acetabulare.
acetabular limbus → acetabular edge.
acetabular lip → acetabular labrum.
acetabular notch Inc. acetabuli/acetabularis.
acetabular reamer *ortho.* (Hüft-)Pfannenfräse *f*.
ac·e·tab·u·lec·to·my [͵æsɪ͵tæbjəˈlektəmɪ] *n ortho.* Azetabulumexzision *f*, Azetabulektomie *f*.
ac·e·tab·u·lo·plas·ty [æsɪˈtæbjələʊ͵plæstɪ] *n ortho.* Azetabuloplastik *f*.
ac·e·tab·u·lum [͵æsɪˈtæbjələm] *n*, *pl* **-la** [-lə] Hüft(gelenks)pfanne *f*, Azetabulum *nt*, Acetabulum *nt*.
ac·e·tal [ˈæsɪtæl] *n chem.* Azetal *nt*, Acetal *nt*, Vollazetal *nt*.
acetal bond Acetalbindung *f*.
ac·et·al·de·hyde [͵æsɪˈtældəhaɪd] *n* Azet-, Acetaldehyd *m*, Äthanal *nt*, Ethanal *nt*.
acetaldehyde dehydrogenase Aldehyddehydrogenase *f*.
acetaldehyde reductase Alkoholdehydrogenase *f abbr.* AD, ADH.
acetal linkage *chem.* Azetalbindung *f*.
ac·et·am·ide [əˈsetəmaɪd] *n* Azetamid *nt*.
ac·et·a·mi·no·phen [͵æsɪtəˈmiːnəfen] *n pharm.* Paracetamol *nt*.
ac·et·an·i·lid [͵æsɪˈtænlɪd] *n* → acetanilide.
ac·et·an·i·lide [͵æsɪˈtænlaɪd] *n* Azet-, Acet-anilid *nt*, Phenylacetamid *nt*.
ac·et·an·i·line [͵æsɪˈtænlɪn, -laɪn] *n* → acetanilide.
ac·e·tan·nin [æsəˈtænɪn] *n* → acetyltannic acid.
ac·et·ar·sol [͵æsɪˈtɑːrsɔl, -əʊl] *n* → acetarsone.
ac·et·ar·sone [͵æsɪˈtɑːrsəʊn] *n pharm.* Azetarsol *f*.
a·ce·tas [əˈsiːtæs] *n* → acetate.
a·ce·tate [ˈæsɪteɪt] *n* Azetat *nt*, Acetat *nt*.
acetate agar *micro.* Azetatagar *m*/*nt*.
acetate kinase Azetatkinase *f abbr.* AK.
acetate replacing factor *old* → lipoic acid.
a·cet·a·zol·a·mide [ə͵setəˈzəʊləmaɪd] *n pharm.* Azetazolamid *nt*.
a·ce·tic [əˈsiːtɪk, əˈset-] *adj* **1.** Essig(säure) betr., Essig-. **2.** sauer.
acetic acid Essigsäure *f*, Äthan-, Ethansäure *f*.
  glacial a. Eisessig *m*.
acetic acid anhydride Essigsäure-, Azetanhydrid *nt*.
acetic acid reaction *lab.* Rivalta-Probe *f*.
acetic aldehyde → acetaldehyde.
acetic anhydride → acetic acid anhydride.
a·ce·ti·fy [əˈsiːtɪfaɪ, əˈset-] **I** *vt* in Essig verwandeln, säuern. **II** *vi* sauer werden.
ac·e·tim·e·ter [͵æsɪˈtɪmɪtər] *n* Säuremesser *m*.
a·ce·to·ac·e·tate [ə͵siːtəʊˈæsɪteɪt, ͵æsɪtəʊ-] *n* Azetoazetat *nt*.
a·ce·to·a·ce·tic acid [͵-əˈsiːtɪk, -əˈsetɪk] *n* Azetessigsäure *f*, β-Ketobuttersäure *f*.
acetoacetic aciduria Azetessigsäureausscheidung *f* im Harn, Diazeturie *f*.
a·ce·to·a·ce·tyl-CoA [͵-əˈsiːtl, -əˈsetl] *n* → acetoacetyl coenzyme A.
acetoacetyl-CoA acyltransferase Acetyl-CoA-Acyltransferase *f*.

acetoacetyl-CoA reductase Azetoazetyl-, Acetoacetyl-CoA-Reduktase *f*.
acetoacetyl-CoA thiolase → acetyl-CoA acetyltransferase.
acetoacetyl coenzyme A Azetoazetyl-, Acetoacetylcoenzym A *nt*, Azetoazetyl- -CoA *nt*.
A·ce·to·bac·ter [ˌ-ˈbæktər] *n micro*. Essig- (säure)bakterien *pl*, Acetobacter *m*.
A·ce·to·bac·te·ra·ce·ae [ˌ-bæktɪˈreɪsiː] *pl micro*. Acetobacteraceae *pl*.
a·ce·to·form [əˈsiːtəfɔːrm] *n* Methenamin *nt*, Hexamin *nt*, Hexamethylentetramin *nt*.
ac·e·to·hex·a·mide [əˌsiːtəʊˈheksəmaɪd, ˌæsɪtəʊ-] *n pharm*. Azetohexamid *nt*.
a·cet·o·in [əˈsetəʊɪn] *n* Acetoin *nt*.
a·ce·to·ki·nase [əˌsiːtəʊˈkaɪneɪz, ˌæsɪtəʊ-, -ˈkɪn-] *n* → acetate kinase.
a·ce·to·lac·tate [ˌ-ˈlækteɪt] *n* Azetolaktat *nt*, Acetolactat *nt*.
acetolactate mutase Azetolaktatmutase *f*.
acetolactate synthase Azetolaktatsynthase *f*.
a·ce·to·lac·tic acid [ˌ-ˈlæktɪk] Azeto-, Acetomilchsäure *f*.
ac·e·tol·y·sis [ˌæsɪˈtɒləsɪs] *n chem*. kombinierte Hydrolyse u. Acetylierung, Azeto-, Acetolyse *f*.
ac·e·tom·e·ter [ˌæsɪˈtɒmɪtər] *n* → acetimeter.
a·ce·to·mor·phine [əˌsiːtəʊˈmɔːrfiːn, ˌæsɪtəʊ-] *n pharm*. Heroin *nt*, Dia(cetyl)morphin *nt*.
ac·e·tone [ˈæsɪtəʊn] *n* Azeton *nt*, Aceton *nt*, Dimethylketon *nt*.
acetone bodies Keto(n)körper *pl*.
a·ce·to·ne·mia [əˌsiːtəˈniːmɪə, ˌæsɪtə-] *n* Azetonämie *f*, Ketonämie *f*.
a·ce·to·ne·mic [ˌ-ˈniːmɪk] *adj* azetonämisch, ketonämisch.
ac·e·ton·gly·cos·u·ria [ˌæsətəʊnˌɡlaɪkəʊˈsjʊərɪə] *n* Acetonglukosurie *f*.
ac·e·to·ni·trile [əˌsiːtəʊˈnaɪtrɪl, ˌæsɪtəʊ-] *n* Azeto-, Acetonitril *nt*.
ac·e·ton·u·ria [ˌ-ˈn(j)ʊərɪə] *n* Acetonurie *f*, Ketonurie *f*.
ac·e·to·phen·a·zine [ˌ-ˈfenəziːn] *n pharm*. Azetophenazin *nt*.
ac·e·to·phe·net·i·din [ˌ-fɪˈnetədiːn] *n pharm*. Phenazetin *nt*, Phenacetin *nt*.
a·ce·to·sal [əˈsiːtəsæl] *n* → acetylsalicylic acid.
a·ce·to·sol·u·ble [əˌsiːtəʊˈsɒljəbl, ˌæsɪtəʊ-] *adj* in Essigsäure löslich, essigsäurelöslich.
ac·e·tous [ˈæsɪtəs] *adj* Essigsäure betr. *od*. bildend, Essigsäure-.
ac·et·phen·ar·sine [ˌæsetfenˈɑːrsiːn] *n* → acetarsone.
ac·et·phe·net·i·din [ˌ-fɪˈnetədiːn] *n pharm*. Phenazetin *nt*, Phenacetin *nt*.
ac·et·py·ro·gall [ˌ-ˈpaɪrəɡæl] *n pharm*. Pyrogallolacetriacitat *nt*.
ac·e·tri·zo·ate [ˌæsɪtraɪˈzəʊeɪt] *n radiol*. Azetrizoat *nt*.
a·ce·tum [əˈsiːtəm] *n, pl* -ta [-tə] 1. Essig *m*, Acetum *nt*. 2. Essig(säure)lösung *f*.
a·cet·u·rate [əˈsetʃəreɪt] *n* N-Acetylglycinat *nt*.
a·ce·tyl [əˈsiːtl, ˈæsətɪl, -tiːl] *n* Azetyl-, Acetyl-(Radikal *nt*).
a·ce·tyl·am·i·no·ben·zene [ˌæsətɪlˌæmɪnəʊˈbenziːn, ˌæsətɪl-] *n* acetanilide.
a·ce·tyl·am·i·no·flu·o·rene [ˌ-ˌæmɪnəʊˈflʊəriːn] *n* Acetylaminofluoren *nt*.
a·cet·y·lase [əˈsetləɪz] *n* → acetyltransferase.
a·cet·y·late [əˈsetleɪt] **I** *vt* azetylieren, acetylieren. **II** *vi* azetyliert werden.
a·cet·y·la·tion [əˌsetəˈleɪʃn] *n* Azetylierung *f*, Acetylierung *f*.

a·ce·tyl·car·ni·tine [ˌæsətɪlˈkɑːrnətiːn, ˌæsətɪl-] *n* Acetylcarnitin *nt*.
acetyl chloride Azetyl-, Acetylchlorid *nt*.
a·ce·tyl·cho·line [ˌ-ˈkəʊliːn] *n abbr*. ACh Azetyl-, Acetylcholin *nt abbr*. ACh.
acetylcholine antagonist Azetylcholinantagonist *m*.
acetylcholine receptor antibodies Acetylcholin-Rezeptor-Antikörper *pl*.
a·ce·tyl·cho·lin·er·gic [ˌ-ˌkəʊləˈnɜːrdʒɪk, -ˌkɑlə-] *adj* azetylcholinerg.
acetylcholinergic synapse azetylcholinerge Synapse *f*.
ac·e·tyl·cho·lin·es·ter·ase [-kəʊlɪˈnestəreɪz] *n abbr*. **AChE** Azetyl-, Acetylcholinesterase *f abbr*. AChE, echte Cholinesterase *f*.
acetylcholinesterase inhibitor (Acetyl-)- Cholinesterasehemmer *m*, -inhibitor *m*.
acetyl-CoA → acetyl coenzyme A.
acetyl-CoA acetyltransferase Acetyl- -CoA-Acetyltransferase *f*, (Acetoacetyl-)Thiolase *f*.
acetyl-CoA acyltransferase Acetyl-CoA- -acyltransferase *f*.
acetyl-CoA carboxylase Acetyl-CoA- -Carboxylase *f*.
acetyl-CoA:α-glucosaminide-N-acetyltransferase Acetyl-CoA:α-Glukosaminid-N-Acetyltransferase *f*.
acetyl-CoA:heparan-α-D-glucosaminide-N-acetyltransferase → acetyl-CoA: α-glucosaminide-N-acetyltransferase.
acetyl-CoA synthetase Acetyl-CoA-Synthetase *f*.
acetyl coenzyme A Azetyl-, Acetylcoenzym A *nt*, Acetyl-CoA *nt*.
ac·e·tyl·cys·te·ine [ˌæsətɪlˈsɪstiːiːn, ˌæsətɪl-] *n pharm*. Acetylcystein *nt*, Acetylzystein *nt*.
4-a·ce·tyl·cyt·i·dine [ˌ-ˈsɪtɪdiːn] *n* 4-Acetylcytidin *nt*.
N⁴-a·ce·tyl·cy·to·sine [ˌ-ˈsaɪtəsiːn, -sɪn] *n* N⁴-Acetylcytosin *nt*.
ac·e·tyl·dig·i·tox·in [ˌ-ˌdɪdʒəˈtɒksɪn] *n pharm*. Acetyldigitoxin *nt*.
a·cet·y·lene [əˈsetlɪn, -iːn] *n* Azetylen *nt*, Acetylen *nt*, Äthin *nt*, Ethin *nt*.
acetylene tretrachloride Tetrachloräthan *nt*, -ethan *nt*.
N-a·ce·tyl·ga·lac·tos·a·mine-4-sulfatase [ˌæsətɪlɡəˌlækˈtəʊsəmiːn, ˌæsətɪl-] *n* N- -Acetylgalactosamine-4-sulfatase *f*.
N-acetylgalactosamine-4-sulfatase deficiency *n* Maroteaux-Lamy-Syndrom *nt*, Morbus Maroteaux-Lamy *m*, Mukopolysaccharidose VI *f abbr*. MPS VI.
N-acetylgalactosamine-6-sulfatase *n* N- -Acetylgalactosamine-6-sulfatase *f*, Chondroitinsulfatsulfatase *f*.
N-acetylgalactosamine-6-sulfatase deficiency Morquio-Syndrom Typ A *nt*.
α-N-a·ce·tyl·ga·lac·tos·a·min·i·dase [ˌ-ɡəˌlæktəʊsəˈmɪnɪdeɪz] *n* α-N-Acetylgalactosaminidase *f*.
β-N-acetylgalactosaminidase β-N-Acetylgalactosaminidase *f*, N-Acetyl-β- -Hexosaminidase A *f*.
N-acetyl-D-glucosamine *n* N-Acetyl-D- -Glukosamin *nt*.
N-a·ce·tyl·glu·co·sa·mine-6-sulfatase [ˌ-ɡluːˈkəʊsəmiːn, -mɪn] *n* N-Acetylglukosamin-6-Sulfatsulfatase *f*.
α-N-a·ce·tyl·glu·co·sa·min·i·dase [ˌ-ɡluːˌkəʊsəˈmɪnɪdeɪz] *n* α-N-Acetylglukosaminidase *f*.
N-acetyl-α-D-glucosaminide-6-sulfatase *n* N-Acetylglukosamin-6-Sulfatsulfatase *f*.
a·ce·tyl·glu·ta·mate [ˌ-ˈɡluːtəmeɪt] *n* Azetyl-, Acetylglutamat *nt*.

acetylglutamate kinase Acetylglutamatkinase *f*.
N-a·ce·tyl·glu·tam·ic acid [ˌ-ɡluːˈtæmɪk] N-Acetylglutaminsäure *f*.
acetyl glyceryl ether phosphoryl choline *abbr*. **AGEPC** Plättchen-aktivierender Faktor *m abbr*. PAF, platelet activating factor *m*, platelet aggregating factor *m*.
N-acetyl-β-hexosaminidase A → β-N- -acetylgalactosaminidase.
a·cet·y·li·za·tion [əˌsetlaɪˈzeɪʃn, -lɪˈz-] *n* → acetylation.
N-a·ce·tyl·man·no·sa·mine [ˌæsətɪlmæˈnəʊsəmiːn, ˌæsətɪl-] *n* N-Acetylmannosamin *nt*.
N-acetylmannosamine kinase N-Acetylmannosaminkinase *f*.
N-a·ce·tyl·mu·ram·ic acid [ˌ-m(j)ʊəˈræmɪk] N-Acetylmuraminsäure *f*.
N-a·ce·tyl·neu·ram·i·nate [ˌ-n(j)ʊəˈræmɪneɪt] *n* N-Acetylneuraminat *nt*.
N-acetylneuraminate lyase N-Acetylneuraminatlyase *f*.
N-acetylneuraminate-9-phosphatase *n* N-Acetylneuraminsäure-9-Phosphatase *f*.
N-acetylneuraminate-9-phosphate synthase N-Acetylneuraminat-9-Phosphat- -Synthase *f*.
N-a·ce·tyl·neur·a·min·ic acid [ˌ-n(j)ʊərəˈmiːnɪk, -əˈmɪn-] *abbr*. **NANA** N-Acetylneuraminsäure *f abbr*. NANA.
N-acetylneuraminic acid-9-phosphate N- -Acetylneuraminsäure-9-Phosphat *nt*.
N-a·ce·tyl·or·ni·thine [ˌ-ˈɔːrnəθiːn] *n* N- -Acetylornithin *nt*.
N-acetylornithine cycle N-Acetylornithin-Zyklus *m*.
acetylornithine deacetylase Acetylornithindeacetylase *f*.
acetylornithine transaminase Acetylornithintransaminase *f*.
acetyl phosphate Azetyl-, Acetylphosphat *nt*.
a·ce·tyl·sal·i·cyl·ic acid [ˌ-ˌsæləˈsɪlɪk] *abbr*. **ASA** Acetylsalicylsäure *f*, Azetylsalizylsäure *f abbr*. ASS.
a·ce·tyl·sul·fa·di·a·zine [ˌ-ˌsʌlfəˈdaɪəziːn] *n* Azetyl-, Acetylsulfadiazin *nt*.
ac·e·tyl·sul·fa·guan·i·dine [ˌ-ˌsʌlfəˈɡwænədɪn, -dɪn] *n* Azetyl-, Acetylsulfaguanidin *nt*.
ac·e·tyl·sul·fa·nil·a·mide [ˌ-ˌsʌlfəˈnɪləmaɪd] *n* Azetyl-, Acetylsulfanilamid *nt*.
ac·e·tyl·sul·fa·thi·a·zole [ˌ-ˌsʌlfəˈθaɪəzəʊl, -əʊl] *n* Azetyl-, Acetylsulfathiazol *nt*.
a·ce·tyl·tan·nic acid [ˌ-ˈtænɪk] Acetylgerbsäure *f*, Acetyltannin *nt*.
ac·e·tyl·tan·nin [ˌ-ˈtænɪn] *n* → acetyltannic acid.
ac·e·tyl·trans·fer·ase [ˌ-ˈtrænsfəreɪz] *n* Azetyl-, Acetyltransferase *f*.
AcG *abbr*. [accelerator globulin] → accelerator factor
ACh *abbr*. → acetylcholine.
A chain (*Insulin*) A-Kette *f*.
ach·a·la·sia [ˌækəˈleɪʒ(ɪ)ə, -zɪə] *n* 1. Achalasie *f*. 2. (Ösophagus-)Achalasie *f*, old Kardiospasmus *m*.
Achard [aˈfɑːr] *A*.'s **syndrome** Achard- -Syndrom *nt*.
Achard-Thiers [tjɛːr] **A.-T. syndrome** Achard-Thiers-Syndrom *nt*.
AChE *abbr*. → acetylcholinesterase.
ache [eɪk] **I** *n* (anhaltender) Schmerz *m*. **II** *vi* (anhaltend) schmerzen, weh tun.
a·chei·lia [əˈkaɪlɪə] *n embryo*. Ach(e)ilie *f*.
a·chei·lous [əˈkaɪləs] *adj embryo*. von Ach(e)ilie betr., ohne Lippen.
a·chei·ria [əˈkaɪrɪə] *n embryo*. Ach(e)irie *f*.
a·chei·ro·po·dia [əˌkaɪrəʊˈpəʊdɪə] *n embryo*. Ach(e)iropodie *f*.

acheirus

a·chei·rus [əˈkaɪrəs] n Ach(e)irus m.
aches and pains inf. Wehwehchen pl.
a·chieve [əˈtʃiːv] vt (Ziel) erreichen, schaffen; (Erfolg) erzielen; erlangen, erringen.
a·chi·lia n → acheilia.
Achilles [əˈkɪliːz]: **A. bursitis** Entzündung f der Bursa tendinis calcanei, Achillobursitis, Bursitis achillea.
A. jerk → A. tendon reflex.
ruptured A. tendon Achillessehnenruptur f, -riß m.
A. tendon Achillessehne f, Tendo calcaneus (Achillis).
A. tendon reflex Achillessehnenreflex m abbr. ASR.
a·chil·lo·bur·si·tis [əˌkiːləʊbɑrˈsaɪtɪs] n Entzündung f der Bursa tendinis calcanei, Achillobursitis, Bursitis achillea.
a·chil·lo·dyn·ia [ˌ-ˈdɪnɪə] n 1. Achillodynie f. 2. → achillobursitis.
ach·il·lor·rha·phy [ækɪˈlɔrəfɪ] n 1. Achillessehnennaht f, Achillorrhaphie f. 2. (operative) Achillessehnenverkürzung f, -raffung f, Achillorrhaphie f.
a·chil·lo·te·not·o·my [əˌkɪləʊtəˈnɒtəmɪ] n Achillessehnendurchtrennung f, Achillotenotomie f.
ach·il·lot·o·my [ækɪˈlɒtəmɪ] n → achillotenotomy.
a·chi·lous adj → acheilous.
ach·ing [ˈeɪkɪŋ] adj schmerzend; weh tun.
a·chi·ria n → acheiria.
a·chi·rus n → acheirus.
a·chlor·hy·dria [ˌeɪklɔːrˈhaɪdrɪə] n Magensäuremangel m, Magenanazidität f, Achlorhydrie f.
a·chlor·hy·dric [ˌ-ˈhaɪdrɪk] adj Achlorhydrie betr. od. zeigend, achlorhydrisch.
achlorhydric anemia Faber-Anämie f, Chloranämie f.
A·cho·le·plas·ma [ˌəkələˈplæzmə] n micro. Acholeplasma f.
A·cho·le·plas·ma·ta·ce·ae [əkələˌplæzməˈteɪsiː] pl micro. Acholeplasmataceae pl.
a·cho·lia [eɪˈkəʊlɪə] n mangelhafte od. fehlende Galle(n)ausscheidung f, Gallenmangel m, Acholie f.
a·chol·ic [eɪˈkɒlɪk] adj Acholie betr., frei von Galle, acholisch.
ach·o·lu·ria [ækəˈlʊərɪə] n Acholurie f.
ach·o·lu·ric [ækəˈlʊərɪk] adj Acholurie betr., ohne Ausscheidung von Gallenpigment im Harn, acholurisch.
acholuric (familial) jaundice hereditäre Sphärozytose f, Kugelzell(en)anämie f, -ikterus m, familiärer hämolytischer Ikterus m, Morbus Minkowski-Chauffard m.
a·chon·dro·gen·e·sis [eɪˌkɒndrəˈdʒenəsɪs] n Achondrogenesis f.
a·chon·dro·pla·sia [ˌ-ˈpleɪʒ(ɪ)ə, -zɪə] n Parrot-Krankheit f, -Syndrom nt, Parrot-Kauffmann-Syndrom nt, Achondroplasie f; Achondroplasia f, fetale Chondrodystrophie f, Chondrodystrophia fetalis.
a·chon·dro·plast [eɪˈkɒndrəplæst] n Chondrodystrophiker(in f) m, Achondroplast m.
a·chon·dro·plas·tic [ˌ-ˈplæstɪk] adj Achondro(dys)plasie betr., von Achondro(dys)plasie betroffen, achondroplastisch.
achondroplastic dwarf Chondrodystrophiker(in f) m, Achondroplast m, chondrodystropherachondroplastischer Zwerg m.
a·chon·dro·plas·ty [ˌ-ˈplæstɪ] n → achondroplasia.
A·cho·ri·on [əˈkɔːrɪɒn] n micro. Trichophyton m.
a·chres·tic [əˈkrestɪk] adj achrestisch.
achrestic anemia achrestische Anämie f.
a·chro·ma·sia [ˌeɪkrəʊˈmeɪʒ(ɪ)ə] n 1. Pigmentmangel m der Haut, Achromasie f. 2. histol. Achromasie f, Achromie f.
ach·ro·mat [ˈeɪkrəmæt, ˈæk-] n 1. → achromatic objective. 2. Farbenblinde(r m) f, Patient(in f) m mit Monochromasie f.
a·chro·mate [ˈækrəmeɪt] n → achromat 2.
Ach·ro·ma·ti·a·ce·ae [ˌækrəʊˌmætəˈeɪsiː], -meɪʃɪ-] pl micro. Achromatiaceae pl.
ach·ro·mat·ic [ˌækrəˈmætɪk, ˌeɪk-] adj 1. unbunt, achromatisch. 2. Achromatin enthaltend. 3. histol. nicht od. schwer anfärbbar.
achromatic lens achromatische Linse f.
achromatic objective achromatisches Objektiv nt, Achromat m.
achromatic vision → achromatopsy.
achro·ma·tin [eɪˈkrəʊmətɪn] n Achromatin nt, Euchromatin nt.
a·chro·ma·tism [eɪˈkrəʊmətɪzəm] n → achromatopsy.
a·chro·mat·o·phil [ˌeɪkrəˈmætəfɪl, ˌæk-, eɪˈkrəʊmətə-] n achromatophiler Organismus m. II adj schwer anfärbend, achromatophil.
a·chro·mat·o·phil·ic [ˌ-ˈfɪlɪk] adj → achromatophil II.
a·chro·ma·top·sia [eɪˌkrəʊməˈtɒpsɪə] n → achromatopsy.
a·chro·ma·top·sy [ˌ-ˈtɒpsɪ] n (totale) Farbenblindheit f, Achromatopsie f, Monochromasie f, Einfarbensehen nt.
a·chro·ma·to·sis [ˌ-ˈtəʊsɪs] n 1. Pigmentmangel m, Achromasie f. 2. histol. fehlendes Färbevermögen nt, Achromatosis f.
a·chro·ma·tous [eɪˈkrəʊmətəs] adj farblos, achromatisch.
a·chro·ma·tu·ria [eɪˌkrəʊməˈt(j)ʊərɪə] n Achromaturie f.
a·chro·mia [eɪˈkrəʊmɪə] n Achromie f, Achromasie f, Achromia f.
a·chro·mic nevus [eɪˈkrəʊmɪk, æˈk-] hypomelanotischer Nävus m, Naevus achromicus/depigmentosus/albus.
A·chro·mo·bac·ter [eɪˈkrəʊməbæktər] n micro. Achromobacter m.
a·chro·mo·cyte [eɪˈkrəʊməsaɪt] n hema. Achromo(retikulo)zyt m, Halbmondkörper m, Schilling-Halbmond m.
a·chro·mo·phil [eɪˈkrəʊməfɪl] n, adj → achromatophil.
a·chro·moph·i·lous [eɪkrəʊˈmɒfɪləs] adj → achromatophil II.
Achucárro [ɑtʃuˈkɑro] n: **A.'s stain** Achucárro-Färbung f.
a·chy·lia [eɪˈkaɪlɪə] n patho. Achylie f, Achylia f.
a·chy·lic anemia [eɪˈkaɪlɪk] idiopathische hypochrome Anämie f.
a·chy·mia [eɪˈkaɪmɪə] n Achymie f, Achymia f.
ach·y·mo·sis [ækɪˈməʊsɪs] n → achymia.
a·cic·u·lar [əˈsɪkjələr] adj nadelförmig.
ac·id [ˈæsɪd] I n 1. chem. Säure f. 2. sauerschmeckende Substanz f. 3. sl. Lysergsäurediäthylamid nt abbr. LSD, Lysergid nt. II adj 4. chem. sauer, säurehaltig, Säure-. 5. (Geschmack) sauer, scharf. 6. fig. ätzend, beißend, bissig.
acid agglutination Säureagglutination f.
ac·id·am·i·nu·ria [æsɪdˌæmɪˈn(j)ʊərɪə] n Aminoazidurie f.
acid anhydride Säureanhydrid nt.
acid-base balance physiol. Säure-Basen-Haushalt m.
acid-base catalysis Säure-Basen-Katalyse f.
acid-base equilibrium → acid-base balance.
acid-base indicator Säure-Basen-Indikator m.
acid-base pair Säure-Basen-Paar nt.
acid-base reaction Säure-Basen-Reaktion f.
acid-base status physiol. Säure-Basen--Status m.
acid catalysis Säurekatalyse f.
acid cell (Magen) Belegzelle f, Parietalzelle f.
acid dye saurer/anionischer Farbstoff m.
acid dyspepsia Dyspepsia acida.
acid elution test hema. Säureelutionstest m.
ac·i·de·mia [æsəˈdiːmɪə] n Azidämie f, dekompensierte Azidose f.
acid-fast adj histol., micro. säurefest.
acid-fast bacteria säurefeste Bakterien pl.
acid-fastness n histol., micro. Säurefestigkeit f.
acid-fast stain säurefeste Färbung f, Färbung f säurefester Bakterien nt.
acid glands Magendrüsen f, Fundus- u. Korpusdrüsen pl, Gll. gastricae propriae.
α₁-acid glycoprotein saures α₁-Glykoprotein nt, α₁-saures Glykoprotein nt.
acid halide Säurehalogenid nt.
acid hydrolase saure Hydrolase f.
acid hydrolysis saure Hydrolyse f.
a·cid·ic [əˈsɪdɪk] adj 1. säurebildend, -reich, -haltig. 2. chem. sauer, säurehaltig, Säure-. 3. silikathaltig.
acidic dye → acid dye.
acidic glycosphingolipid Gangliosid nt, saures Glykosphingolipid nt.
a·cid·i·fi·a·ble [əˈsɪdəfaɪəbl] adj ansäuerbar.
a·cid·i·fi·ca·tion [əˌsɪdəfɪˈkeɪʃn] n 1. Ansäuern nt, Azidifizierung f. 2. (An-)Säuerung f, Azidifikation f.
a·cid·i·fi·er [əˈsɪdəfaɪər] n ansäuernde Substanz f, Säuerungsmittel nt.
a·cid·i·fy [əˈsɪdəfaɪ] I vt (an-)säuern, in Säure verwandeln. II vi sauer werden.
ac·i·dim·e·try [ˌæsɪˈdɪmətrɪ] n 1. Azidimetrie f. 2. Azidometrie f.
acid indigestion (Magen) erhöhte Salzsäureproduktion f, Hyperazidität f, Hyperchlorhydrie f.
acid-induced injury → acid injury.
acid injury Säureverletzung f, -verätzung f, -schädigung f.
acid-insoluble adj säureunlöslich.
a·cid·i·ty [əˈsɪdətɪ] n 1. Säuregrad m, -gehalt m, Azidität f, Acidität f. 2. Säure f, Schärfe f.
acid-labile adj säurelabil.
acid-maltase deficiency Pompe-Krankheit f, generalisierte maligne Glykogenose f, Glykogenose Typ II f.
acid mucopolysaccharides saure Mucopolysaccharide pl.
a·cid·o·gen·ic [əˌsɪdəˈdʒenɪk, ˌæsɪdə-] adj säurebildend, azidogen.
a·cid·o·phil [əˈsɪdəfɪl, ˈæsɪdəʊ-] I n 1. azidophile Zelle od. Struktur f. 2. (Hypophyse) azidophile Zelle f, α-Zelle f. 3. bio. auf saurem Nährboden wachsende Organismen. II adj 4. bio. auf saurem Nährböden wachsend, azido-, acidophil. 5. mit sauren Farbstoffen färbend, azido-, acido-, oxyphil.
acidophil adenoma eosinophiles (Hypophysen-)Adenom nt.
acidophil cell → acidophilic cell.
ac·i·doph·ile [ˈ-faɪl] n, adj → acidophil.
acidophile cell → acidophilic cell.
acidophile granules azidophile Granula pl.
ac·i·do·phil·i·a [ˌ-ˈfiːlɪə] n 1. Eosinophilie f, Eosinophilämie f. 2. eosinophile Beschaffenheit f, Eosinophilie f.
ac·i·do·phil·ic [ˌ-ˈfɪlɪk] adj → acidophil II.
acidophilic adenoma azidophiles/azidophilzelliges (Hypophysen-)Adenom nt.

acidophilic carcinoma azidophilzelliges Karzinom *nt*.
acidophilic cell 1. → acidophil 1. **2.** (*Adenohypophyse*) azidophile Zelle *f*, α-Zelle *f*.
acidophilic erythroblast → acidophilic normoblast.
acidophilic normoblast azidophiler/ orthochromatischer/oxyphiler Normoblast *m*.
ac·i·do·sic [ˌæsɪˈdəʊsɪk] *adj* → acidotic.
ac·i·do·sis [ˌæsɪˈdəʊsɪs] *n* Azidose *f*, Acidose *f*.
ac·i·dos·t·eo·phyte [ˌæsɪˈdɒstɪəʊfaɪt] *n* spitzer Osteophyt *m*.
ac·i·dot·ic [ˌæsɪˈdɒtɪk] *adj* Azidose betr., von Azidose gekennzeichnet, azidotisch, Azidose-.
acid phosphatase *abbr*. **ACP** saure Phosphatase *f abbr*. SP.
acid phosphatase reaction *histol*. Saure-Phosphatase-Reaktion *f*.
acid phosphate saures Phosphat *nt*.
acid phosphomonoesterase → acid phosphatase.
acid reaction *chem*. **1.** saure Reaktion *f*, saures Verhalten *nt*. **2.** Säurenachweis *m*.
acid reflux Säurereflux *m*.
acid salt *chem*. saures Salz *nt*.
acid-soluble *adj* säurelöslich.
acid stability Säurestabilität *f*.
acid-stable *adj* säurestabil.
acid stain saurer Farbstoff *m*.
a-cid-u-lent [əˈsɪdʒələnt] *adj* → acidulous.
a·cid·u·lous [əˈsɪdʒələs] *adj chem*. leicht sauer, säuerlich.
ac·i·dum [ˈæsɪdəm] *n, pl* **-da** [-də] *chem*. Säure *f*.
ac·i·du·ria [ˌæsɪˈd(j)ʊərɪə] *n* Azidurie *f*.
ac·i·du·ric [ˌæsəˈd(j)ʊːrɪk] *adj* → acidophil II.
acid value Säuregehalt *m*.
a·cid·y·la·tion [əˌsɪdəˈleɪʃn] *n* → acylation.
ac·i·nal [ˈæsɪnl] *adj* → acinar.
ac·i·nar [ˈæsɪnər, -nɑːr] *adj* Azinus betr., azinös, azinär.
acinar adenocarcinoma (*Lunge*) azinöses/alveoläres Adenokarzinom *nt*.
acinar cancer → acinar adenocarcinoma.
acinar carcinoma → acinar adenocarcinoma.
acinar cell *histol*. Azinus-, Acinuszelle *f*.
acinar cell carcinoma Azinus-Zell-Karzinom *nt*.
acinar duct *histol*. Schaltstück *nt*.
acinar gland → acinous gland.
ac·i·ne·sia [æsɪˈniːʒ(ɪ)ə] *n* → akinesia.
ac·i·net·ic [æsɪˈnetɪk] *adj* → akinetic.
Ac·i·net·o·bac·ter [æsɪˌnetəˈbæktər] *n* micro. Acinetobacter *m*.
a·cin·ic [əˈsɪnɪk] *adj* → acinar.
acinic cell adenocarcinoma → acinar adenocarcinoma.
acinic cell cancer → acinar adenocarcinoma.
acinic cell carcinoma → acinar adenocarcinoma.
a·cin·i·form [əˈsɪnəfɔːrm] *adj* **1.** beeren-, traubenförmig, azinös. **2.** Kerne enthaltend, mit Kernen gefüllt.
ac·i·ni·tis [æsɪˈnaɪtɪs] *n* (*Drüse*) Azinusentzündung *f*.
ac·i·no·nod·u·lar tuberculosis [ˌæsɪnəʊˈnɒdʒələr] azino-noduläre Lungentuberkulose *f*.
ac·i·nose [ˈæsɪnəʊs] *adj* → acinous.
acinose cancer → acinar adenocarcinoma.
acinose carcinoma → acinar adenocarcinoma.
ac·i·no·tu·bu·lar gland [ˌæsɪnəʊˈt(j)uːbjələr] *histol*. tubuloazinöse/tubuloalveoläre Drüse *f*.

ac·i·nous [ˈæsɪnəs] *adj* → acinar.
acinous adenocarcinoma → acinar adenocarcinoma.
acinous carcinoma → acinar adenocarcinoma.
acinous cell → acinar cell.
acinous gland azinöse/beerenförmige Drüse *f*.
acinous-nodose *adj histol*. azinös-nodös.
ac·i·nus [ˈæsɪnəs] *n, pl* **-ni** [-naɪ] **1.** *histol*. Azinus *m*, Acinus *m*. **2.** *anat*. (Lungen-)Azinus *m*. **3.** *bio*. Beeren- *od*. Traubenkern *m*; Einzelbeere *f*.
a. of sweat gland Schweißdrüsenkörper *m*, Corpus gl. sudoriferae.
AC joint → acromioclavicular joint.
ACL *abbr*. → cruciate ligament (of knee), anterior.
a·clad·i·o·sis [eɪˌklædɪˈəʊsɪs] *n* Akladiose *f*.
ac·me [ˈækmɪ] *n* Höhe-, Kulminationspunkt *m*, Akme *f*.
ac·ne [ˈæknɪ] *n* Finnenausschlag *m*, Akne *f*, Acne *f*.
acne bacillus Propionibacterium acnes, *old* Corynebacterium/Bact. acnes.
acne cosmetica Kosmetika-Akne *f*, Akne/Acne cosmetica.
ac·ne·form [ˈæknɪfɔːrm] *adj* → acneiform.
acneform syphilid akneiformes Syphilid *nt*.
ac·ne·gen [ˈæknɪdʒən] *n* Akne-verursachende Substanz *f*, Aknegen *n*.
ac·ne·gen·ic [ˌ-ˈdʒenɪk] *adj* Akne verursachend *od*. auslösend, aknegen.
ac·ne·i·form [ækˈneɪfɔːrm] *adj* akneähnlich, -förmig, akneiform.
ac·ne·mia [ækˈniːmɪə] *n embryo*., *patho*. Waden(muskel)atrophie *f*, Aknemie *f*.
acne rosacea keratitis Akne-Rosazea-Keratitis *f*, Rosazea-Keratitis *f*.
ac·ni·tis [ækˈnaɪtɪs] *n* Barthélemy'-Krankheit *f*, Aknitis *f*, Acnitis *f*.
ac·o·as·ma [ækəˈæsmə] *n* → acousma.
ac·o·can·ther·in [ækəˈkænθərɪn] *n pharm*. Ouabain *nt*, g-Strophanthin *nt*.
a·con·i·tase [əˈkənɪteɪs] *n* Aconitase *f*, Aconithydratase *f*.
a·con·i·tate hydratase [əˈkɒnɪteɪt] → aconitase.
ac·o·nit·ic acid [ækəˈnɪtɪk] Akonitsäure *f*.
a·con·i·tine [əˈkɒnətiːn, -tɪn] *n* Akonitin *nt*, Aconitin *nt*.
ac·o·nu·re·sis [ækənjəˈriːsɪs] *n* unwillkürlicher Harnabgang *m*.
a·cor [ˈækɔːr] *n* **1.** Säuregrad *m*, -gehalt *m*, Azidität *f*, Acidität *f*. **2.** Säure *f*, Schärfe *f*. **3.** Bitterkeit *f*, Schärfe *f*.
a·co·rea [ækəˈrɪə] *n ophthal*. Akorie *f*.
a·co·ria [əˈkɔːrɪə] *n psychia*. Akorie *f*, Bulimie *f*.
a·cor·tan [əˈkɔːrtæn] *n* Kortikotropin *nt*, -trophin *nt*, Corticotrophin(um) *nt*, (adreno-)corticotropes Hormon *nt abbr*. ACTH, Adrenokortikotropin *nt*.
Acosta [əˈkɒstə]: **A.'s disease** d'Acosta-Syndrom *nt*, (akute) Bergkrankheit *f*, Mal di Puna.
a·cou·asm [əˈkuːæzəm, ˈæku:-] *n* → acousma.
a·cous·ma [əˈkuːzmə] *n, pl* **-mas**, **-mata** [-mətə] *psychia*. Akoasma *nt*.
a·cous·mat·am·ne·sia [əˌkuːzmætæmˈniːʒ(ɪ)ə] *n neuro*. Akusmatamnesie *f*.
a·cous·tic [əˈkuːstɪk] *adj* akustisch, Gehör betr., Gehör-, Schall-, Hör-.
acoustic agnosia Seelentaubheit *f*, psychogene/sensorische Hörstummheit *f*, akustische Agnosie *f*.
acoustic agraphia akustische Agraphie *f*.
a·cous·ti·cal [əˈkuːstɪkl] *adj* → acoustic.
acoustic aphasia Worttaubheit *f*, akustische Aphasie *f*.

acoustic area Area vestibularis.
inferior a. Area vestibularis inferior.
superior a. Area vestibularis superior.
acoustic cells akustische Haarzellen *pl*.
acoustic center Hörzentrum *nt*.
acoustic chamber schalldichter Raum *m*, schalldichte Kammer *f*.
acoustic cortex Hörrinde *f*, akustischer Cortex *m*.
acoustic crest Crista *f* der Bogengangsampulle, Crista ampullaris.
acoustic duct → acoustic meatus, external.
acoustic dysesthesia akustische Überempfindlichkeit *f*, Dysakusis *f*, auditorische/akustische Dysästhesie *f*.
acoustic end-organ akustisches Endorgan *nt*; Cochlea *f*.
acoustic fatigue *HNO* Hörermüdung *f*.
acoustic field Hörfeld *nt*.
acoustic haircells akustische Haarzellen *pl*.
acoustic hallucination akustische Halluzination *f*.
acoustic hyperesthesia *HNO*, *psychia*. Hyperakusis *f*.
acoustic hypesthesia → acoustic hypoesthesia.
acoustic hypoesthesia *HNO* Hörschwäche *f*, Hyp(o)akusis *f*.
acoustic impedance akustische Impedanz *f*, akustischer Widerstand *m*, (Schall-)Impedanz *f*.
acoustic lemniscus Lemniscus lateralis.
acoustic maculae Maculae acusticae/staticae.
acoustic meatus Gehörgang *m*, Meatus acusticus.
external a. äußerer Gehörgang, Meatus acusticus externus.
external a., bony knöcherner Abschnitt des äußeren Gehörgangs, Meatus acusticus externus osseus.
external a., cartilaginous knorpeliger Abschnitt des äußeren Gehörgangs, Meatus acusticus externus cartilagineus.
external a., osseous → external a., bony.
internal a. innerer Gehörgang, Meatus acusticus internus.
internal a., bony/osseous knöcherner Abschnitt des inneren Gehörgangs, Meatus acusticus internus osseus.
acoustic nerve Akustikus *m*, Vestibulokochlearis *m*, VIII. Hirnnerv *m*, N. acusticus/vestibulocochlearis.
acoustic nerve tumor Akustikusneurinom *nt*.
acoustic neurilemoma → acoustic neurinoma.
acoustic neurinoma Akustikusneurinom *nt*.
acoustic neuroma → acoustic neurinoma.
acoustic papilla Organum spirale.
acoustic paralysis kochleäre Schwerhörigkeit *f*.
a·cous·ti·co·fa·cial reflex [əˌkuːstɪkəʊˈfeɪʃl] akustikofazialer Reflex *m*.
a·cous·ti·co·pho·bia [ˌ-ˈfəʊbɪə] *n psychia*. Akustikophobie *f*.
acoustic organ Corti'-Organ *nt*, Organum spirale.
acoustic pore: external a. äußere Öffnung *f* des knöchernen Gehörgangs, Porus acusticus externus.
internal a. Eingang *m* des inneren Gehörgangs, Porus acusticus internus.
acoustic radiation Hörstrahlung *f*, Radiatio acustica.
acoustic reflex Stapediusreflex *m*.
acoustic resistance (Schall-)Impedanz *f*, akustischer Widerstand *m*, akustische Impedanz *f*.

acoustics

a·cous·tics [ə'ku:stɪks] *pl* Akustik *f.*
acoustic schwannoma → acoustic neurinoma.
acoustic shadow (*Ultraschall*) Schallschatten *m.*
acoustic striae Striae medullares ventriculi quarti.
acoustic tubercle Tuberculum acusticum.
acoustic vesicle → auditory vesicle.
ACP *abbr.* **1.** → acid phosphatase. **2.** → acyl carrier protein.
ACP-acyltransferase *n* ACP-Acyltransferase *f.*
ACP-malonyltransferase *n* ACP-Malonyltransferase *f.*
ACPS *abbr.* → acrocephalopolysyndactyly.
ACPS I *abbr.* → acrocephalopolysyndactyly I.
ACPS II *abbr.* → acrocephalopolysyndactyly II.
ACPS III *abbr.* → acrocephalopolysyndactyly III.
ACPS IV *abbr.* → acrocephalopolysyndactyly IV.
ac·quire [ə'kwaɪər] *vt* **1.** erwerben, bekommen; erlangen, erreichen, gewinnen. **2.** (*Wissen*) (er-)lernen, erwerben.
ac·quired [ə'kwaɪərd] *adj* erworben, sekundär.
acquired agammaglobulinemia erworbene Agammaglobulinämie *f.*
acquired anemia erworbene/sekundäre Anämie *f.*
acquired astigmatism *ophthal.* erworbener Astigmatismus *m.*
acquired atelectasis (*Lunge*) erworbene/sekundäre Atelektase *f.*
acquired contracture erworbene Kontraktur *f.*
acquired defect erworbener Defekt *m.*
acquired dysmenorrhea *gyn.* erworbene/sekundäre Dysmenorrhö *f.*
acquired epilepsy erworbene/sekundäre Epilepsie *f.*
acquired hernia erworbene Hernie *f*, erworbener Bruch *m*, Hernia acquisita.
acquired hyperlipoproteinemia sekundäre/symptomatische Hyperlipoproteinämie *f.*
acquired hypogammaglobulinemia erworbene Hypogammaglobulinämie *f.*
acquired ichthyosis erworbene/symptomatische Ichthyosis *f*, Ichthyosis acquisita.
acquired immune deficiency syndrome → acquired immunodeficiency syndrome.
acquired immunity erworbene Immunität *f.*
acquired immunodeficiency syndrome *abbr.* **AIDS** erworbenes Immundefektsyndrom *nt*, acquired immunodeficiency syndrome *abbr.* AIDS.
acquired megacolon erworbenes Megakolon *nt.*
acquired tolerance *immun.* erworbene Immuntoleranz *f.*
ac·qui·si·tion [ˌækwə'zɪʃn] *n* **1.** Erwerb *m*, Anschaffung *f.* **2.** (*Wissen*) Erlernen *nt*, Erfassen *nt*, Aneignung *f.*
ac·quis·i·tus [ə'kwɪsɪtəs] *adj* → acquired.
ac·rag·no·sis [ˌækræg'nəʊsɪs] *n* → acroagnosis.
ac·ral ['ækrəl] *adj* Akren betr., akral, Akren–.
acral-lentiginous melanoma *abbr.* **ALM** akrolentiginöses (malignes) Melanom *nt abbr.* ALM.
acral perfusion Akrendurchblutung *f*, -perfusion *f.*

a·cra·nia [eɪ'kreɪnɪə] *n* Akranie *f*, Acranie *f.*
a·cra·ni·al [eɪ'kreɪnɪəl] *adj* Akranie betr., akranial, acranial.
a·cra·ni·us [eɪ'kreɪnɪəs] *n* Akranius *m*, Acranius *m.*
a·crat·u·re·sis [eɪˌkrætə'ri:sɪs] *n* erschwerte Miktion *f.*
Ac·re·mo·ni·el·la [ˌækrɪˌməʊnɪ'elə] *pl micro.* Acremoniella *pl.*
ac·re·mo·ni·o·sis [ˌækrɪˌməʊnɪ'əʊsɪs] *n* Acremonium-Infektion *f*, Akremoniose *f*, Acremoniose *f*, Cephalosporiose *f.*
Ac·re·mo·ni·um [ˌækrɪ'məʊnɪəm] *n micro.* Acremonium *nt.*
ac·rid ['ækrɪd] *adj* scharf, beißend, reizend.
ac·ri·din ['ækrɪdɪn] *n* → acridine.
ac·ri·dine ['ækrədi:n] *n* Akridin *nt*, Acridin *nt.*
acridine dyes Akridinfarbstoffe *pl.*
acridine orange Akridinorange *nt.*
acridine yellow Akridingelb *nt.*
ac·ri·mo·ny ['ækrəməʊnɪ] *n* Bitterkeit *f*, Schärfe *f.*
a·crit·o·chro·ma·cy [əˌkrɪtəʊ'krəʊməsɪ] *n ophthal.* (totale) Farbenblindheit *f*, Einfarbensehen *nt*, Monochromasie *f*, Achromatopsie *f.*
ac·ro·ag·no·sis [ˌækrəʊæg'nəʊsɪs] *n neuro.* Akroagnosie *f.*
ac·ro·an·es·the·sia [ˌ-ˌænɪs'θɪ:ʒə] *n neuro.* Akroanästhesie *f.*
ac·ro·ar·thri·tis [ˌ-ɑ:r'θraɪtɪs] *n* Gelenkentzündung/Arthritis *f* einer Extremität.
ac·ro·as·phyx·ia [ˌ-æ'sfɪksɪə, -kʃə] *n* **1.** Akroasphyxie *f*, -asphyxia *f.* **2.** → acrocyanosis.
ac·ro·blast ['-blæst] *n* Akroblast *nt.*
ac·ro·brach·y·ceph·a·ly [ˌ-ˌbrækɪ'sefəlɪ] *n* Akrobrachyzephalie *f.*
ac·ro·bys·ti·o·lith [ˌ-'bɪstɪəlɪθ] *n urol.* Vorhaut-, Präputialstein *m*, Postholith *m*, Balanolith *m*, Smegmolith *m.*
ac·ro·bys·ti·tis [ˌ-bɪs'taɪtɪs] *n* Vorhautentzündung *f*, Posthitis *f.*
ac·ro·cen·tric [ˌ-'sentrɪk] *adj* akrozentrisch.
acrocentric chromosome akrozentrisches Chromosom *nt.*
ac·ro·ce·pha·lia [ˌ-sɪ'feɪljə] *n* Spitz-, Turmschädel *m*, Akrozephalie *f*, -cephalie *f*, Oxyzephalie *f*, -cephalie *f*, Hypsizephalie *f*, -cephalie *f*, Turrizephalie *f*, -cephalie *f.*
ac·ro·ce·phal·ic [ˌ-sɪ'fælɪk] **I** *n* Patient(in *f*) *m* mit Akrozephalie. **II** *adj* Akrozephalie betr., von Akrozephalie betroffen *od.* gekennzeichnet, spitz-, turmschädelig, akrozephal, oxyzephal, hypsizephal, turrizephal.
ac·ro·ceph·a·lo·pol·y·syn·dac·ty·ly [ˌ-ˌsefələʊˌpɑlɪsɪn'dæktəlɪ] *n abbr.* **ACPS** Akrozephalopolysyndaktylie *f.*
acrocephalopolysyndactyly I *n abbr.* **ACPS I** Noack-Syndrom *nt.*
acrocephalopolysyndactyly II *n abbr.* **ACPS II** Carpenter-Syndrom *nt.*
acrocephalopolysyndactyly III *n abbr.* **ACPS III** Sakati-Nyhan-Syndrom *nt.*
acrocephalopolysyndactyly IV *n abbr.* **ACPS IV** Goodman-Syndrom *nt.*
ac·ro·ceph·a·lo·syn·dac·tyl·ia [ˌ-ˌsefələʊˌsɪndæk'tɪlɪə] *n* → acrocephalosyndactyly.
ac·ro·ceph·a·lo·syn·dac·ty·lism [ˌ-ˌsefələʊsɪn'dæktəlɪzəm] *n* → acrocephalosyndactyly.
ac·ro·ceph·a·lo·syn·dac·ty·ly [ˌ-ˌsefələʊsɪn'dæktəlɪ] *n* Akrozephalosyndaktylie *f*, Apert-Syndrom *nt.*
acrocephalosyndactyly type III *embryo., ortho.* Chotzen-(Saethre-)Syndrom *nt*, Akrozephalosyndaktylie Typ III *f.*

acrocephalosyndactyly type IV (Klein-)-Waardenburg-Syndrom *nt.*
acrocephalosyndactyly type V Noack--Syndrom *nt.*
ac·ro·ceph·a·lous [ˌ-'sefələs] *adj* → acrocephalic II.
ac·ro·ceph·a·ly [ˌ-'sefəlɪ] *n* → acrocephalia.
ac·ro·chor·don [ˌ-'kɔ:rdən] *n* Stielwarze *f*, Akrochordon *nt*, Acrochordom *nt.*
ac·ro·ci·ne·sis [ˌ-sɪ'ni:sɪs, -saɪ-] *n* pathologische/übermäßige Beweglichkeit *f.*
ac·ro·con·trac·ture [ˌ-kən'træktʃər] *n* Extremitätenkontraktur *f.*
ac·ro·cy·a·no·sis [ˌ-ˌsaɪə'nəʊsɪs] *n* Akroasphyxie *f*, Akrozyanose *f*, Acrocyanosis *f.*
ac·ro·der·ma·ti·tis [ˌ-ˌdɜrmə'taɪtɪs] *n* Akrodermatitis *f.*
ac·ro·der·ma·to·sis [ˌ-ˌdɜrmə'təʊsɪs] *n, pl* **-ses** [-si:z] Akrodermatose *f.*
ac·ro·dol·i·cho·me·lia [ˌ-ˌdɑlɪkəʊ'mi:lɪə] *n* Akrodolichomelie *f.*
ac·ro·dont ['-dɑnt] *n* Akrodont *m.*
ac·ro·dyn·ia [ˌ-'dɪnɪə] *n* Feer'-Krankheit *f*, Rosakrankheit *f*, vegetative Neurose *f* der Kleinkinder, Swift-Syndrom *nt*, Selter-Swift-Feer'-Krankheit *f*, Feer-Selter--Swift-Krankheit *f*, Akrodynie *f*, Acrodynia *f.*
ac·ro·dy·nic erythema [ˌ-'di:nɪk] → acrodynia.
ac·ro·dys·pla·sia [-dɪs'pleɪʒ(ɪ)ə, -zɪə] *n* → acrocephalosyndactyly.
ac·ro·e·de·ma [ˌ-ɪ'di:mə] *n* Akrenödem *nt.*
ac·ro·es·the·sia [ˌ-es'θi:ʒ(ɪ)ə, -zɪə] *n* **1.** erhöhte Empfindlichkeit *f* der Extremitäten. **2.** Extremitätenschmerz *m*, Akroästhesie *f.*
ac·ro·fa·cial dysostosis/syndrome [ˌ-'feɪʃl] *embryo.* Weyers-Syndrom *nt*, Dysostosis acrofacialis.
ac·rog·no·sis [ˌækrɑg'nəʊsɪs] *n neuro.* Akrognosie *f.*
ac·ro·hy·po·ther·my [ˌækrəˌhaɪpə'θɜrmɪ] *n* Akrohypothermie *f.*
ac·ro·ker·a·to·sis [ˌ-ˌkerə'təʊsɪs] *n* Akrokeratose *f.*
ac·ro·ki·ne·sia [ˌ-kɪ'ni:ʒ(ɪ)ə, -zɪə, -kaɪ-] *n* → acrocinesis.
a·cro·le·in [ə'krəʊlɪɪn] *n* Akrolein *nt*, Acrolein *nt*, Acryl-, Acrylaldehyd *m.*
ac·ro·mac·ria [ˌækrə'mækrɪə] *n* → arachnodactyly.
ac·ro·mas·ti·tis [ˌ-mæ'staɪtɪs] *n* Brustwarzenentzündung *f.*
ac·ro·me·ga·lia [ˌ-mɪ'geɪljə] *n* → acromegaly.
ac·ro·me·gal·ic [ˌ-mɪ'gælɪk] *adj* Akromegalie betr., von Akromegalie betroffen, akromegal.
acromegalic gigantism akromegaler Riesenwuchs *m.*
ac·ro·meg·a·lo·gi·gan·tism [ˌ-ˌmegələʊdʒaɪ'gæntɪzəm, -'dʒaɪgænt-] *n* Akromegalogigantismus *m.*
ac·ro·meg·a·loid [ˌ-'megələɪd] *adj* akromegaloid.
ac·ro·meg·a·ly [ˌ-'megəlɪ] *n* Akromegalie *f*, Marie-Krankheit *f*, -Syndrom *nt.*
ac·ro·me·lal·gia [ˌ-mɪ'lældʒ(ɪ)ə] *n* Gerhardt-Syndrom *nt*, Mitchell-Gerhardt--Syndrom *nt*, Weir-Mitchell-Krankheit *f*, Akromelalgie *f*, Erythromelalgie *f*, Erythralgie *f*, Erythermalgie *f.*
ac·ro·me·lic [ˌ-'mi:lɪk] *adj* Gliedmaßenende betr.
acromi- *pref.* → acromio-.
a·cro·mi·al [ə'krəʊmɪəl] *adj* Akromion betr., akromial.
acromial angle Angulus acromialis.
a. of scapula Angulus lateralis (scapulae).

acromial bone Akromion *nt*.
acromial branch: a. of subscapular artery A. subscapularis-Ast *m* zum Akromion, Ramus acromialis a. subscapularis.
a. of thoracoacromial artery A. thoracoacromialis-Ast *m* zum Akromion, Ramus acromialis a. thoraco-acromialis.
acromial bursa Bursa subdeltoidea.
subcutaneous a. Bursa subcutanea acromialis.
acromial extremity of clavicle Extremitas acromialis.
acromial network → acromial rete.
acromial process → acromion.
acromial rete Arteriennetz *nt* des Akromions, Rete acromiale.
ac·ro·mic·ri·a [ˌækrəʊˈmɪkrɪə] *n* Akromikrie *f*.
ac·ro·mik·ri·a *n* → acromicria.
acromio- *pref.* Akromio-.
a·cro·mi·o·cla·vic·u·lar [əˌkrəʊmɪəʊkləˈvɪkjələr] *adj abbr.* **AC, A.C.** Akromion u. Klavikula betr., akromioklavikular.
acromioclavicular articulation äußeres Schlüsselbeingelenk *nt*, Akromioklavikulargelenk *nt*, Schultereckgelenk *nt*, Artic. acromioclavicularis.
acromioclavicular disk Discus articularis acromioclavicularis.
acromioclavicular joint → acromioclavicular articulation.
acromioclavicular ligament Lig. acromioclaviculare.
a·cro·mi·o·cor·a·coid [ˌ-ˈkɔːrəˌkɔɪd, -ˈkɑr-] *adj* Akromion u. Proc. coracoideus betr., korakoakromial.
acromiocoracoid ligament Lig. coracoacromiale.
a·cro·mi·o·hu·mer·al [ˌ-ˈ(h)juːmərəl] *adj* Akromion u. Humerus betr., akromiohumeral.
a·cro·mi·on [əˈkrəʊmɪən] *n, pl* **-mi·a** [-mɪə] Akromion *nt*.
ac·ro·mi·on·ec·to·my [əˌkrəʊmɪəʊˈnektəmɪ] *n ortho.* Akromionresektion *f*, Akromionektomie *f*.
acromion presentation *gyn.* Schulterlage *f*.
acromion process → acromion.
a·cro·mi·o·scap·u·lar [ˌ-ˈskæpjələr] *adj* Akromion u. Skapula betr. *od.* verbindend, akromioskapular.
a·cro·mi·o·tho·rac·ic [ˌ-θɔːˈræsɪk, -θə-] *adj* Akromion u. Thorax betr. *od.* verbindend, akromiothorakal.
ac·ro·neu·ro·sis [ˌækrəʊˌnʊˈrəʊsɪs, -ˌnjʊər-] *n* Akroneurose *f*.
ac·ro·os·te·ol·y·sis [ˌ-ˌɒstɪˈɒləsɪs] *n* Akroosteolyse *f*.
ac·ro·pach·y [ˈpækɪ, əˈkrɑpəkɪ] *n* Marie-Bamberger-Syndrom *nt*, Bamberger-Marie-Syndrom *nt*, Akropachie *f*, hypertrophische-pulmonale Osteoarthropathie *f*.
ac·ro·pach·y·der·ma [ˌ-ˌpækɪˈdɜrmə] *n* Akropachydermie *f*, Pachyakrie *f*.
a. with pachyperiostitis Pachydermoperiostose *f*, Touraine-Solente-Golé-Syndrom *nt*, familiäre Pachydermoperiostose *f*, idiopathische hypertrophische Osteoarthropathie *f*, Akropachydermie *f* mit Pachydermoperiostose, Hyperostosis generalisata mit Pachydermie.
ac·ro·pa·ral·y·sis [ˌ-pəˈræləsɪs] *n* Extremitätenlähmung *f*, Akroparalyse *f*.
ac·ro·par·es·the·sia [ˌ-ˌpærəsˈθiːʒ(ɪ)ə] *n* Akroparästhesie *f*.
acroparesthesia syndrome Akroparästhesie *f*.
a·crop·a·thy [əˈkrɑpəθɪ] *n* Extremitätenerkrankung *f*.

ac·ro·pho·bia [ˌækrəˈfəʊbɪə] *n* Höhenangst *f*, Akrophobie *f*.
ac·ro·pos·thi·tis [ˌ-pɒsˈθaɪtɪs] *n* → acrobystitis.
ac·ro·scle·ro·der·ma [ˌ-ˌsklɪərəˈdɜrmə, -ˌsklɛr-] *n* → acrosclerosis.
ac·ro·scle·ro·sis [ˌ-sklɪˈrəʊsɪs] *n* Akrosklerose *f*, Akrosklerodermie *f*, Acrosclerosis *f*.
ac·ro·so·mal [ˌ-ˈsəʊml] *adj* Akrosom betr., akrosomal.
acrosomal cap → acrosome.
acrosomal granule *embryo.* Akrosombläschen *nt*.
acrosomal head cap → acrosome.
ac·ro·some [ˈsəʊm] *n* (*Spermium*) Kopfkappe *f*, Akrosom *nt*.
acrosome reaction *embryo.* Akrosomreaktion *f*.
ac·ro·sphe·no·syn·dac·tyl·ia [ˌ-ˌsfiːnəʊsɪndækˈtɪlɪə] *n* → acrocephalosyndactyly.
ac·ro·syn·dac·ty·ly [ˌ-sɪnˈdæktəlɪ] *n* Akrosyndaktylie *f*.
ac·ro·ter·ic [ˌ-ˈterɪk] *adj* Akren betr., Akro-.
a·crot·ic [əˈkrɒtɪk] *adj* **1.** (*Prozeß*) oberflächlich. **2.** Akrotie betr., akrot.
ac·ro·tism [ˈækrətɪzəm] *n* Pulslosigkeit *f*, Akrotie *f*, Akrotismus *m*.
ac·ro·troph·o·dyn·ia [ˌækrəʊˌtrɒfəˈdiːnɪə, ˌ-trəʊ-] *n* Akrotrophodynie *f*.
ac·ro·troph·o·neu·ro·sis [ˌ-ˌtrɒfəˌnʊˈrəʊsɪs, -ˌnjʊər-, -ˌtrəʊ-] *n* Akrotrophoneurose *f*.
ac·ryl·al·de·hyde [ˌækrɪlˈældəhaɪd] *n* → acrolein.
a·cryl·a·mide [əˈkrɪləmaɪd, ˌækrəˈlæmaɪd, -mɪd] *n* Akryl-, Acrylamid *nt*.
ac·ry·late [ˈækrɪleɪt] *n* Acrylat *nt*, Akrylat *nt*.
a·cryl·ic [əˈkrɪlɪk] *adj* Acrylat betr., Acrylat-, Acryl-.
acrylic acid Acrylsäure *f*.
acrylic lens Plexiglaslinse *f*.
ac·ry·lo·ni·trile [ˌækrɪləʊˈnaɪtrɪl, -triːl] *n* Acrylnitril *nt*.
7-ACS *abbr.* → 7-amino-cephalosporanic acid.
ACT *abbr.* → anodal closure tetanus.
act [ækt] **I** *n* Tat *f*, Handeln *nt*, Handlung *f*, Maßnahme *f*, Schritt *m*, Tun *nt*, Tätigkeit *f*. **II** *vi* handeln, Maßnahmen ergreifen; tätig sein, wirken. **to ~ as** dienen/fungieren als.
act on *vi chem., techn., med.* (ein-)wirken auf.
ACTH *abbr.* → adrenocorticotropic hormone.
ACTH cells ACTH(-bildende)-Zellen *pl*.
ACTH-RF *abbr.* → adrenocorticotropic hormone releasing factor.
ACTH stimulation test ACTH-Test *m*.
ACTH test → ACTH stimulation test.
ac·ti·di·one [ˌæktəˈdaɪəʊn] *n* Cycloheximid *nt*, Actidion *nt*.
actin- *pref.* → actino-.
ac·tin [ˈæktn] *n* Aktin *nt*, Actin *nt*.
actin-binding protein Aktin-bindendes Protein *nt*.
ac·tin·ic [ækˈtɪnɪk] *adj* Strahlen/Strahlung betr., durch Strahlen/Strahlung bedingt, aktinisch, Strahlen-.
actinic cheilitis Cheilitis actinica.
actinic conjunctivitis *ophthal.* Conjunctivitis actinica/photoelectrica, Keratoconjunctivitis actinica/Ophthalmia photoelectrica.
actinic dermatitis aktinische Dermatitis *f*, Dermatitis actinica.
actinic elastosis aktinische/senile Elastose *f*, basophile Kollagendegeneration *f*, Elastosis actinica/solaris/senilis.

ac·ti·nic·i·ty [æktəˈnɪsətɪ] *n* → actinism.
actinic keratitis Keratitis actinica.
actinic keratosis aktinische/senile Keratose *f*, Keratosis actinica/solaris/senilis, Keratoma senile.
actinic reticuloid *derm.* aktinisches Retikuloid *nt*, aktinische retikuläre Hyperplasie *f*, Aktinoretikulose *f*.
actinic retinitis aktinische Retinitis/Retinopathie *f*.
ac·ti·ni·form [ækˈtɪnɪfɔːrm] *adj* strahlenförmig; ausstrahlend.
ac·ti·nin [ˈæktənɪn] *n* Aktinin *nt*.
ac·ti·nism [ˈæktənɪzəm] *n phys.* Lichtstrahlenwirkung *f*, Aktinität *f*.
ac·tin·i·um [ækˈtɪnɪəm] *n abbr.* **Ac** Aktinium *nt*, Actinium *nt abbr.* **Ac**.
actino- *pref.* Strahl(en)-, Aktino-, Actino-.
Ac·ti·no·ba·cil·lus [ˌæktɪnəʊbəˈsɪləs] *n micro.* Aktinobazillus *m*, Actinobacillus *m*.
ac·ti·no·bi·fi·da [ˌ-ˈbɪfɪdə] *pl micro.* Actinobifida *pl*.
ac·ti·no·chem·is·try [ˌ-ˈkeməstrɪ] *n* Photochemie *f*.
ac·ti·no·cu·ti·tis [ˌ-kjuːˈtaɪtɪs] *n* Strahlendermatitis *f*, aktinische Dermatitis *f*.
ac·ti·no·der·ma·ti·tis [ˌ-dɜrməˈtaɪtɪs] *n* Aktinodermatitis *f*, -dermatose *f*.
ac·tin·o·graph [ækˈtɪnəgræf] *n* **1.** *old* → roentgenogram. **2.** *phys.* Aktinograph *m*.
Ac·ti·no·mad·u·ra [ˌæktɪnəʊˈmædʒərə] *n micro.* Actinomadura *f*.
ac·ti·nom·e·ter [æktəˈnɑmɪtər] *n phys.* Aktinometer *nt*, Pyrheliometer *nt*.
ac·ti·nom·e·try [æktəˈnɑmətrɪ] *n* Strahlungsmessung *f*, Aktinometrie *f*.
ac·ti·no·my·ce·li·al [ˌæktɪnəʊmaɪˈsiːlɪəl] *adj* **1.** Aktinomyzetenmyzel betr. **2.** → actinomycetic.
Ac·ti·no·my·ces [ˌ-ˈmaɪsiːz] *n micro.* Actinomyces *m*.
A. israelii Strahlenpilz *m*, Actinomyces israelii.
ac·ti·no·my·ces [ˌ-ˈmaɪsiːz] *n micro.* Aktinomyzet *m*, Actinomyces *m*.
Ac·ti·no·my·ce·ta·ce·ae [ˌ-maɪsəˈteɪsɪiː] *micro.* Actinomycetaceae *pl*.
Ac·ti·no·my·ce·ta·les [ˌ-maɪsəˈteɪliːz] *pl micro.* Actinomycetales *pl*.
ac·ti·no·my·cete [ˌ-ˈmaɪsiːt, -maɪˈsiːt] *n* → actinomyces.
ac·ti·no·my·ce·tic [ˌ-maɪˈsiːtɪk] *adj* Aktinomyzet(en) betr., Aktinomyzeten-.
ac·ti·no·my·ce·tin [ˌ-maɪˈsiːtn] *n* Aktinomyzetin *nt*.
ac·ti·no·my·ce·to·ma [ˌ-maɪsəˈtəʊmə] *n* Aktinomyzetom *nt*.
ac·ti·no·my·cin [ˌ-ˈmaɪsn] *n* Aktinomyzin *nt*, Actinomycin *nt*.
actinomycin C *n* Aktinomyzin C *nt*, Cactinomycin *nt*.
actinomycin D *n* Aktinomyzin D *nt*, Dactinomycin *nt*.
ac·ti·no·my·co·ma [ˌ-maɪˈkəʊmə] *n* Aktinomykom *nt*.
ac·ti·no·my·co·sis [ˌ-maɪˈkəʊsɪs] *n* Strahlenpilzkrankheit *f*, Aktinomykose *f*, Actinomycosis *f*.
ac·ti·no·my·cot·ic [ˌ-maɪˈkɑtɪk] *adj* Aktinomykose betr., von Aktinomykose betroffen, aktinomykotisch.
actinomycotic appendicitis Appendizitis *f* durch Actinomyces israelii.
actinomycotic mycetoma → actinomycetoma.
ac·ti·no·neu·ri·tis [ˌ-nʊˈraɪtɪs, -njʊə-] *n* Strahlenneuritis *f*.
ac·tin·o·phage [ækˈtɪnəfeɪdʒ] *n* Aktinophage *m*.
ac·ti·no·phy·to·sis [ˌæktɪnəʊfaɪˈtəʊsɪs] *n* **1.** → actinomycosis. **2.** Nokardieninfektion *f*, Nokardiose *f*, Nocardiosis *f*. **3.** *derm.*

actinotherapeutics

Botryomykose *f*, -mykom *nt*, -mykosis *f*, Granuloma pediculatum.
ac·ti·no·ther·a·peu·tics [,-,θerə'pju:tıks] *pl* → actinotherapy.
ac·ti·no·ther·a·py [,-'θerəpı] *n* Bestrahlung(sbehandlung *f*) *f*.
actin strand Aktinstrang *m*.
ac·tion ['ækʃn] *n* **1.** Handeln *nt*, Handlung *f*, Maßnahme(n *pl*) *f*, Aktion *f*. **2.** *physiol.* Tätigkeit *f*, Funktion *f*. **3.** *chem., techn., med.* (Ein-)Wirkung *f*, Wirksamkeit *f* (*on* auf); Vorgang *m*, Prozeß *m*.
a. of the heart Herztätigkeit, -funktion.
action current *physiol.* Aktionsstrom *m*.
action potential Aktionspotential *nt*.
action spectrum *bio., chem.* Aktions-, Wirkungsspektrum *nt*.
action tremor Intentionstremor *m*.
ac·ti·va·ble ['æktıvəbl] *adj* aktivierbar.
ac·ti·vate ['æktıveıt] *vt* **1.** (*a. chem.*) aktivieren, anregen. **2.** *phys.* radioaktiv machen, aktivieren. **3.** *techn.* in Betrieb setzen, aktivieren.
ac·ti·vat·ed atom ['æktəveıtıd] *phys.* angeregtes Atom *nt*.
activated charcoal Aktivkohle *f*, Carbo activatus.
activated ergosterol Ergocalciferol *nt*, Vitamin D₂ *nt*.
ac·ti·va·tion [,æktı'veıʃn] *n* Aktivierung *f*, Anregung *f*.
activation analysis *chem.* Aktivierungsanalyse *f*.
activation energy *chem.* Aktivierungsenergie *f*.
activation factor Faktor XII *m abbr.* F XII, Hageman-Faktor *m*.
activation stage Aktivierungsphase *f*.
activation system Aktivierungssystem *nt*.
ac·ti·va·tor ['æktəveıtər] *n chem., embryo., dent.* Aktivator *m*.
activator ribonucleic acid → activator RNA.
activator RNA Aktivator-RNA *f*, Aktivator-RNS *f*.
ac·tive ['æktıv] *adj* **1.** *bio., med.* aktiv, wirksam, wirkend. **to be ~ against** wirksam sein/helfen gegen. **2.** aktiv, tätig; rege, lebhaft.
active algolagnia Sadismus *m*.
active anaphylaxis *embryo.* aktive Anaphylaxie *f*.
active congestion → active hyperemia.
active electrode aktive/differente Elektrode *f*.
active hyperemia aktive/arterielle Hyperämie *f*.
active immunity aktive Immunität *f*.
active immunization aktive Immunisierung *f*.
active level (of metabolism) *physiol.* Tätigkeitsumsatz *m*.
active movement aktive Bewegung *f*, Willkürbewegung *f*.
active principle *pharm.* aktives Prinzip *nt*, aktiver Bestandteil *m*, Wirkstoff *m*.
active respiration *biochem., physiol.* aktive Atmung *f*, Atmungszustand 3 *nt*.
active scopophilia *psychia., psycho.* Voyeurismus *m*, Voyeurtum *nt*.
active sleep *physiol.* REM-Schlaf *m*, Traumschlaf *m*, paradoxer/desynchronisierter Schlaf *m*.
ac·tiv·i·ty [æk'tıvətı] *n* **1.** (*a. physiol.*) Tätigkeit *f*, Betätigung *f*, Aktivität *f*. **2.** *pharm., bio.* Wirksamkeit *f*; (*a. chem., phys.*) Aktivität *f*, Wirksamkeit *f*.
a. of the heart Herztätigkeit.
ac·to·my·o·sin ['æktə'maıəsın] *n* Aktomyosin *nt*, Actomyosin *nt*.
a·cu·i·ty [ə'kju:ətı] *n* **1.** Schärfe *f*, Klarheit *f*; Scharfsinn *m*, Klugheit *f*. **2.** Sehschärfe *f*, Visus *m*.
a·cu·le·ate [ə'kju:lıt, -lıeıt] *adj* → acuminate.
a·cu·mi·nate [ə'kju:mənıt, -neıt] *adj* spitz, zugespitzt.
acuminate condyloma Feig-, Feuchtwarze *f*, spitzes Kondylom *nt*, Condyloma acuminatum, Papilloma acuminatum/venereum.
acuminate papular syphilid kleinpapulöses/miliares/lichenoides Syphilid *nt*, Lichen syphiliticus.
acuminate wart Feig-, Feuchtwarze *f*, spitzes Kondylom *nt*, Condyloma acuminatum, Papilloma acuminatum/venereum.
ac·u·pres·sure ['ækjʊpreʃər] *n* Akupressur *f*.
ac·u·punc·ture ['ækjʊpʌŋktʃər] **I** *n* Akupunktur *f*. **II** *vt* akupunktieren.
a·cute [ə'kju:t] *adj* **1.** *abbr.* **A** akut, Akut-. **2.** scharf, spitz; (*Schmerz*) scharf, stechend; (*Auge*) scharf; (*Gehör*) fein; akut, brennend; kritisch, bedenklich. **2.** scharfsinnig, klug; raffiniert, schlau.
acute abdomen akutes Abdomen *nt*, Abdomen acutum.
nonsurgical a. konservativ behandelbares akutes Abdomen.
acute abscess akuter Abszeß *m*.
acute acoustic trauma akutes akustisches Trauma *nt*.
acute alcoholism Alkoholrausch *m*, -intoxikation *f*, akuter Alkoholismus *m*.
acute anemia akute Anämie *f*.
acute anterior poliomyelitis (epidemische/spinale) Kinderlähmung *f*, Heine-Medin-Krankheit *f*, Poliomyelitis (epidemica) anterior acuta.
acute appendicitis akute Blinddarmentzündung/Appendizitis *f*, Appendicitis acuta.
acute arthritis akute Arthritis *f*, Arthritis acuta.
acute articular rheumatism → acute rheumatic arthritis.
acute ascending paralysis Landry-Lähmung *f*, -Paralyse *f*, -Typ *m*, Paralysis spinalis ascendens acuta.
acute ascending spinal paralysis 1. Landry-Lähmung *f*, -Paralyse *f*, -Typ *m*, Paralysis spinalis ascendens acuta. **2.** Guillain-Barré-Syndrom *nt*, (Poly-)Radikulonitis *f*, Neuronitis *f*.
acute aseptic meningitis lymphozytäre Meningitis *f*.
acute atrophic paralysis → acute anterior poliomyelitis.
acute bacterial myocarditis (akute) bakterielle Myokarditis *f*.
acute benign pericarditis idiopathische Herzbeutelentzündung/Perikarditis *f*.
acute brain syndrome Delirium *nt*, Delir *nt*.
acute bronchitis akute Bronchitis *f*, Bronchitis acuta.
acute bulbar polioencephalitis akute Bulbärparalyse *f*.
acute catarrhal conjunctivitis *ophthal.* akute Konjunktivitis *f*, Conjunctivitis acuta.
acute catarrhal cystitis akute katarrhalische (Harn-)Blasenentzündung/Zystitis *f*, akuter (Harn-)Blasenkatarrh *m*.
acute catarrhal laryngitis → acute laryngitis.
acute catarrhal rhinitis Nasenkatarrh *m*, Koryza *f*, Coryza *f*, Rhinitis acuta.
acute cholangitis akute Cholangitis *f*.
acute cholecystitis akute Gallenblasenentzündung/Cholezystitis *f*.
acute chorea Sydenham-Chorea *f*, Chorea minor (Sydenham), Chorea juvenilis/rheumatica/infectiosa/simplex.
acute compression triad *card.* Beck-Trias *f*.
acute confusional state Delirium *nt*, Delir *nt*.
acute congestive glaucoma → acute glaucoma.
acute contagious conjunctivitis Koch-Weeks-Konjunktivitis *f*, Konjunktivitis *f* durch Haemophilus aegyptius, akute kontagiöse Konjunktivitis *f*.
acute delirium akutes Delir *nt*, akutes Delirium *nt*, Delirium acutum.
acute dentoalveolar abscess (*Zahn*) akuter Wurzelspitzenabszeß *m*.
acute diffuse serous choroiditis Harada-Syndrom *nt*.
acute disseminated encephalitis/encephalomyelitis Impfenzephalitis *f*, -encephalomyelitis *f*, -enzephalopathie *f*, Vakzinationsenzephalitis *f*, Encephalomyelitis postvaccinalis.
acute disseminated histiocytosis X → acute histiocytosis of the newborn.
acute diverticular inflammation Divertikulitis *f*.
acute epidemic conjunctivitis → acute contagious conjunctivitis.
acute epidemic leukoencephalitis Strümpell-Krankheit *f*.
acute erythremia Di Guglielmo-Krankheit *f*, -Syndrom *nt*, akute Erythrämie/Erythromyelose *f*, akute erythrämische Myelose *f*, Erythroblastose *f* des Erwachsenen.
acute erythremic myelosis → acute erythremia.
acute exudative-proliferative glomerulonephritis exsudative Glomerulonephritis *f*.
acute febrile neutrophilic dermatosis Sweet-Syndrom *nt*, akute febrile neutrophile Dermatose *f*.
acute febrile polyneuritis 1. Landry-Lähmung *f*, -Paralyse *f*, -Typ *m*, Paralysis spinalis ascendens acuta. **2.** Guillain-Barré-Syndrom *nt*, Neuronitis *f*, (Poly-)-Radikuloneuritis *f*.
acute fibrinous pericarditis akute fibrinöse Herzbeutelentzündung/Perikarditis *f*.
acute follicular conjunctivitis *ophthal.* akute follikuläre Konjunktivitis *f*.
acute fulminating meningococcemia Waterhouse-Friderichsen-Syndrom *nt*.
acute gastritis akute Magenschleimhautentzündung/Gastritis *f*, akuter Magenkatarrh *m*.
acute glaucoma akutes Winkelblockglaukom/Engwinkelglaukom *nt*, Glaucoma acutum (congestivum).
acute glomerulonephritis akute Glomerulonephritis *f*.
acute heart failure akute Herzinsuffizienz *f*.
acute hemorrhagic conjunctivitis *ophthal.* akute hämorrhagische Konjunktivitis *f*.
acute hemorrhagic encephalitis akute hämorrhagische Enzephalitis *f*, Encephalitis haemorrhagica acuta.
acute hemorrhagic glomerulonephritis → acute glomerulonephritis.
acute hemorrhagic pancreatitis akut-hämorrhagische Pankreatitis *f*.
acute hepatitis akute Leberentzündung/Hepatitis *f*.
acute histiocytosis of the newborn Abt-Letterer-Siwe-Krankheit *f*, akute/maligne Säuglingsretikulose *f*, maligne generalisierte Histiozytose *f*.

acute hydrocephalus Hydrocephalus acutus.
acute infectious paralysis epidemische Poliomyelitis *f*.
acute inflammation akute Entzündung *f*.
acute intermittent porphyria akute intermittierende Porphyrie *f*, Schwedischer Typ *m* der Porphyrie, Porphyria acuta intermittens.
acute interstitial nephritis akute interstitielle Nephritis *f*.
acute interstitial pneumonitis atypische/primär-atypische Pneumonie *f*.
acute isolated myocarditis idiopathische Myokarditis *f*, Fiedler'-Myokarditis *f*.
acute juvenile cirrhosis chronisch-aktive/chronisch-aggressive Hepatitis *f abbr.* CAH.
acute laryngitis *HNO* akute (katarrhalische) Laryngitis *f*, Laryngitis acuta.
acute laryngotracheobronchitis virus Parainfluenza-2-Virus *nt*, Parainfluenzavirus Typ-2 *nt*.
acute lateral poliomyelitis spinale Form *f* der Kinderlähmung.
acute leukemia *abbr.* **AL** akute/unreifzellige Leukämie *f abbr.* AL.
acute lichenoid pityriasis Mucha-Habermann-Syndrom *nt*, Pityriasis lichenoides et varioliformis acuta (Mucha-Habermann).
acute lymphocytic leukemia *abbr.* **ALL** akute lymphatische Leukämie *f abbr.* ALL.
acute mastoiditis akute Mastoiditis *f*.
acute megacolon akutes/toxisches Megakolon *nt*.
acute miliary tuberculosis akute Miliartuberkulose *f*, Tuberculosis acuta miliaris.
acute myelitis akute Myelitis *f*.
acute myelocytic leukemia *abbr.* **AML** akute myeloische Leukämie *f abbr.* AML, akute nicht-lymphatische Leukämie *f abbr.* ANLL.
acute necrotizing encephalitis akute nekrotisierende Enzephalitis *f*.
acute necrotizing ulcerative gingivitis *abbr.* **ANUG** Plaut-Vincent-Angina *f*, Vincent-Angina *f*, Fusospirillose *f*, Fusospirochätose *f*, Angina ulcerosa/ulceromembranacea.
acute nephritis → acute glomerulonephritis.
a·cute·ness [ə'kju:tnɪs] *n* 1. (*Krankheit*) akutes Stadium *nt*, Heftigkeit *f*, Akutsein *nt*. 2. (*Schmerz*) Intensität *f*, Schärfe *f*. 3. (Sinnes-)Schärfe *f*, Feinheit *f*. 4. Spitze *f*.
a. of hearing Hörschärfe.
a. of sight Sehschärfe.
acute neuropsychologic disorder Delirium *nt*, Delir *nt*.
acute neutrophilic dermatosis → acute febrile neutrophilic dermatosis.
acute nonlymphocytic leukemia *abbr.* **ANLL** → acute myelocytic leukemia.
acute nonspecific lymphadenitis Sinuskatarrh *m*, -histiocytose *f*, akute unspezifische Lymphadenitis *f*.
acute onset akuter Ausbruch *m* (einer Krankheit).
acute osteitis Knochenmark(s)entzündung *f*, Osteomyelitis *f*.
acute pain akuter Schmerz *m*.
acute pancreatitis akute Pankreatitis *f*.
acute parapsoriasis → acute lichenoid pityriasis.
acute parenchymatous hepatitis akute gelbe Leberatrophie *f*.
acute periapical abscess → acute dentoalveolar abscess.
acute pharyngitis Angina catarrhalis.

acute-phase protein/reactant Akute-Phase-Protein *nt abbr.* APP.
acute pleuritis/pleurisy akute Rippenfellentzündung/Pleuritis *f*.
acute pneumonia akute Lungenentzündung/Pneumonie *f*.
acute porphyria → acute intermittent porphyria.
acute posterior ganglionitis Gürtelrose *f*, Zoster *m*, Zona *f*, Herpes zoster.
acute posthemorrhagic anemia (akute) Blutungsanämie *f*, akute (post-)hämorrhagische Anämie *f*.
acute postinfectious polyneuropathy Guillain-Barré-Syndrom *nt*, Neuronitis *f*, (Poly-)Radikuloneuritis *f*.
acute primary hemorrhagic meningoencephalitis Strümpell-Krankheit *f*.
acute process of helix Spina helicis.
acute promyelocytic leukemia (akute) Promyelozytenleukämie *f abbr.* APL, (akute) promyelozytäre Leukämie *f*.
acute purulent bronchitis akut-eitrige Bronchitis *f*.
acute pyelonephritis akute Nierenbeckenentzündung/Pyelonephritis *f*.
acute radiation syndrome akutes Strahlensyndrom *nt*.
acute rejection *chir.* (*Transplantation*) akute Abstoßung(sreaktion *f*) *f*.
acute renal failure *abbr.* **ARF** akutes Nierenversagen *nt*.
acute respiratory disease *abbr.* **ARD** akute Atemwegserkrankung *f*, akute respiratorische Erkrankung *f abbr.* ARE.
acute rheumatic arthritis rheumatisches Fieber *nt abbr.* RF, Febris rheumatica, akuter Gelenkrheumatismus *m*, Polyarthritis rheumatica acuta.
acute rheumatic polyarthritis → acute rheumatic arthritis.
acute rhinitis Nasenkatarrh *m*, Koryza *f*, Coryza *f*, Rhinitis acuta.
acute rickets rachitischer Säuglingsskorbut *m*, Möller-Barlow-Krankheit *f*.
acute schizophrenia akute schizophrene Episode *f*, akute Schizophrenie *f*.
acute situational reaction → acute stress reaction.
acute stress reaction akute Stressreaktion *f*.
acute superior hemorrhagic polioencephalitis Wernicke-Enzephalopathie *f*, -Syndrom *nt*, Polioencephalitis haemorrhagica superior (Wernicke).
acute suppurative tenosynovitis akute eitrige Tenotendovaginitis *f*, Sehnen-(scheiden)phlegmone *f*, Tendosynovitis acuta purulenta.
acute tuberculosis → acute miliary tuberculosis.
acute tubular necrosis *abbr.* **ATN** akute Tubulusnekrose *f*.
acute ulcerative gingivitis → acute necrotizing ulcerative gingivitis.
acute ulceromembranous gingivitis → acute necrotizing ulcerative gingivitis.
acute urticaria akute Urtikaria *f*, Urticaria acuta.
acute vascular purpura Schoenlein-Henoch-Syndrom *nt*, (anaphylaktoide) Purpura Schoenlein-Henoch *f*, rheumatoide/athrombopenische Purpura *f*, Immunkomplexpurpura *f*, -vaskulitis *f*, Purpura anaphylactoides (Schoenlein-Henoch), Purpura rheumatica (Schoenlein-Henoch).
acute vestibular paralysis akuter unilateraler Vestibularisausfall *m*, Vestibularisneuronitis *f*, Neuronitis vestibularis.
acute yellow atrophy akute gelbe Leberdystrophie/-atrophie *f*.

a. of the liver akute gelbe Leberdystrophie/Leberatrophie.
acute yellow dystrophy of the liver → acute yellow atrophy of the liver.
a·cy·a·not·ic [ˌeɪˌsaɪə'nɑtɪk] *adj* azyanotisch.
a·cy·clia [eɪ'saɪklɪə] *n* Kreislaufstillstand *m*.
a·cy·clic [eɪ'saɪklɪk, -'sɪk-] *adj* 1. *chem.* azyklisch, offenkettig; aliphatisch. 2. *physiol.* nicht periodisch, azyklisch.
acyclic compound *chem.* offene Kette *f*.
a·cy·clo·gua·no·sine [eɪˌsaɪklə'gwɑnəsi:n, -sɪn] *n* → acyclovir.
a·cy·clo·vir [eɪ'saɪkləvɪər] *n* Aciclovir *nt*, Acycloguanosin *nt*.
ac·yl ['æsɪl, -i:l] *n* Azyl-, Acyl-(Radikal *nt*).
acyl adenylate Acyladenylat *nt*.
ac·yl·ase ['æsəleɪz] *n* Acylase *f*.
ac·yl·ate ['æsəleɪt] *vt chem.* acylieren, azylieren.
ac·yl·a·tion [ˌæsə'leɪʃn] *n chem.* Acylierung *f*, Azylierung *f*.
acyl carnitine Acylcarnitin *nt*.
acyl carrier protein *abbr.* **ACP** Acyl-Carrier-Protein *nt abbr.* ACP.
ac·yl·cho·line acylhydrolase [ˌæsɪl'kəʊli:n, -'kɑl-] unspezifische/unechte Cholinesterase *f abbr.* ChE, Pseudocholinesterase *f*, Typ II-Cholinesterase *f*, β-Cholinesterase *f*, Butyrylcholinesterase *f*.
acyl-CoA *n* → acyl coenzyme A.
acyl-CoA dehydrogenase Acyl-CoA-dehydrogenase *f*.
acyl-CoA desaturase Acyl-CoA-desaturase *f*.
acyl-CoA synthetase (GDP forming) Acyl-CoA-synthetase *f* (GDP-bildend).
long-chain a. long-chain-Acyl-CoA-synthetase.
medium-chain a. medium-chain-Acyl-CoA-synthetase.
acyl-CoA thioester Acyl-CoA-thioester *m*.
acyl coenzyme A Acylcoenzym A *nt*, Acyl-CoA *nt*.
acyl enzyme Acylenzym *nt*.
ac·yl·glu·co·sa·mine-2-epimerase [ˌ-glu:'kəʊsəmiːn, -mɪn] *n* Acylglucosamin-2-epimerase *f*.
ac·yl·glyc·er·ol [ˌ-'glɪsərɑl, -rɔl] *n* Acylglycerin *nt*, Glycerid *nt*, Neutralfett *nt*.
acylglycerol palmitoyl transferase Acylglycerinpalmitidyltransferase *f*.
N-ac·yl·neu·ra·min·ic acid [ˌ-ˌnjʊərə'mɪnɪk, -ə'miːn-, -ˌnɒ-] Sialinsäure *f*, N-Acylneuraminsäure *f*.
N-ac·yl·sphin·go·sine [ˌ-'sfɪŋgəsi:n, -sɪn] *n* N-Acylsphingosin *nt*, Ceramid *nt*.
acylsphingosine deacylase Acylsphingosindeacylase *f*, Ceramidase *f*.
ac·yl·trans·fer·ase [ˌ-'trænsfəreɪz] *n* Acyltransferase *f*, Transacylase *f*.
a·cys·tia [eɪ'sɪstɪə] *n embryo.* kongenitale Harnblasenaplasie *f*, Acystie *f*.
AD *abbr.* → alcohol dehydrogenase.
ADA *abbr.* → adenosine deaminase.
a·dac·tyl·ia [eɪˌdæk'tɪːlɪə] *n* → adactyly.
a·dac·ty·lism [eɪ'dæktɪlɪzəm] *n* → adactyly.
a·dac·ty·lous [eɪ'dæktɪləs] *adj* Adaktylie betr., von Adaktylie betroffen, zehen- od. fingerlos, adaktyl.
a·dac·ty·ly [eɪ'dæktəlɪ] *n* angeborenes Fehlen von Finger(n) od. Zehe(n), Adaktylie *f*.
ADA deficiency Adenosindesaminasemangel *m*.
Adair-Dighton [ə'deər 'daɪtn]: **A.-D. syndrome** van der Hoeve-Syndrom *nt*.
Adam ['ædəm]: **A.'s apple** Adamsapfel *m*, Prominentia laryngea.

ad·a·man·tine [ˌædəˈmæntiːn, -tɪn, -taɪn] *adj* Zahnschmelz/Adamantin betr.
adamantine layer → adamantine substance of tooth.
adamantine substance of tooth *anat.* (Zahn-)Schmelz *m*, Adamantin *nt*, Substantia adamantina, Enamelum *nt*.
ad·a·man·ti·no·car·ci·no·ma [ˌ-ˌmæntɪnəʊˌkɑːrsəˈnəʊmə] *n* Ameloblastosarkom *nt*.
ad·a·man·ti·no·ma [ˌ-ˌmæntəˈnəʊmə] *n* Adamantinom *nt*, Ameloblastom *nt*.
ad·a·man·to·blast [ˌ-ˈmæntəblæst, -blɑːst] *n old* Zahnschmelzbildner *m*, Adamanto-, Amelo-, Ganoblast *m*.
ad·a·man·to·blas·to·ma [ˌ-ˌmæntəˌblæˈstəʊmə] *n* → adamantinoma.
ad·a·man·to·ma [ædəmænˈtəʊmə] *n* → adamantinoma.
Adams [ˈædəmz]: **A.' disease** → Adams-Stokes disease.
ad·ams·ite [ˈædəmzaɪt] *n* Diphenylaminarsinchlorid *nt*, Adamsit *nt*.
Adams-Stokes [stəʊks]: **A.-S. disease/syncope/syndrome** Adams-Stokes-Anfall *m abbr.* ASA, Adams-Stokes-Synkope *f*, -Syndrom *nt*.
ad·an·son·i·an classification [ædənˈsɑnɪən] *micro.* numerische Taxonomie *f*.
a·dapt [əˈdæpt] **I** *vt* anpassen, adaptieren (*to* an); **~ o.s.** s. anpassen (*to* an). **II** *vi* s. anpassen (*to* an).
a·dapt·a·bil·i·ty [əˌdæptəˈbɪlətɪ] *n* Anpassungsfähigkeit *f*, -vermögen *nt* (*to* an).
a·dapt·a·ble [əˈdæptəbl] *adj* anpassungsfähig (*to* an). **to be ~ to sth.** s. an etw. anpassen können.
ad·ap·ta·tion [ˌædæpˈteɪʃn] *n* Anpassung *f*, Gewöhnung *f*, Adaptation *f*, Adaption *f* (*to* an).
ad·ap·ta·tion·al syndrome [ˌædəpˈteɪʃənl] → adaptation syndrome.
adaptation diseases Adaptationssyndrom *nt*, allgemeines Anpassungssyndrom *nt abbr.* AAS.
adaptation hyperplasia Anpassungs-, Adaptationshyperplasie *f*.
adaptation syndrome Anpassungs-, Adaptationssyndrom *nt*.
a·dapt·a·tive [əˈdæptətɪv] *adj* → adaptive.
adaptative hypertrophy adaptative Hypertrophie *f*.
a·dapt·ed milk [əˈdæptɪd] adaptierte (Säuglings-)Milch *f*.
a·dapt·er [əˈdæptər] *n phys., techn.* Zwischen-, Anschluß-, Einsatz-, Paßstück *nt*, Adapter *m*.
a·dap·tion [əˈdæpʃn] *n* → adaptation.
a·dap·tive [əˈdæptɪv] *adj* anpassungsfähig, adaptiv (*to* an).
adaptive enzyme induzierbares Enzym *nt*.
adaptive immunity erworbene Immunität *f*.
ad·ap·tom·e·ter [æˌdəpˈtɑmɪtər] *n physiol.* Adaptometer *nt*.
ADCC *abbr.* → antibody-dependent cell-mediated/cellular cytotoxicity.
add [æd] **I** *vt* **1.** hinzurechnen, -zählen, addieren (*to* zu). **2.** hinzufügen, dazugeben (*to* zu); *chem.* beimengen, versetzen (*to* mit). **3.** addieren, zusammenzählen. **II** *vi* beitragen (*to* zu).
ad·dict [*n* ˈædɪkt; *v* əˈdɪkt] **I** *n* Süchtige(r *m*) *f*, Suchtkranke(r *m*), Abhängige(r *m*) *f*. **II** *vt* süchtig machen; jdn. gewöhnen (*to* an). **III** *vi* süchtig machen.
ad·dict·ed [əˈdɪktɪd] *adj* süchtig, abhängig (*to* an). **to be/become ~ to heroin/alcohol** heroin-/alkoholabhängig sein/werden.
ad·dic·tion [əˈdɪkʃn] *n* Sucht *f*, Abhängigkeit *f*; Süchtigkeit *f* (*to* nach).
addiction-forming drug → addiction-producing drug.

addiction-producing drug suchterzeugendes Medikament *nt*, Droge *f*.
ad·dic·tive [əˈdɪktɪv] *adj* suchterzeugend. **to be ~** süchtig machen.
addictive drug Suchtmittel *nt*, suchterzeugendes Medikament *nt*.
Addis [ˈædɪs]: **A. count/method/test** Addis(-Hamburger)-Count *m*, Addis-Test *m*.
Addison [ˈædɪsən]: **A.'s anemia** perniziöse Anämie *f*, Biermer-, Addison-Anämie *f*, Morbus Biermer *m*, Perniziosa *f*, Perniciosa *f*, Anaemia perniciosa, Vitamin B_{12}-Mangelanämie *f*.
A.'s disease Addison'-Krankheit *f*, Morbus Addison *m*, Bronze(haut)krankheit *f*, primäre chronische Nebennieren(rinden)insuffizienz *f*.
A.'s planes *anat.* Addison-Ebenen *pl*.
A.'s point Addison'-Punkt *m*.
Addison-Biermer [ˈbɪərmər]: **A.-B. anemia/disease** → Addison's anemia.
ad·di·so·ni·an [ædəˈsəʊnɪən]: **a. anemia** → Addison's anemia.
a. crisis Addison-Krise *f*, akute Nebenniereninsuffizienz *f*.
ad·di·son·ism [ˈædɪsənɪzəm] *n* Addisonismus *m*.
ad·di·tion [əˈdɪʃn] *n* **1.** *mathe.* Addition *f*, Addierung *f*, Zusammenzählen *nt*. **2.** Zusatz *m*, Ergänzung *f*, Hinzufügung *f* (*to* zu). **in ~** zusätzlich (*to* zu). **3.** *chem.* Beimengung *f*; *techn.* Zusatz *m*.
ad·di·tive [ˈædɪtɪv] **I** *n* Zusatz *m*, Additiv *nt*. **II** *adj* zusätzlich, hinzukommend, additiv, Additions-. **to be ~** s. summieren (*in der Wirkung*).
additive effect Additions-, Summationseffekt *m*.
ad·du·cent [əˈd(j)uːsənt] *adj* zur Längsachse hinbewegend, adduzierend.
ad·duct [əˈdʌkt] **I** *n chem.* Addukt *nt*. **II** *vt* zur Längsachse hinbewegen, adduzieren.
ad·duc·tion [əˈdʌkʃn] *n* Hinbewegung *f* zur Längsachse, Adduktion *f*.
adduction contracture Adduktionskontraktur *f*.
ad·duc·tive [əˈdʌktɪv] *adj* → adducent.
ad·duc·tor [əˈdʌktər] *n* → adductor muscle.
adductor brevis (muscle) Adduktor *m* brevis, M. adductor brevis.
adductor canal Schenkel-, Adduktorenkanal *m*, Canalis adductorius.
adductor hallucis (muscle) Adduktor *m* hallucis, M. adductor hallucis.
adductor hiatus Hiatus tendineus/adductorius.
adductor longus (muscle) Adduktor *m* longus, M. adductor longus.
adductor magnus (muscle) Adduktor *m* magnus, M. adductor magnus.
adductor minimus (muscle) Adduktor *m* minimus, M. adductor minimus.
adductor muscle Adduktor *m*, Adduktionsmuskel *m*, M. adductor.
great a. → adductor magnus (muscle).
a. of great toe → adductor hallucis (muscle).
long a. → adductor longus (muscle).
short a. → adductor brevis (muscle).
smallest a. → adductor minimus (muscle).
a. of thumb → adductor pollicis (muscle).
adductor pollicis (muscle) Adduktor *m* pollicis, M. adductor pollicis.
adductor reflex Adduktorenreflex *m*.
adductor tubercle (of femur) Tuberculum adductorium (femoris).
Ade *abbr.* → adenine.
A·den fever [ˈɑːdn, ˈeɪdn] Dengue *nt*, Dengue-Fieber *nt*, Dandy-Fieber *nt*.
Aden ulcer kutane Leishmaniose *f*, Haut-

leishmaniose *f*, Orientbeule *f*, Leishmaniasis cutis.
aden- *pref.* → adeno-.
ad·e·nal·gia [ˌædɪˈnældʒ(ɪ)ə] *n* Drüsenschmerz(en *pl*) *m*, Adenodynie *f*.
ad·e·nase [ˈædəneɪs] *n* → adenine deaminase.
a·den·dric [əˈdendrɪk] *adj* → adendritic.
a·den·drit·ic [ˌædenˈdrɪtɪk] *adj* ohne Dendriten, adendritisch.
ad·e·nec·to·my [ˌædəˈnektəmɪ] *n*, *pl* **-mies** *chir.* Drüsenresektion *f*, Adenektomie *f*.
ad·e·nec·to·pia [ˌædənekˈtəʊpɪə] *n* ektope Drüse *f*.
a·de·nia [əˈdiːnɪə] *n patho.* chronische Lymphknotenvergrößerung *f*.
a·de·nic [əˈdiːnɪk] *adj* Drüse betr., Drüsen-.
a·den·i·form [əˈdenəfɔːrm, -ˈdiːnə-] *adj* drüsenähnlich, -förmig.
ad·e·nine [ˈædənɪn, -niːn, -naɪn] *n abbr.* **A, Ade** 6-Aminopurin *nt*, Adenin *nt abbr.* A, Ade.
adenine arabinoside *abbr.* **ara-A** Vidarabin *nt*, Adenin-Arabinosid *nt abbr.* Ara-A.
adenine deaminase Adenindesaminase *f*.
adenine phosphoribosyl transferase *abbr.* **APRT** Adeninphosphoribosyltransferase *f abbr.* APRT.
ad·e·ni·tis [ædəˈnaɪtɪs] *n* **1.** Drüsenentzündung *f*, Adenitis *f*. **2.** Lymphknotenentzündung *f*, -vergrößerung *f*, Lymphadenitis *f*.
ad·e·ni·za·tion [ædənaɪˈzeɪʃn] *n histol.*, *pathol.* sekundäre Metaplasie *f*.
adeno- *pref.* Drüsen-, Adeno-.
ad·e·no·ac·an·tho·ma [ˌædənəʊˌækənˈθəʊmə] *n* Adenoakanthom *nt*.
ad·e·no·am·e·lo·blas·to·ma [ˌ-ˌæmələʊblæˈstəʊmə] *n* Adenoameloblastom *nt*.
adeno-associated satellite virus → adeno-associated virus.
adeno-associated virus *abbr.* **AAV** adenoassoziiertes Virus *nt abbr.* AAV, Adenosatellitovirus *nt*.
ad·e·no·blast [ˈ-blæst] *n* Adenoblast *m*.
ad·e·no·can·croid [ˌ-ˈkæŋkrɔɪd] *n* Adenokankroid *nt*.
ad·e·no·car·ci·no·ma [ˌ-ˌkɑːrsəˈnəʊmə] *n* Adenokarzinom *nt*, Adenocarcinom *nt*, Ca. adenomatosum *f*.
a. of kidney hypernephroides (Nieren-)-Karzinom *nt*, klarzelliges Nierenkarzinom *nt*, (maligner) Grawitz-Tumor *m*, Hypernephrom *nt*.
ad·e·no·cele [ˈ-siːl] *n* adenomatös-zystischer Tumor *m*, Adenozele *f*.
ad·e·no·cel·lu·li·tis [ˌ-ˌseljəˈlaɪtɪs] *n* Adenozellulitis *f*.
ad·e·no·chon·dro·ma [ˌ-kɑnˈdrəʊmə] *n* Chondroadenom *nt*.
ad·e·no·cyst [ˈ-sɪst] *n* → adenocystoma.
ad·e·no·cys·tic [ˌ-ˈsɪstɪk] *adj* adenoid-zystisch.
adenocystic carcinoma adenoid-zystisches Karzinom *nt*, *old* Zylindrom *nt*, Ca. adenoides cysticum.
ad·e·no·cys·to·ma [ˌ-sɪsˈtəʊmə] *n* Adenokystom *nt*, Kystadenom *nt*, Cystadenom *nt*.
ad·e·no·cyte [ˈ-saɪt] *n* reife Drüsenzelle *f*.
ad·e·no·dyn·ia [ˌ-ˈdiːnɪə] *n* Drüsenschmerz(en *pl*) *m*, Adenodynie *f*.
ad·e·no·ep·i·the·li·o·ma [ˌ-ˌepəˌθiːlɪˈəʊmə] *n* Adenoepitheliom(a) *nt*.
ad·e·no·fi·bro·ma [ˌ-faɪˈbrəʊmə] *n* Adenofibrom(a) *nt*, Fibroadenom *nt*.
ad·e·no·fi·bro·sis [ˌ-faɪˈbrəʊsɪs] *n* Drüsen-, Adenofibrose *f*.
ad·e·nog·e·nous [ædəˈnɑdʒənəs] *adj* von Drüsengewebe (ab-)stammend, adenogen.

ad·e·no·graph·ic [ˌædənəʊˈgræfɪk] *adj* Adenographie betr., adenographisch.
ad·e·nog·ra·phy [ædəˈnɑgrəfɪ] *n* Adenographie *f*.
ad·e·no·hy·poph·y·se·al *adj* → adenohypophysial.
ad·e·no·hy·poph·y·sec·to·my [ˌædənəʊhaɪˌpɑfəˈsɛktəmɪ] *n chir*. Resektion *f* der Adenohypophyse, Adenohypophysektomie *f*.
ad·e·no·hy·poph·y·si·al [ˌ-haɪˌpɑfəˈsiːəl, -ˌhaɪpəˈfiːzɪəl] *adj* Adenohypophyse betr., adenohypophysär, Adenohypophysen-, Hypophysenvorderlappen-, HVL-.
adenohypophysial hormones Hormone *pl* der Adenohypophyse, (Hypenphysen-)Vorderlappenhormone *pl*, HVL--Hormone *pl*.
ad·e·no·hy·poph·y·sis [ˌ-haɪˈpɑfəsɪs] *n* Adenohypophyse *f*, Hypophysenvorderlappen *m abbr*. HVL, Adenohypophysis *f*, Lobus anterior hypophyseos.
ad·e·noid [ˈædnɔɪd] **I** *s pl* → adenoid disease. **II** *adj* **1.** drüsenähnlich, adenoid. **2.** Adenoide betr., adenoid.
ad·e·noi·dal [ˈædənɔɪdl] *adj* → adenoid II.
adenoidal-pharyngeal-conjunctival virus → adenovirus.
adenoid cystic carcinoma adenoidzystisches Karzinom *nt*, *old* Zylindrom *nt*, Ca. adenoides cysticum.
adenoid disease adenoide Vegetationen *pl*, Adenoide *pl*, Rachenmandelhyperplasie *f*.
ad·e·noid·ec·to·my [ˌ-ˈdɛktəmɪ] *n* Adenotomie *f*, Adenoidektomie *f*.
adenoid face Facies adenoidea.
adenoid facies Facies adenoidea.
ad·e·noid·ism [ˈ-dɪzəm] *n* Adenoidismus *m*, adenoides Syndrom *nt*.
ad·e·noid·i·tis [ˌ-ˈdaɪtɪs] *n* Adenoiditis *f*.
adenoid tissue lymphatisches Gewebe *nt*.
adenoid tonsil Rachenmandel *f*, Tonsilla pharyngea(lis)/adenoidea.
adenoid tumor → adenoma.
adenoid vegetation → adenoid disease.
ad·e·no·lei·o·my·o·fi·bro·ma [ˌ-ˌlaɪəʊˌmaɪəʊfaɪˈbrəʊmə] *n* Adenoleiomyofibrom *nt*.
ad·e·no·li·po·ma [ˌ-laɪˈpəʊmə, -lɪ-] *n* Adenolipom *nt*, Lipoadenom *nt*.
ad·e·no·li·po·ma·to·sis [ˌ-laɪˌpəʊməˈtəʊsɪs] *n* Adenolipomatose *f*.
ad·e·no·lym·phi·tis [ˌ-lɪmˈfaɪtɪs] *n* Lymphknotenentzündung *f*, Lymphadenitis *f*.
ad·e·no·lym·pho·cele [ˌ-ˈlɪmfəsiːl] *n* Lymphknotenzyste *f*, Lymphadenozele *f*.
ad·e·no·lym·pho·ma [ˌ-lɪmˈfəʊmə] *n* Warthin-Tumor *m*, Warthin-Albrecht--Arzt-Tumor *m*, Adenolymphom *nt*, Cystadenoma lymphomatosum, Cystadenolymphoma papilliferum.
ad·e·no·ma [ædəˈnəʊmə] *n, pl* **-mas, -ma·ta** [-mətə] Adenom(a) *nt*.
a. of the colon Kolon-, Dickdarmadenom.
ad·e·no·ma·la·cia [ˌædnəʊməˈleɪʃ(ɪ)ə, -sɪə] *n patho*. Drüsenerweichung *f*, Adenomalazie *f*.
ad·e·no·ma·toid [ædəˈnəʊmətɔɪd] *adj* drüsenähnlich, adenomatös.
adenomatoid malformation of the lung kongenitale Zystenlunge *f*.
adenomatoid odontogenic tumor Adenoameloblastom *nt*.
adenomatoid tumor Adenomatoidtumor *m*.
ad·e·no·ma·to·sis [ædəˌnəʊməˈtəʊsɪs] *n* Adenomatose *f*, -matosis *f*.
a. of the colon familiäre Polypose/Polyposis *f*, Polyposis familiaris, Adenomatosis coli.

ad·e·nom·a·tous [ædəˈnɑmətəs] *adj histol., patho*. adenomatös.
adenomatous goiter adenomatöse Struma *f*, Struma adenomatosa.
adenomatous hyperplasia (*Endometrium*) adenomatöse Hyperplasie *f*.
a. of gallbladder → adenomyomatosis of gallbladder.
adenomatous polyp adenomatöser Polyp *m*.
adenomatous polyposis coli → adenomatosis of the colon.
ad·e·no·meg·a·ly [ˌædnəʊˈmegəlɪ] *n* Drüsenvergrößerung *f*, Adenomegalie *f*.
ad·e·no·my·o·ep·i·the·li·o·ma [ˌ-maɪəˌepəˌθiːlɪˈəʊmə] *n* → adenocystic carcinoma.
ad·e·no·my·o·fi·bro·ma [ˌ-ˌmaɪəfaɪˈbrəʊmə] *n* Adenomyofibrom *nt*.
ad·e·no·my·o·ma [ˌ-maɪˈəʊmə] *n* Adenomyom(a) *nt*.
ad·e·no·my·o·ma·to·sis [ˌ-ˌmaɪəməˈtəʊsɪs] *n* Adenomyomatose *f*.
a. of gallbladder Cholecystitis glandularis proliferans.
ad·e·no·my·om·a·tous [ˌ-maɪˈɑmətəs] *adj* adenomyomatös.
ad·e·no·my·o·me·tri·tis [ˌ-ˌmaɪəmɪˈtraɪtɪs] *n* → adenomyosis.
ad·e·no·my·o·sar·co·ma [ˌ-maɪəsɑːrˈkəʊmə] *n* Adenomyosarkom *nt*.
a. of kidney Wilms-Tumor *m*, embryonales Adeno(myo)sarkom *nt*, Nephroblastom *nt*, Adenomyorhabdosarkom *nt* der Niere.
ad·e·no·my·o·sis [ˌ-maɪˈəʊsɪs] *n* Endometriosis uteri interna, *old* Adenomyosis interna.
ad·e·non·cus [ædəˈnɑŋkəs] *n* Drüsenvergrößerung *f*.
ad·e·no·neu·ral [ˌædnəʊˈnjʊərəl, -ˈnʊ-] *adj* Drüse(n) u. Nerv(en) betr.
ad·e·nop·a·thy [ˌædəˈnɑpəθɪ] *n* **1.** Drüsenschwellung *f*, -vergrößerung *f*, Adenopathie *f*. **2.** Lymphknotenschwellung *f*, -vergrößerung *f*, Lymphadenopathie *f*.
ad·e·no·phar·yn·gi·tis [ædnəʊˌfærɪnˈdʒaɪtɪs] *n HNO* Adenopharyngitis *f*.
ad·e·no·phleg·mon [ˌ-ˈflegmən] *n* phlegmonöse Adenitis *f*.
ad·e·noph·thal·mia [ˌædnɑfˈθælmɪə] *n* Entzündung *f* der Meibom'-Drüsen.
ad·e·no·sar·co·ma [ˌædnəʊsɑːrˈkəʊmə] *n* Adenosarkom *nt*.
adenosatellite virus [ˌ-ˈsætlaɪt] → adeno-associated virus.
ad·e·no·scle·ro·sis [ˌ-sklɪəˈrəʊsɪs] *n patho*. Drüsen-, Adenosklerose *f*.
a·den·o·sine [əˈdenəsiːn, -sɪn] *n abbr*. **A** Adenosin *nt abbr*. A.
adenosine 3',5'-cyclic phosphate zyklisches Adenosin-3',5'-phosphat *nt*, cyclo-AMP *abbr*. 3',5'AMP, cAMP.
adenosine deaminase *abbr*. ADA Adenosindesaminase *f abbr*. ADA.
adenosine deaminase deficiency Adenosindesaminasemangel *m*.
adenosine(-5')-diphosphate *n abbr*. **ADP** Adenosin(5')diphosphat *nt abbr*. ADP, Adenosin-5'-pyrophosphat *nt*.
adenosine kinase Adenosinkinase *f*.
adenosine monophosphate *abbr*. **AMP** Adenosinmonophosphat *nt abbr*. AMP, Adenylsäure *f*.
cyclic a. → adenosine 3',5'-cyclic phosphate.
adenosine-3'-phosphate *n* Adenosin-3'--phosphat *nt*.
adenosine-5'-phosphate *n* Adenosin-5'--phosphat *nt*.
adenosine triphosphatase Adenosintriphosphatase *f*, ATPase *f*.

sodium-potassium a. Natrium-Kalium--ATPase *f*, Na$^+$-K$^+$-ATPase *f*.
adenosine(-5')-triphosphate *n abbr*. **ATP** Adenosin(5')triphosphat *nt abbr*. ATP.
ad·e·no·sis [ædəˈnəʊsɪs] *n* **1.** Adenopathie *f*. **2.** Adenomatose *f*. **3.** sklerosierende Adenosis *f*, Korbzellenhyperplasie *f*.
ad·e·no·squa·mous carcinoma [ˌædnəʊ-ˈskweɪməs] adenosquamöses Karzinom *nt*.
a·den·o·syl·ho·mo·cys·te·i·nase [əˌdenəʊsɪlˌhəʊməˈsɪsteɪneɪz] *n* Adenosylhomocysteinase *f*.
S-a·den·o·syl·ho·mo·cys·te·ine [ˌ-həʊməˈsɪstiːn, -ɪn] *n* S-Adenosylhomocystein *nt*.
S-a·den·o·syl·me·thi·o·nine [ˌ-meˈθaɪəniːn, -nɪn] *n* S-Adenosylmethionin *nt*.
S-adenosylmethionine decarboxylase S--Adenosylmethionindecarboxylase *f*.
ad·e·no·tome [ˈædnəʊtəʊm] *n HNO* Adenotom *nt*.
ad·e·not·o·my [ædəˈnɑtəmɪ] *n HNO* Adenotomie *f*, Adenoidektomie *f*.
ad·e·no·ton·sil·lec·to·my [ˌædnəʊˌtɑnsəˈlɛktəmɪ] *n* Adenotonsillektomie *f*.
ad·e·nous [ˈædnəs] *adj* Drüse betr., drüsig, adenös.
ad·e·no·vi·ral [ˌædnəʊˈvaɪrəl] *adj* Adenoviren betr., Adenoviren-, Adenovirus-.
adenoviral pneumonia Adenoviruspneumonie *f*.
Ad·e·no·vir·i·dae [ˌ-ˈvɪraɪdiː] *pl* Adenoviridea *pl*.
ad·e·no·vi·rus [ˌ-ˈvaɪrəs] *n* Adenovirus *nt*.
adenovirus disease Adenoviruserkrankung *f*.
adenovirus infection Adenovirusinfektion *f*.
ad·e·nyl [ˈædnɪl] *n* Adenyl-(Radikal *nt*).
a·den·yl·ate [əˈdɛnlɪt, -eɪt, ˈædnl-] **I** *n* Adenylat *nt*. **II** *vr* adenylieren.
adenylate cyclase *abbr*. **AC** Adenylatcyclase *f abbr*. AC.
adenylate deaminase AMP-Desaminase *f*.
adenylate kinase Adenylatkinase *f*, Myokinase *f*, AMP-Kinase *f*, A-Kinase *f*.
adenyl cyclase → adenylate cyclase.
ad·e·nyl·ic acid [ˌædəˈnɪlɪk] → adenosine monophosphate.
adenylic acid deaminase AMP-Desaminase *f*.
ad·e·nyl·o·suc·ci·nase [ˌædənɪləʊˈsʌksɪneɪs] *n* → adenylosuccinate lyase.
ad·e·nyl·o·suc·ci·nate [ˌ-ˈsʌksɪneɪt] *n* Adenyl(o)succinat *nt*.
adenylosuccinate lyase Adenyl(o)succinatlyase *f*.
adenylosuccinate synthetase Adenyl(o)succinatsynthetase *f*.
ad·e·nyl·py·ro·phos·phate [ˌædnɪlˌpaɪrəˈfɑsfeɪt] *n* → adenosine(-5')-triphosphate.
ad·e·nyl·suc·ci·nate [ˌ-ˈsʌksɪneɪt] *n* → adenylosuccinate.
ad·e·nyl·suc·cin·ic acid [ˌ-sʌkˈsɪnɪk] Adenylbernsteinsäure *f*.
ad·e·ny·lyl [ˈædnɪlɪl] *n* **1.** Adenyl-(Radikal *nt*). **2.** Adenylyl-(Radikal *nt*).
adenylyl cyclase → adenylate cyclase.
ad·e·ny·lyl·trans·fer·ase [ˌædnɪlɪlˈtrænsfəreɪz] *n* Adenylyltransferase *f*.
ad·e·quate stimulus [ˈædəkwɪt] adäquater Reiz *m*.
a·der·mia [eɪˌdɜrmɪə] *n* kongenitaler Hautdefekt *m*, angeborenes Fehlen *nt* der Haut.
a·der·mine [eɪˈdɜrmiːn] *n* Pyridoxin *nt*, Vitamin B$_6$ *nt*.
a·der·mo·gen·e·sis [eɪˌdɜrməˈdʒɛnəsɪs] *n*

embryo. unvollständige Hautentwicklung *f,* Adermogenese *f.*
ADH *abbr.* **1.** → alcohol dehydrogenase. **2.** → antidiuretic hormone.
ad·here [æd'hɪər, əd-] **I** *vt* ver-, ankleben. **II** *vi* **1.** (an-)kleben, (an-)haften (*to* an). **2.** verkleben; verwachsen sein. **3.** (*Regel*) s. halten an, einhalten, befolgen (*to*).
ad·her·ence [æd'hɪərəns, -'her-] *n* **1.** (An-)Kleben *nt,* (An-)Haften *nt,* Adhärenz *f* (*to* an). **2.** (*Vorschrift*) Befolgung *f,* Einhaltung *f* (*to* von). **3.** *micro.* Adhärenz *f,* Adhäsion *f.*
ad·her·ent [æd'hɪərənt, -'her-] *adj* (an-)klebend, (an-)haftend (*to* an); adhärent, verklebt, verwachsen (*to* mit).
adherent denticle *dent.* adhärenter Dentikel *m.*
adherent junction Zonula adherens.
adherent lens Kontaktlinse *f.*
adherent leukoma *ophthal.* adhärentes Leukom *nt,* Leukoma adhaerens.
adherent pericardium adhäsive/verklebende Perikarditis *f,* Pericarditis adhaesiva.
adherent placenta Placenta adhaerens.
adherent tongue Zungenverwachsung *f,* Ankyloglossie *f,* -glosson *nt.*
ad·he·sin [æd'hi:zɪn] *n* Lektin *nt,* Lectin *nt*
ad·he·sion [æd'hi:ʒn, əd-] *n* **1.** → adherence. **2.** *techn., phys.* Adhäsion *f.* **3.** *patho.* Adhäsion *f,* Verklebung *f,* Verwachsung *f* (*to* mit).
adhesion phenomenon *immun.* Immunadhärenz *f.*
ad·he·si·ot·o·my [əd,hi:zɪ'ɑtəmɪ] *n chir.* Adhäsiotomie *f,* Adhäsiolyse *f.*
ad·he·sive [æd'hi:sɪv, əd-] **I** *n* Klebstoff *m,* Binde-, Haftmittel *nt.* **II** *adj* (*a. phys., techn.*) (an-)haftend, klebend, adhäsiv, Adhäsiv-, Adhäsions-, Haft-; Saug-.
adhesive band *chir., patho.* Verwachsungsstrang *m,* Bride *f.*
adhesive bursitis → adhesive peritendinitis.
adhesive capsulitis → adhesive peritendinitis.
adhesive inflammation adhäsive/verklebende Entzündung *f.*
ad·he·sive·ness [æd'hi:sɪvnɪs] *n* **1.** Klebrigkeit *f,* Haftvermögen *nt,* Adhäsion(sfähigkeit *f*) *f.* **2.** (An-)Haften *nt.*
adhesive pericarditis adhäsive/verklebende Perikarditis *f,* Pericarditis adhaesiva.
adhesive peritendinitis schmerzhafte Schultersteife *f,* Periarthritis/Periarthropathia humeroscapularis *abbr.* PHS.
adhesive peritonitis adhäsive/verklebende Peritonitis *f.*
adhesive plaster → adhesive tape 1.
adhesive pleurisy verklebende/adhäsive Pleuritis *f.*
adhesive pleuritis → adhesive pleurisy.
adhesive strangulation of intestines *chir.* Adhäsions-, Brideniieus *m.*
adhesive tape 1. Heftpflaster *nt, inf.* Pflaster *nt.* **2.** Klebeband *nt,* Klebestreifen *m.*
adhesive tendinitis → adhesive peritendinitis.
ADH system ADH-System *nt,* Adiuretin--Vasopressinsystem *nt.*
ad·i·a·bat·ic [,ædɪə'bætɪk, aɪ,daɪə-] *adj phys.* ohne Wärmeaustausch verlaufend, adiabatisch.
ad·i·ad·o·cho·ci·ne·sia [,ædɪ,ædəʊsɪ-'ni:ʒ(ɪ)ə, ,aɪdaɪ,ædəʊkəʊ-] *n* → adiadochokinesia.
ad·i·ad·o·cho·ci·ne·sis [,-sɪ'ni:sɪs, -saɪ-] → adiadochokinesia.
ad·i·ad·o·cho·ki·ne·sia [,-kɪ'ni:ʒ(ɪ)ə, -kaɪ-] *n* Adiadochokinesie *f.*

ad·i·ad·o·cho·ki·ne·sis [,-kɪ'ni:sɪs, -kaɪ-] *n* → adiadochokinesia.
ad·i·ad·o·ko·ki·ne·sia *n* → adiadochokinesia.
ad·i·ad·o·ko·ki·ne·sis [,-kɪ'ni:sɪs, -kaɪ-] *n* → adiadochokinesia.
ad·i·a·spi·ro·my·co·sis [,ædɪəˌspaɪrəmaɪ-'kəʊsɪs, aɪˌdaɪə-] *n* (Lungen-)Adiaspiromykose *f.*
ad·i·a·spore ['spɔ:r, -spəʊr] *n* Adiaspore *f.*
ad·i·a·ther·mal [,-'θɜrml] *adj* wärmeundurchlässig, atherman, adiatherman.
a·di·a·ther·mance [ə,-'θɜrməns] *n* → adiathermancy.
a·di·a·ther·man·cy [ə,-'θɜrmənsɪ] *n* Wärmeundurchlässigkeit *f,* Adiathermanität *f,* Athermanität *f.*
ad·i·cil·lin [ædɪ'sɪlɪn] *n pharm.* Adicillin *nt,* Cephalosporin N *nt,* Penicillin N *nt.*
Adie ['ædɪ]: **A.'s pupil** Adie'-Pupille *f,* Pupillotonie *f.*
A.'s syndrome Adie-Syndrom *nt.*
adip- *pref.* → adipo-.
ad·i·pec·to·my [ædə'pektəmɪ] *n chir.* Fett-(gewebs)entfernung *f,* Lipektomie *f.*
ad·i·phen·ine [ædɪ'feni:n] *n pharm.* Adiphenin *nt.*
a·dip·ic [ə'dɪpɪk] *n, adj* → adipose.
adipic acid Adipinsäure *f.*
adipo- *pref.* Fett-, Adip(o)-, Lip(o)-.
ad·i·po·cele ['ædɪpəʊsi:l] *n* Adipozele *f.*
ad·i·po·cel·lu·lar [,-'seljələr] *adj* aus Bindegewebe u. Fett bestehend, adipozellulär.
ad·i·po·cere [-sɪər] *n* Fettwachs *nt,* Leichenwachs *nt,* Adipocire *f.*
ad·i·po·cyte ['-saɪt] *n* Fett(speicher)zelle *f,* Lipo-, Adipozyt *m.*
ad·i·po·der·mal graft [,-'dɜrml] Hautfettlappen *m.*
ad·i·po·fi·bro·ma [,-faɪ'brəʊmə] *n* Adipofibrom *nt.*
ad·i·po·gen·e·sis [,-'dʒenəsɪs] *n* Fettbildung *f,* Lipogenese *f.*
ad·i·po·gen·ic [,-'dʒenɪk] *adj* **1.** fettbildend, lipogen. **2.** Fettleibigkeit verursachend.
ad·i·pog·e·nous [ædɪ'pɑdʒənəs] *adj* → adipogenic.
ad·i·po·ki·ne·sis [,ædɪpəʊkɪ'ni:sɪs, -kaɪ-] *n* Fettmobilisation *f,* Adipokinese *f.*
ad·i·po·ki·net·ic [,-kɪ'netɪk, -kaɪ-] *adj* Adipokinese betr. *od.* fördernd, adipokinetisch.
adipokinetic hormone lipolytisches Hormon *nt.*
ad·i·po·ki·nin [,-'kaɪnɪn] *n* → adipokinetic hormone.
ad·i·pol·y·sis [ædɪ'pɑləsɪs] *n* Fettspaltung *f,* -abbau *m,* Lipolyse *f.*
ad·i·po·lyt·ic [,ædɪpəʊ'lɪtɪk] *adj* Lipolyse betr. *od.* verursachend, lipolytisch.
ad·i·po·ma [ædɪ'pəʊmə] *n old* → lipoma.
ad·i·pom·e·ter [ædɪ'pɑmɪtər] *n* Adipometer *nt.*
ad·i·po·ne·cro·sis [,ædɪpəʊnɪ'krəʊsɪs] *n* Fettgewebsnekrose *f,* Adiponecrosis *f.*
ad·i·pos·al·gia [,-'sældʒ(ɪ)ə] *n* Adiposalgie *f.*
ad·i·pose ['ædɪpəʊs] **I** *n* (Speicher-)Fett *nt.* **II** *adj* **1.** adipös, fetthaltig, fettig, Fett-. **2.** fett, fettleibig.
adipose arteries of kidney Kapseläste *pl* der Nierenarterie, Aa. capsulares/perirenales.
adipose body: a. of cheek Bichat'-Wangenfettpfropf *m,* Corpus adiposum buccae.
a. of ischiorectal fossa Corpus adiposum fossae ischio-analis.
a. of orbit Fett(gewebs)körper *m* der Orbita, Corpus adiposum orbitae.
adipose capsule Fettkapsel *f.*

a. of kidney Nierenfettkapsel, perirenale Fettkapsel, Capsula adiposa (renis).
adipose cell Fett(speicher)zelle *f.*
adipose degeneration degenerative Verfettung *f,* fettige Degeneration *f,* Degeneratio adiposa.
adipose infiltration Fettinfiltration *f.*
adipose ligament of knee Plica synovialis infrapatellaris.
adipose sarcoma Liposarkom *nt,* Liposarcoma *nt.*
adipose tissue Fettgewebe *nt.*
brown a. braunes Fettgewebe.
white a. → yellow a.
yellow a. weißes *od.* gelbes Fettgewebe.
adipose tissue necrosis → adiponecrosis.
adipose tumor Fett(gewebs)geschwulst *f,* -tumor *m,* Lipom(a) *nt.*
ad·i·po·sis [,ædɪ'pəʊsɪs] *n, pl* **-ses** [-si:z] **1.** → adiposity. **2.** *patho.* (Organ-)Verfettung *f.*
ad·i·po·si·tis [,ædɪpəʊ'saɪtɪs] *n* Entzündung *f* des Unterhautfettgewebes, Pannikulitis *f,* Panniculitis *f.*
ad·i·pos·i·ty [,ædɪ'pɑsətɪ] *n* Fettleibigkeit *f,* Adipositas *f,* Fettsucht *f,* Obesitas *f,* Obesität *f.*
ad·i·po·so·gen·i·tal degeneration/dystrophy/syndrome [ædɪˌpəʊsəʊ'dʒenɪtl] Babinsky-Fröhlich-Syndrom *nt,* Morbus Fröhlich *m,* Dystrophia adiposogenitalis (Fröhlich).
ad·i·po·su·ria [,ædɪpəʊ'sjʊərɪə] *n* Adiposurie *f,* Lipurie *f,* Lipidurie *f.*
a·dip·sa [ə'dɪpsə] *pl* durststillende Mittel *pl.*
a·dip·sia [ə'dɪpsɪə] *n* Durstlosigkeit *f,* Adipsie *f.*
a·dip·sous [ə'dɪpsəs] *adj* durstlöschend, -stillend.
a·dip·sy [ə'dɪpsɪ] *n* → adipsia.
A disk *histol.* A-Band *nt,* A-Streifen *m,* A-Zone *f,* anisotrope Bande *f.*
ad·i·tus ['ædɪtəs] *n, pl* **ad·i·tus, -tus·es** *anat.* Zu-, Eingang *m,* Aditus *m.*
aditus ad antrum Antrum-mastoideum-Eingang *m,* Aditus ad antrum.
ad·ja·cent [ə'dʒeɪsənt] *adj* (an-)grenzend, anstoßend (*to* an), benachbart, Neben-.
ad·join [ə'dʒɔɪn] **I** *vt* (an-)grenzen an. **II** *vi* nebeneinander liegen, an(einander)grenzen.
ad·join·ing [ə'dʒɔɪnɪŋ] *adj* angrenzend, anstoßend, nebeneinanderliegend, Neben-, Nachbar-.
ad·junct ['ædʒʌŋkt] *n* Hilfsmittel *nt,* -maßnahme *f,* Zusatz *m,* Beigabe *f.*
ad·junc·tive [ə'dʒʌŋktɪv, æ-] *adj* helfend, unterstützend, assistierend (*to*).
ad·just [ə'dʒʌst] **I** *vt* **1.** anpassen, angleichen (*to* an), abstimmen (*to* auf). **2.** berichtigen, ändern. **3.** (*Unterschied*) ausgleichen, beseitigen, bereinigen. **4.** *techn.* (ein-, ver-, nach-)stellen, einregeln, richten, regulieren, justieren. **II** *v s.* anpassen (*to* an); techn. s. einstellen lassen.
ad·just·a·ble [ə'dʒʌstəbl] *adj* **1.** nach-, einverstellbar, justier-, regulierbar. **2.** anpassungsfähig.
ad·just·ment [ə'dʒʌstmənt] *n* **1.** Anpassung *f,* Angleichung (*to* an); Ein-, Anpassung *f.* **2.** Berichtigung *f,* Änderung *f.* **3.** *techn.* Ein-, Ver-, Nachstellung *f,* Regulierung *f,* Justierung *f,* Eichung *f.* **4.** *psycho.* optimale Anpassung *f,* Adjustment *nt.* **5.** (*Fraktur*) Einrichtung *f.*
adjustment disorder Anpassungsstörung *f.*
adjustment nystagmus Einstellungsnystagmus *m.*
ad·ju·vant ['ædʒəvənt] **I** *n pharm., immun.* Adjuvans *nt;* Hilfsmittel *nt.* **II** *adj* helfend, förderlich, adjuvant, Hilfs-.

adjuvant chemotherapy adjuvante Chemotherapie f.
adjuvant radiotherapy adjuvante Strahlentherapie f.
Adler ['ɑːdlər; 'ædiər]: **A.'s test** Benzidinprobe f.
A.'s theory psycho. Adler'-Theorie f.
ad·le·ri·an [æd'lıərıən]: **a. psychology** Individualpsychologie f.
a. psychoanalysis → a. psychology.
ad lib abbr. [ad libitum] pharm. nach Belieben.
ad·me·di·al [æd'miːdɪəl] adj nahe der Medianebene (liegend).
ad·me·di·an [æd'miːdɪən] adj in Richtung zur Medianebene.
ad·mi·nic·u·lum [ˌædməˈnɪkjələm] n, pl **-la** [-lə] anat. Sehnenverstärkung f, -verbreiterung f, Adminiculum nt.
ad·min·is·ter [æd'mɪnəstər] vt (Hilfe) leisten; (Medikament) verabreichen (to sb. jdm.).
ad·min·is·tra·tion [ædˌmɪnəˈstreɪʃn] n (Medikament) Verabreichung f.
ad·mis·sion [æd'mɪʃn] n **1.** Einlaß m, Ein-/Zutritt m (to, into zu). **2.** Brit. (Patient) (stationäre) Aufnahme f.
a. to hospital → admission 2.
ad·mit [æd'mɪt] vt **1.** jdn. einlassen, jdm. Zutritt gewähren. **2.** Brit. (Patient) (stationär) aufnehmen (to, into zu). **to be ted to hospital. 3.** (Fehler) zugeben, eingestehen.
ad·mit·tance [æd'mɪtns] n abbr. **A** phys. Scheinleitwert m, Admittanz f.
ad·ner·val [æd'nɜrvl] adj **1.** in der Nähe eines Nerven (liegend). **2.** auf einen Nerven zu, in Richtung auf einen Nerv.
ad·neu·ral [æd'njʊərəl, -'nʊ-] adj → adnerval.
ad·nex·a [æd'neksə] pl Anhangsgebilde pl, Adnexe pl, Adnexa pl.
ad·nex·ec·to·my [ˌædnekˈsektəmɪ] n chir. Adnexektomie f, Adnektomie f.
ad·nex·i·tis [ˌædnekˈsaɪtɪs] n gyn. Entzündung f der Adnexa uteri, Adnexitis f.
a·do·be tick [ə'dəʊbɪ] micro. Argas persicus.
ad·o·les·cence [ædəˈlesəns] n Jugendalter nt, Adoleszenz f.
ad·o·les·cent [ædəˈlesənt] **I** n Jugendliche(r m) f, Heranwachsende(r m) f. **II** adj heranwachsend, heranreifend, jugendlich, adoleszent, Adoleszenten-.
adolescent albuminuria Adoleszenten-, Pubertätsalbuminurie f, -proteinurie f.
adolescent crisis Pupertäts-, Adoleszentenkrise f.
adolescent proteinuria → adolescent albuminuria.
adolescent scoliosis Adoleszentenskoliose f.
a·don·i·din [ə'dɑnədɪn] n Adonidin n.
a·don·in [ə'dɑnɪn, -'dəʊ-] n Adonin nt.
A·don·is vernalis [ə'dɑnɪs, -'dəʊ-] Adoniskraut nt, -röschen nt, Adonis vernalis.
ad·o·nite ['ædənaɪt] n → adonitol.
a·don·i·tol [ə'dɑnətɔl, -təʊl] n Adonit nt, Adonitol nt.
a·dopt [ə'dɑpt] vt **1.** (Kind) adoptieren. **2.** fig. (Methode, Idee) an-, übernehmen, aneignen, adoptieren.
a·dop·tion [ə'dɑpʃn] n **1.** (Kind) Adoption f, Annahme f an Kindes Statt. **2.** fig. An-, Übernahme f, Aneignung f.
ad·o·ral [æd'ɔːrəl, -'ɒr-] adj in der Nähe des Mundes (liegend), zum Mund hin, adoral.
ADP abbr. → adenosine-(5'-)diphosphate.
adren- pref. → adreno-.
ad·re·nal [ə'dreːnl] **I** n Nebenniere f, Gl. suprarenalis/adrenalis. **II** adj Nebenniere betr., adrenal, Nebennieren-.
adrenal adenoma Nebennierenadenom nt.
adrenal agenesis Nebennierenagenesie f.
adrenal apoplexy Nebennierenapoplexie f, Apoplexia adrenalis.
adrenal bleeding Nebennieren(ein)blutung f.
adrenal body → adrenal I.
adrenal capsule → adrenal I.
accessory a.s → adrenal glands, accessory.
adrenal carcinoma Nebennierenkarzinom nt.
adrenal cortex Nebennierenrinde f abbr. NNR, Cortex (gl. suprarenalis).
definitive a. embryo. definitive Nebennierenrinde.
fetal/primitive a. embryo. fetale Nebennierenrinde.
adrenal cortex system Nebennierenrindensystem nt, NNR-System nt.
adrenal-cortical adj → adrenocortical.
adrenal cortical adenoma → adrenocortical adenoma.
adrenal cortical carcinoma → adrenocortical carcinoma.
adrenal cortical insufficiency → adrenocortical insufficiency.
adrenal crisis Addison-Krise f, akute Nebenniereninsuffizienz f.
a·dre·nal·ec·to·mize [əˌdriːnəˈlektəmaɪz] vt eine Adrenalektomie durchführen.
a·dre·nal·ec·to·my [-'lektəmɪ] n Nebennierenentfernung f, -resektion f, Adrenalektomie f, Epinephrektomie f.
adrenal gland Nebenniere f, Gl. suprarenalis/adrenalis.
accessory a.s versprengte Nebennierendrüsen pl, versprengtes Nebennierengewebe nt, Gll. suprarenales/adrenales accessoriae.
adrenal hemorrhage → adrenal bleeding.
adrenal hyperplasia 1. Nebennierenhyperplasie f. **2.** Nebennierenrindenhyperplasie f.
congenital (virilizing) a. → adrenogenital syndrome.
adrenal hypertension adrenale Hypertonie f.
a·dren·a·line [ə'drenlɪn, -liːn] n Adrenalin nt, Epinephrin nt.
a·dren·a·lin·e·mia [əˌdrenəlɪˈniːmɪə] n (Hyper-)Adrenalinämie f.
adrenaline reversal physiol. Adrenalinumkehr f.
a·dren·a·lin·o·gen·e·sis [əˌdrenəlɪnəˈdʒenəsɪs] n Adrenalinbildung f.
adrenal insufficiency 1. Nebenniereninsuffizienz f, Hyp(o)adrenalismus m. **2.** Nebennierenrindeninsuffizienz f, NNR--Insuffizienz f, Hypoadrenokortizismus m, Hypokortikalismus m, Hypokortizismus m.
a·dren·a·lin·u·ria [əˌdrenəlɪˈnjʊərɪə] n Adrenalinausscheidung f im Harn, Adrenalinurie f.
a·dre·nal·i·tis [əˌdrenəˈlaɪtɪs] n Entzündung f der Nebenniere, Adrenalitis f.
adrenal marrow abbr. **AM** Nebennierenmark nt abbr. NNM, Medulla (gl. suprarenalis).
adrenal medulla → adrenal marrow.
adrenal metastasis Nebennierenmetastase f.
a·dren·a·lone [ə'drenələʊn] n pharm. Adrenalon nt.
a·dre·nal·op·a·thy [əˌdrenəˈlɑpəθɪ] n Nebennierenerkrankung f.
adrenal organ embryo. Adrenalorgan nt.
a·dren·a·lo·trop·ic [əˌdrenələʊˈtrɑpɪk] adj auf die Nebenniere einwirkend, adrenalotrop.
adrenal tuberculosis Nebennierentuberkulose f.
adrenal tumor Nebennierentumor m.
adrenal vein Nebennierenvene f, V. suprarenalis.
left a. linke Nebennierenvene, V. suprarenalis sinistra.
right a. rechte Nebennierenvene, V. suprarenalis/adrenalis dextra.
adrenal virilizing syndrome Virilisierung f.
a·dren·ar·che [ˌædrəˈnɑːrkɪ] n Adrenarche f.
ad·re·ner·gic [ˌædrəˈnɜrdʒɪk] **I** n Sympathomimetikum nt. **II** adj adrenerg(isch).
adrenergic block → adrenergic blockade.
adrenergic blockade Adrenorezeptorenblock(ade f) m.
adrenergic blocking → adrenergic blockade.
adrenergic fibers adrenerge Fasern pl.
adrenergic neuron adrenerges Neuron nt.
adrenergic receptor adrenerger Rezeptor m.
α-adrenergic receptor α-adrenerger Rezeptor m, α-Rezeptor m.
β-adrenergic receptor β-adrenerger Rezeptor m, β-Rezeptor m.
adrenergic system adrenerges System nt.
a·dre·nic [ə'drenɪk, -'driː-] adj Nebennieren betr., Nebennieren-, Adren(o)-.
a·dre·nin [ə'driːnɪn] n → adrenaline.
a·dre·nine [ə'driːniːn] n → adrenaline.
ad·re·ni·tis [ˌædrə'naɪtɪs] n → adrenalitis.
adreno- pref. Nebennieren-, Adren(o)-.
a·dre·no·blas·to·ma [əˌdriːnəʊblæsˈtəʊmə] n Adrenoblastom nt.
a·dre·no·cep·tive [-'septɪv] adj adreno(re)zeptiv.
a·dre·no·cep·tor [ˌ-'septər] n Adreno(re)zeptor m, adrenerger Rezeptor m.
a·dre·no·chrome ['-krəʊm] n Adrenochrom nt.
a·dre·no·cor·ti·cal [ˌ-'kɔːrtɪkl] adj Nebennierenrinde betr., adrenokortikal, adrenocortical, Nebennierenrinden-, NNR-.
adrenocortical adenoma Nebennierenrindenadenom nt, NNR-Adenom nt.
adrenocortical atrophy Nebennierenrindenatrophie f, NNR-Atrophie f.
adrenocortical carcinoma Nebennierenrindenkarzinom nt, NNR-Karzinom nt.
adrenocortical hormone Hormon nt der Nebennierenrinde, Nebennierenrindenhormon nt, NNR-Hormon nt.
adrenocortical hyperplasia Nebennierenrindenhyperplasie f, NNR-Hyperplasie f.
adrenocortical insufficiency Nebennierenrindeninsuffizienz f, NNR-Insuffizienz f, Hypoadrenokortizismus m, Hypokortikalismus m, Hypokortizismus m.
acute a. Addison-Krise f, akute Nebenniereninsuffizienz.
chronic a. primäre chronische Nebennieren(rinden)insuffizienz, Bronze(haut)krankheit f, Addison'-Krankheit f, Morbus Addison m.
adrenocortical steroid Adrenocorticosteroid nt.
a·dre·no·cor·ti·co·hy·per·pla·sia [ˌ-ˌkɔːrtɪkəʊˌhaɪpərˈpleɪʒ(ɪ)ə, -ziə] n adrenocortical hyperplasia.
a·dre·no·cor·ti·co·mi·met·ic [ˌ-ˌkɔːrtɪkəʊmɪˈmetɪk, -maɪ-] adj adrenokortikomimetisch.
a·dre·no·cor·ti·co·tro·phic [ˌ-ˌkɔːrtɪkəʊˈtrəʊfɪk, -'trɑ-] adj → adrenocorticotropic.
a·dre·no·cor·ti·co·tro·phin [ˌ-ˌkɔːrtɪkəʊ-

adrenocorticotropic

'trəʊfɪn] n → adrenocorticotropic hormone.
a·dre·no·cor·ti·co·tro·pic [ˌ-ˌkɔːrtɪkəʊ-'trəʊpɪk, -'trɑp-] adj (adreno-)corticotrop, (adreno-)corticotroph.
adrenocorticotropic hormone abbr. ACTH (adreno-)corticotropes Hormon nt abbr. ACTH, (Adreno-)Kortikotropin nt.
adrenocorticotropic hormone releasing factor abbr. **ACTH-RF** Kortikoliberin nt, Corticoliberin nt, corticotropin releasing factor m abbr. CRF, corticotropin releasing hormone m abbr. CRH.
a·dre·no·cor·ti·co·tro·pin [ˌ-ˌkɔːrtɪkəʊ-'trəʊpɪn] n → adrenocorticotropic hormone.
a·dre·no·dox·in [ˌ-'dɑksɪn] n Adrenodoxin nt.
a·dre·no·gen·ic [ˌ-'dʒenɪk] adj durch die Nebenniere(n) verursacht, von ihr ausgelöst od. ausgehend, adrenogen.
a·dre·no·gen·i·tal syndrome [ˌ-'dʒenɪtl] abbr. **AGS** kongenitale Nebennierenrindenhyperplasie f, adrenogenitales Syndrom nt abbr. AGS.
ad·re·nog·e·nous [ædrə'nɑdʒənəs] adj → adrenogenic.
ad·re·no·ki·net·ic [ˌ-kɪ'netɪk, -kaɪ-] adj die Nebenniere stimulierend, adrenokinetisch.
a·dre·no·leu·ko·dys·tro·phy [ˌ-ˌluːkə'dɪstrəfɪ] n abbr. **ALD** Adrenoleukodystrophie f.
a·dren·o·lyt·ic [ˌ-'lɪtɪk] I n Adrenolytikum nt, Sympatholytikum nt. II adj adrenolytisch, sympatholytisch.
a·dre·no·med·ul·lar·y hormone [ˌ-'medəˌlerɪ, -'medʒə-, -mə'dʌlərɪ] Nebennierenmarkhormon nt, NNM-Hormon nt.
a·dre·no·med·ul·lo·tro·pic [ˌ-ˌmedʒθələ-'trəʊpɪk] adj das Nebennierenmark stimulierend, adrenomedullotrop.
a·dre·no·meg·a·ly [ˌ-'megəlɪ] n Nebennierenvergrößerung f, Adrenomegalie f.
a·dre·no·mi·met·ic [ˌ-mɪ'metɪk, -maɪ-] I n Adrenomimetikum nt, Sympathomimetikum nt. II adj sympathikomimetisch, adrenomimetisch.
ad·re·nop·a·thy [ædrə'nɑpəθɪ] n → adrenalopathy.
a·dre·no·pause [ə'driːnəpɔːz] n Adrenopause f.
a·dre·no·pri·val [ˌəˌdriːnəʊ'praɪvl] adj adrenopriv.
a·dre·no·re·cep·tor [ˌ-rɪ'septər] n → adrenoceptor.
a·dre·no·stat·ic [ˌ-'stætɪk] I n Adrenostatikum nt. II adj adrenostatisch.
a·dre·no·ste·rone [ˌ-stɪ'rəʊn, ˌædrɪ'nɑstə-] n Adrenosteron nt.
a·dre·no·tox·in [ˌ-'tɑksɪn] n die Nebennieren schädigende Substanz f, Adrenotoxin nt.
a·dre·no·tro·phic [ˌ-'trəʊfɪk, -'trɑf-] adj → adrenotropic.
a·dre·no·tro·phin [ˌ-'trəʊfɪn, -'trɑf-] n → adrenocorticotropic hormone.
a·dre·no·tro·pic [ˌ-'trəʊpɪk, -'trɑp-] adj adrenotrop.
ad·re·no·tro·pin [ˌ-'trəʊpɪn, -'trɑp-] n → adrenocorticotropic hormone.
ad·sorb [æd'sɔːrb] vt adsorbieren.
ad·sorb·ate [æd'sɔːrbeɪt, -bət] n Adsorbat nt, Adsorptiv nt, adsorbierte Substanz f.
ad·sorb·ent [æd'sɔːrbənt] I n adsorbierende Substanz f, Adsorbens nt, Adsorber m. II adj adsorbierend.
ad·sorp·tion [æd'sɔːrpʃn] n Adsorption f.
adsorption chromatography Adsorptionschromatographie f.

adsorption coefficient Adsorptionskoeffizient m.
adsorption constant → adsorption coefficient.
ad·sorp·tive [æd'sɔːrptɪv] adj → adsorbent II.
ad·ster·nal [æd'stɜrnl] adj in der Nähe des Sternums (liegend), zum Sternum hin.
a·dult [ə'dʌlt, 'ædʌlt] I n Erwachsene(r m) f. II adj 1. erwachsen, Erwachsenen-; ausgewachsen. 2. fig. reif; gereift.
adult celiac disease Erwachsenenform f der Zöliakie, einheimische Sprue f.
adult GM₁-gangliosidosis Erwachsenenform f der GM₁-Gangliosidose.
adult-onset diabetes nicht-insulinabhängiger Diabetes mellitus m, Typ-II-Diabetes mellitus m, non-insulin-dependent diabetes (mellitus) abbr. NIDD(M).
adult paradentitis Paradontose f.
adult periodontitis Paradontose f.
adult respiratory distress syndrome abbr. **ARDS** Schocklunge f, adult respiratory distress syndrome abbr. ARDS.
adult rickets Osteomalazie f, -malacia f, Knochenerweichung f.
adult tuberculosis postprimäre Tuberkulose f.
adult type: a. of amaurotic idiocy Kufs-Syndrom nt, Kufs-Hallervorden-Krankheit f, Erwachsenenform f der amaurotischen Idiotie.
a. of cerebral sphingolipidosis → a. of amaurotic idiocy.
ad·vance [əd'væns, -'vɑːns] I n Fortschritt m, Weiterentwicklung f, Verbesserung f; Voranschreiten nt, Vorwärtsgehen nt. II adj Voraus-, Vorher-, Vor-. III vt 1. (Katheter) vorrücken, schieben. 2. chir., ortho. (Sehne, Muskel etc.) nach vorne verlegen, vorverlegen. 3. (Wachstum) beschleunigen. 4. fördern, vorantreiben, -bringen, weiterbringen. 5. (Meinung) vorbringen, vertreten. II vi fortschreiten, s. entwickeln, Fortschritte machen.
ad·vanced [əd'vænst, -'vɑːnst] adj 1. fortgeschritten, vorgerückt. ~ **stage** fortgeschrittenes Stadium einer Krankheit. 2. fortschrittliche, modern. 3. fortgeschritten, auf hohem Niveau.
ad·vance·ment [əd'vænsmənt, -'vɑːns-] n chir., ortho. (Sehne, Muskel etc.) Vorverlegen nt, Vorverlagerung f.
advancement flap Verschiebelappen m, -plastik f, Vorschiebelappen m, -plastik f.
ad·vent ['ædvent] n Aufkommen nt, Erscheinen nt; Beginn m.
ad·ven·ti·tia [ˌædven'tɪʃ(ɪ)ə] n 1. (Gefäß) Adventitia f, Tunica adventitia. 2. (Organ) Adventitia f, Tunica externa.
ad·ven·ti·tial [ˌædven'tɪʃ(ɪ)əl] adj (Tunica) Adventitia betr., adventitiell, Adventitial-.
adventitial cells Adventitialzellen pl, Makrophagen pl der Gefäßwand.
adventitial coat → adventitia.
a. of uterine tube Tela subserosa tubae uterinae.
adventitial neuritis Entzündung f der Nervenscheide.
ad·ven·ti·tious [ˌædven'tɪʃəs] adj 1. zufällig erworben, (zufällig) hinzukommend, hinzugekommen. 2. zufällig, nebensächlich, Neben-.
adventitious albuminuria akzidentelle Albuminurie/Proteinurie f.
adventitious cyst Pseudozyste f, falsche Zyste f.
adventitious proteinuria → adventitious albuminuria.
ad·verse [æd'vɜrs, 'ædvɜrs] adj ungünstig,

nachteilig (to für); gegensätzlich; widrig entgegenwirkend.
adverse reaction pharm. unerwartete schädigende Nebenwirkung f.
ad·vice [əd'vaɪs] n Rat m, Ratschlag m. **to follow ~** einen Rat befolgen. **to give ~** einen Rat geben. **on the ~ of sb.** auf Anraten von. **to seek/take (medical) ~** (ärztlichen) Rat suchen od. einholen. **to take sb.'s ~** jds. Rat befolgen.
ad·vise [əd'vaɪz] I vt 1. jdm. raten, jdn. beraten, jdm. einen Rat erteilen od. geben (about über; to do etw. zu tun). 2. jdn. unterrichten, informieren, benachrichtigen, in Kenntnis setzen (of von). 3. jdn. warnen (against vor). II vi s. beraten (with mit).
ad·vised [əd'vaɪzd] adj beraten; informiert, unterrichtet.
a·dy·nam·ia [eɪdaɪ'næmɪə, -'neɪm-] n Kraftlosigkeit f, Muskelschwäche f, Adynamie f, Asthenie f.
a·dy·nam·ic [eɪdaɪ'næmɪk] adj kraftlos, schwach, adynamisch.
adynamic ileus paralytischer Ileus m, Ileus paralyticus.
AE abbr. → above-elbow.
AE amputation → above-elbow amputation.
Aeby ['ebɪ:]: **A's muscle** M. depressor labii inferioris.
AE cast → above-elbow cast.
ae·ci·um [ˈiːsɪəm, -'iːʃ-] n, pl **-cia** [-sɪə, -ʃɪə] micro. Azidium nt, Aecidie f.
A·e·des [eɪ'iːdiːz] n micro. Aedes f. **A. aegyptus** Gelbfieberfliege f, A. aegypti.
ae·lu·ro·pho·bia [ˌ-] n → ailurophobia.
AEP abbr. → auditory evoked potential.
ae·qua·tor [ɪ'kweɪtər] n anat. Äquator m, Aequator m, Equator m.
AER abbr. → apical ectodermal ridge.
aer- pref. → aero-.
aer·as·the·nia [eəræs'θiːnɪə] n → aeroneurosis.
aer·ate ['eərɪt, 'eɪəreɪt] vt 1. mit Sauerstoff anreichern, Sauerstoff zuführen. 2. mit Gas/Kohlensäure anreichern. 3. (be-, durch-)lüften.
aer·at·ed ['eərɪtɪd, 'eɪər-] adj 1. mit Luft beladen. 2. mit Gas/Kohlendioxid beladen. 3. mit Sauerstoff beladen, oxygeniert.
aer·a·tion [eə'reɪʃn] n 1. (Be-, Durch-)Lüftung f. 2. Anreicherung f (mit Luft od. Gas). 3. Sauerstoffzufuhr f. 4. physiol. Sauerstoff-Kohlendioxid-Austausch m in der Lunge.
aer·e·mia [eə'riːmɪə] n 1. → aeroembolism. 2. Druckluft-, Caissonkrankheit f.
aer·i·al ['eərɪəl, eɪ'iːrɪəl] adj 1. Luft betr., zur Luft gehörend, luftig, Luft-. 2. aus Luft bestehend, leicht, flüchtig, ätherisch.
aerial conduction HNO Luftleitung f.
aerial mycelium micro. Luftmyzel nt.
aerial sickness Fliegerkrankheit f.
aer·if·er·ous [eə'rɪfərəs] adj gas-, luftleitend, -führend.
aer·i·form ['eərɪfɔːrm, eɪ'iːrə-] adj luft-, gasförmig.
aero- pref. Luft-, Gas-, Aer(o)-.
aer·o·as·the·nia [ˌeəræs'θiːnɪə] n → aeroneurosis.
Aer·o·bac·ter ['bæktər] n micro. Aerobacter nt.
aer·obe ['eərəʊb] n aerobe Zelle f, aerober Mikroorganismus m, Aerobier m, Aerobiont m, Oxybiont m..
aer·o·bic [eə'rəʊbɪk] adj biochem., bio. aerob.
aerobic coverage clin. antibiotische Abdeckung f gegen aerobe Erreger.

aerobic glycolysis *biochem.* aerobe Glykolyse *f*.
aerobic oxidation *biochem.* aerobe Oxidation *f*.
aerobic respiration aerobe Atmung *f*.
aer·o·bi·ol·o·gy [ˌeərəʊbaɪˈɒlədʒɪ] *n* Aerobiologie *f*.
aer·o·bi·o·sis [ˌ-baɪˈəʊsɪs] *n micro.* Aerobiose *f*, Oxibiose *f*.
aer·o·bi·ot·ic [ˌ-baɪˈɒtɪk] *adj micro.* Aerobiose betr., aerobiotisch.
aer·o·cele [ˈ-siːl] *n* Luftzyste *f*, Aerozele *f*, Aerocele *f*.
Aer·o·coc·cus [ˌ-ˈkɒkəs] *n micro.* Aerococcus *m*.
A. **viridans** vergrünende/viridans Streptokokken *pl*, Streptococcus viridans.
ae·ro·col·pos [ˌ-ˈkɒlpəs] *n* Meteorismus *m* der Scheide, Aerokolpos *m*.
aer·o·cys·tog·ra·phy [ˌ-sɪsˈtɒɡrəfɪ] *n* Pneumozystographie *f*.
aer·o·cys·to·scope [ˌ-ˈsɪstəskəʊp] *n* → aerourethroscope.
aer·o·cys·tos·co·py [ˌ-sɪsˈtɒskəpɪ] *n* Pneumozystoskopie *f*.
aer·o·der·mec·ta·sia [ˌ-dɜrmekˈteɪʒ(ɪ)ə] *n* subkutanes Emphysem *nt*, Hautemphysem *nt*.
aer·o·don·tal·gia [ˌ-dɒnˈtældʒ(ɪ)ə] *n* Aero(o)dontalgie *f*.
aer·o·dy·nam·ic [ˌ-daɪˈnæmɪk] *adj* aerodynamisch.
aer·o·dy·nam·ics [ˌ-daɪˈnæmɪks] *pl* Aerodynamik *f*.
aer·o·em·bo·lism [ˌ-ˈembəlɪzəm] *n* Luftembolie *f*, Aeroembolismus *m*.
aer·o·em·phy·se·ma [ˌ-em(p)fəˈziːmə, -(p)faɪ-] *n* Aeroemphysem *nt*.
aer·o·gas·tria [ˌ-ˈɡæstrɪə] *n* (übermäßige) Luftansammlung *f* im Magen, Aerogastrie *f*.
aer·o·gel [ˈ-dʒel] *n* Aerogel *nt*.
aer·o·gen [ˈ-dʒən] *n* luft- *od.* gasbildendes Bakterium *nt*.
aer·o·gen·e·sis [ˌ-ˈdʒenəsɪs] *n* Luft-, Gasbildung *f*.
aer·o·gen·ic [ˌ-ˈdʒenɪk] *adj* gas-, luftbildend.
aerogenic tuberculosis Inhalationstuberkulose *f*.
aer·og·e·nous [eəˈrɒdʒənəs] *adj* → aerogenic.
aer·o·gram [ˈeərəɡræm] *n* Pneumogramm *nt*.
aer·o·med·i·cine [ˌ-ˈmedəsən] *n* Luftfahrtmedizin *f*, Aeromedizin *f*.
aer·om·e·ter [eəˈrɒmɪtər] *n* Aerometer *nt*.
Aer·o·mo·nas [ˌeərəˈməʊnæs] *n micro.* Aeromonas *f*.
aer·o·neu·ro·sis [ˌ-nʊˈrəʊsɪs, -ˈnjʊə-] *n* Aeroneurose *f*, Aeroasthenie *f*.
aero-odontalgia *n* → aerodontalgia.
aero-odontodynia *n* → aerodontalgia.
aero-otitis *n* Aer(o)otitis *f*, Bar(o)otitis *f*, Otitis barotraumatica.
aer·op·a·thy [eəˈrɒpəθɪ] *n* Aeropathie *f*.
aer·o·pause [ˈeərəpɔːz] *n phys.* Aeropause *f*.
aer·o·per·i·to·ne·um [ˌ-ˌperɪtəˈniːəm] *n* Pneumoperitoneum *nt*.
aer·o·per·i·to·nia [ˌ-ˌperɪˈtəʊnɪə] *n* → aeroperitoneum.
aer·o·pha·gia [ˌ-ˈfeɪdʒ(ɪ)ə] *n* (krankhaftes) Luft(ver)schlucken *nt*, Aerophagie *f*.
aer·oph·a·gy [eəˈrɒfədʒɪ] *n* → aerophagia.
aer·o·phil [ˈeərəfɪl] *n* aerophiler Organismus *m*.
aer·o·phil·ic [ˌ-ˈfɪlɪk] *adj* 1. aerophil. 2. → aerobic.
aer·oph·i·lous [eəˈrafɪləs] *adj* → aerophilic.
aer·o·pho·bia [ˌeərəˈfəʊbɪə] *n* Luftscheu *f*, Aerophobie *f*.

aer·o·pi·e·so·ther·a·py [ˌ-paɪˌiːzəʊˈθerəpɪ] *n* Überdrucktherapie *f*, -behandlung *f*.
aer·o·plank·ton [ˌ-ˈplæŋktən] *n* Luft-, Aeroplankton *nt*.
aer·o·ple·thys·mo·graph [ˌ-pləˈθɪzməɡræf] *n* Aeroplethysmograph *m*.
aer·o·si·al·oph·a·gy [ˌ-ˌsaɪəˈlɒfədʒɪ] *n* (krankhaftes) Verschlucken *nt* von Luft u. Speichel, Sialoaerophagie *f*.
aer·o·si·nus·i·tis [ˌ-saɪnəˈsaɪtɪs] *n* Fliegersinusitis *f*, Aerosinusitis *f*, Barosinusitis *f*.
aer·o·sis [eəˈrəʊsɪs] *n* Gasbildung *f* in Geweben *od.* Organen.
aer·o·sol [ˈeərəsɒl] *n* 1. *phys., chem., pharm.* Aerosol *nt*. 2. Sprüh-, Spraydose *f*.
aerosol infection *micro.* Tröpfcheninfektion *f*.
aerosol inhalation Aerosolinhalation *f*.
aer·o·sol·i·za·tion [ˌ-ˌsɒlɪˈzeɪʃn] *n* Vernebeln *nt*.
aerosol keratitis Aerosolkeratitis *f*.
aerosol therapy Aerosoltherapie *f*.
aer·o·stat·ics [ˌ-ˈstætɪks] *pl* Aerostatik *f*.
aer·o·tax·is [ˌ-ˈtæksɪs] *n bio.* Aerotaxis *f*.
aer·o·ti·tis [ˌ-ˈtaɪtɪs] *n* → aero-otitis.
aer·o·tol·er·ant [ˌ-ˈtɒlərənt] *adj micro.* aerotolerant.
aer·o·to·nom·e·ter [ˌ-təʊˈnɒmɪtər] *n* Aerotonometer *nt*.
aer·ot·ro·pism [eəˈrɒtrəpɪzəm] *n micro.* Aerotropismus *m*.
aer·o·u·re·thro·scope [ˌeərəjʊəˈriːθrəskəʊp] *n* Pneumourethroskop *nt*.
aer·o·u·re·thros·co·py [ˌ-jʊərəˈθrɒskəpɪ] *n* Pneumourethroskopie *f*.
aes·cu·lin [ˈeskjəlɪn] *n* Äskulin *nt*.
aesthesi- *pref.* → aesthesio-.
aesthesio- *pref.* Sinnes-, Sensibilitäts-, Gefühls-, Empfindungs-, Ästhesio-.
aes·ti·vo·au·tum·nal fever [ˌestəvɔːɔː-ˈtʌmnəl, eˌstaɪ-] Falciparum-Malaria *f*, Tropen-, Aestivoautumnalfieber *nt*, Malaria tropica.
AFB *abbr.* → aortofemoral bypass.
a·fe·brile [eɪˈfiːbrəl, -ˈfeb-] *adj* fieberfrei, -los, afebril.
a·fe·tal [eɪˈfiːtl] *adj embryo.* ohne einen Fötus.
af·fect [*n* ˈæfekt; *v* əˈfekt] I *n psycho., psychia.* Affekt *m*, Erregung *f*, Gefühlswallung *f*. II *vt* 1. befallen, berühren, (ein-)wirken auf, beeinflussen, beeinträchtigen, in Mitleidenschaft ziehen. 2. angreifen, befallen, affizieren.
affect displacement *psycho.* Affektverschiebung *f*.
af·fect·ed [əˈfektɪd] *adj* 1. befallen (*with* von). 2. betroffen, berührt.
af·fec·tion [əˈfekʃn] *n* 1. Befall *m*, Erkrankung *f*, Affektion *f*. 2. Gemütsbewegung *f*, Stimmung *f*, Affekt *m*. 3. Zuneigung *f*, Liebe *f* (*for, towards* zu). 4. Einfluß *m*, Einwirkung *f*.
af·fec·tive [ˈæfektɪv] *adj* 1. Affekt betr., Gemüts-, Gefühls-. 2. *psycho.* emotional, affektiv, Affekt-.
affective disorder affektive Psychose *f*.
affective personality *psychia.* zyklothymes Temperament *nt*, zyklothyme Persönlichkeit *f*, Zyklothymie *f*.
affective psychosis affektive Psychose *f*.
af·fec·tiv·i·ty [ˌæfekˈtɪvətɪ] *n* Affektivität *f*.
affect spasms Affektkrämpfe *pl*.
af·fen·spal·te [ˈæfənˌspæltɪ] *n* Affenspalte *f*, Sulcus lunatus.
af·fer·ence [ˈæf(ə)rəns] *n* → afferent I.
afference copy *physiol.* Afferenzkopie *f*.
af·fer·ent [ˈæfərənt] I *n physiol.* Afferenz *f*. II *adj* hin-, zuführend, afferent.
afferent arteriole of glomerulus zuführende Glomerulusarterie/-arteriole *f*, Ar-

teriola glomerularis afferens, Vas afferens (glomeruli).
afferent artery of glomerulus → afferent arteriole of glomerulus.
afferent fibers afferente (Nerven-)Fasern *pl*, Neurofibrae afferentes.
af·fe·ren·tia [æfəˈrenʃɪə] *pl* 1. zuführende/afferente Gefäße *pl*. 2. Lymphgefäße *pl*.
afferent loop syndrome *chir.* Syndrom *nt* der zuführenden Schlinge, Afferent-loop-Syndrom *nt*.
afferent nerve afferenter Nerv *m*.
afferent nerve fibers afferente (Nerven-)Fasern *pl*, Neurofibrae afferentes.
afferent neurofibers → afferent nerve fibers.
afferent neuron afferentes Neuron *nt*.
afferent pathway *physiol.* afferente Bahn *f*.
afferent trunk → afferent vessel.
afferent vessel afferentes/zuführendes Gefäß *nt*.
a. of glomerulus → afferent arteriole of glomerulus.
a.s of lymph node Vasa afferentia nodi lymphatici.
af·fin·i·ty [əˈfɪnətɪ] *n, pl* **-ties** 1. *chem.* Affinität *f*, Neigung *f* (*for, to* zu). 2. Verwandtschaft *f* (*durch Heirat*). 3. Verbundenheit *f*, Übereinstimmung *f* (*for, to* mit); Neigung *f* (*for, to* zu). 4. Ähnlichkeit *f*, Wesensverwandtschaft *f*.
affinity chromatography Affinitätschromatographie *f*.
affinity labeling Affinitätsmarkierung *f*.
af·flict [əˈflɪkt] *vt* betrüben, bedrücken, plagen, zusetzen, peinigen.
af·flict·ed [əˈflɪktɪd] *adj* 1. niedergeschlagen, bedrückt, betrübt. 2. befallen, geplagt (*with* mit); leidend (*with* an).
af·flic·tion [əˈflɪkʃn] *n* 1. Gebrechen *nt*; *pl* Beschwerden *pl*. 2. Betrübnis *f*, Niedergeschlagenheit *f*, Kummer *m*.
af·flu·ence [ˈæfloəns] *n* 1. Zustrom *m*. 2. Fülle *f*, Überfluß *m*, Überschuß *m*.
af·flux [ˈæflʌks] *n* 1. Zufluß *m*, Zustrom *m*, Afflux *m*; Blutandrang *m*.
af·flux·ion [əˈflʌkʃn] *n* → afflux.
A fibers A-Fasern *pl*.
a·fi·brin·o·ge·ne·mia [eɪˌfaɪbrɪnədʒəˈniːmɪə] *n* Afibrinogenämie *f*.
af·la·tox·in [ˌæfləˈtɒksɪn] *n bio.* Aflatoxin *nt*.
AFP *abbr.* → alpha-fetoprotein.
a·fraid [əˈfreɪd] *adj* **to be ~** *s.* fürchten, Angst haben (*of* vor).
Af·ri·can [ˈæfrɪkən] I *n* Afrikaner(in *f*) *m*. II *adj* afrikanisch.
Af·ri·can [ˈæfrɪkən]: A. **anemia** Sichelzell(en)anämie *f*, Herrick-Syndrom *nt*.
A. **Coast fever** East-Coast-Fieber *nt*, bovine Piroplasmose/Theileriose *f*.
A. **endomyocardial fibrosis** Endomyokardfibrose *f*, Endomyokardose *f*, Endokardfibroelastose *f*.
A. **hemorrhagic fever** afrikanisches hämorrhagisches Fieber *nt*.
A. **histoplasmosis** afrikanische Histoplasmose *f*.
A. **lymphoma** Burkitt-Lymphom *nt*, -Tumor *m*, epidemisches Lymphom *nt*, B-lymphoblastisches Lymphom *nt*.
A. **red tick** Rhipicephalus everti.
A. **relapsing fever tick** Ornithodorus moubata.
A. **sleeping sickness** → A. trypanosomiasis.
A. **tapeworm** Rinder(finnen)bandwurm *m*, Taenia saginata, Taeniarhynchus saginatus.
A. **tick fever** afrikanisches Zeckenfieber *nt*.

A. trypanosome *micro.* Trypanosoma brucei.
A. trypanosomiasis afrikanische Schlafkrankheit/Trypanosomiasis *f.*
af·ter ['æftər, 'ɑ:f-] **I** *adj* hintere(r, s); nachträglich, Nach-; künftig. **II** *adv* nach(her), danach, darauf, später. **III** *prep* (*zeitlich*) nach; hinter.
af·ter·ac·tion [ˌ-'ækʃn] *n* Nachreaktion *f.*
af·ter·birth ['-bɜrθ] *n gyn.* Nachgeburt *f.*
af·ter·brain ['-breɪn] *n embryo.* Nachhirn *nt*, Metencephalon *nt.*
af·ter·care ['-keər] *n* Nachsorge *f*, -behandlung *f.*
af·ter·cur·rent ['-kɜrent, -kʌr-] *n physiol.* Nachstrom *m.*
after death postmortal, post mortem.
af·ter·dis·charge [-'dɪstʃɑːrdʒ] *n physiol.* Nachentladung *f.*
af·ter·ef·fect [ˌ-ɪ'fekt] *n* Nachwirkung *f*; Folge *f.*
af·ter·im·age [ˌ-'ɪmɪdʒ] *n ophthal., psycho.* Nachbild *nt.*
af·ter·im·pres·sion [ˌ-ɪm'preʃn] *n* → aftersensation.
af·ter·load ['-ləʊd] *n* Nachlast *f*, -belastung *f*, Afterload *f.*
af·ter·load·ed contraction ['-ləʊdɪd] *physiol.* Unterstützungskontraktion *f.*
af·ter·pains [ˌ-'peɪns] *pl gyn.* Nachwehen *pl.*
af·ter·po·ten·tial [ˌ-pə'tenʃl] *n physiol.* Nachpotential *nt.*
af·ter·re·sponse [ˌ-rɪ'spɒns] *n physiol.* Nachantwort *f.*
af·ter·sen·sa·tion [ˌ-sen'seɪʃn] *n physiol., psycho.* Nachempfindung *f.*
af·ter·stain ['-steɪn] *n old* → counterstain I.
af·ter·taste ['-teɪst] *n* Nachgeschmack *m.*
af·ter·treat·ment [ˌ-'triːtmənt] *n* → aftercare.
af·ter·vi·sion [ˌ-'vɪʒn] *n* → afterimage.
af·to·sa [æf'təʊsə] *n* (echte) Maul- u. Klauenseuche *f abbr.* MKS, Febris aphthosa, Stomatitis epidemica, Aphthosis epizootica.
AG *abbr.* → atrial gallop.
Ag *abbr.* 1. → antigen. 2. → argentum.
a·ga·lac·tia [eɪgə'lækʃ(ɪ)ə, -tɪə] *n gyn.* Agalaktie *f.*
a·ga·lac·to·sis [ˌeɪˌgælæk'təʊsɪs] *n* → agalactia.
a·ga·lac·to·su·ria [ˌeɪgəˌlæktə'sjʊərɪə] *n* Agalaktosurie *f.*
a·ga·lac·tous [eɪgə'læktəs] *adj* 1. *gyn.* die Milchsekretion unterdrückend. 2. (*Säugling*) nicht gestillt.
a·gal·or·rhea [əˌgælə'riːə] *n gyn.* Agalaktorrhoe *f.*
a·gam·ete [eɪgə'miːt, eɪ'gæmiːt] *n* Agamet *m.*
a·gam·ic [eɪ'gæmɪk] *adj* → agamous.
a·gam·ma·glob·u·li·ne·mia [eɪˌgæməˌglɒbjələ'niːmɪə] *n* Agammaglobulinämie *f.*
A·ga·mo·coc·ci·di·ida [eɪˌgæməʊˌkɒksə'daɪədə] *pl micro.* Agamococcidiida *pl.*
a·ga·mo·cy·tog·e·ny [ˌ-saɪ'tɒdʒənɪ] *n bio., micro.* Zerfallsteilung *f*, Schizogonie *f.*
A·ga·mo·fi·lar·ia [ˌ-faɪ'leərɪə] *pl micro.* Agamofilaria *f.*
a·ga·mo·gen·e·sis [ˌ-'dʒenəsɪs] *n* ungeschlechtliche/asexuelle Vermehrung/Reproduktion *f*, Agamogenese *f*, Agamogonie *f.*
a·ga·mo·ge·net·ic [ˌ-dʒə'netɪk] *adj* asexuell vermehrend, agamogen(etisch).
a·ga·mog·o·ny [eɪgə'mɒgənɪ] *n* → agamogenesis.
ag·a·mont ['ægəmɒnt] *n* Agamont *m.*
ag·a·mous ['ægəməs] *adj* 1. agam. 2. geschlechtslos, ungeschlechtlich, asexuell.

a·gan·gli·on·ic [eɪˌgæŋglɪ'ɒnɪk] *adj* aganglionär.
aganglionic megacolon aganglionäres/kongenitales Megakolon *nt*, Hirschsprung-Krankheit *f*, Morbus Hirschsprung *m*, Megacolon congenitum.
a·gan·gli·o·no·sis [eɪˌgæŋglɪə'nəʊsɪs] *n* Aganglionose *f.*
a·gar ['ɑːgɑːr, 'ægər, 'eɪ-] *n* Agar *m/nt.*
agar-agar *n* Agar-Agar *m/nt.*
agar culture medium Agarnährboden *m*, Agar *m/nt.*
agar diffusion method/test Agardiffusionsmethode *f*, -test *m.*
a·gar·ic ['ægərɪk, ə'gærɪk] *n bio.* Blätterpilz *m*, -schwamm *m.*
agaric acid → agaricic acid.
a·ga·ric·ic acid [ægə'rɪsɪk] Agaricinsäure *f.*
agar medium *micro.* Agarnährboden *m.*
agar plate *micro.* Agarplatte *f.*
agar slant *micro.* Schrägagar *m/nt.*
agar slant culture *micro.* Schräg(agar)kultur *f.*
a·gas·tria [eɪ'gæstrɪə] *n embryo.* Agastrie *f.*
a·gas·tric [eɪ'gæstrɪk] *adj* ohne Magen, agastrisch.
agastric anemia Anämie *f* nach Magenresektion.
AGCT *abbr.* → antiglobulin consumption test.
age [eɪdʒ] **I** *n* 1. Alter *nt*, Lebensalter *nt*; Altersstufe *f.* 2. Epoche *f*, Ära *f*, Periode *f.* **II** *vi* 3. altern, alt werden. **at the ~ of 65/65 years of ~** im Alter von 65 Jahren, mit 65 Jahren. **what is her ~?/what ~ is she?** wie alt ist sie? **to be of ~** mündig od. volljährig sein. **to come of ~** mündig od. volljährig werden. **at what ~?** in welchem Alter?, mit wieviel Jahren? **the disease occurs at any ~** die Krankheit taucht in jeder Altersgruppe *od.* -stufe auf. 4. altern, ablagern, reifen lassen.
age class → age group.
a·ged [1,1 'eɪdʒɪd; 2 eɪdʒd] **I the ~** *pl* die Alten *pl*, die alten Menschen. **II** *adj* 1. alt, betagt, bejahrt. 2. -jährig, im Alter von ..., ... Jahre alt.
age-dependence *n* Altersabhängigkeit *f.*
age difference Altersunterschied *m.*
age distribution *stat.* Altersverteilung *f.*
age gap Altersunterschied *m.*
age group Jahrgang *m*, Altersstufe *f*, -klasse *f*, -gruppe *f.*
age·ing ['eɪdʒɪŋ] **I** *n* Altern *nt*, Älterwerden *nt.* **II** *adj* alternd, älter werdend.
age involution Altersinvolution *f.*
age limit Altersgrenze *f.*
a·ge·ne·sia [ˌeɪdʒə'niːʒ(ɪ)ə, -sɪə] *n* → agenesis.
a·gen·e·sis [eɪ'dʒenəsɪs] *n, pl* **-ses** [-siːz] 1. Agenesie *f*, Aplasie *f.* 2. Unfruchtbarkeit *f*, Sterilität *f.*
a·ge·net·ic [ˌeɪdʒə'netɪk] *adj* Agenesie betr.
a·gen·i·tal·ism [eɪ'dʒenɪtəlɪzəm] *n* Agenitalismus *m.*
a·gen·o·so·mia [eɪˌdʒenə'səʊmɪə] *n embryo., patho.* Agenosomie *f.*
a·gen·o·so·mus [-'səʊməs] *n embryo., patho.* Patient(in *f*) *m* mit Agenosomie.
a·gent ['eɪdʒənt] **I** *n* 1. *chem., bio., phys., pharm.* Wirkstoff *m*, Mittel *nt*, Agens *nt.* 2. *patho.* Krankheitserreger *m.* 3. (Stell-)Vertreter(in *f*) *m*, Bevollmächtigte(r *m*) *f*, Beauftragte(r *m*) *f.* **II** *adj* wirkend, handelnd, tätig.
AGEPC *abbr.* → acetyl glyceryl ether phosphoryl choline.
age-related *adj* altersbedingt, -bezogen.
a·geu·sia [ə'gjuːzɪə] *n* Geschmacksverlust *m*, -lähmung *f*, Ageusie *f.*
a·geu·sic [ə'gjuːzɪk] *adj* Ageusie betr.
a·geus·tia [ə'gjuːstɪə] *n* → ageusia.

ag·ger ['ædʒər] *n anat.* Vorsprung *m*, Wulst *m*, Agger *m.*
ag·glom·er·ate [*n, adj* ə'glɒmərɪt, -reɪt; *v* -reɪt] **I** *n* Anhäufung *f*, (Zusammen-)Ballung *f*, Agglomerat *nt.* **II** *adj* zusammengeballt, (an-)gehäuft, agglomeriert. **III** *vt* zusammenballen, anhäufen, agglomerieren. **IV** *vi s.* zusammenballen, *s.* anhäufen, agglomerieren.
ag·glom·er·at·ed [ə'glɒmeˌreɪtɪd] *adj* → agglomerate II.
ag·glom·er·a·tion [-'reɪʃn] *n* Zusammenballung *f*, Anhäufung *f*, Agglomeration *f.*
ag·glom·e·rin [ə'glɒmərɪn] *n* Agglomerin *nt.*
ag·glu·tin·a·ble [ə'gluːtɪnəbl] *adj* agglutinierbar, agglutinabel.
ag·glu·ti·nant [ə'gluːtɪnənt] **I** *n* Klebe-, Bindemittel *nt.* **II** *adj* klebend.
ag·glu·ti·nate [*adj* ə'gluːtɪnɪt, -neɪt; *v* -neɪt] **I** *adj* zusammengeklebt, verbunden, agglutiniert. **II** *vt* 1. zusammen-, verkleben, zusammenballen, agglutinieren. 2. an-, zusammenheilen. **III** *vi* zusammenkleben, *s.* verbinden, verklumpen, verkleben, agglutinieren.
ag·glu·ti·nat·ing antibody [ə'gluːtəˌneɪtɪŋ] kompletter/agglutinierender Antikörper *m.*
ag·glu·ti·na·tion [əˌgluːtə'neɪʃn] *n* 1. Zusammen-, Verkleben *nt*, Zusammenballung *f*, Verklumpen *nt*, Agglutination *f.* 2. Zusammen-, Verheilen *nt.*
agglutination assay → agglutination test.
agglutination inhibiting reaction Agglutinationshemmungsreaktion *f abbr.* AHR.
agglutination test Agglutinationsprobe *f*, -test *m*, -reaktion *f.*
heterophil a. 1. Paul-Bunnell-Test. 2. modifizierter Paul-Bunnell-Test mit Pferdeerythrozyten.
latex a. Latex(agglutinations)test.
agglutination titer Agglutinationstiter *m.*
ag·glu·ti·na·tive [ə'gluːtəˌneɪtɪv] *adj* agglutinierend.
agglutinative thrombus hyaliner Thrombus *m.*
ag·glu·ti·na·tor [ə'gluːtəˌneɪtər] *n* 1. agglutinierende Substanz *f.* 2. → agglutinin.
ag·glu·ti·nin [ə'gluːtənɪn] *n* Agglutinin *nt*, Immunagglutinin *nt.*
ag·glu·tin·o·gen [ˌæglə'tɪnədʒən, ə'gluːtɪnə-] *n* Agglutinogen *nt*, agglutinable Substanz *f.*
ag·glu·tin·o·gen·ic [ˌæglɒˌtɪnə'dʒenɪk, əˌgluːtɪnə-] *adj* agglutinin-bildend.
ag·glu·tin·o·phil·ic [ˌ-'fɪlɪk] *adj* leicht agglutinierend.
ag·glu·to·gen·ic [əˌgluːtə'dʒenɪk] *adj* → agglutinogenic.
ag·gra·vate ['ægrəveɪt] *vt* verschlimmern, erschweren, verschärfen, verschlechtern.
ag·gra·vat·ed risk ['ægrəveɪtɪd] erhöhtes Risiko *nt.*
ag·gra·vat·ing ['ægrəveɪtɪŋ] *adj* verschlimmernd, erschwerend, verschärfend, aggravierend.
ag·gra·va·tion [ægrə'veɪʃn] *n* Verschlimmerung *f*, Erschwerung *f*, Verschärfung *f*, Aggravation *f.*
ag·gre·gate [*n, adj* 'ægrɪgɪt, -geɪt; *v* 'ægrɪgeɪt] **I** *n bio., techn.* Anhäufung *f*, Ansammlung *f*, Masse *f*, Aggregat *nt.* **II** *adj* (an-)gehäuft, vereinigt, gesamt, Gesamt-; aggregiert. **III** *vt* aggregieren; anhäufen, -sammeln; vereinigen, verbinden. **IV** *vi s.* (an-)häufen, *s.* ansammeln.
ag·gre·gat·ed follicles ['ægrɪgeɪtɪd] Peyer'-Plaques *pl*, Folliculi lymphatici aggregati.
a. of vermiform appendix Peyer'-Plaques der Appendix vermiformis, Folliculi lym-

phatici aggregati appendicis vermiformis.
aggregated glands → aggregated follicles.
aggregated nodules → aggregated follicles.
ag·gre·ga·tion [ˌægrɪ'geɪʃn] *n* **1.** (An-)Häufung *f*, Ansammlung *f*, Aggregation *f*, Agglomeration *f*. **2.** *chem.* Aggregation *f*. **3.** Aggregat *nt*.
ag·gre·gom·e·ter [ˌægrɪ'gɑmɪtər] *n* Thrombaggregometer *nt*.
ag·gre·gom·e·try [ˌ-'gɑmətrɪ] *n* Thrombaggregometrie *f*.
ag·gres·sin [ə'gresn] *n* Aggressin *nt*.
ag·gres·sion [ə'greʃn] *n* *psycho.* Aggression *f*, Angriffsverhalten *nt* (*on*, *upon* auf).
ag·gres·sive [ə'gresɪv] *adj* **1.** aggressiv, angreifend, angriffslustig, Angriffs-, Aggressions-. **2.** *fig.* dynamisch, aggressiv.
aggressive instinct *psycho.* Todestrieb *m*.
ag·gres·sive·ness [ə'gresɪvnɪs] *n* Angriffslust *f*, Aggressivität *f*.
ag·gres·siv·i·ty [ægrə'sɪvətɪ] *n* → aggressiveness.
ag·ing *n*, *adj* → ageing.
aging process Alterungsprozeß *m*.
ag·i·tate ['ædʒɪteɪt] *vt* **1.** *fig.* beunruhigen, stören, aufregen, aufwühlen. **2.** schütteln, erschüttern, hin u. her bewegen.
ag·i·tat·ed ['ædʒɪteɪtɪd] *adj* aufgeregt, erregt, agitiert.
agitated depression *psychia.* agitierte Depression *f*.
ag·i·ta·tion [ædʒɪ'teɪʃn] *n* **1.** körperliche Unruhe *f*, Agitatio(n) *f*, Agitiertheit *f*. **2.** Erschütterung *f*, Hin- u. Herbewegung *f*. **3.** Aufregung *f*, Erregung *f*, Unruhe *f*.
ag·i·to·graph·ia [ˌædʒɪtəʊ'græfɪə] *n psychia.* Agitographie *f*.
ag·i·to·la·lia [ˌ-'leɪlɪə] *n* → agitophasia.
ag·i·to·pha·sia [ˌ-'feɪʒ(ɪ)ə] *n psychia.* Agitophasie *f*.
a·glos·sia [eɪ'glɑsɪə] *n* Aglossie *f*.
aglossia-adactylia syndrome *embryo.* Aglossie-Adaktylie-Syndrom *nt*, Hypoglossie-Hypodaktylie-Syndrom *nt*.
a·glos·so·sto·mia [eɪˌglɑsə'stəʊmɪə] *n* Aglossostomie *f*.
a·glu·con [ə'glu:kɑn] *n* → aglycon.
a·glu·cone [ə'glu:kəʊn, eɪ-] *n* → aglycon.
a·glu·ti·tion [ˌæglu:'tɪʃn] *n patho.*, *neuro.* Schluckunfähigkeit *f*, Aglutition *f*.
a·gly·ce·mia [əˌglaɪ'si:mɪə, eɪ-] *n* Aglukosämie *f*, Aglykämie *f*.
a·gly·con [ə'glaɪkɑn, eɪ-] *n* Aglukon *nt*, Aglykon *nt*, Genin *nt*.
a·gly·cone [ə'glaɪkəʊn, eɪ-] *n* → aglycon.
a·gly·cos·u·ric [əˌglaɪkəʊ's(j)ʊərɪk, eɪ-] *adj* aglukosurisch, ohne Glukosurie.
ag·ma·ti·nase [æg'mætɪneɪz] *n* Agmatinase *f*.
ag·ma·tine ['ægməti:n] *n* Agmatin *nt*.
ag·na·thia [æg'neɪθɪə] *n* Agnathie *f*.
ag·na·thous ['ægneɪθəs] *adj* Agnathie betr., von Agnathie betroffen, agnath.
ag·na·thus ['ægneɪθəs] *n* Agnathus *m*.
ag·no·gen·ic [ˌægnəʊ'dʒenɪk] *adj* von unbekannter Herkunft *od.* Äthiologie, idiopathisch.
agnogenic myeloid metaplasia idiopathische/primäre myeloische Metaplasie *f*, Leukoerythroblastose *f*, leukoerythroblastische Anämie *f*.
ag·no·sia [æg'nəʊʒ(ɪ)ə, -zɪə] *n* Agnosie *f*.
ag·nos·te·rol [æg'nɑstərɔl, -rəʊl] *n* Agnosterin *nt*.
ag·nos·tic [æg'nɑstɪk] **I** *n* Agnostiker(in *f*) *m*. **II** *adj* Agnosie betr., von Agnosie betroffen, agnostisch.
ag·nos·ti·cal [æg'nɑstɪkl] *adj* → agnostic II.

a·gof·ol·lin [ə'gɑfəlɪn] *n* Estradiol *nt*, Östradiol *nt*.
ag·om·phi·a·sis [ˌægɑm'faɪəsɪs] *n* (völlige) Zahnlosigkeit *f*, Anodontie *f*, Anodontia *f*, Agomphiasis *f*.
a·gom·phi·ous [ə'gɑmfɪəs] *adj* zahnlos.
ag·om·pho·sis [ægɑm'fəʊsɪs] *n* → agomphiasis.
a·go·nad [eɪ'gəʊnæd, -'gɑ-] *n* Patient(in *f*) *m* mit Agonadismus.
a·go·nad·al [eɪ'gɑnædl] *adj* agonadal.
a·go·nad·ism [eɪ'gɑnədɪzəm] *n* Agonadismus *m*.
ag·o·nal ['ægɑnl] *adj* Agonie betr., agonal.
agonal leukocytosis terminale Leukozytose *f*.
ag·o·nist ['ægɑnɪst] *n* **1.** *physiol.*, *pharm.* Agonist *m*. **2.** *anat.* → agonistic muscle.
ag·o·nis·tic [ægɑ'nɪstɪk] *adj* Agonist *od.* Agonismus betr., agonistisch, Agonisten-.
agonistic muscle Antagonist *m*, Gegenmuskel *m*.
ag·o·niz·ing pain ['ægənaɪzɪŋ] qualvolle Schmerzen *pl*.
ag·o·ny ['ægənɪ] *n* **1.** Todeskampf *m*, Agonie *f*. **2.** heftiger unerträglicher Schmerz *m*; Höllenqual(en *pl*) *f*, Pein *f*. **to be in ~** unerträgliche Schmerzen haben, Höllenqualen ausstehen.
ag·o·ra·pho·bia [ˌægərə'fəʊbɪə] *n* Platzangst *f*, Agoraphobie *f*.
a·grafe *n* → agraffe.
a·graffe [ə'græf] *n* Wundklemme *f*, -klammer *f*.
ag·ram·mat·i·ca [ˌægrə'mætɪkæ] *n* → agrammatism.
a·gram·ma·tism [eɪ'græmətɪzəm] *n neuro.* Agrammatismus *m*.
ag·ram·ma·to·lo·gia [eɪˌgræmətə'lɔʊdʒɪə] *n* → agrammatism.
a·gran·u·lar [eɪ'grænjələr] *adj* agranulär.
agranular cortex agranuläre (Hirn-)Rinde *f*, agranulärer Kortex *m*.
agranular isocortex → agranular cortex.
agranular leukocyte → agranulocyte.
agranular reticulum glattes/agranuläres endoplasmatisches Retikulum *abbr.* S-ER.
a·gran·u·lo·cyte [eɪ'grænjələʊsaɪt] *n* agranulärer/lymphoider Leukozyt *m*, Agranulozyt *m*.
a·gran·u·lo·cyt·ic angina [ˌ-'sɪtɪk] → agranulocytosis.
a·gran·u·lo·cy·to·sis [ˌ-saɪ'təʊsɪs] *n* Agranulozytose *f*, maligne/perniziöse Neutropenie *f*.
a·graph·ia [eɪ'græfɪə, ə-] *n* Schreibunfähigkeit *f*, Agraphie *f*.
a·graph·ic [eɪ'græfɪk] *adj* Agraphie betr., agraphisch.
A-G ratio → albumin-globulin ratio.
a·gryp·no·co·ma [əˌgrɪpnə'kəʊmə] *n* Agrypnocoma *f*.
a·gryp·no·dal coma [əˌgrɪp'nəʊdl] akinetischer Mutismus *m*, vigiles Koma *nt*, Coma vigile.
AGS *abbr.* → adrenogenital syndrome.
AGT *abbr.* → antiglobulin test.
a·gue ['eɪgju:] *n* Sumpf-, Wechselfieber *nt*, Malaria *f*.
ague fever → ague.
a·gy·ria [eɪ'dʒaɪrɪə, ə-] *n* Agyrie *f*, Agyrismus *m*.
a·gy·ric [eɪ'dʒaɪrɪk, ə-] *adj* Agyrie betr.
ah *abbr.* → hyperopic astigmatism.
a·hap·to·glo·bi·ne·mia [ə'hæptəʊˌglɒʊbɪ'ni:mɪə] *n* Ahaptoglobulinämie *f*.
A-H conduction time *card.* AH-Intervall *nt*.
AHD *abbr.* → antihyaluronidase.
AHF *abbr.* [antihemophilic factor (A)] → antihemophilic globulin.

AHG *abbr.* → antihemophilic globulin.
A-H interval *card.* AH-Intervall *nt*.
Ahumada-Del Castillo [ahu'mada del kas'tiljo]: **A.-D. syndrome** *gyn.* Argonz-Del Castillo(-Ahumada)-Syndrom *nt*.
A.I. *abbr.* **1.** → apex impulse. **2.** → artificial insemination.
AI *abbr.* **1.** → anaphylatoxin inactivator. **2.** → aortic insufficiency.
Aicardi [ɪ'kɑːrdɪ; ɛkar'di]: **A.'s syndrome** *ped.* Aicardi-Syndrom *nt*.
aich·mo·pho·bia [ˌeɪkmə'fəʊbɪə] *n* Aichmophobie *f*.
A.I.D. *abbr.* → artificial insemination, donor.
aid [eɪd] **I** *n* **1.** Hilfe *f* (*to* für), Hilfeleistung *f* (in bei), Unterstützung *f*, Beistand *m*. **by/with ~ of** mit Hilfe von, mittels. **2.** Helfer(in *f*) *m*, Gehilfe *m*, Gehilfin *f*, Assistent(in *f*) *m*. **3.** Hilfsmittel *nt*, -gerät *nt*. **II** *vt* **4.** unterstützen, beistehen, Hilfe/Beistand leisten, jmd. helfen (*in* bei; *to do* zu tun). **5.** (*Entwicklung*) fördern; etw. erleichtern. **III** *vi* helfen (*in* bei).
AIDS [eɪdz] *abbr.* → aquired immunodeficiency syndrome.
AIDS-associated retrovirus *abbr.* **ARV** → AIDS virus.
Aids-associated virus → AIDS virus.
AIDS-related complex *abbr.* **ARC** AIDS-related-Complex *m* *abbr.* ARC.
AIDS virus human immunodeficiency virus (*nt*) *abbr.* HIV, humanes T-Zell-Leukämie-Virus III *nt* *abbr.* HTLV III, Lymphadenopathie-assoziiertes Virus *nt* *abbr.* LAV, AIDS-Virus *nt*.
A.I.H. *abbr.* → artificial insemination, homologous.
AIHA *abbr.* → autoimmune hemolytic anemia.
ail [eɪl] **I** *vt* schmerzen, weh tun. **II** *vi* kränkeln, kränklich sein.
AILD *abbr.* → angioimmunoblastic lymphadenopathy with dysproteinemia.
ail·ing ['eɪlɪŋ] *adj* kränklich, kränkelnd, leidend.
ail·ment ['eɪlmənt] *n* Krankheit *f*, Erkrankung *f*, Leiden *nt*, Gebrechen *nt*.
ai·lu·ro·pho·bia [aɪˌlʊərə'fəʊbɪə, eɪ-] *n* Angst *f* vor Katzen, Ailurophobie *f*.
aim [eɪm] **I** *n* **1.** Ziel *nt*; Absicht *f*. **2.** *fig.* Zweck *m*, Absicht *f*, Ziel *nt*. **II** *vt* (*Kamera*, *Bestrebungen*) richten (*at* auf). **III** *vi* **3.** zielen (*at* auf). **4.** *fig.* beabsichtigen, abzielen (*at*, *for* auf).
ai·nhum [aɪ'njum] *n* Ainhum(-Syndrom *nt*) *nt*, Dactylosis spontanea.
air [eər] **I** *n* Luft *f*. **II** *adj* pneumatisch, Luft-.
air arthrography *radiol.* Pneumoarthrographie *f*.
air bath Luftbad *nt*, Balneum pneumaticum.
air block *pulmo.* Air-Block-Syndrom *nt*.
air·borne ['eərbɔːrn, -bəʊrn] *adj* durch die Luft übertragen *od.* verbreitet, aerogen.
airborne infection aerogene Infektion *f*.
air cell *histol.* lufthaltiger Hohlraum *m* in Knochen *od.* Geweben, lufthaltige Zelle *f*.
a.s of auditory tube Tubenbuchten *pl*, -zellen *pl*, Cellulae pneumaticae tubae auditivae.
mastoid a.s Warzenfortsatzzellen *pl*, Cellulae mastoideae.
tubal a.s → a.s of auditory tube.
air cleaner Luftreiniger *m*, -filter *m*.
air conduction *abbr.* **AC, A.C.** *physiol.* (*Schall*) Luftleitung *f*.
air-contrast barium enema *radiol.* Doppel-, Bikontrastmethode *f*.
air-cushion sign *radiol.* Klemm'-Zeichen *nt*.

air douche

air douche *HNO* Luftdusche *f.*
air-dried *adj* luftgetrocknet.
air embolism Luftembolie *f.*
air-fluid level *radiol.* (Flüssigkeits-)Spiegel *m.*
air hunger Lufthunger *m,* Kussmaul(-Kien)-Atmung *f.*
air lock Luftschleuse *f.*
air passage Luft-, Atemweg *m.*
air pollution Luftverunreinigung *f,* -verschmutzung *f.*
air pressure Luftdruck *m.*
air-proof ['eərpru:f] **I** *adj* luftdicht. **II** *vt* luftdicht machen.
air pyelography *urol., radiol.* Pneumopyelographie *f.*
air saccules → alveolar saccules.
air sacs → alveolar sacs.
air sickness Fliegerkrankheit *f.*
air sinuses (Nasen-)Nebenhöhlen *pl,* Sinus paranasales.
air·stream ['eərstri:m] *n* Luftstrom *m.*
air supply Luftzufuhr *f.*
air temperature Lufttemperatur *f.*
air thermometer Luftthermometer *nt.*
air·tight ['eətaɪt] *adj* **1.** luftdicht, hermetisch verschlossen. **2.** *fig.* hieb- u. stichfest.
air trapping *radiol.* Lufteinschluß *m.*
air·way ['eəweɪ] *n* **1.** *anat.* Atem-, Luftweg *m.* **2.** Beatmungsrohr *nt,* Tubus *m.*
airway compression Atemwegskompression *f.*
airway obstruction Verlegung *f* der Atemwege, Atemwegsobstruktion *f.*
airway resistance *physiol.* Atemwegswiderstand *m,* Resistance *f.*
airway system Atemwegssystem *nt.*
air vesicles Lungenalveolen *pl,* -bläschen *pl,* Alveoli pulmonis.
AK *abbr.* → above-knee.
Akabori [ækə'bɔ:rɪ]: **A. procedure/reaction** *biochem.* Akabori-Reaktion *f.*
AK amputation Oberschenkelamputation *f,* Amputation *f* durch den Oberschenkel.
aka·mu·shi [ækə'mu:ʃɪ] *n* japanisches Fleckfieber *nt,* Scrub-Typhus *m,* Milbenfleckfieber *nt,* Tsutsugamushi-Fieber *nt.*
akamushi disease → akamushi.
a·kar·y·o·cyte [eɪ'kærɪəsaɪt] *n* kernlose Zelle *f,* Akaryozyt *m.*
a·kar·y·o·mas·ti·gont [,-'mæstɪgənt] *n* micro. Akaryomastigont *m.*
a·kar·y·o·ta [eɪ'kærɪəʊt] *n* → akaryocyte.
a·kar·y·ote [eɪ'kærɪəʊt] *n* → akaryocyte.
a·kat·a·ma·the·sia [eɪˌkætəmə'θi:ʒ(ɪ)ə] *n* Akatamathesie *f.*
a·kat·a·no·e·sis [,-'nəʊɪsɪs] *n* Akatanoese *f.*
ak·a·this·ia [ækə'θɪzɪə] *n* Akathisie *f.*
A-kinase *n* Adenylatkinase *f,* Myokinase *f,* AMP-Kinase *f,* A-Kinase *f.*
a·ki·ne·si·a [eɪkaɪ'ni:ʒ(ɪ)ə, -kɪ-] *n* Bewegungslosigkeit *f,* Bewegungsarmut *f,* Akinese *f,* Akinesie *f.*
a·ki·ne·sis [eɪkaɪ'ni:sɪz] *n* → akinesia.
a·kin·es·the·sia [eɪkɪnəs'θi:ʒ(ɪ)ə] *n* Akinästhesie *f.*
a·ki·net·ic [eɪkaɪ'netɪk] *adj* **1.** Akinese betr. *od.* verursachend, akinetisch, bewegungslos, -arm. **2.** Amitose betr., amitotisch.
akinetic ataxia akinetische Ataxie *f.*
akinetic autism akinetischer Mutismus *m,* vigiles Koma *nt,* Coma vigile.
akinetic epilepsy akinetische Epilepsie *f.*
akinetic mutism → akinetic autism.
a·ki·ya·mi [ækɪ'jæmɪ] *n* Sakushu-Fieber *nt,* Akiyami(-Fieber *nt*) *nt,* Hasamiyami(-Fieber *nt*) *nt.*
a·ko·ria *n* → acoria.
A·kur·ey·ri disease ['ækəreərɪ] epidemische Neuromyasthenie *f,* Encephalomyelitis benigna myalgica.
AL *abbr.* → acute leukemia.
Al *abbr.* → aluminum.
ALA *abbr.* → δ-aminolevulinic acid.
Ala *abbr.* → alanine.
a·la ['eɪlə] *n, pl* **a·lae** ['eɪli:] *bio., anat.* Flügel *m,* Ala *f,* flügelförmige Struktur *f.*
a. of central lobule of cerebellum Ala lobuli centralis (cerebelli).
a. of ilium Becken-, Darmbeinschaufel *f,* Ala ossis ilii.
a. of vomer Ala vomeris.
a·lac·ri·ma [eɪ'lækrɪmə] *n* Alakrimie *f.*
a·lac·ta·sia [eɪlæk'teɪʒ(ɪ)ə, -ziə] *n* Lactasemangel *m,* Alaktasie *f.*
Alajouanine [ˌalaʒua'nin]: **A.'s syndrome** Alajouanine-Syndrom *nt.*
a·la·lia [eɪ'leɪlɪə] *n* Alalie *f,* Alalia *f.*
a·lal·ic [eɪ'lælɪk] *adj* Alalie betr., von Alalie betroffen.
A·land ['ælænd]: **A. eye disease** okulärer Albinismus (Forsius-Eriksson) *m.*
al·a·nine ['ælənɪn, -nɪn] *n abbr.* **Ala** Alanin *nt abbr.* **Ala,** Aminopropionsäure *f.*
alanine aminotransferase *abbr.* **ALT** Alaninaminotransferase *f abbr.* **ALT,** Alanintransaminase *f,* Glutamatpyruvattransaminase *f abbr.* **GPT.**
β-al·a·nin·e·mia [ˌæləni'ni:mɪə] *n* Hyperbetaalaninämie *f,* β-Alaninämie *f.*
β-alanine α-ketoglutarate transaminase → β-alanine transaminase.
β-alanine-oxoglutarate aminotransferase → β-alanine transaminase.
alanine racemase Alaninracemase *f.*
alanine transaminase → alanine aminotransferase.
β-alanine transaminase Aminobuttersäureaminotransferase *f,* β-Alaninaminotransferase *f.*
Alanson ['ælənsən]: **A.'s amputation** *ortho.* Alanson-Amputation *f,* -Technik *f.*
a·lan·tin [ə'læntɪn] *n* Inulin *nt.*
al·a·nyl ['ælənɪl] *n* Alanyl-(Radikal *nt*).
alanyl-tRNA synthetase Alanyl-tRNA-Synthetase *f.*
a·lar [eɪlə] *adj* Ala betr., flügelähnlich, -förmig, Flügel-.
alar bone Flügel-, Keilbein *nt,* Os sphenoidale.
alar cartilage (of nose) Nasenflügelknorpel *m,* Cartilago alaris.
greater a. großer Nasenflügelknorpel, Cartilago alaris major.
lesser a.s kleine Nasenflügelknorpel *pl,* Cartilagines alares minores.
alar chest langer flacher Thorax *m.*
alar folds Plicae alares.
alar lamina → alar plate.
alar ligaments Flügelbänder *pl,* Ligg. alaria.
a. of knee Plicae alares.
alarm reaction *abbr.* **AR** Alarmreaktion *f.*
alar plate *embryo.* Flügelplatte *f,* Lamina alaris.
sensory a. sensible Flügelplatte.
alar process Ala cristae galli.
alar scapula Scapula alata.
alar spine Spina ossis sphenoidalis.
a·la·ryn·ge·al speech [eɪlə'rɪndʒ(ɪ)əl] *HNO* Ösophagussprache *f,* -stimme *f,* -ersatzstimme *f.*
a·las·trim ['æləstrɪm] *n* weiße Pocken *pl,* Alastrim *nt,* Variola minor.
alastrim virus Alastrimvirus *f.*
Albarrán [ælbα'ræn; alba'ran]: **A.'s disease** Ausscheidung *f* von Escherichia coli im Harn.
Albee ['ɔ:lbi:]: **A.'s operation** *gyn.* Albee-Operation *f.*

Albee-Delbet [del'bɛj]: **A.-D. operation** *gyn.* Albee-Delbet-Operation *f.*
Albers-Schönberg ['ælbərs 'ʃønbαrg]: **A.-S. disease** Albers-Schönberg-Krankheit *f,* Marmorknochenkrankheit *f,* Osteopetrosis *f.*
A.-S. marble bones → A.-S. disease.
Albert ['ælbərt]: **A.'s disease** Albert-Krankheit *f,* Entzündung *f* der Bursa tendinis calcanei.
A.'s operation *ortho.* Albert-Operation *f,* Kniegelenksarthrodese *f* nach Albert.
A.'s suture *chir.* Albert-Naht *f.*
al·bi·du·ri·a [ælbɪ'd(j)ʊərɪə] *n* Albidurie *f.*
Albini [æl'bi:nɪ]: **A.'s nodules** Albini'-, Cruveilhier'-Knötchen *pl.*
al·bi·nism ['ælbənɪzəm] *n* **1.** Weißsucht *f,* Albinismus *m.* **2.** Tyrosinase-positiver okulokutaner Albinismus *m.*
al·bi·nis·mus [ælbə'nɪzməs] *n* → albinism.
al·bi·no [æl'baɪnəʊ; *Brit.* -'bi:-] *n* Patient(in *f*) *m* mit Albinismus, Albino *m/f.*
al·bi·noid·ism ['ælbɪ'nɔɪdɪzəm] *n* **1.** Albinoidismus *m.* **2.** Tyrosinase-positiver okulokutaner Albinismus *m.*
al·bi·not·ic [ˌ-'nɑtɪk] *adj* Albinismus betr., von Albinismus betroffen *od.* gekennzeichnet.
albinotic fundus *ophthal.* albinotischer Fundus *m,* Fundus albinoticus.
al·bi·nu·ria [ˌ-'n(j)ʊərɪə] *n* → albiduria.
Albinus [æl'baɪnəs]: **A.' muscle 1.** M. risorius. **2.** M. scalenus medius.
Albright ['ɔ:lbraɪt]: **A.'s disease** → A.'s syndrome.
A.'s dystrophy → A.'s syndrome.
A.'s hereditary osteodystrophy Martin-Albright-Syndrom *nt.*
A.'s syndrome 1. Albright(-McCune)-Syndrom *nt,* McCune-Albright-Syndrom *nt,* polyostotische fibröse Dysplasie *f.* **2.** Martin-Albright-Syndrom *nt.*
Albright-McCune-Sternberg [mə'kju:n'stɑrnbərg] : **A.-M.-S. syndrome** → Albright's syndrome.
al·bu·gin·ea [ælbjuː'dʒɪnɪə] *n* bindegewebige Hodenhülle *f,* Albuginea *f* (testis), Tunica albuginea testis.
a. of ovari Eierstockkapsel *f,* Tunica albuginea ovarii.
al·bu·gin·e·ot·o·my [ˌ-dʒɪnɪ'αtəmɪ] *n chir.* Albugineotomie *f.*
al·bu·gin·e·ous coat [ˌ-'dʒɪnɪəs] → albugineous tunic.
albugineous tunic Tunica albuginea testis/ovarii.
al·bu·gin·i·tis [ˌ-dʒɪ'naɪtɪs] *n* Albuginitis *f.*
al·bu·go [æl'bju:gəʊ] *n ophthal.* weißer Hornhautfleck *m,* Leukom(a) *nt,* Leucoma *nt,* Albugo *f.*
al·bu·men [æl'bju:mən] *n* **1.** Eiweiß *nt,* Albumen *nt.* **2.** → albumin.
al·bu·mim·e·ter [ælbju:'mɪmɪtər] *n* → albuminimeter.
al·bu·min [æl'bju:mɪn] *n* **1.** Albumin *nt.* **2.** Serumalbumin *nt.*
al·bu·mi·nate [æl'bju:mənɪt] *n* Albuminat *nt.*
al·bu·mi·na·tu·ria [ælˌbju:mɪnə'tjʊərɪə] *n* Albuminaturie *f.*
al·bu·mi·ne·mia [ælˌbju:mɪ'ni:mɪə] *n* Albuminämie *f.*
albumin-globulin ratio Albumin-Globulin-Quotient *m,* Eiweißquotient *m.*
al·bu·mi·nim·e·ter [ælˌbju:mɪ'nɪmɪtər] *n* Albuminimeter *nt.*
al·bu·mi·nim·e·try [ˌ-'nɪmətrɪ] *n* Albuminimetrie *f.*
al·bu·mi·no·cho·lia [ælˌbju:mɪnəʊ'kəʊlɪə] *n* Albuminocholie *f.*
al·bu·mi·no·cy·to·log·i·cal [ˌ-saɪtə'lɑdʒɪkl] *adj* albumino-zytologisch.

al·bu·mi·no·cy·to·log·ic dissociation [ˌ-saɪtə'lɑdʒɪk] albuminozytologische Dissoziation *f.*
al·bu·mi·noid [æl'bjuːmɪnɔɪd] **I** *n* Gerüsteiweiß *nt,* Skleroprotein *nt,* Albuminoid *nt.* **II** *adj* eiweißähnlich, -artig, albuminähnlich, -artig, albuminoid.
albuminoid degeneration *pathol.* albuminöse/albuminoide/albuminoid-körnige Degeneration *f,* trübe Schwellung *f.*
albuminoid-granular degeneration → albuminoid degeneration.
albuminoid liver Amyloidleber *f.*
al·bu·mi·nol·y·sis [ælˌbjuːmə'nɑləsɪs] *n* Albuminspaltung *f,* Albuminolyse *f.*
al·bu·mi·nom·e·ter [ˌ-'nɑmɪtər] *n* → albuminimeter.
al·bu·mi·nop·ty·sis [ˌ-'nɑptəsɪs] *n* Albuminoptysis *f.*
al·bu·mi·no·r·rhea [ælˌbjuːmɪnə'riːə] *n* übermäßige Albuminausscheidung *f,* Albuminorrhoe *f.*
al·bu·mi·nous [æl'bjuːmɪnəs] *adj* eiweiß-, albuminhaltig, albuminös.
albuminous cell seröse Drüsenzelle *f.*
albuminous degeneration → albuminoid degeneration.
albuminous swelling → albuminoid degeneration.
albuminous granules zytoplasmatische Granula *pl.*
al·bu·mi·nu·ret·ic [ælˌbjuːmɪnə'retɪk] **I** *n* albuminuretisches Mittel *nt.* **II** *adj* Albuminurie betr. *od.* fördernd, albuminuretisch.
al·bu·min·u·ria [ælˌbjuːmɪ'n(j)ʊərɪə] *n* Eiweißausscheidung *f* im Harn, Albuminurie *f*; Proteinurie *f.*
a. of athletes Sportalbuminurie, -proteinurie.
al·bu·min·u·ric [ˌ-'n(j)ʊərɪk] *adj* Proteinurie betr., proteinurisch, albuminurisch.
albuminuric retinitis Retinitis/Retinopathia albuminurica.
al·bu·ter·ol [æl'bjuːtərɔl, -əʊl] *n pharm.* Salbutamol *m.*
Al·ca·lig·e·nes [ˌælkə'lɪdʒəniːz] *n micro.* Alcaligenes *m.*
al·cap·ton *n* → alkapton.
alcapton bodies Alkaptonkörper *pl.*
al·cap·ton·u·ria *n* → alkaptonuria.
al·cap·ton·u·ric *adj* → alkaptonuric.
Alcock ['ælkɑks, 'ɔl-]: **A.'s canal** Alcock'--Kanal *m,* Canalis pudendalis.
al·co·hol ['ælkəhɔl, -hɒl] *n* **1.** *chem.* Alkohol *m,* Alcohol *m.* **2.** Äthylalkohol *m,* Äthanol *m,* Ethanol *m.* **3.** alkoholische Getränke *pl.*
alcohol abuse Alkoholmißbrauch *m,* -abusus *m.*
alcohol addict Alkoholiker(in *f*) *m,* Alkoholsüchtige(r *m*) *f.*
alcohol addiction → alcoholism.
alcohol amnestic syndrome Alkoholamnesiesyndrom *nt.*
alcohol dehydrogenase *abbr.* **AD, ADH** Alkoholdehydrogenase *f abbr.* AD, ADH.
alcohol dependence → alcoholism.
alcohol diuresis alkoholinduzierte Diurese *f.*
al·co·hol·e·mia [ˌælkəhə'liːmɪə] *n* Alkoholämie *f.*
al·co·hol·ic [ˌælkə'hɑlɪk] **I** *n* Alkoholiker(in *f*) *m,* Alkoholsüchtige(r *m*) *f.* **to be an ~** Alkoholiker *od.* Trinker sein. **II** *adj* **1.** Alkohol betr., alkoholartig *od.* -haltig, alkoholisch, Alkohol-. **2.** alkoholsüchtig.
alcoholic abuse → alcohol abuse.
alcoholic amblyopia *ophthal.* alkoholtoxische Amblyopie *f.*

Alcoholic Anonymous (die) Anonymen Alkoholiker (*pl*).
alcoholic cardiomyopathy alkoholische/ alkohol-toxische Kardiomyopathie *f.*
alcoholic cirrhosis Alkoholzirrhose *f,* Cirrhosis alcoholica.
alcoholic coma Koma *nt* bei Alkoholintoxikation, Coma alcoholicum.
alcoholic delirium Alkoholdelir *nt,* Delirium tremens/alcoholicum.
alcoholic excess Alkoholmißbrauch *m.*
alcoholic fermentation *biochem.* alkoholische Gärung/Fermentation *f.*
alcoholic hepatitis (chronische) Alkoholhepatitis *f,* alkohol-toxische Hepatitis *f.*
alcoholic hyalin *patho.* alkoholisches Hyalin *nt.*
alcoholic hyaline bodies Mallory-Körperchen *pl.*
al·co·hol·ic·i·ty [ˌælkəhə'lɪsətɪ] *n* Alkoholgehalt *m.*
alcoholic myopathy Alkoholmyopathie *f.*
alcoholic neuritis → alcoholic neuropathy.
alcoholic neuropathy alkoholische/alkoholtoxische Neuropathie *f.*
alcoholic pancreatitis alkoholische Pankreatitis *f.*
alcoholic paralysis alkohol-toxische Paralyse *f.*
alcoholic paraplegia alkohol-toxische Paraplegie *f.*
alcoholic patient → alcoholic I.
alcoholic poisoning Alkoholvergiftung *f,* -intoxikation *f.*
alcoholic psychosis *psychia.* Alkoholpsychose *f.*
alhocolic solution alkoholische Lösung *f.*
alcoholic strength Alkoholgehalt *m.*
alcohol intoxication Betrunkenheit *f,* Alkoholrausch *m,* -intoxikation *f.*
al·co·hol·ism ['ælkəhɑlɪzəm] *n* Trunksucht *f,* Alkoholabhängigkeit *f,* Äthylismus *m,* Alkoholismus *m.*
al·co·hol·i·za·tion [ˌælkəˌhɒlə'zeɪʃn] *n* Alkoholisieren *nt,* Alkoholisierung *f.*
al·co·hol·ize ['ælkəhɒlaɪz] *vt* **1.** *chem.* in Alkohol verwandeln, mit Alkohol versetzen *od.* sättigen, alkoholisieren. **2.** jdn. betrunken machen, alkoholisieren.
al·co·hol·om·e·ter [ˌælkəhə'lɑmɪtər] *n* Alkoholometer *nt,* Alkoholmesser *m.*
alcohol-soluble protein Prolamin *nt.*
alcohol thermometer Alkoholthermometer *nt.*
al·co·hol·u·ria [ˌælkəhɒ'l(j)ʊərɪə] *n* Alkoholurie *f.*
alcohol withdrawal Alkoholentzug *m.*
al·co·hol·y·sis [ˌælkə'hɑləsɪs] *n* Alkoholyse *f.*
al·co·sol ['ælkəsɒl, -səʊl] *n* Alkosol *nt.*
al·cu·ro·ni·um chloride [ælkjʊə'rəʊnɪəm] Alcuroniumchlorid *nt.*
ALD *abbr.* → adrenoleukodystrophy.
al·dar·ic acid [æl'dærɪk] Aldar-, Zuckersäure *f.*
al·de·hyde ['ældəhaɪd] *n* **1.** *chem.* Aldehyd *m.* **2.** Azet-, Acetaldehyd *m,* Äthanal *nt,* Ethanal *nt.*
aldehyde dehydrogenase (NAD+) Aldehyddehydrogenase *f.*
aldehyde lyase → aldolase I.
aldehyde oxidase Aldehydoxidase *f.*
al·de·hy·dic [ˌældə'haɪdɪk] *adj* Aldehyd betr., aldehydisch, Aldehyd-.
Alder ['ɑldər; 'ældər]: **A.'s anomaly** Alder-Granulationsanomalie *f,* -körperchen *pl.*
A.'s bodies → A.'s anomaly.
A.'s constitutional granulomatosis → A.'s anomaly.

Alder-Reilly ['raɪlɪ]: **A.-R. anomaly** → Alder's anomaly.
A.-R. bodies Alder-Reilly-Körperchen *pl.*
A.-R. corpuscles Alder-Reilly-Körperchen *pl.*
al·di·mine ['ældɪmiːn] *n* Aldimin *nt.*
al·do·bi·on·ic acid [ˌældəʊbaɪ'ɑnɪk] Aldobionsäure *f.*
al·do·hep·tose [ˌ-'heptəʊs] *n* Aldoheptose *f.*
al·do·hex·ose [ˌ-'heksəʊs] *n* Aldohexose *f.*
al·dol·ase ['-leɪz] *n* **1.** Aldehydlyase *f,* Aldolase *f.* **2.** Fructosediphosphataldolase *f,* -bisphosphataldolase *f,* Aldolase *f abbr.* ALD.
al·dol condensation ['ældɒl, -dɑl] Aldolkondensation *f.*
al·don·ic acid [æl'dɑnɪk] Aldonsäure *f.*
al·do·no·lac·to·nase [ˌældənəʊ'læktəneɪz] *n* Aldonolactonase *f.*
al·do·oc·tose [ˌældəʊ'ɑktəʊs] *n* Aldooctose *f.*
al·do·pen·tose [ˌ-'pentəʊs] *n* Aldopentose *f.*
al·dose ['ældəʊs] *n* Aldose *f,* Aldehydzucker *m.*
aldose 1-epimerase Aldose-1-epimerase *f,* Mutarotase *f.*
aldose reductase Aldosereduktase *f.*
al·do·side ['ældəsaɪd] *n* Aldosid *nt.*
al·dos·ter·one [ˌ-'stɪərəʊn, æl'dɑstərəʊn] *n* Aldosteron *nt.*
aldosterone antagonist Aldosteronantagonist *m.*
aldosterone system Aldosteronsystem *nt.*
al·do·ster·on·ism [ˌ-'stɪərɒnɪzəm] *n* (Hyper-)Aldosteronismus *m.*
al·do·ster·o·no·gen·e·sis [ˌ-ˌstɪərənəʊ'dʒenəsɪs] *n* Aldosteronbildung *f.*
al·do·ster·on·o·ma [ˌ-ˌstɪərə'nəʊmə] *n* aldosteronbildender Tumor *m,* Aldosteronom *nt.*
al·do·ster·o·no·pe·nia [ˌ-ˌstɪərənəʊ'piːnɪə] *n* Aldosteronmangel *m,* Hypoaldosteronismus *m.*
al·do·ster·on·u·ria [ˌ-ˌstɪərə'n(j)ʊərɪə] *n* Aldosteronurie *f.*
al·do·tet·rose [ˌ-'tetrəʊz] *n* Aldotetrose *f.*
al·do·tri·ose [ˌ-'traɪəʊz] *n* Aldotriose *f.*
al·dox·ime [æl'dɑksiːm, -sɪm] *n* Aldoxim *nt.*
Aldrich ['ɔːldrɪtʃ]: **A.'s syndrome** Wiskott--Aldrich-Syndrom *nt.*
Aldrich-Mees [miːz]: **A.-M. lines** Mees--Streifen *pl.*
al·drin ['ɔːldrɪn] *n* Aldrin *nt.*
a·lec·i·thal [eɪ'lesɪθəl] *adj bio.* dotterlos, alezithal.
alecithal ovum *bio.* alezithales Ei *nt.*
A·lep·po [ə'lepəʊ]: **A. boil** Hautleishmaniase *f,* kutane Leishmaniase *f,* Orientbeule *f,* Leishmaniasis cutis.
A. gall Gallapfel *m.*
a·lert [ə'lɜːrt] *adj* **1.** wachsam, aufmerksam. **2.** (*Patient, Kind*) rege, munter, aufgeweckt. **II** *vt* warnen (*to* vor). **to ~ sb. to the risks** jdn. vor den Risiken warnen.
a·lert·ness [ə'lɜːrtnɪs] *n* **1.** Wachsamkeit *f,* Aufmerksamkeit *f.* **2.** Regsamkeit *f,* Munterkeit *f,* Aufgewecktheit *f.*
a·leu·ke·mia [æluː'kiːmɪə] *n* **1.** Leukozytopenie *f.* **2.** → aleukemic leukemia.
a·leu·ke·mic [æluː'kiːmɪk] *adj* aleukämisch.
aleukemic leukemia aleukämische Leukämie *f.*
aleukemic myelosis leukoerythroblastische Anämienämie *f,* idiopathische/primäre myeloische Metaplasie *f,* Leukoerythroblastose *f.*
a·leu·kia [ə'luːkɪə] *n* Aleukie *f*; Leukopenie *f.*

aleukocythemic leukemia

a·leu·ko·cy·the·mic leukemia [ə‚luːkəʊ-saɪ'θiːmɪk] aleukämische Leukämie *f*.
a·leu·ko·cyt·ic [‚-'sɪtɪk] *adj* aleukozytisch, aleukozytär.
a·leu·ko·cy·to·sis [‚-saɪ'təʊsɪs] *n* Aleukozytose *f*; Leukopenie *f*.
a·leu·ri·o·spore [ə'lʊərɪəspəʊər, -spɔːr] *n micro.* Aleurospore *f*, Aleurie *f*.
Alexander [ælɪɡ'zændər]: **A.'s disease/leukodystrophy** Alexander-Syndrom *nt*, -Leukodystrophie *f*.
A.'s operation → Alexander-Adams operation.
Alexander-Adams ['ædəmz]: **A.-A. operation** *gyn.* Alexander-Adams-Operation *f*.
a·lex·i·a [ə'leksɪə, eɪ'l-] *n* Leseunfähigkeit *f*, -unvermögen *nt*, Alexie *f*.
a·lex·ic [ə'leksɪk] *adj* Alexie betr., alektisch.
a·lex·in unit [ə'leksɪn] Komplementeinheit *f*.
a·lex·i·phar·mac [ə‚leksɪ'fɑːrmək] *n, adj old* → alexipharmic.
a·lex·i·phar·mic [‚-'fɑːrmɪk] **I** *n* Gegengift *nt*, -mittel *nt*, Alexipharmakon *nt*, Antidot *nt* (*for, against, to* gegen). **II** *adj* als Gegengift wirkend.
a·lex·i·thy·mia [‚-'θaɪmɪə] *n* Alexithymie *f*.
Alezzandrini [ælɪzæn'driːnɪ]: **A.'s syndrome** Alezzandrini-Syndrom *nt*.
ALG *abbr.* → antilymphocyte globulin.
alg- *pref.* → algesio-.
al·ga ['ælɡə] *n, pl* **-gas, -gae** ['ældʒɪ] *micro.* Alge *f*, Alga *f*.
al·gal ['ælɡəl] *adj* Algen betr., von Algen verursacht, Algen-.
algal fungi *micro.* Algenpilze *pl*, niedere Pilze *pl*, Phykomyzeten *pl*, Phykomyzetes *pl*.
al·gan·es·the·sia [æl‚ɡænes'θiːʒ(ɪ)ə] *n* Aufhebung *f* der Schmerzempfindlichkeit, Schmerzunempfindlichkeit *f*, -losigkeit *f*, Analgesie *f*.
alge- *pref.* → algesio-.
al·ge·fa·cient [ældʒɪ'feɪʃənt] *adj* kühlend; erfrischend.
algesi- *pref.* → algesio-.
al·ge·si·a [æl'dʒiːzɪə] *n* Schmerzempfindlichkeit *f*, -haftigkeit *f*, Algesie *f*; Hyperalgesie *f*.
al·ge·sic [æl'dʒiːzɪk] *adj* schmerzhaft, schmerzend, algetisch.
al·ge·sim·e·ter [ældʒə'sɪmətər] *n* Alge(si)meter *nt*.
al·ge·sim·e·try [‚-'sɪmətrɪ] *n* Alg(es)imetrie *f*.
algesio- *pref.* Schmerz(en)-, Algesi(o)-, Algi(o)-, Alg(o)-.
al·ge·si·o·gen·ic [æl‚dʒiːsɪəʊ'dʒenɪk] *adj* schmerz-verursachend, algogen.
al·ge·si·om·e·ter [æl‚dʒiːsiː'ɒmɪtər] *n* → algesimeter.
al·ge·si·om·e·try [‚-'ɒmətrɪ] *n* → algesimetry.
al·ges·the·sia [‚ældʒes'θiːʒ(ɪ)ə] *n* **1.** Schmerzempfindlichkeit *f*, Algästhesie *f*. **2.** → algesthesis.
al·ges·the·sis [‚-'θiːsɪs] *n* (*Gefühl*) Schmerzempfindung *f*, -wahrnehmung *f*, Algästhesie *f*.
al·get·ic [æl'dʒetɪk] *adj* → algesic.
algi- *pref.* → algesio-.
al·gi·cide ['ældʒəsaɪd] *n* Algizid *nt*.
al·gid ['ældʒɪd] *adj* kühl, kalt.
al·gin ['ældʒɪn] *n* Algin *nt*, Natiumalginat *nt*.
al·gi·nate ['ældʒɪneɪt] *n* Alginat *nt*.
al·gin·ic acid [æl'dʒɪnɪk] Alginsäure *f*.
al·gin·u·re·sis [‚ældʒɪnjə'riːsɪs] *n* Alguria *f*.
algio- *pref.* → algesio-.

al·gi·o·mo·tor [‚ældʒɪəʊ'məʊtər] *adj* alg(i)omotorisch.
al·gi·o·mus·cu·lar [‚-'mʌskjələr] *adj* alg(i)omuskulär.
al·gi·o·vas·cu·lar [‚-'væskjələr] *adj* alg(i)ovaskulär.
algo- *pref.* → algesio-.
al·go·dys·tro·phy [‚ælɡəʊ'dɪstrəfɪ] *n* Algodystrophie(-Syndrom *nt*) *f*.
al·go·gen·e·sia [‚-dʒə'niːʒ(ɪ)ə] *n* Schmerzentstehung *f*.
al·go·gen·e·sis [‚-'dʒenəsɪs] *n* → algogenesia.
al·go·gen·ic [‚-'dʒenɪk] *adj* **1.** Schmerz(en) verursachend, algogen. **2.** Kälte produzierend.
al·go·lag·nia [‚-'læɡnɪə] *n psychia.* Schmerzwollust *f*, Algolagnie *f*.
al·go·men·or·rhea [‚-‚menə'rɪə] *n old* → dysmenorrhea.
al·gom·e·ter [æl'ɡɒmɪtər] *n* → algesimeter.
al·gom·e·try [æl'ɡɒmətrɪ] *n* → algesimetry.
al·go·phil·ia [‚-'fɪlɪə] *n old psychia.* Masochismus *m*, Passivismus *m*.
al·go·pho·bia [‚-'fəʊbɪə] *n psychia.* Algophobie *f*.
al·go·rithm ['-rɪðm] *n mathe., stat.* Algorithmus *m*.
al·go·sis [æl'ɡəʊsɪs] *n* Algose *f*.
al·go·spasm [‚ælɡə'spæzəm] *n* Algospasmus *m*.
al·go·vas·cu·lar [‚-'væskjələr] *adj* → algiovascular.
Alibert [ali'bɛr]: **A.'s disease** Alibert(-Bazin)-Krankheit *f*, (*klassische*) Mycosis fungoides, Mycosis fungoides Alibert-Bazin-Form.
Alice-in-Wonderland syndrome ['ælɪs ɪn ‚wʌndərlænd] *psychia.* Alice-in-Wonderland-Syndrom *nt*.
al·i·cy·clic [‚ælə'saɪklɪk, -'sɪk-] *adj chem.* alizyklisch.
alicyclic compound *chem.* alizyklische Verbindung *f*.
alicyclic hydrocarbon alizyklischer Kohlenwasserstoff *m*.
al·ien·a·tion [‚eɪljə'neɪʃn, ‚eɪlɪə-] *n* **1.** Entfremdung *f* (*from* von); Abwendung *f*, Abneigung *f*. **2.** Entfremdung *f*, Depersonalisation *f*.
a·li·e·nia [eɪlɪ'iːnɪə] *n embryo.* Alienie *f*.
al·i·form ['æləfɔːrm, 'eɪl-] *adj anat.* flügelförmig.
a·lign [ə'laɪn] **I** *vt* **1.** in eine (gerade) Linie bringen, in einer Linie aufstellen, ausrichten (*with* nach). **2.** *phys., techn.* ausrichten, justieren, einstellen, abgleichen. **II** *vi* in eine (gerade) Linie bilden (*with* mit), s. ausrichten (*with* nach).
a·lign·ment [ə'laɪnmənt] *n* **1.** Ausrichten *nt*, Aufstellung *f* in einer (geraden) Linie *f*. **2.** Ausrichtung *f*. **3.** *ortho.* (*Fraktur*) (anatomisch-korrekte) Ausrichtung *f* der Bruchfragmente. **4.** *phys., techn.* Ausrichten *nt*, Justierung *f*, Abgleich(en *nt*) *m*.
alignment chart Nomogramm *nt*.
al·i·ment [*n* 'æləmənt; *v* -‚ment] **I** *n* Nahrung(smittel *nt*) *f*. **II** *vt* jdn. erhalten, unterhalten, versorgen.
al·i·men·tal [‚ælɪ'mentəl] *adj* → alimentary 1.
al·i·men·ta·ry [‚ælɪ'mentərɪ] *adj* **1.** nahrhaft, nährend. **2.** Nahrungs-, Ernährungs-; zum Unterhalt dienend, alimentär. **3.** Verdauungs-, Speise-.
alimentary bolus Bissen *m*, Bolus *m*.
alimentary canal Verdauungskanal *m*, -trakt *m*, Canalis alimentarius/digestivus, Tractus alimentarius.
alimentary diabetes alimentäre Glykosurie *f*.

alimentary duct Brustmilchgang *m*, Milchbrustgang *m*, Ductus thoracicus.
alimentary edema Hungerödem *nt*.
alimentary glycosuria alimentäre Glucosurie/Glykosurie *f*.
alimentary lipemia alimentäre/postprandiale Lipämie *f*.
alimentary osteopathy alimentäre/nutritive Osteopathie *f*, Hungerosteopathie *f*.
alimentary system Verdauungsapparat *m*, Digestitionssystem *nt*, Apparatus digestorius, Systema alimentarium.
alimentary tract → alimentary canal.
al·i·men·ta·tion [‚ælɪmen'teɪʃn] *n* **1.** Ernährung *f*. **2.** Unterhalt *m*.
al·i·men·tol·o·gy [ælɪmen'tɒlədʒɪ] *n* Ernährungslehre *f*.
al·i·men·to·ther·a·py [ælɪ‚mentəʊ'θerəpɪ] *n* diätetische Behandlung *f*.
aline *vt, vi* → align.
a·line·ment *n* → alignment.
al·i·phat·ic [‚ælə'fætɪk] *adj chem.* aliphatisch, offenkettig.
aliphatic compound *chem.* aliphatische Verbindung *f*.
aliphatic hydrocarbon aliphatischer Kohlenwasserstoff *m*.
a·lip·o·gen·ic [əlɪpə'dʒenɪk] *adj chem.* alipogen.
a·lip·oid·ic [əlɪp'ɔɪdɪk] *adj chem.* alipoid.
a·lip·o·trop·ic [əlɪpə'trɒpɪk] *adj biochem.* alipotrop.
al·i·quor·rhea [‚ælɪkwə'rɪə] *n* Aliquorrhoe *f*.
al·i·quot ['ælɪkwɒt, -kwət] **I** *n mathe.* aliquoter Teil *m*, Aliquote *f*. **II** *adj mathe.* ohne Rest teilend, aliquot.
al·i·sphe·noid bone [ælɪ'sfɪnɔɪd] großer Keilbeinflügel *m*, Ala major (ossis sphenoidalis).
a·live [ə'laɪv] *adj* **1.** lebend, lebendig, am Leben. **to keep sb./sth. ~** jdn./etw. am Leben erhalten. **2.** *fig.* lebendig, munter, rege.
a·liz·a·rin [ə'lɪzərɪn] *n chem.* Alizarin *nt*.
alizarin yellow Alizaringelb *nt*.
al·ka·le·mia [‚ælkə'liːmɪə] *n* Alkal(i)ämie *f*.
al·ka·les·cence [‚ælkə'lesəns] *n* Alkaleszenz *f*.
al·ka·les·cent [‚-'lesənt] *adj* alkaleszent.
al·ka·li ['ælkəlaɪ] **I** *n, pl* **-lies, -lis** *chem.* Alkali *nt*. **II** *adj* → alkaline.
al·ka·li·fy ['-lɪfaɪ, æl'kælɪ-] **I** *vt chem.* Alkalien zusetzen, alkalisch/basisch machen, alkalisieren. **II** *vi* (s.) in ein Alkali verwandeln, alkalisieren.
Al·ka·lig·e·nes [‚-'lɪdʒənɪz] *n* → Alcaligenes.
al·ka·lig·e·nous [‚-'lɪdʒɪnəs] *adj* alkalibildend, alkaligen.
alkali metal Alkalimetall *nt*.
al·ka·lim·e·ter [‚-'lɪmɪtər] *n* Alkalimeter *nt*.
al·ka·li·met·ric [‚-lə'metrɪk] *adj chem.* Alkalimetrie betr., alkalimetrisch.
al·ka·lim·e·try [‚-'lɪmətrɪ] *n* Alkalimetrie *f*.
al·ka·line ['ælkəlaɪn, -lɪn] *adj* Alkali(en) enthaltend, alkalisch, basisch, Alkali-.
alkaline earth metal Erdalkalimetall *nt*.
alkaline metal → alkali metal.
alkaline phosphatase *abbr.* **AP, ALP** alkalische Phosphatase *f abbr.* **AP**.
alkaline phosphate alkalisches Phosphat *nt*.
alkaline reaction 1. basische Reaktion *f*, basisches Verhalten *nt*. **2.** Basennachweis *m*.
alkaline reserve *physiol.* Alkalireserve *f*.
al·ka·lin·i·ty [‚-'lɪnətɪ] *n* Alkalität *f*, alkalischer/basischer Zustand *m*, Gehalt *m* an Alkalien.
al·ka·lin·i·za·tion [‚-‚lɪnə'zeɪʃn, -‚laɪnə-, -‚laɪnaɪ-] *n* → alkalization.
al·ka·lin·ize ['-lɪnaɪz] *vt* → alkalify **I**.

al·ka·li·nu·ria [ˌ-lɪ'n(j)ʊərɪə] *n* Alkaliurie *f*.
alkali reserve *physiol.* Alkalireserve *f*.
al·ka·li·za·tion [ˌ-lɪ'zeɪʃn, -laɪ-] *n* Alkalisierung *f*, Alkalisieren *nt*.
al·ka·lize ['-laɪz] *vt* → alkalify I.
al·ka·liz·er ['-laɪzər] *n* alkalisierende Substanz *f*.
al·ka·loid ['-lɔɪd] **I** *n* biochem., bio. Alkaloid *nt*. **II** *adj* alkaliähnlich, alkaloid.
al·ka·lom·e·try [ˌ-'lɑmətrɪ] *n* Alkalometrie *f*.
al·ka·lo·phile ['-ləʊfaɪl] *n micro.* alkalophiler Organismus *m*.
al·ka·lo·sis [ˌ-'ləʊsɪs] *n* Alkalose *f*.
al·ka·lot·ic [ˌ-'lɑtɪk] *adj* Alkalose betr., durch Alkalose gekennzeichnet, alkalotisch, Alkalose(n)-.
al·ka·lu·ria [ˌ-'l(j)ʊərɪə] *n* Alkalurie *f*.
al·kane ['ælkeɪn] *n* Alkan *nt*, Paraffin *nt*.
al·kap·ton [æl'kæptɑn, -tən] *n* Alkapton *f*.
alkapton bodies Alkaptonkörper *pl*.
al·kap·ton·u·ri·a [æl,kæptə'n(j)ʊərɪə] *n* Alkaptonurie *f*.
al·kap·ton·u·ric [ˌ-'n(j)ʊərɪk] *adj* Alkaptonurie betr., von Alkaptonurie betroffen *od.* gekennzeichnet, alkaptonurisch.
al·kene ['ælkiːn] *n* Alken *nt*.
al·kine *n* → alkyne.
al·kyl ['ælkɪl] *n* Alkyl-(Radikal *nt*).
al·kyl·a·mine ['ælkɪləˌmiːn, ˌælkə'læmiːn] *n* Alkylamin *nt*.
al·kyl·ate ['ælkəleɪt] *vt chem.* alkylieren.
al·kyl·at·ing agent ['-leɪtɪŋ] **1.** alkylierendes Agens. **2.** *pharm.* Alkylanz *f*.
al·kyl·a·tion [ˌ-'leɪʃn] *n chem.* Alkylierung *f*.
al·kyl·a·tor ['-leɪtər] *n* → alkylating agent.
al·kyl·ic [æl'kɪlɪk] *adj* Alkylgruppe betr. *od.* enthaltend, Alkyl-.
al·kyne ['ælkaɪn] *n* Alkin *nt*.
ALL *abbr.* → acute lymphatic leukemia.
all- *pref.* → allo-.
all·a·ches·the·sia [ˌælakes'θiːʒ(ɪ)ə] *n* → allesthesia.
al·lan·ti·a·sis [ælən'taɪəsɪs] *n* Wurstvergiftung *f*, Allantiasis *f*.
al·lan·to·cho·ri·on [əˌlæntəʊ'kɔːrɪən] *n embryo.* Allantochorion *nt*.
al·lan·to·en·ter·ic diverticulum [ˌ-en'terɪk] → allantoic diverticulum.
al·lan·to·gen·e·sis [ˌ-'dʒenəsɪs] *n embryo.* Harnsackbildung *f*, Allantogenese *f*.
al·lan·to·ic [ˌælən'təʊɪk] *adj* Allantois betr., allantoisch, Allantois-.
allantoic acid Allantoinsäure *f*.
allantoic circulation *embryo.* Umbilikal-, Nabelschnur-, Allantoiskreislauf *m*.
allantoic cyst Urachuszyste *f*.
allantoic diverticulum *embryo.* Allantoisdivertikel *nt*.
allantoic duct *embryo.* Allantoisgang *m*.
allantoic fluid Allantoisflüssigkeit *f*.
allantoic sac *embryo.* Allantoissack *m*.
allantoic stalk → allantoic duct.
allantoic vein *embryo.* Allantoisvene *f*.
allantoic vesicle → allantoic diverticulum.
al·lan·toid [ə'læntɔɪd] *adj* **1.** *embryo.* allantoisähnlich. **2.** wurstförmig.
allantoid membrane → allantois.
al·lan·toi·do·an·gi·op·a·gus [ælən,tɔɪdəʊˌændʒɪ'ɑpəgəs] *n embryo.* Omphaloangiopagus *m*.
al·lan·to·in [ə'læntəʊɪn] *n* Allantoin *nt*, Glyoxylsäureureid *nt*.
al·lan·to·in·ase [ˌælən'tɔɪneɪs] *n* Allantoinase *f*.
al·lan·to·in·u·ria [əˌlæntəwɪn'(j)ʊərɪə] *n* Allantoinurie *f*.
al·lan·to·is [ə'læntəʊɪs, -tɔɪs] *n, pl* **-to·i·des** [ˌælən'təʊədiːz, ˌælæn-, -tɔɪdɪz] *embryo.* allantoinaler Harnsack *m*, Allantois *f*.

al·lay [ə'leɪ] *vt* **1.** beruhigen, beschwichtigen; (*Angst*) zerstreuen. **2.** (*Schmerz*) lindern, verringern, mildern; (*Durst*) stillen.
al·lel [ə'lel] *n* → allele.
al·lele [ə'liːl] *n genet.* Allel *nt*, Allelomorph *nt*.
al·lel·ic [ə'liːlɪk, -'lel-] *adj* Allel(e) betr., Allelo-, Allelen-.
allelic gene Allel *nt*.
al·le·lism ['æliːlɪzəm] *n* Allelie *f*, Allelomorphismus *m*.
al·le·lo·morph [ə'liːləmɔːrf, -lel-] *n* → allele.
al·le·lo·mor·phic [ˌ-'mɔːrfɪk] *adj* allelomorph, allel.
al·le·lo·morph·ism [ˌ-'mɔːrfɪzəm] *n* → allelism.
al·le·lo·tax·is [ˌ-'tæksɪs] *n embryo.* Allelotaxis *f*.
al·le·lo·tax·y [ə'liːlətæksɪ] *n* → allelotaxis.
Allemann ['ælmæn]: **A.'s syndrome** Allemann-Syndrom *nt*.
Allen ['ælən]: **A.'s test** *chir.* Allen'-Test *m*.
al·ler·gen ['ælərdʒən] *n* Allergen *nt*.
al·ler·gen·ic [ˌ-'dʒenɪk] *adj* Allergie verursachend, als Allergen wirkend, allergen.
al·ler·gic [ə'lərdʒɪk] *adj* Allergie betr., durch Allergie verursacht, von Allergie betroffen, allergisch, überempfindlich (*to* gegen).
allergic alveolitis exogen allergische Alveolitis *f*, Hypersensitivitätspneumonitis *f*.
allergic arthritis allergische Arthritis *f*, Arthritis allergica.
allergic asthma konstitutionsallergisches (Bronchial-)Asthma *nt*.
allergic cold Heuschnupfen *m*, -fieber *nt*.
allergic conjunctivitis allergische/atopische Konjunktivitis *f*, Conjunctivitis allergica; Heuschnupfen *m*, -fieber *nt*.
allergic contact dermatitis allergische Kontaktdermatitis *f*, allergisches Kontaktekzem *nt*.
allergic coryza → allergic cold.
allergic dermatitis 1. → allergic contact dermatitis. **2.** → allergic eczema.
allergic eczema atopische Dermatitis *f*, atopisches/endogenes/exsudatives/neuropathisches/konstitutionelles Ekzem *nt*, Prurigo Besnier, Morbus Besnier, Ekzemkrankheit *f*, neurogene Dermatose *f*.
allergic granulomatosis Churg-Strauss--Syndrom *nt*, allergische granulomatöse Angiitis *f*.
allergic granulomatous angitis → allergic granulomatosis.
allergic inflammation allergische Reaktion/Entzündung *f*.
allergic purpura 1. allergische Purpura *f*, Purpura allergica. **2.** Schoenlein--Henoch-Syndrom *nt*, (anaphylaktoide) Purpura Schoenlein-Henoch *f*, rheumatoide/athrombopenische Purpura *f*, Immunkomplexpurpura *f*, -vaskulitis *f*, Purpura anaphylactoides (Schoenlein--Henoch), Purpura rheumatica (Schoenlein-Henoch).
allergic reaction Überempfindlichkeitsreaktion *f*.
allergic rhinitis allergische Rhinitis *f*, Rhinopathia vasomotorica allergica.
nonseasonal a. perenniale (allergische) Rhinitis.
seasonal a. allergische saisongebundene Rhinitis; Heuschnupfen *m*, -fieber *nt*.
allergic rhinopathy → allergic rhinitis.
allergic shock allergischer/anaphylaktischer Schock *m*, Anaphylaxie *f*.
allergic sinusitis allergische Nebenhöhlenentzündung/Sinusitis *f*.

allergic vascular purpura → allergic purpura 2.
allergic vasculitis Immunkomplexvaskulitis *f*, leukozytoklastische Vaskulitis *f*, Vasculitis allergica, Vasculitis hyperergica cutis, Arteriitis allergica cutis.
allergic vasomotor rhinitis allergische Rhinitis *f*, Rhinopathia vasomotorica allergica.
al·ler·gist ['ælərdʒɪst] *n* → allergologist.
al·ler·gi·za·tion [ˌ-dʒɪ'zeɪʃn] *n* Allergisierung *f*.
al·ler·gize ['-dʒaɪz] *vt* allergisieren.
al·ler·goid ['-gɔɪd] *n* Allergoid *nt*.
al·ler·gol·o·gist [ˌ-'gɑlədʒɪst] *n* Allergologe *m*, -login *f*.
al·ler·gol·o·gy [ˌ-'gɑlədʒɪ] *n* Allergologie *f*.
al·ler·go·sis [ˌ-'gəʊsɪs] *n, pl* **-ses** [-siːz] allergische Erkrankung *f*, Allergose *f*.
al·ler·gy ['ælərdʒɪ] *n, pl* **-gies** Überempfindlichkeit(sreaktion *f*) *f*, Allergie *f* (*to* gegen).
a. to contrast medium Kontrastmittelallergie.
Al·les·che·ria [ˌæləs'kɪərɪə] *n micro.* Allescheria *f*.
al·les·che·ri·a·sis [ˌæləskɪ'raɪəsɪs] *n* Allescheriasis *f*, Allescheriose *f*.
al·les·che·ri·o·sis [ˌ-kɪraɪ'əʊsɪs] *n* → allescheriasis.
al·les·the·sia [ˌæles'θiːʒ(ɪ)ə] *n* Allästhesie *f*, Allachästhesie *f*.
al·le·vi·ate [ə'liːvɪeɪt] *vt* mildern, lindern, (ver-)mindern.
al·le·vi·a·tion [əˌliːvɪ'eɪʃn] *n* **1.** Linderung *f*, Milderung *f*. **2.** Linderungsmittel *nt*, Palliativ *nt*.
al·le·vi·a·tive [ə'liːvɪeɪtɪv, -ətɪv] *adj* lindernd, mildernd, palliativ.
al·le·vi·a·to·ry [ə'liːvɪəˌtɔːriː, -təʊ-] *adj* → alleviative.
al·li·ga·tor skin ['æləgeɪtər] **1.** Fischschuppenkrankheit *f*, Ichthyosis vulgaris. **2.** Saurier-, Krokodil-, Alligatorhaut *f*, Sauriasis *f*.
Allis ['ælɪs]: **A. clamp** Allis-Klemme *f*.
A. forceps → A. clamp.
A. intestinal forceps → A. clamp.
A.'s sign *ortho.* Allis'-Zeichen *nt*.
A. tissue forceps → A. clamp.
Al·li·um ['ælɪəm] *n bio., pharm.* Allium *nt*.
allo- *pref.* all(o)-, Fremd-, All(o)-.
al·lo·al·bu·min [ˌælæl'bjuːmən] *n* Alloalbumin *nt*.
al·lo·an·ti·body [ˌ-'æntɪbɑdɪ] *n* Allo-, Isoantikörper *m*.
al·lo·an·ti·gen [ˌ-'æntɪdʒən] *n* Allo-, Isoantigen *nt*.
al·lo·bar ['-bɑːr] *n* Allobar *nt*.
al·lo·bar·bi·tal [ˌ-'bɑːrbɪtɔl, -tæl] *n pharm.* Allobarbital *nt*.
al·lo·bi·o·sis [ˌ-baɪ'əʊsɪs] *n* Allobiose *f*.
al·lo·cate ['ælkeɪt] *vt* zuteilen, zuweisen (*to*); verteilen (*to* auf).
al·lo·ca·tion [æləˈkeɪʃn] *n* Zuteilung *f*, Zuweisung *f*, Verteilung *f*.
al·lo·cen·tric [ˌæləʊ'sentrɪk] *adj* allozentrisch.
al·lo·chei·ria [ˌæləʊ'kaɪərɪə] *n* Allochirie.
al·lo·ches·the·sia [ˌ-kes'θiːʒ(ɪ)ə] *n* → allesthesia.
al·lo·che·zia [ˌ-'kiːzɪə] *n* Allochezie *f*, -chezia *f*.
al·lo·chi·ral [ˌ-'kaɪrəl] *adj* allochiral.
al·lo·chi·ria [ˌ-'kaɪrɪə] *n* Alloch(e)irie *f*.
al·lo·chro·ma·sia [ˌ-krə'meɪʒ(ɪ)ə] *n* Allochromie *f*, -chromasie *f*.
al·lo·ci·ne·sia [ˌ-sɪ'niːʒ(ɪ)ə, -saɪ-] *n* Allokinesie *f*.
al·lo·col·loid [ˌ-'kɑlɔɪd] *n* Allokolloid *nt*.
al·lo·cor·tex [ˌ-'kɔːrteks] *n* Allocortex *m*.
al·lo·crine ['-kraɪn] *adj* heterokrin.

Allodermanyssus sanguineus

Al·lo·der·ma·nys·sus sanguineus [ˌ-ˌdɜrmə'nɪsəs] *micro.* Allodermanyssus sanguineus.

al·lo·dyn·i·a [ˌ-'diːnɪə] *n* Allodynie *f.*

al·lo·e·rot·i·cism [ˌ-ɪ'rɑtəsɪzəm] *n* Alloerotismus *m.*

al·lo·er·o·tism [ˌ-'erətɪzəm] *n* → alloeroticism.

al·lo·es·the·sia [ˌ-es'θiːʒ(ɪ)ə] *n* → allesthesia.

allo form Diastereo(iso)mer *nt*, Diastomer *nt*, allo-Form *f.*

al·log·a·mous [ə'lɑgəməs] *adj* allogam(isch).

al·log·a·my [ə'lɑgəmɪ] *n* Fremdbefruchtung *f*, Allogamie *f.*

al·lo·ge·ne·ic [ˌæloʊdʒə'niːɪk] *adj* allogenetisch, allogen(isch), homolog.

allogeneic antigen Alloantigen, Allo-, Isoantigen *nt.*

allogeneic graft → allograft 1.

allogeneic transplant → allograft 1.

allogeneic transplantation → allograft 2.

al·lo·gen·ic [ˌ-'dʒenɪk] *adj* → allogeneic.

al·lo·graft ['-ɡræft] *n* 1. allogenes/allogenetisches/homologes Transplantat *nt*, Homo-, Allotransplantat *nt.* 2. allogene/allogenetische/homologe Transplantation *f*, Allo-, Homotransplantation *f.*

allograft reaction Allotransplantatabstoßung(sreaktion *f*) *f.*

al·lo·im·mune [ˌ-ɪ'mjuːn] *adj* alloimmun.

al·lo·i·som·er·ism [ˌ-aɪ'sɑmərɪzəm] *n* Alloisomerie *f.*

al·lo·ker·a·to·plas·ty [ˌ-'kerətoʊplæstɪ] *n ophthal.* Allokeratoplastik *f.*

al·lo·ki·ne·sis [ˌ-kɪ'niːsɪs, -kaɪ-] *n* Allokinese *f.*

al·lo·ki·net·ic [ˌ-kɪ'netɪk] *adj* Allokinese betr., allokinetisch.

al·lo·lac·tose [ˌ-'læktoʊs] *n* Allolaktose *f*, Allolactose *f.*

al·lo·la·lia [ˌ-'leɪlɪə] *n* Allolalie *f.*

al·lom·er·ism [ə'lɑmərɪzəm] *n chem.* Allomerie *f*, Allomerismus *m.*

al·lom·er·i·za·tion [ə,lɑmərɪ'zeɪʃn] *n* Allomerisation *f.*

al·lom·er·ize [ə'lɑməraɪz] *vt* allomerisieren.

al·lo·met·ric [ˌæloʊ'metrɪk] *adj* Allometrie betr., allometrisch.

al·lom·e·try [ə'lɑmətrɪ] *n* Allometrie *f*, Allomorphose *f.*

al·lo·mor·phic [ˌælə'mɔːrfɪk] *adj* allomorph.

al·lo·mor·phism [ˌ-'mɔːrfɪzəm] *n chem.* Allomorphie *f.*

al·lo·path ['-pæθ] *n* Allopath *m.*

al·lo·path·ic [ˌ-'pæθɪk] *adj* Allopathie betr., allopathisch.

al·lop·a·thist [ə'lɑpəθɪst] *n* → allopath.

al·lop·a·thy [ə'lɑpəθɪ] *n* Allopathie *f.*

al·lo·phan·a·mide [ˌælə'fænəmaɪd] *n* Biuret *nt*, Allophanamid *nt.*

al·loph·a·nate [ə'lɑfəneɪt] *n* Allophanat *nt.*

al·lo·phane ['æləfeɪn] *n* Allophan *m.*

al·lo·phan·ic acid [ˌ-'fænɪk] Allophansäure *f.*

al·lo·phore ['-fəʊər] *n* Allophor *nt*, Erythrophor *nt.*

al·loph·thal·mia [ˌæləf'θælmɪə] *n ophthal.* Heterophthalmus *m.*

al·lo·pla·sia [ˌælə'pleɪʒ(ɪ)ə] *n* Allo-, Heteroplasie *f.*

al·lo·plas·mat·ic [ˌ-plæz'mætɪk] *adj* alloplasmatisch.

al·lo·plast ['-plæst] *n* Alloplast(ik *f*) *m.*

al·lo·plas·tic [ˌ-'plæstɪk] *adj* Alloplastik betr., alloplastisch.

al·lo·plas·ty ['-plæstɪ] *n* 1. Alloplastik *f*, Alloendoprothese *f.* 2. (*Operation*) Alloplastik *f.*

al·lo·psy·chic [ˌ-'saɪkɪk] *adj* allopsychisch.

al·lo·psy·cho·sis [ˌ-saɪ'koʊsɪs] *n* Allopsychose *f.*

al·lo·pu·ri·nol [ˌ-'pjʊərənɒl, -nɑl] *n pharm.* Allopurinol *nt.*

al·lo·rhyth·mia [ˌ-'rɪðmɪə] *n* Allo(r)rhythmie *f.*

al·lo·rhyth·mic [ˌ-'rɪðmɪk] *adj* Allorhythmie betr., allo(r)rhythmisch.

all-or-non law Alles-oder-Nichts-Gesetz *nt abbr.* ANG.

al·lor·phine ['ælɔrfiːn] *n* Nalorphin *nt.*

al·lose ['æloʊs] *n* Allose *f.*

al·lo·sen·si·ti·za·tion [ˌælə,sensətaɪ'zeɪʃn, -tɪ-] *n* Allo-, Isosensitivierung *f.*

al·lo·some ['-soʊm] *n bio.* Allosom *nt.*

al·lo·ster·ic [ˌ-'sterɪk, -'stɪər-] *adj* Allosterie betr., allosterisch.

allosteric enzyme allosterisches Enzym *nt.*

allosteric inhibition allosterische Hemmung *f.*

allosteric inhibitor allosterischer Inhibitor *m.*

allosteric modulator allosterischer Modulator/Regulator *m.*

al·lo·ster·ism ['-sterɪzəm] *n chem.* Allosterie *f.*

al·los·ter·y [ə'lɑstərɪ] *n* → allosterism.

al·lot [ə'lɑt] *vt* zuweisen, zuteilen (*to*).

al·lo·therm ['æləθɜrm] *n bio.* 1. heterothermer Organismus *m.* 2. wechselwarmes/ poikilothermes Lebewesen *nt*, Wechselblüter *m.*

al·lot·ment [ə'lɑtmənt] *n* Zuweisung *f*, Zuteilung *f.*

al·lo·tope ['ælətoʊp] *n* Allotop *nt.*

al·lo·to·pia [ˌ-'toʊpɪə] *n* Allo-, Dystopie *f.*

al·lo·top·ic [ˌ-'tɑpɪk] *adj* allotop(isch), dystop(isch).

al·lo·tox·in [ˌ-'tɑksɪn] *n* Allotoxin *nt.*

al·lo·trans·plan·ta·tion [ˌ-trænz,plæn'teɪʃn] *n* → allograft 2.

al·lot·ri·o·geu·sia [ə,lɑtrɪə'gjuːʒ(ɪ)ə] *n* Allotriogeusie *f.*

al·lot·ri·o·geu·stia [ˌ-'gjuːstɪə] *n* → allotriogeusia.

al·lot·rio·ph·a·gy [ə,lɑtrɪ'ɑfədʒɪ] *n* Allotriophagie *f.*

al·lot·ri·os·mia [ˌælətraɪ'ɑsmɪə] *n* Allotriosmie *f*, Heterosmie *f.*

al·lot·ri·u·ria [ə,lɑtrɪ'(j)ʊərɪə] *n* Allotriurie *f.*

al·lo·trope ['ælətroʊp] *n* allotrope Form *f*, Allotrop *nt.*

al·lo·tro·phic [ˌ-'troʊfɪk, -'træf-] *adj* allotroph.

al·lo·tro·pic [ˌ-'troʊpɪk, -'trɑp-] *adj* 1. *chem.* allotrop, allomorph. 2. *psycho.* allotrop.

al·lot·ro·pism [ə'lɑtrəpɪzəm] *n* 1. *chem.* Allotropie *f.* 2. *histol.* Allotropismus *m.*

al·lot·ro·py [ə'lɑtrəpɪ] *n* → allotropism.

al·lo·type [ə'lɑtrəpɪ] *n* Allotyp *m.*

al·lo·typ·ic [ˌælə'tɪpɪk] *adj* allotypisch.

allotypic variation allotypische Variation *f.*

al·lo·ty·py ['ælətaɪpɪ] *n* Allotypie *f.*

al·lox·an [ə'lɑksən] *n* Alloxan *nt*, Mesoxalylharnstoff *m.*

alloxan diabetes Alloxandiabetes *m.*

al·lox·an·tin [ə'lɑksəntɪn] *n* Alloxantin *f.*

al·lox·a·zine [ə'lɑksəziːn] *n* Alloxazin *nt.*

al·lox·u·re·mia [ˌælɑksʊ'riːmɪə] *n* Alloxurämie *f.*

al·lox·u·ria [ælɑk's(j)ʊərɪə] *n* Alloxurie *f.*

al·lox·u·ric [ˌ-'s(j)ʊərɪk] *adj* Alloxurie betr., alloxurisch.

alloxuric base Purinbase *f.*

al·loy ['æloɪ] *n* 1. Metallegierung *f*, Legierung *f.* 2. Mischung *f*, Gemisch *nt.* 3. (Bei-)Mischung *f*, Zusatz *m.*

al·loy·age [ə'lɔɪdʒ] *n* Legieren *nt.*

all-trans retinal Sehgelb *nt*, Xanthopsin *nt*, all-trans-Retinal *nt.*

al·lyl ['ælɪl] *n* Allyl-(Radikal *nt*).

allyl aldehyde Akrolein *nt*, Acrolein *nt*, Acryl-, Allylaldehyd *m.*

al·lyl·mer·cap·to·meth·yl·pen·i·cil·lin [ˌ-mər,kæptoʊ,meθlpenə'sɪlɪn] *n pharm.* Penicillin O *nt*, Allylmercaptomethylpenicillinsäure *f*, Almecillin *f*, Penicillin AT *nt.*

ALM *abbr.* → acral-lentiginous melanoma.

Almeida [al'meɪdə]: **A.'s disease** Lutz-Splendore-Almeida-Krankheit *f*, südamerikanische Blastomykose *f*, Parakokzidioidomykose *f.*

Almén ['almen]: **A.'s test for blood** Almen-Probe *f*, Guajak-Probe *f.*

al·mond ['æl]mənd, 'ɑː-] *n* 1. Mandel(baum *m*) *f.* 2. *anat.* mandelförmige Struktur *f.* 3. Mandelfarbe *f.*

almond milk Mandelmilch *f.*

almond oil Mandelöl *nt.*

bitter a. Bittermandelöl.

sweet a. Mandelöl.

al·mon·er ['ælmənər, 'ɑːl-] *n Brit.* Sozialbetreuer(in *f*)*m* im Krankenhaus.

Al·oe ['æloʊ] *n bot.* Aloe *f.*

aloe ['æloʊ] *n*, *pl* **-oes** *pharm.* Aloe *f.*

al·o·et·ic [ˌæloʊ'etɪk] *adj pharm.* Aloe betr. *od.* enthaltend.

a·lo·gia [ə'loʊdʒ(ɪ)ə] *n neuro.* Alogie *f*, zentrale Aphasie *f.*

al·o·in ['æloʊɪn] *n pharm.* Aloin *nt.*

al·o·pe·cia [ˌælə'piːʃɪə, -sɪə] *n* Kahlheit *f*, Haarausfall *m*, -losigkeit *f*, Alopezie *f*, Alopecia *f.*

a. of the immediate type anagen-dystrophe Alopezie, anagen-dystrophischer Haarausfall, anagen-dystrophisches Effluvium *nt*, Alopezie vom Frühtyp.

a. of the late type telogene Alopezie, telogener Haarausfall, telogenes Effluvium *nt*, Alopezie vom Spättyp.

al·o·pe·cic [ˌælə'piːsɪk] *adj* Alopezie betr., von Alopezie betroffen.

Alouette [alu'et]: **A. amputation/operation** *ortho.* Alouette-Amputation *f*, Hüftgelenksexartikulation *f* nach Alouette.

ALP *abbr.* → alkaline phosphatase.

Alpers ['ælpərs]: **A.' disease/syndrome** Alpers-Syndrom *nt*, Poliodystrophia cerebri progressiva infantilis.

al·pha ['ælfə] *n abbr.* **A**, **α** Alpha *nt abbr.* A, α.

alpha₁-acid glycoprotein α₁-saures Glykoprotein *nt.*

alpha-adrenergic blockade → alpha blockade.

alpha-adrenergic blocking agent → alpha-blocker.

alpha-adrenergic receptor → alpha receptor.

alpha-adrenergic receptor blocking agent/drug → alpha-blocker.

alpha alcoholism α-Alkoholismus *m.*

alpha angle *ophthal.* Alpha-Winkel *m.*

alpha₁-antitrypsin *n* → α₁-antitrypsin.

alpha₁-antitrypsin deficiency → α₁-antitrypsin deficiency.

alpha blockade Alpha(rezeptoren)-blockade *f.*

alpha-blocker *n* Alpha(rezeptoren)-blocker *m*, α-Adrenorezeptorenblocker *m*, Alpha-Adrenorezeptorenblocker *m.*

alpha blocking agent/drug → alpha-blocker.

alpha cell adenocarcinoma (*Pankreas*) A(lpha)-Zelladenom *nt*, -Adenokarzinom *nt.*

alpha cell adenoma → alpha cell adenocarcinoma.

alpha cells 1. (*Pankreas*) A-Zellen *pl*, α-Zellen *pl*. **2.** (*Adenohypophyse*) azidophile Zellen, α-Zellen *pl*.
alpha cell tumor Glukagonom *nt*, Glucagonom(a) *nt*, A-Zell(en)-Tumor *m*.
alpha chain disease Alpha-Kettenkrankheit *f*, α-(Schwere-)Kettenkrankheit *f*, Alpha-Schwerekettenkrankheit *f*.
alpha decay *phys.* α-Zerfall *m*, alpha-Zerfall *m*.
alpha-fetoprotein *n abbr.* **AFP** alpha$_1$-Fetoprotein *nt*, α$_1$-Fetoprotein *nt abbr.* AFP.
alpha fibers α-Fasern *pl*, Aα-Fasern *pl*.
alpha globulin α-Globulin *nt*.
alpha granules α-Granula *pl*.
alpha helix α-Helix *f*.
alpha hemolysin α-Hämolysin *nt*.
alpha-hemolysis *n micro.* Alphahämolyse *f*, α-Hämolyse *f*.
alpha-hemolytic *adj micro.* alphahämolytisch, α-hämolytisch.
alpha-hemolytic streptococci *micro.* alphahämolytische Streptokokken *pl*.
Al·pha·her·pes·vir·i·nae [ælfəˌhɜrpiːzˈvɪərəniː] *pl micro.* Alphaherpesviren *pl*, Alphaherpesvirinae *pl*.
alpha-lipoprotein *n* Lipoprotein *nt* mit hoher Dichte, high density lipoprotein *nt abbr.* HDL, α-Lipoprotein *nt*.
al·pha·lyt·ic [ˌ-ˈlɪtɪk] **I** *n* → alpha-blocker. **II** *adj* Alpharezeptoren blockierend.
alpha$_2$-macroglobulin *n* (α$_2$-)Makroglobulin *nt*.
al·pha·mi·met·ic [ˌ-mɪˈmɛtɪk, -maɪ-] **I** *n* alpharezeptoren-stimulierendes Mittel *nt*, Alphamimetikum *nt*. **II** *adj* alphamimetisch.
alpha motoneuron α-Motoneuron *nt*.
alpha neuron α-Neuron *nt*.
alpha-oxidation *n* alpha-Oxidation *f*, α--Oxidation *f*.
alpha particle *phys.* alpha-Teilchen *nt*, α-Teilchen *nt*.
alpha phase Follikelreifungs-, Proliferationsphase *f*, östrogene Phase *f*.
al·pha·pro·dine [-ˈprəʊdiːn] *n pharm.* Alphaprodin *nt*.
alpha radiation Alphastrahlung *f*, α-Strahlung *f*.
alpha rays α-Strahlen *pl*, Alphastrahlen *pl*, -strahlung *f*.
alpha receptor alphaadrenerger Rezeptor *m*, Alpharezeptor *m*, α-Rezeptor *m*.
alpha rhythm *neuro.* α-Rhythmus *m*, Alpha-, Berger-Rhythmus *m*.
alpha spindle *neuro.* α-Spindel *f*.
alpha staphylolysin α-Staphylolysin *nt*.
alpha streptococci → alpha-hemolytic streptococci.
alpha substance Substantia reticulo-granulo-filamentosa.
alpha-tocopherol *n* α-Tocopherol *nt*, Vitamin E *nt*.
al·pha·vi·rus [ˈælfəvaɪrəs] *n micro.* Alphavirus *nt*.
alpha waves α-Wellen *pl*, alpha-Wellen *pl*.
Al·pine scurvy [ˈælpaɪn, -pɪn] Pellagra *f*, Vitamin-B$_2$-Mangelsyndrom *nt*, Niacinmangelsyndrom *nt*.
Alport [ˈælpɔːrt, ˈɑl-]: **A.'s syndrome** Alport-Syndrom *nt*.
al·pre·no·lol [ælˈprɛnəlɔl, -əʊl] *n pharm.* Alprenolol *nt*.
al·pros·ta·dil [ælˈprɒstədɪl] *n* Alprostadil *nt*, Prostaglandin E1 *nt abbr.* PGE$_1$.
AL protein AL-Protein *nt*, Amyloidprotein-L *nt*.
ALS *abbr.* **1.** → amyotrophic lateral sclerosis. **2.** → antilymphocyte serum.
al·sto·nine [ˈɔːlstəniːn] *n pharm.* Alstonin *nt*.

Alström [ˈælstrəʊm; ˈɑːlstrøm]: **A.'s syndrome** Alström(-Hallgren)-Syndrom *nt*.
ALT *abbr.* → alanine aminotransferase.
al·ter [ˈɔːltər] **I** *vt* (ver-, ab-, um-)ändern, alterieren. **II** *vi s.* (ver-)ändern.
al·ter·a·tion [ˌɔːltəˈreɪʃn] *n* (Ver-, Ab-, Um-)Änderung *f* (*to* an), Alteration *f*.
a. of consciousness Bewußtseinsveränderung.
al·ter·a·tive [ˈɔːltəreɪtɪv, ˈɔːlˈtɛrə-] *adj* verändernd, veränderlich, alterativ.
alterative inflammation alterative Entzündung *f*, Alteration *f*.
al·ter·nans [ˈɔːlˈtɜrnənz] *n* Alternans *m*.
a. of heart → alternans.
al·ter·nate [*adj* ˈɔːltərnət; *v* -ˌneɪt] **I** *adj* alternierend, abwechselnd, wechselweise, wechselseitig. **on ~ days** jeden zweiten Tag. **II** *vt* abwechseln lassen, wechseln, im Wechsel tun. **III** *vi* (s.) (miteinander) abwechseln, alternieren.
alternate anesthesia gekreuzte/alternierende Hemianästhesie *f*, Hemian(a)esthesia cruciata.
alternate cover test *ophthal.* alternierender Abdecktest *m*.
alternate generation Generationswechsel *m*.
alternate hemianesthesia → alternate anesthesia.
alternate hemiplegia → alternate paralysis.
alternate hot and cold bath Wechselbad *nt*.
alternate paralysis Hemiplegia alternans.
al·ter·nat·ing [ˈɔːltərneɪtɪŋ] *adj* abwechselnd, Wechsel-, alternierend.
alternating bath Wechselbad *nt*.
alternating calculus *urol.* Kombinationsstein *m*, kombinierter Harnstein *m*.
alternating current *abbr.* **AC, A.C.** *electr.* Wechselstrom *m*.
alternating hemiplegia gekreuzte Hemiplegie *f*, Hemiplegia alternans/cruciata.
alternating mydriasis alternierende/springende Mydriasis *f*, Mydriasis alternans.
alternating oculomotor hemiplegia Weber-Syndrom *nt*, Hemiplegia alternans oculomotorica.
alternating paralysis → alternate paralysis.
alternating pulse Alternans *m*, Pulsus alternans.
alternating strabismus *ophthal.* alternierendes Schielen *nt*, Strabismus alternans.
al·ter·na·tion [ˌɔːltərˈneɪʃn] *n* **1.** Alternieren *nt*, Abwechslung *f*, Wechsel *m*. **2.** (Strom-)Wechsel *m*.
a. of generations *bio.* Generationswechsel.
a. of patterns *physiol.* Reizmusterwechsel.
al·ter·na·tive [ɔːlˈtɜrnətɪv] **I** *n* Alternative *f* (*to* zu); Wahl *f*, Möglichkeit *f*, Ausweg *m* (*to* für). **II** *adj* alternativ, Alternativ-, Ausweich-, Ersatz-.
alternative complement pathway → alternative pathway.
alternative hypothesis *abbr.* **H$_1$** Alternativhypothese *f abbr.* H$_1$.
alternative inheritance alternative Vererbung *f*.
alternative pathway *hema.* (*Komplement*) alternative Aktivierung *f*.
al·thea [ælˈθiːə] *n pharm.* Althee *f*.
al·ti·tude [ˈæltət(j)uːd] *n* (große) Höhe *f*.
altitude anoxia → altitude disease.
altitude disease (akute) Höhenkrankheit *f*.
altitude erythremia Monge'-Krankheit *f*, chronische Höhenkrankheit *f*.

altitude sickness 1. Höhenkrankheit *f*. **2.** d'Acosta-Syndrom *nt*, akute Bergkrankheit *f*, Mal di Puna.
Altmann [ˈaltman]: **A.'s anilin-acid fuchsin stain** Altmann-Färbung.
A.'s fixative → A.'s fluid.
A.'s fluid Altmann-Lösung *f*.
A.'s granules Altmann-Granula *pl*.
Altmann-Gersh [gerʃ]: **A.-G. method** Altmann-Gersh-Verfahren *nt*.
al·to·fre·quent [ˌæltəʊˈfriːkwənt] *adj* hochfrequent.
al·trose [ˈæltrəʊz] *n* Altrose *f*.
al·tru·ism [ˈæltruːɪzəm] *n* Nächstenliebe *f*, Selbstlosigkeit *f*, Altruismus *m*.
al·tru·ist [ˈæltruːɪst] *n* Altruist(in *f*) *m*.
al·tru·is·tic [ˌæltrəˈwɪstɪk] *adj* altruistisch.
al·um [ˈæləm] *n* **1.** Alumen *nt*, Kalium-Aluminium-Sulfat *nt*. **2.** Alaun *nt*.
alum bath Alaunbad *nt*.
a·lu·men [əˈluːmən] *n* → alum.
alum hematoxylin Hämalaun *nt*.
a·lu·mi·na [əˈluːmɪnə] *n* → aluminium oxide.
a·lu·min·i·um [ˌæljʊˈmɪnɪəm] *n* → aluminum.
aluminium acetate Aluminiumacetat *nt*.
aluminium chloride Aluminiumchlorid *nt*.
aluminium hydrate → aluminium hydroxide.
aluminium hydroxide Aluminiumhydroxid *nt*.
aluminium oxide Aluminiumoxid *nt*.
aluminium phosphate Aluminiumphosphat *nt*.
aluminium sulfate Aluminiumsulfat *nt*.
a·lu·mi·no·sis [əˌluːmɪˈnəʊsɪs] *n* **1.** Aluminose *f*, old Kaolinlunge *f*. **2.** Aluminium(staub)lunge *f*.
a·lu·mi·num [əˈluːmɪnəm] *n abbr.* **Al** Aluminium *nt abbr.* Al, *inf* Alu *nt*.
ALV *abbr.* avian leukemia virus.
al·ve·o·bron·chi·ol·i·tis [ˌælvɪəʊˌbrɒŋkɪəʊˈlaɪtɪs] *n* Alveo(lo)bronchiolitis *f*.
alveol- *pref.* → alveolo-.
al·ve·o·lar [ælˈvɪələr; ˈælvɪˈəʊ-] *adj* **1.** mit Hohlräumen versehen, alveolär. **2.** Zahnod. Lungenalveolen betr., alveolär, Alveolen-, Alveolar-, Alveolo-.
alveolar abscess (*Zahn*) Wurzelspitzenabszeß *m*.
alveolar adenocarcinoma azinöses/alveoläres Adenokarzinom *nt*.
alveolar air Alveolarluft *f*, alveolares Gasgemisch *nt*.
alveolar arch Arcus alveolaris.
mandibular a. Unterkieferzahnreihe *f*, mandibuläre Zahnreihe *f*, Arcus dentalis inferior.
maxillary a. Oberkieferzahnreihe *f*, maxilläre Zahnreihe *f*, Arcus dentalis superior.
alveolar artery: inferior a. Unterkieferschlagader *f*, -arterie *f*, Alveolaris *f* inferior, A. alveolaris inferior.
superior a.ies, anterior vordere Oberkieferschlagadern *pl*, -arterien *pl*, Aa. alveolares superiores anteriores.
superior a., posterior hintere Oberkieferschlagader *f*, -arterie *f*, A. alveolaris superior posterior.
alveolar bone Alveolarknochen *m*.
alveolar border: a. of mandible Arcus alveolaris mandibulae.
a. of maxilla Arcus alveolaris maxillae.
alveolar branch: a.es of infraorbital nerve Oberkieferäste *pl* des N. infraorbitalis, Rami alveolares n. infraorbitalis.
superior a.es of infraorbital nerve, anterior vordere Oberkieferäste *pl* des N. infraorbitalis, Rami alveolares superiores anteriores (n. infraorbitalis).

alveolar bronchioles

superior a. of infraorbital nerve, middle mittlerer Oberkieferast *m* des N. infraorbitalis, Ramus alveolaris superior medius (n. infraorbitalis).
superior a.es of maxillary nerve, posterior hintere Oberkieferäste *pl* des N. maxillaris, Rami alveolares superiores posteriores (n. maxillaris).
alveolar bronchioles Alveolarbronchiolen *pl*, Bronchioli alveolares/respiratorii.
alveolar canals Alveolarkanäle *pl*, Canales alveolares.
a. of maxilla Alveolarkanälchen *pl*, Canales alveolares (maxillae).
alveolar cancer → alveolar carcinoma.
alveolar-capillary block (*Lunge*) Alveo(lo)kapillarblock *m*.
alveolar carcinoma azinöses/alveoläres Adenokarzinom *nt*.
alveolar cavities Zahnfächer *pl*, Alveoli dentales.
alveolar cell Alveolarzelle *f*, Pneumozyt *m*, -cyt *m*.
great a. Nischenzelle, Alveolarzelle/Pneumozyt Typ II.
large a. → great a.
small a. Deckzelle, Alveolarzelle/Pneumozyt Typ I.
squamous a. → small a.
type I a. → small a.
type II a. → great a.
alveolar cell carcinoma/tumor bronchiolo-alveoläres Lungenkarzinom *nt*, Alveolarzellenkarzinom *nt*, Lungenadenomatose *f*, Ca. alveolocellulare/alveolare.
alveolar cyst Alveolar-, Alveolenzyste *f*.
alveolar ducts Alveolargänge *pl*, -duktuli *pl*, Ductus/Ductuli alveolares (pulmonis).
alveolar ductules → alveolar ducts.
alveolar emphysema alveoläres Lungenemphysem *m*.
alveolar epithelial cell → alveolar cell.
alveolar epithelium Alveolenepithel *nt*.
alveolar foramina Forr. alveolaria.
a. of maxilla Forr. alveolaria (maxillae).
alveolar gas → alveolar air.
alveolar gingiva Gingiva alveolaris.
alveolar gland *histol.* alveoläre/säckchenförmige Drüse *f*.
alveolar hydatid alveoläre Echinokokkose *f*.
alveolar hydatid cyst multilokuläre Echinokokkuszyste/Hydatidenzyste *f*.
alveolar hypoventilation (*Lunge*) alveoläre Minderbelüftung/Hypoventilation *f*.
alveolar juga Juga alveolaria.
alveolar macrophage Alveolarmakrophage *m*, -phagozyt *m*.
alveolar margin: a. of mandible Arcus alveolaris mandibulae.
a. of maxilla Arcus alveolaris maxillae.
alveolar nerve: inferior a. Unterkiefernerv *m*, Alveolaris *m* inferior, N. alveolaris inferior.
superior a.s Oberkieferäste *pl* des N. maxillaris u. N. infraorbitalis, Nn. alveolares superiores.
alveolar part of mandible Pars alveolaris mandibulae.
alveolar periosteum Zahnbett *nt*, -halteapparat *m*, Parodont *nt*, Parodontium *nt*.
alveolar phagocyte Alveolarmakrophag *m*, -phagozyt *m*, Staub-, Körnchen-, Rußzelle *f*.
alveolar pores (*Lunge*) Kohn'-Poren *pl*, (Inter-)Alveolarporen *pl*.
alveolar portion of mandible Pars alveolaris mandibulae.
alveolar process of maxilla Alveolarfortsatz *m* des Oberkiefers, Proc. alveolaris maxillae.

alveolar saccules → alveolar sacs.
alveolar sacs Alveolar-, Alveolensäckchen *pl*, Sacculi alveolares.
alveolar septa (of lung) Alveolarsepten *pl*, Interalveolarsepten *pl*.
alveolar ventilation (*Lunge*) alveoläre Ventilation/Belüftung *f*.
alveolar yokes: a. of mandible Juga alveolaria mandibulae.
a. of maxilla Juga alveolaria maxillae.
al·ve·o·late [æl'vɪəleɪt, -lɪt] *adj patho.*, *histol.* (honig-)wabenförmig, zellenförmig, fächerig.
al·ve·o·lec·to·my [ˌælvɪə'lektəmɪ] *n chir.*, *dent.* Alveolektomie *f*.
al·ve·o·li·tis [ˌ-'laɪtɪs] *n* **1.** (*Lunge*) Alveolitis *f*. **2.** *dent.* Entzündung *f* der Zahnalveole, Alveolitis *f*.
alveolo- *pref.* Alveolen-, Alveolar-, Aveolo-.
al·ve·o·lo·cap·il·lar·y block [ælˌvɪəloʊˈkæpəˌlerɪː, -kəˈpɪlərɪ] (*Lunge*) Alveo(lo)kapillarblock *m*.
alveolocapillary membrane alveolokapilläre Membran *f*.
al·ve·o·lo·den·tal [ˌ-'dentl] *adj* Zahn u. Zahnfach betr., alveolodental, dentoalveolär.
alveolodental canals Alveolarkanäle *pl*, Canales alveolares.
alveolodental ligament Wurzelhaut *f*, Desmodont *nt*, Periodontium *nt*.
alveolodental membrane → alveolodental ligament.
alveolodental periostitis Parodontitis *f*, Periodontitis *f*.
al·ve·o·lo·la·bi·al [ˌ-'leɪbɪəl] *adj dent.* Zahnfortsatz u. Lippen betr., alveololabial.
al·ve·o·lo·la·bi·a·lis [ˌ-'leɪbɪ'ælɪs] *n old M.* buccinator.
al·ve·o·lo·pal·a·tal [ˌ-'pælətl] *adj* Zahnfortsatz u. Gaumen betr. *od.* verbindend, alveolopalatal.
al·ve·o·lot·o·my [ˌælvɪə'lɑtəmɪ] *n* Alveolotomie *f*.
al·ve·o·lus [æl'vɪələs] *n*, *pl* **-li** [-laɪ] **1.** Alveole *f*, kleine sackähnliche Ausbuchtung *f*. **2.** Lungenbläschen *nt*, Alveole *f*, Alveolus *m*. **3.** *dent.* Zahnfach *nt*, Alveolus dentalis. **4.** (*Drüse*) Azinus *m*, Acinus *m*.
al·ve·us of hippocampus ['ælvɪəs] Alveus hippocampi.
a·lym·phia [eɪ'lɪmfɪə] *n* Alymphie *f*.
a·lym·pho·cy·to·sis [eɪˌlɪmfəsaɪ'toʊsɪs] *n* Alymphozytose *f*.
a·lym·pho·pla·sia [ˌ-'pleɪʒ(ɪ)ə, -zɪə] *n* Alymphoplasie *f*, -plasia *f*.
Alzheimer ['ɑltshaɪmər] **A.'s cells** Alzheimer'-Zellen *pl*.
A.'s disease Alzheimer'-Krankheit *f*, präsenile Alzheimer-Demenz *f*, Demenz *f* vom Alzheimer-Typ.
A.'s fibers Alzheimer'-Fibrillen *pl*.
A.'s glands senile Drüsen *pl*, Alzheimer'-Drüsen *pl*, Alzheimer'-Plaques *pl*.
A.'s neurofibrillary degeneration Alzheimer'-Fibrillenveränderungen *pl*, Fädchenplaques *pl*.
A.'s plaques → A.'s glands.
A.'s sclerosis → A.'s disease.
AM *abbr.* → adrenal marrow.
Am *abbr.* → americium.
am *abbr.* **1.** → ametropia. **2.** → myopic astigmatism.
am·a·crat·ic [ˌæmə'krætɪk] *adj* → amasthenic.
am·a·crine ['æməkraɪn, eɪ'mæ-] **I** *n* → amacrine cell. **II** *adj* amakrin.
amacrine cell amakrine Zelle *f*, Neurocytus amacrinus.

am·a·krine *n*, *adj* → amacrine.
a·mal·gam [ə'mælgəm] *n* Amalgam *nt*.
a·mal·ga·mate [ə'mælgəmeɪt] **I** *vt* amalgamieren, ein Amalgam bilden *od.* herstellen. **II** *vi* (*a. fig.*) s. vereinigen, verschmelzen.
a·mal·ga·ma·tion [əˌmælgə'meɪʃn] *n* **1.** Amalgamieren *nt*. **2.** Vereinigung *f*, -schmelzung *f*; Zusammenschluß *m*.
amalgam natrium Natriumamalgam *nt*.
Am allotypes [alpha chain marker] Am-Allotypen *pl*.
Am·a·ni·ta [æmə'naɪtə] *n bio.* Amanita *f*.
A. muscaria Fliegenpilz *m*, Amanita muscaria.
A. phalloides grüner Knollenblätterpilz *m*, Amanita phalloides.
Amanita toxin → amanitotoxin.
a·ma·ni·tine [ə'mænɪtiːn] *n* Amanitin *nt*.
a·man·i·to·tox·in [əˌmænɪtoʊ'tɑksɪn] *n* Amanitatoxin *nt*.
a·man·ta·dine [ə'mæntədiːn] *n pharm.* Amantadin *nt*.
amantadine hydrochloride Amantadin-Hydrochlorid *nt*, Amino-Adamantan *nt*, Adamantanamine *nt*.
Am antigens Am-Antigene *pl*.
am·a·ranth ['æmərænθ] *n* Amarant(farbe *f*) *m*.
am·a·ran·thine [æmə'rænθɪn, -θaɪn] *adj* amarant(rot), dunkelrot.
Am·a·ran·thus [æmə'rænθəs] *n* Amarant *m*, Amarant(h)us *m*.
am·a·rine ['æməriːn] *n* Amarin *nt*.
am·a·roi·dal [əmə'rɔɪdl] *adj* (*Geschmack*) leicht bitter.
am·ar·thri·tis [ˌæmɑːr'θraɪtɪs] *n* Polyarthritis *f*.
a·mass [ə'mæs] *vt* an-, aufhäufen, ansammeln.
a·mass·ment [ə'mæsmənt] *n* An-, Aufhäufung *f*, Ansammlung *f*.
am·as·then·ic [ˌæməs'θenɪk] *adj phys.* (*Licht*, *Strahlen*) bündelnd.
a·mas·tia [eɪ'mæstɪə] *n embryo.*, *gyn.* Mammaaplasie *f*, Amastie *f*.
a·mas·ti·gote [eɪ'mæstɪgoʊt] *n micro.* amastigote Form *f*, Leishman-Donovan'-Körperchen *nt*, Leishmania-Form *f*.
amastigote stage → amastigote.
am·a·tho·pho·bia [ˌæməθə'foʊbɪə] *n psychia.* Amathophobie *f*.
Amato [a'maːto] **A.'s bodies** Amato-Körperchen *pl*.
am·au·ro·sis [ˌæmə'roʊsɪs] *n* (totale) Blindheit *f*, Erblindung *f*, Amaurose *f*, Amaurosis *f*.
am·au·rot·ic [ˌ-'rɑtɪk] *adj* Amaurose betr., amaurotisch.
amaurotic cat's eye amaurotisches Katzenauge *nt*.
amaurotic mydriasis *ophthal.* amaurotische Mydriasis *f*.
amaurotic nystagmus okulärer Nystagmus *m*.
a·ma·zia [ə'meɪzɪə] *n* → amastia.
amb- *pref.* → ambi-.
am·be·no·ni·um chloride [ˌæmbɪ'noʊnɪəm] *pharm.* Ambenoniumchlorid *nt*.
am·ber ['æmbər] **I** *n* **1.** Bernstein *m*. **2.** Bernsteinfarbe *f*. **II** *adj* bernsteinfarben, Bernstein-.
amber mutant amber-Mutante *f*.
ambi- *pref.* Beid-, Amb(i)-.
am·bi·dex·ter·i·ty [ˌæmbɪdek'sterətɪ] *n* Beidhändigkeit *f*, Ambidexterie *f*.
am·bi·dex·tral·i·ty [ˌ-dek'strælətɪ] *n* → ambidexterity.
am·bi·dex·trism [ˌ-'dekstrɪzəm] *n* → ambidexterity.
am·bi·dex·trous [ˌ-'dekstrəs] *adj* mit beiden Händen, beidhändig, ambidexter.

am·bi·ent ['æmbɪənt] **I** *n* **1.** Umwelt *f*, Milieu *nt*. **2.** Atmosphäre *f*. **II** *adj* umgebend, Umwelt-, Umgebungs-.
ambient cisterna Cisterna ambiens.
ambient illumination Umgebungsbeleuchtung *f*.
ambient temperature Umgebungstemperatur *f*.
am·bi·gu·i·ty [,æmbɪ'gjuːɪtɪ] *n*, *pl* **-ties** Zwei-, Mehr-, Vieldeutigkeit *f*, Ambiguität *f*; Doppelsinn *m*, Doppelsinnigkeit *f*; Unklarheit *f*.
ambiguo-accessorius-hypoglossal paralysis Jackson-Syndrom *nt*, -Lähmung *f*.
ambiguo-accessorius paralysis *HNO* Schmidt-Syndrom *nt*.
ambiguo-hypoglossal paralysis Tapia-Syndrom *nt*.
ambiguo-spinothalamic paralysis → Avellis' syndrome.
am·big·u·ous [æm'bɪgjʊəs, -jəwəs] *adj* **1.** *anat.* ambiguus, (s.) nach zwei Seiten neigend *od.* strebend. **2.** zwei-, mehr-, vieldeutig, ambig; doppelsinnig; unklar, unbestimmt.
ambiguous nucleus Nc. ambiguus.
am·bi·lat·er·al [,æmbɪ'lætərəl] *adj* beide Seiten betr., ambilateral.
am·bi·o·pia [,-'ɔʊpɪə] *n ophthal.* Doppel-, Doppeltsehen *nt*, Diplopie *f*, Diplopia *f*.
am·bi·sex·trous [,-'sekstrəs] *adj* → ambisexual II.
am·bi·sex·u·al [,-'sekʃəwəl] **I** *n* Bisexuelle(r *m*) *f*. **II** *adj* bisexuell.
am·bi·tend·en·cy [,-'tendənsɪ] *n psychia.* Doppelwertigkeit *f*, Ambitendenz *f*.
am·bi·tion [æm'bɪʃn] *n* **1.** Ehrgeiz *m*. **2.** (ehrgeiziges) Streben *nt*, Wunsch *m*, Begierde *f* (*of* nach; *to do zu tun*).
am·biv·a·lence [æm'bɪvələns] *n psychia.* Doppelwertigkeit *f*, Ambivalenz *f*.
am·biv·a·lent [æm'bɪvələnt] *adj psychia.* ambivalent.
am·bi·ver·sion [,æmbɪ'vɜrʒn] *n psycho.* Ambiversion *f*.
am·bi·vert ['æmbɪvɜrt] *psycho.* **I** *n* ambivertierter Mensch *m*. **II** *adj* ambivertiert.
am·bly·chro·ma·sia [,æmblɪkrəʊ'meɪʒ(ɪ)ə] *n histol.* Amblychromasie *f*.
am·bly·chro·mat·ic [,-krəʊ'mætɪk] *adj histol.* amblychrom(atisch), schwach-färbend.
am·bly·geu·stia [,-'gjuːstɪə] *n* Amblygeusie *f*.
Am·bly·om·ma [,-'ɒmə] *n* Buntzecken *pl*, Amblyomma *nt*.
am·bly·ope ['-ɔʊp] *n* Patient(in *f*) *m* mit Amblyopie *f*, Amblyope(r *m*) *f*.
am·bly·o·pia [,-'ɔʊpɪə] *n* Amblyopie *f*.
am·bly·op·ic [,-'ɒpɪk] *adj* Amblyopie betr., amblyop(isch).
am·bo·cep·tor ['æmbəʊseptər] *n* Ambozeptor *m*.
amboceptor unit Hämolysineinheit *f*.
am·bo·sex·u·al [,-'sekʃəwəl] *n*, *adj* → ambisexual.
am·bra·in ['æmbreɪn, -brəɪn] *n* → ambrin.
am·bre·in ['æmbreɪn, -briːɪn] *n* → ambrin.
am·brin ['æmbrɪn] *n* Ambr(e)in *nt*.
Ambu bag [,æmbjʊ] Ambu-Beutel *m*, -Atembeutel *m*.
am·bu·lance ['æmbjələns] *n* **1.** Kranken-, Rettungswagen *m*, Krankentransporter *m*, Ambulanz *f*. **2.** Feldlazarett *nt*.
ambulance driver Krankenwagenfahrer(in *f*) *m*.
ambulance service Rettungs-, Sanitätsdienst *m*; Rettungswesen *nt*.
am·bu·lant ['æmbjələnt] *adj* beweglich, gehend, gehfähig, Geh-, ambulant, ambulatorisch.

ambulant erysipelas *derm.* Erysipelas migrans.
ambulant plague abortive Pest *f*, Pestis minor.
am·bu·la·tion [,æmbjə'leɪʃn] *n* Gehen *nt*, Laufen *nt*.
am·bu·la·to·ry ['æmbjələtɔːriː, -təʊ-] *adj* → ambulant.
ambulatory care ambulante Betreuung *f*.
ambulatory patient gehfähiger Patient *m*, gehfähige Patientin *f*.
ambulatory plague → ambulant plague.
ambulatory schizophrenia ambulatorische Schizophrenie *f*.
ambulatory typhoid Typhus ambulatorius/levissimus.
am·bus·tion [æm'bʌstʃn] *n* Verbrennung *f*, Verbrühung *f*.
a·me·ba [ə'miːbə] *n*, *pl* **-bas, -bae** [-biː] *micro.* Wechseltierchen *nt*, Amöbe *f*, Amoeba *f*.
am·e·bi·a·sis [,æm'baɪəsɪs] *n* Amöbiasis *f*.
a·me·bic [ə'miːbɪk] *adj* Amöbe(n) betr., durch Amöben verursacht, amöbisch, Amöben-.
amebic abscess Amöbenabszeß *m*.
amebic appendicitis Amöbenappendizitis *f*, Appendizitis *f* durch Entamoeba histolytica.
amebic colitis → amebic dysentery.
amebic dysentery Amöbenruhr *f*, -dysenterie *f*, intestinale Amöbiasis *f*.
amebic granuloma → ameboma.
amebic hepatic abscess Amöbenabszeß *m*.
amebic hepatitis Amöbenhepatitis *f*, Leberamöbiasis *f*.
a·me·bi·ci·dal [ə,miːbə'saɪdl] *adj* amöben(ab-)abtötend, amöbizid.
a·me·bi·cide [ə'miːbəsaɪd] *n* amöbizides Mittel *nt*, Amöbizid *nt*.
amebic liver abscess → amebic hepatic abscess.
amebic pericarditis Amöbenperikarditis *f*.
amebic pneumonia Amöbenpneumonie *f*.
ame·bi·form [ə'miːbəfɔːrm] *adj* → ameboid.
am·e·bi·o·sis [,æmbaɪ'əʊsɪs] *n* → amebiasis.
am·e·bism ['æmɪbɪzəm] *n* **1.** amöboide (Fort-)Bewegung *f*. **2.** Amöbeninfektion *f*.
a·me·bo·flag·el·late [ə,miːbəʊ'flædʒəleɪt] *n micro.* Amöboflagellat *nt*.
ame·boid [ə'miːbɔɪd] *adj bio.* amöbenähnlich *od.* -artig (*in Form od. Bewegung*), amöboid.
ameboid cell amöboide Zelle *f*.
ameboid cell movement amöboide Zellbewegung *f*.
ameboid movement → ameboid cell movement.
ameboid trophozoite Amöbentrophozoit *m*, Magnaform *f*.
am·e·bo·ma [,æmɪ'bəʊmə] *n* Amöbengranulom *nt*, Ameboma *nt*.
a·me·bu·la [ə'miːbjələ] *n*, *pl* **-las, -lae** [-liː] *micro.* (*Amöben*) Minutaform *f*.
a·me·bu·ria [,æmɪ'bjʊərɪə] *n* Amöburie *f*.
a·mei·o·sis [eɪmaɪ'əʊsɪs] *n bio.* Ameiose *f*.
a·mel·a·no·sis [eɪ,melə'nəʊsɪs] *n* Amelanose *f*.
a·mel·a·no·tic [,-'nɒtɪk] *adj* amelanotisch.
amelanotic (malignant) melanoma *abbr.* **AMM** amelanotisches (malignes) Melanom *nt* *abbr.* AMM.
amelanotic nevus amelanotischer Nävus *m*.
a·mel·i·a [ə'melɪə, eɪ'miːlɪə] *n* angeborenes Fehlen *nt* einer *od.* mehrerer Gliedmaße, Amelie *f*, Amelia *f*.

a·me·lic [ə'miːlɪk] *adj* Amelie betr., von Amelie betroffen, amel.
a·mel·io·rate [ə'miːljəreɪt] **I** *vt* verbessern. **II** *vi s.* verbessern, besser werden.
a·mel·io·ra·tion [ə,miːljə'reɪʃn] *n* (*Zustand*) Verbesserung *f* Besserung *f*.
a·mel·io·ra·tive [ə'miːljəreɪtɪv] *adj* (ver-)bessernd.
alveol- *pref.* → alveolo-.
alveolo- *pref.* Zahnschmelz-, Amel(o)-, Adamant(o)-.
am·e·lo·blast ['æməlɔʊblæst] *n old* Zahnschmelzbildner *m*, Adamanto-, Amelo-, Ganoblast *m*.
am·el·o·blas·tic adenomatoid tumor [,-'blæstɪk] Adenoameloblastom *nt*.
ameloblastic fibroma → ameloblastofibroma.
ameloblastic odontoma Odontoadamantinom *nt*, -ameloblastom *nt*, ameloblastisches (Fibro-)Odontom *nt*.
ameloblastic sarcoma Ameloblastosarkom *nt*, Sarcoma ameloblasticum.
am·e·lo·blas·to·fi·bro·ma [,-,blæstəʊfaɪ'brəʊmə] *n* Ameloblastofibrom *nt*.
am·el·o·blas·to·ma [,-'blæs'təʊmə] *n* Ameloblastom *nt*, Adamantinom *nt*.
am·e·lo·gen·e·sis [,-'dʒenəsɪs] *n* Zahnschmelzbildung *f*, Amelogenese *f*.
am·e·lo·gen·ic [,-'dʒenɪk] *adj* **1.** Amelogenese betr. **2.** zahnschmelzbildend, amelogen.
am·e·lus ['æmələs, eɪ'miːe-] *n*, *pl* **-li** [-laɪ, -liː] Mißgeburt *f* mit Amelie, Amelus *m*.
a·me·na·bil·i·ty [ə,miːnə'bɪlətɪ, ə,menə-] *n* Zugänglichkeit *f* (*to* für).
a·me·na·ble [ə'miːnəbl, ə'men-] *adj fig.* zugänglich (*to*); behandelbar (*to* durch), behebbar.
a·me·nia [ə'miːnɪə] *n* → amenorrhea.
a·men·or·rhea [ə,menə'rɪə] *n gyn.* Amenorrhoe *f*, Amenorrhoea *f*.
a. of pregnancy Schwangerschaftsamenorrhoe.
amenorrhea-galactorrhea syndrome Amenorrhoe-Galaktorrhoe-Syndrom *nt*, Galaktorrhoe-Amenorrhoe-Syndrom *nt*.
a·men·or·rhe·al [ə,menə'rɪəl] *adj* Amenorrhoe betr., amenorrhoisch.
a·men·tia [eɪ'menʃ(ɪ)ə] *n* Amenz *f*, Amentia *f*.
A·mer·i·can [ə'merɪkən] **A.** dog tick *micro.* amerikanische Hundezecke *f*, Dermacentor variabilis.
A. hookworm *micro.* Todeswurm *m*, Necator americanus.
A. leishmaniasis amerikanische/mukokutane Leishmaniose *f*, Haut-Schleimhaut-Leishmaniase (Südamerikas) *f*, Leishmaniasis americana.
A. trypanosome *micro.* Trypanosoma cruzei.
A. trypanosomiasis Chagas-Krankheit *f*, amerikanische Trypanosomiasis *f*.
A. wood tick → A. dog tick.
am·er·i·ci·um [,æmə'rɪʃɪəm] *n abbr.* **Am** Amerikum *nt*, Americium *nt abbr.* Am.
Ames ['eɪmz] **A.' test** Ames-Test *m*.
a·met·a·chro·mo·phil [ə,metə'krəʊməfɪl] *adj histol.* orthochromophil.
a·met·a·neu·tro·phil ['-'n(j)uːtrəfɪl] *adj* → ametachromophil.
a·me·thop·ter·in [æmɪ'θæptərɪn] *n pharm.* Amethopterin *nt*, Methotrexat *nt*.
am·e·tria [æ'miːtrɪə, -'met-] *n* Uterusaplasie *f*, Ametrie *f*.
am·e·trom·e·ter [,æmɪ'trɒmətər] *n ophthal.* Ametrometer *nt*.
am·e·tro·pia [,-'trəʊpɪə] *n abbr.* **am** *ophthal.* Ametropie *f*.
am·e·tro·pic [,-'trəʊpɪk, -'trɒp-] *adj* Ame-

AM hormone

tropie betr., von Ametropie betroffen, ametrop(isch).
AM hormone Nebennierenmarkhormon *nt*, NNM-Hormon *nt*.
am·i·an·thoid [æmɪˈænθɔɪd] *adj* asbestähnlich, -förmig.
am·i·an·tho·sis [ˌ-ænˈθəʊsɪs] *n* Asbestose *f*.
Amici [əˈmiːtʃi]: **A.'s disk** Z-Linie *f*, -Streifen *m*, Zwischenscheibe *f*, Telophragma *nt*.
line of A. → A.'s disk.
stria of A. → A.'s disk.
a·mi·cro·bic [eɪmaɪˈkrəʊbɪk, -ˈkrɒb-] *adj* nicht von Mikroben verursacht, amikrobiell.
a·mi·cro·scop·ic [eɪˌmaɪkrəˈskɒpɪk] *adj* submikroskopisch.
a·mic·u·lum of olive [əˈmɪkjələm] Amiculum olivare.
am·i·dase [ˈæmɪdeɪz] *n* Amidase *f*.
am·ide [ˈæmaɪd] *n* Amid *nt*.
amide bond/linkage *chem.* Amidbrücke *f*, -bindung *f*.
amide synthetase Amidsynthetase *f*.
am·i·din [ˈæmɪdɪn] *n* Amylose *f*.
am·i·do·pen·i·cil·la·nic acid [ˌæmɪdiːnəʊˌpenəsəˈlænɪk] Amidopenicillansäure *f*.
am·i·di·no·trans·fer·ase [ˌ-ˈtrænsfəreɪz] *n* Amidinotransferase *f*.
amido- *pref.* Amido-.
a·mi·do·ben·zene [əˌmiːdəʊˈbenziːn, ˌæmɪdəʊ-] *n* Anilin *nt*, Aminobenzol *nt*, Phenylamin *nt*.
a·mi·do·hy·dro·lase [-ˈhaɪdrəleɪz] *n* Amidohydrolase *f*, Desamidase *f*.
amido-ligase *n* Amidoligase *f*.
a·mi·do·py·rine [ˌ-ˈpaɪriːn] *n* → aminopyrine.
Amies [ˈeɪmiːz]: **A. transport medium** Amies-Transportmedium *nt*.
am·i·ka·cin [æmɪˈkæsɪn] *n pharm.* Amikacin *nt*.
a·mil·o·ride [əˈmɪlərɑɪd] *n pharm.* Amilorid *nt*.
a·mim·ia [eɪˈmɪmɪə] *n* Amimie *f*.
am·in·ar·sone [æmɪnˈɑːrsəʊn] *n pharm.* Carbason *nt*, 4-Carbamidophenylarsinsäure *f*.
am·i·nate [ˈæmɪneɪt] *vt chem.* aminieren.
a·mine [əˈmiːn, ˈæmɪn] *n* Amin *nt*.
amine oxidase (copper-containing) Diaminooxidase *f*.
amine oxidase (flavin-containing) Monoamin(o)oxidase *f abbr.* MAO.
amine precursor uptake and decarboxylation cell APUD-, Apud-Zelle *f*.
a·mi·no [əˈmiːnəʊ, ˈæmɪn] *n* Aminogruppe *f*, Amino-(Radikal *nt*), Amino-.
a·mi·no·a·ce·tic acid [əˌmiːnəʊəˈsiːtɪk, -əˈset-] Aminoessigsäure *f abbr.* AS, Glyzin *nt*, Glykokoll *nt*, Glycin *nt abbr.* Gly.
amino acid *abbr.* **AA** Aminosäure *f abbr.* AS.
acidic a. saure Aminosäure.
basic a. basische Aminosäure.
branched chain a. *abbr.* **BCAA** verzweigtkettige Aminosäure.
dispensable a. → non-essential a.
essential a. essentielle Aminosäure.
glucogenic a. glukogene Aminosäure.
ketogenic a. ketogene Aminosäure.
ketoplastic a. ketoplastische Aminosäure.
non-essential a. nicht-essentielle Aminosäure.
nutritionally dispensable a. → non-essential a.
nutritionally indispensable a. → essential a.
rare a. seltene Aminosäure.
standard a. Standardaminosäure.

amino acid activation Aminosäureaktivierung *f*.
amino acid analyzer Aminosäureanalysator *m*.
amino acid arm *biochem.* Aminosäurearm *m*.
amino acid code Aminosäurecode *m*.
amino acid degradation Aminosäureabbau *m*.
a·mi·no·ac·i·de·mia [-ˌæsəˈdiːmɪə] *n* (Hyper-)Aminoazidämie *f*.
amino acid metabolism Aminosäurestoffwechsel *m*, -metabolismus *m*.
am·i·no·ac·i·dop·a·thy [ˌ-æsɪˈdɒpəθi] *n* durch Störung des Aminosäurestoffwechsels hervorgerufene Erkrankung *f*.
amino acid oxidase Aminosäureoxidase *f*.
amino acid oxidation oxidativer Aminosäureabbau *m*, Aminosäureoxidation *f*.
amino acid pool Aminosäurepool *m*.
amino acid receptor Aminosäurerezeptor *m*.
amino acid residue *biochem.* Aminosäurerest *m*.
amino acid sequence Aminosäuresequenz *f*.
amino acid synthesis Aminosäuresynthese *f*.
am·i·no·ac·i·du·ria [ˌ-ˌæsəˈd(j)ʊərɪə] *n* Aminoazidurie *f*.
a·mi·no·ac·yl [əˌmiːnəʊˈæsɪl, -iːl, ˌæmɪnəʊ-] *n* Aminoacyl-(Radikal *nt*).
aminoacyl adenylate Aminoacyladenylat *nt*.
aminoacyl adenylic acid Aminoacyladenylsäure *f*.
a·mi·no·ac·y·lase [ˌ-ˈæsɪleɪs] *n* Aminoacylase *f*, Hippurikase *f*.
aminoacyl binding site A-(Bindungs-)-Stelle *f*, Aminoacyl-(Bindungs)Stelle *f*.
aminoacyl histidine dipeptidase Aminoacylhistidin(di)peptidase *f*, Carnosinase *f*.
aminoacyl site → aminoacyl binding site.
am·i·no·ac·yl·trans·fer·ase [ˌ-ˌæsɪlˈtrænsfəreɪz] *n* Aminoacyltransferase *f*.
aminoacyl-tRNA synthetase Aminoacyl-tRNA-Synthetase *f*.
a·mi·no·a·di·pate [ˌ-ˈædəpeɪt] *n* Aminoadipat *nt*.
aminoadipate semialdehyde Aminoadipatsemialdehyd *m*.
aminoadipate semialdehyde dehydrogenase Aminoadipatsemialdehyddehydrogenase *f*.
aminoadipate transaminase Aminoadipattransaminase *f*.
a·mi·no·a·dip·ic acid [ˌ-əˈdɪpɪk] Aminoadipinsäure *f*.
aminoadipic acid semialdehyde Aminoadipinsäuresemialdehyd *m*.
aminoadipic acid semialdehyde dehydrogenase Aminoadipinsäuresemialdehyddehydrogenase *f*.
aminoadipic acid transaminase Aminoadipinsäuretransaminase *f*.
amino alcohol Aminoalkohol *m*.
a·mi·no·ben·zene [ˌ-ˈbenziːn] *n* Anilin *nt*, Aminobenzol *nt*, Phenylamin *nt*.
p-a·mi·no·ben·zene·sul·fon·a·mide [ˌ-ˌbenziːnsʌlˈfɒnəmaɪd] *n* Sulfanilamid *nt*, *p*-Aminobenzolsulfonamid *nt*.
p-a·mi·no·ben·zene·sul·fon·ic acid [ˌ-ˌbenziːnsʌlˈfɒnɪk] Sulfanilsäure *f*, *p*-Aminobenzolsulfonsäure *f*.
p-a·mi·no·ben·zo·ic acid [ˌ-benˈzəʊɪk] *abbr.* **PAB, PABA** *p*-Aminobenzoesäure *f*, para-Aminobenzoesäure *f*, Paraaminobenzoesäure *f abbr.* **PABA, PAB**.
α-a·mi·no·ben·zyl·pen·i·cil·lin [ˌ-ˌbenzɪlˌpenəˈsɪlɪn] *n pharm.* Ampicillin *nt*, alpha--Aminobenzylpenicillin *nt*.

γ-a·mi·no·bu·tyr·ate [ˌ-ˈbjuːtəreɪt] *n* γ-Aminobutyrat *nt*, gamma-Aminobutyrat *nt*.
aminobutyrate aminotransferase Aminobuttersäureaminotransferase *f*, β-Alaninaminotransaminase *f*.
γ-a·mi·no·bu·tyr·ic acid [ˌ-bjuːˈtɪrɪk] Gammaaminobuttersäure *f abbr.* **GABA**, γ-Amino-*n*-Buttersäure *f*.
ε-a·mi·no·ca·pro·ic acid [ˌ-kəˈprəʊɪk] *abbr.* **EACA** ε--Aminocapronsäure *f*, Epsilon-Aminocapronsäure *f abbr.* **EACS, EACA**.
7-amino-cephalosporanic acid *abbr.* **7-ACS** 7-Amino-cephalosporansäure *f abbr.* 7-ACS.
a·mi·no·cy·cli·tol [əˌmiːnəʊˈsaɪklətɒl, -ˈsɪk-, ˌæmɪnəʊ-] *n pharm.* Aminocyclitol *nt*.
aminocyclitol antibiotic Aminocyclitol--Antibiotikum *nt*.
a·mi·no·di·ni·tro·phe·nol [ˌ-daɪˌnaɪtrəˈfiːnɒl] *n* Dinitroaminophenol *nt*, Pikraminsäure *f*.
2-a·mi·no·eth·a·nol [ˌ-ˈeθənɒl, -nəʊl] *n* Äthanol-, Ethanolamin *nt*, Colamin *nt*, Monoethanolamin *nt*.
a·mi·no·form [əˈmiːnəfɔːrm] *n* Methenamin *nt*, Hexamin *nt*, Hexamethylentetramin *nt*.
a·mi·no·gly·co·side [ˌ-ˈglaɪkəsaɪd] *n* **1.** *chem.* Aminoglykosid *nt*. **2.** *pharm.* Aminoglykosid(-Antibiotikum) *nt abbr.* **AGAB**.
aminoglycoside antibiotic → aminoglycoside 2.
a·mi·no·gram [ˈ-græm] *n biochem.* Aminogramm *nt*.
a·mi·no·het·er·o·cy·clic [ˌ-ˌhetərəʊˈsaɪklɪk] *adj chem.* aminoheterozyklisch.
2-a·mi·no·hex·a·no·ic acid [ˌ-ˌheksəˈnəʊɪk] Norleucin *nt*, α-Amino-*n*-capronsäure *f*.
a·mi·no·hip·pu·rate [ˌ-hɪˈpjʊreɪt, -ˈhɪpjə-] *n* Aminohippurat *nt*.
***p*-aminohippurate clearence** PAH--Clearance *f*.
***p*-a·mi·no·hip·pu·ric acid** [ˌ-hɪˈpjʊrɪk] *abbr.* **PAH, PAHA** *p*-Aminohippursäure *f*, Paraaminohippursäure *f abbr.* **PAH**.
a·mi·no·hy·dro·lase [ˌ-ˈhaɪdrəleɪz] *n* Desaminase *f*, Aminohydrolase *f*.
2-a·mi·no·i·so·va·ler·ic acid [ˌ-ˌaɪsəvəˈlerɪk, -vəˈlɪər-] Valin *nt abbr.* **Val**, α-Aminoisovaleriansäure *f*.
a·mi·no·lev·u·li·nate [ˌ-ˈlevjəlɪneɪt] *n* Aminolävulinat *nt*.
aminolevulinate dehydratase Porphobilinogensynthase *f*.
(5-)aminolevulinate synthase 5-Aminolävulinatsynthase *f*, δ-Aminolävulinatsynthase *f*.
δ-a·mi·no·lev·u·lin·ic acid [ˌ-ˌlevjəˈlɪnɪk] *abbr.* **ALA** δ-Aminolävulinsäure *f abbr.* **ALA, ALS**.
a·mi·no·lip·id [ˌ-ˈlɪpɪd, -ˈlaɪ-] *n* Aminolipid *nt*.
a·mi·no·lip·in [ˌ-ˈlɪpɪn] *n* → aminolipid.
2-a·mi·no·mu·con·ic acid [ˌ-mjuːˈkɒnɪk] 2-Aminomuconsäure *f*.
2-aminomuconic acid semialdehyde 2--Aminomuconsäuresemialdehyd *m*.
2-aminomuconic acid semialdehyde dehydrogenase 2-Aminomuconsäuresemialdehyddehydrogenase *f*.
a·mi·no·ni·trile [ˌ-ˈnaɪtrɪl, -triːl] *n* Aminonitril *nt*.
6-a·mi·no·pen·i·cil·lan·ic acid [ˌ-ˌpenəsəˈlænɪk] *abbr.* **6-APA** 6-Aminopenicillansäure *f abbr.* **6-APA**.
a·mi·no·pep·ti·dase [ˌ-ˈpeptədeɪz] *n* Aminopeptidase *f*.

aminopeptidase (cytosol) Leucinaminopeptidase *f abbr.* LAP, Leucinarylamidase *f.*
a·mi·no·phen·a·zone [ˌɪ-ˈfenəzəʊn] *n* → aminopyrine.
am·i·noph·er·ase [æmɪˈnɑfəreɪs] *n* → aminotransferase.
a·mi·no·phyl·line [əˌmiːnəʊˈfɪliːn, -lɪn] *n pharm.* Aminophyllin *nt.*
a·mi·no·pol·y·pep·ti·dase [ˌ-ˌpɑlɪˈpeptɪdeɪz] *n* → aminopeptidase.
a·mi·no·pro·pi·on·ic acid [ˌ-ˌprəʊpɪˈɑnɪk, -ˈəʊnɪk] *n* → alanine.
a·mi·no·pro·pyl·trans·fer·ase [-ˌprəʊpɪlˈtrænsfəreɪz] *n* Aminopropyltransferase *f.*
am·i·nop·ter·in [æmɪˈnɑptərɪn] *n pharm.* Aminopterin *nt,* 4-Aminofolsäure *f.*
am·i·nop·ter·o·yl·glu·tam·ic acid [æmɪˌnɑptərəwɪlgluːˈtæmɪk] → aminopterin.
2-a·mi·no·pu·rine [əˌmiːnəʊˈpjʊərɪːn, -rɪn] *n abbr.* **AP** 2-Aminopurin *nt abbr.* AP.
6-aminopurine *n* Alanin *nt abbr.* Ala, Aminopropionsäure *f.*
a·mi·no·py·rine [ˌ-ˈpaɪriːn] *n pharm.* Aminophenazon *nt,* Aminopyrin *nt.*
a·mi·no·sac·cha·ride [ˌ-ˈsækəraɪd, -rɪd] *n* Aminozucker *m,* -saccharid *nt.*
a·mi·no·sa·lic·y·late [ˌ-səˈlɪsəleɪt, -lɪt] *n pharm.* Aminosalizylat *nt.*
p-aminosalicylate *n pharm.* Paraaminosalizylat *nt,* p-Aminosalizylat *nt.*
a·mi·no·sal·i·cyl·ic acid [ˌ-sæləˈsɪlɪk] *pharm.* Aminosalizylsäure *f.*
p-aminosalicylic acid *abbr.* **PAS** *pharm.* *p*-Aminosalizylsäure *f,* Paraaminosalizylsäure *f abbr.* PAS.
amino sugar Aminozucker *m.*
am·i·no·su·ria [əˌmiːnəʊˈs(j)ʊərɪə, ˌæmɪnəʊ-] *n* Aminosurie *f,* Aminurie *f.*
amino-terminal *adj chem.* aminoterminal, N-terminal.
a·mi·no·trans·fer·ase [-ˈtrænsfəreɪz] *n* Aminotransferase *f,* Transaminase *f.*
am·i·nu·ria [æmɪˈn(j)ʊərɪə] *n* → aminosuria.
A·mish [ˈɑːmɪʃ, ˈæmɪʃ]: **A. albinism** Yellow-Typ *m* des okulokutanen Albinismus.
am·i·to·sis [ˌæmɪˈtəʊsɪs, ˌeɪmaɪ-] *n* direkte Zellteilung *f,* Amitose *f.*
am·i·tot·ic [-ˈtɑtɪk] *adj* Amitose betr., amitotisch.
AML *abbr.* → acute myeloid leukemia.
AMM *abbr.* → amelanotic (malignant) melanoma.
am·me·ter [ˈæmiːtər] *n* Strom(stärke)messer *m,* Amperemeter *m.*
am·mo·ac·i·du·ria [æməˌæsɪˈd(j)ʊərɪə] *n* kombinierte Ausscheidung *f* von Aminosäuren u. Ammoniak im Urin.
Ammon [ˈæmən]: **A.'s horn** 1. Ammonshorn *nt,* Hippokampus *m,* Hippocampus *m.* 2. (eigentliches) Ammonshorn *nt,* Cornu Ammonis, Pes hippocampi.
A.'s operation *HNO* Tränensacköffnung *f,* -inzision *f,* Dakryozystotomie *f.*
am·mo·ne·mia [ˌæməˈniːmɪə] *n* (Hyper-)Ammonämie *f.*
am·mo·nia [əˈməʊnjə, -nɪə] *n* Ammoniak *nt abbr.* NH₃.
am·mo·ni·ac [əˈməʊnɪæk] *adj* → ammoniacal.
am·mo·ni·a·cal [ˌæməˈnaɪəkl] *adj* Ammoniak enthaltend, ammoniakalisch, Ammoniak-; (*Urin*) nach Ammoniak riechend.
ammoniacal urine → ammoniuria.
ammonia dermatitis Windeldermatitis *f,* posterosives Syphiloid *nt,* Dermatitis ammoniacalis, Dermatitis glutaeale infantum, Erythema glutaeale, Erythema papulosum posterosivum.

ammonia intoxication Ammoniakintoxikation *f.*
ammonia solution Salmiakgeist *m,* wässrige Ammoniaklösung *f.*
diluted a. verdünnter Salmiakgeist.
strong a. konzentrierter Salmiakgeist.
am·mo·ni·o·mag·ne·si·um phosphate [əˈməʊnɪəʊmægˈniːzɪəm, ʒəm, -ʃɪəm] Ammonium-Magnesiumphosphat *nt.*
am·mo·ni·um [əˈməʊnɪəm] *n* Ammoniumion *nt,* -radikal *nt.*
ammonium base, quaternary quartäre Ammonbiumbase *f.*
ammonium bromide Ammoniumbromid *nt.*
ammonium carbonate Ammoniumkarbonat *nt,* Hirschhornsalz *nt.*
ammonium chloride Ammoniumchlorid *nt,* Salmiak *m.*
ammonium ichthyosulfonate *pharm.* Ichthammol *nt,* Ammonium bitumosulfonicum/sulfoichthyolicum.
ammonium nitrate Ammoniumnitrat *nt.*
ammonium oxalate Ammoniumoxalat *nt.*
ammonium phosphate Ammoniumphosphat *nt.*
ammonium salts Ammoniumsalze *pl.*
ammonium sulfoichthyolate → ammonium ichthyosulfonate.
ammonium urate calculus/stone Ammoniumuratstein *m.*
am·mo·ni·u·ria [əˌməʊnɪˈ(j)ʊərɪə] *n* Ammoniakausscheidung *f* im Harn, Ammoniurie *f.*
am·mo·nol·y·sis [æməˈnɑləsɪs] *n biochem.* Ammonolyse *f.*
am·mo·no·tel·ic [əˌməʊnəʊˈtelɪk, -ˈtiː-] *adj bio.* ammonotelisch.
am·ne·mon·ic agraphia [æmnəˈmɑnɪk] Agraphia amnemonica.
am·ne·sia [æmˈniːʒ(ɪ)ə] *n* Erinnerungs-, Gedächtnisstörung *f,* Amnesie *f,* Amnesia *f.*
am·ne·si·ac [æmˈniːzɪæk, -ʒɪæk] **I** *n* Patient(in *f*) *m* mit Amnesie. **II** *adj* Amnesie betr., von Amnesie betroffen, amnesisch, amnestisch.
am·ne·sic [æmˈniːzɪk] *n, adj* → amnesiac.
amnesic aphasia Wortvergessenheit *f,* Wortfindungsstörung *f,* amnestische Aphasie *f.*
amnesic state Amnesiestadium *nt.*
amnesic syndrome → amnestic syndrome.
am·nes·tic [æmˈnestɪk] *adj* 1. → amnesiac II. 2. amnesieverursachend, -erzeugend, amnestisch.
amnestic aphasia → amnesic aphasia.
amnestic apraxia amnestische Apraxie *f.*
amnestic-confabulatory syndrome → amnestic syndrome.
amnestic psychosis → amnestic syndrome.
amnestic syndrome amnestisches Syndrom *nt,* Korsakow-Syndrom *nt,* -Psychose *f.*
amni- *pref.* → amnio-.
am·nic [ˈæmnɪk] *adj* → amniotic.
amnio- *pref.* Amnio(n)-.
am·ni·o·blast [ˈæmnɪəʊblæst] *n embryo.* Amnioblast *m.*
am·ni·o·cele [-ˈsiːl] *n* Nabelschnurbruch *m,* Omphalozele *f,* -cele *f.*
am·ni·o·cen·te·sis [ˌ-senˈtiːsɪs] *n* Fruchtblasenpunktion *f,* Amnionpunktion *f,* Amniozentese *f.*
am·ni·o·cyte [ˈ-saɪt] *n* Amniozyt *m.*
am·ni·o·ec·to·der·mal junction [ˌ-ˌektəˈdɜrməl] *embryo.* amnioektodermale Umschlagsfalte *f.*
am·ni·o·gen·e·sis [ˌ-ˈdʒenəsɪs] *n* Amnionentwicklung *f,* Amniogenese *f.*

am·ni·og·ra·phy [æmnɪˈɑgrəfɪ] *n* Amniographie *f.*
am·ni·on [ˈæmnɪən] *n, pl* **-ni·ons, -ni·a** [-nɪə] Schafshaut *f,* innere Eihaut *f,* Amnion *nt.*
am·ni·on·ic [ˌæmnɪˈɑnɪk] *adj* → amniotic.
amnionic cavity → amniotic cavity.
am·ni·o·ni·tis [ˌæmnɪəˈnaɪtɪs] *n* Amnionentzündung *f,* Amnionitis *f.*
am·ni·or·rhea [ˌæmnɪəˈrɪə] *n* Amniorrhoe *f.*
am·ni·or·rhex·is [ˌ-ˈreksɪs] *n gyn.* Blasensprung *m,* Amnionrupturr *f.*
am·ni·o·scope [ˈ-skəʊp] *n* Amnioskop *nt.*
am·ni·os·co·py [ˌæmnɪˈɑskəpɪ] *n* Fruchtwasserspiegelung *f,* Amnioskopie *f.*
Am·ni·o·ta [ˌæmnɪˈəʊtə] *pl bio.* Amniontiere *pl,* Amnioten *pl.*
am·ni·ote [ˈæmnɪəʊt] *n* Amniot *m.*
am·ni·ot·ic [ˌ-ˈɑtɪk] *adj* Amnion betr., vom Amnion abstammend, amniotisch, Amnio-.
amniotic adhesions → amniotic bands.
amniotic amputation *embryo.,* *ped.* Amputation *f* durch Amnionstränge.
amniotic bands amniotische Stränge *pl,* Simonart'-Bänder *pl.*
amniotic cavity Amnionhöhle *f.*
amniotic corpuscles Amyloidkörperchen *pl,* Corpora amylacea.
amniotic epithelium Amnionepithel *nt.*
amniotic fluid Fruchtwasser *nt,* Amnionflüssigkeit *f,* Aqua/Liquor amnii.
amniotic fluid aspiration Fruchtwasseraspiration *f.*
amniotic fluid embolism Fruchtwasserembolie *f.*
amniotic fluid syndrome Fruchtwasserembolie *f.*
amniotic sac Amnionsack *m,* Fruchtblase *f.*
am·ni·o·tome [ˈæmnɪətəʊm] *n* Amniotom *nt.*
am·ni·ot·o·my [æmnɪˈɑtəmɪ] *n* Amniotomie *f.*
am·o·bar·bi·tal [ˌæməʊˈbɑːrbɪtəl, -tæl] *n pharm.* Amobarbital *nt.*
am·o·di·a·quine [ˌɪ-ˈdaɪəkwɪn] *n pharm.* Amodiaquin *nt.*
A·moe·ba [əˈmiːbə] *n micro.* Amöbe *f,* Amoeba *f.*
a·moe·ba *n* → ameba.
A·moe·bi·da [əˈmiːbɪdə] *pl micro.* Amoebida *pl.*
a·moe·bi·form *adj* → ameboid.
a·moe·boid *adj* → ameboid.
a·moe·bu·la *n* → amebula.
a·mor·phia [əˈmɔːrfɪə] *n* Gestalt-, Formlosigkeit *f,* Amorphsein *f,* Amorphismus *m.*
a·mor·phism [əˈmɔːrfɪzəm] *n* → amorphia.
a·mor·phous [əˈmɔːrfəs] *adj* 1. gestalt-, form-, strukturlos, amorph. 2. *chem.* amorph, nicht kristallin.
amorphous phosphorus roter/amorpher Phosphor *m.*
a·mor·phus [əˈmɔːrfəs] *n embryo.* Amorphus *m.*
Amoss [ˈæmɑs]: **A.' sign** Amoss-Zeichen *nt,* Dreifußzeichen *nt.*
a·mount [əˈmaʊnt] *n* Menge *f;* Maß *nt,* Ausmaß *nt.* **in large ~s** in großen Mengen.
a. of heat *phys.* Wärmemenge.
a. of resistance *phys.* Widerstandswert *m.*
a·mox·i·cil·lin [əˌmɑksəˈsɪlɪn] *n pharm.* Amoxicillin *nt.*
AMP *abbr.* → adenosine monophosphate.
amp. *abbr.* → ampere.
AMP deaminase AMP-Desaminase *f.*
am·per·age [ˈæmpərɪdʒ, æmˈpɪər-] *n* (elektrische) Stromstärke *f.*
am·pere [ˈæmpɪər] *n abbr.* **A, a, amp.** Ampere *nt abbr.* A.

amph(i)-

amph(i)- *pref.* zwei(fach)-, doppel-, amph(i)-.
am·phi·ar·thro·di·al articulation [ˌæmfɪɑːrˈθroʊdɪəl] → amphiarthrosis.
amphiarthrodial joint → amphiarthrosis.
am·phi·ar·thro·sis [ˌ-ɑːrˈθroʊsɪs] *n* Wackelgelenk *nt*, straffes Gelenk *nt*, Amphiarthrose *f*.
am·phi·as·ter ['-æstər] *n histol.* Amphiaster *m*, Diaster *m*.
Am·phib·ia [æmˈfɪbɪə] *pl bio.* Amphibien *pl*, Amphibia *pl*.
am·phib·i·ous [æmˈfɪbɪəs] *adj bio.* amphibisch, Amphibien-.
am·phi·blas·tic [ˌæmfɪˈblæstɪk] *adj bio., histol.* amphiblastisch.
am·phi·blas·tu·la [ˌ-ˈblæstjələ] *n* Amphiblastula *f*.
am·phi·bol·ic [ˌ-ˈbɒlɪk] *adj* zwei-, mehrdeutig, doppelsinnig, schwankend, amphibolisch, amphibol.
amphibolic pathway amphibolischer Stoffwechselweg *m*.
am·phi·chro·ic [ˌ-ˈkroʊɪk] *adj* → amphichromatic.
am·phi·chro·mat·ic [ˌ-kroʊˈmætɪk] *adj* zweifarbig, amphichromatisch.
am·phi·cro·ic [ˌ-ˈkroʊɪk] *adj* → amphichromatic.
am·phi·cyte ['-saɪt] *n* Mantelzelle *f*, Amphizyt *m*.
am·phi·di·ar·thro·sis [ˌ-daɪɑːrˈθroʊsɪs] *n* Amphidiarthrose *f*.
am·phi·gas·tru·la [ˌ-ˈgæstrələ] *n* Amphigastrula *f*.
am·phi·ge·net·ic [ˌ-dʒəˈnetɪk] *adj* amphigen.
am·phi·gon·a·dism [ˌ-ˈgɒnədɪzəm] *n* Amphigonadismus *m*, echter Hermaphroditismus *m*, Hermaphroditismus verus.
am·phig·o·ny [æmˈfɪgəni] *n bio.* sexuelle Fortpflanzung *f*, Amphigonie *f*.
am·phi·kar·y·on [ˌæmfɪˈkærɪɒn] *n histol.* diploider Kern *m*, Amphikaryon *nt*.
am·phi·leu·ke·mic [ˌ-luːˈkiːmɪk] *adj hema.* amphileukämisch.
am·phi·lous ['æmfɪləs] *adj* → amphophil II.
am·phi·mix·is [ˌæmfɪˈmɪksɪs] *n* Amphimixis *f*, Amphimixie *f*.
am·phi·mor·u·la [ˌ-ˈmɔːrələ, -ˈmɑːr-] *n* Amphimorula *f*.
am·phi·nu·cle·us [ˌ-ˈn(j)uːklɪəs] *n* Amphi-, Zentronukleus *m*.
am·phi·path ['-pæθ, -pɑːθ] *n chem.* amphipathische Substanz *f*.
am·phi·path·ic [ˌ-ˈpæθɪk] *adj chem.* amphipathisch.
amphipathic lipid amphipathisches/polares Lipid *nt*.
am·phis·to·ma [æmˈfɪstəmə] *n micro.* Amphistoma *nt*.
am·phi·sto·mi·a·sis [æmˌfɪstəˈmaɪəsɪs] *n* Amphistomiasis *f*.
am·phi·tene ['æmfətiːn] *n bio.* Amphitän *nt*.
am·phit·ri·chous [æmˈtrɪtrəkəs] *adj micro.* amphitrich.
am·phit·y·py [æmˈfɪtəpi] *n* Amphitypie *f*.
am·pho·chro·mat·o·phil [ˌæmfoʊkroʊˈmætəfɪl] *n, adj* → amphophil.
am·pho·chro·mo·phil [ˌ-ˈkroʊməfɪl] *n, adj* → amphophil.
am·pho·cyte ['-saɪt] *n* → amphophil I.
am·pho·di·plo·pia [ˌ-dɪˈploʊpɪə] *n ophthal.* beidseitiges Doppelsehen *nt*, Amphodiplopie *f*.
am·pho·gen·ic [ˌ-ˈdʒenɪk] *adj bio.* amphogen.
am·pho·lyte ['-laɪt] *n* Ampholyt *m*.
am·pho·lyt·ic [ˌ-ˈlɪtɪk] *adj* 1. ampholytisch. 2. amphoter(isch).

am·pho·phil ['-fɪl] I *n* amphophile Zelle *f*, Amphozyt *m*. II *adj* amphophil, amphochrom(at)ophil.
am·pho·phil·ic [ˌ-ˈfɪlɪk] *adj* → amphophil II.
amphophilic cell amphophile Zelle *f*, Amphozyt *m*.
am·phor·ic [æmˈfɔːrɪk] *adj (Schall)* amphorisch.
amphoric murmur Amphorenatmen *nt*.
amphoric rales (*Auskultation*) amphorische Rasselgeräusche *pl*, Amphorenrasseln *nt*.
amphoric resonance Kavernen-, Amphorengeräusch *nt*.
amphoric respiration amphorisches Atmen *nt*, Amphorophonie *f*, Krugatmen *nt*.
am·pho·roph·o·ny [ˌæmfəˈrɒfəni] *n* Amphorophonie *f*.
am·pho·ter·ic [ˌæmfəˈterɪk] *adj chem.* zweisinnig, amphoterisch, amphoter.
amphoteric dye amphoterischer Farbstoff *m*.
amphoteric electrolyte → ampholyte.
am·pho·ter·i·cin B [ˌ-ˈterɪsɪn] *n pharm.* Amphotericin B *nt*.
am·pho·ter·i·ci·ty [ˌ-teˈrɪsətɪ] *n* → amphoterism.
amphoteric reaction *chem.* amphotere Reaktion *f*.
am·pho·ter·ism [æmˈfɒtərɪzəm] *n chem.* Amphoterismus *m*.
am·phot·er·o·di·plo·pia [æmˌfɒtəroʊdɪˈploʊpɪə] *n* Amphodiplopia *f*.
am·phot·er·ous [æmˈfɒtərəs] *adj* → amphoteric.
am·phot·o·ny [æmˈfɒtəni] *n neuro., physiol.* Amphotonie *f*.
am·pho·tro·pic virus [ˌæmfəˈtroʊpɪk, -ˈtrɒp-] amphotropes Virus *nt*.
am·pi·cil·lin [ˌæmpəˈsɪlɪn] *n pharm.* Ampicillin *nt*, alpha-Aminobenzylpenicillin *nt*.
AMP kinase Adenylatkinase *f*, Myokinase *f*, AMP-Kinase *f*, A-Kinase *f*.
am·pli·fi·ca·tion [ˌæmplɪfɪˈkeɪʃn] *n* Verstärkung *f*, Vergrößerung *f*; Erweiterung *f*; Ausdehnung *f*; *phys.* Amplifikation *f*.
amplification cascade Verstärkungskaskade *f*.
amplification factor Verstärkungsfaktor *m*.
am·pli·fi·er ['æmplɪfaɪər] *n phys., techn.* Verstärker *m*.
am·pli·fy ['æmplɪfaɪ] *vt (a. phys.)* verstärken, vergrößern, amplifizieren; erweitern, ausdehnen.
am·pli·fy·ing lens ['æmplɪfaɪɪŋ] Vergrößerungslinse *f*.
am·pli·tude ['æmplɪt(j)uːd] *n* 1. (*a. fig.*) Größe *f*, Weite *f*, Umfang *m*. 2. *phys.* Amplitude *f*, Schwingungs-, Ausschlagsweite *f*.
a. of accommodation *ophthal.* Akkommodationsbreite *f*.
a. of convergence *ophthal.* Konvergenzbreite *f*, -amplitude.
a. of vibration → amplitude 2.
amplitude difference *phys.* Amplitudendifferenz *f*.
am·poule *n* → ampul.
am·pul ['æmp(j)uːl] *n pharm.* bauchiges Gefäß *nt*, Kolben *m*, Ampulle *f*, Ampulla *f*.
am·pule *n* → ampul.
am·pul·la [æmˈpʌlə, -ˈpʊl-] *n, pl* **-lae** [-liː] *anat.* bauchige Auftreibung *f*, Ampulle *f*, Ampulla *f*.
a. of deferent duct Samenleiterampulle, Ampulla ductus deferentis.
a. of lacrimal canaliculus/duct Tränengangsampulle, Ampulla canaliculi/duc-

tus lacrimalis.
a. of (uterine) tube Tubenampulle, Ampulla tubae uterinae.
a. of vas deferens → a. of deferent duct.
am·pul·lar [æmˈpʌlər, -ˈpʊl-] *adj* → ampullary.
ampullar abortion ampullärer Abort *m*, Abort *m* bei Ampullenschwangerschaft.
ampullar nerve: anterior a. N. ampullaris anterior.
inferior a. → posterior a.
lateral a. N. ampullaris lateralis.
posterior a. N. ampullaris posterior.
superior a. → anterior a.
ampullar pregnancy ampulläre Tubargravidität *f*, Graviditas tubaria ampullaris.
am·pul·lar·y [æmˈpʌləri, -ˈpʊl-, ˈæmpəˌleri] *adj* bauchig aufgetrieben *od.* erweitert, ampullär.
ampullary aneurysm sackförmiges Aneurysma *nt*, Aneurysma sacciforme.
ampullary carcinoma Karzinom *nt* der Ampulla hepaticopancreatica.
ampullary crest Crista *f* der Bogengangsampulle, Crista ampullaris.
ampullary crura of semicircular duct Crura membranacea ampullaria (ductus semicirculars).
ampullary edema Ödem *nt* der Apulla hepaticopancreatica, Ampullenödem *nt*.
ampullary limbs of semicircular ducts Crura membranacea ampullaria.
ampullary part of (uterine) tube → ampulla of (uterine) tube.
ampullary stenosis Stenose *f* der Ampulla hepaticopancreatica, Ampullenstenose *f*.
ampullary sulcus Ampullenrinne *f*, Sulcus ampullaris.
am·pul·late [æmˈpʌlɪt, leɪt, ˈæmpə-] *adj* flaschenförmig.
am·pul·li·tis [ˌæmpʊˈlaɪtɪs] *n* 1. Ampullenentzündung *f*, Ampullitis *f*. 2. Entzündung *f* der Samenleiterampulle.
am·pul·lof·u·gal stimulation [ˌæmpoʊˈlɒfjəgəl] *HNO* utrikulofugale Stimulation *f*.
am·pul·lop·et·al stimulation [ˌ-ˈlɒpətəl] *HNO* utrikulopetale Stimulation *f*.
am·pu·tate ['æmpjoʊteɪt] *vt* abnehmen, amputieren.
am·pu·ta·tion [ˌæmpjoʊˈteɪʃn] *n chir.* Abnahme *f*, Amputation *f*.
a. of/through the arm Oberarmamputation.
a. of/through the forearm (hohe) Vorarm-/Unterarmamputation.
a. of/through the leg Unterschenkelamputation.
a. of/through the lower leg → a. of/through the leg.
a. of/through the thigh Oberschenkelamputation.
a. of/through the upper arm Oberarmamputation.
a. at/through the wrist Handgelenkexartikulation *f*, Absetzung *f* im Handgelenk.
amputation neuroma Amputationsneurom *nt*.
amputation saw *ortho.* Amputationssäge *f*.
am·pu·tee [æmpjʊˈtiː] *n* Amputierte(r *m*) *f*.
Amsler ['amslər]: **A.'s chart** *ophthal.* Amsler-Gitter *nt*.
A. test Amsler-Test *m*.
amu *abbr.* → atomic mass unit.
a·mu·sia [eɪˈmjuːzɪə] *n neuro.* Amusie *f*.
Amussat [amyˈsa]: **A.'s incision/operation** Amussat-Schnitt(führung *f*) *m*, -Technik *f*.
A.'s valve Plica spiralis.
am·y·cho·pho·bia [ˌæmɪkoʊˈfoʊbɪə] *n psychia.* Kratzangst *f*, Amychophobie *f*.

a·myc·tic [əˈmɪktɪk] *adj* ätzend, reizend.
a·my·el·en·ce·pha·lia [eɪˌmaɪələnseˈfeɪlɪə] *n embryo.* Amyelenzephalie *f.*
a·my·el·en·ceph·a·lus [ˌ-ˈsefələs] *n embryo.* Amyelenzephalus *m.*
a·my·e·lia [ˌæmaɪˈiːlɪə] *n embryo.* Rückenmark(s)aplasie *f,* Amyelie *f.*
a·my·el·ic [ˌ-ˈelɪk] *adj* Amyelie betr., amyel.
a·my·e·lin·ic [eɪˌmaɪəˈlɪnɪk] *adj* myelinlos, -frei, amyelinisch.
a·my·e·lon·ic [ˌ-ˈlɑnɪk] *adj* **1.** rückenmarkslos, ohne Rückenmark. **2.** knochenmarkslos, ohne Knochenmark.
a·my·e·lot·ro·phy [ˌ-ˈlɑtrəfɪ] *n patho.* Rückenmark(s)atrophie *f,* Amyelotrophie *f.*
a·my·e·lus [əˈmaɪələs] *n embryo.* Amyelus *m.*
a·myg·da·la [əˈmɪgdələ] *n, pl* **-lae** [-liː, -laɪ] *anat.* **1.** mandelförmige Struktur *f,* Amygdala *f.* **2.** Mandelkern(komplex *m*) *m,* Mandelkörper *m,* Nc. amygdalae, Corpus amygdaloideum.
a. of cerebellum Kleinhirnmandel *f,* Tonsilla *f,* Tonsilla cerebelli.
a·myg·da·lase [əˈmɪgdəleɪz] *n* β-Glukosidase *f.*
a·myg·dal·ic acid [əˈmɪgdælɪk] Mandelsäure *f.*
a·myg·da·lin [əˈmɪgdəlɪn] *n* Amygdalin *nt.*
a·myg·da·line [əˈmɪgdəlɪn] *adj* **1.** mandelähnlich, -förmig. **2.** Tonsille(n) betr., Tonsillen-, Mandel-.
a·myg·da·lo·fu·gal fibers, ventral [əˌmɪgdəlɒʊˈfjuːgl] ventrale amygdalofugale Fasern *pl.*
a·myg·da·loid [əˈmɪgdəlɔɪd] *adj* mandelförmig; *anat.* Amygdal-, Mandel-.
a·myg·da·loi·dal [əˌmɪgdəˈlɔɪdl] *adj* → amygdaloid.
amygdaloid area, anterior vordere Zellgruppe *f* des Mandelkerns, Area amygdaloidea anterior.
amygdaloid body → amygdala 2.
amygdaloid complex → amygdala 2.
amygdaloid fossa Gaumenmandel-, Tonsillennische *f,* Fossa tonsillaris.
amygdaloid nucleus → amygdala 2.
amygdaloid tubercle of Schwalbe Area vestibularis.
amyl- *pref.* → amylo-.
am·yl [ˈæmɪl, ˈeɪm-] *n* Amyl-(Radikal *nt*).
am·y·la·ce·ous [æməˈleɪʃəs] *adj* stärkeähnlich, -haltig, Stärke-.
amylaceous bodies Amyloidkörper *pl,* Corpora amylacea.
amyl alcohol Amylalkohol *m.*
am·y·lase [ˈæmɪleɪz] *n* Amylase *f.*
am·y·las·e·mia [ˌæməleɪˈsiːmɪə] *n* Amylasenerhöhung *f,* Amylasämie *f.*
am·y·las·u·ria [ˌæməleɪˈs(j)ʊərɪə] *n* Amylasurie *f.*
am·yl·ene [ˈæmɪliːn] *n* Amylen *nt,* Penten *nt.*
amylene hydrate → amyl alcohol.
am·yl·in [ˈæməlɪn] *n* → amylopectin.
am·yl·ism [ˈæməlɪzəm] *n* Amylalkoholvergiftung *f,* Amylismus *m.*
amyl nitrite Amylnitrit *nt.*
amylo- *pref.* Stärke-, Amyl(o)-.
am·y·lo·bar·bi·tone [ˌæmɪləʊˈbɑːrbɪtəʊn] *n pharm.* Amobarbital *nt.*
am·y·lo·cel·lu·lose [ˌ-ˈseljələʊs] *n* → amylose 2.
am·y·lo·clas·tic [ˌ-ˈklæstɪk] *adj* stärkespaltend, -abbauend.
am·y·lo·co·ag·u·lase [ˌ-kəʊˈægjəleɪs] *n* Amylokoagulase *f.*
am·y·lo·dys·pep·sia [ˌ-dɪsˈpepʃə, -sɪə] *n* Amylodyspepsie *f.*
a·myl·o·gen [əˈmɪlədʒən] *n* → amylose 2.

am·y·lo·gen·e·sis [ˌæmɪləʊˈdʒenəsɪs] *n* Stärkebildung *f.*
am·y·lo·gen·ic [ˌ-ˈdʒenɪk] *adj* stärkebildend, -produzierend, amylogen.
amylo-1,6-glucosidase *n* Amylo-1,6-Glukosidase *f,* Dextrin-1,6-Glukosidase *f.*
amylo-1,6-glucosidase deficiency Cori-Krankheit *f,* Forbes-Syndrom *nt,* hepatomuskuläre benigne Glykogenose *f,* Glykogenose Typ III *f.*
am·y·lo·hy·drol·y·sis [ˌ-haɪˈdrɑləsɪs] *n* Stärkehydrolyse *f,* Amylo(hydro)lyse *f.*
am·y·loid [ˈæmələɪd] **I** *n* Amyloid *nt.* **II** *adj* stärkeähnlich, amyloid.
am·y·loi·dal [æməˈlɔɪdl] *adj* → amyloid II.
amyloid A protein AA-Protein *nt,* Amyloidprotein-A *nt.*
amyloid bodies Amyloidkörper *pl,* Corpora amylacea.
amyloid degeneration amyloide Degeneration *f;* Amyloidose *f.*
amyloid deposit *patho.* Amyloidablagerung *f.*
amyloid kidney Amyloid(schrumpf)niere *f,* Wachs-, Speckniere *f.*
amyloid light chain protein AL-Protein *nt,* Amyloidprotein-L *nt.*
amyloid liver Amyloidleber *f.*
amyloid nephrosis Amyloidnephrose *f.*
am·y·loi·do·sis [æməˌlɔɪˈdəʊsɪs] *n* Amyloidose *f,* amyloide Degeneration *f.*
a. of aging Altersamyloidose, senile Amyloidose.
amyloid struma Amyloidstruma *f.*
amyloid thesaurismosis → amyloidosis.
amyloid tongue Amyloidzunge *f.*
am·y·lol·y·sis [ˌæməˈlɑləsɪs] *n* → amylohydrolysis.
am·y·lo·lyt·ic [ˌæmɪləʊˈlɪtɪk] *adj* Amylo(hydro)lyse betr., stärkespaltend, -auflösend, amylo(hydro)lytisch.
am·y·lo·pec·tin [ˌ-ˈpektɪn] *n* Amylopektin *nt.*
am·y·lo·pec·ti·no·sis [ˌ-ˌpektɪˈnəʊsɪs] *n* Andersen-Krankheit *f,* Amylopektinose *f,* leberzirrhotische retikuloendotheliale Glykogenose *f,* Glykogenose Typ IV *f.*
am·y·lo·plast [ˈ-plæst] *n* Amyloplast *m.*
am·y·lo·plas·tic [ˌ-ˈplæstɪk] *adj* stärkebildend, amyloplastisch.
am·y·lor·rhea [ˌ-ˈrɪə] *n* Amylorrhoe *f.*
am·yl·ose [ˈæmɪləʊz] *n* **1.** Polysaccharid *nt* der Stärkegruppe. **2.** Amylose *f.*
am·y·lo·sis [æmɪˈləʊsɪs] *n* → amyloidosis.
am·y·lo·su·ria [ˌæmɪləʊˈs(j)ʊərɪə] *n* Amylosurie *f.*
am·y·lo·syn·the·sis [ˌ-ˈsɪnθəsɪs] *n* Stärkeaufbau *m,* -synthese *f,* Amylosynthese *f.*
amylo-1:4,1:6-transglucosidase Branchingenzym *nt,* Glucan-verzweigende Glykosyltransferase *f,* 1,4-α-Glucan-branching-Enzym *nt.*
amylo-1:4,1:6-transglucosidase deficiency → amylopectinosis.
am·yl·um [ˈæmɪləm] *n* Stärke *f,* Amylum *nt.*
am·yl·u·ria [æmɪˈl(j)ʊərɪə] *n* Amylurie *f.*
a·my·o·aes·the·sis [eɪˌmaɪəsˈθiːsɪs] *n neuro.* Amyoästhesie *f.*
a·my·o·pla·sia [ˌ-ˈpleɪʒ(ɪ)ə, -ʒɪə] *n* Muskelaplasie *f,* Amyoplasie *f,* -plasia *f.*
a·my·o·sta·sia [ˌ-ˈsteɪʒ(ɪ)ə, -ʃɪə] *n neuro.* Amyostasis *f.*
a·my·o·stat·ic [ˌ-ˈstætɪk] *adj neuro.* amyostatisch.
amyostatic syndrome Wilson-Krankheit *f,* -Syndrom *nt,* Morbus Wilson *m,* hepatolentikuläre/hepatozerebrale Degeneration *f.*
a·my·os·the·nia [eɪˌmaɪəsˈθiːnɪə] *n neuro.* Muskelschwäche *f.*
a·my·os·then·ic [ˌ-ˈθiːnɪk] *adj* Myasthenie betr. *od.* verursachend, von Myasthenie

betroffen, myasthenisch.
a·my·o·tax·ia [eɪˌmaɪəˈtæksɪə] *n* → ataxy.
a·my·o·tax·y [ˌ-ˈtæksɪ] *n* → ataxy.
a·my·o·to·nia [ˌ-ˈtəʊnɪə] *n* Amyotonie *f,* Myatonie *f.*
a·my·o·tro·phia [ˌ-ˈtrəʊfɪə] *n* → amyotrophy.
a·my·o·troph·ic [ˌ-ˈtrɑfɪk, -ˈtrəʊf-] *adj* Amyotrophie betr., amyotrophisch.
amyotrophic lateral sclerosis *abbr.* **ALS** amyotrophische/amyotrophe/myatrophische Lateralsklerose *f abbr.* ALS.
a·my·ot·ro·phy [eɪmaɪˈɑtrəfɪ] *n* Muskelschwund *m,* -atrophie *f,* Amyotrophie *f.*
a·myx·ia [eɪˈmɪksɪə] *n patho.* Schleimarmut *f,* Amyxie *f.*
a·myx·or·rhea [eɪˌmɪksəˈrɪə] *n* Amyxorrhoe *f.*
ANA *abbr.* → antinuclear antibodies.
a·nab·a·sine [əˈnæbəsiːn, -sɪn] *n* Anabasin *nt.*
an·a·bat·ic [ænəˈbætɪk] *adj* (auf-)steigend, s. verstärkend, anabatisch.
an·a·bi·o·sis [ˌænəbaɪˈəʊsɪs] *n bio.* Anabiose *f.*
an·a·bi·ot·ic [ˌ-baɪˈɑtɪk] *adj bio.* Anabiose betr., anabiotisch, scheintod.
anabiotic cell anabiotische Zelle *f.*
an·a·bol·ic [ˌ-ˈbɑlɪk] *adj* Anabolismus betr., aufbauend, anabol, anabolisch.
anabolic agent Anabolikum *nt.*
anabolic pathway anabol(isch)er Stoffwechselweg *m.*
a·nab·o·lism [əˈnæbəlɪzəm] *n* Aufbaustoffwechsel *m,* Anabolismus *m.*
a·nab·o·lite [əˈnæbəlaɪt] *n* Anabolit *m.*
an·a·cat·a·did·y·mus *n* → anakatadidymus.
an·a·cat·es·the·sia *n* → anakatesthesia.
an·a·cho·re·sis [ænəkəˈriːsɪs] *n* **1.** *micro.* Anachorese *f.* **2.** *psychia.* Abkapselung *f,* Anachorese *f.*
an·a·cho·ret·ic [ˌ-kəˈretɪk] *adj micro., psychia.* Anachorese betr., durch Anachorese gekennzeichnet *od.* bedingt, anachoretisch.
anachoretic effect 1. *micro.* Anachorese *f.* **2.** *psychia.* Abkapselung *f,* Anachorese *f.*
an·a·cho·ric [-ˈkɔːrɪk] *adj* → anachoretic.
an·ac·id [ænˈæsɪd] *adj* anazid.
an·a·cid·i·ty [ænəˈsɪdətɪ] *n* Anazidität *f.*
an·a·cli·sis [ænəˈklaɪsɪs] *n ped., psycho.* Anaklisis *f.*
an·a·clit·ic [ˌ-ˈklɪtɪk] *adj ped., psycho.* Anaklisis betr., anaklitisch.
anaclitic depression *psychia.* anaklitische Depression *f,* Anlehnungsdepression *f.*
an·ac·me·sis *n* → anakmesis.
an·a·cou·sia [ænəˈkuːzɪə] *n* → anakusis.
an·a·crot·ic [ˌ-ˈkrɑtɪk] *adj* Anakrotie betr., anakrot.
anacrotic limb anakroter Schenkel *m.*
anacrotic pulse Anakrotie *f,* anakroter Puls *m,* Pulsus anacrotus.
anacrotic wave anakrote Welle *f.*
a·nac·ro·tism [əˈnɑkrətɪzəm] *n* (*Puls*) Anakrotie *f.*
an·a·cu·sis *n* → anakusis.
an·a·de·nia [ˌænəˈdiːnɪə] *n* **1.** Fehlen *nt* von Drüsen, Anadenie *f.* **2.** insuffiziente Drüsenfunktion *f.*
an·a·di·crot·ic pulse [ˌ-daɪˈkrɑtɪk] Anadikrotie *f,* anadikroter Puls *m,* Pulsus anadicrotus.
anadicrotic wave anadikrote Welle *f.*
an·a·did·y·mus [ˌ-ˈdɪdəməs] *n embryo.* Anadidymus *m.*
an·a·dip·sia [ˌ-ˈdɪpsɪə] *n* unstillbarer Durst *m,* Anadipsie *f.*
an·a·dre·nal·ism [ˌ-ˈdriːnlɪzəm] *n* fehlende Nebennierenfunktion *f,* Anadrenalismus *m.*

anadrenia

an·a·dre·nia [ˌ-'driːnɪə] *n* → anadrenalism.
a·nae·mi·a *n* → anemia.
an·aer·obe ['rəʊb, æn'eərəʊb] *n micro.* Anaerobier *m*, Anaerobiont m, Anoxybiont *m*.
an·aer·o·bi·an [ˌ-'rəʊbɪən] I *n* → anaerobe. II *adj* → anaerobic 1.
an·aer·o·bic [ˌ-'rəʊbɪk] *adj* **1.** *micro.* ohne Sauerstoff lebend, anaerob. **2.** *chem.* sauerstoffrei, ohne Sauerstoff.
anaerobic coverage *micro., pharm.* antibiotische Abdeckung *f* gegen anaerobe Erreger.
anaerobic fermentation *biochem.* anaerobe Gärung *f*.
anaerobic pathway *biochem.* anaerober (Stoffwechsel-)Weg *m*.
anaerobic phase *biochem.* anaerobe (Stoffwechsel-)Phase *f*.
anaerobic respiration anaerobe Atmung *f*.
anaerobic stage → anaerobic phase.
an·aer·o·bi·on [ˌ-'rəʊbɪən] *n, pl* **-bi·a** [-bɪə] *old* → anaerobe.
an·aer·o·bi·o·sis [ˌ-rəʊbaɪ'əʊsɪs, ænˌeərəʊ-] *n* Anaerobiose *f*, Anoxybiose *f*.
an·aer·o·bi·ot·ic [ˌ-rəʊbaɪ'ɒtɪk, ænˌeərəʊ-] *adj old* → anaerobic 1.
an·aer·o·gen·ic [æn͵eərəʊ'dʒenɪk, ˌænərəʊ-] *adj* **1.** *micro.* wenig *od.* kein Gas produzierend, anaerogen. **2.** *micro.* die Gasbildung unterdrückend, anaerogen.
an·aer·o·sis [æneər'əʊsɪs] *n patho.* Störung *f* der Atemfunktion.
an·aes·the·sia *n* → anesthesia.
an·a·gen ['ænədʒen] *n* (*Haar*) Wachstums-, Anagenphase *f*.
anagen-dystrophic alopecia/effluvium anagen-dystrophe Alopezie *f*, anagen--dystrophischer Haarausfall *m*, anagen--dystrophisches Effluvium *nt*, Alopezie *f* vom Frühtyp.
anagen hair Anagenhaar *nt*.
Anagnostakis [ə'nægnəstæksɪs]: **A.' operation** *ophthal.* Anagnostakis-Operation *f*.
an·a·go·cy·tic [ænͺægəʊ'saɪtɪk] *adj* Zellwachstum hemmend.
an·a·go·ge [ˌænə'gəʊdʒɪ] *n* → anagogy.
an·a·gog·ic [ˌ-'gɒdʒɪk] *adj psycho.* anagogisch.
an·a·gog·i·cal [ˌ-'gɒdʒɪkl] *adj* → anagogic.
an·a·go·gy [ˌ-'gəʊdʒɪ] *n psycho.* Anagoge *f*.
an·a·kat·a·did·y·mus [ˌ-kætə'dɪdɪməs] *n embryo.* Anakatadidymus *m*.
an·a·kat·es·the·sia [ˌ-kætes'θiːʒ(ɪ)ə] *n* Anakatästhesie *f*.
ak·me·sis [æn'ækmɪsɪs] *n patho., hema.* Reifungshemmung *f*, -stillstand *m*.
an·a·ku·sis [ˌænə'kuːsɪs] *n* (vollständige) Taubheit *f*, Anakusis *f*.
a·nal ['eɪnl] *adj* After/Anus betr., zum After/Anus gehörend, anal, After-, Anal-, Ano-.
anal abscess Analabszeß *m*.
anal anomaly Anusanomalie *f*, -fehlbildung *f*.
anal atresia Analatresie *f*, Atresia ani.
an·al·bu·mi·ne·mia [ænælͺbjuː'niːmɪə] *n* Analbuminämie *f*.
anal canal Analkanal *m*, Canalis analis.
anal carcinoma Afterkrebs *m*, Analkarzinom *nt*.
anal cleft Gesäßspalte *f*, Afterfurche *f*, Crena ani, Rima ani.
anal columns Analsäulen *pl*, -papillen *pl*, Morgagni'-Papillen *pl*, Columnae anales/rectales (Morgagnii).
anal crypts → anal sinuses.
anal cryptitis Entzündung *f* der Morgagni'-Krypten, anale Kryptitis *f*.
an·a·lep·tic [ˌænə'leptɪk] I *n pharm.* Analeptikum *nt*. II *adj* belebend, anregend, stärkend, analeptisch.
anal erotism Analerotik *f*.
anal fascia Fascia diaphragmatis pelvis inferior.
anal fissure Analfissur *f*, Fissura ani.
anal fistula Analfistel *f*, Fistula ani.
anal fold *embryo.* Analfalte *f*.
an·al·ge·sia [ˌænl'dʒiːzɪə] *n* Aufhebung *f* der Schmerzempfindlichkeit, Schmerzunempfindlichkeit *f*, -losigkeit *f*, Analgesie *f*.
an·al·ge·sic [ˌænl'dʒiːzɪk] I *n* schmerzstillendes Medikament *nt*, Schmerzmittel *nt*, Analgetikum *nt*. II *adj* **1.** schmerzstillend, analgetisch. **2.** schmerzunempfindlich.
analgesic cuirasse Hitzig-Zone *f*.
analgesic nephritis → analgesic nephropathy
analgesic nephritis/nephropathy Analgetika-, Phenacetinnephropathie *f*.
analgesic panaris Morvan-Syndrom *nt*, Panaritium analgicum.
analgesic kidney Analgetika-, Phenacetinniere *f*.
analgesic state (*Narkose*) Analg(es)iestadium *nt*, analgetisches Stadium *nt*.
an·al·get·ic [ˌænl'dʒetɪk] *n, adj* → analgesic.
an·al·gia [æn'ældʒɪə] *n* Schmerzlosigkeit *f*, Analgie *f*.
an·al·gic [æn'ældʒɪk] *adj* schmerzunempfindlich.
anal glands zirkumanale Drüsen *pl*, Gll. anales/circumanales.
an·al·ler·gic [ænəl'lɑːdʒɪk] *adj* nicht-allergisch; nicht-allergen (wirkend).
anal membrane *embryo.* Analmembran *f*.
anal mucosa Anal-, Afterschleimhaut *f*.
anal nerves, inferior untere Rektal-, Analnerven *pl*, Nn. anales/h(a)emorrhoidales inferiores, Nn. rectales inferiores.
an·a·log ['ænəlɒg] I *n* → analogue. II *adj phys.* analog.
a·nal·o·gous [ə'næləgəs] *adj* entsprechend, ähnlich, analog (*to, with* mit), ähnlich, gleichartig; vergleichbar (*to, with* mit).
an·a·logue ['ænəlɒg] *n* **1.** Entsprechung *f*, analoger *od.* ähnlicher Fall *m*, Analogon *nt*. **2.** analoges Organ *nt*. **3.** *chem.* analoge Substanz *f*, Analog *nt*, Analogon *nt*.
a·nal·o·gy [ə'nælədʒɪ] *n, pl* **-gies** (*a. chem., bio.*) Analogie *f*, Entsprechung *f*, Ähnlichkeit *f*, Übereinstimmung *f*.
anal orifice → anus.
anal pecten Analkamm *m*, Pecten analis.
an·al·pha·lip·o·pro·tein·e·mia [ænͺælfəͺlɪpəͺprəʊtiː'niːmɪə] *n* Tangier-Krankheit *f*, Analphalipoproteinämie *f*, Hypo-Alpha--Lipoproteinämie *f*.
anal phase *psycho.* anale Phase *f*.
anal pit *embryo.* Aftergrube *f*, Proctodaeum *nt*.
anal plate *embryo.* Analplatte *f*.
anal prolaps Analprolaps *m*, Prolapsus ani.
anal pruritus Afterjucken *nt*, Pruritus ani.
anal reflex Analreflex *m*.
anal region *anat.* Analgegend *f*, -region *f*, Regio analis.
anal retractor *chir.* Analretraktor *m*.
anal sinuses Morgagni'-Krypten *pl*, Analkrypten *pl*, Sinus anales.
anal stage *psycho.* anale Phase *f*.
anal triangle → anal region.
anal trichiasis Trichiasis ani.
anal valves Valvulae anales.
anal verge Analring *m*.
a·nal·y·sand [ə'næləsænd] *n psychia.* Analysand *m*.
a·nal·y·sis [ə'næləsɪs] *n, pl* **-ses** [-siːz] **1.** *chem.* Analyse *f*. **2.** *mathe.* Analysis *f*. **3.** Analyse *f*, Zerlegung *f*, Zergliederung *f*, Aufspaltung *f*; Darlegung *f*, Deutung *f*; Untersuchung *f*; Auswertung *f*. **to make an ~** eine Analyse vornehmen, analysieren. **4.** *psycho.* Psychoanalyse *f*.
a. of specimen Probenanalyse *f*.
a. of variance *abbr.* **ANOVA** *stat.* Varianzanalyse.
an·a·lys·or *n* → analyzer.
an·a·lyst ['ænəlɪst] *n* **1.** Analytiker(in *f*) *m*. **2.** Psychoanalytiker(in *f*) *m*. **3.** Statistiker(in *f*) *m*.
an·a·lyte ['ænəlaɪt] *n* analysierte Substanz *f*.
an·a·lyt·ic [ˌænə'lɪtɪk] *adj* Analyse betr., mittels Analyse, analytisch, Analysen-; psychoanalytisch.
an·a·lyt·i·cal [ˌ-lɪtɪkl] *adj* → analytic.
analytical chemistry → analytic chemistry.
analytical psychology → analytic psychology.
analytic chemistry analytische Chemie *f*, *inf.* Analytik *f*.
analytic psychiatry psychoanalytische Psychiatrie *f*.
analytic psychology analytische Psychologie *f*.
an·a·lyze ['ænəlaɪz] *vt* **1.** analysieren, zergliedern, zerlegen, auswerten; *etw.* genau untersuchen. **2.** eine (Psycho-)Analyse durchführen.
an·a·lyz·er ['ænəlaɪzər] *n* **1.** *phys.* Analysator *m*. **2.** *chem.* Analysator *m*, Autoanalyzer *m*. **3.** *physiol.* Analysator *m*. **4.** Psychoanalytiker(in *f*) *m*.
an·am·ne·sis [ˌænəm'niːsɪs] *n* **1.** Wiedererinnerung *f*, Anamnese *f*. **2.** (*Patient*) Vorgeschichte *f*, Krankengeschichte *f*, Anamnese *f*. **3.** *immun.* immunologisches Gedächtnis *nt*.
an·am·nes·tic [ˌ-'nestɪk] *n* Anamnese betr., anamnestisch, anamnestisch, Anamnese(n)-.
anamnestic reaction/response *immun.* anamnestische Reaktion *f*, Anamnesephänomen *nt*.
an·am·ni·ote [æn'æmnɪəʊt] *n bio.* Anamnier *m*, Anamniot *m*.
an·a·mor·pho·sis [ˌænə'mɔːrfəsɪs, -mɔːr'fəʊsɪs] *n bio.* Anamorphose *f*.
an·an·a·phy·lax·is [ænͺænəfɪ'læksɪs] *n* → antianaphylaxis.
an·an·a·sta·sia [æn͵ænə'steɪʒə] *n neuro.* Anastasie *f*.
an·an·casm [ænən'kæsm] *n psychia.* Anankasmus *m*.
an·an·cas·tia [ænən'kæstɪə] *n* → anancasm.
an·an·cas·tic [ˌ-'kæstɪk] *adj psychia.* zwanghaft, obsessiv-kompulsiv, anankastisch.
an·an·dria [æn'ændrɪə] *n* → aphemia.
an·a·pep·sia [ˌænə'pepsɪə, -ʃə] *n* Anapepsie *f*.
an·a·phase ['ænəfeɪz] *n* Anaphase *f*.
an·a·phia [æn'æfɪə] *n neuro.* Anaphie *f*, Anaphia *f*.
an·a·pho·re·sis [ˌænəfəʊ'riːsɪs] *n* Anaphorese *f*.
an·aph·ro·dis·i·ac [ænͺæfrə'dɪzɪæk] I *n* Anaphrodisiakum *f*. II *adj* den Geschlechtstrieb hemmend.
an·a·phy·lac·tic [ˌænəfɪ'læktɪk] *adj* Anaphylaxie betr., anaphylaktisch.
anaphylactic antibody zytophiler Antikörper *m* der IgE-Klasse.
anaphylactic conjunctivitis allergische/atopische Konjunktivitis *f*, Conjunctivitis allergica; Heuschnupfen *m*, -fieber *nt*.
anaphylactic hypersensitivity anaphylaktische Überempfindlichkeit/Allergie *f*, anaphylaktischer Typ *m* der Überemp-

findlichkeitsreaktion, Überempfindlichkeitsreaktion *f* vom Soforttyp, Typ I der Überempfindlichkeitsreaktion.
anaphylactic rhinitis allergische Rhinitis *f*, Rhinopathia vasomotorica allergica.
anaphylactic shock → anaphylaxis 1.
an·a·phy·lac·tin [ˌænəfɪˈlæktɪn] *n old* → immunoglobulin E.
an·a·phy·lac·to·gen [-ˈlæktədʒən] *n* Anaphylaktogen *nt*.
an·a·phy·lac·to·gen·e·sis [ˌ-ˌlæktəˈdʒenəsɪs] *n* Anaphylaktogenese *f*.
an·a·phy·lac·to·gen·ic [-ˌlæktəˈdʒenɪk] *adj* Anaphylaxie herbeiführend, anaphylaktogen.
an·a·phy·lac·toid [ˌ-ˈlæktɔɪd] *adj* anaphylaxie-ähnlich, anaphylaktoid.
anaphylactoid crisis → anaphylactoid reaction.
anaphylactoid purpura 1. allergische Purpura *f*, Purpura allergica. **2.** Schoenlein-Henoch-Syndrom *nt*, (anaphylaktoide) Purpura Schoenlein-Henoch *f*, rheumatoide/athrombopenische Purpura *f*, Immunkomplexpurpura *f*, -vaskulitis *f*, Purpura anaphylactoides (Schoenlein-Henoch), Purpura rheumatica (Schoenlein-Henoch).
anaphylactoid reaction anaphylaktoide Reaktion *f*.
anaphylactoid shock → anaphylactoid reaction.
an·a·phyl·a·tox·in [ˌænəfɪləˈtɑksɪn] *n* Anaphylatoxin *nt*.
anaphylatoxin inactivator *abbr.* AI Anaphylatoxininaktivator *m abbr.* AI.
an·a·phy·lax·in [ˌænəfɪˈlæksɪn] *n* Immunglobulin E *nt abbr.* IgE.
an·a·phy·lax·is [ˌ-ˈlæksɪs] *n* **1.** allergischer/anaphylaktischer Schock *m*, Anaphylaxie *f*. **2.** → anaphylactic hypersensitivity.
an·a·phy·lo·tox·in [ˌænəfɪləˈtɑksɪn] *n* → anaphylatoxin.
an·a·pla·sia [ænəˈpleɪʒ(ɪ)ə, -zɪə] *n patho.* Anaplasie *f*.
an·a·plas·tia [ænəˈplæstɪə] *n* → anaplasia.
an·a·plas·tic [ænəˈplæstɪk] *adj* Anaplasie betr., anaplastisch.
anaplastic astrocytoma buntes Glioblastom *nt*, Glioblastoma multiforme.
anaplastic carcinoma: large-cell a. großzelliges/großzellig-anaplastisches Bronchialkarzinom *nt*, *inf.* Großzeller *m*.
small-cell a. kleinzelliges/kleinzellig-anaplastisches Bronchialkarzinom *nt*, *inf.* Kleinzeller *m*.
anaplastic cell anaplastische Zelle *f*.
anaplastic seminoma anaplastisches Seminom *nt*.
an·a·ple·ro·sis [ˌænəpləˈroʊsɪs] *n* **1.** Auffüllen *nt*, Ergänzen *nt*, Ersetzen *nt*. **2.** → anaplerotic reaction.
an·a·ple·rot·ic [-ˈrɑtɪk] *adj* anaplerotisch.
anaplerotic reaction anaplerotische Reaktion *f*, Auffüllungsreaktion *f*.
an·ap·no·ther·a·py [ˌænæpnoʊˈθerəpɪ] *n* Inhalationstherapie *f*.
an·ap·tic [ænˈæptɪk] *adj neuro.* anaptisch.
an·ar·thria [ænˈɑːrθrɪə] *n neuro.* Anarthrie *f*.
an·a·sar·ca [ænəˈsɑːrkə] *n* Anasarka *f*.
an·a·sar·cous [ænəˈsɑːrkəs] *adj* Anasarka betr.
an·a·spa·di·as [ænəˈspeɪdɪæs] *n urol.* Anaspadie *f*.
an·a·stal·sis [ænəˈstælsɪs] *n* Anastalsis *f*, Anastaltik *f*.
an·a·stal·tic [ænəˈstæltɪk] *adj* Anastalsis betr., anastaltisch.
an·a·stig·mat·ic [ænəstɪgˈmætɪk] *adj ophtal.* nicht-astigmatisch, anastigmatisch.
anastigmatic lens anastigmatisches/stigmatisches Glas *nt*.
a·nas·to·mose [əˈnæstəmoʊz] *vt, vi* eine Anastomose bilden, anastomosieren.
a·nas·to·mo·sis [əˌnæstəˈmoʊsɪs] *n, pl* **-ses** [-siːz] **1.** *anat.* Anastomose *f*, Anastomosis *f*. **2.** *chir.* Anastomose *f*; Shunt *m*; Fistel *f*.
a·nas·to·mot·ic [əˌnæstəˈmɑtɪk] *adj* Anastomose betr., anastomotisch, Anastomosen-.
anastomotic abscess Anastomosenabszeß *m*.
anastomotic atrial artery anastomosierende Vorhofarterie *f*, Ramus atrialis anastomoticus a. coronariae sinistrae.
anastomotic branch: a. of lacrimal artery with medial meningeal artery Ramus anastomoticus a. lacrimalis cum a. meningea media.
a. of medial meningeal artery with lacrimal artery Ramus anastomoticus a. meningeae mediae cum a. lacrimali.
anastomotic breakdown Anastomoseninsuffizienz *f*.
anastomotic leak Anastomoseninsuffizienz *f*, -leck *nt*, -fistel *f*.
anastomotic obstruction Anastomosenobstruktion *f*.
anastomotic stricture Anastomosenstriktur *f*.
anastomotic ulcer Anastomosenulkus *nt*.
anastomotic vein: inferior a. Labbé'-Vene *f*, V. anastomotica inferior.
superior a. Trolard'-Vene *f*, V. anastomotica superior.
anastomotic vessel Vas anastomoticum.
an·a·tom·ic [ˌænəˈtɑmɪk] *adj* → anatomical.
an·a·tom·i·cal [-ˈtɑmɪkl] *adj* Anatomie betr., anatomisch.
anatomical (dental) crown anatomische (Zahn-)Krone *f*, Corona dentis/anatomica.
anatomical pathology pathologische Anatomie *f*.
anatomical position anatomische Stellung/Lage/Position *f*.
anatomical root (of tooth) anatomische (Zahn-)Wurzel *f*, Radix (dentis) anatomica.
anatomical snuff box Tabatière *f*, Fovea radialis.
anatomical tubercle Wilk'-Krankheit *f*, warzige Hauttuberkulose *f* der Haut, Leichentuberkel *m*, Schlachtertuberkulose *f*, Tuberculosis cutis verrucosa, Verruca necrogenica, Tuberculum anatomicum.
anatomical wart → anatomical tubercle.
an·a·tom·i·co·med·i·cal [ænəˌtɑmɪkoʊˈmedɪkl] *adj* medizinisch-anatomisch.
an·a·tom·i·co·path·o·log·i·cal [ˌ-pæθəˈlɑdʒɪkl] *adj* pathologisch-anatomisch.
an·a·tom·i·co·phys·i·o·log·i·cal [ˌ-ˌfɪzɪəˈlɑdʒɪkl] *adj* physiologisch-anatomisch.
an·a·tom·i·co·sur·gi·cal [ˌ-ˈsɜːrdʒɪkl] *adj* chirurgisch-anatomisch.
a·nat·o·mist [əˈnætəmɪst] *n* Anatom *m*.
a·nat·o·mize [əˈnætəmaɪz] *vt* **1.** anatomieren, sezieren, zerlegen. **2.** *fig.* analysieren, zergliedern.
a·nat·o·my [əˈnætəmɪ] *n, pl* **-mies 1.** Anatomie *f*; Körperbau *m*; anatomische Zerlegung *f*. **2.** *fig.* Zergliederung *f*, Aufbau *m*, Analyse *f*.
an·a·tox·in [ænəˈtɑksɪn] *n* Toxoid *nt*, Anatoxin *nt*.
an·a·troph·ic [ænəˈtrɑfɪk, -ˈtroʊf-] **I** *adj* anatrophische Substanz *f*. **II** *adj* Atrophie verhindernd, anatrophisch.

AnCC *abbr.* → anodal closure contraction.
an·chor [ˈæŋkər] *vt chir., dent., fig.* verankern, befestigen.
an·chor·age [ˈæŋkərɪdʒ] *n chir., dent.* Befestigung *f*, Verankerung *f*, Fixierung *f*.
an·chor·ing villi [ˈæŋkərɪŋ] *histol.* Haftzotten *pl*.
an·cil·lar·y [ˈænsəlerɪː; *Brit.* ænˈsɪlərɪ] *adj* ergänzend, helfend, zusätzlich (*to*), Hilfs-, Zusatz-.
an·cis·troid [ænˈsɪstrɔɪd] *adj* hakenförmig.
an·co·nal [æŋˈkəʊnl] *adj* → anconeal.
an·co·ne·al [æŋˈkəʊnɪəl] *adj* Ell(en)bogen betr., zum Ell(en)bogen gehörend, Ell(en)bogen-.
anconeal bursa Bursa subcutanea olecrani.
a. of triceps muscle Bursa subtendinea m. tricipitis brachii.
anconeal fossa Fossa olecrani.
anconeal process of ulna Ell(en)bogenfortsatz *m*, -höcker *m*, Olekranon *nt*, Olecranon *nt*.
an·co·ne·us (muscle) [æŋˈkəʊnɪəs] Ankoneus *m*, M. anconeus.
lateral a. Caput laterale m. tricipitis brachii.
medial a. Caput mediale m. tricipitis brachii.
an·co·ni·tis [æŋkəˈnaɪtɪs] *n* Entzündung *f* des Ell(en)bogengelenks, Anconitis *f*.
an·crod [ˈæŋkrɑd] *n pharm.* Ancrod *nt*.
ancyl(o)- *pref.* Ankyl(o)-, Ancyl(o)-.
An·cy·los·to·ma [æŋkɪˈlɑstəmə] *n micro.* Ankylostoma *nt*, Ancylostoma *nt*.
A. americanum Todeswurm *m*, Necator americanus.
A. duodenale (europäischer) Hakenwurm *m*, Grubenwurm *m*, Ancylostoma duodenale.
an·cy·lo·sto·mat·ic [ˌæŋkɪləʊstəˈmætɪk] *adj* durch Ancylostoma verursacht.
an·cy·lo·stome [æŋˈkɪləstəʊm] *n* **1.** Ankylostoma *nt*, Ancylostoma *nt*. **2.** Hakenwurm *m*.
an·cy·lo·sto·mi·a·sis [ˌæŋkɪləʊstəʊˈmaɪəsɪs] *n* Hakenwurmbefall *m*, -infektion *f*, Ankylostomiaisis *f*, Ankylostomatosis *f*, Ankylostomatidose *f*.
An·cy·lo·stom·i·dae [ˌ-ˈstɑmədiː] *pl* Hakenwürmer *pl*, Ancylostomidae *pl*.
An·cy·lo·sto·mum [æŋkɪˈlɑstəməm] *n* → Ancylostoma.
an·cy·roid [æŋˈkaɪrɔɪd, ˈæŋkə-] *adj* haken-, ankerförmig.
Anders [ˈændərs]: **A.' disease** Anders'-Krankheit *f*, Adipositas tuberosa simplex.
Andersch [ˈændərʃ]: **A.'s ganglion** unteres Glossopharyngeusganglion *nt*, Ggl. caudalis/inferius n. glossopharyngei.
A.'s nerve N. tympanicus.
Andersen [ˈændərsn]: **A.'s disease** Andersen-Krankheit *f*, Amylopektinose *f*, leberzirrhotische retikuloendotheliale Glykogenose *f*, Glykogenose Typ IV *f*.
A.'s syndrome Andersen-Syndrom *nt*.
A.'s triad → A.'s syndrome.
An·des disease [ˈændɪz] Monge'-Krankheit *f*, chronische Höhenkrankheit *f*.
andr- *pref.* → andro-.
Andral [anˈdral]: **A.'s decubitus** → A.'s sign.
A.'s sign Andral'-Zeichen *nt*.
an·drei·o·ma [ˌændrɪˈəʊmə] *n* → androblastoma 2.
an·dre·o·blas·to·ma [ˌændrɪəʊblæsˈtəʊmə] *n* → androblastoma 2.
andro- *pref.* Mann-, Männer-, Andr(o)-.
an·dro·blas·to·ma [ˌændrəʊblæsˈtəʊmə] *n* **1.** Androblastom *nt*. **2.** Arrhenoblastom *nt*. **3.** Sertoli-Leidig-Zelltumor *m*.

androcyte

an·dro·cyte ['-saɪt] *n* männliche Geschlechts-, Keimzelle *f*, Androzyt *m*.
an·dro·gam·one [ˌ-'gæməʊn] *n* Androgamon *nt*.
an·dro·gen ['-dʒən] *n* männliches Geschlechts-, Keimdrüsenhormon *nt*, Androgen *nt*; androgene Substanz *f*.
androgen binding protein *abbr.* **ABP** androgenbindendes Protein *nt abbr.* ABP.
an·dro·gen·e·sis [ˌ-'dʒenəsɪs] *n* Androgenese *f*.
an·dro·ge·net·ic alopecia in women [ˌ-dʒəˈnetɪk] → androgenetic female alopecia.
androgenetic effluvium androgenetische Alopezie *f*, Haarausfall *m* vom männlichen Typ, männliche Glatzenbildung *f*, androgenetisches Effluvium *nt*, Alopecia androgenetica, Calvities hippocratica.
androgenetic female alopecia weiblicher Typ *m* der Alopecia androgenetica.
androgenetic male alopecia → androgenetic effluvium.
an·dro·gen·ic [ˌ-'dʒenɪk] *adj* androgen.
androgenic hormone → androgen.
an·dro·ge·nic·i·ty [ˌ-dʒəˈnɪsətɪ] *n* Androgenizität *f*.
an·dro·gen·i·za·tion [ˌ-dʒenɪˈzeɪʃn] *n* Vermännlichung *f*, Androgenisation *f*.
an·drog·e·nous [ænˈdrɒdʒənəs] *adj* männliche Nachkommen betr. *od.* erzeugend.
androgen unit Androgeneinheit *f*.
an·dro·gyne ['ændrədʒaɪn, -dʒɪn] *n* weibliche Pseudohermaphrodit *m*.
an·drog·y·nism [ænˈdrɒdʒɪnɪzəm] *n* Androgynie *f*, Pseudohermaphroditismus masculinus.
an·drog·y·noid [ænˈdrɒdʒɪnɔɪd] **I** *n* Pseudohermaphrodit *m*. **II** *adj* Pseudohermaphroditismus masculinus betr.
an·drog·y·nous [ænˈdrɒdʒɪnəs] *adj* androgyn.
an·drog·y·ny [ænˈdrɒdʒɪnɪ] *n* **1.** → androgynism. **2.** Zweigeschlechtlichkeit *f*.
an·droid [ˈændrɔɪd] **I** *n* Android(e) *m*. **II** *adj* einem Mann ähnlich, vermännlicht, android.
an·droi·dal [ænˈdrɔɪdl] *adj* → android II.
android pelvis androides Becken *nt*.
an·drol·o·gy [ænˈdrɒlədʒɪ] *n* Männerheilkunde *f*, Andrologie *f*.
an·dro·ma [ænˈdrəʊmə] *n* → arrhenoblastoma.
an·dro·mer·o·gon [ˌændrəʊˈmerəgɒn] *n* Andromerogon *m*.
an·dro·mer·o·gone [ˌ-ˈmerəgəʊn] *n* → andromerogon.
an·dro·me·rog·o·ny [ˌ-məˈrɒgənɪ] *n* Andromerogonie *f*.
an·dro·mi·met·ic [ˌ-mɪˈmetɪk] *adj* andromimetisch.
an·dro·phile ['-faɪl] *adj* → anthropophilic.
an·droph·i·lous [ænˈdrɒfɪləs] *adj* → anthropophilic.
an·dro·some ['-səʊm] *n* Androsom *nt*.
an·dro·spo·ran·gi·um [ˌ-spəˈrændʒɪəm] *n micro.* Mikrosporangium *nt*.
an·dro·spore ['-spɔʊə, -spɔːr] *n micro.* Mikrospore *f*, Androspore *f*.
an·dro·stane ['-steɪn] *n* Androstan *nt*.
an·dro·stane·di·ol [ˌ-ˈsteɪndɪɒl, -daɪ-] *n* Androstandiol *nt*.
an·dro·stan·o·lone [ˌ-ˈstænəlɒn] *n* Androstanolon *nt*.
an·dro·stene ['-stiːn] *n* Androsten *nt*.
an·dro·stene·di·ol [ˌ-ˈstiːndɪɒl, -daɪ-] *n* Androstendiol *nt*.
an·dro·stene·di·one [ˌ-ˈstiːndɪəʊn, -daɪ-] *n* Androstendion *nt*.
an·dros·ter·one [ænˈdrɒstərəʊn] *n* Androsteron *nt*.
an·ec·dot·al [ænɪkˈdəʊtl] *adj* anekdoten-

haft, anekdotisch, Anekdoten-.
an·e·cho·ic [æneˈkəʊɪk] *adj* echofrei, schalltot.
anechoic chamber schalltoter Raum *m*.
an·ec·ta·sis [ænˈektəsɪs] *n* primäre/kongenitale Atelektase *f*.
Anel ['ænl; aˈnel]: **A.'s lacrimal dilatation** → A.'s operation.
A.'s lacrimal probe *pharm.* Anel-Sonde *f*.
A.'s lacrimal syringe *ophthal.* Anel-Spritze *f*.
A.'s method → A.'s operation.
A.'s operation *ophthal.* Anel-Operation *f*.
A.'s probe → A.'s lacrimal probe.
A.'s syringe → A.'s lacrimal syringe.
an·e·lec·tro·ton·ic zone [ænɪˌlektrəˈtɒnɪk] Polarzone *f*.
an·e·lec·trot·o·nus [ˌænɪlekˈtrɒtənəs] *n physiol.* Anelektrotonus *m*.
a·ne·mia [əˈniːmɪə] *n* Blutarmut *f*, Anämie *f*, Anaemia *f*.
anemia pseudoleukemica infantum von Jaksch-Hayem-Anämie *f*, -Syndrom *nt*, Anaemia pseudoleukaemica infantum *f*.
a·ne·mic [əˈniːmɪk] *adj* Anämie betr., blutarm, anämisch.
anemic anoxia anämische Anoxie *f*.
anemic hypoxia anämische Hypoxie *f*.
anemic infarct ischämischer/anämischer/weißer/blasser Infarkt *m*.
anemic murmur Herzgeräusch *nt* bei Anämie.
anemic pulmonary infarction anämischer Lungeninfarkt *m*.
an·e·mom·e·ter [ænəˈmɒmɪtər] *n* Anemometer *nt*.
a·nem·o·nism [əˈniːmənɪzəm] *n* Anemonismus *m*.
an·e·mo·pho·bia [ˌænɪməʊˈfəʊbɪə] *n* Anemophobie *f*.
an·en·ce·pha·lia [əˌnensɪˈfeɪlɪə] *n* → anencephaly.
an·en·ce·phal·ic [əˌnensɪˈfælɪk] *adj* Anenzephalie betr., hirnlos, anenzephal.
an·en·ceph·a·lous [ˌænənˈsefələs] *adj* hirnlos, anenzephal.
an·en·ceph·a·lus [ˌ-ˈsefələs] *n* Anenzephalus *m*.
an·en·ceph·a·ly [ˌ-ˈsefəlɪ] *n* Hirnlosigkeit *f*, Anenzephalie *f*.
an·en·ter·ous [ænˈentərəs] *adj* darmlos.
an·en·zy·mia [ˌænənˈzɪmɪə, -zaɪ-] *n* Anenzymie *f*.
a·neph·ric [əˈnefrɪk] *adj* ohne Nieren, anephrisch.
an·er·gia [əˈnɜrdʒɪə] *n* → anergy.
an·er·gic [əˈnɜrdʒɪk] *adj* **1.** inaktiv, anerg(isch). **2.** energielos, -arm, anerg(isch) (*to*).
anergic cutaneous leishmaniasis leproide Leishmaniasis *f*, Leishmaniasis cutis/tegumentaria diffusa.
anergic leishmaniasis → anergic cutaneous leishmaniasis.
anergic stupor anergischer Stupor *m*.
an·er·gy [ˈænɜrdʒɪ] *n* **1.** Energielosigkeit *f*, -mangel *m*, Lethargie *f*. **2.** Unempfindlichkeit *f*, Reizlosigkeit *f*, Anergie *f* (*to*).
an·er·oid [ˈænərɔɪd] *adj* keine Flüssigkeit enthaltend, aneroid, Aneroid-.
an·e·ryth·ro·pla·sia [ænɪˌrɪθrəʊˈpleɪʒ(ɪ)ə] *n* Anerythroplasie *f*.
an·e·ryth·ro·plas·tic [ˌ-ˈplæstɪk] *adj* anerythroplastisch.
an·e·ryth·ro·poi·e·sis [ˌ-pɔɪˈiːsɪs] *n* Anerythropo(i)ese *f*.
an·e·ryth·ro·re·gen·er·a·tive [ˌ-rɪˈdʒenəreɪtɪv] *adj hema.* aregenerativ.
an·es·the·ci·ne·sia [əˌnesθəsɪˈniːʒ(ɪ)ə] *n* Anästhekinäsie *f*.
an·es·the·ki·ne·sia [ˌ-kɪˈniːʒ(ɪ)ə] *n* → anesthecinesia.

36

an·es·the·sia [ˌænəsˈθiːʒə] *n* **1.** (Schmerz-, Temperatur-, Berührungs-)Unempfindlichkeit *f*, Anästhesie *f*. **2.** Narkose *f*, Betäubung *f*, Anästhesie *f*.
anesthesia-induced hepatitis anästhetika-induzierte/narkose-induzierte Hepatitis *f*.
anesthesia paralysis postanästhetische Paralyse *f*.
anesthesia-related mortality *stat.* Mortalität *f* unter der Narkose.
anesthesia state Voll-, Allgemeinnarkose *f*, -anästhesie *f*, *inf.* Vollnarkose *f*.
an·es·the·si·ol·o·gist [ˌænəsˌθiːzɪˈɒlədʒɪst] *n* Narkosearzt *m*, -ärztin *f*, Anästhesist(in *f*) *m*.
an·es·the·si·ol·o·gy [ˌ-ˈɒlədʒɪ] *n* Anästhesiologie *f*.
an·es·thet·ic [ˌænəsˈθetɪk] **I** *n* Betäubungs-, Narkosemittel *nt*, Narkotikum *nt*, Anästhetikum *nt*. **to give an ∼**. **II** *adj* Anästhesie betr. *od.* auslösend, anästhetisch, narkotisch, betäubend, Anästhesie-, Narkose-.
anesthetic agent Narkosemittel *nt*, Anästhetikum *nt*.
anesthetic gas Narkosegas *nt*.
anesthetic procedure Anästhesie-, Narkoseverfahren *nt*.
anesthetic-related mortality *stat.* Mortalität *f* unter der Narkose.
an·es·the·tist [əˈnesθɪtɪst; *Brit.* -ˈniːs-] *n* **1.** in Narkoseverfahren ausgebildete Kraft. **2.** *Brit.* → anesthesiologist.
an·es·the·ti·za·tion [əˌnesθɪtaɪˈzeɪʃn] *n* Betäubung *f*, Anästhesierung *f*.
an·es·the·tize [əˈnesθɪtaɪz; *Brit.* -ˈniːs-] *vt* betäuben, narkotisieren, anästhesieren.
an·e·thole [ˈænəθəʊl] *n* Anethol *nt*, p-Propenylanisol *nt*.
a·net·ic [əˈnetɪk] *adj* mildernd, entspannend.
an·eu·ga·my [ænˈjuːgəmɪ] *n* Aneugamie *f*.
an·eu·ploid [ænˈjuːplɔɪd, ˈænjə-] **I** *n* aneuploide Zelle *f*, aneuploides Individuum *m*. **II** *adj* aneuploid.
an·eu·ploi·dy [ˈænjuːplɔɪdɪ, ˈænjə-] *n* Aneuploidie *f*.
an·eu·rin [ˈænjʊrɪn] *n* Thiamin *nt*, Vitamin B₁ *nt*.
an·eu·rine [ˈænjʊriːn] *n* → aneurine.
a·neu·ro·gen·ic [eɪˌnʊərəˈdʒenɪk] *adj* aneurogen.
an·eu·rysm [ˈænjərɪzəm] *n* Aneurysma *nt*.
a. of abdominal aorta Aneurysma der Bauchschlagader, Aneurysma der Aorta abdominalis.
a. of Charcot (and Bouchard) Charcot-Aneurysma.
an·eu·rys·mal [ˌænjəˈrɪzml] *adj* Aneurysma betr., aneurysmatisch, Aneurysma-.
aneurysmal bruit auskultatorisches Geräusch *nt* über einem Aneurysma.
aneurysmal cough Husten *m* bei Aortenaneurysma.
aneurysmal hematoma falsches Aneurysma *nt*, Aneurysma spurium.
aneurysmal murmur Gefäßgeräusch *nt* über einem Aneurysma.
aneurysmal sac Aneurysmasack *m*.
aneurysmal thrill *card.* Aneurysmaschwirren *nt*.
aneurysmal varix Aneurysmaknoten *m*.
an·eu·rys·mat·ic [ˌænjərɪzˈmætɪk] *adj* → aneurysmal.
an·eu·rys·mec·to·my [ˌ-ˈmektəmɪ] *n chir.* Aneurysmaexstirpation *f*, -resektion *f*, Aneurysm(a)ektomie *f*.
an·eu·rys·moid varix [ˈænjərɪzmɔɪd] Aneurysmaknoten *m*.
an·eu·rys·mo·plas·ty [ænjəˈrɪzməplæstɪ] *n chir.* Aneurysmaplastik *f*.

an·eu·rys·mor·rha·phy [ænjərɪz'mɔrəfɪ] *n chir.* Aneurysmorrhaphie *f.*
an·eu·rys·mot·o·my [ænjərɪz'mɑtəmɪ] *n* Aneurysmotomie *f.*
aneurysm rupture Aneurysmaruptur *f.*
ANF *abbr.* 1. → antinuclear factor. 2. → atrial natriuretic factor.
Angelucci [ændʒɪ'luːtʃɪ]: **A.'s syndrome** *ophthal.* Angelucci-Syndrom *nt.*
angi- *pref.* → angio-.
an·gi·al·gia [ændʒɪ'ældʒ(ɪ)ə] *n* Angialgie *f,* Angiodynie *f.*
an·gi·as·the·nia [ˌæs'θiːnɪə] *n* Angiasthenie *f.*
an·gi·ec·ta·sis [ˌ-'ektəsɪs] *n* (Blut-)Gefäßerweiterung *f,* Angiektasie *f,* Angiectasia *f.*
an·gi·ec·tat·ic [ˌ-ek'tætɪk] *adj* Angiektasie betr., angiektatisch.
an·gi·ec·to·my [ˌ-'ektəmɪ] *n chir.* Gefäßentfernung *f,* Angiektomie *f.*
an·gi·ec·to·pia [ˌ-ek'təʊpɪə] *n* Angiektopie *f.*
an·gi·i·tis [ˌ-'aɪtɪs] *n* Gefäßentzündung *f,* Angiitis *f,* Vaskulitis *f,* Vasculitis *f.*
an·gi·na [æn'dʒaɪnə, 'ændʒənə] *n* 1. Halsentzündung *f,* Angina *f.* 2. → angina pectoris.
angina cruris intermittierendes Hinken *nt,* Charcot-Syndrom *nt,* Claudicatio intermittens, Angina cruris, Dysbasia intermittens/angiospastica.
an·gi·nal [æn'dʒaɪnl, 'ændʒənl] *adj* Angina betr., Angina-.
angina pectoris Herzbräune *f,* Stenokardie *f,* Angina pectoris. **variant a.** Prinzmetal-Angina.
angina trachealis Croup *m,* Krupp *m.*
an·gin·i·form [æn'dʒɪnɪfɔːrm] *adj* anginaähnlich, -artig.
an·gi·noid ['ændʒɪnɔɪd] *adj* → anginiform.
an·gin·o·pho·bia [ˌændʒɪnəʊ'fəʊbɪə] *n* Anginophobie *f.*
an·gi·nose ['ændʒɪnəʊs] *adj* Angina pectoris betr., anginös.
anginose scarlatina Scarlatina anginosa.
an·gi·nous ['ændʒɪnəs] *adj* → anginose.
angio- *pref.* (Blut-)Gefäß-, Angio-.
an·gi·o·ar·chi·tec·ton·ics [ˌændʒɪəʊˌɑːrkɪtek'tɑnɪks] *pl* Angioarchitektonik *f.*
an·gi·o·as·the·nia [ˌ-æs'θiːnɪə] *n* → angiasthenia.
an·gi·o·a·tax·ia [ˌ-ə'tæksɪə] *n* Angioataxie *f.*
an·gi·o·blast ['-blæst] *n* 1. Angioblast *m.* 2. *embryo.* Angioblast *nt.*
an·gi·o·blas·tic [ˌ-'blæstɪk] *adj* Angioblast betr., angioblastisch, Angioblasten-.
angioblastic cells *embryo.* angioblastische Zellen *pl.*
angioblastic cyst angioblastische Zyste *f.*
angioblastic meningioma → angioblastoma.
an·gi·o·blas·to·ma [ˌ-blæs'təʊmə] *n* Lindau-Tumor *m,* Angioblastom *nt,* Hämangioblastom *nt.*
an·gi·o·car·di·o·gram [ˌ-'kɑːrdɪəʊgræm] *n* Angiokardiogramm *nt.*
an·gi·o·car·di·o·graph·ic [ˌ-ˌkɑːrdɪəʊ'græfɪk] *adj* angiokardiographisch.
an·gi·o·car·di·og·ra·phy [ˌ-ˌkɑːrdɪ'ɑgrəfɪ] *n* Angiokardiographie *f.*
an·gi·o·car·di·op·a·thy [ˌ-ˌkɑːrdɪ'ɑpəθɪ] *n* Angiokardiopathie *f.*
an·gi·o·car·di·tis [ˌ-kɑːr'daɪtɪs] *n* Angiokarditis *f.*
an·gi·o·cav·ern·ous [ˌ-'kævərnəs] *adj* angiokavernös.
an·gi·o·chon·dro·ma [ˌ-kɑn'drəʊmə] *n* Angiochondrom *nt.*
an·gi·o·cyst ['-sɪst] *n* angioblastische Zyste *f,* Angiozyste *f.*

an·gi·o·derm ['-dɜrm] *n embryo.* Angioblast *nt.*
an·gi·o·di·as·co·py [ˌ-daɪ'æskəpɪ] *n* Angiodiaskopie *f.*
an·gi·o·dyn·ia [ˌ-'diːnɪə] *n* Gefäßschmerzen *pl,* Angialgie *f,* Angiodynie *f.*
an·gi·o·dys·pla·sia [ˌ-dɪs'pleɪʒ(ɪ)ə, -zɪə] *n* Gefäß-, Angiodysplasie *f.*
an·gi·o·dys·tro·phia [ˌ-dɪs'trəʊfɪə] *n* Angiodystrophie *f.*
an·gi·o·dys·tro·phy [ˌ-'dɪstrəfɪ] *n* → angiodystrophia.
an·gi·o·ec·tat·ic [ˌ-ek'tætɪk] *adj* → angiectatic.
an·gi·o·e·de·ma [ˌ-ɪ'diːmə] *n* angioneurotisches Ödem *nt,* Quincke-Ödem *nt.*
an·gi·o·e·dem·a·tous [ˌ-ɪ'demətəs, -'diːm-] *adj* angioödematös.
an·gi·o·el·e·phan·ti·a·sis [ˌ-ˌeləfən'taɪəsɪs] *n* Angioelephantiasis *f.*
an·gi·o·en·do·the·li·o·ma [ˌændʒɪəʊˌendəˌθiːlɪ'əʊmə] *n* Hämangioendotheliom *nt.*
an·gi·o·fi·bro·ma [ˌ-faɪ'brəʊmə] *n* Angiofibrom *nt.*
an·gi·o·fol·lic·u·lar [ˌ-fə'lɪkjələr] *adj* angiofollikular, -follikulär.
angiofollicular mediastinal lymph node hyperplasia benigne Hyperplasie *f* der Mediastinallymphknoten.
an·gi·o·gen·e·sis [ˌ-'dʒenəsɪs] *n* Blutgefäßbildung *f,* Angiogenese *f.*
an·gi·o·gen·ic [ˌ-'dʒenɪk] *adj* Blut *od.* Blutgefäße bildend, angiogenetisch.
angiogenic material *embryo.* angiogenetisches Material *nt.*
an·gi·o·gli·o·ma [ˌ-glaɪ'əʊmə] *n* Angiogliom *nt.*
an·gi·o·gli·o·ma·to·sis [ˌ-ˌglaɪəʊmə'təʊsɪs] *n* Angiogliomatose *f.*
an·gi·o·gram ['-græm] *n* Angiogramm *nt.*
an·gi·o·gran·u·lo·ma [ˌ-ˌgrænjə'ləʊmə] *n* (Häm-)Angiogranulom *nt.*
an·gi·o·graph ['-græf] *n* → angiogram.
an·gi·o·graph·ic [ˌ-'græfɪk] *adj* Angiographie betr., mittels Angiographie, angiographisch, Angiographie-.
angiographic catheter Angiographiekatheter *m.*
an·gi·og·ra·phy [ˌændʒɪ'ɑgrəfɪ] *n radiol.* Gefäßdarstellung *f,* Angiographie *f.*
an·gi·o·he·mo·phil·ia [ˌændʒɪəʊˌhiːmə'fɪlɪə] *n* Angiohämophilie *f,* von Willebrand-Jürgens-Syndrom *nt,* konstitutionelle Thrombopathie *f,* hereditäre/vaskuläre Pseudohämophilie *f.*
an·gi·o·hy·a·li·no·sis [ˌ-ˌhaɪələ'nəʊsɪs] *n* Gefäß, Angiohyalinose *f.*
an·gi·oid ['ændʒɔɪd] *adj* (blut-)gefäßähnlich.
an·gi·o·im·mu·no·blas·tic lymphadenopathy with dysproteinemia [ˌændʒɪəʊˌɪmjʊnə'blæstɪk] *abbr.* **AILD** angio(im)munoblastische Lymphadenopathie *f,* Lymphogranulomatosis X *f.*
an·gi·o·in·va·sive [ˌ-ɪn'veɪsɪv] *adj* gefäß-, angioinvasiv.
an·gi·o·ker·a·to·ma [ˌ-ˌkerə'təʊmə] *n* Blutwarze *f,* Angiokeratom(a) *nt.*
a. of Fordyce Fordyce-Krankheit *f,* Angiokeratoma scroti Fordyce.
a. of scrotum → a. of Fordyce.
an·gi·o·ker·a·to·sis [ˌ-ˌkerə'təʊsɪs] *n* → angiokeratoma.
an·gi·o·ki·ne·sis [ˌ-kɪ'niːsɪs, -kaɪ-] *n* Vasomotorik *f.*
an·gi·o·ki·net·ic [ˌ-kɪ'netɪk, -kaɪ-] *adj* vasomotorisch.
an·gi·o·lei·o·my·o·li·po·ma [ˌ-ˌlaɪəʊˌmaɪəʊlɪ'pəʊmə] *n* Angioleiomyolipom(a) *nt.*
an·gi·o·lei·o·my·o·ma [ˌ-ˌlaɪəʊmaɪ'əʊmə] *n* Angiomyom(a) *nt.*
an·gi·o·leu·ci·tis [ˌ-luː'saɪtɪs] *n* Lymphge-

fäßentzündung *f,* Lymphangitis *f,* Lymphangiitis *f.*
an·gi·o·leu·ki·tis [ˌ-luː'kaɪtɪs] *n* → angioleucitis.
an·gi·o·li·po·lei·o·my·o·ma [ˌ-ˌlaɪpəˌlaɪəʊmaɪ'əʊmə] *n* Angiomyolipom(a) *nt.*
an·gi·o·li·po·ma [ˌ-laɪ'pəʊmə] *n* Angiolipom(a) *nt.*
an·gi·o·lith ['-lɪθ] *n* Gefäßstein *m,* Vaso-, Angiolith *m.*
an·gi·o·lo·gia [ˌ-'lɑdʒɪə] *n* → angiology.
an·gi·ol·o·gy [ˌændʒɪ'ɑlədʒɪ] *n* Gefäßlehre *f,* Angiologie *f.*
an·gi·o·lu·poid [ˌændʒɪəʊ'luːpɔɪd] *n* Angiolupoid *nt,* Brocq-Pautrier-Syndrom *nt.*
an·gi·o·lym·phan·gi·o·ma [ˌ-lɪmˌfændʒɪ'əʊmə] *n* Angiolymphangiom(a) *nt.*
an·gi·o·lym·phi·tis [ˌ-lɪm'faɪtɪs] *n* Lymphgefäßentzündung *f,* Lymphangitis *f,* Lymphangiitis *f.*
an·gi·o·lym·phoid hyperplasia (with eosinophilia) [ˌ-'lɪmfɔɪd] Kimura-Krankheit *f,* -Syndrom *nt,* Morbus Kimura, papulöse Angioplasie *f,* angiolymphoide Hyperplasie *f* mit Eosinophilie (Kimura).
an·gi·o·ma [ændʒɪ'əʊmə] *n, pl* **-ma·ta** [-mətə], **-mas** Gefäßtumor *m,* Angiom(a) *nt.*
an·gi·o·ma·toid tumor [ændʒɪ'əmətɔɪd] → adenomatoid tumor.
an·gi·o·ma·to·sis [ˌændʒɪˌəʊmə'təʊsɪs] *n* Angiomatose *f,* -matosis *f.*
an·gi·om·a·tous [ændʒɪ'ɑmətəs] *adj* angiomatös.
an·gi·o·meg·a·ly [ˌændʒɪəʊ'megəlɪ] *n* Gefäßvergrößerung *f,* -erweiterung *f,* Angiomegalie *f.*
an·gi·o·my·o·li·po·ma [ˌ-ˌmaɪəʊlaɪ'pəʊmə] *n* Angiomyolipom(a) *nt.*
an·gi·o·my·o·ma [ˌ-maɪ'əʊmə] *n* Angiomyom(a) *nt.*
an·gi·o·my·o·neu·ro·ma [ˌ-ˌmaɪənjʊə'rəʊmə, -nɔ-] *n* Angiomyoneurom *nt.*
an·gi·o·my·op·a·thy [ˌ-maɪ'ɑpəθɪ] *n* Angiomyopathie *f.*
an·gi·o·my·o·sar·co·ma [ˌ-ˌmaɪəsɑːr'kəʊmə] *n* Angiomyosarkom(a) *nt.*
an·gi·o·ne·cro·sis [ˌ-nɪ'krəʊsɪs, -ne-] *n* Gefäß(wand)nekrose *f,* Angionekrose *f.*
an·gi·o·ne·o·plasm [ˌ-'niːəplæzəm] *n* (Blut-)Gefäßneubildung *f,* -tumor *m.*
an·gi·o·neu·ral·gia [ˌ-njʊə'rældʒə, -nɔ-] *n* Angioneuralgie *f.*
an·gi·o·neu·rec·to·my [ˌ-njʊə'rektəmɪ, -nɔ-] *n chir.* Gefäß- u. Nervenexzision *f,* Angioneurektomie *f.*
an·gi·o·neu·ro·path·ic [ˌ-ˌnjʊərə'pæθɪk, -ˌnɔ-] *adj* angioneuropathisch.
an·gi·o·neu·rop·a·thy [ˌ-njʊə'rɑpəθɪ, -nɔ-] *n* Angioneuropathie *f.*
an·gi·o·neu·ro·sis [ˌ-njʊə'rəʊsɪs, -nɔ-] *n* Gefäß-, Angio-, Vasoneurose *f.*
an·gi·o·neu·rot·ic [ˌ-njʊə'rɑtɪk, -nɔ-] *adj* angioneurotisch.
angioneurotic anuria angioneurotische Anurie *f.*
angioneurotic edema → angioedema.
angioneurotic hematuria renale Hämaturie *f.*
an·gi·o·neu·rot·o·my [ˌ-njʊə'rɑtəmɪ, -nɔ-] *n chir.* Angioneurotomie *f.*
angio-osteohypertrophy syndrome Klippel-Trénaunay-Syndrom *nt,* Klippel-Trénaunay-Weber-Syndrom *nt,* Osteoangiohypertrophie-Syndrom *nt,* angio-osteo-hypertrophisches Syndrom *nt,* Haemangiectasia hypertrophicans.
an·gi·o·pan·cre·a·ti·tis [ˌ-ˌpæŋkrɪə'taɪtɪs] *n* Entzündung *f* der Pankreasgefäße.
an·gi·o·pa·ral·y·sis [ˌ-pə'ræləsɪs] *n* vaso-

angioparesis

motorische Lähmung f, Angioparalyse f, Angioparese f.
an·gi·o·pa·re·sis [ˌ-pəˈriːsɪs, -ˈpærə-] n → angioparalysis.
an·gi·o·path·ic vertigo [ˌ-ˈpæθɪk] → angiosclerotic vertigo.
an·gi·o·pa·thol·o·gy [ˌ-pəˈθɑlədʒɪ] n Gefäß-, Angiopathologie f.
an·gi·op·a·thy [ændʒɪˈapəθɪ] n Gefäßerkrankung f, Angiopathie f.
an·gi·o·phak·o·ma·to·sis [ˌændʒɪəʊˌfækəməˈtəʊsɪs] n Angiophakomatose f.
an·gi·o·plas·ty [ˈ-plæstɪ] n 1. Angioplastie f. 2. Gefäßplastik f, Angioplastik f.
an·gi·o·poi·e·sis [ˌ-pɔɪˈiːsɪs] n Gefäßbildung f, Angiopo(i)ese f.
an·gi·o·poi·et·ic [ˌ-pɔɪˈetɪk] adj Gefäßbildung betr. od. auslösend, angiopoetisch.
an·gi·o·re·tic·u·lo·en·do·the·li·o·ma [ˌ-rɪˌtɪkjələʊˌendəʊˌθiːlɪˈəʊmə] n Kaposi-Sarkom nt, Morbus Kaposi m, Retikuloangiomatose f, Angioretikulomatose f, idiopathisches multiples Pigmentsarkom Kaposi nt, Sarcoma idiopathicum multiplex haemorrhagicum.
an·gi·or·rha·phy [ændʒɪˈarəfɪ] n Gefäßnaht f, Angiorrhaphie f.
an·gi·o·sar·co·ma [ˌ-ˈsɑːrˈkəʊmə] n Angiosarkom nt.
an·gi·o·scle·ro·sis [ˌ-sklɪˈrəʊsɪs] n Gefäß-(wand)sklerose f, Angiosklerose f.
an·gi·o·scle·rot·ic [ˌ-sklɪˈrɑtɪk] adj Angiosklerose betr., angiosklerotisch.
angiosclerotic gangrene arteriosklerotische Gangrän f, Gangraena arteriosclerotica.
arteriosclerotic vertigo arteriosklerotischer Schwindel m.
an·gi·o·scope [ˈ-skəʊp] n Kapillarmikroskop nt, Angioskop nt.
an·gi·o·sco·to·ma [ˌ-skəˈtəʊmə] n ophthal. Angioskotom nt.
an·gi·o·sco·tom·e·try [ˌ-skəˈtɑmətrɪ] n ophthal. Angioskotometrie f.
an·gi·o·spasm [ˈ-spæzəm] n Gefäßkrampf m, Angiospasmus m, Vasospasmus m.
an·gi·o·spas·tic [ˌ-ˈspæstɪk] adj Angiospasmus betr. od. auslösend, angiospastisch, vasospastisch.
angiospastic anesthesia neuro. angiospastische Anästhesie f.
angiospastic retinopathy angiospastische Retinopathie f, Retinopathia angiospastica.
an·gi·o·ste·no·sis [ˌ-stɪˈnəʊsɪs] n Gefäß-, Angiostenose f.
an·gi·os·te·o·sis [ˌ-ɑstɪˈəʊsɪs] n Gefäßverknöcherung f, -kalzifizierung f.
an·gi·os·to·my [ˈændʒɪˈastəmɪ] n chir. 1. Angiostomie f. 2. Angiostoma nt.
an·gi·o·stron·gy·li·a·sis [ˌændʒɪəʊˌstrandʒɪˈlaɪəsɪs] n Angiostrongyliasis f, Angiostrongylose f.
An·gi·o·stron·gy·lus [ˌ-ˈstrandʒələs] n micro. Angiostrongylus m.
A. cantonensis Rattenlungenwurm m, Angiostrongylus cantonensis.
an·gi·o·te·lec·ta·sis [ˌ-tɪˈlektəsɪs] n, pl **-ses** [-siːz] Gefäßdilatation f.
an·gi·o·ten·sin [ˌ-ˈtensɪn] n Angiotensin nt.
an·gi·o·ten·si·nase [ˌ-ˈtensɪneɪz] n Angiotensinase f.
angiotensin converting enzyme abbr. **ACE** (Angiotensin-)Converting-Enzym nt abbr. ACE.
angiotensin converting enzyme inhibitor Angiotensin-Converting-Enzym-Hemmer m, ACE-Hemmer m.
an·gi·o·ten·sin·o·gen [ˌ-tenˈsɪnədʒən] n Angiotensinogen nt.
an·gi·o·tome [ˈændʒɪətəʊm] n embryo. Angiotom nt, Intersegment nt.
an·gi·ot·o·my [ˌændʒɪˈatəmɪ] n chir. Angiotomie f.
an·gi·o·to·nase [ˌændʒɪəʊˈtəʊneɪz] n → angiotensinase.
an·gi·o·to·nia [ˌ-ˈtəʊnɪə] n Gefäßspannung f, -tonus m, Vasotonus m.
an·gi·o·ton·ic [ˌ-ˈtɑnɪk] adj vasotonisch.
an·gi·o·to·nin [ˌ-ˈtəʊnɪn] n → angiotensin.
an·gi·o·tribe [ˈ-traɪb] n chir. Gefäßquetschklemme f, Angiotriptor m.
an·gi·o·trip·sy [ˈ-trɪpsɪ] n Angiotripsie f, -thrypsie f.
an·gi·o·troph·ic [ˌ-ˈtrɑfɪk, -ˈtrəʊ] adj gefäßernährend, angiotrophisch.
an·gi·tis [ænˈdʒaɪtɪs] n → angiitis.
Angle [ˈæŋgl]: **A.'s classification** Angle'-Klassifikation f.
an·gle [ˈæŋgl] n Winkel m. **at an ~** schräg. **at an ~ of ...** in einem Winkel von ... **at an ~ to** schräg od. im Winkel zu. **at right ~s to** im rechten Winkel zu.
a. of aberration phys. Brechungswinkel.
a. of anomaly ophthal. Anomaliewinkel.
a. of anteversion ortho. (Femur) Anteversionswinkel.
a. of aperture Apertur-, Öffnungswinkel; Apertur f.
a. of chamber Iridokorneal-, Kammerwinkel, Angulus iridocornealis.
a. of convergence ophthal. Konvergenzwinkel.
a. of declination → a. of anteversion.
a. of deviation 1. phys. Brechungswinkel. **2.** phys. (Prisma) Haupt-, Brechungswinkel. **3.** ophthal. Anomaliewinkel.
a. of elevation Elevationswinkel.
a. of incidence Inzidenz-, Einfallswinkel.
a. of inclination Neigung f, Neigungswinkel, Inklination f.
a. of intersection Schnittwinkel.
a. of iris Iridokorneal-, Kammerwinkel, Angulus iridocornealis.
a. of jaw Angulus mandibulae.
a. of mandible Unterkieferwinkel, Angulus mandibulae.
a. of mouth Mundwinkel, Angulus oris.
a. of pelvis Beckenneigung, Inclinatio pelvis.
a. of polarization opt. Polarisationswinkel, Brewster'-Winkel.
a. of reflection phys. Reflektions-, Ausfallswinkel.
a. of refraction Brechungs-, Refraktionswinkel.
a. of rib Angulus costae.
a. of strabismus ophthal. Schielwinkel.
a. of torsion Torsions-, Rotationswinkel.
angle-closure glaucoma akutes Winkelblockglaukom/Engwinkelglaukom nt, Glaucoma acutum (congestivum).
chronic a. chronisches Winkelblockglaukom/Engwinkelglaukom, chronisch-kongestives Glaukom, Glaucoma chronicum congestivum.
intermittent a. intermittierendes Winkelblockglaukom.
latent a. latentes Winkelblockglaukom, Glaucoma prodromale.
angled [ˈæŋgld] adj wink(e)lig, Winkel-.
angle-recession glaucoma sekundäres Glaukom nt nach Contusio bulbi.
an·go·phra·sia [æŋgəʊˈfreɪʒ(ɪ)ə, -zɪə] n Angophrasie f.
an·gor [ˈæŋgər] n → angina.
an·gry [ˈæŋgrɪ] adj **1.** zornig, wütend, verärgert, ärgerlich (at, about auf, über); böse (with, at sb. mit jdm). **2.** entzündet. **3.** brennend.
ang·strom [ˈæŋstrəm] n → Ångström unit.
Ång·ström [ˈæŋstrəm] n → Ångström unit.
Ångström: A.'s law Ångström-Regel f, -Gesetz nt.
A. unit abbr. **A, Å, A.U.** Ångström-Einheit f, Ångström nt abbr. A, Å, A.E.
An·guil·lu·la [æŋˈgwɪljələ] n micro. Anguillula f.
A. intestinalis/stercoralis Zwergfadenwurm m, Kötälchen nt, Strongyloides stercoralis, Anguillula stercoralis.
an·guish [ˈæŋgwɪʃ] n Pein f, Qual f, Schmerz m.
an·guished [ˈæŋgwɪʃt] adj gequält, gepeinigt, von Schmerzen/Angst geplagt.
an·gu·lar [ˈæŋgjələr] adj **1.** wink(e)lig, winkelförmig, Winkel-. **2.** knochig. **3.** fig. linkisch, steif, ungelenk.
angular acceleration Winkel-, Dreh-, Radialbeschleunigung f.
angular aperture phys. Apertur-, Öffnungswinkel m; Apertur f.
angular artery Augenwinkelarterie f, Angularis f, A. angularis.
angular blepharitis ophthal. Augenwinkel-, Lidwinkelblepharitis f, Blepharitis angularis.
angular cheilitis → angular stomatitis.
angular cheilosis → angular stomatitis.
angular conjunctivitis ophthal. Diplobazillenkonjunktivitis f, Conjunctivitis/Blepharoconjunctivitis angularis.
angular convolution Gyrus angularis.
angular curvature Pott-Buckel m, Pott-David-Syndrom nt.
angular fissure Fissura sphenopetrosa.
angular gyrus Gyrus angularis.
angular impression for gasserian ganglion Impressio trigeminalis.
an·gu·lar·i·ty [ˌæŋgjəˈlærətɪ] n, pl **-ties 1.** Wink(e)ligkeit f. **2.** fig. Steifheit f, Ungelenkigkeit f.
angular kyphosis ortho. knickförmige Kyphose f.
angular lever phys. Winkelhebel m.
angular malalignment ortho. (Fraktur) Fehlstellung f mit Achsenabknickung.
angular malunion ortho. (Fraktur) Ausheilung f mit Achsenabknickung.
angular notch of stomach Magenknieeinschnitt m, Inc. angularis ventriculi/gastris.
angular point mathe. Scheitelpunkt m.
angular spine Spina ossis sphenoidalis.
angular stomatitis Perlèche f, Faulecken pl, Mundwinkelcheilitis f, -rhagaden pl, Angulus infectiosus oris/candidamycetica, Cheilitis/Stomatitis angularis.
angular sulcus → angular notch of stomach.
angular vein Augenwinkelvene f, V. angularis.
angular velocity Winkelgeschwindigkeit f.
an·gu·late [ˈæŋgjəlɪt, -leɪt] adj → angular 1.
an·gu·lat·ed [ˈ-leɪtɪd] adj → angular 1.
angulated fracture ortho. abgeknickte Fraktur f, winklige Frakturdislokation f, Dislocatio ad axim.
an·gu·la·tion [ˌ-ˈleɪʃn] n **1.** Abknicken nt. **2.** ortho. (Fraktur) Abknicken nt, Achsenfehlstellung f.
angulation osteotomy ortho. Angulationsosteotomie f.
an·gu·la·to·ry deformity [ˈ-lətɔːriː, -təʊ-] ortho. → angulation 2.
an·gu·lose [ˈ-ləʊs] adj → angular.
an·gu·lous [ˈ-ləs] adj → angular.
an·gu·lus [ˈæŋgjələs] m, pl **-li** [-liː, -laɪ] anat. Winkel m, Angulus m.
an·ha·phia [ænˈhæfɪə] n neuro. Anaphie f, Anaphia f.
an·he·do·nia [ænhɪˈdəʊnɪə] n Anhedonie f.
an·hem·a·to·poi·et·ic anemia [ænˌheməˌtəʊpɔɪˈetɪk] Anämie f durch verminderte od. fehlende Erythrozytenbildung.

an·he·mo·lyt·ic [ˌænˌhiːməˈlɪtɪk] *adj micro.* nichthämolytisch, nichthämolysierend, γ-hämolytisch, gamma-hämolytisch.
anhemolytic streptococci *micro.* gamma--hämolytische/nichthämolysierende Streptokokken *pl.*
an·he·mo·poi·et·ic anemia [ˌænˌhiːməpɔɪˈetɪk] → anhematopoietic anemia.
an·hi·dro·sis [ænhɪˈdrəʊsɪs, -haɪ-] *n* verminderte *od.* fehlende Schweißabsonderung *f*, An(h)idrose *f*, Anhidrosis *f*.
an·hi·drot·ic [ˌ-ˈdrɑtɪk] **I** *n* anhidrotisches Mittel *nt*. **II** *adj* An(h)idrose betr., anhidrotisch.
anhidrotic ectodermal dysplasia *derm.* anhidrotisch ektodermale Dysplasie *f*, ektodermale (kongenitale) Dysplasie *f*, Christ-Siemens-Syndrom *nt*, Guilford--Syndrom *nt*, Jacquet'-Syndrom *nt*, Anhidrosis hypotrichotica/congenita.
an·hy·drase [ænˈhaɪdreɪs] *n* Dehydratase *f*, Hydratase *f*.
an·hy·drate [ænˈhaɪdreɪt] *vt chem.* Wasser entziehen, dehydrieren.
an·hy·dra·tion [ˌænhaɪˈdreɪʃn] *n* 1. Wassermangel *m*, Dehydra(ta)tion *f*, Hypohydratation *f*. 2. Entwässerung *f*, Dehydratation *f*.
an·hy·dre·mia [ˌænhaɪˈdriːmɪə] *n* Wassermangel *m* im Blut, Anhydrämie *f*.
an·hy·dride [ænˈhaɪdraɪd, -drɪd] *n chem.* Anhydrid *nt*.
anhydride bond Anhydridbindung *f*.
an·hy·dro·chlo·ric [ænˌhaɪdrəˈklɔʊrɪk, -ˈklɔː-] *adj* Achlorhydrie betr. *od.* zeigend, achlorhydrisch.
an·hy·dro·hy·drox·y·pro·ges·ter·one [-haɪˌdrɑksɪprəʊˈdʒestərəʊn] *n* Ethisteron *nt*, A.'s cell.
an·hy·drous [ænˈhaɪdrəs] *adj chem.* wasserfrei, anhydriert.
a·ni·ac·i·no·sis [ˌænaɪəsɪˈnəʊsɪs, ˌeɪ-] *n* Niacinmangel *m*.
Anichkov → Anitschkow.
an·ic·ter·ic [ænɪkˈterɪk] *adj* ohne Ikterus (verlaufend), anikterisch.
anicteric hepatitis anikterische Virushepatitis *f*.
anicteric leptospirosis benigne/anikterische Leptospirose *f*.
an·id·e·us [æˈniːdɪəs] *n embryo.* Holoacardius amorphus.
an·i·dro·sis [ˌænɪˈdrəʊsɪs] *n* → anhidrosis.
an·i·drot·ic [ˌænɪˈdrɑtɪk] *n, adj* → anhidrotic.
an·i·ler·i·dine [ænɪˈlerɪdiːn] *n pharm.* Anileridin *nt*.
an·i·lid *n* → anilide.
an·i·lide [ˈænlɪd, -laɪd] *n* Anilid *nt*.
an·i·line [ˈænlɪn, -laɪn] *n* Anilin *nt*, Aminobenzol *nt*, Phenylamin *nt*.
aniline brown Bismarckbraun *nt*.
aniline cancer Anilinkrebs *m*.
aniline tumor → aniline cancer.
a·ni·lin·gus [ˌeɪnəˈlɪŋgəs] *n psychia.* Anilingus *m*.
an·i·lin·ism [ˈænlɪnɪzəm] *n* Anilinvergiftung *f*, Anilinismus *m*.
an·i·lism [ˈænɪlɪzəm] *n* → anilinism.
an·i·ma [ˈænəmə] *n* 1. Seele *f*, Anima *f*. 2. *psychia.* Anima *f*. 3. *pharm.* Wirkstoff *m*, -substanz *f*.
an·i·mal [ˈænɪməl] **I** *n* 1. Tier *nt*, tierisches Lebewesen *nt*. 2. *fig.* Tier *nt*, Bestie *f*. **II** *adj (a. fig.)* animalisch, tierisch.
animal alkaloid Leichengift *nt*, -alkaloid *nt*, Ptomain *nt*.
animal black → animal charcoal.
animal cell tierische/animalische Zelle *f*.
animal fat tierisches Fett *nt*.
animal starch Glykogen *nt*, tierische/animalische Stärke *f*.

animal parasite *micro.* tierischer Parasit *m*, Zooparasit *m*.
animal toxin tierisches Toxin *nt*, Zootoxin *nt*.
animal viruses tierische Viren *pl*.
an·i·mism [ˈænəmɪzəm] *n psychia.* Animismus *m*.
an·i·mus [ˈænɪməs] *n psychia.* Animus *m*.
an·i·on [ˈænaɪən] *n* Anion *nt*, negatives Ion *nt*.
anion exchange hypothesis Hypothese *f* des Anionenaustausches.
anion exchange resin Anionenaustauscher(harz) *nt*, Anresin *nt*.
an·i·on·ic [ˌænaɪˈɑnɪk] *adj* Anion betr., Anione enthaltend, anionisch, Anionen-.
anionic dye anionischer/saurer Farbstoff *m*.
an·i·rid·i·a [ˌænəˈrɪdɪə] *n* Fehlen *nt* der Regenbogenhaut, Aniridie *f*.
anis- *pref.* → aniso-.
an·i·sa·ki·a·sis [ˌænɪsəˈkaɪəsɪs] *n* Heringswurmkrankheit *f*, Anisakiasis *f*.
An·i·sa·kis [ænɪˈsækɪs] *n micro.* Anisakis *m*.
A. marina Heringswurm *m*, Anisakis marina.
an·i·sate [ˈænəseɪt, -sɪt] *n* Anisat *nt*.
an·ise [ˈænɪs] *n* Anis(samen *m*) *m*.
an·is·ei·ko·nia [ˌænəsaɪˈkəʊnɪə] *n ophthal.* Aniseikonie *f*.
an·is·ei·kon·ic lens [ˌ-ˈkɑnɪk] Aniseikonieglas *nt*.
an·i·sin·di·one [ˌænɪsɪnˈdaɪəʊn] *n pharm.* Anisindion *nt*.
an·i·sine [ˈænɪsɪn] *n* Anisin *nt*.
aniso- *pref.* anis(o)-, Anis(o)-.
an·i·so·ac·com·mo·da·tion [ænˌaɪsəəkɑməˈdeɪʃn] *n ophthal.* Anisoakkommodation *f*.
an·i·so·chro·ma·sia [ˌ-krəʊˈmeɪʒɪə] *n* Anisochromasie *f*.
an·i·so·chro·mat·ic [ˌ-krəʊˈmætɪk] *adj* anisochromatisch.
an·i·so·chro·mia [ˌ-ˈkrəʊmɪə] *n* Anisochromie *f*.
an·i·so·co·ria [ˌ-ˈkɔːrɪə, -ˈkoʊr-] *n ophthal.* unterschiedliche Pupillenweite *f*, Pupillendifferenz *f*, Anisokorie *f*.
an·i·so·cy·to·sis [ˌ-saɪˈtəʊsɪs] *n* Anisozytose *f*, -cytose *f*.
an·i·so·dac·ty·ly [ˌ-ˈdæktəlɪ] *n embryo.* Anisodaktylie *f*.
an·i·so·di·a·met·ric [ˌ-daɪəˈmetrɪk] *adj mathe.* anisodiametrisch.
an·i·so·ga·mete [ˌ-gəˈmiːt, -ˈgæmiːt] *n* Aniso-, Heterogamet *m*.
an·i·so·ga·met·ic [ˌ-gəˈmetɪk] *adj* anisogametisch, Anisogameten-.
an·i·sog·a·my [ˌænaɪˈsɑgəmɪ] *n* Aniso-, Heterogamie *f*.
an·i·so·i·co·nia [ænˌaɪsaɪˈkəʊnɪə] *n* → aniseikonia.
an·i·so·kar·y·o·sis [ˌ-kærɪˈəʊsɪs] *n* Anisokaryose *f*, -nukleose *f*.
an·i·so·mas·tia [ˌ-ˈmæstɪə] *n* Anisomastie *f*.
an·i·so·me·lia [ˌ-ˈmiːlɪə] *n embryo.* Anisomelie *f*.
an·i·so·mer·ic [ˌ-ˈmerɪk] *adj chem.* nicht--isomer, anisomer.
an·i·so·met·rope [ˌ-ˈmetrəʊp] *n ophthal.* Patient(in *f*) *m* mit Anisometropie *f*, Anisometroper *m*.
an·i·so·me·tro·pia [ˌ-meˈtrəʊpɪə] *n ophthal.* Anisometropie *f*.
an·i·so·me·trop·ic [ˌ-meˈtrɑpɪk] *adj* Anisometropie betr., anisometrop.
an·i·so·pho·ria [ˌ-ˈfɔːrɪə] *n ophthal.* Höhenschielen *nt*, Anisophorie *f*.
an·i·so·pia [ænɪˈsəʊpɪə] *n ophthal.* ungleiche Sehschärfe *f*, Anisopie *f*.

an·i·so·poi·ki·lo·cy·to·sis [ænˌaɪsəpɔɪˌkɪləʊsaɪˈtəʊsɪs] *n* Anisopoikilozytose *f*.
an·i·so·rhyth·mia [ˌ-ˈrɪðmɪə] *n* Aniso(r)rhythmie *f*.
an·i·sos·mot·ic [ˌænɪsɑsˈmɑtɪk] *adj* anisosmotisch.
an·i·so·spore [ænˈaɪsəspəʊər, -spɔːr] *n* Anisospore *f*.
an·i·so·ton·ic [ˌ-ˈtɑnɪk] *adj* anisoton(isch).
an·i·sot·ro·pal [ænɪˈsɑtrəpəl] *adj* → anisotropic.
an·i·so·trop·ic [ænˌaɪsəˈtrɑpɪk, -ˈtrəʊ-] *adj* doppelbrechend, -refraktär, anisotrop.
anisotropic band *histol.* A-Band *nt*, A-Streifen *m*, A-Zone *f*, anisotrope Bande *f*.
anisotropic disk → anisotropic band.
an·i·sot·ro·pism [æˈnaɪsɑtrəpɪzəm] *n* → anisotropy.
an·i·sot·ro·pous [-ˈsɑtrəpəs] *adj* → anisotropic.
anisotropous disk → anisotropic band.
an·i·sot·ro·py [-ˈsɑtrəpɪ] *n* (optische) Doppelbrechung *f*, Anisotropie *f*.
an·i·sum [əˈnaɪsəm, -ˈniː-] *n* Anis *nt*.
an·i·su·ria [ænɪˈs(j)ʊərɪə] *n* Anisurie *f*.
an·i·trog·e·nous [ænaɪˈtrɑdʒənəs] *adj chem.* nicht-stickstoffhaltig.
Anitschkow [əˈnɪtʃkɑf]: **A.'s body** → A.'s cell.
A.'s cell Anitschkow-Zelle *f*, -Myozyt *m*, Kardiohistiozyt *m*.
A.'s myocyte → A.'s cell.
an·kle [ˈæŋkl] *n* 1. (Fuß-)Knöchel *m*; Knöchelregion *f*, Fessel *f*. 2. oberes Sprunggelenk *nt*, Talokruralgelenk *nt*, Artic. talocruralis. 3. Sprungbein *nt*, Talus *m*.
ankle arthrodesis → ankle fusion.
ankle bone Sprungbein *nt*, Talus *m*.
ankle clonus *neuro.* Fußklonus *m*.
ankle fracture Knöchelbruch *m*, Malleolarfraktur *f*, Fractura malleolaris.
ankle fusion *ortho.* Versteifung/Arthrodese *f* des oberen Sprunggelenks.
ankle jerk → ankle reflex.
ankle joint oberes Sprunggelenk *nt*, Talokruralgelenk *nt*, Artic. talocruralis.
ankle reflex Achillessehnenreflex *m abbr.* ASR.
ankyl(o)- *pref.* Ankyl(o)-.
an·ky·lo·bleph·a·ron [ˌæŋkɪləʊˈblefərɑn] *n ophthal.* Lidverwachsung *f*, Ankyloblepharon *nt*.
an·ky·lo·chei·lia [ˌ-ˈkeɪlɪə] *n* Lippenverwachsung *f*, Ankyloch(e)ilie *f*.
an·ky·lo·col·pos [ˌ-ˈkɑlpəs] *n gyn.* Scheiden-, Vaginalatresie *f*, Atresia vaginalis.
an·ky·lo·dac·ty·ly [ˌ-ˈdæktəlɪ] *n embryo.* Ankylodaktylie *f*.
an·ky·lo·glos·sia [ˌ-ˈglɑsɪə] *n* Zungenverwachsung *f*, Ankyloglossie *f*, -glosson *nt*.
ankyloglossia superior syndrome *embryo.* Ankyloglossum-superior-Syndrom *nt*.
an·ky·lo·pho·bia [ˌ-ˈfəʊbɪə] *n* Ankylophobie *f*.
an·ky·lo·poi·et·ic [ˌ-pɔɪˈetɪk] *adj* versteifend, ankylosierend, Ankylose verursachend.
an·ky·lo·proc·tia [ˌ-ˈprɑkʃɪə] *n old* Afterstruktur *f*.
an·ky·lose [ˈæŋkələʊs] **I** *vt ortho. (Gelenk)* steif machen, versteifen, ankylosieren. **II** *vi ortho.* steif werden, versteifen.
an·ky·losed [ˈæŋkələʊst] *adj ortho. (Gelenk)* versteift.
an·ky·los·ing [ˈæŋkələʊsɪŋ] *adj* versteifend, ankylosierend.
ankylosing spondylitis Bechterew(-Strümpell-Marie)-Krankheit *f*, Marie--Strümpell-Krankheit *f*, Morbus Bechte-

ankylosis   40

rew *m*, Spondylarthritis/Spondylitis ankylopoetica/ankylosans.
an·ky·lo·sis [ˌæŋkə'ləʊsɪs] *n, pl* **-ses** [-siːz] Gelenkversteifung *f*, Ankylose *f*, Ankylosis *f*.
An·ky·los·to·ma *n* → Ancylostoma.
an·ky·lo·sto·mi·a·sis *n* → ancylostomiasis.
an·ky·lot·ic [ˌæŋkə'lɒtɪk] *adj* Ankylose betr., versteift, ankylotisch.
an·ky·lot·o·my [ˌ-'lɒtəmɪ] *n ortho.* Ankylotomie *f*.
an·kyl·u·re·thria [ˌæŋkɪljə'riːθrɪə] *n* Harnröhrenstriktur *f*.
an·ky·roid ['æŋkɪrɔɪd] *adj* haken-, ankerförmig.
an·la·ge ['ɑnlɑːgə] *n, pl* **-gen** [-gən] **1.** *embryo.* (Erb-)Anlage *f*. **2.** *psycho.* Anlage *f*, Prädisposition *f (to* zu).
ANLL *abbr.* [acute nonlymphocytic leukemia] → acute myelocytic leukemia.
Ann Ar·bor [æn'ɑːrbɔr]: **A. A. classification** Ann-Arbor-Klassifizierung *f*.
an·neal [ə'niːl] *vt* **1.** *techn.* ausglühen, vergüten, tempern. **2.** *fig.* härten, stählen.
an·nec·tent [ə'nektənt] *adj* verbindend.
an·ne·lid ['ænəlɪd] *n micro.* Glieder-, Ringelwurm *m*, Annelid *m*.
An·nel·i·da [ə'nelɪdə] *pl micro.* Glieder-, Ringelwürmer *pl*, Anneliden *pl*, Annelida *pl*.
an·nounce [ə'naʊns] *vt* ankündigen, andeuten, anzeigen.
an·nu·lar ['ænjələr] *adj* ringförmig, anulär, zirkulär, Ring-.
annular bands amniotische Stränge *pl*, Simonart'-Bänder *pl*.
annular carcinoma annuläres/zirkulär(wachsend)es Karzinom *nt*.
annular cartilage Ring-, Krikoidknorpel *m*, Cartilago cricoidea.
annular cataract *ophthal.* ringförmige/scheibenförmige Katarakt *f*.
annular hymen *gyn.* ringförmiges Hymen *nt*, Hymen anularis.
annular keratitis Randkeratitis *f*, Keratitis marginalis.
annular lesion anuläre/zirkuläre/ringförmige Schädigung/Läsion *f*.
annular ligament : a. of base of stapes Lig. anulare stapediae.
external a. of ankle Retinaculum mm. peron(a)eorum/fibularium superius.
inferior a. Lig. arcuatum pubis.
internal a. of ankle Retinaculum mm. flexorum (pedis).
a. of radius Lig. anulare radii.
a. of stapes Lig. anulare stapediae.
a.s of trachea Ligg. anularia,trachealia.
annular musculature Ringmuskulatur *f*.
annular pancreas Pancreas an(n)ulare.
annular placenta Ring-, Gürtelplazenta *f*, Placenta anularis.
annular psoriasis *derm.* Psoriasis anularis.
annular radial ligament → annular ligament of radius.
annular scleritis Scleritis anularis.
annular scotoma *ophthal.* Ringskotom *nt*.
annular staphyloma *ophthal.* Ringstaphylom *nt*, Staphyloma anulare.
annular stricture Ringstriktur *f*.
annular syphilid annuläres/zirzinäres Syphilid *nt*.
an·nu·lo·plas·ty [ˌænjələʊ'plæstɪ] *n chir.* Anuloplastik *f*.
an·nu·lor·rha·phy [ˌænjə'lɑrəfɪ] *n chir.* Anulo(r)rhaphie *f*.
an·nu·lo·spi·ral [ˌænjələʊ'spaɪərəl] *adj* anulospiral, anulospiralig.
annulospiral ending anulospiralige Endigung *f*, Anulospiralendigung *f*.
an·nu·lus ['ænjələs] *n, pl* **-lus·es, -li** [-laɪ]

bio., anat. Ring *m*, ringförmige *od.* zirkuläre Struktur *f*, A(n)nulus *m*.
a. of conjunctiva A(n)nulus conjunctivae.
annulus fibrosus Faserring *m*, A(n)nulus *m* fibrosus (disci intervertebralis).
AnOC *abbr.* → anodal opening contraction.
A·no·cen·tor [ˌænəʊ'sentər] *n micro.* Anocentor *m*.
a·no·coc·cyg·e·al [ˌeɪnəkɒk'sɪdʒɪəl] *adj* Anus u. Steißbein betr., anokokzygeal.
anococcygeal body Lig. anococcygeum.
anococcygeal ligament Lig. anococcygeum.
anococcygeal nerve N. anococcygeus.
anococcygeal raphe Lig. anococcygeum.
a·no·cu·ta·ne·ous line [ˌ-kjuː'teɪnɪəs, -jəs] Anokutangrenze *f*, -linie *f*, Linea anocutanea.
an·o·dal [æn'əʊdl] *adj* → anodic.
anodal closure *abbr.* **AC** Anodenschluß *m*, -schließung *f*.
anodal closure clonus *abbr.* **ACCl** Anodenschließungsklonus *m*.
anodal closure contraction *abbr.* **ACC, AnCC** *physiol.* Anodenschließungszuckung *f abbr.* **ASZ, AnSZ**.
anodal closure tetanus *abbr.* **ACT** Anodenschließungstetanus *m*.
anodal current Anodenstrom *m*.
anodal opening clonus *abbr.* **AOCl** Anodenöffnungsklonus *m*.
anodal opening contraction *abbr.* **AOC, AnOC** *physiol.* Anodenöffnungszuckung *f abbr.* **AÖZ, AnÖZ, AOZ**.
an·ode ['ænəʊd] *n* Anode *f*, positive Elektrode *f*, positiver Pol *m*.
anode rays Anodenstrahlen *pl*, -strahlung *f*.
a·no·derm ['ænədɜrm] *n* Anoderm *nt*.
an·od·ic [æ'nɒdɪk, -'nəʊ-] *adj* Anode betr., anodisch, aufsteigend, Anoden-.
an·od·mia [æn'ɒdmɪə] *n* → anosmia.
an·o·don·tia [ˌænə'dɒnʃ(ɪ)ə] *n* (vollständige) Zahnlosigkeit *f*, Anodontie *f*, Anodontia *f*.
an·o·don·tism [ˌænə'dɒntɪzəm] *n* → anodontia.
an·o·dyne ['ænədaɪn] **I** *n* schmerzlinderndes Mittel *nt*, Anodynum *nt*. **II** *adj* schmerzlindernd, -stillend, beruhigend.
an·o·dyn·ia [ˌænə'diːnɪə] *n* Schmerzfreiheit *f*.
a·no·e·sia [ˌænəʊ'iːz(ɪ)ə] *n psychia.* Anoesia *f*.
an·o·et·ic [ˌ-'etɪk] *adj* **1.** *psychia.* Anoesia betr., anoetisch. **2.** unverständlich.
anoia [ə'nɔɪə] *n* → anoesia.
a·nom·a·lo·scope [ə'nɒmələˌskəʊp] *n ophthal.* Anomaloskop *nt*.
a·nom·a·lo·tro·phy [əˌnɒmə'lɒtrəfɪ] *n* Fehlernährung *f*.
a·nom·a·lous [ə'nɒmələs] *adj* regel-, normwidrig, anomal, abnorm; ungewöhnlich.
anomalous complex (*EKG*) abnormaler/pathologischer Komplex *m*.
a·nom·a·ly [ə'nɒmǝlɪ] *n* Anomalie *f*, Abweichung *f* (von der Norm), Unregelmäßigkeit *f*; Ungewöhnlichkeit *f*; Mißbildung *f*.
a. of the middle ear Mittelohrmißbildung, -anomalie.
an·o·mer ['ænəmər] *n chem.* Anomer(es *nt*) *nt*.
an·o·mer·ic [ˌænə'merɪk] *adj* Anomer betr., anomer.
anomeric carbon anomeres Kohlenstoffatom *nt*.
a·no·mia [ə'nəʊmɪə] *n* Anomie *f*.
an·om·ic aphasia [ə'nɒmɪk] Wortvergessenheit *f*, Wortfindungsstörung *f*, amnestische Aphasie *f*.

an·o·nych·ia [ˌænə'nɪkɪə] *n* Anonychie *f*, Anonychosis *f*.
a·non·y·mous [ə'nɒnɪməs] *adj* namenlos, anonym.
anonymous mycobacteria *micro.* nichttuberkulöse/atypische Mykobakterien *pl*.
anonymous veins Vv. brachiocephalicae (dextra et sinistra).
a·no·per·i·ne·al [ˌeɪnəˌperɪ'niːəl] *adj* After/Anus u. Damm/Perineum betr., anoperineal.
A·noph·e·les [ə'nɒfəliːz] *n, pl* **-les** *micro.* Malaria-, Gabel-, Fiebermücke *f*, Anopheles *f*.
a·noph·e·li·cide [ə'nɒfəlɪsaɪd] **I** *n* Anopheles/Anopheliden abtötendes Mittel, Anophelizid *nt*. **II** *adj* Anopheliden abtötend.
a·noph·e·line [ə'nɒfəlɪən, -lɪn] *adj* Anopheliden betr., durch Anopheliden verursacht, Anopheles-, Anopheliden-.
A·noph·e·li·ni [əˌnɒfə'laɪnaɪ] *pl micro.* Anopheliden *pl*.
an·o·pho·ria [ænə'fɔːrɪə] *n ophthal.* latentes Höhenschielen *nt*, Hyperphorie *f*.
an·oph·thal·mia [ˌænɒf'θælmɪə] *n ophthal.* Fehlen *nt* des Augapfels, Anophthalmie *f*, Anophthalmus *m*.
an·oph·thal·mus [ˌænɒf'θælməs] *n* → anophthalmia.
a·no·plas·ty ['eɪnəplæstɪ] *n* After-, Anus-, Anoplastik *f*.
An·o·plu·ra [ænə'plʊərə] *pl micro.* Anoplura *pl*.
a·no·proc·to·plas·ty [eɪnəˌprɒktə'plæstɪ] *n* → anorectoplasty.
an·or·chia [æn'ɔːrkɪə] *n* Fehlen *nt* der Hoden, Anorchie *f*, Anorchidie *f*, Anorchismus *m*.
an·or·chid [æn'ɔːrkɪd] *n* Patient *m* mit Anorchie.
an·or·chid·ic [ənɔːr'kɪdɪk] *adj* Anorchie betr., hodenlos.
an·or·chi·dism [æn'ɔːrkɪdɪzəm] *n* → anorchia.
an·or·chism [æn'ɔːrkɪzəm] *n* → anorchia.
a·no·rec·tal [ˌeɪnə'rektl] *adj* After/Anus u. Mastdarm/Rectum betr., anorektal, Anorektal-.
anorectal abscess anorektaler Abszeß *m*.
anorectal canal *embryo.* Anorektalkanal *m*.
anorectal fistula After-Mastdarm-Fistel *f*, Anus-Rektum-Fistel *f*, Anorektalfistel *f*, Fistula anorectalis.
anorectal junction Anorektalübergang *m*, anorektale Übergangszone *f*/-linie *f*, Linea anorectalis.
anorectal line → anorectal junction.
anorectal spasm Proctalgia fugax.
anorectal syndrome anorektales Syndrom *nt*.
an·o·rec·tic [ˌænə'rektɪk] *pharm.* **I** *n* Appetitzügler *m*, -hemmer *m*, Anorektikum *nt*. **II** *adj* Anorexia betr., appetithemmend, anorektisch.
an·o·rec·ti·tis [ˌeɪnərek'taɪtɪs] *n* Entzündung *f* des Anorektums, Anorektitis *f*.
a·no·rec·to·co·lon·ic [ˌ-ˌrektəkəʊ'lɒnɪk] *adj* Anus, Rektum u. Kolon betr.
a·no·rec·to·plas·ty [ˌ-rektə'plæstɪ] *n chir.* Anus-Rektum-Plastik *f*, Anorektoplastik *f*.
a·no·rec·tum [ˌ-'rektəm] *n* Anorektum *nt*.
an·o·ret·ic [ænə'retɪk] *n, adj* → anorectic.
an·o·rex·ia [ænə'reksɪə] *n* Appetitlosigkeit *f*, Anorexie *f*, Anorexia *f*.
anorexia-cachexia syndrome Anorexie-Kachexie-Syndrom *nt*.
anorexia nervosa (Pubertäts-)Magersucht *f*, Anorexia nervosa/mentalis.

an·o·rex·i·ant [ænə'reksɪənt] *n, adj* → anorexigenic.
an·o·rex·ic [ænə'reksɪk] *n, adj* → anorectic.
an·o·rex·i·gen·ic [ænəˌreksɪ'dʒenɪk] **I** *n* Appetitzügler *m*, -hemmer *m*, Anorektikum *nt*. **II** *adj* Appetitlosigkeit verursachend, appetitzügelnd, -hemmend.
an·or·gas·my [ænɔːr'gæzmɪ] *n psychia.* Anorgasmie *f*.
an·or·thog·ra·phy [ˌænɔːr'θɑgrəfɪ] *n neuro.* Anorthographie *f*.
an·or·tho·pia [ˌ-'θəʊpɪə] *n ophthal.* **1.** Anorthopie *f*. **2.** Schielen *nt*, Strabismus *m*.
an·or·tho·scope [æn'ɔːrθəskəʊp] *n* Anorthoskop *nt*.
a·no·scope ['eɪnəskəʊp] *n* Anoskop *nt*.
a·nos·co·py [eɪ'nɑskəpɪ] *n* Anoskopie *f*.
a·no·scro·tal fascia [ˌeɪnə'skrəʊtl] Fascia perinei superficialis.
a·no·sig·moid·o·scope [ˌeɪnəʊsɪg'mɔɪdəskəʊp] *n* Anosigmoidoskop *nt*.
a·no·sig·moid·o·scop·ic [ˌ-'skɑpɪk] *adj* Anosigmoidoskopie betr., anosigmoidoskopisch.
a·no·sig·moid·os·co·py [eɪnəʊˌsɪgmɔɪ'dɑskəpɪ] *n* Anosigmoidoskopie *f*.
an·os·mat·ic [ænəz'mætɪk] *adj* anosmisch.
an·os·mia [ə'nɑzmɪə] *n neuro.* Fehlen *nt* des Geruchsinnes, Anosmie *f*.
an·os·mic [æn'ɑzmɪk] *adj* **1.** Anosmie betr., anosmisch. **2.** geruchlos.
an·o·so·gno·sia [æˌnəʊsə(g)'nəʊʒ(ɪ)ə] *n neuro.* Anosognosie *f*.
an·os·phra·sia [æˌnɑs'freɪʒ(ɪ)ə, -zɪə] *n* → anosmia.
a·no·spi·nal [eɪnə'spaɪnl] *adj* After/Anus u. Rückenmark betr., anospinal.
anospinal center anospinales Zentrum *nt*, Centrum anospinale.
an·os·te·o·pla·sia [ænˌɑstɪə'pleɪʒ(ɪ)ə] *n* fehlerhafte Knochenbildung *f*, Anosteoplasie *f*.
an·os·to·sis [ˌænɑs'təʊsɪs] *n* fehlerhafte Knochenentwicklung *f*, Anostose *f*.
an·o·tia [æn'əʊʃɪə] *n* Fehlen *nt* der Ohrmuschel, Anotie *f*.
an·o·tro·pia [ˌænə'trəʊpɪə] *n ophthal.* Anotropie *f*.
an·o·tus [æn'əʊtəs] *n embryo.* Anotus *m*.
ANOVA *abbr.* → analysis of variance.
a·no·va·gi·nal [ˌeɪnə'vædʒənl, -və'dʒaɪnl] *adj* After/Anus u. Scheide/Vagina betr. *od.* verbindend, anovaginal.
an·o·var·ia [ˌænəʊ'veərɪə] *n* → anovarism.
an·o·var·i·an·ism [ˌ-'veərɪənɪzəm] *n* → anovarism.
an·o·var·ism [æn'əʊvərɪzəm] *n gyn.* Fehlen *nt* der Eierstöcke, Anovarie *f*.
a·no·ves·i·cal [ˌeɪnə'vesɪkl] *adj* After/Anus u. Harnblase betr. *od.* verbindend, anovesikal.
an·o·vu·lar [æn'ɑvjələr, -'əʊv-] *adj* anovulär, anovulatorisch.
anovular menstruation anovulatorische Menstruation *f*.
an·ov·u·la·tion [ˌænəvjə'leɪʃn] *n gyn.* fehlende Ovulation *f*, Anovulation *f*.
an·ov·u·la·to·ry [æn'ɑvjələtɔːriː, -təʊ-] *adj* → anovular.
anovulatory cycle *gyn.* anovulatorischer Zyklus *m*.
anovulatory menstruation anovulatorische Menstruation *f*.
an·ov·u·lia [ænɑv'jʊəlɪə] *n old* → anovulation.
an·ov·u·lo·men·or·rhea [ænˌɑvjələʊˌmenə'rɪə] *n gyn.* anovulatorischer Zyklus *m*.
an·ox·e·mia [ˌænɑk'siːmɪə] *n* Sauerstoffmangel *m* des Blutes, Anoxämie *f*, Anoxyhämie *f*.
anoxemia test *card.* Hypoxietest *m*.

an·ox·e·mic [ˌ-'siːmɪk] *adj* (*Blut*) sauerstoffarm, anoxämisch.
an·ox·ia [æn'ɑksɪə, ə'nɑk-] *n* Sauerstoffmangel *m*, Anoxie *f*.
a. of the newborn Anoxia neonatorum.
an·ox·ic [æn'ɑksɪk] *adj* Anoxie betr., anoxisch.
anoxic anoxia anoxische Anoxie *f*.
anoxic injury anoxische/anoxie-bedingte Schädigung *f*.
a·nox·y·di·o·sis [æˌnɑksɪ'daɪəʊsɪs] *n* → anaerobiosis.
Anrep ['ænrep]: **A. effect** *card.* Anrep-Effekt *m*.
ANS *abbr.* → autonomic nervous system.
an·sa ['ænsə] *n, pl* **-sae** [-siː] *anat.* Schlinge *f*, Schleife *f*, Ansa *f*.
a. of Vieussen → ansa subclavia.
ansa subclavia Subklaviaschlinge *f*, Ansa subclavia.
an·ser·ine ['ænsəraɪn, -rɪn] **I** *n* Anserin *nt*. **II** *adj* **1.** *anat.* Pes anserinus betr. **2.** *zoo.* Gänse-.
anserine bursa Bursa anserina.
anserine plexus Parotisplexus *m* des N. facialis, Plexus intraparotideus n. facialis.
an·si·form ['ænsɪfɔːrm] *adj anat.* schleifen-, schlingenförmig.
ansiform lobule Lobulus ansiformis.
ant- *pref.* → anti-.
ant·ac·id [ænt'æsɪd] **I** *n* Ant(i)azidum *nt*. **II** *adj* säure(n)neutralisierend, antazid.
an·tag·o·nism [æn'tægənɪzəm] *n* **1.** Antagonismus *m*, Gegensatz *m*, gegeneinander gerichtete Wirkungsweise *f* (*to, against*). **2.** *anat.* Antagonismus *m*, Gegenspiel *nt* (*to, against*). **3.** *pharm.* Antagonismus *m*, Gegenwirkung *f* (*to, against*).
an·tag·o·nist [æn'tægənɪst] *n* **1.** Gegner *m*, Gegenspieler *m*, Widersacher *m*, Antagonist *m* (*to, against*). **2.** *physiol.* Gegenmuskel *m*, -spieler *m*, Antagonist *m* (*to, against*). **3.** *pharm., chem.* Hemmstoff *m*, Antagonist *m* (*to, against*). **4.** *dent.* Antagonist *m* (*to, against*).
an·tag·o·nis·tic [æntægə'nɪstɪk] *adj* antagonistisch (*to* gegen), gegenwirkend, entgegengesetzt wirkend.
an·tag·o·nis·ti·cal [ˌ-'nɪstɪkl] *adj* → antagonistic.
antagonistic muscle Gegenspieler *m*, Gegenmuskel *m*, Antagonist *m*.
antagonistic reflex antagonistischer Reflex *m*.
antagonist inhibition Antagonistenhemmung *f*.
ant·al·ge·sic [æntæl'dʒiːzɪk] *n, adj* → antalgic.
ant·al·gic [ænt'ældʒɪk] **I** *n* Schmerzmittel *nt*, Analgetikum *nt*. **II** *adj* **1.** schmerzlindernd, analgetisch. **2.** schmerzvermeidend.
ant·al·ka·line [ænt'ælkəlaɪn, -lɪn] *adj* lauge(n)neutralisierend.
ant·aph·ro·dis·i·ac [æntˌæfrə'diːzɪæk] **I** *n* Antaphrodisiakum *nt*. **II** *adj* den Sexualtrieb unterdrückend, antaphrodisisch.
ant·ar·thrit·ic [ˌæntɑːr'θrɪtɪk] **I** *n* Antarthritikum *nt*. **II** *adj* Arthritis(beschwerden) mildernd.
ant·asth·mat·ic [ˌæntæz'mætɪk] **I** *n* Antasthmatikum *nt*. **II** *adj* Asthma(beschwerden) mildernd.
ant·a·troph·ic [ˌæntə'trɑfɪk, -'trəʊ-] *adj* ant(i)atrophisch.
ant·a·zo·line [æn'tæzəliːn] *n pharm.* Antazolin *nt*.
ante- *pref.* Ante-.
ante ['æntɪ] **I** *adv* (*zeitlich*) vorher, zuvor; (*räumlich*) vorn, voran. **II** *prep* (*räumlich*

u. zeitlich) vor.
an·te·bra·chi·al [ˌæntɪ'breɪkɪəl, -'bræ-] *adj* Unterarm betr., antebrachial, Unterarm-.
antebrachial fascia Unterarmfaszie *f*, Fascia antebrachii.
antebrachial region Unterarmfläche *f*, -region *f*, Regio/Facies antebrachialis.
anterior a. vordere Unterarmfläche, Regio/Facies antebrachialis anterior.
posterior a. hintere Unterarmfläche, Regio/Facies antebrachialis posterior.
radial a. Radialseite *f* des Unterarms, Regio/Facies antebrachialis radialis.
ulnar a. Ulnarseite *f* des Unterarms, Regio/Facies antebrachialis ulnaris.
volar a. → anterior a.
antebrachial vein, (inter)median Intermedia/Mediana *f* antebrachii, V. intermedia/mediana antebrachii.
an·te·bra·chi·um [ˌ-'breɪkɪəm] *n* Unter-, Vorderarm *m*, Antebrachium *nt*.
an·te·car·di·um [ˌ-'kɑːrdɪəm] *n anat.* Regio epigastrica, Epigastrium *nt*, Magengrube *f*.
an·te·ce·dent [ˌ-'siːdnt] **I** *n* **1.** Vorläufer *m*, Vorstufe *f*, Antezedent *m*. **2.** Vorgeschichte *f*. **II** *adj* voran-, vorhergehend (*to*).
antecedent sign Prodromalsymptom *nt*.
ante ci·bum ['æntɪ 'siːbəm] *abbr.* **ac** *pharm.* vor dem Essen, ante cibum.
an·te·col·ic [ˌæntə'kɑlɪk] *adj* vor dem Kolon (liegend), antekolisch.
an·te·cu·bi·tal fossa [ˌ-'kjuːbɪtl] Ellenbeugengrube *f*, Fossa cubitalis.
an·te·date [ˌn 'æntɪˌdeɪt, v 'æntɪ'deɪt] **I** *n* (Zu-)Rückdatierung *f*. **II** *vt* **1.** (zu-)rückdatieren. **2.** (*Krankheitsverlauf*) beschleunigen.
an·te·flect [ˌ-'flekt] *vt* nach vorne beugen, anteflektieren.
an·te·flexed [ˌ-'flekst] *adj* nach vorne gebeugt, anteflektiert.
an·te·flex·ion [ˌ-'flekʃn] *n* **1.** pathologische Vorwärtsbeugung/Anteflexion *f*. **2.** physiologische Vorwärtsbeugung/Anteflexion *f* des Uterus, Anteflexio uteri.
an·te·grade ['-greɪd] *adj* → anterograde.
antegrade pyelography ante(ro)grade Pyelographie *f*.
antegrade urography *urol., radiol.* antegrade Urographie *f*.
an·te·lo·ca·tion [ˌ-ləʊ'keɪʃn] *n* (*Organ*) Vorwärtsverlagerung *f*.
an·te·mor·tem [ˌ-'mɔːrtəm] *adj* vor dem Tode, ante mortem.
an·te·na·tal [ˌ-'neɪtl] *adj* vor der Geburt (auftretend *od.* entstehend), antenatal, pränatal.
antenatal clinic Schwangerensprechstunde *f*.
antenatal exercises Schwangerschaftsgymnastik *f*.
antenatal hemopoiesis pränatale Blutbildung/Hämopo(i)ese *f*.
an·ten·na [æn'tenə] *n, pl* **-nae** [-niː]; **2. -nas 1.** *bio.* Fühler *m*, Fühlhorn *nt*. **2.** *techn.* Antenne *f*.
an·te·par·tal [æntɪ'pɑːrtl] *adj* vor der Entbindung/Geburt (auftretend *od.* entstehend), vorgeburtlich, antepartal, präpartal.
an·te·par·tum [ˌ-'pɑːrtəm] *adj* → antepartal.
an·te·po·si·tion [ˌ-pə'zɪʃn] *n anat.* Vorwärtsverlagerung *f*, Anteposition *f*.
an·te·pros·tate [ˌ-'prɑsteɪt] *n* Gl. bulbourethralis.
an·te·pros·ta·ti·tis [ˌ-prɑstə'teɪtɪs] *n* Entzündung *f* der Gl. bulbourethralis.
an·te·pul·sion [ˌ-'pʌlʃn] *n* Antepulsion *f*.

antepyretic 42

an·te·py·ret·ic [ˌ-paɪˈriːtɪk] *adj* vor dem Fieberstadium auftretend.
ant·er·gia [ænˈtɜrdʒɪə] *n* **1.** → antagonism. **2.** Widerstand *m*, Resistenz *f*.
ant·er·gic [ænˈtɜrdʒɪk] *adj* → antagonistic.
ant·er·gy [ˈæntɜrdʒɪ] *n* → antergia.
an·te·ri·or [ænˈtɪərɪər] *adj* **1.** *abbr.* **A** vorne liegend, vordere(r, s), anterior, Vorder-, Vor-. **2.** (*zeitlich*) früher (*to* als).
anterior arch of atlas vorderer Atlasbogen *m*, Arcus anterior atlantis.
anterior band of colon freie Kolontänie *f*, T(a)enia libera coli.
anterior basal segment (*Lunge*) vorderes Basalsegment *nt*, Segmentum basale anterius [S VIII].
anterior belly of digastric muscle vorderer Digastrikusbauch *m*, Venter anterior m. digastrici.
anterior border: a. of radius vordere Radiuskante *f*, Margo anterior radii.
 a. of tibia vordere Schienbeinkante *f*, Margo anterior tibiae.
 a. of ulna Ulnarvorderkante *f*, Margo anterior ulnae.
anterior branch: a.es of cervical nerves vordere/ventrale Halsnervenäste *pl*, Rami anteriores/ventrales nn. cervicalium.
 a. of coccygeal nerve vorderer/ventraler Ast *m* des N. coccygeus, Ramus anterior/ventralis n. coccygei.
 a. of great auricular nerve vorderer Ast *m* des N. auricularis magnus, Ramus anterior n. auricularis magni.
 a. of inferior pancreaticoduodenal artery Ramus anterior a. pancreaticoduodenalis inferioris.
 a. of lateral cerebral sulcus Ramus anterior sulci lateralis (cerebri).
 a.es of lumbar nerves vordere/ventrale Äste *pl* der Lumbalnerven, Rami anteriores/ventrales nn. lumbalium.
 a. of medial cutaneous nerve of forearm Ramus anterior n. cutanei antebrachii medialis.
 a. of obturator artery vorderer (End-)Ast *m* der A. obturatoria, Ramus anterior a. obturatoriae.
 a. of obturator nerve vorderer Ast *m* des N. obturatorius, Ramus anterior n. obturatorii.
 a. of recurrent ulnar artery vorderer Ast *m* der A. recurrens ulnaris, Ramus anterior a. recurrentis ulnaris.
 a. of renal artery vorderer Ast *m* der Nierenarterie, Ramus anterior a. renalis.
 a. of right hepatic duct Ramus anterior ductus hepatici dextri.
 a.es of sacral nerves ventrale Äste *pl* der Sakralnerven, Rami anteriores nn. sacralium.
 a. of spinal nerves vorderer Ast *od.* Bauchast *m* der Spinalnerven, Ramus anterior/ventralis nn. spinalium.
 a.es of thoracic nerves Interkostalnerven *pl*, Rami anteriores/ventrales nn. thoracicorum, Nn. intercostales.
 a. of superior thyroid artery vorderer (Drüsen-)Ast *m* der A. thyroidea superior, Ramus glandularis anterior a. thyroideae superioris.
anterior cells vordere Siebbeinzellen *pl*, Sinus anteriores.
anterior chamber cleavage syndrome *ophthal.* Peters-Anomalie *f*, -Syndrom *nt*.
anterior chamber of eye vordere Augenkammer *f*, Camera oculi anterior, Camera anterior (bulbi).
anterior choroiditis *ophthal.* vordere Chorioiditis *f*, Chorioiditis anterior.
anterior column: a. of fauces vorderer Gaumenbogen *m*, Arcus palatoglossus.
 a. of medulla oblongata Pyramis (medullae oblongatae).
 a. of rugae of vagina Columna rugarum anterior.
 a. of spinal cord Vordersäule *f* (des Rückenmarks), Columna anterior/ventralis medullae spinalis.
anterior commissure vordere Kommissur *f*, Commissura anterior cerebri.
 a. of cerebrum → anterior commissure.
 a. of labia vordere Verbindung *f* der großen Schamlippen, Commissura labiorum anterior.
anterior cord syndrome *neuro.* Vorderstrangsyndrom *nt*.
anterior cornual syndrome *neuro.* Vorderhornsyndrom *nt*.
anterior crest of fibula Wadenbein-, Fibulavorderkante *f*, Margo anterior fibulae.
anterior crus: a. of internal capsule vorderer Kapselschenkel *m*, Crus anterius capsulae internae.
 a. of stapes vorderer Steigbügelschenkel *m*, Crus anterius (stapedis).
 a. of superficial inguinal ring Crus mediale anuli inguinalis superficialis.
anterior curvature *ortho.* Kyphose *f*.
anterior divisions of trunks of brachial plexus vordere Äste *pl* der Trunci plexus brachialis, Divisiones anteriores/ventrales truncorum plexus brachialis.
anterior edges of eyelids vordere Lidkanten *pl*, Limbi palpebrales anteriores.
anterior embryotoxon Embryotoxon *nt*, Arcus lipoides juvenilis.
anterior endothelium of cornea inneres Korneaepithel *nt*, Korneaendothel *nt*, Endothelium corneae, Epithelium posterius (corneae).
anterior epithelium of cornea (äußeres) Hornhautepithel *nt*, Epithelium anterius (corneae).
anterior extremity of spleen unterer Milzpol *m*, Extremitas anterior (lienis/splenis).
anterior fontanelle vordere/große Fontanelle *f*, Stirnfontanelle *f*, Fonticulus anterior.
anterior fornix → anterior part of fornix of vagina.
anterior funiculus (**of spinal cord**) Vorderstrang *m* (des Rückenmarks), Funiculus anterior/ventralis medullae spinalis.
anterior gastrotomy *chir.* vordere Gastrotomie *f*.
anterior gray column of spinal cord Vordersäule *f* (der grauen Substanz), Columna anterior/ventralis medullae spinalis.
anterior head of rectus femoris muscle vorderer/gerader Kopf *m* des M. rectus femoris, Caput rectus m. recti femoris.
anterior horn: a. of lateral ventricle Vorderhorn *nt* des Seitenventrikels, Cornu anterius/frontale (ventriculi lateralis).
 a. of spinal cord Vorderhorn *nt* des Rückenmarks, Cornu anterius/ventrale (medullae spinalis).
anterior horn cell Vorderhornzelle *f*.
anterior incisure of ear Inc. anterior (auris).
anterior ligament: a. of colon Taenia omentalis.
 a. of head of rib Lig. capitis costae radiatum.
 a. of malleus vorderes Malleusband *nt*, Lig. mallei anterius.
 a. of radiocarpal joint Lig. radiocarpale palmare.
anterior limb: a. of internal capsule → anterior crus of internal capsule.
 a. of stapes Crus anterius (stapedis).
anterior lobe: a. of cerebellar body Lobus anterior corporis cerebelli.
 a. of cerebellum kranialer (Kleinhirn-)Lappen/Abschnitt *m*, Lobus anterior/cranialis/rostralis cerebelli.
 a. of hypophysis → anterior pituitary.
anterior margin: a. of fibula Fibulavorderrand *m*, Margo anterior fibulae.
 a. of lung vorderer/unterer Lungenrand *m*, Margo anterior/inferior pulmonis.
 a. of nail vorderer freier Nagelrand *m*, Schnitt-, Abnutzungskante *f*, Margo liber unguis.
 a. of parietal bone Margo anterior/frontalis ossis parietalis.
 a. of radius → anterior border of radius.
 a. of testis vorderer/konvexer Hodenrand *m*, Margo anterior testis.
 a. of tibia → anterior border of tibia.
 a. of ulna → anterior border of ulna.
anterior mediastinum vorderer Mediastinalraum *m*, vorderes Mediastinum *nt*, Mediastinum anterius, Cavum mediastinale anterius.
anterior myocardial infarction Vorderwandinfarkt *m*.
anterior nephrectomy *chir.* vordere/transabdominelle Nephrektomie *f*.
anterior neuropore *embryo.* oraler/vorderer Neuroporus *m*.
anterior notch of ear → anterior incisure of ear.
anterior nucleus: dorsal a. of thalamus Nc. anterodorsalis/anterosuperior (thalami).
 medial a. of thalamus Nc. anteromedialis (thalami).
 a.i of thalamus vordere Kerngruppe *pl* des Thalamus, Ncc. anteriores (thalami).
 a. of trapezoid body Nc. corporis trapezoidei anterior.
 ventral a. of thalamus Nc. anteroventralis/anteroinferior (thalami).
anterior part: a. of cerebral peduncle (vorderer) Hirnschenkel *m*, Crus cerebri, Pars anterior/ventralis (pedunculi cerebri).
 a. of fornix of vagina vorderes Scheidengewölbe *nt*, Pars anterior fornicis vaginae.
 a. of trabecular retinaculum vorderer Abschnitt *m* des Hueck'-Bandes, Pars corneoscleralis.
anterior pillar of fornix Gewölbe-, Fornixsäule *f*, -pfeiler *m*, Columna fornicis.
anterior pituitary *abbr.* **AP** Hypophysenvorderlappen *m abbr.* HVL, Adenohypophyse *f*.
anterior pituitary hormone Hormon *nt* der Adenohypophyse, (Hypophysen-)Vorderlappenhormon *nt*, HVL-Hormon *nt*.
anterior pituitary-like substance Choriongonadotropin *nt abbr.* CG.
anterior pituitary system Hypophysenvorderlappensystem *nt*, HVL-System *nt*.
anterior pole: a. of eyeball vorderer Augenpol *m*, Polus anterior bulbi oculi.
 a. of lens vorderer Linsenpol *m*, Polus anterior lentis.
anterior poliomyelitis Poliomyelitis anterior.
 acute a. (epidemische/spinale) Kinderlähmung *f*, Heine-Medin-Krankheit *f*, Poliomyelitis (epidemica) anterior acuta.
anterior posterior bronchus Bronchus anterior posterior.
anterior pouch of Tröltsch Rec. (membranae tympanicae) anterior.
anterior process of malleus vorderer Hammerfortsatz *m*, Proc. anterior mallei.
anterior recess of tympanic membrane vordere Schleimhauttasche *f* des Trommelfells, Rec. (membranae tympanicae) anterior.

anterior region of neck vorderes Halsdreieck *nt*, Regio cervicalis anterior, Trigonum cervicale anterius.
anterior rhinoscopy vordere Rhinoskopie *f*, Rhinoscopia anterior.
anterior rhizotomy *neurochir.* Rhizotomia anterior.
anterior root (of spinal nerves) vordere/motorische Spinalnervenwurzel *f*, *inf.* Vorderwurzel *f*, Radix anterior/motoria/ventralis nn. spinalium.
anterior scleritis Scleritis anterior.
anterior segment (*Lunge*) Vordersegment *nt*, Segmentum anterius [S III].
  inferior a. of kidney Segmentum anterius inferius.
  a. of right lobe of liver Segmentum anterius.
  superior a. of kidney Segmentum anterius superius.
anterior sinuses vordere Siebbeinzellen *pl*, Cellulae/Sinus anteriores.
anterior spinal paralysis (epidemische/spinale) Kinderlähmung *f*, Heine-Medin-Krankheit *f*, Poliomyelitis (epidemica) anterior acuta.
anterior staphyloma Hornhautstaphylom *nt*, Staphyloma anterius.
anterior surface: a. of cornea Hornhautvorderfläche *f*, Facies anterior corneae.
  a. of eyelid äußere/vordere Lidfläche *f*, Facies anterior palpebrarus.
  a. of iris Irisvorderfläche *f*, Facies anterior iridis.
  a. of lens Linsenvorderfläche *f*, Facies anterior lentis.
  a. of sacral bone Facies pelvica (ossis sacri).
  a. of scapula Facies costalis/anterior scapulae.
  a. of uterus Blasenfläche *f* des Uterus, Facies vesicalis uteri.
anterior synechia *ophthal.* vordere Synechie *f*, Synechia anterior.
anterior tibial compartment syndrome Tibialis-anterior-Syndrom *nt*.
anterior tibial sign Tibialis-anterior-Zeichen *nt*.
anterior triangle vorderes Halsdreieck *nt*, Regio cervicalis anterior, Trigonum cervicale anterius.
anterior tubercle: a. of atlas Tuberculum anterius (atlantis).
  a. of cervical vertebrae Tuberculum anterius/caroticum.
  a. of humerus Tuberculum minus (humeri).
  a. of thalamus Tuberculum anterius thalamicum.
anterior urethritis Urethritis anterior.
anterior uveitis *ophthal.* Uveitis anterior.
anterior vein of right ventricle V. ventriculi dextri anterior.
anterior wall: a. of stomach Vorderwand *f* des Magens, Paries anterior ventriculi.
  a. of tympanic cavity vordere Paukenhöhlenwand *f*, Paries caroticus cavitatis tympanicae.
antero- *pref.* vorder-, antero-.
an·ter·o·dor·sal [ˌæntərəʊˈdɔːrsl] *adj* vorne u. dorsal (liegend), anterodorsal.
anterodorsal nucleus of thalamus Nc. anterodorsalis/anterosuperior (thalami).
an·ter·o·ex·ter·nal [ˌ-ɪkˈstɜːrnl] *adj* → anterolateral.
an·ter·o·grade [ˈ-greɪd] *adj* nach vorne gerichtet, nach vorne bewegend, anterograd.
anterograde amnesia anterograde Amnesie *f*.
anterograde block *card.* (*Herz*) anterograder Block *m*.

anterograde conduction *card.* anterograde Erregungsleitung *f*.
an·ter·o·in·fer·i·or [ˌ-ɪnˈfɪərɪər] *adj* vorne u. unten (liegend), anteroinferior.
anteroinferior myocardial infarction Vorderwandspitzeninfarkt *m*.
an·ter·o·in·ter·nal [ˌ-ɪnˈtɜːrnl] *adj* → anteromedial.
an·ter·o·lat·er·al [ˌ-ˈlætərəl] *adj* vorne u. seitlich (liegend), anterolateral.
anterolateral column of spinal cord Seitenstrang *m* (des Rückenmarks), Funiculus lateralis medullae spinalis.
anterolateral cordotomy *neurochir.* Durchtrennung *f* des Tractus spinothalamicus.
anterolateral fontanelle Keilbeinfontanelle *f*, Fonticulus anterolateralis/sphenoidalis.
anterolateral funiculus system Vorderseitenstrangsystem *nt*.
anterolateral myocardial infarction anterolateraler (Myokard-)Infarkt *m*.
anterolateral sulcus: a. of medulla oblongata Vorderseitenfurche *f* der Medulla oblongata, Sulcus anterolateralis/ventrolateralis medullae oblongatae.
  a. of spinal cord Vorderseitenfurche *f* des Rückenmarks, Sulcus anterolateralis/ventrolateralis medullae spinalis.
anterolateral tractotomy *neurochir.* Durchtrennung *f* des Tractus spinothalamicus.
an·ter·o·me·di·al [ˌ-ˈmiːdɪəl, -jəl] *adj* vorne u. medial (liegend), anteromedial.
anteromedial nucleus of thalamus Nc. anteromedialis (thalami).
an·ter·o·me·di·an [ˌ-ˈmiːdɪən] *adj* vorne u. median (liegend), anteromedian.
anteromedian groove: a. of medulla oblongata vordere Mittelfurche *f*, Fissura mediana anterior/ventralis medullae oblongatae.
  a. of spinal cord vordere Rückenmarksfissur *f*, Fissura mediana anterior medullae spinalis.
an·ter·o·pos·te·ri·or [ˌ-pɑˈstɪərɪər] *adj* von vorne nach hinten (verlaufend), anteroposterior.
anteroposterior diameter anteroposteriorer Durchmesser *m*.
anteroposterior radiograph a.p.-Röntgenbild *nt*, a.p.-Aufnahme *f*.
anteroposterior roentgenogram → anteroposterior radiograph.
an·ter·o·sep·tal [ˌ-ˈsɛptəl] *adj* (*Herz*) vor dem Kammerseptum (liegend), anteroseptal.
anteroseptal myocardial infarction anteroseptaler (Myokard-)Infarkt *m*.
an·ter·o·su·pe·ri·or [ˌ-suːˈpɪərɪər] *adj* vorne u. oben (liegend), anterosuperior.
ant·e·rot·ic [æntɪˈrɒtɪk] *n*, *adj* → antaphrodisiac.
an·ter·o·ven·tral [ˌæntərəʊˈvɛntrəl] *adj* vorne u. ventral (liegend), anteroventral.
anteroventral nucleus of thalamus Nc. anteroventralis/anteroinferior (thalami).
an·te·ver·sion [ˌæntɪˈvɜːrʒn] *n* Vorwärtsneigung *f*, Anteversion *f*.
  a. of uterus Vorwärtsneigung/Anteversion der Gebärmutter, Anteversio uteri.
an·te·vert [ˈ-vɜːrt] *vt* nach vorne neigen, antevertieren.
an·te·vert·ed [ˈ-vɜːrtɪd] *adj* nach vorne geneigt, antevertiert.
anteverted hip Coxa antetorta.
an·texed [ænˈtɛkst] *adj* nach vorne gebeugt, anteflektiert.
an·tex·ion [ænˈtɛkʃn] *n* (abnormale) Vorwärtsbeugung *f*.
ant·he·lix [ˌænˈhiːlɪks] *n* → antihelix.

ant·he·lix·plas·ty [æntˌhiːlɪksˈplæstɪ] *n* HNO Anthelixplastik *f*.
ant·hel·min·thic [ˌænθɛlˈmɪnθɪk, ˌænθɛl-] *n, adj* → anthelmintic.
ant·hel·min·tic [ˌ-ˈmɪntɪk] **I** *n* Wurmmittel *nt*, Anthelmintikum *nt*. **II** *adj* gegen Würmer wirkend, wurm(ab)tötend, anthelmintisch.
ant·hem·or·rhag·ic [æntheməˈrædʒɪk] *n, adj* → antihemorrhagic.
an·ther·o·zo·id [ˌænθərəˈzɔɪd, ˈænθərəzɔɪd] *n micro.* Antherozoid *nt*.
ant·her·pet·ic [ˌænθərˈpɛtɪk] *adj* Herpes(infektion) verhindernd *od.* heilend.
an·tho·cy·an·i·din [ˌænθəʊsaɪˈænədɪn] *n* Anthozyanidin *nt*.
an·tho·cy·a·nin [ˌ-ˈsaɪənɪn] *n* Anthozyanin *nt*.
an·tho·pho·bia [ˌ-ˈfəʊbɪə] *n psychia.* Angst *f* vor Blumen, Anthophobie *f*.
an·thra·cene [ˈænθrəsiːn] *n* Anthrazen *nt*, Anthracen *nt*.
an·thrac·ic [ænˈθræsɪk] *adj* Milzbrand/Anthrax betr., Milzbrand-, Anthrax-.
an·thra·coid [ˈænθrəkɔɪd] *adj* **1.** milzbrand-, anthraxähnlich, anthrakoid. **2.** karbunkelähnlich.
an·thra·co·ne·cro·sis [ˌænθrəkəʊnɪˈkrəʊsɪs] *n patho.* Anthrakonekrose *f*.
an·thra·co·sil·i·co·sis [ˌ-kəʊsɪləˈkəʊsɪs] *n* Anthrakosilikose *f*.
an·thra·co·sis [ˌ-ˈkəʊsɪs] *n* Kohlenstaublunge *f*, Anthrakose *f*, Anthracosis pulmonum.
an·thra·cot·ic [ˌ-ˈkɒtɪk] *adj* Kohlenstaublunge/Anthrakose betr., von Anthrakose betroffen, anthrakotisch; durch Kohlestaubpartikel verfärbt.
anthracotic tuberculosis Staublunge *f*, Staublungenerkrankung *f*, Pneumokoniose *f*.
an·thra·lin [ˈænθrəlɪn] *n pharm.* Anthralin *nt*, Dithranol *nt*.
an·thran·i·late synthase [ænˈθrænəleɪt, ˌænθrəˈnɪleɪt, -ɪt] Anthranilatsynthase *f*.
an·thra·nil·ic acid [ˌænθrəˈnɪlɪk] Anthranilsäure *f*, o-Aminobenzoesäure *f*.
an·thra·quin·one [ˌ-kwɪˈnəʊn, -ˈkwɪnəʊn] *n* Anthrachinon *nt*.
an·thra·rob·in [ˌ-ˈrɒbɪn] *n* Anthrarobin *nt*.
an·thrax [ˈænθræks] *n* Milzbrand *m*, Anthrax *m*.
anthrax antiserum *abbr.* **AAS** Milzbrandserum *nt*.
anthrax bacillus Milzbrandbazillus *m*, Bacillus anthracis *f*.
anthrax pneumonia Lungenmilzbrand *m*, Wollsortierer-, Lumpensortierer-, Hadernkrankheit *f*.
anthrax sepsis Milzbrandsepsis *f*.
anthrax spore Milzbrandspore *f*.
anthrax toxin Milzbrandtoxin *nt*.
anthrax vaccine Anthraxvakzine *f*.
an·thro·po·bi·ol·o·gy [ˌænθrəpəʊbaɪˈɒlədʒɪ] *n* Anthropobiologie *f*, biologische Anthropologie *f*.
an·thro·po·cen·tric [ˌ-ˈsɛntrɪk] *adj* anthropozentrisch.
an·thro·po·gen·e·sis [ˌ-ˈdʒɛnəsɪs] *n* Anthropogenese *f*, -genie *f*.
an·thro·pog·e·ny [ˌænθrəˈpɒdʒənɪ] *n* → anthropogenesis.
an·thro·pog·ra·phy [ˌænθrəˈpɒgrəfɪ] *n* Anthropographie *f*.
an·thro·poid [ˈænθrəpɔɪd] *adj* menschenähnlich, anthropoid.
anthropoid apes Menschenaffen *pl*, Anthropoiden *pl*.
anthropoid pelvis anthropoides Becken *nt*.
an·thro·po·ki·net·ics [ˌænθrəpəkɪˈnɛtɪks, -kaɪ-] *pl* Anthropokinetik *f*.

an·thro·po·log·ic [ˌ-'lɑdʒɪk] *adj* Anthropologie betr., anthropologisch.
an·thro·po·log·i·cal [ˌ-'lɑdʒɪkl] *adj* → anthropologic.
an·thro·pol·o·gist [ˌænθrə'pɑlədʒɪst] *n* Anthropologe *m*, -login *f*.
an·thro·pol·o·gy [ˌænθrə'pɑlədʒɪ] *n* Menschenkunde *f*, Anthropologie *f*.
an·thro·pom·e·ter [ˌænθrə'pɑmɪtər] *n* Anthropometer *nt*.
an·thro·po·met·ric [ˌænθrəpə'metrɪk] *adj* Anthropometrie betr., mittels Anthropometrie, anthropometrisch.
an·thro·pom·e·try [ˌænθrə'pɑmətrɪ] *n* Anthropometrie *f*.
an·thro·po·mor·phism [ˌænθrəpə'mɔːrfɪzəm] *n* Anthropomorphismus *m*.
an·thro·po·phil·ic [ˌ-'fɪlɪk] *adj* anthropophil.
an·thro·po·pho·bia [ˌ-'fəʊbɪə] *n psychia.* Menschenscheu *f*, Anthropophobie *f*.
an·thro·pos·o·phy [ˌænθrə'pɑsəfɪ] *n* Anthroposophie *f*.
an·thro·po·zo·o·no·sis [ˌænθrəpəˌzəʊə'nəʊsɪs] *n* Anthropozoonose *f*, Zooanthroponose *f*.
an·thro·po·zo·o·phil·ic [ˌ-ˌzəʊə'fɪlɪk] *adj* anthropozoophil.
ant·hys·ter·ic [ænthɪs'terɪk] *n, adj* → antihysteric.
anti- *pref.* un-, nicht-, Gegen-, Ant(i)-.
an·ti·a·bor·tion·ist [ˌæntɪə'bɔːrʃənɪst, ˌæntaɪ-] *n* Abtreibungsgegner(in *f*) *m*.
anti-acetylcholine receptor antibodies Acetylcholin-Rezeptor-Antikörper *pl*.
anti-AChR *n* → anti-acetylcholine receptor antibodies.
an·ti·a·chro·mo·trich·ia factor [ˌ-eɪkrəʊmə'trɪkɪə] Pantothensäure *f*, Vitamin B₃ *nt*.
an·ti·ac·id [ˌ-'æsɪd] *n* → antacid.
an·ti·ac·ro·dyn·ia factor [ˌ-ˌækrəʊ'dɪnɪə] Pyridoxin *nt*, Vitamin B₆ *nt*.
an·ti·ad·re·ner·gic [ˌ-ˌædrə'nɜrdʒɪk] **I** *n* Adrenalinantagonist *m*, Antiadrenergikum *nt*, Sympatholytikum *nt*. **II** *adj* antiadrenerg, sympatholytisch.
an·ti·ag·glu·ti·nin [ˌ-ə'gluːtnɪn] *n* Antiagglutinin *nt*.
an·ti·al·bu·min [ˌ-æl'bjuːmən] *n* Antialbumin *nt*.
an·ti·a·lex·in [ˌ-ə'leksɪn] *n* → anticomplement.
an·ti·al·ler·gic [ˌ-ə'lɜrdʒɪk] **I** *n* Antiallergikum *nt*. **II** *adj* gegen Allergie gerichtet, antiallergisch.
an·ti·a·lo·pe·cia factor [ˌ-ælə'piːʃɪə] → inositol.
an·ti·a·me·bic [ˌ-ə'miːbɪk] **I** *n* gegen Amöben wirkendes Mittel *nt*, Amöbenmittel *nt*. **II** *adj* gegen Amöben wirkend; amöbentötend, amöbizid.
an·ti·am·y·lase [ˌ-'æmɪleɪz] *n* Antiamylase *f*.
an·ti·an·a·bol·ic [ˌ-ænə'bɑlɪk] *adj* antianabol.
an·ti·an·a·phy·lac·tic [ˌ-ˌænəfɪ'læktɪk] *adj* antianaphylaktisch.
an·ti·an·a·phy·lax·is [ˌ-ˌænəfɪ'læksɪs] *n* Antianaphylaxie *f*.
an·ti·an·dro·gen [ˌ-'ændrədʒən] *n* Antiandrogen *nt*.
an·ti·a·ne·mic [ˌ-ə'niːmɪk] **I** *n* antianämische Substanz *f*. **II** *adj* gegen Anämie gerichtet, antianämisch.
antianemic factor Zyano-, Cyanocobalamin *nt*, Vitamin B₁₂ *nt*.
an·ti·an·ti·bod·y [ˌ-'æntɪbɑdɪ] *n* Anti-Antikörper *m*.
an·ti·an·ti·dote [ˌ-'æntɪdəʊt] *n* Antiantidot *nt*.
anti-antigen antibody Anti-Antigenantikörper *m*.

an·ti·an·ti·tox·in [ˌ-æntɪ'tɑksɪn] *n* Anti-Antitoxin *nt*, Antitoxinantikörper *m*.
an·ti·anx·i·e·ty agent [ˌ-æŋ'zaɪətɪ] angstlösendes Mittel *nt*, Anxiolytikum *nt*.
an·ti·anx·ious [ˌæntɪ'æŋ(k)ʃəs, ˌæntaɪ-] *adj* angstlösend, -lindernd, anxiolytisch.
an·ti·ap·o·plec·tic [ˌ-æpə'plektɪk] *adj* antiapoplektisch.
an·ti·ar·rhyth·mic [ˌ-ə'rɪðmɪk] **I** *n* Antiarrhythmikum *nt*. **II** *adj* antiarrhythmisch.
antiarrhythmic agent/drug → antiarrhythmic I.
an·ti·ar·thrit·ic [ˌ-ɑːr'θrɪtɪk] *n, adj* → antarthritic.
an·ti·asth·mat·ic [ˌ-æz'mætɪk] *n, adj* → antasthmatic.
an·ti·ath·er·o·gen·ic [ˌ-ˌæθərəʊ'dʒenɪk] *adj* antiatherogen.
an·ti·au·tol·y·sin [ˌ-ɔː'tɑləsɪn] *n* Antiautolysin *nt*.
an·ti·bac·te·ri·al [ˌ-bæk'tɪərɪəl] **I** *n* antibakteriell-wirkende Substanz *f*. **II** *adj* gegen Bakterien (wirkend), antibakteriell.
antibacterial chemotherapy antibakterielle Chemotherapie *f*.
antibacterial immunity antibakterielle Immunität *f*.
anti-basement membrane glomerulonephritis Antibasalmembran-Glomerulonephritis *f*.
anti-basement membrane nephritis Anti-Glomerulusbasalmembranantikörper-Nephritis *f*.
an·ti·bech·ic [ˌ-'bekɪk] **I** *n* hustenstillendes Mittel *nt*, Hustenmittel *nt*, Antitussivum *nt*. **II** *adj* hustenlindernd, -stillend, antitussiv.
an·ti·ber·i·ber·i [ˌ-'berɪberɪ] *n* Thiamin *nt*, Vitamin B₁ *nt*.
antiberiberi factor/substance → antiberiberi.
an·ti·bi·o·gram [ˌ-'baɪəgræm] *n* Antibiogramm *nt*.
an·ti·bi·ont [ˌ-'baɪɑnt] *n* Antibiont *m*.
an·ti·bi·o·sis [ˌ-baɪ'əʊsɪs] *n* Antibiose *f*.
an·ti·bi·ot·ic [ˌæntɪbaɪ'ɑtɪk, -bɪ-, ˌæntaɪ-] **I** *n* Antibiotikum *nt*. **II** *adj* antibiotisch.
antibiotic-associated colitis *abbr.* **AAC** antibiotika-assoziierte Kolitis/Colitis *f abbr.* AAC, postantibiotische Enterokolitis *f*.
antibiotic-associated diarrhea/enterocolitis → antibiotic-associated colitis.
antibiotic-induced *adj* durch Antibiotika verursacht *od.* hervorgerufen, antibiotikainduziert.
antibiotic prophylaxis Antibiotikaprophylaxe *f*.
antibiotic resistance Antibiotikaresistenz *f*.
antibiotic-resistant *adj* antibiotikaresistent.
antibiotic sensitivity test Antibiotikasensibilitätstest *m*.
antibiotic therapy Antibiotikatherapie *f*, antibiotische Therapie *f*.
an·ti·bi·o·tin [ˌ-'baɪətɪn] *n* Antibiotin *nt*, Avidin *nt*.
anti-black-tongue factor Niacin *nt*, Nikotin-, Nicotinsäure *f*.
an·ti·blas·tic [ˌ-'blæstɪk] *adj* antiblastisch.
an·ti·bod·y [ˌ-'bɑdɪ] *n, pl* **-bod·ies** *abbr.* **Ab** Antikörper *m abbr.* AK, Ak (to).
  a. to HAV Anti-HAV *nt*, Antikörper gegen HAV.
  a. to HB꜀Ag Anti-HB꜀ *nt*, Antikörper gegen HB꜀Ag.
  a. to HBₑAg Anti-HBₑ *nt*, Antikörper gegen HBₑAg.
  a. to HBₛAg Anti-HBₛ *nt*, Antikörper gegen HBₛAg.
  a. to HDAg Anti-Delta *nt*, Anti-HD *nt*,
Antikörper gegen HDAg.
antibody deficiency disease/syndrome Antikörpermangelsyndrom *nt abbr.* AMS.
antibody-dependent cell-mediated cytotoxicity *abbr.* **ADCC** antikörperabhängige zellvermittelte Zytotoxizität *f*, antibody-dependent cell-mediated/cellular cytotoxicity *abbr.* ADCC.
antibody-dependent cellular cytotoxicity → antibody-dependent cell-mediated cytotoxicity.
antibody excess Antikörperüberschuß *m*.
antibody immunodeficiency Immundefekt *m* mit mangelhafter Antikörperbildung, B-Zell-Immundefekt *m*.
antibody-mediated rejection *immun.* antikörpervermittelte Abstoßung *f*.
antibody test, heterophil 1. Paul-Bunnell-Test *m*. **2.** modifizierter Paul-Bunnell-Test *m* mit Pferdeerythrozyten.
antibody titer Antikörpertiter *m*.
an·ti·bra·chi·um [ˌ-'breɪkɪəm] *n* → antebrachium.
an·ti·bro·mic [ˌ-'brəʊmɪk] **I** *n* de(s)odorierendes/de(s)odorisierendes Mittel *nt*, Desodorans *nt*, Deodorant *nt*. **II** *adj* geruchtilgend, de(s)odorierend, de(s)odorisierend.
an·ti·ca·chec·tic [ˌ-kə'kektɪk] **I** *n* Kachexie verhinderndes *od.* linderndes Mittel *nt*. **II** *adj* Kachexie verhindernd *od.* lindernd.
an·ti·can·cer [ˌ-'kænsər] *adj* antineoplastisch.
anticancer agent antineoplastische Substanz *f*.
anticancer drug → anticancer agent.
anticancer drug therapy zytostatische/antineoplastische Chemotherapie *f*.
an·ti·car·cin·o·gen [ˌ-kɑːr'sɪnədʒən] *n* antikarzinogene Substanz *f*, Antikarzinogen *nt*.
an·ti·car·cin·o·gen·ic [ˌ-kɑrsɪnə'dʒenɪk] *adj* antikarzinogen.
an·ti·car·di·um [ˌ-'kɑːrdɪəm] *n* → antecardium.
an·ti·car·i·o·gen·ic [ˌ-ˌkeərɪə'dʒenɪk] *adj* anticarious.
an·ti·car·i·ous [ˌ-'keərɪəs] *adj chir., dent.* antikariös.
an·ti·cat·a·lyst [ˌ-'kætlɪst] *n* Antikatalysator *m*.
an·ti·cat·a·lyz·er [ˌ-'kætlaɪzər] *n* → anticatalyst.
an·ti·cath·ode [ˌ-'kæθəʊd] *n phys.* Antikathode *f*.
an·ti·ceph·a·lal·gic [ˌ-ˌsefə'lældʒɪk] *adj pharm.* Kopfschmerz(en) heilend *od.* verhindernd.
an·ti·chlo·rot·ic [ˌ-klɔː'rɑtɪk, -kləʊ-] *adj* antichlorotisch.
an·ti·cho·les·ter·e·mic [ˌ-kəˌlestə'riːmɪk] *n* Cholesterinspiegel-senkendes Mittel *nt*, Cholesterinsenker *m*. **II** *adj* Cholesterinspiegel-senkend.
an·ti·cho·les·ter·ol·e·mic [ˌ-kəˌlestərə'liːmɪk] *n, adj* → anticholesteremic.
an·ti·cho·lin·er·gic [ˌ-ˌkəʊlə'nɜrdʒɪk, -ˌkɑl-] **I** *n* Anticholinergikum *nt*, Parasympath(ik)olytikum *nt*. **II** *adj* anticholinerg, parasympatholytisch.
an·ti·cho·lin·es·ter·ase [ˌ-ˌkəʊlə'nestəreɪz, -ˌkɑlə-] *n* (Acetyl-)Cholinesterasehemmer *m*, -inhibitor *m*.
an·tic·i·pate [æn'tɪsəpeɪt] *vt* **1.** erwarten. **2.** vorausberechnen, vorhersehen, ahnen. **3.** zuvorkommen.
an·tic·i·pa·tion [æn-ˌtɪsə'peɪʃn] *n* **1.** Erwartung *f*, Hoffnung *f*. **2.** Vorweg-, Vorausnahme *f*. **3.** (Vor-)Ahnung *f*, Vorgefühl *nt*, Voraussicht *f*.
an·tic·i·pa·tive [æn'tɪsəpeɪtɪv, -pətɪv] *adj* **1.**

→ anticipatory. **2.** ahnungsvoll, vorausahnend; erwartungsvoll.
an·tic·i·pa·to·ry [æn'tɪsəpə,tɔʊrɪ, -,tɔː-] *adj* vorgreifend, vorwegnehmend, erwartend.
anticipatory hypertension Erwartungshypertonie *f*.
anticipatory response Erwartungsreaktion *f*.
an·ti·cli·max [,-'klaɪmæks] *n* Antiklimax *f*.
an·ti·clock·wise [,æntɪ'klɑkwaɪz] *adj*, *adv* gegen den Uhrzeigersinn/die Uhrzeigerrichtung, nach links.
an·tic·ne·mi·on [,æntɪk'niːmɪɑn, -ɔʊn] *n* Schienbein(region *f*) *nt*.
an·ti·co·ag·u·lant [,-kɔʊ'ægjələnt] **I** *n* gerinnungshemmende Substanz *f*, Antikoagulans *nt*, Antikoagulantium *nt*. **II** *adj* gerinnungshemmend, antikoagulierend.
anticoagulant citrate phosphate dextrose solution *hema*. CPD-Stabilisator *m*.
anticoagulant therapy Antikoagulantientherapie *f*.
an·ti·co·ag·u·lat·ed blood [,-kɔʊ'ægjəleɪt-ɪd] mit Antikoagulantien versetztes Blut, antikoaguliertes Blut *nt*.
an·ti·co·ag·u·la·tion [,-kɔʊ,ægjə'leɪʃn] *n* Antikoagulation *f*.
an·ti·co·ag·u·la·tive [,-kɔʊ'ægjəleɪtɪv] *adj* die Blutgerinnung verhindernd, gerinnungshemmend, antikoagulierend.
an·ti·co·don [,-'kɔʊdɑn] *n* Antikodon *nt*, -codon *nt*.
anticodon arm *biochem*. Antikodonarm *m*.
anticodon triplet Antikodontriplett *nt*.
an·ti·col·lag·en·ase [,-'kɑlædʒneɪz] *n* Antikollagenase *f*.
an·ti·co·lon antibody [,-'kɔʊlən] Antikolon-Antikörper *m*.
an·ti·com·ple·ment [,-'kɑmpləmənt] *n* gegen Komplement wirkende Substanz *f*, Antikomplement *nt*.
an·ti·com·ple·men·ta·ry [,-,kɑmplə'mentərɪ] *adj* antikomplementär (wirkend).
anticomplementary serum Antikomplementserum *n*.
an·ti·con·cep·tive [,-kən'septɪv] *adj* empfängnisverhütend, kontrazeptiv, antikonzeptionell.
an·ti·con·cip·i·ens [,-kən'sɪpɪəns] *n* Verhütungsmittel *nt*, Kontrazeptivum *nt*, Antikonzeptivum *nt*.
an·ti·con·vul·sant [,-kən'vʌlsənt] **I** *n* krampflösendes *od*. -verhinderndes Mittel *nt*, Antikonvulsivum *nt*. **II** *adj* krampflösend, -verhindernd, antikonvulsiv.
an·ti·con·vul·sive [,-kən'vʌlsɪv] *n*, *adj* → anticonvulsant.
an·ti·cu·ra·re [,-k(j)ʊə'rɑːrɪ] *n* Kurareantagonist *m*, Antikurare *nt*.
an·ti·cy·tol·y·sin [,-saɪ'tɑləsɪn] *n* Antizytolysin *nt*, -cytolysin *nt*.
an·ti·cy·to·tox·in [,-saɪtə'tɑksɪn] *n* Antizytotoxin *nt*.
anti-D *n hema*. Anti-D(-Antikörper *m*) *nt*.
anti-delta *n* Anti-Delta *nt*, Anti-HD *nt*, Antikörper *m* gegen HDAg.
an·ti·de·pres·sant [,-dɪ'presənt] **I** *n* Antidepressivum *nt*. **II** *adj* Depression(en) verhindernd *od*. lindernd, antidepressiv.
an·ti·di·a·bet·ic [,-daɪə'betɪk] **I** *n* Antidiabetikum *nt*. **II** *adj* antidiabetisch.
antidiabetic agent Antidiabetikum *nt*.
antidiabetic drug → antidiabetic agent.
an·ti·di·a·be·to·gen·ic [,-,daɪəbɪtə'dʒenɪk] **I** *n* Diabetesentwicklung verhindernde Substanz *f*. **II** *adj* Diabetesentwicklung verhindernd, antidiabetogen.

an·ti·di·ar·rhe·al [,-daɪə'rɪəl] **I** *n* Antidiarrhoikum *nt*. **II** *adj* antidiarrhoisch.
antidiarrheal agent → antidiarrheal I.
an·ti·di·ar·rhe·ic [,-daɪə'riːɪk] *n*, *adj* → antidiarrheal.
an·ti·di·ar·rhet·ic [,-daɪə'retɪk] *n*, *adj* → antidiarrheal.
an·ti·dip·ti·cum [,-'dɪptɪkəm] *n* durstverminderndes Mittel *nt*.
an·ti·di·u·re·sis [,-daɪə'riːsɪs] *n* Antidiurese *f*.
an·ti·di·u·ret·ic [,-daɪə'retɪk] **I** *n* Antidiuretikum *nt*. **II** *adj* antidiuretisch.
antidiuretic hormone *abbr*. **ADH** antidiuretisches Hormon *nt abbr*. ADH, Vasopressin *nt*.
antidiuretic phase antidiuretische Phase *f*, antidiuretisches Stadium *nt*.
antidiuretic substance → antidiuretic hormone.
anti-DNA antibody Anti-DNA-Antikörper *m*.
anti-DNase *n* Anti-DNase *f*.
an·ti·do·nor antibody [,-'dɔʊnər] Antispender-Antikörper *m*.
an·ti·dot·al [,-'dɔʊtl] *adj* Antidot betr., als Gegengift wirkend, Gegengift-, Antidot-.
an·ti·dote ['-dɔʊt] **I** *n* Gegengift *nt*, -mittel *nt*, Antidot *nt*, -dotum *nt* (*to, against* gegen). **II** *vt* ein Gegengift verabreichen *od*. anwenden; ein Gift neutralisieren.
an·ti·dot·ic [,-'dɑtɪk] *adj* → antidotal.
an·ti·dot·i·cal [,-'dɑtɪkl] *adj* → antidotal.
an·ti·drom·ic [,-'drɑmɪk] *adj physiol*. gegenläufig, antidrom.
an·ti·dys·en·ter·ic [,-dɪsən'terɪk] **I** *n pharm*. Antidysenterikum *nt*. **II** *adj* Dysenterie verhütend *od*. lindernd *od*. heilend, antidysenterisch.
an·ti·dys·rhyth·mic [,dɪs'rɪðmɪk] *n*, *adj* → antiarrhythmic.
an·ti·e·dem·a·tous [,-ɪ'demətəs, -ɪ'diː-] *n*, *adj* → antiedemic.
an·ti·e·dem·ic [,-ɪ'diːmɪk] **I** *n* Ödem(e) verhütendes *od*. linderndes Mittel *nt*. **II** *adj* Ödem(e) verhindernd *od*. lindernd.
anti-egg white factor Biotin *nt*, Vitamin H *nt*.
an·ti·e·met·ic [,-ə'metɪk] **I** *n* Ant(i)emetikum *nt*. **II** *adj* antiemetisch.
antiemetic agent Ant(i)emetikum *nt*.
an·ti·en·zyme [,-'enzaɪm] *n* Antienzym *nt*, Antiferment *nt*.
an·ti·ep·i·lep·tic [,-epɪ'leptɪk] **I** *n* Antiepileptikum *nt*. **II** *adj* antiepileptisch.
an·ti·e·rot·i·ca [,-ɪ'rɑtɪkə] *pl* An(ti)aphrodisiaka *pl*.
an·ti·es·ter·ase [,-'estəreɪz] *n* Antiesterase *f*.
an·ti·es·tro·gen [,-'estrədʒən] **I** *n* Antiöstrogen *nt*, Östrogenhemmer *m*, -antagonist *m*. **II** *adj* Östrogen(wirkung) hemmend, antiöstrogen, Antiöstrogen-.
an·ti·es·tro·gen·ic [,-,estrə'dʒenɪk] *adj* antiestrogen II.
an·ti·fe·brile [,æntɪ'fiːbrɪl, -feb-, ,æntaɪ-] *adj* → antipyretic.
an·ti·fe·brin [,-'febrɪn] *n* Azet-, Acetanilid *nt*, Phenylacetamid *nt*.
an·ti·fer·ment [,-'fɜrmənt] *n* → antienzyme.
an·ti·fi·bril·la·to·ry [,-'faɪbrɪlətɔːrɪ, -təʊ-] **I** *n* Antifibrillans *nt*, -fibrillantium *nt*. **II** *adj* antifibrillant.
an·ti·fi·bri·nol·y·sin [,-,faɪbrə'nɑləsɪn] *n* Antifibrinolysin *nt abbr*. AFL; Antiplasmin *nt*.
antifibrinolysin test Antifibrinolysintest *m abbr*. AFT.
an·ti·fi·bri·no·lyt·ic [,-,faɪbrənɔʊ'lɪtɪk] *adj* antifibrinolytisch.

antifibrinolytic agent Antifibrinolytikum *nt*.
an·ti·fi·lar·i·al [,-fɪ'leərɪəl] **I** *n* gegen Filarien wirkendes Mittel *nt*, Filarienmittel *nt*. **II** *adj* gegen Filarien wirkend, filarientend.
an·ti·fol ['-fɔʊl] *n* Folsäureantagonist *m*.
an·ti·fo·late [,-'fɔʊleɪt] *n* Folsäureantagonist *m*.
an·ti·freeze ['-friːz] *n chem*., *techn*. Gefrierschutz-, Frostschutzmittel *nt*.
antifreeze protein Anti-Frier-Protein *nt*, Anti-Frost-Protein *nt*.
an·ti·fun·gal [,-'fʌŋgəl] **I** *n* Antimykotikum *nt*. **II** *adj* gegen Pilze/Fungi wirkend, antimykotisch, antifungal.
an·ti·ga·lac·ta·gogue [,-gə'læktəgɔg, -gɑg] *n* → antigalactic I.
an·ti·ga·lac·tic [,-gə'læktɪk] **I** *n* in den Milchfluß verminderndes Mittel *nt*. **II** *adj* den Milchfluß/die Milchabscheidung vermindernd.
anti-GBM antibody → anti-glomerular basement membrane antibody.
anti-GBM antibody disease → anti-basement membrane nephritis.
anti-GBM antibody nephritis → anti-basement membrane nephritis.
anti-GBM glomerulonephritis → anti-basement membrane glomerulonephritis.
an·ti·gen ['æntɪdʒən] *n abbr*. **Ag** Antigen *nt abbr*. AG, Ag.
antigen-antibody complex *abbr*. **AAC** Antigen-Antikörper-Komplex *m abbr*. AAK, Immunkomplex *m abbr*. IK, IC.
antigen-antibody reaction Antigen-Antikörper-Reaktion *f abbr*. AAR.
antigen-binding capacity *abbr*. **ABC** Antigenbindungskapazität *f*, antigen-binding capacity *abbr*. ABC.
antigen binding fragment antigenbindendes Fragment *nt*, Fab(-Fragment *nt*) *nt*.
antigen binding site Antigenbindungsstelle *f*.
antigen-dependent *adj* antigenabhängig.
an·ti·ge·ne·mia [,æntɪdʒə'niːmɪə] *n* Antigenämie *f*.
an·ti·ge·ne·mic [,-'niːmɪk] *adj* Antigenämie betr.
antigen excess Antigenüberschuß *m*.
an·ti·gen·ic [,æntɪ'dʒenɪk] *adj* Antigeneigenschaften besitzend, antigen, Antigen-.
antigenic component antigene Komponente *f*.
antigenic determinant Epitop *nt*, antigene Determinante *f*, Antigendeterminante *f*.
idiotypic a. Idiotyp *m*.
antigenic drift *micro*. Antigendrift *f*, antigenic drift.
antigenic formula Antigenformel *f*.
an·ti·ge·nic·i·ty [,æntɪdʒə'nɪsətɪ] *n* Antigenität *f*.
antigenic pattern Antigenmuster *nt*.
antigenic profile Antigenprofil *nt*.
antigenic property Antigeneigenschaft *f*.
antigenic shift Antigenshift *f*, antigenic shift.
antigenic structure Antigenstruktur *f*.
antigenic variation Antigenwechsel *m*, -variation *f*.
antigen-independent *adj* antigenunabhängig.
antigen matching Antigenmatching *nt*.
antigen presentation *immun*. Antigenpräsentation *f*.
antigen-reactive cell antigen-reaktive Zelle *f*, antigen-reaktiver Lymphozyt *m*.
antigen receptor Antigenrezeptor *m*.
antigen recognition Antigenerkennung *f*.

antigen-responsive cell → antigen-reactive cell.
antigen-sensitive cell → antigen-reactive cell.
antigen-specific *adj* antigenspezifisch.
antigen-stimulated *adj* antigenstimuliert.
antigen unit Antigeneinheit *f*.
antigen-unspecific *adj* antigenunspezifisch.
an·ti·glob·u·lin [ˌæntɪˈglʌbjəlɪn, ˌantaɪ-] *n* Antiglobulin *nt*.
antiglobulin consumption test *abbr*. **AGCT** Antiglobulin-Konsumptionstest *m abbr*. AGKT, AGK-Test *m*.
antiglobulin test *abbr*. **AGT** Antiglobulintest *m*, Coombs-Test *m*.
direct a. direkter Coombs-Test.
indirect a. indirekter Coombs-Test.
anti-glomerular basement membrane antibody (*Niere*) Antibasalmembranantikörper *m*.
anti-glomerular basement membrane antibody disease Anti-Glomerulusbasalmembranantikörper-Nephritis *f*.
an·ti·goi·tro·gen·ic [ˌ-ˌgɔɪtrəˈdʒenɪk] *adj* die Strumaentwicklung hemmend *od.* verhindernd, antistrumigen.
an·ti·gon·a·do·trop·ic [ˌ-ˌgɑnədəʊˈtrɑpɪk, -ˈtrəʊ-] *adj* gonadotrope Hormone hemmend, antigonadotrop.
an·ti·graft antibody [ˈgræft] Antitransplantat-Antikörper *m*.
anti-HAV *n* Anti-HAV *nt*, Antikörper *m* gegen HAV.
anti-HB$_C$ *n* Anti-HB$_C$ *nt*, Antikörper *m* gegen HB$_C$Ag.
anti-HB$_e$ *n* Anti-HB$_e$ *nt*, Antikörper *m* gegen HB$_e$Ag.
anti-HB$_S$ *n* Anti-HB$_S$ *nt*, Antikörper *m* gegen HB$_S$Ag.
anti-HD *n* Anti-Delta *nt*, Anti-HD *nt*, Antikörper *m* gegen HDAg.
an·ti·he·lix [ˌ-ˈhiːlɪks] *n*, *pl* **-lix·es**, **-hel·i·ces** [-ˈhelɪsiːz] Anthelix *f*.
an·ti·hel·min·tic [ˌ-helˈmɪnθɪk] *n*, *adj* → anthelmintic.
an·ti·he·mag·glu·ti·nin [ˌ-ˌhiːməˈgluːtənɪn] *n* Antihämagglutinin *nt*.
an·ti·he·mol·y·sin [ˌ-hɪˈmɑləsɪn] *n* Antihämolysin *nt*.
an·ti·he·mo·ly·tic [ˌ-ˌhiːməˈlɪtɪk, ˌhem-] *adj* gegen Hämolyse wirkend, antihämolytisch.
an·ti·he·mo·phil·ic [ˌ-ˌhiːməˈfɪlɪk, ˌhem-] *adj* antihämophil.
antihemophilic factor (A) *abbr*. **AHF** → antihemophilic globulin.
antihemophilic factor B Faktor IX *m abbr*. F IX, Christmas-Faktor *m*, Autothrombin II *nt*.
antihemophilic factor C Faktor X *m abbr*. F X, Stuart-Prower-Faktor *m*, Autothrombin III *nt*.
antihemophilic globulin *abbr*. **AHG** antihämophiles Globulin *nt abbr*. AHG, Antihämophiliefaktor *m abbr*. AHF, Faktor VIII *m abbr*. F VIII.
antihemophilic human plasma antihämophiles Plasma *nt abbr*. AHP.
an·ti·hem·or·rhag·ic [ˌ-ˌheməˈrædʒɪk] **I** *n* blutstillendes Mittel *nt*, Antihämorrhagikum *nt*, Hämostatikum *nt*, Hämostyptikum *nt*. **II** *adj* blutstillend, antihämorrhagisch, hämostatisch, hämostyptisch.
antihemorrhagic factor Phyllochinone *pl*, Vitamin K *nt*.
antihemorrhagic vitamin → antihemorrhagic factor.
an·ti·hep·a·rin [ˌ-ˈhepərɪn] *n* Plättchenfaktor 4 *m abbr*. PF$_4$, Antiheparin *nt*.
an·ti·het·er·ol·y·sin [ˌ-hetəˈrɑləsɪn] *n* Antiheterolysin *nt*.

an·ti·hi·drot·ic [ˌ-haɪˈdrɑtɪk, -hɪ-] *n*, *adj* → antiperspirant.
an·ti·his·ta·mine [ˌ-ˈhɪstəmiːn, -mɪn] *n* → antihistaminic I.
an·ti·his·ta·min·ic [ˌ-hɪstəˈmɪnɪk] **I** *n* Antihistaminikum *nt*, Antihistamin *nt*, Histaminantagonist *m*. **II** *adj* antihistaminisch.
an·ti·hor·mone [ˌ-ˈhɔːrməʊn] *n* Hormonblocker *m*, -antagonist *m*, Antihormon *nt*.
anti-human globulin test → antiglobulin test.
an·ti·hy·a·lu·ron·i·dase [ˌ-ˌhaɪəlʊˈrɑnɪdeɪz] *n abbr*. **AHD** Antihyaluronidase *f*, Hyaluronidasehemmer *m*, -antagonist *m*.
antihyaluronidase test Antihyaluronidase-Test *m abbr*. AHT.
antihyaluronidase unit Antihyaluronidase-Einheit *f abbr*. AHE.
an·ti·hy·drot·ic [ˌ-haɪdrɪˈɑtɪk] *n*, *adj* → antiperspirant.
an·ti·hy·per·ten·sive [ˌ-ˌhaɪpərˈtensɪv] **I** *n* blutdrucksenkendes Mittel *nt*, Antihypertonikum *nt*, -hypertensivum *nt*. **II** *adj* blutdrucksenkend, antihypertensiv, -hypertonisch.
antihypertensive agent → antihypertensive I.
an·ti·hys·ter·ic [ˌ-hɪsˈterɪk] **I** *n* Antihysterikum *nt*. **II** *adj* Hysterie lindernd *od.* verhütend.
anti-icteric *adj* Ikterus lindernd *od.* verhindernd, antiikterisch.
anti-idiotypic antibody Anti-Idiotypenantikörper *m*.
anti-infectious *n*, *adj* → anti-infective.
anti-infective I *n* infektionsverhinderndes Mittel *nt*, Antiinfektiosum *nt*. **II** *adj* infektionsverhindernd, antiinfektiös.
anti-inflammatory I *n* entzündungshemmendes Mittel *nt*, Entzündungshemmer *m*, Antiphlogistikum *nt*. **II** *adj* entzündungshemmend, antiphlogistisch.
anti-insulin antibody Insulinantikörper *m*.
an·ti·ke·to·gen [ˌ-ˈkiːtəʊdʒən] *n* antiketogene Substanz *f*.
an·ti·ke·to·gen·e·sis [ˌ-ˌkiːtəʊˈdʒenəsɪs] *n* Hemmung *f* der Ketonkörperbildung.
an·ti·ke·to·ge·net·ic [ˌ-ˌkiːtəʊdʒəˈnetɪk] *adj* → antiketogenic.
an·ti·ke·to·gen·ic [ˌ-ˌkiːtəʊˈdʒenɪk] *adj* Ketonkörperbildung hemmend, antiketogen.
an·ti·ke·to·plas·tic [ˌ-ˌkiːtəʊˈplæstɪk] *adj* → antiketogenic.
an·ti·ki·nase [ˌ-ˈkaɪneɪz, -ˈkɪ-] *n* Kinasehemmer *m*, -antagonist *m*, Antikinase *f*.
an·ti·ki·ne·sis [ˌ-kɪˈniːsɪs, -kaɪ-] *n* Antikinese *f*.
an·ti·lac·tase [ˌ-ˈlækteɪz] *n* Laktase-, Lactasehemmer *m*, Antilaktase *f*.
an·ti·leish·man·i·al [ˌ-liːʃˈmænɪəl] **I** *n* gegen Leishmanien wirkendes Mittel *nt*, Leishmanienmittel *nt*. **II** *adj* gegen Leishmanien wirkend; leishmanientötend.
an·ti·lep·rot·ic [ˌ-lepˈrɑtɪk] **I** *n* Antileprotikum *nt*. **II** *adj* gegen Lepra wirkend.
an·ti·leu·ko·ci·din [ˌ-luːˈkɑʊsədɪn] *n* Antileukozidin *nt*, -leukotoxin *nt*.
an·ti·leu·ko·cyt·ic [ˌ-luːkəˈsɪtɪk] *adj* antileukozytär, Antileukozyten-.
an·ti·leu·ko·pro·te·ase [ˌ-ˌluːkəˈprəʊteɪz] *n* Leukoproteasehemmer *m*, Antileukoprotease *f*.
an·ti·leu·ko·tox·in [ˌ-luːkəˈtɑksɪn] *n* → antileukotoxin.
an·ti·lew·is·ite [ˌ-ˈluːɪsaɪt] *n* Dimercaprol *nt*, British antilewisit *nt abbr*. BAL, 2,3-Dimercaptopropanol *nt*.
an·ti·li·pe·mic [ˌ-lɪˈpiːmɪk, -laɪ-] **I** *n* pharm. antilipämisches Substanz *f*, Lipidsenker *m*, Antilipidämikum *f*, Antihyperlipämikum *nt*. **II** *adj* Lipidspiegel senkend, antilipidämisch.
an·ti·lu·et·ic [ˌ-luːˈetɪk] *n*, *adj* → antisyphilitic.
an·ti·lym·pho·cyte antibody [ˌ-ˈlɪmfəsaɪt] Antilymphozyten-Antikörper *m*.
antilymphocyte globulin *abbr*. **ALG** Antilymphozytenglobulin *nt abbr*. ALG.
antilymphocyte serum *abbr*. **ALS** Antilymphozytenserum *nt abbr*. ALS.
an·ti·ly·sin [ˌæntɪˈlaɪsɪn, ˌantaɪ-] *n* Lysinantagonist *m*, Antilysin *nt*.
an·ti·ma·lar·i·al [ˌ-məˈleərɪəl] **I** *n* (Anti-)Malariamittel *nt*. **II** *adj* gegen Malaria wirkend, Antimalaria-.
antimalarial agent/drug → antimalarial I.
an·ti·mere [ˈæntɪmɪər] *n* Antimer(es *nt*) *nt*.
an·ti·mes·en·ter·ic border [ˌæntɪmesənˈterɪk, ˌantaɪ-] dem Mesenterium abgewandte Dünndarmseite *f*.
an·ti·me·tab·o·lite [ˌ-məˈtæbəlaɪt] *n* Antimetabolit *m*.
an·ti·mi·cro·bi·al [ˌ-maɪˈkrəʊbɪəl] **I** *n* antimikrobielles Mittel *nt*; Antibiotikum *nt*. **II** *adj* gegen Mikroorganismen wirkend, antimikrobiell.
antimicrobial agent → antimicrobial I.
antimicrobial chemotherapy antimikrobielle Chemotherapie *f*; Antibiotikatherapie *f*.
an·ti·mi·cro·bic [ˌ-maɪˈkrəʊbɪk] *n*, *adj* old → antimicrobial.
an·ti·mi·cro·so·mal antibody [ˌ-maɪkrəˈsəʊməl] (*Schilddrüse*) mikrosomaler Antikörper *m abbr*. MAK.
an·ti·mi·to·chon·dri·al antibodies [ˌ-maɪtəˈkɑndrɪəl] (Anti-)Mitochondrienantikörper *pl*.
an·ti·mi·tot·ic [ˌ-maɪˈtɑtɪk] **I** *n* Mitosehemmer *m*, Antimitotikum *nt*. **II** *adj* mitosehemmend, antimitotisch.
an·ti·mo·ni·al [ˌ-ˈməʊnɪəl] *adj* Antimon betr. *od.* enthaltend., antimonhaltig, Antimon-.
an·ti·mo·nic [ˌ-ˈməʊnɪk, -ˈmɑnɪk] *adj* fünfwertiges Antimon enthaltend, Antimon-V-.
an·ti·mo·ni·ous [ˌ-ˈməʊnɪəs] *adj* dreiwertiges Antimon enthaltend, Antimon-III-.
an·ti·mo·ni·um [ˌ-ˈməʊnɪəm] *n* → antimony.
an·ti·mo·ny [ˈæntɪməʊnɪ] *n* Antimon *nt*; *chem*. Stibium *nt abbr*. Sb.
antimony chloride Antimonchlorid *nt*.
antimony poisoning Antimonvergiftung *f*.
antimony sodium gluconate Natrium-Stibogluconat *nt*.
anti-Müller-hormone *n embryo*. Anti-Müller-Hormon *nt abbr*. AMH.
an·ti·mus·ca·rin·ic [ˌ-ˌmʌskəˈrɪnɪk, ˌantaɪ-] *adj* gegen Muskarin wirkend, Antimuskarin-.
an·ti·mu·ta·gen [ˌ-ˈmjuːtədʒən] *n* antimutagene Substanz *f*, Antimutagen *nt*.
an·ti·my·co·bac·te·ri·al [ˌ-ˌmaɪkəʊbækˈtɪərɪəl] **I** *n* gegen Mykobakterien wirkendes Mittel *nt*. **II** *adj* gegen Mykobakterien wirkend.
an·ti·my·cot·ic [ˌ-maɪˈkɑtɪk] *adj* gegen Pilze/Fungi wirkend, antimykotisch, antifugal.
an·ti·nar·cot·ic [ˌ-nɑːrˈkɑtɪk] *adj* antinarkotisch.
an·ti·nau·se·ant [ˌ-ˈnɔːzɪənt, -ʃɪ-, -ʒɪ-] **I** *n* gegen Nausea wirkendes Mittel *nt*. **II** *adj* Nausea verhindernd *od.* lindernd.
an·ti·ne·o·plas·tic [ˌ-niːəʊˈplæstɪk] **I** *n* antineoplastische Substanz *f*, Antineoplastikum *nt*. **II** *adj* antineoplastisch.
antineoplastic agent → antineoplastic I.
antineoplastic drug → antineoplastic I.

antineoplastic drug therapy zytostatische/antineoplastische Chemotherapie *f*.
an·ti·ne·phrit·ic [ˌ-nəˈfrɪtɪk] *adj* gegen Nephritis wirkend, antinephritisch.
an·ti·neu·ral·gic [ˌ-nʊˈrældʒɪk, -njʊər-] *adj* antineuralgisch.
antineuralgic agent Antineuralgikum *nt*.
antineuralgic drug → antineuralgic agent.
an·ti·neu·rit·ic [ˌ-n(j)ʊəˈrɪtɪk] *adj* antineuritisch.
antineuritic factor/vitamin Thiamin *nt*, Vitamin B₁ *nt*.
an·ti·neu·ro·tox·in [ˌ-nʊrəˈtɑksɪn, -njʊər-] *n* Neurotoxinantagonist *m*, Antineurotoxin *nt*.
an·ti·neu·tri·no [ˌ-n(j)uːˈtriːnəʊ] *n phys.* Antineutrino *nt*.
an·ti·neu·tron [ˌ-ˈn(j)uːtrən] *n phys.* Antineutron *nt*.
an·ti·nu·cle·ar [ˌ-ˈn(j)uːklɪər] *adj* antinukleär.
antinuclear antibodies *abbr.* **ANA** antinukleäre Antikörper *pl abbr.* ANA.
antinuclear factor *abbr.* **ANF** antinuklearer Faktor *m abbr.* ANF.
an·ti·o·don·tal·gic [ˌ-əʊdanˈtældʒɪk] I *n* Mittel *nt* gegen Zahnschmerz(en), Zahnschmerzmittel *nt*. II *adj* Zahnschmerz(en) lindernd.
an·ti·op·so·nin [ˌ-ˈɑpsənɪn] *n* Opsoninhemmer *m*, Antiopsonin *nt*.
an·ti·ov·u·la·to·ry [ˌ-ˈɑvjələtɔːriː, -təʊ-] *adj* ovulationshemmend, antiovulatorisch.
an·ti·ox·i·dant [ˌ-ˈɑksɪdənt] *n* Antioxydans *nt*.
an·ti·ox·i·dase [ˌ-ˈɑksɪdeɪz] *n* Oxidasehemmer *m*, Antioxidase *f*.
an·ti·ox·y·gen [ˌ-ˈɑksɪdʒən] *n* → antioxidant.
an·ti·par·al·lel [ˌ-ˈpærəlel] *adj* antiparallel.
antiparallel polarity antiparallele Polarität *f*.
an·ti·par·a·lyt·ic [ˌ-pærəˈlɪtɪk] *adj* antiparalytisch.
an·ti·par·a·sit·ic [ˌ-pærəˈsɪtɪk] I *n* gegen Parasiten wirkendes Mittel *nt*, Antiparasitikum *nt*. II *adj* gegen Parasiten wirkend, antiparasitisch.
an·ti·pa·ras·ta·ta [ˌ-pəˈræstətə] *n* Gl. bulbourethralis.
an·ti·par·a·sym·pa·tho·mi·met·ic [ˌ-ˌpærəˌsɪmpəθəʊmɪˈmetɪk, -maɪ-] *adj* antiparasympathomimetisch.
an·ti·par·kin·so·ni·an [ˌ-ˌpɑːrkɪnˈsəʊnɪən] I *n* Antiparkinsonmittel *nt*, Antiparkinsonikum *nt*. II *adj* gegen Parkinson-Krankheit wirkend.
antiparkinsonian agent → antiparkinsonian I.
an·ti·par·ti·cle [ˌ-ˈpɑːrtɪkl] *n phys.* Antiteilchen *nt*.
an·ti·pe·dic·u·lar [ˌ-pɪˈdɪkjələr] *adj* → antipediculotic II.
an·ti·pe·dic·u·lot·ic [ˌ-pɪˌdɪkjəˈlɑtɪk] I *n* Antipedikulosum *nt*, Läusemittel *nt*. II *adj* gegen Läuse wirkend.
an·ti·pel·lag·ra [ˌ-pəˈlægrə] *n* Niacin *nt*, Nikotin-, Nicotinsäure *f*.
antipellagra factor/vitamin → antipellagra.
an·ti·pep·sin [ˌ-ˈpepsɪn] *n* Antipepsin *nt*.
an·ti·pe·ri·od·ic [ˌ-pɪərɪˈɑdɪk] *adj* antiperiodisch.
an·ti·per·i·stal·sis [ˌ-perɪˈstɔːlsɪs, -ˈstæl-] *n* rückläufige Peristaltik *f*, Antiperistaltik *f*.
an·ti·per·i·stal·tic [ˌ-perɪˈstɔːltɪk, -ˈstæl-] I *n* Peristaltik hemmendes Mittel *nt*. II *adj* 1. Antiperistaltik betr. *od.* verursachend, antiperistaltisch. 2. Peristaltik hemmend, antiperistaltisch.
antiperistaltic anastomosis antiperistaltische (Entero-)Anastomose *f*.
anti-pernicious anemia factor Zyano-, Cyanocobalamin *nt*, Vitamin B₁₂ *nt*.
an·ti·per·spi·rant [ˌ-ˈperspɪrənt] I *n* schweißhemmendes Mittel *nt*, Antiperspirant *nt*, -transpirant *nt*, Ant(i)hidrotikum *m*. II *adj* schweißhemmend, ant(i)hidrotisch.
an·ti·phag·o·cyt·ic [ˌ-ˌfægəˈsɪtɪk] *adj* antiphagozytisch, -zytär.
an·ti·phlo·gis·tic [ˌ-fləʊˈdʒɪstɪk] I *n* entzündungshemmendes Mittel *nt*, Entzündungshemmer *m*, Antiphlogistikum *nt*. II *adj* entzündungshemmend, antiphlogistisch.
an·ti·phthi·ri·ac [ˌ-ˈθɪəriæk] *adj pharm.* gegen Läuse wirkend.
an·ti·plas·min [ˌ-ˈplæzmɪn] *n* Antiplasmin *nt*, Antifibrinolysin *nt abbr.* AFL.
an·ti·plas·mo·di·al agent/drug [ˌ-plæzˈməʊdɪəl] gegen Plasmodien wirkendes Mittel *nt*, Antiplasmodikum *nt*.
an·ti·plas·mo·di·an [ˌ-plæzˈməʊdɪən] *adj pharm.* gegen Plasmodien wirkend.
an·ti·plas·tic [ˌ-ˈplæstɪk] I *n pharm.* antiplastische Substanz *f*. II *adj* antiplastisch.
an·ti·plate·let [ˌ-ˈpleɪtlɪt] *adj* gegen Blutplättchen gerichtet, Antithrombozyten-.
antiplatelet antibody Plättchen-, Thrombozytenantikörper *m*.
an·ti·pneu·mo·coc·cal [ˌ-ˌn(j)uːməˈkɑkl] *adj* Pneumokokken hemmend *od.* zerstörend, Anti-Pneumokokken-.
an·ti·pneu·mo·coc·cic [ˌ-ˌn(j)uːməˈkɑksɪk] *adj* → antipneumococcal.
an·tip·o·dal [ænˈtɪpədl] *adj* genau entgegengesetzt, antipodal; antipodisch.
an·ti·port [ˈæntɪpɔːrt, -pəʊrt] *n* Austausch-, Gegen-, Countertransport *m*, Antiport *m*.
an·ti·pre·cip·i·tin [ˌæntɪprɪˈsɪpɪtɪn, ˌantaɪ-] *n* Präzipitinantagonist *m*, Antipräzipitin *nt*.
an·ti·pros·tate [ˌ-ˈprɑsteɪt] *n* Gl. bulbourethralis.
an·ti·pro·te·ase [ˌ-ˈprəʊtɪeɪz] *n* Antiprotease *f*.
an·ti·pro·throm·bin [ˌ-prəʊˈθrɑmbɪn] *adj* gegen Prothrombin wirkend, Antiprothrombin-.
an·ti·pro·to·zo·al [ˌ-ˌprəʊtəˈzəʊəl] I *n* gegen Protozoen wirkendes Mittel *nt*, Antiprotozoenmittel *nt*, Antiprotozoikum *nt*. II *adj* gegen Protozoen wirkend, Antiprotozoen-.
an·ti·pro·to·zo·an [ˌ-ˌprəʊtəˈzəʊən] *n, adj* → antiprotozoal.
an·ti·pru·rit·ic [ˌ-prʊəˈrɪtɪk] I *n* Mittel *nt* gegen Juckreiz, Antipruriginosum *nt*. II *adj* gegen Juckreiz wirkend, antipruriginös.
an·ti·pso·ri·at·ic [ˌ-sɔːrɪˈætɪk] I *n* Mittel *nt* gegen Psoriasis, Antipsorikum *nt*. II *adj* gegen Psoriasis wirkend.
an·ti·psy·chot·ic [ˌ-saɪˈkɑtɪk] *adj* gegen Psychosen wirkend, antipsychotisch.
antipsychotic agent/drug Antipsychotikum *nt*, Neuroleptikum *nt*.
an·ti·py·o·gen·ic [ˌ-paɪəˈdʒenɪk] *adj* Eiterbildung verhindernd, antipyogen.
an·ti·py·re·sis [ˌ-paɪˈriːsɪs] *n* Fieberbekämpfung *f*, Antipyrese *f*.
an·ti·py·ret·ic [ˌ-paɪˈretɪk] I *n* fiebersenkendes Mittel *nt*, Antipyretikum *nt*, Antifebrilium *nt*. II *adj* fiebersenkend, antipyretisch, antifebril.
an·ti·py·rot·ic [ˌ-paɪˈrɑtɪk] I *n* Mittel *nt* zur Behandlung von Brandwunden, Antipyrotikum *nt*. II *adj* gegen Brandwunden wirkend.
an·ti·ra·bies serum [ˌ-ˈreɪbiːz] Tollwut-Immunserum *nt*.
an·ti·ra·chit·ic [ˌ-rəˈkɪtɪk] *adj* antirachitisch.
antirachitic factor Calciferol *nt*, Vitamin D *nt*.
an·ti·re·cep·tor antibody [ˌ-rɪˈseptər] Antirezeptorantikörper *m*.
an·ti·re·flux operation/procedure/surgery [ˌ-ˈriːflʌks] *chir.* Antirefluxoperation *f*, -plastik *f*.
an·ti·re·jec·tion therapy [ˌ-rɪˈdʒekʃn] *chir.* (*Transplantation*) Therapie *f* der Abstoßungsreaktion.
an·ti·ren·net [ˌ-ˈrenɪt] *n* → antirennin.
an·ti·ren·nin [ˌ-ˈrenɪn] *n* Antirennin *nt*.
anti-Rh agglutinin *n* Rh-Agglutinin *nt*, Rhesus-Agglutinin *nt*, Anti-Rh(esus)-Agglutinin *nt*.
an·ti·rheu·mat·ic [ˌ-ruːˈmætɪk] I *n* Rheumamittel *nt*, Antirheumatikum *nt*. II *adj* gegen rheumatische Erkrankungen wirkend, antirheumatisch.
antirheumatic agent/drug → antirheumatic I.
an·ti·rick·ett·si·al [ˌ-rɪˈketsɪəl] I *n* gegen Rickettsien wirkendes Mittel *nt*, Rickettsienmittel *nt*. II *adj* gegen Rickettsien wirkend.
an·ti·schis·to·so·mal [ˌ-ˌʃɪstəˈsəʊml] I *n* gegen Schistosomen wirkendes Mittel *nt*, Schistosomenmittel *nt*. II *adj* gegen Schistosomen wirkend.
an·ti·scor·bu·tic factor/vitamin [ˌ-skɔːrˈbjuːtɪk] Askorbinsäure *f*, Ascorbinsäure *f*, Vitamin C *nt*.
an·ti·seb·or·rhe·ic [ˌ-sebəˈriːɪk] I *n* gegen Seborrhoe wirkendes Mittel *nt*, Antiseborrhoikum *nt*. II *adj* gegen Seborrhoe wirkend, antiseborrhoisch.
an·ti·se·cre·to·ry [ˌ-sɪˈkriːtəri] I *n* antisekretorische/sekretionshemmende Substanz *f*. II *adj* sekretionshemmend, antisekretorisch.
an·ti·sep·sis [ˌ-ˈsepsɪs] *n* Antisepsis *f*, Antiseptik *f*.
an·ti·sep·tic [ˌæntɪˈseptɪk, ˌantaɪ-] *n* antiseptisches Mittel *nt*, Antiseptikum *nt*. II *adj* 1. Verfall *od.* Eiterbildung hemmend, a(nti)septisch. 2. Antisepsis betr., antiseptisch.
antiseptic bath antiseptisches Bad *nt*.
an·ti·sep·ti·cize [ˌ-ˈseptɪsaɪz] *vt* antiseptisch behandeln *od.* machen.
an·ti·se·rum [ˌ-ˈsɪərəm] *n* Immun-, Antiserum *nt*.
antiserum anaphylaxis passive Anaphylaxie *f*.
an·ti·so·cial [ˌ-ˈsəʊʃl] *adj* asozial, gesellschaftsfeindlich.
antisocial behavior antisoziales Verhalten *nt*.
antisocial personality disorder antisoziale Persönlichkeit(sstörung *f*) *f*.
an·ti·spas·mod·ic [ˌ-spæzˈmɑdɪk] I *n* Antispasmodikum *nt*, Spasmolytikum *nt*. II *adj* krampflösend, spasmolytisch.
antispasmodic agent/drug → antispasmodic I.
an·ti·spas·tic [ˌ-ˈspæstɪk] *adj* krampflösend, antispastisch.
an·ti·staph·y·lo·coc·cic [ˌ-ˌstæfɪləˈkɑksɪk] *n* gegen Staphylokokken wirkendes Mittel *nt*. II *adj* gegen Staphylokokken wirkend, Anti-Staphylokokken-.
an·ti·staph·y·lo·he·mol·y·sin [ˌ-ˌstæfɪləhɪˈmɑləsɪn] *n* → antistaphylolysin.
an·ti·staph·y·lol·y·sin [ˌ-stæfəˈlɑləsɪn] *n* Antistaphylolysin *nt abbr.* AStL.
antistaphylolysin reaction Antistaphylolysin-Reaktion *f abbr.* AStR.
antistaphylolysin test Antistaphylolysin-Test *m abbr.* AStT.
antistaphylolysin titer Antistaphylolysin-Titer *m abbr.* AStT.

an·ti·strep·to·coc·cic [ˌ-streptəˈkɑksɪk] **I** *n* gegen Streptokokken wirkendes Mittel *nt*. **II** *adj* gegen Streptokokken wirkend, Anti-Streptokokken-.

an·ti·strep·to·ki·nase [ˌ-ˌstreptəʊˈkaɪneɪz, -ˈkɪ-] *n* Antistreptokinase *f abbr.* ASK.

an·ti·strep·to·ly·sin [ˌ-ˌstreptəˈlaɪsɪn] *n abbr.* **ASL** Antistreptolysin *nt abbr.* ASL.

antistreptolysin O *abbr.* **ASLO, ASO, ASTO** Antistreptolysin O *nt abbr.* ASLO, ASO, ASTO.

antistreptolysin test Antistreptolysin--Test *m abbr.* AST.

antistreptolysin titer Antistreptolysintiter *m,* ASL-, ASO-, AST-Titer *m*.

an·ti·sub·stance [ˌ-ˈsʌbstəns] *n* → antibody.

an·ti·su·dor·al [ˌ-ˈsuːdərəl] *n, adj* → antisudorific.

an·ti·su·dor·if·ic [ˌ-ˌsuːdəˈrɪfɪk] **I** *n* schweißhemmende Substanz *f,* Antiperspirant *nt,* -transpirant *nt,* Ant(i)hidrotikum *nt*. **II** *adj* schweißhemmend, ant(i)hidrotisch.

an·ti·sym·pa·thet·ic [ˌ-ˌsɪmpəˈθetɪk] **I** *n* Sympatholytikum *nt,* Antiadrenergikum *nt*. **II** *adj* sympatholytisch, antiadrenerg.

an·ti·syph·i·lit·ic [ˌ-sɪfəˈlɪtɪk] **I** *n* Mittel *nt* gegen Syphilis, Antiluetikum *nt,* Antisyphilitikum *nt*. **II** *adj* gegen Syphilis wirkend, antiluetisch, antisyphilitisch.

anti-T cell serum Anti-T-Zell(en)serum *nt*.

an·ti·te·tan·ic [ˌ-təˈtænɪk] *adj* antitetanisch, Tetanus-.

antitetanic factor 10 *abbr.* **A.T. 10** *pharm.* Dihydrotachysterin *nt,* -sterol *nt,* A.T. 10 (*nt*).

antitetanic prophylaxis Tetanusprophylaxe *f*.

antitetanic serum *abbr.* **A.T.S.** Tetanusserum *nt*.

an·ti·the·nar eminence [ˌ-ˈθiːnɑr] Kleinfingerballen *m,* Hypothenar *nt,* Eminentia hypothenaris.

an·ti·ther·mic [ˌ-ˈθɜrmɪk] *n, adj* → antipyretic.

an·ti·throm·bin [ˌ-ˈθrɑmbɪn] *n* Antithrombin *nt*.

antithrombin I *abbr.* **AT I** Fibrin *nt*.

antithrombin III *abbr.* **AT III** Antithrombin III *nt abbr.* AT III.

antithrombin III deficiency Antithrombin III-Mangel *m,* AT III-Mangel *m*.

an·ti·throm·bo·ki·nase [ˌ-ˌθrɑmbəˈkaɪneɪz, -ˈkɪ-] *n* Antithrombokinase *f*.

an·ti·throm·bo·plas·tin [ˌ-ˌθrɑmbəˈplæstɪn] *n* Antithromboplastin *nt*.

an·ti·throm·bot·ic [ˌ-θrɑmˈbɑtɪk] **I** *n* Antithrombotikum *nt*. **II** *adj* Thrombose od. Thrombusbildung verhindernd od. erschwerend, antithrombotisch, Anti--Thrombose(n)-.

an·ti·thy·mo·cyte globulin [ˌ-ˈθaɪməsaɪt] *abbr.* **ATG** Antithymozytenglobulin *nt abbr.* ATG.

an·ti·thy·ro·glob·u·lin antibodies [ˌ-ˌθaɪrəˈglɑbjəlɪn] (Anti-)Thyreoglobulinantikörper *pl*.

an·ti·thy·roid [ˌ-ˈθaɪrɔɪd] *adj* gegen die Schilddrüsenfunktion gerichtet *od.* wirkend, antithyr(e)oid, antithyr(e)oidal.

antithyroid antibody (Anti-)Schilddrüsenantikörper *m*.

an·ti·thy·ro·tox·ic [ˌ-ˌθaɪrəʊˈtɑksɪk] *adj* antithyreotoxisch.

an·ti·thy·ro·trop·ic [ˌ-ˌθaɪrəˈtrɑpɪk, -ˈtrəʊ-] *adj* antithyreotrop.

an·ti·ton·ic [ˌ-ˈtɑnɪk] *adj* tonusreduzierend, -mindernd.

an·ti·tox·ic [ˌ-ˈtɑksɪk] *adj* Antitoxin betr., als Antitoxin wirkend, antitoxisch, Antitoxin-.

antitoxic immunity antitoxische Immunität *f*.

antitoxic serum → antitoxin.

an·ti·tox·i·gen [ˌ-ˈtɑksɪdʒən] *n* → antitoxinogen.

an·ti·tox·in [ˌ-ˈtɑksɪn] *n* **1.** *pharm.* Gegengift *nt,* Antitoxin *nt*. **2.** *immun.* (Anti-)Toxinantikörper *m,* Antitoxin *nt*.

an·ti·tox·in·o·gen [ˌ-tɑkˈsɪnədʒən] *n* Antitoxi(no)gen *nt*.

an·ti·tox·i·num [ˌ-tɑkˈsaɪnəm] *n* → antitoxin.

antitoxin unit Antitoxineinheit *f abbr.* A.E.

an·ti·trag·i·cus (muscle) [ˌ-ˈtrædʒɪkəs] M. antitragicus.

an·ti·tra·go·hel·i·cine fissure [ˌ-ˌtreɪgəʊˈheliːsɪn, -sɪn] Antitragus-Helix-Trennfurche *f,* Fissura antitragohelicina.

an·ti·tra·gus [ˌ-ˈtreɪgəs] *n* Antitragus *m*.

antitragus muscle → antitragicus (muscle).

an·ti·trep·o·ne·mal [ˌ-ˌtrepəˈniːməl] **I** *pharm.* gegen Treponemen wirkendes Mittel *nt,* Treponemenmittel *nt*. **II** *adj* gegen Treponemen wirkend, treponemazid.

an·ti·trich·o·mon·al [ˌ-ˌtrɪkəˈmɑnl, -ˈməʊ-, -trɪˈkɑmənl] **I** *n pharm.* gegen Trichomonaden wirkendes Mittel *nt,* Trichomonadenmittel *nt,* Trichomonazid *nt,* Trichomonadizid *nt*. **II** *adj* gegen Trichomonaden wirkend, trichomonazid, trichomonadizid.

an·ti·tris·mus [ˌ-ˈtrɪzməs] *n* Antitrismus *m*.

an·ti·trope [ˈ-trəʊp] *n* antitropes Organ *nt od.* Körperteil *nt*.

an·ti·tro·pic [ˌ-ˈtrɑpɪk, -ˈtrəʊ-] *adj* antitrop.

an·ti·try·pan·o·so·mal [ˌ-trɪˌpænəˈsəʊml] **I** *n pharm.* gegen Trypanosomen wirkendes Mittel *nt,* Trypanosomenmittel *nt*. **II** *adj* gegen Trypanosomen wirkend.

an·ti·tryp·sic [ˌ-ˈtrɪpsɪk] *adj* → antitryptic.

α₁-an·ti·tryp·sin [ˌ-ˈtrɪpsɪn] *n* α₁-Antitrypsin *nt*.

α₁-antitrypsin deficiency/disease alpha₁--Antitrypsinmangel(krankheit *f*) *m*.

an·ti·tryp·tase [ˌ-ˈtrɪpteɪz] *n* Antitryptase *f*.

an·ti·tryp·tic [ˌ-ˈtrɪptɪk] *adj* antitryptisch.

an·ti·tu·ber·cu·lin [ˌ-t(j)uːˈbɜrkjəlɪn] *n* Tuberkulinantikörper *m,* Antituberkulin *nt*.

an·ti·tu·ber·cu·lot·ic [ˌ-t(j)uːˌbɜrkjəˈlɑtɪk] **I** *n pharm.* antituberkulöse Substanz *f,* Tuberkulostatikum *nt,* Antituberkulotikum *nt*. **II** *adj* antituberkulös, tuberkulostatisch.

an·ti·tu·ber·cu·lous [ˌ-t(j)uːˈbɜrkjələs] *adj* → antituberculotic II.

an·ti·tu·bu·lin [ˌ-ˈt(j)uːbjəlɪn] *n* Antitubulin *nt*.

an·ti·tu·mor·i·gen·ic [ˌ-ˌt(j)uːmərɪˈdʒenɪk] *adj* Tumorbildung hemmend, antitumorigen.

an·ti·tus·sive [ˌ-ˈtʌsɪv] **I** *n pharm.* hustenstillendes Mittel *nt,* Hustenmittel *nt,* Antitussivum *nt*. **II** *adj* hustenstillend, antitussiv.

an·ti·ty·phoid [ˌ-ˈtaɪfɔɪd] *adj* Typhus verhindernd, gegen Typhus wirkend, antityphös.

an·ti·ty·ro·si·nase [ˌ-ˈtaɪrəʊsɪneɪz, -ˈtɪrəʊ-] *n* Tyrosinasehemmer *m,* Antityrosinase *f*.

an·ti·ul·cer therapy [ˌ-ˈʌlsər] Ulkustherapie *f*.

an·ti·vac·ci·na·tion·ist [ˌ-ˌvæksɪˈneɪʃənɪst] *n* Impfgegner(in *f*) *m*.

an·ti·ven·ene [ˌ-ˈveniːn] *n* → antivenin.

an·ti·ven·in [ˌ-ˈvenɪn, -ˈviːn] *n* Gegengift *nt,* Antitoxin *nt,* Antivenenum *nt*.

an·ti·ven·om [ˌ-ˈvenəm] *n* → antivenin.

an·ti·ven·om·ous [ˌ-ˈvenəməs] *adj* antitoxisch.

an·ti·ver·tig·i·nous drug [ˌ-vərˈtɪdʒənəs] Antivertiginosum *nt*.

an·ti·vi·ral [ˌ-ˈvaɪrəl] **I** *n pharm.* antivirale/virustatische/viruzide Substanz *f*. **II** *adj* gegen Viren gerichtet, antiviral; virustatisch; viruzid.

antiviral immunity antivirale Immunität *f*.

an·ti·vi·rot·ic [ˌ-vaɪˈrɑtɪk] *n, adj* → antiviral.

an·ti·vi·ta·min [ˌ-ˈvaɪtəmɪn, -ˈvɪte-] *n* Antivitamin *nt,* Vitaminantagonist *m*.

an·ti·zyme [ˈ-zaɪm] *n* Anti(en)zym *nt*.

an·ti·zy·mot·ic [ˌ-zaɪˈmɑtɪk] *adj* enzymhemmend, antienzymatisch.

an·to·don·tal·gic [ˌæntəʊdɑnˈtældʒɪk] *n, adj* → antiodontalgic.

Anton [ˈæntɑn, -tən]: **A.'s symptom** Anton--Zeichen *nt*.

A.'s syndrome 1. Anton-Zeichen *nt*. **2.** Anton-Babinski-Syndrom *nt,* Hemiasomatognosie *f*.

an·tor·phine [ænˈtɑrfiːn] *n* Nalorphin *nt*.

an·tra·cele [ˈæntrəsiːl] *n* → antrocele.

an·tral [ˈæntrəl] *adj* Antrum betr., antral, Antrum-.

antral artery A. sulci centralis.

antral biopsy *chir.* (*Magen*) Antrumbiopsie *f*.

antral carcinoma (*Magen*) Antrumkarzinom *nt*.

antral gastritis Antrumgastritis *f*.

antral lavage *HNO* Kieferhöhlenspülung *f,* -lavage *f*.

an·trec·to·my [ænˈtrektəmɪ] *n chir.* Antrumresektion *f,* Antrektomie *f*.

An·tric·o·la [ænˈtrɪkələ] *n* Antricola *f*.

an·tri·tis [ænˈtraɪtɪs] *n* Antrumentzündung *f,* Antritis *f*.

an·tro·at·ti·cot·o·my [ˌæntrəʊˌætɪˈkɑtəmɪ] *n HNO* Attik(o)antrotomie *f,* Antroattikotomie *f*.

an·tro·buc·cal [ˌ-ˈbʌkəl] *adj* Kieferhöhle u. Mundhöhle betr. *od.* verbindend, antrobukkal.

antrobuccal fistula antrobukkale Fistel *f*.

an·tro·cele [ˈ-siːl] *n* Antrozele *f*.

an·tro·du·o·de·nec·to·my [ˌ-ˌd(j)uːəʊdɪˈnektəmɪ] *n chir.* Antroduodenektomie *f*.

an·tro·dyn·ia [ˌ-ˈdɪnɪə] *n* Antrodynie *f*.

an·tro·nal·gia [ˌ-ˈnældʒ(ɪ)ə] *n* Schmerzen *pl* in der Kieferhöhle, Antronalgie *f*.

an·tro·na·sal [ˌ-ˈneɪzl] *adj* Kieferhöhle u. Nase betr. *od.* verbindend, antronasal.

an·tro·py·lor·ic [ˌ-paɪˈlɔrɪk, -ˈlɑr-] *adj* Antrum pyloricum betr., antropylorisch.

an·tro·scope [ˈæntrəskəʊp] *n* Antroskop *nt*.

an·tros·co·py [ænˈtrɑskəpɪ] *n* Antroskopie *f*.

an·tros·to·my [ænˈtrɑstəmɪ] *n HNO* Antrostomie *f,* Kieferhöhlenfensterung *f*.

an·tro·tome [ˈæntrətəʊm] *n* Antrotom *nt*.

an·trot·o·my [ænˈtrɑtəmɪ] *n HNO* Antrotomie *f*.

an·tro·tym·pan·ic [ˌæntrəʊtɪmˈpænɪk] *adj* Antrum mastoideum u. Paukenhöhle betr. *od.* verbindend, antrotympanisch.

an·tro·tym·pa·ni·tis [ˌ-ˌtɪmpəˈnaɪtɪs] *n HNO* Antrotympanitis *f*.

an·trum [ˈæntrəm] *n, pl* **-tra** [-trə] *anat.* Höhle *f,* Hohlraum *m,* Antrum *nt*.

a. of Highmore Kieferhöhle, Sinus maxillaris.

a. of Willis präpylorischer Magenabschnitt *m,* Antrum (pyloricum).

antrum gastritis → antral gastritis.

a·nu·cle·ar [eɪˈn(j)uːklɪər] *adj bio.,* *phys.* kernlos, anukleär.

anuclear necrosis *patho.* kernlose Nekrose *f*.

a·nu·cle·ate [eɪˈn(j)uːklɪɪt] *adj* → anuclear.

a·nu·cle·at·ed [eɪˈn(j)uːklɪˌeɪtɪd] *adj* entkernt.

ANUG *abbr.* → acute necrotizing ulcerative gingivitis.
an·u·lar carcinoma ['ænjələr] → annular carcinoma.
an·u·lo·plas·ty [ˌænjələʊ'plæstɪ] *n* → annuloplasty.
an·u·lo·spi·ral *adj* → annulospiral.
a·nu·lus *n* → annulus.
an·u·re·sis [ˌænjə'riːsɪs] *n* **1.** Harnverhalt *m*, Anurese *f.* **2.** → anuria.
an·u·ret·ic [ˌænjə'retɪk] *adj* Anurese betr., anuretisch.
a·nu·ria [æn'(j)ʊərɪə] *n* Anurie *f.*
a·nu·ric [æn'(j)ʊərɪk] *adj* Anurie betr., anurisch.
an·u·rous ['ænjərəs, ə'n(j)ʊərəs] *adj* schwanzlos.
a·nus ['eɪnəs] *n, pl* **a·nus·es, ani** ['eɪnaɪ] After *m*, Anus *m.*
a·nus·i·tis [eɪnə'saɪtɪs] *n* After-, Anusentzündung *f*, Anusitis *f.*
an·vil ['ænvɪl] *n* Amboß *m*; *anat.* Incus *m.*
anvil sound Münzenklirren *nt.*
anx·i·e·tas [æŋ'zaɪətæs] *n* **1.** nervöse Unruhe *f.* **2.** → anxiety.
anx·i·e·ty [æŋ'zaɪətɪ] *n, pl* **-ties 1.** Angst *f*, Angstgefühl *nt*, Ängstlichkeit *f*; Unruhe *f*, Besorgnis *f* (*for, about* wegen, um). **2.** *psycho.* Beängstigung *f*, Beklemmung *f.* **3.** Existenzangst *f.*
anxiety attack Angstanfall *m*, Panikattacke *f.*
anxiety disorders Angstneurosen *pl.*
anxiety hysteria *psychia.* hysterische Angst *f*, Angstneurose *f.*
anxiety neurosis → anxiety hysteria.
anxiety reaction → anxiety hysteria.
anxiety state → anxiety hysteria.
anx·i·o·lyt·ic [ˌænzɪə'lɪtɪk] **I** *n* angstlösendes Mittel *nt*, Anxiolytikum *nt.* **II** *adj* angstlösend, anxiolytisch.
anxiolytic agent → anxiolytic I.
anx·ious ['æŋ(k)ʃəs] *adj* **1.** ängstlich, unruhig; besorgt (*for, about* wegen, um). **2.** bestrebt, begierig (*for, to* zu)
an·y·dre·mia [ˌænɪ'driːmɪə] *n* → anhydremia.
AOC *abbr.* → anodal opening contraction.
AOCl *abbr.* → anodal opening clonus.
a·or·ta [eɪ'ɔːrtə] *n, pl* **-tas, -tae** [-tiː] große Körperschlagader *f*, Aorta *f.*
a·or·tal [eɪ'ɔːrtl] *adj* → aortic.
a·or·tal·gia [eɪɔːr'tældʒ(ɪ)ə] *n* Aortenschmerz *m*, Aortalgie *f.*
a·or·tarc·tia [ˌ-'tɑːrkʃɪə] *n* → aortic stenosis.
a·or·tar·tia [ˌ-'tɑːrʃɪə] *n* → aortic stenosis.
a·or·tec·ta·sia [ˌ-tek'teɪʒ(ɪ)ə] *n* → aortectasis.
a·or·tec·ta·sis [ˌ-'tektəsɪs] *n* Aortendilatation *f*, -ektasie *f.*
a·or·tec·to·my [ˌ-'tektəmɪ] *n chir.* Aorten(teil)resektion *f*, Aortektomie *f.*
aor·tic [eɪ'ɔːrtɪk] *adj* Hauptschlagader/Aorta betr., aortal, aortisch, Aorten-, Aorto-.
aortic aneurysm Aortenaneurysma *nt.*
aortic arcade Aortenarkade *f*, Lig. arcuatum medianum.
aortic arch 1. Aortenbogen *m*, Arcus aortae. **2.** ⤷es *pl embryo.* Aortenbögen *pl.*
double a. Aortenringbildung *f*, doppelter Aortenbogen.
right a. Rechtslage *f* des Aortenbogens, Arcus aortae dexter.
aortic arch angiography Aortenbogenangiographie *f.*
aortic arch anomaly Aortenbogenanomalie *f*, -fehlbildung *f.*
aortic arch syndrome Aortenbogensyndrom *nt.*

aortic atresia Aorten(klappen)atresie *f.*
aortic body Glomus aorticum.
aortic body tumor Glomus-aorticum-Tumor *m.*
aortic bulb Aortenbulbus *m*, Bulbus aortae.
aortic catheter Aortenkatheter *m.*
aortic channel *embryo.* Aortenkanal *m.*
aortic coarctation Aortenisthmusstenose *f*, Coarctatio aortae.
   adult type a. Erwachsenenform *f* der Aortenisthmusstenose, infaduktale Aortenisthmusstenose.
   infantile type a. infantile/präduktale Aortenisthmusstenose.
aortic contour *radiol.* Aortenkontur *f.*
aortic diastolic pressure diastolischer Aortendruck *m.*
aortic dissection Aortendissektion *f*, Aneurysma dissecans der Aorta.
aortic glomus Glomus aorticum.
aortic hiatus Hiatus aorticus.
aortic incompetence → aortic regurgitation.
aortic insufficiency *abbr.* **AI** Aorten(klappen)insuffizienz *f.*
aortic isthmus Aortenisthmus *m*, Isthmus aortae.
aortic isthmus stenosis → aortic coarctation.
aortic murmur Aortengeräusch *nt.*
a·or·ti·co·il·i·ac occlusive disease [eɪˌɔːrtɪkəʊ'ɪlɪæk] Leriche-Syndrom *nt*, Aortenbifurkationssyndrom *nt.*
aortic opening Aortenostium *nt*/-öffnung *f* des linken Ventrikels, Ostium aortae.
   a. in/of diaphragm → aortic hiatus.
a·or·ti·co·pul·mo·nar·y [eɪˌɔːrtɪkəʊ'pʌlməˌnerɪ, -nərɪ] *adj* Aorta u. Lungenarterien betr., aort(ik)opulmonal.
aorticopulmonary fenestration → aorticopulmonary window.
aorticopulmonary septal defect → aorticopulmonary window.
aorticopulmonary septum *embryo.* Septum aorticopulmonale.
aorticopulmonary window *card.* Aortikopulmonalfenster *nt*, aortopulmonaler Septumdefekt *m.*
a·or·ti·co·re·nal [ˌ-'riːnl] *adj* Aorta u. Niere(n) betr., aort(ik)orenal.
aorticorenal ganglia Ggll. aorticorenalia.
aortic orifice → aortic opening.
aortic ostium → aortic opening.
aortic paraganglion Zuckerkandl'-Organ *nt*, Paraganglion aorticum abdominale.
aortic plexus vegetativer Plexus *m* der Aorta, Plexus aorticus.
   abdominal a. vegetativer Plexus der Bauchaorta, Plexus aorticus abdominalis.
   thoracic a. vegetativer Plexus der Brustaorta, Plexus aorticus thoracicus.
aortic pressure Aortendruck *m.*
aortic puncture Aortenpunktion *f.*
aortic reflex Depressorreflex *m.*
aortic regurgitation *abbr.* **AR** → aortic insufficiency.
aortic sac *embryo.* Aortensack *m*, -wurzel *f.*
aortic septal defect *card.* Aortikopulmonalfenster *nt*, aortopulmonaler Septumdefekt *m.*
aortic sinus Aortensinus *m*, Sinus aortae.
aortic sinusal aneurysm Aneurysma sinus aortae.
aortic spindle Aortenspindel *f.*
aortic stenosis *abbr.* **AS 1.** Aortenstenose *f.* **2.** Aortenklappenstenose *f*, valvuläre Aortenstenose *f.*
   subvalvular a. infra-/subvalvuläre Aortenstenose.

aortic systolic pressure systolischer Aortendruck *m.*
aortic thrill *card.* Aortenschwirren *nt.*
aortic valve Aortenklappe *f*, Valva aortae.
aortic ventricle of heart linke Herzkammer *f*, linker Ventrikel *m*, Ventriculus sinister cordis.
aortic window *radiol.* Aortenfenster *nt.*
a·or·ti·tis [eɪɔːr'taɪtɪs] *n* Aortenentzündung *f*, Aortitis *f.*
a·or·to·cor·o·nar·y [eɪˌɔːrtə'kɔːrənerɪ, -'kɑr-] *adj* Aorta u. Koronararterien betr., od. verbindend, aortokoronar.
aortocoronary bypass *HTG* aortokoronarer Bypass *m.*
a·or·to·fem·o·ral bypass [ˌ-'femərəl] *abbr.* **AFB** *HTG* aortofemoraler Bypass *m.*
a·or·to·gram [eɪ'ɔːrtəgræm] *n radiol.* Aortogramm *f.*
a·or·tog·ra·phy [eɪɔːr'tɑgrəfɪ] *n radiol.* Kontrastdarstellung *f* der Aorta, Aortographie *f.*
a·or·to·il·i·ac bypass [eɪˌɔːrtə'ɪlɪæk] *HTG* aortoiliakaler Bypass *m.*
a·or·top·a·thy [ˌeɪɔːr'tɑpəθɪ] *n* Aortenerkrankung *f.*
a·or·top·to·sia [ˌeɪɔːrtɑp'təʊsɪə] *n* → aortoptosis.
a·or·top·to·sis [ˌeɪɔːrtɑp'təʊsɪs] *n* Aortensenkung *f*, Aortoptose *f.*
a·or·to·re·nal [eɪˌɔːrtəˈriːnl] *adj* → aorticorenal.
aortorenal bypass aortorenaler Bypass *m.*
a·or·tor·rha·phy [ˌeɪɔːr'tɔrəfɪ] *n chir.* Aortennaht *f*, Aortorrhaphie *f.*
a·or·to·scle·ro·sis [eɪˌɔːrtəsklɪ'rəʊsɪs] *n* Aortensklerose *f*, -verkalkung *f.*
a·or·to·ste·no·sis [ˌ-stɪ'nəʊsɪs] *n* (supravalvuläre) Aortenstenose *f.*
a·or·tot·o·my [eɪɔːr'tɑtəmɪ] *n* Aortotomie *f.*
a·os·mic [eɪ'ɑzmɪk] *adj* → anosmic.
AP *abbr.* → alkaline phosphatase. **2.** → 2-aminopurine. **3.** → anterior pituitary.
6-APA *abbr.* → 6-aminopencillanic acid.
a·pal·les·the·sia [əˌpælɪs'θiːʒ(ɪ)ə] *n* Pallanästhesie *f.*
a·pal·lic [ə'pælɪk] *adj* apallisch.
apallic syndrome apallisches Syndrom *nt.*
a·pan·crea [eɪ'pæŋkrɪə] *n* Pankreasaplasie *f.*
a·pan·cre·at·ic [eɪˌpæŋkrɪ'ætɪk] *adj* ohne Pankreas, apankreatisch.
a·par·a·lyt·ic [eɪˌpærə'lɪtɪk] *adj* aparalytisch.
a·par·a·thy·re·o·sis [eɪˌpærəθaɪrɪ'əʊsɪs] *n* Aparathyreose *f.*
a·par·a·thy·roid·ism [ˌ-'θaɪrɔɪdɪzəm] *n* → aparathyreosis.
a·par·a·thy·ro·sis [ˌ-θaɪ'rəʊsɪs] *n* → aparathyreosis.
a·pa·reu·nia [eɪpə'rjuːnɪə] *n* Apareunie *f.*
ap·ar·thro·sis [ˌæpɑr'θrəʊsɪs] *n* (echtes) Gelenk *nt*, Artic./Junctura synovialis.
ap·a·thet·ic [æpə'θetɪk] *adj* apathisch, gleichgültig, teilnahmslos, indifferent.
ap·a·thet·i·cal [æpə'θetɪkl] *adj* → apathetic.
ap·a·thy ['æpəθɪ] *n* Apathie *f*, Teilnahmslosigkeit *f*, Gleichgültigkeit *f*, Indifferenz *f* (*to* gegenüber).
ap·a·tite ['æpətaɪt] *n* Apatit *nt.*
apatite calculus/stone *urol.* Apatitstein *m.*
a·pa·zone ['æpəzəʊn] *n pharm.* Azapropazon *nt.*
APC *abbr.* → atrial premature contraction.
ape [eɪp] *n bio.* (Menschen-)Affe *f.*
ape fissure Sulcus lunatus.
ape hand Affenhand *f.*
a·pel·lous [ə'peləs] *adj* **1.** *chir.* hautlos, nicht von Haut bedeckt; nicht-vernarbt. **2.** ohne Vorhaut.
a·pep·sia [eɪ'pepsɪə] *n old* Apepsie *f.*

a·per·i·ent [ə'pɪərɪənt] **I** n (mildes) Abführmittel nt, Aperientium nt, Aperiens nt. **II** adj abführend, laxativ.
a·pe·ri·od·ic [ˌeɪpɪrɪ'ɑdɪk] adj aperiodisch, nicht perriodisch.
a·per·i·os·te·al amputation [eɪˌperɪ'ɑstɪəl] ortho. Bunge-Amputation f, aperiostale Amputation f.
a·per·i·stal·sis [ˌ-'stɔːlsɪs, -'stɑl-] n Peristaltikmangel m, -schwäche f, Aperistaltik f, Aperistalsis f.
a·per·i·stal·tic [ˌ-'stɔːltɪk, -'stɑl-] adj aperistaltisch.
a·per·i·tive [ə'perɪtɪv] **I** n → aperient I. **II** adj **1.** appetitanregend. **2.** → aperient II.
Apert [a'peːr]: **A.'s disease** Apert-Syndrom nt, Akrozephalosyndaktylie (Typ Ia) f. **A.'s syndrome** → A.'s disease.
Apert-Crouzon [kru:'zõ]: **A.-C. disease** Apert-Crouzon-Syndrom nt, Akrozephalosyndaktylie Typ IIa f.
ap·er·tur·al ['æpərˌtʃʊərəl] adj Apertur(a) betr., Aperturen-.
ap·er·ture ['-tʃʊər, -tjʊər] n **1.** Öffnung f, Eingang m, Spalt m, Loch nt, Schlitz m. **2.** anat. Apertur f, Apertura f. **3.** phys. Apertur f, (Blenden-)Öffnung f.
a. of frontal sinus Stirnhöhlenmündung f, Apertura sinus frontalis.
a. of glottis Stimmritze f, Rima glottidis.
a. of larynx Kehlkopfeingang, Aditus laryngis.
a. of sphenoid sinus Apertura sinus sphenoidalis.
aperture angle phys. Öffnungswinkel m.
a·pex ['eɪpeks] n, pl **a·pex·es, a·pi·ces** ['eɪpɪsiːz, 'æp-] Spitze f, Gipfel m; Scheitel m; anat. Apex m, Apex m.
a. of arytenoid cartilage Spitze des Aryknorpels, Apex cartilaginis aryt(a)enoideae.
a. of bladder (Harn-)Blasenspitze, Apex vesicae/vesicalis (urinariae).
a. of cochlea Schneckenspitze, Cupula cochleae.
a. of dorsal horn of spinal cord Hinterhornspitze, Apex cornus dorsalis/posterioris medullae spinalis.
a. of head of fibula Apex capitis fibulae.
a. of heart Herzspitze, Apex cordis.
a. of lung Lungenspitze, Apex pulmonis/pulmonalis.
a. of patella untere Patellaspitze, unterer Patellapol m, Apex patellae.
a. of petrous portion of temporal bone Felsenbeinspitze, Apex partis petrosae (ossis temporalis).
a. of posterior horn of spinal cord → a. of dorsal horn of spinal cord.
a. of prostate Prostataspitze, Apex prostatae.
a. of sacrum Kreuzbeinspitze, Apex ossis sacri.
a. of tongue Zungenspitze, Apex linguae.
a. of urinary bladder → a. of bladder.
apex beat Herzspitzenstoß m.
a·pex·car·di·o·gram [ˌeɪpeks'kɑːrdɪəgræm] n Apexkardiogramm nt abbr. APK, APC.
apex cardiogram → apexcardiogram.
a·pex·car·di·og·ra·phy [ˌeɪpeksˌkɑːrdɪ'ɑgrəfɪ] n Apexkardiographie f.
apex cardiography → apexcardiography.
apex impulse abbr. **A.I.** Herzspitzenstoß m.
apex murmur Herzspitzengeräusch nt.
apex pneumonia Spitzenpneumonie f.
Apgar ['æpgɑːr]: **A. scale/score** Apgar-Index m, -Schema nt.
a·pha·cia n → aphakia.
a·pha·cic adj → aphakic.
a·pha·gia [ə'feɪdʒɪə] n Aphagie f.

a·phag·o·prax·ia [əˌfægə'præksɪə] n Unvermögen nt zu Schlucken, Aphagopraxie f.
a·pha·kia [ə'feɪkɪə] n Fehlen nt der Augenlinse, Aphakie f.
a·pha·kic [ə'feɪkɪk] adj Aphakie betr., linsenlos, aphak(isch).
aphakic eye aphakes/linsenloses Auge nt.
aphakic glaucoma Glaukom nt nach Linsenextraktion.
a·pha·lan·gia [æfə'lændʒɪə, eɪ-] n embryo. Phalangenaplasie f, Aphalangie f.
a·phan·i·sis [ə'fænəsɪs] n psychia. Aphanisis f.
a·pha·sia [ə'feɪʒə, -zɪə] n Sprachversagen nt, Aphasie f, Aphemie f.
a·pha·si·ac [ə'feɪzɪæk] n → aphasic I.
a·pha·sic [ə'feɪzɪk] **I** n Patient(in f) m mit Aphasie, Aphasiker(in f) m. **II** adj Aphasie betr., aphasisch.
a·phe·mes·the·sia [əfiːmes'θiːʒ(ɪ)ə] n Leseunfähigkeit f, -unvermögen nt, Alexie f.
a·phe·mi·a [ə'fiːmɪə] n Sprachverlust m, Aphemie f.
aph·e·pho·bia [æfə'fəʊbɪə] n Berührungsangst m, Haphephobie f.
a·pher·e·sis [æfə'riːsɪs] n Apherese f, Pherese f.
a·pho·nia [eɪ'fəʊnɪə] n Stimmlosigkeit f, -verlust m, Aphonie f.
a·phon·ic [eɪ'fɑnɪk, -'fəʊn-] adj stimm-, tonlos, aphon(isch).
a·pho·no·ge·lia [ˌeɪfəʊnəʊ'dʒiːlɪə] n Aphonogelie f.
aph·o·nous ['æfənəs] adj → aphonic.
a·phot·es·the·sia [ˌeɪfəʊtes'θiːʒ(ɪ)ə] n ophthal. Aphotästhesie f.
a·phot·ic [eɪ'fəʊtɪk] adj ohne Licht, dunkel, lichtlos.
a·phra·sia [ə'freɪʒ(ɪ)ə] n Aphrasie f.
aph·ro·di·sia [æfrə'dɪʒ(ɪ)ə] n (übermäßige) sexuelle Erregung f, (krankhaft) gesteigerter Sexualtrieb m, Aphrodisie f.
aph·ro·dis·i·ac [ˌ-'dɪzɪæk] **I** n Aphrodisiakum nt. **II** adj den Geschlechtstrieb anregend/steigernd, aphroditisch, aphrodisisch.
aph·tha ['æfθə] n, pl **-thae** [-θiː] Aphthe f.
aph·thae ['æfθiː] n **1.** pl → aphtha. **2.** rezidivierende aphthöse Stomatitis f.
aph·tho·bul·bous stomatitis [ˌæfθəʊ'bʌlbəs] n aphthous fever.
aph·thoid ['æfθɔɪd] **I** n Aphthoid Pospischill-Feyrter nt, vagantes Aphthoid nt, aphthoide Polypathie f. **II** adj aphthenähnlich, -förmig, aphthoid.
aph·thon·gia [æf'θɑŋdʒɪə] n Aphthongie f.
aph·tho·sis [æf'θəʊsɪs] n, pl **-ses** [-siːz] Aphthose f, Aphthosis f.
aph·thous ['æfθəs] adj Aphthen betr., aphthös, aphthenartig.
aphthous fever micro. (echte) Maul- und Klauenseuche f abbr. **MKS**, Febris aphthosa, Stomatitis epidemica, Aphthosis epizootica.
aphthous stomatitis 1. aphthöse Stomatitis f, Mundfäule f, Gingivostomatitis/Stomatitis herpetica. **2.** rezidivierende aphthöse Stomatitis f.
aphthous ulceration aphthöse Ulzeration f.
aph·tho·vi·rus [ˌæfθəʊ'vaɪrəs] n Aphthovirus nt.
a. of cattle Maul- und Klauenseuche-Virus nt, MKS-Virus nt.
a·phy·lac·tic [eɪfə'læktɪk] adj Aphylaxie betr., aphylaktisch.
a·phy·lax·is [ˌ-'læksɪs] n Aphylaxie f.
ap·i·cal ['eɪpɪkl, 'æp-] adj anat., bio. Spitze f, Apex betr., an der Spitze liegend, apikal, Spitzen-, Apikal-.
apical abscess 1. (Organ-)Spitzenabszeß

m. **2.** Lungenspitzenabszeß m. **3.** (Zahn) Wurzelspitzenabszeß m.
apical body (Spermium) Kopfkappe f, Akrosom nt.
apical branch: a. of left pulmonary artery Ramus apicalis a. pulmonalis sinistrae.
a. of right pulmonary artery Ramus apicalis a. pulmonalis dextrae.
apical bronchus (Lunge) Bronchus m des Spitzensegmentes, Bronchus segmentalis apicalis.
apical complex micro. Apikalkomplex m.
apical dendrite Apikaldendrit m.
apical dental ligament Lig. apicis dentis.
apical ectodermal ridge abbr. **AER** embryo. apikale (Ektoderm-)Randleiste f.
apical foramen (of tooth) Wurzelspitzenöffnung f, For. apicis radicis dentalis.
apical gland of tongue (Blandin-)Nuhn'-Drüse f, Gl. lingualis anterior, Gl. apicis linguae.
apical granuloma Zahngranulom nt, Wurzelspitzengranulom nt.
apical impulse Herzspitzenstoß m.
apical odontoid ligament → apical dental ligament.
apical pericementitis (Zahn) Wurzelspitzenabszeß m.
apical periodontitis Parodontitis apicalis. **chronic a.** → apical granuloma.
apical pneumonia Spitzenpneumonie f.
apical reinfection (Tuberkulose) apikaler Reinfekt m.
apical segment (Lunge) Spitzen-, Apikalsegment nt, Segmentum apicale [S. I].
apical tuberculosis (Lungen-)Spitzentuberkulose f.
a·pi·cec·to·my [eɪpɪ'sektəmɪ, æp-] n HNO Apikektomie f.
a·pi·ce·ot·o·my [ˌ-sɪ'ɑtəmɪ] n → apicotomy.
a·pi·ci·tis [ˌ-'saɪtɪs] n Spitzenentzündung f, Apizitis f, Apicitis f.
A·pi·co·com·plex·a [ˌeɪpɪkəʊkɑm'pleksə] pl micro. Apicocomplexa pl, Sporozoa pl.
a·pi·co·ec·to·my [ˌeɪpɪkəʊ'ektəmɪ, ˌæp-] n dent. (Zahn-)Wurzelspitzenresektion f, Apikoektomie f, Apikotomie f.
a·pi·col·y·sis [eɪpɪ'kɑləsɪs] n chir. (Lunge) Apikolyse f.
a·pi·co·pos·te·ri·or segment [ˌeɪpɪkəʊpə'stɪərɪər, -pəʊ-, ˌæp-] (Lunge) Spitzen- u. Hintersegment nt, apikoposteriores Segment nt, Segmentum apicoposterius [S. I u. II].
a·pi·cos·to·my [ˌæpɪ'kɑstəmɪ, ˌeɪ-] n dent. Apikostomie f.
a·pi·cot·o·my [ˌ-'kɑtəmɪ] n HNO Apikotomie f, Apikoektomie f.
a·pin·e·al·ism [eɪ'pɪnɪəlɪzəm] n Fehlen nt der Zirbeldrüse, Apinealismus m.
a·pi·pho·bia [eɪpɪ'fəʊbɪə, æp-] n psychia. Angst f vor Bienen, Apiphobie f.
a·pi·tu·i·tar·ism [eɪpɪ't(j)uːɪtərɪzəm] n **1.** Hypophysenaplasie f. **2.** Hypophysenvorderlappeninsuffizienz f, HVL-Insuffizienz f, Simmonds-Syndrom nt, Hypopituitarismus m.
a·pla·cen·tal [ˌeɪplə'sentl, ˌæplə-] adj bio. ohne Plazenta, plazentalos, aplazentar.
ap·la·nat·ic [ˌæplə'nætɪk] adj Aplanatie betr., aplanatisch.
aplanatic lens aplanatische Linse f, aplanatisches Glas nt.
a·plan·a·tism [æ'plænətɪzəm] n ophthal. Aplanatie f.
a·pla·sia [ə'pleɪʒ(ɪ)ə] n Aplasie f.
a·plas·tic [eɪ'plæstɪk] adj Aplasie betr., von Aplasie gekennzeichnet, aplastisch.
aplastic anemia aplastische Anämie f. **congenital a.** Fanconi-Anämie, -Syn-

drom *nt*, konstitutionelle infantile Panmyelopathie *f*.
aplastic crisis *hema*. aplastische Krise *f*.
a·pleu·ria [eɪˈplʊərɪə] *n* Rippenaplasie *f*, Apleurie *f*.
ap·ne·a [ˈæpnɪə, æpˈniːə] *n* **1.** Atemstillstand *m*, Apnoe *f*. **2.** → asphyxia.
ap·ne·ic [æpˈniːɪk] *adj* Apnoe betr., apnoisch.
apneic oxygenation Diffusionsatmung *f*.
ap·neu·mat·ic [ˌæpn(j)uːˈmætɪk] *adj* **1.** luftfrei, apneumatisch. **2.** unter Luftausschluß, apneumatisch.
ap·neu·ma·to·sis [ˌæpn(j)uːməˈtəʊsɪs] *n* (*Lunge*) angeborene Atelektase *f*, Apneumatose *f*.
ap·neu·mia [æpˈn(j)uːmɪə] *n* Lungenaplasie *f*, Apneumie *f*.
ap·neu·sis [æpˈn(j)uːsɪs] *n* Apneusis *f*.
ap·o·at·ro·pine [ˌæpəʊˈætrəpiːn, -pɪn] *n pharm*. Apoatropin *nt*.
ap·o·cam·no·sis *n* → apokamnosis.
ap·o·chro·mat [ˈæpkrəʊmeɪt, ˌæpəˈkrəʊ-] *n* Apochromat *m*, apochromatisches Objektiv *nt*.
ap·o·chro·mat·ic [ˌæpəkrəʊˈmætɪk] *adj phys*. apochromatisch.
apochromatic lens apochromatische Linse *f*, apochromatisches Glas *nt*.
apochromatic objective → apochromat.
a·poc·o·pe [əˈpɒkəpɪ] *n chir*. Amputation *f*.
ap·o·cop·tic [ˌæpəˈkɒptɪk] *adj* Amputation betr., Amputations-.
ap·o·crine [ˈæpəkraɪn] *adj histol*. apokrin.
apocrine adenoma tubuläres Adenom *nt* der Vulva, Hidradenom *nt* der Vulva, Hidradenoma papilliferum.
apocrine cell apokrin-sezernierende/apokrine Zelle *f*.
apocrine extrusion apokrine Extrusion *f*.
apocrine gland apokrine Drüse *f*, Gl. apocrinae.
apocrine miliaria Fox-Fordyce-Krankheit *f*, apokrine Miliaria *pl*, Hidradenoma eruptivum, Apocrinitis sudoripara pruriens, Akanthosis circumporalis pruriens.
ap·o·crin·i·tis [æpəkrɪˈnaɪtɪs] *n* eitrige Schweißdrüsenentzündung *f*, Schweißdrüsenabszeß *m*, Hidradenitis suppurativa.
ap·o·dal [ˈæpədəl] *adj* ohne Fuß/Füße, fußlos.
a·po·dia [eɪˈpəʊdɪə, æ-] *n embryo*. angeborene Fußlosigkeit *f*, Apodie *f*.
ap·o·dous [ˈæpədəs] *adj* → apodal.
ap·o·dy [ˈæpədɪ] *n* → apodia.
ap·o·en·zyme [ˌæpəʊˈenzaɪm] *n* Apoenzym *nt*.
ap·o·fer·ri·tin [-ˈferɪtɪn] *n* Apoferritin *nt*.
ap·o·gam·i·a [-ˈgæmɪə] *n* **1.** *bio*. Apogamie *f*. **2.** Jungfernzeugung *f*, Parthenogenese *f*.
a·pog·a·my [əˈpɒgəmɪ] *n* → apogamia.
ap·o·kam·no·sis [ˌæpəkæmˈnəʊsɪs] *n* Apokamnose *f*.
a·po·lar cell [eɪˈpəʊlər] apolare Nervenzelle *f*, apolarer Neurozyt *m*.
apolar neuroblast *embryo*. apolarer Neuroblast *m*.
a·po·lip·o·pro·tein [ˌæpəʊˌlɪpəˈprəʊtiːn, -tiːɪn, -ˌtiːɪn] *n* Apolipoprotein *nt*.
apolipoprotein C-II deficiency (primäre/essentielle) Hyperlipoproteinämie Typ V *f*, fett- u. kohlenhydratinduzierte Hyperlipidämie/Hyperlipoproteinämie *f*, exogen-endogene Hyperlipoproteinämie *f*, kalorisch-induzierte Hyperlipoproteinämie u. Hyperpräbetalipoproteinämie.
ap·o·mix·ia [-ˈmɪksɪə] *n* **1.** *bio*. Apomixis *f*.

2. *bio*. Apogamie *f*. **3.** Jungfernzeugung *f*, Parthenogenese *f*.
ap·o·mix·is [ˌ-ˈmɪksɪs] *n* → apomixia.
ap·o·mor·phine [ˌ-ˈmɔːrfiːn, -fɪn] *n* Apomorphin *nt*.
ap·o·neu·rec·to·my [ˌ-njʊəˈrektəmɪ, -nɔː-] *n* Aponeurosenresektion *f*, Aponeur(os)ektomie *f*.
ap·o·neu·ror·rha·phy [ˌ-njʊəˈrɔːrəfɪ, -nɔː-] *n chir*. Aponeurosennaht *f*, Aponeurorrhaphie *f*.
ap·o·neu·ro·sis [ˌ-njʊəˈrəʊsɪs, -nɔːˈr-] *n*, *pl* **-ses** [-siːz] *anat*. Sehnenhaut *f*, -platte *f*, flächenhafte Sehne *f*, Aponeurose *f*, Aponeurosis *f*.
a. of insertion (*Muskel*) Ansatz-, Insertionsaponeurose.
a. of origin (*Muskel*) Ursprungsaponeurose.
a. of transverse muscle of abdomen Transversusaponeurose, Aponeurosis m. transversus abdominis.
a. of Zinn Aufhängefasern *pl* der Linse, Zonularfasern *pl*, Fibrae zonulares.
ap·o·neu·ro·si·tis [ˌ-njʊərəˈsaɪtɪs, -nɔː-] *n* Aponeurosenentzündung *f*, Aponeurositis *f*.
ap·o·neu·rot·ic [ˌ-njʊəˈrɒtɪk, -nɔːˈr-] *adj* Aponeurose betr., aponeurotisch, aponeurosenähnlich, Aponeurosen-.
aponeurotic fascia tiefe Körperfaszie *f*, Fascia profunda.
aponeurotic membrane → aponeurosis.
aponeurotic reflex Weingrow-Reflex *m*.
ap·o·neu·rot·o·my [ˌ-njʊəˈrɒtəmɪ, -nɔː-] *n chir*. Aponeurosenspaltung *f*, Aponeurotomie *f*.
a·poph·y·sar·y [əˈpɒfɪseriː] *adj* → apophyseal.
apophysary point *neuro*. Trousseau'-Punkt *m*.
ap·o·phys·e·al [əˌpɒfəˈsiːəl, ˌæpəˈfɪzɪəl] *adj* Apophyse(n) betr., apophysär, Apophysen-.
apophyseal fracture traumatische Apophysenlösung *f*, Apophysenabriß *m*.
apophyseal necrosis (aseptische) Apophysennekrose/Apophyseonekrose *f*.
apophyseal point *neuro*. Trousseau'-Punkt *m*.
ap·o·phys·e·op·a·thy [ˌ-fiːzɪˈɒpəθɪ] *n* **1.** Apophysenerkrankung *f*. **2.** Osgood-Schlatter-Krankheit *f*, -Syndrom *nt*, Schlatter-Osgood-Krankheit *f*, -Syndrom *nt*, Apophysitis tibialis adolescentium.
ap·o·phys·i·al *adj* → apophyseal.
ap·o·phys·i·a·ry [æpəˈfɪzɪˌeriː] *adj* → apophyseal.
a·poph·y·sis [əˈpɒfəsɪs] *n*, *pl* **-ses** [-siːz] *anat*. Apophyse *f*, Apophysis *f*.
a·poph·y·si·tis [əˌpɒfɪˈsaɪtɪs] *n* **1.** Apophysenentzündung *f*, Apophysitis *f*. **2.** (aseptische) Apophysennekrose/Apophyseonekrose *f*. **3.** Haglund-Syndrom 1 *nt*, Apophysitis calcanei.
ap·o·plec·tic [æpəˈplektɪk] *adj* Apoplexie betr., apoplektisch.
apoplectic coma Coma apoplecticum.
apoplectic cyst apoplektische Zyste *f*.
apoplectic fit → apoplexy 1.
apoplectic glaucoma hämorrhagisches Glaukom *nt*, Glaucoma haemorrhagicum/apoplecticum.
apoplectic retinitis Verschluß *m* der A. centralis retinae, Zentralarterienthrombose *f*, Apoplexia retinae.
apoplectic stroke → apoplexy 1.
ap·o·plec·ti·form [æpəˈplektɪfɔːrm] *adj* apoplexieartig, -ähnlich, apoplektiform.
apoplectiform deafness Hörsturz *m*, akute Ertaubung *f*.

apoplectiform myelitis apopolektiforme Myelitis *f*, Myelitis apoplectiformis.
apoplectiform myelopathy apoplektiforme Myelopathie *f*, Myelopathia apoplectiformis.
ap·o·plec·toid [æpəˈplektɔɪd] *adj* → apoplectiform.
ap·o·plex·i·a [æpəˈpleksɪə] *n* → apoplexy.
apoplexia uteri Uterusapoplexie *f*, Apoplexia uteri.
ap·o·plex·y [ˈæpəpleksɪ] *n* **1.** Schlaganfall *m*, Gehirnschlag *m*, apoplektischer Insult *m*, Apoplexie *f*, Apoplexia (cerebri) *f*. **2.** Organ(ein)blutung *f*, Apoplexie *f*, -plexia *f*.
a. of the newborn Neugeborenenapoplexie.
ap·o·pro·tein [ˌæpəʊˈprəʊtiːn, -tiːɪn] *n* Apoprotein *nt*.
ap·o·pto·sis [æpəˈtəʊsɪs] *n histol*. Apoptosis *f*.
a·po·ric gland [eɪˈpɔːrɪk, -ˈpəʊ-] Drüse *f* mit innerer Sekretion, endokrine Drüse *f*, Gl. endocrina, Gl. sine ductibus.
ap·o·some [ˈæpəsəʊm] *n* Aposom *nt*.
a·pos·ta·sis [əˈpæstəsɪs] *n* Krankheitsende *nt*, Apostasis *f*.
a·po·stax·is [æpəʊˈstæksɪs] *n* Sickerblutung *f*, leichte Blutung *f*.
ap·o·stem [ˈæpəstem] *n old* → abscess.
a·po·ste·ma [æpəˈstiːmə] *n old* → abscess.
a·po·stem·a·tous cheilitis [æpəˈstemətəs] Volkmann-Cheilitis *f*, -Krankheit *f*, Cheilitis glandularis apostematosa.
ap·o·steme [ˈæpəstiːm] *n old* → abscess.
a·pos·thia [əˈpɒsθɪə] *n* Vorhautaplasie *f*, Aposthie *f*.
a·poth·e·car·y [əˈpɒθəkeərɪ] *n old* → pharmacist.
ap·o·the·ci·um [ˌæpəˈθiːʃɪəm, -sɪ-] *n micro*. Apothezium *nt*.
ap·pa·rat·us [ˌæpəˈrætəs, -ˈreɪtəs] *n*, *pl* **-tus, tus·es 1.** *bio*. System *nt*, Trakt *m*, Apparat *m*; *anat*. Organsystem *nt*, Apparatus *m*. **2.** Apparate *pl*, (*a. fig*.) Maschinerie *f*. **3.** Apparat *m*, Gerät *nt*.
a. of Goormaghtigh juxtaglomerulärer Apparat.
ap·par·ent [əˈpærənt] *adj* **1.** sichtbar, manifest, apparent. **2.** offensichtlich, ersichtlich, klar. **without ~ cause** ohne ersichtlichen Grund.
apparent infection apparente/klinisch-manifeste Infektion *f*.
ap·pear [əˈpɪər] *vi* **1.** erscheinen, auftauchen, s. zeigen, sichtbar werden; (*Ausschlag*) ausbrechen; (*Symptome*) zu Tage treten. **2.** scheinen, den Anschein haben, aussehen.
ap·pear·ance [əˈpɪərəns] *n* **1.** Erscheinung(sbild *nt*) *f*, Phänomen *nt*, äußere (An-)Schein *m*, Erscheinung *f*. **at first ~** beim ersten Anblick. **in ~** anscheinend, dem Anschein nach. **to all ~** allem Anschein nach. **3.** Auftreten *nt*, Vorkommen *nt*; Erscheinen *nt*.
ap·pend·age [əˈpendɪdʒ] *n* Zusatz *m*, Zubehör *nt*; (*a. anat*.) Anhang *m*, Ansatz *m*, Anhängsel *nt*, Fortsatz *m*.
a. of epididymis Nebenhodenhydatide *f*, Appendix epididymidis.
a.s of eye Augenhilfsapparat *m*.
a.s of the skin Hautanhangsgebilde *pl*.
ap·pen·dal·gia [æpənˈdældʒ(ɪ)ə] *n* Schmerzen *pl* in der Blinddarmgegend, Appendalgie *f*.
ap·pen·dec·to·my [ˌ-ˈdektəmɪ] *n chir*. operative Entfernung *f* des Wurmfortsatzes, *inf*. Blinddarmoperation *f*, Appendektomie *f*.
ap·pen·di·cal [əˈpendɪkl] *adj* → appendicular 1.

appendiceal

ap·pen·di·ce·al [ˌæpənˈdɪʃl, əˌpendɪˈsiːəl] *adj* → appendicular 1.
appendiceal abscess appendizitischer Abszeß *m*.
appendiceal carcinoid Appendixkarzinoid *nt*.
appendiceal edema Appendixödem *nt*.
ap·pen·di·cec·to·my [əˌpendəˈsektəmɪ] *n* → appendectomy.
ap·pen·di·cial [ˌæpənˈdɪʃl] *adj* → appendicular 1.
ap·pen·di·ci·tis [əˌpendəˈsaɪtɪs] *n* Wurmfortsatzentzündung *f*, inf. Blinddarmentzündung *f*, Appendizitis *f*, Appendicitis *f*.
ap·pen·di·co·ce·cos·to·my [əˌpendɪkəʊsɪˈkɑstəmɪ] *n chir.* Appendikozäkostomie *f*.
ap·pen·di·co·cele [əˈpendɪkəʊsiːl] *n* Appendikozele *f*.
ap·pen·di·co·en·ter·os·to·my [əˌpendɪkəʊentərˈɑstəmɪ] *n chir.* Appendikoenterostomie *f*.
ap·pen·di·co·li·thi·a·sis [ˌ-lɪˈθaɪəsɪs] *n* Appendikolithiasis *f*.
ap·pen·di·col·y·sis [əˌpendɪˈkɑləsɪs] *n chir.* Appendikolyse *f*.
ap·pen·di·cop·a·thy [ˌ-ˈkɑpəθɪ] *n* (nichtentzündliche) Wurmfortsatzerkrankung *f*, Appendikopathie *f*, Appendicopathia *f*.
ap·pen·di·cos·to·my [ˌ-ˈkɑstəmɪ] *n chir.* Appendikostomie *f*.
ap·pen·di·cu·lar [ˌæpənˈdɪkjələr] *adj* 1. Wurmfortsatz/Appendix betr., Appendic(o)-, Appendik(o)-, Appendix-. 2. Gliedmaße betr. 3. Anhang/Anhängsel betr.
appendicular abscess appendizitischer Abszeß *m*.
appendicular artery Appendixarterie *f*, Appendikularis *f*, A. appendicularis.
appendicular colic Kolik *f od.* kolikartiger Schmerz *m* bei Appendizitis.
appendicular lobe (*Leber*) Riedel'-Lappen *m*.
appendicular lymph nodes Appendixlymphknoten *pl*, Nodi lymphatici appendiculares.
appendicular skeleton Gliedmaßenskelett *nt*, Skeleton appendiculare.
appendicular vein Appendixvene *f*, V. appendicularis.
ap·pen·dix [əˈpendɪks] *n, pl* **-dix·es**, **-dic·es** [-dəsiːz] 1. Anhang *m*, Anhängsel *nt*, Ansatz *m*, Fortsatz *m*; *anat.* Appendix *f*. 2. Wurmfortsatz *m* des Blinddarms, inf. Wurm *m*, Appendix *f* (vermiformis). **to have one's ~ out** s. den Blinddarm herausnehmen lassen.
a. of epididymis → appendage of epididymis.
ap·pen·do·li·thi·a·sis [əˌpendəʊlɪˈθaɪəsɪs] *n* → appendicolithiasis.
ap·per·cep·tion [ˌæpərˈsepʃn] *n* bewußte Wahrnehmung *f*, Apperzeption *f*.
ap·per·cep·tive [ˌ-ˈseptɪv] *adj* Apperzeption betr., apperzeptiv.
ap·per·son·a·tion [æˌpɜrsəˈneɪʃn] *n* → appersonification.
ap·per·son·i·fi·ca·tion [ˌæpərˌsɑnəfɪˈkeɪʃn] *n psychia.* Apersonierung *f*.
ap·pe·tite [ˈæpɪtaɪt] *n* 1. Appetit *m* (*for* auf), Eßlust *f*. **to have an ~** Appetit haben (*for* auf). **to have no ~** keinen Appetit haben (*for* auf). **to have a good ~** einen guten *od.* gesunden Appetit haben. **to have a bad ~** einen schlechten Appetit haben. 2. Verlangen *nt*, Begierde *f*, Gelüst *nt* (*for* nach); Hunger *m* (*for* nach), Neigung *f*, Trieb *m*, Lust *f* (*for* zu).
appetite suppressant Appetitzügler *m*.
ap·pla·na·tion [æplə'neɪʃn] *n* Abflachung *f*, Applanation *f*, Applanatio *f*.

applanation tonometer *ophthal.* Applanationstonometer *nt*.
applanation tonometry *ophthal.* Applanationstonometrie *f*.
ap·pla·nom·e·ter [ˌæpləˈnɑmɪtər] *n* → applanation tonometer.
ap·pla·nom·e·try [ˌ-ˈnɑmətrɪ] *n ophthal.* Applanationstonometrie *f*.
ap·pli·ance [əˈplaɪəns] *n* 1. Vorrichtung *f*, Gerät *nt*, (Hilfs-)Mittel *nt*. 2. Anwenden *nt*, Anwendung *f*, Bedienung *f*.
ap·pli·ca·bil·i·ty [ˌæplɪkəˈbɪlətɪ] *n* Anwendbarkeit *f* (*to* auf), Eignung *f* (*to* für).
ap·pli·ca·ble [ˈæplɪkəbl, əˈplɪkə-] *adj* anwendbar (*to* auf); geeignet, passend (*to* für); angemessen, angebracht (*to*). **not ~** (*in Formularen*) entfällt, nicht zutreffend.
ap·pli·ca·ble·ness [ˈæplɪkəblnɪs] *n* → applicability.
ap·pli·ca·tion [ˌæplɪˈkeɪʃn] *n* 1. Applikation *f* (*to* auf), Anwendung *f*, Verwendung *f*, Gebrauch *m* (*to* auf). **for external ~** zum äußeren Gebrauch. 2. (*Salbe*) Auftragen *nt*; (*Verband*) Anlegen *nt*; (*Medikament*) Verabreichung *f*. 3. Bewerbung *f*, Antrag *m*, Anmeldung *f* (*for* um, für).
application form Antrags-, Bewerbungs-, Anmeldungsbogen *m*.
ap·pli·ca·tor [ˈæplɪkeɪtər] *n* Applikator *m*, Anwendungsgerät *nt*, Aufträger *m*.
ap·plied [əˈplaɪd] *adj* angewandt.
applied anatomy angewandte Anatomie *f*.
applied chemistry angewandte Chemie *f*.
applied research angewandte Forschung *f*, Zweckforschung *f*.
ap·ply [əˈplaɪ] **I** *vt* 1. (*Salbe*) auftragen; (*Pflaster*) anlegen; anbringen, auflegen (*to* an, auf). 2. anwenden (*to* auf), verwenden (*to* für). **to ~ externally** äußerlich anwenden. **II** *vi* 3. gelten (*to* für), zutreffen (*to* auf), betreffen. 4. s. bewerben (*for* um).
ap·point·ment [əˈpɔɪntmənt] *n* Termin *m* (*with* bei); Terminvereinbarung *f*, (geschäftliche) Verabredung *f*. **by ~** nach Vereinbarung, mit (Vor-)Anmeldung.
appointment desk Anmeldung *f*.
ap·po·si·tion [ˌæpəˈzɪʃn] *n* 1. Bei-, Hinzufügung *f*, Bei-, Zusatz *m*. 2. An-, Auflagerung *f*, Apposition *f*.
ap·po·si·tion·al [ˌæpəˈzɪʃnəl] *adj* bei-, zugefügt, an-, aufgelagert, appositionell.
appositional growth appositionelles Wachstum *nt*.
ap·pos·i·tive [əˈpɑzɪtɪv] *adj* → appositional.
ap·prais·al [əˈpreɪzl] *n* (*Verfassung, Lage*) Beurteilung *f*, (Ab-, Ein-)Schätzung *f*.
ap·praise [əˈpreɪz] *vt* beurteilen, (ab-, ein-)schätzen, bewerten. **to ~ the situation** (*falsely*) die Lage (falsch) einschätzen.
ap·pre·ci·a·ble [əˈpriːʃ(ɪ)əbl] *adj* beträchtlich, deutlich, merklich, spürbar.
ap·pre·hend [æprɪˈhend] *vt fig.* begreifen, erfassen, wahrnehmen.
ap·pre·hen·sion [ˌ-ˈhenʃn] *n* 1. Erfassen *nt*, Begreifen *nt*, Apprehension *f*. 2. Auffassungsvermögen *nt*, -gabe *f*, -kraft *f*, Verstand *m*. 3. *psychia.* Besorgnis *f*, Furcht *f*, Apprehension *f*.
ap·pre·hen·sive [ˌ-ˈhensɪv] *adj* 1. empfindlich, empfindsam; reizbar, apprehensiv. 2. *psychia.* besorgt (*for* um), ängstlich, apprehensiv. 3. (leicht) begreifend, auffassungsfähig.
ap·pre·hen·sive·ness [ˌ-ˈhensɪvnɪs] *n* 1. schnelle Auffassungsgabe *f*. 2. → apprehension 3.
ap·proach [əˈprəʊtʃ] **I** *n* 1. Annäherung *f*, (Heran-)Nahen *nt*, (Her-)Anrücken *nt*. 2. Sehweise *f*, Zugang *m*, Approach *m*. 3. *chir.* (operativer) Zugang *m*. 4. Einführung *f* (*to* in), Weg *m*, Zugang *m* (*to* zu). **II** *vt* 5. s. nähern. 6. (*Aufgabe*) herangehen an, anpacken. **III** *vi* 7. s. nähern, näherkommen, heranukommen, (heran-)nahen. 8. *fig.* nahekommen, ähnlich *od.* fast gleich sein, grenzen (*to* an).
ap·proach·a·ble [əˈprəʊtʃəbl] *adj* zugänglich; *fig.* um-, zugänglich.
approach-approach conflict *psycho., psychia.* Appetenz-Appetenz-Konflikt *m*.
approach-avoidance conflict *psycho., psychia.* Appetenz-Aversions-Konflikt *m*.
ap·pro·pri·ate [əˈprəʊprɪət] *adj* 1. geeignet, passend, angebracht, angemessen (*to, for* für). **an ~ diet** eine angepaßte/angemessene Ernährung. **not ~ in pregnancy** nicht geeignet während der Schwangerschaft. 2. entsprechend, zuständig.
ap·prov·al [əˈpruːvl] *n* Zustimmung *f*, Billigung *f*, Einverständnis *nt*; (offizielle) Genehmigung *f*, Zulassung *f* (*of* von, zu).
ap·prove [əˈpruːv] **I** *vt* billigen, anerkennen; genehmigen. **II** *vi* zustimmen, billigen; genehmigen, zulassen (*of*).
ap·proved [əˈpruːvd] *adj* 1. erprobt. 2. genehmigt, zugelassen.
ap·prox·i·mal [əˈprɑksɪməl] *adj* → approximate II.
ap·prox·i·mate [əˈprɑksɪmeɪt] **I** *n* Näherungswert *m*. **II** *adj* annähernd, ungefähr, approximativ, approximal, Näherungs-. **III** *vt* 1. s. nähern, nahekommen, fast erreichen, annähernd gleich sein. 2. *chir.* (*Wundränder*) annähern, zusammenbringen. **IV** *vi* s. nähern (*to*).
ap·prox·i·ma·tion [əˌprɑksəˈmeɪʃn] *n* 1. (*a. mathe., fig.*) (An-)Näherung *f* (*to* an). 2. Näherungswert *m*. 3. *chir.* (*Wundränder*) Annähern *nt*, Annäherung *f*.
approximation method Näherungsverfahren *nt*.
ap·prox·i·ma·tive [əˈprɑksɪmətɪv] *adj* annähernd, approximativ.
a·prac·tic [əˈpræktɪk] *adj* Apraxie betr., apraxisch.
a.p. radiograph → a.p. roentgenogram.
a·prax·i·a [əˈpræksɪə, eɪ-] *n* Apraxie *f*, Apraxia *f*.
a·prax·ic [əˈpræksɪk] *adj* → apractic.
a·prin·dine [əˈprɪndiːn] *n pharm.* Aprindin *nt*.
a·pro·bar·bi·tal [ˌæprəˈbɑːrbɪtəl] *n pharm.* Aprobarbital *nt*.
a·proc·tia [eɪˈprɑkʃɪə] *n embryo.* Anusaplasie *f*, Aproktie *f*.
a.p. roentgenogram a.p.-Röntgenbild *nt*, a.p.-Aufnahme *f*.
a·pron [ˈeɪprən] *n* Schürze *f*.
a·pro·sex·ia [ˌæprəˈseksɪə] *n* Aufmerksamkeitsschwäche *f*, Aprosexie *f*.
a·pros·o·pia [ˌeɪprəˈsəʊpɪə] *n embryo.* Aprosopie *f*.
a·pros·o·pus [eɪˈprɑsəpəs] *n embryo.* Aprosopus *m*.
a·pro·tic [eɪˈprəʊtɪk] *adj chem.* frei von Protonen, aprotisch.
a·pro·ti·nin [eɪˈprəʊtənɪn, æ-] *n* Aprotinin *nt*.
APRT *abbr.* → adenine phosphoribosyl transferase.
ap·sel·a·phe·sia [ˌæpsələˈfiːzɪə] *n neuro.* Verminderung *f* des Tastsinnes, Apsel(h)aphesie *f*.
ap·si·thyr·ia [ˌæpsɪˈθaɪrɪə] *n psychia.* psychogener Stimmverlust *m*, Apsithyrie *f*.
Apt [æpt] *n*: **A. test** *lab.* Apt-Probe *f*.
apt [æpt] *adj* 1. passend, geeignet; treffend. 2. neigen, geneigt sein (*to do* zu tun). 3. begabt (*at* für), geschickt (*at* in), intelligent.

ap·ti·tude ['æptɪt(j)uːd] *n* **1.** Begabung *f*, Befähigung *f* (*for* für), Talent *nt* (*for* für), Geschick *nt*, Eignung *f* (*for* zu). **2.** Neigung *f*, Hang *m* (*for* zu). **3.** Auffassungsgabe *f*, Intelligenz *f*.
aptitude test Eignungs-, Tauglichkeitstest *m*, -prüfung *f*.
ap·ty·a·lia [ˌeɪtaɪ'eɪlɪə, -jə] *n* verminderte *od.* fehlende Speichelsekretion *f*, Aptyalismus *m*, Asialie *f*, Xerostomie *f*.
ap·ty·a·lism [æp'taɪəlɪzəm] *n* → aptyalia.
APUD, Apud ['eɪpəd] *abbr.* [amine precursor uptake and decarboxylation] APUD, Apud.
APUD cell APUD-, Apud-Zelle *f*.
a·pud·o·ma [ˌeɪpə'dəʊmə] *n* Apudom *nt*.
APUD system *old* Helle-Zellen-System *nt*, APUD-, Apud-System *nt*.
a·pu·rin·ic acid [eɪpjə'rɪnɪk] Apurinsäure *f*.
a·pus ['eɪpəs] *n embryo.* Apus *m*.
a·py·e·tous [ə'paɪətəs] *adj* nicht-eitrig, ohne Eiter, aputrid.
a·pyk·no·mor·phous [əˌpɪknə'mɔːrfəs, eɪ-] *adj histol.* apyknomorph.
a·py·og·e·nous [eɪpaɪ'ɒdʒənəs] *adj* nicht durch Eiter verursacht, apyogen.
a·py·ous [eɪ'paɪəs] *adj* ohne Eiter, aputrid.
a·py·ret·ic [ˌeɪpaɪ'retɪk] *adj* fieberfrei, ohne Fieber (verlaufend), apyretisch, afebril.
apyretic tetanus neuromuskuläre Übererregbarkeit *f*, Tetanie *f*.
a·py·rex·ia [ˌ-'reksɪə] *n* Fieberlosigkeit *f*, Apyrexie *f*.
a·py·rim·i·din·ic acid [əˌpaɪrɪmə'dɪnɪk] Apyrimidinsäure *f*.
a·py·ro·gen·ic [eɪˌpaɪrə'dʒenɪk] *adj* nicht fiebererzeugend, apyrogen.
Aq. *abbr.* → aqua.
aq·ua ['ækwə] *n, pl* **aq·uae** ['ækwiː, 'ɑk-], **aq·uas** *abbr.* **Aq. 1.** Wasser *nt*; Aqua *f abbr.* Aq. **2.** *pharm.* (wässrige) Lösung *f*, Aqua *f*.
aq·ua·co·bal·a·min [ˌækwəkəʊ'bæləmɪn] *n* Aquo-, Aquacobalamin *nt*, Vitamin B$_{12b}$ *nt*.
aq·ua·pho·bia [ˌ-'fəʊbɪə] *n psychia.* Angst *f* vor Wasser, Aquaphobie *f*.
aq·ua·punc·ture ['-pʌŋkʃər] *n* subkutane Wasserinjektion *f*.
aq·ue·duct ['-dʌkt] *n anat.* Aquädukt *m*, Aqu(a)eductus *m*.
a. of cochlea Aqu(a)eductus cochleae.
a. of Fallopius Fazialiskanal *m*, Canalis facialis.
a. of mesencephalon Aquädukt, Aqu(a)eductus cerebri/mesencephalici.
a. of midbrain → a. of mesencephalon.
a. of Silvius → a. of mesencephalon.
a. of Sylvius → a. of mesencephalon.
a. of vestibule Endolymphgang *m*, Ductus endolymphaticus.
aq·ue·duc·tus [ˌ-'dʌktəs] *n* → aqueduct.
a·que·ous ['eɪkwəs, 'æk-] **I** *n* Kammerwasser *nt*, Humor aquosus. **II** *adj* wässerig, wäßrig, wasserhaltig, -artig, Wasser-.
aqueous chamber (*Auge*) mit Kammerwasser gefüllter Augenraum.
aqueous humor → aqueous I.
aqueous phase *phys.* wäßrige Phase *f*.
aqueous solution *phys.* wäßrige Lösung *f*.
aqueous vaccine wäßriger Impfstoff *m*.
aq·uo·co·bal·a·min [ˌækwəʊkəʊ'bæləmɪn] *n* → aquacobalamin.
AR *abbr.* **1.** → alarm reaction. **2.** → aortic regurgitation. **3.** → artificial respiration.
Ar *abbr.* → argon.
ara-A *abbr.* [adenine arabinoside] → arabinoadenosine.
ar·a·bic acid ['ærəbɪk] → arabin.
ar·a·bin ['ærəbɪn] *n* Arabin *nt*.
ar·a·bin·o·a·den·o·sine [ˌærəbɪnəʊə'denə-

siːn, -sɪn] *n* Vidarabin *nt*, Adenin-Arabinosid *nt abbr.* Ara-A.
ar·a·bin·o·cyt·i·dine [ˌ-'sɪtəsiːn, -sɪn] *n* → arabinosylcytosine.
a·rab·i·nose [ə'ræbɪnəʊs, 'ærəbə-] *n* Arabinose *f*.
β-a·rab·i·nos·i·dase [əˌræbɪ'nɒsɪdeɪz] *n* β-Arabinosidase *f*.
a·rab·i·no·sis [əˌræbɪ'nəʊsɪs] *n* Arabinoseintoxikation *f*.
a·rab·i·no·su·ria [əˌræbɪnə's(j)ʊərɪə] *n* Arabinosurie *f*.
ar·a·bin·o·syl·a·de·nine [əˌrəbɪnəʊsɪl'ædəniːn] *n* → arabinoadenosine.
a·rab·i·no·syl·cy·to·sine [ˌ-'saɪtəsiːn, -sɪn] *n abbr.* **ara-C** Cytarabin *nt*, Cytosin-Arabinosid *nt abbr.* ara-C.
ar·a·bin·u·lose [ærə'bɪnjələʊs] *n* Arabinulose *f*.
a·rab·i·tol [ə'ræbɪtɒl, -tɔʊl] *n* Arabit *nt*, Arabitol *nt*.
ar·a·bo·py·ra·nose [ˌærəbəʊ'paɪrənəʊz] *n* → arabinose.
ara-C *abbr.* → arabinosylcytosine.
a·rach·ic acid [ə'rækɪk] → arachidic acid.
a·rach·i·date [ə'rækɪdeɪt] *n* Arachidat *nt*, Eicosanoat *nt*.
ar·a·chid·ic acid [ˌærə'kɪdɪk] Arachinsäure *f*, *n*-Eicosansäure *f*.
a·rach·i·don·ate [ə'rækɪˌdəneɪt] *n* Arachidonat *nt*.
arachidonate-5-lipoxygenase *n* Arachidonsäure-5-Lipoxygenase *f*.
arachidonate-12-lipoxygenase *n* Arachidonsäure-12-Lipoxygenase *f*.
ar·a·chi·don·ic acid [ˌærəkɪ'dɒnɪk] Arachidonsäure *f*.
arachidonic acid derivatives Arachidonsäurederivate *pl*, Eicosanoide *pl*.
ar·a·chis oil ['ærəkɪs] Erdnußöl *nt*, Arachisöl *nt*.
a·rach·ne·pho·bia [əˌrækni'fəʊbɪə] *n* → arachnophobia.
A·rach·nia [ə'ræknɪə] *n micro.* Arachnia *f*.
a·rach·nid [ə'ræknɪd] **I** *n* Spinnentier *nt*, Arachnid *m*. **II** *adj* Arachnida betr., spinnenartig.
A·rach·ni·da [ə'ræknɪdə] *pl bio.* Spinnentiere *pl*, Arachnida *pl*.
a·rach·ni·dan [ə'ræknɪdən] *n, adj* → arachnid.
a·rach·nid·ism [ə'ræknɪdɪzəm] *n* Arachnidismus *m*.
a·rach·ni·tis [ˌæræk'naɪtɪs] *n* → arachnoiditis.
a·rach·no·dac·tyl·ia [əˌræknəʊdæk'tɪlɪə] *n* → arachnodactyly.
a·rach·no·dac·ty·ly [ˌ-'dæktəlɪ] *n* **1.** Spinnenfingrigkeit *f*, Arachnodaktylie *f*. **2.** Marfan-Syndrom *nt*, Arachnodaktylie-Syndrom *nt*.
a·rach·no·gas·tria [ˌ-'gæstrɪə] *n* Medusenhaupt *nt*, Caput medusae.
a·rach·noid [ə'ræknɔɪd] **I** *n anat.* Spinnwebenhaut *f*, Arachnoidea *f*. **II** *adj* **1.** spinnenartig, spinnwebartig, spinnennetzähnlich. **2.** Spinnwebenhaut/Arachnoidea betr., arachnoid, arachnoidal, Arachnoidal-.
a. of brain kranielle Spinnwebenhaut, Arachnoidea (mater) encephali/cranialis.
a. of spine spinale Spinnwebenhaut, Arachnoidea (mater) spinalis.
ar·ach·noi·dal [ˌærækˈnɔɪdl] *adj* → arachnoid II.
arachnoidal granulations → arachnoid granulations.
arachnoidal villi Arachnoidalzotten *pl*.
arachnoid canal Cisterna ambiens.
arachnoid cyst Arachnoidalzyste *f*.
ar·ach·noi·dea [ˌæræk'nɔɪdɪə] *n* → arachnoid I.

ar·ach·noi·de·an [ˌ-'nɔɪdɪən] *adj* → arachnoid II.
arachnoid granulations Arachnoidalzotten *pl*, Pacchioni-Granulationen *pl*, Granulationes arachnoideae.
a·rach·noid·ism [ə'ræknɔɪdɪzəm] *n* → arachnidism.
a·rach·noid·i·tis [əˌræknɔɪ'daɪtɪs] *n* Entzündung *f* der Arachnoidea, Arachnoiditis *f*, Arachnitis *f*.
arachnoid membrane → arachnoid I.
arachnoid sheath Arachnoideascheide *f* des N. opticus.
ar·ach·nol·y·sin [ˌæræk'nɒləsɪn] *n* Arachnolysin *nt*.
a·rach·no·pho·bia [əˌræknəʊ'fəʊbɪə] *n psychia.* Angst *f* vor Spinnen, Arachnophobie *f*.
Aran [ə'ræn]: **A.'s law** *ortho.* Aran'-Gesetz *nt*.
Aran-Duchenne [dy'ʃen]: **A.-D. disease** → A.-D. type.
A.-D. muscular atrophy → A.-D. type.
A.-D. type Aran-Duchenne-Krankheit *f*, -Syndrom *nt*, Duchenne-Aran-Krankheit *f*, -Syndrom *nt*, adult-distale Form *f* der spinalen Muskelatrophie, spinale progressive Muskelatrophie *f*.
A·ra·ne·ae [ə'reɪnɪˌiː] *pl bio.* Webspinnen *pl*, Araneae *pl*.
Ar·a·ne·i·da [ærə'nɪədə] *pl* → Araneae.
a·ra·ne·ism [ə'reɪnɪˌɪzəm] *n* → arachnidism.
a·ra·ne·ous [ə'reɪnɪəs] *adj* spinnennetzähnlich.
Arantius [ə'rænʃəs]: **canal of A.** Ductus venosus.
bodies of A. Arantius-Knötchen *pl*, Noduli valvularum semilunarium.
duct of A. Ductus venosus.
A.' ligament Lig. venosum.
nodules of A. → bodies of A.
ventricle of A. 1. Cavum septi pellucidi. **2.** Rautengrube *f*, Fossa rhomboidea.
a·ra·phia [ə'reɪfɪə] *n embryo.* Dysrhaphie *f*.
a·ra·py·ra·nose [ˌærə'paɪrənəʊz] *n* → arabinose.
ARAS *abbr.* → ascending reticular activating system.
ar·bi·trar·y ['ɑːrbɪˌtrerɪ] *adj* willkürlich, nach Ermessen, arbiträr.
ar·bor ['ɑːrbər] *n, pl* **-bo·res** [-'bɔʊriːz] *bio.* Baum *m*.
ar·bo·res·cent [ˌɑːrb'resnt] *adj* baumartig wachsend, verzweigt, Baum-.
arborescent white substance of cerebellum → arbor vitae of vermis.
ar·bor·i·za·tion [ˌɑːrbərɪ'zeɪʃn] *n* (baumartige) Ver-, Aufzweigung *f*, Verästelung *f*, dendritenartige Bildung *f*, Arborisation *f*.
arborization block → arborization heart block.
arborization heart block Arborizations-, Ast-, Verzweigungsblock *m*.
arbor virus → arbovirus.
arbor vi·tae of vermis ['vaɪtɪ] (*Kleinhirn*) Markkörper *m*, Arbor vitae (cerebelli).
ar·bo·vi·ral [ɑːrbə'vaɪrəl] *adj* Arboviren betr., durch Arboviren verursacht, Arboviren-.
arboviral infection Arbovireninfektion *f*, Arbovirose *f*.
ar·bo·vi·rus [ˌ-'vaɪrəs] *n* Arbovirus *nt*, ARBO-Virus *nt*.
arbovirus encephalitis Arbovirus-Enzephalitis *f*.
ARC *abbr.* → AIDS-related complex.
A.R.C. *abbr.* → retinal correspondence, anomalous.
arc [ɑːrk] *n* **1.** (*a. techn.*) Bogen *m*. **2.** *mathe.*

arcate

(Kreis-)Bogen m, Arcus m. **3.** (Licht-)Bogen m.
ar·cate ['ɑːrkeɪt] adj → arcuate.
arc-flash conjunctivitis ophthal. Conjunctivitis actinica/photoelectrica, Keratoconjunctivitis/Ophthalmia photoelectrica.
arch [ɑːrtʃ] **I** n Bogen m, Wölbung f, Gewölbe nt, bogenförmige od. gewölbte Struktur od. Bahn f. **II** vi s. wölben.
a. of aorta Aortenbogen, Arcus aortae.
a. of azygos vein Azygosbogen, Arcus v. azygos.
a. of cricoid (cartilage) Ringknorpelbogen, Arcus cartilaginis cricoideae.
a. of foot Fußgewölbe.
a. of thoracic duct Ductus thoracicus-Bogen, Arcus ductus thoracici.
archae(o)- pref. Archä(o)-, Archi-.
Ar·chae·o·bac·te·ri·a [ˌɑːrkɪoʊbækˈtɪərɪə] pl Archä(o)bakterien pl, Archaebacteria pl.
ar·chae·o·cer·e·bel·lum [ˌ-ˌserəˈbeləm] n Arch(a)eocerebellum nt, Archicerebellum nt.
ar·chae·o·cor·tex [ˌ-ˈkɔːrteks] n Archicortex m, Archipallium nt, Cortex medialis pallii, Arch(a)eocortex m.
ar·cha·ic [ɑːrˈkeɪɪk] adj frühzeitlich, altertümlich, urtümlich, archaisch.
arche- pref. → archae(o)-.
Ar·che·bac·te·ri·a [ˌɑːrkɪbækˈtɪərɪə] pl → Archaeobacteria.
arched crest [ɑːtʃt] Crista arcuata.
ar·che·go·ni·um [ˌɑːrkɪˈgoʊnɪəm] n bio. Archegonium nt.
arch·en·ceph·a·lon [ˌɑːrkenˈsefələn] n Urhirn nt, Archencephalon nt.
arch·en·ter·ic canal [ˌ-ˈterɪk] embryo. Canalis neurentericus.
arch·en·ter·on [ɑːrˈkentərən, -rən] n, pl **-ter·a** [-tərə] Urdarm m, Archenteron nt.
archeo- pref. → archae(o)-.
ar·che·o·cer·e·bel·lum n → archaeocerebellum.
ar·che·o·ci·net·ic adj → archeokinetic.
ar·che·o·ki·net·ic [ˌɑːrkɪoʊkɪˈnetɪk, -kaɪ-] adj archäokinetisch.
ar·che·spore [ˈɑːrkəspɔːr, -spəʊr] n bio. Archespor nt, -sporium nt.
ar·che·spo·ri·um [ˌ-ˈspɔːrɪəm, -ˈspəʊr-] n → archespore.
ar·che·type [ˈ-taɪp] n **1.** Urtyp m, -form f, -bild nt, Archetyp(us m) m. **2.** psychia. Archetypus m.
archi- pref. → archae(o).
ar·chi·blast [ˈ-blæst] n embryo. Archiblast m.
ar·chi·blas·tic [ˌ-ˈblæstɪk] adj archiblastisch.
ar·chi·cer·e·bel·lum [ˌ-ˌserəˈbeləm] n → archaeocerebellum.
ar·chi·cor·tex [ˌ-ˈkɔːrteks] n → archicortex.
ar·chi·cor·ti·cal [ˌ-ˈkɔːrtɪkl] adj Archicortex betr., archikortikal.
ar·chi·cyte [ˈ-saɪt] n befruchtete Eizelle f, Zygote f.
ar·chi·gas·ter [ˌ-ˈgæstər] n → archenteron.
ar·chi·gas·tru·la [ˌ-ˈgæstrələ] n embryo. Archigastrula f.
ar·chi·mor·u·la [ˌ-ˈmɔːrələ, -ˈmɑːr-] n embryo. Archimorula f.
ar·chi·my·ce·tes [ˌ-maɪˈsiːtiːz] pl micro. Urpilze pl, Archimyzeten pl.
ar·chi·neph·ric canal/duct [ˌ-ˈnefrɪk] embryo. Vornierengang m.
ar·chi·neph·ron [ˌ-ˈnefrən] n Archinephron nt.
ar·chi·neu·ron [ˌɑːrkəˈnjʊərɑn, -ˈnʊ-] n Archineuron nt.
ar·chi·pal·li·al [ˌ-ˈpælɪəl] adj Archipallium/

Archicortex betr., archipallial, -kortikal.
ar·chi·pal·li·um [ˌ-ˈpælɪəm] n → archaeocortex.
ar·chi·spore [ˈ-spɔːr, -spəʊr] n → archespore.
ar·chi·stome [ˈ-stəʊm] n embryo. Urdarmöffnung f, Urmund m, Blastoporus m.
ar·chi·tec·ton·ic [ˌ-tekˈtɑnɪk] adj Architektur od. Architektonik betr., architektonisch, baulich; systematisch, strukturell.
ar·chi·tec·ton·ics [ˌ-tekˈtɑnɪks] pl **1.** Architektonik f, Architektur f. **2.** Struktur f, Aufbau m, Anlage f.
ar·chi·tec·ture [ˈ-tektʃər] n (Auf-)Bau m, Struktur f.
ar·cho·cys·to·syr·inx [ˌ-ˌsɪstəˈsɪrɪŋks] n Aftero-Blasen-Fistel f, anovesikale Fistel f.
ar·chop·to·sis [ˌɑːrkəʊˈtəʊsɪs] n old → rectal prolapse.
ar·chor·rha·gia [ˌɑːrkəˈrædʒ(ɪ)ə] n old rektale Blutung f.
arch support ortho. (Schuh-)Einlage f.
ar·ci·form [ˈɑːrsɪfɔːrm] adj bogenförmig, gebogen, gewölbt.
arciform arteries of kidney → arcuate arteries of kidney.
arciform veins of kidney → arcuate veins of kidney.
arc lamp Bogenlampe f.
arc·ta·tion [ɑːrkˈteɪʃn] n Einengung f, Verengerung f.
ar·cu·ate [ˈɑːrkjʊɪt, -ˌweɪt, -jəwət] adj bogenförmig, gewölbt, gebogen.
arcuate artery: a. of foot Bogenarterie f des Fußes, A. arcuata (pedis).
a.ies of kidney (Niere) Bogenarterien pl, Aa. arcuatae renis.
arcuate crest (of arytenoid cartilage) Crista arcuata.
ar·cu·at·ed [ˈɑːrkjʊˌeɪtɪd] adj → arcuate.
arcuate eminence Eminentia arcuata.
arcuate fibers Bogenfasern pl, bogenförmige Verbindungs-/Assoziationsfasern pl, Fibrae arcuatae cerebri.
anterior external a. Fibrae arcuatae externae anteriores.
a. of cerebrum → arcuate fibers.
dorsal external a. Fibrae arcuatae externae posteriores.
internal a. Fibrae arcuatae internae.
posterior external a. → dorsal external a.
ventral external a. → anterior external a.
arcuate ligament: a.s gelbe Bänder pl, Ligg. flava.
external a. of diaphragm → lateral a. (of diaphragm).
internal a. of diaphragm → medial a. (of diaphragm).
a. of knee Lig. popliteum arcuatum.
lateral a. (of diaphragm) Quadratusarkade f, Lig. arcuatum laterale, Arcus lumbocostalis lateralis (Halleri).
medial a. (of diaphragm) Psoasarkade f, Lig. arcuatum mediale, Arcus lumbocostalis medialis (Halleri).
median a. (of diaphragm) Aortenarkade f, Lig. arcuatum medianum.
a. of pubis Lig. arcuatum pubis.
arcuate line: a. of Douglas Linea arcuata Douglasi, Linea arcuata vaginae m. recti abdominis.
highest a. of occipital bone Linea nuchalis suprema.
a. of ilium Linea arcuata ossis ilii.
inferior a. of occipital bone Linea nuchalis inferior.
a. of pelvis Linea terminalis (pelvis).
a. of sheath of rectus abdominis muscle Linea arcuata vaginae m. recti abdominis.
superior a. of occipital bone, (external) Linea nuchalis superior.

supreme a. of occipital bone → highest a. of occipital bone.
arcuate nucleus Ursprungskern m der Fibrae arcuatae externae, Nc. arcuati (medullae oblongatae).
a. of hypothalamus Nc. arcuatus/infundibularis (hypothalami).
a. of medulla oblongata → arcuate nucleus.
arcuate papillae of tongue fadenförmige Papillen pl, Papillae filiformis.
arcuate suture anat. Kranznaht f, Sutura coronalis.
arcuate uterus Uterus arcuatus.
arcuate veins of kidney (Niere) Bogenvenen pl, Vv. arcuatae (renis).
arcuate zone (Ohr) innerer Tunnel m.
arc-weld·er lung [ˈɑːrkweldər] Lungensiderose f, Siderosis pulmonum.
ARD abbr. → acute respiratory disease.
ar·dan·es·the·sia [ɑːrdænesˈθiːʒ(ɪ)ə] n Verlust m der Temperaturempfindung, Therm(o)anästhesie f.
ar·dent [ˈɑːrdnt] adj **1.** heiß, brennend, glühend. **2.** fig. heftig, innig, leidenschaftlich, glühend.
ar·dor [ˈɑːrdər] n **1.** Hitze f, Glut f. **2.** fig. Heftigkeit f, Leidenschaft(lichkeit f) f, Inbrunst f, Glut f.
ARDS abbr. → adult respiratory distress syndrome.
ar·e·a [ˈeərɪə] n, pl **ar·e·as, ar·e·ae** [ˈeərˌiː]: **1.** Gebiet nt, Areal nt, Zone f, Bereich m, Gegend f, Region f; (Ober-)Fläche f. **2.** anat. Area f, anat. (ZNS) Zentrum nt. **3.** mathe. Inhalt m, (Grund-)Fläche f.
a. of facial nerve Area n. facialis.
a. H (of Forel) Forel'-H-Feld nt.
a. H₁ (of Forel) Forel'-H₁-Feld nt.
a. H₂ (of Forel) Forel'-H₂-Feld nt.
a.s of throat Halsregionen pl, Regiones cervicales.
ar·e·ca [əˈriːkə, ˈærɪ-] n Betelnuß f.
A receptor A-Rezeptor m.
a·re·co·line [əˈriːkəliːn, -lɪn, ˈærɪkə-] n pharm. Arekolin f, Arecolinum nt.
a·re·flex·ia [eɪrɪˈfleksɪə] n Reflexlosigkeit f, Fehlen nt normaler Reflexe, Areflexie f.
a·re·gen·er·a·tive [eɪrɪˈdʒenərətɪv, -ˌreɪtɪv] adj aregenerativ; aplastisch.
aregenerative anemia aplastische Anämie f.
chronic congenital a. Blackfan-Diamond-Anämie f, chronische kongenitale aregenerative Anämie f, pure red cell aplasia.
ar·e·na·ceous [ˌærɪˈneɪʃəs] adj → arenose.
Ar·e·na·vir·i·dae [ˌærɪnəˈvɪrɪdiː, -ˈvaɪr-] pl micro. Arenaviren pl, Arenaviridae pl.
ar·e·na·vi·rus [ˌ-ˈvaɪrəs] n Arenavirus nt.
ar·e·noid [ˈærɪnɔɪd] adj → arenose.
ar·e·nose [ˈærɪnəʊs] adj sandig, sandartig.
ar·e·nous [ˈærɪnəs] adj → arenose.
a·re·o·la [əˈriːələ] n, pl **-las, -lae** [-liː] anat. **1.** (kleiner) Hof m, kleiner (Haut-)Bezirk m, Areola f. **2.** histol. Gewebsspalte f, -fissur f.
f. of mammary gland Warzenvorhof m, Areola mammae.
a. of nipple → a. of mammary gland.
a·re·o·lar [əˈrɪələr] adj Areola betr., areolar, zellig, netzförmig.
areolar (central) choroiditis Förster-Chorioiditis f, Areolarchorioiditis f, Chorioiditis areolaris.
areolar gingiva Gingiva areolaris.
areolar glands Montgomery-Knötchen pl, Warzenvorhofdrüsen pl, Gll. areolares.
areolar plexus Venenplexus m der Brustwarze, Plexus venosus areolaris.
areolar tissue lockeres Bindegewebe nt.
areolar venous plexus → areolar plexus.

ar·e·o·li·tis [ˌeərɪəʊˈlaɪtɪs] *n gyn.* Warzenvorhofentzündung *f*, Areolitis *f*.
ar·e·om·e·ter [ˌeərɪˈɒmɪtər] *n phys.* Senk-, Tauch-, Flüssigkeitswaage *f*, Aräometer *nt*.
ar·e·o·met·ric [ˌeərɪəˈmetrɪk] *adj* Aräometrie betr., aräometrisch.
ar·e·om·e·try [ˌeərɪˈɒmətrɪ] *n* Aräometrie *f*.
Arey [ˈeɪrɪ]: **A.'s rule** *gyn.* Arey-Regel *f*.
ARF *abbr.* → acute renal failure.
Arg *abbr.* → arginine.
Ar·gas [ˈɑːɡəs, -ɡæs] *n micro.* Argas *f*.
Ar·gas·i·dae [ɑːrˈɡæsɪdiː] *n micro.* Lederzecken *pl*, Argasidae *pl*.
ar·gen·taf·fin [ɑːrˈdʒentəfɪn] *adj histol.* argentaffin.
ar·gen·taf·fine [ˈ-fiːn] *adj* → argentaffin.
argentaffine cells 1. argentaffine Zellen *pl*. **2.** enterochromaffine/gelbe/argentaffine/enteroendokrine Zellen *pl*, Kultschitzky-Zellen *pl*.
argentaffine granules argentaffine Granula *pl*.
argentaffin fiber Retikulum-, Retikulinfaser *f*, Gitterfaser *f*, argyrophile Faser *f*.
ar·gen·taf·fin·i·ty [ɑːrˌdʒentəˈfɪnətɪ] *n histol.* Argentaffinität *f*.
ar·gen·taf·fi·no·ma [ˌ-fɪˈnəʊmə] *n* Argentaffinom *nt*; Karzinoid *nt*.
argentaffinoma syndrome Flush-, Karzinoidsyndrom *nt*, Biörck-Thorson-Syndrom *nt*.
ar·gen·ta·tion [ɑːrdʒənˈteɪʃn] *n histol.* Versilberung *f*, Silberfärbung *f*.
ar·gen·tic [ɑːrˈdʒentɪk] *adj chem.* silberhaltig.
Ar·gen·tin·e·an [ˌɑːrdʒənˈtɪnɪən]: **A. hemorrhagic fever** Juninfieber *nt*, argentinisches hämorrhagisches Fieber *nt*.
A. hemorrhagic fever virus Juninfiebervirus *nt*.
Ar·gen·tine hemorrhagic fever [ˈɑːrdʒəntaɪn] → Argentinean hemorrhagic fever.
ar·gen·to·phil [ɑːrˈdʒentəfɪl] *adj* → argentaffin.
ar·gen·to·phile [ˈ-faɪl] *adj* → argentaffin.
argentophil fiber Retikulum-, Retikulinfaser *f*, Gitterfaser *f*, argyrophile Faser *f*.
ar·gen·to·phil·ic [ˌ-ˈfɪlɪk] *adj* → argentaffin.
ar·gen·tum [ɑːrˈdʒentəm] *n abbr.* **Ag** Silber *nt*, *chem.* Argentum *nt abbr.* **Ag**.
ar·gil·la [ɑːrˈdʒɪlə] *n* Kaolin *nt*
ar·gil·la·ceous [ɑːrdʒəˈleɪʃəs] *adj* tonhaltig, -artig, Ton-.
ar·gi·nase [ˈɑːrdʒɪneɪz] *n* Arginase *f*.
arginase deficiency → argininemia.
ar·gi·nine [ˈɑːrdʒɪniːn, -naɪn, -nɪn] *n abbr.* **Arg** Arginin *nt abbr.* Arg.
arginine carboxypeptidase Carboxypeptidase N *f*.
arginine decarboxylase Arginindecarboxylase *f*.
arginine kinase Argininkinase *f*.
ar·gi·nin·e·mia [ˌɑːrdʒɪnɪˈniːmɪə] *n* Arginase-Mangel *m*, (Hyper-)Argininämie *f*.
arginine phosphate Arginin(o)phosphat *nt*.
arginine test Arginin-Test *m*.
arginine vasopressin *abbr.* **AVP** Arginin-Vasopressin *nt*, Argipressin *nt*.
ar·gi·ni·no·suc·ci·nase [ˌɑːrdʒənɪnəʊˈsʌksəneɪs] *n* argininosuccinate lyase.
argininosuccinase deficiency → argininosuccinic aciduria.
ar·gi·ni·no·suc·ci·nate [ˌ-ˈsʌksəneɪt] *n* Argininosuccinat *nt*.
argininosuccinate lyase *abbr.* **ASAL, ASL, ASase** Arginin(o)succinatlyase *f abbr.* ASAL, ASL, Arginin(o)succinase *f*.
argininosuccinate lyase deficiency → argininosuccinic aciduria.

argininosuccinate synthetase Arginin(o)succinatsynthetase *f*.
ar·gi·ni·no·suc·cin·ic acid [ˌ-sʌkˈsɪnɪk] *abbr.* **ASA** Argininbernsteinsäure *f*.
argininosuccinic acidemia Argininosukzinämie *f*, -succinämie *f*.
argininosuccinic aciduria Argininbernsteinsäure-Krankheit *f*, -Schwachsinn *m*, Argininosukzinoazidurie *f*, -sukzinurie *f*, -succinurie *f*.
ar·gi·nyl [ˈɑːrdʒənɪl] *n* Arginyl-(Radikal *nt*).
ar·gi·pres·sin [ˌɑːrdʒɪˈpresɪn] *n* → arginine vasopressin.
ar·gon [ˈɑːrɡɒn] *n abbr.* **Ar** Argon *nt abbr.* Ar.
argon laser Argonlaser *m*.
Argonz-Del Castillo [ˈɑːrɡɒnz del kasˈtɪjɒ]: **A.-D. syndrome** → Ahumada-Del Castillo syndrome.
Argyll Robertson [ɑːrˈɡaɪl ˈrɒbərtsən]: **A. R. pupil/sign** Argyll Robertson-Phänomen *nt*, -Zeichen *nt*, -Pupille *f*.
ar·gyr·ia [ɑːrˈdʒɪrɪə] *n* Silberintoxikation *f*, Argyrie *f*, Argyrose *f*.
ar·gy·ri·a·sis [ˌɑːrdʒɪˈraɪəsɪs] *n* → argyria.
ar·gyr·ism [ˈɑːrdʒɪrɪzəm] *n* → argyria.
ar·gyr·o·phil [ˈɑːrdʒɪrəʊfɪl] *adj histol.* argyrophil.
ar·gyr·o·phile [ˈ-faɪl] *adj* → argyrophil.
argyrophil fiber → argentophil fiber.
ar·gyr·o·phil·ia [ˌ-ˈfiːlɪə] *n histol.* Argyrophilie *f*.
ar·gyr·o·phil·ic [ˌ-ˈfɪlɪk] *adj* → argyrophil.
argyrophilic cell argyrophile Zelle *f*.
ar·gyr·oph·i·lous [ˌɑːrdʒəˈrɒfɪləs] *adj* → argyrophil.
ar·gy·ro·sis [ˌɑːrdʒəˈrəʊsɪs] *n* → argyria.
a·rhin·en·ce·pha·lia [ˌeɪraɪnˌensəˈfeɪlɪə, -lɪə] *n* A(r)rhinenzephalie *f*.
a·rhin·ia [əˈraɪnɪə] *n* A(r)rhinie *f*.
a·rhyth·mia [əˈrɪðmɪə] *n* → arrhythmia.
Arias-Stella [ˈeərɪəs ˈstelə]: **A.-S. cells** Arias-Stella-Zellen *pl*.
A.-S. effect → A.-S. phenomenon.
A.-S. phenomenon Arias-Stella-Phänomen *nt*.
A.-S. reaction → A.-S. phenomenon.
a·ri·bo·fla·vin·o·sis [eɪˌraɪbəˌfleɪvəˈnəʊsɪs, -rɪb-] *n* Riboflavinmangel *m*, Ariboflavinose *f*.
a·rise [əˈraɪz] *(arose; arisen) vi* **1.** stammen, herrühren *(from, out of* von); entstehen; s. ergeben *(from, out of* aus). **2.** (Probleme, Fragen) auftauchen, -treten, -kommen, entstehen. **3.** aufstehen, s. erheben.
a·rith·me·tic [*n* əˈrɪθmətɪk; *adj* ˌærɪθˈmetɪk] **I** *n* Arithmetik *f*; Rechnen *nt*. **II** *adj* arithmetisch, rechnerisch, Rechen-.
ar·ith·met·i·cal [ˌærɪθˈmetɪkl] *adj* → arithmetic II.
arithmetic mean arithmetisches Mittel *nt*.
a·rith·mo·ma·nia [əˌrɪθməˈmeɪnɪə] *n* Zählzwang *m*, Arithmomanie *f*.
Ar·i·zo·na [ˌærɪˈzəʊnə] *n micro.* Salmonella arizonae.
ar·ky·o·chrome [ˈɑːrkɪəkrəʊm] *n* arkyochrome Nervenzelle *f*.
ar·ky·o·stich·o·chrome [ˌ-ˈstɪkəkrəʊm] *n* arkyostichochrome Nervenzelle *f*.
Arlt [ˈɑːrlt]: **A.'s recess** Arlt'-Sinus *m*, Maier-Sinus *m*.
A.'s sinus → A.'s recess.
A.'s trachoma Trachom(a) *nt*, ägyptische Körnerkrankheit *f*, trachomatöse Einschlußkonjunktivitis *f*, Conjunctivitis (granulosa) trachomatosa.
arm [ɑːrm] *n* **1.** *anat.* Arm *m*. **to make a long ~** den Arm ausstrecken. **2.** *physiol.* Abzweigung *f*. **3.** *bot.* Ast *m*, Zweig *m*. **4.** *techn.* (Hebel-, Maschinen-)Arm *m*.

ar·ma·men·tar·i·um [ˌɑːrməmənˈteərɪəm] *n* (*Praxis*) Ausrüstung *f*, Einrichtung *f*, Instrumentarium *f*.
Armanni-Ebstein [ɑːrˈmani ˈebstaɪn]:
A.-E. cells Armanni-Ebstein-Zellen *pl*.
A.-E. change → A.-E. lesion.
A.-E. lesion Armanni-Ebstein-Läsion *f*.
A.-E. kidney → A.-E. lesion.
ar·mar·i·um [ɑːrˈmeərɪəm] *n, pl* **-mar·i·a** [-ˈmeərɪə] *n* armamentarium.
ar·ma·ture [ˈɑːrmətʃər] *n* **1.** *phys.* Anker *m*, Läufer *m*, Rotor *m*, Relais *nt*. **2.** Schutz *m*, Verstärkung *f*.
armed tapeworm [ɑːrmd] *micro.* Schweine(finnen)bandwurm *m*, Taenia solium.
arm·less [ˈɑːrmlɪs] *adj* armlos, ohne Arm(e).
arm-like *adj* armförmig, -ähnlich.
ar·mored heart [ˈɑːrmərd] Panzerherz *nt*, Pericarditis calcarea.
ar·mour heart [ˈɑːrmər] → armored heart.
arm pit Achselhöhle *f*.
arm-shaped *adj* armförmig, -ähnlich.
arm splint *ortho.* Armschiene *f*.
Armstrong [ˈɑːrmstrɒŋ]: **A.'s disease** Armstrong'-Krankheit *f*, lymphozytäre Choriomeningitis *f abbr.* LCM.
Arndt [ɑːrnt]: **A.'s law** → Arndt-Schulz law.
Arndt-Gottron [ˈɡɒtrɒn]: **A.-G. syndrome** *derm.* Arndt-Gottron-Syndrom *nt*, Skleromyxödem *nt*.
Arndt-Schulz [ʃʊlts]: **A.-S. law** Arndt-Schulz-Gesetz *nt*.
Arneth [ɑːrˈnet]: **A.'s classification/formula/index** Arneth'-Leukozytenschema *nt*.
A. stages Arneth-Stadien *pl*.
Ar·ni·ca montana [ˈɑːrnɪkə] Bergwohlverleih *m*, Arnika *f*, Arnica montana.
Arnold [ˈɑːrnld]: **A.'s bundle** Arnold'-Bündel *nt*, Tractus frontopontinus.
A.'s canal Arnold-Kanal.
A.'s fold Krause'-Klappe *f*, Valvula sacci lacrimalis inferior.
A.'s ligament oberes Incusband *nt*, Lig. incudis superius.
A.'s nerve Ramus auricularis n. vagi.
Arnold-Chiari [ˈkɪɑːriː]: **A.-C. deformity/malformation/syndrome** Arnold-Chiari-Hemmungsmißbildung *f*, -Syndrom *nt*.
AROA *abbr.* → ocular albinism, autosomal recessive.
a·ro·ma [əˈrəʊmə] *n* Aroma *nt*, Duft *m*, Würze *f*.
a·ro·ma·tase [əˈrəʊməteɪz] *n* Aromatase *f*.
ar·o·mat·ic [əˈrəʊmətɪk] **I** *n* **1.** *chem.* Aromat *m*, aromatische Verbindung *f*. **2.** aromatisches Mittel *nt*, Aromatikum *nt* od. Pflanze *f*, Aromaticum *nt*. **II** *adj* **3.** aromatisch, wohlriechend, würzig, duftig. **4.** *chem.* aromatisch.
aromatic alcohol aromatischer Alkohol *m*, Phenol *nt*.
aromatic character *chem.* aromatischer Charakter *m*.
aromatic compound *chem.* aromatische Verbindung *f*.
aromatic hydrocarbon *chem.* aromatischer Kohlenwasserstoff *m*.
aromatic ring *chem.* aromatischer Ring *m*, aromatische Ringstruktur *f*.
a·ro·ma·ti·za·tion [əˌrəʊmətəˈzeɪʃn] *n* **1.** *chem.* Aromatisierung *f*. **2.** Aromatisieren *nt*, Aromatisierung *f*.
a·ro·ma·tize [əˈrəʊmətaɪz] *vt* **1.** *chem.* aromatisieren. **2.** aromatisieren, Aroma *od.* Duft verleihen, mit Aroma versehen.
around-the-clock *adj* rund um die Uhr, 24stündig.
a·rous·al [əˈraʊzl] *n neuro.* Wachsamkeit *f*, Vigilanz *f*, Vigilität *f*.

arousal reaction physiol. Weckreaktion f.
a·rouse [əˈraʊz] vt (er-)wecken, an-, erregen; (Schmerzen) bereiten, verursachen.
ar·range·ment [əˈreɪndʒmənt] n 1. (An-)Ordnung f, Aufbau m, Formation f, Disposition f. 2. Vereinbarung, Verabredung f, Absprache f, Übereinkunft f. **by ~** nach Absprache, laut Vereinbarung. **to make an ~ with sb.** eine Vereinbarung mit jdm. treffen. 3. ~s pl Vorbereitungen pl. **to make ~s** Vorkehrungen treffen.
ar·ray [əˈreɪ] n Reihe f, Menge f, Anzahl f, Aufgebot f (of an).
ar·rec·tor muscles of hair [æˈrektər] Haaraufrichter pl, Mm. arrectores pilorum.
ar·rest [əˈrest] I n An-, Aufhalten nt, Stillstehen nt, Stillstand m; Hemmung f, Stockung f. II vt 1. an-, aufhalten, zum Stillstand bringen, hemmen, hindern. 2. sperren, feststellen, blockieren, arretieren.
a. of development Entwicklungshemmung.
a. of growth Wachsstumsstillstand.
ar·rest·ed tuberculosis [əˈrestɪd] inaktive/vernarbte/verheilte Tuberkulose f.
Arrhenius [aːˈreɪnɪus]: **A.' doctrine** → A.' theory.
A.' equation Arrhenius'-Gleichung f.
A.' theory Arrhenius'-Theorie f.
ar·rhe·no·blas·to·ma [ˌærənoʊblæsˈtoʊmə, əˌriː-] n 1. Arrhenoblastom nt. 2. Sertoli-Leidig-Zelltumor m.
ar·rhe·no·ma [ˌærɪˈnoʊmə] n → arrhenoblastoma.
ar·rhin·en·ce·pha·lia → arhinencephalia.
ar·rhin·ia n → arhinia.
ar·rhyth·mia [əˈrɪðmɪə] n 1. Arrhythmie f. 2. Herzrhythmusstörung f, Arrhythmie f, Arrhythmia f.
ar·rhyth·mic [əˈrɪðmɪk] adj arrhythmisch.
ar·rhyth·mo·gen·ic [əˌrɪðməˈdʒenɪk] adj Arrhythmie verursachend od. fördernd, arrhythmogen.
ar·rhyth·mo·ki·ne·sis [ˌ-kɪˈniːsɪs, -kaɪ-] n neuro. Arrhythmokinese f.
Arroyo [əˈrɔɪoʊ]: **A.'s sign** [əˈrɔɪoʊ] Arroyo'-Zeichen nt, Asthenokorie f.
ar·sam·bide [ɑːrˈsæmbaɪd] n pharm. Carbason nt, 4-Carbamidophenylarsinsäure f.
ARSB abbr. → arylsulfatase B.
ARSB deficiency → arylsulfatase B deficiency.
ar·se·nate [ˈɑːrsəneɪt, -nɪt] n Arsenat nt.
ar·se·ni·a·sis [ˌɑːrsəˈnaɪəsɪs] n chronische Arsenvergiftung f.
ar·se·nic [n ˈɑːrs(ə)nɪk; adj ɑːrˈsenɪk] I n 1. abbr. **As** Arsen nt abbr. As. 2. Arsentioxid nt, Arsenik nt, Arsenikum nt. II adj fünfwertiges Arsen od. fünfwertige Arsenverbindungen betr. od. enthaltend, Arsen(ik)-, Arsen-V-.
arsenic acid arsenige Säure f, Arsensäure f, Arsensauerstoffsäure f.
ar·sen·i·cal [ɑːrˈsenɪkl] I n arsenhaltige Verbindung f. II adj Arsen(verbindungen) betr., arsenhaltig, Arsen(ik)-.
ar·sen·i·cal·ism [ɑːrˈsenɪkəlɪzəm] n → arseniasis.
arsenical keratosis → arsenical keratosis.
arsenical poisoning Arsenvergiftung f.
arsenic-fast adj arsenresistent.
arsenic keratosis Arsenkeratose f, Arsenwarzen pl.
ar·sen·i·cum [ɑːrˈsenɪkəm] n → arsenic 2.
ar·se·nide [ˈɑːrsənaɪd, -nɪd] n Arsenid nt.
ar·se·ni·ous [ɑːrˈsiːnɪəs] adj → arsenous.
ar·se·nism [ˈɑːrsənɪzəm] n → arseniasis.
ar·se·ni·um [ɑːrˈsiːnɪəm] n → arsenic 1.

ar·sen·i·za·tion [ˌɑːrsenɪˈzeɪʃn] n histol. Arsenbehandlung f.
ar·sen·o·blast [ɑːrˈsenəblæst] n embryo. männl. Vorkern m.
ar·se·no·ther·a·py [ˌɑːrsənoʊˈθerəpɪ] n Arsenbehandlung f, -therapie f.
ar·se·nous [ˈɑːrsənəs] adj dreiwertiges Arsen enthaltend.
arsenous acid arsenige Säure f.
arsenous hydride Arsenwasserstoff m.
ar·sine [ɑːrˈsiːn, ˈɑːrsiːn, -sɪn] n 1. Arsenwasserstoff m, Arsin nt. 2. Arsinderivat nt.
ar·sin·ic acid [ɑːrˈsɪnɪk] Arsinsäure f.
ar·son·ic acid [ɑːrˈsɑnɪk] Arsonsäure f.
ar·te·fact [ˈɑːrtəfækt] n Kunstprodukt nt, artifizielle Veränderung f, Artefakt nt.
ar·te·fac·tu·al [ˌ-ˈfæktʃəwəl] adj Artefakt betr.
ar·ter·al·gia [ˌɑːrtəˈrældʒ(ɪ)ə] n von einer Arterie ausgehender Schmerz m.
ar·ter·ec·to·my [ˌɑːrtəˈrektəmɪ] n → arteriectomy.
ar·ter·e·nol [ɑːrˈtɪərɪnoʊl, ˌɑːrtəˈriːnɒl] n Noradrenalin nt, Norepinephrin nt, Arterenol nt, Levarterenol nt.
arteri- pref. → arterio-.
ar·te·ri·a [ɑːrˈtɪərɪə] n, pl **-ri·ae** [-rɪˌiː] → artery 1.
ar·te·ri·al [ɑːrˈtɪərɪəl] adj Arterien betr., arteriell, arteriös, Arterien-.
arterial anastomosis Arterienanastomose f.
arterial arcade Arterienarkade f, -kaskade f.
arterial arch: a.es of kidney (Niere) Bogenarterien pl, Aa. arcuatae renis.
a. of lower eyelid Arcus palpebralis inferior.
palmar a., deep tiefer Hohlhandbogen m, Arcus palmaris profundus.
palmar a., superficial oberflächlicher Hohlhandbogen m, Arcus palmaris superficialis.
a. of upper eyelid Arcus palpebralis superior.
arterial bleeding arterielle Blutung f.
arterial blood arterielles/sauerstoffreiches Blut nt, Arterienblut nt.
arterial blood gases abbr. **ABG** arterielle Blutgase pl.
arterial blood pressure abbr. **ABP** arterieller (Blut-)Druck m.
arterial bulb Aortenbulbus m, Bulbus aortae.
arterial canal → arterial duct.
arterial catheter Arterienkatheter m.
arterial circle arterieller Anastomosenring m, Circulus arteriosus.
a. of cerebrum → a. of Willis.
greater a. of iris äußeres/ziliares Arteriengeflecht nt der Iris, Circulus arteriosus iridis major.
lesser a. of iris inneres/pupilläres Arteriengeflecht nt der Iris, Circulus arteriosus iridis minor.
major a. of iris → greater a. of iris.
minor a. of iris → lesser a. of iris.
a. of Willis Willis'-Anastomosenkranz m, Circulus arteriosus cerebri, Circulus arteriosus Willisi.
arterial cone Infundibulum nt, Conus arteriosus.
arterial duct Ductus Botalli, Ductus arteriosus.
arterial ectasia Arterienektasie f.
diffuse a. Traubenaneurysma nt, Aneurysma cirsoideum/racemosum.
arterial embolus arterieller Embolus m.
arterial erosion Arterienarrosion f.
arterial flap Arterienlappen m.
arterial gases → arterial blood gases.

arterial grooves → arterial impressions.
arterial hemangioma 1. Kapillarhämangiom nt, Haemangioma capillare. 2. Blutschwamm m, blastomatöses Hämangiom nt, Haemangioma planotuberosum/simplex.
arterial hemorrhage arterielle Blutung f.
arterial high-pressure system arterielles (Hochdruck-)System nt.
arterial hyperemia aktive/arterielle Hyperämie f.
arterial hypertension Bluthochdruck m, arterielle Hypertonie f, Hypertension f.
continued a. Huchard-Krankheit f, Präsklerose f.
arterial hypotension niedriger Blutdruck m, Hypotonie f, Hypotonus m, Hypotonia f, Hypotension f.
arterial hypoxia arterielle Hypoxie f.
ar·te·ri·al·i·za·tion [ɑːrˌtɪərɪəlɪˈzeɪʃn, -laɪ-] n 1. Arterialisierung f, Arterialisation f. 2. Grad m der Sauerstoffsättigung, Arterialisation f. 3. chir. Versorgung f mit arteriellem Blut. 4. Qualität f der Gefäßversorgung, Arterialisation f.
arterial impressions Schädelwandfurchen pl für Meningealarterien, Sulci arteriales.
arterial injury Arterienverletzung f.
arterial lipoidosis → atherosclerosis.
arterial mesocardium embryo. arterielles Mesokard m.
arterial murmur Arteriengeräusch nt.
arterial nephrosclerosis → arterionephrosclerosis.
arterial network: a. of cochlea Arteriengeflecht nt der Cochlea, Glomeruli arteriosi cochleae.
a. of patella patelläres Arteriengeflecht nt, Rete patellare.
arterial obstruction disease → arterial occlusive disease.
arterial occlusion Arterienverschluß m.
arterial occlusive disease (periphere) arterielle Verschlußkrankheit f abbr. AVK.
arterial pressure Arteriendruck m, arterieller Druck m.
diastolic a. diastolischer Arteriendruck, diastolischer arterieller (Blut-)Druck.
mean a. abbr. **MAP** arterieller Mitteldruck.
systolic a. systolischer Arteriendruck, systolischer arterieller (Blut-)Druck.
arterial pulse Arterienpuls m.
arterial reconstruction chir. Arterienrekonstruktion f.
arterial repair chir. operative Arteriennaht f/-versorgung f.
arterial rete Arteriengeflecht nt, Rete arteriosum.
a. of patella patelläres Arteriengeflecht nt, Rete patellare.
arterial sclerosis → arteriosclerosis.
arterial spider Sternnävus m, Spider naevus, Naevus araneus.
arterial sulci → arterial impressions.
arterial supply arterielle Versorgung f.
arterial system → arterial high-pressure system.
arterial tension arterieller Blutdruck m.
arterial thrombus arterieller Thrombus m, Arterienthrombus m.
arterial vein Truncus pulmonalis.
ar·te·ri·ec·ta·sia [ɑːrˌtɪərɪekˈteɪʒ(ɪ)ə] n → arteriectasis.
ar·te·ri·ec·ta·sis [ˌ-ˈektəsɪs] n diffuse Arterienerweiterung f, Arteriektasie f.
ar·te·ri·ec·to·my [ˌ-ˈektəmɪ] n chir. Arterien(teil)resektion f, Arteriektomie f.
ar·te·ri·ec·to·pia [ˌ-ekˈtoʊpɪə] n Arterie(n)ektopie f.
arterio- pref. Arterien-, Arterio-.

ar·te·ri·o·bil·i·ar·y fistula [ɑːrˌtɪərɪəʊ'bɪlɪˌeriː, -'bɪljərɪ] arteriobiliäre Fistel *f*.
ar·te·ri·o·cap·il·lar·y [ˌ-'kæpəˌleriː, -kə'pɪlərɪ] *adj* Arterien u. Kapillaren betr. *od.* verbindend, arteriokapillar.
arteriocapillary sclerosis → arteriosclerosis.
ar·te·ri·o·coc·cyg·e·al gland [ˌ-kɑk'sɪdʒɪəl] Steiß(bein)knäuel *m/nt*, Corpus/Glomus coccygeum.
ar·te·ri·o·di·lat·ing [ˌ-daɪ'leɪtɪŋ] *adj* arterien-, arteriolenerweiternd.
ar·te·ri·o·gen·e·sis [ˌ-'dʒenəsɪs] *n* Arterienbildung *f*, Arteriogenese *f*.
ar·te·ri·o·gram [ɑːr'tɪərɪəgræm] *n radiol.* Arteriogramm *nt*.
ar·te·ri·og·ra·phy [ɑːrˌtɪərɪ'ɑgrəfɪ] *n radiol.* Kontrastdarstellung *f* von Arterien, Arteriographie *f*.
ar·te·ri·o·la [ɑːrˌtɪərɪ'əʊlə] *n, pl* **-lae** [-liː] → arteriole.
ar·te·ri·o·lar [ɑːrtə'rɪələr, ɑːrˌtɪrɪ'əʊlər] *adj* Arteriole(n) betr., arteriolär, Arteriolen-.
arteriolar hyalinosis Arteriolenhyalinose *f*.
arteriolar nephrosclerosis interkapilläre Nephrosklerose *f*, Glomerulosklerose *f*.
hyaline a. benigne Nephrosklerose.
hyperplastic a. Fahr-Volhard-Nephrosklerose, maligne Nephrosklerose.
arteriolar necrosis → arteriolonecrosis.
arteriolar sclerosis → arteriolosclerosis.
arteriolar spasm Arteriolenspasmus *m*, -krampf *m*.
ar·te·ri·ole [ɑːr'tɪərɪəʊl] *n* kleine Arterie *f*, Arteriole *f*, Arteriola *f*.
ar·te·ri·o·lith [ɑːr'tɪərɪəlɪθ] *n* Arterienstein *m*, Arteriolith *m*.
ar·ter·i·o·li·tis [ˌ-'laɪtɪs] *n* Arteriolen(wand)entzündung *f*, Arteriolitis *f*.
ar·te·ri·ol·o·gy [ɑːrˌtɪərɪ'ɑlədʒɪ] *n* Arteriologie *f*.
ar·te·ri·o·lo·ne·cro·sis [ɑːrˌtɪərɪˌəʊləʊnɪ'krəʊsɪs, -ne-] *n* Arteriolennekrose *f*, Arteriolonekrose *f*.
ar·te·ri·o·lo·neph·ro·scle·ro·sis [ˌ-ˌnefrəsklɪ'rəʊsɪs] *n* → arteriolar nephrosclerosis.
ar·te·ri·o·lo·scle·ro·sis [ˌ-sklɪ'rəʊsɪs] *n* Arteriolosklerose *f*.
ar·te·ri·o·lo·scle·rot·ic [ˌ-sklɪ'rɑtɪk] *adj* Arteriolosklerose betr., arteriolosklerotisch.
ar·te·ri·o·ma·la·cia [ɑːrˌtɪərɪəmə'leɪʃ(ɪ)ə] *n* Arterienerweichung *f*.
ar·te·ri·o·mo·tor [ˌ-'məʊtər] *adj* arteriomotorisch.
ar·te·ri·o·my·o·ma·to·sis [ˌ-maɪəmə'təʊsɪs] *n* Myomatose *f* der Arterienwand, Arteriomyomatose *f*.
ar·te·ri·o·ne·cro·sis [ˌ-nɪ'krəʊsɪs, -ne-] *n* Arterionekrose *f*.
ar·te·ri·o·neph·ro·scle·ro·sis [ˌ-ˌnefrəsklɪ'rəʊsɪs] *n* senile Nephrosklerose *f*, Arterionephrosklerose *f*.
ar·te·ri·op·a·thy [ɑːrtərɪ'ɑpəθɪ] *n* Arterienerkrankung *f*, Arteriopathie *f*, -pathia *f*.
ar·te·ri·o·plas·ty [ɑːrˌtɪərɪə'plæstɪ] *n chir.* Arterienplastik *f*.
ar·te·ri·o·re·nal [ˌ-'riːnl] *adj* Arterie(n) u. Niere betr. *od.* verbindend, arteriorenal.
ar·te·ri·or·rha·phy [ɑːrˌtɪərɪ'ɑrəfɪ] *n* Arterienennaht *f*, Arterio(r)rhaphie *f*.
ar·te·ri·or·rhex·is [ɑːrˌtɪərɪ'reksɪs] *n* Arterienruptur *f*, -riß *m*, Arterio(r)rhexis *f*.
ar·te·ri·o·scle·ro·sis [ˌ-sklɪ'rəʊsɪs] *n abbr.* **AS** *inf.* Arterienverkalkung *f*, Arteriosklerose *f*, -sclerosis *f*.
ar·te·ri·o·scle·rot·ic [ˌ-sklɪ'rɑtɪk] *adj* Arteriosklerose betr., arteriosklerotisch.
arteriosclerotic aneurysm arteriosklerotisches Aneurysma *nt*.

arteriosclerotic cardiopathy arteriosklerotische Kardiopathie *f*.
arteriosclerotic gangrene arteriosklerotische Gangrän *f*, Gangraena arteriosclerotica.
arteriolosclerotic kidney arteriolosklerotische Niere *f*.
arteriosclerotic nephritis arteriosklerotische Nephritis *f*.
arteriosclerotic retinopathy arteriosklerotische Retinopathie *f*, Retinopathia arteriosclerotica.
ar·te·ri·o·spasm [ɑːr'tɪərɪəspæzəm] *n* Arterienkrampf *m*, Arteriospasmus *m*.
ar·te·ri·o·spas·tic [ˌ-'spæstɪk] *adj* Arteriospasmus betr. *od.* verursachend, arteriospastisch.
ar·te·ri·o·ste·no·sis [ˌ-stɪ'nəʊsɪs] *n* Arterienstriktur *f*, -stenose *f*.
ar·te·ri·os·te·o·gen·e·sis [ɑːrˌtɪərɪˌɑstɪə'dʒenəsɪs] *n* Arterienkalzifizierung *f*.
ar·te·ri·os·to·sis [ˌ-ɑs'təʊsɪs] *n* Arterienverknöcherung *f*.
ar·te·ri·ot·o·my [ˌ-'ɑtəmɪ] *n chir.* operative Arterieneröffnung *f*, Arteriotomie *f*.
ar·te·ri·ot·o·ny [ˌ-'ɑtənɪ] *n* (intraarterieller) Blutdruck *m*.
ar·te·ri·ous [ɑːr'tɪərɪəs] *adj* → arterial.
ar·te·ri·o·ve·nous [ˌ-'viːnəs] *adj abbr.* **AV, A-V, av** Arterie(n) u. Vene(n) betr. *od.* verbindend, arteriovenös *abbr.* **AV, av.**
arteriovenous anastomosis arteriovenöse Anastomose *f*, AV-Anastomose *f*, Anastomosis arteriolovenularis/arteriovenosa.
glomeriform a. Glomuskörper *m*, glomusförmige Anastomose, Anastomosis arteriovenosa glomeriformis.
arteriovenous aneurysm arteriovenöses Aneurysma *nt*, Aneurysma arteriovenosum.
arteriovenous bridge Brückenanastomose *f*.
arteriovenous difference *abbr.* **avD** arteriovenöse Differenz *f abbr.* avD.
arteriovenous fistula 1. *patho.* arteriovenöse Fistel *f*. **2.** *chir.* arteriovenöser Fistel *f*, arteriovenöser Shunt/Bypass *m*.
congenital a. kongenitale arteriovenöse Fistel.
radiocephalic a. *chir.* A. radialis-V. cephalica-Shunt *m*.
splenic a. 1. arteriovenöse Fistel der A. lienalis. **2.** intrasplenale arteriovenöse Fistel.
traumatic a. (post-)traumatische arteriovenöse Fistel.
arteriovenous malformation *abbr.* **AVM** arteriovenöse Fehlbildung *f*.
arteriovenous pulmonary aneurysm arteriovenöse Lungenfistel *f*.
arteriovenous shunt *chir.* arteriovenöser Shunt/Bypass *m*.
ar·te·ri·o·ven·u·lar anastomosis, glomeriform [ˌ-'venjələr] → arteriovenous anastomosis, glomeriform.
ar·te·ri·tis [ɑːrtə'raɪtɪs] *n* Arterienentzündung *f*, Arteriitis *f*.
arteritis nodosa Kussmaul-Meier-Krankheit *f*, Panarteriitis/Periarteriitis/Polyarteriitis nodosa.
ar·ter·y [ˈɑːrtərɪ] *n, pl* **-ries 1.** *abbr.* **A** *anat.* Schlagader *f*, Pulsader *f*, Arterie *f*, Arteria *f*. **2.** *fig.* Hauptverkehrsader *f*, Schlagader *f*.
a. of angular gyrus A. gyri angularis.
a. of bulb of penis A. bulbi penis.
a. of bulb of vestibule of vagina A. bulbi vestibuli/vaginae.
a. of caudate lobe Lobus caudatus-Arterie, A. lobi caudati.
a. of central sulcus A. sulci centralis.

a.ies of cerebrum (Ge-)Hirnarterien *pl*, -schlagadern *pl*, Aa. cerebrales.
a. of deferent duct Samenleiterarterie, A. ductus deferentis.
a. of ductus deferens → a. of deferent duct.
a. of elastic type Arterie vom elastischen Typ.
a. of labyrinth 1. A. labyrinthi, Ramus meatus acustici interni a. basilaris. **2.** A. labyrinthina.
a.ies of (lower) leg Unterschenkelarterien *pl*.
a.ies of lower limb Beinarterien *pl*.
a.ies of Müller Rankenarterien des Penis, Aa. helicinae (penis).
a. of muscular type Arterie vom muskulären Typ.
a. of postcentral sulcus A. sulci postcentralis.
a. of precentral sulcus A. sulci pr(a)ecentralis.
a. of pterygoid canal A. canalis pterygoidei.
a. of round ligament of uterus A. lig. teretis uteri.
a. of tail of pancreas Pankreasschwanzarterie, A. caudae pancreatis.
arthr- *pref.* Gelenk-, Arthr(o)-.
ar·thrag·ra [ɑːr'θrægrə] *n* Gelenkgicht *f*, Arthragra *f*.
ar·thral [ˈɑːrθrəl] *adj* Gelenk betr., artikulär, Gelenk-, Arthr(o)-.
ar·thral·gia [ɑːr'θrældʒ(ɪ)ə] *n* Gelenkschmerz(en *pl*) *m*, Arthralgie *f*, Arthrodynia *f*.
ar·thral·gic [ɑːr'θrældʒɪk] *adj* Arthralgie betr., arthralgisch.
ar·threc·to·my [ɑːr'θrektəmɪ] *n ortho.* Gelenkresektion *f*, -(teil)entfernung *f*, Arthrektomie *f*.
ar·threm·py·e·sis [ˌɑːrθrempaɪ'iːsɪs] *n* Gelenkeiterung *f*.
ar·thres·the·sia [ɑːrθres'θiːʒ(ɪ)ə] *n* Gelenkempfindung *f*, -sensibilität *f*, Arthrästhesie *f*.
ar·thri·flu·ent abscess [ɑːθrɪ'fluːənt] von einem Gelenk ausgehender Abszeß *m*.
ar·thrit·ic [ɑːr'θrɪtɪk] **I** *n* Patient(in *f*) *m* mit Arthritis, Arthritiker(in *f*) *m*. **II** *adj* Arthritis betr., von Arthritis betroffen, arthritisch.
ar·thrit·i·cal [ɑːr'θrɪtɪkl] *adj* → arthritic II.
arthritic calculus Gichttophus *m*.
arthritic psoriasis Arthritis/Arthropathia psoriatica.
ar·thri·tis [ɑːr'θraɪtɪs] *n* Gelenkentzündung *f*, Arthritis *f*.
arthro- *pref.* Gelenk-, Arthr(o)-.
Ar·thro·bac·ter [ˈɑːrθrəʊbæktər] *n micro.* Arthrobacter *f*.
ar·thro·bac·te·ri·um [ˌ-bæk'tɪərɪəm] *n micro.* Arthrobacterium *nt*.
ar·thro·cele [ˈ-siːl] *n* **1.** Gelenkschwellung *f*, Arthrozele *f*. **2.** Synovialprolaps *m*, Arthrozele *f*.
ar·thro·cen·te·sis [ˌ-sen'tiːsɪs] *n* Gelenkpunktion *f*, Arthrozentese *f*.
ar·thro·chon·dri·tis [ˌ-kɑn'draɪtɪs] *n* Gelenkknorpelentzündung *f*, Arthrochondritis *f*.
ar·thro·cla·sia [ˌ-'kleɪʒ(ɪ)ə] *n ortho.* (operative) Arthrolyse *f*.
ar·thro·clei·sis [ˌ-'klaɪsɪs] *n* → arthrokleisis.
Ar·thro·der·ma [ˌ-'dɜrmə] *n* Arthroderma *f*.
ar·thro·de·sia [ˌ-'diːsɪə] *n* → arthrodesis.
ar·throd·e·sis [ɑːr'θrɑdəsɪs, ˌɑːrθrə'diːsɪs] *n ortho.* operative Gelenkversteifung *f*, Arthrodese *f*.
a. of the wrist Handgelenkversteifung, -arthrodese.

arthrodia 58

ar·thro·dia [ɑːrˈθrəʊdɪə] n → arthrodial articulation.
ar·thro·di·al [ɑːrˈθrəʊdɪəl] adj Arthrodialgelenk betr., arthrodial.
arthrodial articulation Arthrodialgelenk nt, Artic. plana.
arthrodial cartilage → articular cartilage.
arthrodial joint → arthrodial articulation.
ar·thro·dyn·i·a [ˌɑːrθrəˈdiːnɪə] n Gelenkschmerz m, Arthrodynie f, Arthroalgia f.
ar·thro·dys·pla·sia [ˌ-dɪsˈpleɪʒ(ɪ)ə, -zɪə] n Gelenkdysplasie f, Arthrodysplasie f, -dysplasia f.
ar·thro·em·py·e·sis [ˌ-ˌempaɪˈiːsɪs] n Gelenkeiterung f.
ar·thro·en·dos·co·py [ˌ-enˈdɒskəpɪ] n → arthroscopy.
ar·thro·e·rei·sis [ˌɪˈraɪsɪs] n → arthrorisis.
ar·thro·gen·ic [ˌ-ˈdʒenɪk] adj vom Gelenk ausgehend, gelenkbedingt, arthrogen.
arthrogenic contracture gelenkbedingte/arthrogene Kontraktur f.
ar·thro·gram [ˈ-græm] n radiol. Arthrogramm nt.
ar·throg·ra·phy [ɑːrˈθrəɡrəfɪ] n radiol. Kontrastdarstellung f eines Gelenkes, Arthrographie f.
ar·thro·gry·po·sis [ˌɑːrθrəɡrɪˈpəʊsɪs] n operative od. kongenitale Gelenkflexion/-kontraktur f, Arthrogrypose f.
ar·thro·ka·tad·y·sis [ˌ-kəˈtædəsɪs] n Protrusio acetabuli.
ar·thro·klei·sis [ˌ-ˈklaɪsɪs] n 1. operative Gelenkversteifung f, Arthrodese f. 2. Gelenkversteifung f, Ankylose f.
ar·thro·lith [ˈ-lɪθ] n Gelenkstein m, -körper m, Arthrolith m.
ar·thro·li·thi·a·sis [ˌ-lɪˈθaɪəsɪs] n → arthragra.
ar·thro·lo·gia [ˌ-ˈləʊdʒ(ɪ)ə] n → arthrology.
ar·thro·lo·gy [ɑːrˈθrɒlədʒɪ] n Gelenklehre f, Arthrologie f, -logia f.
ar·throl·y·sis [ɑːrˈθrɒləsɪs] n ortho. operative Gelenkmobilisierung f, Arthrolyse f.
ar·thro·men·in·gi·tis [ˌɑːrθrəˌmenɪnˈdʒaɪtɪs] n Entzündung f der Membrana synovialis, Synovitis f, Synoviitis f, Synovialitis f.
ar·throm·e·ter [ɑːrˈθrɒmɪtər] n ortho. Arthrometer nt; Goniometer nt.
ar·throm·e·try [ɑːrˈθrɒmɪtrɪ] n ortho. Arthrometrie f.
ar·thron·cus [ɑːrˈθrɒŋkəs] n Gelenkschwellung f, -tumor m.
ar·thro·neu·ral·gia [ˌɑːrθrənʊˈrældʒə, -njʊər-] n Gelenkneuralgie f.
ar·thro·no·sos [ˌ-ˈnəʊsəs] n → arthropathy.
arthro-onychodysplasia n Nagel-Patella-Syndrom nt, Osteoonychodysplasie f, Osteoonychodysostose f, Onycho-osteodysplasie f.
arthro-ophthalmopathy n Arthro-Ophthalmopathie f.
ar·thro·path·ia [ˌɑːrθrəˈpæθɪə] n → arthropathy.
ar·thro·path·ic [ˌ-ˈpæθɪk] adj Arthropathie betr.
ar·throp·a·thy [ɑːrˈθrɒpəθɪ] n Gelenkerkrankung f, -leiden nt, Arthropathie f, -pathia f.
ar·thro·phy·ma [ˌɑːrθrəˈfaɪmə] n Gelenkschwellung f, -tumor m.
ar·thro·phyte [ˈ-faɪt] n Arthrophyt m.
ar·thro·plas·tic [ˌ-ˈplæstɪk] adj Arthroplastik betr., arthroplastisch.
ar·thro·plas·ty [ˈ-ˌplæstɪ] n 1. Gelenkplastik f, Arthroplastik f. 2. Gelenkprothese f.
ar·thro·pneu·mog·ra·phy [ˌ-n(j)uːˈmɒɡrəfɪ] n Pneumoarthrographie f, Arthropneumografie f.
ar·thro·pneu·mo·roent·gen·og·ra·phy

[ˌ-ˌn(j)uːməˌrentɡənˈɒɡrəfɪ] n → arthropneumography.
ar·thro·pod [ˈ-pɒd] n micro. Arthropode m.
Ar·throp·o·da [ɑːrˈθrɒpədə] pl micro. Gliederfüß(l)er pl, Arthropoden pl.
ar·throp·o·dan [ɑːrˈθrɒpədən] adj → arthropodous.
arthropod-borne virus → arbovirus.
ar·throp·o·dous [ɑːrˈθrɒpədəs] adj Arthropoden betr., durch Arthropoden verursacht, Arthropoden-.
ar·thro·py·o·sis [ˌɑːrθrəpaɪˈəʊsɪs] n Gelenkeiterung f.
ar·thro·rheu·ma·tism [ˌ-ˈruːmətɪzəm] n intraartikuläre Entzündung f.
ar·thro·ri·sis [ˌ-ˈraɪsɪs] n ortho. operative Sperrung/Einschränkung f der Gelenkbeweglichkeit, Arthrorise f.
ar·thro·scin·ti·gram [ˌ-ˈsɪntəɡræm] n radiol. Gelenkszintigramm nt.
ar·thro·scin·tig·ra·phy [ˌ-sɪnˈtɪɡrəfɪ] n radiol. Gelenkszintigraphie f.
ar·thro·scope [ˈ-skəʊp] n Arthroskop nt.
ar·thros·co·py [ɑːrˈθrɒskəpɪ] n Gelenkspiegelung f, Arthroskopie f.
ar·thro·sis [ɑːrˈθrəʊsɪs] n 1. degenerative Gelenkerkrankung f, Arthrose f, Arthrosis f. 2. Gelenk nt, gelenkartige Verbindung f.
ar·thro·spore [ˈɑːrθrəspɔːr, -spəʊr] n micro. Glied(er)-, Arthrospore f.
ar·thros·to·my [ɑːrˈθrɒstəmɪ] n ortho. Arthrostomie f.
ar·thro·syn·o·vi·tis [ˌɑːrθrəˌsɪnəˈvaɪtɪs] n Entzündung f der Gelenkinnenhaut/Membrana synovialis, Synovialitis f, Synovitis f.
ar·thro·tome [ˈ-təʊm] n ortho. Arthrotom nt.
ar·throt·o·my [ɑːrˈθrɒtəmɪ] n ortho. Gelenköffnung f, Arthrotomie f.
ar·thro·trop·ic [ˌɑːrθrəˈtrɒpɪk, -ˈtrəʊp-] adj arthrotrop.
ar·thro·xe·ro·sis [ˌ-zɪˈrəʊsɪs] n degenerative Gelenkerkrankung f, Osteoarthrose f, Gelenk(s)arthrose f, Arthrosis deformans.
Arthus [ˈɑːθəs]: **A. phenomenon/reaction** Arthus-Phänomen nt, -Reaktion f.
A.-type reaction Arthus-Typ m der Überempfindlichkeitsreaktion, Immunkomplex-vermittelte Überempfindlichkeitsreaktion f.
ar·tic·u·lar [ɑːrˈtɪkjələr] adj Gelenk(e) betr., artikulär, Gelenk-, Glieder-.
articular branches of descending genicular artery Kniegelenksäste pl der A. descendens genicularis, Rami articulares a. descendentis genicularis.
articular calculus Gelenkstein m, -konkrement nt.
articular capsule Gelenkkapsel f, Capsula articularis.
cricoarytenoid a. Capsula artic. crico-aryt(a)enoidea.
cricothyroid a. Capsula artic. cricothyroidea.
fibrous a. Membrana fibrosa (capsulae articularis), Stratum fibrosum.
articular cartilage Gelenk(flächen)knorpel m, gelenkflächenüberziehender Knorpel m, Cartilago articularis.
articular cavity Gelenkhöhle f, -raum m, -spalt m, Cavitas articularis.
articular chondrocalcinosis Pseudogicht f, Chondrokalzinose f, Chondrocalcinosis f.
articular chondromatosis Gelenkchondromatose f.
articular circumference Circumferentia articularis.

a. of head of radius → a. of radius.
a. of head of ulna → a. of ulna.
a. of radius Circumferentia articularis (capitis) radii.
a. of ulna Circumferentia articularis (capitis) ulnae.
articular condyle Gelenkkondyle f, Gelenkkopf m.
a. of mandible Gelenkkopf des Unterkiefers, Caput mandibulae.
articular corpuscles Nervenendigungen pl im Gelenk, Corpuscula (nervorum) articularia.
articular crepitus ortho. Gelenkreiben nt.
articular crescent → articular meniscus.
articular discus/disk Gelenkzwischenscheibe f, Diskus m, Discus articularis.
radioulnar a. Discus articularis radioulnaris.
sternoclavicular a. Discus articularis sternoclavicularis.
temporomandibular a. Discus articularis temporomandibularis.
articular dropsy ortho. seröser Gelenkerguß m, Hydarthros(e f) m, Hydrarthros(e f) m, Hydrops articularis.
articular eminence Tuberculum articulare.
articular facet kleine Gelenkfläche f.
articular fossa: inferior a. of atlas untere Gelenkfläche f des Atlas, Facies articularis inferior atlantis.
a. of mandible Fossa mandibularis.
a. of radial head Fovea articularis (capitis radii).
superior a. of atlas obere Gelenkfläche f des Atlas, Facies articularis superior atlantis.
articular fovea Gelenkgrube f.
inferior a. of atlas untere Gelenkfläche f des Atlas, Facies articularis inferior atlantis.
a. of radial head Fovea articularis (capitis radii).
superior a. of atlas obere Gelenkfläche f des Atlas, Facies articularis superior atlantis.
articular fracture Fraktur f gelenkbildender Knochen.
articular gout → arthraga.
articular lip Gelenklippe f, Labrum articulare.
articular meniscus sichel- od. halbmondförmige Gelenkzwischenscheibe f, Meniskus m, Meniscus articularis.
articular muscle an der articularen Gelenkkapsel ansetzender Muskel m, Gelenkmuskel m, Kapselspanner m, M. articularis.
a. of elbow Artikularis m cubiti, M. articularis cubiti.
a. of knee Artikularis m genus, M. articularis genus.
articular network: a. of elbow (joint) Arteriengeflecht nt des Ell(en)bogengelenks, Rete articulare cubiti.
a. of knee Arteriengeflecht nt des Kniegelenks, Rete articulare genus.
articular pit of radial head Fovea articularis (capitis radii).
articular process Gelenkfortsatz m, Proc. articularis.
superior a. of sacrum Proc. articularis superior.
articular rete Gefäßgeflecht nt eines Gelenks, Rete vasculosum articulare.
a. of elbow → articular network of elbow (joint).
a. of knee → articular network of knee.
articular rheumatism → arthritis.
chronic r. rheumatoide Arthritis f, progrediente/primär chronische Polyarthritis f abbr. PCP, PcP.

articular sensation Gelenkempfindung *f*, -sensibilität *f*, Arthrästhesie *f*.
articular sensibility → articular sensation.
articular serum Gelenkschmiere *f*, Synovia *f*.
articular surface Gelenkfläche *f* von Knorpel *od.* Knochen, Facies articularis.
a. of acetabulum Facies lunata (acetabuli).
articular tubercle of temporal bone Tuberculum articulare (ossis temporalis).
articular veins, (temporomandibular) Venen *pl* des Kiefergelenks, Vv. articulares (temporomandibulae).
ar·tic·u·late [*adj* ɑːrˈtɪkjəlɪt; *v* -leɪt] **I** *adj* **1.** *anat.* gelenkig, gegliedert, durch Gelenke verbunden, Gelenk-, Glieder-. **2.** artikuliert, klar *od.* deutlich ausgesprochen, verständlich. **II** *vt* **3.** zusammenfügen, verbinden, durch Gelenke *od.* Glieder verbinden. **4.** artikulieren, (deutlich) aussprechen *od.* ausdrücken. **III** *vi* **5.** ein Gelenk bilden, (durch ein Gelenk) verbunden werden (*with* mit). **6.** artikulieren, deutlich sprechen.
ar·tic·u·lat·ed [-ˌleɪtɪd] *adj* **1.** artikuliert, deutlich u. klar ausgesprochen. **2.** mit Gelenken (versehen), gelenkig; gegliedert. **to be ~ to/with** zusammenhängen mit, ein Gelenk bilden mit.
ar·tic·u·la·tio [ɑːrˌtɪkjəˈleɪʃɪəʊ] *n*, *pl* **-la·ti·o·nes** [-ˌleɪʃɪˈəʊniːz] → articulation 1.
ar·tic·u·la·tion [ɑːrˌtɪkjəˈleɪʃn] *n* **1.** *anat.* Gelenk *nt*, Verbindung(sstelle *f*) *f*, Articulatio *f*. **2.** Zusammen-, Aneinanderfügung *f*, Verbindung *f*. **3.** Artikulation *f*, (deutliche) Aussprache *f*; Artikulieren *nt*, Aussprechen *nt*.
a. of ankle oberes Sprunggelenk, Talokruralgelenk, Artic. talocruralis.
a.s of auditory ossicles Gelenke *od.* gelenkartige Verbindungen der Gehörknöchelchen, Articc. ossiculorum auditorium.
a. of elbow Ell(en)bogengelenk, Artic. cubiti/cubitalis.
a. of head of humerus Schultergelenk, Artic. humeri/glenohumeralis.
a. of head of rib Artic. capitis costae/costalis.
a. of hip Hüftgelenk, Artic. coxae/iliofemoralis.
a. of humerus → a. of head of humerus.
a. of knee Kniegelenk, Artic. genus/genualis.
a. of the pisiform bone Artic. ossis pisiformis.
a. of tubercle of rib Kostotransversalgelenk, Artic. costotransversaria.
ar·tic·u·la·tor [ɑːrˈtɪkjəleɪtər] *n ortho., dent.* Artikulator *m*.
ar·tic·u·la·to·ry [ɑːrˈtɪkjəlætɔːriː, -təʊ-] *adj* Artikulation betr., artikulatorisch.
ar·tic·u·lus [ɑːrˈtɪkjələs] *n*, *pl* **-li** [-laɪ] → articulation 1.
ar·ti·fact [ˈɑːrtəfækt] *n* Kunstprodukt *nt*, artifizielle Veränderung *f*, Artefakt *nt*.
ar·ti·fac·tu·al [ˌ-ˈfæktʃəwəl] *adj* Artefakt betr.
ar·ti·fi·cial [ˌɑːrtɪˈfɪʃl] *adj* artifiziell, künstlich, Kunst-.
artificial abortion induzierter/artifizieller Abort *m*, Schwangerschaftsabbruch *m*, Abortus artificialis.
artificial alimentation künstliche Ernährung *f*.
artificial ankylosis *ortho.* operative Gelenkversteifung *f*, Arthrodese *f*.
artificial anus künstlicher Darmausgang *m*, Kunstafter *m*, Stoma *nt*, Anus praeter (naturalis).

artificial dentition (künstliches) Gebiß *nt*, (Teil-)Gebiß *nt*, Zahnersatz *m*, -prothese *f*.
artificial eye Glasauge *nt*, künstliches Auge *nt*.
artificial fecundation → artificial insemination.
artificial feeding (*Säugling*) Flaschenernährung *f*.
artificial fever künstliches Fieber *nt*.
artificial heart künstliches Herz *nt*, Kunstherz *nt*.
artificial hibernation *anes.* künstlicher Winterschlaf *m*, artifizielle Hibernation *f*.
artificial insemination *abbr.* **A.I.** künstliche Befruchtung *f*, artifizielle Insemination *f abbr.* A.I.
donor a. *abbr.* **A.I.D.** heterologe Insemination, künstliche Befruchtung mit Spendersperma.
homologous a. *abbr.* **A.I.H.** homologe Insemination, künstliche Befruchtung mit Sperma des Ehemannes.
husband a. → homologous a.
artificial kidney künstliche Niere *f*, Hämodialysator *m*.
artificial labor induzierte Geburt *f*.
artificial limb Prothese *f*, Kunstglied *nt*.
artificial lung künstliche Lunge *f*, Oxygenator *m*.
artificial melanin Melanoid *nt*.
artificial pacemaker künstlicher (Herz-)-Schrittmacher *m*.
artificial pneumothorax künstlicher Pneu-(mothorax *m*) *m*.
artificial radioactivity künstliche Radioaktivität *f*.
artificial respiration *abbr.* **AR** künstliche Beatmung *f*.
artificial teeth → artificial dentition.
artificial ventilation künstliche Beatmung *f*.
ARV *abbr.* [AIDS-associated (retro)virus] → AIDS virus.
ar·y·ep·i·glot·tic [ˌærɪˌepɪˈglætɪk] *adj* Aryknorpel u. Kehldeckel/Epiglottis betr., aryepiglottisch.
aryepiglottic fold aryepiglottische Falte *f*, Plica aryepiglottica.
a. of Collier Plica triangularis.
aryepiglottic muscle → aryepiglotticus (muscle).
ar·y·ep·i·glot·ti·cus (muscle) [ˌ-ˌepɪˈglætɪkəs] Aryepiglottikus *m*, M. aryepiglotticus.
ar·y·ep·i·glot·tid·e·an [ˌ-ˌepɪgləˈtɪdɪən] *adj* → aryepiglottic.
aryl- *pref.* Aryl-.
ar·yl·a·mi·dase [ˌærɪlˈæmɪdeɪz] *n* Arylamidase *f*.
ar·yl·a·mine [ˌ-əˈmiːn, -ˈæmɪn] *n* Arylamin *nt*.
arylamine acetyltransferase Arylaminoacetyl(transfer)ase *f*.
ar·yl·a·mi·no·pep·ti·dase [ˌ-əˌmiːnəʊˈpeptɪdeɪz] *n* Arylaminopeptidase *f*.
ar·yl·es·ter·ase [ˌ-ˈestəreɪz] *n* Arylesterase *f*, Arylesterhydrolase *f*.
aryl-ester hydrolase → arylesterase.
ar·yl·form·am·i·dase [ˌ-ˌfɔːrˈmæmɪdeɪz] *n* Arylformamidase *f*, Formylkynureninhydrolase *f*.
aryl-4-hydroxylase *n* Aryl-4-hydroxylase *f*, unspezifische Monooxygenase *f*.
ar·yl·sul·fa·tase [ˌ-ˈsʌlfəteɪz] *n* Arylsulfatase *f*.
arylsulfatase B *abbr.* **ARSB** Arylsulfatase B *f abbr.* ARSB.
arylsulfatase B deficiency Maroteaux--Lamy-Syndrom *nt*, Morbus Maroteaux--Lamy *m*, Mukopolysaccharidose VI *f abbr.* MPS VI.

arylsulfatase test *micro.* Arylsulfatasetest *m*.
ar·y·te·no·ep·i·glot·tic [əˌrɪtnəʊˌepɪˈglætɪk, ˌærəˌtiːnəʊ-] *adj* → aryepiglottic.
ar·y·te·no·ep·i·glot·ti·de·an fold [ˌ-ˌepɪgləˈtiːdɪən] → aryepiglottic fold.
ar·y·te·noid [ˌærɪˈtiːnɔɪd, əˈrɪtnɔɪd] **I** *n* Stell-, Gießbecken-, Aryknorpel *m*, Cartilago aryt(a)enoidea. **II** *adj* Aryknorpel betr., arytänoid.
ar·y·te·noi·dal [ˌærətɪˈnɔɪdl, əˈrɪtnɔɪdl] *adj* → arytenoid II.
arytenoid cartilage → arytenoid I.
ar·y·te·noid·ec·to·my [ˌærɪˌtiːnɔɪˈdektəmɪ] *n chir.* Aryknorpelentfernung *f*, -resektion *f*, Arytänoidektomie *f*.
ar·y·te·noi·de·us obliquus (muscle) [ˌærɪˈtnɔɪdɪəs] Arytänoideus *m* obliquus, M. aryt(a)enoideus obliquus.
arytenoideus transversus (muscle) Arytänoideus *m* transversus, M. aryt(a)enoideus transversus.
ar·y·te·noi·di·tis [əˌrɪtnɔɪˈdaɪtɪs] *n* Aryknorpelentzündung *f*, Arytänoiditis *f*.
arytenoid muscle: oblique a. → arytenoideus obliquus (muscle).
transverse a. → arytenoideus transversus (muscle).
ar·y·te·noi·do·pex·y [ˌærɪtɪˈnɔɪdəʊˌpeksɪ] *n HNO* Kelly-Operation *f*, Kelly-Arytänoidopexie *f*.
arytenoid swellings *embryo.* Arytänoidwülste *pl*.
AS *abbr.* **1.** → aortic stenosis. **2.** → arteriosclerosis.
As *abbr.* **1.** → arsenic 1. **2.** → astigmatism.
ASA *abbr.* **1.** → acetylsalicylic acid. **2.** → argininosuccinic acid.
a·sac·ria [eɪˈseɪkrɪə, -ˈsæk-] *n embryo.* Kreuzbeinaplasie *f*, Asakrie *f*.
ASAL *abbr.* → argininosuccinate lyase.
ASAL deficiency Argininbernsteinsäure--Krankheit *f*, -Schwachsinn *m*, Argininosukzinoazidurie *f*, -sukzinurie *f*, -succinurie *f*.
ASase *abbr.* → argininosuccinate lyase.
ASase deficiency → ASAL deficiency.
ASB *abbr.* → assisted spontaneous breathing.
as·bes·ti·form [æsˈbestɪfɔːrm] *adj* asbestförmig, -artig.
asbestiform degeneration of cartilage *patho.* asbestartige (Knorpel-)Degeneration *f*.
as·bes·tine [æsˈbestɪn, -tiːn] *adj* **1.** asbestartig, Asbest-. **2.** feuerfest, unverbrennbar.
as·bes·tos [æsˈbestəs] *n* Asbest *m*.
asbestos bodies Asbestkörperchen *pl*.
asbestos dust Asbeststaub *m*.
as·bes·to·sis [ˌæsbesˈtəʊsɪs] *n* Asbeststaub-, Bergflachslunge *f*, Asbestose *f*, Asbestosis pulmonum.
asbestosis bodies Asbestkörperchen *pl*.
asbestos-like tinea Asbestgrind *m*, Tinea amiantacea (Alibert), Tinea asbestina, Pityriasis amiantacea, Teigne amiantacé, Keratosis follicularis amiantacea, Impetigo scapida.
asbestos needles Asbestnadeln *pl*.
A-scan *n radiol.* (*Ultraschall*) A-Scan *m*, A-Mode *m*.
as·ca·ri·a·sis [ˌæskəˈraɪəsɪs] *n* Spulwurminfektion *f*, Askariasis *f*, Askari(d)ose *f*, Askaridiasis *f*.
as·car·i·cid·al [ˌæskərɪˈsaɪdl] *adj* askarid(ab)tötend, spulwurmtötend, askarizid.
as·car·i·cide [əˈskærəsaɪd] *n* askarizides Mittel *nt*, Askarizid *nt*.
as·ca·rid [ˈæskərɪd] *n*, *pl* **as·car·i·des** [əˈskærədiːz] *micro.* Ascarid *m*.

Ascaridia

As·ca·rid·ia [ˌæskəˈrɪdɪə] *n micro.* Ascaridia *f.*
as·car·i·di·a·sis [əˌskærɪˈdaɪəsəs] *n* → ascariasis.
As·ca·ri·doi·dea [ˌ-ˈdɔɪdɪə] *pl micro.* Ascaridoidea *pl.*
as·car·i·do·sis [ˌ-ˈdəʊsɪs] *n* → ascariasis.
as·car·i·o·sis [ˌ-ˈəʊsɪs] *n* → ascariasis.
As·ca·ris [ˈæskərɪs] *n micro.* Askaris *f,* Ascaris *f.*
  A. lumbricoides Spulwurm *m,* Ascaris lumbricoides.
  A. vermicularis Madenwurm *m,* Enterobius/Oxyuris vermicularis.
as·ca·ris [ˈæskərɪs] *n, pl* **as·car·i·des** [əˈskærədiːz] *micro.* Spulwurm *m,* Askaris *f,* Ascaris *f.*
as·cend [əˈsend] *vi* (an-, auf-, hinauf-)steigen, nach oben streben, aszendieren.
as·cend·ing [əˈsendɪŋ] *adj* (auf-, an-)steigend, nach oben strebend, aszendierend.
ascending aorta aufsteigende Aorta *f,* aufsteigender Aortenteil *m,* Aorta ascendens, Pars ascendens aortae.
ascending artery A. ascendens/intermesenterica.
ascending branch: anterior a. of left pulmonary artery Ramus anterior ascendens a. pulmonalis sinistrae.
  anterior a. of right pulmonary artery Ramus anterior ascendens a. pulmonalis dextrae.
  a. of deep circumflex iliac artery aufsteigender Ast *m* der A. circumflexa iliaca profunda, Ramus ascendens a. circumflexae iliaca profundae.
  a. of lateral cerebral sulcus Ramus ascendens sulci lateralis (cerebri).
  a. of lateral circumflex femoral artery aufsteigender Ast *m* der A. circumflexa femoris lateralis, Ramus ascendens a. circumflexae femoris lateralis.
  a. of medial circumflex femoral artery aufsteigender Ast *m* der A. circumflexa femoris medialis, Ramus ascendens a. circumflexae femoris medialis.
  posterior a. of left pulmonary artery Ramus posterior ascendens a. pulmonalis sinistrae.
  posterior a. of right pulmonary artery Ramus posterior ascendens a. pulmonalis dextrae.
ascending cholecystitis aufsteigende/aszendierende Gallenblasenentzündung/Cholezystitis *f.*
ascending colon aufsteigendes Colon/Kolon *nt,* Colon ascendens.
ascending current aufsteigender/zentripetaler Strom *m.*
ascending degeneration aufsteigende/retrograde Degeneration *f.*
ascending fibers (*ZNS*) aufsteigende Fasern *pl.*
ascending hemiplegia aufsteigende/aszendierende Hemiplegie *f.*
ascending limb of Henle's loop aufsteigender Schenkel *m* der Henle'-Schleife.
ascending mesocolon Meso *nt* des aufsteigenden Kolons, Mesocolon ascendens.
ascending myelitis aufsteigende/aszendierende Myelitis *f.*
ascending myelopathy aufsteigende/aszendierende Myelopathie *f.*
ascending neuritis → ascending neuropathy.
ascending neuropathy aufsteigende/aszendierende Neuropathie *f.*
ascending paralysis aufsteigende Lähmung *f.*
ascending part: a. of aorta → ascending aorta.

a. of duodenum aufsteigender Duodenumabschnitt *m,* Pars ascendens duodeni.
ascending pathways (*ZNS*) aufsteigende Bahnen *pl.*
ascending pyelography retrograde Pyelographie *f.*
ascending pyelonephritis aufsteigende/aszendierende Pyelonephritis *f.*
ascending ramus of pubis oberer Schambeinast *m,* Ramus superior ossis pubis.
ascending reticular activating system *abbr.* ARAS aufsteigendes retikuläres aktivierendes System *nt abbr.* ARAS.
ascending tract (*ZNS*) aufsteigende Bahn *f.*
ascending urography *urol., radiol.* retrograde Urographie *f.*
as·cent [əˈsent] *n* Aufstieg *m,* Anstieg *m.*
as·cer·tain [ˌæsərˈteɪn] *vt* feststellen, ermitteln, in Erfahrung bringen.
as·cer·tain·a·ble [ˌæsərˈteɪnəbl] *adj* feststellbar, nachweisbar, ermittelbar.
as·cer·tain·ment [æsərˈteɪnmənt] *n* Ermittlung *f,* Feststellung *f.*
asc·hel·minth [ˈæskhelmɪnθ] *n micro.* Schlauch-, Rundwurm *m,* Aschelminth *m,* Nemathelminth *m.*
Asc·hel·min·thes [ˌæskhelˈmɪnθiːz] *pl micro.* Schlauch-, Rundwürmer *pl,* Nemathelminthen *pl,* Aschelminthes *pl.*
Ascher [ˈæʃər]: **A.'s syndrome** Ascher-Syndrom *nt.*
Ascherson [ˈæʃərsən]: **A.'s membrane** *biochem.* Ascherson-Membran *f.*
  A.'s syndrome Ascherson-Syndrom *nt.*
  A.'s vesicle *biochem.* Ascherson-Vesikel *nt,* -Tröpfchen *nt.*
Aschheim-Zondek [ˈæʃhaɪm ˈzandɪk]: **A.-Z. hormone** luteinisierendes Hormon *nt abbr.* LH, Luteinisierungshormon *nt,* Interstitialzellen-stimulierendes Hormon *nt,* interstitial cell stimulating hormone *abbr.* ICSH.
  A.-Z. test *abbr.* AZT *gyn.* Aschheim-Zondek-Reaktion *f abbr.* AZR.
a·schis·to·dac·tyl·ia [eɪˌʃɪstədækˈtɪːlɪə] *n* Verwachsung *f* von Fingern *od.* Zehen, Syndaktylie *f.*
Aschner [ˈæʃnər]: **A.'s phenomenon** Aschner-Versuch *m,* Aschner-Dagnini--Versuch *m,* Bulbusdruckversuch *m.*
  A.'s reflex Aschner-Dagnini-Bulbusreflex *m,* okulokardialer Reflex *m,* Bulbusdruckreflex *m.*
  A.'s sign → A.'s reflex.
  A.'s test → A.'s phenomenon.
Aschner-Dagnini [dægˈnɪniː]: **A.-D. reflex** → Aschner's reflex.
  A.-D. test → Aschner's phenomenon.
Aschoff [ˈæʃɔf]: **A.'s bodies** Aschoff'-Knötchen *pl.*
  A.'s cells Aschoff-Zellen *pl.*
  A.'s node → Aschoff-Tawara's node.
  A.'s nodules → A.'s bodies.
Aschoff-Tawara [təˈwɑːrə]: **A.-T.'s node** Atrioventrikularknoten *m,* AV-Knoten *m,* Aschoff-Tawara'-Knoten *m,* Nodus atrioventricularis.
as·ci·tes [əˈsaɪtiːz] *n* Bauchwassersucht *f,* Aszites *m,* Ascites *m.*
as·cit·ic [əˈsɪtɪk] *adj* Azites betr., aszitisch, Azites-.
ascitic agar Aszitesagar *m/nt.*
ascitic fluid Azites(flüssigkeit *f*) *m.*
as·ci·tog·e·nous [ˌæsɪˈtɑdʒənəs] *adj* asziteserzeugend, -verursachend.
as·co·carp [ˈæskəkɑrp] *n micro.* Askokarp *f,* Ascokarp *f.*
as·co·go·ni·um [ˌ-ˈɡəʊnɪəm] *n micro.* Askogon *nt.*
Ascoli [asˈkoli]: **A.'s reaction** Ascoli-Reaktion *f.*

As·co·my·ce·tae [ˌæskəʊˈmaɪsətiː] *pl* → Ascomycetes.
as·co·my·cete [ˌ-ˈmaɪsiːt, -maɪˈsiːt] *n micro.* Schlauchpilz *m,* Askomyzet *m.*
As·co·my·ce·tes [ˌ-maɪˈsiːtiːz] *pl micro.* Schlauchpilze *pl,* Askomyzeten *pl,* Ascomycetes *pl,* Ascomycotina *pl.*
as·co·my·ce·tous [ˌ-maɪˈsiːtəs] *adj* Schlauchpilz(e) betr., Askomyzeten-.
a·scor·bate [əˈskɔːrbeɪt, -bɪt] *n* Askorbat *nt,* Ascorbat *nt.*
a·scor·be·mia [æskɔːrˈbiːmɪə] *n* Askorbinämie *f.*
a·scor·bic acid [əˈskɔːrbɪk] Askorbinsäure *f,* Ascorbinsäure *f,* Vitamin C *nt.*
a·scor·bu·ria [æskɔːrˈb(j)ʊərɪə] *n* Askorbinsäureausscheidung *f* im Harn, Askorb(in)urie *f.*
as·co·spore [ˈæskəspɔːr, -spəʊr] *n micro.* Askospore *f.*
as·cribe [əˈskraɪb] *vt* zuschreiben, zurückführen (*to* auf).
as·crip·tion [əˈskrɪpʃn] *n* Zuschreibung *f,* Zurückführung (*to* auf).
as·cus [ˈæskəs] *n, pl* **as·ci** [ˈæsaɪ, ˈæski] *micro.* (Sporen-)Schlauch *m,* Askus *m.*
ASD *abbr.* → atrial septal defect.
a·se·cre·to·ry [əˈsiːkrətɔːriː, -təʊ-] *adj* asekretorisch.
a·se·mia [əˈsiːmɪə] *n neuro.* Asemie *f,* Asemia *f,* Asymbolie *f.*
a·sep·sis [əˈsepsɪs, eɪ-] *n, pl* **-ses** [-siːz] **1.** Keimfreiheit *f,* Asepsis *f.* **2.** Herbeiführen von Keimfreiheit, Asepsis *f,* Aseptik *f,* Sterilisation *f,* Sterilisierung *f.*
a·sep·tic [əˈseptɪk, eɪ-] *n* keimfreies Produkt *od.* Nahrungsmittel *nt.* II *adj* **1.** keimfrei, aseptisch; steril. **2.** *patho.* ohne Erregerbeteiligung, aseptisch; avaskulär.
aseptic fever aseptisches Fieber *nt,* Febris aseptica.
a·sep·ti·cism [əˈseptəsɪzəm] *n* keimfreie Wundbehandlung *f,* Aseptik *f.*
aseptic meningitis lymphozytäre Meningitis *f.*
aseptic necrosis aseptische Nekrose *f.*
  a. of bone aseptische/spontane Knochennekrose *f.*
aseptic osteochondrosis *ortho.* aseptische Epiphysennekrose *f,* Chondroosteonekrose *f.*
aseptic wound *ortho.* saubere/aseptische Wunde *f.*
a·sex·u·al [eɪˈsekʃəwəl, -ʃəl, -sjʊəl] *adj* geschlechtslos, ungeschlechtlich, asexual, asexuell, nicht geschlechtlich.
asexual cycle *bio.* asexueller Zyklus *m.*
asexual generation *bio.* ungeschlechtliche/vegetative Fortpflanzung *f.*
a·sex·u·al·i·ty [eɪˌsekʃəˈwælətɪ] *n* Asexualität *f.*
a·sex·u·al·i·za·tion [eɪˌsekʃəwælɪˈseɪʃn] *n* Sterilisation *f;* Kastration *f,* Kastrierung *f.*
asexual reproduction *micro.* ungeschlechtliche/vegetative Fortpflanzung *f.*
asexual stage *micro.* ungeschlechtliche/vegetative Phase *f.*
ash [æʃ] *n* **1.** Asche *f.* **2.** (*Farbe*) Aschgrau *nt.* **3.** *bot.* Esche *f.*
ash·en [ˈæʃən] *adj* kreidebleich, aschfahl, -grau.
ashen-faced *adj* → ashen.
ashen tuber Tuber cinereum.
ashen tubercle → ashen tuber.
Asherman [ˈæʃərmən]: **A.'s syndrome** Asherman-Fritsch-Syndrom *nt.*
Ashley [ˈæʃli]: **A.'s phenomenon** okulokardialer Reflex *m,* Bulbusdruckreflex *m,* Aschner-Dagnini-Bulbusdruckversuch *m.*

ash picture histol. Aschenbild nt, Spodogramm nt.
ash·y dermatitis ['æʃɪ] Erythema dyschromicum perstans.
ashy dermatosis of Ramirez → ashy dermatitis.
a·si·a·lia [ˌeɪsaɪ'eɪliə] n fehlende od. mangelnde Speichelsekretion f, Asialie f, Aptyalismus m.
A·sian ['eɪʒn, 'eɪʃn] I n Asiat(in f) m. II adj asiatisch.
A. influenza asiatische Grippe f.
A. liver fluke hinterindischer Leberegel m, Opisthorchis viverrini.
A·si·at·ic [ˌeɪʒɪ'ætɪk, ˌeɪʃɪ-]: **A. cholera** klassische Cholera f, Cholera asiatica/indica/orientalis/epidemica.
A. schistosomiasis japanische Bilharziose/Schistosomiasis f, Schistosomiasis japonica.
a·sid·ent sign/symptom [ə'saɪnt] Nebensymptom nt.
a·sid·er·o·sis [eɪˌsɪdə'rəʊsɪs] n Eisenmangel m, Asiderose f.
a·sid·er·ot·ic anemia [ˌ-'rɑtɪk] Chlorose f, Chlorosis f.
a·sit·ia [ə'sɪʃɪə] n Asitie f.
as·ji·ke [æs'dʒaɪkiː] n Beriberi f, Vitamin B_1-Mangel(krankheit f) m, Thiaminmangel(krankheit f) m.
Askanazy [aska'naːzi]: **A.'s cells** Hürthle-Zellen pl.
ASL abbr. 1. → antistreptolysin. 2. → argininosuccinate lyase.
ASL deficiency Argininbernsteinsäure-Krankheit f, -Schwachsinn m, Argininosukzinoazidurie f, -sukzinurie f, -succinurie f.
a·sleep [ə'sliːp] adj 1. schlafend. **to be (fast/sound) ~** (fest) schlafen. **to fall ~** einschlafen. 2. (Fuß, Hand) eingeschlafen, taub. 3. schläfrig, träge, untätig.
ASLO abbr. → antistreptolysin O.
Asn abbr. → asparagine.
ASO abbr. → antistreptolysin O.
Asp abbr. → aspartic acid.
as·par·a·gi·nase [æs'pærədʒɪneɪz] n Asparaginase f, Asparaginamidase f.
as·par·a·gine [ə'spærədʒiːn, -dʒɪn] n abbr. Asn Asparagin nt abbr. Asn, Asp-NH_2.
asparagine synthetase Asparaginsynthetase f.
asparagine synthetase (glutamine-hydrolyzing) Asparaginsynthetase (Glutamin hydrolysierend) f.
as·par·a·gi·nyl [æs'pærədʒɪnɪl] n Asparaginyl-(Radikal nt).
a·spar·tame [ə'spɑːrteɪm, 'æspər-] n Aspartam m.
as·par·tase [ə'spɑːrteɪz] n → aspartate ammonia-lyase.
as·par·tate ['-teɪt] n Aspartat nt.
aspartate aminotransferase abbr. **AST** Aspartataminotransferase f abbr. AST, Aspartattransaminase f, Glutamatoxalacetattransaminase f abbr. GOT.
aspartate ammonia-lyase Aspartatammoniaklyase f, Aspartase f.
aspartate carbamoyl transferase → aspartate transcarbamoylase.
aspartate-glutamate carrier Aspartat--Glutamat-Carrier m.
aspartate kinase Aspartatkinase f.
aspartate semialdehyde Aspartatsemialdehyd m.
aspartate semialdehyde dehydrogenase Aspartatsemialdehyddehydrogenase f.
aspartate transaminase → aspartate aminotransferase.
aspartate transcarbamoylase Aspartattranscarbamylase f, Aspartatcarbamyltransferase f, ATCase f.

as·par·thi·one [ə'spɑːrθaɪəʊn] n Asparthion nt.
as·par·tic acid [ə'spɑːrtɪk] abbr. **Asp** Asparaginsäure f abbr. Asp, α-Aminobernsteinsäure f.
as·par·tyl [ə'spɑːrtl, -ˌtiːl] n Aspartyl-(Radikal nt).
β-aspartyl-N-acetylglucosaminidase n β-Aspartyl-N-acetylglucosaminidase f, Aspartylglykosaminidase f.
as·par·tyl·gly·cos·a·min·i·dase [æsˌpɑːrtlˌglaɪˌkəʊsə'mɪnɪdeɪz] n → β-aspartyl-N-acetylglucosaminidase.
as·par·tyl·gly·cos·am·i·nu·ria [ˌ-ˌˌglaɪkəʊsəmɪ'n(j)ʊəriə] n Aspartylglykosaminurie f.
aspartyl phosphate Asparaginsäurephosphat nt, Aspartylphosphat nt.
aspartyl-tRNA-synthetase n Aspartyl-tRNA-Synthetase f.
a·spe·cif·ic [əspɪ'sɪfɪk] adj patho. unspezifisch.
a·spect ['æspekt] n 1. Aussehen nt, Erscheinung f, Anblick m, Form f, Gestalt f. 2. Aspekt m, Seite f, Gesichts-, Blickpunkt m. 3. Seite f, Fläche f, Teil m. 4. Gesichtsausdruck m, Miene f.
as·per·gil·lar [ˌæspər'dʒɪlər] adj Aspergillus betr., durch Aspergillus verursacht, durch Aspergillus bedingt.
as·per·gil·lic acid [ˌ-'dʒɪlɪk] Aspergill(in)säure f.
as·per·gil·lin [ˌ-'dʒɪlɪn] n Aspergillin nt.
as·per·gil·lo·ma [ˌ-dʒɪ'ləʊmə] n Aspergillom nt.
as·per·gil·lo·my·co·sis [ˌ-ˌdʒɪlaɪ'kəʊsɪs] n → aspergillosis.
as·per·gil·lo·sis [ˌ-dʒɪ'ləʊsɪs] n Aspergillusmykose f, Aspergillose f.
as·per·gil·lo·tox·i·co·sis [ˌ-ˌdʒɪləˌtɒksɪ'kəʊsɪs] n → aspergillustoxicosis.
As·per·gil·lus [ˌ-'dʒɪləs] n Kolben-, Gießkannenschimmel m, Aspergillus m.
A. flavus gelbsporiger Kolbenschimmel, Aspergillus flavus.
A. fumigatus rauchgrauer Kolbenschimmel, Aspergillus fumigatus.
A. glaucus grünsporiger Kolbenschimmel, Aspergillus glaucus.
A. niger schwarzer Kolbenschimmel, Aspergillus niger.
as·per·gil·lus [ˌ-'dʒɪləs] n, pl **-li** [-laɪ] Kolben-, Gießkannenschimmel m, Aspergillus m.
aspergillus keratitis Aspergillus-Keratitis f.
as·per·gil·lus·tox·i·co·sis [ˌ-ˌdʒɪləsˌtɒksɪ'kəʊsɪs] n Aspergillustoxikose f.
a·sper·ki·nase [ˌ-'kaɪneɪs, -'kɪ-] n Asperkinase f.
a·sper·ma·tic [ˌeɪspər'mætɪk] adj Aspermie betr., asperm, aspermatisch.
a·sper·ma·tism [eɪ'spɜːrmətɪzəm] n 1. Aspermatie f, Aspermatismus m. 2. Aspermie f.
a·sper·ma·to·gen·e·sis [əˌspɜːrmətə'dʒenəsɪs] n Aspermatogenese f.
a·sper·ma·to·gen·ic sterility [ˌ-'dʒenɪk] urol. aspermatogene Sterilität f.
a·sper·mia [eɪ'spɜːrmiə] n Aspermie f.
a·sper·mic [eɪ'spɜːrmɪk] adj → aspermatic.
as·phyc·tic [æs'fɪktɪk] adj Asphyxie betr., asphyktisch.
as·phyc·tous [æs'fɪktəs] adj → asphyctic.
as·phyg·mia [æs'fɪgmɪə] n vorübergehende Pulslosigkeit f, Asphygmie f.
as·phyx·ia [æs'fɪksɪə] n Asphyxie f.
a. of the newborn Neugeborenenasphyxie, Atemdepressionszustand m des Neugeborenen, Asphyxia neonatorum.
as·phyx·i·al [æs'fɪksɪəl] adj → asphyctic.
as·phyx·i·ant [æs'fɪksɪənt] I n Asphyxie

assign

hervorrufendes Mittel nt. II adj erstickend.
as·phyx·i·ate [æs'fɪksɪeɪt] vt, vi ersticken.
as·phyx·i·at·ing thoracic chondrodystrophy [æs'fɪksɪeɪtɪŋ] Jeune'-Krankheit f, asphyxierende Thoraxdysplasie f.
asphyxiating thoracic dysplasia → asphyxiating thoracic chondrodystrophy.
asphyxiating thoracic dystrophy abbr. **ATD** → asphyxiating thoracic chondrodystrophy.
as·phyx·i·a·tion [æsˌfɪksɪ'eɪʃn] n Erstickungszustand m, Erstickung f.
as·pi·rate [n, adj 'æspərɪt; v -reɪt] **I** n 1. Aspirat nt; Punktat nt. 2. Hauchlaut m, Aspirata f. **II** adj aspiriert. **III** vt 3. ab-, an-, aufsaugen, aspirieren; (Gelenk) punktieren. 4. aspirieren.
as·pi·ra·tion [ˌæspə'reɪʃn] n 1. (Ein-)Atmen nt, Aspiration f. 2. An-, Ab-, Aufsaugen nt, Aspiration f; (Gelenk) Punktion f. 3. patho. Fremdstoffeinatmung f, Aspiration f.
aspiration biopsy Aspirations-, Saugbiopsie f.
fine-needle a. Feinnadelbiopsie.
needle a. Nadelbiopsie.
aspiration biopsy cytology abbr. **ABC** Saug-, Aspirations(biopsie)zytologie f.
aspiration cannula Aspirations-, Punktionskanüle f.
aspiration needle Aspirations-, Punktionsnadel f.
aspiration pneumonia Aspirationspneumonie f.
aspiration pneumonitis Aspirationspneumonie f.
aspiration syringe Aspirations-, Punktionsspritze f.
as·pi·ra·tor ['æspəreɪtər] n Aspirator m.
as·pi·rin ['æspərɪn, -prɪn] n Azetylsalicylsäure f abbr. **ASS**, Acetylsalicylsäure f.
a·sple·nia [ə'spliːniə] n Asplenie f.
asplenia syndrome Ivemark-Syndrom nt.
a·sple·nic [ə'splenɪk, -'spliːn-] adj Asplenie betr., asplenisch.
a·splen·ism [ə'spliːnɪzəm] n → asplenia.
a·spo·ro·gen·ic [ˌeɪspəʊrə'dʒenɪk] adj micro. nichtsporenbildend.
a·spo·rog·e·nous [eɪspə'rɑdʒənəs, -spɔː-] adj → asporogenic.
asporogenous mutant micro. nichtsporenbildende Mutante f.
a·spor·ous [eɪ'spɔːrəs] adj micro. sporenlos.
As·sam fever [æ'sæm] viszerale Leishmaniose/Leishmaniase f, Kala-Azar f, Splenomegalia tropica.
as·sas·sin bugs [ə'sæsɪn] micro. Raubwanzen pl, Reduviiden pl, Reduviidae pl.
as·say [ə'seɪ, æ'seɪ; v æ'seɪ] phys., biochem., chem. **I** n 1. Analyse f, Test m, Probe f, Nachweisverfahren nt, Bestimmung f, Assay m. **to carry out an ~ on a sample** eine Probenbestimmung/-analyse durchführen. 2. Probe(material nt) f. **II** vt analysieren, testen, bestimmen, prüfen, untersuchen, messen.
assay sample Probe(material nt) f.
assay technique Nachweismethode f.
as·sent [ə'sent] **I** n Zustimmung f, Genehmigung f, Einwilligung f (to zu). **to give one's ~** seine Zustimmung geben (to zu). **II** vi zustimmen, einwilligen (to in), genehmigen.
as·sess [ə'ses] vt ab-, einschätzen, (be-)werten, beurteilen.
as·sess·ment [ə'sesmənt] n 1. Ab-, Einschätzung f, Bewertung f, Beurteilung f. 2. (Patient) Untersuchung f.
as·sign [ə'saɪn] vt 1. zuordnen, -weisen,

assignment

-teilen (*to sb.* jdm.); (*Aufgabe*) übertragen, anvertrauen (*to sb.* jdm.). 2. (*Zeitpunkt*) festsetzen, bestimmen.
as·sign·ment [əˈsaɪnmənt] *n* 1. Zuordnung *f*, -weisung *f*, -teilung *f* (*to* zu). 2. Festsetzung *f*, Bestimmung *f*.
as·sim·i·la·ble [əˈsɪmələbl] *adj* assimilierbar.
as·sim·i·late [əˈsɪməleɪt] I *vt* 1. angleichen, anpassen, assimilieren (*to, with* an). 2. *biochem.* umsetzen, assimilieren. 3. *psycho., socio.* aufnehmen, absorbieren, assimilieren. 4. *bio.* assimilieren, aufnehmen, einverleiben. II *vi* s. anpassen, s. angleichen; *socio, psycho.* s. assimilieren.
as·sim·i·la·tion [əˌsɪməˈleɪʃn] *n* 1. (*a. psycho., socio.*) Angleichung *f*, Anpassung *f*, Assimilation *f* (*to* an). 2. *biochem.* Assimilation *f*, Assimilierung *f*. 3. Einverleibung *f*, Aufnahme *f*, Assimilation *f* (*to* in).
assimilation pelvis Assimilationsbecken *nt*.
as·sim·i·la·to·ry [əˈsɪmələˌtɔːriː, -təʊ-] *adj* Assimilation betr., assimilierend, assimilierbar, Assimilierungs-, Assimilations-.
assimilatory product Assimilationsprodukt *nt*, Assimilat *nt*.
as·sist [əˈsɪst] I *vt* 1. helfen, jdm. beistehen, jdn. unterstützen. 2. fördern, unterstützen. 3. teilnehmen (*at* an). II *vi* (aus-)helfen, Hilfe leisten, mitarbeiten, mithelfen (*in* bei).
as·sis·tance [əˈsɪstəns] *n* Hilfe *f*, Beistand *m*; Unterstützung *f*, Beihilfe *f*; Hilfeleistung *f*, Mitarbeit *f*. **to afford/render/give ~ to sb.** bei jdm. Hilfe leisten. **to be of ~** (**to sb.**) jdm. helfen *od.* behilflich sein. **to come to sb.'s ~** jdm. zu Hilfe kommen. **in need of ~** hilfsbedürftig.
as·sis·tant [əˈsɪstənt] I *n* 1. Assistent(in *f*) *m*; Gehilfe *m*, Gehilfin *f*, Mitarbeiter(in *f*) *m*. 2. Hilfe *f*, Hilfsmittel *nt*. II *adj* behilflich (*to*), assistierend, stellvertretend, Hilfs-, Unter-.
assist-control ventilation assistierte Spontanatmung *f*.
as·sist·ed circulation [əˈsɪstɪd] assistierte Zirkulation *f*.
assisted respiration assistierte Beatmung *f*.
assisted spontaneous breathing *abbr.* **ASB** assistierte Spontanatmung *f*.
assisted ventilation assistierte Beatmung *f*.
Assmann [ˈæsmən]: **A.'s focus** Assmann'-Herd *m*, -Frühinfiltrat *nt*.
A.'s tuberculous infiltrate → A.'s focus.
as·so·ci·ate [*n* əˈsəʊʃɪɪt, -ʃɪeɪt; *adj* -ʃɪət, -sɪət, -sɪeɪt; *v* -ʃɪeɪt, -sɪɪt-] I *n* Kollege *m*, Kollegin *f*, Partner(in *f*) *m*, Mitarbeiter(in *f*) *m*. II *adj* (eng) verbunden (*with* mit), angegliedert, zugehörig; verwandt (*with* mit); beigeordnet, Mit-. III *vt* 1. vereinigen, verbinden, angliedern, verknüpfen (*with* mit); anschließen (*with* an). 2. (*a. psycho.*) assoziieren, in Verbindung/Zusammenhang bringen, verknüpfen (*with* mit). 3. *chem.* verknüpfen, verbinden, assoziieren. IV *vi* s. verbinden (*with* mit).
as·so·ci·at·ed antagonists [əˈsəʊʃɪeɪtɪd, -sɪ-] (*Muskel*) assoziierte Antagonisten *pl*.
associated movement Begleitbewegung *f*.
as·so·ci·a·tion [əˌsəʊʃɪˈeɪʃn, -sɪ-] *n* 1. Verbindung *f*, Verknüpfung *f*, Vereinigung *f*, Verkoppelung *f*, Anschluß *m* (*with* an). 2. *psycho.* (Ideen-, Gedanken-)Assoziation *f*, (-)Verknüpfung *f*. 3. *chem.* Assoziation *f* (*von Einzelmolekülen*). 4. Gesellschaft *f*, Verband *m*, Verein(igung *f*) *m*. 5. Zusammenhang *m*, Beziehung *f*.

association area (*ZNS*) Assoziationsfeld *nt*, -areal *nt*.
association cells (*ZNS*) Assoziationszellen *pl*.
association constant Assoziationskonstante *f*.
association (nerve) fibers Assoziationsfasern *pl*, -bahnen *pl*, Neurofibrae associationis.
 interhemispheric a. interhemisphärische Assoziationsfasern.
 long a. lange Assoziationsfasern.
 short a. kurze Assoziationsfasern.
association neurofibers → association (nerve) fibers.
association paralysis (progressive) Bulbärparalyse *f*, Duchenne-Syndrom *nt*.
association test *psycho.* Assoziationsversuch *m*.
as·so·ci·a·tive [əˈsəʊʃɪˌeɪtɪv, -sɪ-, ʃətɪv] *adj* 1. (s.) vereinigend *od.* verbindend, verknüpfend. 2. *psycho.* assoziativ.
associative aphasia assoziative Aphasie *f*, Leitungsaphasie *f*.
associative cortex (*ZNS*) assoziativer Cortex *m*, assoziative Rinde *f*.
associative learning assoziatives Lernen *nt*.
associative thalamus assoziativer Thalamus *m*.
as·sort [əˈsɔːrt] I *vt* 1. einordnen, klassifizieren. 2. sortieren, ordnen, gruppieren, aussuchen, zusammenstellen. II *vi* passen (*with* zu), übereinstimmen (*with* mit).
as·sor·ta·tive [əˈsɔːrtətɪv] *adj* (zu-)ordnend; auswählend.
as·sort·ment [əˈsɔːrtmənt] *n* 1. Sortieren *nt*, Ordnen *nt*; Zusammenstellen *nt*. 2. Zusammenstellung *f*, Sammlung *f*, Auswahl *f* (*of* an).
as·suage [əˈsweɪdʒ] *vt* 1. (*Schmerz*) lindern, mildern. 2. (*Hunger*) stillen, befriedigen. 3. jdn. beruhigen, beschwichtigen.
as·suage·ment [əsweɪdʒmənt] *n* 1. (*Schmerz*) Linderung *f*, Milderung *f*. 2. (*Hunger*) Stillung *f*, Stillen *nt*; Befriedigung *f*. 3. Beruhigungsmittel *nt*. 4. Beruhigung *f*, Beschwichtigung *f*.
as·sume [əˈs(j)uːm] *vt* 1. annehmen, voraussetzen, vermuten. 2. (*Lage*) einnehmen. 3. (*Verantwortung*) übernehmen.
as·sump·tion [əˈsʌmpʃn] *n* Annahme *f*, Voraussetzung *f*, Vermutung *f*. **on the ~ that** unter der Voraussetzung *od*. in der Vermutung, daß.
AST *abbr.* → aspartate aminotransferase.
as·ta·sia [əˈsteɪʒ(ɪ)ə, -zɪə] *n neuro.* Unfähigkeit *f* zu stehen, Astasie *f*.
astasia-abasia *n neuro.* Astasie-Abasie-Syndrom *nt*.
as·tat·ic [əˈstætɪk] *adj* Astasie betr., astatisch.
as·ta·tine [ˈæstətiːn, -tɪn] *n abbr.* **At** Astatin *nt abbr.* At.
as·te·a·tot·ic eczema [ˌæstɪəˈtɒtɪk, əˌstɪə-] → asteatosis.
as·te·a·to·des [ˌ-ˈtəʊdiːz] *n* → asteatosis.
as·te·a·to·sis [ˌ-ˈtəʊsɪs] *n* Exsikkationsekzem *nt*, -dermatitis *f*, asteatotisches/xerotisches Ekzem *nt*, Austrocknungsekzem *nt*, Exsikkationsekzematid *nt*, Asteatosis cutis, Xerosis *f*.
as·ter [ˈæstər] *n* 1. → astrosphere. 2. *bio.* Aster *f*.
a·ste·re·o·cog·no·sy [eɪˌstɪərɪəˈkɒɡnəsɪ] *n* → astereognosis.
a·ster·e·og·no·sis [əˌstɪərɪɒɡˈnəʊsɪs] *n neuro.* taktile Agnosie *f*, Astereognosie *f*, Asterognosis *f*.
as·te·ri·on [æsˈtɪərɪɒn] *n, pl* **-ri·a** [-rɪə] *anat.* Asterion *nt*.
as·te·rix·is [ˌæstəˈrɪksɪs] *n neuro.* Flatter-

tremor *m*, Flapping-Tremor *m*, Asterixis *f*.
a·ster·nal ribs [eɪˈstɜːrnl] falsche Rippen *pl*, Costae spuriae.
a·ster·nia [eɪˈstɜːrnɪə] *n embryo.* Sternumaplasie *f*, Asternie *f*.
as·ter·oid [ˈæstərɔɪd] *adj* stern(en)förmig, asteroid.
asteroid bodies *patho.* Asteroidkörperchen *pl*.
as·the·nia [æsˈθiːnɪə] *n* Kraft-, Energielosigkeit *f*, Schwäche *f*, Asthenie *f*.
as·then·ic [æsˈθenɪk] I *n* Astheniker(in *f*) *m*, Leptosome(r *m*) *f*. II *adj* 1. Asthenie betr., asthenisch, asthenisch. 2. *physiol.* von asthenischem Körperbau, schlankwüchsig, asthenisch.
asthenic type asthenischer Typ *m*, Astheniker *m*.
as·the·no·bul·bo·spi·nal paralysis [æsˌθɪnəʊˌbʌlbəʊˈspaɪnl] Erb-Goldflam-Syndrom *nt*, -Krankheit *f*, Erb-Oppenheim-Goldflam-Syndrom *nt*, -Krankheit *f*, Hoppe-Goldflam-Syndrom *nt*, Myasthenia gravis pseudoparalytica.
as·the·no·co·ria [ˌ-ˈkəʊrɪə] *n ophthal.* Arrojo-Zeichen *nt*, Asthenokorie *f*.
as·then·ope [ˈæsθənəʊp] *n ophthal.* Patient(in *f*) *m* mit Asthenopie, Asthenope(r *m*) *f*.
as·the·no·pho·bia [ˌæsθɪnəʊˈfəʊbɪə] *n ophthal.* Asthenophobie *f*.
as·the·no·pi·a [ˌæsθəˈnəʊpɪə] *n* Schwachsichtigkeit *f*, Asthenopie *f*.
as·the·nop·ic [ˌ-ˈnɒpɪk] *adj* Asthenopie betr., asthenopisch.
as·the·no·sper·mia [ˌæsθɪnəʊˈspɜːrmɪə] *n* Astheno(zoo)spermie *f*.
as·the·no·sper·mic [ˌ-ˈspɜːrmɪk] *adj* Astheno(zoo)spermie betr., asthenosperm.
asth·ma [ˈæzmə] *n* 1. anfallsweise Atemnot *m*, Asthma *nt*. 2. Bronchialasthma *nt*, Asthma bronchiale.
asthma crystals Charcot-Leyden-Kristalle *pl*, Asthmakristalle *pl*.
asth·mat·ic [æzˈmætɪk] I *n* Asthmatiker(in *f*) *m*. II *adj* Asthma betr., asthmatisch, kurzatmig, Asthma-.
asth·mat·i·cal [æzˈmætɪkl] *adj* → asthmatic II.
asthmatic attack Asthmaanfall *m*.
asth·mat·i·form [æzˈmætɪfɔːrm] *adj* asthmaähnlich, -artig, asthmatoid.
asth·mo·gen·ic [ˌæzməʊˈdʒenɪk] I *n* asthmogene Substanz *f*. II *adj* asthmaverursachend, -auslösend, asthmogen.
a·stig·ma·graph [əˈstɪɡməɡræf] *n ophthal.* Astigm(at)ograph *m*.
as·tig·mat·ic [ˌæstɪɡˈmætɪk] *adj* Astigmatismus betr., astigmatisch.
as·tig·mat·i·cal [ˌ-ˈmætɪkl] *adj* → astigmatic.
astigmatic lens Zylinderglas *nt*.
a·stig·ma·tism [əˈstɪɡmətɪzm] *n abbr.* **AS** *ophthal.* Stabsichtigkeit *f*, Astigmatismus *m*.
a. with oblique pencils Astigmatismus mit schrägen Achsen, Astigmatismus obliquus.
a. against the rule inverser Astigmatismus, Astigmatismus gegen die Regel, Astigmatismus inversus.
a. with the rule Astigmatismus nach der Regel, Astigmatismus rectus.
a·stig·ma·tom·e·ter [əˌstɪɡməˈtɒmɪtər] *n ophthal.* Astigm(at)ometer *nt*.
a·stig·ma·tom·e·try [ˌ-ˈtɒmɪtrɪ] *n ophthal.* Astigm(at)ometrie *f*.
as·tig·mat·o·scope [ˌæstɪɡˈmætəskəʊp] *n ophthal.* Astigm(at)oskop *nt*.
a·stig·ma·tos·co·py [əˌstɪɡməˈtɒskəpɪ] *n ophthal.* Astigm(at)oskopie *f*.

a·stig·mia [əˈstɪgmɪə] n → astigmatism.
a·stig·mic [əˈstɪgmɪk] adj → astigmatic.
as·tig·mom·e·ter [ˌæstɪgˈmɑmɪtər] n → astigmatometer.
as·tig·mom·e·try [ˌ-ˈmɑmətrɪ] n → astigmatometry.
as·tig·mo·scope [əˈstɪgməskəʊp] n → astigmatoscope.
as·tig·mos·co·py [əˌstɪgˈmɑskəpɪ] n → astigmatoscopy.
ASTO abbr. → antistreptolysin O.
a·sto·mia [əˈstəʊmɪə] n embryo. angeborenes Fehlen nt des Mundes, Astomie f.
as·to·mous [ˈæstəməs] adj mundlos.
a·sto·mus [əˈstəʊməs] n embryo. Astomus m.
as·trag·a·lar [æˈstrægələr] adj Sprungbein/Talus betr., talar, Sprungbein-, Talus-.
as·tra·ga·lec·to·my [ˌæstrægəˈlɛktəmɪ] n ortho. Talusresektion f.
as·trag·a·lo·cal·ca·ne·an [əˌstrægələʊkælˈkeɪnɪən] adj Sprungbein/Talus u. Fersenbein/Kalkaneus betr., talokalkaneal.
as·trag·a·lo·cru·ral [ˌ-ˈkrʊərəl] adj Sprungbein/Talus u. Unterschenkel(knochen) betr., talokrural.
as·trag·a·loid bone [əˈstrægələɪd] old → astragalus.
as·trag·a·lo·scaph·oid [əˌstrægələʊˈskæfɔɪd] adj Sprungbein/Talus u. Kahnbein/Os naviculare betr., talonavikular.
as·trag·a·lo·tib·i·al [ˌ-ˈtɪbɪəl] adj Sprungbein/Talus u. Schienbein/Tibia betr., talotibial.
as·trag·a·lus [æˈstrægələs] n Sprungbein nt, Talus m.
as·tral [ˈæstrəl] adj 1. bio. Teilungsstern/Aster betr., sternförmig, astral. 2. allg. sternförmig, stellar, Astral-, Stern(en)-.
astral rays histol. Spindelfasern pl.
as·tra·pho·bia [ˌæstrəˈfəʊbɪə] n Gewitterangst f, Astraphobie f.
as·tra·po·pho·bia [ˌæstrəpəˈfəʊbɪə] n → astraphobia.
as·tringe [əˈstrɪndʒ] vt 1. zusammenziehen, -pressen, festbinden. 2. adstringieren, zusammenziehen.
as·trin·gent [əˈstrɪndʒənt] I n Adstringens nt. II adj adstringierend, zusammenziehend.
as·tro·blast [ˈæstrəblæst] n Astroblast m.
as·tro·blas·to·ma [ˌ-blæsˈtəʊmə] n Astroblastom m.
as·tro·cele n → astrocoele.
as·tro·ci·net·ic adj → astrokinetic.
as·tro·coele [ˈæstrəsiːl] n Astrocele f.
as·tro·cyte [ˈæstrəsaɪt] n Sternzelle f, Astrozyt m.
as·tro·cyt·ic glioma [ˌ-ˈsɪtɪk] → astrocytoma.
as·tro·cy·to·ma [ˌ-saɪˈtəʊmə] n Astrozytom nt, -cytoma nt.
as·tro·cy·to·sis [ˌ-saɪˈtəʊsɪs] n Astrozytose f.
as·trog·li·a [æˈstrɒglɪə, ˌæstrəˈglaɪə] n Astroglia f, Makroglia f.
astroglia cell → astrocyte.
as·tro·ki·net·ic [ˌæstrəʊkɪˈnɛtɪk, -kaɪ-] adj bio., histol. astrokinetisch.
as·tro·ma [əˈstrəʊmə] n old → astrocytoma.
as·tro·sphere [ˈæstrəsfɪər] n Astrophäre f, Aster f.
as·tro·stat·ic [ˌ-ˈstætɪk] adj bio., histol. astrostatisch.
as·tro·vi·rus [ˌ-ˈvaɪrəs] n micro. Astrovirus nt.
Astrup [ˈastrup]: **A. procedure** Astrupmethode f, -verfahren nt.
a·sul·fu·ro·sis [əsʌlf(j)əˈrəʊsɪs] n Schwefelmangelkrankheit f.
ASV abbr. → avian sarcoma virus.

a·syl·la·bia [eɪsɪˈleɪbɪə] n neuro. Unvermögen nt zur Silbenerkennung od. -bildung, Asyllabie f.
a·sym·bo·lia [ˌæsɪmˈbəʊlɪə] n neuro. Asymbolie f.
a·sym·bo·ly [əˈsɪmbəlɪ] n → asymbolia.
a·sym·met·ric [eɪsɪˈmɛtrɪk, æ-] adj → asymmetrical.
a·sym·met·ri·cal [eɪsɪˈmɛtrɪkl] adj ungleichmäßig, unsymmetrisch, asymmetrisch.
asymmetrical chondrodystrophy Ollier'-Erkrankung f, -Syndrom nt, Enchondromatose f, Hemichondrodystrophie f, multiple kongenitale Enchondrome pl.
asymmetrical mitosis asymmetrische Mitose f.
asymmetric tonic neck reflex abbr. **ATNR** asymmetrisch-tonischer Nackenreflex/Halsreflex m abbr. ATNR.
a·sym·me·try [eɪˈsɪmətrɪ, æ-] n Asymmetrie f.
a·symp·to·mat·ic [eɪˌsɪm(p)təˈmætɪk] adj symptomlos, -arm, asymptomatisch.
a·symp·tote [ˈæsɪm(p)təʊt] n mathe. Asymptote f.
a·symp·tot·ic [ˌ-ˈtɑtɪk] adj mathe. asymptotisch.
a·symp·tot·i·cal [ˌ-ˈtɑtɪkl] adj asymptotic.
a·syn·ap·sis [eɪsɪˈnæpsɪs] n bio., genet. Asynapsis f.
a·syn·chro·nism [eɪˈsɪŋkrənɪzəm] n Asynchronie f, Asynchronismus m.
a·syn·chro·nous [eɪˈsɪŋkrənəs] adj nicht gleichzeitig, asynchron, Asynchron- (with mit).
asynchronous culture micro. asynchrone Kultur f.
a·syn·chro·ny [eɪˈsɪŋkrənɪ] n → asynchronism.
a·syn·ech·ia [eɪsɪˈnɛkɪə, æ-] n Asynechie f.
a·syn·er·gia [ˌ-ˈnɜrdʒ(ɪ)ə] n → asynergy.
a·syn·er·gic [ˌ-ˈnɜrdʒɪk] adj Asynergie betr., asynergisch.
a·syn·er·gy [eɪˈsɪnərdʒɪ, æ-] n neuro. Asynergie f.
a·sys·to·le [eɪˈsɪstəlɪ, æ-] n Herzstillstand m, Asystolie f.
a·sys·to·li·a [eɪsɪsˈtəʊlɪə] n → asystole.
a·sys·tol·ic [ˌ-ˈtɑlɪk] adj asystolisch.
At abbr. → astatine.
AT I abbr. → antithrombin I.
AT III abbr. → antithrombin III.
A.T. 10 abbr. → antitetanic factor.
a·tac·tic [əˈtæktɪk] adj 1. ungleichmäßig, unregelmäßig, ungeordnet, unkoordiniert, ataktisch. 2. Ataxie betr., durch Ataxie bedingt, ataktisch, ataxisch.
atactic abasia ataktische Abasie f, Abasia atactica.
atactic agraphia absolute/ataktische Agraphie f, Agraphia atactica.
a·tac·ti·form [əˈtæktɪfɔrm] adj ataxieähnlich.
at·a·rac·tic [ˌætəˈræktɪk] I n pharm. Beruhigungsmittel nt, Ataraktikum nt, Ataraxikum nt. II adj Ataraxie betr. od. bewirkend, beruhigend, ataraktisch.
at·a·rax·ia [ˌ-ˈræksɪə] n Unerschütterlichkeit f, (Seelen)Ruhe f, Ataraxie f.
at·a·rax·ic [ˌ-ˈræksɪk] n, adj → ataractic.
at·a·rax·y [ˈætəræksɪ] n → ataraxia.
a·tav·ic [əˈtævɪk, ˈæt-] adj → atavistic.
a·ta·vism [ˈætəvɪzəm] n bio., genet. Atavismus m.
at·a·vis·tic [ætəˈvɪstɪk] adj Atavismus betr., atavistisch.
a·tax·a·pha·sia [əˌtæksəˈfeɪʒ(ɪ)ə] n → ataxiaphasia.
a·tax·ia [əˈtæksɪə] n neuro. Ataxie f, Ataxia f.

a. of gait Gangataxie, lokomotorische Ataxie.
a·tax·i·a·pha·sia [əˌtæksɪəˈfeɪʒ(ɪ)ə] n neuro. Ataxophasie f.
ataxia-teleangiectasia (syndrome) progressive zerebelläre Ataxie f, Louis--Bar-Syndrom nt, Ataxia-Teleangiectasia f, Teleangiektasie-Ataxie-Syndrom nt, Ataxia teleangiectatica.
a·tax·ic [əˈtæksɪk] adj → atactic 2.
ataxic abasia ataktische Abasie f, Abasia ataxica.
ataxic aphasia neuro. motorische Aphasie f, Broca-Aphasie f.
ataxic gait neuro. ataktischer Gang m.
ataxic nystagmus ataxischer Nystagmus m.
ataxic paraplegia ataktische Paraplegie f.
a·tax·i·o·phe·mia [əˌtæksɪəˈfiːmɪə] n → ataxophemia.
a·tax·i·o·pho·bia [ˌ-ˈfəʊbɪə] n → ataxophobia.
a·tax·o·phe·mia [əˌtæksəˈfiːmɪə] n neuro. Ataxophemie f.
a·tax·o·pho·bia [ˌ-ˈfəʊbɪə] n neuro. Ataxophobie f.
a·tax·y [əˈtæksɪ ˈæ-] n → ataxia.
ATCase n → aspartate transcarbamoylase.
ATD abbr. → asphyxiating thoracic dystrophy.
at·el·ec·ta·sis [ˌætəˈlɛktəsɪs] n 1. Atelektase f. 2. Lungenkollaps m, -atelektase f.
at·e·lec·tat·ic [ˌætlɛkˈtætɪk] adj Atelektase betr., atelektatisch, Atelektasen-.
atelectatic rales Entfaltungsknistern nt, -rasseln nt.
a·te·lia [əˈtiːlɪə] n embryo. Atelie f.
at·e·lo·car·dia [ˌætɪləʊˈkɑːrdɪə] n embryo. Atelocardie f.
at·e·lo·ceph·a·lous [ˌ-ˈsɛfələs] adj embryo. atelokephal, -cephal.
at·e·lo·ceph·a·ly [ˌ-ˈsɛfəlɪ] n embryo. Atelokephalie f, -cephalie f.
at·e·lo·chei·lia [ˌ-ˈkaɪlɪə] n embryo. Ateloch(e)ilie f.
at·e·lo·chei·ria [ˌ-ˈkeɪrɪə] n embryo. Ateloch(e)irie f.
at·e·lo·en·ce·pha·lia [ˌ-ɛnsəˈfeɪlɪə, -lɪə] n embryo. Atel(o)enzephalie f, -enkephalie f.
at·e·lo·glos·si·a [ˌ-ˈglɑsɪə] n embryo. Ateloglossie f.
at·e·lo·gna·thi·a [ˌ-ˈnæθɪə, -ˈneɪθ-] n embryo. Atelognathie f.
at·e·lo·my·e·lia [ˌ-maɪˈiːlɪə] n embryo. Atelomyelie f.
at·e·lo·po·dia [ˌ-ˈpəʊdɪə] n embryo. Atelopodie f.
at·e·lo·pro·so·pia [ˌ-prəˈsəʊpɪə] n embryo. Ateloprosopie f.
at·e·lo·ra·chid·ia [ˌ-rəˈkɪdɪə] n embryo. Atelorachidie f.
At·e·lo·sac·cha·ro·my·ces [ˌ-ˌsækərəʊˈmaɪsiːz] n old → Cryptococcus.
at·e·lo·sto·mia [ˌ-ˈstəʊmɪə] n embryo. Atelostomie f.
a·ten·o·lol [əˈtɛnəlɒl, -lɔl] n pharm. Atenolol nt.
ATG abbr. → antithymocyte globulin.
a·the·lia [əˈθiːlɪə] n embryo. angeborenes Fehlen nt der Brustwarze(n), Athelie f.
a·ther·man·cy [æˈθɜrmənsɪ] n phys. Wärmeundurchlässigkeit f, Athermanität f.
a·ther·ma·nous [æˈθɜrmənəs] adj wärmeundurchlässig, nicht durchlässig für Wärmestrahlen, atherman, adiathermal.
a·ther·mic [eɪˈθɜrmɪk] adj ohne Fieber (verlaufend), fieberlos, afebril.
ath·er·o·em·bo·lism [ˌæθərəʊˈɛmbəlɪzəm] n Atheroembolie f.

ath·er·o·em·bo·lus [ˌ-'embələs] *n, pl* **-li** [-laɪ, -liː] Atheroembolus *m*.
ath·er·o·gen·e·sis [ˌ-'dʒenəsɪs] *n* Atherombildung *f*, Atherogenese *f*.
ath·er·o·gen·ic [ˌ-'dʒenɪk] *adj* atherogen.
ath·er·o·ma [ˌæθə'rəʊmə] *n* (*Gefäß*) Atherom *nt*, atherosklerotische Plaque *f*.
ath·er·o·ma·to·sis [ˌæθərəʊmə'təʊsɪs] *n* Atheromatose *f*, Atherosis *f*.
ath·er·om·a·tous [æθə'rɑmətəs] *adj* Atherom betr., in der Art eines Atheroms, atheromatös.
atheromatous cyst (echtes) Atherom *nt*, Grützbeutel *m*, Epidermoid *nt*.
atheromatous degeneration → atheroma.
atheromatous plaque atheromatöses Beet *nt*.
ath·er·o·scle·ro·sis [ˌæθərəʊsklə'rəʊsɪs] *n* Atherosklerose *f*.
ath·er·o·scle·rot·ic aneurysm ['-sklɪ'rɑtɪk] arteriosklerotisches Aneurysma *nt*.
ath·er·o·sis [æθə'rəʊsɪs] *n old* **1.** → atheromatosis. **2.** → atherosclerosis.
ath·e·toid ['æθətɔɪd] *adj* athetosenähnlich, athetoid.
ath·e·to·sic [ˌ-'təʊsɪk] *adj* → athetotic.
ath·e·to·sis [ˌ-'təʊsɪs] *n neuro.* Athetose *f*.
ath·e·tot·ic [ˌ-'tɑtɪk] *adj* Athetose betr., athetotisch.
a·thi·a·min·o·sis [eɪˌθaɪæmɪ'nəʊsɪs] *n* Thiaminmangel *m*.
ath·lete ['æθliːt] *n* Athlet(in *f*) *m*, Sportler(in *f*) *m*.
athlete's foot Athleten-, Sportlerfuß *m*, Fußpilz *m*, Fußpilzerkrankung *f*, Fußmykose *f*, Tinea *f* der Füße, Tinea pedis/pedum, Epidermophytia pedis/pedum.
ath·let·ic [æθ'letɪk] *adj* athletisch, Sport-.
athletic heart Sport-, Sportlerherz *nt*.
athletic proteinuria Marsch-, Anstrengungsproteinurie *f*, -albuminurie *f*.
ath·let·ics [æθ'letɪks] *pl* Sport *m*; Leichtathletik *f*.
athletic type athletischer Typ *m*, Athletiker *m*.
a·threp·sia [ə'θrepsɪə, eɪ-] *n* Säuglingsdystrophie *f*, Marasmus *m*.
ath·rep·sy ['æθrepsɪ] *n* → athrepsia.
a·thy·mia [ə'θaɪmɪə] *n* Athymie *f*.
a·thym·ism [ə'θaɪmɪzəm] *n* Athymie(syndrom *nt*) *f*.
a·thy·mis·mus [ˌeɪθaɪ'mɪsməs] *n* → athymism.
a·thy·re·a [eɪ'θaɪrɪə] *n* **1.** Fehlen *nt* der Schilddrüse, Athyrie *f*. **2.** Schilddrüsenunterfunktion *f*, Hypothyreose *f*, Hypothyr(e)oidismus *m*.
a·thy·re·o·sis [eɪˌθaɪrɪ'əʊsɪs] *n, pl* **-ses** [-siːz] Athyreose *f*.
a·thy·re·ot·ic [ˌ-'ɑtɪk] *adj* → athyrotic.
a·thy·ria [eɪ'θaɪrɪə] *n* **1.** Athyreose *f*. **2.** Schilddrüsenunterfunktion *f*, Hypothyreose *f*, Hypothyr(e)oidismus *m*.
a·thy·roi·da·tion [eɪˌθaɪrɔɪ'deɪʃn] *n* Schilddrüsenunterfunktion *f*, Hypothyreose *f*, Hypothyr(e)oidismus *m*.
a·thy·roid·ism [eɪ'θaɪrɔɪdɪzəm] *n* → athyria.
a·thy·roi·do·sis [eɪˌθaɪrɔɪ'dəʊsɪs] *n* → athyrosis.
a·thy·ro·sis [ˌeɪθaɪ'rəʊsɪs] *n* Athyreose *f*.
a·thy·rot·ic [ˌ-'rɑtɪk] *adj* Athyreose betr., athyreot.
at·lan·tal [æt'læntl] *adj anat.* Atlas betr., Atlas-.
at·lan·tic [æt'læntɪk] *adj* → atlantal.
atlantic part of vertebral artery Atlasabschnitt *m* der A. vertebralis, Pars atlantica (a. vertebralis).
at·lan·to·ax·i·al [ætˌlæntəʊ'æksɪəl] *adj* Atlas u. Axis betr. *od.* verbindend, atlantoaxial.
atlantoaxial articulation → atlantoaxial joint.
atlantoaxial joint: lateral a. unteres Kopfgelenk *nt*, laterales Atlantoaxialgelenk *nt*, Artic. atlanto-axialis lateralis.
medial/median a. mediales Atlantoaxialgelenk *nt*, Artic. atlanto-axialis mediana.
at·lan·to·ep·i·stroph·ic articulation/joint [ˌ-ˌepɪ'strɑfɪk] → atlantoaxial joint, medial/median.
atlanto-occipital *adj* Atlas u. Hinterhauptsbein betr., atlanto-okzipital, atlanto-occipital.
atlanto-occipital articulation → atlanto-occipital joint.
atlanto-occipital fusion *embryo., patho.* Atlasassimilation *f*.
atlanto-occipital joint oberes Kopfgelenk *nt*, Atlantookzipitalgelenk *nt*, Artic. atlanto-occipitalis.
atlanto-occipital ligament: anterior a. 1. Membrana atlanto-occipitale anterior. **2.** Lig. atlanto-occipitale anterius.
deep a. → posterior a.
lateral a. Lig. atlanto-occipitale laterale.
posterior a. Membrana atlanto-occipitalis posterior.
atlanto-occipital membrane: anterior a. 1. Membrana atlanto-occipitalis anterior. **2.** Lig. atlanto-occipitale anterius.
posterior a. Membrana atlanto-occipitalis posterior.
atlanto-odontoid *adj* Atlas u. Dens axis betr. *od.* verbindend, atlanto-odontoid.
at·las ['ætləs] *n, pl* **-las·es 1.** *anat.* erster Halswirbel *m*, Atlas *m*. **2.** (geografischer) Atlas *m*; (Fach-)Atlas *m*.
atlas fracture *ortho.* Atlasfraktur *f*.
at·lo·ax·oid [ætlə'æksɔɪd] *adj* → atlantoaxial.
at·loid ['ætlɔɪd] *adj* → atlantal.
atloido-occipital *adj* atlanto-occipital.
atm *abbr.* → atmosphere 2.
at·mo·graph ['ætməgræf] *n* Atmograph *m*.
at·mol·y·sis [æt'mɑləsɪs] *n* Atmolyse *f*.
at·mom·e·ter [æt'mɑmɪtər] *n* Verdunstungsmesser *m*, Atmometer *nt*, Atmidometer *nt*.
at·mo·sphere ['ætməsfɪər] *n* **1.** Atmosphäre *f*, Lufthülle *f*, Gashülle *f*; Luft *f*. **2.** *abbr.* (*Druck*) Atmosphäre *f* *abbr.* **atm. 3.** *fig.* Atmosphäre *f*; Umgebung *f*; Stimmung *f*.
at·mo·spher·ic [ˌætmə'sfɪərɪk, -'sferɪk] *adj* Atmosphären *od.* Luft betr., atmosphärisch, Atmosphären-, Luft-, Druck-.
at·mos·pher·i·cal [ˌ-'sfɪərɪkl, ˌ-'sfer-] *adj* → atmospheric.
atmospheric nitrogen *chem.* atmosphärischer Stickstoff *m*.
atmospheric pressure atmosphärischer Druck *m*, Luftdruck *m*.
ATN *abbr.* → acute tubular necrosis.
ATNR *abbr.* → asymmetric tonic neck reflex.
at·om ['ætəm] *n* Atom *nt*.
a·tom·ic [ə'tɑmɪk] *adj* **1.** Atom betr., atomar, Atom-. **2.** *fig.* klein, extrem winzig.
a·tom·i·cal [ə'tɑmɪkl] *adj* → atomic 1.
atomic core Atomkern *m*.
atomic energy *phys.* Atom-, Kernenergie *f*.
atomic mass Atommasse *f*, -gewicht *nt*.
atomic mass unit *abbr.* **amu** Atommasseneinheit *f* *abbr.* AME.
atomic nucleus Atomkern *m*.
atomic number *abbr.* **Z** *chem.* Ordnungszahl *f* *abbr.* Z, OZ.
a·tom·ics [ə'tɑmɪks] *pl* Atomphysik *f*.
atomic volume Atomvolumen *nt*.
atomic waste Atommüll *m*.
atomic weight Atomgewicht *nt*.
atomic weight unit *abbr.* **awu** → atomic mass unit.
at·om·i·za·tion [ˌætəmaɪ'zeɪʃn] *n* Zerstäubung *f*, Zerstäuben *nt*, Atomisierung *f*.
at·om·ize ['ætəmaɪz] *vt* **1.** atomisieren, in Atome auflösen *od.* zerkleinern. **2.** *chem.* atomisieren, zerstäuben.
at·om·iz·er ['ætəmaɪzər] *n* Zerstäuber *m*.
atom theory *phys., chem.* Atomtheorie *f*.
a·to·nia [ə'təʊnɪə, eɪ-] *n* → atony.
a·ton·ic [ə'tɑnɪk, eɪ-] *adj* atonisch; schlaff, kraftlos, abgespannt.
atonic astatic diplegia *neuro.* atonisch-astatische Diplegie *f*.
atonic bladder atonische Blase *f*, (Harn-)Blasenatonie *f*.
atonic dyspepsia atonische Dyspepsie *f*.
atonic ectropion *ophthal.* Ektropium paralyticum.
atonic epilepsy atonische Epilepsie *f*.
at·o·nic·i·ty [ætə'nɪsətɪ] *n* **1.** Atonizität *f*. **2.** → atony.
atonic neurogenic bladder neurogene atonische Blase *f*.
atonic pseudoparalysis, congenital Oppenheim-Krankheit *f*, -Syndrom *nt*, Myotonia congenita.
at·o·ny ['ætnɪ] *n* Schwäche *f*, Schlaffheit *f*, Erschlaffung *f*, Tonusmangel *m*, Atonie *f*.
at·o·pen ['ætəpən, -pen] *n* Atopen *nt*.
a·top·ic [eɪ'tɑpɪk, ə-] *adj* **1.** Atopen *od.* Atopie betr., atopisch. **2.** ursprungsfern, an atypischer Stelle liegend *od.* entstehend, (nach außen) verlagert, heterotopisch, ektop(isch). **3.** Ektopie betr., ektopisch.
atopic allergy atopische Allergie *f*.
atopic asthma konstitutionsallergisches (Bronchial-)Asthma *nt*.
atopic cataract *ophthal.* Katarakt *f* bei atopischer Dermatitis.
atopic conjunctivitis allergische/atopische Konjunktivitis *f*, Conjunctivitis allergica; Heuschnupfen *m*, -fieber *nt*.
atopic dermatitis atopische Dermatitis *f*, atopisches/endogenes/exsudatives/neuropathisches/konstitutionelles Ekzem *nt*, Prurigo Besnier, Morbus Besnier, Ekzemkrankheit *f*, neurogene Dermatose *f*.
atopic disease/disorder Atopie *f*.
atopic eczema → atopic dermatitis.
atopic reagin 1. Prausnitz-Küstner-Antikörper *pl*, P-K-Antikörper *pl*. **2.** Reagin *nt*, IgE-Antikörper *m*.
atopic rhinitis perenniale (allergische) Rhinitis *f*.
a·top·og·no·sia [eɪˌtɑpəg'nəʊʒ(ɪ)ə] *n* neuro. Atopognosie *f*.
a·top·og·no·sis [ˌ-'nəʊsɪs] *n* → atopognosia.
at·o·py ['ætəpɪ] *n* **1.** Atopie *f*. **2.** atopische Allergie *f*.
a·tox·ic [eɪ'tɑksɪk] *adj* **1.** ungiftig, nicht-giftig, atoxisch. **2.** nicht durch Gift verursacht.
a·tox·i·gen·ic [eɪˌtɑksə'dʒenɪk] *adj* nicht-toxinbildend.
ATP *abbr.* → adenosine(-5'-)triphosphate.
ATP-ADP carrier ATP-ADP-Carrier *m*.
ATP-ADP cycle ATP-Zyklus *m*.
ATPase *n* Adenosintriphosphatase *f*, ATPase *f*.
ATPase activity ATPase-Aktivität *f*.
ATP-citrate lyase ATP-Citrat-Lyase *f*, citratspaltendes Enzym *nt*.
ATP cycle ATP-Zyklus *m*.
ATP-dependent *adj* ATP-abhängig.
ATP-driven *adj* ATP-getrieben.
ATP-generating *adj* ATP-bildend.

ATP-linked *adj* ATP-gebunden, -abhängig.
ATP-phosphoribosyltransferase ATP--Phosphoribosyltransferase *f.*
ATPS conditions [ambient temperature and pressure, saturated] *physiol.* ATPS--Bedingungen *pl.*
ATP-utilizing *adj* ATP-verbrauchend.
a·trac·tyl·o·side [əˌtræk'tɪləsaɪd] *n* Atractylosid *nt.*
a·trans·fer·ri·ne·mia [eɪˌtrænzferɪ'niːmɪə] *n* Transferrinmangel *m*, Atransferrinämie *f.*
a·trau·mat·ic [eɪtrɔː'mætɪk, -trə-] *adj chir.* nicht-gewebeschädigend, atraumatisch.
atraumatic clamp *chir.* atraumatische Klemme *f.*
atraumatic needle *chir.* atraumatische Nadel *f.*
atraumatic suture atraumatisches Nahtmaterial *nt*, atraumatische Naht *f.*
a·trep·sy [ə'træpsɪ] *n* Säuglingsdystrophie *f*, Marasmus *m.*
a·tre·sia [ə'triːʒ(ɪ)ə] *n* **1.** Fehlen *nt od.* Verschluß *m* einer natürlichen Körperöffnung, Atresie *f*, Atresia *f.* **2.** Involution *f*, Rückbildung(sprozeß *m*) *f.*
 a. of extrahepatic bile ducts Atresie der extrahepatischen Gallenwege.
a·tre·sic [ə'triːzɪk, -sɪk] *adj* → atretic.
a·tret·ic [ə'tretɪk] *adj* Atresie betr., uneröffnet, geschlossen, geschlossen, atretisch.
atretic follicle atretischer Ovarialfollikel *m.*
a·tre·to·ble·pha·ria [əˌtriːtəʊble'færɪə] *n ophthal.* Symblepharon *nt.*
a·tre·to·cys·tia [ˌ-'sɪstɪə] *n* (*Harn*) Blasenatresie *f*, Atretozystie *f.*
a·tre·to·gas·tria [ˌ-'gæstrɪə] *n* Magenatresie *f*, Atretogastrie *f.*
a·tre·to·me·tria [ˌ-'miːtrɪə] *n* Gebärmutter-, Uterusatresie *f*, Atresia uteri, Atretometrie *f.*
a·tre·top·sia [ˌætrɪ'tɑpsɪə] *n* Pupillenatresie *f*, Atresia iridis/pupillae, Atretopsie *f.*
a·tre·tor·rhin·ia [əˌtriːtəʊ'rɪnɪə] *n* Nasen-(gangs)atresie *f*, Atretorrhinie *f.*
a·tre·to·sto·mia [ˌ-'stəʊmɪə] *n* Atresie *f* der Mundöffnung, Atretostomie *f.*
a·tret·u·re·thria [əˌtretjʊə'riːθrɪə] *n* Harnröhren-, Urethraatresie *f*, Atresia urethrae, Atreturethrie *f.*
atri- *pref.* → atrio-.
a·tri·al ['eɪtrɪəl] *adj* Vorhof/Atrium betr., atrial, aurikulär, Vorhof-, Atrio-.
atrial anastomotic artery → anastomotic atrial artery.
atrial appendage (of heart) Herzohr *nt*, Aurikel *nt*, Auricula atrialis.
atrial arrhythmia *card.* Vorhofarrhythmie *f*, atriale Arrhythmie *f.*
atrial artery: left intermediate a. Ramus atrialis intermedius a. coronariae sinistrae.
 right intermediate a. Ramus atrialis intermedius a. coronariae dextrae.
atrial auricle Herzohr *nt*, Auricula atrialis.
atrial auricula → atrial auricle.
atrial beat *card.* Vorhofsystole *f.*
atrial bigeminy *card.* Vorhofbigeminie *f.*
atrial branch: intermediate a. of left coronary artery Ramus atrialis intermedius a. coronariae sinistrae.
 intermediate a. of right coronary artery Ramus atrialis intermedius a. coronariae dextrae.
 a.es of left coronary artery Vorhofäste *pl* der A. coronaria sinistra, Rami atriales a. coronariae sinistrae.
 a.es of right coronary artery Vorhofäste *pl* der A. coronaria dextra, Rami atriales a. coronariae dextrae.
atrial complex *card.* (*EKG*) Vorhofkomplex *m*, P-Welle *f*, P-Zacke *f.*
atrial conduction *card.* intra-atriale Erregungsleitung/Erregungsausbreitung *f.*
atrial contraction Vorhofkontraktion *f.*
 premature a. *abbr.* **PAC** → atrial extrasystole.
atrial diastole Vorhofdiastole *f.*
atrial dissociation *card.* Vorhofdissoziation *f.*
atrial excitation Vorhoferregung *f.*
atrial extrasystole *card.* Vorhofextrasystole *f*, atriale Extrasystole *f.*
atrial fibrillation *card.* Vorhofflimmern *nt*, Delirium cordis.
atrial filling pressure *card.* Vorhoffüllungsdruck *m.*
atrial flutter *card.* Vorhofflattern *nt.*
atrial gallop *abbr.* **AG** *card.* Atrial-, Aurikular-, Vorhofgalopp(rhythmus *m*) *m*, präsystolischer Galopp(rhythmus *m*) *m.*
atrial natriuretic factor *abbr.* **ANF** atrialer natriuretischer Faktor *m abbr.* **ANF**, Atriopeptid *nt*, -peptin *nt.*
atrial natriuretic hormone → atrial natriuretic factor.
atrial natriuretic peptide → atrial natriuretic factor.
atrial premature contraction *abbr.* **APC** *card.* Vorhofextrasystole *f*, atriale Extrasystole *f.*
atrial receptors Vorhofrezeptoren *pl.*
atrial septal defect *abbr.* **ASD** Vorhofseptumdefekt *m*, Atriumseptumdefekt *m abbr.* ASD.
atrial sound Vorhofton *m*, vierter Herzton *m.*
atrial standstill *card.* Vorhofstillstand *m.*
atrial systole *card.* Vorhofsystole *f.*
atrial tachycardia Vorhoftachykardie *f*, atriale Tachykardie *f.*
atrial vein: lateral a. V. lateralis atrii ventriculi lateralis.
 medial a. V. medialis atrii ventriculi lateralis.
atrial veins Vorhofvenen *pl*, Venenäste *pl* der Vorhofwand, Vv. atriales (cordis).
 left a. Vv. atriales sinistrae.
 right a. Vv. atriales dextrae.
a·trich·ia [ə'trɪkɪə] *n* Haarlosigkeit *f*, Fehlen *nt* der Haare, Atrichie *f*, Atrichia *f.*
at·ri·cho·sis [ætrɪ'kəʊsɪs] *n* → atrichia.
at·ri·chous ['ætrɪkəs] *adj* **1.** *micro.* geißellos, atrich. **2.** ohne Haare, haarlos.
atrio- *pref.* Vorhof-, Atrio-.
a·trio·com·mis·su·ro·pex·y [ˌeɪtrɪəʊˌkɑməˈʃʊərəpeksɪ] *n HTG* Atriokommissuropexie *f.*
a·tri·o·dig·i·tal dysplasia [ˌ-'dɪdʒɪtl] Holt--Oram-Syndrom *nt.*
a·tri·o·meg·a·ly [ˌ-'megəlɪ] *n card.* Vorhofdilatation *f*, Atriomegalie *f.*
at·ri·o·nec·tor [ˌ-'nektər] *n* Sinus-, Sinuatrialknoten *m*, SA-Knoten *m*, Keith--Flack'Knoten *m*, Nodus sinuatrialis.
a·tri·o·pep·tide [ˌ-'peptaɪd] *n* → atrial natriuretic factor.
a·tri·o·pep·ti·gen [ˌ-'peptɪdʒən] *n* Atriopeptigen *n.*
a·tri·o·pep·tin [ˌ-'peptɪn] *n* → atrial natriuretic factor.
a·tri·o·sep·tal defect [ˌ-'septəl] → atrial septal defect.
a·tri·o·sep·tos·to·my [ˌ-sep'tɑstəmɪ] *n HTG* Atrioseptostomie *f.*
a·tri·o·sep·to·pex·y [ˌ-'septəʊpeksɪ] *n HTG* Atrioseptopexie *f.*
a·tri·o·sep·to·plas·ty [ˌ-ˌseptəʊ'plæstɪ] *n HTG* Vorhofseptumplastik *f*, Atrioseptoplastik *f.*

a·tri·o·sys·tol·ic murmur [ˌ-sɪs'tɑlɪk] präsystolisches/spät-diastolisches (Herz-)-Geräusch *nt.*
a·tri·ot·o·my [eɪtrɪ'ɑtəmɪ] *n HTG* Vorhoferöffnung *f*, Atriotomie *f.*
a·tri·o·ven·tric·u·lar [ˌeɪtrɪəʊven'trɪkjələr] *adj abbr.* **AV, A-V, av** Vorhof/Atrium u. Kammer/Ventrikel betr. *od.* verbindend, atrioventrikulär. AV, atrioventrikulär, Atrioventrikular-.
atrioventricular band → atrioventricular bundle.
atrioventricular block atrioventrikulärer Block *m*, AV-Block *m.*
 complete a. kompletter/totaler AV--Block, AV-Block III. Grades.
 first degree a. AV-Block I. Grades.
 incomplete a. partieller AV-Block, AV--Block II. Grades.
 partial a. → incomplete a.
 second degree a. → incomplete a.
 third degree a. → complete a.
atrioventricular branches of left coronary artery Vorhof-Kammer-Äste *pl* der A. coronaria sinistra, Rami atrioventriculares a. coronariae sinistrae.
atrioventricular bundle His'-Bündel *nt*, Fasciculus atrioventricularis.
atrioventricular canal *embryo.* Atrioventrikularkanal *m*, AV-Kanal *m.*
 persistent a. persistierender Atrioventrikularkanal/AV-Kanal.
atrioventricular conduction atrioventrikuläre (Erregungs-)Überleitung *f.*
atrioventricular cushion → atrioventricular endocardial cushion.
atrioventricular dissociation *card.* atrioventrikuläre Dissoziation *f.*
atrioventricular endocardial cushion *embryo.* Atrioventrikularkissen *nt.*
atrioventricular extrasystole *card.* nodale Extrasystole *f*, Extrasystole *f* mit Ursprung im AV-Knoten.
atrioventricular groove (Herz-)Kranzfurche *f*, Sulcus coronarius (cordis).
atrioventricular heart block atrioventrikulärer Block *m*, AV-Block *m.*
atrioventricular interval *card.* PQ-Intervall *nt.*
atrioventricular junction *embryo.* atrioventrikulärer Übergang *m.*
atrioventricular nodal artery Ast *m* der rechten *od.* linken Kranzarterie zum AV-Knoten, Ramus nodi atrioventricularis a. coronariae dextrae/sinistrae.
atrioventricular nodal bigeminy *card.* Knotenbigeminie *f.*
atrioventricular nodal rhythm *physiol.* Knotenrhythmus *m*, AV-Rhythmus *m.*
atrioventricular nodal tachycardia AV--Knoten-Tachykardie *f.*
atrioventricular node AV-Knoten *m*, Aschoff--Tawara'-Knoten *m*, Nodus atrioventricularis.
atrioventricular opening (of heart) Vorhof-Kammer-Öffnung *f*, Ostium atrioventriculare.
 left a. Ostium atrioventriculare sinistrum.
 right a. Ostium atrioventriculare dextrum.
atrioventricular rhythm *physiol.* AV--Rhythmus *m*, Knotenrhythmus *m.*
atrioventricular septum (of heart) (*Herz*) Vorhofkammerseptum *nt*, Septum atrioventriculare (cordis).
atrioventricular sulcus → atrioventricular groove.
atrioventricular trunk His'-Bündel *nt*, Fasciculus atrioventricularis.
atrioventricular valve Atrioventrikular-,

Segelklappe *f*, Vorhof-Kammerklappe *f*, Valva atrioventricularis.
left a. Mitralklappe, Mitralis *f*, Bicuspidalis *f*, Valva mitralis, Valvula bicuspidalis, Valva atrioventricularis sinistra.
right a. Trikuspidalklappe, Tricuspidalis *f*, Valva/Valvula tricuspidalis, Valva atrioventricularis dextra.
atrioventricular veins Atrioventrikularvenen *pl*, Vv. atrioventriculares.
a·tri·um ['eɪtrɪəm] *n*, *pl* **-tri·ums, -tria** [-trɪə] 1. *anat.* Vorhof *m*, Atrium *nt*. 2. (Herz-)Vorhof *m*, Kammervorhof *m*, Atrium cordis.
a. of glottis/larynx Kehlkopfvorhof *m*, oberer Kehlkopfinnenraum *m*, Vestibulum laryngis.
a·troph·e·de·ma [ˌətrəʊfɪ'diːmə] *n* angioneurotisches Ödem *nt*, Quincke-Ödem *nt*.
a·tro·phia [ə'trəʊfɪə] *n* → atrophy I.
a·troph·ic [ə'trəʊfɪk, -'trɒf-] *adj* Atrophie betr., von ihr betroffen, durch sie verursacht, atrophisch.
atrophic arthritis 1. atrophische Arthritis *f*. 2. rheumatoide Arthritis *f*, progrediente/primär chronische Polyarthritis *f* *abbr.* PCP, PcP.
atrophic beriberi trockene Form *f* der Beriberi, paralytische Beriberi *f*.
atrophic bronchitis atrophische Bronchitis *f*.
atrophic cirrhosis atrophische Leberzirrhose *f*.
atrophic fracture Spontanfraktur *f* bei Knochenatrophie.
atrophic gastritis chronisch-atrophische Gastritis *f*.
atrophic glossitis (Möller-)Hunter'-Glossitis *f*, atrophische Glossitis *f*.
atrophic-hyperplastic gastritis atrophisch-hyperplastische Gastritis *f*.
atrophic inflammation atrophische/fibroide Entzündung *f*.
atrophic kidney atrophische Niere *f*.
atrophic lung of old age Altersemphysem *nt*, atrophische Alterslunge *f*.
atrophic parapsoriasis *derm.* großherdig--entzündliche Form *f* der Parapsoriasis en plaques, prämaligne Form *f* der Parapsoriasis en plaques, Parapsoriasis en plaques simples.
atrophic pharyngitis Pharyngitis chronica atrophicans.
atrophic rhinitis atrophische Rhinitis *f*, Rhinitis atrophicans.
atrophic senile gingivitis atrophisch-senile Gingivitis *f*.
atrophic spinal paralysis (epidemische/spinale) Kinderlähmung *f*, Heine-Medin--Krankheit *f*, Poliomyelitis (epidemica) anterior acuta.
at·ro·phied ['ætrəfɪːd] *adj* 1. geschrumpft, verkümmert, atrophiert. 2. ausgemergelt, abgezehrt.
at·ro·pho·der·ma [ˌætrəfəʊ'dɜːmə] *n* *derm.* Hautatrophie *f*, Atrophoderma *nt*, -dermia *f*.
a. of Pasini and Pierini Atrophodermia idiopathica Pasini-Pierini.
at·ro·pho·der·ma·to·sis [-ˌdɜːmə'təʊsɪs] *n* Atrophodermatose *f*.
at·ro·pho·der·mia [ˌ-'dɜːmɪə] *n* → atrophoderma.
at·ro·phy ['ætrəfɪ] I *n* Schwund *m*, Rückbildung *f*, Verkümmerung *f*, Atrophie *f*, Atrophia *f*. II *vt* schwinden od. schrumpfen od. atrophieren lassen. atrophieren; aus-, abzehren. III *vi* schwinden, verkümmern, schrumpfen, atrophieren.
a. of the pituitary (gland) Hypophysenatrophie.

'**at·ro·pine** ['ætrəpiːn, -pɪn] *n* *pharm.* Atropin *nt*.
at·ro·pin·ic [ˌ-'pɪnɪk] *adj* atropinartig.
at·ro·pin·ism ['-pɪnɪzəm] *n* Atropinvergiftung *f*.
at·ro·pin·i·za·tion [ˌ-pɪnɪ'zeɪʃn] *n* Behandlung *f* mit Atropin, Atropinisierung *f*.
at·ro·pism ['-pɪzəm] *n* → atropinism.
A.T.S. *abbr.* → antitetanic serum.
at·tach [ə'tætʃ] I *vt* 1. festmachen, befestigen, anheften (*to* an); verbinden (*to* mit); beifügen (*to*); anhaften, verbunden sein (*to* mit). 2. *anat.* (*Muskel*) ansetzen. II *vi* verbunden sein (*to* mit).
at·tached [ə'tætʃt] *adj* 1. verbunden (*to* mit); befestigt (*to* an); festgewachsen. 2. *bio.* festsitzend.
attached craniotomy *neurochir.* osteoplastische Schädeltrepanation/Kraniotomie *f*.
attached denticle adhärenter Dentikel *m*.
attached gingiva Periodontium protectoris, Gingiva *f*.
at·tach·ment [ə'tætʃmənt] *n* 1. Befestigung *f*, Anheftung *f*; Befestigen *nt*, Festmachen *nt*. 2. *anat.* Verbindung *f*; Ansatz *m*, Ansatzstelle *f*, -punkt *m*. 3. *micro.* Adhärenz *f*, Adhäsion *f*, Adsorption *f*. 4. *techn.* Zusatzgerät *nt*, ~**s** *pl* Zubehörteile *pl*.
attachment site *anat.* Ansatzstelle *f*, -punkt *m*.
at·tack [ə'tæk] I *n* 1. Attacke *f*, Anfall *m*. **to avert an ~** einen Anfall vorbeugen, einen Anfall verhüten. 2. *fig.* Angriff *m*, Attakke *f*, (scharfe) Kritik *f*. 3. *chem.* Angriff *m*, Einwirkung *f* (*on* auf). II *vt* 4. angreifen, anfallen, herfallen (*on* über), attakkieren. 5. (*Krankheit*) befallen; *chem.* angreifen. III *vi* angreifen, attackieren.
a. of asthma Asthmaanfall *m*.
a. of nerves Nervenkrise *f*.
at·tain [ə'teɪn] *vt* erreichen, erlangen, erzielen, gelangen zu.
at·tain·ment [ə'teɪnmənt] *n* Erreichen *nt*, Erlangen *nt*; Erlangung *f*; Errungenschaft *f*, (das) Erreichte.
at·tempt [ə'tempt] I *n* Versuch *m* (*to do/doing sth.*) II *vt* versuchen, den Versuch wagen, s. wagen an (*to do/doing sth.*). **to make an ~ to do/doing sth.** versuchen, etw. zu tun.
at·tend [ə'tend] I *vt* 1. pflegen, versorgen; s. kümmern (*to*) um; ärztlich behandeln. **to ~ (on) a patient** einen Kranken behandeln. **the ~ing doctor** der zuständige/behandelnde Arzt. 2. **to be ~ed by/with** einhergehen mit, begleitet von; zur Folge haben, nach s. ziehen. 3. anwesend sein, teilnehmen an; besuchen. II *vi* 4. s. kümmern (*to* um). 5. anwesend sein, teilnehmen an (*at* bei). **to ~ at a birth** bei einer Geburt anwesend sein. **to ~ a lecture** an einer Vorlesung teilnehmen.
at·tend·ance [ə'tendəns] *n* 1. Dienst *m*, Bereitschaft *f*. **a doctor in ~** diensthabender Arzt. 2. Pflege *f*, Versorgung *f*; (ärztliche) Behandlung *f*. **medical ~** ärztliche Behandlung *f*. 3. Anwesenheit *f*, Erscheinen *nt*; Besuch *m* (*beim Arzt*).
at·tend·ant [ə'tendənt] I *n* 1. Begleiterscheinung *f*, Folge *f* (*of*, *on*, *upon*). 2. Aufseher(in *f*) *m*, Wärter(in *f*) *m*. II *adj* 3. verbunden mit, (da-)zugehörig, begleitend; Begleit-. 4. anwesend sein; im Dienst, diensthabend.
at·tend·er [ə'tendər] *n* Besucher(in *f*) *m*.
at·ten·tion [ə'tenʃn] *n* 1. Aufmerksamkeit *f*, selektives Bewußtsein *nt*. **to receive ~** Beachtung finden. 2. (medizinische) Behandlung *od.* Versorgung *od.* Betreuung *f*. **under medical ~** in ärztlicher Behandlung *od.* Versorgung *od.* Betreuung *f*. **to seek medical ~** s. in ärztliche Behandlung begeben.
attention-deficit hyperactivity disorder hyperkinetisches Syndrom *nt* des Kindesalters.
at·ten·u·ant [ə'tenjəwənt] I *n* 1. Verdünnungsmittel *nt*, Verdünner *m*. 2. blutverdünnendes Mittel *nt*. 3. *micro.* attenuierendes Agens *nt*. II *adj* verdünnend, attenuierend.
at·ten·u·ate [*adj* ə'tenjəwɪt; *v* -eɪt] I *adj* 1. verdünnt, vermindert, (ab-)geschwächt, attenuiert. 2. (*Person*) dünn, mager. II *vt* 3. *micro.* (*Virulenz*) vermindern, abschwächen, attenuieren. 4. *chem.* verdünnen; *phys.* dämpfen, herunterregeln, herabsetzen. 5. dünn *od.* schlank machen. III *vi* dünner *od.* schwächer *od.* milder werden.
at·ten·u·at·ed culture [ə'tenjəweɪtɪd] *micro.* attenuierte Kultur *f*.
attenuated vaccine attenuierte Vakzine *f*.
attenuated virus attenuiertes Virus *nt*.
at·ten·u·a·tion [əˌtenjə'weɪʃn] *n* 1. Verdünnen *nt*, Abschwächen *nt*, Vermindern *nt*. 2. *micro.* Attenuierung *f*. 3. *phys.* Dämpfung *f*. 4. (*Person*) Auszehrung *f*, Abmagerung *f*.
at·tic ['ætɪk] *n* *anat.* Kuppelraum *m*, Attikus *m*, Epitympanum *nt*, *Rec.* epitympanicus.
a. of middle ear → attic.
at·ti·ci·tis [ˌætɪ'kaɪtɪs] *n* *HNO* Kuppelraumentzündung *f*, Attizitis *f*.
at·ti·co·an·trot·o·my [ˌætɪkəʊæn'trɒtəmɪ] *n* *HNO* Attik(o)antrotomie *f*, Antroattikotomie *f*.
at·ti·cot·o·my [ˌætɪ'kɒtəmɪ] *n* *HNO* Attikotomie *f*.
at·ti·tude ['ætɪt(j)uːd] *n* 1. (Körper-)Haltung *f*, Stellung *f*. 2. (innere) Haltung *f*; Verhalten *nt*; Einstellung *f*, Standpunkt *m*, Position *f* (*to*, *towards* zu, gegenüber).
at·ti·tu·di·nal reflex [ˌætɪ't(j)uːdɪnl] *physiol.* Stellreflex *m*.
atto- *pref. abbr.* **a** Atto- *abbr.* a.
at·tract [ə'trækt] I *vt* 1. *phys.* anziehen. 2. *fig.* anziehen, anlocken, ansprechen. II *vi* Anziehung(skraft) ausüben.
at·tract·ant [ə'træktənt] *n* Lockstoff *m*, Attraktant *m*.
at·trac·tion [ə'trækʃn] *n* *phys.*, *fig.* Anziehung(skraft *f*) *f*, Attraktion *f*.
a. of affinity chemische Anziehung.
a. of gravity Gravitations-, Schwer-, Anziehungskraft.
attraction sphere Zentroplasma *nt*, Zentrosphäre *f*.
at·trac·tive [ə'træktɪv] *adj* *phys.*, *fig.* anziehend, Anziehungs-.
attractive agent → attractant.
attractive force *phys.* Anziehungskraft *f*.
attractive power → attractive force.
attractive substance → attractant.
at·trib·ute [*n* 'ætrɪbjuːt; *v* ə'trɪbjuːt, -jət] *n* Eigenschaft *f*, Merkmal *nt*, Attribut *nt*. II *vt* zuschreiben, zurückführen (*to* auf).
at·tri·bu·tion [ˌætrə'bjuːʃn] *n* Zuschreibung *f* (*to* zu).
at·trite [ə'traɪt] I *adj* abgenutzt. II *vt* abnutzen, abreiben, verschleißen.
at·trit·ed [ə'traɪtɪd] *adj* → attrite I.
at·tri·tion [ə'trɪʃn] *n* Abrieb *m*, Reibung *f*; (physiologische) Abnutzung *f*, Abreibung *f*, Verschleiß *m*.
a·typ·ia [eɪ'tɪpɪə] *n* (*Krankheitsverlauf*) Regelosigkeit *f*, Atypie *f*.
a·typ·ic [eɪ'tɪpɪk] *adj* → atypical.
a·typ·i·cal [eɪ'tɪpɪkl] *adj* atypisch, untypisch (*for*, *of* für).
atypical achromatopsy → atypical monochromasy.

atypical behavior untypisches od. atypisches Verhalten nt.
atypical bronchopneumonia → atypical pneumonia.
atypical coloboma atypisches Kolobom nt.
atypical facial neuralgia → atypical trigeminal neuralgia.
atypical fibroxanthoma atypisches Fibroxanthom nt, paradoxes Fibrosarkom nt, pseudosarkomatöses Xanthofibrom nt.
atypical hyperplasia atypische Hyperplasie f.
atypical monochromasy atypische/inkomplette Farbenblindheit f.
atypical mycobacteria micro. atypische/nicht-tuberkulöse Mykobakterien pl.
atypical phenylketonuria atypische Phenylketonurie f, Dihydrobiopterinreduktasemangel m, Hyperphenylalaninämie Typ V f.
atypical pneumonia atypische/primär--atypische Pneumonie f.
atypical trigeminal neuralgia atypische Trigeminusneuralgie f.
atypical tuberculosis Mykobakteriose f.
atypical verrucous endocarditis atypische verruköse Endokarditis f, Libman--Sacks-Syndrom nt, Endokarditis--Libman-Sacks, Endocarditis thrombotica.
a·typ·ism [eɪ'taɪpɪzəm] n → atypia.
A.U. abbr. → Angström unit.
Au abbr. 1. → aurum 2. → Australia antigen.
Au antigen → Australia antigen.
audi- pref. → audio-.
au·di·bil·i·ty [ˌɔːdɪ'bɪlətɪ] n Hörbarkeit f, Vernehmbarkeit f.
au·di·ble ['ɔːdɪbl] adj hörbar, vernehmbar, vernehmlich (to für).
au·di·ble·ness ['ɔːdɪblnɪs] n → audibility.
au·di·mu·tism [ɔːdɪ'mjuːtɪzəm] n (motorische) Hörstummheit f, Audimutitas f, fehlende od. verzögerte Sprachentwicklung f.
audio- pref. Gehör-, Hör-, Audi(o)-.
au·di·o·an·al·ge·sia [ˌɔːdɪəʊˌænl'dʒiːzɪə, -ʒə] n Audioanalgesie f.
au·di·o·gen·ic [ˌ-'dʒenɪk] adj 1. durch Schall/Töne verursacht od. ausgelöst, audiogen. 2. laut-, schallbildend.
au·di·o·gram ['-græm] n Audiogramm nt.
au·di·ol·o·gist [ɔːdɪ'ɒlədʒɪst] n Audiologe m, -login f.
au·di·ol·o·gy [ˌ-'ɒlədʒɪ] n Audiologie f.
au·di·om·e·ter [ˌ-'ɒmɪtər] n Audiometer nt.
au·di·o·met·ric [ˌɔːdɪə'metrɪk] adj Audiometer od. Audiometrie betr., mittels Audiometer, audiometrisch.
au·di·om·e·try [ɔːdɪ'ɒmətrɪ] n Audiometrie f.
au·di·o·vis·u·al [ˌɔːdɪə'vɪʒwəl, -ʒʊəl] adj Hören u. Sehen betr., audiovisuell.
au·dit ['ɔːdɪt] n (Über-)Prüfung f, Bilanz f, Revision f, Rechenschaft(slegung f) f; Analyse f.
au·di·tion [ɔː'dɪʃn] n Hörvermögen nt, Hörkraft f; Gehör nt; Hören nt.
au·di·tive ['ɔːdɪtɪv] adj → auditory.
au·di·to·ry ['ɔːdɪt(ə)rɪ, -təʊ-, -tɔː-] adj Gehör od. Hören betr., auditiv, Gehör-, Hör-.
auditory agnosia Seelentaubheit f, psychogene/sensorische Hörstummheit f, akustische Agnosie f.
auditory amnesia → auditory aphasia.
auditory aphasia Worttaubheit f, akustische Aphasie f.
auditory area Area vestibularis.
 inferior a. Area vestibularis inferior.
 superior a. Area vestibularis superior.
auditory artery, internal 1. A. labyrinthi,

Ramus meatus acustici interni a. basilaris. 2. A. labyrinthina.
auditory aura akustische Aura f.
auditory canal Gehörgang m, Meatus acusticus.
 external a. äußerer Gehörgang, Meatus acusticus externus.
 internal a. innerer Gehörgang, Meatus acusticus internus.
auditory cells akustische Haarzellen pl.
auditory center Hörzentrum nt.
auditory cortex Hörrinde f, akustischer Cortex m.
autitory defect Hörstörung f, -defekt m.
auditory dysesthesia akustische Überempfindlichkeit f, Dysakusis f, auditorische/akustische Dysästhesie f.
auditory evoked potential abbr. AEP akustisch evoziertes Potential nt abbr. AEP.
auditory fatique HNO Hörermüdung f.
auditory field Hörfeld nt.
 primary a. primäres Hörfeld.
 secondary a. sekundäres Hörfeld.
auditory foramen: external a. äußerer Gehörgang m, Meatus acusticus externus.
 internal a. innerer Gehörgang m, Meatus acusticus internus.
auditory ganglion Ggl. spirale cochlearis.
auditory haircells akustische Haarzellen pl.
auditory hallucination akustische Halluzination f.
auditory hyperesthesia HNO, psychia. Hyperakusis f.
auditory hyp(o)esthesia HNO Hörschwäche f, Hyp(o)akusis f.
auditory lemniscus Lemniscus lateralis.
auditory meatus: external a. äußerer Gehörgang m, Meatus acusticus externus.
 internal a. innerer Gehörgang m, Meatus acusticus internus.
auditory nerve Akustikus m, Vestibulokochlearis m, VIII. Hirnnerv m, N. acusticus/vestibulocochlearis.
auditory nucleus, large-cell Deiters'-Kern m, Nc. vestibularis lateralis.
auditory ossicles Gehörknöchelchen pl, Ossicula auditus/auditoria.
auditory pathway Hörbahn f.
auditory pit embryo. Ohrgrübchen nt.
auditory placode embryo. Ohrplakode f.
auditory radiation Hörstrahlung f, Radiatio acustica.
auditory saucer embryo. → auditory placode.
auditory sensation Hörempfindung f.
auditory striae Striae medullares ventriculi quarti.
auditory teeth of Huschke Dentes acustici.
auditory threshold Hör(barkeits)schwelle f.
auditory training Hörtraining nt.
auditory triangle Area vestibularis.
auditory tube Ohrtrompete f, Eustach'-Kanal m, -Röhre f, Tuba auditiva/auditoria.
auditory tubercle Tuberculum acusticum.
auditory veins, internal 1. Labyrinthvenen pl, Vv. labyrinthi. 2. Vv. labyrinthinae.
auditory vertigo Ménière'-Krankheit f, Morbus Ménière.
auditory vesicle embryo. Ohrbläschen nt.
Auenbrugger [aʊən'brʊgər]: **A.'s sign** Augenbrugger-Zeichen nt.
Auer ['aʊər]: **A.'s bodies** hema. Auer-Stäbchen pl.
Auerbach ['aʊərbak]: **A.'s ganglia** Ganglien pl der Auerbach'-Plexus.
 A.'s plexus Auerbach'-Plexus m, Plexus myentericus.
aug·ment [ɒg'ment] **I** vt vermehren, ver-

größern, verstärken, steigern. **II** vi s. vermehren, zunehmen, (an-)wachsen.
aug·men·ta·tion [ˌɒgmen'teɪʃn] n Vergrößerung f, -mehrung f, -stärkung f, Wachstum nt, Zunahme f; Zuwachs m.
augmentation factor Wachstumsfaktor m.
aug·men·ta·tive [ɒg'mentətɪv] adj vermehrend, -stärkend, Verstärkungs-.
aug·ment·ed histamine test [ɒg'mentɪd] lab. Histamintest m.
Aujeszky [ɔː'dʒeski:]: **A.'s disease** Pseudowut f, -lyssa f, -rabies f, Aujeszky'--Krankheit f.
 A.'s disease virus Pseudowut-Virus nt.
 A.'s itch → A.'s disease.
au·ra ['ɔːrə] n, pl **-ras**, **-rae** [-riː] 1. Aura f. 2. epileptische Aura f.
au·ral ['ɔːrəl] adj 1. Ohr(en) od. Gehör betr., Ohr(en)-, Gehör-, Hör-; Ton-. 2. Aura betr.
aural aspergillomycosis Ohraspergillose f.
aural aspergillosis → aural aspergillomycosis.
aural aspirator Ohrabsaugeinstrument nt.
aural discharge Ohr(en)fluß m, Ohrenausfluß m, Otorrhoe f.
aural forceps HNO Ohrzängchen nt.
aural fistula Ohrfistel f.
aural polyp Ohrpolyp m.
aural scotoma HNO Skotom nt des Ohres, Scotoma auris.
aural tuberculosis Ohrtuberkulose f.
aural vertigo → auditory vertigo.
au·ra·mine stain ['ɔːrəmiːn, -mɪn] Auraminfärbung f.
au·ran·o·fin [ɔː'rænəfɪn] n pharm. Auranofin nt.
au·ran·ti·a·sis [ˌɔːrən'taɪəsɪs] n Karotin-, Carotingelbsucht f, -ikterus m, Aurantiasis f (cutis), Karotino-, Carotinodermie f, Carotinodermia f, Carotinosis f.
au·ri·a·sis [ɔː'raɪəsɪs] n Auriasis f, Pigmentatio aurosa.
au·ric ['ɔːrɪk] adj Gold betr. od. enthaltend, Gold-.
au·ri·cle ['ɔːrɪkl] n anat. 1. Ohrmuschel f, Aurikel f. 2. Herzohr nt, Auricula atrialis. 3. old → atrium 2.
 a. of heart → auricle 2.
au·ri·co·cer·vi·cal nerve reflex [ˌɔːrɪkəʊ-'sɜːvɪkl] Snellen-Reflex m.
au·ri·co·pal·pe·bral reflex [ˌ-'pælpəbrəl] Kehrer-Reflex m, akustischer Lidreflex m.
au·ric·u·la [ɔː'rɪkjələ] n, pl **-las**, **-lae** [-liː, -laɪ] → auricle.
au·ric·u·lar [ɔː'rɪkjələr] adj 1. Ohr od. ohrförmige Struktur betr., ohrförmig, aurikular, Ohr(en)-, Gehör-, Hör-. 2. old → atrial.
auricular appendage (of heart) → auricle 2.
auricular appendix → auricle 2.
auricular artery: anterior a.ies pl vordere Ohrmuschelaste pl der A. temporalis superficialis, Rami auriculares anteriores a. temporalis superficialis.
 deep a. tiefe Ohrschlagader f, Aurikularis f profunda, A. auricularis profunda.
 left a. linke (Herz-)Kranzarterie, A. coronaria sinistra.
 posterior a. hintere Ohrschlagader f, Aurikularis f posterior, A. auricularis posterior.
 right a. rechte (Herz-)Kranzarterie, A. coronaria dextra.
auricular branch: anterior a.es of superficial temporal artery Ohr(muschel)äste pl der A. temporalis superficialis, Rami auriculares anteriores a. temporalis superficialis.

auricular cartilage

a. of occipital artery Ohrast *m* der A. occipitalis, Ramus auricularis a. occipitalis.
a. of posterior auricular artery Ramus auricularis a. auricularis posterioris.
a. of posterior auricular nerve Ast *m* des N. auricularis posterior zur Ohrmuschelmuskulatur, Ramus auricularis n. auricularis posterioris.
a. of vagus nerve Ohrmuschel- u. Gehörgangsast *m* des N. vagus, Ramus auricularis n. vagi.
auricular cartilage Ohrmuschelknorpel *m*, Knorpelgerüst *nt* der Ohrmuschel, Cartilago auricularis.
auricular complex *card.* (*EKG*) Vorhofkomplex *m*, P-Welle *f*, P-Zacke *f*.
auricular extrasystole *card.* Vorhofextrasystole *f*, atriale Extrasystole *f*.
auricular fibrillation *card.* Vorhofflimmern *nt*.
auricular fissure Fissura tympanomastoidea.
auricular flutter *card.* Vorhofflattern *nt*.
auricular groove, posterior Sulcus auricularis posterior.
auricular hematoma Othämatom *nt*.
auricular hillocks *embryo.* Ohrmuschelhöcker *pl*.
au·ric·u·la·ris (muscle) [ɔːˌrɪkjəˈlɛərɪs, -lɑr-] Ohrmuskel *m*, Aurikularis *m*, M. auricularis.
anterior a. Aurikularis *m* anterior, M. auricularis anterior.
posterior a. Aurikularis *m* posterior, M. auricularis posterior.
superior a. Aurikularis *m* superior, M. auricularis superior.
auricular ligament: anterior a. vorderes Ohrmuschelband *nt*, Lig. auriculare anterius.
posterior a. hinteres Ohrmuschelband *nt*, Lig. auriculare posterius.
superior a. oberes Ohrmuschelband *nt*, Lig. auriculare superius.
auricular muscle → auricularis (muscle).
auricular muscles 1. Ohrmuschelmuskeln *pl*, Mm. auriculares. 2. an der Ohrmuschel ansetzende Muskeln, Ohrmuskeln *pl*.
auricular nerve: anterior a.s Ohrmuscheläste *pl* des N. auriculotemporalis, Nn. auriculares anteriores.
great a. Aurikularis *m* magnus, N. auricularis magnus.
internal a. Ramus posterior n. auricularis magni.
posterior a. Aurikularis *m* posterior, N. auricularis posterior.
auricular notch Inc. anterior auris.
auricular plane of sacral bone Facies auricularis ossis sacri.
auricular standstill *card.* Vorhofstillstand *m*.
auricular surface (of ilium) Facies auricularis ossis ilii.
auricular systole Vorhofsystole *f*.
auricular tachycardia Vorhoftachykardie *f*, atriale Tachykardie *f*.
auricular tubercle Darwin'-Höcker *m*, Tuberculum auriculare.
auricular vein: anterior a.s vordere Ohrvenen *pl*, Vv. auriculares anteriores.
posterior a. hintere Ohrvene *f*, V. auricularis posterior.
au·ric·u·lo·cra·ni·al [ɔːˌrɪkjələʊˈkreɪnɪəl] *adj* aurikulokranial.
auriculo-infraorbital plane *radiol.* Deutsche Horizontale *f*, Frankfurter Horizontale *f*, Ohr-Augen-Ebene *f*.
au·ric·u·lo·tem·po·ral nerve [ˌ-ˈtemprəl] Aurikulotemporalis *m*, N. auriculotemporalis.

auriculotemporal nerve syndrome → auriculotemporal syndrome.
auriculotemporal neuralgia Aurikulotemporalisneuralgie *f*.
auriculotemporal syndrome aurikulotemporales Syndrom *nt*, Frey-Baillarger-Syndrom *nt*, Geschmacksschwitzen *nt*.
au·ric·u·lo·ven·tric·u·lar [ˌ-venˈtrɪkjələr] *adj old* → atrioventricular.
auriculoventricular band His'-Bündel *nt*, Fasciculus atrioventricularis.
auriculoventricular dissociation *card.* atrioventrikuläre Dissoziation *f*.
auriculoventricular extrasystole → atrioventricular extrasystole.
auriculoventricular groove *old* → atrioventricular groove.
auriculoventricular interval *card.* PQ-Intervall *nt*.
auriculoventricular valve *old* → atrioventricular valve.
au·ri·form [ˈɔːrəfɔːrm] *adj* ohrförmig.
au·ri·na·sal [ˌɔːrəˈneɪzl] *adj* Ohr u. Nase betr. *od.* verbindend, aurikulonasal.
au·ri·pig·ment [ˌ-ˈpɪgmənt] *n* Arsentrisulfid *nt*, Rauschgelb *nt*, Auripigment *nt*.
au·ris [ˈɔːrɪs] *n*, *pl* **-res** [-riːz] *anat.* Ohr *nt*, Auris *f*.
au·ri·scope [ˈɔːrəskəʊp] *n* Auriskop *nt*, Otoskop *nt*.
au·ro·chro·mo·der·ma [ˌɔːrəˌkrəʊməˈdɜːrmə] *n derm.* Aurochromodermie *f*.
au·ro·pal·pe·bral reflex [ˌ-ˈpælpəbrəl, -pælˈpiː-] auropalpebraler Reflex *m*.
au·ro·ther·a·py [ˌ-ˈθerəpɪ] *n pharm.*, *ortho.* Gold-, Auro-, Chrysotherapie *f*.
au·ro·thi·o·glu·cose [ˌ-ˌθaɪəʊˈgluːkəʊz] *n* Gold-, Aurothioglukose *f*.
au·ro·thi·o·ma·late disodium [ˌ-ˌθaɪəʊˈmæleɪt, -ˈmeɪl-] Natriumaurothiomalat *nt*, Aurothiomalatnatrium *nt*.
au·rum [ˈɔːrəm] *n abbr.* **Au** *chem.* Gold *nt*, Aurum *nt abbr.* Au.
aus·cult [ˈɔːskʌlt] *vt* → auscultate.
aus·cul·tate [ˈɔːskəlteɪt] *vt* auskultieren, abhören, -horchen.
aus·cul·ta·tion [ˌɔːskəlˈteɪʃn] *n* Auskultation *f*, Abhören *nt*, Abhorchen *nt*.
aus·cul·ta·to·ry [ɔːˈskʌltəˌtɔːriː, -təʊ-] *adj* Auskultation betr., durch Auskultation feststellend *od.* feststellbar, auskultatorisch.
auscultatory gap auskultatorische Lücke *f*.
auscultatory method auskultatorische Blutdruckmessung *f* nach Korotkow.
auscultatory percussion auskultatorische Perkussion *f*.
auscultatory sound Auskultationsgeräusch *nt*.
Austin Flint [ˈɔːstən flɪnt]: **A. F. murmur** *card.* Austin Flint-Geräusch *nt*, Flint-Geräusch *nt*.
A. F. phenomenon → A. F. murmur.
A. F. respiration (*Auskultation*) Kavernenatmen *nt*.
Austin Moore [mʊər]: **A. M. prosthesis** *ortho.* Moore-(Hüft-)Prothese *f*.
Aus·tral·ia antigen [ɔːˈstreɪljə] *abbr.* **Au** Australiaantigen *nt*, Hepatitis B surface-Antigen *nt abbr.* HB$_s$Ag, HB$_s$-Antigen *nt*, Hepatitis B-Oberflächenantigen *nt*.
Aus·tral·ian [ɔːˈstreɪljən]: **A. Q fever** Balkangrippe *f*, Q-Fieber *nt*.
A. tick typhus Queenslandzeckenbißfieber *nt*.
A. X disease *abbr.* **AXD** Murray-Valley-Enzephalitis *f abbr.* MVE, Australian-X Enzephalitis *f*.
A. X disease virus Murray-Valley-Enzephalitis-Virus *nt*.
A. X encephalitis → A. X disease.

aut- *pref.* → auto-.
au·te·cious [ɔːˈtiːʃəs] *adj* → autoecious.
aut·e·col·o·gy [ˌɔːtəˈkɑlədʒɪ] *n* Autökologie *f*.
au·te·me·sia [ˌɔːtɪˈmiːsɪə, -ʃə] *n* idiopathisches Erbrechen *nt*.
au·thor·i·tar·i·an personality [əˌθɔːrɪˈtɛərɪən] autoritäre Persönlichkeit *f*.
au·tism [ˈɔːtɪzəm] *n* 1. Autismus *m*. 2. frühkindlicher Autismus *m*, Kanner-Syndrom *nt*.
au·tis·tic [ɔːˈtɪstɪk] I *n* Patient(in *f*) *m* mit Autismus, Autistiker(in *f*) *m*. II *adj* Autismus betr., autistisch.
autistic disorder Kanner-Syndrom *nt*, frühkindlicher Autismus *m*.
autistic thinking → autism 1.
auto- *pref.* Selbst-, Eigen-, Aut(o)-.
au·to·ac·ti·va·tion [ˌɔːtəʊˌæktəˈveɪʃn] *n* Selbst-, Autoaktivierung *f*.
au·to·ag·glu·ti·na·tion [ˌ-əˌgluːtəˈneɪʃn] *n* Autoagglutination *f*.
au·to·ag·glu·ti·nin [ˌ-əˈgluːtnɪn] *n* Autoagglutinin *nt*.
au·to·ag·gres·sive [ˌ-əˈgresɪv] *adj* autoaggressiv, Autoaggressions-.
autoaggressive disease → autoimmune disease.
au·to·al·ler·gic [ˌ-əˈlɜːrdʒɪk] *adj* → autoimmune.
au·to·al·ler·gy [ˌ-ˈælərdʒɪ] *n* → autoimmunity.
au·to·a·nal·y·sis [ˌ-əˈnæləsɪs] *n psychia.* Auto(psycho)analyse *f*.
au·to·an·a·lyz·er [ˌ-ˈænlaɪzər] *n lab.* Autoanalysator *m*, Autoanalyzer *m*.
au·to·an·am·ne·sis [ˌ-ˌænəmˈniːsɪs] *n* Autoanamnese *f*.
au·to·an·a·phy·lax·is [ˌ-ˌænəfɪˈlæksɪs] *n old* → autoimmunity.
au·to·an·ti·bod·y [ˌ-ˈæntɪbɑdɪ] *n* Autoantikörper *m*.
au·to·an·ti·com·ple·ment [ˌ-ˌæntɪˈkɑmpləmənt] *n* Autoantikomplement *nt*.
au·to·an·ti·gen [ˌ-ˈæntɪdʒən] *n* Autoantigen *nt*.
auto-anti-idiotypic antibodies auto-anti--idiotypische Antikörper *pl*.
au·to·an·ti·sep·sis [ˌ-ˌæntɪˈsepsɪs] *n* physiologische Antisepsis *f*.
au·to·an·ti·tox·in [ˌ-ˌæntɪˈtɑksɪn] *n* Autoantitoxin *nt*.
au·to·ca·tal·y·sis [ˌ-kəˈtæləsɪs] *n* Autokatalyse *f*.
au·to·cat·a·lyst [ˌ-ˈkætəlɪst] *n* Autokatalysator *m*.
au·to·cat·a·lyt·ic [ˌ-ˌkætəˈlɪtɪk] *adj* Autokatalyse betr., von Autokatalyse betroffen *od.* gekennzeichnet, autokatalytisch.
au·to·ca·thar·sis [ˌ-kəˈθɑːrsɪs] *n psychia.* Autokatharsis *f*.
au·to·cath·e·ter·ism [ˌ-ˈkæθɪtərɪzəm] *n* Autokatheterisierung *f*.
au·toch·tho·nal [ɔːˈtɑkθənəl] *adj* autochthonisch.
au·toch·thon·ic [ɔːˌtɑkˈθɑnɪk] *adj* → autochthonisch.
au·toch·tho·nous [ɔːˈtɑkθənəs] *adj* 1. aus s. selbst heraus entstehend, an Ort u. Stelle entstanden, autochthon. 2. eingeboren, bodenständig, autochthon.
autochthonous graft autologes/autogenes Transplantat *nt*, Autotransplantat *nt*.
autochthonous muscles autochthone Muskeln *pl*/Muskulatur *f*.
autochthonous transplantation Autotransplantation *f*, autogene/autologe Transplantation *f*.
au·to·ci·ne·sis [ˌ-səˈniːsɪs] *n* → autokinesis.
au·to·clave [ˈɔːtəkleɪv] I *n* Autoklav *m*. II *vt* autoklavieren.

au·to·cy·tol·y·sin [ˌɔːtəʊsaɪˈtɒləsɪn, -ˌsaɪtəˈlaɪsɪn] *n* → autolysin.
au·to·cy·tol·y·sis [ˌ-saɪˈtɒləsɪs] *n* → autolysis.
au·to·cy·to·lyt·ic [ˌ-ˌsaɪtəˈlɪtɪk] *adj* → autolytic.
au·to·cy·to·tox·in [ˌ-ˌsaɪtəˈtɒksɪn] *n* Auto(zyto)toxin *nt*.
au·to·der·mic graft [ˌ-ˈdɜrmɪk] autologes Hauttransplantat *nt*.
au·to·de·struc·tion [ˌ-dɪˈstrʌkʃn] *n* Selbstzerstörung *f*, Autodestruktion *f*.
au·to·di·ges·tion [ˌ-dɪˈdʒestʃn, -daɪ-] *n* Selbstverdauung *f*, Autodigestion *f*.
au·to·di·ges·tive [ˌ-dɪˈdʒestɪv, -daɪ-] *adj* selbstverdauend, autodigestiv.
au·to·drain·age [ˌ-ˈdreɪnɪdʒ] *n chir*. Autodrainage *f*, interne Drainage *f*.
au·to·ech·o·la·lia [ˌ-ˌekəʊˈleɪlɪə] *n neuro., psychia*. Autoecholalie *f*.
au·toe·cious [ɔːˈtiːʃəs] *adj micro*. wirtstreu, autözisch.
au·to·ec·ze·ma·ti·za·tion [ˌɔːtəʊɪɡˌziːmətɪˈzeɪʃn] *n derm*. Autoekzematisation *f*.
au·to·ep·i·der·mic graft [ˌ-epɪˈdɜrmɪk] → autodermic graft.
au·to·e·rot·ic [ˌ-ɪˈrɒtɪk] *adj* Autoerotik betr., autoerotisch, autoerastisch.
au·to·e·rot·i·cism [ˌ-ɪˈrɒtəsɪzəm] *n* Autoerotik *f*, Autoerotismus *m*, Autoerastie *f*.
au·to·er·o·tism [ˌ-ˈerətɪzəm] *n* → autoeroticism.
au·to·e·ryth·ro·cyte sensitization syndrome [ˌ-ɪˈrɪθrəsaɪt] Erythrozytenautosensibilisierung *f*, schmerzhaftes Ekchymosen-Syndrom *nt*, painful bruising syndrome (*nt*).
au·to·flu·o·res·cence [ˌ-flʊəˈresəns] *n* Autofluoreszenz *f*.
au·to·flu·o·ro·scope [ˌ-ˈflʊərəskəʊp] *n* Autofluoroskop *nt*.
au·tog·a·mous [ɔːˈtæɡəməs] *adj micro*. selbstbefruchtend, autogam.
au·tog·a·my [ɔːˈtæɡəmɪ] *n micro*. Selbstbefruchtung *f*, Autogamie *f*.
au·to·gen·e·ic [ˌɔːtəʊdʒəˈniːɪk] *adj* → autogenous.
au·to·gen·e·sis [ˌ-ˈdʒenəsɪs] *n* Selbstentstehung *f*, Autogenese *f*.
au·to·ge·net·ic [ˌ-dʒəˈnetɪk] *adj* Autogenese betr., autogenetisch.
au·to·gen·ic [ˌ-ˈdʒenɪk] *adj* aus dem Körper entstanden, autogen.
autogenic inhibition autogene Hemmung *f*, Selbsthemmung *f*, Autoinhibition *f*.
autogenic training autogenes Training *f*.
au·tog·e·nous [ɔːˈtædʒənəs] *adj* **1.** von selbst entstehend, autogen. **2.** im Organismus selbst erzeugt, endogen, autogen, autolog.
autogenous graft autologes/autogenes Transplantat *nt*, Autotransplantat *nt*.
autogenous vaccine Eigenimpfstoff *m*, Autovakzine *f*.
au·to·graft [ˈɔːtəʊɡræft] *n* Autotransplantat *nt*, autogenes/autologes Transplantat *nt*.
au·to·graft·ing [ˌ-ˈɡræftɪŋ] *n* Autotransplantation *f*, autogene/autologe Transplantation *f*.
au·tog·ra·phism [ɔːˈtæɡrəfɪzəm] *n* → autography.
au·tog·ra·phy [ɔːˈtæɡrəfɪ] *n* Hautschrift *f*, Dermographie *f*, -graphia *f*, -graphismus *m*.
au·to·he·mag·glu·ti·na·tion [ˌɔːtəʊˌhiːməɡluːtəˈneɪʃn] *n* Autohämagglutination *f*.
au·to·he·mag·glu·ti·nin [ˌ-ˌhiːməˈɡluːtənɪn, -ˌhemə-] *n* Autohämagglutinin *nt*.
au·to·he·mol·y·sin [ˌ-hɪˈmɒləsɪn] *n* Autohämolysin *nt*, hämolysierender Autoantikörper *m*.

au·to·he·mol·y·sis [ˌ-hɪˈmɒləsɪs] *n* Autohämolyse *f*.
autohemolysis test Autohämolysetest *m*, Wärmeresistenztest *m*.
au·to·he·mo·lyt·ic [ˌ-ˌhiːməˈlɪtɪk] *adj* Autohämolyse betr., autohämolytisch.
au·to·he·mo·ther·a·py [ˌ-ˌhiːməˈθerəpɪ] *n* Eigenblutbehandlung *f*, Autohämotherapie *f*.
au·to·he·mo·trans·fu·sion [ˌ-ˌhiːməˈtrænsˈfjuːʒn] *n* Eigenbluttransfusion *f*, Autotransfusion *f*.
au·to·his·to·ra·di·o·graph [ˌ-ˌhɪstəʊˈreɪdɪəʊɡrɑːf] *n* → autoradiograph.
au·to·hyp·no·sis [ˌ-hɪpˈnəʊsɪs] *n* Selbst-, Autohypnose *f*.
au·to·hyp·not·ic [ˌ-hɪpˈnɒtɪk] *adj* Autohypnose betr., autohypnotisch.
au·to·im·mune [ˌ-ɪˈmjuːn] *adj* Autoimmunität betr., autoimmun, Autoimmun-.
autoimmune disease Autoimmunerkrankung *f*, -krankheit *f*, Autoimmunopathie *f*, Autoaggressionskrankheit *f*.
autoimmune hemolytic anemia *abbr*. AIHA autoimmunhämolytische Anämie *f*.
autoimmune hepatitis chronisch-aktive/chronisch-aggressive Hepatitis *f abbr*. CAH.
autoimmune response Autoimmunreaktion *f*.
autoimmune thyroiditis 1. (Auto-)Immunthyr(e)oiditis *f*. **2.** Hashimoto-Thyreoiditis *f*, Struma lymphomatosa.
au·to·im·mu·ni·ty [ˌ-ɪˈmjuːnətɪ] *n* Autoimmunität *f*.
au·to·im·mu·ni·za·tion [ˌ-ˌɪmjənəˈzeɪʃn, -ɪˌmju-] *n* Autoimmunisierung *f*.
au·to·in·fec·tion [ˌ-ɪnˈfekʃn] *n* Selbstinfizierung *f*, Autoinfektion *f*.
au·to·in·fu·sion [ˌ-ɪnˈfjuːʒn] *n* Autoinfusion *f*.
au·to·in·oc·u·la·ble [ˌ-ɪˈnɒkjələbl] *adj micro*. autoinokulierbar.
au·to·in·oc·u·la·tion [ˌ-ɪˌnɒkjəˈleɪʃn] *n micro*. Autoinokulation *f*.
au·to·in·ter·fer·ence [ˌ-ˌɪntərˈfɪərəns] *n micro*. Autointerferenz *f*.
au·to·in·tox·i·cant [ˌɔːtəʊɪnˈtɒksɪkənt] *n* Autotoxin *nt*, Endotoxin *nt*.
au·to·in·tox·i·ca·tion [ˌ-ɪnˌtɒksɪˈkeɪʃn] *n* Selbstvergiftung *f*, Autointoxikation *f*.
au·to·i·sol·y·sin [ˌ-aɪsəʊˈlaɪsɪn, -aɪˈsɒləsɪn] *n* Autoisolysin *nt*.
au·to·ker·a·to·plas·ty [ˌ-ˈkerətəʊplæstɪ] *n ophthal*. autologe Keratoplastik *f*.
au·to·ki·ne·sis [ˌ-kɪˈniːsɪs, -kaɪ-] *n* willkürliche Bewegung *f*, Willkürmotorik *f*, Autokinese *f*.
au·to·ki·net·ic [ˌ-kɪˈnetɪk, -kaɪ-] *adj* Autokinese betr., autokinetisch.
au·to·la·vage [ˌ-ləˈvɑːʒ, -ˈlævɪdʒ] *n chir*. Autolavage *f*.
au·to·le·sion [ˌ-ˈliːʒn] *n* selbstverursachte Verletzung *f*, s. selbst zugefügte Verletzung *f*.
au·to·leu·ko·ag·glu·ti·nin [ˌ-ˌluːkəʊəˈɡluːtənɪn] *n* Autoleukoagglutinin *nt*, agglutinierender Leukozytenautoantikörper *m*.
au·tol·o·gous [ɔːˈtɒləɡəs] *adj* → autogenous.
autologous antibody Autoantikörper *m*, autologer Antikörper *m*.
autologous graft autologes/autogenes Transplantat *nt*, Autotransplantat *nt*.
autologous transfusion → autotransfusion.
autologous transplantation → autografting.
au·tol·y·sate [ɔːˈtɒləseɪt] *n* Autolysat *nt*.
au·to·lyse *vt, vi* → autolyze.
au·to·ly·sin [ˌ-ˈlaɪsɪn, ɔːˈtɒləsɪn] *n* Auto(zyto)lysin *nt*.

au·tol·y·sis [ɔːˈtɒləsɪs] *n* Selbstauflösung *f*, Autolyse *f*; Selbstverdauung *f*, Autodigestion *f*.
au·to·ly·so·some [ˌɔːtəʊˈlaɪsəsəʊm] *n* Autolysosom *nt*.
au·to·lyt·ic [ˌɔːtəˈlɪtɪk] *adj* Autolyse betr., selbstauflösend, autolytisch; selbstverdauend, autodigestiv.
au·to·lyze [ˈɔːtəlaɪz] **I** *vt* eine Autolyse auslösen *od*. verursachen *od*. durchlaufen. **II** *vi* eine Autolyse durchlaufen, s. auflösen.
au·to·mat·ic [ˌ-ˈmætɪk] *adj* **1.** spontan, unwillkürlich, zwangsläufig, automatisch. **2.** selbsttätig, automatisch, selbstgesteuert, Selbst-.
automatic behavior → automatism.
automatic bladder *neuro*. Reflexblase *f*.
automatic epilepsy psychomotorische Epilepsie *f*.
automatic movement automatische/unwillkürliche Bewegung *f*.
au·tom·a·tism [ɔːˈtɒmətɪzəm] *n* automatische/unwillkürliche Handlung *od*. Reaktion *f*, Automatismus *m*.
au·to·mix·is [ˌɔːtəˈmɪksɪs] *n* → autogamy.
au·to·my·so·pho·bia [ˌ-ˌmaɪsəˈfəʊbɪə] *n psychia*. Automysophobie *f*.
au·to·neph·ro·tox·in [ˌ-ˌnefrəˈtɒksɪn] *n* Autonephrotoxin *nt*.
au·to·nom·ic [ˌ-ˈnɒmɪk] *adj* autonom, unabhängig, selbstständig (funktionierend); selbstgesteuert.
au·to·nom·i·cal [ˌ-ˈnɒmɪkl] *adj* → autonomic.
autonomic ataxia vasomotorische Dystonie *f*.
autonomic bladder autonome (Harn-)Blase *f*.
autonomic center vegetatives Zentrum *nt*.
autonomic column of spinal cord intermediolaterale (Rückenmarks-)Säule *f*, Columna autonomica/intermediolateralis medullae spinalis.
autonomic epilepsy autonome Epilepsie *f*, Epilepsie *f* mit autonomen Symptomen.
autonomic ganglia vegetative/autonome Grenzstrangganglien *pl*, Ggll. autonomica/visceralia.
autonomic imbalance → autonomic ataxia.
autonomic innervation vegetative Innervation *f*.
autonomic nerve Eingeweide-, Viszeralnerv *m*, N. autonomicus/visceralis.
autonomic nervous system *abbr*. ANS autonomes/vegetatives Nervensystem *nt abbr*. ANS, Pars autonomica systematis nervosi, Systema nervosum autonomicum.
autonomic nucleus Edinger-Westphal--Kern *m*, Nc. oculomotorius accessorius/autonomicus.
autonomic plexus autonomes/vegetatives Nervengeflecht *nt*, autonomer/vegetativer (Nerven-)Plexus *m*, Plexus autonomicus/visceralis.
autonomic reflex vegetativer Reflex *m*.
autonomic synapse vegetative Synapse *f*.
au·ton·o·mous [ɔːˈtɒnəməs] *adj* → autonomic.
autonomous adenoma autonomes Adenom *nt*.
autonomous bladder autonome (Harn-)Blase *f*.
au·ton·o·my [ɔːˈtɒnəmɪ] *n* Selbständigkeit *f*, Unabhängigkeit *f*, Autonomie *f*.
auto-ophthalmoscope *ophthal*. Auto-ophthalmoskop *nt*.
auto-ophthalmoscopy *n ophthal*. Auto-ophthalmoskopie *f*.

auto-oxidation *n* Autoxydation *f*, Autoxidation *f*.
au·to·path·ic [ˌɔːtəʊˈpæθɪk] *adj* ohne erkennbare Ursache (entstanden), unabhängig von anderen Krankheiten, selbständig, idiopathisch; essentiell, primär, genuin.
au·top·a·thy [ɔːˈtapəθɪ] *n path.* idiopathische Erkrankung *f*, Autopathie *f*.
au·to·pha·gia [ˌɔːtəˈfeɪdʒ(ɪ)ə] *n histol.*, *psycho.* Autophagie *f*.
au·to·phag·ic [ˌ-ˈfædʒɪk] *adj* Autophagie betr., autophagisch.
autophagic vesicle → autophagosome.
au·to·phag·o·some [ˌ-ˈfægəsəʊm] *n* autophagische Vakuole *f*, Autophagosom *nt*.
au·toph·a·gy [ɔːˈtafədʒɪ] *n* → autophagia.
au·to·phil·ia [ˌɔːtəʊˈfiːlɪə] *n old* → narcissism.
au·to·pho·bia [ˌ-ˈfəʊbɪə] *n psychia.* Autophobie *f*.
au·toph·o·ny [ɔːˈtafənɪ] *n* Autophonie *f*.
au·to·plast [ˈɔːtəʊplæst] *n* → autograft.
au·to·plas·tic [ˌ-ˈplæstɪk] **I** *n* → autograft. **II** *adj* Autoplastik betr., autoplastisch.
autoplastic graft → autograft.
au·to·plas·ty [ˈ-plæstɪ] *n chir.* Autoplastik *f*.
au·to·poi·son·ous [ˌ-ˈpɔɪzənəs] *adj* autotoxisch.
au·to·pol·y·mer [ˌ-ˈpɒləmər] *n* Autopolymer *nt*.
au·to·po·lym·er·i·za·tion [ˌ-pəˌlɪmərəˈzeɪʃn, -pəlɪməraɪ-] *n* Autopolymerisation *f*.
au·to·pro·te·ol·y·sis [ˌ-ˌprəʊtɪˈɒləsɪs] *n* Selbstverdauung *f*, Autolyse *f*, Autodigestion *f*.
au·to·pro·throm·bin [ˌ-prəʊˈθrambɪn] *n* Autoprothrombin *nt*.
autoprothrombin I Prokonvertin *nt*, -convertin *nt*, Faktor VII *m abbr.* F V II, Autothrombin I *nt*, Serum-Prothrombin-Conversion-Accelerator *m abbr.* SPCA, stabiler Faktor *m*.
autoprothrombin II Faktor IX *m abbr.* F IX, Christmas-Faktor *m*, Autothrombin II *nt*.
autoprothrombin C Faktor X *m abbr.* F X, Stuart-Prower-Faktor *m*, Autothrombin III *nt*.
au·to·pro·tol·y·sis [ˌ-prəʊˈtɒləsɪs] *n* Autoprotolyse *f*.
au·top·sia [ɔːˈtapsɪə] *n* → autopsy.
au·top·sy [ˈɔːtapsɪ] **I** *n* Leicheneröffnung *f*, Autopsie *f*, Obduktion *f*, Nekropsie *f*. **to conduct** *od.* **carry out an ~** eine Autopsie vornehmen. **to examine/discover at ~** während einer Autopsie untersuchen/feststellen. **2.** *fig.* kritische Analyse *f*. **II** *vt* eine Autopsie vornehmen an.
au·to·psy·chic [ˌɔːtəʊˈsaɪkɪk] *adj* autopsychisch.
au·to·psy·cho·rhyth·mia [ˌ-ˌsaɪkəˈrɪθmɪə] *n psychia.* Autopsychorhythmie *f*.
au·to·psy·cho·sis [ˌ-saɪˈkəʊsɪs] *n psychia.* Autopsychose *f*.
au·to·ra·di·o·gram [ˌ-ˈreɪdɪəʊgræm] *n* → autoradiograph.
au·to·ra·di·o·graph [ˌ-ˈreɪdɪəʊgræf] *n* Autoradiogramm *nt*.
au·to·ra·di·o·graph·ic [ˌ-ˌreɪdɪəʊˈgræfɪk] *adj* autoradiographisch.
au·to·ra·di·og·ra·phy [ˌ-ˌreɪdɪˈɒgrəfɪ] *n* Auto(histo)radiographie *f*.
au·to·re·cep·tor [ˌ-rɪˈsɛptər] *n* Autorezeptor *m*.
au·to·re·du·pli·ca·tion [ˌ-rɪˌd(j)uːplɪˈkeɪʃn] *n* identische Reduplikation *f*, Autoreduplikation *f*.
au·to·reg·u·la·tion [ˌ-ˌregjəˈleɪʃn] *n* Selbst-, Autoregulation *f*, -regulierung *f*, -regelung *f*.

au·to·reg·u·la·to·ry [ˌ-ˈregjələtɔːrɪ, -təʊ-] *adj* autoregulativ, autoregulatorisch.
au·to·re·in·fec·tion [ˌ-riːɪnˈfɛkʃn] *n* **1.** → autoinfection. **2.** autogene Reinfektion *f*.
au·to·re·in·fu·sion [ˌ-riːɪnˈfjuːʒn] *n* Autoreinfusion *f*, Autotransfusion *f*.
au·to·rhyth·mic·i·ty [ˌ-rɪðˈmɪsətɪ] *n* Autorhythmie *f*.
au·to·scope [ˈɔːtəskəʊp] *n* Autoskop *nt*.
au·tos·co·py [ɔːˈtaskəpɪ] *n* Autoskopie *f*.
au·to·sen·si·ti·za·tion [ˌɔːtəʊˌsɛnsɪtɪˈzeɪʃn] *n* Autosensibilisierung *f*, Autoimmunisierung *f*.
au·to·sen·si·tized [ˌ-ˈsɛnsɪtaɪzt] *adj* autosensibilisiert, autoimmun.
au·to·sep·ti·ce·mia [ˌ-ˌsɛptəˈsiːmɪə] *n* Auto-, Endosepsis *f*.
au·to·se·ro·ther·a·py [ˌ-ˌsɪərəʊˈθɛrəpɪ] *n* → autoserum therapy.
au·to·se·rous [ˌ-ˈsɪərəs] *adj* Autoserum betr., autoserös.
au·to·se·rum [ˌ-ˈsɪərəm] *n* Eigen-, Autoserum *nt*.
autoserum therapy Eigenserumbehandlung *f*, Autoserotherapie *f*.
au·to·sex·u·a·lism [ˌ-ˈsɛkʃəwælɪzəm] *n* **1.** → autoerotism. **2.** Narzißmus *m*.
au·to·site [ˈ-saɪt] *n patho.* Autosit *m*.
au·tos·mia [ɔːˈtasmɪə] *n* Autosmie *f*.
au·to·so·mal [ˌɔːtəˈsəʊml] *adj* Autosom(en) betr., autosomal, Autosomen-.
autosomal gene autosomales Gen *nt*.
autosomal heredity autosomale Vererbung *f*.
au·to·so·ma·tog·no·sis [ˌ-ˌsəʊmətəgˈnəʊsɪs] *n* Phantomgefühl *nt*, Autosomatognosie *f*.
au·to·some [ˈ-səʊm] *n* **1.** *genet.* Autosom *nt*, Euchromosom *nt*. **2.** → autophagosome.
autosome aberration autosomale Chromosomenaberration *f*, Autosomenaberration *f*.
autosome abnormality autosomale Chromosomenanomalie *f*, Autosomenanomalie *f*.
au·to·sug·ges·tion [ˌ-sə(g)ˈdʒɛstʃn] *n psychia.* Selbstbeeinflussung *f*, Autosuggestion *f*.
au·to·sug·ges·tive [ˌ-sə(g)ˈdʒɛstɪv] *adj* autosuggestiv.
au·to·syn·the·sis [ˌ-ˈsɪnθəsɪs] *n* Autosynthese *f*.
au·to·ther·a·py [ˌ-ˈθɛrəpɪ] *n* **1.** Selbstheilung *f*, Autotherapie *f*. **2.** Spontanheilung *f*.
au·to·throm·bo·ag·glu·ti·nin [ˌ-ˌθrambəʊəˈgluːtɪnɪn] *n* Autothromboagglutinin *nt*, Plättchenautoagglutinin *nt*.
au·tot·o·my [ɔːˈtatəmɪ] *n* Selbstverstümmelung *f*, Autotomie *f*.
au·to·top·ag·no·sia [ˌ-ˌtapægˈnəʊʒ(ɪ)ə] *n neuro.* Autotopagnosie *f*.
au·to·tox·e·mia [ˌ-takˈsiːmɪə] *n* → autotoxicosis.
au·to·tox·ic [ˌ-ˈtaksɪk] *adj* autotoxisch.
autotoxic cyanosis autotoxische Zyanose *f*, Stokvis-Talma-Syndrom *nt*.
au·to·tox·i·co·sis [ˌ-ˌtaksɪˈkəʊsɪs] *n* Autotoxikose *f*, -intoxikation *f*.
au·to·tox·in [ˌ-ˈtaksɪn] *n* Autotoxin *nt*.
au·to·tox·is [ˌ-ˈtaksɪs] *n* → autotoxicosis.
au·to·trans·fu·sion [ˌ-trænsˈfjuːʒn] *n* Eigenbluttransfusion *f*, Autotransfusion *f*.
au·to·trans·plant [ˌ-ˈtrænsplænt] *n* Autotransplantat *nt*, autogenes/autologes Transplantat *nt*.
au·to·trans·plan·ta·tion [ˌ-ˌtrænsplænˈteɪʃn] *n* Autotransplantation *f*, autogene/autologe Transplantation *f*.
au·to·trep·a·na·tion [ˌ-ˌtrɛpəˈneɪʃn] *n patho.*, *chir.* Autotrepanation *f*.

au·to·troph [ˈ-traf, -trəʊf] *n* autotrophe Zelle *f*, Autotroph *m*.
au·to·troph·ic [ˌ-ˈtrafɪk, -trəʊ-] *adj* Autotrophie betr., autotroph.
autotrophic bacteria autotrophe Bakterien *pl*.
autotrophic cell → autotroph.
autotrophic fixation *biochem.* autotrophe Kohlendioxidfixierung *f*.
au·tot·ro·phy [ɔːˈtatrəfɪ] *n bio.* Autotrophie *f*.
au·to·vac·ci·na·tion [ɔːtəʊˌvæksəˈneɪʃn] *n* Autovakzinebehandlung *f*.
au·to·vac·cine [ˌ-ˈvæksiːn] *n* Eigenimpfstoff *m*, Autovakzine *f*.
au·to·vac·ci·no·ther·a·py [ˌ-væksɪnəʊˈθɛrəpɪ] *n* → autovaccination.
au·tox·e·mia [ˌɔːtakˈsiːmɪə] *n* → autotoxicosis.
au·tox·i·da·tion [ɔːˌtaksɪˈdeɪʃn] *n* Autoxydation *f*, Autoxidation *f*.
au·tox·i·diz·a·ble [ɔːˌtaksɪˈdaɪzəbl] *adj* autoxidierbar.
au·to·zy·gous [ˌɔːtəˈzaɪgəs] *adj genet.* autozygot.
au·tumn [ˈɔːtəm] **I** *n* Herbst *m*. **II** *adj* → autumnal.
au·tum·nal [ɔːˈtʌmnl] *adj* im Herbst vorkommend *od.* auftretend, herbstlich, autumnal, Herbst-, Autumnal-.
autumnal catarrh Heuschnupfen *m*, -fieber *nt*.
autumn fever 1. japanisches Herbstfieber *nt*, (japanisches) Siebentagefieber *nt*, Nanukayami(-Krankheit *f*) *nt*. **2.** Feld-, Ernte-, Schlamm-, Sumpffieber *nt*, Erbsenpflückerkrankheit *f*, Leptospirosis grippotyphosa.
aux·an·o·gram [ˈɔːgzænəgræm] *n micro.* Auxanogramm *nt*.
aux·an·o·graph·ic [ˈɔːgˌzænəˈgræfɪk] *adj micro.* Auxanographie betr., auxanographisch.
auxanographic method *micro.* Auxanographie *f*, Diffusionsmethode *f*.
aux·a·nog·ra·phy [ˌɔːgzəˈnɒgrəfɪ] *n micro.* Auxanographie *f*.
aux·a·nom·e·ter [ˌɔːgzəˈnɒmɪtər] *n micro.* Auxanometer *nt*.
aux·il·ia·ry [ɔːgˈzɪljərɪ, -lərɪ] **I** *n, pl* **-ries** Helfer(in *f*) *m*, Hilfskraft *f*, Assistent(in *f*) *m*. **II** *adj* (mit-)helfend, mitwirkend, Hilfs-; zusätzlich, Ersatz-, Hilfs-, Reserve-.
auxiliary enzyme Hilfsenzym *nt*.
auxiliary nurse Schwesternhelfer(in *f*) *m*.
aux·in [ˈɔːksɪn] *n* Auxin *nt*.
aux·i·om·e·ter [ˌɔːgzɪˈɒmɪtər] *n* **1.** Aux(i)ometer *nt*. **2.** Dynamometer *nt*.
aux·o·car·dia [ˌɔːksəʊˈkɑːrdɪə] *n* **1.** Herzvergrößerung *f*. **2.** (Herz-)Diastole *f*.
aux·o·chrome [ˈ-krəʊm] *n* Auxochrom *nt*.
aux·o·chro·mous [ˌ-ˈkrəʊməs] *adj* auxochrom.
aux·o·cyte [ˈ-saɪt] *n* Auxozyt *m*.
aux·o·hor·mone [ˌ-ˈhɔːrməʊn] *n* Vitamin *nt*.
aux·om·e·ter [ɔːkˈsɒmɪtər] *n* → auxiometer 1.
aux·o·met·ric [ˌɔːksəˈmɛtrɪk] *adj* Auxometrie betr., auxometrisch.
aux·om·e·try [ɔːkˈsɒmɪtrɪ] *n* Messung *f* der Wachstumsgeschwindigkeit, Auxometrie *f*.
aux·o·spore [ˈɔːksəspɔːr, -spəʊr] *n* Auxospore *f*.
aux·o·ton·ic [ˌ-ˈtɒnɪk] *adj* auxoton, auxotonisch.
auxotonic contraction auxotonische Kontraktion *f*.
aux·o·troph [ˈ-traf, -trəʊf] *n* auxotrophe Zelle *f*, Auxotroph *m*.

aux·o·troph·ic [ˌ-'trɑfɪk, -troʊ-] *adj* auxotroph.
auxotrophic cell → auxotroph.
auxotrophic mutant auxotrophe Mutante *f*.
aux·o·type ['-taɪp] *n micro.* Auxotyp *m*.
AV *abbr.* 1. → arteriovenous. 2. → atrioventricular.
A-V *abbr.* 1. → arteriovenous. 2. → atrioventricular.
av *abbr.* 1. → arteriovenous. 2. → atrioventricular.
a·vail·a·ble [ə'veɪləbl] *adj* vorhanden, verfügbar, zur Verfügung stehend; erreichbar sein; erhältlich, lieferbar.
a·vail·a·bil·i·ty [ə,veɪlə'bɪlətɪ] *n* 1. Vorhandensein *nt*, Verfügbarkeit *f*. 2. Erhältlichkeit *f*, Lieferbarkeit *f*.
a·val·vu·lar [eɪ'vælvjələr] *adj* klappenlos, avalvulär.
AV anastomosis → arteriovenous anastomosis.
av·an·tin ['ævæntɪn] *n* Isopropanol *nt*, Isopropylalkohol *m*.
a·vas·cu·lar [eɪ'væskjələr] *adj* ohne Blutgefäße, gefäßlos, avaskulär.
a·vas·cu·lar·i·ty [eɪ,væskjə'lærətɪ] *n* Avaskularität *f*.
a·vas·cu·lar·i·za·tion [eɪ,væskjələrɪ'zeɪʃn, -raɪ-] *n* Unterbindung *f* der Blutzufuhr.
avascular necrosis aseptische/spontane/ avaskuläre Nekrose *f*.
  a. of bone aseptische/spontane Knochennekrose.
  idiopathic a. of the femoral head idiopathische Hüftkopfnekrose des Erwachsenen, avaskuläre/ischämische Femurkopfnekrose.
  a. of lunate Lunatummalazie *f*, Kienböck'-Krankheit *f*.
  a. of scaphoid aseptische/avaskuläre Kahnbeinnekrose.
avascular scar avaskuläre Narbe *f*.
a-v block atrioventrikulärer Block *m*, AV-Block *m*.
AV bundle → atrioventricular bundle.
av bundle → atrioventricular bundle.
A-V conduction *card.* atrioventrikuläre (Erregungs-)Überleitung *f*.
avD *abbr.* → arteriovenous difference.
Avellis [a:'velis]: **A.' paralysis** → A.' syndrome.
  A.' syndrome Avellis-Syndrom *nt*, Avellis-Longhi-Syndrom *nt*, Longhi-Avellis- -Syndrom *nt*.
a·ve·nin [ə'vi:nɪn, 'ævə-] *n* Legumin *nt*.
a·ve·no·lith [ə'vi:nəlɪθ] *n* Avenolith *m*.
av·e·nue ['ævən(j)u:] *n fig.*, *chir.* Zugang *m*, Weg *m* (*of, to* zu).
  a.s *of* Verfahrensweisen *pl*.
av·er·age ['æv(ə)rɪdʒ] **I** *n* Durchschnitt *m*, Mittelwert *m*. **above (the) ~** über dem Durchschnitt, überdurchschnittlich. **below (the) ~** unter dem Durchschnitt, unterdurchschnittlich. **on (an/the) ~** im Durchschnitt, durchschnittlich. **II** *adj* durchschnittlich, Durchschnitts-. **III** *vt* 1. durchschnittlich betragen *od.* ausmachen *od.* haben *od.* erreichen. 2. → average out. **IV** *vi* einen Durchschnitt erzielen.
average out *vt* den Durchschnitt schätzen *od.* ermitteln (*of auf*).
average dose Durchschnittsdosis *f*.
a·ver·sion [ə'vɜrʒn] *n* Widerwille *m*, Abneigung *f*, Abscheu *f* (*to, for, from* vor), Aversion *f* (*to, for, from* gegen).
aversion therapy Aversionstherapie *f*.
a·ver·sive [ə'vɜrsɪv] *adj* Abneigung *od.* Abscheu erweckend *od.* betr., Aversions-.
aversive conditioning/therapy → aversion therapy.

a·vert [ə'vɜrt] *vt fig.* verhüten, verhindern, abwenden.
A·vi·ad·e·no·vi·rus [ˌeɪvɪˌædɪnoʊ'vaɪrəs] *n micro.* Aviadenovirus *nt*.
a·vi·an ['eɪvɪən] *adj* Vögel betr., Vogel-.
avian adenovirus → Aviadenovirus.
avian influenza atypische Geflügelpest *f*, Newcastle disease (*nt*).
avian leukemia virus *abbr.* **ALV** *micro.* Vögel-Leukämie-Virus *nt*, avian leukemia virus *abbr.* ALV.
avian pest → avian influenza.
avian plague *micro.* Hühner-, Geflügelpest *f*.
avian sarcoma Rous-Sarkom *nt*.
avian sarcoma virus *abbr.* **ASV** *micro.* Vögel-Sarkom-Virus *nt*, avian sarcoma virus *abbr.* ASV.
a·vi·a·tion medicine [ˌeɪvɪ'eɪʃn, ˌævɪ-] Luftfahrtmedizin *f*, Aeromedizin *f*.
aviation otitis Aer(o)otitis *f*, Bar(o)otitis *f*, Otitis barotraumatica.
aviation sickness Fliegerkrankheit *f*.
a·vi·a·tor's disease ['eɪvɪeɪtər, 'ævɪ-] (akute) Höhenkrankheit *f*.
av·id ['ævɪd] *adj* (be-)gierig (*for, of* nach).
av·i·din ['ævɪdɪn, ə'vɪdɪn] *n* Avidin *nt*.
a·vid·i·ty [ə'vɪdətɪ] *n* 1. Anziehungs-, Bindungskraft *f*. 2. *chem.* Säure-, Basenstärke *f*. 3. *immun.* Avidität *f*. 4. Gier *f*, Begierde *f* (*for, of* nach).
a·vi·fau·na [ˌeɪvɪ'fɔ:nə, ˌævə-] *n* Vogelwelt *f*, Vogel-, Avifauna *f*. **PQ**-Intervall *nt*.
A-V interval *card.* PQ-Intervall *nt*.
a·vir·u·lence [eɪ'vɪrjələns] *n micro.* Avirulenz *f*.
a·vir·u·lent [eɪ'vɪrjələnt] *adj* nicht-virulent, nicht-ansteckungsfähig, avirulent.
a·vi·ta·min·o·sis [ˌeɪˌvaɪtəmɪ'noʊsɪs, eɪˌvɪ-] *n* Vitaminmangelkrankheit *f*, Avitaminose *f*.
a·vive·ment [avɪv'mɑ̃] *n chir.* Wundrandausschneidung *f*.
AVM *abbr.* → arteriovenous malformation.
A-V nodal bigeminy *card.* Knotenbigemie *f*.
A-V nodal rhythm *physiol.* Knotenrhythmus *m*, AV-Rhythmus *m*.
A-V nodal tachycardia AV-Knoten-Tachykardie *f*.
AV node → atrioventricular node.
Avogadro [ævə'gɑːdroʊ]: **A.'s constant** → A.'s number.
  A.'s law Avogadro'-(Gas-)Gesetz *nt*.
  A.'s hypothesis → A.'s law.
  A.'s number Avogadro'-Zahl *f*.
a·void [ə'vɔɪd] *vt* (ver-)meiden; (*Person, Sache*) ausweichen, aus dem Wege gehen; (*Problem*) umgehen; (*Gefahr*) entgehen, -rinnen.
a·void·ance [ə'vɔɪdns] *n* Vermeidung *f*, Umgehung *f*, Meidung *f* (*of* von).
avoidance-avoidance conflict *psycho.*, *psychia.* Aversions-Aversions-Konflikt *m*.
a·void·ant [ə'vɔɪdnt] *adj* vermeidend, ausweichend.
AVP *abbr.* → arginine vasopressin.
A-V rhythm *physiol.* Knotenrhythmus *m*, AV-Rhythmus *m*.
A-V shunt *chir.* arteriovenöser Shunt *m*.
a·vul·sion [ə'vʌlʃn] *n* Ab-, Ausreißen *nt*, Avulsio *f*.
avulsion fracture Ab-, Ausrißfraktur *f*.
  a. of lateral epicondyle of humerus (Abriß-)Fraktur des Epicondylus lateralis humeri.
  a. of lesser tuberosity (Abriß-)Fraktur des Tuberculum minus humeri.
  a. of medial epicondyle of humerus (Abriß-)Fraktur des Epicondylus medialis humeri.

  a. of ulnar styloid (Abriß-)Fraktur des Proc. styloideus ulnae.
avulsion injury Ausriß-, Abrißverletzung *m*, Ausriß *m*, Abriß *m*.
avulsion trauma → avulsion injury.
a·wake [ə'weɪk] (*v*: **awoke; awoken; awaked**) **I** *adj* wach. **to be/stay ~** wach sein/bleiben. **wide ~** hellwach. **II** *vt* (auf-)wecken. **III** *vi* auf-, erwachen.
a·wak·en [ə'weɪkn] *vt*, *vi* → awake II.
a·wak·en·ing [ə'weɪknɪŋ] **I** *n* (Er-, Auf-)- Wecken *nt*; Auf-, Erwachen *nt*. **frequent/ early ~s from sleep** häufiges/frühes Aufwachen. **II** *adj* erwachend, Weck-.
awakening threshold Weckschwelle *f*.
a·ware [ə'weər] *adj* bewußt, gewahr, unterrichtet (*of* von). **to be/become ~ of sth.** s. einer Sache bewußt sein/werden. **to make sb. ~ of the risks** jdn. auf die Risiken hinweisen.
a·ware·ness [ə'weərnɪs] *n* Kenntnis *f*; Bewußtsein *n*.
a wave *card.* a-Welle *f*, Vorhofwelle *f*.
awu *abbr.* [atomic weight unit] → atomic mass unit.
AXD *abbr.* → Australian X disease.
AXD virus Murray-Valley-Enzephalitis- -Virus *nt*.
Axenfeld ['æksnfɛlt]: **A.'s anomaly** Embryotoxon posterius.
  posterior embryotoxon of A. Embryotoxon posterius.
  A.'s syndrome *ophthal.* Axenfeld-Syndrom *nt*.
a·xen·ic culture [eɪ'zɛnɪk, -'zi:n-] *micro.* Reinkultur *f*.
ax·i·al ['æksɪəl] *adj* Achse betr., axial, achsenförmig, Achsen-.
axial ametropia *ophthal.* Achsenametropie *f*.
axial bond *chem.* axiale Bindung *f*.
axial cataract Spindelstar *m*, Cataracta fusiformis.
axial deviation Achsenabweichung *f*.
axial fiber → axon.
axial filament → axoneme.
axial fusiform cataract → axial cataract.
axial hyperopia *ophthal.* Achsenhyperopie *f*.
axial myopia *ophthal.* Achsenmyopie *f*.
axial neuritis parenchymatöse Neuritis *f*.
axial plane Achsenebene *f*.
axial plate *embryo.* Primitivstreifen *m*.
axial skeleton Rumpfskelett *nt*, Skeleton axiale.
axial stream Axialstrom *nt*.
axial symmetry *mathe.* Achsensymmetrie *f*.
ax·if·u·gal [æk'sɪfjəgl] *adj* in Richtung zur Achse, axifugal.
ax·i·lem·ma [ˌæksɪ'lɛmə] *n* → axiolemma.
ax·il·la [æg'zɪlə, æk's-] *n*, *pl* **-las, -lae** [-liː] Achselhöhle *f*, Achselhöhlengrube *f*, Axilla *f*, Fossa axillaris.
ax·il·lar·y ['æksə,lɛriː, æk'sɪləri] *adj* Achsel(höhle) betr., axillar, Axillar-, Achsel-.
axillary anesthesia *anes.* Axillarisblock *m*, Axillaranästhesie *f*.
axillary aneurysm Aneurysma *nt* der A. axillaris.
axillary arch Langer'-Achselbogen *m*.
axillary artery Achselschlagader *f*, -arterie *f*, Axillaris *f*, A. axillaris.
axillary block (anesthesia) Axillarisblock *m*, Axillaranästhesie *f*.
axillary border of scapula äußerer Skapularand *m*, Margo lateralis scapulae.
axillary dissection *chir.* Axilladissektion *f*, -revision *f*, -ausräumung *f*.
axillary fascia Fascia axillaris.
axillary fold: anterior a. vordere Achselfalte *f*, Plica axillaris anterior.

axillary fossa

posterior a. hintere Achselfalte *f*, Plica axillaris posterior.
axillary fossa → axilla.
axillary glands Achsellymphknoten *pl*, Nodi lymphatici axillares.
axillary line *anat.* Axillarlinie *f*, Linea axillaris.
  anterior a. vordere Axillarlinie, Linea axillaris anterior.
  median a. mittlere Axillarlinie, Linea axillaris media, Linea medio-axillaris.
  posterior a. hintere Axillarlinie, Linea axillaris posterior.
axillary lymph node Achsellymphknoten *m*, Nodus lymphaticus axillaris.
  apical a.s apikale Achsellymphknoten *pl*, Nodi lymphatici (axillares) apicales.
  brachial a.s Oberarmlymphknoten *pl*, Nodi lymphatici (axillares) brachiales.
  deep a.s tiefe Achsellymphknoten *pl*, Nodi lymphatici axillares profundi.
  interpectoral a. Brustwand-, Pektoralislymphknoten, Nodus lymphaticus (axillaris) pectoralis/interpectoralis.
  lateral a.s → brachial a.s.
  pectoral a. → interpectoral a.
  subscapular a.s subskapuläre Lymphknoten *pl*, Nodi lymphatici (axillares) subscapulares.
  superficial a.s oberflächliche Achsellymphknoten *pl*, Nodi lymphatici axillares superficiales.
axillary lymph node dissection → axillary dissection.
axillary lymph node metastasis → axillary metastasis.
axillary margin of scapula → axillary border of scapula.
axillary metastasis Achsellymphknotenmetastase *f*.
axillary nerve Axillaris *m*, N. axillaris.
axillary nodal dissection → axillary dissection.
axillary process of mammary gland Achselfortsatz *m* der Brustdrüse, Proc. axillaris/lateralis gl. mammariae.
axillary recess Rec. axillaris.
axillary region *anat.* Achselgegend *f*, -region *f*, Regio axillaris.
axillary space → axilla.
axillary tail of mammary gland → axillary process of mammary gland.
axillary temperature Achsel(höhlen)-, Axillatemperatur *f*.
axillary triangle Achseldreieck *nt*.
axillary vein Achselvene *f*, V. axillaris.
ax·i·om ['æksɪəm] *n* Axiom *nt*.
ax·i·o·plasm ['æksɪəplæzəm] *n* → axoplasm.
ax·i·o·po·di·um [,-'pəʊdɪəm] *n* → axopodium.
ax·ip·e·tal [æk'sɪpətəl] *adj* zur Achse hin, axipetal.
ax·is ['æksɪs] *n*, *pl* **ax·es** ['æksi:z] **1.** *anat.* zweiter Halswirbel *m*, Axis *m*. **2.** (Körper-, Gelenk-, Organ-)Achse *f*, Axis *m*. **3.** *techn.*, *phys.*, *mathe.* Mittellinie *f*, Achse *f*.
  a. of contraction Kontraktionsrichtung *f*, -achse.
  a. of heart Herzachse *f*.
  a. of lens Linsenachse, Axis lentis.
  a. of pelvis Beckenführungslinie *f*, Beckenachse, Axis pelvis.
axis cylinder → axon.
axis deviation (*EKG*) Achsenabweichung *f*.
axis fracture *ortho.* Axisfraktur *f*.
ax·o·ax·on·ic synapse [,æksæk'sɑnɪk] axo-axonale/axo-axonische Synapse *f*.

ax·o·den·drit·ic synapse [,-den'drɪtɪk] axodendritische Synapse *f*.
ax·o·den·dro·so·mat·ic synapse [,-,dendrəʊsə'mætɪk, -sə'mæ-] axodendrosomatische Synapse *f*.
ax·of·u·gal [æk'sɑfəgəl] *adj* → axifugal.
ax·o·lem·ma ['æksəlemə] *n* Axolemm *nt*.
ax·ol·y·sis [æk'sɑləsɪs] *n patho.* Axolyse *f*.
ax·om·e·ter [æk'sɑmɪtər] *n* → axonometer.
ax·on ['æksɑn] *n* Achsenzylinder *m*, Axon *nt*, Neuraxon *nt*.
ax·on·al ['æksɑnl, -,sɑnl] *adj* Axon betr., axonal, Axo(n)-.
axonal branch Axonzweig *m*, -abzweigung *f*.
axonal degeneration axonale Degeneration *f*.
axonal reaction → axon reaction.
axonal sprouting *patho.* Axon(aus)sprossung *f*.
axonal transport axonaler Transport *m*.
  rapid a. schneller axonaler Transport.
  slow a. langsamer axonaler Transport.
ax·on·a·prax·ia [,æksɑneɪ'præksɪə] *n* Neurapraxie *f*, Neuropraxie *f*.
axon collateral Axonkollaterale *f*.
ax·one ['æksəʊn] *n* → axon.
ax·o·neme ['æksənɪːm] *n* Achsenfaden *m*, Axonem *nt*.
ax·on·ic [æk'sɑnɪk] *adj* → axonal.
ax·o·nom·e·ter [,æksə'nɑmɪtər] *n* Axonometer *nt*.
ax·o·nom·e·try [,-'nɑmɪtrɪ] *n* Parallelperspektive *f*, Axonometrie *f*.
ax·on·ot·me·sis [,æksɑnɑt'miːsɪs] *n* Axonotmesis *f*.
axon reaction *neuro.* retrograde Degeneration *f*, Axonreaktion *f*.
axon reflex Axonreflex *m*.
axon sheath Axonscheide *f*.
axon stream Axonstrom *m*.
ax·op·e·tal [æk'sɑpətəl] *adj* → axipetal.
ax·o·phage ['æksəfeɪdʒ] *n* Axophage *m*.
ax·o·plasm ['æksəplæzəm] *n* Axoplasma *nt*.
ax·o·plas·mic [,-'plæzmɪk] *adj* Axoplasma betr., axoplasmatisch, Axoplasma-.
axoplasmic membrane Axoplasmamembran *f*.
ax·o·po·di·um [,-'pəʊdɪəm] *n*, *pl* **-dia** [-dɪə] Achsenfüßchen *nt*, Axopodium *nt*.
ax·o·so·mat·ic synapse [,-səʊ'mætɪk] axosomatische Synapse *f*.
Ayala [əˈjɑːlə]: **A.'s equation/index** → A.'s quotient.
A.'s quotient *neuro.* Ayala-Quotient *m*, -Gleichung *f*.
Ayer [eər]: **A.'s test** *neuro.* Ayer-Test *m*, -Zeichen *nt*.
Ayer-Tobey ['təʊbɪ]: **A.-T. test** Tobey--Ayer-Test *m*.
Ayerza [aˈjerθa]: **A.'s disease** Ayerza'--Krankheit *f*, primäre Pulmonalsklerose *f*.
A.'s syndrome Ayerza-Syndrom *nt*.
a-zan stain [ɑˈzɑːn] Azan-Färbung *f*, Heidenhain'-Azanfärbung *f*.
a·za·pro·pa·zone [azə'prəʊpəzəʊn] *n pharm.* Azapropazon *nt*.
a·za·ri·bine [eɪzə'rɑɪbiːn] *n pharm.* Azaribin *nt*.
a·za·ser·ine [eɪzə'sɪərɪːn] *n* Azaserin *nt*.
az·at·a·dine [əˈzætədiːn] *n pharm.* Azatadin *nt*.
az·a·thi·o·prine [æzə'θɑɪəpriːn] *n pharm.* Azathioprin *nt*.
az·e·la·ic acid [æzə'leɪɪk] Azelainsäure *f*.
a·ze·o·trop·ic [,eɪzɪə'trɑpɪk] *adj chem.* Azeotropie betr., azeotrop.

a·ze·ot·ro·py [eɪzɪˈɑtrəpɪ] *n chem.* Azeotropie *f*.
az·id *n* → azide.
az·ide ['æzɑɪd, -ɪd, 'eɪ-] *n* Azid *nt*.
az·i·do·thy·mi·dine [,æzɪdəʊ'θɑɪmədiːn, -dɪn] *n abbr.* **AZT** *pharm.* Azidothymidin *nt abbr.* AZT.
az·lo·cil·lin [,æzləʊ'sɪlɪn] *n pharm.* Azlocillin *nt*.
azo- *pref.* Azo-.
az·o·ben·zene [,æzəʊ'benziːn, ,eɪz-] *n* Azobenzol *nt*.
az·o·car·mine [,-'kɑːrmɪn, -mɑɪn] *n* Azokarmin *nt*.
azo compound Azoverbindung *f*.
azo dyes Azofarbstoffe *pl*.
az·o·osper·ma·tism [eɪ,zəʊə'spɜrmətɪzəm] *n* → azoospermia.
az·o·o·sper·mia [,-'spɜrmɪə] *n* Azoospermie *f*.
az·o·o·sper·mic [,-'spɜrmɪk] *adj* Azoospermie betr., azoosperm.
a·zo·pig·ment [,æzəʊ'pɪgmənt] *n* Azopigment *nt*.
A·zo·re·an disease (of the nervous system) [əˈzɔːrɪən, -ˈzɔːr-] Machado--Joseph-Syndrom *nt*, Azorenkrankheit *f*.
az·ote [ˈæzəʊt, eɪˈzəʊt] *n* Stickstoff *m*, Nitrogen *nt*; *chem.* Nitrogenium *nt abbr.* N.
az·o·te·mia [æzəˈtiːmɪə] *n* Azot(h)ämie *f*.
az·o·tem·ic [,-ˈtemɪk, -ˈtiːm-] *adj* Azotämie betr., durch Azotämie verursacht, azotämisch.
azotemic retinitis azotämische Retinitis/Retinopathie *f*.
az·o·ther·mia [-ˈθɜrmɪə] *n* Azothermie *f*.
az·o·tom·e·ter [,-ˈtɑmɪtər] *n chem.* Azotometer *nt*.
az·o·tor·rhea [,æzətəʊˈrɪə] *n* Azotorrhoe *f*.
az·o·tu·ria [æzəˈt(j)ʊərɪə] *n* Azoturie *f*.
az·o·tur·ic [,-ˈt(j)ʊərɪk] *adj* Azoturie betr., azoturisch.
az·ox·y·ben·zene [æ,zɑgsɪˈbenziːn, -benˈziːn] *n* Azoxybenzol *nt*.
AZT *abbr.* **1.** → Aschheim-Zondek test. **2.** → azidothymidine.
A.-Z. test → Aschheim-Zondek test.
az·u·lene [ˈæzəliːn, ˈæzjə-] *n* Azulen *nt*.
az·ure [ˈæzər] *n histol.* Azur(farbstoff *m*) *m*.
azur granules azurophile Granula *pl*.
az·u·ro·phil [ˈæzərəfɪl, əˈzʊərə-] *n* azurophile Zelle *od.* Struktur *f*.
az·u·ro·phile [-fɑɪl, -fɪl] **I** *n* → azurophil. **II** *adj* → azurophilic.
azurophil granules → azur granules.
az·u·ro·phil·ia [,-ˈfɪlɪə] *n histol.*, *hema.* Azurophilie *f*.
az·u·ro·phil·ic [,-ˈfɪlɪk] *adj histol.* azurophil.
az·y·go·gram [ˈæzɪgəgræm, -ˈzɑɪ-] *n radiol.* Azygogramm *nt*.
az·y·gog·ra·phy [,æzɪˈgɑgrəfɪ] *n radiol.* Azygographie *f*.
az·y·gos [ˈæzɪgɑs, əˈzɑɪ-] **I** *n* Azygos *f*, V. azygos. **II** *adj anat.* ungepaart, unpaar.
azygos arteries of vagina Vaginaläste *pl* der A. uterina, Rami vaginales a. uterinae, Aa. azygoi vaginae.
a·zy·go·sperm [eɪˈzɑɪgəspɜrm] *n* → azygospore.
a·zy·go·spore [ˈ-spɔːr, -spʊər] *n bio.* Azygospore *f*.
azygos vein → azygos I.
  left a. Hemiazygos *f*, V. hemiazygos.
az·y·gous, *etc.* → azygos.
azygous ganglion Steiß(bein)knäuel *m/nt*, Corpus/Glomus coccygeum.
a·zym·ia [əˈzɪmɪə, -ˈzɑɪm-] *n* Azymie *f*.

B

B *abbr.* 1. → bel. 2. → boron.
B *abbr.* → beta.
b *abbr.* → barn.
β *abbr.* → beta.
β- *pref. chem.* beta-, β-.
β+ *abbr.* → positron.
BA *abbr.* → blood agar.
Ba *abbr.* → barium.
Baastrup ['baːstrəp]: **B.'s disease/syndrome** *ortho*. Baastrup'-Zeichen *nt*, -Syndrom *nt*, -Krankheit *f*, Arthrosis interspinosa.
Babbitt ['bæbɪt]: **B. metal** Babbitt-Metall *nt*.
Babcock ['bæbkɑk]: **B.'s operation** *chir*. Babcock-Operation *f*, -Krampfaderoperation *f*, -Venenstripping *nt*.
Babès ['baːbeɪ]: **B.' nodes/tubercles** Babès-Knötchen *pl*, Wutknötchen *pl*..
Babès-Ernst ['ɜrnst]: **B.-E. bodies** → B.-E. granules.
B.-E. granules metachromatische Granula *pl*, Babès-Ernst-Körperchen *pl*.
Ba·be·sia [bəˈbiːʒ(ɪ)ə, -zɪə] *n micro*. Babesia *f*.
bab·e·si·a·sis [ˌbæbɪˈsaɪəsɪs, ˌbeɪ-] *n* → babesiosis.
Ba·be·si·el·la [bəˌbiːzɪˈelə] *n* → Babesia.
ba·be·si·o·sis [bəˌbiːzɪˈəʊsɪs] *n* 1. chronische Babesiose *f*. 2. Babesiose *f*, Babesiasis *f*, Piroplasmose *f*.
Babinski [bəˈbɪnskɪ]: **B.'s law** *neuro*. Babinski-Gesetz *nt*, Babinski-Ohr-Phänomen *nt*.
B.'s phenomenon → B.'s toe sign.
B.'s reflex → B.'s toe sign.
B.'s sign 1. Babinski-Zeichen *nt*. 2. → B.'s toe sign.
B.'s syndrome Babinski-Vaquez-Syndrom *nt*.
B.'s test 1. Babinski-Zeichen *nt*. 2. Babinski-Zeichen *nt*, -Reflex *m*, (Groß-)Zehenreflex *m*.
B.'s toe sign Babinski-Zeichen *nt*, -Reflex *m*, (Groß-)Zehenreflex *m*.
Babinski-Fröhlich ['frɛɪlɪk; 'frøːlɪx]: **B.-F. syndrome** Babinski-Fröhlich-Syndrom *nt*, Morbus Fröhlich, Dystrophia adiposogenitalis (Fröhlich).
Babinski-Nageotte [naːʒˈɔt]: **B.-N. syndrome** Babinski-Nageotte-Syndrom *nt*.
Babinski-Vaquez [vaˈke]: **B.-V. syndrome** Babinski-Vaquez-Syndrom *nt*.
Babkin ['bæbkɪn]: **B. reflex** Babkin-Reflex *m*.
ba·by ['beɪbɪ] **I** *n, pl* **-bies** Säugling *m*, Baby *nt*, kleines Kind *nt*. **II** *adj* Baby-, Säuglings-. **from a ~** von frühester Kindheit an. **to be a ~** ein Kind bekommen.
baby boy Sohn *m*, kleiner Junge *m*.
baby farm *inf*. 1. Säuglingsheim *nt*. 2. Heim *nt* fuer ledige schwangere Frauen.
baby food Baby-, Säuglingsnahrung *f*.
baby girl Tochter *f*, kleines Mädchen *nt*.
ba·by·hood ['beɪbɪhʊd] *n* frühe Kindheit *f*, Säuglingsalter *nt*.
ba·by·scales ['beɪbɪskeɪls] *pl* Baby-, Säuglingswaage *f*.
baby skin Aprikosenhaut *f*.
baby tooth Milchzahn *m*, Dens deciduus.
ba·cam·pi·cil·lin [bəˌkæmpɪˈsɪlɪn] *n pharm*. Bacampicillin *nt*.
bac·cate ['bækeɪt] *adj* beerenförmig.
bac·ci·form ['bæksɪfɔːrm] *adj* beerenförmig.
Bachmann ['bækmən]: **B.'s bundle** Bachmann'-Interaurikularbündel *nt*.
Bac·il·la·ce·ae [ˌbæsəˈleɪsiː] *pl micro*. Bacillaceae *pl*.
ba·cil·lar [bəˈsɪlər, ˈbæsɪlər] *adj* → bacillary.
bac·il·la·ry [ˈbæsəˌleriː, bəˈsɪlərɪ] *adj* bazillenen-, stäbchenförmig, -ähnlich, bazilliform, bazillär, Bazillen-.
bacillary dysentery Bakterienruhr *f*, bakterielle Ruhr *f*, Dysenterie *f*.
bacillary layer Schicht *f* der Stäbchen u. Zapfen, Stratum neuroepitheliale retinae.
bac·il·le·mia [ˌbæsəˈliːmɪə] *n* Bazillensepsis *f*, Bazillämie *f*.
bac·il·lif·er·ous [ˌ-ˈlɪfərəs] *adj* bazillen-(über-)tragend.
ba·cil·li·form [bəˈsɪləfɔːrm] *adj* → bacillary.
bac·il·lu·ria [ˌbæsəˈl(j)ʊərɪə] *n* Bazillurie *f*.
Ba·cil·lus [bəˈsɪləs] *n micro*. Bacillus *m*.
B. aerogenes capsulatus Welch-Fränkel--(Gasbrand-)Bazillus, Clostridium perfringens.
B. anthracis Milzbrandbazillus, -erreger *m*, Bacillus anthracis.
B. botulinus Botulinusbazillus, Clostridium botulinum.
B. Calmette-Guérin *abbr*. **BCG** Bacillus Calmette-Guérin *abbr*. BCG.
B. coli Escherich-Bakterium *nt*, Coli--Bakterium *nt*, Escherichia/Bact. coli.
B. enteritidis Gärtner-Bazillus, Salmonella enteritidis.
B. fusiformis Fusobacterium nucleatum/fusiforme/Plaut-Vincenti, Leptotrichia buccalis.
B. leprae Hansen-Bazillus, Leprabazillus, -bakterium *nt*, Mycobacterium leprae.
B. pneumoniae Friedländer-Bakterium *nt*, -Bazillus, Klebsiella pneumoniae, Bact. pneumoniae Friedländer.
B. subtilis Heubazillus, Bacillus subtilis.
B. tetani Tetanus-, Wundstarrkrampfbazillus, -erreger *m*, Clostridium/Plectridium tetani.
B. typhi/typhosus Typhusbazillus, -bacillus, Salmonella typhi.
B. welchii → B. aerogenes capsulatus.
ba·cil·lus [bəˈsɪləs] *n, pl* **-cil·li** [-ˈsɪlaɪ] 1. Bazillus *m*, Bacillus *m*. 2. stäbchenförmiges Bakterium *nt*.
bacillus anthracis toxin Milzbrandtoxin *nt*.
Bacillus Calmette-Guérin *abbr*. **BCG** Bacillus Calmette-Guérin *m abbr*. BCG.

Bacillus Calmette-Guérin vaccine → BCG vaccine.
bac·i·tra·cin [ˌbæsɪˈtreɪsɪn] *n pharm*. Bazitrazin *nt*, Bacitracin *nt*.
back [bæk] **I** *n* 1. *anat*. Rücken *m*, Rückgrat *nt*, Dorsum *nt*. **to be flat on one's ~** bettlägrig sein. 2. Hinter-, Rückseite *f*; (Hand-, Buch-)Rücken *m*. **II** *adv* 3. zurück, rückwärts. **~ and forth** hin u. her, vor u. zurück. 4. (wieder) zurück. 5. (*zeitlich*) zurück, vorher. **III** *vt* unterstützen. **IV** *vi* zurück gehen *od*. fahren, rückwärtsgehen.
back up *vt* unterstützen, den Rücken stärken; (*These*) untermauern.
b. of foot Fußrücken(seite *f*) *m*, Dorsum pedis.
b. of hand Handrücken(seite *f*) *m*, Dorsum manus.
b. of (the) head Hinterkopf *m*, Hinterhaupt *nt*.
back·ache ['bækeɪk] *n* Rückenschmerzen *pl*.
back·al·gia [bækˈældʒ(ɪ)ə] *n* Rückenschmerzen *pl*.
back·bone ['bækbəʊn] *n* 1. *anat*. Rückgrat *nt*, Wirbelsäule *f*, Columna vertebralis. 2. *fig*. Grundgerüst *nt*.
back·cross ['bækkrɔs] **I** *n bio*. Rückkreuzung *f*. **II** *vt bio*. rückkreuzen.
back·flow ['bækfləʊ] *n* Rückfluß *m*, (Zu-)-Rückfließen *nt*.
back·ground ['bækɡraʊnd] *n* 1. (*a. fig*.) Hintergrund *m*, Hintergründe *pl*, Zusammenhänge *pl*, Umstände *pl*; Werdegang *m*. 2. (*soziale*) Verhältnisse *pl*.
background radiation *phys*. Hintergrundstrahlung *f*.
back·ing ['bækɪŋ] *n* 1. Unterstützung *f*, Hilfe *f*. 2. *techn*. Verstärkung *f*; Belag *m*, Überzug *m*. 3. *dent*. Rückenplatte *f*.
back·knee ['bækniː] *n* überstreckbares Knie(gelenk *nt*) *nt*, Hohlknie *nt*, Genu recurvatum.
back muscles Rückenmuskeln *pl*, -muskulatur *f*, Mm. dorsi.
autochthonous b. autochthone Rückenmuskulatur.
deep b. tiefe *od*. tiefere Rückenmuskulatur.
long b. lange Rücken-/Wirbelsäulenmuskulatur.
short b. kurze Rücken-/Wirbelsäulenmuskulatur.
superficial b. oberflächliche Rückenmuskulatur.
back-of-foot reflex Mendel-Bechterew--Reflex *m*, -Zeichen *nt*.
back pain Rückenschmerzen *pl*.
low/lower b. Kreuzschmerzen *pl*.
back radiation (*Schmerz*) Ausstrahlung *f* zum *od*. in den Rücken.
back·side [bækˈsaɪd] *n* 1. Kehr-, Rückseite *f*. 2. *inf*. Hintern *m*, Hinterteil *nt*.
back·slide ['bækslaɪd] *vi forens*. rückfällig werden.

backslider

back·slid·er ['bækslaɪdər] *n forens.* Rückfälliger *m.*
back·ward ['bækwərd] **I** *adj (Entwicklung)* zurück(geblieben), unterentwickelt; rückständig; rückwärts gerichtet. **II** *adv* rückwärts, nach hinten, zurück. **for·ward(s) and ~(s)** hin u. her, vor u. zurück. **to go ~ s.** verschlechtern.
backward curvature *ortho.* Lordose *f.*
backward (heart) failure Rückwärtsversagen *nt*, backward failure (*nt*).
back·wards ['bækwərdz] *adv* → backward II.
bac·lo·fen ['bækləfen] *n pharm.* Baclofen *nt.*
ba·con-rind clot ['beɪkən] *patho.* Speckhautgerinnsel *nt.*
bacon spleen *patho.* Schinkenmilz *f.*
ba·con·y degeneration ['beɪkənɪ] amyloide Degeneration *f*; Amyloidose *f.*
Bact. *abbr.* → Bacterium.
bac·ter·e·mia [ˌbæktə'riːmɪə] *n* Bakteriämie *f.*
bacteri- *pref.* → bacterio-.
bac·te·ria *pl* → bacterium.
bac·te·ri·al [bæk'tɪərɪəl] *adj* Bakterien betr., bakteriell, Bakterien-.
bacterial allergy Überempfindlichkeit *f* gegen Bakterienantigene.
bacterial aneurysm infektiöses Aneurysma *nt.*
bacterial antagonism bakterieller Antagonismus *m*, Bakterienantagonismus *m.*
bacterial antigen Bakterienantigen *nt.*
bacterial arthritis akut-eitrige Gelenkentzündung/Arthritis *f*, Gelenkeiterung *f*, Gelenkempyem *nt*, Pyarthrose *f*, Arthritis purulenta.
bacterial asthma bakteriell-bedingtes Asthma *nt.*
bacterial capsule Bakterienkapsel *f.*
bacterial cast *urol.* Bakterienzylinder *m.*
bacterial cell Bakterienzelle *f.*
bacterial chromosome Bakterienchromosom *nt.*
bacterial colony Bakterienkolonie *f.*
bacterial contamination bakterielle Verseuchung/Kontamination *f.*
bacterial culture Bakterienkultur *f.*
bacterial cystitis bakterielle Blasenentzündung/Cystitis *f.*
bacterial disease bakterielle Erkrankung *f.*
bacterial dissociation bakterielle Dissoziation *f.*
bacterial DNA Bakterien-DNA *f*, Bakterien-DNS *f*, bakterielle DNA *f*, bakterielle DNS *f.*
bacterial endocarditis subakute-bakterielle Endokarditis *f*, Endocarditis lenta.
bacterial filter Bakterienfilter *m.*
bacterial flagellum Bakteriengeißel *f.*
bacterial genetics Bakteriengenetik *f.*
bacterial host Bakterienwirt *m.*
bacterial infection bakterielle Infektion *f.*
bacterial lawn Bakterienrasen *m.*
bacterial myocarditis bakterielle Herzmuskelentzündung/Myokarditis *f.*
bacterial nephritis bakterielle Nephritis *f.*
bacterial pericarditis bakterielle Perikarditis *f.*
bacterial physiology Bakterienphysiologie *f.*
bacterial plaque *dent.* (Zahn-)Plaque *f.*
bacterial pneumonia bakterielle Lungenentzündung/Pneumonie *f.*
bacterial protein Bakterienprotein *nt.*
bacterial rhinitis bakterielle Nasenschleimhautentzündung/Rhinitis *f.*
bacterial satellite Satellitenkolonie *f.*
bacterial sinusitis bakterielle Nebenhöhlenentzündung/Sinusitis *f.*

bacterial spore Bakterienspore *f.*
bacterial strain Bakterienstamm *m.*
bacterial toxin → bacteriotoxin.
bacterial transformation *genet.* Transformation *f.*
bacterial vaccine → bacterin.
bacterial virus → bacteriophage.
bac·te·ri·cho·lia [ˌbæktɪərɪ'kəʊlɪə] *n* Bakterienausscheidung *f* in der Galle, Bakterichoile *f.*
bac·te·ri·cid·al [bæk,tɪərɪ'saɪdl] *adj* bakterientötend, bakterizid.
bac·te·ri·cide [bæk'tɪərɪsaɪd] *n* Bakterizid *nt*, bakterientötender Stoff *m.*
bac·te·ri·cid·in [bæk,tɪərɪ'saɪdn] *n* Bakterizidin *nt*, Bactericidin *nt.*
bac·ter·id ['bæktərɪd] *n* Bakterid *nt.*
bac·te·ri·e·mia [bæk,tɪərɪ'iːmɪə] *n* → bacteremia.
bac·te·ri·form [bæk'tɪərɪfɔːrm] *adj* bakterienähnlich, -förmig.
bac·ter·in ['bæktərɪn] *n* Bakterienimpfstoff *m*, -vakzine *f.*
bacterio- *pref.* Bakterien-, Bakterio-.
bac·te·ri·o·chlo·ro·phyll [bæk,tɪərɪə'klɔːrəfɪl, -'klɔːr-] *n bio.* Bakteriochlorophyll *nt.*
bac·te·ri·o·cid·al [ˌ-'saɪdl] *adj* → bactericidal.
bac·te·ri·o·cid·in [ˌ-'saɪdn] *n* → bactericidin.
bac·te·ri·o·cin [bæk'tɪərɪəsɪn] *n* Bakteriozin *nt*, Bacteriocin *nt.*
bacteriocin-type *n* Bakteriozin-Typ *m*, -Var *m.*
bacteriocin-var *n* → bacteriocin-type.
bac·te·ri·oc·la·sis [bæk,tɪərɪ'ɒkləsɪs] *n* → bacteriolysis.
bac·te·ri·o·gen·ic [bæk,tɪərɪə'dʒenɪk] *adj* durch Bakterien verursacht, bakteriogen, bakteriell, Bakterien-.
bac·te·ri·og·e·nous [bæk,tɪərɪ'ɒdʒənəs] *adj* → bacteriogenic.
bac·te·ri·oid [bæk'tɪərɪɔɪd] **I** *n* Bakterioid *nt*. **II** *adj* bakterienähnlich, -förmig, bakter(i)oid.
bac·te·ri·o·log·ic [bæk,tɪərɪə'lɒdʒɪk] *adj* Bakterien *od.* Bakteriologie betr., bakteriologisch, Bakterien-.
bac·te·ri·o·log·i·cal [ˌ-'lɒdʒɪkl] *adj* → bacteriologic.
bac·te·ri·ol·o·gist [bæk,tɪərɪ'ɒlədʒɪst] *n* Bakteriologe *m*, -login *f.*
bac·te·ri·ol·o·gy [ˌ-'ɒlədʒɪ] *n* Bakteriologie *f*, Bakterienkunde *f.*
bac·te·ri·ol·y·sin [bæk,tɪərɪə'laɪsɪn] *n* Bakteriolysin *nt.*
bac·te·ri·ol·y·sis [bæk,tɪərɪ'ɒləsɪs] *n* Auflösung *f* von Bakterien(zellen), Bakteriolyse *f.*
bac·te·ri·o·lyt·ic [bæk,tɪərɪə'lɪtɪk] *adj* bakterienauflösend, bakteriolytisch.
bacterio-opsonin *n* → bacteriopsonin.
bac·te·ri·o·pex·ia [bæk,tɪərɪə'peksɪə] *n* → bacteriopexy.
bac·te·ri·o·pex·y [ˌ-'peksɪ] *n* Bakteriopexie *f.*
bac·te·ri·o·phage ['-feɪdʒ] *n* Bakteriophage *m*, Phage *m*, bakterienpathogenes Virus *nt.*
bacteriophage plaque *micro.* Plaque *f.*
bacteriophage resistance *micro.* Phagenresistenz *f.*
bac·te·ri·o·pha·gia [ˌ-'feɪdʒ(ɪ)ə] *n* (Twort-)d'Herelle-Phänomen *nt*, Bakteriophagie *f.*
bac·te·ri·oph·a·gy [bæk,tɪərɪ'ɒfədʒɪ] *n* → bacteriophagia.
bac·te·ri·o·pho·bia [bæk,tɪərɪə'fəʊbɪə] *n psychia.* Bakterio-, Bazillophobie *f.*
bac·te·ri·o·phy·to·ma [ˌ-faɪ'təʊmə] *n* bakteriogene Geschwulst(bildung) *f*, Bakteriophytom *nt.*

bac·te·ri·o·plas·min [ˌ-'plæzmɪn] *n* Bakterioplasmin *nt.*
bac·te·ri·o·pre·cip·i·tin [ˌ-prɪ'sɪpətɪn] *n* Bakteriopräzipitin *nt.*
bac·te·ri·o·pro·tein [ˌ-'prəʊtiːn, -tiːɪn] *n* Bakterien-, Bakterioprotein *nt.*
bac·te·ri·op·so·nin [bæk,tɪərɪ'ɒpsənɪn] *n* Bakterienopsonin *nt*, Bakteriopsonin *nt.*
bac·te·ri·o·pur·pu·rin [bæk,tɪərɪə'pɜːrpjərɪn] *n* Bakterien-, Bakteriopurpurin *nt.*
bac·te·ri·o·rho·dop·sin [ˌ-rəʊ'dɒpsɪn] *n* Bakterien-, Bakteriorhodopsin *nt.*
bac·te·ri·o·sis [bæk,tɪərɪ'əʊsɪs] *n* bakterielle Erkrankung *f*, Bakteriose *f.*
bac·te·ri·o·sper·mia [bæk,tɪərɪə'spɜːrmɪə] *n* Bakteriospermie *f.*
bac·te·ri·os·ta·sis [bæk,tɪərɪ'ɒstəsɪs] *n* Bakteriostase *f.*
bac·te·ri·o·stat [bæk'tɪərɪəʊstæt] *n pharm.* bakteriostatisches Mittel *nt*, Bakteriostatikum *nt.*
bac·te·ri·o·stat·ic [ˌ-'stætɪk] **I** *n* → bacteriostat. **II** *adj* bakteriostatisch.
bac·te·ri·o·ther·a·py [ˌ-'θerəpɪ] *n* Bakterien-, Bakteriotherapie *f.*
bac·te·ri·o·tox·e·mia [ˌ-tɒk'siːmɪə] *n* Bakterien-, Bakteriotoxämie *f.*
bac·te·ri·o·tox·ic [ˌ-'tɒksɪk] *adj* bakterienschädigend, -toxisch, bakteriotoxisch.
bac·te·ri·o·tox·in [ˌ-'tɒksɪn] *n* Bakteriengift *nt*, -toxin *nt*, Bakteriotoxin *nt.*
bac·te·ri·o·trop·ic [ˌ-'trɒpɪk, -'trəʊp-] *adj* bakteriotrop.
bac·te·rit·ic [bæktə'rɪtɪk] *adj* durch Bakterien verursacht, bakteriogen, bakteriell.
Bac·te·ri·um [bæk'tɪərɪəm] *n abbr.* **Bact.** *micro.* Bacterium *nt abbr.* Bact.
B. aeruginosum Pseudomonas aeruginosa, Pyozyanus *m.*
B. coli Escherich-Bakterium, Coli-Bakterium *nt*, Escherichia/Bact. coli.
B. pestis Pestbakterium, Yersinia/Pasteurella pestis.
B. sonnei Kruse-Sonne-Ruhrbakterium, E-Ruhrbakterium, Shigella sonnei.
bac·te·ri·um [bæk'tɪərɪəm] *n*, *pl* **-ria** [-rɪə] Bakterie *f*, Bakterium *nt.*
bac·te·ri·u·ria [bæk,tɪərɪ'(j)ʊərɪə] *n* Bakterienausscheidung *f* im Harn, Bakteriurie *f.*
bac·te·ri·u·ric [ˌ-'jʊərɪk] *adj* Bakteriurie betr., bakteriurisch.
bac·te·ro·bi·lia [bæktərəʊ'bɪlɪə] *n* Bakteriocholie *f.*
bac·te·roid ['bæktərɔɪd] **I** *n* Bakteroid *nt*, Bakteroide *f*, Bacteroid *nt*. **II** *adj* bakterienähnlich, -förmig, bakter(i)oid.
Bac·te·roi·da·ce·ae [ˌbæktərɔɪ'deɪsiɪ] *pl micro.* Bacteroidaceae *pl.*
bac·te·roi·dal [ˌbæktə'rɔɪdl] *adj* → bacteroid II.
Bac·te·roi·des [ˌ-'rɔɪdiːz] *n micro.* Bacteroides *f.*
bac·te·roi·des [ˌ-'rɔɪdiːz] *n* Bacteroides *f.*
bac·te·roi·do·sis [ˌ-rɔɪ'dəʊsɪs] *n* Bakteroidesinfektion *f*, Bakteroidose *f*, Bacteroidosis *f.*
bac·ter·u·ria [ˌ-'(j)ʊərɪə] *n* → bacteriuria.
bac·to·pre·nol [ˌbæktəʊ'priːnɒl, -ɒʊl] *n* Bactoprenol *nt*, Undecaprenol *nt.*
bad [bæd] **I** *n* das Schlechte, das Böse; Unglück *nt*. **II** *adj* **1.** schlecht; böse, schlimm, arg, schwer. **2.** falsch, fehlerhaft; schlecht, unbefriedigend. **3.** (*Prognose*) ungünstig, schlecht. **4.** schädlich, ungesund, schlecht (*for* für). **5.** (*Nahrung*) schlecht, verdorben. **6.** (*Schmerz*) schlimm, böse, arg, heftig.
bad breath (übler) Mund-, Atemgeruch *m*, Foetor ex ore, Kakostomie *f*, Halitose *f*, Halitosis *f.*

bad·ly developed ['bædlɪ] unterentwickelt.
BADS syndrome [black locks, oculocutaneous albinism, deafness of the sensorineural type] BADS-Syndrom nt.
Baehr-Löhlein [beər 'ləʊlaɪn; 'løløɪn]: **B.-L. lesion** Löhlein'-Herdnephritis f.
Baelz [beɪltz]: **B.'s disease** Baelz'-Krankheit f, Cheilitis glandularis purulenta superficialis, Myxadenitis labialis.
BAEPS abbr. → brain stem auditory evoked potentials.
Baer [beər]: **B.'s cavity** embryo. von Baer'-Höhle f, -Spalte f.
B.'s law embryo. (von) Baer'-Gesetz nt.
B.'s vesicles gyn. Tertiärfollikel pl, Folliculi ovarici vesiculari.
Baerensprung ['beərənsprʌŋ; 'bɛːrənsprʊŋ]: **B.'s erythrasma** Baerensprung'-Krankheit f, Zwergflechte Baerensprung f, Erythrasma (intertriginosum) nt.
Bäfverstedt ['beɪfərʃtet]: **B.'s syndrome** Bäfverstedt-Syndrom nt, multiples Sarkoid nt, benigne Lymphoplasie f der Haut, Lymphozytom nt, Lymphozytoma cutis, Lymphadenosis benigna cutis.
bag [bæg] **I** n Sack m, Beutel m; Tasche f. **II** vt (auf-)bauschen. **III** vi s. (auf-)bauschen, (an-)schwellen, ausdehnen.
b.s under the eyes Ringe unter den Augen; Tränensäcke pl.
b. of waters inf. Amnionsack m, Fruchtblase f.
ba·gas·sco·sis [bægə'skəʊsɪs] n → bagassosis.
bag·as·so·sis [,-'səʊsɪs] n Bagassosis f.
Bagdad boil/button ['bægdæd, bɑɡ'dæd] Hautleishmaniose f, kutane Leishmaniase f, Orientbeule f, Leishmaniasis cutis.
bag·ging ['bægɪŋ] adj → baggy.
bag·gy ['bægɪ] adj sackartig, -förmig; (Haut) schlaff.
Baillarger [baːjɑ'ʒe]: **external band of B.** äußere Baillarger-Schicht f, äußerer Baillarger-Streifen m, Stria laminae granularis interna (corticis cerebri).
external line/stria/stripe of B. → external band of B.
inner band of B. innere Baillarger-Schicht f, innerer Baillarger-Streifen m, Stria laminae pyramidalis ganglionaris/interna (corticis cerebri).
inner line/stria/stripe of B. → inner band of B.
internal band/line/stria/stripe of B. → inner band of B.
outer band/line/stria/stripe of B. → external band of B.
B.'s sign Baillarger'-Zeichen nt.
Bainbridge ['beɪnbrɪdʒ]: **B. reflex** Bainbridge-Reflex m.
bake [beɪk] **I** vt backen; (aus-)dörren, härten, austrocknen; brennen. **II** vi backen, gebacken werden, dörren, hart werden, zusammen- od. festbacken.
Baker ['beɪkər]: **B.'s cyst** Baker-Zyste f.
bak·ers' yeast ['beɪkər] micro. Back-, Bierhefe f, Saccharomyces cerevisiae.
bak·ing soda ['beɪkɪŋ] Natriumbikarbonat nt.
BAL abbr. → British anti-Lewisite.
balan- pref. → balano-.
bal·ance ['bæləns] **I** n 1. Waage f. 2. Balance f, Gleichgewicht nt, (a. physiol.) Haushalt m. **to keep one's ~** (a. fig.) das Gleichgewicht (be-)halten. **to lose one's ~** das Gleichgewicht od. die Fassung verlieren. 3. Gegengewicht nt (to zu); Ausgleich m (to für); phys. Kompensation f. **II** vt 4. wiegen. 5. (ab-, er-)wägen. 6. (s.) im Gleichgewicht halten, ins Gleichgewicht bringen, ausbalancieren. **III** vi s. im Gleichgewicht halten, s. ausbalancieren; Haltung bewahren.
bal·anced ['bælənst] adj (a. fig.) ausgewogen, ausgeglichen, ausbalanciert, im Gleichgewicht befindlich.
balanced anesthesia anes. Neuroleptanästhesie f, -narkose f.
balanced anesthetic technique → balanced anesthesia.
balanced diet ausgewogene od. balancierte Diät/Ernährung/Kost f.
balance disorder Gleichgewichtsstörung f.
central b. zentrale Gleichgewichtsstörung.
balanced translocation genet. balancierte Translokation f.
balance equation Bilanzgleichung f.
bal·a·neu·tics [bælə'njuːtɪks] pl → balneology.
ba·lan·ic epispadias [bə'lænɪk] urol. glanduläre Epispadie f.
balanic hypospadias urol. glanduläre Hypospadie f.
bal·a·nit·ic epispadias [bælə'nɪtɪk] → balanic epispadias.
balanitic hypospadias → balanic hypospadias.
bal·a·ni·tis [bælə'naɪtɪs] n Eichelentzündung f, Balanitis f.
b. of Zoon Balanitis chronica circumscripta benigna plasmacellularis Zoon, Balanoposthitis (chronica) circumscripta plasmacellularis.
balan- pref. Eichel-, Balan(o)-.
bal·a·no·blen·nor·rhea [,bælənəʊ₁blenə'rɪə] n Balanoblennorrhoe f.
bal·a·no·cele ['-siːl] n urol. Balanozele f.
bal·a·no·chlam·y·di·tis [,-,klæmə'daɪtɪs] n gyn. Balanochlamyditis f.
bal·a·no·plas·ty ['-plæstɪ] n urol. Eichel-, Balanoplastik f.
bal·a·no·pos·thi·tis [,-pɑs'θaɪtɪs] n Entzündung f von Eichel und Vorhaut, Eichel-Vorhautkatarrh m, Balanoposthitis f.
bal·a·no·pos·tho·my·co·sis [,-,pɑsθəʊmaɪ'kəʊsɪs] n Corbus-Krankheit f, gangränöse Balanitis f, Balanitis gangraenosa.
bal·a·no·pre·pu·tial [,-prɪ'pjuːʃl] adj Eichel u. Vorhaut betr. od. verbindend.
bal·a·nor·rha·gia [,-'rædʒ(ɪ)ə] n Balanorrhagie f.
bal·an·or·rhea [,-'rɪə] n eitrige/purulente Balanitis f, Balanorrhoe f; Balanoblennorrhoe f.
bal·an·tid·i·al colitis [bælən'tɪdɪəl] Balantidenkolitis f, Kolitis/Colitis f durch Balantidium coli; Balantidiasis f, Balantidiosis f.
balantidial dysentery → balantidiasis.
bal·an·ti·di·a·sis [,bælənti'daɪəsɪs] n Balantidienruhr f, Balantidiose f, Balantidiasis f.
bal·an·tid·i·o·sis [,bæləntɪdɪ'əʊsɪs] n → balantidiasis.
Bal·an·tid·i·um [,-'tɪdɪəm] n micro. Balantidium nt.
bal·an·ti·do·sis [,-tɪ'dəʊsɪs] n → balantidiasis.
bal·a·nus ['bælənəs] n Eichel f, Glans penis.
bald [bɔːld] **I** adj kahl(köpfig), glatzköpfig; ohne Haare, haarlos. **to go ~** eine Glatze bekommen, kahl werden. **II** vi kahl werden, eine Glatze bekommen.
bald·head ['bɔːldhed] n Glatz-, Kahlkopf m.
bald·head·ed ['-hedɪd] adj kahl, glatzköpfig.
bald·ness ['-nɪs] n Kahlheit f.
bald tongue Möller-Glossitis f, Glossodynia exfoliativa.
Baldy ['bɔːldɪ]: **B.'s hysteropexy/operation** Baldy-Operation f.
Baldy-Franke ['fræŋkə]: **B.-F. operation** Baldy-Franke-Operation f.
Baldy-Webster ['webstər]: **B.-W. hysteropexy/operation** Baldy-Webster-Operation f.
Balfour ['bælfʊər, -fər]: **B. bodies** Aegyptianella pullorum.
Balint ['bælɪnt]: **B.'s syndrome** Balint-Syndrom nt.
Bal·kan nephritis/nephropathy ['bɔːlkən] Balkan-Nephropathie f, -Nephritis f, chronische endemische Nephropathie f.
Ball [bɔːl]: **B.'s valves** Valvulae anales.
ball [bɔːl] **I** n **1.** Ball m, Kugel f, kugelförmiger Körper m; Knäuel m; Klumpen m. **2.** anat. Ballen m. **3.** **~s** pl sl. Hoden pl. **II** vt zusammenballen, zu Kugeln formen. **III** vi s. (zusammen-)ballen.
b. of the eye Augapfel m, Bulbus oculi.
b. of (the) foot (Fuß-)Ballen, Unterseite f der Zehengrundgelenke.
b. of thumb Daumenballen, Thenar nt, Eminentia thenaris.
Ballance ['bæləns]: **B.'s sign** Ballance-Zeichen nt.
ball-and-socket articulation Kugelgelenk nt, Artic. spheroidea.
ball-and-socket joint → ball-and-socket-articulation.
ball-and-stick model chem. Kugel-Stab-Modell nt.
ball bleeding Kugelblutung f.
Baller-Gerold ['bælər 'gerəld]: **B.-G. syndrome** embryo., ortho. Baller-Gerold-Syndrom nt.
Ballet [baˈlɛ]: **B.'s disease** Ophthalmoplegia externa.
B.'s sign ophthal. Ballet'-Zeichen nt.
ball hemorrhage → ball bleeding.
bal·lism ['bælɪzəm] n → ballismus.
bal·lis·mus [bə'lɪzməs] n neuro. Ballismus m.
bal·lis·tic [bə'lɪstɪk] adj 1. neuro. Ballismus betr., ballistisch. 2. phys. ballistisch.
bal·lis·tics [bə'lɪstɪks] pl phys. Ballistik f.
bal·lis·to·car·di·o·gram [,bə-'kɑːrdɪəgræm] n abbr. **BCG** Ballistokardiogramm nt abbr. BKG.
bal·lis·to·car·di·o·graph [,-'kɑːrdɪəgræf] n Ballistokardiograph m.
bal·lis·to·car·di·og·ra·phy [,-ˌkɑːrdɪ'ɑgrəfɪ] n Ballistokardiographie f.
bal·loon [bə'luːn] **I** n Ballon m. **II** adj ballonförmig (aufgetrieben), ballonartig, aufgebläht. **III** vt aufblasen, aufblähen, ausdehnen. **IV** vi s. (auf-)blähen.
balloon angioplasty Ballonangioplastik f.
balloon catheter → balloon-tipped catheter.
balloon cell nevus Ballonzellnävus m.
balloon cells 1. Ballonzellen pl. **2.** derm. ballonierte Naevuszellen pl.
balloon dilatation Ballondilatation f.
bal·loon·ing [bə'luːnɪŋ] n patho. Ballonierung f.
ballooning colliquation → ballooning degeneration.
ballooning degeneration patho. Ballonierung f, ballonierende Degeneration f.
balloon tamponade chir. Ballontamponade f.
balloon-tipped catheter Ballonkatheter m.
bal·lotte·ment [bə'lɑtmənt] n Ballottement nt.
ball reamer ortho. Kugelfräse f.
ball-tip reamer → ball reamer.
ball valve HTG Kugelventilprothese f.

balm

balm [bɑːm] *n* 1. Balsam *m*; *pharm*. Balsamum *nt*. 2. heilendes *od*. linderndes Mittel *nt*.
balm·y ['bɑːmɪ] *adj* balsamisch, heilend, lindernd, Balsam-.
bal·ne·ol·o·gy [ˌbælnɪ'ɒlədʒɪ] *n* Bäderkunde *f*, Heilquellenkunde *f*, Balneologie *f*.
bal·ne·o·ther·a·peu·tics [ˌbælnɪəʊθerə'pjuːtɪks] *pl* → balneotherapy.
bal·ne·o·ther·a·py [ˌ-'θerəpɪ] *n* (Heil-)Bäderbehandlung *f*, Balneotherapie *f*.
bal·ne·um ['bælnɪəm] *n*, *pl* **-nea** [-nɪə] Bad *nt*, Balneum *nt*.
Baló [ber'loʊ; baː'loː]: **B.'s disease** Baló-Krankheit, konzentrische Sklerose *f*, Leucoencephalitis periaxialis concentrica. **concentric sclerosis of B.** → B.'s disease.
bal·sam ['bɔːlsəm] *n* 1. Balsam *m*; *pharm*. Balsamum *nt*. 2. heilende *od*. lindernde Substanz *f*.
b. of copaiba Kopaivabalsam, Balsamum copaivae.
b. of Peru Perubalsam, Balsamum peruvianum.
bal·sam·ic [bɔːl'sæmɪk] *adj* → balmy.
Balser ['bɑːlzər]: **B.'s fatty necrosis** Balser-Nekrose *f*.
Balzer ['bɑːlzər]: **B. type sebaceous adenoma** *derm*. Adenoma sebaceum Balzer.
Bamberger ['bæmbərgər]: **B.'s albuminuria** Bamberger-Albuminurie *f*.
B.'s area Bamberger'-(Dämpfungs-)Feld *nt*.
B.'s disease 1. *neuro*. saltatorischer Reflexkrampf *m*, Bamberger-Krankheit *f*. 2. progressive maligne Polyserositis *f*.
B.'s hematogenic albuminuria → B.'s albuminuria.
B.'s sign Alloch(e)irie *f*.
Bamberger-Marie [ma'riː]: **B.-M. disease/syndrome** Marie-Bamberger-Syndrom *nt*, Bamberger-Marie-Syndrom *nt*, Akropachie *f*, hypertrophische pulmonale Osteoarthropathie *f*.
bam·boo bodies [bæm'buː] Asbestkörperchen *pl*.
bamboo hair Bambus-Haare *pl*, Trichorrhexis-Syndrom *nt*, Trichorrhexis invaginata.
bamboo spine *radiol*. Bambusstabwirbelsäule *f*, Bambusform *f*.
ba·meth·an ['beɪmeθæn] *n pharm*. Bamethan *nt*.
Bancroft ['bæŋkrɒft, -krɑːft]: **B.'s filaria** Bancroft-Filarie *f*, Wuchereria bancrofti.
B.'s filariasis Wuchereria bancrofti-Filariose *f*, Wuchereriasis/Filariasis bancrofti, Bancroftose *f*.
ban·crof·ti·an filariasis ['bæŋkrɒftɪən] → Bancroft's filariasis.
ban·crof·ti·a·sis [ˌbæŋkrɒf'taɪəsɪs] *n* → Bancroft's filariasis.
ban·crof·to·sis [ˌ-'təʊsɪs] *n* → Bancroft's filariasis.
band [bænd] *n* 1. Band *nt*, Schnur *f*, Riemen *m*. 2. *anat*. Band *nt*, Bande *f*, bänderähnliche Struktur *f*. 3. → bandage I.
b. of Broca Broca'-Diagonalband, Bandeletta/Stria diagonalis (Broca).
b.s of Hunter-Schreger *dent*. Schreger'-Hunter'-Linien *pl*.
b. of Reil Reil'-Bündel *nt*.
band·age ['bændɪdʒ] **I** *n* Verband *m*; Binde *f*; Bandage *f*. **II** *vt* verbinden, bandagieren, einen Verband anlegen.
bandage sign Rumpel-Leede-Phänomen *nt*.
band·box resonance ['bændbɒks] hypersonorer Klopfschall *m*.
band cell stabkerniger Granulozyt *m*, *inf*. Stabkerniger *m*..

band form → band cell.
band granulocyte → band cell.
ban·di·coot tick ['bændɪkuːt] *micro*. Haemaphysalis humerosa.
band·ing ['bændɪŋ] *n* 1. *chir*. Bändelung *f*. 2. *genet*. Banding *nt*.
band keratitis bandförmige Keratitis *f*.
Bandl ['bændl]: **B.'s ring** *gyn*. Bandl-Kontraktionsring *m*.
band neutrophil → band cell.
band-shaped keratitis → band keratitis.
ban·dy ['bændɪ] *adj* (*Beine*) krumm.
bandy-leg *n* O-Bein *nt*, Genu varum.
bandy-legged *adj* O-beinig, krummbeinig.
bane [beɪn] *n* Gift *m*, Toxin *nt*.
bane·wort ['beɪnwɜːrt] *n* → belladonna 1.
Bang [bæŋ]: **B.'s bacillus** Bang-Bazillus *m*, Brucella abortus, Bact. abortus Bang.
B.'s disease Bang-Krankheit *f*, Rinderbrucellose *f*.
bang [bæŋ] *n* → bhang.
Bangerter [ˈbæŋərtər]: **B.'s method** *ophthal*. Pleoptik *f*.
bank [bæŋk] **I** *n* Bank *f*; Vorrat *m*, Reserve *f* (*of an*). **II** *vt* (*Blut, Gewebe*) konservieren u. aufbewahren.
Bankart ['bæŋkɑːrt]: **B.'s lesion** Bankart-Läsion *f*.
B.'s operation (for shoulder dislocation) *ortho*. Operation *f* nach Bankart.
B.'s (shoulder) repair → B.'s operation (for shoulder dislocation).
banked (human) blood [bæŋkt] konserviertes (Voll-)Blut *nt*, Blutkonserve *f*.
Bannister ['bænɪstər]: **B.'s disease** Quincke-Ödem *nt*, angioneurotisches Ödem *nt*.
Bannwarth ['bænwɑːrθ]: **B.'s syndrome** Bannwarth-Syndrom *nt*.
Banti ['bænti]: **B.'s disease/syndrome** Banti-Krankheit *f*, -Syndrom *nt*.
B antigen Antigen B *nt*.
BAO *abbr*. → basal acid output.
bar- *pref*. → baro-.
bar [bɑːr] **I** *n* 1. Stange *f*, Stab *m*. 2. Barriere *f*, Schranke *f*, Hindernis *nt* (*to für*). 3. *phys*. Bar *nt* (Einheit des Drucks). 4. *dent*. Verbindung(steile *pl*) *f* einer Zahnprothese. 5. (Farb-)Streifen *m*; (Licht-)Strahl *m*. 6. *chir*. Gewebe- *od*. Hautlappen *m*; Knochenstück *nt*. **II** *vt* (ver-)hindern, hemmen, abhalten (*from von*).
b. of bladder Plica interureterica.
bar·ag·no·sis [ˌbæŋər'nəʊsɪs] *n neuro*. Baragnosis *f*, Abarognosis *f*.
Bárány ['bɑːrɑːnɪ]: **B.'s caloric test** → B.'s test 1.
B.'s pointing test → B.'s test 2.
B.'s sign *neuro*. Bárány-Zeichen *nt*.
B.'s symptom 1. Bárány-Drehstarkreizprüfung *f*. 2. Bárány-Kalorisation *f*.
B.'s syndrome Bárány-Syndrom *nt*, Hemicrania centralis *f*.
B.'s test 1. Bárány-Versuch *m*, -Kalorisation *f*. 2. Bárány-Zeigeversuch *m*.
bar·ba ['bɑːrbə] *n* Bart *m*, Barba *f*.
Bar·ba·dos leg [bɑːr'beɪdəʊz, -dəs] Elephantiasis tropica.
bar·ba·ra·lia·lia [ˌbɑːrbərə'leɪlɪə] *n neuro*. Barbaralalie *f*.
bar·bei·ro [bɑːr'beɪrəʊ, -ruː] *n* brasilianische Schreitwanze *f*, Triatoma megista, Panstrongylus megistus.
Barber ['bɑːrbər]: **B.'s psoriasis** Psoriasis pustulosa Typ Königsbeck-Barber, Psoriasis pustulosa palmaris et plantaris.
bar·ber's itch ['bɑːrbər] 1. Bartflechte *f*, Sycosis barbae/simplex/vulgaris, Folliculitis barbae/simplex. 2. (tiefe) Bartflechte *f*, Tinea barbae, Trichophytia

(profunda) barbae, *old* Sycosis (barbae) parasitaria. 3. Pseudofollikulitis *f*.
barber's rash → barber's itch.
bar·bi·tal ['bɑːrbɪtɒl, -tæl] *n pharm*. Barbital *nt*, Diäthylbarbitursäure *f*, Diethylbarbitursäure *f*.
bar·bi·tal·ism ['bɑːrbɪtɒlɪzəm] *n* → barbituism.
bar·bi·tone ['bɑːrbɪtəʊn] *n Brit*. → barbital.
bar·bi·tu·ism [bɑːr'bɪtʃəwɪzəm] *n pharm*. (chronische) Barbituratvergiftung *f*, Barbitalismus *m*, Barbiturismus *m*.
bar·bi·tu·rate [bɑːr'bɪtʃərɪt, -reɪt] *n* 1. Barbiturat *nt*. 2. *pharm*. Schlaf-, Beruhigungs- *od*. Narkosemittel *nt* auf Barbitursäurebasis, Barbiturat *nt*.
bar·bi·tu·ric acid [ˌbɑːrbɪ't(j)ʊərɪk] Barbitursäure *f*, 4-Hydroxyuracil *nt*, Malonylharnstoff *m*.
bar·bi·tu·rism [bɑːr'bɪtʃərɪzəm] *n* → barbituism.
bar·bo·tage [bɑːrbɒ'tɑːʒ] *n chir.*, *anes*. Barbotage *f*.
Barclay-Baron ['bɑːrklɪ 'bærən]: **B.-B. disease** Dysphagia vallecularis.
Barcroft ['bɑːrkrɒft]: **B.'s apparatus** (Haldane-)Barcroft-Apparat *m*.
Barcroft-Warburg ['vɑːrbʊrk]: **B.-W. apparatus/technique** Warburg-Apparat *m*.
Bard [bɑːr(d)]: **B.'s sign** *neuro.*, *HNO* Bard'-Zeichen *nt*.
Bardet-Biedl [bɑːr'de 'biːdəl]: **B.-B. syndrome** Bardet-Biedl-Syndrom *nt*.
Bard-Pic [pɪk]: **B.-P. syndrome** Bard-Pic-Syndrom *nt*.
bare [beər] **I** *adj* 1. nackt, bloß, unbekleidet; kahl. ~ **to the waist** mit nacktem Oberkörper. 2. barhäuptig. 3. *fig*. nackt, ungeschminkt. **II** *vt* freimachen, entblößen. **to ~ one's arm** den Arm freimachen.
bare area of liver zwerchfellfreie nackte Leberoberfläche *f*, Area nuda (hepatis), Pars affixa hepatis.
bare·foot ['beərfʊt] *adj*, *adv* barfuß, barfüßig, mit bloßen Füßen.
bare·foot·ed ['-fʊtɪd] *adj*, *adv* → barefoot.
bare·leg·ged [ˌ-'leg(ɪ)d] *adj*, *adv* mit bloßen Beinen.
bare·ness ['-nɪs] *n* Nacktheit *f*, Blöße *f*; Kahlheit *f*; Dürftigkeit *f*.
bar·es·the·sia [ˌbæres'θiː(ɪ)ə] *n* Druck-, Gewichtssinn *m*, Barästhesie *f*.
bar·es·the·si·om·e·ter [ˌbærəsˌθiːzɪ'ɑmɪtər] *n neuro*. Druck-, Gewichtssinnmesser *m*, Barästhesiometer *m*.
bar·i·to·sis [ˌbærɪ'təʊsɪs] *n* Barium-, Baryt-, Schwerspatstaublunge *f*, Barytose *f*.
bar·i·um ['beərɪəm, 'bɑːr-] *n abbr*. **Ba** Barium *nt abbr*. Ba.
barium chloride Bariumchlorid *nt*.
barium contrast enema *radiol*. Bariumkonstrasteinlauf *m*.
barium contrast enteroclysis *radiol*. Bariumkonstrastdünndarmeinlauf *m*.
barium enema *radiol*. Bariumeinlauf *m*.
barium meal *radiol*. Bariumbrei *m*.
barium oxide Bariumoxid *nt*.
barium sulfate Bariumsulfat *nt*.
barium technique, double-contrast *radiol*. Bariumdoppelkontrastmethode *f*, Bikonstrastmethode *f*.
bark¹ [bɑːrk] **I** *n* 1. *pharm*. Rinde *f*. 2. *bot*. (Baum-)Rinde *f*, Borke *f*. **II** *vt* abschürfen.
bark² [bɑːrk] *vi inf*. (bellend) husten.
Barkan ['bɑːrkən]: **B.'s operation** *ophthal*. Goniotomie *f*, Trabekulotomie *f*.
bark·ing cough ['bɑːrkɪŋ] bellender Husten *m*.
Barkow ['bɑːrkəʊ]: **cervical colliculus of B.** Crista urethralis femininae.

bar·ley bug ['bɑːrlɪ] *micro.* Acarus hordei.
barley mite → barley bug.
Barlow ['bɑːrləʊ]: **B.'s disease** rachitischer Säuglingsskorbut *m*, Möller-Barlow--Krankheit *f*.
B. syndrome Barlow-Syndrom *nt*, Mitralklappenprolaps-Syndrom *nt*, Klick--Syndrom *nt*, Floppy-Valve-Syndrom *nt*.
barn [bɑːrn] *n abbr.* **b** *phys.* Barn *nt abbr.* b.
Barnes ['bɑːrnz]: **B.'s curve** *gyn.* Barnes'--Krümmung *f*.
B.'s dystrophy Barnes'-Syndrom *nt*.
baro- *pref.* Druck-, Gewicht(s)-, Bar(o)-.
bar·o·ag·no·sis [ˌbærəʊæɡˈnəʊsɪs] *n* → baragnosis.
bar·o·cep·tor [ˌbærəʊˈsɛptər] *n* → baroreceptor.
bar·og·no·sis [bæˌrɑɡˈnəʊsɪs] *n neuro.* Barognosis *f*.
bar·o·ma·crom·e·ter [ˌbærəmæˈkrɑmɪtər] *n* Meß- und Wiegeinstrument *nt* für Säuglinge.
bar·o·met·ric pressure [ˌ-ˈmɛtrɪk] *abbr.* **PB** atmosphärischer Druck *m*, Atmosphärendruck *m*.
baro-otitis *n* → barotitis.
bar·o·phil·ic [ˌ-ˈfɪlɪk] *adj bio.* barophil.
bar·o·re·cep·tor [ˌ-rɪˈsɛptər] *n* Barorezeptor *m*.
baroreceptor reflex Barorezeptor(en)reflex *m*.
bar·o·scope ['-skəʊp] *n lab.* Baroskop *nt*.
bar·o·sen·sor [ˌ-ˈsɛnsər, -sɔːr] *n* Barosensor *m*, -rezeptor *m*.
bar·o·si·nus·i·tis [ˌ-ˌsaɪnəˈsaɪtɪs] *n* Aero-, Barosinusitis *f*.
bar·o·spi·ra·tor [ˌ-ˈspaɪreɪtər] *n* Barospirator *m*.
bar·o·tax·is [ˌ-ˈtæksɪs] *n bio.* Barotaxis *f*.
bar·o·ti·tis [ˌ-ˈtaɪtɪs] *n* Aero(o)titis *f*, Baro(o)titis *f*, Otitis barotraumatica.
bar·o·trau·ma [ˌbærəˈtrɔːmə] *n* **1.** Druckverletzung *f*, Barotrauma *nt*. **2.** *(Ohr)* Barotrauma *nt*.
ba·rot·ro·pism [bəˈrɑtrəpɪzəm] *n bio.* Barotropismus *m*.
Barr [bɑːr]: **B. body** Barr'-Körper *m*, Sex-, Geschlechtschromatin *nt*.
Barraquer [barakˈer]: **B.'s disease** Simons--Syndrom *nt*, Lipodystrophia progressiva/paradoxa.
Barraquer-Simons ['saɪmənz; 'ziːmoːnz]: **B.-S.' syndrome** Barraquer-Simons-Syndrom *nt*, Holländer-Simons-Syndrom *nt*, progressive partielle Lipodystrophie *f*, zephalo-thorakale Lipodystrophie *f*, Lipodystrophia progressiva.
Barré [baˈre]: **B.'s (pyramidal) sign** Barré--Beinhalteversuch *m*.
Barré-Guillain [ɡiˈjẽ]: **B.-G. syndrome** Guillain-Barré-Syndrom *nt*, (Poly-)Radikuloneuritis *f*, Neuronitis *f*.
bar·rel ['bærəl] *n* Faß *nt*, Tonne *f*; *(Spritze)* Zylinder *m*.
barrel chest Faßthorax *m*, faß-/tonnenförmiger Thorax *m*.
barrel-chested *adj* einen Faßthorax haben.
barrel-shaped thorax → barrel chest.
bar·ren ['bærən] *adj* **1.** unfruchtbar, steril, infertil. **2.** *fig.* öde, uninteressant; seicht; dürftig, armselig; unproduktiv, arm *(of* an*)*.
bar·ren·ness ['bærənɪs] *n* **1.** Unfruchtbarkeit *f*, Infertilität *f*, Sterilität *f*. **2.** *fig.* Armut *f (of* an*)*; Unproduktivität *f*.
Barrett ['bærɪt]: **B.'s esophagus** Barrett--Ösophagus *m*.
B.'s syndrome Barrett-Syndrom *nt*.
B.'s ulcer Barrett-Ulkus *nt*.
bar·ri·er ['bærɪər] *n* **1.** Barriere *f*, Schranke

f, Sperre *f*; Hindernis *nt (to für)*. **2.** *phys.* Schwelle *f*.
Bart [bɑːrt]: **B.'s syndrome** *derm.* Bart-Syndrom *nt*.
Barth [bɑːrt]: **B.'s hernia** Barth'-Hernie *f*.
Bartholin [ˌbɑːrˈtəʊlɪn, ˈbɑːrtlɪn]: **B.'s cyst** Bartholin'-Zyste *f*.
B.'s duct Ductus sublingualis major.
B.'s gland Bartholin-Drüse *f*, Gl. vestibularis major.
bar·tho·lin·i·an abscess [bɑːrtəˈlɪnɪən] Bartholin'-Abszeß *m*.
bar·tho·lin·i·tis [ˌbɑːrtəlɪˈnaɪtɪs] *n gyn.* Entzündung *f* der Bartholin'-Drüse, Bartholinitis *f*.
Bartholomew [bɑːrˈθɑləmjuː]: **B.'s rule of fourths** *urol.* Bartholomew'-Viererregel *f*.
Barton ['bɑːrtn]: **B.'s bandage** Barton'--Kinnverband *m*.
B.'s fracture *ortho.* Barton-Fraktur *f*.
B.'s operation *ortho.* Ankyloseoperation *f* nach Barton.
Bar·ton·el·la [ˌbɑːrtəˈnɛlə] *n micro.* Bartonella *f*.
B. bacilliformis Bartonella bacilliformis.
Bartonella anemia Anämie *f* bei Bartonellose.
Bar·ton·el·la·ce·ae [ˌbɑːrtnɛˈleɪsɪiː] *pl micro.* Bartonellaceae *pl*.
bar·ton·el·li·a·sis [ˌ-ˈlaɪəsɪs] *n* → bartonellosis.
bar·ton·el·lo·sis [ˌ-ˈləʊsɪs] *n* Carrión--Krankheit *f*, Bartonellose *f*.
Bartter ['bɑːrtər]: **B.'s syndrome** Bartter--Syndrom *nt*, Hyperplasie *f* des juxtaglomerulären Apparates.
ba·ru·ria [bəˈr(j)ʊərɪə] *n* Barurie *f*.
bar·y·es·the·sia [ˌbæriːsˈθiːʒ(ɪ)ə] *n* → baresthesia.
bar·y·glos·sia [ˌ-ˈɡlɒsɪə] *n neuro.* Baryglossie *f*.
bar·y·la·li·a [ˌ-ˈleɪlɪə] *n neuro.* Barylalie *f*.
bar·y·ma·zia [ˌ-ˈmeɪzɪə] *n gyn.* Brusthypertrophie *f*.
bar·y·pho·nia [ˌ-ˈfəʊnɪə] *n neuro.* Baryphonie *f*.
bar·y·to·sis *n* → baritosis.
ba·sal ['beɪsl] *adj* **1.** an der Basis liegend, Basis betr., basal, Basal-, Grund-; fundamental, grundlegend. **2.** *physiol.* den Ausgangswert bezeichnend *(Temperatur etc.)*.
basal acid output *abbr.* **BAO** *(Magen)* basale Säuresekretion *f*., Basalsekretion *f*, basal acid output *abbr.* BAO.
basal anesthesia Basisnarkose *f*, -anästhesie *f*.
basal artery → basilar artery.
basal artery aneurysm Aneurysma *nt* der A. basilaris.
basal body Basalkörperchen *nt*, -körnchen *nt*, Kinetosom *nt*.
basal body temperature *abbr.* **BBT** basale Körpertemperatur *f*, Basaltemperatur *f*.
basal branch: anterior b. of left pulmonary artery Ramus basalis anterior a. pulmonalis sinistrae.
anterior b. of right pulmonary artery Ramus basalis anterior a. pulmonalis dextrae.
lateral b. of left pulmonary artery Ramus basalis lateralis a. pulmonalis sinistrae.
lateral b. of right pulmonary artery Ramus basalis lateralis a. pulmonalis dextrae.
medial b. of left pulmonary artery Ramus basalis medialis a. pulmonalis sinistrae.
medial b. of right pulmonary artery Ramus basalis medialis a. pulmonalis dextrae.

posterior b. of left pulmonary artery Ramus basalis posterior a. pulmonalis sinstrae.
posterior b. of right pulmonary artery Ramus basalis posterior a. pulmonalis dextrae.
basal cell *(Nase)* Basal-, Ersatzzelle *f*.
basal cell adenoma Basalzell(en)adenom *nt*.
basal cell carcinoma *abbr.* **BCC** Basalzell(en)karzinom *nt*, Carcinoma basocellulare.
basal cell epithelioma Basalzellepitheliom *nt*, Basaliom *nt*, Epithelioma basocellulare.
basal cell nevus Basalzellnävus *m*.
basal cell nevus syndrome Gorlin-Goltz--Syndrom *nt*, Basalzellnävus-Syndrom *nt*, nävoides Basalzell(en)karzinom-Syndrom *nt*, nävoide Basaliome *pl*, Naevobasaliome *pl*, Naevobasaliomatose *f*.
basal cistern Cisterna basalis/interpeduncularis.
basal complex of choroid Bruch'-Membran *f*, Complexus/Lamina basalis (choroideae).
basal corpuscle → basal body.
basal decidua Decidua basalis, Decidua serotina.
basal foot *histol.* Basalfuß *m*.
basal fracture of femoral neck *ortho.* intertrochantäre Oberschenkelfraktur/Femurfraktur *f*.
basal ganglia → basal nucleus 2.
basal granular cells basalgekörnte Zellen *pl*.
basal granule *bio.* Basalkörperchen *nt*.
ba·sal·i·o·ma [ˌbaɪˈsælɪˈəʊmə] *n* **1.** → basal cell carcinoma. **2.** → basal cell epithelioma.
basal joint reflex Mayer-Reflex *m*, Daumenmitbewegungsphänomen *nt*.
basal lamina 1. Basallamina *f*, -membran *f*. **2.** *embryo.* Basal-, Grundplatte *f*, Lamina basalis.
b. of choroid Bruch'-Membran *f*, Complexus/Lamina basalis (choroideae).
b. of ciliary body Lamina basalis (corporis ciliaris).
basal layer: b. of endometrium *inf.* Basalaris *f*, Lamina basalis, Stratum basale endometrii.
b. of epidermis Basal(zell)schicht *f*, Stratum basale epidermidis.
basal membrane Basalmembran *f*, -lamina *f*.
b. of semicircular duct Basalmembran des Bogenganges, Membrana basalis ductus semicircularis.
basal metabolic rate *abbr.* **BMR** *physiol.* Basal-, Grundumsatz *m abbr.* GU.
basal metabolism *physiol.* Grundstoffwechsel *m*, Grundumsatz *m*.
basal neck fracture intertrochantere Oberschenkel-/Femurfraktur *f*.
basal nucleus 1. Olivenkern *m*, Nc. olivaris. **2.** ~*i pl* Basalganglien *pl*, Ncc. basales.
b. of amygdaloid body Nc. basalis corporis amygdaloidei.
b. of Meynert Nc. basalis Meynert.
ba·sa·lo·ma [ˌbeɪsəˈləʊmə] *n* **1.** → basal cell carcinoma. **2.** → basal cell epithelioma.
basal plate 1. Dezidual-, Basalplatte *f*. **2.** *embryo.* Basal-, Grundplatte *f*, Lamina basalis.
motor b. *embryo.* motorische Grundplatte.
b. of neural tube *embryo.* Flügelplatte *f*, Lamina alaris.
b. of spermatozoon *(Spermium)* Basalplatte *f*.

basal-prickle cell acanthoma

basal-prickle cell acanthoma Basal-Stachelzellakanthom *nt*.
basal ridge *dent.* Cingulum *nt*.
basal rings (of alveoli) *(Lungenalveolen)* Basalringe *pl*.
basal segment of lung *(Lunge)* Basalsegment *nt*, Segmentum basale.
 anterior b. vorderes Basalsegment, Segmentum basale anterius [S. VIII].
 lateral b. seitliches Basalsegment, Segmentum basale laterale [S. IX].
 medial b. mediales Basalsegment, medial--basales Segment, Segmentum basale mediale, Segmentum cardiacum [S. VII].
 posterior b. hinteres Basalsegment, Segmentum basale posterius [S. X].
basal skull fracture Schädelbasisbruch *m*, -fraktur *f*.
basal squamous cell carcinoma basosquamöses/intermediäres Karzinom *nt*.
basal tone *physiol.* Basistonus *m*, basaler Tonus *m*.
basal vein Rosenthal'-Vene *f*, Basalis *f*, V. basalis.
 common b. gemeinsame Vene der basalen Lungensegmente, Basalis *f* communis, V. basalis communis.
 inferior b. untere Basalvene, Basalis *f* inferior, V. basalis inferior.
 superior b. obere Basalvene, Basalis *f* superior, V. basalis superior.
base [beɪs] **I** *n* **1.** *anat., fig.* Basis *f*. **2.** Grundfläche *f*; Sockel *m*, Fuß *m*, Unterfläche *f*, -teil *nt*. **3.** *chem.* Base *f*. **4.** *pharm.* Grund-, Hauptbestandteil *m*, Grundstoff *m*. **5.** *(Diskussion)* Ausgangspunkt *m*, Grundlage *f*. **II** *adj* **6.** als Basis dienend, Grund-, Basis-, Ausgangs-. **7.** *(Metall)* unecht, unedel; falsch, minderwertig. **8.** unehelich. **III** *vt* basieren, beruhen *(on* auf). **to be ~d on** basierend/beruhend/ begründet/gestützt auf.
 b. of brain Hirnbasis.
 b. of cerebral peduncle Hirnschenkel *m*, Basis pedunculi cerebri, Crus cerebri, Pars anterior/ventralis pedunculi cerebri.
 b. of cochlea Schneckenbasis, Basis cochleae.
 b. of dorsal horn of spinal cord Hinterhornbasis, Basis cornus dorsalis/posterioris medullae spinalis.
 b. of heart Herzbasis, Basis cordis.
 b. of lung Lungenbasis, Basis pulmonis/ pulmonalis.
 b. of mandible Basis mandibulae.
 b. of modiolus Spindelbasis, Basis modioli.
 b. of posterior horn of spinal cord → b. of dorsal horn of spinal cord.
 b. of prostate Prostatabasis, Basis prostatae.
 b. of skull Schädelbasis, Basis cranii.
 b. of stapes Steigbügelplatte *f*, Basis stapedis.
base anhydride Basenanhydrid *nt*.
base-ball finger ['beɪsbɔːl] *ortho.* Hammerfinger *m*.
base catalysis Basenkatalyse *f*.
 general b. allgemeine Basenkatalyse.
 specific b. spezifische Basenkatalyse.
base composition Basenzusammensetzung *f*.
base deficit *physiol.* Basendefizit *nt*, negativer Basenüberschuß *m*.
bas-e-doid ['bɑːzədɔɪd] *n* Basedoid *nt*.
Basedow ['bɑːzədoʊ]: **B.'s disease** Basedow'-Krankheit *f*, Morbus Basedow.
 B.'s goiter Basedow-Struma *f*, Struma basedowiana.
 B.'s triad → B.'s trias.
 B.'s trias Merseburger Trias *f*.

bas-e-dow-i-form [bɑːzə'doʊfɔːrm] *adj* basedowähnlich, -artig.
base equivalence Basenäquivalenz *f*.
base excess *abbr.* **BE** *physiol.* Basenüberschuß *m*, Basenexzess *m* *abbr.* BE.
 negative b. negativer Basenüberschuß, Basendefizit *nt*.
base fracture *ortho.* Knochenbasisfraktur *f*, Bruch *m* der Knochenbasis.
base-frequency analysis *biochem.* Basenfrequenzanalyse *f*.
base injury Laugenverätzung *f*.
base-line ['beɪslaɪn] **I** *n* Richtlinie *f*, Basisniveau *nt*; Grund-, Ausgangslinie *f*. **II** *adj* wesentlich, elementar, grundlegend.
base-ment ['beɪsmənt] *n* Fundament *nt*, Basis *f*, Basal-.
basement layer → basement membrane.
basement membrane Basalmembran *f*, -lamina *f*.
base pair *biochem.* Basenpaar *nt*.
base pairing *biochem.* Basenpaarung *f*.
base sequence *biochem.* Basensequenz *f*.
base substitution *biochem.* Basensubstitution *f*.
base triplet *biochem.* Basentriplett *nt*.
base units Basiseinheiten *pl*.
ba-si-al-ve-o-lar [ˌbeɪsɪæl'vɪələr] *adj* basialveolär.
ba-si-ar-ach-ni-tis [ˌbeɪsɪˌæræk'naɪtɪs] *n* → basiarachnoiditis.
ba-si-a-rach-noid-i-tis [-ˌəˌræknɔɪ'daɪtɪs] *n* Basalmeningitis *f*, Basiarachnoiditis *f*, -arachnitis *f*.
ba-sic ['beɪsɪk] **I** *the* **~s** *pl* das Wesentliche, Grundlagen *pl*. **II** *adj* **1.** grundlegend, wesentlich, Grund-. **2.** *chem.* basisch, alkalisch.
basic bundles of spinal cord Binnen-, Elementar-, Grundbündel *pl* des Rückenmarks, Intersegmentalfaszikel *pl*, Fasciculi proprii (medullae spinalis).
basic degeneration basophile Degeneration *f*.
basic dimension Grunddimension *f*.
basic dye basischer/kationischer Farbstoff *m*.
basic electrical rhythm *abbr.* **BER** *physiol.* *(Darm)* elektrischer Basisrhythmus *m*.
ba-si-chro-ma-tin [baɪsɪ'kroʊmətɪn] *n* *histol.* Basichromatin *nt*.
ba-si-chro-mi-ole [-ˌ'kroʊmɪoʊl] *n* *histol.* Basichromiole *f*.
basic hydrolysis *chem.* basische Hydrolyse *f*.
ba-sic-i-ty [beɪ'sɪsətɪ] *n* *chem.* **1.** Alkalität *f*, Basizität *f*, Basität *f*. **2.** basischer Zustand *m*.
basic knowledge Grundkenntnisse *pl*, -wissen *nt*.
basic lamella *(Knochen)* Generallamelle *f*.
basic needs Grundbedürfnisse *pl*.
ba-si-cra-ni-al [ˌbeɪsɪ'kreɪnɪəl] *adj* Schädelbasis betr., basilar, basilär, Schädelbasis-.
basicranial flexure *embryo.* Rückenbeuge *f*.
basic research Grundlagenforschung *f*.
basic salt *chem.* basisches Salz *nt*.
basic stain 1. basischer Farbstoff *m*. **2.** basische Färbung *f*.
basic tone *physiol.* *(Schall)* Grundton *m*.
ba-sid-ia *pl* → basidium.
ba-sid-i-o-bo-sis [bəˌsɪdɪəbə'loʊsɪs] *n* Basidiobolose *f*.
Ba-sid-i-o-bo-lus [ˌ-'boʊləs] *n* *micro.* Basidiobolus *m*.
Ba-sid-i-o-my-ce-tes [ˌ-maɪ'siːtiːz] *pl* *micro.* Ständerpilze *pl*, Basidiomyzeten *pl*, -mycetes *pl*.
ba-sid-i-o-my-ce-tous [ˌ-maɪ'siːtəs] *adj* Basidiomyzeten betr., Basidiomyzeten-.

ba-sid-i-o-spore ['-spəʊər, -spɔːr] *n* *micro.* Ständer-, Basidiospore *f*.
ba-sid-i-um [bə'sɪdɪəm] *n*, *pl* **-dia** [-dɪə] *micro.* Sporenständer *m*, Basidie *f*, Basidium *nt*.
ba-si-fa-cial [ˌbeɪsɪ'feɪʃl] *adj* untere Gesichtshälfte betr., basifazial.
ba-sig-e-nous [bə'sɪdʒənəs] *adj* *chem.* basenbildend.
ba-si-hy-al [ˌbeɪsɪ'haɪəl] *n* → basihyoid.
ba-si-hy-oid [ˌ-'haɪɔɪd] *n* Zungenbeinkörper *m*, Corpus ossis hyoidei.
bas-i-lar ['bæsɪlər] *adj* **1.** an der Schädelbasis gelegen, zur (Schädel-)Basis gehörend, basilar, basilär, Schädelbasis-. **2.** → basal.
basilar apophysis Pars basilaris ossis occipitalis.
basilar artery Schädelbasisarterie *f*, Basisarterie *f* des Hirnstamms, Basilaris *f*, A. basilaris.
basilar artery aneurysm A.-basilaris-Aneurysma *nt*.
basilar artery migraine Migräne *f* des Basilarisstromgebietes.
basilar cell → basal cell.
basilar clivus Clivus ossis occipitalis.
basilar crest Crista basilaris.
basilar fissure Fissura spheno-occipitalis.
basilar gliosis basiläre Gliose *f*.
basilar groove → basilar sulcus of pons.
 b. of occipital bone Clivus ossis occipitalis.
 b. of pons → basilar sulcus of pons.
 b. of sphenoid bone Clivus ossis sphenoidalis.
basilar impression Platybasie *f*, basilare Impression *f*.
basilar invagination → basilar impression.
basilar membrane Basalmembran *f*, -lamina *f*.
 b. of cochlear duct Basilarmembran, Membrana basilaris (ductus cochlearis).
basilar meningitis Basalmeningitis *f*.
basilar part of pons ventraler Brückenteil *m*, Pars basilaris/anterior pontis.
basilar plexus Plexus basilaris.
basilar skull fracture Schädelbasisbruch *m*, -fraktur *f*.
basilar spine Tuberculum pharyngeum.
basilar sulcus of pons Brückenfurche *f* für A. basilaris, Sulcus basilaris (pontis).
basilar trunk A. basilaris.
bas-i-lar-y ['bæsəˌlerɪ] *adj* → basilar.
ba-si-lat-er-al [ˌbeɪsɪ'lætərəl] *adj* basal u. lateral (liegend), basilateral.
ba-si-lem-ma [ˌ-'lemə] *n* → basilar membrane.
ba-sil-ic vein [bə'sɪlɪk] Basilika *f*, V. basilica.
 intermedian b. Intermedia/Mediana *f* basilica, V. mediana basilica.
 median b. → intermedian b.
ba-sin ['beɪsn] *n* **1.** Becken *nt*, Schale *f*, Behälter *m*, Basin *nt*. **2.** Becken *nt*, Pelvis *f*.
ba-si-on ['beɪsɪˌɑn] *n* *anat.* Basion *nt*.
ba-sip-e-tal [beɪ'sɪpɪtl] *adj* in Richtung zur Basis hin, basipetal.
ba-si-pha-ryn-ge-al canal [ˌbeɪsɪfə'rɪndʒ(ɪ)əl] Canalis basipharyngeus, Canalis craniovaginalis.
ba-si-phil-ic [ˌ-'fɪlɪk] *adj* → basophil II.
ba-sis ['beɪsɪs] *n*, *pl* **-ses** [-siːz] Basis *f*, Grund *m*, Grundlage *f*, Fundament *nt*. **on the ~** auf der Basis von, auf Grund von. **on the ~ that** davon ausgehend, daß. **to provide/form/lay the ~ for/of sth.** die Grundlage *od.* Basis bilden für etw. **to be treated on an outpatient ~** als ambulanter Patient behandelt werden.
b. of comparison Vergleichsbasis.

ba·si·squa·mous carcinoma [ˌbeɪsɪ'sweɪməs] → basosquamous carcinoma.
ba·si·ver·te·bral [ˌ-'vɜːtəbrəl] *adj* Wirbelkörper betr., Wirbelkörper-.
basivertebral veins Wirbelkörpervenen *pl*, Vv. basivertebrales.
bas·ket ['bæskət; *Brit.* 'bɑːskɪt] *n* Korb *m*.
basket case *sl.* **1.** Arm- u. Beinamputierte(r *m*) *f*. **2.** Nervenbündel *nt*.
basket cell 1. Korbzelle *f*. **2.** Myoepithelzelle *f*.
columnar b. säulenartige Korbzelle.
basket fibers Korbfasern *pl*.
ba·so·cy·to·sis [ˌbeɪsəʊsaɪ'təʊsɪs] *n hema.* Basozytose *f*, Basophilie *f*.
ba·so·e·ryth·ro·cyte [ˌ-ɪ'rɪθrəsaɪt] *n* basophiler Erythrozyt *m*.
ba·so·lat·er·al part of amygdaloid body [ˌ-'lætərəl] untere Kerngruppe *f* des Mandelkerns, Pars basolateralis (corporis amygdaloidei).
ba·so·met·a·chro·mo·phil [ˌ-ˌmetə'krəʊməfɪl] *adj histol.* basometachromophil.
ba·so·phil ['-fɪl] **I** *n* **1.** mit basischen Farbstoffen anfärbbare Zelle *od.* Struktur *f*. **2.** *hema.* basophiler Leukozyt/Granulozyt *m*, *inf.* Basophiler *m*. **3.** (*Adenohypophyse*) basophile Zelle *f*, β-Zelle *f*. **II** *adj* **4.** basophil, mit basischen Farbstoffen anfärbbar. **5.** basophil, aus basophilen Zellen *od.* Strukturen bestehend.
basophil adenoma → basophilic adenoma.
basophil cell → basophilic cell.
basophil chemotactic factor *abbr.* **BCF** *immun.* Basophilen-chemotaktischer Faktor *m abbr.* BCF, basophil chemotactic factor *abbr.* BCF.
ba·so·phile ['-faɪl, -fɪl] *n*, *adj* → basophil.
ba·so·phil·ia [ˌ-'fɪlɪə, -jə] *n* **1.** *hema.* Basozytose *f*. **2.** *hema.* Basophilie *f*. **3.** *histol.* Anfärbbarkeit mit basischen Farbstoffen, Basophilie *f*.
ba·so·phil·ic [ˌ-'fɪlɪk] *adj* → basophil II.
basophilic adenoma basophiles (Hypophysen-)Adenom.
basophilic cell 1. mit basischen Farbstoffen anfärbbare Zelle *f*, basophile Zelle *f*. **2.** (*Adenohypophyse*) basophile Zelle *f*, β--Zelle *f*.
basophilic degeneration basophile Degeneration *f*.
basophilic erythrocyte → basoerythrocyte.
basophilic granulocyte → basophilic leukocyte.
basophilic leukemia Basophilenleukämie *f*, Blutmastzell-Leukämie *f*.
basophilic leukocyte *hema.* basophiler Leukozyt/Granulozyt *m*, *inf.* Basophiler *m*.
basophilic leukocytosis Basophilie *f*, Basozytose *f*.
basophilic leukopenia Basopenie *f*.
basophilic myelocyte basophiler Myelozyt *m*.
basophilic normoblast basophiler Normoblast *m*.
basophilic series → basophil series.
basophil leukopenia Basopenie *f*.
ba·so·phil·o·cyte [ˌbeɪsə'fɪləsaɪt] *n* → basophilic leukocyte.
ba·so·phil·o·cyt·ic leukemia [ˌ-fɪlə'sɪtɪk] → basophilic leukemia.
ba·soph·i·lous [beɪ'sæfələs] *adj* → basophil II.
basophil series *hema.* basophile Reihe *f*.
basophil substance Nissl-Schollen *pl*, -Substanz *f*, -Granula *pl*, Tigroidschollen *pl*.
ba·so·pho·bia [ˌbeɪsə'fəʊbɪə] *n psychia.* krankhafte Angst *f* vorm Laufen, Basophobie *f*.
ba·so·plasm ['-plæzəm] *n histol.* Basoplasma *nt*.
ba·so·squa·mous carcinoma [ˌ-'skweɪməs] basosquamöses/intermediäres Karzinom *nt*.
bass deafness [beɪs] Schwerhörigkeit *f* für niedrige Frequenzen.
Bassen-Kornzweig ['bæsn 'kɔːrnzwaɪg]: **B.-K. syndrome** Bassen-Kornzweig-Syndrom *nt*, Abetalipoproteinämie *f*, A--Beta-Lipoproteinämie *f*.
Bassini [bə'siːnɪ]: **B.'s operation/procedure** Bassini-Operation *f*, Herniotomie *f* nach Bassini.
B.'s suture Bassini-Naht *f*.
Bassler [bə'siːn]: **B.'s sign** *chir.* Bassler-Zeichen *nt*.
bas·tard ['bæstəd] **I** *n* **1.** *bio., genet.* Mischling *m*, Bastard *m*. **2.** uneheliches Kind *nt*. **II** *adj* **3.** unehelich. **4.** *bio., genet.* hybrid, Hybrid-, Bastard-, Mischlings-. **5.** *fig.* nachgemacht, unecht, verfälscht, Bastard-, Pseudo-.
bas·tard·i·za·tion [ˌbæstədaɪ'zeɪʃn] *n bio., genet.* Bastardidierung *f*, Hybridisierung *f*, Hybridisation *f*.
bas·tard·ize ['bæstədaɪz] **I** *vt* entarten lassen, bastardieren, hybridisieren. **II** *vi* entarten.
Bastedo [bæs'tiːdəʊ]: **B.'s sign** *chir.* Bastedo'-Zeichen *nt*.
bat [bæt] *n bio.* Fledermaus *f*.
batch [bætʃ] *n* **1.** Schub *m*; Schwung *m*; Ladung *f*; Stapel *m*. **2.** *pharm.* Charge *f*. **in ~es** schubweise.
batch·wise ['bætʃwaɪz] *adj* schub-, stoß-, chargenweise.
bat ear abstehende Ohrmuschel *f*, abstehendes Ohr *nt*.
bath [bæθ; bɑːθ] **I** *n* **1.** Bad *nt*, Badezimmer *nt*. **2.** (Bade-)Wanne *f*. **3.** Baden *nt*, Bad *nt*. **to take/have a ~** baden, ein Bad nehmen. **4.** *chem.* Bad *nt*. **II** *vt* baden. **III** *vi* baden, ein Bad nehmen.
bathe [beɪð] **I** *vt* **1.** baden. **2.** befeuchten; (*Wunde*) baden, spülen, auswaschen. **II** *vi* ein (Sonnen-)Bad nehmen; baden, schwimmen.
bath·es·the·sia [ˌbæθes'θiːʒ(ɪ)ə] *n* → bathyesthesia.
bath·ing ['beɪðɪŋ] *n* Baden *nt*.
bathing trunk nevus *derm.* Badehosennävus *m*, Schwimmhosennävus *m*.
bath·mo·trop·ic [ˌbæθmə'trɒpɪk, -trəʊ-] *adj* bathmotrop.
bath·mot·ro·pism [bæθ'mɒtrəpɪzəm] *n* Bathmotropie *f*, bathmotrope Wirkung *f*.
bath·o·chrome ['bæθəkrəʊm] *n phys., chem.* Bathochrom *nt*.
bath·o·chrom·y [ˌ-'krəʊmɪ] *n phys., chem.* Bathochromie *f*.
bath·o·pho·bia [ˌ-'fəʊbɪə] *n psychia.* Höhen-, Tiefenangst *f*, Bathophobie *f*.
bath robe Bademantel *m*, Morgenrock *m*.
bath·room ['bæθruːm] *n* **1.** Bad(ezimmer *nt*) *nt*. **2.** Toilette *f*. **to go to/use the ~** auf Toilette gehen.
bath salt Badesalz *nt*.
bath sheet Badetuch *nt*.
bath sponge Badeschwamm *m*.
bath towel Badetuch *nt*.
bath tub (Bade-)Wanne *f*.
bath water Badewasser *nt*.
bath·y·an·es·the·sia [ˌbæθɔʊænəs'θiːʒə] *n neurol.* Verlust *m* der Tiefensensibilität, Bathyanästhesie *f*.
bath·y·car·dia [ˌ-'kɑːdɪə] *n* Bathykardie *f*, Herzsenkung *f*, -tiefstand *m*, Wanderherz *nt*, Kardioptose *f*.

bath·y·chrome *n* → bathochrome.
bath·y·es·the·sia [ˌbæθes'θiːʒ(ɪ)ə] *n neurol.* Tiefensensibilität *f*, Bathyästhesie *f*.
bath·y·gas·try [ˌ-'gæstrɪ] *n* Magensenkung *f*, -tiefstand *m*, Gastroptose *f*.
bath·y·hy·per·es·the·sia [ˌ-ˌhaɪpəres'θiːʒ(ɪ)ə] *n neurol.* Bathyhyperästhesie *f*.
bath·y·hyp·es·the·sia [ˌ-ˌhɪpes'θiːʒ(ɪ)ə] *n neurol.* Bathyhyp(o)ästhesie *f*.
bath·y·pne·a [ˌbæθɪ'(p)niːə] *n* vertiefte Atmung *f*, Bathypnoe *f*.
ba·tra·chi·an position [bə'treɪkɪən] Frosch(schenkel)stellung *f*.
ba·trach·o·pho·bia [bəˌtrækə'fəʊbɪə] *n psychia.* krankhafte Angst *f* vor Fröschen, Batrachophobie *f*.
Batson ['bætsən]: **B.'s (venous) plexus** Venenplexus *pl* der Wirbelsäule, Plexus venosi vertebralis externi et interni.
Batten ['bætn]: **B. disease** → Batten--Mayou disease.
'Batten-Mayou ['meɪjəʊ]: **B.-M. disease** Stock-Vogt-Spielmeyer-Syndrom *nt*, Batten-Spielmeyer-Vogt-Syndrom *nt*, neuronale/juvenile Zeroidlipofuszinose/Ceroidlipofuscinose *f*, juvenile Form *f* der amaurotischen Idiotie.
bat·ter ['bætər] *vt* (heftig u. wiederholt) schlagen, (ver-)prügeln, einschlagen auf; mißhandeln.
bat·tered child syndrome ['bætərd] Syndrom *nt* des geschlagenen Kindes, Battered-child-Syndrom *nt*.
battered parents syndrome Syndrom *nt* der geschlagenen Eltern, Battered--parents-Syndrom *nt*.
bat·ter·y ['bætərɪ] *n*, *pl* **-ter·ies 1.** Gruppe *f*, Reihe *f*, Satz *m*, Batterie *f*. **2.** *psycho.* Persönlichkeitstest(reihe *f*) *m*. **3.** *electr.* Batterie *f*.
b. of experts Expertengruppe *f*.
b. of measurements eine Reihe von Maßnahmen.
b. of tests Testbatterie, Versuchs-, Testreihe, mehrteilige/-stufige Testanordnung *f*.
Battey ['bætɪ]: **B.'s bacillus** Mycobacterium avium/intracellulare, Mycobacterium tuberculosis typus gallinaceus.
Battle ['bætl]: **B.'s incision** Battle-Schnitt *m*.
B.'s sign *ortho.* Battle-Zeichen *nt*, Mastoidknötchen *nt* bei Schädelbasisfraktur.
Battle-Jalaguier-Kammerer ['jɑːlɑːgɪər 'kæmərər]: **B.-J.-K. incision** → Battle's incision.
Baudelocque [bodə'lɒk]: **B.'s diameter** Conjugata externa, Diameter Baudelocque *f*.
Bauhin ['bɔː(h)ɪn]: **B.'s gland** (Blandin-)-Nuhn'-Drüse *f*, Gl. lingualis anterior, Gl. apicis linguae.
B.'s valve Bauhin-Klappe *f*, Ileozäkal-, Ileozökalklappe *f*, Valva ileocaecalis/ilealis.
Baumann ['baʊmən]: **B.'s angle** *ortho.* Baumann'-Winkel *m*.
Baumés [bo'me]: **B.'s scale** Baumé-Skala *f*.
Baumès [bo'mɛ]: **B.'s sign** retrosternaler Schmerz *m* bei Angina pectoris.
B.'s symptom → B.'s sign.
bay [beɪ] *n* **1.** Lorbeer(baum *m*) *m*. **2.** Abteilung *f*, Fach *nt*; (Kranken-)Saal *m*.
Bayard ['beɪəd]: **B.'s ecchymosis** Bayard'--Ekchymosen *pl*.
Bayes [beɪz]: **B.' theorem** *stat.* Bayes--Theorem *nt*.
Bayle [beɪl]: **B.'s disease** *neuro.* progressive Paralyse *f abbr.* PP, Paralysis progressiva.

bay leaf Lorbeerblatt nt.
Bayliss ['beɪlɪs]: **B. effect** Bayliss-Effekt m.
bay-o-net forceps ['beɪənɪt, -net] chir. Bayonettpinzette f.
bayonet needle holder chir. Bayonettnadelhalter m.
bayonet rongeur chir. Bayonettzange f.
bayonet scissors chir. Bayonettschere f.
bay sickness histor. Haff-Krankheit f.
Bazex ['beɪzeks]: **B.'s syndrome** Bazex-Syndrom nt, Akrokeratose f Bazex, paraneoplastische Akrokeratose f, Acrokeratosis paraneoplastica.
Bazin [ba'zɛ̃]: **B.'s disease** Bazin'-Krankheit f, nodöses Tuberkulid nt, Erythema induratum.
BBB abbr. 1. → blood-brain barrier. 2. → bundle-branch block.
B bile B-Galle f, Blasengalle f.
BBT abbr. → basal body temperature.
BC abbr. → biotin carboxylase.
BCAA abbr. → branched chain amino acid.
BCC abbr. → basal cell carcinoma.
BCCP abbr. → biotin carboxyl-carrier protein.
BCDF abbr. → B-cell differentiation factors.
B cell 1. (Pankreas) β-Zelle f, B-Zelle f. 2. (Adenohypophyse) basophile Zelle f, β-Zelle f. 3. hema. B-Lymphozyt m, B-Zelle f.
B cell differentiation factor BSF-2 Humaninterferon-β$_2$ nt.
B-cell differentiation factors abbr. **BCDF** B-Zelldifferenzierungsfaktoren pl.
B-cell growth factors abbr. **BCGF** B-Zellenwachstumsfaktoren pl.
B-cell hyperplasia B-Zellen-Hyperplasie f.
B-cell immunoplastic sarcoma B-Zellen-immunoplastisches Sarkom nt.
B-cell lymphoma B-Zellymphom nt, B-Zellenlymphom nt.
B-cell progenitor B-Zellvorläufer(zelle f) m.
B-cell system B-Zellsystem nt.
B cell tumor (Pankreas) B(eta)-Zelltumor m, Insulinom nt.
BCF abbr. → basophil chemotactic factor.
BCG abbr. 1. → Bacillus Calmette-Guérin. 2. → ballistocardiogram.
BCGF abbr. → B-cell growth factors.
BCG vaccination BCG-Impfung f.
BCG vaccine BCG-Impfstoff m, BCG-Vakzine f.
B chain (Insulin) B-Kette f.
B chromosome überzähliges Chromosom nt.
b.d. abbr. [bis die] pharm. zweimal am Tag.
BE abbr. 1. → base excess. 2. → below-elbow.
Be abbr. → beryllium.
bead [biːd] n Perle f; (Schaum) Bläschen nt; (Schweiß) Tröpfchen nt, Perle f.
bead-ed hair ['biːdɪd] derm. Spindelhaare pl, Monilethrichie f, Monilethrix(-Syndrom nt) f, Aplasia pilorum intermittens.
bead-y ['biːdɪ] adj (Augen) rund u. glänzend.
beady-legged winter horse tick micro. Margaropus winthemi.
beak [biːk] n 1. (Gefäß) Tülle f, Ausguß m; (Katheter) Spitze f. 2. anat., zoo. Fortsatz m, schnabelförmiges Ende nt. 3. Adlernase f. 4. zoo. Schnabel m.
beaked [biːkt, 'biːkɪd] adj 1. mit (einem) Schnabel; schnabelförmig, Schnabel-. 2. vorspringend, spitz. 3. eine Adlernase haben.
beaked pelvis (Becken) Schnabelform f.
beak-er ['biːkər] n Becher m; chem. Becherglas nt.

beaker cell histol. Becherzelle f.
Beale [biːl]: **B.'s (ganglion) cells** Beale'-Ganglienzellen pl.
Beals [biːlz]: **B.' syndrome** Beals-Syndrom nt.
beam [biːm] I n 1. (Licht-)Strahl m, Bündel nt. 2. phys. Peil-, Leit-, Richtstrahl m. 3. Balken m, Stange f, Holm m, Querstange f. II vt 4. mit Balken/Stangen versehen. 5. ausstrahlen. III vi a. fig. strahlen.
b. of rays Strahlenbündel.
Bean [biːn]: **B.'s syndrome** Blaue-Gummiblasen-Nävus-Syndrom nt, Bean-Syndrom nt, blue rubber bleb nevus syndrome (nt).
bean [biːn] n bot. Bohne f.
bean-like ['biːnlaɪk] adj bohnenartig, -förmig.
bear [beər] (**bore**; **borne**) vt 1. (Last, Folgen, Verantwortung) tragen; (Namen) führen; (Gefühle) empfinden; (Spuren) aufweisen, zeigen. 2. (Schmerzen) ertragen, aushalten, (er-)leiden. 3. zur Welt bringen, gebären. 4. (Früchte) tragen. 5. ~ o.s. s. betragen, s. benehmen.
bear down vi (bei der Geburt) pressen.
bear-a-ble ['beərəbl] adj erträglich, zum Aushalten.
Beard [bɪərd]: **B.'s disease** Beard-Syndrom nt, Nervenschwäche f, nervöse Übererregbarkeit f, Neurasthenie f, Neurasthenia f.
beard [bɪərd] n 1. Bart m. 2. zoo. Bartfäden pl, Barteln pl; bot. Grannen pl.
beard-ed ['bɪərdɪd] adj 1. bärtig, einen Bart tragend. 2. zoo. mit Barteln versehen; bot. mit Grannen versehen.
beard-less ['bɪərdlɪs] adj 1. bartlos. 2. fig. (Mann) jugendlich, unreif.
bear-ing ['beərɪŋ] n 1. Betragen nt, Verhalten nt; (Körper-)Haltung f. 2. Einfluß m, Auswirkung f (on auf).
bearing-down gyn. I n Pressen nt. II vt pressen.
bearing-down pain gyn. Senkungsschmerz m.
Bearn-Kunkel [bɑrn 'kʌŋkl]: **B.-K. syndrome** → Bearn-Kunkel-Slater syndrome.
Bearn-Kunkel-Slater ['sleɪtər]: **B.-K.-S. syndrome** Bearn-Kunkel(-Slater)-Syndrom nt, lupoide Hepatitis f.
beat [biːt] (v: **beat; beaten**) I n 1. Pochen nt, Schlagen nt, Klopfen nt. 2. (Puls, Herz) Schlag m. II vt schlagen, (ver-)prügeln. III vi schlagen, pulsieren, pochen, klopfen.
beat frequency Schlagfrequenz f.
Beatty-Bright ['biːtɪ braɪt]: **B.-B. friction sound** Reibegeräusch nt bei Pleuritis, Pleurareiben nt.
Beau [boʊ; bo]: **B.'s disease** Herzinsuffizienz f.
B.'s lines Beau-Furchen pl, -Linien pl.
B.'s syndrome Herzstillstand m, Asystolie f.
beau-ty mark ['bjuːtɪ] Schönheitsfleck m.
Beauvais [boˈvɛ]: **B.' disease** rheumatoide Arthritis f, progrediente/primär chronische Polyarthritis f abbr. PCP, PcP.
Bechterew → Bekhterev.
Beck [bek]: **B.'s gastrotomy** chir. Gastrotomie f nach Beck.
B.'s triad card. Beck-Trias f.
Becker: **B.'s dystrophy** Becker-Muskeldystrophie f.
B.'s nevus Becker-Nävus m, -Melanose f, Melanosis naeviformis.
B.'s muscular dystrophy → B.'s dystrophy.
B.'s phenomenon → B.'s sign.
B.'s sign ophthal. Becker'-Zeichen nt.
Beckmann ['bekmən, -mɑn]: **B.'s apparatus/thermometer** phys. Beckmann-Apparat m, -Thermometer nt.
Beckwith ['bekwɪθ]: **B.'s syndrome** Beckwith-Syndrom nt.
Beckwith-Wiedemann ['viːdəmən]: **B.-W. syndrome** Beckwith-Wiedemann-Syndrom nt, Exomphalos-Makroglossie-Gigantismus-Syndrom nt, EMG-Syndrom nt.
Béclard [beˈklaːr]: **B.'s amputation** Béclard-Amputation f, Hüftgelenksexartikulation f nach Béclard.
B.'s hernia Béclard-Hernie f.
B.'s sign ped. Béclard-Reifezeichen nt.
B.'s triangle Béclard-Dreieck nt.
bec·lo·meth·a·sone [ˌbekloʊˈmeθəsoʊn] n pharm. Beclomet(h)ason nt.
bec·que·rel [bekəˈrel, beˈkrel] n abbr. **Bq** Becquerel nt abbr. Bq.
bed [bed] I n 1. Bett nt; (Feder-)Bett nt; Lager nt. **to be brought to ~** entbunden werden (of von). **to be confined to ~/confinement to ~** bettläg(e)rig sein. **to be in ~** mit dem Bett s.; das Bett hüten. **to die in one's ~** eines natürlichen Todes sterben. **to go to ~** 1. ins Bett gehen. 2. ins Bett gehen (with mit). **to keep one's ~** das Bett hüten. **to make the ~** das Bett machen. **to get/put to ~** jdn. ins/zu Bett bringen. **to take to one's ~** s. (krank) ins Bett legen. 2. anat. Bett nt. 3. techn. Unterlage f, -bau m, Fundament nt, Schicht f. II vt zu Bett bringen, ins Bett legen; (ein-)betten. **to be ~ded** bettlägerig sein.
bed-bath n (Kranken-)Wäsche f im Bett.
bed-bug ['bedbʌg] n (gemeine) Bettwanze f, Cimex lectularius.
bed-case ['bedkeɪs] n bettlägriger Patient m.
bed-clothes ['bedkloʊðs] pl Bettzeug nt.
bed-cov-er ['bedkʌvər] n Bettdecke f.
bed-ding [bedɪŋ] n Bettzeug nt.
bed-lamp ['bedlæmp] n Nachttischlampe f.
Bednar ['bednɑːr]: **B.'s aphthae** Bednar-Aphthen pl.
bed-pan ['bedpæn] n Bettpfanne f.
bed rest 1. Bettruhe f. **to place/keep a patient on complete ~** einem Patienten absolute Bettruhe verordnen. 2. (Bett) verstellbare Rückenstütze f.
bed-rid-den ['bedrɪdn] adj bettläg(e)rig.
bed-room ['bedruːm, -rʊm] n Schlafzimmer nt.
bed-side ['bedsaɪd] n Bettkante f, -rand m. **at the ~** am Krankenbett.
bedside manner Verhalten nt des Arztes am Krankenbett.
Bed-so-nia [bedˈsoʊnɪə] n micro. Chlamydie f, Chlamydia f, PLT-Gruppe f, old Bedsonia f, old Miyagawanella f.
bed-sore ['bedsɔːr, -soʊr] n auf- od. wundgelegene Stelle f, Druckgeschwür nt, Wundliegen nt, Dekubitalulkus nt, Dekubitus m. **to get ~s** s. wund- od. aufliegen.
bed-stand ['bedstænd] n Nachttisch m.
bed table → bedstand.
bed-time [bedtaɪm] n Schlafenszeit f. **to be taken at ~** vor dem Schlafengehen (ein-)nehmen.
bed-wet-ter ['bedwetər] n Bettnässer m.
bed-wet-ting ['bedwetɪŋ] n Bettnässen nt, nächtliches Einnässen nt, Enuresis nocturna.
beef [biːf] n Rindfleisch nt.
beef erythrocytes Rindererythrozyten pl.
beef tapeworm Rinder(finnen)bandwurm m, Taenia saginata, Taeniarhynchus saginatus.
Beer [bɪər]: **B.'s law** Lambert-Beer-Gesetz nt.
beer heart [bɪər] Bierherz nt.

bees·wax ['bi:zwæks] *n* Bienenwachs *nt*.
bee·tle [bi:tl] **I** *n* **1.** Käfer *m*; Küchenschabe *f*. **2.** *pharm.* Stößel *m*. **II** *adj* vorstehend, überhängend. **III** *vi* vorstehen, überhängen.
beetle brows buschige zusammengewachsene Augenbrauen *pl*.
beet sugar [bi:t] Rübenzucker *m*.
be·fore [bɪ'fɔːr, -fəʊr] **I** *adv* (*zeitlich*) vorher, zuvor, früher, bereits, schon; (*räumlich*) vorn, voran. **II** *prep* (*räumlich, zeitlich*) vor.
before death prämortal, ante mortem.
before term *gyn.* (*Geburt*) vorzeitig.
be·gin [bɪ'gɪn] (**began; begun**) *vt, vi* beginnen, anfangen.
be·gin·ner [bɪ'gɪnər] *n* Anfänger(in *f*) *m*, Neuling *m*.
be·gin·ning [bɪ'gɪnɪŋ] *n* **1.** Beginn *m*, Anfang *m*. **at/in the ~** am/im Anfang, zuerst, anfangs. **from the (very) ~** (ganz) von Anfang an. **2.** Anfang *m*, Ursprung *m*. **3. ~s** *pl* (erste) Anfänge *pl*, Anfangsstadium *nt*.
Béguez César [be'gez se'zaːr]: **B. C. disease** Béguez César-Anomalie *f*, Chédiak-Higashi-Syndrom *nt*, Chédiak-Steinbrinck-Higashi-Syndrom *nt*, Béguez César-Anomalie *f*.
be·have [bɪ'heɪv] **I** *vt* **~ o.s.** s. benehmen. **II** *vi* s. verhalten, s. benehmen (*to, towards* gegenüber); (*Kinder*) s. benehmen, s. betragen.
be·hav·ior [bɪ'heɪvjər] *n* **1.** Benehmen *nt*; (*Kinder*) Betragen *nt*; *psycho.* Verhalten *nt* (*to, towards* gegenüber, zu). **2.** *chem., phys., techn.* Verhalten *nt*.
be·hav·ior·al [bɪ'heɪvjərəl] *adj* Verhalten betr., Verhaltens-.
behavioral adaptation Verhaltensanpassung *f*.
behavioral disturbance Verhaltensstörung *f*.
behavioral memory Verhaltensgedächtnis *nt*.
behavioral psychology → behavioristic psychology.
behavioral science Verhaltensforschung *f*.
behavioral scientist Verhaltensforscher(in *f*) *m*.
behavior disorder *psycho.* Verhaltensstörung *f*.
be·hav·ior·ism [bɪ'heɪvjərɪzəm] *n psycho.* Behaviorismus *m*.
be·hav·ior·ist [bɪ'heɪvjərɪst] *psycho.* **I** *n* Behaviorist *m*. **II** *adj* → behavioristic.
be·hav·ior·is·tic [bɪˌheɪvjə'rɪstɪk] *adj psycho.* behavioristisch.
be·hav·ior·is·tic·al [-,'rɪstɪkl] *adj* → behavioristic.
behavioristic psychology behavioristische Psychologie *f*.
behavior modification Verhaltenstherapie *f*.
behavior pattern Verhaltensmuster *nt*, -weise *f*.
behavior reflex erworbener/bedingter Reflex *m*.
behavior therapy *psycho.* Verhaltenstherapie *f*.
behavior trait Verhaltensmerkmal *nt*.
Behçet ['beɪset]: **B.'s disease/syndrome** Behçet-Krankheit *f*, -Syndrom *nt*, bipolare/große/maligne Aphthose *f*, Gilbert-Syndrom *nt*, Aphthose Touraine/Behçet.
be·hen·ic acid [bə'henɪk, -'hiːn-] Behensäure *f*.
be·hind [bɪ'haɪnd] **I** *n inf.* Hinterteil *nt*, Hintern *m*. **II** *adj* zurück, im Rückstand. **III** *prep.* (*räumlich, zeitlich*) hinter. **IV** *adv* hinten, dahinter; nach hinten, zurück.
be·ing ['biːɪŋ] *n* **1.** Sein *nt*, Dasein *nt*, Leben *nt*. **2.** (Lebe-)Wesen *nt*, Geschöpf *nt*. **3.** Wesen *nt*, Natur *f*. **to come into ~** entstehen.

Behla ['beɪlɑ]: **B.'s bodies** Plimmer-Körperchen *pl*.
Behr [ber]: **B.'s disease** Behr'-Krankheit *f*, Optikusatrophie *f*.
Behring ['beɪrɪŋ]: **B.'s law** Behring-Gesetz *nt*.
BEI *abbr.* → butanol-extractable iodine.
Beigel ['baɪgəl]: **B.'s disease** Beigel'-Krankheit *f*, (weiße) Piedra *f*, Trichomycosis nodosa.
bei·kost ['baɪkəʊst] *n ped.* Beikost *f*, -nahrung *f*.
bej·el ['bedʒəl] *n* endemische Syphilis *f*, Bejel *f*.
Békésy ['beɪkəʃi, 'beɪkeɪʃi]: **B. audiometry** Békésy-Audiometrie *f*.
B.'s dispersion theory Dispersions-/Wanderwellentheorie *f* nach Békésy.
B.'s traveling wave theory → B.'s dispersion theory.
Bekhterev ['bektəˌref]: **B.'s arthritis** → B.'s disease.
B.'s disease Bechterew-Krankheit *f*, Morbus Bechterew, Bechterew-Strümpell-Marie-Krankheit *f*, Marie-Strümpell-Krankheit *f*, Spondylarthritis/Spondylitis ankylopoetica/ankylosans.
B.'s nucleus Bechterew-Kern *m*, Nc. vestibularis rostralis/superior.
B.'s reflex 1. Bechterew-Hackenreflex *m*. **2.** Bechterew-Augenreflex *m*. **3.** femoroabdominaler Reflex *m*. **4.** Bechterew-Reflex *m*, paradoxer Pupillenreflex *m*.
B.'s sign 1. Bechterew-Symptom *nt*. **2.** → B.'s reflex 1. **3.** → B.'s reflex 2. **4.** → B.'s reflex 3. **5.** → B.'s reflex 4.
B.'s syndrome Bechterew-Syndrom *nt*.
B.'s test Bechterew-Ischiasphänomen *nt*.
B.'s tract zentrale Haubenbahn *f*, Tractus tegmentalis centralis.
Bekhterev-Mendel ['mendl]: **B.-M. reflex** Mendel-Bechterew-Reflex *m*.
bel [bel] *n abbr.* **B** Bel *nt abbr.* B.
belch [beltʃ] **I** *n* Aufstoßen *nt*, Rülpsen *nt*, Rülpser *m*, Ruktation *f*, Ruktus *m*, Eruktation *f*. **II** *vi* aufstoßen, *inf.* rülpsen.
belch·ing ['beltʃɪŋ] *n* → belch I.
Bell [bel]: **B.'s law** → Bell-Magendie law.
B.'s mania akutes Delir(ium *nt*) *nt*, Delirium acutum.
B.'s nerve N. thoracicus longus.
B.'s palsy/paralysis einseitige Fazialislähmung/-parese *f*, Bell-Lähmung *f*.
B.'s phenomenon *neuro.* Bell-Phänomen *nt*.
B.'s sign → B.'s phenomenon.
B.'s spasm Bell-Spasmus *m*, Fazialiskrampf *m*, Fazialis-Tic *m*, Gesichtszucken *nt*, mimischer Gesichtskrampf *m*, Tic convulsif/facial.
bell [bel] *n* **1.** Glocke *f*, Schelle *f*, Klingel *f*. **2.** Läuten *nt*, Klingeln *nt*, Glockenzeichen *nt*. **3.** *techn.* Glocke *f* (*Stethoskop*) (Schall-)Trichter *m*.
bel·la·don·na [ˌbelə'dɒnə] *n* **1.** Tollkirsche *f*, Belladonna *f*, Atropa belladonna. **2.** *pharm.* → belladonna alkaloids.
belladonna alkaloids Belladonnaalkaloide *pl*.
bel·la·don·nine [ˌ-'dɒniːn, -nɪn] *n pharm.* Belladonnin *n*.
bell curve *stat.* Glockenkurve *f*, Gauss'-Kurve *f*.
Bell-Dally ['dælɪ]: **B.-D. dislocation** *ortho.* Bell-Dally-Dislokation *f*, spontane nicht-traumatische Atlasluxation *f*.
bell gasometer Glockengasometer *nt*.
Bellini [be'liːnɪ]: **B.'s ducts/tubules** Tubuli renales recti.

bell jar *phys.* Glas-, Vakuumglocke *f*.
Bell-Magendie [məˈdʒendɪ; maˈʃɔːˈdi]: **B.-M. law** Bell(-Magendie)-Regel *f*.
bell·met·al resonance ['belmetl] Münzenklirren *nt*.
Bellocq [be'lɒk]: **B.'s procedure** *HNO* Bellocq-Tamponade *f*.
B.'s technique → B.'s procedure.
B.'s tube *HNO* Bellocq-Röhrchen *nt*.
bel·lows ['beloʊz, -əz] *pl* **1.** (*a.* **pair of ~**) Blasebalg *m*. **2.** *inf.* Lunge *f*.
bell-shaped *adj* glockenförmig.
bell-shaped curve *stat.* Glockenkurve *f*, Gauss-Kurve *f*.
bell sound Münzenklirren *nt*.
bel·ly ['belɪ] **I** *n* **1.** Bauch *m*, Abdomen *nt*; Magen u. angrenzende Darmabschnitte. **2.** Muskelbauch *m*, Venter musculi. **3.** *gyn.* Gebärmutter *f*, Uterus *m*. **4.** Vorwölbung *f*; der Bauch *od.* das Innere eines Objekts. **II** *vt, vi* belly out I, II.
belly out I *vt* (an-)schwellen lassen. **II** *vi* bauchig werden, s. (aus-)bauchen, (an-)schwellen.
b. of digastric muscle Digastrikusbauch, Venter m. digastrici.
bel·ly·ache ['belɪeɪk] *n inf.* Bauchschmerzen *pl*, Bauchweh *nt*.
bel·ly·but·ton ['-ˌbʌtn] *n inf.* Nabel *m*.
bel·o·ne·pho·bia [ˌbelənɪ'fəʊbɪə] *n psychia.* krankhafte Furcht *f* vor Nadeln, Belonephobie *f*.
bel·o·noid ['belənɔɪd] *adj* nadel-, griffelförmig.
bel·o·no·ski·as·co·py [ˌbelənəʊskaɪ'æskəpɪ] *n ophthal.* Belonoskiaskopie *f*.
be·low [bɪ'ləʊ] *adv* **1.** unten. **2.** hinab, hinunter, nach unten. **3.** niedriger, tiefer, unter.
below-elbow *adj abbr.* **BE** unterhalb des Ellenbogens (liegend), Unterarm-.
below-elbow amputation (hohe) Vorarm-/Unterarmamputation *f*.
below-elbow cast *ortho.* Unterarmgips(verband *m*) *m*.
below-knee *adj abbr.* **BK** unterhalb des Kniegelenks (liegend), Unterschenkel-.
below-knee amputation *ortho.* (hohe) Unterschenkelamputation *f*.
below-knee cast *ortho.* Unterschenkelgips(verband *m*) *m*.
below-knee prosthesis *ortho.* Unterschenkelprothese *f*.
below-knee stump *ortho.* Unterschenkelstumpf *m*.
Belsey ['belsɪ]: **B. mark IV operation/repair** *chir.* transthorakale Ösophagofundophrenopexie *f* nach Belsey.
belt [belt] *n* **1.** Gürtel *m*; (Anschnall-, Sicherheits-)Gurt *m*. **2.** Gürtel *m*, Gebiet *nt*, Zone *f*.
belt on *vt* an-, umschnallen.
belt-drive ['beltdraɪv] *n techn.* Riemenantrieb *m*.
bem·e·gride ['bemɪgraɪd] *n pharm.* Bemegrid *nt*.
bem·e·ti·zide ['bemətɪzaɪd] *n pharm.* Bemetizid *nt*.
ben·ac·ty·zine [ben'æktɪziːn] *n pharm.* Benactyzin *nt*.
Bence-Jones ['ben(t)s 'dʒəʊnz]: **B.-J. albumin** Bence-Jones-Eiweiß *nt*, -Protein *nt*.
B.-J. albumose → B.-J. albumin.
B.-J. bodies Bence-Jones-Eiweißkörper *pl*.
B.-J. cylinders Sekretkörnchen *pl* der Samenbläschen.
B.-J. myeloma Bence-Jones-Krankheit *f*, -Plasmozytom *nt*, L(eichte)-Ketten-Krankheit *f*.
B.-J. protein Bence-Jones-Protein *nt*, -eiweiß *nt*.

bend

B.-J. proteinuria Bence-Jones-Proteinurie *f*.
B.-J. reaction Bence-Jones-Reaktion *f*.
bend [bend] (*v*: **bent; bent**) **I** *n* Biegung *f*, Krümmung *f*, Kurve *f*. **II** *vt* **1**. um-, durch-, aufbiegen, krümmen. **2**. beugen, neigen. **to ~ one's head** den Kopf neigen. **to ~ one's knee** das Knie beugen. **III** *vi* **3**. s. krümmen, s. (um-, durch-, auf-)biegen. **4**. s. neigen, s. nach unten biegen; eine Biegung/Kurve machen.
bend back *vi* s. zurück- *od.* nach hinten biegen.
bend down *vi* s. beugen, s. neigen, s. bücken.
bend over *vi* s. beugen *od.* neigen über, s. nach vorn beugen.
bend·ing fracture ['bendɪŋ] Biegungsbruch *m*, -fraktur *f*.
bending pressure *phys.* Biegedruck *m*, -beanspruchung *f*, -spannung *f*.
bending resistance *phys.* Biegesteifigkeit *f*.
bending strain → bending pressure.
bending strength → bending resistance.
bending stress → bending pressure.
ben·dro·flu·a·zide [ˌbendrəʊ'fluːəzaɪd] *n* → bendroflumethiazide.
ben·dro·flu·me·thi·a·zide [ˌ-ˌfluːmɪ'θaɪəzaɪd] *n pharm.* Bendroflumethiazid *nt*.
bend·y ['bendɪ] *adj* biegsam.
Benedict ['benədɪkt]: **B.'s solution** Benedict-Zuckerreagenz *nt*.
B.'s test 1. (*for glucose*) Benedict-Glukoseprobe *f*. **2**. (*for urea*) Benedict-Harnstoffprobe *f*.
ben·e·dic·tion hand [benɪ'dɪkʃn] Predigerhand *f*.
Benedict-Roth [rɒθ, rɑθ]: **B.-R. apparatus/ spirometer** Benedict-Roth-Spirometer *nt*.
Benedikt ['benədɪkt]: **B.'s syndrome** *neuro.* Benedikt-Syndrom *nt*, unteres Ruber-Syndrom *nt*, unteres Nc. ruber-Syndrom *nt*, Hirnschenkelhaubensyndrom *nt*.
ben·e·fi·cial [benə'fɪʃl] *adj* **1**. gut, zuträglich, wohltuend, heilsam **2**. nützlich, vorteilhaft, förderlich (*für*).
ben·e·fit ['benəfɪt] **I** *n* **1**. Nutzen *m*, Vorteil *m*, Wirkung *f* (*from* von). **2**. (finanzielle) Unterstützung *f*, Beihilfe *f*, Leistung *f*. **II** *vt* nützen, zugute kommen, fördern. **III** *vi* Nutzen ziehen (*by, from* aus), Vorteil haben (*by, from* von, durch).
be·nign [bɪ'naɪn] *adj* **1**. (*Tumor*) gutartig, benigne, nicht maligne. **2**. nicht rezidivierend, benigne. **3**. (*Verlauf*) günstig, vorteilhaft.
benign albuminuria essentielle Albuminurie/Proteinurie *f*.
be·nig·nan·cy [bɪ'nɪgnənsɪ] *n* Gutartigkeit *f*, Benignität *f*.
benign aneurysm of bone aneurysmatische Knochenzyste *f*.
be·nig·nant [bɪ'nɪgnənt] *adj* → benign.
benign calcified epithelioma verkalktes Epitheliom *nt*, Pilomatrixom *nt*, Pilomatricoma *nt*, Epithelioma calcificans (Malherbe).
benign cholangioma Gallengangsadenom *nt*, benignes Cholangiom *nt*.
benign chondroblastoma Chondroblastom *nt*, Codman-Tumor *m*.
benign croupous angina Angina/Pharyngitis herpetica.
benign cystic teratoma zystisches Teratom *nt*, Dermoidzyste *f* des Ovars, Teratoma coaetaneum.
benign cyst of ovary *gyn.* (*Ovar*) Dermoid(zyste *f*) *nt*, Teratom *nt*.
benign dry pleurisy Bornholmer-Krankheit *f*, epidemische Pleurodynie *f*, Myalgia epidemica.

benign essential tremor hereditärer/essentieller Tremor *m*.
benign familial pemphigus Hailey-Hailey-Syndrom *nt*, -Krankheit *f*, Morbus Hailey-Hailey, Gougerot-Hailey-Hailey-Krankheit *f*, Pemphigus Gougerot-Hailey-Hailey *m*, familiärer gutartiger Pemphigus *m*, Pemphigus chronicus benignus familiaris (Hailey-Hailey), Dyskeratosis bullosa (hereditaria).
benign fibrous histiocytoma of bone nicht-ossifizierendes Fibrom *nt*, fibröser Kortikalisdefekt *m*, fibröser metaphysärer Defekt *m*, benignes fibröses Histiozytom *nt* des Knochens.
benign glycosuria renale Glukosurie/Glycosurie *f*.
benign hypertension benigne Hypertonie *f*.
benign inoculation reticulosis → benign lymphoreticulosis.
be·nig·ni·ty [bɪ'nɪgnətɪ] *n* → benignancy.
benign juvenile melanoma Spindelzellnävus *m*, Spitz-Tumor *m*, Allen-Spitz-Nävus *m*, Spitz-Nävus *m*, Nävus Spitz *m*, Epitheloidzellnävus *m*, benignes juveniles Melanom *nt*.
benign leptospirosis benigne/anikterische Leptospirose *f*.
benign lymphocytic meningitis lymphozytäre Meningitis *f*.
benign lymphogranulomatosis → Boeck's disease.
benign lymphoreticulosis Katzenkratzkrankheit *f*, cat-scratch-disease, benigne Inokulationslymphoretikulose *f*.
benign mastopathia zystische/fibrös-zystische Mastopathie *f*, Mammadysplasie *f*, Mastopathia chronica cystica.
benign mediastinal lymph node hyperplasia benigne Hyperplasie *f* der Mediastinallymphknoten.
benign mesothelioma benignes Mesotheliom *nt*.
benign migratory glossitis Landkartenzunge *f*, Wanderplaques *pl*, Lingua geographica, Exfoliatio areata linguae/dolorosa, Glossitis exfoliativa marginata, Glossitis areata exsudativa.
benign mucosal pemphigoid vernarbendes Pemphigoid *nt*, benignes Schleimhautpemphigoid *nt*, okulärer Pemphigus *m*, Dermatitis pemphigoides mucocutanea chronica.
benign mucous membrane pemphigoid → benign mucosal pemphigoid.
benign myalgic encephalitis → benign myalgic encephalomyelitis.
benign myalgic encephalomyelitis epidemische Neuromyasthenie *f*, Encephalomyelitis benigna myalgica.
benign nephrosclerosis benigne Nephrosklerose *f*.
benign paroxysmal peritonitis familiäres Mittelmeerfieber *nt*, familiäre rekurrente Polyserositis *f*.
benign paroxysmal positional/postural vertigo Lage-, Lagerungsschwindel *m*.
benign polycythemia Gaisböck-Syndrom *nt*, Polycythaemia (rubra) hypertonica.
benign proteinuria → benign albuminuria.
benign stupor *neuro., psychia.* benigner Stupor *m*.
benign synovialoma pigmentierte villonoduläre Synovitis *f abbr.* PVNS, benignes Synovialom *nt*, Riesenzelltumor *m* der Sehnenscheide, Tendosynovitis nodosa.
benign synovioma → benign synovialoma.
benign tertian malaria 1. Vivax-Malaria *f*.

2. Tertiana *f*, Dreitagefieber *nt*, Malaria tertiana.
benign tetanus neuromuskuläre Übererregbarkeit *f*, Tetanie *f*.
benign tumor gutartiger Tumor *m*.
Béniqué [beni'ke]: **B.'s sound** *urol.* Béniqué-Sonde *f*.
Bennett ['benɪt]: **B. agar** Bennett-Agar *m/nt*.
B.'s disease Leukämie *f*, Leukose *f*.
B.'s fracture Bennett'-Luxationsfraktur *f*.
B.'s large corpuscles Nunn-Körperchen *pl*.
B.'s small corpuscles Drysdale-Körperchen *pl*.
ben·ser·a·zide [ben'serəzaɪd] *n pharm.* Benserazid *nt*.
bent humerus [bent] Humerus varus.
ben·ton·ite ['bentənaɪt] *n* Bentonit *nt*.
bentonite flocculation test Bentonit-Flockungstest *m*.
be·numb [bɪ'nʌm] *vt* betäuben, gefühllos machen, erstarren lassen; *fig.* lähmen, betäuben.
be·numbed [bɪ'nʌmd] *adj* betäubt, gefühllos, erstarrt; *fig.* gelähmt. **~ by alcohol** vom Alkohol benommen. **~ by cold** starr vor Kälte.
benz·al·de·hyde [ben'zældəhaɪd] *n* Benzaldehyd *m*.
benz·al·ko·ni·um chloride [ˌbenzæl'kəʊnɪəm] Benzalkoniumchlorid *nt*.
benz·an·thra·cene [ben'zænθrəsiːn] *n* Benzanthracen *nt*.
benz·bro·ma·rone [benz'brəʊmərəʊn] *n pharm.* Benzbromaron *nt*.
ben·zene ['benziːn, ben'ziːn] *n* Benzol *nt*, Benzen *nt*.
benzene compound aromatische Verbindung *f*.
1,3-ben·zene·di·ol [ben ziːn'daɪɒl, -ɑl] *n* Resorcin *nt*, Resorzin *nt*, (*m*-)Dihydroxybenzol *nt*.
1,4-benzenediol *n* Hydrochinon *nt*, Parahydroxybenzol *nt*.
benzene hexachloride Benzolhexachlorid *nt*, Hexachlorcyclohexan *nt abbr.* HCH; Lindan *nt*.
benzene ring *chem.* Benzolring *m*.
benz·es·tro·fol [ben'zestrəfɒl] *n* Estradiol-, Östradiolbenzoat *nt*.
ben·ze·tho·ni·um chloride [ˌbenzɪ'θəʊnɪəm] Benzethoniumchlorid *nt*.
benz·hy·dra·mine hydrochloride [benz'haɪdrəmiːn] *pharm.* Diphenhydraminhydrochlorid *nt*.
ben·zi·dine ['benzɪdiːn, -dɪn] *n* Benzidin *nt*, Diphenyldiamin *nt*.
benzidine test Benzidinprobe *f*.
benz·im·id·az·ole [ˌbenzɪm'ɪdæzəʊl] *n* Benzimidazol *nt*.
2-benzimidazole *n* 2-(α-Hydroxybenzyl)-Benzimidazol *nt abbr.* HBB.
ben·zin *n* → benzine.
ben·zine ['benziːn, ben'ziːn] *n* Benzin *nt*.
ben·zo·a·py·rene [ˌbenzəʊə'paɪriːn] *n* → 3,4-benzpyrene.
ben·zo·ate ['benzəʊeɪt, -ɪt] *n* Benzoat *nt*.
ben·zo·caine ['benzəʊkeɪn] *n pharm.* Benzocain *nt*.
benz·oc·ta·mine [benz'ɒktəmiːn] *n pharm.* Benzoctamin *nt*.
ben·zo·di·az·e·pine [ˌbenzəʊdaɪ'æzəpiːn] *n pharm.* Benzodiazepin *nt*.
ben·zo·gy·nes·tryl [ˌ-gaɪ'nestrɪl] *n* Estradiol-, Östradiolbenzoat *nt*.
ben·zo·ic acid [ben'zəʊɪk] Benzoesäure *f*.
benzoic aldehyde → benzaldehyde.
ben·zoin ['benzəʊɪn] *n* Benzoe *nt*.
ben·zol ['benzɒl, -zəl] *n* → benzene.
ben·zo·lism ['benzəlɪzəm] *n* Benzolvergif-

tung *f*, -intoxikation *f*, -rausch *m*, Benzolismus *m*.
ben·zo·py·rene [ˌbenzəʊˈpaɪriːn] *n* → 3,4-benzpyrene.
ben·zo·thi·a·di·a·zide [ˌbenzəʊˌθaɪəˈdaɪəzaɪd] *n* → benzothiadiazine.
ben·zo·thi·a·di·a·zine [ˌ-ˌθaɪəˈdaɪəziːn] *n pharm.* Benzothiadiazin *nt*.
ben·zo·yl [ˈbenzəʊl, -zəwɪl] *n* Benzoyl-(Radikal *nt*).
ben·zo·yl·a·mi·no·a·ce·tic acid [ˌ-əˌmiːnəʊəˈsiːtɪk, -ˈsetɪk, -ˌæmɪnəʊ-] Hippursäure *f*, Benzoylaminoessigsäure *f*, Benzolglykokoll *nt*.
ben·zo·yl·cho·lin·es·ter·ase [ˌ-ˌkəʊləˈnestəreɪz] *n* unspezifische/unechte Cholinesterase *f abbr.* ChE, Pseudocholinesterase *f*, β-Cholinesterase *f*, Butyrylcholinesterase *f*, Typ II-Cholinesterasse *f*.
ben·zo·yl·gly·cine [ˌ-ˈɡlaɪsiːn, -ɡlaɪˈsiːn] *n* Hippursäure *f*, Benzoylaminoessigsäure *f*, Benzolglykokoll *nt*.
benzoyl peroxide Benzoylperoxid *nt*.
N-benzoyl-L-tyrosyl-p-aminobenzoic acid *abbr.* **BT-PABA** *N*-Benzoyl-L-tyrosyl-*p*-aminobenzoesäure *f abbr.* BT-PABA
3,4-benz·py·rene [benzˈpaɪriːn] *n* 3,4--Benzpyren/Benzo(a)pyren *nt*.
benz·pyr·role [ˌ-ˈpɪrəʊl, -əʊl] *n* 2,3-Benzopyrrol *nt*, Indol *nt*.
benz·quin·a·mide [ˌ-ˈkwɪnəmaɪd] *n pharm.* Benzquinamid *nt*.
benz·thi·a·zide [ˌ-ˈθaɪəzaɪd] *n pharm.* Benzthiazid *nt*.
ben·zyd·a·mine [ˌ-ˈzɪdəmiːn] *n pharm.* Benzydamin *nt*.
ben·zyd·ro·flu·me·thi·a·zide [benˌzɪdrəʊˌfluːmɪˈθaɪəzaɪd] *n* → bendroflumethiazide.
ben·zyl [ˈbenzɪl] *n* Benzyl-(Radikal *nt*).
benzyl alcohol Benzylalkohol *m*, Phenylcarbinol *nt*.
ben·zyl·pen·i·cil·lin [ˌ-ˌpenəˈsɪlɪn] *n pharm.* Benzylpenicillin *nt*, Penicillin G *nt*.
be·phe·ni·um hydroxynaphthoate [bɪˈfiːnɪəm] *pharm.* Bephenium-hydroxy-naphthoat *nt*.
BER *abbr.* → basic electrical rhythm.
BERA *abbr.* → brain stem evoked response audiometry.
Bérard [beˈrar]: **B.'s aneurysm** Bérard-Aneurysma *nt*.
B.'s ligament Bérard'-Band *nt*.
Béraud [beˈro]: **B.'s valve** Krause'-Klappe *f*, Valvula sacci lacrimalis inferior.
ber·be·rine [ˈbɜrbəriːn] *n pharm.* Berberin *nt*.
be·reaved [bɪˈriːvd] *n* der *od.* die Hinterbliebene, die Hinterbliebenen.
be·reave·ment [bɪˈriːvmənt] *n* 1. schmerzlicher Verlust *m* (*durch Tod*), Beraubung *f*. 2. Trauerfall *m*.
ber·ga·mot oil [ˈbɜrɡəmət] Bergamotöl *m*.
Berger [bɛrˈʒe]: **B.'s paresthesia** *neuro.* Berger'-Parästhesie *f*.
B.'s rhythm *neuro.* α-Rhythmus *m*, Alpha-, Berger-Rhythmus *m*.
B.'s sign *ophthal.* Berger-Zeichen *nt*.
B.'s symptom → B.'s sign.
Berger [ˈbɜrɡər]: **B.'s cell** (*Ovar*) Berger-Zelle *f*, Hiluszelle *f*.
B.'s disease → B.'s focal glomerulonephritis.
B.'s effect *neuro.* Berger-Effekt *m*.
B.'s focal glomerulonephritis Berger--Krankheit *f*, -Nephropathie *f*, mesangiale/fokale/fokalbetonte Glomerulonephritis *f*.
B.'s glomerulonephritis → B.'s focal glomerulonephritis.
B.'s interscapular amputation → B.'s method.

B.'s method *ortho.* Amputation *f* nach Berger.
B.'s operation → B.'s method.
B.'s reaction *neuro.* Berger-Reaktion *f*.
Bergeron [bɛrʒəˈrõ]: **B.'s chorea/disease** Bergeron-Krankheit *f*.
Bergey [ˈbɜrɡɪ]: **B.'s classification** *micro.* Bergey'-Klassifikation *f*.
Bergmann [ˈbɜrɡmən]: **B.'s cells** Bergmann'-Stützzellen *pl*.
B.'s chords Striae medullares (ventriculi quarti).
B.'s fibers Bergmann'-Fasern *pl*.
B.'s glia Bergmann'-Glia *f*.
B.'s incision von Bergmann-Inzision *f*.
B.'s supporting cells → B.'s cells.
ber·i·ber·i [ˈberɪˈberɪ] *n* Beriberi *f*, Vitamin B₁-Mangel(krankheit *f*) *m*, Thiaminmangel(krankheit *f*) *m*.
ber·i·ber·ic [berɪˈberɪk] *adj* Beriberi betr., Beriberi-.
ber·ke·li·um [bɜrˈkɪlɪəm] *n abbr.* **Bk** Berkelium *nt abbr.* Bk.
Berlin [ˈbɜrlɪn]: **B.'s disease** Commotio retinae.
B.'s edema Berlin-Netzhautödem *nt*, -Netzhauttrübung *f*.
Ber·lin blue reaction/test [bɜrˈlɪn, ˈbɜrlɪn] Berliner-Blau-Reaktion *f*, Ferriferrocyanid-Reaktion *f*.
ber·lock dermatitis [ˈbɜrlɑk] Berloque--Dermatitis *f*, Kölnisch-Wasser-Dermatitis *f*.
ber·loque dermatitis [ˈbɜrlɑk] → berlock dermatitis.
Bernard [bɛrˈnaːr]: **B.'s canal** Ductus pancreaticus accessorius.
B.'s duct → B.'s canal.
B.'s puncture Bernard'-Zuckerstich *m*.
B.'s syndrome → Bernard-Horner syndrome.
Bernard-Horner [ˈhɔːrnər]: **B.-H. syndrome** Horner-Syndrom *nt*, -Trias *f*, -Symptomenkomplex *m*.
Bernard-Sergent [sɛrˈʒɔ̃]: **B.-S. syndrome** Bernard-Sergent-Syndrom *nt*.
Bernard-Soulier [suˈlje]: **B.-S. disease** → B.-S. syndrome.
B.-S. syndrome *abbr.* **BSS** Bernard-Soulier-Syndrom *nt*.
Bernhardt [ˈbɜrnhaːrt]: **B.'s disease/paresthesia** → Bernhardt-Roth disease.
B.'s formula Bernhardt-Formel *f*.
Bernhardt-Roth [rɑθ]: **B.-R. disease** Bernhardt-Roth-Syndrom *nt*, Meralgia paraesthetica.
B.-R. syndrome → B.-R. disease.
Bernheim [ˈbɜrnhaɪm]: **B.'s syndrome** Bernheim-Syndrom *nt*.
Bernoulli [bɜrˈnuːjɪ]: **B. distribution** *mathe., stat.* Bernouilli-Verteilung *f*.
B. equation Bernoulli-Gleichung *f*.
B. law Bernoulli'-Gesetz *nt*, -Prinzip *nt*.
B. oscillation Bernoulli'-Schwingung *f*.
B. principle → B. law.
B.'s theorem → B. law.
ber·ried [ˈberɪd] *adj* 1. Beeren tragend. 2. beerenförmig, -ähnlich.
Berry [ˈberɪ]: **B.'s ligament** Lig. thyrohyoideum laterale.
ber·ry [ˈberɪ] **I** *n, pl* **-ries** Beere *f*; Beerenfrucht *f*; (*Getreide*) Korn *nt*; Hagebutte *f*. **II** *vi* Beeren pflücken *od.* sammeln; Beeren tragen.
berry aneurysm 1. beerenförmiges Aneurysma *nt*, Beeranaeurysma *nt*. 2. Aneurysma *nt* der A. basilaris.
berry cell *hema.* Morula-, Traubenzelle *f*.
berry-like *adj* beerenähnlich.
Ber·ti·el·la [bɜrtɪˈelə] *n micro.* Bertiella *f*.
Ber·ti·el·li·a·sis [bɜrtɪəˈlaɪəsɪs] *n* Bertiellainfektion *f*, Bertielliasis *f*.

beta decay

Bertin [berˈtɛ̃]: **columns of B.** Bertin'-Säulen *pl*, Columnae renales.
B.'s bones Concha sphenoidalis.
B.'s ligament Bigelow'-Band *nt*, Lig. iliofemorale.
Bertolotti [bɜrtəˈlɑtɪ]: **B.'s syndrome** Bertolotti-Syndrom *nt*.
ber·yl·li·o·sis [bəˌrɪlɪˈəʊsɪs] *n* Berylliumvergiftung *f*, Beryll(i)ose *f*.
be·ryl·li·um [bəˈrɪlɪəm] *n abbr.* **Be** Beryllium *nt abbr.* Be.
beryllium granuloma Berylliumgranulom *nt*.
beryllium poisoning → berylliosis.
be·ryth·ro·my·cin [bəˌrɪθrəˈmaɪsɪn] *n pharm.* Erythromycin B *nt*.
Besnier [besˈnje]: **B.'s prurigo** *derm.* Besnier-Prurigo *f*, Prurigo Besnier.
B. prurigo of pregnancy Prurigo gestationis/gravidarum.
prurigo gestationis of B. → B. prurigo of pregnancy.
Besnier-Boeck [bek]: **B.-B. disease** → Boeck's disease.
Besnier-Boeck-Schaumann [ˈʃɔːmən]: **B.-B.-S. disease** → Boeck's disease.
B.-B.-S. syndrome → Boeck's disease.
Best [best]: **B.'s carmine stain** *histol.* Best'-Karminfärbung *f*.
B.'s disease *ophthal.* Best'-Krankheit *f*.
B.'s macular dystrophy → B.'s disease.
vitelliform degeneration of B. → B.'s disease.
bes·tial [ˈbestʃəl, ˈbiːs-] *adj* 1. tierisch. 2. bestialisch, unmenschlich, brutal.
bes·ti·al·i·ty [ˌbestʃɪˈælətɪ, ˌbiːs-] *n, pl* **-ties** 1. das Tierische. 2. Bestialität *f*, Brutalität *f*, bestialische Grausamkeit *f*. 3. Greueltat *f*. 4. Sodomie *f*.
bes·tial·ize [ˈbestʃəlaɪz, ˈbiːs-] *vt* entmenschlichen, zum Tier machen.
bes·y·late [ˈbesɪleɪt] *n* Benzolsulfonat *nt*.
be·ta [ˈbeɪtə; *Brit.* ˈbiː-] *n abbr.* **B, β** Beta *nt abbr.* B, β.
beta-adrenergic blockade → beta blockade.
beta-adrenergic blocking agent → beta--blocker.
beta-adrenergic blocking drug → beta--blocker.
beta-adrenergic receptor β-adrenerger Rezeptor *m*, β-Rezeptor *m*.
beta-adrenergic receptor blocking agent → beta-blocker.
beta alcoholism β-Alkoholismus *m*.
beta-aminoisobutyric aciduria β-Aminoisobuttersäureausscheidung *f* im Harn.
beta blockade Beta(rezeptoren)blockade *f*.
beta-blocker *n* Betablocker *m*, Beta-Rezeptorenblocker *m*, β-Adrenorezeptorenblocker *m*, Beta-Adrenorezeptorenblocker *m*.
beta-blocking agent → beta-blocker.
beta-blocking drug → beta-blocker.
beta-carotene *n* β-Karotin *nt*, β-Carotin *nt*.
beta cell 1. (*Pankreas*) β-Zelle *f*, B-Zelle *f*. 2. (*Adenohypophyse*) basophile Zelle *f*, β-Zelle *f*.
beta cell adenocarcinoma (*Pankreas*) B(eta)-Zelladenokarzinom *nt*.
beta cell adenoma (*Pankreas*) B(eta)-Zelladenom *nt*.
beta cell tumor (*Pankreas*) B(eta)-Zelltumor *m*, Insulinom *nt*.
beta-cholestanol *n* β-Cholestanol *nt*, Dihydrocholesterin *nt*.
be·ta·cism [ˈbeɪtɪsɪzəm, ˈbiː-] *n neuro.* Betazismus *m*.
beta decay *phys.* β-Zerfall *m*, beta-Zerfall *m*.

beta-endorphin n Beta-Endorphin nt.
beta fibers β-Fasern pl, Aβ-Fasern pl.
beta globulin beta-Globulin nt, β-Globulin nt.
beta granules β-Granula pl.
beta hemolysin β-Hämolysin nt.
beta-hemolysis n micro. β-Hämolyse f, beta-Hämolyse f, Betahämolyse f.
beta-hemolytic adj micro. beta-hämolytisch, β-hämolytisch.
beta-hemolytic streptococci β-hämolytische/beta-hämolytische Streptokokken pl.
Be·ta·her·pes·vir·i·nae [bi:tə‚hɜrpi:z'vɪərəni:] pl micro. Betaherpesvirinae pl.
be·ta·her·pes·vi·rus·es [‚-‚hɜrpi:z'vaɪrəsəs] pl micro. Betaherpesviren pl, Betaherpesvirinae pl.
be·ta·ine ['bi:tə‚i:n, bɪ'teɪɪn] n Betain nt, Trimethylglykokoll nt, Glykokollbetain nt.
betaine-homocysteine methyltransferase Betain-Homocystein-methyltransferase f.
beta-ketobutyric acid Azetessigsäure f, β-Ketobuttersäure f.
beta-lactamase n β-Lactamase f, beta-Lactamase f, β-Laktamase f, beta-Laktamase f.
beta-lactose n Betalaktose f, β-Laktose f.
beta-lipoprotein n Lipoprotein nt mit geringer Dichte, β-Lipoprotein nt, low-density lipoprotein abbr. LDL.
beta-lysin n β-Lysin nt, beta-Lysin nt.
be·ta·meth·a·sone [‚betə'meθəsəʊn, ‚bi:-] n pharm. Betamethason nt.
beta₂-microglobulin n β₂-Mikroglobulin nt, Beta₂-Mikroglobulin nt.
be·ta·naph·thol [‚-'næfθɒl, -θɑl, -'næp-] n Betanaphthol nt.
beta-oxybutyric acid β-Hydroxybuttersäure f.
beta particle phys. β-Teilchen nt, beta-Teilchen nt.
beta phase gestagene Phase f, Sekretions-, Luteal phase f.
beta pleated sheet biochem. Faltblatt(struktur f) nt.
be·ta·qui·nine [‚-'kwaɪnaɪn, -'kwɪ-] n Chinidin nt, Quinidine nt.
beta radiation Betastrahlung f, β-Strahlung f.
beta rays Betastrahlen pl, β-Strahlen pl.
beta rhythm β-Rhythmus m, Betarhythmus m.
beta sheet biochem. Faltblatt(struktur f) nt.
beta staphylolysin β-Staphylolysin nt, beta-Staphylolysin nt.
beta streptococci → beta-hemolytic streptococci.
beta substance Heinz'-Innenkörperchen pl, Heinz-Ehrlich-Körperchen pl.
be·ta·tron ['-trɒn] n phys. Betatron nt.
beta waves β-Wellen pl, beta-Wellen pl.
be·ta·zole ['beɪtəzəʊl] n pharm. Betazol nt.
betazole hydrochloride Betazolhydrochlorid nt.
be·tel cancer ['bi:tl‚ betl] Betelnußkarzinom nt.
betel nut Betel-, Arekanuß f.
be·thane·chol [bɪ'θeɪnkəʊl] n pharm. Bethanechol nt.
Bethesda-Ballerup [bə'θezdə 'bælərʌp]: **B.-B. group** micro. Bethesda-Ballerup--Gruppe f, -Bakterien pl.
bet·ter ['betər] I n das Bessere. **a change for the ~** eine Wende zum Guten. **to change for the ~** besser werden, s. bessern. II adj besser. **to get ~** s. erholen; s. bessern. besser werden. III vt verbessern. IV vi s. (ver-)bessern, besser werden.

be·tween·brain [bɪ'twi:n‚breɪn] n Zwischenhirn nt, Dienzephalon nt, Diencephalon nt.
between-drug comparison Vergleich m zwischen zwei Medikamenten.
Betz [bets]: **B.'s cells** Betz'-Riesenzellen pl. **B.'s cell area** motorischer Cortex m, motorische Rinde(nregion f) f, Motokortex m, -cortex m.
Bevan ['bevən]: **B.'s incision** Bevan-Pararektalschnitt m, -Inzision f.
Bevan-Lewis ['lu:ɪs]: **B.-L. cells** Bevan--Lewis'-Zellen pl.
bev·er·age ['bev(ə)rɪdʒ] n Getränk nt (außer Wasser).
be·yond [bɪ'(j)ɒnd] I adv darüber hinaus, weiter od. jenseits (von), weiter weg. II prep jenseits; außer; über ... hinaus. **~ comprehension** unverständlich. **~ endurance** (Schmerzen) unerträglich.
be·zoar ['bi:zɔ:r, -zəʊr] n patho. Bezoar m.
Bezold [beɪt'sɔ:ld]: **B.'s abscess** HNO Bezold'-Abszeß m.
B.'s ganglion Bezold-Ganglion nt.
B.'s mastoiditis HNO Bezold'-Mastoiditis f.
B.'s perforation HNO Bezold-Mastoidperforation f.
B.'s sign HNO Bezold'-Zeichen nt.
B.'s symptom → B.'s sign.
B.'s triad HNO Bezold'-Trias f.
Bezold-Jarisch ['jɑ:rɪʃ]: **B.-J. reflex** Bezold-Jarisch-Reflex m.
Bf abbr. → blastogenic factor.
B fibers B-Fasern pl.
BFP abbr. → biologic false-positive.
BFU abbr. → burst forming unit.
BG agar → brilliant-green agar.
B-G agar → Bordet-Gengou agar.
bhang [bæŋ] n 1. Haschisch nt, Bhang nt. 2. Hanfpflanze f.
BHF abbr. → Bolivian hemorrhagic fever.
BHIA abbr. → brain-heart infusion agar.
BHN abbr. → Brinell hardness number.
Bi abbr. → bismuth.
bi- pref. 1. zwei-, doppel-, Bi(n)-. 2. → bio-.
bi [baɪ] adj sl. bi, bisexuell.
Bial ['bi:ɑl]: **B.'s reagent** Bial'-Reagens nt.
B.'s test Bial-(Pentose-)Probe f.
Bianchi [bɪ'ɑŋkɪ]: **B.'s nodules** Arantius--Knötchen pl der Aortenklappe, Noduli valvularum semilunarium.
B.'s syndrome neuro. Bianchi-Syndrom nt.
B.'s valve Plica lacrimalis.
bi·ar·tic·u·lar [baɪɑr'tɪkjələr] adj zwei Gelenke betr., biartikular.
bi·ar·tic·u·late [baɪɑ:r'tɪkjəlɛt] adj mit zwei Gelenken versehen, biartikulär.
bi·as ['baɪəs] I n 1. schiefe od. schräge Seite/Fläche/Richtung f. 2. fig. Neigung f, Hang m (toward zu), Vorliebe f (toward für). 3. fig. Vorurteil nt, Befangenheit f. 4. stat. Bias nt. 5. phys. Gittervorspannung f; Gitter(ableit)widerstand m. II adj schräg, schief, diagonal.
bi·ased ['baɪəst] adj voreingenommen, befangen.
bi·ax·i·al joint [baɪ'æksɪəl] biaxiales Gelenk nt.
bi·ba·sic [baɪ'beɪsɪk] adj chem. zweibasisch, -basig, -wertig.
Biber-Haab-Dimmer ['bɪbər 'hɑ:b 'dɪmər]: **B.-H.-D. dystrophy** ophthal. Haab-Dimmer-Dystrophie f.
bib·li·o·film ['bɪblɪəfɪlm] n Mikrofilm m; (Buchseite) Mikrokopie f.
bib·li·o·ma·nia [‚-'meɪnɪə, -jə] n krankhafte Bücherleidenschaft f, Bibliomanie f.
bib·li·o·pho·bia [‚-'fəʊbɪə] n Bibliophobie f.

bib·li·o·ther·a·py [‚-'θerəpɪ] n psychia. Bibliotherapie f.
bib·u·lous ['bɪbjələs] adj 1. aufsaugend, absorbierend. 2. schwammig.
bi·cam·er·al [baɪ'kæmərəl] adj zwei Kammern besitzend, zweikamm(e)rig, Zweikammer-.
bicameral abscess zweigekammerter Abszeß m.
bi·cap·su·lar [baɪ'kæpsələr] adj zwei Kapseln besitzend, bikapsulär.
bi·car·bo·nate [baɪ'kɑ:rbənɪt, -neɪt] n Bikarbonat nt, Bicarbonat nt, Hydrogencarbonat nt.
bicarbonate buffer Bicarbonatpuffer m.
bicarbonate buffer system Bicarbonatpuffersystem nt.
bi·car·bo·nat·e·mia [baɪ‚kɑ:rbəneɪ'ti:mɪə] n (Hyper-)Bikarbonatämie f.
bicarbonate soda Natriumbikarbonat nt.
bi·cel·lu·lar [baɪ'seljələr] adj zweizellig, bizellulär.
bi·ceph·a·lus [baɪ'sefələs] n embryo. Doppelmißbildung f mit zwei Köpfen, Dicephalus m, Dizephalus m, Dikephalus m.
bi·ceps ['baɪseps] I n, pl **-ceps, -ceps·es** zweiköpfiger Muskel m, Bizeps m, M. biceps. II adj zweiköpfig.
biceps brachii (muscle) Bizeps m (brachii), M. biceps brachii.
biceps femoris (muscle) Bizeps m femoris, M. biceps femoris.
biceps femoris reflex Bizeps-Femoris-Reflex m.
biceps jerk → biceps reflex.
biceps muscle → biceps I.
b. of arm → biceps brachii (muscle).
b. of thigh → biceps femoris (muscle).
biceps reflex Bizeps(sehnen)reflex m abbr. BSR.
Bichat [bi:'ʃɑ]: **B.'s band** Bichat-Band nt.
B.'s canal → B.'s foramen.
fissure of B. Fissura transversa cerebralis.
B.'s foramen Cisterna v. magnae cerebri.
B.'s fossa Flügelgaumengrube f, Fossa pterygopalatina.
B.'s membrane Membrana elastica interna.
B.'s tunic Intima f, Tunica intima (vasorum).
bi·chlo·ride [baɪ'klɔ:raɪd, -ɪd] n Bichlorid nt.
bi·chro·mate [baɪ'krəʊmeɪt] n Dichromat nt.
bi·cip·i·tal [baɪ'sɪpɪtl] adj zweiköpfig; Bizeps brachii/femoris betr.
bicipital aponeurosis Bizepsaponeurose f, Aponeurosis m. bicipitis brachii, Aponeurosis bicipitalis.
bicipital bursa Bursa subtendinea m. bicipitis femoris inferior.
bicipital eminence → bicipital tuberosity.
bicipital fascia → bicipital aponeurosis.
bicipital fissure Bizepsrinne f, Sulcus bicipitalis.
lateral b. seitliche Bizepsrinne, Sulcus bicipitalis lateralis/radialis.
medial b. mediale Bizepsrinne, Sulcus bicipitalis medialis/ulnaris.
radial b. → lateral b.
ulnar b. → medial b.
bicipital groove Sulcus intertubercularis (humeri).
lateral b. seitliche Bizepsrinne, Sulcus bicipitalis lateralis/radialis.
medial b. mediale Bizepsrinne, Sulcus bicipitalis medialis/ulnaris.
radial b. → lateral b.
ulnar b. → medial b.
bicipital ridge: anterior b. Crista tuberculi minoris.

external b. Crista tuberculi majoris.
internal b. → anterior b.
posterior b. → external b.
bicipital sulcus → bicipital fissure.
bicipital tuberosity Tuberositas radii.
bi·cip·i·to·fib·u·lar bursa [baɪˌsɪpɪtəʊˈfɪbjələr] → bicipital bursa.
bi·cip·i·to·ra·di·al bursa [ˌ-ˈreɪdɪəl] Bursa bicipitoradialis.
Bickel [ˈbɪkl]: **B.'s ring** lymphatischer Rachenring *m*, Waldeyer'-Rachenring *m*.
bi·clon·al gammopathy [baɪˈkləʊnl] biklonale Gammopathie *f*.
bi·con·cave [baɪˈkænkeɪv, ˌbaɪkɑnˈkeɪv] *adj phys.* bikonkav.
biconcave lens bikonkave Linse *f*, Bikonkavlinse *f*.
bi·con·cav·i·ty [ˌbaɪkənˈkævətɪ] *n* Bikonkavität *f*.
bi·con·vex [baɪˈkɒnveks, ˌbaɪkɑnˈveks] *adj phys.* bikonvex.
bi·con·vex·i·ty [ˌbaɪkənˈveksətɪ] *n* Bikonvexität *f*.
biconvex lens bikonvexe Linse *f*, Bikonvexlinse *f*.
bi·cor·nate [baɪˈkɔːrnaɪt, -nɪt] *adj* → bicornuate.
bicornate uterus Uterus bicornis.
bi·cor·nu·ate [baɪˈkɔːrnjəwɪt, -eɪt] *adj* zweizipfelig.
bi·cus·pid [baɪˈkʌspɪd] **I** *n* Prämolar *m*, vorderer Backenzahn *m*, Dens pr(a)emolaris. **II** *adj* 1. zweizipf(e)lig, bikuspidal, bicuspidal. 2. zweihöckerig.
bi·cus·pi·date [baɪˈkʌspɪdeɪt] *adj* → bicuspid II.
bicuspid tooth → bicuspid I.
bicuspid valve Mitralklappe, Mitralis *f*, Bicuspidalis *f*, Valva mitralis, Valvula bicuspidalis, Valva atrioventricularis sinistra.
bi·cy·cle ergometer [ˈbaɪsɪkl] Fahrradergometer *nt*.
bicycle ergometry Fahrradergometrie *f*.
bi·cy·lin·dri·cal lens [baɪsɪˈlɪndrɪkl] bizylindrische Linse *f*, bizylindrisches Glas *nt*.
b.i.d. *abbr.* [bis in die] *pharm.* zweimal täglich.
bi·dac·ty·ly [baɪˈdæktəlɪ] *n embryo.* Bidaktylie *f*.
Bidder [ˈbɪdər]: **B.'s ganglia** Bidder-, Remak-Haufen *pl*, Bidder(-Remak)-Ganglien *pl*.
bi·der·mo·ma [ˌbaɪdərˈməʊmə] *n embryo., patho.* Bidermom(a) *nt*.
bi·det [bɪˈdeɪ, ˈbiːdeɪ] *n* Bidet *nt*.
bi·di·rec·tion·al [ˌbaɪdɪˈrekʃənl, -daɪ-] *adj* in zwei Richtungen ab- *od.* verlaufend, bidirektional.
bidirectional replication bidirektionale Replikation *nt*.
bi·dis·coi·dal placenta [baɪˈdɪskɔɪdl] Placenta bidiscoidea.
Biederman [ˈbiːdərmən]: **B.'s sign** Biederman-Zeichen *nt*.
Biedl [ˈbiːdl]: **B.'s disease** Bardet-Biedl-Syndrom *nt*.
B.'s syndrome 1. Laurence-Moon-Syndrom *nt.* 2. Laurence-Moon-Bardet-Biedl-Syndrom *nt*, Laurence-Moon-Biedl-Syndrom *nt*, Laurence-Moon-Biedl-Bardet-Syndrom *nt*, dienzephalo-retinale Degeneration *f*.
Bielschowsky [ˌbiːlˈʃɒvskɪ, ˌbel-]: **B.'s disease** Jansky-Bielschowsky-Krankheit *f*, Bielschowsky-Syndrom *nt*, spätinfantile Form *f* der amaurotischen Idiotie.
B.'s phenomenon → B.'s sign.
B.'s sign *ophthal.* Bielschowsky-Zeichen *nt*, -Phänomen *nt*.
B.'s stain Bielschowsky-Silberimprägnierung *f*.

Bielschowsky-Jansky [ˈjanskɪ]: **B.-J. disease** → Bielschowsky disease.
Biemond [bjeˈmɔ̃]: **B.'s syndrome** Biemond(-van Bogaert)-Syndrom *nt*.
bi·en·ni·al [baɪˈenɪəl] *adj* zweijährig, zweijährlich.
Bier [bɪər]: **B.'s amputation** Unterschenkelamputation *f* nach Bier.
B.'s block intravenöse Regionalanästhesie *f abbr.* IVRA.
B.'s hyperemia Bier'-Stauung *f*.
B.'s local anesthesia → B.'s block.
B.'s method 1. Bier'-Stauung *f*. 2. → B.'s block.
B.'s operation → B.'s amputation.
bier [bɪər] *n* (Toten-)Bahre *f*.
Biermer [ˈbɪərmər]: **B.'s anemia/disease** Biermer, Addison-Anämie *f*, Morbus Biermer, perniziöse Anämie *f*, Perniziosa *f*, Perniciosa *f*, Anaemia perniciosa, Vitamin B_{12}-Mangelanämie *f*.
B.'s sign Biermer-Schallwechsel *m*, Gerhardt-Schallwechsel *m*.
Biermer-Ehrlich [ˈeərlɪx]: **B.-E. anemia** → Biermer's anemia.
Biernacki [bjɛərˈnɑːkɪ]: **B.'s sign** Biernacki-Zeichen *nt*.
Biesiadecki [bjɛsjaˈdekɪ]: **B.'s fossa** Fossa iliacosubfascialis.
bi·fer·i·ous pulse [baɪˈfɛrɪəs, -ˈfɪər-] → bisferious pulse.
bi·fid [ˈbaɪfɪd] *adj* zweigeteilt.
Bi·fid·o·bac·te·ri·um [ˌbaɪfɪdəʊbækˈtɪərɪəm] *n micro.* Bifidobacterium *nt*.
B. bifidum Bifidus-Bakterium *nt*, Lactobacillus bifidus, Bifidobacterium bifidum.
bi·fid·o·bac·te·ri·um [ˌ-bækˈtɪərɪəm] *n, pl* -ria [-rɪə] Bifidobakterium *nt*, -bacterium *nt*.
bifid penis *embryo.* Diphallus *m*, Penis duplex.
bifid rib Gabel-, Spaltrippe *f*.
bifid tongue gespaltene Zunge *f*, Lingua bifida.
bifid uterus → bicornate uterus.
bifid uvula Zäpfchen-, Uvulaspalte *f*, Uvula bifida.
bi·fo·cal [beɪˈfəʊkl] **I** *n* 1. ~s *pl* Bifokal-, Zweistärkenbrille *f*. 2. → bifocal lens **II** *adj* zwei Brennpunkte besitzend, bifokal, Zweistärken-, Bifokal-.
bifocal glasses → bifocal I.
bifocal lens Zweistärken-, Bifokallinse *f*, -glas *nt*.
bi·for·myl [baɪˈfɔːrmɪl] *n* Glyoxal *nt*, Oxalaldehyd *m*.
bi·fur·cate [ˈbaɪfərˌkeɪt, baɪˈfərkeɪt] **I** *adj* gegabelt, gabelförmig; in zwei Teile *od.* Äste aufteilend. **II** *vt* (auf-)gabeln, gabelförmig teilen. **III** *vi s.* (auf-)gabeln, s. gabelförmig teilen.
bi·fur·cat·ed [ˈbaɪfərkeɪtɪd] *adj* → bifurcate I.
bifurcated prosthesis *chir.* Bifurkationsprothese *f*.
bifurcate ligament Lig. bifurcatum.
deep b.s Ligg. tarsometatarsalia plantaria.
bi·fur·ca·tion [ˌbaɪfərˈkeɪʃn] *n* Gabelung *f*, Gabel *f*, Zweiteilung *f*, Bifurkation *f*; *anat.* Bifurcatio *f*.
b. of aorta Aortengabel, Bifurcatio aortae.
b. of pulmonary trunk Trunkusbifurkation, Bifurcatio trunci pulmonalis.
b. of trachea Luftröhrengabelung, Trachealbifurkation, Bifurcatio tracheae/trachealis.
bifurcation prosthesis *chir.* Bifurkationsprothese *f*.
big·a·mist [ˈbɪgəmɪst] *n* Bigamist(in *f*) *m*.

big·a·mous [ˈbɪgəməs] *adj* Bigamie betr., in Bigamie lebend, bigamistisch.
big·a·my [ˈbɪgəmɪ] *n, pl* **-mies** Bigamie *f*, Doppelehe *f*.
Bigelow [ˈbɪgɪləʊ]: **B.'s ligament** Bigelow'-Band *nt*, Lig. iliofemorale.
B.'s litholapaxy → B.'s operation.
B.'s operation Litholapaxie *f* nach Bigelow.
B.'s septum Bigelow-Septum *nt*, Schenkelsporn *m*, Calcar femorale.
bi·gem·i·na [baɪˈdʒemɪnə] *pl card.* Bigeminus *m*, Bigeminuspuls *m*, -rhythmus *m*, Pulsus bigeminus.
bi·gem·i·nal pregnancy [baɪˈdʒemɪnl] Zwillingsschwangerschaft *f*.
bigeminal pulse → bigemina.
bigeminal rhythm Bigeminus *m*, Bigeminuspuls *m*, -rhythmus *m*, Pulsus bigeminus.
bi·gem·i·ny [baɪˈdʒemɪnɪ] *n card.* Doppelschlägigkeit *f*, Bigeminie *f*.
bi·is·chi·al diameter [baɪˈɪskɪəl] *gyn.* Querdurchmesser *m* des Beckenausgangs, Diameter transversa des Beckenausgangs.
bi·lat·er·al [baɪˈlætərəl] *adj* 1. von zwei Seiten ausgehend, zwei Seiten betr., zwei-, beidseitig, bilateral, Bilateral-. 2. beide Seiten betr., seitensymmetrisch, beidseitig, Bilateral-.
bilateral deafness beidseitige/bilaterale Schwerhörigkeit *f*.
bilateral hemianopia/hemianopsia *ophthal.* bilaterale/binokuläre Hemianop(s)ie *f*.
bilateral hermaphroditism Hermaphroditismus (verus) bilateralis *m*.
bi·lat·er·al·ism [baɪˈlætərəlɪzəm] *n* Bilateralität *f*, Bilateralsymmetrie *f*.
bilateral oophorectomy *gyn.* beidseitige Eierstockentfernung/Oophorektomie/Ovariektomie *f*.
bilateral paralysis *neuro.* Diplegie *f*, Diplegia *f*.
bilateral paresis *neuro.* Diparese *f*.
bilateral strabismus *ophthal.* alternierendes Schielen *nt*, Strabismus alternans.
bilateral symmetry bilaterale Symmetrie *f*, Bilateralsymmetrie *f*.
bilateral vagotomy *chir.* bilaterale Vagotomie *f*.
bi·lay·er [ˈbaɪleɪər] *n* bimolekulare Schicht *f*, Bilayer *m*.
bilayer structure Bilayerstruktur *f*.
bilayer system Bilayersystem *nt*.
Bilderbeck [ˈbɪldərbek]: **B.'s disease** Feer'-Krankheit *f*, Rosakrankheit *f*, vegetative Neurose *f* der Kleinkinder, Swift-Syndrom *nt*, Selter-Swift-Feer'-Krankheit *f*, Feer-Selter-Swift-Krankheit *f*, Akrodynie *f*, Acrodynia *f*.
bile [baɪl] *n* Galle *f*, Gallenflüssigkeit *f*, Fel *nt*.
bile acid pool Gallensäurepool *m*.
bile acids Gallensäuren *pl*.
bile ascites galliger Aszites *m*; Choleperitoneum *nt*.
bile broth *micro.* Gallebouillon *f*.
bile canaliculi Gallenkanälchen *pl*, -kapillaren *pl*, Canaliculi biliferi.
bile canals, interlobular → bile ducts, interlobular.
bile capillaries 1. Gallekanälchen *pl*, -kapillaren *pl*, Canaliculi biliferi. 2. Cholangiolen *pl*.
bile cast *urol.* Galle(n)zylinder *m*.
bile culture *micro.* Galle(n)kultur *f*.
bile cyst Gallenblase *f*, *inf.* Galle *f*, Vesica fellea/biliaris.
bile drainage *chir.* Gallendrainage *f*.
bile duct Gallengang *m*, Ductus biliferus.

bile duct abscess

common b. *abbr.* **CBD** Hauptgallengang, Choledochus *m*, Ductus choledochus/biliaris.
extrahepatic b.s extrahepatische Gallenwege *pl*.
interlobular b.s interlobuläre Gallengänge *pl*, Ductuli interlobulares (hepatis).
intrahepatic b.s intrahepatische Gallenwege *pl*.
bile duct abscess → biliary abscess.
bile duct adenoma Gallengangsadenom *nt*, benignes Cholangiom *nt*.
bile duct calculus → bile duct stone.
bile duct carcinoma Gallengangskarzinom *nt*, malignes Cholangiom *nt*, Ca. cholangiocellulare.
bile duct drain *chir.* Gallengangsdrain *m*.
bile duct hamartomas Meyenburg'-Komplexe *pl*.
bile duct obstruction *chir.* Gallengangs-, Gallenwegsobstruktion *f*.
  extrahepatic b. extrahepatische Gallengangsobstruktion.
bile duct stone *chir.* Gallengang(s)stein *m*.
bile duct stricture *chir.* Gallengang(s)striktur *f*.
bile duct tumor Gallengangstumor *m*.
bile ductule Cholangiole *f*.
bile fistula → biliary fistula.
bile papilla Vater'-Papille *f*, Papilla duodeni major, Papilla Vateri.
bile peritonitis gallige Peritonitis *f*, Choleperitonitis *f*.
bile pigment 1. Gallenfarbstoff *m*. **2.** ~s *pl* Gallenfarbstoffe *pl*.
bile pigment hemoglobin Choleglobin *nt*, Verdohämoglobin *nt*.
bile reflux Galle(n)reflux *m*.
bile salt agar Gallensalzagar *m/nt*.
bile salts Salze *pl* der Gallensäuren.
bile solubility test *micro.* Galle(n)löslichkeitstest *m*.
bile stasis Galle(n)stauung *f*, -stase *f*.
bile thrombi Galle(n)zylinder *pl*, -thromben *pl*.
Bil·har·zi·a [bɪl'hɑːrzɪə] *n micro.* Pärchenegel *m*, Schistosoma *nt*, Bilharzia *f*.
bil·har·zi·al [bɪl'hɑːrzɪəl] *adj* Schistosoma/Bilharzia betr., durch Schistosoma verursacht, Schistosomen-.
bilharzial appendicitis Appendizitis *f* durch Bilharzienbefall.
bilharzial granuloma Schistosomen-, Schistosomagranulom *nt*.
bil·har·zi·a·sis [ˌbɪlhɑːrˈzaɪəsɪs] *n* Bilharziose *f*, Bilharziase *f*, Schistosomiasis *f*.
bilharzia worm Pärchenegel *m*, Schistosoma *nt*, Bilharzia *f*.
bil·har·zic [bɪl'hɑːrzɪk] *adj* → bilharzial.
bil·har·zi·o·sis [bɪlˌhɑːrzɪ'əʊsɪs] *n* → bilharziasis.
bili- *pref.* Galle(n)-, Bili(o)-.
bil·i·ar·y ['bɪlɪˌerɪ, 'bɪljərɪ] *adj* Galle *od.* Gallenblase *od.* Gallengänge betr., gallig, biliär, biliös, Gallen(gangs)-.
biliary abscess biliärer/biliogener/cholangitischer Leberabszeß *m*.
biliary anastomosis *chir.* Gallengangsanastomose *f*.
biliary aplasia Gallengangsaplasie *f*.
biliary atresia Gallengangsatresie *f*.
biliary calculus Gallenstein *m*, Cholelith *m*, Calculus biliaris/felleus.
biliary canal: interlobular b.s → bile ducts, interlobular.
  intralobular b. → bile ductule.
biliary canaliculi → bile canaliculi.
biliary catheterization Gallengangskatheterisierung *f*.
  transhepatic b. transhepatische Gallengangskatheterisierung *f*.
biliary cirrhosis biliäre (Leber-)Zirrhose *f*,

Hanot-Zirrhose *f*, Cirrhosis biliaris.
  primary b. primär biliäre Zirrhose *abbr.* PBZ, nicht-eitrige destruierende Cholangitis *f*.
  secondary b. sekundär biliäre Zirrhose.
biliary colic Gallenkolik *f*, Colica hepatica.
biliary-cutaneous fistula *patho.* biliokutane Fistel *f*, äußere Gallenfistel *f*, Fistula biliocutanea.
biliary cycle (*Gallensäuren*) enterohepatischer Kreislauf *m*.
biliary drainage 1. Galle(n)abfluß *m*. **2.** *chir.* Gallendrainage *f*, Cholangiodrainage *f*.
  percutaneous transhepatic b. perkutane transhepatische Gallen-/Cholangiodrainage.
biliary duct → bile duct.
biliary duct anastomosis *chir.* Gallengangsanastomose *f*.
biliary ductule → bile ductule.
biliary dyskinesia Gallenblasendyskinesie *f*, Gallendyssynergie *f*, biliäre Dyskinese/Dystonie *f*.
biliary dyssynergia → biliary dyskinesia.
biliary encephalopathy → bilirubin encephalopathy.
biliary-enteric anastomosis → bilidigestive anastomosis.
biliary-enteric bypass → bilidigestive anastomosis.
biliary-enteric fistula *patho.* Gallen--Darm-Fistel *f*, biliodigestive/bilioenterische/biliointestinale Fistel *f*, Fistula biliodigestiva.
biliary excretion Galle(n)ausscheidung *f*.
biliary excretion test Galle(n)ausscheidungstest *m*.
biliary fibrosis Gallengangsfibrose *f*.
biliary fistula *patho.* Galle(n)fistel *f*, biliäre Fistel *f*, Fistula biliaris.
  external b. → biliary-cutaneous fistula.
biliary-gastric fistula Gallen-Magen-Fistel *f*, biliogastrische Fistel *f*.
biliary hypoplasia Gallengangshypoplasie *f*.
biliary-intestinal bypass → bilidigestive anastomosis.
biliary-intestinal fistula → biliary-enteric fistula.
biliary intubation, percutaneous transhepatic → biliary drainage, percutaneous transhepatic.
biliary manometry *chir.* Gallengangsmanometrie *f*.
biliary obstruction Gallengangs-, Gallenwegsobstruktion *f*.
biliary pancreatitis biliäre Pankreatitis *f*.
biliary peritonitis → bile peritonitis.
biliary pressure Gallengangsdruck *m*.
biliary stasis Galle(n)stauung *f*, -stase *f*.
biliary stone → biliary calculus.
biliary stricture *chir.* Gallengangsstriktur *f*.
biliary surgery Gallen(gangs)chirurgie *f*.
biliary system Gallensystem *nt*.
biliary tree Gallengangssystem *nt*.
bil·i·a·tion [ˌbɪlɪ'eɪʃn] *n* Gallensekretion *f*.
bil·i·cy·a·nin [ˌbɪlɪ'saɪənɪn] *n* Bili-, Cholezyanin *nt*.
bil·i·di·ges·tive [ˌbɪlɪ'dʒɛstɪv, -dɪ-] *adj* Gallenblase u. Verdauungstrakt betr. *od.* verbindend, biliodigestiv.
bilidigestive anastomosis *chir.* biliodigestive Anastomose/Fistel *f*, biliodigestiver Bypass/Shunt *m*, biliointestinaler Shunt *m*.
bi·lif·er·ous tubule [bɪ'lɪfərəs] Gallengang(s)kapillare *f*.
bil·i·fla·vin [ˌbɪlɪ'fleɪvɪn, -'flæ-] *n* Biliflavin *nt*.

bil·i·fus·cin [ˌ-'fʌsɪn] *n* Bilifuszin *nt*, -fuscin *nt*.
bil·i·gen·e·sis [ˌ-'dʒenəsɪs] *n* Galle(n)bildung *f*, -produktion *f*, Biligenese *f*.
bil·i·ge·net·ic [ˌ-dʒɪ'netɪk] *adj* **1.** Biligenese betr. **2.** → biligenic.
bil·i·gen·ic [ˌ-'dʒenɪk] *adj* galleproduzierend, -bildend, biligen.
bi·lin [baɪ'lɪn] *n* Bilin *nt*.
bil·ious ['bɪljəs] *adj* **1.** → biliary. **2.** *fig.* reizbar, gereizt, cholerisch.
bilious attack Gallenkolik *f*, Colica hepatica.
bilious colic kolikartige Oberbauchschmerzen *pl* mit Galleerbrechen.
bilious complaint Gallenleiden *nt*, -beschwerden *pl*.
bilious headache Migräne *f*, Migraine *f*.
bil·ious·ness ['bɪljəsnɪs] *n* **1.** Gallenbeschwerden *pl*, -krankheit *f*, Gallenleiden *nt*. **2.** *fig.* Gereiztheit *f*, Reizbarkeit *f*.
bilious vomiting galliges Erbrechen *nt*, Galleerbrechen *nt*, Vomitus biliosus.
bil·i·pra·sin [ˌbɪlɪ'preɪsɪn] *n* Biliprasin *nt*.
bil·i·ra·chia [ˌ-'reɪkɪə] *n* Bilir(h)achie *f*.
bil·i·rha·chia [ˌ-'reɪkɪə] *n* → bilirachia.
bil·i·ru·bin [ˌ'-ruːbɪn] *n* Bilirubin *nt*.
bil·i·ru·bin·ate [ˌ-'ruːbɪneɪt] *n* Bilirubinsalz *nt*, Bilirubinat *nt*.
bilirubin-binding globulin Bilirubin-bindendes Globulin *nt*.
bilirubin-calcium calculus Bilirubinkalkstein *m*, Kalziumbilirubinatstein *m*.
bilirubin-calcium stone → bilirubin-calcium calculus.
bilirubin diglucuronide Bilirubindiglukuronid *nt*.
bil·i·ru·bi·ne·mia [ˌbɪləruːbɪ'niːmɪə] *n* Bilirubinämie *f*.
bilirubin encephalopathy Kernikterus *m*, Bilirubinenzephalopathie *f*.
bil·i·ru·bin·ic [ˌ-ruː'bɪnɪk] *adj* Bilirubin betr., Bilirubin-.
bilirubin sulfate Bilirubinsulfat *nt*.
bilirubin UDP-glucuronyltransferase Glukuronyltransferase *f*.
bil·i·ru·bi·nu·ria [ˌ-ruːbɪ'n(j)ʊərɪə] *n* Bilirubinausscheidung *f* im Harn, Bilirubinurie *f*.
bi·lis ['baɪlɪs] *n* → bile.
bil·i·ver·din [ˌbɪlɪ'vɜrdɪn] *n* Biliverdin *nt*.
bil·i·ver·din·ate [ˌ-'vɜrdɪneɪt] *n* Biliverdinsalz *nt*, Biliverdinat *nt*.
bil·i·ver·din·ic acid [ˌ-vɜr'dɪnɪk] → biliverdin.
bil·i·xan·thin [ˌ-'zænθɪn] *n* Choletelin *nt*, Bilixanthin *nt*.
bil·i·xan·thine [ˌ-'zænθiːn] *n* → bilixanthin.
bill [bɪl] **I** *n* **1.** Rechnung *f*, Liste *f*, Aufstellung *f*; Bescheinigung *f*. **2.** Schnabel *m*, schnabelähnliche Schnauze *f*. **3.** (*Schere*) Schneide *f*. **II** *vt* eine Rechnung ausstellen.
  b. of health Gesundheitsattest *nt*, -paß *m*, -zeugnis *nt*.
Billroth ['bɪlrəʊt]: **B.'s cords** → B.'s strands.
B.'s disease 1. traumatische Meningozele *f*. **2.** Lymphknotenschwellung *f*, -tumor *m*, Lymphom(a) *nt*.
B. hypertrophy idiopathische benigne Pylorushypertrophie *f*, Billroth-Syndrom *nt*.
B.'s operation I Billroth-I-Magenresektion *f*, -Operation *f*.
B.'s operation II Billroth-II-Magenresektion *f*, -Operation *f*.
B.'s strands Milztrabekel *pl*, -stränge *pl*, Trabeculae splenicae.
bi·lo·bate [baɪ'ləʊbeɪt] *adj* bilobär, zweilappig, zweigelappt.
bilobate placenta zweigeteilte Plazenta *f*, Placenta bilobata/bipartita.

bi·lobed placenta ['baɪləʊbt] → bilobate placenta.
bi·lob·u·lar [baɪ'lɒbjələr] *adj* bilobulär.
bi·lob·u·late [baɪ'lɒbjəlɪt] *adj* → bilobular.
bi·loc·u·lar [baɪ'lɑkjələr] *adj* zweikamm(e)rig.
bilocular hydrocele Dupuytren'-Hydrozele *f*.
bilocular stomach *patho.* Sanduhrmagen *m*.
bi·loc·u·late [baɪ'lɑkjəlɪt] *adj* → bilocular.
bi·mal·le·o·lar fracture [baɪməˈlɪələr] bimalleoläre (Knöchel-)Fraktur *f*.
bi·man·u·al [baɪ'mænjʊəl] *adj* mit beiden Händen, bimanuell, beidhändig.
bimanual percussion Finger-Finger-Perkussion *f*.
bimanual version *gyn.* bimanuelle/kombinierte Wendung *f*.
bi·max·il·lar·y [baɪ'mæksəˌlerɪː, -mækˈsɪlərɪ] *adj* Ober- u. Unterkiefer betr., bimaxillär.
Bimberg ['bɪmbɜrg]: **B. bow** *gyn.* Bimberg--Schleife *f*.
bi·met·al [baɪ'metl] **I** *n* Bimetall *nt*. **II** *adj* → bimetallic.
bi·me·tal·lic [ˌbaɪməˈtælɪk] *adj* auf zwei Metalle bezogen, aus zwei Metallen bestehend, bimetallisch.
bimetal thermometer Bimetallthermometer *nt*.
B immunoblast B-Immunoblast *m*.
bi·mod·al [baɪ'məʊdl] *adj* bimodal; *mathe.* zweigipfelig.
bi·mo·lec·u·lar [ˌbaɪməˈlekjələr] *adj* *chem.* aus zwei Molekülen bestehend, bimolekular.
bi·na·ry ['baɪnərɪ, -ˌneriː] *adj* aus zwei Elementen bestehend, binär, binar(isch), zweifach-, Binär-.
binary complex binärer Komplex *m*.
binary compound *chem.* binäre Verbindung *f*.
binary digit → bit.
binary fissure Zweiteilung *f*.
binary symbol Binärzeichen *nt*.
bi·na·sal hemianopia/hemianopsia [baɪ'neɪzl] *ophthal.* binasale Hemianop(s)ie *f*.
bin·au·ral [baɪ'nɔːrəl, 'bɪnɔːrəl] *adj* **1.** beide Ohren betr., mit beiden Ohren, für beide Ohren, binaural, binotisch, beidohrig. **2.** *phys.* zweikanalig, Stereo-.
binaural diplacusis *HNO* binaurale Diplakusis *f*, Diplacusis binauralis.
binaural hearing binaurales/beidohriges Hören *m*.
bind [baɪnd] (*v*: **bound; bound**) **I** *vt* **1.** (an-, um-, fest-)binden; verbinden; (*Bein*) (ver-)binden, (um-)wickeln. **2.** *med.* verstopfen. **3.** *chem.* binden. **4.** *fig.* binden, verpflichten. **II** *vi* **5.** *chem.* binden. **6.** *med.* stopfen. **7.** *fig.* binden(d sein), verpflichten.
bind up *vt* (*Wunde*) verbinden.
bind·er ['baɪndər] *n* **1.** *chem.* Bindemittel *nt*. **2.** Binde *f*. **3.** Einband *m*; Hefter *m*; (Akten-)Deckel *m*.
bind·ing ['baɪndɪŋ] **I** *n* **1.** Binden *nt*; Bindung *f*, bindende Kraft *f*. **2.** *chem.* Bindemittel *nt*. **II** *adj* (an-)bindend, verbindend, Bindungs-; verpflichtend.
binding assay Bindungstest *m*, -assay *m*.
binding capacity Bindungskapazität *f*.
binding constant Assoziationskonstante *f*.
binding energy *chem.* Bindungsenergie *f*.
binding equilibrium *chem.* Bindungsgleichgewicht *nt*.
binding locus → binding site.
binding protein Bindungsprotein *nt*.
binding site *biochem.*, *chem.* Bindungsstelle *f*.
A b. → aminoacyl b.

aminoacyl b. Aminoacylbindungsstelle, A-Bindungsstelle.
antigen b. Antigenbindungsstelle.
complement b. Komplementbindungsstelle.
F$_c$-receptor b. F$_c$-Rezeptorbindungsstelle.
bi·neg·a·tive [baɪ'negətɪv] *adj* *chem.* zweifach negativ.
Binet [bi'neɪ]: **B.'s scale** Binet-Skala *f*.
B.'s test *psycho.* Binet-Simon-Test *m*, -Methode *f*.
Binet-Simon [si'mɔ̃]: **B.-S. scale** Binet--Simon-Skala *f*.
B.-S. test → Binet's test.
Bing [bɪŋ]: **B.'s reflex** Bing-Reflex *m*.
bin·oc·u·lar [bɪ'nɑkjələr, baɪ-] **I** *n* (*oft ~s pl*) Binokular *m*, Binokel *nt*; Brille *f*; Fernglas *nt*; Binokularmikroskop *nt*. **II** *adj* **1.** beide Augen betr. binokular, beidäugig. **2.** binokular, mit zwei Okularen versehen.
binocular accommodation *ophthal.* binokulare Akkommodation *f*.
binocular coordination *neuro.* binokuläre Koordination *f*.
binocular diplopia *ophthal.* binokuläre Diplopie *f*.
binocular fusion *ophthal.* binokuläre Fusion *f*.
binocular hemianopia/hemianopsia *ophthal.* bilaterale/binokuläre Hemianop(s)ie *f*.
binocular microscope binokulares Mikroskop *nt*, Doppelmikroskop *nt*, Binokularmikroskop *nt*.
binocular ophthalmoscope *ophthal.* binokuläres Ophthalmoskop *nt*, Stere(o)ophthalmoskop *nt*.
binocular polyopia Doppel-, Doppeltsehen *nt*, Diplopie *f*, Diplopia *f*.
binocular rivalry *ophthal.* Netzhautrivalität *f*.
binocular strabismus *ophthal.* alternierendes Schielen *nt*, Strabismus alternans.
binocular summation binokulare/binokuläre Summation *f*.
binocular vision binokulares/binokuläres Sehen *nt*.
bi·no·mi·al [baɪ'nəʊmɪəl] **I** *n* *mathe.* zweigliedriger Ausdruck *m*, Binom *nt*. **II** *adj* *mathe.* zweigliedrig, binomisch, Binomial-; *bio.* zweinamig, binominal.
binomial coefficient Binomialkoeffizient *m*.
binomial distribution *stat.* Binomialverteilung *f*.
bi·nom·i·nal [baɪ'nɑmɪnl] *adj* → binomial II.
bin·ot·ic [bɪ'nɑtɪk] *adj* → binaural 1.
bin·ov·u·lar twins [bɪn'ɑvjələr] binovuläre/dissimiläre/dizygote/erbungleiche/heteroovuläre/zweieiige Zwillinge *pl*.
Binswanger ['bɪnswæŋər]: **B.'s dementia/disease/encephalitis/encephalopathy** Binswanger-Enzephalopathie *f*, subkortikale progressive Enzephalopathie *f*, Encephalopathia chronica progressiva subcorticalis.
bi·nu·cle·ar [baɪ'n(j)uːklɪər] *adj* zweikernig.
bi·nu·cle·ate [baɪ'n(j)uːklɪɪt, -eɪt] *adj* → binuclear.
bio- *pref.* Lebens-, Bi(o)-.
bi·o·ac·tive [ˌbaɪəʊˈæktɪv] *adj* biologisch aktiv, bioaktiv.
bi·o·ac·tiv·i·ty [ˌ-ækˈtɪvətɪ] *n* Bioaktivität *f*.
bi·o·a·mine [ˌ-əˈmiːn, -ˈæmɪn] *n* biogenes Amin *nt*, Bioamin *nt*.
bi·o·am·i·ner·gic [ˌ-ˌæmɪˈnɜrdʒɪk] *adj* bioaminerg.
bi·o·as·say [*n* ˌ-əˈseɪ, -ˈæseɪ; *v* -əˈseɪ] **I** *n* Bioassay *m*. **II** *vt* etw. einer Bioassayprüfung unterziehen.
bi·o·a·vail·a·bil·i·ty [ˌ-əˌveɪləˈbɪlətɪ] *n* *pharm.* biologische Verfügbarkeit *f*, Bioverfügbarkeit *f*.
bi·o·a·vail·a·ble [ˌ-əˈveɪləbl] *adj* biologisch verfügbar.
bi·o·be·hav·ior·al [ˌ-bɪˈheɪvjərəl] *adj* biologische Verhaltensforschung betr.
biobehavioral science biologische Verhaltensforschung *f*, biologische Ethologie *f*.
bi·o·blast ['-blæst] *n* **1.** Mitochondrie *f*, -chondrion *nt*, -chondrium *nt*, Chondriosom *nt*. **2.** *bio.* Bioblast *m*.
bi·o·cat·a·lyst [ˌ-ˈkætlɪst] *n* Enzym *nt*.
bi·o·cat·a·lyz·er [ˌ-ˈkætlaɪzər] *n* Enzym *nt*.
bi·o·ce·no·sis [ˌ-sɪˈnəʊsɪs] *n* *bio.* Biozönose *f*.
bi·o·chem·ic [ˌ-ˈkemɪk] *adj* → biochemical II.
bi·o·chem·i·cal [ˌ-ˈkemɪkl] **I** *n* biochemisches Produkt *nt*. **II** *adj* Biochemie betr., biochemisch.
biochemical energetics biochemische Energetik *f*.
biochemical mapping biochemisches Kartieren *nt*, biochemische Kartierung *f*.
bi·o·chem·ist [ˌ-ˈkemɪst] *n* Biochemiker(in *f*) *m*.
bi·o·chem·is·try [ˌ-ˈkemɪstrɪ] *n* physiologische Chemie *f*, Biochemie *f*.
bi·o·che·mor·phol·o·gy [ˌ-ˌkiːmɔːrˈfɑlədʒɪ] *n* Biochemomorphologie *f*.
bi·o·cid·al [ˌ-ˈsaɪdl] *adj* biozid.
bi·o·cide ['baɪəsaɪd] *n* Schädlingsbekämpfungsmittel *nt*, Biozid *nt*.
bi·o·cli·mat·ics [ˌ-klaɪˈmætɪks] *pl* → bioclimatology.
bi·o·cli·ma·to·log·i·cal [ˌ-ˌklaɪmətəˈlɑdʒɪkl] *adj* bioklimatologisch.
bi·o·cli·ma·tol·o·gy [ˌ-ˌklaɪməˈtɑlədʒɪ] *n* Bioklimatologie *f*.
bi·o·coe·no·sis = biocenosis.
bi·o·col·loid [ˌ-ˈkɑlɔɪd] *n* Biokolloid *nt*.
bi·o·com·pat·i·bil·i·ty [ˌ-kəmˌpætəˈbɪlətɪ] *n* Biokompatibilität *f*.
bi·o·com·pat·i·ble [ˌ-kəmˈpætɪbl] *adj* nicht gewebs-/zell-/funktionsschädigend, biokompatibel.
bi·o·cy·ber·net·ics [ˌ-ˌsaɪbərˈnetɪks] *pl* Biokybernetik *f*.
bi·o·cy·cle [ˌ-ˈsaɪkl] *n* biologischer Zyklus *m*, Biozyklus *m*.
bi·o·cy·tin [ˌ-ˈsaɪtɪn] *n* Biocytin *nt*, Biotinyllysin *nt*.
bi·o·de·grad·a·bil·i·ty [ˌ-dɪˈgreɪdəbɪlətɪ] *n* biologische Abbaubarkeit *f*.
bi·o·de·grad·a·ble [ˌ-dɪˈgreɪdəbl] *adj* biologisch abbaubar.
bi·o·deg·ra·da·tion [ˌ-ˌdegrəˈdeɪʃn] *n* biologischer Abbauen *m*.
bi·o·de·grade [ˌ-dɪˈgreɪd] *vi* (s.) biologisch abbauen.
bi·o·de·te·ri·o·ra·tion [ˌ-dɪˌtɪərɪəˈreɪʃn] *n* → biodegradation.
bi·o·dy·nam·ic [ˌ-daɪˈnæmɪk] *adj* Biodynamik betr., biodynamisch, ökologische Landwirtschaft betr.
bi·o·dy·nam·i·cal [ˌ-daɪˈnæmɪkl] *adj* → biodynamic.
bi·o·dy·nam·ics [ˌ-daɪˈnæmɪks, -dɪ-] *pl* Biodynamik *f*.
bi·o·ec·o·log·ic [ˌ-ekəˈlɑdʒɪk, -iːkə-] *adj* bioökologisch.
bi·o·ec·o·log·i·cal [ˌ-ekəˈlɑdʒɪkl, -iːkə-] *adj* → bioecologic.
bi·o·e·col·o·gy [ˌ-ɪˈkɑlədʒɪ] *n* Bioökologie *f*, Ökologie *f*.
bi·o·e·lec·tric [ˌ-ɪˈlektrɪk] *adj* bioelektrisch.
bi·o·e·lec·tri·cal [ˌ-ɪˈlektrɪkl] *adj* → bioelectric.

bioelectrical synapse

bioelectrical synapse (bio-)elektrische Synapse f.
bi·o·e·lec·tric·i·ty [ˌ-ɪlek'trɪsətɪ] n Bioelektrizität f.
bioelectric potential bioelektrisches Potential nt.
bi·o·e·lec·tron·ic [ˌ-ɪlek'trɑnɪk] adj bioelektronisch.
bi·o·e·lec·tron·ics [ˌ-ɪlek'trɑnɪks] pl Bioelektronik f.
bi·o·el·e·ment [ˌ-'eləmənt] n Bioelement nt.
bi·o·en·er·get·ics [ˌ-enər'dʒetɪks] pl biochem. Bioenergetik f.
bi·o·en·gi·neer·ing [ˌ-ˌendʒɪ'nɪərɪŋ] n Biotechnik f, Bioengeneering nt.
bi·o·e·quiv·a·lence [ˌ-ɪ'kwɪvələns] n Bioäquivalenz f.
bi·o·e·quiv·a·lent [ˌ-ɪ'kwɪvələnt] adj bioäquivalent.
bi·o·feed·back [ˌ-'fiːdbæk] n Biofeedback nt.
bi·o·fla·vo·noid [ˌ-'fleɪvənɔɪd, -'flæ-] n Bioflavonoid nt.
bi·o·gen·e·sis [ˌ-'dʒenəsɪs] n Biogenese f.
bi·o·ge·net·ic [ˌ-dʒɪ'netɪk] adj 1. Biogenese betr., biogenetisch. 2. Genetic Engineering betr.
bi·o·ge·net·i·cal [ˌ-dʒɪ'netɪkl] adj → biogenetic.
bi·o·ge·net·ics [ˌ-dʒɪ'netɪks] pl Genmanipulation f, genetische Manipulation f, Genetic engineering nt.
bi·o·gen·ic [ˌ-'dʒenɪk] adj biogen.
biogenic amine → bioamine.
bi·og·e·nous [baɪ'ɑdʒənəs] adj aus Lebewesen entstanden, biogen.
bi·og·e·ny [baɪ'ɑdʒenɪ] n → biogenesis.
bi·o·ge·og·ra·phy [ˌbaɪəʊdʒɪ'ɑgrəfɪ] n Biogeographie f.
bi·o·im·plant [ˌ-'ɪmplænt] n chir. Bioimplantat nt.
bi·o·ki·net·ics [ˌ-kɪ'netɪks, -kaɪ-] pl Biokinetik f.
bio·ki·net·ic zone [ˌ-kɪ'netɪk] biokinetische Zone f.
bi·o·log·ic [ˌbaɪə'lɑdʒɪk] adj → biological II.
bi·o·log·i·cal [baɪə'lɑdʒɪkl] I n pharm. biologisches Präparat nt (Serum, Vakzine etc.). II adj Biologie betr., biologisch.
biological amplifier biologischer Verstärker m.
biological assay → bioassay I.
biological balance biologisches Gleichgewicht nt.
biological child leibliches Kind nt.
biological chemistry → biochemistry.
biological clock physiol. biologische Uhr f, innere Uhr f.
biological engineering → bioengineering.
biological evolution biologische Evolution f, Darwin'-Evolution f.
biological father leiblicher Vater m.
biological half-life (period) biologische Halbwertszeit f.
biological mother leibliche Mutter f.
biological oxidation biologische Oxydation f.
biological parent 1. ~s pl leibliche Eltern pl. **2.** → biological father. **3.** → biological mother.
biological rhythm → biorhythm.
biological system biologisches System nt, Biosystem nt.
biological warfare biologische Kriegsführung f.
biologic false-positive abbr. **BFP** immun. biologisch falsch-positiver Test m, biologisch falsch-positive Reaktion f.
bi·ol·o·gist [baɪ'ɑlədʒɪst] n Biologe m, Biologin f.

bi·ol·o·gy [baɪ'ɑlədʒɪ] n Biologie f.
bi·o·lu·mi·nes·cence [ˌbaɪəʊˌluːmɪ'nesəns] n Biolumineszenz f.
bi·ol·y·sis [baɪ'ɑləsɪs] n Biolyse f.
bi·o·lyt·ic [ˌbaɪə'lɪtɪk] adj 1. Biolyse betr., von Biolyse betroffen, biolytisch. 2. Leben od. Lebewesen zerstörend, biolytisch.
bi·o·mass ['baɪəʊmæs] n Biomasse f.
biomass concentration Biomassenkonzentration f.
bi·o·ma·te·ri·al [ˌ-mə'tɪərɪəl] n Biomaterial nt.
bi·o·math·e·mat·i·cal [ˌ-ˌmæθə'mætɪkl] adj biomathematisch.
bi·o·math·e·mat·ics [ˌ-ˌmæθə'mætɪks] pl Biomathematik f.
bi·ome ['baɪəʊm] n Biom nt.
bi·o·me·chan·i·cal [ˌbaɪəʊmɪ'kænɪkl] adj Biomechanik betr., biomechanisch.
bi·o·me·chan·ics [ˌ-mɪ'kænɪks] pl Biomechanik f.
bi·o·med·i·cal [ˌ-'medɪkl] adj biologisch-medizinisch, medizinisch-biologisch, biomedizinisch.
bi·o·med·i·cine [ˌ-'medəsɪn] n Biomedizin f.
bi·o·mem·brane [ˌ-'membreɪn] n Biomembran nt.
bi·o·mem·bra·nous [ˌ-'membrənəs] adj biomembranös.
bi·o·me·te·or·o·log·i·cal [ˌ-ˌmɪtɪərə'lɑdʒɪkl] adj biometeorologisch.
bi·o·me·te·o·rol·o·gy [ˌ-ˌmɪtɪə'rɑlədʒɪ] n Biometeorologie f, Meteorobiologie f.
bi·o·met·rics [ˌ-'metrɪks] pl → biometry.
bi·om·e·try [baɪ'ɑmətrɪ] n Biometrie f, Biometrik f.
bi·o·mi·cro·scope [ˌ-'maɪkrəskəʊp] n Biomikroskop nt.
bi·o·mi·cros·co·py [ˌ-maɪ'krɑskəpɪ] n 1. Biomikroskopie f. 2. (Auge) Hornhautuntersuchung f, Biomikroskopie f.
bi·o·mol·e·cule [ˌ-'mɑlɪkjuːl] n Biomolekül nt.
bi·o·mo·tor [ˌ-'məʊtər] n anes. Biomotor m.
Bi·om·pha·la·ria [baɪˌɑmfə'leərɪə] n micro. Biomphalaria f.
bi·on ['baɪɑn] n Bion nt.
bi·o·ne·cro·sis [ˌbaɪəʊnɪ'krəʊsɪs, -ne-] n derma., patho. Nekrobiose f, Necrobiosis f.
bi·on·ics [baɪ'ɑnɪks] pl Bionik f.
bi·o·nom·ics [ˌ-'nɑmɪks] pl biologische Ökologie f, Bionomik f.
bi·on·o·my [baɪ'ɑnəmɪ] n Bionomie f.
bio-osmotic adj bioosmotisch.
bi·o·phage ['baɪəfeɪdʒ] n Biophage m.
bi·oph·a·gism [baɪ'ɑfədʒɪzəm] n → biophagy.
bi·oph·a·gous [baɪ'ɑfəgəs] adj biophag.
bi·oph·a·gy [baɪ'ɑfədʒɪ] n Biophagie f.
bi·o·phar·ma·ceu·tics [ˌbaɪəʊˌfɑːrməˈsuːtɪks] pl Biopharmazie f.
bi·o·pho·tom·e·ter [ˌ-fəʊ'tɑmətər] n Biophotometer nt.
bi·o·phys·i·cal [ˌ-'fɪsɪkl] adj Biophysik betr., biophysikalisch.
bi·o·phys·ics [ˌ-'fɪsɪks] pl Biophysik f.
bi·o·phys·i·ol·o·gy [ˌ-fɪzɪ'ɑlədʒɪ] n Biophysiologie f.
bi·o·plasm ['-plæzəm] n Protoplasma nt.
bi·o·plas·mic [ˌ-'plæzmɪk] adj protoplasmatisch.
bi·o·pol·y·mer [ˌ-'pɑlɪmər] n Biopolymer nt.
bi·o·pros·the·sis [ˌ-prɑs'θɪsɪs] n chir. Bioprothese f.
bi·op·sy ['baɪɑpsɪ] (v: **biopsied**) I n Biopsie f. II vt eine Biopsie vornehmen, biopsieren.

biopsy forceps Biopsie-, Probeexzisionszange f, PE-Zange f.
biopsy needle Biopsienadel f.
biopsy specimen forceps → biopsy forceps.
biopsy trephine Biopsiestanze f.
bi·o·psy·chic [ˌ-'saɪkɪk] adj psychobiologisch.
bi·o·psy·chol·o·gy [ˌ-saɪ'kɑlədʒɪ] n Psychobiologie f.
bi·op·ter·in [baɪ'ɑptərɪn] n Biopterin nt.
bi·op·tic [baɪ'ɑptɪk] adj Biopsie betr., bioptisch, Biopsie-.
bi·op·tome ['baɪɑptəʊm] n Bioptom nt, Biopsiesonde f.
bi·or·bit·al [baɪ'ɔːrbɪtl] adj beide Augenhöhlen betr., biorbital.
biorbital angle biorbitaler Winkel m.
bi·o·re·vers·i·ble [ˌ-rɪ'vɜːrsɪbl] adj bioreversibel.
bi·o·rhythm ['-rɪðm] n biologischer Rhythmus m, Biorhythmus m.
bi·o·rhyth·mic [ˌ-'rɪðmɪk] adj biorhythmisch.
bi·os¹ ['baɪɑs] n micro. Bios m.
bi·os² ['baɪɑs] n 1. Inosit nt, Inositol nt. 2. meso-, myo-Inosit m, -Inositol nt.
bios II → biotin.
bi·o·sci·ence ['baɪəʊsaɪəns] n Biowissenschaft f.
bi·os·co·py [baɪ'ɑskəpɪ] n Bioskopie f.
bi·ose ['baɪəʊs] n old Disaccharid nt.
bi·os·mo·sis [baɪɑs'məʊsɪs] n Bi(o)osmose f.
bi·o·spec·trom·e·try [ˌbaɪəʊspek'trɑmətrɪ] n Biospektrometrie f.
bi·o·spec·tros·co·py [ˌ-spek'trɑskəpɪ] n Biospektroskopie f.
bi·o·sphere ['baɪəsfɪər] n Biosphäre f.
bi·o·stat·ics [ˌ-'stætɪks] pl Biostatik f.
bi·o·sta·tis·ti·cian [ˌ-ˌstætə'stɪʃn] n Biostatistiker(in f) m.
bi·o·sta·tis·tics [ˌ-stə'tɪstɪks] pl Biostatistik f.
bi·o·ste·re·o·met·rics [ˌ-ˌsterɪə'metrɪks] pl Biostereometrik f.
bi·o·syn·the·sis [ˌ-'sɪnθəsɪs] n Biosynthese f.
bi·o·syn·thet·ic [ˌ-sɪn'θetɪk] adj Biosynthese betr., biosynthetisch.
biosynthetic pathway Biosyntheseweg m, biosynthetischer (Stoffwechsel-)Weg m.
biosynthetic work biosynthetische Arbeit f.
Biot [biː'oː]: **B.'s breathing/respiration** Biot'-Atmung f.
bi·o·tax·is [baɪəʊ'tæksɪs] n Biotaxis f.
bi·o·tax·y [ˌ-'tæksɪ] n 1. → biotaxis. 2. Taxonomie f.
bi·o·te·lem·e·try [ˌ-tə'lemətrɪ] n Biotelemetrie f.
bi·ot·ic [baɪ'ɑtɪk] adj Leben od. lebende Materie betr., biotisch, Lebens-.
bi·o·tin ['baɪətɪn] n Biotin nt, Vitamin H nt.
biotin carboxylase abbr. **BC**.
biotin carboxyl-carrier protein abbr. **BCCP** Biotin-Carboxyl-Carrier-Protein nt abbr. BCCP.
bi·o·tin·yl·ly·sine [ˌ-tɪnl'laɪsɪn] n → biocytin.
bi·o·tope ['-təʊp] n Lebensraum m, Biotop m/nt.
bi·o·tox·i·ca·tion [ˌ-ˌtæksɪ'keɪʃn] n Biotoxinintoxikation f.
bi·o·tox·i·col·o·gy [ˌ-ˌtæksɪ'kɑlədʒɪ] n Biotoxikologie f.
bi·o·tox·in [ˌ-'tæksɪn] n Biotoxin nt.
bi·o·trans·for·ma·tion [ˌ-ˌtrænsfər'meɪʃn] n Biotransformation f.
bi·o·type ['-taɪp] n Biotyp m, -typus m, -var m.

bi·o·var ['-vɑːr] *n* → biotype.
bi·o·war·fare [‚-'wɔːrfeər] *n* → biological warfare
bi·pa·ren·tal [baɪpə'rentl] *adj* beide Eltern betr., biparental.
bi·pa·ri·e·tal [baɪpə'raɪɪtl] *adj* biparietal.
biparietal diameter *gyn., ped.* biparietaler Durchmesser *m*, Diameter biparietalis.
biparietal suture Pfeilnaht *f*, Sutura sagittalis.
bi·par·tite [baɪ'pɑːrtaɪt] *adj* zweigeteilt, zweiteilig, Zwei(er)-.
bipartite placenta → bilobate placenta.
bipartite uterus Uterus bilocularis/bipartitus/septus.
bi·ped ['baɪped] **I** *n* Zweifüß(l)er *m*, -beiner *m*, Bipede *m*. **II** *adj* zweifüßig, -beinig, bipedisch.
bi·ped·al ['baɪpedl, -pɪdl] *adj* → biped II.
bi·ped·i·cle flap [baɪ'pedɪkl] zweigestielter (Haut-)Lappen *m*.
bi·pen·nate muscle [baɪ'peneɪt] doppeltgefiederter Muskel *m*, M. bipennatus.
bi·per·i·den [baɪ'perɪden] *n pharm.* Biperiden *nt*.
bi·phen·yl [baɪ'fenl, -'fiːnl] *n* Bi-, Diphenyl *nt*.
bi·plane mammogram ['baɪpleɪn] *radiol.* Zwei-Ebenen-Mammogramm *nt*.
bi·po·lar [baɪ'pəʊlər] **I** *n* → bipolar neuron. **II** *adj* zweipolig, bipolar.
bipolar cell → bipolar neuron.
bipolar disorder manisch-depressive Psychose/Krankheit *f*.
bipolar lead *physiol.* (*EKG*) bipolare Ableitung *f*.
bipolar neuroblast *embryo.* bipolarer Neuroblast *m*.
bipolar neuron bipolares Neuron *nt*, bipolare Nervenzelle *f*.
bipolar psychosis → bipolar disorder.
bipolar recording → bipolar lead.
bipolar version → bimanual version.
bi·pos·i·tive [baɪ'pɑzətɪv] *adj chem.* zweifach positiv.
Birbeck ['bɪərbek]: **B.'s granules** Birbeck-Granula *pl*.
Bird [bɜrd]: **B.'s sign** Bird-Zeichen *nt*.
bird-breeder's lung [bɜrd] Vogel-, Taubenzüchterlunge *f*.
bird-fancier's lung → bird-breeder's lung.
bird mite *micro.* Vogelmilbe *f*, Dermanyssus avium.
bird·seed agar ['bɜrdsiːd] Staib-Agar *m/nt*.
bi·re·frac·tive [baɪrɪ'fræktɪv] *adj* → birefringent.
bi·re·frin·gence [baɪ'frɪndʒəns] *n phys.* Doppelbrechung *f*.
bi·re·frin·gent [baɪ'frɪndʒənt] *adj phys.* doppelbrechend, birefraktär.
Birkett ['bɜrket]: **B.'s hernia** Birkett-Hernie *f*, Hernia synovialis.
birth [bɜrθ] *n* **1.** Geburt *f*, Geborenwerden *nt*. **from/since (one's) ~** von Geburt an. **2.** Geburt *f*, Entbindung *f*, Niederkunft *f*, Partus *m*. **at ~** bei/unter der Geburt. **to give ~ (to)** gebären, zur Welt bringen, entbinden.
birth canal *gyn.* Geburtskanal *m*.
birth certificate Geburtsurkunde *f*.
birth·con·trol ['bɜrθkən‚trəʊl] *n* Geburtenregelung *f*, -kontrolle *f*, -beschränkung *f*.
birth-control pill (Antibaby-)Pille *f*.
birth·day ['-deɪ] *n* Geburtstag *m*.
birth defect bei der Geburt vorhandener Defekt *m*, konnataler Defekt *m*.
birth·mark [-mɑːrk] *n* Muttermal *nt*.
birth palsy → birth paralysis.
birth paralysis Geburtslähmung *f*, geburtstraumatische Lähmung *f*.
birth·place ['-pleɪs] *n* Geburtsort *m*.

birth·rate ['-reɪt] *n* Geburtenziffer *f*, -häufigkeit *f*, Natalität *f*.
birth·stool ['-stuːl] *n* Gebärstuhl *m*.
birth-weight ['-weɪt] *n* Geburtsgewicht *nt*.
bis·ac·o·dyl [bɪs'ækədɪl] *n pharm.* Bisacodyl *nt*.
bis·al·bu·mi·ne·mia [bɪsæl‚bjuːmɪ'niːmɪə] *n* Bi(s)albuminämie *f*.
bi·sect [baɪ'sekt, 'baɪsekt] **I** *vt* in zwei Teile (zer-)schneiden *od.* teilen, halbieren. **II** *vi s.* teilen *od.* gabeln.
bi·sec·tion [baɪ'sekʃn] *n* Halbierung *f*, Halbieren *nt*.
bi·sex·u·al [baɪ'sekʃəwəl, -seksjʊəl] **I** *n* Bisexuelle(r *m*) *f*. **II** *adj* **1.** *bio.* doppel-, zweigeschlechtig, zwitterhaft, bisexuell. **2.** (*Sexualität*) bisexuell.
bi·sex·u·al·i·ty [‚baɪseksʃə'wælətɪ] *n* **1.** *bio.* Doppel-, Zweigeschlechtigkeit *f*, Bisexualität *f*. **2.** echter Hermaphroditismus *m*, Hermaphroditis verus. **3.** (*Sexualität*) Bisexualität *f*.
bis·fer·i·ous pulse [bɪs'ferɪəs, -fɪər-] Pulsus bisferiens.
bish·op's cap ['bɪʃəp] Pars superior duodeni.
bis·hy·drox·y·cou·ma·rin [‚bɪshaɪ‚drɒksɪ'kuːmərɪn] *n* Dic(o)umarol *nt*.
bis in die [bɪs ɪn dɪæ] *abbr.* **b.i.d., b.d.** *pharm.* zweimal täglich.
Bis·kra boil ['bɪskrɑː] kutane Leishmaniose *f*, Hautleishmaniose *f*, Orientbeule *f*, Leishmaniasis cutis.
Bismarck ['bɪzmɑːrk]: **B. brown** Bismarckbraun *nt*.
bis·muth ['bɪzməθ] *n abbr.* **Bi** Wismut *nt*, Bismutum *nt abbr.* **Bi**.
bismuth carbonate Wismutkarbonat *nt*. **basic b.** → bismuth subcarbonate.
bismuth gingivitis 1. Gingivitis *f* bei Wismutvergiftung. **2.** → bismuth stomatitis.
bis·muth·ism ['bɪzməθɪzəm] *n* → bismuthosis.
bismuth line Wismutsaum *m*.
bis·muth·o·sis [bɪzmə'θəʊsɪs] *n* (chronische) Wismutvergiftung *f*, Bismutismus *m*, Bismutose *f*.
bismuth stomatitis Wismutstomatitis *f*, Stomatitis bismutica.
bismuth subcarbonate basisches Wismutkarbonat *nt*, Bismutum subcarbonicum.
bismuth subgallate basisches Wismutgallat *nt*, Bismutum subgallicum.
bismuth subnitrate basisches Wismutnitrat *nt*, Bismutum subnitricum.
bismuth subsalicylate Bismutum subsalicylicum.
bismuth sulfite agar Wilson-Blair-Agar *m/nt*, Wismutsulfitagar *m/nt* nach Wilson u. Blair.
bismuth white → bismuth subnitrate.
bi·spe·cif·ic antibody [baɪspɪ'sɪfɪk] hybrider Antikörper *m*.
bi·spher·i·cal lens [baɪ'sferɪkl] bisphärische Linse *f*, bisphärisches Glas *nt*.
2,3-bis·phos·pho·glyc·er·ate [bɪs‚fɑsfəʊ'glɪsəreɪt] *n* 2,3-Diphosphoglycerat *nt*.
bisphosphoglycerate mutase Diphosphoglyceratmutase *f*.
bisphosphoglycerate phosphatase Diphosphoglyceratphosphatase *f*.
bis·phos·pho·glyc·er·o·mu·tase [-‚fɑsfəʊ‚glɪsərəʊ'mjuːteɪz] *n* → bisphosphoglycerate mutase.
bis·tou·ry ['bɪstərɪ] *n chir.* Bistourie *m/nt*.
bi·stra·tal [baɪ'streɪtl] *adj* zweischichtig, -lagig.
bi·sul·fate [baɪ'sʌlfeɪt] *n* Bisulfat *nt*.
bi·sul·fide [baɪ'sʌlfaɪd, -fɪd] *n* Bi-, Disulfid *nt*.
bi·sul·fite [baɪ'sʌlfaɪt] *n* Bisulfit, Hydrogensulfit *nt*.

bit [bɪt] *n* Bit *nt abbr.* bit.
bi·tar·trate [baɪ'tɑːrtreɪt] *n* Bitartrat *nt*.
bite [baɪt] (*v*: **bit; bitten**) **I** *n* **1.** Beißen *nt*; Biß *m*. **2.** Biß(wunde *f*) *m*. **3.** (Insekten-)-Biß *m*, (-)Stich *m*. **4.** Bissen *m*, Happen *m*. **5.** *chem.* Beizen *nt*, Ätzen *nt*. **II** *vt* **6.** beißen. **to ~ one's nails** an den Nägeln kauen. **7.** (*Insekt*) beißen, stechen. **8.** *chem.* beizen, ätzen, zerfressen, angreifen. **III** *vi* **9.** zubeißen. **10.** (*Insekt*) beißen, stechen. **11.** (*Rauch*) beißen, (*Wind*) schneiden.
bi·tem·po·ral diameter [baɪ'temp(ə)rəl] *gyn., ped.* bitemporaler Durchmesser, Diameter bitemporalis.
bitemporal hemianopia/hemianopsia bitemporale Hemianop(s)ie *f*.
bite plane *dent.* Biß-, Okklusionsebene *f*.
bite-shaped *adj* mundgerecht.
bit·ing ['baɪtɪŋ] *adj* (*a. fig.*) beißend, schneidend.
biting lice *micro.* Läuslinge *pl*, Kieferläuse *pl*, Mallophaga *pl*.
bi·tol·ter·ol [baɪ'təʊltərəʊl] *n pharm.* Bitolterol *nt*.
Bitot ['biːtəʊ]: **B.'s patches/spots** Bitot'-Flecken *pl*.
bi·tro·chan·ter·ic [baɪ‚trəʊkən'terɪk] *adj* bitrochantär.
bit·ter ['bɪtər] **I** *n* **1.** Bitterkeit *f*. **2.** (Magen-)Bitter *m*. **II** *adj* (*Geschmack*) bitter; (*Worte, Schicksal*) bitter, schmerzhaft, hart. **III** *vt* bitter machen. **IV** *vi* bitter werden.
bitter almond Bittermandel *f*.
bitter-almond oil Bittermandelöl *nt*.
Bittner ['bɪtnər]: **B.'s agent/milk factor/virus** Mäuse-Mamma-Tumorvirus *nt abbr.* MMTV.
bi·tu·men [baɪ't(j)uːmən, bɪ-, 'bɪtʃʊ-] *n* Bitumen *nt*.
bi·u·rate ['baɪjʊəreɪt] *n* Biurat *nt*.
bi·u·ret [baɪjə'ret, 'baɪjə-] *n* Biuret *nt*, Allophanamid *nt*.
biuret reaction Biuretreaktion *f*.
biuret test → biuret reaction.
bi·va·lence [baɪ'veɪləns, 'bɪvə-] *n chem.* Zweiwertigkeit *f*.
bi·va·len·cy [baɪ'veɪlənsɪ] *n* → bivalence.
bi·va·lent [baɪ'veɪlənt, 'bɪvə-] **I** *n genet.* Bivalent *m*, Chromosomenpaar *nt*, Geminus *m*. **II** *adj* **1.** *chem.* zweiwertig, bi-, divalent. **2.** *genet.* doppelchromosomig, bivalent.
bivalent antibody bivalenter Antikörper *m*.
bi·ven·ter [‚baɪ'ventər] *adj anat.* doppel-, zweibäuchig.
biventer cervicis (muscle) Pars medialis m. semispinalis capitis.
bi·ven·tral [baɪ'ventrəl] **I** *n old* → digastricus (muscle). **II** *adj anat.* zweibäuchig.
biventral lobule Lobulus biventer.
bi·ven·tric·u·lar [baɪven'trɪkjələr] *adj* (*Herz*) beide Kammern betr., biventrikulär.
bi·zarre leiomyoma [bɪ'zɑːr] epitheliales Leiomyom *nt*, Leiomyoblastom *nt*.
Bizzozero [bɪts'ɑːtserəʊ]: **B.'s cells** Blutplättchen *pl*, Thrombozyten *pl*.
B.'s corpuscles → B.'s cells.
B.'s platelets → B.'s cells.
B. red cells Bizzozero-Erythrozyten *pl*.
Bjerrum ['bjerʊm]: **B.'s scotoma** Bjerrum-Zeichen *nt*, -Skotom *nt*.
B. screen Bjerrum-Schirm *m*.
B.'s sign → B. scotoma.
Björk-Schiley ['bjɜrk 'ʃaɪlɪ]: **B.-S. valve** *HTG* Björk-Schiley-Prothese *f*.
Björnstad ['bjɜrnstad]: **B.'s syndrome** Björnstad-Syndrom *nt*.
BK *abbr.* → below-knee.
Bk *abbr.* → berkelium.

BK cast → below-knee cast.
B-K mole syndrome *derm.* BK-mole-Syndrom *nt*, BK-Naevussyndrom *nt*, hereditäres dysplastisches Naevuszellnaevussyndrom *nt*, FAMM-Syndrom *nt.*
Bk virus *micro.* Bk-Virus *nt.*
black [blæk] **I** *n* **1.** Schwarz *nt.* **2.** (*Person*) Schwarze(r *m*) *f*, Farbige(r *m*) *f*, Dunkelhäutige(r *m*) *f.* **II** *adj* **3.** schwarz. **a ~ eye** ein blaues Auge. **to beat s.o. ~ and blue** jdn. grün u. blau schlagen. **to be ~ and blue all over** am ganzen Körper blaue Flecken haben. **4.** (*Person*) schwarz, dunkelhäutig. **III** *vt* → blacken I. **IV** *vi* → blacken II.
black-and-blue *adj* (*Körperstelle*) dunkelblau (verfärbt).
black-and-blue mark blauer Fleck *m*, Hämatom *nt.*
black cancer malignes Melanom *nt abbr.* MM, Melano(zyto)blastom *nt*, Nävokarzinom *nt*, Melanokarzinom *nt*, Melanomalignom *nt*, malignes Nävoblastom *nt.*
black cataract schwarzer Altersstar *m*, Cataracta nigra.
black death 1. Pest *f*, Pestis *f*; *histor.* schwarzer Tod *m.* **2.** Beulen-, Bubonenpest *f*, Pestis bubonica/fulminans/major.
black dermographism schwarzer Dermographismus *m*, Dermographismus niger.
black-en [blækn] **I** *vt* schwärzen, schwarz machen. **II** *vi* schwarz *od.* dunkel werden.
black eye blaues Auge *nt.* **to give s.o. a ~** jdm. ein blaues Auge schlagen.
Blackfan-Diamond ['blækfən 'daıəmənd]: **B.-D. anemia/syndrome** Blackfan-Diamond-Anämie *f*, chronische kongenitale aregenerative Anämie *f*, pure red cell aplasia.
black fever 1. Felsengebirgsfleckfieber *nt*, amerikanisches Zeckenbißfieber *nt*, Rocky Mountain spotted fever (*nt*) *abbr.* RMSF. **2.** viszerale Leishmaniose/Leishmaniase *f*, Kala-Azar *f*, Splenomegalia tropica.
black hairy tongue schwarze Haarzunge *f*, Glossophytie *f*, Melanoglossie *f*, Lingua pilosa/villosa nigra.
black·head ['blækhed] *n* Mitesser *m*, Komedo *m*, Comedo *m.*
black induration *patho.* schiefrige Induration *f.*
black·ish ['blækıʃ] *adj* schwärzlich.
blackish-blue *adj* bläulichschwarz.
black lead Graphit *m.*
black-legged tick *micro.* Ixodes scapularis.
black lung Kohlenstaublunge *f*, Lungenanthrakose *f*, Anthracosis pulmonum.
black measles hämorrhagische Masern *pl.*
black molds *micro.* Schwärzepilze *pl.*
black·out ['blækaʊt] *n* **1.** kurzer plötzlicher Funktionsausfall *m*, Blackout *m/nt.* **2.** *neuro.* (kurze) Ohnmacht *f*, Bewußtlosigkeit *f*, Blackout *m/nt.* **3.** vorübergehender Ausfall *m* des Sehvermögens, Blackout *m/nt.*
black phosphorus schwarzer Phosphor *m.*
black piedra schwarze Haarknötchenkrankheit *f*, Piedra nigra.
black pitted tick *micro.* Rhipicephalus simus.
black sickness → black death 2.
black substance *old anat.* schwarzer Kern *m*, Substantia nigra.
black tongue → black hairy tongue.
black vomit dunkelbraunes Erbrochenes *nt.*
black·wa·ter fever ['blækwɔːtər] Schwarzwasserfieber *nt*, Febris biliosa et haemoglobinurica.
blad·der ['blædər] *n* **1.** *anat., bio.* Blase *f.* **2.** *anat.* Harnblase *f*, Vesica urinaria. **3.** *patho.* Blase *f*, Bläschen *nt*, Bulla *f.*
bladder atony (Harn-)Blasenatonie *f.*
bladder calculus (Harn-)Blasenstein *m*, Zystolith *m*, Calculus vesicae.
bladder carcinoma (Harn-)Blasenkrebs *m*, -karzinom *nt.*
bladder cells *embryo.* Zander-Zellen *pl.*
bladder dilatation Blasen(über)dehnung *f.*
bladder diverticulum (Harn-)Blasendivertikel *nt.*
bladder emptying Blasenentleerung *f.*
bladder evacuation Blasenentleerung *f.*
bladder evacuation reflex Blasenentleerungsreflex *m.*
bladder exstrophy Spaltblase *f*, Blasenekstrophie *f*, -exstrophie *f.*
bladder flap *urol.* (Harn-)Blasenlappen *m.*
bladder inflammation (Harn-)Blasenentzündung *f*, Zystitis *f*, Cystitis *f.*
bladder injury (Harn-)Blasenverletzung *f*, -schädigung *f*, -trauma *nt.*
blad·der·less ['blædərles] *adj bio.* blasenlos, ohne Blase(n).
blad·der·like ['-laık] *adj* blasenähnlich, -artig, blasig.
bladder neck (Harn-)Blasenhals *m*, Cervix vesicae.
bladder outlet obstruction *urol.* Blasenhalsobstruktion *f.*
bladder papilloma (Harn-)Blasenpapillom *nt.*
bladder reflex → bladder evacuation reflex.
bladder stone → bladder calculus.
bladder syringe Blasenspritze *f.*
bladder trauma → bladder injury.
bladder tuberculosis (Harn-)Blasentuberkulose *f.*
bladder wall muscles Blasenwandmuskulatur *f*, Detrusor *m* vesicae, M. detrusor vesicae.
bladder worm Blasenwurm *m*, Zystizerkus *m*, Cysticercus *m.*
blad·der·y ['blædəri] *adj* **1.** blasenähnlich, -artig, blasig. **2.** aufgeblasen.
blade [bleıd] *n* **1.** *anat.* Blatt *nt.* **2.** *techn.* Klinge *f*, Blatt *nt.* **3.** *bot.* Halm *m*, Spreite *f.*
blade holder *chir.* Klingenhalter *m.*
Blalock-Hanlon [bleılak 'hænlən]: **B.-H. operation** Blalock-Hanlon-Operation *f.*
Blalock-Taussig ['tɔːsıg]: **B.-T. anastomosis/operation** Blalock-Taussig-Anastomose *f*, -Operation *f.*
blanch [blæntʃ, blaːntʃ] **I** *vt a. techn.* bleichen. **II** *vi* erbleichen, erblassen, bleich werden (*with* vor).
blanch·er ['blæntʃər, 'blaːn-] *n chem.* Bleichmittel *nt.*
bland [blænd] *adj* **1.** (*Klima*) mild, sanft. **2.** (*Heilmittel*) beruhigend, mild. **3.** (*Kost*) bland, leicht.
bland embolism blande Embolie *f.*
bland embolus blander Embolus *m.*
Blandin [blaːˈdɛ̃, 'blændın]: **B.'s ganglion** Faesebeck-, Blandin'-Ganglion *nt*, Ggl. submandibulare.
B.'s gland Blandin'-Drüse *f*, Zungenspitzendrüse *f*, Gl. lingualis anterior.
bland infarct blander Infarkt *m.*
Blandin-Nuhn [nuːn]: **B.-N.'s gland** → Blandin's gland.
blank [blæŋk] **I** *n* Leere *f*, leere *od.* weiße Stelle *f*, Lücke *f*; Gedächtnislücke *f.* **a ~ in one's memory** Gedächtnis-, Erinnerungslücke. **II** *adj* weiß; unbeschrieben; leer, inhaltslos; (*Gesicht*) ausdruckslos. **his mind went ~** konnte sich an nichts mehr erinnern. **III** *vt* etw. aus- *od.* durchstreichen. **IV** *vi* verwirrt *od.* zerstreut werden, einen Blackout haben.
blank out *vt* → blank III.
blan·ket ['blæŋkıt] *n* (Bett-)Decke *f.*
blank measurement Leermessung *f.*
Blasius ['blaːsıʊs]: **B.' duct** Parotisgang *m*, Stensen'-, Stenon'-Gang *m*, Ductus parotideus.
Blaskovics ['blæskovıtz]: **B. operation** *ophthal.* Blaskovics-Operation *f.*
blast- *pref.* → blasto-.
blast [blæst, blaːst] *n* **1.** Explosion *f*, Detonation *f*; Druckwelle *f.* **2.** *histol., bio.* unreife Zellvorstufe *f*, Blast *m.* **3.** ausgehustete Luft *f.*
blast cell Blast(enzelle *f*) *m.*
blast cell leukemia Stammzellenleukämie *f*, akute undifferenzierte Leukämie *f abbr.* AUL.
blast crisis *hema.* Blastenschub *m*, -krise *f.*
blas·te·ma [blæsˈtiːmə] *n, pl* **-ma·ta** [-mətə] *embryo.* Keimstoff *m*, -gewebe *nt*, Blastem *nt.*
blas·tem·ic [blæsˈtiːmık, -'stɛ-] *adj* Blastem betr.
blas·tid ['blæstıd] *n embryo.* Blastid *m*, Blastide *f.*
blast injury Explosions-, Detonations-, Knalltrauma *nt.*
blasto- *pref.* Keim-, Sproß-, Blast(o)-.
blas·to·cele ['blæstəsiːl] *n embryo.* Furchungs-, Keimhöhle *f*, Blastozöl *nt.*
blas·to·cel·ic [ˌ-'siːlık] *adj* Blastozöl betr.
blas·to·chyle ['-kaıl] *n embryo.* Blastochylus *m.*
blas·to·coel *n* → blastocele.
blas·to·coele *n* → blastocele.
blas·to·coe·lic *adj* → blastocelic.
blas·to·co·nid·i·um [ˌ-kəˈnıdıəm] *n* → blastospore.
blas·to·cyst ['-sıst] *n embryo.* Keimbläschen *nt*, Blastozyste *f.*
blastocyst cavity *embryo.* → blastocele.
blastocyst formation *embryo.* Blastozystenbildung *f*, -entwicklung *f.*
blas·to·cyte ['-saıt] *n embryo.* Blastozyt *m.*
blas·to·cy·to·ma [ˌ-saıˈtəʊmə] *n* → blastoma 1.
Blas·to·den·dri·on [ˌ-ˈdendrıɒn] *n old* → Candida.
blas·to·den·dri·o·sis [ˌ-ˌdendrıˈəʊsıs] *n old* → candidiasis.
blas·to·derm ['-dɜːm] *n embryo.* Keimhaut *f*, Blastoderm *nt.*
blas·to·der·ma [ˌ-ˈdɜːmə] *n* → bastoderm.
blas·to·der·mal [ˌ-ˈdɜːməl] *adj embryo.* Blastoderm betr., vom Blastoderm abstammend, blastodermal.
blas·to·der·mat·ic [ˌ-dɜːrˈmætık] *adj* → blastodermal.
blas·to·der·mic [ˌ-ˈdɜːmık] *adj* → blastodermal.
blastodermic disk *embryo.* Blastodermscheibe *f.*
blastodermic layer Keimzone *f*, -schicht *f.t.*
blas·to·disc ['-dısk] *n* Keimscheibe *f*, -schild *m*, Blastodiskus *m.*
blas·to·gen·e·sis [ˌ-ˈdʒenəsıs] *n* **1.** *embryo.* Keimentwicklung *f*, Blastogenese *f.* **2.** *bio.* asexuelle Vermehrung *f* durch Knospung, Blastogenese *f.* **3.** *hema.* Blastenbildung *f.*
blastogenesis assay gemischte Lymphozytenkultur *f*, Lymphozytenmischkultur *f*, mixed lymphocyte culture *abbr.* MLC, MLC-Assay *m*, MLC-Test *m.*
blas·to·ge·net·ic [ˌ-dʒıˈnetık] *adj* → blastogenic.
blas·to·gen·ic [ˌ-ˈdʒenık] *adj* Keim(zelle) *od.* Keimentwicklung betr., keimgebunden, blastogen.

blastogenic factor *abbr.* **BF** Lymphozytenmitogen *nt*, Lymphozytentransformationsfaktor *m abbr.* LTF.
blas·tog·e·ny [blæs'tɑdʒənɪ] *n bio.*, *embryo.* Blastogenie *f.*
blas·tol·y·sis [blæs'tɑləsɪs] *n* Blastolyse *f.*
blas·to·lyt·ic [ˌblæstə'lɪtɪk] *adj* Blastolyse betr. *od.* auslösend, blastolytisch.
blas·to·ma [blæs'təʊmə] *n*, *pl* **-mas**, **-ma·ta** [-mətə] **1.** Blastom *nt*, Blastozytom *nt.* **2.** (echte) Geschwulst *f*, Neubildung *f*, Tumor *m*, Neoplasma *nt*, Blastom *nt.*
blas·to·ma·toid [blæs'təʊmətɔɪd] *adj* blastomähnlich, blastomatös, blastomös.
blas·to·ma·to·sis [ˌblæstəʊmə'təʊsɪs] *n* **1.** Blastomatose *f.* **2.** Geschwulstbildung *f*, -formation *f*, Tumorbildung *f*, -formation *f.*
blas·to·ma·tous [blæs'təʊmətəs] *adj* → blastomatoid.
blas·to·mere ['blæstəmɪər] *n embryo.* Furchungszelle *f*, Blastomere *f.*
blas·to·me·rot·o·my [ˌ-mɪ'rɑtəmɪ] *n* Blasto(mero)tomie *f.*
blas·to·mo·gen·ic [ˌ-mə'dʒenɪk] *adj* tumorbildend, blastomogen.
blas·to·mog·e·nous [ˌ-'mɑdʒənəs] *adj* blastomogenic.
Blas·to·my·ces [ˌ-'maɪsɪːz] *n micro.* Blastomyces *m.*
blas·to·my·ces [ˌ-'maɪsɪːz] *n*, *pl* **-ce·tes** [-maɪ'siːtɪːz] Hefe-, Sproßpilz *m*, Blastomyzet *m*, Blastomyces *m.*
blas·to·my·cete [ˌ-'maɪsiːt, -maɪ'siːt] *n* → blastomyces.
blas·to·my·ce·tic dermatitis [ˌ-maɪ'siːtɪk] Blastomyzetendermatitis *f*, Dermatitis blastomycotica.
blas·to·my·cin [ˌ-'maɪsn] *n* Blastomyzin *nt.*
Blas·to·my·coi·des immitis [ˌ-maɪ'kɔɪdiːz] *micro.* Coccidioides immitis.
blas·to·my·co·sis [ˌmaɪ'kəʊsɪs] *n* **1.** Blastomycesinfektion *f*, Blastomykose *f*, Blastomykosis *f.* **2.** Erkrankung *f* durch Hefen *od.* hefeähnliche Pilze, Blastomykose *f.*
blas·to·neu·ro·pore [ˌ-'nʊərəpɔːr, -'njʊər-] *n* Blastoneuroporus *m.*
blas·top·a·thy [blæs'tɑpəθɪ] *n* Blastopathie *f.*
blas·toph·tho·ria [ˌblæstɑf'θɔːrɪə] *n embryo.* Keimzelldegeneration *f*, Blastophthorie *f.*
blas·toph·tho·ric degeneration [ˌ-'θɔːrɪk] → blastophthoria.
blas·to·pore ['blæstəpɔːr] *n embryo.* Urdarmöffnung *f*, Urmund *m*, Blastoporus *m.*
blas·to·por·ic canal [ˌ-'pɔːrɪk, -'pɑr-] *embryo.* Canalis neurentericus.
blas·to·sphere ['-sfɪər] *n* → blastula.
blas·to·spore ['-spɔːr, -ˌspɔər] *n micro.* Sproßkonidie *f*, Blastospore *f.*
blas·to·stro·ma [ˌ-'strəʊmə] *n embryo.* Blastostroma *nt.*
blas·tot·o·my [blæs'tɑtəmɪ] *n* → blastomerotomy.
blas·to·zo·oid [ˌblæstə'zəʊɔɪd] *n bio.* Blastozooid *nt.*
blast trauma Explosions-, Detonations-, Knalltrauma *nt.*
blas·tu·la ['blæstʃələ, -stjʊlə] *n*, *pl* **-las**, **-lae** [-liː] *embryo.* Keimblase *f*, Blastula *f.*
blas·tu·lar ['blæstʃələr] *adj* Blastula betr., blastulär, Blastula-.
blas·tu·la·tion [ˌblæstʃə'leɪʃn] *n embryo.* Blastulabildung *f*, -entwicklung *f*, Blastulation *f.*
Blatin [blɑ'tɛ̃] *n*: **B.'s sign/syndrome** Hydatidenschwirren *nt.*
Blat·ta orientalis ['blætə] Küchenschabe *f*,

Kakerlak(e *f*) *m*, orientalische Schabe *f*, Blatta orientalis.
Blat·tar·ia [blə'tɛərɪə] *pl bio.* Schaben *pl*, Blattaria *pl.*
bleach [bliːtʃ] **I** *n* Bleichen *nt*; Bleichmittel *nt.* **II** *vt* bleichen. **III** *vi* bleichen, bleich werden.
bleach·ing ['bliːtʃɪŋ] *n* Bleichen *nt*, Ausbleichen *nt.*
bleaching agent *chem.* Bleichmittel *nt.*
bleaching powder *chem.* Bleichpulver *nt*, Chlorkalk *m*, Calciumhypochlorit *nt.*
blear eye [blɪər] Triefauge *nt*, Lidrandentzündung *f*, Lippitudo *f*, Blepharitis ciliaris/marginalis.
blear-eyed *adj* → bleary-eyed.
blear·y ['blɪərɪ] *adj* **1.** (*Augen, Blick*) trübe, getrübt, verschwommen. **2.** (sehr) müde, ausgelaugt, erschöpft.
bleary-eyed *adj* **1.** mit trüben Augen. **2.** kurzsichtig. **3.** *fig.* begriffsstutzig; einfältig, dumm.
bleb [bleb] *n* **1.** Bläschen *nt*, Blase *f.* **2.** (Haut-)Blase *f*, Bulla *f.*
bleed [bliːd] (*v*: **bled**; **bled**) **I** *vt* zur Ader lassen; (*a. fig.*) schröpfen, bluten lassen. **II** *vi* bluten. **to ~ to death** verbluten.
bleed·er ['bliːdər] *n* **1.** Bluter *m*, Hämophile(r *m*) *f.* **2.** Person *f* die Blut entnimmt; *old* Phlebotomist *m.*
bleeder's joint Blutergelenk *nt*, hämophile Arthritis *f*, Arthropathia haemophilica.
bleed·ing ['bliːdɪŋ] **I** *n* **1.** Bluten *nt*, Blutung *f.* **2.** Aderlaß *m.* **3.** blutendes Gefäß *nt.* **II** *adj* blutend.
b. of the nose Nasenbluten, -blutung, Epistaxis *f.*
bleeding abnormality Blutgerinnungsstörung *f*, -anomalie *f.*
bleeding diathesis Blutungsneigung *f*, hämorrhagische Diathese *f.*
bleeding disorders Blutungsübel *pl*; Blutgerinnungsstörungen *pl.*
bleeding polyp *HNO* angimatöser Polyp *m.*
bleeding tendency Blutungsneigung *f.*
bleeding time Blutungszeit *f.*
blem·ish ['blemɪʃ] **I** *n* (Schönheits-)Fehler *m*, Makel *m*, Verunstaltung *f.* **II** *vt* entstellen, verunstalten.
blend [blend] **I** *n a. bio.* (Ver-)Mischen *nt*, (Ver-)Mischung *f*, Verschmelzung *f.* **II** *vt* vermengen, vermischen, mixen. **III** *vi a. bio.* s. (ver-)mischen.
blenn- *pref.* → blenno-.
blenn·ad·e·ni·tis [ˌblenædɪ'naɪtɪs] *n* Blennadenitis *f.*
blenn·em·e·sis [blen'eməsɪs] *n* Schleimbrechen *nt.*
blenno- *pref.* Schleim-, Blenn(o)-.
blen·no·gen·ic [blenə'dʒenɪk] *adj* schleimbildend, -produzierend, muzinogen.
blen·nog·e·nous [ble'nɑdʒənəs] *adj* → blennogenic.
blen·noid ['blenɔɪd] *adj* schleimähnlich, -förmig, mukoid.
blen·noph·thal·mia [blenɑf'θælmɪə] *n* **1.** Bindehautentzündung *f*, Konjunktivitis *f*, Conjunctivitis *f.* **2.** → blennorrheal conjunctivitis.
blen·nor·rha·gia [blenə'rædʒ(ɪ)ə] *n* **1.** Blennorrhagie *f.* **2.** *old* → gonorrhea.
blen·nor·rhag·ic [ˌ-'rædʒɪk] *adj* Blennorrhagie betr., blennorrhagisch.
blennorrhagic arthritis Gonokokkenarthritis *f*, gonorrhoische Arthritis *f*, Arthritis gonorrhoica.
blen·nor·rhea [ˌ-'rɪə] *n* **1.** Blennorrhö *f*, Blennorrhoe *f.* **2.** *old* → gonorrhea.
blen·nor·rhe·al [ˌ-'rɪəl] *adj* Blennorrhö betr., blennorrhoisch.

blennorrheal conjunctivitis Gonoblennorrhö *f*, Conjunctivitis gonorrhoica.
blen·nos·ta·sis [ble'nɑstəsɪs] *n* Blennostase *f*, -stasis *f.*
blen·no·stat·ic [ˌblenə'stætɪk] *adj* Blennostase betr., blennostatisch.
blen·no·tho·rax [ˌ-'θɔːræks, -'θəʊər-] *n* Blennothorax *m.*
blen·nu·ria [ble'n(j)ʊərɪə] *n* Blennurie *f.*
ble·o·my·cin [bliːə'maɪsɪn] *n pharm.* Bleomycin *nt.*
blephar- *pref.* → blepharo-.
bleph·ar·ad·e·ni·tis [ˌblefərˌædə'naɪtɪs] *n ophthal.* Lidranddrüsenentzündung *f*, Blephar(o)adenitis *f.*
bleph·a·ral ['blefərəl] *adj* Augenlid(er) betr., Lid-, Blephar(o)-.
bleph·a·rec·to·my [blefə'rektəmɪ] *n ophthal.* Lid(knorpel)exzision *f*, Blepharektomie *f.*
bleph·a·re·de·ma [ˌblefərɪ'diːmə] *n* Lidödem *nt.*
bleph·a·rel·o·sis [ˌblefərə'ləʊsɪs] *n ophthal.* Einwärtsstülpung *f* des freien Lidrandes, Entropion *nt*, Entropium *nt.*
bleph·a·rism ['blefərɪzəm] *n* Lidkrampf *m*, Blepharismus *m.*
bleph·a·ri·tis [blefə'raɪtɪs] *n ophthal.* Lidentzündung *f*, Blepharitis *f.*
blepharo- *pref.* (Augen-)Lid-, Blephar(o)-.
bleph·a·ro·ad·e·ni·tis [ˌblefərəˌædə'naɪtɪs] *n* → blepharadenitis.
bleph·a·ro·ad·e·no·ma [ˌ-ædə'nəʊmə] *n ophthal.* Blephar(o)adenom *nt.*
bleph·a·ro·ath·er·o·ma [ˌ-æθə'rəʊmə] *n ophthal.* Blepharoatherom *nt.*
bleph·a·ro·blast ['-blæst] *n* → blepharoplast.
bleph·a·ro·chal·a·sis [ˌ-'kæləsɪs] *n ophthal.* Blepharochalase *f*, -chalasis *f.*
bleph·ar·o·chro·mi·dro·sis [ˌ-krəʊmɪ'drəʊsɪs] *n ophthal.* Blepharochrom(h)idrosis *f.*
bleph·a·roc·lo·nus [blefə'rɑklənəs] *n* Blepharoklonus *m.*
bleph·a·ro·con·junc·ti·vi·tis [ˌblefərəkənˌdʒʌŋ(k)tə'vaɪtɪs] *n ophthal.* kombinierte Lid- u. Bindehautentzündung *f*, Blepharokonjunktivitis *f.*
bleph·ar·o·ker·a·to·con·junc·ti·vi·tis [ˌ-ˌkerətəʊkənˌdʒʌŋ(k)tə'vaɪtɪs] *n ophthal.* Blepharokeratokonjunktivitis *f.*
bleph·ar·o·me·la·no·sis [ˌ-melə'nəʊsɪs] *n ophthal.* Blepharomelanose *f.*
bleph·ar·o·me·las·ma [ˌ-mɪ'læzmə] *pl* Blepharomelasma *f.*
bleph·a·ron ['blefərɑn] *n*, *pl* **-ra** [-rə] (Augen-)Lid *nt*, Palpebra *f*, Blepharon *f.*
bleph·ar·on·cus [blefə'rɑŋkəs] *n* (Augen-)Lidtumor *m*, -schwellung *f.*
bleph·ar·o·pa·chyn·sis [ˌblefərəpə'kɪnsɪs] *n* (Augen-)Lidverdickung *f.*
bleph·ar·o·phi·mo·sis [ˌ-faɪ'məʊsɪs] *n ophthal.* (Augen-)Lidverengerung *f*, -stenose *f*, Blepharophimose *f*, -stenose *f.*
bleph·ar·o·phy·ma [ˌ-'faɪmə] *n* Tumor *m* der Lidhaut.
bleph·a·ro·plast ['-plæst] *n* Basalkörperchen *nt*, Blepharoplast *m.*
bleph·a·ro·plas·tic [ˌ-'plæstɪk] *adj* Basalkörperchen betr., Basalkörperchen-.
bleph·a·ro·plas·ty ['-plæstɪ] *n ophthal.* Lidplastik *f*, Blepharoplastik *f.*
bleph·a·ro·ple·gia [ˌ-'pliːdʒ(ɪ)ə] *n ophthal.* Lidlähmung *f*, Blepharoplegie *f.*
bleph·a·ro·pto·sis [ˌ-'təʊsɪs] *n ophthal.* (Lid-)Ptose *f*, Ptosis *f*, Blepharoptose *f.*
bleph·a·ro·py·or·rhea [ˌ-paɪə'rɪə] *n ophthal.* eitrige Augenentzündung *f*, Blepharopyorrhoe *f.*
bleph·a·ror·rha·phy [blefə'rɑrəfɪ] *n oph-*

blepharospasm

thal., chir. Blepharo(r)rhaphie f, Tarso(r)rhaphie f.
bleph·a·ro·spasm ['blefərəspæzəm] n ophthal. Lidkrampf f, Blepharospasmus m.
bleph·a·ro·spas·mus [ˌ-'spæzməs] n → blepharospasm.
bleph·a·ro·sphinc·ter·ec·to·my [ˌ-sfɪŋktə-'rektəmɪ] n ophthal. Blepharosphinkterektomie f.
bleph·a·ro·stat ['-stæt] n ophthal. Lidhalter m, Blepharostat m.
bleph·a·ro·ste·no·sis [ˌ-stɪ'nəʊsɪs] n → blepharophimosis.
bleph·a·ro·syn·ech·ia [ˌ-sɪ'nekɪə, -'ni:-, -sɪnɪ'kaɪə] n ophthal. Lidverklebung f, -verwachsung f, Blepharosynechie f, -symphysis f, Symblepharon nt.
bleph·a·rot·o·my [blefə'rɒtəmɪ] n ophthal. Blepharotomie f; Tarsotomie f.
Blessig ['blesɪg]: **B.'s cysts/lacunae/spaces** ophthal. Blessig'-Zysten pl.
blind [blaɪnd] **I** n **1.** the ~ pl die Blinden. **2.** Blende f; Jalousie f. **II** adj **3.** blind, Blinden-. **a** ~ **man/woman** ein Blinder/eine Blinde. ~ **from birth** von Geburt an blind. ~ **in one eye** auf einem Auge blind. **4.** fig. blind, verstandnislos (to gegenüber). **5.** (a. anat.) blind endend. **6.** blind (ohne Kenntnisse). **a (double-)~ trial** einfacher (doppelter) Blindversuch m. **7.** matt, nicht poliert. **III** vt **8.** (a. fig.) blenden, blind machen. ~ (a. fig.) blenden. **the right eye was ~ed** das rechte Auge wurde blind. **9.** verdunkeln.
blind·ed study ['blaɪndɪd] stat. Blindstudie f.
blind fistula inkomplette/blinde Fistel f, Fistula incompleta.
blind·fold gait ['blaɪndfəʊld] neuro. Blindgang m.
blind gut Blinddarm m, Zäkum nt, Zökum nt, C(a)ecum nt, Intestinum c(a)ecum.
blind headache Migräne f, Migraine f.
blind·ing disease ['blaɪndɪŋ] → blinding filiarial disease.
blinding filarial disease Onchozerkose f, Onchocercose f, Onchocerciasis f, Knotenfilariose f, Onchocerca-volvulus-Infektion f.
blinding worm Knäuelfilarie f, Onchocerca volvulus.
blind intestine → blind gut.
blind-loop syndrome chir. Blindsack-Syndrom nt, Blind-loop-Syndrom nt, Syndrom nt der blinden Schlinge.
blind·ness ['blaɪnɪs] n **1.** Blindheit f, Erblindung f, hochgradige Sehschwäche f. **2.** totale Blindheit f, Amaurose f, Amaurosis f. **3.** Ausfall m einer Sinneswahrnehmung. **4.** psychogene Blindheit f. **5.** fig. Blindheit f, Verblendung f (to gegenüber).
blind part of retina Pars caeca retinae.
blind rating stat. blinde Auswertung f.
blind spot 1. (Auge) blinder Fleck m, anat. Discus m. optici. **2.** fig. schwacher wunder Punkt m; tote Zone f, toter Winkel m.
blind test Blindversuch m.
blind trial → blind test.
blink [blɪŋk] **I** n Blinzeln nt. **II** vi blinzeln, zwinkern.
blink reflex Korneal-, Blinzel-, Lidreflex m.
blis·ter ['blɪstər] **I** n **1.** (Haut-)Blase f, (-)Bläschen nt, Pustel f. **2.** Brand-, Wundblase f. **3.** Zugpflaster nt. **II** vt Blasen hervorrufen. **III** vi Blasen ziehen od. bekommen.
blister bug Blasenkäfer m, spanische Fliege f, Lytta/Cantharis vesicatoria.
blis·tered ['blɪstərd] adj mit Blasen bedeckt, blasig.
blis·ter·ing ['blɪstərɪŋ] **I** n Blasenbildung f. **II** adj **1.** blasenziehend. **2.** (Hitze) brennend.
bloat [bləʊt] **I** n Magen-, Darmblähung f. **II** vt aufblasen, -blähen. **III** vi auf-, anschwellen.
bloat up vt → bloat II.
bloat out vi → bloat III.
bloat·ed ['bləʊtɪd] adj (an-)geschwollen, aufgebläht, aufgeblasen; (Gesicht) aufgedunsen.
Bloch-Sulzberger [blɒk 'sʌlzbərgər]: **B.-S. disease** → B.-S. syndrome.
B.-S. incontinentia pigmenti → B.-S. syndrome.
B.-S. syndrome Bloch-Sulzberger-Syndrom nt, -Krankheit f, Melanoblastosis Bloch-Sulzberger f, Incontinentia pigmenti Typ Bloch-Sulzberger, Pigmentdermatose Siemens-Bloch f.
block [blɒk] **I** n **1.** Hindernis nt, Blockade f, Sperre f; Blockierung f, Verstopfung f. **2.** (Nerv) Block m, Blockade f. **3.** Leitungs-, Regionalanästhesie f. **4.** psycho. (mentale) Blockierung f, Sperre f. **5.** Block m, Klotz m. **II** vt **6.** (a. fig.) (ver-)hindern, hemmen; blockieren, verstopfen, (ver-, ab-)sperren. **my nose is ~ed** meine Nase ist vestopft. **7.** chem. blockieren; (Säuren) neutralisieren; (Katalysator) inaktivieren.
block up vt blockieren, verstopfen, versperren.
block·ade [blɒ'keɪd] **I** n **1.** Blockade f, Block m. **2.** Sperre f, Hindernis f. **II** vt blockieren, ab-, versperren.
block·age ['blɒkɪdʒ] n **1.** Blockieren nt. **2.** Blockierung f; Verstopfung f; Obstruktion f. **3.** Sperre f, Hindernis f. **4.** psycho. (innere) Blockierung od. Sperre f.
block anesthesia anes. Leitungsanästhesie f, -block m; Regionalanästhesie f.
field b. Feldblock.
nerve b. Nervenblockade, Leitungs-, Regionalanästhesie.
block diagram Blockschaltbild nt, -diagramm nt.
block·er ['blɒkər] n **1.** Blocker m. **2.** → blocking agent.
block·ing ['blɒkɪŋ] **I** n Blocken nt, Blockieren nt. **2.** (innere/mentale) Blockierung f, Sperre f. **II** adj blockierend, blockend.
blocking agent pharm. blockierende Substanz f, Blocker m.
alpha b. Alpha-Adrenorezeptorenblocker, Alpha(rezeptoren)blocker, α--Adrenorezeptorenblocker, .
alpha-adrenergic receptor b. → alpha b.
beta b. Betablocker, Beta-Rezeptorenblocker, β-Adrenorezeptorenblocker, Beta-Adrenorezeptorenblocker.
beta-adrenergic receptor b. → beta b.
calcium b. Kalziumblocker, -antagonist m, Ca-Blocker, Ca-Antagonist f.
cholinergic b. Cholinorezeptorenblocker.
ganglionic b. pharm. Ganglienblocker, Gangioplegikum nt.
histamine receptor-b. Histaminrezeptoren-Antagonist m, -Blocker m, Histaminblocker, Antihistaminikum nt.
neuromuscular b. Muskelrelaxans nt.
blocking antibodies blockierende/inkomplette/nichtagglutinierende Antikörper pl.
blocking drug → blocking agent.
blocking reagent chem. Schutz-, Blockierungsreagenz nt.
block vertebrae Blockwirbel(bildung f) pl.
Blocq [blɒk]: **B.'s disease** neuro. Astasie--Abasie(-Syndrom nt) f.
blood [blʌd] n Blut nt. **to give ~** Blut spenden. **to take ~** Blut entnehmen.

blood agar abbr. **BA** Blutagar m/nt.
glucose cysteine b. Blut-Traubenzucker--Cystein-Agar.
heat b. Kochblutagar, Schokoladenagar.
potato b. Bordet-Gengou-Agar, -Medium nt.
blood agar plate micro. Blutagarplatte f.
blood-air barrier Blut-Gas-Schranke f.
blood albumin Serumalbumin nt.
blood alcohol Blutalkohol m.
blood aspiration Blutaspiration f.
blood bank Blutbank f.
blood bicarbonate Plasmabikarbonat nt.
blood blister Blutblase f.
blood-borne adj durch das Blut übertragen, hämatogen.
blood-borne infection hämatogene Infektion f.
blood-brain barrier abbr. **BBB** Blut-Hirn--Schranke f.
blood calculus Gefäßstein m, Angiolith m.
blood cast urol. Blutzylinder m.
blood cells Blutkörperchen pl, -zellen pl, Hämozyten pl.
packed b. Erythrozytenkonzentrat nt, Erythrozytenkonserve f.
red b. rote Blutkörperchen/-zellen, Erythrozyten pl.
white b. weiße Blutkörperchen/-zellen, Leukozyten pl.
blood-cerebral barrier → blood-brain barrier.
blood-cerebrospinal fluid barrier Blut--Liquor-Schranke f.
blood clot Blutgerinnsel nt, -kuchen m.
red b. roter Abscheidungsthrombus m.
blood clotting Blutgerinnung f, Koagulation f.
blood clotting factor (Blut-)Gerinnungsfaktor m, Koagulationsfaktor m.
blood coagulation Blutgerinnung f.
blood corpuscles → blood cells.
blood count 1. Blutbild nt. **2.** Bestimmung/Auszählung f des Blutbildes.
complete b. abbr. **CBC** → full b.
differential b. Differentialblutbild.
full b. abbr. **FBC** großes Blutbild.
red b. abbr. **RBC** Erythrozytenzahl f abbr. Z_E.
white b. abbr. **WBC** weißes Blutbild, Leukozytenzahl f.
blood crisis Blutkrise f.
blood crystals Hämatoidin(kristalle pl) nt.
blood-CSF barrier → blood-cerebrospinal fluid barrier.
blood culture micro. Blutkultur f.
blood cyst hämorrhagische Zyste f.
blood disk → blood platelet.
blood donation Blutspende f.
blood donor Blutspender(in f) m.
blood dust (of Müller) Blutstäubchen pl, Hämokonien pl, -konia nt.
blood flagellates micro. Blutflagellaten pl.
blood flow Blutfluß m, Durchblutung f, Perfusion f.
blood fluke micro. Pärchenegel m, Schistosoma nt, Bilharzia f.
Japanese b. japanischer Pärchenegel, Schistosoma japonicum.
Manson's b. Schistosoma mansoni.
vesicular b. Blasenpärchenegel, Schistosoma haematobium, Bilharzia haematobia.
blood formation Blutbildung f, Hämatopo(i)ese f, Hämopo(i)ese f.
blood-forming organs blut(zell)bildende Organe pl.
blood gas alteration Blutgasveränderung f.
blood gas analysis Blutgasanalyse f.
blood gas analyzer Blutgasanalysator m.
blood-gas barrier → blood-air barrier.

blood gases Blutgase *pl.*
  arterial b. *abbr.* **ABG** arterielle Blutgase *pl.*
  venous b. *abbr.* **VBG** venöse Blutgase.
blood-gas partition coefficient Blut-Gas--Verteilungskoeffizient *m.*
blood glucose Blutzucker *m,* -glukose *f.*
blood glucose level/value Blutzuckerspiegel *m,* -wert *m,* Glukosespiegel *m.*
Bloodgood ['blʌdgʊd]: **B.'s disease** zystische/fibrös-zystische Mastopathie *f,* Mammadysplasie *f,* Zystenmamma *f,* Mastopathia chronica cystica.
blood group Blutgruppe *f.*
  Duffy b. Duffy-Blutgruppe(nsystem *nt*) *f.*
  Kell b. Kell-Blutgruppe.
  Kidd b. Kidd-Blutgruppe.
  Lewis b. Lewis-Blutgruppe.
  Lutheran b. Lutheran-Blutgruppe.
  MN b. → MNSs b.
  MNSs b. MNSs-Blutgruppe(nsystem *nt*) *f.*
  P b. P-Blutgruppe(nsystem *nt*) *f.*
blood group A Blutgruppe A *f.*
blood group AB Blutgruppe AB *f.*
blood-group antibody Blutgruppenantikörper *m.*
blood-group antigens Blutgruppenantigene *pl.*
blood group B Blutgruppe B *f.*
blood group D Blutgruppe D *f.*
blood group incompatibility Blutgruppenunverträglichkeit *f,* -inkompatibilität *f.*
blood grouping Blutgruppenbestimmung *f.*
blood group protein Blutgruppenprotein *nt.*
blood group specifity Blutgruppenspezifität *f.*
blood group substance Blutgruppenantigen *nt.*
blood group system Blutgruppensystem *nt.*
blood group typing → blood grouping
blood island *embryo.* Blutinsel *f.*
blood lacuna *embryo.* Blutlakune *f.*
blood-less ['blʌdlɪs] *adj* 1. bleich, sehr blaß. 2. blutlos, -leer; leb-, gefühllos, kalt. 3. ohne Blutvergießen, unblutig.
bloodless phlebotomy unblutiger Aderlaß *m.*
blood-let-ting ['blʌdletɪŋ] *n* Aderlaß *m.*
blood level Blutspiegel *m,* -konzentration *f.*
blood loss Blutverlust *m.*
blood macrophage mononukleärer Phagozyt *m,* Monozyt *m.*
blood mast cell Blutmastzelle *f,* basophiler Granulozyt *m.*
blood mole *gyn., patho.* 1. Blutmole *f,* Mola sanguinolenta. 2. Fleischmole *f,* Mola carnosa.
blood pH Blut-pH(-Wert *m*) *m.*
blood picture *lab.* Blutbild *nt.*
blood pigment 1. hämoglobinogenes Pigment *nt.* 2. Blutfarbstoff *m,* Hämoglobin *nt abbr.* **Hb.**
blood plasma Blutplasma *nt,* zellfreie Blutflüssigkeit *f.*
blood plate → blood platelet.
blood platelet Blutplättchen *nt,* Thrombozyt *m.*
blood platelet thrombus Plättchen-, Thrombozytenthrombus *m.*
blood plate thrombus → blood platelet thrombus.
blood poison(ing) Blutvergiftung *f;* Sepsis *f,* Septikämie *f.*
blood pressure *abbr.* **BP** Blutdruck *m.*
  arterial b. *abbr.* **ABP** arterieller (Blut-)Druck.
  arterial mean b. arterieller Mitteldruck.
  basal b. Ruheblutdruck, basaler Blutdruck.
  diastolic b. diastolischer Blutdruck.
  high b. Bluthochdruck *m,* (arterielle) Hypertonie *f,* Hypertension *f,* Hypertonus *m,* Hochdruckkrankheit *f.*
  low b. niedriger Blutdruck *m,* Hypotonie *f,* Hypotonus *m,* Hypotonia *f,* Hypotension *f.*
  mean b. → arterial mean b.
  resting b. → basal b.
  static b. mittlerer Fülldruck, statischer Blutdruck.
  systolic b. systolischer Blutdruck.
  venous b. venöser (Blut-)Druck.
blood pressure gradient Blutdruckgefälle *nt,* -gradient *m.*
blood quotient *hema.* Färbeindex *m abbr.* **FI,** Hämoglobinquotient *m.*
blood sample Blutprobe *f.*
blood sampling Blut(proben)entnahme *f.*
blood serum (Blut-)Serum *nt.*
blood smear Blutausstrich *m.*
blood specimen Blutprobe *f.*
blood sporozoans *micro.* Haemosporidien *pl,* -sporidia *pl.*
blood stream Blutstrom *m,* -kreislauf *m.*
blood substitute Blutersatz *m;* Plasmaersatz *m,* -expander *m.*
blood-suck-er ['blʌdsʌkər] *n bio.* Blutsauger *m.*
blood-suck-ing [,blʌdsʌkɪŋ] *adj bio.* blutsaugend.
blood sugar *abbr.* **BS** Blutzucker *m,* Glukose *f.*
blood supply Blutzufuhr *f,* -versorgung *f.*
blood test Blutuntersuchung *f,* -test *m.*
blood-test *vt* Blut untersuchen *od.* testen.
blood-thymus barrier Blut-Thymus--Schranke *f,* -Barriere *f.*
blood transfusion Bluttransfusion *f,* -übertragung *f.*
blood tumor 1. Aneurysma *nt.* 2. Bluterguß *m,* Hämatom *nt,* Haematoma *f.*
blood type → blood group.
blood-type *vt* die Blutgruppe bestimmen.
blood typing Blutgruppenbestimmung *f.*
blood urea nitrogen *abbr.* **BUN** Blutharnstoffstickstoff *m abbr.* **BUN.**
blood-vascular *adj* Blutgefäße betr.
blood-vascular system Blutgefäßsystem *nt.*
blood vessel Blutgefäß *nt.*
  b.s of retina Netzhautgefäße *pl,* Vasa sanguinea retinae.
  villous b. Zottengefäß *nt.*
blood vessel clamp *chir.* (Blut-)Gefäßklemme *f,* -klammer *f.*
blood volume Blutvolumen *nt.*
  total b. *abbr.* **TBV** totales Blutvolumen *abbr.* **TBV.**
blood vomiting Bluterbrechen *nt,* Hämatemesis *f,* Vomitus cruentus.
blood-y ['blʌdi] *I adj* blutig, bluthaltig, blutbefleckt, Blut-. *II vt* blutig machen, mit Blut beflecken.
bloody ascites hämorrhagischer/blutiger Aszites *m,* Hämaskos *m.*
bloody diarrhea blutiger Durchfall *m,* Blutstuhl *m.*
bloody discharge 1. Blutabsonderung *f,* blutige Sekretion *f.* 2. blutiges Sekret *nt,* blutiger Ausfluß *m.*
bloody stool Blutstuhl *m,* blutiger Stuhl *m;* Hämatochezie *f.*
Bloom [blu:m]: **B.'s syndrome** *derm.* Bloom-Syndrom *nt.*
blotch [blɒtʃ] *n* Hautfleck *m,* Mal *nt.*
blotch-y ['blɒtʃi] *adj* (*Haut*) fleckig.
Blount [blaʊnt]: **B.'s disease** 1. Tibia vara. 2. Blount'-Krankheit *f,* Osteochondrosis deformans tibiae.
  B.'s knee staple Epiphysenklammer *f* nach Blount.
  B.'s operation Epiphyseodese *f* nach Blount.
  B.'s procedure for bone growth asymmetry → B.'s operation.
  B.'s staple → B.'s knee staple.
  B.'s stapling → B.'s operation.
Blount-Barber ['bɑːrbər]: **B.-B. disease** → Blount's disease 2.
blow [bləʊ] (*v:* **blew; blown**) *I n* 1. Schlag *m,* Hieb *m.* 2. (Schicksals-)Schlag *m.* 3. (*Wind*) Brise *f.* 4. (*Nase*) Schneuzen *nt.* 5. Durchblasen *nt* (*mit einem Instrument*). *II vt* 6. wehen, blasen, pusten. 7. (auf-, aus-, durch-)blasen. **to ~ one's nose** s. die Nase putzen, s. schneuzen. 8. sprengen, explodieren lassen, zerstören. *III vi* 9. (*Wind*) blasen, wehen. 10. pusten, blasen. 11. platzen, explodieren, bersten; durchbrennen.
blow through *vt* durchblasen.
blow up *vt* aufblasen.
blow-er ['bləʊər] *n* Gebläse *nt,* Ventilator *m.*
blow fly *bio., micro.* Schmeißfliege *f.*
blow-ing wound ['bləʊɪŋ] offener Pneumothorax *m.*
blown [bləʊn] *adj* geschwollen, vergrößert, aufgedunsen; (*Magen*) (auf-)gebläht, überbläht.
blow-out fracture Blow-out-Fraktur *f,* blow-out fracture (*f*).
blue [blu:] *I n* Blau *nt,* blaue Farbe *f,* blauer Farbstoff *m.* *II adj* 1. blau, Blau-; (*Haut*) bläulich, fahl. 2. traurig, deprimiert, melancholisch. *III vt* blau färben. *IV vi* blau werden; blau anlaufen.
blue asphyxia blaue Apnoe/Asphyxie *f,* Asphyxia livida/cyanotica.
blue atrophy blaue (Haut-)Atrophie *f.*
blue baby *ped.* zyanotischer Säugling *m,* blue baby (*nt*).
blue-black *adj* blauschwarz.
blue blindness Blaublindheit *f,* -schwäche *f,* Tritanop(s)ie *f.*
blue bloater *pulmo.* blue bloater (*m*), BB-Typ *m.*
blue bug *micro.* Argas persicus.
blue cataract Cataracta c(o)erulea.
blue diaper syndrome Blue-diaper-Syndrom *nt.*
blue disease Felsengebirgsfleckfieber *nt,* amerikanisches Zeckenbißfieber *nt,* Rocky Mountain spotted fever (*nt*).*abbr.* **RMSF.**
blue dot cataract → blue cataract.
blue-eyed *adj* blauäugig.
blue fever → blue disease
blue-green algae/bacteria *old* → cyanobacteria.
blue line Bleisaum *m.*
blue navel Cullen-Zeichen *nt,* -Syndrom *nt,* Cullen-Hellendall-Zeichen *nt,* -Syndrom *nt.*
blue-ness ['blu:nɪs] *n* blaue Färbung *f,* blaue Beschaffenheit *f,* Bläue *f.*
blue nevus *derm.* blauer Nävus *m,* Jadassohn-Tièche-Nävus *m,* Naevus caeruleus/coeruleus.
blue phlebitis Pseudoembolie Nicole *f,* Phlegmasia coerulea dolens.
blue pus bacillus *micro.* Pseudomonas aeruginosa, Pyozyaneus *m.*
blue rubber bleb nevus → blue rubber bleb nevus disease.
blue rubber bleb nevus disease/syndrome Bean-Syndrom *nt,* Blaue-Gummiblasen-Nävus-Syndrom *nt,* blue rubber bleb nevus syndrome (*nt*).
blues [blu:z] *pl inf.* Melancholie *f,* Depression *f.*

blue sclerae blaue Skleren *pl.*
blue spot 1. Mongolenfleck *m.* **2. ~s** *pl* Maculae coeruleae, Tâches bleues.
blue stone *chem.* Kupfersulfat *nt.*
blue vision Blausehen *nt,* Zyanop(s)ie *f.*
blue-yellow blindness Blaugelbschwäche *f,* Tritanomalie *f.*
Blum [bluːm]: **B.'s disease/syndrome** hypochlorämische/chloroprive Azotämie *f.*
Blumberg ['blʌmbɜːg]: **B.'s sign** *chir.* Loslaßschmerz *m,* Blumberg-Zeichen *nt,* -Symptom *nt.*
Blumenbach ['bluːmənbax]: **B.'s clivus** Clivus Blumenbachii.
B.'s process Proc. uncinatus ossis ethmoidalis.
Blumenthal ['bluːmənta:l]: **B.'s disease** hema. Erythroleukämie *f.*
blunt [blʌnt] **I** *n* (*Skalpell*) stumpfe Seite *f,* (Klingen-)Rücken *m.* **II** *adj* **1.** stumpf. **2.** *fig.* abgestumpft, unempfindlich (*to gegen*); dumm, beschränkt; grob, barsch. **III** *vt* stumpf machen; *fig.* abstumpfen (*to gegen*); *fig.* abschwächen. **IV** *vi* stumpf werden, s. abstumpfen.
blunt curet *chir.* stumpfe Kürette *f.*
blunt dissection *chir.* stumpfes Präparieren *nt.*
blunt duct adenosis sklerosierende Adenosis *f,* Korbzellenhyperplasie *f.*
blunt hook *chir.* stumpfer Haken *m.*
blunt nerve hook *chir.* stumpfer Nervenhaken *m.*
blunt·ness ['blʌntnɪs] *n* **1.** Stumpfheit *f.* **2.** *fig.* Abgestumpftheit *f* (*to gegen*).
blunt scissors *chir.* stumpfe Schere *f.*
blunt trauma stumpfes Trauma *nt,* stumpfe Verletzung *f.*
blur [blɜː] **I** *n* **1.** undeutlicher/nebelhafter (Sinnes-)Eindruck *m;* Schleier *m/pl* (*vor den Augen*). **2.** Fleck *m,* verwischte Stelle *f;* Makel *m,* Schandfleck *m.* **II** *vt* verwischen, undeutlich/verschwommen machen, trüben; *photo.* verwackeln. **III** *vi* s. verwischen, verschwimmen, eintrüben.
blurred [blɜːd] *adj* unscharf, verschwommen, verwischt, nebelhaft.
blur·ry ['blɜːrɪ] *adj* blurred.
blush [blʌʃ] **I** *n* erröten *nt,* (Scham-)Röte *f.* **II** *vi* erröten, rot werden (*at bei*).
blush·ing ['blʌʃɪŋ] **I** *n* → blush I. **II** *adj* errötend.
B-lymphocyte *n* B-Lymphozyt *m,* B-Lymphocyt *m,* B-Zelle *f.*
B memory cell B-Gedächtniszelle *f.*
BMI *abbr.* → body mass index.
B-mode *n radiol.* (*Ultraschall*) B-Mode *m/ nt,* B-Scan *m.*
BMR *abbr.* → basal metabolic rate.
board ['bəʊəd, bɔːrd] *n* **1.** Brett *nt,* Diele *f;* Balken *m.* **2.** Ausschuß *m,* Kommission *f;* Behörde *f,* Amt *nt.*
b. of examiners Prüfungsausschuß *m.*
b. of health Gesundheitsbehörde *f.*
board-like rigidity *chir.* bretthartes Abdomen *nt.*
Boas ['bəʊæz]: **B.'s algesimeter** Boas-Algesimeter *nt.*
B.' point Boas-Druckpunkt *m.*
B.' test Boas'-Probe *f.*
B.'s test meal Boas(-Ewald)-Probefrühstück *nt.*
boat form [bəʊt] *chem.* Wannenform *f.*
boat-shaped *adj* kahnförmig.
boat-shaped abdomen Kahnbauch *m.*
boat-shaped heart *radiol.* Holzschuhherz *nt,* Aortenkonfiguration *f,* Enten-, Schuhform *f.*
Bochdalek ['bakdælek]: **B.'s duct** *embryo.* Ductus thyroglossalis.
flower spray of B. *anat.* Bochdalek'-Blumenkörbchen *nt.*
B.'s foramen Bochdalek'-Foramen *nt,*

Hiatus pleuroperitonealis.
B.'s ganglion Plexus dentalis superior.
B.'s gap → B.'s foramen.
B.'s hernia *chir.* Bochdalek-Hernie *f.*
B.'s pseudoganglion Plexus dentalis superior.
B.'s sinus → B.'s foramen.
B.'s triangle Bochdalek-Dreieck *nt,* Trigonum lumbocostale.
Bock [bak]: **B.'s ganglion** Ganglion *nt* des Plexus caroticus internus.
B.'s nerve Ramus pharyngealis n. vagi.
Bockhart ['bakhɑːrt]: **B.'s impetigo** Ostiofollikulitis/Ostiofolliculitis/Impetigo Bockhart, Staphyloderma follicularis, Impetigo follicularis Bockhart, Folliculitis staphylogenes superficialis, Folliculitis pustolosa, Staphylodermia Bockhart.
Bodal ['bəʊdl]: **B.'s test** *pharm.* Bodal-Test *m.*
Bodansky [bəʊ'dæntskɪ]: **B. unit** *biochem.* Bodansky-Einheit *f.*
Bodian ['bəʊdɪən]: **B. silver stain** Versilberung *f* nach Bodian.
bod·i·less ['badɪləs] *adj* körperlos; unkörperlich.
bod·i·ly ['badɪlɪ] **I** *adj* körperlich, physisch, Körper-. **II** *adv* **1.** persönlich, in Person. **2.** als Einheit, als Ganzes, geschlossen.
bodily function Körperfunktion *f.*
bodily harm → bodily injury.
bodily illness körperliche Erkrankung *f.*
bodily injury Körperverletzung *f.*
bod·y ['badɪ] **I** *n,* *pl* **bod·ies 1.** Körper *m; anat.* Corpus *m.* **2.** Leiche *f,* Leichnam *m.* **3.** Rumpf *m,* Stamm *m,* Haupt-, Mittelstück *nt;* Haupt(bestand)teil *m.* **5.** *chem.* Substanz *f,* Stoff *m.* **6.** *phys.* Masse *f,* Körper *m.* **7.** Körper(schaft *f) m,* Organ *nt,* Gremium *nt.* **8.** *fig.* das Wesentliche, Substanz *f,* Kern *m.* **II** *adj* körperlich, physisch, Körper-.
b.s of Arantius Arantius-Knötchen *pl,* Noduli valvularum semilunarium.
b. of bladder (Harn-)Blasenkörper, Corpus vesicae.
b. of breast (Brust-)Drüsenkörper, Corpus mammae.
b. of caudate nucleus Caudatuskörper, Corpus nc. caudati.
b. of clavicle Corpus claviculae/claviculare.
b. of clitoris Klitoris-, Clitorisschaft *m,* Corpus clitoridis.
b. of corpus callosum Balkenkörper, Truncus corporis callosi.
b. of epididymis Nebenhodenkörper, Corpus epididymidis.
b. of femur Femurschaft *m,* Corpus femoris.
b. of fibula Fibulaschaft *m,* Corpus fibulae.
b. of fornix Fornixkörper, -stamm, Corpus fornicis.
b. of gall bladder Gallenblasenkörper, Corpus vesicae biliaris.
b. of Highmore Mediastinum testis, Corpus Highmori.
b. of humerus Humerusschaft *m,* Corpus humeri.
b. of hyoid bone Zungenbeinkörper, Corpus ossis hyoidei.
b. of ilium Corpus ossis ilii.
b. of incus Amboßkörper, Corpus incudis.
b. of ischium Sitzbeinkörper, Corpus ossis ischii.
b. of mammary gland → b. of breast.
b. of mandible Corpus mandibulae.
b. of maxilla Corpus maxillae.
b. of nail Corpus unguis.

b. of pancreas Pankreaskörper, Corpus pancreatis.
b. of pelvic bone → b. of pubis.
b. of penis Corpus penis.
b. of pubis Schambeinkörper, Corpus ossis pubis.
b. of radius Radiusschaft *m,* Corpus radii.
b. of Retzius Retzius'-Körperchen *nt.*
b. of rib Rippenkörper, Corpus costae.
b. of sphenoid bone Corpus ossis sphenoidalis.
b. of sternum Brustbeinkörper, Corpus sterni.
b. of stomach Magenkörper, Corpus gastricum/ventriculare.
b. of sweat gland Schweißdrüsenkörper, Corpus gl. sudoriferae.
b. of talus Taluskörper, Corpus tali.
b. of tibia Tibiaschaft *m,* Corpus tibiae/tibiale.
b. of tongue Zungenkörper, Corpus linguae.
b. of ulna Ulnaschaft *m,* Corpus ulnae.
b. of urinary bladder (Harn-)Blasenkörper, Corpus vesicae (urinariae).
b. of uterus Gebärmutter-, Uteruskörper, Corpus uteri.
b. of vertebra Wirbelkörper, Corpus vertebrae/vertebrale.
b. of Vicq d'Azur *old* schwarzer Kern *m,* Substantia nigra.
body cavity Körperhöhle *f.*
body cell Körper-, Somazelle *f.*
body cell mass Körperzellmasse *f.*
body clock innere Uhr *f.*
body fluid Körperflüssigkeit *f.*
body heat Körperwärme *f* -temperatur *f.*
body-image agnosia *neuro.* Autotopagnosie *f.*
body language Körpersprache *f.*
body louse *micro.* Kleiderlaus *f,* Pediculus humanus corporis/humanus/vestimenti.
body mass index *abbr.* **BMI** Quetelet-Index *m,* Körpermasseindex *m,* body mass index *abbr.* BMI.
body odor Körpergeruch *m.*
body orifice Körperöffnung *f.*
body plethysmograph Körperplethysmograph *m.*
body rhythm biologischer Rhythmus *m,* Biorhythmus *m.*
body stalk *embryo.* Bauchstiel *m.*
body surface Körperoberfläche *f.*
body surface area *abbr.* **BSA** *physiol.* Körperoberfläche *f.*
body temperature Körpertemperatur *f.*
basal b. *abbr.* **BBT** basale Körpertemperatur, Basaltemperatur *f.*
body type Konstitutionstyp *m.*
body weight *abbr.* **BW** Körpergewicht *nt* *abbr.* KG.
Boeck [bek]: **B.'s disease/sarcoid** Sarkoidose *f,* Morbus Boeck *m,* Boeck'-Sarkoid *nt,* Besnier-Boeck-Schaumann-Krankheit *f,* Lymphogranulomatosa benigna.
Boerhaave [bəʊr'hɑːviː, bɔːr-]: **B.'s glands** Schweißdrüsen *pl,* Gll. sudoriferae.
B.'s syndrome Boerhaave-Syndrom *nt,* spontane/postemitische/emetogene Ösophagusruptur *m.*
Bogros [bo'gro]: **B.'s space** Bogros'-Raum *m,* Retroinguinalraum *m.*
bo·gus ['bəʊgəs] *adj* gefälscht, unecht, falsch, vorgetäuscht, betrügerisch, Pseudo-, Schein-.
Böhler ['beɪlər, 'bəʊ-; 'bøːlər]: **B.'s salient angle** *ortho.* Böhler'-Tuber-Gelenk-Winkel *m.*
Bohr [bɔːr, bəʊr]: **B. atom** Bohr'-Atom-(modell *nt*) *nt.*
B. effect Bohr-Effekt *m.*
B. equation Bohr'-Formel *f.*

boil [bɔɪl] **I** *n* **1.** *patho.* Eiterbeule *f*, Blutgeschwür *nt*, Furunkel *m*/*nt*. **2.** Kochen *nt*, Sieden *n*. **to be on the ~** kochen. **to bring to the ~** zum Kochen bringen/aufkochen lassen. **to come to the ~** zu kochen anfangen, sieden. **to go off the ~** zu kochen aufhören. **II** *vt* kochen (lassen). **III** *vi* kochen, sieden.
boil away I *vt* verdampfen lassen. **II** *vi* **1.** (weiter-)kochen, sieden. **2.** verdampfen.
boil down I *vt* einkochen. **II** *vi* einkochen, dickflüssig werden.
boil off/out *vt* ab-, auskochen.
boil over *vi* überkochen, überlaufen.
boiled [bɔɪld] *adj* gekocht.
boil·ing [ˈbɔɪlɪŋ] **I** *n* Kochen *nt*, Sieden *nt*. **II** *adj* siedend, kochend, Siede-. **III** *adv* kochen. **~ hot** glühend-, kochendheiß.
boiling heat Siedehitze *f*.
boiling point *abbr.* **b.p.** Siedepunkt *m*.
boiling point elevation Siedepunktserhöhung *f*.
bol *abbr*. → bolus 2.
bole [bəʊl] *n* → bolus 4.
Bo·liv·i·an hemorrhagic fever [bəˈlɪvɪən, bəʊ-] *abbr.* **BHF** bolivianisches hämorrhagisches Fieber *nt* *abbr.* BHF, Madungofieber *nt*.
Bolivian hemorrhagic fever virus *micro*. Madungofiebervirus *nt*.
Boll [bɔʊl]: **B.'s cells** Boll'-Zellen *pl*.
bo·lom·e·ter [bəʊˈlɑmɪtər] *n* *phys*. Bolometer *nt*.
bolt [bəʊlt] **I** *n* Bolzen *m*, Schraube *f* (*mit Mutter*). **II** *vt* verbolzen, mit Bolzen befestigen, fest-, verschrauben.
bolt·ed connection [ˈbəʊltɪd] Schraubverbindung *f*, Verschraubung *f*.
bolted joint → bolted connection.
bolt·head [ˈbəʊlthed] *n* Bolzen-, Schraubenkopf *m*.
bo·lus [ˈbəʊləs] *n* **1.** Bissen *m*, Klumpen *m*, Bolus *m*. **2.** *abbr.* **bol** *pharm*. große Pille *f*, Bolus *f* *abbr* Bol. **3.** Bolus(injektion *f*) *m*. **4.** Tonerde *f*, Bolus(erde *f*) *m*.
bolus alba Kaolin *nt*.
bolus death Bolustod *m*.
bolus injection Bolusinjektion *f*, intravenöse Schnellinjektion *f*.
bom·bard [bɑmˈbɑrd, bəm-] *vt* *phys*., *radiol*. (*mit Strahlen*) beschießen, bombardieren, bestrahlen.
bom·bard·ment [bɑmˈbɑrdmənt, bəm-] *n* *phys*., *radiol*. Bombadierung *f*, Beschießung *f*, Bestrahlung *f*, Bombardment *nt*.
bom·be·sin [ˈbɑmbəsɪn] *n* Bombesin *nt*.
bond [bɑnd] **I** *n* **1.** Verbindung *f*, Band *nt*, Bindung *f*. **2.** *fig*. (Familien-)Bande *f*. **3.** *chem*. Bindung *f*. **4.** *techn*. Bindemittel *nt*. **II** *vt* **5.** *psycho*. Bande knüpfen *od*. herstellen (to mit). **6.** *chem*., *techn*. binden. **III** *vi* *chem*., *techn*. binden.
bond angle *chem*. Bindungswinkel *m*.
bond energy *chem*. Bindungsenergie *f*.
bond·ing [ˈbɑndɪŋ] *n* Verbinden *nt*, Verbindung *f*.
bonding agent Bindemittel *nt*.
bonding structure → bond structure.
bond length *chem*. Bindungslänge *f*.
bond strength Haftfestigkeit *f*.
bond structure *chem*. Bindungsstruktur *f*.
bone [bəʊn] *n* **1.** Knochen *m*, *old form bc*.; *anat*. Os *nt*. **2.** ~s *pl* Gebein (*e pl*) *nt*. **3.** ~s *pl* *inf*. Knochen *pl*, Körper *m*. **4.** *bio*. (Fisch-)Gräte *f*.
b.s of the digits of the foot Ossa digitorum pedis.
b.s of the digits of the hand Ossa digitorum manus.
b.s of the foot Fußknochen *pl*, Ossa pedis.
b.s of the hand Handknochen *pl*, Ossa manus.

b.s of the inferior limb Knochen *pl* der unteren Extremität, Ossa membri inferioris.
b.s of the superior limb Knochen *pl* der oberen Extremität, Ossa membri superioris.
b.s of wrist Handwurzel-, Karpalknochen *pl*, Carpalia *pl*, Ossa carpi.
bone abscess 1. Osteomyelitis *f*. **2.** eitrige Periostitis *f*. **3.** Knochenabszeß *m*.
bone age Knochenalter *nt*.
bone atrophy Knochenatrophie *f*.
acute reflex b. Sudeck'-Dystrophie *f*, Sudeck-Syndrom *nt*, Morbus Sudeck *m*.
bone bank Knochenbank *f*.
bone-block repair *ortho*. Operation *f* nach Eden-Hybinette.
bone-cartilage boundary Knorpel-Knochen-Grenze *f*.
bone cell Knochenzelle *f*, Osteozyt *m*.
bone cement *ortho*. Knochenzement *m*.
bone chip Knochenspan *m*, -chip *m*.
bone chisel *ortho*. Knochenmeißel *m*.
bone conduction *physiol*. Knochenleitung *f*, Osteoakusis *f*, Osteophonie *f*.
cranial b. craniale/osteale Knochenleitung.
craniotympanic b. osteo-/kraniotympanale Knochenleitung.
osteal b. → cranial b.
osteotympanic b. → craniotympanic b.
bone conduction test Knochenleitungstestung *f*.
bone corpuscle Knochenzelle *f*, Osteozyt *m*.
bone crest Knochenleiste *f*, Knochenkamm *m*.
bone cuff *histol*. Knochenmanschette *f*.
perichondral b. perichondrale Knochenmanschette.
bone cyst Knochenzyste *f*.
aneurysmal b. aneurysmatische/hämorrhagische/hämangiomatöse Knochenzyste, aneurysmatischer Riesenzelltumor *m*, benignes Knochenaneurysma *nt*.
hemangiomatous/hemorrhagic b. → aneurysmal b.
juvenile b. juvenile Knochenzyste.
marginal b. (*Gelenk*) Randzyste.
simple b. → solitary b.
solitary b. einfache/solitäre Knochenzyste, Solitärzyste.
subchondral b. subchondrale (Geröll-)Zyste.
unicameral b. → solitary b.
bone deformity Knochendeformität *f*.
bone density *ortho*., *radiol*. Knochendichte *f*.
bone dysplasia Knochendysplasie *f*.
bone fibers Sharpey'-Faser *f*.
bone file *ortho*. Knochenfeile *f*.
bone fracture Knochenbruch *m*, -fraktur *f*, Fractura *f*, *inf*. Bruch *m*, Fraktur *f*.
bone fragment Knochenfragment *nt*.
bone graft *ortho*. **1.** Knochentransplantat *nt*. **2.** Knochentransplantation *f*.
bone grafting *ortho*. Knochentransplantation *f*.
bone ground substance Knochengrundsubstanz *f*.
bone growth Knochenwachstum *nt*.
bone holder *ortho*. Knochenhaltezange *f*, -faßzange *f*, Repositionszange *f*.
bone-holding clamp/forceps Knochenhaltezange *f*, -faßzange *f*.
bone hook *ortho*. Knochenhaken *m*.
bone hunger *patho*. Knochenhunger *m*.
bone infarct Knocheninfarkt *m*.
bone infection Knocheninfektion *f*.
bone inflammation Knochenentzündung *f*, Ostitis *f*.

bone island Knocheninsel *f*, solitäre Enostose *f*.
bone lacuna Knochenzellhöhle *f*, -lakune *f*.
bone·let [ˈbəʊnlɪt] *n* Knöchelchen *nt*, kleiner Knochen *m*.
bone lever *ortho*. Knochenhebel *m*.
bone marrow Knochenmark *nt*, Medulla ossium.
fatty b. → yellow b.
gelatinous b. weißes Knochenmark, Gallertmark.
primary b. *embryo*. primäres Knochenmark.
red b. rotes blutbildendes Knochenmark, Medulla ossium rubra.
secondary b. *embryo*. sekundäres Knochenmark.
yellow b. gelbes fetthaltiges Knochenmark, Fettmark, Medulla ossium flava.
bone marrow abscess Knochenmarkabszeß *m*.
bone marrow aplasia Knochenmarkaplasie *f*.
bone marrow biopsy Knochenmarkbiopsie *f*.
bone marrow cavity Markhöhle, Cavitas medullaris.
bone marrow culture Knochenmarkskultur *f*.
bone marrow giant cell Knochenmarksriesenzelle *f*, Megakaryozyt *m*.
bone marrow necrosis Knochenmarknekrose *f*.
bone marrow puncture Knochenmarkpunktion *f*.
bone marrow smear Knochenmarkausstrich *m*.
bone marrow toxicity Knochenmarkschädlichkeit *f*, -toxizität *f*.
bone marrow transplantation Knochenmarktransplantation *f*.
bone matrix Knochenmatrix *f*, Osteoid *nt*, organische Knochengewebsgrundsubstanz *f*.
bone metastasis Knochenmetastase *f*, ossäre Metastase *f*.
osteoclastic b. osteoklastische Knochenmetastase.
osteoplastic b. osteoplastische Knochenmetastase.
bone necrosis Knochen-, Osteonekrose *f*.
aseptic b. aseptische Knochennekrose.
avascular b. avaskuläre Knochennekrose.
chemical b. chemische Knochennekrose.
epiphyseal ischemic b. aseptische Epiphysennekrose, Chondroosteonekrose.
post-traumatic b. → traumatic b.
radiation b. Strahlenosteonekrose *f*, Osteoradionekrose *f*.
thermal b. thermische Knochennekrose.
traumatic b. (post-)traumatische Knochennekrose *f*.
bone pain Knochenschmerz(en *pl*) *m*, Ostealgie *f*, Osteodynie *f*.
bone plate *ortho*. (Knochen-)Platte *f*.
bone remodelling *histol*. Knochenumbau *m*.
bone rongeur *ortho*. Knochenfaßzange *f*, -haltezange *f*.
bone saw *ortho*. Knochensäge *f*.
bone scan *radiol*. **1.** Knochenszintigraphie *f*, -scan *m*; Skelettszintigraphie *f*. **2.** Knochenszintigramm *nt*, -scan *m*.
bone scanning → bone scan 1.
bone sclerosis Knochensklerosierung *f*, -sklerose *f*, Osteosklerose *f*.
bone screw *ortho*. Knochenschraube *f*.
self-tapping b. selbstschneidende Knochenschraube.
bone sensibility *neuro*. Vibrationsempfindung *f*, Pallästhesie *f*.

bone skin Knochenhaut *f*, Periost *nt*.
bone spur Knochensporn *m*.
bone structure Knochenbau *m*.
bone suture *anat*. Knochennaht *f*.
bone tissue Knochengewebe *nt*.
bone trabeculae Knochenbälkchen *pl*, -trabekel *pl*.
bone tuberculosis Knochentuberkulose *f*, Knochen-Tb *f*.
bone tumor Knochengeschwulst *f*, -tumor *m*.
Bonhoeffer ['bɑnhefər]: **B.'s sign/symptom** *psychia*. Bonhoeffer-Zeichen *nt*.
Bonnet [bɔ'nɛ]: **B.'s capsule** Bonnet-Kapsel *f*.
B.'s operation *ophthal*. Bonnet-Operation *f*, -Enukleation *f*.
B.'s position Bonnet-Position *f*.
B.'s sign *neuro*. Bonnet-Zeichen *nt*.
Bonnet-Dechaume-Blanc [de'ʃom blɑ̃]: **B.-D.-B. syndrome** Bonnet-Dechaume-Blanc-Syndrom *nt*.
Bonnevie-Ullrich [bɔn'vi 'ʊlrɪx]: **B.-U. syndrome** Bonnevie-Ullrich-Syndrom *nt*, Pterygium-Syndrom *nt*.
Bonnier [bɔn'je]: **B.'s syndrome** Bonnier-Syndrom *nt*.
bont tick [bɑnt] *micro*. Amblyomma hebraeum.
bon·y ['bəʊnɪ] *adj* 1. knochig, knochenähnlich, knöchern, ossär, Knochen-. 2. (*Person*) (stark-)knochig. 3. (knochen-)dürr, dünn, nur Haut u. Knochen.
bony ankylosis *ortho*. knöcherne Gelenkversteifung/Ankylose *f*, Ankylosis ossea.
bony callus (Knochen-)Kallus *m*, Callus *m*.
bony canal of ear Canalis semicircularis osseus.
bony cavity of nose knöcherne Nasenhöhle *f*, Cavitas/Cavum nasi/nasalis osseum.
bony crepitus *ortho*. Knochenreiben *nt*, Crepitus *m*.
bony deformity Knochendeformität *f*.
bony excrescence Knochenvorsprung *m*.
bony extension *ortho*. Knochenzug *m*, -extension *f*.
bony focus (*Entzündung*) Knochenherd *m*.
bony hard palate harter Gaumen *m*, Palatum durum.
bony labyrinth (*Innenohr*) knöchernes/ossäres Labyrinth *nt*, Labyrinthus osseus.
bony lesion *ortho*. Knochenläsion *f*, -schädigung *f*.
bony metastasis → bone metastasis.
bony outgrowth Knochenvorsprung *m*.
bony palate knöcherner Gaumen *m*, Palatum osseum.
bony part: b. of auditory tube knöcherner Tubenabschnitt *m*, Pars ossea tubae auditivae.
b. of nasal septum knöcherner Abschnitt *m* des Nasenseptums, Pars ossea septi nasi.
bony pelvis knöchernes Becken *nt*, Beckenring *m*.
bony rib Rippenknochen *m*, knöcherne Rippe *f*.
bony ridge Knochenkamm *m*, -leiste *f*.
bony septum of nose → bony part of nasal septum.
bony sequestrum *ortho*. Knochensequester *nt*.
bony spur Knochensporn *m*.
bony suture *anat*. Naht *f*, Knochennaht *f*, Verwachsungslinie *f*, Sutura *f*.
bony syndactyly ossäre Syndaktylie *f*.
bony traction *ortho*. Knochenzug *m*, -extension *f*.
bony union *ortho*. (*Fraktur*) knöcherne Vereinigung *f*, knöcherne Konsolidierung *f*.

Böök [beɪk]: **B.'s syndrome** Böök-Syndrom *nt*, PHC-Syndrom *nt*.
boom [buːm] **I** *n* Dröhnen *nt*, Brummen *nt*. **II** *vi* dröhnen, brummen.
Bo·oph·i·lus [bəʊ'ɑfɪləs] *n micro*. Boophilus *nt*.
boost [buːst] **I** *n* 1. Erhöhung *f*, Steigerung *f*; Belebung *f*, Auftrieb *f*. 2. *phys*. Verstärkung *f*. **II** *vt* 3. verstärken, fördern, beleben, Auftrieb geben, steigern. 4. *phys*. Druck erhöhen, unter erhöhten Druck setzen; *electr*. (*Spannung*) verstärken, anheben.
boost·er ['buːstər] *n* 1. *immun*. Auffrischung(simpfung *f*) *f*, Verstärkung(sreaktion *f*) *f*. 2. *techn*. Verstärker *m*, Verstärkung *f*.
booster dose Boosterdosis *f*.
booster response immunologisches Gedächtnis *nt*.
booster shot Auffrischung(simpfung *f*) *f*.
boot [buːt] *n* Stiefel *m*, Schuh *m*.
bo·rac·ic acid [bə'ræsɪk, bɔ-] → boric acid.
bo·rate ['bɔːrɪt, -reɪt, 'bəʊ-] *n* Borat *nt*.
bo·rax ['bɔːræks, 'bəʊr-] *n* Borax *nt*, Natriumtetraborat *nt*.
bor·bo·ryg·mus [ˌbɔːrbə'rɪgməs] *n, pl* **-mi** [-maɪ] Borborygmus *m*.
bor·der ['bɔːrdər] **I** *n* Rand *m*, Saum *m*, Grenze *f*; Kante *f*, Leiste *f*. **II** *vt* (um-)säumen, begrenzen, einfassen. **III** *vi* (*a. fig.*) (an-)grenzen (*on, upon* an).
b. of acetabulum Acetabulumrand, Limbus acetabuli, Margo acetabularis.
b. of uterus Uterusrand, Margo uteri.
border cells 1. (*Innenohr*) Grenzzellen *pl*. 2. (*Magen*) Beleg-, Parietalzellen *pl*.
border contrast *physiol*. Grenzkontrast *m*.
border line (*a. fig.*) Grenzlinie *f*; Grenze *f*.
bor·der·line ['bɔːrdərlaɪn] **I** *n* Patient(in *f*) *m* mit Borderline-Psychose. **II** *adj* 1. (*a. fig.*) auf od. an der Grenze. 2. unbestimmt, unentschieden.
borderline case Grenzfall *m*, borderline case *m*.
borderline hypertension labile Hypertonie *f*.
borderline leprosy Borderline-Lepra *f abbr*. BL, dimorphe Lepra *f*, Lepra dimorpha.
borderline personality disorder Borderline-Persönlichkeit(sstörung *f*) *f*.
borderline rays *radiol*. Bucky-Strahlen *pl*, Grenzstrahlen *pl*.
borderline schizophrenia latente Schizophrenie *f*, Borderline-Psychose *f*, Borderline-Schizophrenie *f*.
borderline tumor Borderline-Tumor *m*.
border zone Grenzzone *f*, -schicht *f*.
Bor·de·tel·la [ˌbɔːrdɪ'telə] *pl micro*. Bordetella *f*.
B. pertussis Keuchhustenbakterium *nt*, Bordet-Gengou-Bakterium *nt*, Bordetella/Haemophilus pertussis.
Bordet-Gengou [bɔr'dɛ ʒɑ̃ːn'gu]: **B.-G. agar** Bordet-Gengou-Agar *m/nt*, -Medium *nt*.
B.-G. bacillus → Bordetella pertussis.
B.-G. culture medium → B.-G. agar.
B.-G. medium → B.-G. agar.
B.-G. phenomenon Bordet-Gengou-Reaktion *f*, -Phänomen *nt*.
B.-G. potato blood agar → B.-G. agar.
B.-G. reaction → B.-G. phenomenon.
bore [bɔːr, bɔr] **I** *n* Bohrung *f*; Innendurchmesser *m*; Kaliber *nt*. **II** *vt* (aus-, durch-)bohren, s. durchbohren durch. **III** *vi* (auf-, aus-)bohren, Bohrungen machen.
bore·dom ['bɔːrdəm, 'bəʊr-] *n* Lang(e)weile *f*, Langweiligkeit *f*.
bor·ic acid ['bɔːrɪk, 'bəʊr-] Borsäure *f*.

bor·ing ['bəʊərɪŋ, 'bɔːr-] **I** *n* Bohren *nt*, Bohrung *f*. **II** *adj* bohrend, Bohr-.
boring pain bohrender Schmerz *m*.
bo·rism ['bəʊərɪzəm, 'bɔːr-] *n* Borvergiftung *f*, Borismus *m*.
Börjeson ['bɔːrjəsən; 'bœrjəsən]: **B.'s syndrome** Börjeson-Forssman-Lehmann-Syndrom *nt*.
Börjeson-Forssman-Lehmann ['fɔərsmæn 'leɪmən]: **B.-F.-L. syndrome** → Börjeson's syndrome.
born [bɔːrn] **I** *adj* 1. geboren. **to be ~** geboren werden. **I was ~ in 1955** ich bin/wurde 1955 geboren. **when were you ~?** wann sind Sie geboren? **newly ~ baby** Neugeborene(s) *nt*. 2. *fig*. (*Idee*) entstehen. **II** *ptp* → bear.
borne [bɔːrn] **I** *adj* übertragen, weitergegeben. **II** *pret* → bear.
Bor·ne·o camphor ['bɔːrnɪəʊ] → borneol.
bor·ne·ol ['bɔːrnɪɒl, -əʊl] *n* Borneol *nt*, Borneokampfer *m*.
Born·holm disease ['bɔːrnhɒlm] Bornholmer Krankheit *f*, epidemische Pleurodynie *f*, Myalgia epidemica.
bor·nyl alcohol ['bɔːrnɪl, -nɪl] → borneol.
bo·ron ['bɔːrɑn, 'bəʊr-] *n abbr*. **B** Bor *nt abbr*. B.
Bor·rel·ia [bə'relɪə, -'riːlɪə, -jə] *n micro*. Borrelia *f*.
bor·rel·ia [bə'relɪə, -'riːlɪə, -jə] *n micro*. Borrelia *f*.
bor·rel·i·o·sis [bəˌrelɪ'əʊsɪs] *n* Borrelieninfektion *f*, Borreliose *f*.
Borst-Jadassohn [bɔːrst 'jɑːdɑzɔn]: **intraepidermal epithelioma B.-J.** intraepidermales Epitheliom Borst-Jadassohn *nt*.
bosch yaws [bɑʃ] südamerikanische Hautleishmaniose *f*, kutane Leishmaniase *f* Südamerikas, Chiclero-Ulkus *m*.
bos·om ['bʊzəm] *n* 1. Brust *f*, Brustregion *f*. 2. (*weibliche*) Brüste *pl*, Busen *m*.
boss [bɒs, bɑs] *n* (An-)Schwellung *f*, Beule *f*, Höcker *m*.
bos·se·lat·ed ['bɑsəleɪtɪd] *adj* mit Beulen/Höckern besetzt.
bos·se·la·tion [bɑsə'leɪʃn] *n* 1. kleine Beule *f*, kleiner Höcker *m*. 2. Beulen-, Höckerbildung *f*.
Bostock ['bɒstɒk]: **B.'s catarrh/disease** Heuschnupfen *m*, -fieber *nt*.
Boston ['bɑstən, 'bɒs-]: **B. brace** *ortho*. Bostonkorsett *nt*.
B. exanthem Boston-Exanthem *nt*, Pseudorubeolae *pl*.
B.'s sign Boston-Zeichen *nt*.
Botallo [bɒ'tɑlɔ]: **B.'s duct** Ductus Botalli, Ductus ateriosus.
B.'s foramen *embryo*. For. ovale cordis.
ligament of B. Lig. arteriosum.
bo·tan·ic [bə'tænɪk] *adj* → botanical **II**.
bo·tan·i·cal [bə'tænɪkl] **I** *n pharm*. Pflanzenheilmittel *nt*. **II** *adj* Pflanzen- od. Botanik betr., botanisch, Pflanzen-.
bot·a·nist ['bɑtnɪst] *n* Botaniker(in *f*) *m*.
bot·a·ny ['bɑtnɪ] *n* Pflanzenkunde *f*, Botanik *f*.
bo·thrid·i·um [bəʊ'θrɪdɪəm] *n, pl* **-dia** [-dɪə] *micro*. Bothridium *nt*.
both·ri·o·ceph·a·li·a·sis [ˌbɑθrɪəʊˌsefə'laɪəsəs] *n* Fischbandwurminfektion *f*, Diphyllobothriose *f*, Diphyllobothriasis *f*, Bothriozephalose *f*, Bothriocephalosis *f*.
Both·ri·o·ceph·a·lus [ˌ-'sefələs] *n micro*. Diphyllobothrium *nt*, Bothriocephalus *m*, Dibothriocephalus *m*.
both·ri·um ['bɑθrɪəm] *n, pl* **-ri·ums, -ria** [-rɪə] *micro*. Sauggrube *f*, Bothrium *nt*.
bot·ry·oid ['bɑtrɪɔɪd] *adj* traubenförmig.
bot·ry·oi·dal [bɑtrɪ'ɔɪdl] *adj* → botryoid.
botryoid sarcoma Sarkoma botryoides.

bot·ry·o·my·co·sis [ˌbɑtrɪəmaɪ'kəʊsɪs] *n derm.* Botryomykose *f*, -mykom *nt*, -mykosis *f*, Granuloma pediculatum.
bot·ry·o·my·cot·ic [ˌ-maɪ'kɑtɪk] *adj* Botryomykosis betr., von Botryomykosis betroffen, botryomykotisch.
Böttcher ['bœtçər]: **B.'s cells** Böttcher-Zellen *pl*.
B.'s crystals Böttcher-Kristalle *pl*.
bot·tle ['bɑtl] **I** *n* Flasche *f*. **to bring up on the ~** mit der Flasche großziehen. **II** *vt* (in Flaschen) abfüllen.
bottle up *vt fig. psycho.* (*Gefühle*) in s. aufstauen, in s. hineinfressen, unterdrücken.
bot·tled ['bɑtld] *adj* in Flaschen (ab-)gefüllt.
bottle-fed baby Flaschenkind *nt*.
bottle-feed *vt* aus der Flasche ernähren.
bottle nose Säufer-, Trinkernase *f*.
bottle-nosed *adj* rot-, schnapsnasig.
bottle sound Amphorenatmen *nt*.
bottle warmer Flaschenwärmer.
bot·tom ['bɑtəm] **I** *n* **1.** Boden *m*, Grund *m*, unterster Teil *m*, (unteres) Ende *nt*, Fuß *m*. **2.** Unterseite *f*, untere Seite *f*. **3.** Gesäß *nt, inf.* Hintern *m, inf.* Po *m*. **4.** Grundlage *f*. **II** *adj* untere(r, s), unterste(r, s), schlechteste(r, s), niedrigste(r, s), Tiefst-.
b. of internal acoustic meatus Boden des inneren Gehörganges, Fundus meatus acustici interni.
bot·u·li·form ['bɑtʃəlɪfɔːrm, bə't(j)uːl-] *adj* wurstförmig.
bot·u·lin ['bɑtʃəlɪn] *n* Botulinustoxin *nt*.
bot·u·li·nal [bɑtʃə'laɪnl] *adj* Clostridium botulinum *od.* Botulinustoxin betr., Botulinus-.
botulinal antitoxin Botulinusantitoxin *nt*, antitoxisches Botulinusserum *nt*.
bo·tu·line ['bɑtʃəlaɪn] *n* → botulin.
bot·u·li·no·gen·ic [bɑtʃəˌlɪnə'dʒenɪk] *adj* Botulinustoxin enthaltend *od.* bildend, botulinogen.
bot·u·li·num antitoxin [ˌ-'laɪnəm] → botulinal antitoxin.
bot·u·li·nus antitoxin [ˌ-'laɪnəs] → botulinal antitoxin.
botulinus toxin → botulin.
bot·u·lism ['bɑtʃəlɪzəm] *n* Vergiftung *f* durch Botulinustoxin, Botulismus *m*.
botulism antitoxin → botulinal antitoxin.
bot·u·lis·mo·tox·in [bɑtʃəˌlɪzmə'tɑksɪn] *n* → botulin.
bot·u·lo·gen·ic [bɑtʃələʊ'dʒenɪk] *adj* → botulinogenic.
bou·ba ['buːbə] *n* Frambösie *f*, Pian *f*, Parangi *f*, Yaws *f*, Framboesia tropica.
Bouchard [buːˈʃɑːr]: **B.'s coefficient** Bouchard-Index *m*.
B.'s disease myopathische Magendilatation *f*.
B.'s nodes/nodules Bouchard-Knoten *pl*.
bouche de tapir [buːʃ də taˈpiːr] *patho.* Tapirlippe *f*, -schnauze *f*.
Bouchet-Gsell [buːˈʃɛ gsɛl]: **B.-G. disease** Schweinehüterkrankheit *f*, Bouchet-Gsell-Krankheit *f*, Leptospirosis pomona.
bou·gie ['buːdʒɪ, -ʒɪ] *n chir.* Dehnsonde *f*, Bougie *m*.
bou·gie·nage [buːʒɪˈnɑːʒ] *n chir.* Bougieren *nt*, Bougierung *f*.
bou·gi·nage *n* → bougienage.
Bouillaud [buːˈjoː]: **B.'s disease** Bouillaud'-Krankheit *f*, rheumatische Endokarditis *f*.
B.'s sign Bouillaud'-Zeichen *nt*.
B.'s syndrome rheumatische Endo- u. Perikarditis *f*, Bouillaud-Syndrom *nt*.
bouil·lon ['buːljɒn, -jən; buːˈjõ] *n* **1.** Fleischbrühe *f*, Bouillon *f*. **2.** *micro.* Nährbrühe

f, -bouillon *f*, Bouillon *f*.
Bouin ['buːẽ]: **B.'s fixative** Bouin'-Lösung *f*, -Flüssigkeit *f*.
B.'s fluid → B.'s fixative.
B.'s solution → B.'s fixative.
bou·lim·ia *n* → bulimia.
bound [baʊnd] *adj* **1.** *chem.* gebunden. **2.** gebunden, verpflichtet, eingeschränkt.
bound·a·ry ['baʊndərɪ] *n, pl* **-ries 1.** Grenze *f*, Grenzlinie *f*, Rand *m*. **2.** *phys., mathe.* Be-, Abgrenzung *f*; Rand *m*; Umfang *m*.
boundary line Grenzlinie *f*.
boundary membrane Grenzmembran *f*.
bound·ing mydriasis ['baʊndɪŋ] *ophthal.* alternierende/springende Mydriasis *f*, Mydriasis alternans.
bound water gebundenes Wasser *nt*.
bouquet fever [buːˈkeɪ, buː-; buˈkɛ] Dengue *nt*, Dengue-Fieber *nt*, Dandy-Fieber *nt*.
Bourgery [burʒəˈriː]: **B.'s ligament** Lig. popliteum obliquum.
Bourneville [burnˈviːl]: **B.'s disease** Morbus Bourneville *m*, Bourneville-Syndrom *nt*, tuberöse (Hirn-)Sklerose *f*, Epiloia *f*.
Bourneville-Pringle ['prɪŋgl]: **B.-P. disease/syndrome** Bourneville-Pringle-Syndrom *nt*, Pringle-Bourneville-Syndrom *nt*, -Phakomatose *f*.
bout [baʊt] *n* (*Krankheit*) Anfall *m*, Episode *f*.
bou·ton·neuse (fever) [buːtəˈnuːz; butɔ-ˈnøz] Boutonneusefieber *nt*, Fièvre boutonneuse *f*.
bou·ton·nière deformity [buːtəˈnɪər; butɔ-ˈnjɛːr] *ortho.* Knopflochdeformität *f*.
bouton terminal [buːˈtõ] *pl* **boutons terminaux** synaptische Endknöpfchen *pl*, Boutons terminaux.
Bouveret [buvəˈrɛ]: **B.'s disease** Bouveret-Syndrom *nt*, paroxysmale Tachykardie *f*.
B.'s sign Bouveret-Zeichen *nt*.
B.'s syndrome → B.'s disease.
bo·vine ['baʊvaɪn, -viːn] *bio.* **I** *n* Rind *nt*. **II** *adj* bovin, Rinder-.
bovine babesiosis *micro.* Texas-Fieber *nt*.
bovine brucellosis Rinderbrucellose *f*, Bang-Krankheit *f*.
bovine heart Ochsenherz *nt*, Bukardie *f*, Cor bovinum.
bovine malaria Texas-Fieber *nt*.
bovine theileriasis East-Coast-Fieber *nt*, bovine Piroplasmose/Theileriose *f*.
bovine theileriosis → bovine theileriasis.
bovine tuberculosis Rindertuberkulose *f*.
Bowditch ['baʊdɪtʃ]: **B.'s law** Bowditch-Effekt *m*, Alles-oder-Nichts-Gesetz *nt* der Herzkontraktion.
bow·el ['baʊəl] **I** *n* **1.** (*meist* ~s *pl*) Darm *m*; Eingeweide *pl*, Gedärm *nt*. **to open/move the ~s** abführen. **to have open ~s** regelmäßig(en) Stuhlgang haben. **2.** das Innere *od.* die Mitte eines Objekts. **II** *vt* disembowel.
bowel anastomosis *chir.* Darm-, Enteroanastomose *f*.
bowel cleansing Darmreinigung *f*.
mechanical b. mechanische Darmreinigung.
bowel disease Darmerkrankung *f*.
inflammatory b. entzündliche Darmerkrankung.
bowel distension Darm(über)blähung *f*.
bowel diverticulum Darmdivertikel *nt*.
bowel evacuation → bowel movement 1.
bowel flora Darmflora *f*.
bowel habits Stuhlgewohnheiten *pl*, -frequenz *f*.
bowel injury Darmverletzung *f*, -schädigung *f*.

bowel motility Darmmotilität *f*.
bowel movement 1. Darmentleerung *f*, Stuhlgang *m*, Defäkation *f*. **2.** Stuhl *m*, Kot *m*, Fäzes *pl*, Faeces *pl*, Fäkalien *pl*.
bowel obstruction *chir.* Darmverlegung *f*, -obstruktion *f*, -verschluß *m*; Ileus *m*.
strangulated b. Strangulationsileus *m*.
bowel perforation *chir.* Darmdurchbruch *m*, -perforation *f*.
bowel preparation *chir.* (präoperative) Darmvorbereitung *f*.
bowel sounds *abbr.* **BS** Darmgeräusche *pl*.
high-pitched b. hochgestellte Darmgeräusche *pl*, klingendes Preßstrahlgeräusch *nt*.
bowel trauma → bowel injury.
bowel wall biopsy Darmwandbiopsie *f*.
Bowen ['baʊən]: **B.'s carcinoma** Bowen-Karzinom *nt*.
B.'s disease Bowen-Krankheit *f*, -Dermatose *f*, Morbus Bowen, Dyskeratosis maligna.
B.'s precancerous dermatitis/dermatosis → B.'s disease.
bow·en·oid ['baʊənɔɪd] *adj patho.* bowenoid.
bowl [baʊl] *n* **1.** Schüssel *f*, Schale *f*, Napf *m*. **2.** (Wasch-)Becken *nt*; (Toiletten-)-Schüssel *f*. **3.** schalenförmige Vertiefung *od.* Einsenkung *f*, Höhlung *f*.
bow-leg ['baʊleg] O-Bein *nt*, Genu varum.
bow-leg·ged ['baʊleg(ɪ)d] *adj* O-beinig.
Bowman ['baʊmən]: **B.'s capsule** Bowman'-Kapsel *f*, Capsula glomeruli.
B.'s glands Bowman'-Spüldrüsen *pl*, Gll. olfactoriae.
B.'s lamina → B.'s membrane.
B.'s layer → B.'s membrane.
B.'s membrane Bowman'-Membran *f*, vordere Basalmembran *f*, Lamina elastica anterior *f*, Lamina limitans anterior (corneae).
B.'s muscle Ziliaris *m*, Ziliarmuskel *m*, Ciliaris *m*, M. ciliaris.
B.'s probe Bowman-Sonde *f*.
B.'s space (*Niere*) Bowman'-Raum *m*.
box [bɑks] *n* **1.** Kiste *f*, Kasten *m*; Schachtel *f*; Dose *f*, Büchse *f*. **2.** Behälter *m*, Gefäß *nt*, Gehäuse *nt*, Hülse *f*.
boxe-note *n* hypersonorer Klopfschall *m* (*bei Lungenemphysem*).
box·er's ear ['bɑksər] Blumenkohl-, Boxerohr *nt*.
boxer's encephalopathy Boxerencephalopathie *f*, Encephalopathia traumatica.
boxer's fracture Boxer-Fraktur *f*.
boy [bɔɪ] *n* Junge *m*, Knabe *m*; *inf.* Sohn *m*.
Boyden ['bɔɪdn]: **B.'s sphincter** M. sphincter ductus choledochi.
Boyer [bwaˈjɛ]: **B.'s bursa** Boyer-Schleimbeutel *m*.
B.'s cyst Boyer-Zyste *f*.
boy·hood ['bɔɪhʊd] *n* Knabenzeit *f*, Kindheit *f*, Jugend(zeit *f*) *f*.
Boyle [bɔɪl]: **B.'s law** Boyle-Mariotte'-Gesetz *nt*.
Bozeman ['baʊzmən]: **B.'s catheter** → Bozeman-Fritsch catheter.
B.'s operation *gyn.* Bozeman-Operation *f*, Hysterozystokleisis *f*.
B.'s position Bozeman-Lagerung *f*.
Bozeman-Fritsch [frɪtʃ]: **B.-F. catheter** Bozeman-Fritsch-Katheter *m*.
BP *abbr.* → blood pressure.
b.p. *abbr.* → boiling point.
Bq *abbr.* → becquerel.
Br *abbr.* → bromine.
brace [breɪs] **I** *n* **1.** *ortho.* Schiene *f*, Schienenapparat *m*; Korsett *nt*; Orthese *f*. **2.** *ortho.* (Gips-, Kunststoff-)Schale *f*,

brachi-

Hülse *f.* **3.** *dent.* ~s *pl* Zahnklammer *f*, -spange *f.* **4.** *techn.* Halter *m*, Strebe *f*, Stütze *f*, Bügel *m*, Band *nt.* **II** *vt* verstreben, -steifen, -ankern, stützen, klammern.
brachi- *pref.* → brachio-.
bra·chi·al ['breɪkɪəl, -jəl] *adj* Arm betr., zum Arm gehörend, brachial, Arm-.
brachial anesthesia *anes.* Brachialisblock *m*.
brachial artery (Ober-)Armschlagader *f*, -arterie *f*, Brachialis *f*, A. brachialis.
 deep b. tiefe Armschlagader, Brachialis *f* profunda, A. profunda brachii.
 superficial b. oberflächliche Armschlagader, Brachialis *f* superficialis, A. brachialis superficialis.
brachial fascia Oberarmfaszie *f*, Fascia brachii/brachialis.
bra·chi·al·gia [ˌbreɪkɪ'ældʒ(ɪ)ə, ˌbræk-] *n* Brachialgie *f*, -algia *f*.
brachial glands kubitale Lymphknoten *pl*, Nodi lymphatici cubitales.
bra·chi·a·lis (muscle) [ˌbreɪkɪ'eɪlɪs, ˌbræk-] Brachialis *m*, M. brachialis.
brachial lymph nodes Oberarmlymphknoten *pl*, Nodi lymphatici (axillares) brachiales.
brachial muscle → brachialis (muscle).
brachial palsy → brachial paralysis.
brachial paralysis *neuro.* Armplexuslähmung *f*, Lähmung *f* des Plexus brachialis.
 lower (arm type of) b. untere Armplexuslähmung, Klumpke'-Lähmung, Klumpke-Déjérine-Lähmung.
 upper (arm type of) b. obere Armplexuslähmung, Erb'-Duchenne-Lähmung, Erb'-Lähmung.
brachial plexus Armgeflecht *nt*, -plexus *m*, Plexus brachialis.
brachial region: anterior b. Oberarmvorderfläche *f*, vordere Oberarmregion *f*, Regio/Facies brachialis anterior.
 posterior b. Oberarmhinterfläche *f*, hintere Oberarmregion *f*, Regio/Facies brachialis posterior.
brachial surface: anterior b. → brachial region, anterior.
 posterior b. → brachial region, posterior.
brachial syndrome Thoracic-outlet-Syndrom *nt*, Engpaß-Syndrom *nt*.
brachial triangle Achseldreieck *nt*.
brachial veins Oberarmvenen *pl*, Begleitvenen *pl* der A. brachialis, Vv. brachiales.
brachio- *pref.* Arm-, Brachi(o)-.
bra·chi·o·car·pal [ˌbreɪkɪəʊ'kɑːrpl] *adj* Unterarm *od.* Radius u. Handwurzel betr.
brachiocarpal articulation proximales Handgelenk *nt*, Artic. radiocarpalis.
brachiocarpal joint → brachiocarpal articulation.
bra·chi·o·ce·phal·ic [ˌ-sə'fælɪk] *adj* Arm u. Kopf betr. *od.* verbindend, brachiocephal, brachiocephal.
brachiocephalic arteritis Martorell'-Krankheit *f*, -Syndrom *nt*, Takayasu'-Krankheit *f*, -Syndrom *nt*, Pulslos-Krankheit *f*, pulseless disease.
brachiocephalic artery → brachiocephalic trunk.
brachiocephalic trunk Truncus brachiocephalicus.
brachiocephalic vein: left b. Brachiocephalica *f* sinistra, V. brachiocephalica sinistra.
 right b. Brachiocephalica *f* dextra, V. brachiocephalica dextra.
bra·chi·o·cru·ral [ˌ-'kruərəl] *adj* Arm(e) u. Bein(e) betr., brachiokrural, -crural.
bra·chi·o·cu·bi·tal [ˌ-'kjuːbɪtl] *adj* Oberarm u. Ell(en)bogen *od.* Unterarm betr.

brachiocubital ligament Lig. collaterale ulnare.
bra·chi·o·cyl·lo·sis [ˌ-sɪ'ləʊsɪs] *n* → brachiocyrtosis.
bra·chi·o·cyr·to·sis [ˌ-sɪər'təʊsɪs] *n* Armdeformität *f*, -verkrüppelung *f*.
bra·chi·o·ra·di·al [ˌ-'reɪdɪəl] *adj* Oberarm *od.* Humerus u. Radius betr., humeroradial.
brachioradial articulation Humeroradialgelenk *nt*, Artic. humeroradialis.
bra·chi·o·ra·di·a·lis (muscle) [ˌ-ˌreɪdɪ'eɪlɪs] Brachioradialis *m*, M. brachioradialis.
brachioradial joint → brachioradial articulation.
brachioradial ligament Lig. collaterale radiale.
brachioradial muscle → brachioradialis (muscle).
brachioradial reflex Radius-, Radiusperiostreflex *m abbr*. RPR.
brach·i·ose ['brækɪəʊz] *n* Isomaltose *f*, Dextrinose *f*.
bra·chi·ot·o·my [breɪkɪ'ɒtəmɪ] *n gyn.* Brachiotomie *f*.
bra·chi·o·ul·nar [ˌbreɪkɪəʊ'ʌlnər] *adj* Oberarm *od.* Humerus u. Ulna betr., humeroulnar.
brachioulnar articulation Humeroulnargelenk *nt*, Artic. humeroulnaris.
brachioulnar joint → brachioulnar articulation.
bra·chi·um ['breɪkɪəm, 'bræk-] *n*, *pl* **-chia** [-kɪə] *anat.* Arm *m*; Oberarm *m*; armähnliche Struktur *f*, Brachium *nt*.
 b. of caudal colliculus Brachium colliculi caudalis/inferioris.
 b. of cranial colliculus Brachium colliculi cranialis/rostralis/superioris.
 b. of inferior colliculus → b. of caudal colliculus.
 b. of rostral colliculus → b. of cranial colliculus.
 b. of superior colliculus → b. of cranial colliculus.
Brachmann-de Lange ['brækmən də 'læŋɪ]: **B.d.L. syndrome** Lange-Syndrom *nt*, Cornelia de Lange-Syndrom *nt*, Brachmann-de-Lange-Syndrom *nt*, Amsterdamer Degenerationstyp *m*.
Bracht [brɑːkt; braxt]: **B.'s maneuver** *gyn.* Bracht'-Handgriff *m*.
brachy- *pref.* Kurz-, Brachy-.
brach·y·ba·sia [brækɪ'beɪsɪə] *n neuro.* Brachybasie *f*.
brach·y·ba·so·pha·lan·gia [ˌ-ˌbeɪsəʊfə'lændʒ(ɪ)ə] *n patho.* Brachybasophalangie *f*.
brach·y·car·dia [ˌ-'kɑːrdɪə] *n* → bradycardia.
brach·y·ce·pha·lia [ˌ-sɪ'feɪljə] *n* → brachycephaly.
brach·y·ce·phal·ic [ˌ-sɪ'fælɪk] *adj* Brachyzephalie betr., von Brachyzephalie betroffen, kurz-, rundköpfig, brachykephal, -zephal.
brach·y·ceph·a·lism [ˌ-'sefəlɪzəm] *n* → brachycephaly.
brach·y·ceph·a·lous [ˌ-'sefələs] *adj* → brachycephalic.
brach·y·ceph·a·ly [ˌ-'sefəlɪ] *n* Rund-, Breit-, Kurzköpfigkeit *f*, Brachyzephalie *f*, -kephalie *f*; Breit-, Kurzkopf *m*, Brachyzephalus *m*.
brach·y·chei·lia [ˌ-'kaɪlɪə] *n embryo.* Brachych(e)ilie *f*.
brach·y·chei·ria [ˌ-'kaɪrɪə] *n patho.* Kurzhändigkeit *f*, Brachych(e)irie *f*.
bra·chych·i·ly [brə'kɪkəlɪ] *n* → brachycheilia.
brach·y·chron·ic [ˌbrækɪ'krɒnɪk] *adj* (*Krankheitsverlauf*) akut.

brach·y·cne·mic [ˌ-'(k)niːmɪk] *adj* → brachyknemic.
brach·y·cra·ni·al [ˌ-'kreɪnɪəl] *adj* → brachycranic.
brach·y·cra·nic [ˌ-'kreɪnɪk] *adj* kurzköpfig.
brach·y·dac·ty·ly [ˌ-'dæktəlɪ] *n patho.* Kurzfingrigkeit *f*, -zehigkeit *f*, Brachydaktylie *f*.
brach·y·e·soph·a·gus [ˌ-ɪ'sɒfəgəs] *n patho.* Brachyösophagus *m*.
brach·y·gna·thia [ˌbrækɪ(g)'neɪθɪə] *n patho.* Brachygnathie *f*.
brach·y·hy·per·pha·lan·gia [ˌbrækɪˌhaɪpərfə'lændʒ(ɪ)ə] *n patho.* Brachyhyperphalangie *f*.
brach·y·hy·po·pha·lan·gia [ˌ-ˌhaɪpəʊfə'lændʒ(ɪ)ə] *n patho.* Brachyhypophalangie *f*.
brach·y·kne·mic [ˌ-'niːmɪk] *adj* kurzbeinig.
brach·y·mes·o·pha·lan·gia [ˌ-ˌmezəfə'lændʒ(ɪ)ə] *n patho.* Brachymesophalangie *f*.
brach·y·met·a·car·pal·ism [ˌ-ˌmetə'kɑːrpəlɪzəm] *n* → brachymetacarpia.
brach·y·met·a·car·pia [ˌ-ˌmetə'kɑːrpɪə] *n patho.* Brachymetakarpie *f*.
brach·y·met·a·tar·sia [ˌ-ˌmetə'tɑːrsɪə] *n patho.* Brachymetatarsie *f*.
brach·y·pel·lic pelvis [ˌ-'pelɪk] transversovales Becken *nt*.
brach·y·pha·lan·gia [ˌ-fə'lændʒ(ɪ)ə] *n patho.* Brachyphalangie *f*.
brach·y·syn·dac·ty·ly [ˌ-sɪn'dæktəlɪ] *n embryo.* Brachysyndaktylie *f*.
brach·y·tel·e·pha·lan·gia [ˌ-ˌteləfə'lændʒ(ɪ)ə] *n patho.* Brachytelephalangie *f*.
brach·y·ther·a·py [ˌ-'θerəpɪ] *n radiol.* Brachytherapie *f*.
brac·ing ['breɪsɪŋ] **I** *n* Verstreben *nt*, Verstärken *nt*, Verankern *nt*; Verstrebung *f*, Verstärkung *f*. **II** *adj* belebend, stärkend, erfrischend, stimulierend, anregend.
bracing climate Reizklima *nt*.
brack·et ['brækɪt] *n* Halter *m*, Träger *m*, Stütze *f*, Stützarm *m*.
brady- *pref.* brady-, Brady-.
brad·y·a·cu·sia [ˌbrædɪə'kuːsɪə] *n HNO* Bradyakusie *f*, -akusis *f*.
brad·y·ar·rhyth·mia [ˌ-ə'rɪðmɪə] *n* (*Herz*) Bradyarrhythmie *f*.
brad·y·ar·thria [ˌ-'ɑːrθrɪə] *n* → bradylalia.
brad·y·car·dia [ˌ-'kɑːrdɪə] *n card.* Bradykardie *f*.
brad·y·car·di·ac [ˌ-'kɑːrdɪæk] **I** *n* Bradykardie-verursachendes Mittel *nt.* **II** *adj* Bradykardie betr. *od.* verursachend, von Bradykardie gekennzeichnet, bradykard(isch), bradykardisierend.
bradycardia-Tachykardie syndrome Bradykardie-Tachykardie-Syndrom *nt*.
brad·y·car·dic [ˌ-'kɑːrdɪk] *n*, *adj* → bradycardiac.
brad·y·ci·ne·sia [ˌ-sɪ'niːʒ(ɪ)ə] *n* → bradykinesia.
brad·y·crot·ic [ˌ-'krɒtɪk] *adj* pulsreduzierend, -verlangsamend, bradykrot.
brad·y·di·as·to·le [ˌ-daɪ'æstəlɪ] *n card.* verlangsamte Diastole *f*, Bradydiastolie *f*.
brad·y·e·coi·a [ˌ-ɪ'kɔɪə] *n neuro.* partielle Schwerhörigkeit *f*.
brad·y·es·the·sia [ˌ-es'θiːʒ(ɪ)ə] *n neuro.* Bradyästhesie *f*.
brad·y·gen·e·sis [ˌ-'dʒenəsɪs] *n embryo.* Entwicklungsverzögerung *f*, Bradygenese *f*.
brad·y·glos·sia [ˌ-'glɒsɪə] *n* → bradylalia.
brad·y·ki·ne·sia [ˌ-kɪ'niːʒ(ɪ)ə, -kaɪ-] *n neuro.* Bewegungsverlangsamung *f*, Bradykinesie *f*.
brad·y·ki·net·ic [ˌ-kɪ'netɪk, -kaɪ-] *adj neuro.* bradykinetisch.

brad·y·kin·in [ˌ-'kɪnɪn, -'kaɪ-] *n* Bradykinin *nt*.
brad·y·ki·nin·o·gen [ˌ-kɪ'nɪnədʒən, -kaɪ-] *n* Kallidin *nt*, Lysyl-Bradykinin *nt*.
brad·y·la·lia [ˌ-'leɪlɪə] *n neuro.* verlangsamtes Sprechtempo/Sprechen *nt*, Skandieren *nt*, Bradylalie *f*, -arthrie *f*, -glossie *f*, -phasie *f*.
brad·y·lex·ia [ˌ-'leksɪə] *n neuro.* verlangsamtes Lesen/Lesetempo *nt*, Bradylexie *f*.
brad·y·lo·gia [ˌ-'ləʊdʒ(ɪ)ə] *n* → bradylalia.
brad·y·men·or·rhea [ˌ-menə'riːə] *n gyn.* verlängerte Menstruation *f*, Bradymenorrhoe *f*.
brad·y·me·tab·o·lism [ˌ-mə'tæbəlɪzəm] *n* Bradymetabolismus *m*.
brad·y·pep·sia [ˌ-'pepsɪə] *n* verlangsamte Verdauung *f*.
brad·y·pha·gia [ˌ-'feɪdʒ(ɪ)ə] *n neuro.* verlangsamtes Essen *nt*, Bradyphagie *f*.
brad·y·pha·sia [ˌ-'feɪʒ(ɪ)ə] *n* 1. → bradylalia. 2. → bradyphemia.
brad·y·phe·mia [ˌ-'fiːmɪə] *n neuro.* verlangsamte Sprache *f*, Bradyphemie *f*, -phasie *f*.
brad·y·phra·sia [ˌ-'freɪʒ(ɪ)ə] *n neuro.* Bradyphrasie *f*.
brad·y·phre·nia [ˌ-'friːnɪə] *n neuro.* Bradyphrenie *f*.
brad·y·pne·a [ˌ-'(p)niə] *n* verlangsamte Atmung *f*, Bradypnoe *f*.
brad·y·pra·gia [ˌ-'preɪʒɪə] *n neuro.* Bradypragie *f*.
brad·y·rhyth·mia [ˌ-'rɪðmɪə] *n* → bradycardia.
brad·y·sper·ma·tism [ˌ-'spɜrmətɪzəm] *n andro.* Bradyspermie *f*.
brad·y·sphyg·mia [ˌ-'sfɪgmɪə] *n card.* Pulsverlangsamung *f*, Bradysphygmie *f*.
brad·y·stal·sis [ˌ-'stɔːlsɪs, -'stæl-] *n* verlangsamte Peristaltik *f*, Bradystaltik *f*.
brad·y·tach·y·car·dia [ˌ-ˌtækɪ'kɑːrdɪə] *n card.* Bradykardie-Tachykardie(-Syndrom *nt*) *f*.
brad·y·tel·e·o·ci·ne·sia [ˌ-ˌtelɪəʊsɪ'niːʒ(ɪ)ə] *n* → bradyteleokinesis.
brad·y·tel·e·o·ki·ne·sis [ˌ-ˌtelɪəʊkɪ'niːsɪs, -kaɪ-] *n neuro.* Bradyteleokinese *f*.
brad·y·to·cia [ˌ-'təʊsɪə] *n gyn.* Wehenschwäche *f*, Bradytokie *f*.
brad·y·tro·phia [ˌ-'trəʊfɪə] *n* Bradytrophie *f*.
brad·y·troph·ic [ˌ-'trɒfɪk, -'trəʊ-] *adj* bradytroph.
brad·y·u·ria [ˌ-'(j)ʊərɪə] *n urol.* verlangsamte Harnentleerung *f*, Bradyurie *f*.
bra·dy·zo·ite [ˌ-'zəʊaɪt] *n micro.* Bradyzoit *m*.
Bragard ['brægərd] *B.'s sign neuro., ortho.* Bragard'-Zeichen *nt*.
Braille [breɪl] *B.'s method/system* Brailleschrift *f*, Blindenschrift *f*.
braille [breɪl] *n* Braille's method.
Brailsford-Morquio ['breɪlsfɔːrd mɔːr-'kiːəʊ] *B.-M. disease* Morquio(-Ullrich)-Syndrom *nt*, Morquio-Brailsford-Syndrom *nt*, spondyloepiphysäre Dysplasie *f*, Mukopolysaccharidose Typ IV *f abbr.* MPS IV.
Brain [breɪn] *B.'s reflex* Brain-Reflex *m*.
brain [breɪn] *n* 1. Gehirn *nt; anat.* Encephalon *nt*, Cerebrum *nt*. 2. (*a.* ∼s *pl*) Verstand *m*, Hirn *nt*, 'Köpfchen' *nt*, Intelligenz *f*, Intellekt *m*.
brain abscess Hirnabszeß *m*.
otogenic b. otogener Hirnabszeß.
brain aneurysm Hirn(arterien)aneurysma *nt*.
brain atrophy Hirnatrophie *f*.
brain axis → brain stem.
brain bleeding Hirnblutung *f*.

brain calculus Hirnkonkrement *nt*, Enzephalolith *m*.
brain-case ['breɪnkeɪs] *n* (Ge-)Hirnschädel *m*, Neurokranium *nt*, Neurocranium *nt*.
brain cell Nervenzelle *f*, Neuron *nt*.
brain center Hirnzentrum *nt*.
brain concussion Gehirnerschütterung *f*, Kommotionssyndrom *nt*, Commotio cerebri.
brain contusion Hirnprellung *f*, -kontusion *f*, Contusio cerebri.
brain damage Hirnschaden *m*, Hirnschädigung *f*, Enzephalopathie *f*.
brain-damaged *adj* hirngeschädigt.
brain-dead *adj* hirntod.
brain death Hirntod *m*.
brain edema Hirnödem *nt*.
brain fever *inf.* idiopathische Enzephalitis *f*.
brain-heart infusion agar *abbr.* **BHIA** Hirn-Herz-Dextrose-Medium *nt*.
brain-heart infusion medium → brain--heart infusion agar.
brain hemorrhage Hirnblutung *f*.
brain injury Gehirnverletzung *f*, -trauma *nt*.
brain metastasis Hirnmetastase *f*.
brain-pan ['breɪnpæn] *n* → braincase.
brain perfusion Hirndurchblutung *f*, -perfusion *f*.
brain-pow·er ['breɪnpaʊər] *n* 1. Intelligenz *f*, Geisteskraft *f*. 2. Kapazität *f*, Spezialist *m*.
brain purpura Hirnpurpura *f*, Purpura cerebri.
brain sand Hirnsand *m*, Acervulus *m* (cerebri).
brain-sick *adj inf.* geisteskrank, verrückt.
brain stem Hirnstamm *m*, Truncus cerebri/encephali.
brain stem auditory evoked potentials *abbr.* **BAEPS** auditorisch evozierte Hirnstammpotentiale *pl*.
brain-stem center Hirnstammzentrum *nt*.
brain stem electric responses *abbr.* **BSER** brain stem electric responses *pl abbr.* BSER.
brain stem evoked response audiometry *abbr.* **BERA** Messung *f* akustisch evozierter Hirnstammpotentiale, brain stem evoked response audiometry *abbr.* BERA.
brain stem function Hirnstamm-, Stammhirnfunktion *f*.
brain stem lesion Hirnstammläsion *f*.
brain stem potential Hirnstammpotential *nt*.
brain stem reflex Hirnstamm-, Stammhirnreflex *m*.
brain-storm ['breɪnstɔːrm] I *n* 1. (plötzlicher) Einfall *m od.* Idee *f*, Geistesblitz *m*. 2. *psychia.* Anfall *m* von Geistesstörung *od.* -verwirrung. 3. Brainstorming *nt*. II *vt* ein Problem einem Brainstorming unterziehen. III *vi* Brainstorming betreiben *od.* praktizieren.
brain sugar Zerebrose *f*, D-Galaktose *f*.
brain swelling Hirnschwellung *f*.
brain syndrome: acute b. Delirium *nt*, Delir *nt*.
organic b. psychoorganisches Syndrom *nt*, (hirn-)organisches Psychosyndrom *nt*.
brain trauma Gehirnverletzung *f*, -trauma *nt*.
brain tumor (Ge-)Hirntumor *m*.
brain vesicles *embryo.* Hirnbläschen *pl*.
primary b. primäre Hirnbläschen.
secondary b. sekundäre Hirnbläschen.
brain-wash ['breɪnwɒʃ] I *n* Gehirnwäsche *f*. II *vt* jdn. einer Gehirnwäsche unterziehen.

brain-wash·ing ['breɪnwɒʃɪŋ] *n* → brainwash I.
brain wave 1. (*meist* ∼s *pl*) Hirnströme *pl*. 2. → brainstorm 1.
brain·y ['breɪnɪ] *adj inf.* gescheit, intelligent, klug.
brake [breɪk] I *n techn.* Bremse *f*. II *adj techn.* Brems-. III *vt, vi* bremsen.
brak·ing ['breɪkɪŋ] I *n* Bremsen *nt*. II *adj* Brems-.
braking radiation *phys.* Bremsstrahlung *f*.
bran [bræn] *n* Kleie *f*.
bran bath Kleiebad *nt*.
branch [bræntʃ, brɑːntʃ] I *n* (*a. fig.*) Zweig *m*, Ast *m*, Verzweigung *f*; *anat.* Ramus *m*. II *adj* Zweig-, Neben-. III *vi* 1. (her-)stammen (*from* von). 2. übergehen, auslaufen (*into* in).
branch off/out *vi* s. ausdehnen, s. vergrößern; s. verzweigen *od.* verästeln, s. gabeln.
b.es of amygdaloid body A. choroidea--Äste *pl* zum Corpus amygdaloideum, Rami corporis amygdaloidei.
b.es of anterior perforated substance A. choroidea anterior-Äste *pl* zur Capsula interna, Rami substantiae perforatae anterioris.
b. to cauda of caudate nucleus Ast der A. communicans posterior zur Cauda nuclei caudati, Ramus caudae nuclei caudati a. communicantis posterioris.
b. for dorsal corpus callosum Corpus callosum-Ast der A. occipitalis medialis, Ramus corpus callosi dorsalis a. occipitalis medialis.
b.es of globus pallidus A. choroidea-Äste *pl* zum Globus pallidus, Rami globi pallidi.
b.es of hepatic artery A. hepatica propria--Äste *pl*, Rami a. hepaticae propriae.
b.es of internal capsule A. choroidea-Äste *pl* zum hinteren Teil der Capsula interna, Rami capsulae internae.
b.es to isthmus of faucium of lingual nerve Rami isthmi faucium n. lingualis, Rami fauciales n. lingualis.
b.es of lateral geniculate body A. choroidea-Äste *pl* zum seitlichen Kniehöcker, Rami corporis geniculati lateralis.
b. for oculomotor nerve A. communicans posterior-Ast der III. Hirnnerv, Ramus n. oculomotorii a. communicantis posterioris.
b.es of optical tract A. choroidea-Äste *pl* zum Tractus opticus, Rami tractus optici.
b.es of proper hepatic artery → b.es of hepatic artery.
b.es of red nucleus A. choroidea-Äste *pl* zum Nc. ruber, Rami nc. rubri.
b.es of substantia nigra A. choroidea-Äste *pl* zur Substantia nigra, Rami substantiae nigrae.
b.es of tuber cinereum A. choroidea-Äste *pl* zum Tuber cinereum, Rami tuberis cinerei.
b.es to tympanic membrane of auriculotemporal nerve Trommelfelläste *pl* des N. auriculotemporalis, Rami membranae tympani n. auriculotemporalis.
b.es of vertebral peduncles Mittelhirnäste *pl* der A. cerebri posterior, Rami pedunculares a. cerebri posterioris.
branched ['bræntʃd] *adj* verästelt, verzweigt.
branched chain *chem.* verzweigte Kette *f*.
branched-chain *adj chem.* verzweigtkettig.
branched-chain amino acid *abbr.* **BCAA** verzweigtkettige Aminosäure *f*.

branched-chain amino acid transaminase

branched-chain amino acid transaminase branched-chain-Aminosäuretransaminase *f*.
branched-chain α-keto acid decarboxylase → branched-chain 2-keto acid dehydrogenase.
branched-chain 2-keto acid dehydrogenase branched-chain-2-Ketosäuredehydrogenase *f*.
branched-chain ketoacidemia → branched-chain ketoaciduria.
branched-chain ketoaciduria Ahornsirup-Krankheit *f*, -Syndrom *nt*, Valin-Leucin-Isoleucinurie *f*, Verzweigtkettendecarboxylase-Mangel *m*.
branched-chain ketoaminoacidemia → branched-chain ketoaciduria.
branched-chain ketonuria → branched-chain ketoaciduria.
branch·er deficiency ['bræntʃər] Andersen-Krankheit *f*, Amylopektinose *f*, leberzirrhotische retikuloendotheliale Glykogenose *f*, Glykogenose Typ IV *f*.
brancher deficiency glycogenosis → brancher deficiency
brancher enzyme Branchingenzym *nt*, Glucan-verzweigende Glykosyltransferase *f*, 1,4-α-Glucan-branching-Enzym *nt*.
brancher glycogen storage disease → brancher deficiency
bran·chi·al ['bræŋkɪəl] *adj embryo*. Kiemen(bögen) betr., von Kiemen(bögen) ausgehend, branchial, branchiogen, Kiemenbogen-.
branchial arch *embryo*. Kiemen-, Schlund-, Pharyngialbogen *m*.
branchial arch muscle Kiemenbogenmuskel *m*, -muskulatur *f*.
branchial arch nerve *embryo*. Kiemenbogennerv *m*.
branchial cleft Schlundfurche *f*, Kiemenspalte *f*.
branchial cleft cyst laterale Halszyste *f*, branchiogene Zyste *f*.
branchial cyst → branchial cleft cyst.
branchial fissures *embryo*. Kiemenspalten *pl*.
branchial fistula branchiogene Fistel *f*.
branchial groove → branchial cleft.
branchial pouch Schlundtasche *f*.
branch·ing ['bræntʃɪŋ] I *n* Verzweigung *f*, Verästelung *f*. II *adj s*. verweigend, *s*. verästelnd
branching enzyme → brancher enzyme
branching factor → brancher enzyme
bran·chi·o·ge·net·ic [,bræŋkɪəʊdʒə'netɪk] *adj* → branchiogenous.
branchiogenetic cyst → branchial cleft cyst.
bran·chi·o·gen·ic [,-'dʒenɪk] *adj embryo*. Kiemen(bögen) betr., von Kiemen(bögen) ausgehend, branchiogen.
bran·chi·og·e·nous [,bræŋkɪ'ɑdʒənəs] *adj embryo*. aus einer Kiemenspalte od. einem Kiemenbogen entstanden, branchiogen.
branchiogenous cyst → branchial cleft cyst.
bran·chi·o·ma [bræŋkɪ'əʊmə] *n patho*. branchiogene Geschwulst *f*, branchiogener Tumor *m*, Branchiom(a) *nt*.
Brandt-Andrews [brænt 'ændru:z]: **B.-A. maneuver/method** *gyn*. Brandt-Andrews-Handgriff *m*.
bran·dy nose ['brændɪ] Kartoffel-, Säuferfer-, Pfund-, Knollennase *f*, Rhinophym *nt*, Rhinophyma *nt*.
Branham ['brænhæm]: **B.'s bradycardia/sign** *card*. Nicoladoni-Branham-Zeichen *nt*, Branham-Zeichen *nt*, Nicoladoni-Isreal-Branham-Zeichen *nt*, -Phänomen *nt*.

Bran·ha·mel·la [,brænhə'melə] *n micro*. Branhamella *f*, Moraxella (Branhamella) *f*.
B. catarrhalis Moraxella (Branhamella) catarrhalis.
bran·ny ['brænɪ] *adj* aus Kleie, kleiehaltig, -artig, kleiig.
branny tetter (Kopf-)Schuppen *pl*, Pityriasis simplex capitis.
brash [bræʃ] *n patho*. Sodbrennen *nt*, Pyoris *f*.
brass [bræs, brɑːs] *n* 1. Messing *nt*. 2. Bronze *f*.
brass chill → brass-founder's fever.
brass eye Chalkitis *f*.
brass-founder's ague → brass-founder's fever.
brass-founder's fever Bronzegieß(er)fieber *nt*.
bras·sid·ic acid [brə'sɪdɪk] Brassidinsäure *f*.
brass·y cough ['bræsɪ, 'brɑːsɪ] blecherner Husten *m*.
Brauch-Romberg [braʊx 'rɑmbɜrg]: **B.-R. symptom** → Romberg's symptom 1.
Braun [braʊn]: **B.'s anastomosis** *chir*. Braun'-(Fußpunkt-)Anastomose *f*.
B.'s canal *embryo*. Canalis neurentericus.
B.'s hook Braun'-Haken *m*.
B.'s ring *gyn*. Bandl-Kontraktionsring *m*.
B.'s splint *ortho*. Braun-Schiene *f*.
Braune ['braʊnɪ]: **B.'s canal** *gyn*. Geburtskanal *m*.
B.'s muscle M. puborectalis.
Bravais ['bræveɪ, brɑ'vɛ]: **B.-jacksonian epilepsy** Jackson-Epilepsie *f*.
Braxton-Hicks ['brækstən hɪks]: **B.-H. version** *gyn*. Braxton-Hicks-Version *f*, Hicks-Version *f*.
bra·zier's chill ['breɪʒər] → brass-founder's fever.
Bra·zil·ian [brə'zɪljən]: **B. blastomycosis** Lutz-Splendore-Almeida-Krankheit *f*, brasilianische/südamerikanische Blastomykose *f*, Parakokzidioidomykose *f*, Granuloma paracoccidioides.
B. ophthalmia *ophthal*. Hornhauterweichung *f*, Keratomalazie *f*.
B. pemphigus brasilianischer Pemphigus *m*, brasilianischer Pemphigus foliaceus *m*, Pemphigus brasiliensis, Fogo Salvagem.
B. spotted fever Felsengebirgsfleckfieber *nt*, amerikanisches Zeckenbißfieber *nt*, Rocky Mountain spotted fever (*nt*) abbr. RMSF.
bread [bred] *n* 1. Brot *nt*. 2. Lebensunterhalt *m*. **to earn one's ~** sein Brot *od*. seinen Lebensunterhalt verdienen.
bread flour Gluten-, Klebermehl *nt*.
bread·stuff ['bredstʌf] *n* 1. Brotgetreide *nt*, -mehl *nt*. 2. Brot *nt*.
breadth ['bredθ] *n* 1. Breite *f*, Weite *f*. 2. *fig*. Ausdehnung *f*, Größe *f*, Spannweite *f*, Umfang *m*.
b. of accommodation *ophthal*. Akkommodationsbreite.
break [breɪk] (*v*: broke; broken) I *n* 1. Bruch *m*, (Ab-, Zer-, Durch-, Entzwei-)Brechen *nt*, Bruchstelle *f*, Riß *m*, Spalt *m*, Lücke *f*, Zwischenraum *m*, Öffnung *f*. 3. Pause *f*. **without a ~** ununterbrochen. 4. *fig*. Bruch *m* (*from*, *with* mit). II *vt* 5. ab-, auf-, durchbrechen, (er-, zer-)brechen. **to ~ s.o.'s head** jdm. den Schädel einschlagen. **to ~ one's leg** s. das Bein brechen. 6. zerreißen, -schlagen, -trümmern, kaputtmachen. 7. *phys*. (Strahlen) abfangen, dämpfen, abschwächen. 8. ab-, unterbrechen, trennen, aufheben. 9. *electr*. unterbrechen; ab-, ausschalten. 10. (*Gesetz*) bre-

chen, (*Vorschrift*) übertreten. III *vi* 11. brechen; zerbrechen, zerspringen, -reißen, platzen, kaputtgehen. 12. (*Wunde*) aufgehen, (auf-)platzen, (-)springen, (-)reißen. 13. (*Gesundheit*) nachlassen, abnehmen; (*psychisch, physisch*) zusammenbrechen. 14. (*Stimme*) mutieren, im Stimmbruch sein. 15. (*in Tränen*) ausbrechen.
break away I *vt* ab-, losbrechen, wegreißen (*from* von). II *vi* los-, abbrechen, absplittern (*from* von).
break down I *vt* 1. ein-, nieder-, abreißen, abbrechen; zerlegen. 2. *fig*. aufgliedern, aufschlüsseln, analysieren. 3. *chem*. aufspalten, auflösen, abbauen. II *vi* 4. (*a. fig*.) zusammenbrechen, versagen. 5. zerbrechen, in die Brüche gehen, eine Panne haben.
break off *vt, vi* abbrechen (*from* von).
break open I *vt* aufbrechen. II *vi* aufspringen, -platzen.
break out I *vt* heraus-, aus-, losbrechen. II *vi* (*Krankheit*) ausbrechen (*in, with* in). **~ in a rash** einen Ausschlag bekommen. **~ in tears** in Tränen ausbrechen.
break through I *vt* durchbrechen; (*Problem*) überwinden. II *vi* durchbrechen, hervorkommen, den Durchbruch schaffen.
break up I *vt* abbrechen, aufheben, beendigen, schließen. II *vi* zerbrechen, zerteilen, *s*. auflösen; (*physisch, psychisch*) zusammenbrechen.
break·a·ble ['breɪkəbl] *adj* zerbrechlich.
break·age ['breɪkɪdʒ] *n* (Zer-)Brechen *nt*, Bruch *m*; Bruchstelle *f*.
break·bone fever ['breɪkbəʊn] Dengue *nt*, Dengue-Fieber *nt*, Dandy-Fieber *nt*.
break·down ['breɪkdaʊn] *n* 1. Zusammenbruch *m*. 2. Schaden *m*, Störung *f*. 3. *fig*. Aufgliederung *f*, Aufschlüsselung *f*, Analyse *f*. 4. *chem*. Aufspaltung *f*, Auflösung *f*, Abbau *m*.
b. of suture *chir*. Nahtinsuffizienz *f*.
breakdown strength *phys*. Durchschlagsfestigkeit *f*.
breakdown voltage *phys*. Durchschlagsspannung *f*.
break·fast ['brekfəst] I *n* Frühstück *nt*. **for ~** zum Frühstück. **to have ~** frühstücken. II *vi* frühstücken. **to ~** s.th. *etw*. zum Frühstück haben.
breakfast food Frühstücksnahrung *f*.
break·ing ['breɪkɪŋ] *n* Brechen *m*, Bruch *m*.
b. of the voice Stimmbruch *m*, -wechsel *m*, Mutatio(n) *f*.
breaking current *phys*. Öffnungs(induktions)strom *m*.
breaking factor *phys*. Bruchfaktor *m*.
breaking load *phys*. Bruchlast *f*.
breaking point *phys., techn*. Bruch-, Zerreißgrenze *f*. **to have reached/be at ~ *fig*.** kurz vor dem (physischen *od*. psychischen) Zusammenbruch stehen, am Ende seiner Kraft sein.
breaking strain → breaking tension
breaking strength *phys*. Bruch-, Reißfestigkeit *f*.
breaking stress → breaking tension.
breaking tension *phys*. Bruchbeanspruchung *f*, Zerreißspannung *f*.
breaking test *phys*. Bruchprobe *f*.
break·out ['breɪkaʊt] *n* (*Krankheit*) Ausbruch *m*.
break·through ['breɪkθru:] *n* (*a. fig*.) Durchbruch *m*.
break·up ['breɪkʌp] *n* 1. Auflösung *f*, Aufspaltung *f*. 2. *chem*. Zerlegung *f*, Spaltung *f*. 3. (*physischer od. psychischer*) Zerfall/Zusammenbruch *m*. 4. (*Ehe, Gesundheit*) Zerrüttung *f*.

breast [brest] *n* 1. (weibliche) Brust *f*, *anat.* Mamma *f.* **to give the ~ to a baby** einem Kind die Brust geben, ein Kind stillen. 2. Brustdrüse *f*, Gl. mammaria. 3. Brust(kasten *m*) *f*, Pectus *nt*, Thorax *m.*
breast abscess Brust(drüsen)abszeß *m.*
breast anlage *embryo.* Brustanlage *f.*
breast biopsy Brust(drüsen)biopsie *f.*
breast·bone ['brestbəʊn] *n* Brustbein *nt*, Sternum *nt.*
breast cancer → breast carcinoma.
breast carcinoma Brust(drüsen)krebs *m*, -karzinom *nt*, Mammakarzinom *nt*, *inf.* Mamma-Ca *nt*, Ca. mammae.
 colloid b. verschleimendes/muzinöses Brust(drüsen)karzinom.
 cribriform b. kribriformes Brust(drüsen)karzinom.
 ductal b. Milchgangskarzinom.
 ductal b. with productive fibrosis, infiltrating → scirrhous b.
 familial b. familiäres/familiär-gehäuftes Brust(drüsen)karzinom.
 inflammatory b. inflammatorisches Brust(drüsen)karzinom.
 intraductal b. intraduktales/intraduktalwachsendes Brust(drüsen)karzinom.
 lobular b. lobuläres Brust(drüsen)karzinom.
 medullary b. medulläres Brust(drüsen)karzinom.
 minimal b. Minimalkrebs, -karzinom, intraduktales *od.* lobuläres Carcinoma in situ.
 mucinous b. → colloid b.
 papillary b. papilläres Brust(drüsen)karzinom.
 scirrhous b. szirrhöses Brust(drüsen)karzinom, Szirrhus *m*, Carcinoma solidum simplex der Brust.
 tubulary b. tubuläres Brust(drüsen)karzinom.
breast-feed *vt*, *vi* stillen, die Brust geben.
breast-feeding *n* Brustfütterung *f*, -ernährung *f*, Stillen *nt.*
breast fibroadenoma Fibroadenom *nt* der Brust(drüse).
 giant b. Riesenfibroadenom *nt* der Brust(drüse).
breast-height *n* Brusthöhe *f.*
breast-high *adj* brusthoch, -tief.
breast milk Brust-, Frauen-, Muttermilch *f.*
breast pang Herzbräune *f*, Stenokardie *f*, Angina pectoris.
breast parenchyma Brust(drüsen)parenchym *nt.*
breast primordium *embryo.* Brustkeim *m.*
breast-preserving procedure/technique *gyn.* brusterhaltende Technik/Operation *f.*
breast resection, segmental *gyn.* Segment-, Quadrantenresektion *f*, Lumpektomie *f*, Tylektomie *f.*
breast tumor Brust(drüsen)tumor *m*, -geschwulst *f.*
breath [breθ] *n* 1. Atem(luft *f*) *m.* **to catch one's ~** Atem holen, verschnaufen. **to draw ~** Atem holen. **to have bad ~** Mundgeruch haben, aus dem Mund riechen. **to hold one's ~** den Atem anhalten. **to gasp for ~** nach Luft schnappen. **out of ~** außer Atem, atemlos. **short of ~** kurzatmig. 2. Atmung *f*, Atmen *nt*, Atemzug *m.* **to take a deep ~** tief Luft einatmen. **his ~ is failing** seine Atmung wird schwächer. 3. Atempause *f.*
breath·a·ble ['bri:ðəbl] *adj* 1. atem-, inhalierbar. 2. (*Material*) luftdurchlässig, atmungsaktiv.
breath·a·lyze ['breθəlaɪz] *forens.* I *vt* (ins Röhrchen) blasen *od.* pusten lassen. II *vi* (ins Röhrchen) blasen *od.* pusten.
breath·a·lyz·er ['breθəlaɪzər] *n forens.* (Atem-)Alkoholtestgerät *nt*, Röhrchen *nt.*
breathe [bri:ð] I *vt* 1. atmen, ein- u. ausatmen. 2. erschöpfen, den Atem nehmen, zum Keuchen bringen. II *vi* 3. atmen, luftholen, ein- u. ausatmen. **to ~ heavily** schwer atmen, keuchen. **to ~ one's last** sterben, seinen letzten Atemzug tun. 4. Atem holen, (s.) verschnaufen. 5. (*Material, Haut*) atmen, luftdurchlässig *od.* atmungsaktiv sein.
breathe in *vi* einatmen.
breathe out *vi* ausatmen.
breathe·a·ble *adj* → breathable.
breath·er ['bri:ðər] *n* 1. Atem-, Verschnaufpause *f.* 2. Person, die (schwer etc.) atmet. 3. Strapaze *f.* 4. *techn.* Entlüfter *m.* 5. *techn.* (Be-)Atmungshilfe *f.*
breath-holding *n* (un-)willkürliches Luftanhalten *nt.*
breath·ing ['bri:ðɪŋ] *n* 1. Atmen *nt*, Atmung *f.* 2. Atemzug *m.* 3. Atem-, Verschnaufpause *f.*
breathing apparatus Atem-, Sauerstoffgerät *nt.*
breathing cycle Atmungszyklus *m.*
breathing exercise(s) Atemübung(en *pl*) *f*, -gymnastik *f.*
breathing difficulties Atembeschwerden *pl.*
breathing mechanics Atem-, Atmungsmechanik *f.*
breathing reserve *physiol.* Atemreserve *f.*
breathing work *physiol.* Atmungsarbeit *f.*
breath·less ['breθlɪs] *adj* 1. nicht atmend, einen Atemstillstand anzeigen, tot. 2. atemlos, außer Atem, keuchend, luftschnappend, dyspnoisch.
breath·less·ness ['-nɪs] *n* 1. *med.* Dyspnoe *f*, Atemnot *f*, Kurzatmigkeit *f.* 2. Atemlosigkeit *f.*
breath sounds *abbr.* **BS** Atemgeräusche *pl.*
 bronchial b. Bronchialatmen *nt*, bronchiale Atemgeräusche.
 bronchovesicular b. bronchivesikuläres Atmen *nt*, bronchivesikuläre Atemgeräusche.
 vesicular b. Vesikulär-, Bläschenatmen *nt*, vesikuläre Atemgeräusche.
breath·tak·ing ['breθteɪkɪŋ] *adj* den Atem nehmend, schlimm, fruchtbar, schrecklich.
breath test (Atem-)Alkoholtest *m.*
B receptor B-Rezeptor *m.*
Breda ['breda]: **B.'s disease** Frambösie *f*, Framboesia tropica, Pian *f*, Parangi *f*, Yaws *f.*
breech [bri:tʃ] *n* 1. Hinterteil *nt*, Gesäß *nt.* 2. → breech delivery.
breech birth → breech delivery.
breech delivery *gyn.* Steißgeburt *f*, Geburt *f* aus Beckenendlage/Steißlage.
breech presentation *gyn.* Beckenendlage *f* *abbr.* **BEL**; Steißlage *f.*
 complete b. vollkommene Steiß-Fuß-Lage.
 double b. → complete b.
 frank b. einfache Steißlage.
 incomplete b. unvollkommene Steißlage.
 single b. → frank b.
breed [bri:d] (*v:* bred; bred) I *n bio.* Rasse *f*, Zucht *f*, Brut *f.* II *vt* 1. erzeugen, hervorbringen, gebären. 2. *micro.* züchten. 3. *fig.* hervorrufen, verursachen, führen zu. 4. auf-, erziehen, ausbilden. III *v s.* fortpflanzen, s. vermehren, brüten.
breed·ing ['bri:dɪŋ] *n* 1. Fortpflanzung *f*, Vermehrung *f.* 2. Züchten *nt*, (Auf-)Zucht *f*, Züchtung *f.*

breeding ground Brutstätte *f*, -platz *m*; *bact.* Nährboden *m.*
breg·ma ['breɡmə] *n*, *pl* **-ma·ta** [-mətə] *anat.* 1. Bregma *nt*, Vorderkopf *m.* 2. Bregma *nt.*
breg·mat·ic [breɡ'mætɪk] *adj* Bregma betr.
bregmatic bone Os parietale.
bregmatic fontanelle vordere/große Fontanelle *f*, Stirnfontanelle *f*, Fonticulus anterior.
breg·ma·to·mas·toid suture [ˌbreɡmətəʊ-'mæstɔɪd] Sutura parietomastoidea.
Breisky ['braɪskɪ]: **B.'s disease** Breisky-Krankheit *f*, Kraurosis/Craurosis vulvae.
brems·strah·lung ['brɛmzʃtra:luŋ] *n phys.* Bremsstrahlung *f.*
Brennemann ['brenəmən]: **B.'s syndrome** Brennemann-Syndrom *nt.*
Brenner ['brenər]: **B.'s tumor** Brenner-Tumor *m.*
Breschet [breˈʃɛ]: **B.'s bones** Ossa suprasternalia.
 B.'s canals Breschet-Kanäle *pl*, Diploekanäle *pl*, Canales diploici.
 B.'s hiatus Breschet-Hiatus *m*, Schneckenloch *nt*, Helicotrema *nt.*
 B.'s sinus Sinus sphenoparietalis.
 B.'s veins Breschet-Venen *pl*, Diploevenen *pl*, Vv. diploicae.
Brescia-Cimino ['breʃa 'simino]: **B.-C. fistula/shunt** *chir.* (Brescia-)Cimino-Shunt *m.*
Bretonneau [brətɔ'no]: **B.'s angina/disease** Diphtherie *f*, Diphtheria *f.*
Breus [brɔs]: **B. mole** *gyn.* Breus-Mole *f.*
brevi- *pref.* Kurz-, Brevi-.
Brev·i·bac·te·ri·um [ˌbrevɪbæk'tɪərɪəm] *n micro.* Brevibacterium *nt.*
brev·i·col·lis [ˌ-'kɒlɪs] *n* Kurz-, Froschhals *m.*
Brewer ['brʊər]: **B.'s infarcts** (*Niere*) Brewer-Infarkt(herde *pl*) *m.*
 B.'s point Brewer-Punkt *m.*
brew·ers' yeast ['brʊər] *micro.* Back-, Bierhefe *f*, Saccharomyces cerevisiae.
Brewster ['bru:stər]: **B.'s law** *opt.* Polarisationswinkel *m*, Brewster-Winkel *m.*
Bricker ['brɪkər]: **B.'s ileal conduit** → B.'s operation.
 B.'s ileoureterostomy → B.'s operation.
 B.'s operation Bricker-Operation *f*, -Plastik *f*, -Blase *f*, Ileum-Conduit *m/nt*, Ileum-, Dünndarmblase *f.*
 B.'s ureteroileostomy → B.'s operation.
Brickner ['brɪknər]: **B.'s sign** *neuro.* Brickner-Zeichen *nt.*
brick-pox ['brɪkpɒks] *n* Backsteinblattern *pl.*
bridge [brɪdʒ] I *n* 1. Brücke *f*, Steg *m.* 2. (zeitliche) Überbrückung *f.* 3. *anat.* (Nasen-)Brücke *f.* 4. *dent.* (Zahn-)Brücke *f.* 5. *ophthal.* (Brillen-)Steg *m.* 6. *chem.* Brücke *f.* II *vt* (*a. fig.*) überbrücken; eine Brücke bauen über.
 b. of nose *anat.* (Nasen-)Brücke.
 b. of Varolius (*ZNS*) Brücke, Pons (Varolii/cerebri).
bridge·a·ble ['brɪdʒəbl] *adj* überbrückbar.
bridge coloboma Brückenkolobom *nt.*
bridge corpuscle Haftplatte *f*, Desmosom *nt.*
bridge·work ['brɪdʒwɜːk] *n dent.* (Zahn-)Brücke *f.*
bridg·ing ['brɪdʒɪŋ] *n* Überbrückung *f.*
bri·dle stricture ['braɪdl] Bridenstriktur *f.*
bri·dou [bri'du] *n* Perlèche *f*, Faulecken *pl*, Mundwinkelcheilitis *f*, -rhagaden *pl*, Cheilitis/Stomatitis angularis, Angulus infectiosus oris/candidamycetica.
brief [bri:f] *adj* 1. kurz, vorübergehend,

briefing

kurzlebig, von kurzer Dauer. 2. (*Bericht*) kurz(gefaßt), knapp. **in ~** kurz.
brief·ing ['briːfɪŋ] *n* **1.** (genaue) Instruktion(en *pl*) *od.* Anweisung(en *pl*) *f*. **2.** Lagebericht *m*, Lagebesprechung *f*.
Bright [braɪt]: **B.'s disease 1.** Nierenerkrankung *f*. **2.** Bright-Krankheit *f*, chronische Nephritis *f*, Glomerulonephritis *f*.
bright [braɪt] *adj* **1.** hell, glänzend, leuchtend, strahlend (*with* von, vor). **2.** (*Geräusch*) hell, metallisch. **3.** *fig.* lebhaft, munter; intelligent, klug.
bright·en ['braɪtn] **I** *vt* **1.** heller machen; aufhellen. **2.** jdn. aufheitern, aufmuntern. **II** *vi* **3.** aufhellen, hell(er) werden, s. klären. **4.** lebhafter werden, s. beleben. **5.** (*Prognose*) günstiger werden.
bright-eyed *adj* mit glänzenden *od.* strahlenden Augen; helläugig.
bright·ness ['braɪtnɪs] *n* **1.** Helligkeit *f*, Klarheit *f*, Glanz *m*. **2.** Intelligenz *f*, Klugheit *f*. **3.** Aufgewecktheit *f*, Lebhaftigkeit *f*.
bright pain heller Schmerz *m*.
Brill [brɪl]: **B.'s disease** → Brill-Zinsser disease.
bril·liant ['brɪljənt] *adj* **1.** glänzend, strahlend, leuchtend, glitzernd. **2.** *fig.* brillant, hervorragend.
brilliant cresyl blue *histol.* Brillantkresylblau *nt*.
brilliant green Brillantgrün *nt*.
brilliant-green agar Brillantgrün(-Gallen)-Agar *m*/*nt*.
brilliant-green bile salt agar → brilliant-green agar.
brilliant vital red Brillantrot *nt*.
brilliant yellow Brillantgelb *nt*.
Brill-Symmers ['sɪmərs]: **B.-S. disease** Brill-Symmers-Syndrom *nt*, Morbus Brill-Symmers *m*, zentroplastisch-zentrozytisches (malignes) Lymphom *nt*, großfollikuläres Lymphoblastom/Lymphom *nt*.
Brill-Zinsser ['zɪnsər]: **B.-Z. disease** Brill(-Zinsser)-Krankheit *f*.
brim [brɪm] *n* **1.** (Gefäß-)Rand *m*. **2.** *anat.* Beckenrand *m*, Apertura pelvis/pelvica superior.
brim·stone liver ['brɪmstəʊn] *patho.* Feuersteinleber *f*.
brine [braɪn] *n* Lake *f*, Salzbrühe *f*, Sole *f*; Salzwasser *nt*.
Brinell [brɪ'nel]: **B. hardness number** *abbr.* **BHN** *phys.* Brinell-Härte *f abbr.* HB.
bring [brɪŋ] (**brought; brought**) *vt* **1.** (mit-) bringen, überbringen, -mitteln, herbeibringen, -schaffen. **2.** jdn. veranlassen (*to do* zu tun); jdn überzeugen *od.* überreden. **3.** bewirken, (mit s.) bringen.
bring about *vt* bewirken, verursachen, veranlassen, anregen.
bring around *vt* (*Person*) wieder zu Bewußtsein bringen.
bring forth *vt, vi* gebären, zur Welt bringen.
bring on *vt* (*Krankheit*) herbeiführen, verursachen, auslösen.
bring round *vt* → bring around.
bring to *vt* (*Bewußtlosen*) wiederbeleben, wieder zu Bewußtsein bringen.
bring up *vt* **1.** (*Kind*) auf-, großziehen, erziehen. **2.** (etw.) erbrechen; (*Säugling*) spucken.
bri·no·lase ['braɪnəleɪs] *n* Brinolase *f*.
Brinton ['brɪntn]: **B.'s disease** entzündlicher Schrumpfmagen *m*, Brinton-Krankheit *f*, Magenzirrhus *m*, Linitis plastica.
brin·y ['braɪnɪ] *adj* salzig, salz-, solehaltig.
Brion-Kayser [briˈɔ̃ 'kaɪzər]: **B.-K. disease** Paratyphus *m*.

Briquet [briˈkɛ]: **B.'s syndrome** Briquet-Syndrom *nt*.
brise·ment [briːzˈmɑ̃] *n ortho.* operative Gelenkmobilisierung *f*, Brisement *nt*.
brisk [brɪsk] **I** *adj* **1.** flott, flink, rasch. **2.** *med.* (*Diurese*) forsiert, stark. **3.** lebhaft, rege. **4.** frisch, anregend, belebend. **II** *vt*, *vi* → brisk up.
brisk up I *vt* beleben, anregen. **II** *vi* s. beleben, aufmuntern.
brisk reflexes gute Reflexe *pl*.
brisk walk flotter/schneller Spaziergang *m*.
Brissaud [briˈso]: **B.'s dwarf** Brissaud-Zwerg *m*.
B.'s reflex Brissaud-Reflex *m*.
B.'s scoliosis ischialgie-bedingte Skoliose *f*.
Brissaud-Marie [maˈri]: **B.-M. syndrome** Brissaud-Syndrom *nt*.
Brissaud-Sicard [siˈkaːr]: **B.-S. syndrome** Brissaud-Sicard-Syndrom *nt*.
bris·tle ['brɪsl] **I** *n* Borste *f*; (Bart-)Stoppel *f*. **II** *vt* (*Haare*) aufrichten. **III** *vi* → bristle up.
bristle up *vi* (*Haare*) s. sträuben.
bris·tly ['brɪslɪ] *adj* borstig, stachelig, stoppelig, Stoppel-.
Brit·ish ['brɪtɪʃ]: **B. anti-Lewisite** *abbr.* **BAL** Dimercaprol *nt*, British anitisit *nt abbr.* BAL, 2,3-Dimercaptopropanol *nt*.
B. dog tick *micro.* **1.** Ixodes canisuga. **2.** Rhipicephalus sanguineus.
B. thermal unit *abbr.* **B.T.U.** British thermal unit *abbr.* B.T.U., britische Wärmeeinheit *f*.
Britten-Davidson ['brɪtn 'deɪvɪdsən]: **B.-D. model** Britten-Davidson-Modell *nt*.
brit·tle ['brɪtl] *adj* **1.** spröde, zerbrechlich, brüchig. **2.** *fig.* scharf, hart, schneidend.
brittle bones 1. Osteogenesis imperfecta, Osteopsathyrosis *f*. **2.** Osteoporose *f*, -porosis *f*.
brittle bone syndrome → brittle bones.
brittle diabetes insulinabhängiger Diabetes (mellitus) *m*, Typ 1 Diabetes (mellitus).
brit·tle·ness ['brɪtlnɪs] *n* Sprödigkeit *f*, Zerbrechlichkeit *f*, Brüchigkeit *f*.
broach [brəʊtʃ] *n chir.* Stecheisen *nt*, Ahle *f*, Pfriem *m*, Räumahle *f*.
broad [brɔːd] *adj* **1.** breit, weit, ausgedehnt. **2.** hell. **3.** (*Akzent*) stark; (*Wissen*) breit. **4.** (*Hinweis*) deutlich, klar. **5.** allgemein. **6.** tolerant, großzügig.
Broadbent ['brɔːdbent]: **B.'s sign** Broadbent-Zeichen *nt*.
B.'s inverted sign Broadbent-Aneurysmazeichen *nt*.
broad-beta disease (primäre/essentielle) Hyperlipoproteinämie Typ III *f*, Hypercholesterinämie *f* mit Hypertriglyzeridämie, Broad-Beta-Disease (*nt*), Hyperpoproteinämie *f* mit breiter Betabande.
broad-beta proteinemia → broad-beta disease.
broad-breasted *adj* breitbrüstig.
broad-chested *adj* breitbrüstig.
broad condyloma breites Kondylom *nt*, Condyloma latum/syphiliticum.
broad·en ['brɔːdn] **I** *vt* breiter machen, verbreitern; (*a. fig.*) erweitern, ausdehnen. **II** *vi* breiter werden, s. erweitern *od.* verbreitern (*into* zu).
broad-faced ['brɔːdfeɪst] *adj* breit-, mondgesichtig.
broad fascia Fascia lata.
broad fish tapeworm *micro.* (breiter) Fischbandwurm *m*, Grubenkopfbandwurm *m*, Diphyllobothrium latum; Bothriocephalus latus.

broad foot Spreizfuß *m*, Pes transversus.
broad·ish ['brɔːdɪʃ] *adj* ziemlich *od.* relativ breit. **a ~ face** ein relativ breites Gesicht, Mondgesicht *nt*.
broad ligament: b. of liver sichelförmiges Leberband *nt*, Lig. falciforme (hepatis).
b. of lung Lig. pulmonale.
b. of uterus breites Mutter-/Uterusband *nt*, Lig. latum uteri.
broad ligament abscess parametraner Abszeß *m*.
broad ligament pregnancy ektopische Schwangerschaft *f* im Lig. latum uteri.
broad marginal confrontation method *HTG* Jaboulay-Methode *f*, Jaboulay-Brian-Methode *f*.
broad-minded *adj* (*Person*) tolerant, offen, liberal, unvoreingenommen.
broad nose Breitnase *f*.
broad-spectrum *adj* **1.** wirksam gegen eine Vielzahl von Mikroorganismen, Breitsprektum-. **2.** vielfältig anwendbar *od.* einsetzbar.
broad-spectrum antibiotic *pharm.* Breitspektrum-, Breitbandantibiotikum *nt*.
broad tapeworm → broad fish tapeworm.
Broca ['brəʊkə; brɔˈka]: **B.'s amnesia** Broca-Amnesie *f*.
B.'s aphasia *neuro.* motorische Aphasie *f*, Broca-Aphasie *f*.
B.'s area motorisches Sprachzentrum *nt*, motorische/frontale Broca'-(Sprach-)-Region *f*, Broca'-Feld *nt*.
band of B. → diagonal band of B.
B.'s center → B.'s area.
B.'s convolution → B.'s gyrus.
B.'s diagonal band → diagonal band of B.
diagonal band of B. Broca'-Diagonalband *nt*, Bandaletta/Stria diagonalis (Broca).
B.'s fissure Broca-Fissur *f*.
B.'s formula Broca-Formel *f*.
B.'s gyrus Broca-Windung *f*, -Gyrus *m*.
B.'s (motor) speech area/field/region → B.'s area.
B.'s parolfactory area Area subcallosa/parolfactoria.
pilaster of B. *anat.* Linea aspera.
B.'s plane Sehebene *f*.
B.'s region Broca-Windung *f*, -Gyrus *m*.
Brock [brɒk]: **B.'s infundibulotomy** *HTG* Brock-Operation *f*, transventrikuläre Infundibulektomie *f*.
B.'s operation *HTG* **1.** Brock-Operation *f*, transventrikuläre Valvotomie *f*. **2.** → B.'s infundibulotomy.
B.'s syndrome Mittellappensyndrom *nt*.
Brockenbrough ['brɒknbrəʊ]: **B.'s sign** Brockenbrough-Zeichen *nt*.
Brocq [brɔk]: **B.'s disease** Brocq'-Krankheit *f*, Parapsoriasis en plaques, chronische superfizielle Dermatitis *f*.
Broders ['brəʊdərs]: **B.' classification/index** *patho.* Broders-Index *m*.
Brodie ['brəʊdɪ]: **B.'s abscess** Brodie'-(Knochen-)Abszeß *m*.
B.'s bursa 1. Bursa subtendinea m. gastrocnemii medialis. **2.** Bursa m. semimembranosi.
B.'s disease 1. chronische hypertrophische Synovitis *f* des Kniegelenks. **2.** hysterische Arthralgie *f*.
B.'s knee chronisch hypertrophische Synovitis *f* des Kniegelenks.
B.'s ligament Brodie'-Band *nt*.
B.'s sign *urol.* Brodie-Zeichen *nt*.
Brodmann ['brɒdmən]: **B.'s areas** Brodmann'-Felder *pl*, -Areae *pl*.
Broesike ['briːzɪkɪ; 'brøːsɪkə]: **B.'s fossa** Broesike'-Raum *m*, Fossa parajejunalis.
bro·ken ['brəʊkn] **I** *adj* **1.** zerbrochen; (*Knochen*) gebrochen. **2.** (*Gesundheit*,

Ehe) zerrüttet. **3.** (*körperlich od. seelisch*) gebrochen. **4.** (*Schlaf*) unterbrochen. **II** *ptp* → break.
broken dose fraktionierte Dosis *f*, Dosis refracta.
broken-down *adj* **1.** verbraucht, erschöpft; kaputt. **2.** (*Nerven*) zerrüttet; (*seelisch*) gebrochen; (*gesundheitlich*) am Ende, verbraucht.
broken heart (tiefe) Trauer/Depression *f*, Verzweiflung *f*, Hoffnungslosigkeit *f*.
broken-hearted *adj* gebrochen, verzweifelt, bekümmert; deprimiert.
bro·mate ['brəʊmeɪt] *n chem.* Bromat *nt*.
bro·mat·ed ['brəʊmeɪtɪd] *adj* → brominated.
bro·ma·ther·a·py [brəʊmə'θerəpɪ] *n* → bromatotherapy.
bro·ma·tol·o·gy [ˌ-'tɒlədʒɪ] *n* Bromatik *f*, Bromatographie *f*, Bromatologie *f*.
bro·ma·to·ther·a·py [ˌbrəʊmətəʊ'θerəpɪ] *n* Broma(to)therapie *f*; Diätetik *f*.
bro·ma·to·tox·in [ˌ-'tɒksɪn] *n* Lebensmittel-, Bromatotoxin *nt*.
bro·ma·tox·ism [brəʊmə'tɒksɪzəm] *n* Lebensmittelvergiftung *f*.
bro·maz·e·pam [brəʊ'mæzɪpæm] *n pharm.* Bromazepam *nt*.
brom·cre·sol green [brɒm'kriːsəl] Bromkresolgrün *nt*.
bromcresol purple Bromkresolpurpur *nt*.
bro·me·lain ['brəʊmɪleɪn] *n* Bromelain *nt*.
bro·me·lin ['brəʊməlɪn, brəʊ'miː-] *n* Bromelin *nt*.
brom·hex·ine [brəʊm'heksiːn] *n* Bromhexin *nt*.
brom·hi·dro·sis [brəʊmɪ'drəʊsɪs] *n* Brom(h)idrosis *f*.
bro·mic ['brəʊmɪk] *adj* fünfwertiges Brom betr. *od.* enthaltend.
bro·mide ['brəʊmaɪd, -mɪd] *n* Bromid *nt*.
bromide acne Bromakne *f*.
bro·mi·dro·sis [brəʊmɪ'drəʊsɪs] *n* → bromhidrosis.
bro·mi·nat·ed ['brəʊmɪˌneɪtɪd] *adj* bromhaltig, bromiert.
bro·mine ['brəʊmiːn, -mɪn] *n abbr.* **Br** Brom *nt abbr.* **Br**.
bro·min·ism ['brəʊmɪnɪzəm] *n* → bromism.
bro·mism ['brəʊmɪzəm] *n* chronische Brom(id)vergiftung *f*, Bromismus *m*.
brom·i·so·val·um [brəʊmˌaɪsəʊ'væləm] *n pharm.* Bromisoval *n*.
bro·min·ized ['brəʊmɪnaɪzd] *adj* → brominated.
bro·mo·ben·zene [ˌbrəʊməʊ'benziːn] *n* Brombenzol *nt*.
bro·mo·chlo·ro·tri·flu·o·ro·eth·ane [ˌ-ˌklɔːrətraɪˌflʊərə'eθeɪn] *n anes.* Halothan *nt*, Fluothan *nt*.
bro·mo·crip·tine [ˌ-'krɪptiːn] *n pharm.* Bromocriptin *nt*.
5-bro·mo·de·ox·y·u·ri·dine [ˌ-ˌdɪˌɒksɪ'jʊərɪdiːn, -dɪn] *n abbr.* **BUDR** 5-Brom(o)desoxyuridin *nt abbr.* BUDR.
bro·mo·der·ma [ˌ-'dɜːmə] *n derm.* Bromodermie *f*, -derma *nt*.
bro·mo·form ['-fɔːm] *n* Bromoform *nt*, Tribrommethan *nt*.
bro·mo·ma·nia [ˌ-'meɪnɪə] *n pharm., psychia.* Bromomanie *f*.
bro·mo·phe·nol blue [ˌ-'fiːnəl, -nɒl] → bromphenol blue.
bro·mop·nea [brəʊmɒp'niːə] *n* (übler) Mund-/Atemgeruch *m*, Halitose *f*, Halitosis *f*, Kakostomie *f*, Foetor ex ore.
bro·mo·sul·fo·phthal·e·in [brəʊmə,sʌlfəʊ'θæliːɪn] *n* → bromsulphalein.
bromosulfophthalein test Bromosulfalein-, Bromosulfophthalein-, Bromosulphthalein-, Bromthaleintest *m*, BSP--Test *m*.
5-bro·mo·u·ra·cil [ˌ-'jʊərəsɪl] *n abbr.* **BU** 5-Bromuracil *nt abbr.* (5-)BU.
bro·mo·vi·nyl·de·ox·y·u·ri·dine [ˌ-,vaɪnlˌdɪˌɒksɪ'jʊərɪdiːn, -dɪn] *n abbr.* **BVDU** *pharm.* Bromovinyldesoxyuridin *nt abbr.* BVDU.
brom·per·i·dol [brəʊm'perɪdəl, -dɒl] *n pharm.* Bromperidol *nt*.
brom·phen·ir·a·mine [ˌ-fe'nɪrəmiːn] *n pharm.* Brompheniramin *nt*.
brom·phe·nol [brəʊm'fiːnəl, -nɒl] *n* Bromphenol *nt*.
bromphenol blue Bromphenolblau *nt*.
brom·sul·fo·phthal·e·in [ˌ-ˌsʌlfəʊ'θæliːɪn] *n* → bromsulphalein.
bromsulfophthalein test → bromosulfophthalein test.
brom·sul·phal·e·in [brəʊmsʌl'fæliːɪn] *n abbr.* **BSP** Bromosulfalein *nt*, Bromosulphthalein *nt*, Bromthalein *nt*, Bromsulfophthalein *nt abbr.* BSP.
bromsulphalein test → bromosulfophthalein test.
brom·thy·mol blue [brəʊm'θaɪmɒl, -mal] Bromthymolblau *nt*.
bro·mum ['brəʊmʊm] *n* → bromine.
bro·u·rat·ed ['brəʊmjəreɪtɪd] *adj* Brom *od.* Bromsalze enthaltend; bromiert.
brom·u·ret ['brəʊmjəret] *n* → bromide.
bronch- *pref.* → broncho-.
bronch·ad·e·ni·tis [brɒŋkædɪ'naɪtɪs] *n* Bronch(o)adenitis *f*.
bron·chi·al ['brɒŋkɪəl] *adj* Bronchus *od.* Bronchialsystem betr., bronchial, Broncho-, Bronchial-.
bronchial adenoma Bronchialadenom *nt*.
bronchial allergy → bronchial asthma.
bronchial arteries, (anterior) → bronchial branches of internal thoracic artery.
bronchial asthma Bronchialasthma *nt*, Asthma bronchiale.
bronchial branches: b. of internal thoracic artery Bronchialäste *pl* der A. thoracica interna, Rami bronchiales a. thoracicae internae.
intrasegmental b. Rami bronchiales segmentorum.
b. of thoracic aorta Bronchienäste *pl* der Aorta thoracica, Bronchialarterien *pl*, Aa. bronchiales, Rami bronchiales aortae thoracicae.
b. of vagus nerve Vagusäste *pl* zum Lungenhilus, Rami bronchiales n. vagi.
bronchial breathing Bronchialatmen *nt*, bronchiales Atemgeräusch *nt*.
bronchial bud *embryo.* Bronchusknospe *f*.
bronchial calculus Bronchialstein *m*, Broncholith *m*, Calculus bronchialis.
bronchial carcinoid Bronchialkarzinoid *nt*.
bronchial carcinoma → bronchogenic carcinoma.
bronchial cast *patho.* Bronchialausguß *m*.
bronchial constriction → bronchoconstriction.
bronchial crisis Bronchialkrise *f*.
bronchial cylindroma Bronchialzylindrom *nt*.
bronchial cyst bronchogene Zyste *f*.
bronchial dissimination *patho.* bronchogene Aussaat *f*.
bronchial fistula Bronchusfistel *f*.
bronchial fremitus Bronchialfremitus *m*, Fremitus bronchialis.
bronchial glands Bronchialdrüsen *pl*, Gll. bronchiales.
bronchial hemorrhage Bluthusten *nt*, -spucken *nt*, Hämoptoe *f*, Hämoptyse *f*, Hämoptysis *f*.

bronchial lavage Bronchiallavage *f*, -spülung *f*, Bronchuslavage *f*, -spülung *f*.
bronchial mucosa Bronchialschleimhaut *f*, Tunica mucosa bronchiorum.
bronchial murmur Bronchialatmen *nt*, bronchiales Atemgeräusch *nt*.
bronchial musculature Bronchialmuskulatur *f*.
bronchial occlusion Bronchus-, Bronchienverschluß *m*.
bronchial pneumonia Bronchopneumonie *f*, lobuläre Pneumonie *f*.
bronchial polyp Bronchialpolyp *m*.
bronchial rales → bronchial murmur.
bronchial respiration Bronchialatmen *nt*, bronchiales Atmen *nt*.
bronchial spasm → bronchospasm.
bronchial stenosis → bronchostenosis.
bronchial stone → bronchial calculus.
bronchial stricture Bronchusstriktur *f*.
bronchial suture *chir.* Bronchusnaht *f*, Bronchorrhaphie *f*.
bronchial system Bronchialbaum *m*, -system *nt*, Arbor bronchialis.
bronchial tree → bronchial system.
bronchial tuberculosis Bronchustuberkulose *f*.
bronchial veins Bronchialvenen *pl*, Vv. bronchiales.
bronchial voice → bronchophony.
bron·chi·arc·tia [ˌbrɒŋkɪ'ɑːkʃɪə] *n* → bronchostenosis.
bron·chic cells ['brɒŋkɪk] Lungenalveolen *pl*, Alveoli pulmonis.
bron·chi·ec·ta·sia [ˌbrɒŋkɪek'teɪʒ(ɪ)ə, -zɪə] *n* → bronchiectasis.
bron·chi·ec·ta·sic [ˌ-'ektɪzɪk] *adj* → bronchiectatic.
bron·chi·ec·ta·sis [ˌ-'ektəsɪs] *n* Bronchiektase *f*, Bronchiektasie *f*.
bron·chi·ec·tat·ic [ˌ-ek'tætɪk] *adj* Bronchiektas(i)e betr., von Bronchiektas(i)e gekennzeichnet, bronchiektatisch.
bronchiectatic cavity Bronchiektase(n)höhle *f*.
bron·chi·lo·quy [brɒŋ'kɪləkwɪ] *n* → bronchophony.
bron·chi·o·cele ['brɒŋkɪəʊsiːl] *n* Bronchiolenerweiterung *f*, -dilatation *f*.
bron·chi·o·cri·sis [ˌ-'kraɪsɪs] *n* Bronchiokrise *f*.
bron·chi·o·gen·ic [ˌ-'dʒenɪk] *adj* → bronchogenic.
bronchiogenic carcinoma → bronchogenic carcinoma.
bron·chi·o·lar adenocarcinoma [ˌbrɒŋkɪ'əʊlər, brɒŋ'kaɪə-] → bronchiolar carcinoma.
bronchiolar carcinoma bronchiolo-alveoläres Lungenkarzinom *nt*, Alveolarzellenkarzinom *nt*, Lungenadenomatose *f*, Ca. alveolocellulare/alveolare.
bron·chi·o·lec·ta·sis [ˌbrɒŋkɪəʊ'lektəsɪs] *n* Bronchiolenerweiterung *f*, Bronchiolektas(i)e *f*.
bron·chi·ol·i·tis [ˌ-'laɪtɪs] *n* **1.** Bronchiolenentzündung *f*, Bronchiolitis *f*, Bronchitis capillaris. **2.** Bronchopneumonie *f*, lobuläre Pneumonie *f*; Herd-, Fokalpneumonie *f*.
bron·chi·ole ['brɒŋkɪəʊl] *n* Bronchiole *f*, Bronchiolus *m*.
bron·chi·o·lo·al·ve·o·lar adenocarcinoma [ˌbrɒŋkɪəʊləʊæl'vɪələr] → bronchioloalveolar carcinoma.
bronchioloalveolar carcinoma bronchiolo-alveoläres Lungenkarzinom *nt*, Alveolarzellenkarzinom *nt*, Lungenadenomatose *f*, Ca. alveolocellulare/alveolare.
bron·chi·o·lus [brɒŋ'kaɪələs, brɒŋ-] *n, pl* **-li** [-laɪ] → bronchiole.

bronchionectasia

bron·chi·o·nec·ta·sia [ˌbraŋkɪəʊnekˈteɪʒ(ɪ)ə] n → bronchiolectasis.
bron·chi·o·spasm [ˌ-spæzəm] n → bronchospasm.
bron·chi·o·ste·no·sis [ˌ-stɪˈnəʊsɪs] n → bronchostenosis.
bron·chis·mus [braŋˈkɪzməs] n → bronchospasm.
bron·chit·ic [braŋˈkɪtɪk] I n Patient(in f) m mit Bronchitis, Bronchitiker(in f) m. II adj Bronchitis betr., bronchitisch.
bronchitic asthma bronchitisches/katarrhalisches Asthma nt, Asthmabronchitis f.
bron·chi·tis [braŋˈkaɪtɪs] n Entzündung f der Bronchialschleimhaut, Bronchitis f.
broncho- pref. Bronchien-, Broncho-, Bronchi-, Bronchus-.
bron·cho·ad·e·ni·tis [ˌbraŋkəʊˌædəˈnaɪtɪs] n → bronchadenitis.
bron·cho·al·ve·o·lar [ˌ-ælˈvɪələr] adj bronchoalveolär, bronchiolo-alveolär.
bronchoalveolar carcinoma bronchiolo--alveoläres Lungenkarzinom nt, Alveolarzellenkarzinom nt, Lungenadenomatose f, Ca. alveolocellulare/alveolare.
bron·cho·al·ve·o·li·tis [ˌ-ˌælvɪəˈlaɪtɪs] n Bronch(o)alveolitis f.
bron·cho·as·per·gil·lo·sis [ˌ-ˌæspərdʒɪˈləʊsɪs] n Bronchial-, Bronchoaspergillose f.
bron·cho·blas·to·my·co·sis [ˌ-ˌblæstəʊmaɪˈkəʊsɪs] n Bronchoblastomykose f.
bron·cho·blen·nor·rhea [ˌ-ˌblenəˈrɪə] n Bronchoblennorrhoe f.
bron·cho·can·di·di·a·sis [ˌ-ˌkændɪˈdaɪəsɪs] n Bronchialcandidose f, -moniliasis f.
bron·cho·cav·ern·ous [ˌ-ˈkævərnəs] adj bronchokavernös.
bron·cho·cele [ˈ-siːl] n (lokalisierte) Bronchuserweiterung f, -dilatation f, Bronchozele f.
bron·cho·con·stric·tion [ˌ-kənˈstrɪkʃn] n Broncho-, Bronchuskonstriktion f.
bron·cho·con·stric·tor [ˌ-kənˈstrɪktər] I n bronchokonstriktive Substanz f. II adj bronchokonstriktiv.
bron·cho·dil·a·ta·tion [ˌ-ˌdaɪləˈteɪʃn, -dɪ-] n Bronchodilatation f, -erweiterung f.
bron·cho·di·la·tion [ˌ-daɪˈleɪʃn, -dɪ-] n Bronchodilation f.
bron·cho·dil·a·tor [ˌ-ˈdaɪlətər, -ˈdɪ-] I n pharm. Bronchodilatator m, -spasmolytikum nt. II adj bronchodila(ta)torisch.
bron·cho·e·de·ma [ˌ-ɪˈdiːmə] n Ödem nt der Bronchialschleimhaut, Bronchialödem nt.
bron·cho·e·goph·o·ny [ˌ-ɪˈgafənɪ] n (Auskultation) Ziegenmeckern nt, Kompressionsatmen nt, Ägophonie f.
bron·cho·e·soph·a·ge·al [ˌ-ɪˌsafəˈdʒiːəl] adj Bronchus u. Ösophagus betr. od. verbindend, bronchoösophageal.
bronchoesophageal fistula bronchoösophageale Fistel f.
bronchoesophageal muscle → bronchoesophageus (muscle).
bron·cho·e·soph·a·ge·us (muscle) [ˌ-ɪsəˈfædʒ(ɪ)əs, -ɪˌsafəˈdʒiːəs] M. broncho-(o)esophageus.
bron·cho·e·soph·a·gos·co·py [ˌ-ɪˌsafəˈgaskəpɪ] n Bronchoösophagoskopie f.
bron·cho·fi·ber·scope [ˈ-faɪbərskəʊp] n flexibles Bronchoskop nt, Glasfaserbronchoskop nt.
bron·cho·fi·ber·sco·py [ˌ-faɪˈbərskəpɪ] n Bronchofiberendoskopie f.
bron·cho·fi·bros·co·py [ˌ-faɪˈbraskəpɪ] n → bronchofiberscopy.
bron·cho·gen·ic [ˌ-ˈdʒenɪk] adj von den Bronchien ausgehend, bronchogen.
bronchogenic adenocarcinoma bronchogenes Adenokarzinom nt.
bronchogenic carcinoma 1. Bronchialkrebs m, -karzinom nt. **2.** Lungenkrebs m, -karzinom nt.
small-cell b. kleinzelliges Bronchialkarzinom.
bronchogenic cyst bronchogene Zyste f.
bronchogenic spread bronchogene Aussaat f.
bron·cho·gram [ˈbraŋkəʊgræm] n radiol. Bronchogramm nt.
bron·cho·graph·ic [ˌ-ˈgræfɪk] adj Bronchographie betr., mittels Bronchographie, bronchographisch.
bron·chog·ra·phy [branˈkagrəfɪ] n radiol. Bronchographie f.
bron·cho·lith [ˈbraŋkəʊlɪθ] n Bronchialstein m, Broncholith m, Calculus bronchialis.
bron·cho·li·thi·a·sis [ˌ-lɪˈθaɪəsɪs] n Broncholithiasis f.
bron·cho·ma·la·cia [ˌ-məˈleɪʃ(ɪ)ə] n patho. Bronchomalazie f.
bron·cho·me·di·as·ti·nal trunk [ˌ-miːdɪəˈstaɪnl]: **left b.** Truncus bronchomediastinalis sinister.
right b. Truncus bronchomediastinalis dexter.
bron·cho·mon·i·li·a·sis [ˌ-mənəˈlaɪəsɪs] n → bronchocandidiasis.
bron·cho·mo·tor [ˌ-ˈməʊtər] adj bronchomotorisch.
bron·cho·my·co·sis [ˌ-maɪˈkəʊsɪs] n Bronchomykose f.
bron·cho·no·car·di·o·sis [-nəʊˌkɑːrdɪˈəʊsɪs] n Nocardieninfektion f der Bronchien.
broncho-oidiosis n → bronchocandidiasis.
bron·cho·pan·cre·at·ic fistula [ˌ-ˌpæŋkrɪˈætɪk, -ˌpæŋ-] Bronchus-Pankreas-Fistel f, bronchopankreatische Fistel.
bron·chop·a·thy [braŋˈkapəθɪ] n Bronchialerkrankung f, Bronchopathie f.
bron·choph·o·ny [braŋˈkafənɪ] n Bronchialstimme f, Bronchophonie f.
bron·cho·plas·ty [ˈbraŋkəʊplæstɪ] n chir. Bronchusplastik f.
bron·cho·ple·gia [ˌ-ˈpliːdʒ(ɪ)ə] n Bronchoplegie f, Bronchuslähmung f.
bron·cho·pleu·ral [ˌ-ˈplʊərəl] adj Bronchien u. Pleura betr. od. verbindend, bronchopleural.
bronchopleural fistula bronchopleurale Fistel f, Fistula bronchopleuralis.
bron·cho·pleu·ro·pneu·mo·nia [ˌ-ˌplʊərəʊn(j)uːˈməʊnɪə] n kombinierte Bronchopneumonie f u. Pleuritis, Bronchopleuropneumonie f.
bron·cho·pneu·mo·nia [ˌ-n(j)uːˈməʊnɪə] n Bronchopneumonie f, lobuläre Pneumonie f; Herd-, Fokalpneumonie f.
bron·cho·pneu·mon·ic [ˌ-n(j)uːˈmanɪk] adj Bronchopneumonie betr., von Bronchopneumonie betroffen, durch sie verursacht, bronchopneumonisch.
bronchopneumonic aspergillosis bronchopulmonale Aspergillose f.
bronchopneumonic focus bronchopneumonischer Herd m.
bron·cho·pneu·mo·ni·tis [ˌ-ˌn(j)uːməˈnaɪtɪs] n → bronchopneumonia.
bron·cho·pneu·mop·a·thy [ˌ-n(j)uːˈmapəθɪ] n Erkrankung f von Bronchien u. Lunge(ngewebe), Bronchopneumopathie f.
bron·cho·pul·mo·nar·y [ˌ-ˈpʌlməˌnerɪ, -ˈpʊl-] Lunge u. Bronchien betr., bronchopulmonal, Bronchopulmonal-.
bronchopulmonary cyst bronchopulmonale Zyste f.
bronchopulmonary dysplasia bronchopulmonale Dysplasie f.
bronchopulmonary lymph nodes Hiluslymphknoten pl, Nodi lymphatici bronchopulmonales/hilares.
bronchopulmonary segments Lungensegmente pl, Segmenta bronchopulmonalia.
bronchopulmonary spirochetosis → bronchospirochetosis.
bron·cho·ra·di·og·ra·phy [ˌ-ˌreɪdɪˈagrəfɪ] n radiol. Bronchoradiographie f.
bron·chor·rha·gia [ˌ-ˈrædʒ(ɪ)ə] n Bronchial-, Bronchusblutung f, Bronchorrhagie f.
bron·chor·rha·phy [branˈkarəfɪ] n HTG. Bronchusnaht f, Bronchorrhaphie f.
bron·chor·rhea [ˌbraŋkəʊˈrɪə] n Bronchorrhoe f.
bron·cho·scope [ˈ-skəʊp] n Bronchoskop nt.
bron·cho·scop·ic [ˌ-ˈskapɪk] adj Bronchoskop od. Bronchoskopie betr., bronchoskopisch.
bronchoscopic spirometry → bronchospirometry.
bron·chos·co·py [branˈkaskəpɪ] n Bronchoskopie f.
bron·cho·si·nus·i·tis [ˌbraŋkəʊˌsaɪnəˈsaɪtɪs] n Sino-, Sinubronchitis f, sinubronchiales/sinupulmonales Syndrom nt.
bron·cho·spasm [ˌ-spæzəm] n Bronchial-, Bronchospasmus m.
bron·cho·spi·ro·chet·o·sis [ˌ-ˌspaɪrəkɪˈtəʊsɪs] n hämorrhagische Bronchitis f, Bronchitis haemorrhagica, Bronchospirochaetosis Castellani.
bron·cho·spi·rog·ra·phy [ˌ-ˌspaɪˈragrəfɪ] n Bronchospirographie f.
bron·cho·spi·rom·e·ter [ˌ-spaɪˈramɪtər] n Bronchospirometer nt.
bron·cho·spi·rom·e·try [ˌ-spaɪˈramɪtrɪ] n Bronchospirometrie f.
bron·cho·stax·is [ˌ-ˈstæksɪs] n Blutung f aus der Bronchuswand/Bronchialschleimhaut, Bronchostaxis f.
bron·cho·ste·no·sis [ˌ-stɪˈnəʊsɪs] n Bronchuseinengung f, -stenose f, Bronchostenosis f.
bron·chos·to·my [branˈkastəmɪ] n chir. Bronchostomie f.
bron·cho·tome [ˈbraŋkətəʊm] n chir. Bronchotom nt.
bron·chot·o·my [branˈkatəmɪ] n chir. Bronchotomie f.
bron·cho·tra·che·al [ˌbraŋkəʊˈtreɪkɪəl] adj Bronchien u. Trachea betr. od. verbindend, bronchotracheal, tracheobronchial.
bron·cho·ve·sic·u·lar [ˌ-vəˈsɪkjələr] adj → bronchoalveolar.
bronchovesicular breathing bronchovesikuläres/vesikobronchiales Atmen/Atmungsgeräusch nt.
bronchovesicular respiration → bronchovesicular breathing.
bron·chus [ˈbraŋkəs] n, pl **-chi** [-kaɪ] Luftröhrenast m, Bronchus m.
Brönsted [ˈbrønsted]: **B.'s theory** chem. Brönstedt-Theorie f.
Brönsted-Lowry [ˈlaʊrɪ]: **B.-L. concept** Brönstedt-Lowry-Konzept nt.
bron·to·pho·bia [ˌbrantəˈfəʊbɪə] n psychia. Gewitterangst f, Brontophobie f.
bronze [branz] I n 1. Bronze f; Bronzelegierung f. 2. Bronzefarbe f. II adj bronzen, bronzefarben, Bronze-. III vt (Haut) bräunen. IV vi (Haut) bräunen, braun werden.
bronzed [branzt] adj (sonnen-)gebräunt, braun.
bronzed diabetes Hämochromatose f, Bronzediabetes m, Siderophilie f, Eisenspeicherkrankheit f.

bronzed disease Addison'-Krankheit f, Morbus Addison m, Bronze(haut)krankheit f, primäre chronische Nebennieren(rinden)insuffizienz f.
bronze diabetes → bronzed diabetes.
bronzed skin Bronze-Haut f.
brood ['bru:d] I n bio. Brut f, Wurf m. II adj brütend, Brut-. III vt (a. fig.) ausbrüten. IV vi brüten; fig. brüten (on, over über).
brood body micro. Brutkörper m.
brood cell Mutterzelle f.
brood-er ['bru:dər] n 1. Brutkasten m. 2. fig. Grübler m.
brood-y ['bru:dɪ] adj 1. grüblerisch, nachdenklich. 2. inf. to be ~ den Wunsch nach einem Kind haben. 3. (Henne) brütig.
Brooke [brʊk]: **B.'s disease** 1. Keratosis follicularis contagiosa (Morrow--Brooke). 2. Brooke'-Krankheit f, Trichoepitheliom nt, multiple Trichoepitheliome pl, Trichoepithelioma papulosum multiplex, Epithelioma adenoides cysticum.
B.'s tumor → B.'s disease 2.
broth [brɒθ, brɔθ] n 1. Suppe f, (Kraft-, Fleisch-)Brühe f. 2. micro. Nährbrühe f, (Nähr-)Bouillon f.
broth culture Bouillonkultur f.
broth-dilution test micro. Reihenverdünnungstest m.
microtiter b. Mikrodilutionsverfahren nt.
broth·er ['brʌðər] I n Bruder m. II adj Bruder-. ~s and sisters Geschwister pl.
brother complex psychia. Bruder-, Kainkomplex m.
broth·er·ly ['brʌðərlɪ] adj brüderlich.
brow [braʊ] n 1. Stirn f. 2. (Augen-)Braue f.
Brown [braʊn]: **B. dermatome** Brown-Dermatom nt.
B.'s syndrome ophthal. Brown-Syndrom nt.
brown [braʊn] I n Braun nt, braune Farbe f, brauner Farbstoff m. II adj braun; (Gesichtsfarbe) bräunlich, (Haar) brünett. III vt (Haut) bräunen. IV vi braun werden, bräunen.
brown algae bio. Braunalgen pl.
brown atrophy patho. braune Atrophie f.
b. of liver braune Leberatrophie.
brown bread 1. Schwarzbrot nt. 2. Mischbrot nt. 3. Vollkornbrot nt.
brown cataract brauner Altersstar m, Cataracta brunescens.
brown colon Dickdarmmelanose f, braunes Kolon nt, Melanosis coli.
brown dog tick micro. Rhipicephalus sanguineus.
Browne [braʊn]: **B. operation** urol. Browne-Operation f.
brown edema braunes Lungenödem nt.
brown fat braunes Fettgewebe nt.
brown-i-an movement ['braʊnɪən] Brown'-Molekularbewegung f.
brownian-Zsigmondy movement [sɪg'mɒndɪ] brownian movement.
brown induration patho. braune Induration f.
Browning ['braʊnɪŋ]: **B.'s vein** Browning'-Vene f.
brown lung Baumwollfieber nt, Baumwoll(staub)pneumokoniose f, Byssinose f.
Brown-Séquard [se'ka:r]: **B.-S. disease** → B.-S.'s paralysis.
B.-S.'s paralysis Brown-Séquard-Lähmung f, -Syndrom nt.
B.-S.'s sign → B.-S.'s paralysis.
B.-S.'s syndrome → B.-S.'s paralysis.
brown-skinned adj braun(häutig).
brown striae Retzius'-Streifung f.
Brown-Symmers ['sɪmərs]: **B.-S. disease** Brown-Symmers'-Krankheit f.
brown tumor (Knochen) 1. brauner Tumor m. 2. brauner Riesenzelltumor m.
brow pang 1. Supraorbitalneuralgie f. 2. Halbseitenkopfschmerz m, halbseitiger/einseitiger Kopfschmerz m, Hemikranie f, Hemicrania f.
brow presentation gyn. Stirnlage f.
Bruce [bru:s]: **B.'s tract** Bruce'-Faserbündel nt, Fasciculus septomarginalis.
Bruce and Muir [mjʊər]: **tract of B. a. M.** → Bruce's tract.
Bru·cel·la [bru:'selə] n micro. Brucella f.
B. abortus Bang'-Bazillus m, Brucella abortus, Bact. abortus Bang.
B. melitensis Maltafieber-Bakterium nt, Brucella/Bact. melitensis.
B. suis Brucella suis, Bact. abortus suis.
bru·cel·la [bru:'selə] n Brucella f.
Brucella agar Brucellenagar m/nt.
Bru·cel·la·ce·ae [,bru:sə'leɪsɪi:] pl micro. Brucellaceae pl.
bru·cel·lar [bru:'selər] adj Brucellen betr., durch Brucellen verursacht, Brucellen-.
bru·cel·lin [bru:'selɪn] n micro. Brucellin nt.
bru·cel·lo·sis [bru:sə'ləʊsɪs] n 1. Brucellose f. 2. Malta-, Mittelmeerfieber nt.
Bruch [brʊk; brʊx]: **B.'s glands** ophthal. Bruch'-Drüsen pl, -Follikel pl.
B.'s layer Bruch'-Membran f, Complexus/Lamina basalis (choroideae).
B.'s membrane → B.'s layer.
bru·cine ['bru:si:n, -sɪn] n Brucin nt.
Brücke ['brykə]: **B.'s fibers** Brücke'-Fasern pl, -Muskel m, Fibrae longitudinales/meridionales m. ciliaris.
B.'s lines Brücke'-Bänder pl.
B.'s muscle → B.'s fibers.
B.'s reagent Brücke-Reagenz nt.
Brudzinski [bru:d'zɪnskɪ]: **B.'s reflex** → B.'s sign 2.
B.'s sign 1. Brudzinski'-Nackenzeichen nt, Brudzinski'-Zeichen nt. 2. Brudzinski'-Kontralateralreflex m, Brudzinski'-Zeichen nt, Brudzinski-kontralateraler Reflex m.
Bruening ['brynɪŋ]: **B. (pneumatic) otoscope** Bruening'-Otoskop nt.
B. pneumatic speculum Bruening-Ohrtrichter m, -Ohrspekulum nt.
Brug [brʊg]: **B.'s filaria** → Brugia malayi.
B.'s filariasis Brugia malayi-Filariose f, Brugiose f, Filariasis malayi.
Brug·ia ['brʊgɪə, 'bru:dʒɪə] n micro. Brugia f.
B. malayi Malayenfilarie f, Brugia/Wuchereria malayi.
B. pahangi Brugia pahangi.
Brugsch [brʊgʃ]: **B.'s syndrome** Brugsch--Syndrom nt.
bruise [bru:z] I n 1. Quetschung f, Prellung f. 2. blauer Fleck m, Bluterguß m. II vt quetschen, Prellungen zufügen, jdn. grün u. blau schlagen. III vi eine Prellung od. einen Bluterguß bekommen.
bruit [bru:t] n Geräusch nt.
b. de canon card. Kanonenschlag m, Bruit de canon.
b. de diable Nonnensausen nt, -geräusch nt, Kreiselgeräusch nt, Bruit de diable.
b. de moulin Mühlradgeräusch nt, Bruit de moulin.
Brunhilde [brʊn'hɪldə]: **B. virus** Brunhilde-Stamm m, -Virus nt, Poliovirus Typ I
Brunn [brʊn]: **B.'s epithelial nests** (von) Brunn'-Epithelnester pl.
Brunner ['brʊnər]: **B.'s glands** Brunner'--Drüsen pl, Duodenaldrüsen pl, Gll. duodenales (Brunneri).
brun·ner·o·ma [,brʊnə'rəʊmə] n Adenom nt der Brunner'-Drüsen, Brunneriom nt.
brun·ne·ro·sis [,-'rəʊsɪs] n Hyperplasie f der Brunner'-Drüsen, Brunnerosis f.
bru·no·ni·an movement [bru:'nəʊnɪən] → brownian movement.
Bruns [bru:nz]: **B.' ataxia (of gait)** Bruns'--Gangataxie f.
B.' disease Bruns'-Krankheit f.
B.' sign neuro. Bruns-Syndrom nt.
B.' syndrome → B.' sign.
Brunschwig ['bru:nswɪg]: **B.'s operation** 1. gyn., chir. Brunschwig-Operation f. 2. chir. Pankreatoduodenektomie f, Duodenopankreatektomie f.
B.'s pancreatoduodenectomy → B.'s operation 2.
B.'s total pelvic exenteration → B.'s operation 1.
Bruns·wick bird plague ['brʌnzwɪk] Hühner-, Geflügelpest f.
Brunton ['brʌntn]: **B.'s otoscope** Brunton--Otoskop nt.
brush [brʌʃ] I n 1. Bürste f; Pinsel m. 2. Bürsten m zu geben sth. a ~ etw. (ab-)bürsten. 3. phys. Strahlen-, Lichtbündel nt. vt 4. (ab-)bürsten; pinseln. **to ~ one's teeth/hair** s. die Zähne putzen/s. das Haar bürsten. 5. fegen, kehren; wischen.
brush away vt ab-, wegbürsten, wegwischen.
brush off vt ab-, wegbürsten, wegwischen.
b.es of Ruffini Ruffini'-Endorgane pl.
brush biopsy Bürstenabstrich m.
brush border histol. Bürstensaum m, Kutikulasaum m.
brush burn Verbrennung f durch Reibung(shitze).
Brushfield ['brʌʃfi:ld]: **B.'s spots** ophthal. Brushfield-Flecken pl.
Brushfield-Wyatt ['waɪət]: **B.-W. disease/syndrome** Brushfield-Wyatt-Syndrom nt.
bru·tal ['bru:tl] adj 1. brutal, grausam, unmenschlich, roh. 2. (Sprache) derb, ungehobelt. 3. (Kritik) hart, scharf. 4. tierisch, viehisch.
bru·tal·i·ty [bru:'tælətɪ] n, pl -ties Brutalität f, Grausamkeit f, Rohheit f.
bru·tal·ize ['bru:tlaɪz] vt 1. gewalttätig machen, brutalisieren. 2. brutal od. unmenschlich behandeln.
Bruton [bru:tn]: **B.'s agammaglobulinemia** Bruton-Typ m der Agammaglobulinämie, infantile X-chromosomale Agammaglobulinämie f, kongenitale (geschlechtsgebundene) Agammaglobulinämie f.
B.'s disease → B.'s agammaglobulinemia.
brux [brʌks] vt mit den Zähnen knirschen.
brux·ism ['brʌksɪzəm] n (unwillkürliches) Zähneknirschen nt, Bruxismus m.
brux·o·ma·nia [,brʌksəʊ'meɪnɪə, -jə] n Bruxomanie f.
Bryant ['braɪənt]: **B.'s line** Bryant'-Linie f.
B.'s sign ortho. Bryant-Zeichen n.
B.'s traction ortho. Bryant-Extension f, vertikale Überkopfextension f, Overheadtraction f.
B.'s triangle ortho. Bryant-Dreieck nt, Iliofemoraldreieck nt.
BS abbr. **1.** → blood sugar. **2.** → bowel sounds. **3.** → breath sounds.
BSA abbr. → body surface area.
BS agar → bismuth sulfite agar.
B-scan n radiol. (Ultraschall) B-Scan m, B-Mode nt/m.
BSER abbr. → brain stem electric responses.
BSER audiometry → brain stem evoked response audiometry.
BSP abbr. → bromsulphalein.
BSP test → bromosulfophthalein test.

BT-PABA

BT-PABA *abbr.* → *N*-benzoyl-L-tyrosyl-*p*--aminobenzoic acid.
BTPS condition [body temperature and pressure, saturated] *physiol.* BTPS-Bedingungen *pl.*
B.T.U. *abbr.* → British thermal unit.
BU *abbr.* → 5-bromouracil.
bub·ble ['bʌbl] **I** *n* **1.** (Gas-, Luft-, Seifen-)-Blase *f*, (-)Bläschen *nt.* **2.** Blasenbildung *nt*; Sprudeln *nt*, Strudeln *nt*, Perlen *nt.* **II** *vt* Blasen verursachen *od.* machen. **III** *vi* Blasen bilden; sprudeln, schäumen, perlen.
bubble bath Schaumbad *nt.*
bubble oxygenator Bubble-Oxygenator *m.*
bub·bly ['bʌblɪ] *adj* **1.** sprudelnd, schäumend; blasenartig, -förmig, blasig. **2.** *fig. inf.* sprühend, temperamentvoll.
bu·bo ['b(j)uːbəʊ] *n, pl* **-boes** *patho.* entzündlich-vergrößerter Lymphknoten *m*, Bubo *m.*
bu·bon [by'bõ] *n* → bubo.
bu·bon·al·gia [b(j)uːbəˈnældʒ(ɪ)ə] *n* Leistenschmerz *m.*
bu·bon·ic [b(j)uːˈbɒnɪk] *adj* Bubonen betr., Beulen-, Bubonen-.
bubonic plague Beulen-, Bubonenpest *f*, Pestis bubonica/fulminans/major.
bu·bon·o·cele [b(j)uːˈbɒnəsiːl] *n* inkompletter Leistenbruch *m*, Bubonozele *f.*
bu·bon·u·lus [b(j)uːˈbɒnjələs] *n* **1.** *derm.* Bubonulus *m.* **2.** *derm.* Lymphangiitis dorsalis penis, Bubonulus *m.*
bu·car·dia [b(j)uːˈkɑːrdɪə] *n card.* Ochsenherz *nt*, Bukardie *f*, Cor bovinum.
buc·ca ['bʌkə] *n anat.* Wange *f*, Bucca *f*, Mala *f.*
buc·cal ['bʌkəl] *adj* Wange betr., bukkal, buccal, Wangen-, Bukkal-.
buccal artery Backenschlagader *f*, A. buccalis.
buccal branches of facial nerve Wangenäste *pl* des N. facialis, Rami buccales n. facialis.
buccal cavity Vestibulum oris.
buccal fat pad Bichat'-Fettpropf *m*, Wangenfettpropf *m*, Corpus adiposum buccae (Bichati).
buccal glands Speicheldrüsen *pl* der Wangenschleimhaut, Bukkaldrüsen *pl*, Gll. buccales.
buccal lymph node Wangenlymphknoten *m*, Nodus (lymphaticus) buccinatorius.
buccal mucosa Wangenschleimhaut *f.*
buccal nerve Buccalis *m*, N. buccalis.
buccal region *anat.* Wangengegend *f*, -region *f*, Regio buccalis.
buccal teeth Backenzähne *pl.*
buc·ci·na·tor ['bʌksəneɪtər] *n* → buccinator muscle.
buccinator artery → buccal artery.
buccinator fascia → buccopharyngeal fascia.
buccinator lymph node → buccal lymph node.
buccinator muscle Wangenmuskel *m*, Bukzinator *m*, Buccinator *m*, M. buccinator.
buccinator nerve → buccal nerve.
buc·co·cer·vi·cal [bʌkəˈsɜːrvɪkl] *adj* **1.** Wange u. Hals betr., bukkozervikal. **2.** (*Zahn*) bukkozervikal. **3.** → buccogingival.
buc·co·gin·gi·val [ˌ-ˈdʒɪndʒəvəl, -dʒɪnˈdʒaɪ-] *adj* **1.** Wange u. Zahnfleisch/Gingiva betr., bukkogingival. **2.** (*Zahn*) bukkogingival.
buc·co·glos·so·phar·yn·gi·tis [ˌ-ˌglɒsəʊˌfærɪnˈdʒaɪtɪs] *n* Bukkoglossopharyngitis *f.*

buc·co·la·bi·al [ˌ-ˈleɪbɪəl] *adj* Wange u. Lippe(n) betr., bukkolabial.
buc·co·lin·gual [ˌ-ˈlɪŋgwəl] *adj* **1.** Wange u. Zunge betr., bukkolingual. **2.** (*Zahn*) bukkolingual.
buc·co·max·il·lar·y [ˌ-ˈmæksəˌlerɪ, -mækˈsɪlərɪ] *adj* Wange u. Oberkiefer/Maxilla betr., bukkomaxillär.
buccomaxillary fistula bukkomaxilläre Fistel *f.*
buc·co·na·sal membrane [ˌ-ˈneɪzl] *embryo.* Oronasal-, Bukkonasalmembran *f*, Membrana bucconasalis.
buc·co·pha·ryn·ge·al [ˌ-fəˈrɪndʒ(ɪ)əl] *adj* Wange *od.* Mund u. Rachen/Pharynx betr., bukkopharyngeal.
buccopharyngeal fascia **1.** Fascia buccopharyngea. **2.** Fascia buccopharyngealis.
buccopharyngeal membrane **1.** *embryo.* Rachen-, Buccopharyngealmembran *f.* **2.** Fascia pharyngobasilaris.
buccopharyngeal muscle → buccopharyngeus (muscle).
buc·co·pha·ryn·ge·us (muscle) [ˌ-fəˈrɪndʒ(ɪ)əs, -ˌfærɪnˈdʒiːəs] *old* M. buccopharyngeus, Pars buccopharyngea m. constrictoris pharyngis superioris.
buc·cu·la ['bʌkjələ] *n, pl* **-lae** [-liː] Doppelkinn *nt.*
Buck [bʌk]: **B.'s extension** → B.'s traction.
B.'s fascia Buck'-Faszie *f*, tiefe Penisfaszie *f*, Fascia penis profunda.
B.'s traction *ortho.* Buck-Extension *f.*
buck·et-han·dle deformity/fracture/tear ['bʌkɪt] *ortho.* (*Meniskus*) Korbhenkelriß *m.*
buck·led aorta ['bʌkəlt] *radiol.* Pseudocoarctatio aortae.
Buckley ['bʌkli]: **B.'s syndrome** Buckley--Syndrom *nt*, Hyperimmunglobinämie E *f.*
Bucky ['bʌkɪ]: **B.'s diaphragm** *radiol.* Bucky-Blende *f*, Streustrahlenraster *nt.*
B.'s rays *radiol.* Bucky-Strahlen *pl*, Grenzstrahlen *pl.*
Bucky-Potter ['pɒtər]: **B.-P. diaphragm** → Bucky's diaphragm.
bu·cli·zine ['bjuːklɪziːn] *n pharm.* Buclizin *nt.*
bu·clo·sa·mide [bʌkˈləʊsəmaɪd] *n pharm.* Buclosamid *nt.*
bu·cry·late ['bjuːkrɪleɪt] *n* Isobutyl-2--cyan(o)acrylat *nt.*
bud [bʌd] **I** *n* **1.** *anat., embryo.* Knospe *f*, Anlage *f.* **2.** *bio.* Knospe *f*, Auge *nt*; Keim *m.* **3.** *fig.* Keim *m*, Anfangsstadium *nt.* **II** *vi* knospen, keimen.
Budd [bʌd]: **B.'s cirrhosis** Budd-Zirrhose *f.*
B.'s disease → B.'s cirrhosis.
B.'s jaundice *old* akute gelbe Leberatrophie *f.*
B.'s syndrome → Budd-Chiari syndrome.
Budd-Chiari [kɪˈɑːrɪ]: **B.-C. disease** → B.-C. syndrome.
B.-C. syndrome Budd-Chiari-Syndrom *nt*, Endophlebitis hepatica obliterans.
bud·ding ['bʌdɪŋ] *n* **1.** Knospenbildung *f*, -treiben *nt.* **2.** *micro.* Sprossung *f*, Knospung *f*, Budding *nt.*
Budge [bʌdʒ]: **B.'s center** **1.** Budge'-Zentrum *nt*, ziliospinales Zentrum *nt*, Centrum ciliospinale. **2.** Centrum genitospinale.
Budin [byˈdɛ̃]: **B.'s rule** *ped.* Budin'-Regel *f.*
bud·less ['bʌdlɪs] *adj* knospenlos.
bud-like [-laɪk] *adj* knospenähnlich, -artig.
bud mutation *genet.* Sport *m*, Knospen-, Sproßmutation *f.*
BUDR *abbr.* → 5-bromodeoxyuridine.
Buerger ['bɜːrgər]: **B.'s disease** Winiwarter-Buerger-Krankheit *f*, Morbus Winiwarter-Buerger *m*, Endangiitis/Thrombangiitis/Thrombendangiitis obliterans.
B.'s symptom Buerger'-Zeichen *nt.*
bu·fa·di·en·o·lides [bjuːfədaɪˈenəʊlaɪdz] *pl* Bufadienolide *pl.*
bu·fa·gen·ins [-ˈdʒenɪns] *pl* Bufagenine *pl.*
bu·fa·gins [-ˈdʒɪnz] *pl* Bufagenine *pl.*
bu·fa·lin [-ˈlɪn] *n* Bufalin *nt.*
bu·fan·o·lide [bjuːˈfænəlaɪd] *n* Bufanolid *nt.*
bu·fa·tri·en·o·lides [bjuːfətraɪˈenəʊlaɪdz] *pl* Bufatrienolide *pl.*
bu·fen·o·lides [bjuːˈfenəlaɪdz] *pl* Bufenolide *pl.*
buf·fa·lo hump ['bʌfələʊ] Stiernacken *m*, -höcker *m*, Büffelnacken *m*, -höcker *m.*
buffalo neck → buffalo hump.
buff·er ['bʌfər] **I** *n chem.* Puffer *m*; Pufferlösung *f.* **2.** (*a. fig.*) Puffer *m.* **II** *vt* (*a. chem.*) puffern, als Puffer wirken gegen.
buffer action Pufferwirkung *f.*
buffer base Pufferbase *f.*
buffer capacity Pufferkapazität *f.*
buff·ered ['bʌfərd] *adj chem.* gepuffert.
buff·er·ing capacity ['bʌfərɪŋ] Pufferkapazität *f.*
buffering power Puffervermögen *nt*, -kapazität *f.*
buffer pair *biochem.* Pufferpaar *nt.*
buffer range Pufferbereich *m.*
buffer salt Puffersalz *nt.*
buffer solution Pufferlösung *f.*
buffer system Puffersystem *nt.*
  bicarbonate b. Bicarbonatpuffersystem.
  phosphate b. Phosphatpuffersystem.
  proteinate b. Protein(at)puffersystem.
buff·y coat ['bʌfɪ] *hema.* Leukozytenmanschette *f*, buffy coat.
buffy crust → buffy coat.
bu·for·min [bjuːˈfɔːrmɪn] *n pharm.* Buformin *nt.*
bu·fo·tal·in [ˌbjuːfəˈtælɪn, -ˈteɪl-] *n* Bufotalin *nt.*
bu·fo·te·nin [ˌ-ˈtenɪn] *n* Bufotenin *nt.*
bu·fo·tox·in [ˌ-ˈtɒksɪn] *n* Bufotoxin *nt.*
bug [bʌg] *n* **1.** Wanze *f*; Insekt *nt.* **2.** Infekt *nt.* **3.** *inf.* Bazillus *m*, Erreger *m.*
Buhl [buːl]: **B.'s desquamative pneumonia** käsige Pneumonie *f.*
B.'s disease *ped.* Buhl'-Krankheit *f.*
build [bɪld] (*v*: **built**; **built**) **I** *n* **1.** Körperbau *m*, Statur *f*, Figur *f.* **2.** Form *f*, Gestalt *f.* **II** *vt* (er-, auf-)bauen, errichten; konstruieren, herstellen.
build on *vt* anbauen, erweitern, verlängern, vergrößern.
build up *vt* **1.** (*Muskeln*) (langsam) aufbauen; vergrößern, (ver-)stärken; **to ~ one's health** seine Gesundheit stärken *od.* kräftigen. **2.** (*Dosis*) erhöhen, steigern. **II** *vi* s. bilden, entstehen, s. aufbauen; zunehmen.
build·er ['bɪldər] *n chem.* Aufbausubstanz *f.*
build·ing ['bɪldɪŋ] *n* Aufbau *m*, Er-, Aufbauen *nt*, Errichten *nt*, Entstehen *nt.*
building block (*a. techn., fig.*) Baustein *m.*
building block molecule Bausteinmolekül *nt.*
build-up *adj* verstärkt, verbreitet, erweitert; gepolstert.
build-up ['bɪldʌp] *n* **1.** Aufbau *m.* **2.** *fig.* Zuwachs *m*, Zunahme *f*, Anwachsen *nt*, Ansammlung *f.*
build-up shoes Schuhe *pl* mit überhoher Sohle, orthopädische Schuhe *pl.*
built [bɪlt] *adj* geformt, gebaut, entwickelt. **II** *pret, ptp* → build.
bulb [bʌlb] **I** *n* **1.** *anat.* Bulbus *m*; knollenod. zwiebelförmiger Vorsprung *m.* **2.** *bot.* Knolle *f*, Zwiebel *f.* **3.** knollenförmiger Körper *m*; (Glas-)Ballon *m*, (Glüh-)Bir-

ne f, (Thermometer) Kolben m. **II** vi anschwellen.
bulb out vi → bulb II.
b. of aorta Aortenbulbus, Bulbus aortae.
b. of corpus spongiosum → b. of penis.
b. of eye Augapfel m, Bulbus oculi.
b. of heart embryo. Bulbus cordis.
b.s of Krause Krause'-Endkolben pl, Corpuscula bulboidea.
b. of occipital horn of lateral ventricle Bulbus cornus occipitalis/posterioris (ventriculi lateralis).
b. of penis Bulbus penis.
b. of posterior horn of lateral ventricle → b. of occipital horn of lateral ventricle.
b. of urethra → b. of penis.
b. of vestibule of vagina Schwellkörper des Scheidenvorhofes, Bulbus vestibuli (vaginae).
bul·bar ['bʌlbər, -bɑːr] adj **1.** Bulbus betr., bulbär, Bulbär-, Bulbus-. **2.** Medulla oblongata betr., bulbär. **3.** → bulbed.
bulbar anesthesia neuro. Sensibilitätsverlust m bei Brückenschädigung.
bulbar apoplexy Apoplexia bulbaris.
bulbar colliculus Harnröhrenschwellkörper m, Corpus spongiosum penis.
bulbar conjunctiva Bindehaut f des Augapfels, Tunica conjunctiva bulbaris.
bulbar fascia Tenon'-Kapsel f, Vagina bulbi.
bulbar myelitis Entzündung f der Medulla oblongata.
bulbar palsy → bulbar paralysis.
bulbar paralysis (progressive) Bulbärparalyse f, Duchenne-Syndrom nt.
acute b. akute Bulbärparalyse.
asthenic b. Myasthenia gravis pseudoparalytica.
infectious b. Pseudowut f, -lyssa f, -rabies f, Aujeszky'-Krankheit f.
progressive b. (progressive) Bulbärparalyse, Duchenne-Syndrom nt.
progressive b. in children familiäre progressive Bulbärparalyse, Fazio-Londe--Syndrom nt.
bulbar poliomyelitis bulbopontine Form f der Kinderlähmung.
bulbar sheath → bulbar fascia.
bulbed [bʌlbd] adj knollen-, zwiebelförmig od. -artig, knollig, wulstig.
bul·bi·form ['bʌlbɪfɔːrm] adj knollen-, zwiebelförmig, bulbiform, bulboid, bulbös.
bul·bi·tis [bʌl'baɪtɪs] n urol. Entzündung f des Bulbus penis, Bulbitis f.
bul·bo·a·tri·al [ˌbʌlbəʊ'eɪtrɪəl] adj embryo. Bulbus cordis u. Atrium betr., bulboatrial.
bul·bo·cav·er·no·sus (muscle) [ˌ-ˌkævər-'nəʊsəs] → bulbospongiosus (muscle).
bul·bo·cav·ern·ous glands [ˌ-'kævərnəs] → bulbourethral glands.
bulbocavernous muscle → bulbospongiosus (muscle).
bulbocavernous reflex neuro. Bulbocavernosus-Reflex m.
bul·bo·gas·trone [ˌ-'gæstrəʊn] n Bulbogastron nt.
bul·boid ['bʌlbɔɪd] adj → bulbiform.
bulboid corpuscles Krause'-Endkolben pl, Corpuscula bulboidea.
bul·bo·mim·ic reflex [ˌ-'mɪmɪk] bulbomimischer Reflex m, Mondonesi-Reflex m.
bul·bo·pon·tine sulcus [ˌ-'pɒntaɪn, -tiːn] Sulcus bulbopontinus.
bul·bo·re·tic·u·lo·spi·nal tract [ˌ-rɪˌtɪkjələʊ'spaɪnl] Tractus bulboreticulospinalis.
bul·bo·sa·cral system [ˌ-'sækrəl, -'seɪ-] parasympathisches (Nerven-)System nt, Parasympathikus m, parasympathischer

Teil m des vegetativen Nervensystems, Pars parasympathetica systematis nervosi autonomici.
bul·bo·spi·nal inspiratory neuron [ˌ-'spaɪnl] bulbospinal inspiratorisches Neuron nt, I_BS-Neuron n.
bulbospinal paralysis Erb-Goldflam--Syndrom nt, -Krankheit f, Erb-Oppenheim-Syndrom nt, -Krankheit f, Hoppe-Goldflam-Syndrom nt, Myasthenia gravis pseudoparalytica.
bul·bo·spon·gi·o·sus (muscle) [ˌ-ˌspʌndʒɪ-'əʊsəs] Bulbospongiosus m, M. bulbospongiosus/bulbocavernosus.
bul·bo·tha·lam·ic tract [ˌ-θə'læmɪk] Tractus bulbothalamicus.
bul·bo·trun·cus [ˌ-'trʌŋkəs] n embryo. Bulbotruncus m.
bul·bo·u·re·thral [ˌ-jʊə'riːθrəl] adj Bulbus penis betr., bulbourethral, Bulbourethral-.
bulbourethral artery A. bulbi penis.
bulbourethral glands Cowper'-Drüsen pl, Bulbourethraldrüsen pl, Gll. bulbourethrales (Cowperi).
bul·bous ['bʌlbəs] adj → bulbiform.
bulbous nose Kartoffel-, Säufer-, Pfund-, Knollennase f, Rhinophym nt, Rhinophyma nt.
bul·bo·ven·tric·u·lar [ˌ-ven'trɪkjələr] adj bulboventrikulär.
bulboventricular flange → bulboventricular fold.
bulboventricular fold embryo. Bulboventrikularfalte f.
bulboventricular part of heart tube embryo. bulboventrikulärer Abschnitt m des Herzschlauchs.
bulboventricular sulcus embryo. bulboventrikuläre Furche f, Sulcus bulboventricularis.
bul·bus ['bʌlbəs] n, pl **-bi** [-baɪ, -biː] anat. **1.** → bulb 1. **2.** Markhirn nt, verlängertes Mark nt, Medulla oblongata, Bulbus m (medullae spinalis), Myelencephalon nt.
bulge [bʌldʒ] **I** n **1.** Wölbung f, Ausbuchtung f, Bauch m, Anschwellung f, Beule f, Wulst m. **2.** Anschwellen nt, Zunahme f. **II** vi **3.** (an-)schwellen, s. wölben; s. (aus-)bauchen, s. vorbuchten; (Augen) hervorstehen, -treten, -quellen. **4.** platzen od. gefüllt sein (with vor), voll sein (with von, mit), gefüllt sein (with mit).
bulge out vi → bulge 3.
bulged [bʌldʒd] adj → bulgy.
bulg·ing ['bʌldʒɪŋ] adj → bulgy.
bulg·y ['bʌldʒɪ] adj (her-)vorstehend, -tretend, -quellend; geschwollen, prall gefüllt.
bu·lim·i·a [b(j)uː'lɪmɪə, -'liː-] n **1.** Heißhunger m, Eß-, Freßsucht f, Hyperorexie f, Bulimie f. **2.** Bulimia nervosa f, Bulimarexie f, Freß-Kotzsucht f, Eß-Brechsucht f.
bu·lim·ic [b(j)uː'lɪmɪk, -'liː-] adj Bulimie betr., von Bulimie betroffen, bulimisch.
bulk [bʌlk] **I** n **1.** Umfang m, Volumen nt, Ausmaß nt, Größe f; Masse f. **2.** massige od. korpulente Gestalt f. **3.** Ballaststoffe pl; ballaststoffreiche Nahrung f. **4.** der größere Teil, Hauptteil m, -masse f. **II** vt (An-)Schwellung verursachen, schwerer od. dicker werden, anwachsen. **III** vi s. vergrößern, anschwellen, s. (auf-)blähen, s. ausbauchen, s. ausweiten.
bulk·age ['bʌlkɪdʒ] n Balaststoffe pl.
bulk fiber Ballaststoffe pl.
bulk·i·ness ['bʌlkɪnɪs] n **1.** Massige nt, Massigkeit f, Wuchtigkeit f. **2.** (Person) Beleibtheit f, Dicke f, Unförmigkeit f, Korpulenz f.
bulk modulus of elasticity abbr. **K** Volumenelastizitätsmodul m abbr. **K**.

bulk nutrient Hauptnahrungsmittel nt, Hauptnährstoff m.
bulk·y ['bʌlkɪ] adj **1.** voluminös, sperrig, massig. **2.** (Gestalt) korpulent, massig, dick, wuchtig.
bull [bʊl] n **1.** bio. Bulle f, Stier m; Männchen nt. **2.** inf. Bulle f, großer starkgebauter Mann m.
bul·la ['bʊlə] n, pl **-lae** [-liː, -laɪ] **1.** derm. Blase f, Bulla f. **2.** anat. blasenähnliche Struktur f, Höhle f, Bulla f.
bul·late ['bʊlet, -ɪt, 'bʌl-] adj **1.** derm. mit Blasen besetzt, mit Blasenbildung einhergehend, bullös. **2.** aufgebläht, aufgeblasen, bullös.
Buller ['bʊlər] B.'s **bandage/shield** ophthal. Buller'-Augenschutz m, -Schild nt.
bul·let ['bʊlɪt] n (Gewehr-)Kugel f.
Bul·lis fever ['bʊlɪs] Bullis-Fieber nt, Lone-Star-Fieber nt.
bull neck (Diphtherie) Cäsarenhals m, Collum proconsulare.
bull-necked adj stiernackig.
bul·lo·sis [bʊ'ləʊsɪs] n derm. Bullosis f, Epidermolysis bullosa.
bul·lous ['bʊləs, 'bʌl-] adj Bullae betr., durch Bullae gekennzeichnet, bullös, (groß-)blasig.
bullous concha anat. Concha bullosa.
bullous congenital ichthyosiform erythroderma Erythrodermia congenitalis ichthyosiformis bullosa.
bullous emphysema bullöses (Lungen-)-Emphysem nt.
bullous fever Metzger-, Fleischerpemphigus m, Pemphigus acutus febrilis gravis.
bullous myringitis bullöse Trommelfellentzündung/Myringitis f, Myringitis bullosa.
bullous pemphigoid bullöses Pemphigoid nt, Alterspemphigus m, Parapemphigus m.
localized b. lokalisiertes bullöses Pemphigoid.
bullous syphilid bullöses Syphilid nt; Pemphigus syphiliticus.
bullous urticaria bullöse Urtikaria f, Urticaria bullosa/vesiculosa.
bu·met·a·nide [bjuː'metənaɪd] n pharm. Bumetanid.
Bumke ['buːmkə] B.'s **pupil/symptom** neuro. Bumke-Zeichen nt.
bump·er fracture ['bʌmpər] Stoßstangenfraktur f.
BUN abbr. → blood urea nitrogen.
bunch [bʌntʃ] **I** n **1.** Umfang m, Bund m. **2.** phys. (Strahlen-)Bündel nt. **3.** inf. (Menschen-)Traube f. **4.** Buckel m, Höcker m, Schwellung f, Beule f. **II** vt bündeln, zusammenfassen.
bunch·y ['bʌntʃɪ] adj **1.** buschig, büschelig; traubenförmig. **2.** (her-)vorstehend, -tretend, -quellend; bauschig; angeschwollen.
bun·dle ['bʌndl] n **I** n (a. anat.) Bündel nt.
by ~s bündelweise. **2.** inf. (Nerven-)Bündel nt. **II** vt bündeln.
b. of His His'-Bündel nt, Fasciculus atrioventricularis.
b. of rays phys. Strahlenbündel.
b. of Stanley Kent → b. of His.
b. of Vicq d'Azur Vicq d'Azyr'-Bündel, Fasciculus mamillothalamicus.
bundle branch: left b. linker Tawara--Schenkel m, linker Schenkel m des Reiz-/Erregungsleitungssystems, Crus sinistrum fasciculi atrioventricularis.
right b. rechter Tawara-Schenkel m, rechter Schenkel m des Reiz-/Erregungsleitungssystems, Crus dextrum fasciculi atrioventricularis.

bundle-branch block

bundle-branch block *abbr.* **BBB** *card.* Schenkelblock *m.*
  left b. *abbr.* **LBBB** Linksschenkelblock *abbr.* LSB.
  right b. *abbr.* **RBBB** Rechtsschenkelblock *abbr.* RSB.
bundle-branch heart block → bundle--branch block.
bundle repair *neurochir.*, *ortho.* interfaszikuläre Nervennaht *f.*
bundle-sheath cells Zellen *pl* der Bündelschicht.
Bunge ['buŋə]: **B.'s amputation** *ortho.* Bunge-Amputation *f,* aperiostale Amputation *f.*
  B.'s law *ped.* Bunge'-Regel *nt.*
  B.'s spoon *ophthal.* Bunge'-Augenlöffel *m.*
Büngner ['bɪŋnər; 'bʏŋ-]: **B.'s bands** Büngner'-Bänder *pl.*
bun·ion ['bʌnjən] *n ortho.* chronisch entzündeter Großzehenballen *m.*
Bunnel ['bʌnl]: **B. figure-of-eight suture** Achternaht *f* ohne Ausziehdraht.
  B.'s suture *chir.* 1. Ausziehnaht *f,* Bunnell-Naht *f* mit Ausziehdraht. 2. Sehnennaht *f* mit Ausziehdraht. 3. → B. figure--of eight suture.
Bunsen ['bʌnsən]: **B. burner** Bunsenbrenner *m.*
  B. coefficient *abbr.* α Bunsen-Löslichkeitskoeffizient *m abbr.* α.
Bunsen-Roscoe ['rɒskəʊ]: **B.-R. law** Bunsen-Roscoe-Gesetz *nt.*
Bun·ya·vir·i·dae [bʌnjə'vɪrədiː, -'vaɪr-] *pl micro.* Bunyaviren *pl,* Bunyaviridae *pl.*
Bun·y·a·vi·rus [,-'vaɪrəs] *n micro.* Bunyavirus *nt.*
bunyavirus encephalitis California-Enzephalitis *f abbr.* CE.
buoy·ant ['bɔɪənt, 'buːjənt] *adj* schwimmend, tragend; schwebend, Schwebe-.
buoyant density Schwebedichte *f.*
buph·thal·mia [,b(j)uf'θælmɪə, bəf-] *n* → buphthalmos.
buph·thal·mos [,-'θælməs] *n ophthal.* Ochsenauge *nt,* Glaukom *nt* der Kinder, Hydrophthalmus *m,* Buphthalmus *m.*
buph·thal·mus [,-'θælməs] *n* → buphthalmos.
bu·piv·a·caine [b(j)u'pɪvəkeɪn] *n pharm.* Bupivacain *nt.*
bu·pre·nor·phine [,b(j)uprɪ'nɔːrfiːn] *n pharm.* Buprenorphin *nt.*
bur [bɜr] *n dent.* (Zahn-)Bohrer *m.*
Burdach [bʊrdæk; 'bʊrdax]: **column of B.** → B.'s tract.
  fasciculus of B. → B.'s tract.
  B.'s fibers Burdach-Fasern *pl.*
  B.'s fissure Burdach-Spalte *f.*
  B.'s nucleus Burdach'-Kern *m,* Nc. cuneatus.
  B.'s tract Burdach'-Strang *m,* Fasciculus cuneatus (medullae spinalis).
Burd·wan fever ['bɜrdwən] viszerale Leishmaniose/Leishmaniase *f,* Kala-Azar *f,* Splenomegalia tropica.
bu·ret [bjʊə'ret] *n chem.* Bürette *f.*
bu·rette *n* → buret.
Burger ['bɜrgər]: **B.'s sign** Burger-Zeichen *nt,* Heryng-Zeichen *nt.*
Bürger-Grütz ['bʏrgər grʏts]: **B.-G. disease/syndrome** Bürger-Grütz-Syndrom *nt,* (primäre/essentielle) Hyperlipoproteinämie Typ I *f,* fettinduzierte/exogene Hypertriglyzeridämie *f,* fettinduzierte/exogene Hyperlipämie *f,* Hyperchylomikronämie *f,* familiärer C-II-Apoproteinmangel *m.*
Burgess [bɜrdʒɪs]: **B.' operation/technique** *chir.* Unterschenkelamputation *f* nach Burgess.

Burkitt ['bɜrkɪt]: **B.'s lymphoma/tumor** Burkitt-Lymphom *nt,* -Tumor *m,* epidemisches Lymphom *nt,* B-lymphoblastisches Lymphom *nt.*
burn [bɜrn] (*v:* burnt; burnt) **I** *n* **1.** Verbrennen *nt.* **2.** Brandwunde *f,* Verbrennung *f;* Verbrennungskrankheit *f.* **II** *vt* ab-, verbrennen, versengen, durch Feuer *od.* Hitze beschädigen. **III** *vi* **3.** (ver-)brennen, anbrennen, versengen. **4.** (*a. fig., Wunde*) brennen. **5.** *chem.* verbrennen, oxydieren. **6.** in den Flammen umkommen, verbrennen; verbrannt werden, den Feuertod erleiden.
burn away I *vt* (*Haut*) wegbrennen. **II** *vi* (vor s. hin) brennen; herunterbrennen; verbrennen.
burn out *vt* **1.** ausbrennen. **2. to ~ o.s. out** s. (gesundheitlich) ruinieren, s. kaputtmachen.
burn·able ['bɜrnəbl] **I** *n* Brennstoff *m,* -material *nt.* **II** *adj* brennbar.
burn care *ortho.* Verbrennungsversorgung *f,* -behandlung *f.*
burned-out pancreas *patho.* ausgebrannes Pankreas *nt.*
bur·ner ['bɜrnər] *n* Brenner *m.*
Burnett ['bɜrnɪt, bɜr'net]: **B.'s syndrome** Milchalkalisyndrom *nt,* Burnett-Syndrom *nt.*
burn·ing ['bɜrnɪŋ] **I** *n* Brennen *nt;* Überhitzung *f.* **II** *adj* brennend; glühend.
burning feet syndrome Gopalan-Syndrom *nt,* Syndrom *nt* der brennenden Füße, heiße Greisenfüße *pl,* Burning-feet--Syndrom *nt.*
burning pain brennender Schmerz *m.*
burning tongue Zungenbrennen *nt,* Glossopyrosis *f,* -pyrie *f.*
burn injury Verbrennungsverletzung *f,* Verbrennung *f.*
burn patient Verbrennungspatient(in *f*) *m,* Patient(in *f*) *m* mit Verbrennung(sverletzung).
Burns [bɜrnz]: **B.' falciform process** → B.' ligament.
  B.' ligament 1. Margo falciformis (hiatus saphenus). **2.** Cornu superius hiatus saphenus.
burn shock Verbrennungsschock *m.*
burn unit Verbrennungsstation *f,* -einheit *f.*
burn wound Brandwunde *f,* Verbrennung *f.*
burn·y ['bɜrnɪ] *adj* brennend, stechend.
Burow ['bʊrəʊ]: **B.'s triangle** *chir.* Burow--Dreieck *nt.*
  B.'s vein Burow'-Vene *f.*
burp [bɜrp] **I** *n* Aufstoßen *nt,* Rülpsen *nt;* Rülpser *m;* *inf.* (*Säugling*) 'Bäuerchen' *nt.* **II** *vt* (*Säugling*) ein 'Bäuerchen' machen lassen. **III** *vi* aufstoßen, rülpsen; (*Säugling*) ein 'Bäuerchen' machen.
burr [bɜr] *n dent.* (Zahn-)Bohrer *m.*
burr cell Stechapfelform *f,* Echinozyt *m.*
burr erythrocyte → burr cell.
bur·row ['bʌrəʊ, 'bʌrəʊ] **I** *n* **1.** *derm.* Hautgang *m.* **2.** *patho.*, *chir.* Fistel *f.* **II** *v s.* (ein-)bohren, einen Gang graben *od.* bohren (*into* in).
burst out *vi* hervor-, herausbrechen, ausbrechen.
burst through *vi* durch-, ausbrechen.
bur·row·ing hairs ['bʌrəʊɪŋ, 'bʌrəʊ-] Pili incarnati/recurvati; Pseudofolliculitis barbae.
burrowing phagedenic ulcer Meleney--Geschwür *nt,* Pyoderma gangraenosum, Dermatitis ulcerosa, Pyodermia ulcerosa serpiginosa.
bur·sa ['bɜrsə] *n,* *pl* **-sae** [-siː] **1.** *anat.*, *bio.*

Beutel *m,* Tasche *f,* Aussackung *f,* Bursa *f.* **2.** Schleimbeutel *m,* Bursa synovialis.
  b. of Achilles (tendon) Bursa tendinis calcanei (Achillis).
  b. of anterior tibial muscle Bursa subtendinea m. tibialis anterioris.
  b. of calcaneal tendon → b. of Achilles (tendon).
  b. of Fabricius *bio.* Bursa Fabricii.
  b. of iliopsoas muscle Bursa subtendinea iliaca.
  b. of lateral head of gastrocnemius muscle Bursa subtendinea m. gastrocnemii lateralis.
  b. of latissimus dorsi muscle Bursa subtendinea m. latissimi dorsi.
  b. of medial head of gastrocnemius muscle Bursa subtendinea m. gastrocnemii medialis.
  b. of piriformis muscle Bursa m. piriformis.
  b. of popliteal muscle Bursa m. poplitei, Rec. subpopliteus.
  b. of quadratus femoris muscle Bursa subtendinea iliaca.
  b. of semimembranosus muscle Bursa m. semimembranosi.
  b. of tensor veli palatini muscle Bursa m. tensoris veli palatini.
bursa-equivalent *n hema.* Bursa-Äquivalent *nt.*
bur·sal ['bɜrsl] *adj* Schleimbeutel/Bursa betr., Schleimbeutel-.
bursal cyst Schleimbeutel(retentions)zyste *f.*
bursal synovitis → bursitis.
bur·sec·to·my [bɜr'sɛktəmɪ] *n ortho.* Schleimbeutelentfernung *f,* -resektion *f,* Bursektomie *f.*
bur·si·tis [bɜr'saɪtɪs] *n ortho.* Schleimbeutelentzündung *f,* Bursitis *f.*
bur·so·lith ['bɜrsəlɪθ] *n ortho.* Bursolith *m.*
bur·sop·a·thy [bɜr'sɒpəθɪ] *n* Schleimbeutelerkrankung *f,* Bursopathie *f.*
bur·sot·o·my [bɜr'sɒtəmɪ] *n chir.* Schleimbeuteleröffnung *f,* Bursotomie *f.*
burst [bɜrst] (*v:* burst; burst) **I** *n* **1.** Bersten *nt,* Platzen *nt.* **2.** (plötzliches) Ausbrach *m,* Anstieg *m.* **3.** Bruch *m,* Riß *m.* **4.** *phys.* (Strom-)Stoß *m,* Impuls *m.* **II** *vt* (auf-)sprengen, (-)platzen, (-)brechen, zum Platzen bringen. **III** *vi* **5.** bersten, (zer-, auf-)platzen, aufspringen. **6.** zerbrechen, zersplittern. **7.** ausbrechen (*into* in). **to ~ into tears** in Tränen ausbrechen.
burst open I *vt* aufbrechen, -stechen. **II** *vi* aufplatzen.
burst forming unit *abbr.* **BFU** *immun.* burst forming unit (*f*) *abbr.* BFU.
burst fracture *ortho.* (Wirbelkörper) Berstungsbruch *m,* -fraktur *f.*
burst·ing fracture ['bɜrstɪŋ] → burst fracture.
Burton ['bɜrtn]: **B.'s line/sign** Bleisaum *m.*
Bu·ru·li ulcer ['bʊərəlɪ] Buruli-Ulkus *nt.*
Bury ['bɛrɪ]: **B.'s disease** Erythema elevatum diutinum, Erythema microgyratum persistens, Erythema figuratum perstans, Erythema elevatum et diutinum.
Buschke ['bʊʃkə]: **B.'s disease** → Busse--Buschke disease.
  B.'s scleredema Buschke-Sklerödem *nt,* Scleroedema adultorum (Buschke), Scleroedema Buschke.
Buschke-Löwenstein ['lɛɪvənstaɪn]: **B.-L. tumor** Buschke-Löwenstein-Tumor *m,* -Kondylom *nt,* Condylomata gigantea.
Buschke-Ollendorff ['ɔlənˌdɔrf]: **B.-O. syndrome** Buschke-Ollendorff-Syndrom *nt,* Dermatofibrosis lenticularis disseminata mit Osteopoikilie.
bush·y ['bʊʃɪ] *adj* buschig.
bush yaws [bʊʃ] südamerikanische Haut-

leishmaniase *f*, kutane Leishmaniase *f* Südamerikas, Chiclero-Ulkus *nt*.
bushy chorion Zotten-, Chorionplatte *f*, Chorion frondosum.
Busquet [buːsˈkeɪ; bysˈkɛ]: **B.'s disease** Busquet'-Krankheit *f*.
Busse [ˈbʊsə]: **B.'s saccharomyces** *micro*. Cryptococcus neoformans.
Busse-Buschke [ˈbʊʃkə]: **B.-B. disease** Busse-Buschke-Krankheit *f*, europäische Blastomykose *f*, Kryptokokkose *f*, Kryptokokkus-Mykose *f*, Cryptococcus-Mykose *f*, Cryptococcose *f*, Torulose *f*.
bust [bʌst] *n* Büste *f*, (weibliche) Brust *f od.* Busen *m*.
bu·sul·fan [bjuːˈsʌlfæn] *n pharm*. Busulfan *nt*.
bu·sul·phan *n* → busulfan.
bu·tal·bi·tal [bjuːˈtælbɪtæl] *n pharm*. Butalbital *nt*.
bu·ta·mi·rate [bjuːtəˈmaɪreɪt] *n pharm*. Butamirat *nt*.
bu·tane [ˈbjuːteɪn] *n* (*n*-)Butan *nt*.
1,4-bu·tane·di·o·ic acid [ˌbjuːteɪndaɪˈəʊɪk] Bernsteinsäure *f*.
bu·ta·nil·i·caine [ˌbjuːtəˈnɪlɪkeɪn] *n pharm. anes*. Butanilicain *nt*.
bu·ta·no·ic acid [ˌbjuːtəˈnəʊɪk] → butyric acid.
***n*-bu·ta·nol** [ˈbjuːtnɒl, -ɑl] *n n*-Butanol *nt*.
butanol-extractable iodine *abbr*. **BEI** Butanol-extrahierbares Jod/Iod *nt abbr*. BEJ, BEI.
bu·thet·a·mate [bjuːˈθetəmeɪt] *n pharm*. Butetamat *nt*.
bu·thi·a·zide [bjuːˈθaɪəzaɪd] *n pharm*. Butizid *nt*, Thiabutazid *nt*.
Bütschli [ˈbɪtʃlɪ]: **B.'s nuclear spindle** Kern-, Mitosespindel *f*.
butt [bʌt] **I** *n* **1**. Kopfstoß *m*. **2**. *inf*. Hintern *m*. **II** *vt* jdn. einen (Kopf-)Stoß versetzen. **III** *vi* mit dem Kopf stoßen.
Butter [ˈbʌtər]: **B.'s cancer** Karzinom *nt* der Flexura coli dextra.
but·ter [ˈbʌtər] **I** *n* **1**. Butter *f*. **2**. butterähnliche Substanz *f*. **II** *vt* buttern, mit Butter bestreichen.
b. of arsenic Arsentrioxid *nt*, Arsenik *nt*, Arsenikum *nt*.

b. of zinc Zinkchlorid *nt*.
butter bacillus Clostridium butyricum.
but·ter·fat [ˈbʌtərfæt] *n* Butterfett *nt*.
but·ter·fly fracture [ˈbʌtərflaɪ] **1**. Schmetterlings-, Butterflyfraktur *f*. **2**. (*Becken*) Schmetterlingsbruch *m*, doppelseitiger vorderer Ringbruch *m*.
butterfly-shaped vertebra *radiol., ortho*. Schmetterlingswirbel *m*.
but·ter·milk [ˈ-mɪlk] *n* Buttermilch *f*.
but·ter·y [ˈbʌtərɪ] *adj* butterartig, -ähnlich, butterig, Butter-.
butter yellow Butter-, Dimethylgelb *nt*, *p*-Dimethylaminoazobenzol *nt abbr*. DAB.
but·tock [ˈbʌtək] *n* **1**. Gesäßbacke *f*. **2**. ~s *pl* Gesäß *nt*, Hinterbacken *pl*, Clunes *pl*, Nates *pl*.
but·ton [ˈbʌtn] *n* **1**. (Kleider-)Knopf *m*; (Klingel-, Licht-, Druck-, Schalt-)Knopf *m*, Drucktaste *f*. **2**. *anat., chir*. knopfähnliche Struktur *f*, Knopf *m*. **3**. *bot*. Knospe *f*, Auge *nt*.
but·ton·hole [ˈbʌtnhəʊl] *n* **1**. Knopfloch *nt*. **2**. → buttonhole incision.
buttonhole deformity 1. *ortho*. Knopflochdeformität *f*. **2**. → buttonhole mitral stenosis.
buttonhole incision *chir*. Knopflochschnitt *m*.
buttonhole iridectomy *ophthal*. periphere Iridektomie *f*.
buttonhole mitral stenosis (*Mitralis*) Knopflochstenose *f*, Fischmaulstenose *f*.
but·tress plate [ˈbʌtrɪs] *ortho*. Abstützplatte *f*.
bu·tyl [ˈbjuːtl, -tɪl] *n* Butyl-(Radikal *nt*).
butyl alcohol Butylalkohol *m*, *n*-Butanol *m*.
bu·tyl·ene [ˈbjuːtliːn] *n* Butylen *nt*, Buten *nt*.
bu·tyl·mer·cap·tan [ˌbjuːtɪlmərˈkæptæn] *n* Butylmercaptan *nt*.
bu·tyr·a·ceous [ˌbjuːtəˈreɪʃəs] *adj chem*. butterartig, -haltig.
bu·tyr·ate [ˈbjuːtəreɪt] *n* Butyrat *nt*.
butyrate kinase Butyratkinase *f*.
bu·tyr·ic acid [bjuːˈtɪrɪk] Buttersäure *f*, Butansäure *f*.

bu·tyr·o·cho·lin·es·ter·ase [ˌbjuːtɪərəʊˌkəʊləˈnestəreɪz] *n* unspezifische/unechte Cholinesterase *f abbr*. ChE, Pseudocholinesterase *f*, β-Cholinesterase *f*, Butyrylcholinesterase *f*, Typ II-Cholinesterasse *f*.
bu·ty·roid [ˈbjuːtərɔɪd] *adj chem*. butterähnlich.
bu·ty·rom·e·ter [bjuːtəˈrɑmɪtər] *n chem*. Butyrometer *nt*.
bu·ty·ro·phe·none [ˌbjuːtɪərəʊˈfiːnəʊn] *n pharm*. Butyrophenon *nt*.
bu·ty·ro·scope [bjuːˈtɪərəskəʊp] *n* → butyrometer.
bu·tyr·ous [ˈbjuːtərəs] *adj* **1**. → butyraceous. **2**. → butyroid.
bu·ty·ryl·cho·line esterase [ˈbjuːtərɪlˈkəʊliːn] → butyrocholinesterase.
bu·yo cheek cancer [ˈbaɪəʊ] Betelnußkarzinom *nt*.
Buzzard [ˈbʌzərd]: **B.'s maneuver** Buzzard-Kunstgriff *m*.
buzz·ing [ˈbʌzɪŋ] *n* Brummen *nt*, Summen *nt*, Surren *nt*, Schwirren *nt*.
BVDU *abbr*. → bromovinyldeoxyuridine.
B virus Herpes-B-Virus *nt*, Herpesvirus similae.
BW *abbr*. → body weight.
Bwam·ba [ˈbwɑmbə]: **B. fever** Bwamba-Fieber *nt*.
B. fever virus Bwamba-Virus *nt*.
B. virus → B. fever virus.
by·pass [ˈbaɪpæs, -pɑːs] **I** *n* **1**. *chir*. Umgehungsplastik *f*, -anastomose *f*, Bypass *m*; Shunt *m*. **2**. *techn*. Umleitung *f*, Umgehung *f*; Nebenleitung *f*, Bypass *m*. **3**. *phys*. Nebenschluß *m*, Shunt *m*. **II** *vt* umgehen; ab-, um-, vorbeileiten, shunten.
bypass operation *chir*. Bypassoperation *f*.
by-product *n* Neben-, Abfall-, Sekundärprodukt *nt*.
bys·si·no·sis [ˌbɪsəˈnəʊsɪs] *n pulmo*. Baumwollfieber *nt*, Baumwoll(staub)pneumokoniose *f*, Byssinose *f*.
bys·si·not·ic [-ˈnɑtɪk] **I** *n* Patient(in *f*) *m* mit Byssinose, Byssinotiker(in *f*) *m*. **II** *adj* Byssinose betr.
Bywaters [ˈbaɪwɔːtərs]: **B.' syndrome** Crush-, Bywaters-Syndrom *nt*.

C

C *abbr.* **1.** → calorie 2. **2.** → capacitance 2. **3.** → carbon. **4.** → cathodal. **5.** → cathode. **6.** → centigrade. **7.** → clearance 1. **8.** → compliance 1. **9.** → concentration 1. **10.** → contraction. **11.** → coulomb. **12.** → cysteine. **13.** → cytidine. **14.** → cytosine. **15.** → heat capacity. **16.** → thermal conductance.

c *abbr.* **1.** → calorie 1. **2.** → centi-. **3.** → heat capacity, specific. **4.** → molar concentration.

c. *abbr.* → circa.

CA *abbr.* **1.** → cancer. **2.** → carbonic anhydrase. **3.** → carcinoma. **4.** → cardiac arrest. **5.** → chronological age. **6.** → coronary artery. **7.** → cytosine arabinoside.

Ca *abbr.* **1.** → calcium. **2.** → cancer. **3.** → carcinoma. **4.** → cathodal. **5.** → cathode.

ca. *abbr.* → circa.

Ca antagonist Kalzium-, Calciumantagonist *m*.

cab·i·net ['kæbɪnət] *n* Medikamenten-, Akten-, Laborschrank *m*, (Wand-)Schränkchen *nt*; Vitrine *f*.

Cabot ['kæbət]: **C.'s ring bodies** *hema.* Cabot'-Ringe *pl*.

ca·ca·o [kəˈkɑːoʊ, -ˈkeɪoʊ] *n* **1.** Kakaobaum *m*. **2.** Kakaobohne *f*.

cacao bean → cacao 2.

cacao butter *pharm.* Kakaobutter *f*, Butyrum cacao.

Ca-carrier *n* Ca-Carrier *m*, Calcium-Carrier *m*.

cac·a·tion [kæˈkeɪʃn] *n* Darmentleerung *f*, Stuhlgang *m*, Defäkation *f*.

CaCC *abbr.* → cathodal closure contraction.

Cacchi-Ricci ['kætʃi 'ritʃi]: **C.-R. disease** Cacchi-Ricci-Syndrom *nt*, Schwammniere *f*.

Ca-channel *n* → calcium channel.

ca·chec·tic [kəˈkektɪk] *adj* Kachexie betr., von Kachexie betroffen, ausgezehrt, kachektisch.

cachectic edema kachektisches Ödem *nt*.

cachectic fever viszerale Leishmaniose/Leishmaniase *f*, Kala-Azar *f*, Splenomegalia tropica.

ca·chec·tin [kəˈkektɪn] *n* Tumor-Nekrose--Faktor *m abbr.* TNF, Cachectin *nt*.

ca·chet [kæˈʃeɪ, 'kæʃeɪ] *n pharm.* (Oblaten-)Kapsel *f*.

ca·chex·ia [kəˈkeksɪə] *n* Auszehrung *f*, Kachexie *f*, Cachexia *f*.

ca·chex·i·al fever [kəˈkeksɪəl] → cachectic fever

ca·chex·y [kəˈkeksɪ] *n* → cachexia.

cach·in·na·tion [kækəˈneɪʃn] *n psychia.* lautes unangebrachtes Lachen/Gelächter *nt*.

cac·o·cho·li·a [ˌkækoʊˈkoʊlɪə, -ˈkɑl-] *n patho.* Kakocholie *f*.

cac·o·chy·lia [ˌ-ˈkaɪlɪə] *n* **1.** *patho.* Kakochylie *f*. **2.** Verdauungsstörung *f*, Indigestion *f*.

cac·o·dyl ['-dɪl] *n* Kakodyl *nt*, Dimethylarsin *nt*.

cac·o·dyl·ate [ˌ-ˈdɪleɪt] *n* Kakodylat *nt*.

cac·o·dyl·ic acid [ˌ-ˈdɪlɪk] Kakodylsäure *f*, Dimethylarsinsäure *f*.

cac·o·gen·e·sis [ˌ-ˈdʒenəsɪs] *n embryo.* fehlerhafte Entwicklung *f*, Kakogenese *f*.

cac·o·gen·ic [ˌ-ˈdʒenɪk] *adj embryo.* Kakogenese betr., kakogen.

cac·o·geu·sia [ˌ-ˈgjuːʒ(ɪ)ə] *n* übler/schlechter Geschmack *m*, Kakogeusie *f*.

cac·o·me·lia [ˌ-ˈmiːlɪə, -ˈmel-] *n embryo.* angeborene Extremitätenfehlbildung *f*, Kakomelie *f*.

cac·o·rhyth·mic [ˌ-ˈrɪðmɪk] *adj cardio.* kakorhythmisch.

ca·cos·mia [kəˈkɑzmɪə] *n* Kakosmie *f*.

ca·cot·ro·phy [kəˈkɑtrəfɪ] *n patho.* Fehl-, Mangelernährung *f*.

cac·tin·o·my·cin [ˌkæktɪnəˈmaɪsɪn] *n pharm.* Cactinomycin *nt*, Aktinomyzin C *nt*.

cac·u·men [kəˈkjuːmən] *n, pl* **-mi·na** [-mɪnə] (Organ-)Spitze *f*.

ca·cu·mi·nal [kəˈkjuːmɪnəl] **I** *n* Kakuminal(laut *m*) *m*. **II** *adj* eine Spitze betr., Spitzen-, Kakuminal-.

CAD *abbr.* [coronary artery disease] → coronary heart disease.

ca·dav·er [kəˈdævər] *n* Leiche *f*, Leichnam *m*; Kadaver *m*.

cadaver donor *chir.* Leichenspender *m*.

ca·dav·er·ic [kəˈdævərɪk] *adj* Leiche betr., leichenhaft, Leichen-, Kadaver-.

cadaveric alkaloid Leichengift *nt*, -alkaloid *nt*, Ptomain *nt*.

cadaveric ecchymoses Leichenflecken *pl*.

cadaveric rigidity Leichen-, Totenstarre *f*, Rigor mortis.

cadaveric transplant Leichen-, Kadavertransplantat *nt*.

cadaveric transplantation Kadavertransplantation *f*, Transplantation *f* von Leichenorganen.

ca·dav·er·ine [kəˈdævəriːn] *n* Kadaverin *nt*, Cadaverin *nt*, Pentamethylendiamin *nt*, 1,5-Diaminopentan *nt*.

ca·dav·er·ous [kəˈdævərəs] *adj* **1.** → cadaveric. **2.** leichenblaß; ausgezehrt, -gemergelt, kachektisch.

ca·dence [ˈkeɪdns] *n* **1.** (Sprech-)Rhythmus *m*. **2.** (Takt-)Schlag *m*, Rhythmus *m*. **3.** (Stimme) Tonfall *m*, Modulation *f*, Kadenz *f*.

ca·den·cy [ˈkeɪdnsɪ] *n, pl* **-cies** → cadence.

cad·mi·o·sis [kædmɪˈoʊsɪs] *n pulmo.* Pneumokoniose *f* durch Kadmiumstaub.

cad·mi·um [ˈkædmɪəm] *n abbr.* **Cd** Kadmium *nt*, Cadmium *nt* *abbr.* Cd.

ca·du·ca [kəˈduːkə] *n* Schwangerschaftsendometrium *nt*, Dezidua *f*, Decidua *f*, Caduca *f*, Decidua membrana, Membrana deciduae.

ca·du·ce·us [kəˈd(j)uːsɪəs, -sjəs, -ʃəs] *n, pl* **-cei** [-sɪaɪ, -sjaɪ] Äskulapstab *m*.

ca·du·ci·ty [kəˈd(j)uːsətɪ] *n* **1.** Gebrechlichkeit *f (im Alter)*, (Alters-)Schwäche *f*; Senilität *f*. **2.** Vergänglichkeit *f*.

cae·cal [ˈsiːkl] *adj* blind endend; zökal, zäkal, zum Zäkum gehörend; Blinddarm-.

cae·cum [ˈsiːkəm] *n, pl* **-ca** [-kə] *anat.* **1.** blind endende Aussackung *f*, Blindsack *m*. **2.** Blinddarm *m*, Zäkum *nt*, Zökum *nt*, C(a)ecum *nt*, Intestinum c(a)ecum.

cae·si·um *n* → cesium.

café au lait spots [ˈkæfeɪ oʊ leɪ] Milchkaffeeflecken *pl*, Café au lait-Flecken *pl*.

caf·fein *n* → caffeine.

caf·feine [kæˈfiːn, 'kæf-, 'kæfiːn] *n* Koffein *nt*, Coffein *nt*, Methyltheobromin *nt*, 1,3,7-Trimethylxanthin *nt*.

caffeine contracture Koffeinkontraktur *f*.

caf·fein·ism [kæˈfiːnɪzəm, 'kæfi(ə)nɪz-] *n* chronische Koffeinintoxikation *f*, Koffeinismus *m*.

Caffey [ˈkæfɪ]: **C.'s disease/syndrome** Caffey-Silverman-Syndrom *nt*, Caffey-de Toni-Syndrom *nt*, Caffey-Smith-Syndrom *nt*, Hyperostosis corticalis infantilis.

Caffey-Silverman [ˈsɪlvərmæn]: **C.-S. syndrome** → Caffey's disease.

cage [keɪdʒ] *n* **1.** Käfig *m*. **2.** (Knochen-, Stahl-)Gerüst *nt*.

caged-ball valve [keɪdʒt] *HTG* Kugelventilprothese *f*.

Cahn-Ingold-Prelog [kɑːn ˈɪŋgəld ˈpreləg]: **C.-I.-P. convention/system** Cahn-Ingold-Prelog-System *nt*, RS-System *nt*.

cain complex [keɪn] *psychia.* Bruder-, Kainkomplex *m*.

cais·son disease/sickness [ˈkeɪsn, -sɑn] Druckluft-, Caissonkrankheit *f*.

Cajal [kaˈhal]: **C.'s cells** Cajal-Zellen *pl*. **C.'s cell stain** Cajal-Silberimprägnierung *f*.
horizontal cells of C. → C.'s cells.
interstitial nucleus of C. Cajal'-Kern *m*, -Zellen *pl*, Nc. interstitialis.
C.'s method → C.'s cell stain.

caj·e·pu·tol [ˈkædʒəpjuːtɒl] *n* Cineol *nt*, Eukalyptol *nt*.

caj·o·pu·tol *n* → cajeputol.

cake [keɪk] *n* **1.** Kuchen *m*, Torte *f*; Fladen(-Brot *nt*) *m*. **2.** festgeformte Masse *f*, Klumpen *m*, Brocken *m*. **a ~ of soap/ice** ein Stück Seife/ein Broken od. Stück Eis. **3.** Kruste *f*, (Schmutz-)Schicht *f*. **4.** *phys.* Filterkuchen *m*. **II** *vt* verkrusten, mit einer Kruste überziehen. **III** *vi* (zusammen-, ver-)klumpen, s. zusammenballen, zusammenbacken.

caked breast [keɪkt] *gyn.* Stauungsmastitis *f*.

cake kidney *patho.* Kuchen-, Klumpenniere *f*.

cak·ey [ˈkeɪkɪ] *adj* klumpend, klumpig, verklumpt.

caky *adj* → cakey.

Cal *abbr.* → calorie 2.

cal *abbr.* → calorie 1.

Cal·a·bar ['kæləbɑːr]: **C. bean** Calabarbohne *f*.
C. edema → C. swelling.
C. swelling Calabar-Beule *f*, -Schwellung *f*, Kamerum-Schwellung *f*, Loiasis *f*, Loiase *f*.
cal·ca·ne·al [kæl'keɪnɪəl] *adj* Fersenbein betr., kalkaneal, Fersenbein-, Kalkaneus-.
calcaneal apophysitis *ortho.* Haglund-Syndrom *nt*, Apophysitis calcanei.
calcaneal bone Fersenbein *nt*, Kalkaneus *m*, Calcaneus *m*.
calcaneal branches: c. of fibular artery Kalkaneusäste *pl* der A. fibularis, Rami calcanei a. fibularis/peroneae.
lateral c. of sural nerve Außenknöcheläste *pl* des N. suralis, Rami calcanei laterales n. suralis.
medial c. of tibial nerve Innenknöcheläste *pl* des N. tibialis, Rami calcanei mediales n. tibialis.
c. of posterior tibial artery Kalkaneusäste *pl* der A. tibialis posterior, Rami calcanei a. tibialis posteroris.
calcaneal bursa Bursa tendinis calcanei (Achillis).
subcutaneous c. Bursa subcutanea calcanea.
calcaneal fracture *ortho.* Fersenbeinbruch *m*, -fraktur *f*, Kalkaneusfraktur *f*.
calcaneal network → calcaneal rete.
calcaneal osteochondrosis *ortho.* → calcaneal apophysitis.
calcaneal process of cuboid (bone) Proc. calcaneus (ossis cuboidei).
calcaneal region *anat.* Ferse *f*, Fersenregion *f*, Calx *f*, Regio calcanea.
calcaneal rete Arteriennetz *nt* am Kalkaneus, Rete calcaneum.
calcaneal spur *ortho.* Fersen-, Kalkaneussporn *m*.
calcaneal sulcus Sulcus calcanei.
calcaneal tendon Achillessehne *f*, Tendo calcaneus/Achillis.
calcaneal tuber Fersenbeinhöcker *m*, Tuber calcanei.
calcaneal tubercle Tuberculum calcanei.
calcaneal tuberosity Fersenbeinhöcker *m*, Tuber calcanei.
cal·ca·ne·an [kæl'keɪnɪən] *adj* → calcaneal.
cal·ca·ne·i·tis [,kæl,keɪnɪ'aɪtɪs] *n ortho.* Fersenbein-, Kalkaneusentzündung *f*, Kalkaneitis *f*.
calcaneo- *pref.* Ferse(nbein)-, Kalkaneo-.
cal·ca·ne·o·a·poph·y·si·tis [kæl,keɪnɪəə-,pəfə'saɪtɪs] *n* → calcaneal apophysitis.
cal·ca·ne·o·a·strag·a·loid [,-ə'stræləgɔɪd] *adj* Fersen- u. Sprungbein betr., talokalkaneal.
cal·ca·ne·o·cu·boid [,-'kjuːbɔɪd] *adj* Fersen- u. Würfelbein betr., kalkaneokuboidal.
calcaneocuboid articulation Kalkaneokuboidgelenk *nt*, Artic. calcaneocuboidea.
calcaneocuboid joint → calcaneocuboid articulation.
calcaneocuboid ligament Lig. calcaneocuboideum.
dorsal c. Lig. calcaneocuboideum dorsale.
plantar c. Lig. calcaneocuboideum plantare.
cal·ca·ne·o·dyn·ia [,-'diːnɪə] *n ortho.* Fersenschmerz(en *pl*) *m*, Kalkaneodynie *f*.
cal·ca·ne·o·fib·u·lar [,-'fɪbjələr] *adj* Fersen- u. Wadenbein betr., kalkaneofibular.
calcaneofibular ligament Lig. calcaneofibulare.
cal·ca·ne·o·na·vic·u·lar [,-nə'vɪkjələr] *adj* Fersen- u. Kahnbein betr., kalkaneonavikular.
calcaneonavicular ligament Lig. calcaneonaviculare.
plantar c. Lig. calcaneonaviculare plantare.
cal·ca·ne·o·plan·tar [,-'plæntər] *adj* Fersenbein u. Fußsohle betr., kalkaneoplantar.
cal·ca·ne·o·scaph·oid [,-'skæfɔɪd] *adj* → calcaneonavicular.
cal·ca·ne·o·tib·i·al [,-'tɪbɪəl] *adj* Fersen- u. Schienbein betr., kalkaneotibial.
calcaneotibial ligament Pars tibiocalcanea lig. mediale.
cal·ca·ne·um [kæl'keɪnɪəm] *n, pl* **-nea** [-nɪə] → calcaneus.
cal·ca·ne·us [kæl'keɪnɪəs] *n, pl* **-nei** [-nɪaɪ] **1.** Fersenbein *nt*, Kalkaneus *m*, Calcaneus *m*. **2.** Hackenfuß *m*, Pes calcaneus.
cal·ca·no·dyn·ia [,kælkənəʊ'diːnɪə] *n* → calcaneodynia.
cal·car avis ['kælkɑr] Calcar avis.
cal·car·e·ous [kæl'keərɪəs] *adj* kalkartig, kalkig, Kalk-.
calcareous cataract Kalkstar *m*, Cataracta calcarea.
calcareous infiltration Kalkinfiltration *f*.
cal·ca·rine ['kælkəraɪn] *adj* **1.** Calcar avis betr. **2.** stachelförmig.
calcarine branch of medial occipital artery A. occipitalis medialis-Ast *m* zum Sulcus calcarinus, Ramus calcarinus a. occipitalis medialis.
calcarine complex Calcar avis.
calcarine fissure → calcarine sulcus.
calcarine sulcus Spornfurche *f*, Kalkarina *f*, Fissura calcarina, Sulcus calcarinus.
cal·car·i·u·ria [kæl,keərɪ'(j)ʊərɪə] *n* Kalkariurie *f*.
cal·car·oid ['kælkərɔɪd] *adj* kalziumähnlich.
cal·ce·mia [kæl'siːmɪə] *n* erhöhter Kalziumgehalt *m* des Blutes, Hyperkalz(i)ämie *f*.
cal·ci·bil·ia [kælsɪ'bɪlɪə] *n* Kalzibilie *f*.
cal·cic ['kælsɪk] *adj* Kalk od. Kalzium betr. od. enthaltend, Kalk-, Kalzium-.
cal·ci·co·sil·i·co·sis [,kælsɪkəʊ,sɪlə'kəʊsɪs] *n pulmo.* Kalzikosilikose *f*.
cal·ci·co·sis [kælsɪ'kəʊsɪs] *n pulmo.* Kalzikosis *f*.
cal·ci·di·ol [,-'daɪɒl, -ɒʊl] *n* 25-Hydroxycholecalciferol *nt*, Calcidiol *nt*.
cal·ci·a·mes [kæl'sɪfəmiːz] *n* → calcium hunger.
cal·cif·e·di·ol [,kælsɪfə'daɪɒl, -ɒʊl] *n* → calcidiol.
cal·cif·er·ol [kæl'sɪfərɒl, -rəl] *n* **1.** Calciferol *nt*, Vitamin D *nt*. **2.** Ergocalciferol *nt*, Vitamin D_2 *nt*.
cal·cif·er·ous [kæl'sɪfərəs] *adj* Kalzium(karbonat) enthaltend *od.* bildend, kalkhaltig.
cal·cif·ic [kæl'sɪfɪk] *adj* kalkbildend.
cal·ci·fi·ca·tion [,kælsəfɪ'keɪʃn] *n* **1.** Kalkbildung *f*. **2.** *patho.* Verkalkung *f*, Kalkeinlagerung *f*, Kalzifikation *f*, Kalzifizierung *nt*.
calcification lines Retzius'-Streifung *f*.
calcific bursitis Bursitis/Tendinitis scapulohumeralis.
cal·ci·fied cartilage ['kælsɪfaɪd] verkalkter/kalzifizierter Knorpel *m*.
calcified epithelioma → calcifying epithelioma of Malherbe.
calcified fetus *embryo.* Steinkind *nt*, Lithopädion *nt*.
calcified thrombus Phlebolith *m*.
cal·ci·fy ['kælsɪfaɪ] *vt, vi* verkalken, Kalk(e) ablagern *od.* ausscheiden, kalzifizieren.

cal·ci·fy·ing epithelioma of Malherbe ['kælsəfaɪɪŋ] Pilomatrikom *nt*, -matrixom *nt*, verkalkendes Epitheliom Malherbe *nt*, Epithelioma calcificans Malherbe.
cal·ci·na·tion [kælsɪ'neɪʃn] *n chem.* Kalzinierung *f*, Kalzination *f*.
cal·cine ['kælsaɪn] *chem.* **I** *vt* kalzinieren. **II** *vi* kalziniert werden.
cal·ci·no·sis [kælsɪ'nəʊsɪs] *n patho.* Kalzinose *f*, Calcinosis *f*.
cal·ci·nur·ic diabetes [,-'n(j)ʊərɪk] vermehrte Kalziumausscheidung *f* im Harn, Hyperkalzurie *f*, Hyperkalziurie *f*.
cal·ci·o·ki·ne·sis [,kælsɪəʊki'niːsɪs, -kaɪ-] *n* Kalziummobilisation *f*.
cal·ci·o·ki·net·ic [,-kɪ'netɪk, -kaɪ-] *adj* kalziummobilisierend.
cal·ci·pec·tic [kælsə'pektɪk] *adj* Kalzipexie betr. *od.* verursachend.
cal·ci·pe·nia [,-'piːnɪə] *n* Kalziummangel *m*, Kalzipenie *f*.
cal·ci·pex·ic [,-'peksɪk] *adj* → calcipectic.
cal·ci·pex·is [,-'peksɪs] *n* → calcipexy.
cal·ci·pex·y [,-'peksɪ] *n* Kalzipexie *f*.
cal·ci·phil·ia [,-'fɪlɪə] *n* Kalziphilie *f*.
cal·ci·phy·lac·tic [,-fɪ'læktɪk] *adj* Kalziphylaxie betr., von Kalziphylaxie betroffen, kalziphylaktisch.
cal·ci·phy·lax·is [,-fɪ'læksɪs] *n* Kalziphylaxie *f*.
cal·ci·priv·ia [,-'prɪvɪə] *n* Kalziumentzug *m*, -mangel *m*.
cal·ci·priv·ic [,-'prɪvɪk] *adj* durch Kalziummangel hervorgerufen *od.* bedingt, kalzipriv.
cal·ci·to·nin [,-'təʊnɪn] *n* Kalzitonin *nt*, Calcitonin *nt*, Thyreocalcitonin *nt*.
cal·ci·tri·ol [kæl'sɪtrɒl, -ɒl] *n* 1,25-Dihydroxycholecalciferol *nt*, Calcitriol *nt*.
cal·ci·um ['kælsɪəm] *n abbr.* **Ca** Kalzium *nt*, Calcium *nt abbr.* Ca.
calcium antagonist Kalziumblocker *m*, -antagonist *m*, Ca-Blocker *m*, Ca-Antagonist *m*.
calcium-ATPase (system) Calcium-ATPase(-System *nt*) *f*, Ca-ATPase *f*.
calcium balance Kalziumhaushalt *m*.
calcium-blocking agent → calcium antagonist.
calcium bromide Kalziumbromid *nt*.
calcium carbonate Kalziumkarbonat *nt*.
calcium carbonate calculus/stone Kalziumkarbonatstein *m*.
calcium channel Kalziumkanal *m*, Ca-Kanal *m*.
calcium channel blocker → calcium antagonist.
calcium chloride Kalziumchlorid *nt*.
calcium citrate Kalziumcitrat *nt*.
calcium compounds kalziumhaltige Verbindungen *pl*, Kalziumverbindungen *pl*.
calcium deficiency Kalziummangel *m*.
calcium fluoride Kalziumfluorid *nt*.
calcium folinate Kalziumfolinat *nt*.
calcium gluconate Kalziumgluconat *nt*.
calcium gout 1. Profichet'-Krankheit *f*, -Syndrom *nt*, Kalkgicht *f*, Calcinosis circumscripta. **2.** → Calcinosis.
calcium hunger *patho.* Kalziumhunger *m*.
calcium lactate Kalziumlaktat *nt*.
calcium oxalate Kalziumoxalat *nt*.
calcium oxalate calculus/stone Kalziumoxalatstein *m*.
calcium phosphate Kalziumphosphat *nt*.
calcium phosphate calculus/stone Kalziumphosphatstein *m*.
calcium pump Kalziumpumpe *f*, Ca-Pumpe *f*.
calcium pyrophosphate dihydrate *abbr.* **CPPD** Calciumpyrophosphatdihydrat *nt abbr.* CPPD.

calcium pyrophosphate dihydrate (crystal deposition) disease

calcium pyrophosphate dihydrate (crystal deposition) disease Chondokalzinose f, Pseudogicht f, Calciumpyrophosphatdihydratablagerung f, CPPD-Ablagerung f.
calcium sulfate Kalziumsulfat nt.
calcium thesaurismosis → calcinosis.
calcium urate Kalziumurat nt.
calcium urate calculus/stone Kalziumuratstein m.
cal·ci·u·ria [ˌkælsə'(j)ʊərɪə] n Kalziurie f.
cal·cu·la·ble ['kælkjələbl] adj 1. kalkulierbar, berechen-, bestimm-, ermittelbar. 2. zuverläßig, verlässlich.
cal·cu·lar·y ['kælkjəˌlerɪː, -lərɪ] adj Kalkulus betr., kalkulös, Stein-.
cal·cu·late ['-leɪt] I vt be-, ausrechnen; (ab-)schätzen, veranschlagen, kalkulieren. II vi rechnen, eine Berechnung/Kalkulation anstellen; etw. einschätzen.
cal·cu·lat·ed ['-leɪtɪd] adj 1. berechnet, kalkuliert, ermittelt, geschätzt. 2. (Plan) durchdacht; beabsichtigt.
calculated risk kalkuliertes Risiko nt.
cal·cu·la·tion [ˌ-'leɪʃn] n Aus-, Berechnung f; Kalkulation f, Schätzung f.
cal·cu·lo·gen·e·sis [ˌkælkjələʊ'dʒenəsɪs] n Kalkulus-, Steinbildung f.
cal·cu·lo·sis [kælkjə'ləʊsɪs] n patho. Steinleiden nt, Lithiasis f, Calculosis f.
cal·cu·lous ['kælkjələs] adj Stein(bildung) betr., kalkulös, Stein-.
calculous concrement Gelenkstein m, -konkrement nt.
cal·cu·lus ['kælkjələs] n, pl **-li** [-laɪ] Steinchen nt, Konkrement nt, Stein m, Kalkulus m, Calculus m.
calculus cirrhosis sekundär biliäre Leberzirrhose f bei Cholilithiasis.
Caldani [kæl'dɑːnɪ]: **C.'s ligament** Lig. coracoclaviculare.
Caldwell ['kɔldwel]: **C. projection/view** radiol. Caldwell-Projection f, -Technik f.
Caldwell-Luc [lʌk]: **C.-L. operation** HNO Caldwell-Luc-Operation f.
Caldwell-Moloy ['mɔlɔɪ]: **C.-M. classification** Caldwell-Moloy-Einteilung f, -Klassifikation f.
cal·e·fa·cient [kælə'feɪʃənt] adj (er-)wärmend.
calf [kæf, kɑːf] n, pl **calves** [-vz] 1. Wade f, anat. Sura f. 2. bio. Kalb nt.
calf bone Wadenbein nt, Fibula f.
cal·i·ber ['kælɪbər] n (Innen-)Durchmesser m, Kaliber nt.
cal·i·brate ['kælɪbreɪt] vt eichen, kalibrieren, standardisieren.
cal·i·bra·ter n → calibrator.
cal·i·bra·tion [ˌkælɪ'breɪʃn] n Eichen nt, Kalibrierung f, Kalibrieren nt.
cal·i·bra·tor ['kælɪbreɪtər] n lab. Standard-(lösung f) m, Eichmaterial nt.
cal·i·ce·al [ˌkælə'sɪəl] adj Kalix/Kelch betr., Kelch-.
caliceal diverticulum (Niere) Kelchdivertikel nt.
cal·i·cec·ta·sis [ˌ-'sektəsɪs] n urol. Nierenkelchdilatation f, Kalikektasie f.
cal·i·cec·to·my [ˌ-'sektəmɪ] n urol. operative Nierenkelchentfernung f, Kalikektomie f.
ca·lic·i·form cell [kə'lɪsəfɔːrm] Becherzelle f.
caliciform papillae Wallpapillen pl, Papillae vallatae.
cal·i·cine ['kælɪsɪn] adj Kelch/Kalix betr., kelchähnlich, -förmig.
Cal·i·ci·vi·rus [ˌkælɪsɪ'vaɪrəs] n micro. Caliciviren pl.
cal·i·ci·vi·rus·es [ˌ-'vaɪrəsəs] pl micro. Caliciviren pl, Caliciviridae pl.

cal·i·co·plas·ty ['kælɪkəʊplæstɪ] n urol. Kalikoplastik f.
cal·i·cot·o·my [kælɪ'katəmɪ] n urol. Kalikotomie f.
ca·lic·u·lus [kə'lɪkjələs] n, pl **-li** [-laɪ] anat. kleiner Kelch m, kleine kelchartige Struktur f, Caliculus m.
ca·li·ec·ta·sis [ˌkælɪ'ektəsɪs] n → calicectasis.
ca·li·ec·to·my [ˌ-'ektəmɪ] n → calicectomy.
cal·i·for·nia [ˌkælə'fɔːrnɪə, -jə]: **C. black-legged tick** Ixodes pacificus.
C. disease Posada-Mykose f, Wüstenfieber nt, Kokzioidomykose f, Coccioidomycose f, Granuloma coccioides.
C. encephalitis abbr. CE California-Enzephalitis f abbr. CE.
C. encephalitis virus micro. California(-Enzephalitis)-Virus nt.
C. virus → C. encephalitis virus.
cal·i·for·ni·um [ˌ-'fɔːrnɪəm] n abbr. **Cf** Californium nt abbr. Cf.
ca·li·o·plas·ty ['kælɪəplæstɪ] n → calicoplasty.
ca·li·or·rha·phy ['kælɪɑrəfɪ] n urol. Kali(k)orrhaphie f.
ca·li·ot·o·my [kælɪ'atəmɪ] n → calicotomy.
cal·i·pers ['kælɪpərs] pl Greif-, Tastzirkel m, Taster m.
ca·lix ['keɪlɪks, 'kæ-] n, pl **cal·i·ces** [-lɪsɪːz] anat. Kelch m, kelchförmige Struktur f, Calix m.
call [kɔːl] I n 1. Ruf m, Schrei m (for nach). a ~ **for help** ein Hilferuf. 2. (kurzer) Besuch m; (Arzt) Konsultation f. **to make a** ~ (**at the hospital/on sb.**) aufsuchen; jdn. besuchen, jdm. einen Besuch abstatten. 3. **on** ~ dienstuend, -habend, im Dienst. 4. (Telefon-)Anruf m. **to give s.o. a** ~ jdn. anrufen. **to make a** ~ telefonieren. II vt 5. jdn. (herbei-)rufen, jdn. kommen lassen. 6. jdn. telefonisch anrufen. 7. befehlen, anordnen. 8. jdn. wecken. 9. **to be** ~**ed** heißen. **What's she** ~**ed**? Wie heißt sie? **a lady** ~**ed Reuter** eine Dame namens Reuter. III vi 10. rufen, schreien. **to** ~ **for help** um Hilfe rufen. 11. jdn. (kurz) besuchen. 12. telefonieren.
call for vi 1. jdn. rufen, jdn./etw. kommen lassen; verlangen (nach). 2. verlagen, erfordern.
call in I vt 1. jdn. zu Rate ziehen, hinzuziehen, konsultieren. 2. jdn. heineinrufen. II vi (kurz) besuchen.
call on vi jdn. (kurz) besuchen.
call out vi rufen, schreien. **to** ~ **for help** um Hilfe rufen.
CALLA abbr. → common acute lymphoblastic leukemia antigen.
Callander ['kæləndər]: **C.'s amputation** ortho. Oberschenkelamputation f nach Callander.
Calleja [kal'jeha]: **C.'s islands/islets** Calleja-Inseln pl, Cajal-Inseln pl.
cal·ler ['kɔːlər] n 1. Besucher(in f) m. 2. Anrufer(in f) m.
Call-Exner [kɔːl; kal 'eksnər]: **C.-E. bodies** Call-Exner-Körperchen pl.
cal·lic·re·in [ˌkælɪk'riːɪn] n Kallikrein nt.
Cal·liph·o·ra [kə'lɪfərə] n micro. Calliphora f.
Cal·li·phor·i·dae [ˌkælə'fɔːrəˌdiː] pl micro. Schmeiß-, Goldfliegen pl, Calliphoridae pl.
cal·lo·sal [kæ'ləʊsl] adj Balken/Corpus callosum betr., Balken-.
callosal agenesis Balkenmangel m, Agenesis corporis callosi.
callosal convolution Gyrus cinguli/cingulatus.
callosal fibers Balkenfasern pl.
callosal fissure Sulcus corporis callosi.

callosal gyrus Gyrus cinguli/cingulatus.
callosal sulcus Sulcus corporis callosi.
cal·los·i·tas [kæ'lasɪtəs] n → callus 1.
cal·los·i·ty [kæ'lasətɪ] n 1. → callus 1. 2. fig. Gefühllosigkeit f (to gegenüber).
cal·lo·so·mar·gin·al artery [kəˌləʊsəʊ-'mɑːrdʒɪnl] A. callosomarginalis.
callosomarginal fissure Sulcus cinguli/cingulatus.
callosomarginal sulcus Sulcus cinguli/cingulatus.
cal·lo·sum [kæ'ləʊsəm, kə-] n, pl **-sa** [-sə] anat. Balken m, Corpus callosum.
cal·lous ['kæləs] I adj 1. schwielig, verhärtet, verhornt, kallös. 2. fig. gefühllos, herzlos (to gegenüber). II vt 3. schwielig/ kallös machen, verhärten. 4. fig. gefühllos machen. III vi 5. schwielig/kallös werden, s. verhärten. 6. fig. gefühllos werden, abstumpfen (to gegenüber).
cal·lus ['kæləs] n, pl **-lus·es**, **cal·li** ['kælaɪ] 1. Hornschwiele f, Kallus m, Callositas f, Callus m. 2. (Knochen-)Kallus m, Callus m.
callus ulcer Ulcus callosum.
calm [kɑːm] I n Ruhe f, Stille f. II adj ruhig, still. III vt beruhigen, besänftigen. IV vi s. beruhigen.
calm down vt, vi → calm III, IV.
calm·a·tive ['kɑːmətɪv, 'kælmə-] I n pharm. Beruhigungsmittel nt, Sedativum nt. II adj beruhigend, sedativ.
Calmette [kal'met]: **C.'s conjunctival reaction** → C.'s test.
C.'s ophthalmic reaction → C.'s test.
C.'s test Calmette'-Konjunktivaltest m.
C.'s vaccine BCG-Impfstoff m, BCG-Vakzine f.
Calmette-Guérin [ge'rɛ̃]: **C.-G. bacillus** Bacillus Calmette-Guérin m abbr. BCG.
calm·ness ['kɑːmnɪs] n → calm I.
cal·mod·u·lin [kæl'madjəlɪn] n Kalmodulin nt, Calmodulin nt.
cal·o·mel ['kæləmel, -məl] n Kalomel nt, Calomel nt, Quecksilber-I-Chlorid nt.
calomel electrode Kalomelelektrode f.
cal·or ['kælər, 'keɪ-] n patho. Calor m.
ca·lor·ic [kə'lɔrɪk, 'kælərɪk] I n Wärme f. II adj 1. Wärme betr., Kalorien-, Wärme-, Energie-. 2. Kalorie(n) betr., kalorisch. **the** ~ **contents of food** der Kaloriengehalt der Nahrung. 3. (Nahrung, Diät) kalorienreich.
caloric equivalent Energieeäquivalent nt, kalorisches Äquivalent nt.
caloric nystagmus physiol., neuro. kalorischer/thermischer Nystagmus m.
caloric quotient kalorischer Quotient m.
caloric requirement Kalorienbedarf m.
caloric response physiol. thermische Reizantwort f.
caloric test Bárány-Versuch m, -Kalorisation f.
caloric value Kalorienwert m.
ca·lo·rie ['kælərɪ] n 1. abbr. **c**, **cal** phys. (Standard-)Kalorie f, (kleine) Kalorie f, Gramm-Kalorie f abbr. cal. 2. abbr. **C**, **Cal** (große) Kalorie f, Kilokalorie f abbr. Kcal, Cal. 3. Kalorie f, kalorischer Wert eines Nahrungsmittels.
calorie-conscious adj kalorienbewußt.
ca·lor·i·fa·cient [kəˌlarɪ'feɪʃnt] adj (Nahrung) wärmeerzeugend.
cal·o·rif·ic [ˌkælə'rɪfɪk] adj wärme-erzeugend, Wärme-, Kalori-.
calorific capacity phys. spezifische Wärme f.
ca·lor·i·ge·net·ic [kəˌlɔːrədʒə'netɪk, ˌkælərə-] adj → calorigenic.
ca·lor·i·gen·ic [ˌ-'dʒenɪk] adj Wärme od. Energie entwickelnd, Wärme- od. Energiebildung fördernd, kalorigen.

cal·o·rim·e·ter [ˌkæləˈrɪmətər] *n* Kalorimeter *nt*.
cal·o·ri·met·ric [ˌkælərəˈmetrɪk, kəˌlɔːr-] *adj* Kalorimetrie betr., mittels Kalorimetrie, kalorimetrisch.
cal·o·ri·met·ri·cal [ˌ-ˈmetrɪkl] *adj* → calorimetric.
cal·o·rim·e·try [ˌkæləˈrɪmətrɪ] *n* Wärmemessung *f*, Kalorimetrie *f*.
ca·lor·i·trop·ic [ˌkælərəˈtrɑpɪk, kəˌlɔːr-] *adj* thermotrop.
cal·o·ry *n* → calorie.
Calot [kaˈlo]: **C.'s triangle** Calot'-Dreieck *nt*.
cal·se·ques·trin [ˌkælsəˈkwestrɪn] *n* Calsequestrin *nt*.
cal·var·i·a [kælˈveərɪə] **I** *sing* → calvarium. **II** *pl* → calvarium.
cal·var·i·al [ˌ-ˈveərɪəl] *adj* Schädeldach/Calvaria betr., Schädeldach-, Kalotten-.
cal·var·i·um [ˌ-ˈveərɪəm] *n*, *pl* **-var·i·a** [-rɪə] knöchernes Schädeldach *nt*, Kalotte *f*, Calvaria *f*.
Calvé [kalˈve]: **C.'s disease** Calvé-Syndrom *nt*, -Krankheit *f*, Vertebra plana osteonecrotica.
Calvé-Perthes [ˈpertiːz, ˈperθ-]: **C.-P. disease** PerthesKrankheit *f*, Perthes-Legg--Calvé-Krankheit *f*, Morbus Perthes *m*, Legg-Calvé-Perthes(-Waldenström)--Krankheit *f*, Osteochondropathia deformans coxae juvenilis, Coxa plana (idiopathica).
Calvin [ˈkælvɪn]: **C. cycle** *biochem.* Calvin--Zyklus *m*.
cal·vi·ti·es [kælˈvɪʃɪˌiːz] *n* Kahlheit *f*, Haarausfall *m*, -losigkeit *f*, Alopezie *f*, Alopecia *f*.
cal·vous [ˈkælvəs] *adj derm.* kahl(köpfig), glatzköpfig.
calx [kælks] *n*, *pl* **calx·es, cal·ces** [ˈkælsiːz] **1.** *chem.* Kalk *m*, Kalziumoxid *nt*. **2.** *anat.* Ferse *f*, Fersenregion *f*, Calx *f*, Regio calcanea.
cal·y·ce·al *adj* → caliceal.
calyceal diverticulum → caliceal diverticulum.
cal·y·cec·ta·sis *n* → calicectasis.
cal·y·cec·to·my *n* → calicectomy.
cal·y·cine *adj* → calicine.
cal·y·cle [ˈkælɪkl] *n* → caliculus.
cal·y·co·plas·ty *n* → calicoplasty.
cal·y·cot·o·my *n* → calicotomy.
ca·lyc·u·lus *n* → caliculus.
ca·ly·ec·ta·sis [kæləˈektəsɪs] *n* → calicectasis.
Ca·lym·ma·to·bac·te·ri·um [kəˌlɪmətəʊbækˈtɪərɪəm] *n micro.* Calymmatobacterium *nt*.
C. granulomatis Donovan-Körperchen *nt*, Calymmatobacterium/Donovania granulomatis.
ca·ly·o·plas·ty [ˈkælɪəplæstɪ] *n* → calicoplasty.
ca·ly·or·rha·phy [ˌkælɪˈɔrəfɪ] *n* → caliorrhaphy.
ca·ly·ot·o·my [ˌ-ˈɑtəmɪ] *n* → calicotomy.
ca·lyx *n* → calix.
cam·bi·um [ˈkæmbɪəm] *n*, *pl* **-ums, -bia** [-bɪə] (*Knochen*) Kambiumschicht *f*.
cambium layer (*Periost*) Kambiumschicht *f*.
cam·el·oid anemia [ˈkæməlɔɪd] *hema.* hereditäre Elliptozytose *f*, Ovalozytose *f*, Kamelozytose *f*, Elliptozytenanämie *f*.
cameloid cell *hema.* Elliptozyt *m*, Ovalozyt *m*.
cam·er·a [ˈkæm(ə)rə] *n*, *pl* **-er·as, -er·ae** [-əri] **1.** *anat.* Kammer *f*, Camera *f*. **2.** Kamera *f*, Fotoapparat *m*, Film-, Fernsehkamera *f*.

Camerer [ˈkæmərər]: **C.'s law** *bio.* Camerer'-Regel *f*.
cam·i·sole [ˈkæmɪsəʊl] *n psychia.* Zwangsjacke *f*.
cam·o·mile [ˈkæməmaɪl, -mɪl] *n* echte Kamille *f*, Chamomilla *f*, Matricaria chamomilla/officinalis.
camomile tea Kamillentee *m*.
cAMP *abbr.* → cyclic AMP.
cam·paign [kæmˈpeɪn] **I** *n* (Abwehr-)-Kampf *m*, Bekämpfungsaktion *f*, Schutzaktion *f* (*against* gegen). **II** *vi* kämpfen (*against* gegen).
Camper [ˈkæmpər]: **C.'s angle** Camper'--Gesichtswinkel *m*.
C.'s chiasm Camper'-Kreuzung, Chiasma tendinum (digitorum manus).
C.'s ligament Urogenitaldiaphragma *nt*, Diaphragma urogenitale.
C.'s plane Camper-Ebene *f*, Nasoaurikularebene *f*.
CAMP factor [Christie, Atkins, Munch--Petersen] *micro.* CAMP-Faktor *m*.
camp fever [kæmp] *micro.* epidemisches/klassisches Fleckfieber *nt*, Läusefleckfieber *nt*, Fleck-, Hunger-, Kriegstyphus *m*, Typhus exanthematicus.
cam·phol [ˈkæmfəl, -fɒl, -fəʊl] *n* → camphyl alcohol.
cam·phor [ˈkæmfər] *n* Kampfer *m*, Campfer *m*, Camphora *f*.
cam·phor·a·ceous [kæmfəˈreɪʃəs] *adj* kampferähnlich.
cam·phor·at·ed [ˈkæmfəreɪtɪd] *adj* kampferhaltig, mit Kampfer versetzt.
cam·phor·ism [ˈkæmfərɪzəm] *n* Kampferintoxikation *f*, Camphorismus *m*.
camphor oil Kampferöl *nt*.
cam·phyl alcohol [ˈkæmfɪl] *n* Borneokampfer *m*, Borneol *nt*, Borneolum *nt*.
cam·pim·e·ter [kæmˈpɪmətər] *n ophthal.* Kampimeter *nt*.
cam·pim·e·try [kæmˈpɪmətrɪ] *n ophthal.* Kampimetrie *f*.
cam·po·spasm [ˈkæmpəspæzəm] *n* → camptocormia.
cam·pot·o·my [kæmˈpɑtəmɪ] *n neurochir.* Campotomie *f*.
CAMP test *micro.* CAMP-Test *m*.
camp·to·cor·mia [ˌkæm(p)təˈkɔrmɪə] *n ortho.* Kamptokormie *f*.
camp·to·cor·my [ˌ-ˈkɔrmɪ] *n* → camptocormia.
camp·to·dac·tyl·ia [ˌ-dækˈtiːlɪə] *n* → camptodactyly.
camp·to·dac·tyl·ism [ˌ-ˈdæktɪlɪzəm] *n* → camptodactyly.
camp·to·dac·ty·ly [ˌ-ˈdæktəlɪ] *n ortho.* Kamptodaktylie *f*, Kamp(t)omelie *f*.
camp·to·me·lia [ˌ-ˈmiːlɪə, -jə] *n* Kamp(t)omelie *f*.
camp·to·mel·ic [ˌ-ˈmelɪk] *adj* Kamptomelie betr., kamp(t)omel *f*.
camptomelic syndrome Kamptomelie--Syndrom *nt*.
camp·to·spasm [ˈ-spæzəm] *n* → camptocormia.
Cam·py·lo·bac·ter [ˌkæmpɪləˈbæktər] *n micro.* Campylobacter *m*.
Campylobacter enteritis Campylobacter--Enteritis *f*.
cam·py·lo·bac·te·ri·o·sis [ˌ-ˌbæktɪərɪˈəʊsɪs] *n* Campylobacteriose *f*.
Campylobacter medium *micro.* Campylobactermedium *nt*.
cam·py·lo·dac·ty·ly [ˌ-ˈdæktəlɪ] *n* → camptodactyly.
Camurati-Engelmann [cæməˈrɑːti ˈeŋgəlmən]: **C.-E. disease** (Camurati-)Engelmann-Erkrankung *f*, -Syndrom *nt*, Osteopathia hyperostotica multiplex infantilis.

Can·a·da balsam [ˈkænədə] Kanadabalsam *nt*, Balsamum canadense.
Canada-Cronkhite [ˈkrɑŋkaɪt]: **C.-C. syndrome** Cronkhite-Canada-Syndrom *nt*.
ca·nal [kəˈnæl] (*v:* **canal(l)ed**) **I** *n* Gang *m*, Röhre *f*, Kanal *m*; *anat.* Canalis *m*. **II** *vt* kanalisieren.
c. of Arantius Ductus venosus.
c. of Corti (*Ohr*) innerer Tunnel *m*.
c. of Cuvier *embryo.* Cuvier'-Gang, -Kanal.
c. of epididymis Nebenhodengang, Ductus epididymidis.
c.s of Hering Hering'-Kanälchen *pl*.
c. of Nuck Proc. vaginalis peritonei.
c. of Oken Wolff'-Gang, Urnierengang, Ductus mesonephricus.
c.s of Rivinius Ductus sublinguales minores.
c. of Stenon Parotisgang *m*, Stensen'-, Stenon'-Gang *m*, Ductus parotideus.
c. of Stilling Cloquet'-Kanal, Canalis hyaloideus.
c. of stomach Magenstraße *f*, Canalis gastricus/ventricularis.
c. for tensor tympani muscle Semicanalis m. tensoris tympani.
can·a·lic·u·lar [ˌkænəˈlɪkjələr] *adj anat.* Kanälchen betr., kanälchenähnlich, kanalikulär.
canalicular abscess kanalikulärer Brustdrüsenabzeß *m*.
canalicular ducts Milchgänge *pl*, Ductus lactiferi.
canalicular phase *embryo.* (*Lunge*) Phase *f* des Gangwachstums.
can·a·lic·u·li·tis [kænəˌlɪkjəˈlaɪtɪs] *n ophthal.* Entzündung *f* der Tränenkanälchen, Kanalikulitis *f*.
can·a·lic·u·li·za·tion [kænəˌlɪkjəlaɪˈzeɪʃn] *n* Kanälchenbildung *f*.
can·a·lic·u·lo·rhi·nos·to·my [ˌkænəˌlɪkjələraɪˈnɑstəmɪ] *n ophthal.* Kanalikulorhinostomie *f*.
can·a·lic·u·lus [ˌkænəˈlɪkjələs] *n*, *pl* **-li** [-laɪ] *anat.* kleiner Kanal *m*, Kanälchen *nt*, Canaliculus *m*.
c. of chorda tympani Chordakanal, Canaliculus chordae tympani.
c. of cochlea Canaliculus cochleae.
ca·nal·i·za·tion [kəˌnælɪˈzeɪʃn, ˌkænl-] *n* Kanalbildung *f*, Kanalisation *f*, Kanalisierung *f*.
can·al·ize [ˈkænlaɪz, kəˈnælaɪz] *vt* kanalisieren.
Canavan [ˈkænəvæn]: **C.'s disease/sclerosis** Canavan-Syndrom *nt*, (Canavan-)van Bogaert-Bertrand-Syndrom *nt*, frühinfantile spongiöse Dystrophie *f*.
can·a·van·ase [kəˈnævəneɪz] *n old* → arginase.
can·a·van·ine [ˌkænəˈvæniːn, kəˈnævə-] *n* Canavanin *nt*.
Canavan-van Bogaert-Bertrand [væn bərˈtrɑ̃]: **C.-v.B.-B. disease** → Canavan's disease.
can·cel·late [ˈkænsəleɪt, -lɪt] *adj* **1.** *anat.* spongiös, schwammig, schwammartig. **2.** *histol.* gitterförmig, -ähnlich.
can·cel·lat·ed [ˌ-ˈleɪtɪd] *adj* → cancellate.
cancelled bone Spongiosa *f*, Substantia spongiosa/trabecularis (ossium).
can·cel·lous [ˈkænsələs] *adj* → cancellate 1.
cancellous bone → cancellated bone.
cancellous osteoma spongiöses Osteom *m*, Osteoma spongiosum.
cancellous screw *ortho.* Spongiosaschraube *f*.
cancellous tissue → cancellated bone.
can·cel·lus [kænˈseləs] *n anat.* gitterförmige Struktur *f*.

can·cer ['kænsər] *n abbr.* **CA, Ca 1.** Krebs *m*, maligner Tumor *m*, Malignom *nt*. **2.** → carcinoma. **3.** Sarkom *nt*, Sarcoma *nt abbr.* Sa.
can·cer·ate ['kænsəreɪt] *vi* kanzerös werden, einen Krebs bilden.
can·cer·a·tion [,kænsə'reɪʃn] *n* Krebsbildung *f*, Kanzerisierung *f*.
cancer bodies 1. Plimmer-Körperchen *nt*. **2.** Russell'-Körperchen *pl*.
cancer-causing *adj* krebserregend, -auslösend, -erzeugend, onkogen, karzinogen, kanzerogen.
cancer cell Krebs-, Tumorzelle *f*.
cancer chemotherapy zytostatische/antineoplastische Chemotherapie *f*.
can·cer·e·mia [kænsə'riːmɪə] *n patho.* Kanzerämie *f*.
cancer en cuirasse Panzerkrebs *m*, Cancer en cuirasse.
can·cer·i·ci·dal [,kænsərɪ'saɪdl] *adj* krebszerstörend.
can·cer·i·gen·ic [,-'dʒenɪk] *adj* → cancer-causing.
cancer in situ Oberflächenkarzinom *nt*, präinvasives/intraepitheliales Karzinom *nt*, Carcinoma in situ.
can·cer·i·za·tion [,-'zeɪʃn] *n* → canceration.
can·cer·o·ci·dal [,kænsərəʊ'saɪdl] *adj* → cancericidal.
can·cer·o·gen·ic [,-'dʒenɪk] *adj* → cancer-causing.
can·cer·o·pho·bia [,-'fəʊbɪə] *n* → cancerphobia.
can·cer·ous ['kænsərəs] *adj* Krebs betr., krebsig, krebsbefallen, -artig, kanzerös, karzinomatös.
cancerous cachexia Kachexie *f* bei Malignomerkrankung.
cancer patient Krebspatient(in *f*) *m*, Patient(in *f*) *m* mit Krebserkrankung.
can·cer·pho·bia [,kænsər'fəʊbɪə] *n* Krebsangst *f*, Kanzerophobie *f*, Karzinophobie *f*.
cancer-related *adj* durch Krebs(erkrankung) bedingt *od.* verursacht.
cancer risk Krebsrisiko *nt*.
cancer surgery Tumor-, Krebschirurgie *f*, Chirurgie *f* maligner Tumoren.
can·cri·form ['kæŋkrəfɔːrm] *adj* krebsähnlich, -förmig.
can·croid ['kæŋkrɔɪd] **I** *n* Kankroid *nt*. **II** *adj* krebsähnlich, kankroid.
can·del·a [kæn'delə, -'diː-] *n abbr.* **cd** *phys.* Candela *f abbr.* cd.
can·de·la·brum cell [,kændə'lɑːbrəm, -'leɪ-] *histol.* Armleuchterzelle *f*.
Can·di·da ['kændɪdə] *n micro.* Candida *f*, Monilia *f*, Oidium *nt*.
C. albicans Candida albicans, *old* Monilia/Oidium albicans.
candida antigen Candidaantigen *nt*.
Candida esophagitis Candida-Ösophagitis *f*.
candida granuloma → candidal granuloma.
candida intertrigo → candidal intertrigo.
can·di·dal ['kændɪdəl] *adj* Candida betr., durch Candida verursacht, Kandida-, Candida-.
candidal granuloma Candida-, Soorgranulom *nt*.
candidal intertrigo Candidose *f* der Körperfalten, Candida-Intertrigo *f*.
candidal vulvovaginitis Candida-Vulvovaginitis *f*.
can·di·date ['kændɪdeɪt, -dət] *n* Anwärter(in *f*) *m*, Kandidat(in *f*) *m* (*for* für); Prüfling *m*; Versuchs-, Testperson *f*, Proband(in *f*) *m*.

can·di·de·mia [,kændə'diːmɪə] *n* Candidämie *f*.
can·di·di·a·sis [,-'daɪəsɪs] *n* Kandida-, Candida-, Soormykose *f*, Candidiasis *f*, Candidose *f*, Moniliasis *f*, Moniliose *f*.
c. of the oral mucosa Mundsoor, Candidose der Mundschleimhaut.
can·di·did ['kændədɪd] *n* Candidid *nt*, Candida-Mykid *nt*.
can·di·din ['kændədɪn] *n* Candidin *nt*.
can·di·do·sis [,kændɪ'dəʊsɪs] *n* → candidiasis.
can·di·du·ria [,-'d(j)ʊərɪə] *n* Candidaausscheidung *f* im Harn, Candidurie *f*.
can·died ['kændɪd] *adj* gezuckert, überzuckert, kandiert; *pharm.* dragiert.
can·dle ['kændl] *n* **1.** (Wachs-)Kerze *f*. **2.** → candela.
candle-meter *n phys.* Lux *nt abbr.* lx.
cane [keɪn] *n* (Rohr-, Geh-)Stock *m*.
cane-cutter's cramp Heizerkrampf *m*.
cane-field fever Zuckerrohrfieber, Zuckerplantagenleptospirose *f*, cane-field fever (*nt*).
cane sugar Rüben-, Rohrzucker *m*, Saccharose *f*.
ca·nic·o·la fever [kə'nɪkjələ] **1.** Kanikola-, Canicolafieber *nt*, Leptospirosis canicola. **2.** Stuttgarter-Hundeseuche *f*.
ca·nine ['keɪnaɪn] **I** *n* **1.** Eck-, Reißzahn *m*, Dens caninus. **2.** *bio.* Hund. **II** *adj* **3.** Dens caninus betr. **4.** *bio.* Hunde-, Hunds-.
canine fossa Fossa canina.
canine laugh sardonisches Lachen *nt*, Risus sardonicus.
canine leishmaniasis Mittelmeerform *f* der viszeralen Leishmaniose.
canine leptospirosis → canicola fever.
canine muscle *anat.* M. levator anguli oris.
canine spasm sardonisches Lachen *nt*, Risus sardonicus.
canine tooth → canine 1.
canine typhus → canicola fever.
ca·ni·nus [keɪ'naɪnəs, kə-] *n anat.* M. levator anguli oris.
ca·ni·ti·es [kə'nɪʃɪ,iːz] *n derm.* Grau-, Weißhaarigkeit *f*, Canities *f*, Poliosis *f*.
can·na·bi·di·ol [,kænəbɪ'daɪəʊl, -ɒl] *n* Cannabidiol *nt*.
can·nab·i·noid [kə'næbɪnɔɪd, 'kænəbɪ-] *n* Cannabinoid *nt*.
can·nab·i·nol [kə'næbɪnɒl, -nəl] *n* Cannabinol *nt*.
can·na·bis (sa·ti·va) ['kænəbɪs] *n* **1.** (indischer) Hanf *m*, Cannabis (sativa). **2.** (*Rauschgift*) Kannabis *m*, Cannabis *m*, Marihuana *nt*, Haschisch *nt*.
can·na·bism ['kænəbɪzəm] *n* **1.** Cannabisintoxikation *f*. **2.** Haschischsucht *f*, Cannabisabusus *m*, Cannabismus *m*.
can·nel·lat·ed ['kænəleɪtɪd] *adj* geriffelt, gerieft, gerillt, kanneliert.
can·nel·lat·ed → cannelated.
can·ni·bal ['kænɪbl] *n* **1.** Menschenfresser *m*, Kannibale *m*, Anthropophage *m*. **2.** *bio.* Kannibale *m*.
can·ni·bal·ic [,kænɪ'bælɪk] *adj* kannibalisch.
can·ni·bal·ism ['kænɪbəlɪzəm] *n* Kannibalismus *m*.
can·ni·bal·is·tic [,-'lɪstɪk] *adj* kannibalisch.
Cannizzaro [kænɪ'zɑːrəʊ]: **C.'s reaction** Cannizzaro-Reaktion *f*.
Cannon ['kænən]: **C.'s point** Cannon-Böhm-Punkt *m*.
C.'s ring C.'s point.
C.'s theory Cannon-Notfallreaktion *f*.
can·non-ball pulse ['kænənbɔːl] **1.** Corrigan-Puls *m*, Pulsus celer et altus. **2.** Wasserhammerpuls *m*.

cannon beat ['kænən] → cannon sound.
cannon sound Kanonenschlag *m*, Bruit de canon.
can·nu·la ['kænjələ] *n, pl* **-las, -lae** [-liː] Hohlnadel *f*, Kanüle *f*.
can·nu·lar ['kænjələr] *adj* röhrenförmig.
can·nu·late ['kænjə,leɪt, -lɪt] **I** *adj* → cannular. **II** *vt* eine Kanüle legen *od.* einführen, kanülieren.
can·nu·la·tion [,kænjə'leɪʃn] *n* Kanüleneinführung *f*, -legen *nt*, Kanülierung *f*.
can·nu·li·za·tion [,kænjəlɪ'zeɪʃn] *n* → cannulation.
cant [kænt] *n* Schräge *f*, Neigung *f*, geneigte Fläche *f*.
Cantelli [kæn'teli]: **C.'s sign** Cantelli-Zeichen *nt*, Puppenaugenphänomen *nt*.
can·ter·ing rhythm ['kæntərɪŋ] Galopp *m*, Galopprhythmus *m*.
can·thal ['kænθəl] *adj* Augenwinkel betr.
canthal hypertelorism *ophthal.* Telekanthus *m*.
canthal ligament Lig. palpebrale laterale.
can·tha·ri·a·sis [kænθə'raɪəsɪs] *n micro.* Kanthariasis *f*.
can·thar·i·dal [kæn'θærɪdl] *adj micro.* Kanthariden betr., Kantharidin-.
can·thar·i·des [kæn'θærɪdiːz] *pl* Blasen-, Pflasterkäfer *pl*, spanische Fliegen *pl*, Kantharidin *pl*, Cantharides *pl*.
can·thar·i·din [kæn'θærədɪn] *n* Kantharidin *nt*, Cantharidin *f*.
can·thec·to·my [kæn'θektəmɪ] *n ophthal.* Kanthektomie *f*.
can·thi·tis [kæn'θaɪtɪs] *n ophthal.* Augenwinkelentzündung *f*, Kanthitis *f*.
can·thol·y·sis [kæn'θɒləsɪs] *n ophthal.* Kantholyse *f*.
can·tho·plas·ty ['kænθəplæstɪ] *n ophthal.* Kanthoplastik *f*.
can·thor·rha·phy [kæn'θɒrəfɪ] *n ophthal.* Kantho(r)rhaphie *f*.
can·thot·o·my [kæn'θɒtəmɪ] *n ophthal.* Kanthotomie *f*.
can·thus ['kænθəs] *n, pl* **-thi** [-θaɪ] Augenwinkel *m*, Kanthus *m*, Canthus *m*.
C antigen *hema.* Antigen C *nt*.
Cantor ['kæntər, -tɔr]: **C. tube** Cantor-Sonde *f*.
ca·nu·la *n* → cannula.
ca·nu·lar *adj* → cannular.
CaOC *abbr.* → cathodal opening contraction.
CaOCl *abbr.* → cathodal opening clonus.
caou·tchouc ['kaʊtʃʊk] *n* Naturgummi *nt*, Kautschuk *m*.
caoutchouc pelvis *patho.* Gummibecken *nt*.
CAP *abbr.* **1.** → catabolite gene-activator protein. **2.** → cyclic AMP receptor protein.
cap [kæp] *n* **1.** *anat.* Kniescheibe *f*, Patella *f*. **2.** haubenähnliche Struktur *f*, Kappe *f*. **3.** *dent.* (Ersatz-)Krone *f*. **4.** (Schutz-, Verschluß-)Kappe *f*, Deckel *m*. **5.** Mütze *f*, Kappe *f*; (Schwestern-)Haube *f*. **6.** *inf.* (Drogen-)Kapsel *m*. **II** *vt* **7.** (mit einer Kappe) bedecken *od.* überziehen; verschließen, zumachen. **8.** (*Schicht*) liegen auf *od.* über, überlagern. **9.** (*Deckel, Kappe*) abnehmen, -ziehen.
ca·pa·bil·i·ty [,keɪpə'bɪlətɪ] *n, pl* **-ties 1.** Kompetenz *f*, (Leistungs-)Fähigkeit *f*, Tüchtigkeit *f*. **2.** ~s *pl* Potential *nt* (*of sth.* zu etw.).
ca·pa·ble ['keɪpəbl] *adj* **1.** (leistungs-)fähig, tüchtig, kompetent. **2.** geeignet, tauglich (*for* zu). **3.** fähig, imstande (*of doing* zu tun); zulassend.
ca·pa·cious [kə'peɪʃəs] *adj* geräumig, weit; *fig.* aufnahmefähig.

ca·pac·i·tance [kəˈpæsɪtəns] *n* **1.** Speichervermögen *nt*, -fähigkeit *f*, Kapazität *f*. **2.** *abbr*. **C** (elektrische) Kapazität *f*.
capacitance vessel Kapazitätsgefäß *nt*.
ca·pac·i·ta·tion [kəˌpæsɪˈteɪʃn] *n embryo*. Kapazitation *f*.
ca·pac·i·tive [kəˈpæsɪtɪv] *adj electr*. kapazitiv.
capacitive current kapazitiver Strom *m*.
capacitive load kapazitive Belastung *f*.
capacitive reactance kapazitiver Widerstand *m*, Kapazitanz *f*.
ca·pac·i·tor [kəˈpæsɪtər] *n electr*. Kondensator *m*.
ca·pac·i·ty [kəˈpæsətɪ] **I** *n, pl* **-ties 1.** Kapazität *f*, Fassungsvermögen *nt*, Volumen *nt*, (Raum-)Inhalt *m*. **filled to ~** randvoll, ganz voll. **to have a ~ of** ein Volumen von ... haben. **2.** Auffassungsgabe *f*, -vermögen *m*. **3.** (Leistungs-)Fähigkeit *f*, (-)Vermögen *nt*. **4.** *chem*. Bindungskapazität *f*. **5.** *phys. old* → capacitance. **6.** Eigenschaft *f*, Funktion *f*. **II** *adj* maximal, Höchst-, Maximal-.
c. for learning Lernfähigkeit.
CAPD *abbr*. → continuous ambulatory peritoneal dialysis.
Capdepont [kapdəˈpõ]: **C.'s disease** Glaszähne *pl*, Capdepont-Zahndysplasie *f*, -Syndrom *nt*, Stainton-Syndrom *nt*, Dentinogenesis imperfecta hereditaria.
Capgras [ˈkapgrɑ]: **C.' phenomenon/syndrome** *psychia*. Capgras-Syndrom *nt*.
cap·il·lar·ec·ta·sia [ˌkæpɪˌlerəkˈteɪʒ(ɪ)ə] *n* Kapillarektasie *f*.
Cap·il·lar·ia [ˌ-ˈleərɪə] *n micro*. Capillaria *f*.
cap·il·lar·i·a·sis [ˌkæpɪləˈraɪəsɪs] *n micro*. **1.** Capillaria-Infektion *f*, Capillariasis *f*. **2.** intestinale Capillariasis *f*, Capillariasis philippinensis.
cap·il·lar·i·os·co·py [ˌkæpəˌlerɪˈɑskəpɪ] *n* → capillaroscopy.
cap·il·lar·i·tis [kəpɪləˈraɪtɪs] *n* Kapillarenentzündung *f*, Kapillaritis *f*.
cap·il·lar·i·ty [ˌkæpɪˈlærətɪ] *n phys*. Kapillarität *f*, Kapillarwirkung *f*.
cap·il·la·rop·a·thy [ˌkæpɪləˈrɑpəθɪ] *n* Kapillarerkrankung *f*.
cap·il·la·ros·co·py [ˌ-ˈrɑskəpɪ] *n* Kapillarmikroskopie *f*, Kapillaroskopie *f*.
cap·il·lar·y [ˈkæpəˌlerɪ, kəˈpɪlərɪ] **I** *n, pl* **-ries 1.** Haargefäß *nt*, Kapillare *f*, Vas capillare. **2.** Kapillarröhre *f*, -gefäß *nt*. **3.** Lymphkapillare, Vas lymphocapillare. **II** *adj* haarfein, -förmig, kapillar, kapillär; *phys*. Kapillarität betr.; *anat*. Kapillare(n) betr., Kapillar-.
capillary action *phys*. → capillarity.
capillary angioma → capillary hemangioma.
capillary apoplexy kapilläre Apoplexie *f*.
capillary attraction *phys*. → capillarity.
capillary bed Kapillarbett *nt*, -stromgebiet *nt*, -netz *nt*.
capillary bronchiectasis Bronchiolenerweiterung *f*, -dilatation *f*.
capillary bronchitis Bronchopneumonie *f*, lobuläre Pneumonie *f*; Herd-, Fokalpneumonie *f*.
capillary buds Kapillarsprossen *pl*.
capillary circulation Kapillarkreislauf *m*, -zirkulation *f*.
capillary density Kapillardichte *f*, Kapillarisierung *f*.
capillary embolism Kapillarembolie *f*.
capillary embolus Kapillarembolus *m*.
capillary endothelium Kapillarendothel *nt*.
capillary fracture Haarbruch *m*, Knochenfissur *f*.
capillary fragility Kapillarfragilität *f*.

capillary fragility test Kapillarresistenzprüfung *f*.
capillary hemangioma 1. Kapillarhämangiom *nt*, Haemangioma capillare. **2.** Blutschwamm *m*, blastomatöses Hämangiom *nt*, Haemangioma planotuberosum/simplex.
capillary hemorrhage Kapillarblutung *f*.
capillary loop Kapillarschlinge *f*.
capillary lymphangioma kapilläres/einfaches Lymphangiom *nt*, Lymphangioma capillare/simplex.
capillary membrane Kapillarmembran *f*.
capillary pericytes Rouget-Zellen *pl*.
capillary permeability Kapillardurchlässigkeit *f*, -permeabilität *f*.
capillary pressure Kapillardruck *m*.
capillary pulse Kapillarpuls *m*, Quincke'-Zeichen *nt*.
capillary resistance test → capillary fragility test.
capillary system Kapillarbett *nt*, -stromgebiet *nt*, -netz *nt*.
villous c. villöses Kapillarbett, -system *nt*.
capillary tube → capillary 2.
capillary vessel Kapillargefäß *nt*, Vas capillare.
cap·il·li·ti·um [ˌkæpəˈlɪʃɪəm] *n micro*. Kapillitium *nt*.
cap·il·lo·mo·tor [ˌkæpɪləˈməʊtər] *adj* kapillomotorisch.
ca·pil·lus [kəˈpɪləs] *n, pl* **-li** [-laɪ, -liː] (Kopf-)Haar *nt*, Capillus *m*.
cap·i·stra·tion [ˌkæpɪˈstreɪʃn] *n ped., urol*. Phimose *f*.
cap·i·tate [ˈkæpɪteɪt] **I** *n* Kapitatum *nt*, Os capitatum. **II** *adj bio., anat*. kopfförmig.
capitate bone → capitate I.
cap·i·tat·ed [ˈkæpɪteɪtɪd] *adj* → capitate II.
capitate eminence → capitulum 2.
capitate papillae Wallpapillen *pl*, Papillae vallatae.
cap·i·ta·tum [ˌkæpɪˈteɪtəm] *n, pl* **-ta·ta** [-ˈteɪtə] *n* Kapitatum *nt*, Os capitatum.
cap·i·tel·lum [ˌ-ˈteləm] *n, pl* **-la** [-lə] → capitulum 2.
ca·pit·u·lar [kəˈpɪtʃələr] *adj* Knochenkopf *od*. -köpfchen/Capitulum betr., kapitulär.
capitular articulation (of rib) Rippenkopfgelenk *nt*, Artic. capitis costae/costalis.
capitular joint (of rib) → capitular articulation (of rib).
capitular ligament, volar Lig. metacarpeum transversum profundum.
ca·pit·u·lum [kəˈpɪtʃələm] *n, pl* **-la** [-lə] **1.** Knochenkopf *m*, -köpfchen *nt*, Kapitulum *nt*, Capitulum *nt*. **2.** Humerusköpfchen *nt*, Capitulum humeri.
c. of humerus → capitulum 2.
capitulum ulnae syndrome *ortho*. Caput-ulnae-Syndrom *nt*.
Caplan [ˈkæplæn]: **C.'s nodules/syndrome** Caplan-Syndrom *nt*, Caplan-Colinet-Petry-Syndrom *nt*, Silikoarthritis *f*.
cap·line bandage [ˈkæpləɪn] *ortho*. Kopfmütze(nverband *m*) *f*.
cap·ne·ic [ˈkæpnɪːɪk] *adj* kapnoisch.
Cap·no·cy·toph·a·ga [ˌkæpnəʊsaɪˈtɑfəgə] *n micro*. Capnocytophaga *f*.
cap·no·phil·ic [ˌkæpnəˈfɪlɪk] *adj micro*. kohlendioxidliebend, kapnophil.
cap·ping [ˈkæpɪŋ] *n immun*. Capping *nt*.
Capps [ˈkæps]: **C.'s reflex** Capps-Reflex *m*. **C.'s sign 1.** Capps-Zeichen *nt*. **2.** Capps-Reflex *m*.
cap·rate [ˈkæpreɪt] *n* Kaprat *nt*, Caprat *nt*.
cap·re·o·my·cin [ˌkæprɪəˈmaɪsɪn] *n pharm*. Capreomycin *nt*.
ca·pril·o·quism [kəˈprɪləkwɪzəm] *n* (*Auskultation*) Ziegenmeckern *nt*, Kompressionsatmen *nt*, Ägophonie *f*.

cap·rin [ˈkæprɪn] *n* Caprin *nt*.
cap·rine [ˈkæpraɪn] *n* Norleucin *nt*, α-Amino-*n*-capronsäure *f*.
cap·ri·zant [ˈkæprɪzænt] *adj* (*Puls*) schnellend.
cap·ro·ate [ˈkæprəweɪt] *n* Kaproat *nt*, Caproat *nt*.
ca·pro·ic acid [kəˈprəʊɪk] Kapron-, Capronsäure *f*, Butylessigsäure *f*, Hexansäure *f*.
cap·ro·yl [ˈkæprəwɪl, -wiːl] *n* Caproyl-, Hexyl-(Radikal *nt*).
cap·ro·yl·a·mine [ˌkæprəwɪləˈmiːn, -ˈæmɪn] *n n*-Hexylamin *nt*.
cap·ry·late [ˈkæprəleɪt] *n* Kaprylat *nt*, Caprylat *nt*.
ca·pryl·ic acid [kəˈprɪlɪk, kæ-] Kapryl-, Caprylsäure *f*, Oktansäure *f*.
CAPS *abbr*. → carbamoyl-phosphate synthetase (ammonia).
CAPS deficiency → carbamoyl phosphate synthetase deficiency.
cap·sa·i·cin [kæpˈseɪəsɪn] *n* Capsaicin *nt*.
cap·sid [ˈkæpsɪd] *n micro*. Kapsid *nt*.
capsid protein Kapsidprotein *nt*.
cap·si·tis [kæpˈsaɪtɪs] *n ophthal*. Entzündung *f* der Glaskörperkapsel, Kapsitis *f*.
cap·so·mer [ˈkæpsəmər] *n micro*. Kapsomer *nt*.
cap·so·mere [ˈ-mɪər] *n* → capsomer.
cap·sot·o·my [kæpˈsɑtəmɪ] *n* → capsulotomy.
cap·su·lar [ˈkæpsələr] *adj* **1.** Kapsel betr., kapsulär, kapselartig, -förmig, Kapsel-. **2.** → capsulate.
capsular abscess *ortho*. (*Gelenk*) Kapselphlegmone *f*.
capsular antigen Kapselantigen *nt*, K-Antigen *nt*.
capsular artery: inferior c. untere Nebennierenarterie *f*, Suprarenalis *f* inferior, A. suprarenalis inferior.
middle c. mittlere Nebennierenarterie *f*, Suprarenalis *f* media, A. suprarenalis/adrenalis media.
capsular branches of renal artery Kapseläste *pl* der Nierenarterie, Aa. capsulares/perirenales.
capsular cataract Kapselstar *m*, Cataracta capsularis.
capsular cirrhosis (of liver) Glisson'-Zirrhose *f*.
capsular contracture kapsuläre Kontraktur *f*.
capsular decidua Decidua capsularis/reflexa.
capsular fibers Kapselfasern *pl*, Fasern *pl* der inneren Kapsel.
capsular glaucoma Kapselhäutchenglaukom *nt*, Glaucoma capsulare.
capsular hyalinosis (Milz-)Kapselhyalinose *f*.
capsular ligament: c.s *pl* Kapselbänder *pl*, Ligg. capsularia.
internal c. Lig. capitis femoris.
capsular membrane Gelenkkapsel *f*, Capsula articularis.
capsular nephritis Nephritis *f* mit Entzündung der Bowman-Kapsel.
capsular space (*Niere*) Bowman'-Raum *m*.
capsular swelling *micro*. Neufeld-Reaktion *f*, Kapselquellungsreaktion *f*.
capsular thrombosis syndrome Capsula-interna-Thrombose-Syndrom *nt*.
capsular veins Vv. capsulares.
cap·su·late [ˈkæpsəleɪt, -lɪt, -sjʊ-] *adj* eingekapselt, verkapselt.
cap·su·lat·ed [ˌ-leɪtɪd] *adj* → capsulate.
cap·su·la·tion [ˌkæpsəˈleɪʃn] *n pharm*. Verkapseln *nt*, Verkaps(e)lung *f*.
cap·sule [ˈkæpsəl, -s(j)uːl] **I** *n* **1.** *bio*. Kapsel

capsule cell

f, Hülle *f*, Schale *f*. **2.** *anat.* (Organ-)Kapsel *f*, Capsula *f*. **3.** *pharm.* (Arznei-)Kapsel *f*. **4.** *micro.* (Schleim-)Kapsel *f*. **5.** *patho.* Tumorkapsel *f*. **6.** (*Flasche*) (Metall-)Kapsel *f*. **II** *adj* klein u. kompakt, Kurz-. **III** *vt* ein-, verkapseln.
c. of ganglion Gangllienkapsel, Capsula ganglii/ganglionica.
c. of heart Herzbeutel *m*, Perikard *nt*, Pericardium *nt*.
c. of lens Linsenkapsel, Capsula lentis.
c. of pancreas Pankreaskapsel, Capsula pancreatis.
c. of prostate Prostatakapsel, Capsula prostatica.
capsule cell Mantelzelle *f*, Amphizyt *m*.
cap·sul·ec·to·my [kæpsə'lektəmɪ] *n chir.* operative (Teil-)Entfernung *f* einer Organkapsel, Kapsulektomie *f*.
capsule forceps *chir.* Kapselfaßzange *f*.
capsule polysaccharide *micro.* Kapselpolysaccharid *nt*.
capsule stain *micro.* Kapselfärbung *f*.
capsule swelling reaction *micro.* Neufeld-Reaktion *f*, Kapselquellungsreaktion *f*.
cap·su·li·tis [kæpsə'laɪtɪs] *n* Kapselentzündung *f*, Kapsulitis *f*.
cap·sul·ize ['kæpsəlaɪz, -sjʊ-] *vt* ein-, verkapseln.
cap·su·lo·len·tic·u·lar [ˌkæpsjələʊlen'tɪkjələr] *adj ophthal.* (*Auge*) Linse u. Linsenkapsel betr., kapsulolentikulär.
cap·su·lo·lig·a·men·tal contracture [ˌ-lɪgə'mentl] kapsulär-ligamentäre Kontraktur *f*.
cap·su·lo·ma [kæpsə'ləʊmə] *n* kapsulärer *od.* subkapsulärer Nierentumor *m*.
cap·su·lo·plas·ty ['kæpsjələʊplæstɪ] *n ortho.* Kapselplastik *f*.
cap·su·lo·pu·pil·lar·y membrane [ˌ-'pjuːpɪlərɪ, -ˌleriː] *embryo.* Membrana pupillaris.
cap·su·lor·rha·phy [kæpsə'lɒrəfɪ] *n chir.*, *ortho.* Kapselnaht *f*, Kapsulorrhaphie *f*.
cap·sul·o·tome ['kæpsjələtəʊm] *n ophthal.* Kapselmesser *nt*, Kapsulotom *nt*.
cap·su·lot·o·my [kæpsjə'lɒtəmɪ] *n chir.*, *ophthal.*, *ortho.* Kapseleröffnung *f*, -spaltung *f*, Kapsulotomie *f*.
capsulotomy scissors *chir.*, *ortho.* Kapselschere *f*.
cap·to·pril ['kæptəprɪl] *n pharm.* Captopril *nt*.
cap·ture beat ['kæptʃər] *card.* Capture beat (*m*).
cap·ut ['keɪpʊt, 'kæp-] *n*, *pl* **ca·pi·ta** ['kæpɪtə] *anat.* **1.** Kopf *m*, Caput *nt*. **2.** kopfförmige Struktur *f*.
caput-epiphysis angle *ortho.* (*Femur*) Kopf-Epiphysen-Winkel *m*.
car·a·mel ['kærəməl, -mel] *n pharm.* Karamel *m*, gebrannter Zucker *m*.
ca·ra·te [kə'rɑːtɪ] *n* Carate *f*, Pinta *f*, Mal del Pinto.
car·a·way ['kærəweɪ] *n* Kümmel *m*.
caraway oil Kümmelöl *nt*.
car·ba·chol ['kɑːrbəkɒl, -kal] *n* Karbachol *nt*, Carbachol *nt*, Carbamoylcholinchlorid *nt*.
car·ba·mate ['kɑːrbəmeɪt, kɑːr'bæmeɪt] *n* Carbamat *nt*.
car·ba·maz·e·pine [kɑːrbə'mæzəpiːn] *n pharm.* Carbamazepin *nt*.
car·bam·ic acid [kɑːr'bæmɪk] Carbaminsäure *f*, Carbamidsäure *f*.
carbamic acid ethyl ester Urethan *nt*, Carbaminsäureäthylester *nt*.
car·ba·mide ['kɑːrbəmaɪd, -mɪd, kɑːr'bæm-] *n* Harnstoff *m*, Karbamid *nt*, Carbamid *nt*, Urea *f*.
carb·am·i·no·he·mo·glo·bin [kɑːrb,æmɪ-

nəʊ'hiːməˌgləʊbɪn] *n* Carbaminohämoglobin *nt*, Carbhämoglobin *nt*.
car·ba·mo·ate ['kɑːbəməʊeɪt] *n* → carbamate.
car·bam·o·yl [kɑːr'bæməwɪl, -iːl] *n* Carbam(o)yl-(Radikal *nt*).
N-car·ba·mo·yl·as·par·tate [ˌkɑːrbəməʊɪlæs'pɑːrteɪt] *n* N-Carbam(o)ylaspartat *nt*.
carbamoylaspartate dehydrase Dihydroorotase *f*.
carbamoyl phosphate Carbam(o)ylphosphat *nt*.
carbamoyl-phosphate synthetase (ammonia) *abbr.* **CAPS** Carbam(o)ylphosphatsynthetase (Ammoniak) *f abbr.* CAPS.
carbamoyl phosphate synthetase deficiency Carbam(o)ylphosphatsynthetasemangel *m*, kongenitale Hyperammonämie Typ I *f*.
carbamoyl-phosphate synthetase (glutamine) Carbam(o)ylphosphatsynthetase (Glutamin) *f*.
carbamoyl phosphoric acid Carbam(o)ylphosphorsäure *f*.
car·ba·mo·yl·trans·fer·ase [ˌ-'trænsfəreɪz] *n* Carbam(o)yltransferase *f*, Transcarbam(o)ylase *f*.
car·ba·mo·yl·u·rea [ˌ-jə'rɪə] *n* Biuret *nt*, Allophanamid *nt*.
car·ba·myl ['kɑːrbəmɪl] *n* → carbamoyl.
car·ba·myl·cho·line [ˌkɑːrbəmɪl'kəʊliːn, -'kal-] *n* Carbamylcholin *nt*.
carbamylcholine chloride → carbachol.
carb·an·i·on [kɑːrb'ænaɪən, -aɪan] *n chem.* Carbanion *nt*.
car·ba·ril *n* → carbaryl.
car·bar·sone [ˈkɑːrbəsəʊn] *n pharm.* Carbason *nt*, 4-Carbamidophenylarsinsäure *f*.
car·ba·ryl ['kɑːrbərɪl] *n* Carbaryl *nt*.
car·baz·o·chrome [kɑːr'bæzəkrəʊm] *n pharm.* Carbazochrom *nt*.
car·baz·o·tate [kɑːr'bæzəteɪt] *n* Pikrat *nt*.
car·ben·i·cil·lin [ˌkɑːrbenə'sɪlɪn] *n pharm.* Carbenicillin *nt*, α-Carboxypenicillin *nt*.
car·ben·ox·o·lone [kɑːr'bɛn'ɒksələʊn] *n pharm.* Carbenoxolon *nt*.
carb·he·mo·glo·bin [kɑːrb'hiːməgləʊbɪn] *n* → carbaminohemoglobin.
car·bide ['kɑːrbaɪd, -bɪd] *n* Karbid *nt*.
car·bi·do·pa [kɑːrbɪ'dəʊpə] *n pharm.* Carbidopa *nt*.
car·bi·ma·zole [kɑːr'bɪməzəʊl] *n pharm.* Carbimazol *nt*.
car·bi·nol ['kɑːrbɪnɒl, -nɑl] *n* Methanol *nt*, Methylalkohol *m*.
car·bin·ox·a·mine [kɑːrbɪn'ɒksəmiːn] *n pharm.* Carbinoxamin *nt*.
car·bo ['kɑːrbəʊ] *n* Kohle *f*, Carbo *m*.
car·bo·cho·line [ˌkɑːrbəʊ'kəʊliːn] *n* → carbachol.
car·bo·chrom·en *n* → carbocromen.
car·bo·cro·men [ˌ-'krəʊmiːn] *n pharm.* Carboc(h)romen *nt*.
car·bo·cy·clic [ˌ-'saɪklɪk, -sɪk-] *adj chem.* karbo-, carbozyklisch.
car·bo·di·im·ide [ˌ-daɪ'ɪmaɪd] *n* Carbodiimid *nt*.
car·bo·gas·e·ous [ˌ-'gæsɪəs] *adj* mit Kohlendioxid beladen.
car·bo·gen ['kɑːrbədʒən] *n chem.* Carbogen *nt*.
car·bo·he·mia [ˌ-'hiːmɪə] *n physiol.* (*Blut*) Kohlendioxidüberschuß *m*, Karbo-, Carbohämie *f*.
car·bo·he·mo·glo·bin [ˌ-'hiːməˌgləʊbɪn] *n* → carbaminohemoglobin.
car·bo·hy·drase [ˌ-'haɪdreɪz] *n* Karbo-, Carbohydrase *f*.
car·bo·hy·drate [ˌ-'haɪdreɪt, -drɪt] *n* Kohle(n)hydrat *nt abbr.* KH, Saccharid *nt*.

carbohydrate breakdown *biochem.* Kohlenhydratabbau *m*.
carbohydrate broth Kohlenhydrat(nähr)bouillon *f*.
carbohydrate catabolism Kohlenhydratkatabolismus *m*.
carbohydrate-induced hyperlipemia 1. (primäre/essentielle) Hyperlipoproteinämie Typ III *f*, Hypercholesterinämie *f* mit Hypertriglyzeridämie, Broad-Beta-Disease (*nt*), Hyperlipoproteinämie *f* mit breiter Betabande. **2.** (primäre/essentielle) Hyperlipoproteinämie Typ IV *f*, endogene/kohlenhydratinduzierte Hyperlipidämie/Triglyzeridämie *f*, familiäre Hypertriglyzeridämie *f*.
carbohydrate-induced hypertriglyceridemia (primäre/essentielle) Hyperlipoproteinämie Typ III *f*, Hypercholesterinämie *f* mit Hypertriglyzeridämie, Broad-Beta-Disease (*nt*), Hyperlipoproteinämie *f* mit breiter Betabande.
carbohydrate malabsorption Kohlenhydratmalabsorption *f*.
carbohydrate metabolism Kohlenhydratstoffwechsel *m*, -metabolismus *m*.
carbohydrate synthesis Kohlenhydratsynthese *f*.
car·bo·hy·dra·tu·ria [ˌ-ˌhaɪdrə't(j)ʊərɪə] *n* (übermäßige) Kohlenhydratausscheidung *f* im Harn, Karbo-, Carbohydraturie *f*.
car·bo·late [ˈkɑːbəleɪt] *n* Phenolat *nt*.
car·bol·fuch·sin paint [ˌkɑːrbal'f(j)ʊksɪn, -'fjuːʃɪn] *derm.* Castellani-Lösung *f*.
carbolfuchsin solution → carbolfuchsin paint.
carbolfuchsin stain *histol.* Karbolfuchsinfärbung *f*.
carbol-gentian violet stain Karbolgentianaviolettfärbung *f*.
car·bol·ic acid [kɑːr'bɑlɪk] Phenol *nt*, Karbolsäure *f*, Monohydroxybenzol *nt*.
car·bol·ism ['kɑːrbəlɪzəm] *n* Phenolvergiftung *f*, -intoxikation *f*, Karbolismus *m*.
car·bo·li·za·tion [kɑːrbəlaɪ'zeɪʃn] *n* Behandlung *f* mit Phenol, Karbolisierung *f*, Phenolisierung *f*.
car·bo·lize ['kɑːrbəlaɪz] **I** *vt* mit Phenol behandeln. **II** *vi* mit Phenol behandelt werden.
car·bo·lu·ria [kɑːrbə'l(j)ʊərɪə] *n* Phenolausscheidung *f* im Harn, Karbolurie *f*, Phenolurie *f*.
car·bon ['kɑːrbən] *n abbr.* **C** Kohlenstoff *m*; *chem.* Carboneum *nt abbr.* C.
car·bo·na·ceous [kɑːrbə'neɪʃəs] *adj chem.* Kohle(nstoff) enthaltend, kohlenstoffhaltig, -artig.
carbon arc Kohlenstofflichtbogen *m*, Bogenentladung *f*/Lichtbogen *m* zwischen Kohlenstoffelektroden.
car·bon·ate [*n* 'kɑːrbənət, -nɪt; *v* -neɪt] **I** *n* Karbonat *nt*, Carbonat *nt*. **II** *vt* **1.** karbonisieren, mit Kohlensäure *od.* Kohlendioxid versetzen. **2.** in Karbonat umwandeln, karbinosieren.
c. of soda Soda *nt*, kohlensaures Natron *nt*, Natriumkarbonat.
carbonate dehydratase → carbonic anhydrase.
car·bon·at·ed water ['kɑːrbəneɪtɪd] Sodawasser *nt*.
carbon atom, asymmetric *chem.* asymmetrisches Kohlenstoffatom *nt*.
carbon-carbon bond Kohlenstoff-Kohlenstoff-Bindung *f*.
carbon compound Kohlenstoffverbindung *f*.
carbon cycle *biochem.* Kohlenstoffkreislauf *m*.
carbon dioxide *abbr.* CO_2 Kohlendioxid *nt abbr.* CO_2.

carbon dioxide acidosis *physiol.* respiratorische Azidose *f.*
carbon dioxide bath Kohlendioxidbad *nt.*
carbon dioxide cycle → carbon cycle.
carbon dioxide fixation *biochem.* Kohlendioxidfixierung *f.*
carbon dioxide laser Kohlendioxidlaser *m*, CO$_2$-Laser *m.*
carbon dioxide narcosis Kohlensäurenarkose *f.*
carbon dioxide partial pressure *abbr.* Pco$_2$, pCO$_2$ Kohlendioxidpartialdruck *m*, CO$_2$-Partialdruck *m abbr.* Pco$_2$, pCO$_2$.
carbon dioxide snow Trockeneis *nt*, Kohlendioxidschnee *m*, gefrorenes Kohlendioxid *nt.*
carbon dioxide tension *physiol.* Kohlendioxidspannung *f.*
carbon disulfide poisoning Schwefelkohlenstoffvergiftung *f.*
carbon dust *electr.* Kohlenstaub *m.*
car·bo·ne·mia [ˌkɑːrbəˈniːmɪə] *n* → carbohemia.
carbon fiber Kohlenstoffaser *f*, C-Faser *f.*
car·bon·ic [kɑːrˈbɒnɪk] *adj chem.* Kohlenstoff *od.* Kohlensäure *od.* Kohlendioxid betr., Kohlen-.
carbonic acid Kohlensäure *f.*
carbonic anhydrase *abbr.* CA Kohlensäureanhydrase *f*, Karbonatdehydratase *f*, Carboanhydrase *f abbr.* CA, CAH.
carbonic anhydrase inhibitor Carboanhydrasehemmstoff *m*, -inhibitor *m.*
carbonic anhydride → carbon dioxide.
car·bon·if·er·ous [ˌkɑːrbəˈnɪfərəs] *adj chem.* Kohle(nstoff) enthaltend *od.* erzeugend, kohlenstoffhaltig, kohlehaltig.
car·bon·i·za·tion [ˌkɑːrbənaɪˈzeɪʃn] *n chem.* Karbonisation *f*, Karbonisieren *nt*, Verkohlung *f.*
car·bon·ize [ˈkɑːrbənaɪz] *chem.* I *vt* verkohlen, karbonisieren. II *vi* verkohlen. ~ **at a low temperature** schwelen.
carbon monoxide *abbr.* CO Kohlenmonoxid *nt abbr.* CO, Kohlenoxid *nt*; Kohlensäureanhydrid *nt.*
carbon monoxide hemoglobin → carboxyhemoglobin.
carbon monoxide poisoning Kohlenmonoxidvergiftung *f*, CO-Vergiftung *f.*
carbon skeleton *chem.* Kohlenstoffgerüst *nt.*
19-carbon steroids C-19-Steroide *pl.*
carbon tetrachloride Kohlenstofftetrachlorid *nt*, Tetrachlorkohlenstoff *m.*
car·bo·nu·ria [ˌkɑːrbəˈn(j)ʊərɪə] *n physiol.* Karbonurie *f*, Carbonurie *f.*
car·bon·yl [ˈkɑːrbənɪl] *n* Karbonyl-, Carbonyl-(Radikal *nt*).
car·box·y·bi·o·tin [kɑːrˌbɒksɪˈbaɪətɪn] *n* Carboxybiotin *nt.*
car·box·y·dis·mu·tase [ˌ-ˈdɪsmjuːteɪz] *n* Karboxy-, Carboxydismutase *f.*
car·box·y·es·ter·ase [ˌ-ˈestəreɪz] *n* Carboxyesterase *f.*
γ-car·box·y·glu·ta·mate [ˌ-ˈgluːtəmeɪt] *n* γ--Carboxyglutamat *nt.*
car·box·y·he·mo·glo·bin [ˌ-ˈhiːməˌgloʊbɪn] *n abbr.* CO-Hb Carboxyhämoglobin *nt abbr.* CO-Hb, Kohlenmonoxidhämoglobin *nt.*
car·box·y·he·mo·glo·bi·ne·mia [ˌ-ˌhiːməˌgloʊbəˈniːmɪə] *n* Carboxyhämoglobinämie *f.*
car·box·yl [kɑːrˈbɒksɪl] *n* Karboxyl-, Carboxyl-(Radikal *nt*).
car·box·yl·ase [kɑːrˈbɒksɪleɪz] *n* Carboxylase *f*, Carboxilase *f.*
α-carboxylase *n* Pyruvatcarboxylase *f abbr.* PC.

car·box·yl·ate [kɑːrˈbɒksɪleɪt] *n* Karboxylat *nt*, Carboxylat *nt.*
car·box·yl·a·tion [kɑːrˌbɒksɪˈleɪʃn] *n chem.* Karboxylierung *f*, Carboxylierung *f.*
car·box·yl·es·ter·ase [kɑːrˌbɒksɪlˈestəreɪz] *n* Carboxylesterase *f.*
car·box·yl·ic acid [ˌkɑːrbɑkˈsɪlɪk] Karbon-, Carbonsäure *f.*
carboxylic ester hydrolase → carboxylesterase.
car·box·yl·trans·fer·ase [kɑːrˌbɒksɪlˈtrænsfəreɪz] *n abbr.* CT Carboxyltransferase *f abbr.* CT, Transcarboxylase *f.*
car·box·y·ly·ase [kɑːrˌbɒksɪˈlaɪeɪz] *n* Carboxylyase *f.*
car·box·y·meth·yl·cel·lu·lose [ˌ-ˌmeθlˈseljələʊs] *n* Carboxymethylcellulose *f*, CM--Cellulose *f.*
car·box·y·my·o·glo·bin [ˌ-ˌmaɪəˈgloʊbɪn] *n* Carboxymyoglobin *nt.*
α-car·box·y·pen·i·cil·lin [ˌ-ˌpenəˈsɪlɪn] *n* → carbenicillin.
car·box·y·pep·ti·dase [ˌ-ˈpeptɪdeɪz] *n* Carboxypeptidase *f.*
carboxypeptidase A Carboxypeptidase A *f.*
carboxypeptidase B Carboxypeptidase B *f.*
carboxypeptidase N Carboxypeptidase N *f.*
car·box·y·pol·y·pep·ti·dase [ˌ-ˌpɒlɪˈpeptɪdeɪz] *n* 1. → carboxypeptidase. 2. → carboxypeptidase A.
car·box·y·some [kɑːrˈbɒksɪsoʊm] *n* Carboxysom *nt.*
carboxy-terminal *adj biochem.* carboxyterminal, C-terminal.
6-car·box·y·u·ra·cil [kɑːrˌbɒksɪˈjʊərəsɪl] *n* Orotsäure *f*, 6-Carboxyuracil *nt.*
car·boy [ˈkɑːrbɔɪ] *n* Korbflasche *f*; *lab.* (Glas-)Ballon (*für* Säuren).
car·bro·mal [kɑːrˈbroʊml] *n pharm.* Carbromal *nt.*
car·bun·cle [ˈkɑːrbʌŋkl] *n* Karbunkel *m*, Carbunculus *m.*
car·bun·cu·lar [kɑːrˈbʌŋkjələr] *adj* karbunkelähnlich, karbunkulär, karbunkulös.
car·bun·cu·loid [kɑːrˈbʌŋkjəlɔɪd] *adj* → carbuncular.
car·bun·cu·lo·sis [kɑːrˌbʌŋkjəˈloʊsɪs] *n* Karbunkulose *f.*
car·bu·ta·mide [kɑːrˈbjuːtəmaɪd] *n pharm.* Carbutamid *nt.*
car·bu·ter·ol [kɑːrˈbjuːtərɒl] *n pharm.* Carbuterol *nt.*
car·case [ˈkɑːrkəs] *n* → carcass.
car·cass [ˈkɑːrkəs] *n* 1. (Tier-)Kadaver *m*, Aas *nt.* 2. (Menschen-)Leiche *f*, Leichnam *m.*
Carcassonne [karkaˈsɔn]: **C.'s ligament** Lig. puboprostaticum.
C.'s perineal ligament präurethrales Band *nt*, Carcassonne'-, Waldeyer'-Band *nt*, Lig. transversum perinei.
perineal ligament of C. → C.'s perineal ligament.
carcin- *pref.* → carcino-.
car·ci·ne·mia [ˌkɑːrsəˈniːmɪə] *n* → cancerous cachexia.
carcino- *pref.* Krebs-, Karzinom-, Karzin(o)-.
car·ci·no·em·bry·on·ic antigen [ˌkɑːrsɪnəʊˈembrɪənɪk] *n abbr.* CEA carcinoembryonales Antigen *nt abbr.* CEA.
car·cin·o·gen [kɑːrˈsɪnədʒən, ˈkɑːrsənoʊ-] *n* krebserregende/karzinogene Substanz *f*, Karzinogen *nt*, Kanzerogen *nt*, Krebsentstehung *f*, Karzino-, Kanzerogenese *f.*
car·ci·no·gen·e·sis [ˌ-ˈdʒenəsɪs] *n patho.* Krebsentstehung *f*, Karzino-, Kanzerogenese *f.*
car·ci·no·gen·ic [ˌkɑːrsɪnəˈdʒenɪk] *adj*

krebserregend, -erzeugend, -auslösend, onkogen, kanzerogen, karzinogen.
car·ci·no·ge·nic·i·ty [ˌ-dʒəˈnɪsətɪ] *n* Karzinogenität *f.*
car·ci·noid [ˈkɑːrsɪnɔɪd] *n* Karzinoid *nt.*
c. of the appendix Appendixkarzinoid.
c. of the ileum Ileumkarzinoid.
carcinoid adenoma of bronchus Bronchialkarzinoid *nt.*
carcinoid flush Karzinoidflush *m.*
carcinoid syndrome Flush-, Karzinoidsyndrom *nt*, Biörck-Thorson-Syndrom *nt.*
carcinoid tumor → carcinoid.
c. of bronchus Bronchialkarzinoid *nt.*
car·ci·nol·o·gy [kɑːrsəˈnɑlədʒɪ] *n old* → oncology.
car·ci·nol·y·sis [kɑːrsəˈnɑləsɪs] *n* Karzinolyse *f.*
car·ci·no·lyt·ic [ˌkɑːrsənoʊˈlɪtɪk] *adj* karzinolytisch.
car·ci·no·ma [ˌkɑːrsəˈnoʊmə] *n*, *pl* **-mas, -ma·ta** [-mətə] *abbr.* CA, Ca Karzinom *nt*, *inf.* Krebs *m*, Carcinoma *nt abbr.* Ca.
c. of the ampulla of Vater Karzinom der Ampulla hepaticopancreatica.
c. of the body of uterus *gyn.* Korpuskarzinom, Gebärmutterkörperkrebs, Ca. corporis uteri.
c. of the choledochal duct Choledochuskarzinom, Karzinom des Ductus choledochus.
c. of the common bile duct → c. of the choledochal duct.
c. of the cystic duct Zystikuskarzinom, Ca. des Ductus cysticus.
c. en cuirasse Panzerkrebs, Cancer en cuirasse.
c. of the fallopian tube *gyn.* Tubenkarzinom.
c. of the head of pancreas (Pankreas-)Kopfkarzinom.
c. of the lip Lippenkrebs, -karzinom.
c. of the papilla of Vater Papillenkarzinom, Karzinom der Papilla Vateri.
c. of the scrotum Skrotumkarzinom, Ca. scroti.
c. of the sigmoid colon Sigmakarzinom.
c. of the stomach Magenkrebs, -karzinom.
c. of the tail of pancreas (Pankreas-)-Schwanzkarzinom.
c. of the tongue Zungenkrebs, -karzinom.
c. of the uterine cervix Gebärmutterhalskrebs, -karzinom, Kollum-, Zervixkarzinom, Ca. cervicis uteri.
carcinoma en cuirasse Panzerkrebs *m*, Cancer en cuirasse.
carcinoma growing in situ in situ wachsendes Karzinom *nt.*
carcinoma in situ Oberflächenkarzinom *nt*, präinvasives/intraepitheliales Karzinom *nt*, Carcinoma in situ *abbr.* CIA.
carcinoma simplex of breast szirrhöses Brust(drüsen)karzinom *nt*, Szirrhus *m*, Carcinoma solidum simplex der Brust.
car·ci·no·ma·toid [ˌ-ˈnɑmətɔɪd] *adj* karzinomähnlich, -förmig, karzinomatös.
car·ci·no·ma·to·pho·bia [ˌkɑːrsəˌnoʊmətoʊˈfoʊbɪə] *n* Krebsangst *m*, Kanzerophobie *f*, Karzinophobie *f.*
car·ci·no·ma·to·sis [ˌkɑːrsəˌnoʊməˈtoʊsɪs] *n* Karzinomatose *f*, Karzinose *f.*
car·ci·no·ma·tous [ˌkɑːrsəˈnɑmətəs] *adj* Karzinom betr., krebsig, karzinomartig, karzinomatös.
carcinomatous lymphangiosis Lymphangiosis carcinomatosa.
carcinomatous meningitis Meningealkarzinose *f*, Meningitis carcinomatosa.
carcinomatous metastasis Krebs-, Karzinommetastase *f.*

carcinomatous myelopathy

carcinomatous myelopathy paraneoplastische Myelopathie *f*.
carcinomatous myopathy Lambert-Eaton-Syndrom *nt*, pseudomyasthenisches Syndrom *nt*.
car·ci·no·phil·ia [ˌkɑːrsɪnəʊˈfɪlɪə] *n* Karzinophilie *f*.
car·ci·no·phil·ic [ˌ-ˈfɪlɪk] *adj* karzinophil.
car·ci·no·pho·bia [ˌ-ˈfəʊbɪə] *n* → carcinomatophobia.
car·ci·no·sar·co·ma [ˌ-sɑːrˈkəʊmə] *n* Karzinosarkom *nt*, Carcinosarcoma *nt*.
car·ci·no·sis [kɑːrsəˈnəʊsɪs] *n* → carcinomatosis.
car·ci·no·stat·ic [ˌkɑːrsɪnəʊˈstætɪk] *adj* das Karzinomwachstum hemmend, karzinostatisch.
car·ci·nous [ˈkɑːrsnəs] *adj* → carcinomatous.
carcinous pericarditis Perikard-, Herzbeutelkarzinose *f*.
Carden [ˈkɑːrdən]: C.'s amputation/disarticulation *ortho*. Kniegelenksexartikulation *f* nach Carden.
car·di·a [kɑːrdɪə] *n*, *pl* **-di·as**, **-di·ae** [-dɪˌiː] *anat*. **1.** Mageneingang *m*, -mund *m*, Kardia *f*, Cardia *f*, Pars cardiaca gastris/ventriculi. **2.** Ösophagus(ein)mündung *f*, Ostium cardiacum.
cardi- *pref*. → cardio-.
car·di·ac [ˈkɑːrdɪæk] **I** *n* **1.** Herzkranke(r *m*) *f*, Herzpatient(in *f*) *m*. **2.** *pharm*. Herzmittel *nt*, Kardiakum *nt*. **II** *adj* **3.** Herz betr., kardial, Herz-. **4.** Magenmund/Kardia betr.
cardiac activity Herztätigkeit *f*.
cardiac albuminuria → cardiac proteinuria.
cardiac aneurysm Herzwand-, Kammerwand-, Ventrikelaneurysma *nt*, Aneurysma cordis.
cardiac anomaly Herzfehlbildung *f*, -anomalie *f*.
cardiac antrum subphrenischer Ösophagusabschnitt *m*, Antrum cardiacum.
cardiac arrest *abbr*. CA Herzstillstand *m*.
cardiac asthma Herzasthma *nt*, Asthma cardiale.
cardiac atrophy Herz(muskel)atrophie *f*.
cardiac beat Herzschlag *m*, -aktion *f*, -zyklus *m*.
cardiac branch: cervical c.es of vagus nerve, inferior untere Vagusäste *pl* zum Plexus cardiacus, Rami cardiaci cervicales inferiores n. vagi.
cervical c.es of vagus nerve, superior obere Vagusäste *pl* zum Plexus cardiacus, Rami cardiaci cervicales superiores n. vagi.
inferior c.es of recurrent laryngeal nerve → cervical c.es of vagus nerve, inferior.
c. of right pulmonary artery Ramus cardiacus a. pulmonalis dextrae, Ramus basalis medialis a. pulmonalis dextrae.
thoracic c.es of vagus nerve thorakale Herzäste *pl* des N. vagus, Rami cardiaci thoracici n. vagi.
cardiac bronchus Bronchus segmentalis basalis medialis, Bronchus cardiacus.
cardiac calculus Herzkonkrement *nt*, Kardiolith *m*.
cardiac catheterization Herzkatheterismus *m*, -katheterisierung *f*.
cardiac catheter Herzkatheter *m*.
cardiac center kreislaufregulatorisches Zentrum *nt*.
cardiac cirrhosis Stauungsinduration *f* der Leber, Cirrhose cardiaque.
cardiac conducting system Erregungsleitungssystem *nt* des Herzens, kardiales Erregungsleitungssystem *nt*, Systema conducens cordis.

cardiac conduction system → cardiac conducting system
cardiac contusion Herzprellung *f*, Contusio cordis.
cardiac crisis *neuro*. Herzkrise *f*.
cardiac cycle Herzzyklus *m*.
cardiac death Herztod *m*.
cardiac decompensation Herzdekompensation *f*, kardiale Dekompensation *f*.
cardiac decompression Herzdekompression *f*.
cardiac denervation kardiale Denervierung *f*, Herzdenervierung *f*.
cardiac depressor nerve: left c. linker Aortennerv *m*, N. depressor sinister.
right c. rechter Aortennerv *m*, N. depressor dexter.
cardiac depressor reflex Depressorreflex *m*.
cardiac disease Herzerkrankung *f*, -krankheit *f*, -leiden *nt*.
cardiac dropsy Herzbeutelwassersucht *f*, Hydroperikard *nt*, -perikardium *nt*, Hydrokardie *f*, Hydrops pericardii.
cardiac dullness Herzdämpfung *f*.
cardiac dynamics *physiol*. Herzdynamik *f*.
cardiac dyspnea kardiale Dyspnoe *f*.
cardiac edema kardiales Ödem *nt*.
cardiac failure *abbr*. CF Herzinsuffizienz *f*, -versagen *nt*, Herzmuskelschwäche *f*, Myokardinsuffizienz *f*, Insufficientia cordis.
cardiac ganglia Wrisberg'-Ganglien *pl*, Ggll. cardiaca.
cardiac glands Cardia-, Kardiadrüsen *pl*.
cardiac glycoside Herzglykosid *nt*.
cardiac hemoptysis kardiale Hämoptyse *f*.
cardiac hypertrophy Herzhypertrophie *f*.
cardiac impression: c. of liver Impressio cardiaca hepatis.
c. of lung Herzmulde *f* der Lunge, Impressio cardiaca.
cardiac incisure: c. of left lung Inc. cardiaca pulmonis sinistri.
c. of stomach Inc. cardiaca (gastris/ventriculi).
cardiac index *abbr*. CI Herzindex *m abbr*. HI.
cardiac infarction Herz(muskel)infarkt *m*, Myokardinfarkt *m*, *inf*. Infarkt *m*.
cardiac insufficiency Herzinsuffizienz *f*, -versagen *nt*, Herzmuskelschwäche *f*, Myokardinsuffizienz *f*, Insufficientia cordis.
congestive c. dekompensierte Herzinsuffizienz.
cardiac jelly *embryo*. Herzgallerte *f*.
cardiac liver Stauungsinduration *f* der Leber, Cirrhose cardiaque.
cardiac loop *embryo*. Herzschleife *f*.
cardiac lymphatic ring Lymphknotenring *m* der Kardia, A(n)nulus lymphaticus cardiae.
cardiac malformation Herzfehlbildung *f*, -malformation *f*.
cardiac massage Herzmassage *f*.
cardiac monitoring Überwachung *f* der Herzfunktion.
cardiac murmur *card*. Herzgeräusch *nt*.
cardiac muscle Herzmuskel *m*, Herzmuskelgewebe *nt*; Myokard *nt*.
cardiac muscle abscess Herzmuskelabszeß *m*.
cardiac muscle fiber Herzmuskelfaser *f*.
cardiac muscle necrosis Herzmuskel-, Myokardnekrose *f*.
cardiac nerve: (cervical) c., inferior N. cardiacus cervicalis inferior.
(cervical) c., middle N. cardiacus cervicalis medius.

118

(cervical) c., superior N. cardiacus cervicalis superior.
thoracic c.s Nn. cardiaci thoracici.
cardiac neuralgia *old* → angina pectoris.
cardiac neurosis Herzneurose *f*.
cardiac notch: c. of left lung → cardiac incisure of left lung.
c. of stomach → cardiac incisure of stomach.
cardiac opening → cardiac orifice.
cardiac orifice Speiseröhren-, Ösophagus(ein)mündung *f*, Ostium cardiacum, Cardia *f*.
cardiac output 1. Herzzeitvolumen *nt abbr*. HZV. **2.** Herzminutenvolumen *nt abbr*. HMV.
cardiac-output hypertension Minutenvolumenhochdruck *m*.
cardiac pacemaker 1. *physiol*. Herzschrittmacher *m*. **2.** *card*. künstlicher Herzschrittmacher *m*, Pacemaker *m*.
artificial c. → cardiac pacemaker 2.
cardiac performance Herzleistung *f*.
cardiac perfusion Herzdurchblutung *f*, -perfusion *f*.
cardiac pericardium Epikard *nt*, viszerales Perikard *nt*, Lamina visceralis pericardii, Epicardium *nt*.
cardiac plexus vegetatives Herzgeflecht *nt*, -plexus *m*, Plexus cardiacus.
anterior c. vorderer kleinerer Abschnitt des Herzplexus, Plexus cardiacus superficialis.
deep c. hinterer größerer Abschnitt des Herzplexus, Plexus cardiacus profundus.
great c. → deep c.
superficial c. → anterior c.
cardiac polyp Herzpolyp *m*.
cardiac power Herzleistung *f*.
cardiac primordia *embryo*. Herzanlagen *pl*.
cardiac proteinuria kardial-bedingte Albuminurie/Proteinurie *f*.
cardiac region Herzgegend *f*, -region *f*.
cardiac reserve *card*. Reservekraft *f*.
cardiac rupture Herzmuskelriß *m*, -ruptur *f*, Myokardruptur *f*.
cardiac scar Herzmuskelschwiele *f*.
cardiac segment of inferior pulmonary lobe medial-basales Segment *nt* des Lungenunterlappens, Segmentum cardiacum, Segmentum basale mediale [S. VII].
cardiac shock kardialer/kardiogener/kardiovaskulärer Schock *m*, Kreislaufschock *m*.
cardiac skeleton Herzskelett *nt*.
cardiac sound Herzton *m*.
abnormal c. Herzgeräusch *nt*.
fourth c. IV. Herzton, Vorhofton.
cardiac standstill *card*. Herzstillstand *m*, Asystolie *f*.
cardiac surgery Herzchirurgie *f*.
open c. Chirurgie am offenen Herzen, offene Herzchirurgie.
cardiac syncope kardiale Synkope *f*.
cardiac tachyarrhythmia Tachyarrhythmie *f*.
cardiac tamponade Perikard-, Herz(beutel)tamponade *f*.
cardiac transplant Herztransplantat *nt*.
cardiac transplantation Herztransplantation *f*.
heterotopic c. heterotope Herztransplantation.
orthotopic c. orthotope Herztransplantation.
cardiac tumor Herztumor *m*.
cardiac valve replacement Herzklappenersatz *m*.
cardiac valves Herzklappen *pl*.
cardiac valvular disease Herzklappenerkrankung *f*.

cardiac valvular injury Herzklappenverletzung f.
cardiac vein: c.s pl Herzvenen pl, Venen pl des Herzens, Vv. cordis.
 anterior c.s vordere Herzvenen pl, Vv. cordis/cardiacae anteriores.
 great c. große Herzvene f, Cordis f magna, V. cordis/cardiaca magna.
 middle c. mittlere Herzvene f, Cordis f media, V. cordis/cardiaca media.
 small c. kleine Herzvene f, Cordis f parva, V. cordis/cardiaca parva.
 smallest c.s Thebesi'-Venen pl, kleinste Herzvenen pl, Vv. cordis/cardiacae minimae.
cardiac vertigo kardialer Schwindel m.
cardiac vessel injury Herzgefäßverletzung f.
cardiac work Herzarbeit f.
car·di·a·gra ['kɑːrdɪəgrə] n Herzbräune f, Stenokardie f, Angina pectoris.
car·di·al·gia [kɑːrdɪ'ældʒ(ɪ)ə] n 1. Herzschmerz(en pl) m, Kardiodynie f, Kardialgie f. 2. Magenschmerzen pl; Sodbrennen nt; Kardialgie f.
cardia region Kardiaregion f.
car·di·as·the·nia [kɑːrdɪæs'θiːnɪə] n Herzschwäche f.
car·di·asth·ma [ˌkɑːrdɪ'æzmə] n → cardiac asthma.
car·di·cen·te·sis [ˌ-sen'tiːsɪs] n → cardiocentesis.
car·di·ec·ta·sis [ˌ-'ektəsɪs] n Herzdilatation f, -erweiterung f, Kardiektasie f.
car·di·ec·to·my [ˌ-'ektəmɪ] n chir. Kardiaresektion f, Kardiektomie f.
car·di·ec·to·py [ˌ-'ektəpɪ] n Herz-, Kardi(o)ektopie f.
car·di·nal ['kɑːrdɪnl] I n 1. Scharlachrot nt. 2. → cardinal number. II adj 3. hauptsächlich, grundlegend, kardinal, Haupt-, Grund-, Kardinal-. 4. scharlachrot.
cardinal ligament Kardinalband nt, Lig. cardinale uteri.
cardinal number mathe. Kardinal-, Grundzahl f.
cardinal numeral → cardinal number.
cardinal point Kardinalpunkt m.
cardinal symptom Primär-, Haupt-, Leit-, Kardinalsymptom nt.
cardinal vein: anterior c.s embryo. vordere Kardinalvenen pl, Vv. cardinales anteriores.
 common c. embryo. Kardinalvenenstamm m, V. cardinalis communis.
 posterior c.s embryo. hintere Kardinalvenen pl, Vv. cardinales posteriores.
cardio- pref. 1. Herz-, Kardia-, Kardio-, Cardio-. 2. Kardia-, Kardio-.
car·di·o·ac·cel·er·a·tor [ˌkɑːrdɪəʊæk'selərəɪtər] n die Herzarbeit-beschleunigendes Mittel nt.
car·di·o·ac·tive [ˌ-'æktɪv] adj die Herzfunktion beeinflußend od. stimulierend.
car·di·o·an·gi·og·ra·phy [ˌ-ændʒɪ'ɑgrəfɪ] n Angiokardiographie f.
car·di·o·an·gi·ol·o·gy [ˌ-ændʒɪ'ɑlədʒɪ] n Kardioangiologie f.
car·di·o·a·or·tic [ˌ-eɪ'ɔːrtɪk] adj Herz u. Aorta betr., kardioaortal, aortokardial.
Car·di·o·bac·te·ri·um [ˌ-bæk'tɪərɪəm] n micro. Cardiobacterium nt.
cardio-cardiac reflex kardio-kardialer Reflex m.
car·di·o·cele ['kɑːrdɪəsiːl] n Kardiozele f.
car·di·o·cen·te·sis [ˌ-sen'tiːsɪs] n Herzpunktion f, Kardiozentese f, -centese f.
car·di·o·cha·la·sia [ˌ-kə'leɪzɪə] n chir. Kardiochalasie f.
car·di·o·ki·net·ic [ˌ-sɪ'netɪk] adj, n → cardiokinetic.
car·di·o·cir·cu·la·to·ry [ˌ-'sɜːrkjələtəˌriː,

-təʊ-] adj Herz u. Kreislauf betr., Herz-Kreislauf-.
car·di·o·cir·rho·sis [ˌ-sɪ'rəʊsɪs] n → cardiac cirrhosis.
car·di·oc·la·sis [kɑːrdɪ'ɑkləsɪs] n → cardiorrhexis.
car·di·o·di·a·phrag·mat·ic [ˌkɑːrdɪədaɪəˌfræg'mætɪk] adj Herz u. Zwerchfell betr., phreniko-, phrenokardial.
cardiodiaphragmatic angle Herz-Zwerchfell-Winkel m.
car·di·o·di·la·tin [ˌ-'daɪlətɪn] n Cardiodilatin nt.
car·di·o·di·la·tor [ˌ-'daɪleɪtər] n chir. Kardia-, Kardiodila(ta)tor m.
car·di·o·di·o·sis [ˌ-daɪ'əʊsɪs] n chir. Kardiadilatation f.
car·di·o·dy·nam·ics [ˌ-daɪ'næmɪks] pl Herz-, Kardiodynamik f.
car·di·o·dyn·ia [ˌ-'diːnɪə] n → cardialgia 1.
car·di·o·e·soph·a·ge·al [ˌ-ɪˌsɑfə'dʒiːəl] adj Magenmund/Kardia u. Speiseröhre/Ösophagus betr. od. verbindend, ösophagokardial.
cardioesophageal junction ösophagogastrale/gastroösophageale Übergangszone f.
car·di·o·fa·cial syndrome [ˌ-'feɪʃl] kardiofaziales Syndrom nt.
car·di·o·gen·e·sis [ˌ-'dʒenəsɪs] n embryo. Herzentwicklung f, Kardiogenese f.
car·di·o·gen·ic [ˌ-'dʒenɪk] adj 1. aus dem Herz stammend, vom Herzen ausgehend, kardiogen. 2. embryo. Kardiogenese betr., kardiogen.
cardiogenic area embryo. kardiogene Zone f.
cardiogenic plate embryo. kardiogene Platte f, Herzanlage f.
cardiogenic shock → cardiac shock.
car·di·o·gram ['-græm] n Kardiogramm nt.
car·di·o·graph ['-græf] n Kardiograph m.
car·di·o·graph·ic [ˌ-'græfɪk] adj kardiographie betr., kardiographisch.
car·di·og·ra·phy [kɑːrdɪ'ɑgrəfɪ] n Kardiographie f.
car·di·o·he·mo·throm·bus [ˌkɑːrdɪəˌhiːmə'θrɑmbəs] n → cardiothrombus.
car·di·o·he·pat·ic [ˌ-hɪ'pætɪk] adj Herz u. Leber betr., hepatokardial, hepatokardial.
cardiohepatic angle/triangle Ebstein-Winkel m, Herz-Leber-Winkel m.
car·di·o·hep·a·to·meg·a·ly [ˌ-ˌhepətəʊ'megəlɪ] n Kardiohepatomegalie f.
car·di·oid ['kɑːrdɪɔɪd] adj herzähnlich, -förmig.
car·di·o·in·hib·i·tor [ˌkɑːrdɪəʊɪn'hɪbɪtər] n pharm. kardioinhibitorisches Mittel nt.
car·di·o·in·hib·i·to·ry [ˌ-ɪn'hɪbətəˌriː, -təʊ-] adj die Herztätigkeit hemmend, kardioinhibitorisch.
car·di·o·ki·net·ic [ˌ-kɪ'netɪk] I n stimulierendes Herzmittel nt, Kardiokinetikum nt. II adj die Herztätigkeit stimulierend, kardiokinetisch.
car·di·o·ky·mo·graph·ic [ˌ-kaɪmə'græfɪk] adj Kardiokymographie betr., kardiokymographisch.
car·di·o·ky·mog·ra·phy [ˌ-kaɪ'mɑgrəfɪ] n Kardiokymographie f.
car·di·o·lip·in [ˌ-'lɪpɪn] n Cardiolipin nt, Diphosphatidylglycerin nt.
car·di·o·lith ['-lɪθ] n Herzkonkrement nt, Kardiolith m.
car·di·ol·o·gist [kɑːrdɪ'ɑlədʒɪst] n Kardiologe m, -login f.
car·di·ol·o·gy [ˌ-'ɑlədʒɪ] n Kardiologie f.
car·di·ol·y·sis [ˌ-'ɑləsɪs] n HTG Herzlösung f, -mobilisierung f, Kardiolyse f.
car·di·o·ma·la·cia [ˌkɑːrdɪəʊmə'leɪʃ(ɪ)ə] n

patho. Kardiomalazie f.
car·di·o·me·ga·lia [ˌ-mɪ'geɪlʒə] n → cardiomegaly.
car·di·o·meg·a·ly [ˌ-'megəlɪ] n patho. Herzvergrößerung f, Kardiomegalie f.
car·di·om·e·ter [kɑːrdɪ'ɑmɪtər] n Kardiometer nt.
car·di·om·e·try [ˌ-'ɑmətrɪ] n Kardiometrie f.
car·di·o·mo·til·i·ty [ˌkɑːrdɪəʊməʊ'tɪlətɪ] n Herzbeweglichkeit f, -motilität f.
car·di·o·mus·cu·lar [ˌ-'mʌskjələr] adj Herzmuskel/Myokard betr., kardiomuskulär, Herzmuskel-, Myokard-.
car·di·o·my·o·li·po·sis [ˌ-maɪəlɪ'pəʊsɪs] n patho. fettige Herzmuskeldegeneration f.
car·di·o·my·op·a·thy [ˌ-maɪ'ɑpəθɪ] n abbr. CM Myokardiopathie f. MKP, Kardiomyopathie f, Cardiomyopathie f abbr. CM.
car·di·o·my·o·pex·y [ˌ-'maɪəpeksɪ] n chir. Kardiomyopexie f.
car·di·o·my·ot·o·my [ˌ-maɪ'ɑtəmɪ] n chir. Kardiomyotomie f, Ösophagokardiomyotomie f, Heller-Operation f.
car·di·o·na·trin [ˌ-'neɪtrɪn] n atrialer natriuretischer Faktor m abbr. ANF, Atriopeptid nt, -peptin nt.
car·di·o·ne·cro·sis [ˌ-nɪ'krəʊsɪs, -ne-] n Herz(muskel)nekrose f.
car·di·o·nec·tor [ˌ-'nektər] n Erregungsleitungssystem nt des Herzens, Systema conducens cordis.
car·di·o·neph·ric [ˌ-'nefrɪk] adj Herz u. Nieren betr., kardiorenal, renokardial.
car·di·o·neu·ral [ˌ-'njʊərəl, -'nʊ-] adj Herz u. Nervensystem betr., kardioneural.
car·di·o·neu·ro·sis [ˌ-njʊə'rəʊsɪs, -nʊ-] n → cardiac neurosis.
cardio-omentopexy n chir. Kardioomentopexie f.
car·di·o·path ['kɑːrdɪəpæθ] n Herzkranke(r m) f.
car·di·o·path·ia [ˌkɑːrdɪə'pæθɪə] n → cardiopathy.
car·di·o·path·ic [ˌ-'pæθɪk] adj Herzerkrankung betr., von einer Herzerkrankung betroffen, kardiopathisch.
cardiopathic amyloidosis kardiopathische Amyloidose f.
car·di·op·a·thy [kɑːrdɪ'ɑpəθɪ] n Herzerkrankung f, -leiden nt, Kardiopathie f.
car·di·o·per·i·car·di·o·pex·y [ˌkɑːrdɪəʊˌperɪ'kɑːrdɪəpeksɪ] n chir. Kardioperikardiopexie f.
car·di·o·per·i·car·di·tis [ˌ-ˌperɪkɑːr'daɪtɪs] n kombinierte Herz- u. Herzbeutelentzündung f, Kardioperikarditis f.
car·di·o·pho·bia [ˌ-'fəʊbɪə] n Herzangst f, Kardiophobie f.
car·di·o·phre·nia [ˌ-'friːnɪə] n DaCosta-Syndrom nt, Effort-Syndrom nt, Phrenikokardie f, neurozirkulatorische Asthenie f, Soldatenherz nt.
car·di·o·phren·ic angle [ˌ-'frenɪk] Herz-Zwerchfell-Winkel m.
car·di·o·plas·ty ['-plæstɪ] n chir. Kardia-, Kardioplastik f, Ösophagogastroplastik f.
car·di·o·ple·gia [ˌ-'pliːdʒ(ɪ)ə] n (künstlich induzierter) Herzstillstand m, Kardioplegie f.
car·di·o·ple·gic [ˌ-'pliːdʒɪk, -'pledʒ-] adj kardioplegisch.
cardioplegic solution kardioplege Lösung f.
car·di·o·pneu·mat·ic [ˌ-nju:'mætɪk, -nʊ-] adj Herz u. Atmung betr., kardiorespiratorisch.
car·di·o·pneu·mo·graph [ˌ-'nju:məgræf, -nʊ-] n Kardiopneumograph m.
car·di·o·pneu·mon·o·pex·y [ˌ-nju:'mɑnə-

cardioptosia

peksı, -no-] *n HTG* Kardiopneumopexie *f.*
car·di·op·to·sia [ˌkɑːrdɪɑpˈtəʊsɪə] *n* → cardioptosis.
car·di·op·to·sis [kɑːrdɪˈɑptəsɪs] *n* Herzsenkung *f,* -tiefstand *m,* Wanderherz *nt,* Kardioptose *f.*
car·di·o·pul·mo·nar·y [ˌkɑːrdɪəʊˈpʌlməˌnerɪ, -nərɪ] *adj* Herz u. Lunge(n) betr. *od.* verbindend, kardiopulmonal, Herz--Lungen-.
cardiopulmonary bypass *HTG* kardiopulmonaler Bypass *m,* Herz-Lungen-Bypass *m.*
cardiopulmonary murmur → cardiorespiratory murmur.
cardiopulmonary resuscitation *abbr.* **CPR** kardiopulmonale Reanimation/Wiederbelebung *f.*
cardiopulmonary transplantation Herz--Lungen-Transplantation *f.*
car·di·o·punc·ture [ˌ-ˈpʌŋ(k)tʃər] *n* → cardiocentesis.
car·di·o·py·lor·ic [ˌ-paɪˈlɔːrɪk, -ˈlɑr-, -pɪ-] *adj* Kardia u. Pylorus betr.
car·di·o·re·nal [ˌ-ˈriːnl] *adj* Herz u. Nieren betr., kardiorenal, renokardial.
car·di·o·res·pi·ra·to·ry murmur [ˌ-rɪˈspaɪrətɔːriː, -ˈrespɪrətɔːriː, -təʊ-] kardiorespiratorisches Geräusch *nt.*
car·di·or·rha·phy [kɑːrdɪˈɔrəfɪ] *n HTG* Herzmuskelnaht *f,* Kardiorrhaphie *f.*
car·di·or·rhex·is [ˌkɑːrdɪəʊˈreksɪs] *n* Herz(wand)ruptur *f,* -riß *m,* Kardiorrhexis *f.*
car·di·o·scle·ro·sis [ˌkɑːrdɪəʊsklɪˈrəʊsɪs] *n* Herz(muskel)sklerose *f,* -fibrose *f,* Kardiosklerose *f.*
car·di·o·scope [ˈ-skəʊp] *n* Kardioskop *nt.*
car·di·o·se·lec·tive [ˌ-sɪˈlektɪv] *adj* kardioselektiv.
car·di·o·spasm [ˈ-spæzəm] *n* Ösophagus-, Kardiaachalasie *f,* Kardiospasmus *m,* Kardiakrampf *m.*
car·di·o·sphyg·mo·gram [ˌ-ˈsfɪgməgræm] *n* Kardiosphygmogramm *nt.*
car·di·o·sphyg·mo·graph [ˌ-ˈsfɪgməgræf] *n* Kardiosphygmograph *m.*
car·di·o·splen·o·pex·y [ˌ-ˈspliːnəpeksɪ] *n chir.* Kardiosplenopexie *f.*
car·di·o·ste·no·sis [ˌ-stɪˈnəʊsɪs] *n* Kardiastenose *f.*
car·di·o·ta·chom·e·ter [ˌ-tæˈkɑmɪtər] *n* Kardiotachometer *f.*
car·di·o·ta·chom·e·try [ˌ-tæˈkɑmətrɪ] *n* Kardiotachometrie *f.*
car·di·o·ther·a·py [ˌ-ˈθerəpɪ] *n* Behandlung *f* von Herzerkrankungen/-leiden.
car·di·o·throm·bus [ˌ-ˈθrɑmbəs] *n* Herzthrombus *m.*
car·di·o·thy·ro·tox·i·co·sis [ˌ-θaɪrəˌtɑksɪˈkəʊsɪs] *n* Kardiopathie *f* bei Thyreotoxikose, Thyreokardiopathie *f.*
car·di·o·to·co·gram [ˌ-ˈtəʊkəgræm] *n abbr.* **CTG** *gyn.* Kardiotokogramm *nt,* Cardiotokogramm *nt abbr.* CTG.
car·di·o·to·co·graph [ˌ-ˈtəʊkəgræf] *n gyn.* Kardiotokograph *m.*
car·di·o·to·co·gra·phy [ˌ-təʊˈkɑgrəfɪ] *n gyn.* Kardiotokographie *f.*
car·di·o·to·kog·ra·phy *n* → cardiotocography.
car·di·ot·o·my [kɑːrdɪˈɑtəmɪ] *n* 1. Herzeröffnung *f,* -schnitt *m,* Kardiotomie *f.* 2. → cardiomyotomy.
car·di·o·ton·ic [ˌkɑːrdɪəʊˈtɑnɪk] **I** *n* stärkendes Herzmittel *nt,* Kardiotonikum *nt,* Cardiotonicum *nt.* **II** *adj* herzstärkend, -tonisierend, kardiotonisch.
car·di·o·tox·ic [ˌ-ˈtɑksɪk] *adj* herzschädigend, kardiotoxisch.
car·di·o·val·vot·o·my [ˌ-vælˈvɑtəmɪ] *n* cardiovalvutomy.

car·di·o·val·vu·lar [ˌ-ˈvælvjələr] *adj* Herzklappen betr., Herzklappen-.
car·di·o·val·vu·li·tis [ˌ-ˌvælvjəˈlaɪtɪs] *n* Herzklappenentzündung *f.*
car·di·o·val·vu·lot·o·my [ˌ-ˌvælvjəˈlɑtəmɪ] *n HTG* Herzklappenspaltung *f,* Kardiovalvulotomie *f.*
car·di·o·vas·cu·lar [ˌ-ˈvæskjələr] *adj abbr.* **CV** Herz u. Kreislauf *od.* Blutgefäße betr., kardiovaskulär, Herz-Kreislauf-, Kreislauf-.
cardiovascular center (Herz-)Kreislaufzentrum *nt.*
cardiovascular collapse Herz-Kreislauf--Kollaps *m,* kardiovaskulärer Kollaps *m.*
cardiovascular disease Herz-Kreislauf--Erkrankung *f,* kardiovaskuläre Erkrankung *f.*
  functional c. DaCosta-Syndrom *nt,* Effort-Syndrom *nt,* Phrenikokardie *f,* neurozirkulatorische Asthenie *f,* Soldatenherz *nt.*
cardiovascular receptor kardiovaskulärer Rezeptor *m.*
cardiovascular response kardiovaskuläre Reizantwort/Reaktion/Anpassung *f.*
cardiovascular shock → cardiac shock.
cardiovascular status kardiovaskulärer Status *m.*
cardiovascular syphilis kardiovaskuläre Syphilis *f.*
cardiovascular system *abbr.* **CVS** Herz--Kreislauf-System *nt,* (Blut-)Kreislauf *m,* kardiovaskuläres System *nt,* Systema cardiovasculare.
cardiovascular vertigo kardiovaskulärer Schwindel *m.*
car·di·o·vas·col·o·gy [ˌ-væˈsɑlədʒɪ] *n* → cardioangiology.
car·di·o·ver·sion [ˈkɑːrdɪəvɜːrʒn] *n* Kardioversion *f.*
car·di·o·ver·ter [ˈ-vɜːrtər] *n* Defibrillator *m.*
car·di·tis [kɑːrˈdaɪtɪs] *n* Herzentzündung *f,* Karditis *f,* Carditis *f.*
care [keər] **I** *n* 1. (Zahn-, Haut-)Pflege *f;* (Kranken-, Säuglings-)Pflege *f,* Betreuung *f,* Behandlung *f.* **to be under the ~ of a doctor** in ärztlicher Behandlung sein. **to come under medical ~** in ärztliche Behandlung kommen. **to take ~ of** aufpassen auf, etw./jdn. pflegen, s. kümmern um. 2. Schutz *m,* Fürsorge *f,* Obhut *f.* 3. Besorgnis *f,* Kummer *m,* Sorge *f.* 4. Sorgfalt *f,* Aufmerksamkeit *f,* Eifer *m.* **to take ~** vorsichtig sein. **II** *vi* s. sorgen (*about* über, um); s. kümmern (*about* um).
care for *vi* 1. s. kümmern um; (jdn.) versorgen, pflegen, betreuen. (**well**) **~d-for** (*Person*) gut versorgt, gepflegt. 2. Interesse haben für; s. etw. machen aus.
care·ful [ˈkeərfəl] *adj* 1. vorsichtig, achtsam. 2. gründlich, gewissenhaft, sorgfältig. 3. achtsam, behutsam, umsichtig, rücksichtsvoll (*of, about, in*).
care·ful·ness [ˈkeərfəlnɪs] *n* Vorsicht *f;* Gründlichkeit *f,* Sorgfalt *f;* Sorgsamkeit *f,* Umsichtigkeit *f.*
care·giv·er [ˈkeərgɪvər] *n psycho.* Betreuer(in *f*) *m,* Vormund *m,* (Für-)Sorgeberechtigte(r *f*) *m.*
care unit spezialisierte Pflegeeinheit/-station *f.*
  coronary c. *abbr.* **CCU** kardiologische Wach-/Intensivstation.
  intensive c. *abbr.* **ICU** Intensiv-, Wachstation.
  neonatal intensive c. Neugeborenenintensivstation.
Carey Coombs [ˈkeərɪ kuːmz]: **C. C. murmur** *card.* Coombs-Geräusch *nt.*
Carhart [ˈkɑːrhɑːrt]: **C.'s dip** *HNO* Carhart-Senke *f.*

120

C.'s test *HNO* Schwellenschwundtest *m,* Carhart-Test *m.*
car·i·cin [ˈkeərəsɪn] *n* Papain *nt.*
car·ies [ˈkeərɪːz, -rɪːz] *n* 1. Knochenkaries *f,* -fraß *m,* -schwund *m,* Karies *f.* 2. *dent.* (Zahn-)Karies *f,* Zahnfäule *f,* -fäulnis *f,* Caries dentium.
ca·ri·na [kəˈraɪnə, -ˈriː-] *n, pl* **-nae, -nas** [-niː] *anat., bio.* Kiel *m,* kielförmige Struktur *f,* Carina *f.*
  c. of trachea Karina *f,* Carina tracheae.
car·i·nate abdomen [ˈkærəneɪt] Kahnbauch *m.*
car·i·o·gen·e·sis [ˌkeərɪəˈdʒenəsɪs] *n dent., ortho.* Kariesentstehung *f,* -bildung *f,* Kariogenese *f.*
car·i·o·gen·ic [ˌ-ˈdʒenɪk] *adj* Kariesbildung fördernd *od.* auslösend, kariogen.
car·i·ous [ˈkeərɪəs] *adj dent., ortho.* von Karies betroffen *od.* befallen, angefault, zerfressen, kariesähnlich, kariös.
carious osteitis Knochenmark(s)entzündung *f,* Osteomyelitis *f.*
car·i·so·pro·date [kɑːrˌaɪsəˈprəʊdeɪt] *n* → carisoprodol.
car·i·so·pro·dol [ˌ-ˈprəʊdɑl, -dɔl] *n pharm.* Carisoprodol *nt.*
Carlens [ˈkɑːrlənz]: **C.'s catheter** *anes.* Carlens-Tubus *m.*
Carleton [ˈkɑːrltən]: **C.'s spots** Carleton--Flecken *pl.*
Carls·bad salt [ˈkɑːrlzbæd] Karlsbader Salz *nt.*
Carman [ˈkɑːrmən]: **C.'s sign** *radiol.* Carman-Meniskus *m.*
car·min·a·tive [kɑːrˈmɪnətɪv, ˈkɑːrməˌneɪtɪv] *pharm.* **I** *n* Mittel *nt* gegen Blähungen, Karminativum *nt,* Carminativum *nt.* **II** *adj* gegen Blähungen wirkend, karminativ.
car·mine [ˈkɑːrmɪn, -maɪn] *n* Karmin *nt.*
carmine red Karminrot *nt.*
car·min·ic acid [kɑːrˈmɪnɪk] Karminsäure *f.*
car·min·o·phil [kɑːrˈmɪnəfɪl] **I** *n* karminophile Substanz/Struktur/Zelle *f.* **II** *adj* mit Karmin färbend, karminophil.
car·min·o·phile [ˈ-faɪl] *adj* → carminophil II.
car·mi·noph·i·lous [kɑːrmɪˈnɑfɪləs] *adj* → carminophil II.
car·mi·num [kɑːrˈmaɪnəm] *n* → carmine.
car·mus·tine [ˈkɑːrməstiːn] *n pharm.* Carmustin *nt.*
car·ne·ous [ˈkɑːrnɪəs] *adj patho.* fleischig.
carneous mole *gyn.* Fleischmole *f,* Mola carnosa.
Carnett [ˈkɑːrnet]: **C.'s sign** *chir.* Carnett--Zeichen *nt.*
car·ni·fi·ca·tion [ˌkɑːrnɪfɪˈkeɪʃn] *n patho.* Karnifikation *f.*
car·ni·tine [ˈkɑːrnɪtiːn] *n* Karnitin *nt,* Carnitin *nt.*
carnitine acyltransferase Carnitinacyltransferase *f.*
carnitine deficiency Karnitin-, Carnitinmangel(krankheit *f*) *m.*
carnitine palmitoyl transferase Carnitinpalmitoyltransferase *f.*
carnitine palmitoyl transferase deficiency Carnitinpalmitoyltransferasemangel *m.*
Car·niv·o·ra [kɑːrˈnɪvərə] *pl bio.* Fleischfresser *pl,* Karnivoren *pl,* Carnivora *pl.*
car·ni·vore [ˈkɑːrnəvɔːr, -vəʊr] *n bio.* Fleischfresser *m,* Karnivor(e) *m,* Kreophage *m.*
car·niv·o·rous [kɑːrˈnɪvərəs] *adj bio.* fleischfressend, karnivor.
car·no·si·nase [ˈkɑːrnəsɪneɪz] *n* Aminoacylhistidin(di)peptidase *f,* Carnosinase *f.*

carnosinase deficiency → carnosinemia.
car·no·sine ['kɑːrnəsiːn, -sɪn] *n* Karnosin *nt*, Carnosin *nt*, β-Alanin-L-Histidin *nt*.
car·no·si·ne·mia [ˌkɑːrnəsɪ'niːmɪə] *n* Karnosinämie(-Syndrom *nt*) *f*, Carnosinämie(-Syndrom *nt*) *f*.
car·no·si·nu·ria [ˌ-ˈn(j)ʊərɪə] *n* Karnosinurie *f*, Carnosinurie *f*.
Carnot [kar'no]: **C.'s reflex** Carnot-Reflex *m*.
Caroli [karɔ'li]: **C.'s disease/syndrome** Caroli-Syndrom *nt*.
car·o·ten·ase ['kærəʊtneɪz] *n* Karotinase *f*.
car·o·tene ['kærətiːn] *n chem.* Karotin *nt*, Carotin *nt*.
α-carotene *n* α-Karotin *nt*.
β-carotene *n* β-Karotin *nt*.
β-carotene-15,15'-dioxygenase *n* Karotinase *f*.
γ-carotene *n* γ-Karotin *nt*.
car·o·te·ne·mia [kærətɪ'niːmɪə] *n* Karotinämie *f*, Carotinämie *f*.
ca·rot·e·no·der·ma [kəˌratnəʊ'dɜrmə] *n* Karotingelbsucht *f*, -ikterus *m*, Carotingelbsucht *f*, -ikterus *m*, Karotinodermie *f*, Carotinodermie *f*, Xanthodermie *f*, Aurantiasis cutis.
ca·rot·e·no·der·mia [ˌ-ˈdɜrmɪə] *n* → carotenoderma.
ca·rot·e·noid [kə'rɑtnɔɪd] **I** *n* Karotinoid *nt*, Carotinoid *nt*. **II** *adj* karotinoid.
carotenoid pigment Karotinoidpigment *nt*.
car·o·te·no·sis [kærətɪ'nəʊsɪs] *n* → carotenemia.
ca·rot·ic [kə'rɑtɪk] *adj* 1. → carotid. 2. benommen, stuporös.
ca·rot·i·co·tym·pan·ic arteries [kəˌrɑtɪkəʊtɪm'pænɪk] Paukenhöhlenäste *pl* der A. carotis interna, Aa. caroticotympanicae.
caroticotympanic canaliculi Canaliculi caroticotympanici.
caroticotympanic canals → caroticotympanic canaliculi.
caroticotympanic nerves Nn. caroticotympanici.
caroticotympanic tubules → caroticotympanic canaliculi.
ca·rot·id [kə'rɑtɪd] **I** *n* Halsschlagader *f*, Karotis *f*, A. carotis. **II** *adj* Karotis betr., Karotis-.
carotid angiogram Karotisangiogramm *nt*.
carotid angiography Karotisangiographie *f*.
carotid artery: common c. Halsschlagader *f*, gemeinsame Kopfschlagader *f*, Karotis *f* communis, A. carotis communis.
external c. äußere Kopfschlagader *f*, Karotis *f* externa, A. carotis externa.
internal c. innere Kopfschlagader *f*, Karotis *f* interna, A. carotis interna.
carotid bifurcation Karotisgabel(ung *f*) *f*, Bifurcatio carotidis.
carotid body → carotid glomus.
carotid body tumor Glomus-caroticum-Tumor *m*.
carotid bruit *card.* Strömungsgeräusch *nt* über der A. carotis.
carotid bulbus → carotid sinus.
carotid canal Karotiskanal *m*, Canalis caroticus.
carotid ganglion Ganglion *nt* des Plexus caroticus internus.
inferior c. Schmiedel'-Ganglion.
superior c. oberes Karotisganglion.
carotid gland → carotid glomus.
carotid glomus Karotisdrüse *f*, Paraganglion *nt* der Karotisgabel, Paraganglion/Glomus caroticum.
carotid groove of sphenoid bone Sulcus caroticus (ossis sphenoidalis).
carotid nerve: external c.s Nn. carotici externi.
internal c. N. caroticus internus.
carotid occlusive disease Karotisstenose *f*.
carotid plexus vegetatives Geflecht *nt* der A. carotis interna, Plexus caroticus internus.
common c. vegetatives Geflecht der A. carotis communis, Plexus caroticus communis.
external c. vegetatives Geflecht der A. carotis externa, Plexus caroticus externus.
internal c. → carotid plexus.
carotid pulse Karotispuls *m*.
carotid pulse curve Carotis-, Karotispulskurve *f abbr.* CPK.
carotid sheath Karotisscheide *f*, Vagina carotica (fasciae cervicalis).
carotid sinus Karotis-, Carotissinus *m*, Bulbus/Sinus caroticus.
carotid sinus branch of glossopharyngeal nerve → carotid sinus nerve.
carotid sinus nerve Karotissinusnerv *m*, Hering'-Blutdruckzügler *m*, Ramus sinus carotici n. glossopharyngei.
carotid sinus reflex 1. Karotissinisreflex *m*. 2. Karotissinussyndrom *nt*, hyperaktiver Karotissinusreflex *m*, Charcot--Weiss-Baker-Syndrom *nt*.
carotid sinus syncope/syndrome → carotid sinus reflex 2.
carotid sinus test Karotissinusdruckversuch *m*.
carotid stenosis Karotisstenose *f*.
carotid sulcus Sulcus caroticus.
carotid triangle Karotisdreieck *nt*, Trigonum caroticum.
inferior c. Trigonum musculare/omotracheale.
carotid trigone → carotid triangle.
carotid tubercle Tuberculum caroticum/anterius.
carotid vein, external V. retromandibularis.
carotid wall of tympanic cavity vordere Paukenhöhlenwand *f*, Paries caroticus.
ca·rot·i·dyn·ia [kəˌrɑtɪ'dɪnɪə] *n* Karotidodynie *f*.
car·o·tin ['kærətɪn] *n* → carotene.
car·o·ti·ne·mia *n* → carotenemia.
car·o·ti·no·sis [ˌkærətɪ'nəʊsɪs] *n* → carotenemia.
ca·rot·o·dyn·ia [kəˌrɑtə'dɪnɪə] *n* Karotidodynie *f*.
car·pal ['kɑːrpəl] **I** ~s *pl* → carpal bones. **II** *adj* Handwurzel(knochen) betr., karpal, Handwurzel(knochen)-, Karpal-, Karpo-.
carpal arch: anterior c. palmares Arteriengeflecht *nt* der Handwurzel.
dorsal c. dorsales Arteriengeflecht *nt* der Handwurzel, Rete carpale dorsale.
palmar c. → anterior c.
posterior c. → dorsal c.
carpal articulations Interkarpalgelenke *pl*, Articc. intercarpales.
carpal bone: central c. Os centrale.
first c. Os trapezium.
fourth c. Os hamatum.
great c. Os capitatum.
intermediate c. Os lunatum.
radial c. Os scaphoideum.
second c. Os trapezoideum.
third c. Os capitatum.
ulnar c. Os triquetrum.
carpal bones Handwurzel-, Karpalknochen *pl*, Carpalia *pl*, Ossa carpi.
carpal branch: dorsal c. of radial artery dorsaler Handwurzelast *m* der A. radialis, Ramus carpalis dorsalis a. radialis.
dorsal c. of ulnar artery dorsaler Handwurzelast *m* der A. ulnaris, Ramus carpalis dorsalis a. ulnaris.
palmar c. of radial artery palmarer Handwurzelast *m* der A. radialis, Ramus carpalis palmaris a. radialis.
palmar c. of ulnar artery palmarer Handwurzelast *m* der A. ulnaris, Ramus carpalis palmaris a. ulnaris.
carpal canal Handwurzelkanal *m*, -tunnel *m*, Karpalkanal *m*, -tunnel *m*, Canalis carpi/carpalis.
car·pa·le [kɑːr'peɪlɪ] *n, pl* -**lia** [-lɪə] → carpal bones.
carpal joints → carpal articulations.
carpal ligament: dorsal c.s Ligg. intercarpalia dorsalia.
radiate c. Lig. carpi radiatum.
carpal network, dorsal → carpal rete, dorsal.
carpal region *anat.* Handwurzel *f*, Handwurzelgegend *f*, -region *f*, Regio carpalis.
anterior c. Vorder-/Beugeseite *f* der Handwurzel, Regio carpalis anterior.
posterior c. Rück-/Streckseite *f* der Handwurzel, Regio carpalis posterior.
carpal rete, dorsal Arteriennetz *nt* des Handwurzelrückens, Rete carpale dorsale.
carpal retinaculum Retinaculum flexorum (manus), Lig. carpi transversum.
carpal sulcus Sulcus carpi.
carpal tunnel → carpal canal.
carpal tunnel syndrome *abbr.* **CTS** Karpaltunnelsyndrom *nt*.
car·pec·to·my [kɑːr'pektəmɪ] *n ortho.* Karpalknochenresektion *f*, Karpektomie *f*.
Carpenter ['kɑːrpəntər]: **C. syndrome** Carpenter'-Syndrom *nt*, Akrozephalo-(poly)syndaktylie II *f*.
car·pho·lo·gia [ˌkɑːrfə'ləʊdʒ(ɪ)ə] *n* → carphology.
car·phol·o·gy [kɑːr'fɑlədʒɪ] *n psychia., neuro.* Flockenlesen *nt*, Floccilatio *f*, Floccilegium *nt*, Karphologie *f*, Krozidismus *m*.
carpo- *pref.* Handwurzel(knochen)-, Karpal-, Karpo-.
car·po·car·pal [ˌkɑːrpə'kɑːrpəl] *adj* karpokarpal, intra-, interkarpal.
Carpoe ['kɑːrpəʊ, kɑːr'pəʊ]: **C.'s rhinoplasty** *HNO* Indische Methode/Rhinoplastik *f*.
car·po·go·ni·um [ˌkɑːrpə'gəʊnɪəm] *n micro.* Karpogon *nt*.
car·po·met·a·car·pal [ˌ-ˌmetə'kɑːrpl] *adj abbr.* **CMC** Handwurzel u. Mittelhand betr., karpometakarpal.
carpometacarpal articulation Karpometakarpalgelenk *nt*, CM-Gelenk *nt*, Artic. carpometacarpalis.
first c. → c. of thumb.
c. of thumb Sattelgelenk/Karpometakarpalgelenk des Daumens, Artic. carpometacarpalis pollicis.
carpometacarpal joint *abbr.* **CMCJ** → carpometacarpal articulation.
first c. → carpometacarpal articulation of thumb.
carpometacarpal ligaments Ligg. carpometacarpalia.
anterior c. → palmar c.
dorsal c. Ligg. carpometacarpalia dorsalia.
palmar c. Ligg. carpometacarpalia palmaria.
posterior c. → dorsal c.
volar c. → palmar c.
car·po·pe·dal contraction [ˌ-ˈpiːdl, -ˈped-] → carpopedal spasm.
carpopedal spasm Karpopedalspasmus *m*.

carpophalangeal

car·po·pha·lan·ge·al [ˌ-fəˈlændʒɪəl] *adj* karpophalangeal.
car·pop·to·sis [ˌkɑːrpəpˈtəʊsɪs] *n neuro.* Fall-, Kußhand *f*.
car·po·spore [ˈkɑːrpəspəʊər] *n micro.* Karpospore *f*.
car·pro·fen [kɑːrˈprəʊfen] *n pharm.* Carprofen *nt*.
car·pus [ˈkɑːrpəs] *n, pl* **-pi** [-paɪ] Handwurzel *f*, Handwurzelgelenk *nt*, Karpus *m*, Carpus *m*.
Carrel [kəˈrel; kaˈrel]: **C.'s method 1.** Carrel'-Naht *f*. **2.** *ortho.* Wundbehandlung *f* nach Dakin-Carrel.
C. treatment → C.'s method 2.
Carrel-Dakin [ˈdeɪkɪn]: **C.-D. fluid** verdünnte Natriumhypochloritlösung *f*.
C.-D. treatment → Carrel method 2.
car·ri·er [ˈkærɪər] *n* **1.** *biochem., physiol.* Träger(substanz *f*) *m*, Carrier *m*. **2.** *micro.* (Über-)Träger *m*, Infektions-, Keimträger *m*, Vektor *m*; Carrier *m*. **3.** *genet.* Träger *m*. **4.** *chir.* Halter *m*, Träger *m*; Nadel *f*. **5.** *techn.* Träger *m*, Transport *m*. **6.** Überbringer *m*, Bote *m*, Träger *m*. **7.** Transportbehälter *m*.
carrier cell Freßzelle *f*, Phagozyt *m*, Phagocyt *m*.
carrier-free *adj radiol., biochem.* (*Radioisotop*) rein, pur.
carrier gas *phys.* Trägergas *nt*.
carrier lipid *biochem.* Träger-, Carrierlipid *nt*.
carrier-mediated (active) transport trägervermittelter/carriervermittelter (aktiver) Transport *m*.
carrier molecule Träger-, Carriermolekül *nt*.
carrier protein Träger-, Carrierprotein *nt*.
carrier state → carrier 2.
Carrión [kærɪˈɑn]: **C.'s disease** Carrión-Krankheit *f*, Bartonellose *f*.
car·ri·on [ˈkærɪən] **I** *n* Aas *nt*, Kadaver *m*; faules/verdorbenes Fleisch *nt*. **II** *adj* **1.** faulig, aasig. **2.** aasfressend.
car·rot [ˈkærət] *n* Karotte *f*, Möhre *f*, Mohrrübe *f*, Gelbe Rübe *f*.
Carr-Price [ˈkɑːr ˈpraɪs]: **C.-P. reaction/test** Carr-Price-Reaktion *f*.
car·ry [ˈkærɪ] *vt* **1.** tragen, (über-)bringen; (*Nachricht*) (über-)bringen, weitergeben. **2.** transportieren, befördern. **3.** etw. mit s./bei s. haben, mitführen. **4.** (*Gewicht*) (aus-)halten, tragen. **5.** *gyn.* schwanger sein, ein Kind austragen. **6.** (zu-)führen; (*Schall*) (weiter-)leiten, übertragen (*to* zu). **7.** (*Krankheit*) weiter-, übertragen, verbreiten. **8.** *a. fig.* (unter-)stützen; unterhalten, ernähren. **9.** *fig.* zur Folge haben.
carry out *vt* aus-, durchführen. **to ~ an analysis/a diagnosis/an examination** eine Analyse/Diagnose/Untersuchung durchführen.
carry over *vi* bleiben, fort-, andauern, weiterbestehen, anhalten.
carry through *vt* **1.** (*Aufgabe*) vollenden, -bringen, ausführen. **2.** jdm. durchhelfen, jdn. durchbringen.
Carry-Blair [ˈkærɪ ˈbleər]: **C.-B. transport medium** Carry-Blair-Transportmedium *nt*.
car·ry·cot [ˈkærɪkɑt] *n* (Baby-)Tragetasche *f*.
car·ry·ing [ˈkærɪŋ] **I** *n* Tragen *nt*; Beförderung *f*, Transport *m*. **II** *adj* tragend, Trage-.
carry-over *n* (*Wirkung, Zustand*) Fortdauer *f od.* Weiterbestehen *nt*.
car·te·o·lol [ˈkɑːrtɪəlɑl] *n pharm.* Carteolol *nt*.

Carter [ˈkɑːrtər]: **C.'s black mycetoma** *derm.* Carter-Krankheit *f*, Madurafuß *m* durch Madurella mycetomi.
C.'s fever Rückfallfieber *nt* durch Borrelia carteri.
C.'s mycetoma → C.'s black mycetoma.
car·ti·lage [ˈkɑːrtlɪdʒ] *n* Knorpel *m*, Knorpelgewebe *nt*; *anat.* Cartilago *f*.
c. of acoustic meatus Gehörgangsknorpel, Cartilago meatus acustici.
c. of auditory tube Tuben-, Ohrtrompetenknorpel, Cartilago tubae auditoriae
c. of auricle Ohrmuschelknorpel, Knorpelgerüst *nt* der Ohrmuschel, Cartilago auricularis.
c. of nasal septum Septum-, Scheidewandknorpel, Cartilago septi nasi.
c. of pharyngotympanic tube Cartilago tubae auditoriae.
cartilage bone Ersatzknochen *m*.
cartilage breakdown Knorpelabbau *m*.
cartilage breakdown zone *histol.* Eröffnungszone *f*.
cartilage capsule Knorpelkapsel *f*.
cartilage cell Knorpelzelle *f*, Chondrozyt *m*.
cartilage cell space → cartilage lacuna.
cartilage chip *ortho.* Knorpelspan *m*, -chip *m*.
cartilage clamp → cartilage-holding forceps.
cartilage corpuscle → cartilage cell.
cartilage forceps → cartilage-holding forceps.
cartilage ground substance Knorpelgrundsubstanz *f*, Chondroid *nt*.
cartilage-holding forceps *ortho.* Knorpelfaßzange *f*.
cartilage lacuna Knorpelzellmulde *f*, -höhle *f*, -lakune *f*.
cartilage matrix Knorpelmatrix *f*, -grundsubstanz *f*.
cartilage neoplasia Knorpelgeschwulst *f*, -tumor *m*, -neoplasie *f*.
cartilage plate 1. Epiphysen(fugen)knorpel *m*, epiphysäre Knorpelzone *f*, Cartilago epiphysialis. **2.** epiphysäre Wachstumszone *f*, Epiphysenfuge *f*.
cartilage proliferation Knorpelproliferation *f*.
cartilage territory → chondrone.
car·ti·lag·in [ˈkɑːrtlædʒɪn] *n* → chondrogen.
car·ti·la·gin·e·ous [kɑːrtləˈdʒɪnɪəs, -njəs] *adj* → cartilaginous.
car·ti·la·gin·i·fi·ca·tion [ˌkɑːrtləˌdʒɪnɪfɪˈkeɪʃn] *n* Verknorpeln *nt*, Knorpelbildung *f*.
car·ti·la·gin·i·form [-ˈdʒɪnəfɔːrm] *adj* knorpelförmig, -ähnlich, chondroid.
car·ti·lag·i·noid [kɑːrtɪˈlædʒənɔɪd] *adj* → cartilaginiform.
car·ti·lag·i·nous [ˌ-ˈlædʒɪnəs] *adj* aus Knorpel bestehend, knorpelig, verknorpelt, kartilaginär, Knorpel-.
cartilaginous articulation Synchondrose *f*, Symphyse *f*, Junctura cartilaginea.
cartilaginous joints Articc. cartilagineae.
cartilaginous neurocranium → chondrocranium.
cartilaginous ossification Ersatzknochenbildung *f*, indirekte Ossifikation/ Osteogenese *f*, chondrale Ossifikation/ Osteogenese *f*, Osteogenesis cartilaginea.
cartilaginous part: c. of auditory tube Knorpeliger Tubenabschnitt *m*, Pars cartilaginea tubae auditivae.
c. of nasal septum knorpeliger Abschnitt *m* der Nasenscheidewand, Pars cartilaginea septi nasi.
cartilaginous perisplenitis Perisplenitis pseudocartilaginea.

cartilaginous tissue Knorpelgewebe *nt*, Knorpel *m*.
car·ti·la·go [ˌkɑːrtəˈleɪgəʊ] *n, pl* **-la·gi·nes** [-ˈlædʒəniːz] → cartilage.
cart·wheel structure [ˈkɑːrt,(h)wiːl] *histol.* Radspeichenstruktur *f*.
car·un·cle [ˈkærənkl, kəˈrʌŋkl] *n anat.* Karunkel *f*, Caruncula *f*.
ca·run·cu·la [kəˈrʌŋkjələ] *n, pl* **-lae** [-liː, -laɪ] → caruncle.
Carus [ˈkærəs]: **C.'** circle/curve *gyn.* Carus'-Krümmung *f*.
Carvallo [kɑːrˈvajo]: **C.'s sign** *card.* Carvallo'-Zeichen *nt*.
car·vone [ˈkɑːrvəʊn] *n* Carvon *nt*.
cary(o)- *pref.* (Zell-)Kern-, Kary(o)-, Nukle(o)-, Nucle(o)-.
car·y·o·chrome cells [ˈkeərɪəkrəʊm] karyochrome (Nerven-)Zelle *f*.
car·ze·nide [ˈkɑːrzɪnaɪd] *n pharm.* Carzenid *nt*.
Casal [kaˈsal]: **C.'s collar/necklace** *derm.* Casal'-Halsband *nt*, -Kragen *m*, -Kollier *nt*.
cas·cade [kæsˈkeɪd] *n* mehrstufiger Prozeß *m*, Kaskade *f*.
cascade stomach Kaskadenmagen *m*.
case [keɪs] **I** *n* **1.** (Krankheits-)Fall *m*; Patient(in *f*) *m*. **2.** (*Person*) Fall *m*; Angelegenheit *f*, Sache *f*. **a typical ~** ein typischer Fall (*of* von). **3.** Fall *m*, Vorkommnis *nt*, Fall *m*, Lage *f*, Umstand *m*. **in ~ of emergency** im Notfall. **in any ~** auf jeden Fall; jedenfalls. **in no ~** unter keinen Umständen, auf keinen Fall; keinesfalls. **5.** Behälter *m*; Kiste *f*, Kasten *m*, Kästchen *nt*, Schachtel *f*, Etui *nt*, (Schutz-)Hülle *f*, Überzug *m*; Gehäuse *nt*; *chir.* Besteckkasten *m*. **II** *vt* einhüllen (*in* in), umgeben (*in* mit).
c. of conscience Gewissensfrage *f*.
ca·se·ate [ˈkeɪsɪeɪt] *vt patho.* verkäsen.
ca·se·at·ing [ˈkeɪsɪeɪtɪŋ] *adj patho.* verkäsend, verkäst.
caseating pneumonia käsige/verkäsende Pneumonie *f*.
ca·se·a·tion [ˌkeɪsɪˈeɪʃn] *n* **1.** *patho.* Verkäsung *f*, Verkäsen *nt*. **2.** *biochem.* Caseinausfällung *f*.
caseation necrosis → caseous degeneration.
case book Buch *nt* mit od. Sammlung *f* von Fallbeschreibungen u. -beispielen.
case-control study Fallkontrollstudie *f*.
case history 1. Fall-, Krankengeschichte *f*. **2.** Fallbeispiel *nt*, typisches Beispiel *nt*. **3.** *socio., psycho.* Vorgeschichte *f* (*eines Falles*).
ca·sein [ˈkeɪsiːn, -siːɪn, keɪˈsiːn] *n* **1.** Kasein *nt*, Casein *nt*. **2.** *Brit.* → paracasein.
casein agar Caseinagar *m/nt*.
ca·sein·o·gen [keɪˈsiːnədʒən, ˌkeɪsɪˈn-] *Brit.* → casein 1.
case-load [ˈkeɪsləʊd] *n* Patientenanzahl *f*, -menge *f*, Anzahl/Menge *f* behandelter Patienten.
ca·se·og·e·nous [keɪsɪˈɑdʒənəs] *adj* (*a. patho.*) verkäsend.
ca·se·ous [ˈkeɪsɪəs] *adj* (*a. patho.*) käsig, käseartig, -ähnlich, -förmig, verkäst.
caseous abscess verkäsender Abszeß *m*.
caseous degeneration verkäsende Degeneration/Nekrose *f*, Verkäsung *f*.
caseous lymphadenitis Pseudotuberkulose *f*.
caseous necrosis → caseous degeneration.
caseous nephritis verkäsende Nephritis *f*, Nephritis caseosa.
caseous osteitis tuberkulöser Knochenfraß *m*.
caseous pneumonia käsige/verkäsende Pneumonie *f*.

caseous tonsillitis Angina/Tonsillitis lacunaris.
caseous tubercle *patho.* verkäsender Tuberkel *m*.
case study 1. → case history 1. **2.** Fallstudie *f*.
case·work ['keɪswɜrk] *n socio.* Einzelfallhilfe *f*, -arbeit *f*, soziale Einzelarbeit *f*, Case-work *nt*.
case·work·er ['keɪswɜrkər] *n socio.* Sozialarbeiter(in *f*) *m*.
case·worm ['keɪswɜrm] *n micro.* Echinokokkus *m*, Echinococcus *m*.
cas·ing ['keɪsɪŋ] *n* **1.** Gehäuse *nt*; (Schutz-)Hülle *f*, Verkleidung *f*, Mantel *m*. **2.** Rahmen *m*, Gerüst *nt*.
Casoni [kə'səʊnɪ]: **C.'s (intradermal/skin) reaction/test** Casoni-Test *m*.
Casselberry ['kæslberɪ]: **C.'s position** *chir.* Casselberry-Lagerung *f*.
Casser ['kɑːser]: **C.'s fontanelle** hintere Seitenfontanelle *f*, Warzenfontanelle *f*, Fonticulus mastoideus/posterolateralis.
 C.'s ligament Lig. mallei laterale.
 C.'s muscle Lig. mallei laterale.
cas·se·ri·an [kə'sɪərɪən]: **c. fontanelle** hintere Seitenfontanelle *f*, Warzenfontanelle *f*, Fonticulus mastoideus/posterolateralis.
 c. ligament Lig. mallei laterale.
 c. muscle Lig. mallei laterale.
Casserio [kə'sɪərɪəʊ] → Casser.
Casserius [kə'sɪərɪəs] → Casser.
cas·sette [kə'set, kæ-] *n* (Film-, Band-)Kassette *f*.
cast [kæst, kɑːst] (*v:* **cast; cast**) **I** *n* **1.** Guß *m*; Gußform *f*; (*a. dent.*) Abguß *m*, Abdruck *m*; Modell *nt*, Form *f*. **2.** *ortho.* fester Verband *m*, Stützverband *m*. **3.** *ortho.* Gips(verband) *m*. **4.** *ophthal.* (leichtes) Schielen *nt*, Strabismus *m*. **to have a ~ in one eye** schielen. **5.** Schattierung *f*, (Farb-)Ton *m*. **6.** *urol.* (Harn-)Zylinder *m*. **II** *vt* **7.** *bio.* werfen, gebären. **8.** (aus-, ab-)werfen; (*Haare, Zähne*) verlieren. **9.** einen Abguß/Abdruck herstellen *od.* formen. **10.** (*Blick*) werfen, (*Auge*) richten (*at, on, upon* auf); (*Licht*) werfen (*on* auf). **III** *vi s.* formen (lassen), geformt werden.
Castellani [kæstə'lænɪ]: **C.'s bronchitis** Bronchospirochaetosis Castellani *f*, hämorrhagische Bronchitis *f*, Bronchitis haemorrhagica.
 C.'s disease → C.'s bronchitis.
 C.'s paint *derm.* Castellani-Lösung *f*.
 C.'s test Castellani-Agglutinin-Absättigung *f*.
Castellani-Low [ləʊ]: **C.-L. sign/symptom** Castellani-Low-Zeichen *nt*.
cast immobilization *ortho.* Immobilisation *f* im Gipsverband.
cast·ing ['kæstɪŋ, 'kɑːstɪŋ] *n* **1.** Guß *m*, Gießen *nt*. **2.** (*a. dent.*) Abguß *m*, Gußstück *nt*; Form *f*, Modell *nt*. **3.** (*Haut, Schuppen*) Abwerfen *nt*; (*Haare*) Ausfallen *nt*.
Castle ['kæsl, 'kɑːsl]: **C.'s factor 1.** hä-
intrinsic-Faktor *m*, intrinsic factor. **2.** Zyano-, Cyanocobalamin *nt*, Vitamin B$_{12}$ *nt*.
Castleman [kæsəlmən]: **C.'s lymphocytoma** Castleman-Tumor *m*, -Lymphozytom *nt*, hyalinisierende plasmazelluläre Lymphknotenhyperplasie *f*.
cas·tor bean tick ['kæstər, 'kɑs-] *micro.* Holzbock *m*, Ixodes ricinus.
castor oil Rizinusöl *nt*.
cas·trate ['kæstreɪt] **I** *n* Kastrat *m*. **II** *vt* kastrieren, entmannen.
castrate cell *patho.* Kastrationszelle *f*.
cas·tra·tion [kæs'treɪʃn] *n* Kastrierung *f*, Kastration *f*.
castration anxiety *psychia.* Kastrationsangst *m*.

castration cell *patho.* Kastrationszelle *f*.
castration complex *psychia.* Kastrationsangst *f*.
cas·u·al·ty ['kæʒəltɪː, 'kæʒjʊəl-] *n* **1.** Unfall *m*. **2.** (Unfall-)Verletzung *f*. **3.** Verletzte(r *m*) *f*, Verwundete(r *m*) *f*, Opfer *nt*. **4.** *inf.* Unfallstation *f*, Notaufnahme *f*.
cas·u·is·tics [kæʒʊ'ɪstɪks] *pl* Kasuistik *f*.
CAT *abbr.* → computerized axial tomography.
cat [kæt] *n* Katze *f*.
ca·tab·a·sis [kə'tæbəsɪs] *n* (*Krankheit*) Nachlassen *nt*, Abklingen *nt*, Katabasis *f*.
cat·a·bat·ic [kætə'bætɪk] *adj* (*Krankheit*) nachlassend, zurückgehend, abklingend.
cat·a·bi·o·sis [‚-baɪ'əʊsɪs] *n* Katabiose *f*.
cat·a·bi·ot·ic [‚-baɪ'ɒtɪk] *adj* Katabiose betr., katabiotisch.
cat·a·bol·ic [‚-'bɒlɪk] *adj* Katabolismus betr., katabol(isch).
catabolic enzyme kataboles/katabolisches Enzym *nt*.
catabolic pathway katabolischer Stoffwechselweg *m*.
ca·tab·o·lin [kə'tæbəlɪn] *n* → catabolite.
ca·tab·o·lism [kə'tæbəlɪzəm] *n* Abbaustoffwechsel *m*, Katabolismus *m*, Katabolie *f*.
ca·tab·o·lite [kə'tæbəlaɪt] *n* Katabolit *m*.
catabolite gene-activator protein *abbr.* **CAP** Cyclo-AMP-Rezeptorprotein *nt* *abbr.* CRP, Katabolit-Gen-Aktivatorprotein *nt* *abbr.* CAP.
catabolite repression Katabolitenrepression *f*.
ca·tab·o·lize [kə'tæbəlaɪz] *vt, vi* abbauen, katabolisieren.
cat·a·crot·ic [‚kætə'krɒtɪk] *adj card.* (*Pulswelle*) katakrot.
catacrotic pulse Katakrotie *f*, katakroter Puls *m*, Pulsus catacrotus.
catacrotic wave katakrote Welle *f*.
ca·tac·ro·tism [kə'tækrətɪzəm] *n card.* (*Pulswelle*) Katakrotie *f*.
cat·a·di·crot·ic [‚kætədaɪ'krɒtɪk] *adj card.* (*Pulswelle*) katadikrot.
catadicrotic pulse Katadikrotie *f*, katadikroter Puls *m*, Pulsus catadicrotus.
catadicrotic wave katadikrote Welle *f*.
cat·a·di·cro·tism [‚-'daɪkrətɪzəm] *n card.* (*Pulswelle*) Katadikrotie *f*.
cat·a·did·y·mus [‚-'dɪdəməs] *n embryo.* Katadidymus *m*.
cat·a·di·op·tric [‚-daɪ'ɒptrɪk] *adj phys.* kombiniert reflektorisch u. refraktär, katadioptrisch.
cat·a·gen ['kætədʒən] *n* Katagen *nt*.
cat·a·gen·e·sis [‚-'dʒenəsɪs] *n histol.* Involution *f*, Re(tro)gression *f*.
cat·a·lase ['kætəleɪz] *n* Katalase *f*.
catalase-negative *adj* katalasenegativ.
catalase-positive *adj* katalasepositiv.
catalase test *micro.* Katalase-Test *m*.
cat·a·lep·sis [‚kætə'lepsɪs] *n* → catalepsy.
cat·a·lep·sy ['-lepsɪ] *n psychia.* Katalepsie *f*.
cat·a·lep·tic [‚-'leptɪk] **I** *n psychia.* Kataleptiker(in *f*) *m*. **II** *adj* Katalepsie betr., von Katalepsie betroffen, kataleptisch.
cat·a·lep·ti·form [‚-'leptɪfɔːrm] *adj* katalepsieähnlich, kataleptoid, kataleptiform.
cat·a·lep·toid [‚-'leptɔɪd] *adj* → cataleptiform.
cat·a·lo·gia [‚-'ləʊdʒ(ɪ)ə] *n psychia.* Verbigeration *f*.
ca·tal·y·sis [kə'tæləsɪs] *n*, *pl* **-ses** [-siːz] *chem.* Katalyse *f*.
cat·a·lyst ['kætlɪst] *n* Katalysator *m*, Akzelerator *m*.
cat·a·lyt·ic [‚kætə'lɪtɪk] *adj* Katalyse betr., katalytisch, Katalyse-.

catalytic subunit *biochem.* katalytische Untereinheit *f*.
cat·a·ly·za·tor [kætlɪ'zeɪtər] *n* → catalyst.
cat·a·lyze ['kætlaɪz] *vt* katalysieren, beschleunigen.
cat·a·lyz·er ['kætlaɪzər] *n* → catalyst.
cat·a·me·nia [kætə'miːnɪə] *n gyn.* Regelblutung *f*, Menstruation *f*, Menses *pl*.
cat·a·me·ni·al [‚-'miːnɪəl, -njəl] *adj* Menstruation betr., Menstruations-.
cat·a·men·o·gen·ic [‚-‚menə'dʒenɪk] *adj* menstruationsauslösend.
cat·am·ne·sis [‚kætæm'niːsɪs] *n* Katamnese *f*.
cat·am·nes·tic [‚-'nestɪk] *adj* Katamnese betr., katamnestisch.
cat·a·pha·sia [kætə'feɪʒ(ɪ)ə] *n* → catalogia.
cat·a·pho·re·sis [‚-fə'riːsɪs] *n* Kataphorese *f*.
cat·a·pho·ret·ic [‚-fə'retɪk] *adj* Kataphorese betr. kataphoretisch.
cat·a·pho·ria [‚-'fɔːrɪə] *n ophthal.* Kataphorie *f*.
cat·a·phy·lax·is [‚-fɪ'læksɪs] *n immun.* Kataphylaxie *f*.
cat·a·pla·sia [‚-'pleɪʒ(ɪ)ə] *n histol., patho.* Kataplasie *f*.
cat·a·pla·sis [kə'tæpləsɪs] *n* → cataplasia.
cat·a·plasm ['-plæzəm] *n pharm.* Breiumschlag *m*, -packung *f*, Kataplasma *nt*.
cat·a·plas·ma [‚-'plæzmə] *n* → cataplasm.
cat·a·plec·tic [‚-'plektɪk] *adj* Kataplexie betr., von ihr betroffen, kataplektisch.
cat·a·plex·is [‚-'pleksɪs] *n* → cataplexy.
cat·a·plex·y ['-pleksɪ] *n psychia.* Lachschlag *m*, Schrecklähmung *f*, Tonusverlustsyndrom *nt*, Kataplexie *f*, Gelolepsie *f*, Geloplegie *f*.
cat·a·ract ['-rækt] *n ophthal.* grauer Star *m*, Katarakt *f*, Cataracta *f*.
cat·a·rac·ta [‚-'ræktə] *n* → cataract.
cataract extraction *ophthal.* Kataraktextraktion *f*.
 extracapsular c. extrakapsuläre Kataraktextraktion.
 intracapsular c. intrakapsuläre Kataraktextraktion.
cataract lens Kataraktglas *nt*.
cat·a·rac·to·gen·ic [kætə‚ræktə'dʒenɪk] *adj* die Starentwicklung fördernd *od.* auslösend, kataraktogen.
cataract-oligophrenia syndrome Marinesco-Sjögren-Syndrom *nt*.
cat·a·rac·tous [‚kætə'ræktəs] *adj* Katarakt betr., von Katarakt betroffen, Katarakt-, Star-.
ca·tarrh [kə'tɑːr] *n* katarrhalische Entzündung *f*, Katarrh *m*.
ca·tarrh·al [kə'tɑːrəl] *adj* Katarrh betr., katarrhalisch.
catarrhal appendicitis katarrhalische Appendizitis *f*, Appendicitis catarrhalis.
catarrhal asthma bronchitisches/bronchialrhalisches Asthma *n*, Asthmabronchitis *f*.
catarrhal bronchitis Bronchialkatarrh *m*, katarrhalische Bronchitis *f*, Bronchitis catarrhalis.
catarrhal cholecystitis katarrhalische Gallenblasenentzündung/Cholezystitis *f*.
catarrhal conjunctivitis Bindehautkatarrh *m*, Conjunctivitis catarrhalis.
 chronic c. chronische katarrhalische Konjunktivitis *f*, Conjunctivitis catarrhalis chronica.
catarrhal cystitis Desquamationskatarrh *m*, Cystitis catarrhalis.
catarrhal dysentery Sprue *f*.
catarrhal-erosive gastroduodenitis katarrhalisch-erosive Gastroduodenitis *f*.
catarrhal gastritis katarrhalische Gastritis *f*, Magenkatarrh *m*.

catarrhal gingivitis Gingivitis catarrhalis/simplex.
catarrhal inflammation → catarrh.
catarrhal jaundice (Virus-)Hepatitis A *f abbr.* HA, epidemische Hepatitis *f*, Hepatitis epidemica.
catarrhal ophthalmia katarrhalische/muköse Ophthalmie *f*.
catarrhal pharyngitis Angina catarrhalis.
catarrhal pneumonia Bronchopneumonie *f*, lobuläre Pneumonie *f*; Herd-, Fokalpneumonie *f*.
catarrhal sinusitis katarrhalische Nebenhöhlenentzündung/Sinusitis *f*.
catarrhal stage (*Entzündung*) katarrhalische Phase *f*, Katarrh(al)phase *f*.
catarrhal stomatitis katarrhalische Stomatitis *f*, Stomatitis catarrhalis/simplex.
catarrhal tonsillitis katarrhalische Tonsillitis *f*, Tonsillitis/Angina catarrhalis.
catarrhal ulcerative keratitis katarrhalisch-ulzerative Keratitis *f*.
cat·a·stal·sis [ˌkætəˈstɔːlsɪs, -stæl-] *n* Katastaltik *f*, Katastalsis *f*.
cat·a·stal·tic [ˌ-ˈstɔːltɪk, -stæl-] **I** *n* Hemmer *m*, Hemmstoff *m*, Inhibitor *m*. **II** *adj* hemmend, inhibitorisch.
cat·a·state [ˈ-steɪt] *n* → catabolite.
cat·a·stat·ic [ˌ-ˈstætɪk] *adj* → catabolic.
cat·a·stroph·ic reaction [ˌ-ˈstrɒfɪk] *psychia.* Katastrophenreaktion *f*.
cat·a·thy·mia [ˌ-ˈθaɪmɪə] *n psychia.* Katathymie *f*.
cat·a·thy·mic [ˌ-ˈθaɪmɪk] *adj* Katathymie betr., katathym.
cat·a·to·nia [ˌ-ˈtəʊnɪə] *n* → catatonic schizophrenia.
cat·a·ton·ic [ˌ-ˈtɒnɪk] **I** *n psychia.* Katatoniker(in *f*) *m*, Patient(in *f*) *m* mit Katatonie. **II** *adj* katatonisch.
catatonic dementia katatone Demenz *f*.
catatonic schizophrenia *psychia.* katatone Schizophrenie *f*, Katatonie *f*.
cat·a·tri·crot·ic [ˌ-traɪˈkrɒtɪk] *adj card.* (*Pulswelle*) katatrikrot.
catatricrotic pulse Katatrikrotie *f*, katatrikroter Puls *m*, Pulsus catatricrotus.
cat·a·tri·cro·tism [ˌ-ˈtraɪkrətɪzəm] *n card.* (*Pulswelle*) Katatrikrotie *f*.
cat-bite disease [kæt] → cat-bite fever.
cat-bite fever Katzenbißfieber *nt*.
catch·ment area [ˈkætʃmənt] (*Krankenhaus*) Einzugs-, Versorgungsgebiet *nt*.
cat·e·chin [ˈkætɪtʃɪn, -kɪn] *n* Catechin *m*, Catechol *nt*.
cat·e·chol [ˈkætɪkɒl, -kəl] *n* **1.** → catechin. **2.** Brenzkatechin *nt*, -catechin *nt*.
cat·e·chol·a·mine [ˌkætəˈkəʊləmiːn, -ˈkəʊl-] *n* Katecholamin *nt*, (Brenz-)Katechinamin *nt*.
catecholamine-O-methyltransferase *n abbr.* **COMT** Catecholamin-O-methyltransferase *f abbr.* COMT.
catecholamine receptor → catecholaminergic receptor.
cat·e·chol·a·min·er·gic [ˌ-ˌkɒləmɪˈnɜːdʒɪk] *adj* katecholaminerg(isch).
catecholaminergic neuron katecholaminerges Neuron *nt*.
catecholaminergic receptor katecholaminerger Rezeptor *m*.
catecholaminergic system katecholaminerges System *nt*.
catechol oxidase *o*-Diphenoloxidase *f*, Catecholoxidase *f*, Polyphenoloxidase *f*.
cat·e·chu·ic acid [ˌ-ˈtʃuːɪk, -ˈk(j)uːɪk] → catechin.
cat·e·go·rize [ˈkætɪɡəraɪz] *vt* kategorisieren, klassifizieren, nach Kategorien einteilen *od.* ordnen.
cat·e·go·ri·za·tion [ˌkætəɡərɪˈzeɪʃn, -ɡəʊ-] *n* Klassifizierung *f*, Kategorisierung *f*.

cat·e·go·ry [ˈkætɪɡərɪ, -ˌɡəʊrɪ] *n*, *pl* **-ries** Kategorie *f*, Gruppe *f*, Art *f*, Klasse *f*. **to fall into the high-risk ~** zur Risikogruppe gehören.
cat·e·lec·trot·o·nus [ˌkætəlekˈtrɒtnəs] *n neuro.* Katelektrotonus *m abbr.* KET.
cat·e·nate [ˈkætɪneɪt] *vt* verketten, aneinanderreihen, -knüpfen.
cat·e·nat·ed dimer [ˈkætneɪtɪd] *biochem.* Catena-Dimer *nt*.
cat·e·noid [ˈkætənɔɪd] *adj* kettenförmig, -ähnlich, Ketten-.
ca·ten·u·late [kəˈtenjələt, -leɪt] *adj* → catenoid.
cat·er·pil·lar cell [ˈkætə(r)pɪlər] Anitschkow-Zelle *f*, -Myozyt *m*, Kardiohistiozyt *m*.
caterpillar dermatitis Raupendermatitis *f*.
caterpillar-hair ophthalmia Ophthalmia nodosa/pseudotuberculosa.
caterpillar ophthalmia → caterpillar-hair ophthalmia.
cat·gut [ˈkætɡət] *n chir.* Katgut *nt*, Catgut *nt*.
catgut suture → catgut.
ca·thaer·e·sis *n* → catheresis.
ca·thar·sis [kəˈθɑːrsɪs] *n*, *pl* **-ses** [-siːz] **1.** *psychia.* seelische Reinigung *f*, Läuterung *f*, Abreaktion *f*, Katharsis *f*. **2.** Reinigung *f*, Säuberung *f*; Abführung *f*.
ca·thar·tic [kəˈθɑːrtɪk] **I** *n pharm.* Abführmittel *nt*, Kathartikum *nt*, Laxans *nt*, Purgans *nt*, Purgativ(um *nt*) *nt*. **II** *adj pharm.* abführend, kathartisch, purgierend, Abführ-. **2.** *psychia.* Katharsis betr., kathartisch.
ca·thar·ti·cal [kəˈθɑːrtɪkl] *adj* → carthartic II.
ca·thep·sin [kəˈθepsɪn] *n* Kathepsin *nt*, Cathepsin *nt*.
ca·ther·e·sis [kəˈθerəsɪs] *n* (arzneimittelbedingte) Schwäche *f*.
cath·e·ret·ic [ˌkæθɪˈretɪk] *adj* **1.** schwächend. **2.** schwach ätzend.
cath·e·ter [ˈkæθɪtər] *n* Katheter *m*.
catheter angiography Katheterangiographie *f*.
catheter arteriography Katheterarteriographie *f*.
catheter aspiration Katheteraspiration *f*.
catheter blockade Katheterblockade *f*.
catheter clamp Katheterklemme *f*.
catheter dilatation Katheterdilatation *f*.
catheter drainage Katheterdrainage *f*.
percutaneous c. perkutane Katheterdrainage.
catheter embolization Katheterembolisation *f*.
catheter fever Katheter-, Urethral-, Harnfieber *nt*, Febris urethralis.
catheter forceps Kathetereinführzange *f*.
cath·e·ter·ism [ˈkæθɪtərɪzəm] *n* → catheterization.
cath·e·ter·ize [ˈkæθɪtəraɪz] *vt* einen Katheter einführen/legen, katheterisieren, abthetern.
cath·e·ter·i·za·tion [ˌkæθɪtəraɪˈzeɪʃn] *n* Katheterisierung *f*, Katheterismus *m*.
catheter kinking Katheterabknickung *f*, -abknicken *nt*.
cath·e·ter·o·stat [ˈkæθɪtərəstæt, kæˈθiːtərəʊ-] *n* Katheterständer *m*.
catheter patency Katheterdurchgängigkeit *f*.
catheter sepsis Kathetersepsis *f*.
catheter tip Katheterspitze *f*.
ca·thex·is [kəˈθeksɪs] *n*, *pl* **-thex·es** [-ˈθeksɪz] *psychia.* Kathexis *f*.
cath·i·so·pho·bia [ˌkæθɪsəʊˈfəʊbɪə] *n* Akathisie *f*.
cath·o·dal [ˈkæθədl] *adj abbr.* **C, Ca** *electr.*

Kathode betr., kathodisch, katodisch, Kathoden-.
cathodal closure clonus *abbr.* **CCCl** *physiol.* Kathodenschließungsklonus *m*.
cathodal closure contraction *abbr.* **CCC, CaCC** Kathodenschließungszuckung *f abbr.* KSZ, KaSZ.
cathodal closure tetanus *abbr.* **CCTe** *physiol.* Kathodenschließungstetanus *m*.
cathodal opening clonus *abbr.* **COCl, CaOCl** *physiol.* Kathodenöffnungsklonus *m*.
cathodal opening contraction *abbr.* **COC, CaOC** Kathodenöffnungszuckung *f abbr.* KÖZ, KaÖZ.
cathodal opening tetanus *abbr.* **COTe** *physiol.* Kathodenöffnungstetanus *m*.
cath·ode [ˈkæθəʊd] *n abbr.* **C, Ca** *electr.* Kathode *f abbr.* K.
cathode ray oscilloscope *abbr.* **CRO** Kathodenstrahloszilloskop *nt*.
cathode rays Kathodenstrahlen *pl*, -strahlung *f*.
cathode-ray tube *abbr.* **CRT** Kathodenstrahlröhre *f*.
ca·thod·ic [kæˈθɒdɪk, -ˈθəʊ-, kə-] *adj* → cathodal.
cath·o·lyte [ˈkæθəlaɪt] *n phys.* Katholyt *m*.
cat·i·on [ˈkætˌaɪən, -ən] *n* Kation *nt*.
cation exchange Kationenaustausch *m*.
cation exchanger Kationenaustauscher *m*.
cation exchange resin Kationenaustauscherharz *nt*, Katresin *nt*.
cat·i·on·ic [ˌkætaɪˈɒnɪk] *adj* Kation betr. *od.* enthaltend, kationisch, Kationen-.
cationic dye basischer/kationischer Farbstoff *m*.
cat·lin [ˈkætlɪn] *n chir.* zweischneidiges Amputationsmesser *nt*.
cat·ling [ˈkætlɪŋ] *n* catlin.
cat liver fluke *micro.* Katzenleberegel *m*, Opisthorchis felineus.
cat louse *micro.* Felicula subrustrata.
ca·top·tric [kəˈtɒptrɪk] *adj phys.* katoptrisch.
ca·top·trics [kəˈtɒptrɪks] *pl phys.* Katoptrik *f*.
cat-scratch disease/fever Katzenkratzkrankheit *f*, cat scratch disease (*nt*), benigne Inokulationslymphoretikulose *f*, Miyagawanellose *f*.
cat's cry syndrome → cri-du-chat syndrome.
cat's eye amaurosis *ophthal.* amaurotisches Katzenauge *nt*.
Cattell [kəˈtel]: **C.'s sign** *chir.* (*Pankreas*) Cattell'-Zeichen *nt*.
cat·tle plague [ˈkætl] Rinderpest *f*.
cattle tick *micro.* Rinderzecke *f*, Boophilus annulatus.
Ca·tu virus [ˈkæt(j)uː] *micro.* Catuvirus *nt*.
cau·da [ˈkaʊdə, ˈkɔːdə] *n*, *pl* **-dae** [-diː] *anat.* Schwanz *m*, Schweif *m*, Kauda *f*, Cauda *f*.
cauda equina *inf.* Kauda *f*, Cauda *f* equina.
cauda equina syndrome Kauda-Syndrom *nt*, Cauda-equina-Syndrom *nt*.
cau·dal [ˈkɔːdl] *adj* **1.** fuß-, schwanzwärts (gelegen), kaudal, caudal. **2.** Cauda equina betr., Kauda-, Kaudal-.
caudal analgesia → caudal anesthesia.
caudal anesthesia *anes.* Kaudalanästhesie *f*.
continuous c. Dauerkaudalanästhesie, kontinuierliche Kaudalanästhesie.
caudal artery mittlere Kreuzbeinarterie *f*, Sakralis *f* mediana, A. sacralis mediana.
caudal block → caudal anesthesia.
caudal branch of vestibular nerve unterer Teil *m* des N. vestibularis, Pars caudalis inferior n. vestibularis.

caudal canal Kauda(l)kanal *m*.
caudal colliculus unterer/hinterer Hügel *m* der Vierhügelplatte, Colliculus inferior.
caudal dysplasia syndrome sakrokokzygeale Agenesie *f*, Syndrom *nt* der kaudalen Regression.
caudal fovea Fovea caudalis/inferior.
caudal ganglion: c. of glossopharyngeal nerve unteres Glossopharyngeusganglion *nt*, Ggl. caudalis/inferius n. glossopharyngei.
c. of vagus nerve unteres Vagusganglion *nt*, Ggl. caudalis/inferius n. vagi.
caudal lobe of cerebellum kaudaler (Kleinhirn-)Lappen *m*, kaudaler (Kleinhirn-)Abschnitt *m*, Lobus caudalis/posterior cerebelli.
caudal neuropore *embryo*. hinterer/kaudaler Neuroporus *m*.
caudal pancreatectomy *chir*. distale Pankreatektomie *f*, Linksresektion *f*.
caudal regression syndrome → caudal dysplasia syndrome.
caudal retinaculum Retinaculum caudale.
caudal vertebrae → coccygeal vertebrae.
cau·date ['kɔːdeɪt] *adj bio*. einen Schwanz besitzend, geschwänzt; schwanzförmig.
caudate branches of anterior choroidal artery Rami caudae nuclei caudati.
cau·dat·ed ['kɔːdeɪtɪd] *adj* → caudate.
caudate eminence (of liver) → caudate process (of liver).
caudate lobe (of liver) Spieghel'-Leberlappen *m*, Lobus caudatus.
caudate nucleus Schweifkern *m*, Nc. caudatus.
caudate process (of liver) Proc. caudatus (hepatis).
caudate vertebrae → coccygeal vertebrae.
cau·da·to·len·tic·u·lar [kɔːˌdeɪtəʊlenˈtɪkjələr] *adj* Nc. caudatus u. Nc. lenticularis betr., kaudatolentikulär.
cau·da·tum [kɔːˈdeɪtəm] *n* Schweifkern *m*, Nc. caudatus.
cau·dec·to·my [kɔːˈdektəmɪ] *n neurochir*. Kaudektomie *f*.
cau·do·ceph·a·lad [ˌkɔːdəʊˈsefəlæd] *adj* kaudozephal, -kephal.
cau·do·len·tic·u·lar [ˌ-ˈlentɪkjələr] *adj* → caudatolenticular.
cau·li·flow·er ear ['kɔːləflaʊər, 'kɑl-] Blumenkohl-, Boxerohr *nt*.
caus·al ['kɔːzl] *adj* Ursache betr., auf die Ursache gerichtet, ursächlich, kausal, Kausal-; verursachend.
cau·sal·gia [kɔːˈzældʒ(ɪ)ə] *n neuro*. Kausalgie *f*.
causal treatment Kausalbehandlung *f*.
caus·a·tive ['kɔːzətɪv] *adj* verursachend, begründend, kausal (*of*).
cause [kɔːz] **I** *n* 1. Ursache *f*; Grund *m*, Anlaß *m*, Veranlaßung *f* (*for* zu). 2. Sache *f*, Angelegenheit *f*, Frage *f*. **II** *vt* 3. verursachen, hervorrufen, bewirken. 4. veranlassen.
caus·tic ['kɔːstɪk] **I** *n* 1. Ätz-, Beizmittel *nt*, Kaustikum *nt*. 2. → caustic curve. 3. → caustic surface. **II** *adj* kaustisch, ätzend, beißend, brennend.
caustic burn Verätzung *f*.
caustic curve *phys*. kaustische Kurve *f*, Brennlinie *f*.
caus·tic·i·ty [kɔːsˈtɪsətɪ] *n* Ätz-, Beizkraft *f*.
caustic potash Ätzkali *nt*, Kaliumhydroxid *nt*.
caustic soda Ätznatron *nt*, kaustische Soda *f*, Natriumhydroxid *nt*.
caustic substance → caustic 1.

caustic surface *phys*. Brennfläche *f*.
cau·ter·ant ['kɔːtərənt] *n*, *adj* → caustic.
cau·ter·i·za·tion [ˌkɔːtəraɪˈzeɪʃn] *n* (Aus-)Brennen *nt*, Kauterisation *f*, Kauterisieren *nt*, Kaustik *f*.
cau·ter·ize ['kɔːtəraɪz] *vt* (aus-)brennen, (ver-)ätzen, kauterisieren.
cau·ter·y ['kɔːtərɪ] *n* 1. → cauterization. 2. Brenneisen *nt*, Kauter *m*. 3. → caustic 1.
cautery snare *chir*. Diathermieschlinge *f*.
ca·va ['kɑːvə, 'keɪ-] *n* 1. Kava *f*, V. cava. 2. *pl* → cavum.
cav·a·gram ['kævəɡræm] *n* → cavogram.
ca·val ['keɪvəl, 'kɑː-] *adj* Vene cava betr., Kava-.
caval valve Eustachio'-, Sylvius'-Klappe *f*, Valvula v. cavae inferioris.
cav·a·scope ['kævəskəʊp] *n* Kavernoskop *nt*.
cave [keɪv] **I** *n* Höhle *f*. **II** *vt* aushöhlen.
ca·ve·o·la (intercellularis) [keɪvɪˈəʊlə] *histol*. Caveola *f* (intercellularis).
cav·ern ['kævərn] **I** *n* 1. (pathologischer) Hohlraum *m*, Kaverne *f*, Caverna *f*. 2. *anat*. Hohlraum *m*, Höhle *f*, Kaverne *f*, Caverna *f*. **II** *vt* aushöhlen.
cavern out *vt* aushöhlen.
c.s of cavernous bodies Schwellkörperkavernen *pl*, Cavernae corporum cavernosorum.
c.s of corpora cavernosa → c.s of cavernous bodies.
c.s of corpus spongiosum → c.s of spongy body.
c.s of spongy body Kavernen *pl* des Harnröhrenschwellkörpers, Cavernae corporis spongiosi.
ca·ver·na [kəˈvɜrnə] *n*, *pl* -**nae** [-niː] → cavern.
cavern formation *patho*. Kavernenbildung *f*.
cav·er·ni·tis [kævərˈnaɪtɪs] *n urol*. Entzündung *f* der Penisschwellkörper, Kavernitis *f*, Cavernitis *f*.
cav·er·no·ma [kævərˈnəʊmə] *n* → cavernous hemangioma.
cav·er·no·scope ['kævərnəskəʊp] *n* Kavernoskop *nt*.
cav·er·nos·co·py [ˌkævərˈnɒskəpɪ] *n* Kavernoskopie *f*.
cav·er·no·si·tis [ˌkævərnəˈsaɪtɪs] *n* → cavernitis.
cav·er·nos·to·my [ˌkævərˈnɒstəmɪ] *n chir*. Kavernostomie *f*.
cav·er·not·o·my [ˌ-ˈnɒtəmɪ] *n chir*. Kaverneneröffnung *f*, Speleo-, Kavernotomie *f*.
cav·ern·ous ['kævərnəs] *adj* 1. *anat*. Hohlräume enthaltend, kavernös. 2. *patho*. Kavernen enthaltend, porös, kavernös, schwammig. 3. (*Augen*) tiefliegend; (*Wangen*) eingefallen, hohl. 4. (*Atmung*) amphorisch.
cavernous angioma → cavernous hemangioma.
cavernous body: c. of clitoris Klitorisschwellkörper *m*, Corpus cavernosum clitoridis.
c. of penis (Penis-)Schwellkörper *m*, Corpus cavernosum penis.
cavernous-carotid aneurysm Karotis--Kavernosus-Aneurysma *nt*, -Fistel *f*.
cavernous groove of sphenoid bone Sulcus caroticus (ossis sphenoidalis).
cavernous hemangioma kavernöses Hämangiom *nt*, Kavernom *nt*, Haemangioma tuberonodosum.
cavernous lymphangioma 1. kavernöses Lymphangiom *nt*, Lymphangioma cavernosa. 2. Zystenhygrom *nt*, Hygroma/Lymphangioma cysticum.
cavernous malformation of portal vein *patho*. kavernöse Malformation/Fehlbildung *f* der Pfortader.
cavernous nerves: c. of clitoris Schwellkörpernerven *pl* der Klitoris, Nn. cavernosi clitoridis.
c. of penis Schwellkörpernerven *pl* des Penis, Nn. cavernosi penis.
cavernous part: c. of internal carotid artery Sinus cavernosus-Abschnitt *m* der A. carotis interna, Pars cavernosa (a. carotidis internae).
c. of (male) urethra spongiöser Urethraabschnitt *m*, Pars spongiosa (urethrae masculinae).
cavernous plexus Sinus cavernosus-Plexus *m*, Plexus cavernosus.
c. of clitoris Plexus cavernosus clitoridis.
c. of concha Venenplexus der Nasenmuschel, Plexus cavernosi concharum.
c. of penis Plexus cavernosus penis.
cavernous rales (*Auskultation*) Kavernenjauchzen *nt*, -juchzen *nt*.
cavernous resonance Kavernen-, Amphorengeräusch *nt*.
cavernous respiration (*Auskultation*) Kavernenatmen *nt*.
cavernous rhonchi → cavernous rales.
cavernous sinus Sinus cavernosus.
cavernous sinus branch of internal carotid artery Karotis interna-Ast *m* zum Sinus cavernosus, Ramus sinus cavernosi.
cavernous sinus fistula Sinus-cavernosus-Fistel *f*.
cavernous sinus syndrome Sinus-cavernosus-Syndrom *nt*.
cavernous sinus thrombosis Sinus-cavernosus-Thrombose *f*.
cavernous tumor → cavernous hemangioma.
cavernous veins (of penis) Schwellkörpervenen *pl*, Vv. cavernosae (penis).
cav·il·la [kəˈvɪlə] *n anat*. Keilbein *nt*, Os sphenoidale.
CA virus → croup-associated virus.
cav·i·ta·ry ['kævɪterɪ] *adj* → cavernous.
cavitary myelitis Syringomyelitis *f*.
cavitary tuberculosis kavernöse Tuberkulose *f*.
cav·i·tas ['kævɪtæs] *n*, *pl* **cav·i·ta·tes** [kævɪˈteɪtiːz] → cavity 2.
cav·i·tate ['kævɪteɪt] *vi* aushöhlen.
cav·i·ta·tion [kævɪˈteɪʃn] *n* 1. *patho*., *dent*. Höhlen-, Hohlraum-, Kavernenbildung *f*, Aushöhlung *f*. 2. → cavity 2.
ca·vi·tis [keɪˈvaɪtɪs] *n* Entzündung *f* der V. cava inferior *od*. superior.
cav·i·ty ['kævɪtɪ] *n*, *pl* -**ties** 1. Hohlraum *m*, (Aus-)Höhlung *f*. 2. *anat*. Höhle *f*, Höhlung *f*, Raum *m*, Cavitas *f*, Cavum *nt*. 3. *dent*. Loch *nt* (*im Zahn bei Karies*).
c. of concha Cavum/Cavitas conchalis.
c.ies of corpora cavernosa Schwellkörperkavernen *pl*, Cavernae corporum cavernosorum.
c.ies of corpus spongiosum Kavernen *pl* des Harnröhrenschwellkörpers, Cavernae corporis spongiosi.
c. of middle ear Paukenhöhle *f*, Cavum tympani, Cavitas tympanica.
c. of septum pellucidum Cavum septi pellucidi.
cavity carcinoma Kavernenkarzinom *nt*.
cavity hemorrhage *pulmo*. Kavernenblutung *f*.
ca·vog·ra·phy [keɪˈvɒɡrəfɪ] *n radiol*. Kontrastdarstellung *f* der V. cava, Kavographie *f*.
ca·vum ['keɪvəm] *n*, *pl* -**va** [-və] → cavity.
c. of septum pellucidum Cavum septi pellucidi.
cav·us ['keɪvəs] *n ortho*. Hohlfuß *m*, Pes cavus.

Cazenave

Cazenave [kazə'naːv]: **C.'s vitiligo** Pelade *f*, kreisrunder Haarausfall *m*, Alopecia areata, Area Celsi.
C band *genet.* (*Chromosom*) C-Bande *f*.
C banding *genet.* C-Banding *nt*.
CBC *abbr.* → complete blood count.
CBD *abbr.* [common bile duct] → common duct.
CBF *abbr.* → cerebral blood flow.
CBG *abbr.* **1.** → corticosteroid-binding globulin. **2.** → cortisol-binding globulin.
C bile C-Galle *f*.
C3b INA *abbr.* → C3b inactivator.
C3b inactivator *abbr.* **C3b INA** *immun.* C3b-Inaktivator *m abbr.* C3b-INA, Faktor I *m*.
CBS *abbr.* → chronic brain syndrome.
CCA *abbr.* → chimpanzee coryza agent.
CCA virus → chimpanzee coryza agent.
CCC *abbr.* → cathodal closure contraction.
CCCI *abbr.* → cathodal closure clonus.
C cells 1. (*Pankreas*) γ-Zellen *pl*, C-Zellen *pl*, C-Zellen *pl*. **2.** (*Schilddrüse*) parafollikuläre Zellen *pl*, C-Zellen *pl*. **3.** chromophobe Zellen *pl*.
CCK *abbr.* → cholecystokinin.
CCM *abbr.* → congestive cardiomyopathy.
C3 convertase *immun.* C3-Konvertase *f*, 4-2-Enzym *nt*.
C5 convertase *immun.* C5-Konvertase *f*.
CCTe *abbr.* → cathodal closure tetanus.
CCU *abbr.* → coronary care unit.
C$_4$-cycle *n biochem.* C$_4$-Zyklus *m*, Hatch-Slack-Zyklus *m*.
C.D. *abbr.* → curative dose.
Cd *abbr.* → cadmium.
cd *abbr.* → candela.
C.D.$_{50}$ *abbr.* → curative dose, median.
CD4 cell/lymphocyte CD4-Zelle *f*, CD4--Lymphozyt *m*, T4$^+$-Zelle *f*, T4$^+$-Lymphozyt *m*.
CD8 cell/lymphocyte CD8-Zelle *f*, CD8--Lymphozyt *m*, T8$^+$-Zelle *f*, T8$^+$-Lymphozyt *m*.
CDH *abbr.* → congenital dislocation of the hip.
cDNA *abbr.* → complementary DNA.
CDP *abbr.* → cytidine-(5'-)diphosphate.
CE *abbr.* **1.** → California encephalitis. **2.** → contractile element.
Ce *abbr.* → cerium.
CEA *abbr.* → carcinoembryonic antigen.
CE angle → caput-epiphysis angle.
ce·bo·ceph·a·lus [ˌsiːbəʊ'sefələs] *n embryo.* Kebo-, Zebo-, Cebozephalus *m*.
ce·bo·ceph·a·ly [ˌ-'sefəlɪ] *n embryo.* Affenkopf *m*, Kebo-, Zebo-, Cebozephalie *f*.
cec- *pref.* → ceco-.
ce·cal ['siːkəl] *adj* blind endend; zökal, zäkal, zum Zäkum gehörend; Blinddarm-.
cecal appendage → cecal appendix.
cecal appendix Wurmfortsatz *m* des Blinddarms, *inf.* Wurm *m*, Appendix *f* (vermiformis).
cecal artery: anterior c. vordere Blinddarmarterie *f*, A. c(a)ecalis anterior.
 posterior c. hintere Blinddarmarterie *f*, A. c(a)ecalis posterior.
cecal bud Zäkumknospe *f*, -anlage *f*.
cecal folds zäkale Peritonealfalten *pl*, Plicae c(a)ecales.
cecal foramen For. c(a)ecum (ossis frontalis).
 c. of frontal bone → cecal foramen.
 c. of tongue For. caecum linguae.
cecal hernia Hernie *f* mit Blinddarm im Bruchsack.
cecal recess Retrozäkalgrube *f*, Rec. retroc(a)ecalis.
cecal swelling → cecal bud.
cecal vascular fold Plica c(a)ecalis vascularis.

cecal volvulus Zäkalvolvulus *m*.
ce·cec·to·my [sɪ'sektəmɪ] *n chir.* Blinddarm-, Zäkumresektion *f*, Zäkektomie *f*, Typhlektomie *f*.
ce·ci·tis [sɪ'saɪtɪs] *n* Zäkumentzündung *f*, Typhlitis *f*.
ceco- *pref.* Blinddarm-, Zäko-, Zäkum-.
ce·co·cele ['siːkəʊsiːl] *n chir.* Zäkozele *f*.
ce·co·cen·tral [ˌ-'sentrəl] *adj* → centrocecal.
cecocentral scotoma *ophthal.* zentrozäkales Skotom *nt*.
ce·co·col·ic [ˌ-'kɒlɪk] *adj* Zäkum u. Kolon betr., zäkokolisch.
ce·co·co·lon [ˌ-'kəʊlən] *n* Zäkokolon *nt*.
ce·co·co·lo·pex·y [ˌ-'kəʊləpeksɪ] *n chir.* Zäkokolopexie *f*.
ce·co·co·los·to·my [ˌ-kəʊ'lɒstəmɪ] *n chir.* Zäkum-Kolon-Fistel *f*, Zäkokolostomie *f*, Kolozäkostomie *f*.
ce·co·fix·a·tion [ˌ-fɪk'seɪʃn] *n* → cecopexy.
ce·co·il·e·os·to·my [ˌ-ˌɪlɪ'ɒstəmɪ] *n chir.* Zäkum-Ileum-Fistel *f*, Zäkoileostomie *f*, Ileozäkostomie *f*.
ce·co·pex·y ['-peksɪ] *n chir.* Zäkumfixation *f*, -anheftung *f*, Zäkopexie *f*, Typhlopexie *f*.
ce·co·pli·ca·tion [ˌ-plɪ'keɪʃn] *n chir.* Zäkoplikation *f*.
ce·co·rec·tos·to·my [ˌ-rek'tɒstəmɪ] *n chir.* Zäkum-Rektum-Fistel *f*, Zäkorektostomie *f*.
ce·cor·rha·phy [sɪ'kɒrəfɪ] *n chir.* Zäkumnaht *f*, Zäkorrhaphie *f*.
ce·co·sig·moi·dos·to·my [ˌsiːkəʊˌsɪgˌmɔɪ'dɒstəmɪ] *n chir.* Zäkum-Sigma-Fistel *f*, Zäkosigmoidostomie *f*.
ce·cos·to·my [sɪ'kɒstəmɪ] *n chir.* Zäkumfistel *f*, -fistelung *f*, Zäko-, Typhlostomie *f*.
ce·cot·o·my [sɪ'kɒtəmɪ] *n chir.* Zäkumeröffnung *f*, Zäko-, Typhlotomie *f*.
ce·cum ['siːkəm] *n, pl* **-ca** [-kə] *anat.* **1.** blind endende Aussackung *f*, Blindsack *m*. **2.** Blinddarm *m*, Zäkum *nt*, Zökum *nt*, C(a)ecum *nt*, Intestinum c(a)ecum.
Ce·de·cea [sɪ'diːsɪə] *n micro.* Cedecea *f*.
CEE *abbr.* → Central European encephalitis.
Ceelen ['siːlən]: **C.'s disease** Ceelen-Gellerstedt-Syndrom *nt*, primäre/idiopathische Lungenhämosiderose *f*.
Ceelen-Gellerstedt ['gelərstet]: **C.-G. syndrome** Ceelen-Gellerstedt-Syndrom *nt*, primäre/idiopathische Lungenhämosiderose *f*.
CEE virus *micro.* CEE-Virus *nt*, FSME--Virus *nt*.
cef·a·clor ['siːfəklɔːr, -kləʊr] *n pharm.* Cefaclor *nt*.
cef·a·drox·il [ˌsefə'drɒksɪl] *n pharm.* Cefadroxil *nt*.
cef·a·lex·in [ˌ-'leksɪn] *n pharm.* Cefalexin *nt*.
cef·a·man·dole [ˌ-'mændəʊl] *n pharm.* Cefamandol *nt*.
cef·az·o·lin [sə'fæzəlɪn] *n pharm.* Cefazolin *nt*.
ce·fo·per·a·zone [ˌsiːfəʊ'perəzəʊn] *n pharm.* Cefoperazon *nt*.
ce·fo·tax·ime [ˌ-'tæksiːm] *n pharm.* Cefotaxim *nt*.
ce·fox·i·tin [sə'fɒksətɪn] *n pharm.* Cefoxitin *nt*.
cef·ta·zi·dime ['seftəzɪdiːm] *n pharm.* Ceftazidim *nt*.
cef·ti·zox·ime [ˌseftɪ'zɒksiːm] *n pharm.* Ceftizoxim *nt*.
cef·tri·a·xone [seftraɪ'æksəʊn] *n pharm.* Ceftriaxon *nt*.
cef·u·rox·ime [sefə'rɒksiːm] *n pharm.* Cefuroxim *nt*.

Cegka ['se(g)kə, 'sedʒ-]: **C.'s sign** Cejka--Zeichen *nt*.
ce·la·ri·um [sə'leərɪəm] *n* Mesothel *nt*.
Cel·e·bes vibrio ['seləbiːz, sə'liːbiːz] *micro.* Vibrio El-Tor *nt*, Vibrio cholerae biovar eltor.
celi- *pref.* → celio-.
ce·li·ac ['siːlɪæk] *adj anat.* Bauch(höhle) betr., Bauch(höhlen)-.
celiac angiography/arteriography Angiographie *f* des Truncus c(o)eliacus u. seiner Äste, Zöliakographie *f*.
celiac axis *anat.* Truncus c(o)eliacus.
celiac branches of vagus nerve Vagusäste *pl* zum Plexus c(o)eliacus, Rami c(o)eliaci n. vagi.
celiac crisis *ped.* Zöliakiekrise *f*.
celiac disease Zöliakie *f*, gluteninduzierte Enteropathie *f*.
celiac ganglia Ggll. c(o)eliaca.
celiac lymph nodes Lymphknoten *pl* des Truncus coeliacus, Nodi lymphatici viscerales coeliaci.
celiac nerves → celiac branches of vagus nerve.
celiac plexus 1. Sonnengeflecht *nt*, Plexus solaris, Plexus coeliacus. **2.** lymphatischer Plexus coeliacus.
celiac syndrome → celiac disease.
celiac trunk Truncus c(o)eliacus.
ce·li·al·gia [siːlɪ'ældʒɪə] *n* Abdominal-, Bauch-, Leibschmerzen *pl*, Abdominalgie *f*.
ce·li·ec·to·my [ˌ-'ektəmɪ] *n chir.* (Teil-)Entfernung *f* eines Bauchorgans.
celio- *pref.* Bauch(höhlen)-, Abdominal-, Zölio-.
ce·li·o·cen·te·sis [ˌsiːlɪəsen'tiːsɪs] *n chir.* Bauch(höhlen)punktion *f*, Zöliozentese *f*, -centese *f*.
ce·li·o·col·pot·o·my [ˌ-kal'pɒtəmɪ] *n gyn.* Kolpozöliotomie *f*, Coeliotomia vaginalis.
ce·li·o·dyn·ia [ˌ-'diːnɪə] *n* → celialgia.
ce·li·o·en·ter·ot·o·my [ˌ-ˌentə'rɒtəmɪ] *n chir.* (trans-)abdominale Enterotomie *f*, Laparoenterotomie *f*.
ce·li·o·gas·tros·to·my [ˌ-gæs'trɒstəmɪ] *n chir.* Zölio-, Laparogastrostomie *f*.
ce·li·o·gas·trot·o·my [ˌ-gæs'trɒtəmɪ] *n chir.* (trans-)abdominale Gastrotomie *f*, Zölio-, Laparogastrotomie *f*.
ce·li·o·hys·ter·ec·to·my [ˌ-ˌhɪstə'rektəmɪ] *n* **1.** *gyn.* transabdominale Hysterektomie *f*, Laparohysterektomie *f*, Hysterectomia abdominalis. **2.** *gyn.* Hysterectomia c(a)esarea.
ce·li·o·hys·ter·ot·o·my [ˌ-ˌhɪstə'rɒtəmɪ] *n gyn.* transabdominelle Hysterotomie *f*, Abdomino-, Laparo-, Zöliohysterotomie *f*.
ce·li·o·ma [siːlɪ'əʊmə] *n* Bauchhöhlentumor *m*.
ce·li·o·my·o·mec·to·my [ˌsiːlɪəˌmaɪə'mektəmɪ] *n gyn.* (trans-)abdominale Myomektomie *f*, Laparomyomektomie *f*.
ce·li·o·my·o·mot·o·my [ˌ-ˌmaɪə'mɒtəmɪ] *n gyn.* transabdominale Myomotomie *f*, Laparomyomotomie *f*.
ce·li·o·my·o·si·tis [ˌ-ˌmaɪə'saɪtɪs] *n* Bauchmuskelentzündung *f*.
ce·li·o·par·a·cen·te·sis [ˌ-ˌpærəsen'tiːsɪs] *n chir.* Stichinzision/Parazentese *f* der Bauchhöhle; Zöliozentese *f*.
ce·li·or·rha·phy [siːlɪ'ɒrəfɪ] *n chir.* Bauchdecken-, Bauchwandnaht *f*, Zöliorrhaphie *f*.
ce·li·o·sal·pin·gec·to·my [ˌsiːlɪəˌsælpɪn'dʒektəmɪ] *n gyn.* transabdominale Salpingektomie *f*, Zölio-, Laparosalpingektomie *f*.
ce·li·o·sal·pin·got·o·my [ˌ-ˌsælpɪn'gɒtəmɪ]

n gyn. transabdominelle Salpingotomie *f*, Zölio-, Laparosalpingotomie *f*.
ce·li·o·scope ['siːlɪəskəʊp] *n* Zölio-, Laparoskop *nt*.
ce·li·os·co·py [ˌsiːlɪ'ɒskəpɪ] *n* Bauch(höhlen)spiegelung *f*, Zölio-, Laparoskopie *f*.
ce·li·ot·o·my [ˌ-'ɒtəmɪ] *n chir.* **1.** Bauch-(höhlen)eröffnung *f*, Zölio-, Laparotomie *f*. **2.** Bauch(decken)schnitt *m*.
celiotomy incision Bauchdeckenschnitt *m*.
ce·li·tis [sɪ'leɪtɪs] *n patho.* (intra-)abdominelle Entzündung *f*.
cell [sel] *n* **1.** *bio., histol.* Zelle *f*. **2.** *phys.* (Speicher-)Zelle *f*, Element *nt*; *techn.* Schaltzelle *f*. **3.** Zelle *f*, Kammer *f*; Fach *nt*.
c.s of **Claudius** Claudius'-(Stütz-)Zellen *pl*.
c.s of **Müller** Müller'-Stützzellen *pl*, -Stützfasern *pl*.
c. of van **Gehuchten** Neuron *nt* vom Golgi--Typ.
cell aggregation Zellaggregation *f*, -verband *m*.
cell aggregate → cell aggregation.
cell antibody Zellantikörper *m*.
cell atrophy Zellatrophie *f*.
cell attachment Zellkontakt *m*, Junktion *f*.
cell axis Zellachse *f*.
cell biology *bio.* Zell-, Zyto-, Cytobiologie *f*.
cell blockade *micro.* Virusinterferenz *f*.
cell body 1. *bio.* Zelleib *m*, -körper *m*. **2.** Zelleib *m* der Nervenzelle, Perikaryon *nt*.
cell-bound antibody zellgebundener Antikörper *m*.
cell budding *micro.* Zellsprossung *f*, -knospung *f*.
cell center Zentrosom *nt*, Zentriol *nt*, Zentralkörperchen *nt*.
cell clone Zellklon *m*.
cell coat *bio.* Zellhülle *f*.
cell contact → cell attachment.
cell count Zellzählung *f*.
red c. *abbr.* RCC **1.** Erythrozytenzahl *f abbr.* Z_E. **2.** Bestimmung *f* der Erythrozytenzahl.
white c. *abbr.* WCC **1.** Leukozytenzahl *f*. **2.** Bestimmung *f* der Leukozytenzahl.
cell culture Zellkultur *f*.
human diploid c. *abbr.* HDCC humane diploide Zell(en)kultur, human diploid cell culture *abbr.* HDCC.
monkey kidney c. Affennierenzellkultur.
cell cycle Zellzyklus *m*.
cell death Zelltod *m*, -untergang *m*, Zytonekrose *f*.
cell differentiation Zelldifferenzierung *f*.
cell disintegration Zellzerfall *m*.
cell dispersion Zellsuspension *f*, -dispersion *f*.
cell division Zellteilung *f*.
differential c. differentielle Zellteilung.
direct c. direkte Zellteilung, Amitose *f*.
meiotic c. → reduction c.
mitotic c. mitotische Zellteilung, Mitose *f*.
reduction c. **1.** Reduktionsteilung, Meiose *f*. **2.** erste Reifeteilung.
cell elongation Zellverlängerung *f*.
cell enlargement Zellvergrößerung *f*.
cell envelope Zellhülle *f*, -umhüllung *f*.
cell extract Zellextrakt *f*.
cell-fixed antibody → cell-bound antibody.
cell-free *adj* zellfrei.
cell-free system zellfreies System *nt*.
cell fusion Zellverschmelzung *f*, -fusion *f*.
cell host *micro.* Wirtszelle *f*.
Cel·lia ['siːlɪə] *n micro.* Malaria-, Gabel-, Fiebermücke *f*, Anopheles *f*.
cel·li·form ['selɪfɔːrm] *adj* → cell-like.

cel·lif·u·gal [se'lɪf(j)əɡəl] *adj* → cellulifugal.
cell immunity Zell-, Gewebsimmunität *f*.
cell inclusion Zelleinschluß *m*.
cel·lip·e·tal [se'lɪpətəl] *adj* → cellulipetal.
cell layer Zellschicht *f*.
cell-like *adj* zellähnlich, -förmig.
cell line Zellinie *f*, -reihe *f*, Zell-Linie *f*.
continuous c. permanente Zellinie.
diploid c. diploide Zellinie.
cell lysis Zell-, Zytolyse *f*.
cell mass, intermediate *embryo.* Nephrotom *nt*.
cell matrix Zellmatrix *f*.
cell-mediated hypersensitivity *immun.* T--zellvermittelte Überempfindlichkeitsreaktion *f*, Tuberkulin-Typ/Spät-Typ/Typ IV *m* der Überempfindlichkeitsreaktion.
cell-mediated immunity. CMI zellvermittelte/zelluläre Immunität *f*.
cell-mediated lympholysis (assay) *abbr.* CML zellvermittelte Lympho(zyto)lyse *f*.
cell-mediated reaction → cell-mediated hypersensitivity.
cell membrane Zellmembran *f*, -wand *f*, Plasmalemm *nt*.
cell metabolism Zellstoffwechsel *m*, -metabolismus *m*.
cell migration Zellwanderung *f*.
cell movement Zellbewegung *f*.
ameboid c. amöboide Zellbewegung.
cell necrosis Zell-, Zytonekrose *f*.
cell nucleus Zellkern *m*, Nukleus *m*, Nucleus *m*.
cel·lo·bi·ase [ˌseləʊ'baɪeɪs] *n* β-Glukosidase *f*.
cel·lo·bi·ose [ˌ-'baɪəʊs] *n* Cellobiose *f*, Cellose *f*.
cel·lo·bi·u·ron·ic acid [ˌ-baɪjʊə'rɒnɪk] Cellobiuronsäure *f*.
cel·lo·hex·ose [ˌ-'heksəʊs] *n* Cellohexose *f*.
cel·loi·din [səˈlɔɪdɪn] *n* Zelloidin *nt*, Celloidin *nt*.
cel·lo·phane ['seləfeɪn] *n* Zello-, Cellophan *nt*.
cellophane rales (*Auskultation*) trockenes Knisterrasseln *nt*.
cel·lose ['seləʊs] *n* → cellobiose.
cel·lo·tet·rose [ˌseləʊ'tetrəʊs] *n* Cellotetrose *f*.
cel·lo·tri·ose [ˌ-'traɪəʊs] *n* Cellotriose *f*.
cell permeability Zellpermeabilität *f*.
cell physiology Zell-, Zytophysiologie *f*.
cell plasma Zell-, Zytoplasma *nt*.
cell plate *micro.* Zellplatte *f*.
cell population Zellpopulation *f*.
cell respiration innere Atmung *f*, Zell-, Gewebeatmung *f*.
cell sap = cytosol.
cell-surface antibody Oberflächenantikörper *m*.
cell-surface antigen (Zell-)Oberflächenantigen *nt*.
cell-surface marker *immun.* Zelloberflächenmarker *m*.
cell suspension Zellaufschwemmung *f*, -suspension *f*.
cell tropism Zelltropismus *m*.
cell turgor Zellturgor *m*.
cell turnover *histol.* Zellmauserung *f*.
cel·lu·la ['seljʊlə] *n, pl* -lae [-liː] *anat.* kleine Zelle *f*, Cellula *f*.
cel·lu·lar ['seljʊlər] *adj* Zelle betr., aus Zellen bestehend, zellulär, zellular, zellig, Zell-, Zyto-, Cyto-.
cellular cancer medulläres Karzinom *nt*, Ca. medullare.
cellular cartilage parenchymatöser/zellulärer Knorpel *m*.
cellular defence (system) zelluläre Abwehr *f*, zelluläres Abwehrsystem *nt*.

cellular edema zelluläres Ödem *nt*, Zellödem *nt*.
cellular fission Zellteilung *f*, -spaltung *f*.
cellular fuel Zellbrennstoff *m*.
cellular hyalin zelluläres Hyalin *nt*.
cellular hydrops Zellhydrops *m*.
cellular immunity → cell-mediated immunity.
cellular immunodeficiency zellulärer Immundefekt *m*, T-Zell-Immundefekt *m*.
cellular infiltration Zellinfiltration *f*.
cellular injury Zellschädigung *f*.
cel·lu·lar·i·ty [seljə'leərətɪ] *n* Zellreichtum *m*.
cellular layer Zellschicht *f*.
cellular metabolism Zellstoffwechsel *m*, -metabolismus *m*.
cellular nevus Nävuszell(en)nävus *m abbr.* NZN, Naevus naevocellularis.
cellular oncogene zelluläres Onkogen *nt*.
cellular pathologist Zell-, Zytopathologe *m*, -login *f*.
cellular pathology Zell-, Zytopathologie *f*.
cellular pleomorphism Zellpleomorphismus *m*.
cellular polymorphism Zellpolymorphie *f*.
cellular polyp adenomatöser Polyp *m*.
cel·lu·lase ['seljəleɪs] *n* Cellulase *f*.
cel·lule ['seljuːl] *n* → cellula.
cel·lu·lic·i·dal [seljə'lɪsɪdl] *adj* zell(en)zerstörend, zellentötend, zytozoid.
cel·lu·lif·u·gal [ˌ-'lɪf(j)əɡəl] *adj* vom Zellleib weg(führend).
cel·lu·lin ['seljəlɪn] *n* → cellulose.
cel·lu·lip·e·tal [ˌ-'lɪpətəl] *adj* zum Zelleib hin(führend).
cel·lu·li·tis [seljə'laɪtɪs] *n* Entzündung *f* des Unterhautbindegewebes, Zellulitis *f*, Cellulitis *f*.
cel·lu·lo·neu·ri·tis [seljələʊnjʊə'raɪtɪs, -nʊ-] *n* Nervenzell-, Neuronenentzündung *f*, Neuronitis *f*.
cel·lu·lo·san ['seljələʊsæn] *n* Hemizellulose *f*, -cellulose *f*.
cel·lu·lose ['seljələʊs] *n* Zellulose *f*, Cellulose *f*.
cellulose degeneration amyloide Degeneration *f*; Amyloidose *f*.
cellulose synthase Cellulosesynthase *f*.
cel·lu·lo·tox·ic [ˌseljələʊ'tɒksɪk] *adj* **1.** zellschädigend, zytotoxisch. **2.** durch Zytotoxin(e) hervorgerufen, zytotoxisch.
cel·lu·lous ['seljələs] *adj* aus Zellen bestehend, zellulär.
cell wall Zellwand *f*.
cell wall antigen Zellwandantigen *nt*.
ce·lom = coelom.
ce·lo·ma [sɪ'ləʊmə] *n* → coelom.
ce·lom·ic *adj* → coelomic.
ce·lo·nych·ia [ˌsiːləʊ'nɪkɪə] *n derm.* Löffel-, Hohlnagel *m*, Koilonychie *f*.
ce·lo·phle·bi·tis [ˌ-flɪ'baɪtɪs] *n patho.* Entzündung *f* der V. cava inferior *od.* superior.
ce·los·chi·sis [sɪ'lɒskəsɪs] *n embryo.* Bauchwandspalte *f*, Zeloschisis *f*, Gastroschisis *f*.
cel·o·scope ['siːləskəʊp] *n* **1.** → cavernoscope. **2.** → celioscopy.
ce·los·co·py [sɪ'lɒskəpɪ] *n* **1.** → cavernoscopy. **2.** → celioscopy.
ce·lo·so·mia [ˌsiːlə'səʊmɪə] *n embryo.* Zelosomie *f*.
ce·lo·thel ['θel] *n* Mesothel *nt*.
ce·lo·the·li·o·ma [ˌ-θiːlɪ'əʊmə] *n* Mesotheliom(a) *nt*.
ce·lo·the·li·um [ˌ-'θiːlɪəm] *n* Mesothel *nt*.
ce·lot·o·my [sɪ'lɒtəmɪ] *n chir.* Hernien-, Bruchoperation *f*, Herniotomie *f*.

CELO virus [chicken, embryo, lethal, orphan] CELO-Virus *nt*.
ce·lo·vi·rus [ˌsiːləʊˈvaɪrəs] *n* → CELO virus.
Celsius [ˈselsɪəs, -ʃɪəs]: **C. scale** Celsiusskala *f*.
C. thermometer Celsiusthermometer *nt*.
Celsus [ˈselsəs]: **C.' alopecia** Pelade *f*, kreisrunder Haarausfall *m*, Alopecia areata, Area Celsi.
C.' area → C.' alopecia.
C.' kerion Celsus'-Kerion *nt*, Kerion Celsi.
C.' vitiligo → C.' alopecia.
ce·ment [sɪˈment] **I** *n* **1.** Zement *m*. **2.** Klebstoff *m*, Kleister *m*, Kitt *m*, Bindemittel *nt*, -substanz *f*; Gips *m*. **3.** *dent.* (Zahn-)Zement *m*, Cementum *nt*, Substantia ossea dentis. **4.** *dent.* Präparat *nt* für Zahnfüllungen, Zement *m*. **II** *vt* zementieren; (ein-, ver-)kitten, leimen.
ce·men·ta·tion [ˌsɪmənˈteɪʃn] *n ortho., dent.* (Ein-)Zementieren *nt*, (Ver-)Kitten *nt*, (Ein-)Zementierung *f*.
cement cell Zementzelle *f*, Zementozyt *m*.
cement gun *ortho.* (Knochen-)Zementspritze *f*.
ce·men·ti·fi·ca·tion [sɪˌmentɪfɪˈkeɪʃn] *n* → cementogenesis.
ce·ment·i·fy·ing fibroma [sɪˈmentɪfaɪɪŋ] → cementoblastoma.
ce·ment·ing substance [sɪˈmentɪŋ] → cement substance.
ce·men·ti·tis [ˌsɪmənˈtaɪtɪs] *n dent.* Zementitis *f*.
cement line Kittlinie *f*.
ce·men·to·blast [sɪˈmentəblæst] *n dent.* Zementbildner *m*, -zelle *f*, Zementoblast *m*.
ce·men·to·blas·to·ma [-ˌblæsˈtəʊmə] *n dent.* Zementfibrom *nt*, Zement(o)blastom *nt*.
ce·men·to·cla·sia [-ˈkleɪʒ(ɪ)ə] *n dent.* Zementoklasie *f*.
ce·men·to·clast [ˈklæst] *n* Zementoklast *m*, Odontoklast *m*, -clast *m*.
ce·men·to·cyte [ˈ-saɪt] *n* Zementzelle *f*, Zementozyt *m*.
ce·men·to·gen·e·sis [ˌ-ˈdʒenəsɪs] *n dent.* Zementbildung *f*, Zementogenese *f*.
ce·men·to·ma [sɪˌmenˈtəʊmə] *n dent.* Zementom *nt*.
ce·men·to·per·i·os·ti·tis [sɪˌmentəˌperɪəsˈtaɪtɪs] *n dent.* Parodontitis *f*, Periodontitis *f*.
ce·men·to·sis [sɪmənˈtəʊsɪs] *n dent.*, HNO Zementhyperplasie *f*, Hyperzementose *f*.
cement substance *histol.* Kittsubstanz *f*.
ce·men·tum [sɪˈmentəm] *n* → cement 3.
cementum hyperplasia → cementosis.
ce·nen·ceph·a·lo·cele [ˌsɪnənˈsefələʊsiːl] *n* Zönenzephalozele *f*.
ce·nes·the·sia [ˌsɪnesˈθiːʒ(ɪ)ə] *n* Zönästhesie *f*.
ce·nes·the·sic [ˌ-ˈθiːsɪk] *adj* Zönästhesie betr., zönästhestisch.
ce·nes·the·si·op·a·thy [ˌ-θiːzɪˈɒpəθɪ] *n* Zönästhesiopathie *f*.
ce·nes·thet·ic [ˌ-ˈθetɪk] *adj* → cenesthesic.
ce·nes·thop·a·thy [ˌ-ˈθɒpəθɪ] *n* → cenesthesiopathy.
ce·no·bi·um [sɪˈnəʊbɪəm] *n micro.* Schleimkolonie *f*, Zönobium *nt*.
cen·o·cyte [ˈsenəsaɪt] *n bio.* Zönozyt *m*, -zyte *f*.
cen·sor [ˈsensər] *n psychia.* Zensor *m*.
cent. *abbr.* → centigrade.
cen·ter [ˈsentər] **I** *n* **1.** *phys., mathe., fig.* Zentrum *nt*, Mittelpunkt *m*; Dreh-, Angelpunkt *m*, Achse *f*. **2.** *anat.* Zentrum *nt*, Zentrale *f*, Zentralstelle *f*. **3.** *physiol.* (ZNS-)Zentrum *nt*, Centrum *nt*. **II** *vt* **4.** (*a. fig.*) in den Mittelpunkt stellen **5.** *techn.* zentrieren, auf den Mittelpunkt *od.* das Zentrum ausrichten/einstellen. **6.** *fig.* konzentrieren, richten (*on* auf). **III** *vi* **7.** im Mittelpunkt stehen. **8.** s. konzentrieren *od.* richten (*in, on* auf), s. drehen (*round* um). **9.** s. (an einer Stelle) ansammeln *od.* aufhäufen, (ver-)sammeln (*at, about, around, on* um).
c. of attraction *phys.* Anziehungsmittelpunkt.
c. of cerebellum Kleinhirnmark *nt*, Corpus medullare cerebelli.
c. of gravity *phys.* **1.** Schwerpunkt. **2.** Gleichgewichtspunkt.
c. of gyration *phys.* Drehpunkt.
c. for horizontal gaze movements Zentrum für horizontale Blickbewegungen.
c. of mass *phys.* Massenträgheitszentrum.
c. of motion *phys.* Drehpunkt.
c. for vertical gaze movements Zentrum für vertikale Blickbewegungen.
cen·ter·ing [ˈsentərɪŋ] *n* Zentrieren *nt*, Einmitten *nt*.
Centers for Disease Control *abbr.* **CDC** Centers for Disease Control *abbr.* CDC (*US-amerikanisches Gesundheitsamt*).
cen·tes·i·mal [senˈtesəməl] *adj* hundertste(r, s), hundertteilig, zentesimal, Zentesimal-.
cen·te·sis [senˈtiːsɪs] *n* Punktion *f*, Zentese *f*.
centi- *pref. abbr.* **c** Zenti-, Centi- *abbr.* c.
cen·ti·grade [ˈsentɪɡreɪd] *adj abbr.* **C, cent.** hundertgradig, -teilig.
centigrade scale 1. hundertteilige Skala *f*. **2.** Celsius-Skala *f*.
centigrade thermometer Celsiusthermometer *nt*.
cen·ti·gram [ˈ-ɡræm] *n abbr.* **cg** Zentigramm *nt*.
cen·ti·gramme *n Brit.* → centigram.
cen·ti·gray [ˈ-ɡreɪ] *n abbr.* **cGy** Centigray *nt abbr.* cGy.
cen·ti·li·ter [ˈ-liːtər] *n abbr.* **cl** Zentiliter *m/nt abbr.* cl.
cen·ti·me·ter [ˈ-miːtər] *n abbr.* **cm** Zenti-, Centimeter *m/nt abbr.* cm.
cen·tral [ˈsentrəl] *adj* **1.** zentral *od.* in der Mitte (liegend), zentrisch, Zentral-, Mittel-, Haupt-. **2.** *anat.* das ZNS betr; das Zentrum eines Wirbels betr., zentral. **3.** *phys.* (*Kraft*) von einem Punkt ausgehend, auf einen Punkt gerichtet.
Central African tick fever zentralafrikanisches Zeckenfieber *nt*.
central amaurosis *ophthal.* zentrale Amaurose *f*, Amaurosis centralis.
central anesthesia *neuro.* zentrale/zentral-bedingte Anästhesie *f*.
central angiospastic retinitis → central angiospastic retinopathy.
central angiospastic retinopathy Retinitis/Chorioretinopathia centralis serosa.
central anosmia *neuro.* zentrale Anosmie *f*.
central aphasia *neuro.* Total-, Globalaphasie *f*.
central apparatus *histol., bio.* Zentralapparat *m*.
central artery: anterolateral c.ies Aa. centrales/thalamostriatae anterolaterales.
anteromedial c.ies Aa. centrales/thalamostriatae anteromediales.
long c. A. centralis longa, A. recurrens.
posterolateral c.ies Aa. centrales posterolaterales.
posteromedial c.ies Aa. centrales posteromediales.
c. of retina zentrale Netzhautschlagader *f*, -arterie *f*, A. centralis retinae.
short c. A. centralis brevis.
c.ies of spleen (*Milz*) Zentralarterien *pl*.
central ataxia *neuro.* zentrale Ataxie *f*.
central body Zentralkörperchen *nt*, Zentriol *nt*.
central bone Os centrale.
central bradycardia *card.* zentrale Bradykardie *f*.
central bulb *histol.* Zentralkolben *m*.
central callus *ortho.* zentraler/innerer Kallus *m*.
central canal: c.s of modiolus longitudinale Spindel-/Modioluskanälchen *pl*, Canales longitudinales modioli.
c. of spinal cord Zentralkanal *m* des Rückenmarks, Canalis centralis (medullae spinalis).
c. of Stilling → c. of vitreous body.
c. of vitreous body Cloquet'-Kanal *m*, Canalis hyaloideus.
central cataract *ophthal.* Zentralstar *m*, Cataracta centralis.
central cell *histol.* Hauptzelle *f*.
central chondroma echtes/zentrales Chondrom *nt*, Enchondrom *nt*.
central chondrosarcoma *patho.* zentrales Chondrosarkom *nt*, Enchondrosarkom *nt*.
central choroiditis zentrale Chorioiditis *f*, Chorioiditis centralis.
central chromatolysis zentrale/retrograde Chromatolyse *f*.
central columella of cochlea Schneckenachse *f*, -spindel *f*, Modiolus *f*.
central complex *biochem.* zentraler/ternärer Komplex *m*.
central convolution: anterior c. Gyrus pr(a)ecentralis.
posterior c. Gyrus postcentralis.
central convulsion *neuro.* zentrale Konvulsion *f*.
central core disease (of muscle) Central-Core-Disease (*nt*), -Krankheit *f*.
central cyanosis zentrale Zyanose *f*.
central deafness zentrale Hörstörung/Schwerhörigkeit *f*.
central disk-shaped retinopathy *ophthal.* Kuhnt-Junius-Krankheit *f*, scheibenförmige/disziforme senile feuchte Makuladegeneration *f*.
central dislocation of the hip *ortho.* zentrale Luxation *f* des Femurkopfes, zentrale Hüftgelenksluxationsfraktur *f*.
central emetic *pharm.* zentrales Emetikum *nt*.
Central European encephalitis *abbr.* **CEE** zentraleuropäische Zeckenenzephalitis *f*, Frühsommer-Enzephalitis *f abbr.* FSE, Frühsommer-Meningo-Enzephalitis *f abbr.* FSME, Central European encephalitis *abbr.* CEE.
Central European encephalitis virus *micro.* CEE-Virus *nt*, FSME-Virus *nt*.
Central European tick-borne fever → Central European encephalitis.
central fever zentrales Fieber *nt*.
central fibroma of bone desmoplastisches Fibrom *nt*.
central fibrosarcoma zentrales Fibrosarkom *nt*.
central fissure → central sulcus of cerebrum.
central fovea of retina Sehgrube *f*, Fovea centralis (retinae).
central ganglioneuroma zentrales Ganglioneurom *nt*, Ganglioglio(m)a *nt*.
central gray zentrales Höhlengrau *nt*, Substantia grisea centralis.
central gyrus: anterior c. Gyrus pr(a)ecentralis.
posterior c. Gyrus postcentralis.
central implantation *gyn., embryo.* oberflächliche/superfizielle Einnistung/Implantation *f*.

central line → central venous catheter.
central lobule of cerebellum Zentralläppchen *nt*, Lobulus centralis (cerebelli).
central myelitis zentrale Myelitis *f*, Myelitis centralis.
central necrosis zentrale Nekrose *f*, Zentralnekrose *f*.
central nervous system *abbr.* **CNS** Zentralnervensystem *nt abbr.* ZNS, Gehirn u. Rückenmark *nt*, Systema nervosum centrale, Pars centralis systematis nervosi.
central neuritis parenchymatöse Neuritis *f*.
central nucleus: c. of amygdaloid body Nc. centralis corporis amygdaloidei.
 lateral c. of thalamus Nc. centralis lateralis (thalami).
 medial c. of thalamus Nc. centralis medialis (thalami).
 superior c. Nc. centralis superior.
 c. of ventral column of spinal cord Nc. centralis.
central nystagmus zentraler Nystagmus *m*.
central osteitis 1. Knochenmark(s)entzündung *f*, Osteomyelitis *f*. 2. Endostentzündung *f*, Endostitis *f*.
central pain zentraler Schmerz *m*.
central paralysis zentrale Lähmung *f*.
central part of lateral ventricle mittlerer/zentraler Seitenhornabschnitt *m*, Pars centralis (ventriculi lateralis cerebri).
central pillar of cochlea Schneckenachse *f*, -spindel *f*, Modiolus *f*.
central pit Sehgrube *f*, Fovea centralis.
central point *mathe.* Mittelpunkt *m*.
central pontine myelinoclasis/myelinolysis zentrale pontine Myelinolyse *f*.
central pulse wave transmission time zentrale Pulswellenlaufzeit *f*.
central region of brain Zentralregion *f*.
central scotoma *ophthal.* Zentralskotom *nt*, zentrales Skotom *nt*.
central serous retinopathy → central angiospastic retinopathy.
central shivering pathway zentrale Zitterbahn *f*.
central softening of thrombus *patho.* puriforme Erweichung *f*.
central spindle Zentralspindel *f*.
central sulcus: c. of cerebrum Rolando'-Fissur *f*, Zentralfurche *f* des Großhirns, Sulcus centralis (cerebri).
 c. of insula Sulcus centralis insulae.
central superior nodes obere Mesenteriallymphknoten *pl*, Nodi lymphatici mesenterici superiores, Nodi superiores centrales.
central tendon: c. of diaphragm Zentralfläche *f* des Zwerchfells, Centrum tendineum.
 c. of perineum Sehnenplatte *f* des Damms, Centrum tendineum perinei.
central tract of thymus zentraler Thymusstrang *m*, Tractus centralis thymis.
central understanding of speech zentrales Sprachverstehen/Sprachverständnis *nt*.
central vein Zentralvene *f*.
 c.s of hepatic lobules → c.s of liver.
 c.s of liver Zentralvenen *pl*, Vv. centrales (hepatis).
 c. of retina Zentralvene der Netzhaut, V. centralis retinae.
 c. of suprarenal gland Zentralvene der Nebenniere, V. centralis glandulae suprarenalis.
central venous alimentation zentralvenöse Ernährung *f*.
central venous catheter zentraler Venenkatheter *m*, zentraler Venenkatheter *m*.

central venous feeding zentralvenöse Ernährung *f*.
central venous nutrition *abbr.* **CVN** zentralvenöse Ernährung *f*.
central venous pressure *abbr.* **CVP** zentralvenöser Druck *m abbr.* ZVD, zentraler Venendruck *m*.
central vertigo zentraler Schwindel *m*.
central vision direktes/zentrales Sehen *nt*.
cen·tre *n Brit.* → center.
cen·tren·ce·phal·ic [ˌsentrənsɪ'fælɪk] *adj* zentrenzephal.
centrencephalic epilepsy zentrenzephale Epilepsie *f*.
centrencephalic system (*ZNS*) zentrenzephales System *nt*.
centri- *pref.* Zentrum-, Zentri-, Zentro-, Zentral-.
cen·tri·ac·i·nar emphysema [ˌsentrɪ'æsɪnər] zentro-/zentriazinäres (Lungen-)Emphysem *nt*.
cen·tric ['sentrɪk] *adj* 1. zum Zentrum gehörend, im Zentrum/Mittelpunkt befindlich, zentral, zentrisch. 2. *anat., physiol.* zu einem Nervenzentrum gehörend, vom Nervenzentrum stammend *od.* kommend.
cen·tri·cal ['sentrɪkl] *adj* → centric.
centric fusion *genet.* Robertson-Translokation *f*.
cen·trif·u·gal [sen'trɪfjəgl] **I** *n* Zentrifuge *f*, (Trenn-)Schleuder *f*. **II** *adj* 1. vom Zentrum wegstrebend, vom Zentrum wegleitend *od.* -gerichtet, zentrifugal. 2. *physiol.* vom ZNS wegführend, zentrifugal, ableitend, efferent.
centrifugal current absteigender/zentrifugaler Strom *m*.
centrifugal force Zentrifugal-, Zentrifugations-, Fliehkraft *f*.
cen·trif·u·gal·i·za·tion [senˌtrɪfjəgəlɪ'zeɪʃn] *n* → centrifugation.
cen·trif·u·gal·ize [sen'trɪfjəgəlaɪz] *vt* → centrifuge II.
centrifugal nerve efferenter/zentrifugaler Nerv *m*.
cen·trif·u·gate [sen'trɪfjəgɪt, -geɪt] *vt* → centrifuge II.
cen·trif·u·ga·tion [senˌtrɪfjə'geɪʃn] *n* Zentrifugierung *f*, Zentrifugieren *nt*.
cen·tri·fuge ['sentrɪfjuːdʒ] **I** *n* Zentrifuge *f*, (Trenn-)Schleuder *f*. **II** *vt* zentrifugieren, schleudern.
cen·tri·lob·u·lar [ˌsentrɪ'lɑbjələr] *adj histol.* zentrilobulär.
centrilobular emphysema zentrilobuläres (Lungen-)Emphysem *nt*.
cen·tri·ole ['sentrɪəʊl] *n* Zentriol *nt*.
cen·trip·e·tal [sen'trɪpɪtl] *adj* zum Zentrum *od.* ZNS hinstrebend, zentripetal; *physiol.* afferent.
centripetal current aufsteigender/zentripetaler Strom *m*.
centripetal force Zentripetalkraft *f*.
centripetal nerve afferenter/zentripetaler Nerv *m*.
centripetal obesity Stammfettsucht *f*.
centro- *pref.* → centri-.
cen·tro·ac·i·nar cells [ˌsentrəʊ'æsɪnər, -nɑr] (*Pankreas*) zentroazinäre Zellen *pl*.
centroacinar emphysema → centriacinar emphysema.
cen·tro·blast ['blæst, -blɑst] *n* Germino-, Zentroblast *m*.
cen·tro·blas·tic-centrocytic malignant lymphoma [-'blæstɪk] zentroblastisch-zentrozytischen (malignes) Lymphom *nt*, Brill-Symmers-Syndrom *nt*, Morbus Brill-Symmers, großfollikuläres Lymphom/Lymphoblastom *nt*.
centroblastic malignant lymphoma zentroblastisches Lymphom *nt*.

cephalic artery

cen·tro·ce·cal [ˌ-'siːkl] *adj ophthal.* zentrozäkal.
centrocecal scotoma *ophthal.* zentrozäkales Skotom *nt*.
cen·tro·cyte ['-saɪt] *n* Germino-, Zentrozyt *m*.
cen·tro·cyt·ic malignant lymphoma [ˌ-'sɪtɪk] zentrozytisches (malignes) Lymphom *nt*, lymphozytisches Lymphosarkom *nt*.
cen·tro·des·mose [ˌ-'dezməʊs] *n micro.* Zentrodesmose *f*.
cen·tro·des·mus [ˌ-'dezməs] *n* → centrodesmose.
cen·tro·lec·i·thal [ˌsentrəʊ'lesɪθəl] *adj bio.* zentrolezithal.
centrolecithal ovum *bio.* zentrolezithales Ei *nt*.
cen·tro·lob·u·lar [ˌ-'lɑbjələr] *adj* → centrilobular.
cen·tro·me·di·an nucleus of Lyus [ˌ-'miːdɪən] Nc. centromedianus thalami.
centromedian nucleus of thalamus → centromedian nucleus of Lyus
cen·tro·mere ['-mɪər] *n* Zentromer *nt*, Kinetochor *f*.
cen·tro·mer·ic [ˌ-'merɪk, -'mɪər-] *adj* Zentromer betr., zentromer.
centromeric banding *genet.* C-Banding *nt*.
cen·tro·nu·cle·ar myopathy [ˌ-'n(j)uːklɪər] zentronukleäre Myopathie *f*.
centro-osteosclerosis *n* → centrosclerosis.
cen·tro·phe·nox·ine [ˌ-fɪ'nɑksiːn] *n pharm.* Centrophenoxin *nt*.
cen·tro·plasm ['-plæzəm] *n histol.* Zentroplasma *f*.
cen·tro·plast ['-plæst] *n micro.* Zentroplast *m*.
cen·tro·scle·ro·sis [ˌ-sklɪ'rəʊsɪs] *n ortho.* (*Knochen*) Markhöhlensklerose *f*.
cen·tro·some ['-səʊm] *n* 1. Zentrosom *nt*, Zentriol *nt*, Zentralkörperchen *nt*. 2. Mikrozentrum *nt*, Zentrosphäre *f*.
cen·tro·sphere ['-sfɪər] *n* 1. Zentroplasma *nt*, Zentrosphäre *f*. 2. → centrosome 1.
cen·tro·stal·tic [ˌ-'stæltɪk] *adj* zentrostaltisch.
cen·tro·stri·a·tal fibers [ˌ-ˌstraɪ'eɪtl] zentrostriatale Fasern *pl*, Fibrae centrostriatales.
CEP *abbr.* → congenital erythropoietic porphyria.
cephal- *pref.* → cephalo-.
ceph·a·lad ['sefəlæd] *adj anat.* kopfwärts.
ceph·a·lal·gia [ˌsefə'lældʒ(ɪ)ə] *n* Kopfschmerz(en *pl*) *m*, Kephalgie *f*, Zephalgie *f*, Cephalgia *f*, Cephalalgia *f*, Cephal(a)ea *f*, Kephal(a)ea *f*, Kephalalgie *f*, Kephalodynie *f*.
ceph·a·lea [ˌ-'lɪə] *n* → cephalalgia.
ceph·al·e·de·ma [ˌsefəlɪ'diːmə] *n* Kephal-, Zephalödem *nt*.
ceph·al·e·mat·o·cele [ˌsefəlɪ'mætəsɪːl] *n* → cephalhematocele.
ceph·al·e·ma·to·ma [ˌsefəlɛ'məʊmə] *n* → cephalhematoma.
ceph·a·lex·in [ˌsefə'leksɪn] *n pharm.* Cefalexin *nt*.
ceph·al·gia [sɪ'fældʒ(ɪ)ə] *n* → cephalalgia.
ceph·al·he·mat·o·cele [ˌsefəlhɪ'mætəsɪːl] *n* Kephalhämatozele *f*.
ceph·al·he·ma·to·ma [ˌ-ˌhiːmə'təʊmə] *n* Kopfblutgeschwulst *f*, Kephalhämatom *nt*.
ceph·al·hy·dro·cele [ˌ-'haɪdrəsɪːl] *n* Kephalohydrozele *f*.
ce·phal·ic [sɪ'fælɪk; *Brit.* keː-] *adj* Kopf(region) betr., kopfwärts, kranial, kephalisch, Kopf-, Schädel-.
cephalic artery → carotid artery, common.

cephalic flexure

cephalic flexure *embryo.* Scheitelbeuge *f.*
cephalic-medullary angle Hirnstamm-Hirnbasis-Winkel *m.*
cephalic phase (*Verdauung*) vagale/zephale Phase *f.*
cephalic presentation *gyn.* Kopf-, Schädellage *f.*
cephalic reflexes Hirnnervenreflexe *pl.*
cephalic tetanus → cephalotetanus.
cephalic vein Cephalica *f*, V. cephalica.
accessory c. Cephalica *f* accessoria, V. cephalica accessoria.
intermediate/median c. Cephalica *f* intermedia/mediana, V. mediana cephalica.
cephalic vesicles *embryo.* Hirnbläschen *pl.*
ceph·a·lin ['sefəlın] *n* Kephalin *nt*, Cephalin *nt.*
cephalin-cholesterol flocculation test Hanger-Flockungstest *m*, Kephalin-Cholesterin-Test *m.*
ceph·a·li·tis [sefə'laıtıs] *n* Gehirnentzündung *f*, Enzephalitis *f*, Encephalitis *f.*
ceph·a·li·za·tion [ˌsefəlı'zeıʃn] *n embryo.* Zephalization *f*, Kephalisation *f.*
cephalo- *pref.* Kopf-, Schädel-, Kephal(o)-, Zephal(o)-.
ceph·a·lo·cau·dal [ˌsefəloʊ'kɔːdl] *adj* kraniokaudal.
cephalocaudal axis Körperlängsachse *f.*
cephalocaudal folding *embryo.* kraniokaudale Krümmung *f.*
ce·phal·o·cele ['sefəloʊsiːl] *n* Kephalo-, Zephalozele *f.*
ceph·a·lo·cen·te·sis [ˌ-sen'tiːsıs] *n chir.* Zephalozentese *f*, -centese *f.*
ceph·a·lo·dac·ty·ly [ˌ-'dæktəlı] *n embryo.* Zephalodaktylie *f.*
ceph·a·lo·dym·ia [ˌ-'dımıə] *n embryo.* Kephalo-, Zephalodymie *f.*
ceph·a·lod·y·mus [sefə'lodıməs] *n* Kephalo-, Zephalodymus *m.*
ceph·a·lo·dyn·ia [sefəloʊ'diːnıə] *n* → cephalalgia.
ceph·a·lo·gen·e·sis [ˌ-'dʒenəsıs] *n embryo.* Kopfentwicklung *f*, Kephalo-, Kraniogenese *f.*
ceph·a·lo·gram ['-græm] *n* Kephalogramm *nt.*
ceph·a·lo·he·mat·o·cele [ˌ-hı'mætəsiːl] *n* → cephalhematoma.
ceph·a·lo·he·ma·to·ma [ˌ-ˌhiːmə'toʊmə] *n* → cephalhematoma.
ceph·a·lo·ma [sefə'loʊmə] *n old* medulläres Karzinom *nt*, Ca. medullare.
ceph·a·lo·med·ul·la·ry angle [ˌsefəloʊ-'medəlerɪ; -'meˈdʌlərɪ] → cephalic-medullary angle.
ceph·a·lo·meg·a·ly [ˌ-'megəlı] *n* Kopfvergrößerung *f*, Kephalomegalie *f.*
ceph·a·lom·e·lus [sefə'lomıləs] *n embryo.* Zephalo-, Kephalomelus *m.*
ceph·a·lo·men·in·gi·tis [sefəloʊˌmenın-'dʒaıtıs] *n* Hirnhautentzündung *f*, Meningitis cerebralis.
ceph·a·lom·e·ter [sefə'lamıtər] *n* Schädelmesser *m*, Kephalometer *nt.*
ceph·a·lo·met·ric radiograph [ˌsefəloʊ-'metrık] → cephalogram.
cephalometric roentgenogram → cephalogram.
ceph·a·lom·e·try [sefə'lamətrı] *n* Schädelmessung *f*, Kephalometrie *f.*
ceph·a·lo·mo·tor [ˌsefələ'moʊtər] *adj* Kopfbewegungen betr., den Kopf bewegend, kephalomotorisch.
ceph·a·lo·nia [sefə'loʊnıə] *n* Kephalonie *f.*
ceph·a·lop·a·gus [sə'lapəgəs] *n embryo.* Kranio-, Kephalopagus *m.*
ceph·a·lop·a·thy [ˌ-'lapəθı] *n* Kopfkrankung *f*, Kephalopathie *f.*
ceph·a·lo·pha·ryn·ge·us [ˌsefələfə'rındʒı-əs] *n* M. constrictor pharyngis superior.
ceph·a·lo·ple·gia [ˌ-'pliːdʒ(ı)ə] *n neuro.* Kephaloplegie *f.*
ceph·a·lo·spor·an·ic acid [ˌ-spɔː'rænık] Cephalosporansäure *f.*
ceph·a·lo·spor·in [ˌ-'spɔːrın, -'spoʊ-] *n pharm.* Cephalo-, Zephalo-, Kephalosporin *nt.*
ceph·a·lo·spor·i·nase [ˌ-'spoʊrıneız] *n* Cephalosporinase *f.*
cephalosporin C Cephalosporin C *nt.*
cephalosporin N Adicillin *nt*, Cephalosporin N *nt*, Penicillin N *nt.*
ceph·a·lo·spo·ri·o·sis [ˌ-ˌspoʊrı'oʊsıs] *n* Cephalosporiuminfektion *f*, Cephalosporiose *f.*
Ceph·a·lo·spo·ri·um [ˌ-'spoʊrıəm] *n micro.* Cephalosporium *nt.*
ceph·a·lo·stat ['-stæt] *n* → cephalometer.
ceph·a·lo·tet·a·nus [ˌ-'tetənəs] *n* Kopftetanus *m*, Tetanus capitis.
ceph·a·lo·thin ['sefəloʊθın] *n pharm.* Kephalothin *nt*, Cephalotin *nt.*
ceph·a·lo·tho·rac·ic [ˌ-θə'ræsık] *adj* Kopf u. Thorax betr., kraniothorakal, kephalothorakal, thorakokranial.
ceph·a·lo·tho·ra·co·il·i·op·a·gus [ˌ-θɔːrə-kəʊɪlı'apəgəs] *n embryo.* Kephalothorakoiliopagus *m.*
ceph·a·lo·tho·ra·cop·a·gus [ˌ-θɔːrə'kapə-gəs] *n embryo.* Kephalothorakopagus *m.*
ceph·a·lo·tri·gem·i·nal angiomatosis [ˌ-traı'dʒemınl] Sturge-Weber(-Krabbe)-Krankheit *f*, -Syndrom *nt*, enzephalofaziale Angiomatose *f*, Neuroangiomatosis encephalo-oculo-cutanea, Angiomatosis encephalo-oculo-cutanea, Angiomatosis encephalotrigeminalis.
ceph·a·lo·tome ['-toʊm] *n* Kephalotom *nt.*
ceph·a·lot·o·my [sefə'latəmı] *n embryo.* Kephalotomie *f.*
ceph·a·lo·tribe ['sefəloʊtraıb] *n gyn.* Kephalotrib *m*, -tripter *m.*
ceph·a·lo·trip·sy ['-trıpsı] *n gyn.* Kephalotripsie *f*, -thrypsie *f.*
ceph·a·pi·rin [sefə'paırın] *n pharm.* Cefapirin *nt.*
ceph·ra·dine ['sefrədiːn] *n pharm.* Cefradin *nt.*
ce·ra ['sıərə] *n* Wachs *nt.*
ce·ra·ceous [sı'reıʃəs] *adj* wachsähnlich, -artig.
ce·ram·ic [sə'ræmık] **I** *n* **1.** *chem.* Metalloxid *nt.* **2.** keramisches Material *nt*, Keramik *f.* **II** *adj* keramisch.
cer·am·i·dase [sə'ræmıdeız] *n* Acylsphingosindeacylase *f*, Ceramidase *f.*
ceramidase deficiency Farber'-Krankheit *f*, disseminierte Lipogranulomatose *f.*
cer·a·mide ['serəmaıd] *n* Zeramid *nt*, Ceramid *nt.*
ceramide cholinephosphotransferase Ceramidcholinphosphotransferase *f.*
ceramide glucoside Gluko-, Glucocerebrosid *nt.*
ceramide lactoside Lactosyl-*N*-acylsphingosin *nt.*
ceramide lactosidosis Lactosylceramidose *f*, neutrale β-Galaktosidase-Defekt *m.*
ceramide trihexosidase Ceramidtrihexosidase *f*, α-(D)-Galaktosidase A *f.*
ceramide trihexosidase deficiency Fabry-Syndrom *nt*, Morbus Fabry *m*, hereditäre Thesaurismose Ruiter-Pompen-Weyers *f*, Ruiter-Pompen-Weyers-Syndrom *nt*, Thesaurismosis hereditaria lipoidica, Angiokeratoma corporis diffusum (Fabry), Angiokeratoma universale.
ceramide trihexoside Trihexosylceramid *nt.*
ce·rane ['sıəreın, 'ser-] *n* Hexacosan *nt.*
cer·a·sin ['serəsın] *n* Zerasin *nt*, Cerasin *nt.*
ce·rate ['sıəreıt] *n pharm.* Wachssalbe *f*, Cerat *nt*, Ceratum *nt.*
cer·a·tec·to·my [serə'tektəmı] *n ophthal.* Hornhautvorwölbung *f*, -staphylom *nt*, Keratektasie *f*, Kerektasie *f.*
cer·a·tin ['serətın] *n* Hornstoff *m*, Keratin *nt.*
cer·a·to·cri·coi·de·us (muscle) [ˌserətoʊ-kraı'kɔıdıəs] Zeratokrikoideus *m*, M. ceratocricoideus.
cer·a·to·cri·coid ligament [ˌ-'kraıkɔıd] Lig. ceratocricoideum.
ceratocricoid muscle → ceratocricoideus (muscle).
cer·a·to·glos·sus [ˌ-'glasəs] *n* M. chondroglossus.
cer·a·to·pha·ryn·ge·al muscle [ˌ-fə'rın-dʒ(ı)əl] → ceratopharyngeus (muscle).
cer·a·to·pha·ryn·ge·us (muscle) [ˌ-fə'rın-dʒ(ı)əs] Pars ceratopharyngea m. constrictoris pharyngis medii.
Cer·a·to·pog·on·i·dae [ˌ-pə'ganədıː] *pl micro.* Gnitzen *pl*, Ceratopogonidae *pl.*
cer·a·tum [sə'reıtəm] *n* → cerate.
cer·car·ia [sər'keərıə] *n*, *pl* **-car·i·ae** ['keərıˌiː] *micro.* Schwanzlarve *f*, Zerkarie *f*, Cercaria *f.*
cer·car·i·al [sər'keərıəl] *adj* Zerkarie(n) betr., durch Zerkarien hervorgerufen, Zerkarien-.
cercarial dermatitis Schwimmbadkrätze *f*, Weiherhippel *m*, Bade-, Schistosomen-, Zerkariendermatitis *f.*
cer·ca·ri·ci·dal [sərˌkærə'saıdl] *adj* zerkarien(ab)tötend, zerkarizid.
cer·ca·ri·en·hul·len·re·ak·tion [sərˌkærı-ənˌhʌlənrı'ækʃn] *n micro.* Zerkarienhüllenreaktion *f*, Cercarien-Hüllen-Reaktion *f abbr.* CHR.
cer·clage [sɜːr'klaːʒ] *n chir., gyn.* Zerklage *f*, Cerclage *f.*
c. of fractured bone Knochencerclage *f.*
cerclage wire Cerclagedraht *m.*
cer·co·cys·tis [ˌsɜːrkoʊ'sıstıs] *n micro.* Zystizerkoid *nt*, Cysticercoid *nt.*
cer·coid ['sɜːrkɔıd] *n micro.* Zerkoid *nt.*
Cer·com·o·nas [sɜːr'kamənəs] *n micro.* Cercomonas *f.*
Cer·cos·po·ra [sɜːr'kaspərə] *n micro.* Cercospora *f.*
ce·re·al ['sıərıəl] **I** *n* Getreidepflanze *f*, Kornfrucht *f*, Zerealie *f*; Getreide *nt.* **II** *adj* Getreide-.
cerebell- *pref.* → cerebello-.
cer·e·bel·lar [serə'belər] *adj* Kleinhirn/Cerebellum betr., zum Zerebellum gehörend, zerebellar, zerebellär, Kleinhirn-, Cerebello-.
cerebellar abscess Kleinhirnabszeß *m.*
cerebellar apoplexy 1. Kleinhirnapoplexie *f*, Apoplexia cerebelli. **2.** Kleinhirn(ein)blutung *f.*
cerebellar artery: inferior c., anterior vordere untere Kleinhirnarterie *f*, Cerebelli *f* inferior anterior, A. inferior anterior cerebelli.
inferior c., posterior hintere untere Kleinhirnarterie *f*, Cerebelli *f* inferior posterior, A. inferior posterior cerebelli.
superior c. obere Kleinhirnarterie *f*, Cerebelli *f* superior, A. superior cerebelli.
cerebellar ataxia *neuro.* zerebelläre Ataxie *f.*
hereditary c. Nonne-Marie-Krankheit *f*, (Pierre) Marie-Krankheit *f*, zerebellare Heredoataxie, Heredoataxia cerebellaris.
cerebellar cortex Kleinhirnrinde *f*, Cortex cerebellaris.
cerebellar cyst Kleinhirnzyste *f.*
cerebellar degeneration Kleinhirndegeneration *f.*

cerebellar epilepsy zerebellare Epilepsie f.
cerebellar fissures Kleinhirnfurchen pl, Fissurae cerebelli.
cerebellar folia Kleinhirnwindungen pl, Folia cerebelli.
cerebellar fossa of occipital bone Fossa cerebellaris.
cerebellar gait neuro. zerebellärer Gang m.
cerebellar gliosis Kleinhirngliose f, zerebelläre Gliose f.
cerebellar glomeruli Glomeruli cerebellaria.
cerebellar hemisphere Kleinhirnhälfte f, -hemisphäre f, Hemisph(a)erium cerebelli.
cerebellar notch: anterior c. Inc. cerebelli anterior.
posterior c. Inc. cerebelli posterior.
cerebellar peduncle Kleinhirnstiel m, Pedunculus cerebellaris.
caudal c. unterer Kleinhirnstiel, Pedunculus cerebellaris caudalis/inferior.
cranial c. oberer Kleinhirnstiel, Pedunculus cerebellaris rostralis/superior.
inferior c. → caudal c.
middle c. mittlerer Kleinhirnstiel, Pedunculus cerebellaris medius/pontinus.
pontine c. → middle c.
rostral c. → cranial c.
superior c. → cranial c.
cerebellar plate embryo. Kleinhirnplatte f.
cerebellar syndrome Kleinhirnsyndrom nt.
cerebellar tonsil Kleinhirnmandel f, Tonsilla f, Tonsilla cerebelli.
cerebellar tracts Kleinhirnbahnen pl.
c. of lateral funiculus Kleinhirnseitenstrangbahnen.
cerebellar veins Kleinhirnvenen pl, Vv. cerebelli.
cer·e·bel·lif·u·gal [ˌserəbəˈlɪfjəgəl] adj → cerebellofugal.
cer·e·bel·lip·e·tal [ˌ-ˈlɪpətəl] adj → cerebellopetal.
cer·e·bel·li·tis [ˌ-ˈlaɪtɪs] n Kleinhirnentzündung f, Zerebellitis f, Cerebellitis f.
cerebello- pref. Kleinhirn-, Zerebello-, Cerebello-.
cer·e·bel·lof·u·gal [ˌ-ˈlɑfjəgəl] adj zerebellofugal.
cerebellofugal fibers zerebellofugale Fasern pl.
cer·e·bel·lo·med·ul·lar·y [ˌserəˌbeloʊˈmedəˌleri:, -ˈmedʒə-] adj Kleinhirn/Cerebellum u. Medulla oblongata betr. od. verbindend, zerebellomedullär.
cerebellomedullary cistern Cisterna magna/cerebellomedullaris.
cerebellomedullary malformation syndrome Arnold-Chiari-Hemmungsmißbildung f, -Syndrom nt.
cerebello-olivary adj Kleinhirn u. Olive betr. od. verbindend, zerebello-olivär.
cer·e·bel·lop·e·tal [serəbəˈlɑpətəl] adj zerebellopetal.
cer·e·bel·lo·pon·tile [ˌserəˌbeloʊˈpɑnti:l] adj Kleinhirn u. Brücke/Pons betr. od. verbindend, zerebellopontin, Kleinhirn--Brücken-.
cerebellopontine angle Kleinhirn--Brücken-Winkel m, Angulus pontocerebellaris.
cer·e·bel·lo·pon·tine [ˌ-ˈpɑnti:n] adj → cerebellopontile.
cerebellopontine angle → cerebellopontile angle.
cerebellopontine angle syndrome Kleinhirnbrückenwinkel-Syndrom nt, Cushing-Syndrom II nt.

cerebellopontine angle tumor Akustikusneurinom nt.
cer·e·bel·lo·ru·bral tract [ˌ-ˈruːbrəl] zerebellorubrale Bahn f, Tractus cerebellorubralis.
cer·e·bel·lo·ru·bro·spi·nal tract [ˌ-ˌruːbroʊˈspaɪnl] zerebellorubrospinale Bahn f.
cer·e·bel·lo·spi·nal [ˌ-ˈspaɪnl] adj Kleinhirn/Cerebellum u. Rückenmark/Medulla spinalis betr. od. verbindend, zerebellospinal.
cerebellospinal tract zerebellospinale Bahn f, Tractus cerebellospinalis.
cer·e·bel·lo·tha·lam·ic tract [ˌ-θəˈlæmɪk] dentatothalamic tract.
cer·e·bel·lum [serəˈbeləm] n, pl -lums, -la [-lə] Kleinhirn nt, Zerebellum nt, Cerebellum nt.
cerebr- pref. → cerebro-.
ce·re·bral [səˈriːbrəl, ˈserə-] adj Gehirn betr., zerebral, cerebral, (Ge-)Hirn-, Zerebral-, Zerebro-.
cerebral abscess Hirnabszeß m.
cerebral activity (Ge-)Hirntätigkeit f.
cerebral adiposity zerebrale Fettsucht/ Adipositas f.
cerebral agraphia neuro. zerebrale Agraphie f.
cerebral amaurosis ophthal. zerebrale/ zentrale Blindheit/Amaurose f.
cerebral anesthesia neuro. zerebrale/zerebral-bedingte Anästhesie f.
cerebral aneurysm Hirn(arterien)aneurysma nt.
congenital c. 1. kongenitales Hirn(arterien)aneurysma. 2. Aneurysma im Bereich des Circulus arteriosus.
cerebral angiography Zerebralangiographie f.
cerebral anthrax zerebraler Milzbrand m.
cerebral apophysis Zirbel-, Pinealdrüse f, Pinea f, Corpus pineale, Gl. pinealis, Epiphyse f, Epiphysis cerebri.
cerebral apoplexy 1. Schlaganfall m, Gehirnschlag m, apoplektischer Insult m, Apoplexie f, Apoplexia (cerebri) f. 2. Hirnblutung f.
cerebral aqueduct Aquädukt m, Aqu(a)eductus cerebri/mesencephalici.
cerebral arteriography Zerebralarteriographie f.
cerebral arteriosclerosis Arteriosklerose f der Hirnarterien, Zerebralarterienskelrose f, zerebrale Arterien-/Gefäßsklerose f.
cerebral artery: c.ies pl (Ge-)Hirnarterien pl, Aa. cerebrales.
anterior c. vordere Gehirnarterie f, Cerebri f anterior, A. cerebri anterior.
middle c. mittlere Gehirnarterie f, Cerebri f media, inf. Media f, A. cerebri media.
posterior c. hintere Gehirnarterie f, Cerebri f posterior, A. cerebri posterior.
cerebral artery aneurysm Hirn(arterien)aneurysma nt.
cerebral ataxia neuro. zerebrale Ataxie f.
cerebral atrophy (Groß-)Hirnatrophie f.
circumscribed c. Pick'-(Hirn-)Atrophie f, -Krankheit f, -Syndrom nt.
cerebral beriberi Wernicke-Korsakoff--Syndrom nt.
cerebral bleeding (Groß-)Hirnblutung f, (Ein-)Blutung f ins Großhirn.
massive c. Hirnmassenblutung.
cerebral blood flow abbr. **CBF** Hirndurchblutung f.
cerebral calculus Hirnkonkrement nt, Enzephalolith m.
cerebral circulation Gehirnkreislauf m, -durchblutung f.

cerebral claudication Claudicatio intermittens cerebralis.
cerebral commissure, posterior hintere Kommissur f, Commissura epithalamica, Commissura posterior cerebri.
cerebral compression Hirnkompression f, -quetschung f.
cerebral concussion Gehirnerschütterung f, Kommotionssyndrom nt, Commotio cerebri.
cerebral contusion Hirnprellung f, -kontusion f, Contusio cerebri.
cerebral cortex (Groß-)Hirnrinde f, -mantel m, Kortex m, Pallium nt, Cortex cerebralis.
cerebral cortex reflex Haab-Reflex m, Rindenreflex m der Pupille.
cerebral cortical infarction Hirnrindeninfarkt m.
cerebral cranium Hirnschädel m, Neurocranium nt, Cranium cerebrale.
cerebral crisis Schlaganfall m, Gehirnschlag m, apoplektischer Insult m, Apoplexie f, Apoplexia (cerebri) f.
cerebral death Hirntod m, biologischer Tod m.
cerebral decompression Schädeldekompression f; Entlastungstrepanation f.
cerebral diabetes Cerebroseausscheidung f im Harn.
cerebral dysrhythmia neuro. (EEG) diffuse/paroxysmale Dysrhythmie f.
cerebral edema Hirnödem nt.
cerebral electrotherapy abbr. **CET** zerebrale Elektrotherapie f, Elektroschlaftherapie f.
cerebral embolism zerebrale Embolie f, Embolie f einer Zerebralarterie.
cerebral fatique zentrale/psychische Ermüdung f.
cerebral fissure, lateral → cerebral sulcus, lateral.
cerebral flexure → cephalic flexure.
cerebral fossa: lateral c. Fossa lateralis cerebralis.
c. of occipital bone Fossa cerebralis.
cerebral function (Ge-)Hirnfunktion f.
cer·e·bral·gia [serəˈbrældʒ(ɪ)ə] n Kopfschmerz(en pl) m, Kephalgie f, Kephalgie f, Cephalgia f, Cephalalgia f, Cephal(a)ea f, Kephal(a)ea f, Kephalalgie f, Kephalodynie f.
cerebral gigantism Sotos-Syndrom nt.
cerebral hemisphere Großhirnhälfte f, -hemisphäre f, Endhirnhälfte f, -hemisphäre f, Hemisph(a)erium cerebralis.
primitive c. embryo. primitive Großhirnhemisphäre.
cerebral hemorrhage → cerebral bleeding.
cerebral hernia Hirnbruch m, -hernie f, Hernia cerebralis.
cerebral hyperesthesia zerebrale Hyperästhesie f.
cerebral infarction Hirninfarkt m.
hemorrhage c. hämorrhagischer Hirninfarkt.
cerebral injury Gehirnverletzung f, -trauma nt.
cerebral layer of retina Stratum cerebrale, Pars nervosa (retinae).
cerebral lipidosis → cerebral sphingolipidosis.
cerebral lobes Hirnlappen pl, Lobi cerebrales.
cerebral malaria zerebrale Malaria f, Malaria cerebralis.
cerebral meningitis Hirnhautentzündung f, Meningitis cerebralis.
cerebral metabolism Hirnstoffwechsel m, -metabolismus m.

cerebral metastasis (Groß-)Hirnmetastase f.
cerebral nerve → cranial nerve.
cerebral palsy Zerebralparese f.
 infantile c. abbr. **ICP** infantile Zerebralparese f, zerebrale Kinderlähmung f.
cerebral paralysis Zerebralparalyse f; Zerebralparese f.
cerebral paraplegia zerebrale Paraplegie f.
cerebral part: c. of hypophysis Neurohypophyse f, Hypophysenhinterlappen m abbr. **HHL**, Neurohypophysis f, Lobus posterior hypophyseos.
 c. of internal carotid artery intraduraler/zerebraler Abschnitt m der A. carotis interna, Pars cerebralis (a. carotidis internae).
 c. of retina → cerebral layer of retina.
cerebral peduncle Hirnstiel m, Pedunculus cerebralis/cerebri.
cerebral poliomyelitis Polioenzephalitis f, Polioencephalitis f.
cerebral porosis Porenzephalie f.
cerebral purpura Hirnpurpura f, Purpura cerebri.
cerebral respiration Corrigan-Atmung f.
cerebral spasm Zerebralspasmus m.
cerebral sphingolipidosis zerebrale Lipidose/Sphingolipidose f.
cerebral stratum of retina → cerebral layer of retina.
cerebral sulcus, lateral Sylvius'-Furche f, Sulcus lateralis.
cerebral swelling Hirnschwellung f.
cerebral tetanus Kopftetanus m, Tetanus capitis.
cerebral toxic pericapillary bleeding Hirnpurpura f, Purpura cerebri.
cerebral tracts (Groß-)Hirnbahnen pl.
cerebral trauma Gehirnverletzung f, -trauma nt.
cerebral tuberculosis 1. tuberkulöse Meningitis f, Meningitis tuberculosa. **2.** zerebrales Tuberkulom nt.
cerebral vein: c.s pl Großhirnvenen pl, Vv. cerebri.
 anterior c.s Begleitvenen pl der A. cerebri anterior, Vv. anteriores cerebri.
 deep c.s tiefe Hirnvenen pl, Vv. profundae cerebri.
 great c. Galen-Vene f, Cerebri f magna, V. magna cerebri.
 inferior c.s Hirnbasisvenen pl, Vv. inferiores cerebri.
 internal c.s innere Hirnvenen pl, Vv. internae cerebri.
 middle c., deep Begleitvene f der A. cerebri media, Cerebri f media profunda, V. media profunda cerebri.
 middle c.s, superficial Vv. mediae superficiales cerebri.
 superficial c.s oberflächliche Hirnvenen pl, Vv. superficiales cerebri.
 superior c.s obere Hirnmantelvenen pl, Vv. superiores cerebri.
cerebral vertigo zerebraler Schwindel m.
cerebral vesicles embryo. Hirnbläschen pl.
ce·re·bri·form [sə'ri:brəfɔ:rm] adj hirnähnlich.
cerebriform cancer/carcinoma medulläres Karzinom nt, Ca. medullare.
cerebriform tongue Faltenzunge f, Lingua plicata/scrotalis.
cer·e·brif·u·gal [ˌserə'brɪfjəgəl] adj vom Gehirn weg(führend), cerebrifugal.
cer·e·brip·e·tal [ˌ-'brɪpətəl] adj zum Gehirn hin(führend), cerebripetal.
cer·e·bri·tis [ˌ-'braɪtɪs] n Großhirnentzündung f, Zerebritis f, Cerebritis f.
cerebro- pref. (Ge-)Hirn-, Zerebral-, Zerebro-, Cerebro-.

cer·e·bro·a·troph·ic hyperammonemia [ˌserəbrəʊə'trɒfɪk, sə,ri:brə-] Rett-Syndrom nt.
cer·e·bro·car·di·ac [ˌ-'kɑ:rdɪˌæk] adj Großhirn u. Herz betr., zerebrokardial.
cer·e·bro·cer·e·bel·lar [ˌ-ˌserə'belər] adj Großhirn/Cerebrum u. Kleinhirn/Cerebellum betr. od. verbindend, zerebrozerebellar, -zerebellär.
cer·e·bro·ga·lac·tose [ˌ-gə'læktəʊs] n Cerebrogalaktose f.
cer·e·bro·ga·lac·to·side [ˌ-gə'læktəsaɪd] n Cerebrogalaktosid nt.
cer·e·bro·hep·a·to·re·nal syndrome [ˌ-ˌhepətəʊ'ri:nl] zerebrohepatorenales Syndrom nt, ZHR-Syndrom nt, Zellweger-Syndrom nt.
cer·e·bro·hy·phoid [ˌ-'haɪfɔɪd] adj hirngewebsähnlich, -artig.
cer·e·broid ['serəbrɔɪd, sə'rɪ:-] adj hirnsubstanzähnlich, zerebroid.
cer·e·bro·ma [ˌserə'brəʊmə] n **1.** patho. Hirntumor m, -geschwulst f, Enzephalom nt. **2.** → cerebriform cancer.
cer·e·bro·mac·u·lar degeneration [ˌserəbrəʊ'mækjələr] abbr. **CMD** zerebromakuläre/zerebroretinale Degeneration f.
cer·e·bro·ma·la·cia [ˌ-mə'leɪʃ(ɪ)ə] n Hirnerweichung f, Zerebromalazie f, Cerebromalacia f.
cer·e·bro·med·ul·lar·y [ˌ-'medəˌleri:, -'medʒə-] adj → cerebrospinal.
cerebromedullary tube embryo. Neuralrohr nt.
cer·e·bro·me·nin·ge·al [ˌ-mɪ'nɪndʒɪəl] adj Gehirn/Cerebrum u. Hirnhäute betr. od. verbindend, zerebromeningeal, meningozerebral.
cer·e·bro·men·in·gi·tis [ˌ-ˌmenɪn'dʒaɪtɪs] n Meningoenzephalitis f, -encephalitis f, Enzephalo-, Encephalomeningitis f.
cer·e·bron ['serəbrɒn] n Zerebron nt, Phrenosin nt.
cer·e·bron·ic acid [ˌserə'brɒnɪk] Cerebronsäure f.
cerebro-ocular adj Großhirn/Cerebrum u. Auge betr., zerebro-okular.
cer·e·bro·path·ia [ˌserəbrəʊ'pæθɪə] n → cerebropathy.
cer·e·brop·a·thy [serə'brɒpəθi] n Hirnerkrankung f, Enzephalopathie f, Zerebropathie f, Cerebropathia f, Cerebropathia f.
cer·e·bro·pon·tile [ˌserəbrəʊ'pɒntaɪl, -tl] adj Großhirn/Cerebrum u. Brücke/Pons betr., zerebropontin.
cer·e·bro·pu·pil·lar·y reflex [ˌ-'pju:pəˌleri:, -ləri] Haab-Reflex m, Rindenreflex m der Pupille.
cer·e·bro·ra·chid·i·an [ˌ-rə'kɪdɪən] adj → cerebrospinal.
cer·e·bro·ret·i·nal angiomatosis [ˌ-'retnəl] Netzhautangiomatose f, (von) Hippel-Lindau-Syndrom nt, Angiomatosis retinae cystica.
cerebroretinal degeneration → cerebromacular degeneration.
cer·e·bro·scle·ro·sis [ˌ-sklɪ'rəʊsɪs] n Hirn-, Zerebralsklerose f.
cer·e·bro·scope ['serəbrəʊskəʊp] n Enzephaloskop nt.
cer·e·bros·co·py [ˌserə'brɒskəpi] n Enzephaloskopie f.
cer·e·brose ['serəbrəʊz] n Zerebrose f, D-Galaktose f.
cer·e·bro·side ['serəbrəʊsaɪd] n Zerebrosid nt, Cerebrosid nt.
cerebroside β-galactosidase Galaktosylceramidase f, Galactocerebrosid-β-galaktosidase f.
cerebroside β-glucosidase Glukozerebrosidase f, Gluko-, Glucocerebrosidase f.

cerebroside lipidosis/lipoidosis → cerebrosidosis 2.
cerebroside sulfatase Zerebrosid-, Cerebrosidsulfatase f.
cer·e·bro·si·do·sis [ˌserəˌbrəʊsaɪ'dəʊsɪs] n **1.** Zerebrosidspeicherkrankheit f, Zerebrosidose f, Cerebrosidose f. **2.** Gaucher'-Erkrankung f, -Krankheit f, -Syndrom nt, Morbus Gaucher m, Glukozerebrosidose f, Zerebrosidlipidose f, Glykosylzeramidlipidose f, Lipoidhistiozytose f vom Kerasintyp.
cer·e·bro·sis [ˌserə'brəʊsɪs] n organische/degenerative Hirnerkrankung f, Enzephalose f.
cer·e·bro·spi·nal [ˌserəbrəʊ'spaɪnl] adj Gehirn/Cerebrum u. Rückenmark/Medulla spinalis betr. od. verbindend, zerebro-, cerebrospinal.
cerebrospinal axis → central nervous system.
cerebrospinal fever → cerebrospinal meningitis, epidemic.
cerebrospinal fluid abbr. **CSF** Hirnflüssigkeit f, Gehirn- u. Rückenmarksflüssigkeit f, Liquor m, Liquor cerebrospinalis.
cerebrospinal fluid otorrhea Otoliquorrhoe f.
cerebrospinal meningitis abbr. **C.S.M.** kombinierte Hirnhaut- u. Rückenmarkshautentzündung f, Meningitis cerebrospinalis.
 epidemic c. Meningokokkenmeningitis f, Meningitis cerebrospinalis epidemica.
cerebrospinal nervous system → central nervous system.
cerebrospinal pressure Liquordruck m.
cerebrospinal rhinorrhea nasale Liquorrhoe f, Liquorrhoe f aus der Nase.
cerebrospinal syphilis 1. Lues cerebrospinalis. **2.** luische Spinalparalyse Erb f.
cerebrospinal system → central nervous system.
cer·e·bro·spi·nant [ˌ-'spaɪnənt] **I** n auf Gehirn u. Rückenmark einwirkende Substanz f. **II** adj auf Gehirn u. Rückenmark einwirkend.
cer·e·bros·to·my [ˌserə'brɒstəmi] n neurochir. Zerebrostomie f.
cer·e·bro·su·ria [ˌserəbrəʊ's(j)ʊərɪə] n Cerebroseausscheidung f im Harn.
cer·e·brot·o·my [ˌserə'brɒtəmi] n neurochir. Hirnschnitt m, Zerebrotomie f.
cer·e·bro·vas·cu·lar [ˌserəbrəʊ'væskjələr] adj Hirngefäße betr., zerebrovaskulär.
cerebrovascular accident abbr. **CVA** Hirnschlag m, Schlaganfall m, apoplektischer Insult m, Apoplexie f, Apoplexia cerebri.
cerebrovascular disease zerebrovaskuläre Verschlußkrankheit f.
cerebrovascular insufficiency zerebrovaskuläre Insuffizienz f.
cerebrovascular occlusive disease → cerebrovascular disease.
cer·e·brum ['serəbrəm, sə'ri:brəm] n, pl **-brums, -bra** [-brə] Großhirn nt, Zerebrum nt, Cerebrum nt.
cere·cloth ['sɪərklɒθ, -klɑθ] n Wachstuch nt.
ce·re·sin ['serəsɪn] n chem. Erdwachs nt, Zeresin nt.
ce·ri·um ['sɪərɪəm] n abbr. **Ce** Cerium nt abbr. **Ce**.
ce·roid ['sɪrɔɪd] n histol. Zeroid nt, Ceroid nt.
ce·ro·tin ['serətɪn] n → ceryl alcohol.
cer·ti·fi·a·ble [sɜrtə'faɪəbl] adj **1.** zu bescheinigen(d). **2.** (Krankheit) meldepflichtig. **3.** psychia. in einem Zustand, der die Zwangseinweisung in eine Anstalt rechtfertigt; inf. verrückt.

cer·tif·i·cate [n sər'tɪfɪkɪt; v -keɪt] **I** n **1.** Bescheinigung f, Attest nt, Schein m, Zertifikat nt. **2.** Gutachten nt. **3.** (Schul-)Zeugnis nt. **II** vt etwas bescheinigen; (Bescheinigung, Zeugnis) ausstellen od. geben.
cer·ti·fi·ca·tion [ˌsərtəfɪ'keɪʃn, sərˌtɪfə-] n **1.** Ausstellen nt einer Bescheinigung, Bescheinigen nt. **2.** (Krankheit) Meldung f. **3.** Zwangseinweisung f in eine Anstalt. **4.** → certificate 1.
cer·ti·fied ['sərtəfaɪd] adj **1.** (Patient) für geisteskrank erklärt. **2.** bescheinigt, beglaubigt.
cer·ti·fy ['sərtəfaɪ] **I** vt **1.** bescheinigen, versichern, attestieren; beglaubigen, beurkunden. **2.** (Krankheit) (an-)melden. **3.** (Patient) für geisteskrank erklären. **4.** (Patient) zwangseinweisen. **II** vi ~ to etw. bezeugen, attestieren.
ce·ru·le·an [sə'ruːlɪən] adj blau.
cerulean cataract ophthal. Cataracta c(o)erulea.
ce·ru·lo·plas·min [səˌruːlə'plæzmɪn] n Zörulo-, Zärulo-, Coerulo-, Caeruloplasmin nt, Ferroxidase I f.
ce·ru·men [sɪ'ruːmən] n Ohr(en)schmalz nt, Zerumen nt, Cerumen nt.
ce·ru·mi·nal [sɪ'ruːmɪnl] adj Ohr(en)schmalz/Cerumen betr., Zeruminal-, Ceruminal-.
ceruminal impaction Ohr(en)schmalz-, Zeruminalpfropf m, Cerumen obturans.
ce·ru·mi·nol·y·sis [sɪˌruːmɪ'nɑləsɪs] n HNO Zeruminolyse f.
ce·ru·mi·no·lyt·ic [sɪˌruːmɪnə'lɪtɪk] **I** n zerumenauflösendes Mittel nt. **II** adj zerumenauflösend, zeruminolytisch.
ce·ru·mi·no·ma [sɪˌruːmɪ'nəʊmə] n HNO Tumor m der Ohrschmalzdrüsen, Zeruminom nt.
ce·ru·mi·no·sis [ˌ-'nəʊsɪs] n übermäßige Ohrschmalzabsonderung f.
ce·ru·mi·nous [sɪ'ruːmɪnəs] adj → ceruminal.
ceruminous glands Ohrschmalz-, Zeruminaldrüsen pl, Gll. ceruminosae.
cer·vi·cal ['sɜːvɪkl, -viːk-; Brit. ˌsɜːr'vaɪkl] adj **1.** Hals/Cervix betr., zervikal, Hals-, Zervikal-, Nacken-. **2.** Gebärmutterhals/Cervix uteri betr., zervikal, Gebärmutterhals-, Zervix-, Cervix-.
cervical achalasia hohe/zervikale/krikopharyngeale Achalasie f.
cervical adhesions gyn. Zervixverwachsungen pl, -verklebungen pl.
cervical ansa Hypoglossusschlinge f, Ansa cervicalis.
deep c. tiefer Ast m der Hypoglossusschlinge, A. cervicalis profunda.
superficial c. oberflächlicher Ast m der Hypoglossusschlinge, Ansa cervicalis superficialis.
cervical artery: ascending c. aufsteigende Halsschlagader f, -arterie f, Cervicalis f ascendens, A. cervicalis ascendens.
deep c. tiefe Halsschlagader f, -arterie f, Cervicalis f profunda, A. cervicalis profunda.
descending c.s, deep Hinterhauptsäste pl der A. occipitalis, Rami occipitales a. occipitalis.
superficial c. oberflächliche Halsarterie f, Cervicalis f superficialis, Ramus superficialis a. transversae colli.
transverse c. quere Halsschlagader f, -arterie f, Transversa f colli, A. transversa (colli).
cervical atresia Zervixatresie f, Atresia cervicalis.
cervical branch of facial nerve Halsast m des N. facialis, Ramus colli/cervicalis n. facialis.
cervical canal (of uterus) Zervikalkanal m, Canalis cervicis uteri.
cervical carcinoma (of uterus) Gebärmutterhalskrebs m, -karzinom nt, Kollum-, Zervixkarzinom nt, Ca. cervicis uteri.
cervical collar ortho. Halskrawatte f.
cervical colliculus: c. of Barkow Crista urethralis femininae.
c. of female urethra → c. of Barkow.
cervical compression syndrome → cervical disc syndrome.
cervical cord → cervical part of spinal cord.
cervical cord injury/trauma Halsmarkverletzung f, -trauma nt.
cervical cyst Halszyste f.
lateral c. seitliche Halszyste.
median c. mediane Halszyste.
cervical cytology gyn. Zervixzytologie f.
cervical disc syndrome zervikales Bandscheibensyndrom nt.
cervical diverticulum Halsdivertikel nt.
cervical dysphagia oropharyngeale Dysphagie f.
cervical dysplasia → cervical intraepithelial neoplasia.
cervical dystocia gyn. Zervixdystokie f.
cervical ectropion gyn. Portioektropion nt, -ektropium nt, -ektopie f, Ektopia portionis.
cervical enlargement (of spinal cord) anat. Intumescentia cervicalis.
cervical esophagus → cervical part of esophagus.
cervical fascia Halsfaszie f, Fascia cervicalis.
deep c. Fascia nuchae.
cervical fibromatosis Fibromatosis colli.
cervical fistula 1. branchiogene Fistel f. 2. Halsfistel f.
median c. mediane Halsfistel.
cervical flexure embryo. Nackenbeuge f.
cervical forceps gyn. Portiofaßzange f.
cervical fusion ortho. operative Versteifung f der Halswirbelsäule, Halswirbelfusion f.
cervical fusion syndrome Klippel-Feil-Syndrom nt.
cervical ganglion: inferior c. unterer Teil m des Ggl. cervicothoracicum.
middle c. mittleres Halsganglion nt, Ggl. cervicale medium.
superior c. oberes Halsganglion nt, Ggl. cervicale superius.
c. of uterus Frankenhäuser'-Ganglion nt.
cervical glands (of uterus) Zervixdrüsen pl, Gll. cervicales (uteri).
cervical hydrocele Hydrocele colli.
cervical hygroma (Zysten-)Hygrom nt des Halses, Hygroma/Lymphangioma cysticum colli.
cervical intraepithelial neoplasia abbr. CIN gyn. zervikale Plattenepitheldysplasie f, cervicale intraepitheliale Neoplasie f abbr. CIN.
cervical ligament: anterior c. Membrana tectoria.
lateral c. Kardinalband nt, Lig. cardinale uteri.
posterior c. Nackenband nt, Lig. nuchae.
c. of sinus tarsi Lig. talocalcaneum interosseum.
cervical lymph nodes Hals-, Zervikallymphknoten pl, Nodi lymphatici cervicales.
anterior c. vordere Halslymphknoten pl, Nodi lymphatici cervicales anteriores.
deep c. tiefe Halslymphknoten pl, Nodi lymphatici cervicales profundi.
deep anterior c. tiefe vordere Halslymphknoten pl, Nodi lymphatici cervicales anteriores profundi.
deep lateral c. tiefe seitliche Halslymphknoten pl, Nodi lymphatici cervicales laterales profundi.
lateral c. seitliche Halslymphknoten pl, Nodi lymphatici cervicales laterales.
prelaryngeal c. prälaryngeale Lymphknoten pl, Nodi lymphatici pr(a)elaryngeales.
superficial c. oberflächliche Halslymphknoten pl, Nodi lymphatici cervicales superficiales.
superficial anterior c. vordere oberflächliche Halslymphknoten pl, Nodi lymphatici cervicales anteriores superficiales.
superficial lateral c. seitliche oberflächliche Halslymphknoten pl, Nodi lymphatici cervicales laterales superficiales.
cervical mucosa gyn. Zervixschleimhaut f.
cervical mucus Zervixschleim m.
cervical muscles Halsmuskeln pl, -muskulatur f, Mm. colli/cervicis.
cervical nerve: c.s pl Hals-, Zervikalnerven pl, Nn. cervicales.
descending c. Radix inferior ansae cervicalis.
transverse c. Transversus m colli, N. transversus colli.
cervical nucleus, lateral Nc. lateralis cervicalis.
cervical part: c. of esophagus Halsabschnitt m der Speiseröhre, Pars cervicalis (o)esophagi.
c. of internal carotid artery Halsabschnitt m der A. carotis interna, Pars cervicalis a. carotidis internae.
c. of spinal cord Hals-, Zervikalsegmente pl, Halsmark nt, Halsabschnitt m des Rückenmarks, Cervicalia pl, Pars cervicalis (medullae spinalis).
c. of thoracic duct Halsabschnitt m des Ductus thoracicus, Pars cervicalis ductus thoracici.
c. of trachea Halsabschnitt m der Luftröhre, Pars cervicalis tracheae.
c. of vertebral artery Halsabschnitt m der A. vertebralis, Pars transversaria/cervicalis (a. vertebralis).
cervical pleura Pleurakuppel f, Cupula pleurae.
cervical plexus Halsgeflecht nt, -plexus m, Plexus cervicalis.
cervical polyp gyn. Zervixpolyp m.
cervical pregnancy Zervixschwangerschaft f, -gravidität f, Einnistung f im Zervikalkanal.
cervical region: c.s pl Halsregionen pl, Regiones cervicales.
anterior c. vorderes Halsdreieck nt, Regio cervicalis anterior, Trigonum cervicale anterius.
lateral c. hinteres Halsdreieck nt, Regio cervicalis lateralis, Trigonum cervicale posterius.
posterior c. Nackengegend f, -region f, Regio cervicalis posterior, Regio nuchalis.
cervical rib Halsrippe f, Costa cervicalis.
cervical rib syndrome ortho., neuro. Skalenus-Syndrom nt, Scalenus-anterior-Syndrom nt, Naffziger-Syndrom nt.
cervical segments of spinal cord Hals-, Zervikalsegmente pl, Halsmark nt, Halsabschnitt m des Rückenmarks, Cervicalia pl, Pars cervicalis (medullae spinalis).
cervical septum, intermediate Septum cervicale intermedium.
cervical sinus embryo. Sinus cervicalis.
cervical smear gyn. (Zervix-)Abstrich m.

cervical spine

cervical spine Halswirbelsäule f abbr. HWS.
cervical spine fracture Halswirbelsäulenfraktur f.
cervical spine injury/trauma Halswirbelsäulenverletzung f, -trauma nt.
cervical sympathectomy zervikale Sympathektomie f.
cervical syndrome ortho., neuro. Zervikalsyndrom nt.
post-traumatic c. posttraumatisches Zervikalsyndrom.
cervical tension syndrome posttraumatisches Halswirbelsäulensyndrom nt.
cervical triangle: anterior c. → cervical region, anterior.
posterior c. → cervical region, lateral.
cervical vein: deep c. tiefe Halsvene f, Begleitvene f der A. cervicalis profunda, V. cervicalis profunda.
transverse c.s Begleitvenen pl der A. transversa colli, Vv. transversae cervicis/colli.
cervical vertebra Halswirbel m abbr. HW, Vertebra cervicalis.
cer·vi·cec·to·my [ˌsɜrvɪ'sɛktəmɪ] n gyn. Zervixresektion f.
cer·vi·ci·tis [ˌ-'saɪtɪs] n gyn. Zervixentzündung f, Zervizitis f, Cervicitis f.
cer·vi·co·ax·il·lar·y [ˌsɜrvɪkəʊ'æksɪlerɪː, -æk'sɪlərɪ] adj Hals/Cervix u. Axilla betr., zervikoaxillär.
cer·vi·co·bas·i·lar ligament [ˌ-'bæsɪlər] Membrana tectoria.
cer·vi·co·bra·chi·al·gia [ˌ-ˌbrækɪ'ældʒɪə, -ˌbreɪ-] n neuro. Zervikobrachialgie f.
cer·vi·co·bra·chi·al neuralgia [ˌ-'breɪkɪəl, -'bræ-] neuro. zervikobrachiale Neuralgie f.
cervicobrachial plexus Plexus brachialis et cervicalis.
cervicobrachial syndrome → cervical rib syndrome.
cer·vi·co·breg·mat·ic diameter [ˌ-breg'mætɪkɪ] gyn., ped. Diameter cervicobregmatica.
cer·vi·co·col·pi·tis [ˌ-kɑl'paɪtɪs] n gyn. Entzündung f von Zervix u. Vagina, Zervikokolpitis f, -vaginitis f.
cer·vi·co·dor·sal [ˌ-'dɔːrsl] adj Hals/Cervix u. Rücken/Dorsum betr., zervikodorsal.
cer·vi·co·dyn·ia [ˌ-'diːnɪə] n Nacken-, Halsschmerz(en pl) m, Zervikodynie f.
cer·vi·co·fa·cial [ˌ-'feɪʃl] adj Hals/Cervix u. Gesicht betr., zervikofazial.
cervicofacial actinomycosis zervikofaziale Aktinomykose f.
cervico-occipital adj Hals/Cervix u. Hinterhaupt/Occiput betr., zerviko-okzipital.
cervico-ocular pathway physiol. zerviko--okuläre Reflexbahn f.
cervico-oculo-acustic syndrome Wildervanck-Syndrom nt, zerviko-okulo-akustisches Syndrom nt.
cer·vi·co·pex·y ['-peksɪ] n gyn. Zervikopexie f.
cer·vi·co·plas·ty ['-plæstɪ] n 1. (plastische) Hals-/Nackenchirurgie f. 2. gyn. Zervixplastik f.
cer·vi·co·scap·u·lar [ˌ-'skæpjələr] adj Hals/Cervix u. Schulterblatt/Scapula betr., zervikoskapular.
cer·vi·co·tho·rac·ic ganglion [ˌ-θɔː'ræsɪk, -'θəʊ-] Ggl. cervicothoracicum/stellatum.
cer·vi·cot·o·my [ˌsɜrvɪ'kɑtəmɪ] n gyn. Zervixschnitt m, Zervixdurchtrennung f, Zerviko-, Trachelotomie f.
cer·vi·co·u·ter·ine ganglion [ˌsɜrvɪkəʊ'juːtərɪn, -təraɪn] → cervical ganglion of uterus.
cer·vi·co·vag·i·nal [ˌ-'vædʒənl, -və'dʒaɪnl] adj gyn. Zervix u. Scheide/Vagina betr.,

od. verbindend, zervikovaginal, vaginozervikal.
cer·vi·co·vag·i·ni·tis [ˌ-ˌvædʒə'naɪtɪs] n → cervicocolpitis.
cer·vi·co·ves·i·cal [ˌ-'vesɪkl] adj gyn., urol. Zervix u. (Harn-)Blase betr. od. verbindend, zervikovesikal, vesikozervikal.
cer·vix ['sɜrvɪks] n, pl **-vix·es** [-ˌvɪksɪz], **-vices** ['sɜrvɪˌsiːz, sɜr'vaɪ-] 1. Hals m, halsförmige Struktur f, Nacken m, Zervix f, Cervix f, Kollum nt, Collum nt. 2. Gebärmutter-, Uterushals m, Zervix f, Cervix uteri.
c. of uterus → cervix 2.
cervix forceps gyn. Portiofaßzange f.
cervix-holding forceps → cervix forceps.
ce·ryl alcohol ['sɪrəl] Cerylalkohol m.
ce·sar·e·an hysterectomy [sɪ'zeərɪən] gyn. Hysterectomia c(a)esarea.
cesarean operation → cesarean section.
cesarean section abbr. **CS** gyn. Kaiserschnitt m, Schnittentbindung f, inf. Sectio f, Sectio caesarea.
classic c. klassische Schnittentbindung, Sectio caesarea classica.
corporeal c. → classic c.
extraperitoneal c. abdominale extraperitoneale Schnittentbindung, Sectio caesarea abdominalis extraperitonealis.
transperitoneal c. abdominale interperitoneale Schnittentbindung, Sectio caesarea abdominalis interperitonealis.
vaginal c. vaginaler Kaiserschnitt, Sectio caesarea vaginalis.
CESD abbr. → cholesterol ester storage disease.
ce·si·um ['siːzɪəm] n abbr. **Cs** Cäsium nt, Caesium nt abbr. Cs.
cesium chloride Cäsiumchlorid nt.
cessation [se'seɪʃn] n Aufhören nt, Einstellung f, Einstellen nt; Ende nt, Stillstand m.
c. of breathing Atmungsstillstand, Apnoe f.
c. of growth Wachstumsstillstand.
Cestan [sɛs'tɑ̃]: **C.'s syndrome** Cestan-Paralyse f, Cestan-Chenais-Syndrom nt.
Cestan-Chenais [ʃ(ə)'nɛ]: **C.-C. syndrome** → Cestan's syndrome.
Cestan-Raymond [rɛ'mɔ̃]: **C.-R. syndrome** Raymond-Cestan-Syndrom nt.
C1 esterase inhibitor → C1 inhibitor.
ces·to·ci·dal [ˌsestəʊ'saɪdl] adj cestoden(ab)tötend, zestozid, zestozid.
Ces·to·da [ses'təʊdə] pl micro. Bandwürmer pl, Zestoden pl, Cestoda pl, Cestodes pl.
ces·tode ['sestəʊd] **I** n Bandwurm m, Zestode f. **II** adj → cestoid.
ces·to·di·a·sis [ˌsestə'daɪəsɪs] n Bandwurm-, Zestodeninfektion f.
ces·toid ['sestɔɪd] adj bandwurmähnlich, -artig, zestodenartig.
Ces·toi·dea [ses'tɔɪdɪə] pl micro. Cestoidea pl.
CET abbr. → cerebral electrotherapy.
ce·ta·ce·um [sɪ'teɪʃɪəm, -sɪəm] n pharm. Walrat m/nt, Cetaceum nt.
cet·al·ko·ni·um chloride [setæl'kəʊnɪəm] pharm. Cetalkoniumchlorid nt.
ce·ta·nol ['setənɒl, -nɔl] n Cetylalkohol m.
ce·tri·mide ['siːtrɪmaɪd] n → cetrimonium bromide.
cet·ri·mo·ni·um bromide [setrɪ'məʊnɪəm] pharm. Cetrimoniumbromid nt.
ce·tyl alcohol ['siːtɪl, 'setɪl] Cetyl-, Palmitylalkohol m.
ce·tyl·pyr·i·din·i·um chloride [ˌsiːtɪlˌpɪrə'dɪnɪəm] pharm. Cetylpyridiniumchlorid nt.
ce·vi·tam·ic acid [siːvɪ'tæmɪk, sev'-] Askor-

binsäure f, Ascorbinsäure f, Vitamin C nt.
CF abbr. **1.** → cardiac failure. **2.** → chemotactic factor. **3.** → Christmas factor. **4.** → citrovorum factor. **5.** → complement fixation. **6.** → cystic fibrosis (of the pancreas).
Cf abbr. **1.** → californium. **2.** [colicinogenic factor] → colicinogen.
CF antibody → complement-fixing antibody.
CF antigen → complement-fixing antigen.
CF1 (ATPase) → chloroplast ATPase.
CFC abbr. → colony forming cell.
CFF abbr. → critical flicker frequency.
C fibers C-Fasern pl.
CFR abbr. → complement fixation reaction.
CFS-brain barrier Hirn-Liquor-Schranke f.
C.F.T. abbr. → complement-fixation test.
CFU abbr. → colony forming unit.
CFU-C abbr. → colony forming unit in culture.
CG abbr. → chorionic gonadotropin.
cg abbr. → centigram.
CGD abbr. → chronic granulomatous disease (of childhood).
cGMP abbr. → cyclic GMP.
cGy abbr. → centigray.
Chaddock ['tʃædɒk]: **C. reflex/sign** Chaddock-Zeichen nt, -Reflex m.
chafe [tʃeɪf] **I** n wunde/aufgeriebene (Haut-)Stelle f. **II** vt (Haut) auf-, durchreiben, auf-, durchscheuern, wundreiben. **III** vi (s.) durchreiben, (s.) wundreiben.
Chagas ['ʃɑːgəs]: **C.' disease** Chagas-Krankheit f, amerikanische Trypanosomiasis f.
Chagas-Cruz [kruːz]: **C.-C. disease** → Chagas' disease.
cha·gas·ic myocarditis [ʃə'gæsɪk] Chagas--Myokarditis f.
cha·go·ma [ʃə'gəʊmə] n Chagom nt.
Cha·gres fever ['tʃɑːgres] Chagres-Fieber nt.
Chagres virus Chagres-Virus nt.
chain [tʃeɪn] **I** n **1.** (a. techn.) Kette f; (bio)chem., micro. Kette f. **2.** fig. Kette f, Reihe f. **II** vi eine Kette bilden.
c. of infection Infektionskette.
α chain α-Kette f.
β chain β-Kette f.
chain elongation Kettenverlängerung f.
chain growth Kettenwachstum nt.
chain-initiation codon Initial-, Initiations-, Starterkodon nt.
chain isomerism Kettenisomerie f.
chain-react vi eine Kettenreaktion durchlaufen.
chain reaction phys., chem., fig. Kettenreaktion f.
chain reflex Reflexkette f.
chain-smoke vi kettenrauchen.
chain-smoker n Kettenraucher(in f) m.
chain termination Kettenabbruch m.
chain-termination codon (Ketten-)Abbruchs-, Terminationskodon nt.
chain-termination mutant Kettenabbruchs-, Terminationsmutante f.
chair [tʃeər] n **1.** Stuhl m, Sessel m. **2.** Lehrstuhl (of für); Vorsitz m.
chair form chem. Sesselform f.
CHAI virus (cytopathic, human autointerfering) micro. CHAI-Virus nt.
cha·la·sia [kə'leɪzɪə] n **1.** Chalasie f, Chalasia f. **2.** gastroösophagealer Reflux m.
cha·la·sis [kə'leɪsɪs] n → chalasia.
cha·las·to·der·mia [ˌkəˌlæstə'dɜrmɪə] n → chalazodermia.
cha·la·za [kə'leɪzə] n → chalazion.
cha·la·zi·on [kə'leɪzɪən, keɪ'leɪ-] n, pl **-zia**

[-zɪə] *ophthal.* Hagelkorn *nt*, Chalazion *nt*.
chalazion clamp *ophthal.* Chalzionpinzette *f*.
chalazion forceps *ophthal.* Chalazionpinzette *f*.
chalazion knife *ophthal.* Chalazionmesser *nt*.
cha·la·zo·der·mia [kə,leɪzəʊˈdɜrmɪə] *n derm.* Fall-, Schlaffhaut *f*, Cutis-laxa--Syndrom *nt*, generalisierte Elastolyse *f*, Zuviel-Haut-Syndrom *nt*, Dermatochalasis *f*, Dermatolysis *f*, Dermatomegalie *f*, Chalazodermie *f*, Chalodermie *f*.
chal·ci·tis [kælˈsaɪtɪs] *n* → chalkitis.
chal·co·sis [kælˈkəʊsɪs] *n* Chalkose *f*, Chalcosis *f*.
chal·ice [ˈtʃælɪs] *n anat.* Becher *m*, Kelch *m*.
chalice cell Becherzelle *f*.
chal·i·co·sis [,kælɪˈkəʊsɪs] *n* Kalkstaublunge *f*, Chalikose *f*, Chalicosis *f* (pulmonum).
chalk [tʃɔːk] *n* Kreide *f*, Kalk(stein *m*) *m*.
chal·ki·tis [kælˈkaɪtɪs] *n ophthal.* Chalkitis *f*.
chalk stone Gelenkstein *m*, -konkrement *nt*.
chalk·y [ˈtʃɔːkɪ] *adj* Kreide/Kalk enthaltend, wie Kreide, kreidig, kalkig, kalkhaltig, Kalk-.
chalky bones Marmorknochenkrankheit *f*, Albers-Schönberg-Krankheit *f*, Osteopetrosis *f*.
chalky gout Gicht *f* mit Tophibildung.
chal·one [ˈkæləʊn] *n* Chalon *nt*, Statin *nt*.
cha·lyb·e·ate [kəˈlɪbɪət] **I** *n* eisenhaltiges Medikament *nt*, **II** *adj* eisen-, stahlhaltig.
cham·ae·ce·phal·ic [,kæmɪsɪˈfælk] *adj* flachköpfig, chamäzephal, -kranial.
cham·ae·ceph·a·ly [,-ˈsefəlɪ] *n* Flachköpfigkeit *f*, Chamäzephalie *f*, -kranie *f*.
cham·ae·pros·o·py [,-ˈprɒsəpɪ, -prəˈsəʊpɪ] *n* Breitgesichtigkeit *f*, Chamäprosopie *f*.
cham·ber [ˈtʃeɪmbər] *n* **1.** *anat.* Kammer *f*, Camera *f*. **2.** *techn.* Kammer *f*. **3.** Kammer *f*, (Empfangs-)Raum *m*; Kammer *f*, Körperschaft *f*.
c. of (the) heart Herzkammer *f*.
Chamberlain [ˈtʃeɪmbərlɪn]: **C.'s line** Chamberlain-Linie *f*.
Chamberland [ˈtʃeɪmbərlænd]: **C. filter** Chamberlandfilter *m*.
Chamberlen [ˈtʃeɪmbərlən]: **C. forceps** *gyn.* Chamberlen-Zange *f*.
cham·e·ce·phal·ic *adj* → chamaecephalic.
cham·e·ceph·a·ly *n* → chamaecephaly.
cham·e·pros·o·py *n* → chamaeprosopy.
cham·o·mile [ˈkæməmaɪl, -miːl] *n* echte Kamille *f*, Chamomilla *f*, Matricaria chamomilla/officinalis.
Chance [tʃæns, tʃɑːns]: **C. fracture** *ortho.* Chance-Fraktur *f*.
chan·cre [ˈʃæŋkər] *n* **1.** primäres Hautgeschwür *nt* (*bei Geschlechtskrankheiten*), Schanker *m*. **2.** harter Schanker *m*, Hunter-Schanker *m*, syphilitischer Primäraffekt *m*, Ulcus durum.
chan·cri·form [ˈʃæŋkrɪfɔːrm] *adj* schankerähnlich, -förmig, schankriform, schankrös.
chancriform pyodermia *derm.* Pyodermia chancriformis.
chancriform syndrome primär-extrapulmonale Kokzidioidomykose *f*.
chan·croid [ˈʃæŋkrɔɪd] *n* Chankroid *nt*, weicher Schanker *m*, Ulcus molle.
chan·croi·dal [ʃæŋˈkrɔɪdl] *adj* Chankroid betr., Chankroid-.
chancroidal bubo schankröser/virulenter Bubo *m*.
chancroidal ulcer → chancroid.

chancroid ulcer → chancroid.
chan·crous [ˈʃæŋkrəs] *adj* schankerähnlich, schankrös.
Chandler [ˈtʃændlər, ˈtʃɑːn-]: **C.'s disease** *ortho.* idiopathische Hüftkopfnekrose *f* des Erwachsenen, avaskuläre/ischämische Femurkopfnekrose *f* (des Erwachsenen).
change [tʃeɪndʒ] **I** *n* **1.** (Ver-)Änderung *f*; (*a. chem.*) Wandel *m*, (Ver-, Um-)Wandlung *f*; Wechsel *m*. ~ **for the better** Fortschritt *m*, (Ver-)Besserung *f*. ~ **for the worse** Rückschritt *m*, Verschlechterung *f*, Verschlimmerung *f*. **2.** (Aus-)Tausch *m*. **II** *vt* **3.** (ver-, um-)ändern; (*a. chem.*) umwandeln (*in, into* in); umformen, verwandeln (*in, into* zu). **to ~ color** die Farbe wechseln; blaß werden, erröten. **4.** (*techn.*) (aus-)wechseln, aus-, vertauschen. **to ~ one's clothes** s. umziehen. **5.** (*Bettwäsche*) wechseln; (*Säugling*) trockenlegen, die Windeln wechseln. **III** *vi* **6.** s. (ver-)ändern, wechseln. **to ~ for the better** besser werden, s. bessern. **to ~ for the worse** schlimmer werden, s. verschlimmern, s. verschlechtern. **7.** s. verwandeln (*into* in); übergehen (*to, into* in).
change over *vt* umwandeln, umstellen, -formen, verwandeln (*to* zu).
c. of air Luftveränderung *f*.
c. of dressing Verbandswechsel *m*.
c. of life 1. Menopause *f*. **2.** Klimakterium *nt*.
c. of personality Persönlichkeits-, Wesensveränderung *f*.
c. of position Lageveränderung *f*.
c. of sound Biermer-, Gerhardt-Schallwechsel *m*.
c. of voice Stimmbruch *m*, -wechsel, Mutatio(n *f*) *f*.
change·a·bil·i·ty [,tʃeɪndʒəˈbɪlətɪ] *n* **1.** Unbeständigkeit *f*, Veränderlichkeit *f*. **2.** Wankelmut *m*, Wechselhaftigkeit *f*.
change·a·ble [ˈtʃeɪndʒəbl] *adj* **1.** (*Person*) unbeständig, schwankend, wankelmütig. **2.** veränderlich, wechselhaft, wechselnd.
change·a·ble·ness [ˈ-nɪs] *n* → changeability.
change·ful [ˈtʃeɪndʒfəl] *adj* veränderlich, unbeständig, inkonstant.
change·less [ˈ-lɪs] *adj* unveränderlich, beständig, konstant.
change-over *n* Umstellung *f* (*from...to* von...auf), vollständiger Wechsel (*to* zu).
chang·ing [ˈtʃeɪndʒɪŋ] **I** *n* Wechsel *m*, Veränderung *f*. **II** *adj* wechselnd, veränderlich.
changing room Umkleideraum *m*.
chan·nel [ˈtʃænl] (*v:* channel(l)ed) **I** *n* **1.** Kanal *m*, Rinne *f*, Röhre *f*, (röhrenförmiger) Gang *m*. **2.** *phys.* Kanal *m*, Frequenz *f*. **3.** *bio.* (*Protein*) Tunnel *m*. **4.** *techn.* Nut *f*, Furche *f*. **5.** *fig.* Weg *f*, Bahn *f*; Richtung *f*, Kurs *m*. **II** *vt* **6.** rinnenförmig aushöhlen, furchen, bahnen. **7.** *techn.* nuten, furchen. **8.** *fig.* kanalisieren.
channel protein Kanal-, Tunnelprotein *nt*.
Chaoul [ʃaʊl]: **C. therapy** Chaoul'-Nachbestrahlung *f*.
chapped [tʃæpt] *adj* (*Haut*) rissig, schrundig, aufgesprungen.
char·ac·ter [ˈkærɪktər] *n* **1.** Charakter *m*, Wesen *n*, Art *f*. **2.** Charakteristikum *nt*, Merkmal *nt*, (charakteristisches) Kennzeichen *nt*, Eigenschaft *f*. **3.** Persönlichkeit *f*, Charakter *m*.
character analysis Charakteranalyse *f*.
character disorder Persönlichkeitsstörung *f*.
char·ac·ter·is·tic [,kærɪktəˈrɪstɪk] **I** *n* Charakteristikum *nt*, Merkmal *nt*, (charakteristisches) Kennzeichen *nt*, Eigenschaft *f*.

II *adj* charakteristisch, bezeichnend, typisch (*of* für).
char·ac·ter·is·ti·cal [,-ˈrɪstɪkl] *adj* → characteristic II.
characteristic symptom charakteristisches Symptom *nt*.
char·ac·ter·i·za·tion [,kærɪkt(ə)rəˈzeɪʃn, -raɪ-] *n* Charakterisierung *f*.
char·ac·ter·ize [ˈkærɪktəraɪz] *vt* charakterisieren, kennzeichnen, beschreiben, schildern.
char·ac·ter·less [ˈkærɪktərlɪs] *adj* **1.** *psycho.* charakterlos, ohne Charakter. **2.** (*Symptom*) nichtssagend, verschwommen, uncharakteristisch.
character neurosis *psycho., psychia.* Charakterneurose *f*, Kernneurose *f*.
char·bon [ʃarˈbɔ̃] *n* Milzbrand *m*, Anthrax *m*.
char·coal [ˈtʃɑːrkəʊl] *n* Holzkohle *f*.
charcoal agar Holzkohleagar *m/nt*.
charcoal-yeast extract agar *micro.* Aktivkohle-Hefeextrakt-Agar *m/nt*, charcoal--yeast extract agar.
Charcot [ʃarˈko]: **aneurysm of C.** Charcot--Aneurysma *nt*.
aneurysm of C. (and Bouchard) Charcot--Aneurysma *nt*.
C.'s arthropathy → **C.'s disease 2.**
C.'s cirrhosis primäre biliäre Zirrhose *f abbr.* PBZ, nicht-eitrige destruierende Cholangitis *f*.
C.'s disease 1. *neuro.* Charcot-Krankheit *f*, myatrophische/amyotroph(isch)e Lateralsklerose *f abbr.* ALS. **2.** Charcot-Gelenk *nt*, -Krankheit *f*, tabische Arthropathie *f*, Arthropathia tabica.
C.'s fever intermittierendes Fieber *nt* bei Cholelithiasis.
C.'s foot *ortho., neuro.* Charcot-Fuß *m*.
C.'s gait Charcot-Gang *m*.
C.'s intermittent fever → **C.'s fever.**
C.'s joint → **C.'s disease 2.**
C.'s sclerosis → **C.'s disease 1.**
C.'s sign → Charcot-Zeichen *nt*, -Steppergang *m*. **2.** Charcot-Zeichen *nt*, -Predigerhand *f*.
C.'s syndrome 1. → **C.'s disease 1. 2.** *chir.* intermittierendes Fieber *nt* bei Cholelithiasis. **3.** *card.* Charcot-Syndrom *nt*, intermittierendes Hinken *nt*, Angina cruris, Claudicatio intermittens, Dysbasia intermittens/angiospastica.
C.'s triad 1. *neuro.* Charcot'-Trias *f*. **2.** *chir.* (*Galle*) Charcot'-Trias *f*, -Symptomenkomplex *m*.
C.'s vertigo Kehlkopf-, Larynxschwindel *m*, Vertigo laryngica.
Charcot-Böttcher [ˈbœtʃər]: **C.-B. crystalloids** Boettcher-Kristalle *pl*.
Charcot and Bouchard [buˈʃɑːr]: **aneurysm of C.a.B.** Charcot-Aneurysma *nt*.
Charcot-Leyden [ˈlaɪdən]: **C.-L. crystals** Charcot-Leyden-Kristalle *pl*, Asthmakristalle *pl*.
Charcot-Marie [maˈriː]: **C.-M. atrophy/type** Charcot-Marie-Krankheit *f*, -Syndrom *nt*, Charcot-Marie-Tooth-Hoffmann--Krankheit *f*, -Syndrom *nt*.
Charcot-Marie-Tooth [tuːθ]: **C.-M.-T. atrophy/disease** → Charcot-Marie atrophy.
C.-M.-T. type *abbr.* CMT → Charcot-Marie atrophy.
Charcot-Neumann [ˈnɔʏman]: **C.-N. crystals** → Charcot-Leyden crystals.
Charcot-Rubin [ˈruːbɪn]: **C.-R. crystals** → Charcot-Leyden crystals.
Charcot-Weiss-Baker [vaɪs ˈbeɪkər]: **C.-W.-B. syndrome** *card.* Charcot-Weiss--Baker-Syndrom *nt*, Karotissinussyndrom *nt*, hyperaktiver Karotissinusreflex *m*.

charge

charge [tʃɑːrdʒ] **I** n 1. electr. Ladung f. **to be on ~** aufgeladen werden. 2. fig. Last f, Belastung f. 3. Gebühr f, Unkosten pl. 4. Verantwortung f, Leitung f, Aufsicht f (of für). **to be in ~ of** die Verantwortung haben für; leiten. **the person in ~** der/die Verantwortliche, die verantwortliche Person. **to take ~** die Leitung/Aufsicht übernehmen. 5. Mündel nt, Schützling m; Patient(in f) m. **the patient in/under his ~** der ihm anvertraute Patient. **II** vt 6. techn. beschicken, (an-)füllen; (Batterie) (auf-)laden. 7. chem. sättigen (with mit). 8. **to ~ sb. with sth.** jdn. mit etw. beauftragen. 9. berechnen. 10. anklagen, beschuldigen.
charged ['tʃɑːrdʒt] adj (a. fig.) geladen; (Batterie) (auf-)geladen.
charged molecule geladenes Molekül nt.
charge gradient Ladungsgradient m.
charge number chem. Ordnungszahl nt abbr. Z, OZ.
charg·er ['tʃɑːrdʒər] n electr. Ladegerät nt.
charg·ing ['tʃɑːrdʒɪŋ] n 1. techn. Beschickung f. 2. electr. (Auf-)Ladung f. 3. Beladung f.
char·la·tan ['ʃɑrlətn] n Quacksalber m, Kurpfuscher m.
char·la·tan·ism ['ʃɑrlətnɪzəm] n Kurpfuscherei f, Quacksalberei f.
char·la·tan·ry ['ʃɑrlətnrɪ] n → charlatanism.
Charles ['tʃɑːrlz]: **C.' law** phys. Gay-Lussac'-Gesetz nt.
char·ley horse ['tʃɑːrlɪ] inf. Muskelkater m.
Charlin ['ʃɑːrlɪn]: **C.'s syndrome** neuro. Charlin-Syndrom nt.
Charlouis [ʃɑr'lwɪ]: **C.' disease** Frambösie f, Framboesia tropica, Pian f, Parangi f, Yaws f.
Charnley ['tʃɑːrnlɪ]: **C. hip arthroplasty** ortho. Charnley-Prothese f. **C. hip prosthesis** → C. hip arthroplasty.
Charrière [ʃɑr'jɛːr]: **C. scale** Charrière-Scheibe f, -Skala f.
chart [tʃɑːrt] **I** n 1. Tabelle f; graphische Darstellung f, Skala f, Diagramm nt, Schaubild nt. 2. (Fieber-)Kurve f, Kurve(nblatt nt) f. **II** vt 3. graphisch darstellen, eintragen. 4. in eine Kurve einzeichnen od. auftragen.
chas·ma ['kæzmə] n anat. Riß m, Spalte f, Kluft f.
chas·mus ['kæzməs] n → chasma.
Chassaignac [ʃɑsɛ'njak]: **C.'s space** Chassaignac-Raum m. **C.'s tubercle** Tuberculum caroticum/anterius vertebra cervicalis VI.
Chassard-Lapiné [ʃɑˈsɑːr lapiˈne]: **C.-L. maneuver** radiol. Chassard-Lapiné-Methode f.
Chauffard [ʃoˈfɑːr]: **C.'s point** Chauffard-Punkt m. **C.'s syndrome** Chauffard-Ramon-Still-Syndrom nt, Still-Syndrom nt, juvenile Form f der chronischen Polyarthritis.
Chauffard-Still [stɪl]: **C.-S. syndrome** → Chauffard's syndrome.
chaul·mau·gra oil → chaulmoogra oil.
chaul·moo·gra oil [tʃɒlˈmuːgrə] Chaulmugraöl nt, Chaulmoograöl nt.
chaul·moo·gric acid [tʃɒlˈmuːgrɪk] Chaulmugrasäure f.
chaul·mu·gra oil → chaulmoogra oil.
Chaussé [ʃoˈse]: **C. view** radiol., HNO Aufnahme f nach Chaussé.
Chaussier [ʃosˈje]: **C.'s areola** Chaussier-Areola f. **C.'s line** Chaussier'-Linie f. **C.'s sign** Chaussier'-Zeichen nt.
Chauveau [ʃoˈvo]: **C.'s bacillus/bacterium** Clostridium chauvoei.

CHD abbr. → coronary heart disease.
ChE abbr. → cholinesterase.
Cheadle ['tʃiːdl]: **C.'s disease** rachitischer Säuglingsskorbut m, Möller-Barlow-Krankheit f.
check [tʃɛk] **I** n 1. Check m, Untersuchung f, (Über-, Nach-)Prüfung f, Kontrolle f. **to keep a ~ (up)on sth./sb.** jdn./etw. unter Kontrolle halten od. kontrollieren od. überwachen. **to make a ~ on sb./sth.** jdn./etw. überprüfen; bei jdm./etw. eine Kontrolle durchführen. **to give sth. a ~** etw. nachsehen, überprüfen. 2. (Person, Sache) Hindernis nt, Hemmnis nt (on für). **to act as a ~ (up)on sth.** etw. unter Kontrolle halten. **without a ~** ungehindert. 3. (plötzlicher) Stillstand m, (An-)Halten nt; Einhalt m; Rückschlag m. 4. Kontrollzeichen nt, Häkchen n (auf Listen). **II** vt 5. checken, kontrollieren, (über-, nach-)prüfen; vergleichen (against mit); (Liste) abhaken, ankreuzen. 6. stoppen, auf-, anhalten, zum Halten od. Stillstand od. Stehen bringen, hemmen. 7. in Schranken halten, unter Kontrolle bringen, zügeln. 8. reduzieren, herabsetzen, verringern, drosseln. **III** vi 9. genau entsprechen, übereinstimmen (with mit). 10. etw. nach-, überprüfen (upon).
check on vi → check upon.
check out vt 1. → check 5. 2. s. erkundigen nach, s. informieren über.
check over vt checken, kontrollieren, (über-, nach-)prüfen.
check upon vi über-, nachprüfen, untersuchen; recherchieren.
check·a·ble ['tʃɛkəbl] adj kontrollier-, nachprüfbar.
check·list ['tʃɛklɪst] n Kontroll-, Vergleichs-, Checkliste f.
check mark → check 4.
check-over n (gründliche) Untersuchung f, Überprüfung f, Kontrolle f.
check-up n 1. → check-over. 2. Check-up m; (umfangreiche) Vorsorgeuntersuchung f. **to have a ~/to go for a ~** einen Check-up machen lassen.
check x-ray Kontroll(röntgen)aufnahme f.
Chédiak-Higashi [ʃediˈak hɪˈgæʃɪ]: **C.-H. anomaly/disease** → C.-H. syndrome. **C.-H. syndrome** abbr. CHS Béguez César-Anomalie f, Chédiak-Higashi-Syndrom nt, Chédiak-Steinbrinck-Higashi-Syndrom nt, Béguez César-Anomalie f.
Chédiak-Steinbrinck-Higashi ['staɪnbrɪŋk]: **C.-S.-H. anomaly/syndrome** → Chédiak-Higashi syndrome.
cheek [tʃiːk] n 1. Backe f, Wange f; anat. Bucca f, Mala f. 2. inf. (Po-)Backe f.
cheek area Wangengegend f, -region f, Regio buccalis.
cheek·bone ['tʃiːkboʊn] n Jochbein nt, Os zygomaticum.
cheek region → cheek area.
cheek teeth Backenzähne pl.
cheese [tʃiːz] n 1. Käse m. 2. ped. inf. halbverdaute Milch, die von Säuglingen ausgespuckt wird.
cheese mite micro. Tyrophagus longior.
cheese poisoning Käsevergiftung f, Tyrotoxikose f.
chees·y ['tʃiːzɪ] adj käsig, käseartig, verkäsend.
cheesy abscess verkäsender Abszeß m.
cheesy bronchitis käsige Bronchitis f.
cheesy degeneration verkäsende Degeneration/Nekrose f, Verkäsung f.
cheesy necrosis → cheesy degeneration.
cheesy nephritis → caseous nephritis.
cheesy pneumonia käsige/verkäsende Pneumonie f.

136

che·gre flea ['tʃiːgər] micro. Sandfloh m, Tunga/Dermatophilus penetrans.
cheil- pref. → cheilo-.
chei·lal·gia [kaɪˈlældʒ(ɪ)ə] n Lippenschmerz(en pl) m, Ch(e)ilalgie f.
chei·lec·to·my [kaɪˈlɛktəmɪ] n 1. HNO Lippenexzision f, Cheilektomie f. 2. ortho. Cheilektomie f.
chei·lec·tro·pi·on [ˌkaɪlɛkˈtroʊpɪən] n HNO Cheilektropion nt.
chei·li·on ['kaɪlɪən] n Mundwinkelpunkt m, Cheilion nt.
chei·li·tis [kaɪˈlaɪtɪs] n Lippenentzündung f, Cheilitis f.
cheilitis glandularis Cheilitis glandularis. **superficial suppurative type c.** Baelz'-Krankheit f, Cheilitis glandularis purulenta superficialis, Myxadenitis labialis.
cheilo- pref. Lippe(n-), Cheil(o-).
chei·lo·an·gi·os·co·py [ˌkaɪloʊˌændʒɪˈɑskəpɪ] n Cheiloangioskopie f.
chei·lo·car·ci·no·ma [ˌkaɪloʊˌkɑːrsɪˈnoʊmə] n Lippenkrebs m, -karzinom nt.
chei·lo·gna·tho·pal·a·tos·chi·sis [ˌ-ˌneɪθoʊˌpæləˈtɑskəsɪs] n Wolfsrachen m, Lippen-Kiefer-Gaumen-Spalte f, Cheilognathopalatoschisis f.
chei·lo·gna·tho·pros·o·pos·chi·sis [ˌ-ˌneɪθəˌprɑsəˈpɑskəsɪs] n → cheilognathopalatoschisis.
chei·lo·gna·thos·chi·sis [ˌ-neɪˈθɑskəsɪs] n Lippen-Kiefer-Spalte f, Cheilognathoschisis f.
chei·lo·gna·tho·u·ra·nos·chi·sis [ˌ-ˌneɪθoʊˌjʊərəˈnɑskəsɪs] n → cheilognathopalatoschisis.
chei·lo·pha·gia [ˌ-ˈfeɪdʒ(ɪ)ə] n psychia. Lippenbeißen nt, Cheilophagie f.
chei·lo·plas·ty ['-ˌplæstɪ] n chir. Lippenplastik f, Cheiloplastik f.
chei·lor·rha·phy [kaɪˈlɔrəfɪ] n chir. Lippennaht f, Cheilorrhaphie f.
chei·los·chi·sis [kaɪˈlɑskəsɪs] n Lippenspalte f, Hasenscharte f, Cheiloschisis f.
chei·lo·sis [kaɪˈloʊsɪs] n (Lippen-)Rhagaden pl, Cheilosis f.
chei·lo·sto·mat·o·plas·ty [ˌkaɪloʊˈstoʊmætəplæstɪ] n chir. Lippen-Mund-Plastik f, Cheilostomatoplastik f.
chei·lot·o·my [kaɪˈlɑtəmɪ] n chir. Lippeninzision f, Cheilotomie f.
cheir- pref. → cheiro-.
cheir·ag·ra [kaɪˈrægrə] n Ch(e)iragra f.
cheir·al·gia [kaɪˈrældʒ(ɪ)ə] n Handschmerz m, Ch(e)iralgie f, Ch(e)iralgia f.
cheir·ar·thri·tis [ˌkaɪrɑːrˈθraɪtɪs] n Entzündung f von Hand- u. Fingergelenken.
cheiro- pref. Hand-, Cheir(o-), Chir(o-).
chei·ro·bra·chi·al·gia [ˌkaɪroʊˌbrækɪˈældʒ(ɪ)ə, -ˌbreɪkɪ-] n Ch(e)irobrachialgie f.
chei·ro·cin·es·the·sia [ˌ-ˌsɪnəsˈθiːʒ(ɪ)ə] n cheirokinesthesia.
chei·ro·kin·es·the·sia [ˌ-kɪnəsˈθiːʒ(ɪ)ə] n Ch(e)irokinästhesie f.
chei·ro·kin·es·thet·ic [ˌ-kɪnəsˈθɛtɪk] adj Ch(e)irokinästhesie betr., ch(e)irokinästhetisch.
chei·rol·o·gy [kaɪˈrɑlədʒɪ] n Daktylologie f (Finger- u. Gebärdensprache der Taubstummen).
chei·ro·meg·a·ly [ˌkaɪroʊˈmɛgəlɪ] n Tatzenhand f, Ch(e)iromegalie f.
chei·ro·plas·ty ['-ˌplæstɪ] n chir. (plastische) Handchirurgie f, Ch(e)iroplastik f.
chei·ro·po·dal·gia [ˌ-poʊˈdældʒ(ɪ)ə] n Schmerzen pl in Händen u. Füßen, Ch(e)iropodalgie f, -podalgia f.
chei·ro·pom·pho·lyx [ˌ-ˈpɑm(p)fəlɪks] n derm. Ch(e)iropompholyx m.
chei·ro·scope ['-skoʊp] n ophthal. Cheiroskop nt.
chei·ro·spasm ['-spæzəm] n Handmuskel-

Schreibkrampf *m*, Chirospasmus *m*, Cheirismus *m*.
che·late ['ki:leɪt] **I** *n* Chelat *nt*. **II** *vt* ein Chelat bilden.
chelate complex Chelatkomplex *m*.
che·lat·ing agent ['ki:leɪtɪŋ] Chelat-, Komplexbildner *m*.
che·la·tion [ki:'leɪʃn] *n* Chelatbildung *f*, Chelation *f*.
chel·i·don ['kelɪdɑn] *n* Ellenbogengrube *f*, Fossa cubitalis.
che·loid ['ki:lɔɪd] *n* Wulstnarbe *f*, Keloid *nt*.
che·lo·ma [kɪ'ləʊmə] *n* → cheloid.
chem- *pref.* → chemi-.
chem·a·bra·sion [ˌkemə'breɪʒn] *n chir.* Chemoabrasion *f*, -abradierung *f*.
chem·ex·fo·li·a·tion [ˌ-eksˌfəʊlɪ'eɪʃn] *n* → chemabrasion.
chemi- *pref.* Chemie-, Chemo-.
chem·i·a·try ['kemɪətrɪ] *n histor.* Iatrochemie *f*, Chemiatrie *f*.
chemic- *pref.* → chemi-.
chem·i·cal ['kemɪkl] **I** *n* **1.** Chemikalie *f*, chemische Substanz *f*, chemisches Produkt *nt*. **2.** ~s *pl inf.* Rauschgift *nt*, bewußtseinsverändernde Drogen *pl*. **II** *adj* Chemie betr., chemisch, Chemo-.
chemical affinity chemische Anziehung(skraft *f*) *f*.
chemical agent chemisches Agens *nt*, chemische Verbindung *f*.
chemical antidote chemisches Antidot *nt*.
chemical architectonics Chemoarchitektonik *f*.
chemical attractant *bio.* chemischer Lockstoff *m*, Attraktant *m*.
chemical attraction chemische Anziehung *f*.
chemical bond chemische Bindung *f*.
chemical burn chemische Verbrennung *f*, Verätzung *f*.
chemical cautery → chemocautery.
chemical composition chemische Zusammensetzung *f*; chemisches Präparat *nt*.
chemical compound chemische Verbindung *f*.
chemical conjunctivitis chemische Konjunktivitis *f*.
chemical coupling *biochem.* chemische Kopplung *f*.
chemical coupling hypothesis Hypothese *f* der chemischen Kopplung.
chemical dependency Drogenabhängigkeit *f*, -sucht *f*, Alkoholabhängigkeit *f*, -sucht *f*.
chemical dermatitis allergische Kontaktdermatitis *f* durch Chemikalien.
chemical diabetes *old* pathologische Glukosetoleranz *f*.
chemical energy chemische Energie *f*.
chemical equation chemische (Reaktions-)Gleichung *f*.
chemical equivalent chemisches Grammäquivalent *nt*.
chemical evolution chemische Evolution *f*.
chemical fiber Chemie-, Kunstfaser *f*.
chemical formula chemische Formel *f*.
chemical gastritis Ätzgastritis *f*, Gastritis corrosiva.
chemical injury Verletzung *f* durch Chemikalien; Verätzung *f*.
chemical labeling chemische Markierung *f*.
chemical laboratory Chemielabor *nt*.
chemical messenger chemischer Bote *m*, chemische Botensubstanz *f*, Chemotransmitter *m*.
chemical mutagen *genet.* chemisches Mutagen *nt*.
chemical osteonecrosis chemische Knochennekrose/Osteonekrose *f*.

chemical peritonitis Reizperitonitis *f*.
chemical pneumonia chemische Pneumonie *f*.
chemical prophylaxis → chemoprophylaxis.
chemical reaction chemische Reaktion *f*. **scalar c.** skalare/ungerichtete (chemische) Reaktion. **vectorial c.** vektorielle/gerichtete (klinische) Reaktion.
chemical senses chemische Sinne *pl* (*Geschmacks-* u. *Geruchssinn*).
chemical sterilization chemische Sterilisation *f*, Sterilisation *f* durch Chemikalien.
chemical stimulus chemischer Reiz *m*.
chemical sympathectomy pharmakologische Sympathektomie *f*.
chemical synapse chemische Synapse *f*.
chemico- *pref.* → chemi-.
chem·i·co·bi·o·log·i·cal [ˌkemɪkəʊˌbaɪə-'lɑdʒɪkl] *adj* Biochemie betr., biochemisch.
chem·i·co·cau·ter·y [ˌ-'kɔːtərɪ] *n* → chemocautery.
chem·i·co·phys·i·cal [ˌ-'fɪzɪkl] *adj* Chemie und Physik betr., physikalische Chemie betr., physikochemisch, chemisch-physikalisch.
chem·i·co·phys·i·o·log·ic [ˌ-ˌfɪzɪə'lɑdʒɪk] *adj* Chemie u. Physiologie betr., chemophysiologisch.
chem·i·lum·i·nes·cence [ˌkemɪˌluːmə'nesəns] *n* → chemoluminescence.
chem·i·os·mo·sis [ˌ-ɑz'məʊsɪs] *n* → chemosmosis.
chem·i·os·mot·ic [ˌ-ɑz'mɑtɪk] *adj* → chemosmotic.
chemiosmotic coupling *biochem.* chemiosmotische Kopplung *f*.
chemiosmotic (coupling) hypothesis Hypothese *f* der chemiosmotischen Kopplung, chemiosmotische Hypothese *f*.
chem·i·o·tax·is [ˌkemɪəʊ'tæksɪs] *n* → chemotaxis.
chem·i·o·ther·a·py [ˌ-'θerəpɪ] *n* → chemotherapy.
chem·ism ['kemɪzəm] *n* Chemismus *m*.
chem·i·sorp·tion [ˌkemə'zɔːrpʃn] *n* Chemosorption *f*.
chem·ist ['kemɪst] *n* **1.** Chemiker(in *f*) *m*. **2.** *Brit.* Apotheker(in *f*) *m*, Drogist(in *f*) *m*.
chem·is·try ['kemɪstrɪ] *n, pl* **-tries 1.** Chemie *f*. **2.** chemische Eigenschaften/Reaktionen/Phänomene *pl*.
chemo- *pref.* → chemi-.
che·mo ['kiːməʊ, 'keməʊ] *n inf.* → chemotherapy.
che·mo·ar·chi·tec·ton·ics [ˌkiːməʊˌɑːrkɪtek'tɑnɪks, ˌkeməʊ-] *pl* → chemical architectonics.
che·mo·at·trac·tant [ˌ-ə'træktənt] *n* → chemotactic factor.
che·mo·au·to·troph [ˌ-'ɔːtətrəf, -trəʊf] *n* chemoautotropher Organismus *m*, Chemoautotroph *m*.
che·mo·au·to·troph·ic [ˌ-ˌɔːtə'trɑfɪk, -trəʊ-] *adj* chemoautotroph.
chemoautotrophic bacteria chemoautotrophe Bakterien *pl*.
che·mo·bi·ot·ic [ˌ-baɪ'ɑtɪk] *n pharm.* Kombination *f* von Antibiotikum u. Chemotherapeutikum.
che·mo·cau·ter·y [ˌ-'kɔːtərɪ] *n chir.* Chemokauterisation *f*, -kaustik *f*.
che·mo·ce·pha·lia [ˌ-sɪ'feɪlɪə] *n* → chamaecephaly.
che·mo·ceph·a·ly [ˌ-'sefəlɪ] *n* → chamaecephaly.
che·mo·cep·tor [ˌ-'septər] *n* → chemoreceptor.

chemosensitivity

che·mo·co·ag·u·la·tion [ˌ-kəʊˌægjə'leɪʃn] *n chir.* Chemokoagulation *f*.
che·mo·dec·to·ma [ˌ-dek'təʊmə] *n* Chemodektom *nt*, nicht-chromaffines Paragangliom *nt*.
che·mo·dif·fer·en·ti·a·tion [ˌ-dɪfəˌrentʃɪ-'eɪʃn] *n embryo.* Chemodifferenzierung *f*.
che·mo·em·bo·li·za·tion [ˌ-ˌembəlɪ'zeɪʃn, -laɪ-] *n* Embolisation *f* durch Chemikalien, Chemoembolisation *f*.
che·mo·het·er·o·troph [ˌ-'hetərətrɑf, -trəʊf] *n* chemoheterotropher Organismus *m*, Chemoheterotroph *m*.
che·mo·het·er·o·troph·ic [ˌ-ˌhetərə'trɑfɪk, -'trəʊ-] *adj* chemoheterotroph.
chemoheterotrophic bacteria chemoheterotrophe Bakterien *pl*.
che·mo·hor·mo·nal [ˌ-hɔːr'məʊnl] *adj* chemohormonal.
che·mo·im·mu·nol·o·gy [ˌ-ˌɪmjə'nɑlədʒɪ] *n* Immun(o)chemie *f*.
che·mo·ki·ne·sis [ˌ-kɪ'niːsɪs, -kaɪ-] *n* Chemokinese *f*.
che·mo·ki·net·ic [ˌ-kɪ'netɪk, -kaɪ-] *adj* chemokinetisch.
che·mo·lith·o·troph [ˌ-'lɪθətrɑf, -trəʊf] *n* chemolithotropher Organismus *m*, Chemolithotroph *m*.
che·mo·lith·o·troph·ic [ˌ-ˌlɪθə'trɑfɪk, -'trəʊ-] *adj* chemolithotroph.
chemolithotrophic bacteria chemolithotrophe Bakterien *pl*.
chemolithotrophic cell chemolithotrophe Zelle *f*.
che·mo·lum·i·nes·cence [ˌ-ˌluːmɪ'nesəns] *n* Chemi-, Chemolumineszenz *f*.
che·mol·y·sis [kɪ'mɑləsɪs] *n* Chemolyse *f*.
che·mo·me·chan·i·cal [ˌkiːməʊmə'kænɪkl, ˌkem-] *adj* chemomechanisch.
che·mo·mor·pho·sis [ˌ-mɔːr'fəʊsɪs] *n genet.* Chemomorphose *f*.
che·mo·nu·cle·ol·y·sis [ˌ-ˌn(j)uːklɪ'ɑləsɪs] *n ortho., neurochir.* (Chemo-)Nukleolyse *f*.
chemo-organotroph *n* chemoorganotropher Organismus *m*, Chemoorganotroph *m*.
chemo-organotrophic *adj* chemoorganotroph.
chemo-organotrophic bacteria chemoorganotrophe Bakterien *pl*.
chemo-organotrophic cell chemoorganotrophe Zelle *f*.
che·mo·pal·li·dec·to·my [ˌ-ˌpælɪ'dektəmɪ] *n neurochir.* Chemopallidektomie *f*.
che·mo·pal·li·do·thal·a·mec·to·my [ˌ-ˌpælɪdəʊˌθæləˈmektəmɪ] *n neurochir.* Chemopallidothalamektomie *f*.
che·mo·phys·i·ol·o·gy [ˌ-ˌfɪzɪ'ɑlədʒɪ] *n* physiologische Chemie *f*, Biochemie *f*.
che·mo·pro·phy·lax·is [ˌ-ˌprəʊfɪ'læksɪs] *n pharm.* Chemoprophylaxe *f*, Infektionsprophylaxe *f* durch Chemotherapeutika.
che·mo·re·cep·tion [ˌ-rɪ'sepʃn] *n* Chemo(re)zeption *f*.
che·mo·re·cep·tive [ˌ-rɪ'septɪv] *adj* chemorezeptiv.
chemoreceptive cell chemorezeptive Zelle *f*.
che·mo·re·cep·tor [ˌ-rɪ'septər] *n* Chemo(re)zeptor *m*.
chemoreceptor reflex Chemorezeptorenreflex *m*.
chemoreceptor tumor Chemodektom *nt*.
che·mo·re·flex [ˌ-'riːfleks] *n* Chemoreflex *m*.
che·mo·re·sist·ance [ˌ-rɪ'zɪstəns] *n* Chemoresistenz *f*.
che·mo·sen·si·tive [ˌ-'sensətɪv] *adj* chemosensitiv, chemoempfindlich.
che·mo·sen·si·tiv·i·ty [ˌ-ˌsensə'tɪvətɪ] *n* Chemosensibilität *f*.

che·mo·sen·sor [ˌ-'sensɔr, -sər] *n* Chemosensor *m*.
che·mo·sen·so·ry [ˌ-'sensəri] *adj* chemosensorisch.
che·mo·se·ro·ther·a·py [ˌ-ˌsiərə'θerəpi] *n* kombinierte Chemo- u. Serumtherapie *f*.
che·mo·sis [kɪ'məʊsɪs] *n ophthal*. Chemosis *f*.
che·mos·mo·sis [ˌkiːmɑz'məʊsɪs, ˌkem-] *n* Chem(i)osmose *f*.
che·mos·mot·ic [ˌ-ɑz'mɑtɪk] *adj* Chem(i)osmose betr., chem(i)osmotisch.
chem·o·sorp·tion [ˌkiːməʊ'sɔːrpʃn, ˌkem-] *n* → chemisorption.
che·mo·sphere ['-sfɪər] *n* Chemosphäre *f*.
che·mo·stat ['-stæt] *n micro*. Chemostat *m*.
che·mo·sur·ger·y [ˌ-'sɜrdʒəri] *n* Chemochirurgie *f*.
che·mo·syn·the·sis [ˌ-'sɪnθəsɪs] *n* Chemosynthese *f*.
che·mo·syn·thet·ic [ˌ-sɪn'θetɪk] *adj* Chemosynthese betr., chemosynthetisch.
chemosynthetic bacteria chemosynthetische Bakterien *pl*.
chemosynthetic cell chemosynthetische Zelle *f*.
che·mo·tac·tic [ˌ-'tæktɪk] *adj* Chemotaxis betr., durch Chemotaxis, chemotaktisch.
chemotactic factor *abbr*. **CF** Chemotaktin *nt*, chemotaktischer Faktor *m*.
che·mo·tac·tin [ˌ-'tæktɪn] *n* → chemotactic factor.
che·mo·tax·in [ˌ-'tæksɪn] *n* → chemotactic factor.
che·mo·tax·is [ˌ-'tæksɪs] *n* Chemotaxis *f*.
che·mo·thal·a·mec·to·my [ˌ-θælə'mektəmi] *n neurochir*. Chemothalamektomie *f*.
che·mo·ther·a·peu·tic [ˌ-ˌθerə'pjuːtɪk] *adj* Chemotherapie betr., mittels Chemotherapie, chemotherapeutisch.
chemotherapeutic agent Chemotherapeutikum *nt*.
che·mo·ther·a·peu·ti·cal [ˌ-ˌθerə'pjuːtɪkl] *adj* → chemotherapeutic.
chemotherapeutic index therapeutische Breite *f*, therapeutischer Index *m*.
che·mo·ther·a·peu·tics [ˌ-ˌθerə'pjuːtɪks] *pl* → chemotherapy.
che·mo·ther·a·py [ˌ-'θerəpi] *n* Chemotherapie *f*.
che·mot·ic [kɪ'mɑtɪk] *adj ophthal*. Chemosis betr., chemotisch.
che·mo·trans·mit·ter [ˌkiːməʊtrænz'mɪtər, ˌkem-] *n* chemischer Bote *m*, chemische Botensubstanz *f*, Chemotransmitter *m*.
che·mo·troph ['-trɑf, '-trəʊf] *n* chemotropher Organismus *m*, Chemotroph *m*.
che·mo·troph·ic [ˌ-'trɑfɪk, '-trəʊf-] *adj* chemotroph.
chemotrophic bacteria chemotrophe Bakterien *pl*.
chemotrophic cell chemotrophe Zellen *pl*.
che·mo·trop·ic [ˌ-'trɑpɪk] *adj* Chemotropismus betr., chemotrop.
che·mot·ro·pism [kɪ'mɑtrəpɪzəm] *n* Chemotropismus *m*.
che·mo·type ['-taɪp] *n micro*. Chemotyp *m*, -var *m*.
che·mo·var ['-vɑːr] *n* → chemotype.
Cheneau [ʃe'nəʊ]: **C.** brace Cheneau-Korsett *nt*.
Cheney ['tʃeɪni]: **C.'s syndrome** *radio., ortho*. Cheney-Syndrom *nt*.
che·nic acid ['kiːnɪk] → chenodeoxycholic acid.
che·no·de·ox·y·cho·late [ˌkiːnəʊdiˌɑksɪ'kəʊleɪt, ˌken-] *n* Chenodesoxycholat *nt*.
che·no·de·ox·y·cho·lic acid [ˌ-dɪˌɑksɪ'kəʊlɪk, -'kɑl-] Chenodesoxycholsäure *f*.
che·no·de·ox·y·cho·lyl·gly·cine [ˌ-dɪˌɑksɪˌkəʊlɪl'glaɪsiːn] *n* Glykochenodesoxycholsäure *f*.
che·no·de·ox·y·cho·lyl·tau·rine [ˌ-dɪˌɑksɪˌkɑlɪl'tɔːriːn, -rɪn] *n* Taurochenodesoxycholsäure *f*.
che·no·di·ol [ˌ-'daɪɑl, -ɑl] *n* → chenodeoxycholic acid.
che·no·po·di·um oil [ˌ-'pəʊdiəm] *pharm*. Wurmsamenöl *nt*.
Chenuda [tʃə'nuːdə]: **C. virus** Chenuda-Virus *nt*.
Chernez ['tʃernez; ʃer'ne]: **C. incision** *gyn*. Chernez-Schnitt *m*.
cher·ry angiomas ['tʃeri] senile Angiome/Hämangiome *pl*, Alters(häm)angiome *pl*.
cherry-red spot Tay-Fleck *m*.
che·ru·bic facies [tʃə'ruːbɪk] *patho*. cherubinisches Engelsgesicht *nt*.
cher·ub·ism ['tʃerəbɪzəm] *n* Cherubismus *m*, Cherubinismus *m*.
chest [tʃest] *n* **1.** Brust *f*, Brustkorb *m*, Thorax *m*; Oberkörper *m*, Brustteil *nt*. **2.** Kiste *f*, Kasten *m*; Kommode *f*.
chest·ed ['tʃestɪd] *adj* -brüstig. **to be ~** es auf der Lunge haben, lungenleidend sein.
Chester ['tʃestər]: **C.'s disease (of bone)** → Chester-Erdheim disease (of bone).
Chester-Erdheim ['ɜrdhaɪm]: **C.-E. disease (of bone)** Chester(-Erdheim)-Erkrankung *f*, -Syndrom *nt*, Knochenxanthomatose *f*.
chest film → chest x-ray.
chest injury Brustkorbverletzung *f*, -trauma *nt*, Thoraxverletzung *f*, -trauma *nt*. **blunt c.** stumpfes Thoraxtrauma. **penetrating c.** perforierendes Thoraxtrauma.
chest lead (*EKG*) Brustwandableitung *f*.
chest organs Brustorgane *pl*, Organe *pl* des Brustraumes.
chest pain Brustschmerzen *pl*, Schmerzen *pl* im Brustkorb.
chest physiotherapy Atemgymnastik *f*.
chest trauma → chest injury.
chest tube *chir*. Thoraxdrain *m*.
chest wall Brust-, Thoraxwand *f*.
chest wall cancer sekundäres Brustwandkarzinom *nt*.
chest x-ray *abbr*. **cxr** Thorax(röntgen)aufnahme *f*.
chest·y ['tʃesti] *adj* **1.** einen ausgeprägten breiten Brustkorb *od*. Busen haben. **2.** (*Husten*) tiefsitzend; bronchitisch; verschleimt.
chew [tʃuː] **I** *n* Kauen *nt*; das Gekaute. **II** *vt* (zer-)kauen. **III** *vi* kauen.
chew·ing [tʃuːɪŋ] *n* Kauen *nt*, Kauvorgang *m*.
chewing surface (of tooth) (*Zahn*) Kaufläche *f*.
Cheyne ['tʃeɪn]: **C.'s nystagmus** → Cheyne-Stokes nystagmus.
Cheyne-Stokes ['stəʊks]: **C.-S. asthma** Herzasthma *nt*.
C.-S. breathing Cheyne-Stokes-Atmung *f*, periodische Atmung *f*.
C.-S. nystagmus Cheyne-Stokes-Nystagmus *m*.
C.-S. psychosis Cheyne-Stokes-Psychose *f*.
C.-S. respiration → C.-S. breathing.
C.-S. sign → C.-S. breathing.
CHF *abbr*. → congestive heart failure.
Chiari [kiˈɑːri]: **C.'s disease** Budd-Chiari-Syndrom *nt*, Endophlebitis hepatica obliterans.
C.'s network → C.'s reticulum.
C.'s operation for congenital hip dislocation → C.'s osteotomy.
C.'s osteotomy *ortho*. Beckenosteotomie *f* nach Chiari.
C.'s reticulum *card*. Chiari-Netzwerk *nt*.
C.'s syndrome → C.'s disease.

Chiari-Arnold ['ɑrnɔlt]: **C.-A. syndrome** Arnold-Chiari-Hemmungsmißbildung *f*, -Syndrom *nt*.
Chiari-Budd [bʌd]: **C.-B. syndrome** Budd-Chiari-Syndrom *nt*, Endophlebitis hepatica obliterns.
Chiari-Frommel ['frɔməl]: **C.-F. disease/syndrome** Chiari-Frommel-Syndrom *nt*, Laktationsatrophie *f* des Genitals.
chi·asm ['kaɪæzəm] *n* → chiasma.
c. of digits of hand Camper'-Kreuzung *f*, Chiasma tendinum (digitorum manus).
chi·as·ma [kaɪ'æzmə] *n, pl* **-mas, -ma·ta** [-mətə] **1.** *anat.* (x-förmige) (Über-)Kreuzung *f*, Chiasma *nt*. **2.** *genet*. Überkreuzung *f* von Chromosomen, Chiasma *nt*.
chi·as·mal [kaɪ'æzməl] *adj* → chiasmatic.
chiasma stage *genet*. Chiasmastadium *nt*.
chiasma syndrome Chiasma-Syndrom *nt*.
chi·as·mat·ic [ˌkaɪəz'mætɪk, kaɪˌæz-] *adj* kreuzförmig.
chiasmatic branch of posterior communicating artery Ramus chiasmaticus a. communicantis posterioris.
chiasmatic cistern Cisterna chiasmatica.
chiasmatic recess Rec. opticus.
chiasmatic sulcus Chiasma opticus-Rinne *f*, Sulcus pr(a)echiasmatis/pr(a)echiasmaticus.
chiasmatic syndrome Chiasma-Syndrom *nt*.
chi·as·ma·ty·py [kaɪ'æzmətaɪpi] *n genet*. Crossing-over *nt*, Crossover *nt*.
chi·as·mic [kaɪ'æzmɪk] *adj* → chiasmatic.
chi·as·mom·e·ter [kaɪəz'mɑmɪtər] *n* → chiastometer.
chi·as·tom·e·ter [kaɪæz'tɑmɪtər] *n ophthal*. Chiasmo-, Chiastometer *nt*.
Chi·ba needle ['tʃiːbə, tʃiː'bɑː] *radiol*. Chiba-Nadel *f*.
Chi·ca·go classification [ʃɪ'kɑːɡəʊ] *genet*. Chicago-Einteilung *f*, -Klassifikation *f*.
Chicago disease Gilchrist-Krankheit *f*, nordamerikanische Blastomykose *f*.
chick [tʃɪk] *n* Küken *nt*, junger Vogel *m*.
chick egg Hühnerei *nt*.
embryonated c. *micro*. bebrütetes/angebrütetes/embryoniertes Hühnerei *nt*.
chick embryo Hühnerembryo *m*.
chick·en ['tʃɪkɪn] *n* Huhn *nt*; Hühnchen *nt*, Küken *nt*; Hühnerfleisch *nt*.
chicken breast Kiel-, Hühnerbrust *f*, Pectus gallinatum/carinatum.
chicken-breasted *adj* hühnerbrüstig, mit Hühnerbrust.
chicken fat clot/thrombus *patho*. Speckhautgerinnsel *nt*.
chicken louse → chicken mite.
chicken mite *micro*. Vogelmilbe *f*, Dermanyssus avium/gallinae.
chicken pest *micro*. Hühner-, Geflügelpest *f*.
chick·en·pox ['tʃɪkənˌpɑks] *n* Wind-, Wasserpocken *pl*, Varizellen *pl*, Varicella *f*.
chickenpox virus Varicella-Zoster-Virus *nt abbr*. **VZV**.
Chick-Martin [tʃɪk 'mɑːrtn]: **C.-M. test** *micro*. Chick-Martin-Test *m*.
chick-pea ['tʃɪkpiː] *n* Kichererbse *f*.
chi·cle·ro ulcer [tʃɪ'kleərəʊ] südamerikanische Hautleishmaniase *f*, kutane Leishmaniase *f* Südamerikas, Chiclero-Ulkus *m*.
chi·cle ulcer ['tʃɪkl] → chiclero ulcer.
chief [tʃiːf] **I** *n* **1.** Hauptteil *m*. **2.** Chef(in *f*) *m*, Vorgesetzte(r *m*) *f*; Leiter(in *f*) *m*. **II** *adj* oberste(r, s), höchste(r, s), erste(r, s), wichtigste(r, s), Haupt-, Ober-.
chief agglutinin *immun*. Haupt-, Majoragglutinin *nt*.
chief cell 1. Hauptzelle *f*. **2.** Pinealozyt *m*.

3. chromaffine Zelle *f.* 4. chromophobe Zelle *f.*
c. of pineal → chief cell 2.
chief complaint Primär-, Haupt-, Leitsymptom *nt*, führendes Symptom *nt.*
chief vector *mathe., phys.* Hauptvektor *m.*
Chievitz ['tʃɪwɪts]: **C.'s layer** *embryo.* Chievitz-Schicht *f.*
C.'s organ *embryo.* Chievitz-Organ *nt.*
chig·ger ['tʃɪɡər] *n micro.* Trombicula-Larve *f*, Chigger *m.*
chig·o *n* → chigoe.
chig·oe ['tʃɪɡəʊ, -ɡə] *n micro.* Sandfloh *m*, Tunga/Dermatophilus penetrans.
chigoe flea → chigoe.
chik·un·gun·ya [ˌtʃɪkən'ɡʌnjə] *n* Chikungunya-Fieber *nt.*
chikungunya virus *micro.* Chikungunya-Virus *nt.*
chil- *pref.* → cheilo-.
Chilaiditi [kɪlə'diːtɪ]: **C.'s sign/syndrome** Chilaiditi-Syndrom *nt*, Interpositio coli/hepatodiaphragmatica.
chi·lal·gia [kaɪ'læld(ɪ)ə] *n* → cheilalgia.
chil·blain ['tʃɪlbleɪn] *n* Frostbeule *f*, Erythema pernio, Pernio *m.*
chilblain lupus Lupus pernio.
Child [tʃaɪld]: **C.'s classification** Child-Klassifikation *f.*
C.'s operation/procedure *chir.* Child-Methode *f*, -Operation *f*, subtotale distale/linksseitige Pankreatektomie *f*, subtotale Pankreaslinksresektion *f.*
child [tʃaɪld] *n, pl* **child·ren** ['tʃɪldrən] 1. Kind *nt*; Kleinkind *nt*; Baby *nt*, Säugling *m*; Nachkomme *m.* **with ~** schwanger. **from a ~** von Kindheit an. 2. *fig.* unreife *od.* kindliche *od.* kindische Person *f.*
child abuse Kindesmißhandlung *f.*
child-battering *n* (körperliche) Kindesmißhandlung *f.*
child-bear·ing ['tʃaɪldˌbeərɪŋ] **I** *n* Schwangerschaft *u.* Geburt *f*; Gebären *nt*, Niederkunft *f.* **II** *adj* gebärfähig. **of ~ age** im gebärfähigen Alter.
child·bed ['tʃaɪldbed] *n* Kind-, Wochenbett *nt*, Puerperium *nt.*
childbed fever *patho.* Kindbett-, Wochenbettfieber *nt*, Puerperalfieber *nt*, -sepsis *f*, Febris puerperalis.
child benefit Kindergeld *nt.*
child·birth ['tʃaɪldbɜːθ] *n* Geburt *f*, Niederkunft *f*, Entbindung *f.* **a difficult ~** eine schwierige Geburt.
child-care ['tʃaɪldkeər] *n* Kinderbetreuung *f*, -fürsorge *f.*
child custody elterliches Sorgerecht *nt* (*für ein Kind*).
child-free ['tʃaɪldfriː] *adj* kinderlos (*aus freier Entscheidung*).
child guidance heilpädagogische Betreuung *f.*
child·hood ['tʃaɪldˌhʊd] *n* Kindheit *f.* **from ~** von Kindheit an.
childhood (type) tuberculosis Primärtuberkulose *f.*
child·ish ['tʃaɪldɪʃ] *adj* 1. kindisch, unreif, infantil. 2. kindlich, infantil.
child·ish·ness ['-nɪs] *n* 1. Kindlichkeit *f.* 2. kindisches Gehabe *nt*, Kinderei *f.*
child labor Kinderarbeit *f.*
child·less ['tʃaɪldles] *adj* kinderlos.
child·less·ness ['tʃaɪldlesnɪs] *n* Kinderlosigkeit *f.*
child·like ['tʃaɪldlaɪk] *adj* → childish 2.
child neglect Kindesvernachlässigung *f.*
child-proof ['tʃaɪldpruːf] *adj* kindersicher.
childproof bottle Arzneiflasche *f* mit kindersicherem Verschluß.
child psychiatry Kinderpsychiatrie *f.*
child psychologist Kinderpsychologe *m*, -psychologin *f.*

child psychology Kinderpsychologie *f.*
child-resistent *adj* kindersicher.
child-resistant closure kindersicherer Verschluß *m.*
child welfare Kinderfürsorge *f.*
chi·lec·to·my *n* → cheilectomy.
chi·lec·tro·pi·on *n* → cheilectropion.
Chil·e saltpeter ['tʃiːlɪ] Chilesalpeter *m*, Natriumnitrat *nt.*
chi·li·tis *n* → cheilitis.
chill [tʃɪl] **I** *n* 1. Frösteln *nt*, Kältegefühl *nt*, (Fieber-)Schauer *m.* 2. (*a. fig.*) Kühle *f*, Kälte *f.* 3. (*a. ~s pl*) Schüttelfrost *m.* 4. *Brit.* Erkältung *f.* **to catch a ~** *s.* erkälten. **II** *adj* 5. kühl, kalt. 6. *fig.* unfreundlich, frostig. **III** *vt* (*Lebensmittel*) (ab-)kühlen, kalt machen. **IV** *vi* 7. abkühlen. 8. zittern, frösteln.
chills and fever Schüttelfrost *m.*
chill·y [tʃɪlɪ] *adj* (*a. fig.*) kalt, frostig, kühl; fröstelnd. **to feel ~** frösteln.
chilo- *pref.* → cheilo-.
chi·lo·gna·tho·pal·a·tos·chi·sis *n* → cheilognathopalatoschisis.
chi·lo·gna·tho·pros·o·pos·chi·sis *n* → cheilognathoprosoposchisis.
chi·lo·gna·thos·chi·sis *n* → cheilognathoschisis.
chi·lo·gna·tho·u·ra·nos·chi·sis *n* → cheilognathouranoschisis.
chi·lo·mas·ti·gi·a·sis [ˌkeɪləʊˌmæstɪˈɡaɪəsɪs] *n micro.* Chilomastixinfektion *f*, Chilomastosis *f*, Chilomastigiasis *f.*
Chi·lo·mas·tix [ˌ-'mæstɪks] *n micro.* Chilomastix *f.*
chi·lo·mas·tix·i·a·sis [ˌ-ˌmæstɪk'saɪəsɪs] *n* → chilomastigiasis.
chi·lo·pha·gia *n* → cheilophagia.
chi·lo·plas·ty *n* → cheiloplasty.
Chi·lop·o·da [kaɪ'lɒpədə] *pl micro.* Chilopoda *pl.*
chi·lo·po·di·a·sis [kaɪləpə'daɪəsəs] *n* Chilopodainfektion *f*, Chilopodiasis *f.*
chi·lor·rha·phy *n* → cheilorrhaphy.
chi·los·chi·sis *n* → cheiloschisis.
chi·lo·sis *n* → cheilosis.
chi·lo·sto·mat·o·plas·ty *n* → cheilostomatoplasty.
chi·lot·o·my *n* → cheilotomy.
chi·mae·ra *n* → chimera.
chi·me·ra [kaɪ'mɪərə] *n embryo.* Chimäre *f.*
chi·mer·ic plasmid [kaɪ'merɪk] *genet.* Rekombinationsplasmid *nt.*
chim·ney sweep's cancer ['tʃɪmnɪ] Kaminkehrer-, Schornsteinfegerkrebs *m.*
chim·pan·zee coryza agent [ˌtʃɪmpæn'ziː] *abbr.* **CCA** *old micro.* RS-Virus *nt*, Respiratory-Syncytial-Virus *nt.*
chi·myl alcohol ['kaɪmɪl] Chimylalkohol *m.*
chin [tʃɪn] *n* Kinn *nt*, Kinnvorsprung *m*, *anat.* Mentum *nt.*
Chi·na clay ['tʃaɪnə] Kaolin *nt.*
chin·a·crine ['kɪnəkriːn, 'krɪn-] *n* Quinacrin *nt*, Chinacrin *nt.*
chin area Kinngegend *f*, -region *f*, Regio mentalis.
Chi·nese liver fluke [tʃaɪ'niːz] *micro.* chinesischer Leberegel *m*, Clonorchis/Opisthorchis sinensis.
Chinese restaurant syndrome *abbr.* **CRS** Chinarestaurant-Syndrom *nt.*
chin jerk → chin reflex.
chin muscle Kinnmuskel *m*, Mentalis *m*, M. mentalis.
chin reflex Masseter-, Unterkieferreflex *m.*
chin region → chin area.
chi·on·a·blep·sia [ˌkaɪənə'blepsɪə] *n* Schneeblindheit *f*, Chion(o)ablepsie *f.*
chip [tʃɪp] **I** *n* 1. (Metall-, Holz-)Splitter *m*, Span *m.* 2. *chir., ortho.* (Knochen-, Knor-pel-)Span *m*, (-)Chip *m.* 3. *techn.* (Mikro-, Computer-)Chip *m.* **II** *vt* 4. (mit Axt *od.* Meißel) behauen. 5. (*Splitter*) abraspeln. 6. *sl.* (gelegentlich) Rauschgift einnehmen. **III** *vi* abbröckeln, abbrechen.
chir- *pref.* → cheiro-.
chi·rag·ra *n* → cheiragra.
chi·ral ['kaɪrəl] *adj* chiral.
chi·ral·i·ty [kaɪ'rælətɪ] *n chem.* Händigkeit *f*, Chiralität *f*; Stereoisomerie *f.*
chi·rar·thri·tis *n* → cheirarthritis.
chiro- *pref.* → cheiro-.
chi·ro·bra·chi·al·gia *n* → cheirobrachialgia.
chi·ro·cin·es·the·sia [ˌkaɪrəʊsɪnəs'θiːʒ(ɪ)ə] *n* → cheirokinesthesia.
chi·ro·kin·es·the·sia *n* → cheirokinesthesia.
chi·rol·o·gy [kaɪ'rɒlədʒɪ] *n* Daktylologie *f* (*Finger- u. Gebärdensprache der Taubstummen*).
chi·ro·meg·a·ly *n* → cheiromegaly.
chi·ro·plas·ty *n* → cheiroplasty.
chi·ro·po·dal·gia *n* → cheiropodalgia.
chi·rop·o·dist [kɪ'rɒpədɪst, kaɪ-, ʃɪ-] *n* Fußpfleger(in *f*) *m*, Pediküre *f*, Podologe *m*, -login *f.*
chi·rop·o·dy [-'rɒpədɪ] *n* Fußpflege *f*, Pediküre *f.*
chi·ro·pom·pho·lyx *n* → cheiropompholyx.
chi·ro·prac·tic [ˌkaɪrəʊ'præktɪk] *n* 1. Manipulationstherapie *f*, Chiropraktik *f.* 2. chiropractor.
chi·ro·prac·tor [ˌ-'præktər] *n* Chiropraktiker(in *f*) *m*, -praktor *m.*
chi·ro·prax·is [ˌ-'præksɪs] *n* → chiropractic.
chi·ro·scope *n* → cheiroscope.
chi·ro·spasm *n* → cheirospasm.
chi·rur·geon [kaɪ'rɜːdʒən] *n old* → surgeon.
chi·rur·ger·y [kaɪ'rɜːdʒərɪ] *n old* → surgery.
chi·rur·gic [kaɪ'rɜːdʒɪk] *adj old* → surgical.
chis·el ['tʃɪzəl] **I** *n ortho.* Meißel *m*, Stemmeisen *nt*, (Stech-)Beitel *m.* **II** *vt* (aus-)meißeln, mit einem Meißel bearbeiten. **III** *vi* meißeln.
chis·eled ['tʃɪzəld] *adj* 1. (aus-)gemeißelt, geformt. 2. (*Gesichtszüge*) scharfgeschnitten.
chisel fracture *ortho.* (*Radiusköpfchen*) Meißelfraktur *f.*
chi-squared distribution ['kaɪˌskweəd] *stat.* Chi-Quadrat-Verteilung *f*, χ^2-Verteilung *f.*
chi-square distribution → chi-squared distribution.
chi-square test *stat.* Chi-Quadrat-Test *m*, χ^2-Test *m.*
chi·tin ['kaɪtɪn] *n* Chitin *nt.*
chi·tin·ase ['kaɪtɪneɪz] *n* Chitinase *f*, Chitodextrinase *f.*
chi·tin·ous ['kaɪtɪnəs] *adj* chitinhaltig, -ähnlich.
chitinous degeneration amyloide Degeneration *f*; Amyloidose *f.*
chitin synthase Chitinsynthase *f.*
chi·to·bi·ose [kaɪtəʊ'baɪəʊs] *n* Chitobiose *f.*
chi·to·dex·trin·ase [ˌ-'dekstrɪneɪz] *n* → chitinase.
chi·to·sa·mine [kaɪ'təʊsəmiːn] *n* Glukosamin *nt*, Aminoglukose *f.*
chi·tose ['kaɪtəʊz] *n* Chitose *f.*
chi·to·tri·ose [kaɪtəʊ'traɪəʊs] *n* Chitotriose *f.*
chla·my·de·mia [klæmɪ'diːmɪə] *n* Chlamydämie *f.*
Chla·myd·ia [klə'mɪdɪə] *n micro.* Chlamydie *f*, Chlamydia *f*, PLT-Gruppe *f.*

chlamydia

chla·myd·ia [klə'mɪdɪə] *n, pl* **-mid·i·ae** [-'mɪdɪ,i:] → Chlamydia.
Chla·myd·i·a·ce·ae [klə,mɪdɪ'eɪsɪi:] *pl micro*. Chlamydiaceae *pl*.
chla·myd·i·al [klə'mɪdɪəl] *adj* Chlamydien betr., durch Chlamydien bedingt *od*. hervorgerufen, Chlamydien-.
chlamydial disease → chlamydiosis.
Chla·myd·i·al·es [klə'mɪdɪæli:z] *pl micro*. Chlamydiales *pl*.
chlamydial infection → chlamydiosis.
chlamydial pneumonia/pneumonitis Chlamydienpneumonie *f*.
chla·myd·i·o·sis [klə,mɪdɪ'əʊsɪs] *n* Chlamydienerkrankung *f*, -infektion *f*, Chlamydiose *f*.
chla·myd·o·spore [klə'mɪdəspəʊər, -spɔ:r] *n micro*. Chlamydospore *f*.
chlamydospore agar (*Candida*) Chlamydosporenagar *m/nt*.
Chlam·y·do·zo·a·ce·ae [,klæmɪdəʊ,zəʊ-'eɪsɪi:] *pl* → Chlamydiaceae.
Chlam·y·do·zo·on [,klæmɪdəʊ'zəʊən] *n* → Chlamydia.
CH length → crown-heel length.
chlo·as·ma [kləʊ'æzmə] *n derm*. Chloasma *nt*.
chlor- *pref*. Chlor(o)-.
chlor·a·ce·tic acid [,klɔ:rə'si:tɪk, -'set-, ,kləʊər-] → chloroacetic acid.
chlor·ac·ne [klɔʊər'æknɪ, klɔ:r-] *n derm*. Chlorakne *f*, Chlorarylakne *f*, Akne/Acne chlorica.
chlo·ral ['klɔ:rəl, 'kləʊr-] *n* 1. Chloral *nt*, Trichlorazetaldehyd *m*. 2. → chloral hydrate.
chloral hydrate Chloralhydrat *nt*, Chloralum hydratum.
chlo·ral·ism ['klɔʊərəlɪzəm, 'klɔ:r-] *n* Chloralvergiftung *f*, Chloralismus *m*; Chloralomanie *f*.
chlo·ral·i·za·tion [,klɔʊərəlɪ'zeɪʃn, ,klɔ:r-] *n* 1. → chloralism. 2. *old* Chloralnarkose *f*, -betäubung *f*.
chlor·am·bu·cil [klɔʊr'æmbjəsɪl, klɔ:r-] *n pharm*. Chlorambucil *nt*.
chlo·ra·mine T [klɔʊ'ræmi:n, 'kləʊr-, klɔ:-'ræmi:n] Chloramin T *nt*.
chlor·am·phen·i·col [,-'æm'fenɪkɒl] *n pharm*. Chloramphenicol *nt*.
chloramphenicol acetyltransferase Chloramphenicolacetyltransferase *f*.
chlo·ra·ne·mia [,-ə'ni:mɪə] *n* → chlorosis.
chlo·rate ['klɔ:reɪt, -ɪt, 'kləʊ-] *n* Chlorat *nt*.
chlor·a·za·nil [kləʊ'ræzənɪl, klɔ:-] *n pharm*. Chlorazanil *nt*.
chlor·benz·ox·a·mine [,kləʊr,ben'zɒksəmɪn, -mi:n, ,klɔ:r-] *n pharm*. Chlorbenzoxamin *nt*.
chlor·benz·ox·y·eth·a·mine [,-ben,zɒksɪ'eθəmi:n] *n* → chlorbenzoxamine.
chlor·bu·tol [-'bju:tɒl] *n* → chlorobutanol.
chlor·dan ['klɔʊrdæn] *n* → chlordane.
chlor·dane ['klɔʊrdeɪn] *n* Chlordan *nt*.
chlor·di·az·e·pox·ide [,klɔʊrdaɪæzə'pɒksaɪd, ,klɔ:r-] *n pharm*. Chlordiazepoxid *nt*.
chlor·e·mia [kləʊ'ri:mɪə] *n* 1. → chlorosis. 2. erhöhter Chloridgehalt *m* des Blutes, Hyperchlorämie *f*.
chlor·gua·nide [,klɔʊr'gwænaɪd, ,klɔ:r-] *n pharm*. Proguanil *nt*.
chlor·hex·i·dine [,-'heksədi:n] *n pharm*. Chlorhexidin *nt*.
chlor·hy·dria [,-'haɪdrɪə] *n* (Hyper-)Chlorhydrie *f*.
chlo·ric ['klɔʊrɪk, 'klɔ:-] *adj* Chlor betr. *od*. enthaltend, Chlor-.
chlo·ride ['-raɪd] *n* Chlorid *nt*.
chloride channel Chloridkanal *m*, Cl⁻-Kanal *m*.
chloride shift Hamburger-Phänomen *nt*, Chloridverschiebung *f*.

chlo·ri·dim·e·ter [,klɔʊrɪ'dɪmɪtər] *n* Chloridi-, Chloridometer *nt*.
chlo·ri·dim·e·try [,-'dɪmətrɪ] *n* Chloridbestimmung *f*, Chloridi-, Chloridometrie *f*.
chlo·ri·dom·e·ter [,-'dɒmɪtər] *n* → chloridimeter.
chlor·id·or·rhea [,klɔʊraɪdə'rɪə] *n* Chlorverlustdiarrhoe *f*, Chlorid-Diarrhoe *f*.
chlor·i·du·ria [,klɔʊrɪ'd(j)ʊərɪə] *n* übermäßige Chloridausscheidung *f* im Harn, Chloridurie *f*, Chlorurese *f*.
chlo·ri·nat·ed ['klɔʊrɪneɪtɪd, 'klɔ:-] *adj* chlorhaltig.
chlorinated lime Chlorkalk *m*, Calcaria chlorata.
chlo·rine ['klɔ:ri:n, -ɪn, 'kləʊr-] *n abbr*. **Cl** Chlor *nt abbr*. Cl.
chlorine acne → chloracne.
chlorine water Chlorwasser *nt*, Aqua chlorata.
chlo·rite ['-raɪt] *n* Chlorit *nt*.
chlor·mad·i·none [,-'mædɪnəʊn] *n pharm*. Chlormadinon *nt*.
chlor·meth·az·a·none [,-meθ'æzənəʊn] *n* → chlormezanone.
chlor·meth·yl [,-'meθl] *n* → methyl chloride.
chlor·mez·a·none [,-'mezənəʊn] *n pharm*. Chlormezanon *nt*.
chloro- *pref*. Chlor(o)-.
chlo·ro·a·ce·tic acid [,klɔ:rəʊə'si:tɪk, ,kləʊrəʊ-] Chloressigsäure *f*.
chlo·ro·a·ne·mia [,-ə'ni:mɪə] *n* → chlorosis.
Chlo·ro·bac·te·ri·a·ce·ae [,-bæk,tɪərɪ'eɪsɪi:] *pl micro*. Chlorobacteriaceae *pl*.
Chlo·ro·bi·a·ce·ae [,-baɪ'eɪsɪi:] *pl* → Chlorobacteriaceae.
chlo·ro·blast ['-blæst] *n* Erythroblast *m*, Erythrozytoblast *m*.
chlo·ro·bu·ta·nol [,-'bju:tnɒl, -nəʊl] *n pharm*. Chlor(o)butanol *nt*.
chlo·ro·cre·sol [,-'kri:sɒl, -sɒl] *n pharm*. Chlorkresol *nt*, Chlorocresol *nt*.
chlo·ro·eth·ane [,-'eθeɪn] *n* Äthyl-, Ethylchlorid *nt*, Monochloräthan *nt*, -ethan *nt*.
chlo·ro·eth·yl·ene [,-'eθəli:n] *n* Vinylchlorid *nt abbr*. VC.
chlo·ro·form ['-fɔ:rm] *n* Chloroform *nt*, Trichlormethan *nt*.
chlo·ro·form·ism ['-fɔ:rmɪzəm] *n* 1. Chloroformvergiftung *f*, Chloroformismus *m*; Chloroformomanie *f*. 2. Chloroformnarkose *f*.
chlo·ro·gua·nide [,-'gwænaɪd] *n pharm*. Proguanil *nt*.
chlo·ro·he·min [,-'hi:mɪn] *n* Teichmann-Kristalle *pl*, salzsaures Hämin *nt*, Hämin(kristalle *pl*) *nt*, Chlorhämin(kristalle *pl*) *nt*, Chlorhämatin *nt*.
chlo·ro·leu·ke·mia [,-lu:'ki:mɪə] *n* → chloroma.
chlo·ro·lym·pho·sar·co·ma [,-,lɪmfəsɑ:r-'kəʊmə] *n patho*. Chlorolymphosarkom *nt*, -lymphom *nt*.
chlo·ro·ma [klə'rəʊmə] *n patho*. Chlorom *nt*, Chloroleukämie *f*, Chlorsarkom *nt*.
chloroma tous sarcoma [kləʊ'rɑmətəs] → chloroma.
chlo·rom·e·try [kləʊ'rɑmətrɪ] *n* Chlorbestimmung *f*, -messung *f*, Chlorometrie *f*.
chlo·ro·my·e·lo·ma [,klɔʊrəmaɪə'ləʊmə, ,klɔ:r-] *n* 1. *patho*. Chlormyelom *nt*, -myelose *f*, -myeloblastom *nt*. 2. → chloroma.
chlo·ro·pe·nia [,-'pi:nɪə] *n* Chloridmangel *m*, Hypochlorämie *f*, Chloropenie *f*.
chlo·ro·pex·ia [,-'peksɪə] *n* Chlorbindung *f*, -fixierung *f*, Chloropexie *f*.
chlo·ro·phe·nol [,-'fi:nɒl, -nəl] *n* Chlorphenol *nt*.
p-chlorophenol *n* p-Chlor(o)phenol *nt*.
chlo·ro·phen·o·thane [,-'fenəθeɪn] *n* Chlo-

rophenothan *nt*, Penticidum *nt*, Dichlordiphenyltrichloräthan *nt abbr*. DDT.
chlo·ro·phyl(l) ['klɔ:rəfɪl, 'kləʊ-] *n* Blattgrün *nt*, Chlorophyll *nt*.
chlo·ro·phyl·lase [,-'fɪleɪs] *n* Chlorophyllase *f*.
chlo·ro·phyl·lin ['-fɪlɪn] *n* Chlorophyllin *nt*.
chlo·ro·pia [kləʊ'rəʊpɪə] *n* → chloropsia.
chlo·ro·plast ['klɔ:rəplæst, 'kləʊ-[*n bio*. Chloroplast *m*.
chloroplast ATPase *abbr*. **CF1 (ATPase)** Chloroplasten-ATPase *f*, CF1-ATPase *f abbr*. CF1.
chlo·ro·plas·tid [,-'plæstɪd] *n* → chloroplast.
chlo·ro·pri·vic [,-'praɪvɪk] *adj* chloropriv.
chlo·rop·sia [kləʊ'rɑpsɪə] *n ophthal*. Grünsehen *nt*, Chlorop(s)ie *f*.
chlo·ro·quine ['klɔʊrəkwaɪn, -kwi:n, 'klɔ:r-] *n pharm*. Chloroquin *nt*.
chlo·ro·sis [klə'rəʊsɪs] *n hema*. Chlorose *f*, Chlorosis *f*.
chlo·ro·thi·a·zide [,kləʊrə'θaɪəzaɪd, ,klɔ:r-] *n pharm*. Chlorothiazid *nt*.
chlo·ro·thy·mol [,-'θaɪmɒl, -məʊl] *n* (4-)-Chlorthymol *nt*.
chlo·rot·ic [klə'rɒtɪk] *adj* Chlorose betr., von Chlorose betroffen, chlorotisch.
chlorotic anemia → chlorosis.
chlo·ro·tri·an·i·sene [,kləʊrətraɪ'ænɪsi:n, ,klɔ:r-] *n pharm*. Chlorotrianisen *nt*.
chlo·rous ['klɔ:rəs, 'kləʊ-] *adj chem*. dreiwertiges Chlor enthaltend, chlorig.
chlorous acid chlorige Säure *f*.
chlo·ro·vin·yl·di·chlo·ro·ar·sine [,kləʊrə-,vaɪnldaɪ,klɔʊrə'ɑ:rsi:n, ,klɔ:r-] *n* Lewisit *nt*.
chlor·phen·ox·a·mine [kləʊrfe'nɒksəmi:n, klɔ:r-] *n pharm*. Chlorphenoxamin *nt*.
chlor·phen·ter·mine [,-'fentərmi:n] *n pharm*. Chlorphentermin *nt*.
chlor·prom·a·zine [,-'prɒməzi:n] *n pharm*. Chlorpromazin *nt*.
chlor·prop·a·mide [,-'prɒpəmaɪd, -'prəʊ-] *n pharm*. Chlorpropamid *nt*.
chlor·pro·thix·ene [,-prəʊ'θɪksi:n] *n pharm*. Chlorprothixen *nt*.
chlor·quin·al·dol [,-'kwɪnældɒl, -dəʊl] *n pharm*. Chlorquinaldol *nt*.
chlor·tet·ra·cy·cline [,-,tetrə'saɪklaɪn, -klɪn] *n pharm*. Chlortetracyclin *nt*.
chlor·thal·i·done [,-'θælɪdəʊn] *n pharm*. Chlortalidon *nt*.
chlor·then·ox·a·zin(e) [,-,θe'nɒksəzi:n, -zɪn] *n pharm*. Chlorthenoxazin *nt*.
chlor·thy·mol [,-'θaɪmɒl, -məʊl] *n* → chlorothymol.
chlor·um ['klɔʊrəm, 'klɔ:r-] *n* → chlorine.
chlor·u·re·sis [,kləʊrjə'ri:sɪs, ,klɔ:r-] *n* → chloriduria.
chlor·u·ret·ic [,-jə'retɪk] *adj* Chlor(id)ausscheidung fördernd, chloruretisch, chloriduretisch.
chlor·u·ria [,-'(j)ʊərɪə] *n* → chloriduria.
chlor·zox·a·zone [,-'zɒksəzəʊn] *n pharm*. Chlorzoxazon *nt*.
cho·a·na ['kəʊənə] *n, pl* **-nae** [-ni:] *anat*. Trichter *m*, Choane *f*, Choana *f*.
cho·a·nal ['kəʊənəl] *adj* Choane(n) betr., Choanal-.
choanal atresia Choanalatresie *f*.
choanal polyp HNO Choanalpolyp *m*.
cho·a·noid ['kəʊənɔɪd] *adj* trichterförmig.
cho·a·no·cyte ['kəʊənəʊsaɪt] *n bio*. Choanozyt *m*, -zyte *f*.
cho·a·no·mas·ti·gote (stage) [,-'mæstɪgəʊt] *micro*. choanomastigote Form *f*, jugendliche Crithidia-Form *f*.
choc·o·late ['tʃɒk(ə)lət] I *n* 1. Schokolade(ngetränk *nt*) *f*. 2. Schokoladenbraun *nt*. II *adj* 3. Schokoladen-. 4. schokoladen-, dunkelbraun.

chocolate agar Kochblut-, Schokoladenagar m/nt.
chocolate cyst gyn. Schokoladen-, Teerzyste f.
Chodzko ['tʃatskəʊ]: **C.'s reflex** Chodzko-Reflex m.
choice [tʃɔɪs] n **1.** Wahl f, Auswahl f. **to have the ~** die Wahl haben. **to have no ~ about doing/but to do** keine andere Wahl haben als. **to make a ~** wählen, eine Wahl treffen. **to take one's ~** s. etw. aussuchen. **2.** (das) Beste od. Bessere. **drug of ~** das bevorzugte Medikament; das Mittel der Wahl. **treatment of ~** die bevorzugte Behandlung, die Behandlung der Wahl.
Choix fever [wa] Felsengebirgsfleckfieber nt, amerikanisches Zeckenbißfieber nt, Rocky Mountain spotted fever (nt) abbr. RMSF.
choke [tʃəʊk] I n **1.** Würgen nt, Ersticken nt. **2. the ~s** pl (Caissonkrankheit) Chokes pl. **3.** Erdrosseln nt. II vt **4.** (er-, ab-)würgen, den Hals einschnüren; ersticken, erdrosseln. **5.** (Tränen) zurückhalten. **6.** phys. (Strom) drosseln. **7.** verstopfen. III vi **8.** ersticken (on an). **9.** würgen. **10.** einen Erstickungsanfall haben. **11.** s. verstopfen.
choke off vt abwürgen, stoppen, drosseln.
choke up vt verstopfen; (Stimme) ersticken.
choke-damp ['tʃəʊkdæmp] n chem. Grubengas n, Kohlendioxyd nt.
choked disk [tʃəʊkt] ophthal. Papillenödem nt, Stauungspapille f.
chokes [tʃəʊks] pl (Caissonkrankheit) Chokes pl.
chok·ing ['tʃəʊkɪŋ] adj erstickend.
choking air stickige Luft f.
chol- pref. → cholo-.
cho·la·gog·ic [ˌkɒləˈgɒdʒɪk, ˌkələ-] adj den Gallefluß anregend, galletreibend, cholagog.
cho·la·gogue ['-gɒg] I n **1.** pharm. galletreibendes Mittel nt, Cholagogum nt. **2.** → cholecystagogue. II adj → cholagogic.
cho·lal·ic acid [kəʊˈlælɪk] → cholyltaurine.
cho·lal·ic [kəʊˈlælɪk, -ˈleɪ-] adj Galle betr., Gallen-, Chol-.
cho·lane [ˈkəʊleɪn, ˈkɑl-] n Cholan nt.
chol·an·e·re·sis [ˌkəʊˌlænəˈriːsɪs, ˌkəʊlænˈerəsɪs[n Cholanarese f.
cholangi- pref. → cholangio-.
chol·an·gei·tis [ˌkəʊlænˈdʒaɪtɪs] n → cholangitis.
chol·an·gi·ec·ta·sis [kəˌlændʒɪˈektəsɪs] n Gallengangserweiterung f, -dilatation f, Cholangioektasie f.
cholangio- pref. Gallengangs-, Cholangi(o)-.
chol·an·gi·o·ad·e·no·ma [kəʊˌlændʒɪəˌædɪˈnəʊmə] n Gallengangsadenom nt, benignes Cholangiom nt.
chol·an·gi·o·car·ci·no·ma [ˌ-ˌkɑːrsəˈnəʊmə] n Gallengangskarzinom nt, malignes Cholangiom nt, chlorangiozelluläres Karzinom nt, Ca. cholangiocellulare.
chol·an·gi·o·cel·lu·lar carcinoma [ˌ-ˈseljələr] → cholangiocarcinoma.
chol·an·gi·o·cho·le·cys·to·cho·le·doch·ec·to·my [kəʊˌlændʒɪəˌsɪstəˌkəʊlədəˈkektəmɪ] n chir. Cholangiocholecystocholedochektomie f.
chol·an·gi·o·du·o·de·nos·to·my [ˌ-d(j)uːəˈdɪˈnɑstəmɪ] n chir. Gallengang-Duodenum-Fistel f, Cholangioduodenostomie f.
chol·an·gi·o·en·ter·os·to·my [ˌ-entəˈrɑstəmɪ] n chir. Gallengang-Darm-Fistel f, Cholangioenterostomie f.
chol·an·gi·o·fi·bro·sis [ˌ-faɪˈbrəʊsɪs] n Gallengangsfibrose f, Cholangiofibrose f.
chol·an·gi·o·gas·tros·to·my [ˌ-gæsˈtrɑstəmɪ] n chir. Gallen-Magen-Fistel f, Cholangiogastrostomie f.
chol·an·gi·og·e·nous [kəʊˌlændʒɪˈɒdʒənəs] adj von den Gallengängen ausgehend, cholang(i)ogen.
chol·an·gi·o·gram [kəˈlændʒɪəɡræm] n chir., radiol. Cholangiogramm nt.
chol·an·gi·og·ra·phy [kəˌlændʒɪˈɒgrəfɪ] n chir., radiol. Kontrastdarstellung f der Gallengänge, Cholangiographie f.
cholangiography catheter Cholangiographiekatheter m.
chol·an·gi·o·hep·a·ti·tis [kəʊˌlændʒɪəˌhepəˈtaɪtɪs] n Cholangiohepatitis f.
chol·an·gi·o·hep·a·to·ma [ˌ-ˌhepəˈtəʊmə] n patho. Cholangiohepatom(a) nt, Hepatocholangiokarzinom nt.
chol·an·gi·o·je·ju·nos·to·my [ˌ-dʒɪdʒuːˈnɑstəmɪ] n chir. Gallengang-Jejunum-Fistel f, Cholangiojejunostomie f.
chol·an·gi·o·lar [kəʊlænˈdʒɪələr] adj Cholangiole betr., Cholangiolen-.
chol·an·gi·ole [kəʊˈlændʒɪəʊl] n Cholangiole f.
chol·an·gi·o·lit·ic hepatitis [kəʊˌlændʒɪəʊˈlɪtɪk] → cholestatic hepatitis.
chol·an·gi·o·li·tis [ˌ-ˈlaɪtɪs] n Cholangiolenentzündung f, Cholangiolitis f.
chol·an·gi·o·ma [kəʊˌlændʒɪˈəʊmə] n Gallengangstumor m, Cholangiom nt.
chol·an·gi·o·pan·cre·a·tog·ra·phy [kəʊˌlændʒɪəˌpæŋkrɪəˈtægrəfɪ] n chir., radiol. Cholangiopankreat(ik)ographie f.
chol·an·gi·os·co·py [kəʊˌlændʒɪˈɒskəpɪ] n Gallenwegsendoskopie f, Cholangioskopie f.
chol·an·gi·os·to·my [ˌ-ˈɒstəmɪ] n chir. **1.** Gallengangsfistelung f, Cholangiostomie f. **2.** Gallengangsfistel f, Cholangiostomie f.
chol·an·gi·ot·o·my [ˌ-ˈɒtəmɪ] n chir. Gallengangseröffnung f, Cholangiotomie f.
chol·an·git·ic [ˌkəʊlænˈdʒɪtɪk] adj Cholangitis betr., von Cholangitis betroffen, cholangitisch.
cholangitic abscess biliärer/biliogener/cholangitischer Leberabszeß m.
cholangitic hepatitis → cholestatic hepatitis.
chol·an·gi·tis [ˌ-ˈdʒaɪtɪs] n Gallengangsentzündung f, Cholangitis f.
cho·lan·ic acid [kəʊˈlænɪk] Cholansäure f.
cho·la·no·poi·e·sis [ˌkəʊlənəʊpɔɪˈiːsɪs] n Gallen(säuren)bildung f.
cho·las·cos [kəʊˈlæskɒs] n **1.** Cholaskos nt, Choleperitoneum f. **2.** biliärer Aszites m.
cho·late [ˈkəʊleɪt] n Cholat nt.
cholate synthetase Cholatsynthetase f.
cholate thiokinase → cholate synthetase.
chole- pref. → cholo-.
cho·le·bil·i·ru·bin [ˌkəʊləˌbɪləˈruːbɪn, ˌkɒlə-] n Cholebilirubin nt.
cho·le·cal·cif·er·ol [ˌ-kælˈsɪfərɒl, -rəl] n Cholecalciferol nt, -kalziferol nt, Colecalciferol nt, Vitamin D_3 nt.
cho·le·chrome ['-krəʊm] n Gallenpigment nt, -farbstoff m.
cho·le·chro·mo·poi·e·sis [ˌ-ˌkrəʊməpɔɪˈiːsɪs] n Gallenpigmentbildung f, -synthese f.
cho·le·cy·a·nin [ˌ-ˈsaɪənɪn] n Bili-, Cholezyanin nt.
cho·le·cyst ['-sɪst] n Gallenblase f, inf. Galle f, Vesica fellea/biliaris.
cho·le·cys·ta·gog·ic [ˌ-ˌsɪstəˈgɒdʒɪk] adj die Gallenblase anregend, cholekinetisch.
cho·le·cys·ta·gogue [ˌ-ˈsɪstəgɒg] n pharm. Cholekinetikum nt, Cholezystagogum nt.

cholecystogogic

cho·le·cys·tal·gia [ˌ-sɪsˈtældʒ(ɪ)ə] n Gallenblasenschmerz m, Cholezystalgie f.
cho·le·cys·tat·o·ny [ˌ-sɪsˈtætənɪ] n Gallenblasenatonie f, Cholezystatonie f.
cho·le·cys·tec·ta·sia [ˌ-ˌsɪstekˈteɪʒ(ɪ)ə] n Gallenblasenausweitung f, -ektasie f, Cholezystektasie f.
cho·le·cys·tec·to·my [ˌ-sɪsˈtektəmɪ] n chir. Gallenblasenentfernung f, Cholezystektomie f.
cho·le·cys·ten·dy·sis [ˌ-sɪsˈtendəsɪs] n → cholecystotomy.
cho·le·cys·ten·ter·ic [ˌ-ˌsɪstenˈterɪk] adj → cholecystointestinal.
cho·le·cys·ten·ter·a·nas·to·mo·sis [ˌ-sɪsˌtentərəʊəˌnæstəˈməʊsɪs] n → cholecystenterostomy.
cho·le·cys·ten·ter·or·rha·phy [ˌ-sɪsˌtentəˈrɔrəfɪ] n chir. Cholezyst(o)entero(r)rhaphie f.
cho·le·cys·ten·ter·os·to·my [ˌ-sɪsˌtentəˈrɑstəmɪ] n chir. Gallenblasen-Darm-Fistel f, -Anastomose f, Cholezyst(o)enteroanastomose f, -enterostomie f.
cho·le·cyst·gas·tros·to·my [ˌ-sɪstgæsˈtrɑstəmɪ] n → cholecystogastrostomy.
cho·le·cys·tic [ˌ-ˈsɪstɪk] adj Gallenblase betr., Gallenblasen-, Cholezyst(o)-.
cho·le·cys·tis [ˌ-ˈsɪstɪs] n → cholecyst.
cho·le·cys·ti·tis [ˌ-sɪsˈtaɪtɪs] n Gallenblasenentzündung f, Cholezystitis f, -cystitis f.
cho·le·cyst·ne·phros·to·my [ˌ-ˌsɪstneˈfrɑstəmɪ] n → cholecystopyelostomy.
cholecysto- pref. Gallenblasen-, Cholezyst(o)-.
cho·le·cys·to·chol·an·gi·o·gram [ˌ-ˌsɪstəkəʊˈlændʒɪəgræm] n chir., radiol. Cholezyst(o)cholangiogramm nt.
cho·le·cys·to·cho·lan·gi·og·ra·phy [ˌ-ˌsɪstəkəˌlændʒɪˈɒgrəfɪ] n chir., radiol. Cholezyst(o)cholangiographie f.
cho·le·cys·to·co·lon·ic [ˌ-ˌsɪstəkəʊˈlɒnɪk] adj Gallenblase u. Kolon betr. od. verbindend, Gallenblasen-Kolon-, Cholezystokolo-.
cholecystocolonic fistula 1. patho. Gallenblasen-Kolon-Fistel f. **2.** chir. Gallenblasen-Kolon-Fistel f, Cholezystokolostomie f.
cho·le·cys·to·co·los·to·my [ˌ-ˌsɪstəkəˈlɒstəmɪ] n chir. Gallenblasen-Kolon-Fistel f, Cholezystokolostomie f.
cho·le·cys·to·du·o·de·nal fistula [ˌ-ˌd(j)uːəˈdiːnl] **1.** patho. Gallenblasen-Duodenum-Fistel f, Fistula cholecystoduodenalis. **2.** chir. Gallenblasen-Duodenum-Fistel f, Cholezystoduodenostomie f.
cho·le·cys·to·du·o·de·nos·to·my [ˌ-ˌsɪstəˌd(j)uːədɪˈnɑstəmɪ] n chir. Gallenblasen-Duodenum-Fistel f, Cholezystoduodenostomie f.
cho·le·cys·to·en·ter·ic [ˌ-ˌsɪstænˈterɪk] adj → cholecystointestinal.
cholecystoenteric fistula → cholecystointestinal fistula.
cho·le·cys·to·en·ter·os·to·my [ˌ-ˌsɪstəentəˈrɑstəmɪ] n → cholecystenterostomy.
cho·le·cys·to·gas·tric [ˌ-ˌsɪstəˈgæstrɪk] adj Gallenblase u. Magen betr. od. verbindend, Gallenblasen-Magen-.
cholecystogastric fistula 1. patho. Gallenblasen-Magen-Fistel f, Fistula cholecystogastrica. **2.** chir. Gallenblasen-Magen-Fistel f, Cholezystogastrostomie f.
cho·le·cys·to·gas·tros·to·my [ˌ-ˌsɪstəgæsˈtrɑstəmɪ] n chir. Gallenblasen-Magen-Fistel f, Cholezystogastrostomie f, -gastroanastomose f.
cho·le·cys·to·gog·ic [ˌ-ˌsɪstəˈgɒdʒɪk] adj → cholecystagogic.

cho·le·cys·to·gram [ˌ-'sɪstəgræm] *n chir.*, *radiol.* Cholezystogramm *nt.*
cho·le·cys·tog·ra·phy [ˌ-sɪs'tɑgrəfɪ] *n chir.*, *radiol.* Kontrastdarstellung *f* der Gallenblase, Cholezystographie *f.*
cho·le·cys·to·il·e·os·to·my [ˌ-ˌsɪstəˌɪlɪ'ɑstəmɪ] *n chir.* Gallenblasen-Ileum-Fistel *f,* Cholezystoileostomie *f.*
cho·le·cys·to·in·tes·ti·nal [ˌ-ˌsɪstəɪn'testənl] *adj* Gallenblase u. Darm betr. od. verbindend, cholezystointestinal, Gallenblasen-Darm-.
cholecystointestinal fistula 1. *patho.* Gallenblasen-Darm-Fistel *f,* cholezystointestinale Fistel *f,* Fistula cholecystointestinalis. **2.** *chir.* Gallenblasen-Darm-Fistel *f,* Cholecystoenterostomie *f.*
cho·le·cys·to·je·ju·nos·to·my [ˌ-ˌsɪstədʒɪdʒuː'nɑstəmɪ] *n chir.* Gallenblasen-Jejunum-Fistel *f,* Cholezystojejunostomie *f.*
cho·le·cys·to·ki·net·ic [ˌ-ˌsɪstəkɪ'netɪk] *adj* → cholecystagogic.
cholecystokinetic agent → cholecystagogue.
cho·le·cys·to·ki·nin [ˌ-ˌsɪstə'kaɪnɪn] *n abbr.* CCK Cholezystokinin *nt abbr.* CCK, Pankreozymin *nt abbr.* PZ.
cho·le·cys·to·li·thi·a·sis [ˌ-ˌsɪstəlɪ'θaɪəsɪs] *n chir.*, *patho.* Cholezystolithiasis *f.*
cho·le·cys·to·lith·o·trip·sy [ˌ-ˌsɪstə'lɪθətrɪpsɪ] *n chir.* Cholezystolithotripsie *f.*
cho·le·cys·to·my [ˌ-'sɪstəmɪ] *n* → cholecystotomy.
cho·le·cys·to·ne·phros·to·my [ˌ-ˌsɪstəne'frɑstəmɪ] *n* → cholecystopyelostomy.
cho·le·cys·top·a·thy [ˌ-sɪs'tɑpəθɪ] *n* Gallenblasenerkrankung *f,* Cholezystopathie *f.*
cho·le·cys·to·pex·y [ˌ-'sɪstəpeksɪ] *n chir.* Gallenblasenanheftung *f,* -fixierung *f,* Cholecystopexie *f.*
cho·le·cys·top·to·sis [ˌ-sɪstə'təʊsɪs] *n* Gallenblasensenkung *f,* Cholezystoptose *f,* Choloptose *f.*
cho·le·cys·to·py·e·los·to·my [ˌ-ˌsɪstəpaɪə'lɑstəmɪ] *n chir.*, *urol.* Gallenblasen-Nierenbecken-Fistel *f,* Cholezystopyelostomie *f,* -nephrostomie *f.*
cho·le·cys·tor·rha·phy [ˌ-sɪs'tɔrəfɪ] *n* Gallenblasennaht *f,* Cholezysto(r)rhaphie *f.*
cho·le·cys·to·so·nog·ra·phy [ˌ-ˌsɪstəsə'nɑgrəfɪ] *n* Gallenblasensonographie *f.*
cho·le·cys·tos·to·my [ˌ-sɪs'tɑstəmɪ] *n chir.* (Anlegen *nt* einer) Gallenblasenfistel *f,* Cholezystostomie *f.*
cho·le·cys·tot·o·my [ˌ-sɪs'tɑtəmɪ] *n chir.* Gallenblaseneröffnung *f,* Cholezystotomie *f.*
choledoch- *pref.* → choledocho-.
cho·le·doch ['kəʊlɪdɑk] **I** *n* → choledochus. **II** *adj* → choledochal.
cho·le·doch·al [ˈkəʊləˌdɑkl, kəˈdɛkl] *adj* Choledochus betr, Choledocho-, Choledochus-.
choledochal calculus *chir.* Choledochusstein *m,* Choledocholith *m.*
choledochal cyst Choledochuszyste *f.*
type III c. → choledochocele.
type IV c. polyzystische Choledochuszyste.
choledochal diverticulum Choledochusdivertikel *nt.*
choledochal duct → choledochus.
choledochal stone → choledochal calculus.
cho·led·o·chec·to·my [kəʊˌledəʊ'kektəmɪ] *n chir.* Choledochusresektion *f,* -exzision *f,* Choledochektomie *f.*
cho·led·o·chen·dy·sis [ˌ-'kendəsɪs] *n* → choledochotomy.
cho·le·do·chi·arc·tia [ˌ-ˌkaɪ'ærktɪə] *n* Cho-

ledochusstenose *f.*
chol·e·do·chi·tis [ˌ-'kaɪtɪs] *n patho.* Choledochusentzündung *f,* Choledochitis *f.*
choledocho- *pref.* Choledochus-, Choledocho-.
cho·led·o·cho·cele [kəˈledəkəsiːl] *n* intraduodenale Papillenzyste *f,* Choledochozele *f.*
cho·led·o·cho·chol·e·do·chos·to·my [ˌ-kəˌledəˈkɑstəmɪ] *n chir.* Choledochocholedochostomie *f,* -anastomose *f.*
cho·led·o·cho·du·o·de·nos·to·my [ˌ-d(j)uːədɪ'nɑstəmɪ] *n chir.* Choledochus-Duodenum-Fistel *f,* Choledochoduodenostomie *f.*
cho·led·o·cho·en·ter·os·to·my [ˌ-ˌentə'rɑstəmɪ] *n chir.* Choledochus-Darm-Fistel *f,* Choledochoenterostomie *f,* -enteroanastomose *f.*
cho·led·o·cho·gas·tros·to·my [ˌ-gæs'trɑstəmɪ] *n chir.* Choledochus-Magen-Fistel *f,* Choledochogastrostomie *f.*
cho·led·o·cho·gram ['-græm] *n chir.*, *radiol.* Choledochogramm *nt.*
cho·led·o·chog·ra·phy [kəˌledə'kɑgrəfɪ] *n chir.*, *radiol.* Kontrastdarstellung *f* des Ductus choledochus, Choledochographie *f.*
cho·led·o·cho·hep·a·tos·to·my [kəˌledəkəˌhepə'tɑstəmɪ] *n chir.* Choledochus-Leber-Fistel *f,* Choledochohepatostomie *f.*
cho·led·o·cho·il·e·os·to·my [ˌ-ɪlɪ'ɑstəmɪ] *n chir.* Choledochus-Ileum-Fistel *f,* Choledochoileostomie *f.*
cho·led·o·cho·je·ju·nos·to·my [ˌ-dʒɪˌdʒuː'nɑstəmɪ] *n chir.* Choledochus-Jejunum-Fistel *f,* Choledochojejunostomie *f.*
cho·led·o·cho·lith [ˌ-'ledəkəlɪθ] *n* Choledochusstein *m,* Choledocholith *m.*
cho·led·o·cho·li·thi·a·sis [ˌ-lɪ'θaɪəsɪs] *n* Choledocholithiasis *f.*
cho·led·o·cho·li·thot·o·my [ˌ-lɪ'θɑtəmɪ] *n chir.* Choledochussteinentfernung *f,* Choledocholithotomie *f.*
cho·led·o·cho·lith·o·trip·sy [ˌ-'lɪθətrɪpsɪ] *n chir.* Choledocholithotripsie *f.*
cho·led·o·cho·li·thot·ri·ty [ˌ-lɪ'θɑtrətɪ] *n* → choledocholithotripsy.
cho·led·o·cho·plas·ty [ˌ-'plæstɪ] *n chir.* Choledochusplastik *f.*
cho·led·o·chor·rha·phy [kəˌledə'kɔrəfɪ] *n chir.* Choledocho(r)rhaphie *f,* Choledochusnaht *f.*
cho·led·o·cho·scope [kəˈledəkəskəʊp] *n* Choledochoskop *nt.*
cho·led·o·chos·co·py [kəˌledə'kɑskəpɪ] *n* Choledochoskopie *f.*
cho·led·o·chos·to·my [ˌ-'kɑstəmɪ] *n chir.* Choledochostomie *f.*
cho·led·o·chot·o·my [ˌ-'kɑtəmɪ] *n chir.* Choledochuseröffnung *f,* Choledochotomie *f.*
cho·led·o·chous [kəˈledəkəs] *adj* galle(n)haltig, -führend.
cho·led·o·chus [kəˈledəkəs] *n, pl* **-chi** [-kaɪ, -kiː]* Hauptgallengang *m,* Choledochus *m,* Ductus choledochus/biliaris.
choledochus cyst → choledochal cyst.
cho·le·glo·bin [ˌkəʊlə'gləʊbɪn, ˌkɑl-] *n* Choleglobin *nt,* Verdohämoglobin *nt.*
cho·le·he·mia [ˌ-'hiːmɪə] *n* → cholemia.
cho·le·ic [kəˈliːɪk, kəʊ-] *adj* Galle betr., Galle(n)-, Chole(e)-.
cho·le·lith ['kəʊləlɪθ, 'kɑl-] *n* Gallenstein *m,* -konkrement *nt,* Cholelith *m,* Calculus biliaris/felleus.
cho·le·li·thi·a·sis [ˌ-lɪ'θaɪəsɪs] *n* Gallensteinleiden *nt,* Cholelithiasis *f.*
cho·le·lith·ic [ˌ-'lɪθɪk] *adj* Gallenstein(e) betr., Cholelithen-, Cholelith(o)-.
cho·le·li·thot·o·my [ˌ-lɪ'θɑtəmɪ] *n chir.* Gallensteinentfernung *f,* Cholelithotomie *f.*

cho·le·lith·o·trip·sy [ˌ-'lɪθətrɪpsɪ] *n chir.* Gallensteinzertrümmerung *f,* Cholelithotripsie *f.*
cho·le·li·thot·ri·ty [ˌ-lɪ'θɑtrətɪ] *n* → cholelithotripsy.
cho·le·me·sis [kəˈlemɪsɪs] *n* Galleerbrechen *nt,* Cholemesis *f.*
cho·le·mia [kəʊ'liːmɪə] *n* Cholämie *f.*
cho·lem·ic [kəʊ'liːmɪk] *adj* Cholämie betr., cholämisch.
cholemic nephrosis cholämische Nephrose *f.*
cholemic tubulopathy (*Niere*) cholämische Tubulopathie *f.*
cho·le·mim·e·try [ˌkəʊlə'mɪmɪtrɪ, ˌkɑl-] *n* Cholämimetrie *f.*
cho·le·path·ia [ˌ-'pæθɪə] *n* Gallenwegserkrankung *f,* -leiden *nt,* Cholepathie *f.*
cho·le·per·i·to·ne·um [ˌ-ˌperɪtə'niːəm] *n* galliger Aszites *m,* Choleperitoneum *nt,* Choleaskos *m.*
cho·le·per·i·to·ni·tis [ˌ-ˌperɪtə'naɪtɪs] *n* gallige Peritonitis *f,* Choleperitonitis *f.*
cho·le·poi·e·sis [ˌ-pɔɪ'iːsɪs] *n* Galle(n)bildung *f,* Cholepoese *f.*
cho·le·poi·et·ic [ˌ-pɔɪ'etɪk] *adj* Galle(n)bildung betr., gallebildend, cholepoetisch.
cho·le·pra·sin [ˌ-'præsɪn] *n* Choleprasin *nt.*
chol·er·a ['kɑlərə] *n* Cholera *f.*
cholera bacillus Komma-Bazillus *m,* Vibrio cholerae/comma.
chol·er·a·gen ['kɑlərədʒən] *n* Choleraenterotoxin *nt,* Choleragen *nt.*
chol·e·ra·ic [ˌkɑlə'reɪɪk] *adj* Cholera betr., Cholera-.
choleraic diarrhea Sommerdiarrhö *f.*
cholera morbus Sommercholera *f,* Cholera aestiva.
cholera nostras Brechdurchfall *m,* -ruhr *f,* einheimische/unechte Cholera *f,* Cholera nostras.
chol·er·a·phage ['kɑlərəfeɪdʒ] *n micro.* Choleraphage *m.*
cholera-red reaction Cholera-Rotreaktion *f abbr.* CRR, Nitrosoindolreaktion *f.*
cholera toxin → choleragen.
cholera vaccine Cholera-Impfstoff *m,* -Vakzine *f.*
cho·le·re·sis [ˌkɑlə'riːsɪs, ˌkəʊ-] *n* Gallensekretion *f,* Cholerese *f.*
cho·le·ret·ic [ˌ-'retɪk] **I** *n* Choleretikum *nt.* **II** *adj* die Cholerese betr. od. stimmulierend, choleretisch.
choleretic agent → choleretic I.
chol·er·ic ['kɑlərɪk, kəˈlerɪk] *adj* aufbrausend, jähzornig, cholerisch.
chol·er·i·form ['kɑlərɪfɔːrm, kəˈlerɪ-] *adj* choleraähnlich, -förmig, choleriform.
chol·er·i·gen·ic [ˌkɑlərɪ'dʒenɪk] *adj* Cholera verursachend, Cholera-.
chol·er·i·ge·nous [kɑlə'rɪdʒənəs] *adj* → choleragenic.
chol·er·ine ['kɑləriːn] *n* Choleradiarrhö *f,* Cholerine *f.*
chol·er·oid ['kɑlərɔɪd] *adj* → choleriform.
chol·er·rha·gia [kəʊlə'rædʒ(ɪ)ə] *n* (übermäßiger) Gallenfluß *m,* Cholerrhagie *f.*
cho·le·scin·ti·gram [kəʊlə'sɪntɪgræm, kɑlə-] *n chir.*, *radiol.* Gallenwegsszintigramm *nt,* Cholezintigramm *nt.*
chol·e·scin·tig·ra·phy [ˌ-sɪn'tɪgrəfɪ] *n chir.*, *radiol.* Gallenwegsszintigraphie *f,* Choleszintigraphie *f.*
cho·les·tane [kəˈlestiːn, kəʊ'lestiːn] *n* Cholestan *nt.*
cho·les·ta·nol [kəˈlestənɔl, -nəʊl] *n* Cholestanol *nt,* Dihydrocholesterin *nt.*
cho·les·ta·sia [ˌkəʊlə'steɪʒ(ɪ)ə, -ʃə, ˌkɑl-] *n* → cholestasis.
cho·les·ta·sis [ˌ-'steɪsɪs, -'stæ-] *n* Galle(n)stauung *f,* Cholestase *f,* Cholostase *f.*

cho·le·stat·ic [ˌ-'stætɪk] *adj* Cholestase betr., von Cholestase gekennzeichnet, cholestatisch.
cholestatic hepatitis cholestatische Hepatitis *f*, Hepatitis *f* bei Gallestauung.
cholestatic jaundice cholestatische Gelbsucht *f*, cholestatischer Ikterus *m*.
cho·les·te·a·to·ma [kəˌlestɪə'təʊmə] *n* HNO Perlgeschwulst *f*, Cholesteatom *nt*.
cho·les·te·a·tom·a·tous [ˌ-'tɑmətəs] *adj* HNO Cholesteatom betr., cholesteatomatös.
cho·le·ste·a·to·sis [ˌ-'təʊsɪs] *n* Cholesteatose *f*, -tosis *f*.
cho·les·ter·e·mia [kəˌlestə'riːmɪə] *n* → cholesterolemia.
cho·les·ter·in [kə'lestərɪn] *n* → cholesterol.
cho·les·ter·in·e·mia [kə'lestərɪ'niːmɪə] *n* → cholesterolemia.
cho·les·ter·i·no·sis [ˌ-'nəʊsɪs] *n* → cholesterosis.
cho·les·ter·i·nu·ria [ˌ-'n(j)ʊərɪə] *n* → cholesteroluria.
cho·les·ter·o·gen·e·sis [kəˌlestərəʊ'dʒenəsɪs] *n* Cholesterinbildung *f*, -synthese *f*.
cho·les·ter·o·der·ma [ˌ-'dɜrmə] *n* derm. Xanthosis *f*, Xanthodermie *f*.
cho·les·ter·ol [kə'lestərəʊl, -rɒl] *n* Cholesterin *nt*, Cholesterol *nt*.
cholesterol acyltransferase Cholesterin-acyltransferase *f*.
cho·les·ter·ol·ase [kəʊ'lestərəʊleɪz] *n* → cholesterol esterase.
cholesterol calculus Cholesterinstein *m*.
cho·les·ter·ol·e·mia [kəˌlestərəʊ'liːmɪə] *n* erhöhter Cholesteringehalt *m* des Blutes, Hypercholesterinämie *f*.
cho·les·ter·ol·er·e·sis [kəˌlestərəʊl'erəsɪs] *n* (verstärkte) Cholesterinausscheidung *f*.
cholesterol ester Cholesterinester *m*.
cholesterol esterase Cholesterinase *f*, Cholesterinesterase *f*, Cholesterase *f*, Cholesterinesterhydrolase *f* abbr. CHE.
cholesterol ester storage disease abbr. CESD Cholesterinesterspeicherkrankheit *f*.
cho·les·ter·ol·es·ter·sturz [ˌ-'estərsturz] *n* Cholesterinestersturz *m*, Estersturz *m*.
cholesterol granuloma Cholesteringranulom *nt*.
cholesterol lipoidosis Hand-Schüller--Christian-Krankheit *f*, Schüller-Hand--Christian-Krankheit *f*, Schüller-Krankheit *f*.
cho·les·ter·ol·o·poi·e·sis [kəˌlestərəlɔʊpɔɪ'iːsɪs] *n* (*Leber*) Cholesterinbildung *f*, -synthese *f*.
cho·les·ter·ol·o·sis [kəˌlestərə'ləʊsɪs] *n* → cholesterosis.
cholesterol-pigment-calcium calculus/stone Cholesterinpigmentkalkstein *m*.
cholesterol stone Cholesterinstein *m*.
cholesterol sulfatase Sterylsulfatase *f*.
cholesterol thesaurismosis → cholesterol lipoidosis
cho·les·ter·ol·u·ria [ˌ-'l(j)ʊərɪə] *n* Cholesterinausscheidung *f* im Harn, Cholesterinurie *f*.
cho·les·ter·o·sis [kəˌlestə'rəʊsɪs] *n* Cholesterinose *f*.
cho·let·e·lin [kə'letlɪn] *n* Choletelin *nt*, Bilixanthin *nt*.
cho·le·ther·a·py [ˌkəʊlə'θerəpɪ, ˌkɑl-] *n* Behandlung *f* mit Gallensalzen.
cho·le·u·ria [ˌ-'(j)ʊərɪə] *n* → choluria.
cho·le·ver·din [ˌ-'vɜrdɪn] *n* Biliverdin *nt*.
cho·lic acid ['kəʊlɪk, 'kɑl-] Cholsäure *f*.
cho·line ['kəʊliːn, 'kɑl-] *n* Cholin *nt*, Bilineurin *nt*, Sinkalin *nt*.
choline acetylase → choline acetyltransferase

choline acetyltransferase Cholinacetyl(transfer)ase *f*.
choline acetyltransferase I Azetyl-, Acetylcholinesterase *f* abbr. AChE, echte Cholinesterase *f*.
choline esterase I → choline acetyltransferase I.
choline esterase II → cholinesterase.
choline kinase Cholinkinase *f*.
choline phosphatase Phospholipase D *f*, Lecithinase D *f*.
choline phosphatidyl → choline phosphoglyceride.
choline phosphoglyceride Phosphatidylcholin *nt*, Cholinphosphoglycerid *nt*, Lecithin *nt*, Lezithin *nt*.
choline phosphokinase → choline kinase.
cho·line·phos·pho·trans·fer·ase [ˌkəʊliːnˌfɑsfəʊ'trænsfəreɪz, ˌkɑl-] *n* Cholinphosphotransferase *f*.
cho·lin·er·gic [ˌkəʊliː'nɜrdʒɪk, ˌkɑ-] I *n* Parasympathikomimetikum *nt*, Cholinergikum *nt*. II *adj* cholinerg(isch).
cholinergic blockade Cholinorezeptor(en)blockade *f*.
cholinergic blocker Cholinorezeptorenblocker *m*.
cholinergic crisis cholinerge/cholinergische Krise *f*.
cholinergic fibers cholinerge (Nerven-)Fasern *pl*.
cholinergic neuron cholinerges Neuron *nt*.
cholinergic receptor → cholinoceptor.
cholinergic system cholinerges System *nt*.
cholinergic urticaria Anstrengungs-, Schwitzurtikaria *f*, cholinergische Urtikaria *f*, Urticaire par effort.
choline salicylate *pharm.* Cholinsalicylat *nt*.
cho·lin·es·ter ['kəʊlɪnestər] *n* Cholinester *m*.
cho·lin·es·ter·ase [ˌkəʊlɪ'nestəreɪz] *n* abbr. ChE unspezifische/unechte Cholinesterase *f* abbr. ChE, Pseudocholinesterase *f*, Typ II-Cholinesterase *f*, β-Cholinesterase *f*, Butyrylcholinesterase *f*.
cholinesterase inhibitor Cholinesterasehemmer *m*, -inhibitor *m*.
choline theophyllinate *pharm.* Cholintheophyllinat *nt*.
cho·li·no·cep·tive [ˌkəʊlɪnəʊ'septɪv] *adj* cholino(re)zeptiv.
cho·li·no·cep·tor [ˌ-'septər] *n* Cholino(re)zeptor *m*, cholinerger Rezeptor *m*.
cho·li·no·lyt·ic [ˌ-'lɪtɪk] I *n* Cholinolytikum *nt*. II *adj* cholinolytisch.
cho·li·no·mi·met·ic [ˌ-'mɪmetɪk, -maɪ-] *adj* cholinomimetisch, parasympath(ik)omimetisch.
cholinomimetic agent *pharm.* Cholinomimetikum *nt*.
cho·li·no·re·cep·tor [ˌ-rɪ'septər] *n* → cholinoceptor.
cholo- *pref.* Galle(n)-, Chole-, Chol(o)-.
chol·o·chrome ['kəʊləkrəʊm, 'kɑl-] *n* Gallenpigment *nt*.
chol·o·cy·a·nin [ˌ-'saɪənɪn] *n* Bili-, Cholezyanin *nt*.
cho·lo·cyst ['-sɪst] *n* Cisterna chyli.
chol·o·gen·ic [ˌ-'dʒenɪk] *adj* → cholepoietic.
chol·o·ge·net·ic [ˌ-dʒə'netɪk] *adj* → cholepoietic.
cho·lo·he·mo·tho·rax [ˌ-ˌhiːmə'θɔːræks, -ˌhem-] *n* Cholehämothorax *m*.
chol·o·lith ['-lɪθ] *n* → cholelith.
chol·o·li·thi·a·sis [ˌ-lɪ'θaɪəsɪs] *n* → cholelithiasis.
chol·o·lith·ic [ˌ-'lɪθɪk] *adj* → cholelithic.
cho·lo·lyl-CoA synthetase ['-lɪl] Cholatsynthetase *f*.

chol·o·poi·e·sis [ˌ-pɔɪ'iːsɪs] *n* → cholepoiesis.
chol·or·rhe·a [ˌ-'riːə] *n* übermäßiger Gallefluß *m*, Cholorrhoe *f*.
cho·los·co·py [kə'lɑskəpɪ] *n* → cholangioscopy.
cho·lo·tho·rax [ˌkəʊlə'θɔːræks, ˌkɑl-] *n* Cholethorax *m*.
chol·u·ria [kəʊ'l(j)ʊərɪə] *n* Ausscheidung *f* von Galle(n)farbstoffen im Harn, Cholurie *f*.
chol·ur·ic [kəʊ'lʊərɪk] *adj* Cholurie betr., cholurisch.
cho·lyl·gly·cine [ˌkəʊlɪl'glaɪsiːn] *n* Glykocholsäure *f*.
cho·lyl·tau·rine [ˌ-'tɔːriːn] *n* Taurocholsäure *f*.
chondr- *pref.* → chondro-.
chon·dral ['kɒndrəl] *adj* Knorpel betr., knorp(e)lig, kartilaginär, chondral.
chon·dral·gia [kɒn'dræld͡ʒ(ɪ)ə] *n* → chondrodynia.
chon·dral·lo·pla·sia [ˌkɒndræləʊ'pleɪʒ(ɪ)ə, -zɪə] *n* Chondr(o)alloplasie *f*, Chondrodystrophie *f*.
chon·drec·to·my [kɒn'drektəmɪ] *n* ortho. Knorpelresektion *f*, Chondrektomie *f*.
chon·dric ['kɒndrɪk] *adj* → chondral.
chon·dri·fi·ca·tion [ˌkɒndrəfɪ'keɪʃn] *n* Knorpelbildung *f*, Chondrogenese *f*; Verknorpeln *nt*.
chon·dri·fy ['kɒndrɪfaɪ] *vi* verknorpeln, s. in Knorpel umwandeln.
chon·dri·gen ['kɒndrɪdʒən] *n* → chondrogen.
chon·drin ['kɒndrɪn] *n* Knorpelleim *m*, Chondrin *nt*.
chon·dri·o·some ['kɒndrɪəʊsəʊm] *n* Mitochondrie *f*, -chondrion *nt*, -chondrium *nt*, Chondriosom *nt*.
chon·dri·tis [kɒn'draɪtɪs] *n* Knorpelentzündung *f*, Chondritis *f*.
chondro- *pref.* Knorpel-, Chondr(o)-.
chon·dro·ad·e·no·ma [ˌkɒndrəʊˌædə'nəʊmə] *n* Chondroadenom *nt*.
chon·dro·an·gi·o·ma [ˌ-ˌændʒɪ'əʊmə] *n* Chondroangiom *nt*.
chon·dro·blast ['-blæst] *n* knorpelbildende Zelle *f*, Chondroblast *m*, -plast *m*.
chon·dro·blas·tic osteosarcoma [ˌ-'blæstɪk] → chondrosarcomatous osteosarcoma.
chon·dro·blas·to·ma [ˌ-blæs'təʊmə] *n* Chondroblastom *nt*, Codman-Tumor *m*.
chon·dro·cal·ci·no·sis [ˌ-ˌkælsə'nəʊsɪs] *n* Chondrokalzinose *f*, Pseudogicht *f*, CPPD-Ablagerung *f*, Calciumpyrophosphatdihydratablagerung *f*, Chondrocalcinosis *f*.
chon·dro·car·ci·no·ma [ˌ-ˌkɑːrsə'nəʊmə] *n* patho. Chondrokarzinom *nt*.
chon·dro·clast ['-klæst] *n* Knorpelfreßzelle *f*, Chondroklast *m*.
chon·dro·cos·tal [ˌ-'kɒstl] *adj* Rippenknorpel betr., chondrokostal, kostochondral, Rippenknorpel-.
chon·dro·cra·ni·um [ˌ-'kreɪnɪəm] *n, pl* -niums, -nia [-nɪə] *embryo.* Knorpelschädel *m*, Primordialkranium *nt*, Chondrokranium *nt*, -cranium *nt*.
chon·dro·cyte ['-saɪt] *n* Knorpelzelle *f*, Chondrozyt *m*, -cyt *m*.
chon·dro·der·ma·ti·tis [ˌ-ˌdɜːrmə'taɪtɪs] *n* patho. Dermatochondritis *f*, Chondrodermatitis *f*.
chon·dro·dyn·ia [ˌ-'diːnɪə] *n* Knorpelschmerz *m*, Chondrodynie *f*, -dynia *f*, Chondralgie *f*.
chon·dro·dys·pla·sia [ˌ-dɪs'pleɪʒ(ɪ)ə, -zɪə] *n* **1.** Knorpelbildungsstörung *f*, Chondrodysplasie *f*, -dysplasia *f*. **2.** → chondrodystrophy.

chondrodystrophia

chon·dro·dys·tro·phia [ˌ-dɪsˈtrəʊfɪə] *n* → chondrodystrophy.
chon·dro·dys·troph·ic [ˌ-dɪsˈtrafɪk, -ˈtrəʊ-] *adj* Chondrodystrophie betr., von Chondrodystrophie betroffen, chondrodystroph, -dystrophisch.
chondrodystrophic dwarf Chondrodystrophiker *m*, Achondroplast *m*.
chondrodystrophic micromelia chondrodystrophe Mikromelie *f*, Micromelia chondromalacia.
chon·dro·dys·tro·phy [ˌ-ˈdɪstrəfɪ] *n* Chondrodystrophie *f*, -dystrophia *f*, Chondr(o)alloplasie *f*.
chon·dro·ec·to·der·mal [ˌ-ˌektəˈdɜrml] *adj embryo.* chondroektodermal.
chondroectodermal dysplasia Ellis-van Creveld-Syndrom *nt*, Chondroektodermaldysplasie *f*, chondroektodermale Dysplasie *f*.
chon·dro·en·do·the·li·o·ma [ˌ-ˌendəʊˌθiːlɪˈəʊmə] *n patho.* Chondroendotheliom *nt*.
chon·dro·ep·i·phys·e·al [ˌ-ˌepɪˈfiːzɪəl, -ɪˌpɪfəˈsiːəl] *adj* Epiphysen(fugen)knorpel betr., chondroepiphysär.
chon·dro·e·piph·y·si·tis [ˌ-ɪˌpɪfəˈsaɪtɪs, -ˌepɪfɪˈsaɪ-] *n ortho.* Entzündung *f* des Epiphysenknorpels, Chondroepiphysitis *f*.
chon·dro·fi·bro·ma [ˌ-faɪˈbrəʊmə] *n patho.* Chondrofibrom *nt*, chondromyxoides Fibrom *nt*.
chon·dro·gen [ˈkandrəʊˌdʒən] *n* Chondrogen *nt*.
chon·dro·gen·e·sis [ˌ-ˈdʒenəsɪs] *n* Knorpelbildung *f*, Chondrogenese *f*.
chon·dro·gen·ic [ˌ-ˈdʒenɪk] *adj* knorpelbildend, -formend, chondrogen.
chon·drog·e·nous [kanˈdrɑdʒənəs] *adj* → chondrogenic.
chon·drog·e·ny [ˈkanˌdrɑdʒənɪ] *n* → chondrogenesis.
chon·dro·glos·sus (muscle) [ˌkandrəʊˈɡlɑsəs] Chondroglossus *m*, M. chondroglossus.
chon·dro·hy·po·pla·sia [ˌ-ˌhaɪpəˈpleɪʒ(ɪ)ə, -ʒɪə] *n* abortive Form *f* der Chondrodysplasie, Chondrohypoplasie *f*.
chon·droid [ˈkɑndrɔɪd] **I** *n* Knorpelgrundsubstanz *f*, Chondroid *nt*. **II** *adj* knorpelähnlich, -förmig, chondroid.
chondroid chordoma *patho.* chondroides Chordom *nt*.
chon·dro·it·ic [ˌkɑndrəˈwɪtɪk] *adj* Knorpel betr., aus Knorpel bestehend, knorpelig, knorpelähnlich, -förmig, chondroid.
chon·droi·tin sulfatase [kɑnˈdrɔɪtɪn] Chondroitinsulfatsulfatase *f*, N-Acetylgalaktosamin-6-sulfatsulfatase *f*.
chondroitin sulfate Chondroitinsulfat *nt*.
chondroitin-4-sulfate → chondroitin sulfate A.
chondroitin-6-sulfate → chondroitin sulfate C.
chondroitin sulfate A Chondroitinsulfat A *nt*, Chondroitin-4-Sulfat *nt*.
chondroitin sulfate B Chondroitinsulfat B *nt*, Dermatansulfat *nt*.
chondroitin sulfate C Chondroitinsulfat C *nt*, Chondroitin-6-Sulfat *nt*.
chon·dro·li·po·ma [ˌkandrəʊlaɪˈpəʊmə, -lɪ-] *n patho.* Chondrolipom *nt*.
chon·drol·y·sis [kanˈdrɑləsɪs] *n patho.* Knorpelauflösung *f*, Chondrolyse *f*.
chon·dro·ma [kanˈdrəʊmə] *n patho.* Knorpelgeschwulst *f*, -tumor *m*, Chondrom(a) *nt*.
chon·dro·ma·la·cia [ˌkɑndrəʊməˈleɪʃ(ɪ)ə] *n patho.* Knorpelerweichung *f*, Chondromalazie *f*, -malacia *f*.
c. of the patella → chondromalacia patellae.
chondromalacia patellae *ortho.* Büdinger-Ludloff-Läwen-Syndrom *nt*, Chondromalacia patellae.
chon·dro·ma·to·sis [ˌ-məˈtəʊsɪs] *n ortho.* multiple Chondrome *pl*, Chondromatose *f*.
chon·drom·a·tous [kanˈdrɑmətəs] *adj* Chondrom betr., chondromatös.
chon·dro·mere [ˈkɑndrəmɪər] *n embryo.* Chondromer *m*.
chon·dro·met·a·pla·sia [ˌ-ˌmetəˈpleɪʒ(ɪ)ə, -ʒɪə] *n patho.* Chondrometaplasie *f*.
chon·dro·mu·cin [ˌ-ˈmjuːsɪn] *n* → chondromucoid.
chon·dro·mu·coid [ˌ-mjuːˈkɔɪd] *n* Chondromukoid *nt*.
chon·dro·mu·co·pro·tein [ˌ-ˌmjuːkəˈprəʊtiːn, -tiːɪn] *n* Chondromukoprotein *nt*, Chondroglycoprotein *nt*.
chon·dro·my·o·ma [ˌ-maɪˈəʊmə] *n patho.* Chondromyom *nt*.
chon·dro·myx·o·fi·bro·sar·co·ma [ˌ-ˌmɪksəˌfaɪbrəʊsɑːrˈkəʊmə] *n patho.* Chondromyxofibrosarkom *nt*.
chon·dro·myx·oid fibroma [ˌ-ˈmɪksɔɪd] → chondrofibroma.
chon·dro·myx·o·ma [ˌ-mɪkˈsəʊmə] *n patho.* Chondromyxom *nt*.
chon·dro·myx·o·sar·co·ma [ˌ-ˌmɪksəsɑːrˈkəʊmə] *n patho.* Chondromyxosarkom *nt*.
chon·dro·ne·cro·sis [ˌ-nɪˈkrəʊsɪs, -ne-] *n* Knorpel-, Chondronekrose *f*.
chondro-osseous *adj* aus Knochen- u. Knorpelgewebe bestehend, chondro-ossär, osteochondral.
chondro-osteoarthritis *n* Chondroosteoarthritis *f*.
chondro-osteodystrophy *n* Chondroosteodystrophie *f*, Osteochondrodystrophie *f*.
chondro-osteoma *n* Osteochondrom *nt*, (osteo-)kartilaginäre Exostose *f*.
chondro-osteosarcoma *n patho.* Chondroosteosarkom *nt*.
chon·dro·path·ia [ˌ-ˈpæθɪə] *n* → chondropathy.
chon·drop·a·thy [kanˈdrɑpəθɪ] *n patho., ortho.* (degenerative) Knorpelerkrankung *f*, Chondropathie *f*, -pathia *f*.
chon·dro·pha·ryn·ge·al muscle [ˌkandrəʊfəˈrɪndʒ(ɪ)əl] *n* chondropharyngeus (muscle) l.
chon·dro·pha·ryn·ge·us (muscle) [ˌ-fəˈrɪndʒ(ɪ)əs] **1.** Pars chondropharyngea. **2.** M. constrictor pharyngis medius.
chon·dro·phyte [ˈ-faɪt] *n patho., ortho.* Chondrophyt *m*.
chon·dro·pla·sia [ˌ-ˈpleɪʒ(ɪ)ə, -ʒɪə] *n histol.* Chondroplasie *f*.
chon·dro·plast [ˈ-ˌplæst] *n* → chondroblast.
chon·dro·plas·ty [ˈ-ˌplæstɪ] *n chir.* Knorpel-, Chondroplastik *f*.
chon·dro·po·ro·sis [ˌ-pəˈrəʊsɪs] *n histol.* Chondroporose *f*.
chon·dro·pro·teid [ˌ-ˈprəʊtiːd, -tiːɪd] *n* → chondroprotein.
chon·dro·pro·tein [ˌ-ˈprəʊtiːn, -tiːɪn] *n* Chondroprotein *nt*.
chon·dro·sa·mine [kanˈdrəʊsəmiːn, -mɪn] *n* Chondrosamin *nt*, D-Galaktosamin *nt*.
chon·dro·sar·co·ma [ˌkandrəsɑːrˈkəʊmə] *n patho.* Knorpel-, Chondrosarkom *nt*, Chondroma sarcomatosum, Enchondroma malignum.
chon·dro·sar·co·ma·to·sis [ˌ-sɑːrˌkəʊməˈtəʊsɪs] *n patho.* Chondrosarkomatose *f*.
chon·dro·sar·co·ma·tous [ˌ-sɑːrˈkɑmətəs] *adj* Chondrosarkom betr., chondrosarkomatös.
chondrosarcomatous osteosarcoma chondroblastisches/chondrosarkomatöses Osteosarkom *nt*.
chon·dro·sep·tum [ˌ-ˈseptəm] *n* knorpeliger Abschnitt *m* des Nasenseptums, Pars cartilaginea septi nasi.
chon·dro·sin [ˈkandrəsɪn] *n* Chondrosin *nt*.
chon·dro·sis [kanˈdrəʊsɪs] *n patho.* Chondrose *f*, Chondrosis *f*.
chon·dro·skel·e·ton [ˌkandrəˈskelətən] *n* Knorpelskelett *nt*.
chon·dro·some [ˈ-ˌsəʊm] *n* → chondriosome.
chon·dros·te·o·ma [kanˌdrɑstɪˈəʊmə] *n* → chondro-osteoma.
chon·dro·ster·nal [ˌkandrəʊˈstɜrnl] *adj* Brustbein u. Rippenknorpel betr., sternochondral, sternokostal.
chondrosternal articulations Sternokostalgelenke *pl*, Articc. sternocostales.
chondrosternal joints → chondrosternal articulations.
chondrosternal ligament Lig. sternocostale.
chon·dro·ster·no·plas·ty [ˌ-ˈstɜrnəplæstɪ] *n ortho.* Chondrosternoplastik *f*.
chon·dro·tome [ˈ-ˌtəʊm] *n ortho.* Knorpelmesser *nt*, Chondrotom *nt*.
chon·drot·o·my [kanˈdrɑtəmɪ] *n ortho.* Knorpeldurchtrennung *f*, -durchschneidung *f*, -einschnitt *m*, Chondrotomie *f*.
chon·dro·trop·ic hormone [ˌkandrəˈtrɑpɪk] Wachstumshormon *nt*, somatotropes Hormon *nt abbr.* STH, Somatotropin *nt*.
chon·dro·xiph·oid [ˌ-ˈzɪfɔɪd, -zaɪ-] *adj* Schwertfortsatz betr., chondroxiphoid.
chondroxiphoid ligaments Ligg. costoxiphoidea.
cho·ne·chon·dro·ster·non [ˌkəʊnɪˌkandrəʊˈstɜrnən] *n ortho.* Trichterbrust *m*, Pectus excavatum/infundibulum/recurvatum.
Chopart [ʃɔˈpaːr]: **C.'s amputation** Chopart-Amputation *f*, -Exartikulation *f*.
C.'s articulation Chopart'-Gelenklinie *f*, Artic. tarsi transversa.
C.'s joint → C.'s articulation.
C.'s mediotarsal amputation → C.'s amputation.
C.'s operation → C.'s amputation.
cho·ran·gi·o·ma [kəˌrændʒɪˈəʊmə] *n* → chorioangioma.
chord [kɔːrd] *n* → chorda.
chor·da [ˈkɔːrdə] *n, pl* **-dae** [-diː] *anat.* Schnur *f*, Strang *m*, Band *nt*, Chorda *f*.
chorda dorsalis *embro.* Chorda dorsalis.
chor·dal [ˈkɔːrdl] *adj* **1.** Chorda betr., chordal. **2.** Chorda dorsalis betr.
chordal canal *embryo.* Chordakanal *m*.
Chor·da·ta [kɔːrˈdeɪtə, -ˈdɑː-] *pl bio.* Achsentiere *pl*, Chordata *pl*.
chorda tympani Chorda tympani.
chorda tympani canal Chordakanal *m*, Canaliculus chordae tympani.
chorda tympani nerve → chorda tympani.
chor·dec·to·my [kɔːrˈdektəmɪ] *n HNO* Stimmband(teil)resektion *f*, -ausschneidung *f*, Chordektomie *f*.
chor·dee [kɔːrˈdiː, kəʊr-] *n* **1.** Gryposis penis. **2.** Penis lunatus.
chor·di·tis [kɔːrˈdaɪtɪs] *n* **1.** *HNO* Stimmbandentzündung *f*, Chorditis *f* (vocalis). **2.** *urol.* Samenstrangentzündung *f*, Funikulitis *f*, Funiculitis *f*.
chor·do·blas·to·ma [ˌkɔːrdəʊblæsˈtəʊmə] *n patho.* Chordoblastom *nt*.
chor·do·car·ci·no·ma [ˌ-kɑːrsɪˈnəʊmə] *n* → chordoma.
chor·do·ep·i·the·li·o·ma [ˌ-ˌepəˌθiːlɪˈəʊmə] *n* → chordoma.
chor·do·ma [kɔːrˈdəʊmə] *n patho.* Chordom *nt*, Notochordom *nt*.

chor·do·pex·y ['kɔːrdəpeksɪ] *n HNO* Stimmbandfixierung *f*, Chordopexie *f*.
chor·do·sar·co·ma [ˌ-sɑːr'koʊmə] *n* → chordoma.
chor·dot·o·my [kɔːr'dɑtəmɪ] *n neurochir.* Chordotomie *f*.
cho·rea [kəˈrɪə, kɔː-, koʊ-] *n neuro.* Chorea *f*.
 c. in pregnancy Schwangerschaftschorea, Chorea gravidarum.
cho·re·al [kəˈrɪəl, kɔː-, koʊ-] *adj* → choreic.
cho·re·at·ic [ˌkɔːrɪ'ætɪk, ˌkoʊ-] *adj* → choreic.
cho·re·ic [kəˈriːɪk, kɔː-, koʊ-] *adj* Chorea betr., von Chorea betroffen, choreaartig, choreatisch, Chorea-, Choreo-.
cho·re·i·form [kəˈrɪəfɔːrm] *adj* choreaähnlich, choreiform, choreatiform.
choreo- *pref.* Choreo-, Chorea-.
cho·re·o·ath·e·toid [ˌkɔːrɪə'æθətɔɪd] *adj neuro.* choreoathetoid.
cho·re·o·ath·e·to·sis [ˌ-æθə'toʊsɪs] *n neuro.* Choreathetose *f*.
cho·re·oid ['kɔːrɪɔɪd] *adj* → choreiform.
cho·ri·al ['kɔːrɪəl] *adj* Chorion betr., chorial, Chorio(n)-.
cho·ri·o·ad·e·no·ma [ˌkɔːrɪoʊædə'noʊmə, ˌkoʊ-] *n patho.* Chorioadenom *nt*.
cho·ri·o·al·lan·to·ic culture [ˌ-ˌælən'toʊɪk] *micro.* Chorioallantoiskultur *f*.
chorioallantoic membrane → chorioallantois.
chorioallantoic placenta Placenta chorio--allantoica.
cho·ri·o·al·lan·to·is [ˌ-ə'læntoʊɪs, -tɔɪs] *n* Chorioallantois *f*, Chorioallantoismembran *f abbr* CAM.
cho·ri·o·am·ni·on·ic placenta [ˌ-ˌæmnɪ-'ɑnɪk] Placenta chorio-amniotica.
cho·ri·o·am·ni·o·ni·tis [ˌ-ˌæmnɪə'naɪtɪs] *n gyn.* Chorioamnionitis *f*.
cho·ri·o·an·gi·o·fi·bro·ma [ˌ-ˌændʒɪoʊfaɪ-'broʊmə] *n patho., gyn.* Chorioangiofibrom *nt*.
cho·ri·o·an·gi·o·ma [ˌ-ˌændʒɪ'oʊmə] *n patho., gyn.* Chorioangiom *nt*.
cho·ri·o·blas·to·ma [ˌ-blæs'toʊmə] *n* → choriocarcinoma.
cho·ri·o·blas·to·sis [ˌ-blæs'toʊsɪs] *n gyn.* Chorioblastose *f*.
cho·ri·o·cap·il·la·ris [ˌ-ˌkæpɪ'leərɪs] *n* Choriocapillaris *f*, Lamina choroidocapillaris.
cho·ri·o·cap·il·lar·y lamina/layer [ˌ-'kæpɪˌlerɪ, -kə'pɪlərɪ] → choriocapillaris.
cho·ri·o·car·ci·no·ma [ˌ-kɑːrsɪ'noʊmə] *n patho., gyn.* Chorioblastom *nt*, (malignes) Chorio(n)epitheliom *nt*, Chorionkarzinom *nt*, fetaler Zottenkrebs *m*.
cho·ri·o·ep·i·the·li·o·ma [ˌ-epəˌθɪlɪ'oʊmə] *n* → choriocarcinoma.
cho·ri·o·gen·e·sis [ˌ-'dʒenəsɪs] *n gyn., embryo.* Chorionentwicklung *f*, Choriogenese *f*.
cho·ri·oid ['kɔːrɪɔɪd, 'koʊr-] *n* → choroid I.
cho·ri·oi·dal [kɔːrɪ'ɔɪdl, koʊr-] *adj* → choroidal.
cho·ri·oi·dea [kɔːrɪ'ɔɪdɪə, koʊr-] *n* → choroid I.
chorioid plexus bleeding/hemorrhage (*ZNS*) Plexusblutung *f*.
cho·ri·o·ma [kɔːrɪ'oʊmə] *n* Choriom *nt*.
cho·ri·o·mam·mo·tro·pin [ˌkoʊrɪoʊˌmæmə'troʊpɪn, ˌkɔːrɪ-] *n* humanes Plazenta--Laktogen *nt abbr.* HPL, Chorionsomatotropin *nt*.
cho·ri·o·men·in·gi·tis [ˌ-ˌmenɪn'dʒaɪtɪs] *n* Choriomeningitis *f*.
cho·ri·on ['kɔːrɪɑn, 'koʊ-] *n* **1.** *embryo.* Zottenhaut *f*, mittlere Eihaut *f*, Chorion *nt*. **2.** *bio.* äußere Eihaut/Membran *f*, Chorion *nt*. **3.** *old* Endometrialstroma *nt*.

cho·ri·on·ep·i·the·li·o·ma [ˌkoʊrɪɑnˌepə-ˌθɪlɪ'oʊmə] *n* → choriocarcinoma.
cho·ri·on·ic [kɔːrɪ'ɑnɪk, koʊ-] *adj* Zottenhaut/Chorion betr., chorional, chorial, Chorion-.
chorionic carcinoma → choriocarcinoma.
chorionic cavity *embryo.* Chorionhöhle *f*, extraembryonales Zölom *nt*.
chorionic epithelioma → choriocarcinoma.
chorionic epithelium Chorionepithel *nt*.
chorionic gonadotropin *abbr.* **CG** Choriongonadotropin *nt abbr.* CG.
 human c. *abbr.* **HCG, hCG** humanes Choriongonadotropin *abbr.* HCG.
chorionic plate Zotten-, Chorionplatte *f*, Chorion frondosum.
chorionic sac → chorion sac.
chorionic somatomammotropine humanes Plazenta-Laktogen *nt abbr.* HPL, Chorionsomatotropin *nt*.
chorionic villi Chorionzotten *pl*.
cho·ri·o·ni·tis [kɔːrɪə'naɪtɪs, koʊ-] *n gyn.* Chorionentzündung *f*, Chorionitis *f*.
chorion laeve Zottenglatze *f*, Chorion laeve.
chorion sac 1. *embryo.* Zottenhaut *f*, mittlere Eihaut *f*, Chorion *nt*. **2.** *bio.* äußere Eihaut/Membran *f*, Chorion *nt*.
cho·ri·o·ret·i·nal [ˌkoʊrɪoʊ'retnəl, ˌkɔː-] *adj* Aderhaut/Choroidea u. Netzhaut/Retina betr., chorioretinal.
cho·ri·o·ret·i·ni·tis [ˌ-ˌretə'naɪtɪs] *n ophthal.* Entzündung *f* von Aderhaut u. Netzhaut, Chorioretinitis *f*.
cho·ri·o·ret·i·nop·a·thy [ˌ-ˌretə'nɑpəθɪ] *n ophthal.* Erkrankung *f* von Ader- u. Netzhaut, Chorioretinopathie *f*.
cho·ri·o·vi·tel·line placenta [ˌ-vaɪ'telɪn, vɪ-] Placenta choriovitellina.
cho·ris·mate mutase [kəˈrɪzmeɪt] Chorisminsäuremutase *f*.
chorismate synthase Chorisminsäuresynthase *f*.
cho·ris·mic acid [kəˈrɪzmɪk] Chorisminsäure *f*.
cho·ris·ta [kəˈrɪstə] *n patho., embryo.* Choristie *f*.
cho·ris·to·blas·to·ma [kəˌrɪstoʊblæs'toʊmə] *n* **1.** → Choristoblastom *nt*. **2.** → choristoma.
cho·ris·to·ma [ˌkɔːrɪ'stoʊmə] *n patho., embryo.* Choristom(a) *nt*, Chorestom *nt*.
cho·roid ['kɔːrɔɪd, 'koʊr-] **I** *n* Aderhaut *f*, Chor(i)oidea *f*. **II** *adj* Chorion od. Corium betr., Chorion-.
cho·roi·dal [kəˈrɔɪdl] *adj* Aderhaut/Choroidea betr., Aderhaut-.
choroidal artery, (anterior) A. choroidea (anterior).
choroidal atrophy, progressive → choroideremia.
choroidal branches: c. of lateral ventricle A. choroidea-Äste *pl* zum Plexus choroideus des Seitenventrikels, Rami choroidei ventriculi lateralis.
 c. of third ventricle A. choroidea-Äste *pl* zum Plexus choroideus des III. Ventrikels, Rami choroidei ventriculi tertii.
choroidal cataract Uveitiskatarakt *f*, Cataracta chorioidealis.
choroidal fissure Fissura choroidea.
choroidal taenia T(a)enia choroidea.
choroid branch: c. of fourth ventricle A. choroidea-Ast *pl* zum Plexus des IV. Ventrikels, Ramus choroideus ventriculi quarti.
 medial c.es of posterior cerebral artery A. cerebri posterior-Äste *pl* zum III. Ventrikel, Rami choroidei mediales a. cerebri posterioris.
 lateral c.es of posterior cerebral artery →

posterolateral c.es of posterior cerebral artery.
 posterolateral c.es of posterior cerebral artery A. cerebri posterior-Äste *pl* zum Seitenventrikel, Rami choroidei posteriores laterales a. posterioris cerebri.
cho·roi·de·a [kəˈrɔɪdɪə] *n* → choroid I.
cho·roi·dec·to·my [ˌkɔːrɔɪ'dektəmɪ, ˌkoʊ-] *n neurochir.* Choroidektomie *f*.
cho·roid·e·re·mia [ˌkɔːrɔɪdə'riːmɪə, ˌkoʊ-] *n ophthal.* Chorioideremie *f*, Degeneratio chorioretinalis progressiva.
choroid fissure 1. *embryo.* Augenbecherspalte *f*. **2.** Fissura choroidea.
choroid glomus Glomus choroideum.
cho·roid·i·tis [ˌkɔːrɔɪ'daɪtɪs, ˌkoʊ-] *n ophthal.* Aderhautentzündung *f*, Chor(i)oiditis *f*.
cho·roi·do·cap·il·la·ris [kəˌrɔɪdoʊˌkæpɪ-'leərɪs] *n* → choriocapillaris.
cho·roi·do·cyc·li·tis [ˌ-sɪk'laɪtɪs] *n ophthal.* Chor(i)oidozyklitis *f*.
cho·roi·do·i·ri·tis [ˌ-aɪ'raɪtɪs] *n ophthal.* Entzündung *f* von Aderhaut u. Iris, Chor(i)oidoiritis *f*.
cho·roi·dop·a·thy [ˌkoʊrɔɪ'dɑpəθɪ, ˌkɔː-] *n* **1.** → choroiditis. **2.** → choroidosis.
cho·roi·do·ret·i·ni·tis [kəˌrɔɪdoʊretə'naɪtɪs] *n* → chorioretinitis.
cho·roi·do·sis [ˌkɔːrɔɪ'doʊsɪs, ˌkoʊ-] *n ophthal.* (degenerative) Aderhauterkrankung *f*, Chorioidose *f*.
choroid plexus Plexus choroideus.
 c. of fourth ventricle Plexus choroideus des IV. Ventrikels, Plexus choroideus ventriculi quarti.
 inferior c. → c. of fourth ventricle.
 c. of lateral ventricle Plexus choroideus des Seitenventrikels, Plexus choroideus ventriculi lateralis.
 c. of third ventricle Plexus choroideus des III. Ventrikels, Plexus choroideus ventriculi tertii.
choroid vein: inferior c. untere Choroidalvene *f*, Choroidea *f* inferior, V. choroidea inferior.
 superior c. obere Choroidalvene *f*, Choroidea *f* superior, V. choroidea superior.
Chotzen ['ʃoʊtsən, 'kɔː-]: **C. syndrome** *embryo., ortho.* Chotzen-(Saethre-)Syndrom *nt*, Akrozephalosyndaktylie Typ III *f*.
Christensen ['krɪstənsən]: **C.'s urea agar** *micro.* Harnstoffagar *m/nt* nach Christensen.
Christian ['krɪstʃən]: **C.'s disease/syndrome 1.** Hand-Schüller-Christian-Krankheit *f*, Schüller-Hand-Christian-Krankheit *f*, Schüller-Krankheit *f*. **2.** → Christian-Weber disease.
Christiansen-Douglas-Haldane ['krɪstʃənsən 'dʌɡləs 'hɔldeɪn]: **C.-D.-H. effect** Christiansen-Douglas-Haldane-Effekt *m*, Haldane-Effekt *m*.
Christian-Weber ['vaɪbər]: **C.-W. disease** (Pfeiffer-)Weber-Christian-Syndrom *nt*, rezidivierende fieberhafte nicht-eitrige Pannikulitis *f*, Panniculitis nodularis nonsuppurativa febrilis et recidivans.
Christmas ['krɪsməs]: **C. factor** *abbr.* **CF** Faktor IX *m abbr.* F IX, Christmas-Faktor *m*, Autothrombin II *nt*.
 C. disease Hämophilie B *f*, Christmas--Krankheit *f*, Faktor IX-Mangel(krankheit *f*) *m*.
Christopher ['krɪstəfər]: **C.'s spots** Maurer-Tüpfelung *f*, -Körnelung *f*.
Christ-Siemens [krɪst 'siːmənz]: **C.-S. syndrome** → Christ-Siemens-Touraine syndrome.
Christ-Siemens-Touraine [tuˈreːn]: **C.-S.-T. syndrome** Christ-Siemens-Syn-

chrom-

drom *nt*, Guilford-Syndrom *nt*, Jacquet'--Syndrom *nt*, (anhidrotisch) ektodermale Dysplasie *f*, ektodermale kongenitale Dysplasie *f*, Anhidrosis hypotrichotica/congenita.
chrom- *pref.* → chromo-.
chro·maf·fin [krəʊˈmæfɪn, ˈkrəʊmə-] *adj histol*. chromaffin, chromaphil, phäochrom.
chomaffin body Paraganglion *nt*.
chromaffin cells chromaffine/phäochrome Zellen *pl*.
chromaffin-cell tumor Phäochromozytom *nt*.
chro·maf·fine [krəʊˈmæfiːn, ˈkrəʊmə-] *adj* → chromaffin.
chromaffine paraganglia sympathische Paraganglien *pl*.
chro·maf·fin·i·ty [ˌkrəʊməˈfɪnəti] *n histol*. Chromaffinität *f*.
chro·maf·fi·no·blas·to·ma [krəʊˌmæfɪnəʊblæsˈtəʊmə] *n patho*. Chromaffinoblastom *nt*, Argentaffinom *nt*.
chro·maf·fi·no·ma [krəʊməfɪˈnəʊmə] *n patho*. chromaffiner Tumor *m*, Chromaffinom *nt*.
chro·maf·fi·nop·a·thy [ˌ-ˈnɑpəθɪ] *n patho*. Erkrankung *f* des chromaffinen Systems, Chromaffinopathie *f*.
chromaffin system chromaffines System *nt*.
chromaffin tissue chromaffines Gewebe *nt*.
chromaffin tumor Paragangliom(a) *nt*.
chro·ma·phil [ˈkrəʊməfɪl] *adj* → chromaffin.
chrom·ar·gen·taf·fin [ˌkrəʊmɑːrˈdʒentəfɪn] *adj histol*. chromargentaffin.
chromat- *pref.* → chromato-.
chro·mate [ˈkrəʊmeɪt] I *n* Chromat *nt*. II *vt* chromieren, verchromen; mit Chromsalzlösung behandeln.
chro·mat·ic [krəʊˈmætɪk] *adj* 1. Farbe betr., chromatisch, Farben-. 2. → chromatinic.
chromatic aberration chromatische Aberration *f*, Newton-Aberration *f*.
chromatic audition *neuro*., *HNO* Auditio chromatica/colorata.
chromatic granules Nissl-Schollen *pl*, -Substanz *f*, -Granula *pl*, Tigroidschollen *pl*.
chro·ma·tic·i·ty diagram [ˌkrəʊməˈtɪsəti] *phys*. Farbendreieck *nt*.
chromatic spectrum Spektrum *nt* des sichtbaren Lichtes.
chromatic vision → chromatopsia.
chro·ma·tid [ˈkrəʊmətɪd] *n* Chromatid *nt*, Chromatide *f*.
chromatid segment Chromatidabschnitt *m*.
chro·ma·tin [ˈkrəʊmətɪn] *n* 1. Chromatin *nt*. 2. Heterochromatin *nt*.
chromatin fiber Chromatinfaden *m*.
chro·ma·tin·ic [ˌkrəʊməˈtɪnɪk] *adj* Chromatin betr., aus Chromatin bestehend, Chromatin-.
chromatinic body Nukleoid *m*, Karyoid *m*, (Bakterien-)Chromosom *nt*.
chromatin-negative *adj bio., genet.* chromatinnegativ.
chromatin nucleolus Karyosom *nt*.
chro·ma·ti·nol·y·sis [krəʊmətɪˈnɑləsɪs] *n* → chromatolysis.
chro·mat·i·nor·rhex·is [krəʊˌmætɪnəˈreksɪs] *n histol*. Chromatinauflösung *f*, -fragmentation *f*, Chromat(in)orrhexis *f*.
chromatin-positive *adj bio, genet*. chromatinpositiv.
chromatin reservoir Karyosom *nt*..
chro·ma·tism [ˈkrəʊmətɪzəm] *n* 1. pathologische Pigmentablagerung/Pigmentierung *f*. 2. → chromatic aberration.
chromato- *pref.* Farb-, Chromat(o)-.
chro·mat·o·blast [krəˈmætəblæst] *n histol*. Chromatoblast *m*.
chro·ma·ci·ne·sis [ˌkrəʊmətəʊsɪˈniːsɪs] *n* → chromatokinesis.
chro·ma·to·der·ma·to·sis [ˌ-ˌdɜːrməˈtəʊsɪs] *n derm*. Chromatodermatose *f*, -dermatosis *f*, Chromatose *f*, Pigmentanomalie *f*.
chro·ma·tog·e·nous [krəʊməˈtɑdʒənəs] *adj* farb(stoff)bildend, chromatogen, chromogen.
chro·mat·o·gram [krəˈmætəgræm, ˈkrəʊmətə-] *n* Chromatogramm *nt*.
chro·mat·o·graph [krəˈmætəgræf] I *n* Chromatograph *m*. II *vt* mittels Chromatographie analysieren, chromatographieren.
chro·mat·o·graph·ic [krəˌmætəˈgræfɪk, ˌkrəʊmətə-] *adj* Chromatographie betr., mittels Chromatographie, chromatographisch.
chromatographic analysis → chromatography.
chro·ma·tog·ra·phy [ˌkrəʊməˈtɑgrəfɪ] *n* Chromatographie *f*.
chro·ma·toid [ˈkrəʊmətɔɪd] I *n histol*. Chromatoid *nt*. II *adj* → chromatoidal.
chro·ma·toid·al [krəʊməˈtɔɪdl] *adj histol*. chromatoid.
chromatoidal body Chromidialkörperchen *nt*.
chro·ma·to·ki·ne·sis [ˌkrəʊmətəʊkɪˈniːsɪs, -kaɪ-] *n histol*. Chromatokinese *f*.
chro·ma·tol·y·sis [ˌkrəʊməˈtɑləsɪs] *n histol*. Chromatinauflösung *f*, Chromatino-, Chromatolyse *f*, Tigrolyse *f*.
chro·ma·to·lyt·ic [ˌkrəʊmətəʊˈlɪtɪk] *adj* Chromatolyse betr., chromatinauflösend, chromatolytisch.
chro·ma·tom·e·ter [ˌkrəʊməˈtɑmɪtər] *n* 1. Chromometer *nt*, Kolorimeter *nt*. 2. Chromatoptometer *nt*, Chromoptometer *nt*.
chro·ma·top·a·thy [ˌ-ˈtɑpəθɪ] *n* → chromatodermatosis.
chro·ma·to·pec·tic [ˌkrəʊmətəˈpektɪk] *adj* → chromopectic.
chro·ma·to·pex·is [ˌ-ˈpeksɪs] *n* → chromopexy.
chro·ma·to·phil [ˈ-fɪl] *n*, *adj* → chromophil.
chro·ma·to·phile [ˈ-fɪl] *n*, *adj* → chromophil.
chro·ma·to·phil·ia [ˌ-ˈfɪlɪə] *n histol*. Chromatophilie *f*.
chro·ma·to·phil·ic [ˌ-ˈfɪlɪk] *adj* → chromophil II.
chro·ma·toph·i·lous [ˌkrəʊməˈtɑfɪləs] *adj* → chromophil II.
chro·ma·to·pho·bia [ˌkrəʊmətəˈfəʊbɪə] *n* → chromophobia.
chro·ma·to·phore [ˈ-fɔːr, -fəʊr] *n* 1. Chromatophor *m*. 2. → chromophore.
chromatophore nevus of Naegeli Franceschetti-Jadassohn-Syndrom *nt*, Naegeli-Syndrom *nt*, Naegeli-Bloch--Sulzberger-Syndrom *nt*, retikuläre Pigmentdermatose *f*, Melanophorennaevus *m*, familiärer Chromatophorennaevus *m*, Incontinentia pigmenti Typ Franceschetti-Jadassohn.
chro·ma·to·phor·o·trop·ic [ˌ-ˌfɔːrəˈtrɑpɪk, -ˈtrəʊp-] *adj histol*. chromatophorotrop.
chro·ma·to·plasm [ˈ-plæzəm] *n histol*. Chromatoplasma *nt*.
chro·ma·top·sia [krəʊməˈtɑpsɪə] *n* Farbensehen *nt*, Chromatop(s)ie *f*, Chromopsie *f*.
chro·ma·top·tom·e·ter [ˌ-tɑpˈtɑmɪtər] *n* → chromatometer 2.

chro·ma·top·tom·e·try [ˌ-tɑpˈtɑmətrɪ] *n ophthal*. Chromatoptometrie *f*, Chromoptometrie *f*.
chro·mat·o·scope [krəˈmætəskəʊp] *n* Chromatoskop *nt*, Chromoskop *nt*.
chro·ma·tos·co·py [ˌkrəʊməˈtɑskəpɪ] *n* 1. *ophthal*. Chromatoskopie *f*, Chromoskopie *f*. 2. Chromodiagnostik *f*, Chrom(at)oskopie *f*.
chro·ma·to·sis [ˌ-ˈtəʊsɪs] *n* 1. *histol*. Pigmentierung *f*. 2. → chromatodermatosis.
chro·ma·tot·ro·pism [ˌ-ˈtɑtrəpɪzəm] *n* Chromatotropismus *m*.
chro·ma·tu·ria [ˌ-ˈt(j)ʊərɪə] *n* (pathologische) Harnverfärbung *f*, Chromaturie *f*.
chrome [krəʊm] I *n* 1. → chromium. 2. Kalium-, Natriumdichromat *nt*. II *vt* chromate II.
chrom·es·the·sia [ˌkrəʊmesˈθiːʒ(ɪ)ə, -zɪə] *n neuro*. Chromästhesie *f*.
chrome ulcer Chromatgeschwür *nt*, -ulkus *nt*.
chrome yellow Chromgelb *nt*, Bleichromat *nt*.
chrom·hi·dro·sis [ˌkrəʊmɪˈdrəʊsɪs, -haɪ-, -hɪ-] *n derm*. Chrom(h)idrosis *f*.
chro·mic [ˈkrəʊmɪk] *adj* Chrom betr., Chrom-.
chromic acid Chromsäure *f*.
chromic anhydride → chromic acid.
chromic catgut *chir*. Chromcatgut *nt*.
chro·mi·cized catgut [ˈkrəʊməsaɪzd] *chir*. Chromcatgut *nt*.
chro·mid·i·al substance [krəʊˈmɪdɪəl] rauhes/granuläres endoplasmatisches Retikulum *nt abbr*. R-ER.
chro·mid·i·um [krəʊˈmɪdɪəm] *n*, *pl* **-dia** [-dɪə] *histol*. Chromidium *nt*, Chromidie *f*.
chro·mi·dro·sis [krəʊmɪˈdrəʊsɪs] *n* → chromhidrosis.
chro·mi·um [ˈkrəʊmɪəm] *n abbr*. **Cr** Chrom *nt abbr*. Cr.
chromo- *pref.* Farb(en)-, Chrom(o)-.
chromo bacteria pigmentbildende/chromogene Bakterien *pl*.
Chro·mo·bac·te·ri·um [ˌkrəʊməʊbækˈtɪərɪəm] *n micro*. Chromobacterium *nt*.
chro·mo·blast [ˈ-blæst] *n embryo*. Chromoblast *m*.
chro·mo·blas·to·my·co·sis [ˌ-ˌblæstəʊmaɪˈkəʊsɪs] *n* → chromomycosis.
chro·mo·cen·ter [ˈ-sentər] *n* Karyosom *nt*.
chro·mo·cho·los·co·py [ˌ-kəˈlɑskəpɪ] *chir*. Chromocholoskopie *f*.
chro·mo·cys·tos·co·py [ˌ-sɪsˈtɑskəpɪ] *urol*. Chromozystoskopie *f*.
chro·mo·cyte [ˈ-saɪt] *n histol*. pigmenthaltige/pigmentierte Zelle *f*, Chromozyt *m*.
chro·mo·di·ag·no·sis [ˌ-daɪəgˈnəʊsɪs] *n* Chromodiagnostik *f*.
chro·mo·gen [ˈ-dʒən] *n* 1. *chem*. Chromogen *nt*. 2. *bio*. chromogener Organismus *m*.
chro·mo·gen·e·sis [ˌ-ˈdʒenəsɪs] *n* Farbstoffbildung *f*, Chromogenese *f*.
chro·mo·gen·ic [ˌ-ˈdʒenɪk] *adj* farbstoffbildend, chromogen.
chromogenic bacteria pigmentbildende/chromogene Bakterien *pl*.
chro·mo·i·som·er·ism [ˌ-ɪˈsɑmərɪzəm] *n chem*. Chromoisomerie *f*.
chro·mo·lip·oid [ˌ-ˈlɪpɔɪd, -ˈlaɪ-] *n* Lipochrom *nt*, Lipoidpigment *nt*.
chro·mol·y·sis [krəʊˈmɑləsɪs] *n* → chromatolysis.
chro·mo·mere [ˈkrəʊməmɪər] *n* 1. *histol*. Chromomer *nt*. 2. Granulomer *nt*.
chro·mom·e·ter [krəʊˈmɑmɪtər] *n* → chromatometer 1.
chro·mo·my·co·sis [ˌkrəʊməmaɪˈkəʊsɪs] *n* Chromo(blasto)mykose *f*.

chro·mo·nar ['-nɑːr] *n pharm.* Carbocromen *nt.*
chro·mone ['krəʊməʊn] *n* **1.** Kumarin *nt*, Cumarin *nt.* **2.** Kumarinderivat *nt.*
chro·mo·ne·ma [ˌkrəʊməˈniːmə] *n, pl* **-ne·ma·ta** [-ˈniːmətə] Chromonema *f.*
chro·mo·neme ['-niːm] *n* → chromonema.
chro·mo·nu·cle·ic acid [ˌ-nʊˈkliːɪk, -ˈkleɪ-; -ˈn(j)uːkliːɪk] Desoxyribonukleinsäure *f abbr.* DNS, DNA.
chro·mo·par·ic [ˌ-ˈpærɪk] *adj* → chromogenic.
chro·mop·a·thy [krəʊˈmɑpəθɪ] *n* → chromatodermatosis.
chro·mo·pec·tic [ˌkrəʊməˈpektɪk] *adj* Chromopexie betr. *od.* fördernd, pigmentbindend, -fixierend.
chro·mo·pex·ic [ˌ-ˈpeksɪk] *adj* → chromopectic.
chro·mo·pex·is [ˌ-ˈpeksɪs] *n* → chromopexy.
chro·mo·pex·y ['-peksɪ] *n* Pigmentfixierung *f*, -bindung *f*, Chromopexie *f.*
chro·mo·phage ['-feɪdʒ] *n histol.* Chromophage *m.*
chro·mo·phil ['-fɪl] **I** *n* chromophile Struktur *od.* Zelle *f.* **II** *adj* chromophil, chromatophil.
chromophil corpuscles → chromophilous bodies
chro·mo·phile ['-faɪl, -fɪl] *n, adj* → chromophil.
chro·mo·phil·ic [ˌ-ˈfɪlɪk] *adj* → chromophil II.
chromophilic granules → chromophilous bodies
chro·moph·i·lous [krəʊˈmɑfɪləs] *adj* → chromophil II.
chromophilous bodies Nissl-Schollen *pl*, -Substanz *f*, -Granula *pl*, Tigroidschollen *pl.*
chromophil substance → chromophilous bodies
chro·mo·phobe ['krəʊməfəʊb] **I** *n* **1.** chromophobe Zelle *od.* Struktur *f.* **2.** (*Adenohypophyse*) chromophobe Zelle *f*, γ-Zelle *f.* **II** *adj* schwer anfärbbar, chromophob.
chromophobe adenoma chromophobes (Hypophysen-)Adenom *nt.*
chromophobe cell → chromophobe I.
chro·mo·pho·bia [ˌ-ˈfəʊbɪə] *n histol.* Chromophobie *f.*
chro·mo·pho·bic [ˌ-ˈfəʊbɪk] *adj* → chromophobe II.
chromophobic adenoma → chromophobe adenoma
chromophobic cell → chromophobe I.
chro·mo·phore ['-fɔːr, -fəʊr] *n* Farbradikal *nt*, Chromophor *nt.*
chro·mo·phor·ic [ˌ-ˈfɔːrɪk, -ˈfɑr-] *adj* **1.** farbgebend, chromophor. **2.** *bio.* farbtragend, chromophor.
chro·moph·o·rous [krəʊˈmɑfərəs] *adj* → chromophoric.
chro·mo·pho·to·ther·a·py [ˌkrəʊməˌfəʊtəˈθerəpɪ] *n* Chromophototherapie *f*, Buntlichttherapie *f.*
chro·mo·plasm ['-plæzəm] *n* → chromatin.
chro·mo·plast ['-plæst] *n bio.* Chromoplast *m.*
chro·mo·plas·tid [ˌ-ˈplæstɪd] *n bio.* Chromoplastid *m.*
chro·mo·pro·te·in [ˌ-ˈprəʊtiːn, -tiːɪn] *n* Chromoprotein *nt*, -proteid *nt.*
chro·mo·pro·tein·u·ric nephrosis [ˌ-ˌprəʊtɪˈn(j)ʊərɪk] *patho.* chromoproteinurische Nephrose *f*, Chromoproteinniere *f*; Crush-Niere *f.*
chro·mop·sia [krəʊˈmɑpsɪə] *n* → chromatopsia.
chrom·op·tom·e·ter [ˌkrəʊmɑpˈtɑmətər] *n* → chromatometer 2.

chro·mo·ret·i·nog·ra·phy [ˌkrəʊməretɪˈnɑɡrəfɪ] *n ophthal.* Chromoretinographie *f.*
chro·mo·scope ['-skəʊp] *n* → chromatoscope.
chro·mos·co·py [krəʊˈmɑskəpɪ] *n* → chromatoscopy.
chro·mo·so·mal [ˌkrəʊməˈsəʊml] *adj* Chromosom(en) betr., chromosomal, Chromosomen-.
chromosomal anomaly Chromosomenanomalie *f.*
chromosomal mutation Chromosomenmutation *f.*
 numerical c. numerische Chromosomenmutation.
 structural c. strukturelle Chromosomenmutation.
chromosomal resistance *micro., pharm.* chromosomale Resistenz *f.*
chromosomal sex chromosomales/genetisches Geschlecht *nt.*
chro·mo·some ['krəʊməsəʊm] *n* **1.** Chromosom *nt.* **2.** *bio.* (Bakterien-)Chromosom *nt*, Nukleoid *m*, Karyoid *m.*
chromosome aberration Chromosomenaberration *f.*
 autosome c. Autosomenaberration, autosomale Chromosomenaberration.
 genetical c. genetische Chromosomenaberration.
 sex c. Heterosomenaberration, gonosomale Chromosomenaberration.
chromosome abnormality Chromosomenanomalie *f*, -aberration *f.*
 autosome c. autosomale Chromosomenanomalie.
 genetic c. genetische Chromosomenanomalie.
 sex c. gonosomale Chromosomenanomalie.
 structural c. Strukturanomalie.
chromosome anomaly Chromosomenanomalie *f.*
chromosome arm Chromosomenarm *m.*
chromosome band Chromosomenbande *f.*
chromosome banding Chromosomenbanding *nt.*
chromosome complement Chromosomensatz *m.*
 aneuploid c. aneuploider Chromosomensatz.
 diploid c. diploider Chromosomensatz.
 haploid c. haploider Chromosomensatz.
chromosome pairing Chromosomenpaarung *f.*
chromosome puff *genet.* Puff *m.*
chro·mo·tox·ic [ˌkrəʊməˈtɑksɪk] *adj* Hämoglobin zerstörend, durch Hämoglobinzerstörung hervorgerufen, chromotoxisch.
chro·mo·trich·ia [ˌ-ˈtrɪkɪə] *n derm.* Haarfarbe *f*, -färbung *f*, pigmentiertes Haar *nt*, Chromotrichie *f*, -trichia *f.*
chro·mo·trop·i·cal factor [ˌ-ˈtrɪkɪəl] *p*-Aminobenzoesäure *f*, para-Aminobenzoesäure *f*, Paraaminobenzoesäure *f abbr.* PABA, PAB.
chro·mo·trop·ic [ˌ-ˈtrɑpɪk] *adj* chromotrop.
chro·mo·u·re·ter·os·co·py [ˌ-jəˌriːtəˈrɑskəpɪ] *n* → chromocystoscopy.
chron- *pref.* → chrono-.
chro·nax·ia [krəʊˈnæksɪə] *n* → chronaxy.
chro·nax·ie ['krəʊnæksɪ] *n* → chronaxy.
chro·nax·im·e·ter [ˌkrəʊnækˈsɪmətər] *n physiol.* Chronaxi(e)meter *nt.*
chro·nax·im·e·try [ˌ-ˈsɪmətrɪ] *n physiol.* Chronaxi(e)metrie *f.*
chro·nax·is [krəʊˈnæksɪs] *n* → chronaxy.
chro·nax·y ['krəʊnæksɪ, krəʊˈnæk-] *n physiol.* Kennzeit *f*, Chronaxie *f.*

chronic glomerulonephritis

chron·ic ['krɑnɪk] *adj s.* langsam entwickelnd, langsam verlaufend, (an-)dauernd, anhaltend, langwierig, chronisch, Dauer-.
chronic abscess chronischer/kalter Abszeß *m.*
chronic acholuric jaundice → chronic familial icterus.
chronic active/aggressive hepatitis chronisch-aktive/chronisch-aggressive Hepatitis *f abbr.* CAH.
chron·i·cal ['krɑnɪkl] *adj* → chronic.
chronic alcoholic hepatitis chronische Alkoholhepatitis *f*, alkohol-toxische Hepatitis *f.*
chronic alcoholism chronischer Alkoholismus *m.*
chronic appendicitis chronische Blinddarmreizung/Appendizitis *f*, Appendicitis chronica.
chronic arthritis chronische Gelenkentzündung/Arthritis *f*, Arthritis chronica.
chronic atrophic gastritis chronisch-atrophische Magenschleimhautentzündung *f*, Gastritis *f.*
chronic brain syndrome *abbr.* **CBS** chronisch-organisches Psychosyndrom *nt*, chronisches psychoorganisches Syndrom *nt.*
chronic bronchitis chronische Bronchitis *f*, Bronchitis chronica.
chronic carrier *micro.* Dauerträger *m*, -ausscheider *m.*
chronic catarrhal laryngitis chronische katarrhalische Laryngitis *f.*
chronic cholecystitis chronische Gallenentzündung/Cholezystitis *f.*
chronic chorea Erbchorea *f*, Chorea Huntington, Chorea chronica progressiva hereditaria.
chronic cicatrizing enteritis → Crohn's disease.
chronic circumscribed plasmocytic balanoposthitis Balanitis chronica circumscripta benigna plasmacellularis (Zoon).
chronic cystic gastritis chronisch-zystische Gastritis *f.*
chronic cystic mastitits → cystic disease of the breast.
chronic cystitis chronische Blasenentzündung/Zystitis *f*, Cystitis chronica.
chronic desquamative gingivitis chronisch desquamative Gingivitis *f.*
chronic destructive interstitial nephritis chronisch interstitielle destruierende Nephritis *f.*
chronic diffuse alopecia in women weiblicher Typ *m* der Alopecia androgenetica.
chronic eczema lichenifiziertes Ekzem *nt.*
chronic endemic fluorosis chronische Fluorvergiftung *f*, Fluorose *f.*
chronic eosinophilic pneumonia eosinophile Pneumonie *f*, eosinophiles Lungeninfiltrat *nt.*
chronic familial icterus hereditäre Sphärozytose *f*, Kugelzell(en)anämie *f*, Kugelzell(en)ikterus *m*, familiärer hämolytischer Ikterus *m*, Morbus Minkowski--Chauffard.
chronic familial jaundice → chronic familial icterus.
chronic fatty degeneration pneumonia chronisch verfettende Pneumonie *f.*
chronic fibrous thyroiditis eisenharte Struma Riedel *f*, Riedel-Struma *f*, chronische hypertrophische Thyreoiditis *f.*
chronic follicular gastritis chronisch-follikuläre Gastritis *f.*
chronic glaucoma Simplex-, Weitwinkelglaukom *nt*, Glaucoma simplex.
chronic glomerulonephritis chronische Glomerulonephritis *f.*

chronic granulocytic leukemia → chronic myelocytic leukemia.
chronic granulomatous disease (of childhood) abbr. **CGD** (progressive) septische Granulomatose f, kongenitale Dysphagozytose f.
chronic heart failure chronische Herzinsuffizienz f.
chronic hemorrhagic villous synovitis pigmentierte villonoduläre Synovitis f abbr. PVNS, benignes Synovialom nt, Riesenzelltumor m der Sehnenscheide, Tendosynovitis nodosa, Arthritis villonodularis pigmentosa.
chronic hepatitis chronische Leberentzündung/Hepatitis f.
chronic hyperplastic rhinitis chronische hyperplastische Rhinitis/Rhinopathie f, Rhinitis hyperplastica/hypertrophicans, Rhinopathia chronica hyperplastica.
chronic hypertrophic bronchitis chronisch-hypertrophische Bronchitis f, Bronchitis hypertrophicans.
chronic hypertrophic emphysema panazinäres/panlobuläres/diffuses Lungenemphysem nt.
chronic hypocomplementemic glomerulonephritis membranoproliferative Glomerulonephritis f.
chronic idiopathic hypotension Shy-Drager-Syndrom nt.
chronic idiopathic jaundice Dubin-Johnson-Syndrom nt.
chronic idiopathic xanthomatosis Hand-Schüller-Christian-Krankheit f, Schüller-Hand-Christian-Krankheit f, Schüller-Krankheit f.
chronic inflammation chronische Entzündung f.
chronic inflammatory arthritis rheumatoide Arthritis f, progrediente/primär chronische Polyarthritis f abbr. PCP, PcP.
chronic interstitial cystitis chronisch interstitielle (Harn-)Blasenentzündung/Zystitis f, Cystitis intermuralis/interstitialis.
chronic interstitial hepatitis → cirrhosis of liver.
chronic interstitial nephritis chronisch-interstitielle Nephritis f.
chronic interstitial salpingitis patho., gyn. chronisch interstitielle Salpingitis f.
chro·nic·i·ty [krəˈnɪsətɪ] n langsamer schleichender Verlauf m (einer Krankheit); chronischer Zustand m, Chronizität f.
chronic leukemia abbr. **CL** chronische/reifzellige Leukämie f abbr. CL.
chronic lichenoid pityriasis Pityriasis lichenoides chronica.
chronic lymphadenoid thyroiditis Hashimoto-Thyreoiditis f, Struma lymphomatosa.
chronic lymphocytic leukemia abbr. **CLL** chronische lymphatische Leukämie f abbr. CLL, chronische lymphozytische Leukämie f, chronische Lymphadenose f.
chronic lymphocytic thyroiditis Hashimoto-Thyreoiditis f, Struma lymphomatosa.
chronic malaria chronische Malaria f.
chronic mastoiditis HNO chronische Mastoiditis f.
chronic mountain sickness Monge'-Krankheit f, chronische Höhenkrankheit f.
chronic myelocytic leukemia abbr. **CML** chronische myeloische Leukämie f abbr. CML, chronische granulozytäre Leukämie f, chronische Myelose f.

chronic nephritis → chronic glomerulonephritis.
chronic neuropsychologic disorder → chronic brain syndrome.
chronic nonleukemic myelosis idiopathische/primäre myeloische Metaplasie f, Leukoerythroblastose f, leukoerythroblastische Anämie f.
chronic nonsuppurative destructive cholangitis primär biliäre Zirrhose abbr. PBZ, nicht-eitrige destruierende Cholangitis f.
chronic nonsuppurative osteitis nicht-eitrige Osteomyelitis f, sklerosierende Osteomyelitis f, Garré'-Osteomyelitis f, -Krankheit f, Osteomyelitis sicca Garré.
chronic nonsuppurative osteomyelitis → chronic nonsuppurative osteitis.
chronic obstructive airways disease abbr. **COAD** → chronic obstructive lung disease.
chronic obstructive lung disease abbr. **COLD** chronisch-obstruktive Lungenerkrankung/Atemwegserkrankung f.
chronic obstructive pulmonary disease abbr. **COPD** → chronic obstructive lung disease.
chronic organic brain syndrome → chronic brain syndrome.
chronic osteitis chronische Knochenentzündung f, Ostitis chronica.
chronic pain chronischer Schmerz m, chronische Schmerzen pl.
chronic pancreatitis chronische Bauchspeicheldrüsenentzündung/Pankreatitis f.
chronic parapsoriasis → chronic lichenoid pityriasis.
chronic peptic esophagitis Refluxösophagitis f.
chronic pericarditis chronische Herzbeutelentzündung/Perikarditis f.
chronic persistent/persisting hepatitis chronisch-persistierende Hepatitis f abbr. CPH.
chronic pharyngitis Pharyngitis chronica.
chronic pneumonia chronische Lungenentzündung/Pneumonie f.
chronic progressive hereditary chorea → chronic chorea.
chronic progressive nonhereditary chorea senile Chorea f, nicht-hereditäre Chorea f.
chronic pyelonephritis chronische Nierenbeckenentzündung/Pyelonephritis f, chronisch interstitielle destruierende Nephritis f.
chronic recurrent pancreatitis chronisch-rezidivierende Pankreatitis f.
chronic rejection chir. chronische Abstoßung(sreaktion f) f.
chronic relapsing osteomyelitis patho. chronisch-rezidivierende Osteomyelitis f.
chronic respiratory disease abbr. **CRD** chronische Atemwegserkrankung.
chronic rhinitis chronische Rhinitis/Rhinopathie f.
chronic rhinopharyngitis chronische Rhinopharyngitis f.
chronic sinusitis HNO chronische (Nasen-)Nebenhöhlenentzündung/Sinusitis f.
chronic sleeping sickness westafrikanische Schlafkrankheit/Trypano(so)miasis f.
chronic stroke Monge'-Krankheit f, chronische Höhenkrankheit f.
chronic subcortical encephalitis Binswanger-Enzephalopathie f, subkortikale progressive Enzephalopathie f, Encephalopathia chronica progressiva subcorticalis.
chronic subglottic laryngitis chronische

subglottische Laryngitis f, Chorditis vocalis inferior, Laryngitis subglottica chronica.
chronic superficial dermatitis Brocq'-Krankheit f, chronische superfizielle Dermatitis f, Parapsoriasis en plaques.
chronic superficial gastritis chronische Oberflächengastritis f.
chronic suppurative osteitis sklerosierende/nicht-eitrige Osteomyelitis f, Garré'-Osteomyelitis f, -Krankheit f, Osteomyelitis sicca Garré.
chronic suppurative pericementitis Alveolarpyorrhoe f, Parodontitis marginalis.
chronic thyroiditis eisenharte Struma Riedel f, Riedel-Struma f, chronische hypertrophische Thyreoiditis f.
chronic tonsillitis HNO chronische Tonsillitis f.
chronic tophaceous gout ortho. chronisches Gichtstadium nt.
chronic ulcer chronisches Geschwür nt.
chronic urticaria chronische Urtikaria f, Urticaria chronica.
chronic vertigo chronischer Schwindel m, Status vertiginosus.
chronic villous arthritis chronisch villöse Arthritis f, Arthritis chronica villosa.
chrono- pref. Zeit-, Chron(o)-.
chron·o·bi·o·log·ic [ˌkrɒnəʊˌbaɪəˈlɒdʒɪk, ˌkrɒn-] adj Chronobiologie betr., chronobiologisch.
chron·o·bi·o·log·i·cal [ˌ-ˌbaɪəˈlɒdʒɪkl] adj → chronobiologic.
chron·o·bi·ol·o·gy [ˌ-baɪˈɒlədʒɪ] n Chronobiologie f.
chron·og·no·sis [ˌkrɒnɒɡˈnəʊsɪs] n Zeitgefühl nt, Chronognosie f.
chron·o·graph [ˈkrɒnəɡræf] n Chronograph m.
chron·o·log·i·cal [ˌ-ˈlɒdʒɪkl] adj chronologisch; zeitlich; kalendarisch.
chronological age abbr. **CA** kalendarisches Alter nt.
chronological order chronologische Reihenfolge f.
chron·o·log·ic disorientation [ˌ-ˈlɒdʒɪk] neuro. zeitliche Desorientiertheit f.
chro·nol·o·gize [krəˈnɒlədʒaɪz] vt chronologisieren, nach dem zeitlichen Verlauf ordnen.
chron·om·e·ter [krəˈnɒmɪtər] n Zeitmesser m, Chronometer nt.
chron·o·met·ric [ˌkrɒnəˈmɛtrɪk] adj chronometrisch.
chron·o·met·ri·cal [ˌ-ˈmɛtrɪkl] adj → chronometric.
chron·om·e·try [krəˈnɒmɪtrɪ] n Zeitmessung f, Chronometrie f.
chron·o·phar·ma·col·o·gy [ˌkrɒnəˌfɑːməˈkɒlədʒɪ] n Chronopharmakologie f.
chron·o·pho·bia [ˌ-ˈfəʊbɪə] n psychia. Zeitfurcht f, Chronophobie f.
chron·o·pho·to·graph [ˌ-ˈfəʊtəɡræf] n radiol. Chronophotographie f.
chron·o·phys·i·ol·o·gy [ˌ-ˌfɪzɪˈɒlədʒɪ] n Chronophysiologie f.
chron·o·scope [ˈ-skəʊp] n Chronoskop nt.
chron·o·trop·ic [ˌ-ˈtrɒpɪk, -ˈtrəʊ-] adj chronotrop.
chro·not·ro·pism [krəˈnɒtrəpɪzəm] n Chronotropie f, -tropismus m, chronotrope Wirkung f.
chrys- pref. → chryso-.
chrys·a·ro·bin [ˌkrɪsəˈrəʊbɪn] n pharm. Chrysarobin nt.
chry·si·a·sis [krɪˈsaɪəsɪs] n 1. derm. Chrysiasis f, Auriasis f. 2. → chrysoderma.
chryso- pref. Gold-, Chrys(o)-, Aur(o)-.
chrys·o·der·ma [ˌkrɪsəˈdɜːmə] n derm. Chrysoderma nt, Chrysosis f.

chrys·oi·din ['krɪsɔɪdɪn] *n pharm., histol.* Chrysoidin *nt.*
Chrys·o·my·ia [krɪsə'maɪ(j)ə] *pl micro.* Chrysom(y)ia *pl.*
Chrys·ops ['krɪsɑps] *n micro.* Blindbremse *f,* Chrysops *f.*
Chrys·o·spor·i·um [ˌkrɪsə'spɔʊrɪəm] *n micro.* Chrysosporium *nt.*
chrys·o·ther·a·py [ˌ-'θerəpɪ] *n* Gold-, Chryso-, Aurotherapie *f.*
CHS *abbr.* → Chédiak-Higashi syndrome.
chthon·o·pha·gia [ˌθɑnə'feɪdʒ(ɪ)ə] *n psychia.* Erdeessen *nt,* Geophagie *f.*
chtho·noph·a·gy [θə'nɑpədʒɪ] *n* → chthonophagia.
Churg-Strauss [tʃɑrg straʊs]: **C.-S. syndrome** Churg-Strauss-Syndrom *nt,* allergische granulomatöse Angiitis *f.*
Chvostek ['vɑstek]: **C.'s sign** *neuro.* Chvostek-Zeichen *nt.*
C.'s symptom → C.'s sign.
C.'s test → C.'s sign.
Chvostek-Weiss ['vaɪs]: **C.-W. sign** → Chvostek's sign.
chyl·an·gi·ec·ta·sia [kaɪˌlændʒɪek'teɪʒ(ɪ)ə] *n* → chyle cyst.
chyl·an·gi·o·ma [kaɪˌlændʒɪ'əʊmə] *n patho.* Chylangiom(a) *nt.*
chy·la·que·ous [kaɪ'lækwɪəs] *adj* wäßrig--chylös.
chyle [kaɪl] *n* Milchsaft *m,* Chylus *m.*
chyle bladder Cisterna chyli.
chyle cistern Cisterna chyli.
chyl·ec·ta·sia [kaɪlek'teɪʒ(ɪ)ə] *n* → chyle cyst.
chyle cyst Chyluszyste *f,* Chyl(angi)ektasie *f.*
chyl·e·mia [kaɪ'liːmɪə] *n* Chylämie *f.*
chyle stasis Chylusstauung *f.*
chy·li·fa·cient [ˌkaɪlə'feɪʃənt] *adj* chylusbildend.
chy·li·fac·tion [ˌkaɪlə'fækʃn] *n biochem.* Chylusbildung *f,* primäre Fettassimilation *f.*
chy·li·fac·tive [ˌ-'fæktɪv] *adj* → chylifacient.
chy·lif·er·ous [kaɪ'lɪf(ə)rəs] *adj* **1.** → chylifacient. **2.** chylus(ab)führend.
chyliferous duct Brustmilchgang *m,* Milchbrustgang *m,* Ductus thoracicus.
chyliferous vessel (*Darm*) Lymphkapillare *f.*
chy·li·fi·ca·tion [ˌkaɪlɪfɪ'keɪʃn] *n* → chylifaction.
chy·li·form ['kaɪləfɔːrm] *adj* chylusähnlich, -artig, chylös.
chyliform ascites → chyloperitoneum.
chy·lo·cele ['-siːl] *n* **1.** Chylus-, Chylozele *f,* -cele *f.* **2.** Elephantiasis scroti.
chy·lo·cyst ['-sɪst] *n* Cisterna chyli.
chy·lo·der·ma [ˌ-'dɜrmə] *n patho.* Elephantiasis *f,* Chyloderma *nt.*
chy·loid ['kaɪlɔɪd] *adj* chylusähnlich, chylös.
chy·lo·me·di·as·ti·num [ˌkaɪləˌmɪdɪə'staɪnəm] *n patho.* Chylomediastinum *nt.*
chy·lo·mi·cron [ˌ-'maɪkrɑn] *n, pl* **-crons,** **-cra** [-krə] Chylo-, Lipomikron *nt,* Chyluströpfchen *nt,* -kügelchen *nt.*
chy·lo·mi·cro·ne·mia [ˌ-ˌmaɪkrə'niːmɪə] *n patho.* (Hyper-)Chylomikronämie *f.*
chy·lo·per·i·car·di·tis [ˌ-ˌperɪkɑː'daɪtɪs] *n patho.* Chyloperikarditis *f.*
chy·lo·per·i·car·di·um [ˌ-ˌperɪ'kɑːrdɪəm] *n patho.* Chyloperikard *nt.*
chy·lo·per·i·to·ne·um [ˌ-ˌperɪtə'nɪəm] *n patho.* Chyloperitoneum *nt,* Chylaskos *m,* Chylaszites *m.*
chy·lo·phor·ic [ˌ-'fɔːrɪk] *adj* chylus(ab)führend.
chy·lo·pleu·ra [ˌ-'plʊərə] *n* → chylothorax.
chy·lo·pneu·mo·tho·rax [ˌ-ˌn(j)uːmə'θəʊræks] *n patho.* Chylopneumothorax *m.*
chy·lo·poi·e·sis [ˌ-pɔɪ'iːsɪs] *n* Chylusbildung *f,* Chylopoese *f.*
chy·lo·poi·et·ic [ˌ-pɔɪ'etɪk] *adj* Chylopoese betr., chylusbildend, chylopoetisch.
chy·lor·rhe·a [ˌ-'rɪə] *n patho.* **1.** Chylorrhö *f,* Chylorrhoe *f.* **2.** chylöser Durchfall *m,* Chylorrhö *f,* Chylorrhoe *f.*
chy·lo·tho·rax [ˌ-'θɔʊræks] *n patho.* Chylothorax *m.*
chy·lous ['kaɪləs] *adj* Chylus betr., aus Chylus bestehend, chylusähnlich, -artig, chylös, Chylus-, Chyl(o)-.
chyious arthritis *ortho.* Filarienarthritis *f.*
chylous ascites → chyloperitoneum.
chylous diarrhea → chylorrhea 2.
chylous hydrocele Chylozele *f,* Hydrocele chylosa.
chylous hydrothorax → chylothorax.
chylous stasis Chylusstauung *f.*
chylous urine chylöser Urin *m;* Chylurie *f.*
chy·lu·ria [kaɪ'l(j)ʊərɪə] *n* Chylurie *f,* Chylolipurie *f,* Galakturie *f.*
chy·lus ['kaɪləs] *n* → chyle.
chy·mase ['kaɪmeɪz] *n* Chymase *f.*
chy·mi·fi·ca·tion [ˌkaɪməfɪ'keɪʃn] *n* Chymifikation *f,* Chymusbildung *f.*
chy·mo·pa·pa·in [ˌkaɪməʊpə'peɪɪn] *n* Chymopapain *nt.*
chy·mo·poi·e·sis [ˌ-pɔɪ'iːsɪs] *n* Chymusbildung *f,* Chymopoese *f.*
chy·mo·sin ['kaɪməsɪn] *n* Chymosin *nt,* Labferment *nt,* Rennin *nt.*
chy·mo·sin·o·gen [ˌ-'sɪnədʒən] *n* Prochymosin *nt,* Prorennin *nt.*
chy·mo·tryp·sin [ˌ-'trɪpsɪn] *n* Chymotrypsin *nt.*
chy·mo·tryp·sin·o·gen [ˌ-trɪp'sɪnədʒən] *n* Chymotrypsinogen *nt.*
chy·mous ['kaɪməs] *adj* Chymus betr., chymusartig, chymös.
chy·mus ['kaɪməs] *n* → chyme.
CI *abbr.* → cardiac index.
C.I. *abbr.* → color index.
Ci *abbr.* → curie.
Ciaccio ['tʃætʃəʊ]: **C.'s glands** Nebennierendrüsen *pl,* Gll. lacrimales accessoriae.
C.'s method *histol.* Ciaccio-Lipoidfärbung *f.*
C.'s stain → C.'s method.
ci·bo·pho·bia [ˌsaɪbəʊ'fəʊbɪə] *n psychia.* Cibophobie *f.*
cic·a·trec·to·my [ˌsɪkə'trektəmɪ] *n chir.* Narbenausschneidung *f,* -exzision *f.*
cic·a·tri·cial [ˌ-'trɪʃl] *adj* Narbe betr., narbig, vernarbend, zikatriziell, Narben-.
cicatricial alopecia narbige Alopezie *f,* Alopecia cicatricans.
cicatricial contracture *ortho.* Narbenkontraktur *f.*
cicatricial ectropion *ophthal.* Ektropium cicatriceum.
cicatricial keloid Narbenkeloid *nt.*
cicatricial kidney Narbenniere *f,* narbige Schrumpfniere *f.*
cicatricial pemphigoid vernarbendes Pemphigoid *nt,* benignes Schleimhautpemphigoid *nt,* okulärer Pemphigus *m,* Dermatitis pemphigoides mucocutanea chronica.
cicatricial pull *chir., ortho.* Narbenzug *m.*
cicatricial scoliosis *ortho.* Narbenskoliose *f.*
cicatricial stenosis narbige Stenose *f.*
cicatricial stricture Narbenstriktur *f.*
cic·a·tri·cle ['sɪkətrɪkl] *n gyn.* Cicatricula *f.*
cic·a·tri·cot·o·my [ˌsɪkətrɪ'kɑtəmɪ] *n chir.* Narbendurchtrennung *f,* -revision *f.*
cic·a·tri·sot·o·my [ˌ-trɪ'sɑtəmɪ] *n* → cicatricotomy.
cic·a·trix ['sɪkətrɪks] *n, pl* **cic·a·tri·ces** [sɪkə'traɪsiːz] Narbe *f,* Narbengewebe *nt,* Cicatrix *f.*
cic·a·tri·zant [ˌ-'traɪzənt] **I** *n* die Narbenbildung förderndes Mittel *nt.* **II** *adj* die Narbenbildung fördernd *od.* auslösend.
cic·a·tri·za·tion [ˌ-trɪ'zeɪʃn] *n* Narbenbildung *f,* Vernarben *nt,* Synulosis *m.*
cic·a·trize ['sɪkətraɪz] **I** *vt* vernarben lassen. **II** *vi* vernarben, mit Narbenbildung verheilen.
ci·clo·pir·ox [ˌsaɪkləʊ'pɪərɑks] *n pharm.* Ciclopirox *nt.*
cic·u·tine ['sɪkjətiːn] *n* Cicutin *nt,* Cicutinum *nt,* Koniin *nt,* Coniin *nt,* Coniinum *nt.*
cic·u·tism ['sɪkjətɪzəm] *n* Wasserschierlingvergiftung *f,* Cicutismus *m.*
cic·u·tox·in [ˌsɪkjə'tɑksɪn] *n* Cicutoxin *nt.*
CIE *abbr.* → counterimmunoelectrophoresis.
ci·gua·te·ra [ˌsiːgwə'terə] *n* Ciguatera *f.*
cig·u·a·tox·in [ˌ-'tɑksɪn] *n* Ciguatoxin *nt.*
cil·ia ['sɪlɪə] *pl* **1.** *sing* → cilium. **2.** (Augen-)Wimpern *pl,* Zilien *pl,* Cilia *pl.*
cil·i·a·ris (**muscle**) [sɪlɪ'eərɪs] Ziliarmuskel *m,* Ciliaris *m,* M. ciliaris.
cil·i·a·rot·o·my [ˌsɪlɪə'rɑtəmɪ] *n ophthal.* Ziliarkörperdurchtrennung *f,* Ziliarotomie *f.*
cil·i·ar·y ['sɪlɪerɪ, 'sɪlɪərɪ] *adj* Wimpernhaare/Cilien *od.* Ziliarkörper betr., ziliar, ciliar, Wimper-, Ziliar-, Cilio-.
ciliary apparatus → ciliary body.
ciliary arteries Ziliararterien *pl,* Aa. ciliares.
anterior c. vordere Ziliararterien, Aa. ciliares anteriores.
(posterior) c., long lange (hintere) Ziliararterien, Aa. ciliares posteriores longae.
(posterior) c., short kurze (hintere) Ziliararterien, Aa. ciliares posteriores breves.
ciliary beat Zilienschlag *m.*
ciliary blepharitis Triefauge *nt,* Lidrandentzündung *f,* Lippitudo *f,* Blepharitis ciliaris/marginalis.
ciliary body Strahlenkörper *m,* -apparat *m,* Ziliarkörper *m,* -apparat *m,* Ciliarkörper *m,* -apparat *m,* Corpus ciliare.
ciliary canals Fontana-Räume *pl,* Spatia anguli iridocornealis.
ciliary cartilage Lidknorpel *m,* Tarsus *m* (palpebrae).
ciliary crown Strahlenkranz *m* des Ziliarkörpers, Corona ciliaris.
ciliary disk Orbiculus ciliaris.
ciliary folds Plicae ciliares.
ciliary ganglion Schacher'-Ganglion *nt,* Ziliarganglion *nt,* Ggl. ciliare.
ciliary glands of conjunctiva Moll'-Drüsen *pl,* Gll. ciliares.
ciliary margin of iris äußerer/ziliarer Irisrand *m,* Margo ciliaris (iridis).
ciliary membrane Zilienmembran *f.*
ciliary muscle → ciliaris (muscle).
ciliary nerves: long c. lange Ziliarnerven *pl,* Nn. ciliares longi.
short c. kurze Ziliarnerven *pl,* Nn. ciliares breves.
ciliary part of retina Ziliarabschnitt *m* der Retina, Pars ciliaris retinae.
ciliary processes Ziliarfortsätze *pl,* Procc. ciliares.
ciliary reflex Ziliarreflex *m.*
ciliary ring → ciliary disk.
ciliary staphyloma Staphyloma ciliare.
ciliary veins Ziliarvenen *pl,* Vv. ciliares.
anterior c. vordere Ziliarvenen *pl,* Vv. ciliares anteriores.
posterior c. hintere Ziliarvenen *pl,* Vv. vorticosae, Vv. choroideae oculi.
ciliary zonule Zinn'-(Strahlen-)Zone *f,* Zonula ciliaris.

Ciliata

Cil·i·a·ta [ˌsɪlɪˈeɪtə] n Ziliaten pl, Wimpertierchen pl, Ciliata pl.
cil·i·ate [ˈsɪlɪət, -lɪeɪt] bio. **I** n Wimpertierchen nt, Wimperinfusiorium nt, Ziliat m, Ciliat m. **II** adj mit Zilien/Wimpern(haaren) versehen, zilientragend, bewimpert.
cil·i·at·ed [ˈsɪlɪeɪtɪd] adj → ciliate II.
ciliated cell histol. zilientragende Zelle f.
ciliated epithelium Flimmerepithel nt.
cil·i·ec·to·my [ˌsɪlɪˈektəmɪ] n ophthal. **1.** operative (Teil-)Entfernung f des Ziliarkörpers, Ziliektomie f, Zyklektomie f. **2.** Lidrandresektion f, Ziliektomie f.
cil·i·o·gen·e·sis [ˌsɪlɪəʊˈdʒenəsɪs] n histol. Zilienbildung f, -entwicklung f.
cil·i·o·late [ˈsɪlɪəlɪt, -leɪt] adj → ciliate II.
Cil·i·oph·o·ra [sɪlɪˈɑfərə] pl micro. Ciliophora pl.
cil·i·o·ret·i·nal [ˌsɪlɪəˈretɪnl] adj Ziliarkörper u. Retina betr., zilioretinal.
cil·i·o·scle·ral [ˌ-ˈsklɪərəl] adj Ziliarkörper u. Sklera betr., zilioskleral.
cil·i·o·spi·nal center [ˌ-ˈspaɪnl] Budge'-Zentrum nt, ziliospinales Zentrum nt, Centrum ciliospinale.
ciliospinal reflex ziliospinaler Reflex m.
cil·i·ot·o·my [sɪlɪˈɑtəmɪ] n ophthal. Ziliarnervendurchtrennung f, Ziliotomie f.
cil·i·um [ˈsɪlɪəm] n, pl **cil·i·a** [ˈsɪlɪə], **-ums 1.** Augenlid nt. **2.** (Kino-)Zilie f.
cil·lo [ˈsɪləʊ] n → cillosis.
cil·lo·sis [sɪˈləʊsɪs] n neuro. spastisches Oberlidzittern nt, Cillosis f.
ci·met·i·dine [səˈmetədiːn] n pharm. Cimetidin nt.
Ci·mex [ˈsaɪmeks] n micro. Bettwanze f, Cimex m.
C. hemipterus tropische Bettwanze, Cimex hemipterus.
C. lectularius gemeine Bettwanze, Cimex lectularius.
C. pipistrella Fledermauswanze, Cimex pipistrella.
C. rotundatus → C. hemipterus.
ci·mex [ˈsaɪmeks] n, pl **ci·mi·ces** [ˈsɪməsiːz] → Cimex.
Ci·mic·i·dae [saɪˈmɪsədiː] pl micro. Cimicidae pl.
cim·i·co·sis [sɪməˈkəʊsɪs] n Cimicosis f, Cimiciasis f.
Cimino [ˈsɪmənəʊ]: **C. shunt** (Brescia-)-Cimino-Shunt m.
CIN abbr. → cervical intraepithelial neoplasia.
C1 inactivator → C1 inhibitor.
cin·an·es·the·sia [ˌsɪnænəsˈθiːʒə] n neuro. Verlust f der Bewegungsempfindung, Kinanästhesie f.
cin·cho·na (bark) [sɪŋˈkəʊnə] pharm. Fieber-, Chinarinde f.
cin·chon·i·dine [sɪŋˈkɑnədiːn] n pharm. Cinchonidin nt.
cin·cho·nine [ˈsɪŋkəniː] n pharm. Cinchonin nt.
cin·cho·nin·ic acid [sɪŋkəˈnɪnɪk] pharm. Cinchoninsäure f.
cin·cho·nism [ˈsɪŋkənɪzəm] n pharm. Chininvergiftung f, Cinchonismus m, Chinismus m.
cin·cho·phen [ˈsɪŋkəfen] n pharm. Cinchophen nt.
cin·cli·sis [sɪŋˈklaɪsɪs] n Cinclisis f.
cinc·ture sensation [ˈsɪŋktʃər] neuro. Gürtelgefühl nt, Zonästhesie f.
cine- pref. Cine-, Kine-.
cin·e·an·gi·o·car·di·og·ra·phy [ˌsɪnəˌændʒɪəʊˌkɑːrdɪˈɑgrəfɪ] n radiol. Kineangiokardiographie f.
cin·e·an·gi·o·graph [ˌ-ˈændʒɪəgræf] n radiol. Kineangiograph m.
cin·e·an·gi·og·ra·phy [ˌ-ændʒɪˈɑgrəfɪ] n radiol. Kineangiographie f.

cin·e·den·sig·ra·phy [ˌ-denˈsɪgrəfɪ] n radiol. Kinedensigraphie f.
cine-esophagography n radiol. Kinematographie f der Speiseröhre, Kineösophagographie f.
cin·e·flu·o·rog·ra·phy [ˌ-fluəˈrɑgrəfɪ] n → cineradiography.
cin·e·gas·tros·co·py [ˌ-gæsˈtrɑskəpɪ] n Kinegastroskopie f.
cin·e·mat·ic amputation [ˌ-ˈmætɪk] chir., ortho. plastische Amputation f, Kineplastik f.
cin·e·mat·ics [ˌ-ˈmætɪks] pl Bewegungslehre f, Kinematik f.
cin·e·mat·i·za·tion [ˌ-mætɪˈzeɪʃn] n chir., ortho. plastische Amputation f, Kineplastik f.
cin·e·ma·tog·ra·phy [ˌ-məˈtɑgrəfɪ] n cineradiography.
cin·e·mat·o·ra·di·og·ra·phy [ˌ-ˌmætəˌreɪdɪˈɑgrəfɪ] n → cineradiography.
cin·e·mi·crog·ra·phy [ˌ-maɪˈkrɑgrəfɪ] n Kinemikrographie f.
cin·e·ol [ˈsɪnɪˌɑl, -əʊl] n Eukalyptol nt, Zineol nt, Cineol nt.
cin·e·pha·ryn·go·e·soph·a·go·gram [ˌsɪnəfəˌrɪŋgəʊəˈsɑfəgəgræm] n. Kinematogramm nt von Pharynx u. Ösophagus.
cin·e·phle·bog·ra·phy [ˌ-flɪˈbɑgrəfɪ] n radiol. Kinephlebographie f.
cin·e·pho·to·mi·crog·ra·phy [ˌ-ˌfəʊtəmaɪˈkrɑgrəfɪ] n cinemicrography.
cin·e·plas·tic amputation [ˌ-ˈplæstɪk] → cineplasty.
cin·e·plas·tics [ˌ-ˈplæstɪks] pl → cineplasty.
cin·e·plas·ty [ˈ-plæstɪ] n chir., ortho. plastische Amputation f, Kineplastik f.
cin·e·ra·di·og·ra·phy [ˌ-ˌreɪdɪˈɑgrəfɪ] n radiol. (Röntgen-)Kinematographie f, Kineradiographie f.
ci·ne·rea [sɪˈnɪərɪə] n graue Gehirn- u. Rückenmarkssubstanz f, graue Substanz f, Substantia grisea.
ci·ne·re·al [sɪˈnɪərɪəl] adj **1.** aschfarben, grau. **2.** anat. (ZNS) graue Substanz betr.
cin·e·roent·gen·o·flu·o·rog·ra·phy [ˌ-ˌrentgənəfluəˈrɑgrəfɪ] n → cineradiography.
cin·e·roent·gen·og·ra·phy [ˌ-rentgəˈnɑgrəfɪ] n → cineradiography.
cin·es·al·gia [sɪnəsˈældʒ(ɪ)ə] n neuro., ortho. Muskelschmerzen pl bei Bewegung, Kines(i)algie f.
ci·net·o·plasm [sɪˈnetəplæzəm] n Kinetoplasma nt.
ci·net·o·plas·ma [ˌsɪnətəʊˈplæzmə] n cinetoplasm.
cin·e·u·rog·ra·phy [ˌsɪnəjəˈrɑgrəfɪ] n radiol. Kineurographie f.
cin·gu·lar branch of callosomarginal artery [ˈsɪŋgjələr] Ast m der A. calloso marginalis zum Sulcus cinguli, Ramus cingularis a. callosomarginalis.
cin·gu·late convolution [ˈsɪŋgjəlɪt, -leɪt] Gyrus cinguli/cingulatus.
cingulate gyrus → cingulate convolution.
cingulate sulcus Sulcus cinguli/cingulatus.
cin·gule [ˈsɪŋgjuːl] n → cingulum.
cin·gu·lec·to·my [sɪŋgjəˈlektəmɪ] n neurochir. Zingulektomie f.
cin·gu·lot·o·my [ˌ-ˈlɑtəmɪ] n neurochir. Zingulotomie f.
cin·gu·lum [ˈsɪŋgjələm] n, pl **-la** [-lə] **1.** anat. Gürtel m, gürtelförmige Struktur f, Cingulum nt. **2.** (ZNS) Cingulum nt (cerebri). **3.** dent. Cingulum nt.
cin·gu·lum·ot·o·my [ˌsɪŋgələmˈɑtəmɪ] n → cingulotomy.
C1 INH abbr. → C1 inhibitor.

C1-INH deficiency → C1 inhibitor deficiency.
C1 inhibitor abbr. **C1 INH** immun. C1-Inaktivator m abbr. C1-INH, C1-Esterase-Inhibitor m.
C1 inhibitor deficiency hereditäres Angioödem nt, hereditäres Quincke-Ödem nt.
cin·na·mene [ˈsɪnəmiːn] n Styrol nt, Vinylbenzol nt.
cin·na·mon [ˈsɪnəmən] **I** n **1.** Zimt m, Kaneel m. **2.** Zimtfarbe f. **II** adj zimtfarben, -braun, -farbig.
cinnamon oil Zimtöl nt.
cin·nar·i·zine [sɪˈnærɪziːn] n pharm. Cinnarizin nt.
cin·nip·i·rine [sɪˈnɪpɪriːn] n → cinnarizine.
ci·nol·o·gy [sɪˈnɑlədʒɪ] n Bewegungslehre f, Kinesiologie f.
ci·nom·e·ter [sɪˈnɑmɪtər] n Bewegungsmesser m, Kinesi(o)meter nt.
cin·o·plasm [ˈsɪnəplæzəm] n Kinetoplasma nt.
ci·o·nec·to·my [ˌsaɪəˈnektəmɪ] n HNO Zäpfchenentfernung f, Uvularesektion f, Uvulektomie f.
ci·o·ni·tis [ˌ-ˈnaɪtɪs] n HNO Zäpfchenentzündung f, Uvulitis f, Kionitis f.
ci·on·op·to·sis [ˌ-nɑpˈtəʊsɪs] n HNO Zäpfchensenkung f, Uvuloptose f.
ci·o·nor·rha·phy [ˌ-ˈnɔrəfɪ] n HNO Zäpfchennaht f, Uvulo-, Staphylorrhaphie f.
ci·o·no·tome [saɪˈɑnətəʊm] n HNO Zäpfchenmesser nt, Uvulotom nt.
ci·o·not·o·my [saɪəˈnɑtəmɪ] n HNO Zäpfchenspaltung f, Uvulotomie f.
cir·ca [ˈsɜrkə] adv abbr. **c., ca.** zirka, ungefähr, etwa abbr. ca.
cir·ca·di·an [sɜrˈkeɪdɪən, -ˈkæ-, ˌsɜrkəˈdiːən] adj über den ganzen Tag (verteilt), tagesrhythmisch, zirkadian, circadian.
circadian periodicity Zirkadianperiodik f.
circadian rhythm zirkadianer Rhythmus m, 24-Stunden-Rhythmus m, Tagesrhythmus m.
cir·ci·nate [ˈsɜrsəneɪt] adj **1.** zirzinär. **2.** kreis-, ringförmig, zirkulär. **3.** rund, rundlich.
circinate psoriasis derm. Psoriasis anularis.
circinate retinitis → circinate retinopathy.
circinate retinopathy Retinitis/Retinopathia circinata.
cir·cle [ˈsɜrkl] **I** n **1.** Kreis m; Kreisfläche f, -umfang m, -inhalt m. **2.** Kreis m, Ring m, kreis- od. ringförmige Formation f; anat. Circulus m. **3.** fig. Zyklus m, Kreislauf m. **4.** Zirkel m, (Personen-)Kreis m. **II** vt umringen, umgeben; um-, einkreisen.
c. of Haller → c. of Zinn.
c. of Willis Willis'-Anastomosenkranz m, Circulus arteriosus cerebri, Circulus arteriosus Willisi.
c. of the year Jahreszyklus m.
c. of Zinn Haller'-, Zinn'-Gefäßkranz m, Circulus vasculosus n. optici.
cir·clet [ˈsɜrklɪt] n kleiner Kreis m; Ring m, Reif m.
cir·cling disease [ˈsɜrklɪŋ] Listeriose f.
cir·cuit [ˈsɜrkɪt] n **1.** Kreislauf m, Umlauf m; Kreisbewegung f. **2.** techn. elektrischer Strom-/Schaltkreis m. **in** ~ angeschlossen. **to open/close the** ~ den Stromkreis öffnen/ schließen. **to put in** ~ anschließen. **3.** phys. magnetischer Kreis m. **4.** Umfang m, Umkreis m. **in** ~ im Umfang. **5.** Runde f, Rundgang m, -reise f. **II** vt umkreisen.
circuit breaker techn. Stromkreisunterbrecher m.
cir·cu·lar [ˈsɜrkjələr] adj **1.** rund, ring-, kreisförmig, zirkulär, Kreis-, Rund-. **2.** zyklisch, periodisch, wiederkehrend. **3.** umständlich.

circular amputation *chir., ortho.* Amputation *f* mit Zirkelschnitt.
circular bandage Zirkulärverband *m*.
circular cone *mathe.* Kreiskegel *m*.
circular cut *chir., ortho.* Zirkelschnitt *m*.
circular dichroism *phys.* Zirkulardichroismus *m*.
circular fibers of ciliary muscle Müller'-Muskel *m*, Fibrae circulares m. ciliaris.
circular folds (of Kerckring) Kerckring'-Falten *pl*, Plicae circulares.
circular function *mathe.* Kreisfunktion *f*.
circular hymen *gyn.* ringförmiges Hymen *nt*, Hymen anularis.
circular incision Zirkelschnitt *m*.
circular layer: c. of drumhead → c. of tympanic membrane.
 c. of muscular tunic of colon zirkuläre Muskelschicht *f* des Kolons, Stratum circulare tunicae muscularis coli.
 c. of muscular tunic of rectum zirkuläre Muskelschicht *f* des Rektums, Stratum circulare tunicae muscularis recti.
 c. of muscular tunic of small intestine zirkuläre Muskelschicht *f* des Dünndarms, Stratum circulare tunicae muscularis intestini tenuis.
 c. of muscular tunic of stomach zirkuläre Muskelschicht *f* des Magens, Stratum circulare tunicae muscularis gastris.
 c. of tympanic membrane zirkuläre Trommelfellfasern *pl*, Stratum circulare membranae tympani.
circular motion Kreisbewegung *f*.
circular permutation *biochem.* zirkuläre Permutation *f*.
circular psychosis manisch-depressive Psychose/Krankheit *f*.
circular sulcus of insula Ringfurche *f* der Insel, Sulcus circularis insulae.
circular vection *physiol., micro.* Zirkularvektion *f*.
cir·cu·late ['sɜrkjəleɪt] **I** *vt* in Umlauf setzen *od.* bringen, zirkulieren lassen. **II** *vi* zirkulieren, umlaufen.
cir·cu·lat·ing ['-leɪtɪŋ] *adj* zirkulierend, umlaufend, im Umlauf/Kreislauf befindlich, in Umlauf.
cir·cu·la·tion [,-'leɪʃn] *n* 1. Zirkulation *f*, Kreislauf *m*. 2. *physiol.* (Blut-)Kreislauf *m*, (-)Zirkulation *f*. **to release into the ~** ins Blut/in den Blutkreislauf abgeben.
cirulation volume zirkulierendes Blutvolumen *nt*.
cir·cu·la·tive ['-leɪtɪv, -lətɪv] *adj* → circulatory.
cir·cu·la·to·ry ['-lətɔʊri, -tɔː-] *adj* (Blut-)Kreislauf betr., zirkulierend, umlaufend, Kreis-, Zirkulations-, (Blut-)Kreislauf-.
circulatory arrest Kreislaufstillstand *m*.
circulatory center Kreislaufzentrum *nt*.
circulatory collapse Kreislaufkollaps *m*.
circulatory disturbance Kreislaufstörung *f*.
circulatory shock Kreislaufschock *m*.
circulatory system *physiol.* (Blut-)Kreislauf *m*, (-)System *nt*.
cir·cum·a·nal glands [,sɜrkəm'eɪnl] zirkumanale Drüsen *pl*, Gll. anales/circumanales.
cir·cum·a·re·o·lar incision [,-ə'rɪələr] *gyn.* Warzenhofrandschnitt *m*, periareolärer Schnitt *m*.
cir·cum·ar·tic·u·lar [,-ɑːr'tɪkjələr] *adj* um ein Gelenk herum (liegend), periartikulär.
cir·cum·ax·il·lar·y [,-æksəleriː, -æk'sɪlərɪ] *adj* periaxillär.
cir·cum·bul·bar [,-'bʌlbɑːr, -bər] *adj* peribulbär.
cir·cum·cise ['-saɪz] *vt* 1. *urol.* eine Beschneidung durchführen, beschneiden. 2. *chir.* umschneiden.
cir·cum·ci·sion [,-'sɪʒn] *n* 1. *urol.* Beschneidung *f*, Zirkumzision *f*. 2. *chir.* Umschneidung *f*, Zirkumzision *f*, Circumcisio *f*.
cir·cum·cor·ne·al [,-'kɔːrnɪəl] *adj* zirkum-, perikorneal.
cir·cum·duc·tion [,-'dʌkʃn] *n* Kreisbewegung *f*, Zirkumduktion *f*.
cir·cum·fer·ence [sər'kʌmfərəns] *n* Umkreis *m*, (Kreis-)Umfang *m*; Ausdehnung *f*, Peripherie *f*, Zirkumferenz *f*, *anat.* Circumferentia *f*.
 c. of head of radius Circumferentia articularis radii.
cir·cum·fer·en·tial [sər,kʌmfə'renʃl] *adj* Umfang/Peripherie betr., peripher(isch), Umfangs-.
circumferential cartilage 1. Labrum glenoidale. 2. Labrum acetabulare.
circumferential implantation *gyn., embryo.* oberflächliche/superfizielle Einnistung/Implantation *f*.
circumferential lamella (*Knochen*) Generallamelle *f*.
cir·cum·flex ['sɜrkəmfleks] *adj anat.* (*Nerv, Blutgefäß*) gekrümmt, gebogen.
circumflex artery Kranzarterie *f*, A. circumflexa.
 deep c., internal Ramus profundus a. circumflexae femoris medialis.
 femoral c., lateral äußere Oberschenkel-/Femurkranzarterie, Circumflexa *f* femoris lateralis, A. circumflexa femoris lateralis.
 femoral c., medial innere Oberschenkel-/Femurkranzarterie, Circumflexa *f* femoris medialis, A. circumflexa femoris medialis.
 humeral c., anterior vordere Kranzarterie des Humerus, Circumflexa *f* humeri anterior, A. circumflexa humeri anterior.
 humeral c., posterior hintere Kranzarterie des Humerus, Circumflexa *f* humeri posterior, A. circumflexa humeri posterior.
 iliac c., deep tiefe Hüftkranzarterie *f*, Zirkumflexa iliaca profunda, A. circumflexa iliaca profunda.
 iliac c., superficial oberflächliche Hüftkranzarterie *f*, Circumflexa *f* iliaca superficialis, A. circumflexa iliaca superficialis.
 c. of scapula Kranzschlagader *f* des Schulterblattes, Circumflexa *f* scapulae, A. circumflexa scapulae.
circumflex branch: c. of left coronary artery Ramus circumflexus a. coronariae sinistrae.
 fibular c. of posterior tibial artery Ramus circumflexus fibularis a. tibialis posterioris.
circumflex nerve Axillaris *m*, N. axillaris.
circumflex vein: anterior c. of humerus V. circumflexa anterior humeralis.
 posterior c. of humerus V. circumflexa posterior humeralis.
 c. of scapula V. circumflexa scapulae.
cir·cum·flu·ent [sər'kʌmfluːənt] *adj* umgebend, umfließend.
cir·cum·in·su·lar [,sɜrkəm'ɪns(j)ələr] *adj* (*ZNS*) periinsular.
cir·cum·in·tes·ti·nal [,-ɪn'testənl, -,ɪntes-'taɪnl] *adj* um den Darm herum (liegend), zirkum-, periintestinal, perienteral.
cir·cum·ja·cent [,-'dʒeɪsnt] *adj* umgebend, umliegend.
cir·cum·len·tal [,-'lentəl] *adj* um die Linse herum (liegend), zirkumlental, perilentikulär.
cir·cum·neu·tral [,-'n(j)uːtrəl] *adj* (*PH-Wert*) fast neutral.

cir·cum·nu·cle·ar [,-'n(j)uːklɪər] *adj* um einen Kern herum (liegend), zirkum-, perinukleär.
cir·cum·oc·u·lar [,-'ɑkjələr] *adj ophthal.* um das Auge herum (liegend), periokulär, -okular, -ophthalmisch.
cir·cum·o·ral [,-'ɔːrəl, -'əʊr-] *adj* um den Mund herum (liegend), zirkum-, perioral.
circumoral cyanosis zirkumorale/periorale Zyanose *f*.
cir·cum·or·bit·al [,-'ɔːrbɪtl] *adj* um die Orbita herum (liegend), zirkum-, periorbital.
cir·cum·re·nal [,-'riːnl] *adj* um die Niere herum (liegend), zirkum-, perirenal.
cir·cum·scribe ['-skraɪb] *vt* 1. umfahren, umschreiben, eine Linie ziehen um. 2. ein-, beschränken.
cir·cum·scribed ['-skraɪbd] *adj* auf einen Bereich beschränkt, umschrieben, begrenzt, zirkumskript.
circumscribed albinism *derm.* partieller/umschriebener Albinismus *m*, Piebaldismus *m*, Albinismus circumscriptus.
circumscribed edema Quincke-Ödem *nt*, angioneurotisches Ödem *nt*.
circumscribed gangrene umschriebene Gangrän *f*.
circumscribed myxedema prätibiales Myxödem *nt*, Myxoedema circumscriptum tuberosum, Myxoedema praetibiale symmetricum.
circumscribed neurodermatitis Vidal'-Krankheit *f*, Lichen Vidal *m*, Lichen simplex chronicus (Vidal), Neurodermitis circumscriptus.
circumscribed peritonitis örtlich umschriebene Bauchfellentzündung *f*, Peritonitis circumscripta.
circumscribed precancerous melanosis of Dubreuilh Dubreuilh-Krankheit *f*, -Erkrankung *f*, Dubreuilh-Hutchinson-Krankheit *f*, -Erkrankung *f*, prämaligne Melanose *f*, melanotische Präkanzerose *f*, Lentigo maligna, Melanosis circumscripta praeblastomatosa/praecancerosa (Dubreuilh).
circumscribed scleroderma zirkumskripte Sklerodermie *f*, lokalisierte Sklerodermie *f*, Sclerodermia circumscripta, Morphoea *f*, Morphaea *f*.
cir·cum·stance ['-stæns] *n* 1. Umstand *m*. 2. **~s** *pl* Umstände *pl*, Verhältnisse *pl*, (Sach-)Lage *f*. **in/under no ~** auf keinen Fall, unter keinen Umständen. **in certain ~s** unter Umständen, eventuell. **in/under the ~s** unter diesen Umständen. **to carry out in/under difficult ~s** unter schwierigen Bedingungen durchführen. 3. **~s** *pl* (Lebens-)Verhältnisse *pl*, (-)Lage *f*. **in easy/poor/reduced ~s** in gesicherten/ärmlichen/bescheidenen Verhältnissen. **the social ~s** die soziale Verhältnisse.
cir·cum·stan·tial [,-'stænʃl] *adj* 1. ausführlich, detailliert. **a ~ report**. 2. nebensächlich, von untergeordneter Bedeutung. 3. durch die Umstände bedingt.
cir·cum·stan·ti·al·i·ty [,-,stænʃɪ'ælətɪ] *n* 1. Ausführlichkeit *f*. 2. Detail *nt*, Einzelheit *f*.
cir·cum·stan·ti·ate [,-'stænʃɪeɪt] *vt* genau u. ausführlich beschreiben; (*Theorie*) mit Beweisen untermauern *od.* belegen.
cir·cum·ton·sil·lar abscess [,-'tɑnsɪlər] *HNO* Peritonsillarabszeß *m*.
cir·cum·val·late papillae [,-'vælet] Wallpapillen *pl*, Papillae vallatae.
circumvallate placenta Placenta circumvallata.
cir·cum·vas·cu·lar [,-'væskjələr] *adj* um ein Gefäß herum (liegend), zirkum-, perivaskulär.

circumventricular organs

cir·cum·ven·tric·u·lar organs [ˌ-ven'trɪkjələr] zirkumventrikuläre Organe *pl*.
cir·cum·vo·lute [sər'kəmvəluːt, ˌsɑrkəm'vəulu:t] *adj* gewunden, verdreht.
cir·rho·gen·ic [sɪrəʊ'dʒenɪk] *adj* → cirrhogenous.
cir·rhog·e·nous [sɪ'rɑdʒənəs] *adj* Zirrhoseentstehung fördernd *od.* auslösend, zirrhogen.
cir·rhon·o·sus [sɪ'rɑnəsəs] *n patho., ped.* Cirrhonosis *f*.
cir·rho·sis [sɪ'rəʊsɪs] *n*, *pl* **-ses** [-siːz] **1.** Zirrhose *f*, Cirrhosis *f*. **2.** → c. of liver.
c. of liver Leberzirrhose, Cirrhosis hepatis.
c. of lung Lungenzirrhose, diffuse interstitielle Lungenfibrose *f*.
c. of stomach → cirrhotic gastritis.
cir·rhot·ic [sɪ'rɑtɪk] **I** *n* Patient(in *f*) *m* mit Zirrhose, Zirrhotiker(in *f*) *m*. **II** *adj* Zirrhose betr., von Zirrhose betroffen, zirrhös, zirrhotisch, Zirrhose(n)-.
cirrhotic gastritis Magenzirrhus *m*, entzündlicher Schrumpfmagen *m*, Brinton--Krankheit *f*, Linitis plastica.
cirrhotic inflammation atrophische/fibroide Entzündung *f*.
cirrhotic patient → cirrhotic I.
cir·rus ['sɪrəs] *n*, *pl* **-ri** [-raɪ] *micro.* Zirrus *m*.
cir·sec·to·my [sər'sektəmɪ] *n chir.* Varizen(teil)entfernung *f*, -resektion *f*, -exzision *f*, Cirsektomie *f*.
cir·so·cele ['sɜrsəsiːl] *n* Krampfaderbruch *m*, Cirsozele *f*, -cele *f*, Varikozele *f*, Hernia varicosa.
cir·sod·e·sis [sər'sɑdəsɪs] *n chir.* Varizenumstechung *f*, -ligatur *f*, Cirsodesis *f*.
cir·soid ['sɜrsɔɪd] *adj* trauben-, knotenförmig, krampfaderknotenähnlich.
cirsoid aneurysm Traubenaneurysma *nt*, Aneurysma cirsoideum/racemosum.
cirsoid placenta Placenta cirsoidea.
cir·som·pha·los [sər'sɑmfələs] *n* Medusenhaupt *nt*, Cirsomphalus *m*, Caput medusae.
cis- *pref.* cis-.
cis [sɪs] *adj chem.* diesseits, cis.
cis configuration *chem., genet.* cis-Konfiguration *f*.
cis-pla·tin ['sɪsplətɪn] *n pharm.* Cisplatin *nt*.
cis-platinum *n* → cisplatin.
11-cis retinal 11-cis-Retinal *nt*.
cis·sa [ˈsɪsə] *n* → citta.
cis·tern ['sɪstərn] *n anat.* Flüssigkeitsreservoir *nt*, Zisterne *f*, Cisterna *f*.
c. of chiasma Cisterna chiasmatica.
c. of fossa of Sylvius → c. of lateral cerebral fossa.
c. of lateral cerebral fossa Cisterna fossae lateralis cerebri.
c. of nuclear envelope perinukleäre Zisterne, perinukleärer Spaltraum *m*, Cisterna caryothecae/nucleolemmae.
c. of Sylvius → c. of lateral cerebral fossa.
cis·ter·na [sɪs'tɜrnə] *n*, *pl* **-nae** [-niː] → cistern.
cis·ter·nal [sɪs'tɜrnl] *adj* Zisterne(n) betr., Zisternen-.
cisternal puncture Subokzipital-, Zisternen-, Hirnzisternenpunktion *f*.
cis·ter·no·graph·ic [ˌsɪstərnəʊ'græfɪk] *adj radiol.* zisternographisch.
cis·ter·nog·ra·phy [ˌsɪstər'nɑgrəfɪ] *n radiol.* Zisterno-, Cisternographie *f*.
cis-trans isomer cis-trans-Isomer *nt*.
cis-trans isomerism cis-trans Isomerie *f*, geometrische Isomerie *f*.
cis-trans test *genet.* cis-trans-Test *m*.
cis·tron ['sɪstrən] *n genet.* Cistron *nt*.
cis·ves·tism [sɪs'vestɪzəm] *n psychia.* Cisvestismus *m*.

cis·ves·ti·tism [sɪs'vestɪtɪzəm] *n* → cisvestism.
Citelli [tʃɪ'telɪ]: **C.'s syndrome** Citelli-Syndrom *nt*.
cit·rase ['sɪtreɪz] *n* → citrate lyase.
cit·ra·tase ['sɪtrəteɪz] *n* → citrate lyase.
cit·rate ['sɪtreɪt, 'saɪ-] *n* Zitrat *nt*, Citrat *nt*.
citrate agar Zitrat-, Citratagar *m/nt*.
citrate aldolase → citrate lyase.
citrate cleavage enzyme ATP-Citrat--Lyase *f*, citratspaltendes Enzym *nt*.
cit·rat·ed ['sɪtreɪtɪd, 'saɪ-] *adj* zitrathaltig.
citrated plasma Zitrat-, Citratplasma *nt*.
citrate lyase Zitrataldolase *f*, -lyase *f*, Citrataldolase *f*, -lyase *f*.
citrate medium *micro.* Zitratnährboden *m*.
citrate phosphate dextrose *abbr.* **CPD** *hema.* CPD-Stabilisator *m*.
citrate-pyruvate cycle Zitrat-Pyruvat-Zyklus *m*, Citrat-Pyruvat-Zyklus *m*.
citrate (si-)synthase Zitratsynthase *f*.
cit·re·ous ['sɪtrɪəs] *adj* zitronengelb.
cit·ric acid ['sɪtrɪk] Zitronensäure *f*.
citric acid cycle Krebs-, Zitronensäure-, Zitratzyklus *m*, Tricarbonsäurezyklus *m*.
cit·ri·des·mo·lase [ˌsɪtrə'dezməleɪz] *n* → citrate lyase.
Cit·ro·bac·ter [ˌ-'bæktər] *n micro.* Citrobacter *f*.
ci·trog·e·nase [sɪ'trɑdʒəneɪz] *n* → citrate (si-)synthase.
ci·trov·o·rum factor [sɪ'trəvərəm] *abbr.* **CF** N^{10}-Formyl-Tetrahydrofolsäure *f*, Citrovorum-Faktor *m*, Leukovorin *nt*, Leucovorin *nt*.
cit·rul·line ['sɪtrəliːn] *n* Zitrullin *nt*, Citrullin *nt*.
cit·rul·lin·e·mia [ˌsɪtrəlɪ'niːmɪə] *n* Citrullinämie *f*, Argininbernsteinsäure-synthetase-mangel *m*.
citrulline ureidase Citrullinureidase *f*.
cit·rul·lin·u·ria [ˌ-'n(j)ʊərɪə] *n* **1.** erhöhte Citrullinausscheidung *f* im Harn, Citrullinurie *f*. **2.** → citrullinemia.
cit·ta ['sɪtə] *n gyn.* Heißhunger *m* der Schwangeren.
cit·to·sis [sɪ'təʊsɪs] *n* → citta.
Civatte [si'vat]: **C.'s disease** → poikiloderma of C.
poikiloderma of C. *derm.* Civatte'-Krankheit *f*, -Poikilodermie *f*.
civ·et liver fluke ['sɪvɪt] *micro.* hinterindischer Leberegel *m*, Opisthorchis viverrini.
Civinini [ˌtʃɪvɪ'niːnɪ]: **C.'s canal** → chorda tympani canal.
C.'s ligament Lig. pterygospinale.
C.'s process Proc. pterygospinosus.
C.'s spine → C.'s process.
CJD *abbr.* → Creutzfeldt-Jakob disease.
C-J disease → Creutzfeldt-Jakob disease.
CK *abbr.* → creatine kinase.
CL *abbr.* → chronic leukemia.
Cl *abbr.* → chlorine.
cl *abbr.* → centiliter.
clad·i·o·sis [ˌklædɪ'əʊsɪs] *n derm.* Kladiose *f*, Cladiosis *f*.
Clado [klɑ'do]: **C.'s anastomosis** *anat.* Clado'-Anastomose *f*.
C.'s band *gyn.* Clado'-Band *nt*.
C.'s ligament → C.'s band.
C.'s point *chir.* Clado'-Punkt *m*.
Cla·dor·chis watsoni [klæ'dɔːrkɪs] *micro.* Watsonius watsoni.
clad·o·spo·ri·o·sis [ˌklædəˌspəʊrɪ'əʊsɪs] *n* Cladosporiumerkrankung *f*, Cladosporiose *f*, -sporiosis *f*.
Clad·o·spo·ri·um [ˌ-'spəʊrɪəm] *n micro.* Cladosporium *nt*.
C. carrionii Cladosporium carrionii.
C. mansoni Cladosporium mansoni.

C. werneckii Cladosporium werneckii.
clair·voy·ance [kleər'vɔɪəns] *n* Hellsehen *nt*, Präkognition *f*.
clam digger's itch [klæm] Schwimmbadkrätze *f*, Weiherhippel *m*, Bade-, Schistosomen-, Zerkariendermatitis *f*.
clam·my ['klæmɪ] *adj* (*Haut*) feuchtkalt, klamm.
clamp [klæmp] **I** *n chir., techn.* Klemme *f*, Klammer *f*. **II** *vt* (ein-)spannen, (fest-, ab-)klemmen, mit Klammer(n) befestigen, (ver-, an-)klammern.
clamp current Klemmstrom *m*.
clap [klæp] *n* **the ~** *inf.* → gonorrhea.
clap·o·tage [klapɔ'taːʒ] *n* Plätschergeräusch *nt* (*des Magens*), Clapotement *nt*.
cla·pote·ment [klapɔt'mɑ̃] *n* → clapotage.
Clapton ['klæptn]: **C.'s line** Clapton-Linie *f*.
Clara ['klɑːrə]: **C. cells** Clara-Zellen *pl*.
cla·rif·i·cant [klæ'rɪfɪkənt] *n chem.* Klärsubstanz *f*, Klär(ungs)mittel *nt*.
clar·i·fi·ca·tion [ˌklærəfɪ'keɪʃn] *n* **1.** *chem.* (Ab-)Klären *nt*, (Ab-)Klärung *f*. **2.** *fig.* (Er-, Auf-)Klärung *f*, Klarstellung *f*.
clar·i·fi·er ['klærɪfaɪər] *n* → clarificant.
clar·i·fy ['klærɪfaɪ] **I** *vt* **1.** *chem.* (ab-)klären, reinigen. **2.** *fig.* (auf-, er-)klären, klarstellen. **II** *vi* **3.** *chem.* s. klären, klar werden; s. absetzen. **4.** *fig.* s. (auf-)klären.
clar·i·ty ['klærətɪ] *n* Klarheit *f*.
Clark [klɑːrk]: **C.'s electrode** Clark-Elektrode *f*.
C. I Diphenylarsinchlorid *nt*, Clark I *nt*.
C. II Diphenylarsincyanid *nt*, Clark II *nt*.
Clarke [klɑːrk]: **C.'s cells** Clarke'-Zellen *pl*.
C.'s column Clarke'-Säule *f*, -Kern *m*, Columna thoracica, Nc. thoracicus.
dorsal nucleus of C. → C.'s column.
C.'s nucleus → C.'s column.
C.'s ulcer 1. knotiges/solides/noduläres/nodulo-ulzeröses Basaliom *nt*, Basalioma exulcerans, Ulcus rodens. **2.** *gyn.* Zervikalulkus *nt*.
Clarke-Hadfield ['hædfiːld]: **C.-H. syndrome** Mukoviszidose *f*, zystische (Pankreas-)Fibrose *f*, Fibrosis pancreatica cystica.
clas·mat·o·cyte [klæz'mætəsaɪt] *n* Makrophag(e) *m*.
clas·ma·to·sis [ˌklæzmə'təʊsɪs] *n histol.* Klasmatose *f*.
clas·mo·cy·to·ma [ˌklæzməsaɪ'təʊmə] *n* Retikulosarkom *nt*, Retikulumzell(en)sarkom *nt*, Retothelsarkom *nt*.
clasp [klæsp, klɑːsp] **I** *n* **1.** Klammer *f*, Klemme *f*; Haken *m*, Spange *f*. **2.** Umklammerung *f*, fester (Hand-)Griff *m*. **II** *vt* (um-)klammern, ein-, zuhaken, mit Haken befestigen *od.* schließen; festschnallen, fassen.
clasp-knife effect → clasp-knife phenomenon.
clasp-knife phenomenon *neuro.* Taschenmesserphänomen *nt*, Klappmesserphänomen *nt*.
clasp-knife rigidity → clasp-knife phenomenon.
class. *abbr.* **1.** → classic, classical. **2.** → classification. **3.** → classified.
class [klæs, klɑːs] **I** *n* **1.** Gruppe *f*, Kategorie *f*, Klasse *f*. **2.** *socio.* (Gesellschafts-)Klasse *f*, (Bevölkerungs-)Schicht *f*. **3.** *bio.* Klasse *f*, Gruppe *f*, Art *f*. **II** *vt* klassifizieren, (in Klassen) einteilen *od.* einordnen *od.* einstufen.
class I antigen *immun.* MHC-Klasse I--Antigen *nt*.
class II antigen *immun.* MHC-Klasse II--Antigen *nt*.
clas·sic ['klæsɪk] *abbr.* **class.** **I** *n* Klassiker *m*; klassisches Werk *nt*, Standardwerk *nt*. **II** *adj* **1.** erstklassig, ausgezeichnet. **2.**

klassisch, maßgeblich, als Standard/Maßstab/Richtlinie/Norm geltend od. dienend. the ~ reference book. 3. klassisch, traditionell, konventionell, herkömmlich. the ~ method die klassische od. konventionelle Methode. 4. elementar, grundlegend, wesentlich; typisch. the ~(al) symptoms of a disease.
clas·si·cal ['klæsɪkl] adj abbr. **class.** → classic II.
classical conditioning klassische Konditionierung f.
classical genetics klassische Genetik f.
classical hemophilia Hämophilie A f, klassische Hämophilie f, Faktor-VIII-Mangel m.
classical hysteria klassische Hysterie f, klassisches Konversionssyndrom nt.
classical phenylketonuria Fölling-Krankheit f, -Syndrom nt, Morbus Fölling m, Phenylketonurie f abbr. PKU, Brenztraubensäureschwachsinn m, Oligophrenia phenylpyruvica.
classical seminoma patho. klassisches Seminom nt.
classical thermodynamics klassische Thermodynamik f, Gleichgewichtsthermodynamik f.
classic apraxia ideokinetische/ideomotorische Apraxie f.
classic cholera klassische Cholera f, Cholera asiatica/indica/orientalis/epidemica.
classic complement pathway → classic pathway.
classic galactosemia (hereditäre/kongenitale) Galaktosämie f, Galaktoseintoleranz f.
classic migraine klassische Migräne f.
classic pathway immun. (*Komplement*) klassischer Aktivierungsweg m.
classic typhus epidemisches/klassisches Fleckfieber nt, Läusefleckfieber nt, Fleck-, Hunger-, Kriegstyphus m, Typhus exanthematicus.
clas·si·fi·a·ble ['klæsɪfaɪəbl] adj klassifizierbar.
clas·si·fi·ca·tion [ˌklæsəfɪ'keɪʃn] n abbr. **class.** 1. Klassifizieren nt, (*in Klassen*) Einordnen od. Einstufen nt. Einteilen nt. 2. Klassifikation f, Klassifizierung f, Einordnung f, -teilung f. 3. bio. Einordnung f.
clas·si·fi·ca·to·ry [klæ'sɪfɪkəˌtɔːriː, -ˌtəʊ-, 'klæsə-] adj klassifizierend, Klassifikations-.
clas·si·fied ['klæsɪfaɪd] adj abbr. **class.** klassifiziert, (in Klassen od. Gruppen) eingeteilt.
clas·si·fy ['klæsɪfaɪ] vt klassifizieren, einteilen (*into* in); (ein-)gruppieren, kategorisieren; einstufen (*into* in).
class I MHC antigen MHC-Klasse I-Antigen nt.
class II MHC antigen MHC-Klasse II-Antigen nt.
clas·tic ['klæstɪk] adj 1. (in Fragmente) zerfallend, brüchig. 2. (*Modell*) zerlegbar.
clas·to·gen ['klæstədʒən] n Klastogen nt.
clas·to·gen·ic [ˌ-'dʒenɪk] adj klastogen.
clas·to·thrix ['-θrɪks] n derm. Trichorrhexis nodosa.
clath·rate ['klæθreɪt] n chem. Klathrat nt.
clathrate compound → clathrate.
Clauberg ['klaʊbɑrg]: **C.'s (culture) medium** Clauberg-Nährboden m.
C.'s test micro. Clauberg-Test m.
C.'s unit old Clauberg-Einheit f, Kaninchen-Einheit f abbr. K.E.
Claude [kloːd]: **C.'s hyperkinesis sign** Claude'-(Hyperkinese-)Zeichen nt.
C.'s syndrome neuro. Claude-Syndrom nt, unteres Ruber-Syndrom nt, unteres Syndrom nt des Nc. ruber.
Claude Bernard-Horner [bɛr'naːr 'hɔːrnər]: **C. B.-H. syndrome** Horner-Syndrom nt, -Trias f, -Symptomenkomplex m.
clau·di·cant ['klɔːdɪkənt] I n Patient(in f) m mit Claudicatio. II adj Claudicatio betr., von ihr betroffen; hinkend.
clau·di·ca·tion [ˌklɔːdɪ'keɪʃn] n Hinken nt, Claudikation f, Claudicatio f.
clau·di·ca·to·ry ['klɔːdɪkətɔːriː, -təʊ-] adj Claudicatio (intermittens) betr.
Claudius ['klɔːdɪəs]: **cells of C.** Claudius'-Zellen pl, Stützzellen pl.
C.' fossa Claudius'-Grube f, Fossa ovarica.
supporting cells of C. → cells of C.
claus·tral ['klɔːstrəl] adj Claustrum betr.
claus·tro·phil·ia [ˌklɔːstrə'fɪlɪə] n psychia. Klaustrophilie f, -manie f.
claus·tro·pho·bia [ˌ-'fəʊbɪə] n psychia. Angst f vor geschlossenen Räumen, Platzangst f, Klaustro-, Claustrophobie f.
claus·tro·pho·bic [ˌ-'fəʊbɪk] adj Klaustrophobie betr., klaustrophobisch, -phob.
claus·trum ['klɔːstrəm, 'klaʊ-] n, pl **-tra** [-trə] Claustrum nt.
clau·su·ra [klɔː'sʊərə] n Fehlen nt od. Verschluß m einer natürlichen Körperöffnung, Atresie f, Atresia f.
cla·va ['kleɪvə, 'klɑː-] n, pl **-vae** ['kleɪviː, 'klɑːvaɪ] Tuberculum gracile f.
cla·vate ['kleɪveɪt] adj keulenförmig.
clavate papillae pilzförmige Papillen pl, Papillae fungiformes.
Clav·i·ceps purpurea ['klævɪseps] micro. Claviceps purpurea f.
Clav·i·cip·i·ta·ce·ae [ˌ-ˌsɪpɪ'teɪsɪiː] pl micro. Clavicipitaceae pl.
Clav·i·cip·i·ta·les [ˌ-ˌsɪpɪ'teɪliːz] pl micro. Clavicipitales pl.
clav·i·cle ['klævɪkl] n Schlüsselbein nt, Klavikel f, Klavikula f, Clavicula f.
clavicle aplasia Schlüsselbeinaplasie f.
clavicle hypoplasia Schlüsselbeinhypoplasie f.
clav·i·cor·a·co·ax·il·lar·y aponeurosis [ˌklævɪˌkɔːrəkoʊ'æksəˌlerɪː, -ˌæk'sɪlərɪ] Fascia clavipectoralis.
clav·i·cot·o·my [klævɪ'kɑtəmɪ] n ortho. Schlüsselbeindurchtrennung f, -resektion f, Clavikotomie f, Kleidotomie f.
cla·vic·u·la [klə'vɪkjələ] n, pl **-lae** [-liː] → clavicle.
cla·vic·u·lar [klə'vɪkjələr] adj Schlüsselbein/Klavikula betr., klavikular, Schlüsselbein-, Klavikula-, Clavicula-.
clavicular branch of thoracoacromial artery A. thoracoacromialis-Ast m zur Klavikula, Ramus clavicularis a. thoracoacromialis.
clavicular incisure of sternum → clavicular notch of sternum.
clavicular notch of sternum Inc. clavicularis (sterni).
clavicular region Schlüsselbeinregion f, Regio clavicularis.
clavicular sign Higouménakis-Zeichen nt.
cla·vic·u·lus [klə'vɪkjələs] n, pl **-li** [-laɪ] histol. Sharpey-Faser f.
clav·i·form ['klævɪfɔːrm] adj keulenförmig.
clav·i·pec·to·ral [ˌ-'pektərəl] adj Schlüsselbein/Klavikula u. Thorax od. Brust betr.
clavipectoral fascia Fascia clavipectoralis.
clavipectoral triangle Trigonum clavipectorale.
clavipectoral trigone → clavipectoral triangle.
clav·u·lan·ic acid [klævjə'lænɪk] pharm. Clavulansäure f.
cla·vus ['kleɪvəs, 'klɑː-] n, pl **-vi** [-vaɪ, -viː] Hühnerauge nt, Leichdorn m, Klavus m, Clavus m.
claw [klɔː] 1. bio. Kralle f, Klaue f; (*Krebs*) Schere f. 2. Kratzwunde f. 3. techn. Haken m, Greifer m.
claw foot ortho. Klauenfuß m, Klauenhohlfuß m, Krallenhohlfuß m.
claw hand ortho. Klauen-, Krallenhand f.
claw toe ortho. Krallenzeh(e f) m.
clay [kleɪ] n Ton(erde f) m, Lehm m, Mergel m.
clay-bank ['kleɪbæŋk] adj lehmfarben, gelblich-braun.
Claybrook ['kleɪbrʊk]: **C.'s sign** Claybrook'-Zeichen nt.
clay-colored adj claybank.
clay·ey ['kleɪiː] adj lehmig, tonig, Ton-, Lehm-.
clay·ey·ness n → clayiness.
clay·i·ness ['kleɪɪnɪs] n Klebrigkeit f (*wie von Lehm*).
clay·pipe cancer ['kleɪpaɪp] Pfeifenraucherkrebs m.
clay soil → clay.
Cl⁻ channel physiol. Chloridkanal m, Cl⁻-Kanal m.
clean [kliːn] I adj 1. sauber, rein; frisch. 2. (*Wunde*) sauber, rein; aseptisch, keimfrei; sterilisiert. 3. unverfälscht, (*Substanz*) unvermischt, rein. ~ **air/water**. 4. (*Schnitt*) glatt, eben. 5. unbedingt, uneingeschränkt, vollkommen, -ständig. 6. sl. clean, nicht mehr drogenabhängig. 7. nicht radioaktiv. 8. ebenmäßig, fair. II adv 9. anständig, fair. 10. sauber, rein(lich). 11. inf. völlig, gänzlich, glatt, rein. III vt säubern, reinigen, putzen; waschen.
clean down vt abwaschen, gründlich waschen.
clean·a·bil·i·ty [ˌkliːnə'bɪlətɪ] n Waschbarkeit f.
clean·a·ble ['kliːnəbl] adj waschbar, gut zu reinigen.
clean-cut adj 1. scharfgeschnitten, klar. 2. klar umrissen, deutlich. 3. eindeutig, klar. a ~ case.
clean features klare Gesichtszüge pl.
clean·er ['kliːnər] n Reiniger m; (Fenster-) Putzer m; Reinemachefrau f; Reinigungsmittel nt; Reinigungsmaschine f.
clean·ing ['kliːnɪŋ] n the ~ to do the ~ saubermachen, reinigen, putzen.
cleaning lady Reinemachefrau f.
clean·li·ness ['klenlɪnɪs] n Sauberkeit f, Reinlichkeit f.
clean·ly [adj 'klenlɪ; adv 'kliːnlɪ] I adj reinlich, sauber. II adv reinlich.
clean·ness ['kliːnnɪs] n Sauberkeit f, Reinheit f.
cleanse [klenz] vt säubern, reinigen (*of, from* von; *with* mit).
cleans·er ['klenzər] n Reiniger m; Reinigungsmittel nt.
clean-shaven adj glattrasiert.
cleans·ing tissue ['klenzɪŋ] Reinigungstuch nt.
clean wound chir. saubere/aseptische Wunde f.
clear [klɪər] I adj 1. (*Licht, Augen*) klar, hell; (*Stimme*) rein, hell; (*Kopf*) klar, hell; (*Haut*) klar; (*Lunge*) frei; (*Flüssigkeit*) klar, durchsichtig, rein; (*Farbe*) unvermischt. 2. (*Zugang*) offen, frei, unbehindert (*of* von). 3. klar, deutlich. a ~ **case** ein klarer od. eindeutiger Fall von. 4. deutlich, unmißverständlich. II adv 5. hell, klar; deutlich. 6. gänzlich, glatt, ganz. **to cut a piece ~ off.** III vt 7. (weg-, ab-)räumen, wegschaffen, beseitigen; freimachen. **to ~ the airways.** 8. (*Flüssigkeit*) klären, klarmachen. 9. klarstel-

clear adenoma

len, klar *od.* verständlich machen. **10.** s. räuspern. **to ~ one's throat. 11.** abbauen, ausscheiden, reinigen; (*Darm*) entleeren. **IV** *vi* **12.** s. klären, klar *od.* heller werden. **13.** heilen.
clear away *vt* wegschaffen, -räumen, Platz schaffen.
clear off *vt* → clear away.
clear up *vt* **1.** (auf-, er-)klären. **2.** aufräumen.
clear adenoma → clear cell adenoma.
clear·age ['klɪərɪdʒ] *n* → clearance 2.
clear·ance ['klɪərəns] *n* **1.** *abbr.* **C** *physiol.* Clearance *f abbr.* C. **2.** Verschwinden *nt*, Schwund *m*. **3.** Beseitigung *f*, Freimachung *f*, Räumung *f*; Reinigung *f*, Klärung *f*.
clear carcinoma → clear cell carcinoma.
clear cell adenocarcinoma 1. → clear cell carcinoma of kidney. **2.** *patho.* Mesonephrom(a) *nt*.
clear cell adenoma hellzelliges Adenom *nt*.
clear cell carcinoma hellzelliges Karzinom *nt*, Klarzell(en)karzinom *nt*, Ca. clarocellulare.
c. of kidney hypernephroides (Nieren-)-Karzinom, klarzelliges Nierenkarzinom, (maligner) Grawitz-Tumor *m*, Hypernephrom *nt*.
clear cell chondrosarcoma *patho.* hellzelliges Chondrosarkom *nt*.
clear-cell hidradenoma noduläres Hidradenom *nt*, Hidradenoma solidum.
clear cell myoepithelioma *patho.* hellzelliges Myoepitheliom *nt*.
clear cells Helle-Zellen *pl*, Hell-, Klarzellen *pl*.
clear-cut *adj* **1.** scharfgeschitten, klar umrissen. **2.** eindeutig, deutlich. **a ~ case of** ein klarer Fall von.
clear·er ['klɪərər] *n lab.* Klärmittel *nt*, -substanz *f*; Reinigungs-, Klärapparat *m od.* -gerät *nt*.
clear-eyed *adj* **1.** mit scharfen Augen. **2.** *fig.* klar-, scharfsichtig.
clear·head·ed ['klɪərhedɪd] *adj* klardenkend.
clear·ing ['klɪərɪŋ] *n* **1.** Verschwinden *nt*, Schwund *m*. **2.** (Aus-, Auf-)Räumen *nt*, Säuberung *f*.
clearing agent *lab.* Klärmittel *nt*, -substanz *f*.
clear layer of epidermis Stratum lucidum epidermidis.
clear·ness ['klɪərnɪs] *n* Klarheit *f*, Deutlichkeit *f*; Reinheit *f*; (Bild-)Schärfe *f*.
clear-sighted *adj* → clear-eyed.
cleav·a·ble ['kli:vəbl] *adj* teilbar, spaltungs-, teilungsfähig.
cleav·age ['kli:vɪdʒ] *n* **1.** (*a. fig.*) Spaltung *f*, (Auf-)Teilung *f*. **2.** Spalt *m*. **3.** *embryo.* (Zell-)Teilung *f*, Furchung(steilung *f*) *f*. **4.** *chem.* Spaltung *f*.
cleavage cavity *embryo.* Furchungs-, Keimhöhle *f*, Blastozöl *nt*.
cleavage cell *embryo.* Furchungszelle *f*, Blastomere *f*.
cleavage division *embryo.* (Zell-)Teilung *f*, Furchung(steilung *f*) *f*.
cleavage fracture *ortho.* **1.** Abscher-, Abschälungsfraktur *f*, flake fracture (*f*). **2.** Abscherfraktur *f* des Capitulum humeri.
cleavage lines (*Haut*) Spaltlinien *pl*.
cleavage nucleus *embryo.* Zygotenkern *m*.
cleavage product Spaltprodukt *nt*.
cleave [kli:v] (**cleft, cleaved, clove; cleft, cleaved, cloven**) **I** *vt* **1.** (zer-)spalten, (zer-)teilen. **2.** (*Luft, Wasser*) durchdringen, -schneiden. **3.** (ab-, zer-, durch-)trennen. **II** *vi* **4.** s. teilen, s. (auf-)spalten. **5.** durchschneiden (*through*).

cleaved follicular center cell [kli:vd] Germino-, Zentrozyt *m*.
cleav·er ['kli:vər] *n* Hackbeil *nt*, Hackmesser *nt*.
Cleeman ['kli:mən]: **C.'s sign** *ortho.* Cleeman'-Zeichen *nt*.
cleft [kleft] **I** *n* Spalt(e *f*) *m*, Furche *f*, Fissur *f*. **II** *adj* gespalten, geteilt, (auseinander-)-klaffend. **III** *pret, ptp* → cleave.
cleft foot Spaltfuß *m*.
cleft formation *patho.* Spaltbildung *f*.
cleft hand Spalthand *f*.
cleft jaw Kieferspalte *f*, Gnathoschisis *f*.
cleft lip Hasenscharte *f*, Lippenspalte *f*, Cheiloschisis *f*.
cleft palate Gaumenspalte *f*, Palato-, Uranoschisis *f*, Palatum fissum.
cleft spine Spondyloschisis *f*, R(h)achischisis posterior.
cleft tongue gespaltene Zunge *f*, Lingua bifida.
cleft vertebra Spaltwirbel *m*, Wirbelspalt *m*, Spina bifida.
cleid- *pref.* → cleido-.
clei·dag·ra [klaɪ'dægrə] *n patho.* Schlüsselbeingicht *f*, Kleidagra *f*, Cleidagra *f*.
clei·dal ['klaɪdəl] *adj* → clavicular.
cleido- *pref.* Schlüsselbein-, Klavikula(r)-, Kleido-.
clei·do·cos·tal [‚klaɪdəʊ'kɒstl] *adj* Schlüsselbein u. Rippe(n) betr., kostoklavikular, -klavikulär.
clei·do·cra·ni·al [‚-'kreɪnɪəl] *adj* Schlüsselbein u. Kopf betr., kleidokranial.
cleidocranial dysostosis/dysplasia Dysplasia/Dysostosis cleidocranialis, Scheuthauer-Marie-Syndrom *nt*.
clei·do·mas·toid [‚-'mæstɔɪd] *adj* Schlüsselbein u. Proc. mastoideus betr.
clei·dor·rhex·is [‚-'reksɪs] *n* → clavicotomy.
clei·dot·o·my [klaɪ'dɒtəmɪ] *n* → clavicotomy.
clei·sag·ra [klaɪ'sægrə] *n* → cleidagra.
clei·si·o·pho·bia [‚klaɪsɪə'fəʊbɪə] *n old* → claustrophobia.
clei·thro·pho·bia [‚klaɪθrə'fəʊbɪə] *n old* → claustrophobia.
clem·a·stine ['klemәstiːn] *n pharm.* Clemastin *nt*.
clem·i·zole ['klemɪzəʊl] *n pharm.* Clemizol *nt*.
clemizole penicillin G *pharm.* Clemizol-Penicillin G *nt*, Clemizol-Benzylpenicillin *nt*.
clench [klentʃ] **I** *n* Zusammenpressen *nt*; fester Griff *m*. **II** *vt* **1.** (*Fäuste*) ballen; (*Lippen*) fest zusammenpressen; (*Zähne*) zusammenbeißen; (*Nerven*) anspannen. **2.** (fest) zugreifen *od.* -packen. **III** *vi* s. fest zusammenpressen; s. anspannen.
clench·ing ['klentʃɪŋ] *n* (*Lippen, Kiefer*) Zusammenpressen *nt*.
clep·to·ma·nia [‚kleptə'meɪnɪə, -njə] *n psychia.* krankhafter Stehltrieb *m*, Kleptomanie *f*.
clep·to·ma·ni·ac [‚-'meɪnɪ‚æk] *psychia.* **I** *n* Kleptomane -manin *f*. **II** *adj* an Kleptomanie leidend, kleptomanisch.
Clevenger ['klevəndʒər]: **C.'s fissure** Sulcus temporalis inferior.
clew [klu:] *n* → clue.
click [klɪk] **I** *n* **1.** Klicken *nt*, Knacken *nt*, Knipsen *nt*, Ticken *nt*. **2.** *card.* Click *m*. **3.** (*Zunge*) Schnalzlaut *m*, Schnalzer *m*. **4.** Einschnappen *nt*, Einrasten *nt*. **II** *vt* **5.** klicken *od.* knacken lassen; knipsen lassen. **6.** schnalzen. **III** *vi* **7.** klicken, knacken, ticken; zu-, einschnappen, einrasten. **8.** schnalzen.
click syndrome *card.* Click-Syndrom *nt*, Klick-Syndrom *nt*.

clid- *pref.* → cleido-.
cli·dag·ra *n* → cleidagra.
cli·dal ['klaɪdəl] *adj* → clavicular.
cli·din·i·um bromide [klɪ'dɪnɪəm] *pharm.* Clidiniumbromid *nt*.
clido- *pref.* → cleido-.
cli·do·cos·tal *adj* → cleidocostal.
cli·do·cra·ni·al *adj* → cleidocranial.
clidocranial dysostosis → cleidocranial dysostosis.
cli·en·tele [‚klaɪən'tel, ‚kliːən-, ‚kliːɑ̃ːn'tel] *n* Klientel *f*, Klienten *pl*; Patienten(kreis *m*) *pl*; Kunden *pl*.
cli·mac·te·ri·al [klaɪ‚mæk'tɪərɪəl] *adj* Klimakterium betr., klimakterisch.
cli·mac·ter·ic [klaɪ'mæktərɪk, ‚klaɪmæk-'terɪk] **I** *n* **1.** *physiol.* Klimakterium *nt*, Klimax *f*, Wechseljahre *pl*. **2.** kritische *od.* entscheidende Phase *f*, Krise *f*. **II** *adj* **3.** kritisch, entscheidend, Krisen-. **4.** s. steigernd *od.* zuspitzend. **5.** → climacterial.
cli·mac·ter·i·cal [‚klaɪmæk'terɪkl] *adj* kritisch, entscheidend, Krisen-.
climacteric arthritis *ortho.*, *gyn.* klimakterische Arthropathie *f*, Arthropathia ovaripriva.
climacteric melancholia Involutionspsychose *f*.
climacteric syndrome Menopausensyndrom *nt*.
cli·mac·te·ri·um [‚-'tɪərɪəm] *n, pl* **-ria** [-rɪə] → climacteric 1.
cli·mate ['klaɪmɪt] *n* **1.** Klima *nt*. **2.** *fig.* Klima *nt*, Atmosphäre *f*.
cli·mat·ic [klaɪ'mætɪk] *adj* klimatisch, Klima-.
climatic bubo Lymphogranuloma inguinale/venereum *nt abbr.* LGV, Lymphopathia venerea, Morbus Durand-Nicolas-Favre *m*, klimatischer Bubo *m*, vierte Geschlechtskrankheit *f*, Poradenitis inguinalis.
cli·ma·to·log·ic [‚klaɪmətə'lɒdʒɪk] *adj* klimatologisch.
cli·ma·to·log·i·cal [‚-'lɒdʒɪkl] *adj* → climatologic.
cli·ma·tol·o·gy [‚klaɪmə'tɒlədʒɪ] *n* Klimatologie *f*, Klimakunde *f*.
cli·ma·to·ther·a·peu·tics [‚klaɪmətəʊ‚θerə-'pjuːtɪks] *pl* → climatotherapy.
cli·ma·to·ther·a·py [‚-'θerəpɪ] *n* Klimatherapie *f*, -behandlung *f*.
cli·max ['klaɪmæks] **I** *n* **1.** Höhepunkt *m*, Gipfel *m*, Akme *f*. **2.** *physiol.* Höhepunkt *m*, Orgasmus *m*, Klimax *f*. **3.** → climacteric 1. **II** *vt* auf den Höhepunkt bringen, steigern. **III** *vi* den Höhepunkt erreichen, s. steigern.
climb [klaɪm] **I** *n* (*a. fig.*) (An-)Steigen *nt*, Anstieg *m*. **II** *vt* (*a. fig.*) klettern auf. **III** *vi* (*a. fig.*) ansteigen, klettern.
climb·ing fibers ['klaɪmɪŋ] *histol.* Kletterfasern *pl*.
clime [klaɪm] *n* → climate.
clin. *abbr.* → clinical.
clin·da·my·cin [‚klɪndə'maɪsɪn] *n pharm.* Clindamycin *nt*.
cling·ing fibers [klɪŋɪŋ] → climbing fibers.
clin·ic ['klɪnɪk] **I** *n* **1.** Poliklinik *f*, Ambulanz *f*, Ambulatorium *nt*. **2.** Sprechstunde *f*; Beratungs- *od.* Therapiegruppe *f*. **to have a ~** eine Sprechstunde abhalten. **3.** Gemeinschaftspraxis *f*. **4.** (spezialisiertes) (Kranken-)Haus *nt*, Klinik *f*. **5.** Bedside-Teaching *nt*, Unterweisung *f* (*von Studenten*) am Krankenbett. **II** *adj* → clinical.
clin·i·cal ['klɪnɪkl] *adj abbr.* **clin. 1.** klinisch, Klinik/Krankenhaus betr., klinisches (Krankheits-)Bild betr., zum Krankenzimmer gehörend. **2.** *fig.* nüchtern, sachlich, unpersönlich, objektiv.

clinical chemistry klinische Chemie *f*.
clinical course (*Krankheit*) klinischer Verlauf *m*, Befund *m*.
clinical crown → clinical dental crown.
clinical death klinischer Tod *m*.
clinical dental crown klinische (Zahn-)-Krone *f*, Corona clinica.
clinical diagnosis klinische Diagnose *f*.
clinical-diagnostic *adj* klinisch-diagnostisch.
clinical examination klinische Untersuchung *f*.
clinical finding klinischer Befund *m*.
clinical improvement klinische Besserung *f*.
clinical medicine 1. klinische Medizin *f*. **2.** klinischer Studienabschnitt *m*, klinisches Studium *nt*.
clinical microscopy klinische Mikroskopie *f*.
clinical pathology klinische Pathologie *f*.
clinical picture klinisches (Krankheits-)-Bild *nt*, Befund *m*.
clinical psychology klinische Psychologie *f*.
clinical root (of tooth) klinische Zahnwurzel *f*, Radix (dentis) clinica.
clinical setting klinisches Gesamtbild *nt*, klinischer Gesamteindruck *m*.
clinical sign (klinischer) Befund *m*.
clinical spectrometry Biospektrometrie *f*.
clinical spectroscopy Biospektroskopie *f*.
clinical staging klinisches Staging *nt*.
clinical status klinischer Status *m*.
clinical study 1. klinische Studie *f*. **2. ~ies** *pl* klinischer Abschnitt *m* des Medizinstudiums.
clinical test klinischer Test *m*.
clinical thermometer Fieberthermometer *nt*.
clinical trial *stat.* klinische Studie *f*.
cli·ni·cian [klɪˈnɪʃn] *n* Kliniker *m*.
clin·i·co·an·a·tom·i·cal [ˌklɪnɪkəʊænəˈtɒmɪkl] *adj* klinisch-anatomisch.
clin·i·co·path·o·log·ic [ˌ-ˌpæθəˈlɒdʒɪk] *adj* klinisch-pathologisch.
clin·i·co·path·o·log·i·cal [ˌ'lɒdʒɪkl] *adj* → clinicopathologic.
clin·i·co·pa·thol·o·gy [ˌ-pəˈθɒlədʒɪ] *n* klinische Pathologie *f*.
cli·no·ceph·a·lism [ˌklaɪnəˈsefəlɪzəm] *n* → clinocephaly.
cli·no·ceph·a·ly [ˌ-ˈsefəlɪ] *n embryo.* Sattelkopf *m*, Klinokephalie *f*, -zephalie *f*.
cli·no·dac·tyl·ism [ˌ-ˈdæktəlɪzəm] *n* → clinodactyly.
cli·no·dac·ty·ly [ˌ-ˈdæktəlɪ] *n embryo.* Klinodaktylie *f*.
cli·nog·ra·phy [klaɪˈnɒgrəfɪ] *n* graphische Darstellung *f* klinischer Befunde.
cli·noid [ˈklaɪnɔɪd] *adj anat.* bettförmig, klinoid.
clinoid process Proc. clinoideus.
  anterior c. Proc. clinoideus anterior.
  medial c. Proc. clinoideus medius.
  posterior c. Proc. clinoideus posterior.
cli·nom·e·ter [klaɪˈnɒmɪtər] *n* → clinoscope.
cli·no·scope [ˈklaɪnəskəʊp] *n ophthal.* Klinoskop *nt*.
cli·no·stat·ic [ˌ-ˈstætɪk] *adj* im Liegen (auftretend), klinostatisch.
cli·no·ther·a·py [ˌ-ˈθerəpɪ] *n* Behandlung *f* durch Bettruhe, Klinotherapie *f*.
cli·o·quin·ol [klaɪəˈkwɪnɒl] *n pharm.* Clioquinol *nt*.
clip [klɪp] **I** *n* Klemme *f*, Klammer *f*; Spange *f*; *chir.* Klipp *m*, Clip *m*. **II** *vt* (an-)-klammern, (mit einer Klammer *od.* Klemme) befestigen, einen Clip befestigen *od.* anbringen.
clip-applying forceps *chir.* Clipzange *f*.

clip forceps *chir.* Clipzange *f*.
clip-introducing forceps *chir.* Clipzange *f*.
clis·e·om·e·ter [ˌklɪsɪˈɒmɪtər] *n* Klisiometer *nt*.
cli·sis [ˈklaɪsɪs] *n* Neigung *f*, Tendenz *f*.
cli·tel·lum [klaɪˈteləm] *n, pl* **-la** [-lə] *micro.* Clitellum *nt*.
clith·ro·pho·bia [ˌklɪθrəˈfəʊbɪə] *n old* → claustrophobia.
clit·o·ral [ˈklɪtərəl, ˈklaɪ-] *adj* Klitoris betr., Klitoris-.
clit·o·rec·to·my [klɪtəˈrektəmɪ] *n* → clitoridectomy.
clit·o·ri·dauxe [ˌklɪtərɪˈdɔːksɪ] *n* → clitorism 1.
clit·o·rid·e·an [klɪtəˈrɪdɪən, klaɪ-] *adj* → clitoral.
clit·o·ri·dec·to·my [ˌklɪtərɪˈdektəmɪ] *n gyn.* Klitorisresektion *f*, -entfernung *f*, Klitorisektomie *f*, Klitoridektomie *f*.
clit·o·ri·di·tis [ˌ-ˈdaɪtɪs] *n* → clitoritis.
clit·o·ri·dot·o·my [ˌ-ˈdɒtəmɪ] *n gyn.* **1.** Klitorisinzision *f*, -spaltung *f*, Klitorotomie *f*. **2.** weibliche Beschneidung *f*, Klitoridotomie *f*.
clit·o·ri·meg·a·ly [ˌ-ˈmegəlɪ] *n* Klitorisvergrößerung *f*.
clit·o·ris [ˈklɪtərɪs, ˈklaɪ-, klɪˈtɔːrɪs, -ˈtəʊr-] *n* Kitzler *m*, Klitoris *f*, Clitoris *f*.
clitoris crisis *neuro.* Klitoriskrise *f*.
clit·o·rism [ˈklɪtərɪzəm, ˈklaɪ-] *n gyn.* **1.** Klitorishypertrophie *f*, Klitorismus *m*. **2.** schmerzhafte Klitorisschwellung/-erektion *f*, Klitorismus *m*.
clit·o·ri·tis [klɪtəˈraɪtɪs, klaɪ-] *n gyn.* Klitorisentzündung *f*, Klitoritis *f*.
clit·o·ro·meg·a·ly [ˌklɪtərəˈmegəlɪ, ˌklaɪ-] *n* → clitorimegaly.
clit·o·ro·plas·ty [ˈ-plæstɪ] *n gyn.* Klitorisplastik *f*.
clit·o·rot·o·my [klɪtəˈrɒtəmɪ] *n gyn.* → clitoridotomy 1.
cli·val [ˈklaɪvəl] *adj* Klivus betr., Klivus-.
cli·vus [ˈklaɪvəs] *n, pl* **-vi** [-vaɪ] *anat.* Abhang *m*, Klivus *m*, Clivus *m*; Clivus Blumenbachii.
clivus branch of internal carotid artery Ramus clivi.
CLL *abbr.* → chronic lymphocytic leukemia.
C.L.O. *abbr.* → cod-liver oil.
clo·a·ca [kləʊˈeɪkə] *n, pl* **-cae** [-siː] **1.** *embryo., bio.* Kloake *f*, Cloaca *f*. **2.** *patho.* Kloake *f*, Fistelgang *m* bei Osteomyelitis.
clo·a·cal [kləʊˈeɪkl] *adj* Kloake betr., Kloaken-.
cloacal exstrophy *urol.* Kloakenekstrophie *f*, -exstrophie *f*.
cloacal fold *embryo.* Kloakenfalte *f*.
cloacal membrane *embryo.* Kloakenmembran *f*.
clo·a·co·gen·ic [ˌkləʊeɪkəʊˈdʒenɪk] *adj patho., embryo.* kloakogen.
clo·ba·zam [ˈkləʊbəzæm] *n pharm.* Clobazam *nt*.
clock [klɒk] *n* **1.** Uhr *f*. **(a)round the ~** rund um die Uhr; 24 Stunden (lang); ununterbrochen. **2.** Kontroll-, Stoppuhr *f*. **3.** *bio.* innere Uhr *f*.
clock hour volle Stunde *f*.
clock·wise [ˈklɒkwaɪz] *adj* im Uhrzeigersinn, rechtsläufig, -drehend.
clockwise rotation Drehung *f* im Uhrzeigersinn; Rechtsdrehung *f*.
clo·cor·to·lone [kləˈkɔːrtələʊn] *n pharm.* Clocortolon *nt*.
clo·dron·ic acid [kləˈdrɒnɪk] *pharm.* Clodronsäure *f*.
clo·faz·i·mine [kləʊˈfæzɪmiːn] *n pharm.* Clofazimin *nt*.
clo·fi·brate [kləʊˈfaɪbreɪt] *n pharm.* Clofibrat *nt*.

clog [klɒg] **I** *vt* **1.** verstopfen. **2.** hemmen, hindern. **II** *vi s.* verstopfen; klumpig werden, s. zusammenballen.
clog up *vt* → clog 1.
clo·mi·phene [ˈkləʊmɪfiːn] *n pharm.* Clomiphen *nt*.
clomiphene test Clomiphen-Test *m*.
clo·mip·ra·mine [kləʊˈmɪprəmiːn] *n pharm.* Clomipramin *nt*.
clon·al [ˈkləʊnl] *adj* Klon betr., klonal, Klon-.
clo·nal·i·ty [kləʊˈnælətɪ] *n* Fähigkeit *f* zur Klonierung/Klonbildung.
clonal-selection hypothesis/theory Klon-Selektions-Hypothese *f*, -Theorie *f*.
clo·na·ze·pam [kləʊˈneɪzəpæm] *n pharm.* Clonazepam *nt*.
clone [kləʊn] **I** *n* Klon *m*, Clon *nt*. **II** *vt* klonen.
clon·ic [ˈklɒnɪk, ˈkləʊ-] *adj* Klonus betr., klonisch, Klonus-.
clonic contraction klonische Kontraktion *f*.
clonic convulsion klonische Konvulsion *f*.
clon·i·co·ton·ic [ˌklɒnɪkəʊˈtɒnɪk] *adj* klonisch-tonisch.
clonic spasm → clonus.
clon·i·dine [ˈklɒnɪdiːn, ˈkləʊ-] *n pharm.* Clonidin *nt*.
clon·ing [ˈkləʊnɪŋ] *n* Klonierung *f*, Klonbildung *f*.
clo·no·gen·ic [ˌkləʊnəʊˈdʒenɪk] *adj immun.* die Klonbildung anregend, klonogen.
clo·nor·chi·a·sis [ˌkləʊnɔːrˈkaɪəsɪs] *n* Klonorchiasis *f*, Clonorchiose *f*, Clonorchiasis *f*, Opisthorchiasis *f*.
clo·nor·chi·o·sis [kləʊˌnɔːrkaɪˈəʊsɪs] *n* → chlonorchiasis.
Clo·nor·chis si·nen·sis [kləʊˈnɔːrkɪs, klɑn-] *micro.* chinesischer Leberegel *m*, Clonorchis/Opisthorchis sinensis.
clon·o·spasm [ˈklɒnəspæzəm, ˈkləʊn-] *n* → clonus.
clo·no·type [ˈ-taɪp] *n immun.* Klonotyp *m*.
clo·nus [ˈkləʊnəs] *n physiol.* Klonus *m*, Clonus *m*.
clo·pa·mide [kləʊˈpæmaɪd] *n pharm.* Clopamid *nt*.
clo·pen·thix·ol [ˌkləʊpənˈθɪksəʊl] *n pharm.* Clopenthixol *nt*.
clo·pred·nol [kləʊˈprednəʊl] *n pharm.* Cloprednol *nt*.
Cloquet [klɒˈkeɪ, klɔˈkɛ]: **C.'s canal** Cloquet'-Kanal *m*, Canalis hyaloideus.
C.'s fascia Cloquet-Faszie *f*.
C.'s hernia Cloquet-Hernie *f*, Hernia femoralis pectinea.
C.'s ligament Cloquet'-Band *nt*, Vestigium proc. vaginalis.
C.'s node Cloquet-Drüse *f*, Rosenmüller--Cloquet-Drüse *f*, Rosenmüller-Drüse *f*.
round ligament of C. Lig. capitis costae intraarticulare.
C.'s septum Cloquet-Septum *nt*, Septum femorale.
C.'s space Cloquet-Raum *m*.
clor·az·e·pate [klɔːˈræzɪpeɪt] *n pharm.* Clorazepat *nt*.
close [*n, v* kləʊz; *adj* kləʊs] **I** *n* **1.** Ende *nt*, (Ab-)Schluß *m*. **2.** Schließen *nt*, Schließung *f*. **II** *adj* **3.** (*Struktur*) fest, dicht. **4.** dicht, nah. **~ together** nah(e) beieinander. **~ to** in der Nähe von, nahe *od.* dicht bei; (*zeitlich*) nahe bevorstehend; *fig.* (jdm.) nahestehend. **5.** (*Person*) vertraut, eng, nah; (*Ähnlichkeit*) stark, groß. **6.** eingehend, genau, gründlich. **~ investigation** *f*. **7.** lückenlos, stichhaltig, streng logisch. **8.** geschlossen, zu; eingeschlossen *od.* umgeben von. **9.** fest-, engsitzend, enganliegend. **10.** (*Haar*) kurz. **11.** stickig, schwül,

close-by 156

drückend. **12.** *fig.* (*Person*) verschlossen, verschwiegen. **III** *vt* **13.** (ab-, zu-, ver-)schließen, zumachen. **to ~ in layers** *chir.* (*Wunde*) schichtweise verschließen. **14.** verstopfen, blockieren; versperren. **15.** *psycho.* s. verschließen. **16.** *techn.* (Stromkreis) schließen. **17.** beenden, (ab-)schließen. **IV** *vi* **18.** geschlossen werden. **19.** *allg.* s. schließen; (*Wunde*) heilen, zugehen. **20.** aufhören, enden, zu Ende gehen.
close about *vi* umgeben, -schließen, s. schließen um.
close up *vi* (*Wunde*) s. schließen, zugehen, heilen.
close-by *adj* in der Nähe, nahe, angrenzend, benachbart.
closed [kloʊzd] *adj* **1.** geschlossen, zu. **2.** (*Person*) verschlossen. **3.** ge-, versperrt. **4.** in s. geschlossen, autark.
closed amputation *chir.*, *ortho.* geschlossene Amputation *f*, Amputation *f* mit Lappendeckung.
closed anesthesia *anes.* geschlossene Narkose/Anästhesie *f*; geschlossenes Narkosesystem *nt*.
closed-angle glaucoma *patho.* akutes Winkelblockglaukom/Engwinkelglaukom *nt*, Glaucoma acutum (congestivum).
closed chain *chem.* geschlossene Kette *f*, Ringform *f*.
closed-chain compound *chem.* Ringverbindung *f*.
closed dislocation *ortho.* einfache/geschlossene Luxation *f*.
closed form *chem.* geschlossene Form *f*.
closed fracture *ortho.* einfache/geschlossene/unkomplizierte Fraktur *f*.
closed-loop obstruction *chir.* Adhäsionsileus/Strangulationsileus *m* einer Darmschleife.
closed pneumothorax geschlossener Pneu(mothorax *m*) *m*.
closed reduction *ortho.* geschlossene Reposition *f*.
closed rhinolalia *HNO* geschlossenes Näseln *nt*, Hyporhinolalie *f*, Rhinolalia clausa.
closed system geschlossenes System *nt*.
close-fitting *adj* eng-, festsitzend, enganliegend.
close-lipped *adj* → close-mouthed.
close-mouthed *adj fig.* verschlossen, verschwiegen, schweigsam.
close-ness ['kloʊsnɪs] *n* **1.** Dichte *f*, Festigkeit *f*. **2.** Nähe *f*; *fig.* Vertrautheit *f*. **3.** Gründlich-, Genauigkeit *f*. **4.** Schwüle *f*, stickige Luft *f*. **5.** Verschlossenheit *f*, Verschwiegenheit *f*.
clos-et ['klɑzɪt] *n* **1.** (Wand-)Schrank *m*. **2.** (Wasser-)Klosett *nt*.
close vision Nahsehen *nt*, Nahsicht *f*.
clos-ing contraction ['kloʊzɪŋ] Schließungskontraktion *f*.
closing pressure Verschlußdruck *m*.
closing volume Verschlußvolumen *nt*.
clos-trid-i-al [klɑ'strɪdiəl] *adj* Clostridien betr., durch sie verursacht, Clostridien-.
clostridial bacteremia Clostridienbakteriämie *f*.
clostridial cellulitis Clostridien-Cellulitis *f*.
clostridial myonecrosis Gasbrand *m*, -gangrän *f*, -ödem *nt*, malignes Ödem *nt*.
clostridial spores *micro.* Clostridiensporen *pl*.
clos-trid-i-o-pep-ti-dase A [klɑˌstrɪdiə'peptɪdeɪz] Clostridium-histolyticum-kollagenase *f*, Clostridiopeptidase A *f*.
clostridiopeptidase B Clostridium-histolyticum-proteinase B *f*, Clostridiopeptidase B *f*, Clostripain *nt*.

Clos-trid-i-um [klɑ'strɪdiəm] *n micro.* Clostridium *nt*.
C. botulinum Botulinusbazillus *m*, Clostridium botulinum, *old* Bact./Bacillus botulinus.
C. novyi Clostridium novyi/oedematiens.
C. novyi type B Bacillus gigas Zeissler, Clostridium novyi typ B.
C. novyi type C Clostridium bubalorum Prévot, Clostridium novyi typ C.
C. perfringens Welch-Fränkel-(Gasbrand-)Bazillus *m*, Clostridium perfringens.
C. septicum Pararauschbrandbazillus *m*, Clostridium septicum.
C. tetani Tetanusbazillus *m*, -erreger *m*, Wundstarrkrampfbazillus *m*, -erreger *m*, Clostridium/Plectridium tetani.
C. welchii *Brit.* → C. perfringens.
clos-trid-i-um [klɑ'strɪdiəm] *n*, *pl* **-dia** [-dɪə] Klostridie *f*, Clostridie *f*, Clostridium *nt*.
clostridium botulinum toxin Clostridium botulinum-Toxin *nt*.
clo-sure ['kloʊʒər] *n* **1.** *allg.* Schließung *f*, (Zu-, Ab-)Schließen *nt*; Stillegung *f*. **2.** (*Wunde*) Verschließen *nt*. **3.** Verschluß *m*.
c. in (**anatomic**) **layers** *chir.* schichtweiser Wundverschluß, Etagennaht *f*.
clot [klɑt] **I** *n* **1.** Klumpen *m*, Klümpchen *nt*. **2.** (Blut-, Fibrin-)Gerinnsel *nt*. **II** *vt* zum Gerinnen bringen. **III** *vi* **3.** gerinnen; (*Blut*) koagulieren. **4.** Klumpen bilden; (*Milch*) dick werden.
cloth [klɔθ, klɑθ] *n*, *pl* **cloths** Tuch *nt*, Gewebe *nt*; Lappen *m*.
clothes [kloʊ(ð)z] *pl* Kleider *pl*, Kleidung *f*; (Bett-)Wäsche *f*.
clothes louse *micro.* Kleiderlaus *f*, Pediculus humanis corporis/humanus/vestimenti.
cloth-ing ['kloʊðɪŋ] *n* (Be-)Kleidung *f*.
clo-trim-a-zole [kloʊ'trɪməzoʊl] *n pharm.* Clotrimazol *nt*.
clot-ta-ble fibrinogen ['klɑtəbl] *lab.* gerinnbares/gerinnungsfähiges Fibrinogen *nt*.
clot-ted ['klɑtɪd] *adj* **1.** geronnen. **2.** klumpig. **3.** (*Haar*) verklebt.
clot-ting ['klɑtɪŋ] *n* (Blut-, Fibrin-)Gerinnung *f*, Koagulation *f*; Klumpenbildung *f*.
clotting factors (Blut-)Gerinnungsfaktoren *pl*.
clotting time (Blut-)Gerinnungszeit *f*.
reptilase c. Reptilasezeit.
thrombin c. (Plasma-)Thrombinzeit *abbr.* TT, TZ, Antithrombinzeit *abbr.* ATZ.
clot-ty ['klɑti] *adj* klumpig.
cloud [klaʊd] **I** *n* **1.** (Staub-, Rauch-)Wolke *f*. **2.** dunkle *od.* trübe Stelle *f*, Schatten *m*; (*Flüssigkeit*) Trübung *f*, Wolke *f*. **II** *vt* (*a. fig.*) trüben. **III** *vi* (*a. fig.*) s. trüben, s. verdunkeln; (*Glas*) s. beschlagen.
c. of electrons *phys.* Elektronenwolke, -schwarm *m*.
cloud chamber *phys.* Nebelkammer *f*.
cloud-ed ['klaʊdɪd] *adj* **1.** trübe, bewölkt. (*Flüssigkeit*) trübe, getrübt, wolkig; (*Glas*) beschlagen. **2.** *fig.* (*Verstand*) getrübt, verwirrt, konfus, wirr.
cloud-i-ness ['klaʊdnɪs] *n* Trübung *f*; Undeutlichkeit *f*, Verschwommenheit *f*; Schleier *m*.
cloud-ing ['klaʊdɪŋ] *n* Verschwommenheit *f*, Verschattung *f*; (*Verstand*) (Ein-)Trübung *f*, Umwölkung *f*.
c. of consciousness Bewußtseinseintrübung.
cloud track *phys.* Nebelspur *f*.
cloud-y ['klaʊdi] *adj* **1.** bewölkt, trübe; (*Flüssigkeit*) wolkig, trübe, unklar. **2.** *fig.* unscharf, undeutlich, verschwommen.

cloudy swelling *patho.* albuminöse/albuminoide/albuminoid-körnige Degeneration *f*, trübe Schwellung *f*.
cloudy urine trüber/getrübter Urin *m*, Urina jumentosa.
Clough-Richter [klʌf 'rɪktər]: **C.-R.'s syndrome** Clough-Syndrom *nt*, Clough-Richter-Syndrom *nt*, Kältehämagglutinationskrankheit *f*.
Clouston ['klaʊstən]: **C.'s syndrome** Clouston-Syndrom *nt*, hydrotisch ektodermale Dysplasie *f*.
clo-ver-leaf arrangement ['kloʊvərˌli:f] *biochem.* Kleeblattformation *f*.
clo-ver mite ['kloʊvər] *micro.* Bryobia praetiosa.
Cloward ['klaʊərd]: **C.'s method for spinal fusion** *ortho.* Cloward-Operation *f*.
C.'s technique → C.'s method for spinal fusion.
clown-ism ['klaʊnɪzəm] *n psychia.* Clownismus *m*.
clox-a-cil-lin [klɑksə'sɪlɪn] *n pharm.* Cloxacillin *nt*.
clox-y-quin ['klɑksəkwɪn] *n pharm.* Cloxiquin *nt*.
clubbed ['klʌbt] *adj* **1.** keulenförmig. **2.** klumpig, Klump-. **3.** (*Finger*) schlegelförmig; (*Fuß*) klumpfüßig.
clubbed digits → clubbed fingers.
clubbed fingers Trommelschlegelfinger *pl*, Digiti hippocratici.
club-bing ['klʌbɪŋ] *n* (*Finger, Zehe*) Trommelschlegelbildung *f*.
club-foot ['klʌbfʊt] *n ortho.* (angeborener) Klumpfuß *m*, Pes equinovarus (excavatus et adductus).
club-foot-ed ['klʌbfʊtɪd] *adj* klumpfüßig.
club fungi *micro.* Ständerpilze *pl*, Basidiomyzeten *pl*, -mycetes *pl*.
club hair Kolben-, Telogenhaar *nt*.
club-hand ['klʌbhænd] *n ortho.*, *neuro.* Klumphand *f*, Manus vara.
club-shaped *adj* keulenförmig.
clue [klu:] *n* **1.** Hinweis *m* (*for, to* auf); Anhaltspunkt *m* (*for, to* für). **2.** Knäuel *m/nt*.
clue cells *gyn.*, *patho.* Clue-Zellen *pl*.
clump [klʌmp] **I** *n* **1.** Klumpen *m*; Haufen *m*, Masse *f*. **2.** *immun.* Verklumpung *f*, Zusammenballung *f*, Agglutination *f*. **II** *vi* s. zusammenballen, verklumpen, verkleben, agglutinieren.
clump foot → clubfoot.
clump-ing ['klʌmpɪŋ] *n* **1.** Verklumpen *nt*, Zusammenballen *nt*, Agglutination *f*. **2.** → clump 2.
clumping factor Clumping-Faktor *m*.
clump kidney Kuchen-, Klumpenniere *f*.
clump-y ['klʌmpi] *adj* verklumpt, verklebt, agglutiniert.
clu-ne-al cleft ['klu:niəl] Gesäßspalte *f*, Afterfurche *f*, Crena ani, Rima ani.
cluneal nerves: inferior c. untere Clunialnerven *pl*, Rami clunium/glut(a)eales inferiores.
middle c. mittlere Clunialnerven *pl*, Rami clunium/glut(a)eales medii.
superior c. obere Clunialnerven *pl*, Rami clunium/glut(a)eales superiores.
clu-nes ['klu:ni:z] *pl anat.* Gesäß(backen *pl*), Hinterbacken *pl*, Clunes *pl*, Nates *pl*.
clus-ter ['klʌstər] **I** *n* **1.** *bot.* Traube *f*, Büschel *m*. **2.** Haufen *m*, Anhäufung *f*, Ansammlung *f*. **II** *vi* **3.** s. versammeln, eine Gruppe *od.* Gruppen bilden, s. (zusammen-)drängen (*around* um). **4.** traubenod. büschelartig wachsen.
clus-tered ['klʌstərd] *adj* büschel- *od.* traubenförmig, gebündelt.
cluster headache (Bing-)Horton-Syn-

drom *nt*, Erythroprosopalgie *f*, Histaminkopfschmerz *m*, -kephalgie *f*, cluster headache.
clut·ter·ing ['klʌtərɪŋ] *n neuro., psychia.* nervöses verwirrtes Sprechen *nt*.
Clutton ['klʌtn]: **C.'s joint** Clutton-Krankheit *f*, -Gelenk *nt*, -Syndrom *nt*.
cly·sis ['klaɪsɪs] *n, pl* **-ses** [-siːz] Infusionslösung *f*, -flüssigkeit *f*, Nährlösung *f*, -flüssigkeit *f*.
clys·ma ['klɪzmə] *n, pl* **-ma·ta** [-mətə] Einlauf *m*, Klistier *nt*, Klysma *nt*, Clysma *nt*.
clys·ter ['klɪstər] **I** *n* → clysma. **II** *vt* → clysterize.
clys·ter·ize ['klɪstəraɪz] *vt* jdm. einen Einlauf geben.
CM *abbr.* → cardiomyopathy.
Cm *abbr.* → curium.
cm *abbr.* → centimeter.
CMC *abbr.* → carpometacarpal.
CM-cellulose → carboxymethylcellulose.
CMCJ *abbr.* [carpometacarpal joint] → carpometacarpal articulation.
CMC joint → carpometacarpal articulation.
CMD *abbr.* → cerebromacular degeneration.
CMI *abbr.* → cell-mediated immunity.
CML *abbr.* **1.** → cell-mediated lympholysis. **2.** → chronic myelocytic leukemia.
CMP *abbr.* → cytidine monophosphate.
CMT *abbr.* → Charcot-Marie-Tooth atrophy.
CMV *abbr.* → cytomegalovirus.
CMVIG *abbr.* → cytomegalovirus immune globulin.
cne·mi·al ['niːmɪəl] *adj* Schienbein betr., Schienbein-.
Cne·mi·do·cop·tes [ˌniːmɪdəʊˈkɑptiːz] *pl micro.* Knemidokoptes *pl*.
cne·mis ['niːmɪs] *n* Unterschenkel *m*; Schienbein *nt*, Tibia *f*; Schienbeinregion *f*.
cne·mi·tis [niːˈmaɪtɪs] *n* Schienbein-, Tibiaentzündung *f*.
cni·da ['naɪdə] *n, pl* **-dae** [-diː] *bio.* Nesselkapsel *f*, Nematozyste *f*, Knide *f*.
cni·do·blast ['naɪdəblæst] *n micro.* Nesselzelle *f*.
cni·do·cil ['-sɪl] *n micro.* Knidozil *nt*.
cni·do·cyst ['-sɪst] *n* → cnida.
CNS *abbr.* → central nervous system.
CNS disease ZNS-Erkrankung *f*, Erkrankung *f* des zentralen Nervensystems.
CNS metastasis ZNS-Metastase *f*, Metastase *f* ins ZNS.
CNV *abbr.* → contingent negative variation.
CO *abbr.* → carbon monoxide.
Co *abbr.* → cobalt.
CO₂ *abbr.* → carbon dioxide.
co·ac·er·vate [kəʊˈæsərvɪt, -veɪt, ˌkəʊəˈsɜrvɪt] *n* Koazervat *nt*.
co·ac·er·va·tion [kəʊˌæsərˈveɪʃn] *n* Koazervatbildung *f*.
co·act [kəʊˈækt] *vt* zusammenarbeiten, -wirken.
co·ac·tion [kəʊˈækʃn] *n* Zusammenarbeit *f*, -wirken *nt*.
co·ac·tive [kəʊˈæktɪv] *adj* zusammenwirkend.
COAD *abbr.* [chronic obstructive airways disease] → chronic obstructive lung disease.
co·ad·ap·ta·tion [kəʊˌædəpˈteɪʃn] *n* Koadaptation *f*.
co·ag·glu·ti·na·tion [kəʊəˌgluːtəˈneɪʃn] *n* Koagglutination *f*.
co·ag·glu·ti·nin [kəʊəˈgluːtnɪn] *n* Koagglutinin *nt*.
co·ag·u·la·bil·i·ty [kəʊˌægjələˈbɪlɪti] *n* Gerinnbarkeit *f*, Koagulierbarkeit *f*, Koagulabilität *f*.

co·ag·u·la·ble [kəʊˈægjələbl] *adj* gerinnbar, gerinnungsfähig, koagulierbar, koagulabel.
co·ag·u·lant [kəʊˈægjələnt] **I** *n* gerinnungsförderndes Mittel *nt*, Koagulans *nt*. **II** *adj* Koagulation bewirkend *od.* beschleunigend *od.* verursachend, gerinnungs-, koagulationsfördernd.
co·ag·u·lase [kəʊˈægjəleɪz] *n* Koagulase *f*, Coagulase *f*.
coagulase-negative *adj* koagulasenegativ.
coagulase-positive *adj* koagulasepositiv.
coagulase test Koagulasetest *m*.
co·ag·u·late [kəʊˈægjəleɪt] **I** *vt* gerinnen *od.* koagulieren lassen. **II** *vi* gerinnen, koagulieren.
co·ag·u·lat·ed protein [kəʊˈægjəleɪtɪd] koaguliertes Protein *nt*.
co·ag·u·la·tion [kəʊˌægjəˈleɪʃn] *n* **1.** Gerinnung *f*, Koagulation *f*. **2.** Blutgerinnung *f*. **3.** → coagulum.
coagulation cascade Gerinnungs-, Koagulationskaskade *f*.
coagulation defect *hema.* (Blut-)Gerinnungsstörung *f*.
coagulation factors (Blut-)Gerinnungsfaktoren *pl*.
coagulation necrosis *patho.* Koagulationsnekrose *f*.
coagulation status *lab.* Gerinnungsstatus *m*.
coagulation test *lab.* Gerinnungstest *m*.
coagulation thrombus Gerinnungs-, Schwanzthrombus *m*, roter Thrombus *m*.
coagulation time (Blut-)Gerinnungszeit *f*.
co·ag·u·la·tive [kəʊˈægjəleɪtɪv, -lətɪv] *adj* gerinnungsfördernd, -verursachend, koagulationsfördernd.
co·ag·u·lop·a·thy [kəʊˌægjəˈlɑpəθi] *n* (Blut-)Gerinnungsstörung *f*, Koagulopathie *f*.
co·ag·u·la·tor [kəʊˈægjəleɪtər] *n chir.* Koagulator *m*.
co·ag·u·lum [kəʊˈægjələm] *n, pl* **-la** [-lə] (Blut-)Gerinnsel *nt*, Koagel *nt*, Koagulum *nt*.
coal [kəʊl] *n* (Stein-, Holz-)Kohle *f*.
coal-black *adj* kohl(raben)schwarz.
coal dust Kohlenstaub *m*.
co·a·lesce [ˌkəʊəˈles] **I** *vt* verbinden, verschmelzen, vereinigen. **II** *vi* zusammenwachsen, verschmelzen (*into* in), s. verbinden *od.* vereinigen.
co·a·les·cence [ˌ-ˈlesn(t)s] *n* Verschmelzen *nt*, Vereinigen *nt*, Verschmelzung *f*, Vereinigung *f*, Zusammenwachsen *nt*.
co·a·les·cent [ˌ-ˈlesnt] *adj* verschmelzend, zusammenwachsend, s. vereinigend.
coal miner's lung *pulmo.* Kohlenstaublunge *f*, Lungenanthrakose *f*, Anthracosis pulmonum.
coal miner's phthisis → coal miner's lung.
coal oil Petroleum *nt*.
coal pigment Kohle(n)pigment *nt*.
coal tar Steinkohlenteer *m*.
co·apt [kəʊˈæpt] *vt* (*Wundränder*) annähern; (*Frakturenden*) annähern, einrichten.
co·ap·ta·tion [ˌkəʊæpˈteɪʃn] *n* (*Wundränder*) Annähern *nt*; *ortho.* Einrichten *nt*.
co·arct [kəʊˈɑːrkt] *vt* zusammen-, aneinanderpressen.
co·arc·tate [kəʊˈɑːrkteɪt, -tɪt] **I** *adj* zusammen-, aneinandergepreßt. **II** *vt* → coarct.
co·arc·ta·tion [ˌkəʊɑːrkˈteɪʃn] *n* Verengung *f*, Verengerung *f*, Striktur *f*, Koarktation *f*; *anat.* Coarctatio *f*.
c. of aorta Aortenisthmusstenose *f*, Coarctatio aortae *f*.
co·arc·tot·o·my [ˌ-ˈtɑtəmi] *n chir.* Strikturendurchtrennung *f*, Koarktotomie *f*.

coarse [kɔːrs, kəʊərs] *adj* **1.** grob, grobkörnig. **2.** (*Haut, Stimme*) rauh. **3.** (*Tremor*) grobschlägig. **4.** *fig.* grob, derb, roh. **5.** (*Einstellung*) grob, ungenau.
coarse-grained *adj* **1.** grobfaserig, -körnig. **2.** *fig.* grob, derb.
coars·en [ˈkɔːrsn, ˈkəʊər-] **I** *vt* grob *od.* rauh machen. **II** *vi* grob *od.* rauh werden.
coarse·ness [ˈkɔːrsnɪs, ˈkəʊərs-] *n* **1.** Rauheit *f*, Grobfaserig-, Grobkörnigkeit *f*. **2.** *fig.* Derb-, Grob-, Rohheit *f*.
coarse tremor grobschlägiger Tremor *m*.
CoA(-SH) *abbr.* → coenzyme A.
coast erysipelas [kəʊst] Onchozerkose *f*, Onchocercose *f*, Onchocerciasis *f*, Knotenfilariose *f*, Onchocerca-volvulus-Infektion *f*.
coat [kəʊt] **I** *n* **1.** Haut *f*, Fell *nt*, Hülle *f*. **2.** Mantel *m*, (Arzt-)Kittel *m*. **3.** Überzug *m*, Beschichtung *f*, Schicht *f*, Decke *f*. **II** *vt* **4.** beschichten, überziehen. **5.** bedecken, umhüllen (*with* mit).
coat·ed [ˈkəʊtɪd] *adj* **1.** beschichtet, überzogen (*with* mit); *pharm.* dragiert. **2.** (*Zunge*) belegt. **3.** imprägniert; gestrichen. **4.** bekleidet.
coated tablet Dragée *nt*, Pille *f*.
coated tongue belegte Zunge *f*.
coated vesicle *histol.* Stachelsaumbläschen *nt*.
coat·ing [ˈkəʊtɪŋ] *n* Schicht *f*, Beschichtung *f*, Deckschicht *f*; (*Zunge*) Belag *m*; *pharm.* Überzug *m*.
coat protein Hüllprotein *nt*.
CoA-transferase *n* Coenzym A-Transferase *f*, CoA-Transferase *f*.
Coats [kəʊts]: **C.'s disease/retinitis** Coats-Syndrom *nt*, Morbus Coats *m*, Retinitis exsudativa externa.
co·bal·a·min [kəʊˈbæləmɪn] *n* Kobalamin *nt*, Cobalamin *nt*.
co·balt [ˈkəʊbɔːlt] *n abbr.* **Co** Kobalt *nt*, Cobalt *nt abbr.* Co.
cobalt 60 Kobalt 60 *nt abbr.* Co-60, ⁶⁰Co.
cobalt irradiation *radiol.* Kobaltbestrahlung *f*.
co·bal·tous chloride [kəʊˈbɔːltəs] *pharm.* Kobalt-II-chlorid *nt*.
cobalt radiation *radiol.* Kobaltbestrahlung *f*.
co·bam·ic acid [kəʊˈbæmɪk] Cobamsäure *f*.
co·bam·ide [kəʊˈbæmaɪd] *n* Cobamid *nt*.
Cobb [kɑb]: **C. method** *ortho.* (*Skoliose*) Bestimmung *f* des Krümmungswinkels nach Cobb, Cobb-Methode *f*.
cob·bler's chest [ˈkɑblər] Schusterbrust *f*.
cob·ble·stone mucosa [ˈkɑbəlstəʊn] *patho.* (*Schleimhaut*) Pflastersteinrelief *nt*.
co·bin·am·ide [kəʊˈbɪnəmaɪd] *n* Cobinamid *nt*.
co·bin·ic acid [kəʊˈbɪnɪk] Cobinsäure *f*.
co·bra venom cofactor [ˈkəʊbrə] *immun.* C3-Proaktivator *m*, Faktor B *m*.
co·byr·ic acid [kəʊˈbɪrɪk] Cobyrsäure *f*.
co·byr·in·a·mide [kəʊbɪˈrɪnəmaɪd] *n* → cobyric acid.
co·byr·in·ic acid [ˌ-ˈrɪnɪk] Cobyrinsäure *f*.
cobyrinic hexa-amide → cobyric acid.
COC *abbr.* → cathodal opening contraction.
co·ca [ˈkəʊkə] *n* **1.** *bot.* Koka *f*, Coca *f*. **2.** Kokablätter *pl*, Folia cocae.
co·cain *n* → cocaine.
co·caine [kəʊˈkeɪn, ˈkəʊ-] *n* Kokain *nt*, Cocain *nt*.
cocaine abusus → cocainism 1.
cocaine intoxication → cocainism 2.
co·cain·ism [kəʊˈkeɪnɪzəm, ˈkəʊkə-] *n* **1.** Kokainmißbrauch *m*, -abusus *m*, -abhängigkeit *f*, Kokainismus *m*, Cocainis-

cocainization

mus *m*. 2. chronische Kokainvergiftung *f*, Kokainismus *m*, Cocainismus *m*.
co·cain·i·za·tion [kəʊˌkeɪnɪ'zeɪʃn, -naɪ-] *n anes*. Kokainisierung *f*, Cocainisierung *f*.
co·cain·ize [kəʊ'keɪnaɪz, 'kəʊkə-] *vt* mit Kokain(lösung) betäuben, kokainisieren.
co·car·box·y·lase [kəʊkɑːr'bɑksəleɪz] *n old* → thiamine pyrophosphate.
co·car·cin·o·gen [kəʊkɑːr'sɪnədʒən] *n* Kokarzinogen *nt*.
co·car·ci·no·gen·e·sis [kəʊˌkɑːrsnəʊ'dʒenəsɪs] *n* Kokarzinogenese *f*.
coc·cal ['kɑkəl] *adj* Kokken betr., kokkenähnlich, -förmig, Kokken-.
Coc·cid·i·a [kɑk'sɪdɪə] *pl micro*. Kokzidien *pl*, Coccidia *pl*.
coc·cid·i·al [kɑk'sɪdɪəl] *adj* Kokzidien betr., durch sie verursacht, Kokzidien-.
coccidial disease → coccidiosis.
coc·cid·i·an [kɑk'sɪdɪən] **I** *n* → coccidium. **II** *adj* → coccidial.
coc·cid·i·oi·dal [kɑkˌsɪdɪ'ɔɪdl] *adj* Kokzidioido-, Kokzidioiden-.
coccidioidal granuloma 1. → coccidioidomycosis. **2.** sekundäre/progressive Kokzidioidomykose *f*, Sekundärform *f* der Kokzidioidomykose.
coccidioidal meningitis Kokzidioidenmeningitis *f*.
Coc·cid·i·oi·des [ˌ-'ɔɪdiːz] *n* Kokzidioidespilz *m*, Coccidioides *m*.
coc·cid·i·oi·din [ˌ-'ɔɪdɪn] *n* Kokzidioidin *nt*, Coccidioidin *nt*.
coccidioidin skin test Kokzidioidin-(Haut)-Test *m*.
coccidioidin test → coccidioidin skin test.
coc·cid·i·oi·do·ma [kɑkˌsɪdɪɔɪ'dəʊmə] *n* Kokzidioidom *nt*.
coc·cid·i·oi·do·my·co·sis [kɑkˌsɪdɪˌɔɪdɑmaɪ'kəʊsɪs] *n* Wüstenfieber *nt*, Posada-Mykose *f*, Kokzidioidomykose *f*, Coccidioidomycose *f*, Granuloma coccidioides.
coc·cid·i·oi·do·sis [kɑkˌsɪdɪɔɪ'dəʊsɪs] *n* → coccidioidomycosis.
coc·cid·i·o·sis [kɑkˌsɪdɪ'əʊsɪs] *n* Kokzidienbefall *m*, -erkrankung *f*, Kokzidiose *f*, Coccidiosis *f*.
coc·cid·i·um [kɑk'sɪdɪəm] *n*, *pl* **-dia** [-dɪə] *micro*. Kokzidie *f*, Coccidium *nt*.
coc·ci·gen·ic [ˌkɑksə'dʒenɪk] *adj* durch Kokken bedingt *od*. hervorgerufen, kokkenbedingt, Kokken-.
coc·ci·nel·la [ˌ-'nelə] *n* → cochineal.
coc·ci·nel·lin [ˌ-'nelɪn] *n* Karmin *nt*.
cocco- *pref*. Beeren-, Trauben-, Kokken-.
coc·co·gen·ic [ˌkɑkə'dʒenɪk] *adj* → coccigenic.
coc·cog·e·nous [kə'kɑdʒənəs] *adj* → coccigenic.
coc·coid ['kɑkɔɪd] *adj* kokkenähnlich, kokkoid.
coc·cu·lin ['kɑkjəlɪn] *n* Pikrotoxin *nt*, Cocculin *nt*.
coc·cus ['kɑkəs] *n*, *pl* **-ci** [-saɪ, -siː] Kokke *f*, Kokkus *m*, Coccus *m*.
coc·cy·al·gia [ˌkɑksə'ældʒ(ɪ)ə] *n* → coccygodynia.
coc·cy·dyn·ia [ˌ-'dɪnɪə] *n* → coccygodynia.
coc·cy·gal·gia [ˌ-'gældʒ(ɪ)ə] *n* → coccygodynia.
coc·cyg·e·al [kɑk'sɪdʒɪəl] *adj* Steißbein/Os coccygis betr., kokzygeal, coccygeal, Steißbein-, Kokzygo-.
coccygeal artery mittlere Kreuzbeinarterie *f*, Sakralis *f* mediana, A. sacralis mediana.
coccygeal body → coccygeal glomus.
coccygeal bone → coccyx.
coccygeal dimple → coccygeal foveola.
coccygeal eminence Cornu sacrale.
coccygeal fistula Steißbeinfistel *f*, Fistula coccygealis.
coccygeal foveola Steißbeingrübchen *nt*, Foveola coccygea.
coccygeal gland → coccygeal glomus.
coccygeal glomus Steiß(bein)knäuel *m/nt*, Corpus/Glomus coccygeum.
coccygeal horn Cornu coccygeum.
coccygeal ligament, superior Lig. iliofemorale.
coccygeal muscle → coccygeus (muscle).
coccygeal nerve kokzygealer Spinalnerv *m*, Kokzygeus *m*, N. coccygeus.
coccygeal part of spinal cord → coccygeal segments of spinal cord.
coccygeal plexus Steißbein-, Kokzygealplexus *m*, Plexus coccygeus.
coccygeal segments of spinal cord Steißbein-, Kokzygealsegmente *pl*, Steißbeinabschnitt *m* des Rückenmarks, Coccygea *pl*, Pars coccygea (medullae spinalis).
coccygeal vertebrae Steiß(bein)wirbel *pl*, Vertebrae coccygeae.
coc·cy·gec·to·my [ˌkɑksə'dʒektəmɪ] *n chir*. Steißbeinresektion *f*, Kokzygektomie *f*.
coc·cy·ge·o·pu·bic diameter [kɑkˌsɪdʒɪəʊ'pjuːbɪk] *gyn*. Distantia pubococcygea.
coc·cy·ge·us (muscle) [kɑk'sɪdʒɪəs] Steißbeinmuskel *m*, Kokzygeus *m*, M. coccygeus.
coc·cy·go·dyn·ia [ˌkɑksɪgəʊ'dɪnɪə] *n* Steißbeinschmerz *m*, Kokzygodynie *f*, Coccygodynie *f*.
coc·cy·got·o·my [ˌkɑksə'gɑtəmɪ] *n chir*. Steißbeinlösung *f*, Kokzygotomie *f*.
coc·cy·o·dyn·ia [ˌkɑksɪəʊ'dɪnɪə] *n* → coccygodynia.
coc·cyx ['kɑksɪks] *n*, *pl* **-cy·ges** [-'saɪdʒiːz, -sɪdʒiːz] Steißbein *nt*, Coccyx *f*, Os coccygis.
Cochin-China diarrhea ['kəʊtʃɪn 'tʃaɪnə] tropische Sprue *f*.
coch·i·neal [ˌkɑtʃə'niːl, 'kɑtʃəniːl] *n* Koschenille(rot *nt*) *f*, Cochenille(rot *nt*) *f*.
coch·le·a ['kɑklɪə, 'kəʊ-] *n*, *pl* **-le·ae** [-liː, -liaɪ] *anat*. **1.** spiral- *od*. schneckenförmige Struktur *f*, Cochlea *f*. **2.** (Gehörgangs-, Innenohr-)Schnecke *f*, Kochlea *f*, Cochlea *f*.
coch·le·ar ['kɑklɪər, 'kəʊ-] *adj anat*. schneckenförmig; (Innenohr-)Schnecke/Cochlea betr., kochlear.
cochlear area (of internal acoustic meatus) Area cochleae.
cochlear artery → cochlear branch of labyrinthine artery.
cochlear articulation Ellipsoid-, Eigelenk *nt*, Artic. ellipsoidea.
cochlear branch of labyrinthine artery Kochleaast *m* der A. labyrinthina, Ramus cochlearis a. labyrinthinae.
cochlear canal → cochlear duct.
cochlear canaliculus Canaliculus cochleae.
cochlear duct (häutiger) Schneckengang *m*, Ductus cochlearis.
cochlear ganglion Corti'-Ganglion *nt*, Ggl. cochleare, Ggl. spirale cochlearis.
cochlear haircells Corti'-Haarzellen *pl*.
coch·le·ar·i·form [kɑklɪ'ærəfɔːrm, kəʊ-] *adj* löffelförmig.
cochleariform process Proc. cochleariformis.
cochlear implant *HNO* Cochlear implant (*nt*).
cochlear joint → cochlear articulation.
cochlear labyrinth Schneckenlabyrinth *nt*, Labyrinthus cochlearis.
cochlear microphonics (kochleäres) Mikrophonpotential *nt*.

158

cochlear nerve Hörnerv *m*, Cochlearis *m*, Pars cochlearis n. vestibulocochlearis, N. cochlearis.
cochlear nucleus: c.i *pl* Cochleariskerne *pl*, Ncc. cochleares.
anterior c. vorderer Cochleariskern *m*, Nc. cochlearis anterior.
dorsal c. hinterer Cochleariskern *m*, Nc. cochlearis posterior.
posterior c. → dorsal c.
ventral c. → anterior c.
cochlear potentials → cochlear microphonics.
cochlear presbyacusis, conductive *HNO* kochleärer Leitungstyp *m* der Presbyakusis.
cochlear recess (of vestibule) Rec. cochlearis (vestibuli).
cochlear root of vestibulocochlear nerve unterer/kochlearer Anteil *m* des N. vestibulocochlearis, Pars inferior n. vestibulocochlearis.
cochlear window rundes Fenster *nt*, Fenestra cochleae/rotunda.
coch·le·i·tis [kɑklɪ'aɪtɪs] *n HNO* Entzündung *f* der Innenohrschnecke, Kochleitis *f*, Cochl(e)itis *f*.
coch·le·o·neu·ral deafness [ˌkɑklɪəʊ'njʊərəl, -'nʊ-] *HNO* kochleoneurale Schwerhörigkeit *f*.
cochleo-orbicular reflex → cochleopalpebral reflex.
coch·le·o·pal·pe·bral reflex [ˌ-'pælpəbrəl] **1.** auropalpebraler Reflex *m*. **2.** Kochleopalpebralreflex *m*.
coch·le·o·pu·pil·lar·y reflex [ˌ-'pjuːpəˌlerɪː, -lərɪ] Kochleopupillarreflex *m*.
coch·le·o·sta·pe·di·al reflex [ˌ-stə'piːdɪəl] Stapediusreflex *m*.
coch·le·o·top·ic [ˌ-'tɑpɪk] *adj* kochleotop.
coch·le·o·ves·tib·u·lar [ˌ-ve'stɪbjələr] *adj* kochleovestibulär.
cochleovestibular neuritis Neuritis cochleovestibularis.
coch·li·tis [kɑk'laɪtɪs] *n* → cochleitis.
cock [kɑk] *n* **1.** *bio*. Hahn *m*; Männchen *nt*. **2.** *techn*. (Wasser-, Gas-, Absperr-)Hahn *m*. **3.** *sl*. Penis *m*.
Cockayne [kɑ'keɪn]: **C.'s disease/syndrome** Cockayne-Syndrom *nt*.
Cockayne-Touraine [tuː'rɛn]: **C.-T. syndrome** Cockayne-Touraine-Syndrom *nt*, Epidermolysis bullosa (hereditaria) dystrophica dominans, Epidermolysis bullosa hyperplastica.
cock's comb *anat*. Hahnenkamm *m*, Crista galli.
cock·roach ['kɑkrəʊtʃ] *n* (Küchen-)Schabe *f*, Kakerlak(e *f*) *m*.
cock·tail ['kɑkteɪl] *n* Cocktail *m*, Mixgetränk *nt*.
COCI *abbr*. → cathodal opening clonus.
co·coa ['kəʊkəʊ] **I** *n* **1.** Kakao *m*, Kakaopulver *nt*, -getränk *nt*, -bohne *f*. **2.** Mittelbraun *nt*. **II** *adj* kakaofarben, mittelbraun; kakao-, Kakao-.
cocoa bean Kakaobohne *f*.
cocoa brown Mittelbraun *nt*.
cocoa butter Kakaobutter *f*, Butyrum cacao.
co·con·scious [kəʊ'kɑntʃəs] *adj psychia*. nebenbewußt.
co·con·scious·ness [kəʊ'kɑntʃəsnɪs] *n psychia*. Nebenbewußtsein *nt*.
co·con·trac·tion [kəʊkən'trækʃn] *n* Kokontraktion *f*.
co·co·nut butter ['kəʊkənʌt] Kokosbutter *f*.
coc·tion ['kɑkʃn] *n* Kochen *nt*, Sieden *nt*.
coc·to·la·bile [ˌkɑktəʊ'leɪbl, -baɪl] *adj* kochlabil, -unbeständig, siedelabil, -unbeständig.

coc·to·sta·bile [ˌ-'steɪbl, -baɪl] *adj* koch-, siedestabil, -fest.
coc·to·sta·ble [ˌ-'steɪbl] *adj* → coctostabile.
co·cul·ti·va·tion [kəʊˌkʌltə'veɪʃn] *n* Kokultivation *f*, Kokultivierung *f*.
code [kəʊd] **I** *n* **1.** Kodex *m*, Regeln *pl*, Normen *pl*. **2.** *techn., genet.* Code *m*, Kode *m*. **II** *vt* codieren, kodieren, verschlüsseln, in einen Code umsetzen.
co·deine ['kəʊdi:n] *n* Kodein *nt*, Codein *nt*, Methylmorphin *nt*.
code number Code-, Kennziffer *f*.
code word Code-, Schlüsselwort *nt*.
cod fish vertebra [kɑd] *radiol., ortho.* Fischwirbel *m*.
cod·ing ['kəʊdɪŋ] **I** *n* Verschlüsseln *nt*, Codieren *nt*, Codierung *f*; *stat.* Chiffrieren *nt*. **II** *adj* kodierend.
coding sequence kodierende Sequenz *f*, Codesequenz *f*.
coding triplet kodierendes Triplett *nt*.
coding unit *biochem.* kodierende Einheit *f*, Codeeinheit *f*.
cod-liver oil *abbr.* **C.L.O.** (Dorsch-)Lebertran *m*.
Codman ['kɑdmən]: **C.'s sign** Codman-Zeichen *nt*.
C.'s triangle *radiol., ortho.* Codman-Dreieck *nt*.
C.'s tumor Chondroblastom *nt*, Codman--Tumor *m*.
co·dom·i·nance [kəʊ'dɑmɪnəns] *n genet.* Kodominanz *f*.
co·dom·i·nant [kəʊ'dɑmɪnənt] *adj genet.* kodominant.
codominant genes kodominante Gene *pl*.
codominant inheritance kodominante Vererbung *f*.
co·don ['kəʊdɑn] *n genet.* Kodon *nt*, Codon *nt*.
codon-anticodon complex Codon-Anticodon-Komplex *m*.
codon specifity Codonspezifität *f*.
codon triplet Codontriplett *nt*.
Coe [kəʊ]: **C. virus** Coe-Virus *nt*, Coxsackievirus A21 *nt*.
coe·cum ['si:kəm] *n*, *pl* **-ca** [-kə] → cecum.
co·ef·fi·cient [ˌkəʊə'fɪʃənt] **I** *n* **1.** *phys.* Koeffizient *m*. **2.** mitwirkende Kraft *f*, Faktor *m*. **II** *adj* mit-, zusammenwirkend.
c. of correlation *stat.* Korrelationskoeffizient.
c. of friction Reibungskoeffizient.
c. of variation *abbr.* **CV** Variationskoeffizient.
c. of velocity Geschwindigkeitskoeffizient.
c. of viscosity Viskositätskoeffizient.
coe·len·ter·on [sɪ'lentərɑn] *n embryo.* Urdarm *m*, Archenteron *nt*.
coe·li·ac *adj* → celiac.
coe·lo·blas·tu·la [ˌsi:lə'blæstʃələ] *n embryo.* Zöloblastula *f*.
coe·lom ['si:lɑm] *n*, *pl* **-loms, coe·lo·ma·ta** [sɪ'ləʊmətə] *embryo.* Zölom *nt*, Zölomhöhle *f*, Coeloma *nt*.
coe·lo·ma ['si:ləʊmə] *n* → coelom.
coe·lom·ic [sɪ'lɑmɪk, -'ləʊ-] *adj embryo.* Zölom betr., Zölom-.
coelomic cavity → coelom.
coelomic epithelium *embryo.* Zölomepithel *nt*.
coe·lo·thel ['si:ləθel] *n* Mesothel *nt*.
coe·nes·the·sia *n* → cenesthesia.
coe·no·cyte *n* → cenocyte.
coe·nu·rus [sɪ'n(j)ʊərəs] *n*, *pl* **-ri** [-raɪ, -ri:] *micro.* Zönurus *m*, Coenurus *m*.
co·en·zyme [kəʊ'enzaɪm] *n* Koenzym *nt*, Coenzym *nt*.
coenzyme I *old* → nicotinamide-adenine dinucleotide.

coenzyme II *old* → nicotinamide-adenine dinucleotide phosphate.
coenzyme A *abbr.* **CoA(-SH)** Coenzym A *nt abbr.* CoA(-SH).
coenzyme B₁₂ Coenzym B_{12} *nt*, 5'-Desoxyadenosylcobalamin *nt*.
coenzyme Q *old* → ubiquinone.
coenzyme R Biotin *nt*, Vitamin H *nt*.
co·erce [kəʊ'ɜrs] *vt* **1.** einschränken. **2.** zwingen, nötigen (*into doing* zu tun); erwingen.
co·er·cion [kəʊ'ɜrʃn] *n* **1.** Einschränkung *f*. **2.** Zwang *m*; Nötigung *f*.
co·er·cive [kəʊ'ɜrsɪv] **I** *n* Zwangsmittel *nt*. **II** *adj* Zwangs-, zwingend, nötigend; *phys.* koerzitiv.
coeur en sabot [kɜr ɑ̃ sa'bo] *card.* (*Herz*)Holzschuhform *f*.
co·ex·ist [ˌkəʊɪg'zɪst] *vi* gleichzeitig/nebeneinander auftreten *od.* bestehen *od.* leben, koexistieren.
co·ex·ist·ance [ˌ-'zɪstəns] *n* Nebeneinanderbestehen *nt*, -leben *nt*, Koexistenz *f*.
co·ex·ist·ent [ˌ-'zɪstənt] *adj* gleichzeitig/nebeneinander bestehend *od.* auftretend *od.* lebend, koexistent.
co·fac·tor ['kəʊfæktər] *n biochem.* Ko-, Cofaktor *m*.
c. of thromboplastin Proakzelerin *nt*, Proaccelerin *nt*, Acceleratorglobulin *nt*, labiler Faktor *m*, Faktor V *nt abbr.* F V.
cofactor V Prokonvertin *nt*, -convertin *nt*, Faktor VII *m abbr.* F V II, Autothrombin I *nt*, Serum-Prothrombin-Conversion-Accelerator *m abbr.* SPCA, stabiler Faktor *m*.
co·fer·ment ['kəʊfɜrmənt] *n* → coenzyme.
cof·fee ['kɑfi] **I** *n* **1.** Kaffee *m*; Kaffeegetränk *nt*, -bohne *f*. **2.** eine Tasse Kaffee. **3.** Kaffeebraun *nt*, Mittel- bis Dunkelbraun *nt*. **II** *adj* kaffeebraun, -farben.
coffee-colored *adj* → coffee II.
coffee-ground vomit kaffeesatzartiges Erbrechen *nt*, Kaffeesatzerbrechen *nt*.
coffee poisoning Koffeinvergiftung *f*, -intoxikation *f*, Koffeinismus *m*.
cof·fin lid crystals ['kɑfɪn, 'kɔ-] *urol.* Sargdeckelkristalle *pl*.
Coffin-Lowry ['kɑfɪn, 'kɔ-, 'laʊrɪ]: **C.-L. syndrome** → Coffin-Siris syndrome.
Coffin-Siris ['sɪrɪs]: **C.-S. syndrome** Coffin--Lowry-Syndrom *nt*.
Cogan ['kəʊgən]: **C.'s disease/syndrome** *ophthal.* Cogan-Syndrom *nt*.
cog·ni·tion [kɑg'nɪʃn] *n* **1.** Wahrnehmung *f*, Erkennen *nt*, Verstehen *nt*, Kognition *f*. **2.** Erkenntnis *f*, Wissen *nt*, Kenntnis *f*.
cog·ni·tive ['kɑgnɪtɪv] *adj* auf Erkenntnis beruhend, erkenntnismäßig, kognitiv.
cognitive behavior therapy kognitive Verhaltenstherapie *f*.
cognitive development geistige Entwicklung *f*.
cognitive learning kognitives Lernen *nt*.
cognitive therapy → cognitive behavior therapy.
cog·nize ['kɑgnaɪz] *vt* erkennen, verstehen, begreifen.
cogwheel phenomenon ['kɑg(h)wi:l] *neuro.* Zahnradphänomen *nt*.
cogwheel rigidity → cogwheel phenomenon.
cogwheel sign → cogwheel phenomenon.
co·hab·it [kəʊ'hæbɪt] *vi* (unverheiratet) zusammenleben.
co·hab·it·ant [kəʊ'hæbɪtənt] *n* Lebensgefährte *m*, -gefährtin *f*.
co·hab·i·ta·tion [kəʊˌhæbɪ'teɪʃn] *n* **1.** Zusammenleben *nt*. **2.** Beischlaf *m*, Koitus *m*, Geschlechtsverkehr *m*, Kohabitation *f*, Cohabitatio *f*.
CO-Hb *abbr.* → carboxyhemoglobin.

co·here [kəʊ'hɪər] *vi* **1.** zusammenhängen, -kleben, verbunden sein. **2.** *phys.* kohärent sein. **3.** *fig.* übereinstimmen, eine Einheit bilden (*with* mit). **4.** *fig.* in (logischem) Zusammenhang stehen, zusammenhängen.
co·her·ence [kəʊ'hɪərəns, -'her-] *n* **1.** (*a. fig.*) Zusammenhalt *m*. **2.** *phys.* Kohärenz *f*. **3.** Übereinstimmung (*with* mit). **4.** (logischer) Zusammenhang *m*.
co·her·en·cy [kəʊ'hɪərənsɪ] *n* → coherence.
co·her·ent [kəʊ'hɪərənt, -'her-] *adj* **1.** zusammenhängend, -klebend, verbunden. **2.** *phys.* kohärent. **3.** übereinstimmend. **4.** (logisch) zusammenhängend.
co·he·sion [kəʊ'hi:ʒn] *n* **1.** *phys.* Anziehung(skraft *f*) *f*, Kohäsion *f*. **2.** Zusammenhalt *m*; Bindekraft *f*.
co·he·sive [kəʊ'hi:sɪv] *adj* auf Kohäsion beruhend, zusammenhaltend, -hängend, kohäsiv, Binde-, Kohäsions-.
cohesive agent Bindemittel *nt*.
cohesive force → cohesiveness.
co·he·sive·ness [kəʊ'hi:sɪvnɪs] *n* **1.** Kohäsions-, Bindekraft *f*. **2.** Festigkeit *f*.
Cohn [kəʊn]: **C.'s solution** Cohn-Nährlösung *f*.
C.'s test *ophthal.* Cohn-Test *m*.
Cohnheim ['kəʊnhaɪm]: **C.'s areas** Cohnheim'-Felderung *f*, Säulchenfelderung *f*.
C.'s artery Endarterie *f*, Cohnheim'-Arterie *f*.
C.'s fields → C.'s areas.
C.'s theory Cohnheim'-Emigrationstheorie *f*, -Entzündungstheorie *f*.
co·ho·ba·tion [ˌkəʊhəʊ'beɪʃn] *n* Redestillieren *nt*, Redestillation *f*.
co·hort ['kəʊhɔrt] *n socio.*, *stat.* Kohorte *f*.
cohort study Kohortenstudie *f*.
coil [kɔɪl] **I** *n* **1.** *gyn.* Spirale *f*, (Intrauterin-)Pessar *nt*. **2.** *techn.* Spirale *f*, Spule *f*, Rolle *f*; (elektrische) Wicklung *f*. **II** *v* aufrollen, (auf-)wickeln; spiralenförmig winden *od.* umschlingen. ~ **o.s. up** s. zusammenrollen. **III** *v* s. winden, s. zusammenrollen.
coil up → coil III.
c. of sweat gland Schweißdrüsenkörper *m*, Corpus gl. sudoriferae.
coil gland knäuelförmige Drüse *f*, Gl. eccrina.
co·in·cide [ˌkəʊɪn'saɪd] *vi* **1.** (*zeitlich od. räumlich*) zusammenfallen, -treffen (*with* mit). **2.** übereinstimmen (*with* mit).
co·in·ci·dence [kəʊ'ɪnsɪdəns] *n* **1.** (*räumliches od. zeitliches*) Zusammenfallen *nt*, -treffen *nt*. **2.** Übereinstimmung *f*. **3.** Zufall *m*.
co·in·ci·dent [kəʊ'ɪnsɪdənt] *adj* **1.** (*räumlich od. zeitlich*) zusammenfallend, -treffend (*with* mit). **2.** übereinstimmend.
co·in·ci·den·tal [kəʊˌɪnsɪ'dentl] *adj* zufällig.
coin-counting [kɔɪn] *n psychia., neuro.* Münzenzählen *nt*, Pillendrehen *n*.
coin lesion (*Lunge*) Rundherd *m*.
co·in·stan·ta·ne·ous [ˌkəʊɪnstən'teɪnɪəs] *adj* gleichzeitig, simultan.
coin test Münzklirren *nt*.
co·i·so·gen·ic [kəʊˌaɪsə'dʒenɪk] *adj* → congenic.
co·i·tal ['kəʊɪtəl] *adj* Koitus betr., koital, Koitus-.
Coiter ['kɔɪtər]: **C.'s muscle** M. corrugator supercilii.
co·i·tion [kəʊ'ɪʃn] *n* → coitus.
co·i·to·pho·bia [ˌkəʊɪtə'fəʊbɪə] *n psychia.* Angst *f* vorm Beischlaf, Koitophobie *f*.
co·i·tus ['kəʊɪtəs] *n* Geschlechtsverkehr *m*, Beischlaf *m*, Koitus *m*, Coitus *m*.
coitus interruptus Koitus/Coitus interruptus.

colamine

co·la·mine ['kɒʊləmiːn, kəʊ'læmɪn] *n* (Mono-)Äthanolamin *nt*, Ethanolamin *nt*.
col·chi·cine ['kɒltʃəsiːn, -sɪn, 'kɒlkə-] *n* Kolchizin *nt*, Colchicin *nt*.
COLD *abbr.* → chronic obstructive lung disease.
cold [kəʊld] **I** *n* **1.** Kälte *f*. **2.** Erkältung *f*, Schnupfen *m*. **to have a ~** erkältet sein; (einen) Schnupfen haben. **a heavy/bad ~** eine schwere Erkältung. **to get/catch/take (a) ~** s. eine Erkältung zuziehen, s. erkälten. **II** *adj* **3.** kalt, kühl. **4.** frierend. **5.** *fig.* kühl, kalt; unfreundlich; sachlich; gefühl-, teilnahmslos (*to* gegen); gefühlskalt. **6.** kalt, tot, leblos. **7.** *inf.* bewußtlos. **c. in the head** akuter Nasenkatarrh *m*, Coryza *f*, Rhinitis acuta.
cold abscess 1. chronischer/kalter Abszeß *m*. **2.** tuberkulöser Abszeß *m*.
cold adaptation Kälteadaptation *f*.
cold agglutination Kälteagglutination *f*.
cold agglutinin Kälteagglutinin *nt*.
cold agglutinin disease Kälteagglutininkrankheit *f*.
cold agglutinin pneumonia atypische/primär-atypische Pneumonie *f*.
cold agglutinin syndrome → cold agglutinin disease.
cold allergy Kälteallergie *f*, -überempfindlichkeit *f*.
cold antibody Kälteantikörper *m*.
cold-blooded *adj* **1.** *bio.* wechselwarm, kaltblütig, poikilo-, hetero-, allotherm. **2.** *inf.* kälteempfindlich. **3.** *fig.* kaltblütig, gefühllos.
cold body Leiche *f*, Leichnam *m*.
cold cautery Kryokauter *m*.
cold gangrene trockene Gangrän *f*.
cold hemagglutinin Kältehämagglutinin *nt*.
cold hemagglutinin disease → cold agglutinin disease.
cold hemolysin Kältehämolysin *nt*; Donath-Landsteiner-Antikörper *m*.
cold intolerance Kälteintoleranz *f*.
cold ischemia kalte Ischämie *f*.
cold light Kaltlicht *nt*.
cold·ness ['kəʊldnɪs] *n* Kälte *f*.
cold nodule (*Schilddrüse*) kalter Knoten *m*.
cold pack kalter Wickel/Umschlag *m*.
cold-pack *vt* einen kalten Wickel *od.* Umschlagen machen.
cold point Kaltpunkt *m*.
cold pressure test Hines-Brown-Test *m*, Cold-pressure-Test *m*, CP-Test *m*.
cold-reactive antibody Kälteantikörper *m*.
cold receptor Kaltrezeptor *m*.
cold room Kühlraum *m*.
cold sensation Kaltempfindung *f*.
cold sensitive cells kaltsensitive Zellen *pl*.
cold sensor Kaltsensor *m*.
cold shock 1. kalter Schock *m*. **2.** Kälteschock *m*.
cold sore(s) Herpes simplex (febrilis); *inf.* Fieberbläschen *pl*.
cold spot *physiol.* Kaltpunkt *m*.
cold stress Kältebelastung *f*, -stress *m*.
cold sweat kalter Schweiß *m*.
cold turkey *inf.* radikale Entziehungskur *f*. **to go ~** eine (radikale) Entziehungskur durchmachen.
cold-turkey *inf.* **I** *adj* abrupt u. vollständig. **~ withdrawal from drugs.** **II** *vt, vi* (radikal) entziehen.
cold urticaria Kälteurtikaria *f*, Urticaria *f* e frigore.
cold vasodilation Kältevasodilatation *f*, Lewis-Reaktion *f*.
cold viruses → common cold viruses.
Cole [kəʊl] **C.'s recess** *radio.* Cole-Rezessus *m*.
C.'s sign *radiol.* Cole'-Zeichen *nt*.
cole- *pref.* → coleo-.
Cole-Cecil ['sesəl] **C.-C. murmur** *card.* Cole-Cecil-Geräusch *nt*.
col·ec·ta·sia [ˌkɒʊlek'teɪʒ(ɪ)ə, -ʃɪə] *n* Dickdarm-, Kolonerweiterung *f*, Kolektasie *f*.
col·ec·to·my [kə'lektəmɪ, kɒʊ-] *n* *chir.* Dickdarmentfernung *f*, -exstirpation *f*, Kolonentfernung *f*, -exstirpation *f*, Kolektomie *f*.
col·e·i·tis [kɒlɪ'aɪtɪs, kəʊlɪ-] *n* *gyn.* Scheidenentzündung *f*, Vaginitis *f*, Kolpitis *f*.
coleo- *pref.* Scheiden-, Kolpo-, Vaginal-, Vagino-.
col·e·o·cele ['kɒʊlɪəsiːl, 'kɒ-] *n* → colpocele 1.
col·e·o·cys·ti·tis [ˌ-sɪs'taɪtɪs] *n* *old* → colpocystitis.
co·le·op·to·sis [kɒʊlɪəp'təʊsɪs] *n* → coloptosis.
col·e·ot·o·my [kɒʊlɪ'ɒtəmɪ] *n* *gyn.* Scheiden-, Vaginalschnitt *m*, Kolpo-, Kolpotomie *f*.
co·les ['kəʊliːz] *n* (männliches) Glied *nt*, Penis *m*, Phallus *m*, Membrum virile.
co·les·ti·pol [kəʊ'lestɪpɒl] *n* *pharm.* Colestipol *nt*.
co·li·bac·il·le·mia [ˌkɒʊlɪˌbæsɪ'liːmɪə] *n* Kolibakteriämie *f*, -bazillämie *f*.
co·li·bac·il·lo·sis [ˌ-ˌbæsɪ'ləʊsɪs] *n* Infektion *f* mit Escherichia coli, Kolibazillose *f*, -bazilleninfektion *f*.
co·li·bac·il·lu·ria [ˌ-ˌbæsɪl'(j)ʊərɪə] *n* Escherichia coli-Ausscheidung *f* im Harn, Kolibazillurie *f*, Kolibazillenausscheidung *f*, Koliurie *f*.
co·li·ba·cil·lus [ˌ-bə'sɪləs] *n* → coli bacillus.
coli bacillus Escherich-Bakterium *nt*, Colibakterium *nt*, -bazillus *m*, Kolibazillus *m*, Escherichia/Bact. coli.
col·ic ['kɒlɪk] **I** *n* Kolik *f*. **II** *adj* **1.** Kolon betr., kolisch, Kolon-, Kol(o)-, Col(o)-. **2.** → colicky.
colic artery: left c. linke Kolonschlagader *f*, Colica *f* sinistra, A. colica sinistra.
middle c. mittlere Kolonschlagader *f*, Colica *f* media, A. colica media.
right c. rechte Kolonschlagader *f*, Colica *f* dextra, A. colica dextra.
right c., inferior A. ileocolica.
superior c., accessory → middle c.
colic branch of ileocolic artery Ramus colicus a. ileocolicae.
colic flexure Kolon-, Colonflexur *f*, Flexura coli.
hepatic c. → right c.
left c. linke Kolonflexur, Flexura lienalis coli, Flexura coli sinistra.
right c. rechte Kolonflexur, Flexura hepatica coli, Flexura coli dextra.
splenic c. → left c.
colic impression of liver Kolonabdruck *m* auf der Leberoberfläche, Impressio colica (hepatis).
col·i·cin ['kɒlɪsɪn, 'kɒʊl-] *n* Kolizin, Colicin *nt*.
col·i·cin·o·gen [kɒlɪ'sɪnədʒən, kəʊl-] *n* Kolizinogen *nt*, Colicinogen *nt*, Col-Faktor *m*, kolizinogener/colicinogener Faktor *m*.
col·i·cin·o·gen·ic factor [ˌ-ˌsɪnə'dʒenɪk] *abbr. Cf* → colicinogen.
col·i·ci·nog·e·ny [ˌ-sɪ'nɒdʒənɪ] *n* Kolizinogenie *f*, Colicinogenie *f*.
colic intussusception Dickdarm-, Koloninvagination *f*.
col·ick·y ['kɒlɪkɪ] *adj* **1.** kolikartig, Kolik-. **2.** Kolik verursachend *od.* auslösend.
colicky pain kolikartiger Schmerz *m*.
colic omentum großes (Bauch-)Netz *nt*, Omentum majus.
col·i·co·ple·gia [ˌkɒlɪkəʊ'pliːdʒ(ɪ)ə] *n* kombinierte Bleikolik u. -lähmung, Kolikoplegie *f*.
colic plexus: left c. A. colica sinistra-Abschnitt *m* des Plexus mesentericus inferior.
middle c. A. colica media-Abschnitt *m* des Plexus mesentericus superior.
right c. A. colica dextra-Abschnitt *m* des Plexus mesentericus superior.
colic taeniae Kolontänien *pl*, Taeniae coli.
colic vein: intermediate c. mittlere Kolonvene *f*, V. colica intermedia/media.
left c. linke Kolonvene *f*, V. colica sinistra.
middle c. → intermediate c.
right c. rechte Kolonvene *f*, V. colica dextra.
co·li·cys·ti·tis [ˌkɒlɪsɪs'taɪtɪs] *n* Zystitis *f* durch Escherichia coli, Kolizystitis *f*.
co·li·cys·to·py·e·li·tis [ˌ-ˌsɪstəˌpaɪə'laɪtɪs] *n* Zystopyelitis *f* durch Escherichia coli, Kolizystopyelitis *f*.
co·li·form ['kɒlɪfɔːrm, 'kəʊ-] **I** *n* → coliform bacteria. **II** *adj* koliähnlich, -form, coliform.
coliform bacilli → coliform bacteria.
coliform bacteria coliforme Bakterien *pl*, Koli-, Colibakterien *pl*.
co·li·my·cin [ˌkɒlɪ'maɪsɪn] *n* → colistin.
co·lin·e·ar·i·ty [kəʊˌlɪnɪ'ærətɪ] *n* Kolinearität *f*, Colinearität *f*.
co·li·ne·phri·tis [ˌkɒlɪne'fraɪtɪs] *n* Nephritis *f* durch Escherichia coli, Kolinephritis *f*.
col·i·phage ['kɒləfeɪdʒ] *n* *micro.* Koli-, Coliphage *m*.
co·li·pli·ca·tion [ˌkɒʊlɪplaɪ'keɪʃn] *n* → coloplication.
co·li·punc·ture [ˌ-'pʌŋktʃər] *n* → colocentesis.
co·lis·tin [kə'lɪstɪn] *n* *pharm.* Colistin *nt*, Polymyxin E *nt*.
co·li·tis [kə'laɪtɪs] *n* Dickdarm-, Kolonentzündung *f*, Kolitis *f*, Colitis *f*.
co·li·tose ['kɒlɪtəʊs] *n* Kolitose *f*, Colitose *f*.
co·li·tox·e·mia [ˌkɒʊlɪtak'siːmɪə] *n* Kolitoxämie *f*.
co·li·tox·i·co·sis [ˌ-ˌtɑksɪ'kəʊsɪs] *n* Kolitoxikose *f*.
co·li·tox·in [ˌ-'taksɪn] *n* Koli-, Colitoxin *nt*.
co·li·u·ria [ˌ-'(j)ʊərɪə] *n* → colibacilluria.
col·lab·o·rate [kə'læbəreɪt] *vi* zusammen-, mitarbeiten (*on* bei; *with s.o.* mit jdm.).
col·lab·o·ra·tion [kəˌlæbə'reɪʃn] *n* Zusammenarbeit *f*, -arbeiten *nt*, in Zusammenarbeit mit. **to work in ~** zusammenarbeiten.
col·lab·o·ra·tive [kə'læbəreɪtɪv, -rətɪv] *adj* zusammenarbeitend, Gemeinschafts-.
col·lab·o·ra·tor [kə'læbəreɪtər] *n* Mitarbeiter(in *f*) *m*.
col·la·cin ['kɒləsɪn] *n* Kollazin *nt*.
col·la·gen ['kɒlədʒən] *n* Kollagen *nt*.
col·la·gen·ase [kə'lædʒəneɪz] *n* Kollagenase *f*.
col·la·ge·na·tion [ˌkɒlədʒə'neɪʃn] *n* → collagenization.
collagen fiber Kollagenfaser *f*.
collagen fibril Kollagenfibrille *f*.
collagen disease → collagenosis.
collagen disorder *patho.* Störung *f* des Kollagenstoffwechsels.
col·la·gen·ic [kə'lædʒenɪk] *adj* **1.** → collagenous. **2.** → collagenogenic.
collagenic fiber Kollagenfaser *f*.
col·la·ge·ni·za·tion [kəˌlædʒənɪ'zeɪʃn] *n* **1.** Kollagenbildung *f*, -synthese *f*. **2.** Kollagenisierung *f*.
col·lag·e·no·blast [kə'lædʒənəʊblæst] *n* kollagenproduzierender Fibroblast *m*.

col·lag·e·no·cyte ['-saɪt] *n* → collagenoblast.
col·lag·e·no·gen·ic [ˌ-'dʒenɪk] *adj* Kollagensynthese betr; kollagenproduzierend.
col·lag·e·nol·y·sis [kəˌlædʒə'nɑləsɪs] *n* Kollagenabbau *m*, -auflösung *f*, Kollagenolyse *f*.
col·lag·e·no·lyt·ic [kəˌlædʒənəʊ'lɪtɪk] *adj* kollagenauflösend, -abbauend, kollagenolytisch.
col·la·gen·o·sis [ˌkɑlədʒə'nəʊsɪs] *n* Kollagenkrankheit *f*, Kollagenose *f*, Kollagenopathie *f*.
col·lag·e·nous [kə'lædʒənəs] *adj* aus Kollagen bestehend, Kollagen formend *od.* produzierend, Kollagen-.
collagenous fiber Kollagenfaser *f*.
collagen sugar Aminoessigsäure *f abbr.* AS, Glyzin *nt*, Glycin *nt*, Glykokoll *nt abbr.* Gly.
collagen-vascular disease → collagenosis.
col·lapse [kə'læps] **I** *n* 1. (physischer *od.* psychischer) Zusammenbruch *m*, Kollaps *m*. 2. (*a. fig.*) Einsturz *m*, Zusammenbruch *m*; Fehlschlag *m*. **II** *vt* (*Organ*) kollabieren lassen. **III** *vi* 5. (psychisch *od.* physisch) zusammenbrechen, einen Kollaps erleiden, kollabieren. 6. (*Organ*) kollabieren. 7. (*a. fig.*) zusammenbrechen, einstürzen; scheitern.
col·laps·ing pulse [kə'læpsɪŋ] 1. Corrigan--Puls *m*, Pulsus celer et altus. 2. Wasserhammerpuls *m*.
col·lar [kɑlər] *n* Kragen *m*; Halsband *nt*; Halskrause *f*.
c. of pearls syphilitisches Leukoderm *nt*, Halsband *nt* der Venus.
c. of venus → c. of pearls.
collar and cuff *ortho.* Collar-and-Cuff(-Verband *m*) *m*.
collar bone Schlüsselbein *nt*, Klavikel *f*, Klavikula *f*, Clavicula *f*.
collar-button abscess Kragenknopfabszeß *m*.
collar-button ulcers *radiol.* Kragenknopfulzerationen *pl*, -relief *nt*.
collar cell → choanocyte.
col·las·tin [kə'læstɪn] *n patho.* Kollastin *nt*.
col·lat·er·al [kə'lætərəl] **I** *n anat.* Kollaterale *f*. **II** *adj* 1. seitlich, außen (liegend), kollateral, Seiten-, Kollateral-. 2. nebeneinander(liegend), benachbart, parallel, kollateral. 3. zusätzlich, Zusatz-; begleitend, Begleit-, Neben-. 4. gleichzeitig (auftretend). 5. indirekt.
collateral artery Kollateralarterie *f*, A. collateralis.
middle c. mittlere Kollateralarterie, Collateralis *f* media, A. collateralis media.
radial c. radiale Kollateralarterie, Collateralis *f* radialis, A. collateralis radialis.
ulnar c., inferior untere ulnare Kollateralarterie, A. collateralis ulnaris inferior.
ulnar c., superior obere ulnare Kollateralarterie, A. collateralis ulnaris superior.
collateral branch of posterior intercostal arteries Kollateralast *m* der Aa. intercostales posteriores, Ramus collateralis (aa. intercostalium posteriorum).
collateral bronchiectasis *pulmo.* kollaterale Bronchiektasie *f*.
collateral circulation Kollateralkreislauf *m*.
collateral eminence of lateral ventricle Eminentia collateralis (ventriculi lateralis).
collateral fissure Sulcus collateralis.
collateral ganglia prävertebrale Ganglien *pl*.
collateral hyperemia kollaterale Hyperämie *f*.

collateral ligament Seitenband *nt*, Kollateralband *nt*, Lig. collaterale.
carpal c., radial Lig. collaterale carpi radiale.
carpal c., ulnar Lig. collaterale carpi ulnare.
fibular c. Lig. collaterale fibulare.
c.s of interphalangeal articulations of foot Ligg. collateralia articc. interphalangealium pedis.
c.s of interphalangeal articulations of hand Ligg. collateralia articc. interphalangealium manus.
c.s of metacarpophalangeal articulations Ligg. collateralia articc. metacarpophalangealium.
c.s of metatarsophalangeal articulations Ligg. collateralia articc. metatarsophalangealium.
radial c. Lig. collaterale radiale.
radial c. of carpus → carpal c., radial.
tibial c. inneres/mediales Knieseitenband, Lig. collaterale tibiale.
ulnar c. Lig. collaterale ulnare.
ulnar c. of carpus → carpal c., ulnar.
collateral sulcus Sulcus collateralis.
collateral trigone of lateral ventricle Trigonum collaterale ventriculi lateralis.
collateral vessel Kollateralgefäß *nt*, Vas collaterale.
col·lect [kə'lekt] **I** *vt* 1. (ein-, an-, auf-)sammeln, zusammentragen. 2. *fig.* (~ o.s.) s. sammeln *od.* fassen. **II** *vi* 3. s. (ver-)sammeln, zusammenkommen. 4. s. (an-)sammeln, s. (an-)häufen. 5. sammeln.
col·lect·ed [kə'lektɪd] *adj* 1. gesammelt. 2. *fig.* gesammelt, gefaßt, ruhig.
col·lect·ing [kə'lektɪŋ] **I** *n* Sammeln *nt*. **II** *adj* Sammel-.
collecting lens *phys.* Sammellinse *f*.
collecting lymph nodes Sammellymphknoten *pl*.
collecting phase Sammelphase *f*.
collecting trunk Sammelgefäß *nt*.
collecting tubes (*Niere*) Sammelröhrchen *pl*.
collecting tubule Sammelrohr *nt*, -röhrchen *nt*.
col·lec·tion [kə'lekʃn] *n* 1. (Ein-, An-)Sammeln *nt*; Beschaffung *f*, Zusammentragen *nt*. 2. (An-)Sammlung *f*. 3. *fig.* Fassung *f*, Gefaßtheit *f*.
c. of statistics statistische Erhebung(en *pl*) *f*.
Colles ['kɑlɪs, 'kɑli:z]: **C.' fascia** Fascia diaphragmatis urogenitalis inferior.
C.' fracture *ortho.* Colles-Fraktur *f*.
C.' ligament Lig. inguinale reflexum.
reverse C.' fracture *ortho.* Smith-Fraktur *f*.
C.' space Colles'-Raum *m*.
triangular ligament of C. Fascia diaphragmatis urogenitalis inferior.
Collet [kɑ'lɛ]: **C.'s syndrome** → Collet--Sicard syndrome.
Collet-Sicard [si'kɑ:r]: **C.-S. syndrome** *neuro.* Collet-Syndrom *nt*, Sicard-Syndrom *nt*.
col·lic·u·lec·to·my [kəˌlɪkjə'lektəmɪ] *n urol.* Resektion *f* des Samenhügels, Kollikulektomie *f*.
col·lic·u·li·tis [ˌ-'laɪtɪs] *n urol.* Samenhügelentzündung *f*, Kollikulitis *f*, Colliculitis *f*.
col·lic·u·lus [kə'lɪkjələs] *n, pl* -li [-laɪ, -li:] *anat.* kleiner Hügel *od.* Vorsprung *m*, Colliculus *m*.
c. of arytenoid cartilage Colliculus cartilaginis arytaenoideae.
colliculus-seminalis hypertrophy *urol.* Colliculus-seminalis-Hypertrophie *f*.
col·lie-itch mite ['kɑlɪ] *micro.* Rhizoglyphus parasiticus.

colloid osmotic pressure

Collier ['kɑljər]: **aryepiglottic fold of C.** Plica triangularis.
C.'s tract mediales Längsbündel *nt*, Fasciculus longitudinalis medialis.
col·lier's lung ['kɑljər] Kohlenstaublunge *f*, Lungenanthrakose *f*, Anthracosis pulmonum.
col·li·ga·tive ['kɑlɪɡeɪtɪv] *adj phys.* kolligativ.
colligative properties *phys.* kolligative Eigenschaften *pl*.
col·li·ma·tion [kɑlɪ'meɪʃn] *n phys.* Kollimation *f*.
col·li·ma·tor ['-meɪtər] *n phys.* Kollimator *m*, Kollineator *m*.
Collip ['kɑlɪp]: **C. unit** Collip-Einheit *f*.
col·li·qua·tion [ˌkɑlɪ'kweɪʃn, -ʃn] *n histol.*, *patho.* Einschmelzung *f*, Verflüssigung *f*, Kolliquation *f*.
col·liq·ua·tive ['kɑlɪkweɪtɪv, kə'lɪkwətɪv] *adj histol.*, *patho.* mit Verflüssigung einhergehend, kolliquativ, Kolliquations-.
colliquative degeneration → colliquative necrosis.
colliquative diarrhea profuse/kolliquative Diarrhö *f*.
colliquative necrosis *patho.* Kolliquationsnekrose *f*.
Collis ['kɑlɪs]: **C. gastroplasty** *chir.* Magenplastik *f* nach Collis.
col·li·sion tumor [kə'lɪʒn] *patho.* Kollisionstumor *m*.
col·lo·chem·is·try [kɑlə'kemɪstrɪ] *n* Kolloidchemie *f*.
col·lo·di·a·phys·e·al [ˌ-ˌdaɪə'fɪːzɪəl] *adj* Hals/Collum u. Schaft/Diaphyse betr., kollodiaphysär.
collodiaphyseal angle Schenkelhalsschaftwinkel *m*, Kollodiaphysenwinkel *m*, Collo-Diaphysen-Winkel *m*, Collum--Corpus-Winkel *m*, CD-Winkel *m*.
col·lo·di·on [kə'ləʊdɪən] *n* Kollodium *nt*, Collodium *nt*, Zellulosedinitrat *nt*.
collodion baby *ped.* Kollodiumbaby *nt*.
col·loid ['kɑlɔɪd] **I** *n* 1. *chem.* Kolloid *nt*, kolloiddisperses System *nt*. 2. *histol.* Kolloid *nt*. 3. → colloidal solution. **II** *adj* → colloidal.
colloid adenoma (*Schilddrüse*) Kolloidadenom *nt*, makrofollikuläres Adenom *nt*.
col·loi·dal [kə'lɔɪdl, kɑ-] *adj* kolloidal, kolloid.
colloidal solution Kolloidlösung *f*, kolloidale Lösung *f*.
colloid cancer → colloid carcinoma.
colloid carcinoma Gallertkrebs *m*, -karzinom *nt*, Schleimkrebs *m*, -karzinom *nt*, Kolloidkrebs *m*, -karzinom *nt*, Ca. colloides/gelatinosum/mucoides/mucosum.
colloid chemistry Kolloidchemie *f*.
colloid corpuscles Amyloidkörper *pl*, Corpora amylacea.
colloid cyst Kolloidzyste *f*.
colloid degeneration kolloide Degeneration *f*.
c. of choroid Chorioiditis gutta senilis, Altersdrusen *pl*.
colloid goiter Kolloid-, Gallertstruma *f*, Struma colloides.
nodular c. knotige Kolloidstruma, Struma colloides nodosa.
col·loi·din [kə'lɔɪdɪn] *n* Kolloidin *nt*, Colloidin *nt*.
colloid nodule Kolloidknoten *m*.
col·loi·do·cla·sia [kəˌlɔɪdəʊ'kleɪʒ(ɪ)ə] *n* → colloidoclasis.
col·loi·doc·la·sis [ˌ-'kleɪsɪs] *n patho.* Kolloidoklasie *f*.
colloid osmotic hemolysis kolloidosmotische Hämolyse *f*.
colloid osmotic pressure kolloidosmotischer Druck *m abbr.* KOD.

colloid solution

colloid solution Kolloidlösung f, kolloidale Lösung f.
colloid tumor Myxom(a) nt.
col·lox·y·lin [kəˈlɑksəlɪn] n Schießbaumwolle f, Nitrozellulose f.
col·lum [ˈkɑləm] n, pl **-la** [-lə] anat. 1. Hals m, Collum nt. 2. halsförmige Struktur f, Hals m, Kollum nt, Collum nt, Cervix f, Zervix f.
col·lu·nar·i·um [ˌkɑljəˈnɛərɪəm] n, pl **-nar·ia** [-ˈnɛərɪə] HNO Nasendusche f, -spülung f, Collunarium nt.
col·lu·to·ri·um [ˌkɑləˈtɔːrɪəm, -ˈtəʊr-] n → collutory.
col·lu·to·ry [ˈkɑlətɔːriː, -təʊ-] n, pl **-ries** Mundwasser nt, Collutorium nt.
col·lyr·i·um [kəˈlɪərɪəm] n, pl **-riums, -ria** [-rɪə] Augenwasser nt, Collyrium nt.
col·o·bo·ma [ˌkɑləˈbəʊmə] n, pl **-mas, -ma·ta** [-mətə] ophthal. Kolobom nt, Coloboma(a) nt.
  c. of choroid Aderhautkolobom.
  c. of ciliary body Kolobom des Ziliarkörpers.
  c. of fundus Funduskolobom.
  c. of iris Iriskolobom.
  c. of lens Linsenkolobom.
  c. of optic disk Sehnervenkolobom.
  c. of optic nerve → c. of optic disk.
  c. at optic nerve entrance Kolobom am Sehnerveneintritt.
  c. of retina Netzhautkolobom.
  c. of vitreous Glaskörperkolobom.
col·o·bo·ma·tous [ˌ-ˈbəʊmətəs] adj kolobomartig, kolobomatös.
co·lo·ce·cos·to·my [ˌkɑʊləsɪˈkɑstəmɪ, ˌkɑ-] n → cecocolostomy.
co·lo·cen·te·sis [ˌ-senˈtiːsɪs] n chir. Kolonpunktion f, Kolozentese f.
co·lo·cho·le·cys·tos·to·my [ˌ-ˌkɑʊləsɪsˈtɑstəmɪ] n chir. Gallenblasen-Kolon-Fistel f, Cholezystokolostomie f.
co·lo·cly·sis [ˌ-ˈklaɪsɪs] n Kolonspülung f.
co·lo·clys·ter [ˌ-ˈklɪstər] n Dickdarm-, Koloneinlauf m, Kolonklysma nt.
co·lo·co·los·to·my [ˌ-kəˈlɑstəmɪ] n chir. Kolokolostomie f.
co·lo·cu·ta·ne·ous fistula [ˌ-kjuːˈteɪnɪəs] äußere Dickdarm-/Kolonfistel f, kolokutane Fistel.
col·o·cynth [ˈkɑləsɪnθ] n Koloquinte f, Bitterapfel m.
col·o·cyn·thi·dism [ˌ-ˈsɪnθɪdɪzəm] n Colocynthidismus m.
col·o·cyn·thin [ˌ-ˈsɪnθɪn] n Colocynthin nt.
col·o·cyn·this [ˌ-ˈsɪnθɪs] n → colocynth.
co·lo·en·ter·ic fistula [ˌkɑʊlæenˈtɛrɪk, ˌkɑ-] patho. Dickdarm-Darm-Fistel f, innere Dickdarmfistel f.
co·lo·en·ter·i·tis [ˌ-ˌentəˈraɪtɪs] n Entzündung f von Dünn- u. Dickdarm, Enterokolitis f, Enterocolitis f.
co·lo·fix·a·tion [ˌ-fɪkˈseɪʃn] n chir. Kolonanheftung f, -fixation f, Kolo-, Colofixation f.
co·lo·hep·a·to·pex·y [ˌ-ˈhepətəpeksɪ] n chir., patho. Kolohepatopexie f.
co·lo·il·e·al [ˌ-ˈɪlɪəl] adj Ileum u. Kolon betr. od. verbindend, ileokolisch.
coloileal fistula Kolon-Ileum-Fistel f, ileokolische Fistel f.
co·lol·y·sis [kəˈlɑləsɪs] n chir. Kolonlösung f, Kololyse f.
Co·lo·ra·do tick fever [kəˈlʌmbɪən] Felsengebirgsfleckfieber nt, amerikanisches Zeckenbißfieber nt, Rocky Mountain spotted fever (nt) abbr. RMSF.
co·lon [ˈkəʊlɑn] n Kolon nt, Colon nt, Intestinum colon.
co·lon·al·gia [ˌkəʊləˈnældʒ(ɪ)ə] n Dickdarm-, Kolonschmerz m, Kolonalgie f.
colon bacillus → colibacillus.

colon carcinoma Kolon-, Dickdarmkarzinom nt, -krebs m.
colon cut-off sign radiol. Colon-cut-off-Zeichen nt.
co·lon·ic [kəʊˈlɑnɪk] adj Kolon betr., Kolon-, Dickdarm-.
colonic anastomosis chir. Kolonanastomose f.
colonic atresia Kolonatresie f.
colonic crypt Kolon-, Dickdarmkrypte f.
colonic dilatation Kolondilatation f.
  toxic c. toxische Kolondilatation, toxisches Megakolon nt.
colonic disease Dickdarm-, Kolonerkrankung f.
colonic diverticulosis Dickdarm-, Kolondivertikulose f.
colonic diverticulum Dickdarm-, Kolondivertikel nt.
colonic evacuation reflex Darmentleerungsreflex m.
colonic fistula Dickdarm-, Kolonfistel f.
  external c. äußere Dickdarm-/Kolonfistel, kolokutane Fistel.
  inner c. innere Dickdarm-/Kolonfistel.
colonic inflammation → colitis.
colonic injury Dickdarm-, Kolonverletzung f, -trauma nt.
colonic interposition 1. chir. Koloninterposition f, -zwischenschaltung f. 2. chir. Koloninterponat nt.
colonic ischemia Kolonischämie f.
colonic motility Kolonmotilität f.
colonic mucosa Kolonschleimhaut f.
colonic obstruction → colon obstruction.
  false c. Ogilvie-Syndrom nt, Pseudo-Obstruktionsileus m.
colonic perforation chir. Dickdarm-, Kolonperforation f.
  free c. freie Kolonperforation.
colonic polyp Dickdarm-, Kolonpolyp m.
colonic resection chir. Kolon(teil)entfernung f, Kolonresektion f.
colonic stricture chir. Kolonstriktur f.
colonic trauma → colonic injury.
colon injury → colonic injury.
colon interposition → colonic interposition.
co·lo·ni·tis [ˌkɑʊləˈnaɪtɪs, ˌkɑlə-] n → colitis.
col·o·ni·za·tion [ˌkɑlənɪˈzeɪʃn] n 1. Kolonisierung f, Besiedlung f. 2. Einnisten nt, Innidation f.
colon motility Kolonmotilität f.
Co·lon·na [kəˈlɑnə]: **C.'s operation** ortho. 1. Colonna-Operation f. 2. Colonna-Codivilla-Operation f.
colon obstruction chir. Dickdarmobstruktion f, -obstruktionsverschluß m, Kolonobstruktion f, -obstruktionsverschluß m.
co·lo·nop·a·thy [ˌkəʊləˈnɑpəθɪ, ˌkɑl-] n Dickdarm-, Kolonerkrankung f.
co·lo·nor·rha·gia [ˌkəʊləˈnærdʒ(ɪ)ə, ˌkɑl-] n Dickdarm-, Kolonblutung f, Kolorrhagie f.
co·lo·nor·rhea [ˌ-ˈrɪə] n → colorrhea.
co·lon·o·scope [kəʊˈlɑnəskəʊp] n Kolon-, Kolonoskop nt.
co·lon·os·co·py [kəʊləˈnɑskəpɪ] n Dickdarmspiegelung f, -endoskopie f, Kolonspiegelung f, -endoskopie f, Koloskopie f, Kolonoskopie f.
colon resection → colonic resection.
colon tube Dickdarmsonde f, -rohr nt.
col·o·ny [ˈkɑlənɪ] n, pl **-nies** bio., bact. Kolonie f.
colony forming cell abbr. **CFC** koloniebildende Zelle f, colony forming cell abbr. CFC.
colony forming unit abbr. **CFU** immun. colony forming unit (f) abbr. CFU.
colony forming unit in culture abbr.

CFU-C immun. colony forming unit in culture (f) abbr. CFU-C.
colony-stimulating factor abbr. **CSF** kolonie-stimulierender Faktor m, Colony-stimulating-Faktor m abbr. CSF.
co·lop·a·thy [kəˈlɑpəθɪ] n → colonopathy.
co·lo·pex·ia [ˌkəʊləˈpeksɪə] n → colopexy.
co·lo·pex·ot·o·my [ˌ-pekˈsɑtəmɪ] n chir. Kolopexotomie f.
co·lo·pex·y [ˈ-peksɪ] n chir. Kolonanheftung f, Kolopexie f, Colopexia f.
co·loph·o·ny [kəˈlɑfənɪ] n Kolophonium nt, Colophonium nt.
co·lo·pli·ca·tion [ˌkəʊləplaɪˈkeɪʃn] n chir. Koloplikation f, Coloplicatio f.
co·lo·proc·tec·to·my [ˌ-prɑkˈtektəmɪ] n chir. Resektion f von Kolon u. Rektum, Koloproktektomie f, Proktokolektomie f.
co·lo·proc·ti·tis [ˌ-prɑkˈtaɪtɪs] n Entzündung f von Kolon u. Rektum, Koloproktitis f, Proktokolitis f.
co·lo·proc·tos·to·my [ˌ-prɑkˈtɑstəmɪ] n → colorectostomy.
co·lop·to·sia [ˌkəʊlɑpˈtəʊsɪə] n → coloptosis.
co·lop·to·sis [ˌ-ˈtəʊsɪs] n patho. Dickdarm-, Kolonsenkung f, Koloptose f, Coloptosis f.
co·lo·punc·ture [ˌkəʊləˈpʌŋktʃər] n → colocentesis.
col·or [ˈkʌlər] I n 1. Farbe f, Farbstoff m. 2. Haut-, Gesichtsfarbe f, Teint m; dunkle Hautfarbe f; (Gesichts-)Röte f. **to change ~** erröten; blaß werden. **to have ~** gesund aussehen. **to have little ~** blaß aussehen. **to lose ~** erbleichen, blaß werden. II vt färben. III vi 3. s. (ver-)färben, Farbe annehmen. 4. erröten, rot werden.
col·or·a·bil·i·ty [ˌkʌlərəˈbɪlətɪ] n Färbbarkeit f.
col·or·a·ble [ˈkʌlərəbl] adj färbbar.
color adaptation chromatische Adaptation f.
Col·o·ra·do tick fever [ˌkɑləˈreɪdəʊ, -ˈrɑːd-] abbr. **CTF** Colorado-Zeckenfieber nt, amerikanisches Gebirgszeckenfieber nt.
Colorado tick fever virus Colorado tick fever-Virus nt, Colorado-Zeckenfiebervirus nt, CTF-Virus nt.
color amblyopia ophthal. Farbenamblyopie f.
color anomaly ophthal. → color blindness 1.
color anomia ophthal. Farbenanomie f.
col·or·ant [ˈkʌlərənt] n Farbe f, Farbstoff m, Färbemittel nt.
col·or·a·tion [ˌkʌləˈreɪʃn] n 1. Färben nt, Kolorieren nt. 2. Farbgebung f, -zusammenstellung f. 3. bio. Färbung f.
color-blind adj 1. farbenblind. 2. fig. blind (to für).
color blindness 1. Farbenfehlsichtigkeit f, -anomalie f, Chromatodysop(s)ie f, Dyschromatop(s)ie f. 2. totale Farbenblindheit f, Achromatop(s)ie f, Monochromasie f.
color cell histol. pigmenthaltige/pigmentierte Zelle f, Chromozyt m.
color constancy Farb(en)konstanz f.
col·o·rec·tal [ˌkɑləˈrektl, ˌkəʊ-] adj Kolon u. Rektum betr. od. verbindend, kolorektal.
colorectal cancer/carcinoma kolorektales Karzinom nt.
colorectal resection chir. Teilresektion f von Kolon u. Rektum, kolorektale Resektion f.
co·lo·rec·ti·tis [ˌkəʊlərekˈtaɪtɪs] n → coloproctitis.
co·lo·rec·tos·to·my [ˌ-rekˈtɑstəmɪ] n chir.

Kolon-Rektum-Anastomose *f*, -Fistel *f*, Kolorektostomie *f*.
col·o·rec·tum [ˌkaləˈrektəm] *n* Kolon u. Rektum, Kolorektum *nt*.
col·ored [ˈkʌlərd] **I** *n* Farbige(r *m*) *f*. the ~ Farbige *pl*. **II** *adj* **1.** bunt, farbig, Bunt-, Farb-. **2.** (*Person*) farbig, dunkelhäutig.
colored corpuscles rote Blutzellen *pl*, -körperchen *pl*, Erythrozyten *pl*.
colored vision 1. → color vision. **2.** → chromatopsia.
color filter *photo*. Farbfilter *m*.
color hearing *neuro*. → chromesthesia.
color hemianopsia *ophthal*. Farbenhemianopsie *f*, Hemiachromatopsie *f*, Hemichromatopsia *f*.
col·or·if·ic [ˌkʌləˈrɪfɪk] *adj* farbgebend, Farb-.
col·or·im·e·ter [ˌ-ˈrɪmɪtər] *n* Farb(en)messer *m*, Kolorimeter *nt*, Chromatometer *nt*.
col·or·i·met·ric [ˌkʌlərɪˈmetrɪk] *adj* → colorimetrical.
col·or·i·met·ri·cal [ˌ-ˈmetrɪkl] *adj* Kolorimetrie betr., kolorimetrisch.
colorimetric analysis → colorimetry.
col·or·im·e·try [ˌkʌləˈrɪmətrɪ] *n* Farbvergleich *m*, -messung *f*, Kolori-, Colorimetrie *f*.
color index *abbr*. **C.I.** Färbeindex *m abbr*. FI, Hämoglobinquotient *m*.
col·or·ing [ˈkʌlərɪŋ] *n* **1.** (Ein-)Färben *nt*. **2.** Färbemittel *nt*, Farbstoff *m*, Farbe *f*. **3.** Gesichts-, Hautfarbe *f*, Teint *m*.
col·or·less [ˈkʌlərlɪs] *adj* farblos; *fig*. neutral, unparteiisch.
colorless corpuscle weiße Blutzelle *f*, weißes Blutkörperchen *nt*, Leukozyt *m*.
col·or·less·ness [ˈkʌlərlɪsnɪs] *n* Farblosigkeit *f*; *fig*. Neutralität *f*.
color mixture Farbmischung *f*.
 additive c. additive Farbmischung.
 subtractive c. subtraktive Farbmischung.
color reaction *chem*. Farbreaktion *f*.
co·lor·rha·gia [ˌkəʊləˈrædʒ(ɪ)ə] *n* → colonorrhagia.
co·lor·rha·phy [kəʊˈlɒrəfɪ] *n chir*. Dickdarm-, Kolonnaht *f*, Kolorrhaphie *f*.
co·lor·rhea [ˌkəʊləˈrɪə] *n* Schleimabgang *m* aus dem Kolon.
color scotoma *ophthal*. Farbskotom *nt*.
color sense Farbsinn *m*.
color-specific *adj* farbspezifisch.
color spectrum (*Licht*) sichtbares Spektrum *nt*, Spektrum *nt* des sichtbaren Lichtes.
color triangle Farbendreieck *nt*.
color valency Farbvalenz *f*.
color vision Farbensehen *nt*, Chromatop(s)ie *f*, Chromopsie *f*.
color-vision deficit *ophthal*. Farbsinnesstörung *f*.
col·o·scope [ˈkaləskəʊp] *n* → colonoscope.
co·los·co·py [kəˈlaskəpɪ] *n* → colonoscopy.
co·lo·sig·moi·dos·to·my [ˌkəʊləˌsɪgmɔɪˈdastəmɪ] *n chir*. Kolon-Sigma-Fistel *f*, -Anastomose *f*, Kolosigmoidostomie *f*.
co·los·to·my [kəˈlastəmɪ] *n chir*. **1.** Dickdarm-, Kolonfistelung *f*, Kolostomie *f*. **2.** Dickdarm-, Kolonfistel *f*, Kolostoma *nt*, Kolostomie *f*.
colostomy bag Kolostomabeutel *m*.
co·los·tric [kəˈlastrɪk] *adj* Kolostrum betr., Kolostrum-.
co·los·tror·rhea [kəˌlastrəˈrɪə] *n gyn*. Kolostrumdiarrhoe *f*.
co·los·trous [kəˈlastrəs] *adj* kolostrumhaltig.
co·los·trum [kəˈlastrəm] *n* Vormilch *f*, Kolostrum *nt*, Colostrum *nt*.

colostrum bodies/corpuscles Donné--Körperchen *pl*, Kolostrumkörperchen *pl*.
co·lot·o·my [kəˈlatəmɪ] *n chir*. Dickdarmeröffnung *f*, -durchtrennung *f*, Koloneröffnung *f*, -durchtrennung *f*, Kolotomie *f*.
co·lo·vag·i·nal [ˌkəʊləˈvædʒɪnl] *adj* Dickdarm/Kolon u. Scheide/Vagina betr. *od*. verbindend, kolovaginal.
colovaginal fistula *patho*. Dickdarm--Scheiden-Fistel *f*, kolovaginale Fistel *f*.
co·lo·ves·i·cal [ˌ-ˈvesɪkl] *adj* Dickdarm/Kolon u. Harnblase betr. *od*. verbindend, kolovesikal.
colovesical fistula *patho*. (Harn-)Blasen--Kolon-Fistel *f*, Fistula vesicocolica.
colp- *pref*. → colpo-.
col·pal·gia [kalˈpældʒ(ɪ)ə] *n gyn*. Scheidenschmerz *m*, Kolpalgie *f*, Vaginodynie *f*.
col·pa·tre·sia [ˌkalpəˈtriːʒ(ɪ)ə] *n* Scheiden-, Vaginalatresie *f*, Atresia vaginalis.
col·pec·ta·sia [kalpekˈteɪʒ(ɪ)ə] *n* → colpectasis.
col·pec·ta·sis [kalˈpektəsɪs] *n gyn*. Scheidenerweiterung *f*, Kolpektasie *f*.
col·pec·to·my [kalˈpektəmɪ] *n gyn*. Exzision *f* der Scheidenwand, Kolpektomie *f*.
col·peu·rys·is [kalˈpjʊərəsɪs] *n* → colpectasis.
col·pis·mus [kalˈpɪzməs] *n* Scheiden-, Vaginalkrampf *m*, Vaginismus *m*.
col·pi·tis [kalˈpaɪtɪs] *n gyn*. Scheidenentzündung *f*, Kolpitis *f*, Vaginitis *f*.
colpo- *pref*. Scheiden-, Kolp(o)-, Vaginal-.
col·po·cele [ˈkalpəsiːl] *n gyn*. **1.** Scheidenbruch *m*, Kolpozele *f*, Hernia vaginalis. **2.** → colpoptosis.
col·po·ce·li·o·cen·te·sis [ˌ-ˌsiːlɪəsenˈtiːsɪs] *n chir*., *gyn*. transvaginale Bauch(höhlen)punktion *f*, Kolpozöliozentese *f*.
col·po·ce·li·ot·o·my [ˌ-sɪlɪˈatəmɪ] *n gyn*. Kolpozöliotomie *f*, Coeliotomia vaginalis.
col·po·clei·sis [ˌ-ˈklaɪsɪs] *n gyn*. operativer Scheidenverschluß *m*, Kolpokleisis *f*, -klisis *f*.
col·po·cys·ti·tis [ˌ-sɪsˈtaɪtɪs] *n* Entzündung *f* von Harnblase u. Scheide, Kolpozystitis *f*.
col·po·cys·to·cele [ˌ-ˈsɪstəsiːl] *n* Kolpozystozele *f*.
col·po·cys·to·plas·ty [ˌ-ˈsɪstəplæstɪ] *n* Kolpozystoplastik *f*.
col·po·cys·tot·o·my [ˌ-sɪsˈtatəmɪ] *n gyn*. transvaginale Zystotomie *f*, Scheiden--Blasen-Schnitt *m*, Kolpozystotomie *f*.
col·po·cys·to·u·re·ter·o·cys·tot·o·my [ˌ-ˌsɪstəjʊəˌriːtərəsɪsˈtatəmɪ] *n gyn*., *urol*. Kolpozystoureterozystotomie *f*.
col·po·cys·to·u·re·ter·ot·o·my [ˌ-ˌsɪstəjʊəriːtəˈratəmɪ] *n gyn*., *urol*. Kolpozystoureteroterotomie *f*.
col·po·cy·to·gram [ˌ-ˈsaɪtəgræm] *n gyn*. Kolpozytogramm *nt*.
col·po·cy·tol·o·gy [ˌ-saɪˈtalədʒɪ] *n* Vaginal-, Kolpozytologie *f*.
col·po·dyn·ia [ˌ-ˈdiːnɪə] *n* → colpalgia.
col·po·hy·per·pla·sia [ˌ-ˌhaɪpərˈpleɪʒ(ɪ)ə, -zɪə] *n gyn*. Scheiden(schleimhaut)hyperplasie *f*, Kolpohyperplasie *f*.
col·po·hys·ter·ec·to·my [ˌ-ˌhɪstəˈrektəmɪ] *n gyn*. transvaginale Gebärmutterentfernung/Hysterektomie *f*, Kolpohysterektomie *f*, Hysterektomia vaginalis.
col·po·hys·ter·o·pex·y [ˌ-ˈhɪstərəpeksɪ] *n gyn*. transvaginale Hysteropexie *f*, Kolpohysteropexie *f*.
col·po·mi·cro·scope [ˌ-ˈmaɪkrəskəʊp] *n* Kolpomikroskop *nt*.
col·po·mi·cros·co·py [ˌ-maɪˈkraskəpɪ] *n gyn*. Kolpomikroskopie *f*.

col·po·my·co·sis [ˌ-maɪˈkəʊsɪs] *n* Scheiden-, Vaginalmykose *f*.
col·po·my·o·mec·to·my [ˌ-maɪəˈmektəmɪ] *n gyn*. transvaginale Myomektomie *f*, Kolpomyomektomie *f*.
col·po·pa·thy [kalˈpapəθɪ] *n* Scheiden-, Vaginalerkrankung *f*, Kolpo-, Vaginopathie *f*.
col·po·per·i·ne·o·plas·ty [ˌkalpəˌperɪˈnɪəplæstɪ] *n gyn*. Scheidendammplastik *f*, Kolpoperineoplastik *f*, Vaginoperineoplastik *f*.
col·po·per·i·ne·or·rha·phy [ˌ-ˌperɪnɪˈɔrəfɪ] *n gyn*. Scheidendammnaht *f*, Kolpoperineorrhaphie *f*, Vaginoperineorrhaphie *f*.
col·po·pex·y [ˈkalpəpeksɪ] *n gyn*. Scheidenanheftung *f*, Kolpo-, Vaginopexie *f*.
col·po·plas·ty [ˈ-plæstɪ] *n* Scheiden-, Vaginal-, Kolpo-, Vaginoplastik *f*.
col·po·poi·e·sis [ˌ-pɔɪˈiːsɪs] *n gyn*. künstliche Scheidenbildung *f*, Kolpopoese *f*.
col·pop·to·sis [ˌ-(p)ˈtəʊsɪs] *n gyn*. Scheidenvorfall *m*, Kolpoptose *f*.
col·po·rec·to·pex·y [ˌkalpəˈrektəpeksɪ] *n chir*., *gyn*. Kolporektopexie *f*.
col·por·rha·gia [ˌ-ˈreɪdʒ(ɪ)ə] *n* vaginale Blutung *f*, Scheidenblutung *f*, Kolporrhagie *f*.
col·por·rha·phy [kalˈpɔrəfɪ] *n gyn*. **1.** Scheiden-, Vaginalnaht *f*, Kolporrhaphie *f*, Colporrhaphia *f*. **2.** Scheidenraffung *f*, Kolporrhaphie *f*, Colporrhaphia *f*.
col·por·rhex·is [ˌkalpəˈreksɪs] *n* Scheidenriß *m*, Kolporrhexis *f*.
col·po·scope [ˈ-skəʊp] *n* Kolposkop *nt*.
col·po·scop·ic [ˌ-ˈskapɪk] *adj* Kolposkop *od*. Kolposkopie betr., kolposkopisch.
col·pos·co·py [kalˈpaskəpɪ] *n* Kolposkopie *f*.
col·po·spasm [ˈkalpəspæzəm] *n* Scheiden-, Vaginalkrampf *m*.
col·po·stat [ˈ-stæt] *n gyn*., *radiol*. Kolpostat *m*.
col·po·ste·no·sis [ˌ-stɪˈnəʊsɪs] *n gyn*. Scheidenverengerung *f*, Kolpostenose *f*.
col·po·ste·not·o·my [ˌ-stɪˈnatəmɪ] *n gyn*. Kolpostenotomie *f*.
col·pot·o·my [kalˈpatəmɪ] *n gyn*. Scheiden-, Vaginalschnitt *m*, Kolpo-, Vaginotomie *f*.
col·po·u·re·ter·o·cys·tot·o·my [ˌkalpəjʊəˌriːtərəʊsɪsˈtatəmɪ] *n gyn*., *urol*. Kolpoureterozystotomie *f*.
col·po·u·re·ter·ot·o·my [ˌ-jʊəˌriːtəˈratəmɪ] *n gyn*., *urol*. Kolpoureterotomie *f*.
col·po·xe·ro·sis [ˌ-zɪˈrəʊsɪs] *n gyn*. Scheidenxerose *f*.
col·u·mel·la [ˌkal(j)əˈmelə] *n*, *pl* **-lae** [-liː, -laɪ] **1.** *anat*. kleine Säule *f*, Columella *f*. **2.** *micro*. Kolumella *f*, Columella *f*.
col·umn [ˈkaləm] *n* **1.** Säule *f*, Pfeiler *m*. **2.** *anat*. säulenförmige Struktur *f*, zylindrische Formation *f*, Columna *f*. **3.** *fig*. (Rauch-, Quecksilber-, Luft-, Wasser-)Säule *f*.
c.s of Bertin Bertin'-Säulen *pl*, Columnae renales.
c. of Burdach Burdach'-Strang *m*, Fasciculus cuneatus (medullae spinalis).
c. of fornix Gewölbe *f*, Fornixsäule *f*, -pfeiler, Columna fornicis.
c. of Lissauer Lissauer'-(Rand-)Bündel *nt*, Tractus dorsolateralis.
c. of mercury Quecksilbersäule *f*.
c.s of Morgagni Analsäulen *pl*, -papillen *pl*, Morgagni'-Papillen *pl*, Columnae anales/rectales.
c. of spinal cord Rückenmarkssäulen *pl*.
c. of Spitzka-Lissauer Lissauer'-(Rand-)-Bündel *nt*, Tractus dorsolateralis.
c.s of vaginal rugae Längswülste *pl* der

columna

Vagina(l)wand, Columnae rugarum (vaginae).
co·lum·na [kəˈlʌmnə] *n, pl* **-nas, -nae** [-niː, -naɪ] → column 2.
co·lum·nal [kəˈlʌmnəl] *adj* → columnar.
co·lum·nar [kəˈlʌmnər] *adj* säulenförmig, -artig, zylindrisch, Säulen-.
columnar cartilage Säulenknorpel *m*.
columnar cell hochprismatische Epithelzelle *f*.
columnar epithelium hochprismatisches (Zylinder-)Epithel *nt*.
columnar layer Basal(zell)schicht *f*, Stratum basale epidermidis.
column chromatography Säulenchromatographie *f*.
co·ly·pep·tic [ˌkɒʊlɪˈpeptɪk] *adj* verdauungshemmend.
co·ma [ˈkəʊmə] *n, pl* **-mas, -mae** [-miː] 1. tiefe Bewußtlosigkeit *f*, Koma *nt*, Coma *nt*. **to be in a ~** im Koma liegen. **to fall/go into (a) ~** ins Koma fallen, komatös werden. 2. Apathie *f*, Stumpfheit *f*. 3. *phys.*, *ophthal.* Asymmetriefehler *m*, Linsenfehler *m*, Koma *nt*, Coma *nt*.
coma cast (*Harn*) Komazylinder *m*.
co·ma·tose [ˈkɒmətəʊs, ˈkəʊmə-] *adj* 1. komatös, in tiefer Bewußtlosigkeit. 2. apathisch, stumpf, torpid, träge, schlaff.
com·bat [ˈkʌmbæt, ˈkʌm-; *v* kəmˈbæt] **I** *n* Kampf *m*. **II** *vt* bekämpfen. **III** *vi* kämpfen.
com·bi·na·tion [ˌkʌmbəˈneɪʃn] **I** *n* 1. Verbinden *nt*, Vereinigung *f*; Verbindung *f*, Kombination *f*; Zusammenstellung *f*. **in ~ with** zusammen *od.* gemeinsam mit. 2. *chem.* Verbindung *f*. 3. *techn.* Kombination *f*. 4. Verbindung *f*, Gemeinschaft *f* (*von Personen*). **II** *adj* Kombinations-.
combination beat *card.* Kombinationssystole *f*.
combination calculus *urol.* Kombinationsstein *m*, kombinierter Harnstein *m*.
combination chemotherapy kombinierte Chemotherapie *f*.
combination therapy Kombinationsbehandlung *f*, -therapie *f*.
combination tumor *patho.* Kombinationstumor *m*.
com·bi·na·tive [ˈkʌmbəneɪtɪv, kəmˈbaɪnə-] *adj* verbindend, Verbindungs-.
combine [*n* kəmˈbaɪn; *v* kəm-, ˈkʌmbaɪn] **I** *n* (*a. fig.*) Vereinigung *f*, Verbindung *f*. **II** *vt* kombinieren, vereinigen, zusammensetzen; verbinden. **III** *vi* 1. zusammenschließen; (*a. chem.*) s. verbinden. 2. zusammenwirken.
com·bined [kəmˈbaɪnd] *adj* vereinigt, kombiniert; *chem.* verbunden.
combined aphasia *neuro.* kombinierte Aphasie *f*.
combined fat-induced and carbohydrate--induced hyperlipemia (primäre/essentielle) Hyperlipoproteinämie *f* Typ V, fett- u. kohlenhydratinduzierte Hyperlipidämie/Hyperlipoproteinämie *f*, exogen-endogene Hyperlipoproteinämie *f*, kalorisch-induzierte Hyperlipoproteinämie *f*, Hyperchylomikronämie u. Hyperpräbetalipoproteinämie.
combined hemorrhoids intermediäre Hämorrhoiden *pl*.
combined immunodeficiency (syndrome) kombinierter Immundefekt *m*.
combined pregnancy kombinierte uterine u. extrauterine Schwangerschaft *f*.
combined sclerosis → combined system disease.
combined system disease Lichtheim--Syndrom *nt*, Dana-Lichtheim-Krankheit *f*, Dana-(Lichtheim-Putnam-)Syn-

drom *nt*, funikuläre Spinalerkrankung/Myelose *f*.
combined version *gyn.* bimanuelle/kombinierte Wendung *f*.
com·bin·ing site [kəmˈbaɪnɪŋ] Antigenbindungsstelle *f*.
com·bus·ti·bil·i·ty [kəmˌbʌstəˈbɪlətɪ] *n* Brennbarkeit *f*, Entzündlichkeit *f*.
com·bus·ti·ble [kəmˈbʌstɪbl] **I** *n* Brennstoff *m*, -material *nt*. **II** *adj* brennbar, entflammbar, (leicht) entzündbar.
com·bus·tion [kəmˈbʌstʃn] *n* 1. Verbrennung *f*. 2. *biochem.* Veratmung *f*, biologische Verbrennung *f*. 3. *chem.* Verbrennung *f*, Oxidation *f*.
come [kʌm] **I** *n* Kommen *nt*. **II** *vi* 1. kommen; erscheinen, auftreten. **to ~ and go** kommen u. gehen. 2. (her-)kommen, abstammen (*of*, *from* von). 3. werden, s. entwickeln. **to ~ all right** in Ordnung kommen. 4. kommen, s. entwickeln, s. ereignen.
come about *vi* geschehen, passieren.
come across *vi* (zufällig) stoßen auf, treffen auf.
come around *vi* das Bewußtsein wiedererlangen, wieder zu s. kommen.
come at *vi* 1. etw. herausfinden, feststellen, erkennen, entdecken. 2. (*Problem*) angehen.
come back *vi* 1. wieder einfallen (*to s.o.* jdm.). 2. s. wieder erinnern. 3. zurückkommen, -gehen.
come by *vi* kriegen, s. eine Verletzung *od.* Krankheit zuziehen.
come down *vi* 1. erkranken, krank werden (*with* an). 2. (*Temperatur*) sinken, (he-)runtergehen.
come in *vi* aufkommen, in Mode kommen. **~ useful** s. als nützlich erweisen, (sehr) gelegen kommen.
come on *vi* 1. Fortschritte machen, vorankommen; wachsen. 2. (*Schmerzen, Symptome*) anfangen, beginnen, einsetzen.
come out *vi* 1. s. zeigen, herauskommen, zum Vorschein kommen, (*Ausschlag*) ausbrechen. **to ~ in a sweat** im Schweiß ausbrechen. **to ~ in a rash** einen Ausschlag bekommen. 2. (*Haare*) ausfallen, ausgehen. 3. (*Fakten*) bekanntwerden, ans Licht kommen.
come over *vi* 1. (*Übelkeit*) befallen, überkommen. 2. vorbei-, herüberkommen, (kurz) besuchen *od.* vorbeischauen.
come round *vi* 1. → come around. 2. → come over 2. 3. s. wieder beruhigen, wieder vernünftig werden.
come through *vi* (*Patient*) durchkommen; (*Krankheit*) überstehen.
come to *vi* → come around.
come up *vi* (*Essen*) wieder hochkommen, erbrochen werden.
come upon *vi* 1. → come on. 2. → come across.
com·e·do [ˈkɒmɪdəʊ] *n, pl* **-dos, -do·nes** [-ˈdəʊniːz] *derm.* Komedo *m*, Comedo *m*; *inf.* Mitesser *m*.
comedo carcinoma → comedocarcinoma.
com·e·do·car·ci·no·ma [ˌkɒmɪdəʊkɑːsɪˈnəʊmə] *n gyn.* (*Brust*) Komedokarzinom *nt*.
com·e·do·mas·ti·tis [ˌ-mæsˈtaɪtɪs] *n gyn.* Komedomastitis *f*.
comedo nevus Naevus comedonicus, Naevus comedo-follicularis.
co·mes [ˈkəʊmɪz] *n pl* **com·i·tes** [ˈkɒmɪtiːz] *anat.* Begleitgefäß *nt*, Begleitvene *f*.
co·mes·ti·ble [kəˈmestɪbl] **I** *~s pl* Lebensmittel *pl*. **II** *adj* eß-, genießbar.
com·fort [ˈkʌmfərt] **I** *n* 1. Trost *m*, Beruhi-

gung *f*. **to give ~ to** Trost zusprechen *od.* spenden. 2. Komfort *m*, Bequemlichkeit *f*. **II** *vt* trösten.
com·fort·a·ble [ˈkʌmftəbl, ˈkʌmfərtəbl] *adj* 1. bequem, komfortabel. **to make s.o./o.s. ~** es jdm./s. bequem machen. **the patient had a ~ night** der Patient hatte eine ruhige Nacht. **her condition is ~** sie ist wohlauf. **are you ~?** liegen *od.* sitzen Sie bequem?; haben Sie es bequem?. **to feel ~** s. wohl fühlen. 2. wohltuend, angenehm.
com·for·ter [ˈkʌmfərtər] *n* 1. Steppdecke *f*. 2. *Brit.* Schnuller *m*.
com·fort·less [ˈkʌmfərtlɪs] *adj* unbequem.
com·i·tant squint [ˈkʌmɪtənt] → comitant strabismus.
comitant strabismus *ophthal.* Begleitschielen *nt*, Strabismus comitans.
com·ma bacillus [ˈkɒmə] Komma-Bazillus *m*, Vibrio cholerae/comma.
com·mand input [kəˈmænd, -mɑːnd] *techn.* Führungsgröße *f*.
comma tract of Schultze Schultze'-Komma *nt*, Fasciculus interfascicularis/semilunaris.
com·mence [kəˈmens] *vt, vi* beginnen, anfangen.
com·mence·ment [kəˈmensmənt] *n* Anfang *m*, Beginn *m*.
com·men·sal [kəˈmensəl] *micro.* **I** *n* Kommensale *m*, Paraphage *m*. **II** *adj* kommensal.
com·men·sal·ism [kəˈmensəlɪzəm] *n micro.* Mitessertum *nt*, Kommensalismus *m*.
com·men·su·ra·bil·i·ty [kəˌmens(j)ərəˈbɪlətɪ] *n* 1. Vergleichbarkeit *f*, Kommensurabilität *f*. 2. richtiges Verhältnis.
com·men·su·ra·ble [kəˈmensərəbl] *adj* (*a. mathe., phys.*) 1. vergleichbar, kommensurabel (*with* mit). 2. im richtigen Verhältnis (zueinander stehend), angemessen.
com·men·su·rate [kəˈmensərɪt, -ʃər-] *adj* 1. entsprechend (*to, with* mit); angemessen. 2. gleich groß, von gleichem Umfang, von gleicher Dauer. 3. → commensurable.
com·mer·cial [kəˈmɜːrʃl] *adj* 1. kommerziell, Handels-, Geschäfts-; kaufmännisch. 2. für den Handel bestimmt, Handels-; (*Präparat*) handelsüblich. 3. *chem.* nicht ganz rein, technisch, kommerziell.
commercial formula *ped.* industrielle/künstliche Säuglingsnahrung *f*.
com·mi·nute [ˈkɒmɪn(j)uːt] **I** *adj* → comminuted. **II** *vt* 1. pulverisieren, zermahlen, zerstoßen, zerreiben. 2. zerkleinern, zersplittern.
com·mi·nut·ed [ˈkɒmən(j)uːtɪd] *adj* 1. zerkleinert, zersplittert. 2. zerrieben, gemahlen, pulverisiert.
comminuted fracture *ortho.* Trümmer-, Splitterbruch *m*, Kommunitivfraktur *f*, Fractura communituta.
com·mi·nu·tion [ˌkɒmɪˈn(j)uːʃn] *n* 1. *ortho.* Zersplitterung *f*, Zertrümmerung *f*, Zerkleinerung *f*. 2. Zerreibung *f*, Pulverisierung *f*. 3. Abnutzung *f*.
com·mis·su·ra [ˌkɒmɪˈʃʊərə, -s(j)ʊərə] *n, pl* **-rae** [-riː] *anat.* commissure.
com·mis·su·ral [kəˈmɪʃərəl, ˌkɒməˈʃʊərəl] *adj* Kommissur betr., kommissural, Kommissuren-.
commissural cells Kommissurenzellen *pl*.
commissural cheilitis Perlèche *f*, Fauleckcen *pl*, Mundwinkelcheilitis *f*, -rhagade *pl*, Angulus infectiosus oris/candidamycetica, Cheilitis/Stomatitis angularis.
commissural fibers → commissural nerve fibers.
commissural nerve fibers Kommissurenfasern *pl*, Neurofibrae commissurales.

commissural neurofibers → commissural nerve fibers.
commissural nucleus Nc. commissuralis.
commissural plate *embryo.* Kommissurenplatte *f.*
com·mis·sure ['kɑməʃʊər] *n* Naht *f*, Verbindung(sstelle *f*) *f*; *anat.* Kommissur *f*, Commissura *f*.
 c. of caudal colliculi Commissura colliculorum inferiorum.
 c. of cranial colliculi → c. of rostral colliculi.
 c. of epithalamus hintere Kommissur, Commissura epithalamica, Commissura posterior cerebri.
 c. of fornix Fornix-, Hippocampuskommissur, Commissura hippocampi/fornicis.
 c. of habenula Commissura habenularis/habenularum.
 c. of inferior colliculi → c. of caudal colliculi.
 c. of lips Commissura labiorum.
 c. of rostral colliculi Commissura colliculorum superiorum.
 c. of superior colliculi → c. of rostral colliculi.
com·mis·sur·or·rha·phy [ˌ-ʃʊəfɪ] *n HTG* Kommissurenraffung *f*, Kommissurorrhaphie *f.*
com·mis·sur·ot·o·my [ˌ-ʃʊə'rɑtəmɪ] *n HTG* Kommissurenschnitt *m*, Kommissurotomie *f.*
com·mit [kə'mɪt] *vt* 1. jdn. einweisen (*to* in). 2. (*Verbrechen*) begehen, verüben. **to ~ suicide** Selbstmord begehen. 3. jdn. verpflichten(*to* zu); **~ o.s.** s. verpflichten (*to* zu). 4. anvertrauen, übergeben (*to*).
com·mit·ment [kə'mɪtmənt] *n* 1. Einlieferung *f*, Einweisung *f* (*to* in); (Zwangs-)-Einweisung *f* in eine Heilanstalt. 2. Begehung *f*, Verübung *f.* 3. Verpflichtung *f* (*to* zu). **to undertake a ~** eine Verpflichtung eingehen. 4. Überantwortung *f*, Übertragung (*to* an).
com·mit·tal [kə'mɪtl] *n* → commitment 1.
com·mit·ted progenitor [kə'mɪtɪd] determinierte Vorläuferzelle *f.*
com·mon ['kɑmən] *adj* 1. häufig (anzutreffend), weitverbreitet, geläufig, normal, gewöhnlich. 2. gemeinsam, gemeinschaftlich; öffentlich, allgemein, Gemein-. 3. *bio.* gemein. 4. üblich, allgemein (gebräuchlich). **to be ~ with** üblich bei.
common acne Akne/Acne vulgaris.
common acute lymphoblastic leukemia antigen *abbr.* **CALLA** common ALL-Antigen *nt abbr.* CALLA.
common atrium *embryo.* Cor triloculare biventriculare.
common bedbug (gemeine) Bettwanze *f*, Cimex lectularius.
common bile duct *abbr.* **CBD** → common duct.
common cold (banale) Erkältung *f*, Erkältungskrankheit *f*, Schnupfen *m.*
common cold viruses Schnupfenviren *pl.*
common digital nerves Nn. digitales communes.
common duct Choledochus *m*, Ductus choledochus.
common duct bile Choledochusgalle *f*, A-Galle *f.*
common duct exploration *chir.* Choledochusrevision *f.*
common duct stones → choledocholithiasis.
common flea Menschenfloh *m*, Pulex irritans.
common integument äußere Haut *f*, Integumentum commune.
common-intermediate principle *biochem.*

Prinzip *nt* des gemeinsamen Zwischenprodukts.
common limb of membranous semicircular ducts Crus membranaceum commune.
common male alopecia → common male baldness.
common male baldness 1. androgenetische Alopezie *f*, Haarausfall *m* vom männlichen Typ, männliche Glatzenbildung *f*, androgenetisches Effluvium *nt*, Alopecia androgenetica, Calvities hippocratica. 2. Alopecia hereditaria, Hypotrichia hereditaria capitis.
common migraine einfache Migräne *f.*
common roundworm *micro.* Spulwurm *m*, Ascaris lumbricoides.
common salt Kochsalz *nt*, Natriumchlorid *nt.*
common sense gesunder Menschenverstand *m.* **in ~** vernünftigerweise.
common-sense *adj* vernünftig, verständig; (*Meinung*) gesund.
common sensibility Zönästhesie *f.*
common sheath: c. of tendons of peroneal muscle gemeinsame Sehnenscheide *f* der Peronäussehnen, Vagina tendinum mm. peron(a)eorum/fibularium communis.
 c. of testis and spermatic cord Fascia spermatica interna.
common variable agammaglobulinemia → common variable unclassificable immunodeficiency.
common variable hypogammaglobulinemia → common variable unclassificable immunodeficiency.
common variable immunodeficiency → common variable unclassifiable immunodeficiency.
common variable unclassifiable immunodeficiency *immun.* variabler nicht--klassifizierbarer Immundefekt *m.*
common verruca *derm.* gemeine/gewöhnliche Warze *f*, Stachelwarze *f*, Verruca vulgaris.
common wart → common verruca.
com·mo·tion [kə'məʊʃn] *n* 1. kontinuierliche *od.* wiederkehrende *od.* andauernde Erschütterung *f.* 2. *psycho.* seelische/innere Erregung/Verwirrung/Aufregung *f.* 3. Gehirnerschütterung *f*, Kommotionssyndrom *nt*, Commotio cerebri.
com·mu·ni·ca·bil·i·ty [kəˌmjuːnɪkə'bɪlətɪ] *n* 1. Übertragbarkeit *f.* 2. Mitteilbarkeit *f.* 3. Mitteilsamkeit *f*, Redseligkeit *f.*
com·mu·ni·ca·ble [kə'mjuːnɪkəbl] *adj* 1. (*Krankheit*) übertragbar, ansteckend. 2. mitteilbar. 3. kommunikativ, mitteilsam, redselig.
communicable disease übertragbare/ansteckbare Krankheit *f.*
com·mu·ni·ca·ble·ness [kə'mjuːnɪkəblnɪs] *n* → communicability.
com·mu·ni·cate [kə'mjuːnɪkeɪt] **I** *vt* 1. mitteilen (*sth. to s.o.* jdm. etw.); über-, vermitteln. 2. (*Krankheit*) übertragen (*to* auf). **II** *vi* kommunizieren, s. austauschen, in Verbindung stehen (*with* mit); s. in Verbindung setzen (*with* mit).
com·mu·ni·cat·ed insanity [kə'mjuːnɪkeɪtɪd] *psychia.* induziertes Irresein *nt*, Folie à deux.
com·mu·ni·cat·ing [kə'mjuːnɪkeɪtɪŋ] *adj* Verbindungs-.
communicating artery Verbindungsarterie *f*, A. communicans.
 anterior c. (of cerebrum) vordere Verbindungsarterie, Communicans *f* anterior, A. communicans anterior.
 posterior c. (of cerebrum) hintere Verbindungsarterie, Communicans *f* posterior, A. communicans posterior.

communicating branch Verbindungsast *m*, Ramus communicans.
 c.es of auriculotemporal nerve with facial nerve Rami communicantes n. auriculotemporalis cum n. faciali.
 c. of ciliary ganglion with nasociliary nerve sensorische Wurzel *f* des Ggl. ciliare, Ramus communicans ggl. ciliaris cum n. nasociliaris, Radix sensoria/nasociliaris ggl. ciliare.
 c. of common fibular nerve Ramus communicans fibularis/peron(a)eus n. fibularis/peron(a)ei communis.
 c. of facial nerve with glossopharyngeal nerve Ramus communicans n. facialis cum n. glossopharyngeo.
 c. of facial nerve with tympanic plexus Ramus communicans n. facialis cum plexu tympanico.
 c. of fibular artery Verbindungsast der A. fibularis zur A. tibialis posterior, Ramus communicans a. peron(a)eae/fibularis.
 c. of glossopharyngeal nerve with auricular branch of vagus nerve Ramus communicans n. glossopharyngei cum ramo auriculari n. vagi.
 gray c. Ramus communicans griseus.
 c. of intermediate nerve with tympanic plexus Ramus communicans n. intermedii cum plexu tympanico.
 c. of intermediate nerve with vagus nerve Ramus communicans n. intermedii cum n. vago.
 c. of lacrimal nerve with zygomatic nerve Ramus communicans n. lacrimalis cum n. zygomatico.
 c. of lingual nerve with chorda tympani Ramus communicans n. lingualis cum chorda tympani.
 c.es of lingual nerve with hypoglossal nerve Rami communicantes n. lingualis cum n. hypoglosso.
 c. of median nerve with ulnar nerve Ramus communicans n. mediani cum n. ulnari.
 c. of nasociliary nerve with ciliary ganglion Ramus communians n. nasociliaris cum ganglione ciliari.
 c. of otic ganglion with auriculotemporal nerve Ramus communicans ganglii otici cum n. auriculotemporali.
 c. of otic ganglion with chorda tympani Ramus communicans ganglii otici cum chorda tympani.
 c. of otic ganglion with medial pterygoid nerve Ramus communicans ganglii otici cum n. pterygoideo mediali.
 c. of otic ganglion with meningeal branches of mandibular nerve Ramus communicans ganglii otici cum ramo meningeo n. mandibularis.
 c.es of spinal nerves Verbindungsäste *pl* der Spinalnerven zum Grenzstrang, Rami communicantes n. spinalium.
 c.es of submandibular ganglion with lingual nerve Rami communicantes ganglii submandibularis cum n. linguali.
 c. of superior laryngeal nerve with recurrent laryngeal nerve Ramus communicans n. laryngealis superioris cum n. laryngeali recurrenti.
 ulnar c. of radial nerve Ramus communicans ulnaris n. radialis.
 c. of vagus nerve with hypoglossal nerve Ramus communicans n. vagi cum n. glossopharyngeo.
 c. of vestibular nerve with cochlear nerve Verbindungsast *m* des N. vestibularis mit N. cochlaeris, Ramus communicans cochlearis.
 white c. Ramus communicans albus.
communicating hydrocele Hydrocele communicans.

communicating hydrocephalus Hydrocephalus communicans.
communicating veins Verbindungs-, Perforansvenen *pl*, Vv. perforantes.
com·mu·ni·ca·tion [kə͵mjuːnɪ'keɪʃn] *n* 1. *phys.*, *infect.* Übertragung *f* (*to* auf). 2. Mitteilung *f* (*to* an); Verbindung *f*, (Meinungs-, Gedanken-)Austausch *m*, Verständigung *f*, Kommunikation *f*. **in ~ with** in Verbindung stehen mit.
c. of power Kraftübertragung.
com·mu·ni·ty [kə'mjuːnətɪ] *n*, *pl* **-ties** 1. (soziale, politische etc.) Gemeinschaft *f*; *bio.* Gemeinschaft *f*. 2. **the ~ die** Öffentlichkeit, die Gesellschaft, die Allgemeinheit. 3. Gemeinde *f*. 4. Staat *m*.
community care Gemeindepflege *f*.
community center Gemeindezentrum *nt*.
community nurse Gemeindeschwester *f*.
Comolli [kə'məʊlɪ; ko'moli]: **C.'s sign** *ortho.* Comolli'-Zeichen *nt*.
com·pact [*n* 'kɒmpækt; *adj* 'kɒm-, kəm-'pækt; *v* kəm'pækt] **I** *n* kompakte Masse *f*. **II** *adj* 1. kompakt, dicht, fest, hart, geballt, massiv. 2. (*Figur*) gedrungen. **III** *vt* kompakt machen, zusammendrücken, -pressen, verdichten.
com·pac·ta [kəm'pæktə] *n* Kompakta *f*, Compacta *f*, Lamina/Pars compacta, Stratum compactum endometrii.
compact bone Kompakta *f*, Substantia compacta.
com·pact·ed·ness [kəm'pæktədnɪs] *n* → compactness.
compact layer of endometrium → compacta.
com·pact·ness [kəm'pæktnɪs] *n* Kompaktheit *f*.
compact osteoma *patho.* kompaktes Osteom *m*, Osteoma eburneum.
compact part (of substantia nigra) Pars compacta.
compact substance of bone → compact bone.
compact tissue → compact bone.
com·pa·ra·bil·i·ty [͵kɒmpərə'bɪlətɪ] *n* Vergleichbarkeit *f*.
com·pa·ra·ble ['kɒmpərəbl, kəm'peər-] *adj* vergleichbar (*to*, *with* mit); gleichartig, entsprechend.
com·pa·ra·ble·ness ['-nɪs] *n* → comparability.
com·par·a·scope [kəm'pærəskəʊp] *n* Vergleichsmikroskop *nt*.
com·par·a·tive [kəm'pærətɪv] *adj* vergleichend, Vergleichs-; verhältnismäßig, relativ.
comparative anatomy vergleichende Anatomie *f*.
comparative medicine vergleichende Medizin *f*.
comparative pathology vergleichende Pathologie *f*.
comparative percussion vergleichende Perkussion *f*.
comparative psychology vergleichende Psychologie *f*.
comparative study Vergleichsstudie *f*.
com·pare [kəm'peər] **I** *n* Vergleich *m*. **beyond/without ~** unvergleichlich. **II** *vt* 1. vergleichen (*with*, *to* mit); gleichsetzen, -stellen (*to* mit). 2. miteinander vergleichen, nebeneinanderstellen. **III** *vi* s. vergleichen (lassen) (*with* mit).
com·par·i·son [kəm'pærɪsn] *n* Vergleich *m* (*to* mit). **by ~** vergleichsweise, im Vergleich dazu. **in ~** im Vergleich (*with* mit, zu). **to make/draw a ~** einen Vergleich ziehen. **to stand/bear ~** einen Vergleich standhalten (*with* mit).
com·par·o·scope *n* → camparascope.

com·part·ment [kəm'pɑːrtmənt] **I** *n* Abteilung *f*, Abschnitt *m*, Fach *nt*, Kammer *f*, Raum *m*. **II** *vt* auf-, unterteilen.
com·part·men·tal [͵kɒmpɑːrt'mentl, kəm-] *adj* aufgeteilt; fach-, felderartig.
com·part·men·tal·i·za·tion [kəmpɑːrt͵mentlaɪ'zeɪʃn] *n* → compartment formation.
com·part·men·ta·tion [kəm͵pɑːrtmən'teɪʃn] *n* → compartment formation.
compartment formation Kompartmentierung *f*, Kompart(i)mentbildung *f*.
compartment syndrome *ortho.* Kompartmentsyndrom *nt*.
com·pat·i·bil·i·ty [kəm͵pætə'bɪlətɪ] *n* Verträglichkeit *f*, Vereinbarkeit *f*, Kompatibilität *f* (*with* mit).
com·pat·i·ble [kəm'pætɪbl] *n* vereinbar, verträglich, zusammenpassend, austauschbar, kompatibel (*with* mit).
com·pat·i·ble·ness [kəm'pætɪblnɪs] *n* → compatibility.
com·pen·sate ['kɒmpənseɪt] **I** *vt* 1. (*a. psycho.*, *techn.*) ausgleichen, aufheben, kompensieren. 2. (finanziell) entschädigen (*for* für). **II** *vi psycho.* kompensieren.
com·pen·sat·ed acidosis ['kɒmpənseɪtɪd] *physiol.* kompensierte Azidose *f*.
compensated alkalosis *physiol.* kompensierte Alkalose *f*.
compensated glaucoma Simplex-, Weitwinkelglaukom *nt*, Glaucoma simplex.
com·pen·sat·ing ['kɒmpənseɪtɪŋ] *adj* ausgleichend, kompensierend, Ausgleichs-, Kompensations-.
compensating emphysema → compensatory emphysema.
com·pen·sa·tion [͵kɒmpən'seɪʃn] *n* 1. (*a. chem.*, *techn.*) Ausgleich *m*, Aufhebung *f*, Kompensation *f*. 2. *psycho.* Kompensation *f*, Kompensieren *nt*. 3. Entschädigung *f*, (Rück-)Erstattung *f*.
com·pen·sa·tion·al [͵-'seɪʃənl] *adj* Kompensations-, Ausgleichs-, Ersatz-.
compensation neurosis Renten-, Unfall-, Entschädigungsneurose *f*, Rentenbegehren *nt*, -tendenz *f*, traumatische Neurose *f*, tendenziöse Unfallreaktion *f*.
com·pen·sa·tive ['-͵seɪtɪv, kəm'pensə-] *adj* 1. ausgleichend, kompensierend, kompensatorisch. 2. entschädigend, Entschädigungs-.
com·pen·sa·to·ry [kəm'pensətɔːriː, -͵təʊ-] *adj* → compensative.
compensatory atrophy *patho.* kompensatorische Atrophie *f*.
compensatory circulation → collateral circulation.
compensatory emphysema kompensatorisches (Lungen-)Emphysem *nt*.
compensatory hyperemia kompensatorische Hyperämie *f*.
compensatory hypertrophy *patho.* Arbeits-, Aktivitätshypertrophie *f*.
compensatory mechanism kompensatorischer Mechanismus *m*, Kompensationsmechanismus *m*.
compensatory pause *card.* kompensatorische Pause *f*.
compensatory scoliosis *ortho.* kompensatorische Skoliose *f*.
com·pete [kəm'piːt] *vi* s. gegenseitig Konkurrenz machen (*for* um); konkurrieren (*with* mit); kämpfen (*for* um, *against* gegen).
com·pe·tence ['kɒmpətəns] *n* 1. Fähigkeit *f*, Tüchtigkeit *f*, Kompetenz *f*. 2. *embryo.*, *micro.* Kompetenz *f*. 3. *physiol.* (regelrechte) Funktion(sfähigkeit) *f*; (*Herzklappen*) (vollständiger) Schluß *m*. 4. *immun.* Immunkompetenz *f*.
competence factor Kompetenzfaktor *m*.

com·pe·ten·cy ['kɒmpətənsɪ] *n* → competence.
com·pe·tent ['kɒmpətənt] *adj* 1. *bio.* funktionsfähig. 2. fähig (*to do* zu tun). 3. fach-, sachkundig, kompetent, qualifiziert.
com·pe·ti·tion [͵kɒmpɪ'tɪʃn] *n* 1. *bio.* Existenzkampf *m*. 2. Konkurrenz(kampf *m*) *f*, Wettstreit *m*, -kampf *m*, Wettbewerb *m* (*for* um).
com·pet·i·tive [kəm'petɪtɪv] *adj* 1. *bio.*, *chem.* kompetitiv. 2. konkurrierend, Konkurrenz-, Wettbewerbs-.
competitive antagonist *biochem.* kompetitiver Antagonist *m*; Antimetabolit *m*.
competitive binding assay *lab.* kompetitiver Bindungstest/-assay *m*.
competitive inhibition *biochem.* kompetitive Hemmung *f*.
com·pla·cence [kəm'pleɪsəns] *n* → complacency.
com·pla·cen·cy [kəm'pleɪsənsɪ] *n*, *pl* **-cies** Selbstzufriedenheit *f*, Selbstgefälligkeit *f*.
com·pla·cent [kəm'pleɪsənt] *adj* selbstzufrieden, selbstgefällig.
com·plain [kəm'pleɪn] *vi* s. beklagen, s. beschweren (*of*, *about* über); klagen (*of* über).
com·plaint [kəm'pleɪnt] *n* 1. Leiden *nt*, Erkrankung *f*, Beschwerden *pl*; Symptom *nt*. **a rare ~** eine seltende Krankheit. 2. Klage *f*, Beschwerde *f* (*about* über).
com·ple·ment [*n* 'kɒmplɪmənt; *v* -͵ment] **I** *n* 1. Ergänzung *f* (*to*), Vervollkommnung *f* (*to*). 2. Komplementär-, Gegenfarbe *f* (*to* zu). 3. *immun.* Komplement *n*, Komplement *nt*. **II** *vt* ergänzen, vervollkommnen.
complement activation *immun.* Komplementaktivierung *f*.
com·ple·men·tal [͵kɒmplə'mentl] *adj* → complementary.
complemental inheritance komplementäre Vererbung *f*.
com·ple·men·ta·ry [͵-'ment(ə)rɪ] *adj* ergänzend, komplementär, Ergänzungs-, Komplementär-.
complementary antibody komplementärer Antikörper *m*.
complementary base *biochem.* Komplementärbase *f*.
complementary color → complement 2.
complementary DNA *abbr.* **cDNA** komplementäre DNA *f abbr.* cDNA, komplementäre DNS *f*.
complementary genes Komplementärgene *pl*.
complementary opposition sign Grasset-Zeichen *nt*, Hoover-Zeichen *nt*, Phänomen *nt* der komplementären Opposition.
complementary strand Komplementärstrang *m*.
com·ple·men·ta·tion [͵kɒmpləmən'teɪʃn] *n genet.*, *micro.* Komplementation *f*.
complementation test Komplementierungstest *m*.
complement binding reaction → complement fixation reaction.
complement components Komplementkomponenten *pl*, -faktoren *pl*.
complement deviation Neisser-Wechsberg-Phänomen *nt*.
complement factor Komplementfaktor *m*.
complement fixation *abbr.* **CF** *immun.* Komplementbindung *f*.
complement fixation reaction *abbr.* **CFR** *immun.* Komplementbindungsreaktion *f abbr.* **KBR**.
complement fixation test *abbr.* **C.F.T.** → complement fixation reaction.
Treponema pallidum c. Treponema-pallidum-Komplementbindungstest *m*.

complement-fixing *adj* komplementbindend.
complement-fixing antibody komplementbindender Antikörper *m*.
complement-fixing antigen komplementbindendes Antigen *nt*.
complement inactivation Komplementinaktivierung *f*.
complement receptor Komplement-bindender Rezeptor *m*.
complement system Komplementsystem *nt*.
complement unit Komplementeinheit *f*.
com·plete [kəm'pli:t] **I** *adj* 1. ganz, vollständig, komplett, völlig, vollzählig, total, Gesamt-. 2. fertig, abgeschlossen, beendet. **II** *vt* 3. vervollständigen, komplettieren. 4. abschließen, beenden, zu Ende bringen, fertigstellen.
complete abortion kompletter/vollständiger Abort *m*, Abortus completus.
complete achromatopsy *physiol., ophthal.* (totale) Farbenblindheit *f*, Achromatop(s)ie *f*, Monochromasie *f*.
complete agglutinin → complete antibody.
complete antibody kompletter/agglutinierender Antikörper *m*.
complete antigen *immun.* komplettes Antigen *nt*, Vollantigen *nt*.
complete blood count *abbr.* **CBC** großes Blutbild *nt*.
complete cast *ortho.* zirkulärer Gips(verband *m*) *m*.
complete cataract *ophthal.* kompletter/vollständiger Star *m*, Totalstar *m*, Cataracta totalis.
complete colectomy *chir.* totale Kolonexstirpation/Kolektomie *f*.
complete coloboma *ophthal.* totales Kolobom *nt*.
complete combustion *phys.* vollständige Verbrennung *f*.
complete dislocation *ortho.* komplette Luxation/Dislokation *f*.
complete epispadias *urol.* komplette Epispadie *f*.
complete fistula komplette Fistel *f*, Fistula completa.
complete fracture *ortho.* vollständige Fraktur *f*, (Knochen-)Durchbruch *m*, Fractura perfecta.
complete hemianopia/hemianopsia *ophthal.* komplette Hemianop(s)ie *f*.
complete hernia *chir.* kompletter/vollständiger Bruch *m*, Hernia completa.
complete hysterectomy *gyn.* totale Gebärmutterentfernung/Hysterektomie *f*, Hysterectomia totalis.
complete imperfect albinism *derm.* Tyrosinase-positiver okulokutaner Albinismus *m*.
complete iridectomy *ophthal.* komplette/totale/vollständige Iridektomie *f*.
com·plete·ness [kəm'pli:tnɪs] *n* Vollständigkeit *f*, Vollkommen-, Komplettheit *f*.
complete medium *micro.* Voll(nähr)medium *nt*.
complete monochromasy → complete achromatopsy.
complete perfect albinism *derm.* Tyrosinase-negativer okulokutaner Albinismus *m*.
complete recovery vollständige *od.* komplette Wiederherstellung/Heilung/Erholung *f*; *chir.* Restitutio ad integrum.
complete remission *abbr.* **CR** *oncol.* Vollremission *f*, komplette Remission *f abbr.* CR.
complete syndactyly *ortho., embryo.* komplette Syndaktylie *f*.
complete transposition of great arteries → complete transposition of great vessels.
complete transposition of great vessels *card., ped.* Transposition *f* der großen Arterien/Gefäße *abbr.* TGA.
com·ple·tion [kəm'pli:ʃn] *n* 1. Vervollständigung *f*, Komplettierung *f*. 2. Beendigung *f*, Vollendung *f*, Fertigstellung *f*, Abschluß *m*.
completion test *psycho.* Lücken-, Intelligenztest *m*.
com·plex [*n* 'kɒmpleks; *adj, v* kəm'pleks] **I** *n* 1. Komplex *m*, Gesamtheit *f*, (das) Gesamte; (Gebäude-)Komplex *m*. 2. *psycho.* Komplex *m*; Zwangsidee *f*, -vorstellung *f*. 3. *biochem., chem.* Komplex *m*. **II** *adj* 4. zusammengesetzt. 5. komplex, vielschichtig, kompliziert, differenziert. **III** *vt, vi chem.* einen Komplex bilden (*with mit*).
com·plex·ing agent [kəm'pleksɪŋ] *chem.* Komplexbildner *m*.
com·plex·ion [kəm'plekʃn] *n* 1. (Haut-, Gesichts-)Farbe *f*, Teint *m*. 2. Aspekt *m*, Zug *m*, Blick-, Gesichtspunkt *m*.
com·plex·ioned [kəm'plekʃnd] *adj* von (dunkler etc.) Haut- *od.* Gesichtsfarbe, mit (blassem etc.) Teint.
com·plex·i·ty [kəm'pleksətɪ] *n, pl* **-ties** 1. Komplexität *f*, Kompliziertheit *f*, Vielschichtigkeit *f*. 2. (das) Komplexe.
complex lipid kompliziertes/verseifbares Lipid *nt*.
complex odontoma *patho.* komplexes Odontom *nt*.
complex symmetry *micro.* komplexe Symmetrie *f*.
com·pli·ance [kəm'plaɪəns] *n* 1. *physiol, phys. abbr.* **C** Weit-, Dehnbarkeit *f*, Compliance *f abbr.* C. 2. Einverständnis *nt* (*with in*); Befolgung *f*, Einhaltung *f*, Compliance *f*.
com·pli·ca·cy ['kɒmplɪkəsɪ] *n, pl* **-cies** 1. Kompliziertheit *f*. 2. **⁓cies** *pl* Komplikationen *pl*.
com·pli·cate ['kɒmplɪkeɪt] **I** *adj* kompliziert. **II** *vt* komplizieren.
com·pli·cat·ed ['kɒmplɪkeɪtɪd] *adj* kompliziert, komplex, mit anderen Erkrankungen/Verletzungen assoziiert.
complicated cataract *ophthal.* komplizierter Star *m*, Cataracta complicata.
complicated dislocation *ortho.* komplizierte Luxation *f*.
complicated fracture Fraktur *f* mit Weichteilverletzung.
complicated labor komplizierte Geburt *f*.
com·pli·ca·tion [ˌ-'keɪʃn] *n* Komplikation *f*; Kompliziertheit *f*. **to experience/encounter/have ⁓s** auf Komplikationen stoßen.
com·plu·et·ic reaction [kɒmplu:'etɪk] Wassermann-Test *m*, -Reaktion *f abbr.* WaR, Komplementbindungsreaktion *f* nach Wassermann.
com·ply [kəm'plaɪ] *vi* 1. (*eine Anordnung*) einhalten, befolgen (*with*). 2. (*einem Wunsch*) nachkommen; erfüllen (*with*).
com·po·nent [kəm'pəʊnənt, kɒm-] **I** *n* Bestandteil *m*, Teil *m*, Komponente *f*. **II** *adj* einen (Bestand-)Teil bildend, zusammensetzend, Teil-.
c.s of complement Komplementkomponenten *pl*, -faktoren *pl*.
component A of prothrombin Proakzelerin *nt*, Proaccelerin *nt*, Acceleratorglobulin *nt*, labiler Faktor *m*, Faktor V *m abbr.* F V.
component part (Bestand-)Teil *m*.
com·pose [kəm'pəʊz] *vt* 1. **⁓ o.s.** s. beruhigen, s. sammeln, s. fassen. 2. zusammenstellen, -setzen. **be ⁓d of** zusammengesetzt/bestehend aus. 3. ver-, abfassen, entwerfen.
com·posed [kəm'pəʊzd] *adj* ruhig, gefasst, gelassen.
com·pos·ed·ness [kəm'pəʊzɪdnɪs, -z(d)nɪs] *n* Ruhe *f*, Gelassenheit *f*. **to lose one's ⁓** aus der Fassung geraten, die Beherrschung verlieren. **to regain one's ⁓** s. wieder fassen, seine Selbstbeherrschung wiederfinden.
com·pos·ing [kəm'pəʊzɪŋ] *adj* beruhigend, Beruhigungs-.
com·pos·ite [kəm'pɒzɪt] **I** *n* Zusammensetzung *f*, Mischung *f*, Kompositum *nt*. **II** *adj* zusammengesetzt (*of aus*); gemischt.
composite articulation Artic. composita/complexa.
composite flap *chir.* zusammengesetzter/kombinierter (Haut-)Lappen *m*.
composite graft *chir.* gemischtes Transplantat *nt*, Mehrorgantransplantat *nt*, composite graft (*nt/f*).
composite joint → composite articulation.
composite odontoma *patho.* komplexes Odontom *nt*.
composite transplant → composite graft.
com·po·si·tion [ˌkɒmpə'zɪʃn] *n* 1. Zusammensetzung *f*, Aufbau *m*, Struktur *f*; Beschaffenheit *f*, Komposition *f*. 2. Ver-, Abfassen *nt*; Entwurf *m*. 3. Zusammensetzung *f*, Bildung *f*.
composition tumor *patho.* Kompositionstumor *m*.
com·po·sure [kəm'pəʊʒər] *n* → composedness.
com·pound [*n* 'kɒmpaʊnd; *adj* 'kɒm-, kɒm'paʊnd; *v* kəm'paʊnd, 'kɒm-] **I** *n* 1. Zusammensetzung *f*, Mischung *f*. 2. *chem.* Verbindung *f*. 3. *pharm.* Kombination(spräparat *nt*) *f*, Kompositum *nt*, Compositum *nt*. **II** *adj* zusammengesetzt, aus mehreren Komponenten bestehend; (*Fraktur*) kompliziert. **III** *vt* 4. zusammensetzen, -stellen, kombinieren, verbinden, (ver-)mischen. **to be ⁓ed of** s. zusammensetzen aus. 5. herstellen, bilden. 6. verstärken, intensivieren, verschlimmern, vergrößern.
compound A 11-Dehydrocorticosteron *nt*, Kendall-Substanz A *f*.
compound aneurysm kombiniertes Aneurysma *nt*.
compound articulation Artic. composita/complexa.
compound astigmatism *ophthal.* Astigmatismus compositus.
compound B Kortiko-, Corticosteron *nt*, Compound B Kendall.
compound cyst multilokuläre Zyste *f*.
compound dislocation *ortho.* offene Luxation *f*.
compound E → cortisone.
compound eye *bio.* Facetten-, Netzauge *nt*.
compound F → cortisol.
compound flap → composite flap.
compound fracture *ortho.* offene/komplizierte Fraktur *f*, offener/komplizierter (Knochen-)Bruch *m*, Wundfraktur *f*, Fractura complicata.
compound gland zusammengesetzte Drüse *f*.
compound granular cell Gitterzelle *f*.
compound joint → compound articulation.
compound lipid Heterolipid *nt*.
compound melanocytoma *derm.* Spitz--Tumor *m*, Nävus Spitz, spindelzelliger Nävus *m*, benignes juveniles Melanom *nt*.
compound microscope Verbundmikroskop *nt*.
compound nevus *derm.* Kombinationsnävus *m*, Compound-Nävus *m*.

compound protein

compound protein → conjugated protein.
com·pre·hend [ˌkʌmprɪ'hend] vt 1. begreifen, erfassen, verstehen. 2. umfassen, einschließen.
com·pre·hen·si·ble [ˌ-'hensɪbl] adj begreiflich, verständlich, faßbar.
com·pre·hen·sion [ˌ-'henʃn] n 1. Begriffs-, Wahrnehmungsvermögen nt, Fassungskraft f, Auffassungsgabe f, Verstand m, Verständnis nt (of für). 2. Begreifen nt, Verstehen nt (of). to be quick/slow of ~ schnell/langsam begreifen. 3. bewußte Wahrnehmung f, Apperzeption f.
com·press [n 'kʌmpres; v kəm'pres] I n Kompresse f, (feuchter) Umschlag m. II vt 1. zusammendrücken, -pressen. 2. (Arterie) stauen. 3. phys., techn. komprimieren, verdichten.
com·pressed [kəm'prest] adj 1. zusammengedrückt, -gepreßt, -gedrängt. 2. phys., techn. komprimiert, verdichtet. 3. bio. schmal.
compressed air Preß-, Druckluft f.
compressed-air disease Druckluft-, Caissonkrankheit f.
compressed-air illness → compressed-air disease.
compressed-air sickness → compressed-air disease.
com·press·i·bil·i·ty [kəmˌpresə'bɪlətɪ] n, pl -ties Zusammendrückbarkeit f; techn. phys. Komprimier-, Verdichtbarkeit f.
com·press·i·ble [kəm'presɪbl] adj zusammendrückbar; phys., techn. komprimier-, verdichtbar.
com·pres·sion [kəm'preʃn] n Zusammenpressen nt, -drücken nt; phys., techn. Kompression f, Verdichtung f; Druck m.
c. of the brain Hirnkompression, -quetschung f.
c. of the trachea Luftröhren-, Trachea(l)kompression.
compression atelectasis pulmo. Kompressionsatelektase f.
compression atrophy Druckatrophie f.
compression bandage Druck-, Kompressionsverband m.
compression fracture ortho. Kompressionsbruch m, -fraktur f, Stauchungsbruch m, -fraktur f.
compression myelitis → compression myelopathy.
compression myelopathy Kompressionsmyelopathie f.
compression paralysis Druck-, Kompressionslähmung f.
compression plate ortho. Zugplatte f.
compression pressure techn. Verdichtungsdruck m.
compression screw ortho. Zugschraube f.
compression syndrome Crush-Syndrom nt, -Niere f, Bywaters-Krankheit f, Quetschungs-, Verschüttungs-, Muskelzerfallsyndrom nt, myorenales/tubulovaskuläres Syndrom nt.
com·pres·sive [kəm'presɪv] adj zusammendrückend, -pressend, Preß-, Druck-.
compressive strength phys. Druckfestigkeit f.
compressive stress Druckspannung f.
com·pres·sor [kəm'presər] n 1. anat. Preß-, Schließmuskel m, Kompressor m, M. compressor. 2. Kompressorium nt; Gefäß-, Arterienklemme f. 3. techn. Kompressor m, Verdichter m.
c. of naris → compressor naris (muscle).
com·pres·so·ri·um [ˌkʌmpre'sɔːrɪəm] n, pl -ria [-rɪə] → compressor 2.
compressor muscle of naris → compressor naris (muscle).
compressor naris (muscle) Kompressor m naris, M. compressor naris, Pars trans-

versa m. nasalis.
com·prise [kəm'praɪz] vt 1. s. zusammensetzen od. bestehen aus. 2. umfassen.
com·pro·mise ['kʌmprəmaɪz] I n Kompromiß m; Zugeständnis nt. **to make a ~** einen Kompromiß schließen. II vt 1. (Gesundheit) gefährden, beeinträchtigen. 2. durch einen Kompromiß beilegen od. schlichten. III vi einen Kompromiß schließen, s. vergleichen (on über).
Compton ['kʌmptən]: **C. effect** Compton-Effekt m.
C. electron Compton-Elektron nt.
C. scattering Quanten-, Compton-Streuung f.
com·pul·sion [kəm'pʌlʃn] n psycho., psychia. (innerer) Zwang m, unwiderstehlicher Drang m. **under ~** unter Zwang od. Druck, gezwungen, zwangsweise.
compulsion neurosis Zwangsneurose f, Anankasmus m, anankastisches Syndrom nt, obsessiv-kompulsive Reaktion f.
com·pul·sive [kəm'pʌlsɪv] adj psycho., psychia. zwanghaft, zwingend, kompulsiv, Zwangs-, Kompulsiv-.
compulsive neurosis → compulsion neurosis.
compulsive personality zwanghafte/anankastische Persönlichkeit(sstörung f) f, Zwangscharakter m.
com·pul·so·ry [kəm'pʌlsərɪ] adj 1. zwangsweise, gezwungen, Zwangs-. 2. obligatorisch, verbindlich, zwingend vorgeschrieben, Pflicht-.
compulsory measures Zwangsmaßnahmen pl.
com·pu·ta·tion [ˌkʌmpjuː'teɪʃn] n 1. (Be-, Aus-, Er-)Rechnen nt, Kalkulieren nt. 2. Berechnung f, Kalkulation f, Schätzung f.
com·pute [kəm'pjuːt] I n → computation. II vt (be-, aus-, er-)rechnen; schätzen, veranschlagen (at auf). III vi rechnen.
com·put·ed tomography [kəm'pjuːtɪd] abbr. CT → computerized axial tomography.
com·put·er [kəm'pjuːtər] n 1. Computer m, Rechner m. 2. Rechner m, Kalkulator m.
computer-assisted tomography → computerized axial tomography.
computer-controlled adj computergesteuert.
computer diagnostics Computerdiagnostik f.
computer forecast stat. Hochrechnung f.
computer graphics Computergrafik f.
com·put·er·ize [kəm'pjuːtəraɪz] vt mit Hilfe eines Computers errechnen, mit Hilfe eines Computers durchführen.
com·put·er·ized [kəm'pjuːtəraɪzd] adj mit Hilfe eines Computers, unter Einsatz eines Computers, computergestützt.
computerized axial tomography abbr. CAT radiol. Computertomographie f abbr. CT, CAT.
computerized tomography abbr. CT → computerized axial tomography.
computer language Computersprache f.
computer-operated adj computergesteuert.
computer prediction stat. Hochrechnung f.
computer science Informatik f.
computer scientist Informatiker(in f) m.
computer simulation Computersimulation f.
computer-supported adj computergestützt.
computer system Rechenanlage f.
COMT abbr. → catecholamine-O-methyltransferase.
ConA abbr. → concanavalin A.

co·nal artery ['kəʊnl]: **left c.** Ast m der linken Herzkranzarterie zum Conus arteriosus, Ramus coni arteriosi a. coronariae sinistrae.
right c. Ast m der rechten Herzkranzarterie zum Conus arteriosus, Ramus coni arteriosi a. coronariae dextrae.
co·nar·i·um [kəʊ'neərɪəm] n, pl -ria [-rɪə] anat. Zirbeldrüse f, Corpus pineale.
co·na·tion [kəʊ'neɪʃn] n psycho., psychia. Willenstrieb m, Antrieb m, Begehren nt.
co·na·tive ['kəʊnətɪv] adj psycho., psychia. triebhaft, Willens-, Begehrens-, Trieb-.
con·ca·na·va·lin A [ˌkʌnkə'nævəlɪn] n abbr. **ConA** Concanavalin A nt abbr. ConA.
con·cat·e·nate [kən'kætənɪt] I adj (kettenartig) verknüpft, Kaskaden-. II vt verketten, verknüpfen.
con·cat·e·na·tion [kənˌkætə'neɪʃn] n Verkettung f, Verknüpfung f; Kette f.
Concato [kən'kætəʊ]: **C.'s disease** progressive maligne Polyserositis f.
con·cave [n 'kʌnkeɪv; v kən'keɪv] I n konkave (Ober-)Fläche f, (Aus-)Höhlung f. II adj nach innen gewölbt, vertieft, hohl, konkav, Konkav-, Hohl-. III vt konkav formen, aushöhlen.
concave cavity of temporal bone Fossa mandibularis (ossis temporalis).
concave lens konkave Linse f, Konkavlinse f, (Zer-)Streuungslinse f.
con·cav·i·ty [kən'kævətɪ] n 1. Konkavität f, konkave Beschaffenheit f, Krümmung f (nach innen). 2. → concave 1.
con·ca·vo·con·cave lens [kʌnˌkeɪvəʊkən'keɪv] konkavokonkave/bikonkave Linse f, Bikonkavlinse f.
con·ca·vo·con·vex lens [ˌ-kən'veks] konkavokonvexe Linse f.
con·cealed [kən'siːld] adj verborgen, verdeckt; nicht-palpierbar.
concealed hemorrhage innere Blutung f.
concealed hernia chir. nicht-palpierbare Hernie f.
con·ceive [kən'siːv] vt 1. (Kind) empfangen, schwanger werden. 2. begreifen, s. vorstellen, s. denken. II vi schwanger werden, empfangen.
con·cen·trate ['kʌnsəntreɪt] I n chem. Konzentrat nt. II adj chem. konzentriert. III vt 1. konzentrieren; (Gedanken) richten (on auf). 2. chem. (Lösung) konzentrieren, anreichern. 3. konzentrieren, sammeln, zusammenballen, -drängen. IV vi 4. s. konzentrieren (on auf). 5. s. sammeln, s. zusammendrängen, s. zusammenballen. 6. chem. s. konzentrieren, s. anreichern.
con·cen·trat·ed ['-treɪtɪd] adj chem. konzentriert.
con·cen·tra·tion [ˌ-'treɪʃn] n 1. chem. abbr. C Konzentration f, Anreicherung f. **at/in a high ~** in hoher Konzentration. **at/in a low ~** in niedriger Konzentration. **a fall in ~** Konzentrationsabfall m. **a rise in ~** Konzentrationsanstieg. 2. Konzentration f, Konzentrierung f, angespannte Aufmerksamkeit f, (geistige) Sammlung f. 3. Zusammenballung f, -drängung f, (An-)Sammlung f, Konzentration f, Konzentrierung f.
concentration ability physiol. (Niere) Konzentrationsvermögen nt.
concentration culture Anreicherungskultur f.
concentration gradient Konzentrationsgradient m.
concentration work Arbeit f gegen einen Konzentrationsgradienten.
con·cen·tra·tive ['-treɪtɪv, kən'sentrə-] adj konzentrierend.
con·cen·tric [kən'sentrɪk] adj konzentrisch.

con·cen·tri·cal [kənˈsentrɪkl] *adj* → concentric.
concentric atrophy *patho.* konzentrische Atrophie *f*.
concentric corpuscles Hassall'-Körperchen *pl*.
concentric hypertrophy *patho.* konzentrische Hypertrophie *f*.
con·cen·tric·i·ty [ˌkɒnsənˈtrɪsətɪ] *n* Konzentrität *f*.
concentric lamella Havers'-(Knochen-)-Lamelle *f*.
concentric periaxial encephalitis/leukoencephalitis → concentric sclerosis of Baló.
concentric sclerosis of Baló Baló-Krankheit *f*, konzentrische Sklerose *f*, Leucoencephalitis periaxialis concentrica.
con·cept [ˈkɒnsept] I *n* Auffassung *f*, Begriff *m*, Konzeption *f*. II *vt inf.* planen, ausdenken, ersinnen.
con·cep·tion [kənˈsepʃn] *n* 1. *gyn.* Empfängnis *f*, Befruchtung *f*, Konzeption *f*, Conceptio *f*. 2. Vorstellung *f*, Auffassung *f*; Konzeption *f*, Idee *f* (*of* von). 3. Auffasungsvermögen *nt*, Begreifen *nt*, Erfassen *nt*. 4. Entwurf *m*, Konzept *nt*, Plan *m*.
con·cep·tive [kənˈseptɪv] *adj* 1. *gyn.* Konzeption betr., konzeptions-, empfängnisfähig, Empfängnis-, Konzeptions-. 2. begreifend, empfänglich, Begriffs-.
con·cep·tu·al [kənˈseptʃʊəl] *adj* begrifflich, Begriffs-.
con·cern [kənˈsɜːn] I *n* 1. Angelegenheit(en *pl*) *f*, Sache *f*, Anliegen *nt*. 2. Sorge *f*, Besorgnis *f* (*at, about, for* wegen, um). 3. Interesse *nt* (*about, for, in,* für); Teilnahme *f* (*about, for, in,* an). 4. Bedeutung *f*, Wichtigkeit *f*. II *vt* 5. betreffen, angehen. 6. beschäftigen. **to ~ o.s. with** s. befassen mit. 7. beunruhigen. **to be ~d about/at** s. Sorgen machen um/wegen. 8. handeln von.
con·cerned [kənˈsɜːnt] *adj* 1. besorgt (*at, about, for* um); beunruhigt (*at, about, for* wegen). 2. betroffen. **the department ~d** die zuständige Abteilung. 3. verwickelt (*in* in); beteiligt (*in* an). 4. beschäftigt (*with* mit).
con·cert·ed [kənˈsɜːtɪd] *adj* (aufeinander) abgestimmt, gemeinsam, konzertiert.
concerted inhibition konzertierte Hemmung/Inhibition *f*.
concerted proton transfer konzertierte Protonenübertragung *f*.
con·cha [ˈkɒŋkə] *n, pl* **-chae** [-kiː] *anat.* Muschel *f*, muschelförmige Struktur *f*, Concha *f*.
c. of auricle Ohrmuschelhöhlung *f*, Concha (auricularis).
c. of cranium knöchernes Schädeldach *nt*, Kalotte *f*, Calvaria *f*.
con·chal [ˈkɒŋkəl] *adj* Concha betr., muschelförmig.
conchal cartilage Ohrmuschelknorpel *m*, Knorpelgerüst *nt* der Ohrmuschel, Cartilago auricularis.
conchal crest: c. of maxilla Crista conchalis maxillae.
c. of palatine bone Crista conchalis ossis palatini.
con·chi·tis [kɒŋˈkaɪtɪs] *n* Conchaentzündung *f*, Konchitis *f*, Conchitis *f*.
con·choi·dal bodies [kɒŋˈkɔɪdl] Schaumann'-Körperchen *pl*.
con·cho·scope [ˈkɒŋkəskəʊp] *n HNO* Konchoskop *nt*.
con·cho·tome [ˈkɒŋkətəʊm] *n HNO* Konchotom *nt*.
con·cho·to·my [kɒŋˈkɒtəmɪ] *n HNO* Muschelresektion *f*, Konchotomie *f*, Turbinektomie *f*.

con·cli·na·tion [ˌkɒŋklɪˈneɪʃn] *n ophthal.* Konklination *f*, Inzykloverganz *f*.
con·clude [kənˈkluːd] I *vt* 1. be- *od.* abschließen (*with* mit); beenden. 2. folgern, schließen (*from* aus); zu dem Schluß kommen. II *vi* 3. enden, aufhören (*with* mit). 4. s. entschließen (*to do* zu tun).
con·clu·sion [kənˈkluːʒn] *n* 1. Abschluß *m*, Schluß *m*, Ende *nt*. 2. (Schluß-)Folgerung *f*. **to come to the ~** zu dem Schluß gelangen (*that* daß). **to draw a ~** einen Schluß ziehen. **to make a ~** zusammenfassend. **Schlüsse ziehen** (*about, from, on* aus). 3. Entscheidung *f*, Beschluß *m*. **to reach a ~** eine Entscheidung treffen.
con·clu·sive [kənˈkluːsɪv] *adj* 1. überzeugend, schlüssig. **~ evidence** eindeutige Beweise. 2. abschließend.
con·com·i·tance [kənˈkɒmɪtəns] *n* 1. Begleiterscheinung *f*. 2. Zusammenbestehen *nt*, gleichzeitiges Vorhandensein *nt*.
con·com·i·tan·cy [kənˈkɒmɪtənsɪ] *n* → concomitance.
con·com·i·tant [kənˈkɒmɪtənt] I *n* Begleiterscheinung *f*. II *adj* begleitend, gleichzeitig, Begleit-.
concomitant immunity begleitende Immunität *f*, Prämunition *f*.
concomitant strabismus *ophthal.* Begleitschielen *nt*, Strabismus concomitans.
concomitant symptom Begleit-, Nebensymptom *nt*.
con·cord·ance [kənˈkɔːdəns, kən-] *n embryo.* Konkordanz *f*.
con·cord·ant [kənˈkɔːdnt] *adj* übereinstimmend, konkordat (*to, with* mit).
con·cre·ment [ˈkɒŋkrəmənt] *n* Stein *m*, Konkrement *nt*.
con·cres·cence [kənˈkresns] *n histol.*, *embryo.* Verwachsen *nt*, Zusammenwachsen *nt*, Verschmelzung *f*, Verwachsung *f*.
con·crete [ˈkɒŋkriːt, ˈkɒŋ-, kɒŋˈkriːt] I *n* feste *od.* kompakte Masse *f*. II *adj* 1. fest, dicht, kompakt. 2. konkret, faßbar, wahrnehmbar, fest umrissen. III *vt* 3. zu einer kompakten Masse formen *od.* verbinden. 4. konkretisieren, verdeutlichen, veranschaulichen. IV *vi* s. zu einer kompakten Masse vereinigen, fest werden.
con·cre·tio [kənˈkriːʃɪəʊ] *n* → concretion
con·cre·tion [-ˈkriːʃn] *n* 1. Verschmelzung *f*, Vereinigung *f*. 2. *patho.* Zusammenwachsen *nt*, Verwachsung *f*, Concretio *f*. 3. Verhärtung *f*, Häufung *f*, Knoten *m*. 4. → concrement. 5. → concrete I.
con·cur [kənˈkɜː] *vi* 1. zusammenwirken. 2. zusammenfallen, -treffen. 3. übereinstimmen (*with s.o.* mit jdm.; *in sth.* in etw.).
con·cur·rence [kənˈkɜːrəns, -ˈkʌr-] *n* 1. Mitwirkung *f*; Zusammenwirken *nt*. 2. Zusammentreffen *nt*. 3. Übereinstimmung *f*. 4. *mathe.* Schnittpunkt *m*.
con·cur·ren·cy [-ˈkɜːrənsɪ] *n* → concurrence.
con·cur·rent [-ˈkɜːrənt] I *n* Begleitumstand *m*. II *adj* 1. gemeinsam, vereint; mit-, zusammenwirkend. 2. übereinstimmend (*with* mit). 3. gleichzeitig *od.* nebeneinander (bestehend) (*with* mit); zusammenfallend (*with* mit); mit- *od.* bei-, nebeneinander (*with* mit); *mathe.* s. schneidend.
con·cuss [kənˈkʌs] *vt* erschüttern. **to be ~ed** eine Gehirnerschütterung erleiden.
con·cus·sion [kənˈkʌʃn] *n* Erschütterung *f*, Kommotion *f*, Commotio *f*.
c. of/on the brain Gehirnerschütterung, Kommotionssyndrom *nt*, Commotio cerebri.
c. of the labyrinth Labyrintherschütterung, Commotio labyrinthi.
c. of the spinal cord Rückenmarkserschütterung, Commotio (medullae) spinalis.

c. of the retina Commotio retinae.
concussion myelitis → concussion myelopathy.
concussion myelopathy traumatische Myelopathie *f*.
concussion syndrome Kommotions-Syndrom *nt*.
con·cus·sive [kənˈkʌsɪv] *adj* erschütternd.
con·demn [kənˈdem] *vt* 1. (*a. juristisch*) verurteilen (*as* als; *for* wegen); verdammen, mißbilligen. 2. für ungeeignet *od.* (gesundheits-)schädlich erklären. 3. für unheilbar (krank) erklären.
con·dem·na·tion [ˌkɒndemˈneɪʃn] *n* (*a. juristische*) Verurteilung *f*; Mißbilligung *f*, Tadel *m*.
con·den·sa·bil·i·ty [kənˌdensəˈbɪlətɪ] *n phys.* Kondensierbarkeit *f*.
con·den·sa·ble [kənˈdensəbl] *adj phys.* kondensierbar.
con·den·sate [kənˈdenseɪt, ˈkɒndən-] *n phys.* Kondensat *nt*, Kondensationsprodukt *nt*.
con·den·sa·tion [ˌkɒndenˈseɪʃn] *n* 1. *chem.* Kondensation *f*, Verdichtung *f*. 2. *phys.* Kondensation *f*, Verflüssigung *f*. 3. *phys.* Kondensat *nt*, Kondensationsprodukt *nt*. 4. Verdichtung *f*; Zusammendrängung *f*, Anhäufung *f*.
condensation reaction *chem.* Kondensierungsreaktion *f*.
con·dense [kənˈdens] I *vt* 1. *chem., techn.* kondensieren, komprimieren, verdichten. 2. *phys.* kondensieren, niederschlagen. II *vi* kondensieren, s. niederschlagen, s. verflüssigen, s. verdichten.
con·densed [kənˈdenst] *adj* kondensiert; verdichtet, komprimiert; konzentriert.
condensed milk kondensierte Milch *f*, Kondens-, Dosenmilch *f*.
condensed state *histol.* (*Mitochondrien*) kondensierter Zustand *m*.
con·dens·er [kənˈdensər] *n* 1. *phys.* Kondensator *m*; Verflüssiger *m*; Kondensator *m*. 2. Kondensor(linse *f*) *m*, Sammellinse *f*. 3. *dent.* Stopfer *m*.
condenser diaphragm *phys.* Kondensorblende *f*.
con·dens·ing agent [kənˈdensɪŋ] kondensierendes Agens/Reagenz *nt*, Kondensierungsreagenz *nt*.
condensing enzyme *old* → citrate (si-)-synthase.
condensing lens → condenser 2.
condensing osteitis nicht-eitrige Osteomyelitis *f*, sklerosierende Osteomyelitis *f*, Garré-Osteomyelitis *f*, -Krankheit *f*, Osteomyelitis sicca Garré.
con·di·ment [ˈkɒndɪmənt] *n* Gewürz(stoff *m*) *nt*, Würze *f*.
con·di·tion [kənˈdɪʃn] I *n* 1. Bedingung *f*, Voraussetzung *f*. **on ~ that** vorausgesetzt, daß; unter der Bedingung, daß. **on no ~** keinesfalls, auf keinen Fall. 2. ~s *pl* Verhältnisse (*pl*), Bedingungen *pl*, Umstände *pl*. 3. (physischer *od.* psychischer) Zustand *m*, Verfassung *f*, Befinden *nt*; *sport.* Kondition *f*, Form *f*. **in good ~** in guter Verfassung, gesund. **in bad ~** in schlechter Verfassung, krank. 4. Leiden *nt*, Beschwerden *pl*. 5. Lage *f*. II *vt* 6. bestimmen, festsetzen, (s. aus-)bedingen (*that* daß). 7. in Form bringen. 8. die Voraussetzung sein für. 9. (*a. psycho.*) konditionieren (*to, for* auf).
c.s of milieu Milieubedingungen *pl*.
con·di·tion·al [kənˈdɪʃnəl] *adj* bedingt (*on, upon* durch); abhängig (*on, upon* von); vorbehaltlich, mit Vorbehalt.
conditional-lethal mutant *genet., micro.* konditionell letale Mutante *f*.
con·di·tioned [kənˈdɪʃnd] *adj* 1. bedingt,

abhängig. **2.** in gutem Zustand, in guter Verfassung. **3.** *pyscho.* konditioniert.
conditioned hemolysis Immunhämolyse *f.*
conditioned reflex *abbr.* **CR** erworbener/bedingter Reflex *m.*
conditioned response *psycho.* konditionierte Reaktion *f.*
conditioned stimulus *abbr.* **CS** bedingter Reiz *m,* conditioned stimulus *abbr.* CS.
con·di·tion·ing [kənˈdɪʃənɪŋ] *n physiol., psycho.* Konditionierung *f.*
conditioning therapy *psycho.* Verhaltenstherapie *f.*
con·dom [ˈkʌndəm, ˈkɒn-] *n* Kondom *nt/m,* Präservativ *nt.*
con·duce [kənˈd(j)uːs] *vi* dienlich *od.* förderlich sein, beitragen (*towards, to* zu).
con·du·cive [kənˈd(j)uːsɪv] *adj* dienlich, förderlich (*to*); nützlich (*to* für). **~ to health** gesundheitsfördernd. **~ to conception** empfängsfördernd.
con·duct [*n* ˈkɒndʌkt; *v* kənˈdʌkt] **I** *n* **1.** Leitung *f,* Verwaltung *f.* **2.** *fig.* Benehmen *nt,* Betragen *nt,* Verhalten *nt,* Führung *f.* **II** *vt* **3.** führen, geleiten, begleiten. **4.** leiten, verwalten. **5. ~ o.s.** s. benehmen, s. verhalten, s. betragen. **6.** *phys.* leiten. **III** *vi phys.* leiten, als Leiter wirken.
con·duct·ance [kənˈdʌktəns] *n phys.* elektrische Leitfähigkeit *f,* Wirkleitwert *m,* Konduktanz *f.*
conduct disorder Anpassungsstörung *f* im Sozialverhalten.
con·duct·i·bil·i·ty [kənˌdʌktəˈbɪləti] *n* → conductivity.
con·duct·i·ble [kənˈdʌktɪbl] *adj phys., physiol.* leitfähig, leitend, Leit-, Leitungs-.
con·duct·ing [kənˈdʌktɪŋ] *adj* → conductible.
conducting system *physiol.* (Erregungs-)Leitungssystem *nt.*
  cardiac c. Erregungsleitungssystem des Herzens, Systema conducens cordis.
  c. of heart → cardiac c.
con·duc·tion [kənˈdʌkʃn] *n* **1.** *phys., physiol.* Leitung *f.* Leitvermögen *nt.* **2.** Leitung *f,* Führung *f.*
conduction anesthesia *anes.* Leitungsanästhesie *f,* -block *m;* Regionalanästhesie *f.*
conduction aphasia *neuro.* Leitungsaphasie *f,* assoziative Aphasie *f.*
conduction block *card.* (*Herz*) Leitungsblock *m.*
conduction deafness *HNO* Schalleitungsstörung *f,* -schwerhörigkeit *f,* Mittelohrschwerhörigkeit *f,* -taubheit *f.*
conduction disturbance *card.* (*Herz*) Leitungsstörung *f.*
conduction system → conducting system.
  cardiac c. → conducting system, cardiac.
  c. of heart → conducting system, cardiac.
conduction time *card.* Überleitungszeit *f,* Intervall *nt.*
conduction velocity Leit(ungs)geschwindigkeit *f.*
con·duc·tive [kənˈdʌktɪv] *adj* → conductible.
conductive cochlear presbyacusis *HNO* kochleärer Leitungstyp *m* der Presbyakusis *f.*
conductive deafness → conduction deafness.
conductive heat Leitungs-, Konduktionswärme *f.*
con·duc·tiv·i·ty [ˌkɒndʌkˈtɪvəti] *n phys., physiol.* Leitfähigkeit *f,* Leitvermögen *nt,* Konduktivität *f.*
con·duc·tor [kənˈdʌktər] *n* **1.** *phys., electr.* Leiter *m.* **2.** *chir.* (Führungs-)Hohlsonde *f.*

con·duit [ˈkɒnd(w)ɪt, -d(j)uːɪt] *n* **1.** Rohr *nt,* Röhre *f,* Kanal *m.* **2.** *urol., chir.* Conduit *nt/m.*
con·du·ran·go [ˌkɒndəˈræŋɡəʊ] *n pharm.* Condurango *nt.*
con·dy·lar [ˈkɒndɪlər] *adj* Kondylus betr., kondylär.
condylar articulation Ellipsoid-, Eigelenk *nt,* Artic. ellipsoidea/condylaris.
condylar axis Kondylenachse *f.*
condylar canal Kondylkanal *m,* Canalis condylaris.
condylar cord Kondylenachse *f.*
condylar fossa Fossa condylaris.
condylar fracture *ortho.* Kondylenbruch *m,* -fraktur *f.*
  comminuted c. of the femur Femurgelenktrümmerfraktur.
  lateral c. Fraktur des Epicondylus lateralis humeri.
  c. of the lateral condyle of humerus → lateral c.
  medial c. Fraktur des Epicondylus medialis humeri.
  c. of the medial condyle of humerus → medial c.
condylar joint → condylar articulation.
condylar process Unterkieferköpfchen *nt,* Proc. condylaris.
con·dy·lar·thro·sis [ˌkɒndəlɑːrˈθrəʊsɪs] *n* → condylar articulation.
con·dyle [ˈkɒndaɪl] *n* Gelenkkopf *m,* Knochenende *nt,* Kondyle *f,* Condylus *m.*
  c. of femur Femurkondyle, Condylus femoris.
  c. of humerus Humeruskondyle, Condylus humeri.
  c. of mandible Unterkieferköpfchen *nt,* Proc. condylaris mandibulae.
  c. of tibia Tibiakondyle, Condylus tibiae.
con·dy·lec·to·my [ˌkɒndəˈlɛktəmi] *n chir.* Kondylenresektion *f,* Kondylektomie *f.*
con·dy·loid [ˈkɒndɪlɔɪd] *adj* knöchelähnlich, kondylenähnlich, -förmig.
condyloid articulation → condylar articulation.
condyloid canal → condylar canal.
condyloid fossa → condylar fossa.
condyloid joint → condylar articulation.
condyloid process → condylar process.
  inferior c. of vertebrae unterer Gelenkfortsatz *m* der Wirbelkörper, Proc. articularis inferior, Zygapophysis inferior.
  superior c. of vertebrae oberer Gelenkfortsatz *m* der Wirbelkörper, Proc. articularis superior, Zygapophysis superior.
condyloid surface of tibia obere Gelenkfläche *f* des Schienbeins, Facies articularis superior tibiae.
con·dy·lo·ma [ˌkɒndəˈləʊmə] *n, pl* **-mas, -ma·ta** [-mətə] *derm.* **1.** Kondylom *nt,* Condyloma *nt.* **2.** (spitze) Feigwarze *f,* Feuchtwarze *f,* spitzes Kondylom, Condyloma acuminatum, Papilloma acuminatum/venereum. **3.** breites Kondylom, Condyloma latum/syphiliticum.
con·dy·lo·ma·toid [ˌ-ˈləʊmətɔɪd] *adj derm.* kondylomähnlich.
con·dy·lo·ma·to·sis [ˌ-ləʊməˈtəʊsɪs] *n derm.* Kondylomatose *f.*
con·dy·lom·a·tous [ˌ-ˈlɒmətəs] *adj derm.* kondylomatös.
con·dy·lot·o·my [ˌ-ˈlɒtəmi] *n ortho.* Kondylendurchtrennung *f,* -spaltung *f,* Kondylotomie *f.*
cone [kəʊn] *n* **1.** *anat.* kegel-, zapfenförmiges Gebilde *nt,* Zapfen *m,* Konus *m,* Conus *m.* **2. ~s** *pl* → cone cells. **3.** *mathe.* *fig.* Kegel *m,* kegelförmiger Gegenstand *m; techn.* Konus *m; bot.* Zapfen *m.*
cone achromatopsy *ophthal.* Zapfen(farben)blindheit *f.*

cone biopsy Konusbiopsie *f.*
cone cells (*Auge*) Zapfen(zellen *pl*) *pl.*
coned [kəʊnd] *adj* kegel-, zapfenförmig; zapfentragend.
cone monochromasy → cone achromatopsy.
cone-nose (bugs) → cone-nosed bugs.
cone-nosed bugs *micro.* Raubwanzen *pl,* Reduviiden *pl,* Reduviidae *pl.*
cone-shaped *adj* zapfen-, kegelförmig.
co·nex·us [kəˈnɛksəs, kɑ-] *n anat.* Co(n)nexus *m.*
con·fab·u·la·tion [kənˌfæbjəˈleɪʃn, kɒn-] *n neuro., psychia.* Konfabulation *f,* Confabulatio *f.*
con·fec·tion [kənˈfɛkʃn] *n* **1.** Zuckerwerk *nt,* Konfekt *nt.* **2.** *pharm.* mit Zucker, Honig *od.* Syrup zubereitete Medikamente, Latwerge *f.*
con·fer [kənˈfɜːr] *vt* weiter-, übertragen, verleihen.
con·fig·u·ra·tion [kənˌfɪɡjəˈreɪʃn] *n* **1.** *chem.* Konfiguration *f,* räumliche Anordnung *f.* **2.** Konfiguration *f,* (Auf-)Bau *m,* (äußere) Form *f,* Gestalt *f;* Struktur *f.* **3.** *mathe.* (geometrische) Figur *f.* **4.** *psycho.* Gestalt *f.*
con·fig·u·ra·tion·al [ˌ-ˈreɪʃnəl] *adj* Konfiguration betr.
configurational formula *chem.* Raumformel *f,* stereochemische Formel *f.*
configurational isomerism Raum-, Stereoisomerie *f.*
con·fig·u·ra·tive [kənˈfɪɡjərətɪv, -jəˌreɪt-] *adj* → configurational.
con·fine [*n* ˈkɒnfaɪn; *v* kənˈfaɪn] **I** *n* (*a. fig.*) Rand *m,* Schwelle *f,* Grenze *f.* **II** *vt* **1.** begrenzen, be-, einschränken, **to ~ o.s. to** s. beschränken auf. **2.** (*Bewegungsfreiheit*) einschränken. **3. to be ~d of (a child)** entbinden, entbunden werden (von), niederkommen (mit).
con·fined [kənˈfaɪnd] *adj* **1.** begrenzt, beschränkt (*to* auf); beengt. **2.** in den Wehen liegen. **3.** gebunden *od.* gefesselt sein (*to* an). **~ to bed** ans Bett gefesselt, bettlägerig. **~ to a wheelchair** an den Rollstuhl gefesselt.
con·fine·ment [kənˈfaɪnmənt] *n* **1.** Ein-, Beschränkung *f* (*to* auf); Ein-, Beengung *f;* Beengtheit *f.* **2.** Gefesseltsein *nt* (*to* an). **~ to bed** Bettlägerigkeit *f.* **3.** Niederkunft *f,* Entbindung *f.*
con·firm [kənˈfɜːrm] *vt* **1.** bestätigen. **2.** jdn. in etw. bestärken *od.* bestätigen (*s.o. in sth.*).
con·fir·ma·tion [ˌkɒnfərˈmeɪʃn] *n* Bestätigung *f;* (Be-)Stärkung *f,* Bekräftigung *f.*
con·firm·a·tive [kənˈfɜːrmətɪv] *adj* bestätigend, Bestätigungs-.
con·firm·a·to·ry [kənˈfɜːrmətɔːri, -təʊ-] *adj* → confirmative.
con·firmed [kənˈfɜːrmd] *adj* **1.** bestätigt, genehmigt. **2.** bestärkt, bekräftigt. **3.** chronisch. **4.** eingefleischt, unverbesserlich.
con·flict [*n* ˈkɒnflɪkt; *v* kənˈflɪkt] **I** *n* **1.** (innerer/seelischer) Konflikt *m.* **2.** Konflikt *m,* Auseinandersetzung *f,* Kontroverse *f.* **II** *vi* in Konflikt stehen, im Widerspruch *od.* Gegensatz stehen (*with* zu); kollidieren (*with* mit).
con·flict·ing [kənˈflɪktɪŋ] *adj* widersprüchlich.
conflict research Konfliktforschung *f.*
con·flu·ence [ˈkɒnfluəns] *n* **1.** *anat.* Konflux *m,* Konfluenz *f,* Confluens *m.* **2.** *patho.* Zusammenfließen *nt,* Konfluieren *nt,* Konfluenz *f.*
  c. of sinuses Confluens sinuum.
con·flu·ent [ˈkɒnfluənt] *adj* zusammenfließend, -laufend, konfluierend.
confluent and reticulate papillomatosis

Gougerot-Carteaud-Syndrom *nt*, Papillomatosis confluens et reticularis.
con·fo·cal [kən'fəʊkl] *adj phys.* mit dem selben Brennpunkt, konfokal.
con·form [kən'fɔːrm] **I** *vt* angleichen, anpassen (*to* an). **II** *vi* s. angleichen, s. anpassen (*to* an); s. richten (*to* nach); übereinstimmen (*to* mit).
con·for·ma·tion [ˌkɑnfɔːr'meɪʃn] *n* **1.** *chem.* räumliche Anordnung *f*, Konformation *f*. **2.** Bau *m*, Form *f*, Gestalt *f*, Struktur *f*; Gestaltung *f*. **3.** Anpassung *f*, Angleichung *f* (*to* an).
β-conformation *n biochem.* β-Konformation *f*.
con·for·ma·tion·al [ˌ-'meɪʃnl] *adj* Konformation betr., Konformations-.
conformational coupling *biochem.* Konformationskopplung *f*.
conformational coupling hypothesis Hypothese *f* der Konformationskopplung, Hypothese *f* der Kopplung über Konformationsänderung.
conformational formula Konformationsformel *f*.
conformational isomerism Konformationsisomerie *f*.
con·for·mer [kən'fɔːrmər] *n* Konformationsisomer *nt*.
con·form·i·ty [kən'fɔːrmətɪ] *n* **1.** Übereinstimmung *f* (*with* mit). **in ~ with** in Übereinstimmung mit, übereinstimmend mit. **2.** Anpassung *f* (*to* an).
con·front [kən'frʌnt] *vt* **1.** gegenüberstellen, konfrontieren (*with* mit). **2.** vergleichen. **3.** (*Schwierigkeiten*) gegenübertreten, begegnen, s. stellen.
con·fron·ta·tion [ˌkɑnfrən'teɪʃn] *n* Gegenüberstellung *f*; Auseinandersetzung *f*, Konfrontation *f*.
con·fuse [kən'fjuːz] *vt* **1.** jdn. konfus machen *od.* verwirren *od.* durcheinander bringen (*with* mit). **2.** (miteinander) verwechseln (*with* mit).
con·fused [kən'fjuːzd] *adj* **1.** verlegen, bestürzt. **2.** (*Person, Gedanken*) konfus, verworren, wirr. **3.** (*Gedanken, Sprache*) undeutlich, verworren.
con·fu·sion [kən'fjuːʒn] *n* **1.** (geistige) Verwirrung *f*, Desorientierung *f*, Desorientiertheit *f*. **2.** Wirrwarr *m*, Unklarheit *f*; Durcheinander *nt*, Unordnung *f*. **3.** Bestürzung *f*, Verlegenheit *f*. **in (a state of) ~** verwirrt, bestürzt, verlegen.
con·fu·sion·al [kən'fjuːʒnl] *adj* Verwirrung/Konfusion betr. *od.* verursachend, verwirrend, Konfusions-.
confusion colors *ophthal.* Verwechslungsfarben *pl*.
con·geal [kən'dʒiːl] **I** *vt* erstarren *od.* hart werden lassen; (*Blut*) gerinnen lassen. **II** *vi* erstarren, hart *od.* starr *od.* fest werden; (*Blut*) gerinnen; gefrieren.
con·geal·a·ble [kən'dʒiːləbl] *adj* gerinnbar, gefrierbar.
con·geal·ment [kən'dʒiːlmə] *n* **1.** Erstarren *nt*, Fest-, Hartwerden *nt*, Gefrieren *nt*, Gerinnen *nt*. **2.** erstarrte *od.* geronnene Masse *f*.
con·ge·la·tion [ˌkɑndʒə'leɪʃn] *n* **1.** *patho.* Erfrierung(serscheinung *f*) *f*, Kongelation *f*, Congelatio *f*. **2.** → congealment.
congelation urticaria Kälteurtikaria *f*, Urticaria e frigore.
con·ge·ner ['kɑndʒənər] *n bio.* Gattungsverwandte(r *m*) *f*; Art-, Stammverwandte(r *m*) *f*, Artgenosse *m*..
con·ge·ner·ic [ˌkɑndʒə'nerɪk] *adj* → congenerous.
con·gen·er·ous [kən'dʒenərəs] *adj* **1.** (*Funktion*) gleichartig. **2.** *bio.* art-, gattungs-, stammverwandt (*to* with).

con·gen·ial [kən'dʒiːnɪəl] *adj* **1.** gleichartig, kongenial, (geistes-)verwandt (*with* mit). **2.** zuträglich (*to* für).
con·gen·i·tal [kən'dʒenɪtl, kən-] *adj* angeboren, kongenital; *patho.* congenitus, congenitalis.
congenital abducens-facial paralysis Möbius-Syndrom *nt*, -Kernaplasie *f*.
congenital absence of heart *patho.* Akardie *f*.
congenital adrenal hyperplasia kongenitale Nebennierenrindenhyperplasie *f*, adrenogenitales Syndrom *nt abbr.* AGS.
congenital afibrinogenemia kongenitale Afibrinogenämie *f*.
congenital agammaglobulinemia *hema.* Bruton-Typ *m* der Agammaglobulinämie, infantile X-chromosomale Agammaglobulinämie *f*, kongenitale (geschlechtsgebundene) Agammaglobulinämie *f*.
congenital aleukia → congenital leukopenia.
congenital alopecia kongenitale Alopezie *f*, Alopecia congenitalis, Atrichia congenita.
congenital alveolar dysplasia Atemnotsyndrom *nt* des Neugeborenen *abbr.* ANS, Respiratory-distress-Syndrom *nt* des Neugeborenen *abbr.* RDS.
congenital amputation kongenitale/intrauterine Amputation *f*.
congenital anemia of the newborn *hema.*, *ped.* fetale Erythroblastose *f*, Erythroblastosis fetalis.
congenital astigmatism *ophthal.* kongenitaler/angeborener Astigmatismus *m*.
congenital atelectasis (*Lunge*) angeborene/kongenitale Atelektase *f*.
congenital atonic pseudoparalysis Oppenheim-Krankheit *f*, -Syndrom *nt*, Myotonia congenita.
congenital baldness → congenital alopecia.
congenital bowleg angeborenes/kongenitales O-Bein *nt*, Crus varum congenitum.
congenital bronchiectasis kongenitale Bronchiektas(i)e *f*.
congenital cataract angeborener Star *m*, Cataracta congenita.
congenital chloride diarrhea *ped.* familiäre Chlorverlustdiarrhö *f*, Chlorid-Diarrhö-Syndrom *nt*.
congenital cholesteatoma okkultes/kongenitales Cholesteatom *nt*.
congenital cloaca *embryo.*, *patho.* Cloaca congenitalis/persistens.
congenital clubfoot angeborener Klumpfuß *m*, Pes equinovarus (excavatus et adductus).
congenital contracture *ortho.* kongenitale/angeborene Kontraktur *f*.
congenital conus *ophthal.* Fuchs'-Kolobom *nt*.
congenital cystic disease of the lung *patho.* kongenitale Zystenlunge *f*.
congenital deafness kongenitale/angeborene Schwerhörigkeit/Taubheit *f*.
congenital defect Geburtsfehler *m*, kongenitaler Defekt *m*.
congenital dislocation *ortho.* angeborene/konnatale Luxation *f*.
c. of the hip *abbr.* **CDH** kongenitale Hüftgelenkluxation, anthropologische Luxation, Luxatio congenita coxae.
c. of the knee joint kongenitale/angeborene Kniegelenkluxation.
c. of the patella angeborene/kongenitale Patellaluxation.
congenital dyskeratosis Zinsser-Cole-Engman-Syndrom *nt*, kongenitale Dyskeratose *f*, Dyskeratosis congenita, Polydysplasia ectodermica Typ Cole-Rauschkolb-Toomey.
congenital dysphagocytosis progressive septische Granulomatose *f*, kongenitale Dysphagozytose *f*.
congenital dysplasia of the hip kongenitale Hüftdysplasie *f*, Dysplasia coxae congenita.
congenital ectodermal defect *derm.* anhidrotisch ektodermale Dysplasie *f*, ektodermale (kongenitale) Dysplasie *f*, Christ-Siemens-Syndrom *nt*, Guilford-Syndrom *nt*, Jacquet'-Syndrom *nt*, Anhidrosis hypotrichotica/congenita.
congenital epulis Epulis congenita/connata.
congenital erythropoietic porphyria *abbr.* **CEP** kongenitale erythropoetische Porphyrie *f*, Günther'-Krankheit *f*, Porphyria erythropo(i)etica congenita.
congenital facial diplegia Möbius-Syndrom *nt*, -Kernaplasie *f*.
congenital familial icterus hereditäre Sphärozytose *f*, Kugelzell(en)anämie *f*, Kugelzell(en)ikterus *m*, kongenitaler hämolytischer Ikterus *m*, Morbus Minkowski-Chauffard *m*.
congenital fracture kongenitale Fraktur *f*, intrauterin erworbene Fraktur *f*.
congenital generalized fibromatosis kongenitale generalisierte Fibromatose *f*.
congenital glaucoma *ophthal.* Ochsenauge *nt*, angeborenes Glaukom *nt*, Hydrophthalmus *m* (congenitus), Buphthalmus *m* (congenitus), Glaucoma infantile.
congenital goiter angeborene/kongenitale Struma *f*, Neugeborenenstruma *f*, Struma connata.
congenital hemolytic icterus/jaundice → congenital familial icterus.
congenital hepatic fibrosis *patho.* kongenitale hereditäre Leberfibrose *f*.
congenital hereditary nystagmus → congenital nystagmus.
congenital hernia angeborene/kongenitale Hernie *f*, Hernia congenita.
congenital hydrocele angeborene/kongenitale Hydrozele *f*.
congenital hydrocephalus kongenitaler/primärer Hydrozephalus *m*, Hydrocephalus congenitalis.
congenital hydrops Hydrops congenitus/fetus universalis, Hydrops fetalis.
congenital hyperbilirubinemia → congenital familial icterus.
congenital hypogammaglobulinemia → congenital agammaglobulinemia.
congenital ichthyosiform erythroderma Erythrodermia congenitalis ichthyosiformis bullosa.
congenital ichthyosis *derm.* Ichthyosis congenita/congenitalis, Hyperkeratosis congenita/congenitalis.
congenital instinct angeborener Trieb *m*, Naturtrieb *m*, Instinkt *m*.
congenital lactase malabsorption Lactase-Mangel *m*, Laktase-Mangel *m*, kongenitale/hereditäre Laktoseintoleranz *f*.
congenital leukoderma *derm.* Weißsucht *f*, Albinismus *m*.
congenital leukokeratosis *derm.* weißer Schleimhautnävus *m*, Naevus spongiosus albus mucosae.
congenital leukopathia → congenital leukoderma.
congenital leukopenia kongenitale Leukozytopenie/Neutropenie *f*.
congenital lipomatosis of pancreas Shwachman-Syndrom *nt*, Shwachman-Blackfan-Diamond-Oski-Khaw-Syndrom *nt*.

congenital lymphedema → congenital trophedema.
cogenital malformation kongenitale Mißbildung/Fehlbildung/Malformation *f*.
congenital megacolon aganglionäres/kongenitales Megakolon *nt*, Hirschsprung-Krankheit *f*, Morbus Hirschsprung *m*, Megacolon congenitum.
congenital methemoglobinemia enzymopathische/hereditäre Methämoglobinämie *f*.
congenital multiple arthrogryposis Guérin-Stern-Syndrom *nt*, Arthrogryposis multiplex congenital.
congenital myotonia Thomsen-Syndrom *nt*, Myotonia congenita/hereditaria.
congenital myxedema Kretinismus *m*.
congenital nephritis kongenitale Nephritis *f*.
congenital neutropenia → congenital leukopenia.
congenital nonhemolytic jaundice Crigler-Najjar-Syndrom *nt*, idiopathische Hyperbilirubinämie *f*.
congenital nystagmus angeborener/kongenitaler Nystagmus *m*.
congenital oculofacial paralysis Möbius--Syndrom *nt*, -Kernaplasie *f*.
congenital pancytopenia Fanconi-Anämie *f*, -Syndrom *nt*, konstitutionelle infantile Panmyelopathie *f*.
congenital paramyotonia Eulenburg--Syndrom *nt*, -Krankheit *f*, Paramyotonia congenita.
congenital photosensitive porphyria → congenital erythropoietic porphyria.
congenital progressive lipodystrophy Lawrence-Syndrom *nt*, lipatrophischer Diabetes *m*.
congenital pseudarthrosis *ortho.* kongenitale Pseudarthrose *f*.
congenital pyloristenosis/pylorostenosis *ped.*, *chir.* kongenitale Pylorusstenose *f*, Pylorustenose *f* der Säuglinge.
congenital rubella syndrome kongenitale Röteln *pl*, kongenitale Röteln-Syndrom *nt*.
congenital scoliosis *ortho.* kongenitale/angeborene Skoliose *f*.
congenital stenosis of mitral valve Duroziez-Syndrom *nt*, -Erkrankung *f*, angeborene Mitral(klappen)stenose.
congenital sucrose-isomaltose malabsorption Saccharase-Isomaltase-Mangel *m*.
congenital sutural alopecia Hallermann--Streiff(-Francois)-Syndrom *nt*, Dyskephaliesyndrom *nt* von Francois, Dysmorphia mandibulo-oculo-facialis.
congenital syphilis angeborene/kongenitale Syphilis *f*, Lues connata/congenita, Syphilis connata/congenita.
c. of bone kongenitale Knochensyphilis, Osteochondritis syphylitica, Wegner'--Krankheit *f*.
congenital torticollis angeborener Schiefhals *m*, kongenitaler Torticollis *m*.
congenital toxoplasmosis *ped.* konnatale Toxoplasmose *f*.
congenital trophedema (hereditäres) Trophödem *nt*, Milroy-Syndrom *nt*, Meige-Syndrom *nt*, Nonne-Milroy--Meige-Syndrom *nt*.
congenital virilizing adrenal hyperplasia → congenital adrenal hyperplasia.
con·gest [kən'dʒest] **I** *vt* ansammeln, anhäufen, zusammendrängen, stauen; verstopfen, blockieren; (mit Blut) überfüllen. **II** *vi* s. ansammeln, s. stauen; verstopfen.
con·gest·ed [kən'dʒestɪd] *adj* 1. überfüllt (*with* von); zusammengedrängt. 2. (mit Blut) überfüllt, voll, gestaut, Stauungs-.
congested kidney Stauungsniere *f*.
congested liver Stauungsleber *f*.
congested lung Stauungslunge *f*.
con·ges·tion [kən'dʒestʃn] *n* 1. Stau(ung *f*) *m*, Stockung *f*; Ansammlung *f*, Anhäufung *f*, Andrang *m*. 2. (Blut-)Stauung *f*, Kongestion *f*, Congestio.
c. of liver Leberstauung.
con·ges·tive [kən'dʒestɪv] *adj* Kongestion betr., kongestiv, Stauungs-.
congestive bronchitis Stauungsbronchitis *f*.
congestive cardiomyopathy *abbr.* **CCM** kongestive Kardiomyopathie *f abbr.* CCM, dilatative Kardiomyopathie *f abbr.* DCM.
congestive cirrhosis (of liver) Stauungsinduration *f* der Leber, Cirrhose cardiaque.
congestive gastritis Stauungsgastritis *f*.
congestive glaucoma akutes Winkelblockglaukom/Engwinkelglaukom *nt*, Glaucoma acutum (congestivum).
congestive headache Stauungskopfschmerz *m*.
congestive heart failure *abbr.* **CHF** dekompensierte Herzinsuffizienz *f*.
congestive hemorrhage Stauungsblutung *f*.
congestive splenomegaly Banti-Syndrom *nt*.
con·glo·bate [kən'gləʊbeɪt, 'kɑŋ-] **I** *adj* zusammengeballt, kugelig, konglobiert. **II** *vt* zusammenballen, konglobieren (*into* zu). **III** *vi* s. zusammenballen, konglobieren (*into* zu).
conglobate acne Akne/Acne conglobata.
con·glo·ba·tion [ˌkɑnɡləʊ'beɪʃn, ˌkɑŋ-] *n* Zusammenballung *f*, Konglobation *f*.
con·globe [kən'gləʊb, kɑŋ-] *vt, vi* → conglobate II, III.
con·glom·er·ate [*n*, *adj* kən'glɑmərɪt, kɑŋ-; *v* -reɪt] **I** *n* Konglomerat *nt*. **II** *adj* zusammenballt, geknäuelt. **III** *vt* zusammenballen, anhäufen, ansammeln. **VI** *vi* s. zusammenballen, s. anhäufen *od*. ansammeln.
con·glom·er·at·ic [-ˌglɑmə'rætɪk] *adj* Konglomerat betr., konglomeratisch, Konglomerat-.
con·glom·er·a·tion [-ˌglɑmə'reɪʃn] *n* (An-)Häufung *f*, (An-)Sammlung *f*, Gemisch *nt*; (Zusammen-)Ballung *f*.
con·glu·ti·nant [kən'ɡluːtnənt, kɑŋ-] *adj* (*Wundränder*) zusammenklebend, (an-)-haftend.
con·glu·ti·na·tion [-ˌɡluːtə'neɪʃn] *n* 1. *hema.*, *immun.* Konglutination *f*, Conglutinatio *f*. 2. Verklebung *f*, Verwachsung *f*, Adhäsion *f*.
conglutination-agglutination thrombus Konglutinations-, Abscheidungsthrombus *m*, weißer/grauer Thrombus *m*.
conglutination reaction Konglutinationsreaktion *f*, cin *m*.
con·glu·ti·nin [-'gluːtnɪn] *n immun.* Konglutinin *nt*.
con·glu·ti·no·gen [-'gluːtɪnədʒən] *n immun.* Konglutinogen *nt*.
Con·go-Crimean hemorrhagic fever ['kɑŋɡəʊ] Kongo-Krim-Fieber *nt*, hämorrhagisches Krim-Fieber *nt*.
Congo-Crimean hemorrhagic fever virus *micro.* Krimfieber-Virus *nt*, C-CHF-Virus *nt*.
Con·go·lian red fever [kɑŋ'ɡəʊlɪən] endemisches/murines Fleckfieber *nt*, Ratten-, Flohfleckfieber *nt*.
Congo red Kongorot *nt*.
Congo red fever endemisches/murines Fleckfieber *nt*, Ratten-, Flohfleckfieber *nt*.
Congo red stain *histol.* Kongorotfärbung *f*.
con·gru·ence ['kɑŋɡruːəns, kən'ɡruː-] *n* 1. *phys.*, *stat.* Deckungsgleichheit *f*, Übereinstimmung *f*, Kongruenz *f* (*with* mit). 2. Übereinstimmung *f*.
con·gru·en·cy ['-ɡruːənsɪ] *n* → congruence.
con·gru·ent ['-ɡruːənt] *adj* 1. *phys.*, *stat.* übereinstimmend, deckungsgleich, kongruent. 2. übereinstimmend *od.* vereinbar (*to*, *with* mit); passend (*to*, *with* zu); entsprechend.
con·gru·i·ty [kən'ɡruːətɪ, kɑŋ-, kɑŋ-] *n* congruence 1.
con·gru·ous ['kɑŋɡrəwəs] *adj* → congruent.
con·ic ['kɑnɪk] *adj* → conical.
con·i·cal ['kɑnɪkl] *adj* konisch, zapfen-, kegelförmig.
conical cornea *ophthal.* Hornhautkegel *m*, Keratokonus *m*.
con·i·cal·ness ['-nɪs] *n* → conicity.
conical papillae (of Soemmering) konische Papillen *pl*, Papillae concicae.
co·nic·i·ty [kə'nɪsətɪ] *n* Kegelform *f*, Konizität *f*.
co·nid·i·al [kə'nɪdɪəl] *adj micro.* Konidien betr., konidientragend, Konidien-.
co·nid·i·o·phore [kə'nɪdɪəfəʊər] *n micro.* Konidienträger *m*, Konidiophor *nt*.
co·nid·i·o·spore ['-spəʊər, -spɔːr] *n micro.* Konidiospore *f*.
co·nid·i·um [kə'nɪdɪəm] *n*, *pl* **-dia** [-dɪə] *micro.* Konidie *f*, Conidium *nt*.
co·ni·form ['kəʊnɪfɔːrm, 'kɑn-] *adj* kegelförmig.
co·ni·ine ['kəʊniːɪn] *n pharm.* Cicutin *nt*, Cicutinum *nt*, Koniin *nt*, Coniin *nt*, Coniinum *nt*.
co·ni·o·fi·bro·sis [ˌkəʊnɪəʊfaɪ'brəʊsɪs] *n pulmo.* Koniofibrose *f*, Coniofibrosis *f*.
co·ni·om·e·ter [ˌkəʊnɪ'ɑmɪtər] *n* Konio-, Konimeter *nt*.
co·ni·o·phage ['kəʊnɪəʊfeɪdʒ] *n histol.*, *patho.* 1. Staubfreßzelle *f*, Koniophage *m*. 2. Alveolarmakrophage *m*, -phagozyt *m*.
co·ni·o·sis [kəʊnɪ'əʊsɪs] *n patho.* Staub(ablagerungs)krankheit *f*, Koniose *f*.
Co·ni·o·spor·i·um [ˌkəʊnɪəʊ'spəʊrɪəm] *n micro.* Coniosporium *nt*.
co·ni·o·spo·ro·sis [ˌ-spə'rəʊsɪs] *n* Koniosporose *f*.
co·ni·ot·o·my [kəʊnɪ'ɑtəmɪ] *n chir.*, *HNO* Koniotomie *f*, Konikotomie *f*, (Inter-)Krikothyreotomie *f*.
co·ni·o·tox·i·co·sis [ˌkəʊnɪəʊˌtaksɪ'kəʊsɪs] *n pulmo.* Koniotoxikose *f*.
con·i·za·tion [ˌkəʊnɪ'zeɪʃn, kɑn-] *n* 1. *chir.* Konisation *f*. 2. *gyn.* Portio-, Zervixkonisation *f*.
con·join [kən'dʒɔɪn] **I** *vt* verbinden, vereinigen. **II** *vi* s. verbinden, s. vereinigen.
con·joined [kən'dʒɔɪnd] *adj* verbunden, verknüpft, vereinigt.
conjoined twins *embryo.* Doppelmißbildung *f*.
con·joint [kən'dʒɔɪnt] *adj* verbunden, verknüpft; gemeinsam.
conjoint tendon Falx inguinalis, Tendo conjunctivus.
con·ju·gal ['kɑndʒəɡəl] *adj* Ehe(gatten) betr., ehelich, Ehe-, Gatten-.
con·ju·gant ['kɑndʒəɡənt] *n bio.*, *genet.* Konjugant *m*.
con·ju·gate [*n*, *adj* 'kɑndʒəɡɪt, -ˌɡeɪt; *v* -ˌɡeɪt] **I** *n* 1. → conjugate diameter (of pelvis). 2. *chem.* Konjugat *nt*. **II** *adj* 3. gepaart, (paarweise) verbunden, paarig. 4. *chem.* konjugiert. **III** *vt chem.* konjugie-

ren. **IV** *vi* **5.** *bio.* s. paaren. **6.** konjugieren, s. konjugieren lassen.
conjugate acid konjugierte Säure *f.*
conjugate base konjugierte Base *f.*
con·ju·gat·ed [ˈkɒndʒəgeɪtɪd] *adj chem.* konjugiert; konjugierte Doppelbindungen enthaltend.
conjugated antigen *immun.* konjugiertes Hapten *nt.*
conjugated bilirubin direktes/konjugiertes/gepaartes Bilirubin *nt.*
conjugate deviation *ophthal.* konjugierte/assoziierte Augenabweichung *f*, Déviation conjuguée.
conjugated eye movement konjugierte Augenbewegung *f.*
conjugated hapten → conjugated antigen.
conjugated hyperbilirubinemia konjugierte Hyperbilirubinämie *f*, Erhöhung *f* des konjugierten Bilirubins.
conjugate diameter (of pelvis) Beckenlängsdurchmesser *m*, Conjugata *f* (pelvis), Diameter conjugata (pelvis).
anatomic c. Conjugata anatomica.
Baudelocque's c. → external c.
diagonal c. Conjugata diagonalis.
external c. Conjugata externa, Diameter Baudelocque.
internal c. → anatomic c.
obstetric c. Conjugata anatomica vera obstetrica.
true c. → anatomic c.
conjugated protein zusammengesetztes Protein *nt.*
conjugate nystagmus konjugierter Nystagmus *m.*
conjugate paralysis Konjugationslähmung *f.*
conjugate transfer *micro.* Konjugationstransfer *m.*
con·ju·ga·tion [ˌkɒndʒəˈgeɪʃn] *n* **1.** Verbindung *f*, Vereinigung *f*, Verschmelzung *f.* **2.** *genet.*, *micro.* Konjugation *f.* **3.** *chem.* Konjugation *f.*
conjugation process *bio.*, *biochem.* Konjugationsprozeß *m.*
con·junc·tion [kənˈdʒʌŋkʃn] *n* **1.** Verbindung *f*, Vereinigung *f.* **in ~ with** in Verbindung mit. **2.** Zusammentreffen *nt.*
con·junc·ti·va [ˌkɒndʒʌŋkˈtaɪvə] *n*, *pl* **-vas**, **-vae** [-viː] (Augen-)Bindehaut *f*, Konjunktiva *f*, Conjunctiva *f*, Tunica conjunctiva.
con·junc·ti·val [ˌ-ˈtaɪvl] *adj* Bindehaut/Conjunctiva betr., konjunktival, Bindehaut-, Konjunktival-.
conjunctival arteries: anterior c. vordere Bindehautarterien *pl*, Aa. conjunctivales anteriores.
posterior c. hintere Bindehautarterien *pl*, Aa. conjunctivales posteriores.
conjunctival edema *ophthal.* Bindehaut-, Konjunktivalödem *nt.*
conjunctival fornix: inferior c. untere Umschlagsfalte *f* der Konjunktiva, Fornix conjunctivae inferior.
superior c. obere Umschlagsfalte *f* der Konjunktiva, Fornix conjunctivae superior.
conjunctival glands Krause-Drüsen *pl*, Konjunktivaldrüsen *pl*, Gll. conjunctivales.
conjunctival reaction *derm.*, *immun.* Konjunktivalprobe *f*, -test *m*, Ophthalmoreaktion *f*, -test *m.*
conjunctival reflex Konjunktivalreflex *m.*
conjunctival ring A(n)nulus conjunctivae.
conjunctival sac Bindehautsack *m*, Saccus conjunctivalis.
conjunctival swab *ophthal.* Bindehaut-, Konjunktivalabstrich *m.*
conjunctival test → conjunctival reaction.

conjunctival veins Bindehautvenen *pl*, Vv. conjunctivales.
con·junc·tive [kənˈdʒʌŋktɪv] *adj* **1.** verbunden, verknüpft. **2.** verbindend, Verbindungs-, Binde-. **3.** *mathe.* konjunktiv.
con·junc·ti·vi·plas·ty [kənˈdʒʌŋktəvɪplæstɪ] *n* → conjunctivoplasty.
con·junc·ti·vi·tis [kənˌdʒʌŋktəˈvaɪtɪs] *n ophthal.* Bindehautentzündung *f*, Konjunktivitis *f*, Conjunctivitis *f.*
con·junc·ti·vo·dac·ry·o·cys·to·rhi·nos·to·my [kənˌdʒʌŋktɪvəʊˌdækrɪəʊˌsɪstəraɪˈnɒstəmɪ] *n HNO* Konjunktivodakryozystorhinostomie *f.*
con·junc·ti·vo·dac·ry·o·cys·tos·to·my [ˌ-ˌdækrɪəʊˌsɪsˈtɒstəmɪ] *n HNO* Konjunktivodakryozystostomie *f.*
con·junc·ti·vo·ma [kənˌdʒʌŋktɪˈvəʊmə] *n patho.* Bindehaut-, Konjunktivaltumor *m*, Conjunctivoma *nt.*
con·junc·ti·vo·plas·ty [ˌkəndʒʌŋkˈtaɪvəplæstɪ] *n HNO* Bindehautplastik *f.*
con·junc·ti·vo·rhi·nos·to·my [kənˌdʒʌŋktɪvəʊraɪˈnɒstəmɪ] *n HNO* Konjunktivorhinostomie *f.*
Conn [kɒn]: **C.'s syndrome** primärer Hyperaldosteronismus *m*, Conn-Syndrom *nt.*
con·na·tal [ˈkɒneɪtl, kəˈn-] *adj* angeboren, bei der Geburt vorhanden, konnatal.
con·nate [ˈkɒneɪt, kəˈneɪt] *adj* → connatal.
con·nect [kəˈnekt] **I** *vt* **1.** (*a. fig.*) verbinden, verknüpfen (*to*, *with* mit); *fig.* in Verbindung od. Zusammenhang bringen; jdn. (telefonisch) verbinden. **2.** *techn.* (an-)koppeln, anschließen (*to* an); verbinden, anhängen. **II** *vi* eine Verbindung haben (*to*, *with* zu); in Verbindung treten od. stehen.
con·nect·ed [kəˈnektɪd] *adj* **1.** verbunden, in Verbindung stehen (*with* zu); eine Beziehung haben (*with* zu); verknüpft. **2.** verwandt (*with* mit). **3.** *techn.* ver-, gekoppelt; angeschlossen.
con·nect·ing [kəˈnektɪŋ] *adj* verbindend, Verbindungs-, Anschluß-, Binde-.
connecting filament Ooblast *m.*
connecting link Binde-, Zwischenglied *nt.*
connecting segment Verbindungsstück *nt.*
connecting stalk *embryo.* Haftstiel *m.*
connecting tubules (*Niere*) Zwischenstücke *pl.*
connecting villi *embryo.* Haftzotten *pl.*
con·nec·tion [kəˈnekʃn] *n* **1.** (*a. techn.*) Verbindung *f* (*with* mit); Anschluß *m* (*to*, *with* an, zu); Verbindung(sstück *nt*) *f*, Bindeglied *nt.* **2.** Zusammenhang *m*, Beziehung *f.* **in this ~** in diesem Zusammenhang. **3.** (persönliche) Beziehung *f.* **4.** Geschlechtsverkehr *m.*
con·nec·tive [kəˈnektɪv] **I** *n* Bindung *f*, Verbindung(sstück *nt*) *f.* **II** *adj* verbindend, Verbindungs-, Binde-.
connective tissue Bindegewebe *nt*, Binde- u. Stützgewebe *nt.*
areolar c. lockeres Bindegewebe.
collagenous c. kollagenfaseriges Bindegewebe.
dense fiber parallel c. straffes parallelfaseriges Bindegewebe.
dense (fibrous) c. straffes Bindegewebe
dense interwoven c. straffes geflechtartiges Bindegewebe.
embryonic c. Mesenchym *nt*, embryonales Bindegewebe.
endoganglionic c. endoganglionäres Bindegewebe.
gelatinous c. gallertartiges/gallertiges Bindegewebe.
interstitial c. interstitielles Bindegewebe.
loose (fibrous) c. lockeres Bindegewebe.
mucous c. → gelatinous c.
reticular c. retikuläres Bindegewebe.

consciousness

connective tissue callus *ortho.*, *patho.* bindegewebiger (Knochen-)Kallus *m.*
connective tissue capsule Bindegewebskapsel *f.*
connective tissue cell Bindegewebszelle *f.*
connective tissue cleft Bindegewebsspalt *m.*
connective tissue hyalin *patho.* bindegewebiges Hyalin *nt.*
connective tissue massage Bindegewebsmassage *f.*
connective tissue membrane Bindegewebsmembran *f.*
connective tissue nevus Bindegewebsnävus *m.*
connective tissue scar Bindegewebsnarbe *f*, -schwiele *f.*
connective tissue sheath bindegewebige Scheide/Umhüllung *f*, Bindegewebsscheide *f*, -umhüllung *f.*
c. of Key and Retzius Endoneurium *nt.*
connective tissue tumor Bindegewebstumor *m.*
connective tissue tunic Bindegewebshülle *f.*
Connell [ˈkɒnəl]: **C. suture** *chir.* Connell-Naht *f.*
con·nex·on [kəˈneksən] *n* Connexon *nt.*
con·nex·us [kəˈneksəs] *n anat.* Co(n)nexus *f.*
con·nu·bi·al [kəˈn(j)uːbɪəl] *adj* ehelich, Ehe-.
co·noid [ˈkəʊnɔɪd] **I** *n bio.* Konoid *nt.* **II** *adj* kegelförmig.
co·noi·dal [kəʊˈnɔɪdl] *adj* → conoid **II**.
conoid ligament Lig. conoideum.
conoid tubercle Tuberculum conoideum.
con·oph·thal·mus [ˌkəʊnɒfˈθælməs] *n ophthal.* Hornhautstaphylom *nt*, Konophthalmus *m.*
Conor and Bruch [ˈkɒnər brɒk; bruːx]: **C. a. B.'s disease** Boutonneuse-Fieber *nt*, Fièvre boutonneuse.
con·qui·nine [ˈkɒŋkwɒniːn, -nɪn] *n* Chinidin *nt*, Quinidine *nt.*
Conradi [kɒnˈraːdɪ]: **C.'s disease** Conradi-Syndrom *nt*, Conradi-Hünermann-(Raap-)Syndrom *nt*, Chondrodysplasia/Chondrodystrophia calcificans congenita.
C.'s line Conradi-Linie *f.*
C.'s syndrome → C.'s disease.
Conradi-Drigalski [drɪˈgælskɪ]: **C.-D. agar** Drigalski-Conradi-Nährboden *m.*
Conradi-Hünermann [ˈhyːnərman]: **C.-H. syndrome** → Conradi's disease.
con·san·guine [kɒnˈsæŋgwɪn] *adj* → consanguineous.
con·san·guin·e·al [ˌkɒnsæŋˈgwɪnɪəl] *adj* → consanguineous.
con·san·guin·e·ous [ˌ-ˈgwɪnɪəs] *adj* blutsverwandt.
con·san·guin·i·ty [ˌ-ˈgwɪnətɪ] *n* Blutsverwandtschaft *f*, Konsanguinität *f.*
con·science [ˈkɒnʃəns] *n* Gewissen *nt.*
con·sci·en·tious [ˌkɒnʃɪˈenʃəs, ˌkɒnsɪ-] *adj* **1.** gewissenhaft. **2.** Gewissens-. **on ~ grounds** aus Gewissensgründen.
con·scious [ˈkɒnʃəs] *adj* **1.** (*Patient*) bei Bewußtsein. **2.** bewußt, bei Bewußtsein gegenwärtig. **diet-~/weight-~** gewichtsbewußt. **to be/become ~ of** s. einer Sache bewußt sein/werden. **3.** bewußt, absichtlich, wissentlich.
con·scious·ness [ˈ-nɪs] *n* **1.** s. Bewußtsein *nt*, Wissen *nt* (*of* von, um). **2.** Denken *nt*, Empfinden *nt*. **3.** Bewußtsein(szustand *m*) *nt.* **to lose ~** das Bewußtsein verlieren, ohnmächtig werden. **to regain ~** das Bewußtsein wieder erlangen, wieder zu s. kommen.

conscious perception bewußte Wahrnehmung f, Apperzeption f.
con·sec·u·tive [kən'sekjətɪv] adj aufeinanderfolgend, Folge-; (Zahlen) fortlaufend.
consecutive aneurysm diffuses Aneurysma nt.
con·sec·u·tive·ness [kən'sekjətɪvnɪs] n Aufeinanderfolge f.
consecutive symptom Folgeerscheinung f.
con·sen·su·al [kən'senʃʊəl, -'senʃəwəl, -'senʃəl] adj 1. gleichsinnig, übereinstimmend, konsensuell. 2. physiol. unwillkürlich, Reflex-.
consensual light reflex konsensueller Lichtreflex m.
consensual reaction 1. → consensual reflex. 2. konsensuelle Reaktion f.
consensual reflex gekreuzter/diagonaler/konsensueller Reflex m.
con·sen·sus [kən'sensəs] n, pl **-sus·es** (allgemeine) Übereinstimmung f.
con·sent [kən'sent] I n Zustimmung f (to zu); Einwilligung f (to in); Einverständnis(erklärung f) f (to zu). **by mutual ~** in gegenseitigem Einverständnis. **to give (written) ~** (schriftliche) Einwilligung geben. **to obtain ~** Einverständnis einholen. II vi zustimmen (to zu); einwilligen (to in); s. bereit erklären (to do zu tun).
con·se·quence ['kɒnsɪkwens] n 1. Konsequenz f, Folge f, Resultat nt, Auswirkung f (of). **in ~** folglich, daher. **in ~ of** infolge (von). **in ~ of which** infolgedessen. **to take the ~s** die Folgen tragen. 2. Tragweite f, Wichtigkeit f. **of ~s** wichtig (to für). **of no ~s** ohne Bedeutung, unbedeutend (to für).
con·se·quent ['kɒnsɪkwent] I n Folge f. II adj 1. resultierend od. s. ergebend (on, upon aus). 2. konsequent, logisch richtig.
con·se·quent·ly ['kɒnsɪkwentlɪ] adv folglich, daher, infolgedessen; als Folge.
con·serv·a·tive [kən'sɜrvətɪv] adj 1. erhaltend, bewahrend, konservierend, konservativ. 2. (Therapie) zurückhaltend, vorsichtig, konservativ.
conservative replication genet. konservative Replikation f.
conservative treatment konservative Behandlung f.
con·serve [kən'sɜrv] vt konservieren; erhalten, bewahren.
con·sol·i·dant [kən'sɒlɪdənt] I n pharm. Konsolidierungsmittel nt. II adj (Heilung) fördernd, festigend, konsolidierend.
con·sol·i·da·tion [kən,sɒlɪ'deɪʃn] n 1. (Ver-)Stärkung f, Festigung f. 2. Konsolidierung f, Festigung f; Ausheilung f; Induration f.
con·so·lute ['kɒnsəluːt] adj (vollständig) mischbar.
con·so·nant ['kɒnsənənt] n Konsonant m, Mitlaut m.
con·so·nan·tal [,kɒnsə'næntl] adj konsonantisch, Konsonanten-.
con·so·na·ting ['kɒnsəneɪtɪŋ] adj mitklingend, konsonierend.
consonating rales pulmo. metallische Rasselgeräusche pl, metallisches Rasseln nt.
con·stan·cy ['kɒnstənsɪ] n Konstanz f, Beständigkeit f, Unveränderlichkeit f; Bestand m, Dauer f.
con·stant ['kɒnstənt] I n mathe., phys., fig. Konstante f, konstante od. feste Größe f. II adj 1. unveränderlich, konstant, gleichbleibend. 2. (an-)dauernd, ständig, stetig, konstant. 3. mathe., phys. konstant.
c. of friction Reibungskoeffizient.
c. of gravitation Gravitationskonstante.
constant current konstanter Gleichstrom m.

constant field equation Goldman-Gleichung f, Goldman-Hodgkin-Katz-Gleichung f.
constant region biochem. C-Region f, konstante Region f.
con·sti·pate ['kɒnstəpeɪt] vt verstopfen, konstipieren, obstipieren.
con·sti·pat·ed ['kɒnstəpeɪtɪd] adj verstopft, konstipiert, obstipiert.
con·sti·pa·tion [,kɒnstə'peɪʃn] n (Stuhl-)Verstopfung f, Obstipation f, Konstipation f.
con·stit·u·ent [kən'stɪtʃuːənt] I n Bestandteil m; chem., mathe., phys. Komponente f. II adj einzeln, einen Teil bildend, Teil-.
constituent part → constituent I.
con·sti·tu·tion [,kɒnstɪ't(j)uːʃn] n 1. Zusammensetzung f, (Auf-)Bau m, Struktur f, Beschaffenheit f. 2. med., psycho. Konstitution f, körperliche/seelische Struktur f od. Verfassung f; (Person) Gesamterscheinungsbild nt. 3. chem. Konstitution f, Anordnung f (der Atome im Molekül).
con·sti·tu·tion·al [,kɒnstɪ't(j)uːʃənl] I n inf. Spaziergang m. II adj 1. konstitutionell, anlagebedingt, konstitutionsmäßig, naturgegeben. 2. gesundheitsfördernd. 3. grundlegend, wesentlich; Struktur-, Konstitutions-.
constitutional disease konstitutionelle/anlagebedingte Erkrankung/Krankheit f.
constitutional emphysema Altersemphysem nt, konstitutionelles/seniles Lungenemphysem nt.
constitutional formula Strukturformel f.
constitutional hemolytic anemia → congenital familial icterus.
constitutional hepatic dysfunction Meulengracht(-Gilbert)-Krankheit f, -Syndrom nt, intermittierende Hyperbilirubinämie Meulengracht f, Icterus juvenilis intermittens Meulengracht.
constitutional hyperbilirubinemia → constitutional hepatic dysfunction.
constitutional infantile panmyelopathy Fanconi-Anämie f, -Syndrom nt, konstitutionelle infantile Panmyelopathie f.
constitutional isomerism Strukturisomerie f.
constitutional reaction konstitutionelle Reaktion f.
constitutional symptom Allgemeinsymptom nt.
constitutional thrombopathy 1. (von) Willebrand-Jürgens-Syndrom nt, konstitutionelle Thrombopathie f, hereditäre/vaskuläre Pseudohämophilie f, Angiohämophilie f. 2. Glanzmann-Naegeli-Syndrom nt, Thrombasthenie f.
constitutional type Konstitutionstyp m.
constitutional ulcer symptomatisches Ulkus nt.
con·sti·tu·tive ['kɒnstɪt(j)uːtɪv, kən'stɪtʃətɪv] adj 1. → constituent II. 2. grundlegend, wesentlich, bestimmend, konstitutiv. 3. phys., chem., konstitutiv. 4. gestaltend, aufbauend.
constitutive enzyme konstitutives Enzym nt.
constitutive mutant konstitutive Mutante f.
con·strict [kən'strɪkt] vt 1. (Muskel) zusammenziehen; verengen, einschnüren. 2. (a. fig.) behindern, be-, einschränken; einengen.
con·strict·ed [-'strɪktɪd] adj zusammengezogen; (a. fig.) ver-, eingeengt, be-, eingeschränkt.
con·stric·tion [-'strɪkʃn] n 1. Zusammenziehen nt, Einschnüren nt, Verengen nt. 2. Einengung f, Einschnürung f, Konstrik-

tion f, Striktur f. 3. Beschränkung f, Beengtheit f, Enge f.
con·stric·tive [-'strɪktɪv] adj zusammenziehend, einschnürend, konstriktiv; fig. einengend, beschränkend.
constrictive endocarditis Löffler-Endokarditis f, -Syndrom nt, Endocarditis parietalis fibroplastica.
constrictive pericarditis card. konstriktive Perikarditis f, Pericarditis constrictiva.
con·stric·tor [-'strɪktər] n zusammenziehender od. verengender Muskel m, Konstriktor m, Constrictor m, M. constrictor.
c. of pharynx → constrictor pharyngis (muscle).
constrictor muscle of pharynx → constrictor pharyngis (muscle).
constrictor pharyngis inferior (muscle) Konstriktor/Constrictor m pharyngis inferior, M. constrictor pharyngis inferior.
constrictor pharyngis medius (muscle) Konstriktor/Constrictor m pharyngis medius, M. constrictor pharyngis medius.
constrictor pharyngis (muscle) Konstriktor/Constrictor m pharyngis, M. constrictor pharyngis.
constrictor pharyngis superior (muscle) Konstriktor/Constrictor m pharyngis superior, M. constrictor pharyngis superior.
con·struc·tion·al apraxia [kən'strʌkʃənl] neuro. konstruktive Apraxie f.
con·struc·tive [kən'strʌktɪv] adj 1. aufbauend, schöpferisch, konstruktiv. 2. physiol. anabol, anabolisch.
con·sult [kən'sʌlt] I vt 1. konsultieren, zu Rate ziehen, um Rat fragen (about um). 2. (in einem Buch) nachschlagen. II vi (s.) beraten, beratschlagen (about über).
con·sult·ant [kən'sʌltənt] n 1. beratender Arzt m, Konsiliararzt m od. -ärztin f, Konsiliarius m. 2. Facharzt m od. -ärztin f (an einem Krankenhaus). 3. Berater(in f) m; Gutachter(in f) m.
con·sul·ta·tion [,kɒnsəl'teɪʃn] n ärztliche Beratung f, Konsultation f, Konsilium f.
consultation hour Sprechstunde f.
con·sump·tion [kən'sʌmpʃn] n 1. Verbrauch m, Konsumption f. 2. Auszehrung f, Konsumption f. 3. old Schwindsucht f.
consumption coagulopathy 1. hema. Verbrauchskoagulopathie f. 2. disseminierte intravasale Koagulation f abbr. DIC, disseminierte intravasale Gerinnung f abbr. DIG.
con·sump·tive [kən'sʌmptɪv] I n old Schwindsüchtige(r m) f. II adj verbrauchend, verzehrend, konsumptiv, Verbrauchs-; auszehrend.
con·tact ['kɒntækt] I n 1. (a. fig.) Kontakt m, Fühlung f, Berührung f, Verbindung f. **to come into ~ with** in Berührung kommen mit. **to make ~ with** in Kontakt kommen mit; Verbindung herstellen mit. 2. infect. Kontaktperson f. 3. electr. Kontakt m, Anschluß m. II vt s. in Verbindung setzen mit, Kontakt aufnehmen mit, s. wenden an.
contact acid chem. Kontaktsäure f.
contact acne Kontaktakne f, Akne/Acne vinenata.
contact allergen Kontaktallergen nt.
contact allergy Kontaktallergie f.
con·tac·tant [kən'tæktənt] n Kontaktallergen nt.
contact area Kontaktfläche f.
contact brush electr. Kontaktbürste f.

contact catalysis heterogene Katalyse f, Kontaktkatalyse f.
contact dermatitis 1. Kontaktdermatitis f, Kontaktekzem nt. **2.** allergische Kontaktdermatitis f, allergisches Kontaktekzem nt.
  allergic c. allergische Kontaktdermatitis, allergisches Kontaktekzem.
  photoallergic c. Photokontaktallergie f, photoallergische (Kontakt-)Dermatitis, photoallergisches Ekzem.
contact eczema derm. Kontaktekzem nt, -dermatitis f.
contact electricity Kontakt-, Berührungselektrizität f.
contact factor Faktor XII m abbr. F XII, Hageman-Faktor m.
contact glasses → contact lens.
contact hemolysis Kontakthämolyse f.
contact hypersensitivity Kontaktallergie f.
contact infection Kontaktinfektion f.
contact inhibition Kontakt-, Dichtehemmung f.
contact lens Kontaktlinse f, -glas nt, Haftglas nt, -schale f, Kontaktschale f.
  corneal c. Korneallinse.
  hard c. harte Kontaktlinse.
  scleral c. Sklerallinse.
  soft c. weiche Kontaktlinse.
contact metastasis Kontaktmetastase f.
contact receptor Kontaktrezeptor m.
contact surface Kontaktfläche f.
contact urticaria Kontakturtikaria f.
con·ta·gion [kən'teɪdʒən] n **1.** (Krankheits-)Übertragung f durch Kontakt. **2.** übertragbare/kontagiöse Krankheit f. **3.** kontagiöses Partikel nt, Kontagion nt, Kontagium nt.
con·ta·gi·os·i·ty [kən,teɪdʒɪ'ɒsətɪ] n Übertragbarkeit f, Ansteckungsfähigkeit f, Kontagiosität f.
con·ta·gious [kən'teɪdʒəs] adj (direkt) übertragbar, ansteckend, kontagiös, Kontagions-.
contagious aphtha micro. (echte) Maul- u. Klauenseuche f abbr. MKS, Febris aphthosa.
contagious disease → communicable disease.
contagious ecthyma Orf f, atypische Schafpocken pl, Steinpocken pl, Ecthyma contagiosum, Stomatitis pustulosa contagiosa.
contagious pustular dermatitis → contagious ecthyma.
contagious pustular stomatitis → contagious ecthyma.
con·ta·gium [kən'teɪdʒ(ɪ)əm] n, pl **-gia** [-dʒ(ɪ)ə] kontagiöses Partikel nt, Kontagion nt, Kontagium nt.
con·tam·i·nant [kən'tæmɪnənt] n verschmutzende/verunreinigende Substanz f; phys. Verseuchungsstoff m.
con·tam·i·nate [kən'tæmɪneɪt] vt verunreinigen, verschmutzen, vergiften, infizieren, verseuchen, kontaminieren.
con·tam·i·nat·ed wound [kən'tæmɪneɪtɪd] ortho. kontaminierte Wunde f.
con·tam·i·na·tion [kən,tæmɪ'neɪʃn] n **1.** Verseuchung f, Verunreinigung f; Vergiftung f, Kontamination f; Giftstoffe pl. **2.** neuro., psychia. Verschmelzung f, Kontamination f.
con·tent ['kɒntent] n **1.** (a. ~s pl) (Raum-)Inhalt m, Fassungsvermögen nt, Volumen nt. **2.** fig. Gehalt m (of an); Inhalt m, Substanz f.
con·ti·gu·i·ty [,kɒntɪ'gjuːətɪ] n, pl **-ties 1.** Aneinandergrenzen nt, Angrenzen nt (to an); Berührung f (to mit), Kontiguität f. **2.** (räumliches od. zeitliches) Zusammentreffen nt, Zusammenfallen nt, Kontiguität f.
con·tig·u·ous [kən'tɪgjəwəs] adj angrenzend, anstoßend (to an); berührend; nahe (to an); benachbart.
con·ti·nence ['kɒntɪnəns] n **1.** Kontinenz f. **2.** (sexuelle) Enthaltsamkeit f, Zurückhaltung f, Mäßigung f.
con·ti·nen·cy ['kɒntɪnənsɪ] n → continence.
con·ti·nent ['kɒntɪnənt] adj **1.** kontinent. **2.** (sexuell) enthaltsam, zurückhaltend.
con·tin·gent negative variation [kən'tɪndʒənt] abbr. **CNV** neuro., HNO späte kortikale Gleichspannungspotentiale pl, contingent negative variation abbr. CNV.
con·tin·ued [kən'tɪnjuːd] adj anhaltend, fortgesetzt, fortlaufend, stetig, unaufhörlich, kontinuierlich.
continued arterial hypertension Huchard-Krankheit f, Präsklerose f.
continued fever kontinuierliches Fieber nt, Kontinua f, Continua f, Febris continua.
con·ti·nu·i·ty [,kɒntə'n(j)uːətɪ] n Stetigkeit f, ununterbrochener Fortdauer f, Fortbestehen nt, ununterbrochener Zusammenhang m, Kontinuität f.
con·tin·u·ous [kən'tɪnjəwəs] adj ununterbrochen, fortlaufend, fortwährend, andauernd, stetig, ständig, unaufhörlich, kontinuierlich.
continuous ambulatory peritonal dialysis abbr. **CAPD** kontinuierliche ambulante Peritonealdialyse f.
continuous arrhythmia card. absolute Arrhythmie f, Arrhythmia absoluta/perpetua.
continuous capillary geschlossene Kapillare f, Typ 1-Kapillare f.
continuous current konstanter Gleichstrom m.
continuous drip Dauertropf(infusion f) m.
continuous fever → continued fever.
continuous instillation Dauertropf(infusion f) m.
continuous murmur kontinuierliches Geräusch nt.
continuous phase phys. äußere/dispergierende Phase f, Dispergens nt, Dispersionsmedium nt, -mittel nt.
continuous positive airway pressure (breathing) abbr. **CPAP** CPAP-(Be-)Atmung f, kontinuierliche (Be-)Atmung f gegen erhöhten Druck.
continuous positive pressure breathing abbr. **CPPB** → continuous positive airway pressure (breathing).
continuous positive pressure ventilation abbr. **CPPV** kontinuierliche assistierte Überdruck(be)atmung f.
continuous spectrum kontinuierliches Spektrum nt.
continuous suture chir. fortlaufende Naht f.
continuous tremor kontinuierlicher Tremor m.
continuous variation kontinuierliche Variation f.
con·tin·u·um model [kən'tɪnjəwəm] phys. Kontinuum-Modell n.
con·tour ['kɒntʊər] I n Umriß m, Umrißlinie f, Kontur f. II vt **1.** die Konturen zeichnen od. andeuten, konturieren. **2.** (Zahn, Knochen) remodellieren.
con·tour·ing [kən'tʊərɪŋ] n (Zahn, Knochen) Konturieren nt, Konturierung f, (Re-)Modellieren nt.
contour lines dent. Owen'-Linien pl.
contra- pref. Contra-, Gegen-, Wider-.
con·tra·cep·tion [,kɒntrə'sepʃn] n Empfängnisverhütung f, Konzeptionsverhütung f, Antikonzeption f, Kontrazeption f.
con·tra·cep·tive [,-'septɪv] I n empfängnisverhütendes Mittel nt, Verhütungsmittel nt, Kontrazeptivum nt. II adj empfängnisverhütend, kontrazeptiv, antikonzeptionell.
contraceptive device gyn. (mechanisches) Verhütungsmittel nt, Kontrazeptivum nt.
contraceptive diaphragm gyn. Diaphragma(pessar nt) nt.
con·tra·clock·wise [,-'klɒkwaɪz] adj gegen den Uhrzeigersinn/die Uhrzeigerrichtung, nach links.
con·tract [n, adj 'kɒntrækt; v kən'trækt] I n Vertrag m, Kontrakt m. II vt **1.** (Muskel) zusammenziehen, verkürzen, verringern, kontrahieren; (Pupille) verengen; verkleinern. **2.** (Krankheit) s. zuziehen. **3.** einen Vertrag schließen; (Verpflichtung) eingehen. III vi **4.** (Muskel) s. zusammenziehen, (s.) kontrahieren; (Pupille) s. verengen; s. verkleinern, (ein-)schrumpfen. **5.** einen Vertrag schließen, s. vertraglich verpflichten.
con·tract·ed [kən'træktɪd] adj **1.** zusammengezogen, (ein-)geschrumpft, kontrahiert, Schrumpf-. **2.** ge-, verkürzt. **3.** fig. engstirnig, beschränkt. **4.** (Stirn) gerunzelt. **5.** vereinbart.
contracted kidney patho. Schrumpfniere f.
contracted pelvis verengtes Becken nt.
con·tract·i·bil·i·ty [kən,træktə'bɪlətɪ, kən-] n → contractility.
con·tract·i·ble [-'træktɪbl] adj → contractile.
con·trac·tile [-'træktɪ, -tɪl] adj zusammenziehbar, kontraktil, kontraktionsfähig.
contractile element abbr. **CE** physiol. kontraktiles Element nt abbr. CE.
contractile force Kontraktionskraft f.
contractile protein kontraktiles Protein nt.
contractile tension Kontraktionsspannung f.
contractile tissue kontraktiles od. kontraktionsfähiges Gewebe nt.
contractile vein Drosselvene f.
con·trac·til·i·ty [,kɒntræk'tɪlətɪ] n Fähigkeit f zur Kontraktion, Kontraktilität f.
con·tract·ing [kən'træktɪŋ] adj (s.) zusammenziehend.
con·trac·tion [kən'trækʃn] n **1.** abbr. **C** Kontraktion f, Zusammenziehung f; (Muskel-)Kontraktion f, Zuckung f; Kontrahieren nt; (Pupille) Verengen nt; Schrumpfen nt. **2.** patho. → contracture. **3.** gyn. Wehe f, Kontraktion f. **4.** Zuziehung f (einer Krankheit).
contraction period Anspannungsphase f.
contraction velocity Kontraktionsgeschwindigkeit f.
con·trac·ture [kən'træktʃər] n physiol., patho. Kontraktur f.
con·tra·fis·sure [,kɒntrə'fɪʃər] n ortho. Contre-coup-Fraktur f.
con·tra·in·ci·sion [,-'sɪʒn] n chir. Gegenöffnung f, Kontrainzision f.
con·tra·in·di·cant [,-'ɪndɪkənt] adj kontraindizierend.
con·tra·in·di·cat·ed [,-'ɪndɪkeɪtɪd] adj nicht anwendbar, nicht zur Anwendung empfohlen, kontraindiziert.
con·tra·in·di·ca·tion [,-ɪndɪ'keɪʃn] n Gegenanzeige f, Gegen-, Kontraindikation f.
con·tra·lat·er·al [,-'lætərəl] adj **1.** auf der entgegengesetzten Seite (liegend), gegenseitig, kontralateral. **2.** neuro. gekreuzt, kontralateral.
contralateral hemiplegia kontralaterale Hemiplegie f.

contralateral reflex/sign Brudzinski-Zeichen *nt*, Brudzinski-Kontralateralreflex *m*, Brudzinski-kontralateraler Reflex *m*.
con·trast [*n* 'kɒntræst; *v* kən'træst] **I** *n* **1.** Kontrast *m*, (starker) Gegensatz *m*, (auffallender) Unterschied *m* (*between* zwischen; *to*, *with* zu). **to form a ~ to** einen Kontrast bilden zu. **in ~ to/with** im Gegensatz zu. **2.** *radiol.* (Bild-)Kontrast *m*. **II** *vi* kontrastieren (*with* mit); (*Farben*) s. abheben (*with* von); im Gegensatz/in Kontrast stehen (*with* zu).
contrast agent → contrast medium.
contrast bath *heilgymn.* Wechselbad *nt*.
contrast color Kontrastfarbe *f*.
contrast dye 1. → contrast medium. **2.** *histol.* Kontrastfärbemittel *nt*.
contrast enema *radiol.* Bariumkontrasteinlauf *m*.
contrast enhancement *physiol.* Kontrastverschärfung *f*.
contrast formation Kontrastbildung *f*.
con·tra·stim·u·lant [ˌkɒntrə'stɪmjələnt] **I** *n pharm.* Beruhigungsmittel *nt*. **II** *adj* kontrastimulierend; beruhigend.
con·trast·ing [kən'træstɪŋ] *adj* kontrastierend, kontrastiv, Kontrast-.
contrasting colors kontrastierende Farben *pl*, Kontrastfarben *pl*.
con·tras·tive [kən'træstɪv] *adj* → contrasting.
contrast medium *radiol.* Kontrastmittel *nt abbr.* KM, Röntgenkontrastmittel *nt abbr.* RKM.
contrast radiography *radiol.* Röntgenkontrastdarstellung *f*.
contrast roentgenography → contrast radiography.
contrast stain 1. Kontrastfärbemittel *nt*. **2.** Kontrastfärbung *f*.
con·trast·y [kən'træstɪ, 'kɒn-] *adj* kontrastreich, reich an Kontrasten.
con·tra·sup·pres·sor cell [ˌkɒntrəsə'presər] Kontrasuppressorzelle *f*.
con·tre·coup ['kɒntrəku:] *n chir.*, *ortho.* Contre-coup *m*, Contre-coup-Verletzung *f*, -Mechanismus *m*.
contrecoup contusion Contre-coup-Hirnprellung *f*.
con·trol [kən'trəʊl] **I** *n* **1.** Kontrolle *f*, Herrschaft *f* (*of*, *over* über). **to be in ~ of/to have ~ of** etw. leiten, verwalten; jdn. beaufsichtigen. **to be under ~** unter Kontrolle sein. **to bring/get under ~** unter Kontrolle bringen. **to be/get out of ~** außer Kontrolle sein/geraten. **to have ~ over** beherrschen, die Kontrolle haben über. **to have sth. under ~** etw. unter Kontrolle haben; etw. beherrschen. **to keep under ~** unter Kontrolle haben, fest in der Hand haben. **to lose ~ over/of** die Kontrolle über. Gewalt verlieren über. **to lose ~ of o.s.** die (Selbst)Beherrschung verlieren. **2.** Selbstbeherrschung *f*; Körperhaltung *f*. **3.** Kontrolle *f*, Aufsicht *f*, Überwachung *f* (*of*, *over* über); Leitung *f*, Verwaltung *f* (*of*). **4.** *techn.* Steuerung *f*, Bedienung *f*; Regler *m*, Schalter *m*; Regelung *f*, Regulierung *f*. **5.** Kontrolle *f*, Anhaltspunkt *m*; Vergleichs-, Kontrollwert *m*, Kontrollversuch *m*, -person *f*, -gruppe *f*. **II** *vt* **6.** in Schranken halten, eindämmen, Einhalt gebieten, bekämpfen, im Rahmen halten. **to ~ o.s.** s. beherrschen. **7.** beherrschen, unter Kontrolle haben/bringen; bändigen. **8.** kontrollieren, überwachen, beaufsichtigen. **9.** leiten, lenken, führen, verwalten; (*a. techn.*) regeln, steuern, regulieren.
control circuit *techn.* Kontroll-, Regler-, Steuerkreis *m*.
control curve Kontrollkurve *f*.
control experiment Kontroll-, Gegenversuch *m*, Kontrollexperiment *nt*, -studie *f*.
control group Kontrollgruppe *f*.
con·trol·la·ble [kən'trəʊləbl] *adj* **1.** kontrollierbar, zu kontrollieren. **2.** *techn.* regulier-, steuerbar.
con·trolled [kən'trəʊld] *adj* beherrscht, kontrolliert; *techn.* geregelt.
controlled drain *chir.* Dochtdrain *m*.
controlled respiration → controlled ventilation.
controlled system *techn.* Regelstrecke *f*.
controlled variable *techn.* Regelgröße *f*.
controlled ventilation kontrollierte Beatmung *f*.
con·trol·ler [kən'trəʊlər] *n techn.* Regler *m*.
con·trol·ling element [kən'trəʊlɪŋ] *techn.* Stellglied *m*.
controlling signal *techn.* Kontrollsignal *nt*, -größe *f*, Steuersignal *nt*, -größe *f*, Stellsignal *nt*, -größe *f*.
control substance *biochem.* Steuer-, Kontrollsubstanz *f*.
control system *techn.* Kontroll-, Steuersystem *nt*.
control system technology *techn.* Regeltechnik *f*.
control system theory Regelungstheorie *f*, -lehre *f*.
control theory → control system theory.
con·tund [kən'tʌnd] *vt* → contuse.
con·tuse [kən't(j)u:z] *vt* quetschen, Prellungen zufügen, jdn. grün u. blau schlagen.
con·tused wound [kən't(j)u:zd] Quetschwunde *f*.
con·tu·sion [kən't(j)u:ʒn] *n* Prellung *f*, Quetschung *f*, Kontusion *f*, Contusio *f*.
contusion cataract *ophthal.* Kontusionskatarakt *f*, -star *m*.
contusion glaucoma sekundäres Glaukom *nt* nach Contusio bulbi.
contusion pneumonia (post-)traumatische Pneumonie *f*.
con·u·lar ['kɒnjʊlər] *adj* konusförmig.
co·nus ['kəʊnəs] *n*, *pl* -**ni** [-ni:, -naɪ] *anat.* kegel-, zapfenförmiges Gebilde *nt*, Zapfen *m*, Konus *m*.
conus artery: left c. Ast *m* der linken Herzkranzarterie zum Conus arteriosus, Ramus coni arteriosi a. coronariae sinistrae.
right/third c. Ast *m* der rechten Herzkranzarterie zum Conus arteriosus, Ramus coni arteriosi a. coronariae dextrae.
conus branch: (left) c. of left coronary artery A. coronaria sinistra-Ast *m* zum Conus arteriosus, Ramus coni arteriosi a. coronariae sinistrae.
(right) c. of right coronary artery A. coronaria dextra-Ast *m* zum Conus arteriosus, Ramus coni arteriosi a. coronariae dextrae.
conus cordis *embryo.* Conus cordis.
conus cushion *embryo.* Conuswulst *m*.
conus swelling → conus cushion.
con·va·lesce [ˌkɒnvə'les] *vi* genesen, gesund werden.
con·va·les·cence [ˌkɒnvə'lesəns] *n* Genesung *f*, Rekonvaleszenz *f*.
convalescence serum → convalescent human serum.
con·va·les·cent [ˌkɒnvə'lesənt] **I** *n* Genesende(r *m*) *f*, Rekonvaleszent(in *f*) *m*. **II** *adj* Genesung betr., genesend, rekonvaleszent, Genesungs-, Rekonvaleszenten-.
convalescent carrier Rekonvaleszenzausscheider *m*.
convalescent home Erholungs-, Genesungsheim *nt*.
convalescent human serum Rekonvaleszentenserum *nt*.
convalescents' serum → convalescent human serum.

con·vec·tion [kən'vekʃn] *n* Konvektion *f*.
con·vec·tion·al [kən'vekʃnəl] *adj* Konvektions-.
con·vec·tive [kən'vektɪv] *adj* Konvektion betr., mittels Konvektion, konvektiv, Konvektions-.
convective heat Strömungswärme *f*, -hitze *f*, Konvektionswärme *f*, -hitze *f*.
convective heat transfer coefficient *abbr.* h_c konvektive Wärmeübergangszahl *f abbr.* h_c.
convective transport konvektiver Transport *m*.
con·verge [kən'vɜrdʒ] *vi* (*a. mathe.*, *phys.*) zusammenlaufen, -streben (*at* in, an); s. (einander) nähern (*to*, *towards*); konvergieren (*at* in); konvergent verlaufen.
con·ver·gence [kən'vɜrdʒəns] *n* (*a. fig.*, *phys.*, *mathe*) Annäherung *f*, Zusammenstreben *nt*, Zusammenlaufen *nt*, Konvergenz *f* (*to*, *towards* an).
convergence movement Konvergenzbewegung *f*.
convergence nystagmus Konvergenznystagmus *m*, konvergierender Nystagmus *m*.
convergence principle Konvergenzprinzip *nt*.
convergence response Naheinstellungs-, Konvergenzreaktion *f*.
con·ver·gen·cy [kən'vɜrdʒənsɪ] *n* → convergence.
con·ver·gent [kən'vɜrdʒənt] *adj* zusammenlaufend, -strebend, s. (einander) nähernd, konvergent, konvergierend.
convergent evolution *bio.* konvergente Evolution *f*.
convergent rays konvergente/konvergierende Strahlen *pl*.
convergent strabismus Einwärtsschielen *nt*, Isotropie *f*, Strabismus convergens/internus.
con·ver·ging [kən'vɜrdʒɪŋ] *adj* → convergent.
converging lens → convex lens.
converging meniscus Konkavokonvexlinse *f*.
con·ver·sa·tion·al speech [ˌkɒnvər'seɪʃənl] Umgangssprache *f*.
con·ver·sion [kən'vɜrʒn, -ʃn] *n* **1.** Ver-, Umwandlung *f* (*into* in); Umstellung *f* (*to* auf); Konversion *f*. **2.** *chem.*, *phys.* Umsetzung *f*; *electr.* Umformung *f*; *mathe.* Umrechnung *f* (*into* in). **3.** *psycho.* Konversion *f*. **4.** *micro.* lysogene Konversion *f*, Phagenkonversion *f*.
conversion disorder *psycho.* Konversionsreaktion *f*, -neurose *f*, -hysterie *f*, hysterische Reaktion/Neurose *f*.
conversion hysteria → conversion disorder.
conversion hysteric neurosis → conversion disorder.
conversion-neurotic pain konversionsneurotischer Schmerz *m*.
conversion reaction → conversion disorder.
conversion table Umrechnungstabelle *f*.
conversion type → conversion disorder.
con·vert [kən'vɜrt] **I** *vt* **1.** (*a. chem.*, *physiol.*) um-, verwandeln (*into* in); umstellen (*to* auf); konvertieren. **2.** *electr.* umformen (*into* zu); *techn.* verwandeln (*into* in); *mathe.* umrechnen (*into* in). **II** *vi* s. verwandeln (lassen) (*into* in); umgewandelt werden.
con·ver·tase [kən'vɜrteɪz] *n* Convertase *f*.
con·vert·i·bil·i·ty [kənˌvɜrtə'bɪlətɪ] *n* (*a. chem.*, *physiol.*) Umwandelbarkeit *f*, Konvertibilität *f*.
con·vert·i·ble [kən'vɜrtɪbl] *adj* um-, ver-

wandelbar, konvertibel; *mathe.* umrechenbar.
con·vert·i·ble·ness ['-nɪs] *n* → convertibility.
con·ver·tin [kən'vɜrtɪn] *n* Prokonvertin *nt*, -convertin *nt*, Faktor VII *m abbr.* F V II, Autothrombin I *nt*, Serum-Prothrombin-Conversion-Accelerator *m abbr.* SPCA, stabiler Faktor *m*.
con·vex [kɑn'veks, kən-] I *n* konvexer Körper *m*, konvexe Fläche *f.* II *adj* nach außen gewölbt, konvex.
con·vex·i·ty [kən'veksətɪ] *n* 1. Konvexität *f*, konvexe Beschaffenheit *f*, Wölbung *f* (nach außen). 2. → convex I.
convex lens konvexe Linse *f*, Konvexlinse *f*, Sammellinse *f*.
convex margin of testis konvexer/vorderer Hodenrand *m*, Margo anterior testis.
convex mirror Konvexspiegel *m*.
con·vex·o·ba·sia [kɑn‚veksoʊ'beɪsɪə] *n patho.*, *ortho.* Konvexobasie *f*, basiläre Impression *f*, Basilarimpression *f*.
convexo-concave *adj* konvex-konkav, Konvexokonkav-.
convexo-concave lens Konvexokonkavlinse *f*.
convexo-convex lens Konvexokonvexlinse *f*.
con·vo·lute ['kɑnvəluːt] I *adj* (zusammen-, übereinander-)gerollt. II *vt* aufrollen, (auf-)wickeln, zusammenrollen. III *vi* s. aufrollen, s. (auf-)wickeln, s. zusammenrollen.
con·vo·lut·ed ['kɑnvəluːtɪd] *adj* (ein-)gerollt, gewunden, spiralig, knäuelig, knäuelförmig.
convoluted part of renal cortex (*Niere*) Rindenlabyrinth *nt*, Pars convoluta.
convoluted T-cell lymphoma T-Zellenlymphom *nt* vom convoluted-cell-Typ.
con·vo·lu·tion [‚-'luːʃn] *n* 1. *anat.* (Gehirn-)Windung *f*, Gyrus *m*. 2. *histol.* Knäuel *m*, Konvolut *nt*. 3. *techn.* Windung *f*, Knäuel *nt*, Konvolut *nt*.
c.s of cerebellum Kleinhirnwindungen *pl*, Gyri/Folia cerebelli.
c.s of cerebrum (Groß-)Hirnwindungen *pl*, Gyri cerebrales.
con·vo·lu·tion·al [‚-'luːʃnl] *adj* (Gehirn-)Windung betr., Konvolutions-.
convolutional atrophy *neuro.*, *patho.* Pick'-(Hirn-)Atrophie *f*, -Krankheit *f*, -Syndrom *nt*.
con·vo·lu·tion·ar·y [‚-'luːʃənɛriː] *adj* → convolutional.
con·vul·sant [kən'vʌlsənt] I *n* krampfauslösendes Mittel *nt*, Konvulsivum *nt*. II *adj* krampf-, konvulsionsauslösend.
con·vul·sion [-'vʌlʃn] *n* Krampf *m*, Zuckung *f*, Konvulsion *f*.
con·vul·si·vant [-'vʌlsɪvənt] *n*, *adj* → convulsant.
con·vul·sive [-'vʌlsɪv] *adj* Konvulsion betr., krampfartig, krampfend, konvulsiv, konvulsivisch.
convulsive state *neuro.* Epilepsie *f*, Epilepsia *f*.
convulsive tic *neuro.* Bell-Spasmus *m*, Fazialiskrampf *m*, Fazialis-Tic *m*, Gesichtszucken *nt*, mimischer Gesichtskrampf *m*, Tic convulsiv/facial.
coo·ing murmur ['kuːɪŋ] musikalisches (Herz-)Geräusch *nt*.
cool [kuːl] I *n* Kühle *f*, Frische *f*. II *adj* 1. kühl, frisch; kühl(end), Kühle aushaltend; erfrischend. 2. fieberfrei. 3. *fig.* kühl, ruhig, beherrscht, gelassen; kalt, abweisend. III *vt* 4. (ab-)kühlen, kalt werden lassen. 5. abkühlen, erfrischen. IV *vi* kühl werden, s. abkühlen.
Cooley ['kuːlɪ]: **C.'s anemia/disease** Cooley-Anämie *f*, homozygote β-Thalassämie *f*, Thalassaemia major.
Coolidge ['kuːlɪdʒ]: **C. tube** *radiol.* Coolidge-Röhre *f*.
cool·ing ['kuːlɪŋ] I *n* Kühlung *f*, Abkühlung *f*. II *adj* abkühlend; kühlend, erfrischend, Kühl-.
Coombs [kuːms]: **C.' murmur** *card.* Coombs-Geräusch *nt*.
C. test *immun.* Antiglobulintest *m*, Coombs-Test *m*.
C. test, direct direkter Coombs-Test.
C. test, indirect indirekter Coombs-Test.
Coombs-positive *adj immun.* Coombs-positiv.
Coombs-negative *adj immun.* Coombs-negativ.
Cooper ['kuːpər, 'kʊpər]: **C.'s fascia** Fascia cremasterica.
C.'s hernia 1. Hey-Hernie *f*, Hernia encystica. 2. Hesselbach-Hernie *f*, Cooper-Hernie *f*.
inguinal ligament of C. → C.'s ligament 1.
C.'s irritable breast Cooper-Syndrom *nt*, -Neuralgie *f*, -Mastodynie *f*, Neuralgia mammalis.
C.'s irritable testis Cooper'-Hodenneuralgie *f*.
C.'s ligament 1. Cooper'-Band *nt*, Lig. pectineale. 2. Chorda obliqua.
C.'s suspensory ligaments Ligg. suspensoria mammaria.
co·op·er·ate [koʊ'ɑpəreɪt] *vi* kooperieren, zusammenarbeiten, -wirken (*with* mit jdm.; *in sth.* bei etw.).
co·op·er·a·tion [koʊ‚ɑpə'reɪʃn] *n* Kooperation *f*, Zusammenarbeit *f*, Mitwirkung *f*.
co·op·er·a·tive [koʊ'ɑpərətɪv, -'ɑprə-, -reɪtɪv] *adj* (*a. physiol.*) kooperativ, kooperierend, zusammenarbeitend, -wirkend.
cooperative bond *chem.* kooperative Bindung *f*.
co·op·er·a·tiv·i·ty [koʊ‚ɑpərə'tɪvətɪ] *n biochem.* Kooperativität *f*.
Coopernail ['kuːpərneɪl, 'koʊ-]: **C.'s sign** *ortho.* Coopernail'-Zeichen *nt*.
co·or·di·nate [*n*, *adj* koʊ'ɔːrdnɪt; *v* -neɪt] I *n mathe.* Koordinate *f*. II *adj* koordiniert, (aufeinander) abgestimmt; bei-, nebengeordnet, gleichrangig, -wertig; *mathe.* Koordinaten-. III *vt* koordinieren, aufeinander abstimmen; bei-, nebenordnen, gleichschalten. IV *vi* s. aufeinander abstimmen.
co·or·di·nat·ed induction [koʊ'ɔːrdɪneɪtɪd] *biochem.* koordinierte Induktion *f*.
coordinated reflex koordinierter Reflex *m*.
coordinated regulation *biochem.* koordinierte Regulation *f*.
coordinate repression *biochem.* koordinierte Repression *f*.
coordinate system *mathe.* Koordinatensystem *nt*.
co·or·di·na·tion [koʊ‚ɔːrdə'neɪʃn] *n* (*a. physiol.*) Koordination *f*, Koordinierung *f*, Abstimmung *f* (aufeinander), (harmonisches) Zusammenwirken *nt*, Übereinstimmung *f*.
coordination bond *chem.* Koordinationsbindung *f*.
coordination position *chem.* Koordinationsstelle *f*.
co·pai·ba [koʊ'peɪbə, -'paɪ-] *n pharm.* Kopaivabalsam *m*, Balsamum copaivae.
CO₂ partial pressure Kohlendioxidpartialdruck *m*, CO_2-Partialdruck *m abbr.* Pco_2, pCO_2.
COPD *abbr.* [chronic obstructive pulmonary disease] → chronic obstructive lung disease.

Cope [koʊp]: **C.'s clamp** *chir.* Cope'-Klemme *f*.
C.'s sign *chir.* Psoaszeichen *nt*, Cope-Zeichen *nt*.
cope [koʊp] *vi* 1. kämpfen, s. messen, es aufnehmen (*with* mit). 2. gewachsen sein; fertig werden (*with* mit); bewältigen, meistern.
co·pe·pod ['koʊpəpɑd] *n micro.* Kopepod *m*.
Co·pep·o·da [koʊ'pepədə] *pl micro.* Ruderfußkrebse *pl*, Kopepoden *pl*, Copepoda *pl*.
co·pi·ous ['koʊpɪəs] *adj* reichlich, ausgiebig, massenhaft, kopiös.
co·pi·ous·ness ['-nɪs] *n* Reichtum *m*, Fülle *f*, Überfluß *m*.
CO poisoning Kohlenmonoxidvergiftung *f*, CO-Vergiftung *f*, CO-Intoxikation *f*.
co·pol·y·mer [koʊ'pɑlɪmər] *n* Ko-, Copolymer *nt*.
co·po·lym·er·ase [‚koʊpə'lɪmərɛɪz, koʊ-'pɑlɪmə-] *n* Copolymerase *f*.
cop·per ['kɑpər] I *n* 1. *abbr.* **Cu** Kupfer *nt*, *chem.* Cuprum *nt abbr.* Cu. 2. Kupferbehälter *m*, -gefäß *nt*. 3. Kupferrot *nt*. II *adj* 4. kupfern, Kupfer-. 5. kupferrot. III *vt techn.* verkupfern.
copper cataract *ophthal.* Kupferstar *m*, Chalcosis lentis.
copper colic Darmkolik *f* bei Kupfervergiftung.
copper line Kupfersaum *m*.
copper nose Kartoffel-, Säufer-, Pfund-, Knollennase *f*, Rhinophym *nt*, Rhinophyma *f*.
copper red Kupferrot *nt*.
copper sulfate Kupfersulfat *nt*, *old* Kupfervitriol *nt*.
cop·per·y ['kɑpərɪ] *adj* kupferig, kupferhaltig-, artig, -farbig.
Coppet [kɔ'pɛ]: **C.'s law** *phys.*, *chem.* Coppet'-Regel *f*.
copr- *pref.* → copro-.
cop·ra·cra·sia [‚kɑprə'kreɪsɪə] *n* Stuhl-, Darminkontinenz *f*, Incontinentia alvi.
cop·ra·go·gue ['-gɔg, -gɑg] *n pharm.* Kopragogum *nt*.
copra mite ['kɑprə, 'koʊ-] *micro.* Tyrophagus castellani.
co·pre·cip·i·tin [‚kɑprɪ'sɪpətɪn] *n hema.* Koprazipitin *nt*.
cop·rem·e·sis [kɑp'remɪsɪs] *n* Koterbrechen *nt*, Kopremesis *f*.
copro- *pref.* Kot-, Fäkal-, Kopro-, Stuhl-, Sterko-.
cop·ro·an·ti·bod·y [‚kɑprə'æntɪbɑdɪ] *n immun.* Koproantikörper *m*.
cop·ro·lag·nia [‚-'lægnɪə] *n psycho.* Koprolagnie *f*.
cop·ro·la·lia [‚-'leɪlɪə] *n psycho.*, *psychia.* Kotsprache *f*, Koprolalie *f*, -phrasie *f*.
cop·ro·lith ['-lɪθ] *n* Kotstein *m*, Koprolith *m*.
cop·ro·ma [kɑp'roʊmə] *n* Kotgeschwulst *f*, Fäkulom *nt*, Koprom *nt*, Sterkorom *nt*.
cop·ro·pha·gia [‚kɑprə'feɪdʒ(ɪ)ə] *n* → coprophagy.
co·proph·a·gous [kə'prɑfəgəs] *adj* 1. *bio.* s. von Kot ernährend, koprophag. 2. *psychia.* Kot essend, koprophag.
co·proph·a·gy [kə'prɑfədʒɪ] *n* 1. *bio.* Kotfressen *nt*, Koprophagie *f*. 2. *psychia.* Kotessen *nt*, Koprophagie *f*.
cop·ro·phil ['kɑprəfɪl] *n micro.* koprophiler Organismus *m*.
cop·ro·phile ['-fɪl] I *n* → coprophil. II *adj* → coprophilic.
cop·ro·phil·ia [‚-'fɪlɪə] *n psychia.* Koprophilie *f*.
cop·ro·phil·ic [‚-'fɪlɪk] *adj* 1. *psychia.* kotlie-

coprophilous

bend, koprophil. **2.** *bio.*, *micro.* in Mist/Dung lebend, koprophil.
co·proph·i·lous [kə'prɒfıləs] *adj* → coprophilic.
cop·ro·pho·bia [,kɒprə'fəʊbıə] *n psychia.* Kotangst *f*, Koprophobie *f*.
cop·ro·phra·sia [,-'freıʒ(ı)ə, -zıə] *n* → coprolalia.
cop·ro·por·phyr·ia [,-pɔːr'fıərıə] *n* Koproporphyrie *f*.
cop·ro·por·phy·rin [,-'pɔːrfərın] *n* Koproporphyrin *nt*.
cop·ro·por·phy·rin·o·gen [,-,pɔːrfı'rınədʒən] *n* Koproporphyrinogen *nt*.
coproporphyrinogen oxidase Koproporphyrinogenoxidase *f*.
cop·ro·por·phy·rin·u·ria [,-,pɔːrfərı'n(j)ʊərıə] *n* Koproporphyrinurie *f*.
co·pros·ta·nol [kə'prɒstənəl, -nəʊl] *n* Koprostanol *nt*.
co·pros·ta·sis [kə'prɒstəsıs] *n* Kotstauung *f*, -verhaltung *f*, Fäkal-, Koprostase *f*.
co·pros·ter·in [kə'prɒstərın] *n* → coprostanol.
co·pros·ter·ol [kə'prɒstərɒl, -rəʊl] *n* → coprostanol.
cop·ro·zo·ic [,kɒprə'zəʊık] *adj micro.* in Kot lebend, koprozoisch.
cop·u·late ['kɒpjəleıt] *vi* **1.** koitieren. **2.** *bio.* s. paaren, s. begatten, kopulieren.
cop·u·la·tion [,kɒpjə'leıʃn] *n* **1.** → coitus. **2.** *bio.* Paarung *f*, Begattung *f*, Kopulation *f*.
cop·y DNA ['kɒpı] → complementary DNA.
cor [kɔːr, kəʊr] *n* Herz *nt*; *anat.* Cor *nt*, Cardia *f*.
cor·a·cid·i·um [,kɒrə'sıdıəm] *n*, *pl* **-dia** [-dıə] *micro.* Wimper-, Flimmerlarve *f*, Korazidium *nt*, Coracidium *nt*.
coraco- *pref.* Korako-.
cor·a·co·a·cro·mi·al [,kɒrəkəʊə'krəʊmıəl] *adj* Proc. coracoideus u. Akromion betr., korakoakromial.
coracoacromial ligament Lig. coracoacromiale.
cor·a·co·bra·chi·al [,-'breıkıəl] *adj* Proc. coracoideus u. Oberarm betr., korakobrachial.
coracobrachial bursa Bursa m. coracobrachialis.
cor·a·co·bra·chi·a·lis (muscle) [-,breıkı'eılıs] Korakobrachialis *m*, M. coracobrachialis.
coracobrachial muscle → coracobrachialis (muscle).
cor·a·co·cla·vic·u·lar [,-klə'vıkjələr] *adj* Proc. coracoideus u. Schlüsselbein betr., korakoklavikulär.
coracoclavicular fascia → clavipectoral fascia.
coracoclavicular ligament Lig. coracoclaviculare.
external c. Lig. trapezoideum.
internal c. Lig. conoideum.
cor·a·co·cos·tal fascia [,-'kɒstl, -'kɔstl] → clavipectoral fascia.
cor·a·co·hu·mer·al [,-'(h)juːmərəl] *adj* Proc. coracoideus u. Humerus betr., korakohumeral.
coracohumeral ligament Lig. coracohumerale.
cor·a·coid ['kɒrəkɔıd, 'kɑr-] **I** *n* → coracoid process. **II** *adj* rabenschnabelförmig, korakoid; Proc. coracoideus betr.
coracoid bursa Bursa subtendinea m. subscapularis.
cor·a·coi·di·tis [,kɒrəkɔı'daıtıs] *n ortho.* Korakoiditis *f*.
coracoid ligament of scapula Lig. transversum scapulae superius.
coracoid process Rabenschnabelfortsatz *m*, Proc. coracoideus.
cor·a·co·ra·di·a·lis [,kɒrəkəʊ,reıdı'eılıs] *n anat.* Caput breve m. bicipitis brachii.
cor·al calculus ['kɒrəl, 'kɑ-] *urol.* Korallenstein *m*, Hirschgeweihstein *m*, (Becken-)Ausgußstein *m*.
cor·al·li·form cataract [kə'rælıfɔːrm] Korallenstar *m*, Cataracta coralliformis.
cor·asth·ma [kɔːr'æzmə] *n* Heufieber *nt*, -schnupfen *m*.
Corbus ['kɔːrbəs]: **C.' disease** Corbus'-Krankheit *f*, gangränöse Balanitis *f*, Balanitis gangraenosa.
cord [kɔːrd] *n* **1.** *anat.* schnur- od. strangähnliche Struktur *f*, Strang *m*, Band *nt*, Chorda *f*. **2.** Leine *f*, Kordel *f*, Strang *m*, Schnur *f*.
c. of Nuck Proc. vaginalis peritonei, Proc. vaginalis testis.
cor·date [kɔːrdeıt] *adj* herzförmig.
cordate pelvis Kartenherzbecken *nt*.
cord bladder *neuro.* Reflexblase *f*.
cord blood Nabelschnurblut *nt*.
cord·ec·to·my [kɔːr'dektəmı] *n* **1.** *chir.* Bandausschneidung *f*, -exzision *f*. **2.** *HNO* Chordektomie *f*.
cord factor Cordfaktor *m*, Trehalose-6,6'-dimykolat *nt*.
cor·di·al [kɔːrdʒəl, -dıəl] **I** *n pharm.* belebendes Mittel *nt*, Stärkungsmittel *nt*. **II** *adj* **1.** belebend, stärkend. **2.** herzlich, freundlich, warm, aufrichtig.
cor·di·form [kɔːrdəfɔːrm] *adj* herzförmig.
cordiform ligament of diaphragm Centrum tendineum.
cordiform pelvis Kartenherzbecken *nt*.
cord injury Rückenmarksverletzung *f*.
cor·di·tis [kɔːr'daıtıs] *n neuro.* Samenstrangentzündung *f*, Funikulitis *f*, Funiculitis *f*.
cor·do·pex·y ['kɔːrdəpeksı] *n HNO* Chordopexie *f*.
cor·dot·o·my [kɔːr'dɒtəmı] *n*, *pl* **-mies 1.** *HNO* Stimmlippendurchtrennung *f*, Chordotomie *f*. **2.** *neurochir.* Durchschneidung/Durchtrennung *f* der Schmerzbahn im Rückenmark, Chordotomie *f*.
cord paralysis Stimmbandlähmung *f*.
cord swelling Rückenmarksschwellung *f*.
core- *pref.* → coreo-.
core [kɔːr, kəʊr] *n* **1.** (*a. fig.*) Kern *m*; das Innerste *nt*; Mark *nt*. **2.** (Eiter-)Pfropf *m*. **3.** *electr.* (*Elektromagnet*) Kern *m*. **4.** *micro.* (*Virus*) Core (*nt/m*), Innenkern *m*. **5.** *bot.* Kerngehäuse *nt*. **6.** *phys.* Reaktorkern *m*, Core *nt*.
cor·e·clei·sis *n* → coreclisis.
cor·e·cli·sis [kɔːrı'klaısıs] *n ophthal.* **1.** Pupillenverschluß *m*, -okklusion *f*. **2.** Iriseinklemmung *f*, Korenklisis *f*, Iridenkleisis *f*, Iridenklisis *f*.
cor·ec·ta·sia [,kəʊrek'teıʒ(ı)ə] *n* → corectasis.
cor·ec·ta·sis [kəʊr'ektəsıs] *n* (pathologische) Pupillenerweiterung *f*, -dilatation *f*, Korektasie *f*.
cor·ec·tome [kəʊr'ektəʊm] *n ophthal.* Iridektomiemesser *nt*, Korektom *nt*, Iridektom *nt*.
cor·ec·to·me·di·al·y·sis [kəʊr,ektəʊmıdı'æləsıs] *n ophthal.* periphere Iridektomie *f*.
cor·ec·to·my [kəʊr'ektəmı] *n ophthal.* Iris(teil)entfernung *f*, Irisresektion *f*, Iridektomie *f*, Korektomie *f*.
cor·ec·to·pia [,kəʊrek'təʊpıə] *n ophthal.* Pupillenverlagerung *f*, -ektopie *f*, Korektopie *f*, Ectopia/Ectopia pupillae.
cor·e·di·al·y·sis [,kəʊrıdaı'æləsıs] *n ophthal.* Irislösung *f*, Iridodialyse *f*, -dialysis *f*.
cor·e·di·as·ta·sis [,-daı'æstəsıs] *n* Pupillenerweiterung *f*, -dilatation *f*, Korediastasis *f*; Mydriasis *f*.
co·re·duc·tant [kəʊrı'dʌktənt] *n* Ko-, Coreduktant *m*.
co·rel·y·sis [kəʊ'reləsıs] *n ophthal.* (operative) Irislösung *f*, Iridolyse *f*, Korelyse *f*; Synechiotomie *f*.
co·re·mi·um [kəʊ'riːmıəm] *n*, *pl* **-mia** [-mıə] *micro.* Koremium *nt*.
cor·e·mor·pho·sis [,kəʊrımɔːr'fəʊsıs] *n ophthal.* operative Pupillenbildung *f*, Koremorphose *f*.
cor·en·cli·sis [,kəʊren'klaısıs] *n ophthal.* operative Iriseinklemmung *f*, Korenklisis *f*, Iridenkleisis *f*, Iridenklisis *f*.
coreo- *pref.* Pupillen-, Iris-, Irido-, Kore(o)-.
cor·e·om·e·ter [,kəʊrı'ɒmıtər] *n ophthal.* Pupillenmesser *m*, Pupillo-, Koriometer *nt*.
cor·e·om·e·try [,-'ɒmıtrı] *n ophthal.* Pupillenmessung *f*, Pupillo-, Koriometrie *f*.
cor·e·o·plas·ty ['kəʊrıəʊplæstı] *n ophthal.* Pupillen-, Irisplastik *f*.
cor·e·pex·y [kəʊrı'peksı] *n* → corepraxy.
core polysaccharide *micro.* Kernpolysaccharid *nt*.
cor·e·prax·y [,-'præksı] *n ophthal.* Koreopraxie *f*.
co·re·press·or [,kəʊrı'presər] *n biochem.* Ko-, Corepressor *m*.
core protein *micro.* Coreprotein *nt*.
CO_2 response *physiol.* CO_2-Antwort *f*.
cor·e·ste·no·ma [,kəʊrestı'nəʊmə] *n ophthal.* (pathologische) Pupillenverengung *f*, -konstriktion *f*.
core temperature (of body) Körperkerntemperatur *f*.
co·re·to·me·di·al·y·sis [,kəʊrətəʊmıdı'æləsıs] *n* → corectomedialysis.
co·ret·o·my [kəʊ'retəmı] *n ophthal.* Irisdurchtrennung *f*, -ausschneidung *f*, Iridotomie *f*, Koretotomie *f*.
Cori ['kɔːrı, 'kəʊ-]: **C. cycle** Cori-Zyklus *m*. **C.'s disease** Cori-Krankheit *f*, Forbes-Syndrom *nt*, hepatomuskuläre benigne Glykogenose *f*, Glykogenose Typ III *f*.
C.'s ester Cori-Ester *m*, Glukose-1-phosphat *nt*.
co·ri·um ['kɔːrıəm, 'kəʊr-] *n*, *pl* **-ria** [-rıə] *anat.* Lederhaut *f*, Korium *nt*, Corium *nt*, Dermis *f*.
corn [kɔːrn] *n* **1.** Hühnerauge *nt*, Leichdorn *m*, Klavus *m*, Clavus *m*. **2.** (Samen-, Getreide-)Korn *nt*.
cor·ne·a ['kɔːrnıə] *n*, *pl* **-ne·as, -ne·ae** [-nı,iː] *anat.* (Augen-)Hornhaut *f*, Kornea *f*, Cornea *f*.
cor·ne·al ['kɔːrnıəl] *adj* Hornhaut/Cornea betr., Hornhaut-, Kornea-.
corneal astigmatism *ophthal.* Hornhautastigmatismus *m*, kornealer Astigmatismus *m*.
corneal burn Hornhaut-, Korneaverbrennung *f*.
corneal dystrophy *ophthal.* Hornhautdystrophie *f*.
granular c. granuläre/bröckelige Hornhautdystrophie, Typ Groenouw I *m*.
macular c. makuläre/fleckförmige Hornhautdystrophie, Typ Groenouw II *m*.
corneal ectasia *ophthal.* Hornhautvorwölbung *f*, -staphylom *nt*, Keratektasie *f*.
corneal endothelium inneres Korneaepithel *nt*, Korneaendothel *nt*, Endothelium posterius (corneae).
corneal epithelium (äußeres) Hornhautepithel *nt*, Epithelium anterius (corneae).
corneal lens Korneallinse *f*.
corneal margin Limbus corneae.
corneal pannus *ophthal.* Pannus corneae.

corneal reflex 1. *neuro.* Korneal-, Blinzel-, Lidreflex *m.* 2. *ophthal.* Hornhautreflex *m*, -reflexion *f.*
corneal staphyloma Hornhautstaphylom *nt*, Staphyloma corneae.
corneal ulcer Hornhautgeschwür *nt*, -ulkus *nt*, Ulcus corneae.
catarrhal c. Ulcus corneae catarrhalia/marginalia.
serpiginous c. Ulcus corneae serpens.
corneal vertex Hornhautscheitel *m*, Vertex corneae.
cor·ne·i·tis [kɔːrnɪˈaɪtɪs] *n ophthal.* Hornhautentzündung *f*, Keratitis *f.*
Cornelia de Lange [kɔːrˈniːljə də ˈlɑːŋə]: **C.d.L. syndrome** Cornelia de Lange-Syndrom *nt*, Brachmann-de-Lange-Syndrom *nt*, Lange-Syndrom *nt*, Amsterdamer Degenerationstyp *m.*
cor·ne·o·bleph·a·ron [ˌkɔːrnɪoʊˈblefərən] *n ophthal.* Verwachsung/Verklebung *f* von Hornhaut u. Lid(rand).
cor·ne·o·i·ri·tis [ˌ-aɪˈraɪtɪs] *n* Entzündung *f* von Hornhaut/Kornea u. Iris, Korneoiritis *f*, Iridokeratitis *f.*
cor·ne·o·ret·i·nal potential [ˌ-ˈretɪnəl] *physiol., HNO* Korneoretinalpotential *nt.*
cor·ne·o·scle·ra [ˌ-ˈsklɪərə] *n* Kornea u. Sklera, Korneosklera *f.*
cor·ne·o·scle·ral [ˌ-ˈsklɪərəl] *adj* Kornea u. Sklera betr., korneoskleral.
corneoscleral junction Perikornealring *m*, Limbus corneae.
corneoscleral part of trabecular retinaculum vorderer Abschnitt *m* des Hueck'-Bands, Pars corneoscleralis.
cor·ne·ous [ˈkɔːrnɪəs] *adj* hornartig, hornig.
Corner-Allen [ˈkɔːrnər ˈælən]: **C.-A. test** Corner-Allen-Test *m.*
C.-A. unit Corner-Allen-Einheit *f.*
Cornet [ˈkɔːrnet]: **C.'s forceps** Cornet-Pinzette *f.*
cor·nic·u·late [kɔːrˈnɪkjəlɪt, -leɪt] *adj* hornförmig, gehörnt.
corniculate cartilage Santorini-Knorpel *m*, Cartilago corniculata.
corniculate tubercle Tuberculum corniculatum.
cor·nic·u·lum [kɔːrˈnɪkjələm] *n* → corniculate cartilage.
cor·ni·fi·ca·tion [ˌkɔːrnəfɪˈkeɪʃn] *n* Verhornung *f*, Verhornen *nt*, Keratinisation *f.*
cor·ni·fied [ˈkɔːrnəfaɪd] *adj* verhornt, verhornend.
Corning [ˈkɔːrnɪŋ]: **C.'s anesthesia/method** *anes.* Spinalanästhesie *f*, inf. Spinale *f.*
corn·meal agar [ˈkɔːrnmiːl] Maismehlagar *m/nt.*
cor·noid [ˈkɔːrnɔɪd] *adj* hornartig, -förmig.
corn smut *micro.* Maisbrand *m*, Ustilago maydis.
cor·nu [ˈkɔːrn(j)uː] *n*, *pl* **-nua** [-n(j)uːə] *anat.* Horn *nt*, hornförmige Struktur *f*, Cornu *nt.*
c. of coccyx Cornu coccygeum.
c. of sacrum Cornu sacrale.
cor·nu·al [ˈkɔːrn(j)əwəl] *adj anat.* Horn/Cornu betr.
cor·nu·ate [ˈkɔːrn(j)əweɪt] *adj* → cornual.
co·ro·di·as·ta·sis [ˌkɔʊrədaɪˈæstəsɪs] *n* → corediastasis.
co·ro·na [kəˈroʊnə] *n*, *pl* **-nas, -nae** [-niː] *anat.* Kranz *m*, kranzförmige Struktur *f*, Corona *f.*
c. of glans (penis) Randwulst *m* der Eichel, Peniskorona *f*, Corona glandis.
cor·o·nal [kəˈroʊnl, ˈkɔːrən, ˈkɑr-] *adj* 1. *anat.* Schädelkranz od. Kranznaht betr., koronal, Kranz-. 2. *dent.* Zahnkrone betr., koronal, Kronen-.
coronal cavity Kronenabschnitt *m* der Zahn-/Pulpahöhle, Cavitas coronae.
coronal cells → corona radiata cells.
cor·o·na·le [ˌkɔːrəˈnæli, -ˈneɪ-] *n* Stirnbein *nt*, Os frontale.
coronal margin: c. of frontal bone Margo parietalis ossis frontalis.
c. of parietal bone Margo frontalis ossis parietalis.
coronal plane *anat.* Frontalebene *f.*
coronal pulp → coronal cavity.
coronal suture *anat.* Kranznaht *f*, Sutura coronalis.
corona radiata 1. (*ZNS*) Stabkranz *m*, Corona radiata. 2. (*Ovum*) von Bischoff'-Korona *f*, Corona radiata (folliculi ovarici).
corona radiata cells *embryo.* Corona-radiata-Zellen *pl.*
cor·o·na·ria [ˌkɔːrəˈneərɪə] *n* → coronary artery.
cor·o·na·rism [ˈkɔːrənærɪzəm] *n* 1. → coronary insufficiency. 2. Herzbräune *f*, Stenokardie *f*, Angina pectoris.
cor·o·na·ri·tis [ˌkɔːrənəˈraɪtɪs] *n* → coronary arteritis.
cor·o·nar·y [ˈkɔːrənəri, ˈkɑr-] **I** *n*, *pl* **-naries** 1. Koronararterie *f*, (Herz-)Kranzarterie *f*, (Herz-)Kranzgefäß *nt*, Koronarie *f*, A. coronaria. 2. → coronary occlusion. 3. → coronary thrombosis. **II** *adj* 4. kranz-, kronenähnlich od. -förmig. 5. *anat.* Kranz-/Koronararterien betr., koronar, Koronar(arterien)-.
coronary angiography *radiol.* Koronarangiographie *f*, Koronarographie *f.*
coronary angle *anat.* Angulus frontalis (ossis parietalis).
coronary arteriography → coronary angiography.
coronary arteriosclerosis Koronar(arterien)sklerose *f.*
coronary arteritis Entzündung *f* der Herzkranzgefäße, Koronararterienentzündung *f*, Koron(i)itis *f*, Koronarangiitis *f.*
coronary artery *abbr.* CA 1. (Herz-)Kranzarterie *f*, (Herz-)Kranzgefäß *nt*, Koronararterie *f*, Koronarie *f*, A. coronaria. 2. Kranzarterie *f*, Kranzgefäß *nt*, A. coronaria.
descending c., posterior Ramus interventricularis superior.
c. of heart → coronary artery 1.
left c. of heart linke (Herz-)Kranzarterie, A. coronaria sinistra.
left c. of stomach linke Magen(kranz)arterie, Gastrica *f* sinistra, A. gastrica sinistra.
right c. of heart rechte (Herz-)Kranzarterie, A. coronaria dextra.
right c. of stomach rechte Magen(kranz)arterie, Gastrica *f* dextra, A. gastrica dextra.
coronary artery bypass *HTG* aorto-koronarer Bypass *m.*
coronary artery disease *abbr.* CAD → coronary heart disease.
coronary artery injury Koronararterienverletzung *f.*
coronary artery sclerosis Koronar(arterien)sklerose *f.*
coronary blood flow → coronary perfusion.
coronary bypass *HTG* aorto-koronarer Bypass *m.*
coronary care unit *abbr.* CCU kardiologische Wach-/Intensivstation *f.*
coronary cataract *ophthal.* Kranzstar *m*, Cataracta coronaria.
coronary chemoreflex koronarer Chemoreflex *m.*
coronary circulation Koronarkreislauf *m.*
coronary dilatator *pharm.* Koronardilatator *m.*
coronary dilator → coronary dilatator.
coronary disease of the hip *ortho.* idiopathische Hüftkopfnekrose *f* des Erwachsenen, avaskuläre/ischämische Femurkopfnekrose *f* (des Erwachsenen).
coronary failure akute Koronarinsuffizienz *f.*
coronary heart disease *abbr.* CHD koronare Herzkrankheit *f abbr.* KHK, koronare Herzerkrankung *f abbr.* KHE, stenosierende Koronarsklerose *f*, degenerative Koronarerkrankung *f.*
coronary insufficiency Koronarinsuffizienz *f.*
acute c. akute Koronarinsuffizienz.
coronary ligament: c. of liver Lig. coronarium.
c. of radius Lig. anulare radii.
coronary occlusion Koronar(arterien)verschluß *m.*
coronary perfusion Koronardurchblutung *f*, -perfusion *f.*
coronary plexus: anterior c. of heart Plexus coronarius cordis anterior.
gastric c. Magenplexus *pl*, Plexus gastrici.
posterior c.es of heart Plexus coronarius cordis posterior.
coronary reflex Koronar(arterien)reflex *m.*
coronary reserve Koronarreserve *f.*
coronary sclerosis Koronar(arterien)sklerose *f.*
coronary sinus Sinus coronarius.
coronary sulcus (of heart) (Herz-)Kranzfurche *f*, Sulcus coronarius.
coronary thrombosis Koronar(arterien)thrombose *f.*
coronary valve Thebesius'-(Sinus-)Klappe *f*, Sinusklappe *f*, Valva/Valvula sinus coronarii.
coronary vasodilatator *pharm.* Koronardilatator *m.*
coronary vasodilator → coronary vasodilatator.
coronary vein: left c. V. coronaria sinistra.
right c. V. coronaria dextra.
corona veneris Stirnband *nt* der Venus, Corona veneris.
Cor·o·na·vir·i·dae [ˌkɔːrənəˈvɪrədiː, -ˈvaɪr-] *pl micro.* Coronaviridae *pl.*
Cor·o·na·vi·rus [ˌ-ˈvaɪrəs] *n micro.* Coronavirus.
cor·o·na·vi·rus [ˌ-ˈvaɪrəs] *n* → Coronavirus.
coronavirus infection Coronavirus-, Coronavireninfektion *f.*
co·ro·ne [kəˈroʊni] *n* → coronoid process of mandible.
cor·o·ner [ˈkɔːrənər, ˈkɑr-] *m forens.* Coroner *m.*
cor·o·noid [ˈkɔːrənɔɪd] *adj* kronenförmig.
cor·o·noi·dec·to·my [ˌkɔːrənɔɪˈdektəmi] *n HNO* Resektion *f* des Proc. coronoideus mandibulae.
coronoid fossa (of humerus) Fossa coronoidea.
coronoid head of pronator teres muscle Caput ulnare m. pronatoris teretis.
coronoid process: c. of mandible Kronenfortsatz *m* des Unterkiefers, Proc. coronoideus mandibulae.
c. of ulna Proc. coronoideus ulnae.
co·ro·plas·ty [ˈkɔːrəplæsti] *n* → coreoplasty.
co·ros·co·py [kəˈraskəpi] *n ophthal.* Retinoskopie *f*, Skiaskopie *f.*
co·rot·o·my [kəˈratəmi] *n* → corectomy.
cor·po·ral [ˈkɔːrp(ə)rəl] *adj* → corporeal.
cor·po·re·al [kɔːrˈpɔːrɪəl, ˈpəʊr-] *adj anat.* Körper/Corpus betr., körperlich, leiblich, Körper-, Korpus-, Corpus-.

corporeal adhesions

corporeal adhesions *gyn.* Korpusverwachsungen *pl*, -verklebungen *pl*.
corps [kɔːr, kaʊr] *n, pl* **corps** [kɔːrz, kaʊrz]
1. Körperschaft *f*, Corps *nt*, Korporation *f*. 2. → corpus.
corpse [kɔːrps] *n* Leiche *f*, Leichnam *m*.
corpse fat Fett-, Leichenwachs *nt*, Adipocire *f*.
cor·pu·lence ['kɔːrpjələns] *n* Beleibtheit *f*, Korpulenz *f*.
cor·pu·len·cy ['kɔːrpjələnsɪ] *n* → corpulence.
cor·pu·lent ['kɔːrpjələnt] *adj* beleibt, korpulent.
cor pulmonale *card.* Cor pulmonale.
cor·pus ['kɔːrpəs] *n, pl* **-po·ra** [-pərə] *anat.* Körper *m*, Corpus *m*.
  c. of caudate nucleus Caudatuskörper, Corpus nc. caudati.
  c. of uterus Gebärmutter-, Uteruskörper, Corpus uteri.
corpus albicans Corpus albicans.
corpus callosum Balken *m*, Commissura magna cerebri, Corpus callosum.
corpus carcinoma *gyn.* Korpuskarzinom *nt*, Gebärmutterkörperkrebs *m*, Ca. corporis uteri.
cor·pus·cle ['kɔːrpəsl, -pʌsl] *n* 1. *anat.* Körperchen *nt*, Korpuskel *nt*, Corpusculum *nt*. 2. *chem., phys.* Masse-, Elementarteilchen *nt*, Korpuskel *nt*.
cor·pus·cu·lar [kɔːrˈpʌskjələr] *adj* Korpuskeln betr., aus Korpuskeln bestehend, korpuskular, Korpuskular-, Teilchen-.
corpuscular radiation *phys.* Teilchen-, Partikel-, Korpuskelstrahlung *f*.
cor·pus·cu·lum [kɔːrˈpʌskjələm] *n, pl* **-la** [-lə] → corpuscle 1.
corpus fibrosum Corpus albicans.
corpus luteum Gelbkörper *m*, Corpus luteum.
  cystic c. zystisches Corpus luteum.
corpus luteum cyst Corpus-luteum-Zyste *f*.
corpus luteum deficiency syndrome Corpus-luteum-Insuffizienz *f*.
corpus luteum hormone Gelbkörperhormon *nt*, Corpus-luteum-Hormon *nt*, Progesteron *nt*.
corpus luteum hormone unit Progesteron-Einheit *f*.
cor·rect [kəˈrekt] *I adj* 1. korrekt, richtig, fehlerfrei, zutreffend, wahr. 2. genau. **II** *vt* 3. korrigieren, verbessern, berichtigen. 4. *chem., phys.* ausgleichen, neutralisieren. 5. jdn. zurechtweisen *od.* tadeln, jdn. bestrafen (*for* wegen).
cor·rec·tion [kəˈrekʃn] *n* 1. Korrektur *f*, Korrektion *f*, (Fehler-)Verbesserung *f*, Richtigstellung *f*. 2. *mathe., phys.* Korrektionskoeffizient *m*. 3. *chem., phys.* Ausgleich *m*, Neutralisierung *f*. 4. Zurechtweisung *f*, Tadel *m*; Bestrafung *f*.
cor·rec·tive [kəˈrektɪv] **I** *n* 1. Abhilfe *f*; Heil-, Gegenmittel *nt*, Korrektiv *nt* (*of, to* gegen). 2. → corrigent I. **II** *adj* 3. korrigierend, verbessernd, berichtigend, Korrektur-, Verbesserungs-. 4. (*a. chem.*) korrektiv, ausgleichend, neutralisierend.
corrective osteotomy *ortho.* Korrekturosteotomie *f*.
corrective saccade *physiol.* Korrektursakkade *f*.
cor·rect·ness [kəˈrektnɪs] *n* Korrektheit *f*, Richtigkeit *f*.
cor·re·late ['kɔːrəleɪt, 'kɑr-] **I** *adj* korrelativ, übereinstimmend, aufeinander bezüglich, wechselseitig, einander bedingend. **II** *vt* korrelieren, zueinander in Beziehung setzen, in Übereinstimmung bringen (*with* mit); aufeinander abstimmen. **III** *vi* korrelieren, (s.) entsprechen, übereinstimmen (*with* mit); s. aufeinander beziehen, miteinander in Wechselbeziehung stehen.
cor·re·lat·ed ['-leɪtɪd] *adj* → correlate I.
correlated state dynamisches Gleichgewicht *nt*, Fließgleichgewicht *nt*.
cor·re·la·tion [,-ˈleɪʃn] *n* Korrelation *f*, Wechselbeziehung *f*, -wirkung *f*, Zusammenhang *m*; Übereinstimmung (*with* mit).
correlation coefficient Korrelationskoeffizient *m*.
correlation ratio *stat.* Korrelationsverhältnis *nt*.
correlation rule Korrelationsregel *f*.
cor·rel·a·tiv [kəˈrelətɪv] *adj* korrelativ, aufeinander abgestimmt, in Wechselbeziehung stehend, s. gegenseitig ergänzend.
Correra [kɔˈrerə]: **C.'s line** *radiol.* Correra-Linie *f*.
cor·re·spond·ence [,kɔːrəˈspɑndəns] *n* Übereinstimmung *f* (*to, with* mit); (*Netzhaut*) Korrespondenz *f*.
cor·re·spond·ing [,-ˈspɑndɪŋ] *adj* einander entsprechend *od.* zugeordnet, funktionell zusammengehörend, in Verbindung stehend, korrespondierend (*with* mit).
corresponding points *opthal.* korrespondierende Netzhautpunkte *pl*.
Corrigan ['kɔrɪɡən]: **C.'s disease** Aorteninsuffizienz *f*.
  C.'s line *card.* Corrigan-Linie *f*.
  C.'s pulse Corrigan-Puls *m*, Pulsus celer et altus.
  C.'s respiration Corrigan-Atmung *f*.
  C.'s sign 1. → C.'s line. 2. → C.'s respiration.
cor·ri·gent ['kɔːrɪdʒənt] **I** *n pharm.* (Geschmacks-)Korrigens *nt*, Corrigentium *nt*. **II** *adj* korrigierend, verbessernd, mildernd.
cor·rin ['kɑrɪn, 'kɔ-] *n* Corrin *nt*.
cor·rode [kəˈrəʊd] **I** *vt* 1. *chem., techn.* anfressen, zerfressen, angreifen, ätzen, korrodieren. 2. *fig.* zerfressen, zerstören. **II** *vi* 3. *chem., techn.* korrodieren, korrodierend wirken, ätzen, fressen (*into* an); rosten. 4. zerstört werden, verfallen.
cor·roid [ˈkɔrɔɪd] *n* Corroid *nt*, Corrinoid *nt*.
cor·ro·sion [kəˈrəʊʒn] *n* 1. *chem., techn.* Korrosion *f*. 2. *techn.* Korrosionsprodukt *nt*; Rost *m*. 3. *fig.* Untergrabung *f*.
cor·ro·sive [kəˈrəʊsɪv] **I** *n chem., techn.* Ätz-, Korrosionsmittel *nt*, (ver-)ätzende Substanz *f*. **II** *adj* 1. *chem., techn.* korrodierend, zersetzend, angreifend, ätzend, Korrosions-. 2. *fig.* nagend, quälend; ätzend.
corrosive burn Verätzung *f*.
corrosive gastritis Ätzgastritis *f*, Gastritis corrosiva.
corrosive injury Verätzung *f*.
corrosive ulcer Noma *f*, Wangenbrand *m*, Wasserkrebs *m*, infektiöse Gangrän *f* des Mundes, Cancer aquaticus, Chancrum oris, Stomatitis gangraenosa.
cor·ru·ga·tor supercilii (muscle) [ˈkɔːrəˌɡeɪtər] Korrugator *m* supercilii, M. corrugator supercilii.
cor·set [ˈkɔːrsɪt] *n ortho.* (Stütz-)Korsett *nt*.
corset cancer *patho.* Panzerkrebs *m*, Cancer en cuirasse *f*.
cor·tex [ˈkɔːrteks] *n, pl* **-ti·ces** [-tɪsiːz] 1. *anat.* Rinde *f*, äußerste Schicht *f*, Kortex *m*, Cortex *m*. 2. (*a. bot.*) Rinde *f*, Schale *f*.
  c. of lens Linsenrinde, Cortex lentis.
  c. of ovari Eierstockrinde, Cortex ovarii.
  c. of suprarenal gland Nebennierenrinde *abbr.* NNR, Cortex gl. suprarenalis.
cor·tex·o·lone [kɔːrˈteksəloʊn] *n* Cortexolon *nt*.
cor·tex·one [kɔːrˈteksoʊn] *n* (11-)Desoxycorticosteron *nt abbr.* DOC, Desoxykortikosteron *nt*, Cortexon *nt*.
Corti [ˈkɔːrtɪ]: **C.'s arch** Corti-Bogen *m*.
  canal of C. → C.'s tunnel.
  C.'s cells Corti-Haarzellen *pl*.
  C.'s fibers → C.'s pillars.
  C.'s ganglion Corti'-Ganglion *nt*, Ggl. spirale cochleae.
  C.'s membrane Corti-Membran *f*, Membrana tectoria ductus cochlearis.
  C.'s organ Corti'-Organ *nt*, Organum spirale.
  pillar cells of C. → C.'s pillars.
  C.'s pillars (*Ohr*) Pfeilerzellen *pl*, Corti'-Pfeilerzellen *pl*.
  pillars of C.'s organ → C.'s pillars.
  C.'s rods → C.'s pillars.
  C.'s tunnel (*Ohr*) innerer Tunnel *m*.
cor·ti·ad·re·nal [,kɔːrtɪəˈdriːnl] *adj* → corticoadrenal.
cortic- *pref.* → cortico-.
cor·ti·cal [ˈkɔːrtɪkl] *adj* Rinde/Cortex betr., kortikal, Rinden-, Kortiko-, Cortico-.
cortical adenoma Nierenrindenadenom *nt*.
cortical afferents kortikale Afferenzen *pl*, kortikopetale Fasern *pl*.
cortical aphasia *neuro.* kortikale Aphasie *f*.
cortical apraxia *neuro.* motorische Apraxie *f*.
cortical area (*ZNS*) Rindenfeld *nt*, -areal *nt*, Area *f*.
cortical atrophy Rindenatrophie *f*.
cortical audiometry *neuro., HNO* Kortexaudiometrie *f*, EEG-Audiometrie *f*.
cortical blindness *ophthal.* Rindenblindheit *f*.
cortical bone Kortikalis *f*, Substantia corticalis *f* (*ossium*).
cortical cataract *ophthal.* Rindenstar *m*, Cataracta corticalis.
cortical cords *embryo.* Rindenstränge *pl*.
cortical deafness *HNO* kortikale Schwerhörigkeit *f*.
cortical efferents kortikale Efferenzen *pl*, kortikofugale Fasern *pl*.
cortical encephalitis Encephalitis corticalis.
cortical epilepsy Rindenepilepsie *f*, Epilepsia corticalis.
cortical field → cortical area.
cortical hormone Nebennierenrindenhormon *nt*, NNR-Hormon *nt*.
cor·ti·ca·lis screw [kɔːrtɪˈkeɪlɪs] *ortho.* Kortikalisschraube *f*.
cortical labyrinth (*Niere*) Rindenlabyrinth *nt*.
cortical layer Rindenschicht *f*.
cortical lobules of kidney (Nieren-)Rindenläppchen *nt*, Lobuli corticales.
cortical map Hirnrindenkarte *f*.
cortical neuron Cortexneuron *nt*.
cortical nucleus of amygdaloid body Nc. corticalis corporis amygdaloidei.
cortical osteitis Knochenhaut-, Periostentzündung *f*, Periostitis *f*.
cortical paralysis kortikale Lähmung *f*.
cortical part: c. of middle cerebral artery End-/Rindenabschnitt *m* der A. cerebri media, Pars terminalis/corticalis a. cerebri mediae.
  c. of posterior cerebral artery End-/Rindenabschnitt *m* der A. cerebri posterior, Pars terminalis/corticalis a. cerebri posterioris.
cortical plate *embryo.* Rindenplatte *f*.
cortical potential *neuro.* Rindenpotential *nt*.

evoked c. evoziertes Rindenpotential.
fast c.s mittlere neurogene Potentiale *pl*, schnelle Rindenpotentiale *pl*.
late c.s späte kortikale Gleichspannungspotentiale *pl*, contingent negative variation *abbr*. CNV.
cortical reaction *embryo*. kortikale Reaktion *f*.
cortical region (*ZNS*) Rindenbezirk *m*, -region *f*.
   basal c. basale Rindenregion.
   orbital c. orbitale Rindenregion.
   premotor c. prämotorische Rindenregion.
cortical sinus Intermediärsinus *m*.
cortical substance: c. of bone → cortical bone.
   c. of cerebellum Kleinhirnrinde *f*, Cortex cerebellaris.
   c. of kidney Nierenrinde *f*, Cortex renalis.
   c. of lens Linsenrinde *f*, Cortex lentis.
   c. of lymph node Lymphknotenrinde *f*, Cortex nodi lymphatici.
   c. of suprarenal gland Nebennierenrinde *f abbr*. NNR, Cortex gl. suprarenalis.
cor·ti·cec·to·my [kɔːrtəˈsektəmɪ] *n neurochir*. Kortikektomie *f*, Tupektomie *f*.
cor·ti·cif·u·gal [ˌ-ˈsɪfjəgl] *adj* → corticofugal.
cor·ti·cip·e·tal [ˌ-ˈsɪpətl] *adj* → corticopetal.
cortico- *pref.* Rinden-, Kortex-, Kortik(o)-.
cor·ti·co·ad·re·nal [ˌkɔːrtɪkəʊəˈdriːnl] *adj* Nebennierenrinde betr., adrenokortikal, Nebennierenrinden-, NNR-.
cor·ti·co·af·fer·ent [ˌ-ˈæfərənt] *adj* kortikoafferent, kortikofugal.
cor·ti·co·bul·bar [ˌ-ˈbʌlbər, -bɑːr] *adj* Hirnrinde/Cortex u. Medulla oblongata *od*. Hirnstamm betr. *od*. verbindend, kortikobulbär.
corticobulbar fibers → corticonuclear fibers.
corticobulbar tract → corticonuclear tract.
cor·ti·co·cer·e·bel·lar [ˌ-ˌserəˈbelər] *adj* Großhirnrinde/Cortex u. Kleinhirn/Cerebellum betr. *od*. verbindend, kortikozerebellar.
corticocerebellar tracts kortikozerebellare Fasern/Bahnen *pl*.
cor·ti·co·cer·e·bral [ˌ-ˈserəbrəl] *adj* (Groß-)Hirnrinde betr., Großhirnrinden-, Kortiko-.
cor·ti·co·di·en·ce·phal·ic [ˌ-ˌdaɪənsəˈfælɪk] *adj* Großhirnrinde u. Zwischenhirn/Diencephalon betr. *od*. verbindend, kortikodienzephal.
cor·ti·co·ef·fer·ent [ˌ-ˈefərənt] *adj* kortikoefferent, kortikofugal.
cor·ti·co·fu·gal [ˌ-ˈfjuːgl] *adj* kortikofugal.
corticofugal fibers → cortical efferents.
cor·ti·co·hy·po·tha·lam·ic tract [ˌ-ˌhaɪpəʊθəˈlæmɪk] Tractus corticohypothalamicus.
cor·ti·coid [ˈkɔːrtɪkɔɪd] *n* Kortikoid *nt*, Corticoid *nt*.
cor·ti·co·lib·er·in [ˌkɔːrtɪkəʊˈlɪbərɪn] *n* → corticotropin releasing factor.
cor·ti·co·me·di·al part of amygdaloid body [ˌ-ˈmiːdɪəl] kortikomediale Kerngruppe *f* des Mandelkerns, Pars corticomedialis/olfactoria (corporis amygdaloidei).
cor·ti·co·med·ul·lar·y [ˌ-məˈdʌlərɪ, -ˈmedəˌleri, -ˈmedʒə-] *adj* Rinde/Cortex u. Mark/Medulla betr., kortikomedullär, corticomedullär, Mark-, Rinden-.
corticomedullary border of kidney → corticomedullary junction (of kidney).
corticomedullary junction (of kidney) (*Niere*) Mark-Rinden-Grenze *f*, kortikomedulläre Übergangszone *f*.
cor·ti·co·mes·en·ce·phal·ic [ˌ-ˌmesənsəˈfælɪk, -kəˈf-] *adj* Großhirnrinde u. Mittelhirn/Mesencephalon betr. *od*. verbindend, kortikomesencephal.
cor·ti·co·ni·gral fibers [ˌ-ˈnaɪgrəl] kortikonigräre Fasern *pl*, Fibrae corticonigrales.
cor·ti·co·nu·cle·ar fibers [ˌ-ˈn(j)uːklɪər] kortikonukleäre/kortikobulbäre Fasern *pl*, Fibrae corticonucleares.
corticonuclear tract kortikobulbäre Bahn *f*, Tractus corticonuclearis.
cor·ti·cop·e·tal [kɔːrtɪˈkɒpətəl] *adj* kortikopetal.
corticopetal fibers → cortical afferents.
cor·ti·co·pon·tine [ˌkɔːrtɪkəʊˈpɒntaɪn, -tiːn] *adj* Hirnrinde/Cortex u. Brücke/Pons betr. *od*. verbindend, kortikopontin.
corticopontine fibers Großhirn-Brückenfasern *pl*, kortikopontine Fasern *pl*, Fibrae corticopontinae.
corticopontine tract *old* → corticopontine fibers.
cor·ti·co·pon·to·cer·e·bel·lar fibers [ˌ-ˌpɒntəʊˌserəˈbelər] kortikopontozerebellare Fasern *pl*.
cor·ti·co·pu·pil·lar·y reflex [ˌ-ˈpjuːpəˌleriː, -lərɪ] Haab-Reflex *m*, Rindenreflex *m* der Pupille.
cor·ti·co·re·tic·u·lar fibers [ˌ-rɪˈtɪkjələr] kortikoretikuläre Fasern *pl*, Fibrae corticoreticulares.
cor·ti·co·ru·bral fibers [ˌ-ˈruːbrəl] kortikorubrale Fasern *pl*, Fibrae corticorubrales.
corticorubral tract → corticorubral fibers.
cor·ti·co·spi·nal [ˌ-ˈspaɪnl] *adj* Hirnrinde/Cortex u. Rückenmark/Medulla spinalis betr. *od*. verbindend, kortikospinal.
corticospinal fibers kortikospinale Fasern *pl*, Pyramidenbahnfasern *pl*, Fibrae corticospinales.
corticospinal tract Pyramidenbahn *f*, Tractus corticospinalis/pyramidalis.
   anterior c. direkte/vordere Pyramidenbahn, Tractus pyramidalis/corticospinalis anterior.
   crossed c. → lateral c.
   direct c. → anterior c.
   lateral c. seitliche/gekreuzte Pyramidenbahn, Tractus corticospinalis/pyramidalis lateralis.
   ventral c. → anterior c.
cor·ti·co·ster·oid [ˌ-ˈsterɔɪd, -ˈstɪər-] *n* Kortiko-, Corticosteroid *nt*.
corticosteroid-binding globulin *abbr*. **CBG** Transkortin *nt*, -cortin *nt*, Cortisol-bindendes Globulin *nt abbr*. CBG.
corticosteroid-binding protein → corticosteroid-binding globulin.
corticosteroid-induced glaucoma Kortison-, Cortisonglaukom *nt*.
cor·ti·cos·ter·one [ˌkɔːrtɪˈkɒstərəʊn] *n* Kortiko-, Corticosteron *nt*, Compound B Kendall.
cor·ti·co·stri·a·tal fibers [ˌkɔːrtɪkəʊstraɪˈeɪtl] kortikostriatale Fasern *pl*, Fibrae corticostriatales.
cortico-striatal-spinal degeneration Creutzfeldt-Jakob-Erkrankung *f abbr*. CJE, Creutzfeldt-Jakob-Syndrom *nt*, Jakob-Creutzfeldt-Erkrankung *f*, Jakob-Creutzfeldt-Syndrom *nt*.
cor·ti·co·stri·a·to·spi·nal atrophy [ˌ-ˌstraɪətəʊˈspaɪnl] → cortico-striatal-spinal degeneration.
cor·ti·co·tec·tal fibers [ˌ-ˈtektəl] kortikotektale Fasern *pl*, Fibrae corticotectales.
corticotectal tract Tractus corticotectalis.
cor·ti·co·teg·men·tal fibers [ˌ-ˈtegmentl] kortikotegmentale Fasern *pl*, Fibrae corticotegmentales.

cor·ti·co·tha·lam·ic [ˌ-θəˈlæmɪk] *adj* Hirnrinde/Cortex u. Thalamus betr. *od*. verbindend, kortikothalamisch.
corticothalamic fibers kortikothalamische Fasern *pl*, Fibrae corticothalamicae.
cor·ti·co·trope [ˈ-trəʊp] *n* → corticotroph (cell).
cor·ti·co·troph (cell) [ˈ-trəʊf] ACTH-produzierende Zelle *f* der Adenohypophyse.
cor·ti·co·troph·ic [ˌ-ˈtrɒfɪk] *adj* → corticotropic.
cor·ti·co·tro·phin [ˌ-ˈtrɒfɪn] *n* → corticotropin.
corticotroph-lipotroph (cell) → corticotroph (cell).
cor·ti·co·trop·ic [ˌ-ˈtrɒpɪk] *adj* auf die Nebennierenrinde einwirkend, kortikotrop, adrenokortikotrop.
cor·ti·co·tro·pin [ˌ-ˈtrəʊpɪn] *n* Kortikotropin *nt*, -trophin *nt*, Corticotrophin(um) *nt*, (adreno-)corticotropes Hormon *nt abbr*. ACTH, Adrenokortikotropin *nt*.
corticotropin releasing factor *abbr*. **CRF** Kortikoliberin *nt*, Corticoliberin *nt*, corticotropin releasing factor (*m*) *abbr*. CRF, corticotropin releasing hormone (*nt*) *abbr*. CRH.
corticotropin releasing hormone *abbr*. **CRH** → corticotropin releasing factor.
cor·ti·lymph [ˈkɔːrtɪlɪmf] *n* Tunnellymphe *f*.
cor·ti·sol [ˈkɔːrtɪsɒl, -səʊl] *n* Kortisol *nt*, Cortisol *nt*, Hydrocortison *nt*.
cortisol-binding globulin *abbr*. **CBG** Transkortin *nt*, -cortin *nt*, Cortisol-bindendes Globulin *nt abbr*. CBG.
cortisol dehydrogenase Cortisoldehydrogenase *f*, 11-β-Hydroxysteroiddehydroxygenase *f*.
cor·ti·sone [ˈkɔːrtɪzəʊn] *n* Kortison *nt*, Cortison *nt*.
co·run·dum [kəˈrʌndəm] *n* Korund *m*.
cor·us·ca·tion [ˌkɔːrəˈskeɪʃn, ˌkar-] *n neuro*., *psychia*. (Auf-)Blitzen *nt*; Funkeln *nt*.
cor villosum *patho*. Zottenherz *nt*, Cor villosum *nt*.
Corvisart [kɔrviˈsaːr]: **C.'s disease** *card*. Fallot'-Tetralogie *f* mit Arcus aortae dexter, Corvisart-(Fallot-)Komplex *m*.
C.'s facies Corvisart-Gesicht *nt*.
cor·ym·bi·form [kəˈrɪmbəfɔːrm] *adj* gehäuft, gruppiert, korymbiform.
cor·ym·bose [ˈkɔːrɪmbəʊs, kəˈrɪm-] *adj* → corymbiform.
corymbose syphilid Bombensyphilid *nt*, korymbiformes Syphilid *nt*.
Cor·y·ne·bac·te·ri·a·ce·ae [ˌkɔːrənɪbækˌtɪərɪˈeɪsɪˌiː] *pl micro*. Corynebacteriaceae *pl*.
Cor·y·ne·bac·te·ri·um [ˌ-bækˈtɪərɪəm] *n micro*. Corynebacterium *nt*.
   C. diphtheriae Diphtheriebazillus *m*, -bakterium *nt* (Klebs-)Löffler-Bazillus *m*, Corynebacterium/Bact. diphtheriae.
   C. pseudodiphtheriticum Löffler'-Pseudodiphtheriebazillus *m*, Corynebacterium pseudodiphtheriticum.
   C. pseudotuberculosis Preisz-Nocard-Bazillus *m*, Corynebacterium pseudotuberculosis.
cor·y·ne·bac·te·ri·um [ˌ-bækˈtɪərɪəm] *n*, *pl* **-ria** [-rɪə] *micro*. 1. Korynebakterium *nt*, Corynebacterium *nt*. 2. koryneformes Bakterium *nt*, Diphtheroid *nt*.
co·ryn·e·form [kəˈrɪnəfɔːrm] *adj micro*. keulenförmig, koryneform.
coryneform bacterium → corynebakterium 2.
co·ry·za [kəˈraɪzə] *n* (Virus-)Schnupfen *m*, Nasenkatarrh *m*, Koryza *f*, Coryza *f*, Rhinitis acuta.
coryza virus Rhinovirus *nt*.
cos·met·ic [kazˈmetɪk] **I** *n* kosmetisches

cosmetic dermatitis

Mittel *nt*, Kosmetikum *nt*. **II** *adj* **1.** kosmetisch, Schönheits-. **2.** *fig.* kosmetisch, (nur) oberflächlich.
cosmetic dermatitis allergische Kontaktdermatitis *f* durch Kosmetika, Dermatitis cosmetica.
cosmetic operation kosmetische Operation *f*.
cosmetic surgery kosmetische Chirurgie *f*, Schönheitschirurgie *f*.
cos·mic ['kazmɪk] *adj* das Weltall betr., kosmisch.
cos·mi·cal ['kazmɪkl] *adj* → cosmic.
cosmic rays *phys.* kosmische Strahlung *f*, Höhenstrahlung *f*.
cos·mo·pol·i·tan relapsing fever [ˌkazmə-'palɪtn] epidemisches (europäisches) Rückfallfieber *nt*, Läuserückfallfieber *nt*.
cos·ta ['kastə] *n*, *pl* **-tae** [-tiː] **1.** *anat.* Rippe *f*, Costa *f*, Os costale. **2.** *micro.* Randfaden *m*.
cos·tal ['kastl, 'kɒstl] *adj* Rippe(n) betr., kostal, Rippen-, Kostal-.
costal angle *anat.* Angulus costae.
costal arch Rippenbogen *m*, Arcus costalis.
costal arch reflex Rippenbogenreflex *m*.
costal bone knöchernes Rippenteil *nt*, Os costale.
costal branch of internal thoracic artery, lateral seitlicher Rippenast *m* der A. thoracica interna, Ramus costalis lateralis (a. thoracicae internae).
costal cartilage Rippenknorpel *m*, Cartilago costalis.
costal chondritis 1. → costochondritis. **2.** Tietze-Syndrom *nt*.
costal fossa Fovea costalis.
inferior c. Fovea costalis inferior.
superior c. Fovea costalis superior.
transverse c. Fovea costalis proc. transversi.
c. of transverse process → transverse c.
costal fovea Fovea costalis.
inferior c. Fovea costalis inferior.
superior c. Fovea costalis superior.
transverse c. Fovea costalis proc. transversi.
cos·tal·gia [kas'tældʒ(ɪ)ə] *n* Rippenschmerz *m*, Kostalgie *f*.
costal groove Rippenfurche *f*, Sulcus costae.
costal incisures of sternum Incc. costales.
costal notches of sternum Incc. costales.
costal pit Fovea costalis interior.
c. of transverse process Fovea costalis proc. transversi.
costal pleura Rippenfell *nt*, Pleura costalis.
costal pleurisy Rippenfellentzündung *f*.
costal process Lendenwirbelquerfortsatz *m*, Proc. costalis.
costal respiration Brustatmung *f*.
costal sulcus → costal groove.
costal surface of scapula Rippenfläche *f* der Skapula, Facies costalis/scapulae anterior.
costal tuberosity of clavicle Impressio lig. costoclavicularis.
cos·ta·tec·to·my [ˌkastə'tɛktəmɪ] *n* → costectomy.
cos·tec·to·my [kas'tɛktəmɪ] *n chir., ortho.* Rippenresektion *f*, -exzision *f*, Kostektomie *f*.
Costen ['kastn] **C.'s syndrome** Costen-Syndrom *nt*, temporomandibuläres Syndrom *nt*.
cos·ti·car·ti·lage [ˌkastɪ'kaːrtlɪdʒ] *n* → costal cartilage.
cos·ti·cer·vi·cal [ˌ-'sɜrvɪkəl] *adj* Rippe(n)/Costa(e) u. Hals/Cervix betr. *od.* verbindend, kostozervikal.

cos·ti·form ['-fɔːrm] *adj* rippenförmig.
co·stim·u·la·tor [kəʊ'stɪmjəleɪtər] *n biochem., genet.* Kostimulator *m*.
cos·ti·spi·nal [ˌkastɪ'spaɪnl] *adj* Rippe(n) u. Wirbelsäule betr. *od.* verbindend, kostospinal, spinokostal.
cos·tive ['kastɪv, 'kɔs-] *adj* Verstopfung/Obstipation betr. *od.* verursachend, verstopft, obstipiert, konstipiert.
cos·tive·ness ['-nɪs] *n* → constipation.
costo- *pref.* Rippen-, Kosto-.
cos·to·cen·tral [ˌkastə'sɛntrəl] *adj* Rippen u. Wirbelkörper betr., kostozentral, kostovertebral.
costocentral articulation Artic. capitis costae/costalis.
costocentral joint → costocentral articulation.
costocentral ligament: anterior c. Lig. capitis costae radiatum.
intraarticular c. Lig. capitis costae intraarticulare.
cos·to·cer·vi·cal (arterial) axis [ˌ-'sɜrvɪkl] Truncus costocervicalis *abbr.* TCC.
costocervical trunk Truncus costocervicalis *abbr.* TCC.
cos·to·chon·dral [ˌ-'kandrəl] *adj* Rippenknorpel betr., kostochondral, Rippenknorpel-.
costochondral articulations *anat.* Articc. costochondrales.
costochondral joints → costochondral articulations.
costochondral separation *ortho.* kostochondraler Abriß *m*.
costochondral syndrome kostochondrales Syndrom *nt*.
cos·to·chon·dri·tis [ˌ-kan'draɪtɪs] *n* Rippenknorpelentzündung *f*, Kostochondritis *f*.
cos·to·cla·vic·u·lar [ˌ-klə'vɪkjələr] *adj* Rippen u. Schlüsselbein betr., kostoklavikulär, -klavikular.
costoclavicular ligament Lig. costoclaviculare.
costoclavicular line Parasternallinie *f*, Linea parasternalis.
costoclavicular synchondrosis → costoclavicular ligament.
costoclavicular syndrome Kostobrachial-, Kostoklavikularsyndrom *nt*.
cos·to·col·ic ligament [ˌ-'kalɪk] Lig. phrenicocolicum.
cos·to·cor·a·coid [ˌ-'kɔːrəkɔɪd] *adj* Rippen u. Proc. coracoideus betr., kostokorakoid.
costocoracoid ligament Lig. transversum scapulae superius.
cos·to·di·a·phrag·mat·ic recess/sinus [ˌ-ˌdaɪəfræg'mætɪk] Kostodiaphragmalsinus *m*, -spalte *f*, Sinus phrenicocostalis, Rec. costodiaphragmaticus.
cos·to·gen·ic [ˌ-'dʒɛnɪk] *adj* von einer Rippe (ab-)stammend.
cos·to·in·fe·ri·or [ˌ-ɪn'fɪərɪər] *adj* die unteren Rippen betr.
cos·to·me·di·as·ti·nal recess [ˌ-ˌmiːdɪə-'staɪnl] Kostomediastinalsinus *m*, -spalte *f*, Rec. costomediastinalis.
cos·to·pec·to·ral reflex [ˌ-'pɛktərəl] Pektoralis-major-Reflex *m*.
cos·to·phren·ic [ˌ-'frɛnɪk] *adj* Rippen/Costae u. Zwerchfell betr., kostophrenisch, kostodiaphragmal.
costophrenic angle Rippen-Zwerchfell--Winkel *m*.
costophrenic septal lines Kerley-B-Linien *pl*.
cos·to·pleu·ral [ˌ-'plʊərəl] *adj* Rippen/Costae u. Pleura betr., kostopleural.
cos·to·scap·u·lar [ˌ-'skæpjələr] *adj* Rippen/Costae u. Schulterblatt/Scapula

betr., kostoscapular.
cos·to·scap·u·la·ris [ˌ-ˌskæpjə'lɛərɪs] *n* M. serratus anterior.
cos·to·ster·nal [ˌ-'stɜrnl] *adj* Rippen u. Brustbein betr., sternokostal, kostosternal.
costosternal articulations Brustbein-Rippen-Gelenk *pl*, Sternokostalgelenke *pl*, Articc. sternocostales.
costosternal joints → costosternal articulations.
costosternal ligaments, radiate Ligg. sternocostalia radiata.
cos·to·ster·no·plas·ty [ˌ-'stɜrnəplæstɪ] *n ortho.* Rippen-Sternum-Plastik *f*, Kostosternoplastik *f*.
cos·to·su·pe·ri·or [ˌ-suː'pɪərɪər] *adj* die oberen Rippen betr.
cos·to·tome ['-təʊm] *n chir., ortho.* Rippenmesser *nt*, Kostotom *nt*.
cos·tot·o·my [kas'tatəmɪ] *n chir., ortho.* Rippendurchtrennung *f*, Kostotomie *f*.
cos·to·trans·verse [ˌ-træns'vɜrs, -'trænsvɜrs] *adj* zwischen Rippen u. Querfortsatz liegend, kostotransversal.
costotransverse articulation Artic. costotransversaria.
cos·to·trans·ver·sec·to·my [ˌ-ˌtrænzvər-'sɛktəmɪ] *n ortho., chir.* Kostotransversektomie *f*.
costotransverse foramen For. costotransversarium.
costotransverse joint → costotransverse articulation.
costotransverse ligament Lig. costotransversarium/costotransversum.
lateral c. Lig. costotransversarium laterale.
superior c. Lig. costotransversarium superius.
cos·to·ver·te·bral [ˌ-'vɜrtəbrəl] *adj* Rippen u. Wirbel betr., kostovertebral.
costovertebral angle *abbr.* CVA Kostovertebralwinkel *m*.
costovertebral articulations Kostovertebralgelenke *pl*, Articc. costovertebrales.
lateral c. Kostotransversalgelenk, Artic. costotransversaria.
medial c. Artic. capitis costae/costalis.
costovertebral joints → costovertebral articulations.
costovertebral ligament Lig. capitis costae radiatum.
cos·to·xiph·oid [ˌ-'zɪfɔɪd] *adj* Rippen u. Proc. xiphoideus betr.
costoxiphoid ligaments Ligg. costoxiphoidea.
co·sub·strate [kəʊ'sʌbstreɪt] *n biochem.* Co-, Kosubstrat *nt*.
co·syn·tro·pin [ˌkəʊsɪn'trəʊpɪn] *n* Kosyntropin *nt*, Tetracosactid *nt*, β¹-24-Kortikotropin *nt*.
cot [kat] *n* Kinderbett(chen *nt*) *nt*.
Cotard [kə'taːr] **C.'s syndrome** Cotard-Syndrom *nt*.
cot death *ped.* plötzlicher Kindstod *m*, Krippentod *m*, sudden infant death syndrome (*nt*) *abbr.* SIDS, Mors subita infantum.
COTe *abbr.* → cathodal opening tetanus.
co·throm·bo·plas·tin [ˌkəʊˌθrambəʊ'plæstɪn] *n* Prokonvertin *nt*, -convertin *nt*, Faktor VII *m abbr.* F V II, Autothrombin I *nt*, Serum-Prothrombin-Conversion-Accelerator *m abbr.* SPCA, stabiler Faktor *m*.
co·ti·nine ['katənɪːn] *n* Cotinin *nt*.
co·trans·duc·tion [ˌkəʊtrænz'dʌkʃn] *n biochem., genet.* Ko-, Cotransduktion *f*.
co·trans·mit·ter [ˌ-'mɪtər] *n* Cotransmitter *m*.
co·trans·port [kəʊ'trænspɔːrt, -pəʊrt] *n*

physiol. gekoppelter Transport *m*, Co-transport *m*, Symport *m*.
Cotrel ['kɑtrel]: **C. brace** Cotrel-Korsett *nt*.
C. cast *ortho.* EDF-Gips [Extension, Derotation, Flexion] *m*, Cotrel-Gips(verband *m*) *m*.
co-trimoxazole *n pharm.* Cotrimoxazol *nt*.
Cotte [kɔt]: **C.'s operation** *neurochir.*, *ortho.* Cotte-Operation *f.*
Cotting ['kɑtɪŋ]: **C.'s operation** *derm.*, *ortho.* Cotting-Operation *f.*
cot·ton ['kɑtn] **I** *n* **1.** Baumwolle *f*; Baumwollpflanze *f.* **2.** Baumwollstoff *m*, -gewebe *nt*, -garn *nt*, -kleidung *f.* **II** *adj* baumwollen, Baumwoll-.
cotton applicator *chir.* Watteträger *m.*
cotton-dust asthma Baumwollfieber *nt*, Baumwoll(staub)pneumokoniose *f*, Byssinose *f.*
cotton effect Cotton-Effekt *m.*
cotton-mill fever → cotton-dust asthma.
cot·ton-pox ['kɑtnpɑks] *n* Alastrim *nt*, weiße Pocken *pl*, Variola minor.
cotton probe → cotton wool probe.
cotton wool *Brit.* (Verbands-)Watte *f.*
cotton wool exudates → cotton wool spots.
cotton wool patches → cotton wool spots.
cotton wool probe *chir.* Watteträger *m.*
cotton wool spots *ophthal.* Cotton-wool--Herde *pl.*
Cotugno [koʊ'tuːnjoʊ]: **C.'s disease** → Cotunnius' disease.
Cotunnius [koʊ'tʊniəs]: **C.' aqueduct/canal 1.** Cotunnius-Kanal *m*, Aqu(a)eductus vestibuli. **2.** Canaliculus cochleae.
C.' disease Cotunnius-Syndrom *nt*, Ischiassyndrom *nt.*
C.'s liquid Cotunnius-Flüssigkeit *f*, Perilymphe *f*, -lympha *f*, Liquor Cotunnii.
nerve of C. N. nasopalatinus.
C.' space Cotunnius'-Raum *m.*
cot value *genet.* Cot-Wert *m.*
cot·y·le·don [ˌkɑtə'liːdn] *n* **1.** Zottenbaum *m*, -büschel *nt*, Plazentalappen *m*, Cotyledo *f*, Kotyledo *f*, Kotyledone *f.* **2.** *bio.* Keimblatt *nt* (*der Samenpflanzen*), Cotyledo *f*, Kotyledone *f.*
cot·y·le·don·ar·y placenta [ˌ-'liːdneriː] Placenta cotyledonaria.
cot·y·loid ['kɑtlɔɪd] *adj anat.*, *bio.* **1.** schalenförmig. **2.** Azetabulum betr., azetabular, azetabulär.
cotyloid cavity Hüft(gelenks)pfanne *f*, Azetabulum *nt*, Acetabulum *nt.*
cotyloid incisure → cotyloid notch.
cotyloid ligament Labrum acetabulare.
cotyloid notch Inc. acetabuli/acetabularis.
cough [kɔf, kɑf] **I** *n* **1.** Husten *m*; Tussis *f.* **to have a ~** Husten haben. **2.** Husten *nt.* **II** *vt* (ab-, aus-)husten. **III** *vi* husten.
cough out/up → cough II. **to ~ up blood** Blut husten.
cough drop Hustenbonbon *nt*, -pastille *f.*
cough·ing bout ['kɔfɪŋ, 'kɑf-] Hustenanfall *m.*
coughing center Hustenzentrum *nt.*
coughing reflex Hustenreflex *m.*
cough lozenge → cough drop.
cough plate *micro.* Hustenplatte *f.*
cough syncope Hustenschlag *m*, -synkope *f.*
cough syrup Hustensaft *m*, -sirup *m.*
Coulomb ['kuːlɑm, kuː'lɑm, -loʊm]: **C.'s law** Coulomb'-Gesetz *nt.*
cou·lomb *n abbr.* **C** Coulomb *nt abbr.* C.
Coul·ter counter ['koʊltər] *lab.* Coulter--Counter *m.*
cou·ma·rin ['kuːmərɪn] *n* **1.** Kumarin *nt*, Cumarin *nt.* **2.** Kumarinderivat *nt.*
Councilman ['kaʊnsəlmən]: **C.'s bodies/lesions** *patho.* Councilman-Körperchen *pl.*
coun·sel ['kaʊnsəl] **I** *n* **1.** Rat(schlag *m*) *m*; Beratung *f*, Beratschlagung *f*; Entschluß *m*, Absicht *f*, Plan *m.* **2.** (Rechts-)Anwalt *m*, (-)Berater *m*, (-)Beistand *m.* **II** *vt* jdn. raten, jdm. einen Rat geben *od.* erteilen.
coun·sel·ing ['kaʊnsəlɪŋ] *n* Beratung *f.*
count [kaʊnt] **I** *n* **1.** (Ab-, Auf-, Aus-)Zählung *f*, Zählen *nt*, (Be-)Rechnung *f.* **2.** Ergebnis *nt*, (An-)Zahl *f*, Menge *f.* **II** *vt* **3.** (ab-, auf-, aus-)zählen, (be-)rechnen. **4.** mitzählen, berücksichtigen, mitrechnen. **III** *vi* rechnen.
coun·ter¹ ['kaʊntər] *n* Zähler *m*, Zählvorrichtung *f*, Zählgerät *nt.*
coun·ter² ['kaʊntər] **I** *n* Gegenteil *nt.* **II** *adj* entgegengesetzt, Gegen-. **III** *vt* entgegenwirken.
coun·ter·act [ˌkaʊntər'ækt] *vt* entgegenwirken, -arbeiten; kompensieren, neutralisieren; bekämpfen.
coun·ter·ac·tion [ˌ-'ækʃn] *n* Gegenwirkung *f*; Neutralisierung *f*; Bekämpfung *f*, Gegenmaßnahme *f.*
coun·ter·ac·tive [ˌ-'æktɪv] *adj* entgegenwirkend, Gegen-.
coun·ter·at·trac·tion [ˌ-ə'trækʃn] *n phys.* entgegengesetzte Anziehungskraft *f.*
coun·ter·bal·ance [*n* '-ˌbælənts; *v* ˌ-'bælənts] (*a. fig.*, *techn.*) **I** *n* Gegengewicht (*to zu*). **II** *vt* ein Gegengewicht bilden zu, ausgleichen, aufwiegen.
coun·ter·blow ['-bloʊ] *n* (*a. fig.*) Gegenschlag *m.*
coun·ter·check [*n* '-tʃek; *v* ˌ-'tʃek] **I** *n* **1.** Gegenwirkung *f.* **2.** Gegen-, Nachkontrolle *f.* **II** *vt* **3.** entgegenwirken. **4.** gegen-, nachprüfen, kontrollieren.
coun·ter·clock·wise [ˌ-'klɑkwaɪz] *adj* gegen den Uhrzeigersinn/die Uhrzeigerrichtung, nach links.
coun·ter·cur·rent ['-kɜrənt] *n* Gegenstrom *m*, -strömung *f.*
countercurrent diffusion Gegenstromdiffusion *f.*
countercurrent distribution *phys.* Gegenstromverteilung *f.*
countercurrent exchange Gegenstromaustausch *m.*
countercurrent immunoelectrophoresis → counterimmunoelectrophoresis.
countercurrent mechanism *phys.* Gegenstromprinzip *nt.*
countercurrent principle *phys.* Gegenstromprinzip *nt.*
countercurrent system Gegenstromsystem *nt.*
coun·ter·ef·fect [ˌ-ɪ'fekt] *n* Gegenwirkung *f.*
coun·ter·e·lec·tro·pho·re·sis [ˌ-ə ˌlektroʊfə'riːsɪs] *n* → counterimmunoelectrophoresis.
coun·ter·ex·ten·sion [ˌ-ɪk'stenʃn] *n* → counterextraction.
coun·ter·im·mu·no·e·lec·tro·pho·re·sis [ˌ-ˌɪmjənoʊəˌlektroʊfə'riːsɪs] *n abbr.* **CIE** Gegen(immuno)elektrophorese *f.*
coun·ter·in·ci·sion [ˌ-ɪn'sɪʒn] *n chir.* Gegenschnitt *m*, -inzision *f.*
coun·ter·ir·ri·tant [ˌ-'ɪrətənt] **I** *n pharm.* Gegenreizmittel *nt.* **II** *adj* einen Gegenreiz hervorrufend.
coun·ter·ir·ri·ta·tion [ˌ-ɪrə'teɪʃn] *n* Gegenreiz *m*, -reizung *f.*
coun·ter·meas·ure ['-meʒər] *n* Gegenmaßnahme *f.*
coun·ter·o·pen·ing [ˌ-'oʊp(ə)nɪŋ] *n chir.* Gegenöffnung *f*, -punktion *f.*
coun·ter·poi·son ['-pɔɪzən] *n* Gegengift *nt*, Gegenmittel *nt*, Antitoxin *nt*, Antidot *nt.*
coun·ter·pres·sure ['-preʃər] *n* Gegendruck *m.*
coun·ter·pul·sa·tion [ˌ-pʌl'seɪʃn] *n card.* Gegenpulsation *f.*
coun·ter·punc·ture ['-pʌŋ(k)tʃər] *n* → counteropening.
coun·ter·stain [*n* '-steɪn; *v* ˌ-'steɪn] **I** *n* Gegen-, Kontrastfärbung *f.* **II** *vt* gegenfärben.
coun·ter·trac·tion [ˌ-'trækʃn] *n ortho.* Gegenzug *m*, -extension *f.*
coun·ter·trans·fer·ence [ˌ-trænz'fɜrəns] *n psycho.*, *psychia.* Gegenübertragung *f.*
coun·ter·trans·port [ˌkaʊntər'trænspɔrt, -pɔrt] *n* Austausch-, Gegen-, Countertransport *m*, Antiport *m.*
coun·ter·weigh [ˌ-'weɪ] *vt* → counterbalance II.
coun·ter·weight ['-weɪt] *n* (*a. fig.*) Gegengewicht *nt* (*to zu*).
count·ing cell ['kaʊntɪŋ] → counting chamber.
counting chamber *lab.* Zählkammer *f.*
counts per minute *abbr.* **c.p.m.** *radiol.* counts per minute *abbr.* c.p.m.
counts per second *abbr.* **c.p.s.** *radiol.* counts per second *abbr.* c.p.s.
coup [kuː] *n* Schlag *m*, Hieb *m.*
cou·ple ['kʌpl] **I** *n* Paar *nt*; Ehepaar *nt.* **a ~ of** zwei; ein paar, einige. **a ~ of times** ein paarmal. **II** *vt* **1.** *bio.* paaren. **2.** (zusammen-)koppeln, verbinden; *techn.* (ver-, an-)kuppeln. **III** *vi bio.* s. paaren.
cou·pled ['kʌpəld] *adj* **1.** (*a. fig.*) gepaart, verbunden (*with* mit). **2.** *techn.* gekoppelt; ge-, verkoppelt.
coupled beat *card.* Bigeminus *m.*
coupled pulse → coupled rhythm.
coupled reactions gekoppelte Reaktionen *pl.*
coupled rhythm Bigeminus *m*, Bigeminuspuls *m*, -rhythmus *m*, Pulsus bigeminus.
coupled transport → cotransport.
cou·pling ['kʌplɪŋ] *n* **1.** Verbindung *f*, Vereinigung *f.* **2.** *bio.* Paarung *f.* **3.** *techn.* Kopplung *f*, Kupplung *f.*
coupling factor *biochem.* Kopplungsfaktor *m.*
cour·ba·ture ['kʊrbətʊər; *French* kurba'tyːr] *n* **1.** Muskelziehen *nt*, -schmerz(en *pl*) *m.* **2.** Druckluft-, Caissonkrankheit *f.*
course [kɔrs, kɔərs] *n* **1.** (natürlicher) (Ver-)Lauf *m*, Ablauf *m*, (Fort-)Gang *m.* **in the ~ of** im (Ver-)Lauf, während. **in (the) ~ of time** im Laufe der Zeit. **~ of a disease** Krankheitsverlauf *m.* **2.** Lebenslauf *m*, -bahn *f*, -karriere *f.* **3.** Zyklus *m*, Reihe *f*, Folge *f.* **4.** Kurs *m*, Lehrgang *m.* **5.** Kur *f*, Behandlungszyklus *m.* **to undergo a ~ of treatment** s. einer (längeren) Behandlung unterziehen. **6.** Reihenfolge *f*, Aufeinanderfolge *f.* **7.** *fig.* Verfahren *nt*, Methode *f*, Kurs *m.* **8.** Monatsblutung *f*, Periode *f*, Regel *f*, Menses *pl*, Menstruation *f.*
c. of action Vorgehen(sweise *f*) *nt.*
Courvoisier [kʊrvwa'sje]: **C.'s gallbladder** Courvoisier'-Gallenblase *f.*
C.'s law Courvoisier'-Regel *f.*
C.'s sign Courvoisier'-Zeichen *nt.*
Courvoisier-Terrier [tɛ'rje]: **C.-T. syndrome** Courvoisier-Zeichen *nt.*
Couvelaire [kuve'lɛːr]: **C. syndrome/uterus** Couvelaire-Uterus *m*, -Syndrom *nt*, Uterusapoplexie *f*, uteroplazentare Apoplexie *f*, Apoplexia uteroplacentaris.
cou·ver·cle [kuː'vɜrkl] *n hema.*, *patho.* extraversales Blutgerinnsel *nt.*
co·val·ence [koʊ'veɪləns] *n chem.* Kovalenz *f.*
co·va·len·cy [koʊ'veɪlənsɪ] *n* → covalence.
co·va·lent [koʊ'veɪlənt] *adj chem.* kovalent.

covalent activation *biochem.* kovalente Aktivierung *f.*
covalent bond *chem.* Atombindung *f*, kovalente Bindung *f.*
covalent catalysis kovalente Katalyse *f.*
covalent modification kovalente Modifikation *f.*
covalent structure *chem.* Primärstruktur *f.*
co·var·i·ance [kəʊ'veərɪəns] *n stat.* Kovarianz *f.*
cov·er ['kʌvər] **I** *n* **1.** (*a. fig.*) Decke *f*; Ab-, Bedeckung *f*; Deckel *m.* **2.** Hülle *f*, Umhüllung *f*, Mantel *m*; Überzug *m.* **3.** → coverage. **4.** *techn.* Schutzmantel *m*, -haube *f*, -kappe *f.* **5.** Schutz *m* (*from* vor, gegen). **II** *vt* **6.** zu-, bedecken (*with* mit). **.ed with** voll mit. **7.** um-, einhüllen, bedecken, überziehen (*in*, *with*); einwickeln. **8.** *~ o.s. a. fig.* (s.) schützen (*from*, *against* vor, gegen). **9.** umfassen, beinhalten, enthalten, behandeln. **10.** *stat.* erfassen. **11.** *bio.* decken, bespringen.
cov·er·age ['kʌv(ə)rɪdʒ] *n* **1.** *pharm.* (antibiotische) Abdeckung *f.* **2.** *stat.* Erfassung *f.*
cover cell → covering cell.
cov·ered ['kʌvərd] *adj* be-, gedeckt, überzogen.
covered perforation *chir.* gedeckte Perforation *f.*
cov·er·glass ['kʌvərglæs] *n* Deckglas *nt.*
cov·er·ing ['kʌvərɪŋ] **I** *n* Umhüllung *f.* **II** *adj* (be-)deckend, Deck-, Schutz-, Hüll-.
covering cell Hüll-, Mantel-, Deckzelle *f.*
covering epithelium Deckepithel *nt*, oberflächenbildendes Epithel *n.*
cov·er·slip ['kʌvərslɪp] *n* → coverglass.
cover test *ophthal.* Abdecktest *m.*
cover-uncover test *ophthal.* Abdeck-Aufdecktest *m.*
Cowden ['kaʊdən]: **C.'s disease/syndrome** multiple Hamartome-Syndrom *nt*, Cowden-Krankheit *f*, -Syndrom *nt.*
Cowdry ['kaʊdrɪ]: **C. bodies** Cowdry-Körper *pl.*
Cowen ['kaʊən]: **C.'s sign** Cowen-Zeichen *nt.*
Cowper ['kuːpər, 'kaʊ-]: **C.'s gland** Cowper'-Drüse *f*, Bulbourethraldrüse *f*, Gl. bulbourethralis.
C.'s cyst Cowper-Zyste *f*, Retentionszyste *f* der Gl. bulbourethralis.
C.'s ligament Cowper'-Band *nt.*
pubic ligament of C. Leistenband *nt*, Lig. inguinale, Arcus inguinale.
cow·pe·ri·an duct [kaʊ'pɪərɪən, kuː-] Ductus gl. bulbourethralis.
cow·per·i·tis [kaʊpəˈraɪtɪs] *n urol.* Entzündung *f* der Cowper-Drüse, Cowperitis *f.*
cow·pox [ˈkaʊpɒks] *n* Kuhpocken *pl.*
cowpox virus *micro.* Kuhpockenvirus *nt.*
cow's milk anemia [kaʊ] *hema., ped.* Kuhmilchanämie *f.*
Cox [kɒks]: **C. vaccine** Cox-Vakzine *f.*
cox·a [ˈkɒksə] *n*, *pl* **cox·ae** [ˈkɒksiː] Hüfte *f*, Hüftregion *f*, Coxa *f*, Regio coxalis.
coxa adducta → coxa vara.
coxa flexa → coxa vara.
cox·al bone [ˈkɒksəl] *adj* Hüftbein *nt*, -knochen *m*, Os coxae/pelvicum.
cox·al·gia [kɒkˈsældʒ(ɪ)ə] *n* **1.** Hüft(gelenk)schmerz *m*, Koxalgie *f*, Coxalgia *f.* **2.** → coxarthrosis. **3.** → coxitis.
cox·al·gic pelvis [kɒkˈsældʒɪk] Koxitisbecken *nt.*
coxa plana Perthes-Krankheit *f*, Morbus Perthes *m*, Perthes-Legg-Calvé-Krankheit *f*, Legg-Calvé-Perthes'-(Waldenström)-Krankheit *f*, Osteochondropathia deformans coxae juvenilis, Coxa plana *n.* (idiopathica).

cox·ar·thri·a [kɒksˈɑːrθrɪə] *n* → coxitis.
cox·ar·thri·tis [ˌkɒksɑːrˈθraɪtɪs] *n* → coxitis.
cox·ar·throp·a·thy [kɒksɑːrˈθrɒpəθɪ] *n* Hüftgelenk(s)erkrankung *f*, Koxarthropathie *f.*
cox·ar·thro·sis [kɒksɑːrˈθrəʊsɪs] *n* Koxarthrose *f*, Coxarthrosis *f*, Arthrosis deformans coxae, Malum coxae senile.
coxa valga Coxa valga.
coxa vara Coxa vara.
adolescent c. Lösung *f* der Femurepiphyse, Epiphyseolysis/Epiphysiolysis capitis femoris, Coxa vara adolescentium.
Cox·i·el·la [kɒksɪˈelə] *n micro.* Coxiella *f.*
cox·i·tis [kɒkˈsaɪtɪs] *n* Hüftgelenk(s)entzündung *f*, Koxitis *f*, Coxitis *f*, Kox-, Coxarthritis *f.*
cox·o·dyn·ia [ˌkɒksəʊˈdiːnɪə] *n* → coxalgia 1.
cox·o·fem·o·ral [ˌ-ˈfemərəl] *adj* Hüfte u. Oberschenkel betr., koxofemoral.
coxofemoral articulation Hüftgelenk *nt*, Artic. coxae/iliofemoralis.
coxofemoral joint → coxofemoral articulation.
cox·o·tu·ber·cu·lo·sis [ˌ-t(j)uːˌbɜːrkjəˈləʊsɪs] *n* **1.** Hüftgelenktuberkulose *f.* **2.** tuberkulöse Hüftgelenkentzündung/Koxitis *f*, Coxitis tuberculosa.
Cox·sack·ie encephalitis [kɒkˈsækɪ] Coxsackie-Enzephalitis *f.*
Coxsackie virus → coxsackievirus.
cox·sack·ie·vi·rus [kɒkˈsækɪvaɪrəs] *n micro.* Coxsackievirus *nt.*
co·zy·mase [kəʊˈzaɪmeɪs] *n* Nicotinamid-adenin-dinucleotid *nt* abbr. NAD, Diphosphopyridinnucleotid *nt* abbr. DPN, Cohydrase I *f*, Coenzym I *nt.*
C3PA *abbr.* → C3 proactivator.
C3PAase *abbr.* C3 proactivator convertase.
C3PA convertase → C3 proactivator convertase.
CPAP *abbr.* → continuous positive airway pressure (breathing).
CPAP breathing → continuous positive airway pressure (breathing).
C₄-pathway *n biochem.* Hatch-Slack-Zyklus *m*, C₄-Zyklus *m.*
CPD *abbr.* → citrate phosphate dextrose.
CPE *abbr.* → cytopathic effect.
C peptide C-Peptid *nt.*
CPK *abbr.* [creatine phosphokinase] → creatine kinase.
c.p.m. *abbr.* → counts per minute.
CPPB *abbr.* [continuous positive pressure breathing] → continuous positive airway pressure (breathing).
CPPD *abbr.* → calcium pyrophosphate dihydrate.
CPPD crystal deposition disease → CPPD disease.
CPPD disease Chrondokalzinose *f*, Pseudogicht *f*, Calciumpyrophosphatdihydrataablagerung *f*, CPPD-Ablagerung *f.*
CPPV *abbr.* → continuous positive pressure ventilation.
CPR *abbr.* → cardiopulmonary resuscitation.
C3 proactivator *abbr.* **C3PA** *immun.* C3--Proaktivator *m*, Faktor B *m.*
C3 proactivator convertase *abbr.* **C3PAase** *immun.* C3-Proaktivatorkonvertase *f*, Faktor D *m.*
C-protein *n* C-Protein *n.*
c.p.s. *abbr.* → counts per second.
CR *abbr.* **1.** → complete remission. **2.** → conditioned reflex.
Cr *abbr.* **1.** → chromium. **2.** → creatine. **3.** → creatinine.
crab hand [kræb] *derm.* Erysipeloid *nt*, Rotlauf *m*, Schweinerotlauf *m*, Pseudoerysipel *nt*, Rosenbach'-Krankheit *f*, Erythema migrans.
crab louse *micro.* Filzlaus *f*, Phthirus pubis, Pediculus pubis.
Crabtree [ˈkræbtriː]: **C. effect** Crabtree--Effekt *m.*
crack [kræk] **I** *n* **1.** Krach *m*, Knall *m*, Knacks *m*, Knacken *nt.* **2.** Sprung *m*, Riß *m.* **3.** *ortho.* Haarbruch *m*, Knochenfissur *f.* **4.** Spalt(e *f*) *m*, Schlitz *m*, Ritz(e *f*) *m.* **5.** *forens.* Crack *nt.* **II** *vt* zerbrechen, (zer-)spalten, (zer-)sprengen. **III** *vi* **6.** krachen, knallen, knacken. **7.** (zer-)springen, (zer-)platzen, (zer-)bersten, (zer-)brechen, rissig werden, (auf-)reißen, einen Sprung bekommen.
cracked heel [krækt] grübchenförmige Keratolysen *pl*, Keratoma (plantaris) sulcatum.
cracked-pot resonance → cracked-pot sound.
cracked-pot sound Geräusch *nt* des gesprungenen Topfes, Bruit du pot fêlé.
cranial c. Macewen-Zeichen *nt*, Schädelschettern *nt.*
crack·le [ˈkrækl] **I** *n* Knistern *nt*, Rasseln *nt*, Krachen *nt*, Prasseln *nt*, Knattern *nt.* **II** *vt* knistern od. rasseln od. krachen lassen. **III** *vi* knistern, rasseln, prasseln, krachen, knattern.
crack·ling rales [ˈkræklɪŋ] *pulmo.* Knisterrasseln *nt.*
cra·dle [ˈkreɪdl] *n* **1.** Wiege *f.* **2.** Bettbügel *m*, Reifenbahre *f.*
cradle cap Milchschorf *m*, frühexsudatives Ekzematoid *nt*, konstitutionelles Säuglingsekzem *nt*, Eccema infantum, Crusta lactea.
Crafoord [ˈkrɑːfɔːrd]: **C.'s clamp** *chir.* Crafoord-Klemme *f.*
Craig [kreɪg]: **C. splint** *ortho.* Craig-Schiene *f.*
Cramer [ˈkreɪmər]: **C.'s splint** *ortho.* Cramer-Schiene *f.*
cramp [kræmp] **I** *n* (Muskel-)Krampf *m*, Crampus *m*, Krampus *m*; Spasmus *m.* **II** *vt* Krämpfe verursachen *od.* auslösen.
cramp·ing [ˈkræmpɪŋ] *adj* krampfartig, krampfend.
cramping pain krampfender/krampfartiger Schmerz *m.*
Crampton [ˈkræmptən]: **C.'s line** Crampton-Linie *f.*
C.'s muscle Brücke'-Fasern *pl*, -Muskel *m*, Fibrae longitudinales/meridionales m. ciliaris.
C.'s test Crampton-Test *m.*
Crandall [ˈkrændl]: **C.'s syndrome** Crandall-Syndrom *nt.*
crani- *pref.* → cranio-.
cra·ni·al [ˈkreɪnɪəl] *adj* kopfwärts, kranial; Schädel betr., Schädel-.
cranial arachnoid (*Gehirn*) Spinnwebenhaut *f*, Arachnoidea (mater) encephali/cranialis.
cranial arteritis (senile) Riesenzellarteriitis *f*, Horton-Riesenzellarteriitis *f*, -Syndrom *nt*, Arteriitis cranialis/gigantocellularis/temporalis.
cranial base Schädelbasis *f*, Basis cranii.
external c. äußere Schädelbasis, Basis cranii externa.
internal c. innere Schädelbasis, Basis cranii interna.
cranial bones Schädelknochen *pl*, Cranialia *pl*, Ossa cranii.
cranial cavity Schädel-, Hirnhöhle *f*, Cavitas cranii.
cranial colliculus oberer/vorderer Hügel *m* der Vierhügelplatte, Colliculus superior.

cranial conduction *physiol.* Knochenleitung *f*.
cranial diameter Schädeldurchmesser *m*.
cranial flexure *embryo.* Scheitelbeuge *f*.
cranial fontanelles Schädelfontanellen *pl*, Fonticuli cranii.
cranial fossa Schädelgrube *f*, Fossa cranii/cranialis.
 anterior c. vordere Schädelgrube, Fossa cranii/cranialis anterior.
 middle c. mittlere Schädelgrube, Fossa cranii/cranialis media.
 posterior c. hintere Schädelgrube, Fossa cranii/cranialis posterior.
cranial index Schädelindex *m*.
cranial lobe of cerebellum kranialer (Kleinhirn-)Lappen *m*, kranialer (Kleinhirn-)Abschnitt *m*, Lobus anterior cerebelli.
cranial meningocele Hirnhautbruch *m*, kraniale Meningozele *f*.
cranial nerve Kopf-, Hirnnerv *m*, N. cranialis/encephalicus.
 eighth c. Vestibulokochlearis *m*, VIII. Hirnnerv, N. vestibulocochlearis [VIII].
 eleventh c. Akzessorius *m*, XI. Hirnnerv, N. accessorius [XI].
 fifth c. Trigeminus *m*, V. Hirnnerv, N. trigeminus [V].
 first c. Riechnerv, Olfaktorius *m*, I. Hirnnerv, N. olfactorius [I].
 fourth c. Trochlearis *m*, IV. Hirnnerv, N. trochlearis [IV].
 ninth c. Glossopharyngeus *m*, IX. Hirnnerv, N. glossopharyngeus [IX].
 second c. Sehnerv, Optikus *m*, II. Hirnnerv, N. opticus [II].
 seventh c. Fazialis *m*, VII. Hirnnerv, N. facialis/intermediofacialis [VII].
 sixth c. Abduzens *m*, VI. Hirnnerv, N. abducens [VI].
 tenth c. Vagus *m*, X. Hirnnerv, N. vagus [X].
 third c. Okulomotorius *m*, III. Hirnnerv, N. oculomotorius [III].
 twelfth c. Hypoglossus *m*, XII. Hirnnerv, N. hypoglossus [XII].
cranial nerve ganglia Hirnnervenganglien *pl*.
cranial nerve nuclei Hirnnervenkerne *pl*, Nuclei nn. cranialium/encephalicorum.
cranial puncture → cisternal puncture.
cranial roots of accessory nerve obere Akzessoriuswurzeln *pl*, Radices craniales n. accessorii, Pars vagalis n. accessorii.
cranial sinuses Durasinus *pl*, Hirnsinus *pl*, Sinus *pl* der Dura mater encephali, Sinus venosi durales, Sinus durae matris.
cranial sutures Schädelnähte *pl*, Suturae cranii/craniales.
cranial synchondroses kraniale Synchondrosen *pl*, Synchondrosen der Schädelknochen, Synchondroses cranii/craniales.
cranial vault Schädeldach *nt*, Kalotte *f*.
Cra·ni·a·ta [ˌkreɪnɪ'eɪtə] *pl* Wirbeltiere *pl*, Vertebraten *pl*, Vertebrata *pl*.
cra·ni·ec·to·my [kreɪnɪ'ektəmɪ] *n ortho., neurochir.* Kraniektomie *f*.
cranio- *pref.* Schädel-, Kranio-.
cra·ni·o·au·ral [ˌkreɪnɪəʊ'ɔːrəl] *adj* Schädel/Cranium u. Ohr betr., kranioaural.
cra·ni·o·buc·cal pouch [ˌ-'bʌkəl] *embryo.* Rathke'-Tasche *f*.
cra·ni·o·car·di·ac reflex [ˌ-'kɑːrdɪæk] kraniokardialer Reflex *m*.
cra·ni·o·car·po·tar·sal dysplasia/dystrophy [ˌ-ˌkɑːpəʊ'tɑːrsl] Freeman-Sheldon-Syndrom *nt*, kranio-karpo-tarsales Dysplasie-Syndrom *nt*, Dysplasia cranio-carpo-tarsalis.

cra·ni·o·cau·dal [ˌ-'kɔːdl] *adj* kraniokaudal.
cra·ni·o·cele ['-siːl] *n* Kraniozele *f*, Enzephalozele *f*.
cra·ni·o·cer·e·bral [ˌ-'serəbrəl] *adj* Schädel/Cranium u. Großhirn/Cerebrum betr., kraniozerebral.
cra·ni·ocl·a·sis [kreɪnɪ'ɒkləsɪs] *n gyn.* Kranioklasie *f*, Kraniotomie *f*; Enzephalotomie *f*.
cra·ni·o·clast ['kreɪnɪəklæst] *n gyn.* Kranioklast *m*.
cra·ni·o·clas·ty ['-klæstɪ] *n* → cranioclasis.
cra·ni·o·clei·do·dys·os·to·sis [ˌ-ˌklaɪdəʊdɪsɒs'təʊsɪs] *n* → cleidocranial dysostosis.
cra·ni·o·di·a·phys·e·al dysplasia [ˌ-ˌdaɪə'fiːzɪəl] kraniodiaphysäre Dysplasie *f*.
cra·ni·o·did·y·mus [ˌ-'dɪdəməs] *n embryo.* Kraniodidymus *m*.
cra·ni·o·fa·cial [ˌ-'feɪʃl] *adj* Schädel/Cranium u. Gesicht betr., kraniofazial.
craniofacial dysjunction fracture LeFort III-Fraktur *f*.
craniofacial dysostosis Crouzon-Syndrom *nt*, Dysostosis cranio-facialis.
cra·ni·og·ra·phy [kreɪnɪ'ɒgrəfɪ] *n* Kraniographie *f*.
cra·ni·ol·o·gy [kreɪnɪ'ɒlədʒɪ] *n* Schädellehre *f*, Kraniologie *f*.
cra·ni·o·ma·la·cia [ˌkreɪnɪəmə'leɪʃ(ɪ)ə] *n* Schädel(knochen)erweichung *f*, Kraniomalazie *f*.
cra·ni·o·me·nin·go·cele [ˌ-mɪ'nɪŋgəsiːl] *n* Kraniomeningozele *f*.
cra·ni·o·meta·phy·se·al dysplasia [ˌ-mɪ'tæfəsɪəl, -ˌmetə'fɪzɪəl] kraniometaphysäre Dysplasie *f*.
cra·ni·om·e·ter [ˌkreɪnɪ'ɒmɪtər] *n* Schädelmesser *m*, Kraniometer *nt*.
cra·ni·o·met·ric [ˌkreɪnɪə'metrɪk] *adj* Kraniometrie betr., kraniometrisch.
cra·ni·o·met·ri·cal [ˌ-'metrɪkl] *adj* → craniometric.
cra·ni·om·e·try [ˌkreɪnɪ'ɒmətrɪ] *n* Schädelmessung *f*, Kraniometrie *f*.
cra·ni·op·a·gus [ˌ-'ɑːpəgəs] *n, pl* **-gi** [-gaɪ, -dʒaɪ] *embryo.* Kephalo-, Zephalo-, Kraniopagus *m*.
cra·ni·op·a·thy [ˌ-'ɒpəθɪ] *n* Schädel(knochen)erkrankung *f*, Kraniopathie *f*.
cra·ni·o·pha·ryn·ge·al duct [ˌkreɪnɪəʊfə-'rɪndʒɪəl] → craniopharyngeal pouch.
craniopharyngeal duct tumor → craniopharyngioma.
craniopharyngeal pouch *embryo.* Rathke'-Tasche *f*.
cra·ni·o·pha·ryn·gi·o·ma [ˌ-fəˌrɪndʒɪ'əʊmə] *n patho.* Kraniopharyngiom *nt*, Erdheim-Tumor *m*.
cra·ni·o·plas·ty ['-plæstɪ] *n ortho., neurochir.* Schädelplastik *f*, Kranioplastik *f*.
cra·ni·o·punc·ture ['-pʌŋ(k)tʃər] *n* Schädelpunktur *f*.
cra·ni·or·rha·chid·i·an [ˌ-rə'kɪdɪən] *adj* → craniospinal.
cra·ni·or·rha·chis·chi·sis [ˌ-rə'kɪskəsɪs] *n embryo.* (angeborene) Schädel- und Wirbelsäulenspalte *f*, Kraniorrhachischisis *f*.
cra·ni·o·sa·cral [ˌ-'seɪkrəl] *adj* **1.** kraniosakral. **2.** parasympathisches (Nerven-)System betr.
craniosacral system parasympathisches (Nerven-)System *nt*, Parasympathikus *m*, parasympathischer Teil *m* des vegetativen Nervensystems, Pars parasympathetica systematis nervosi autonomici.
cra·ni·os·chi·sis [ˌkreɪnɪ'ɒskəsɪs] *n, pl* **-ses** [-siːz] angeborene Schädelspalte *f*, Kranioschisis *f*, Cranium bifidum.
cra·ni·o·scle·ro·sis [ˌkreɪnɪəʊsklɪ'rəʊsɪs] *n* Schädelknochenverdickung *f*, Kranio-

sklerose *f*, Leontiasis cranii.
cra·ni·os·co·py [kreɪnɪ'ɒskəpɪ] *n* Kranioskopie *f*.
cra·ni·o·spi·nal [ˌkreɪnɪəʊ'spaɪnl] *adj* Schädel/Cranium u. Wirbelsäule betr., kraniospinal.
craniospinal ganglia Spinalganglien *pl* der Hirn- u. Rückenmarksnerven, Ggll. craniospinalia/encephalospinalia/sensoria.
cra·ni·o·ste·no·sis [ˌ-stɪ'nəʊsɪs] *n* Kraniostenose *f*.
cra·ni·os·to·sis [ˌkreɪnɪ'ɒstəsɪs] *n, pl* **-ses** [-siːz] kongenitale (Schädel-)Nahtverknöcherung *f*, Kraniostose *f*.
cra·ni·o·syn·os·to·sis [ˌkreɪnɪəʊˌsɪnɒs'təʊsɪs] *n, pl* **-ses** [-siːz] vorzeitiger (Schädel-)Nahtverschluß *m*, Kraniosynostose *f*.
craniosynostosis-radial aplasia syndrome *embryo., ortho.* Baller-Gerold-Syndrom *nt*.
cra·ni·ot·a·bes [ˌ-'teɪbiːz] *n* Kraniotabes *f*.
cra·ni·o·tome ['-təʊm] *n ortho., neurochir.* Kraniotom *nt*.
cra·ni·ot·o·my [ˌkreɪnɪ'ɒtəmɪ] *n* **1.** *ortho., neuro.* Schädeleröffnung *f*, Kraniotomie *f*, Trepanation *f*. **2.** → cranioclasis.
cra·ni·o·to·nos·co·py [ˌkreɪnɪəʊtə'nɒskəpɪ] *n* auskultatorische Schädelperkussion *f*.
cra·ni·o·to·pog·ra·phy [ˌ-tə'pɒgrəfɪ] *n* Schädel-, Kraniotopographie *f*.
cra·ni·o·try·pe·sis [ˌ-trə'piːsɪs] *n ortho., neurochir.* Schädeltrepanation *f*.
cra·ni·o·tym·pan·ic [ˌ-tɪm'pænɪk] *adj* Schädel/Cranium u. Paukenhöhle/Tympanum betr., kraniotympanal.
cra·ni·o·ver·te·bral [ˌ-'vɜːrtəbrəl] *adj* Kopf u. Wirbel betr., kraniovertebral.
craniovertebral articulation oberes Kopfgelenk *nt*, Atlantookzipitalgelenk *nt*, Artic. atlanto-occipitalis.
craniovertebral joint → craniovertebral articulation.
cra·ni·tis [kreɪ'naɪtɪs] *n* Schädelknochenentzündung *f*.
cra·ni·um ['kreɪnɪəm] *n, pl* **-nia** [-nɪə] Schädel *m*, Kranium *nt*, Cranium *nt*.
cranium bifidum Spaltschädel *m*, Cranium bifidum.
cranium bifidum occultum Cranium bifidum occultum.
crap·u·lence ['kræpjələns] *n* Unmäßigkeit *f*, übermäßiger Nahrungs- *od.* Alkoholgenuß *m*.
crap·u·len·cy ['kræpjələnsɪ] *n* → crapulence.
crap·u·lent ['kræpjələnt] *adj* durch übermäßige Nahrungs-/Alkoholaufnahme bedingt *od.* hervorgerufen; betrunken; unmäßig.
crap·u·lous ['kræpjələs] *adj* → crapulent.
crash [kræʃ] **I** *n* **1.** Unfall *m*, Zusammenstoß *m*. **2.** Krachen *nt*. **II** *vt* **3.** zertrümmern, zerschmettern. **4.** einen Unfall haben (mit). **III** *vi* (krachend) zerbersten, zerbrechen, zerschmettert werden.
crash cart Notfall-, Reanimationswagen *m*.
cras·sa·men·tum [kræsə'mentəm] *n* **1.** Blutgerinnsel *m*, -kuchen *m*. **2.** coagulum.
cra·ter ['kreɪtər] *n patho.* (*Ulkus*) Krater *m*.
cra·ter·i·form ['kreɪtərɪfɔːrm] *adj* kraterförmig, trichterförmig.
cra·ter·i·za·tion [kreɪtəraɪ'zeɪʃn] *n chir., ortho.* kraterförmige Ausschneidung *f*, Kraterbildung *f*.
cra·vat [krə'væt] *n* → cravat bandage.
cravat bandage Krawatte(nverband *m*) *f*.
CRD *abbr.* → chronic respiratory disease.
C-reactive protein *abbr.* **CRP** C-reaktives Protein *nt abbr.* CRP.

cream

cream [kriːm] I *n* 1. *pharm.* Creme *f*, Krem *f*. 2. (*Milch*) Rahm *m*, Sahne *f*. II *adj* creme(farben).
c. of tartar *chem.* Weinstein *m*.
cream-colored *adj* creme(farben).
cream-faced *adj* bleich, blaß.
crease [kriːs] *n* (Haut-)Falte *f*.
cre·a·sote *n* → creosote.
cre·a·tine ['kriːətiːn, -tɪn] *n abbr.* **Cr** Kreatin *nt*, Creatin *nt*, α-Methylguanidinoessigsäure *f*.
creatine kinase *abbr.* **CK** Kreatin-, Creatinkinase *f abbr.* CK, Kreatin-, Creatinphosphokinase *f abbr.* CPK.
cre·a·tin·e·mia [kriətɪ'niːmɪə] *n* vermehrter Kreatingehalt *m* des Blutes, Kreatinämie *f*, Creatinämie *f*.
creatine phosphate Kreatin-, Creatinphosphat *nt abbr.* CP, Phosphokreatin *nt*.
creatine phosphokinase *abbr.* **CPK** → creatine kinase.
creatine phosphotransferase → creatine kinase.
cre·at·i·nine [kri'ætəniːn, -nɪn] *n abbr.* **Cr** Kreatinin *nt*, Creatinin *nt*.
creatinine clearance Kreatinin-, Creatininclearance *f*.
creatinine coefficient Creatinin-, Kreatininkoeffizient *m*.
cre·a·tin·u·ria [,kriətɪ'n(j)ʊərɪə] *n* vermehrte Kreatinausscheidung *f* im Harn, Kreatinurie *f*, Creatinurie *f*.
cre·a·tor·rhea [,kriətə'rɪə] *n* Kreatorrhö *f*.
cre·a·to·tox·ism [,-'taksɪzəm] *n* Fleischvergiftung *f*.
crèche [kreʃ, kreɪʃ] *n* (Kinder-)Krippe *f*.
Credé [krɛ'de]: **C.'s antiseptic** Silbernitrat *nt*.
C.'s maneuver → C.'s method.
C.'s method 1. Credé'-Prophylaxe *f*, Credéisieren *nt*. 2. Credé'-Handgriff *m*.
creep·ing ['kriːpɪŋ] I *n* Kriechen *nt*, Wandern *m*. II *adj a. fig.* kriechend, schleichend; kribbelnd.
creeping disease *micro.* creeping disease (*nt*), Hautmaulwurf *m*, Larva migrans, Myiasis linearis migrans.
creeping eruption/myiasis → creeping disease.
creeping ulcer 1. Ulcus serpens. 2. Ulcus corneae serpens. 3. Ulcus molle serpiginosum.
C region *biochem.* konstante Region *f*, C-Region *f*.
cre·mas·ter [krɪ'mæstər] *n* → cremaster muscle.
cre·mas·ter·ic [,kremə'sterɪk] *adj* M. cremaster betr., Kremaster-.
cremasteric artery Kremasterarterie *f*, Cremasterica *f*, A. cremasterica.
cremasteric coat of testis → cremaster muscle.
cremasteric fascia Fascia cremasterica.
cremasteric reflex Hoden-, Kremaster-, Cremasterreflex *m abbr.* CrR.
cremaster muscle Kremaster *m*, M. cremaster.
cre·mate ['kriːmeɪt] *vt* (*Leichnam*) verbrennen, einäschern.
cre·ma·tion [krɪ'meɪʃn] *n* (*Leichnam*) Verbrennung *f*, Einäscherung *f*, Feuerbestattung *f*.
cre·ma·to·ri·um [,kriːmə'tɔːrɪəm, -'təʊ-, ,krem-] *n, pl* **-ri·ums, -ria** [-rɪə] Krematorium *nt*.
crem·no·cele ['kremnəsiːl] *n chir.* Hernia labialis.
cre·mor ['kriːmər] *n pharm.* Creme *f*, Cremor *m*.
cre·na ['kriːnə, 'krenə] *n, pl* **-nae** [-niː] *anat.* Furche *f*, Spalte *f*, Rinne *f*, Crena *f*.

cre·nate ['kriːneɪt] *adj* → crenated.
cre·nat·ed ['kriːneɪtɪd] *adj* gekerbt, gefurcht.
crenated erythrocyte Stechapfelform *f*, Echinozyt *m*.
crenate margin of spleen oberer Milzrand *m*, Margo superior lienis/splenis.
cre·na·tion [krɪ'neɪʃn] *n* 1. Kerbung *f*, Furchung *f*. 2. → crenated erythrocyte.
cren·a·ture ['krenətʃər, 'kriː-] *n* → crenation 1.
cren·o·cyte ['krenəsaɪt, 'kriːn-] *n* → crenated erythrocyte.
cre·o·sol ['kriːəsɒl, -sɑl] *n* Kreosol *nt*, Creosol *nt*.
cre·o·sote ['krɪəsəʊt] *n* Kreosot *nt*, Kreosotum *nt*.
crep·i·tant ['krepɪtənt] *adj* 1. (*Lunge*) knisternd, rasselnd; knarrend. 2. knisternd, knackend.
crepitant rales (*Lunge*) feinblasiges Knisterrasseln *nt*.
crep·i·tate ['krepɪteɪt] *vt* knacken, knistern, rasseln, knarren.
crep·i·ta·tion [krepɪ'teɪʃn] *n* 1. Knistern *nt*, Knarren *nt*. 2. (*Lunge*) Knistern *nt*, Knisterrasseln *nt*, Krepitation *f*, Crepitatio *f*, Crepitus *m*. 3. *ortho.* (*Fraktur*) Reiben *nt*, Reibegeräusch *nt*, Krepitation *f*, Crepitatio *f*, Crepitus *m*.
crep·i·tus ['krepɪtəs] *n* → crepitation.
crepitus indux Crepitatio indux.
crepitus redux Crepitatio redux.
cre·scen·do murmur ['krɪ'ʃendəʊ, -'sen-] Crescendogeräusch *nt*, Geräusch *nt* mit Crescendocharakter.
crescendo-decrescendo murmur Crescendo-Decrescendo-Geräusch *nt*.
cres·cent ['kresənt] I *n* 1. *histol.* Halbmond *m*, halbmondförmige Struktur *f*. 2. ⌐s *pl* (*Malaria*) Sichelkeime *pl*. II *adj* halbmond-, (mond-)sichelförmig.
c. of Giannuzzi (von) Ebner'-Halbmond, Giannuzzi'-Halbmond, Heidenhain'-Halbmond, seröser Halbmond.
crescent body 1. → crescent of Giannuzzi. 2. Halbmondkörper *m*, Schilling-Halbmond *m*, Achromo(retikolo)zyt *m*.
crescent cell 1. ⌐s *pl* → crescent of Giannuzzi. 2. Sichelzelle *f*.
crescent cell anemia Sichelzell(en)anämie *f*, Herrick-Syndrom *nt*.
cres·cen·tic [krɪ'sentɪk] *adj* halbmond-, (mond-)sichelförmig.
crescent-shaped *adj* halbmondförmig, (mond-)sichelförmig.
cre·sol ['kriːsɒl, -sɑl] *n* Kresol *nt*.
cresol red Kresolrot *nt*.
crest [krest] *n* 1. Leiste *f*, Kamm *m*, Grat *m*. 2. *anat.* (Knochen-)Leiste *f*, Crista *f*. 3. *fig.* Scheitel-, Höchstwert *m*, Spitze *f*; Gipfel *m*, Scheitelpunkt *m*.
c. of cochlear window Randleiste des runden Fensters, Crista fenestrae cochleae.
c. of greater tubercle Crista tuberculi majoris.
c. of ilium Darmbeinkamm, Crista iliaca.
c. of lesser tubercle Crista tuberculi minoris.
c. of little head of rib Crista capitis costae.
c.s of nail matrix Nagelbettleisten *pl*, Cristae matricis unguis.
c. of neck of rib Crista colli costae.
c. of palatine bone Crista palatina.
c. of supinator muscle Crista m. supinatoris.
c. of vestibule Crista vestibuli.
crest·ed ['krestɪd] *adj* mit einer Leiste/einem Kamm *etc.* versehen.
crest factor *phys.* Scheitelfaktor *m*.
crest-like *adj* kammartig, leistenförmig.
CREST syndrome [calcinosis cutis, Raynaud's phenomenon, esophageal dysfunction, sclerodactyly, and telangiectasia] CREST-Syndrom *nt*.
crest voltage *electr.* Spitzenspannung *f*.
cres·yl blue (brilliant) ['kresɪl, 'kriːs-] Kresylblau *nt*, Brillantkresylblau *nt*.
cre·syl·ic acid [krɪ'sɪlɪk] → cresol.
cre·tin ['kriːtn] *n* an Kretinismus leidender Patient, Kretin *m*.
cretin dwarf hypothyreotischer Zwerg *m*.
cre·tin·ism ['kriːtnɪzəm] *n* Kretinismus *m*.
cre·tin·is·tic [kriːtə'nɪstɪk] *adj* → cretinous.
cre·tin·oid ['kriːtnɔɪd] *adj* kretinoid.
cretinoid idiocy → cretinism.
cre·tin·ous ['kriːtnəs] *adj* Kretinismus betr., kretinhaft.
Creutzfeldt-Jakob ['krɔʏtsfelt 'jaːkɔp]: **C.-J. disease** *abbr.* **CJD** Creutzfeldt-Jakob-Erkrankung *f abbr.* CJE, Creutzfeldt-Jakob-Syndrom *nt*, Jakob-Creutzfeldt-Erkrankung *f*, Jakob-Creutzfeldt-Syndrom *nt*.
C.-J. syndrome → C.-J. disease.
crev·ice ['krevɪs] *n* Spalt(e *f*) *m*, (schmaler) Riß *m*, Ritze *f*.
CRF *abbr.* → corticotropin releasing factor.
CRH *abbr.* [corticotropin releasing hormone] → corticotropin releasing factor.
crib death [krɪb] → cot death.
crib·rate ['krɪbreɪt, -rɪt] *adj* siebartig durchlöchert.
cri·bra·tion [krɪ'breɪʃn] *n* 1. (Durch-)Sieben *nt*. 2. siebartige Beschaffenheit *f*.
crib·ri·form ['krɪbrəfɔːrm] *adj anat.* siebförmig, kribriform.
cribriform area of renal papilla siebartige Oberfläche *f* der Nierenpapillen, Area cribrosa.
cribriform bone *old* Siebbein *nt*, Os ethmoidale.
cribriform carcinoma kribriformes Karzinom *nt*, Ca. cribriforme/cribrosum.
cribriform fascia 1. Fascia cribrosa. 2. Septum femorale.
cribriform hymen *gyn.* Hymen cribriformis.
cribriform lamina Fascia cribrosa.
c. of ethmoid bone Siebbeinplatte *f*, Lamina cribrosa ossis ethmoidalis.
c. of transverse fascia Septum femorale.
cribriform membrane Fascia cribrosa.
cribriform plate of ethmoid bone → cribriform lamina of ethmoid bone.
cribriform tissue lockeres Bindegewebe *nt*.
crib·rous lamina of sclera ['krɪbrəs] Siebplatte *f* der Sklera, Lamina cribrosa sclerae.
crib·rum ['kraɪbrəm, 'krɪb-] *n, pl* **-rums, -ra** [-brə] → cribriform lamina of ethmoid bone.
Crichton-Browne ['kraɪtn braʊn]: **C.-B.'s sign** *neuro.* Crichton-Browne-Zeichen *nt*.
cri·co·ar·y·te·noid [,kraɪkəʊˌærɪ'tiːnɔɪd, -ə'rɪtnɔɪd] *adj* krikoarytänoid.
cri·co·ar·y·te·noi·de·us [,-ˌærɪtɪ'nɔɪdɪəs] *n* → cricoarytenoideus muscle.
cricoarytenoideus lateralis (muscle) *inf.* Lateralis *m*, Cricoarytänoideus *m* lateralis, M. cricoaryt(a)enoideus lateralis.
cricoarytenoideus muscle Cricoarytänoideus *m*, M. cricoaryt(a)enoideus.
cricoarytenoideus posterior (muscle) *inf.* Postikus *m*, Cricoarytänoideus *m* posterior, M. cricoaryt(a)enoideus posterior.
cricoarytenoid ligament, posterior *old* hinteres Krikoarytnoidband *nt*, Lig. cricoaryt(a)enoideum.
cricoarytenoid muscle → cricoarytenoideus (muscle).

cri·co·e·soph·a·ge·al tendon [ˌ-ˌɪˌsɑfəˈdʒiːəl, -ˌɪsəˈfædʒɪəl] Tendo crico-(o)esophageus.
cri·coid [ˈkraɪkɔɪd] *anat.* I *n* Ring-, Krikoidknorpel *m*, Cartilago cricoidea. II *adj* ringförmig, krikoid, cricoid, Kriko-.
cricoid cartilage → cricoid I.
cri·coi·dec·to·my [ˌkraɪkɔɪˈdektəmɪ] *n chir.*, HNO Ringknorpelexzision *f*, Krikoidektomie *f*.
cri·co·pha·ryn·ge·al [ˌkraɪkəʊfəˈrɪndʒɪəl, -ˌfærɪnˈdʒiːəl] *adj* Ringknorpel/Cartilago cricoidea u. Rachen/Pharynx betr., krikopharyngeal.
cricopharyngeal achalasia hohe/zervikale/krikopharyngeale Achalasie *f*.
cricopharyngeal achalasia syndrome Asherson-Syndrom *nt*.
cricopharyngeal ligament Santorini'-Band *nt*, Lig. cricopharyngeum.
cricopharyngeal muscle → cricopharyngeus (muscle).
cricopharyngeal myotomy *chir.* operative Durchtrennung *f* des M. cricopharyngeus, krikopharyngeale Myotomie *f*.
cri·co·pha·ryn·ge·us (muscle) [ˌ-fəˈrɪndʒɪəs] *old* M. cricopharyngeus, Pars cricopharyngea m. constrictoris pharyngis inferioris.
cri·co·thy·re·ot·o·my [ˌ-ˌθaɪrɪˈɑtəmɪ] *n chir.* Krikothyreotomie *f*.
cri·co·thy·ro·ar·y·te·noid ligament [ˌ-ˌθaɪrəʊˌærɪˈtiːnɔɪd, -əˈrɪtnɔɪd] Conus elasticus, Membrana cricovocalis.
cri·co·thy·roid [ˌ-ˈθaɪrɔɪd] *adj* Ringknorpel u. Schilddrüse *od.* Schildknorpel betr. *od.* verbindend, krikothyroid(al), krikothyreoid.
cricothyroid artery Ramus cricothyroideus (a. thyroideae superioris).
cricothyroid branch of superior thyroid artery → cricothyroid artery.
cri·co·thy·roi·de·us (muscle) [ˌ-θaɪˈrɔɪdɪəs] Krikothyroideus *m*, M. cricothyroideus.
cricothyroid ligament Lig. cricothyroideum.
  lateral c. *old* → cricothyroarytenoid ligament.
  median c. Lig. cricothyroideum medianum.
cricothyroid membrane → cricothyroarytenoid ligament.
cricothyroid muscle → cricothyroideus (muscle).
cri·co·thy·roid·ot·o·my [ˌ-ˌθaɪrɔɪˈdɑtəmɪ] *n* → cricothyrotomy.
cri·co·thy·rot·o·my [ˌ-θaɪˈrɑtəmɪ] *n chir.* Krikothyroidotomie *f*.
cri·cot·o·my [kraɪˈkɑtəmɪ] *n chir.* Ringknorpelspaltung *f*, Krikotomie *f*.
cri·co·tra·che·al [ˌkraɪkəʊˈtreɪkɪəl] *adj* Ringknorpel/Cartilago cricoidea u. Luftröhre/Trachea betr. *od.* verbindend, krikotracheal.
cricotracheal ligament Lig. cricotrachealе.
cricotracheal separation *ortho.* krikotrachealer Abriß *m*.
cri·co·tra·che·ot·o·my [ˌ-ˌtreɪkɪˈɑtəmɪ] *n chir.* Krikotracheotomie *f*.
cri·co·vo·cal membrane [ˌ-ˈvəʊkl] → cricothyroarytenoid ligament.
cri-du-chat syndrome [kri dy ʃa] Katzenschreisyndrom *nt*, Cri-du-chat-Syndrom *nt*.
Crigler-Najjar [ˈkrɪɡlər ˈnadʒar]: **C.-N. disease** Crigler-Najjar-Syndrom *nt*, idiopathische Hyperbilirubinämie *f*.
  C.-N. jaundice/syndrome → C.-N. disease.
Crile [kraɪl]: **C.'s clamp** Crile-Klemme *f*.
Cri·me·an-Congo hemorrhagic fever [kraɪˈmɪən] → Crimean hemorrhagic fever.
Crimean-Congo hemorrhagic fever virus → Crimean hemorrhagic fever virus.
Crimean hemorrhagic fever Kongo--Krim-Fieber *nt*, hämorrhagisches Krim--Fieber *nt*.
Crimean hemorrhagic fever virus Krimfieber-Virus *nt*, C-CHF-Virus *nt*.
crim·i·nal abortion [ˈkrɪmənl] illegaler/krimineller Schwangerschaftsabbruch *f*, Abortus criminalis.
cri·nis [ˈkraɪnɪs] *n, pl* **-nes** [-niːz] Haar *nt*, Crinis *m*.
crip·ple [ˈkrɪpl] I *n* (Körper-)Behinderter *m*; Krüppel *m*. II *vt* zum Krüppel machen; lähmen. III *vi* humpeln, hinken.
crip·pled [ˈkrɪpəld] *adj* verkrüppelt; gelähmt.
cri·sis [ˈkraɪsɪs] *n, pl* **-ses** [-siːz] Krise *f*, Krisis *f*, Crisis *f*.
crisis intervention Krisenintervention *f*.
cris·pa·tion [krɪsˈpeɪʃn] *n physiol., neuro.* leichtes Muskelzucken *nt*.
cris·ta [ˈkrɪstə] *n, pl* **-tae** [-tiː] *anat.* (Knochen-)Leiste *f*, Kamm *m*, Grat *m*, Crista *f*.
  c. of pubis Crista pubis.
crista galli Hahnenkamm *m*, Crista galli.
cris·tate margin of spleen [ˈkrɪsteɪt] → crenate margin of spleen.
crista type mitochondrium Mitochondrium *nt* vom Crista-Typ.
Critchett [ˈkrɪtʃet]: **C.'s operation** *ophthal.* Critchett-Schieloperation *f*.
cri·te·ri·on [kraɪˈtɪərɪən] *n, pl* **-ri·ons, -ria** [-rɪə] Maßstab *m*, (Unterscheidungs-)Merkmal *nt*, Kriterium *nt*.
  c. of malignancy *patho.* Malignitätskriterium *nt*.
Cri·thid·ia [krɪˈθɪdɪə] *pl micro.* Crithidien *pl*, Crithidia *f*.
cri·thid·i·al [krɪˈθɪdɪəl] *adj micro.* crithidial, Crithidien-.
crit·i·cal [ˈkrɪtɪkəl] *adj* 1. kritisch, entscheidend; gefährlich, bedenklich, ernst. 2. kritisch, prüfend; mißbilligend.
critical angle *phys.* kritischer Einfallswinkel *m*, Grenzwinkel *m*.
critical care unit Intensiv-, Wachstation *f*.
critical closing pressure kritischer Verschlußdruck *m*.
critical condition kritischer Zustand *m*.
critical constants *phys.* kritische Konstanten *pl*.
critical flicker frequency *abbr.* **CFF** *physiol.* Flimmerfusionsfrequenz *f*, kritische Flimmerfrequenz *f*, critical flicker frequency *abbr.* CFF.
critical load Grenzbelastung *f*.
critical mass *phys.* kritische Masse *f*.
critical micelle concentration *phys.* kritische Mizellenkonzentration *f*.
critical point → critical temperature.
critical pressure *phys.* kritischer Druck *m*.
critical temperature *phys.* kritische Temperatur *f*.
CRL *abbr.* → crown-rump length.
C.R. length → crown-rump length.
CRO *abbr.* → cathode ray oscilloscope.
cro·ci·dis·mus [krɑsɪˈdɪzməs] *n neuro., psychia.* Flockenlesen *nt*, Floccilatio *f*, Floccilegium *nt*, Karphologie *f*, Krozidismus *m*, Crocidismus *m*.
croc·o·dile skin [ˈkrɑkədaɪl] 1. Fischschuppenkrankheit *f*, Ichthyosis vulgaris. 2. Saurier-, Krokodil-, Alligatorhaut *f*, Sauriasis *f*.
crocodile tears syndrome Krokodilstränenphänomen *nt*, gustatorisches Weinen *nt*.
crocodile tongue Faltenzunge *f*, Lingua plicata/scrotalis.

Crohn [krəʊn]: **C.'s disease** Crohn'-Krankheit *f*, Morbus Crohn *m*, Enteritis regionalis, Ileocolitis regionalis/terminalis, Ileitis regionalis/terminalis.
cro·mo·gly·cate [ˌkrəʊməˈɡlaɪkeɪt] *n pharm.* Cromoglykat *nt*.
cro·mo·gly·cic acid [ˌ-ˈɡlaɪsɪk] → cromolyn.
cro·mo·lyn [ˈ-lɪn] *n pharm.* Cromoglicin-, Cromoglycinsäure *f*, Cromolyn *nt*.
Cronkhite-Canada [ˈkrɑŋkaɪt ˈkænədə]: **C.-C. syndrome** Cronkhite-Canada-Syndrom *nt*.
Crooke [krʊk]: **C.'s cells** Crooke-Zellen *pl*.
  C.'s change Crooke-Degeneration *f*.
  C.'s hyaline change → C.'s change.
  C.'s hyaline degeneration → C.'s change.
Crooke-Russell [ˈrʌsl]: **C.-R. change** Crooke-Degeneration *f*.
Crosby [ˈkrɑzbɪ]: **C.'s capsule** Crosby-Sonde *f*.
Cross [krɔs, kras]: **C. syndrome** Cross--McKusick-Breen-Syndrom *nt*.
cross [krɔːs, kras] I *n* 1. *allg.* Kreuz *nt*, Kreuz(chen *nt*) *n*. 2. Kreuzung(spunkt *m*) *f*. 3. *bio.* Kreuzung *f*, Kreuzungsprodukt *nt* (*between* zwischen). 4. *fig.* Mittel-, Zwischending *nt*. II *adj* 5. quer (liegend *od.* verlaufend); Quer-; schräg, Schräg-; *s.* kreuzend, *s.* schneidend. 6. *bio.* Kreuzungs-. 7. *stat.* Querschnitts-. III *vt* 8. über-, durchqueren, -schreiten; *fig.* überschreiten; *s.* kreuzen mit; ankreuzen; (*Plan*) durchkreuzen. 9. *bio.* kreuzen. IV *vi* 10. *s.* kreuzen, *s.* schneiden; quer liegen *od.* verlaufen. 11. *bio. s.* kreuzen (lassen). 12. *bio.* Gene austauschen.
cross agglutination *hema.* Kreuzagglutination(sreaktion *f*) *f*.
cross agglutinin → cross-reacting agglutinin.
cross-arm flap Cross-arm-Plastik *f*.
cross-birth [ˈkrɔsbɑrθ, ˈkras-] *n obst.* (*Fetus*) Querlage *f*.
cross-bite [ˈ-baɪt] *n dent.* Kreuzbiß *m*.
cross-bred [ˈ-bred] I *n* Hybride *f*/*m*, Kreuzung *f*, Mischling *m*. II *adj* gekreuzt, hybrid.
cross-breed [ˈ-briːd] I *n* → crossbred I. II *vt, vi* kreuzen.
cross-breed·ing [ˈ-briːdɪŋ] *n* 1. Hybridisierung *f*, Hybridisation *f*. 2. Hybridisation, Bastardisierung *f*.
cross-bridge *n chem.* Querbrücke *f*.
cross-clamp *vt chir.* (vollständig) abklemmen.
cross-cultural psychiatry transkulturelle Psychiatrie *f*.
cross dialysis parabiotische Dialyse *f*.
crossed [krɔst] *adj* gekreuzt.
crossed adductor jerk → crossed adductor reflex.
crossed adductor reflex gekreuzter Adduktorenreflex *m*.
crossed anesthesia *neuro.* gekreuzte/alternierende Hemianästhesie *f*, Hemian(a)esthesia cruciata.
crossed diplopia *ophthal.* gekreuzte/heteronyme/temporale Diplopie *f*.
crossed embolism paradoxe/gekreuzte Embolie *f*.
crossed eyes → cross-eye.
crossed hemianesthesia → crossed anesthesia.
crossed hemianopia gekreuzte/heteronyme Hemianop(s)ie *f*.
crossed hemianopsia → crossed hemianopia.
crossed hemiplegia gekreuzte Hemiplegie *f*, Hemiplegia alternans/cruciata.
crossed jerk → crossed reflex.
crossed knee jerk → crossed knee reflex.

crossed knee reflex

crossed knee reflex gekreuzter Patellar-(sehnen)reflex *m*.
crossed metastasis gekreuzte Metastase *f*.
crossed paralysis 1. Hemiplegia alternans. 2. Hemiplegia cruciata.
crossed reflex gekreuzter/diagonaler/konsensueller Reflex *m*.
cross-eye *n ophthal*. Einwärtsschielen *nt*, Esotropie *f*, Strabismus convergens/internus.
cross-eyed *adj ophthal*. (nach innen) schielend. **to be ~** schielen.
cross-face anastomosis faziofaziale Anastomose *f*.
cross-fertilization *n bio*. Kreuzbefruchtung *f*.
cross-fertilize *vi* s. kreuzweise befruchten.
cross-finger flap Cross-finger-Plastik *f*.
cross flap Cross-over-Plastik *f*.
cross-hatch ['krɔːʃætʃ, 'krɑs-] *n* Quer-, Kreuzschraffierung *f*.
cross-immunity *n* Kreuzimmunität *f*.
cross infection Kreuzinfektion *f*.
cross·ing ['krɔːsɪŋ, 'krɑs-] *n* 1. Kreuzen *nt*, Kreuzung *f*. 2. Durch-, Überquerung *f*.
c. of the tendons Camper'-Kreuzung, Chiasma tendinum (digitorum manus).
crossing over *vi bio*. Gene austauschen.
crossing-over *n genet*. Chiasmabildung *f*, Faktorenaustausch *m*, Crossing-over *nt*.
cross-leg flap Cross-leg-Plastik *f*.
cross-link *n* → cross linkage
cross linkage *chem*. Quervernetzung *f*, -verbindung *f*.
cross-linker *n chem*. Vernetzer *m*.
cross-match *vt* eine Kreuzprobe machen *od*. durchführen, *inf*. kreuzen.
cross-match ['krɔːsmætʃ, 'krɑs-] *n* Kreuzprobe *f*.
cross matching 1. → crossmatch. 2. Durchführung *f* einer Kreuzprobe, Crossmatching *nt*.
Cross-McKusick-Breen [mə'kjuːzɪk briːn]: **C.M.-B. syndrome** Cross-McKusick-Breen-Syndrom *nt*.
cross·o·ver ['-əʊvər] *n* 1. → crossing 2. 2. → crossing-over.
crossover flap *chir*. Crossover-Plastik *f*.
cross-react *vt* kreuzreagieren, eine Kreuzreaktion geben.
cross-reacting *adj* kreuzreagierend.
cross-reacting agglutinin kreuzreagierendes Agglutinin *nt*.
cross-reacting antibody kreuzreagierender Antikörper *m*.
cross-reacting antigen kreuzreagierendes Antigen *nt*.
cross-reaction *n* Kreuzreaktion *f*.
cross-reactive *adj* kreuzreaktiv, -reagierend.
cross-reactive protein *abbr*. **CRP** kreuzreagierendes Protein *nt*.
cross-reactivity *n* Kreuzreaktivität *f*.
cross-refer *vt* (durch einen Querverweis) verweisen (*to* auf).
cross-reference *n* Kreuz-, Querverweis *m*.
cross-resistance *n* Kreuzresistenz *f*.
cross section 1. Querschnitt *m*; Querschnittszeichnung *f*. 2. *fig*. Querschnitt *m* (*of* durch).
cross-section I *adj* Querschnitts-. **II** *vt* quer durchschneiden; einen Querschnitt machen durch; im Querschnitt darstellen.
cross-sectional *adj* → cross-section I.
cross-sectional area Querschnittsfläche *f*.
cross-sectional pulse Querschnitts-, Volumenpuls *m*.
cross-sensitivity *n immun*. Kreuzsensibilität *f*.

cross-sensitization *n immun*. Kreuzsensibilisierung *f*.
cross-sensitizing *adj immun*. kreuzsensibilisierend.
cross-stitch *n* Kreuzstich *m*.
cross-striation *n* Querstreifung *f*.
cross·way ['-weɪ] *n anat*. (Nerven-)Kreuzung *f*.
cro·ta·lo·tox·in [ˌkrəʊtələʊ'tɒksɪn] *n* Crotalotoxin *nt*.
cro·ta·mine ['krəʊtəmiːn] *n* Crotamin *nt*.
cro·tam·i·ton [krəʊ'tæmɪtən] *n pharm*. Crotamiton *nt*.
cro·teth·a·mide [krəʊ'teθəmaɪd] *n pharm*. Crotethamid *nt*.
cro·tin ['krəʊt(ɪ)n] *n* Krotin, Crotin *nt*.
cro·ton·ic acid [krəʊ'tɒnɪk, -'tɒn-] Kroton-, Crotonsäure *f*.
cro·ton·ism ['krəʊtənɪzəm] *n* Krotonölvergiftung *f*, Crotonismus *m*.
cro·ton oil ['krəʊtn] Kroton-, Crotonöl *nt*.
cro·tox·in [krəʊ'tɒksɪn] *n* Crotoxin *nt*.
croup [kruːp] *n* 1. Krupp *m*, Croup *m*. 2. echter/diphtherischer Krupp *m*. 3. falscher Krupp *m*, Pseudokrupp *m*.
croup-associated virus *micro*. Parainfluenza 2-Virus *nt*, Parainfluenzavirus Typ 2 *nt*.
croup·ous ['kruːpəs] *adj* 1. → croupy. 2. pseudomembranös, entzündlich-fibrinös.
croupous bronchitis kruppöse/(pseudo-)-membranöse Bronchitis *f*, Bronchitis crouposa/fibrinosa/plastica/pseudomembranacea.
croupous conjunctivitis kruppöse/pseudomembranöse Konjunktivitis *f*, Bindehautkrupp *m*, Conjunctivitis pseudomembranacea.
croupous cystitis diphtherische/kruppöse (Harn-)Blasenentzündung/Zystitis *f*.
croupous inflammation → croupy inflammation.
croupous laryngitis kruppöse Laryngitis *f*.
croupous membrane Pseudomembran *f*.
croupous nephritis akute Glomerulonephritis *f*.
croupous pharyngitis kruppöse/pseudomembranöse Pharyngitis *f*.
croupous pneumonia Lobär-, Lappenpneumonie *f*.
croupous rhinitis pseudomembranöse/fibrinöse Rhinitis *f*, Rhinitis pseudomembranacea.
croupous sore throat Angina crouposa.
croup·y ['kruːpɪ] *adj* kruppartig, -ähnlich, kruppös.
croupy inflammation kruppöse Entzündung *f*.
Crouzon [kruːˈzɔ̃]: **C.'s disease/syndrome** Crouzon-Syndrom *nt*, Dysostosis cranio-facialis.
crow·ing convulsion ['krəʊɪŋ] falscher Krupp *m*, Pseudokrupp *m*, subglottische Laryngitis *f*, Laryngitis subglottica.
crown [kraʊn] *n* 1. *anat*. Scheitel *m*, Wirbel *m* (des Kopfes), Corona *f*. 2. anatomische Krone, Corona dentis/anatomica. 3. *dent*. Zahn-, *a*. höchster Punkt *m*, Gipfel *m*. 5. *fig*. Höhepunkt *m*, Krönung *f*. **II** *vt dent*. überkronen.
c. of the head Corona capitis.
crown cavity → coronal cavity.
crown-heel length Scheitel-Fersen-Länge *f abbr*. SFL.
crown part of pulp → coronal pulp.
crown-rump length *abbr*. **CRL** Scheitel-Steiß-Länge *f abbr*. SSL.
CRP *abbr*. 1. → C-reactive protein. 2. → cross-reactive protein. 3. → cyclic AMP receptor protein.

CRS *abbr*. → Chinese restaurant syndrome.
CRST syndrome [calcinosis cutis, Raynaud's phenomenon, sclerodactyly, and telangiectasia] CRST-Syndrom *nt*.
CRT *abbr*. → cathode-ray tube.
cru·cial ['kruːʃl] *adj* 1. old → cruciate. 2. kritisch, entscheidend (*to*, *vor* für).
cru·ci·ate ['kruːʃɪət, -ʃɪeɪt] *adj* kreuzförmig.
cruciate eminence → cruciform eminence.
cruciate ligament kreuzförmiges Band *nt*, Kreuzband *nt*, Lig. cruciforme/cruciatum.
c. of ankle Y-Band *nt*, Retinaculum mm. extensorum pedis inferius.
anterior c. (of knee) *abbr*. **ACL** vorderes (Kniegelenks-)Kreuzband, Lig. cruciatum anterius (genus).
c. of atlas Lig. cruciforme atlantis.
c.s of knee Kreuzbänder *pl*, Ligg. cruciata genus/genualia.
posterior c. (of knee) *abbr*. **PCL** hinteres (Kniegelenks-)Kreuzband, Lig. cruciatum posterius (genus).
cruciate muscle Muskel *m* mit gekreuzten Fasern, M. cruciatus.
cruciate paralysis → crossed paralysis.
cru·ci·ble ['kruːsəbl] *n* (Schmelz-)Tiegel *m*.
cru·ci·form ['kruːsəfɔːrm] *adj* kreuzförmig.
cruciform eminence Eminentia cruciformis.
cruciform ligament → cruciate ligament.
c. of atlas → cruciate ligament of atlas.
crude [kruːd] *adj* 1. roh, ungekocht; unbehandelt, -bearbeitet, Roh-. 2. *fig*. roh, grob, derb; primitiv; unreif, unfertig.
crude fiber Ballaststoffe *pl*.
crude tubercle *patho*. verkäsender Tuberkel *m*.
crude urine wässriger Harn/Urin *m*.
cru·or ['kruːɔːr] *n* Blutgerinnsel *nt*, -kuchen *m*, -klumpen *m*, Kruor *m*, Cruor sanguinis.
cru·ral ['krʊərəl] *adj* (Unter-)Schenkel *od*. schenkelähnliche Struktur betr., krural, (Unter-)Schenkel-.
crural aponeurosis → crural fascia.
crural arch *anat*. Leistenband *nt*, Arcus inguinalis, Lig. inguinale.
crural canal Canalis femoralis.
c. of Henle Schenkel-, Adduktorenkanal *m*, Canalis adductorius.
crural fascia oberflächliche Unterschenkelfaszie *f*, Fascia cruris.
crural hernia *chir*. Schenkelhernie *f*, -bruch *m*, Merozele *f*, Hernia femoralis/cruralis.
crural ligament Leistenband *nt*, Lig. inguinale, Arcus inguinale.
crural plexus vegetativer Plexus *m* der A. femoralis, Plexus femoralis.
crural region Unterschenkel(region *f*) *m*, Regio/Facies cruralis.
anterior c. Unterschenkelvorderseite *f*, Regio/Facies cruralis anterior.
posterior c. Unterschenkelrückseite *f*, Regio/Facies cruralis posterior.
crural ring Eingang *m* des Canalis femoralis, A(n)nulus femoralis.
crural septum Cloquet-Septum *nt*, Septum femorale.
crural surface: anterior c. → crural region, anterior.
posterior c. → crural region, posterior.
cru·re·us ['krʊərɪəs] *n anat*. M. vastus intermedius.
cruro- *pref*. Unterschenkel-, Schenkel-.
cru·ro·ta·lar [ˌkrʊərəʊ'teɪlər] *adj* Unterschenkel u. Sprungbein betr., talokrural.
crurotalar articulation oberes Sprungge-

lenk *nt*, Talokruralgelenk *nt*, Artic. talocruralis.
crurotalar joint → crurotalar articulation.
crus [krʌs, kruːs] *n*, *pl* **cru·ra** ['kruərə] *anat.* Schenkel *m*, Unterschenkel *m*, schenkelähnliche Struktur *f*, Crus *nt*.
c.ra of anthelix Antihelixschenkel *pl*, Crura antihelicis.
c. of clitoris Klitoris-, Clitorisschenkel, Crus clitoridis.
c.ra of fornix Fornixschenkel *pl*, Crura fornicis.
c. of helix Helixanfang *m*, Crus helicis.
c. of penis Schwellkörperschenkel, Crus penis.
crush [krʌʃ] **I** *n* (Zer-)Quetschen *nt*. **II** *vt* **1.** zerquetschen, -drücken, -malmen. **2.** auspressen, -drücken. **III** *vi* zerquetscht *od.* zerdrückt werden.
crush fracture *ortho.* (Wirbelkörper-)Kompressionsfraktur *f*.
crush injury Quetschung *f*, Quetschungsverletzung *f*.
crush kidney Crush-Niere *f*, Chromoproteinniere *f*, chromoproteinurische Niere *f*.
crush syndrome → compression syndrome.
crust [krʌst] **I** *n* Kruste *f*, Borke *f*, Grind *nt*, Schorf *m*, Crusta *f*. **II** *adj* → crusted. **III** *vi* verkrusten, eine Kruste/ein Grind bilden.
crus·ta ['krʌstə] *n*, *pl* **-tae** [-tiː, -taɪ] → crust I.
crust·ed ['krʌstɪd] *adj* mit einer Kruste überzogen, verkrustet, krustig.
crusted ringworm *derm.* Erb-, Flechten-, Kopf-, Pilzgrind *m*, Favus *m*, Tinea (capitis) favosa, Dermatomycosis favosa.
crusted scabies Scabies *f*, norwegische Skabies *f*, Scabies crustosa/norvegica.
crusted tetter Eiter-, Grind-, Krusten-, Pustelflechte *f*, feuchter Grind *m*, Impetigo contagiosa/vulgaris.
crutch [krʌtʃ] *n ortho.* Krücke *f*. **to go on ~es** auf/an Krücken gehen.
Crutchfield ['krʌtʃfiːld]: **C. clamp/tongs** *ortho.* Crutchfield-Zange *f*, -Klammer *f*.
crutch palsy Krückenlähmung *f*.
crutch paralysis → crutch palsy.
Cruveilhier [kryvɛ'je]: **C.'s articulation** oberes Kopfgelenk *nt*, Atlantookzipitalgelenk *nt*, Artic. atlanto-occipitalis.
C.'s atrophy → C.'s disease.
C.'s disease Cruveilhier'-Krankheit *f*, spinale progressive Muskelatrophie *f*.
C.'s fascia Fascia perinei superficialis.
C.'s fossa Fossa scaphoidea (ossis sphenoidalis).
glenoid ligaments of C. Ligg. plantaria articc. metatarsophalangearum.
C.'s joint → C.'s articulation.
C.'s ligaments Ligg. plantaria.
navicular fossa of C. Fossa scaphoidea (ossis sphenoidalis).
C.'s nodules Cruveilhier-, Albini'-Knötchen *pl*.
C.'s paralysis → C.'s disease.
C.'s plexus Cruveilhier'-Plexus *m*.
C.'s sign Medusenhaupt *nt*, Cirsomphalus *m*, Caput medusae.
Cruveilhier-Baumgarten ['baumgartən]:
C.-B. cirrhosis → C.-B. syndrome.
C.-B. disease Cruveilhier-Baumgarten-Krankheit *f*.
C.-B. murmur *card.* Cruveilhier-Baumgarten-Geräusch *nt*.
C.-B. syndrome Cruveilhier(-von)-Baumgarten-Syndrom *nt*.
Cruz [kruːz]: **C.'s trypanosomiasis** → Cruz-Chagas disease.
Cruz-Chagas ['tʃagas]: **C.-C. disease** Chagas-Krankheit *f*, amerikanische Trypanosomiasis *f*.
cry- *pref.* → cryo-.
cry [kraɪ] **I** *n* **1.** Schrei *m*, Ruf *m*. **2.** Geschrei *nt*. **a ~ for help** ein Hilferuf. **3.** Weinen *nt*. **II** *vt* weinen. **III** *vi* **4.** schreien, (laut) rufen, verlangen (*for* nach). **5.** weinen; heulen, jammern (*for* um; *over* wegen).
cry·al·ge·sia [ˌkraɪæl'dʒiːzɪə, -ʒə] *n* Kälteschmerz *m*, Kryalgesie *f*.
cry·an·es·the·sia [ˌ-ænəs'θiːʒə] *n* Kryanästhesie *f*.
cry·es·the·sia [ˌ-es'θiːʒ(ɪ)ə] *n* **1.** Kälteempfindung *f*, Kryästhesie *f*. **2.** Kälteüberempfindlichkeit *f*, Kryästhesie *f*.
crym(o)- *pref.* → cryo-.
cry·mo·an·es·the·sia [ˌkraɪməuˌænəs'θiː-ʒə] *n* Kälte-, Kryoanästhesie *f*.
cry·mo·dyn·ia [ˌ-'dɪnɪə] *n* → cryalgesia.
cry·mo·phil·ic [ˌ-'fɪlɪk] *adj* → cryophilic.
cry·mo·phy·lac·tic [ˌ-fɪ'læktɪk] *adj* → cryophylactic.
cry·mo·ther·a·peu·tics [ˌ-θerə'pjuːtɪks] *pl* → cryotherapy.
cry·mo·ther·a·py [ˌ-'θerəpɪ] *n* → cryotherapy.
cryo- *pref.* Kälte-, Frost-, Kry(o)-, Psychro-.
cry·o·an·al·ge·sia [ˌkraɪəuˌænl'dʒiːzɪə, -ʒə] *n* Kryoanalgesie *f*.
cry·o·an·es·the·sia [ˌ-ænəs'θiːʒə] *n* → cryomoanesthesia.
cry·o·bank ['-bæŋk] *n* Kryobank *f*.
cry·o·bi·ol·o·gy [ˌ-baɪ'ɒlədʒɪ] *n* Kryobiologie *f*.
cry·o·car·di·o·ple·gia [ˌ-ˌkɑːrdɪəu'pliːdʒ(ɪ)ə] *n* Kryokardioplegie *f*.
cry·o·cau·ter·y [ˌ-'kɔːtərɪ] *n* Kryokauter *m*.
cry·o·con·i·za·tion [ˌ-ˌkəunə'zeɪʃn, -ˌkʌn-] *n gyn.* Kryokonisation *f*.
cry·ode ['kraɪəud] *n* → cryoprobe.
cry·o·ex·trac·tion [ˌ-ɪk'strækʃn] *n ophthal.* Kryoextraktion *f*.
cry·o·ex·trac·tor [ˌ-ɪk'stræktər] *n ophthal.* Kryoextraktor *m*.
cry·o·fi·brin·o·gen [ˌ-faɪ'brɪnədʒən] *n* Kryofibrinogen *nt*.
cry·o·fi·brin·o·gen·e·mia [ˌ-faɪˌbrɪnədʒə'niːmɪə] *n* Kryofibrinogenämie *f*.
cry·o·gam·ma·glob·u·lin [ˌ-ˌgæmə'glɒbjəlɪn] *n* → cryoglobulin.
cry·o·gen ['-dʒən] *n* Kältemittel *nt*, -mischung *f*.
cry·o·gen·ic [ˌ-'dʒenɪk] *adj* kälteerzeugend, kryogen.
cryogenic block → crymoanesthesia.
cry·o·glob·u·lin [ˌ-'glɒbjəlɪn] *n* Kälte-, Kryoglobulin *nt*.
cry·o·glob·u·lin·e·mia [ˌ-ˌglɒbjəlɪ'niːmɪə] *n* Kryoglobulinämie *f*.
cry·o·hy·poph·y·sec·to·my [ˌ-haɪˌpɒfə'sek-təmɪ] *n neurochir.* Kryohypophysektomie *f*.
cry·om·e·ter [kraɪ'ɒmɪtər] *n phys.* Kryometer *nt*.
cry·o·pal·li·dec·to·my [ˌkraɪəupælɪ'dektə-mɪ] *n neurochir.* Kryopallidektomie *f*.
cry·op·a·thy [kraɪ'ɒpəθɪ] *n* Kryopathie *f*.
cry·o·pex·y ['kraɪəpeksɪ] *n ophthal.* Kryo(retino)pexie *f*.
cry·o·phile ['-faɪl] *n micro.* kälteliebender/psychrophiler Mikroorganismus *m*.
cry·o·phil·ic [ˌ-'fɪlɪk] *adj micro.* kälteliebend, psychrophil.
cry·o·phy·lac·tic [ˌ-fɪ'læktɪk] *adj micro.* kälteresistent, -beständig.
cry·o·pre·cip·i·tate [ˌ-prɪ'sɪpɪtət, -teɪt] *n* Kryopräzipitat *nt*.
cry·o·pre·cip·i·ta·tion [ˌ-prɪˌsɪpə'teɪʃn] *n* Kryopräzipitation *f*.
cry·o·pres·er·va·tion [ˌ-ˌprezə'veɪʃn] *n* Kälte-, Kryokonservierung *f*.
cry·o·probe ['-prəub] *n* Kältesonde *f*, -stab *m*, Kryosonde *f*, -stab *m*, Kryode *f*.
cry·o·pros·ta·tec·to·my [ˌ-ˌprɒstə'tektəmɪ] *n urol.* Kryoprostatektomie *f*.
cry·o·pro·tec·tive [ˌ-prə'tektɪv] *adj* vor Kälte(schaden) schützend.
cry·o·pro·tein [ˌ-'prəutiːn, -tiːn] *n* Kälte-, Kryoprotein *nt*.
cry·o·scope ['-skəup] *n* Kryoskop *nt*.
cry·o·scop·i·cal [ˌ-'skɒpɪkl] *adj* Kryoskopie betr., kryoskopisch.
cry·os·co·py [kraɪ'ɒskəpɪ] *n chem.* Kryoskopie *f*.
cry·o·stat ['kraɪəstæt] *n* Kryostat *m*.
cry·o·sur·ger·y [ˌ-'sɜːrdʒ(ə)rɪ] *n* Kälte-, Kryochirurgie *f*.
cry·o·sur·gi·cal [ˌ-'sɜːrdʒɪkl] *adj* Kryochirurgie betr., kryochirurgisch.
cry·o·thal·a·mec·to·my [ˌ-ˌθælə'mektəmɪ] *n* → cryothalamotomy.
cry·o·thal·a·mot·o·my [ˌ-ˌθælə'mɒtəmɪ] *n neurochir.* Kryothalamotomie *f*.
cry·o·ther·a·py [ˌ-'θerəpɪ] *n* Kälte-, Kryotherapie *f*.
cry·o·tol·er·ant [ˌ-'tɒlərənt] *adj* kälteunempfindlich, -widerstandsfähig, -tolerant.
crypt [krɪpt] *n anat.* seichte (Epithel-)Grube *f*, Krypte *f*, Crypta *f*.
c.s of Fuchs Iriskrypten *pl*.
c.s of Haller → c.s of Littre.
c.s of iris Iriskrypten *pl*.
c.s of Littre Vorhaut-, Präputialdrüsen *pl*, Tyson'-Drüsen *pl*, präputiale (Talg-)Drüsen *pl*, Gll. pr(a)eputiales.
c.s of Morgagni Morgagni'-Krypten *pl*, Analkrypten *pl*, Sinus anales.
c.s of palatine tonsil Fossulae tonsillares tonsillae palatinae.
c.s of pharyngeal tonsil Fossulae tonsillares tonsillae pharyngeae.
c.s of Tyson → c.s of Littre.
cryp·ta ['krɪptə] *n*, *pl* **-tae** [-tiː] → crypt.
crypt abscess Kryptenabszeß *m*.
crypt·an·am·ne·sia [krɪptˌænəm'niːʒ(ɪ)ə, -zɪə] *n* → cryptomnesia.
cryp·tec·to·my [krɪp'tektəmɪ] *n chir.* Kryptenexzision *f*.
cryp·tes·the·sia [krɪptes'θiːʒ(ɪ)ə] *n* Hellsehen *nt*, Präkognition *f*.
cryp·tic ['krɪptɪk] *adj* verborgen, versteckt, kryptisch.
cryp·ti·tis [krɪp'taɪtɪs] *n* Kryptenentzündung *f*, Kryptitis *f*.
cryp·to·ceph·a·lus [ˌkrɪptəu'sefələs] *n embryo.* Kryptozephalus *m*.
Cryp·to·coc·ca·ce·ae [ˌ-kə'keɪsɪˌiː] *pl micro.* Cryptococcaceae *pl*.
cryp·to·coc·cal [ˌ-'kɒkəl] *adj* Kryptokokken betr., durch Kryptokokken hervorgerufen, Kryptokokken-, Cryptococcus-.
cryptococcal meningitis Kryptokokkenmeningitis *f*.
cryp·to·coc·co·ma [ˌ-kə'kəumə] *n* Kryptokokkengranulom *nt*, Torulom *nt*.
cryp·to·coc·co·sis [ˌ-kə'kəusɪs] *n* europäische Blastomykose *f*, Busse-Buschke-Krankheit *f*, Cryptococcus-Mykose *f*, Kryptokokkose *f*, Cryptococcose *f*, Torulose *f*.
Cryp·to·coc·cus [ˌ-'kɒkəs] *n micro.* Kryptokokkus *m*, Cryptococcus *m*.
cryp·to·crys·tal·line [ˌ-'krɪstlɪn, -laɪn] *adj* kryptokristallin.
cryp·to·did·y·mus [ˌ-'dɪdəməs] *n embryo.* Kryptodidymus *m*.
cryp·to·gam ['-gæm] *n bio.* Sporenpflanze *f*, Kryptogame *f*.
cryp·to·gam·ic [ˌ-'gæmɪk] *adj bio.* kryptogam(isch).
cryp·tog·a·mous [krɪp'tɒgəməs] *adj* → cryptogamic.

cryptogamy

cryp·tog·a·my [krɪp'tɒgəmɪ] *n* Kryptogamie *f*.
cryp·to·ge·net·ic [ˌkrɪptədʒə'netɪk] *adj* → cryptogenic.
cryp·to·gen·ic [ˌ-'dʒenɪk] *adj* kryptogen, kryptogenetisch.
cryptogenic cirrhosis kryptogene (Leber-)Zirrhose *f*.
cryptogenic epilepsy idiopathische/essentielle/endogene/kryptogenetische/genuine Epilepsie *f*.
cryptogenic infection kryptogene Infektion *f*.
cryp·to·lith ['-lɪθ] *n* Kryptenstein *m*, Kryptolith *m*.
cryp·to·men·or·rhea [ˌ-menə'rɪə] *n gyn.* Kryptomenorrhoe *f*.
cryp·to·mer·ic [ˌ-'merɪk] *adj genet.* kryptomer.
cryp·tom·e·rism [krɪp'tɒmərɪzəm] *n genet.* Kryptomerie *f*.
cryp·to·mer·o·ra·chis·chi·sis [ˌkrɪptəˌmerərə'kɪskəsɪs] *n* Spina bifida occulta.
cryp·tom·ne·sia [krɪpˌtɒm'niːʒə] *n* Kryptomnesie *f*.
cryp·tom·o·nad [-'tɒmənæd] *n micro.* Kryptomonade *f*.
Cryp·tom·o·nas [-'tɒmənəs, -næs] *n micro.* Cryptomonas *f*.
cryp·toph·thal·mia [-tɑf'θælmɪə] *n* → cryptophthalmos.
cryp·toph·thal·mos [-tɑf'θælməs] *n embryo., ophthal.* verborgenes Auge *nt*, Kryptophthalmus *m*.
cryp·toph·thal·mus [-tɑf'θælməs] *n* → cryptophthalmos.
cryptophthalmus syndrome Fraser-Syndrom *nt*, Kryptophthalmus-Syndrom *nt*.
cryp·tor·chid [-'tɔːrkɪd] **I** *n* Patient *m* mit Kryptorchismus. **II** *adj* Kryptorchismus betr., kryptorchid.
cryp·tor·chi·dec·to·my [-ˌtɔːrkɪ'dektəmɪ] *n chir.* Hodenentfernung/Orchidektomie *f* bei Kryptorchismus.
cryp·tor·chi·dism [-'tɔːrkədɪzəm] *n* Hodenretention *f*, Kryptorchismus *m*, Retentio/ Maldescensus testis.
cryp·tor·chi·do·pex·y [-ˌtɔːrkɪdə'peksɪ] *n urol.* Hodenfixation *f*, -fixierung *f*, Orchio-, Orchidopexie *f*.
cryp·tor·chi·dy [-'tɔːrkədɪ] *n* → cryptorchidism.
cryp·tor·chism [-'tɔːrkɪzəm] *n* → cryptorchidism.
cryp·to·scope ['krɪptəskəʊp] *n radiol.* Fluoroskop *nt*.
cryp·tos·co·py [krɪp'tɒskəpɪ] *n radiol.* (Röntgen-)Durchleuchtung *f*, Fluoroskopie *f*.
cryp·to·spo·rid·i·o·sis [ˌkrɪptəspəˌrɪdɪ'əʊsɪs, -spəʊ-] *n* Kryptosporidiose *f*, Cryptosporidiosis *f*.
Cryp·to·spo·rid·i·um [ˌ-spə'rɪdɪəm, -spəʊ-] *n micro.* Cryptosporidium *nt*.
cryp·to·tia [krɪp'təʊʃɪə] *n embryo.* Kryptotie *f*.
cryp·to·xan·thin [ˌkrɪptə'zænθiːn, -θɪn] *n* Kryptoxanthin *nt*.
crys·tal ['krɪstl] **I** *n* Kristall *m*; Kristall(glas *nt*) *nt*. **II** *adj* → crystalline. **III** *vt* kristallisieren.
crystal lattice *phys.* Kristallgitter *nt*.
crys·tal·lin ['krɪstəlɪn] *n biochem.* Kristallin *nt*.
crys·tal·line ['krɪstliːn, -laɪn] *adj* **1.** kristallartig, kristallinisch, kristallin, kristallen, Kristall-. **2.** *fig.* kristallklar, kristallen.
crystalline capsule Linsenkapsel *f*, Capsula lentis.
cristalline humor 1. Humor vitreus. **2.** Glaskörper *m*, Corpus vitreum.

crystalline lens *anat.* (Augen-)Linse *f*, Lens *f* (cristallina).
crystalline salt Ionenkristall *m*.
crys·tal·liz·a·ble ['krɪstlaɪzəbl] *adj* kristallisierbar.
crystallizable fragment *abbr.* **Fc** kristallisierbares Fragment *nt*, Fc-Fragment *nt*.
crys·tal·li·za·tion [ˌkrɪstlə'zeɪʃn, -laɪ-] *n* Kristallisierung *f*, Kristallisieren *nt*, Kristallisation *f*, Kristallbildung *f*.
crys·tal·lize ['krɪstlaɪz] *vt, vi* (aus-)kristallisieren.
crys·tal·lo·graph·ic model [ˌkrɪstlə'græfɪk] *chem.* kristallographisches Modell *nt*.
crys·tal·log·ra·phy [ˌkrɪstə'lɒgrəfɪ] *n phys.* Kristallographie *f*.
crys·tal·loid ['krɪstlɔɪd] **I** *n* Kristalloid *nt*. **II** *adj* kristallähnlich, kristalloid.
crys·tal·lu·ria [krɪstə'l(j)ʊərɪə] *n* Kristallausscheidung *f* im Harn, Kristallurie *f*.
crystal rash *derm.* Sudamina *pl*, Miliaria cristallina.
crystal synovitis *ortho.* Synovitis *f* durch Ablagerung kristalliner Substanzen.
crystal violet Kristallviolett *nt*, Methylrosaliniumchlorid *nt*.
CS *abbr.* **1.** → cesarean section. **2.** → conditioned stimulus.
Cs *abbr.* → cesium.
CsCl gradient method CsCl-Gradientenmethode *f*, Cäsiumchloridgradientenmethode *f*.
CSF *abbr.* **1.** → cerebrospinal fluid. **2.** → colony-stimulating factor.
CSF-brain barrier Hirn-Liquor-Schranke *f*.
CSF otorrhea Otoliquorrhoe *f*.
CSF pressure Liquordruck *m*.
CSF rhinorrhea nasale Liquorrhoe *f*, Liquorrhoe *f* aus der Nase.
C-shaped scoliosis *ortho.* C-förmige Skoliose *f*.
Csillag ['sɪlag]: **C.'s disease** Weißfleckenkrankheit *f*, White-Spot-Disease (*nt*), Lichen sclerosus et atrophicus, Lichen albus.
C.S.M. *abbr.* → cerebrospinal meningitis.
C-substance → C-Substanz *f*.
CT *abbr.* **1.** → carboxyltransferase. **2.** [computed/computerized tomography] → computerized axial tomography.
Cte·no·ce·phal·i·des [ˌtenəʊsɪ'fælədiːz, ˌtiː-] *pl micro.* Ctenocephalides *pl.*
C-terminal *adj chem.* carboxy-terminal, C-terminal.
CTF *abbr.* → Colorado tick fever.
CTF virus → Colorado tick fever virus.
CTG *abbr.* → cardiotocogram.
CTL *abbr.* [cytotoxic T-lymphocyte] → cytotoxic T-cell.
CTP *abbr.* → cytidine(-5'-)triphosphate.
CTS *abbr.* → carpal tunnel syndrome.
Cu *abbr.* → copper 1.
Cu·ban itch ['kjuːbən] → cottonpox.
cu·bic ['kjuːbɪk] *adj* **1.** Kubik-, Raum-. **2.** kubisch, würfelförmig, gewürfelt.
cu·bi·cal ['kjuːbɪkl] *adj* → cubic.
cubical epithelium → cuboidal epithelium.
cubic capacity Fassungsvermögen *nt*.
cubic content Kubik-, Rauminhalt *m*.
cubicle ['kjuːbɪkl] *n* (Umkleide-, Untersuchungs-)Kabine *f*.
cubic measure Körper-, Raum-, Kubikmaß *nt*.
cubic meter Kubik-, Raum-, Festmeter *m/nt*.
cubic symmetry kubische Symmetrie *f*.
cu·bi·tal ['kjuːbɪtl] *adj* **1.** Ell(en)bogen(gelenk) betr., kubital, Ell(en)bogen-. **2.** Unterarm *od.* Ulna betr., ulnar, Unterarm-, Ulna-.

cubital articulation Ell(en)bogengelenk *nt*, Artic. cubiti/cubitalis.
cubital bursa, interosseous Bursa cubitalis interossea.
cubital fossa Ellenbeugengrube *f*, Fossa cubitalis.
cubital joint → cubital articulation.
cubital lymph nodes kubitale Lymphknoten *pl*, Nodi lymphatici cubitales.
cubital nerve Ulnaris *m*, N. ulnaris.
cubital network, articular → cubital rete, articular.
cubital region: anterior c. vordere Ell(en)bogengegend/-region *f*, Regio/Facies cubitalis anterior.
posterior c. hintere Ell(en)bogengegend/ -region *f*, Regio/Facies cubitalis posterior.
cubital rete, articular Arteriengeflecht *nt* des Ell(en)bogengelenks, Rete articulare cubiti.
cubital tunnel syndrome *ortho., neuro.* Kubitaltunnelsyndrom *nt*.
cubital vein, (inter)median Intermedia/ Mediana *f* cubiti, V. mediana cubiti.
cubito- *pref.* Ell(en)bogen-, Unterarm-, Kubito-.
cu·bi·to·ra·di·al [ˌkjuːbɪtəʊ'reɪdɪəl] *adj* Ulna u. Radius betr., radioulnar.
cubitoradial articulation: inferior c. unteres Speichen-Ellen-Gelenk *nt*, unteres Radioulnargelenk *nt*, Artic. radioulnaris distalis.
superior c. oberes Speichen-Ellen-Gelenk *nt*, oberes Radioulnargelenk *nt*, Artic. radioulnaris proximalis.
cubitoradial bursa Bursa cubitalis interossea.
cubitoradial joint: inferior c. → cubitoradial articulation, inferior.
superior c. → cubitoradial articulation, superior.
cu·bi·to·ul·nar [ˌ-'ʌlnər] *adj* Ell(en)bogen u. Ulna betr., kubitoulnar.
cubitoulnar ligament Lig. collaterale ulnare.
cu·bi·tus ['kjuːbɪtəs] *n* **1.** Ell(en)bogengelenk *nt*, Ell(en)bogen *m*, Artic. cubiti/cubitalis. **2.** Unterarm *m*. **3.** *old* → ulna.
cubitus valgus Cubitus valgus.
cubitus varus Cubitus varus.
cu·boid ['kjuːbɔɪd] **I** *n* Würfelbein *nt*, Kuboid *nt*, Os cuboideum. **II** *adj* würfelförmig, kuboid.
cu·boi·dal [kjuː'bɔɪdl] *adj* → cuboid II.
cuboidal epithelium isoprismatisches/kubische Epithel *nt*.
cuboid bone → cuboid I.
cuboid cell isoprismatische/kubische Epithelzelle *f*.
cuboideo- *pref.* Würfelbein-.
cu·boi·de·o·met·a·tar·sal ligaments, short [kjuːˌbɔɪdɪəʊˌmetə'tɑːrsl] Ligg. tarsometatarsalia plantaria.
cu·boi·de·o·na·vic·u·lar ligament [ˌ-nə'vɪkjələr]: **dorsal c.** Lig. cuboideonaviculare dorsale.
oblique/plantar c. Lig. cuboideonaviculare plantare.
cu·boi·do·dig·i·tal reflex [kjuːˌbɔɪdəʊ'dɪdʒɪtl] *neuro.* Mendel-Bechterew-Reflex *m*.
cu·bo·na·vic·u·lar ligament [ˌkjuːbəʊnə'vɪkjələr] → cuboideonaviculare ligament, oblique/plantar.
cu·bo·scaph·oid ligament, plantar [ˌ-'skæfɔɪd] → cuboideonavicular ligament, oblique/plantar.
cuff [kʌf] *n* (aufblasbare) Manschette *f*, Cuff *m*.
cul-de-sac [ˌkʌldɪ'sæk] *n, pl* **culs-de-sac** Sackgasse *f*; *anat.* blind endende Aus- *od.* Einbuchtung *f*.

cul·do·cen·te·sis [ˌkʌldəsen'tiːsɪs] *n gyn.* Kuldozentese *f.*
cul·do·scope ['-skəʊp] *n gyn.* Kuldoskop *nt.*
cul·dos·co·py [kʌl'dɑskəpɪ] *n gyn.* Kuldoskopie *f*, Douglas(s)kopie *f.*
cul·dot·o·my [kʌl'dɑtəmɪ] *n gyn.* Kuldotomie *f.*
Cu·lex ['kjuːleks] *n*, *pl* **-li·ces** [-ləsiːz] *micro.* Kulexmücke *f*, Culex *m.*
cu·lic·i·cide [kjuː'lɪsəsaɪd] *n* → culicide.
Cu·lic·i·dae [-'lɪsədiː] *pl micro.* Stechmücken *pl*, Moskitos *pl*, Culicidae *pl.*
cu·li·ci·dal [kjuːlə'saɪdl] *adj* Stechmücken/Culicidae abtötend.
cu·li·cide ['-saɪd] *n* Stechmücken-abtötendes Mittel *nt.*
Cu·li·ci·nae [ˌ-'saɪniː] *pl micro.* Culicinae *pl.*
Cu·li·ci·ni [ˌ-'saɪnaɪ] *pl micro.* Culicini *pl.*
Cu·li·coi·des [ˌ-'kɔɪdiːz] *pl* Bartmücken *pl*, Culicoides *pl.*
Cu·li·se·ta [ˌ-'siːtə] *n micro.* Culiseta *f.*
Cullen ['kʌlʃən] **C.'s sign** Cullen(-Hellendall)-Zeichen *nt*, -Syndrom *nt.*
cul·men (of cerebellum) ['kʌlmən] *n* Gipfel *m* des Kleinhirnwurms, Culmen *nt* (cerebelli).
cul·ti·va·tion [ˌkʌltə'veɪʃn] *n bio., micro.* Züchtung *f*, Kultivierung *f.*
cul·tur·a·ble ['kʌltʃ(ə)rəbl] *adj micro.* züchtbar, kulturfähig, kultivierbar.
cul·tur·al ['kʌltʃərl] *adj socio.* Kultur betr., kulturell; *bio.* Kultur-.
cultural shock Kulturschock *m.*
cul·ture ['kʌltʃər] **I** *n* 1. Kultur *f.* 2. Züchtung *f*, Zucht *f*, Kultur *f.* **II** *vt* züchten, eine Kultur anlegen von.
cul·tured ['kʌltʃərd] *adj* kultiviert; gezüchtet, Zucht-, Kultur-.
culture dish Petrischale *f.*
culture filtrate Kulturfiltrat *nt.*
culture flask Kulturgefäß *nt.*
culture fluid Kulturflüssigkeit *f.*
culture medium Kultursubstrat *nt*, (künstlicher) Nährboden *m.*
  agar c. Agarnährboden, Agar *m/nt.*
  Bordet-Gengou c. Bordet-Gengou-Agar *m/nt*, -Medium *nt.*
  Clauberg's c. Clauberg-Nährboden.
  Czapek-Dox c. *micro.* Czapek-Dox-Nährlösung *f*, -Medium *nt.*
  differential c. *micro.* Differentialnährboden, -medium *nt.*
  enriched c. angereichertes Medium *nt.*
  gelatin c. Gelatinenährboden, -medium *nt.*
  litmus-milk c. *micro.* Lackmus-Milchbouillon *f*, -Milchmedium *nt.*
  Löffler's blood c. Löffler-Serum(nährboden *m*) *nt.*
  Löwenstein-Jensen c. Löwenstein-Jensen--Nährboden, -Medium *nt.*
  organ c. Organkultur.
  Petragnani c. Petragnani-Medium *nt.*
  selective c. Selektivnährboden, -medium *nt.*
  Wilson-Blair c. Wilson-Blair-Agar *m/nt*, Wismutsulfitagar *m/nt* nach Wilson u. Blair.
culture plate Kulturplatte *f.*
culture solution Nährlösung *f.*
culture-specific syndrome kulturspezifisches Syndrom *nt.*
culture tube Kulturröhrchen *nt.*
culture vessel *micro.* Kulturgefäß *nt.*
cu·ma·rin ['k(j)uːmərɪn] *n* → coumarin.
cu·mu·late [*adj* 'kjuːmjəlɪt, -leɪt; *v* -leɪt] **I** *adj* (an-, auf-)gehäuft, kumuliert. **II** *vt* kumulieren, (an-, auf-)häufen, ansammeln. **III** *vi* kumulieren, s. (an-, auf-)häufen, s. sammeln.

cu·mu·la·tion [ˌ-'leɪʃn] *n* (An-)Häufung *f*, Kumulation *f*, Anreicherung *f.*
cu·mu·la·tive ['-lətɪv, -leɪtɪv] *adj* s. (an-)häufend, anwachsend, kumulativ; Gesamt-.
cumulative dose *radiol.* kumulierte (Strahlen-)Dosis *f.*
cumulative effect Gesamtwirkung *f.*
cumulative gene Polygen *nt.*
cumulative inhibition kumulative Hemmung *f.*
cumulative radiation dose → cumulative dose.
cu·mu·lus ['kjuːmjələs] *n*, *pl* **-li** [-laɪ, -liː] 1. Haufen *m*, (An-)Häufung *f.* 2. *anat.* kleiner Hügel *m*, Cumulus *m.*
cumulus cells *embryo.* Cumulus-oophorus-Zellen *pl*, Cumuluszellen *pl.*
cumulus oophorus cells → cumulus cells.
cu·ne·ate ['kjuːnɪət, -nɪeɪt] *adj anat.* keilförmig.
cuneate fasciculus: c. of medulla oblongata Fasciculus cuneatus medullae oblongatae.
  c. of spinal cord Burdach'-Strang *m*, Fasciculus cuneatus medullae spinalis.
cuneate funiculus → cuneate fasciculus of spinal cord.
cuneate lobe → cuneus.
cuneate nucleus Burdach'-Kern *m*, Nc. cuneatus.
  accessory/lateral c. Monakow'-Kern, Nc. cuneatus accessorius.
cuneate tubercle Tuberculum cuneatum.
cu·ne·i·form [kjʊ'nɪ(ə)fɔːrm] *anat.* **I** *n* Keilbein *nt*, Os cuneiforme. **II** *adj* keilförmig.
cuneiform bone Keilbein *nt*, Os cuneiforme.
  external c. → lateral c.
  first c. → medial c.
  inner c. → medial c.
  intermediate c. mittleres Keilbein, Os cuneiforme intermedium.
  lateral c. äußeres Keilbein, Os cuneiforme laterale.
  medial c. inneres Keilbein, Os cuneiforme mediale.
  middle c. → intermediate c.
  outer c. → lateral c.
  second c. → intermediate c.
  third c. → lateral c.
cuneiform cartilage Wrisberg'-Knorpel *m*, Cartilago cuneiformis.
cuneiform cataract *ophthal.* (*Linse*) periphere Speichentrübungen *pl*, Cataracta cuneiformis.
cuneiform lobe Lobulus biventer.
cuneiform nucleus Nc. cuneiformis (mesencephalicus).
cuneiform tubercle Wrisberg'-Höckerchen *nt*, -knötchen *nt*, Tuberculum cuneiforme.
cuneo- *pref.* Keilbein-.
cu·ne·o·cer·e·bel·lar tract [ˌkjuːnɪəʊˌserə-'belər] Tractus cuneocerebellaris.
cu·ne·o·cu·boid [ˌ-'kjuːbɔɪd] *adj* Keilbein/Os cuneiforme u. Würfelbein/Os cuboideum betr., kuneokuboid.
cuneocuboid articulation Artic. cuneocuboidea.
cuneocuboid joint → cuneocuboid articulation.
cuneocuboid ligament Lig. cuneocuboideum.
  dorsal c. Lig. cuneocuboideum dorsale.
  interosseous c. Lig. cuneocuboideum interosseum.
  plantar c. Lig. cuneocuboideum plantare.
cu·ne·o·met·a·tar·sal ligaments, interosseous [ˌ-ˌmetə'tɑːrsl] Ligg. cuneometatarsalia interossea.
cu·ne·o·na·vic·u·lar [ˌ-nə'vɪkjələr] *adj*

Keilbein/Os cuneiforme u. Kahnbein/Os naviculare betr., kuneonavikular.
cuneonavicular articulation Artic. cuneonavicularis.
cuneonavicular joint → cuneonavicular articulation.
cuneonavicular ligaments Ligg. cuneonaviculare.
  dorsal c. Ligg. cuneonavicularia dorsalia.
  plantar c. Ligg. cuneonavicularia plantaria.
cu·ne·o·scaph·oid [ˌ-'skæfɔɪd] *adj* → cuneonavicular.
cu·ne·us ['kjuːnɪəs] *n*, *pl* **-nei** [-nɪaɪ] *anat.* Keil *m*, Cuneus *m.*
cu·nic·u·lus [kjuː'nɪk(j)ələs] *n*, *pl* **-li** [-liː, -laɪ] *derm.* (*Skabies*) Milbengang *m.*
cu·ni·form ['kjuːnəfɔːrm] *n*, *adj* → cuneiform.
cun·ni·linc·tion [ˌkʌnə'lɪŋkʃn] *n* → cunnilingus.
cun·ni·linc·tus [ˌ-'lɪŋktəs] *n* → cunnilingus.
cun·ni·lin·gus [ˌ-'lɪŋgəs] *n* Kunnilingus *m*, Cunnilingus *m.*
cun·nus ['kʌnəs] *n anat.* weibliche Scham *f*, Vulva *f*, Cunnus *m*, Pudendum femininum.
cup [kʌp] **I** *n* 1. Tasse *f*; Becher *m*, Napf *m*, Schale *f*, Kelch *m.* 2. schalen- od. becherförmiger Gegenstand *m.* 3. *bio.* Kelch *m.* 4. Körbchen *nt* (*des Büstenhalters*). 5. Schröpfkopf *m*, -glas *nt.* **II** *vt* 6. schröpfen. 7. (*Hand*) hohlmachen.
cup·board ['kʌpbərd] *n* Schrank *m.*
cup·ful ['kʌpfʊl] *n* eine Tasse(voll).
cu·po·la ['kjuːpələ] *n* → cupula.
cupped [kʌpt] *adj* ausgehöhlt, hohl.
cup pessary *gyn.* Portiokappe *f.*
cup·ping ['kʌpɪŋ] *n* Schröpfen *nt.*
cupping glass Schröpfkopf *m*, -glas *nt.*
cup reamer *ortho.* (Hüft-)Pfannenfräse *f.*
cu·pre·mia [k(j)uː'priːmɪə] *n erhöhter* Kupfergehalt *m* des Blutes, Kuprämie *f.*
cu·pric ['k(j)uːprɪk] *adj* zweiwertiges Kupfer enthaltend, Cupri-, Kupfer-II-.
cupric sulfate → copper sulfate.
cu·pri·u·ria [ˌk(j)uprɪ'(j)ʊərɪə] *n* Kupferausscheidung *f* im Harn, Kupriurie *f.*
cu·prous ['k(j)uːprəs] *adj* einwertiges Kupfer enthaltend, Cupro-, Kupfer-I-.
cu·pru·re·sis [ˌk(j)uprə'riːsɪs] *n* vermehrte Kupferausscheidung *f* im Harn, Kuprurese *f.*
cu·pru·ret·ic [ˌ-'retɪk] *adj* Kupferausscheidung betr. od. fördernd, kupruretisch.
cu·pu·la ['kjuːp(j)ələ] *n*, *pl* **-lae** [-liː] *anat.* Kuppel *f*, Cupula *f.*
  c. of ampullary crest Ampullenkuppel, Cupula cristae ampullais.
  c. of cochlea Schneckenspitze *f*, Cupula cochleae.
  c. of pleura Pleurakuppel, Cupula pleurae.
cu·pu·lar ['kjuːp(j)ələr] *adj* becher-, kelchförmig, -artig.
cupular caecum (of cochlear duct) blindes Ende *nt* des Ductus cochlearis, C(a)ecum cupulare (ductus cochlearis).
cupular space oberer Teil *m* des Kuppelraums, Pars cupularis (rec. epitympanici).
cu·pu·late ['kjuːp(j)əleɪt, -lɪt] *adj* → cupular.
cu·pu·li·form ['-fɔːrm] *adj* → cupular.
cu·pu·lo·gram ['-græm] *n physiol.* Kupulogramm *nt.*
cu·pu·lo·li·thi·a·sis [ˌ-lɪ'θaɪəsɪs] *n physiol., HNO* Kupulolithiasis *f.*
cu·pu·lom·e·try [ˌkʌp(j)ə'lɑmətrɪ] *n physiol.* Kupulometrie *f.*
cur·a·bil·i·ty [ˌkjʊərə'bɪlətɪ] *n* Heilbarkeit *f*, Kurabilität *f.*
cur·a·ble ['kjʊərəbl] *adj* heilbar, kurabel.

cu·ra·re [k(j)ʊəˈrɑːrɪ] *n* Kurare *nt*, Curare *nt*.
cu·ra·re·mi·met·ic [k(j)ʊəˌrɑːrɪmɪˈmetɪk, -maɪ-] *adj* curareähnlich wirkend, curaremimetisch.
cu·ra·ri *n* → curare.
cu·ra·ri·form [k(j)ʊəˈrɑːrɪfɔːrm] *adj* curareähnlich.
cu·ra·ri·za·tion [k(j)uːˌrɑːrɪˈzeɪʃn] *n* Behandlung *f* mit Curare, Kurarisierung *f*.
cu·ra·rize [k(j)uːˈrɑːraɪz] *vt* mit Curare behandeln, kurarisieren.
cur·a·tive [ˈkjʊərətɪv] **I** *n* Heilmittel *nt*. **II** *adj* heilend, auf Heilung ausgerichtet, heilungsfördernd, kurativ, Heil(ungs)-.
curative dose *abbr.* **C.D.** Dosis curativa *abbr.* D.C., D$_{cur}$.
median c. *abbr.* **C.D.$_{50}$** mittlere Dosis curativa *abbr.* D.C.$_{50}$.
curative ratio therapeutische Breite *f*, therapeutischer Index *m*.
curative resection *chir.* kurative Resektion *f*.
curative treatment kurative Behandlung *f*.
cur·cu·ma [ˈkɜrkjʊmə] *n bot., pharm.* Gelbwurz *f*, Kurkume *f*.
cur·cu·min [ˈkɜrkjəmɪn] *n* Kurkumin *nt*.
curd [kɜrd] *n* geronnene/dicke Milch *f*, Quark *m*.
cure [kjʊər] **I** *n* **1.** Kur *f*, Heilverfahren *nt*, Behandlung *f* (*for* gegen). **2.** Behandlungsverfahren *nt*, -schema *nt*, Therapie *f*. **3.** (*Krankheit*) Heilung *f*. **4.** (Heil-)Mittel *nt* (*for* gegen). **5.** *fig.* Mittel *nt*, Abhilfe *f*, Rezept *nt* (*for* gegen). **6.** Haltbarmachung *f*. **7.** *techn.* (Aus-)Härtung *f*; Vulkanisieren *nt*. **II** *vt* **8.** jdn. heilen, kurieren (*of* von); (*Krankheit*) heilen. **9.** haltbar machen. **10.** aushärten; vulkanisieren. **III** *vi* **11.** Heilung bringen, heilen. **12.** eine Kur machen, kuren.
cu·ret *n*, *vt* → curette.
cu·ret·ment [kjʊəˈretmənt] *n* → curettage.
cu·ret·tage [kjʊəˈretɪdʒ, ˌkjʊərəˈtɑːʒ] *n chir.* Ausschabung *f*, Auskratzung *f*, Kürettage *f*, Kürettement *nt*, Curettage *f*.
cu·rette [kjʊəˈret] **I** *n chir.* Kürette *f*. **II** *vt* (*mit einer Kürette*) ausschaben, auskratzen, kürettieren.
cu·rette·ment [kjʊəˈretmənt] *n* → curettage.
Curie [ˈkjʊərɪ, kjʊəˈriː]: **C.'s law** Curie'-Gesetz *nt*, -Regel *f*.
C.'s therapy Curie-Therapie *f*.
cu·rie [ˈkjʊərɪ, kjʊəˈriː] *n abbr.* **Ci** Curie *nt abbr.* Ci.
cu·ri·um [ˈkʊərɪəm] *n abbr.* **Cm** *chem.* Curium *nt abbr.* Cm.
Curling [ˈkɜrlɪŋ]: **C. factor** Griseofulvin *nt*.
C.'s ulcer Curling-Ulkus *nt*.
cur·ling esophagus [ˈkɜrlɪŋ] *radiol.* Korkenzieherösophagus *m*.
cur·rant jelly clot [ˈkɜrənt, ˈkʌr-] *hema., patho.* Kruorgerinnsel *nt*, Cruor sanguinis.
currant jelly stool *patho.* Stuhl *m* mit Frischblutauflagerung.
currant jelly thrombus → currant jelly clot.
cur·rent [ˈkɜrənt, ˈkʌr-] **I** *n* **1.** (*a. fig.*) Strom *m*, Strömung *f*; *electr.* Strom *m*. **against/with the ~** gegen den/mit dem Strom. **2.** *fig.* Trend *m*, Tendenz *f*. **II** *adj* **3.** gegenwärtig, aktuell, jetzig, laufend. **4.** üblich, gebräuchlich, verbreitet.
c. of injury Verletzungsstrom.
current density Stromdichte *f*.
current distribution Stromverteilung *f*.
current pulse Stromstoß *m*.
current state *techn.* Istwert *m*.
current-voltage curve Stromspannungskurve *f*.

cur·ric·u·lum [kəˈrɪkjələm] *n*, *pl* **-lums**, **-la** [-lə] Studien-, Lehrplan *m*, Kurrikulum *nt*, Curriculum *nt*.
curriculum vi·tae [ˈvaɪtiː, ˈviːtaɪ] *abbr.* **cv** Lebenslauf *m*.
Curschmann [ˈkʊrʃmən]: **C.'s disease** Zuckergußleber *f*, Perihepatitis chronica hyperplastica.
C.'s spirals *patho.* Curschmann-Spiralen *pl.*
cur·sive epilepsy [ˈkɜrsɪv] Dromolepsie *f*, Epilepsia cursiva.
Curtius [ˈkʊərt(s)ɪəs]: **C.' syndrome** Curtius-Syndrom *nt*, Hemihypertrophie *f*.
cur·va·tu·ra [ˌkɜrvəˈtjʊərə] *n*, *pl* **-rae** [-riː] *anat.* → curvature 1.
cur·va·ture [ˈkɜrvətʃər, -ˌtʃʊ(ə)r, -ˌtjʊər] *n* **1.** Krümmung *f*, Wölbung *f*; *anat.* Kurvatur *f*, Curvatura *f*. **2.** Magenkrümmung *f*, -kurvatur *f*, Curvatura gastrica/ventricularis.
c. of stomach → curvature 2.
curvature ametropia *ophthal.* Krümmungsametropie *f*.
curvature hyperopia *ophthal.* Krümmungshyperopie *f*.
curvature myopia *ophthal.* Krümmungsmyopie *f*.
curve [kɜrv] **I** *n* (*a. mathe.*) Kurve *f*; Krümmung *f*, Biegung *f*, Bogen *m*, Rundung *f*, Wölbung *f*. **II** *vt* biegen, wölben, krümmen. **III** *vi* einen Bogen/eine Biegung machen, sich biegen, s. runden.
c. of Ellis and Garland Ellis-Damoiseau'-Linie *f*.
curved [kɜrvd] *adj* gekrümmt, gebogen, geschwungen, gewölbt, Bogen-.
curved applicator *chir.* gebogener Watteträger *m*.
curved line: **highest c. of occipital bone** Linea nuchalis suprema.
c. of ilium Linea arcuata ossis ilii.
inferior c. of ilium Linea glut(a)ealis inferior.
inferior c. of occipital bone Linea nuchalis inferior.
middle c. of ilium Linea glut(a)ealis anterior.
superior c. of ilium Linea glut(a)ealis posterior.
superior c. of occipital bone, (external) Linea nuchalis superior.
supreme c. of occipital bone → highest c. of occipital bone.
curved scissors *chir.* gebogene Schere *f*.
Cushing [ˈkʊʃɪŋ]: **C.'s basophilism** → C.'s syndrome 1.
C.'s disease zentrales Cushing-Syndrom *nt*, Morbus Cushing *m*.
C.'s effect → C.'s phenomenon.
medicamentous C.'s syndrome medikamentöses Cushing-Syndrom *nt*.
C.'s phenomenon Cushing-Effekt *m*, -Phänomen *nt*.
C.'s reaction → C.'s phenomenon.
C.'s suture *chir.* Cushing-Naht *f*.
C.'s syndrome 1. Cushing-Syndrom *nt*. **2.** Kleinhirnbrückenwinkel-Syndrom *nt*, Cushing-Syndrom II *nt*.
C.'s ulcer Cushing-Ulkus *nt*.
cush·in·goid [ˈkʊʃɪŋɡɔɪd] *adj* Cushing-ähnlich, cushingoid.
cush·ion [ˈkʊʃn] **I** *n* **1.** Kissen *nt*; (*a. fig.*) Polster *nt*. **2.** *techn.* Puffer *m*, Dämpfer *m*, Polster *nt*. **II** *vt* polstern, dämpfen, puffern, abfedern.
cusp [kʌsp] *n* **1.** Spitze *f*, Zipfel *m*; *anat.* Cuspis. **2.** Herzklappenzipfel *m*, Klappensegel *nt*, Cuspis *m*. **3.** Zahnhöcker *m*, Cuspis dentis, Cuspis coronae (dentis).
cus·pate [ˈkʌspeɪt, -pɪt] *adj* → cuspid II.

cus·pat·ed [ˈkʌspeɪtɪd] *adj* → cuspid II.
cusped [kʌspt] *adj* → cuspid II.
cus·pid [ˈkʌspɪd] **I** *n* Eck-, Reißzahn *m*, Dens caninus. **II** *adj* mit Zipfel(n) *od.* Höcker(n) versehen, spitz (zulaufend).
cus·pi·date [ˈkʌspədeɪt] *adj* → cuspid II.
cus·pi·dat·ed [ˈ-deɪtɪd] *adj* → cuspid II.
cuspid tooth → cuspid I.
cus·pis [ˈkʌspɪs] *n*, *pl* **-pi·des** [-pɪdiːz] *anat.* → cusp.
Custer [ˈkʌstər]: **C. cells** Custer-Zellen *pl.*
cut [kʌt] **I** *n* **1.** Schnitt *m*. **2.** Schnittwunde *f*, -verletzung *f*. **3.** (Haar-)Schnitt *m*. **4.** (*a. techn.*) Schnittfläche *f*; Ein-, Anschnitt *m*. **5.** Gesichtsschnitt *m*. **6.** *electr.* Unterbrechung *f*, Sperre *f*, Ausfall *m*. **II** *adj* **7.** beschnitten, (zu-, auf-)geschnitten, Schnitt-. **8.** *bot.* (ein-)gekerbt. **III** *vt* **9.** (an-, be-, zer-)schneiden, ab-, durchschneiden, einen Schnitt machen in. **to ~ one's finger** sich in den Finger schneiden. **to ~ to pieces** zerstückeln, -trennen. **10.** (*a.* **to ~ one's teeth**) zahnen, Zähne bekommen. **11.** verletzen. **12.** *chem., techn.* verdünnen; verwässern. **13.** (*Strom*) abstellen. **14.** reduzieren, senken, vermindern, kürzen. **IV** *vi* **15.** schneiden, bohren, stechen (*in, into* in). **16.** (*Kragen*) einschneiden. **17.** (*Zähne*) durchbrechen. **18.** s. schneiden, s. kreuzen.
cut down I *vt* verringern, reduzieren, einschränken; herabsetzen, drosseln (*by* um; *to* auf). **II** *vi* s. einschränken (*on sth.*).
cut into *vi* (ein-)schneiden in.
cut off *vt* **1.** abschneiden, -trennen, unterbinden; amputieren. **2.** *techn.* ab-, ausschalten, -drehen; unterbrechen. **3.** *fig.* (*Beziehung*) abbrechen; trennen, isolieren, absondern (*from* von).
cut open *vt* aufschneiden.
cut out *vt* **1.** *inf.* etw. unterlassen, aufhören mit, etw. bleiben *od.* sein lassen. **2.** (her-)ausschneiden.
cut through *vt* durchschneiden.
cut up *vt* **1.** zerschneiden. **2.** zerlegen. **3. to be ~** gekränkt *od.* betrübt sein.
cu·ta·ne·o·mu·co·ve·al syndrome [kjuːˌteɪnɪoˌmjuːkoʊˈviːəl] Behçet-Krankheit *f*, -Syndrom *nt*, bipolare/große/maligne Aphthose *f*, Gilbert-Syndrom *nt*, Aphthose Touraine/Behçet.
cu·ta·ne·ous [kjuːˈteɪnɪəs] *adj* Haut/Cutis betr., kutan, dermal, Haut-, Derm(a)-.
cutaneous afferent Hautafferenz *f*.
cutaneous amputation *chir.* Amputation *f* mit Hautlappendeckung.
cutaneous amyloidosis Hautamyloidose *f*.
cutaneous anthrax Hautmilzbrand *m*.
cutaneous blastomycosis Hautblastomykose *f*, kutane Blastomykose *f*.
cutaneous branch Hautast *m*, Ramus cutaneus.
anterior c.es of femoral nerve vordere Hautäste *pl* des N. femoralis, Rami cutanei anteriores n. femoralis.
anterior c. of iliohypogastric nerve vorderer Hautast des N. iliohypogastricus, Ramus cutaneus anterior n. iliohypogastrici.
anterior c. of intercostal nerves vorderer Hautast der Interkostalnerven, Ramus cutaneus anterior (pectoralis/abdominalis) nn. intercostalium.
crural c.es of saphenous nerve, medial Hautäste *pl* des N. saphenus zum medialen Unterschenkel, Rami cutanei cruris mediales n. sapheni.
lateral c. of iliohypogastric nerve seitlicher Hautast des N. iliohypogastricus, Ramus cutaneus lateralis n. iliohypogastrici.

lateral c. of intercostal nerves seitlicher Hautast der Interkostalnerven, Ramus cutaneus lateralis (pectoralis/abdominalis) nn. intercostalium.
lateral c. of posterior intercostal arteries Ramus cutaneus lateralis aa. intercostalium posteriorum.
c. of obturator nerve Hautast des N. obturatorius, Ramus cutaneus n. obturatorii.
cutaneous candidiasis kutane Kandidamykose/Kandidose/Candidose/Candidamykose *f*.
cutaneous cyst dermale/kutane Zyste *f*, Hautzyste *f*.
cutaneous diphtheria Hautdiphtherie *f*, Diphtheria cutanea.
cutaneous dropsy Ödem *nt*, Oedema *nt*.
cutaneous emphysema Hautemphysem *nt*, Emphysema subcutaneum.
cutaneous fungus *micro.* Dermatophyt *m*.
cutaneous glands Hautdrüsen *pl*, Gll. cutis.
cutaneous horn *derm.* Hauthorn *nt*, Cornu cutaneum, Keratoma giganteum.
cutaneous larva migrans Hautmaulwurf *m*, Larva migrans, Myiasis linearis migrans, creeping disease (*nt*).
cutaneous layer of tympanic membrane (Platten-)Epithel *nt* der Trommelfellaußenseite, Kutisschicht *f*, Stratum cutaneum membranae tympani.
cutaneous leishmaniasis kutane Leishmaniose/Leishmaniase *f*, Hautleishmaniose *f*, Orientbeule *f*, Leishmaniasis cutis.
 anergic c. → diffuse c.
 diffuse c. leproide Leishmaniasis, Leishmaniasis cutis/tegumentaria diffusa.
 South American c. südamerikanische Hautleishmaniase, kutane Leishmaniase Südamerikas, Chiclero-Ulkus *nt*.
cutaneous leprosy tuberkuloide Lepra *f abbr.* TL, Lepra tuberculoides.
cutaneous lymphoplasia Bäfverstedt-Syndrom *nt*, benigne Lymphoplasie *f* der Haut, multiples Sarkoid *nt*, Lymphozytom *nt*, Lymphocytoma cutis, Lymphadenosis benigna cutis.
cutaneous muscle in die Haut einstrahlender Muskel *m*, M. cutaneous.
cutaneous necrosis Hautnekrose *f*.
cutaneous nerve Hautnerv *m*, N. cutaneus.
 dorsal c. of foot, intermediate mittlerer Hautnerv des Fußrückens, N. cutaneus dorsalis intermedius.
 dorsal c. of foot, lateral lateraler Hautnerv des Fußrückens, N. cutaneus dorsalis lateralis.
 dorsal c. of foot, medial medialer Hautnerv des Fußrückens, N. cutaneus dorsalis medialis.
 femoral c., lateral seitlicher Hautnerv des Oberschenkels, N. cutaneus femoris lateralis.
 femoral c., posterior hinterer Hautnerv des Oberschenkels, N. cutaneus femoralis posterior.
 lateral c. of arm, inferior seitlicher Hautnerv des (Unter-)Arms, N. cutaneus brachii lateralis inferior.
 lateral c. of arm, superior seitlicher Hautnerv des (Ober-)Arms, N. cutaneus brachii lateralis superior.
 lateral c. of calf → sural c., lateral.
 lateral c. of forearm seitlicher Hautnerv des Unterarms, N. cutaneus antebrachii lateralis.
 lateral c. of thigh → femoral c., lateral.
 medial c. of arm medialer Hautnerv des Oberarms, N. cutaneus brachii medialis.
 medial c. of calf → sural c., medial.
 medial c. of forearm medialer Hautnerv des Unterarms, N. cutaneus antebrachii medialis.
 perforating c. N. cutaneus perforans.
 posterior c. of arm hinterer Hautnerv des Oberarms, N. cutaneus brachii posterior.
 posterior c. of arm, lateral N. cutaneus brachii lateralis posterior.
 posterior c. of forearm hinterer Hautnerv des Unterarms, N. cutaneus antebrachii posterior.
 posterior c. of thigh → femoral c., posterior.
 sural c., lateral seitlicher Hautnerv der Wade, N. cutaneus surae lateralis.
 sural c., medial medialer Hautnerv der Wade, N. cutaneus surae medialis.
cutaneous papilloma Stielwarze *f*, Akrochordon *nt*, Acrochordon *nt*.
cutaneous porphyria Porphyria cutanea.
cutaneous pupillary reflex → cutaneous pupil reflex.
cutaneous pupil reflex ziliospinaler Reflex *m*.
cutaneous reaction Haut-, Kuti-, Dermoreaktion *f*.
cutaneous receptor Hautrezeptor *m*.
cutaneous schistosomiasis *derm.* Schwimmbadkrätze *f*, Weiherhippel *m*, Bade-, Schistosomen-, Zerkariendermatitis *f*.
cutaneous sebum Hauttalg *m*, Sebum cutaneum.
cutaneous sensation kutane Sensibilität *f*.
cutaneous sensory organs Hautsinnesorgane *pl*.
cutaneous syndactyly *embryo.* kutane Syndaktylie *f*.
cutaneous tag Stielwarze *f*, Akrochordon *nt*, Acrochordon *nt*.
cutaneous test Hauttest *m*.
cutaneous tuberculosis Hauttuberkulose *f*, Tuberculosis cutis.
cutaneous ureterostomy *urol.* Harnleiter-Haut-Fistel *f*, Ureterokutaneostomie *f*.
cutaneous vein Hautvene *f*, V. cutanea.
 ulnar c. Basilika *f*, V. basilica.
cu·ti·cle ['kjuːtɪkl] *n* **1.** *anat.* Häutchen *nt*, hauchdünner Überzug *m* von Epithelzellen, Kutikula *f*, Cuticula *f*. **2.** Nagelhäutchen *nt*, Eponychium *nt*.
cu·tic·u·la [kjuːˈtɪkjələ] *n*, *pl* **-lae** [-liː] *anat.* → cuticle 1.
cu·tic·u·lar [kjuːˈtɪkjələr] *adj* Kutikula betr., kutikular.
cuticular layer kutikulare Schicht *f*.
 c. of tympanic membrane → cutaneous layer of tympanic membrane.
cu·ti·re·ac·tion [ˌkjuːtɜrɪˈækʃn] *n* → cutaneous reaction.
cutireaction test Hauttest *m*.
cu·tis ['kjuːtɪs] *n*, *pl* **-tis·es**, **-tes** [-tiːz] *anat.* Haut *f*, Kutis *f*, Cutis *f*.
cutis graft Kutislappen *m*.
cutis laxa Fall-, Schlaffhaut *f*, Cutis-laxa-Syndrom *nt*, generalisierte Elastolyse *f*, Zuviel-Haut-Syndrom *nt*, Dermatolysis *f*, Dermatochalasis *f*, Dermatomegalie *f*, Chalazodermie *f*, Chalodermie *f*.
cutis plate *neuro.* Dermatom *nt*.
cut surface Schnittfläche *f*.
cut·ter ['kʌtər] *n* Schneidewerkzeug *nt*, -maschine *f*; Fräser *m*, Tiefbohrer *m*.
cut·ting ['kʌtɪŋ] **I** *n* **1.** (Aus-, Ab-, Be-)Schneiden *nt*. **2.** Herabsetzung *f*, (Ver-)Minderung *f*, Senkung *f*, Reduzierung *f*. **II** *adj* **3.** schneidend, Schnitt-, Schneide-. **4.** scharf; (*a. fig.*) beißend, spitz.
cutting edge (*Zahn*) Schneidekante *f*, Margo incisalis.
 c. of nail vorderer/freier Nagelrand *m*, Schnitt-, Abnutzungskante *f*, Margo liber unguis.
cu·vet *n* → cuvette.
cu·vette [k(j)uːˈvet] *n* Küvette *f*.
Cuvier [ˈkjuːvɪɛr; kyˈvje]: **C.'s canal** *embryo.* Cuvier'-Gang *m*, -Kanal *m*.
 C.'s ducts/sinuses *embryo.* Kardinalvenen *pl*.
CV *abbr.* **1.** → cardiovascular. **2.** → coefficient of variation.
cv *abbr.* → curriculum vitae.
CVA *abbr.* **1.** → cerebrovascular accident. **2.** → costovertebral angle.
C virus → coxsackievirus.
CVN *abbr.* → central venous nutrition.
CVP *abbr.* → central venous pressure.
CVS *abbr.* → cardiovascular system.
c wave *card.* c-Welle *f*.
cxr *abbr.* → chest x-ray.
Cy *abbr.* → cyanogen.
cyan- *pref.* → cyano-.
cy·an·al·co·hol [saɪənˈælkəhɑl] *n* → cyanohydrin.
cy·an·a·mide [saɪˈænəmaɪd, -mɪd] *n* **1.** Karbamin-, Carbaminsäurenitril *nt*, Zyanamid *nt*, Cyanamid *nt*. **2.** Calciumcyanamid *nt*.
cy·a·nate [ˈsaɪəneɪt, -nɪt] *n* Zyanat *nt*, Cyanat *nt*.
cy·an·eph·i·dro·sis [ˌsaɪənˌefɪˈdroʊsɪs] *n* → cyanhidrosis.
cy·an·he·mo·glo·bin [ˌ-ˈhiːməɡloʊbɪn, -ˈhemə-] *n* Zyan-, Cyanhämoglobin *nt*, Hämoglobincyanid *nt*.
cy·an·hi·dro·sis [ˌ-haɪˈdroʊsɪs] *n* Blaufärbung *f* des Schweißes, Zyan-, Cyanhidrosis *f*.
cy·an·hy·dric acid [ˌ-ˈhaɪdrɪk] Zyanwasserstoffsäure *f*, Blausäure *f*.
cy·an·ic acid [saɪˈænɪk] Zyan-, Cyansäure *f*.
cy·a·nid [ˈsaɪənɪd] *n* → cyanide.
cy·a·nide [ˈsaɪənaɪd, -nɪd] *n* Zyanid *nt*, Cyanid *nt*.
cyanide methemoglobin → cyanmethemoglobin.
cyanide poisoning Zyanidvergiftung *f*.
cy·an·met·he·mo·glo·bin [ˌsaɪənˌmet'hiːməɡloʊbɪn, -ˈhemə-] *n abbr.* **HbCN** Zyan-, Cyanmethämoglobin *nt*, Methämoglobincyanid *nt*.
cyanmethemoglobin method Zyanhämoglobinmethode *f*.
cy·an·met·my·o·glo·bin [ˌ-metˌmaɪəˈɡloʊbɪn] *n* Zyan-, Cyanmetmyoglobin *nt*, Metmyoglobinzyanid *nt*.
cyano- *pref.* Zyan(o)-, Cyan(o)-, Blau-.
cy·a·no·ac·et·y·lene [ˌsaɪənoʊəˈsetɪliːn, -ɪn] *n* Cyanoacetylen *nt*.
β-cy·a·no·al·a·nine [ˌ-ˈæləniːn, -nɪn] *n* β-Cyanoalanin *nt*.
cy·a·no·al·co·hol [ˌ-ˈælkəhɑl] *n* → cyanohydrin.
Cy·a·no·bac·te·ria [ˌ-bækˈtɪərɪə] *pl micro. old* blau-grüne Algen *pl*, Cyanobacteria *pl*.
cy·a·no·chro·ic [ˌ-ˈkroʊɪk] *adj* → cyanotic.
cy·an·och·rous [saɪəˈnɑkrəs] *adj* → cyanotic.
cy·a·no·co·bal·a·min [ˌsaɪənoʊkoʊˈbæləmɪn] *n* Zyano-, Cyanocobalamin *nt*, Vitamin B$_{12}$ *nt*.
cy·a·no·der·ma [ˌ-ˈdɜrmə] *n* → cyanosis.
cy·a·no·form [saɪˈænəfɔrm] *n* Zyano-, Cyanoform *nt*.
cy·an·o·gen [saɪˈænədʒən] *n abbr.* **Cy** Zyanogen *nt*, Cyanogen *nt*.
cyanogen bromide *chem.* Bromcyan *nt*.
cyanogen chloride Chlorcyan *nt*.
cy·a·no·guan·i·din [ˌsaɪənoʊˈɡwænɪdɪn, -dɪn, -ˈɡwɑːnɪ-, saɪˌænoʊ-] *n* Zyano-, Cyanoguanidin *nt*, Dicyandiamid *nt*.

cyanohydrin

cy·a·no·hy·drin [ˌ-'haɪdrɪn] n Zyan(o)alkohol m.
cy·an·o·phil [saɪ'ænəfɪl] **I** n zyanophile Zelle f od. Struktur f. **II** adj → cyanophilous.
cy·an·o·phile ['-faɪl] n → cyanophil I.
cy·a·noph·i·lous [saɪə'nɑfɪləs] adj histol. zyanophil.
Cy·a·no·phy·ce·ae [ˌsaɪənə'faɪsɪˌiː] pl → Cyanobacteria.
cy·a·nop·ia [ˌsaɪə'nəʊpɪə] n → cyanopsia.
cy·a·nop·sia [ˌ-'nɑpsɪə] n Blausehen nt, Zyanop(s)ie f.
cy·a·nop·sin [ˌ-'nɑpsɪn] n Zyanopsin nt.
cy·a·nose ['saɪənəʊs] n → cyanosis.
cy·a·nosed ['saɪənəʊsd] adj → cyanotic.
cy·a·no·sis [ˌsaɪə'nəʊsɪs] n Blausucht f, Zyanose f, Cyanosis f.
cy·a·not·ic [ˌ-'nɑtɪk] adj Zyanose betr., mit Zyanose einhergehend, zyanotisch.
cyanotic atrophy patho. zyanotische Atrophie f, Sauerstoffmangelatrophie f.
c. of liver Stauungsinduration f der Leber, Cirrhose cardiaque.
cyanotic induration patho. zyanotische Induration f.
cy·a·nu·ria [ˌ-'n(j)ʊərɪə] n patho. Zyanurie f.
cy·a·nu·ric acid [ˌ-'n(j)ʊərɪk] Zyanur-, Cyanursäure f.
cy·ber·net·ic [ˌsaɪbər'netɪk] adj kybernetisch.
cy·ber·net·ics [ˌ-'netɪks] pl Kybernetik f.
CYC abbr. → cyclophosphamide.
cycl- pref. → cyclo-.
cyc·la·mate ['saɪkləmeɪt, 'sɪk-] n Zyklamat nt, Cyclamat nt.
cy·clam·ic acid [saɪ'klæmɪk] Cyclohexansulfaminsäure f, N-Cyclohexylsulfaninsäure f.
cyc·la·min ['sɪkləmɪn] n Cyclamin nt.
cy·clan·de·late [saɪ'klændɪleɪt] n pharm. Cyclandelat nt.
cy·clase ['saɪkleɪs] n Zyklase f, Cyclase f.
cy·cle ['saɪkl] **I** n **1.** Zyklus m, Kreis(lauf m) m; (a. phys.) Periode f. **in ~s** periodisch **2.** chem. Ring m. **II** vt periodisch wiederholen. **III** vi periodisch wiederkehren.
cyc·lec·to·my [sɪk'lektəmɪ, saɪ-] n ophthal. **1.** Ziliarkörperentfernung f, Ziliektomie f, Zyklektomie f. **2.** operative Teilentfernung f des Lidrandes, Ziliektomie f.
cy·clen·ce·pha·lia [ˌsaɪklənsɪ'feɪlɪə, ˌsɪk-] n → cyclencephaly.
cy·clen·ceph·a·lus [ˌ-'sefələs] n embryo. Zyklenzephalus m.
cy·clen·ceph·a·ly [ˌ-'sefəlɪ] n embryo. Zykl(o)enzephalie f.
cy·clic ['saɪklɪk, 'sɪk-] adj **1.** zyklisch, periodisch, Kreislauf-. **2.** chem. zyklisch, ringförmig, Ring-, Zyklo-.
cyclic adenosine monophosphate → cyclic AMP.
cy·cli·cal ['saɪklɪkl, 'sɪk-] adj → cyclic.
cyclic albuminuria zyklische/intermittierende Albuminurie f.
cyclic AMP abbr. **cAMP** zyklisches Adenosin-3',5'-Phosphat nt, Zyklo-AMP nt, Cyclo-AMP nt abbr. cAMP, 3'-5'AMP.
cyclic AMP receptor protein abbr. **CAP, CRP** Cyclo-AMP-Rezeptorprotein nt abbr. CRP, Katabolit-Gen-Aktivatorprotein nt abbr. CAP.
cyclic compound chem. Ringverbindung f.
cyclic endoperoxide zyklisches Endoperoxid nt.
cyclic GMP abbr. **cGMP** zyklisches Guanosin-3',5'-Phosphat nt abbr. 3',5'-GMP, zyklisches GMP nt, Zyklo--GMP nt, Cyclo-GMP nt abbr. cGMP.
cyclic guanosine monophosphate → cyclic GMP.

cyclic hydrocarbon ringförmiger/zyklischer Kohlenwasserstoff m.
cyclic neutropenia periodische/zyklische Leukozytopenie f, periodische/zyklische Neutropenie f.
cy·cli·cot·o·my [ˌsaɪklɪ'kɑtəmɪ, sɪk-] n → cyclotomy.
cyclic phosphorylation biochem. zyklische Phosphorylierung f.
cyclic vomiting periodisches/zyklisches/rekurrierendes Erbrechen nt.
cyc·li·tis [sɪk'laɪtɪs, saɪ-] n Ziliarkörperentzündung f, Zyklitis f, Cyclitis f.
cy·cli·za·tion [ˌsaɪklə'zeɪʃn, ˌsɪk-] n chem. Ringschluß m, -bildung f, Zyklisierung f.
cy·clize ['saɪklaɪz, 'sɪ-] vt chem. zyklisieren, cyclisieren.
cyclo- pref. **1.** Kreis-, Zykl(o)-, Cycl(o)-. **2.** Ziliarkörper-.
cy·clo·bar·bi·tal [ˌsaɪkləʊ'bɑːrbətɔl] n pharm. Cyclobarbital nt.
cy·clo·bar·bi·tone [ˌ-'bɑːrbətəʊn] n → cyclobarbital.
cy·clo·ceph·a·lia [ˌ-sɪ'feɪlɪə] n → cyclopia.
cy·clo·ceph·a·lus [ˌ-'sefələs] n → cyclops.
cy·clo·ceph·a·ly [ˌ-'sefəlɪ] n → cyclopia.
cy·clo·cer·a·ti·tis [ˌ-serə'taɪtɪs] n → cyclokeratitis.
cy·clo·cho·roid·i·tis [ˌ-kɔːrɔɪ'daɪtɪs] n ophthal. Zyklochorioiditis f.
cy·clo·cry·o·ther·a·py [ˌ-ˌkraɪə'θerəpɪ] n ophthal. Zyklokryotherapie f.
cy·clo·di·al·y·sis [ˌ-daɪ'æləsɪs] n ophthal. Zyklodialyse f.
cy·clo·di·a·ther·my [ˌ-'daɪəθɜːrmɪ] n ophthal. Zyklodiathermie f.
cy·clo·duc·tion [ˌ-'dʌkʃn] n ophthal. Zykloduktion f.
cy·clo·e·lec·trol·y·sis [ˌ-ɪlek'trɑləsɪs] n ophthal. Zykloelektrolyse f.
cy·clo·hex·ane·hex·ol [ˌ-ˌheksein'heksɔl, -sɒl] n Inosit nt, Inositol nt.
cy·clo·hex·ane·sul·fam·ic acid [ˌ-ˌheksein-sʌl'fæmɪk] → cyclamic acid.
cy·clo·hex·a·nol [ˌ-'heksənɔl, -nɒl] n Zyklo-, Cyclohexanol nt.
cy·clo·hex·ene [ˌ-'heksiːn] n Zyklo-, Cyclohexen nt.
cy·clo·hex·i·mide [ˌ-'heksəmaɪd, -mɪd] n Cycloheximid nt, Actidion nt.
cy·clo·hex·yl·sul·fam·ic acid [ˌ-ˌheksɪlsʌl-'fæmɪk] → cyclamic acid.
cy·cloid ['saɪklɔɪd] psychia. **I** n zykloider Patient m. **II** adj zykloid.
cycloid disorder → cyclothymia.
cycloid personality → cyclothymia.
cy·clo·i·som·er·ase [ˌsaɪkləʊaɪ'sɑmereɪz] n Zyklo-, Cycloisomerase f.
cy·clo·ker·a·ti·tis [ˌ-kerə'taɪtɪs] n ophthal. Entzündung f von Ziliarkörper u. Hornhaut, Zyklokeratitis f.
cy·clo·li·gase [ˌ-'laɪgeɪz] n Zyklo-, Cycloligase f.
cy·clo·mas·top·a·thy [ˌ-mæs'tɑpəθɪ] n old → cystic disease of the breast.
cy·clo·ox·y·gen·ase [ˌ-'ɑksɪdʒəneɪz] n Zyklo-, Cyclooxigenase f.
cy·clo·pen·ta·mine [ˌ-'pentəmiːn] n pharm. Cyclopentamin nt.
cy·clo·pen·tane [ˌ-'penteɪn] n Zyklo-, Cyclopentan nt.
cy·clo·pen·ta·none [ˌ-'pentənəʊn] n Zyklo-, Cyclopentanon nt.
cy·clo·pen·ta·no·phen·an·threne [ˌ-pen-ˌtiːnəʊfɪ'nænθriːn] n Cyclopentanophenanthren nt.
cy·clo·pen·thi·a·zide [ˌ-pen'θaɪəzaɪd] n pharm. Cyclopenthiazid nt.
cy·clo·pen·to·late [ˌ-'pentəleɪt] n pharm. Cyclopentolat nt.
cy·clo·pho·ria [ˌ-'fɔːrɪə] n ophthal. Zyklophorie f.

cy·clo·phor·om·e·ter [ˌ-fə'rɑmɪtər] n ophthal. Zyklophorometer nt.
cy·clo·phos·pha·mide [ˌ-'fɑsfəmaɪd] n abbr. **CYC** pharm. Cyclophosphamid nt.
cy·clo·pho·to·co·ag·u·la·tion [ˌ-ˌfəʊtəʊ-kəʊˌægjə'leɪʃn] n ophthal. Zyklophotokoagulation f.
cy·clo·phre·nia [ˌ-'friːnɪə] n psychia. manisch-depressive Psychose f, Zyklophrenie f.
Cy·clo·phyl·li·dea [ˌ-'fɪliːdiː] pl micro. Cyclophyllidea f.
cy·clo·pia [saɪ'kləʊpɪə] n embryo. Zyklopie f, Zyklozephalie f.
cy·clo·ple·gia [ˌsaɪkləʊ'pliːdʒ(ɪ)ə] n ophthal. Akkommodationslähmung f, Zykloplegie f.
cy·clo·ple·gic [ˌ-'pliːdʒɪk] **I** n pharm. Zykloplegie-verursachende Substanz f. **II** adj Zykloplegie betr. od. verursachend, zykloplegisch.
cy·clo·pro·pane [ˌ-'prəʊpeɪn] n Zyklo-, Cyclopropan nt.
cy·clops ['saɪklɒps] n embryo. Zyklop m, Zyklozephalus m, Synophthalmus m.
cy·clo·ro·ta·to·ry [ˌ-'rəʊtəˌtɔːriː, -təʊ-] adj zyklorotatorisch.
cy·clo·ser·ine [ˌ-'seriːn] n pharm. Cycloserin nt.
cy·clo·sis [saɪ'kləʊsɪs] n, pl **-ses** [-siːz] bot. (Zyto-)Plasmazirkulation f, Zyklosis f.
cy·clo·spasm [ˌsaɪkləspæzm] n ophthal. Akkommodationskrampf m, Zyklospasmus m.
cy·clo·spor·in A [ˌ-'spɔːrɪn] → cyclosporine.
cy·clo·spor·ine [ˌ-'spɔːriːn] n Cyclosporin (A) nt.
cy·clo·thi·a·zide [ˌ-'θaɪəzaɪd] n pharm. Cyclothiazid nt.
cy·clo·thyme ['-θaɪm] n psychia. zyklothymer Patient(in f) m, Zyklothyme(r m) f.
cy·clo·thy·mia [ˌ-'θaɪmɪə] n psychia. zyklothymes Temperament nt, zyklothyme Persönlichkeit f, Zyklothymie f.
cy·clo·thym·i·ac [ˌ-'θaɪmɪæk] adj → cyclothymic.
cy·clo·thy·mic [ˌ-'θaɪmɪk] adj Zyklothymie betr., mit Symptomen der Zyklothymie, zyklothym.
cyclothymic personality (disorder) → cyclothymia.
cy·clo·tome ['-təʊm] n ophthal. Zyklotom nt.
cy·clot·o·my [saɪ'klɑtəmɪ] n ophthal. Ziliarmuskeldurchtrennung f, Zyklotomie f.
cy·clo·tron ['saɪklətrɑn] n Zyklotron nt.
cy·clo·tro·pia [ˌ-'trəʊpɪə] n ophthal. Zyklotropie f, Strabismus rotatorius.
cy·clo·zo·on·o·sis [ˌ-zəʊ'ɑnəsɪs, ˌzəʊə'nəʊ-sɪs] n micro. Zyklozoonose f.
CYE agar micro. Aktivkohle-Hefeextrakt-Agar m/nt, charcoal-yeast extract agar.
cy·e·si·og·no·sis [saɪˌɪsɪəg'nəʊsɪs] n gyn. Schwangerschaftsnachweis m, -feststellung f.
cy·e·sis [saɪ'iːsɪs] n, pl **-ses** [-siːz] Schwangerschaft f, Gravidität f, Graviditas f.
cyl·i·cot·o·my [sɪlə'kɑtəmɪ] n → cyclotomy.
cyl·in·der ['sɪlɪndər] n Zylinder m; Walze f, Rolle f.
cy·lin·dric [sɪ'lɪndrɪk] adj walzen-, zylinderförmig, zylindrisch, Zylinder-.
cy·lin·dri·cal [sɪ'lɪndrɪkl] adj → cylindric.
cylindrical lens Zylinderglas nt.
cylindric bronchiectasis zylindrische Bronchiektasi(e)e f.
cylindric cell hochprismatische Epithelzelle f.
cy·lin·dri·form [sɪ'lɪndrəfɔːrm] adj → cylindric.

cy·lin·dro·ad·e·no·ma [sɪˌlɪndrəʊˌædə-'nəʊmə] *n* → cylindroma.
cyl·in·droid ['sɪlɪndrɔɪd] **I** *n urol.* Zylindroid *nt*, Pseudozylinder *m*. **II** *adj* zylinderähnlich, zylindroid.
cylindroid aneurysm zylindrisches Aneurysma *nt*, Aneurysma cylindricum.
cyl·in·dro·ma [ˌ-'drəʊmə] *n* **1.** Zylindrom *nt*, Cylindroma *nt*, Spiegler-Tumor *m*; (*Kopfhaut*) Turbantumor *m*. **2.** adenoidzystisches Karzinom *nt*, Ca. adenoides cysticum.
cyl·in·drom·a·tous carcinoma [ˌ-'drɑmətəs] → cylindroma 2.
cyl·in·dru·ria [ˌ-'drʊərɪə] *n* Ausscheidung *f* von Harnzylindern, Zylindrurie *f*.
cyl·lo·sis [sɪ'ləʊsɪs] *n* **1.** *ortho.* Fußdeformität *f*. **2.** *ortho.* (angeborener) Klumpfuß *m*, Pes equinovarus (excavatus et adductus).
cy·mar·in [saɪ'mɑːrɪn, 'sɪ-] *n pharm.* Cymarin *nt*, k-Strophantin-α *nt*.
cy·mar·ose [saɪ'mærəʊz] *n* Cymarose *f*.
cym·ba ['sɪmbə] *n anat., bio.* bootförmige Struktur *f*, Cymba *f*.
cym·bi·form ['sɪmbɪfɔːrm] *adj* bootförmig.
cym·bo·ce·pha·lia [ˌsɪmbəʊsɪ'feɪljə] *n* → cymbocephaly.
cym·bo·ce·phal·ic [ˌ-sɪ'fælɪk] *adj* Zymbo-/Skaphozephalie betr., zymbozephal, -kephal, skaphozephal, -kephal.
cym·bo·ceph·a·lous [ˌ-'sefələs] *adj* → cymbocephalic.
cym·bo·ceph·a·ly [ˌ-'sefəlɪ] *n embryo.* Kahn-, Leistenschädel *m*, Skaphokephalie *f*, -zephalie *f*, Zymbozephalie *f*.
cy·mo·graph ['saɪməgræf] *n* Kymograph *m*.
cy·nan·che [sɪ'næŋkɪ] *n* Halsentzündung *f*; Angina *f*.
cy·nan·thro·py [saɪ'nænθrəpɪ, sɪ-] *n psychia.* Kynanthropie *f*.
cyn·ic spasm ['sɪnɪk] sardonisches Lachen *nt*, Risus sardonicus.
cy·no·dont ['saɪnədɑnt] *n* Eck-, Reißzahn *m*, Dens caninus.
cyn·o·pho·bia [ˌsaɪnə'fəʊbɪə] *n psychia.* krankhafte Angst *f* vor Hunden, Kynophobie *f*.
cy·o·pho·ria [saɪə'fɔːrɪə] *n* Schwangerschaft *f*, Gravidität *f*, Graviditas *f*.
cy·pi·o·nate [saɪpɪəneɪt] *n* Zyklopentanpropionat *nt*.
cy·pro·hep·ta·dine [ˌsaɪprəʊ'heptədiːn, ˌsɪ-] *n pharm.* Cyproheptadin *nt*.
cy·pro·ter·one [saɪ'prəʊtərəʊn] *n pharm.* Cyproteron *nt*.
Cyriax ['sɪərɪæks, 'saɪ]: **C.'s syndrome** Cyriax-Syndrom *nt*.
cyr·to·sis [sɜr'təʊsɪs] *n* **1.** Kyphose *f*. **2.** Knochendeformierung *f*, -verdrehung *f*.
Cys *abbr.* → cysteine.
Cys-Cys *abbr.* → cystine.
cyst- *pref.* → cysto-.
cyst [sɪst] *n* **1.** *anat., patho.* sackartige Geschwulst *f*, Zyste *f*, Cyste *f*, Kyste *f*, Kystom *nt*. **2.** *micro.* Zyste *f*. **3.** *bio.* Zyste *f*, Ruhezelle *f*, Kapsel *f*, Hülle *f*.
cyst·ad·e·no·car·ci·no·ma [sɪstˌædnəʊˌkɑːrsɪ'nəʊmə] *n patho.* Cyst-, Kyst-, Zystadenokarzinom *nt*, Cystadenocarcinoma *nt*.
cyst·ad·e·no·fi·bro·ma [-ˌædnəʊfaɪ'brəʊmə] *n patho.* Cyst-, Kyst-, Zystadenofibrom *nt*, Cystadenofibroma *nt*.
cyst·ad·e·no·ma [-ædə'nəʊmə] *n* Cyst-, Kyst-, Zystadenom *nt*, Adenokystom *nt*, zystisches Adenom *nt*, Zystom *nt*, Kystom *nt*, Cystadenoma *nt*.
cyst·ad·e·no·sar·co·ma [-ˌædnəʊsɑːr'kəʊmə] *n patho.* Cyst-, Kyst-, Zystadenosarkom *nt*, Cystadenosarcoma *nt*.

cys·tal·gia [sɪs'tældʒ(ɪ)ə] *n urol.* (Harn-)Blasenschmerz *m*, (Harn-)Blasenneuralgie *f*, Zystalgie *f*.
cys·ta·thi·o·nase [ˌsɪstə'θaɪəneɪz] *n* → cystathionine γ-lyase.
cys·ta·thi·o·nine [ˌ-'θaɪəniːn, -nɪn] *n* Zysta-, Cystathionin *nt*.
cystathionine γ-lyase Cystathionin-γ-Lyase *f*, Cystathionase *f*.
cystathionine β-synthase Cystathionin-β-Synthase *f*.
cys·ta·thi·o·nin·u·ria [ˌ-ˌθaɪənɪ'n(j)ʊərɪə] *n* Cystathioninurie *f*.
cys·ta·tro·phia [ˌ-'trəʊfɪə] *n urol.* (Harn-)Blasenatrophie *f*, Zystatrophie *f*.
cys·tau·che·ni·tis [ˌsɪstɔːkɪ'naɪtɪs] *n urol.* (Harn-)Blasenhalsentzündung *f*, Zystokollitis *f*, Cystitis colli.
cys·tau·che·not·o·my [ˌ-'nɑtəmɪ] *n urol.* (Harn-)Blasenhalsinzision *f*.
cyst·du·o·de·nos·to·my [sɪstˌd(j)uːədɪ'nɑstəmɪ] *n* → cystoduodenostomy.
cys·te·am·ine [ˌsɪstɪ'æmɪn, 'sɪstɪəmiːn] *n* Cysteamin *nt*.
cys·tec·ta·sia [sɪstek'teɪʒ(ɪ)ə] *n* → cystectasy.
cys·tec·ta·sy [sɪs'tektəsɪ] *n urol.* **1.** (Harn-)Blasenerweiterung *f*, (Harn-)Blasendilatation *f*, Zystektasie *f*. **2.** Gallenblasenerweiterung *f*, -dilatation *f*, Cholezystektasie *f*.
cys·tec·to·my [sɪs'tektəmɪ] *n* **1.** *chir.* Zystenentferung *f*, -ausschneidung *f*, Zystektomie *f*. **2.** *urol.* (Harn-)Blasenentfernung *f*, Zystektomie *f*.
cys·te·ic acid ['sɪstiːɪk] Cysteinsäure *f*.
cys·te·ine ['sɪstiːɪn] *n abbr.* **C, Cys** Zystein *nt*, Cystein *nt*, abbr. C, Cys.
cysteine aminotransferase Cysteinaminotransferase *f*, -transaminase *f*.
cysteine dioxigenase Cysteindeoxigenase *f*.
cysteine enzyme Cysteinenzym *nt*.
cysteine reductase (NADH) Cysteinreduktase *f* (NADH).
cysteine sulfinic acid Cysteinsulfinsäure *f*.
cysteine synthase Cysteinsynthase *f*.
cysteine transaminase → cysteine aminotransferase.
cys·te·in·yl [ˌsɪstɪ'ɪnl] *n* Cysteinyl-(Radikal *nt*).
cys·ten·ceph·a·lus [ˌsɪstən'sefələs] *n embryo.* Zystenzephalus *m*.
cyst·gas·tros·to·my [sɪstgæs'trɑstəmɪ] *n* → cystogastrostomy.
cys·tic ['sɪstɪk] *adj* **1.** Zyste betr., zystisch, blasenartig, Zysten-. **2.** Gallen- *od.* Harnblase betr., (Harn-)Blasen-, Gallenblasen-, Zysto-.
cystic acne Akne/Acne cystica.
cystic adenoma → cystadenoma.
cystic angiomatosis of bone *ortho., patho.* skelettale Hämangiomatose/Lymphangiomatose *f*, Angiomatose/Lymphangiektasie *f* des Knochens.
cystic artery Gallenblasenarterie *f*, Zystika *f*, Cystica *f*, A. cystica.
cystic bile (Gallen-)Blasengalle *f*.
cystic bronchiectasis zystische Bronchiektas(i)e *f*, Bronchiektasie *f* mit Zystenbildung.
cystic cystitis zystische (Harn-)Blasenentzündung *f*, Cystitis cystica.
cystic defect of bone, ganglionic intraossäres Ganglion *nt*, juxtaartikuläre Knochenzyste *f*.
cystic degeneration *patho.* zystische Degeneration *f*.
cystic disease: c. of the breast zystische/fibrös-zystische Mastopathie *f*, Mammadysplasie *f*, Zystenmamma *f*, Mastopa-

thia chronica cystica.
c. of the liver kongenitale Leberzyste(n *pl*) *f*, Zystenleber *f*.
c. of the lung Zystenlunge *f*.
c. of the lung, congenital *patho.* kongenitale Zystenlunge *f*.
c. of renal medulla familiäre juvenile Nephronophthisis *f*, hereditäre idiopathische Nephronophthisis *f*.
cystic duct Gallenblasengang *m*, Zystikus *m*, Cysticus *m*, Ductus cysticus.
cystic duct obstruction *chir.* Zystikusverschluß *m*, -obstruktion *f*, Ductus-cysticus-Verschluß *m*.
cystic duct stone *chir.* Zystikusstein *m*, (Gallen-)Stein *m* im Ductus cysticus.
cystic emphysema zystisches Lungenemphysem *nt*.
cys·ti·cer·coid [ˌsɪstə'sɜrkɔɪd] *n micro.* Zystizerkoid *nt*, Cysticercoid *nt*.
cys·ti·cer·co·sis [ˌ-sɜr'kəʊsɪs] *n* Zystizerkose *f*, Cysticercose *f*.
Cys·ti·cer·cus [ˌ-'sɜrkəs] *n micro.* Cysticercus *m*.
C. bovis Cysticercus bovis, Finne *f* des Rinderfinnenbandwurms.
C. cellulosae Cysticercus cellulosae, Finne *f* des Schweinefinnenbandwurms.
cys·ti·cer·cus [ˌ-'sɜrkəs] *n, pl* **-cer·ci** [-'sɜrsaɪ] *micro.* Blasenwurm *m*, Zystizerkus *m*, Cysticercus *m*.
cysticercus disease → cysticercosis.
cystic fibroma zystisches Fibrom *nt*, Fibroma cysticum.
cystic fibrosis (of the pancreas) *abbr.* **CF** Mukoviszidose *f*, zystische (Pankreas-)Fibrose *f*, Fibrosis pancreatica cystica.
cystic goiter zystische Struma *f*.
cystic hernia Blasenhernie *f*, -bruch *m*, -vorfall *m*, Zystozele *f*, Cystocele *f*.
cystic hygroma Zystenhygrom *nt*, Hygroma/Lymphangioma cysticum.
c. of the neck Zystenhygrom des Halses, Hygroma/Lymphangioma cysticum colli.
cystic hyperplasia zystische Hyperplasie *f*.
c. of the breast → cystic mastopathia.
cystic kidney Zystenniere *f*.
congenital c. kongenitale Zystenniere.
cystic lung Zystenlunge *f*.
cystic lymphangioma → cystic hygroma.
cystic mastopathia zystische/fibrös-zystische Mastopathie *f*, Zystenmamma *f*, Mammadysplasie *f*, Mastopathia chronica cystica.
cystic medial necrosis Erdheim-Gsell-Syndrom *nt*, Gsell-Erdheim-Syndrom *nt*, Medionecrosis *f* Erdheim-Gsell.
cystic mole *gyn.* Blasenmole *f*, Mola hydatidosa.
cystic node Lymphknoten *m* am Gallenblasenhals, Nodus cysticus.
cys·ti·co·li·thec·to·my [ˌsɪstɪkəʊlɪ'θektəmɪ] *n chir.* Zystikussteinentfernung *f*, Zystikolithektomie *f*.
cys·ti·co·lith·o·trip·sy [ˌ-'lɪθətrɪpsɪ] *n chir.* Zystikolithotripsie *f*.
cys·ti·cor·rha·phy [sɪstɪ'kɔrəfɪ] *n chir.* Zystikusnaht *f*, Zystikorrhaphie *f*.
cystic osteofibromatosis Jaffé-Lichtenstein-Krankheit *f*, Jaffé-Lichtenstein-Uehlinger-Syndrom *nt*, fibröse (Knochen-)Dysplasie *f*, nicht-ossifizierendes juveniles Osteofibrom *nt*, halbseitige von Recklinghausen-Krankheit *f*, Osteodystrophia fibrosa unilateralis.
cys·ti·cot·o·my [sɪstɪ'kɑtəmɪ] *n chir.* Zystikuseröffnung *f*, Zystikotomie *f*.
cystic plexus vegetativer Plexus *m* der A. cystica.
cystic polyp zystischer Polyp *m*; gestielte Zyste *f*.

cystic teratoma *gyn.* (*Ovar*) Dermoid(zyste *f*) *nt*, (zystisches) Teratom *nt*, Teratoma coaetaneum.
cystic tumor zystischer Tumor *m*.
cystic ureteritis zystische Harnleiterentzündung/Ureteritis *f*, Ureteritis cystica.
cystic vein Gallenblasenvene *f*, V. cystica.
cystid(o)- *pref.* → cysto-.
cys·ti·do·ce·li·ot·o·my [ˌsɪstɪdəʊˌsɪlɪˈatəmɪ] *n* → cystidolaparotomy.
cys·ti·do·lap·a·rot·o·my [ˌ-ˌlæpəˈratəmɪ] *n urol.* transabdomineller Blasenschnitt *m*.
cys·ti·do·tra·chel·ot·o·my [ˌ-ˌtrækəˈlatəmɪ, -ˌtreɪ-] *n* → cystauchenotomy.
cys·ti·fel·le·ot·o·my [ˌsɪstəfelɪˈatəmɪ] *n chir.* Gallenblaseneröffnung *f*, Cholezystotomie *f*.
cys·tif·er·ous [sɪsˈtɪfərəs] *adj* → cystigerous.
cys·ti·form [ˈsɪstəfɔːrm] *adj* zystenförmig, -ähnlich.
cys·tig·er·ous [sɪsˈtɪdʒərəs] *adj* zystenhaltig, zystisch.
cys·tine [ˈsɪstiːn, -tɪn] *n abbr.* **Cys-Cys** Zystin *n*, Cystin *nt*, Dicystein *nt*.
cystine calculus Zystinstein *m*.
cystine disease → cystinosis.
cys·ti·ne·mia [sɪstəˈniːmɪə] *n* Zystin-, Cystinämie *f*.
cystine stone → cystine calculus.
cystine storage disease → cystinosis.
cystine-tellurite agar Cystin-Tellurit-Medium *nt*.
cys·ti·no·sis [ˌsɪstəˈnəʊsɪs] *n* Zystinspeicherkrankheit *f*, Zystinose *f*, Cystinose *f*, Lignac-Syndrom *nt*, Aberhalden-Fanconi-Syndrom *nt*.
cys·ti·nu·ria [ˌ-ˈn(j)ʊərɪə] *n* Zystin-, Cystinurie *f*.
cys·ti·nu·ric [ˌ-ˈ(j)ʊərɪk] *adj* Zystinurie betr., zystinurisch.
cys·tiph·or·ous [sɪsˈtɪfərəs] *adj* → cystigerous.
cys·tir·rha·gia [ˌsɪstəˈrædʒ(ɪ)ə] *n* → cystorrhagia.
cys·tir·rhea [ˌ-ˈrɪə] *n* → cystorrhea.
cys·tis [ˈsɪstɪs] *n, pl* **-ti·des** [-tədiːz] Zyste *f*, Blase *f*; *anat.* blasenförmiges (Hohl-)Organ *nt*.
cys·ti·stax·is [ˌsɪstəˈstæksɪs] *n* Sickerblutung *f* aus der (Harn-)Blasenschleimhaut.
cys·ti·tis [sɪsˈtaɪtɪs] *n* (Harn-)Blasenentzündung *f*, Zystitis *f*, Cystitis *f*.
cys·ti·tome [ˈsɪstətəʊm] *n ophthal.* Kapselfliete *f*, Zystitom *nt*.
cys·tit·o·my [sɪsˈtɪtəmɪ] *n ophthal.* (Linsen-)Kapselinzision *f*, Zystitomie *f*.
cysto- *pref.* Harnblasen-, Blasen-, Zyst(o)-.
cys·to·ad·e·no·ma [ˌsɪstəˌædəˈnəʊmə] *n* → cystadenoma.
cys·to·car·ci·no·ma [ˌ-ˌkɑːrsɪˈnəʊmə] *n patho.* Zystokarzinom *nt*, Cystocarcinoma *nt*.
cys·to·cele [ˈsɪstəsiːl] *n* (Harn-)Blasenhernie *f*, -bruch *m*, -vorfall *m*, Zystozele *f*, Cystocele *f*.
cys·to·chro·mos·co·py [ˌ-krəʊˈmaskəpɪ] *n urol.* Chromozystoskopie *f*.
cys·to·co·los·to·my [ˌ-kəˈlastəmɪ] *n* **1.** *urol.* Blasen-Kolon-Fistel *f*, Zystokolostomie *f*. **2.** *chir.* Gallenblasen-Kolon-Fistel *f*, Cholezystokolostomie *f*.
cys·to·di·aph·a·nos·co·py [ˌ-daɪˌæfəˈnaskəpɪ] *n urol.* Zystodiaphanoskopie *f*.
cys·to·di·ver·tic·u·lum [ˌ-ˌdaɪvərˈtɪkjələm] *n* (Harn-)Blasendivertikel *nt*.
cyst·o·du·od·e·nos·to·my [ˌ-ˌd(j)uːədɪˈnastəmɪ] *n chir.* Zystduodenostomie *f* ins Duodenum, Zyst(o)duodenostomie *f*.
cys·to·dyn·ia [ˌ-ˈdiːnɪə] *n* (Harn-)Blasenschmerz *m*, Zystodynie *f*.
cys·to·e·lyt·ro·plas·ty [ˌ-əˈlɪtrəplæstɪ] *n chir.* operative Blasen-Scheiden-Versorgung *f*, -Naht *f*.
cys·to·en·ter·ic [ˌ-enˈterɪk] *adj* Harnblase u. Darm betr. *od.* verbindend, zystoenterisch, vesikointestinal.
cystoenteric anastomosis (Harn-)Blasen-Darm-Anastomose *f*, (Harn-)Blasen-Darm-Fistel *f*, zystoenterische/vesikointestinale Anastomose *f*.
cys·to·en·ter·o·cele [ˌ-ˈentərəsiːl] *n chir.* Zystoenterozele *f*.
cys·to·en·ter·os·to·my [ˌ-entəˈrastəmɪ] *n chir.* Zystendrainage *f* in den Darm, Zystoenterostomie *f*.
cys·to·e·pip·lo·cele [ˌ-ɪˈpɪpləsiːl] *n chir.* Zystoepiplozele *f*.
cys·to·ep·i·the·li·o·ma [ˌ-epəˌθɪːlɪˈəʊmə] *n patho.* Zystoepitheliom *nt*, Cystoepithelioma *nt*.
cys·to·fi·bro·ma [ˌ-faɪˈbrəʊmə] *n patho.* Zystofibrom *nt*, Cystofibroma *nt*.
cys·to·gas·tros·to·my [ˌ-gæsˈtrastəmɪ] *n chir.* Zystendrainage *f* in den Magen, Zyst(o)gastrostomie *f*.
cys·to·gram [ˈgræm] *n radiol.* Zystogramm *nt*.
cys·tog·ra·phy [sɪsˈtagrəfɪ] *n radiol.* Kontrastdarstellung *f* der Harnblase, Zystographie *f*.
cys·to·he·pat·ic triangle [ˌsɪstəhɪˈpætɪk] Calot'-Dreieck *nt*.
cys·toid [ˈsɪstɔɪd] **I** *n* zystenähnliche Struktur *f*, Pseudozyste *f*. **II** *adj patho.* zystenähnlich, -artig, zystoid.
cystoid degeneration (of retina) *ophthal.* Blessig-Zyste *f*.
cys·to·je·ju·nos·to·my [ˌsɪstədʒɪˌdʒuːˈnastəmɪ] *n chir.* Zystendrainage *f* ins Jejunum, Zystojejunostomie *f*.
cys·to·lith [ˈ-lɪθ] *n* Blasenstein *m*, Zystolith *m*, Calculus vesicae.
cys·to·li·thec·to·my [ˌ-lɪˈθektəmɪ] *n urol.* Blasensteinschnitt *m*, -operation *f*, -entfernung *f*, Zystolithektomie *f*.
cys·to·li·thi·a·sis [ˌ-lɪˈθaɪəsɪs] *n urol.* Blasensteinleiden *nt*, Zystolithiasis *f*.
cys·to·li·thot·o·my [ˌ-lɪˈθatəmɪ] *n* → cystolithectomy.
cys·to·ma [sɪsˈtəʊmə] *n* → cystadenoma.
cys·tom·e·ter [sɪsˈtamɪtər] *n urol.* Zysto(mano)meter *nt*.
cys·to·met·ro·gram [ˌsɪstəˈmetrəgræm] *n urol.* Zystometrogramm *nt*.
cys·to·me·trog·ra·phy [ˌ-məˈtragrəfɪ] *n urol.* Zystometrographie *f*.
cys·tom·e·try [sɪsˈtamətrɪ] *n urol.* Zysto(mano)metrie *f*.
cys·to·mor·phous [ˌsɪstəˈmɔːrfəs] *adj* zysten-, blasenförmig.
cys·to·my·o·ma [ˌ-maɪˈəʊmə] *n patho.* zystisches Myom *nt*, Cystomyoma *nt*.
cys·to·myx·o·ad·e·no·ma [ˌ-ˌmɪksædəˈnəʊmə] *n patho.* Cystomyxoadenoma *nt*.
cys·to·myx·o·ma [ˌ-mɪkˈsəʊmə] *n patho.* muzinöses Zystadenom *nt*, Cystomyxoma *nt*.
cys·to·ne·phro·sis [ˌ-nɪˈfrəʊsɪs] *n patho.* Zystenniere *f*, Zystonephrose *f*.
cys·to·neu·ral·gia [ˌ-njʊəˈrældʒ(ɪ)ə, -nʊ-] *n* (Harn-)Blasenneuralgie *f*.
cys·to·pa·ral·y·sis [ˌ-pəˈræləsɪs] *n* → cystoplegia.
cys·to·pex·y [ˈ-peksɪ] *n urol.* (Harn-)Blasenanheftung *f*, Zystopexie *f*.
cys·toph·o·rous [sɪsˈtafərəs] *adj* zystenhaltig, zystisch.
cys·toph·thi·sis [sɪsˈtafθəsɪs] *n* (Harn-)Blasentuberkulose *f*.
cys·to·plas·ty [ˈ-plæstɪ] *n urol.* (Harn-)Blasenplastik *f*, Zystoplastik *f*.
cys·to·ple·gia [ˌ-ˈpliːdʒ(ɪ)ə] *n* (Harn-)Blasenlähmung *f*, Zystoplegie *f*.
cys·to·proc·tos·to·my [ˌ-prakˈtastəmɪ] *n urol., chir.* Blasen-Enddarm-Fistel *f*, Zystorektostomie *f*, Vesikorektostomie *f*.
cys·top·to·sis [ˌsɪstapˈtəʊsɪs] *n urol.* (Harn-)Blasenvorfall *m* in die Harnröhre.
cys·to·py·e·li·tis [ˌ-paɪəˈlaɪtɪs] *n urol.* Entzündung *f* von Harnblase u. Nierenbecken, Zystopyelitis *f*.
cys·to·py·e·log·ra·phy [ˌ-paɪəˈlagrəfɪ] *n radiol., urol.* Kontrastdarstellung *f* von Harnblase u. Nierenbecken, Zystopyelographie *f*.
cys·to·py·e·lo·ne·phri·tis [ˌ-ˌpaɪələʊnɪˈfraɪtɪs] *n urol.* Zystopyelonephritis *f*.
cys·to·ra·di·og·ra·phy [ˌ-ˌreɪdɪˈagrəfɪ] *n radiol., urol.* Kontrastdarstellung *f* der Harnblase, Zystoradiographie *f*.
cys·to·rec·tos·to·my [ˌ-rekˈtastəmɪ] *n* → cystoproctostomy.
cys·tor·rha·gia [ˌ-ˈrædʒ(ɪ)ə] *n* (Harn-)Blasenblutung *f*, Blutung *f* aus der Harnblase, Zystorrhagie *f*.
cys·tor·rha·phy [sɪsˈtarəfɪ] *n* (Harn-)Blasennaht *f*, Zystorrhaphie *f*.
cys·tor·rhe·a [ˌsɪstəˈrɪə] *n urol.* Schleimabsonderung *f* aus der Harnblase.
cys·to·sar·co·ma (phyllodes/phylloides) [ˌ-sɑːrˈkəʊmə] *gyn., patho.* Cystosarcoma phyllo(i)des.
cys·tos·chi·sis [sɪsˈtaskəsɪs] *n patho.* Blasenspalte *f*, Zystoschisis *f*.
cys·to·scope [ˈsɪstəskəʊp] *n urol.* Blasenspiegel *m*, Zystoskop *nt*.
cys·to·scop·ic [ˌ-ˈskapɪk] *adj* Zystoskopie betr., mittels Zystoskop(ie), zystoskopisch.
cystoscopic urography *urol., radiol.* retrograde Urographie *f*.
cys·tos·co·py [sɪsˈtaskəpɪ] *n urol.* (Harn-)Blasenspiegelung *f*, Zystoskopie *f*.
cys·to·spasm [ˈsɪstəspæzəm] *n* (Harn-)Blasenkrampf *m*, Zystospasmus *m*.
cys·to·sper·mi·tis [ˌ-spərˈmaɪtɪs] *n urol.* Samenblasenentzündung *f*, Spermatozystitis *f*, Vesikulitis *f*, Vesiculitis *f*.
cys·to·stax·is [ˌ-ˈstæksɪs] *n* → cystistaxis.
cys·tos·to·my [sɪsˈtastəmɪ] *n* **1.** *chir.* künstliche Blasenfistel *f*, Zystostoma *nt*. **2.** Blasenfistelanlegung *f*, Zystostomie *f*.
cys·to·tome [ˈ-təʊm] *n* **1.** *urol.* Blasenmesser *nt*, Zystotom *nt*. **2.** → cystitome.
cys·tot·o·my [sɪsˈtatəmɪ] *n* **1.** *urol.* (Harn-)Blasenschnitt *m*, Zystotomie *f*. **2.** *chir.* Zysteneröffnung *f*, -schnitt *m*, Zystotomie *f*.
cys·to·tra·che·lot·o·my [ˌsɪstəˌtrækəˈlatəmɪ, -ˌtreɪ-] *n* → cystauchenotomy.
cys·to·u·re·ter·i·tis [ˌ-jʊəˌriːtəˈraɪtɪs] *n urol.* Entzündung *f* von Harnblase u. Harnleiter, Zystoureteritis *f*.
cys·to·u·re·ter·o·gram [ˌ-jʊəˈriːtərəgræm] *n radiol., urol.* Zystoureterogramm *nt*.
cys·to·u·re·ter·og·ra·phy [ˌ-jʊəˌriːtəˈragrəfɪ] *n radiol., urol.* Kontrastdarstellung *f* von Harnblase u. Harnleiter, Zystoureterographie *f*.
cys·to·u·re·ter·o·py·e·li·tis [ˌ-jʊəˌriːtərəˌpaɪəˈlaɪtɪs] *n urol.* Zystoureteropyelitis *f*.
cys·to·u·re·ter·o·py·e·lo·ne·phri·tis [ˌ-jʊəˌriːtərəˌpaɪələʊnɪˈfraɪtɪs] *n urol.* Zystoureteropyelonephritis *f*.
cys·to·u·re·thri·tis [ˌ-ˌjʊərəˈθraɪtɪs] *n urol.* Entzündung *f* von Harnblase u. Harnröhre, Zystourethritis *f*.
cys·to·u·re·thro·cele [ˌ-jəˈriːθrəsiːl] *n urol., gyn.* Zystourethrozele *f*.
cys·to·u·re·thro·gram [ˌ-jəˈriːθrəgræm] *n urol., radiol.* Zystourethrogramm *nt*.
cys·to·u·re·throg·ra·phy [ˌ-jʊərəˈθragrəfɪ]

n radiol., urol. Kontrastdarstellung *f* von Harnblase u. Harnröhre, Zystourethrographie *f*, Urethrozystographie *f*.
cys·to·u·re·thro·scope [,-jə'ri:θrəskəʊp] *n urol.* Zystourethroskop *nt*, Urethrozystoskop *nt*.
cys·to·u·re·thros·co·py [,-jʊərə'θrɒskəpɪ] *n urol.* Zystourethroskopie *f*, Urethrozystoskopie *f*.
cys·tous ['sɪstəs] *adj* Zyste betr., zystisch, blasenartig, Zysten-.
cyst Roux-en-Y jejunostomy *chir.* Zystojejunostomie *f* mit Roux-Y-Schlinge.
cyst stage Zystenstadium *nt*.
cyt- *pref.* → cyto-.
cyt·ar·a·bine ['sɪtærəbi:n] *n* → cytosine arabinoside.
cyth·e·mol·y·sis [,sɪθɪ'mɒləsɪs, ,saɪθe-] *n* Erythrozytenauflösung *f*, -zerstörung *f*, -abbau *m*, Hämolyse *f*, Hämatozytolyse *f*.
cyth·er·o·ma·nia [,sɪθərə'meɪnɪə, -jə] *n psychia.* Mannstollheit *f*, Nymphomanie *f*, Andromanie *f*, Hysteromanie *f*.
cyt·i·dine ['sɪtɪdi:n, -dɪn] *n abbr.* **C** Zytidin *nt*, Cytidin *nt abbr.*C.
cytidine deaminase Zytidin-, Cytidindesaminase *f*.
cytidine(-5'-)diphosphate *n abbr.* **CDP** Zytidin(-5'-)diphosphat *nt*, Cytidin(-5'-)diphosphat *nt abbr.* CDP.
cytidine diphosphate choline Zytidin-, Cytidindiphosphatcholin *nt*.
cytidine monophosphate *abbr.* **CMP** Zytidinmonophosphat *nt*, Cytidinmonophosphat *nt abbr.* CMP, Cytidylsäure *f*.
cytidine(-5'-)triphosphate *n abbr.* **CTP** Zytidin(-5'-)triphosphat *nt*, Cytidin(-5'-)triphosphat *nt abbr.* CTP.
cy·ti·dyl·ate [,saɪtə'dɪleɪt, ,sɪtə-] *n* Cytidylat *nt*.
cyt·i·dyl·ic acid [,sɪtɪ'dɪlɪk, ,saɪtɪ-] → cytidine monophosphate.
cyt·i·sine ['sɪtəsi:n, -sɪn] *n* Zytisin *nt*, Cytisin *nt*.
cyt·i·sism ['sɪtəsɪzəm] *n* Cytisinvergiftung *f*, Vergiftung *f* durch Goldregen, Zytisismus *m*.
cyto- *pref.* Zell-, Zyt(o)-, Cyt(o)-.
cy·to·an·a·lyz·er [,saɪtəʊ'ænlaɪzər] *n* Zell-, Zytoanalysator *m*.
cy·to·ar·chi·tec·ton·ic [,-,ɑ:rkɪtek'tɒnɪk] *adj* Zytoarchitektur *nt*. -architektonik betr., zytoarchitektonisch.
cytoarchitectonic field zytoarchitektonisches Feld *nt*.
cy·to·ar·chi·tec·ton·ics [,-,ɑ:rkɪtek'tɒnɪks] *pl* → cytoarchitecture.
cy·to·ar·chi·tec·tu·ral [,-,ɑ:rkɪ'tektʃərəl] *adj* → cytoarchitectonic.
cy·to·ar·chi·tec·ture [,-'ɑ:rkɪtektʃər] *n* Zytoarchitektur *f*, -architektonik *f*.
cy·to·bi·ol·o·gy [,-baɪ'ɒlədʒɪ] *n* Zell-, Zyto-, Cytobiologie *f*.
cy·to·blast ['-blæst -blɑ:st] *n* **1.** Zellkern *m*, Zyto-, Cytoblast *m*. **2.** → cytotrophoblast.
cy·to·cen·trum [,-'sentrəm] *n* **1.** Zentrosom *nt*, Zentriol *nt*, Zentralkörperchen *nt*. **2.** Mikrozentrum *nt*, Zentrosphäre *f*.
cy·to·chem·ism [,-'kemɪzəm] *n* Zytochemismus *m*.
cy·to·chem·is·try [,-'kemɪstrɪ] *n* Zytochemie *f*, Histopochemie *f*.
cy·to·chrome ['-krəʊm] *n* Zyto-, Cytochrom *nt*.
cytochrome a₃ → cytochrome (c) oxidase.
cytochrome aa₃ → cytochrome (c) oxidase.
cytochrome b₅ reductase Cytochrom b_5-Reduktase *f*.
cytochrome (c) oxidase Cytochrom a_3 *nt*, Cytochrom(c)oxidase *f*, Ferrocytochrom-c-Sauerstoff-Oxidoreduktase *f*; *old* Warburg'-Atmungsferment *f*.
cytochrome P₄₅₀ reductase NADPH-Cytochromreduktase *f*, Cytochrom-P_{450}-Reduktase *f*.
cytochrome system Atmungskette *f*.
cy·to·ci·dal [,-'saɪdl] *adj* zellzerstörend, -abtötend, zytozid.
cy·to·cide ['-saɪd] *n* zytozides Mittel *nt*.
cy·to·ci·ne·sis [,-sɪ'ni:sɪs, -saɪ-] *n* → cytokinesis.
cy·toc·la·sis [saɪ'tɒkləsɪs] *n* Zellzerstörung *f*, -fragmentierung *f*, Zytoklasis *f*.
cy·to·clas·tic [,saɪtə'klæstɪk] *adj* zytoklastisch.
cy·to·cu·prein [,-'ku:prɪən] *n* Hyperoxid-, Superoxiddismutase *f abbr.* SOD, Hämocuprein *nt*, Erythrocuprein *nt*.
cy·tode ['saɪtəʊd] *n histol.* Zytode *f*.
cy·to·den·drite [saɪtə'dendraɪt] *n* Dendrit *m*.
cy·to·di·ag·no·sis [,-daɪəg'nəʊsɪs] *n* Zell-, Zytodiagnostik *f*.
cy·to·di·ag·nos·tic [,-daɪəg'nɒstɪk] *adj* Zytodiagnostik betr., zytodiagnostisch.
cy·to·di·er·e·sis [,-daɪ'erəsɪs] *n* Zellteilung *f*, Zytodiärese *f*.
cy·to·dif·fer·en·ti·a·tion [,-,dɪfə,rentʃɪ'eɪʃn] *n* Zell-, Zytodifferenzierung *f*.
cy·to·fla·vin [,-'fleɪvɪn, -'flæ-] *n* Zytoflavin *nt*.
cy·tog·a·my [saɪ'tɒgəmɪ] *n* Zytogamie *f*.
cy·to·gene ['saɪtədʒi:n] *n* Zytogen *nt*, Plasmagen *nt*.
cy·to·gen·e·sis [,-'dʒenəsɪs] *n* Zellbildung *f*, -entwicklung *f*, Zytogenese *f*.
cy·to·ge·net·ic [,-dʒə'netɪk] *adj* Zytogenetik betr., mittels Zytogenetik, zytogenetisch.
cy·to·ge·net·i·cal [,-dʒə'netɪkl] *adj* → cytogenetic.
cy·to·ge·net·ics [,-dʒə'netɪks] *pl* Zell-, Zyto-, Cytogenetik *f*.
cy·to·gen·ic [,-'dʒenɪk] *adj* **1.** Zytogenese betr., zytogen. **2.** zell(en)bildend, zytogen.
cytogenic anemia perniziöse Anämie *f*, Biermer-Anämie *f*, Addison-Anämie *f*, Morbus Biermer *m*, Perniciosa *f*, Perniziosa *f*, Anaemia perniciosa, Vitamin B_{12}-Mangelanämie *f*.
cy·tog·e·nous [saɪ'tɒdʒənəs] *adj* → cytogenic.
cy·tog·e·ny [saɪ'tɒdʒənɪ] *n* → cytogenesis.
cy·to·glu·co·pe·nia [,saɪtə,glu:kəʊ'pi:nɪə] → cytoglycopenia.
cy·to·gly·co·pe·nia [,-,glaɪkəʊ'pi:nɪə] *n* intrazellulärer Glukosemangel *m*.
cy·tog·o·ny [saɪ'tɒgənɪ] *n bio.* Zytogonie *f*.
cy·to·gram ['saɪtəgræm] *n histol., patho.* Zytogramm *nt*.
cy·to·his·to·gen·e·sis [,-,hɪstə'dʒenəsɪs] *n* Zytohistogenese *f*.
cy·to·his·to·log·ic [,-,hɪstə'lɒdʒɪk] *adj* zytohistologisch.
cytohistologic diagnosis → cytologic diagnosis.
cy·to·his·tol·o·gy [,-hɪs'tɒlədʒɪ] *n* Zytohistologie *f*.
cy·to·hor·mone [,-'hɔ:rməʊn] *n* Zell-, Zytohormon *nt*.
cy·to·hy·a·lo·plasm [,-'haɪələplæzəm] *n* zytoplasmatische Matrix *f*, Grundzytoplasma *nt*, Hyaloplasma *nt*.
cy·toid ['saɪtɔɪd] *adj* zellähnlich, -artig, -förmig.
cy·to·kal·i·pe·nia [,saɪtə,kælɪ'pi:nɪə] *n* intrazellulärer Kaliummangel *m*.
cy·to·kine ['-kaɪn] *n* Zytokin *nt*.
cy·to·ki·ne·sis [,-kɪ'ni:sɪs, kaɪ-] *n* Zell(leib)teilung *f*, Zyto-, Cytokinese *f*.

cy·to·ki·nin [,-'kaɪnɪn] *n* Zyto-, Cytokinin *nt*.
cy·to·lem·ma [,-'lemə] *n bio.* äußere Zellmembran *f*, Zytolemm *nt*.
cy·to·lip·in H [,-'lɪpɪn] Lactosyl-*N*-acylsphingosin *nt*.
cy·to·log·ic [,-'lɒdʒɪk] *adj* Zytologie betr., zytologisch.
cy·to·log·i·cal [,-'lɒdʒɪkl] *adj* → cytologic.
cytologic diagnosis zytologische/zytostologische Diagnostik *f*, Zytodiagnostik *f*.
cy·tol·o·gist [saɪ'tɒlədʒɪst] *n* Zytologe *m*, Zytologin *f*.
cy·tol·o·gy [saɪ'tɒlədʒɪ] *n* **1.** Zell(en)lehre *f*, -forschung *f*, Zyto-, Cytologie *f*. **2.** → cytodiagnosis.
cy·to·lymph ['saɪtəlɪmf] *n* zytoplasmatische Matrix *f*, Grundzytoplasma *nt*, Hyaloplasma *nt*.
cy·tol·y·sate [saɪ'tɒlɪseɪt] *n* Zytolysat *nt*.
cy·tol·y·sin [saɪ'tɒləsɪn] *n* Zytolysin *nt*.
cy·tol·y·sis [saɪ'tɒləsɪs] *n* Zellauflösung *f*, -zerfall *m*, Zytolyse *f*.
cy·to·ly·so·some [,saɪtə'laɪsəsəʊm] *n* **1.** autophagische Vakuole *f*, Autophagosom *nt*. **2.** Zytolysosom *nt*.
cy·to·lyt·ic [,-'lɪtɪk] *adj* Zytolyse betr. od. auslösend, zytolytisch.
cy·to·ma [saɪ'təʊmə] *n patho.* Zelltumor *m*, Zytom *nt*.
cy·to·me·gal·ic inclusion cell [,-mə'gælɪk] Zytomegaliezelle *f*.
cytomegalic inclusion disease Zytomegalie(-Syndrom) *nt*, Zytomegalievirusinfektion *f*, zytomegale Einschlußkörperkrankheit *f*.
cytomegalic inclusion disease virus → cytomegalovirus.
cy·to·meg·a·lo·vi·rus [,-,megələ'vaɪrəs] *n abbr.* **CMV** Zyto-, Cytomegalievirus *nt abbr.* CMV.
cytomegalovirus hepatitis Zytomegalievirushepatitis *f*, CMV-Hepatitis *f*.
cytomegalovirus immune globulin *abbr.* **CMVIG** Zytomegalievirusimmunoglobulin *nt*.
cytomegalovirus infection → cytomegalic inclusion disease.
cytomegalovirus mononucleosis Zytomegalievirusmononukleose *f*, CMV-Mononukleose *f*, Paul-Bunnel-negative infektiöse Mononukleose *f*.
cytomegalovirus pneumonia Zytomegalieviruspneumonie *f*, CMV-Pneumonie *f*.
cy·to·mem·brane [,-'membreɪn] *n* Zell-, Zytomembran *f*, Zellwand *f*, Plasmalemm *nt*.
cy·to·mere ['-mɪər] *n micro.* Zytomer *nt*.
cy·to·met·a·pla·sia [,-,metə'pleɪʒ(ɪ)ə, -zɪə] *n* Zell-, Zytometaplasie *f*.
cy·tom·e·ter [saɪ'tɒmɪtər] *n* Zytometer *nt*.
cy·tom·e·try [saɪ'tɒmɪtrɪ] *n* Zellmessung *f*, Zytometrie *f*.
cy·to·mor·phol·o·gy [,saɪtəmɔ:r'fɒlədʒɪ] *n* Zell-, Zytomorphologie *f*.
cy·to·mor·pho·sis [,-mɔ:r'fəʊsɪs, -'mɔ:rfə-] *n* Zytomorphose *f*.
cy·to·ne·cro·sis [,-nɪ'krəʊsɪs, -ne-] *n* Zelltod *m*, -untergang *m*, -nekrose *f*, Zytonekrose *f*.
cy·to·path·ic [,-'pæθɪk] *adj* zellschädigend, zytopathisch.
cytopathic effect *abbr.* **CPE** zytopathischer Effekt *m abbr.* CPE.
cy·to·path·o·gen·e·sis [,-,pæθə'dʒenəsɪs] *n* Zytopathogenese *f*.
cy·to·path·o·ge·net·ic [,-,pæθədʒə'netɪk] *adj* zytopathogenetisch.
cy·to·path·o·gen·ic [,-,pæθə'dʒenɪk] *adj* zytopathogen.

cytopathogenic virus *micro.* zytopathogenes Virus *nt.*
cy·to·path·o·ge·nic·i·ty [ˌ-ˌpæθədʒə'nɪsətɪ] *n* Zytopathogenität *f.*
cy·to·path·o·log·ic [ˌ-pæθə'lɑdʒɪk] *adj* Zytopathologie betr., zytopathologisch.
cy·to·path·o·log·i·cal [ˌ-pæθə'lɑdʒɪkl] *adj* → cytopathologic.
cy·to·pa·thol·o·gist [ˌ-pə'θɑlədʒɪst] *n* Zellpathologe *m*, -login *f*, Zytopathologe *m*, -login *f.*
cy·to·pa·thol·o·gy [ˌ-pə'θɑlədʒɪ] *n* Zell-, Zytopathologie *f.*
cy·to·pem·phis [ˌ-'pemfɪs] *n* → cytopempsis.
cy·to·pem·psis [ˌ-'pempsɪs] *n* Vesikulartransport *m*, Zytopempsis *f.*
cy·to·pe·nia [ˌ-'piːnɪə] *n hema.* Zell(zahl)verminderung *f*, Zytopenie *f.*
cy·to·phag·o·cy·to·sis [ˌ-ˌfægəsaɪ'təʊsɪs] *n* → cytophagy.
cy·toph·a·gous [saɪ'tɑfəɡəs] *adj* zellfressend, zytophag.
cy·toph·a·gy [saɪ'tɑfədʒɪ] *n* Zytophagie *f.*
cy·to·phil·ic [ˌsaɪtə'fɪlɪk] *adj* zytophil.
cytophilic antibody zytophiler Antikörper *m.*
cy·to·pho·tom·e·ter [ˌ-fəʊ'tɑmɪtər] *n* Zytophotometer *nt.*
cy·to·pho·to·met·ric [ˌ-ˌfəʊtə'metrɪk] *adj* Zytophotometrie betr., mittels Zytophotometrie, zytophotometrisch.
cy·to·pho·tom·e·try [ˌ-fəʊ'tɑmətrɪ] *n* Zytophotometrie *f*, Mikrospektrophotometrie *f.*
cy·to·phy·lac·tic [ˌ-fɪ'læktɪk] *adj* zytophylaktisch.
cy·to·phy·lax·is [ˌ-fɪ'læksɪs] *n* Zytophylaxie *f.*
cy·to·phys·ics [ˌ-'fɪzɪks] *pl* Zell-, Zytophysik *f.*
cy·to·phys·i·ol·o·gy [ˌ-fɪzɪ'ɑlədʒɪ] *n* Zell-, Zytophysiologie *f.*
cy·to·pig·ment ['-pɪɡmənt] *n* Zell-, Zytopigment *nt.*
cy·to·plasm ['-plæzəm] *n* (Zell-)Protoplasma *nt*, Zyto-, Cytoplasma *nt.*
cy·to·plas·mic [ˌ-'plæzmɪk] *adj* Zytoplasma betr., aus Zytoplasma bestehend, zytoplasmatisch, Zytoplasma-.
cytoplasmic cycle *micro.* zytoplasmatischer Zyklus *m.*
cytoplasmic granules zytoplasmatische Granula *pl.*
cytoplasmic inheritance zytoplasmatische/extranukleäre Vererbung *f.*
cytoplasmic membrane → cytomembrane.
cytoplasmic receptor zytoplasmatischer Rezeptor *m.*
cytoplasmic streaming (Zyto-)Plasmazirkulation *f*, Zyklosis *f.*
cy·to·poi·e·sis [ˌ-pɔɪ'iːsɪs] *n* Zellbildung *f*, Zytopoese *f.*
cy·to·proct ['-prɑkt] *n bio.* Zellafter *m*, Zytopyge *nt.*
cy·to·py·ge [ˌ-'paɪdʒɪ] *n* → cytoproct.
cy·tor·rhex·is [ˌ-'reksɪs] *n* Zellzerfall *m*, Zytorrhexis *f.*
cy·tos·co·py [saɪ'tɑskəpɪ] *n* Zytoskopie *f.*
cy·to·sine ['saɪtəsiːn, -sɪn] *n abbr.* **C** Zytosin *nt*, Cytosin *nt.*
cytosine arabinoside *abbr.* **CA** Cytarabin *nt*, Zytosin-, Cytosinarabinosid *nt*, Ara-C *nt.*
cytosine deaminase Cytosindesaminase *f.*
cy·to·skel·e·ton [ˌsaɪtə'skelɪtn] *n* Zell-, Zytoskelett *nt.*
cy·to·sol ['-sɒl, -sɑl] *n* Zytosol *nt.*
cytosol aminopeptidase Arylaminopeptidase *f.*
cytosol pool Zytosolpool *m.*
cy·to·some ['-səʊm] *n* **1.** Zellkörper *m*, Zytosoma *nt.* **2.** Zytosom *nt.*
cy·tos·ta·sis [saɪ'tɑstəsɪs] *n* Zytostase *f.*
cy·to·stat·ic ['saɪtə'stætɪk] **I** *n* Zytostatikum *nt.* **II** *adj* zytostatisch.
cytostatic agent → cytostatic I.
cytostatic chemotherapy zytostatische/antineoplastische Chemotherapie *f.*
cy·to·stome ['-stəʊm] *n micro.* Zellmund *m*, Zytostom *nt.*
cy·to·tac·tic [ˌ-'tæktɪk] *adj* Zytotaxis betr., zytotaktisch.
cy·to·tax·is [ˌ-'tæksɪs] *n* Zytotaxis *f.*
cy·to·tox·ic [ˌ-'tɑksɪk] *adj* zellschädigend, -vergiftend, zytotoxisch.
cytotoxic antibiotic zytotoxisches Antibiotikum *nt.*
cytotoxic antibody zytotoxischer Antikörper *m.*
cytotoxic chemotherapy zytotoxische Chemotherapie *f.*
cytotoxic hypersensitivity *immun.* Überempfindlichkeitsreaktion *f* vom zytotoxischen Typ, Typ II *m* der Überempfindlichkeitsreaktion.
cy·to·tox·ic·i·ty [ˌ-tɑk'sɪsətɪ] *n* Zytotoxizität *f.*
cytotoxic reaction zytotoxische Reaktion *f.*
cytotoxic T-cell zytotoxische T-Zelle *f*, zytotoxischer T-Lymphozyt *m*, T-Killerzelle *f.*
cytotoxic T-lymphocyte *abbr.* **CTL** → cytotoxic T-cell.
cy·to·tox·in [ˌ-'tɑksɪn] *n* Zytotoxin *nt.*
cy·to·troph·o·blast [ˌ-'trɑfəblæst, -'trəʊf-] *n* Zytotrophoblast *m*, Langhans'-Zellschicht *f.*
cytotrophoblast shell Zytotrophoblasthülle *f.*
cy·to·trop·ic [ˌ-'trɑpɪk, -'trəʊp-] *adj* auf Zellen gerichtet, zytotrop.
cytotropic antibody zytophiler Antikörper *m.*
cy·tot·ro·pism [saɪ'tɑtrəpɪzəm] *n* Zytotropismus *m.*
cy·tu·ria [saɪ'tʊərɪə] *n* Zellausscheidung *f* im Harn, Zyturie *f.*
Czapek ['tʃapek]: **C. solution agar** → Czapek-Dox agar.
Czapek-Dox [dɑks]: **C.-D. agar** *micro.* Czapek-Dox-Nährlösung *f*, -Medium *nt.*
C.-D. culture medium → C.-D. agar.
C.-D. medium → C.-D. agar.
Czermak ['tʃermak]: **globular spaces of C.** → C.'s spaces.
C.'s lines → C.'s spaces.
C.'s spaces Czermak-Räume *pl*, Interglobularräume *pl*, Spatia interglobularia.
Czerny ['tʃernɪ]: **C.'s suture 1.** Czerny-Naht *f.* **2.** Czerny-Pfeilernaht *f.*
Czerny-Lembert [lem'bɛːr]: **C.-L. suture** Czerny-Lembert-Naht *f.*

D

D *abbr.* 1. → debye. 2. → deuterium. 3. → dielectric constant. 4. → diffusing capacity. 5. → diffusion coefficient. 6. → diopter.
d *abbr.* → deci-.
Δ *abbr.* → delta 1.
δ *abbr.* 1. → delta 1. 2. → standard deviation.
DA *abbr.* → diphenylchlorarsine.
D.A. *abbr.* → developmental age.
dA *abbr.* → deoxyadenosine.
Daae [deɪ]: **D.'s disease** Bornholmer Krankheit *f*, epidemische Pleurodynie *f*, Myalgia epidemica.
DaCosta [dəˈkɒstə]: **D.'s syndrome** Effort-Syndrom *nt*, DaCosta-Syndrom *nt*, neurozirkulatorische Asthenie *f*, Soldatenherz *nt*, Phrenikokardie *f*.
d'Acosta [dəˈkɒstə]: **d'A.'s disease** d'Acosta-Syndrom *nt*, (akute) Bergkrankheit *f*, Mal di Puna.
dacry- *pref.* → dacryo-.
dac·ry·ad·e·nal·gia [ˌdækrɪˌædɪˈnældʒ(ɪ)ə] *n* → dacryoadenalgia.
dac·ry·ad·e·ni·tis [ˌ-ˌædəˈnaɪtɪs] *n* → dacryoadenitis.
dac·ry·ag·o·ga·tre·sia [ˌ-ˌægəʊgəˈtriːʒ(ɪ)ə] *n* HNO, patho. Tränenröhrchenverschluß *m*, -atresie *f*.
dac·ry·a·gogue [ˈdækrɪəgɒg, -gag] **I** *n* 1. *pharm.* tränentreibende Substanz *f*, Dakryagogum *nt*. 2. Tränenröhrchen *nt*, Canaliculus lacrimalis. **II** *adj* tränentreibend.
dac·ry·cys·tal·gia [ˌ-sɪsˈtældʒ(ɪ)ə] *n* → dacryocystalgia.
dac·ry·cys·ti·tis [ˌ-sɪsˈtaɪtɪs] *n* → dacryocystitis.
dac·ry·el·co·sis [ˌ-elˈkəʊsɪs] *n* → dacryohelcosis.
dacryo- *pref.* Tränen-, Dakry(o)-, Dacry(o)-.
dac·ry·o·ad·e·nal·gia [ˌdækrɪəʊˌædɪˈnældʒ(ɪ)ə] *n* Tränendrüsenschmerz *m*, Schmerz *m* in einer Tränendrüse, Dakryoadenalgie *f*.
dac·ry·o·ad·e·nec·to·my [ˌ-ˌædəˈnektəmɪ] *n* chir., ophthal. Tränendrüsenentfernung *f*, Dakry(o)adenektomie *f*.
dac·ry·o·ad·e·ni·tis [ˌ-ˌædəˈnaɪtɪs] *n* Tränendrüsenentzündung *f*, Dakryoadenitis *f*.
dac·ry·o·blen·nor·rhea [ˌ-ˌblenəˈriːə] *n* ophthal. chronischer Tränenfluß *m* bei Tränendrüsenentzündung, Dakryoblennorrhoe *f*.
dac·ry·o·can·a·lic·u·li·tis [ˌ-ˌkænəˌlɪkjəˈlaɪtɪs] *n* Tränenröhrchenentzündung *f*, Dakryokanalikulitis *f*, -canaliculitis *f*.
dac·ry·o·cele [ˈ-siːl] *n* → dacryocystocele.
dac·ry·o·cyst [ˈ-sɪst] *n* Tränensack *m*, Saccus lacrimalis.
dac·ry·o·cys·tal·gia [ˌ-sɪsˈtældʒ(ɪ)ə] *n* Tränensackschmerz *m*, Dakryozystalgie *f*.
dac·ry·o·cys·tec·ta·sia [ˌ-ˌsɪstekˈteɪʒ(ɪ)ə] *n* Tränensackdilatation *f*, -erweiterung *f*, Dakryozystektasie *f*.

dac·ry·o·cys·tec·to·my [ˌ-sɪsˈtektəmɪ] *n* chir., ophthal. Tränensackentfernung *f*, -resektion *f*, Dakryozystektomie *f*.
dac·ry·o·cys·tis [ˌ-ˈsɪstɪs] *n* → dacryocyst.
dac·ry·o·cys·ti·tis [ˌ-sɪsˈtaɪtɪs] *n* Tränensackentzündung *f*, Dakryozystitis *f*, -cystitis *f*.
dac·ry·o·cys·ti·tome [ˌ-ˈsɪstətəʊm] *n* ophthal. Dakryozystitom *nt*.
dac·ry·o·cys·tit·o·my [ˌ-sɪsˈtɪtəmɪ] *n* ophthal. Tränenröhrcheninzision *f*, -schnitt *m*, Dakryozystitomie *f*.
dac·ry·o·cys·to·blen·nor·rhea [ˌ-ˌsɪstəˌblenəˈriːə] *n* ophthal. chronisch exsudative/eitrige Tränensackentzündung *f*, Tränensackeiterung *f*, Dakryozystoblennorrhoe *f*.
dac·ry·o·cys·to·cele [ˌ-ˈsɪstəsiːl] *n* Tränensackbruch *m*, Dakryo(zysto)zele *f*.
dac·ry·o·cys·to·eth·moi·dos·to·my [ˌ-ˌsɪstəˌeθmɔɪˈdɒstəmɪ] *n* ophthal. Dakryozystoethmoidostomie *f*.
dac·ry·o·cys·to·gram [ˌ-ˈsɪstəgræm] *n* ophthal., radiol. Dakryozystogramm *nt*.
dac·ry·o·cys·tog·ra·phy [ˌ-sɪsˈtɒgrəfɪ] *n* ophthal., radiol. Kontrastdarstellung *f* der Tränenwege, Dakryozystographie *f*.
dac·ry·o·cys·top·to·sis [ˌ-sɪstəpˈtəʊsɪs] *n* ophthal. Dakryozystoptose *f*.
dac·ry·o·cys·to·rhi·no·ste·no·sis [ˌ-ˌsɪstəˌraɪnəʊstɪˈnəʊsɪs] *n* Verschluß *m*/Stenose *f* des Ductus nasolacrimalis, Dakryozystorhinostenose *f*.
dac·ry·o·cys·to·rhi·nos·to·my [ˌ-ˌsɪstəraɪˈnɒstəmɪ] *n* ophthal. Toti-Operation *f*, Dakryo(zysto)rhinostomie *f*.
dac·ry·o·cys·to·ste·no·sis [ˌ-ˌsɪstəstɪˈnəʊsɪs] *n* Tränensackschrumpfung *f*, -stenose *f*, Dakryozystostenose *f*.
dac·ry·o·cys·tos·to·my [ˌ-sɪsˈtɒstəmɪ] *n* ophthal. Dakryozystostomie *f*.
dac·ry·o·cys·to·tome [ˌ-ˈsɪstətəʊm] *n* Tränensackmesserchen *nt*, Dakryozystotom *nt*.
dac·ry·o·cys·tot·o·my [ˌ-sɪsˈtɒtəmɪ] *n* ophthal. Tränensackeröffnung *f*, -inzision *f*, Dakryozystotomie *f*.
dac·ry·o·gen·ic [ˌ-ˈdʒenɪk] *adj* tränenflußanregend.
dac·ry·o·hel·co·sis [ˌ-helˈkəʊsɪs] *n* Geschwür *nt* des Tränensacks od. Tränenröhrchens, Dakryo(h)elkose *f*.
dac·ry·o·hem·or·rhea [ˌ-heməˈriːə] *n* ophthal. Absonderung *f* blutiger/bluthaltiger Tränen, blutiger Tränenfluß *m*, Dakryohämorrhoe *f*.
dac·ry·o·lith [ˈdækrɪəlɪθ] *n* Tränenstein *m*, Dakryolith *m*.
dac·ry·o·li·thi·a·sis [ˌ-lɪˈθaɪəsɪs] *n* Dakryolithiasis *f*.
dac·ry·o·ma [dækrɪˈəʊmə] *n* 1. Dakryom *nt*, Dakryoma *nt*. 2. → dacryops 2.
dac·ry·ops [ˈdækrɪɒps] *n* 1. übermäßiger Tränenfluß *m*, wässrige Augen *pl*. 2. Retentionszyste *f* der Tränendrüse, Dakryops *m*.

dac·ry·o·py·or·rhea [ˌdækrɪəˌpaɪəˈrɪə] *n* ophthal. eitriger Tränenfluß *m*, Dakryopyorrhoe *f*.
dac·ry·o·py·o·sis [ˌ-paɪˈəʊsɪs] *n* Tränensack- od. Tränenröhrchen(ver)eiterung *f*, Eiterung *f* der Tränenwege, Dakryopyosis *f*.
dac·ry·o·rhi·no·cys·tot·o·my [ˌ-ˌraɪnəsɪsˈtɒtəmɪ] *n* → dacryocystorhinostomy.
dac·ry·or·rhea [ˌ-ˈriːə] *n* übermäßiger Tränenfluß *m*, Tränenträufeln *nt*, Dakryorrhoe *f*, Epiphora *f*.
dac·ry·o·scin·tig·ra·phy [ˌ-sɪnˈtɪgrəfɪ] *n* Tränenwegs-, Dakryoszintigraphie *f*.
dac·ry·o·si·nus·i·tis [ˌ-saɪnəˈsaɪtɪs] *n* Entzündung *f* von Tränenröhrchen u. Sinus ethmoidalis, Dakryosinusitis *f*.
dac·ry·o·so·le·ni·tis [ˌ-ˌsəʊləˈnaɪtɪs] *n* Tränenröhrchenentzündung *f*, Dakryosolenitis *f*.
dac·ry·o·ste·no·sis [ˌ-stɪˈnəʊsɪs] *n* Tränengangsstenose *f*, Dakryostenose *f*.
dac·ry·o·syr·inx [ˌ-ˈsɪrɪŋks] *n* 1. Tränenröhrchen *nt*, Canaliculus lacrimalis. 2. Tränengang(s)fistel *f*.
dac·ti·no·my·cin [ˌdæktɪnəˈmaɪsn] *n* pharm. Dactinomycin *nt*, Actinomycin D *nt*.
dactyl- *pref.* → dactylo-.
dac·tyl [ˈdæktl] *n anat.* Digitus *m*, Zehe *f*, Finger *m*.
dac·ty·lal·gia [dæktəˈlældʒ(ɪ)ə] *n* Fingerschmerz *m*, Daktylalgie *f*, Daktylodynie *f*.
dac·tyl·e·de·ma [ˌdæktlɪˈdiːmə] *n* 1. Fingerschwellung *f*, -ödem *nt*. 2. Zehenschwellung *f*, -ödem *nt*.
dac·tyl·ia [dækˈtɪlɪə, -jə] *n* → dactylium.
dac·tyl·i·on [dækˈtɪlɪən] *n* → dactylium.
dac·ty·li·tis [dæktəˈlaɪtɪs] *n* Fingerentzündung *f*, Zehenentzündung *f*, Daktylitis *f*.
dac·tyl·i·um [dækˈtɪlɪəm] *n* Verwachsung *f* von Fingern od. Zehen, Syndaktylie *f*.
dactylo- *pref.* Finger-, Zehen-, Daktyl(o)-.
dac·ty·lo·camp·so·dyn·ia [ˌdæktɪləʊˌkæmpsəˈdiːnɪə] *n neuro., ortho.* schmerzhafte Finger- od. Zehenverkrümmung *f*, Daktylokampsodynie *f*.
dac·tyl·o·dyn·ia [ˌ-ˈdiːnɪə] *n* → dactylalgia.
dac·tyl·o·gram [ˈ-græm] *n* Fingerabdruck *m*, Daktylogramm *nt*.
dac·ty·log·ra·phy [dæktɪˈlɒgrəfɪ] *n* Daktylographie *f*.
dac·ty·lo·gry·po·sis [ˌdæktɪləgraɪˈpəʊsɪs, -grɪ-] *n* (permanente) Finger- od. Zehenverkrümmung *f*, -beugung *f*, Daktylogrypose *f*.
dac·ty·lol·o·gy [ˌdæktɪˈlɒlədʒɪ] *n* Daktylologie *f* (*Finger- u. Gebärdensprache der Taubstummen*).
dac·ty·lol·y·sis [ˌ-ˈlɒləsɪs] *n* operative od. spontane Finger- od. Zehenamputation *f*.
dac·ty·lo·meg·a·ly [ˌdæktɪləˈmegəlɪ] *n* übermäßige Größe *f* von Fingern od. Zehen, Daktylomegalie *f*, Makrodaktylie *f*, Megalodaktylie *f*.

dactylophasia

dac·ty·lo·pha·sia [ˌi-'feɪʒ(ɪ)ə] *n* → dactylology.
dac·ty·los·co·py [dæktə'lɒskəpɪ] *n* Daktyloskopie *f*.
dac·ty·lo·spasm ['dæktɪləspæzəm] *n* Fingerkrampf *m*, -spasmus *m*, Zehenkrampf *m*, -spasmus *m*, Daktylospasmus *m*.
dac·ty·lus ['dæktɪləs] *n* → dactyl.
DADDS *abbr.* → diacetyl diaminodiphenylsulfone.
dADP *abbr.* → deoxyadenosine diphosphate.
DAF *abbr.* → decay accelerating factor.
D.A.H. *abbr.* [disordered action of the heart] → DaCosta's syndrome.
dah·lin ['dɑ:lɪn] *n* Inulin *nt*
dai·ly ['deɪlɪ] *adj* täglich, Tages-.
daily dose Tagesdosis *f abbr.* TD.
daily output Tagesleistung *f*; (*Urin*) Tagesmenge *f*.
Dakin ['deɪk(ɪ)n]: **D.'s antiseptic** → D.'s fluid.
D.'s fluid verdünnte Natriumhypochloritlösung *f*.
D.'s (modified) solution → D.'s fluid.
Dakin-Carrel [kɑ'rel]: **D.-C. method/treatment** *ortho.* Wundbehandlung *f* nach Dakin-Carrel.
Dale [deɪl]: **D.'s phenomenon/reaction** Dale'-Versuch *m*.
Dalen-Fuchs ['dɑ:lən f(j)u:ks; fʊks]: **D.-F. nodules** *ophthal.* Dalen'-Flecken *pl*, Dalen-Fuchs-Knötchen *pl*.
Dall [dɔ:l]: **D.'s principle** Dall'-Prinzip *nt*.
Dalrymple ['dælrɪmpl]: **D.'s disease** Entzündung *f* von Ziliarkörper u. Hornhaut, Zyklokeratitis *f*.
D.'s sign Dalrymple'-Zeichen *nt*.
Dalton ['dɔ:ltn]: **D.'s law** Dalton'-Gesetz *nt* (*der Partialdrücke*).
dal·ton ['dɔ:ltn] *n* Dalton *nt*, Atommasseneinheit *f*.
Dalton-Henry ['henrɪ]: **D.-H. law** Dalton-Henry-(Absorptions-)Gesetz *nt*, Henry-Dalton-Gesetz *nt*.
dal·ton·ism ['dɔ:ltnɪzəm] *n ophthal.* 1. Farbenblindheit *f*, Daltonismus *m*. 2. Rot-Grün-Blindheit *f*, Daltonismus *m*.
dam·age ['dæmɪdʒ] I *n* 1. Schaden *m*, Schädigung *f*, Beschädigung *f* (*to* an). **to do ~** to beschädigen. 2. Schadensersatz *m*. **to pay ~s** Schadensersatz zahlen. **to seek ~s** auf Schadensersatz klagen. II *vt* beschädigen. III *vi* Schaden nehmen, beschädigt werden.
dam·aged ['dæmɪdʒd] *adj* beschädigt, defekt.
dam·ag·ing ['dæmədʒɪŋ] *adj* schädlich, schädigend, nachteilig (*to* für).
Damoiseau [damwa'zo]: **D.'s curve/sign** Ellis-Damoiseau'-Linie *f*.
dAMP *abbr.* → deoxyadenosine monophosphate.
damp [dæmp] I *n* Feuchtigkeit *f*. II *adj* feucht. III *vt* 1. be-, anfeuchten. 2. *phys.* dämpfen. IV *vi* feucht werden.
damped [dæmpt] *adj* (*a. phys.*) gedämpft.
damped oscillation *phys.* gedämpfte Schwingung *f*.
damp·er ['dæmpər] *n* (*a. fig.*, *techn.*) Dämpfer *m*.
damp·ing ['dæmpɪŋ] *n* Dämpfen *nt*, Dämpfung *f*.
damp·ish ['dæmpɪʃ] *adj* etw. feucht.
damp·ness ['dæmpnɪs] *n* Feuchtigkeit *f*.
damp-proof *adj* feuchtigkeitsbeständig.
Dana [deɪnə]: **D.'s operation** *neuro.* Dana-Operation *f*, Rhizotomia posterior.
da·na·zol ['deɪnəzɒl, -zəl] *n pharm.* Danazol *nt*.
Danbolt-Closs ['dænbəʊlt klɒs; klɒs]: **D.-C. syndrome** Danbolt-Syndrom *nt*,

Danbolt-Closs-Syndrom *nt*, Akrodermatitis/Acrodermatitis enteropathica.
Dance [dæns, dɑ:ns]: **D.'s sign** *chir.* Dance-Zeichen *nt*.
danc·ing chorea ['dænsɪŋ, dɑ:nsɪŋ] → dancing disease.
dancing disease Chorea festinans.
dancing spasm Bamberger-Krankheit *f*, saltatorischer Reflexkrampf *m*.
dan·druff ['dændrʌf] *n* → dandruff.
dan·druff ['dændrəf] *n* 1. (Kopf-, Haar-)Schuppe(n *pl*) *f*. 2. *derm.* Pityriasis simplex capitis.
Dandy ['dændɪ]: **D. operation 1.** Dandy-Operation *f*, Ventrikulo(zisterno)stomie *f* des III. Ventrikels. **2.** Dandy-Operation *f*, subokzipitale Trigeminusdurchtrennung *f*.
dan·dy fever ['dændɪ] Dengue *nt*, Dengue-Fieber *nt*, Dandy-Fieber *nt*.
Dandy-Walker ['wɔ:kər]: **D.-W. deformity/syndrome** Dandy-Walker-Syndrom *nt*, -Krankheit *f*.
Dane [deɪn]: **D. particle** Hepatitis-B-Virus *nt abbr.* HBV.
Danforth ['dænfɔʊrθ]: **D.'s sign** Danforth-Symptom *nt*.
dan·ger ['deɪndʒər] I *n* Gefahr (*to* für). **to be in ~ of one's life** in Lebensgefahr schweben. **to be out of ~** außer Gefahr sein; über dem Berg sein. II *adj* Gefahren-.
d. of infection Infektionsgefahr.
danger area → danger zone.
dan·ger·ous ['deɪndʒ(ə)rəs] *adj* gefährlich (*to*, *for* für), gefahrvoll.
d. to life lebensgefährlich.
danger zone *physiol.* Gefahrenzone *f*, -bereich *m*, Zone *f* der unvollständigen Kompensation.
dan·gle foot ['dæŋgl] Fallfuß *m*.
Danlos [dænlɑs]: **D.' disease/syndrome** Ehlers-Danlos-Syndrom *nt*.
DANS *abbr.* → 5-dimethylamino-1-naphthalenesulfonic acid.
dan·syl chloride ['dænsɪl] *biochem.* Dansylchlorid *nt*.
dan·tro·lene ['dæntrəli:n] *n pharm.* Dantrolen *nt*.
dantrolene sodium *pharm.* Dantrolen-Natrium *nt*.
Dan·u·bi·an endemic familial nephropathy [dæn'ju:bɪən] Balkan-Nephropathie *f*, -Nephritis *f*, chronische endemische Nephropathie *f*.
Danysz ['dænɪzəm od 'dænɪʃ]: **D.'s effect/phenomenon** *immun.* Danysz-Phänomen *nt*.
DAP *abbr.* → diaminopimelic acid.
daph·nism ['dæfnɪzəm] *n* Daphnismus *m*.
DA pregnancy test Schwangerschaftslatexagglutinationshemmtest *m*.
dap·sone ['dæpsəʊn] *n pharm.* Dapson *nt*, Diaminodiphenylsulfon *nt abbr.* DDS.
Darier ['dærɪeɪ; dɑ'rje]: **D.'s disease** Darier'-Krankheit *f*, Dyskeratosis follicularis (vegetans), Porospermosis follicularis vegetans, Porospermosis cutanea, Keratosis vegetans.
D.'s sign Darier'-Zeichen *nt*.
Darier-Roussy [ru'si]: **D.-R. sarcoid** Darier-Roussy-Sarkoid *nt*.
Darier-White [(h)waɪt]: **D.-W. disease** → Darier's disease.
dark [dɑ:rk] I *n* Dunkel *nt*, Dunkelheit *f*; dunkle Farbe *f*; Schatten *m*. II *adj* dunkel.
dark adaptation *physiol.* Dunkeladaptation *f*, -anpassung *f*.
dark-blue *adj* dunkelblau.
dark·en ['dɑ:rkn] I *vt* 1. verdunkeln, dunkel machen. 2. dunkel *od.* dunkler färben; schwärzen. 3. *fig.* (*Sinn*) trüben, verdunkeln. 4. (*Augen*) blind machen; (*Sehkraft*) vermindern. II *vi* 5. dunkel werden, s. verdunkeln. 6. s. dunkel *od.* dunkler färben. 7. (*a. fig.*) s. trüben.
dark-eyed *adj* dunkeläugig.
dark-field *adj* Dunkelfeld-.
darkfield condenser Dunkelfeldkondensor *m*.
dark-field microscope Dunkelfeldmikroskop *nt*.
dark-field microscopy Dunkelfeldmikroskopie *f*.
dark hair dunkles *od.* brünettes Haar *nt*.
dark-haired *adj* dunkelhaarig.
dark·ish ['dɑ:rkɪʃ] *adj* etw. dunkel; schwärzlich.
dark·ness ['dɑ:rknɪs] *n* 1. Dunkelheit *f*, Finsternis *f*. 2. Blindheit *f*. 3. dunkle Färbung *f*. 4. *fig.* Unwissenheit *f*.
dark phase *of* dark reactions.
dark reactions *bio.* Dunkelreaktionen *pl*, -phase *f*.
dark-room ['dɑ:rkru:m, -rʊm] *n photo.* Dunkelkammer *f*.
Darkshevich [dɑ:rk'ʃevɪtʃ]: **D.'s fibers** Darkschewitsch'-Fasern *pl*.
D.'s nucleus Darkschewitsch'-Kern *m*, Nc. Darkschewitsch.
dark-skinned ['dɑ:rkskɪnd] *adj* dunkelhäutig.
Darling ['dɑ:rlɪŋ]: **D.'s disease** Darling'-Krankheit *f*, Histoplasmose *f*, retikuloendotheliale Zytomykose *f*.
d'Arsonval ['dɑ:rsnvæl, -vɔl]: **d'A. current** Tesla-Strom *m*, Hochfrequenzstrom *m*.
dar·tos ['dɑ:rtɑs] *n* Muskelhaut *f* des Skrotums, M. dartos.
dartos fascia of scrotum → dartos.
dartos muscle → dartos.
Darwin [dɑ:rwɪn]: **D.'s ear** Darwin-Ohr *nt*.
D.'s tubercle Darwin'-Höcker *m*, Tuberculum auriculare.
dar·win·i·an [dɑ:r'wɪnɪən]: **d. apex** Apex auricularis.
d. ear Darwin-Ohr *nt*.
d. evolution biologische Evolution *f*, Darwin'-Evolution *f*.
d. theory Darwinismus *m*.
d. tubercle Darwin'-Höcker *m*, Tuberculum auriculare.
Dar·wi·nism ['dɑ:rwənɪzəm] *n bio.* Darwinismus *m*.
da·ta ['deɪtə, 'dætə] *pl* 1. Daten *pl*, Angaben *pl*, Unterlagen *pl*, Einzelheiten *pl*. 2. *phys.*, *techn.* Meß-, Versuchswerte *pl*, -daten *pl*. 3. (Computer-)Daten *pl*.
data bank Datenbank *f*.
data base → data bank.
data collection Datenerfassung *f*.
data exchange Datenaustausch *m*.
data processing Datenverarbeitung *f*.
data protection Datenschutz *m*.
date [deɪt] I *n* 1. Datum *nt*, Tag *m*; Zeitpunkt *m*. 2. **out of ~** veraltet, überholt. **up to ~** zeitgemäß, modern. **to bring up to ~** auf den neuesten Stand bringen. II *vt* datieren. III *vi* datiert sein (*from* von).
d. of birth Geburtsdatum.
date fever Dengue *nt*, Dengue-Fieber *nt*, Dandy-Fieber *nt*.
dATP *abbr.* → deoxyadenosine triphosphate.
da·tu·ra [də't(j)ʊərə] *n bot.* Stechapfel *m*, Datura stramonium.
da·tu·rine [də't(j)ʊəri:n, -rɪn] *n* Hyoscyamin *nt*, Hyoszyamin *nt*.
da·tu·rism [də't(j)ʊərɪzəm] *n* Stechapfelvergiftung *f*, Daturismus *m*.
daugh·ter ['dɔ:tər] *n* (a. *fig.*) Tochter *f*.
daughter cell *histol.* Tochterzelle *f*.
daughter chromatid Tochterchromatide *f*.

daughter chromosome Tochterchromosom *nt*.
daughter colony *micro.* Tochterkolonie *f*.
daughter cyst Tochterzyste *f*, sekundäre Zyste *f*.
daughter yaw Tochterpapel *f*, daughter yaw.
daughter molecule Tochtermolekül *nt*.
daughter nucleus Tochterkern *m*.
dau·no·my·cin [dɔːnəˈmaɪsɪn] *n* → daunorubicin.
dau·no·ru·bi·cin [ˌ-ˈruːbəsɪn] *n pharm.* Daunorubicin *nt*, Daunomycin *nt*, Rubidomycin *nt*.
Dav·ai·ne·i·dae [ˌdævəˈnɪədiː] *pl micro.* Davaineidae *pl.*
David [ˈdaˈvid]: **D.'s disease** Wirbeltuberkulose *f*, Spondylitis tuberculosa.
Davidoff [ˈdeɪvɪdɑf; ˈdavidɔf]: **D.'s cell** Paneth'-(Körner-)Zelle *f*, Davidoff-Zelle *f*.
Davidsohn [ˈdeɪvɪdsəʊn]: **D. differential absorption test** *immun.* modifizierter Paul-Bunnell-Test *m* nach Davidsohn.
D.'s sign *HNO* Davidsohn'-Zeichen *nt*.
Daviel [daˈvjel]: **D.'s operation** *ophthal.* Daviel-Operation *f*, -Linsenextraktion *f*.
Davis [ˈdeɪvɪs]: **D.' graft** *chir.* Davis-Hautinsel *f*, -Hauttransplantat *nt*.
Dawbarn [ˈdɔːbɑːrn]: **D.'s sign** *ortho.* Dawbarn-Zeichen *nt*.
Dawson [ˈdɔːsən]: **D.'s encephalitis** subakute sklerosierende Panenzephalitis *f abbr.* SSPE, Einschlußkörperchenenzephalitis *f* Dawson, subakute sklerosierende Leukenzephalitis *f* van Bogaert.
Day [deɪ]: **D.'s factor** Fol(in)säure *f*, Folacin *nt*, Pteroylglutaminsäure *f*, Vitamin B$_c$ *nt*.
D.'s test Day'-Probe *f*.
day [deɪ] *n* Tag *m*; (festgesetzter) Tag *m*, Termin *m*. **the ~ after** tags darauf, am nächsten Tag; der nächste Tag. **all ~** den ganzen Tag. **before ~** vor Tagesanbruch. **the ~ before** tags zuvor, am vorhergehende Tag. **from ~ to ~** von Tag zu Tag, zusehends. **twice a ~** zweimal täglich/am Tage.
day blindness Nykt(er)alopie *f*, Tagblindheit *f*.
day-book [ˈdeɪbʊk] *n* Tagebuch *nt*.
day-care center Tagesstätte *f*, -heim *nt*.
day-dream [ˈdeɪdriːm] *n* Tag-, Wachtraum *m*. **II** *vi* (mit offenen Augen) träumen.
day-dream·er [ˈdeɪdriːmər] *n* Träumer(in *f*) *m*.
day hospital Tagesklinik *f*.
day·lamp [ˈdeɪlæmp] *n* Tageslichtlampe *f*.
day length Tageslänge *f*.
day·light [ˈdeɪlaɪt] *n* 1. Tageslicht *nt*. **by/in ~** bei Tage(eslicht). 2. Tagesanbruch *m*. **at ~** bei Tagesanbruch.
daylight vision → day vision.
day nursery (Kinder-)Tagesstätte *f*, -heim *nt*.
day sight *ophthal.* Nachtblindheit *f*, Hemeralopie *f*.
day terrors *ped.* Tagangst *f*, Pavor diurnus.
day·time [ˈdeɪtaɪm] **I** *n* Tag *m*. **in the ~** tagsüber, während des Tages. **II** *adv* am Tag(e), Tages-.
day-to-day *adj* (all-)täglich, Alltags-. **on a ~ basis** tageweise.
day vision Tages(licht)sehen *nt*, photopisches Sehen *nt*.
daze [deɪz] **I** *n* (*a. fig.*) Betäubung *f*, Lähmung *f*, Benommenheit *f*. **II** *vt* 1. (*a. fig.*) betäuben, lähmen. 2. blenden, verwirren.
dazed [deɪzd] *adj* 1. betäubt, benommen. 2. geblendet, verwirrt.

daz·zle [ˈdæzl] **I** *n* Blenden *nt*; Leuchten *nt*, blendender Glanz *m*. **II** *vt* 1. blenden. 2. *fig.* verwirren, verblüffen.
daz·zling [ˈdæzlɪŋ] *adj* 1. (*a. fig.*) blendend, glänzend; strahlend. 2. verwirrend.
dB *abbr.* → decibel.
db *abbr.* → decibel.
DBA *abbr.* → dibenzanthracene.
D.C. *abbr.* → direct current.
dC *abbr.* → deoxycytidine.
dCDP *abbr.* → deoxycytidine diphosphate.
D cells D-Zellen *pl*, δ-Zellen *pl*.
D-cell tumor → delta cell tumor.
DCI *abbr.* → dichloroisoproterenol.
dCMP *abbr.* → deoxycytidine monophosphate.
DC potential Gleichspannungs-, Bestandspotential *nt*.
dCTP *abbr.* → deoxycytidine triphosphate.
DD *abbr.* → differential diagnosis.
DDS *abbr.* [diaminodiphenylsulfone] → dapsone.
DDT *abbr.* → dichlorodiphenyltrichloroethane.
de·a·ce·tyl·la·nat·o·side [diˌæsətɪlləˈnætəsaɪd] *n* Desacetyllanatosid *nt*.
deacetyllanatoside C → deslanoside.
de·a·cid·i·fi·ca·tion [dɪəˌsɪdɪfɪˈkeɪʃn] *n chem.* Entsäuern *nt*, Entsäuerung *f*; Neutralisieren *nt*, Neutralisierung *f*.
de·a·cid·i·fy [dɪəˈsɪdɪfaɪ] *vt* entsäuern; neutralisieren.
de·ac·ti·va·tion [dɪˌæktɪˈveɪʃn] *n* Inaktivieren *nt*, Inaktivierung *f*.
de·ac·yl·ase [diˈæsɪleɪz] *n* Deacylase *f*.
de·ac·yl·ate [diˈæsɪleɪt] *vt chem.* deacylieren.
de·ac·yl·a·tion [dɪˌæsɪˈleɪʃn] *n chem.* Deacylierung *f*.
dead [ded] **I** *pl* **the ~** die Toten. **II** *adj* 1. tot, gestorben; leblos. 2. totenähnlich, tief. **a ~ sleep**. 3. abgestorben, nekrotisch; gefühllos, taub. 4. *fig.* unzugänglich, unempfindlich, taub (*to* für). 5. *fig.* gefühllos, gleichgültig (*to* gegenüber). 6. veraltet, überlebt. 7. *techn.* außer Betrieb; (*Batterie*) leer. 8. ohne Ausgang, blind (enden). 9. (*Ton*) dumpf; (*Augen, Farben*) matt, stumpf, glanzlos. **III** *adv* absolut, völlig, total. **~ tired** todmüde. **~ asleep** im tiefsten Schlaf.
dead-beat [ˈdedbiːt] *adj phys.* aperiodisch (gedämpft).
dead body Leiche *f*, Leichnam *m*.
dead·en [ˈdedn] *vt* 1. dämpfen, (ab-)schwächen; (*Schmerz*) mildern. 2. (*Nerv*) abtöten; (*Gefühl*) abstumpfen (*to* gegenüber). 3. schalldicht machen.
dead end blindes Ende *nt*; (*a. fig.*) Sackgasse *f*.
dead-end *adj* ohne Ausgang, blind (endend).
dead-end host *micro.* Fehlendwirt *m*.
de·a·den·yl·ate [dɪəˈdenlɪt, -eɪt, -ˈædnl-] *vt chem.* deadenylieren.
dead fetus syndrome Dead-fetus-Syndrom *nt*.
dead·house [ˈdedhaʊs] *n* Leichenschauhaus *nt*; Leichenhalle *f*.
dead·li·ness [ˈdedlɪnɪs] *n* tödliche Wirkung *f*; *fig.* vernichtende Wirkung *f*.
dead·ly [ˈdedlɪ] *adj* tödlich, todbringend, zum Tode führend; totenähnlich, Todes-; *fig.* vernichtend.
deadly nightshade Tollkirsche *f*, Atropa belladonna.
deadly pallor Todes-, Leichenblässe *f*.
dead matter tote Materie *f*.
dead·ness [ˈdednɪs] *n* 1. Leblosigkeit *f*. 2. (*a. fig.*) Gefühllosigkeit *f*, Gleichgültigkeit *f*, Taubheit *f* (*to* gegenüber).

dead space *anat., physiol.* Totraum *m*.
anatomical d. anatomischer Totraum.
functional d. → physiological d.
physiological d. physiologischer/funktioneller Totraum.
dead space ventilation *physiol.* Totraumventilation *f*.
dead time *physiol.* Totzeit *f*.
DEAE-cellulose *n* → diethylaminoethylcellulose.
deaf [def] **I** *pl* **the ~** die Tauben. **II** *adj* 1. taub, gehörlos; schwerhörig, hörgeschädigt. **~ in one ear** taub auf einem Ohr. 2. *fig.* taub (*to* gegen); unzugänglich (*to* für).
deaf aid Hörgerät *nt*, -apparat *m*, -hilfe *f*.
deaf-and-dumb *adj* → deaf-mute II.
deaf-and-dumb alphabet Fingeralphabet *nt* (*der Taubstummen*).
deaf-and-dumb language Taubstummensprache *f*.
deaf·en [ˈdefn] *vi* 1. taub machen. 2. (*fig.*) betäuben (*with* durch). 3. (*Schall*) (ab-)dämpfen.
deaf·en·ing [ˈdefnɪŋ] *n* Ertaubung *f*, Taubwerden *nt*, Ertauben *nt*.
de·af·fer·en·ta·tion [dɪˌæfərənˈteɪʃn] *n neurochir., patho.* Deafferenzierung *f*.
deaf-mute I *n* Taubstumme(r *m*) *f*. **II** *adj* taubstumm, Taubstummen-.
deaf-muteness *n* Taubstummheit *f*, Mutisurditas *f*, Surdomutitas *f*.
deaf-mutism *n* → deaf-muteness.
deaf·ness [ˈdefnɪs] *n* 1. Taubheit *f*, Gehörlosigkeit *f*, Anakusis *f*, Kophosis *f*; Schwerhörigkeit *f*. 2. (*a. fig.*) Taubheit *f* (*to* gegenüber).
de·al·ba·tion [dælˈbeɪʃn] *n* Bleichen *nt*, Ausbleichen *f*.
de·al·co·hol·i·za·tion [dɪˌælkəˌhɒlɪˈzeɪʃn] *n chem.* Alkoholentzug *m*, -entfernung *f*, Dealkoholisierung *f*.
de·al·kyl·a·tion [dɪˌælkəˈleɪʃn] *n chem.* Dealkylierung *f*.
de·al·ler·gi·za·tion [dɪˌælɜːdʒɪˈzeɪʃn] *n* Desensibilisierung *f*, Deallergisierung *f*.
de·am·i·dase [dɪˈæmɪdeɪz] *n* Desamidase *f*, Amidohydrolase *f*.
de·am·i·da·tion [dɪˌæmɪˈdeɪʃn] *n* → deamidization.
de·am·i·di·za·tion [dɪˌæmɪdaɪˈzeɪʃn] *n chem.* Desamidierung *f*.
de·am·i·nase [dɪˈæmɪneɪz] *n* Desaminase *f*, Aminohydrolase *f*.
de·am·i·na·tion [dɪˌæmɪˈneɪʃn] *n chem.* Desaminierung *f*.
de·am·i·ni·za·tion [dɪˌæmɪnəˈzeɪʃn] *n* → deamination.
de·a·nol [ˈdɪənɒl] *n pharm.* Deanol *nt*, β-Dimethylaminoethylalkohol *m*, 2-Dimethylaminoethanol *nt*.
de·a·qua·tion [dɪəˈkweɪʃn] *n chem.* Wasserentzug *m*, -entfernung *f*, Dehydrierung *f*.
de·ar·te·ri·a·li·za·tion [dɪɑːrˌtɪərɪəlaɪˈzeɪʃn] *n* Dearterialisation *f*.
death [deθ] *n* Tod *m*, Exitus *m*; Todesfall *m*; (Ab-)Sterben *nt*. **after ~** postmortal, post mortem. **before ~** prämortal, ante mortem.
d. by accident Tod durch Unfall, Unfalltod.
d. by asphyxia Tod durch Ersticken, Ersticken *nt*.
d. from drowning Tod durch Ertrinken, Ertrinken *nt*.
death agony Todeskampf *m*.
death-bed [ˈdeθbed] *n* Sterbe-, Totenbett *nt*. **to be on one's ~** im Sterben liegen.
death benefit Sterbegeld *nt*.
death certificate Totenschein *m*, Sterbeurkunde *f*.

death cup *bot.* Grüner Knollenblätterpilz *m*, Amanita phalloides.
death·day ['deθdeɪ] *n* Todestag *m*.
death instinct *psycho.* Todestrieb *m*.
death in utero intrauteriner Fruchttod *m*; Totgeburt *f*.
death·like ['deθlaɪk] *adj* → deadly.
death·ly ['deθlɪ] *adj* → deadly.
death phase *micro.* Absterbephase *f*.
death·place ['deθpleɪs] *n* Sterbeort *m*.
death rate Sterbe-, Sterblichkeitsziffer *f*, -rate *f*, Mortalität *f*, Zahl *f* der Todesfälle.
death rattle Todesröcheln *nt*.
death rigor Leichen-, Totenstarre *f*, Rigor mortis.
death·watch ['deθwɒtʃ] *n* Totenwache *f*.
Deaver ['diːvər]: **D.'s incision** *chir.* Deaver-Inzision *f*.
De·bar·y·o·my·ces [ˌdɪbærɪəˈmaɪsiːz] *n micro.* Debaryomyces *m*.
de·bil·i·tate [dɪˈbɪləteɪt] *vt* schwächen, entkräften.
de·bil·i·ta·tion [dɪˌbɪləˈteɪʃn] *n* Schwächung *f*, Entkräftung *f*.
de·bil·i·ty [dɪˈbɪlətɪ] *n* 1. Schwäche *f*, Kraftlosigkeit *f*. 2. Schwäche-, Erschöpfungszustand *m*.
de·bouch [dɪˈbuːʃ, -ˈbaʊtʃ] *vi* (ein-)münden (*into* in); s. ergießen.
de·bouch·ment ['-mənt] *n* (Ein-)Mündung *f*.
de·branch·er deficiency [dɪˈbræntʃər] Cori-Krankheit, Forbes-Syndrom *nt*, hepatomuskuläre benigne Glykogenose, Glykogenose Typ III.
debrancher enzyme Amylo-1,6-Glukosidase *f*, Dextrin-1,6-Glukosidase *f*.
debrancher glycogen storage disease → debrancher deficiency.
de·branch·ing enzyme (glycogen) [dɪˈbræntʃɪŋ] → debrancher enzyme.
Debré-Sémélaigne [dəˈbre semeˈlɛːɲ]: **D.-S. syndrome** Debré-Sémélaigne-Syndrom *nt*.
de·bride [dɪˈbriːd, deɪ-] *vt* (*Wunde*) reinigen, eine Wundtoilette durchführen.
de·bride·ment ['-mənt] *n* Wundtoilette *f*, -reinigung *f*, Débridement *nt*.
de·bris [dɪˈbriː, ˈdeɪbrɪ, 'deb-] *n* (nekrotische) Zelltrümmer *pl*, -reste *pl*, Gewebstrümmer *pl*, -reste *pl*.
de·bulk·ing [dɪˈbʌlkɪŋ] *n chir.* partielle Geschwulstverkleinerung *f*, Debulking *nt*.
de·bye [dɪˈbaɪ] *n abbr.* **D** *phys.* Debye *nt abbr.* D.
deca- *pref.* Deka-, Deca-.
de·cal·ci·fi·ca·tion [dɪˌkælsəfɪˈkeɪʃn] *n* 1. *patho.* Dekalzifizierung *f*, Dekalzifikation *f*. 2. Entkalkung *f*, Entkalken *nt*.
de·cal·ci·fy [dɪˈkælsəfaɪ] *vt* 1. dekalzifizieren. 2. entkalken.
dec·a·meth·o·ni·um [ˌdekəmɪˈθəʊnɪəm] *n* Deka-, Decamethonium *nt*.
decamethonium bromide Deka-, Decamethoniumbromid *nt*.
decamethonium iodide Deka-, Decamethoniumjodid *nt*.
dec·ane ['dekeɪn] *n chem.* Dekan *nt*, Decan *nt*.
de·can·nu·la·tion [dɪˌkænjəˈleɪʃn] *n* Kanülenentfernung *f*, Dekanülierung *f*, Décanulement *nt*.
de·cant [dɪˈkænt] *vt* dekantieren.
de·can·ta·tion [ˌdiːkænˈteɪʃn] *n* Dekantieren *nt*, Dekantation *f*.
de·ca·pac·i·ta·tion [ˌdiːkəˌpæsɪˈteɪʃn] *n embryo.* Dekapazitation *f*.
decapacitation factor *embryo.* Dekapazitationsfaktor *m*.
dec·a·pep·tide [ˌdekəˈpeptaɪd] *n* Deka-, Decapeptid *nt*.

de·cap·i·ta·tion [dɪˌkæpɪˈteɪʃn] *n* Dekapitation *f*, Dekapitierung *f*.
de·cap·i·ta·tor [dɪˈkæpɪteɪtər] *n gyn.* Dekapitationsinstrument *nt*, -haken *m*.
de·cap·su·la·tion [dɪˌkæps(j)əˈleɪʃn] *n* 1. *chir.* (Organ-)Kapselentfernung *f*, Dekapsulation *f*. 2. *urol.* Nierenkapselentfernung *f*, Dekapsulation *f*.
de·car·box·yl·ase [ˌdiːkɑːrˈbɒksəleɪz] *n* Dekarboxylase *f*, Decarboxylase *f*.
de·car·box·yl·ate [ˌ-ˈbɒksəleɪt] *vt chem.* dekarboxylieren, decarboxylieren.
de·car·box·yl·at·ed dopa [ˌ-ˈbɒksəleɪtɪd] → dopamine.
de·car·box·yl·a·tion [ˌ-ˌbɒksəˈleɪʃn] *n chem.* Dekarboxylierung *f*, Decarboxylierung *f*.
de·cay [dɪˈkeɪ] **I** *n* 1. *fig.* Ver-, Zerfall *m*, Verschlechterung *f*; (Alters-)Schwäche *f*. 2. Zerfall *m*; Verwesung *f*, Auflösung *f*, Zersetzung *f*; Fäule *f*, Fäulnis *f*; (*Zähne*) Karies *nt*. 3. *phys.* (*Radium*) Zerfall *m*. **II** *vi* 4. *fig.* ver-, zerfallen, schwach werden, schwinden, zugrunde gehen. 5. zerfallen; verwesen, s. auflösen, s. zersetzen, (ver-)faulen; (*Zähne*) kariös werden. 6. (*Radium*) zerfallen.
decay accelerating factor *abbr.* **DAF** *immun.* decay accelerating factor (*m*) *abbr.* DAF.
decay constant Zerfallskonstante *f*.
decay density *phys.* Zerfallsdichte *f*.
decay product *phys.* Zerfallsprodukt *nt*.
de·cayed [dɪˈkeɪd] *adj* 1. (*Zähne*) kariös. 2. verfallen, faul, verwest, schlecht.
de·cease [dɪˈsiːs] **I** *n* Tod *m*, Ableben *nt*. **II** *vi* (ver-)sterben, verscheiden.
de·ceased [dɪˈsiːst] **I** *pl* **the ~** der/die Verstorbene *od.* Tote; die Verstorbenen *od.* Toten. **II** *adj* ver-, gestorben.
de·cel·er·ate [dɪˈseləreɪt] **I** *vt* 1. verzögern, verlangsamen. 2. (*Geschwindigkeit*) herabsetzen, abbremsen. **II** *vi* 3. s. verlangsamen. 4. abbremsen, seine Geschwindigkeit verringern.
de·cel·er·a·tion [dɪˌseləˈreɪʃn] *n* 1. Verlangsamung *f*, Verzögerung *f*, Geschwindigkeitsabnahme *f*. 2. *gyn.* Dezeleration *f*.
deceleration injury/trauma *ortho.* Dezelerationstrauma *nt*.
de·cen·ter [dɪˈsentər] *vt ophthal.* dezentrieren.
de·cer·e·bra·tion [dɪˌserəˈbreɪʃn] *n* Enthirnung *f*, Dezerebration *f*, Decerebration *f*, Dezerebrierung *f*.
decerebration rigidity Enthirnungs-, Dezerebrierungsstarre *f*.
de·cer·e·brize [dɪˈserəbraɪz] *vt* enthirnen, dezerebrieren.
de·chlo·ri·da·tion [dɪˌklɔːrɪˈdeɪʃn, -ˌklɔːr-] *n* Chlorid-, Salzentzug *m*, Dechloridation *f*, Dechloridierung *f*.
de·chlo·ri·na·tion [dɪˌklɔːrɪˈneɪʃn, -ˌklɔːr-] *n* → dechloridation.
deci- *pref. abbr.* **d** Zehntel-, Dezi-, Deci-.
dec·i·bel ['desəbel] *n abbr.* **dB, db** Dezibel *nt abbr.* dB.
de·cid·ua [dɪˈsɪdʒəwə] *n, pl* **-uas, -uae** [-dʒwiː] Schwangerschaftsendometrium *nt*, Dezidua *f*, Decidua *f*, Caduca *f*, Decidua membranacea, Membrana deciduae.
de·cid·u·al [dɪˈsɪdʒəwəl] *adj* Dezidua betr., dezidual, decidual, Dezidua-, Decidua-.
decidual cells Deziduazellen *pl*.
decidual endometritis *gyn.* Endometritis decidualis, Dezidualitis *f*, Deciduitis *f*.
decidual membrane → decidua.
decidual plate Dezidual-, Basalplatte *f*.
decidual reaction → decidua reaction.
decidual septa Deziduasepten *pl*.
decidua reaction *embryo.* deziduale Reaktion *f*.

de·cid·u·ate placenta [dɪˈsɪdʒəweɪt] Placenta deciduata.
de·cid·u·a·tion [dɪˌsɪdʒəˈweɪʃn] *n gyn.* Abstoßung/Desquamation *f* der Lamina functionalis.
de·cid·u·i·tis [dɪˌsɪdʒəˈwaɪtɪs] *n gyn.* Deziduaentzündung *f*, Deziduitis *f*, Decidu(al)itis *f*, Endometritis decidualis.
de·cid·u·o·cel·lu·lar carcinoma [dɪˌsɪdʒəwəʊˈseljələr] Chorioblastom *nt*, (malignes) Chorionepitheliom *nt*, fetaler Zottenkrebs *m*, Chorionkarzinom *nt*.
deciduocellular sarcoma *old* → deciduocellular carcinoma.
de·cid·u·o·ma [dɪˌsɪdʒəˈwəʊmə] *n gyn., patho.* Deziduom *nt*.
de·cid·u·o·sar·co·ma [dɪˌsɪdʒəwəʊsɑːrˈkəʊmə] *n old* → deciduocellular carcinoma.
de·cid·u·ous [dɪˈsɪdʒəwəs] *adj* nicht bleibend, aus-, abfallend; *fig.* vergänglich.
deciduous dentition Milchzähne *pl*, -gebiß *nt*, Dentes decidui.
deciduous membrane → decidua.
deciduous placenta → deciduate placenta.
deciduous tooth Milchzahn *m*, Dens deciduus.
dec·i·gram ['desɪɡræm] *n abbr.* **dg** Dezigramm *nt abbr.* dg.
dec·i·li·ter [-ˈliːtər] *n abbr.* **dl** Deziliter *m/nt abbr.* dl.
dec·i·mal ['desɪml] **I** *n* 1. → decimal fraction. 2. Dezimalzahl *f*. **II** *adj* auf der Zahl 10 beruhend, dezimal, Dezimal-.
decimal fraction *mathe.* Dezimalbruch *m*.
dec·i·mal·i·za·tion [ˌdesɪməlaɪˈzeɪʃn] *n* Dezimalisierung *f*.
dec·i·mal·ize ['desɪməlaɪz] *vt* dezimalisieren, auf das Dezimalsystem umstellen.
decimal system Dezimalsystem *nt*.
dec·i·me·ter ['desɪmiːtər] *n abbr.* **dm** Dezimeter *m/nt abbr.* dm.
deck plate [dek] *embryo.* Deckplatte *f*.
deck·plat·te ['dɛkplatə] *n* → deck plate.
de·clar·a·tive (long-term) memory [dɪˈklærətɪv] deklaratives Langzeitgedächtnis *nt*.
dec·li·na·tion [ˌdeklɪˈneɪʃn] *n* 1. Neigung *f*, Schräglage *f*. 2. Abweichung *f* (*from* von). 3. *fig.* Verfall *m*, Niedergang *m*. 4. *ophthal., phys.* Deklination *f*.
de·cline [dɪˈklaɪn] **I** *n* 1. Neigung *f*, Senkung *f*. 2. Niedergang *m*, Verfall *m*. 3. Verschlechterung *f*, Abnahme *f*, Rückgang *m*, Verfall *m* (*of, in*); Siechtum *nt*. **II** *vt* neigen, senken. **III** *vi* 4. s. neigen, s. senken, abfallen. 5. s. neigen, zur Neige gehen. 6. verfallen, in Verfall geraten. 7. s. verschlechtern, abnehmen, zurückgehen; (*körperlich*) verfallen.
de·clive [dɪˈklaɪv] *n anat.* Declive *nt*.
de·cli·vis [dɪˈklaɪvɪs] *n* → declive.
de·coct [dɪˈkɒkt] *vt* abkochen, absieden.
de·coc·tion [dɪˈkɒkʃn] *n* 1. (Ab-)Kochen *nt*, Absieden *nt*. 2. *pharm.* Absud *m*, Dekokt *nt*, Decoctum *nt*, Decoctio *f*.
de·coc·tum [dɪˈkɒktəm] *n* → decoction 2.
de·code [dɪˈkəʊd] *vt* entschlüsseln, dechiffrieren, dekodieren, decodieren.
de·cod·ing [dɪˈkəʊdɪŋ] *n* Entschlüsseln *nt*, Ablesen *nt*, Dechiffrieren *nt*, Dekodieren *nt*, Dekodierung *f*.
de·col·la·tion [ˌdiːkɒˈleɪʃn] *n gyn.* Dekapitation *f*, Dekapitierung *f*.
de·col·or [dɪˈkʌlər] *vt* → decolorize.
de·col·or·ant [dɪˈkʌlərənt] **I** *n* Bleichmittel *nt*. **II** *adj* entfärbend, bleichend.
de·col·or·a·tion [ˌdiːkʌləˈreɪʃn] *n* Entfärben *nt*, Bleichen *nt*.
de·col·or·i·za·tion [dɪˌkʌlərɪˈzeɪʃn] *n* → decoloration.

de·col·or·ize [dɪ'kʌlǝraɪz] *vt* entfärben, bleichen, dekolorieren.
de·com·pen·sate [dɪ'kɑmpǝnseɪt] *vi* entgleisen, dekompensieren.
de·com·pen·sat·ed [dɪ'kɑmpǝnseɪtɪd] *adj* nicht ausgeglichen, entgleist, dekompensiert.
de·com·pen·sa·tion [ˌdɪkɑmpǝn'seɪʃn] *n* 1. Dekompensation *f*. 2. Herzdekompensation *f*, kardiale Dekompensation *f*.
de·com·pose [ˌdikǝm'pǝʊz] I *vt chem., phys.* spalten, scheiden, zerlegen. 2. zersetzen. II *vi* 3. zerfallen, s. auflösen (*into* in). 4. s. zersetzen, verwesen, zer-, verfallen.
de·com·posed [ˌ-'pǝʊst] *adj* verfallen, verfault, verwest, schlecht.
de·com·po·si·tion [dɪˌkɑmpǝ'zɪʃn] *n* 1. *chem.* Zerlegung *f*, (Auf-)Spaltung *f*, Zerfall *m*, Abbau *m*. 2. Verwesung *f*, Fäulnis *f*, Zersetzung *f*, Auflösung *f*.
de·com·press [ˌdɪkǝm'pres] *vt techn.* von (hohem) Druck entlasten, dekomprimieren.
de·com·pres·sion [ˌ-'preʃn] *n* 1. *techn.* Druckabfall *m*, Dekompression *f*. 2. Druckentlastung *f*, Dekompression *f*.
d. of heart/pericardium Herzdekompression.
d. of spinal cord *neurochir., ortho.* Rückenmark(s)dekompression.
decompression chamber Dekompressionskammer *f*.
decompression hyperemia Entlastungshyperämie *f*.
decompression sickness Druckluft-, Caissonkrankheit *f*.
de·con·ges·tant [ˌ-'dʒestǝnt] I *n pharm.* abschwellendes Mittel *nt*, Dekongestionsmittel *nt*. II *adj* abschwellend.
de·con·ges·tive [ˌ-'dʒestɪv] *adj* abschwellend.
de·con·ju·ga·tion [dɪˌkɑndʒǝ'geɪʃn] *n* Dekonjugation *f*.
de·con·tam·i·nate [ˌdɪkǝn'tæmɪneɪt] *vt* entgiften, entgasen, entseuchen, entstrahlen, dekontaminieren.
de·con·tam·i·na·tion [ˌ-ˌtæmɪ'neɪʃn] *n* Entgiftung *f*, Entgasung *f*, Entseuchung *f*, Entstrahlung *f*, Dekontaminierung *f*, Dekontaminierung *f*.
de·cor·ti·ca·tion [dɪˌkɔːrtɪ'keɪʃn] *n chir.* operative Entrindung *f*, Rindenentfernung *f*, Dekortikation *f*.
d. of lung Dekortikation von Pleuraschwarten.
de·crease [*n* 'dɪkriːs; *v* dɪ'kriːs] I *n* Abnahme *f*, Verminderung *f*, Verringerung *f*, Verkleinerung *f*, Verkürzung *f*, Reduzierung *f*, Rückgang *m*; Nachlassen *nt*, Abnehmen *nt*. II *vt* vermindern, verringern, verkleinern, verkürzen, herabsetzen, reduzieren. III *vi* abnehmen, nachlassen, zurückgehen, s. vermindern, s. verringern, s. verkleinern, s. verkürzen, s. reduzieren.
dec·re·ment ['dekrǝmǝnt] *n* 1. Abnahme *f*, Verringerung *f*. 2. *phys.* Amplitudenabnahme *f*, Dekrement *nt*. 3. *patho.* Decrementum *nt*, Stadium decrementis.
de·crep·it [dɪ'krepɪt] *adj* alters-/schwach, (körperlich) heruntergekommen, hinfällig, dekrepit.
de·crep·i·tate [dɪ'krepɪteɪt] *chem.* I *vt* (*Salz*) verknistern. II *vi* dekrepitieren.
de·crep·i·ta·tion [dɪ'krepɪteɪʃn] *n chem.* 1. Verknistern *nt*. 2. Dekrepitation *f*.
de·crep·i·tude [dɪ'krepɪt(j)uːd] *n* Altersschwäche *f*, Hinfälligkeit *f*.
de·cru·des·cence [dɪkrǝ'desǝns] *n* (*Symptom*) Abnahme *f*, Dekrudeszenz *f*.

de·crus·ta·tion [dɪkrǝ'steɪʃn] *n chir.* Krustenentfernung *f*, -beseitigung *f*, Dekrustieren *nt*.
de·cu·ba·tion [dɪkjǝ'beɪʃn] *n* Dekubation *f*, Dekubationsperiode *f*.
de·cu·bi·tal [dɪ'kjuːbɪtl] *adj* Dekubitus betr., dekubital, Dekubital-, Dekubitus-.
decubital gangrene Wundliegen *nt*, Dekubitalulkus *nt*, -geschwür *nt*, Dekubitus *m*, Decubitus *m*.
decubital ulcer → decubitus 1.
de·cu·bi·tus [dɪ'kjuːbɪtǝs] *n, pl* **-tus** 1. Wundliegen *nt*, Dekubitalulkus *nt*, -geschwür *nt*, Dekubitus *m*, Decubitus *m*. 2. Hinlegen *nt*; Liegen *nt*.
decubitus ulcer → decubitus 1.
de·cus·sate [*adj* dɪ'kʌseɪt, -ɪt, 'dekǝ-; *v* -seɪt] I *adj* s. (über-)kreuzend, s. schneidend; gekreuzt. II *vt* (über-)kreuzen III *vi* s. (über-)kreuzen, s. schneiden.
de·cus·sa·tio [ˌdekǝ'seɪʃɪǝʊ, ˌdiːkǝ-] *n, pl* **-ti·o·nes** [-saɪʃɪ'ǝʊniːz] → decussation.
de·cus·sa·tion [ˌ-'seɪʃn] *n* (Über-)Kreuzung *f*; *anat.* Decussatio *f*.
d. of cranial cerebellar peduncles große Haubenkreuzung *f*, Kreuzung der oberen Kleinhirnstiele, Wernekinck'-Kreuzung *f*, Decussatio pedunculorum cerebellarium cranialium/superiorum.
d. of fillet → d. of medial lemnisci.
d. of medial lemnisci mediale Schleifenkreuzung *f*, Decussatio lemniscorum medialium, Decussatio sensoria.
d. of optic nerve Sehnervenkreuzung, Chiasma opticum.
d. of pyramids Pyramiden(bahn)kreuzung, Decussatio pyramidum/motoria.
d. of superior cerebellar peduncles → d. of cranial cerebellar peduncles.
d.s of tegmentum Haubenkreuzungen *pl*, Decussationes tegmenti/tegmentales.
d. of trochlear nerves Decussatio nn. trochlearium, Decussatio trochlearis.
de·dif·fer·en·ti·a·tion [dɪˌdɪfǝˌrenʃɪ'eɪʃn] *n patho.* Entdifferenzierung *f*; Anaplasie *f*.
deep [diːp] *adj* 1. (*Wasser, Wunde*) tief; breit; niedrig (gelegen). 2. (*Haut*) subkutan; (*Farben*) satt, dunkel; (*Stimme*) dunkel; (*Schlaf*) tief; (*Atemzug*) tief; (*Interesse*) groß, stark; (*Wissen*) fundiert; (*Forschung*) eingehend, gründlich. 3. *psycho.* unbewußt. 4. vertieft, versunken. ~ **in thought** in Gedanken versunken.
deep artery of penis tiefe Penisarterie *f*, Profunda *f* penis, A. profunda penis.
deep branch: d. of lateral plantar nerve tiefer Ast *m* des N. plantaris lateralis, Ramus profundus n. plantaris lateralis.
d. of medial circumflex femoral artery tiefer Ast *m* der A. circumflexa femoris medialis, Ramus profundus a. circumflexae femoris medialis.
d. of medial plantar nerve tiefer Ast *m* der A. plantaris medialis, Ramus profundus a. plantaris medialis.
d. of radial nerve tiefer Radialisast *m*, Ramus profundus n. radialis.
d. of superior gluteal artery tiefer Ast *m* der A. glut(a)ea superior, Ramus profundus a. glut(a)eae superioris.
d. of transverse cervical artery A. dorsalis scapulae, Ramus profundus a. transversae cervicis/colli.
d. of ulnar nerve tiefer Ulnarisast *m*, Ramus profundus n. ulnaris.
deep breathing vertiefte Atmung *f*, Bathypnoe *f*.
deep cortex (*Lymphknoten*) thymusabhängiges Areal *nt*, T-Areal *nt*, thymusabhängige/parakortikale Zone *f*.

deep·en ['diːpǝn] I *vt* 1. tief(er) machen, vertiefen; verbreitern. 2. *fig.* verstärken, steigern, vergrößern, vertiefen. 3. (*Farben*) dunkler machen; (*Stimme*) senken. II *vi* 4. tiefer werden, s. vertiefen; s. verbreitern. 5. *fig.* s. steigern, s. verstärken. 6. (*Farben*) dunkler werden, (nach-)dunkeln; (*Stimme*) tieferwerden.
deep fascia tiefe Körperfaszie *f*, Fascia profunda.
d. of arm Oberarmfaszie *f*, Fascia brachii/brachialis.
d. of back Fascia thoracolumbalis.
d. of forearm Unterarmfaszie *f*, Fascia antebrachii.
d. of penis tiefe Penisfaszie, Buck'-Faszie, Fascia penis profunda.
d. of perineum Urogenitaldiaphragma *nt*, Diaphragma urogenitale.
d. of thigh Oberschenkelfaszie *f*, Fascia lata (femoris).
deep-freeze *vt* tiefkühlen, einfrieren.
deep freezer Tiefkühlgerät *nt*, Gefriergerät *nt*.
deep head of flexor pollicis brevis muscle Caput profundum.
deep head of triceps brachii muscle Caput mediale m. tricipitis brachii.
deep keratitis interstitielle/parenchymatöse Keratitis *f*, Keratitis interstitialis/parenchymatosa.
deep lamina/layer of levator (muscle) of upper eyelid tiefes Blatt *nt* der Levatorsehne, Lamina profunda m. levatoris palpebrae superioris.
deep lymph nodes of upper limb tiefe Armlymphknoten *pl*, Nodi lymphatici profundi (membri superioris).
deep muscles tiefe Muskeln *pl od.* Muskulatur *f*.
deep mycosis tiefe Mykose *f*, Systemmykose *f*.
deep pain Tiefenschmerz *m*.
deep part: d. of external sphincter (muscle) of anus Pars profunda.
d. of parotid gland Pars profunda gl. parotideae.
deep portion of parotid gland → deep part of parotid gland.
deep psychology Psychoanalyse *f*.
deep punctate keratitis Keratitis profunda punctata.
deep pustular keratitis Keratitis pustiliformis profunda.
deep reflex Sehnenreflex *m*.
deep-seated *adj* (*a. fig.*) tiefsitzend.
deep sensation → deep sensibility.
deep sensibility Tiefensensibilität *f*, Bathyästhesie *f*.
deep-set *adj* tiefliegend.
deep sleep tiefer Schlaf *m*, Tiefschlaf *m*.
deep vein V. profunda.
d.s of clitoris tiefe Klitorisvenen *pl*, Vv. profundae clitoridis.
d.s of head tiefe Kopfvenen *pl*.
ds of inferior limbs Vv. profundae membri inferioris.
d.s of penis tiefe Penisvenen *pl*, Vv. profundae penis.
d.s of superior limbs Vv. profundae membri superioris.
deep vein thrombosis *abbr.* **DVT** tiefe Venenthrombose *f abbr.* TVT.
deep-voiced *adj* tief.
deer fly [dɪǝr] *micro.* Chrysops discalis.
deer-fly disease → deer-fly fever.
deer-fly fever Tularämie *f*, Hasen-, Nagerpest *f*, Lemming-Fieber *nt*, Ohara-, Francis-Krankheit *f*.
Deetjen ['deɪtjǝn]: **D.'s bodies** Blutplättchen *pl*, Thrombozyten *pl*.
de·fat·i·ga·tion [dɪˌfætɪ'geɪʃn] *n* (extreme)

defatted

Ermüdung f, Übermüdung f, Erschöpfung f.
de·fat·ted [dɪ'fætɪd] *adj* fettarm, fettfrei, entfettet.
def·e·cate ['defɪkeɪt] **I** *vt (Flüssigkeit)* klären, reinigen. **II** *vi* 1. Stuhl(gang) haben, den Darm entleeren, defäkieren, defäzieren. 2. s. klären, s. reinigen.
def·e·ca·tion [,defɪ'keɪʃn] *n* 1. Reinigung f, Klärung f. 2. Darmentleerung f, Stuhlgang m, Defäkation f.
defecation reflex Defäkationsreflex m.
de·fect ['dɪfekt, dɪ'fekt] *n* 1. Defekt m, Fehler m, Schaden m, schadhafte Stelle f (*in* an). 2. Mangel m, Schwäche f, Unvollkommenheit f. 3. (geistiger *od.* psychischer) Defekt m; (körperliches) Gebrechen n.
de·fec·tive [dɪ'fektɪv] **I** *n* Kranke(r m) f; Krüppel m; Schwachsinnige(r m) f. **II** *adj* 1. mangelhaft, unzulänglich. 2. schadhaft, defekt. 3. (*geistig od. psychisch*) defekt; schwachsinnig.
defective bacteriophage *micro.* defekter Phage m.
defective interfering virus particles *micro.* defekte interferierende Viruspartikel *pl*, DI-Partikel *pl*.
de·fec·tive·ness ['-nɪs] *n* Mangelhaftigkeit f, Unzulänglichkeit f; Schadhaftigkeit f.
defective phage → defective bacteriophage.
defective virus *micro.* defektes Virus nt.
de·fem·i·ni·za·tion [dɪ,femənaɪ'zeɪʃn] *n gyn.* Entweiblichung f, Defeminisierung f.
de·fence *n Brit.* → defense.
de·fend [dɪ'fend] *vt* verteidigen (*from*, *against* gegen); schützen (*from*, *against* vor).
de·fense [dɪ'fens] *n* Verteidigung f, Schutz m, Abwehr f. **in ~ of** zum Schutze von. **in ~ of life** in Notwehr.
defense behavior Abwehrverhalten nt.
de·fense·less [dɪ'fenslɪs] *adj* schutz-, wehr-, hilflos.
defense mechanism 1. *psycho.* Abwehrmechanismus m. 2. *physiol.* Abwehrapparat m, -mechanismus m.
defense reaction → defense mechanism.
defense reflex 1. Abwehrreflex m. 2. Fluchtreflex m.
de·fen·sive [dɪ'fensɪv] *adj* schützend, abwehrend, Abwehr-, Schutz-.
defensive function Abwehrtätigkeit f, -funktion f.
defensive system Abwehrsystem nt.
 cellular d. zelluläre Abwehr f, zelluläres Abwehrsystem.
 humoral d. humorale Abwehr f, humorales Abwehrsystem.
 nonspecific d. unspezifisches Abwehrsystem.
 specific d. spezifisches Abwehrsystem.
def·er·ens canal ['defərənz] → deferent duct.
def·er·ent ['defərənt] *adj anat.* ableitend, (hin-)abführend, deferens.
deferent duct Samenleiter m, Ductus deferens.
 vestigial d. Ductus deferens vestigialis.
def·er·en·tec·to·my [,defərən'tektəmɪ] *n urol.* (Teil-)Entfernung f des Samenleiters, Deferentektomie f, Vasektomie f, Vasoresektion f.
def·er·en·tial [,defə'renʃl] *adj* Samenleiter betr., Samenleiter-, Ductus-deferens-.
deferential artery Samenleiterarterie f, A. ductus deferentis.
deferential plexus Ductus-deferens-Geflecht nt, Plexus deferentialis.

def·er·en·ti·tis [defərən'taɪtɪs] *n urol.* Samenleiterentzündung f, Deferentitis f.
de·fer·ox·a·mine [,dɪfər'ɒksəmi:n] *n pharm.* Deferoxamin nt, Desferrioxamin nt.
de·ferred shock [dɪ'fɜrd] verzögerter Schock m.
def·er·ves·cence [,dɪfər'vesəns] *n* Entfieberung f, Defereszenz f.
def·er·ves·cent [,-'vesənt] **I** *n* Antipyretikum nt. **II** *adj* fiebersenkend, antipyretisch.
defervescent stage Stadium nt des Fieberabfalls, Stadium decrementi/defervescentiale.
de·fi·bril·la·tion [dɪ,fɪbrə'leɪʃn] *n card.* Defibrillation f.
de·fi·bril·la·tor [dɪ,fɪbrɪ'leɪtər] *n card.* Defibrillator m.
de·fi·bri·nat·ed [dɪ'faɪbrɪneɪtɪd] *adj* fibrinfrei, defibriniert.
defibrinated blood defibriniertes/fibrinfreies Blut nt.
de·fi·bri·na·tion [dɪ,faɪbrɪ'neɪʃn] *n* Defibrinieren nt, Defibrination nt.
defibrination syndrome *hema.* Defibrinations-, Defibrinisierungssyndrom nt.
de·fi·cien·cy [dɪ'fɪʃənsɪ] *n* 1. Mangel m, Defizit nt (*of* an); Fehlen nt (*of* von). 2. Unzulänglichkeit f, Mangelhaftigkeit f.
deficiency anemia Mangelanämie f, nutritive/alimentäre Anämie f.
deficiency disease Mangelkrankheit f.
deficiency symptom Mangelerscheinung f, -symptom nt.
de·fi·cient [dɪ'fɪʃənt] *adj* 1. Mangel leidend (*in* an). **to be ~ in** ermangeln, arm sein an. 2. mangelhaft, fehlend, mangelnd, mangelhaft.
def·i·cit ['defəsɪt; dɪ'fɪsɪt] *n* Mangel m (*in* an); Defizit nt; Verlust m, Ausfall m.
de·fin·a·ble [dɪ'faɪnəbl] *adj* definier-, bestimm-, erklärbar.
de·fine [dɪ'faɪn] *vt* 1. definieren, bestimmen, festlegen, erklären. 2. ab-, be-, umgrenzen, klar *od.* scharf abzeichnen lassen.
def·i·nite ['defənɪt] *adj* 1. eindeutig, klar, präzise, exakt, fest; genau festgelegt, bestimmt. 2. klar umrissen, festumrissen. 3. definitiv, endgültig, bestimmt.
def·i·ni·tion [defə'nɪʃn] *n* 1. Definition f; Definierung f, genaue Bestimmung f. 2. Begriffsbestimmung f. 2. Exaktheit f, Genauigkeit f. 3. Trennschärfe f; Bildschärfe f; Präzision f.
de·fin·i·tive [dɪ'fɪnɪtɪv] *adj* 1. *bio., embryo.* voll entwickelt, vollständig ausgeprägt, definitiv. 2. definitiv, endgültig. 3. bestimmend, beschreibend. 4. maßgeblich (*on* für); Standard-.
definitive callus *ortho.* Intermediärkallus m.
definitive choanae *embryo.* definitive Choanen pl.
definitive host *micro.* Endwirt m.
definitive kidney *embryo.* Nachniere f, Metanephros m.
definitive notochord *embro.* Chorda dorsalis.
de·flect [dɪ'flekt] **I** *vt* ablenken, ableiten; (*Licht*) beugen. **II** *vi* abweichen; (*Zeiger*) ausschlagen (*from* von).
de·flec·tion [dɪ'flekʃn] *n* Aus-, Ablenkung f, Abweichung f, Ableitung f, Deflexion f; (*Zeiger*) Ausschlag m; (*Licht*) Beugung f.
de·flec·tive [dɪ'flektɪv] *adj* ablenkend; beugend.
def·lo·rate ['defləreɪt] *vt* → deflower.
def·lo·ra·tion [,deflə'reɪʃn] *n* Entjungferung f, Defloration f.

de·flow·er [dɪ'flaʊər] *vt* entjungfern, deflorieren.
de·flow·er·ing [dɪ'flaʊərɪŋ] *n* → defloration.
de·form [dɪ'fɔrm] *vt* 1. (*a. techn.*) deformieren, verformen. 2. deformieren, verunstalten, entstellen. 3. umformen, umgestalten.
de·form·a·bil·i·ty [dɪ,fɔrmə'bɪlətɪ] *n* Verformbarkeit f.
de·form·a·ble [dɪ'fɔrməbl] *adj techn.* verformbar.
de·for·ma·tion [dɪ,fɔr'meɪʃn, ,defər-] *n* 1. (*a. techn.*) Deformation f, Verformung f. 2. Deformität f, Deformation f, Entstellung f, Verunstaltung f. 3. Umgestaltung f, Umformung f.
deformation phase *physiol.* Umformungsphase f, -zeit f.
de·formed [dɪ'fɔrmd] *adj* 1. (*a. techn.*) deformiert, verformt. 2. deformiert, verunstaltet, entstellt, mißgestaltet. 3. (*Charakter*) verdorben, abartig.
de·form·ing spondylopathy/spondylosis [dɪ'fɔrmɪŋ] *ortho.* Spondylosis/Spondylopathia deformans.
de·form·i·ty [dɪ'fɔrmətɪ] *n, pl* **-ties** 1. Deformität f, Deformation f, Verunstaltung f, Mißbildung f. 2. Mißgestalt f. 3. Verdorbenheit f, Abartigkeit f.
de·for·myl·ase [dɪ'fɔrmɪleɪz] *n* Deformylase f.
de·gen·er·a·cy [dɪ'dʒenərəsɪ] *n* 1. Degeneration f, Degeneriertheit f, Entartung f. 2. Degenerieren nt.
de·gen·er·ate [*n, adj* dɪ'dʒenərɪt; *v* -reɪt] **I** *n* degenerierter Mensch m. **II** *adj* degeneriert, zurückgebildet, verfallen; entartet. **III** *vi* degenerieren (*into* zu); s. zurückbilden, verfallen; entarten (*into* zu).
de·gen·er·at·ed [dɪ'dʒenəreɪtɪd] *adj* → degenerate II.
degenerated adenoma *patho.* entartetes Adenom nt.
de·gen·er·ate·ness [dɪ'dʒenərɪtnɪs] *n* → degeneracy.
de·gen·er·a·tion [dɪ,dʒenə'reɪʃn] *n* 1. Degeneration f, Entartung f. 2. *patho.* Degeneration f, Verfall m, Verkümmerung f, Rückbildung f, Entartung f.
de·gen·er·a·tive [dɪ'dʒenərətɪv, -reɪt-] *adj* degenerierend, degenerativ, Degenerations-; entartend.
degenerative arthritis degenerative Gelenkerkrankung f, Osteo-, Gelenkarthrose f, Arthrosis deformans.
 d. of hip joint Koxarthrose f, Coxarthrosis f, Arthrosis deformans coxae, Malum coxae senile.
degenerative atrophy degenerative Atrophie f.
degenerative chorea Erbchorea f, Chorea Huntington, Chorea chronica progressiva hereditaria.
degenerative condition degenerative Erkrankung f.
degenerative inflammation degenerative Entzündung f.
degenerative myopia *ophthal.* bösartige/maligne Myopie f.
degenerative nephritis Nephrose f, Nephrosis f.
degenerative neuralgia degenerative Neuralgie f.
degenerative osteoarthritis of hip joint → degenerative arthritis of hip joint.
degenerative rheumatism degenerativer Rheumatismus m.
degenerative spondylarthritis *ortho.* Spondylarthrose f.
de·germ [dɪ'dʒɜrm] *vt* → disinfect.

de·ger·mi·nate [dɪ'dʒɜrmənert] *vt* → disinfect.
de·glu·ti·ble [dɪ'glʊtɪbl] *adj* (ver-)schluckbar.
de·glu·ti·tion [ˌdɪglʊ'tɪʃn] *n* Schluckakt *m*, (Ver-)Schlucken *nt*, Hinunterschlucken *nt*, Deglutition *f*.
deglutition apnea Apnoe *f* während des Schluckaktes, Deglutitionsapnoe *f*.
deglutition center Schluckzentrum *nt*.
deglutition pneumonia Aspirationspneumonie *f*.
deglutition reflex Schluckreflex *m*.
Degos [dɪ'gəʊ; dɑ'go]: **D.' disease/syndrome** Köhlmeier-Degos-Syndrom *nt*, Degos-Delort-Tricot-Syndrom *nt*, tödliches kutaneointestinales Syndrom *nt*, Papulosis maligna atrophicans (Degos), Papulosis atrophicans maligna, Thrombangitis cutaneaintestinalis disseminata.
deg·ra·da·tion [ˌdegrə'deɪʃn] *n* **1.** *chem.* Abbau *m*, Zerlegung *f*, Degradierung *f*. **2.** *bio.* Degeneration *f*, Entartung *f*. **3.** Verschlechterung *f*; Verminderung *f*, Schwächung *f*, Herabsetzung *f*.
deg·ra·da·tive pathway ['degrədeɪtɪv] *biochem.* Abbauweg *m*.
de·grade [dɪ'greɪd] **I** *vt* **1.** schwächen, herabsetzen, vermindern. **2.** *chem.* zerlegen, abbauen. **II** *vi* **3.** *chem.* zerfallen. **4.** *bio.* degenerieren, entarten. **5.** *s.* verschlechtern; schwach *od.* schwächer werden, (Kräfte) nachlassen.
de·gran·u·la·tion [ˌdiːgrænjʊ'leɪʃn] *n* Degranulation *f*, Degranulierung *f*.
de·gree [dɪ'griː] *n* **1.** Grad *m*, Stufe *f*. **by ~s** nach u. nach, stufenweise. **2.** *mathe.*, *phys.* Grad *m*. **an angle of 45 ~s** ein Winkel von 45 Grad. **twenty ~s Celsius** zwanzig Grad Celsius. **3.** (Verwandtschafts-)Grad *m*. **4.** (*a. fig.*) Grad *m*, Ausmaß *nt*. **5.** (akademischer) Grad *m*.
d. of dissociation Dissoziationsgrad.
d. of doctor Doktorwürde *f*, Doktorgrad.
d.s of freedom Freiheitsgrade *pl*.
d. of purity Reinheitsgrad.
d. of saturation Sättigungsgrad.
d. of specialization Spezialisierungsgrad.
de·gus·ta·tion [ˌdɪgʌ'steɪʃn] *n* **1.** Geschmackssinn *m*. **2.** Schmecken *nt*.
de·hal·o·gen·ase [dɪ'hælədʒɪneɪz] *n* Dehalogenase *f*.
de·hisce [dɪ'hɪs] *vi* aufspringen, aufplatzen, (auseinander-)klaffen.
de·his·cence [dɪ'hɪsəns] *n* (Wunde) Klaffen *nt*, Auseinanderweichen *nt*, Dehiszenz *f*.
de·his·cent [dɪ'hɪsənt] *adj* aufplatzend, aufspringend, (auseinander-)klaffend.
de·hu·mid·i·fi·er [ˌdi(h)juː'mɪdəfaɪər] *n* Entfeuchter *m*.
de·hu·mid·i·fy [ˌdi(h)juː'mɪdəfaɪ] *vt* entfeuchten, Feuchtigkeit entziehen.
de·hy·drase [dɪ'haɪdreɪz] *n* **1.** *old* → dehydratase. **2.** *old* → dehydrogenase.
de·hy·dra·tase [dɪ'haɪdrəteɪz] *n* Dehydratase *f*, Hydratase *f*.
de·hy·drate [dɪ'haɪdreɪt] **I** *vt* Wasser entfernen *od.* entziehen, entwässern, dehydrieren; (vollständig) trocknen. **II** *vi* Wasser verlieren *od.* abgeben, dehydrieren.
de·hy·drat·ed alcohol [dɪ'haɪdreɪtɪd] absoluter Alkohol *m*, Alcoholus absolutus.
de·hy·dra·tion [ˌdɪhaɪ'dreɪʃn] *n* **1.** *chem.* Dehydrierung *f*, Wasserstoffabspaltung *f*. **2.** Dehydration *f*, Wasserentzug *m*; Entwässerung(stherapie *f*) *f*. **3.** *patho.* Wassermangel *m*, Dehydration *f*, Dehydratation *f*, Hypohydratation *f*.
dehydration fever *ped.* Durstfieber *nt*.
de·hy·dro·an·dros·ter·one [dɪˌhaɪdrəæn'drɑstərəʊn] *n old* → dehydroepiandrosterone.
de·hy·dro·a·scor·bic acid [ˌ-ə'skɔːrbɪk] Dehydroascorbinsäure *f*.
de·hy·dro·bil·i·ru·bin [ˌ-'bɪləruːbɪn] *n* Biliverdin *nt*.
de·hy·dro·cho·late [ˌ-'kəʊleɪt] *n* Dehydrocholat *nt*.
7-de·hy·dro·cho·les·ter·ol [ˌ-kə'lestərəʊl, -rɒl] *n* 7-Dehydrocholesterin *nt*, Provitamin D₃ *nt*.
de·hy·dro·cho·lic acid [ˌ-'kəʊlɪk, -'kɒl-] Dehydrocholsäure *f*.
11-de·hy·dro·cor·ti·cos·ter·one [ˌ-ˌkɔːrtɪ-'kɑstərəʊn] *n* 11-Dehydrocorticosteron *nt*, Kendall-Substanz A *f*.
de·hy·dro·ep·i·an·dros·ter·one [ˌ-ˌepiæn-'drɑstərəʊn] *n abbr.* **DHEA** Dehydroepiandrosteron *nt abbr.* DHEA, Dehydroisoandrosteron *nt*.
dehydroepiandrosterone sulfate *abbr.* **DHEAS** Dehydroepiandrosteronsulfat *nt abbr.* DHEAS.
de·hy·dro·gen·ase [dɪ'haɪdrədʒəneɪz] *n* Dehydrogenase *f*, Dehydrase *f*.
de·hy·dro·gen·ate [dɪ'haɪdrədʒəneɪt] *vt chem.* Wasserstoff entziehen/abspalten, dehydrogenieren, dehydrieren.
de·hy·dro·gen·a·tion [dɪˌhaɪdrədʒə'neɪʃn] *n chem.* Wasserstoffentzug *m*, -abspaltung *f*, Dehydrogenierung *f*, Dehydrierung *f*.
de·hy·dro·gen·ize [dɪ'haɪdrədʒənaɪz] *vt* → dehydrogenate.
de·hy·dro·i·so·an·dros·ter·one [ˌ-ˌaɪsəæn-'drɑstərəʊn] *n* → dehydroepiandrosterone.
de·hy·dro·mor·phine [ˌ-'mɔːrfiːn] *n* Pseudomorphin *nt*, Dehydromorphin *nt*.
de·hy·dro·pep·ti·dase [ˌ-'peptɪdeɪz] *n* Aminoacylase *f*, Hippurikase *f*.
(5-)de·hy·dro·qui·nate dehydratase [ˌ-'kwaɪneɪt] (5-)Dehydrochinäuredehydratase *f*.
(5-)dehydroquinate synthase Dehydrochinasäuresynthase *f*.
5-de·hy·dro·quin·ic acid [ˌ-'kwɪnɪk] 5-Dehydrochinasäure *f*.
de·hy·dro·ret·i·nal [ˌ-'retnəl] *n* Dehydroretinal *nt*, Retinal₂ *nt*.
(3-)de·hy·dro·ret·i·nol [ˌ-'retnɒl, -nɑl] *n* (3-)Dehydroretinol *nt*, Vitamin A₂ *nt*.
3-de·hy·dro·sphin·ga·mine [ˌ-'sfɪŋgəmiːn, -mɪn] *n* 3-Dehydrosphinganin *nt*.
de·hy·drox·yl·a·tion [dɪhaɪ'drɑksɪ'leɪʃn] *n chem.* Dehydroxylierung *f*.
de·i·o·dase [dɪ'aɪədeɪz] *n* Dejodase *f*, Dejodinase *f*.
de·io·di·na·tion [dɪˌaɪədɪ'neɪʃn] *n chem.* Dejodierung *f*, Dejodinierung *f*.
de·i·on·i·za·tion [dɪˌaɪənaɪ'zeɪʃn] *n chem.* De-, Entionisierung *f*.
Deiters ['daɪtərs]: **D.' cells 1.** Deiters'--Stützzellen *pl*. **2.** (*ZNS*) Deiters'-Zellen *pl*.
D.' nucleus Deiters'-Kern *m*, Nc. vestibularis lateralis.
D.' supporting cells → D.' cells 1.
D.' tract Held'-Bündel *nt*, Tractus vestibulospinalis.
déjà entendue [deɪ'ʒɑ; de'ʒa ɑ̃tɑ̃'dy] Déjà--entendu-Erlebnis *nt*.
déjà éprouvé [epruː've] Déjà-éprouvé-Erlebnis *nt*.
déjà fait [fɛ] Déjà-fait-Erlebnis *nt*.
déjà pensé [pɑ̃'se] Déjà-pensé-Erlebnis *nt*.
déjà raconté [rækɔ̃'te] Déjà-raconté-Erlebnis *nt*.
déjà vécu [ve'ky] Déjà-vécu-Erlebnis *nt*.
déjà voulu [vuː'ly] Déjà-voulu-Erlebnis *nt*.
déjà vu ['vy] Déjà-vu-Erlebnis *nt*.
de·jec·ta [dɪ'dʒektə] *pl* Exkremente *pl*.

de·jec·tion [dɪ'dʒekʃn] *n* **1.** Niedergeschlagenheit *f*, Mutlosigkeit *f*, Melancholie *f*. **2.** Stuhlgang *m*, Defäkation *f*. **3.** Stuhl *m*, Kot *m*, Fäzes *pl*.
Déjérine [deʒe'rin]: **aberrant fibers of D.** → D.'s fibers.
D.'s disease → Déjérine-Sottas atrophy.
D.'s fibers Déjérine-Fasern *pl*, Fibrae aberrantes.
D.'s hand phenomenon → D.'s reflex.
D.'s reflex Déjérine-Handreflex *m*.
D.'s sign *neuro.* Déjérine-Zeichen *nt*.
D.'s type amyotrophische/amyotrophe/ myatrophische Lateralsklerose *f abbr.* ALS.
Déjérine-Klumpke ['klʊmpkə]: **D.-K. paralysis/syndrome** untere Armplexuslähmung *f*, Klumpke'-Lähmung *f*, Klumpke--Déjérine-Syndrom *nt*.
Déjérine-Landouzy [lɑ̃duː'si]: **D.-L. atrophy/dystrophy/type** fazio-skapulo-humerale Muskeldystrophie *f*, Landouzy-Déjérine-Krankheit *f*, -Syndrom *nt*, -Typ *m*.
Déjérine-Lichtheim ['lɪçthaɪm]: **D.-L. phenomenon** Déjérine-Lichtheim-Phänomen *nt*, Déjérine-Phänomen *nt*.
Déjérine-Roussy [ruː'si]: **D.-R. syndrome** *neuro.* Déjérine-Roussy-Syndrom *nt*, Thalamussyndrom *nt*.
Déjérine-Sottas [sɔ'tɑ]: **D.-S. atrophy/disease/syndrome** Déjérine-Sottas-Krankheit *f*, -Syndrom *nt*, hypertrophische Neuropathie (Déjérine-Sottas) *f*, hereditäre motorische u. sensible Neuropathie Typ III *f abbr.* HMSN.
Déjérine-Thomas ['tɑmɑs]: **D.-T. atrophy** Déjérine-Thomas-Syndrom *nt*, olivopontozerebelläre Atrophie *f*.
deka- *pref.* → deca-.
de·lac·ri·ma·tion [dɪˌlækrə'meɪʃn] *n ophthal.* übermäßige Tränensekretion *f*, übermäßiger Tränenfluß *m*.
de·lac·ta·tion [dɪlæk'teɪʃn] *n ped.*, *gyn.* Abstillen *nt*, Ablaktation *f*, Ablactatio *f*.
de·lam·i·na·tion [dɪˌlæmɪ'neɪʃn] *n* Delamination *f*.
de Lange [də 'lɑŋə]: **d.L. syndrome** Lange--Syndrom *nt*, Cornelia de Lange-Syndrom *nt*, Brachmann-de-Lange-Syndrom *nt*, Amsterdamer Degenerationstyp *m*.
de·lay [dɪ'leɪ] **I** *n* Aufschub *m*, Verzögerung *f*; Verspätung *f*. **II** *vt* **1.** ver-, aufschieben, verzögern. **2.** hemmen, aufhalten.
de·layed [dɪ'leɪd] *adj* verzögert, verschleppt, verspätet; ver-, aufgeschoben; Spät-.
delayed allergy → delayed-type hypersensitivity.
delayed apoplexy Spätapoplexie *f*, verzögerte traumatische Apoplexie *f*.
delayed compliance *physiol.* Streßrelaxation *f*, delayed-Compliance *f*.
reverse d. reverse Streßrelaxation, reverse delayed-Compliance *f*.
delayed complication Spätkomplikation *f*.
delayed conduction *card.* AV-Block I. Grades *m*.
delayed dentition verspätete/verzögerte Zahnung *f*, Dentitio tarda.
delayed development of speech fehlende *od.* verzögerte Sprachentwicklung *f*, (motorische) Hörstummheit *f*, Audimutitas *f*.
delayed epilepsy Spätepilepsie *f*, Epilepsia tarda/tardiva.
delayed graft/grafting verzögerte/aufgeschobene Hautdeckung/Transplantation *f*.

delayed hypersensitivity

delayed hypersensitivity *abbr.* **DH** → delayed-type hypersensitivity.
delayed menstruation verzögerte Menstruation *f*, Menstruatio tarda.
delayed pain zweiter/verzögerter Schmerz *m*.
delayed reflex verzögerter Reflex *m*.
delayed shock verzögerter Schock *m*.
delayed suture verzögerte Wundnaht *f*.
delayed-type hypersensitivity *abbr.* **DTH** T-zellvermittelte Überempfindlichkeitsreaktion *f*, Tuberkulin-Typ *od.* Spät-Typ *od.* Typ IV *m* der Überempfindlichkeitsreaktion *f*.
delayed union (of fracture) *ortho.* verzögerte Frakturheilung *f*.
Delbet [dɛl'be]: **D.'s sign** *chir.* Delbet-Zeichen *nt*.
Del Castillo [del kas'tijo]: **D. syndrome** del Castillo-Syndrom *nt*, Castillo-Syndrom *nt*, Sertoli-Zell-Syndrom *nt*, Sertoli-cell-only-Syndrom *nt*, Germinal(zell)aplasie *f*.
DeLee [də'li:]: **D.'s operation** *gyn.* (de) Lee-Spiegelhandgriff *m*.
del·e·te·ri·ous [ˌdeliˈtɪərɪəs] *adj* (gesundheits-)schädlich, zerstörend, deletär; giftig.
de·le·tion [dɪˈliːʃn] *n* (Aus-)Streichung *f*, (Aus-)Löschung *f*; *genet.* Deletion *f*.
Del·hi sore ['deli] kutane Leishmaniose/Leishmaniase *f*, Hautleishmaniose *f*, Orientbeule *f*, Leishmaniasis cutis.
de·lib·er·ate hyperventilation [dɪˈlɪbərɪt] forcierte Atmung *f*, willkürliche Hyperventilation *f*.
de·lim·it [dɪˈlɪmɪt] *vt* → delimitate.
de·lim·i·tate [dɪˈlɪmɪteɪt] *vt* ab-, begrenzen.
de·lim·i·ta·tion [dɪˌlɪmɪˈteɪʃn] *n* Ab-, Begrenzung *f*.
de·lim·i·ta·tive [dɪˈlɪmɪteɪtɪv] *adj* ab-, begrenzend.
de·lin·quent [dɪˈlɪŋkwənt] **I** *n* Straffällige(r *m*) *f*, Delinquent(in *f*) *m*. **II** *adj* straffällig.
del·i·quesce [ˌdelɪˈkwes] *vi chem.* 1. zerfließen, zergehen. 2. weg-, zerschmelzen.
del·i·ques·cence [-ˈkwesəns] *n chem.* 1. Zerfließen *nt*. 2. Weg-, Zerschmelzen *nt*.
del·i·ques·cent [-ˈkwesənt] *adj* 1. *chem.* zerfließend. 2. zerschmelzend.
de·lir·i·ant [dɪˈlɪərɪənt] **I** *n* 1. deliranter Patient *m*, delirante Patientin *f*, Delirende(r *m*) *f*. 2. Delirium verursachende *od.* auslösende Substanz *f*. **II** *adj* Delirium verursachend *od.* auslösend.
de·lir·i·ous [dɪˈlɪərɪəs] *adj* an Delirium leidend, mit Symptomen des Delirs, delirant, delirös.
de·lir·i·um [dɪˈlɪərɪəm] *n, pl* -**lir·i·ums, -lir·ia** [-ˈlɪərɪə] Delirium *nt*, Delir *nt*.
delirium alcoholicum Alkoholdelir *nt*, Delirium tremens/alcoholicum.
delirium tremens 1. → delirium alcoholicum. 2. Entzugssyndrom *nt*, -delir *nt*, Delirium tremens.
del·i·tes·cence [ˌdelɪˈtesəns] *n* 1. Inkubationszeit *f*, -periode *f*. 2. plötzliches Verschwinden *nt* von Symptomen *od.* Effloreszenzen.
de·liv·er [dɪˈlɪvər] *vt* 1. *gyn.* (*eine Frau*) entbinden; (*Kind*) gebären, zur Welt bringen. 2. *gyn.* (*Plazenta*) manuell lösen. 3. *ophthal.* (*Linse*) entbinden.
de·liv·er·y [dɪˈlɪvərɪ] *n* 1. *gyn.* Geburt *f*, Entbindung *f*, Partus *m*. 2. *gyn.* (*Plazenta*) manuelle Lösung *f*. 3. *ophthal.* (*Linse*) Entbindung *f*.
delivery date rule *gyn.* Naegele-Regel *f*.
delivery room Kreißsaal *m*.
de·lo·mor·phic [ˌdiːləʊˈmɔːrfɪk] *adj* → delomorphous.

de·lo·mor·phous [ˌ-ˈmɔːrfəs] *adj histol.* delomorph.
de·louse [diˈlaʊs] *vt* entlausen.
de·lous·ing [diˈlaʊsɪŋ] *n* Entlausen *nt*, Entlausung *f*.
del·ta ['deltə] *n* 1. *abbr.* **Δ, δ** Delta *nt* *abbr.* Δ, δ. 2. Delta *nt*, Dreieck *nt*.
delta agent Deltaagens *nt*, Hepatitis-Delta-Virus *nt* *abbr.* HDV.
delta alcoholism δ-Alkoholismus *m*.
delta antigen (Hepatitis-)Deltaantigen *nt* *abbr.* HDAg.
delta cell adenocarcinoma (*Pankreas*) D-Zelladenokarzinom *nt*, Delta-Zelladenokarzinom *nt*.
delta cell adenoma (*Pankreas*) Delta-Zelladenom *nt*, D-Zelladenom *nt*.
delta cells 1. (*Pankreas*) D-Zellen *pl*, δ-Zellen *pl*. 2. (*Adenohypophyse*) basophile Zellen *pl*, β-Zellen *pl*.
delta cell tumor D-Zell(en)-Tumor *m*, Somatostatinom *nt*.
del·ta·cor·ti·sone [ˌdeltəˈkɔːrtəzəʊn] *n pharm.* Prednison *nt*.
delta hepatitis Hepatitis D *f*, Deltahepatitis *f*.
delta rhythm δ-Rhythmus *m*, Deltarhythmus *m*.
delta staphylolysin δ-Staphylolysin *nt*, delta-Staphylolysin *nt*.
delta virus Deltaagens *nt*, Hepatitis-Delta-Virus *nt* *abbr.* HDV.
delta waves *physiol.* Deltawellen *pl*, delta-Wellen *pl*, δ-Wellen *pl*.
del·toid ['deltɔɪd] **I** *n* Deltamuskel *m*, Deltoideus *m*, M. deltoideus. **II** *adj* 1. M. deltoideus betr. 2. deltaförmig, dreieckig.
del·toi·dal [delˈtɔɪdl] *adj* → deltoid 2.
deltoid artery → deltoid branch of deep brachial artery.
deltoid branch: d. of deep brachial artery M. deltoideus-Ast *m* der A. profunda brachii, Ramus deltoideus a. profundae brachii.
d. of thoracoacromial artery A. thoracoacromialis-Ast *m* zum M. deltoideus, Ramus deltoideus a. thoracoacromialis.
deltoid bursa Bursa subacromialis.
deltoid crest → deltoid tuberosity of humerus.
deltoid eminence → deltoid tuberosity of humerus.
del·toi·de·us (muscle) [delˈtɔɪdɪəs] → deltoid I.
deltoid fascia Fascia deltoidea.
deltoid impression (of humerus) Tuberositas deltoidea (humeri).
deltoid ligament Deltaband, Innenknöchelband, Lig. deltoideum, Lig. mediale (artic. talocruralis).
d. of ankle (joint) → deltoid ligament.
d. of elbow Lig. collaterale ulnare.
deltoid muscle → deltoid I.
deltoid region *anat.* Deltoidgegend *f*, -region *f*, Regio deltoidea.
deltoid ridge → deltoid tuberosity of humerus.
deltoid tubercle → deltoid tuberosity of humerus.
deltoid tuberosity of humerus Tuberositas deltoidea (humeri).
de·lu·sion [dɪˈluːʒn] *n* 1. *psychia.* Wahn *m*, Wahnidee *f*. 2. Wahn *m*, Selbsttäuschung *f*, Verblendung *f*, Irrtum *m*, Irrglauben *m*. 3. Illusion *f*, Täuschung *f*.
d. of grandeur expansiver Wahn, Größenwahn, Megalomanie *f*.
d. of negation nihilistischer Wahn.
d. of persecution persekutorischer Wahn, Verfolgungswahn.
d. of poverty Verarmungswahn.
d. of reference Beziehungswahn.

de·lu·sion·al [dɪˈluːʒnl] *adj* eingebildet, wahnhaft, Wahn-.
delusional disorders → delusional paranoid disorders.
delusional idea *psychia.* Wahnidee *f*.
delusional paranoid disorders paranoide Syndrome *pl*, Paranoia *f*.
de·lu·sive [dɪˈluːsɪv] *adj* 1. → delusional. 2. täuschend, irreführend, trügerisch.
de·lu·so·ry [dɪˈluːsərɪ] *adj* 1. → delusional. 2. → delusive 2.
de·mand pacemaker [dɪˈmænd, -ˈmɑːnd] *card.* Demand-Herzschrittmacher *m*, Demand-Pacemaker *m*.
de·mar·cate ['diːmɑːrkeɪt] *vt* abgrenzen, trennen, demarkieren (*from* gegen, von).
de·mar·cat·ed ['diːmɑːrkeɪtɪd] *adj patho.* abgegrenzt, demarkiert.
demarcated gangrene demarkierte Gangrän *f*.
de·mar·ca·tion [ˌdiːmɑːrˈkeɪʃn] *n* Abgrenzung *f*, Demarkation *f*; Abgrenzen *nt*, Demarkieren *nt*.
demarcation current *patho.* Verletzungsstrom *m*.
demarcation potential Demarkationspotential *nt*.
demarcation tissue *patho.* Demarkationsgewebe *nt*.
de·mar·ka·tion *n* → demarcation.
Demarquay [demarˈkeɪ]: **D.'s sign/symptom** *patho.* Demarquay-Zeichen *nt*.
de·mas·cu·lin·i·za·tion [dɪˌmæskjələnɪˈzeɪʃn] *n* Demaskulinisation *f*.
de·mas·cu·lin·iz·ing [dɪˈmæskjəlɪnaɪzɪŋ] *adj* demaskulinisierend.
dem·e·clo·cy·cline [ˌdeməkləʊˈsaɪkliːn] *n pharm.* Demeclocyclin *nt*, Demethylchlortetracyclin *nt*.
dem·e·col·cine [ˌdeməˈkɒlsiːn] *n pharm.* Demecolcin *nt*, N-desacetyl-N-methylcolchicin *nt*.
de·ment·ed [dɪˈmentɪd] *adj* 1. an Demenz leidend, dement. 2. wahnsinnig, verrückt.
de·men·tia [dɪˈmenʃɪə] *n* 1. geistiger Verfall *m*, *inf.* Verblödung *f*, Demenz *f*, Dementia *f*. 2. *old* Wahnsinn *m*.
dementia pugilistica Boxerenzephalopathie *f*, Encephalopathia traumatica.
de·meth·yl·a·tion [dɪˌmeθəˈleɪʃn] *n chem.* Demethylierung *f*.
de·meth·yl·chlor·tet·ra·cy·cline [dɪˌmeθəlˌklɔːrˌtetrəˈsaɪkliːn] *n abbr.* **DMCT** → demeclocycline.
demi- *pref.* Halb-, Demi-, Semi-.
dem·i·lune ['demɪluːn] **I** *n histol.* Halbmond *m*, Mondsichel *f*. **II** *adj* halbmond-, (mond)sichelförmig.
d. of Giannuzzi → demilune body.
d. of Heidenhain → demilune body.
demilune body (von) Ebner'-Halbmond *m*, Giannuzzi'-Halbmond *m*, Heidenhain'-Halbmond *m*, seröser Halbmond *m*.
demilune cells → demilune body.
de·min·er·al·i·za·tion [dɪˌmɪn(ə)rəlaɪˈzeɪʃn] *n* Demineralisation *f*.
de·min·er·al·ize [dɪˈmɪn(ə)rəlaɪz] *vt* entsalzen, demineralisieren.
dem·o·dec·tic [deməˈdektɪk] *adj* durch Demodex hervorgerufen.
demodectic blepharitis *ophthal.* Blepharitis *f* durch Demodex folliculorum.
Dem·o·dex ['deməˌdeks, ˈdiːm-] *n micro.* Demodex *f*.
D. folliculorum Haarbalgmilbe *f*, Demodex folliculorum.
Dem·o·dic·i·dae [ˌdemɪˈdɪkɪdiː] *pl micro.* Demodicidae *pl*.
dem·o·dic·i·do·sis [ˌdemɪˌdɪsɪˈdəʊsɪs] *n derma.* Demodikose *f*, Demodicidose *f*, Pityriasis folliculorum, Akne rosacea demodes.

dem·o·di·co·sis [ˌdeməd」'kəʊsɪs] n → demodicidosis.
dem·o·gram ['deməgræm, 'diːmə-] n Demogramm nt.
dem·o·graph·ic [ˌ-'græfɪk] adj Demographie betr., mittels Demographie, demographisch.
de·mog·ra·phy [dɪ'mɑgrəfɪ] n Demographie f.
dem·on·strate ['demənstreɪt] vt demonstrieren, darlegen, zeigen, veranschaulichen, anschaulich machen.
dem·on·stra·tion [ˌdemən'streɪʃn] n 1. Demonstrierung f, Demonstration f, (anschauliche) Darstellung f, Veranschaulichung f, praktisches Beispiel nt. 2. Beweis m (of für).
de·mon·stra·tive [də'mɑnstrətɪv] adj 1. beweisend, überzeugend, anschaulich (zeigend). 2. auffällig, betont, demonstrativ.
dem·on·stra·tor ['demənstreɪtər] n 1. Assistent(in f) m, Demonstrator m. 2. Beweis(mittel nt) m.
de·mo·pho·bia [deməˈfəʊbɪə] n psychia. Angst f vor Menschenansammlungen, Demophobie f.
De Morgan [də'mɔːrgən]: **D.M.'s spots** senile (Häm-)Angiome pl, Alters(häm)angiome pl.
de·mor·phin·i·za·tion [dɪˌmɔːrfənaɪˈzeɪʃn] n schrittweiser Morphinentzug m.
Demours [də'mʊr]: **D.' membrane** hintere Basalmembran f, Descemet'-Membran f, Lamina elastica posterior Descemeti, Lamina limitans posterior (corneae).
dem·ox·e·pam [demˈɒksɪpæm] n pharm. Demoxepam nt.
de·mu·co·sa·tion [ˌdɪmjuːkə'zeɪʃn] n chir. Schleimhautentfernung f, -exzision f.
de·mul·cent [dɪ'mʌlsənt] I n pharm. Demulcens nt. II adj (reiz-)lindernd.
de Musset [də my'ze]: **d.M.'s sign** (de) Musset-Zeichen nt.
de·my·e·li·nate [dɪ'maɪəlɪneɪt] vt entmarken, demyelinisieren.
de·my·e·li·nat·ing disease [dɪ'maɪəlɪneɪtɪŋ] Entmarkungskrankheit f, demyelinisierende Erkrankung/Krankheit f.
demyelinating encephalopathy demyelinisierende Enzephalopathie f.
de·my·e·li·na·tion [ˌdɪmaɪəlɪ'neɪʃn] n Entmarkung f, Demyelinisation f, Demyelinisierung f, Myelinverlust m.
de·my·e·lin·i·za·tion [dɪˌmaɪəlɪnə'zeɪʃn] → demyelination.
de·na·tur·ant [dɪ'neɪtʃərənt] n denaturierendes Mittel nt, Denaturierungs-, Vergällungsmittel nt.
de·na·tur·a·tion [dɪˌneɪtʃə'reɪʃn] n chem. 1. Denaturierung f, Denaturieren nt. 2. Vergällen nt, Denaturieren nt.
de·na·ture [dɪ'neɪtʃər] vt chem. 1. denaturieren. 2. vergällen, denaturieren.
de·na·tured [dɪ'neɪtʃərd] adj 1. denaturiert. 2. vergällt, denaturiert.
denatured alcohol vergällter/denaturierter Alkohol m.
denatured protein denaturiertes Protein nt.
den·drax·on [den'dræksɑn] n Endbäumchen nt, Telodendron nt.
den·dric ['dendrɪk] → dendritic.
den·dri·form ['dendrəfɔːrm] adj verzweigt, verästelt, dendritisch.
dendriform keratitis Keratitis dendrica, Herpes-simplex-Keratitis f.
dendriform ulcer Ulcus dendriticum.
den·drite ['dendraɪt] n Dendrit m.
den·drit·ic [den'drɪtɪk] adj anat. Dendrit betr., verästelt, dendritisch.
den·drit·i·cal [den'drɪtɪkl] adj → dendritic.

dendritic axon dendritisches Axon nt, Dendrit m.
dendritic calculus urol. Korallenstein m, Hirschgeweihstein m, (Becken-)Ausgußstein m.
dendritic cancer papilläres Karzinom nt, Ca. papillare/papilliferum.
dendritic cell 1. dendritische Retikulumzelle f. 2. interdigitierende Retikulumzelle f.
follicular d. → dendritic cell 1.
dendritic keratitis → dendriform keratitis.
dendritic process dendritischer Fortsatz m, Dendrit m.
dendritic stem Dendritenstamm m.
dendritic stone Korallenstein m, Hirschgeweihstein m, (Becken-)Ausgußstein m.
dendritic synovitis Synovitis/Synovialitis villosa.
dendritic tree Dendritenbaum m.
dendritic ulcer Ulcus dendriticum.
den·dro·den·drit·ic synapse [ˌdendrəʊden'drɪtɪk] dendrodendritische Synapse f.
den·droid ['dendrɔɪd] adj → dendriform.
den·dron ['dendrən] n, pl **-drons, -dra** [-drə] → dendrite.
de·ner·vate [dɪ'nɜrveɪt] vt denervieren.
de·ner·vat·ed [dɪ'nɜrveɪtɪd] adj denerviert.
denervated bladder neuro. autonome Blase f.
den·gue ['deŋgeɪ, -gɪ] n Dengue nt, Dengue-Fieber nt, Dandy-Fieber nt.
dengue fever → dengue.
dengue hemorrhagic fever Dengue--hämorrhagisches Fieber nt.
dengue shock syndrome Dengue--Schocksyndrom nt.
dengue virus Dengue-Virus nt.
de·ni·al [dɪ'naɪəl] n 1. psychia. Verleugnung f. 2. Verweigerung f, Ablehnung f.
den·i·da·tion [denɪ'deɪʃn] n gyn. Abstoßung/Desquamation f der Lamina functionalis während der Menstruation.
Denis Browne ['denɪs braʊn]: **D. B. method** ortho. funktionelle Schienenbehandlung f nach Denis Browne.
D. B. operation urol. Browne-Operation f.
D. B. procedure → D. B. method.
D. B. splint ortho. (Denis) Browne-Schiene f.
den·i·tra·tion [daɪnaɪ'treɪʃn] n → denitrification.
den·i·tri·fi·ca·tion [dɪˌnaɪtrəfɪ'keɪʃn] n chem. Denitrifizierung f, Denitrifikation f, Denitrierung f.
de·ni·tri·fy [dɪ'naɪtrəfaɪ] vt chem. denitrifizieren, denitrieren.
de·ni·tro·gen·a·tion [dɪˌnaɪtrɔdʒɪ'neɪʃn] n Denitrogenisierung f, Denitrogenisation f.
Denman ['denmən]: **D.'s method/spontaneous evolution/version** gyn. Denman-Spontanentwicklung f.
de·nom·i·na·tor [dɪ'nɑməneɪtər] n mathe. Nenner m.
Denonvilliers [dənɒvɪl'je]: **D.' aponeurosis** rektovaginale Scheidewand f, rektovaginales Septum nt, Septum rectovaginale f.
D.' fascia → D.' aponeurosis.
D.' ligament Lig. puboprostaticum.
D.' operation HNO Denonvilliers'-Operation f.
dens [denz] n, pl **den·tes** ['dentiːz] anat. 1. Zahn m, Dens m; zahnähnlicher Teil/Fortsatz m. 2. → dens axis.
dens axis Zahn m des II. Halswirbels, Dens (axis).
dense [dens] adj 1. dicht. 2. fig. beschränkt, begriffsstutzig. 3. photo. (Negativ) überbelichtet.
dense·ness ['densnɪs] n → density.

den·si·fy ['densəfaɪ] I vt verdichten. II vi s. verdichten.
den·sim·e·ter [den'sɪmɪtər] n → densitometer 1.
den·si·met·ric analysis [ˌdensɪ'metrɪk] → densitometry.
den·si·tom·e·ter [ˌdensɪ'tɑmɪtər] n 1. Densi(to)meter nt, Dichtemesser m. 2. Densitometer nt, Densograph m.
den·si·tom·e·try [ˌdensɪ'tɑmɪtrɪ] n Dichtemessung f, -bestimmung f, Densi(to)metrie f.
den·si·ty ['densətɪ] n 1. (a. phys., chem.) Dichte f, Dichtheit f. 2. fig. Beschränktheit f, Begriffsstutzigkeit f. 3. photo. (Negativ) Schwärzung f.
density distribution Dichteverteilung f.
density gradient Dichtegradient m.
density-gradient centrifugation Dichtegradienten-, Zonenzentrifugation f.
density inhibition Kontakt-, Dichtehemmung f.
dent- pref. → dento-.
dent·ag·ra [den'tægrə, 'dentəgrə] n → dentalgia.
den·tal ['dentl] I n Dental(laut m) m; Alveolar(laut m) m. II adj 1. Zahn od. Zähne betr., dental, zahnärztlich, zahnheilkundlich, Zahn-. 2. von den Zähnen ausgehend, dentogen.
dental abscess (Zahn) Wurzelspitzenabszeß m.
dental alveoli Zahnfächer pl, Alveoli dentales.
d. of mandible Alveoli dentales mandibulae.
d. of maxilla Alveoli dentales maxillae.
dental arch Zahnreihe f, -bogen m, Arcus dentalis.
inferior d. Unterkieferzahnreihe, mandibuläre Zahnreihe, Arcus dentalis inferior.
superior d. Oberkieferzahnreihe, maxilläre Zahnreihe, Arcus dentalis superior.
dental artery: anterior d.s vordere Oberkieferschlagadern pl, -arterien pl, Aa. alveolares superiores anteriores.
inferior d. Unterkieferschlagader f, -arterie f, Alveolaris f inferior, A. alveolaris inferior.
dental assistant Zahnarzthelfer(in f) m.
dental branches: d. of anterior superior alveolar arteries Zahnäste pl der oberen vorderen Alveolararterien, Rami dentales aa. alveolarium superiorum anteriorum.
d. of inferior alveolar artery Zahnäste pl der A. alveolaris inferioris, Rami dentales a. alveolaris inferioris.
inferior d. of inferior dental plexus Zahnwurzeläste pl des Plexus dentalis inferior, Rami dentales inferiores (plexus dentalis inferioris).
d. of posterior superior alveolar artery Zahnäste pl der oberen hinteren Alveolararterie, Rami dentales a. alveolaris superioris posterioris.
superior d. of superior dental plexus Zahnwurzeläste pl des Plexus dentalis superior, Rami dentales superiores (plexus dentalis superioris).
dental calculus Zahnstein m, Calculus dentalis/dentis.
dental canal: inferior d. Unterkieferkanal m, Canalis mandibulae.
posterior d.s Alveolarkanälchen pl, Canales alveolares (maxillae).
dental canaliculi Canaliculi dentales.
dental care Zahn-, Mundpflege f.
dental caries (Zahn-)Karies f, Zahnfäule f, Caries dentium.
dental cavity Zahn-, Pulpahöhle f, Cavitas dentis/pulparis.

dental cement

dental cement (Zahn-)Zement *m*, Cementum *nt*, Substantia ossea dentis.
dental clinic Zahnklinik *f*.
dental crown (Zahn-)Krone *f*, Corona dentis.
  anatomical d. anatomische Krone, Corona dentis/anatomica.
  clinical d. klinische Krone, Corona clinica.
dental cusp Zahnhöcker *m*, Cuspis dentis, Cuspis coronae (dentis).
dental cuticle Schmelzoberhäutchen *nt*, Cuticula dentis.
dental cyst odontogene Zyste *f*.
dental dysplasia dentoalveoläre Dysplasie *f*.
dental enamel Zahnschmelz *m*, Adamantin *nt*, Substantia adamantina, Enamelum *nt*.
dental floss Zahnseide *f*.
dental fluorosis Dentalfluorose *f*.
dental formula Zahn-, Gebißformel *f*.
dental fovea of atlas Fovea dentis (atlantis).
dental germ 1. Zahnanlage *f*. **2.** Zahnkeim *m*.
den·tal·gia [den'tældʒ(ɪ)ə] *n* Zahnschmerz(en *pl*) *m*, Dentalgie *f*, Dentalgia *f*, Dentagra *f*.
dental granuloma Zahngranulom *nt*, Wurzelspitzengranulom *nt*.
dental hygiene Zahnhygiene *f*, Mundpflege *f*.
dental laboratoy Zahnlabor *nt*.
dental lamella *embryo.* Zahnleiste *f*.
dental ligament, apical Lig. apicis dentis.
dental mirror Mundspiegel *m*.
dental neck Zahnhals *m*, Cervix dentis.
dental nerve, inferior Unterkiefernerv *m*, Alveolaris *m* inferior, N. alveolaris inferior.
dental papilla *embryo.* mesenchymale Zahnpapille *f*, Papilla dentis.
dental plaque *dent.* Zahnbelag *m*, Plaque *f*.
dental plate → dental prosthesis.
dental plexus: inferior d. Plexus dentalis inferior.
  superior d. Plexus dentalis superior.
dental process Alveolarfortsatz *m* des Oberkiefers, Proc. alveolaris maxillae.
dental prosthesis künstliches Gebiß *nt*, Zahnersatz *m*, -prothese *f*, (Teil-)Gebiß *nt*.
dental prosthetics Zahntechnik *f*, Zahnersatzkunde *f*, zahnärztliche Prothetik *f*.
dental pulp (Zahn-)Pulpa *f*, Pulpa dentis.
dental reflector Zahnspiegel *m*.
dental root (Zahn-)Wurzel *f*, Radix dentis.
dental silk Zahnseide *f*.
dental stone → dental calculus.
dental surgeon Zahn- u. Kieferchirurg(in *f*) *m*.
dental surgery Zahn- u. Kieferchirurgie *f*.
dental technician Zahntechniker(in *f*) *m*, Dentist(in *f*) *m*.
dental tophus → dental calculus.
dental treatment Zahnbehandlung *f*.
dental trepanation/trephination *dent.* Trepanation *f*.
dental tubercle Tuberculum coronae/dentis.
den·tate ['denteɪt] *adj* mit Zähnen versehen, gezähnt.
dentate band → dentate gyrus 1.
den·ta·tec·to·my [ˌdentə'tektəmɪ] *n* neurochir. Dentatektomie *f*.
den·tat·ed ['denteɪtɪd] *adj* → dentate.
dentate fascia Fascia dentata hippocampi, Gyrus dentatus.
detate fissure Fissura hippocampi, Sulcus hippocampalis/hippocampi.

dentate gyrus 1. Gyrus dentatus, Fascia dentata hippocampi. **2.** Gyrus fasciolaris.
dentate ligaments of spinal cord Ligg. denticulata.
dentate line Anokutanlinie *f*, Linea anocutanea.
dentate margin Anokutanlinie *f*, Linea anocutanea.
dentate nucleus Dentatum *nt*, Nc. dentatus.
dentate suture *anat.* Zackennaht *f*, Sutura serrata.
den·ta·to·ru·bral fasciculus [ˌdenˌteɪtəʊ-'ruːbrəl] → dentorubral fasciculus.
dentatorubral fibers dentatorubrale Fasern *pl*, Fibrae dentatorubrales.
den·ta·to·tha·lam·ic tract [denˌteɪtəʊθə-'læmɪk] *old* Kleinhirn-Thalamus-Trakt *m*, *old* Tractus cerebellothalamicus, Tractus dentatothalamicus.
den·ta·tum [den'teɪtəm] *n* → dentate nucleus.
denti- *pref.* → dento-.
den·ti·buc·cal [ˌdentɪ'bʌkl] *adj* Zähne u. Wange betr., dento-, odontobukkal.
den·ti·cle ['dentɪkl] *n* **1.** *anat.* Zähnchen *nt*, Denticulus *nt*. **2.** Dentinkörnchen *nt*, Dentikel *m*.
den·tic·u·late [den'tɪkjəlɪt, -leɪt] *adj* mit kleinen Zähnchen versehen, gezähnt, gezackt.
den·tic·u·lat·ed [den'tɪkjəleɪtɪd] *adj* → denticulate.
denticulate hymen *gyn.* Hymen dentatus.
denticulate ligaments Ligg. denticulata.
den·ti·fi·ca·tion [ˌdentəfɪ'keɪʃn] *n* → dentinogenesis.
den·ti·form ['dentɪfɔːrm] *adj* zahnförmig, dentiform.
den·ti·frice ['-frɪs] *n* Zahnreinigungsmittel *nt*, -pulver *nt*, Zahnsteinentfernungsmittel *nt*, -pulver *nt*, Dentifricium *nt*.
den·ti·la·bi·al [ˌ-'leɪbɪəl] *adj* Zähne u. Lippen betr., dentolabial, odontolabial.
den·ti·lin·gual [ˌ-'lɪŋgwəl] **I** *n* Dentilingual(laut *m*) *m*. **II** *adj* Zähne u. Zunge betr., dentolingual, odontolingual.
den·tim·e·ter [den'tɪmɪtər] *n* *dent.* Dentimeter *nt*.
den·tin [dentn, -tɪn] *n* *anat.* Zahnbein *nt*, Dentin *nt*, Dentinum *nt*, Substantia eburna (dentis).
den·ti·nal [dentɪnəl] *adj* Dentin betr., dentinal, Zahnbein-.
dentinal canals Canaliculi dentales.
dentinal dysplasia Capdepont-Zahndysplasie *f*, -Syndrom *nt*, Glaszähne *pl*, Stainton-Syndrom *nt*, Dentinogenesis imperfecta hereditaria.
dentinal sheath Neumann'-Scheide *f*.
dentinal tubule Dentinkanälchen *nt*.
dentin cell → dentinoblast.
den·tine ['dentiːn] *n* → dentin.
den·ti·no·blast ['dentɪnəblæst] *n* Dentinoblast *m*, Odontoblast *m*.
den·ti·no·blas·to·ma [ˌ-blæs'təʊmə] *n* → dentinoma.
den·ti·no·gen·e·sis [ˌ-'dʒenəsɪs] *n* Zahnbein-, Dentinbildung *f*, Dentinogenese *f*.
den·ti·no·gen·ic [ˌ-'dʒenɪk] *adj* Dentin bildend *od.* produzierend, dentinogen.
den·ti·noid ['dentɪnɔɪd] **I** *n* unverkalkte Dentinmatrix *f*, Prädentin *nt*, Dentinoid *nt*. **II** *adj* dentinähnlich, -förmig, dentinoid.
den·ti·no·ma [ˌdentɪ'nəʊmə] *n* Dentinom *nt*.
den·tin·os·te·oid [ˌdentɪn'ɒstɪɔɪd] *n* benigner Dentin-Osteoid-Mischtumor *m*, Dentinosteom *nt*.
den·ti·num [den'taɪnəm] *n* → dentin.
den·tip·a·rous [den'tɪpərəs] *adj* mit Zäh-

nen versehen, Zähne tragend, gezähnt.
den·tist ['dentɪst] *n* Zahnarzt *m*, -ärztin *f*.
den·tis·try ['dentɪstrɪ] *n* **1.** Zahn(heil)kunde *f*, Zahnmedizin *f*, Dentologie *f*, Odontologie *f*. **2.** Ausübung/Praxis *f* der Zahnheilkunde *od.* des zahnärztlichen Berufes. **3.** zahnärztliche bzw. -chirurgische Leistungen *pl*.
den·ti·tion [den'tɪʃn] *n* **1.** Zahnen *nt*, Zahndurchbruch *m*, Dentition *f*, Dentitio *f*. **2.** Zahnreihe *f*, (natürliches) Gebiß *nt*.
dento- *pref.* Zahn-, Dent(i)-, Dent(o)-, Odont(o)-.
den·to·al·ve·o·lar [ˌdentəʊæl'vɪələr] *adj* Zahn(fach) betr., dentoalveolär.
dentoalveolar abscess (akuter) Wurzelspitzenabszeß *m*.
dentoalveolar articulation Gomphosis *f*, Artic. dentoalveolaris.
dentoalveolar dysplasia dentoalveoläre Dysplasie *f*.
dentoalveolar joint → dentoalveolar articulation.
den·to·fa·cial orthopedics [ˌ-'feɪʃl] Kieferorthopädie *f*.
dentofacial surgery Gesichts- u. Kieferchirurgie *f*.
den·toid ['dentɔɪd] *adj* zahnförmig, -artig, dentoid, odontoid.
dentoid process of axis Dens axis.
den·to·li·va [ˌdentə'laɪvə] *n* (*ZNS*) Olive *f*, Oliva *f*.
den·to·ma [den'təʊmə] *n* → dentinoma.
den·to·ru·bral fasciculus [ˌdentəʊ'ruːbrəl] dentorubrales Bündel *nt*, Fasciculus dentorubralis.
dentorubral tract Tractus dentorubralis.
den·to·sur·gi·cal [ˌ-'sɜːrdʒɪkl] *adj* zahnchirurgisch.
den·ture ['dentʃər] *n* (künstliches) Gebiß *nt*, (Teil-)Gebiß *nt*, Zahnersatz *m*, -prothese *f*.
denture cell → dentinoblast.
denture prosthetics Zahntechnik *f*, Zahnersatzkunde *f*, zahnärztliche Prothetik *f*.
Denucé [deny'se]: **D.'s ligament** Lig. quadratum.
de·nu·cle·at·ed [dɪ'n(j)uːklɪeɪtɪd] *adj* entkernt, kernlos, denukleiert.
de·nu·da·tion [ˌdɪnjuː'deɪʃn, ˌdenjə-] *n* *patho.* Denudation *f*.
Den·ver classification ['denvər] *genet.* Denver-System *nt*, -Klassifikation *f*.
Denver shunt Denver-Shunt *m*.
de·o·dor·ant [dɪ'əʊdərənt] **I** *n* de(s)odorierendes/de(s)odorisierendes Mittel *nt*, Desodorans *nt*, Deodorant *nt*. **II** *adj* geruch(s)tilgend, de(s)odorierend, de(s)odorisierend.
de·o·dor·ize [dɪ'əʊdəraɪz] *vt*, *vi* de(s)odorieren, de(s)odorisieren.
de·o·dor·iz·er [dɪ'əʊdəraɪzər] *n* → deodorant I.
de·or·sum·duc·tion [dɪˌɔːrsəm'dʌkʃn] *n* *ophthal.* Abwärtswendung *f* eines Auges, Infraduktion *f*.
de·or·sum·ver·gence [ˌ-'vɜːrdʒəns] *n* *ophthal.* Infravergenz *f*.
de·or·sum·ver·sion [ˌ-'vɜːrʒn] *n* *ophthal.* Abwärtswendung *f* beider Augen, Infraversion *f*.
de·os·si·fi·ca·tion [dɪˌɒsɪfɪ'keɪʃn] *n* *patho.* (*Knochen*) Demineralisation *f*.
de·ox·i·da·tion [dɪˌɒksɪ'deɪʃn] *n* *chem.* Sauerstoffentfernung *f*, -entzug *m*, Desoxidation *f*.
de·ox·i·dize [dɪ'ɒksədaɪz] *vt* Sauerstoff entziehen, desoxidieren.
deoxy- *pref.* Desoxy-.
de·ox·y·a·den·o·sine [dɪˌɒksɪə'denəsiːn, -sɪn] *n* *abbr.* **dA** Desoxyadenosin *nt* abbr. dA, Adenindesoxyribosid *nt*.

deoxyadenosine diphosphate *abbr.* **dADP** Desoxyadenosindiphosphat *nt abbr.* dADP.
deoxyadenosine monophosphate *abbr.* **dAMP** Desoxyadenosinmonophosphat *nt abbr.* dAMP, Desoxyadenylsäure *f*.
deoxyadenosine triphosphate *abbr.* **dATP** Desoxyadenosintriphosphat *nt abbr.* dATP.
5'-de·ox·y·a·den·o·syl·co·bal·a·min [ˌ-ə-ˌdenəsɪlkəʊˈbæləmɪn] *n* Coenzym B$_{12}$ *nt*, 5'-Desoxyadenosylcobalamin *nt*.
de·ox·y·a·den·yl·ate [ˌ-əˈdenlɪt, -eɪt, ˈædnl-] *n* Desoxyadenylat *nt*.
de·ox·y·ad·e·nyl·ic acid [ˌ-ædəˈnɪlɪk] → deoxyadenosine monophosphate.
de·ox·y·cho·late [ˌ-ˈkəʊleɪt] *n* Desoxycholat *nt*.
deoxycholate agar *micro.* Natriumdesoxycholatagar *m/nt* nach Leifson, Leifson-Agar *m/nt*.
deoxycholate citrate agar *micro.* Desoxycholat-Zitrat-Agar *m/nt* nach Leifson.
de·ox·y·cho·lic acid [ˌ-ˈkəʊlɪk, -ˈkɑl-] Desoxycholsäure *f*.
de·ox·y·cho·lyl·gly·cine [ˌ-ˌkəʊlɪlˈɡlaɪsiːn] *n* Glycindesoxycholat *nt*.
de·ox·y·cho·lyl·tau·rine [ˌ-ˌkəʊlɪlˈtɔːriːn, -rɪn] *n* Taurindesoxycholat *nt*.
11-de·ox·y·cor·ti·cos·ter·one [ˌ-ˌkɔːrtɪˈkɑstərəʊn, -ˈkəʊs-] *n abbr.* **DOC** (11-)-Desoxycorticosteron *nt abbr.* DOC, Desoxykortikosteron *nt*, Cortexon *nt*.
deoxycorticosterone acetate *abbr.* **DOCA** Desoxycorticosteronazetat *nt abbr.* DOCA.
11-de·ox·y·cor·ti·sol [dɪˌɑksɪˈkɔːrtɪsɒl, -səʊl] *n* 11-Desoxycortisol *nt*.
de·ox·y·cy·ti·dine [ˌ-ˈsaɪtədiːn] *n abbr.* **dC** Desoxycytidin *nt abbr.* dC, *old* Cytidin *nt*.
deoxycytidine diphosphate *abbr.* **dCDP** Desoxycytidindiphosphat *nt abbr.* dCDP.
deoxycytidine monophosphate *abbr.* **dCMP** Desoxycytidinmonophosphat *nt abbr.* dCMP, Desoxycytidylsäure *f*.
deoxycytidine triphosphate *abbr.* **dCTP** Desoxycytidintriphosphat *nt abbr.* dCTP.
de·ox·y·cy·ti·dyl·ate [ˌ-ˌsaɪtəˈdɪleɪt] *n* Desoxycytidylat *nt*.
de·ox·y·cy·ti·dyl·ic acid [ˌ-ˌsaɪtəˈdɪlɪk] → deoxycytidine monophosphate.
de·ox·y·gen·ate [dɪˈɑksɪdʒəneɪt] *vt* Sauerstoff entziehen, desoxygenieren.
de·ox·y·ge·nat·ed blood [dɪˈɑksɪdʒəneɪtɪd] venöses/sauerstoffarmes Blut *nt*.
deoxygenated hemoglobin → deoxyhemoglobin.
de·ox·y·gen·a·tion [dɪˌɑksɪdʒəˈneɪʃn] *n chem.* Sauerstoffentzug *m*, Desoxygenierung *f*, Desoxygenation *f*.
de·ox·y·gua·no·sine [dɪˌɑksɪˈɡwɑnəsiːn, -sɪn] *n abbr.* **dG** Desoxyguanosin *nt abbr.* dG.
deoxyguanosine diphosphate *abbr.* **dGDP** Desoxyguanosindiphosphat *nt abbr.* dGDP.
deoxyguanosine monophosphate *abbr.* **dGMP** Desoxyguanosinmonophosphat *nt abbr.* dGMP, Desoxyguanylsäure *f*.
deoxyguanosine triphosphate *abbr.* **dGTP** Desoxyguanosintriphosphat *nt abbr.* dGTP.
de·ox·y·guan·y·late [ˌ-ˈɡwɑnleɪt] *n* Desoxyguanylat *nt*.
de·ox·y·gua·nyl·ic acid [ˌ-ˌɡwɑˈnɪlɪk] → deoxyguanosine monophosphate.
de·ox·y·he·mo·glo·bin [ˌ-ˈhiːməɡləʊbɪn, -ˈhemə-] *n* reduziertes/desoxygeniertes Hämoglobin *nt*, Desoxyhämoglobin *nt*.

6-deoxy-L-mannose *n* Isodulcit *nt*, (L-)Rhamnose *f*, 6-Desoxy-L-mannose *f*.
de·ox·y·my·o·glo·bin [ˌ-ˈmaɪəɡləʊbɪn] *n* Desoxymyoglobin *nt*.
de·ox·y·nu·cle·o·tid·yl transferase (terminal) [ˌ-ˌn(j)uːkliəˈtaɪdl] → DNA nucleotidylexotransferase.
de·ox·y·pen·tose·nu·cle·ic acid [ˌ-ˌpentəʊsnˌjuːˈkliːɪk, -ˈkleɪ-] → deoxyribonucleic acid.
de·ox·y·ri·bo·nu·cle·ase [ˌ-ˌraɪbəʊˈn(j)uːkleɪs] *n abbr.* **DNAase, DNase, DNase** Desoxyribonuclease *f*, DNase *f*, DNSase *f*, DNAase *f*.
deoxyribonuclease I Desoxyribonuclease I *f*, DNase I *f*, neutrale Desoxyribonuclease *f*.
deoxyribonuclease II Desoxyribonuclease II *f*, DNase II *f*, saure Desoxyribonuclease *f*.
de·ox·y·ri·bo·nu·cle·ic acid [ˌ-ˌraɪbəʊn(j)uːˈkliːɪk, -ˈkleɪ-] *n abbr.* **DNA** Desoxyribonukleinsäure *f abbr.* DNS, DNA.
bacterial d. Bakterien-DNA *f*, Bakterien-DNS *f*, bakterielle DNA *f*, bakterielle DNS *f*.
chromosomal d. chromosomale DNA *f*, chromosomale DNS *f*.
double-helical d. Doppelhelix-, Duplex-, Doppelstrang-DNA *f abbr.* dsDNA, Doppelhelix-, Duplex-, Doppelstrang-DNS *f abbr.* dsDNS.
double-stranded d. *abbr.* **dsDNA** → double-helical d.
duplex d. → double-helical d.
extrachromosomal d. extrachromosomale DNA *f*, extrachromosomale DNS *f*.
extranuclear d. extranukleäre DNA *f*, extranukleäre DNS *f*.
mitochondrial d. mitochondriale DNA *f abbr.* mtDNA, mitochondriale DNS *f abbr.* mtDNS.
mt d. → mitochondrial d.
nuclear d. Kern-DNA *f*, Kern-DNS *f*.
regulatory d. spacer-DNA *f*, Regulator-DNA *f*, Regulator-DNS *f*.
satellite d. Satelliten-DNA *f*, Satelliten-DNS *f*.
single-stranded d. *abbr.* **ssDNA** Einzelstrang-DNA *f abbr.* ssDNA, Einzelstrang-DNS *f abbr.* ssDNS.
starter d. Starter-DNA *f*, Starter-DNS *f*.
viral d. Virus-DNA *f*, Virus-DNS *f*, virale DNA *f*, virale DNS *f*.
de·ox·y·ri·bo·nu·cle·o·pro·tein [ˌ-ˌraɪbəʊˌn(j)uːkliəʊˈprəʊtiːn, -tiːɪn] *n abbr.* **DNP** Desoxyribonukleoprotein *nt*.
de·ox·y·ri·bo·nu·cle·o·side [ˌ-ˌraɪbəʊˈn(j)uːkliəsaɪd] *n* Desoxyribonukleosid *nt*, nucleosid *nt*, Desoxyribosid *nt*.
deoxyribonucleoside diphosphate *abbr.* **dRDP** Desoxyribonukleosiddiphosphat *nt abbr.* dRDP.
deoxyribonucleoside monophosphate *abbr.* **dRMP** Desoxyribonukleosidmonophosphat *nt abbr.* dRMP.
deoxyribonucleoside triphosphate *abbr.* **dRTP** Desoxyribonukleosidtriphosphat *nt abbr.* dRTP.
de·ox·y·ri·bo·nu·cle·o·tide [ˌ-ˌraɪbəʊˈn(j)uːkliətaɪd] *n* Desoxyribonukleotid *nt*, -nucleotide *nt*.
de·ox·y·ri·bose [ˌ-ˈraɪbəʊs] *n* Desoxyribose *f*.
deoxy sugar Desoxyzucker *m*.
de·ox·y·thy·mi·dine [ˌ-ˈθaɪmɪdiːn] *n abbr.* **dT** Desoxythymidin *nt abbr.* dT, *old* Thymidin *nt*.
deoxythymidine diphosphate *abbr.* **dTDP** Desoxythymidindiphosphat *nt abbr.* dTDP.
deoxythymidine monophosphate *abbr.*

dTMP Desoxythymidinmonophosphat *nt abbr.* dTMP, Desoxythymidylsäure *f*.
deoxythymidine triphosphate *abbr.* **dTTP** Desoxythymidintriphosphat *nt abbr.* dTTP.
de·ox·y·thy·mi·dyl·ate [ˌ-ˌθaɪməˈdɪleɪt] *n* Desoxythymidylat *nt*.
de·ox·y·thy·mi·dyl·ic acid [ˌ-ˌθaɪməˈdɪlɪk] → deoxythymidine monophosphate.
de·ox·y·vi·rus [ˌ-ˈvaɪrəs] *n* → DNA-viruses.
de·pend [dɪˈpend] *vi* 1. anhängen, abhängig sein *(on, upon* von); angewiesen sein *(on, upon auf)*. 2. s. verlassen *(on, upon auf)*.
de·pend·a·bil·i·ty [dɪˌpendəˈbɪlətɪ] *n* Zuverlässigkeit *f*, Verläßlichkeit *f*.
de·pend·a·ble [dɪˈpendəbl] *adj* zuverlässig, verläßlich.
de·pend·ance *n* → dependence.
de·pend·an·cy *n* → dependence 1.
de·pend·ant *n, adj* → dependent.
de·pend·ence [dɪˈpendəns] *n* 1. Abängigkeit *f (on, upon* von). 2. *psychia.* (Substanz-)Abhängigkeit *f*, Sucht *f*, Dependence *f*. 3. Vertrauen *nt (on, upon auf, in)*.
de·pend·en·cy [dɪˈpendənsɪ] *n* → dependence 1.
de·pend·ent [dɪˈpendənt] **I** *n* 1. Abhängige(r *m*) *f*; (Familien-)Angehörige(r *m*) *f*. 2. (Sucht-)Abhängige(r *m*) *f*, Süchtige(r *m*) *f*. **II** *adj* 3. abhängig *(on, upon* von); angewiesen *(on, upon auf)*. 4. vertrauend *(on, upon auf)*.
dependent form *biochem.* D-Form *f*.
de·pend·o·vi·rus·es [dɪˈpendəʊvaɪrəsəs] *pl micro.* Dependoviren *pl*.
de·per·son·al·i·za·tion [dɪˌpɜrsnəlaɪˈzeɪʃn] *n psychia.* Depersonalisation *f*.
depersonalization disorder (neurotisches) Depersonalisationssyndrom *nt*.
depersonalization neurosis/syndrome → depersonalization disorder.
de Pezzer [də peˈzeː]: **d.P.'s catheter** Pezzer-Katheter *m*.
dephospho-glycogen synthase Dephosphoglykogensynthase *f*.
dephospho-phosphorylase kinase Dephosphophosphorylasekinase *f*.
de·phos·pho·ry·late [dɪˈfɑsfəreɪlt] *vt biochem.* dephosphorylieren.
de·phos·pho·ry·la·tion [dɪˌfɑsfɔːrəˈleɪʃn] *n biochem.* Phosphorylierung *f*.
de·pig·men·ta·tion [dɪˌpɪɡmənˈteɪʃn] *n* Pigmentverlust *m*, -mangel *m*, -schwund *m*, Depigmentierung *f*.
dep·i·late [ˈdepəleɪt] *vt* enthaaren, depilieren.
dep·i·la·tion [depəˈleɪʃn] *n* Enthaarung *f*, Depilation *f*.
de·pil·a·to·ry [dɪˈpɪlətɔːriː, -təʊ-] **I** *n* Enthaarungsmittel *nt*, Depilatorium *nt*. **II** *adj* enthaarend.
depilatory agent → depilatory I.
depilatory cream Enthaarungscreme *f*.
de·plete [dɪˈpliːt] *vt* 1. leeren, leer machen *(of* von). 2. Flüssigkeit entziehen.
de·ple·tion [dɪˈpliːʃn] *n* 1. Entleerung *f*. 2. Flüssigkeitsentzug *m*, Depletion *f*. 3. Flüssigkeitsarmut *f*, Depletion *f*.
de·ple·tion·al hyponatremia [dɪˈpliːʃnl] Verlusthyponat(r)ämie *f*.
de·plum·ing mite [dɪˈpluːmɪŋ] *micro.* Knemidokoptes gallinae.
de·po·lar·i·za·tion [dɪˌpəʊləraɪˈzeɪʃn] *n phys., physiol.* Depolisarisierung *f*, Depolarisation *f*.
depolarization phase *physiol.* Depolarisationsphase *f*.
de·po·lar·ize [dɪˈpəʊləraɪz] *vt* depolarisieren.

depolarizer

de·po·lar·iz·er [dɪ'pəʊləraɪzər] *n pharm.* depolarisierendes Muskelrelaxans *nt*.
de·po·lar·iz·ing afterpotential [dɪ'pəʊləraɪzɪŋ] depolarisierendes Nachpotential *nt*.
de·po·lym·er·ase [dɪpə'lɪməreɪz, dɪ'pɒlɪmə-] *n* Depolymerase *f*.
de·po·lym·er·i·za·tion [dɪpə'lɪməraɪ'zeɪʃn, dɪˌpɒlɪmerɪ'zeɪʃn] *n chem.* Depolymerisieren *nt*, Depolymerisation *f*.
de·po·lym·er·ize [dɪpə'lɪməraɪz, dɪ'pɒlɪmə-] *vt, vi* depolymerisieren.
de·pos·it [dɪ'pɒzɪt] **I** *n* (Boden-)Satz *m*, Niederschlag *m*, Sediment *nt*, Ablagerung *f*. **II** *vi* s. absetzen, s. ablagern, s. niederschlagen.
de·pot ['depəʊ] *n physiol.* Depot *nt*, Speicher *m*; Speicherung *f*, Ablagerung *f*.
depot fat Depot-, Speicherfett *nt*.
depot lipid → depot fat.
dep·ra·va·tion [ˌdeprə'veɪʃn] *n* **1.** (*Zustand*) Verschlechterung *f*, Depravation *f*. **2.** *psychia.* (*sittlicher u. moralischer*) Verfall *m*, Depravation *f*.
de·prav·i·ty [dɪ'prævətɪ] *n* → depravation.
de·press [dɪ'pres] *vt* **1.** (*Person*) deprimieren, nieder-, bedrücken. **2.** (*Taste*) (nieder-, herunter-)drücken. **3.** (*Leistungsfähigkeit*) herabsetzen; (*Funktion*) dämpfen; (*Körperkraft*) schwächen.
de·pres·sant [dɪ'presnt] **I** *n* Beruhigungsmittel *nt*, Sedativ(um) *nt*. **II** *adj* **1.** dämpfend, hemmend. **2.** beruhigend, sedativ.
de·pressed [dɪ'prest] *adj* **1.** deprimiert, niedergeschlagen, bedrückt. **2.** eingedrückt; *bio.* abgeflacht, abgeplattet.
depressed (skull) fracture Schädelimpressionsfraktur *f*.
de·press·ing [dɪ'presɪŋ] *adj* deprimierend, bedrückend.
de·pres·sion [dɪ'preʃn] *n* **1.** Depression *f*, Niedergeschlagenheit *f*, Schwermut *f*, Tief *nt*. **2.** Vertiefung *f*, Mulde *f*, Einsenkung *f*, Eindruck *m*. **3.** (Herunter-, Nieder-)Drücken *nt*. **4.** Schwächung *f*, Herabsetzung *f*; (*Funktion*) Dämpfung *f*. **5.** Entkräftung, Schwäche *f*.
d. of consciousness Bewußtseinseintrübung *f*, -störung *f*.
d. of optic disk Pupillenexkavation *f*, Excavatio pupillae/disci n. optici.
de·pres·sive [dɪ'presɪv] **I** *n* eine an Depression leidende Person. **II** *adj* **1.** deprimierend. **2.** *psycho.* depressiv, schwermütig, an Depression(en) leidend.
depressive delusion depressiver Wahn *m*.
depressive neurosis *psychia.* Dysthymie *f*.
depressive reaction → depressive neurosis.
de·pres·sor [dɪ'presər] *n* **1.** (Ab-)Senker *m*, Herab-, Herunterdrücker *m*, Herab-/Herunterzieher *m*; *anat.* Depressor *m*, M. depressor. **2.** → depressor nerve. **3.** Spatel *m*. **4.** *pharm.* Depressor(substanz *f*) *m*. **5.** *biochem., genet.* Depressor(substanz *f*) *m*.
depressor anguli oris (muscle) Depressor *m* anguli oris, M. depressor anguli oris, *old* M. triangularis.
depressor center Depressorenzentrum *nt*.
depressor labii inferioris (muscle) Depressor *m* labii inferioris, M. depressor labii inferioris.
depressor muscle *old* Herabzieher *m*, Depressor *m*, M. depressor.
d. of angle of mouth → depressor anguli oris (muscle).
d. of lower lip → depressor labii inferioris (muscle).
d. of septum → depressor septi (muscle).
superciliary d. → depressor supercilii (muscle).

depressor nerve depressorischer Nerv *m*.
depressor reflex Depressorreflex *m*.
depressor septi (muscle) Depressor *m* septi, M. depressor septi.
depressor supercilii (muscle) Depressor *m* supercilii/glabellae, M. depressor supercilii.
de·priv·al [dɪ'praɪvl] *n* → deprivation.
dep·ri·va·tion [ˌdeprə'veɪʃn] *n* **1.** Entzug *m*, Entziehung *f*, Beraubung *f*, Deprivation *f*. **2.** *psychia.* Mangel *m*, Deprivation *f*.
deprivation disease → deficiency disease.
de·pro·tein·i·za·tion [dɪprəʊˌtɪnə'zeɪʃn, -ˌtiːɪnɪ-] *n* Eiweißentfernung *f*, Deproteinierung *f*.
de·pro·tein·ize [dɪ'prəʊtɪnaɪz, -tiːɪn-] *vt* Eiweiß entfernen, deproteinieren.
depth [depθ] *n* **1.** Tiefe *f*. **2.** (*Wissen, Farben, Ton, Gefühle*) Tiefe *f*.
d. of field → d. of focus.
d. of focus *photo.* Tiefenschärfe *f*, Schärfentiefe *f*.
depth dose *radiol.* Tiefendosis *f*.
depth gauge *chir., ortho.* Tiefenmesser *m*, -lehre *f*, -meßgerät *nt*.
depth interview *psycho.* Tiefeninterview *nt*.
depth perception Tiefenwahrnehmung *f*, -perzeption *f*.
depth psychology Tiefenpsychologie *f*.
dep·u·rant ['depjərənt] **I** *n* **1.** Abführmittel *nt*, Depurans *nt*. **2.** Reinigungsmittel *nt*, Depurantium *nt*. **II** *adj* reinigend.
dep·u·rate ['depjəreɪt] *vt chem.* reinigen.
dep·u·ra·tive ['depjəreɪtɪv] **I** *n* Reinigungsmittel *nt*. **II** *adj* reinigend.
dep·u·ra·tor ['depjəreɪtər] *n* Reinigungsmittel *nt*.
de·qua·lin·i·um chloride [dɪkwə'lɪniən] *pharm.* Dequaliniumchlorid *nt*.
de Quervain [də ker've]: **d.Q.'s disease** de Quervain'-Krankheit *f*, Tendovaginitis stenosans de Quervain.
d.Q.'s thyroiditis de Quervain-Thyreoiditis *f*, subakute nicht-eitrige Thyreoiditis *f*, granulomatöse Thyreoiditis *f*, Riesenzellthyreoiditis *f*.
der·a·del·phus [ˌderə'delfəs] *n embryo.* Deradelphus *m*.
der·an·en·ce·pha·lia [derˌænensɪ'feɪljə, -lɪə] *n embryo.* Deranenzephalie *f*.
der·an·en·ceph·a·ly [-ˌ-'sefəlɪ] *n* → deranencephalia.
de·range·ment [dɪ'reɪndʒmənt] *n* **1.** Unordnung *f*, Durcheinander *nt*. **2.** Geistesgestörtheit *f*, -störung *f*.
Dercum ['dɜːkəm]: **D.'s disease** Dercum'-Krankheit *f*, Lipalgie *f*, Adiposalgie *f*, Adipositas/Lipomatosis dolorosa.
de·re·al·i·za·tion [dɪˌrɪələ'zeɪʃn] *n psychia.* Derealisation *f*.
de·re·ism [dɪ'riːɪzəm, deɪ'reɪ-] *n psychia.* dereistisches/autistisches Denken *nt*, Dereismus *m*.
de·re·is·tic [ˌdɪrɪ'ɪstɪk] *adj* Dereismus betr., dereistisch.
dereistic thinking → dereism.
der·en·ce·pha·lia [ˌderensɪ'feɪljə, lɪə] *n* → derencephaly.
der·en·ceph·a·lo·cele [-ˌ-'sefələsiːl] *n embryo.* Derenzephalozele *f*.
der·en·ceph·a·lus [ˌ-ˈsefələs] *n embryo.* Derenzephalus *m*.
der·en·ceph·a·ly [-ˌ-'sefəlɪ] *n embryo.* Derenzephalie *f*.
de·re·pres·sion [ˌdiːrɪ'preʃn] *n genet., biochem.* Derepression *f*.
der·i·vant ['derɪvənt] *n, adj* → derivative.
der·i·va·tion [ˌderə'veɪʃn] *n* **1.** Ab-, Herleitung *f* (*from* von). **2.** Herkunft *f*, Abstammung *f*, Ursprung *m*.
de·riv·a·tive [dɪ'rɪvətɪv] **I** *n* **1.** *embryo.*,

histol., chem. Abkömmling *m*, Derivat *nt*. **2.** *pharm.* Derivantium *nt*. **3.** Ab-, Herleitung *f*; *etw.* Ab- *od.* Hergeleitetes. **II** *adj* **4.** abgeleitet (*from* von). **5.** sekundär.
de·rive [dɪ'raɪv] **I** *vt* **1.** herleiten, übernehmen (*from* von). **2.** *chem., mathe.* ableiten. **II** *vi* **3.** (ab-, her-)stammen (*from* von, aus); ausgehen (*from* von). **4.** s. her- *od.* ableiten (*from* von).
de·rived [dɪ'raɪvd] *adj* → derivative II.
derived protein Eiweiß-, Proteinderivat *nt*.
derm(a)- *pref.* → dermato-.
der·ma ['dɜːmə] *n* **1.** Haut *f*, Derma *nt*, Cutis *f*. **2.** Lederhaut *f*, Dermis *f*, Corium *nt*.
der·ma·bra·sion [ˌdɜːmə'breɪʒn] *n derm.* Dermabrasion *f*, Dermabrasio *f*.
Der·ma·cen·tor ['dɜːməsentər] *n micro.* Dermacentor *m*.
der·ma·gra·phy [dɜːr'mægrəfɪ] *n* → dermatographism.
der·mal ['dɜːml] *adj* **1.** Lederhaut/Dermis betr., dermal, Dermis-. **2.** Haut/Derma betr., dermal, kutan, Haut-, Derm-.
dermal cyst dermale/kutane Zyste *f*, Hautzyste *f*.
dermal-fat graft Hautfettlappen *m*.
der·mal·gia [dɜːr'mældʒ(ɪ)ə] *n* → dermatalgia.
dermal graft Dermislappen *m*.
dermal leishmanoid Post-Kala-Azar-Hautleishman(o)id *nt*, Post-Kala-Azar-Dermatose *f*, Post-Kala-Azar dermale Leishmaniose *f*, Post-Kala-Azar dermale Leishmanoide *f*.
dermal melanocytoma blauer Nävus *m*, Jadassohn-Tièche-Nävus *m*, Naevus caeruleus/coeruleus.
dermal nevus (intra-)dermaler/koriarer Nävus *m*.
dermal papillae Hautpapillen *pl*, Papillae dermatis/corii.
dermal ridges Hautleisten *pl*, Cristae cutis.
dermal sensation kutane Sensibilität *f*.
dermal tuberculosis Hauttuberkulose *f*, Tuberculosis cutis.
der·ma·my·i·a·sis [ˌdɜːməmaɪ'aɪəsɪs] *n derm.* Dermatomyiasis *f*.
Der·ma·nys·si·dae [ˌ-ˈnɪsədiː] *pl micro.* Dermanyssidae *pl*.
Der·ma·nys·sus [ˌ-ˈnɪsəs] *n micro.* Dermanyssus *m*.
D. gallinae Vogelmilbe *f*, Dermanyssus avium/gallinae.
der·ma·skel·e·ton [ˌ-ˈskelɪtn] *n bio.* Außen-, Ekto-, Exoskelett *nt*.
dermat- *pref.* → dermato-.
der·ma·tal·gia [ˌdɜːmə'tældʒ(ɪ)ə] *n* Hautschmerz *m*, Schmerzhaftigkeit *f* der Haut, Dermatalgie *f*, Dermatodynie *f*.
der·ma·tan sulfate Dermatansulfat *nt*, Chondroitinsulfat B *nt*.
der·mat·ic [dɜːr'mætɪk] *adj* → dermal.
der·ma·ti·tis [ˌdɜːmə'taɪtɪs] *n* Hautentzündung *f*, Dermatitis *f*.
dermatitis herpetiformis Duhring'-Krankheit *f*, Dermatitis herpetiformis Duhring, Morbus Duhring-Brocq *m*, Hidroa bullosa/herpetiformis/pruriginosa, Hidroa mitis et gravis.
dermato- *pref.* Haut-, Dermat(o)-.
der·ma·to·al·lo·plas·ty [ˌdɜːmətəʊ'æləplæstɪ] *n* → dermatohomoplasty.
der·ma·to·ar·thri·tis [ˌ-ɑːr'θraɪtɪs] *n* Hauterkrankung *f* bei gleichzeitiger Arthritis.
der·ma·to·au·to·plas·ty [ˌ-'ɔːtəplæstɪ] *n chir.* autologe Haut(lappen)plastik *f*, Hautautoplastik *f*, -autotransplantation *f*, Dermatoautoplastik *f*.
Der·ma·to·bia hominis [ˌdɜːmə'təʊbɪə

micro. Dasselfliege *f*, Dermatobia hominis.
der·ma·to·bi·al myiasis [ˌ-'təʊbɪəl] → dermatobiasis.
der·ma·to·bi·a·sis [ˌdɜrmətəʊ'baɪəsɪs] *n derm.* Dasselbeule *f*, furunkuloide Myiasis *f*, Beulenmyiasis *f*, Dermatobiasis *f*.
der·ma·to·can·di·di·a·sis [ˌ-ˌkændɪ'daɪəsɪs] *n* kutane Kandidose/Candidose/Kandidamykose/Candidamykose *f*.
der·ma·to·cel·lu·li·tis [-'seljə'laɪtɪs] *n hema.* Dermatozellulitis *f*, -cellulitis *f*.
der·ma·to·chal·a·sis [ˌ-'kæləsɪs] *n* Fall-, Schlaffhaut *f*, Cutis-laxa-Syndrom *nt*, generalisierte Elastolyse *f*, Zuviel-Haut--Syndrom *nt*, Dermatochalasis *f*, Dermatolysis *f*, Dermatomegalie *f*, Chalazodermie *f*, Chalodermie *f*.
der·ma·to·cha·la·zia [ˌ-kə'leɪzɪə] *n* → dermatochalasis.
der·ma·to·co·ni·o·sis [ˌ-ˌkəʊnɪ'əʊsɪs] *n* Staubdermatose *f*, Dermatokoniose *f*.
der·ma·to·con·junc·ti·vi·tis [ˌ-kənˌdʒʌŋ(k)tə'vaɪtɪs] *n* Dermatokonjunktivitis *f*.
der·ma·to·cyst ['-sɪst] *n* → dermal cyst.
der·ma·to·dyn·ia [ˌ-'diːnɪə] *n* → dermatalgia.
der·ma·to·dys·pla·sia [ˌ-ˌdɪs'pleɪʒ(ɪ)ə, -zɪə] *n* Hautdysplasie *f*.
der·ma·to·fi·bro·ma [ˌ-faɪ'brəʊmə] *n* Haut-, Dermatofibrom *nt*, Dermatofibroma *nt*.
der·ma·to·fi·bro·sar·co·ma [ˌ-ˌfaɪbrəsɑː'kəʊmə] *n* Dermatofibrosarkom *nt*, Dermatofibrosarcoma *nt*.
dermatofibrosarcoma protuberans Dermatofibrosarcoma protuberans.
der·ma·to·gen·ic [ˌ-'dʒenɪk] *adj* von der Haut ausgehend, durch sie bedingt, dermatogen.
dermatogenic cataract Katarakt *f* bei Dermatosen, Cataracta syndermatotica.
dermatogenic contracture dermatogene Kontraktur *f*.
dermatogenic torticollis dermatogener/kutaner Schiefhals/Torticollis *m*.
dermatogenic wryneck → dermatogenic torticollis.
der·mat·o·graph [dɜr'mætəgræf] *n* Dermograph *m*.
der·ma·to·graph·ic [ˌdɜrmətə'græfɪk] *adj* Dermographismus betr., durch ihn charakterisiert, dermographisch.
der·ma·tog·ra·phism [dɜrmə'tɑgrəfɪzəm] *n derm.* Hautschrift *f*, Dermographie *f*, Dermographia *f*, Dermographismus *m*.
der·ma·tog·ra·phy [dɜrmə'tɑgrəfɪ] *n* → dermatographism.
der·ma·to·het·er·o·plas·ty [ˌdɜrmətə'hetərəplæstɪ] *n chir.* heterologe Haut(lappen)-plastik *f*, Dermatoheteroplastik *f*.
der·ma·to·ho·mo·plas·ty [ˌ-'həʊməplæstɪ] *n* homologe Haut(lappen)plastik *f*, Dermatohomoplastik *f*.
der·ma·to·log·ic [ˌ-'lɑdʒɪk] *adj* Dermatologie betr., dermatologisch.
der·ma·to·log·i·cal [ˌ-'lɑdʒɪkl] *adj* → dermatologic.
der·ma·tol·o·gist [ˌdɜrmə'tɑlədʒɪst] *n* Hautarzt *m*, -ärztin *f*, Dermatologe *m*, -login *f*.
der·ma·tol·o·gy [ˌ-'tɑlədʒɪ] *n* Dermatologie *f*.
der·ma·tol·y·sis [ˌ-'tɑləsɪs] *n* → dermatochalasis.
der·ma·to·lyt·ic bullous dermatosis [ˌdɜrmətə'lɪtɪk] Epidermolysis bullosa dystrophica.
der·ma·to·mal [dɜrmə'təʊml] *adj* → dermatomic.
der·mat·o·mat·ic [dɜrmətə'mætɪk] *adj* dermatomic.

der·ma·tome ['dɜrmətəʊm] *n* 1. *embryo.* Dermatom *nt*. 2. *neuro.* Hautsegment *nt* eines Spinalnerven, Dermatom *nt*. 3. *chir.* Dermatom *nt*.
der·ma·to·meg·a·ly [ˌdɜrmətə'megəlɪ] *n* → dermatochalasis.
der·ma·to·mere [dɜr'mætəmɪər, 'dɜrmətə-] *n embryo.* Dermatomer *nt*.
der·ma·to·mic [dɜrmə'tɑmɪk] *adj neuro.* Dermatom betr., Dermatom-.
dermatomic area → dermatome 2.
der·ma·to·my·ces [ˌdɜrmətə'maɪsiːz] *n* → dermatophyte.
der·ma·to·my·co·sis [ˌ-maɪ'kəʊsɪs] *n* Pilzerkrankung *f* der Haut, Dermatomykose *f*, Dermatomycosis *f*.
der·ma·to·my·i·a·sis [ˌ-maɪ'aɪəsɪs] *n* → dermamyiasis.
der·ma·to·my·o·ma [ˌ-maɪ'əʊmə] *n* Dermatoleiomyom *nt*.
der·ma·to·my·o·si·tis [ˌ-maɪə'saɪtɪs] *n* Lilakrankheit *f*, Dermatomyositis *f*.
der·ma·to·neu·ro·sis [ˌ-njʊə'rəʊsɪs, -nʊ-] *n* Dermato-, Dermoneurose *f*.
der·ma·to·path·ia [ˌ-'pæθɪə] *n* → dermatopathy.
der·ma·to·path·ic [ˌ-'pæθɪk] *adj* dermatopathisch, dermopathisch.
dermatopathic lymphadenopathy *derm.* Pautrier-Woringer-Syndrom *nt*, dermatopathische Lymphopathie/Lymphadenitis *f*, lipomelanotische Retikulose *f*.
der·ma·top·a·thy [ˌdɜrmə'tɑpəθɪ] *n* Hauterkrankung *f*, -leiden *nt*, Dermatopathie *f*, Dermopathie *f*.
Der·ma·toph·i·lus [ˌ-'tɑfɪləs] *n micro.* Dermatophilus *m*.
der·ma·to·pho·bia [ˌdɜrmətə'fəʊbɪə] *n psychia.* krankhafte Angst *f* vor Hautkrankheiten, Dermatophobie *f*.
der·ma·to·phy·lax·is [ˌ-fɪ'læksɪs] *n* Hautschutz *m*, Dermatoprophylaxe *f*, Dermophylaxie *f*.
der·mat·o·phyte [dɜr'mætəfaɪt, 'dɜrmətə-] *n* Dermatophyt *m*.
der·ma·to·phyt·ic [ˌdɜrmətə'fɪtɪk] *adj* durch Dermatophyten hervorgerufen.
dermatophytic onychomycosis *derm.* Onychomykose *f*, Tinea unguium.
der·ma·to·phy·tid [ˌ-'faɪtɪd, dɜrmə'tɑfətɪd] *n* Dermatophytid *nt*.
der·ma·to·phy·to·sis [ˌ-faɪ'təʊsɪs] *n* Dermatophytose *f*, -phytosis *f*, -phytie *f*.
der·ma·to·plas·tic [ˌ-'plæstɪk] *adj* Dermatoplastik betr., dermatoplastisch.
der·ma·to·plas·ty [ˌ-'plæstɪ] *n chir.* Haut-(lappen)plastik *f*, Dermatoplastik *f*.
der·ma·to·pol·y·neu·ri·tis [ˌ-ˌpɑlɪnjʊə'raɪtɪs, -nʊ-] *n* Feer'-Krankheit *f*, Rosakrankheit *f*, vegetative Neurose *f* der Kleinkinder, Swift-Syndrom *nt*, Selter--Swift-Feer'-Krankheit *f*, Feer-Selter--Swift-Krankheit *f*, Akrodynie *f*, Acrodynia *f*.
der·ma·tor·rha·gia [ˌ-'rædʒ(ɪ)ə] *n* Haut-(ein)blutung *f*, Dermatorrhagie *f*, Dermorrhagie *f*.
der·ma·tor·rhex·is [ˌ-'reksɪs] *n* Dermatorrhexis *f*.
der·ma·to·scle·ro·sis [ˌ-sklɪə'rəʊsɪs] *n* Darrsucht *f*, Sklerodermie *f*, Skleroderm *nt*, Sklerodermia *f*.
der·ma·to·sis [dɜrmə'təʊsɪs] *n, pl* **-ses** [-sɪz] *derm.* Hauterkrankung *f*, -krankheit *f*, krankhafte Hautveränderung *f*, Dermatose *f*, Dermatosis *f*.
der·ma·to·skel·e·ton [ˌdɜrmətə'skelɪtn] *n bio.* Außen-, Ekto-, Exoskelett *nt*.
der·ma·to·ther·a·py [ˌ-'θerəpɪ] *n* Behandlung/Therapie *f* von Hautkrankheiten, Dermatotherapie *f*.

der·ma·to·trop·ic [ˌ-'trɑpɪk, -'trəʊp-] *adj* dermatotrop, dermotrop.
der·ma·to·zo·i·a·sis [ˌ-zəʊ'aɪəsɪs] *n* → dermatozoonosis.
der·ma·to·zo·on [ˌ-'zəʊɑn] *n* Hautparasit *m*, -schmarotzer *m*, Dermatozoon *nt*.
der·ma·to·zo·o·no·sis [ˌ-zəʊə'nəʊsɪs] *n* Dermatozoonose *f*.
der·ma·tro·phia [dɜrmə'trəʊfɪə] *n* → dermatrophy.
der·mat·ro·phy [dɜr'mætrəfɪ] *n* Hautatrophie *f*, Dermatrophie *f*.
der·mic ['dɜrmɪk] *adj* → dermal.
dermic graft → dermal graft.
der·mis ['dɜrmɪs] *n* Lederhaut *f*, Dermis *f*, Corium *nt*.
der·mi·tis [dɜr'maɪtɪs] *n* → dermatitis.
dermo- *pref.* → dermato-.
der·mo·blast ['dɜrməblæst] *n embryo.* Dermoblast *m*.
der·mo·cy·ma [ˌ-'saɪmə] *n embryo.* Dermocykema *f*.
der·mo·cy·mus [ˌ-'saɪməs] *n* → dermocyma.
der·mo·graph·ia [ˌ-'græfɪə] *n* → dermographism.
der·mog·ra·phism [dɜr'mɑgrəfɪzəm] *n* → dermatographism.
der·mog·ra·phy [dɜr'mɑgrəfɪ] *n* → dermatographism.
der·moid ['dɜrmɔɪd] **I** *n* 1. Dermoid(zyste *f*) *nt*. 2. *gyn.* (*Ovar*) Dermoid(zyste *f*) *nt*, Teratom *nt*. **II** *adj* hautähnlich, -artig, dermoid, dermatoid.
dermoid cyst → dermoid I.
der·moi·dec·to·my [ˌdɜrmɔɪ'dektəmɪ] *n chir.* Dermoidentfernung *f*, -exzision *f*, Dermoidektomie *f*.
dermoid tumor → dermoid I.
der·mol·y·sis [dɜr'mɑləsɪs] *n* → dermatochalasis.
der·mo·lyt·ic bullous dermatosis [ˌdɜrmə'lɪtɪk] Epidermolysis bullosa dystrophica.
der·mom·e·ter [dɜr'mɑmɪtər] *n* Dermometer *nt*.
der·mom·e·try [dɜr'mɑmɪtrɪ] *n* Dermometrie *f*.
der·mo·my·o·tome [ˌdɜrmə'maɪətəʊm] *n embryo.* Dermomyotom *nt*.
der·mo·ne·crot·ic [ˌ-nɪ'krɑtɪk] *adj* dermonekrotisch.
der·mo·neu·ro·trop·ic [ˌ-ˌnjʊərə'trɑpɪk, -'trəʊp-] *adj* dermoneurotrop.
der·mo·path·ic [ˌ-'pæθɪk] *adj* → dermatopathic.
der·mop·a·thy [dɜr'mɑpəθɪ] *n* → dermatopathy.
der·mo·phyte ['dɜrməfaɪt] *n* → dermatophyte.
der·mo·plas·ty ['-plæstɪ] *n* → dermatoplasty.
der·mo·re·ac·tion [ˌ-rɪ'ækʃn] *n* Haut-, Dermoreaktion *f*.
der·mo·skel·e·ton [ˌ-'skelɪtn] *n* → dermatoskeleton.
der·mo·syn·o·vi·tis [ˌ-ˌsɪnə'vaɪtɪs] *n* Dermosynovitis *f*.
der·mo·tox·in [ˌ-'tɑksɪn] *n* Dermotoxin *nt*.
der·mo·trop·ic [ˌ-'trɑpɪk, -'trəʊp-] *adj* → dermatotropic.
der·mo·tu·ber·cu·lin reaction [ˌ-t(j)uː'bɜrkjəlɪn] Pirquet-Reaktion *f*, -Test *m*.
der·mo·vas·cu·lar [ˌ-'væskjələr] *adj* Haut(blut)gefäße betr., dermovaskulär.
der·o·did·y·mus [derə'dɪdəməs] *n embryo.* Derodidymus *m*.
de·ro·ta·tion osteotomy [dɪrəʊ'teɪʃn] *ortho.* Derotationsosteotomie *f*.
DES *abbr.* → diethylstilbestrol.
de·sal·i·nate [dɪ'sælɪneɪt] *vt* entsalzen.
de·sal·i·na·tion [dɪˌsælɪ'neɪʃn] *n* Salzentzug *m*, Entsalzung *f*, Desalination *f*.

desalinator

de·sal·i·na·tor [dɪ'sælɪneɪtər] *n* Entsalzungsanlage *f*.
de·sal·i·ni·za·tion [dɪˌsælɪnaɪ'zeɪʃn] *n* → desalination.
de·sal·i·nize [dɪ'sælɪnaɪz] *vt* → desalinate.
de·salt [dɪ'sɔːlt] *vt* → desalinate.
De Sanctis-Cacchione [də 'sæŋktɪs kækɪ-'əʊnɪ]: **D.-C. syndrome** De Sanctis--Cacchione-Syndrom *nt*.
de·sat·u·ra·tion [dɪˌsætʃə'reɪʃn] *n chem.* Einführung *f* einer Mehrfachbindung, Desaturierung *f*.
desaturation reaction Desaturierungsreaktion *f*.
Desault [de'so]: **D.'s apparatus/bandage/ dressing** Desault-Verband *m*.
  D.'s ligature Desault'-Ligatur *f*.
  D.'s plaster bandage Desault-Gipsverband *m*.
  D.'s sign *ortho.* Desault'-Zeichen *nt*.
Descartes [deɪ'kɑːrt; de'kart]: **D.' law** Descartes'-Brechungsgesetz *nt*.
Descemet [desə'meɪ; desə'mɛ]: **D.'s membrane** Descemet'-Membran *f*, hintere Basalmembran *f*, Lamina elastica posterior Descemeti, Lamina limitans posterior (corneae).
des·ce·me·ti·tis [desəmɪ'taɪtɪs] *n ophthal.* Entzündung *f* der Descemet'-Membran, Descemetitis *f*.
des·ce·met·o·cele [desə'metəsiːl] *n ophthal.* Descemetozele *f*, Keratozele *f*.
de·scend [dɪ'send] **I** *vt* hinuntergehen, -steigen, herabsteigen, -steigen. **II** *vi* 1. herab-, heruntergehen, hinuntergehen, -steigen, -sinken; abfallen. 2. ab-, herstammen (*from* von).
de·scend·ant [dɪ'sendənt] *n* Nachkomme *m*, Abkömmling *m*, Deszendent *m*.
de·scend·ing aorta [dɪ'sendɪŋ] absteigende Aorta *f*, Aorta descendens, Pars descendens aortae.
descending branch: anterior d. of left pulmonary artery Ramus anterior descendens a. pulmonalis sinistrae.
  anterior d. of right pulmonary artery Ramus anterior descendens a. pulmonalis dextrae.
  d. of lateral circumflex femoral artery absteigender Ast *m* der A. circumflexa femoris lateralis, Ramus descendens a. circumflexae femoris lateralis.
  d. of occipital artery Ramus descendens a. occipitalis.
  posterior d. of left pulmonary artery Ramus posterior descendens a. pulmonalis sinistrae.
  posterior d. of right pulmonary artery Ramus posterior descendens a. pulmonalis dextrae.
descending cholecystitis absteigende/deszendierende Gallenblasenentzündung/Cholezystitis *f*.
descending colon absteigendes Kolon *nt*, Colon descendens.
descending current absteigender/zentrifugaler Strom *m*.
descending degeneration absteigende/deszendierende Degeneration *f*.
descending fibers absteigende Fasern *pl*.
descending inhibition absteigende Hemmung *f*.
descending limb of Henle's loop (*Niere*) absteigender Schenkel *m* der Henle'--Schleife.
descending mesocolon Mesokolon *nt* des Colon descendens, Mesocolon descendens.
descending myelitis absteigende/deszendierende Myelitis *f*.
descending myelopathy absteigende/deszendierende Myelopathie *f*.
descending neuritis → descending neuropathy.
descending neuropathy absteigende/deszendierende Neuropathie *f*.
descending part: d. of aorta → descending aorta.
  d. of duodenum absteigender Duodenumabschnitt *m*, Pars descendens duodeni.
descending ramus of pubis unterer Schambeinast *m*, Ramus inferior ossis pubis.
descending tract absteigende Bahn *f*.
descending urography *urol., radiol.* Ausscheidungsurographie *f*.
de·scent [dɪ'sent] *n* 1. Herab-, Hinunter-, Heruntergehen *nt*, -steigen *nt*, -sinken *nt*; Senkung *f*. 2. *patho., embryo.* Vorfall *m*, Deszensus *m*, Descensus *m*. 3. Abstammung *f*, Herkunft *f*.
  d. of testicle/testis Hodendeszensus, Descensus testis.
Deschamps [de'ʃã]: **D.' needle** Deschamps--Nadel *f*.
de·scrip·tive [dɪ'skrɪptɪv] *adj* beschreibend, schildernd, darstellend, erläuternd, deskriptiv; anschaulich.
descriptive anatomy beschreibende/systematische Anatomie *f*.
de·scrip·tive·ness ['-nɪs] *n* Anschaulichkeit *f*.
descriptive psychiatry beschreibende Psychiatrie *f*.
descriptive science beschreibende/deskriptive Wissenschaft *f*.
de·sen·si·ti·za·tion [dɪˌsensɪtə'zeɪʃn] *n* 1. *immun.* Desensibilisierung *f*, Hyposensibilisierung *f*. 2. *psychia.* Desensibilisierung *f*.
desensitization therapy *psychia.* Desensibilisierungstherapie *f*.
de·sen·si·tize [dɪ'sensɪtaɪz] *vt* 1. *immun.* desensibilisieren, hyposensibilisieren, unempfindlich *od.* immun machen (*to* gegen). 2. *psychia.* desensibilisieren. 3. *phys.* lichtunempfindlich machen, desensibilisieren.
des·ert fever ['dezərt] 1. Wüstenfieber *nt*, Posada-Mykose *f*, Kokzioidomykose *f*, Coccioidomycose *f*, Granuloma coccioides. 2. San Joaquin-Valley-Fieber *nt*, Wüsten-, Talfieber *nt*, Primärform *f* der Kokzidioidomykose.
desert rheumatism → desert fever 2.
des·fer·ri·ox·a·mine [desˌferɪ'ɑksəmiːn] *n* → deferoxamine.
des·ic·cant ['desɪkənt] **I** *n* (Aus-)Trockenmittel *nt*, Desikkans *nt*, Exsikkans *nt*. **II** *adj* (aus-)trocknend, exsikkativ.
des·ic·cate ['desɪkeɪt] *vt, vi* (aus-)trocknen, (aus-)dörren.
des·ic·cat·ed milk ['desɪkeɪtɪd] Trockenmilch *f*.
des·ic·ca·tion [ˌdesɪ'keɪʃn] *n* (Aus-)Trocknen *nt*, (Aus-)Trocknung *f*, Exsikkation *f*, Exsikkose *f*.
desiccation keratitis Keratitis/Keratopathia e lagophthalmo.
des·ic·ca·tive ['desɪkeɪtɪv] *n, adj* → desiccant.
des·ic·ca·tor ['desɪkeɪtər] *n* 1. *chem.* Exsikkator *m*, Desikkator *m*. 2. Trockenapparat *m*.
des·ip·ra·mine [də'zɪprəmiːn] *n pharm.* Desipramin *m*.
de·sire [dɪ'zaɪər] **I** *n* Wunsch *m*, Verlangen *nt*, Drang *m*, Begehren *nt*, Begierde *f* (*for* nach). **II** *vt* wünschen, verlangen, begehren, wollen.
de·sired [dɪ'zaɪərd] *adj* er-, gewünscht; ersehnt.
desired state *techn.* Sollwert *m*.

Desjardins [deʒar'dɛ̃]: **D.' point** Desjardins'-Punkt *m*.
des·lan·o·side [des'lænəsaɪd] *n pharm.* Deslanosid *nt*, Desacetyllanatosid C *nt*.
desm- *pref.* → desmo-.
des·mal·gia [dez'mældʒ(ɪ)ə] *n ortho.* Bandschmerzen *nt*, Schmerzen *pl* in einem Band/Ligament, Desmalgie *f*, Desmodynie *f*.
des·mec·ta·sia [dezmek'teɪʒ(ɪ)ə] *n* → desmectasis.
des·mec·ta·sis [dez'mektəsɪs] *n ortho.* Bänderdehnung *f*, -ektasie *f*, Desmektasie *f*.
des·mi·tis [dez'maɪtɪs] *n ortho.* Bänderentzündung *f*, Desmitis *f*.
desmo- *pref.* Bänder-, Desm(o)-.
des·mo·cra·ni·um [ˌdezmə'kreɪnɪəm] *n embryo.* Mesenchymschädel *m*, Desmokranium *nt*, Desmocranium *nt*.
des·mo·cyte ['-saɪt] *n* juvenile Bindegewebszelle *f*, Fibroblast *m*.
des·mo·cy·to·ma [ˌ-saɪ'təʊmə] *n patho.* Bindegewebsgeschwulst *f*, Fibrom(a) *nt*.
des·mo·don·ti·um [ˌ-'dɑnʃəm] *n* Wurzelhaut *f*, Desmodontium *f*, Periodontium *nt*.
des·mo·dyn·ia [ˌ-'diːnɪə] *n* → desmalgia.
des·mo·en·zyme [ˌ-'enzaɪm] *n* Desmoenzym *nt*.
des·mog·e·nous [dez'mɑdʒənəs] *adj* von einem Band ausgehend; auf bindegewebiger Grundlage, desmogen.
des·mo·he·mo·blast [dezmə'hiːməblæst] *n* Mesenchym *nt*, embryonales Bindegewebe *nt*.
des·moid ['dezmɔɪd] **I** *n* Desmoid *nt*. **II** *adj* 1. fibrös, fibroid, desmoid. 2. bindegewebsartig, bandartig, sehnenartig, desmoid.
desmoid tumor → desmoid I.
des·mo·lase ['dezməleɪz] *n* Desmolase *f*.
des·mo·ma [dez'məʊmə] *n* → desmoid I.
des·mo·ne·o·plasm [ˌdezmə'nɪəplæzəm] *n* Bindegewebstumor *m*, -neoplasma *nt*.
des·mop·a·thy [dez'mɑpəθɪ] *n* Sehnen-, Bändererkrankung *f*, Desmopathie *f*.
des·mo·pla·sia [ˌdezmə'pleɪʒ(ɪ)ə, -zɪə] *n* Desmoplasie *f*.
des·mo·plas·tic fibroma [ˌ-'plæstɪk] desmoplastisches Fibrom *nt*.
desmoplastic nevus *derm.* desmoplastischer Nävus *m*.
des·mo·pres·sin [ˌ-'presɪn] *n pharm.* Desmopressin *nt*.
des·mor·rhex·is [ˌ-'reksɪs] *n* Sehnen-, Bandruptur *f*, Bänderriß *m*, Desmorrhexis *f*.
des·mo·sine ['dezməsɪn] *n* Desmosin *nt*.
des·mo·sis [dez'məʊsɪs] *n* Bindegewebserkrankung *f*.
des·mo·some ['dezməsəʊm] *n* Haftplatte *f*, Desmosom *nt*, Macula adhaerens.
des·mos·ter·ol [des'mɑstərɔl, -əʊl] *n* Desmosterin *nt*.
des·mot·o·my [dez'mɑtəmɪ] *n ortho.* Sehnen-, Band-, Bänderdurchtrennung *f*, Desmotomie *f*.
des·mo·tro·pism [dez'mɑtrəpɪzəm] *n chem.* Tautomerie *f*.
des·o·nide ['dezənaɪd] *n pharm.* Desonid *nt*.
de·sorb [dɪ'zɔːrb] *vt* desorbieren.
de·sorp·tion [dɪ'zɔːrpʃn] *n* Desorption *f*.
des·ox·i·met·a·sone [desˌɑksɪ'metəsəʊn] *n pharm.* Desoximetason *nt*.
desoxy- *pref.* → deoxy-.
des·ox·y·cor·ti·cos·ter·one [ˌdesɑksɪˌkɔːrtɪ'kɑstərəʊn] *n* → 11-deoxycorticosterone.
des·ox·y·cor·tone [ˌ-'kɔːrtəʊn] *n* → 11-deoxycorticosterone.

des·ox·y·eph·e·drine [ˌ-'efɪdriːn, -ɪ'fedrɪn] *n pharm.* Methamphetamin *nt.*
des·ox·y·phe·no·bar·bi·tal [ˌ-ˌfiːnə'bɑːrbɪtɒl, -tæl] *n pharm.* Primidon *nt.*
des·ox·y·ri·bo·nu·cle·ase [ˌ-ˌraɪboʊ'n(j)uːkleɪs] *n* → deoxyribonuclease.
des·ox·y·ri·bo·nu·cle·ic acid [ˌ-ˌraɪboʊn(j)uː'kliːɪk, -kleɪ-] → deoxyribonucleic acid.
des·ox·y·ri·bose [ˌ-'raɪboʊs] *n* → deoxyribose.
desoxy-sugar *n* Desoxyzucker *m.*
de·spi·ral·i·za·tion [dɪˌspaɪrəlɪ'zeɪʃn] *n* Entspiralisierung *f,* -spiralisation *f.*
des·qua·mate ['deskwəmeɪt] *vi* s. (ab-)schuppen, s. häuten.
des·qua·ma·tion [ˌdeskwə'meɪʃn] *n* (Ab-)Schuppung *f,* Abschilferung *f,* Desquamation *f.*
des·qua·ma·tive ['deskwəmeɪtɪv, dɪ'skwæmətɪv] *adj* abschuppend, abschilfernd, desquamativ, Desquamations-, Desquamativ-.
desquamative and regenerative phase Desquamations-Regenerations-Phase *f.*
desquamative catarrhal cystitis *urol.* Desquamationskatarrh *m,* Cystitis catarrhalis.
desquamative gingivitis Gingivitis desquamativa.
desquamative phase *gyn.* Desquamationsphase *f.*
desquamative pneumonia käsige Pneumonie *f.*
des·qua·ma·to·ry ['deskwəmə ˌtɔːriː, -ˌtəʊ-, dɪ'skwæmə-] *adj* → desquamative.
dest. *abbr.* (destillatus) → distilled.
de·stroy [dɪ'strɔɪ] *vt* 1. zerstören, zertrümmern, vernichten, ruinieren, unbrauchbar machen. 2. töten, umbringen; (*Tier*) einschläfern.
de·stroy·ing angel [dɪ'strɔɪɪŋ] *bio.* grüner Knollenblätterpilz *m,* Amanita phalloides.
de·struc·tion [dɪ'strʌkʃn] *n* 1. Zerstörung *f,* Destruktion *f.* 2. Tötung *f;* (*Tier*) Einschläferung *f.*
de·struc·tive [dɪ'strʌktɪv] *adj* zerstörend, zerstörerisch, zerrüttend, verderblich, schädlich, destruktiv, destruierend. ~ **to health** gesundheitsschädlich.
destructive arthropathy destruierende Arthropathie *f.*
destructive distillation Zersetzungs-, Trockendestillation *f.*
destructive emphysema *pulmo.* chronisch-destruktives (Lungen-)Emphysem *nt.*
de·sulf·hy·drase [dɪsʌlf'haɪdreɪz] *n* Desulfhydrase *f,* Desulfurase *f.*
de·sul·fu·rase [dɪ'sʌljəreɪz] *n* → desulfhydrase.
de·syn·chro·nized sleep [dɪ'sɪŋkrənaɪzd] *physiol.* paradoxer/desynchronisierter Schlaf *m,* REM-Schlaf *m,* Traumschlaf *m.*
DET *abbr.* → diethyltryptamine.
de·tach [dɪ'tætʃ] I *vt* 1. (ab-, los-)trennen, (los-)lösen, losmachen. 2. absondern, freimachen. II *vi* s. (los-)lösen, s. absondern (*from* von).
de·tached craniotomy [dɪ'tætʃt] *neurochir.* osteoklastische Schädeltrepanation *f;* Kraniektomie *f.*
detached iris *ophthal.* Irisablösung *f* vom Ziliarrand, Iridodialyse *f,* -dialysis *f.*
detached retina → detachment of retina.
de·tach·ment [dɪ'tætʃmənt] *n* 1. (Ab-)Trennung *f,* (Los-)Lösung *f* (*from* von). 2. *fig.* (innerer) Abstand *m,* Distanz *f,* Losgelöstsein *nt;* Objektivität *f.* 3. Gleichgültigkeit *f* (*from* gegenüber).

d. of retina *ophthal.* Netzhautablösung, Ablatio retinae, Amotio retinae.
de·tect [dɪ'tekt] *vt* entdecken, feststellen, (heraus-)finden, ermitteln; wahrnehmen.
de·tect·a·ble [dɪ'tektəbl] *adj* → detectible.
de·tect·i·ble [dɪ'tektɪbl] *adj* feststellbar.
de·tec·tion [dɪ'tekʃn] *n* Entdeckung *f,* Feststellung *f;* Wahrnehmung *f;* Aufdeckung *f.*
detection threshold *physiol.* Wahrnehmungsschwelle *f.*
de·tec·tor [dɪ'tektər] *n* Detektor *m.*
de·terge [dɪ'tɜrdʒ] *vt ortho.* (*Wunde*) reinigen.
de·ter·gent [dɪ'tɜrdʒənt] I *n* 1. Netzmittel *nt,* Detergens *nt.* 2. (*Wunde*) Reinigungsmittel *nt,* Detergens *nt.* 3. Reinigungsmittel *nt,* Waschmittel *nt,* Detergens *nt.* II *adj* reinigend.
de·te·ri·o·rate [dɪ'tɪəriəreɪt] I *vt* verschlechtern, verschlimmern, beeinträchtigen. II *vi* 1. (*Zustand*) s. verschlechtern, s. verschlimmern, schlechter werden. 2. verfallen, herunterkommen.
de·te·ri·o·ra·tion [dɪˌtɪəriə'reɪʃn] *n* (*Zustand*) Verschlechterung *f,* Verschlimmerung *f,* Deterioration *f,* Deteriorisierung *f.*
de·ter·mi·nant [dɪ'tɜrmɪnənt] I *n* 1. *bio., mathe.* Determinante *f.* 2. entscheidender od. ausschlaggebender Faktor *m.* II *adj* entscheidend, bestimmend, determinant, determinierend.
de·ter·mi·nate [dɪ'tɜrmɪnət] *adj* determiniert, fest(gelegt), bestimmt, entschieden.
determinate cleavage determinierte Furchung(steilung *f*) *f.*
de·ter·mi·na·tion [dɪˌtɜrmɪ'neɪʃn] *n* 1. Entscheidung *f,* Entschluß *m;* Beschluß *m.* 2. Bestimmung *f,* Ermittlung *f,* Determinierung *f;* Festlegung *f,* -setzung *f.* 3. Entschlossenheit *f.* 4. *embryo.* Determination *f.*
de·ter·mi·na·tive [dɪ'tɜrmɪnətɪv, -neɪt-] *adj* 1. determinativ, bestimmend, eingrenzend, festlegend, determinativ, Bestimmungs-. 2. entscheidend.
de·ter·mine [dɪ'tɜrmɪn] I *vt* 1. bestimmen, festlegen, -setzen, determinieren. 2. feststellen, ermitteln, ermitteln. 3. beschließen, entscheiden. II *vi* s. entschließen (*on* zu); s. entscheiden (*on* für).
de·ter·mined [dɪ'tɜrmɪnt] *adj* 1. entschlossen. 2. entschieden; bestimmt, festgelegt, determiniert.
de·ter·min·ism [dɪ'tɜrmənɪzəm] *n* Determinismus *m.*
det·o·nate ['detneɪt] I *vt* detonieren/explodieren lassen, zur Detonation bringen. II *vi* detonieren, explodieren.
det·o·na·tion [detə'neɪʃn] *n* Detonation *f,* Explosion *f.*
de Toni-Fanconi [də 'tɒʊni fæn'kɒʊni]: **d.T.-F. syndrome** Debré-de Toni-Fanconi--Syndrom *nt.*
de·tor·sion [dɪ'tɔːrʃn] *n chir.* Detorsion *f,* Derotation *f.*
de·tox·i·cate [dɪ'tɒksɪkeɪt] *vt* → detoxify.
de·tox·i·ca·tion [dɪˌtɒksɪ'keɪʃn] *n* → detoxification.
de·tox·i·fi·ca·tion [dɪˌtɒksɪfɪ'keɪʃn] *n* Entgiftung *f,* Detoxikation *f,* Desintoxikation *f.*
de·tox·i·fy [dɪ'tɒksɪfaɪ] *vt* entgiften.
det·ri·ment ['detrəmənt] *n* Nachteil *m,* Schaden *m* (*to* für). **(to be) a ~ to health** gesundheitsschädlich (sein).
det·ri·men·tal [ˌdetrə'mentl] *adj* nachteilig, schädlich (*to* für).
de·tri·tion [dɪ'trɪʃn] *n* Abreibung *f,* Abnutzung *f,* Abnutzung *f.*

de·tri·tus [dɪ'traɪtəs] *n, pl* **de·tri·tus** *patho.* (Gewebs-, Zell-)Trümmer *pl,* Geröll *nt,* Schutt *m,* Detritus *m.*
de·trun·ca·tion [dɪˌtrʌŋ'keɪʃn] *n gyn.* Dekapitation *f.*
de·tru·sor (muscle) [dɪ'truːsər] *n* Detrusor *m,* M. detrusor.
d. of bladder → detrusor vesicae (muscle).
detrusor urinae (muscle) → detrusor vesicae (muscle).
detrusor vesicae (muscle) Blasenwandmuskulatur *f,* Detrusor *m* vesicae, M. detrusor vesicae.
de·tu·ba·tion [diːtjuː'beɪʃn] *n* Extubation *f,* Extubieren *nt.*
de·tu·mes·cence [ˌdɪt(j)uː'mesəns] *n* Abschwellen *nt,* Detumeszenz *f.*
deut- *pref.* → deuterio-.
deu·ten·ceph·a·lon [d(j)uːtn'sefələn] *n old* → diencephalon.
deu·ter·a·nom·al [ˌd(j)uːtərə'naməl] *n ophthal.* Deuteranomale(r *m*) *f.*
deu·ter·a·nom·a·lous [ˌ-ə'namələs] *adj ophthal.* Deuteranomalie betr., von ihr betroffen, deuteranomal.
deu·ter·a·nom·a·ly [ˌ-ə'naməli] *n ophthal.* Grünschwäche *f,* Deuteranomalie *f.*
deu·ter·an·ope ['-ənoʊp] *n ophthal.* Deuteranope(r *m*) *f.*
deu·ter·a·no·pia [ˌ-ə'noʊpiə] *n ophthal.* Grünblindheit *f,* Rot-Grün-Dichromasie *f,* Deuteranop(s)ie *f.*
deu·ter·a·nop·ic [ˌ-ə'nɒpɪk] *adj ophthal.* Deuteranop(s)ie betr., von ihr betroffen, deuteranop.
deu·ter·a·nop·sia [ˌ-ə'nɒpsiə] *n* → deuteranopia.
deu·te·ri·on [d(j)uː'tɪəriən] *n* → deuteron.
deu·te·ri·um [d(j)uː'tɪəriəm] *n ophthal.* **D, ²H** schwerer Wasserstoff *m,* Deuterium *nt abbr.* D, ²H.
deuterium oxide *abbr.* **D₂O** schweres Wasser *nt,* Deuteriumoxid *nt abbr.* D₂O.
deutero- *pref.* Zweite(r, s), Zweit-, Deuter(o)-, Deut(o)-.
deu·ter·o·he·min [ˌd(j)uːtərə'hiːmɪn, -'hem-] *n* Deuterohämin *nt.*
deu·ter·o·he·mo·phil·ia [ˌ-ˌhemə'fɪliə, -ˌhiːm-] *n hema.* Deuterohämophilie *f.*
Deu·ter·o·my·ces [ˌ-'maɪsiːz] *pl* → Deuteromycetes.
Deu·ter·o·my·ce·tae [ˌ-maɪ'siːtiː] *pl* → Deuteromycetes.
deu·ter·o·my·cete [ˌ-'maɪsiːt] *n micro.* unvollständiger Pilz *m,* Deuteromyzet *m,* -mycet *m.*
Deu·ter·o·my·ce·tes [ˌ-maɪ'siːtiːz] *pl micro.* unvollständige Pilze *pl,* Deuteromyzeten *pl,* Deuteromycetes *pl,* Deuteromycotina *pl,* Fungi imperfecti.
deu·ter·on ['d(j)uːtərən] *n* Deuteriumkern *m,* Deuteron *nt,* Deuton *nt.*
deu·ter·o·path·ic [ˌd(j)uːtərə'pæθɪk] *adj* Deuteropathie betr., deuteropathisch; (*Krankheit, Symptom*) sekundär, zusätzlich.
deu·te·rop·a·thy [d(j)uː'tɒrəpəθi] *n* Sekundärleiden *nt,* -erkrankung *f,* Deuteropathie *f,* zusätzliches/sekundäres Symptom *nt.*
deu·ter·o·plasm ['d(j)uːtərəplæzəm] *n* → deutoplasm.
deu·ter·o·por·phy·rin [ˌ-'pɔːrfɪrɪn] *n* Deuteroporphyrin *nt.*
deu·ter·o·some ['-səʊm] *n* Deuterosom *nt.*
Deu·ter·o·sto·mia [ˌ-'stəʊmiə] *pl bio.* Zweitmünder *pl,* Rückenmarkstiere *pl,* Deuterostomier *pl,* Deuterostomia *f.*
deu·ter·o·to·cia [ˌ-'təʊsiə] *n bio.* Deuterotokie *f.*
deu·ter·ot·o·ky [d(j)uːtə'rɒtəki] *n* → deuterotocia.

deutiodide

deu·ti·o·dide [d(j)u:'taɪədaɪd] n Dijodid nt, Diiodid nt.
deuto- pref. → deutero-.
deu·to·chlo·ride [ˌd(j)u:tə'klɔ:raɪd, -ɪd] n Bichlorid nt.
deu·to·i·o·dide [ˌ-'aɪədaɪd] n → deutiodide.
deu·tom·er·ite [d(j)u:'tɑmәraɪt] n micro. Deutomerit m.
deu·ton ['d(j)u:tɑn] n → deuteron.
deu·to·neph·ron [ˌd(j)u:tə'nefrɑn] n Urniere f, Wolff'-Körper m, Mesonephron nt, Mesonephros m.
deu·to·plasm ['-plæzəm] n Nahrungsdotter m, Deuto-, Deuteroplasma nt.
Deutschländer ['dɔʏtʃlɛntər]: **D.'s disease 1.** Deutschländer-Fraktur f, Marschfraktur f. **2.** Metatarsal(knochen)tumor m.
DEV abbr. → duck embryo vaccine.
de·vas·a·tion [dɪvəˈseɪʃn] n old → devascularization.
de·vas·cu·lar·i·za·tion [dɪˌvæskjələrɪˈzeɪʃn, -raɪ-] n patho., chir. Devaskularisation f, Devaskularisierung f.
devascularization injury devaskularisierende Verletzung f.
de·vel·op [dɪ'veləp] **I** vt **1.** (Theorie, Verfahren, Geist etc.) entwickeln (into, in zu). **2.** (Krankheit) s. zuziehen. **3.** fördern, entwickeln. **II** vi s. entwickeln, s. bilden (from aus; into zu); entstehen, werden.
de·vel·op·a·ble [dɪ'veləpəbl] adj entwicklungsfähig.
de·vel·oped [dɪ'veləpd] adj ausgebildet.
de·vel·op·er [dɪ'veləpər] n **1.** photo. Entwickler(flüssigkeit f) m. **2.** ped. Spätentwickler m.
de·vel·op·ing [dɪ'veləpɪŋ] adj wachsend, entstehend, Entwicklungs-.
developing bath photo. Entwicklungsbad nt.
de·vel·op·ment [dɪ'veləpmənt] n **1.** Entwicklung f. **2.** Werden nt, Entstehen nt, Wachstum nt, Bildung f.
de·vel·op·men·tal [dɪˌveləp'mentl] adj Entwicklungs-.
developmental age abbr. **D.A.** Entwicklungsalter nt abbr. **EA.**
developmental anomaly Entwicklungsanomalie f, -störung f.
developmental psychology Entwicklungspsychologie f.
de·vi·ance ['dɪviəns] n von der Norm abweichendes Verhalten nt, Devianz f.
de·vi·ant ['dɪviənt] **I** n psycho. vom normalen Verhalten abweichendes Individuum nt. **II** adj vom normalen Verhalten abweichend, deviant; dissozial.
de·vi·ate [n, adj 'dɪvɪɪt; v -eɪt] **I** n → deviant **I. II** adj → deviant **II. III** vt ablenken. **IV** vi abweichen, abgehen (from von).
de·vi·a·tion [ˌdɪvɪ'eɪʃn] n **1.** Abweichung f, Abweichen nt (from von). **2.** phys. Ablenkung f; Abweichung f. **3.** stat. Abweichung f (vom Mittelwert), Deviation f. **4.** ophthal. Schielen nt, Strabismus m.
d. to the left Linksverschiebung f.
d. to the right Rechtsverschiebung f.
de·vi·a·tion·al nystagmus [ˌdɪvɪ'eɪʃnl] Endstellungs-, Pseudonystagmus m.
Devic [də'vɪk]: **D.'s disease** Devic-Syndrom nt, Krankheit f, Neuromyelitis optica.
de·vice [dɪ'vaɪs] n **1.** Vorrichtung f, Einrichtung f, Gerät nt. **2.** Plan m, Projekt nt, Vorhaben nt. **3.** Entwurf m, Muster nt, Zeichnung f.
dev·il's grip ['devl] Bornholmer Krankheit f, epidemische Pleurodynie f, Myalgia epidemica.
de·vi·om·e·ter [dɪvɪ'ɑmɪtər] n ophthal. Schielmesser nt, Deviometer nt.
de·vis·cer·a·ton [dɪvɪsə'reɪʃn] n chir. Eingeweideentfernung f, Deviszeration f.

de·vi·tal·i·za·tion [dɪˌvaɪtəlaɪˈzeɪʃn, -lɪ-] n **1.** patho. Abtöten nt, Devitalisation f, Devitalisierung f. **2.** dent. (Zahnpulpa) Devitalisation f, Abtöten nt, Devitalisierung f. **3.** fig. Schwächung f.
de·vi·tal·ize [dɪ'vaɪtəlaɪz] vt abtöten, devitalisieren; fig. schwächen.
dev·o·lu·tion [ˌdevə'lu:ʃn] n Devolution f.
Dev·on·shire colic ['devənʃɪər, -ʃər] Bleikolik f, Colica saturnina.
Dewar ['d(j)u:ər]: **D. flask** Dewar-Gefäß nt.
dew point [d(j)u:] phys. Taupunkt m.
dex·a·meth·a·sone [ˌdeksə'meθəzoʊn] n pharm. Dexamethason nt.
dexamethasone suppression test Dexamethason-(Kurz-)Test m.
dex·et·i·mide [dek'setɪmaɪd] n pharm. Dexetimid nt.
dex·i·o·car·dia [ˌdeksɪə'kɑ:rdɪə] n → dextrocardia.
dex·pan·the·nol [deks'pænθɪnɔl] n pharm. Dexpanthenol n.
dex·ter ['dekstər] adj rechte(r, s), rechts-(seitig), dexter.
dex·ter·i·ty [deks'terətɪ] n **1.** Geschicklichkeit f, Gewandtheit f. **2.** → dextrality.
dex·ter·ous ['dekst(ə)rəs] adj **1.** geschickt, gewandt. **2.** rechtshändig.
dextr- pref. → dextro-.
dex·tral ['dekstrəl] **I** n Rechtshänder(in f) m. **II** adj **1.** rechtshändig. **2.** → dexter.
dex·tral·i·ty [deks'trælətɪ] n Rechtshändigkeit f, Dextr(e)ralität f.
dex·tran ['dekstrən, -træn] n Dextran nt.
dex·tran·ase ['dekstrəneɪz] n Dextranase f.
dex·trane ['dekstreɪn] n → dextran.
dex·tran·o·mer [deks'trænəmər] n pharm. Dextranomer nt.
dex·trin ['dekstrɪn] n Dextrin nt, Dextrinum nt.
dex·trin·ase ['dekstrɪneɪz] n Dextrinase f.
α-dextrinase n α-Dextrinase f, Oligo-1,6--α-Glukosidase f.
dextrin-1,6-glucosidase n Amylo-1,6-Glukosidase f, Dextrin-1,6-Glukosidase f.
dex·trin·ose ['dekstrɪnoʊz] n Isomaltose f, Dextrinose f.
dex·tri·no·sis [ˌdekstrə'noʊsɪs] n Glykogenspeicherkrankheit f, Glykogenthesaurismose f, Glykogenose f.
dex·trin·u·ria [ˌdekstrə'n(j)ʊərɪə] n Dextrinausscheidung f im Harn, Dextrinurie f.
dextro- pref. Rechts-, Dextr(o)-.
dex·tro ['dekstroʊ] adj → dextrorotatory.
dex·tro·am·phet·a·mine [ˌdekstræm'fetəmi:n, -mɪn] n pharm. Dextroamphetamin nt.
dex·tro·car·dia [ˌ-'kɑ:rdɪə] n patho. Rechtsverlagerung f des Herzens, Dextrokardie f.
dex·tro·car·di·o·gram [ˌ-'kɑ:rdɪəgræm] n Elektrokardiogramm nt der rechten Herzhälfte, Dextrokardiogramm nt.
dex·tro·car·di·og·ra·phy [ˌ-ˌkɑ:rdɪ'ɑgrəfɪ] n Dextrokardiographie f.
dex·tro·cer·e·bral [ˌ-'serəbrəl] adj physiol. dextrozerebral.
dex·tro·cli·na·tion [ˌ-klaɪ'neɪʃn] n → dextrocycloduction.
dex·tro·com·pound [ˌ-'kɑmpaʊnd] n chem. rechtsdrehende Verbindung f.
dex·tro·cy·clo·duc·tion [ˌ-ˌsaɪklə'dʌkʃn] n ophthal. Dextrozykloduktion f.
dex·tro·cy·clo·ver·sion [ˌ-ˌsaɪklə'vɜrʒn] n ophthal. Dextrozykloversion f.
dex·tro·duc·tion [ˌ-'dʌkʃn] n ophthal. Dextroduktion f.
dex·tro·gas·tria [ˌ-'gæstrɪə] n Rechtsverlagerung f des Magens, Dextrogastrie f.
dex·tro·glu·cose [ˌ-'glu:koʊz] n → dextrose.

dex·tro·gram ['-græm] n card. Dextrogramm nt.
dex·tro·gy·ral [ˌ-'dʒaɪrəl] adj → dextrorotatory.
dex·tro·gy·ra·tion [ˌ-dʒaɪ'reɪʃn] n → dextrorotation.
dex·tro·man·u·al [ˌ-'mænjəwəl] adj rechtshändig.
dex·tro·meth·or·phan [ˌ-meθ'ɔ:rfæn] n pharm. Dextromethorphan n.
dex·tro·mor·am·ide [ˌ-mɔ:r'æmaɪd] n pharm. Dextromoramid n.
dex·trop·e·dal [deks'trɑpədəl] adj rechtsfüßig.
dex·tro·po·si·tion [ˌdekstrəpə'zɪʃn] n Rechtsverlagerung f, Dextroposition f, Dextropositio f.
d. of aorta Rechtsverlagerung der Aorta, Dextropositio aortae.
dex·tro·pro·pox·y·phene [ˌ-proʊ'pɑksəfi:n] n pharm. Dextropropoxyphen nt.
dex·tro·ro·ta·ry [ˌ-'roʊtərɪ] adj → dextrorotatory.
dex·tro·ro·ta·tion [ˌ-roʊ'teɪʃn] n chem. Rechtsdrehung f, Dextrorotation f.
dex·tro·ro·ta·to·ry [ˌ-'roʊtətɔ:rɪ, -toʊ-] adj chem. rechtsdrehend, dextrorotatorisch, dextrogyral.
dex·trose ['dekstroʊs] n Traubenzucker m, D-Glucose f, Glukose f, Dextrose f, Glykose f.
dex·tro·su·ria [ˌdekstrə's(j)ʊərɪə] n old → glucosuria.
dex·tro·thy·rox·ine sodium [ˌ-θaɪ'rɑksi:n] n pharm. Dextrothyroxin-Natrium nt.
dex·tro·tor·sion [ˌ-'tɔ:rʃn] n **1.** patho. Verdrehung/Torsion f nach rechts, Dextrotorsion f. **2.** ophthal. → dextrocycloduction.
dex·tro·trop·ic [ˌ-'trɑpɪk, -'troʊp-] adj rechtsdrehend, nach rechts drehend.
dex·trous ['dekstrəs] adj → dexterous.
dex·trous·ness ['-nɪs] n dexterity.
dex·tro·ver·sion [ˌdekstrə'vɜrʒn] n **1.** Rechtsdrehung f, Dextroversion f. **2.** ophthal. Dextroversion f. **3.** card. Dextroversio cordis.
dex·tro·vert·ed [ˌ-'vɜrtɪd] adj nach rechts gedreht, dextrovertiert.
D form biochem. D-Form f.
DFP abbr. → diisopropyl fluorophosphate.
DG abbr. → diacylglycerine.
dG abbr. → deoxyguanosine.
dg abbr. → decigram.
dGDP abbr. → deoxyguanosine diphosphate.
dGMP abbr. → deoxyguanosine monophosphate.
dGTP abbr. → deoxyguanosine triphosphate.
DH abbr. [delayed hypersensitivity] → delayed-type hypersensitivity.
DHA abbr. → docosahexaenoic acid.
DHE abbr. → dihydroergotamine.
DHEA abbr. → dehydroepiandrosterone.
DHEAS abbr. → dehydroepiandrosterone sulfate.
DHEA sulfate → dehydroepiandrosterone sulfate.
d'Herelle [de'rɛl]: **d'H. phenomenon** Bakteriophage f, d'Herelle-Phänomen nt, Twort-d'Herelle-Phänomen nt.
DHFR abbr. → dihydrofolate reductase.
dho·bie mark dermatitis ['doʊbi:] Wäscherkrätze f.
DHPG abbr. (9-[1,3-dihydroxy-2-propoxy--methyl] guanine) → ganciclovir.
DHPR abbr. → dihydropteridine reductase.
DHPR deficiency → dihydropteridine reductase deficiency.
DHS abbr. → dynamic hip screw.

DHT *abbr.* → dihydrotestosterone.
DHU *abbr.* → dihydrouridine.
DHU arm *biochem.* DHU-Arm *m*, Dihydrouridinarm *m*.
DI *abbr.* → diabetes insipidus.
di- *pref.* Zwei-, Zweifach-, Di-, Bi-.
dia- *pref.* Zwischen-, Dia-.
di·a·be·tes [daɪə'biːtɪs, -tiːz] *n* **1.** Diabetes *m*. **2.** → diabetes mellitus.
diabetes insipidus *abbr.* **DI** Diabetes insipidus.
  central d. zentraler Diabetes insipidus, Diabetes insipidus centralis/neurohormonalis.
  nephrogenic d. renaler/nephrogener Diabetes insipidus, Diabetes insipidus renalis.
diabetes mellitus *abbr.* **DM** Zuckerkrankheit *f*, Zuckerharnruhr *f*, Diabetes mellitus.
  growth-onset d. → insulin-dependent d.
  insulin-dependent d. *abbr.* **IDD, IDDM** insulinabhängiger Diabetes (mellitus), Typ-I-Diabetes (mellitus), Insulinmangeldiabetes.
  juvenile(-onset) d. → insulin-dependent d.
  juvenile-onset d. of adult *abbr.* **JODA** Typ-I-Diabetes mellitus des Erwachsenen, juvenile-onset diabetes of adult *abbr.* JODA.
  ketosis-prone d. → insulin-dependent d.
  ketosis-resistant d. → non-insulin-dependent d.
  maturity-onset d. → non-insulin-dependent d.
  maturity-onset d. of youth *abbr.* **MODY** Typ-II-Diabetes mellitus bei Jugendlichen, maturity-onset diabetes of youth *abbr.* MODY.
  non-insulin-dependent d. *abbr.* **NIDD, NIDDM** nicht-insulinabhängiger Diabetes mellitus, Typ-II-Diabetes mellitus, non-insulin-dependent diabetes (mellitus) *abbr.* NIDD(M).
di·a·bet·ic [daɪə'betɪk] **I** *n* Diabetiker(in *f*) *m*. **II** *adj* **1.** Diabetes betr., zuckerkrank, diabetisch, Diabetes-. **2.** durch Diabetes bedingt *od.* ausgelöst *od.* verursacht, diabetisch; diabetogen.
diabetic acidosis diabetische/diabetogene Azidose *f*.
diabetic amaurosis diabetische/diabetogene Blindheit/Amaurose *f*.
diabetic angiopathy diabetische Angiopathie *f*.
diabetic arthropathy diabetische Arthropathie *f*.
diabetic bullosis Bullosis diabeticorum.
diabetic cataract Zuckerstar *m*, Cataracta diabetica.
diabetic coma diabetisches/hyperglykämisches Koma *nt*, Kussmaul-Koma *nt*, Coma diabeticum/hyperglycaemicum.
diabetic dermopathy diabetische Derm(at)opathie *f*, Diabetid *nt*.
diabetic fetopathy diabetische Embryopathie/Fetopathie *f*, Embryopathia/Fetopathia diabetica.
diabetic gangrene diabetische Gangrän *f*.
diabetic glomerulosclerosis Kimmelstiel-Wilson-Syndrom *nt*, diabetische Glomerulosklerose *f*.
diabetic iritis *ophthal.* diabetische Iritis *f*.
diabetic ketoacidosis diabetische Ketoazidose *f*.
diabetic microangiopathy diabetische Mikroangiopathie *f*.
diabetic nephrosclerosis → diabetic glomerulosclerosis.
diabetic neuropathy diabetische Neuropathie *f*.

diabetic puncture Bernard'-Zuckerstich *m*.
diabetic retinitis → diabetic retinopathy.
diabetic retinopathy diabetische Retinopathie *f*, Retinopathia diabetica.
  exudative d. Retinopathia diabetica exsudativa.
  hemorrhagic proliferating d. Retinopathia diabetica haemorrhagica proliferans.
  hypertensive angiospastic d. Retinopathia diabetica hypertensiva (angiospastica).
  simple d. Retinopathia diabetica simplex.
diabetic vulvitis diabetische Vulvitis/Vulvovaginitis *f*, Vulvitis/Vulvovaginitis diabetica.
di·a·be·tid [daɪə'biːtɪd] *n* → diabetic dermopathy.
di·a·be·to·gen·ic [daɪəˌbetə'dʒenɪk] *adj* Diabetes verursachend *od.* auslösend, diabetogen.
di·a·be·tog·e·nous [daɪəbɪ'tɑdʒənəs] *adj* durch Diabetes bedingt, diabetogen; diabetisch.
di·a·be·to·graph [daɪə'biːtəgræf] *n* Diabetograph *m*.
di·a·be·tom·e·ter [daɪəbɪ'tɑmɪtər] *n* Diabetometer *nt*.
di·a·bro·sis [daɪə'broʊsɪs] *n patho.* perforierende Ulzeration *f*, Diabrose *f*, Diabrosis *f*.
di·a·brot·ic [daɪə'brɑtɪk] **I** *n* korrosives Mittel *nt*. **II** *adj* ulzerierend, korrodierend.
di·ac·e·tate [daɪ'æsɪteɪt] *n* Diazetat *nt*, Diacetat *nt*.
di·ac·e·te·mia [daɪæsɪ'tiːmɪə] *n* Diazetämie *f*.
di·a·ce·tic acid [daɪə'siːtɪk, -'set-] Azetessigsäure *f*, β-Ketobuttersäure *f*.
di·a·cet·ic·ac·i·du·ri·a [ˌdaɪəˌsetɪkˌæsɪ'd(j)ʊərɪə] *n* → diaceturia.
di·ac·e·to·nu·ri·a [daɪˌæsɪtoʊ'n(j)ʊərɪə] *n* → diaceturia.
di·ac·e·tu·ri·a [daɪæsɪ't(j)ʊərɪə] *n* Azetessigsäureausscheidung *f* im Harn, Diazeturie *f*.
di·ac·e·tyl [daɪ'æsɪtl] *n* Diazetyl *nt*, Diacetyl *nt*.
di·ac·e·tyl·cho·line [daɪˌæsɪtl'koʊliːn, -'kal-] *n pharm., anes.* Succinylcholinchlorid *nt*, Suxamethoniumchlorid *nt*.
diacetyl diaminodiphenylsulfone *abbr.* **DADDS** *pharm.* Diacetyldiaminodiphenylsulfon *nt abbr.* DADDS.
di·ac·e·tyl·mor·phine [daɪˌæsɪtl'mɔːrfiːn] *n pharm.* Heroin *nt*, Dia(cetyl)morphin *nt*.
di·ac·e·tyl·tan·nic acid [ˌ-'tænɪk] Acetylgerbsäure *f*, Acetyltannin *nt*.
di·a·cho·re·ma [daɪəkə'riːmə] *n* **1.** Ausscheidung *f*, Exkrement *nt*, Excrementum *nt*. **2.** Stuhl *m*, Kot *m*, Exkremente *pl*, Fäzes *pl*, Faeces *pl*.
di·a·cho·re·sis [ˌ-kə'riːsɪs] *n* Darmentleerung *f*, Miktion *f*, Defäkation *f*.
di·ac·id [daɪ'æsɪd] *chem.* **I** *n* zweibasische Säure *f*. **II** *adj* zweibasisch.
di·a·cla·sia [daɪə'kleɪʒ(ɪ)ə] *n* → diaclasis.
di·ac·la·sis [daɪ'æklæsɪs] *n* **1.** *ortho.* Osteoklase *f*, Osteoklasie *f*. **2.** *patho.* vermehrte Osteoklastentätigkeit *f*, Osteoklasie *f*, Osteoklase *f*.
di·a·con·dy·lar fracture [daɪə'kɑndɪlər] transkondyläre Fraktur *f*.
di·ac·ri·nous [daɪ'ækrɪnəs] *adj histol.* diakrin.
di·ac·ri·sis [daɪ'ækrəsɪs] *n* **1.** → diagnosis. **2.** *patho.* Diakrisie *f*, Diacrisis *f*.
di·a·crit·ic [daɪə'krɪtɪk] *adj* **1.** → diagnostic II. **2.** unterscheidend, diakritisch.
di·ac·tin·ic [ˌdaɪæk'tɪnɪk] *adj phys.* aktinische Strahlen durchlassend, diaktin, diaktinisch.
di·ac·yl·glyc·er·in [ˌdaɪæsɪl'glɪsərɪn] *n*

abbr. **DG** Diacylglycerin *nt abbr.* DG, *old* Diglycerid *nt*.
di·ac·yl·glyc·er·ol [ˌ-'glɪsərɔl, -rɑl] *n* → diacylglycerine.
diacylglycerol acyltransferase Diacylglycerinacyltransferase *f*.
diacylglycerol lipase Lipoproteinlipase *f abbr.* LPL.
di·ad ['daɪæd] *n genet.* Dyade *f*.
di·a·der·mic [daɪə'dɜrmɪk] *adj* durch die Haut hindurch (wirkend), perkutan.
di·ad·o·cho·ci·ne·sia [daɪˌædəkoʊsɪ'niːʒ(ɪ)ə] *n* → diadochokinesia.
di·ad·o·cho·ci·net·ic [ˌ-sɪ'netɪk] *adj* → diadochokinetic.
di·ad·o·cho·ki·ne·sia [ˌ-kɪ'niːʒ(ɪ)ə, -kaɪ-] *n* Diadochokinese *f*.
di·ad·o·cho·ki·ne·sis [ˌ-kɪ'niːsɪs, -kaɪ-] *n* → diadochokinesia.
di·ad·o·cho·ki·net·ic [ˌ-kɪ'netɪk] *adj* Diadochokinese betr., diadochokinetisch.
di·ag·nose [daɪəg'noʊz] **I** *vt* diagnostizieren. **II** *vi* eine Diagnose stellen.
di·ag·no·sis [ˌdaɪəg'noʊsɪs] *n*, *pl* **-ses** [-siːz] **1.** Diagnose *f*, Diagnostik *f*. **2.** Diagnostik *f*.
  d. by exclusion Ausschlußdiagnose.
di·ag·nos·tic [daɪəg'nɑstɪk] **I** *n* **1.** Symptom *nt*, charakteristisches Merkmal *nt*. **2.** Diagnose *f*. **II** *adj* Diagnose *od.* Diagnostik betr., diagnostisch.
diagnostic aid diagnostisches Hilfsmittel *nt*.
diagnostic anesthesia diagnostische Anästhesie *f*.
di·ag·nos·ti·cate [ˌdaɪəg'nɑstɪkeɪt] *vt, vi* → diagnose.
di·ag·nos·tics [ˌdaɪəg'nɑstɪks] *pl* Diagnostik *f*.
diagnostic serology Sero-, Serumdiagnostik *f*.
diagnostic tool → diagnostic aid.
di·ag·o·nal [daɪ'æg(ə)nl] **I** *n mathe.* Diagonale *f*. **II** *adj* schräg(laufend), diagonal, Diagonal-.
diagonal band of Broca Broca'-Diagonalband *nt*, Bandaletta/Stria diagonalis (Broca).
diagonal conjugate *anat., gyn.* Conjugata diagonalis.
diagnostic biopsy diagnostische Biopsie *f*, Probebiopsie *f*.
di·a·gram ['daɪəgræm] **I** *n* Diagramm *nt*, graphische Darstellung *f*, Schema *nt*; Schau-, Kurvenbild *nt*. **II** *vt* graphisch darstellen, in ein Diagramm eintragen.
di·a·ki·ne·sis [ˌdaɪəkɪ'niːsɪs, -kaɪ-] *n* Diakinese *f*.
di·al·de·hyde [daɪ'ældəhaɪd] *n* Dialdehyd *nt*.
di·al·yl·bis·nor·tox·i·fer·in dichloride [daɪˌælɪlbɪsnɔːr'tɑksɪferɪn] Alcuroniumchlorid *nt*.
di·a·lu·rate [daɪ'ælʊreɪt] *n* Dialurat *nt*.
di·a·lu·ric acid [daɪə'lʊərɪk] Dialursäure *f*.
di·al·y·sance [daɪə'laɪsəns, daɪ'ælɪsəns] *n* Dialysierfähigkeit *f*, Dialysance *f*.
di·al·y·sate [daɪ'æləseɪt] *n* Dialysat *nt*.
di·al·y·sis [daɪ'æləsɪs] *n, pl* **-ses** [-siːz] Dialyse *f*.
dialysis catheter Dialysekatheter *m*.
dialysis dementia → dialysis encephalopathy (syndrome).
dialysis disequilibrium syndrome Dysäquilibriumsyndrom *nt*, zerebrales Dialysesyndrom *nt*.
dialysis encephalopathy (syndrome) chronisch-progressive dialysebedingte Enzephalopathie *f*, Dialyseenzephalopathie *f*.
dialysis fluid Dialyseflüssigkeit *f*, Dialysierflüssigkeit *f*.

dialysis shunt Dialyseshunt *m*.
dialysis unit Dialysestation *f*, -einheit *f*.
di·a·lyt·ic [ˌdaɪəˈlɪtɪk] *adj* dialytisch.
dialytic parabiosis parabiotische Dialyse *f*.
di·a·lyz·a·ble [ˈdaɪəlaɪzəbl] *adj* dialysierbar, dialysabel.
di·al·y·zate [daɪˈæləzeɪt] *n* → dialysate.
di·a·lyze [ˈdaɪəlaɪz] *vt* mittels Dialyse trennen, dialysieren.
di·a·lyz·er [ˈdaɪəlaɪzər] *n* Dialysator *m*.
di·a·mag·net·ic [daɪəmægˈnetɪk] *adj phys.* diamagnetisch.
di·a·mag·net·ism [daɪəˈmægnətɪzəm] *n phys.* Diamagnetismus *m*.
di·am·e·ter [daɪˈæmɪtər] *n* Durchmesser *m*, Diameter *m*. **in ~** im Durchmesser.
di·am·e·tral [daɪˈæmɪtrəl] *adj* → diametric 1.
di·a·met·ric [ˌdaɪəˈmetrɪk] *adj* **1.** Diameter betr., diametrisch. **2.** *fig.* diametral, genau entgegengesetzt.
di·a·met·ri·cal [ˌ-ˈmetrɪkl] *adj* → diametric.
di·a·mide [ˈdaɪəmaɪd, daɪˈæmɪd] *n* **1.** Diamid *nt*. **2.** Hydrazin *nt*, Diamid *nt*.
di·am·ine [ˈdaɪəmiːn, daɪˈæmɪn] *n* Diamin *nt*.
diamine oxidase Diaminooxidase *f*, Histaminase *f*.
di·am·i·no·ac·ri·dine [daɪˌæmɪnəʊˈækrɪdiːn, -dɪn] *n* Proflavin *nt*, Diaminoacridin *nt*.
p-di·am·i·no·di·phen·yl [ˌ-daɪˈfenl] *n* Benzidin *nt*, Diphenyldiamin *nt*.
di·am·i·no·di·phen·yl·sul·fone [ˌ-daɪˌfenlˈsʌlfəʊn] *n abbr.* **DDS** *m* dapsone.
di·am·i·no·pim·e·late [ˌ-ˈpɪməleɪt, -lɪt] *n* Diaminopimelat *nt*.
diaminopimelate decarboxylase Diaminopimelatdecarboxylase *f*.
diaminopimelate epimerase Diaminopimelatepimerase *f*.
di·am·i·no·pi·mel·ic acid [ˌ-pəˈmelɪk, -ˈmiːl-] *abbr.* **DAP** Diaminopimelinsäure *f*.
di·am·i·nu·ria [daɪəmɪˈn(j)ʊərɪə] *n* Diaminurie *f*.
di·am·ni·ot·ic [ˌdaɪæmnɪˈɒtɪk] *adj embryo.* diamniotisch.
Diamond-Blackfan [ˈdaɪ(ə)mənd ˈblækfæn]: **D.-B. syndrome** Blackfan-Diamond-Anämie *f*, chronische kongenitale aregenerative Anämie *f*, pure red cell aplasia.
dia·mond pyramid hardness [ˈdaɪ(ə)mənd] *phys.* Vickers-Pyramidendruckhärte *f*.
diamond-shaped murmur Crescendo--Decrescendo-Geräusch *nt*.
di·a·mor·phine [ˌdaɪəˈmɔːrfiːn] *n* → diacetylmorphine.
Di·an·a complex [daɪˈænə] *psychia.* Diana--Komplex *m*.
di·a·pause [ˈdaɪəpɔːz] *n bio., embryo.* Diapause *f*.
di·a·pe·de·sis [ˌdaɪəpɪˈdiːsɪs] *n histol.* Wanderung *f*, Emigration *f*, Diapedese *f*.
di·a·pe·det·ic [ˌ-ˈdetɪk] *adj* Diapedese betr., Diapedese-.
di·a·per [ˈdaɪ(ə)pər] *n* Windel *f*.
diaper dermatitis *derm., ped.* Windeldermatitis *f*, Dermatitis pseudosyphilitica papulosa, Dermatitis ammoniacalis, Dermatitis glutaealis infantum, Erythema papulosum posterosivum, Erythema glutaeale.
diaper erythema → diaper dermatitis.
diaper rash → diaper dermatitis.
di·a·pha·ne·i·ty [dɪˌæfəˈniːɪtɪ, ˌdaɪəfə-] *n* (Strahlen-, Licht-)Durchlässigkeit *f*, Transparenz *f*, Diaphanie *f*.
di·aph·a·nog·ra·phy [daɪˌæfəˈnɒgrəfɪ] *n* Diaphanographie *f*.

di·aph·a·nom·e·ter [ˌ-ˈnɒmɪtər] *n* Diaphanometer *nt*.
di·aph·a·nom·e·try [ˌ-ˈnɒmətrɪ] *n* Diaphanometrie *f*.
di·aph·a·no·scope [daɪˈæfənəʊskəʊp] *n* Diaphanoskop *nt*.
di·aph·a·nos·co·py [daɪˌæfəˈnɒskəpɪ] *n* Diaphanoskopie *f*, Durchleuchten *nt*, Diaphanie *f*, Transillumination *f*.
di·aph·o·rase [daɪˈæfəreɪz] *n* Diaphorase *f*, Lipoamiddehydrogenase *f*.
di·a·pho·re·sis [ˌdaɪəfəˈriːsɪs] *n* Schweißsekretion *f*, Schwitzen *nt*, Diaphorese *f*.
di·a·pho·ret·ic [ˌ-ˈretɪk] **I** *n* schweißtreibendes Mittel *nt*, *old* Diaphoretikum *nt*, Sudoriferum *nt*. **II** *adj* schweißtreibend, diaphoretisch.
di·a·phragm [ˈdaɪəfræm] *n* **1.** *anat.* Zwerchfell *nt*, Scheidewand *f*, Diaphragma *nt*. **2.** *phys.* (halbdurchlässige) Scheidewand *od.* Membran *f*, Blende *f*. **3.** *gyn.* (Scheiden-)Diaphragma *nt*.
d. of mouth M. mylohyoideus.
d. of sella turcica Diaphragma sellae.
di·a·phrag·ma [daɪəˈfrægmə] *n, pl* **-ma·ta** [-mətə] → diaphragm 1.
di·a·phrag·mal·gia [ˌdaɪəfrægˈmældʒ(ɪ)ə] *n* Zwerchfellschmerz *m*, Diaphragmalgie *f*, Diaphragmodynie *f*.
di·a·phrag·mat·ic [ˌ-ˈmætɪk] *adj* Diaphragma *od.* Zwerchfell betr., diaphragmatisch.
diaphragmatic arch: external d. Lig. arcuatum laterale.
internal d. Lig. arcuatum mediale.
diaphragmatic arteries untere Zwerchfellarterien *pl*, Aa. phrenicae inferiores.
superior d. obere Zwerchfellarterien *pl*, Aa. phrenicae superiores.
diaphragmatic breathing Zwerchfellatmung *f*.
diaphragmatic crura Zwerchfellschenkel *pl*.
diaphragmatic defect Zwerchfelldefekt *m*.
diaphragmatic eventration Zwerchfellhochstand *m*.
diaphragmatic excursion Zwerchfellbewegung *f*.
diaphragmatic flutter Zwerchfellflattern *nt*.
diaphragmatic hernia Zwerchfellhernie *f*, Hernia diaphragmatica.
diaphragmatic hiatus Hiatus diaphragmaticus (sellae).
diaphragmatic injury Zwerchfellverletzung *f*, -trauma *nt*.
diaphragmatic muscle *old* → diaphragm 1.
diaphragmatic nerve Phrenikus *m*, N. phrenicus.
diaphragmatic paralysis Zwerchfelllähmung *f*, -paralyse *f*.
diaphragmatic phenomenon Litten-Phänomen *nt*.
diaphragmatic pleura Zwerchfellpleura *f*, Pleura diaphragmatica.
diaphragmatic pleurisy basale Brustfellentzündung/Pleuritis *f*, Pleuritis diaphragmatica.
diaphragmatic plexus Plexus phrenicus.
diaphragmatic respiration Zwerchfellatmung *f*.
diaphragmatic surface of heart Zwerchfellfläche *f* des Herzens, Facies diaphragmatica/inferior (cordis).
diaphragmatic trauma Zwerchfellverletzung *f*, -trauma *nt*.
di·a·phrag·ma·ti·tis [daɪəˌfrægməˈtaɪtɪs] *n* → diaphragmitis.
di·a·phrag·mat·o·cele [ˌ-ˈfrægˈmætəsiːl] *n* → diaphragmatic hernia.

di·a·phrag·mi·tis [ˌ-frægˈmaɪtɪs] *n* Zwerchfellentzündung *f*, Diaphragmatitis *f*, Diaphragmitis *f*.
di·a·phrag·mo·dyn·ia [ˌ-ˌfrægməˈdiːnɪə] *n* → diaphragmalgia.
diaphragm pessary *gyn.* Diaphragmapessar *nt*, Diaphragma *nt*.
diaphragm phenomenon Litten-Phänomen *nt*.
di·aph·y·sar·y [daɪˈæfɪzerɪ] *adj* → diaphyseal.
di·a·phys·e·al [daɪəˈfiːzɪəl] *adj* Knochenschaft/Diaphyse betr., diaphysär, Diaphysen-.
diaphyseal aclasis *ortho.* multiple kartilaginäre Exostosen *pl*, hereditäre multiple Exostosen *pl*, multiple Osteochondrome *pl*, Ecchondrosis ossificans.
diaphyseal dysplasia (Camurati-) Engelmann-Erkrankung *f*, -Syndrom *nt*, Osteopathia hyperostotica multiplex infantilis.
diaphyseal fracture Schaftbruch *m*, Diaphysenfraktur *f*.
diaphyseal sclerosis → diaphyseal dysplasia.
di·a·phys·ec·to·my [daɪəfɪzˈektəmɪ] *n ortho.* Diaphysenentfernung *f*, -resektion *f*, Diaphysektomie *f*.
di·a·phys·i·al *adj* → diaphyseal.
diaphysial center diaphysärer Knochenkeim *m*.
di·aph·y·sis [daɪˈæfəsɪs] *n, pl* **-ses** [-siːz] Knochenschaft *m*, -mittelstück *nt*, Diaphyse *f*, Diaphysis *f*.
di·a·phys·i·tis [daɪəfɪˈzaɪtɪs] *n* Diaphysenentzündung *f*, Diaphysitis *f*.
di·a·pi·re·sis [ˌdaɪəpaɪˈriːsɪs] *n* → diapedesis.
di·a·pla·cen·tal [ˌdaɪəpləˈsentəl] *adj* durch die Plazenta hindurch, diaplazentär, diaplazentar.
di·a·plex·us [daɪəˈpleksəs] *n* Plexus choroideus ventriculi tertii.
di·a·poph·y·sis [daɪəˈpɒfəsɪs] *n anat.* Proc. articularis superior.
di·a·py·e·sis [daɪəpaɪˈiːsɪs] *n* Eiterung *f*.
di·ar·rhe·a [daɪəˈrɪə] *n* Durchfall *m*, Diarrhoe *f*, Diarrhoea *f*, Diarrhö(e) *f*.
di·ar·rhe·al [daɪəˈrɪəl] *adj* Diarrhoe betr., von ihr betroffen *od.* gekennzeichnet, diarrhoisch, Durchfall-, Diarrhoe-.
diarrheal illness Durchfallerkrankung *f*.
di·ar·rhe·ic [daɪəˈrɪɪk] *adj* → diarrheal.
di·ar·rhe·o·gen·ic [daɪəˌrɪəˈdʒenɪk] *adj* Diarrhoe auslösend *od.* verursachend.
di·ar·thric [daɪˈɑːrθrɪk] *adj* zwei Gelenke betr., diarthrisch, diartikulär.
di·ar·thro·di·al articulation [ˌdaɪɑːrˈθrəʊdɪəl] echtes Gelenk *nt*, Diarthrose *f*, Artic./Junctura synovialis.
diarthrodial cartilage Gelenk(flächen)knorpel *m*, gelenkflächenüberziehender Knorpel *m*, Cartilago articularis.
diarthrodial joint → diarthrodial articulation.
di·ar·thro·sis [daɪɑːrˈθrəʊsɪs] *n, pl* **-ses** [-siːz] → diarthrodial articulation.
di·ar·tic·u·lar [daɪɑːrˈtɪkjələr] *adj* → diarthric.
di·as·chi·sis [daɪˈæskəsɪs] *n neuro.* Diaschisis *f*.
di·a·scope [ˈdaɪəskəʊp] *n derm.* Glasplättchen *nt*, -spatel *m*, Diaskop *nt*.
di·as·co·py [daɪˈæskəpɪ] *n* **1.** *radiol.* Durchleuchtung *f*, Diaskopie *f*, Transillumination *f*. **2.** *derm.* Diaskopie *f*.
di·a·sos·tic [daɪəˈsɒstɪk] *adj* **1.** Hygiene betr., auf Hygiene beruhend, der Gesundheit dienend, hygienisch. **2.** Hygiene betr., sauber, frei von Verschmutzung, hygienisch.

di·as·pi·ro·nec·ro·bi·o·sis [daɪˌæspɪərəʊˌnekrəbaɪˈəʊsɪs] *n* disseminierte Nekrobiose *f.*
di·as·pi·ro·ne·cro·sis [daɪˌæspɪərəʊnɪˈkrəʊsɪs] *n* → diaspironecrobiosis.
di·a·stal·sis [ˌdaɪəˈstælsɪs] *n* Diastalsis *f*, Diastaltik *f.*
di·a·stal·tic [ˌ-ˈstæltɪk] *adj* **1.** Diastalsis betr., diastaltisch. **2.** reflektorisch, Reflex-.
di·a·stase [ˈ-steɪz] *n* Diastase *f.*
di·a·sta·sic [ˌ-ˈsteɪsɪk] *adj* → diastatic.
di·as·ta·sis [daɪˈæstəsɪs] *n, pl* **-ses** [-siːz] **1.** *physiol.* Diastase *f.* **2.** *patho.* Auseinanderklaffen *nt*, -weichen *nt*, Diastase *f*, Diastasis *f.* **3.** *card.* Diastase *f*, Diastasis cordis.
di·as·tas·u·ria [daɪəsteɪˈs(j)ʊərɪə] *n* Amylaseausscheidung *f* im Harn, Amylasurie *f.*
di·a·stat·ic [ˌdaɪəˈstætɪk] *adj* **1.** *biochem., physiol.* Diastase betr., Diastase(n)-. **2.** *patho.* Diastasis betr., diastatisch.
di·a·stem [ˈdaɪəstem] *n* → diastema.
di·a·ste·ma [ˌdaɪəˈstiːmə] *n, pl* **-ma·ta** [-mətə] **1.** *anat.* Lücke *f*, Spalte *f.* **2.** (angeborene) Zahnlücke *f*, Diastema *nt.* **3.** *histol.* Diastema *f.*
di·a·ste·ma·to·cra·nia [daɪəˌstɪmətəˈkreɪnɪə] *n embryo.* Diastematokranie *f*, Diastematocrania *f.*
di·a·ste·ma·to·my·e·lia [ˌ-maɪˈiːlɪə] *n embryo.* Diastematomyelie *f.*
di·a·ste·ma·to·py·e·lia [ˌ-paɪˈiːlɪə] *n embryo.* Diastematopyelie *f.*
di·as·ter [ˈdaɪæstər] *n histol.* Diaster *f.*
di·a·ster·e·o·i·so·mer [daɪəˌsterɪəʊˈaɪsəmər, -ˌstɪər-] *n* → diastereomer.
di·a·ster·e·o·i·so·mer·ic [ˌ-ˌaɪsəˈmerɪk] *adj chem.* diastereo(iso)mer.
di·a·ster·e·o·i·so·mer·ism [ˌ-ˌaɪˈsɑmərɪzəm] *n* Diastereo(iso)merie *f*, Diastomerie *f.*
di·a·ster·e·o·mer [ˌdaɪəˈsterɪəmər, -ˈstɪər-] *n* Diastereo(iso)mer *nt*, Diastomer *nt*, allo-Form *f.*
di·a·ster·e·o·mer·ic [ˌ-merɪk] *adj* → diastereoisomeric.
di·as·to·le [daɪˈæstəli] *n* Diastole *f.*
di·as·tol·ic [ˌdaɪəˈstɑlɪk] *adj* Diastole betr., diastolisch, Diastolen-.
diastolic blood pressure diastolischer (Blut-)Druck *m.*
diastolic murmur diastolisches (Herz-)Geräusch *nt*, Diastolikum *nt.*
 early d. frühdiastolisches (Herz-)Geräusch.
 late d. *card.* präsystolisches/spät-diastolytisches (Herz-)Geräusch.
diastolic pressure → diastolic blood pressure.
diastolic thrill *card.* diastolisches Schwirren *nt.*
di·as·to·my·e·lia [daɪˌæstɔmaɪˈiːlɪə] *n* → diastematomyelia.
di·a·stroph·ic [ˌdaɪəˈstrɑfɪk] *adj (Knochen)* verkrümmt, gebogen, diastrophisch.
diastrophic dwarf diastrophischer Zwerg *m.*
di·as·tro·phism [daɪˈæstrəfɪzəm] *n (Knochen)* Verkrümmung *f*, Verbiegung *f.*
di·a·tax·ia [ˌdaɪəˈtæksɪə] *n neuro.* Diataxie *f.*
di·a·te·la [ˌ-ˈtiːlə] *n anat.* Tela choroidea ventriculi tertii.
di·a·ther·mal [ˌ-ˈθɜrml] *adj* → diathermic.
di·a·ther·man·ous [ˌ-ˈθɜrmənəs] *adj* wärmedurchlässig, diatherman.
di·a·ther·mic [ˌ-ˈθɜrmɪk] *adj* Diathermie betr., diatherm.
di·a·ther·mo·co·ag·u·la·tion [ˌ-ˌθɜrməkəʊˌæɡjəˈleɪʃn] *n* chirurgische Diathermie *f*, Elektrokoagulation *f.*

di·a·ther·my [ˈ-θɜrmɪ] *n* Diathermie *f.*
di·ath·e·sis [daɪˈæθəsɪs] *n, pl* **-ses** [-siːz] angeborene *od.* erworbene Neigung/Bereitschaft/Disposition *f*, Diathese *f*, Diathesis *f.*
di·a·thet·ic [daɪəˈθetɪk] *adj* Diathese betr., Diathese-.
di·a·to·ma·ceous earth [ˌdaɪətəˈmeɪʃəs] Diatomeenerde *f*, Kieselgur *nt.*
di·a·tom·ic [ˌdaɪəˈtɑmɪk] *adj chem.* **1.** aus zwei Atomen bestehend, diatomar. **2.** zweibasisch.
diatomic oxygen molekularer Sauerstoff *m.*
di·a·tri·zo·ate [daɪətraɪˈzəʊeɪt] *n radiol.* Diatrizoat *nt.*
di·aux·ie [daɪˈɔːksɪ] *n micro. (Bakterien)* zweiphasisches Wachstum *m*, Diauxie *f.*
di·az·e·pam [daɪˈæzəpæm] *n pharm.* Diazepam *nt.*
diazo- *pref.* Diazo-.
di·az·o·ben·zene [daɪˌæzəʊˈbenziːn] *n* Diazobenzol *nt.*
di·az·o·ben·zene-sul·fon·ic acid [daɪˌæzəʊˌbenziːnsʌlˈfɑnɪk] Diazobenzolsulfonsäure *f.*
diazo compound Diazoverbindung *f.*
di·a·zo·ma [daɪəˈzəʊmə] *n, pl* **-ma·ta** [-mətə] Zwerchfell *nt*, Diaphragma *nt.*
diazo reaction Ehrlich-Diazoreaktion *f.*
di·az·o·ti·za·tion [daɪˌæzətɪˈzeɪʃn] *n chem.* Diazotierung *f.*
di·az·o·tize [daɪˈæzətaɪz] *vt chem.* diazotieren, eine Diazogruppe einführen.
di·az·ox·ide [ˌdaɪæzˈɑksaɪd] *n pharm.* Diazoxid *nt.*
di·ba·sic [daɪˈbeɪsɪk] *adj chem.* zweibasisch.
dibasic acid zweibasische *od.* zweiwertige Säure *f.*
dibasic phosphate sekundäres Phosphat *nt.*
di·benz·an·thra·cene [daɪˌbenzˈænθrəsiːn] *n abbr.* **DBA** Dibenzanthrazen *nt.*
di·benz·e·pin [daɪˈbenzəpɪn] *n pharm.* Dibenzepin *nt.*
di·ben·zo·thi·a·zine [daɪˌbenzəʊˈθaɪəziːn, -zɪn] *n pharm.* Phenothiazin *nt.*
di·benz·ox·az·e·pine [daɪˌbenzɑksˈæzəpiːn] *n pharm.* Dibenzoxazepin *nt.*
di·both·ri·o·ceph·a·li·a·sis [daɪˌbɒθrɪəʊˌsefəˈlaɪəsɪs] *n* → diphyllobothriasis.
Di·both·ri·o·ceph·a·lus [ˌ-ˈsefələs] *n* → Diphyllobothrium.
di·bra·chia [daɪˈbreɪkɪə] *n embryo.* Dibrachie *f.*
di·bra·chi·us [daɪˈbreɪkɪəs] *n embryo.* Dibrachius *m.*
di·bro·mide [daɪˈbrəʊmaɪd] *n* Dibromid *nt.*
di·bu·caine [daɪˈbjuːkeɪn] *n pharm., anes.* Dibucain *nt.*
dibucaine number *abbr.* **DN** Dibucain-Zahl *f.*
dibucaine test Dibucain-Test *m.*
di·bu·to·line sulfate [daɪˈbjuːtliːn] *pharm.* Dibutolinsulfat *nt.*
DIC *abbr.* → disseminated intravascular coagulation.
di·cac·o·dyl [daɪˈkækədɪl] *n* Kakodyl *nt*, Dimethylarsin *m.*
di·car·bon·ate [daɪˈkɑrbəneɪt, -nɪt] *n* Bikarbonat *nt*, Bicarbonat *nt*, Hydrogencarbonat *nt.*
di·car·box·yl·ate carrier [daɪkɑːrˈbɑksəleɪt] Dicarboxylatcarrier *m.*
di·car·box·yl·ic acid [ˌ-kɑːrˈbɑkˈsɪlɪk] Dikarbonsäure *f*, Dicarbonsäure *f.*
di·cen·tric chromosome [daɪˈsentrɪk] dizentrisches Chromosom *n.*
di·ceph·a·lous [daɪˈsefələs] *adj embryo.* dizephal, dikephal.

di·ceph·a·lus [daɪˈsefələs] *n embryo.* Doppelmißbildung *f* mit zwei Köpfen, Dicephalus *m*, Dizephalus *m*, Dikephalus *m.*
di·ceph·a·ly [daɪˈsefəlɪ] *n embryo.* Dikephalie *f*, Dizephalie *f*, Dicephalie *f.*
di·chei·lia [daɪˈkeɪlɪə] *n embryo.* Dich(e)ilie *f.*
di·chei·ria [daɪˈkeɪrɪə] *n embryo.* Dich(e)irie *f.*
di·chei·rus [daɪˈkaɪrəs] *n embryo.* Dich(e)irus *m.*
di·chi·lia *n* → dicheilia.
di·chi·ria *n* → dicheiria.
di·chi·rus *n* → dicheirus.
di·chlo·ride [daɪˈklɔːraɪd, -rɪd, -ˈklɔər-] *n* Dichlorid *nt.*
di·chlo·ro·di·eth·yl sulfide [daɪˌklɔːrəʊdaɪˈeθəl] Gelbkreuz *nt*, Senfgas *nt*, Lost *nt*, Dichlordiäthylsulfid *nt.*
di·chlo·ro·di·fluor·o·meth·ane [daɪˌklɔːrədaɪˌflʊərəˈmeθeɪn] *n* Dichlordifluormethan *nt.*
di·chlo·ro·di·phen·yl·tri·chlor·o·eth·ane [daɪˌklɔːrədaɪˌfenltraɪˌklɔːrəʊˈeθeɪn] *n abbr.* **DDT** Dichlordiphenyltrichloräthan *nt abbr.* **DDT.**
di·chlo·ro·i·so·pro·ter·e·nol [daɪˌklɔːrəˌaɪsprəʊˈterɪnɔl] *n abbr.* **DCI** *pharm.* Dichlorisoproterenol *nt.*
di·chlo·ro·phen [daɪˈklɔːrəfen] *n pharm.* Dichlorophen *nt.*
di·chlo·ro·tet·ra·flu·o·ro·eth·ane [daɪˌklɔːrəˌtetrəˌflʊərəˈeθeɪn] *n* Dichlortetrafluoräthan *nt.*
di·chlor·o·vos [daɪˈklɔːrəvɑs] *n* → dichlorvos.
di·chlor·vos [daɪˈklɔːrvɑs] *n* Dichlorvos *nt abbr.* DDVP.
di·chog·e·ny [daɪˈkɑdʒənɪ] *n embryo.* Dichogenie *f.*
di·cho·ri·al twins [daɪˈkɔːrɪəl] → dizygotic twins.
di·cho·ri·on·ic twins [daɪkɔːrɪˈɑnɪk, -ˌkəʊ-] → dizygotic twins.
di·chot·ic [daɪˈkɑtɪk] *adj* → dichotomous.
di·chot·o·mi·za·tion [daɪˌkɑtəmaɪˈzeɪʃn] *n* → dichotomy.
di·chot·o·mize [daɪˈkɑtəmaɪz] *vt* aufspalten, gabeln.
di·chot·o·mous [dɪˈkɑtəməs] *adj* zweiteilig, zweigeteilt, dichotom(isch).
di·chot·o·my [daɪˈkɑtəmɪ] *n* (Auf-)Spaltung *f*, (Zwei-)Teilung *f*, gabelartige Verzweigung *f*, Dichotomie *f.*
di·chro·ic [daɪˈkrəʊɪk] *adj* **1.** *phys.* dichroitisch. **2.** → dichromatic.
di·chro·ism [ˈdaɪkrəʊɪzəm] *n phys.* Dichroismus *m.*
di·chro·it·ic [ˌdaɪkrəʊˈɪtɪk] *adj* **1.** → dichroic 1. **2.** → dichromatic.
di·chro·ma·sy [daɪˈkrəʊməsɪ] *n ophthal.* Di-, Bichromasie *f*, Dichromatopsie *f.*
di·chro·mat [ˈdaɪkrəʊmæt] *n ophthal.* Patient(in *f*) *m* mit Dichromasie, Dichromate(r *m*) *f.*
di·chro·mate [daɪˈkrəʊmeɪt] *n* Dichromat *nt.*
di·chro·mat·ic [ˌdaɪkrəˈmætɪk] *adj* **1.** Dichromasie betr., dichromat. **2.** *phys.* zweifarbig, dichromatisch.
dichromatic vision → dichromasy.
di·chro·ma·tism [daɪˈkrəʊmətɪzəm] *n* **1.** *ophthal.* → dichromasy. **2.** *phys.* Zweifarbigkeit *f*, Dichromasie *f*, Dichromatismus *m.*
di·chro·ma·top·sia [daɪkrəʊməˈtɑpsɪə] *n* → dichromasy.
di·chro·mic [daɪˈkrəʊmɪk] *adj* zwei Farben betr., dichrom(isch).
di·chro·mo·phil [daɪˈkrəʊməfɪl] *adj histol.* dichromophil.
di·chro·moph·i·lism [daɪkrəˈmɑfəlɪzəm] *n histol.* Dichromophilie *f.*

Dick

Dick [dɪk]: **D. method/reaction** → D. test.
 D. test Dick-Test m, -Probe f.
 D. test toxin Scharlachtoxin nt, erythrogenes Toxin nt.
 D. toxin → D. test toxin.
Dickens ['dɪkɪns]: **D. shunt** Pentosephosphatzyklus m, Phosphogluconatweg m.
di·clo·fen·ac [daɪ'kləʊfənæk] n pharm. Diclofenac nt.
di·clox·a·cil·lin [daɪˌklaksə'sɪlɪn] n pharm. Dicloxacillin nt.
di·co·ria [daɪ'kaʊrɪə] n → diplocoria.
di·cou·ma·rin [daɪ'k(j)u:mərɪn] n → dicumarol.
di·cro·ce·li·a·sis [ˌdaɪkrəsɪ'laɪəsɪs] n Dicrocoeliuminfektion f, -befall m, Dicrocoeliasis f.
Di·cro·coe·li·um [ˌdaɪkrə'sɪlɪəm] n micro. Dicrocoelium nt.
 D. dendriticum/lanceolatum kleiner Leberegel m, Lanzettegel m, Dicrocoelium dendriticum/lanceolatum.
di·crot·ic [daɪ'kratɪk] adj phys. dikrot.
dicrotic pulse Dikrotie f, dikroter Puls m, Pulsus dicrotus.
dicrotic wave phys. dikrote Welle f.
di·cro·tism ['daɪkrətɪzəm] n phys. Dikrotie f.
dic·ty·o·ki·ne·sis [ˌdɪktɪəkɪ'ni:sɪs, -kaɪ-] n histol. Diktyokinese f.
dic·ty·o·ma n → diktyoma.
dic·ty·o·some ['dɪktɪəsəʊm] n Diktyosom nt.
di·cu·ma·rol [daɪ'k(j)u:mərəl, -ral] n Dic(o)umarol nt.
di·cy·clic [daɪ'zaɪklɪk] adj dizyklisch.
di·cys·te·ine [daɪ'sɪstɪi:n] n Zystin nt, Cystin nt, Dicystein nt.
di·dac·ty·lism [daɪ'dæktlɪzəm] n embryo. Didaktylie f.
di·dac·ty·lous [daɪ'dæktɪləs] adj embryo. didaktyl.
did·y·mal·gia [ˌdɪdə'mældʒ(ɪ)ə] n Hodenschmerz(en pl) m, Hodenneuralgie f, Orchialgie f.
did·y·mi·tis [ˌdɪdə'maɪtɪs] n Hodenentzündung f, Orchitis f, Didymitis f.
did·y·mo·dyn·ia [ˌdɪdəməʊ'di:nɪə] n → didymalgia.
did·y·mous ['dɪdəməs] adj doppelt, gepaart, Zwillings-, Doppel-.
did·y·mus ['dɪdəməs] n **1.** Hoden m, Testis m, Didymus m. **2.** embryo. Zwilling m, Zwillingsmißbildung f, Didymus m.
die [daɪ] vi sterben. **to ~ of old age** an Altersschwäche sterben. **to ~ of hunger** verhungern. **to ~ of thirst** verdursten.
di·echo·scope [daɪ'ekəskəʊp] n physiol. Diechoskop nt.
di·e·cious [daɪ'i:ʃəs] adj bio. diözisch.
diel·drin ['di:ldrɪn] n Dieldrin nt.
Dieffenbach ['di:fənbax]: **D.'s amputation** ortho. Oberschenkelamputation f nach Dieffenbach.
 D.'s method/operation HNO Dieffenbach--Methode f, -Verfahren nt, -Verschiebeplastik f.
di·e·lec·tric [ˌdaɪɪ'lektrɪk] I n Dielektrikum nt. II adj dielektrisch, nichtleitend, isolierend.
dielectric constant abbr. **D** Dielektrizitätskonstante f abbr. D, Dielektrizitätszahl f.
di·e·lec·trol·y·sis [ˌdaɪɪlek'traləsɪs] n Dielektrolyse f, Iontophorese f.
di·en·ce·phal·ic [ˌdaɪensə'fælɪk] adj Zwischenhirn/Diencephalon betr., dienzephal, Diencephalon-.
diencephalic epilepsy autonome Epilepsie f, Epilepsie f mit autonomen Symptomen.
diencephalic syndrome dienzephales (Abmagerungs-)Syndrom nt.

diencephalic-telencephalic border Zwischenhirn-Endhirn-Grenze f.
di·en·ceph·a·lo·hy·po·phys·i·al [ˌdaɪənˌsefələʊˌhaɪpə'fi:zɪəl] adj Dienzephalon u. Hypophyse betr., dienzephalohypophysial.
di·en·ceph·a·lon [ˌdaɪən'sefələn] n Zwischenhirn nt, Dienzephalon nt, Diencephalon nt.
diencephalon vesicle embryo. Zwischenhirnbläschen nt.
di·en·es·trol [ˌdaɪɪn'estral, -ɔl] n pharm. Dienestrol nt.
Di·ent·a·moe·ba [daɪˌentə'mi:bə] n micro. Dientamoeba f.
 D. fragilis Dientamoeba fragilis.
di·ent·a·me·ba diarrhea [daɪˌentə'mi:bə] Dientamoeba fragilis-Diarrhö f.
di·er·e·sis [daɪ'erəsɪs] n, pl **-ses** [-si:z] chir. (Zer-)Teilen nt, Trennen nt.
di·et ['daɪət] I n **1.** Nahrung f, Kost f, Ernährung f, Diät f. **2.** Schon-, Krankenkost f, Diät f. **to be/go on a ~** eine Diät machen, Diät leben (müssen), auf Diät gesetzt sein. **to put sb. on a ~** jdm. eine Diät verordnen, jdn. auf Diät setzen. II vt jdn. auf Diät setzen. III vi Diät halten, Diät leben.
di·e·tar·y ['daɪəteri] I n Diätzettel m, -vorschrift f. II adj diätetisch, Diät-, Ernährungs-.
dietary amenorrhea gyn. Notstandsamenorrhoe f, ernährungsbedingte/nutritive Amenorrhoe f.
dietary cure Diätkur f.
dietary fiber Ballaststoffe pl, ballaststoffreiche Nahrung f.
di·e·tet·ic [daɪə'tetɪk] adj Diät betr., diätetisch, Diät-, Ernährungs-.
di·e·tet·i·cal [daɪə'tetɪkl] adj → dietetic.
dietetic albuminuria diätetische Albuminurie/Proteinurie f.
dietetic neuritis Beriberi f, Vitamin B_1--Mangel(krankheit f) m, Thiaminmangel(krankheit f) m.
dietetic proteinuria → dietetic albuminuria.
di·e·tet·ics [daɪə'tetɪks] pl Diät-, Ernährungslehre f, Diätetik f.
dietetic treatment diätetische Behandlung f.
di·eth·a·nol·a·mine [daɪˌeθə'nɑləmi:n] n Diäthanolamin nt.
di·eth·yl·a·mine [daɪˌeθələ'mi:n, -'æmɪn] n Diäthylamin nt.
di·eth·yl·am·i·no·eth·yl·cel·lu·lose [daɪˌeθələˌmi:nəʊˌeθəl'seljələʊs, -ˌæmɪnəʊ-] n Diäthylaminoäthylcellulose f, DEAE--Cellulose f.
di·eth·yl·bar·bi·tu·ric acid [daɪˌeθəlˌbɑrbə'tʊərɪk] pharm. Barbital nt, Diäthylbarbitursäure f, Diethylbarbitursäure f.
di·eth·yl·ene·di·a·mine [-daɪˌeθəli:n'daɪəmi:n] n pharm. Piperazin nt, Diäthylendiamin nt.
di·eth·yl·ene dioxide [daɪ'eθəli:n] → dioxane.
di·eth·yl ether [daɪ'eθəl] Äther m, Ether m, Diäthyläther m, Diethylether m.
diethyl-p-nitrophenyl thiophosphate Parathion nt, E 605 nt.
di·eth·yl·stil·bes·trol [daɪˌeθəlˌstɪl'bestrəl, -rəʊl] n abbr. **DES** pharm. Diäthylstilböstrol nt, Diethylstilbestrol nt abbr. DES.
di·eth·yl·trypt·a·mine [-'trɪptəmi:n] n abbr. **DET** pharm. Diäthyltryptamin nt, Diethyltryptamin nt abbr. DET.
di·e·ti·cian [daɪə'tɪʃn] n dietitian.
di·e·ti·tian [daɪɪ'tɪʃn] n Diätetiker(in f) m.
diet kitchen Diätküche f.
Dietl ['di:tl]: **D.'s crisis** Dietl-Krise f, -Syndrom nt.

diet list Diät(fahr)plan m.
di·e·to·ther·a·py [ˌdaɪətəʊ'θerəpi] n Diäto-, Ernährungstherapie f.
diet restriction Kost-, Diätbeschneidung f, -beschränkung f.
Dieulafoy [djølɑ'fwa]: **D.'s erosion** Dieulafoy-Erosion f, -Ulkus nt.
 D.'s triad Dieulafoy'-Trias f.
di·fen·ox·in [ˌdaɪfen'ɑksɪn] n pharm. Difenoxin nt.
dif·fer ['dɪfər] vi **1.** s. unterscheiden, verschieden sein, abweichen (from von). **2.** nicht übereinstimmen (from, with mit); anderer Meinung sein (from, with als).
dif·fer·ence ['dɪf(ə)rəns] I n **1.** Unterschied m (between-, in (zwischen)). **2.** mathe. Differenz f. **3.** Auseinandersetzung f, Differenz f. II vt unterscheiden (from von; between zwischen).
 d. in leg length Beinlängendifferenz f.
 d. in length Längenunterschied, -differenz.
 d. of opinion Meinungsverschiedenheit f.
difference equation mathe. Differenzgleichung f.
difference spectrum phys. Differenzspektrum nt.
dif·fer·ent ['dɪf(ə)rənt] adj andere(r, s); verschieden (from, to von), anders (from, to als); verschieden(artig), unterschiedlich.
dif·fer·en·tial [dɪfə'renʃl] I n **1.** Unterscheidungsmerkmal nt. **2.** mathe. Differential nt. II adj **3.** unterschiedlich, verschieden; unterscheidend, Unterscheidungs-; charakteristisch. **4.** mathe., phys. Differential-.
differential centrifugation Differentialzentrifugation f.
differential diagnosis abbr. **DD** Differentialdiagnose f abbr. DD.
differential limen abbr. **DL** Unterschieds-, Differentialschwelle f, Differenzlimen nt abbr. DL.
differential medium micro. Differentialnährboden m, -medium nt.
differential response physiol. dynamische/phasische Antwort f, Differentialantwort f.
differential sensor physiol. Differentialsensor m, D-Sensor m, D-Fühler m.
differential stain Differentialfärbung f.
differential study Differentialstudie f.
differential threshold → differential limen.
dif·fer·en·ti·ate [dɪfə'renʃɪeɪt] I vt **1.** unterscheiden (from von); einen Unterschied machen zwischen. **2.** mathe., bio., histol. differenzieren. II vi **3.** s. unterscheiden, differenzieren, s. unterschiedlich entwickeln (from von). **4.** differenzieren, einen Unterschied machen, unterscheiden (between zwischen).
dif·fer·en·ti·a·tion [dɪfəˌrenʃɪ'eɪʃn] n **1.** (a. mathe., bio.) Differenzierung f, Unterscheidung f. **2.** histol. Differenzierung f, Differenzieren nt.
differentiation antigen immun. Differenzierungsantigen nt.
dif·fi·cult ['dɪfɪkʌlt, -kəlt] adj **1.** schwer, schwierig (of für). **2.** (Person) schwierig.
difficult breathing erschwerte Atmung f, Atemnot f, Dyspnoe f.
difficult menstruation schmerzhafte Regelblutung/Menorrhoe f, Dysmenorrhoe f, Menorrhalgie f.
difficult respiration → difficult breathing.
dif·fi·cul·ty ['dɪfɪkʌltɪ, -kəltɪ] n Schwierigkeit f; Problem nt; Hindernis nt; schwierige Lage f; Beschwerden pl.
 d. in breathing Atembeschwerden pl.
dif·flu·ence ['dɪflu:əns] n phys. Verflüssigen nt.

dif·fract [dɪˈfrækt] *vt phys.* beugen, brechen.
dif·frac·tion [dɪˈfrækʃn] *n phys.* Beugung *f*, Diffraktion *f*.
diffraction pattern *phys.* Beugungsmuster *nt*.
diffraction spot *phys.* Beugungsfleck *m*.
dif·frac·tive [dɪˈfræktɪv] *adj phys.* beugend.
dif·fu·sate [dɪˈfjuːzeɪt] *n* Dialysat *nt*.
dif·fuse [dɪˈfjuːz] **I** *adj* **1.** *chem., phys.* verzerstreut, unscharf, diffus. **2.** *fig.* diffus, ungeordnet, verschwommen; weitschweifig. **II** *vt* **3.** *chem., phys.* zerstreuen, diffundieren, unscharf *od.* diffus reflektieren. **4.** (*a. fig.*) verbreiten; ausgießen, ausschütten. **III** *vi* **5.** *chem., phys.* diffundieren, s. zerstreuen, s. vermischen. **6.** (*a. fig.*) s. verbreiten *od.* ausbreiten.
diffuse abscess Phlegmone *f*.
diffuse aneurysm diffuses Aneurysma *nt*.
diffuse angiokeratoma Fabry-Syndrom *nt*, Morbus Fabry *m*, Thesaurismosis hereditaria lipoidica, hereditäre Thesaurismose Ruiter-Pompen-Weyers *f*, Ruiter-Pompen-Weyers-Syndrom *nt*, Angiokeratoma corporis diffusum (Fabry), Angiokeratoma universale.
diffuse choroiditis diffuse Chorioiditis *f*, Chorioiditis diffusa.
diffuse cutaneous leishmaniasis leproide Leishmaniasis *f*, Leishmaniasis cutis/tegumentaria diffusa.
diffuse deep keratitis Keratitis profunda.
diffuse emphysema diffuses/panazinäres/panlobuläres Lungenemphysem *nt*.
diffuse gliosis diffuse Gliose *f*.
diffuse glomerulonephritis diffuse Glomerulonephritis *f*.
diffuse goiter diffuse Schilddrüsenhyperplasie/Struma *f*, Struma diffusa.
diffuse histiocytic lymphoma 1. zentroblastisches Lymphom *nt*. **2.** zentrozytisches (malignes) Lymphom *nt*, lymphozytisches Lymphosarkom *nt*.
diffuse idiopathic skeletal hyperostosis *abbr.* **DISH** diffuse idiopathische skelettäre/ossäre Hyperostose *f*.
diffuse infantile familial sclerosis Krabbe-Syndrom *nt*, Globoidzellen-Leukodystrophie *f*, Galaktozerebrosidlipidose *f*, Galaktozerebrosidose *f*, Angiomatosis encephalo-cutanea, Leukodystrophia cerebri progressiva hereditaria.
diffuse-infiltrating *adj* diffus-infiltrierend.
diffuse inflammation diffuse Entzündung *f*.
diffuse inflammatory sclerosis of Schilder Schilder'-Krankheit *f*, Encephalitis periaxialis diffusa.
diffuse intravascular coagulation → disseminated intravascular coagulation.
diffuse leprosy of Lucio Lucio-Phänomen *nt*.
diffuse light diffuses Licht *nt*, Streulicht *nt*.
diffuse lymphoma Lymphosarkom *nt*.
diffuse myelitis diffuse Myelitis *f*.
diffuse palmoplantar keratoderma Morbus Unna-Thost *m*, Keratosis palmoplantaris diffusa circumscripta, Keratoma palmare et plantare hereditarium, Ichthyosis palmaris et plantaris (Thost).
diffuse periaxial encephalitis → diffuse inflammatory sclerosis of Schilder.
diffuse peritonitis generalisierte Bauchfellentzündung *f*, Peritonitis diffusa.
diffuse pleurisy diffuse Brustfellentzündung *f*/Pleuritis *f*.
diffuse scleroderma diffuse/progressive/systemische Sklerodermie *f*, systemische Sklerose *f*, Systemsklerose *f*, Sclerodermia diffusa/progressiva.

diffuse sclerosis 1. → diffuse inflammatory sclerosis of Schilder. **2.** → diffuse systemic sclerosis.
diffuse systemic sclerosis systemische Sklerose *f*, Systemsklerose *f*, progressive/diffuse/systemische Sklerodermie *f*, Sclerodermia diffusa/progressiva.
diffuse toxic goiter Basedow'-Krankheit *f*, Morbus Basedow *m*.
diffuse well-differentiated lymphocytic lymphoma *abbr.* **DWDL** diffuse well-differentiated lymphocytic lymphoma *abbr.* DWDL.
diffuse well-differentiated lymphoma zentrozytisches (malignes) Lymphom *nt*, lymphozytisches Lymphosarkom *nt*.
dif·fus·i·bil·i·ty [dɪˌfjuːzəˈbɪlətɪ] *n chem., phys.* Diffusionsvermögen *nt*.
dif·fus·i·ble [dɪˈfjuːzəbl] *adj* diffusionsfähig.
dif·fus·ing capacity [dɪˈfjuːzɪŋ] *abbr.* **D** *phys.* Diffusionskapazität *f*.
dif·fu·sion [dɪˈfjuːʒn] *n* **1.** *chem., phys.* Diffusion *f*. **2.** (*a. fig.*) Aus-, Verbreitung *f*. **3.** Dialyse *f*. **4.** Immundiffusion *f*.
diffusion anoxia Diffusionsanoxie *f*.
diffusion barrier Diffusionsbarriere *f*.
diffusion capacity → diffusing capacity.
diffusion coefficient *abbr.* **D** Diffusionskoeffizient *m abbr.* D.
 Krogh's d. Krogh'-Diffusionskoeffizient.
diffusion conductivity Diffusionsleitfähigkeit *f*.
diffusion constant → diffusion coefficient.
diffusion equation Diffusionsgleichung *f*.
diffusion equilibrium Diffusionsgleichgewicht *nt*.
diffusion factor *micro.* Hyaluronidase *f*.
diffusion hypoxia Diffusionshypoxie *f*.
diffusion method *micro.* Auxanographie *f*.
diffusion path Diffusionsstrecke *f*.
diffusion potential Diffusionspotential *nt*.
diffusion pressure Diffusionsdruck *m*.
diffusion resistance Diffusionswiderstand *m*.
diffusion respiration Diffusionsatmung *f*.
dif·fu·sive [dɪˈfjuːsɪv] *adj* (*a. fig.*) s. verbreitend; Diffusions-.
dif·fu·sive·ness [-nɪs] *n* Diffusionsvermögen *nt*, -fähigkeit *f*.
dif·fu·siv·i·ty [dɪfjuːˈsɪvətɪ] *n* → diffusion coefficient.
di·flor·a·sone [daɪˈflɔːrəsəʊn] *n pharm.* Diflurason *nt*.
di·flu·cor·to·lone [daɪfluːˈkɔːrtləʊn] *n pharm.* Diflucortolon *nt*.
di·flu·ni·sal [daɪˈfluːnɪsæl] *n pharm.* Diflunisal *nt*.
di·gal·lic acid [daɪˈgælɪk] Gerbsäure *f*, Tannin *nt*, Acidus tannicum.
di·ga·met·ic [daɪgəˈmetɪk] *adj micro.* digametisch, heterogametisch.
di·gas·tric [daɪˈgæstrɪk] **I** *n* Digastrikus *m*, M. digastricus. **II** *adj* zweibäuchig, digastrisch; M. digastricus betr., Digastrikus-.
digastric branch of facial nerve N. facialis-Ast *m* zum hinteren Digastrikusbauch, Ramus digastricus (n. facialis).
digastric fossa Fossa digastrica.
digastric fovea Fossa digastrica.
digastric impression Fossa digastrica.
digastric incisure of temporal bone Inc. mastoidea.
digastric muscle → digastric I.
digastric nerve → digastric branch of facial nerve.
digastric triangle Unterkieferdreieck *nt*, Trigonum submandibulare.
di·gas·tri·cus (muscle) [daɪˈgæstrɪkəs] → digastric I.
di·gen·e·sis [daɪˈdʒenəsɪs] *n bio.* Generationswechsel *m*, Digenese *f*, Digenesis *f*.

digital artery

di·ge·net·ic [daɪdʒəˈnetɪk] *adj bio.* digen.
DiGeorge [dɪˈdʒɔːrdʒ]: **D. syndrome** Di-George-Syndrom *nt*, Schlundtaschensyndrom *nt*, Thymusaplasie *f*.
di·gest [daɪˈdʒest, dɪ-] **I** *vt* **1.** verdauen, abbauen, digerieren; verdauen helfen. **2.** *chem.* digerieren, aufspalten, -lösen. **3.** *fig.* verdauen, (innerlich) verarbeiten. **4.** *fig.* ordnen, klassifizieren. **II** *vi* verdauen, digerieren; s. verdauen lassen, verdaulich sein. **to ~ well** leicht verdaulich sein.
di·gest·ant [-ˈdʒestənt] *n* → digestive I.
di·gest·er [-ˈdʒestər] *n* → digestive I.
di·gest·i·bil·i·ty [-ˌdʒestəˈbɪlətɪ] *n* Verdaulichkeit *f*.
di·gest·i·ble [-ˈdʒestəbl] *adj* durch Verdauung abbaubar, verdaulich, -bar, digestierbar.
di·ges·tion [-ˈdʒestʃn] *n* **1.** Verdauung *f*, Digestion *f*; Verdauungstätigkeit *f*. **to have a good/bad ~** eine gute/schlechte Verdauung haben. **2.** *fig.* (innerliche) Verarbeitung *f*, Verdauung *f*. **3.** *fig.* Ordnen *nt*, Klassifizierung *f*.
di·ges·tive [-ˈdʒestɪv] **I** *n* die Verdauung förderndes *od.* anregendes Mittel *nt*, Digestionsmittel *nt*, Digestivum *nt*. **II** *adj* Verdauung betr. *od.* fördernd, durch sie bedingt, verdauungsfördernd, digestiv, Verdauungs-, Digestions-.
digestive albuminuria diätetische Albuminurie/Proteinurie *f*.
digestive apparatus Verdauungsapparat *m*, Digestitionssystem *nt*, Apparatus digestorius, Systema alimentarium.
digestive canal → digestive tract.
digestive enzyme Verdauungsenzym *nt*.
digestive fever leichter Temperaturanstieg *m* während der Verdauung.
digestive glycosuria alimentäre Glukosurie/Glycosurie *f*.
digestive juice Verdauungssaft *m*.
digestive leukocytosis Verdauungsleukozytose *f*, postprandiale Leukozytose *f*.
digestive proteinuria → digestive albuminuria.
digestive system → digestive apparatus.
digestive tract Verdauungskanal *m*, -trakt *m*, Canalis alimentarius/digestivus, Tractus alimentarius.
digestive tube → digestive tract.
Dighton-Adair [ˈdaɪtn əˈdeər]: **D.-A. syndrome** van der Hoeve-Syndrom *nt*.
dig·it [ˈdɪdʒɪt] *n* **1.** Finger *m*, Zeh(e *f*) *m*, Digitus *m*. **2.** *mathe.* Ziffer *f*, Digit *nt*.
dig·it·al [ˈdɪdʒɪtl] *adj* **1.** Finger betr., mit dem Finger, fingerähnlich, digital, Finger-. **2.** *mathe.* in Ziffern dargestellt, mittels Ziffern, diskret, digital, Digital-.
digital artery Zehen- *od.* Fingerarterie *f*.
 collateral d.s → palmar d.s, proper.
 common d.s of foot plantare Mittelfußarterien *pl*, Aa. metatarsales plantares.
 dorsal d.s of foot Zehenrückenarterien *pl*, dorsale Zehenarterien *pl*, Aa. digitales dorsales pedis.
 dorsal d.s of hand dorsale Fingerarterien *pl*, Aa. digitales dorsales manus.
 palmar d.s, common gemeinsame palmare Fingerarterien *pl*, Aa. digitales palmares communes.
 palmar d.s, proper eigene palmare Fingerarterien *pl*, Aa. digitales palmares propriae.
 plantar d.s, common gemeinsame plantare Zehenarterien *pl*, Aa. digitales plantares communes.
 plantar d.s, proper eigene plantare Zehenarterien *pl*, Aa. digitales plantares propriae.
 volar d.s, common → palmar d.s, common.
 volar d.s, proper → palmar d.s, proper.

digital computer Digitalrechner *m*.
digital examination digitale Untersuchung *f*.
digital fossa 1. Fossa malleoli lateralis. 2. Fossa trochanterica.
digital impressions Impressiones digitatae/gyrorum.
dig·i·tal·in [ˌdɪdʒɪ'tælɪn, 'dɪdʒɪtəlɪn] *n* 1. *pharm.* Digitalin(um) *nt*. 2. *pharm.* Digitalinum verum.
Dig·i·tal·is [ˌdɪdʒɪ'tælɪs, -'teɪl-] *n* 1. *bio.* Fingerhut *m*, Digitalis *f*. 2. *pharm.* Digitalis purpurea folium.
D. feruginea rostfarbener Fingerhut, Digitalis feruginea.
D. lanata wolliger Fingerhut, Digitalis lanata.
D. lutea gelber Fingerhut, Digitalis lutea.
D. purpurea purpurroter Fingerhut, Digitalis purpurea.
digitalis glycoside *pharm.* Digitalisglykosid *nt*, Herzglykosid *nt*.
digitalis leaf → Digitalis 2.
dig·i·tal·ism ['dɪdʒɪtlɪzəm] *n* Digitalisvergiftung *f*, -intoxikation *f*, Digitalismus *m*.
digitalis poisoning → digitalism.
digitalis therapy → digitalization.
digitalis unit Digitaliseinheit *f*.
dig·i·tal·i·za·tion [ˌdɪdʒɪˌtælɪ'zeɪʃn, ˌdɪdʒɪtlaɪ'zeɪʃn] *n* Digitalistherapie *f*, Digitalisierung *f*.
dig·i·tal·ize ['dɪdʒɪtlaɪz, ˌdɪdʒɪ'tælaɪz] *vt* 1. mit Digitalis behandeln, digitalisieren. 2. → digitize.
digital joints Interphalangealgelenke *pl*, IP-Gelenke *pl*, Articc. interphalangeales.
digital nerve Finger- *od.* Zehennerv *m*.
dorsal d.s, radial → dorsal d.s of radial nerve.
dorsal d.s, ulnar → dorsal d.s of ulnar nerve.
dorsal d.s of foot dorsale Zehennerven *pl*, Nn. digitales dorsales pedis.
dorsal d.s of lateral surface of great toe and of medial surface of second toe Nn. digitales dorsales hallucis lateralis et digiti secundi medialis.
dorsal d.s of radial nerve dorsale Fingeräste *pl* des N. radialis, Nn. digitales dorsales n. radialis.
dorsal d.s of ulnar nerve dorsale Fingeräste *pl* des N. ulnaris, Nn. digitales dorsales n. ulnaris.
palmar d.s of median nerve, common palmare Fingeräste *pl* des N. medianus, Nn. digitales palmares communes n. mediani.
palmar d.s of median nerve, proper Endäste *pl* der Fingeräste des N. medianus, Nn. digitales palmares proprii n. mediani.
palmar d.s of ulnar nerve, common palmare Fingeräste *pl* des N. ulnaris, Nn. digitales palmares communes n. ulnaris.
palmar d.s of ulnar nerve, proper Endäste *pl* der palmaren Fingeräste des N. ulnaris, Nn. digitales palmares proprii n. ulnaris.
plantar d.s of lateral plantar nerve, common Nn. digitales plantares communes n. plantaris lateralis.
plantar d.s of lateral plantar nerve, proper Nn. digitales plantares proprii n. plantaris lateralis.
plantar d.s of medial plantar nerve, common Nn. digitales plantares communes n. plantaris medialis.
plantar d.s of medial plantar nerve, proper Nn. digitales plantares proprii n. plantaris medialis.
dig·i·tal·oid ['dɪdʒɪtælɔɪd] *adj* digitalisähnlich, digitaloid.
dig·i·tal·ose [ˌdɪdʒɪ'tæləʊs, -'teɪ-] *n* Digitalose *f*.
digital reflex *neuro.* Fingerbeugereflex *m*, Trömner-Reflex *m*, -Fingerzeichen *nt*, Knipsreflex *m*.
digital subtraction angiography *abbr.* **DSA** *radiol.* digitale Subtraktionsangiographie *f abbr.* DSA.
digital vein Finger- *od.* Zehenvene *f*.
common d.s of foot Vv. digitales communes pedis.
dorsal d.s of foot Venen *pl* des Zehenrückens, Vv. digitales dorsales pedis, Vv. digitales pedis dorsales.
palmar d.s palmare Fingervenen *pl*, Vv. digitales palmares.
plantar d.s Venen *pl* der Zehenbeugeseite, Vv. digitales plantares.
dig·i·tate ['dɪdʒɪteɪt] *adj* 1. *bio.* mit Fingern *od.* fingerähnlichen Fortsätzen, gefingert. 2. fingerähnlich, -förmig.
dig·i·tat·ed ['-teɪtɪd] *adj* → digitate.
digitate warts Verrucae digitatae.
dig·i·ta·tio [dɪdʒɪ'teɪʃɪəʊ] *n*, *pl* **-ti·o·nes** [-teɪʃɪ'əʊniːz] → digitation.
dig·i·ta·tion [ˌdɪdʒɪ'teɪʃn] *n anat.* fingerförmiger Fortsatz *m*, Digitation *f*, Digitatio *f*.
dig·i·ti·form ['dɪdʒɪtəfɔːrm] *adj* fingerähnlich, -förmig.
dig·i·tin ['dɪdʒɪtɪn] *n* → digitonin.
dig·i·tize ['dɪdʒɪtaɪz] *vt* (*EDV*) in Ziffern darstellen, digitalisieren.
dig·i·tog·e·nin [ˌdɪdʒɪ'tɒdʒənɪn, ˌdɪdʒɪtəʊ'dʒenɪn] *n pharm.* Digitogenin *nt*.
dig·i·to·nin [ˌdɪdʒɪ'təʊnɪn] *n pharm.* Digitonin *nt*.
digitonin reaction *lab.* Digitoninreaktion *f*.
dig·i·tox·i·gen·in [ˌdɪdʒə,tɒksɪ'dʒenɪn] *n pharm.* Digitoxigenin *nt*.
dig·i·tox·in [ˌdɪdʒɪ'tɒksɪn] *n pharm.* Digitoxin *nt*.
dig·i·tox·ose [ˌdɪdʒɪ'tɒksəʊs] *n* Digitoxose *f*.
di·glos·sia [daɪ'glɒsɪə] *n embryo.* Lingua bifida.
di·glyc·er·ide [daɪ'glɪsəraɪd] *n old* → diacylglycerine.
diglyceride lipase Lipoproteinlipase *f abbr.* LPL.
dig·ox·i·gen·in [dɪdʒˌɒksɪ'dʒenɪn] *n pharm.* Digoxigenin *nt*.
dig·ox·in [dɪdʒ'ɒksɪn, daɪ'gɒksɪn] *n pharm.* Digoxin *nt*.
Di Guglielmo [dɪ guˈljelmo]: **D.G. disease/ syndrome** Di Guglielmo-Krankheit *f*, -Syndrom *nt*, akute Erythrämie *f*, akute erythrämische Myelose *f*, Erythroblastose *f* des Erwachsenen, akute Erythromyelose *f*.
di·het·er·o·zy·gote [daɪˌhetərə'zaɪgəʊt] *n genet.* Dihybride *f*, Dihybrid *m*.
di·het·er·o·zy·gous [ˌ-'zaɪgəs] *adj genet.* dihybrid.
di·hy·brid [daɪ'haɪbrɪd] **I** *n* → diheterozygote. **II** *adj* → diheterozygous.
di·hy·dral·a·zine [daɪhaɪ'drælozɪːn- zɪn] *n pharm.* Dihydralazin *nt*.
di·hy·drate [daɪ'haɪdreɪt] *n* Dihydrat *nt*.
di·hy·dric alcohol [daɪ'haɪdrɪk] zweiwertiger Alkohol *m*.
di·hy·dro·bi·op·ter·in [daɪˌhaɪdrəʊbaɪ'ɒptərɪn] *n* Dihydrobiopterin *nt*.
dihydrobiopterin reductase Dihydrobiopterinreduktase *f*.
dihydrobiopterin reductase deficiency atypische Phenylketonurie *f*, Dihydrobiopterinreduktasemangel *m*, Hyperphenylalaninämie Typ V *f*.
dihydrobiopterin synthetase Dihydrobiopterinsynthetase *f*.
dihydrobiopterin synthetase deficiency → dihydrobiopterin reductase deficiency.
di·hy·dro·cal·cif·er·ol [ˌ-kæl'sɪfərɒl, -rɑl] *n* Dihydrocalciferol *nt*, Vitamin D_4 *nt*.
di·hy·dro·cho·les·ter·ol [ˌ-kə'lestərəʊl, -rɒl] *n* Cholestanol *nt*, Dihydrocholesterin *nt*.
di·hy·dro·co·deine [ˌ-'kəʊdiːn, -dɪən] *n pharm.* Dihydrocodein *nt*.
di·hy·dro·co·de·i·none [ˌ-kəʊ'dɪənəʊn] *n pharm.* Hydrocodon *nt*.
di·hy·dro·cor·ti·sol [ˌ-'kɔːrtəsɒl, -səʊl] *n pharm.* Dihydrokortisol *nt*, Dihydrocortisol *nt*.
di·hy·dro·di·pi·co·lin·ate [ˌ-daɪˌpɪkə'lɪneɪt] *n* Dihydrodipicolinat *nt*.
dihydrodipicolinate synthase Dihydrodipicolinatsynthase *f*.
(2,3-)di·hy·dro·di·pi·co·lin·ic acid [ˌ-daɪpɪkə'lɪnɪk] (2,3-)Dihydrodipicolinsäure *f*.
di·hy·dro·er·go·cor·nine [ˌ-ˌɜːrgəʊ'kɔːrniːn, -nɪn] *n pharm.* Dihydroergocornin *nt*.
di·hy·dro·er·go·cris·tine [ˌ-ˌɜːrgə'krɪstiːn, -tɪn] *n pharm.* Dihydroergocristin *nt*.
di·hy·dro·er·got·a·mine [ˌ-ɜːr'gɒtəmiːn, -mɪn] *n abbr.* **DHE** *pharm.* Dihydroergotamin *nt abbr.* DHE.
di·hy·dro·er·go·tox·ine [ˌ-ˌɜːrgə'tɒksiːn, -sɪn] *n pharm.* Dihydroergotoxin *nt*.
di·hy·dro·fo·late reductase [ˌ-'fəʊleɪt] *abbr.* **DHFR** Dihydrofolatreduktase *f abbr.* DHFR.
dihydrofolate reductase deficiency Dihydrofolatreduktasemangel *m*, DHFR-Mangel *m*.
di·hy·dro·fo·lic acid [ˌ-'fəʊlɪk, -'fɑl-] Dihydrofolsäure *f*.
dihydrofolic acid reductase → dihydrofolate reductase.
di·hy·dro·fol·lic·u·lin [ˌ-fə'lɪkjəlɪn, -fɑ-] *n* Estradiol *nt*, Östradiol *nt*.
di·hy·dro·lip·o·am·ide dehydrogenase [ˌ-'lɪpə'æmaɪd, -ɪd] Dihydrolipoyltransacetylase *f*.
dihydrolipoamide dehydrogenase Dihydrolipoyldehydrogenase *f*, Lipoamiddehydrogenase *f*.
dihydrolipoamide succinyltransferase Dihydrolipoylsuccinyltransferase *f*.
di·hy·dro·li·po·ic acid [ˌ-lɪ'pəʊɪk] Dihydroliposäure *f*.
di·hy·dro·lip·o·yl dehydrogenase [ˌ-'lɪpəwɪl] → dihydrolipoamide dehydrogenase.
dihydrolipoyl transacetylase → dihydrolipoamide acetyltransferase.
di·hy·dro·mor·phi·none [ˌ-'mɔːrfɪnəʊn] *n pharm.* Hydromorphon *nt*, Dihydromorphinon *nt*.
di·hy·dro·or·o·tase [ˌ-'ɔːrəteɪz] *n* Dihydroorotase *f*.
di·hy·dro·o·rot·ic acid [ˌ-ɔː'rɒtɪk] Dihydroorotsäure *f*.
di·hy·dro·pter·i·dine reductase [ˌ-'terɪdiːn, -dɪn] *abbr.* **DHPR** Dihydropteridinreduktase *f abbr.* DHPR.
di·hy·dro·ret·i·nal [ˌ-'retnæl] *n* Dihydroretinal *nt*.
di·hy·dro·ret·i·nol [ˌ-'retnɑl, -ɒl] *n* Dihydroretinol *nt*, Retinol$_2$ *nt*, Vitamin A$_2$ *nt*.
di·hy·dro·strep·to·my·cin [ˌ-ˌstreptəʊ'maɪsn] *n pharm.* Dihydrostreptomycin *nt abbr.* DSM.
di·hy·dro·ta·chys·te·rol [ˌ-tæ'kɪstərɒl, -rəʊl] *n pharm.* Dihydrotachysterin *nt*, -sterol *nt*, A.T. 10 (*nt*).
di·hy·dro·tes·tos·ter·one [ˌ-tes'tɒstərəʊn] *n abbr.* **DHT** *pharm.* Dihydrotestosteron *nt abbr.* DHT.
di·hy·dro·thee·lin [ˌ-'θiːlɪn] *n* Estradiol *nt*, Östradiol *nt*.
5,6-di·hy·dro·u·ra·cil [ˌ-'jʊərəsɪl] *n* 5,6-Dihydrouracil *nt*.

dihydrouracil dehydrogenase Dihydrouracildehydrogenase f.
di·hy·dro·u·ri·dine [ˌ-'juərɪdiːn, -dɪn] n abbr. **DHU** Dihydrouridin nt abbr. DHU.
di·hy·drox·y·ac·e·tone [ˌdaɪhaɪˌdrɑksɪ'æsɪtəʊn] n Dihydroxyazeton nt, -aceton nt.
dihydroxyacetone phosphate Dihydroxyacetonphosphat nt, Phosphodihydroxyaceton nt.
dihydroxyacetone phosphate acyltransferase Dihydroxyacetonphosphatacyltransferase f.
di·hy·drox·y·ac·id dehydratase [ˌ-'æsɪd] Dihydroxysäuredehydratase f.
2,5-di·hy·drox·y·ben·zo·ic acid [ˌ-ben'zəʊɪk] Gentisinsäure f, Dihydroxybenzoesäure f.
(1,25-)di·hy·drox·y·cho·le·cal·cif·er·ol [ˌ-ˌkəʊləkæl'sɪfərɒl, -rɑl] n (1,25-)Dihydroxycholecalciferol nt.
di·hy·drox·y·flu·o·rane [ˌ-'flʊəræn] n Fluorescein nt, -zein nt, Resorcinphthalein nt.
2,5-di·hy·drox·y·phen·yl·a·ce·tic acid [ˌ-ˌfenlə'siːtɪk] Homogentisinsäure f, 2,5--Dihydroxyphenylessigsäure f.
3,4-di·hy·drox·y·phen·yl·al·a·nine [-ˌfenɪl'æləniːn] n → dopa.
2,6-di·hy·drox·y·pu·rine [ˌ-'pjʊəriːn, -rɪn] n 2,6-Dihydroxypurin nt, Xanthin nt.
di·i·o·dide [daɪ'aɪədaɪd] n Dijodid nt, Diiodid nt.
3,5-di·i·o·do·thy·ro·nine [daɪˌaɪədəʊ'θaɪrəniːn, -nɪn] n 3,5-Dijodthyronin nt.
(3,5-)di·i·o·do·ty·ro·sine [ˌ-'taɪrəsiːn, -sɪn] n (3,5-)Dijodtyrosin nt.
di·i·so·cy·a·nate asthma [daɪˌaɪsə'saɪəneɪt, -nɪt] Isozyanatasthma nt.
di·i·so·pro·pyl fluorophosphate [daɪˌaɪsəʊ'prəʊpɪl] abbr. **DFP** Diisopropylfluorphosphat nt abbr. DFP, Fluostigmin nt.
di·kar·y·on [daɪ'kæriən] n micro. Dikaryon nt.
di·kar·y·ote [daɪ'kæriəʊt] n bio. Dikaryo(n)t m.
di·ke·tone [daɪ'kiːtəʊn] n chem. Diketon nt.
di·ke·to·pi·per·a·zine [daɪˌkiːtəʊpaɪ'perəziːn, -'pɪpərəziːn] n Diketopiperazin nt.
dik·ty·o·ma [dɪktɪ'əʊmə] n patho. Diktyom nt.
di·lac·er·a·tion [daɪˌlæsə'reɪʃn] n 1. Zerreißung f. 2. ophthal. Dilazeration f.
Di·lan·tin gingivitis/hyperplasia [daɪ'læntɪn] → diphenylhydantoin gingivitis.
di·lat·a·bil·i·ty [daɪˌleɪtə'bɪləti] n phys. Dehnbarkeit f, (Aus-)Dehnungsvermögen nt.
di·lat·a·ble [daɪ'leɪtəbl] adj (aus-)dehnbar, dilatierbar, dilatabel.
di·la·tan·cy [daɪ'leɪtnsɪ] n phys. Fließverfestigung f, Dilatanz f.
di·lat·ant [daɪ'leɪtnt] adj phys. dilatant.
dil·a·ta·tion [ˌdɪlə'teɪʃn, ˌdaɪlə-] n 1. phys. Dilatation f, (Aus-)Dehnung f. 2. (pathologische od. künstliche) Erweiterung f, Dilatation f.
dilatation catheter Dilatationskatheter m.
dil·a·ta·tor ['dɪləteɪtə(r), 'daɪ-] n 1. chir. Dilatator m, Dilatorium nt. 2. anat. Dilatator m, M. dilatator/dilator. 3. pharm. Dilatans nt, Dilatorium nt.
dilatator muscle → dilatator 2.
dilatator naris (muscle) Dilatator m naris, Pars alaris m. nasalis, M. dilatator naris.
dilatator pupillae (muscle) Pupillenöffner m, Dilatator m pupillae, M. dilator/dilatator pupillae.
di·late [daɪ'leɪt] I vt dilatieren, (aus-)dehnen, (aus-)weiten, erweitern. II vi dilatieren, s. (aus-)dehnen, s. (aus-)weiten, s. erweitern.
di·la·ter [daɪ'leɪtər, 'daɪ-] n → dilatator.

di·lat·ing catheter [daɪ'leɪtɪŋ, 'daɪ-] Dilatationskatheter m.
dilating pains gyn. Schmerzen pl während der Eröffnungsphase.
di·la·tion [daɪ'leɪʃn, dɪ-] n → dilatation.
dilation catheter Dilatationskatheter m.
dil·a·tom·e·ter [ˌdɪlə'tɒmɪtər, ˌdaɪ-] n chem., phys. Dilatometer nt.
di·la·tor [daɪ'leɪtər, dɪ-, 'daɪ-] n → dilatator.
d. of naris → dilatator naris (muscle).
d. of pupil → dilatator pupillae (muscle).
dilator muscle → dilatator 2.
d. of naris → dilatator naris (muscle).
d. of pupil → dilatator pupillae (muscle).
di·la·zep ['dɪləzep] n pharm. Dilazep f.
dill oil [dɪl] pharm. Dillöl nt.
dil·ti·a·zem [dɪl'taɪəzem] n pharm. Diltiazem nt.
dil·u·ent ['dɪljəwənt, -jʊənt] I n Verdünner m, Verdünnungsmittel nt, Diluens nt, Diluent m. II adj verdünnend.
di·lute [dɪ'l(j)uːt, daɪ-] I adj verdünnt. II vt verdünnen, verwässern, strecken, diluieren.
di·lut·ed [dɪ'l(j)uːtɪd, daɪ-] adj → dilute I.
di·lu·tion [dɪ'l(j)uːʃn, daɪ-] n Verdünnung f; verdünnte Lösung f, Dilution f.
di·lu·tion·al hyponatremia [dɪ'l(j)uːʃnl, daɪ-] Verdünnungshyponatr(i)ämie f.
dilution anemia Verdünnungsanämie f; Hydrämie f, Hydroplasmie f.
dilution coagulopathy Verdünnungskoagulopathie f.
dilution coefficient Verdünnungskoeffizient m.
dilution test Verdünnungstest m.
dim [dɪm] I adj 1. schwach, trüb; (halb-)dunkel; dämmerig. 2. undeutlich, verschwommen; (Farben) matt, blaß; (Augen) matt, trüb; (Augenlicht) schwach; (Erinnerung) verschwommen. II vt verdunkeln, abblenden, dämpfen; (a. fig.) trüben. III vi trübe od. dunkler od. matt werden; (a. fig.) s. trüben.
Di·mas·tig·a·moe·ba [daɪˌmæstɪgə'miːbə] n micro. Naegleria nt.
di·me·di·ate placenta [daɪ'miːdɪət] Placenta duplex.
di·me·lia [daɪ'miːlɪə] n embryo. Dimelie f.
di·me·lus [daɪ'miːləs] n embryo. Dimelus m.
di·men·hy·dri·nate [daɪˌmen'haɪdrəneɪt] n pharm. Dimenhydrinat nt.
di·men·sion [daɪ'menʃn, dɪ-] n 1. Ausdehnung f, Abmessung f, Maß nt, Dimension f. 2. (a. fig.) Ausmaß nt, Größe f, Grad nt, Dimension f. 3. ⚲s pl phys. Dimension f.
di·men·sion·less [daɪ'menʃnləs, dɪ-] adj 1. phys. dimensionslos. 2. winzig, klein.
di·mer ['daɪmər] n chem., micro. Dimer nt, Dimeres f.
di·mer·cap·rol [ˌdaɪmər'kæprɒl, -rəʊl] n Dimercaprol nt, British antilewisit nt abbr. **BAL**, 2,3-Dimercaptopropanol nt.
di·mer·ic [daɪ'merɪk] adj 1. chem. zweiteilig, zweigliedrig. 2. dimerous f.
di·mer·i·za·tion [ˌdaɪmeraɪ'zeɪʃn] n Dimerisierung f.
dim·er·ous ['dɪmərəs] adj bio. zweiteilig, dimer.
di·met·a·crine [daɪ'metəkriːn] n pharm. Dimetacrin nt.
di·meth·i·cone [daɪ'meθɪkəʊn] n pharm. Dimeticon nt.
di·meth·in·dene [daɪ'meθɪndiːn] n pharm. Dimetinden nt.
di·meth·is·ter·one [daɪmeθ'ɪstərəʊn] n pharm. Dimethisteron nt.
2,5-dimethoxy-4-methylamphetamine n abbr. **DOM** pharm. 2,5-Dimethoxy-4-methylamphetamin nt abbr. DOM.
3,4-di·me·thox·y·phen·yl·eth·yl·am·ine [daɪmɪˌθɑksɪˌfenlˌeθɪl'æmɪn] n abbr.

DMPE pharm. 3,4-Dimethyloxyphenylessigsäure f abbr. DMPE.
di·me·thox·y·phen·yl penicillin [daɪmɪˌθɑksɪ'fenl] pharm. Methizillin nt, Methicillin nt.
di·meth·yl·a·cet·a·mide [daɪˌmeθələ'setəmaɪd, -ˌæsɪ'tæmaɪd] n abbr. **DMAC** Dimethylacetamid nt abbr. DMAC.
N^2,N^2-di·meth·yl·ad·e·nine [ˌ-'ædənɪn, -niːn] n N^2,N^2-Dimethyladenin nt.
(3,3-)di·meth·yl·al·lyl·py·ro·phos·phor·ic acid [ˌ-ˌælɪlˌpaɪrəʊfɑs'fɔːrɪk] (3,3-)Dimethylallylpyrophosphorsäure f.
di·meth·yl·al·lyl·trans·fer·ase [ˌ-ˌælɪl'trænsfəreɪz] n Dimethylallyltransferase f.
di·meth·yl·a·mine [ˌ-ə'miːn, -'æmɪn] n Dimethylamin nt.
p-di·meth·yl·a·mi·no·az·o·ben·zene [ˌ-əˌmiːnəʊˌæzəʊ'benziːn, -ˌæmɪnəʊ-] n Butter-, Dimethylgelb nt, p-Dimethylaminoazobenzol nt abbr. **DAB**.
5-dimethylamino-1-naphthalenesulfonic acid abbr. **DANS** 5-Dimethylamino-1--naphthalinsulfonsäure f abbr. DANS.
1,3-di·meth·yl·am·yl·a·mine [ˌ-ˌæmɪlə'miːn, -'æmɪn] n 1,3-Dimethylamylamin nt, Methylhexanamin nt.
di·meth·yl·ar·sin·ic acid [ˌ-ɑːr'sɪnɪk] Kakodylsäure f, Dimethylarsinsäure f.
7,12-di·meth·yl·benz(a)·an·thra·cene [daɪˌmeθəlˌbenz(ə)'ænθrəsiːn] n abbr. **DMBA** 7,12-Dimethylbenzanthracen nt abbr. DMBA.
di·meth·yl·ben·zene [ˌ-'benziːn] n Xylol nt, Dimethylbenzol nt.
5,6-di·meth·yl·ben·zim·id·az·ole [ˌ-ˌbenzɪmɪ'dæzəʊl, -ˌbenzə'mɪdəzəʊl] n 5,6-Dimethylbenzimidazol nt.
di·meth·yl·car·bi·nol [ˌ-'kɑːrbɪnɒl, -nɑl] n Isopropanol nt, Isopropylalkohol m.
β,β-di·meth·yl·cys·te·ine [ˌ-'sɪstiːɪn, -sɪstɪˌiːn] n pharm. D-Penicillamin nt, D-β,β--Dimethylcystein nt, β-Mercaptovalin nt.
di·meth·yl·gly·cine [ˌ-'glaɪsɪn, -glaɪ'siːn] n Dimethylglycin nt.
N^2,N^2-di·meth·yl·gua·nine [ˌ-'gwɑniːn] n N^2,N^2-Dimethylguanin nt.
di·meth·yl·ke·tone [ˌ-'kiːtəʊn] n Azeton nt, Aceton nt, Dimethylketon nt.
dimethyl morphine Thebain nt.
dimethyl phthalate abbr. **DMP** Dimethylphthalat nt abbr. DMP.
dimethyl sulfate Dimethylsulfat nt.
dimethyl sulfoxide abbr. **DMSO** Dimethylsulfoxid nt abbr. DMSO.
di·meth·yl·the·tin [ˌ-'θiːtɪn] n Dimethylthetin nt.
dimethylthetin homocysteine methyltransferase Dimethylthetin-Homocystein-Methyltransferase f.
di·meth·yl·thi·am·bu·tene [ˌ-'θaɪæm'bjuːtiːn] n pharm. Dimethylthiambuten nt.
di·meth·yl·tryp·ta·mine [ˌ-'trɪptəmiːn, -mɪn] n abbr. **DMT** pharm. Dimethyltryptamin nt abbr. DMT.
dimethyl tubocurarine Dimethyltubocurarin(ium) nt.
dimethyl tubocurarine chloride pharm. Dimethyltubocurarinium-chlorid nt.
di·me·tria [daɪ'miːtrɪə] n gyn. Uterus duplex/didelphys.
di·mid·i·ate hermaphroditism [daɪ'mɪdɪeɪt] Hermaphroditismus (verus) dimidiatus/lateralis.
di·min·ish [dɪ'mɪnɪʃ] I vt 1. verringern, (ver-)mindern; verkleinern. 2. reduzieren, herabsetzen; (ab-)schwächen. II vi 3. s. vermindern, s. verringern, weniger werden. 4. abnehmen.
di·min·ished thirst [dɪ'mɪnɪʃd] (pathologisch) verminderter Durst m, Hypodipsie f.

diminution

dim·i·nu·tion [ˌdɪməˈn(j)uːʃn] n (Ver-)Minderung f, Verringerung f; Verkleinerung f; Herabsetzung f; Abnahme f; Reduktion f.
dim light Dämmerlicht nt.
Dimmer [ˈdɪmər]: **D.'s keratitis** ophthal. Dimmer-Keratitis f, Keratitis nummularis.
dim·ness [ˈdɪmnɪs] n Trübheit f; Halbdunkel nt; Undeutlichkeit f, Verschwommenheit f, Unschärfe f; Mattheit f, Glanzlosigkeit f.
di·mor·phic [daɪˈmɔːrfɪk] adj → dimorphous.
dimorphic fungus micro. dimorpher Pilz m.
di·mor·phism [daɪˈmɔːrfɪzəm] n Dimorphie f, Dimorphismus m.
di·mor·phous [daɪˈmɔːrfəs] adj zweigestaltig, dimorph; in zwei verschiedenen Formen auftretend.
dimorphous leprosy dimorphe Lepra f, Borderline-Lepra f abbr. BL, Lepra dimorpha.
dim·ple [ˈdɪmpl] **I** n 1. Grübchen nt. 2. Delle f, Vertiefung f. **II** vi Grübchen bekommen, s. einbeulen.
dim·pled [ˈdɪmpld] adj mit Grübchen.
di·ni·trate [daɪˈnaɪtreɪt] n Dinitrat nt.
di·ni·tro·a·mi·no·phe·nol [daɪˌnaɪtrəʊəˌmiːnəʊˈfiːnəʊl, -nɒl] n Dinitroaminophenol nt, Pikraminsäure f.
di·ni·tro·ben·zene [ˌ-ˈbenziːn, -benˈziːn] n abbr. **DNB** Dinitrobenzol nt abbr. DNB.
di·ni·tro·cel·lu·lose [ˌ-ˈseljələʊs] n Dinitrozellulose f, Schießbaumwolle f, Nitrozellulose f.
(2,4-)di·ni·tro·chlo·ro·ben·zene [ˌ-ˌklɔːrəˈbenziːn] n abbr. **DNCB** (2,4-)Dinitrochlorbenzol nt abbr. DNCB.
di·ni·tro·cre·sol [ˌ-ˈkriːsɒl, -sal] n → dinitro-o-cresol.
(2,4-)di·ni·tro·fluor·o·ben·zene [ˌ-ˌflʊərəʊˈbenziːn, -ˈflʊər-] n abbr. **DNFB** (2,4-)Dinitrofluorbenzol nt abbr. DNFB, Sanger-Reagenz nt.
dinitro-o-cresol n Dinitro-o-Kresol nt abbr. DNK.
di·ni·tro·phe·nol [ˌ-ˈfiːnɒl, -nal] n abbr. **DNP** Dinitrophenol nt abbr. DNP.
Di·nob·del·la [daɪnɒbˈdelə] n micro. Dinobdella f.
Din·o·flag·el·la·ta [ˌdaɪnəˌflædʒəˈleɪtə] pl micro. Dinoflagellaten pl, Dinoflagellata pl.
di·no·flag·el·late [ˌ-ˈflædʒəleɪt] n micro. Dinoflagellat m.
Di·no·fla·gel·li·da [ˌ-fləˈdʒelɪdə] pl → Dinoflagellata.
di·no·prost [ˈ-prɒst] n Dinoprost nt, Prostaglandin F₂α nt abbr. PGF₂α.
di·no·pros·tone [ˌ-ˈprɒstəʊn] n Dinoproston nt, Prostaglandin E₂ nt abbr. PGE₂.
di·nu·cle·o·tide [daɪˈn(j)uːklɪətaɪd] n Dinukleotid nt.
Di·oc·to·phy·ma renale [daɪˌɒktəˈfaɪmə] micro. Nierenwurm m, Riesenpalisadenwurm m, Eustrongylus gigas, Dioctophyma renale.
di·oc·tyl calcium sulfosuccinate [daɪˈɒktɪl] n docusate calcium.
dioctyl sodium sulfosuccinate → docusate sodium.
di·oe·cious adj → diecious.
di·ol·a·mine [daɪˈɒləmiːn] n → diethanolamine.
di·op·sim·e·ter [daɪɒpˈsɪmɪtər] n ophthal. Gesichtsfeldmesser m.
di·op·ter [daɪˈɒptər] n abbr. **D** Dioptrie f abbr. dpt, old Brechkrafteinheit f abbr. BKE.
di·op·tom·e·ter [daɪɒpˈtɒmɪtər] n ophthal. Refraktionsmesser m, Dioptometer nt.
di·op·tom·e·try [daɪəpˈtɒmətrɪ] n ophthal. Refraktionsmessung f, Dioptometrie f.
di·op·tric [daɪˈɒptrɪk] **I** n → diopter. **II** adj Dioptrie betr., dioptrisch; (licht-)brechend.
dioptric aberration phys. sphärische Aberration f.
di·op·tri·cal [daɪˈɒptrɪkl] adj → dioptric II.
dioptric apparatus dioptrischer Apparat m.
di·op·trics [daɪˈɒptrɪks] pl phys. Brechungs-, Refraktionslehre f, Dioptrik f.
di·op·trom·e·ter [daɪəpˈtrɒmɪtər] n → dioptometer.
di·op·trom·e·try [daɪəpˈtrɒmɪtrɪ] n → dioptometry.
di·op·try [ˈdaɪəptrɪ] n → diopter.
di·ose [ˈdaɪəʊs] n Diose f, Glykolaldehyd m.
di·ox·ane [daɪˈɒkseɪn] n (1,4-)Dioxan nt, Diäthylendioxid nt.
di·ox·id [daɪˈɒksaɪd, -ɪd] n Dioxid nt.
di·ox·in [daɪˈɒksɪn] n Dioxin nt.
di·ox·y·gen [daɪˈɒksɪdʒən] n molekularer Sauerstoff m.
di·ox·y·gen·ase [daɪˈɒksɪdʒəneɪz] n Sauerstofftransferase f, Dioxygenase f.
dip [dɪp] **I** n 1. (Unter-, Ein-)Tauchen nt. 2. (Tauch-)Bad nt, Lösung f. 3. Neigung f, Senkung f, Gefälle nt; Sinken nt. 4. gyn. Dip m. 5. card. Dip m. **II** vt 6. (ein-)tauchen (in in). 7. färben, in eine Farblösung tauchen. **III** vi 8. untertauchen, eintauchen; sinken. 9. s. senken, s. neigen.
DI particles micro. defekte interferierende Viruspartikel pl, DI-Partikel pl.
di·pep·ti·dase [daɪˈpeptɪdeɪz] n Dipeptidase f.
di·pep·tide [daɪˈpeptaɪd] n Dipeptid nt.
di·pep·ti·dyl carboxypeptidase [daɪˈpeptədɪl] (Angiotensin-)Converting-Enzym nt abbr. ACE.
Di·pet·a·lo·ne·ma [daɪˌpetləʊˈniːmə] n micro. Dipetalonema f.
di·pet·a·lo·ne·mi·a·sis [daɪˌpetləʊnɪˈmaɪəsɪs] n Mansonelliasis f.
di·phal·lia [daɪˈfælɪə] n embryo. Diphallie f.
di·phal·lus [ˈdaɪfæləs] n embryo. Diphallus m.
di·phase [ˈdaɪfeɪz] adj zwei-, diphasisch, Zweiphasen-.
di·pha·sic [daɪˈfeɪzɪk] adj → diphase.
diphasic complex card. (EKG) diphasischer Komplex m.
diphasic meningoencephalitis zentraleuropäische Zeckenenzephalitis f, Frühsommer-Enzephalitis f abbr. FSE, Frühsommer-Meningoenzephalitis f abbr. FSME, Central European encephalitis abbr. CEE.
diphasic milk fever → diphasic meningoencephalitis.
di·pheb·u·zol [daɪˈfebjəzɒl, -əʊl] n pharm. Phenylbutazon nt.
di·phen·a·di·one [daɪˌfenəˈdaɪəʊn] n pharm. Diphenadion nt.
di·phen·hy·dra·mine [ˌdaɪfenˈhaɪdrəmiːn] n pharm. Diphenhydramin nt.
diphenhydramine hydrochloride pharm. Diphenhydraminhydrochlorid nt.
di·phe·nol oxidase [daɪˈfiːnɒl, -nɒl] o-Diphenoloxidase f, Cathecholoxidase f, Polyphenoloxidase f.
di·phen·ox·y·late [ˌdaɪfenˈɒksɪleɪt] n pharm. Diphenoxylat nt.
di·phen·yl [daɪˈfenl] n Bi-, Diphenyl nt.
di·phen·yl·a·mine [daɪˌfenləˈmiːn, -ˈæmɪn] n Diphenylamin nt.
di·phen·yl·a·mine·ar·sine chloride [ˌ-əˌmiːnˈɑːrsiːn, -sɪn, -ˌæmɪn] Diphenylaminsinchlorid nt, Adamsit m.
di·phen·yl·chlor·ar·sine [ˌ-ˌklɔːˈrɑːrsiːn, -sɪn, -ˌklɔː-] n abbr. **DA** Diphenylarsinchlorid nt, Clark I nt.
di·phen·yl·cy·an·ar·sine [ˌ-ˌsaɪənˈɑːrsiːn, -sɪn] n Diphenylarsincyanid nt, Clark II nt.
di·phen·yl·hy·dan·to·in [ˌ-haɪˈdæntəwɪn] n pharm. Diphenylhydantoin nt, Phenytoin nt.
diphenylhydantoin gingivitis/hyperplasia Zahnfleischhyperplasie f bei Phenytointherapie.
di·phen·yl·pyr·a·line [ˌ-ˈpɪərəliːn] n pharm. Diphenylpyralin nt.
di·phos·gene [daɪˈfɒzdʒiːn] n Diphosgen nt.
di·phos·pha·ti·dyl·glyc·er·ol [daɪˌfɒsfəˌtaɪdlˈɡlɪsərɒl, -rəl] n Diphosphatidylglycerin nt, Cardiolipin nt.
1,3-di·phos·pho·glyc·er·ate [daɪˌfɒsfəʊˈɡlɪsəreɪt] n abbr. **1,3-DPG** 1,3-Diphosphoglycerat nt abbr. 1,3-DIPG, 3-Phosphoglyceroylphosphat nt, Negelein-Ester nt.
2,3-diphosphoglycerate n abbr. **2,3-DPG** 2,3-Diphosphoglycerat nt abbr. 2,3-DIPG, Greenwald-Ester m.
diphosphoglycerate mutase Diphosphoglyceratmutase f.
diphosphoglycerate phosphatase Diphosphoglyceratphosphatase f.
di·phos·pho·pyr·i·dine nucleotide [ˌ-ˈpɪrɪdiːn, -dɪn] abbr. **DPN** old → nicotinamide-adenine dinucleotide.
di·phos·pho·thi·a·min [ˌ-ˈθaɪəmɪn] n Thiaminpyrophosphat nt. TPP, old Cocarboxylase f.
di·phos·pho·trans·fer·ase [ˌ-ˈtrænsfəreɪz] n Diphosphotransferase f, Pyrophosphokinase f, Pyrophosphotransferase f.
diph·the·ria [dɪfˈθɪərɪə, dɪp-] n Diphtherie f, Diphtheria f.
diphtheria anatoxin Diphtherie-Anatoxin nt, Diphtherie(formol)toxoid nt.
diphtheria antitoxin Diphtherieantitoxin nt.
diphtheria bacillus Diphtheriebazillus m, -bakterium nt, (Klebs-)Löffler-Bazillus m, Corynebacterium/Bact. diphtheriae.
diph·the·ri·al [dɪfˈθɪərɪəl, dɪp-] adj → diphtheric.
diphtheria-like adj → diphtheroid II.
diphtheria toxin Diphtherietoxin nt.
diagnostic d. → d. for Schick test.
d. for Schick test Schick-Test-Toxin.
diphtheria toxoid → diphtheria anatoxin.
diph·ther·ic [dɪfˈθerɪk, dɪp-] adj Diphtherie betr., durch sie verursacht, diphtherisch, Diphtherie-.
diphtheric conjunctivitis Conjunctivitis diphtherica.
diphtheric inflammation diphtherische Entzündung f, pseudomembranös-nekrotisierende Entzündung f.
diphtheric paralysis (post-)diphtherische Lähmung f.
diph·the·rit·ic [ˌdɪfθəˈrɪtɪk] adj → diphtheric.
diphtheritic croup echter/diphtherischer Krupp m.
diphtheritic cystitis diphtherische/kruppöse (Harn-)Blasenentzündung/Zystitis f.
diphtheritic enteritis Enteritis diphtherica.
diphtheritic laryngitis Kehlkopfdiphtherie f, Laryngitis diphtherica.
diphtheritic membrane diphtherische Pseudomembran f.
diphtheritic myocarditis diphtherische Myokarditis f, Myokarditis f bei Diphtherie.

diphtheritic paralysis → diphtheric paralysis.
diphtheritic pharyngitis Rachendiphtherie f.
diph·the·roid ['dɪfθərɔɪd] **I** n **1.** coryneformes Bakterium nt. **2.** old → Propionibacterium. **3.** Pseudodiphtherie f, Diphtheroid nt. **II** adj diphtherieähnlich, diphtheroid.
diph·the·ro·tox·in [ˌdɪfθərəʊ'tɑksɪn] n → diphtheria toxin.
diph·thong ['dɪfθɑŋ, 'dɪp-] n Doppellaut m, Diphthong m.
diph·thon·gia [dɪf'θɒŋ(g)ɪə, -'θɑŋ-] n Diphthon(g)ie f, Diplophonie f.
di·phyl·lo·both·ri·a·sis [daɪˌfɪləʊbɒθ'raɪəsɪs] n Fischbandwurminfektion f, Diphyllobothriose f, Diphyllobothriasis f, Bothriozephalose f, Bothriocephalosis f.
Di·phyl·lo·both·ri·i·dae [ˌ-bəθ'raɪədiː] pl micro. Diphyllobothriidae pl.
Di·phyl·lo·both·ri·um [ˌ-'bɑθrɪəm] n micro. Diphyllobothrium nt, Bothriocephalus m, Dibothriocephalus m.
D. latum (breiter) Fischbandwurm m, Grubenkopfbandwurm m, Diphyllobothrium latum, Bothriocephalus latus.
D. taenioides → D. latum.
diphyllobothrium anemia Anämie f durch/bei Fischbandwurmbefall.
diph·y·o·dont ['dɪfɪədɒnt] adj diphyodont.
diph·y·o·don·tia [ˌdɪfɪə'dɒnʃɪə] n doppelte Zahnung f, Zahnwechsel m, Diphyodontie f.
di·pic·o·lin·ic acid [daɪpɪkəʊ'lɪnɪk] Dipicolinsäure f.
dipicolinic acid synthetase Dipicolinsäureresynthetase f.
di·pip·a·none [daɪ'pɪpənəʊn] n pharm. Dipipanon nt.
di·piv·e·frin [dɪ'pɪfəfrɪn, daɪ-] n pharm. Dipivefrin nt.
DIPJ abbr. → DIP joint.
DIP joint Endgelenk von Finger od. Zehe, distales Interphalangealgelenk nt, DIP-Gelenk nt, Artic. interphalangealis distalis.
dipl- pref. → diplo-.
dip·la·cu·sia [ˌdɪplə'k(j)uːzɪə] n → diplacusis.
dip·la·cu·sis [ˌ-k(j)uːsɪs] n Doppelhören nt, Diplakusis f, Diplacusis f.
di·ple·gia [daɪ'pliːdʒ(ɪ)ə] n neuro. doppelseitige Lähmung f, Diplegie f, Diplegia f.
di·ple·gic [daɪ'pliːdʒɪk] adj Diplegie betr., von ihr betroffen od. gekennzeichnet, diplegisch.
diplo- pref. Doppel-, Dipl(o)-.
dip·lo·al·bu·min·u·ria [ˌdɪplæl'bjuːmɪ'n(j)ʊərɪə] n kombinierte pathologische u. physiologische Albuminurie f.
dip·lo·ba·cil·lus [ˌ-bə'sɪləs] n, pl **-cil·li** [-'sɪlaɪ] micro. Diplobazillus m, Diplobakterium nt.
d. of Morax-Axenfeld → diplococcus of Morax-Axenfeld.
dip·lo·bac·te·ri·um [ˌ-bæk'tɪərɪəm] n, pl **-ri·a** [-rɪə] micro. Diplobakterium.
dip·lo·blas·tic [ˌ-'blæstɪk] adj embryo. (Keimblatt) zweiblättrig.
dip·lo·car·dia [ˌ-'kɑːrdɪə] n embryo. Diplokardie f.
dip·lo·ceph·a·lus [ˌ-'sɛfələs] n → dicephalus.
dip·lo·ceph·a·ly [ˌ-'sɛfəlɪ] n → dicephaly.
dip·lo·chei·ria [ˌ-'kaɪrɪə] n → dicheiria.
dip·lo·chi·ria [ˌ-'kaɪrɪə] n → dicheiria.
dip·lo·coc·cal [ˌ-'kɑkəl] adj Diplokokken betr., durch sie verursacht, Diplokokken-.
dip·lo·coc·coid [ˌ-'kɑkɔɪd] adj diplokokkenähnlich.

Dip·lo·coc·cus [ˌ-'kɑkəs] n micro. Diplococcus m.
D. gonorrhoeae Gonokokkus m, Gonococcus m, Neisseria gonorrhoeae.
D. intracellularis Meningokokkus m, Neisseria meningitidis.
D. lanceolatus → D. pneumoniae.
D. pneumoniae Fränkel-Pneumokokkus m, Pneumokokkus m, Streptococcus/Diplococcus pneumoniae.
dip·lo·coc·cus [ˌ-'kɑkəs] n, pl **-ci** [-siː, -saɪ, -kiː, -kaɪ] micro. Diplokokkus m, Diplococcus m.
d. of Morax-Axenfeld Diplobakterium nt Morax-Axenfeld, Moraxella (Moraxella) lacunata.
d. of Neisser Gonokokkus, Neisseria gonorrhoeae.
dip·lo·co·ria [ˌ-'kɔːrɪə, -kəʊ-] n ophthal. Dikorie f, Diplokorie f.
dip·lo·ë ['dɪpləʊɪ] n Diploë f, Spongiosa f des Schädeldaches.
dip·lo·et·ic [ˌdɪpləʊ'ɛtɪk] adj Diploë betr., diploisch, Diploë-.
dip·lo·gen·e·sis [ˌ-'dʒɛnəsɪs] n embryo. Diplogenese f.
Dip·lo·go·nop·o·rus [ˌ-gəʊ'nɑpərəs] n micro. Diplogonoporus m.
di·plo·ic [dɪ'pləʊɪk] adj **1.** → diploetic. **2.** doppelt, zweifach.
diploic canals Breschet-, Diploekanäle pl, Canales diploici.
diploic vein Diploëvene f, Breschet'-Vene f, V. diploica.
frontal ~ V. diploica frontalis.
occipital ~ V. diploica occipitalis.
temporal ~, anterior V. diploica temporalis anterior.
temporal ~, posterior V. diploica temporalis posterior.
dip·loid ['dɪplɔɪd] **I** n diploide Zelle f, diploides Individuum nt. **II** adj mit doppeltem Chromosomensatz, diploid.
dip·loi·dy ['dɪplɔɪdɪ] n genet. Diploidie f.
dip·lo·kar·y·on [ˌdɪplə'kærɪən] n Diplokaryon nt.
dip·lo·mo·nad [ˌ-'mɑnæd] n micro. Diplomonade f.
Dip·lo·mo·nad·i·da [ˌ-mə'nædɪdə] pl micro. Diplomonadida pl.
Dip·lo·mon·a·di·na [ˌ-ˌmɑnə'daɪnə] pl micro. Diplomonadina pl.
dip·lo·my·e·lia [ˌ-maɪ'iːlɪə] n embryo. Diplomyelie f.
dip·lon ['dɪplɑn] n → deuteron.
dip·lo·neu·ral [ˌdɪplə'njʊərəl, -nʊ-] adj (Muskel) zweifach innerviert, diploneural.
dip·lo·pa·gus [dɪp'lɑpəgəs] n embryo. Diplopagus m.
dip·lo·phase ['dɪpləfeɪz] n bio. Diplophase f, diploide Phase f.
dip·lo·pho·nia [ˌ-'fəʊnɪə] n → diphthongia.
di·plo·pia [dɪ'pləʊpɪə] n ophthal. Doppel-, Doppeltsehen nt, Diplopie f, Diplopia f.
di·plo·pi·om·e·ter [dɪˌpləʊpɪ'ɑmɪtər] n ophthal. Diplopiemesser m.
dip·lo·po·dia [ˌdɪplə'pəʊdɪə] n embryo. Diplopodie f.
dip·lo·scope ['-skəʊp] n ophthal. Diploskop nt.
dip·lo·so·ma·tia [ˌ-səʊ'meɪʃɪə] n embryo. Diplosomie f.
dip·lo·some ['-səʊm] n Diplosom nt.
dip·lo·so·mia [ˌ-'səʊmɪə] n → diplosomatia.
dip·lo·tene ['-tiːn] n Diplotän nt.
di·po·dia [daɪ'pəʊdɪə] n → diplopodia.
di·po·lar [daɪ'pəʊlər] adj zweipolig, dipolar, bipolar.
dipolar ion Zwitterion nt, dipolares Ion nt.
di·pole ['daɪpəʊl] n **1.** phys. Dipol m. **2.**

chem. dipolares Molekül nt, Dipol m.
dipole moment phys. Dipolmoment nt.
dipole vector Dipolvektor m.
dipped speech [dɪpt] neuro. verwaschene Sprache/Artikulation f.
di·pros·o·pus [daɪ'prɒsəpəs] n embryo. Diprosopus m.
dip·se·sis [dɪp'siːsɪs] n **1.** Durst m. **2.** krankhafter/pathologischer Durst m, krankhaftes Durstgefühl nt.
dip·sia ['dɪpsɪə] n Durst m.
dip·so·gen ['dɪpsədʒən] n durststeigerndes od. -auslösendes Mittel nt.
dip·so·gen·ic [ˌ-'dʒɛnɪk] adj durstverursachend, -auslösend, -steigernd.
dip·so·ma·nia [ˌ-'meɪnɪə, -jə] n inf. Quartalsaufen nt, periodische Trunksucht f, Dipsomanie f.
dip·so·ma·ni·ac [ˌ-'meɪnɪæk] n inf. Quartalsäufer(in f) m, Dipsomane m, -manin f.
dip·so·sis [dɪp'səʊsɪs] n extremer/krankhafter Durst m, krankhaftes Durstgefühl nt.
Dip·ter·a ['dɪptərə, -trə] pl bio. Zweiflügler pl, Diptera pl.
di·py·gus [daɪ'paɪgəs, 'dɪpɪgəs] n embryo. Dipygus m.
dip·y·li·di·a·sis [ˌdɪpəlɪ'daɪəsɪs] n Infektion f od. Befall m durch Dipylidium caninum, Dipylidiasis f.
Dip·y·lid·i·um [ˌdɪpə'lɪdɪəm] n micro. Dipylidium nt.
D. caninum Gurkenkernbandwurm m, Dipylidium caninum.
di·py·rid·a·mole [daɪpaɪ'rɪdəməʊl] n pharm. Dipyridamol nt.
di·rect [dɪ'rɛkt, daɪ-] **I** adj **1.** direkt, gerade; unmittelbar, persönlich. **2.** klar, eindeutig; offen, ehrlich. **II** vt **3.** richten, lenken (to an; towards auf). **4.** leiten, regeln, führen; anordnen, bestimmen; befehlen. **as ~ed** wie verordnet.
direct away from vt jdn./etw. ablenken von.
direct access direkter Zugriff m, Direktzugriff m.
direct antagonists (Muskel) direkte Antagonisten pl.
direct astigmatism ophthal. Astigmatismus m nach der Regel, Astigmatismus rectus.
direct auscultation direkte Auskultation f.
direct bilirubin direktes/konjugiertes/gepaartes Bilirubin nt.
direct calorimetry direkte Kalorimetrie f.
direct current abbr. **D.C.** electr. Gleichstrom m.
direct diplopia ophthal. direkte/gleichseitige/ungekreuzte/homonyme Diplopie f, Diplopia simplex.
direct fracture ortho. direkte Fraktur f, direkter Bruch m.
direct generation bio. ungeschlechtliche/vegetative Fortpflanzung f.
direct hernia chir. innerer/direkter/gerader Leistenbruch m, Hernia inguinalis interna/medialis/directa.
direct image virtuelles/scheinbares Bild nt.
di·rec·tion [dɪ'rɛkʃn, daɪ-] n **1.** Richtung f. **2.** fig. Tendenz f, Strömung f, Richtung f. **3.** Leitung f, Führung f, Aufsicht f. **4.** Anweisung f, Anleitung f, (An-)Weisung f, Vorschrift f, Anordnung f. **by/at ~ of** auf Anweisung von.
d. of rotation Drehrichtung, -sinn m.
d.s for use Gebrauchsanweisung, -anleitung.
di·rec·tion·al [dɪ'rɛkʃnəl, daɪ-] adj gerichtet, Richtungs-.
directional hearing Richtungshören nt.

di·rec·tion·al·i·ty [dɪˌrekʃəˈnælətɪ, daɪ-] *n phys.* Ausrichtung *f*.

di·rec·tive [dɪˈrektɪv, daɪ-] **I** *n* (An-)Weisung *f*, Vorschrift *f*, Anordnung *f*. **II** *adj* leitend, lenkend, richtungsgebend.

direct laryngoscopy direkte Kehlkopfspiegelung/Laryngoskopie *f*, Autoskopie *f*.

direct metaplasia direkte Metaplasie *f*.
direct metastasis direkte Metastase *f*.
direct ophthalmoscopy direkte Ophthalmoskopie *f*.

di·rec·tor [dɪˈrektər, daɪ-] *n* **1.** Direktor(in *f*) *m*, Leiter(in *f*) *m*. **2.** *chir.* Führungs-(hohl)sonde *f*.

direct oxidase Oxygenase *f*.
direct percussion direkte Perkussion *f*.
direct rays Primärstrahlen *pl*.
direct transfusion direkte Transfusion *f*.
direct veins, lateral direkte Seitenvenen *pl*, Vv. directae laterales.
direct vision direktes/zentrales Sehen *nt*.

Di·ro·fi·lar·ia [ˌdaɪrəʊfɪˈleərɪə] *n micro.* Dirofilaria *nt*.
D. immitis Herzwurm *m*, Dirofilaria immitis.

di·ro·fil·a·ri·a·sis [-ˌfɪləˈraɪəsɪs] *n* Dirofilarieninfektion *f*, Dirofilariasis *f*.

dirt [dɜːt] *n* Schmutz *m*, Dreck *m*; Kot *m*.

dirt·y [ˈdɜːtɪ] **I** *adj* **1.** schmutzig, verschmutzt, Schmutz-. **2.** (*Wunde*) infiziert, septisch. **3.** *fig.* schmutzig, unanständig; niederträchtig. **II** *vt* be-, verschmutzen. **III** *vi* schmutzig werden.

dirty wound 1. verschmutzte Wunde *f*. **2.** infizierte/septische Wunde *f*.

dis·a·bil·i·ty [ˌdɪsəˈbɪlətɪ] *n* **1.** Leiden *nt*, Gebrechen *nt*, Behinderung *f*. **2.** Arbeits-, Erwerbsunfähigkeit *f*, Invalidität *f*.

dis·a·ble [dɪsˈeɪbl] *vt* verkrüppeln, behindern.

dis·a·bled [dɪsˈeɪbld] **I** *the ~ pl* die Behinderten. **II** *adj* **1.** (*körperlich od. geistig*) behindert; verkrüppelt. **2.** arbeits-, erwerbsunfähig, invalid(e). **3.** unbrauchbar, untauglich.

dis·a·ble·ment [dɪsˈeɪbəlmənt] *n* **1.** (*körperliche od. geistige*) Behinderung *f*. **2.** Arbeits-, Erwerbsunfähigkeit *f*, Invalidität *f*. **3.** → disability *f*.

di·sac·cha·ri·dase [daɪˈsækərɪdeɪz] *n* Disaccharidase *f*.
disaccharidase deficiency Disaccharidasemangel *m*.
intestinal d. → disaccharide intolerance *f*.

di·sac·cha·ride [daɪˈsækəraɪd, -rɪd] *n* Zweifachzucker *m*, Disaccharid *nt*.
disaccharide intolerance Disaccharidintoleranz *f*.
type I d. Saccharase-Isomaltase-Mangel *m*.
type II d. Lactase-Mangel *m*, Laktase-Mangel *m*, kongenitale/hereditäre Laktoseintoleranz *f*.

di·sac·cha·rid·u·ria [daɪˌsækəraɪˈd(j)ʊərɪə] *n* Disaccharidausscheidung *f* im Harn, Disaccharidurie *f*.

di·sac·cha·rose [daɪˈsækərəʊs] *n* → disaccharide.

dis·a·cid·i·fy [dɪsəˈsɪdəfaɪ] *vt* (*Säure*) neutralisieren, entfernen.

dis·ap·pear·ing bone (disease) [dɪsəˈpɪərɪŋ] *ortho.* Gorham-(Staut-)Erkrankung *f*.

dis·ar·tic·u·late [dɪsɑːˈtɪkjəleɪt] *vt* **1.** zergliedern, trennen. **2.** *ortho.* exartikulieren.

dis·ar·tic·u·la·tion [dɪsɑːˌtɪkjəˈleɪʃn] *n* **1.** Zergliederung *f*. **2.** *ortho.* Exartikulation *f*.
d. of the knee Kniegelenk(s)exartikulation.

dis·as·sim·i·late [dɪsəˈsɪməleɪt] *vt* → dissimilate.

dis·as·sim·i·la·tion [dɪsəˌsɪməˈleɪʃn] *n* → dissimilation.

disazo- *pref.* → diazo-.

DISC *abbr.* → ductal in situ-carcinoma.

disc- *pref.* → disco-.

disc [dɪsk] *n* → disk.

dis·cec·to·my [dɪsˈektəmɪ] *n* → diskectomy.

disc electrophoresis *lab.* Diskelektrophorese *f*.

dis·charge [*n* ˈdɪstʃɑːdʒ; *v* dɪsˈtʃɑːdʒ] **I** *n* **1.** *patho., physiol.* Ausfluß *m*, Absonderung *f*, Ausscheidung *f*, Sekret *nt*. **2.** Aus-, Abfluß *m*; Abgabe *f*; Freisetzung *f*, Ausstoßen *nt*; (*a. electr.*) Entladung *f*. **3.** (*Patient*) Entlassung *f*. **II** *vt* **4.** *patho., physiol.*, absondern, ausscheiden. **5.** (*Patient*) entlassen (*from* aus). **6.** ausströmen; ab-, ablassen; *electr.* entladen. **III** *vi* **7.** eitern. **8.** s. ergießen; abfließen; ausströmen lassen; s. entladen.

discharge pattern *physiol.* Entladungsmuster *nt*.

discharge potential *physiol.* Entladungspotential *nt*.

dis·ci·form [ˈdɪsɪfɔːm] *adj* scheibenförmig, disziform.

disciform degeneration of macula retinae *ophthal.* Kuhnt-Junius-Krankheit *f*, scheibenförmige/disziforme senile feuchte Makuladegeneration *f*.

disciform keratitis scheibenförmige Keratitis *f*, Keratitis disciformis.

disciform macular degeneration → disciform degeneration of macula retinae.

disciform retinitis → disciform degeneration of macula retinae.

dis·cis·sion [dɪˈsɪʃn] *n* **1.** *chir.* operative Spaltung/Eröffnung/Durchtrennung *f*, Diszision *f*, Discisio *f*. **2.** → d. of cataract.
d. of cataract *ophthal.* Eröffnung der Linsenkapsel, Diszision, Discisio cataractae.

dis·ci·tis [dɪsˈkaɪtɪs] *n* **1.** Diskusentzündung *f*, Diszitis *f*, Discitis *f*. **2.** *ortho.* Bandscheibenentzündung *f*, Diszitis *f*, Discitis *f*.

dis·cli·na·tion [ˌdɪsklɪˈneɪʃn] *n ophthal.* Disklination *f*.

disco- *pref.* Scheiben-, Bandscheiben-, Disk(o)-, Disc(o)-.

dis·co·blas·tic [ˌdɪskəʊˈblæstɪk] *adj embryo.* Diskoblastula betr., diskoblastisch.

dis·co·blas·tu·la [ˌ-ˈblæstələ] *n embryo.* Diskoblastula *f*.

dis·co·gas·tru·la [ˌ-ˈgæstrələ] *n embryo.* Diskogastrula *f*.

dis·co·ge·net·ic [ˌ-dʒəˈnetɪk] *adj* → discogenic.

dis·co·gen·ic [ˌ-ˈdʒenɪk] *adj* von den Bandscheiben ausgehend, durch sie verursacht, diskogen, Bandscheiben-.

dis·co·gram *n* → diskogram.

dis·cog·ra·phy *n* → diskography.

dis·coid [ˈdɪskɔɪd] **I** *n pharm.* scheibenförmige Tablette *f*. **II** *adj* scheibenförmig, diskoid, diskoidal, disziform.

dis·coi·dal [dɪsˈkɔɪdl] *adj* → discoid II.

dis·coid·ec·to·my [ˌdɪskɔɪdˈektəmɪ] *n* → diskectomy.

discoid meniscus *ortho.* (*Kniegelenk*) diskoider Meniskus *m*, Scheibenmeniskus *m*.
congenital d. → discoid meniscus.
lateral d. → discoid meniscus.

discoid placenta *gyn.* diskoide/scheibenförmige Plazenta *f*, Placenta discoidea.

discoid psoriasis *derm.* Psoriasis discoidea.

dis·col·or [dɪsˈkʌlər] **I** *vt* **1.** verfärben. **2.** entfärben, bleichen, dekolorieren. **II** *vi* **3.** s. verfärben. **4.** die Farbe verlieren, verblassen.

dis·col·or·a·tion [dɪsˌkʌləˈreɪʃn] *n* **1.** Verfärbung *f*. **2.** Entfärbung *f*, Bleichung *f*, Farbverlust *m*. **3.** Fleck *m*, entfärbte *od.* farblose Stelle *f*.

dis·com·fort [dɪsˈkʌfərt] *n* **1.** (körperliche) Beschwerde *f*. **2.** Unannehmlichkeit *f*, Verdruß *m*; Sorge *f*, Qual *f*.

discomfort threshold *physiol.* Unbehaglichkeitsschwelle *f*.

dis·con·tin·u·ance [ˌdɪskənˈtɪnjuːəns] *n* Unterbrechung *f*; Abbruch *m*, Einstellung *f*, Aufgabe *f*, Aufhören *nt*.

dis·con·tin·u·a·tion [ˌdɪskənˌtɪnjuːˈeɪʃn] *n* → discontinuance.

dis·con·tin·ue [ˌdɪskənˈtɪnjuː] *vt* unterbrechen, aussetzen; abbrechen, einstellen, aufgeben, aufhören.

dis·con·ti·nu·i·ty [ˌdɪskəntɪˈn(j)uːətɪ] *n* **1.** Zusammenhang(s)losigkeit *f*. **2.** Unterbrechung *f*, Diskontinuität *f*.

dis·con·tin·u·ous [dɪskənˈtɪnjəwəs] *adj* unzusammenhängend; unterbrochen, mit Unterbrechungen; (*a. mathe., phys.*) diskontinuierlich.

discontinuous capillary diskontinuierliche Kapillare *f*, Typ 3-Kapillare *f*.

discontinuous phase *phys.* disperse/innere Phase *f*, Dispersum *nt*.

discontinuous variation diskontinuierliche Variation *f*.

dis·co·p·a·thy [dɪsˈkɒpəθɪ] *n ortho.* Bandscheibenerkrankung *f*, -schaden *m*, Diskopathie *f*.

dis·co·pla·cen·ta [ˌdɪskəpləˈsentə] *n gyn.* diskoide/scheibenförmige Plazenta *f*, Placenta discoidea.

dis·cord [ˈdɪskɔːrd] *n physiol.* Mißklang *m*, Dissonanz *f*.

dis·cord·ance [dɪsˈkɔːrdəns] *n genet.* Diskordanz *f*.

dis·cor·dant [dɪsˈkɔːrdənt] *adj* gegenteilig, -sinnig, unterschiedlich, nicht übereinstimmend, diskordant.

dis·co·ria *n* → dyscoria.

dis·crep·ance [dɪˈskrepəns] *n* → discrepancy.

dis·crep·an·cy [dɪˈskrepənsɪ] *n* **1.** Widerspruch *m*, Unstimmigkeit *f*, Diskrepanz *f*. **2.** Zwiespalt *m*.

dis·crep·ant [dɪˈskrepənt] *adj* **1.** s. widersprechend, abweichend.

dis·crete [dɪˈskriːt] *adj* getrennt, einzeln; aus einzelnen Teilen bestehend; unstetig; *mathe., phys.* diskret.

dis·crim·i·na·bil·i·ty [dɪˌskrɪmənəˈbɪlətɪ] *n* Unterscheidbarkeit *f*, Diskriminierbarkeit *f*.

dis·crim·i·nant [dɪˈskrɪmənənt] *n mathe.* Diskriminante *f*.

dis·crim·i·nate [*adj* dɪˈskrɪmənət; *v* -neɪt] **I** *adj* unterscheidend, Unterschiede machend. **II** *vt* unterscheiden; absondern, abtrennen (*from* von). **III** *vi* unterscheiden, einen Unterschied machen (*between* zwischen). **to ~ against s.o.** jdn. benachteiligen *od.* diskriminieren.

dis·crim·i·na·tion [dɪˌskrɪməˈneɪʃn] *n* Unterscheidung *f* (*between* zwischen); Diskriminierung *f*, Diskriminieren *nt*.

discrimination curve *physiol.* (*Gehör*) Diskriminationskurve *f*.

discrimination loss *physiol.* (*Gehör*) Diskriminationsverlust *m*.

dis·crim·i·na·tive [dɪˈskrɪmənətɪv, -neɪ-] *adj* unterscheidend, Unterschiede machend, charakteristisch, diskriminierend.

dis·crim·i·na·tor [dɪˈskrɪmənətər] *n radiol.* Diskriminator *m*.

dis·crim·i·na·to·ry [dɪ'skrɪmənətɔːriː, -təʊ-] *adj* → discriminative.
dis·cus ['dɪskəs] *n, pl* **-cus·es, dis·ci** ['dɪs(k)aɪ] → disk 1.
dis·di·ad·o·cho·ki·ne·sia *n* → dysdiadochokinesia.
dis·ease [dɪ'ziːz] **I** *n* Krankheit *f*, Erkrankung *f*, Leiden *nt*; Morbus *m*. **II** *vt* krank machen.
 d.s of childhood Kinderkrankheiten *pl*, Erkrankungen *pl* des Kindesalters.
 d.s of civilization Zivilisationskrankheiten *pl*.
 d.s of old age Alterskrankheiten *pl*, Erkrankungen *pl* des Alters.
dis·eased [dɪ'ziːzd] *adj* krank, erkrankt, Krankheits-; krankhaft.
disease process Krankheitsprozeß *m*, -verlauf *m*.
dis·em·bow·el [ˌdɪsem'baʊəl] *vt chir.* Eingeweide entfernen.
dis·em·bow·el·ment [ˌ-'baʊəlmənt] *n chir.* Eingeweideentfernung *f*, Eviszeration *f*.
dis·en·gage [ˌdɪsen'geɪdʒ] **I** *vt* **1.** los-, freimachen, befreien (*from* von). **2.** befreien, entbinden (*from* von). **II** *vi s.* frei machen, loskommen (*from* von).
dis·en·gage·ment [ˌ-'geɪdʒmənt] *n* **1.** Befreiung *f* (*from* von). **2.** *gyn.* Entbindung *f*, Entbinden *nt* (*from* von). **3.** *chem.* Entbindung *f*, Freiwerden *nt*.
dis·e·qui·lib·ri·um [dɪsˌekwə'lɪbrɪəm] *n* gestörtes Gleichgewicht *nt*, Ungleichgewicht *nt*.
dis·es·the·sia *n* → dysesthesia.
dis·ger·mi·no·ma *n* → dysgerminoma.
DISH *abbr.* → diffuse idiopathic skeletal hyperostosis.
dish [dɪʃ] *n* (flache) Schüssel *f*, Schale *f*.
dis·ha·bit·u·a·tion [dɪshəˌbɪtʃə'weɪʃn] *n physiol.* Dishabituation *f*.
dis·har·mon·ic diplacusis [dɪshɑːr'mɒnɪk] *HNO* Diplacusis disharmonica, Parakusis dysharmonica.
dis·har·mo·ny [dɪs'hɑːrmənɪ] *n* Disharmonie *f*.
dis·in·fect [ˌdɪsɪn'fekt] *vt hyg.* keimfrei machen, desinfizieren.
dis·in·fect·ant [ˌ-'fektənt] *hyg.* **I** *n* Desinfektionsmittel *nt*, Desinfektans *nt*, Desinfiziens *nt*. **II** *adj* desinfizierend, keim(ab)tötend.
dis·in·fec·tion [ˌ-'fekʃn] *n hyg.* Entseuchung *f*, Entkeimung *f*, Desinfektion *f*, Desinfizierung *f*.
dis·in·fec·tor [ˌ-'fektər] *n hyg.* Desinfektionsapparat *m*, Desinfektor *m*.
dis·in·fest [ˌ-'fest] *vt hyg.* von Ungeziefer befreien, entwesen.
dis·in·fes·ta·tion [ˌ-fes'teɪʃn] *n hyg.* Entwesung *f*, Desinfestation *f*.
dis·in·hi·bi·tion [dɪsˌɪn(h)ɪ'bɪʃn] *n physiol., psycho.* Enthemmung *f*, Disinhibition *f*.
dis·in·sec·tion [ˌdɪsɪn'sekʃn] *n* → disinsectization.
dis·in·sec·ti·za·tion [ˌ-ˌsektɪ'zeɪʃn] *n hyg.* Ungezieferbekämpfung *f*, Dis-, Desinsektion *f*.
dis·in·sec·tor [ˌ-'sektər] *n hyg.* Dis-, Desinsektor *m*.
dis·in·ser·tion [ˌ-'sɜrʃn] *n* **1.** *ortho.* Sehnenabriß *m* am Ansatz. **2.** *ophthal.* periphere Netzhautablösung *f*.
dis·in·te·grate [dɪs'ɪntəgreɪt] **I** *vt* auflösen, aufspalten. **II** *vi* ver-, zerfallen, s. (in seine Bestandteile) auflösen, s. aufspalten.
dis·in·te·gra·tion [dɪsˌɪntə'greɪʃn] *n* **1.** Auflösung *f*, Aufspaltung *f*, Zerfall *m*. **2.** *patho., physiol., psycho.* Zerfall *m*, Disintegration *f*.
disintegration constant *phys.* Zerfallskonstante *f*.

dis·in·vag·i·na·tion [dɪsɪnˌvædʒə'neɪʃn] *n chir.* Desinvagination *f*.
dis·joint ['dɪsdʒɔɪnt] *vt* **1.** auseinandernehmen, zerlegen, zerstückeln, zergliedern. **2.** *ortho.* verrenken, ausrenken. **3.** → disarticulate.
dis·junc·tion [dɪs'dʒʌŋ(k)ʃn] *n* **1.** Trennung *f*, Absonderung *f*. **2.** *genet.* (Chromosomen-)Disjunktion *f*. **3.** *ophthal.* Disjunktion *f* der Koordination.
disk- *pref.* → disco-.
disk [dɪsk] *n* **1.** *allg.* Scheibe *f*; *anat.* Diskus *m*, Discus *m*. **2.** Bandscheibe *f*, Intervertebral-, Zwischenwirbelscheibe *f*, Discus intervertebralis.
disk diffusion test *micro., pharm.* Plattendiffusionstest *m*.
dis·kec·to·my [dɪs'kektəmɪ] *n ortho., neurochir.* Bandscheiben(teil)entfernung *f*, -resektion *f*, Diskektomie *f*; Nukleotomie *f*.
disk electrophoresis Disk-Elektrophorese *f*.
dis·ki·form ['dɪskəfɔːrm] *adj* → disciform
dis·ki·tis [dɪs'kaɪtɪs] *n* → discitis.
disk kidney scheibenförmige Niere *f*, Scheibenniere *f*.
disko- *pref.* → disco-.
dis·ko·gram ['dɪskəgræm] *n radiol.* Diskogramm *nt*.
dis·kog·ra·phy [dɪs'kɒgrəfɪ] *n radiol.* Kontrastdarstellung *f* einer Bandscheibe, Diskographie *f*.
disk oxygenator Scheibenoxygenator *m*.
disk prolapse *ortho., neurochir.* Bandscheibenvorfall *m*, -prolaps *m*, -hernie *f*.
 pendulating d. pendelnder Bandscheibenprolaps.
 sequestrated d. sequestrierter/freier Bandscheibenprolaps.
disk removal *n* → diskectomy.
disk-shaped cataract ringförmige/scheibenförmige Katarakt *f*.
disk-shaped placenta diskoide/scheibenförmige Plazenta *f*, Placenta discoidea.
disk syndrome Bandscheibensyndrom *nt*.
dis·lo·cate ['dɪsləʊkeɪt, dɪs'ləʊ-] *vt* **1.** verrücken, verschieben. **2.** *ortho.* aus-, verrenken, ausgliedern, luxieren, dislozieren.
dis·lo·ca·tio [ˌdɪsləʊ'keɪʃɪəʊ] *n* → dislocation.
dis·lo·ca·tion [ˌ-'keɪʃn] *n* **1.** Verlagerung *f*, Lageanomalie *f*, -atypie *f*, Dislokation *f*. **2.** *genet.* (Chromosomen-)Dislokation *f*. **3.** *ortho.* Verrenkung *f*, Ausrenkung *f*, Luxation *f*; Dislokation *f*. **4.** *ortho.* Fragmentverschiebung *f*, Dislokation *f*, Dislocatio *f*.
 d.s of the carpus Handwurzelluxationen *pl*.
 d. of the elbow Ellenbogen(gelenk)luxation.
 d. of the hip Hüftgelenk(s)luxation.
 d. of the knee joint Kniegelenk(s)luxation.
 d. of the lens *ophthal.* Linsenluxation.
 d. of the lunate Lunatumluxation.
 d. of the patella Patellaluxation.
dislocation fracture Luxationsfraktur *f*, Verrenkungsbruch *m*.
dis·mem·ber [dɪs'membər] *vt* **1.** zergliedern, zerstückeln. **2.** (*Arm, Bein*) amputieren.
dis·mem·ber·ment [dɪs'membərmənt] *n* **1.** Zerstückelung *f*, Zergliederung *f*. **2.** *ortho.* Gliedmaßen(teil)amputation *f*.
dis·mu·tase ['dɪsmjuːteɪz] *n* Dismutase *f*.
dis·mu·ta·tion [ˌdɪsmjuː'teɪʃn] *n bio., chem.* Dismutation *f*.
di·so·mic [daɪ'səʊmɪk] *adj genet.* Disomie betr., disom.
di·so·mus [daɪ'səʊməs] *n embryo.* Disomus *m*.

di·so·my ['daɪsəʊmɪ] *n* **1.** *genet.* Disomie *f*. **2.** *embryo.* Duplicitas completa, Disomie *f*.
di·so·pyr·a·mide [ˌdaɪsəʊ'pɪrəmɪd] *n pharm.* Disopyramid *nt*.
dis·or·der [dɪs'ɔːrdər] **I** *n* **1.** Unordnung *f*, Durcheinander *nt*; Systemlosigkeit *f*. **2.** pathologischer Zustand *m*, (krankhafte) Störung *f*, Erkrankung *f*, Krankheit *f*. **II** *vt* **3.** in Unordnung bringen, durcheinander bringen. **4.** eine Erkrankung hervorrufen.
 d. of sound conduction Schalleitungsstörung.
 d. of sound perception Schallwahrnehmungsstörung.
dis·or·dered [dɪs'ɔːrdərd] *adj* **1.** durcheinander, ungeordnet. **2.** gestört, krank, erkrankt.
disordered action of the heart *abbr.* **D.A.H.** → DaCosta's syndrome.
dis·or·gan·i·za·tion [dɪsˌɔːrgənə'zeɪʃn] *n patho.* Desorganisation *f*.
dis·or·gan·ized schizophrenia [dɪs'ɔːrgənaɪzd] hebephrene Schizophrenie *f*, Hebephrenie *f*.
dis·o·ri·ent [dɪs'ɔːrɪent] *vt* jdn. verwirren, desorientieren.
dis·o·ri·en·tate [dɪs'ɔːrɪenteɪt] *vt* → disorient.
dis·o·ri·en·tat·ed [dɪs'ɔːrɪenteɪtɪd] *adj* verwirrt, desorientiert.
dis·o·ri·en·ta·tion [dɪsˌɔːrɪen'teɪʃn] *n* Verwirrtheit *f*, Desorientiertheit *f*.
dis·ox·i·da·tion [dɪsˌɒksə'deɪʃn] *n* → deoxidation.
dis·par ['dɪspær] *adj* → disparate.
dis·pa·rate ['dɪspərət, dɪ'spær-] *adj* ungleich(artig), grundverschieden, unvereinbar, dispar, disparat.
dis·pa·rate·ness ['-nɪs] *n* → disparity.
disparate points *ophthal.* disparate Netzhautpunkte *pl*.
dis·par·i·ty [dɪ'spærətɪ] *n* **1.** Verschiedenheit *f*, Unvereinbarkeit *f*, Disparität *f*. **2.** *ophthal.* Disparation *f*.
disparity angle Disparitätswinkel *m*.
dis·pen·sa·ble [dɪ'spensəbl] *adj* entbehrlich.
dis·pen·sa·ry [dɪ'spensərɪ] *n* **1.** Poliklinik *f*, Ambulanz *f*. **2.** Arzneimittelausgabe(stelle *f*) *f*; Krankenhausapotheke *f*.
dis·pen·sa·to·ry [dɪ'spensətɔːriː, -təʊ-] *n* Arzneiverordnungsbuch *nt*, Dispensatorium *nt*.
dis·pense [dɪ'spens] *vt* **1.** austeilen, verteilen. **2.** *pharm.* Arzneimittel zubereiten u. abgeben, dispensieren.
dis·pens·er [dɪ'spensər] *n* **1.** *pharm.* Spender *m*. **2.** Automat *m*, Spender *m*.
dis·pens·ing [dɪ'spensɪŋ] *adj pharm.* dispensierend.
dispensing chemist *Brit.* Apotheker(in *f*) *m*.
di·sper·my ['daɪspɜrmɪ] *n embryo.* Doppelbefruchtung *f*, Dispermie *f*.
dis·per·sal [dɪ'spɜrsl] *n* → dispersion 1.
dis·per·sant [dɪ'spɜrsənt] *n* **1.** Dispersionsmittel *nt*, Dispergens *nt*. **2.** Dispergiermittel *nt*, Dispergator *m*.
dis·perse [dɪ'spɜrs] *vt* **1.** (ver-, zer-)streuen, verteilen, verbreiten; auflösen; (*Licht*) streuen. **2.** *phys.* dispergieren, zerstreuen, (fein) verteilen. **II** *vi s.* zerstreuen *od.* auflösen; s. verteilen.
dis·persed phase [dɪ'spɜrsd] → disperse phase.
disperse medium Dispersionsmedium *nt*.
disperse phase *phys.* disperse/innere Phase *f*, Dispersum *nt*.
disperse system disperses System *nt*, Dispersion *f*.

dis·pers·ing electrode [dɪ'spɜrsɪŋ] inaktive/indifferente/passive Elektrode *f*.
dispersing lens Streulinse *f*.
dis·per·sion [dɪ'spɜrʒn, -ʃn] *n* 1. (Zer-, Ver-)Streuung *f*, Zerlegung *f*, Verteilung *f*, Dispersion *f*. 2. *phys*. Dispersion *f*, Suspension *f*, disperses System *nt*. 3. *pharm*. Dispersion *f*.
dispersion colloid Dispersionskolloid *nt*.
dispersion medium → dispersion phase.
dispersion phase *phys*. äußere/dispergierende Phase *f*, Dispergens *nt*, Dispersionsmedium *nt*, -mittel *nt*.
dispersion system → disperse system.
dis·per·sive [dɪ'spɜrsɪv] *adj* (ver-, zer-)streuend, verteilend, dispergierend, Dispersions-.
dispersive medium → disperse medium.
dispersive replication *genet*. dispersive Replikation *f*.
dis·per·soid [dɪ'spɜrsɔɪd] *n* Dispersionskolloid *nt*.
dis·per·son·al·i·za·tion [dɪsˌpɜrsnəlaɪ'zeɪʃn] *n* → depersonalization.
di·spi·ra [daɪ'spaɪrə] *n* → dispireme.
di·spi·rem [daɪ'spaɪrəm] *n* → dispireme.
di·spi·reme [daɪ'spaɪriːm] *n* Doppelknäuel *nt*, Dispirem *nt*.
dis·place [dɪs'pleɪs] *vt* 1. verschieben, -lagern, -rücken. 2. (*a. psycho.*) verdrängen. 3. (*a. chem.*) ersetzen. 4. jdn. entlassen *od.* ablösen.
dis·placed fracture [dɪs'pleɪsd] dislozierte Fraktur *f*, Fraktur *f* mit Dislokation der Bruchenden.
dis·place·ment [dɪs'pleɪsmənt] *n* 1. Verlagerung *f*, Verschiebung *f*, Verrückung *f*. 2. (*a. psycho.*) Verdrängung *f*. 3. *ortho*. (*Fraktur*) Fragmentverschiebung *f*, Dislokation *f*, Dislocatio *f*. 4. Ablösung *f*, Entlassung *f*. 5. *psycho*. Affektverlagerung *f*. 6. Ersatz *m*; Ersetzen *nt*.
displacement analysis *lab*. kompetitiver Bindungstest/-assay *m*.
displacement osteotomy *ortho*. Umstellungsosteotomie *f*.
displacement reaction *chem*. Verdrängungsreaktion *f*.
displacement velocity *chem*. Verschiebungsgeschwindigkeit *f*.
dis·po·si·tion [dɪspə'zɪʃn] *n* Veranlagung *f*, Disposition *f*.
dis·pro·por·tion [dɪsprə'pɔːrʃn] *n* Mißverhältnis *nt*.
dis·pro·por·tion·ate [dɪsprə'pɔːrʃənɪt] *adj* 1. unverhältnismäßig (groß *od.* klein), in keinem Verhältnis stehend, disproportioniert. 2. unangemessen; übertrieben. 3. unproportioniert.
disproportionate dwarfism disproportionierter Zergwuchs *m*.
dis·rupt [dɪs'rʌpt] *vt* auseinanderbrechen, zerbrechen; auseinanderreißen, zerreißen; (zer-)spalten. II *vi* auseinanderbrechen; zerreißen.
dis·rup·tion [dɪs'rʌpʃn] *n* 1. Zerbrechung *f*; Zerreißung *f*. 2. Zerrissenheit *f*, Spaltung *f*. 3. Bruch *m*; Riß *m*. 4. *embryo*. Disruption *f*.
dis·rup·tive [dɪs'rʌptɪv] *adj* 1. zerbrechend; zerreißend. 2. zerrüttend. 3. *phys*. disruptiv.
disruptive strength *phys*. Durchschlagfestigkeit *f*.
disruptive voltage *phys*. Durchschlagsspannung *f*.
Disse ['dɪsiː; 'dɪsə]: **D.'s space** Disse'-Raum *m*, perisinusoidaler Raum *m*.
dis·sect [dɪ'sekt, daɪ-] *vt* 1. zergliedern, zerlegen; spalten. 2. *anat., patho., chir.* zergliedern, zerlegen, sezieren, präparieren.
dis·sect·ing [dɪ'sektɪŋ, daɪ-] *adj* dissezierend, trennend, spaltend, Sezier-.
dissecting aneurysm dissezierendes Aneurysma *nt*, Aneurysma dissecans.
dissecting cellulitis of scalp profunde dekalvitierende Follikulitis *f*, Perifolliculitis capitis abscedens et suffodiens.
dissecting metritis Metritis dissecans.
dissecting scissors *chir*. Präparierschere *f*.
dis·sec·tion [dɪ'sekʃn, daɪ-] *n* 1. Zergliederung *f*, Zerlegung *f*; (genaue) Analyse *f*. 2. *anat., patho.* Zergliedern *nt*, Zerlegen *nt*, Sezieren *nt*. 3. *anat., patho.* Leicheneröffnung *f*, Sektion *f*, Obduktion *f*. 4. *chir.* Präparieren *nt*, Darstellen *nt*; Ausräumung *f*, Resektion *f*, Dissektion *f*. 5. *chir., patho.* Präparat *nt*.
dis·sec·tor [dɪ'sektər, daɪ-] *n anat., patho.* Dissektor *m*.
dis·sem·i·nat·ed [dɪ'semənettɪd] *adj* verbreitet, verstreut, disseminiert.
disseminated choroiditis *ophthal*. hintere/disseminierte Chorioiditis *f*, Chorioiditis disseminata.
disseminated condensing osteopathy Osteopoikilose *f*, -poikilie *f*, Osteopathia condensans disseminata.
disseminated cutaneous gangrene Dermatitis gangraenosa infantum, Ecthyma gangraenosum/terebrans.
disseminated inflammation disseminierte Entzündung *f*.
disseminated intravascular coagulation *abbr*. **DIC** 1. disseminierte intravasale Koagulation *f abbr*. DIC, disseminierte intravasale Gerinnung *f abbr*. DIG. 2. Verbrauchskoagulopathie *f*.
disseminated intravascular coagulation syndrome → disseminated intravascular coagulation 1.
disseminated lipogranulomatosis Farber'-Krankheit *f*, disseminierte Lipogranulomatose *f*.
disseminated metastatic disease disseminierte Metastasierung *f*.
disseminated myelitis disseminierte Myelitis *f*.
disseminated neuritis Polyneuritis *f*.
disseminated neurodermatitis atopische Dermatitis *f*, atopisches/endogenes/exsudatives/neuropathisches/konstitutionelles Ekzem *nt*, Prurigo Besnier, Morbus Besnier *m*, Ekzemkrankheit *f*, neurogene Dermatose *f*.
disseminated pruritic angiodermatitis ekzematoidartige Purpura *f*, epidemische purpurisch-lichenoide Dermatitis *f*, disseminierte pruriginöse Angiodermatitis *f*.
disseminated sclerosis *patho*. multiple Sklerose *f abbr*. MS, Polysklerose *f*, Sclerosis multiplex, Encephalomyelitis disseminata.
disseminated tuberculosis 1. disseminierte Tuberkulose *f*. 2. Miliartuberkulose *f*, miliare Tuberkulose *f*, Tuberculosis miliaris.
disseminated xanthoma disseminiertes Xanthom *nt*, Xanthoma disseminatum.
dis·sem·i·na·tion [dɪˌsemɪ'neɪʃn] *n* 1. Aussäung *f*, Verbreitung *f*. 2. *patho*. Aussaat *f*, Streuung *f*, Dissemination *f*. 3. *micro*. Dissemination *f*.
dis·sert [dɪ'sɜrt] *vi* → dissertate.
dis·ser·tate ['dɪsərteɪt] *vi* einen Vortrag halten, eine Abhandlung schreiben (*on* über).
dis·ser·ta·tion [ˌdɪsər'teɪʃn] *n* 1. (wissenschaftliche) Abhandlung *f*; Dissertation *f*. 2. (wissenschaftlicher) Vortrag *m*.
dis·sim·i·lar [dɪ'sɪmɪlər] *adj* ungleich(artig), unähnlich (*to*); verschieden (*to* von).
dis·sim·i·lar·i·ty [dɪˌsɪmɪ'lærətɪ] *n* 1. Ungleichheit *f*, Ungleichartigkeit *f*, Unähnlichkeit *f*, Verschiedenheit *f*. 2. Unterschied *m*.
dissimilar twins → dizygotic twins.
dis·sim·i·late [dɪ'sɪmɪleɪt] I *vt* 1. unähnlich machen. 2. *physiol*. abbauen, dissimilieren. II *vi* 3. unähnlich werden. 4. *physiol*. dissimilieren, s. abbauen.
dis·sim·i·la·tion [dɪˌsɪmɪ'leɪʃn] *n* 1. Verlust *m od*. Beseitigung *f* der Ähnlichkeit, Entähnlichung *f*. 2. *physiol*. Dissimilation *f*, Katabolismus *m*, Abbau *m*.
dis·si·mil·i·tude [ˌdɪsɪ'mɪlɪt(j)uːd] *n* → dissimilarity.
dis·sim·u·la·tion [dɪˌsɪmjə'leɪʃn] *n* Verbergen *nt od*. Verheimlichen *nt* von Krankheitssymptomen, Dissimulation *f*.
dis·so·ci·a·ble [dɪ'səʊʃ(ɪ)əbl] *adj* 1. (ab-)trennbar; unvereinbar. 2. *chem*. dissoziierbar.
dis·so·ci·ate [dɪ'səʊʃɪeɪt, -sɪ-] I *vt* 1. (ab-)trennen, auf-, loslösen, absondern (*from* von). 2. *chem*. dissoziieren. II *vi* 3. s. (ab-)trennen, s. auf- *od*. loslösen. 4. *chem*. dissoziieren, (in Ionen) zerfallen.
dis·so·ci·at·ed anesthesia [dɪ'səʊʃɪeɪtɪd, -sɪ-] *neuro*. dissoziierte Sensibilitätsstörung *f*.
dissociated nystagmus dissoziierter Nystagmus *m*.
dis·so·ci·a·tion [dɪˌsəʊʃɪ'eɪʃn, -sɪ-] *n* 1. (Ab-)Trennung *f*, Auf-, Loslösung *f*. 2. *chem., psycho.* Dissoziation *f*.
dissociation anesthesia → dissociated anesthesia.
dissociation constant *abbr*. **K** *chem*. Dissoziationskonstante *f abbr*. K.
apparent d. *abbr*. K' apparente Dissoziationskonstante *abbr*. K'.
basic d. basische Dissoziationskonstante.
concentration d. → apparent d.
proton d. Protonendissoziationskonstante.
thermodynamic/true d. thermodynamische/wahre Dissoziationskonstante.
dissociation curve Dissoziations-, Bindungskurve *f*.
dis·so·ci·a·tive disorder [dɪ'səʊʃɪeɪtɪv, -sɪ-] *psychia*. dissoziative Störung *f*.
dissociative reaction → dissociative disorder.
dis·so·lu·tion [ˌdɪsə'luːʃn] *n* 1. (Auf-)Lösen *nt*. 2. Verflüssigen *nt*, Verflüssigung *f*. 3. *chem*. Zersetzung *f*; (Auf-)Lösung *f*. 4. Lösung *f*, Lockerung *f*. 5. Tod *m*.
dis·solve [dɪ'zɑlv] I *vt* 1. (auf-)lösen; *chem*. zersetzen. 2. schmelzen, verflüssigen. II *vi* s. auflösen; zerfallen.
dis·sol·vent [dɪ'zɑlvənt] I *n* Lösungsmittel *nt*, Solvens *nt*, Dissolvens *nt*. II *adj* (auf-)lösend; zersetzend.
dis·sym·met·ric [ˌdɪsɪ'metrɪk] *adj* → dissymmetrical.
dis·sym·met·ri·cal [ˌ-'metrɪkl] *adj* 1. unsymmetrisch, asymmetrisch. 2. *chem*. enantiomorph.
dis·sym·me·try [dɪ'sɪmətrɪ] *n* Asymmetrie *f*.
dist. *abbr*. → distilled.
dis·tal ['dɪstl] *adj* vom Mittelpunkt/von der Körpermitte entfernt liegend, distal.
distal convolution (*Niere*) distales Konvolut *nt*.
distal ileitis Crohn'-Krankheit *f*, Morbus Crohn *m*, Enteritis regionalis, Ileocolitis regionalis/terminalis, Ileitis regionalis/terminalis.
distal pancreatectomy *chir*. distale Pankreatektomie *f*, Linksresektion *f*.
subtotal d. subtotale distale/linksseitige Pankreatektomie *f*, subtotale Linksre-

sektion *f*, Child-Operation *f*, subtotale Pankrealinksresektion.
distal part of adenohypophysis Prähypophyse *f*, Pars distalis adenohypophyseos.
distal phalanx distales Glied *nt*, Endglied *nt*, -phalanx *f*, Nagelglied *nt*, Phalanx distalis.
distal tingling on percussion Tinel--Hoffmann'-Klopfzeichen *nt*.
distal tubule (*Niere*) Mittelstück *nt*, distaler Tubulus *m*.
dis·tance ['dɪstəns] *n* **1.** Entfernung *f* (*from* von); Distanz *f*, Zwischenraum *m*, Abstand *m* (*between* zwischen); Entfernung *f*, Strecke *f*. **2.** *fig.* Abstand *m*, Distanz *f*, Zurückhaltung *f*. **3.** (zeitlicher) Abstand *m*, Zeitraum *m*.
d. between the eyes Augenabstand.
d. of vision Sehweite *f*.
dis·tant ['dɪstənt] *adj* **1.** (*a. zeitl.*) entfernt, fern, weit (*from* von); auseinanderliegend. **2.** (*Verwandtschaft*) entfernt. **3.** *fig.* distanziert, kühl, zurückhaltend.
distant flap Fernplastik *f*.
dis·tan·tial aberration [dɪs'tænʃəl] *phys.* Fernaberration *f*, distantielle Aberration *f*.
distant metastasis Fernmetastase *f*.
distant vision Fernsehen *nt*, -sicht *f*.
dis·tend [dɪ'stend] **I** *vt* (aus-)dehnen; (auf-)blähen. **II** *vi* s. (aus-)dehnen; s. (auf-)blähen.
dis·tend·ed [dɪ'stendɪd] *adj* (aus-)gedehnt, erweitert; aufgetrieben, (auf-)gebläht.
distended abdomen geblähtes/überblähtes Abdomen *nt*.
dis·ten·si·bil·i·ty [dɪˌstensə'bɪlətɪ] *n* Dehnbarkeit *f*, Ausdehnungsfähigkeit *f*.
dis·ten·si·ble [dɪ'stensɪbl] *adj* (aus-)dehnbar, ausdehnungsfähig.
dis·ten·sion [dɪ'stenʃn] *n* **1.** (Aus-)Dehnung *f*. **2.** (Auf-)Blähung *f*.
distension stimulus Dehnungsreiz *m*, -stimulus *m*.
dis·ten·tion *n* → distension.
distention cyst Retentionszyste *f*.
dis·tich·ia [dɪs'tɪkɪə] *n* → distichiasis.
dis·ti·chi·a·sis [ˌdɪstə'kaɪəsɪs] *n ophthal.* Distichiasis *f*.
dis·til [dɪ'stɪl] *vt, vi* → distill.
dis·till [dɪ'stɪl] **I** *vt* (ab-, heraus-)destillieren (*from* aus). **II** *vi* destillieren; (allmählich) kondensieren.
distill off/out *vt* ausdestillieren.
dis·till·a·ble [dɪ'stɪləbl] *adj* destillierbar.
dis·til·late ['dɪstlɪt, -eɪt, dɪ'stɪlɪt] *n* Destillat *nt* (*from* aus).
dis·til·la·tion [ˌdɪstə'leɪʃn] *n* **1.** Destillation *f*, Destillieren *nt*. **2.** Destillat *nt*. **3.** Extrakt *m*, Auszug *m*.
dis·tilled [dɪ'stɪld] *adj abbr.* **dest., dist.** destilliert.
distilled oil ätherisches Öl *nt*.
distilled water destilliertes Wasser *nt*, Aqua destillata.
dis·till·er [dɪ'stɪlər] *n* Destillations-, Destillierapparat *m*.
Dis·to·ma ['dɪstəmə] *n micro.* Distoma *nt*, Distomum *nt*.
D. felineum Katzenleberegel *m*, Opisthorchis felineus.
D. haematobium Blasenpärchenegel *m*, Schistosoma haematobium.
D. hepaticum großer Leberegel *m*, Fasciola hepatica.
D. sinensis chinesischer Leberegel *m*, Clonorchis/Opisthorchis sinensis.
dis·to·ma·to·sis [ˌdaɪˌstəʊmə'təʊsɪs] *n* → distomiasis.
dis·to·mia [dɪs'təʊmɪə] *n embryo.* Distomie *f*.

dis·to·mi·a·sis [ˌdaɪstəʊ'maɪəsɪs] *n* Distomainfektion *f*, Distomatose *f*, Distomiasis *f*.
Dis·to·mum ['dɪstəməm] *n* → Distoma.
di·sto·mus [daɪ'stəʊməs] *n embryo.* Distomus *m*.
dis·tor·tion [dɪ'stɔːrʃn] *n* **1.** *ortho.* Verstauchung *f*, Distorsion *f*, Distorsio *f*. **2.** *phys.* Verzerrung *f*, Verzeichnung *f*, Distorsion *f*.
dis·trac·tion [dɪ'strækʃn] *n* **1.** Zerstreuung *f*, Ablenkung *f*. **2.** Zerstreutheit *f*; Verwirrung *f*. **3.** *ortho.* Distraktion *f*.
dis·tress [dɪ'stres] **I** *n* **1.** (körperliche *od.* geistige) Qual *f*, Pein *f*, Schmerz *m*. **2.** Leid *nt*, Kummer *m*, Sorge *f*; Not *f*, Elend *nt*; Notlage *f*, Notstand *m*. **II** *vt* **3.** quälen, peinigen. **4.** bedrücken, beunruhigen.
dis·tri·bu·tion [ˌdɪstrə'bjuːʃn] *n* **1.** Verteilung *f*, Austeilung *f*. **2.** *phys.* Verteilung *f*, Verzweigung *f*. **3.** Verbreitung *f*, Ausbreitung *f*. **4.** *mathe.* Verteilung *f*.
distribution coefficient Verteilungskoeffizient *m*.
distribution curve Verteilungskurve *f*.
distribution function *mathe.* Verteilungsfunktion *f*.
distribution pattern Verteilungsmuster *nt*.
distribution shock Verteilungsschock *m*.
distribution volume Verteilungsvolumen *nt*.
dis·tri·chi·a·sis [ˌdɪstrə'kaɪəsɪs] *n derm.* Districhiasis *f*.
dis·trict ['dɪstrɪkt] *n* Distrikt *m*, (Verwaltungs-, Stadt-)Bezirk *m*, Kreis *m*; Viertel *nt*; Gegend *f*, Gebiet *nt*.
district nurse Gemeindeschwester *f*.
dis·turb [dɪ'stɜːrb] **I** *vt* (*a. electr., techn.*) stören; behindern, beeinträchtigen; beunruhigen; in Unordnung bringen. **II** *vi* stören.
dis·turb·ance [dɪ'stɜːrbəns] *n* **1.** (*a. electr., techn.*) Störung *f*; Behinderung *f*, Beeinträchtigung *f*; Beunruhigung *f*; Durcheinanderbringen *nt*. **2.** *psycho.* (seelische) Erregung *f*; (geistige) Verwirrung *f*; Verhaltensstörung *f*.
d. of balance Gleichgewichtsstörung *f*.
d. of circulation Kreislaufstörung *f*.
d. in conduction Erregungsleitungsstörung.
d. of equilibrium Gleichgewichtsstörung *f*.
d.s of memory Gedächtnisstörungen *pl*.
d. of micturition Blasenentleerungsstörung.
d. of orientation Orientierungsstörung.
d. of sound conduction Schalleitungsstörung.
d. of speech Sprachstörung *f*.
dis·turbed [dɪ'stɜːrbd] **I** *the* ~ *pl* (verhaltens-)gestörte Personen *pl*. **II** *adj* **1.** (geistig) gestört; verhaltensgestört. **2.** beunruhigt (*at, by* über).
dis·turb·ing [dɪ'stɜːrbɪŋ] *adj* störend; beunruhigend (*to* für).
di·sul·fate [daɪ'sʌlfeɪt] *n* Disulfat *nt*.
di·sul·fide [daɪ'sʌlfaɪd, -fɪd] *n* Disulfid *nt*.
disulfide bond Disulfidbindung *f*.
disulfide bridge *chem.* Disulfidbrücke *f*.
di·sul·fi·ram [ˌdaɪsʌl'fɪərəm] *n pharm.* Disulfiram *nt*, Tetraäthylthiuramidsulfid *nt*.
dis·use atrophy [dɪs'juːs] Inaktivitätsatrophie *f*.
disuse osteoporosis Inaktivitätsosteoporose *f*.
di·syn·ap·tic [daɪsɪ'næptɪk] *adj* disynaptisch.
di·ter·pene [daɪ'tɜːrpiːn] *n* Diterpen *nt*.
di·thi·ol [daɪ'θaɪəl, -al] *n* Dithiol *nt*.
dith·ra·nol ['dɪθrənəl] *n pharm.* Anthralin *nt*, Dithranol *nt*.

Dittrich ['dɪtrɪk; -trɪç]: **D.'s plugs** *patho.* Dittrich-Pfröpfe *pl*.
D.'s stenosis *radiol.* infundibuläre Pulmonal(is)stenose *f*.
di·u·re·sis [ˌdaɪə'riːsɪs] *n, pl* **-ses** [-siːz] (übermäßige) Harnausscheidung *f*, Harnfluß *m*, Diurese *f*.
di·u·ret·ic [ˌdaɪə'retɪk] **I** *n pharm.* harntreibendes Mittel *nt*, Diuretikum *nt*. **II** *adj* Diurese betr., harntreibend, diuresefördernd, -anregend, diuretisch.
di·u·ria [daɪ'(j)ʊərɪə] *n urol.* Diurie *f*.
di·ur·nal [daɪ'ɜrnl] *adj* am Tage, tagsüber, täglich, Tag(es)-; diurnal, tageszyklisch.
diurnal epilepsy Epilepsia diurna.
diurnal rhythm Tagesrythmus *m*, tageszyklischer/tagesperiodischer Rhythmus *m*.
di·va·ga·tion [ˌdaɪvə'geɪʃn] *n psychia.* Weitschweifigkeit *f*, Divagation *f*.
di·va·lent [daɪ'veɪlənt] *adj chem.* zweiwertig, divalent.
di·verge [dɪ'vɜːrdʒ, daɪ-] **I** *vt* ablenken. **II** *vi* **1.** (*a. mathe., phys.*) divergieren, auseinanderstreben, -laufen, -gehen. **2.** abweichen (*from* von).
di·ver·gence [dɪ'vɜːrdʒəns, daɪ-] *n* **1.** *bio., mathe., ophthal., phys.* Auseinanderstreben *nt*, -laufen *nt*, -gehen *nt*, Divergenz *f*. **2.** Abweichung *f* (*from* von).
divergence principle Divergenzprinzip *nt*.
di·ver·gen·cy [dɪ'vɜːrdʒənsɪ, daɪ-] *n* → divergence.
di·ver·gent [dɪ'vɜːrdʒənt, daɪ-] *adj* **1.** (*a. mathe., bio., phys.*) auseinanderstrebend, -laufend, -gehend, divergent, divergierend. **2.** abweichend.
divergent evolution *bio.* divergente/aufspaltende Evolution *f*.
divergent rays divergente/divergierende Strahlen *pl*.
divergent squint → divergent strabismus.
divergent strabismus *ophthal.* Auswärtsschielen *nt*, Exotropie *f*, Strabismus divergens.
di·verg·ing lens [dɪ'vɜːrdʒɪŋ, daɪ-] konkave Linse *f*, Konkavlinse *f*, (Zer-)Streuungslinse *f*.
diverging meniscus Konvexokonkavlinse *f*.
div·er's palsy/paralysis ['daɪvər] Druckluft-, Caissonkrankheit *f*.
di·ver·tic·u·lar [ˌdaɪvər'tɪkjələr] *adj* Divertikel betr., divertikelähnlich, Divertikel-.
diverticular abscess Divertikelabszeß *m*.
diverticular bleeding Divertikelblutung *f*.
diverticular carcinoma Divertikelkarzinom *nt*.
diverticular disease (*Darm*) durch Divertikel *od.* Divertikulitis *od.* Divertikulose hervorgerufener Symptomenkomplex.
diverticular hemorrhage Divertikelblutung *f*.
diverticular hernia *chir.* Hernie *f* mit Meckel'-Divertikel im Bruchsack.
diverticular inflammation → diverticulitis.
di·ver·tic·u·lar·i·za·tion [ˌdaɪvərˌtɪkjəˌlærɪ'zeɪʃn] *n* Divertikelbildung *f*.
di·ver·tic·u·lec·to·my [ˌ-'lektəmɪ] *n chir.* Divertikelresektion *f*, -entfernung *f*, -abtragung *f*, Divertikulektomie *f*.
di·ver·tic·u·li·tis [ˌ-'laɪtɪs] *n* Divertikelentzündung *f*, Divertikulitis *f*.
di·ver·tic·u·lo·pe·xy [ˌdaɪvərtɪkjələ'peksɪ] *n chir.* Divertikelanheftung *f*, -fixierung *f*, Divertikulopexie *f*.
di·ver·tic·u·lo·sis [ˌdaɪvərˌtɪkjə'ləʊsɪs] *n* Divertikulose *f*.
d. of the colon Kolon-, Dickdarmdivertikulose.

diverticulum

d. of the common bile duct polyzystische Choledochuszysten pl.
d. of the gallbladder Cholecystitis glandularis proliferans.
d. of the small intestine Dünndarmdivertikulose.
di·ver·tic·u·lum [ˌdaɪvərˈtɪkjələm] n, pl **-la** [-lə] anat. Divertikel nt, Diverticulum nt.
d.la of ampulla (of deferent duct) Ampullendivertikel pl, -säckchen pl, Diverticula ampullae (ductus deferentes).
di·vide [dɪˈvaɪd] I vt **1.** teilen; zerteilen, spalten (into in); (ab-)trennen, scheiden (from von). **2.** ver-, aus-, aufteilen (among, between unter). **3.** einteilen, gliedern (into, in in). **4.** mathe. dividieren, teilen (by durch). II vi **5.** s. teilen; s. aufteilen, s. auflösen, zerfallen (into in). **6.** s. trennen (from von). **7.** s. gliedern (lassen) (into in). **8.** mathe. s. dividieren od. teilen lassen (by durch).
di·vid·ed [dɪˈvaɪdɪd] adj **1.** (a. fig.) geteilt; Teil-. **2.** getrennt. **3.** zu-, aufgeteilt, verteilt.
divided dose fraktionierte Dosis f, Dosis refracta.
di·vid·er [dɪˈvaɪdər] n Trennwand f, Raumaufteiler m.
di·vid·ing [dɪˈvaɪdɪŋ] adj (ab-)trennend, Trennungs-.
dividing nucleus bio. Teilungskern m.
div·ing goiter [ˈdaɪvɪŋ] Tauchkropf m.
diving reflex Tauchreflex m.
di·vi·nyl [daɪˈvaɪnl] n Divinyl nt.
di·vis·i·bil·i·ty [dɪˌvɪzəˈbɪlətɪ] n Teilbarkeit f.
di·vis·i·ble [dɪˈvɪzəbl] adj teilbar.
di·vi·sion [dɪˈvɪʒn] n **1.** Teilung f; Zerteilung f, Spaltung f (into in); Abtrennung f (from von). **2.** Ver-, Aus-, Aufteilung f (among, between unter). **3.** Einteilung f, Gliederung f (into in). **4.** mathe. Division f, Teilen nt. **5.** Trenn-, Scheide-, Grenzlinie f; Trennwand f. **6.** Abschnitt m, Teil m; Fach nt, Kategorie f, Gruppe f; Abteilung f. **7.** bio. (Unter-)Klasse f, (Unter-)Abteilung f.
di·vi·sion·al [dɪˈvɪʒnəl] adj Trenn-, Scheide-; Abteilungs-.
di·vulse [daɪˈvʌls, dɪ-] vt gewaltsam trennen, auseinanderreißen.
di·vul·sion [dɪˈvʌlʃn, daɪ-] n gewaltsame Trennung f, Auseinanderreißen nt.
Dixon Mann [ˈdɪksən mæn]: **D. M.'s sign** Mann-Zeichen m.
di·zy·got·ic [ˌdaɪzaɪˈgɑtɪk] adj zweieiig, dizygot.
dizygotic twins binovuläre/dissimiläre/dizygote/erbungleiche/heteroovuläre/zweieiige Zwillinge pl.
di·zy·gous [daɪˈzaɪgəs] adj → dizygotic.
diz·zi·ness [ˈdɪzɪnɪs] n **1.** (subjektiver) Schwindel m, Schwind(e)ligkeit f. **2.** Schwindelanfall m. **3.** Benommenheit f.
diz·zy [ˈdɪzɪ] I adj **1.** schwind(e)lig. **2.** verwirrt, benommen. **3.** wirr, konfus. II vi schwind(e)lig machen; verwirren.
djen·kol·ic acid [dʒenˈkɑlɪk, -dʒeŋ-] Djenkolsäure f.
DL abbr. → differential limen.
dl abbr. → deciliter.
DLE abbr. → lupus erythematosus, discoid.
DM abbr. → diabetes mellitus.
dm abbr. → decimeter.
DMAC abbr. → dimethylacetamide.
DMBA abbr. → 7,12-dimethylbenz(a)anthracene.
DMCT abbr. [demethylchlortetracycline] → demeclocycline.
DMP abbr. → dimethyl phthalate.
DMPE abbr. → 3,4-dimethoxyphenylethylamine.

DMSO abbr. → dimethyl sulfoxide.
DMT abbr. → dimethyltryptamine.
DN abbr. → dibucaine number.
DNA abbr. → deoxyribonucleic acid.
DNAase abbr. → deoxyribonuclease.
DNA-containing viruses micro. DNA-Viren pl, DNS-Viren pl.
DNA-directed DNA polymerase DNA--abhängige DNA-Polymerase f, DNA--abhängige DNS-Polymerase f, DNS--Nukleotidyltransferase f, DNS-Polymerase f I, Kornberg-Enzym nt.
DNA-directed RNA polymerase DNA--abhängige RNA-Polymerase f, DNS--abhängige RNS-Polymerase f, Transkriptase f.
DNA gyrase DNA-Gyrase f, DNS-Gyrase f.
DNA helix Watson-Crick-Modell nt, Doppelhelix f.
DNA ligase DNA-Ligase f, DNS-Ligase f, Polynukleotidligase f, Polydesoxyribonukleotidsynthase f (ATP) f.
DNA nucleotidylexotransferase DNS--Nukleotidylexotransferase f, DNA-Nukleotidylexotransferase f, terminale Desoxynukleotidyltransferase f abbr. TdT.
DNA nucleotidyltransferase → DNA-directed DNA polymerase.
DNA polymerase DNS-Polymerase f, DNA-Polymerase f.
DNA polymerase I → DNA-directed DNA polymerase.
DNA polymerase II RNS-abhängige DNS-Polymerase f, RNA-abhängige DNA-Polymerase f, reverse Transkriptase f abbr. RT.
DNAse abbr. → deoxyribonuclease.
DNase abbr. → deoxyribonuclease.
DNA-specific adj DNA-spezifisch.
DNA-specific inhibitor DNA-spezifischer Inhibitor m.
DNA template DNA-Matrize f.
DNA viruses micro. DNA-Viren pl, DNS-Viren pl.
DNB abbr. → dinitrobenzene.
DNCB abbr. → (2,4-)dinitrochlorobenzene.
DNFB abbr. → (2,4-)dinitrofluorobenzene.
DNP abbr. **1.** → deoxyribonucleoprotein. **2.** → dinitrophenol.
D₂O abbr. → deuterium oxide.
do [du:] (did; done) I vt tun, machen; ausführen, vollbringen, leisten; tätigen; etw. anfertigen; (Verbrechen) begehen; (Essen) zubereiten.**to ~ a test/examination** einen Test/eine Untersuchung machen. II vi **1.** handeln, vorgehen, tun; s. verhalten. **2. ~ well 1.** weiter-, voran-, vorwärtskommen (with bei mit). **2.** gedeihen, s. gut erholen; gesund sein.
do away vt etw. beseitigen od. abschaffen od. vernichten (with). **2. to ~ with o.s.** s. umbringen.
do in vt to fell/be done in inf. geschafft od. fertig od. erledigt sein.
do out vt saubermachen, säubern; aufräumen.
do up vt (Kleider) zumachen, -knöpfen.
do with vi (sehr gut) brauchen können.
do without vi auskommen od. s. behelfen ohne.
do·a·ble [ˈduːəbl] adj machbar, ausführbar.
Dobie [ˈdəʊbɪ]: **D.'s line/layer** Z-Linie f, Z-Streifen m, Zwischenscheibe f, Telophragma nt.
do·bu·ta·mine [dəʊˈbjuːtəmiːn] n pharm. Dobutamin nt.
DOC abbr. → 11-deoxycorticosterone.
DOCA abbr. → deoxycorticosterone acetate.

doc·o·sa·hex·a·e·no·ic acid [ˌdɑkəsəˌheksərˈnəʊɪk] abbr. **DHA** Docosahexensäure f.
doc·tor [ˈdɑktər] n **1.** Arzt m, Ärztin f, Doktor(in f) m. **2.** Doktor m (of... der...).
doc·to·rand [ˈdɑktərænd] n Doktorand(in f) m.
doc·tor·ate [ˈdæktərɪt] n Doktorat nt, Doktorwürde f, -titel m.
doctor-patient-relationship Arzt-Patient--Beziehung f.
doc·tor·ship [ˈdɑktərʃɪp] n → doctorate.
doc·trine [ˈdɑktrɪn] n Doktrin f, Lehre f, Lehrmeinung f.
doc·u·sate calcium [ˈdɑkjəseɪt] pharm. Docusat-Kalzium nt, Kalziumdioctylsulfosukzinat nt.
docusate sodium pharm. Docusat-Natrium nt, Natriumdioctylsulfosukzinat nt.
do·dec·a·dac·ty·li·tis [dəʊˌdekəˌdæktəˈlaɪtɪs] n → duodenitis.
do·dec·a·dac·ty·lon [ˌ-ˈdæktɪlɑn] n → duodenum.
do·dec·a·no·ic acid [ˌ-ˈnəʊɪk] Laurinsäure f, n-Dodecansäure f.
Döderlein [ˈdeːdərlaɪn; ˈdød-]: **D.'s bacillus** Döderlein'-Stäbchen pl.
Doerfler-Stewart [ˈdœrflər ˈst(j)uːərt]: **D.-S. test** HNO Doerfler-Stewart-Test m.
dog button [dɑg] pharm. Brechnuß f, Nux vomica.
Dogiel [dɔʒiˈel]: **D.'s cells** Dogiel-Zellen pl. **D.'s corpuscles** Dogiel-Körperchen pl.
dog·ma [ˈdɑgmə] n Grundsatz m, (starrer) Lehrsatz m, Dogma nt.
dog nose Gundu-, Goundou-Syndrom nt.
dog tapeworm 1. Blasenbandwurm m, Hundebandwurm m, Echinococcus granulosus, Taenia echinococcus. **2.** → double-pored d.
double-pored d. Gurkenkernbandwurm m, Dipylidium caninum.
dog tick micro. **1.** Hundezecke f, Haemaphysalis leachi. **2.** → American d. **3.** → British d.
American d. amerikanische Hundezecke, Dermacentor variabilis.
British d. 1. Ixodes canisaga. **2.** Rhipicephalus sanguineus.
brown d. Rhipicephalus sanguineus.
Pacific coast d. Dermacentor occidentalis. **Döhle** [ˈdiːlɪ; ˈdøːlə]: **D.'s bodies** Döhle'-(Einschluß-)Körperchen pl.
D.'s disease Aortensyphilis f, Mesaortitis luetica, Aortitis syphilitica.
D.'s furrows/grooves Döhle'-Furchen pl.
D.'s inclusion bodies → **D.'s bodies**.
Döhle-Heller [ˈhelər]: **D.-H. aortitis/disease** Döhle'sche Krankheit.
Doléris [dɔleˈriː]: **D.' operation** gyn. Doléris--Operation f.
dolicho- pref. lang-, dolicho-.
dol·i·cho·ce·pha·lia [ˌdɑlɪkəʊsɪˈfeɪljə] n → dolichocephaly.
dol·i·cho·ce·phal·ic [ˌ-sɪˈfælɪk] adj embryo. langköpfig, dolichokephal, -zephal.
dol·i·cho·ceph·a·lism [ˌ-ˈsefəlɪzəm] n → dolichocephaly.
dol·i·cho·ceph·a·lous [ˌ-ˈsefələs] adj → dolichocephalic.
dol·i·cho·ceph·a·ly [ˌ-ˈsefəlɪ] n embryo. Langköpfigkeit f, Langschädel m, Dolichokephalie f, -zephalie f.
dol·i·cho·co·lon [ˌ-ˈkəʊlən] n embryo. Dolichokolie f.
dol·i·cho·cra·ni·al [ˌ-ˈkreɪnɪəl] adj → dolichocephalic.
dol·i·cho·fa·cial [ˌ-ˈfeɪʃl] adj embryo. langgesichtig, dolichofazial.
dol·i·chol [ˈdɑlɪkɑl, -kəl] n Dolichol nt.
dol·i·cho·pel·lic [ˌdɑlɪkəʊˈpelɪk] adj → dolichopelvic.

dolichopellic pelvis longitudinal-ovales Becken nt.
dol·i·cho·pel·vic [ˌ-'pelvɪk] adj embryo., gyn. dolichopelvisch.
dol·i·cho·pro·sop·ic [ˌ-prə'sɑpɪk, -'səʊp-] adj → dolichofacial.
dol·i·cho·sten·o·me·lia [ˌ-ˌstenə'miːlɪə] n Spinnenfingrigkeit f, Dolichostenomelie f, Arachnodaktylie f.
dol·i·chyl phosphate ['dɑləkɪl] Dolichylphosphat nt.
doll's eye reflex [dɑl] → doll's eye sign.
doll's eye sign Cantelli-Zeichen nt, Puppenaugenphänomen nt.
doll's head phenomenon → doll's eye sign.
Döllinger ['delɪŋər; 'dœlɪŋ-]: **D.'s tendinous ring** anat. Döllinger-Sehnenring m.
Dolman ['dɑlmən]: **D.'s test** ophthal. Dolman-Test m.
do·lor ['doʊlər] n, pl **do·lo·res** [də'lɔːrɪs] patho. Schmerz m, Dolor m.
do·lo·rif·ic [ˌdoʊlə'rɪfɪk] adj schmerz(en)auslösend, -verursachend.
do·lo·rim·e·try [ˌdoʊlə'rɪmətrɪ] n Schmerzmessung f.
do·lor·o·gen·ic [dəˌlɔʊrə'dʒenɪk] adj → dolorific.
dolorogenic zone Triggerzone f.
DOM abbr. → 2,5-dimethoxy-4-methylamphetamine.
do·main [doʊ'meɪn] n 1. biochem. Domäne f, domain. 2. fig. Bereich m, Gebiet nt, Domäne f.
dome [doʊm] n 1. Wölbung f. 2. Kuppel f, kuppelförmige Bildung f, Gewölbe nt.
  d. of diaphragm Zwerchfellkuppel.
  d. of pleura Pleurakuppel.
domed [doʊmd] adj → dome-shaped.
dome-shaped adj kuppelförmig, gewölbt.
do·mes·tic [dəˈmestɪk] adj häuslich, Haus-, Haushalts-, Familien-, Privat-.
domestic accident Unfall m im Haushalt, häuslicher Unfall m.
dom·i·cil·i·ary [ˌdɑmə'sɪlɪərɪ] adj Haus-, Wohnungs-.
domiciliary treatment Hausbehandlung f.
domiciliary visit Hausbesuch m.
dom·i·nance ['dɑmɪnəns] n 1. (Vor-)Herrschaft f, (Vor-)Herrschen nt. 2. bio., genet., physiol. Dominanz f.
dom·i·nant ['dɑmɪnənt] I n genet. Dominante f. II adj 1. dominant, dominierend, (vor-)herrschend; überwiegend. 2. genet. Dominanz betr., (im Erbgang) dominierend, dominant.
dominant gene dominantes Gen nt.
dominant hemisphere neuro. dominierende/dominante Hemisphäre f.
dominant heredodegenerative deafness dominant hereditär-degenerative Schwerhörigkeit f.
dominant inheritance dominante Vererbung f.
dom·i·nate ['dɑmɪneɪt] I vt (be-)herrschen, dominieren. II vi (vor-)herrschen, dominieren.
do·mi·phen ['doʊmɪfen] n pharm. Domiphen nt.
dom·per·i·done [dɑm'perɪdoʊn] n pharm. Domperidon nt.
do·nate [doʊ'neɪt, 'doʊ-] vt (Blut) spenden; stiften, schenken.
Donath-Landsteiner ['doʊnæθ 'lændstaɪnər; doːnaːt 'lantʃtaɪnər]: **D.-L. cold autoantibody** Donath-Landsteiner-Antikörper m.
  D.-L. phenomenon Donath-Landsteiner-Phänomen nt.
  D.-L. test Donath-Landsteiner-Reaktion f.
do·na·tion [doʊ'neɪʃn] n 1. (Blut, Organ) Spende f. 2. Spende f, Stiftung f, Schenkung f.
do·na·tor ['doʊneɪtər] n → donor.
Donders ['dɑndər]: **D.' glaucoma** ophthal. Offenwinkel-, Weitwinkel-, Simplexglaukom nt, Glaucoma simplex.
  D.'s law ophthal. Donders-Gesetz nt (der konstanten Orientierung).
  D.' pressure Donders-Druck m.
  D.' rings Donders-Ringe pl.
  D.' space Donders-Raum m.
  D.' test Donders-Test m.
Donnan ['dɑnən]: **D.'s equilibrium** (Gibbs-)-Donnan-Gleichgewicht nt.
  D.'s factor Donnan-Faktor m.
Donné [dɔ'ne]: **D.'s bodies/corpuscles** Donné-Körperchen pl, Kolostrumkörperchen pl.
Donohue ['dɑnəjuː]: **D.'s disease/syndrome** Leprechaunismus(-Syndrom nt) m.
do·nor ['doʊnər] n 1. (Blut-, Organ-)Spender(in f) m. 2. chem. Donor m, Donator m. 3. Stifter(in f) m, Schenker(in f) m.
donor antigen Spenderantigen nt.
donor blood Spenderblut nt.
donor card Organspenderausweis m.
donor cell Spenderzelle f.
donor insemination heterologe Insemination f, künstliche Befruchtung f mit Spendersperma.
donor organ Spenderorgan nt.
donor-recipient matching immun. Spender-Empfänger-Matching nt.
donor serum Spenderserum nt.
donor-specific transfusion abbr. **DST** spenderspezifische Transfusion f.
Donovan ['dɑnəvən]: **D.'s body** Donovan-Körperchen nt, Calymmatobacterium granulomatis, Donovania granulomatis.
Don·o·va·nia granulomatis [ˌdɑnə'væniə] micro. → Donovan's body.
don·o·va·no·sis [dɑnəvæ'noʊsɪs] n Lymphogranuloma inguinale/venereum nt abbr. **LGV**, Lymphopathia venerea, Morbus Durand-Nicolas-Favre m, klimatischer Bubo m, vierte Geschlechtskrankheit f, Poradenitis inguinalis.
DOPA abbr. [3,4-dihydroxyphenylalanine] → dopa.
do·pa ['doʊpə] n abbr. **DOPA** 3,4-Dihydroxyphenylalanin nt, Dopa nt, DOPA nt.
dopa decarboxylase Dopadecarboxylase f, DOPA-decarboxylase f.
do·pa·mine ['doʊpəmiːn] n Dopamin nt, Hydroxytyramin nt.
dopamine β-hydroxylase → dopamine β-monooxygenase.
dopamine β-monooxygenase Dopamin-β-monooxygenase f, Dopamin-β-hydroxylase f.
do·pa·mi·ner·gic [ˌdoʊpəmɪ'nɜrdʒɪk] adj von Dopamin aktiviert od. übertragen, durch Dopaminfreisetzung wirkend, dopaminerg.
dopaminergic neuron dopaminerges Neuron nt.
dopaminergic system dopaminerges System nt.
dopamine system Dopaminsystem nt.
dopa-oxydase → Monophenolmonooxygenase f, Monophenyloxidase f.
do·pase ['doʊpeɪz] n → dopa-oxydase.
Doppler ['dɑplər]: **D. effect** Doppler-Effekt m, -Prinzip nt.
  D. phenomenon → D. effect.
  D. principle → D. effect.
  D. shift Doppler-Verschiebung f.
  D. ultrasonography Doppler-Sonographie f.
Dorendorf ['doːrəndɔrf]: **D.'s sign** card. Dorendorf'-Zeichen nt.
dor·man·cy ['dɔːrmənsɪ] n 1. Schlaf m, Schlafzustand m. 2. micro. Wachstumsruhe f, Dormanz f.
dor·mant ['dɔːrmənt] adj 1. schlafend. 2. micro. ruhend, dormant. 3. fig. verborgen, latent.
dor·nase ['dɔːrneɪz] n Dornase f.
Dorno ['dɔːrnoʊ]: **D.'s rays** Dorno-Strahlung f.
Dorothy Reed ['dɑrəθɪ riːd]: **D. R. cell** Sternberg(-Reed)-Riesenzelle f.
dors- pref. → dorso-.
dor·sad ['dɔːrsæd] adj anat. zum Rücken hin, rückenwärts, dorsad.
dor·sal ['dɔːrsl] adj rückseitig, zum Rücken/zur Rückseite hin (liegend), zum Rücken gehörig, dorsal, Rück(en)-, Dorsal-.
dorsal aortae embryo. dorsale Aorten pl.
dorsal artery: d. of clitoris A. dorsalis clitoridis.
  d. of foot Fußrückenarterie f, -schlagader f, Dorsalis f pedis, A. dorsalis pedis.
  d. of nose Nasenrückenarterie f, A. dorsalis nasi, A. nasalis externa.
  d. of penis dorsale Penisarterie f, Dorsalis f penis, A. dorsalis penis.
  d.s of tongue Zungenrückenarterien pl, Rami dorsales linguae a. lingualis.
dorsal border: d. of radius Radiushinterrand m, Margo posterior radii.
  d. of ulna Ulnahinterrand m, Margo posterior ulnae.
dorsal branch: d.es of cervical nerves hintere/dorsale Halsnervenäste pl, Rami dorsales/posteriores nn. cervicalium.
  d. of coccygeal nerve hinterer Ast m des N. coccygeus, Ramus dorsalis/posterior n. coccygei.
  d. of lumbar arteries Rückenast m der Lumbalarterien, Ramus dorsalis aa. lumbalium.
  d.es of lumbar nerves Rückenäste pl der Lendennerven, Rami dorsales/posteriores nn. lumbalium.
  d. of posterior intercostal arteries hinterer Ast m der hinteren Interkostalarterien, Ramus dorsalis aa. intercostalium posteriorum.
  d. of posterior intercostal veins Rückenast m der hinteren Interkostalvenen, Ramus dorsalis vv. intercostalium posteriorum.
  d.es of sacral nerves dorsale/hintere Äste pl der Sakralnerven, Rami dorsales/posteriores nn. sacralium.
  d. of spinal nerves hinterer Ast m od. Rückenast m der Spinalnerven, Ramus dorsalis/posterior nn. spinalium.
  d. of subcostal artery Rückenast m der A. subcostalis, Ramus dorsalis a. subcostalis.
  d.es of superior intercostal artery Rückenäste pl der A. intercostalis suprema, Rami dorsales a. intercostalis supremae.
  d.es of thoracic nerves Rückenäste pl der Brust-/Thorakalnerven, Rami dorsales/posteriores nn. thoracicorum.
  d. of ulnar nerve dorsaler (Haupt-)Ast m des N. ulnaris, Ramus dorsalis n. ulnaris.
dorsal column Hintersäule f (der grauen Substanz), Columna dorsalis/posterior (medullae spinalis).
  d. of spinal cord → dorsal column.
dorsal column nuclei Hinterstrangkerne pl.
dorsal column system Hinterstrangsystem nt, Lemniscussystem nt.
dorsal decubitus Rückenlage f.
dorsal divisions of trunks of brachial plexus hintere Äste pl der Trunci plexus brachialis, Divisiones dorsales/posteriores truncorum plexus brachialis.

dorsal fascia, deep Fascia thoracolumbalis.
dorsal funiculus (of spinal cord) Hinterstrang *m*, Funiculus dorsalis/posterior (medullae spinalis).
dor·sal·gia [dɔːrˈsældʒ(ɪ)ə] *n* Rückenschmerz(en *pl*) *m*, Dorsalgie *f*, Dorsodynie *f*.
dorsal hernia *chir.* Lendenbruch *m*, Hernia lumbalis.
dorsal horn Hinterhorn *nt* (des Rückenmarks), Cornu dorsale/posterius (medullae spinalis).
 d. of spinal cord → dorsal horn.
dorsal horn neuron Hinterhornneuron *nt*.
dorsal margin of radius → dorsal border of radius.
dorsal mesentery *embryo.* dorsales Mesenterium *nt*.
dorsal mesocardium *embryo.* dorsales Mesokard *nt*.
dorsal mesocolon *embryo.* dorsales Mesokolon *nt*.
dorsal mesoduodenum *embryo.* dorsales Mesoduodenum *nt*.
dorsal mesogastrium *embryo.* dorsales Mesogastrium *nt*.
dorsal nerve: d. of clitoris N. dorsalis clitoridis.
 d. of penis N. dorsalis penis.
 d. of scapula Dorsalis *m* scapulae, N. dorsalis scapulae.
dorsal nucleus → d. of Clarke.
 anterior d. Nc. dorsalis anterior.
 d. of Clarke Clarke'-Säule *f*, Clarke-Stilling'-Säule *f*, Stilling'-Kern, Nc. thoracicus, Columna thoracica.
 d. of glossopharyngeal nerve Nc. dorsalis n. glossopharyngei.
 posterior d. Nc. dorsalis posterior.
 d.i of thalamus dorsale Thalamuskerne *pl*, Ncc. dorsales (thalami).
 d. of trapezoid body dorsaler Trapezkern *m*, Nc. dorsalis corporis trapezoidei.
 d. of vagus nerve hinterer Kern *m* des N. vagus, hinterer Vaguskern *m*, Nc. dorsalis n. vagi, Nc. vagalis dorsalis.
dorsal pancreas *embryo.* dorsales Pankreas *nt*.
dorsal part: d. of cerebral peduncle Pars dorsalis/posterior pedunculi cerebri.
 d. of lateral geniculate body Kern *m* des lateralen Kniehöckers, Nc. corporis geniculati lateralis.
 d. of medial geniculate body Kern *m* des medialen Kniehöckers, Nc. corporis geniculati medialis.
 d. of pons Tegmentum pontis, Pars posterior pontis.
dorsal phthisis Wirbeltuberkulose *f*, Spondylitis tuberculosa.
dorsal plate *embryo.* Deckplatte *f*.
dorsal position Rückenlage *f*.
dorsal regions *anat.* Rückenfelder *pl*, -regionen *pl*, Regiones dorsales.
dorsal rhizotomy *neurochir.* Rhizotomia posterior.
dorsal root hintere/sensible Spinal(nerven)wurzel *f*, Radix dorsalis/posterior/sensoria nn. spinalium.
 d. of spinal nerves → dorsal root.
dorsal root ganglion (sensorisches) Spinalganglion *nt*, Ggl. spinale/sensorium.
dorsal spine Wirbelsäule *f*, Rückgrat *nt*, Columna vertebralis.
dorsal surface of scapula Skapularückfläche *f*, Facies posterior scapulae.
dorsal sympathectomy dorsale Sympathektomie *f*.
dorsal thalamus dorsaler Thalamusabschnitt *m*, Thalamus dorsalis.

dorsal tubercle (of radius) Tuberculum dorsale (radii).
dorsal vein: d. of corpus callosum dorsale Balkenvene *f*, V. dorsalis corporis callosi.
 deep d. of clitoris V. dorsalis profunda clitoridis.
 deep d. of penis tiefe Penisrückenvene *f*, V. dorsalis profunda penis.
 superficial d.s of clitoris oberflächliche hintere Klitorisvenen *pl*, Vv. dorsales superficiales clitoridis.
 superficial d.s of penis oberflächliche Penisrückenvenen *pl*, Vv. dorsales superficiales penis.
dorsal vertebrae Thorakal-, Brustwirbel *pl abbr* BW, Vertebrae thoracicae.
dorsi- *pref.* → dorso-.
dor·si·duct [ˈdɔːrsɪdʌkt] *vt* nach hinten *od.* zum Rücken ziehen.
dor·si·flex [ˈ-fleks] *vt* nach rückwärts beugen, dorsalflektieren.
dor·si·flex·ion [ˌ-ˈflekʃn] *n* Beugung *f* nach rückwärts/in Richtung der Rückseite, Dorsalflexion *f*.
dor·si·flex·or [ˈ-fleksər] *n* dorsal flektierender Muskel *m*.
 d.s of foot (*Fuß*) Dorsalflexoren *pl*.
dor·si·lat·er·al [ˌ-ˈlætərəl] *adj* → dorsolateral.
dor·si·lum·bar [ˌ-ˈlʌmbər, -bɑːr] *adj* → dorsolumbar.
dor·si·me·di·an [ˌ-ˈmiːdɪən] *adj* → dorsomedial.
dor·si·spi·nal [ˌ-ˈspaɪnl] *adj* Rücken u. Wirbelsäule betr., dorsospinal.
dor·si·ven·tral [ˌ-ˈventrəl] *adj* vom Rücken zum Bauch hin, dorsoventral.
dorso- *pref.* Dorso(-)-, Dorsi-.
dor·so·an·te·ri·or [ˌdɔːrsəʊænˈtɪərɪər] *adj* gyn. dorsoanterior.
dor·so·cu·boi·dal reflex [ˌ-kjuːˈbɔɪdl] *neuro.* Mendel-Bechterew-Reflex *m*.
dor·so·dyn·ia [ˌ-ˈdiːnɪə] *n* → dorsalgia.
dor·so·lat·er·al [ˌ-ˈlætərəl] *adj* hinten u. auf der Seite (liegend), dorsolateral.
dorsolateral fasciculus → dorsolateral tract.
dorsolateral fissure of cerebellum Fissura dorsolateralis/posterolateralis (cerebelli).
dorsolateral groove: d. of medulla oblongata → dorsolateral sulcus of medulla oblongata.
 d. of spinal cord → dorsolateral sulcus of spinal cord.
dorsolateral nucleus (of ventral column of spinal cord) Nc. posterolateralis.
dorsolateral plate *embryo.* Flügelplatte *f*, Lamina alaris.
dorsolateral sulcus: d. of medulla oblongata Hinterseitenfurche *f* der Medulla oblongata, Sulcus posterolateralis medullae oblongatae.
 d. of spinal cord Hinterseitenfurche *f* des Rückenmarks, Sulcus posterolateralis medullae spinalis.
dorsolateral tract Lissauer'-(Rand-)Bündel *nt*, Tractus dorsolateralis.
dor·so·lum·bar [ˌdɔːrsəʊˈlʌmbər, -bɑːr] *adj* Rücken u. Lenden betr., dorsolumbal.
dor·so·me·di·al [ˌ-ˈmiːdɪəl] *adj anat.* hinten u. in der Mitte (liegend), dorsomedial.
dorsomedial nucleus: d. of thalamus Nc. medialis dorsalis (thalami).
 d. of ventral column of spinal cord Nc. posteromedialis.
dor·so·me·di·an [ˌ-ˈmiːdɪən] *adj* → dorsomedial.
dor·so·pos·te·ri·or [ˌ-pɒˈstɪərɪər] *adj gyn.* dorsoposterior.
dor·so·sa·cral position [ˌ-ˈsækrəl, -ˈseɪ-] *chir.* Steinschnittlage *f*.

dor·so·ven·tral [ˌ-ˈventrəl] *adj* → dorsiventral.
dor·sum [ˈdɔːrsəm] *n, pl* **-sa** [-sə] *anat.* Rücken *m*, Rückseite *f*, Dorsum *nt*.
 d. of foot Fußrücken, Dorsum pedis, Regio dorsalis pedis.
 d. of hand Handrücken(seite), Dorsum manus.
 d. of nose Nasenrücken, Dorsum nasi.
 d. of penis Penisrücken, Dorsum penis.
 d. of tongue Zungenrücken, Dorsum linguae.
dorsum pedis reflex *neuro.* Mendel-Bechterew-Reflex *m*.
dorsum sellae Dorsum sellae.
dos·age [ˈdəʊsɪdʒ] *n pharm.* 1. Dosierung *f*, Verabreichung *f*. 2. Dosis *f*, Menge *f*; Portion *f*.
dosage compensation *genet.* Dosiskompensation *f*.
dosage-meter *n* → dosimeter.
dose [dəʊs] I *n* 1. *pharm.* Dosis *f*, Gabe *f*. 2. *radiol.* (Strahlen-)Dosis *f*. 3. Dosis *f*, Portion *f*. II *vt* 4. *pharm.* dosieren, in Dosen verabreichen 5. jdm. eine Dosis verabreichen, Arznei geben.
dose-dependent *adj* dosisabhängig.
dose distribution *radiol.* Dosisverteilung *f*.
dose-effect curve Dosis-Wirkungs-Kurve *f*.
dose-response curve → dose-effect curve.
do·sim·e·ter [dəʊˈsɪmɪtər] *n radiol.* Dosismesser *m*, Dosimeter *nt*.
do·si·met·ric [ˌdəʊsəˈmetrɪk] *adj radiol.* Dosimetrie betr., dosimetrisch.
do·sim·e·try [dəʊˈsɪmɪtrɪ] *n radiol.* Strahlendosismessung *f*, Dosimetrie *f*.
do·sis [ˈdəʊsɪs] *n* → dose I.
dos·si·er [ˈdɒsɪeɪ, -sɪər] *n* (Kranken-)Akten *pl*, Dossier *nt*.
dot [dɒt] *n histol.* Punkt *m*, Pünktchen *nt*, Tüpfelchen *nt*.
dot·age [ˈdəʊtɪdʒ] *n* (*geistige*) Altersschwäche *f*, Senilität *f*.
do·tard·ness [ˈdəʊtədnɪs] *n* → dotage.
Dott [dɒt]: **D.'s operation** Dott'-Operation *f*.
dot·ted tongue [ˈdɒtɪd] Stippchenzunge *f*.
dou·ble [ˈdʌbl] I *n* das Doppelte, das Zweifache; Gegenstück *nt*, Doppel *nt*. II *adj* 1. doppelt, zweifach, Doppel-. 2. doppelseitig. 3. verdoppelt, Doppelt-. II *vt* 4. verdoppeln, verzweifachen. 5. doppelt legen *od.* falten, zusammenfalten. IV *vi* s. verdoppeln.
double athetosis *neurol.* Athetose double/duplex.
double-barrel colostomy *chir.* doppelläufiger Dickdarmafter *m*.
double-blind experiment Doppelblindstudie *f*, -experiment *nt*; *pharm., psycho.* Doppelblindversuch *m*.
double-blind hypothesis *psychia.* Double-Blind-Hypothese *f*.
double-blind test → double-blind experiment.
double-blind trial → double-blind experiment.
double bond Doppelbindung *f*.
double-bond character *chem.* Doppelbindungscharakter *m*.
double-channel catheter doppelläufiger Katheter *m*.
double-check I *n* (genaue) Nachprüfung *f*. II *vt, vi* (genau) nachprüfen.
double chin Doppelkinn *nt*.
double-chinned *adj* mit Doppelkinn.
double-congenital athetosis → double athetosis.
double-contrast arthrography *radiol.* Doppelkontrastarthrographie *f*.

double-contrast barium technique → double-contrast radiography.
double-contrast radiography *radiol.* Doppelkontrast-, Bikontrastmethode *f*.
double-current catheter doppelläufiger Katheter *m*.
double-diffusion in one dimension *immun.* Oakley-Fulthorpe-Technik *f*, eindimensionale Immun(o)diffusion *f* nach Oakley-Fulthorpe.
double-diffusion in two dimensions *immun.* Ouchterlony-Technik *f*, zweidimensionale Immun(o)diffusion *f* nach Ouchterlony.
double disharmonic hearing Doppelhören *nt*, Diplakusis *f*, Diplacusis *f*.
double displacement mechanism/reaction *biochem.* doppelte Verdrängungsreaktion *f*, Ping-Pong-Mechanismus *m*, -Reaktion *f*.
double-edged *adj* (*Messer*) zweischneidig.
double exposure *photo.* 1. Doppelbelichtung *f*. 2. doppelt belichtetes Foto *nt*.
double fracture Zweietagenfraktur *f*.
double-helical DNA → double-stranded DNA.
double helix Watson-Crick-Modell *nt*, Doppelhelix *f*.
double hemiplegia → diplegia.
double insanity *psychia.* induziertes Irresein *nt*, Folie à deux.
double knot doppelter Knoten *m*.
double-loop hernia retrograde Hernie *f*, Hernie en W.
double-lumen catheter doppelläufiger Katheter *m*.
double malformation *embryo.* Doppelmißbildung *f*.
double monster *embryo., patho.* Doppelmißbildung *f*, Duplicitas *f*, Monstrum duplex.
double-mouthed uterus Uterus biforis.
double pedicle flap zweigestielter (Haut-)Lappen *m*.
double penis *embryo.* Diphallus *m*, Penis duplex.
double pneumonia doppelseitige Pneumonie *f*.
double refraction of flow *phys.* Strömungsdoppelbrechung *f*.
double salt *chem.* Doppelsalz *nt*.
double-shock sound Bruit de rappel.
double-strand break Doppelstrangbruch *m*.
double-stranded *adj abbr.* **ds** *genet.* doppelsträngig *abbr.* ds, Doppelstrang-.
double-stranded DNA Doppelhelix-, Duplex-, Doppelstrang-DNA *f abbr.* dsDNA, Doppelhelix-, Duplex-, Doppelstrang-DNS *f abbr.* dsDNS.
double-stranded RNA Doppelstrang-RNA *f abbr.* dsRNA, Doppelstrang-RNS *f abbr.* dsRNS.
dou·blet ['dʌblɪt] *n* 1. Doppellinse *f*, Duplet(t) *nt*. 2. Paar *nt*. 3. Duplikat *nt*.
double tongue gespaltene Zunge *f*, Lingua bifida.
double vision *ophthal.* Doppeltsehen *nt*, Diplopie *f*, Diplopia *f*.
doub·ling dose ['dʌblɪŋ] *radiol.* Verdopplungsdosis *f*.
doubling time *abbr.* **t_D** *micro.* Verdopplungszeit *f*.
douche [du:ʃ] I *n* 1. Dusche *f*, Brause *f*. 2. (Aus-)Spülung *f*. 3. Spülapparat *m*, Irrigator *m*, Dusche *f*. II *vt* 4. (ab-)duschen. 5. (aus-)spülen. III *vi* 6. s. duschen. 7. eine Spülung machen, spülen.
dough-nut kidney ['dəʊnət, -nʌt] Ringniere *f*.
Douglas ['dʌgləs]: **D.' abscess** Douglas-Abszeß *m*, Abszeß *m* im Douglas'-Raum.

D.' bag *chir.* Douglas(-Sieb)-Plastik *f*.
D.'s cul-de-sac Douglas'-Raum *m*, Excavatio recto-uterina.
D.' fold 1. → **D.' ligament**. 2. → **D.' line**.
D.' ligament Douglas-Falte *f*, -Ligament *nt*, Plica rectouterina.
D.' line Douglas-Linie *f*, Linea arcuata vaginae m. recti abdominis.
D.' mechanism → **D.' spontaneous evolution**.
D.' method → **D.' spontaneous evolution**.
pouch of D. → **D.'s cul-de-sac**.
semicircular line of D. → **D.' line**.
D.'s space → **D.'s cul-de-sac**.
D.' spontaneous evolution *gyn.* Douglas-Selbstentwicklung *f*, -Wendung *f*.
doug·las·cele ['dʌgləsi:l] *n* Douglas-Hernie *f*, Douglasozele *f*, Enterocele vaginalis posterior.
doug·la·si·tis [dʌglə'saɪtɪs] *n* Entzündung *f* des Douglas'-Raums, Douglasitis *f*.
dow·el ['daʊəl] *n chir., dent.* Pflock *m*, Dübel *m*.
Down [daʊn]: **D.'s disease/syndrome** Down-Syndrom *nt*, Trisomie 21(-Syndrom *nt*) *f*, Mongolismus *m*, Mongoloidismus *m*.
down [daʊn] I *n* 1. *fig.* Abstieg *m*, Rückgang *m*. 2. Tiefpunkt *m*, -stand *m*. 3. Depression *f*, Tiefpunkt *f*. 4. → downer. 5. *embryo., ped.* Flaum *m*, Wollhaar(kleid *nt*) *nt*, Lanugo *f*. II *adj* 6. nach unten/abwärts (gerichtet *od.* laufend), Abwärts-; unten (befindlich). 7. deprimiert, niedergeschlagen. III *adv* 8. (*Temperatur*) gefallen (*by* um); her-, hinunter, nach unten, unten. 9. bettlägerig.
down·er ['daʊnər] *n inf.* Beruhigungsmittel *nr*, Sedativum *nt*.
Downey ['daʊnɪ]: **D.'s cells** *hema.* Downey-Zellen *pl*, monozytoide Zellen *pl*, Pfeiffer'-Drüsenfieber-Zellen *pl*.
down·heart·ed [daʊn'hɑ:rtɪd] *adj* niedergeschlagen, entmutigt, deprimiert.
down·most ['daʊnməʊst] *adj* unterste(r, s), niedrigste(r, s).
down·y ['daʊnɪ] *adj* mit Flaum bedeckt, aus Flaum bestehend, flaumig.
dox·a·bram ['dɒksəpræm] *n pharm.* Doxabram *nt*.
dox·e·pin ['dɒksəpɪn] *n pharm.* Doxepin *nt*.
dox·o·ru·bi·cin [ˌdɒksə'ru:bəsɪn] *n pharm.* Doxorubicin *nt*, Adriamycin *nt*.
dox·y·cy·cline [ˌdɒksə'saɪkli:n, -lɪn] *n pharm.* Doxycyclin *nt*.
dox·yl·a·mine [dɒk'sɪləmi:n] *n pharm.* Doxylamin *nt*.
Doyen [dwa'jē]: **D.'s raspatory** *ortho.* Doyen-Raspatorium *nt*.
Doyne [dɔɪn]: **D.'s familial honeycomb choroiditis** *ophthal.* Altersdrusen *pl*, Chorioiditis guttata senilis.
D.'s familial honeycomb degeneration → **D.'s familial honeycomb choroiditis**.
D.'s honeycomb choroidopathy → **D.'s familial honeycomb choroiditis**.
D.'s honeycomb degeneration → **D.'s familial honeycomb choroiditis**.
1,3-DPG *abbr.* → 1,3-diphosphoglycerate.
2,3-DPG *abbr.* → 2,3-diphosphoglycerate.
DPN *abbr.* [diphosphopyridine nucleotide] *old* → nicotinamide-adenine dinucleotide.
D.R. *abbr.* → reaction of degeneration.
dr *abbr.* → dram.
drachm [dræm] *n* → dram.
drac·on·ti·a·sis [ˌdrækən'taɪəsɪs] *n* → dracunculiasis.
dra·cun·cu·lar [drə'kʌŋkjələr] *adj* Dracunculus betr., durch Dracunculus verursacht.
dra·cun·cu·li·a·sis [drəˌkʌŋkjʊ'laɪəsɪs] *n* Medinawurminfektion *f*, Guineawurm-

infektion *f*, Drakunkulose *f*, Drakontiase *f*, Dracunculosis *f*, Dracontiasis *f*.
Dra·cun·cu·loi·dea [ˌ-'lɔɪdɪə] *pl micro.* Dracunculoidea *pl*.
dra·cun·cu·lo·sis [ˌ-'ləʊsɪs] *n* → dracunculiasis.
Dra·cun·cu·lus [drə'kʌŋkjələs] *n micro.* Dracunculus *m*.
D. medinensis Medina-, Guineawurm *m*, Dracunculus/Filaria medinensis.
draft [dræft, drɑ:ft] *n* 1. Skizze *f*, Entwurf *m*, Konzept *nt*. 2. (Luft-)Zug *m*. 3. *pharm.* (abgemessene) Dosis *f* einer Arzneimittellösung.
dra·gée [dræ'ʒeɪ] *n pharm.* Dragée *nt*.
drag·on worm ['drægən] → Dracunculus medinensis.
drain [dreɪn] I *n* 1. Ableitung *f*; Ableiten *nt*, Abfließen *nt*, Ablaufen *nt*, Drainieren *nt*, Drainage *f*, Dränage *f*. 2. *chir.* Drain *m*, Drän *m*. 3. Entwässerung *f*, Trockenlegung *f*, Dränage *f*. II *vt* 4. drainieren, dränieren, durch Drain(s) ableiten. 5. *abod.* austrocknen lassen. 6. *fig.* jdn. ermüden, jds. Kräfte aufzehren. 7. filtrieren. III *vi* austrocknen.
drain off/away I *vt* eine Flüssigkeit ableiten *od.* abließen lassen. II *vi* ablaufen, abfließen.
drain·age ['dreɪnɪdʒ] *n* 1. Drainage *f*, Dränage *f*, Ableitung *f* (*von Wundflüssigkeit*); Abfluß *m*. 2. Drainieren *nt*, Dränieren *nt*, Ableiten *nt*; Abfließen *nt*, Ablaufen *nt*.
d. of the middle ear Mittelohr-, Paukendrainage *f*.
drainage bronchus Drainagebronchus *m*.
drainage tube Drainagerohr *nt*.
dram [dræm] *n abbr.* **dr** *pharm.* Drachme *f*, Dram *m*.
drape [dreɪp] *chir.* I *n* (Abdeck-)Tuch *nt*. II *vt* abdecken.
Draper ['dreɪpər]: **D.'s law** Draper-Gesetz *nt*.
drap·e·to·ma·nia [ˌdræpɪtəʊ'meɪnɪə, -jə] *n psychia.* Wandersucht *f*, Drapetomanie *f*.
dras·tic ['dræstɪk] I *n* starkes Abführmittel *nt*, Drastikum *nt*. II *adj* 1. (*Abführmittel*) drastisch, stark. 2. drastisch, durchgreifend, gründlich, rigoros.
draught [dræft, drɑ:ft] *n* → draft.
draw·er phenomenon [drɔ:r] *ortho.* Schubladenphänomen *nt*, -zeichen *nt*.
anterior d. vorderes Schubladenphänomen.
posterior d. hinteres Schubladenphänomen.
drawer sign → drawer phenomenon.
drawer test → drawer phenomenon.
draw·ing pain ['drɔ:ɪŋ] ziehender Schmerz *m*.
dRDP *abbr.* → deoxyribonucleoside diphosphate.
dream [dri:m] (*v* dreamed; dreamt) I *n* Traum *m*; Traumzustand *m*. **to have a ~ about** träumen von. II *vt* 1. träumen. 2. erträumen, ersehnen. III *vi* träumen (*about, of* von); verträumt sein.
dream up *vt* s. ausdenken, phantasieren.
dream analysis Traumanalyse *f*.
dream·er ['dri:mər] *n* Träumer(in *f*) *m*.
dream·i·ness ['dri:mɪnɪs] *n* Verträumtheit *f*; Traumzustand *m*.
dream·ing ['dri:mɪŋ] *adj* verträumt, träumerisch, (wach) träumend, Traum-.
dreaming sleep REM-Traumschlaf *m*, paradoxer/desynchronisierter Schlaf *m*.
dream·less ['dri:mlɪs] *adj* traumlos, ohne Träume.
dream·like ['dri:mlaɪk] *adj* traumhaft, -ähnlich, -artig.
dream pain Schlafschmerz *m*, Hypnalgie *f*.

dream·y ['driːmɪ] *adj* 1. verträumt, träumerisch, (wach) träumend. 2. → dreamlike.
Dreiding ['draɪdɪŋ]: **D. model** *chem.* Dreiding-Modell *nt.*
drep·a·no·cyte ['drepənəʊsaɪt] *n hema.* Sichelzelle *f*, Drepanozyt *m.*
drep·a·no·cy·te·mia [ˌ-saɪ'tiːmɪə] *n* → drepanocytic anemia.
drep·a·no·cyt·ic [ˌ-'sɪtɪk] *adj* Sichelzellen betr., Sichelzell(en)-.
drepanocytic anemia Sichelzell(en)anämie *f*, Herrick-Syndrom *nt.*
drep·a·no·cy·to·sis [ˌ-saɪ'təʊsɪs] *n hema.* Drepanozytose *f.*
Dresbach ['drezbæk, -bax]: **D.'s anemia/syndrome** Dresbach-Syndrom *nt*, hereditäre Elliptozytose *f*, Ovalozytose *f*, Kamelozytose *f*, Elliptozytenanämie *f.*
dress [dres] **I** *n* Kleidung *f.* **II** *vt* 1. an-, bekleiden, anziehen. 2. *ortho.* (*Wunde*) verbinden, behandeln, einen Verband anlegen.
dres·sing ['dresɪŋ] *n* 1. Verbinden *nt*, Verband anlegen *nt.* 2. Verband *m.* 3. Verbandsmaterial *nt.*
dressing cart Verbandswagen *m.*
dressing change Verbandswechsel *m.*
dressing trolley Verbandswagen *m.*
Dressler ['dreslər]: **D.'s syndrome** *card.* Dressler-Myokarditis *f*, -Syndrom *nt*, Postmyokardinfarktsyndrom *nt abbr.* PMI.
drib·ble ['drɪbl] **I** *vt* (herab-)tröpfeln lassen, träufeln. **II** *vi* tröpfeln, träufeln.
dried milk [draɪd] ~ dry milk.
dried plasma Trockenplasma *nt.*
drift [drɪft] *n* 1. Treiben *nt*; Abdrift *f*, Abtrieb *m.* 2. *genet., immun.* Drift *f.*
Drigalski-Conradi [drɪ'gælskɪ, kɔn'raːdɪ]: **D.-C. agar** Drigalski-Conradi-Nährboden *m.*
drill [drɪl] **I** *n* Bohrmaschine *f*, -gerät *nt*, (Drill-)Bohrer *m.* **II** *vt* 1. bohren; durchbohren. 2. (*Zahn, Knochen*) an-, ausbohren. **III** *vi* bohren.
drill bit Bohrspitze *f.*
drill chuck Bohr-, Spannfutter *nt.*
drill gauge Bohrlehre *f.*
drill guide Bohrbüchse *f*, -führung *f.*
drill·ing ['drɪlɪŋ] *n* Bohren *nt*, Bohrung *f.*
drink [drɪŋk] **I** *n* 1. Getränk *nt*; alkoholisches Getränk *nt.* **to have/take a ~** etw. trinken. **to give s.o. a ~** jmd. etw. zu trinken geben. 2. Schluck *m.* **a ~ of water** ein Schluck Wasser. **II** *vt* trinken. **III** *vi* trinken; ein Trinker sein.
drink·a·ble ['drɪŋkəbl] *adj* trinkbar; genießbar.
drink·er ['drɪŋkər] *n* Trinker(in *f*) *m.*
drink·ing ['drɪŋkɪŋ] **I** *n* Trinken *nt*; gewohnheitsmäßiges Trinken *nt.* **II** *adj* trinkend, Trink-.
drinking test *ophthal.* Wasser(belastungs)versuch *m*, Wasserstoß *m.*
drinking water Trinkwasser *nt.*
drip [drɪp] **I** *n* (Dauer-)Tropfinfusion *f*, Dauertropf *m*, *inf.* Tropf *m.* **II** *vt* tröpfeln *od.* tropfen lassen. **III** *vi* (herab-)tröpfeln, (herab-)tropfen (*from* von).
drip-feed *vt* parenteral/künstlich ernähren.
drip-feed ['drɪpfiːd] *n* → dripfeeding.
drip-feed·ing ['drɪpˌfiːdɪŋ] *n* parenterale/künstliche Ernährung *f.*
drive [draɪv] *n* 1. *psycho.* Antrieb *m*, Drang *m*, Trieb *m.* 2. *physiol.* Antrieb *m.* 3. Schwung *m*, Elan *m*, Energie *f*, Dynamik *f.*
driv·ing ['draɪvɪŋ] *adj* (an-)treibend, Treib-, Trieb-, Antriebs-.
driving force Antrieb *m*, Antriebskraft *f*, treibende Kraft *f.*

dRMP *abbr.* → deoxyribonucleoside monophosphate.
dro·code ['drəʊkəʊd] *n* → dihydrocodeine.
drom·e·dar·y curve ['drɒmɪderɪ, 'drʌm-] Dromedarkurve *f*, zweigipf(e)lige Kurve *f.*
drom·o·gram ['drɒməgræm] *n physiol.* Dromogramm *nt.*
drom·o·graph ['-græf] *n physiol.* Dromograph *m.*
drom·o·ma·nia [ˌ-'meɪnɪə, -jə] *n psychia.* krankhafter Lauftrieb *m*, Dromomanie *f.*
dro·mo·stan·o·lone [ˌ-'stænələʊn] *n pharm.* Dromostanolon *nt.*
drom·o·trop·ic [ˌ-'trɒpɪk] *adj physiol.* dromotrop.
dro·mot·ro·pism [drə'mɒtrəpɪzəm] *n physiol.* Dromotropie *f*, dromotrope Wirkung *f.*
dro·mot·ro·py [drə'mɒtrəpɪ] *n* → dromotropism.
drop [drɒp] **I** *n* 1. Tropfen *m.* 2. ~s *pl pharm.* Tropfen *pl.* 3. Fall *m*, Fallen *nt*; Sturz *m.* 4. (Ab-)Fall *m*, Sturz *m.* **II** *vt* (herab)tropfen *od.* (herab-)tröpfeln lassen. **III** *vi* 5. (herab-)tropfen, herabtröpfeln. 6. (herab-, herunter-)fallen (*from* von; *out of* aus). 7. (nieder-)sinken, fallen; umfallen, zu Boden sinken. 8. (ab-)sinken, s. senken; fallen, sinken, heruntergehen.
drop attack *neuro.* Drop-Anfall *m*, drop attack (*f*).
dro·per·i·dol [drəʊ'perɪdɒl, -dəl] *n pharm.* Droperidol *nt.*
drop finger *ortho.* Hammerfinger *m.*
drop foot Fallfuß *m.*
drop-foot gait *neuro.* Steppergang *m.*
drop hand *ortho., neuro.* Fall-, Kußhand *f.*
drop heart Herzsenkung *f*, -tiefstand *m*, Wanderherz *nt*, Kardioptose *f.*
drop·let ['drɒplɪt] *n* Tröpfchen *nt.*
droplet infection Tröpfcheninfektion *f.*
dropped beat [drɒpt] *card.* Kammersystolenausfall *m*, dropped beat (*m*).
dropped-beat pulse intermittierender Puls *m*, Pulsus intermittens.
drop·per ['drɒpər] *n pharm.* Tropfenzähler *m*, -glas *nt*, Tropfer *m.*
drop·si·cal ['drɒpsɪkl] *adj* Hydrops betr., hydroptisch.
dropsical nephritis nephrotisches Syndrom *nt*; Nephrose *f.*
drop·sy ['drɒpsɪ] *n* Hydrops *m.*
d. of amnion *gyn.* Hydramnion *nt.*
d. of belly Aszites *m*, Ascites *m.*
d. of brain Wasserkopf *m*, Hydrozephalus *m*, Hydrocephalus *m.*
d. of chest Hydrothorax *m.*
d. of head ~ d. of brain.
Dro·soph·i·la [drəʊ'sɒfɪlə, drɒ-] *n micro.* Drosophila *f.*
D. melanogaster Taufliege *f*, Drosophila melanogaster.
drown [draʊn] **I** *vt* ertränken. **to ~ o.s.** s. ertränken. **II** *vi* ertrinken.
drown·ing ['draʊnɪŋ] *n* Ertrinken *nt.*
drow·si·ness ['draʊzɪnɪs] *n* Schläfrigkeit *f*, Benommenheit *f.*
drow·sy ['draʊsɪ] *adj* 1. schläfrig, benommen; verschlafen. 2. einschläfernd.
dRTP *abbr.* → deoxyribonucleoside triphosphate.
drug [drʌg] **I** *n* 1. Arzneimittel *nt*, Arznei *f*, Medikament *nt.* 2. Droge *f*, Rauschgift *nt.* **to be on ~s** rauschgiftsüchtig sein. 3. Betäubungsmittel *nt*, Droge *f.* **II** *vt* 4. jdm. Medikamente geben; unter Drogen setzen. 5. betäuben. **III** *vi* Drogen *od.* Rauschgift nehmen.
drug abuse 1. Arzneimittel-, Medikamentenmißbrauch *m.* 2. Drogenmißbrauch *m.*

drug addict 1. Drogenabhängige(r *m*) *f*, -süchtige(r *m*) *f.* 2. Arzneimittel-, Medikamentensüchtige(r *m*) *f.*
drug-addicted *adj* 1. drogen-, rauschgiftsüchtig. 2. arzneimittel-, medikamentensüchtig.
drug addiction 1. Drogen-, Rauschgiftsucht *f.* 2. Arzneimittel-, Medikamentensucht *f.*
drug allergy Arzneimittelallergie *f*, -überempfindlichkeit *f.*
drug alopecia Alopecia medicamentosa.
drug clinic Drogenklinik *f.*
drug dependence 1. Drogen-, Rauschgiftabhängigkeit *f.* 2. Arzneimittel-, Medikamentenabhängigkeit *f.*
drug-dependent *adj* 1. drogen-, rauschgiftabhängig. 2. medikamenten-, arzneimittelabhägig.
drug disease durch Arzneimittel hervorgerufene Erkrankung/Krankheit *f.*
drug eruption *derm.* Arzneimitteldermatitis *f*, -exanthem *nt*, Dermatitis medicamentosa.
fixed d. fixes Arzneimittelexanthem.
drug-fast *adj* ~ drug-resistant.
drug fever arzneimittelinduziertes/medikamenteninduziertes Fieber *nt.*
drug·gist ['drʌgɪst] *n* Apotheker(in *f*) *m.*
drug hypersensitivity Arzneimittelallergie *f*, -überempfindlichkeit *f.*
drug-induced alopecia Alopecia medicamentosa.
drug-induced coma arzneimittelinduziertes Koma *nt.*
drug-induced diuresis arzneimittelinduzierte Diurese *f.*
drug-induced hepatitis arzneimittelinduzierte Hepatitis *f.*
drug-induced jaundice Arzneimittel-, Drogenikterus *m.*
drug-induced lupus medikamentenbedingter Lupus erythematodes visceralis.
drug-induced rhinitis arzneimittelinduzierte Rhinopathie *f*, Rhinopathia medicamentosa.
drug interactions Arzneimittelwechselwirkungen *pl.*
drug prophylaxis medikamentöse Infektionsprophylaxe *f.*
drug psychosis Drogenpsychose *f.*
drug rash ~ drug eruption.
drug resistance Arzneimittelresistenz *f.*
drug-resistant *adj* arzneimittelresistent.
drug therapy Arzneimittel-, Medikamententherapie *f*, medikamentöse Therapie *f.*
drug toxicity Arzneimitteltoxizität *f.*
drug treatment medikamentöse Behandlung *f.*
drum [drʌm] *n* 1. (*a. techn.*) Trommel *f*, Walze *f*, Zylinder *m*, trommelförmiger Behälter *m.* 2. *inf.* Paukenhöhle *f*, Tympanon *nt*, Tympanum *nt*, Cavum tympani, Cavitas tympanica. 3. *inf.* Trommelfell *nt*, Membrana tympanica.
drum·head ['drʌmhed] *n* → drum membrane.
drum membrane Trommelfell *nt*, Membrana tympanica.
Drummond ['drʌmənd]: **D.'s sign** *card.* Drummond'-Zeichen *nt.*
drum·stick ['drʌmstɪk] *n histol.* Drumstick *m*, Trommelschlegel *m.*
drumstick fingers Trommelschlegelfinger *pl*, Digiti hippocratici.
drunk·en·ness ['drʌŋkənɪs] *n* 1. (Be-)Trunkenheit *f*, Alkoholrausch *m*, -intoxikation *f.* 2. Trunksucht *f.*
dru·sen ['druːzn] *pl* 1. *micro.* (Strahlenpilz-)Drusen *pl.* 2. *ophthal.* Drusen *pl.* 3. *opthal.* Altersdrusen *pl*, Chorioiditis guttata senilis.

dry [draɪ] **I** adj **1.** trocken, Trocken-; ausgedörrt, dürr, ausgetrocknet. **2.** fig. nüchtern, trocken; kühl, gelassen. **II** vt **3.** trocknen, trocken machen; abtrocknen (on an). **4.** austrocknen. **III** vi trocknen, trocken werden; ein-, aus-, vertrocknen.
dry up vt, vi austrocknen.
dry abscess trockener Abszeß m.
dry beriberi trockene Form f der Beriberi, paralytische Beriberi f.
dry bronchitis trockene Bronchitis f, Bronchitis f ohne Auswurf, Bronchitis sicca.
dry caries trockener Knochenfraß/Knochenschwund m, trockene Knochenkaries f, Caries sicca.
dry cholera Cholera sicca.
dry colostomy chir. trockene Kolostomie f.
dry cough trockener Husten m.
dry distillation chem. trockene Destillation f, Trockendestillation f.
dry gangrene trockene Gangrän f.
dry heat trockene Hitze f.
dry hernia Hernie f ohne Bruchwasser, Hernia sicca.
dry ice Trockeneis nt, Kohlendioxidschnee m, gefrorenes Kohlendioxid nt.
dry·ing agent ['draɪɪŋ] chem. Trockenmittel nt.
drying-out n inf. Trockenlegen nt, (Alkohol-)Entzug m, Desintoxikation f.
drying oven Trockenofen m, -schrank m.
drying rack Trockengestell n, -ständer m.
dry joint ortho. chronisch villöse Arthritis f, Arthritis chronica villosa.
dry labor gyn. Xerotokie f.
dry milk Trockenmilch f, Milchpulver nt.
dry necrosis trockene Nekrose f.
dry·ness ['draɪnɪs] n trockener Zustand m; trockener Zustand m.
dry nurse Säuglingsschwester f.
dry-nurse vt (Säugling) pflegen.
dry pack trockene Packung f.
dry pannus ophthal. Pannus sicca.
dry pericarditis trockene Perikarditis f, Pericarditis sicca.
dry pleurisy/pleuritis trockene Rippenfellentzündung/Pleuritis f, Pleuritis sicca.
dry rales (Lunge) trockene Rasselgeräusche pl.
Drysdale ['draɪzdeɪl]: **D.'s corpuscles** Drysdale-Körperchen pl.
dry synovitis Synovitis/Synovialitis sicca.
dry weight Trockengewicht nt.
ds abbr. → double-stranded.
DSA abbr. → digital subtraction angiography.
dsDNA abbr. → deoxyribonucleic acid, double-stranded .
D sensor D-Sensor m, -Fühler m, Differentialsensor m.
dsRNA abbr. [double-stranded ribonucleic acid] → double-stranded RNA.
DST abbr. → donor-specific transfusion.
D-S test → Doerfler-Stewart test.
dT abbr. → deoxythymidine.
dTDP abbr. → deoxythymidine diphosphate.
DTH abbr. → delayed-type hypersensitivity.
dTMP abbr. → deoxythymidine monophosphate.
D.T.P. sign [distal tingling on percussion] Tinel-Hoffmann'-Klopfzeichen nt.
dTTP abbr. → deoxythymidine triphosphate.
D₁ tumor Vipom nt, VIPom nt, VIP-produzierendes Inselzelladenom nt, D₁-Tumor m.
du·al ['d(j)uːəl] adj doppelt, zweifach, dual, Doppel-, Zwei-, Dual-.

du·al·ism ['d(j)uːəlɪzəm] n Dualismus m.
du·al·is·tic [ˌd(j)uːə'lɪstɪk] adj dualistisch.
du·al·i·ty [d(j)uː'ælətɪ] n Zwei-, Doppelheit f, Dualität f.
du·al·ize ['d(j)uːəlaɪz] vt verdoppeln, verzweifachen, dualisieren.
dual logarithm abbr. **ld** dualer Logarithmus m abbr. ld, Logarithmus dualis.
Duane [dweɪn, duː'eɪn]: **D.'s syndrome** ophthal. Duane-Syndrom nt, Stilling--Türk-Duane-Syndrom nt.
D.'s test ophthal. Duane-Test m.
Dubini [du'biːnɪ]: **D.'s chorea/disease** Dubini-Syndrom nt, Chorea electrica.
Dubin-Johnson ['djuːbɪn 'dʒɒnsən]: **D.-J. syndrome** Dubin-Johnson-Syndrom nt.
Dubin-Sprinz [sprɪnz]: **D.-S. disease/syndrome** → Dubin-Johnson syndrome.
DuBois [dy'bwa]: **D.'s formula** DuBois'--Formel f.
Dubois [dy'bwa]: **D.' abscesses/disease** Dubois-Abszesse pl.
DuBois-Reymond [rɛ'mɔ̃ː]: **D.-R.'s law** Du Bois-Reymond-Gesetz nt.
Dubreuil-Chambardel [dy'brœj ʃabaːr'del]: **D.-C. syndrome** Dubreuil-Chambardel-Syndrom nt.
Dubreuilh [dy'brœj]: **circumscribed precancerous melanosis of D.** prämaligne Melanose f, melanotische Präkanzerose f, Dubreuilh-Krankheit f, -Erkrankung f, Dubreuilh-Hutchinson-Krankheit f, -Erkrankung f, Lentigo maligna, Melanosis circumscripta praeblastomatosa/praecancerosa Dubreuilh.
precancerous melanosis of D. → circumscribed precancerous melanosis of D.
Duchenne [dy'ʃen]: **D. atrophy** Duchenne--Krankheit f, -Muskeldystrophie f, Duchenne-Typ m der progressiven Muskeldystrophie, pseudohypertrophe pelvifemorale Form f, Dystrophia musculorum progressiva Duchenne.
D.'s disease 1. → Duchenne-Aran disease. **2.** Duchenne-Syndrom nt, progressive Bulbärparalyse f. **3.** Rückenmark(s)schwindsucht f, -darre f, Duchenne-Syndrom nt, Tabes dorsalis. **4.** → D. atrophy.
D. gait Hüfthinken nt, Trendelenburg--(Duchenne-)Hinken nt.
D.'s muscular dystrophy → D. atrophy.
D.'s paralysis 1. → D.'s disease 2. **2.** Duchenne-Erb paralysis. **3.** → D. atrophy.
D.'s sign Duchenne-Zeichen nt.
D.'s syndrome → D.'s disease 2.
D.'s type → D. atrophy.
Duchenne-Aran [ə'ræn]: **D.-A. disease** Aran-Duchenne-Krankheit f, -Syndrom nt, Duchenne-Aran-Krankheit f, -Syndrom nt, adult-distale Form f der spinalen Muskelatrophie f, spinale progressive Muskelatrophie f.
D.-A. muscular atrophy → D.-A. disease.
D.-A. type → D.-A. disease.
Duchenne-Erb [ɜrb; ɛːrb]: **D.-E. paralysis/syndrome** Erb-Duchenne-Lähmung f, Erb'-Lähmung f, obere Armplexuslähmung f.
Duchenne-Griesinger ['griːzɪŋər]: **D.-G. disease** Duchenne-Griesinger-Syndrom nt.
Duchenne-Landouzy [læn'duːzɪ; lɑduˈziː]: **D.-L. dystrophy/type** fazioskapulohumerale Form f der Dystrophia musculorum progressiva, Duchenne-Landouzy-Atrophie f.
duck embryo vaccine [dʌk] abbr. **DEV** Entenembryo(tollwut)vakzine f.
Duckworth ['dʌkwɜrθ]: **D.'s phenomenon/sign** card. Duckworth-Phänomen nt.
Ducrey [du'kreɪ]: **D.'s bacillus** micro.

Ducrey'-Streptobakterium nt, Streptobazillus m des weichen Schankers, Haemophilus ducreyi, Coccobacillus ducreyi.
duct [dʌkt] n **1.** Röhre f, Kanal m, Leitung f. **2.** anat. Gang m, Kanal m, Ductus m.
d. of Arantius Ductus venosus.
d. of bulbourethral gland Ausführungsgang der Gl. bulbourethralis, Ductus gl. bulbo-urethralis.
d. of epididymis Nebenhodengang, Ductus epididymidis.
d. of epoophoron Gartner'-Gang, Längsgang des Epoophorons, Ductus epoophoronis longtitudinalis.
d. of His Ductus thyroglossalis.
d.s of Luschka Luschka'-Gänge pl.
d. of Müller Müller'-Gang, Ductus paramesonephricus.
d. of Pecquet Brustmilchgang, Milchlymphgang, Ductus thoracicus.
d. of Stenon Parotisgang, Stensen'-, Stenon'-Gang, Ductus parotideus.
d. of Vater Ductus thyroglossalis.
d. of Wolff Wolff'-Gang, Urnierengang, Ductus mesonephricus.
duc·tal ['dʌktl] adj Gang/Ductus betr., duktal, Gang-.
ductal breast papilloma gyn., patho. Milchgangspapillom nt.
ductal cancer/carcinoma → duct cancer.
ductal drainage Gangdrainage f.
ductal ectasia Gangektasie f, Duktektasie f.
ductal in situ-carcinoma abbr. **DISC** gyn., patho. (Brust) duktales in-situ-Carcinoma nt abbr. DISC.
ductal stenosis Gangstenose f.
duct cancer/carcinoma duktales Karzinom nt, Gangkarzinom nt, Ca. ductale.
duct epithelium histol. Gangepithel nt.
duc·tile ['dʌktl, -tɪl] adj dehn-, streckbar, duktil; (aus-)ziehbar; biegsam, geschmeidig.
duc·til·i·ty [dʌk'tɪlətɪ] n Dehn-, Streckbarkeit f, Duktilität f; (Aus-)Ziehbarkeit f.
duc·tion ['dʌkʃn] n ophthal. Duktion f.
duct·less ['dʌktlɪs] adj histol. ohne Ausführungsgang.
ductless glands endokrine od. unechte Drüsen pl, Gll. endocrinae, Gll. sine ductibus.
duc·tog·ra·phy [dʌk'tɑgrəfɪ] n gyn., radiol. Duktographie f; Galaktographie f.
duct papilloma gyn. (Brustdrüse) intraduktales Papillom nt.
duc·tu·lar ['dʌktjələr] adj Kanälchen/Ductulus betr.
ductular cell adenoma patho. duktales (Pankreas-)Adenom nt.
duct·ule ['dʌkt(j)uːl] n anat. kleiner Gang m, Kanälchen f, Ductulus m.
duc·tus ['dʌktəs] n, pl **duc·tus** → duct 2.
ductus arteriosus Ductus Botalli, Ductus arteriosus.
patent d. offener/persistierender Ductus arteriosus Botalli, Ductus arteriosus Botalli apertus/persistens.
ductus venosus Arantius'-Kanal m, Ductus venosus.
Duddell ['dʌdəl]: **D.'s membrane** hintere Basalmembran f, Descemet'-Membran f, Lamina elastica posterior Descemeti, Lamina limitans posterior (corneae).
Duffy ['dʌfɪ]: **D. blood group (system)** Duffy--Blutgruppe f, -Blutgruppensystem nt.
Dugas ['duːgæz]: **D.' sign** ortho. Dugas-Zeichen nt.
D.' test ortho. Dugas-Test m.
Duhamel [d(j)uː'mel; dya'mel]: **D. operation** chir. Duhamel-Operation f.
Duhring ['d(j)ʊərɪŋ]: **D.'s disease** Duhring'-

Dührssen

-Krankheit *f*, Dermatitis herpetiformis Duhring, Morbus Duhring-Brocq *m*, Hidroa bullosa/herpetiformis/pruriginosa, Hidroa mitis et gravis.
Dührssen ['dɪrsən; 'dy:rsən]: **D.'s incisions** *gyn.* Dührssen-Inzisionen *pl.*
Duke [d(j)u:k]: **D.'s method/test** *hema.* Duke-Methode *f*, Bestimmung *f* der Blutungszeit nach Duke.
Dukes [d(j)u:ks]: **D.' classification** *patho.* Dukes-Klassifikation *f*, -Einteilung *f*.
D.' disease Dukes'-Krankheit *f*, Dukes--Filatoff-Krankheit *f*, Filatow-Dukes--Krankheit *f*, vierte Krankheit *f*, Parascarlatina *f*, Rubeola scarlatinosa.
D.' system → D.' classification.
dul·cite ['dʌlsaɪt] *n* Dulcit *nt*, Galactid *nt*.
dul·ci·tol ['dʌlsɪtɒl, -tal] *n* → dulcite.
dul·cose ['dʌlkəʊs] *n* → dulcite.
dul·ness *n* → dullness.
dull [dʌl] **I** *adj* **1.** (*Messer*) stumpf; (*Schmerz*) dumpf; (*Schall*) dumpf, abgeschwächt; (*Spiegel*) blind; (*Farben*) matt, stumpf, glanzlos; (*Licht*) trüb. **2.** teilnahmslos, abgestumpft, gleichgültig. **3.** träge, langsam, schwerfällig; schwer von Begriff. **4.** gelangweilt; langweilig. **II** *vt* **5.** *fig.* abstumpfen. **6.** (ab-)schwächen; mildern, dämpfen; (*Schmerz*) betäuben. **III** *vi* **7.** (*a. fig.*) stumpf werden, abstumpfen. **8.** träge werden. **9.** s. abschwächen.
dull·ness ['dʌlnɪs] *n* **1.** Stumpfheit *f*; (*Schmerz*, *Schall*) Dumpfheit *f*; Blindheit *f*; Mattheit *f*; Trübheit *f*. **2.** Teilnahmslosigkeit *f*, Abgestumpftheit *f*, Gleichgültigkeit *f*; Dummheit *f*. **3.** Trägheit *f*, Schwerfälligkeit *f*. **4.** Langweiligkeit *f*.
dull pain dumpfer Schmerz *m*.
Dulong-Petit [dy'lɔ̃ p(ə)'ti]: **D.-P. law** Dulong-Petit-Gesetz *nt*.
dumb [dʌm] **I** *n* die ~ *pl* die Stummen. **II** *adj* **1.** stumm, ohne Sprache. **2.** sprachlos, stumm.
dumb·bell crystals ['dʌmbel] *urol.* hantelförmige Harnkristalle *pl*, Hantelformen *pl*.
dumb·ness ['dʌmnɪs] *n* **1.** Stummheit *f*. **2.** Sprachlosigkeit *f*.
Dum·dum fever ['dʌmdʌm] viszerale Leishmaniose/Leishmaniase *f*, Kala--Azar *f*, Splenomegalia tropica.
dum·my ['dʌmɪ] *n* Plazebo *nt*, Placebo *nt*.
dump·ing ['dʌmpɪŋ] *n* → dumping syndrome.
dumping syndrome Dumpingsyndrom *nt*.
early postprandial d. Frühdumping *nt*, postalimentäres Frühsyndrom *nt*.
late postprandial d. Spätdumping *nt*, postalimentäres Spätsyndrom *nt*, reaktive Hypoglykämie *f*.
Duncan ['dʌŋkən]: **D.'s disease** → D.'s syndrome.
D.'s mechanism *gyn.* Duncan-Mechanismus *m*.
D. placenta Duncan-Plazenta *f*.
D.'s syndrome Duncan-Syndrom *nt*.
D.'s ventricle Cavum septi pellucidi.
duoden- *pref.* → duodeno-.
du·o·de·nal [ˌd(j)u:əʊ'di:nl, d(j)u:'ædnəl] *adj* Zwölffingerdarm/Duodenum betr., vom Duodenum stammend, duodenal, Duodenal-, Duodenum-.
duodenal ampulla Ampulla duodeni.
duodenal anastomosis *chir.* Duodenumanastomose *f*.
duodenal artery A. pancreaticoduodenalis inferior.
duodenal atresia Duodenal-, Duodenumatresie *f*.
duodenal branches: d. of anterior pancreaticoduodenal artery Duodenumäste *pl* der A. pancreaticoduodenalis anterior, Rami duodenales a. pancreaticoduodenalis anterioris.
d. of superior pancreaticoduodenal artery Duodenumäste *pl* der A. pancreaticoduodenalis superior, Rami duodenales a. pancreaticoduodenalis superioris.
duodenal bulb Bulbus duodeni, Pars superior duodeni.
duodenal cap **1.** → duodenal ampulla. **2.** → duodenal bulb.
duodenal C-loop duodenale C-Schlinge *f*.
duodenal-cutaneous fistula *patho.* äußere/kutane Duodenumfistel *f*.
duodenal diverticulum Duodenum-, Duodenaldivertikel *nt*.
periampullary d. periampulläres Duodenaldivertikel.
duodenal fistula *patho.* Duodenal-, Duodenumfistel *f*.
external d. → duodenal-cutaneous fistula.
duodenal flexure Zwölffingerdarmkrümmung *f*, Duodenalflexur *f*, Flexura duodeni.
inferior d. untere Duodenalflexur, Flexura duodeni inferior.
superior d. obere Duodenalflexur, Flexura duodeni superior.
duodenal fold Peritonealfalte *f* des Duodenums, Plica duodenalis.
inferior d. Plica duodenalis inferior, Plica duodenomesocolica.
longitudinal d.s Plicae longitudinales duodeni.
superior d. Duodenojejunalfalte, Plica duodenalis superior, Plica duodenojejunalis.
duodenal fossa: inferior d. → duodenal recess, inferior.
superior d. → duodenal recess, superior.
duodenal glands Brunner'-Drüsen *pl*, Duodenaldrüsen *pl*, Gll. duodenales.
duodenal impression (of liver) Duodenumabdruck *m* auf der Leberoberfläche, Impressio duodenalis (hepatis).
duodenal opening of stomach → duodenal orifice of stomach.
duodenal orifice of stomach Ostium pyloricum.
duodenal papilla Duodenalpapille *f*, Papilla duodeni.
major d. Vater'-Papille, Papilla duodeni major, Papilla Vateri.
minor d. kleine Duodenalpapille, Papilla duodeni minor.
duodenal perforation Duodenumperforation *f*.
duodenal recess duodenale Bauchfelltasche *f*, Rec. duodenalis.
inferior d. Rec. duodenalis inferior.
superior d. Treitz'-Grube *f*, Rec. duodenalis superior.
duodenal repair *chir.* Versorgung *f* od. Verschluß *m* einer Duodenumverletzung.
duodenal retractor *chir.* Duodenumspreizer *m*.
duodenal ulcer Zwölffingerdarmgeschwür *nt*, Duodenalulkus *nt*, Ulcus duodeni.
duodenal veins Duodenumvenen *pl*, Vv. duodenales.
du·o·de·nec·to·my [ˌd(j)u:ədɪ'nektəmɪ] *n chir.* Zwölffingerdarmentfernung *f*, Duodenum(teil)entfernung *f*, -resektion *f*, Duodenektomie *f*.
du·o·de·ni·tis [ˌd(j)u:ədɪ'naɪtɪs] *n* Entzündung *f* der Duodenalschleimhaut, Duodenitis *f*.
duodeno- *pref.* Duodeno-, Duodenal-, Duodenum-.
du·o·de·no·cho·lan·ge·i·tis [ˌd(j)u:ə,dɪ:nəʊkəʊˌlændʒɪ'aɪtɪs] *n* Duodeno(entero)cholangitis *f*.
du·o·de·no·chol·an·gi·tis [ˌ-kəʊlæn'dʒaɪtɪs] *n* → duodenocholangeitis.
du·o·de·no·cho·le·cys·tos·to·my [ˌ-kəʊləsɪ'stɒstəmɪ] *n chir.* Duodenum-Gallenblasen-Fistel *f*, -Fistelung *f*, Duodenocholezystostomie *f*, Duodenozystostomie *f*.
du·o·de·no·cho·led·o·chot·o·my [ˌ-kəʊˌledəʊ'kɒtəmɪ] *n chir.* Duodenocholedochotomie *f*.
du·o·de·no·col·ic [ˌ-'kɒlɪk] *adj* Duodenum u. Kolon betr. *od.* verbindend, koloduodenal.
du·o·de·no·cys·tos·to·my [ˌ-sɪ'stɒstəmɪ] *n* → duodenocholecystostomy.
du·o·de·no·du·o·de·nos·to·my [ˌ-ˌd(j)u:ədɪ'nɒstəmɪ] *n chir.* Duodenoduodenostomie *f*.
du·o·de·no·en·ter·os·to·my [ˌ-ˌentə'rɒstəmɪ] *n chir.* Duodenoenterostomie *f*.
du·od·e·no·gram [d(j)u:'ɒdnəgræm] *n radiol.* Kontrastaufnahme *f* des Duodenums, Duodenogramm *nt*.
du·o·de·no·he·pat·ic [d(j)u:ə,di:nəʊhɪ'pætɪk] *adj* Zwölffingerdarm/Duodenum u. Leber/Hepar betr., hepatoduodenal, Hepatoduodenal-.
duodenohepatic ligament Lig. hepatoduodenale.
du·o·de·no·il·e·os·to·my [ˌ-ɪlɪ'ɒstəmɪ] *n chir.* Duodenoileostomie *f*.
du·o·de·no·je·ju·nal [ˌ-dʒɪ'dʒu:nl] *adj* Zwölffingerdarm/Duodenum u. Leerdarm/Jejunum betr. *od.* verbindend, duodenojejunal, Duodenojejunal-.
duodenojejunal angle → duodenojejunal flexure.
duodenojejunal flexure Duodenojejunalflexur *f*, Flexura duodenojejunalis.
duodenojejunal fold Duodenojejunalfalte *f*, Plica duodenalis superior, Plica duodenojejunalis.
duodenojejunal fossa → duodenal recess, superior.
duodenojejunal hernia *chir.* Treitz'-Hernie *f*, Hernia duodenojejunalis.
duodenojejunal recess → duodenal recess, superior.
du·o·de·no·je·ju·nos·to·my [ˌ-dʒɪˌdʒu:'nɒstəmɪ] *n chir.* Duodenojejunostomie *f*.
du·o·de·nol·y·sis [d(j)u:ədɪ'nɒləsɪs] *n chir.* Duodenolyse *f*, Duodenummobilisation *f*.
du·o·de·no·mes·o·col·ic fold [d(j)u:ə,di:nəʊˌmezə'kɒlɪk, -ˌkəʊ-, -ˌmi:zə-] Plica duodenalis inferior, Plica duodenomesocolica.
du·o·de·no·pan·cre·a·tec·to·my [ˌ-ˌpæŋkrɪə'tektəmɪ] *n chir.* Duodenopankreatektomie *f*.
du·o·de·no·plas·ty [d(j)u:ə'di:nəʊplæstɪ] *n chir.* Duodenal-, Duodenumplastik *f*.
du·o·de·no·re·nal ligament [d(j)u:ə,di:nəʊ'ri:nl] Lig. duodenorenale.
du·o·de·nor·rha·phy [d(j)u:ədɪ'nɒrəfɪ] *n chir.* Duodenal-, Duodenumnaht *f*, Duodenorrhaphie *f*.
du·o·de·no·scope [d(j)u:'di:nəskəʊp] *n* Duodenoskop *nt*.
du·o·de·nos·co·py [ˌd(j)u:ədɪ'nɒskəpɪ] *n* Zwölffingerdarmendoskopie *f*, Duodenoskopie *f*.
du·o·de·nos·to·my [ˌ-'nɒstəmɪ] *n chir.* Anlage *f* einer äußeren Duodenalfistel, Duodenostomie *f*.
du·o·de·not·o·my [ˌ-'nɒtəmɪ] *n chir.* Zwölffingerdarmeröffnung *f*, Duodenal-, Duodenumeröffnung *f*, Duodenotomie *f*.
du·o·de·num [ˌd(j)u:əʊ'di:nəm, d(j)u:'ɒdnəm] *n*, *pl* **-nums**, **-na** [-nə] Zwölffingerdarm *m*, Duodenum *nt*, Intestinum duodenum.

du·o·vi·rus [d(j)uːəˈvaɪrəs] *n micro.* Rotavirus *nt.*
Duplay [duːˈpleɪ; dyˈplɛ]: **D.'s bursitis/disease** Duplay-Bursitis *f*, Entzündung/Bursitis *f* der Bursa subdeltoidea.
  D.'s operation *urol.* Duplay-Operation *f.*
  D.'s syndrome → D.'s bursitis.
du·plex [ˈd(j)uːpleks] *adj* doppelt, zweifach, Doppel-.
duplex DNA → double-stranded DNA.
duplex placenta Placenta duplex.
duplex structure Doppelhelix-, Duplexstruktur *f.*
duplex uterus Uterus duplex.
du·pli·ci·tas [d(j)uːˈplɪsɪtæs] *n* 1. *embryo.* Doppelmißbildung *f*, Duplicitas *f*, Monstrum duplex. 2. *anat.* Verdoppelung *f*, Duplikatur *f.*
du·pli·cate [*n, adj* ˈd(j)uːplɪkɪt; *v* -keɪt] I *n* Duplikat *nt*, Zweitausfertigung *f*; Kopie *f*. II *adj* 1. doppelt, zweifach, Doppel-. 2. genau gleich *od.* entsprechend. III *vt* ein Duplikat anfertigen, duplizieren, verdoppeln; kopieren.
du·pli·ca·tion [ˌd(j)uːplɪˈkeɪʃn] *n* 1. → duplicate I. 2. Vervielfältigung *f*, Verdoppelung *f.* 3. *genet.* Duplikation *f.* 4. *anat.* Verdoppelung *f*, Doppelbildung *f*, Duplikatur *f.*
du·pli·ca·ture [ˈd(j)uːplɪkətʃʊər, -tʃər] *n anat.* Verdoppelung *f*, Doppelbildung *f*, Duplikatur *f.*
du·plic·i·ty [d(j)uːˈplɪsɪtɪ] *n* 1. *fig.* Doppelzüngigkeit *f*, Falschheit *f.* 2. doppeltes/zweifaches Vorhandensein *nt*, Duplizität *f.*
Dupré [dyˈpre]: **D.'s disease/syndrome** Meningismus *m.*
Dupuy-Dutemps [dyˈpɥi dyˈtɑ̃]: **D.-D.' operation** *ophthal.* Dupuy-Dutemps-Operation *f.*
Dupuytren [dypɥəˈtrɑ̃]: **D.'s amputation** *ortho.* Schultergelenk(s)exartikulation *f* nach Dupuytren.
  D.'s contraction/contracture → D.'s disease.
  D.'s disease Dupuytren'-Kontraktur *f*, -Erkrankung *f.*
  D.'s disease of the foot Ledderhose-Syndrom *nt*, Morbus Ledderhose *m*, plantare Fibromatose *f*, Plantaraponeurosenkontraktur *f*, Dupuytren'-Kontraktur *f* der Plantarfaszie, Fibromatosis plantae.
  D.'s fascia Palmaraponeurose *f*, Aponeurosis palmaris.
  D.'s fracture 1. distale Fibulafraktur *f*, Außenknöchelfraktur *f.* 2. *ortho.* Galeazzi-Fraktur *f.*
  D.'s hydrocele Dupuytren'-Hydrozele *f.*
  D.'s operation → D.'s amputation.
  D.'s sign *ortho.* Dupuytren'-Zeichen *nt.*
  D.'s suture *chir.* Dupuytren'-Naht *f*, kontinuierliche Lembert-Naht *f.*
du·ra [ˈd(j)ʊərə] *n* → dura mater.
du·ral [ˈd(j)ʊərəl] *adj* Dura mater betr., dural, Dura-.
dural endothelioma Meningiom(a) *nt*, Meningeom(a) *nt.*
dural metastasis Durametastase *f.*
dural pocket Duratasche *f.*
dural psammoma *patho.* Durapsammom *nt.*
dural sac Duralsack *m.*
dural sheath Durascheide *f* des N. opticus.
dura mater [ˈmeɪtər] äußere Hirn- u. Rückenmarkshaut, Dura *f*, Dura mater.
  d. of brain harte Hirnhaut, *inf.* Dura, Dura mater cranialis/encephali, Pachymeninx *f.*
  d. of spinal cord harte Rückenmarkshaut, *inf.* Dura, Dura mater spinalis.

du·ra·ma·tral [d(j)ʊərəˈmeɪtrəl] *adj* → dural.
Durand-Nicolas-Favre [dyˈrɑ̃ nikɔˈla faːvrə]: **D.-N.-F. disease** Morbus Durand--Nicolas-Favre *m*, klimatischer Bubo *m*, vierte Geschlechtskrankheit *f*, Lymphogranuloma inguinale/venereum *abbr.* LGV, Lymphopathia venerea, Poradenitis inguinalis.
Duran-Reynals [ˈreɪnlz]: **D.-R. factor** *micro.* Hyaluronidase *f.*
  D.-R. permeability/spreading factor → D.-R. factor.
du·ra·plas·ty [ˈd(j)ʊərəplæstɪ] *n neurochir.* Duraplastik *f.*
Dürck [dɜrk; dʏrk]: **D.'s granulomas/nodes** *patho.* Dürck-Granulome *pl.*
Duret [dyˈre]: **D.'s lesion** Duret-Berner--Blutung *f.*
du·ro·ar·ach·ni·tis [d(j)ʊərəʊˌærækˈnaɪtɪs] *n* Entzündung *f* von Dura mater u. Arachnoidea, Duroarachnitis *f.*
Duroziez [dyrɔzˈje]: **D.'s disease** Duroziez-Syndrom *nt*, -Erkrankung *f*, angeborene Mitralklappenstenose *f.*
  D.'s murmur/sign/symptom *card.* Duroziez-Doppelgeräusch *nt.*
dust [dʌst] I *n* Staub *m*; Pulver *nt*, Puder *m*, Mehl *nt*; Bestäubungsmittel *nt.* II *vt* (be-)stäuben, bepudern.
dust asthma stauballergisches Asthma *nt.*
dust-borne *adj* durch Staubpartikel übertragen.
dust cell Staub-, Körnchen-, Rußzelle *f*, Alveolarmakrophage *m*, Phagozyt *m.*
dust corpuscles Blutstäubchen *pl*, Hämokonien *pl*, -konia *pl.*
dust-free [ˈdʌstfriː] *adj* staubfrei.
dust-proof *adj* staubdicht.
dusty [ˈdʌstɪ] *adj* 1. staubig, voller Staub, mit Staub bedeckt. 2. staubartig. 3. sandfarben.
Dutton [ˈdʌtn]: **D.'s disease** Dutton(-Rückfall)-Fieber *nt*, Rückfallfieber *nt* durch Borrelia duttoni.
  D.'s relapsing fever → D.'s disease.
  D.'s spirochete *micro.* Borrelia/Spirochaeta duttoni.
Duverney [dyverˈnɛj]: **D.'s fissure** Incisura cartilaginis meatus acustici externi.
  D.'s foramen Winslow'-Foramen *nt*, -Loch *nt*, For. epiploicum/omentale.
  D.'s fracture Duverney-Fraktur *f.*
  D.'s glands Cowper'-Drüsen *pl*, Bulbourethraldrüsen *pl*, Gll. bulbourethrales.
  D.'s muscle Pars lacrimalis m. orbicularis oculi.
DVT *abbr.* → deep vein thrombosis.
dwarf [dwɔːrf] I *n, pl* **dwarfs, dwarves** Zwerg(in) *f) m*, Nanus *m.* II *adj* zwergenhaft, Zwerg-. III *vt* 1. verkümmern lassen, im Wachstum hindern. 2. verkleinern; zusammenschrumpfen lassen. IV *vi* verkümmern; zusammenschrumpfen.
dwarf·ish [ˈdwɔːrfɪʃ] *adj* 1. zwergenhaft, winzig. 2. unter-, unentwickelt.
dwarf·ish·ness [-nɪs] *n* → dwarfism.
dwarf·ism [ˈdwɔːrfɪzəm] *n* Zwergwuchs *m*, Zwergwüchsigkeit *f*, Nan(n)osomie *f*, Nan(n)ismus *f.*
dwarf kidney *patho.* Zwergniere *f.*
dwarf pelvis Zwergbecken *nt*, Pelvis nana.
dwarf tapeworm *micro.* Zwergbandwurm *m*, Hymenolepis nana.
DWDL *abbr.* → diffuse well-differentiated lymphocytic lymphoma.
Dwyer [ˈdwaɪər]: **D.'s method/operation** *ortho.* Skolioseoperation *f* nach Dwyer.
  D.'s technique (of interbody fusion) → D.'s method.
Dy *abbr.* → dysprosium.
dy·ad [ˈdaɪæd] *n genet.* Dyade *f.*

dy·as·ter [ˈdaɪæstər] *n histol.* Amphiaster *m*, Diaster *m.*
dy·dro·ges·ter·one [ˌdaɪdrəʊˈdʒestərəʊn] *n pharm.* Dydrogesteron *nt.*
dye [daɪ] I *n* 1. Farbstoff *m*, Färbeflüssigkeit *f*, -mittel *nt.* 2. Tönung *f*, Färbung *f*, Farbe *f.* II *vt* färben. III *vi* s. färben lassen.
dye-dilution curve Indikator-, Farbstoffverdünnungskurve *f.*
dye-dilution method Indikator-, Farbstoffverdünnungsmethode *f.*
dye·ing [ˈdaɪɪŋ] *n* Färben *nt.*
dy·er [ˈdaɪər] *n* Farbstoff *m*, Färbemittel *nt.*
dye-stuff [ˈdaɪstʌf] *n* → dyer.
Dyggve-Melchior-Clausen [ˈdɪgvə ˈmelkjɔːr ˈklaʊzən]: **D.-M.-C. syndrome** Dyggve-Melchior-Clausen-Syndrom *nt.*
Dyke-Davidoff [daɪk ˈdeɪvɪdəf; ˈdavɪdɔf]: **D.-D. syndrome** Dyke-Davidoff-Syndrom *nt.*
dynam- *pref.* → dynamo-.
dy·nam·ic [daɪˈnæmɪk] I *n* Schwung *m*, treibende Kraft *f*, Triebkraft *f*, Dynamik *f.* II *adj* dynamisch.
dy·nam·i·cal [daɪˈnæmɪkl] *adj* → dynamic II.
dynamic block Liquorblock(ade *f) m.*
dynamic coefficient Viskositätskoeffizient *m.*
dynamic compliance (of lung) dynamische Compliance *f.*
dynamic engram dynamisches Engramm *nt.*
dynamic equilibrium Fließgleichgewicht *nt*, dynamisches Gleichgewicht *nt.*
dynamic hip screw *abbr.* **DHS** *ortho.* dynamische Hüftschraube *f abbr.* DHS.
dynamic ileus *chir.* spastischer Ileus *m.*
dynamic murmur dynamisches Herzgeräusch *nt.*
dynamic psychiatry psychoanalytische Psychiatrie *f.*
dynamic response *physiol.* dynamische/phasische Antwort *f*, Differentialantwort *f.*
dy·nam·ics [daɪˈnæmɪks] *pl* Dynamik *f*, Kraftlehre *f.*
dynamic viscosity *abbr.* η absolute/dynamische Viskosität *f abbr.* η.
dynamic work dynamische Arbeit *f.*
dynamo- *pref.* Kraft-, Dynamo(o)-.
dy·na·mo·gen·e·sis [ˌdaɪnəməʊˈdʒenəsɪs] *n* Kraftentwicklung *f*, Dynamogenese *f.*
dy·na·mo·gen·ic [ˌ-ˈdʒenɪk] *adj physiol.* dynamogen.
dynamogenic zone dynamogene/ergotrope Zone *f.*
dy·na·mog·e·nous [ˌdaɪnəˈmɒdʒənəs] *adj* → dynamogenic.
dy·na·mog·e·ny [ˌ-ˈmɒdʒənɪ] *n* → dynamogenesis.
dy·nam·o·graph [daɪˈnæməgræf] *n* Dynamograph *m.*
dy·na·mog·ra·phy [ˌdaɪnəˈmɒgrəfɪ] *n* Dynamographie *f.*
dy·na·mom·e·ter [ˌ-ˈmɒmɪtər] *n* Kraftmesser *m*, Dynamometer *nt.*
dy·nam·o·scope [daɪˈnæməskəʊp] *n* Dynamoskop *nt.*
dy·na·mos·co·py [ˌdaɪnəˈmɒskəpɪ] *n* Dynamoskopie *f.*
dyne [daɪn] *n old phys.* Dyn *nt*, Dyne *f.*
dy·ne·in [ˈdaɪnɪ(ɪ)n] *n* Dynein *nt.*
dy·nor·phin [daɪˈnɔːrfɪn] *n* Dynorphin *nt.*
dys- *pref.* Dys-.
dys·a·cou·sia [dɪsəˈkuːzɪ(ɪ)ə] *n* → dysacusis.
dys·a·cou·sis [dɪsəˈkuːsɪs] *n* → dysacusis.
dys·a·cous·ma [dɪsəˈkuːzmə] *n* → dysacusis.
dys·a·cu·sis [dɪsəˈkuːsɪs] *n HNO* 1. Störung *f* der Gehörempfindung, Gehörab-

dysadaptation

nahme *f*, Dysakusis *f*. **2.** akustische Überempfindlichkeit *f*, Dysakusis *f*, auditorische/akustische Dysästhesie *f*.

dys·ad·ap·ta·tion [dɪsˌædæpˈteɪʃn] *n* → dysaptation.

dys·ad·re·nal·ism [dɪsəˈdriːnlɪzəm] *n* Fehlfunktion *f* der Nebenniere(n), Dysadrenalismus *m*.

dys·a·dre·no·cor·ti·cism [dɪsəˌdriːnəˈkɔːrtəsɪzəm] *n* → dysadrenalism.

dys·an·ag·no·sia [dɪsˌænægˈnəʊsɪə] *n* neuro. Dysanagnosie *f*.

dys·an·ti·graph·ia [dɪsˌæntɪˈgræfɪə] *n* neuro. Dysantigraphie *f*.

dys·a·phia [dɪsˈæfɪə] *n* neuro. Tastsinnstörung *f*, Dysaphie *f*.

dys·ap·ta·tion [ˌdɪsæpˈteɪʃn] *n* ophthal. mangelhafte Adaptation(sfähigkeit *f*) *f*, Dysadaptation *f*.

dys·ar·thria]dɪsˈɑːrθrɪə] *n* neuro. Dysarthrie *f*.

dys·ar·thro·sis [ˌdɪsɑːrˈθrəʊsɪs] *n* **1.** → dysarthria. **2.** ortho. Gelenkdeformität *f*, -fehlbildung *f*, Dysarthrose *f*, Dysarthrosis *f*.

dys·au·to·no·mia [dɪsˌɔːtəˈnəʊmɪə] *n* Riley-Day-Syndrom *nt*, Dysautonomie *f*.

dys·bar·ism [dɪsˈbærɪzəm] *n* patho. Dysbarismus *m*.

dys·ba·sia [dɪsˈbeɪzɪə, -ʒə] *n* neuro. Gehstörung *f*, Dysbasie *f*, Dysbasia *f*.

dys·be·ta·lip·o·pro·tein·e·mia [dɪsˌbeɪtəˌlɪpəˌprəʊtɪˈniːmɪə] *n* (primäre/essentielle) Hyperlipoproteinämie *f* Typ III, Hypercholesterinämie *f* mit Hypertriglyzeridämie, Broad-Beta-Disease (*nt*), Hyperlipoproteinämie *f* mit breiter Betabande.

dys·bo·lism [ˈdɪsbəlɪzəm] *n* patho. abnormer Stoffwechsel *m*, Dysbolismus *m*.

dys·bu·lia [dɪsˈbjuːlɪə] *n* psychia. Störung *f* der Willensbildung, Willenshemmung *f*, Dysbulie *f*, Dysbulia *f*.

dys·cal·cu·lia [dɪskælˈkjuːlɪə] *n* neuro. Dyskalkulie *f*.

dys·ce·pha·lia [dɪssɪˈfeɪlɪə] *n* → dyscephaly.

dys·ceph·a·ly [dɪsˈsefəlɪ] *n* embryo. Dyszephalie *f*, Dyskephalie *f*.

dys·chei·ria [dɪsˈkaɪrɪə] *n* neuro. Dysch(e)irie *f*.

dys·che·sia *n* → dyschezia.

dys·che·zia [dɪsˈkiːzɪə] *n* erschwerte/gestörte Defäkation *f*, Dyschezie *f*.

dys·chi·ria [dɪsˈkaɪrɪə] *n* → dyscheiria.

dys·cho·lia [dɪsˈkəʊlɪə] *n* patho. Störung *f* der Galle(n)zusammensetzung, Dyscholie *f*.

dys·chon·dro·pla·sia [dɪsˌkɑndrəˈpleɪʒ(ɪ)ə, -zɪə] *n* Ollier'Erkrankung *f*, -Syndrom *nt*, Enchondromatose *f*, multiple kongenitale Enchondrome *pl*, Hemichondrodystrophie *f*. **d. with hemangiomas** Maffucci-Kast-Syndrom *nt*.

dys·chon·dros·te·o·sis [ˌdɪskɑnˌdrɑstɪˈəʊsɪs] *n* ortho. Léri-Weill-Syndrom *nt*.

dys·chro·ma·sia [dɪskrəʊˈmeɪʒ(ɪ)ə] *n* → dyschromatopsia.

dys·chro·ma·top·sia [dɪsˌkrəʊməˈtɑpsɪə] *n* ophthal. Farbenfehlsichtigkeit *f*, Dyschromatopsie *f*, Chromatodysopsie *f*.

dys·chro·mia [dɪsˈkrəʊmɪə] *n* derm. Dyschromie *f*, Dyschromia *f*.

dys·chy·lia [dɪsˈkaɪlɪə] *n* patho. Dyschylie *f*.

dys·ci·ne·sia [dɪsɪˈniːʒ(ɪ)ə] *n* → dyskinesia.

dys·col·me·sis *n* → dyskoimesis.

dys·co·ria [dɪsˈkəʊrɪə] *n* **1.** ophthal. Entrundung *f* u. Verlagerung der Pupille, Dyskorie *f*. **2.** neuro. abnorme Pupillenreaktion *f*, Dyskorie *f*.

dys·cor·ti·cism [dɪsˈkɔːrtəsɪzəm] *n* Störung *f* der Nebennierenrindenfunktion, Dyskortizismus *m*.

dys·cra·nia [dɪsˈkreɪnɪə] *n* embryo. Dyskranie *f*.

dys·cra·sia [dɪsˈkreɪʒ(ɪ)ə] *n* **1.** Dyskrasie *f*. **2.** old → disease I.

dys·cra·sic [dɪsˈkreɪsɪk] *adj* → dyscratic.

dys·crat·ic [dɪsˈkrætɪk] *adj* Dyskrasie betr., dyskrasisch, dyskratisch.

dys·cri·nia [dɪsˈkrɪnɪə] *n* Dyskrinie *f*.

dys·cri·nism [ˈdɪskrənɪzəm] *n* → dyscrinia.

dys·di·ad·o·cho·ci·ne·sia [dɪsdaɪˌædəkəʊsɪˈniːʒ(ɪ)ə] *n* → dysdiadochokinesia.

dys·di·ad·o·cho·ci·net·ic [ˌ-sɪˈnetɪk] *adj* → dysdiadochokinetic.

dys·di·ad·o·cho·ki·ne·sia [ˌ-kɪˈniːʒ(ɪ)ə, kaɪ-] *n* neuro. gestörte Diadochokinese *f*, Dysdiadochokinese *f*.

dys·di·ad·o·cho·ki·net·ic [ˌ-kɪˈnetɪk] *adj* Dysdiadochokinese betr., dysdiadochokinetisch.

dys·dip·sia [dɪsˈdɪpsɪə] *n* neuro. Dysdipsie *f*.

dys·e·coi·a [dɪsɪˈkɔɪə] *n* → dysacusis.

dys·em·bry·o·ma [dɪsˌembrɪˈəʊmə] *n* embryo. Dysembryom *nt*, embryonales Teratom *nt*.

dys·em·bry·o·pla·sia [dɪsˌembrɪəʊˈpleɪʒ(ɪ)ə, -zɪə] *n* embryo. embryonale/pränatale Fehlbildung/Malformation *f*, Dysembryoplasie *f*.

dys·e·mia [dɪsˈiːmɪə] *n* fehlerhafte Blutzusammensetzung *f*, Dysämie *f*, Blutdyskrasie *f*.

dys·en·ce·pha·lia [dɪsensɪˈfeɪlɪə, -lɪə] *n* embryo., neuro. Dysenzephalie *f*.

dys·en·ter·ic [dɪsnˈterɪk] *adj* Dysenterie betr., dysenterisch, Dysenterie-.

dysenteric diarrhea dysenterieähnliche Diarrhoe *f*.

dys·en·ter·i·form [dɪsˈentərɪfɔːrm] *adj* dysenterieähnlich, dysenteriform.

dys·en·ter·y [ˈdɪsntərɪ] *n* Ruhr *f*, Dysenterie *f*, Dysenteria *f*.

dys·e·qui·lib·ri·um [dɪsˌɪkwəˈlɪbrɪəm] *n* Ungleichgewicht *nt*, Dysäquilibrium *nt*.

dys·er·e·the·sia [dɪserɪˈθiːʒ(ɪ)ə] *n* neuro. Beeinträchtigung *f* der Reizempfindlichkeit, Dyseräthesie *f*.

dys·er·e·thism [dɪsˈerɪθɪzəm] *n* → dyserethesia.

dys·er·gia [dɪˈsɜːrdʒ(ɪ)ə] *n* neuro. Dysergie *f*.

dys·e·ryth·ro·poi·et·ic anemia [dɪsɪˌrɪθrəpɔɪˈetɪk] Anämie *f* mit Erythrozytenbildungsstörung.

dys·es·the·sia [dɪsesˈθiːʒ(ɪ)ə] *n* Dysästhesie *f*.

dys·es·thet·ic [dɪsesˈθetɪk] *adj* Dysästhesie betr., dysästhetisch.

dys·fi·brin·o·gen [dɪsfaɪˈbrɪnədʒən] *n* nicht-gerinnbares Fibrinogen *nt*, Dysfibrinogen *nt*.

dys·fi·brin·o·ge·ne·mia [ˌdɪsfaɪˌbrɪnədʒəˈniːmɪə] *n* Dysfibrinogenämie *f*.

dys·fi·brin·o·ge·ne·mic [ˌ-ˈniːmɪk] *adj* Dysfibrinogenämie betr., dysfibrinogenämisch.

dys·fi·brous layer of cerebral cortex [dɪsˈfaɪbrəs] Lamina dysfibrosa.

dys·func·tion [dɪsˈfʌŋkʃn] *n* Funktionsstörung *f*, Dysfunktion *f*.

dys·gam·ma·glob·u·li·ne·mia [dɪsˌgæməˌglɑbjəlɪˈniːmɪə] *n* immun. Dysgammaglobulinämie *f*.

dys·ge·ne·sia [dɪsdʒɪˈniːʒ(ɪ)ə] *n* → dysgenesis.

dys·gen·e·sis [dɪsˈdʒenəsɪs] *n* patho., embryo. Fehlentwicklung *f*, fehlerhafte Entwicklung *f*, Dysgenesie *f*, Dysgenesia *f*.

dys·gen·ic [dɪsˈdʒenɪk] *adj* dysgenisch.

dys·gen·ics [dɪsˈdʒenɪks] *pl* Dysgenik *f*.

dys·gen·i·tal·ism [dɪsˈdʒenɪtlɪzəm] *n* Fehlentwicklung *f* der Geschlechtsorgane, Dysgenitalismus *m*.

dys·ger·mi·no·ma [dɪsdʒɜːrmɪˈnəʊmə] *n* gyn., patho. Seminom *nt* des Ovars, Dysgerminom(a) *nt*.

dys·geu·sia [dɪsˈgjuːʒ(ɪ)ə] *n* neuro. Störung *f* des Geschmackempfindens, Dysgeusie *f*.

dys·glob·u·li·ne·mia [dɪsˌglɑbjəlɪˈniːmɪə] *n* Dysglobulinämie *f*.

dys·gna·thia [dɪsˈnæθɪə, -ˈneɪ-] *n* Kieferfehlentwicklung *f*, Dysgnathie *f*.

dys·gnath·ic [dɪsˈnæθɪk, -ˈneɪ-] *adj* Dysgnathie betr., dysgnath.

dys·gno·sia [dɪsˈnəʊʒ(ɪ)ə] *n* Intelligenzdefekt *m*, Störung *f* der geistigen Leistungsfähigkeit, Dysgnosie *f*.

dys·gon·ic [dɪsˈgɑnɪk] *adj* micro. dysgonisch.

dys·gram·ma·tism [dɪsˈgræmətɪzəm] *n* neuro. Dysgrammatismus *m*.

dys·gran·u·lar [dɪsˈgrænjələr] *adj* histol. dysgranulär.

dys·graph·ia [dɪsˈgræfɪə] *n* neuro. Schreibstörung *f*, Dysgraphie *f*.

dys·hem·a·to·poi·e·sia [dɪsˌhemətəpɔɪˈiːʒ(ɪ)ə] *n* → dyshematopoiesis.

dys·hem·a·to·poi·e·sis [ˌ-pɔɪˈiːsɪs] *n* fehlerhafte Blutbildung/Hämopoese *f*, Dyshämopoese *f*.

dys·hem·a·to·poi·et·ic [ˌ-pɔɪˈetɪk] *adj* Dyshämopoese betr., dyshämopoetisch.

dys·he·mo·poi·e·sis [dɪsˌhiːməpɔɪˈiːsɪs] *n* → dyshematopoiesis.

dys·he·mo·poi·et·ic [ˌ-pɔɪˈetɪk] *adj* → dyshematopoietic.

dys·hi·dria [dɪsˈhɪdrɪə] *n* → dyshidrosis.

dys·hi·dro·sis [dɪshaɪˈdrəʊsɪs, -hɪ-] *n* **1.** Störung *f* der Schweißdrüsentätigkeit, Dys(h)idrosis *f*, Dyshidrie *f*. **2.** derm. Dys(h)idrose *f*, Dyshidrosis *f*, Dyshidrose-Syndrom *nt*, dyshidrotisches Ekzem *nt*, Pompholyx *f*.

dys·hi·drot·ic eczema [dɪshaɪˈdrɑtɪk] dyshidrotisches Ekzem *nt*.

dys·hor·mo·no·gen·e·sis [dɪsˌhɔːrmənəˈdʒenəsɪs] *n* fehlerhafte Hormonbildung/Hormonsynthese *f*, Dyshormonogenese *f*.

dys·hy·dro·sis *n* → dyshidrosis.

dys·id·ria [dɪsˈɪdrɪə] *n* → dyshidrosis.

dys·id·ro·sis [dɪsɪdˈrəʊsɪs, dɪsaɪ-] *n* → dyshidrosis.

dys·junc·tion *n* → disjunction.

dys·junc·tive nystagmus [dɪsˈdʒʌŋktɪv] dissoziierter Nystagmus *m*.

dys·kar·y·o·sis [dɪsˌkærɪˈəʊsɪs] *n* patho. Dyskaryose *f*.

dys·kar·y·ot·ic [dɪsˌkærɪˈɑtɪk] *adj* Dyskaryose betr., von ihr betroffen, dyskaryotisch.

dys·ker·a·to·ma [dɪsˌkerəˈtəʊmə] *n* derm. dyskeratotischer Tumor *m*, Dyskeratom(a) *nt*.

dys·ker·a·to·sis [dɪsˌkerəˈtəʊsɪs] *n* derm. Verhornungsstörung *f*, Dyskeratose *f*, Dyskeratosis *f*.

dyskeratosis follicularis, isolated derm. warziges Dyskeratom *nt*, Dyskeratoma segregans/verrucosum/lymphadenoides, Dyskeratosis follicularis isolata, Dyskeratosis segregans.

dys·ker·a·tot·ic [dɪsˌkerəˈtɑtɪk] *adj* Dyskeratose betr., von ihr betroffen, dyskeratotisch.

dys·ki·ne·sia [dɪskɪˈniːʒ(ɪ)ə, -kaɪ-] *n* motorische Fehlfunktion *f*, Dyskinesie *f*, Dyskinesia *f*.

dys·ki·net·ic [dɪskɪˈnetɪk] *adj* Dyskinesie betr., dyskinetisch.

dys·koi·me·sis [dɪskɔɪ'miːsɪs] *n neuro.* Einschlafstörung *f*, Dyskoimesis *f*.
dys·la·lia [dɪs'leɪlɪə, -'læl-] *n HNO, neuro.* Stammeln *nt*, Dyslalie *f*.
dys·lex·ia [dɪs'leksɪə] *n neuro.* Lesestörung *f*, Leseschwäche *f*, Dyslexie *f*, Legasthenie *f*.
dys·lip·i·do·sis [dɪslɪpə'dəʊsɪs] *n, pl* **-ses** [-siːz] *patho.* Fettstoffwechselstörung *f*, Dyslipidose *f*.
dys·li·poi·do·sis [dɪsˌlaɪpɔɪ'dəʊsɪs] *n, pl* **-ses** [-siːz] → dyslipidosis.
dys·li·po·pro·tein·e·mia [dɪsˌlaɪpəˌprəʊtɪ'niːmɪə, -ˌlɪp-] *n patho.* Dyslipoproteinämie *f*.
dys·lo·gia [dɪs'ləʊdʒ(ɪ)ə] *n* **1.** *neuro.* Dyslogie *f*, Dyslogia *f*. **2.** *HNO* Dyslogie *f*, Dyslogia *f*.
dys·ma·ture [dɪsmə't(j)ʊər, -'tʃʊər] *adj* **1.** *patho.* unreif, dysmatur. **2.** *ped.* unreif, hypotroph, hypoplastisch.
dys·ma·tu·ri·ty [dɪsmə't(j)ʊərətɪ, -'tʃʊər-] *n* **1.** *patho.* Reifestörung *f*, Dysmaturität *f*. **2.** *ped.* pränatale Dystrophie *f*, Dysmaturität *f*.
dys·meg·a·lop·sia [dɪsˌmegə'lɑpsɪə] *n ophthal.* Dysmegalopsie *f*.
dys·me·lia [dɪs'miːlɪə] *n embryo., patho.* Gliedmaßenfehlbildung *f*, Dysmelie *f*.
dysmelia syndrome Dysmelie-Syndrom *nt*, Thalidomid-Embryopathie *f*, Contergan-Syndrom *nt*.
dys·men·or·rhea [dɪsˌmenə'rɪə] *n* schmerzhafte Regelblutung/Menorrhoe *f*, Dysmenorrhoe *f*, Menorrhalgie *f*.
dys·men·or·rhe·al [-ˌrɪəl] *adj gyn.* Dysmenorrhoe betr., dysmenorrhoisch.
dys·men·tia [dɪs'menʃɪə] *n neuro.* (temporäre) Intelligenzstörung *f*, (temporärer) Intelligenzdefekt *m*.
dys·met·a·bol·ic [dɪsmetə'bɑlɪk] *adj* Dysmetabolismus betr., dysmetabolisch.
dys·me·tab·o·lism [dɪsmə'tæbəlɪzəm] *n* Stoffwechselstörung *f*, fehlerhafter Stoffwechsel *m*, Dysmetabolismus *m*.
dys·me·tria [dɪs'metrɪə] *n neuro.* Dysmetrie *f*.
dys·me·trop·sia [dɪsmɪ'trɑpsɪə] *n ophthal.* Dysmetropsie *f*.
dys·mim·ia [dɪs'mɪmɪə] *n neuro.* Störung *f* der Mimik/Gestik, Dysmimie *f*.
dys·mne·sia [dɪs'niːʒ(ɪ)ə] *n neuro.* Gedächtnisstörung *f*, Dysmnesie *f*.
dys·mne·sic [dɪs'niːzɪk] *adj* Dysmnesie betr., dysmnestisch.
dysmnesic psychosis → dysmnesic syndrome.
dysmnesic syndrome amnestisches Syndrom *nt*, Korsakow-Syndrom *nt*, -Psychose *f*.
dys·mor·phia [dɪs'mɔːrfɪə] *n* → dysmorphism.
dys·mor·phism [dɪs'mɔːrfɪzəm] *n embryo.* Gestaltanomalie *f*, Deformität *f*, Fehlbildung *f*, Dysmorphie *f*, Dysmorphia *f*.
dys·mor·pho·pho·bia [dɪsˌmɔːrfə'fəʊbɪə] *n psychia.* Dysmorphophobie *f*.
dys·mor·phop·sia [dɪsmɔːr'fɑpsɪə] *n ophthal.* Dysmorphopsie *f*.
dys·mo·til·i·ty [ˌdɪsməʊ'tɪlətɪ] *n patho.* Dysmotilität *f*.
dys·my·e·li·na·tion [dɪsˌmaɪələ'neɪʃn] *n patho.* Dysmyelinogenese *f*.
dys·my·o·to·nia [dɪsˌmaɪə'təʊnɪə] *n* Muskeldystonie *f*, muskuläre Dystonie *f*.
dys·o·don·ti·a·sis [dɪsəʊdɑntɪ'aɪəsɪs] *n dent.* **1.** Fehlentwicklung *f* der Zahnanlage, Dysodontie *f*. **2.** verzögerte/erschwerte/fehlerhafte Zahnung *f*, Dysodontie *f*.
dys·on·to·gen·e·sis [dɪsˌɑntə'dʒenəsɪs] *n embryo.* Störung *f* der Fruchtentwicklung, Dysontogenese *f*.

dys·on·to·ge·net·ic [ˌ-dʒə'netɪk] *adj* Dysontogenese betr., dysontogenetisch.
dys·o·pia [dɪs'əʊpɪə] *n ophthal.* Sehstörung *f*, Dysop(s)ie *f*, Dysdopsia *f*.
dys·op·sia [dɪs'ɑpsɪə] *n* → dysopia.
dys·o·rex·ia [dɪsə'reksɪə] *n neuro.* Dysorexie *f*.
dys·or·ga·no·pla·sia [dɪsˌɔːrgənə'pleɪʒ(ɪ)ə, -ʒɪə] *n embryo.* Organfehlentwicklung *f*, Dysorganoplasie *f*.
dys·or·ia [dɪs'ɔːrɪə] *n patho.* Störung *f* der Gefäßpermeabilität, Dyshorie *f*, Dysorie *f*, Dysorose *f*.
dys·or·ic [dɪs'ɔːrɪk] *adj* Dysorie betr., dysorisch.
dys·os·mia [dɪs'ɑzmɪə] *n neuro.* Störung *f* des Geruchssinns, Dysosmie *f*, Dysosphresie *f*.
dys·os·te·o·gen·e·sis [dɪsˌɑstɪə'dʒenəsɪs] *n ortho.* fehlerhafte/gestörte Knochenentwicklung *f*, Dysosteogenese *f*; Dysostose *f*.
dys·os·to·sis [dɪsɑs'təʊsɪs] *n* fehlerhafte/gestörte Knochenentwicklung/Knochenbildung *f*, Dysostose *f*, Dysostosis *f*.
dys·pa·reu·nia [dɪspə'ruːnɪə] *n gyn.* schmerzhafter Geschlechtsverkehr/Koitus *m*, Dyspareunie *f*, Algopareunie *f*.
dys·pep·sia [dɪs'pepsɪə] *n patho.* Dyspepsie *f*, Dyspepsia *f*.
dys·pep·tic [dɪs'peptɪk] *adj* Dyspepsie betr., von ihr betroffen, dyspeptisch.
dys·per·ma·tism [dɪ'spɜːrmətɪzəm] *n* → dysspermatism.
dys·pha·gia [dɪs'feɪdʒ(ɪ)ə] *n* Schluckstörung *f*, Dysphagie *f*, Dysphagia *f*.
dys·pha·gy ['dɪsfədʒɪ] *n* → dysphagia.
dys·pha·sia [dɪs'feɪʒ(ɪ)ə, -ʒɪə] *n neuro.* Dysphasie *f*, Dysphasia *f*.
dys·phe·mia [dɪs'fiːmɪə] *n neuro.* Dysphemie *f*.
dys·pho·nia [dɪs'fəʊnɪə] *n HNO* Stimmstörung *f*, Stimmbildungsstörung *f*, Dysphonie *f*, Dysphonia *f*.
dys·phon·ic [dɪs'fɑnɪk] *adj* Dysphonie betr., dysphonisch.
dys·pho·ret·ic [dɪsfə'retɪk] *adj* **1.** → dysphoric. **2.** Dysphorie auslösend.
dys·pho·ria [dɪs'fɔːrɪə, -'fɔːr-] *n* Verstimmung *f*, Mißstimmung *f*, Übellaunigkeit *f*, Gereiztheit *f*, Dysphorie *f*.
dys·pho·ri·ant [dɪs'fɔːrɪənt] *adj* → dysphoretic.
dys·phor·ic [dɪs'fɔːrɪk, -'fɑr-] *adj* Dysphorie betr., übellaunig, gereizt, verstimmt, dysphorisch.
dys·phra·sia [dɪs'freɪʒ(ɪ)ə, -zɪə] *n neuro.* Dysphrasie *f*.
dys·phy·lax·ia [dɪsfɪ'læksɪə] *n neuro.* Durchschlafstörung *f*, Dysphylaxie *f*.
dys·pla·sia [dɪs'pleɪʒ(ɪ)ə] *n patho.* Fehlbildung *f*, Fehlentwicklung *f*, Mißgestalt *f*, Dysplasie *f*, Dysplasia *f*.
d. of cervix *gyn.* zervikale Plattenepitheldysplasie *f*, cervicale intraepitheliale Neoplasie *f abbr.* CIN.
dysplasia oculodentodigitalis syndrome Meyer-Schwickerath-Weyers-Syndrom *nt*, okulodentodigitales Syndrom *nt*.
dys·plas·tic [dɪs'plæstɪk] *adj* Dysplasie betr., von ihr gekennzeichnet, dysplastisch.
dysplastic kidney dysplastische Niere *f*, Nierendysplasie *f*.
dysplastic nevus *derm.* dysplastischer Nävus *m*.
dysp·nea [dɪsp'nɪə] *n* erschwerte Atmung *f*, Atemnot *f*, Kurzatmigkeit *f*, Dyspnoe *f*.
d. of exertion Belastungsdyspnoe.
dysp·ne·ic [dɪsp'nɪɪk] *adj* Dyspnoe betr., dyspnoisch.

dysp·noe·a *n* → dyspnea.
dys·poi·e·sis [dɪspɔɪ'iːsɪs] *n* Bildungsstörung *f*, Dyspo(i)ese *f*.
dys·pon·der·al [dɪs'pɑndərəl] *adj* Dysponderosis betr., durch sie hervorgerufen.
dysponderal amenorrhea *gyn.* Amenorrhoe *f* bei Über- od. Untergewicht.
dys·pon·de·ro·sis [dɪsˌpɑndə'rəʊsɪs] *n* Störung *f* des Körpergewichts, Dysponderosis *f*.
dys·prax·ia [dɪs'præksɪə] *n neuro.* (leichte) Apraxie *f*, Dyspraxie *f*.
dys·pro·si·um [dɪs'prəʊsɪəm, -ʃɪ-] *n abbr.* Dy Dysprosium *nt abbr.* Dy.
dys·pro·tein·e·mia [dɪsˌprəʊtɪ'niːmɪə] *n patho.* Dysproteinämie *f*.
dys·pro·tein·em·ic [ˌ-'niːmɪk] *adj* Dysproteinämie betr., dysproteinämisch.
dys·raph·ia [dɪs'reɪfɪə] *n embryo.* Dysrhaphie *f*.
dys·ra·phism ['dɪsrəfɪzəm] *n* → dysrhaphia.
dys·re·flex·ia [dɪsrɪ'fleksɪə] *n neuro.* Reflexstörung *f*, Dysreflexie *f*.
dys·rha·phia *n* → dysraphia.
dys·rha·phism *n* → dysraphia.
dys·rhyth·mia [dɪs'rɪðmɪə] *n* Rhythmusstörung *f*, Dysrhythmie *f*.
dys·se·ba·cea *n* → dyssebacia.
dys·se·ba·cia [ˌdɪsɪ'beɪʃɪə] *n derm.* Dyssebacea *f*, Dyssteatosis *f*.
dys·som·nia [dɪ'sɑmnɪə] *n* Schlafstörung *f*, Dyssomnie *f*.
dys·sper·ma·tism [dɪ'spɜːrmətɪzəm] *n* Dysspermatismus *m*.
dys·sper·ma·to·gen·ic sterility [dɪsˌspɜːrmətə'dʒenɪk] *urol.* dysspermatogene Sterilität *f*.
dys·sper·mia [dɪ'spɜːrmɪə] *n* → dysspermatism.
dys·sta·sia [dɪ'steɪʒ(ɪ)ə] *n neuro.* Dysstasie *f*, Dysstasia *f*.
dys·syl·la·bia [dɪsɪ'leɪbɪə] *n neuro.* Silbenstottern *nt*, Dyssyllabie *f*.
dys·sym·bo·lia [dɪsɪm'bəʊlɪə] *n neuro.* Dyssymbolie *f*.
dys·sym·bo·ly [dɪ'sɪmbəlɪ] *n* → dyssymbolia.
dys·syn·er·gia [dɪsɪn'ɜːrdʒ(ɪ)ə] *n neuro.* **1.** Synergiestörung *f*, Dyssynergie *f*, Dyssynergia *f*. **2.** Ataxie *f*, Ataxia *f*.
dys·sys·to·le [dɪ'sɪstəlɪ] *n card.* gestörte/abnormale Systole *f*.
dys·ta·sia [dɪs'teɪʒ(ɪ)ə] *n* → dysstasia.
dys·tax·ia [dɪs'tæksɪə] *n neuro.* leichte/partielle Ataxie *f*, Dystaxia *f*.
dys·thy·mia [dɪs'θaɪmɪə] *n psychia.* Dysthymie *f*.
dys·thy·mic [dɪs'θaɪmɪk] *adj psychia.* depressiv, dysthym.
dysthymic disorder → dysthymia.
dys·thy·re·o·sis [ˌdɪsθaɪrɪ'əʊsɪs] *n patho.* fehlerhafte/mangelnde Schilddrüsenentwicklung *f*, Störung *f* der Schilddrüsenfunktion, Dysthyreose *f*.
dys·thy·roid·ism [dɪs'θaɪrɔɪdɪzəm] *n* → dysthyreosis.
dys·to·cia [dɪs'təʊʃ(ɪ)ə] *n gyn.* abnormaler/gestörter/erschwerter Geburtsverlauf *m*, Dystokie *f*.
dys·to·nia [dɪs'təʊnɪə] *n patho.* mangelhafter/fehlerhafter Spannungszustand/Tonus *m*, Dystonie *f*.
dys·ton·ic [dɪs'tɑnɪk] *adj* Dystonie betr., dyston, dystonisch.
dys·to·pia [dɪs'təʊpɪə] *n patho.* Verlagerung *f*, Dystopie *f*, Dystopia *f*, Heterotopie *f*.
dys·top·ic [dɪs'tɑpɪk] *adj* verlagert, dystop, heterotop.
dys·to·py ['dɪstəpɪ] *n* → dystopia.
dys·tro·phia [dɪs'trəʊfɪə] *n* → dystrophy.

dys·troph·ic [dɪsˈtrɑfɪk, -ˈtrəʊf-] *adj* Dystrophie betr., dystroph(isch).
dystrophic gait watschelnder Gang *m*, Watschelgang *m*, Watscheln *nt*.
dys·troph·o·neu·ro·sis [dɪsˌtrɑfənjʊəˈrəʊsɪs] *n patho.* nutritive/alimentäre Trophoneurose *f*.
dys·tro·phy [ˈdɪstrəfɪ] *n patho.* Dystrophie *f*, Dystrophia *f*.
dys·tro·py [ˈdɪstrəpɪ] *n* Dystropie *f*.
dys·u·re·sia [dɪsjəˈriːzɪə] *n* → dysuria.
dys·u·ria [dɪsˈjʊərɪə] *n urol.* schmerzhafte Miktion *f*, Fehl-, Schwerharnen *nt*, Dysurie *f*, Dysuria *f*.
dys·u·ri·ac [dɪsˈjʊərɪæk] *n* Patient(in *f*) *m* mit Dysurie, Dysuriker(in *f*) *m*.
dys·u·ric [dɪsˈjʊərɪk] *adj* Dysurie betr., dysurisch.
dys·u·ry [ˈdɪsjʊərɪ] *n* → dysuria.
dys·ver·sion [dɪsˈvɜrʒn] *n* Dysversion *f*.
dys·vi·ta·min·o·sis [ˌdɪsvɪtəmɪˈnəʊsɪs] *n* Dysvitaminose *f*.
dys·zo·o·sper·mia [dɪszəʊəˈspɜrmɪə] *n embryo.* Dyszoospermie *f*.

E

E *abbr.* → extinction coefficient, molar.
E' *abbr.* → volume elasticity coefficient.
E$_1$ *abbr.* → estrone.
E$_2$ *abbr.* → estradiol.
E$_3$ *abbr.* → estriol.
E$_4$ *abbr.* → estetrol.
E *abbr.* → absorption coefficient, molar.
e$^+$ *abbr.* → positron.
ϵ *abbr.* **1.** → emissivity. **2.** → extinction coefficient.
η *abbr.* → dynamic viscosity.
EA *abbr.* **1.** → early antigen. **2.** → enteral alimentation.
EACA *abbr.* → epsilon-aminocaproic acid.
EAC rosette assay [erythrocyte, antibody, complement] *immun.* EAC-Rosettentest *m*.
Eadie-Hofstee ['iːdɪ 'hɑfstiː]: **E.-H. plot** Eadie-Hofstee-Darstellung *f*.
EAE *abbr.* → experimental allergic encephalomyelitis.
EAG *abbr.* → electroatriogram.
Eagle ['iːgəl]: **E. syndrome** Eagle-Syndrom *nt*.
EAHF complex [eczema, asthma, hay fever] EAHF-Komplex *m*, Ekzem-Asthma-Heufieber-Komplex *m*.
Eales ['iːlz]: **E.' disease** *ophthal.* Eales-Krankheit *f*, -Erkrankung *f*, Periphlebitis retinae.
E antigen *hema.* Antigen E *nt*.
EAP *abbr.* → epiallopregnanolone.
ear [ɪər] *n* **1.** Ohr *nt*; *anat.* Auris *f*. **2.** Gehör *nt*, Ohr *nt*. **3.** Öse *f*, Öhr *nt*.
ear·ache ['ɪəreɪk] *n* Ohr(en)schmerzen *pl*, Otalgie *f*.
ear block *HNO* Tubenblockade *f*.
ear bones Mittelohrknochen *pl*, Gehörknöchelchen *pl*, Ossicula auditoria/auditus.
ear concha Ohrmuschel *f*; *anat.* Concha auricularis.
ear crystals *physiol.* Ohrkristalle *pl*, Otokonien *pl*, -lithen *pl*, -conia *pl*, Statokonien *pl*, -lithen *pl*, -conia *pl*.
ear drops Ohrentropfen *pl*.
ear·drum ['ɪərdrʌm] *n* **1.** Paukenhöhle *f*, Tympanum *nt*, Tympanum *nt*, Cavum tympani, Cavitas tympanica. **2.** Trommelfell *nt*, Membrana tympanica.
eared [ɪərd] *adj* **1.** -ohrig, mit Ohren. **2.** mit Ösen versehen.
ear·flap ['ɪərflæp] *n* Ohrschützer *m*.
ear·lap ['ɪərlæp] *n* **1.** → earflap. **2.** → ear lobule. **3.** → external ear.
ear·lobe ['ɪərləʊb] *n* → ear lobule.
ear lobule Ohrläppchen *nt*, Lobulus auricularis.
ear·ly ['ɜrlɪ] **I** *adj* früh, (früh-)zeitig, vorzeitig; zu früh, Früh-. **II** *adv* früh(zeitig); bald.
early abortion *gyn.* Frühabort *m*, früher Abort *m*.
early antigen *abbr.* **EA** *immun.* (*EBV*) Frühantigen *nt*, Early-Antigen *nt* *abbr.* EA.

early cancer 1. *patho.* Frühkarzinom *nt*, early cancer (*m*). **2.** → e. of stomach.
e. of stomach Frühkarzinom des Magens, Magenfrühkarzinom.
early carcinoma of stomach → early cancer of stomach.
early deceleration *gyn.* Frühdezeleration *f*, Frühtief *nt*, frühe Dezeleration *f*, Dip I *m*.
early diagnosis Frühdiagnose *f*.
early diastolic dip *card.* frühdiastolischer Dip *m*, Dip-Phänomen *nt*.
early diastolic murmur frühdiastolisches (Herz-)Geräusch *nt*.
early erythroblast → early normoblast.
early gastric cancer → early cancer of stomach.
early infantile autism frühkindlicher Autismus *m*, Kanner-Syndrom *nt*.
early infiltration *patho.* Frühinfiltration *f*.
early-inspiritory neuron *physiol.* frühinspiratorisches Neuron *nt*, e-I-Neuron *nt*.
early invasion *patho.* Frühinvasion *f*.
early juvenile type of cerebral sphingolipidosis Jansky-Bielschowsky-Krankheit *f*, Bielschowsky-Syndrom *nt*, spätinfantile Form *f* der amaurotischen Idiotie.
early latent syphilis Frühlatenz *f*, Syphilis/Lues latens seropositiva.
early normoblast basophiler Normoblast *m*.
early operation *chir.* Frühoperation *f*.
early post-traumatic epilepsy frühe (post-)traumatische Epilepsie *f*.
early protein *micro.* (*Virus*) Frühprotein *nt*.
early receptor potential *abbr.* **ERP** frühes/primäres Rezeptorpotential *nt*, early receptor potential *abbr.* ERP.
early satiety *chir.* Syndrom *nt* des zu kleinen Restmagens.
early syphilis Frühsyphilis *f*.
early systemic dissemination *patho.* Frühgeneralisation *f*.
ear-minded *adj psycho.* auditiv.
ear muscle Ohrmuskel *m*.
ear, nose and throat *abbr.* **ENT** Hals-, Nasen-, Ohrenheilkunde *f* *abbr.* HNO, Otorhinolaryngologie *f*.
ear ossicles Gehörknöchelchen *pl*, Ossicula auditus/auditoria.
ear·pick ['ɪərpɪk] *n* Ohrlöffel *m*.
ear·piece ['ɪərpiːs] *n* **1.** Ohrenklappe *f*. **2.** (*Stethoskop*) Ohrstück *nt*. **3.** (Brillen-)Bügel *m*.
ear pit *embryo.* Ohrgrübchen *nt*.
ear plane *radiol.* Deutsche Horizontale *f*, Frankfurter Horizontale *f*, Ohr-Augen-Ebene *f*.
ear·plug ['ɪərplʌg] *n* Wattepfropf *m*.
ear protector Ohrenschützer *m*, -schutz *nt*.
ear speculum Ohrtrichter *m*, -spekulum *nt*.
earth [ɜrθ] *n* **1.** Erde *f*, Erdball *m*; Erde *f*,

(Erd-)Boden *m*. **2.** *chem.* Erde *f*. **3.** *phys.* Erde *f*, Erdung *f*, Masse *f*.
ear tick *micro.* Otobius megnini.
ear trumpet Hörrohr *nt*.
ear·wax ['ɪərwæks] *n physiol.* Ohr(en)schmalz *nt*, Zerumen *nt*, Cerumen *nt*.
ease [iːz] **I** *n* **1.** Erleichterung *f*, Befreiung *f* (*from* von). **to give s.o.** ~ jdm. Erleichterung verschaffen. **2.** Mühelosigkeit *f*, Leichtigkeit *f*. **with** ~ mühelos, leicht. **II** *vt* erleichtern; (*Schmerz*) lindern; beruhigen; (*Druck*) verringern; lockern, entspannen. **III** *vi* Erleichterung *od.* Entspannung *od.* Linderung verschaffen.
ease off/up *vi* nachlassen, s. entspannen.
ease·ful ['iːzfəl] *adj* erleichternd.
East African sleeping sickness [iːst] → East African trypanosomiasis.
East African trypanosomiasis ostafrikanische Trypanosomiasis/Schlafkrankheit *f*.
East Coast fever East-Coast-Fieber *nt*, bovine Piroplasmose/Theileriose *f*.
East·ern equine encephalitis ['iːstərn] *abbr.* **EEE** östliche Pferdeenzephalitis *f*, Eastern equine encephalitis/encephalomyelitis *abbr.* EEE.
Eastern equine encephalitis virus *micro.* Eastern equine encephalitis/encephalomyelitis-Virus *nt*, EEE-Virus *nt*.
Eastern equine encephalomyelitis → Eastern equine encephalitis.
Eastern equine encephalomyelitis virus → Eastern equine encephalitis virus.
Eastern schistosomiasis japanische Schistosomiasis/Bilharziose *f*, Schistosomiasis japonica.
eas·y breathing ['iːzɪ] → eupnea.
easy death leichter/schmerzloser Tod *m*, Euthanasie *f*.
easy respiration → eupnea.
eat·a·ble ['iːtəbl] **I** ~*s pl* Lebens-, Nahrungsmittel *pl*. **II** *adj* eß-, genießbar.
eat·ing habits ['iːtɪŋ] Eßgewohnheiten *pl*.
Eaton ['iːtn]: **E. agent** Eaton-agent *nt*, Mycoplasma pneumoniae.
E. agent pneumonia Mycoplasma-pneumoniae-Pneumonie *f*, Mykoplasmapneumonie *f*.
Eaton-Lambert ['læmbərt]: **E.-L. syndrome** Lambert-Eaton-Rooke-Syndrom *nt*, myoasthenisches Syndrom *nt*.
Ebbecke [ə'bek; 'ebəkɪ]: **E.'s reaction** *derm.* Hautschrift *f*, Dermographie *f*, Dermographia *f*, Dermographismus *m*.
Ebbinghaus ['ɛbɪŋhaʊs]: **E. test** *psycho.* Ebbinghaus-Lückentest *m*.
Eberth ['eɪbərt; 'eːb-]: **E.'s bacillus** Typhusbazillus *m*, -bacillus *m*, Salmonella typhi.
E.'s lines Eberth-Linien *pl*.
E-ber·thel·la typhi [ˌiːbər'θelə, ˌeɪb-] *micro. old* → Eberth's bacillus.
EBNA *abbr.* → Epstein-Barr nuclear antigen.
Ebner ['ebnər; 'eːb-]: **E.'s glands** (von) Ebner'-Drüsen *pl*, (von) Ebner-Spüldrüsen *pl*.

Ebola

E·bo·la [ɪ'bəʊlə]: E. disease → E. fever.
E. fever Ebolaviruskrankheit f, Ebola-Fieber nt, Ebola hämorrhagisches Fieber nt.
E. hemorrhagic fever → E. fever.
E. virus micro. Ebola-Virus nt, Sudan-Zaire-Virus n.
E. virus disease → E. fever.
E. virus fever → E. fever.
e·bo·na·tion [iːbəʊ'neɪʃn] n ortho. (Knochen-)Fragmententfernung f.
e·bri·e·ty [ɪ'braɪətɪ] n einfacher/unkomplizierter Alkoholrausch m, Trunkenheit f, Ebrietas f.
Ebstein ['ebstaɪn]: **E.'s angle** Ebstein-Winkel m, Herz-Leber-Winkel m. **E.'s anomaly/disease card.** Ebstein-Anomalie f, -Syndrom nt.
e·bul·lient [ɪ'bʌljənt, -'bʊl-] adj 1. siedend, aufwallend. 2. überfließend, überkochend; sprudelnd, überschäumend.
eb·ul·lism ['ebjəlɪzəm] n patho. Ebullismus m, Aeroembolismus m.
e·bur ['ebər] n 1. Elfenbein nt. 2. patho. elfenbeinähnliches Gewebe nt.
e·bur·nat·ed vertebra ['ebərneɪtɪd] ortho. Elfenbeinwirbel m.
e·bur·nat·ing osteoma ['ebərneɪtɪŋ] ortho. kompaktes Osteom nt, Osteoma eburnum.
e·bur·na·tion [ebər'eɪʃn] n ortho. Osteosklerose f, Eburnisation f, Eburneation f, Eburnifikation f, Eburnisierung f.
e·bur·ne·ous [ɪ'bɜrnɪəs] adj elfenbeinartig, -ähnlich.
EBV abbr. → Epstein-Barr virus.
EBV antigen → Epstein-Barr virus antigen.
EB virus → Epstein-Barr virus.
EC abbr. → enterochromaffin.
ECAO virus [enteric, cytopathic, avian, orphan] micro. ECAO-Virus nt.
ec·ao·vi·rus ['ekəʊəvaɪrəs] n → ECAO virus.
é·car·teur [eɪkɑːr'tɜr; ekar'tœr] n chir. (Wund-)Haken m; Wundspreizer m, -sperrer m.
e·cau·date [ɪ'kɔːdeɪt] adj schwanzlos, ohne Schwanz.
ec·bol·ic [ek'bɒlɪk] **I** n 1. wehenförderndes Mittel nt, Wehenmittel nt. 2. Abortivum nt. **II** adj 3. wehenfördernd. 4. abtreibend, abortiv.
ec·bo·line ['ekbəliːn] n → ergotoxine.
ECBO virus [enteric, cytopathic, bovine, orphan] micro. ECBO-Virus nt.
ec·bo·vi·rus [ekbə'vaɪrəs] n → ECBO virus.
EC cells → enterochromaffin cells.
ec·cen·tric [ɪk'sentrɪk] **I** n 1. Exzentriker(in f) m. 2. techn. Exzenter m. 3. mathe. exzentrische Figur f. **II** adj 4. fig. exzentrisch; überspannt, verschroben; ausgefallen, ungewöhnlich. 5. mathe., techn., bio. exzentrisch, nicht zentral; ohne gemeinsamen Mittelpunkt; nicht durch den Mittelpunkt gehend.
ec·cen·tri·cal [ɪk'sentrɪkl] adj → eccentric II.
eccentric atrophy patho. exzentrische Atrophie f.
eccentric hypertrophy patho. exzentrische Hypertrophie f.
eccentric vision indirektes/periphäres Sehen nt.
ec·cen·tro·chon·dro·pla·sia [ɪk,sentrəʊ-,kɒndrəʊ'pleɪʒ(ɪ)ə, -zɪə] n → eccentro-osteochondrodysplasia.
eccentro-osteochondrodysplasia n Mukopolysaccharidose f Typ IV abbr. MPS IV, Morquio(-Ullrich)-Syndrom nt, Morquio-Brailsford-Syndrom nt, spondyloepiphysäre Dysplasie f.
ec·chon·dro·ma [ekɒn'drəʊmə] n ortho. peripheres Chondrom nt, Ekchondrom nt.
ec·chon·dro·sis [ekɒn'drəʊsɪs] n → ecchondroma.
ec·chon·dro·tome [e'kɒndrətəʊm] n chir. Knorpelmesser nt, Chondrotom nt.
ec·chy·mo·ma [ekɪ'məʊmə] n Ekchymom nt.
ec·chy·mo·sis [ekɪ'məʊsɪs] n, pl **-ses** [-siːz] kleinflächige Hautblutung f, Ekchymose f, Ecchymosis f.
ec·chy·mot·ic [ekɪ'mɒtɪk] adj Ekchymosen betr., Ekchymose(n)-.
ec·co·prot·ic [ekəʊ'prɒtɪk] **I** n pharm. Abführmittel nt, Kathartikum nt, Laxans nt, Purgans nt, Purgativ(um) nt. **II** adj 1. abführend, kathartisch, purgierend, Abführ-. 2. psychia. Katharsis betr., kathartisch.
ECCO virus [enteric, cytopathic, cat, orphan] micro. ECCO-Virus nt.
ec·co·vi·rus [ekəʊ'vaɪrəs] n → ECCO virus.
ec·crine ['ekrɪn, -raɪn, -riːn] adj nach außen absondernd, ekkrin.
eccrine acrospiroma noduläres Hidradenom nt, Hidradenoma solidum.
eccrine extrusion ekkrine Extrusion f, Krinozytose f.
eccrine gland ekkrine Drüse f, Gl. eccrina.
eccrine poroma ekkrines Porom nt, Poroakanthom nt.
eccrine spiradenoma patho. ekkrines Spiradenom nt.
ec·cri·sis ['ekrəsɪs] n 1. Ausscheidung f von Abfallstoffen. 2. Abfall(produkt nt) m. 3. → excrement.
ec·cy·e·sis [eksaɪ'iːsɪs] n, pl **-ses** [-siːz] → extrauterine pregnancy.
ec·dem·ic [ek'demɪk] adj epidem. ekdemisch.
ec·der·on ['ekdərɒn] n → epidermis.
ECDO virus [enteric, cytopathic, dog, orphan] micro. ECDO-Virus nt.
ec·do·vi·rus [ekdəʊ'vaɪrəs] n → ECDO virus.
ec·dy·sone ['ekdɪzəʊn] n Ekdyson nt, Ecdyson nt.
ECF abbr. 1. → eosinophil chemotactic factor. 2. → extracellular fluid.
ECF-A abbr. → eosinophil chemotactic factor of anaphylaxis.
ECG abbr. → electrocardiogram.
E·chid·noph·a·ga [ekɪd'nafəgə] pl micro. Echidnophaga pl.
ech·i·nate ['ekɪneɪt] n → echinulate.
E·chi·no·chas·mus [ɪ,kaɪnəʊ'kæzməs] n micro. Echinochasmus m.
e·chi·no·coc·cal [,-'kɒkl] adj Echinokokken betr., durch sie verursacht, Echinokokken-.
echinococcal cystic disease → echinococcosis.
e·chi·no·coc·ci·a·sis [,-kɒ'kaɪəsɪs] n → echinococcosis.
e·chi·no·coc·co·sis [,-kɒ'kəʊsɪs] n Echinokokkenkrankheit f, -infektion f, Echinokokkose f, Hydatidose f.
e·chi·no·coc·cot·o·my [,-kɒ'kɒtəmɪ] n chir. Echinokokkenzystenentfernung f, -exzision f.
E·chi·no·coc·cus [,-'kɒkəs] n micro. Echinokokkus m, Echinococcus m.
E. granulosus Blasenbandwurm m, Hundebandwurm m, Echinococcus granulosus, Taenia echinococcus.
E. multilocularis Echinococcus multilocularis.

echinococcus cyst Echinokokkenblase f, -zyste f, Hydatide f.
echinococcus disease → echinococcosis.
e·chi·no·cyte [ɪ'kaɪnəsaɪt] n hema. Stechapfelform f, Echinozyt m.
e·chi·noph·thal·mia [ɪ,kaɪnɒf'θælmɪə] n ophthal. Echinophthalmie f.
E·chi·no·rhyn·chus [ɪ,kaɪnə'rɪŋkəs] n micro. Echinorhynchus m.
Ech·i·nos·to·ma [ekɪ'nɒstəmə] n micro. Echinostoma m.
e·chi·no·sto·mi·a·sis [ɪ,kaɪnəstə'maɪəsɪs] n Echinostomainfektion f, Echinostomiasis f.
e·chin·u·late [ɪ'kɪnjəlɪt, -leɪt] adj mit Stacheln versehen, stach(e)lig.
ech·o ['ekəʊ] **I** n Echo nt, Widerhall m. **II** vi echoen, widerhallen (with von).
ech·o·a·cou·sia [,ekəʊə'kuːʒɪə] n HNO Echohören nt, Echoakusis f, Diplacusis echoica.
ech·o·car·di·o·gram [,-'kɑːrdɪəgræm] n Echokardiogramm nt.
ech·o·car·di·o·graph·ic [,-,kɑːrdɪə'græfɪk] adj Echokardiographie betr., mittels Echokardiographie, echokardiographisch.
ech·o·car·di·og·ra·phy [,-,kɑːrdɪ'ɒɡrəfɪ] n Echokardiographie f, Ultraschallkardiographie f abbr. UKG.
echo diplacusis → echoacousia.
ech·o·en·ceph·a·lo·gram [,-en'sefələʊgræm] n Echoenzephalogramm nt.
ech·o·en·ceph·a·lo·graph [,-en'sefələʊgræf] n Echoenzephalograph m.
ech·o·en·ceph·a·log·ra·phy [,-en,sefə'lɒgrəfɪ] n Echoenzephalographie f.
ech·o·gen·ic [,-'dʒenɪk] adj radiol. echogen.
ech·o·gram ['-græm] n radiol. Echogramm nt, Sonogramm nt.
ech·o·graph ['-græf] n radiol. Sonograph m.
ech·o·graph·ia [,-'græfɪə] n neuro. Echographie f.
e·chog·ra·phy [e'kɒɡrəfɪ] n radiol. Ultraschalldiagnostik f, Echographie f, Sonographie f.
ech·o·ic [e'kəʊɪk] adj echoartig, echoisch, Echo-.
echoic memory akustisches/echoisches Gedächtnis nt.
ech·o·ki·ne·sia [,ekəʊkɪ'niːʒ(ɪ)ə] n psychia. Echokinese f, Echopraxie f.
ech·o·ki·ne·sis [,-kɪ'niːsɪs, -kaɪ-] n → echokinesia.
ech·o·la·lia [,-'leɪlɪə] n psychia. Echolalie f, Echophrasie f.
ech·o·lu·cent [,-'luːsnt] adj schalldurchlässig.
ech·o·ma·tism [e'kɒmətɪzəm] n psychia. Echoerscheinungen pl, Echomatismus m.
ech·o·mim·ia [ekəʊ'mɪmɪə] n psychia. Echomimie f.
ech·o·mo·tism [,-'məʊtɪzəm] n → echokinesia.
e·chop·a·thy [e'kɒpəθɪ] n → echomatism.
ech·o·pho·no·car·di·og·ra·phy [,ekəʊ,fəʊnəkɑːrdɪ'ɒɡrəfɪ] n Echophonokardiographie f, Ultraschallphonokardiographie f.
e·choph·o·ny [e'kɒfənɪ] n Echophonie f.
ech·o·phra·sia [ekəʊ'freɪʒ(ɪ)ə, -zɪə] n → echolalia.
ech·o·prax·ia [,-'præksɪə] n → echokinesia.
ech·o·prax·is [,-'præksɪs] n → echolalia.
echo speech → echolalia.
ech·o·thi·o·phate [,-'θaɪəfeɪt] n pharm. Ecotiophat nt.
echothiophate iodide Ecotiopatiodid nt.
ECHO virus [enteric, cytopathic, human, orphan] ECHO-Virus nt, Echovirus nt.

ech·o·vi·rus [ˌ-'vaɪrəs] *n* → ECHO virus.
Eck [ek]: **E. fistula** Eck-Fistel *f*.
Ecker ['ekər]: **E.'s fissure** Fissura petrooccipitalis.
ec·lamp·sia [ɪ'klæmpsɪə] *n gyn*. Eklampsie *f*, Eclampsia *f*.
ec·lamp·sism [ɪ'klæmpsɪzəm] *n gyn*. Präeklampsie *f*, Eklampsismus *m*.
ec·lamp·tic [ɪ'klæmptɪk] *adj* Eklampsie betr., eklamptisch.
eclamptic retinopathy Retinopathia eclamptica gravidarum.
eclamptic toxemia *gyn*. Schwangerschaftstoxikose *f*, Gestose *f*.
ec·lamp·tism [ɪ'klæmptɪzəm] *n gyn*. eklamptischer Symptomenkomplex *m*.
ec·lamp·to·gen·ic [ɪˌklæmptə'dʒenɪk] *adj* Eklampsie verursachend, eklamptogen.
eclamptogenic toxemia → eclamptic toxemia.
ec·lamp·tog·en·ous [ɪˌklæmp'tɒdʒənəs] *adj* → eclamptogenic.
e·clipse [ɪ'klɪps] *n micro*. Eklipse *f*.
e·clipsed conformation [ɪ'klɪpsd] *chem*. ekliptische Konformation *f*.
eclipse period/phase → eclipse.
ec·mne·sia [ek'niːʒ(ɪ)ə] *n neuro., psychia*. Ekmnesie *f*.
ECMO *abbr*. → extracorporeal membrane oxygenation.
ECMO virus [enteric, cytopathic, monkey, orphan] *micro*. ECMO-Virus *nt*.
ec·mo·vi·rus [ekmə'vaɪrəs] *n* → ECMO virus.
eco- *pref*. Umwelt-, Öko-.
e·co·bi·ot·ic [ˌekəʊbaɪ'ɒtɪk, ˌiːkəʊ-] *adj* ökobiotisch.
e·co·ca·tas·tro·phe [ˌ-kə'tæstrəfɪ] *n* Öko-, Umweltkatastrophe *f*.
e·co·cide ['-saɪd] *n* Umweltzerstörung *f*.
e·co·cli·mate [ˌ-'klaɪmɪt] *n* Standort-, Biotop-, Ökoklima *nt*.
e·co·cli·mat·ic [ˌ-klaɪ'mætɪk] *adj* ökoklimatisch.
ECoG *abbr*. → electrocorticogram.
e·co·ge·net·ics [ˌ-dʒə'netɪks] *pl* Ökogenetik *f*.
e·co·log·i·cal [ˌ-'lɒdʒɪkl] *adj* ökologisch.
ecological awareness Umweltbewußtsein *nt*, Ökobewußtsein *nt*.
ecological balance ökologisches Gleichgewicht *nt*.
ecological chemistry Ökochemie *f*.
ecological system → ecosystem.
e·col·o·gist [ɪ'kɒlədʒɪst] *n* Ökologe *m*, -login *f*.
e·col·o·gy [ɪ'kɒlədʒɪ] *n* Ökologie *f*.
e·co·ma·nia [ˌekə'meɪnɪə, -jə, ˌiːkə-] *n psychia*. Oikomanie *f*.
e·con·a·zole [ɪ'kɒnəzəʊl] *n pharm*. Econazol *nt*.
e·co·nom·ic [ˌekə'nɒmɪk, ˌiːkə-] *adj* (volks-)wirtschaftlich, ökonomisch, Wirtschafts-.
e·co·nom·i·cal [ˌ-'nɒmɪkl] *adj* wirtschaftlich, sparsam. **to be ~** haushalten *od*. sparsam umgehen (*with* mit).
Economo [eɪ'kɒnəməʊ]: **E.'s disease/encephalitis** (von) Economo-Krankheit *f*, -Enzephalitis *f*, europäische Schlafkrankheit *f*, Encephalitis epidemica/lethargica.
e·con·o·my [ɪ'kɒnəmɪ] *n* 1. Wirtschaftlichkeit *f*, Sparsamkeit *f*, Einsparung *f*. 2. Wirtschaft *f*, Wirtschaftssystem *nt*, -lehre *f*.
e·co·par·a·site [ˌekəʊ'pærəsaɪt, ˌiːkə-] *n* → ectoparasite.
e·co·pho·bia [ˌ-'fəʊbɪə] *n psychia*. Oikophobie *f*.
e·co·phys·i·ol·o·gy [ˌ-fɪzɪ'ɒlədʒɪ] *n* Ökophysiologie *f*.

e·co·spe·cies ['-spiːʃɪːz] *n* Ökospezies *f*.
e·co·sphere ['-sfɪər] *n* Ökosphäre *f*.
e·cos·tate [ɪ'kɒsteɪt, -tɪt] *adj* ohne Rippen, rippenlos.
e·co·sys·tem ['ekəʊsɪstəm, 'iːkəʊ-] *n* Ökosystem *nt*, ökologisches System *nt*.
ec·o·tax·is [ˌ-'tæksɪs] *n hema*. Öko-, Oikotaxis *f*.
ec·o·type ['-taɪp] *n bio*. Ökotypus *m*, Ökotyp *m*.
é·cou·teur [ekuˈtœːr] *n psychia*. Écouteur *m*.
ec·pho·ria [ekˈfɔːrɪə, -ˈfəʊ-] *n neuro*. Ekphorie *f*.
ec·phy·a·di·tis [ˌekfaɪəˈdaɪtɪs] *n* Wurmfortsatzentzündung *f*, *inf*. Blinddarmentzündung *f*, Appendizitis *f*, Appendicitis *f*.
ec·phy·ma [ekˈfaɪmə] *n derm*. Auswuchs *m*, Höcker *m*, Ekphyma *nt*.
ECPO virus [enteric, cytopathic, porcine, orphan] *micro*. ECPO-Virus *nt*.
ec·po·vi·rus [ekpəʊˈvaɪrəs] *n* → ECPO virus.
é·crase·ment [ekrazˈmɑ̃] *n chir*. Écrasement *nt*.
é·cra·seur [ekraˈzœːr] *n chir*. Écraseur *m*.
ECS *abbr*. **1.** → electrocerebral silence. **2.** → extracellular space.
ECSO virus [enteric, cytopathic, swine, orphan] *micro*. ECSO-Virus *nt*.
ec·so·vi·rus [eksəˈvaɪrəs] *n* → ECSO virus.
ec·sta·size ['ekstəsaɪz] **I** *vt* in Ekstase versetzen. **II** *vi* in Ekstase geraten.
ec·sta·sy ['ekstəsɪ] *n* Ekstase *f*, krankhafte Erregung *f*, Status raptus.
ec·stat·ic [ekˈstætɪk] *adj* Ekstase betr., ekstatisch.
ec·stro·phy ['ekstrəfɪ] *n* → exstrophy.
ECT *abbr*. [electroconvulsive therapy] → electroshock therapy.
ect- *pref*. → ecto-.
ec·ta·co·lia [ektəˈkəʊlɪə] *n patho*. Dickdarm-, Kolonektasie *f*, Kolektasie *f*.
ec·tad ['ektæd] *adj anat*. nach außen, (nach) auswärts.
ec·tal ['ektl] *adj* oberflächlich, äußerlich, an der Oberfläche (liegend).
ec·ta·sia [ekˈteɪʒ(ɪ)ə] *n patho*. Ausdehnung *f*, -weitung *f*, Ektasie *f*, Ektasia *f*.
ec·ta·sis ['ektəsɪs] *n* → ectasia.
ec·ta·sy ['ektəsɪ] *n* → ectasia.
ec·tat·ic [ekˈtætɪk] *adj* erweitert, (aus-)gedehnt, ektatisch.
ectatic aneurysm ektatisches Aneurysma *nt*.
ect·eth·moid [ekˈteθmɔɪd] *n anat*. Labyrinthus ethmoidalis.
ec·thy·ma [ekˈθaɪmə] *n derm*. Ekthym *nt*, Ekthyma *nt*, Ecthyma *nt*.
ecthyma gangrenosum Ekthyma/Ecthyma gangraenosum, Ekthyma/Ecthyma terebrans infantum, Ecthyma cachecticorum, Ecthyma gangraenosum terebrans.
ec·thy·ma·ti·form [ekθaɪˈmætɪfɔːrm] *adj* ekthymähnlich, -artig, ekthymatös.
ec·thy·ma·tous syphilid [ekˈθaɪmətəs] pustulöses Syphilid *nt*.
ec·thy·mi·form [ekˈθaɪməfɔːrm] *adj* → ecthymatiform.
ecto- *pref*. Ekt(o)-, Exo-.
ec·to·an·ti·gen [ˌektəʊˈæntɪdʒən] *n* Ekto-, Exoantigen *nt*.
ec·to·bi·ol·o·gy [ˌ-baɪˈɒlədʒɪ] *n* Ektobiologie *f*.
ec·to·blast ['-blæst] *n* → ectoderm.
ec·to·car·di·a [ˌ-ˈkɑːrdɪə] *n embryo*. Herzektopie *f*, Ektokardie *f*, Ectopia cordis, Kardiozele *f*, Hernia cordis.
ec·to·cer·vi·cal [ˌ-ˈsɜːrvɪkl, sɜːˈvaɪkl] *adj* Ektozervix betr., ektozervikal, Ektozervix-.

ec·to·cer·vix [ˌ-ˈsɜːrvɪks] *n* Ektozervix *f*, Portio vaginalis cervicis.
ec·to·cho·roi·dea [ˌ-kəˈrɔɪdɪə] *n anat*. Lamina suprachoroidea.
ec·to·co·lon [ˌ-ˈkəʊlən] *n patho*. Dickdarm-, Kolondilatation *f*.
ec·to·cu·nei·form [ˌ-kjuːˈnɪəfɔːrm] *n anat*. Os cuneiforme laterale.
ec·to·cyt·ic [ˌ-ˈsɪtɪk] *adj* außerhalb der Zelle (liegend), ekto-, exozytär.
ec·to·dac·ty·ly-ectodermal dysplasia-clefting syndrome [ˌ-ˈdæktəlɪ] EEC-Syndrom *nt*.
ec·to·derm ['-dɜːrm] *n embryo*. äußeres Keimblatt *nt*, Ektoblast *nt*, Ektoderm *nt*.
ec·to·der·mal [ˌ-ˈdɜːrml] *adj* Ektoderm betr., vom Ektoderm abstammend, ektodermal.
ectodermal dysplasia Ektodermaldysplasie *f*, Dysplasia ectodermalis.
 anhidrotic e. Christ-Siemens-Touraine-Syndrom *nt*, anhidrotisch ektodermale Dysplasie *f*, ektodermale kongenitale Dysplasie *f*, Anhidrosis hypotrichotica polydysplastica.
 congenital e. → anhidrotic e.
 hypohidrotic e. → anhidrotic e.
ectodermal placode *embryo*. Ektodermplakode *f*.
ec·to·der·ma·to·sis [ˌ-dɜːrməˈtəʊsɪs] *n* → ectodermosis.
ec·to·der·mic [ˌ-ˈdɜːrmɪk] *adj* → ectodermal.
ec·to·der·mo·sis [ˌ-dɜːrˈməʊsɪs] *n embryo., patho*. Ektodermose *f*, Ektodermatose *f*.
ec·to·en·zyme [ˌ-ˈenzaɪm] *n* Ekto-, Exoenzym *nt*.
ec·to·eth·moid [ˌ-ˈeθmɔɪd] *n* → ectethmoid.
ec·to·gen·ic [ˌ-ˈdʒenɪk] *adj* → exogenous.
ec·tog·e·nous [ekˈtædʒənəs] *adj* → exogenous.
ectogenous infection exogene Infektion *f*.
ec·to·glia [ekˈtæglɪə] *n* Ektoglia *f*.
ec·to·glob·u·lar [ˌektəʊˈglɒbjələr] *adj hema*. exo-, extraglobulär.
ec·tog·o·ny [ekˈtægənɪ] *n micro*. Ektogonie *f*, Metaxenie *f*.
ec·to·hor·mone [ˌektəʊˈhɔːrməʊn] *n* Ektohormon *nt*.
ec·to·lec·i·thal [ˌ-ˈlesɪθəl] *adj bio*. ektolezithal.
ec·tol·y·sis [ekˈtɒləsɪs] *n histo*. Ektoplasmaauflösung *f*, Ektolyse *f*.
ec·to·mere [ˈektəmɪər] *n embryo*. Ektomere *f*.
ec·to·mes·o·blast [ˌ-ˈmesəblæst] *n embryo*. Ektomesoblast *nt*.
ec·to·morph ['-mɔːrf] *n psychia*. Ektomorpher *m*, Longitypus *m*.
ec·to·mor·phic [ˌ-ˈmɔːrfɪk] *adj* ektomorph.
ec·to·my ['ektəmɪ] *n chir*. Herausschneiden *nt*, (Total-)Entfernung *f*, Ektomie *f*.
ec·to·nu·cle·ar [ˌektəʊˈn(j)uːklɪər] *adj* außerhalb des Zellkerns (liegend), ekto-, exonukleär.
ec·top·a·gus [ekˈtæpəgəs] *n embryo*. Ektopagus *m*.
ec·to·par·a·site [ˌektəʊˈpærəsaɪt] *n micro*. Außen-, Ektoparasit *m*, Ektosit *f*.
ec·to·pec·to·ra·lis [ˌ-pektəˈreɪlɪs, -ˈreɪ-] *n anat*. M. pectoralis major.
ec·to·phyte ['-faɪt] *n bio*. Ektophyt *m*.
ec·to·pia [ekˈtəʊpɪə] *n* angeborene Gewebs- *od*. Organverlagerung *f*, Ektopie *f*, Ektopia *f*, Ectopia *f*, Extraversion *f*, Eversion *f*.
ec·top·ic [ekˈtæpɪk] *adj* 1. ursprungsfern, an atypischer Stelle liegend *od*. entstehend, (nach außen) verlagert, heterotopisch, ektop(isch). 2. Ektopie betr., ektopisch.

ectopic ACTH syndrome Syndrom *nt* der ektopischen ACTH-Bildung.
ectopic anus *embryo.* Analatresie *f*, Atresia ani.
ectopic beat *card.* ektope/ektopische Erregung(sbildung *f*) *f*.
ectopic center → ectopic focus.
ectopic focus *physiol.* ektopes Zentrum *nt*, ektopischer Fokus *m*.
ectopic hyperparathyroidism paraneoplastischer Hyperparathyreoidismus *m*, Pseudohyperparathyreoidismus *m*.
ectopic ossification ektope/ektopische Knochenbildung/Verknöcherung/Ossifikation *f*.
ectopic pacemaker ektoper/ektopischer Schrittmacher *m*.
ectopic pancreas heterotopes//ektopes Pankreas(gewebe *nt*) *nt*, Pankreasektopie *f*, -heteropie *f*.
ectopic pregnancy → extrauterine pregnancy.
ectopic rhythm ektope/ektopische Erregungsbildung *f*.
ectopic tachycardia heterotope Tachykardie *f*.
ec·to·plasm ['εktəplæzəm] *n* Ekto-, Exoplasma *nt*.
ec·to·plas·mat·ic [ˌ-plæzˈmætɪk] *adj* Ektoplasma betr., ektoplasmatisch.
ec·to·plas·mic [ˌ-ˈplæzmɪk] *adj* → ectoplasmatic.
ec·to·plast ['-plæst] *n* Zellmembran *f*, -wand *f*, Plasmalemm *nt*.
ec·to·plas·tic [ˌ-ˈplæstɪk] *adj* → ectoplasmatic.
ec·to·pter·y·goid [ˌ-ˈterɪɡɔɪd] *n anat.* M. pterygoideus lateralis.
ec·to·py [ˈεktəpɪ] *n* → ectopia.
ec·to·site [ˈεktəsaɪt] *n* → ectoparasite.
ec·to·skel·e·ton [ˌ-ˈskelɪtn] *n bio.* Exoskelett *nt*.
ec·to·sphere ['-sfɪər] *n* Ekto-, Exosphäre *f*.
ec·to·spore ['-spoʊər, -spɔːər] *n micro.* Exo-, Ektospore *f*.
ec·tos·te·al [εkˈtɒstɪəl] *adj* Knochenaußenfläche *f* betr., auf der Knochenaußenfläche (liegend).
ec·to·syl·vi·an gyrus, posterior [ˌεktoʊˈsɪlvɪən] Gyrus ectosylvius posterior.
ec·to·sym·bi·ont [ˌ-ˈsɪmbaɪɒnt] *n bio.* Ekto-, Exosymbiont *m*.
ec·to·therm ['-θɜrm] *n* ektothermer Organismus *m*.
ec·to·therm·ic [ˌ-ˈθɜrmɪk] *adj* Ektothermie betr., ektothermisch.
ec·to·ther·my [ˌ-ˈθɜrmɪ] *n* Ektothermie *f*.
ec·to·thrix ['-θrɪks] *n micro.* Ektothrix *nt*.
ec·to·tox·in [ˌ-ˈtɒksɪn] *n* Exo-, Ektotoxin *nt*.
ec·to·trop·ic virus [ˌ-ˈtrɒpɪk] *micro.* ektotropes Virus *nt*.
ec·to·zo·al [ˌ-ˈzoʊəl] *adj* Ektozoen betr., durch sie ausgelöst *od.* verursacht, Ektozoen-.
ec·to·zo·on [ˌ-ˈzoʊɒn] *n, pl* -zoa [-ˈzoʊə] *bio.* tierischer Ektoparasit *m*, Ektozoon *nt*.
ectr(o)- *pref.* Ektr(o)-.
ec·tro·chei·ry [ˌεktrəˈkaɪrɪ] *n embryo.* Ektroch(e)irie *f*.
ec·tro·chi·ry *n* → ectrocheiry.
ec·tro·dac·tyl·ia [ˌ-dækˈtɪlɪə] *n* → ectrodactyly.
ec·tro·dac·ty·lism [ˌ-ˈdæktəlɪzəm] *n* → ectrodactyly.
ec·tro·dac·ty·ly [ˌ-ˈdæktəlɪ] *n embryo.* Ektrodaktylie *f*.
ec·trog·e·ny [εkˈtrɒdʒənɪ] *n embryo.* angeborener Mangel *od.* Defekt *m*, angeborene Mißbildung *f*, angeborenes Fehlen *nt*, Ektrogenie *f*.

ec·tro·me·lia [ˌεktroʊˈmiːlɪə] *n embryo.* Ektromelie *f*.
ec·tro·mel·ic [ˌ-ˈmelɪk] *adj embryo.* von Ektromelie betroffen, ektromel.
ec·trom·e·lus [εkˈtrɒmɪləs] *n embryo.* Ektromelus *m*.
ec·tro·met·a·car·pia [ˌεktrəˌmetəˈkɑːrpɪə] *n embryo.* Ektrometakarpie *f*.
ec·tro·met·a·tar·sia [ˌ-ˌmetəˈtɑːrsɪə] *n embryo.* Ektrometatarsie *f*.
ec·tro·pha·lan·gia [ˌ-fəˈlændʒ(ɪ)ə] *n embryo.* Ektrophalangie *f*.
ec·tro·pi·on [εkˈtroʊpɪən, pɪɒn] *n* **1.** *ophthal.* Ektropion *nt*, Ektropium *nt*. **2.** *gyn.* Auswärtskehrung *f*, Umstülpung *f*, Ektropium *nt*, Ektopia portionis.
ec·tro·pi·o·nize [εkˈtroʊpɪənaɪz] *vt ophthal. (Lid)* umstülpen, nach außen wenden, ektropionieren.
ec·tro·pi·um [εkˈtroʊpɪəm] *n* → ectropion.
ec·trop·o·dy [εkˈtrɒpədɪ] *n embryo.* Ektropodie *f*.
ec·tro·syn·dac·tyl·ia [ˌεktrəsɪndækˈtɪlɪə] *n* → ectrosyndactyly.
ec·tro·syn·dac·ty·ly [ˌ-sɪnˈdæktəlɪ] *n embryo.* Ektrosyndaktylie *f*.
ECW *abbr.* → extracellular water.
ec·ze·ma [ˈεksəmə, ˈεɡzə-, ɪɡˈziː-] *n derm.* Ekzem *nt*, Ekzema *nt*, Eczema *nt*, Eccema *nt*.
eczema herpeticum *derm.* Kaposi-Dermatitis *f*, varizelliforme Eruption Kaposi *f*, Ekzema/Eccema herpeticatum, Pustulosis acuta varioliformis/varicelliformis.
eczema intertrigo *derm.* Wundsein *nt*, (Haut-)Wolf *m*, Intertrigo *f*, Dermatitis intertriginosa.
eczema margination Tinea inguinalis, Epidermophytia inguinalis, Eccema marginatum, Ekzema marginatum Hebra.
ec·zem·a·ti·za·tion [ɪɡˌziːmətɪˈzeɪʃn, -ˌzem-] *n derm.* Ekzematisation *f*.
ec·zem·a·to·gen·ic [ɪɡˌziːmətoʊˈdʒenɪk, -ˌzem-] *adj* ekzemverursachend, -auslösend, ekzematogen.
ec·zem·a·toid [ɪɡˈziːmətɔɪd, -ˈzem-] *adj* ekzemähnlich, ekzematoid.
ec·zem·a·tous [ɪɡˈziːmətəs, -ˈzem-] *adj* ekzematös.
eczematous conjunctivitis *ophthal.* Conjunctivitis scrofulosa/phlyctaenulosa, Keratoconjunctivitis scrofulosa/phlyctaenulosa.
eczematous dermatitis → eczema.
E.D. *abbr.* → effective dose.
E.D.₅₀ *abbr.* → effective dose, median.
e·dath·a·mil [ɪˈdæθəmɪl] *n* → edetate.
Eddowes [ˈεdoʊz]: **E.' disease/syndrome** Eddowes-Spurway-Syndrom *nt*, Eddowes-Syndrom *nt*.
Edebohls [ˈεdəboʊlz]: **E.' position** Simon-Lage *f*.
e·de·ma [ɪˈdiːmə] *n, pl* -mas, -ma·ta [-mətə] Ödem *nt*, Oedema *nt*.
e. of lung Lungenödem *nt*.
e. of optic disk Papillenödem *nt*, Stauungspapille *f*.
e·dem·a·tig·e·nous [ˌɪˌdeməˈtɪdʒənəs] *adj* → edematogenic.
e·dem·a·ti·za·tion [ˌɪˌdemətɪˈzeɪʃn] *n* Ödematisierung *f*.
e·dem·a·to·gen·ic [ˌɪˌdemətoʊˈdʒenɪk] *adj* ödemerzeugend, -verursachend, ödematogen.
e·dem·a·tous [ɪˈdemətəs] *adj* Ödem betr., ödematös.
edematous necrosis *patho.* Quellungsnekrose *f*.
edematous pancreatitis Zöpfel-Ödem *nt*, Pankreasödem *nt*.

Eden-Hybinette [ˈiːdn haɪbəˈnet]: **E.-H. operation** *ortho.* Operation *f* nach Eden-Hybinette.
e·den·tate [ɪˈdenteɪt] *adj* → edentulous.
e·den·tu·late [ɪˈdentʃəleɪt, -lɪt] *adj* → edentulous.
e·den·tu·lous [ɪˈdentʃələs] *adj* ohne Zähne, zahnlos.
ed·e·tate [ˈedəteɪt] *n* EDTA-Salz *nt*, Edetat *nt*.
e·det·ic acid [ɪˈdetɪk] → ethylenediaminetetraacetic acid.
EDF brace (elongation, derotation, flexion) *ortho.* EDF-Korsett *nt* (Extension, Derotation, Flexion).
EDF cast *ortho.* EDF-Gips(verband *m*) *m*, Cotrel-Gips(verband *m*) *m*.
edge [edʒ] **I** *n* **1.** (*Messer*) Schneide *f*. **2.** Rand *m*, Saum *m*; Kante *f*; Grenze *f*, Grenzlinie *f*. **II** *vt* **3.** schärfen, schleifen, scharf machen. **4.** umranden, umsäumen; begrenzen.
edged [edʒd] *adj* **1.** scharf, schneidend, -schneidig. **2.** -kantig. **3.** eingefaßt; -randig, -gerändert.
ed·i·ble [ˈedɪbl] *n, adj* → eatable.
Edinger [ˈedɪŋɡər; ˈedɪŋər]: **E.'s nucleus** Edinger-Westphal nucleus.
Edinger-Westphal [ˈvestfɑːl]: **E.-W. nucleus** Edinger-Westphal-Kern *m*, Nc. oculomotorius accessorius/autonomicus.
e·dis·y·late [ɪˈdɪsəleɪt] *n* 1,2-ethanedisulfonate.
Edman [ˈedmən]: **E. degradation** *biochem.* Edman-Abbau *m*.
E. method *biochem.* Edman-Methode *f*.
E.'s reagent *biochem.* Phenylisothiocyanat *nt abbr.* PITC, Edman-Reagenz *nt*.
sequential E. method sequentielle Edman-Methode *f*.
subtractive E. method subtraktive Edman-Methode *f*.
Edridge-Green [ˈedrɪdʒ ɡriːn]: **E.-G. lamp** Edridge-Green-Lampe *f*.
ed·ro·pho·ni·um [ˌedrəˈfoʊnɪəm] *n pharm.* Edrophonium *nt*.
Edsall [ˈedsæl]: **E.'s disease** Hitzekrampf *m*, -tetanie *f*.
EDTA *abbr.* → ethylenediaminetetraacetic acid.
ed·u·cate [ˈedʒəkeɪt, ˈedjuː-] *vt* erziehen, unterrichten, (aus-)bilden.
ed·u·ca·tion [ˌedʒəˈkeɪʃn, edjuː-] *n* **1.** Erziehung *f*, (Aus-)Bildung *f*. **2.** Bildung *f*, Bildungsstand *m*. **3.** Bildungs-, Schulwesen *nt*. **4.** (Aus-)Bildungsgang *m*.
ed·uce [ɪˈd(j)uːs] *vt chem.* ausziehen, extrahieren.
e·duct [ˈiːdʌkt] *n chem.* Auszug *m*, Edukt *nt*.
e·duc·tion [ɪˈdʌkʃn] *n* **1.** *chem.* Ausziehen *nt*, Extrahieren *nt*. **2.** → educt.
e·dul·co·rant [ɪˈdʌlkərənt] *adj* süßend.
e·dul·co·rate [ɪˈdʌlkəreɪt] *vt* süßen.
Edwards [ˈedwərdz]: **E.' syndrome** *genet.* Edwards-Syndrom *nt*, Trisomie 18-Syndrom *nt*.
Ed·ward·si·el·la [ˌedˌwɔːrdsɪˈelə] *n micro.* Edwardsiella *f*.
EEC syndrome EEC-Syndrom *nt*.
EEE *abbr.* → Eastern equine encephalitis.
EEE virus *micro.* Eastern equine encephalitis/encephalomyelitis-Virus *nt*, EEE-Virus *nt*.
EEG *abbr.* → electroencephalogram.
eel·worm [ˈiːlwɜrm] *n micro.* Spulwurm *m*, Ascaris lumbricoidis.
EF *abbr.* → elongation factor.
EFA *abbr.* → fatty acid, essential.
ef·fect [ɪˈfekt] **I** *n* **1.** Wirkung *f*, Effekt *m*; Auswirkung *f* (*on, upon* auf). **2.** Folge *f*, Wirkung *f*, Ergebnis *nt*, Resultat *nt*. **of no**

~/without ~ ohne Erfolg; ohne Wirkung; erfolg-, wirkungslos. **to take ~ wirken. to have a good ~ on** eine Wirkung haben *od.* wirken auf. **to be of ~** wirken. **3.** *electr.* induzierte Leistung *f*, Sekundärleistung *f.* **II** *vt* **4.** be-, erwirken, herbeiführen. **5.** ausführen, erledigen, vollbringen, tätigen, leisten.
ef·fec·tive [ɪˈfektɪv] *adj* **1.** wirksam, wirkend, wirkungsvoll, effektiv. **to be ~** wirken, wirksam werden. **to be ~ wirken** (*on* auf). **2.** tatsächlich, wirklich, effektiv.
effective dose *abbr.* **E.D.** Effektivdosis *f abbr.* ED, Dosis effectiva/efficax *abbr.* DE, Wirkdosis *f abbr.* WD.
median e. *abbr.* ED$_{50}$ mittlere effektive Dosis *abbr.* ED$_{50}$, mittlere wirksame Dosis *abbr.* WD$_{50}$, Dosis effectiva media.
effective half-live (period) effektive Halbwertzeit *f*.
ef·fec·tive·ness [ɪˈfektɪvnɪs] *n* Wirksamkeit *f*, Effektivität *f*; Wirkung *f*, Effekt *m*.
effective output tatsächliche/effektive Leistung *f*.
effective renal blood flow *abbr.* **ERBF** effektiver renaler Blutfluß *m abbr.* ERBF.
effective renal plasma flow *abbr.* **ERPF** effektiver renaler Plasmafluß *m abbr.* ERPF.
effective resistance *electr.* Wirkwiderstand *m*.
effective temperature *physiol.* Effektivtemperatur *f*.
ef·fec·tiv·i·ty [ɪfekˈtɪvətɪ] *n* → effectiveness.
ef·fec·tor [ɪˈfektər] *n physiol., biochem.* Effektor *m*.
effector cell Effektorzelle *f*.
effector hormone Effektorhormon *nt*.
effector organ Effektor-, Erfolgsorgan *nt*.
ef·fec·tu·al [ɪˈfektʃ(əw)əl] *adj* **1.** wirksam, effektiv. **to be ~** wirken. **2.** wirklich, tatsächlich.
ef·fec·tu·al·i·ty [ɪˌfektʃəˈwælətɪ] *n* Wirksamkeit *f*, Effektivität *f*.
ef·fec·tu·al·ness [ɪˈfektʃ(əw)əlnɪs] *n* → effectuality.
ef·fec·tu·ate [ɪˈfektʃəweɪt] *vt* bewerkstelligen, bewirken, ausführen.
ef·fec·tu·a·tion [ɪˌfektʃəˈweɪʃn] *n* Bewerkstelligung *f*, Bewirkung *f*; Ausführung *f*.
ef·fem·i·na·cy [ɪˈfemɪnəsɪ] *n* → effemination.
ef·fem·i·nate [*n, adj* ɪˈfemənɪt; *v* -neɪt] *psycho.* **I** *n* Weichling *m*, femininer Mensch *m*. **II** *adj* **1.** weiblich, unmännlich, effeminiert. **2.** verweichlicht, weich. **III** *vt* weiblich *od.* weibisch machen. **IV** *vi* weiblich *od.* weibisch werden, s. weiblich fühlen *od.* verhalten, effeminieren; verweichlichen.
ef·fem·i·nate·ness [ɪˈfemɪneɪtnɪs] *n* → effemination.
ef·fem·i·na·tion [ɪˌfemɪˈneɪʃn] *n psycho.* Feminisierung *f*, Verweiblichung *f*, Effemination *f*.
ef·fer·ence [ˈefərəns] *n* → efferent I.
efference copy Efferenzkopie *f*.
ef·fer·ent [ˈefərənt] **I** *n physiol.* Efferenz *f*. **II** *adj* zentrifugal, efferent; weg-, herausführend, heraus-, ableitend.
efferent arteriole of glomerulus abführende/efferente Glomerulusarterie *f*, abführende/efferente Glomerulusarteriole *f*, Arteriola glomerularis efferens, Vas efferens (glomeruli).
efferent artery of glomerulus → efferent arteriole of glomerulus.
efferent fibers → efferent neurofibers.
ef·fer·en·tial [efəˈrenʃl] *adj* → efferent II.
efferent loop syndrome *chir.* Efferent-loop-Syndrom *nt*, Syndrom *nt* der abführenden Schlinge.

efferent nerve efferenter Nerv *m*.
efferent nerve fibers → efferent neurofibers.
efferent neurofibers efferente (Nerven-)Fasern *pl*, Neurofibrae efferentes.
efferent neuron efferentes Neuron *nt*.
efferent trunk → efferent vessel.
efferent vessel ableitendes/efferentes Gefäß *nt*.
e. of glomerulus → efferent arteriole of glomerulus.
e.s of lymph node efferente Lymphknotengefäße *pl*, Vasa efferentia nodi lymphatici.
ef·fer·vesce [efərˈves] *vi* (auf-)brausen, sprudeln, schäumen.
ef·fer·ves·cent [efərˈvesənt] *adj* sprudelnd, schäumend; übersprudelnd, -schäumend.
ef·fi·ca·cious [efɪˈkeɪʃəs] *adj* wirksam, wirkungsvoll, effektiv.
ef·fi·ca·cious·ness [efɪˈkeɪʃəsnɪs] *n* Wirksamkeit *f*, Effektivität *f*.
ef·fi·ca·cy [ˈefɪkəsɪ] *n* → efficaciousness.
ef·fi·cien·cy [ɪˈfɪʃənsɪ] *n* **1.** (Leistungs-)Fähigkeit *f*, Effizienz *f*. **2.** Wirksamkeit *f*, Effizienz *f*. **3.** *phys.* Wirkungsgrad *m*, Nutzleistung *f*, Effizienz *f*. **4.** Wirtschaftlichkeit *f*, Rationalität *f*, Effizienz *f*.
ef·fi·cient [ɪˈfɪʃənt] *adj* effizient; (leistungs-)fähig, leistungsstark; wirksam; wirtschaftlich, rationell.
ef·flo·resce [efləˈres] *vi* **1.** *chem.* ausblühen, auskristallisieren, auswittern. **2.** *derm.* aufblühen, s. entfalten.
ef·flo·res·cence [efləˈresəns] *n derm.* Hautblüte *f*, Effloreszenz *f*.
ef·flo·res·cent [efləˈresənt] *adj* **1.** *chem.* effloreszierend, ausblühend. **2.** *derm.* (auf-)blühend.
ef·flu·vi·um [ɪˈfluːvɪəm] *n, pl* **-via** [-vɪə] **1.** Ausfall *m*, Entleerung *f*, Erguß *m*, Effluvium *nt*. **2.** Haarausfall *m*, Effluvium (capillorum). **3.** Ausdünstung *f*, Effluvium *nt*. **4.** *phys.* Ausfluß *m*.
ef·fort [ˈefərt] *n* Anstrengung *f*, Bemühung *f*, Versuch *m*; Leistung *f*.
effort proteinuria Marschproteinurie *f*, -albuminurie *f*, Anstrengungsproteinurie *f*, -albuminurie *f*.
effort syndrome Effort-Syndrom *nt*, DaCosta-Syndrom *nt*, neurozirkulatorische Asthenie *f*, Soldatenherz *nt*, Phrenikokardie *f*.
ef·fuse [*adj* ɪˈfjuːs; *v* ɪˈfjuːz] **I** *adj micro.* (*Kolonie*) ausgebreitet. **II** *vt* (*Flüssigkeit*) aus-, vergießen; (*Gas*) ausströmen lassen. **III** *vi* auslaufen, -fließen; ausströmen.
ef·fu·sion [ɪˈfjuːʒn] *n* **1.** *patho.* Erguß *m*, Flüssigkeitsansammlung *f*. **2.** Ergußflüssigkeit *f*, Exsudat *nt*, Transsudat *nt*. **3.** (*Flüssigkeit*) Ausgießen *nt*, Vergießen *nt*; (*Gas*) Ausströmen *nt*.
e·ga·grop·i·lus [egəˈgrɑpɪləs] *n* Haarball *m*, Trichobezoar *m*.
e·gest [ɪˈdʒest] *vt physiol.* ausscheiden.
e·ges·ta [ɪˈdʒestə] *pl* Ausscheidungen *pl*, Egesta *pl*.
e·ges·tion [ɪˈdʒestʃn] *n* Abgabe *f* unverdaulicher Stoffe, Ausscheidung *f*, Egestion *f*.
EGF *abbr.* → epidermal growth factor.
egg [eg] *n* **1.** Ei *nt*, Ovum *nt*. **2.** → egg cell. **3.** Ei *nt*, eiförmige Struktur *f*.
egg albumin Ovalbumin *nt*.
egg cell Eizelle *f*, Oozyt *m*, Ovozyt *m*, Ovum *nt*.
egg envelope → egg membrane.
egg membrane Eihaut *f*.
egg-shaped *adj* eiförmig.
egg-shell [ˈegʃel] **I** *n* **1.** Eierschale *f*. **2.** Eierschalenfarbe *f*. **II** *adj* **3.** zerbrechlich, dünn. **4.** eierschalenfarben.
egg white Eiklar *nt*, Eiweiß *nt*.
e·glan·du·lar [ɪˈglændʒələr] *adj* → eglandulous.
e·gland·u·lous [ɪˈglændʒələs] *adj* ohne Drüsen, drüsenlos, aglandulär.
Egli [ˈeglɪ]: **E.'s glands** Uterschleimdrüsen *pl*, Gll. mucosae ureteris.
e·go [ˈiːgəʊ, ˈegəʊ] *n, pl* **e·gos** **1.** *psycho.* Ich *nt*, Selbst *nt*, Ego *nt*. **2.** Selbstgefühl *nt*.
e·go·bron·choph·o·ny [ˌiːgəʊbranˈkɑfənɪ, ˌegəʊ-] *n* (*Auskultation*) Ziegenmeckern *nt*, Kompressionsatmen *nt*, Ägophonie *f*.
e·go·cen·tric [ˌ-ˈsentrɪk] **I** *n* egozentrischer Mensch *m*, Egozentriker(in *f*) *m*. **II** *adj* egozentrisch.
e·go·cen·trism [ˌ-ˈsentrɪzəm] *n* (übertriebene) Ich- *od.* Selbstbezogenheit *f*, Egozentrik *f*.
ego-ideal *n psycho.* Ego-Ideal *nt*, Ich-Ideal *nt*.
e·go·ism [ˈiːgəʊɪzəm, ˈegəʊ-] *n psycho.* Ich-, Selbstsucht *f*, Egoismus *m*.
e·go·ist [ˈiːgəʊɪst, ˈegəʊ-] *n* Egoist(in *f*) *m*.
e·go·is·tic [ˌiːgəʊˈɪstɪk, ˌegəʊ-] *adj* egoistisch, selbstsüchtig.
e·go·is·ti·cal [ˌ-ˈɪstɪkl] *adj* → egoistic.
e·go·ma·nia [ˌ-ˈmeɪnɪə, -jə] *n psychia.* krankhafte Selbstsucht *f*, Egomanie *f*.
e·goph·o·ny [ɪˈgɑfənɪ] *n* egobronchophony.
e·go·tism [ˈiːgətɪzəm, ˈegə-] *n psycho.* Selbstüberhebung *f*, krankhafte Selbstgefälligkeit *f*, Egotismus *m*.
e·go·trop·ic [ˌiːgəʊˈtrɑpɪk, ˌegəʊ-] *adj* → egocentric II.
Egyptian [ɪˈdʒɪpʃn]: **E. chlorosis** Anämie *f* bei Ankylostomabefall, ägyptische/tropische Chlorose *f*.
E. conjunctivitis *ophthal.* Trachom(a) *nt*, ägyptische Körnerkrankheit *f*, trachomatöse Einschlußkonjunktivitis *f*, Conjunctivitis (granulosa) trachomatosa.
E. hematuria Blasenbilharziose *f*, Schistosomiasis urogenitalis.
E. ophthalmia → E. conjunctivitis.
E$_h$ *abbr.* → redox potential.
EHEC *abbr.* → Escherichia coli, enterohemorrhagic.
Ehlers-Danlos [ˈeɪlərz ˈdænləs]: **E.-D. disease/syndrome** Ehlers-Danlos-Syndrom *nt*.
Ehrenritter [ˈeːrənrɪtər]: **E.'s ganglion** Ehrenritter'-Ganglion *nt*, Ggl. superius n. glossopharyngei.
Ehrlich [ˈeərlɪx, ˈeːrlɪç]: **E.'s aldehyde reagent** Ehrlich-Aldehydreagenz *f*.
E.'s anemia aplastische Anämie *f*.
E.'s diazo reaction Ehrlich-Diazoreaktion *f*.
E.'s diazo reagent Ehrlich-Diazoreagenz *nt*.
E.'s inner bodies *hema.* Heinz(-Ehrlich)-Innenkörper *pl*.
E.'s side-chain theory Ehrlich-Seitenkettentheorie *f*.
E.'s test 1. Ehrlich-Reaktion *f*, -Aldehydprobe *f*. **2.** Ehrlich-Reaktion *f*, -Diazoreaktion *f*.
Ehr·lich·ia [eərˈlɪkɪə] *n micro.* Ehrlichia *f*.
EIA *abbr.* → enzyme immunoassay.
Eichhorst [ˈaɪkhɔːrst, ˈaɪçhɔrst]: **E.'s neuritis** interstitielle Neuritis *f*.
Eicken [ˈaɪkn]: **E.'s method** *HNO* Eicken-Hypopharyngoskopie *f*.
ei·co·nom·e·ter [aɪkəʊˈnɑmɪtər] *n* → eikonometer.
ei·co·sa·no·ate [aɪˌkəʊsəˈnəʊeɪt] *n* Eicosanoat *nt*, Arachidat *nt*.

n-ei·co·sa·no·ic acid [,aɪkəsə'nəʊɪk] Arachinsäure *f*, n-Eicosansäure *f*.
ei·co·sa·noid [aɪ'kəʊsənɔɪd] *n* Arachidonsäurederivat *nt*, Eicosanoid *nt*.
ei·co·sa·tri·e·no·ic acid [aɪˌkəʊsətraɪɪ'nəʊɪk] Eicosatriensäure *f*.
ei·det·ic [aɪ'detɪk] I *n* Eidetiker(in *f*) *m*. II *adj* eidetisch.
ei·dop·tom·e·try [eɪdəp'tɑmətrɪ] *n* ophthal. Eidoptometrie *f*.
EIEC *abbr*. → Escherichia coli, enteroinvasive.
eighth nerve [eɪtθ, eɪθ] Akustikus *m*, Vestibulokochlearis *m*, VIII. Hirnnerv *m*, N. acusticus/vestibulocochlearis.
eighth nerve tumor Akustikusneurinom *nt*.
Ei·ke·nel·la corrodens [aɪkə'nelə] *micro*. Eikenella corrodens *f*.
ei·ko·nom·e·ter [aɪkə'nɑmɪtər] *n* ophthal. Eikonometer *nt*.
ei·loid ['aɪlɔɪd] *adj* spiralförmig, spiralig.
Ei·me·ria [aɪ'mɪərɪə] *n* micro. Eimeria *f*.
e-I neuron → early-inspiritory neuron.
Einhorn ['aɪnhɔːrn]: **E.'s saccharimeter** Einhorn'-Gärungsröhrchen *nt*.
ein·stein·i·um [aɪn'staɪnɪəm] *n abbr*. **Es** Einsteinium *nt abbr*. Es.
Einthoven ['aɪnthəʊvən]: **E.'s law** Einthoven-Regel *f*, -Gleichung *f*.
E.'s method → standard E.'s triangle.
standard E.'s triangle Standardableitung *f* nach Einthoven, Einthoven-Dreieck *f*.
Eisenmenger ['aɪsənmeŋər]: **E.'s complex/disease/syndrome/tetralogy** Eisenmenger-Komplex *m*, -Syndrom *nt*, -Tetralogie *f*.
ei·sod·ic [aɪ'sɑdɪk] *adj* zuführend, afferent.
e·jac·u·late [*n* ɪ'dʒækjəlɪt; *v*-leɪt] I *n* (ausgespritzte) Samenflüssigkeit *f*, Ejakulat *nt*, Ejaculat *nt*. II *vt* Samenflüssigkeit ausspritzen, ejakulieren. III *vi* einen Samenerguß haben, ejakulieren.
e·jac·u·la·tion [ˌɪdʒækjə'leɪʃn] *n* Samenerguß *m*, Ejakulation *f*.
ejaculation center Erektions-, Ejakulationszentrum *nt*.
e·jac·u·la·to·ry [ɪ'dʒækjələˌtɔːrɪː, -ˌtəʊ-] *adj* Ejakulations-.
ejaculatory duct Ausspritzungs-, Ejakulationsgang *m*, Ductus ejaculatorius.
e·jac·u·lum [ɪ'dʒækjələm] *n* → ejaculate I.
e·ject [ɪ'dʒekt] *vt* (*a. techn*.) auswerfen, ausstoßen.
e·jec·tion [ɪ'dʒekʃn] *n* 1. Ausstoßen *nt*, Auswerfen *nt*, Ejektion *f*. 2. Ausstoß *m*, Auswurf *m*.
ejection clicks *card*. Austreibungsgeräusche *pl*, -töne *pl*.
ejection fraction (*Herz*) Auswurf-, Austreibungs-, Ejektionsfraktion *f*.
ejection murmur Austreibungs-, Ejektionsgeräusch *nt*.
ejection period (*Herz*) Austreibungsphase *f*.
ejection sounds → ejection clicks.
ejection velocity Auswurfgeschwindigkeit *f*.
e·jec·tive [ɪ'dʒektɪv] *adj* Ausstoß(ungs)-, Austreibungs-, Auswurf-.
Ekbom ['ɛkbɑm]: **E. syndrome** Ekbom-Syndrom *nt*, Wittmaack-Ekbom-Syndrom *nt*, Syndrom *nt* der unruhigen Beine.
EKG *abbr*. → electrocardiogram.
EKY *abbr*. → electrokymogram.
el·a·id·ic acid [elə'ɪdɪk] Elaidinsäure *f*.
e·lai·o·ma [ɪlɪ'əʊmə] *n* → eleoma.
e·lai·om·e·ter [ɪleɪ'ɑmɪtər] *n* → eleometer.
E·lap·i·dae [ɪ'læpədiː] *pl bio*. Elapidae *pl*, Elapinae *f*.
e·las·tance [ɪ'læstəns] *n physiol*. Elastance *f abbr*. E.

e·las·tase [ɪ'læsteɪz] *n* Elastase *f*, Elastinase *f*, Pankreaselastase *f*, Pankreopeptidase E *f*.
e·las·tic [ɪ'læstɪk] I *n* Gummi *nt*, Gummiband *nt*, -ring *m*. II *adj* 1. elastisch, dehnbar, biegsam, nachgebend, federnd. 2. *phys*. (elastisch) verformbar, ausdehnungs-, expansionsfähig. 3. Gummi-.
e·las·ti·ca [ɪ'læstɪkə] *n* 1. Naturgummi *nt*, Kautschuk *m*. 2. *anat*. Elastika *f*, Tunica elastica. 3. Media *f*, Tunica media.
elastic artery Arterie *f* vom elastischen Typ.
elastica stain *histol*. Elasticafärbung *f*.
elastica-van Gieson stain *abbr*. **E.v.G.** *histol*. Elastica-van Gieson-Färbung *f*, E. v. G-Färbung *f*.
elastic bandage elastische Binde *f*.
elastic cartilage elastischer Knorpel *m*, Cartilago elastica.
elastic cone (of larynx) Conus elasticus (laryngis), Membrana cricovocalis.
elastic deformation *phys*. elastische Verformung *f*.
elastic element *phys*. elastisches Element *nt*.
parallel e. *abbr*. **PE** parallelelastisches Element *abbr*. PE.
series e. *abbr*. **SE** serienelastisches Element *abbr*. SE.
elastic fiber elastische Faser *f*.
e·las·ti·cin [ɪ'læstəsɪn] *n* → elastin.
e·las·tic·i·ty [ɪlæ'stɪsɪtɪ] *n* Dehnbarkeit *f*, Biegsamkeit *f*, Federkraft *f*, Elastizität *f*.
elastic lamina: external e. *histol*. Elastica *f* externa, Membrana elastica externa.
internal e. *histol*. Elastica *f* interna, Membrana elastica interna.
elastic limit *phys*. Elastizitätsgrenze *f*.
elastic membrane elastische Membran *f*.
external e. *histol*. Elastica *f* externa, Membrana elastica externa.
internal e. *histol*. Elastica *f* interna, Membrana elastica interna.
elastic modulus *phys*. Elastizitätsmodul *m*, -koeffizient *m*.
elastic pulse elastischer Puls *m*.
elastic resistance elastischer Widerstand *m*.
elastic skin → Ehlers-Danlos disease.
elastic stocking Gummistrumpf *m*, Stützstrumpf *m*.
elastic tension elastische Spannung *f*.
elastic tissue elastisches Bindegewebe *nt*, Bindegewebe *nt* mit vorwiegend elastischen Fasern.
elastic tunic Elastika *f*, Tunica elastica.
elastic vessel → elastic artery.
e·las·tin [ɪ'læstɪn] *n* Gerüsteiweißstoff *m*, Elastin *nt*.
e·las·tin·ase [ɪ'læstɪneɪz] *n* → elastase.
e·las·to·fi·bro·ma [ɪˌlæstəfaɪ'brəʊmə] *n patho*. Elastofibrom *nt*.
e·las·to·gel [ɪ'læstədʒel] *n* Elastogel *nt*.
e·las·toid [ɪ'læstɔɪd] *n patho*. Elastoid *nt*.
elastoid degeneration 1. Elastose *f*, Elastosis *f*. **2.** amyloide Degeneration *f* elastischer Fasern.
e·las·toi·din [ɪ'læstɔɪdɪn] *n* Elastoidin *nt*.
e·las·toi·do·sis [ɪˌlæstɔɪ'dəʊsɪs] *n derm*. Elastoidose *f*, Elastoidosis *f*.
e·las·tol·y·sis [ɪlæs'tɑlasɪs] *n derm*., *patho*. Elastolyse *f*, Elastolysis *f*.
e·las·to·lyt·ic [ɪˌlæstə'lɪtɪk] *adj* elastolytisch.
e·las·to·ma [ɪlæs'təʊmə] *n derm*. Elastom *nt*, Elastoma *nt*.
e·las·to·mer(es) *nt*.
e·las·tom·e·ter [ɪlæs'tɑmɪtər] *n* Elastometer *nt*.

e·las·tom·e·try [ɪlæs'tɑmətrɪ] *n* Elastometrie *f*.
e·las·to·mu·cin [ɪˌlæstə'mjuːsɪn] *n* Elastomuzin *nt*, -mucin *nt*.
e·las·tor·rhex·is [ɪlæstə'reksɪs] *n patho*. Elastorrhexis *f*.
e·las·tose [ɪ'læstəʊs] *n* Elastose *f*.
e·las·to·sis [ɪlæs'təʊsɪs] *n* 1. *patho*. (Gefäß-)Elastose *f*. 2. *derm*. (Haut-)Elastose *f*, Elastosis *f*.
e·las·tot·ic [ɪlæs'tɑtɪk] *adj* Elastose betr., Elastosen-.
e·la·tion [ɪ'leɪʃn] *n psycho*. Hochstimmung *f*, Begeisterung *f*.
el·bow ['elbəʊ] *n* 1. Ell(en)bogen *m*; *anat*. Cubitus *m*. 2. Ell(en)bogengelenk *nt*, Artic. cubiti/cubitalis. 3. L-förmige Kurve *od*. Biegung *f*, Knick *m*, Krümmung *f*, Knie *nt*.
elbow disarticulation *ortho*. Ellenbogen-(gelenk)exartikulation *f*.
elbow dislocation *ortho*. Ellbogen(gelenk)luxation *f*.
elbowed catheter ['elbəʊd] gebogener (Blasen-)Katheter *m*.
elbow joint → elbow 2.
elbow reflex Trizepssehnenreflex *m abbr*. TSR.
elbow region Ell(en)bogengegend *f*, -region *f*, Regio/Facies cubitalis.
anterior e. vordere Ell(en)bogenregion, Regio/Facies cubitalis anterior.
posterior e. hintere Ell(en)bogenregion, Regio/Facies cubitalis posterior.
elbow room *fig*. Bewegungsfreiheit *f*, Spielraum *m*.
el·co·sis [el'kəʊsɪs] *n* Geschwür(s)leiden *nt*, Helkosis *f*.
el·drin ['eldrɪn] *n* Rutin *nt*, Rutosid *nt*.
ele- *pref*. → ele(o)-.
e·lec·tive [ɪ'lektɪv] *adj* auswählend, elektiv, Wahl-, Elektiv-.
elective culture Elektivkultur *f*; Anreicherungskultur *f*.
elective mutism elektiver Mutismus *m*.
elective procedure *chir*. Wahl-, Elektiveingriff *m*, -operation *f*.
elective surgical procedure elective procedure.
E·lec·tra complex [ɪ'lektrə] *psychia*. Elektra-Komplex *m*.
e·lec·tric [ɪ'lektrɪk] *adj* elektrisch, Elektro-, Elektrizitäts-, Strom-.
e·lec·tri·cal [ɪ'lektrɪkl] *adj* → electric.
electrical alternans *physiol*. elektrische Alternans *m*.
electrical axis *physiol*. elektrische Achse *f*.
electrical burn elektrische/elektro-thermische Verbrennung *f*.
electrical capacitance elektrische Kapazität *f*.
electrical charge elektrische Ladung *f*.
electrical conductivity elektrische Leitfähigkeit/Konduktivität *f*.
electrical eye Photozelle *f*, photoelektrische Zelle *f*.
electrical excitation elektrische Erregung *f*.
electrical field elektrisches Feld *nt*.
electrical flux elektrischer Induktionsfluß *m*.
electrical gradient elektrischer Gradient *m*.
electrical impulse elektrischer Impuls *m*.
electrical nystagmus elektrischer Nystagmus *m*.
electrical phosphene *neuro*., *ophthal*. elektrisches Phosphen *nt*.
electrical resistance elektrischer Widerstand *m*.

electrical synapse *bio.* elektrische Synapse *f.*
electrical vector elektrischer Vektor *m.*
electric anesthesia → electroanesthesia.
electric attraction elektrische Anziehung *f.*
electric bath hydroelektrisches Bad *nt.*
electric blanket Heizkissen *nt.*
electric burn → electrical burn.
electric cataract Blitzstar *m*, Cataracta electrica.
electric cautery → electrocautery.
electric chorea Dubini-Syndrom *nt*, Chorea electrica.
electric circuit elektrischer Strom-, Schaltkreis *m.*
electric coagulation → electrocoagulation.
electric convulsive therapy → electroshock therapy.
electric current elektrischer Strom *m.*
electric discharge elektrische Entladung *f.*
electric energy elektrische Energie *f.*
electric irritability *physiol.* elektrische Erregbarkeit *f.*
e·lec·tric·i·ty [ɪlekˈtrɪsətɪ] *n* 1. Elektrizität *f*; Strom *m.* 2. Elektrizitätslehre *f.*
electric ophthalmia *ophthal.* Conjunctivitis actinica/photoelectrica, Keratoconjunctivitis/Ophthalmia photoelectrica.
electric response audiometry *abbr.* ERA HNO Electric-Response-Audiometrie *f abbr.* ERA, Evoked-Response-Audiometrie *f.*
electric shock 1. elektrischer Schlag *m*, Stromschlag *m.* 2. *physiol.* Elektroschock *m.*
electric shock therapy → electroshock therapy.
electric shock treatment → electroshock therapy.
electric tension elektromotorische Kraft *f abbr.* EMK.
e·lec·tri·fi·ca·tion [ɪˌlektrəfɪˈkeɪʃn] *n* 1. Elektrisierung *f.* 2. (*Behandlung*) Elektrisierung *f*, Elektrisieren *nt.*
e·lec·tri·fy [ɪˈlektrəfaɪ] *vt* 1. elektrisieren, elektrisch (auf-)laden; jdm. einen elektrischen Schlag versetzen. 2. mit elektrischem Strom behandeln, elektrisieren.
electro- *pref.* Elektro-, Elektrizitäts-, Elektronen-.
e·lec·tro·a·cous·tic [ɪˌlektroəˈkuːstɪk] *adj* elektroakustisch.
e·lec·tro·ac·u·punc·ture [ɪˌ-ˈækjʊpʌŋktʃər] *n* Elektroakupunktur *f.*
e·lec·tro·aer·o·sol [ɪˌ-ˈeərəsɒl] *n* Elektroaerosol *nt.*
e·lec·tro·af·fin·i·ty [ɪˌlektroəˈfɪnətɪ] *n* Elektro(nen)affinität *f.*
e·lec·tro·an·al·ge·si·a [ɪˌ-ˌænlˈdʒiːzɪə] *n* Elektroanalgesie *f.*
e·lec·tro·a·nal·y·sis [ɪˌ-əˈnæləsɪs] *n* Elektroanalyse *f.*
e·lec·tro·an·es·the·sia [ɪˌ-ˌænəsˈθiːʒə] *n anes.* Elektroanästhesie *f.*
e·lec·tro·a·tri·o·gram [ɪˌ-ˈeɪtrɪəɡræm] *n abbr.* EAG *card.* Elektroatriogramm *nt abbr.* EAG.
e·lec·tro·ax·o·nog·ra·phy [ɪˌ-ˌæksəˈnɒɡrəfɪ] *n neuro.* (Elektro-)Axonographie *f.*
e·lec·tro·bi·ol·o·gy [ɪˌ-baɪˈɒlədʒɪ] *n* Elektrobiologie *f.*
e·lec·tro·bi·os·co·py [ɪˌ-baɪˈɒskəpɪ] *n* Elektrobioskopie *f.*
e·lec·tro·car·di·o·gram [ɪˌ-ˈkɑːrdɪəɡræm] *n abbr.* ECG, EKG Elektrokardiogramm *nt abbr.* EKG.
e·lec·tro·car·di·o·graph [ɪˌ-ˈkɑːrdɪəɡræf] *n* Elektrokardiograph *m.*
e·lec·tro·car·di·o·graph·ic [ɪˌ-ˌkɑːrdɪəˈɡræfɪk] *adj* Elektrokardiographie betr., mittels Elektokardiographie, elektrokardiographisch.
electrocardiographic complex *card.* EKG-Komplex *m.*
e·lec·tro·car·di·og·ra·phy [ɪˌ-ˌkɑːrdɪˈɒɡrəfɪ] *n* Elektrokardiographie *f.*
e·lec·tro·car·di·o·pho·no·gram [ɪˌ-ˌkɑːrdɪəˈfəʊnəɡræm] *n* Elektrokardiophonogramm *nt.*
e·lec·tro·car·di·o·pho·no·graph [ɪˌ-ˌkɑːrdɪəˈfəʊnəɡræf] *n* Elektrokardiophonograph *m.*
e·lec·tro·car·di·o·scope [ɪˌ-ˈkɑːrdɪəskəʊp] *n* Elektrokardioskop *nt*, (Oszillo-)Kardioskop *nt.*
e·lec·tro·car·di·os·co·py [ɪˌ-ˌkɑːrdɪˈɒskəpɪ] *n* Elektrokardioskopie *f*, (Oszillo-)Kardioskopie *f.*
e·lec·tro·ca·tal·y·sis [ɪˌ-kəˈtæləsɪs] *n* elektrische Katalyse *f*, Elektrokatalyse *f.*
e·lec·tro·cau·ter·i·za·tion [ɪˌ-ˌkɔːtəraɪˈzeɪʃn] *n* → electrocautery 2.
e·lec·tro·cau·ter·y [ɪˌ-ˈkɔːtərɪ] *n* 1. Elektrokauter *m*, Elektrokaustiknadel *f.* 2. Elektrokauterisation *f*, -kaustik *f.*
e·lec·tro·ce·re·bral silence [ɪˌ-səˈriːbrəl, -ˈserə-] *abbr.* ECS *neuro.* Null-Linien-EEG *nt*, isoelektrisches Elektroenzephalogramm *nt.*
e·lec·tro·chem·i·cal [ɪˌ-ˈkemɪkl] *adj* Elektrochemie betr., elektrochemisch.
electrochemical cell *phys.* elektrochemische Zelle *f.*
electrochemical equivalent elektrochemisches Äquivalent *nt.*
electrochemical gradient elektrochemischer Gradient *m.*
electrochemical potential elektrochemisches Potential *nt.*
e·lec·tro·chem·is·try [ɪˌ-ˈkemɪstrɪ] *n* Elektrochemie *f.*
e·lec·tro·cho·le·cys·tec·to·my [ɪˌ-ˌkɒləsɪsˈtektəmɪ] *n chir.* elektrochirurgische Cholezystektomie *f*, Elektrocholezystektomie *f.*
e·lec·tro·chro·ma·tog·ra·phy [ɪˌ-ˌkrəʊməˈtɒɡrəfɪ] *n* → electrophoresis.
e·lec·tro·co·ag·u·la·tion [ɪˌ-kəʊˌæɡjəˈleɪʃn] *n* Elektrokoagulation *f*, Kaltkaustik *f.*
e·lec·tro·coch·le·o·gram [ɪˌ-ˈkɒklɪəɡræm] *n* Elektrokochleogramm *nt abbr.* ECochG.
e·lec·tro·coch·le·o·graph [ɪˌ-ˈkɒklɪəɡræf] *n* Elektrokochleograph *m.*
e·lec·tro·coch·le·o·graph·ic audiometry [ɪˌ-ˌkɒklɪəˈɡræfɪk] → electrocochleography.
e·lec·tro·coch·le·og·ra·phy [ɪˌ-ˌkɒklɪˈɒɡrəfɪ] *n* Elektrokochleographie *f.*
e·lec·tro·con·duc·tive [ɪˌ-kənˈdʌktɪv] *adj* stromleitend.
e·lec·tro·con·trac·til·i·ty [ɪˌ-ˌkɒntrækˈtɪlətɪ] *n* Elektrokontraktilität *f.*
e·lec·tro·con·vul·sive shock [ɪˌ-kənˈvʌlsɪv] → electroshock therapy.
electroconvulsive therapy *abbr.* ECT → electroshock therapy.
electroconvulsive treatment → electroshock therapy.
e·lec·tro·cor·ti·co·gram [ɪˌ-ˈkɔːrtɪkəɡræm] *n abbr.* ECoG Elektrokortikogramm *nt abbr.* ECoG.
e·lec·tro·cor·ti·cog·ra·phy [ɪˌ-ˌkɔːrtɪˈkɒɡrəfɪ] *n* Elektrokortikographie *f.*
e·lec·tro·cute [ɪˈlektrəkjuːt] *vt* 1. durch elektrischen Strom töten. 2. auf dem elektrischen Stuhl hinrichten.
e·lec·tro·cu·tion [ɪˌlektrəˈkjuːʃn] *n* 1. Tod *m* durch elektrischen Strom. 2. Hinrichtung *f* durch elektrischen Strom.
e·lec·tro·cys·tog·ra·phy [ɪˌlektrəsɪsˈtɒɡrəfɪ] *n urol.* Elektrozystographie *f*, Elektrourographie *f.*
e·lec·trode [ɪˈlektrəʊd] *n* Elektrode *f.*
electrode equation Elektrodengleichung *f.*
electrode potential Elektrodenspannung *f*, Elektrodenpotential *nt.*
e·lec·tro·der·mal [ɪˌlektrəˈdɜːrml] *adj* elektrodermal.
e·lec·tro·der·ma·tome [ɪˌ-ˈdɜːrmətəʊm] *n* Elektrodermatom *nt.*
e·lec·tro·des·ic·ca·tion [ɪˌ-ˌdesɪˈkeɪʃn] *n* Elektrodesikkation *f*, -dehydratation *f.*
e·lec·tro·di·ag·no·sis [ɪˌ-ˌdaɪəɡˈnəʊsɪs] *n* Elektrodiagnostik *f.*
e·lec·tro·di·ag·nos·tic [ɪˌ-ˌdaɪəɡˈnɒstɪk] *adj* Elektrodiagnostik betr., elektrodiagnostisch.
e·lec·tro·di·ag·nos·tics [ɪˌ-ˌdaɪəɡˈnɒstɪks] *pl* → electrodiagnosis.
electrodiagnostic studies → electrodiagnosis.
e·lec·tro·di·al·y·sis [ɪˌ-daɪˈæləsɪs] *n* Elektrodialyse *f.*
e·lec·tro·di·a·lyze [ɪˌ-ˈdaɪəlaɪz] *vt* elektrodialysieren.
e·lec·tro·di·a·lyz·er [ɪˌ-ˈdaɪəlaɪzər] *n* Elektrodialysator *m.*
e·lec·tro·di·a·phane [ɪˌ-ˈdaɪəfeɪn] *n* Diaphanoskop *nt.*
e·lec·tro·di·aph·a·no·scope [ɪˌ-daɪˈæfənəskəʊp] *n* → electrodiaphane.
e·lec·tro·di·aph·a·nos·co·py [ɪˌ-daɪˌæfəˈnɒskəpɪ] *n* Durchleuchten *nt*, Transillumination *f*, Diaphanie *f*, Diaphanoskopie *f.*
e·lec·tro·dy·nam·ic [ɪˌ-daɪˈnæmɪk] *adj* elektrodynamisch.
e·lec·tro·dy·nam·ics [ɪˌ-daɪˈnæmɪks] *pl phys.* Elektrodynamik *f.*
e·lec·tro·en·ceph·a·lo·gram [ɪˌ-enˈsefələɡræm] *n abbr.* EEG Elektronenzephalogramm *nt abbr.* EEG.
e·lec·tro·en·ceph·a·lo·graph [ɪˌ-enˈsefələɡræf] *n* Elektroenzephalograph *m.*
e·lec·tro·en·ceph·a·lo·graph·ic dysrhythmia [ɪˌ-enˌsefələˈɡræfɪk] *neuro.* (*EEG*) diffuse/paroxysmale Dysrhythmie *f.*
e·lec·tro·en·ceph·a·log·ra·phy [ɪˌ-enˌsefəˈlɒɡrəfɪ] *n* Elektroenzephalographie *f.*
e·lec·tro·en·dos·mo·sis [ɪˌ-ˌendəzˈməʊsɪs] *n* Elektroendosmose *f.*
e·lec·tro·ex·ci·sion [ɪˌ-ekˈsɪʒn] *n chir.* elektrochirurgische Exzision *f*, Elektroexzision *f.*
e·lec·tro·fo·cus·ing [ɪˌ-ˈfəʊkəsɪŋ] *n* Elektrofokussierung *f*, isoelektrische Fokussierung *f.*
e·lec·tro·gas·tro·gram [ɪˌ-ˈɡæstrəɡræm] *n* Elektrogastrogramm *nt.*
e·lec·tro·gas·tro·graph [ɪˌ-ˈɡæstrəɡræf] *n* Elektrogastrograph *m.*
e·lec·tro·gas·tro·g·ra·phy [ɪˌ-ˌɡæsˈtrɒɡrəfɪ] *n* Elektrogastrographie *f.*
e·lec·tro·gen·ic [ɪˌ-ˈdʒenɪk] *adj* elektrogen.
electrogenic transport elektrogener Transport *m.*
e·lec·tro·gram [ɪˈlektrəɡræm] *n* Elektrogramm *nt*, Elektrometerdiagramm *nt.*
e·lec·tro·graph [ɪˈlektrəɡræf] *n* 1. → electrogram. 2. registrierendes Elektrometer *nt*, Elektrograph *m.*
e·lec·trog·ra·phy [ɪˌlekˈtrɒɡrəfɪ] *n* Elektrographie *f.*
e·lec·tro·gus·tom·e·try [ɪˌlektrəɡʌsˈtɒmətrɪ] *n physiol.* Elektrogustometrie *f.*
e·lec·tro·he·mo·sta·sis [ɪˌ-hɪˈmɒstəsɪs] *n* Blut(ungs)stillung *f* mittels Elektrokaustik.
e·lec·tro·hys·ter·o·gram [ɪˌ-ˈhɪstərəɡræm] *n* Elektrohysterogramm *nt.*
e·lec·tro·hys·ter·o·graph [ɪˌ-ˈhɪstərəɡræf] *n* Elektrohysterograph *m.*

electrohysterography

e·lec·tro·hys·te·rog·ra·phy [ˌhɪstə'rɒgrəfɪ] *n* Elektrohysterographie *f.*
e·lec·tro·im·mu·no·dif·fu·sion [ˌ-ˌɪmjənəʊdɪ'fjuːʒn, -ɪˌmjuː-] *n* Elektroimmun(o)diffusion *f.*
e·lec·tro·ki·net·ic [ˌ-kɪ'netɪk, -kaɪ-] *adj* elektrokinetisch.
e·lec·tro·ki·net·ics [ˌ-kɪ'netɪks, -kaɪ-] *pl phys.* Elektrokinetik *f.*
e·lec·tro·ky·mo·gram [ˌ-'kaɪməgræm] *n abbr.* **EKY** Elektrokymogramm *nt abbr.* EKY, EKyG.
e·lec·tro·ky·mo·graph·ic [ˌ-kaɪmə'græfɪk] *adj* elektrokymographisch.
e·lec·tro·ky·mog·ra·phy [ˌ-kaɪ'mɒgrəfɪ] *n radiol.* Elektrokymographie *f,* Fluorokardiographie *f.*
e·lec·tro·lep·sy ['-lepsɪ] *n* → electric chorea.
e·lec·tro·li·thot·ri·ty [ˌ-lɪ'θɒtrətrɪ] *n urol.* elektrische Steinauflösung *f,* Elektrolitholyse *f;* Elektrolithotripsie *f.*
e·lec·trol·y·sis [ɪlek'trɒləsɪs] *n* **1.** *chem., phys.* Elektrolyse *f.* **2.** *derm.* (therapeutische) Elektrolyse *f,* Elektro-, Galvanopunktur *f,* Elektrostixis *f.*
e·lec·tro·lyte [ɪ'lektrəlaɪt] *n* Elektrolyt *m.*
electrolyte deficit Elektrolytmangel *m,* -defizit *nt.*
electrolyte intoxication Elektrolytintoxikation *f.*
e·lec·tro·lyt·ic [ˌ-'lɪtɪk] *adj* Elektrolyse betr., elektrolytisch.
e·lec·tro·lyt·i·cal [ˌ-'lɪtɪkl] *adj* → electrolytic.
electrolytic cell *phys.* Elektrolysezelle *f.*
electrolytic dissociation elektrolytische Dissoziation *f.*
e·lec·tro·lyz·a·ble [ˌ-'laɪzəbl] *adj* elektrolysierbar.
e·lec·tro·lyze ['-laɪz] *vt* mittels Elektrolyse zersetzen, elektrolysieren.
e·lec·tro·mag·net [ˌ-'mægnɪt] *n* Elektromagnet *m.*
e·lec·tro·mag·net·ic [ˌ-mæg'netɪk] *adj* Elektromagnet(ismus) betr., elektromagnetisch.
electromagnetic field elektromagnetisches Feld *nt.*
electromagnetic flowmeter elektromagnetischer Flußmesser *m.*
electromagnetic interaction elektromagnetische Wechselwirkung *f.*
electromagnetic radiation elektromagnetische Strahlung *f.*
e·lec·tro·mag·net·ics [ˌ-mæg'netɪks] *pl* → electromagnetism.
electromagnetic spectrum elektromagnetisches Spektrum *nt.*
electromagnetic waves elektromagnetische Wellen *pl.*
e·lec·tro·mag·net·ism [ˌ-'mægnɪtɪzəm] *n* Elektromagnetismus.
e·lec·tro·ma·nom·e·ter [ˌ-mə'nɒmɪtər] *n* Elektromanometer *nt.*
e·lec·tro·mas·sage [ˌ-mə'sɑːʒ, -sɑːdʒ] *n* Elektromassage *f.*
e·lec·tro·me·chan·i·cal [ˌ-mə'kænɪkl] *adj* elektromechanisch.
e·lec·tro·me·chan·ics [ˌ-mə'kænɪks] *pl* Elektromechanik *f.*
e·lec·trom·e·ter [ɪlek'trɒmɪtər] *n* Elektrometer *nt.*
e·lec·tro·met·ric [ɪˌlektrəʊ'metrɪk] *adj* elektrometrisch.
e·lec·trom·e·try [ɪlek'trɒmətrɪ] *n chem.* Elektrometrie *f.*
e·lec·tro·mo·tive [ɪˌlektrə'məʊtɪv] *adj* elektromotorisch.
electromotive force *abbr.* **EMF, emf** elektromotorische Kraft *f abbr.* EMK.
e·lec·tro·my·o·gram [ˌ-'maɪəgræm] *n* Elektromyogramm *nt.*
e·lec·tro·my·o·graph [ˌ-'maɪəgræf] *n* Elektromyograph *m.*
e·lec·tro·my·og·ra·phy [ˌ-maɪ'ɒgrəfɪ] *n abbr.* **EMG** Elektromyographie *f abbr.* EMG.
e·lec·tron [ɪ'lektrɒn] **I** *n* Elektron *nt.* **II** *adj* Elektronen-.
electron acceptor Elektronenakzeptor *m.*
e·lec·tro·nar·co·sis [ɪˌlektrəʊnɑːr'kəʊsɪs] *n* Elektronarkose *f.*
electron beam Elektronenstrahl *m.*
electron carrier Elektronen(über)träger *m.*
electron-carrying *adj* elektronen(über)tragend.
electron cascade Elektronenkaskade *f.*
electron-dense *adj histol.* elektronendicht.
electron-dense granules *histol.* elektronendichte Granula *pl.*
electron density *phys.* Elektronendichte *f.*
electron donor *chem.* Elektronendonor *m.*
e·lec·tro·neg·a·tive [ɪˌlektrəʊ'negətɪv] *adj* Elektronegativität betr., elektronegativ, negativ elektrisch.
e·lec·tro·neg·a·tiv·i·ty [ˌ-negə'tɪvətɪ] *n* Elektronegativität *f.*
electron equivalent Elektronenäquivalent *nt.*
e·lec·tro·neu·rog·ra·phy [ˌ-njʊə'rɒgrəfɪ] *n* → electroneuronography.
e·lec·tro·neu·rol·y·sis [ˌ-njʊə'rɒləsɪs] *n* Elektroneurolyse *f.*
e·lec·tro·neu·ro·my·og·ra·phy [ˌ-ˌnjʊərəmaɪ'ɒgrəfɪ] *n* Elektroneuromyographie *f.*
e·lec·tro·neu·ro·nog·ra·phy [ˌ-njʊərə'nɒgrəfɪ] *n abbr.* **ENoG** Elektroneurographie *f,* Elektroneuronographie *f abbr.* ENoG.
e·lec·tro·neu·tral·i·ty [ˌ-n(j)uː'trælətɪ] *n* Elektroneutralität *f.*
electron flow Elektronenfluß *m.*
e·lec·tron·ic [ɪlek'trɒnɪk] *adj* Elektron(en) *od.* Elektronik betr., elektronisch, Elektronen-, Elektro-.
electronic configuration Elektronenkonfiguration *f.*
electronic data processing elektronische Datenverarbeitung *f abbr.* EDV.
electronic interaction Elektronenwechselwirkung *f.*
electronic number Elektronenzahl *f.*
e·lec·tron·ics [ɪlek'trɒnɪks] *pl* Elektronik *f.*
electron microscope Elektronenmikroskop *m.*
electron-microscopic(al) *adj* mit Hilfe eines Elektronenmikroskops (sichtbar), elektronenmikroskopisch.
electron microscopy Elektronenmikroskopie *f.*
electron-pair acceptor *chem.* Elektronenpaarakzeptor *m.*
electron-pair donor *chem.* Elektronenpaardonor *m.*
electron paramagnetic resonance *abbr.* **EPR** → electron spin resonance.
electron paramagnetic resonance spectroscopy → electron spin resonance spectroscopy.
electron sheII *phys.* Elektronenschale *f.*
electron spin Elektronenspin *m.*
electron spin resonance *abbr.* **ESR** Elektronenspinresonanz *f abbr.* ESR.
electron spin resonance spectroscopy Elektronenspinresonanzspektroskopie *f,* ESR-Spektroskopie *f,* paramagnetische Resonanzspektroskopie *f.*
electron-transfering *adj* elektronenübertragend.
electron-transfering protein elektronenübertragendes Protein *nt.*
electron transport Elektronentransport *m.*
light-induced e. lichtinduzierter Elektronentransport.
microsomal e. mikrosomaler Elektronentransport.
photoinduced e. photoinduzierter Elektronentransport.
photosynthetic e. photosynthetischer Elektronentransport
electron-transport chain *biochem.* Elektronentransportkette *f,* elektronenübertragende Kette *f.*
electron-transport cycle Elektronentransportzyklus *m.*
electron-transport system *biochem.* Elektronentransportsystem *nt.*
electron volt *abbr.* **eV, ev** Elektronenvolt *nt abbr.* eV.
e·lec·tro·nys·tag·mo·gram [ɪˌlektrəʊnɪs'tægməgræm] *n* Elektronystagmogramm *nt.*
e·lec·tro·nys·tag·mo·graph [ˌ-nɪs'tægməgræf] *n* Elektronystagmograph *m.*
e·lec·tro·nys·tag·mog·ra·phy [ˌ-nɪstæg'mɒgrəfɪ] *n abbr.* **ENG** Elektronystagmographie *f abbr.* ENG.
e·lec·tro·oc·u·lo·gram [ˌ-'ɒkjələgræm] *n abbr.* **EOG** Elektrookulogramm *nt abbr.* EOG.
e·lec·tro·oc·u·log·ra·phy [ˌ-ɒkjə'lɒgrəfɪ] *n* Elektrookulographie *f.*
electro-olfactogram *n abbr.* **EOG** Elektroolfaktogramm *nt abbr.* EOG.
e·lec·tro·op·tic [ˌ-'ɒptɪk] *adj* Elektrooptic betr., elektrooptisch.
e·lec·tro·op·ti·cal [ˌ-'ɒptɪkl] *adj* → electrooptic.
e·lec·tro·op·tics [ˌ-'ɒptɪks] *pl* Elektrooptik *f.*
e·lec·tro·os·mose [ˌ-'ɒzməʊs] *n* → electroosmosis.
e·lec·tro·os·mo·sis [ˌ-ɒz'məʊsɪs] *n* Elektroosmose *f.*
e·lec·tro·os·mot·ic [ˌ-ɒz'mɒtɪk] *adj* elektroosmotisch.
e·lec·tro·pher·o·gram [ˌ-'ferəgræm] *n* Elektropherogramm *nt,* Pherogramm *nt.*
e·lec·tro·phile ['-faɪl] *n chem.* elektrophile Substanz *f od.* Gruppe *f.*
e·lec·tro·phil·ic [ˌ-'fɪlɪk] *adj chem.* Elektronen suchend, elektrophil.
e·lec·tro·pho·re·gram [ˌ-'fɔːrəgræm] *n* → electropherogram.
e·lec·tro·pho·re·sis [ˌ-fə'riːsɪs] *n* Elektrophorese *f.*
e·lec·tro·pho·ret·ic [ˌ-fə'retɪk] *adj* Elektrophorese betr., mittels Elektrophorese, elektrophoretisch.
electrophoretic pattern Elektrophoresemuster *nt.*
e·lec·tro·pho·ret·o·gram [ˌ-fə'retəgræm] *n* → electropherogram.
e·lec·troph·o·rus [ɪlek'trɒfərəs] *n phys.* Elektrophor *m.*
e·lec·tro·pho·tom·e·ter [ɪˌlektrəfəʊ'tɒmɪtər] *n* Elektrophotometer *nt.*
e·lec·tro·pho·to·ther·a·py [ˌ-ˌfəʊtə'θerəpɪ] *n* Elektrophototherapie *f.*
e·lec·tro·phren·ic respiration [ˌ-'frenɪk] *abbr.* **EPR** elektrophrenische (Be-)Atmung *f.*
e·lec·tro·phys·i·o·log·ic [ˌ-ˌfɪzɪə'lɒdʒɪk] *adj* Elektrophysiologie betr., elektrophysiologisch.
e·lec·tro·phys·i·o·log·i·cal [ˌ-ˌfɪzɪə'lɒdʒɪkl] *adj* → electrophysiologic.
e·lec·tro·phys·i·ol·o·gy [ˌ-ˌfɪzɪ'ɒlədʒɪ] *n* Elektrophysiologie *f.*
e·lec·tro·plate ['-pleɪt] *vt* galvanisieren, elektroplattieren.

e·lec·tro·plat·ing ['-pleɪtɪŋ] *n* Galvanisieren *nt*, Elektroplattieren *nt*.
e·lec·tro·plex·y ['-pleksɪ] *n* elektrischer Schock *m*, Elektroschock *m*.
e·lec·tro·pos·i·tive [,-'pɑzɪtɪv] *adj* elektropositiv, positiv elektrisch.
e·lec·tro·pos·i·tiv·i·ty [,-,pɑzɪ'tɪvətɪ] *n* Elektropositivität *f*.
e·lec·tro·punc·ture [,-'pʌŋktʃər] *n* Elektropunktur *f*.
e·lec·tro·ra·di·om·e·ter [,-reɪdɪ'ɑmɪtər] *n* Elektroradiometer *nt*.
e·lec·tro·re·sec·tion [,-rɪ'sekʃn] *n chir.* Elektroresektion *f*.
e·lec·tro·ret·i·no·gram [,-'retnəgræm] *n abbr.* ERG Elektroretinogramm *nt abbr.* ERG.
e·lec·tro·ret·i·no·graph [,-'retnəgræf] *n* Elektroretinograph *m*.
e·lec·tro·ret·i·nog·ra·phy [,-retɪ'nɑgrəfɪ] *n* Elektroretinographie *f*.
e·lec·tro·scope [ɪ'lektrəskəʊp] *n phys., physiol.* Elektroskop *nt*.
e·lec·tro·scop·ic [,-'skɑpɪk] *adj* elektroskopisch.
electro-secretion coupling *physiol.* Elektrosekretionskopplung *f*.
e·lec·tro·shock ['-ʃɑk] *n* **1.** elektrischer Schock *m*, Elektroschock *m*. **2.** → electroshock therapy. **3.** *card.* Elektroschock *m*.
electroshock therapy *abbr.* **EST** Elektroschock-, Elektrokrampftherapie *f abbr.* EKT, Elektrokrampfbehandlung *f*.
e·lec·tro·sleep ['-sliːp] *n* zerebrale Elektrotherapie *f*, Elektroschlaftherapie *f*.
e·lec·tros·mo·sis [ɪ,lektrɑz'məʊsɪs] *n* → electroosmosis.
e·lec·tro·spec·tro·gram [ɪ,lektrəʊ'spektrəgræm] *n* Elektrospektrogramm *nt*.
e·lec·tro·spec·tro·gra·phy [,-spek'trɑgrəfɪ] *n* Elektrospektrographie *f*.
e·lec·tro·spi·no·gram [,-'spaɪnəgræm] *n* Elektrospinogramm *nt*.
e·lec·tro·spi·nog·ra·phy [,-spaɪ'nɑgrəfɪ] *n* Elektrospinographie *f*.
e·lec·tro·stat·ic [,-'stætɪk] *adj* Elektrostatik betr., elektrostatisch.
electrostatic attraction *phys.* elektrostatische Anziehung *f*.
electrostatic force *phys.* elektrostatische Kraft *f*.
electrostatic lens elektrostatische Linse *f*.
electrostatic repulsion *phys.* elektrostatische Abstoßung *f*.
e·lec·tro·stat·ics [,-'stætɪks] *pl* Elektrostatik *f*.
e·lec·tro·stim·u·la·tion [,-stɪmjə'leɪʃn] *n* elektrische Reizung *f*, Elektrostimulation *f*.
e·lec·tro·stri·a·to·gram [,-straɪ'eɪtəgræm] *n* Elektrostriatogramm *nt*.
e·lec·tro·stric·tion [,-'strɪkʃn] *n phys.* Elektrostriktion *f*.
e·lec·tro·sur·ger·y [,-'sɜrdʒərɪ] *n* Elektrochirurgie *f*.
e·lec·tro·sur·gi·cal [,-'sɜrdʒɪkl] *adj* Elektrochirurgie betr., elektrochirurgisch.
electrosurgical incision elektrochirurgische Inzision *f*.
e·lec·tro·syn·the·sis [,-'sɪnθəsɪs] *n* Elektrosynthese *f*.
e·lec·tro·tac·tic [,-'tæktɪk] *adj* Elektrotaxis betr., elektrotaktisch.
e·lec·tro·tax·is [,-'tæksɪs] *n* Elektrotaxis *f*.
e·lec·tro·tha·na·sia [,-θə'neɪʒɪə] *n* → electrocution.
e·lec·tro·ther·a·peu·tic bath [,-θerə'pjuːtɪk] hydroelektrisches Bad *nt*.
e·lec·tro·ther·a·peu·tics [,-,θerə'pjuːtɪks] *pl* Elektrotherapie *f*.

e·lec·tro·ther·a·pist [,-'θerəpɪst] *n* Elektrotherapeut(in *f*) *m*.
e·lec·tro·ther·a·py [,-'θerəpɪ] *n* → electrotherapeutics.
e·lec·tro·tome ['-təʊm] *n* elektrisches Skalpell *nt*, Elektrotom *nt*.
e·lec·trot·o·my [ɪlek'trɑtəmɪ] *n chir.* Elektrotomie *f*.
e·lec·tro·ton·ic [ɪ,lektrə'tɑnɪk] *adj* Elektrotonus betr., elektrotonisch.
electrotonic coupling *physiol.* elektrotonische Kopplung *f*.
electrotonic current elektrotonischer Strom *m*.
electrotonic junction offener Zellkontakt *m*, Nexus *m*.
electrotonic potential elektrotonisches Potential *nt*.
electrotonic spread *physiol.* elektrotonische Ausbreitung *f*.
e·lec·trot·o·nus [ɪlek'trɑtnəs] *n* Elektrotonus *m*.
e·lec·trot·ro·pism [ɪlek'trɑtrəpɪzəm] *n* Elektrotropismus *m*.
e·lec·tro·ul·tra·fil·tra·tion [ɪ,lektrəʊ,ʌltrəfɪl'treɪʃn] *n* Elektroultrafiltration *f*.
e·lec·tro·u·re·ter·o·gram [,-jʊə'riːtərəgræm] *n urol.* Elektroureterogramm *nt*.
e·lec·tro·u·re·te·rog·ra·phy [,-jʊə,riːtə'rɑgrəfɪ] *n urol.* Elektroureterographie *f*.
e·lec·tro·va·go·gram [,-'veɪgəʊgræm] *n* (Elektro-)Vagogramm *nt*.
e·lec·tro·va·lence [,-'veɪləns] *n* **1.** *chem.* Elektronenwertigkeit *f*, Elektrovalenz *f*. **2.** *chem.* Ionenbindung *f*.
e·lec·tro·va·len·cy [,-'veɪlənsɪ] *n* → electrovalence.
e·lec·tro·ver·sion [,-'vɜrʒn] *n card.* Elektrokonversion *f*, Elektroversion *f*, Elektroreduktion *f*, Synchrondefibrillation *f*, Kardioversion *f*.
e·lec·tro·vert ['-vɜrt] *vt card.* eine Elektrokonversion durchführen.
e·lec·tu·ar·y [ɪ'lektʃʊerɪ] *n pharm.* **1.** Latwerge *f*, Electuarium *nt*. **2.** Linctus *m*.
el·e·doi·sin [elɪ'dɔɪsɪn] *n pharm.* Eledoisin *nt*.
el·e·i·din [ɪ'liːɪdɪn] *n* Eleidin *nt*.
Elek ['iːlek]: **E. test** *micro.* Elek-Plattentest *m*.
Elek-Ouchterlony ['ɒktərləʊnɪ]: **E.-O. test** Elek-Ouchterlony-Test *m*.
el·e·ment ['eləmənt] *n* **1.** Element *nt*; Bauteil *nt*, Baustein *m*; Grundbestandteil *m*. **2.** *mathe., phys.* Element *nt*; *electr.* Element *nt*, Zelle *f*; *chem.* Grundstoff *m*. **3.** ~s *pl* Grundlagen *pl*.
el·e·men·tal [elə'mentl] *adj* elementar, ursprünglich; wesentlich, grundlegend, Elementar-, Ur-.
elemental diet Elementardiät *f*, bilanzierte synthetische Diät *f*.
el·e·men·ta·ry [elə'ment(ə)rɪ] *adj* **1.** → elemental. **2.** elementar, einfach, simpel. **3.** *chem., mathe., phys.* elementar, Elementar-. **4.** rudimentär, unterentwickelt.
elementary bodies 1. Einschluß-, Elementarkörperchen *pl*. **2.** Blutplättchen *pl*, Thrombozyten *pl*.
elementary cell *embryo.* Furchungszelle *f*, Blastomere *f*.
elementary charge *chem., phys.* Elementarladung *f*.
elementary granule *histol.* Elementargranulum *nt*.
elementary membrane Einheits-, Elementarmembran *f*.
elementary particle *phys.* Elementarteilchen *nt*.
eleo- *pref.* Öl-, Oleo-.
e·le·o·ma [elɪ'əʊmə] *n patho.* Elaiom *nt*, Oleom *nt*, Oleogranulom *nt*, Oleoskle-

rom *nt*, Paraffinom *nt*.
el·e·om·e·ter [elɪ'ɑmɪtər] *n* Oleometer *nt*.
el·e·o·tho·rax [elɪəʊ'θɔːræks] *n histor.* Oleothorax *m*.
el·e·phan·ti·ac [elə'fæntɪæk] *adj* → elephantiasic.
el·e·phan·ti·as·ic [elə,fæntɪ'æsɪk] *adj* Elephantiasis betr., Elephantiasis-.
el·e·phan·ti·a·sis [eləfən'taɪəsɪs] *n* **1.** *patho.* Elephantiasis *f*. **2.** Elephantiasis tropica.
el·e·phant leg ['eləfənt] → elephantiasis 2.
el·e·phan·toid [elə'fæntɔɪd] *adj* elephantoid.
el·e·vate ['eləveɪt] *vt* erhöhen; (auf-, hoch-)heben; (*Stimme, Blick*) erheben; (*Niveau*) heben, verbessern.
el·e·vat·ed ['eləveɪtɪd] *adj* erhöht; gehoben; hoch, Hoch-.
el·e·va·tion [elə'veɪʃn] *n* Erhöhung *f*, Elevation *f*, (Auf-, Hoch-)Heben *nt*, Anhebung *f*; (*Niveau*) Hebung *f*, Verbesserung *f*.
el·e·va·tor ['eləveɪtər] *n* **1.** *anat.* Heber *m*, Hebemuskel *m*, Levator *m*, M. levator. **2.** *chir.* Elevatorium *nt*. **3.** Lift *m*, Fahrstuhl *m*, Aufzug *m*.
el·e·venth nerve [ɪ'levənθ] Akzessorius *m*, XI. Hirnerv *m*, N. accessorius [XI].
el·fin facies syndrome ['elfɪn] Williams-Beuren-Syndrom *nt*.
e·lic·it·ing stimulus [ɪ'lɪsɪtɪŋ] auslösender Reiz *m*.
e·lim·i·na·ble [ɪ'lɪmənəbl] *adj* ausscheidbar, eliminierbar.
e·lim·i·nate [ɪ'lɪməneɪt] *vt* **1.** beseitigen, entfernen, ausmerzen, eliminieren (*from* aus). **2.** *chem., pharm.* ausscheiden, eliminieren.
e·lim·i·na·tion [ɪ,lɪmə'neɪʃn] *n* **1.** Beseitigung *f*, Entfernung *f*, Ausmerzung *f*, Eliminierung *f*. **2.** *chem., pharm.* Ausscheidung *f*, Elimination *f*. **3.** *mathe.* Elimination *f*.
e·lin·gu·a·tion [ɪlɪŋ'gweɪʃn] *n chir.* Zungen(teil)amputation *f*, Glossektomie *f*.
ELISA *abbr.* → enzyme-linked immunosorbent assay.
e·lix·ir [ɪ'lɪksər] *n pharm.* Elixier *nt*.
el·ko·sis [el'kəʊsɪs] *n* Geschwür(s)leiden *nt*, Helkosis *f*.
Elliot ['elɪət, 'eljət]: **E.'s operation** *ophthal.* Elliot-Trepanation *f*.
E.'s position Elliot-Lagerung *f*.
E.'s sign *ophthal.* Elliot-Skotom *nt*.
el·lip·sis [ɪ'lɪpsɪs] *n psychia.* Ellipsis *f*.
el·lip·soid [ɪ'lɪpsɔɪd] *n* **1.** *anat.* spindel- od. ellipsenförmige Struktur *f*. **2.** (*Milz*) Ellipsoid *nt*, Schweigger-Seidel'-Hülse *f*. **3.** *mathe., phys.* Ellipsoid *nt*. **II** *adj* → ellipsoidal.
el·lip·soi·dal [ɪlɪp'sɔɪdl, elɪp-] *adj* ellipsenförmig, -ähnlich, ellipsoid, elliptisch.
ellipsoidal articulation Ellipsoid-, Eigelenk *nt*, Artic. ellipsoidea/condylaris.
ellipsoidal joint → ellipsoidal articulation.
ellipsoid arterioles → ellipsoid 2.
el·lip·tic [ɪ'lɪptɪk] *adj* → elliptical.
el·lip·ti·cal [ɪ'lɪptɪkl] *adj* Ellipse betr., elliptisch, ellipsenförmig.
elliptical recess (of vestibule) Rec. ellipticus (vestibuli).
el·lip·to·cy·ta·ry [ɪ,lɪptə'saɪtərɪ] *adj* Elliptozyten betr., elliptozytär, Elliptozyten-.
elliptocytary anemia → elliptocytosis.
el·lip·to·cyte [ɪ'lɪptəsaɪt] *n hema.* Elliptozyt *m*, Ovalozyt *m*.
el·lip·to·cyt·ic anemia [,-'sɪtɪk] → elliptocytosis.
el·lip·to·cy·to·sis [,-saɪ'təʊsɪs] *n hema.* Dresbach-Syndrom *nt*, hereditäre Elliptozytose *f*, Ovalozytose *f*, Kamelozytose *f*, Elliptozytenanämie *f*.

elliptocytotic

el·lip·to·cy·tot·ic [,-saɪ'tɒtɪk] *adj* Elliptozytose betr., Elliptozytose-.
elliptocytotic anemia → elliptocytosis.
Ellis ['elɪs]: **E.' curve** Ellis-Damoiseau'-Linie *f*.
  E.' line → E.' curve.
  E.' sign Ellis-Zeichen *nt*.
Ellis and Garland ['gɑːrlənd]: **curve of E. a. G.** → Ellis' curve.
Ellis-Garland: E.-G. line → Ellis' curve.
Ellis-van Creveld [væn 'kreɪfeld]: **E.-v.C. syndrome** Ellis-van Creveld-Syndrom *nt*, Chondroektodermaldysplasie *f*, chondroektodermale Dysplasie *f*, Chondrodysplasia ectodermica.
Ellman ['elmən]: **E.'s reagent** Ellman'-Reagenz *nt*, 5,5'-Dithiobis-2-nitrobenzoesäure *f*.
Ellsworth-Howard ['elzwɜrθ 'haʊərd]: **E.-H. test** Ellsworth-Howard-Test *m*, Phosphaturietest *m*.
Eloesser [e'lesər]: **E. flap** Eloesser-Plastik *f*.
  E. procedure Eloesser-Operation *f*.
e·lon·gate [ɪ'lɔːŋgeɪt, 'iːlɑŋ-] **I** *adj* → elongated. **II** *vt* verlängern; strecken, dehnen. **III** *vi* s. verlängern, länger werden.
e·lon·gat·ed [ɪ'lɔːŋgeɪtɪd, 'iːlɑŋ-] *adj* verlängert; (aus-)gestreckt, länglich.
e·lon·ga·tion [ɪlɔːŋ'geɪʃn, iːlɑŋ-] *n* **1.** Verlängerung *f*; Dehnung *f*, Streckung *f*. **2.** *patho*. Elongation *f*, Elongatio *f*. **3.** *phys*. Elongation *f*.
elongation factor *abbr*. **EF** *biochem*. Verlängerungs-, Elongationsfaktor *m abbr*. EF.
elongation phase *biochem*. Elongationsphase *f*.
Eisberg ['elsbɜrg]: **E.'s test** *HNO* Elsberg-Test *m*.
Elschnig ['elʃnɪg]: **E.'s bodies/pearls** *ophthal*. Elschnig-Körperchen *pl*.
Elsner ['elsnər]: **E.'s asthma** Stenokardie *f*, Angina pectoris, Herzbräune *f*.
El Tor vibrio *micro*. Vibrio El-Tor *nt*, Vibrio cholerae biovar eltor.
el·u·ent [ɪ'luːənt] *n* eluent.
el·u·ate ['eljəwɪt, -eɪt] *n phys*., *chem*. Eluat *nt*.
eluate factor Pyridoxin *nt*, Vitamin B_6 *nt*.
el·u·ent ['eljəwənt, -juːənt] *n* Eluant *nt*.
e·lu·sive ulcer [ɪ'luːsɪv] Fenwick-Ulkus *nt*, Hunner-Ulkus *nt*, Hunner-Fenwick-Ulkus *nt*, Fenwick-Hunner-Ulkus *nt*.
e·lute [ɪ'luːt] *vt phys*., *chem*. auswaschen, (her-)auspülen, eluieren.
e·lu·tion [ɪ'luːʃn] *n phys*., *chem*. Auswaschen *nt*, (Her-)Ausspülen *nt*, Eluieren *nt*, Elution *f*.
elution curve *phys*., *chem*. Auswasch-, Elutionskurve *f*.
e·lu·tri·ate [ɪ'luːtrɪeɪt] *vt* (aus-)schlemmen.
e·lu·tri·a·tion [ɪˌluːtrɪ'eɪʃn] *n* (Aus-)Schlemmen *nt*.
Ely ['iːlɪ]: **E.'s sign/test** Ely-Zeichen *nt*.
EMA *abbr*. → ethylmalonic-adipic aciduria.
e·ma·ci·ate [ɪ'meɪʃɪeɪt] **I** *adj* → emaciated. **II** *vt* **1.** ab-, auszehren, ausmergeln. **2.** *chem*. auslaugen.
e·ma·ci·at·ed [ɪ'meɪʃɪeɪtɪd] *adj* **1.** abgemagert, ab-, ausgezehrt, ausgemergelt. **2.** *chem*. ausgelaugt.
e·ma·ci·a·tion [ɪˌmeɪʃɪ'eɪʃn] *n* **1.** Auszehrung *f*, (extreme) Abmagerung *f*, Emaciatio *f*. **2.** *chem*. Auslaugung *f*.
em·a·nate ['emənet] **I** *vt* ausströmen, ausstrahlen. **II** *vi* **1.** entmannen, ausstrahlen (*from* von). **2.** ausgehen, stammen (*from* von).
em·a·na·tion [emə'neɪʃn] *n* **1.** Ausströmen *nt*. **2.** Ausströmung *f*, Ausstrahlung *f*, Emanation *f*.

em·a·na·to·ri·um [ˌemənə'tɔʊrɪəm, -tɔː-] *n* Inhalationsraum *m*, Emanatorium *nt*.
em·a·no·ther·a·py [ˌemənəʊ'θerəpɪ] *n* Emantionstherapie *f*.
e·mas·cu·late [*adj* ɪ'mæskjəlɪt; *v* -leɪt] **I** *adj* → emasculated. **II** *vt* **1.** entmannen, kastrieren. **2.** verweichlichen. **3.** schwächen.
e·mas·cu·lat·ed [ɪ'mæskjəleɪtɪd] *adj* **1.** entmannt, kastriert. **2.** weibisch, unmännlich. **3.** verweichlicht.
e·mas·cu·la·tion [ɪˌmæskjə'leɪʃn] *n* **1.** Entmannung *f*, Kastrierung *f*, Kastration *f*, Emaskulation *f*. **2.** Verweichlichung *f*. **3.** (Ab-)Schwächung *f*.
EMB agar → eosin-methylene blue agar.
em·balm [em'bɑːm] *vt* **1.** (ein-)balsamieren, salben, einreiben. **2.** *hyg*. mit Konservierungsstoffen behandeln.
em·balm·ment [em'bɑːmənt] *n* (Ein-)Balsamieren *nt*, (Ein-)Balsamierung *f*.
Embden-Mayerhof ['embdən 'maɪərhɒf]: **E.-M. pathway** Embden-Mayerhof-Weg *m*.
Embden-Mayerhof-Parnas ['parnəs]: **E.-M.-P. pathway** → Embden-Mayerhof pathway.
em·bed [em'bed] *vt* **1.** (*a. histol*.) (ein-)betten; (ein-)lagern. **2.** (fest) umschließen, um-, einhüllen.
em·bed·ded denticle [em'bedɪd] interstitieller Dentikel *m*.
em·bed·ding [em'bedɪŋ] *n histol*., *patho*. Einbetten *nt*, Einbettung *f*.
em·bo·la·lia [embə'leɪlɪə] *n* → embolalia.
em·bo·le ['embəlɪ] *n* emboly.
em·bo·lec·to·my [embə'lektəmɪ] *n chir*. operative Embolusentfernung *f*, intraluminale Desobliteration *f*, Embolektomie *f*.
embolectomy catheter Embolektomiekatheter *m*.
em·bo·lia [em'bəʊlɪə] *n* → emboly.
em·bol·ic [em'bɒlɪk] *adj* Embolus *od*. Embolie betr., embolisch, Embolie-, Embolus-.
embolic abscess embolischer Abszeß *m*.
embolic aneurysm embolisches Aneurysma *nt*.
embolic apoplexy embolische Apoplexie *f*, embolischer Hirninfarkt *m*.
embolic disease → embolism.
embolic gangrene embolische Gangrän *f*.
embolic infarct embolischer Infarkt *m*.
embolic pneumonia (post-)embolische Pneumonie *f*.
embolic therapy → embolization 2.
em·bol·i·form [em'bɒlɪfɔrm] *adj anat*. **1.** keilförmig. **2.** embolusähnlich, pfropfenförmig, emboliform.
emboliform nucleus Nc. emboliformis (cerebelli).
em·bo·lism ['embəlɪzəm] *n* Embolie *f*, Embolia *f*.
em·bo·li·za·tion [ˌembəlɪ'zeɪʃn] *n* **1.** *patho*. Embolusbildung *f*, -entstehung *f*. **2.** *chir*. (therapeutische) Embolisation *f*; Katheterembolisation *f*.
em·bo·lize ['embəlaɪz] *vt chir*. embolisieren.
em·bo·lo·la·lia [ˌembəʊləʊ'leɪlɪə] *n psychia*. Embololalie *f*, Embolophrasie *f*.
em·bo·lo·my·co·sis [ˌ-maɪ'kəʊsɪs] *n patho*. Embolomykose *f*.
em·bo·lo·my·cot·ic [ˌ-maɪ'kɒtɪk] *adj* Embolomykose betr., embolomykotisch.
embolomycotic aneurysm embolomykotisches Aneurysma *nt*.
em·bo·lo·phra·sia [-'freɪʒ(ɪ)ə, -zɪə] *n* → embololalia.
em·bo·lus ['embələs] *n*, *pl* **-li** [-laɪ, -liː] Embolus *m*.
em·bo·ly ['embəlɪ] *n embryo*. Embolie *f*.

em·bouche·ment [ãˈbuʃmã] *n* Gefäßeinmündung *f* in ein anderes Gefäß.
em·brace reflex [ɪm'breɪs, em-] *neuro*., *ped*. Moro-Reflex *m*.
em·bro·cate ['embrəkeɪt] *vt* (*Salbe*) einreiben.
em·bro·ca·tion [embrə'keɪʃn] *n* **1.** Einreibung *f*. **2.** Einreibemittel *nt*, Embrocatio *f*.
em·bry·ec·to·my [embrɪ'ektəmɪ] *n gyn*. Embryektomie *f*.
em·bry·o ['embrɪəʊ] **I** *n*, *pl* **-os** Embryo *m*. **II** *adj* → embryonic. **in ~ *fig*.** im Werden, im Entstehen.
em·bry·o·blast ['embrɪəʊblæst] *n* Embryoblast *m*.
embryoblast pole Embryoblastenpol *m*.
em·bry·o·car·di·a [ˌ-'kɑːrdɪə] *n* **1.** *patho*. Embryokardie *f*, Status embryocardicus. **2.** *card*. Pendel-, Ticktack-Rhythmus *m*, Embryokardie *f*.
em·bry·oc·to·ny [embrɪ'aktənɪ] *n* Fetusschädigung *f*, -abtötung *f*, Foetizid *m*, Fetizid *m*.
em·bry·o·gen·e·sis [ˌembrɪəʊ'dʒenəsɪs] *n* Embryogenese *f*, Embryogenie *f*.
em·bry·o·ge·net·ic [ˌ-dʒə'netɪk] *adj* → embryogenic 1.
em·bry·o·gen·ic [ˌ-'dʒenɪk] *adj* **1.** Embryogenese betr., embryogen. **2.** einen Embryo bilden, embryogen.
em·bry·og·e·ny [ˌembrɪ'ɑdʒənɪ] *n* → embryogenesis.
em·bry·oid ['embrɪɔɪd] **I** *n* Embryoid *nt*. **II** *adj* embryoähnlich, embryoid.
em·bry·o·log·ic [ˌembrɪə'lɒdʒɪk] *adj* → embryological.
em·bry·o·log·i·cal [ˌ-'lɒdʒɪkl] *adj* embryologisch.
em·bry·ol·o·gist [ˌembrɪ'ɑlədʒɪst] *n* Embryologe *m*, -login *f*.
em·bry·ol·o·gy [ˌ-'ɑlədʒɪ] *n* Embryologie *f*.
em·bry·o·ma [ˌ-'əʊmə] *n* embryonaler Tumor *m*, Embryom(a) *nt*.
e. of kidney → embryonal nephroma.
em·bry·o·mor·phous [ˌembrɪə'mɔːrfəs] *adj* embryomorph.
em·bry·o·nal ['embrɪənl, ˌembrɪ'əʊnl] *adj* → embryonic.
embryonal adenomyosarcoma → embryonal nephroma.
embryonal adenosarcoma → embryonal nephroma.
embryonal carcinoma 1. embryonales Karzinom *nt*, Ca. embryonale. **2.** embryonales Hodenkarzinom *nt*.
embryonal carcinosarcoma → embryonal nephroma.
embryonal knot Embryoknoten *m*.
embryonal leukemia *hema*. Stammzellenleukämie *f*, akute undifferenzierte Leukämie *f abbr*. AUL.
embryonal nephroma Wilms-Tumor *m*, embryonales Adeno(myo)sarkom *nt*, Nephroblastom *nt*, Adenomyorhabdosarkom *nt* der Niere.
embryonal nuclear cataract *ophthal*. Cataracta centralis pulverulenta.
embryonal period Embryonalperiode *f*.
embryonal sarcoma → embryonal nephroma.
embryonal teratoma embryonales/solides/malignes Teratom *nt*, Teratoma embryonale.
embryonal tumor → embryoma.
em·bry·o·nary ['embrɪənrɪ] *adj* → embryonic.
em·bry·o·nate ['embrɪəneɪt] *adj* → embryonated.
em·bry·o·nat·ed ['embrɪəneɪtɪd] *adj* **1.** Embryo(nen) enthaltend. **2.** befruchtet. **3.** *micro*. bebrütet, angebrütet, embryoniert.

embryonated egg *micro.* embryoniertes/bebrütetes Hühnerei *nt.*
em·bry·o·na·tion [ˌembrɪəˈneɪʃn] *n* Embryonenbildung *f.*
em·bry·on·ic [ˌembrɪˈɒnɪk] *adj* Embryo od. Embryonalstadien betr., vom Embryonalstadium stammend, embryonal, embryonisch, Embryo-, Embryonal-.
embryonic area → embryonic disk.
embryonic cell *embryo.* Furchungszelle *f*, Blastomere *f.*
embryonic determination embryonale Determination *f.*
embryonic development Embryonalentwicklung *f.*
embryonic disk Keimscheibe *f*, -schild *m*, Blastodiskus *m.*
embryonic ectoderm embryonales Ektoderm *nt.*
embryonic hepatoma Lebermischtumor *m*, Hepatoblastom *nt.*
embryonic layer Keimschicht *f.*
embryonic membrane Embryonal-, Keimhülle *f.*
embryonic period Embryonalperiode *f.*
embryonic pole embryonaler Pol *m.*
embryonic sac *embryo.* Blastozyste *f.*
embryonic shield → embryonic disk.
embryonic tumor → embryoma.
embryonic ventricle of heart embryonale Herzkammer *f*, embryonaler Ventrikel *m.*
em·bry·on·i·form [ˌembrɪˈɒnɪfɔːrm] *adj* → embryoid II.
em·bry·o·noid [ˈembrɪənɔɪd] *adj* → embryoid II.
em·bry·o·path·ia [ˌembrɪəˈpæθɪə] *n* → embryopathy.
em·bry·o·path·ic cataract [ˌ-ˈpæθɪk] *ophthal.* Linsentrübung/Katarakt *f* bei Embryopathie.
em·bry·o·pa·thol·o·gy [ˌ-pəˈθɒlədʒɪ] *n* Embryopathologie *f.*
em·bry·op·a·thy [embrɪˈɒpəθɪ] *n* Embryopathie *f*, Embryopathia *f.*
em·bry·o·plas·tic [ˌembrɪəˈplæstɪk] *adj* Embryobildung betr., embryoplastisch.
embryoplastic tumor embryoplastischer Tumor *m.*
em·bry·o·scope [ˈ-skəʊp] *n* Embryoskop *nt.*
em·bry·o·tome [ˈ-təʊm] *n gyn.* Embryotom *nt.*
em·bry·ot·o·my [ˌembrɪˈɒtəmɪ] *n chir.* Embryotomie *f*, -tomia *f*, Dissectio fetus.
em·bry·o·tox·ic [ˌembrɪəˈtɒksɪk] *adj* den Embryo schädigend, embryotoxisch.
em·bry·o·tox·on [ˌ-ˈtɒksən] *n* **1.** *ped.* Embryotoxon *nt.* **2.** *ophthal.* Embryotoxon *nt*, Arcus lipoides juvenilis.
embryo transfer Embryo(nen)transfer *m*, Embryonenübertragung *f abbr.* ET, Embryonenimplantation *f.*
embryo transplant → embryo transfer.
em·bry·o·troph [ˈ-trɒf, -trɔf] *n bio.*, *embryo.* Keimlingsnahrung *f*, Embryotrophe *f.*
em·bry·o·troph·ic [ˌ-ˈtrɒfɪk, -ˈtrəʊ-] *adj* embryotrophisch.
em·bry·ot·ro·phy [ˌembrɪˈɒtrəfɪ] *n bio.*, *embryo.* Keim-, Embryoernährung *f*, Embryotrophie *f.*
em·bry·ous [ˈembrɪəs] *adj* → embryonic.
EMC *abbr.* [encephalomyocarditis] → EMC syndrome.
EMC syndrome Enzephalomyokarditis *f*, Encephalomyocarditis *f abbr.* EMC, EMC-Syndrom *nt.*
e·med·ul·late [iˈmedleɪt, iˈmedʒə-] *vt* (Knochen-)Mark entfernen *od.* extrahieren.
e·mei·o·cy·to·sis *n* → emiocytosis.

e·merge [ɪˈmɜːdʒ] *vi* **1.** auftauchen. **2.** *fig.* s. herausstellen, s. zeigen, auftauchen; hervorgehen, herauskommen (*from* aus). **3.** ausbrechen; auftreten, in Erscheinung treten, zum Vorschein kommen. **4.** s. entwickeln, entstehen.
e·mer·gence [ɪˈmɜːdʒəns] *n* **1.** Auftauchen *nt*, Aufkommen *nt*; Hervortreten *nt*, Entstehung *f.* **2.** *pharm.* Emergence *f.*
e·mer·gen·cy [ɪˈmɜːdʒənsɪ] **I** *n* Notfall *m*; Not(lage *f*) *f.* **in case of ~, in an ~** im Notfall. **II** *adj* Not-, Behelfs-, Hilfs-. **for ~ use only** nur für den Notfall.
emergency call Notruf *m.*
emergency door/exit Notausgang *m.*
emergency measure Not(stands)maßnahme *f.*
emergency medicine Notfallmedizin *f.*
emergency operation Not(fall)operation *f*, Not-OP *f.*
emergency reaction Notfallreaktion *f.*
emergency situation Not(fall)situation *f.*
emergency theory Cannon-Notfallreaktion *f.*
emergency treatment Not(fall)behandlung *f.*
emergency ward Notaufnahme *f.*
e·mer·gent [ɪˈmɜːdʒənt] *adj* **1.** Not(fall) betr., Not-, Behelfs-, Hilfs-. **2.** ausbrechend, auftretend, in Erscheinung tretend, zum Vorschein kommend. **3.** s. entwickelnd, entstehend.
Emerson [ˈemərsən] *n:* **E. effect** Emerson-Effekt *m.*
e·me·sia [ɪˈmiːʒ(ɪ)ə] *n* → emesis.
em·e·sis [ˈeməsɪs] *n* (Er-)Brechen *nt*, Emesis *f.*
e·met·ic [əˈmetɪk] **I** *n pharm.* Brechmittel *nt*, Emetikum *nt.* **II** *adj* Brechreiz *od.* Erbrechen auslösend, emetisch.
em·e·tine [ˈemətiːn, -tɪn] *n* Emetin *nt.*
em·e·to·ca·thar·tic [ˌemətəʊkəˈθɑːrtɪk] **I** *n pharm.* kombiniertes Abführ- u. Brechmittel *nt*, Emetokathartikum *nt.* **II** *adj* emetisch u. kathartisch.
em·e·to·gen·ic [ˌ-ˈdʒenɪk] *adj* durch Erbrechen bedingt *od.* ausgelöst, emetogen.
EMF *abbr.* **1.** → electromotive force. **2.** → erythrocyte maturation factor.
emf *abbr.* → electromotive force.
EMG *abbr.* → electromyography.
EMG syndrome → exomphalus-macroglossia-gigantism syndrome.
em·i·gra·tion [ˌemɪˈgreɪʃn] *n immun.*, *hema.* Emigration *f*; Diapedese *f.*
emigration theory Cohnheim-Emigrationstheorie *f*, -Entzündungstheorie *f.*
em·i·nence [ˈemɪnəns] *n* Vorsprung *m*, Erhöhung *f*, Höcker *m*; *anat.* Eminentia *f.*
e. of concha Eminentia conchae.
e. of maxilla Tuber maxillare, Eminentia maxillaris.
e. of scapha Eminentia scaphae.
e. of triangular fossa Agger perpendicularis, Eminentia fossae triangularis auriculae.
e. of triquetral fossa → e. of triangular fossa.
em·i·nent [ˈemɪnənt] *adj* (her-)vorragend, vorstehend, -springend, -tretend.
em·i·o·cy·to·sis [ˌemɪəʊsaɪˈtəʊsɪs] *n* Eme(i)ozytose *f.*
em·is·sar·i·um [ˌemɪˈseərɪəm] *n, pl* **-ria** [-rɪə] → emissary 1.
em·is·sar·y [ˈemɪˌserɪ, -sərɪ] *n, pl* **-sar·ies 1.** Emissarium *nt*, V. emissaria. **2.** (*Schädel*) Venenaustrittsstelle *f.*
emissary vein → emissary 1.
e·mis·sion [ɪˈmɪʃn] *n* **1.** Ausstoß *m*; Aus-, Abstrahlung *f*; Absonderung *f*, Ausscheidung *f*; *phys.* Emission *f*, Aussendung *f.* **2.** Aus-, Verströmen *nt.* **3.** *physiol.*

unwillkürliche Ejakulation *f*; Ausfluß *m.*
emission electron *phys.* Emissionselektron *nt.*
em·is·siv·i·ty [ˌeməˈsɪvətɪ] *n abbr.* ∊ *phys.* Emissionskoeffizient *m abbr.* ε.
EMIT *abbr.* → enzyme-multiplied immunoassay technique.
e·mit [ɪˈmɪt] *vt* ausstoßen; (*Wärme*) ab-, ausstrahlen; aus-, verströmen; absondern, ausscheiden; *phys.* emittieren, aussenden.
em·men·a·gogue [əˈmenəgɒg, -gɑg, əˈmiːnə-] *n pharm.* Emmenagogum *nt.*
em·men·ia [əˈmenɪə, əˈmiːn-] *n* Monatsblutung *f*, Periode *f*, Regel *f*, Menses *pl*, Menstruation *f.*
em·men·ic [əˈmenɪk, əˈmiːn-] *adj* Menstruation betr., menstrual, Menstruations-, Regel-.
Emmet [ˈemət]: **E.'s operation** *gyn.* Emmet-Operation *f*, Trachelorrhaphie *f.*
em·me·trope [ˈemɪtrəʊp] *n ophthal.* Normalsichtige(r *m*) *f*, Emmetrope(r *m*) *f.*
em·me·tro·pia [ˌemɪˈtrəʊpɪə] *n ophthal.* Normalsichtigkeit *f*, Emmetropie *f abbr.* E.
em·me·trop·ic [ˌemɪˈtrɒpɪk, -ˈtrəʊp-] *adj ophthal.* Emmetropie betr., normalsichtig, emmetrop.
Em·mon·sia [ɪˈmɒnsɪə] *n micro.* Emmonsia *f.*
Em·mon·si·el·la capsulata [ɪmɒnsaɪˈelə] *micro.* Emmonsiella capsulata *f.*
em·o·din [ˈemədɪn] *n* Emodin *nt.*
e·mol·lient [ɪˈmɒljənt] **I** *n pharm.* erweichendes Mittel *nt*, Emolliens *nt*, Emollientium *nt.* **II** *adj* lindernd, beruhigend, weichmachend.
e·mo·tion [ɪˈməʊʃn] *n* Gefühl *nt*, Gefühlsregung *f*, Gemütsbewegung *f*, Emotion *f.*
e·mo·tion·a·ble [ɪˈməʊʃnəbl] *adj* erregbar.
e·mo·tion·al [ɪˈməʊʃnl] *adj* Gefühl *od.* Gemüt betr., emotional, emotionell, gefühlmäßig, -betont, seelisch, Gefühls-, Gemüts-.
emotional amenorrhea *gyn.* emotional-bedingte Amenorrhoe *f.*
emotional brain limbisches System *nt.*
emotional dependence psychische Abhängigkeit *f.*
emotional disorder Geistesstörung *f*, -krankheit *f.*
emotional disturbance 1. seelische Erregung *f.* **2.** Verhaltensstörung *f.*
e·mo·tion·al·ist [ɪˈməʊʃnlɪst] *n* Gefühlsmensch *m.*
e·mo·tion·al·i·ty [ɪˌməʊʃəˈnælətɪ] *n* emotionale Verhaltensweise *f*, Emotionalität *f.*
emotional leukocytosis Streßleukozytose *f.*
emotional outbreak Gefühlsausbruch *m.*
emotional overlay *psycho.* psychogene Überlagerung *f.*
emotional sweatening emotionales Schwitzen *nt.*
e·mo·tion·less [ɪˈməʊʃnlɪs] *adj* emotions-, gefühllos; ausdrucklos, ungerührt.
e·mo·tive [ɪˈməʊtɪv] *adj* emotiv, gefühlsbedingt; gefühlsbetont; gefühlvoll.
em·path·ic [emˈpæθɪk] *adj* einfühlend, empathisch.
em·pa·thize [ˈempəθaɪz] **I** *vt* s. einfühlen in. **II** *vi* Einfühlungsvermögen haben *od.* zeigen.
em·pa·thy [ˈempəθɪ] *n* Einfühlung(svermögen *nt*) *f*, Empathie *f.*
em·per·i·po·le·sis [emˌperɪpəʊˈliːsɪs] *n immun.* Emperipolesis *f.*
em·phrax·is [emˈfræksɪs] *n* (*Gefäß*) Verstopfung *f*, Blockierung *f*, Emphraxis *f.*
em·phy·se·ma [emfəˈsiːmə] *n* **1.** Aufblä-

emphysematous

hung *f*, Emphysem *nt*, Emphysema *nt*. 2. → e. of lung.
e. of lung Lungenemphysem, -blähung *f*, Emphysema pulmonum.
em·phy·sem·a·tous [ˌemfə'semətəs, -'siː-] *adj* emphysematig, emphysematös.
emphysematous asthma emphysematöses Asthma *nt*.
emphysematous bulla Emphysemblase *f*.
emphysematous cholecystitis emphysematöse Gallenblasenentzündung/Cholezystitis *f*, Cholecystitis emphysematosa.
emphysematous gangrene *patho.* Gasbrand *m*, -gangrän *f*, -ödem *nt*, -ödemerkrankung *f*, malignes Ödem *nt*, Gasphlegmone *f*, Gangraena emphysematosa.
emphysematous (pulmonary) sclerosis emphysematöse Lungensklerose *f*.
em·pir·ic [em'pırık] **I** *n* Empiriker(in *f*) *m*. **II** *adj* auf Erfahrung beruhend, empirisch, Erfahrungs-.
em·pir·i·cal [em'pırıkl] *adj* → empiric II.
empirical formula *chem.* empirische Formel *f*.
em·pir·i·cism [em'pırəsızəm] *n* Empirie *f*, Erfahrungsmethode *f*.
empiric treatment empirische Behandlung *f*.
em·plas·trum [em'plæstrəm] *n pharm.* Pflaster *nt*, Emplastrum *nt*.
em·pros·thot·o·nos [ˌempros'θɑtənəs] *n neuro., psychia.* Emprosthotonus *m*, Episthotonus *m*.
em·pros·thot·o·nus *n* → emprosthotonos.
emp·ty ['emptı] **I** *adj* leer. **~ of ohne. to take on an ~ stomach** auf nüchternen Magen nehmen. **II** *vt* 1. (aus-, ent-)leeren, leer machen. 2. leeren, (aus-)gießen (*into* in). **III** *vi* 3. leer werden, s. leeren. 4. (*Vene*) münden (*into* in). 5. (*Blase/Darm*) s. entleeren.
emp·ty·ing phase ['emptɪɪŋ] Entleerungsphase *f*.
empty intestine Jejunum *nt*, Intestinum jejunum.
empty sella syndrome *radiol.* Syndrom *nt* der leeren Sella.
emp·ty·sis ['emtəsıs] *n* 1. Aushusten *nt*, Abhusten *nt*, Expektoration *f*, Expektorieren *nt*. 2. Bluthusten *nt*, -spucken *nt*, Hämoptoe *f*, Hämoptyse *f*, Hämoptysis *f*.
empty weight Eigen-, Leergewicht *nt*.
em·py·e·ma [empaı'iːmə] *n, pl* **-mas, -ma·ta** [-mətə] Empyem *nt*, Empyema *nt*.
e. of the chest Pyothorax *m*, Thorax-, Pleuraempyem, eitrige Pleuritis *f*.
e. of the pericardium eitrige Perikarditis *f*, Pericarditis purulenta, Pyoperikard *nt*.
em·py·e·mic [empaı'iːmık] *adj* Empyem betr., empyemartig, empyematös, Empyem-.
em·py·o·cele [e'mpaıəsiːl] *n* 1. Empyozele *f*. 2. *ped.* Empyomphalus *m*.
em·py·reu·mat·ic [ˌempaıruː'mætık] *adj chem.* empyreumatisch.
e·mul·gent artery [ı'mʌldʒənt] Nierenarterie *f*, -schlagader *f*, Renalis *f*, A. renalis.
e·mul·si·ble [ı'mʌlsɪbl] *adj* → emulsifiable.
e·mul·si·fi·a·ble [ı'mʌlsəfaıəbl] *adj* emulgierbar.
e·mul·si·fi·ca·tion [ıˌmʌlsəfı'keıʃn] *n* Emulgieren *nt*, Emulgierung *f*.
e·mul·si·fi·er [ı'mʌlsəfaıə] *n* Emulgator *m*.
e·mul·si·fy [ı'mʌlsəfaı] *vt, vi* emulgieren.
e·mul·si·fy·ing agent [ı'mʌlsəfaıɪŋ] → emulsifier.
e·mul·sion [ı'mʌlʃn] *n* Emulsion *f*; *pharm.* Emulsio *f*.
emulsion colloid → emulsoid.

e·mul·sive [ı'mʌlsıf] *adj* emulgierend, Emulsions-.
e·mul·soid [ı'mʌlsɔıd] *n* Emulsionskolloid *nt*, Emulsoid *nt*.
e·mul·sum [ı'mʌlsəm] *n, pl* **-sa** [-sə] → emulsion.
ENA *abbr.* → extractable nuclear antigens.
e·nal·a·pril [ı'næləprıl] *n pharm.* Enalapril *nt*.
e·nam·el [ı'næml] **I** *n* 1. Email(le *f*) *nt*, Schmelzglas *nt*. 2. *techn.* Lack *m*, Glasur *f*, Schmelz *m*. 3. *anat.* (Zahn-)Schmelz *m*, Adamantin *nt*, Substantia adamantina, Enamelum *nt*. **II** *adj* 4. Email-, Emaillier-. 5. (Zahn-)Schmelz-. **III** *vt* emaillieren, glasieren, lackieren.
enamel cell → enameloblast.
enamel drop → enameloma.
e·nam·el·o·blast [ı'næmələʊblæst] *n* Adamanto-, Amelo-, Ganoblast *m*.
e·nam·e·lo·blas·to·ma [ˌ-blæs'təʊmə] *n* Adamantinom *nt*, Ameloblastom *nt*.
e·nam·e·lo·ma [ˌɪnæmə'ləʊmə] *n* Schmelzperle *f*, Enamelom *nt*.
enamel organ *embryo.* Schmelzorgan *nt*, Zahnglocke *f*.
enamel pearl → enameloma.
enamel prisms Schmelzprismen *pl*.
e·nam·e·lum [ı'næmıləm] *n* → enamel 3.
en·an·them [ı'nænθəm] *n* → enanthema.
en·an·the·ma [ˌɪnæn'θiːmə] *n, pl* **-ma·ta** [-mətə] Schleimhautausschlag *m*, Enanthem *nt*.
en·an·them·a·tous [ˌɪnæn'θemətəs] *adj* Enanthem betr., enanthematös, Enanthem-.
en·an·ti·o·bi·o·sis [ˌɪnæntɪəʊbaɪ'əʊsıs] *n bio.* Enantiobiose *f*.
en·an·ti·o·mer ['-mər] *n* optisches Isomer *nt*, Spiegelbildisomer *nt*, Enantiomer *nt*.
en·an·ti·om·er·ism [ˌɪnæntɪ'ɑmərızəm] *n* optische Isomerie *f*, Spiegelbildisomerie *f*, Enantiomerie *f*.
en·an·ti·o·morph [ı'næntɪəʊmɔːrf] *n* → enantiomer.
en·an·ti·o·mor·phic [ˌ-'mɔːrfık] *adj* Enantiomerie betr., enantiomer, spiegelbildisomer.
en·an·ti·o·mor·phism [ˌ-'mɔːrfızəm] *n* → enantiomerism.
en·ar·thro·di·al [ˌenɑːr'θrəʊdɪəl] *adj* Nußgelenk/Enarthrose betr., enarthrotisch.
enarthrodial articulation Nußgelenk *nt*, Enarthrose *f*, Artic. cotylica, Enarthrosis sph(a)eroidea.
enarthrodial joint → enarthrodial articulation.
en·ar·thro·sis [ˌenɑːr'θrəʊsıs] *n, pl* **-ses** [-siːz] → enarthrodial articulation.
en bloc [ɑ̃ blɒk] *adv* im ganzen, als Ganzes, en bloc.
en bloc excision *chir.* En-Bloc-Exzision *f*.
en bloc resection *chir.* En-Bloc-Resektion *f*.
en·can·this [en'kænθıs] *n ophthal.* Augenwinkelgeschwulst *f*, Enkanthis *f*.
en·cap·su·late [ın'kæpsəleıt, -sjəʊ-] **I** *vt* ein-, verkapseln. **II** *vi* s. verkapseln.
en·cap·su·lat·ed [ın'kæps(j)əleıtıd] *adj* verkapselt, eingekapselt.
encapsulated nerve ending sensibles Endorgan *nt*, Terminal-, Nervenendkörperchen *nt*, Corpusculum nervosum terminale.
en·cap·su·la·tion [ınˌkæps(j)ə'leıʃn] *n* Ver-, Einkapseln *nt*.
en·cap·sule [ın'kæpsəl, -sjʊl] *vt, vi* → encapsulate.
en·cap·suled [ın'kæpsjuːld] *adj* → encapsulated.
en·car·di·tis [enkɑːr'daıtıs] *n* → endocarditis.

en·case [en'keıs] *vt* umhüllen, umschließen; einschließen.
en·case·ment [en'keısmənt] *n* Umhüllung *f*, -schließung *f*; Einschließung *f*.
en·cas·ing cell [en'keısıŋ] Deck-, Mantel-, Hüllzelle *f*.
en·ceinte [ɑ̃'sɛ̃ːt] *adj* schwanger.
en·ce·li·i·tis [enˌsılı'aıtıs] *n patho.* Entzündung *f* eines Intraabdominalorgans.
en·ce·li·tis [ensı'laıtıs] *n* → enceliitis.
encephal- *pref.* → encephalo-.
en·ceph·a·lal·gia [enˌsefə'lældʒ(ı)ə] *n* Kopfschmerz(en *pl*) *m*, Kopfweh *nt*, Kephalgie *f*, Kephalalgie *f*, Kephal(a)ea *f*, Cephalgia *f*, Cephalalgia *f*, Cephal(a)ea *f*, Kephalodynie *f*, Zephalgie *f*, Zephalalgie *f*.
en·ceph·a·lat·ro·phy [enˌsefə'lætrəfı] *n* Gehirnatrophie *f*.
en·ceph·al·aux·e [ˌ-'lɔːksı] *n* Gehirnhypertrophie *f*.
en·ceph·a·le·mia [ˌ-'liːmıə] *n* Hirnstauung *f*.
en·ce·phal·ic [ˌensı'fælık, ˌenkə-] *adj* Gehirn/Encephalon betr., enzephal, Hirn-, Gehirn-, Encephal(o)-, Enzephal(o)-.
encephalic angioma Hirnarterienangiom *nt*.
encephalic nerves Kopf-, Hirnnerven *pl*, Nn. craniales/encephalici.
encephalic trunk Hirnstamm *m*, Truncus cerebri/encephali.
encephalic vesicles *embryo.* Hirnbläschen *pl*.
en·ceph·a·lin [ın'sefəlın, en'kefə-] *n* → enkephalin.
en·ceph·a·lit·ic [enˌsefə'lıtık] *adj* Enzephalitis betr., von ihr betroffen, enzephalitisch, Enzephalitis-.
en·ceph·a·li·tis [ˌ-'laıtıs] *n* Gehirnentzündung *f*, Enzephalitis *f*, Encephalitis *f*.
encephalitis B japanische B-Enzephalitis *f* *abbr.* JBE, Encephalitis japonica B.
encephalitis C St. Louis-Enzephalitis *f* *abbr.* SLE.
encephalitis viruses *micro.* Enzephalitisviren *pl*, enzephalitis-verursachende Viren *pl*.
en·ceph·a·lit·o·gen [ˌ-'lıtədʒən] *n* enzephalitis-verursachendes Agens *nt*.
en·ceph·a·lit·o·gen·ic [ˌ-lıtə'dʒenık] *adj* enzephalitis-verursachend, -auslösend.
En·ce·phal·i·to·zo·on [enˌsı fælıtə'zəʊən] *n micro.* Encephalitozoon *nt*.
en·ce·phal·i·to·zo·no·sis [ˌ-zəʊə'nəʊsıs] *n* Encephalitozoon-Infektion *f*, Encephalitozoonosis *f*, -zoonose *f*.
en·ceph·a·li·za·tion [enˌsefələ'zeıʃn] *n* Enzephalisierung *f*, Enzephalisation *f*.
encephalization factor *abbr.* K Enzephalisierungs-, Enzephalisationsfaktor *m* *abbr.* K.
encephalo- *pref.* Gehirn-, Enzephal(o)-, Encephal(o)-.
encephalo-arteriography *n radiol.* Enzephaloarteriographie *f*, Hirnangiographie *f*.
en·ceph·a·lo·cele [en'sefələsiːl] *n* Hirnbruch *m*, Enzephalozele *f*, Hernia cerebri.
en·ceph·a·lo·cys·to·cele [ˌ-'sıstəsiːl] *n* Enzephalozystozele *f*.
en·ceph·a·lo·di·al·y·sis [ˌ-daı'æləsıs] *n* Gehirnerweichung *f*.
en·ceph·a·lo·dyn·ia [ˌ-'diːnıə] *n* Kopfschmerz(en *pl*) *m*, Kephalgie *f*, Zephalgie *f*, Cephalgia *f*, Cephalalgia *f*, Cephal(a)ea *f*, Kephal(a)ea *f*, Kephalalgie *f*, Kephalodynie *f*.
en·ceph·a·lo·dys·pla·sia [ˌ-dıs'pleıʒ(ı)ə, -zıə] *n embryo.* angeborene Gehirnfehlbildung *od.* -anomalie *f*.

en·ceph·a·lo·fa·cial angiomatosis [‚-'feɪʃl] Sturge-Weber(-Krabbe)-Krankheit *f*, -Syndrom *nt*, enzephalofaziale Angiomatose *f*, Neuroangiomatosis encephalofacialis, Angiomatosis encephalo-oculo--cutanea, Angiomatosis encephalotrigeminalis.
en·ceph·a·lo·gram [en'sefələgræm] *n radiol.* Enzephalogramm *nt*.
en·ceph·a·log·ra·phy [en‚sefə'lagrəfɪ] *n radiol.* Enzephalographie *f*.
en·ceph·a·loid [en'sefəlɔɪd] **I** *n* medulläres Karzinom *nt*, Ca. medullare. **II** *adj* gehirn- *od.* gehirnsubstanzähnelnd, gehirnähnlich, enzephaloid.
encephaloid cancer/carcinoma → encephaloid I.
en·ceph·a·lo·lith [en'sefələlɪθ] *n* Hirnkonkrement *nt*, Enzephalolith *m*.
en·ceph·a·lo·ma [‚ensəfə'ləʊmə] *n* 1. *patho.* Hirntumor *m*, -geschwulst *f*, Enzephalom *nt*. 2. → encephaloid I.
en·ceph·a·lo·ma·la·cia [en‚sefələmə'leɪʃ(ɪ)ə] *n patho., neuro.* (Ge-)Hirnerweichung *f*, Enzephalo-, Encephalomalazie *f*, Encephalomalacia *f*.
en·ceph·a·lo·men·in·gi·tis [‚-menɪn'dʒaɪtɪs] *n* Entzündung *f* von Gehirn u. Hirnhäuten, Enzephalo-, Encephalomeningitis *f*, Meningoenzephalitis *f*, -encephalitis *f*.
en·ceph·a·lo·me·nin·go·cele [‚-mɪ'nɪŋgəsi:l] *n* Enzephalomeningozele *f*, Meningoenzephalozele *f*.
en·ceph·a·lo·me·nin·gop·a·thy [‚-mɪnɪŋ'ɡɑpəθɪ] *n* Erkrankung *f* von Gehirn u. Hirnhäuten, Enzephalomeningopathie *f*, Meningoenzephalopathie *f*.
en·ceph·a·lo·mere ['-mɪər] *n embryo.* Neuromer *nt*.
en·ceph·a·lom·e·ter [en‚sefə'lamɪtər] *n* Enzephalometer *nt*.
en·ceph·a·lo·my·e·li·tis [en‚sefələʊmaɪə'laɪtɪs] *n* Entzündung *f* von Gehirn u. Rückenmark, Enzephalomyelitis *f*, Encephalomyelitis *f*.
en·ceph·a·lo·my·el·o·cele [‚-maɪ'eləsi:l] *n* Enzephalomyelozele *f*.
en·ceph·a·lo·my·e·lo·men·in·gi·tis [‚-‚maɪəlɔʊ‚menɪn'dʒaɪtɪs] *n* Enzephalomyelomeningitis *f*.
en·ceph·a·lo·my·e·lo·neu·rop·a·thy [‚-‚maɪələʊnjʊə'rɑpəθɪ] *n* Erkrankung *f* von Gehirn, Rückenmark u. peripheren Nerven, Enzephalomyeloneuropathie *f*.
en·ceph·a·lo·my·e·lon·ic axis [‚-maɪə'lɔnɪk] Zentralnervensystem *nt abbr.* ZNS, Gehirn u. Rückenmark *nt*, Systema nervosum centrale, Pars centralis systematis nervosi.
en·ceph·a·lo·my·e·lop·a·thy [‚-maɪə'lɑpəθɪ] *n* Erkrankung *f* von Gehirn u. Rückenmark, Enzephalomyelopathie *f*.
en·ceph·a·lo·my·e·lo·ra·dic·u·li·tis [‚-‚maɪələʊrə‚dɪkjə'laɪtɪs] *n* Entzündung *f* von Gehirn, Rückenmark u. Spinalnervenwurzeln, Enzephalomyeloradikulitis *f*.
en·ceph·a·lo·my·e·lo·ra·dic·u·lo·neu·ri·tis [‚-‚maɪələʊrə‚dɪkjələʊnjʊə'raɪtɪs] *n* Guillain-Barré-Syndrom *nt*, (Poly-)Radikuloneuritis *f*, Neuronitis *f*.
en·ceph·a·lo·my·e·lo·ra·dic·u·lop·a·thy [‚-‚maɪələʊrə‚dɪkjələ'lɑpəθɪ] *n* Erkrankung *f* von Gehirn, Rückenmark u. Spinalnervenwurzeln, Enzephalomyeloradikulopathie *f*.
en·ceph·a·lo·my·o·car·di·tis [‚-‚maɪəkɑ:r'daɪtɪs] *n abbr.* **EMC** Enzephalomyokarditis *f*, Encephalomyocarditis *f abbr.* EMC, EMC-Syndrom *nt*.
en·ceph·a·lon [ɪn'sefəlɑn, -lən, en'kefə-] *n*, *pl* **-la** [-lə] Gehirn *nt*, Enzephalon *nt*, Encephalon *nt*.
encephalo-ophthalmic dysplasia Reese--Syndrom *nt*, Krause-Reese-Syndrom *nt*, Dysplasia encephalo-ophthalmica.
en·ceph·a·lo·path·ia [en‚sefələʊ'pæθɪə] *n* → encephalopathy.
en·ceph·a·lo·path·ic [‚-'pæθɪk] *adj* Enzephalopathie betr., enzephalopathisch.
en·ceph·a·lop·a·thy [en‚sefə'lɑpəθɪ] *n* Enzephalopathie *f*, Encephalopathia *f*.
en·ceph·a·lo·punc·ture [en‚sefələʊpʌŋ(k)tʃər] *n* Hirnpunktion *f*.
en·ceph·a·lo·py·o·sis [‚-paɪ'əʊsɪs] *n* eitrige/purulente Hirnentzündung *f*, Hirneiterung *f*.
en·ceph·a·lo·ra·chid·i·an [‚-rə'kɪdɪən] *adj* 1. Gehirn/Encephalon u. Rückenmark/Medulla spinalis betr. *od.* verbindend, enzephalospinal. 2. Großhirn/Cerebrum u. Rückenmark/Medulla spinalis betr. *od.* verbindend, zerebro-, cerebrospinal.
en·ceph·a·lo·ra·dic·u·li·tis [‚-rə‚dɪkjə'laɪtɪs] *n* Entzündung *f* von Gehirn u. Spinalnervenwurzeln, Enzephaloradikulitis *f*.
en·ceph·a·lor·rha·gia [‚-'rædʒ(ɪ)ə] *n* 1. Hirn(ein)blutung *f*, Enzephalorrhagie *f*. 2. apoplektischer Insult *m*, Apoplexie *f*, Apoplexia cerebri.
en·ceph·a·los·chi·sis [en‚sefə'lɑskəsɪs] *n embryo.* Enzephaloschisis *f*.
en·ceph·a·lo·scle·ro·sis [en‚sefələʊsklɪə'rəʊsɪs] *n* Hirnsklerose *f*, Enzephalosklerose *f*.
en·ceph·a·lo·scope [en'sefələskəʊp] *n* Enzephaloskop *nt*.
en·ceph·a·los·co·py [en‚sefə'lɑskəpɪ] *n* Enzephaloskopie *f*.
en·ceph·a·lo·sep·sis [en‚sefələ'sepsɪs] *n* Gehirngangrän *f*.
en·ceph·a·lo·sis [en‚sefə'ləʊsɪs] *n* organische/degenerative Hirnerkrankung *f*, Enzephalose *f*.
en·ceph·a·lo·spi·nal [en‚sefələʊ'spaɪnl] *adj* 1. Gehirn/Encephalon u. Rückenmark/Medulla spinalis betr. *od.* verbindend, enzephalospinal. 2. Großhirn/Cerebrum u. Rückenmark/Medulla spinalis betr. *od.* verbindend, zerebro-, cerebrospinal.
encephalospinal axis Zentralnervensystem *nt abbr.* ZNS, Gehirn u. Rückenmark *nt*, Systema nervosum centrale, Pars centralis systematis nervosi.
encephalospinal ganglia Spinalganglien *pl* der Hirn- u. Rückenmarksnerven, Ggll. craniospinalia/encephalospinalia/sensoria.
en·ceph·a·lo·thlip·sis [en‚sefələʊ'θlɪpsɪs] *n* Hirnkompression *f*.
en·ceph·a·lo·tome [en'sefələtəʊm] *n gyn., neurochir.* Enzephalotom *nt*.
en·ceph·a·lot·o·my [en‚sefə'lɑtəmɪ] *n* 1. *neurochir.* operativer Hirnschnitt *m*, Enzephalotomie *f*. 2. *gyn.* Enzephalotomie *f*, Kraniotomie *f*.
en·ceph·a·lo·tri·gem·i·nal angiomatosis [‚-traɪ'dʒemɪnl] → encephalofacial angiomatosis.
En·ces·to·da [ense'stəʊdə] *pl micro.* Bandwürmer *pl*, Zestoden *pl*, Cestoda *pl*, Cestodes *pl*.
en·chon·dral [en'kɑndrəl, en-] *adj* → endochondral.
en·chon·dro·ma [‚enkɑn'drəʊmə] *n* echtes/zentrales (Osteo-)Chondrom *nt*, Enchondrom *nt*.
en·chon·dro·ma·to·sis [en‚kɑndrəmə'təʊsɪs] *n* Ollier'-Erkrankung *f*, -Syndrom *nt*, Enchondromatose *f*, multiple kongenitale Enchondrome *pl*, Hemichondrodystrophie *f*.
en·chon·dro·ma·tous [‚enkɑn'drɑmətəs] *adj* Enchondrom betr., enchondromartig, enchondromatös.
en·chon·dro·sar·co·ma [en‚kɑndrəsɑ:r'kəʊmə] *n patho.* zentrales Chondrosarkom *nt*, Enchondrosarkom *nt*.
en·chon·dro·sis [enkɑn'drəʊsɪs] *n* 1. Enchondrose *f*, Enchondrosis *f*. 2. → enchondroma.
en·chy·le·ma [enkaɪ'li:mə] *n histol.* Plasmasaft *m*, Enchylem(a) *nt*.
en·cia·vo·ma [enklə'vəʊmə] *n patho.* Speicheldrüsenmischtumor *m*.
en·clit·ic [en'klɪtɪk] *adj gyn.* enklitisch.
en·code [ɪn'kəʊd] *vi* verschlüsseln, kodieren, codieren.
en·code·ment [ɪn'kəʊdmənt] *n* Verschlüsselung *f*, Chiffrierung *f*, Kodierung *f*, Codierung *f*.
en·cop·re·sis [enkɑ'pri:sɪs] *n* Einkoten *nt*, Enkopresis *f*.
en·cra·ni·al [en'kreɪnɪəl] *adj* → endocranial.
en·cra·ni·us [en'kreɪnɪəs] *n embryo.* Enkranius *m*.
en·cy·e·sis [ensaɪ'i:sɪs] *n gyn.* (regelrechte intrauterine) Schwangerschaft *f*.
en·cy·o·py·e·li·tis [ensaɪə‚paɪə'laɪtɪs] *n gyn.* Schwangerschaftspyelitis *f*.
en·cyst [en'sɪst] **I** *vt* einkapseln, enzystieren. **II** *vi s.* einkapseln, enzystieren.
en·cys·ta·tion [ensɪs'teɪʃn] *n* → encystment.
en·cyst·ed [en'sɪstɪd] *adj* verkapselt, enzystiert.
encysted calculus verkapselter Blasenstein *m*.
encysted hernia *chir.* Hey-Hernie *f*, Hernia encystica.
encysted peritonitis 1. Peritonitis encapsulans. 2. Bauchfell-, Peritonealabszeß *m*.
en·cyst·ment [en'sɪstmənt] *n* Ver-, Einkapseln *nt*; Ver-, Einkapselung *f*, Enzystierung *f*.
end- *pref.* → endo-.
end [end] **I** *n* 1. (*örtlich, zeitlich*) Ende *nt*. 2. Ende *nt*, Spitze *f*; Rest *m*, Endstück *nt*, Stummel *m*. 3. Tod *m*. 4. Ergebnis *nt*, Resultat *nt*. **II** *vt* 5. beenden. 6. töten, umbringen. **III** *vi* enden, aufhören.
end·an·ge·i·tis *n* → endangiitis.
en·dan·ger [en'deɪndʒər] *vi* in Gefahr bringen, gefährden.
en·dan·gered [en'deɪndʒərd] *adj* gefährdet, in Gefahr; *bio.* vom Aussterben bedroht.
en·dan·gi·i·tis [‚endændʒɪ'aɪtɪs] *n* Entzündung *f* der Gefäßinnenwand, Endang(i)itis *f*, Endango(i)itis *f*.
en·dan·gi·um [en'dændʒɪəm] *n* Gefäßinnenwand *f*, Endangium *nt*, Intima *f*, Tunica intima (vasorum).
end·a·or·ti·tis [‚endeɪɔ:r'taɪtɪs] *n* Entzündung *f* der Aortenintima, Endaortitis *f*.
end·ar·ter·ec·to·my [‚endɑ:rtə'rektəmɪ] *n chir.* Ausschälplastik *f*, Endarteriektomie *f*, Intimektomie *f*.
end·ar·te·ri·al [‚endɑ:r'tɪərɪəl] *adj* in einer Arterie (liegend), end-, intraarteriell.
end·ar·te·ri·tis [‚endɑ:rtə'raɪtɪs] *n* Entzündung *f* der Arterienintima, Endarter(i)itis *f*, Endoarter(i)itis *f*.
end·ar·te·ri·um [‚endɑ:r'tɪərɪəm] *n* Arterienintima *f*.
end artery Endarterie *f*.
end·au·ral [end'ɔ:rəl] *adj* im Ohr (liegend), endaural.
end·brain ['endbreɪn] *n* 1. Endhirn *nt*, Telenzephalon *nt*, -cephalon *nt*. 2. → endbrain vesicle.
endbrain vesicle *embryo.* Endhirnbläschen *nt*, Telencephalon *nt*.

end-brush

end-brush *n histol.* Endbäumchen *nt*, Telodendron *nt*.
end-bud *n embryo.* End-, Schwanzknospe *f*.
end bulb Endkörperchen *nt*, -kolben *m*.
  e. of Krause Krause'-Endkolben *pl*, Corpuscula bulboidea.
end-chon-dral [end'kɑndrəl] *adj* → endochondral.
end colostomy *chir.* endständiger Dickdarmafter *m*, endständiges Kolostoma *nt*.
end-diastolic *adj* enddiastolisch.
end-diastolic pressure enddiastolischer (Füllungs-)Druck *m*.
end-diastolic volume enddiastolisches Füllungsvolumen *nt*.
en-deic-tic [en'daɪktɪk] *adj* Symptom(e) betr., auf Symptomen beruhend, kennzeichnend, bezeichnend, symptomatisch (*of* für).
en-de-mia [en'diːmɪə] *n* Endemie *f*, endemische Krankheit *f*.
en-de-mi-al [en'diːmɪəl] *adj* → endemic II.
en-dem-ic [en'demɪk] I *n* → endemia. II *adj* endemisch.
en-dem-i-cal [en'demɪkl] *adj* → endemic II.
endemic disease → endemia.
endemic goiter endemische Struma *f*, Jodmangelstruma *f*.
endemic hematuria Urogenitalbilharziose *f*, (Harn-)Blasenbilharziose *f*, Schistosomiasis urogenitalis.
endemic hemoptysis parasitäre Hämoptoe/Hämoptyse *f*.
en-de-mic-i-ty [ˌendə'mɪsətɪ] *n* 1. Endemie *f*. 2. *bio.* Endemismus *m*.
endemic neuritis Beriberi *f*, Vitamin B₁-Mangel(krankheit *f*) *m*, Thiaminmangel(krankheit *f*) *m*.
endemic osteoarthritis Kaschin-Beck-Krankheit *f*, -Syndrom *nt*.
endemic paralytic vertigo *neuro.* Vertigo epidemica.
endemic poliomyelitis endemische Poliomyelitis *f*.
endemic polyneuritis → endemic neuritis.
endemic relapsing fever endemisches Rückfallfieber *nt*, Zeckenrückfallfieber *nt*.
endemic syphilis Bejel *f*, endemische Syphilis *f*.
endemic typhus endemisches/murines Fleckfieber *nt*, Ratten-, Flohfleckfieber *nt*.
en-de-mism ['endəmɪzəm] *n* → endemicity.
en-de-mo-ep-i-dem-ic [ˌendɪməʊepɪ'demɪk] I *n* Endemoepidemie *f*. II *adj* endemoepidemisch.
end-er-gon-ic [ˌendər'gɑnɪk] *adj chem.* energieverbrauchend, endergon(isch).
endergonic reaction endergone/endergonische Reaktion *f*.
en-der-mat-ic [endər'mætɪk] *adj* → endermic.
en-der-mic [en'dɜrmɪk] *adj* in der Haut (befindlich), in die Haut (eingeführt), endermal, intrakutan.
en-der-mism [en'dɜrmɪzəm] *n pharm.* endermale/intrakutane Medikation *f*.
en-der-mo-sis [endər'məʊsɪs] *n* Endermose *f*.
end-feet *pl* synaptische Endknöpfchen *pl*, Boutons terminaux.
end-flake *n* → end-plate.
end-group analysis *biochem.* Endgruppenanalyse *f*, -bestimmung *f*.
end-ing ['endɪŋ] *n* 1. *histol.* Endigung *f*. 2. Ende *nt*, Schluß *m*; Beendigung *f*, Abschluß *m*. 3. Tod *m*, Ende *nt*.

end-less ['endlɪs] *adj* endlos, ohne Ende, unendlich, Endlos-.
endless chain geschlossene *od.* endlose Kette *f*.
end-nuclei *pl* Ncc. terminationis.
Endo ['endəʊ]: **E. agar** Endoagar *m/nt*.
  E.'s fuchsin agar Endo-Fuchsinagar *m/nt*.
  E.'s medium → E. agar.
endo- *pref.* Intra-, End(o)-.
en-do-ab-dom-i-nal [ˌendəʊæb'dɑmɪnl] *adj* innerhalb des Abdomens (liegend), endo-, intraabdominal.
endoabdominal fascia Fascia transversalis.
endo-amylase *n* α-Amylase *f*, Endoamylase *f*.
en-do-an-eu-rys-mo-plas-ty [ˌænjə'rɪzməplæstɪ] *n* → endoaneurysmorrhaphy.
en-do-an-eu-rys-mor-rha-phy [ˌænjərɪz'mɑrəfɪ] *n chir.* Endoaneurysmorrhaphie *f*.
en-do-an-gi-i-tis [ˌændʒɪ'aɪtɪs] *n* → endangiitis.
en-do-a-or-ti-tis [ˌeɪɔːr'taɪtɪs] *n* → endoaortitis.
en-do-ap-pen-di-ci-tis [ˌəˌpendə'saɪtɪs] *n* Endoappendizitis *f*.
en-do-ar-te-ri-tis [ˌɑːrtə'raɪtɪs] *n* → endarteritis.
en-do-aus-cul-ta-tion [ˌɔːskəl'teɪʃn] *n* Endoauskultation *f*.
en-do-bi-o-sis [ˌbaɪ'əʊsɪs] *n micro., bio.* Endobiose *f*.
en-do-bi-ot-ic [ˌbaɪ'ɑtɪk] *adj micro., bio.* endobiotisch.
en-do-blast ['blæst] *n* → entoderm.
en-do-blas-tic ['blæstɪk] *adj* → entodermal.
en-do-bron-chi-al ['brɑŋkɪəl] *adj* innerhalb eines Bronchus (liegend), endo-, intrabronchial, Endobronchial-.
endobronchial anesthesia Endobronchialanästhesie *f*, -narkose *f*.
endobronchial catheter Endobronchialkatheter *m*.
endobronchial intubation endobronchiale Intubation *f*.
endobronchial tube Endobronchialtubus *m*.
en-do-bron-chi-tis [ˌbrɑn'kaɪtɪs] *n* Endobronchitis *f*.
en-do-cap-il-lar-y glomerulonephritis [ˌkə'pɪlərɪ] endokapilläre Glomerulonephritis *f*.
en-do-car-di-ac [ˌ'kɑːrdɪæk] *adj* → endocardial 2.
en-do-car-di-al [ˌ'kɑːrdɪəl] *adj* 1. im Herzinnern (liegend), endokardial. 2. Endokard betr., endokardial.
endocardial biopsy Endokardbiopsie *f*.
endocardial candidiasis Candida-Endokarditis *f*.
endocardial cushion *embryo.* Endokardkissen *nt*.
  atrioventricular e. Atrioventrikularkissen.
  truncoconal e. Trunkoconalkissen.
endocardial cushion defect Endokardkissendefekt *m*.
endocardial fibroelastosis Endokardfibroelastose *f*, Fibroelastosis endocardii.
endocardial fibrosis Endokardfibrose *f*.
endocardial sclerosis Endokardfibroelastose *f*, Fibroelastosis endocardii.
endocardial thrombus Endokardialthrombus *m*.
endocardial tube *embryo.* Endokardschlauch *m*.
en-do-car-di-op-a-thy [ˌkɑːrdɪ'ɑpəθɪ] *n* Endokarderkrankung *f*, Endokardopathie *f*.
en-do-car-dit-ic [ˌkɑːr'dɪtɪk] *adj* Endokarditis betr., endokarditisch, Endokarditis-.

en-do-car-di-tis [ˌkɑːr'daɪtɪs] *n* Endokardentzündung *f*, Endokarditis *f*, Endocarditis *f*.
en-do-car-di-um [ˌ'kɑːrdɪəm] *n, pl* **-dia** [-dɪə] innerste Herzwandschicht *f*, Endokard *nt*, Endocardium *nt*.
en-do-cel-lu-lar [ˌ'seljələr] *adj* innerhalb einer Zelle (liegend), intrazellulär.
en-do-cer-vi-cal [ˌ'sɜrvɪkl, -sə:'vaɪkl] *adj gyn.* im Zervikalkanal (liegend), endozervikal, Endozervix-.
endocervical carcinoma *gyn.* Zervixhöhlenkarzinom *nt*.
en-do-cer-vi-ci-tis [ˌsɜrvə'saɪtɪs] *n gyn.* Endozervixentzündung *f*, Endozervizitis *f*, -cervicitis *f*, Endometritis cervicis.
en-do-cer-vix [ˌ'sɜrvɪks] *n* 1. Halskanal *m* der Zervix, Zervikalkanal *m*, Endozervix *f*. 2. Schleimhaut(auskleidung *f*) *f* des Zervikalkanals, Endozervix *f*.
en-do-chon-dral [ˌ'kɑndrəl] *adj* in Knorpel entstehend *od.* liegend *od.* auftretend, endochondral, enchondral, intrakartilaginär.
endochondral bone Ersatzknochen *m*.
endochondral ossification en(do)chondrale Knochenbildung/Verknöcherung *f*, Ossifikation/Osteogenese *f*.
en-do-coch-le-ar potential [ˌ'kɑklɪər, -'kəʊ-] kochleäres Bestandspotential *nt*.
en-do-co-li-tis [ˌkə'laɪtɪs] *n* Entzündung *f* der Kolonschleimhaut, katarrhalische Kolitis *f*, Endokolitis *f*.
en-do-col-pi-tis [ˌkɑl'paɪtɪs] *n gyn.* Entzündung *f* der Scheidenschleimhaut, Endokolpitis *f*.
en-do-com-men-sal [ˌkə'mensəl] *n micro.* Endokommensale *m*.
en-do-cor-pus-cu-lar [ˌkɔːr'pʌskjələr] *adj* endo-, intrakorpuskulär.
en-do-cra-ni-al [ˌ'kreɪnɪəl] *adj* 1. im Schädel/Cranium (liegend), endokranial, intrakranial, -kraniell. 2. Endokranium betr., endokranial, Endokranium-.
en-do-cra-ni-tis [ˌkreɪ'naɪtɪs] *n* Endokranitis *f*, Pachymeningitis externa.
en-do-cra-ni-um [ˌ'kreɪnɪəm] *n, pl* **-nia** [-nɪə] Endokranium *nt*, -cranium *nt*, Dura mater encephali.
en-do-cri-nal [ˌendə'kraɪnl, -'krɪnl] *adj* → endocrine II.
en-do-crine ['krɪn, -kraɪn] I *n* 1. → endocrine gland. 2. innere Sekretion *f*, Inkretion *f*. II *adj* Endokrinum betr., mit innerer Sekretion, endokrin.
endocrine-active *adj* endokrin-aktiv.
endocrine atrophy endokrine/endokrinogene Atrophie *f*.
endocrine cells of gut basalgekörnte Zellen *pl*.
endocrine exophthalmus endokriner Exophthalmus *m*.
endocrine fracture Fraktur *f* bei Endokrinopathie.
endocrine gigantism endokriner/endokrinbedingter Riesenwuchs *m*.
endocrine gland Drüse *f* mit innerer Sekretion, endokrine Drüse *f*, Gl. endocrina, Gl. sine ductibus.
endocrine hypertension endokrine Hypertonie *f*, endokrinbedingter Hochdruck *m*.
endocrine-inactive *adj* endokrin-inaktiv.
endocrine ophthalmopathy endokrine Ophthalmopathie *f*, endokrine Orbitopathie *f*.
endocrine osteoporosis endokrine/hormonale Osteoporose *f*.
endocrine part of pancreas endokrines Pankreas(teil *nt*) *nt*, Langerhans'-Inseln *pl*, Inselorgan *nt*, Pars endocrina pancreatis.

endocrine polyglandular syndrome *abbr.* **EPS** multiple endokrine Adenopathie *f abbr.* **MEA**, multiple endokrine Neoplasie *f abbr.* **MEN**, pluriglanduläre Adenomatose *f.*
endocrine system → endocrinium.
en·do·crin·ic [ˌ-ˈkrɪnɪk] *adj* → endocrine II.
en·do·crin·i·um [ˌ-ˈkrɪnɪəm] *n* endokrines System *nt,* Endokrin(i)um *nt.*
en·do·crin·o·log·ic sex [ˌ-ˌkrɪnəˈlɑdʒɪk, -ˌkraɪ-] endokrinologisches/phänotypisches Geschlecht *nt.*
en·do·cri·nol·o·gist [ˌ-krɪˈnɑlədʒɪst, -kraɪ-] *n* Endokrinologe *m,* -login *f.*
en·do·cri·nol·o·gy [ˌ-krɪˈnɑlədʒɪ, -kraɪ-] *n* Endokrinologie *f.*
en·do·cri·nop·a·thy [ˌ-krɪˈnɑpəθɪ] *n* Endokrinopathie *f.*
en·do·crin·o·ther·a·py [ˌ-krɪnəˈθerəpɪ] *n* Endokrinotherapie *f;* Hormontherapie *f.*
en·do·crin·o·trop·ic [ˌ-krɪnəˈtrɑpɪk, -ˈtroʊp-] *adj* endokrinotrop.
en·doc·ri·nous [enˈdɑkrɪnəs] *adj* → endocrine II.
en·do·cyc·lic [ˌendoʊˈsɪklɪk] *adj chem.* endozyklisch.
en·do·cyst [ˈ-sɪst] *n micro.* Endozyste *f.*
en·do·cys·ti·tis [ˌ-sɪsˈtaɪtɪs] *n urol.* Entzündung *f* der Blasenschleimhaut, Endozystitis *f,* -cystitis *f.*
en·do·cyte [ˈ-saɪt] *n* Endozyt *m.*
en·do·cy·to·sis [ˌ-saɪˈtoʊsɪs] *n* Endozytose *f.*
en·do·de·ox·y·ri·bo·nu·cle·ase [ˌ-dɪˌɑksɪˌraɪboʊˈn(j)uːkleɪz] *n* Endodesoxyribonuklease *f.*
en·do·derm [ˈ-dɜrm] *n* → entoderm.
en·do·der·mal [ˌ-ˈdɜrml] *adj* → entodermal.
endodermal cell endodermale Zelle *f.*
en·do·der·mic [ˌ-ˈdɜrmɪk] *adj* → entodermal.
en·do·don·ti·um [ˌ-ˈdɑnʃɪəm] *n* Zahnpulpa *f,* Pulpa dentis.
en·do·en·ter·i·tis [ˌ-entəˈraɪtɪs] *n* Entzündung *f* der Darmschleimhaut, Endoenteritis *f.*
en·do·en·zyme [ˌ-ˈenzaɪm] *n* Endoenzym *nt,* intrazelluläres Enzym *nt.*
en·do·ep·i·der·mal [ˌ-epɪˈdɜrml] *adj* innerhalb der Epidermis (liegend), intra-, endoepidermal.
en·do·ep·i·the·li·al [ˌ-epɪˈθiːlɪəl] *adj* innerhalb des Epithels (liegend), intra-, endoepithelial.
endoepithelial gland endoepitheliale/intraepitheliale Drüse *f.*
en·do·er·gic [ˌ-ˈɜrdʒɪk] *adj* endoerg(isch).
en·do·e·soph·a·gi·tis [ˌ-ɪˌsɑfəˈdʒaɪtɪs] *n* Entzündung *f* der Ösophagusschleimhaut, Endoösophagitis *f.*
en·do·gam·ic [ˌ-ˈgæmɪk] *adj* → endogamous.
en·dog·a·mous [enˈdɑgəməs] *adj micro.* endogam.
en·dog·a·my [enˈdɑgəmɪ] *n micro.* Endogamie *f.*
en·do·gan·gli·on·ic [ˌendoʊˌgæŋglɪˈɑnɪk] *adj* innerhalb eines Ganglions (liegend), intra-, endoganglionär.
en·do·gas·trec·to·my [ˌ-gæsˈtrektəmɪ] *n chir.* operative Entfernung *f* der Magenschleimhaut, Endogastrektomie *f.*
en·do·gas·tric [ˌ-ˈgæstrɪk] *adj* im Magen (liegend), endo-, intragastral.
en·do·gas·tri·tis [ˌ-gæsˈtraɪtɪs] *n* Magenschleimhautentzündung *f,* Endogastritis *f;* Gastritis *f.*
en·do·ge·net·ic [ˌ-dʒəˈnetɪk] *adj* → endogenous.
en·do·gen·ic [ˌ-ˈdʒenɪk] *adj* → endogenous.

endogenic toxicosis Selbstvergiftung *f,* Autointoxikation *f.*
en·dog·e·nous [enˈdɑdʒənəs] *adj* 1. im Innern entstehend *od.* befindlich, nicht von außen zugeführt, endogen. 2. aus innerer Ursache, von innen kommend, anlagebedingt, endogen.
endogenous cycle *micro.* endogener Zyklus *m.*
endogenous depression *psychia.* endogene Depression *f.*
endogenous eczema *derm.* endogenes/atopisches/exsudatives/neuropathisches/konstitutionelles Ekzem *nt,* atopische Dermatitis *f,* Ekzemkrankheit *f,* Eccema endogenicum.
endogenous infection endogene Infektion *f.*
endogenous pigment endogenes Pigment *nt,* Endopigment *nt.*
endogenous pyrogen *abbr.* **EP** endogenes Pyrogen *nt abbr.* **EP.**
endogenous reinfection endogene Reinfektion *f.*
endogenous retrovirus endogenes Retrovirus *nt.*
endogenous syndactyly endogene Syndaktylie *f.*
endogenous tubulopathy (*Niere*) endogene Tubulopathie *f.*
en·dog·e·ny [enˈdɑdʒənɪ] *n micro.* Endogenese *f,* Endogenie *f.*
en·do·glo·bar [ˌendoʊˈgloʊbər] *adj* → endoglobular.
en·do·glob·u·lar [ˌ-ˈglɑbjələr] *adj hema.* endo-, intraglobulär; intrakorpuskulär; intraerythrozytär.
en·do·her·ni·or·rha·phy [ˌ-ˌhɜrnɪˈɔrəfɪ] *n chir.* Endoherniorrhaphie *f.*
en·do·her·ni·ot·o·my [ˌ-ˌhɜrnɪˈɑtəmɪ] *n* → endoherniorrhaphy.
en·do·in·tox·i·ca·tion [ˌ-ɪnˌtɑksɪˈkeɪʃn] *n* Endo(toxin)intoxikation *f,* Autointoxikation *f.*
en·do·lab·y·rin·thi·tis [ˌ-ˌlæbərɪnˈθaɪtɪs] *n HNO* Endolabyrinthitis *f.*
en·do·la·ryn·ge·al [ˌ-ˌlɪˈrɪndʒ(ɪ)əl] *adj* innerhalb des Kehlkopfes (liegend), endo-, intralaryngeal.
En·do·li·max nana [ˌ-ˈlaɪmæks] *micro.* Endolimax nana *f.*
en·do·lu·mi·nal [ˌ-ˈluːmənl] *adj* endo-, intraluminal.
en·do·lymph [ˈendəlɪmf] *n* Endolymphe *f,* Endolympha *f.*
en·do·lym·pha [ˌ-ˈlɪmfə] *n* → endolymph.
en·do·lym·phat·ic [ˌ-lɪmˈfætɪk] *adj* Endolymphe betr., endolymphatisch.
endolymphatic duct Endolymphgang *m,* Ductus endolymphaticus.
endolymphatic hydrops Ménière'-Krankheit *f,* Morbus Ménière *m.*
endolymphatic labyrinth häutiges/membranöses Labyrinth *nt,* Labyrinthus membranaceus.
endolymphatic sac Saccus endolymphaticus.
en·dol·y·sin [enˈdɑləsɪn] *n* Endolysin *nt.*
en·dol·y·sis [enˈdɑləsɪs] *n histol.* Endolyse *f.*
en·do·mas·toid·i·tis [ˌendoʊˌmæstɔɪˈdaɪtɪs] *n HNO* Endomastoiditis *f.*
en·do·me·tri·al [ˌ-ˈmiːtrɪəl] *adj* Endometrium betr., endometrial, Endometrium-.
endometrial atrophy Endometriumatrophie *f.*
endometrial carcinoma Endometriumkarzinom *nt,* Ca. endometriale.
endometrial cyst Endometriumzyste *f.*
endometrial hyperplasia Endometriumhyperplasie *f,* Hyperplasia endometrii..
endometrial stroma Endometriumstroma *nt.*

en·do·me·tri·oid [ˌ-ˈmiːtrɪɔɪd] *adj* endometriumähnlich, endometrioid.
en·do·me·tri·o·ma [ˌ-miːtrɪˈoʊmə] *n gyn.* Endometriom *nt.*
en·do·me·tri·o·sis [ˌ-ˌmiːtrɪˈoʊsɪs] *n gyn.* Endometriose *f,* Endometriosis (externa) *f.*
en·do·me·tri·tis [ˌ-mɪˈtraɪtɪs] *n gyn.* Entzündung *f* der Gebärmutterschleimhaut, Endometriumentzündung *f,* Endometritis *f.*
en·do·me·tri·um [ˌ-ˈmiːtrɪəm] *n, pl* **-tria** [-trɪə] Gebärmutter-, Uterusschleimhaut *f,* Endometrium *nt,* Tunica mucosa uteri.
en·do·mi·to·sis [ˌ-maɪˈtoʊsɪs] *n* Endomitose *f.*
en·do·mi·tot·ic [ˌ-maɪˈtɑtɪk] *adj* Endomitose betr., endomitotisch.
en·do·mor·phic [ˌ-ˈmɔrfɪk] *adj* endomorph.
en·do·mor·phy [ˈ-mɔrfɪ] *n* Endomorphie *f.*
En·do·my·ces [ˌ-ˈmaɪsiːz] *n micro.* Endomyces *m.*
En·do·my·ce·ta·les [ˌ-ˌmaɪsəˈteɪliːz] *pl micro.* Endomycetales *pl.*
en·do·my·o·car·di·al [ˌ-ˌmaɪoʊˈkɑːrdɪəl] *adj* Endokard u. Myokard betr., endomyokardial, Endomyokard-.
endomyocardial fibrosis Endomyokardfibrose *f,* Endokardfibroelastose *f,* Endomyokardose *f.*
en·do·my·o·car·di·tis [ˌ-ˌmaɪoʊkɑːrˈdaɪtɪs] *n* Entzündung *f* von Endokard u. Myokard, Endomyokarditis *f.*
en·do·my·si·um [ˌ-ˈmiːzɪəm, -ʒɪəm] *n, pl* **-my·si·a** [-zɪə, -ʒɪə] Hüllgewebe *nt* der Muskelfaser, Endomysium *nt.*
en·do·na·sal [ˌ-ˈneɪzl] *adj* in der Nasenhöhle (liegend), endo-, intranasal.
en·do·neu·ral membrane [ˌ-ˈnjʊərəl, -ˈnɜr-] Schwann'-Scheide *f,* Neuri-, Neurolemm *nt,* Neurilemma *nt.*
endoneural sheath Endoneuralscheide *f.*
en·do·neu·ri·al [ˌ-ˈnjʊərɪəl, -ˈnɜr-] *adj* Endoneurium betr., Endoneurium-.
en·do·neu·ri·tis [ˌ-njʊəˈraɪtɪs, -nɜr-] *n* Endoneuriumentzündung *f,* Endoneuritis *f.*
en·do·neu·ri·um [ˌ-ˈnjʊərɪəm, -ˈnɜr-] *n, pl* **-ri·a** [-rɪə] Endoneurium *nt.*
en·do·neu·rol·y·sis [ˌ-njʊəˈrɑləsɪs, -nɜr-] *n neurochir.* interfaszikuläre Neurolyse *f,* Endoneurolyse *f.*
en·do·nu·cle·ar [ˌ-ˈn(j)uːklɪər] *adj histol.* im Zellkern (liegend), endonuklear, -nukleär, intranukleär.
en·do·nu·cle·ase [ˌ-ˈn(j)uːkliːeɪz] *n* Endonuklease *f,* -nuclease *f.*
en·do·par·a·site [ˌ-ˈpærəsaɪt] *n bio., micro.* Endo-, Entoparasit *m,* Endosit *m,* Binnen-, Innenparasit *m.*
en·do·pel·vic [ˌ-ˈpelvɪk] *adj* im Becken (liegend), endopelvin, intrapelvin.
endopelvic fascia viszerale Beckenfaszie *f,* Fascia endopelvina, Fascia pelvis visceralis.
en·do·pep·ti·dase [ˌ-ˈpeptɪdeɪz] *n* Endopeptidase *f,* Protei(n)ase *f.*
en·do·per·i·car·di·ac [ˌ-perɪˈkɑːrdɪæk] *adj* im Perikard (liegend), endo-, intraperikardial.
en·do·per·i·car·di·al [ˌ-perɪˈkɑːrdɪəl] *adj* Endokard u. Perikard betr., endoperikardial, Endoperikard-.
en·do·per·i·car·di·tis [ˌ-ˌperɪkɑːrˈdaɪtɪs] *n* Entzündung *f* von Endokard u. Perikard, Endoperikarditis *f.*
en·do·per·i·myo·car·di·tis [ˌ-ˌperɪˌmaɪoʊkɑːrˈdaɪtɪs] *n* Entzündung *f* von Endo-, Myo- u. Perikard, Endoperimyokarditis *f,* Endomyoperikarditis *f,* Pankarditis *f.*
en·do·per·i·neu·ri·tis [ˌ-ˌperɪnjʊəˈraɪtɪs,

endoperitoneal

-nʊ-] *n* Entzündung *f* von Endoneurium u. Perineurium, Endoperineuritis *f*.
en·do·per·i·to·ne·al [ˌperɪtəʊˈniːəl] *adj* innerhalb des Peritoneums (liegend), endo-, intraperitoneal.
en·do·per·ox·ide [ˌ-pəˈrɒksaɪd] *n* Endoperoxid *nt*.
en·do·phle·bi·tis [ˌ-flɪˈbaɪtɪs] *n* Entzündung *f* der Veneninnenwand, Endophlebitis *f*.
en·doph·thal·mi·tis [endəfθælˈmaɪtɪs] *n ophthal*. Endophthalmitis *f*, Endophthalmie *f*, Endophthalmia *f*.
en·do·phyte [ˈendəfaɪt] *n bot*. pflanzlicher Endoparasit *m*, Endophyt *m*.
en·do·phyt·ic [ˌ-ˈfɪtɪk] *adj* **1.** *bot.* Endophyt betr., endophytisch. **2.** *patho.* nach innen wachsend, endophytisch.
en·do·plasm [ˈendəʊplæzəm] *n* Endo(zyto)plasma *nt*, Entoplasma *nt*.
en·do·plas·mic [ˌ-ˈplæzmɪk] *adj* Endoplasma betr., im Endoplasma liegend, endoplasmatisch.
endoplasmic reticulum *abbr.* **ER** endoplasmatisches Retikulum *nt abbr*. ER.
agranular e. → smooth e.
granular e. → rough e.
rough e. *abbr.* **R-ER** rauhes/granuläres endoplasmatisches Retikulum *abbr.* R-ER, Ergastoplasma *nt*.
smooth e. *abbr.* **S-ER** glattes/agranuläres endoplasmatisches Retikulum *abbr.* S-ER.
en·do·plas·tic [ˌ-ˈplæstɪk] *adj* → endoplasmic.
en·do·pol·y·ploid [ˌ-ˈpɒlɪplɔɪd] *adj* Endopolyploidie betr., endopolyploid.
en·do·pol·y·ploi·dy [ˌ-ˈpɒlɪplɔɪdɪ] *n* **1.** Endopolyploidie *f*. **2.** → endomitosis.
en·do·pros·the·sis [ˌ-prɒsˈθiːsɪs] *n ortho., chir*. Endoprothese *f*.
en·do·ra·di·og·ra·phy [ˌ-reɪdɪˈɒgrəfɪ] *n* Endoradiographie *f*.
en·do·ra·di·o·sonde [ˌ-ˈreɪdɪəʊsɒnd] *n* Endoradiosonde *f*; Intestinalsender *m*.
en·do·re·du·pli·ca·tion [ˌ-rɪˌd(j)uːplɪˈkeɪʃn] *n genet*. Endoreduplikation *f*.
end-organ *n* **1.** sensibles Endorgan *nt*, Terminal-, Nervenendkörperchen *nt*, Corpusculum nervosum terminale. **2.** motorisches Endorgan *nt*, motorische Endplatte *f*.
en·do·rhi·ni·tis [ˌ-raɪˈnaɪtɪs] *n* Entzündung *f* der Nasenschleimhaut, Endorhinitis *f*.
en·dor·rha·chis [ˌ-ˈreɪkɪs] *n* äußeres Blatt *nt* der Dura mater spinalis, Endorrhachis *f*.
en·do·ri·bo·nu·cle·ase [ˌ-ˌraɪbəʊˈn(j)uːklɪeɪz] *n* Endoribonuklease *f*, -nuclease *f*.
en·dor·phin [enˈdɔːrfɪn] *n* Endorphin *nt*, Endomorphin *nt*.
en·do·sal·pin·gi·o·sis [ˌendəʊˌsælpɪndʒɪˈəʊsɪs] *n* → endosalpingosis.
en·do·sal·pin·gi·tis [ˌ-ˌsælpɪnˈdʒaɪtɪs] *n gyn*. Entzündung *f* der Tubenschleimhaut, Endosalpingitis *f*.
en·do·sal·pin·go·ma [ˌ-ˌsælpɪnˈgəʊmə] *n gyn*. Tubenadenomyom *nt*, Endosalpingom *nt*.
en·do·sal·pin·go·sis [ˌ-ˌsælpɪnˈgəʊsɪs] *n gyn*. **1.** Tubenendometriose *f*, Endometriosis tubae. **2.** Eierstock-, Ovarialendometriose *f*, Endometriosis ovarii.
en·do·sal·pinx [ˌ-ˈsælpɪŋks] *n, pl* **-sal·pin·ges** [-sælˈpɪndʒiːz] Tubenmukosa *f*, -schleimhaut *f*, Endosalpinx *f*, Tunica mucosa tubae uterinae.
en·do·sarc [ˈensɑːrk] *n micro.* Protozoenendoplasma *nt*.
en·do·scope [ˈ-skəʊp] *n* Endoskop *nt*.
en·do·scop·ic [ˌ-ˈskɒpɪk] *adj* Endoskop *od*.

Endoskopie betr., mittels Endoskop *od*. Endoskopie, endoskopisch.
endoscopic biopsy endoskopische Biopsie *f*.
endoscopic polypectomy endoskopische Polypenabtragung/Polypektomie *f*.
endoscopic retrograde cholangiography *abbr.* **ERC** endoskopische retrograde Cholangiographie *f abbr.* ERC.
endoscopic retrograde cholangiopancreatography *abbr.* **ERCP** endoskopische retrograde Cholangiopankreatographie *f abbr.* ERCP.
endoscopic retrograde pancreatography *abbr.* **ERP** endoskopische retrograde Pankreatographie *f abbr.* ERP.
endoscopic sclerotherapy endoskopische Sklerosierung/Sklerotherapie *f*.
en·dos·co·py [enˈdɒskəpɪ] *n* Spiegelung *f*, Endoskopie *f*.
en·do·se·cre·to·ry [ˌendəʊsɪˈkriːtərɪ] *adj* endosekretorisch; endokrin.
en·do·sep·sis [ˌ-ˈsepsɪs] *n patho*. Endosepsis *f*.
en·do·site [ˈ-saɪt] *n* → endoparasite.
en·do·skel·e·ton [ˌ-ˈskelɪtn] *n* Innen-, Endo-, Entoskelett *nt*.
en·dos·mom·e·ter [ˌendazˈmɒmɪtər] *n* Endosmometer *nt*.
en·dos·mo·sis [ˌendazˈməʊsɪs] *n phys*. Endosmose *f*.
en·dos·mot·ic [ˌendazˈmɒtɪk] *adj* Endosmose betr., endosmotisch.
en·do·some [ˈendəsəʊm] *n* Endosom *nt*.
en·do·sperm [ˈ-spɜːrm] *n bio*. Endosperm *nt*.
en·do·spore [ˈ-spɔːr, -spəʊr] *n micro*. Endospore *f*.
en·do·spo·ri·um [ˌ-ˈspɔːrɪəm] *n micro*. Endospor *nt*, Endosporium *nt*.
en·dos·te·al [enˈdɒstɪəl] *adj* **1.** Endost betr., endostal. **2.** im Knochen liegend *od*. auftretend, endostal, intraossär.
endosteal fibrosarcoma endostales Fibrosarkom *nt*.
en·dos·te·i·tis [enˌdɒstɪˈaɪtɪs] *n ortho*. Endostentzündung *f*, Endostitis *f*.
en·dos·te·o·ma [enˌdɒstɪˈəʊmə] *n* Endostom *nt*.
en·dos·te·um [enˈdɒstɪəm] *n, pl* **-tea** [-tɪə] innere Knochenhaut *f*, Endost *nt*, Endosteum *nt*.
en·dos·ti·tis [ˌendasˈtaɪtɪs] *n* → endosteitis.
en·dos·to·ma [ˌendasˈtəʊmə] *n* → endosteoma.
en·do·sym·bi·ont [ˌendəʊˈsɪmbɪˌɒnt] *n* Endosymbiont *m*.
en·do·sym·bi·o·sis [ˌ-ˌsɪmbɪˈəʊsɪs] *n* Endosymbiose *f*.
en·do·ten·din·e·um [ˌ-tenˈdɪnɪəm] *n* Endotenon *nt*, Endotendineum *nt*.
en·do·ten·on [ˌ-ˈtenən] *n* → endotendineum.
en·do·the·li·al [ˌ-ˈθiːlɪəl] *adj* Endothel betr., aus Endothel bestehend, endothelial, Endothel-.
endothelial cancer → endothelioma.
endothelial cell endothelial(e)zelle *f*.
endothelial cyst endotheliale Zyste *f*.
en·do·the·li·al·i·za·tion [ˌ-ˈθiːlɪˌælɪˈzeɪʃn] *n* Endothelialisierung *f*.
endothelial myeloma → Ewing's sarcoma.
endothelial pore Endothelpore *f*, -fenster *nt*.
endothelial tissue → endothelium.
endothelial tube *histol*. Endothelrohr *nt*.
endothelial window Endothelfenster *nt*.
en·do·the·li·i·tis [ˌ-θiːlɪˈaɪtɪs] *n* Endotheliumentzündung *f*, Endotheli(i)tis *f*.
en·do·the·li·o·blas·to·ma [ˌ-θiːlɪəblæsˈtəʊmə] *n* Endothelioblastom *nt*.

en·do·the·li·o·cho·ri·al [ˌ-θiːlɪəˈkɔːrɪəl] *adj histol.* endotheliochorial.
endotheliochorial placenta Placenta endotheliochorialis.
en·do·the·li·o·cyte [ˌ-ˈθiːlɪəsaɪt] *n hema*. Endotheliozyt *m*.
en·do·the·li·o·cy·to·sis [ˌ-ˌθiːlɪəsaɪˈtəʊsɪs] *n* Endotheliozytose *f*.
en·do·the·li·oid [ˌ-ˈθiːlɪɔɪd] *adj* endothelähnlich, endothelioid, Endothelioid-.
endothelioid cells *hema*. Endothelioidzellen *pl*.
en·do·the·li·ol·y·sin [ˌ-θiːlɪˈɒləsɪn] *n* Endotheliolysin *nt*.
en·do·the·li·o·lyt·ic [ˌ-ˈθiːlɪəˈlɪtɪk] *adj* endothelzerstörend, -auflösend, endotheliolytisch.
en·do·the·li·o·ma [ˌ-ˈθiːlɪˈəʊmə] *n* Endotheliom *nt*.
en·do·the·li·o·ma·to·sis [ˌ-ˌθiːlɪəməˈtəʊsɪs] *n* Endotheliomatose *f*.
en·do·the·li·o·my·o·ma [ˌ-ˌθiːlɪəmaɪˈəʊmə] *n old* Gefäß-, Angioleiomyom(a) *nt*.
en·do·the·li·o·sar·co·ma [ˌ-ˌθiːlɪəsɑːrˈkəʊmə] *n* Kaposi-Sarkom *nt*, Morbus Kaposi *m*, Retikuloangiomatose *f*, Angioretikulomatose *f*, idiopathisches multiples Pigmentsarkom Kaposi *nt*, Sarcoma idiopathicum multiplex haemorrhagicum.
en·do·the·li·o·sis [ˌ-ˈθiːlɪˈəʊsɪs] *n* Endotheliose *f*, Retikuloendotheliose *f*.
en·do·the·li·o·tox·in [ˌ-ˌθiːlɪəˈtɒksɪn] *n* Endotheliotoxin *nt*.
en·do·the·li·o·trop·ic [ˌ-ˌθiːlɪəˈtrɒpɪk, -ˈtrəʊp-] *adj* endotheliotrop.
en·do·the·li·um [ˌ-ˈθiːlɪəm] *n, pl* **-lia** [-lɪə] Endothel *nt*, Endothelium *nt*.
en·do·therm [ˈendəθɜːrm] *n* endothermer Organismus *m*.
en·do·ther·mal [ˌ-ˈθɜːrml] *adj* → endothermic.
endothermal reaction *chem*. endotherme Reaktion *f*.
en·do·ther·mic [ˌ-ˈθɜːrmɪk] *adj* Wärme von außen aufnehmend, wärmebindend, endotherm.
endothermic reaction → endothermal reaction.
en·do·tho·rac·ic [ˌ-θɔːˈræsɪk, -θəʊ-] *adj* im Thorax (liegend), endo-, intrathorakal.
endothoracic fascia endothorakale Faszie *f*, Fascia endothoracica.
en·do·thrix [ˈ-θrɪks] *n micro., derm*. Endothrix *nt*.
en·do·tox·e·mia [ˌ-tɑkˈsiːmɪə] *n* endogene Toxämie *f*, Endotoxämie *f*.
en·do·tox·ic bacterium [ˌ-ˈtɑksɪk] *micro*. endotoxinbildendes Bakterium *nt*.
en·do·tox·i·co·sis [ˌ-ˌtɑksɪˈkəʊsɪs] *n* Endotoxikose *f*.
endotoxic shock Endotoxinschock *m*.
en·do·tox·in [ˌ-ˈtɑksɪn] *n* Endotoxin *nt*.
endotoxin poisoning Endotoxinvergiftung *f*.
endotoxin shock → endotoxic shock.
en·do·tra·che·al [ˌ-ˈtreɪkɪəl] *adj* in der Luftröhre (liegend), endo-, intratracheal.
endotracheal anesthesia Endotrachealanästhesie *f*, -narkose *f*.
endotracheal catheter Endotrachealkatheter *m*.
endotracheal intubation endotracheale Intubation *f*.
endotracheal tube Endotrachealtubus *m*.
en·do·tra·che·i·tis [ˌ-ˌtreɪkɪˈaɪtɪs] *n* Entzündung *f* der Trachea(l)schleimhaut, Endotracheitis *f*.
en·do·tra·che·li·tis [ˌ-ˌtreɪkəˈlaɪtɪs] *n* → endocervicitis.
en·do·u·re·thral [ˌ-jʊəˈriːθrəl] *adj* in der Harnröhre (liegend), endo-, intraurethral.

en·do·u·ter·ine [ˌ-ˈjuːtərɪn, -raɪn] *adj* in der Gebärmutter (liegend), endo-, intrauterin.
en·do·vac·ci·na·tion [ˌ-ˌvæksɪˈneɪʃn] *n hyg.* Schluckimpfung *f*, Endovakzination *f*.
en·do·vas·cu·li·tis [ˌ-væskjəˈlaɪtɪs] *n* → endangiitis.
en·do·ve·ni·tis [ˌ-vɪˈnaɪtɪs] *n* → endophlebitis.
en·do·ve·nous [ˌ-ˈviːnəs] *adj* innerhalb einer Vene (liegend), intravenös.
end·piece [ˈendpiːs] *n* Endstück *n*.
  e. of spermatozoon Endstück des Spermiums.
end-plate *n histol.* Endplatte *f*.
end-plate current *physiol.* Endplattenstrom *m*.
end-plate potential *abbr.* **EPP** *physiol.* Endplattenpotential *nt abbr* EPP.
end point Endpunkt *m*.
end-point nystagmus → end-position nystagmus.
end-position nystagmus Endstellungs-, Pseudonystagmus *m*.
end product Endprodukt *nt*.
end-product inhibition Endprodukt-, Rückkopplungshemmung *f*, feedback- -Hemmung *f*.
end-product repression *biochem.* Endproduktrepression *f*.
end stage Endstadium *nt*.
end-stage liver disease terminale Leberinsuffizienz *f*.
end-stage renal disease *abbr.* **ESRD** terminale Niereninsuffizienz *f*.
end-systolic *adj* endsystolisch.
end-systolic volume endsystolisches (Rest-)Volumen *nt*.
end-tidal *adj* (*Lunge*) endexspiratorisch.
end-to-end anastomosis *chir.* End-zu- -End-Anastomose *f*, terminoterminale Anastomose *f*.
end-to-side anastomosis *chir.* End-zu- -Seit-Anastomose *f*, terminolaterale Anastomose *f*.
en·dur·a·ble [ɪnˈdʊərəbl, -ˈdjʊər-] *adj* erträglich, auszuhalten.
en·dur·ance [ɪnˈdʊərəns, -ˈdjʊər-] **I** *n* **1.** Durchhaltevermögen *nt*, Ausdauer *f*, Geduld *f*. **2.** Erdulden *nt*, Aushalten *nt*, Ertragen *nt*. **3.** Belastung *f*, Strapaze *f*. **II** *adj* Dauer-, Belastungs-.
endurance capacity Dauerleistungsfähigkeit *f*.
endurance limit Dauerleistungsgrenze *f*, Belastungsgrenze *f*.
endurance test Belastungstest *m*.
endurance training Ausdauertraining *nt*.
en·dure [ɪnˈdʊər, -ˈdjʊər] **I** *vt* (Er-)leiden, aushalten, ertragen, erdulden. **II** *vi* an-, fortdauern; durchhalten.
end-weave anastomosis (*Sehne*) Durchflechtungsanastomose *f*.
en·dy·ma [ˈendəmə] *n* → ependyma.
ene·di·ol [iːnˈdaɪɒl, -əʊl] *n* Endiol *nt*.
en·e·ma [ˈenəmə] *n, pl* **-mas**, **-ma·ta** [-mətə] Einlauf *m*, Klistier *nt*, Klysma *nt*, Clysma *nt*.
en·e·ma·tor [ˈenəmeɪtər] *n* Klistierspritze *f*.
en·er·get·ic [ˌenərˈdʒetɪk] *adj* **1.** energiegeladen, voller Energie. **2.** energisch.
en·er·get·i·cal [ˌ-ˈdʒetɪkl] *adj* → energetic.
en·er·get·ics [ˌ-ˈdʒetɪks] *pl* Energetik *f*.
en·er·ge·tis·tic [ˌ-dʒɪˈtɪstɪk] *adj* Energetik betr., energetisch.
en·er·gid [ˈenərdʒɪd, -dʒɪd] *n* Energide *f*.
en·er·gize [ˈenərdʒaɪz] *vt phys.* erregen, Antrieb geben, laden.
en·er·gized [ˈenərdʒaɪzd] *adj* energiereich, -geladen.
en·er·giz·er [ˈenərdʒaɪzər] *n* Energiespender *m*.
en·er·gom·e·ter [enərˈgɒmɪtər] *n* Pulsmesser *m*, Energometer *nt*.
en·er·gy [ˈenərdʒɪ] *n* **1.** *chem.*, *phys.* Energie *f*, Kraft *f*. **2.** (Tat-)Kraft *f*, Schwung *m*, Energie *f*.
  e. of motion Bewegungsenergie, kinetische Energie.
energy balance *physiol.* Energiehaushalt *m*, -bilanz *f*.
energy charge Energiegehalt *m*, -inhalt *m*, -ladung *f*.
energy conservation Energieerhaltung *f*.
energy consumption Energieverbrauch *m*.
energy conversion Energieumwandlung *f*.
energy coupling Energiekopplung *f*.
energy cycle Energiekreislauf *m*.
energy-dependend *adj* energieabhängig.
energy diagram Energiediagramm *nt*.
energy equivalent Energieäquivalent *nt*, kalorisches Äquivalent *nt*.
energy-independent *adj* energieunabhängig.
energy level Energieniveau *nt*.
energy metabolism Energiestoffwechsel *m*.
energy peak Energiegipfel *m*, -peak *m*.
energy-poor *adj* energiearm.
energy-providing *adj* energieliefernd.
energy-requiring *adj* energieverbrauchend.
energy-rich *adj* energiereich.
energy-rich bond energiereiche Bindung *f*.
energy-rich compound energiereiche Verbindung *f*.
energy-rich linkage → energy-rich bond.
energy source Energiequelle *f*.
energy-transducing *adj* energietransformierend.
energy transfer Energieübertragung *f*, -transfer *m*.
energy transformation Energieumwandlung *f*, -tranformation *f*.
energy turnover Energieumsatz *m abbr* EU.
energy unit Energieeinheit *f*.
energy-yielding *adj* energieliefernd.
en·er·vate [ˈenərveɪt] **I** *adj* → enervated. **II** *vt* **1.** entkräften, schwächen. **2.** *chir.*, *neuro.* enervieren, denervieren.
en·er·vat·ed [ˈenərveɪtɪd] *adj* **1.** entkräftet, geschwächt. **2.** *chir.*, *neuro.* enerviert, denerviert.
en·er·va·tion [enərˈveɪʃn] *n* **1.** Entkräftung *f*, Schwächung *f*. **2.** Schwäche *f*, Entkräftung *f*. **3.** *chir.*, *neuro.* Enervation *f*, Denervation *f*; Enervierung *f*, Denervierung *f*; Enervieren *nt*, Denervieren *nt*.
E neuron *physiol.* E-Neuron *nt*, spätexspiratorisches Neuron *nt*.
en·flu·rane [ˈenflʊəreɪn] *n* Enfluran *nt*, Ethrane *nt*.
ENG *abbr.* → electronystagmography.
en·gage·ment [enˈgeɪdʒmənt] *n* **1.** Beschäftigung *f*, Stelle *f*, (An-)Stellung *f*; Beschäftigung *f*, Tätigkeit *f*. **2.** *gyn.* (Frucht-)Einstellung *f* in der Beckeneingangsebene.
en·gas·tri·us [enˈgæstrɪəs] *n embryo.* Engastrius *m*.
Engelmann [ˈeŋəlmən; ˈɛŋəlmən]: **E.'s disease** Engelmann-Erkrankung *f*, Camurati-Engelmann-Erkrankung *f*, -Syndrom *nt*, Osteopathia hyperostotica multiplex infantilis.
  E.'s disk H-Bande *f*, H-Streifen *m*, H-Zone *f*, helle Zone *f*, Hensen'-Zone *f*.
Engel-Recklinghausen [ˈeŋəl ˈrɛklɪŋhaʊsn; ˈɛŋ-]: **E.-R. disease** Engel-(von) Recklinghausen-Syndrom *nt*, (von) Recklinghausen-Krankheit *f*, Osteodystrophia fibrosa cystica generalisata, Ostitis fibrosa cystica (generalisata).
Englisch [ˈeŋlɪʃ]: **E.'s sinus** Sinus petrosus inferior.
Eng·lish [ˈɪŋ(g)lɪʃ]: **E. chamomile** echte Kamille *f*, Chamomilla *f*, Matricaria chamomilla/officinalis.
  E. disease Rachitis *f*.
  E. position *gyn.* Sims-Lage *f*.
en·globe [enˈgləʊb] *vt* phagozytieren.
Engman [ˈeŋmən]: **E.'s disease** Engman-Krankheit *f*, infektiöse ekzematoide Dermatitis *f*.
en·gorged [enˈgɔːrdʒt] *adj patho.* prall, gefüllt, (an-)geschwollen.
en·gorge·ment [enˈgɔːrdʒmənt] *n patho.* **1.** *patho.* (An-)Schwellung *f*. **2.** Anschoppung *f*, Engorgement *nt*.
en·gram [ˈengræm] *n physiol.* Gedächtnisspur *f*, Engramm *nt*; Erinnerungsbild *nt*.
en·gulf·ment [enˈgʌlfmənt] *n micro.* (*Virus*) Penetration *f*.
en·hance [enˈhæns, -ˈhɑːns] *vt* verstärken, vergrößern, erhöhen, steigern, (an-)heben.
en·hance·ment [enˈhænsmənt, -ˈhɑːns-] *n* **1.** Steigerung *f*, Erhöhung *f*, Vergrößerung *f*. **2.** *pharm.*, *immun.*, *radiol.* Enhancement *nt*.
en·hanc·er sequence [enˈhænsər, -ˈhɑːns-] *genet.* Enhancer-, Verstärkersequenz *f*.
en·hex·y·mal [enˈheksɪməl] *n pharm.* Hexobarbital *nt*.
en·keph·a·lin [enˈkefəlɪn] *n* Enkephalin *nt*.
en·keph·a·lin·er·gic [enˌkefəlɪˈnɜːrdʒɪk] *adj* enkephalinerg(isch).
ENL *abbr.* → erythema nodosum leprosy.
en·large [ɪnˈlɑːrdʒ] **I** *vt* (*Organ*, *Kenntnisse*) erweitern; verbreitern; *photo.* vergrößern. **II** *vi* s. erweitern, s. ausdehnen, s. vergrößern; anschwellen; *photo.* s. vergrößern lassen.
en·larged [ɪnˈlɑːrdʒd] *adj* vergrößert, ausgedehnt, erweitert.
enlarged spleen Milzvergrößerung *f*, -schwellung *f*, -tumor *m*, Splenomegalie *f*, -megalia *f*.
en·large·ment [ɪnˈlɑːrdʒmənt] *n* Erweiterung *f*, Vergrößerung *f*, Ausdehnung *f*; (*a. anat.*) Schwellung *f*, Auftreibung *f*.
en·larg·er [ɪnˈlɑːrdʒər] *n photo.* Vergrößerungsgerät *nt*, -apparat *m*.
en·larg·ing follicle [ɪnˈlɑːrdʒɪŋ] (*Ovar*) Sekundärfollikel *m*, wachsender Follikel *m*.
ENoG *abbr.* → electroneuronography.
e·nol [ˈɪnɒl] *n* Enol *nt*.
e·no·lase [ˈen(ə)leɪz] *n* Enolase *f abbr.* ENO.
enol ester Enolester *m*.
enol form *chem.* Enolform *f*.
enol-keto tautomerism Keto-Enol-Tautomerie *f*.
en·oph·thal·mia [enɒfˈθælmɪə] *n* → enophthalmos.
en·oph·thal·mos [enɒfˈθælmɒs] *n ophthal.* Zurücksinken *nt* des Augapfels, Enophthalmie *f*, Enophthalmus *m*.
en·oph·thal·mus *n* → enophthalmos.
en·os·to·sis [enəsˈtəʊsɪs] *n ortho.* Enostose *f*.
en·o·yl [ˈiːnəʊɪl] *n* Enoyl-(Radikal *nt*).
enoyl-ACP hydratase Enoyl-ACP-hydratase *f*.
enoyl-ACP reductase (NADPH) Enoyl- -ACP-reduktase (NADPH) *f*.
enoyl-CoA hydratase Enoyl-CoA-hydratase *f*, Enoyl-hydra(ta)se *f*.
enoyl-CoA isomerase Enoyl-CoA-isomerase *f*.
enoyl hydrase → enoyl-CoA hydratase.

en pas·sant synapse [ã pa'sã] Parallelkontakt *m*, Bouton en passage.
en·rich [en'rɪtʃ] *vt micro.* anreichern, den Nährwert erhöhen.
en·riched medium [en'rɪtʃt] angereichertes Medium *nt.*
en·rich·ment [en'rɪtʃmənt] *n micro.* Anreicherung *f.*
enrichment culture Anreicherungskultur *f.*
Enroth ['enraθ]: **E.'s sign** Enroth-Zeichen *nt.*
en·sheath·ing callus [en'ʃi:ðɪŋ] Kallusscheide *f.*
en·si·form ['ensəfɔ:rm] *adj anat.* schwertförmig.
ensiform appendix *anat.* Schwertfortsatz *m*, Proc. xiphoideus.
ensiform cartilage → ensiform appendix.
en·si·ster·num [ˌensɪs'tɜrnəm] *n* → ensiform appendix.
en·som·pha·lus [en'sɑmfələs] *n embryo.* Ensomphalus *m.*
en·stro·phe ['enstrəʊfɪ] *n* → entropion.
ENT *abbr.* → ear, nose and throat.
ent- *pref.* → ento-.
ent·am·e·bi·a·sis [ˌentæmɪ'baɪəsɪs] *n* Entamoebainfektion *f*, Entamöbose *f.*
Ent·a·moe·ba [entə'mi:bə] *n micro.* Entamoeba *f.*
E. histolytica Ruhramöbe *f*, Entamoeba histolytica/dysenteriae.
en·ta·sia [en'teɪzɪə] *n neuro.* tonischer Krampf/Spasmus *m.*
en·ta·sis ['entəsɪs] *n* → entasia.
ent·ep·i·con·dyle [ˌentˌepɪ'kɑndaɪl, -dl] *n anat.* innere/mediale Humerusepikondyle *f*, Epicondylus medialis humeri.
enter- *pref.* → entero-.
en·ter·ad·en [en'terədən] *n* Darmdrüse *f.*
en·ter·ad·e·ni·tis [ˌentərˌædɪ'naɪtɪs] *n* Darmdrüsenentzündung *f.*
en·ter·al ['entərəl] *adj* Darm betr., im Darm (liegend), durch den Darm, enteral, intestinal, Darm-, Intestinal-, Enter(o)-.
enteral alimentation *abbr.* **EA** enterale Ernährung *f.*
enteral contents Darminhalt *m.*
enteral diarrhea Diarrhö *f* bei Enteritis, enteritische Diarrhö *f.*
enteral feeding → enteral alimentation.
enteral nutrition → enteral alimentation.
en·ter·al·gia [entə'rældʒ(ɪ)ə] *n* Darmschmerz(en *pl*) *m*, -neuralgie *f*, Enteralgie *f*; Leibschmerz(en *pl*) *m.*
en·ter·am·ine [en'teɪzɪə] *n* Serotonin *nt*, 5-Hydroxytryptamin *nt.*
en·ter·ec·ta·sis [ˌ-'ektəsɪs] *n* Darm(über)blähung *f.*
en·ter·ec·to·my [ˌ-'ektəmɪ] *n chir.* Darm(teil)entfernung *f*, -resektion *f*, Enterektomie *f*; Eingeweideresektion *f.*
en·ter·e·pip·lo·cele [ˌ-ɪ'pɪpləsi:l] *n* → enteroepiplocele.
en·ter·ic [en'terɪk] **I** ∼ *pl* → enteric bacteria. **II** *adj* (Dünn-)Darm betr., enterisch, Dünndarm-, Darm-, Entero-.
enteric alimentation → enteral alimentation.
enteric bacteria Entero-, Darmbakterien *pl.*
enteric cyst → enterocystoma.
enteric fever 1. enterische Salmonellose *f*, Salmonellenenteritis *f.* **2.** Bauchtyphus *m*, Typhus (abdominalis) *m*, Febris typhoides *f.*
enteric intussusception Dünndarminvagination *f.*
enteric nervous system Darmnervensystem *nt.*
enteric plexus enterischer Plexus *m*, Plexus entericus.

enteric virus → enterovirus.
en·ter·i·tis [entə'raɪtɪs] *n* Darm(wand)entzündung *f*, Dünndarmentzündung *f*, Enteritis *f.*
enteritis necroticans Darmbrand *m*, Enteritis necroticans.
entero- *pref.* Darm-, Eingeweide-, Enter(o)-.
en·ter·o·a·nas·to·mo·sis [ˌentərəʊəˌnæstə'məʊsɪs] *n chir.* Darmanastomose *f*, Enteroanastomose *f*, Enteroenterostomie *f.*
en·ter·o·an·the·lone [ˌ-'ænθɪləʊn] *n* → enterogastrone.
En·ter·o·bac·ter [ˌ-'bæktər] *n micro.* Enterobacter *m.*
En·ter·o·bac·te·ri·a·ce·ae [ˌ-bækˌtɪərɪ'eɪsɪ-i:] *pl micro.* Enterobacteriaceae *pl.*
en·ter·o·bi·a·sis [ˌ-'baɪəsɪs] *n* Enterobiusinfektion *f*, Madenwurminfektion *f*, -befall *m*, Enterobiasis *f*, Enterobiose *f*, Oxyuriasis *f.*
en·ter·o·bil·i·a·ry [ˌ-'bɪlɪˌerɪ:, -'bɪljərɪ] *adj* Dünndarm u. Gallenwege betr., enterobiliär.
En·ter·o·bi·us [entə'rəʊbɪəs] *n micro.* Enterobius *m.*
E. vermicularis Madenwurm *m*, Enterobius/Oxyuris vermicularis.
en·ter·o·bro·sia [ˌentərəʊ'brəʊʒɪə] *n* Darmperforation *f.*
en·ter·o·bro·sis [ˌ-'brəʊsɪs] *n* → enterobrosia.
en·ter·o·cele ['-si:l] *n* **1.** *anat.* Bauchhöhle *f*, Cavitas abdominalis. **2.** *chir.* Darmbruch *m*, Enterozele *f.* **3.** *gyn.* Enterozele *f*, Hernia vaginalis enterocele *f.*
en·ter·o·cen·te·sis [ˌ-sen'ti:sɪs] *n chir.* Darmpunktion *f*, Enterozentese *f.*
en·ter·o·cho·le·cys·tos·to·my [ˌ-ˌkɑləsɪs'tɑstəmɪ] *n chir., patho.* Dünndarm-Gallenblasen-Fistel *f*, -Fistelung *f.*
en·ter·o·cho·le·cys·tot·o·my [ˌ-ˌkɑləsɪs'tɑtəmɪ] *n chir.* Enterocholezystotomie *f.*
en·ter·o·chro·maf·fin [ˌ-'krəʊməfɪn] *adj abbr.* **EC** enterochromaffin *abbr.* EC.
enterochromaffin cells enterochromaffine/argentaffine/gelbe/enteroendokrine Zellen *pl*, Kultschitzky-Zellen *pl.*
enterochromaffin system enterochromaffines System *nt.*
en·ter·o·ci·ne·sia [ˌ-sɪ'ni:ʒ(ɪ)ə] *n* Peristaltik *f.*
en·ter·o·clei·sis [ˌ-'klaɪsɪs] *n* **1.** *chir.* Deckung *f* einer Darmperforation, Darm(wand)verschluß *m*, Enterokleisis *f.* **2.** *patho.* Darmverschluß *m*, Enterokleisis *f.*
en·te·roc·ly·sis [entə'rɑkləsɪs] *n* **1.** Dünndarmeinlauf *m*, hoher Einlauf *m*, Enteroklysma *nt.* **2.** (*Nährlösung*) Enteroklysma *nt.*
en·ter·o·coc·ce·mia [ˌentərəʊkɑk'si:mɪə] *n* Enterokokkensepsis *f.*
en·ter·o·coc·cus [ˌ-'kɑkəs] *n, pl* **-ci** [-kaɪ, -ki:, -saɪ] *micro.* Enterokokkus *m*, Enterokokke *f*, Enterococcus *m.*
en·ter·o·coel *n* → enterocoele.
en·ter·o·coe·le ['-si:l] *n embryo.* Enterozöl *nt*, Enterozoelom *nt.*
en·ter·o·coe·lom [ˌ-'si:ləm] *n* → enterocoele.
en·ter·o·col·ec·to·my [ˌ-kə'lektəmɪ, -kəʊ-] *n chir.* Enterokolektomie *f.*
enterocolic fistula *patho.* (Dünn-)Darm-Kolon-Fistel *f*, enterokolische Fistel *f*, Fistula enterocolica.
en·ter·o·co·li·tis [ˌ-kə'laɪtɪs] *n* Entzündung *f* von Dünn- u. Dickdarm, Enterokolitis *f*, Enterocolitis *f.*
en·ter·o·co·los·to·my [ˌ-kə'lɑstəmɪ] *n chir.* Dünndarm-Dickdarm-Fistel *f*, -Anasto-

mose *f*, Enterokolostomie *f.*
en·ter·o·cu·ta·ne·ous [ˌ-kju:'teɪnɪəs] *adj* Darm u. Haut betr. *od.* verbindend, enterokutan.
enterocutaneous fistula *patho.* enterokutane Fistel *f*, äußere Darmfistel *f.*
en·ter·o·cyst ['-sɪst] *n* → enterocystoma.
en·ter·o·cys·to·cele [ˌ-'sɪstəsi:l] *n* Enterozystozele *f.*
en·ter·o·cys·to·ma [ˌ-sɪs'təʊmə] *n* enterogene Zyste, Dottergangszyste *f*, Enterozyste; Enterozystom *nt*, -kystom *nt.*
en·ter·o·cyte ['-saɪt] *n* Saumzelle *f*, Enterozyt *m.*
en·ter·o·dyn·ia [ˌ-'di:nɪə] *n* → enteralgia.
en·ter·o·en·do·crine cells [ˌ-'endəkraɪn, -krɪn] → enterochromaffin cells.
en·ter·o·en·ter·ic fistula [ˌ-en'terɪk] *patho.* enteroenterische Fistel *f.*
en·ter·o·en·ter·os·to·my [ˌ-ˌentə'rɑstəmɪ] *n* → enteroanastomosis.
en·ter·o·e·pip·lo·cele [ˌ-ɪ'pɪpləsi:l] *n chir.* Darmnetzbruch *m*, Enter(o)epiplozele *f.*
en·ter·o·gas·tric reflex [ˌ-'gæstrɪk] enterogastrischer Reflex *m.*
en·ter·o·gas·tri·tis [ˌ-gæ'straɪtɪs] *n* Magen-Darm-Katarrh *m*, Gastroenteritis *f.*
en·ter·o·gas·trone [ˌ-'gæstrəʊn] *n* Enterogastron *nt*, (Entero-)Anthelon *nt.*
en·ter·og·e·nous [entə'rɑdʒənəs] *adj* im (Dünn-)Darm entstehend *od.* entstanden, enterogen.
enterogenous cyanosis autotoxische Zyanose *f*, Stokvis-Talma-Syndrom *nt.*
enterogenous cyst → enterocystoma.
en·ter·o·glu·ca·gon [ˌentərəʊ'glu:kəgən] *n* Enteroglukagon *nt*, intestinales Glukagon *nt.*
en·ter·o·gram ['-græm] *n* Enterogramm *nt.*
en·ter·o·graph ['-græf] *n* Enterograph *m.*
en·te·rog·ra·phy [entə'rɑgrəfɪ] *n* Enterographie *f.*
en·ter·o·he·pat·ic circulation [ˌentərəʊhɪ'pætɪk] enterohepatischer Kreislauf *m.*
en·ter·o·hep·a·ti·tis [ˌ-ˌhepə'taɪtɪs] *n* Entzündung *f* von Leber u. Darm, Enterohepatitis *f.*
en·ter·o·hep·a·to·cele [ˌ-'hepətəsi:l] *n chir., ped.* Enterohepatozele *f.*
en·ter·o·hy·dro·cele [ˌ-'haɪdrəsi:l] *n* Enterohydrozele *f.*
en·ter·oi·dea [entə'rɔɪdɪə] *pl* fiebrige Enteritiden *pl.*
en·ter·o·in·tes·ti·nal [ˌentərəʊɪn'testənl, -ɪntes'taɪnl] *adj* intestino-intestinal.
en·ter·o·ki·nase [ˌ-'kaɪneɪz, -'kɪn-] *n* Enterokinase *f*, -peptidase *f.*
en·ter·o·ki·ne·sia [ˌ-kɪ'ni:ʒ(ɪ)ə, kaɪ-] *n* Peristaltik *f.*
en·ter·o·ki·net·ic [ˌ-kɪ'netɪk] *adj* enterokinetisch, peristaltisch.
en·ter·o·lith ['-lɪθ] *n* Darmstein *m*, Enterolith *m.*
en·ter·o·li·thi·a·sis [ˌ-lɪ'θaɪəsɪs] *n* Enterolithiasis *f.*
en·ter·ol·y·sis [entə'rɑləsɪs] *n chir.* Darmlösung *f*, Lösung *f* von Darmverwachsungen, Enterolyse *f.*
en·ter·o·me·ga·lia [ˌentərəʊmɪ'geɪlɪə] *n* → enteromegaly.
en·ter·o·meg·a·ly [ˌ-'megəlɪ] *n* Darmvergrößerung *f*, Enteromegalie *f*, Megaenteron *nt.*
en·ter·o·mere ['-mɪər] *n embryo.* Enteromer *nt.*
en·ter·o·mer·o·cele [ˌ-'merəsi:l] *n chir.* Schenkelbruch *m*, -hernie *f*, Merozele *f*, Hernia femoralis/curalis.
En·ter·o·mon·a·di·na [ˌ-ˌmɑnə'daɪnə] *pl micro.* Enteromonadina *pl.*
En·ter·o·mo·nas [ˌ-'məʊnæs, -'mɑ-] *n micro.* Enteromonas *m.*

en·ter·o·my·co·der·mi·tis [ˌ-ˌmaɪkədɜr-'maɪtɪs] *n* → endoenteritis.
en·ter·o·my·co·sis [ˌ-maɪ'kəʊsɪs] *n* Darm-, Enteromykose *f*.
en·ter·on ['entərɒn, -rən] *n anat.* Darm *m*, Enteron *nt*; Dünndarm *m*; Verdauungstrakt *m*.
en·ter·o·ni·tis [ˌentərəʊ'naɪtɪs] *n* → enteritis.
entero-oxyntin *n* Enterooxyntin *nt*.
en·ter·o·pa·re·sis [ˌ-pə'riːsɪs] *n* Darmlähmung *f*, Enteroparese *f*, -paralyse *f*.
en·ter·o·path·ic acrodermatitis [ˌ-'pæθɪk] Akrodermatitis/Acrodermatitis enteropathica.
en·ter·o·path·o·gen [ˌ-'pæθədʒən] *n* enteropathogener Mikroorganismus *m*.
en·ter·o·path·o·gen·ic [ˌ-pæθə'dʒenɪk] *adj* Darmerkrankungen hervorrufend *od.* auslösend, enteropathogen.
en·te·rop·a·thy [entə'rɒpəθɪ] *n* Darmerkrankung *f*, Enteropathie *f*.
en·ter·o·pep·ti·dase [ˌentərəʊ'peptɪdeɪz] *n* → enterokinase.
en·ter·o·pex·y ['-peksɪ] *n chir.* Darmheftung *f*, Enteropexie *f*.
en·ter·o·plas·ty ['-plæstɪ] *n chir.* Darm-, Enteroplastik *f*.
en·ter·o·ple·gia [ˌ-'pliːdʒ(ɪ)ə] *n chir.* adynamischer/paralytischer Ileus *m*.
en·ter·op·to·sia [ˌentərɒp'təʊsɪə] *n* → enteroptosis.
en·ter·op·to·sis [ˌentərɒp'təʊsɪs] *n chir., patho.* Darm-, Eingeweidesenkung *f*, Enteroptose *f*, Splanchnoptose *f*.
en·ter·o·pty·chia [ˌentərəʊ'taɪkɪə] *n* → enteroptychy.
en·ter·op·ty·chy [ˌ-'taɪkɪ] *n chir.* Darmplikatur *f*, -plikation *f*.
en·ter·o·re·nal [ˌ-'riːnl] *adj* Darm u. Niere betr. *od.* verbindend, entero-, intestinorenal.
en·ter·or·rha·gia [ˌ-'rædʒ(ɪ)ə] *n* Darmblutung *f*, Enterorrhagie *f*.
en·ter·or·rha·phy [entərɒ'rɒrəfɪ] *n chir.* Darmnaht *f*, Enterorrhaphie *f*.
en·ter·or·rhea [ˌentərəʊ'rɪə] *n* Durchfall *m*, Diarrhoe *f*, Diarrhoea *f*, Diarrhö(e) *f*.
en·ter·or·rhex·is [ˌ-'reksɪs] *n* Darmriß *m*, -ruptur *f*, Enterorrhexis *f*.
en·ter·o·scope ['-skəʊp] *n* Darmendoskop *nt*, Enteroskop *nt*.
en·ter·o·sep·sis [ˌ-'sepsɪs] *n* Enterosepsis *f*.
en·ter·o·spasm ['-spæzəm] *n* Darmkrampf *m*, Spasmus/Krampf *m* der Darmmuskulatur, Enterospasmus *m*.
en·ter·o·sta·sis [ˌ-'steɪsɪs, -'stæ-] *n* Enterostase *f*.
en·ter·o·stax·is [ˌ-'stæksɪs] *n patho.* Sickerblutung *f* aus der Darmschleimhaut.
en·ter·o·ste·no·sis [ˌ-stɪ'nəʊsɪs] *n* Darmverengung *f*, -stenose *f*, Enterostenose *f*.
en·ter·os·to·my [ˌentə'rɒstəmɪ] *n* 1. *chir.* operative (Dünn-)Darmausleitung *f*, Enterostomie *f*. 2. *chir.* Enterostoma *nt*. 3. → enteroanastomosis.
en·ter·o·tome ['entərətəʊm] *n chir.* Enterotom *nt*.
en·te·rot·o·my [entə'rɒtəmɪ] *n chir.* Darmschnitt *m*, -eröffnung *f*, Enterotomie *f*.
en·ter·o·tox·e·mia [ˌentərəʊtɒk'siːmɪə] *n patho.* Enterotox(in)ämie *f*.
en·ter·o·tox·ic [ˌ-'tɒksɪk] *adj* Enterotoxin betr. *od.* enthaltend, enterotoxisch.
en·ter·o·tox·i·ca·tion [ˌ-ˌtɒksɪ'keɪʃn] *n* → enterotoxism.
en·ter·o·tox·i·gen·ic [ˌ-ˌtɒksɪ'dʒenɪk] *adj* enterotoxinbildend, enterotoxigen.
en·ter·o·tox·in [ˌ-'tɒksɪn] *n* Enterotoxin *nt*.
en·ter·o·tox·ism [ˌ-'tɒksɪzm] *n* Entero(in)toxikation *f*; Autointoxikation *f*.

en·ter·o·trop·ic [ˌ-'trɒpɪk, -'trəʊp-] *adj* enterotrop.
en·ter·o·vag·i·nal [ˌ-'vædʒənl] *adj* Darm u. Scheide/Vagina betr. *od.* verbindend, enterovaginal.
enterovaginal fistula *patho.* Darm-Scheiden-Fistel *f*, enterovaginale Fistel *f*.
en·ter·o·ves·i·cal [ˌ-'vesɪkl] *adj* Darm u. Harnblase betr. *od.* verbindend, enterovesikal.
enterovesical fistula *patho.* Darm-(Harn-)Blasen-Fistel *f*, Darm-Blasen-Fistel *f*, enterovesikale Fistel *f*.
en·ter·o·vi·ral [ˌ-'vaɪrəl] *adj* Enteroviren betr., enteroviral, Enteroviren-.
en·ter·o·vi·rus [ˌ-'vaɪrəs] *n micro.* Enterovirus *nt*.
enterovirus 72 Hepatitis-A-Virus *nt abbr.* HAV.
en·ter·o·zo·on [ˌ-'zəʊɒn] *n, pl* **-zoa** [-'zəʊə] *micro.* tierischer Darmparasit *m*, Enterozoon *nt*.
en·thal·py ['enθælpɪ, en'θæl-] *n* Enthalpie *f abbr.* H.
en·the·sis [enθɪsɪs] *n* 1. *anat.* Muskel-, Sehnenansatz *m*, -insertion *f*. 2. *chir.* alloplastische Deckung *f*, Alloplastik *f*.
en·the·si·tis [enθɪ'saɪtɪs] *n* Entzündung *f* eines Muskel- *od.* Sehnenansatzes.
en·the·sop·a·thy [enθɪ'sɒpəθɪ] *n ortho.* Insertionstendopathie *f*, Enthes(i)opathie *f*.
en·thla·sis ['enθləsɪs] *n ortho. (Schädel)* Impressionsfraktur *f*.
en·tire [en'taɪər] *adj* 1. ganz, völlig, vollkommen, vollzählig, vollständig, komplett; ganz, unvermindert, Gesamt-. 2. ganz, unversehrt, unbeschädigt. 3. *micro. (Kolonie)* glatt, rund.
en·ti·ty ['entɪtɪ] *n* Entität *f*.
Entner-Doudoroff ['entnər 'duːdərɒf]: **E.-D. fermentation/pathway** *biochem.* Entner-Doudoroff-Abbau *m*.
ento- *pref.* End(o)-, Ent(o)-.
en·to·blast [entəʊblæst] *n* 1. → entoderm. 2. Zellnukleolus *m*.
en·to·cele ['-siːl] *n chir.* innere Hernie *f*, Hernia interna.
en·to·cho·roi·dea [ˌ-kə'rɔɪdɪə] *n anat.* Choroidocapillaris *f*, Lamina choroidocapillaris.
en·to·cor·nea [ˌ-'kɔːrnɪə] *n anat.* hintere Basalmembran *f*, Descemet'-Membran *f*, Lamina elastica posterior Descemeti, Lamina limitans posterior (corneae).
en·to·cra·ni·al [ˌ-'kreɪnɪəl] *adj* → endocranial.
en·to·cra·ni·um [ˌ-'kreɪnɪəm] *n* → endocranium.
en·to·cu·ne·i·form [ˌ-kjuː'nɪəfɔːrm, 'kjuːnɪə-] *n anat.* Os cuneiforme mediale.
en·to·derm ['-dɜrm] *n embryo.* inneres Keimblatt *nt*, Entoderm *nt*.
en·to·der·mal [ˌ-'dɜrml] *adj* Entoderm betr., vom Entoderm abstammend, entodermal.
entodermal cell endodermale Zelle *f*.
en·to·der·mic [ˌ-'dɜrmɪk] *adj* → entodermal.
en·to·mere ['-mɪər] *n embryo.* Entomer *nt*.
en·to·mo·log·i·cal [ˌ-mə'lɒdʒɪkl] *adj* entomologisch.
en·to·mol·o·gist [ˌ-'mɒlədʒɪst] *n* Insektologe *m*, -login *f*, Entomologe *m*, -login *f*.
en·to·mol·o·gy [ˌ-'mɒlədʒɪ] *n* Insektenkunde *f*, Entomologie *f*.
en·to·mo·pho·bia [ˌentəʊməʊ'fəʊbɪə] *n psychia.* Insektenangst *f*, Entomophobie *f*.
En·to·moph·thor·a [ˌ-'mɒfθərə] *n micro.* Entomophthora *f*.
En·to·moph·tho·ra·ce·ae [ˌ-ˌmɒfθə'reɪsiː] *pl micro.* Entomophthoraceae *pl*.

En·to·moph·tho·ra·les [ˌ-ˌmɒfθə'reɪliːz] *pl micro.* Entomophthorales *pl*.
en·to·moph·tho·ro·my·co·sis [ˌ-ˌmɒfθərəʊmaɪ'kəʊsɪs] *n* Entomophthora-Mykose *f*, Entomophthorose *f*.
en·to·par·a·site [ˌ-'pærəsaɪt] *n* → endoparasite.
en·to·pe·dun·cu·lar nucleus [ˌ-pɪ'dʌŋkjələr] Nc. endopeduncularis.
ent·oph·thal·mia [entɒf'θælmɪə] *n* → endophthalmia.
en·to·phyte ['entəfaɪt] *n* → endophyte.
en·to·plasm ['-plæzəm] *n* → endoplasm.
ent·op·tic [ent'ɒptɪk] *adj ophthal.* im Augeninnern (entstanden *od.* liegend), entoptisch.
ent·op·to·scope [en'tɒptəskəʊp] *n ophthal.* Entoptoskop *nt*.
ent·op·tos·co·py [ˌentɒp'tɒskəpɪ] *n ophthal.* Entoptoskopie *f*.
ent·or·ga·nism [ent'ɔːrgænɪzəm] *n* → endoparasite.
en·to·rhi·nal region [ˌentəʊ'raɪnl] Regio entorhinalis.
en·to·sarc ['-sɑːrk] *n* → endosarc.
en·tos·to·sis [entəs'təʊsɪs] *n* → enostosis.
ent·ot·ic [ent'ɒtɪk, -'əʊ-] *adj* im Ohr entstanden *od.* liegend, entotisch, endaural.
en·to·zo·on [ˌentəʊ'zəʊɒn] *n, pl* **-zoa** [-'zəʊə] *micro.* tierischer Endoparasit *m*, Entozoon *nt*.
ENTP *abbr.* → excitatory nerve-terminal potential.
en·train·ing agent/signal [en'treɪnɪŋ] *physiol.* Zeitgeber *m*.
en·trap·ment neuropathy [en'træpmənt] Nervenschädigung *f* durch Einklemmung, Nervenkompressionssyndrom *nt*.
en·trip·sis [en'trɪpsɪs] *n pharm.* Einreibung *f*, Einsalbung *f*, Inunktion *f*, Inunctio *f*.
en·tro·pi·on [en'trəʊpɪɒn, -ɪən] *n ophthal.* Einwärtsstülpung *f* des freien Lidrandes, Entropion *nt*, Entropium *nt*.
en·tro·pi·on·ize [en'trəʊpɪənaɪz] *vt* nach innen wenden, umstülpen, entropionieren.
en·tro·pi·um [en'trəʊpɪəm] *n* → entropion.
en·tro·py ['entrəpɪ] *n abbr.* S *phys., mathe.* Entropie *f abbr.* S.
entropy change *chem.* Entropieänderung *f*.
e·nu·cle·ate [ɪ'n(j)uːklɪeɪt] *vt chir.* ausschälen, enukleieren.
e·nu·cle·a·tion [ɪˌn(j)uːklɪ'eɪʃn] *n* 1. *chir.* Ausschälung *f*, Enukleation *f*. 2. *genet.* Enukleation *f*, Enukleation *f*.
enucleation scissors *ophthal.* Enukleationsschere *f*.
enucleation spoon *ophthal.* Enukleationslöffel *m*.
en·u·re·sis [ˌenjə'riːsɪs] *n* Einnässen *nt*, Bettnässen *nt*, Enuresis *f*.
en·u·ret·ic [ˌ-'retɪk] **I** *n* Enuretiker(in *f*) *m*; *ped.* Bettnässer(in *f*) *m*. **II** *adj* Enuresis betr.
en·vel·op [*n* en'veləp, 'envə-; *v* en'veləp] **I** *n* → envelope. **II** *vt (a. anat.)* (ein-)hüllen (in *in*).
en·ve·lope ['envələʊp] *n* 1. *anat.* Hülle *f*, Schale *f*. 2. *micro.* (Virus-)Hülle *f*, Envelope *nt/m*. 3. Umhüllung *f*; (Brief-)Umschlag *m*.
en·vel·oped virus ['envələʊpd] *micro.* umhülltes/behülltes Virus *nt*.
en·vel·op·ment [en'veləpmənt] *n* Ein-, Umhüllung *f*, Hülle *f*.
en·ve·no·ma·tion [enˌvenə'meɪʃn] *n* Envenomisation *f*.
en·vi·ron·ment [en'vaɪ(r)ənmənt] *n* Umgebung *f*; Umwelt *f*; Milieu *nt*.
en·vi·ron·men·tal [enˌvaɪ(r)ən'mentl] *adj* Umgebungs-, Umwelt-, Milieu-.

environmental conditions Umweltbedingungen pl.
environmental factor Umweltfaktor m, -einfluß m.
environmental load Umweltbelastung f.
environmental medicine Umweltmedizin f.
environmental physiology Umweltphysiologie f.
environmental psychology Umweltpsychologie f.
environmental stimuli Umweltreize pl, extero(re)zeptive/äußere Reize pl.
environmental temperature Umgebungstemperatur f.
en·vy ['envɪ] **I** n Neid m (of auf). **II** vt jdn. beneiden.
en·zo·ot·ic disease [enzəʊ'ɒtɪk] Enzoonose f.
enzootic hepatitis Rift-Valley-Fieber nt.
en·zy·got·ic [ˌenzaɪ'ɡɒtɪk] adj eineiig, monozygot.
enzygotic twins eineiige/erbgleiche/identische/monozygote/monovuläre Zwillinge pl.
en·zy·mat·ic [ˌenzɪ'mætɪk] adj Enzym(e) betr., durch Enzyme bewirkt, enzymatisch, Enzym-.
enzymatic adaptation induzierte Enzymsynthese f, Enzyminduktion f.
enzymatic cleavage enzymatische Spaltung f.
enzymatic débridement chir. enzymatisches Débridement nt.
enzymatic hydrolysis enzymatische Hydrolyse f.
enzymatic pancreatitis tryptische Pankreatitis f, Pankreasnekrose f.
enzymatic splitting enzymatische Spaltung f.
en·zyme ['enzaɪm] n Enzym nt, old Ferment nt.
enzyme activity Enzymaktivität f.
enzyme antagonist Enzymantagonist m, Antienzym nt.
enzyme-bound adj enzymgebunden.
enzyme-catalyzed adj enzymkatalysiert.
enzyme-cofactor complex Enzym-Cofaktor-Komplex m, Holoenzym nt.
enzyme conformation Enzymkonformation f.
enzyme immunoassay abbr. **EIA** Enzymimmunoassay m abbr. EIA.
enzyme induction Enzyminduktion f.
enzyme inhibition Enzymhemmung f.
enzyme inhibitor Enzymhemmstoff m, -inhibitor m.
enzyme-inhibitor complex Enzym-Inhibitor-Komplex m.
enzyme kinetics Enzymkinetik f.
enzyme-linked immunosorbent assay abbr. **ELISA** Enzyme-linked-immunosorbent-Assay m abbr. ELISA.
enzyme-multiplied immunoassay technique abbr. **EMIT** Enzyme-multiplied-immunoassay-Technique (f) abbr. EMIT.
enzyme pattern Enzymmuster nt.
enzyme profile Enzymprofil nt.
enzyme repression biochem. Enzymrepression f.
enzyme-substrate complex Enzym-Substrat-Komplex m.
enzyme-substrate-inhibitor complex Enzym-Substrat-Inhibitor-Komplex m.
enzyme unit Enzymeinheit f.
en·zy·mic [en'zaɪmɪk] adj → enzymatic.
en·zy·mol·y·sis [ˌenzaɪ'mɒləsɪs, -zɪ-] n enzymatische Spaltung f.
en·zy·mop·a·thy [ˌenzaɪ'mɒpəθɪ] n Enzymopathie f.
EOG abbr. **1.** → electrooculogram. **2.** → electro-olfactogram.

e·o·sin ['iːəsɪn] n Eosin nt.
eosin-methylene blue agar micro. Eosin--Methylenblau-Agar m/nt, EMB-Agar m/nt, EMB-Nährboden m.
e·o·sin·o·blast [ɪə'sɪnəblæst] n hema. Eosino(philo)blast m.
e·o·sin·o·cyte [ɪə'sɪnəsaɪt] n → eosinophil 2.
e·o·sin·o·pe·nia [ɪəˌsɪnə'piːnɪə] n hema. Eosinopenie f.
e·o·sin·o·phil [ɪə'sɪnəfɪl] **I** n **1.** eosinophile Struktur od. Zelle f. **2.** eosinophiler Leukozyt/Granulozyt m, inf. Eosinophiler m. **II** adj → eosinophilic.
eosinophil adenoma eosinophiles (Hypophysen-)Adenom nt.
eosinophil chemotactic factor abbr. **ECF 1.** Eosinophilen-chemotaktischer Faktor m abbr. ECF. **2.** → e. of anaphylaxis.
e. of anaphylaxis abbr. **ECF-A** Eosinophilen-chemotaktischer Faktor m der Anaphylaxie abbr. ECF-A.
e·o·sin·o·phile [ɪə'sɪnəfaɪl] **I** n → eosinophil I. **II** adj → eosinophilic.
eosinophil granules eosinophile Granula pl.
e·o·sin·o·phil·ia [ɪəˌsɪnə'fɪlɪə, -ljə] n **1.** Eosinophilie f, Eosinophilämie f. **2.** eosinophile Beschaffenheit f, Eosinophilie f.
e·o·sin·o·phil·ic [ˌ-'fɪlɪk] adj **1.** histol. mit Eosin färbend, eosinophil. **2.** hema. eosinophile Leukozyten od. Eosinophilie betr., eosinophil.
eosinophilic adenoma eosinophiles (Hypophysen-)Adenom nt.
eosinophilic cell adenocarcinoma eosinophilzelliges Adenokarzinom nt.
eosinophilic endomyocardial disease Löffler-Endokarditis f, -Syndrom nt, Endocarditis parietalis fibroplastica.
eosinophilic erythroblast → eosinophilic normoblast.
eosinophilic gastroenteritis eosinophile Gastroenteritis f.
eosinophilic granulocyte → eosinophil 2.
eosinophilic granuloma 1. eosinophiles (Knochen-)Granulom nt. **2.** Heringswurmkrankheit f, Anisakiasis f.
eosinophilic leukemia Eosinophilenleukämie f.
eosinophilic leukocyte → eosinophil 2.
eosinophilic leukopenia Eosinopenie f.
eosinophilic meningitis/meningoencephalitis eosinophile Meningitis/Meningoenzephalitis f.
eosinophilic myelocyte eosinophiler Myelozyt m.
eosinophilic normoblast azidophiler/orthochromatischer Normoblast m.
eosinophilic pneumonia eosinophilzellige Pneumonie f.
eosinophilic series → eosinophil series.
e·o·sin·o·phil·o·cyt·ic leukemia [ɪəˌsɪnoˌfɪlə'sɪtɪk] Eosinophilenleukämie f.
e·o·sin·o·phi·lo·sis [ˌ-fɪ'ləʊsɪs] n → eosinophilia 1.
e·o·sin·o·phil·o·tac·tic [ˌ-ˌfɪlə'tæktɪk] adj → eosinotactic.
e·o·si·noph·i·lous [ˌiəsɪ'nɒfɪləs] adj → eosinophilic.
eosinophil series hema. eosinophile Reihe f.
e·o·sin·o·tac·tic [ɪəˌsɪnə'tæktɪk] adj hema. eosinotaktisch.
e·o·sin·o·tax·is [ˌ-'tæksɪs] n hema. Eosinotaxis f.
EP abbr. **1.** → endogenous pyrogen. **2.** → evoked potential.
ep·ac·me [ep'ækmɪ] n Epakme f.
e·pac·tal [ɪ'pæktəl] **I** ˌs pl → epactal bones. **II** adj überzählig.
epactal bones Nahtknochen pl, Ossa suturalia.

epactal cartilages akzessorische Nasenknorpel pl, Cartilagines nasales accessoriae.
ep·ar·sal·gia [epɑːr'sældʒ(ɪ)ə] n Schmerzen pl bei Überbelastung, Eparsalgie f, Eparsalgia f.
ep·ar·te·ri·al bronchus [ˌepɑːr'tɪərɪəl] Bronchus m des rechten Oberlappens, Bronchus lobaris superior dexter, Ramus bronchialis eparterialis.
ep·ax·i·al [ep'æksɪəl] adj hinter od. über einer Achse, epaxial.
EPC abbr. → external pneumatic compression.
EPEC abbr. → Escherichia coli, enteropathogenic.
ep·en·ceph·al [ˌepən'sefəl] n → epencephalon.
ep·en·ceph·a·lon [ˌ-'sefəˌlɒn, -lən] n, pl **-lons, -la** [-lə] embryo. Nachhirn nt, Metenzephalon nt, -encephalon nt.
ep·en·dop·a·thy [ˌ-'dɒpəθɪ] n → ependymopathy.
ep·en·dy·ma [ə'pendɪmə] n Ependym nt.
ep·en·dy·mal [ə'pendɪml] adj Ependym betr., aus Ependym bestehend, ependymal, Ependym-.
ependymal canaliculi Ependymkanälchen pl.
ependymal cell → ependymocyte.
ependymal cyst Ependymzyste f, ependymale Zyste f.
ependymal fiber Ependymfaser f.
ep·en·dy·mar·y [ə'pendəˌmerɪ] adj → ependymal.
ep·en·dy·mi·tis [ə,pendɪ'maɪtɪs] n Ependymentzündung f, Ependymitis f.
ep·en·dy·mo·blast [ə'pendɪməʊblæst] n Ependymoblast m, embryonale Ependymzelle f.
e·pen·dy·mo·blas·to·ma [ˌ-blæs'təʊmə] n Ependymoblastom nt.
ep·en·dy·mo·cyte ['-saɪt] n Ependymzelle f, Ependymozyt m.
e·pen·dy·mo·cy·to·ma [ˌ-saɪ'təʊmə] n → ependymoma.
e·pen·dy·mo·ma [ə,pendɪ'məʊmə] n Ependymom nt, Ependymozytom nt, Ependym(o)gliom nt, Ependym(o)epitheliom nt, Pfeilerzellgliom nt.
e·pen·dy·mop·a·thy [ə,pendɪ'mɑpəθɪ] n Ependymerkrankung f, Ependymopathie f.
ep·er·sal·gia [epər'sældʒ(ɪ)ə] n → eparsalgia.
Ep·e·ryth·ro·zo·on [epɪ,rɪθrə'zəʊən] n micro. Eperythrozoon nt.
ep·e·ryth·ro·zo·o·no·sis [ˌ-,zəʊə'nəʊsɪs] n Eperythrozooninfektion f, Eperythrozoonose f.
eph·apse ['efæps] n Ephapse f.
eph·ap·tic [ɪ'fæptɪk] adj ephaptisch.
ephaptic transmission ephaptische Übertragung f.
ep·har·mo·ny [ep'hɑːrmənɪ] n Epharmonie f, Epharmose f.
e·phe·bic [ɪ'fiːbɪk] adj Jugend od. Pubertät(speriode) betr., ephebisch, Pubertäts-.
e·phe·bo·gen·e·sis [ɪ,fiːbə'dʒenəsɪs] n Ephebogenese f.
e·phe·drine [ɪ'fedrɪn, 'efɪdriːn] n pharm. Ephedrin nt.
e·phel·i·des [ɪ'felɪdiːz] pl Sommersprossen pl, Epheliden pl, Lentigo aestiva.
e·phe·lis [ɪ'felɪs] n → ephelides.
e·phem·e·ra [ɪ'femərə] n **1.** kurzlebige/vorübergehende Erscheinung f. **2.** bio. Eintagsfliege f. **3.** Eintagsfieber nt, Ephemera f, Febricula f, Febris herpetica/ephemera.
e·phem·er·al [ɪ'femərəl] adj kurzlebig, flüchtig, transient.

ephemeral fever Eintagsfieber *nt*, Ephemera *f*, Febricula *f*, Febris herpetica/ ephemera.
epi- *pref.* Epi-, Ep-, Eph-.
ep·i·al·lo·preg·nan·o·lone [ˌepɪˌæləʊpregˈnænəloʊn] *n abbr.* **EAP** Epiallopregnanolon *nt abbr.* EAP.
ep·i·an·dros·ter·one [ˌ-ænˈdrɒstərəʊn] *n* Epi-, Isoandrosteron *nt*.
ep·i·bi·ont [ˌ-ˈbaɪɒnt] *n bio.* Epibiont *m*.
ep·i·bi·o·sis [ˌ-baɪˈəʊsɪs] *n bio.* Epibiose *f*.
ep·i·blast [ˈ-blæst] *n* → ectoderm.
epiblast cell epiblastische Ektodermzelle *f*.
ep·i·blas·tic [ˌ-ˈblæstɪk] *adj* epiblastisch; ektodermal.
ep·i·bleph·a·ron [ˌ-ˈblefərən] *n embryo.* Epiblepharon *nt*.
e·pib·o·le *n* → epiboly.
e·pib·o·ly [ɪˈpɪbəlɪ] *n embryo.* Umwachsung *f*, Epibolie *f*.
ep·i·bul·bar [epɪˈbʌlbər] *adj* auf dem Augapfel (liegend), epibulbär.
ep·i·can·thal [ˌ-ˈkænθl] *adj* Lidfalte/Epikanthus betr., epikanthal, Epikanthus-.
epicanthal fold → epicanthus.
ep·i·can·thic [ˌ-ˈkænθɪk] *adj* → epicanthal.
ep·i·can·thine [ˌ-ˈkænθaɪn] *adj* → epicanthal.
ep·i·can·thus [ˌ-ˈkænθəs] *n, pl* **-thi** [-θaɪ, -θiː] Mongolenfalte *f*, Epikanthus *m*, Plica palpebronasalis.
ep·i·car·cin·o·gen [ˌ-kɑːrˈsɪnədʒən] *n* Epikarzinogen *nt*.
ep·i·car·di·a [ˌ-ˈkɑːrdɪə] *n* Epikardia *f*.
ep·i·car·di·ac [ˌ-ˈkɑːrdɪæk] *adj* → epicardial.
ep·i·car·di·al [ˌ-ˈkɑːrdɪəl] *adj* 1. Epikard betr., epikardial. 2. Epikardia betr., epikardial.
epicardial ridge *embryo.* Herzwulst *m*.
ep·i·car·di·ec·to·my [ˌ-ˌkɑːrdɪˈektəmɪ] *n HTG* Epikardresektion *f*, Epikardektomie *f*.
ep·i·car·di·um [ˌ-ˈkɑːrdɪəm] *n, pl* **-dia** [-dɪə] Epikard *nt*, viszerales Perikard *nt*, Epicardium *nt*, Lamina visceralis pericardii.
ep·i·chord·al [ˌ-ˈkɔːrdl] *adj* epichordal.
ep·i·cho·ri·on [ˌ-ˈkɔːrɪən] *n embryo.* Epichorion *nt*.
ep·i·cil·lin [ˌ-ˈsɪlɪn] *n pharm.* Epicillin *nt*.
ep·i·con·dy·lal·gia [ˌ-ˌkɒndɪˈlældʒ(ɪ)ə] *n ortho.* Epikondylenschmerz *m*, Epikondylalgie *f*.
ep·i·con·dy·lar [ˌ-ˈkɒndɪlər] *adj* → epicondylian.
epicondylar crest: lateral e. Crista supracondylaris lateralis.
medial e. Crista supracondylaris medialis.
epicondylar fracture: lateral e. Fraktur *f* des Epicondylus lateralis humeri.
medial e. Fraktur *f* des Epicondylus medialis humeri.
ep·i·con·dyle [ˌ-ˈkɒndaɪl, -dl] *n* Gelenkhöcker *m*, Epikondyle *f*, Epicondylus *m*.
e. of femur Femurepikondyle, Epicondylus femoris.
e. of humerus Humerusepikondyle, Epicondylus humeri.
ep·i·con·dyl·i·an [ˌ-kənˈdiːlɪən] *adj* Epikondyle betr., epikondylär, Epikondylen-.
ep·i·con·dyl·ic [ˌ-kənˈdɪlɪk] *adj* → epicondylian.
ep·i·con·dy·li·tis [ˌ-ˌkɒndɪˈlaɪtɪs] *n ortho.* Epikondylenentzündung *f*, Epikondylitis *f*, Epicondylitis *f*.
ep·i·con·dy·lus [ˌ-ˈkɒndɪləs] *n, pl* **-li** [-laɪ] → epicondyle.
ep·i·cor·a·coid [ˌepɪˈkɔːrəkɔɪd] *adj* epikorakoid.
ep·i·cor·ne·a·scle·ri·tis [ˌ-ˌkɔːrnɪəsklɪəˈraɪ-

tɪs] *n ophthal.* Epikorneaskleritis *f*.
ep·i·cos·tal [ˌ-ˈkɒstl, -ˈkɔːstl] *adj* auf einer Rippe (liegend), epikostal.
ep·i·cra·ni·al [ˌ-ˈkreɪnɪəl] *adj* auf dem Schädel (liegend), epikranial.
epicranial aponeurosis Kopfhautaponeurose *f*, Galea aponeurotica, Aponeurosis epicranialis.
epicranial muscle → epicranius (muscle).
ep·i·cra·ni·um [ˌ-ˈkreɪnɪəm] *n* Epikranium *nt*, Epicranium *nt*.
ep·i·cra·ni·us (muscle) [ˌ-ˈkreɪnɪəs] Epikranius *m*, M. epicranius.
ep·i·cri·sis [ˈ-kraɪsɪs] *n* 1. *patho.* Epikrise *f*. 2. *med.* Schlußbeurteilung *f*, Epikrise *f*.
ep·i·crit·ic [ˌ-ˈkrɪtɪk] *adj* 1. Epikrise betr., epikritisch. 2. *physiol.* epikritisch.
epicritic sensibility epikritische Sensibilität *f*.
ep·i·cys·ti·tis [ˌepɪsɪsˈtaɪtɪs] *n urol.* Epizystitis *f*.
ep·i·cys·tot·o·my [ˌ-sɪsˈtɒtəmɪ] *n urol.* suprapubischer Blasenschnitt *m*, suprapubische Zystotomie *f*, Epizystotomie *f*.
ep·i·cyte [ˈ-saɪt] *n* 1. *histol.* Deckzelle *f*, Epizyt *m*; Podozyt *m*. 2. *bio.* äußerste Ektoplasmaschicht *f* von Protozoen.
ep·i·dem·ic [epɪˈdemɪk] **I** *n* epidemische Krankheit/Erkrankung *f*, Epidemie *f*. **II** *adj* epidemieartig auftretend, epidemisch.
epidemic acne *derm.* Keratosis follicularis contagiosa (Morrow-Brooke).
epidemic arthritic erythema Rattenbißkrankheit *f*, Rattenbißfieber II *nt*, atypisches Rattenbißfieber *nt*, Haverhill-Fieber *nt*, Bakterienrattenbißfieber *nt*, Streptobazillenrattenbißfieber *nt*, Erythema arthriticum epidemicum.
epidemic benign dry pleurisy → epidemic pleurodynia.
epidemic cerebrospinal meningitis Meningokokkenmeningitis *f*, Meningitis cerebrospinalis epidemica.
epidemic conjunctivitis Koch-Weeks--Konjunktivitis *f*, Konjunktivitis *f* durch Haemophilus aegyptius, akute kontagiöse Konjunktivitis *f*.
epidemic diaphragmatic pleurisy → epidemic pleurodynia.
epidemic diarrhea of newborn infektiöse Säuglingsenteritis/Säuglingsdyspepsie *f*.
epidemic disease → epidemic I.
epidemic encephalitis 1. → Economo's encephalitis. 2. epidemische Enzephalitis *f*, Encephalitis epidemica.
epidemic erythema Feer'-Krankheit *f*, Rosakrankheit *f*, vegetative Neurose *f* der Kleinkinder, Swift-Syndrom *nt*, Selter-Swift-Feer'-Krankheit *f*, Feer--Selter-Swift-Krankheit *f*, Akrodynie *f*, Acrodynia *f*.
epidemic gangrene → ergotism.
epidemic hemoglobinuria epidemische Hämoglobinurie *f*.
epidemic hemorrhagic fever hämorrhagisches Fieber *nt* mit renalem Syndrom *abbr.* HFRS, koreanisches hämorrhagisches Fieber *nt*, akute hämorrhagische Nephrosonephritis *f*, Nephropathia epidemica.
epidemic hepatitis (Virus-)Hepatitis A *f abbr.* HA, epidemische Hepatitis *f*, Hepatitis epidemica.
epidemic infantile paralysis → epidemic poliomyelitis.
epidemic jaundice → epidemic hepatitis.
epidemic keratoconjunctivitis *ophthal.* epidemische Keratokonjunktivitis *f*, Keratoconjunctivitis epidemica.
epidemic keratoconjunctivitis virus Adenovirus Typ 8 *nt*.

epidemic myalgia → epidemic pleurodynia.
epidemic myalgic encephalomyelitis → epidemic neuromyasthenia.
epidemic neuromyasthenia epidemische Neuromyasthenie *f*, Encephalomyelitis benigna myalgica.
epidemic parotiditis → epidemic parotitis.
epidemic parotitis Mumps *m/f*, Ziegenpeter *m*, Parotitis epidemica.
epidemic pleurodynia Bornholmer--Krankheit *f*, epidemische Pleurodynie *f*, Myalgia epidemica.
epidemic poliomyelitis epidemische Poliomyelitis *f*.
epidemic relapsing fever epidemisches (europäisches) Rückfallfieber *nt*, Läuserückfallfieber *nt*.
epidemic stomatitis (echte) Maul- u. Klauenseuche *f abbr.* MKS, Febris aphthosa, Stomatitis epidemica, Aphthosis epizootica.
epidemic transient diaphragmatic spasm → epidemic pleurodynia.
epidemic typhus epidemisches/klassisches Fleckfieber *nt*, Läuseflechfieber *nt*, Fleck-, Hunger-, Kriegstyphus *m*, Typhus exanthematicus.
epidemic vertigo *neuro.* Vertigo epidemica.
epidemic vomiting epidemisches Erbrechen *nt*, Bradley-Krankheit *f*.
ep·i·de·mi·ol·o·gist [epɪˌdiːmɪˈɒlədʒɪst] *n* Epidemiologe *m*, -login *f*.
ep·i·de·mi·ol·o·gy [epɪˌdiːmɪˈɒlədʒɪ] *n* Epidemiologie *f*.
ep·i·derm [ˈepɪdɜːrm] *n* → epidermis.
ep·i·der·ma [ˌ-ˈdɜːrmə] *n* → epidermis.
ep·i·der·mal [ˌ-ˈdɜːrml] *adj* 1. Oberhaut/ Epidermis betr., epidermal, Epidermis-, Epiderm(o)-. 2. epidermisähnlich, epidermoid.
epidermal cyst → epidermoid I.
epidermal growth factor *abbr.* **EGF** epidermaler Wachstumsfaktor *m*, epidermal growth factor *abbr.* EGF.
epidermal inclusion cyst epidermale Einschlußzyste *f*.
epidermal nevus epidermaler Nävus *m*.
epidermal ridges Hautleisten *pl*, Cristae cutis.
ep·i·der·mat·ic [ˌ-dɜːrˈmætɪk] *adj* → epidermal 1.
ep·i·der·ma·ti·tis [ˌ-ˌdɜːrməˈtaɪtɪs] *n* Epidermisentzündung *f*, Epidermatitis *f*, Epidermitis *f*.
ep·i·der·mat·o·plas·ty [ˌ-dɜːrˈmætəplæstɪ] *n chir.* Epidermisplastik *f*.
ep·i·der·mic [ˌ-ˈdɜːrmɪk] *adj* → epidermal 1.
epidermic cell Epidermiszelle *f*.
epidermic-dermic nevus Junktions-, Grenz-, Abtropfungs-, Übergangsnävus *m*, junktionaler Nävus *m*.
epidermic graft *chir.* Reverdin-Läppchen *nt*, -Lappen *m*, Epidermisläppchen *nt*, -lappen *m*.
ep·i·der·mis [epɪˈdɜːrmɪs] *n* Oberhaut *f*, Epidermis *f*.
ep·i·der·mi·tis [ˌ-dɜːrˈmaɪtɪs] *n* → epidermatitis.
ep·i·der·mi·za·tion [ˌ-ˌdɜːrmɪˈzeɪʃn] *n chir.* Epidermistransplantation *f*, Hauttransplantation *f*.
ep·i·der·mo·dys·pla·sia verruciformis [ˌ-ˌdɜːrmədɪsˈpleɪʒ(ɪ)ə, -ziə] *derm.* Epidermodysplasia verruciformis, Lewandowsky-Lutz-Syndrom *nt*.
ep·i·der·moid [ˌ-ˈdɜːrmɔɪd] **I** *n* Epidermoid *nt*, Epidermal-, Epidermis-, Epidermoidzyste *f*, (echtes) Atherom *nt*, Talgreten-

epidermoid cancer/carcinoma 260

tionszyste f. II adj epidermisähnlich, epidermoid.
epidermoid cancer/carcinoma Plattenepithelkarzinom nt, Ca. planocellulare/platycellulare.
epidermoid cyst → epidermoid I.
epidermoid inclusion cyst epidermale Einschlußzyste f.
ep·i·der·mol·y·sis [,-dər'mɑləsɪs] n derm. Epidermolysis f.
epidermolysis bullosa: acquired e. derm. Epidermolysis bullosa acquisita.
junctional e. derm. Herlitz-Syndrom nt, kongenitaler nicht-syphilitischer Pemphigus m, Epidermolysis bullosa (hereditaria) letalis, Epidermolysis bullosa atrophicans generalisata gravis Herlitz.
epidermolysis bullosa dystrophica: albopapuloid e. derm. Pasini-Syndrom nt, Pasini-Pierini-Syndrom nt, Epidermolysis bullosa albopapuloidea.
dominant e. Cockayne-Touraine-Syndrom nt, Epidermolysis bullosa (hereditaria) dystrophica dominans, Epidermolysis bullosa hyperplastica.
hyperplastic e. → dominant e.
epidermolysis bullosa simplex, localized Weber-Cockayne-Syndrom nt, Epidermolysis bullosa simplex Weber-Cockayne, Epidermolysis bullosa manuum et pedum aestivalis.
ep·i·der·mo·lyt·ic [,epɪdərmə'lɪtɪk] adj Epidermolysis betr., epidermolytisch.
epidermolytic hyperkeratosis 1. Erythrodermia congenitalis ichthyosiformis bullosa. **2.** Sauriasis f, Ichthyosis hystrix, Hyperkeratosis monstruosa.
ep·i·der·mo·my·co·sis [,-dərməmar'koʊsɪs] n derm. Dermatophytose f, -phytosis f, -phytie f, Epidermomykose f.
ep·i·der·moph·y·tid [,epɪdər'mɑfətɪd] n Epidermophytid nt, Dermatophytid nt.
Ep·i·der·moph·y·ton [,-'mɑfətən] n micro. Epidermophyton nt.
ep·i·der·moph·y·to·sis [,-,mɑfə'toʊsɪs] n derm. Epidermophytie f; Dermatophytie f.
ep·i·did·y·mal [epɪ'dɪdəməl] adj Epididymis betr., epididymal, Nebenhoden-, Epididymis-.
epididymal branches of testicular artery Rami epididymales a. testicularis.
ep·i·did·y·mec·to·my [,-,dɪdə'mektəmɪ] n urol. Nebenhodenentfernung f, Epididymektomie f.
ep·i·did·y·mid·ec·to·my [,-,dɪdəmɪ'dektəmɪ] n → epididymectomy.
ep·i·did·y·mis [epɪ'dɪdəmɪs] n, pl **-did·y·mi·des** [-dɪ'dɪmɪdiːz] Nebenhoden m, Epididymis f, Parorchis m.
ep·i·did·y·mis·o·plas·ty [,-'dɪdəmɪsoʊplæstɪ] n → epididymoplasty.
ep·i·did·y·mi·tis [,-dɪdə'maɪtɪs] n urol. Nebenhodenentzündung f, Epididymitis f.
ep·i·did·y·mo·def·er·en·tec·to·my [,epɪ,dɪdəmoʊ,defərən'tektəmɪ] n → epididymovasectomy.
ep·i·did·y·mo·def·er·en·tial [,-defə'renʃl] adj Nebenhoden u. Samenleiter betr.
ep·i·did·y·mo·def·er·en·ti·tis [,-,defərən'taɪtɪs] n urol. Entzündung f von Nebenhoden u. Samenstrang, Epididymodeferentitis f, -funikulitis f.
epididymo-orchitis n urol. Entzündung f von Nebenhoden u. Hoden, Epididymoorchitis f.
ep·i·did·y·mo·plas·ty ['-plæstɪ] n urol. Nebenhoden-, Epididymisplastik f.
ep·i·did·y·mot·o·my [epɪ,dɪdə'mɑtəmɪ] n urol. Epididymotomie f.
ep·i·did·y·mo·vas·ec·to·my [epɪ,dɪdəmoʊvæ'sektəmɪ] n urol. Nebenhodenentfernung f mit (teilweiser) Samenstrangresektion, Epididymovasektomie f.
ep·i·did·y·mo·vas·os·to·my [,-væs'ɑstəmɪ] n urol. Epididymovasostomie f.
ep·i·du·ral [,epɪ'dʊrəl, -'djʊər-] I n → epidural anesthesia. II adj auf der Dura mater (liegend), epi-, extra-, supradural, Epidural-.
epidural abscess epiduraler/extraduraler Abszeß m, Epiduralabszeß m.
epidural aerocele epidurale Pneumozele f.
epidural analgesia Epiduralanalgesie f.
epidural anesthesia Epidural-, Periduralanästhesie f, inf. Epidurale f, inf. Periduralе f.
continous/fractional e. kontinuierliche Epiduralanästhesie.
lumbar e. Lumbalanästhesie.
epidural bleeding extradurale Blutung f, Epiduralblutung f.
epidural block → epidural anesthesia.
epidural cavity → epidural space.
epidural empyema epidurales Empyem nt.
epidural hematoma Epiduralhämatom nt, epidurales/extradurales Hämatom nt.
epidural hemorrhage → epidural bleeding.
epidural meningitis epidurale Pachymeningitis f, Pachymeningitis externa.
epidural space Epiduralraum m, -spalt m, Spatium epidurale/peridurale.
ep·i·du·rog·ra·phy [,epɪdjʊə'rɑgrəfɪ] n radiol. Kontrastdarstellung f des Epiduralraums, Epidurographie f.
ep·i·fas·cial [,-'fæʃ(ɪ)əl] adj auf einer Faszie (liegend), epifaszial.
ep·i·gas·tral·gia [,-gæ'strældʒ(ɪ)ə] n Oberbauchschmerz(en pl) m, Epigastralgie f.
ep·i·gas·tric [,-'gæstrɪk] adj Oberbauch/Epigastrium betr., epigastrisch.
epigastric angle epigastrischer Winkel m, Rippenbogenwinkel m, Angulus infrasternalis.
epigastric artery: external e. tiefe Hüftkranzarterie f, Zirkumflexa f iliaka profunda, A. circumflexa iliaca profunda.
inferior e. untere Bauchdeckenarterie f, Epigastrica f inferior, A. epigastrica inferior.
superficial e. oberflächliche Bauchdeckenarterie f, Epigastrica f superficialis, A. epigastrica superficialis.
superior e. obere Bauchdeckenarterie f, Epigastrica f superior, A. epigastrica superior.
epigastric aura neuro. epigastrische Aura f.
epigastric fold epigastrische Falte f, Plica umbilicalis lateralis.
epigastric fossa Magengrube f, Fossa epigastrica.
epigastric fullness epigastrisches Völlegefühl nt, Völlegefühl nt im Oberbauch.
epigastric hernia chir. epigastrische Hernie f, Hernia epigastrica, Epigastrozele f.
epigastric incision Mittel-, Medianschnitt m.
epigastric lymph nodes, inferior Lymphknoten pl der A. epigastrica inferior, Nodi lymphatici parietales epigastrici inferiores.
epigastric pain → epigastralgia.
epigastric plexus Sonnengeflecht nt, Plexus solaris, Plexus coeliacus.
epigastric pulse Puls m über der Aorta abdominalis, Pulsus abdominalis.
epigastric reflex epigastrischer Reflex m.
epigastric region → epigastrium.
epigastric vein: inferior e. untere Bauchwandvene f, V. epigastrica inferior.
superficial e. oberflächliche Bauchwandvene f, V. epigastrica superficialis.
superior e.s obere Bauchwandvenen pl, Vv. epigastricae superiores.
epigastric zone → epigastrium.
ep·i·gas·tri·um [,-'gæstrɪəm] n anat. Oberbauch(gegend f) m, Epigastrium nt, Regio epigastrica.
ep·i·gas·tri·us [,-'gæstrɪəs] n embryo. Epigastrius m.
ep·i·gas·tro·cele [,-'gæstrəsiːl] n → epigastric hernia.
ep·i·gen·e·sis [,-'dʒenəsɪs] n Epigenese f.
ep·i·ge·net·ic [,-dʒə'netɪk] adj Epigenese betr., epigenetisch.
ep·i·ge·net·ics [,-dʒə'netɪks] pl Epigenetik f.
ep·i·gen·i·tal tubules [,-'dʒenɪtl] Epigenitalis f, Tubuli epigenitalis.
ep·i·glot·tal [,-'glɑtl] adj → epiglottic.
epiglottal swelling embryo. Epiglottiswulst m.
ep·i·glot·tec·to·my [,-glɑ'tektəmɪ] n → epiglottidectomy.
ep·i·glot·tic [,-'glɑtɪk] adj Kehldeckel/Epiglottis betr., epiglottisch, Kehldeckel-, Epiglottis-.
epiglottic cartilage 1. → epiglottis. **2.** knorpeliges Kehldeckelskelett nt, Cartilago epiglottica.
epiglottic petiole Epiglottis-, Kehldeckelstiel m, Petiolus epiglottidis.
epiglottic tubercle Epiglottishöckerchen nt, Tuberculum epiglotticum.
epiglottic vallecula Vallecula epiglottica.
ep·i·glot·tid·e·an [,-glɑ'tiːdɪən] adj → epiglottic.
ep·i·glot·ti·dec·to·my [,-,glɑtɪ'dektəmɪ] n HNO Kehldeckelentfernung f, -resektion f, Epiglottisentfernung f, -resektion f, Epiglottidektomie f, Epiglottektomie f.
ep·i·glot·ti·di·tis [,-,glɑtɪ'daɪtɪs] n HNO Kehldeckel-, Epiglottisentzündung f, Epiglottiditis f, Epiglottitis f.
ep·i·glot·tis [,-'glɑtɪs] n Kehldeckel m, Epiglottis f.
ep·i·glot·ti·tis [,-glɑ'taɪtɪs] n → epiglottiditis.
e·pig·na·thus [ɪ'pɪgnəθəs] n embryo., patho. Epignathus m.
e·pig·o·nal [ɪ'pɪgənəl] adj embryo. epigonal, epigonad.
ep·i·hy·al [epɪ'haɪəl] adj → epihyoid.
epihyal ligament Lig. stylohyoideum.
ep·i·hy·oid [,-'haɪɔɪd] adj auf od. über dem Zungenbein (liegend), epihyal, epihyoid.
ep·i·la·mel·lar [,-lə'melər] adj auf od. über der Basalmembran (liegend), epilamellär.
ep·i·late ['epɪleɪt] vt Haare entfernen, enthaaren, epilieren, depilieren.
ep·i·la·tion [epɪ'leɪʃn] n Enthaarung f, Haarentfernung f, Epilation f, Epilierung f, Depilation f.
ep·i·lem·ma [epɪ'lemə] n → endoneurium.
ep·i·lep·sia [,-'lepsɪə] n → epilepsy.
ep·i·lep·sy ['-lepsɪ] n neuro. Epilepsie f, Epilepsia f.
ep·i·lep·tic [,-'leptɪk] neuro. I n Patient(in f) m mit Epilepsie, Epileptiker(in f) m. II adj Epilepsie betr., durch Epilepsie hervorgerufen, an Epilepsie leidend, epileptisch, Epilepsie-.
epileptic attack neuro. epileptischer Anfall m.
epileptic aura neuro. epileptische Aura f.
epileptic dementia epileptische Demenz f.
epileptic seizure neuro. epileptischer Anfall m.
epileptic state Status epilepticus.
epileptic stupor neuro. postkonvulsiver Stupor m.

ep·i·lep·ti·form [ˌepɪˈleptɪfɔːrm] *adj neuro.* epilepsieartig, epileptiform, epileptoid.
epileptiform convulsion epileptiformer Krampf(anfall *m*) *m*.
epileptiform neuralgia Trigeminusneuralgie *f*, Neuralgia trigeminalis.
ep·i·lep·to·gen·ic [ˌ-leptəˈdʒenɪk] *adj neuro.* einen epileptischen Anfall auslösend, epileptogen.
epileptogenic zone epileptogene Zone *f*.
ep·i·lep·tog·e·nous [ˌ-lepˈtadʒənəs] *adj* → epileptogenic.
epileptogenous zone → epileptogenic zone.
ep·i·lep·toid [ˌ-ˈleptɔɪd] *adj* → epileptiform.
ep·i·lep·tol·o·gist [ˌ-lepˈtalədʒɪst] *n neuro.* Epilepsiespezialist *m*, Epileptologe *m*, -login *f*.
ep·i·lep·tol·o·gy [ˌ-lepˈtalədʒɪ] *n neuro.* Epilepsieforschung *f*, Epileptologie *f*.
ep·i·loi·a [ˌ-ˈlɔɪə] *n* Bourneville-Syndrom *nt*, Morbus Bourneville *m*, tuberöse (Hirn-)Sklerose *f*, Epiloia *f*.
ep·i·man·dib·u·lar [ˌ-mænˈdɪbjələr] *adj* auf *od.* über der Mandibula (liegend), epimandibulär.
ep·i·mas·ti·gote [ˌ-ˈmæstɪɡəʊt] *n micro.* epimastigote Form *f*, Crithidia-Form *f*.
epimastigote stage → epimastigote.
ep·i·mem·bra·nous glomerulonephritis [epɪˈmembrənəs] membranöse Glomerulonephritis *f*.
ep·i·men·or·rha·gia [ˌ-ˌmenəˈreɪdʒ(ɪ)ə] *n gyn.* Epimenorrhagie *f*.
ep·i·men·or·rhea [ˌ-ˌmenəˈrɪə] *n gyn.* Epimenorrhea *f*.
ep·i·mer [ˈepəmər] *n chem.* Epimer *nt*.
ep·i·mer·ase [ˈepɪmereɪz] *n* Epimerase *f*.
ep·i·mere [ˈepɪmɪər] *n embryo.* Epimer *nt*.
ep·i·mer·i·za·tion [ˌepɪmərɪˈzeɪʃn] *n chem.* Epimerisierung *f*.
ep·i·mes·trol [ˌ-ˈmestrəʊl] *n pharm.* Epimestrol *nt*.
ep·i·mor·pho·sis [ˌ-mɔːrˈfəʊsɪs] *n bio., patho.* Epimorphose *f*.
ep·i·my·o·car·di·al mantle [ˌ-ˌmaɪəˈkɑːrdɪəl] *embryo.* Myoepikardmantel *m*.
ep·i·mys·i·ot·o·my [ˌ-ˌmɪsɪˈatəmɪ] *n chir.* Durchtrennung *f* der Muskelscheide, Epimysiotomie *f*.
ep·i·my·si·um [ˌ-ˈmɪzɪəm, -ˈmɪʒ-] *n, pl* -mysia [-ˈmɪzɪə, -ˈmɪʒ-] Muskelscheide *f*, Epimysium *nt*, Perimysium externum.
ep·i·ne·phrec·to·my [ˌ-nɪˈfrektəmɪ] *n old* → adrenalectomy.
ep·i·neph·rine [ˌ-ˈnefrɪn, -riːn] *n* Adrenalin *nt*, Epinephrin *nt*.
ep·i·neph·ri·ne·mia [ˌ-ˌnefrɪˈniːmɪə] *n* (Hyper-)Adrenalinämie *f*.
epinephrine reversal Adrenalinumkehr *f*.
ep·i·ne·phri·tis [ˌ-nɪˈfraɪtɪs] *n old* → adrenalitis.
ep·i·ne·phro·ma [ˌ-nɪˈfrəʊmə] *n old* → renal cell carcinoma.
ep·i·neph·ros [ˌ-ˈnefrɒs, -rɒs] *n* Nebenniere *f*, Epinephros *nt*, Epinephron *nt*, Gl. adrenalis/suprarenalis.
ep·i·neu·ral [ˌ-ˈnjʊərəl, -ˈnʊ-] *adj* auf einem Wirbelbogen (liegend), epineural.
ep·i·neu·ri·al [ˌ-ˈnʊrɪəl, -ˈnjʊər-] *adj* Epineurium betr., epineurial.
epineurial repair *ortho., neurochir.* Epineurialnaht *f*, primäre (End-zu-End-)Nervennaht *f*.
ep·i·neu·ri·um [ˌ-ˈnʊrɪəm, -ˈnjʊər-] *n, pl* -ria [-rɪə] Epineurium *nt*.
ep·i·o·nych·i·um [epɪəˈniːkɪəm] *n* Nagelhäutchen *nt*, Eponychium *nt*.
ep·i·or·chi·um [epɪˈɔːrkɪəm] *n* Epiorchium *nt*, Lamina visceralis tunicae vaginalis testis.

ep·i·ot·ic [ˌ-ˈatɪk] *adj* auf *od.* über dem Ohr (liegend), epiotisch.
ep·i·pas·tic [ˌ-ˈpæstɪk] *pharm.* **I** *n* Streupulver *nt*, Puder *m*. **II** *adj* als Puder verwendbar.
ep·i·per·i·car·di·al [ˌ-ˌperɪˈkɑːrdɪəl] *adj* auf dem Perikard (liegend), um das Perikard herum, epiperikardial.
ep·i·pha·ryn·ge·al [ˌ-fəˈrɪndʒ(ɪ)əl, -ˌfærɪnˈdʒiːəl] *adj* Nasenrachen/Epipharynx betr., epi-, nasopharyngeal, Nasenrachen-, Epipharyng(o)-, Epipharynx-, Nasopharynx-.
ep·i·phar·yn·gi·tis [ˌ-ˌfærɪnˈdʒaɪtɪs] *n* Epipharynx-, Nasopharynxentzündung *f*, Epipharyngitis *f*, Nasopharyngitis *f*.
ep·i·phar·ynx [ˌ-ˈfærɪŋks] *n* Nasenrachen *m*, Epi-, Naso-, Rhinopharynx *m*, Pars nasalis pharyngis.
ep·i·phe·nom·e·non [ˌ-fɪˈnamənən] *n* Begleiterscheinung *f*, Begleitsymptom *nt*, Epiphänomen *nt*.
e·piph·o·ra [ɪˈpɪfərə] *n ophthal.* Tränenträufeln *nt*, Dakryorrhoe *f*, Epiphora *f*.
ep·i·phre·nal [epɪˈfriːnl] *adj* → epiphrenic.
ep·i·phren·ic [ˌ-ˈfrenɪk] *adj* auf *od.* über dem Zwerchfell (liegend), epiphrenisch, epiphrenal.
epiphrenic diverticulum *chir.* (*Ösophagus*) epiphrenisches/epiphrenales/parahiatales Divertikel *nt*.
ep·i·phys·e·al [ˌ-ˈfɪzɪəl, ɪˌpɪfəˈsiːəl] *adj* Epiphyse betr., zur Epiphyse gehörend, epiphysär, Epiphysen-, Epiphyseo-.
epiphyseal cartilage Epiphysen(fugen)knorpel *m*, epiphysäre Knorpelzone *f*, Cartilago epiphysialis.
epiphyseal disk → epiphyseal plate 1.
epiphyseal dysplasia *ortho.* Epiphysendysplasie *f*, epiphysäre Dysplasie *f*.
multiple e. multiple epiphysäre Dysplasie Ribbing-Müller *f*.
epiphyseal fracture traumatische Epiphysenlösung *f*, Epiphysenfraktur *f*.
epiphyseal growth plate → epiphyseal plate 1.
epiphyseal ischemic necrosis *ortho.* aseptische Epiphysennekrose *f*, Osteochondrose *f*, -chondrosis *f*, Chondroosteonekrose *f*.
epiphyseal line Epiphysenlinie *f*, Epiphysenfugennarbe *f*, Linea epiphysialis.
epiphyseal plate 1. epiphysäre Wachstumszone *f*, Epiphysenfuge *f*. 2. → epiphyseal cartilage.
epiphyseal syndrome Pellizzi-Syndrom *nt*, Macrogenitosomia praecox.
ep·i·phys·e·od·e·sis *n* → epiphysiodesis.
ep·i·phys·i·al *adj* → epiphyseal.
epiphysial aseptic necrosis aseptische Epiphysennekrose *f*.
epiphysial center epiphysärer Knochenkeim *m*.
epiphysial line → epiphyseal line.
ep·i·phys·i·od·e·sis [ˌ-ˌfɪzɪˈadəsɪs] *n ortho.* Epiphyseodese *f*.
ep·i·phys·i·oid [ˌ-ˈfɪzɪɔɪd] *adj* epiphysenähnlich.
ep·i·phys·i·ol·y·sis [ˌ-ˌfɪzɪˈaləsɪs] *n ortho.* Epiphysenlösung *f*, Epiphysiolyse *f*.
ep·i·phys·i·om·e·ter [ˌ-ˌfɪzɪˈamɪtər] *n ortho.* Epiphysiometer *nt*.
ep·i·phys·i·op·a·thy [ˌ-ˌfɪzɪˈapəθɪ] *n* 1. *ortho.* Epiphysenerkrankung *f*, Epiphysiopathie *f*. 2. *neuro., neurochir.* Epiphysenerkrankung *f*, Epiphysiopathie *f*.
e·piph·y·sis [ɪˈpɪfəsɪs] *n, pl* -ses [-siːz] 1. (Knochen-)Epiphyse *f*, Epiphysis *f*. 2. Zirbeldrüse *f*, Corpus pineale, Gl. pinealis, Epiphyse *f*, Epiphysis cerebri.
e·piph·y·si·tis [ɪˌpɪfəˈsaɪtɪs] *n ortho.* Epiphysenentzündung *f*, Epiphysitis *f*.

e. of calcaneus Sever'-Krankheit *f*, Apophysitis/Apophyseose calcanei.
ep·i·phyte [ˈepɪfaɪt] *n* 1. *bio.* pflanzlicher Schmarotzer/Parasit *m*, Epiphyt *m*. 2. *derm.* Hautschmarotzer *m*, Epi(dermo)phyt *m*.
ep·i·phyt·ic [epəˈfɪtɪk] *adj* Epiphyt betr., epiphytisch.
ep·i·pi·al [epɪˈpaɪəl] *adj* auf der Pia mater (liegend), epipial.
epipl(o)- *pref.* Netz-, Oment(o)-, Epipl(o)-.
e·pip·lo·cele [ɪˈpɪpləsiːl] *n chir.* Netzbruch *m*, Epiplozele *f*.
ep·i·plo·ec·to·my [ˌepɪpləˈektəmɪ] *n chir.* Omentumresektion *f*, Omentektomie *f*, Epiploektomie *f*.
e·pip·lo·en·ter·o·cele [ɪˌpɪpləˈentərəʊsiːl] *n* Epiploenterozele *f*, Omentoenterozele *f*.
ep·i·plo·ic [epɪˈpləʊɪk] *adj* großes Netz/Epiploon betr., epiploisch, omental, Oment(o)-.
epiploic abscess epiploischer Abszeß *m*, Abszeß *m* des Bauchnetzes.
epiploic appendages Appendices epiploicae/omentales.
epiploic appendagitis Entzündung *f* der Appendices epiploicae.
epiploic appendices → epiploic appendages.
epiploic branches: e. of left gastroepiploic artery Netzbeuteläste *pl* der A. gastroepiploica sinistra, Rami epiploici/omentales a. gastroepiploicae/gastro-omentalis sinistrae.
e. of left gastroomental artery → e. of left gastroepiploic artery.
e. of right gastroepiploic artery Netzbeuteläste *pl* der A. gastroepiploica dextra, Rami epiploici/omentales a. gastroepiploicae/gastro-omentalis dextrae.
e. of right gastroomental artery → e. of right gastroepiploic artery.
epiploic foramen Winslow'-Foramen *nt*, -Loch *nt*, For. epiploicum/omentale.
epiploic sac Netzbeutel *m*, Bauchfelltasche *f*, Bursa omentalis.
epiploic vein: left e. Begleitvene *f* der A. gastroepiploica sinistra, V. gastroepiploica/gastro-omentalis sinistra.
right e. Begleitvene *f* der A. gastroepiploica dextra, V. gastroepiploica/gastro-omentalis dextra.
e·pip·lo·i·tis [ɪˈpɪpləwaɪtɪs] *n* (Bauch-)Netzentzündung *f*, Omentitis *f*, Epiploitis *f*.
e·pip·lo·me·ro·cele [ɪˌpɪpləˈmerəsiːl] *n chir.* Epiplomerozele *f*.
ep·i·plom·phal·o·cele [epɪplamˈfæləsiːl] *n chir.* Epiplomphalozele *f*.
e·pip·lo·on [ɪˈpɪpləwan] *n, pl* -loa [-ləwə] 1. (Bauch-)Netz *nt*, Omentum *nt*, Epiploon *nt*. 2. großes Netz *nt*, Omentum majus.
e·pip·lo·pex·y [ɪˈpɪpləpeksɪ] *n chir.* Omentopexie *f*, Epiplopexie *f*.
e·pip·lo·plas·ty [ɪˈpɪpləplæstɪ] *n chir.* Netz-, Omentum-, Omentoplastik *f*.
e·pip·lor·rha·phy [ɪˌpɪpˈlɔːrəfɪ] *n chir.* (Bauch-)Netznaht *f*, Omentorrhaphie *f*.
ep·i·py·gus [epɪˈpaɪɡəs] *n embryo.* Epipygus *m*.
ep·i·scle·ra [ˌ-ˈsklɪərə] *n* Episklera *f*, Lamina episcleralis.
ep·i·scle·ral [ˌ-ˈsklɪərəl] *adj* 1. Episklera betr., episkleral, Episkleral-. 2. auf der Lederhaut/Sclera liegend, episkleral.
episcleral arteries Skleraäste *pl* der Aa. ciliares anteriores, Aa. episclerales.
episcleral lamina → episclera.
episcleral space Tenon'-Raum *m*, Spatium episclerale.

episcleral veins

episcleral veins Episkleralvenen *pl*, Vv. episclerales.
ep·i·scle·ri·tis [ˌ-sklɪəˈraɪtɪs] *n ophthal*. Episkleraentzündung *f*, Episkleritis *f*.
ep·i·scle·ro·ti·tis [ˌ-ˌsklɪərəˈtaɪtɪs] *n* → episcleritis.
episi(o)- *pref.* Episi(o)-, Vulva-, Vulvo-.
e·pi·si·o·per·i·ne·o·plas·ty [əˌpɪzɪəˌperɪˈnɪəplæstɪ] *n gyn*. Episioperineoplastik *f*.
e·pi·si·o·per·i·ne·or·rha·phy [ˌ-ˌperɪnɪˈɔrəfɪ] *n gyn*. Vulva-Damm-Naht *f*, Episioperineorrhaphie *f*.
e·pi·si·o·plas·ty [ˈplæstɪ] *n gyn*. Vulvaplastik *f*, Episioplastik *f*.
e·pi·si·or·rha·phy [əˌpɪzɪˈɔrəfɪ] *n gyn*. 1. Schamlippennaht *f*, Episiorrhaphie *f*. 2. Naht *f* einer Episiotomie, Episiorrhaphie *f*.
e·pi·si·o·ste·no·sis [əˌpɪzɪəstɪˈnəʊsɪs] *n gyn*. Episiostenose *f*.
e·pi·si·ot·o·my [əˌpɪzɪˈɒtəmɪ] *n gyn*. (Scheiden-)Dammschnitt *m*, Episiotomie *f*.
ep·i·sode [ˈepɪsəʊd] *n* 1. *psychia*. vorübergehende rückbildungsfähige Störung *f*, Episode *f*. 2. Anfall *m*, Attacke *f*, Episode *f*.
ep·i·sod·ic [ˌepɪˈsɒdɪk] *adj* episodisch, episodenhaft.
ep·i·sod·i·cal [ˌ-ˈsɒdɪkl̩] *adj* → episodic.
episodic amnesia amnestische Episode *f*.
episodic memory episodisches (Langzeit-)Gedächtnis *nt*.
episodic pain episodischer/episodenartiger Schmerz *m*.
ep·i·some [ˈ-səʊm] *n* Episom *nt*.
ep·i·spa·dia [ˌ-ˈspeɪdɪə] *n* → epispadias.
ep·i·spa·di·ac [ˌ-ˈspeɪdɪæk] *adj* → epispadial.
ep·i·spa·di·al [ˌ-ˈspeɪdɪəl] *adj* Epispadie betr., epispadial, epispadisch, Epispadie-.
ep·i·spa·di·as [ˌ-ˈspeɪdɪəs] *n embryo., urol*. obere Harnröhrenspalte *f*, Epispadie *f*, Fissura urethrae superior.
ep·i·spi·nal [ˌ-ˈspaɪnl̩] *adj* auf der Wirbelsäule *od*. dem Rückenmark (liegend), epispinal.
ep·i·sple·ni·tis [ˌ-splɪˈnaɪtɪs] *n* Milzkapselentzündung *f*, Episplenitis *f*.
e·pis·ta·sis [ɪˈpɪstəsɪs] *n* 1. *genet*. Epistasis *f*, Epistasie *f*, Epistase *f*. 2. *lab*. (*Urin*) Schaum- *od*. Häutchenbildung *f*.
e·pis·ta·sy [ɪˈpɪstəsɪ] *n* → epistasis.
ep·i·stat·ic [epɪˈstætɪk] *adj* Epistasis betr., epistatisch.
ep·i·stax·is [ˌ-ˈstæksɪs] *n* Nasenbluten *nt*, -blutung *f*, Epistaxis *f*.
ep·i·ster·nal [ˌ-ˈstɜːnl̩] *adj* auf *od*. über dem Sternum (liegend), episternal, suprasternal.
episternal bones Ossa suprasternalia.
e·pis·thot·o·nus [epɪsˈθɒtənəs] *n neuro., psychia*. Episthotonus *m*, Emprosthotonus *m*.
ep·i·stro·phe·us [epɪˈstrəʊfɪəs] *n* Epistropheus *m*, Axis *m*, II. Halswirbel *m*.
ep·i·tar·sus [ˌ-ˈtɑːrsəs] *n ophthal*. angeborenes Pterygium *nt*, Epitarsus *m*.
ep·i·tax·y [ˌ-ˈtæksɪ] *n* Epitaxie *f*.
ep·i·ten·din·e·um [ˌ-tenˈdɪnɪəm] *n* Epitendineum *nt*, Epitenon *nt*.
ep·i·te·non [ˌ-ˈtenɒn] *n* → epitendineum.
ep·i·tha·lam·ic [ˌ-θəˈlæmɪk] *adj* 1. oberhalb des Thalamus (liegend), epithalamisch. 2. Epithalamus betr., epithalamisch, Epithalamus-.
epithalamic commissure hintere Kommissur *f*, Commissura epithalamica, Commissura posterior cerebri.
ep·i·thal·a·mus [ˌ-ˈθæləməs] *n, pl* **-mi** [-maɪ] Epithalamus *m*.
ep·i·tha·lax·ia [ˌ-θəˈlæksɪə] *n* (Schleimhaut-)Epithelabschuppung *f*, (Schleimhaut-)Epitheldesquamation *f*, Epithalaxis *f*.
epitheli- *pref.* → epithelio-.
ep·i·the·li·al [epɪˈθiːlɪəl, -jəl] *adj* Epithel betr., aus Epithel bestehend, epithelial, Epithel-.
epithelial body Nebenschilddrüse *f*, Epithelkörperchen *nt*, Parathyr(e)oidea *f*, Gl. parathyroidea.
epithelial cancer Karzinom *nt, inf.* Krebs *m*, Carcinoma *nt abbr.* Ca.
epithelial cast (*Harn*) Epithelien-, Epithelzylinder *m*.
epithelial cell Epithelzelle *f*.
  alveolar e. Alveolarzelle *f*, Pneumozyt *m*, -cyt *m*.
  follicular e. Follikelzelle *f*.
epithelial cyst 1. epitheliale Zyste *f*. 2. Epidermoid *nt*, Epidermal-, Epidermis-, Epidermoidzyste *f*, (echtes) Atherom *nt*, Talgretentionszyste *f*.
epithelial hyalin *patho.* epitheliales Hyalin *nt*.
ep·i·the·li·al·i·za·tion [ˌ-ˌθiːlɪəlaɪˈzeɪʃn̩] *n patho.* Epithelialisierung *f*, Epithelisation *f*.
ep·i·the·li·al·ize [ˌ-ˈθiːlɪəlaɪz] *vt* mit Epithel überziehen, epithelisieren.
epithelial interferon β-Interferon *nt abbr.* IFN-β.
epithelial lamina Ependymüberzug *m* des Plexus choroideus, Lamina epithelialis.
epithelial layer of tympanic membrane (*Trommelfell*) epitheliale Schicht *f*, Kutisschicht *f*, Stratum cutaneum membranae tympani.
epithelial nests of von Brunn (von) Brunn'-Epithelnester *pl*.
epithelial nevus epidermaler Nävus *m*.
epithelial punctate keratitis Keratitis superficialis punctata.
epithelial rests of Malassez Malassez'-Epithelreste *pl*.
epithelial tissue → epithelium.
epithelial tumor → epithelioma.
ep·i·the·li·i·tis [epɪˌθiːlɪˈaɪtɪs] *n* Epithelentzündung *f*, Epithel(i)tis *f*.
epithelio- *pref.* Epithel-, Epithelium-, Epitheli(o)-.
ep·i·the·li·o·cho·ri·al [epɪˌθiːlɪəˈkɔːrɪəl] *adj* epitheliochorial.
epitheliochorial placenta Placenta epitheliochorialis.
ep·i·the·li·o·fi·bril [ˌ-ˈfaɪbrəl] *n* Tonofibrille *f*.
ep·i·the·li·o·glan·du·lar [ˌ-ˈɡlændʒələr] *adj* Drüsenepithel betr., Drüsenepithel-.
ep·i·the·li·oid [epɪˈθiːlɪɔɪd] *adj* epithelähnlich, epitheloid.
epithelioid cell 1. epitheloide Zelle *f*. 2. Pinealozyt *m*.
epithelioid cell granuloma epitheloidzelliges Granulom *m*.
epithelioid cell nevus Spitz-Tumor *m*, -Nävus *m*, Allen-Spitz-Nävus *m*, Epitheloidzellnävus *m*, Spindelzellnävus *m*, benignes juveniles Melanom *nt*.
epithelioid cell tubercle Epitheloidzelltuberkel *m*.
epithelioid leiomyoma epitheliales Leiomyom *nt*, Leiomyoblastom *nt*.
epithelioid sarcoma Epitheloidsarkom *nt*.
ep·i·the·li·ol·y·sis [epɪˌθiːlɪˈɒləsɪs] *n* Epitheliolyse *f*.
ep·i·the·li·o·lyt·ic [ˌ-ˌθiːlɪəˈlɪtɪk] *adj* Epitheliolyse betr. *od*. verursachend, epitheliolytisch.
ep·i·the·li·o·ma [ˌ-ˌθiːlɪˈəʊmə] *n* 1. epithelialer Tumor *m*, epitheliale Geschwulst *f*, Epitheliom *nt*, Epithelioma *nt*. 2. Karzinom *nt, inf.* Krebs *m*, Carcinoma *nt abbr.* Ca.
ep·i·the·li·o·ma·tous [ˌ-ˌθiːlɪˈəʊmətəs] *adj* Epitheliom betr., epitheliomatös, epitheliomartig.
ep·i·the·li·o·sis [ˌ-ˌθiːlɪˈəʊsɪs] *n* 1. *ophthal*. Epitheliosis *f*. 2. *micro*. Epitheliosis *f*. 3. *gyn*. Epitheliosis *f*.
ep·i·the·li·um [epɪˈθiːlɪəm, -jəm] *n, pl* **-li·ums, -li·a** [-lɪə, -jə] Deckgewebe *nt*, Epithel-, Epithelialgewebe *nt*, Epithel *nt*, Epithelium *nt*.
  e. of lens Linsenepithel, Epithelium lentis.
  e. of semicircular duct Bogengangsepithel, Epithelium ductus semicirculares.
ep·i·the·li·za·tion [ˌ-ˌθiːlɪˈzeɪʃn̩] *n* → epithelialization.
ep·i·the·lize [ˌ-ˈθiːlaɪz] *vt* → epithelialize.
e·pith·e·sis [ɪˈpɪθəsɪs] *n* 1. *ortho*. operative Korrektur *f* einer Extremitätendeformität. 2. Epithese *f*.
ep·i·tope [ˈepɪtəʊp] *n immun*. antigene Determinante *f*, Epitop *nt*.
ep·i·tox·oid [ˌepɪˈtɒksɔɪd] *n* Epitoxoid *nt*.
ep·i·trich·i·um [ˌ-ˈtrɪkɪəm] *n embryo*. Periderm *nt*, Epitrichium *nt*.
ep·i·troch·le·a [ˌ-ˈtrɒklɪə] *n anat*. innere/mediale Humerusepikondyle *f*, Epitrochlea *f*, Epicondylus medialis humeri.
ep·i·tu·ber·cu·lo·sis [ˌ-tə̩ˌbɜːrkjʊˈləʊsɪs] *n radio., ped.* Epituberkulose *f*.
ep·i·tym·pan·ic [ˌ-tɪmˈpænɪk] *adj* 1. oberhalb der Paukenhöhle liegend, epitympanisch, epitympanal. 2. Epitympanum betr., epitympanisch, epitympanal.
epitympanic recess → epitympanum.
ep·i·tym·pa·num [ˌ-ˈtɪmpənəm] *n* Kuppelraum *m*, Attikus *m*, Epitympanum *nt*, Epitympanon *nt*, Rec. epitympanicus.
ep·i·typh·li·tis [ˌepɪtɪfˈlaɪtɪs] *n* 1. Wurmfortsatzentzündung *f, inf.* Blinddarmentzündung *f*, Appendizitis *f*, Appendicitis *f*. 2. Paratyphlitis *f*.
ep·i·ty·phlon [ˌ-ˈtaɪflɒn] *n anat*. Wurmfortsatz *m, inf.* Blinddarm *m*, Appendix vermiformis.
ep·i·zo·ic [ˌ-ˈzəʊɪk] *adj* Epizoen betr., epizoisch.
ep·i·zo·on [ˌ-ˈzəʊɒn] *n, pl* **-zoa** [-zəʊə] Hautschmarotzer *m*, -parasit *m*, Epizoon *nt*.
ep·i·zo·ot·ic [ˌ-zəʊˈɒtɪk] *adj* epizootisch.
epizootic aphthae (echte) Maul- u. Klauenseuche *f abbr.* MKS, Febris aphthosa, Stomatitis epidemica, Aphthosis epizootica.
epizootic disease Epizootie *f*.
epizootic stomatitis → epizootic aphthae.
ep·o·nych·i·al [epəˈnɪkɪəl] *adj* Eponychium betr., eponychial.
ep·o·nych·i·um [ˌepəˈnɪkɪəm] *n, pl* **-nych·i·a** [-ˈnɪkɪə] 1. Nagelhäutchen *nt*, Eponychium *nt*. 2. Nagelhaut *f*, Cuticula *f*, Perionychium *nt*, Perionyx *m*.
ep·o·nym [ˈepɒnɪm] *n* Eponym *nt*.
ep·o·nym·ic [ˌepəˈnɪmɪk] **I** *n* → eponym. **II** *adj* nach Person benannt, Eponym-.
e·pon·y·mous [əˈpɒnəməs] *adj* → eponymic II.
ep·o·oph·o·rec·to·my [epəʊˌɒfəˈrektəmɪ] *n gyn*. Epoophorektomie *f*.
ep·o·oph·o·ron [ˌ-ˈɒfərɒn] *n* Nebeneierstock *m*, Rosenmüller'-Organ *nt*, Parovarium *nt*, Epoophoron *f*.
ep·o·pro·sten·ol [ˌ-ˈprɒstənɒl, -nɔl] *n* Prostazyklin *nt*, -cyclin *nt*, Prostaglandin I$_2$ *f abbr*. PGI$_2$.
ep·ox·ide [eˈpɒksɪd, ɪˈp-] *n* Epoxid *nt*.
EPP end-plate potential.
EPR *abbr.* 1. [electron paramagnetic resonance] → electron spin resonance. 2. → electrophrenic respiration.

EPR spectroscopy [electron paramagnetic resonance spectroscopy] → electron spin resonance spectroscopy.
EPS *abbr.* 1. → endocrine polyglandular syndrome. 2. → exophthalmos-producing substance.
EPSC *abbr.* → excitatory postsynaptic current.
ep·si·lon alcoholism ['epsɪlɒn] ε-Alkoholismus *m*, Dipsomanie *f*, periodisches Trinken *nt*, *inf.* Quartalsaufen *nt*.
epsilon-aminocaproic acid *abbr.* EACA ε-Aminocapronsäure *f*, Epsilon-Aminocapronsäure *f abbr.* EACS, EACA.
epsilon angle *ophthal.* Epsilon-Winkel *m*.
epsilon staphylolysin *micro.* ε-Staphylolysin *nt*.
Epsom salt ['epsəm] Bittersalz *nt*, Magnesiumsulfat *nt*.
EPSP *abbr.* → excitatory postsynaptic potential.
Epstein ['epstain]: **E.'s disease** Diphtheroid *nt*, diphtheroide Erkrankung *f*.
E.'s nephrosis/syndrome nephrotisches Syndrom *nt*, Nephrose *f*.
Epstein-Barr [bɑːr]: **E.-B. nuclear antigen** *abbr.* EBNA Epstein-Barr nukleäres Antigen *nt abbr.* EBNA, Epstein-Barr nuclear antigen.
E.-B. virus *abbr.* EBV *micro.* Epstein-Barr-Virus *nt abbr.* EBV, EB-Virus *nt*.
E.-B. virus antigen Epstein-Barr-Virus-Antigen *nt*, EBV-Antigen *nt*.
e·pu·lis [ɪ'pjuːlɪs] *n, pl* **-li·des** [-ləˌdiːz] 1. *HNO, dent.* Epulis *f*. 2. *ortho.* peripheres verknöcherndes Fibrom *nt*.
e. of the newborn Epulis congenita/connata.
ep·u·lo·fi·bro·ma [ˌepjələʊfaɪ'brəʊmə] *n HNO* Epulofibrom *nt*, Epulis fibromatosa/fibrosa.
ep·u·loid ['epjəlɔɪd] *adj* epulisähnlich, -artig, epuloid.
ep·u·lo·sis [epjə'ləʊsɪs] *n* Vernarben *nt*, Vernarbung *f*, Narbenbildung *f*, Synulosis *f*.
ep·u·lot·ic [epjə'lɒtɪk] *adj* Vernarbung betr. *od.* fördernd, vernarbend.
e·qual ['iːkwəl] *adj* 1. gleich. **to be ~ to** gleichen, gleich sein. 2. (*Fläche*) plan, eben. 3. gleichmäßig, -förmig.
e·qual·i·ty [ɪ'kwɒlətɪ] *n* Gleichheit *f*; *mathe.* Gleichförmigkeit *f*.
e·qual·i·za·tion [ˌiːkwəlaɪ'zeɪʃn] *n* Ausgleich *m*; Gleichstellung *f*, -machung *f*.
e·qual·ize ['iːkwəlaɪz] I *vt* ausgleichen; gleichstellen, -machen. II *vi sport.* ausgleichen, Ausgleich schaffen.
e·qual·iz·ing ['iːkwəlaɪzɪŋ] *adj* Ausgleichs-.
e·quate [ɪ'kweɪt] I *vt* gleichmachen; ausgleichen; (*a. mathe.*) gleichsetzen (*to* mit). II *vi* gleichen.
e·qua·tion [ɪ'kweɪʃn, -ʒn] *n* 1. *mathe., chem.* Gleichung *f*. 2. Angleichung *f*, Ausgleich *m*.
e·qua·tion·al [ɪ'kweɪʒənl, -ʃə-] *adj* Gleichungs-; *electr.* Ausgleichs-.
equation formula Gleichungsformel *f*.
e·qua·tor [ɪ'kweɪtər] *n* Äquator *m*, *anat.* Aequator *m*, Equator *m*.
e. of eyeball Augapfeläquator, Aequator/Equator bulbi oculi.
e. of lens Linsenrand *m*, Aequator/Equator lentis.
e·qua·to·ri·al [ˌiːkwə'tɔːrɪəl, -'təʊ-, ˌekwə-] *adj* äquatorial, Äquator-, Äquatorial-.
equatorial bond *chem.* äquatoriale Bindung *f*.
equatorial plane Äquatorialebene *f*.
equatorial plate Äquatorialplatte *f*.
equatorial staphyloma Staphyloma aequatoriale.

e·qui·an·es·thet·ic [ˌiːkwɪˌænəs'θetɪk] *adj* äquianästhetisch.
e·qui·an·gu·lar [ˌ-'æŋgjələr] *adj mathe.* gleichwink(e)lig.
e·qui·axed ['-ækst] *adj* gleichachsig.
e·qui·ax·i·al [ˌ-'æksɪəl] *adj* → equiaxed.
e·qui·ca·lor·ic [ˌ-kə'lɒrɪk, -lɔːr-] *adj* äquiкалорisch, isokalorisch.
e·qui·dis·tant [ˌ-'dɪstənt] *adj* gleichweit entfernt, äquidistant (*from* von).
e·qui·lat·er·al [ˌ-'lætərəl, ˌek-] *mathe.* I *n* gleichseitige Figur *f*. II *adj* gleichseitig.
e·quil·i·brate [ɪ'kwɪləbreɪt, ˌikwə'laɪbreɪt] *vt* ins Gleichgewicht bringen, im Gleichgewicht halten, äquilibrieren.
e·quil·i·bra·tion [ɪˌkwɪlə'breɪʃn, ˌikwəlɪ-'breɪʃn] *n* 1. → equilibrium. 2. Aufrechterhaltung *od.* Herstellung *f* des Gleichgewichts, Äquilibration *f*.
e·qui·lib·ri·um [ˌikwə'lɪbrɪəm, ˌekwə-] *n, pl* **-ri·ums, -ria** [-rɪə] Gleichgewicht *nt*, Äquilibrium *nt*, Equilibrium *nt*. **in ~** im Gleichgewicht (*with* mit). **to keep** *od.* **maintain one's ~** das Gleichgewicht halten. **to lose one's ~** das Gleichgewicht verlieren.
equilibrium constant Gleichgewichtskonstante *f*.
equilibrium dialysis *immun.* Gleichgewichtsdialyse *f*.
equilibrium potential Gleichgewichtspotential *nt*.
equilibrium process Gleichgewichtsprozeß *m*.
equilibrium reaction Gleichgewichtsreaktion *f*.
equilibrium thermodynamics klassische Thermodynamik *f*, Gleichgewichtsthermodynamik *f*.
e·qui·mo·lar [ˌikwə'məʊlər, ˌek-] *adj chem.* äquimolar.
e·qui·mo·lec·u·lar [ˌ-mə'lekjələr, -] *adj chem.* äquimolekular.
e·quine ['iːkwaɪn, 'ek-] *adj* Pferde betr., Pferde-.
equine encephalitis → equine encephalomyelitis.
equine encephalomyelitis Encephalitis/Encephalomyelitis equina *f*.
equine gait *neuro.* Steppergang *m*.
equine smallpox Pferdepocken *pl*, Variola equina.
e·qui·no·pho·bia [ˌikwaɪnə'fəʊbɪə] *n psychia.* krankhafte Angst *f* vor Pferden, Equinophobie *f*.
e·qui·no·val·gus [ˌ-'vælgəs] *n ortho.* Pes equinovalgus.
e·qui·no·va·rus [ˌ-'værəs] *n ortho.* Klumpfuß *m*, Pes equinovarus (excavatus et adductus).
e·qui·nus [ɪ'kwaɪnəs] *n ortho.* Spitzfuß *m*, Pes equinus.
e·quip [ɪ'kwɪp] *vt* ausrüsten, ausstatten (*with* mit); einrichten.
e·quip·ment [ɪ'kwɪpmənt] *n* Ausrüstung *f*, Ausstattung *f*; Einrichtung *f*; Gerät(e *pl*) *nt*, Anlage(n *pl*) *f*, Maschine(n *pl*) *f*.
e·qui·pon·der·ant [ˌikwə'pɒndərənt, ˌek-] *adj* gleich schwer.
e·qui·pon·der·ate [ˌ-'pɒndəreɪt] I *vt* im Gleichgewicht halten. II *vi* gleich schwer sein (*to, with* mit).
e·qui·po·ten·tial [ˌ-pə'tenʃl] *adj* äquipotential, -potentiell.
e·qui·po·ten·ti·al·i·ty [ˌ-pəˌtenʃɪ'ælətɪ] *n* Äquipotenz *f*.
equipotential line *phys.* Äquipotentiallinie *f*.
e·quiv·a·lence [ɪ'kwɪvələns] *n* Gleichwertigkeit *f*, Äquivalenz *f*.
e·quiv·a·len·cy [ɪ'kwɪvələnsɪ] *n* → equivalence.
e·quiv·a·lent [ɪ'kwɪvələnt] I *n* 1. Äqui-

valent *nt* (*of* für); Entsprechung *f*, Gegenstück *nt* (*of* zu). 2. *chem.* Grammäquivalent *nt*. II *adj* 3. gleichwertig, entsprechend, äquivalent (*to*). 4. gleichbedeutend (*to* mit). 5. *chem., mathe., phys.* äquivalent.
e·quiv·o·cal symptom [ɪ'kwɪvəkəl] unspezifisches Symptom *nt*.
ER *abbr.* → endoplasmic reticulum.
Er *abbr.* → erbium.
ERA *abbr.* → electric response audiometry.
e·rase [ɪ'reɪs] *vt chir.* ausschaben, auskratzen, ausräumen, abkratzen.
e·ra·sion [ɪ'reɪʒn, -ʃn] *n chir.* Ausschabung *f*, Ausräumung *f*, Auskratzung *f*.
Erb [ɑrb]: **E.'s atrophy** → E.'s disease.
E.'s disease Erb'-Muskelatrophie *f*, -Muskeldystrophie *f*, -Syndrom *nt*, Dystrophia musculorum progressiva Erb.
E.'s palsy 1. → E.'s disease. 2. → Erb-Duchenne paralysis.
E.'s paralysis 1. → E.'s disease. 2. → Erb-Duchenne paralysis. 3. → E.'s spastic paraplegia.
E.'s phenomenon Erb-Zeichen *nt*.
E.'s point Erb'-Punkt *m*.
E.'s sclerosis → Erb-Charcot disease.
E.'s sign 1. → Erb-Zeichen *nt*. 2. → Erb-Westphal sign.
E.'s spastic paraplegia luische Spinalparalyse Erb *f*.
E.'s syndrome Erb-Goldflam-Syndrom *nt*, -Krankheit *f*, Erb-Oppenheim-Goldflam-Syndrom *nt*, -Krankheit *f*, Hoppe-Goldflam-Syndrom *nt*, Myasthenia gravis pseudoparalytica.
E.'s syphilitic spastic paraplegia → E.'s spastic paraplegia.
Erb-Charcot [ʃɑr'koː]: **E.-C. disease** Erb-Charcot-Syndrom *nt*, -Krankheit *f*, spastische Spinalparalyse *f*.
Erb-Duchenne [dy'ʃɛn]: **E.-D. paralysis** obere Armplexuslähmung *f*, Erb'-Lähmung *f*, Erb-Duchenne-Lähmung *f*.
ERBF *abbr.* → effective renal blood flow.
Erb-Goldflam ['gɒltflam]: **E.-G. disease** Erb-Goldflam-Syndrom *nt*, -Krankheit *f*, Erb-Oppenheim-Goldflam-Syndrom *nt*, -Krankheit *f*, Hoppe-Goldflam-Syndrom *nt*, Myasthenia gravis pseudoparalytica.
er·bi·um ['ɑrbɪəm] *n abbr.* Er Erbium *nt abbr.* Er.
Erb-Landouzy [læn'duːzɪ; lɑdu'zɪ]: **E.-L. disease** Erb-Landouzy-Déjérine-Syndrom *nt*, fazioskapulohumeraler Typ *m* der Muskeldystrophie.
Erb-Westphal ['vɛstfɑːl]: **E.-W. sign** Erb-Westphal-Zeichen *nt*, Erb-Zeichen *nt*.
ERC *abbr.* → endoscopic retrograde cholangiography.
ERCP *abbr.* → endoscopic retrograde cholangiopancreatography.
Erdheim ['ɛrdhaɪm]: **E.'s cystic medial necrosis** → Erdheim-Gsell medial necrosis.
E. tumor Erdheim-Tumor *m*, Kraniopharyngiom *nt*.
Erdheim-Gsell [gsɛl]: **E.-G. medial necrosis** Erdheim-Gsell-Syndrom *nt*, Gsell-Erdheim-Syndrom *nt*, Medionecrosis *f* Erdheim-Gsell.
e·rect [ɪ'rekt] I *adj* 1. gerade, aufrecht, aufgerichtet. **to stand ~** gerade *od.* aufrecht stehen. 2. (*Penis*) erigiert, steif. II *vt* 3. aufrichten, hoch-, aufstellen. **to ~ o.s.** s. aufrichten. 4. errichten, (er-, auf-)bauen, montieren.
e·rec·tile [ɪ'rektil, -tɪl, -taɪl] *adj* 1. erigibel, schwellfähig, erektionsfähig, erektil. 2. aufrichtbar, aufgerichtet.
erectile tissue erektiles Gewebe *nt*.

erectile tumor kavernöses Hämangiom *nt*, Kavernom *nt*, Haemangioma tuberonodosum.
erect image virtuelles/scheinbares Bild *nt*.
e·rec·tion [ɪ'rekʃn] *n* **1.** Auf-, Errichtung *f*; (Auf-, Er-)Bauen *nt*, Aufstellen *nt*, Errichten *nt*; Montage *f*. **2.** *physiol.* Erektion *f*.
erection center → ejaculation center.
e·rec·tor (muscle) [ɪ'rektər] Aufrichtemuskel *m*, Erektor *m*, M. erector.
e. of penis Ischiokavernosus *m*, -cavernosus *m*, M. ischiocavernosus.
e. of spine → erector spinae (muscle).
erector spinae (muscle) Erektor *m* spinae, Sakrospinalis *m*, *old* M. sacrospinalis, M. erector spinae.
erect position aufrechte Körperhaltung *f*, Orthostase *f*.
er·e·mo·phil·ia [ˌerəmou'filɪə] *n psychia*. Eremophilie *f*.
er·e·mo·pho·bia [ˌ-'foubɪə] *n psychia*. Eremophobie *f*.
er·e·thism ['erəθɪzəm] *n* (krankhaft) gesteigerte Erregbarkeit *f*, Übererregbarkeit *f*, Erethismus *m*, Erethie *f*.
er·e·this·mic [erə'θɪzmɪk] *adj* → erethistic.
er·e·this·tic [erə'θɪstɪk] *adj* (über-)erregt, (über-)erregbar, reizbar, gereizt, erethisch.
er·e·thit·ic [erə'θɪtɪk] *adj* → erethistic.
e·reu·tho·pho·bia [ɪˌruːθo'foubɪə] *n* → erythrophobia 1.
ERF *abbr*. → excitatory receptive field.
ERG *abbr*. → electroretinogram.
erg- *pref*. → ergo-.
erg [ɜrg] *n old* Erg *nt*.
er·ga·sia [ər'geɪʒ(ɪ)ə] *n psychia*. (geistige) Arbeit *f*, Ergasie *f*.
er·ga·sio·ma·nia [ərˌgeɪsɪou'meɪnɪə, -jə] *n psychia*. Arbeitswut *f*, Beschäftigungsdrang *m*, Ergasiomanie *f*.
er·ga·sio·pho·bia [ˌ-'foubɪə] *n psychia*. pathologische Arbeitsscheu *f*, Ergasiophobie *f*.
er·gas·to·plasm [ər'gæstəplæzəm] *n* rauhes/granuläres endoplasmatisches Retikulum *abbr*. R-ER, Ergastoplasma *nt*.
ergo- *pref*. Arbeits-, Erg(o)-.
er·go·ba·sine [ˌɜrgou'beɪsɪn] *n* → ergometrine.
er·go·cal·cif·er·ol [ˌ-kæl'sɪfərəl, -rɔl] *n* Ergocalciferol *nt*, Vitamin D₂ *nt*.
er·go·car·di·o·gram [ˌ-'kɑːrdɪəgræm] *n* Ergokardiogramm *nt*.
er·go·car·di·og·ra·phy [ˌ-ˌkɑːrdɪ'ɑgrəfɪ] *n* Ergokardiographie *f*.
er·go·cor·nine [ˌ-'kɔːrniːn, -nɪn] *n pharm*. Ergocornin *nt*.
er·go·cris·tine [ˌ-'krɪstiːn, -stɪn] *n pharm*. Ergocristin *nt*.
er·go·cryp·tine [ˌ-'krɪptiːn] *n pharm*. Ergokryptin *f*, -cryptin *nt*.
er·go·dy·nam·o·graph [ˌ-daɪ'næməgræf] *n physiol*. Ergodynamograph *m*.
er·go·es·the·si·o·graph [ˌ-es'θiːzɪəgræf] *n physiol*. Ergoästhesiograph *m*.
er·go·gen·ic [ˌ-'dʒenɪk] *adj physiol*. die Arbeitsleistung erhöhend.
er·go·gram ['-græm] *n physiol*. Ergogramm *nt*.
er·go·graph ['-græf] *n physiol*. Ergograph *m*.
er·go·graph·ic [ˌ-'græfɪk] *adj* Ergographie *od*. Ergograph betr., ergographisch.
er·gog·ra·phy [ər'gɑgrəfɪ] *n physiol*. Ergographie *f*.
er·gom·e·ter [ər'gɑmɪtər] *n* Ergometer *nt*.
ergometer work Ergometerarbeit *f*.
er·go·met·ric [ˌɜrgo'metrɪk] *adj* Ergometer *od*. Ergometrie betr., ergometrisch.
er·go·met·rine [ˌ-'metriːn, -'mɪt-, -trɪn] *n*

pharm. Ergometrin *nt*, Ergonovin *nt*, Ergobasin *nt*.
er·gom·e·try [ər'gɑmətrɪ] *n* Ergometrie *f*.
er·go·nom·ics [ˌɜrgə'nɑmɪks] *pl* Ergonomie *f*, Ergonomik *f*.
er·go·no·vine [ˌ-'nouviːn, -vɪn] *n* → ergometrine.
er·go·plasm ['-plæzəm] *n* → ergastoplasm.
er·go·some ['-soum] *n* Poly(ribo)som *nt*, Ergosom *nt*.
er·go·stat ['ɜrgəstæt] *n physiol*. Ergostat *m*.
er·gos·te·rin [ər'gɑstərɪn] *n* → ergosterol.
er·gos·te·rol [ər'gɑstərɔl, -rɑl] *n* Ergosterol *nt*, Ergosterin *nt*, Provitamin D₂ *nt*.
er·go·stet·rine [ˌɜrgou'stetriːn, -rɪn] *n* → ergometrine.
er·got·a·mine [ər'gɑtəmiːn, -mɪn] *n pharm*. Ergotamin *nt*.
er·got·am·i·nine [ˌɜrgɑt'æməniːn] *n pharm*. Ergotaminin *nt*.
er·go·ther·a·py [ˌɜrgə'θerəpɪ] *n* Beschäftigungstherapie *f*, Ergotherapie *f*.
er·go·thi·o·ne·ine [ˌ-ˌθaɪou'niːɪn] *n* Ergothionein *nt*.
er·got·ism ['ɜrgətɪzəm] *n* Vergiftung *f* durch Mutterkornalkaloide, Ergotismus *m*.
er·go·to·cine [ˌɜrgou'tousiːn] *n* → ergometrine.
er·go·tox·ine [ˌ-'tɑksiːn, -sɪn] *n pharm*. Ergotoxin *nt*.
ergot poisoning ['ɜrgət] → ergotism.
er·go·trop·ic [ˌɜrgou'trɑpɪk, -'trou-] *adj physiol*. leistungssteigernd, kraftentfaltend, ergotrop.
ergotropic hormone ergotropes Hormon *nt*.
ergotropic zone ergotrope/dynamogene Zone *f*.
Erichsen ['erɪksən]: **E.'s sign** Erichsen-Zeichen *nt*.
Erlanger-Gasser ['ɜrlæŋər 'gæsər]: **E.-G. classification** Erlanger-Gasser-Einteilung *f*, -Klassifikation *f*.
Erlenmeyer ['erlənmaɪər, 'er-]: **E. flask** Erlenmeyer-Kolben *m*.
E. flask deformity *ortho*., *radiol*. Erlenmeyer-Kolben-Phänomen *nt*.
ERO *abbr*. → evoked response olfactometry.
e·rode [ɪ'roud] *vt* erodieren, auswaschen; ätzen; weg-, zer-, anfressen; *fig*., *techn*. verschleißen.
e·rod·ent [ɪ'roudnt] *adj* → erosive.
e·rog·e·ne·i·ty [ɪˌrɑdʒə'niːətɪ] *n* erogene Beschaffenheit *f*, Erogenität *f*.
er·o·gen·ic [erə'dʒenɪk] *adj* → erogenous.
e·rog·e·nous [ɪ'rɑdʒənəs] *adj* erogen, erotogen.
erogenous zones erogene Zonen *pl*.
E rosette assay *immun*. E-Rosettentest *m*.
e·ro·sion [ɪ'rouʒn] *n* **1.** oberflächlicher (Schleim-)Hautdefekt *m*, Erosion *f*. **2.** Abtragung *f*, Auswaschung *f*; Ätzung *f*; Zerfressung *f*; angefressene Stelle *f*, Erosion *f*. **3.** *techn*., *fig*. Verschleiß *m*.
e·ro·sive [ɪ'rousɪv] *adj* zerfressend, ätzend, erosiv.
erosive balanitis erosive Balanitis *f*, Balanitis erosiva.
erosive gastritis erosive Gastritis *f*, Gastritis erosiva.
e·rot·ic [ɪ'rɑtɪk] *adj* erotisch.
e·rot·i·cism [ɪ'rɑtəsɪzəm] *n* → erotism.
e·rot·i·co·ma·nia [ɪˌrɑtɪkou'meɪnɪə, -jə] *n* → erotomania.
erotic pyromania *psychia*. Pyrolagnie *f*.
er·o·tism ['erətɪzəm] *n* **1.** Erotik *f*. **2.** Erotismus *m*, Erotizismus *m*.
e·ro·to·gen·e·sis [ɪˌroutə'dʒenəsɪs] *n* Erotogenese *f*.

e·ro·to·gen·ic [ˌ-'dʒenɪk] *adj* → erogenous.
erotogenic zone erogene Zone *f*.
e·ro·to·ma·nia [ˌ-'meɪnɪə, -jə] *n psychia*. **1.** Liebestollheit *f*, Erotomanie *f*, Hypererosie *f*. **2.** Liebeswahn *m*, Erotomanie *f*.
e·ro·to·pho·bia [ˌ-'foubɪə] *n psychia*. Erotophobie *f*.
ERP *abbr*. **1.** → early receptor potential. **2.** → endoscopic retrograde pancreatography. **3.** → event-related potential.
ERPF *abbr*. → effective renal plasma flow.
er·rat·ic [ɪ'rætɪk] *adj* **1.** (*Schmerzen*) erratisch; (*im Körper*) umherwandernd. **2.** (*Bewegung*) ungleichmäßig, unregelmäßig, regellos, ziellos. **3.** unstet, sprunghaft, launenhaft, unberechenbar.
er·ror ['erər] *n* **1.** Fehler *m*, Irrtum *m*, Versehen *nt*. **2.** *mathe*., *stat*. Fehler *m*, Abweichung *f*. **3.** *biochem*. Fehler *m*, Abweichung *f*, Defekt *m*.
ERT *abbr*. → estrogen replacement therapy.
e·ruct [ɪ'rʌkt] *vi* → eructate.
e·ruc·tate [ɪ'rʌkteɪt] *vi* aufstoßen; *inf*. rülpsen.
e·ruc·ta·tion [ɪrʌk'teɪʃn] *n* Aufstoßen *nt*, *inf*. Rülpsen *nt*, Ruktation *f*, Eruktation *f*.
e·rupt [ɪ'rʌpt] *vi* **1.** ausbrechen, hervorbrechen (*from* aus); eruptieren. **2.** (*Zähne*) durchbrechen, durchkommen.
e·rup·tion [ɪ'rʌpʃn] *n* **1.** Ausbruch *m*, Hervortreten *nt*, Hervorbrechen *nt*, Eruption *f*. **2.** *dent*. (*Zähne*) Durchbruch *m*. **3.** *derm*. (*Ausschlag*) Ausbruch *m*, Eruption *f*. **4.** *derm*. Ausschlag *m*, Eruption *f*, Eruptio *f*.
e·rup·tive [ɪ'rʌptɪv] *adj* **1.** ausbrechend, eruptiv. **2.** *derm*. von Ausschlag begleitet, eruptiv.
eruptive fever 1. Zeckenbißfieber *nt*. **2.** mit Exanthem einhergehendes Fieber *nt*, Febris exanthematica.
eruptive hemangioma eruptives Hämangiom *nt*.
ERV *abbr*. → expiratory reserve volume.
Er·win·ia [ɜr'wɪnɪə] *n micro*. Erwinia *f*.
er·y·sip·e·las [erɪ'sɪpələs] *n derm*. Wundrose *f*, Rose *f*, Erysipel *nt*, Erysipelas *nt*, Streptodermia cutanea lymphatica.
er·y·sip·el·a·tous [ˌerəsɪ'pelətəs] *adj* **1.** Erysipel betr., Erysipel-. **2.** erysipelähnlich, erysipeloid.
er·y·sip·e·loid [erɪ'sɪpəlɔɪd] **I** *n derm*. Erysipeloid *nt*, Rotlauf *m*, Schweinerotlauf *m*, Pseudoerysipel *nt*, Rosenbach'-Krankheit *f*, Erythema migrans *f*. **II** *adj* erysipelähnlich, erysipeloid.
Er·y·sip·e·lo·thrix [erə'sɪpəlouθrɪks] *n micro*. Erysipelothrix *f*.
E. insidiosa/rhusiopathiae Schweinerotlauf-Bakterium *nt*, Erysipelothrix insidiosa/rhusiopathiae.
er·y·sip·e·lo·tox·in [erəˌsɪpəlou'tɑksɪn] *n* Erysipelotoxin *nt*.
er·y·the·ma [erə'θiːmə] *n derm*. (entzündliche) Hautrötung *f*, Erythem *nt*, Erythema *nt*.
erythema chronicum migrans *derm*. Wanderröte *f*, Erythema chronicum migrans.
erythema infectiosum *ped*., *derm*. Ringelröteln *pl*, fünfte Krankheit *f*, Morbus quintus *m*, Sticker'-Krankheit *f*, Megalerythem *nt*, Erythema infectiosum, Megalerythema epidemicum/infectiosum.
erythema nodosum Knotenrose *f*, Erythema nodosum.
erythema nodosum leprosy *abbr*. **ENL** Erythema nodosum leprosum *abbr*. ENL.
er·y·them·a·tous [erə'θemətəs, -'θiːmə-]

adj derm. Erythem betr., durch ein Erythem gekennzeichnet, erythematös.
erythrematous syphilid *derm.* makulöses Syphilid *nt*, Roseola syphilitica.
er·y·the·mo·gen·ic [erəˌθiːməˈdʒenɪk] *adj derm.* erythemauslösend, -verursachend.
erythr- *pref.* → erythro-.
er·y·thral·gia [erɪˈθrældʒ(ɪ)ə] *n* Erythralgie *f*.
er·y·thras·ma [erɪˈθræzmə] *n derm.* Baerensprung'-Krankheit *f*, Erythrasma *nt*.
e·ryth·re·de·ma [ɪˌrɪθrəˈdiːmɪə] *n* Feer'-Krankheit *f*, Rosakrankheit *f*, vegetative Neurose *f* der Kleinkinder, Swift-Syndrom *nt*, Selter-Swift-Feer'-Krankheit *f*, Feer-Selter-Swift-Krankheit *f*, Akrodynie *f*, Acrodynia *f*.
erythredema polyneuropathy → erythredema.
er·y·thre·mia [erɪˈθriːmɪə] *n hema.* Osler'-Krankheit *f*, Osler-Vaquez-Krankheit *f*, Vaquez-Osler-Syndrom *nt*, Morbus Vaquez-Osler *m*, Polycythaemia (rubra) vera, Erythrämie *f*.
er·y·thre·mic [erɪˈθriːmɪk] *adj* Erythrämie betr., erythrämisch.
e·ryth·re·mo·mel·al·gia [ɪˌrɪθrəməʊmɪˈlældʒ(ɪ)ə] *n* → erythromelalgia.
e·ryth·rism [ɪˈrɪθrɪzəm, ˈerɪθrɪzəm] *n* 1. Erythrismus *m*. 2. Rothaarigkeit *f*, Rutilismus *m*, Erythrismus *m* Erythrotrichie *f*.
er·y·thris·tic [erɪˈθrɪstɪk] *adj* 1. Erythrismus betr., von Erythrismus gekennzeichnet, erythristisch. 2. rothaarig.
e·ryth·ri·tol [ɪˈrɪθrətɒl, -təl] *n* Erythrit *nt*, Erythroglucin *nt*, Erythrol *nt*, Tetrahydroxybutan *nt*.
erythritol tetranitrate → erythrityl tetranitrate.
e·ryth·ri·tyl tetranitrate [ɪˈrɪθrətɪl] *pharm.* Erythrityltetranitrat *nt*.
erythro- *pref.* Rot-, Erythr(o)-, Erythrozyten-.
e·ryth·ro·blast [ɪˈrɪθrəblæst] *n* Erythroblast *m*, Erythrozytoblast *m*.
e·ryth·ro·blas·te·mia [ˌ-blæsˈtiːmɪə] *n hema.* Erythroblastämie *f*, Erythroblastose *f*.
e·ryth·ro·blas·tic [ˌ-ˈblæstɪk] *adj derm.* Erythroblasten betr.
erythroblastic anemia: e. of childhood Cooley-Anämie *f*, homozygote β-Thalassämie *f*, Thalassaemia major.
  familial e. (familiäre) Erythroblastenanämie *f*, Thalassaemia minor.
  primary e. → e. of childhood.
e·ryth·ro·blas·to·ma [ˌ-blæsˈtəʊmə] *n hema.* Erythroblastom *nt*.
e·ryth·ro·blas·to·ma·to·sis [ˌ-blæstəməˈtəʊsɪs] *n hema.* Erythroblastomatose *f*.
e·ryth·ro·blas·to·pe·nia [ˌ-blæstəˈpɪnɪə] *n hema.* Erythroblastopenie *f*.
e·ryth·ro·blas·to·sis [ˌ-blæsˈtəʊsɪs] *n hema.* Erythroblastose *f*, Erythroblastämie *f*.
e·ryth·ro·blas·tot·ic [ˌ-blæsˈtɒtɪk] *adj* Erythroblastose betr., Erythroblasten(n)-.
e·ryth·ro·ca·tal·y·sis *n* → erythrokatalysis.
e·ryth·ro·chro·mia [-ˈkrəʊmɪə] *n hema.* Rotfärbung *f*, rötliche Verfärbung *f*, Erythrochromie *f*.
er·y·throc·la·sis [erəˈθrækləsɪs] *n hema.* Erythrozytenfragmentierung *f*, Erythroklasie *f*.
e·ryth·ro·clas·tic [ɪˌrɪθrəˈklæstɪk] *adj hema.* Erythroklasie betr., erythroklastisch.
e·ryth·ro·cu·prein [ˌ-ˈk(j)uːpriːɪn] *n* Superoxiddismutase *f abbr.* SOD, Hämocuprein *nt*, Erythrocuprein *nt*.
e·ryth·ro·cy·a·no·sis [ˌ-saɪəˈnəʊsɪs] *n derm.*

Erythrozyanose *f*, Erythrocyanosis *f*.
e·ryth·ro·cyte [ɪˈrɪθrəsaɪt] *n* rote Blutzelle *f*, rotes Blutkörperchen *nt*, Erythrozyt *m*.
erythrocyte agglomeration Erythrozytenagglomeration *f*.
erythrocyte agglutination Erythrozytenagglutination *f*.
erythrocyte agglutinogen Erythrozytenagglutinogen *nt*.
erythrocyte aggregation Erythrozytenaggregation *f*.
erythrocyte anomaly Erythrozytenanomalie *f*.
erythrocyte antigen Erythrozytenantigen *nt*.
erythrocyte autosensitization syndrome Erythrozytenautosensibilisierung *f*, schmerzhafte Ekchymosen-Syndrom *nt*, painful bruising syndrome (*nt*).
erythrocyte color coefficient *hema.* Erythrozytenfärbekoeffizient *m*, Färbekoeffizient *m*.
erythrocyte color index *hema.* Erythrozytenfärbeindex *m*, Färbeindex *m*.
erythrocyte count Erythrozytenzahl *f*, Erythrozytenzählung *f*.
erythrocyte enzymes Erythrozytenenzyme *pl*.
erythrocyte fragility *physiol.* Erythrozytenresistenz *f*.
  mechanical f. mechanische Erythrozytenresistenz.
  osmotic f. osmotische Erythrozytenresistenz.
erythrocyte fragility test Erythrozytenresistenztest *m*.
erythrocyte ghost Blutkörperchenschatten *m*, Erythrozytenghost *m*.
erythrocyte maturation Erythrozytenreifung *f*.
erythrocyte maturation factor *abbr.* **EMF** *old* → cyanocobalamin.
erythrocyte membrane Erythrozytenmembran *f*.
erythrocyte mosaicism *embryo.* Erythrozytenmosaizismus *m*.
erythrocyte number Erythrozytenzahl *f*.
erythrocyte progenitor Erythrozytenvorläufer(zelle *f*) *m*.
erythrocyte pyruvate kinase deficiency Pyruvatkinasemangel *m*.
erythrocyte resistance Erythrozytenresistenz *f*.
erythrocyte rosette assay *immun.* E-Rosettentest *m*.
erythrocyte sedimentation rate *abbr.* **ESR** Blutkörperchensenkung *f abbr.* BKS, Blutkörperchensenkungsgeschwindigkeit *f abbr.* BSG, *inf.* Blutsenkung *f*.
erythrocyte sedimentation reaction → erythrocyte sedimentation rate.
erythrocyte series → erythrocytic series.
e·ryth·ro·cy·the·mia [ɪˌrɪθrəsaɪˈθiːmɪə] *n* 1. Erythrozythämie *f*, Erythrozytose *f*. 2. Polyzythämie *f*, Polycythaemia. 3. → erythremia.
e·ryth·ro·cyt·ic [ˌ-ˈsɪtɪk] *adj* Erythrozyten betr., erythrozytär, Erythrozyten-, Erythrozyto-, Erythro-.
erythrocytic cycle *micro.* erythrozytärer Zyklus *m*, erythrozytäre Phase *f*.
erythrocytic leukemia → erythroleukemia.
erythrocytic phase → erythrocytic cycle.
erythrocytic series *hema.* erythrozytäre Reihe *f*.
e·ryth·ro·cy·to·blast [ˌ-ˈsaɪtəblæst] *n* → erythroblast.
e·ryth·ro·cy·tol·y·sin [ˌ-saɪˈtɒlɪsɪn] *n* Erythro(zyto)lysin *nt*, Hämolysin *nt*.
e·ryth·ro·cy·tol·y·sis [ˌ-saɪˈtɒlɪsɪs] *n hema.*

1. Erythrozytenauflösung *f*, Erythro(zyto)lyse *f*. 2. Erythro(zyto)lyse *f*, Hämolyse *f*.
e·ryth·ro·cy·tom·e·ter [ˌ-saɪˈtɒmɪtər] *n* Erythrozytometer *nt*.
e·ryth·ro·cy·tom·e·try [ˌ-saɪˈtɒmətrɪ] *n* Erythrozytometrie *f*.
erythrocyto-opsonin *n* Hämopsonin *nt*.
e·ryth·ro·cy·to·pe·nia [ˌ-saɪtəˈpɪnɪə] *n* → erythropenia.
e·ryth·ro·cy·toph·a·gous [ˌ-saɪˈtɒfəgəs] *adj* Erythrophagozytose betr., erythrophagisch.
e·ryth·ro·cy·toph·a·gy [ˌ-saɪˈtɒfədʒɪ] *n* Erythrophagozytose *f*, Erythrophagie *f*.
e·ryth·ro·cy·to·poi·e·sis [ˌ-ˌsaɪtəpɔɪˈiːsɪs] *n* → erythropoiesis.
e·ryth·ro·cy·tor·rhex·is [ˌ-saɪtəˈreksɪs] *n hema.* Erythro(zyto)rrhexis *f*.
e·ryth·ro·cy·tos·chi·sis [ˌ-saɪˈtɒskəsɪs] *n hema.* Erythro(zyto)schisis *f*.
e·ryth·ro·cy·to·sis [ˌ-saɪˈtəʊsɪs] *n hema.* Erythrozytose *f*, Erythrozythämie *f*.
e·ryth·ro·cy·tu·ria [ˌ-saɪˈt(j)ʊərɪə] *n* Erythrozytenausscheidung *f* im Harn, Erythrozyturie *f*; Hämaturie *f*.
e·ryth·ro·de·gen·er·a·tive [ˌ-dɪˈdʒenərətɪv, -ˌreɪtɪv] *adj* erythrodegenerativ.
e·ryth·ro·der·ma [ˌ-ˈdɜrmə] *n derm.* 1. Erythroderma *nt*, Erythrodermie *f*, Erythrodermia *f*, Erythrodermatitis *f*. 2. → exfoliative dermatitis.
e·ryth·ro·der·ma·ti·tis [ˌ-dɜrməˈtaɪtɪs] *n* → erythroderma 1.
e·ryth·ro·der·mia [ˌ-ˈdɜrmɪə] *n* → erythroderma 1.
e·ryth·ro·der·mic psoriasis [ˌ-ˈdɜrmɪk] *derm.* psoriatische Erythrodermie *f*, Erythrodermia psoriatica, Psoriasis erythrodermica.
e·ryth·ro·dex·trin [ˌ-ˈdekstrɪn] *n* Erythrodextrin *nt*, e-Dextrin *nt*.
e·ryth·ro·don·tia [ˌɪrɪθrəˈdɒnʃɪə] *n* Erythrodontie *f*.
e·ryth·ro·gen·e·sis [ˌ-ˈdʒenəsɪs] *n* Erythrozytenbildung *f*, Erythrogenese *f*.
e·ryth·ro·gen·ic [ˌ-ˈdʒenɪk] *adj* 1. erythrozytenbildend, erythro(zyto)gen. 2. Erythem erzeugend, erythrogen.
erythrogenic toxin *micro.* Scharlachtoxin *nt*, erythrogenes Toxin *nt*.
e·ryth·ro·gone [ˈgəʊn] *n hema.* Promegaloblast *m*.
e·ryth·ro·go·ni·um [ˌ-ˈgəʊnɪəm] *n* → erythrogone.
e·ryth·ro·he·pat·ic protoporphyria [ˌ-hɪˈpætɪk] *derm.* erythrohepatische/erythropoetische Protoporphyrie *f*, protoporphyrinämische Lichtdermatose *f*, Protoporphyria erythropoetica.
er·y·throid [ˈerɪθrɔɪd] *adj (Farbe)* rötlich.
erythroid cell Zelle *f* der erythrozytären Reihe.
e·ryth·ro·ka·tal·y·sis [ɪˈrɪθrəkəˈtæləsɪs] *n hema.* Erythrozytenabbau *m*, Erythrokatalyse *f*.
e·ryth·ro·ker·a·to·der·mia [ˌ-ˌkerətəʊˈdɜrmɪə] *n derm.* Erythrokeratodermie *f*.
erythrokeratodermia variabilis Mendes da Costa-Syndrom *nt*, Erythrokeratodermia figurata variabilis (Mendes da Costa), Keratitis rubra figurata.
e·ryth·ro·ki·net·ics [ˌ-kɪˈnetɪks] *pl hema.* Erythro(zyten)kinetik *f*.
e·ryth·ro·leu·ke·mia [ˌ-luːˈkiːmɪə] *n hema.* Erythroleukämie *f*.
e·ryth·ro·leu·ko·blas·to·sis [ˌ-ˌluːkəblæsˈtəʊsɪs] *n* Icterus neonatorum gravis.
e·ryth·ro·leu·ko·sis [ˌ-luːˈkəʊsɪs] *n* Erythroleukose *f*.
er·y·throl·y·sin [erəˈθrælɪsɪn] *n* → erythrocytolysin.

er·y·throl·y·sis [erə'θrɑləsɪs] *n* → erythrocytolysis.
er·y·throl ['erəθrɔl, ɪ'riːθ-, -rəʊl] *n* → erythritol.
e·ryth·ro·lose [ɪ'rɪθrələʊz] *n* Erythrolose *f*.
erythrol tetranitrate *pharm*. Erythrityltetranitrat *nt*.
e·ryth·ro·mel·al·gia [ɪ,rɪθrəmel'ældʒ(ɪ)ə] *n derm*. Gerhardt-Syndrom *nt*, Mitchell-Gerhardt-Syndrom *nt*, Weir-Mitchell-Krankheit *f*, Erythromelalgie *f*, Erythralgie *f*, Erythermalgie *f*, Acromelalgie *f*.
e·ryth·ro·me·lia [,-'miːlɪə] *n derm*. Erythromelie *f*.
er·y·throm·e·ter [erɪ'θrɑmɪtər] *n* 1. *derm*. Erythrometer *nt*. 2. → erythrocytometer.
er·y·throm·e·try [erɪ'θrɑmətrɪ] *n* 1. *derm*. Erythrometrie *f*. 2. → erythrocytometry.
e·ryth·ro·my·cin [ɪ,rɪθrə'maɪsɪn] *n pharm*. Erythromycin *nt*.
er·y·thron ['erɪθrɑn] *n hema*. Erythron *nt*, Erythrozytenorgan *nt*.
e·ryth·ro·ne·o·cy·to·sis [ɪ,rɪθrə,nɪəsaɪ'təʊsɪs] *n hema*. Erythroneozytose *f*.
e·ryth·ro·nor·mo·blas·tic anemia [,-,nɔːrmə'blæstɪk] *old* → hypochromic anemia.
e·ryth·ro·par·a·site [,-'pærəsaɪt] *n micro*. Erythroparasit *m*.
er·y·throp·a·thy [erɪ'θrɑpəθɪ] *n hema*. Erythro(zyto)pathie *f*.
e·ryth·ro·pe·nia [ɪ,rɪθrə'piːnɪə] *n hema*. Erythrozytenmangel *m*, Erythro(zyto)penie *f*.
e·ryth·ro·phage ['-feɪdʒ] *n hema*. Erythro(zyto)phage *m*.
e·ryth·ro·pha·gia [,-'feɪdʒ(ɪ)ə] *n* → erythrocytophagy.
e·ryth·ro·phag·o·cy·to·sis [,-,fægəʊsaɪ'təʊsɪs] *n* → erythrocytophagy.
er·y·throph·a·gous [erɪ'θrɑfəgəs] *adj* → erythrocytophagous.
e·ryth·ro·phil [ɪ'rɪθrəfɪl] **I** *n* erythrophile Zelle *f od*. Substanz *f*. **II** *adj* → erythrophilic.
e·ryth·ro·phil·ic [ɪ,rɪθrə'fɪlɪk] *adj histol*. erythrophil.
er·y·throph·i·lous [erɪ'θrɑfɪləs] *adj* → erythrophilic.
e·ryth·ro·pho·bia [ɪ,rɪθrə'fəʊbɪə] *n psychia*. 1. Errötungsfurcht *f*, Erythrophobie *f*. 2. Rotangst *f*, Erythrophobie *f*.
e·ryth·ro·pho·bic [,-'fəʊbɪk] *adj histol*. erythrophob.
e·ryth·ro·phore ['-fɔːr, -fəʊər] *n* Allophor *nt*, Erythrophor *m*.
e·ryth·ro·phyll ['-fɪl] *n* Erythrophyll *nt*.
er·y·throp·ia [erɪ'θrɑpɪə] *n* → erythropsia.
e·ryth·ro·pla·kia [ɪ,rɪθrə'pleɪkɪə] *n derm*. Erythroplakie *f*, Erythroplakia *f*.
e·ryth·ro·pla·sia [,-'pleɪʒ(ɪ)ə, -zɪə] *n derm*. Erythroplasie *f*.
e. of Queyrat Erythroplasie Queyrat, Queyrat-Syndrom *nt*.
e·ryth·ro·poi·e·sis [,-pɔɪ'iːsɪs] *n* Erythro(zyto)genese *f*, Erythrozytenbildung *f*, Erythropo(i)ese *f*.
e·ryth·ro·poi·et·ic [,-pɔɪ'etɪk] *adj* Erythropo(i)ese betr. *od*. stimulierend, erythropo(i)etisch.
erythropoietic porphyria erythropoetische Porphyrie *f*, Porphyria erythropo(i)etica.
congenital e. → erythropoietic uroporphyria.
erythropoietic protoporphyria → erythrohepatic protoporphyria.
erythropoietic stimulating factor *abbr*. **ESF** → erythropoietin.
erythropoietic uroporphyria kongenitale erythropoetische Porphyrie *f*, Günther'-Krankheit *f*, Morbus Günther *m*, Porphyria erythropo(i)etica congenita, Porphyria congenita Günther.
e·ryth·ro·poi·e·tin [,-'pɔɪətɪn] *n* Erythropo(i)etin *nt*, erythropoetischer Faktor *m*, Hämato-, Hämopoietin *nt*.
e·ryth·ro·pros·o·pal·gia [,-,prɑsə'pældʒ(ɪ)ə] *n* Histaminkopfschmerz *m*, -kephalgie *f*, Horton-Syndrom *nt*, -Neuralgie *f*, Bing-Horton-Syndrom *nt*, -Neuralgie *f*, Cephalaea histaminica, Erythroprosopalgie *f*, cluster headache (*nt*).
er·y·throp·sia [erɪ'θrɑpsɪə] *n ophthal*., *physiol*. Rotsehen *nt*, Erythrop(s)ie (*f*).
er·y·throp·sin [,erɪ'θrɑpsɪn] *n* Sehpurpur *nt*, Rhodopsin *nt*.
e·ryth·ro·pyk·no·sis [ɪ,rɪθrəpɪk'nəʊsɪs] *n hema*. Erythropyknose *f*.
e·ryth·ror·rhex·is [,-'reksɪs] *n* → erythrocytorrhexis.
er·y·throse ['erɪθrəʊs] *n biochem*. Erythrose *f*.
e·ryth·ro·sed·i·men·ta·tion [ɪ,rɪθrə,sedɪmen'teɪʃn] *n* Erythrozytensenkung *f*, -sedimentation *f*.
erythrose-4-phosphate *n* Erythrose-4-phosphat *nt*.
erythrose-4-phosphoric acid Erythrose-4-phosphorsäure *f*.
e·ryth·ro·sin [ɪ'rɪθrəsɪn] *n* Erythrosin *nt*.
er·y·thro·sis [erɪ'θrəʊsɪs] *n derm*. Erythrose *f*, Erythrosis *f*.
e·ryth·ro·sta·sis [ɪ,rɪθrə'steɪsɪs] *n hema*. Erythrostase *f*.
e·ryth·ro·thi·o·ne·ine [,-,θaɪə'niːɪn] *n* → ergothioneine.
e·ryth·ru·lose [ɪ'rɪθrəlɔʊs] *n* Erythrulose *f*.
er·y·thru·ria [erɪ'θr(j)ʊərɪə] *n patho*. Ausscheidung *f* von rötlichem Harn, Erythrurie *f*.
ES *abbr*. → extracellular space.
Es *abbr*. → einsteinium.
es·cape [ɪ'skeɪp] **I** *n* 1. (*Gas*) Entweichen *nt*, Ausströmen *nt*; (*Flüssigkeit*) Ausfließen *nt*, Auslaufen *nt*. 2. Entkommen *nt*, Entrinnen *nt*, Flucht *f* (*from* aus, vor). **II** *vi* 3. (*Gas*) entweichen, ausströmen; (*Flüssigkeit*) auslaufen. 4. entkommen, entwischen, flüchten (*from* aus); fliehen (*from* vor).
escape beat → escaped beat.
escape contraction → escaped beat.
es·caped beat [ɪ'skeɪpd] *card*. Ersatzsystole *f*, escaped beat (*m*).
escaped contraction → escaped beat.
escape reflex Fluchtreflex *m*.
escape rhythm *cardio*. Ersatzrhythmus *m*.
es·cap·ism [ɪ'skeɪpɪzəm] *n psycho*. Wirklichkeitsflucht *f*, Eskapismus *m*.
es·cap·ist [ɪ'skeɪpɪst] *psycho*. **I** *n* Eskapist(in *f*) *m*. **II** *adj* eskapistisch.
es·char ['eskɑːr, -kər] *n* (Verbrennungs-, Gangrän-)Schorf *m*, Eschar *f*.
es·cha·rot·ic [eskə'rɑtɪk] **I** *n* Ätzmittel *nt*, Kaustikum *nt*, Escharotikum *nt*. **II** *adj* (ver-)ätzend, korrodierend.
es·cha·rot·o·my [ekskə'rɑtəmɪ] *n chir*. Escharotomie *f*.
Escherich ['eʃərɪk]: **E.'s bacillus** → Escherichia coli.
Esch·e·rich·ia [,eʃə'rɪkɪə] *n micro*. Escherichia *f*.
E. coli Escherich-Bakterium *nt*, Colibakterium *nt*, -bazillus *m*, Kolibazillus *m*, Escherichia/Bact. coli.
E. coli, enterohemorrhagic *abbr*. **EHEC** enterohämorrhagisches Escherichia coli *abbr*. EHEC.
E. coli, enteroinvasive *abbr*. **EIEC** enteroinvasives Escherichia coli *abbr*. EIEC.
E. coli, enteropathogenic *abbr*. **EPEC** enteropathogenes Escherichia coli *abbr*. EPEC.
E. coli, enterotoxicogenic *abbr*. **ETEC** enterotoxisches Escherichia coli *abbr*. ETEC.
es·cin ['eskɪn] *n pharm*. Aescin *nt*.
es·cu·lent ['eskjələnt] **I** *n* Nahrungsmittel *nt*. **II** *adj* eßbar, genießbar.
es·cu·lin ['eskjəlɪn] *n pharm*. Äskulin *nt*.
es·er·ine ['esəriːn, -rɪn] *n* Eserin *nt*, Physostignin *nt*.
ESF *abbr*. [erythropoietic stimulating factor] → erythropoietin.
Esmarch ['esmɑːrk; 'ɛsmɑrç]: **E.'s bandage/tourniquet/wrap** Esmarch-Binde *f*.
es·march ['esmɑːrk] *n* → Esmarch's bandage.
e·so·cat·a·pho·ria [,esəʊkætə'fɔːrɪə] *n ophthal*. Esokataphorie *f*.
e·so·de·vi·a·tion [,esədɪvɪ'eɪʃn] *n* 1. → esophoria. 2. → esotropia.
esoph·a· *pref*. → esophago-.
e·soph·a·gal·gia [ɪ,sɑfə'gældʒ(ɪ)ə] *n* → esophagodynia.
e·soph·a·ge·al [ɪ,sɑfə'dʒiːəl, ,ɪsə'fædʒɪəl] *adj* Speiseröhre/Ösophagus betr., ösophageal, oesophageal, ösophagisch, Speiseröhren-, Ösophag(o)-, Ösophagus-.
esophageal achalasia (Ösophagus-)Achalasie *f*, *old* Kardiospasmus *m*.
esophageal agenesis Ösophagusagenesie *f*.
esophageal anomaly Ösophagusfehlbildung *f*, -anomalie *f*.
esophageal aplasia Ösophagusaplasie *f*.
esophageal arteries, inferior Ösophagusäste *pl* der A. gastrica sinistra, Rami (o)esophageales a. gastricae sinistrae.
esophageal atresia Ösophagusatresie *f*.
esophageal branches of inferior thyroid artery Ösophagusäste *pl* der A. thyroidea inferior, Rami (o)esophageales a. thyroideae inferioris.
e. of left gastric artery → esophageal arteries, inferior.
e. of recurrent laryngeal nerve Ösophagusäste *pl* des N. laryngeus recurrens, Rami (o)esophageales n. laryngei recurrentis.
e. of thoracic aorta Ösophagusäste *pl* der Brustaorta, Rami (o)esophageales aortae thoracicae.
esophageal cancer/carcinoma Speiseröhrenkrebs *m*, -karzinom *nt*, Ösophaguskrebs *m*, -karzinom *nt*.
esophageal cardiogram *card*. Ösophagealableitung *f*, -kardiogramm *nt*, Ösophaguskardiogramm *nt*.
esophageal dilatation *chir*. Speiseröhrendehnung *f*, -dilatation *f*, Ösophagusdehnung *f*, -dilatation *f*.
esophageal diverticulum Speiseröhren-, Ösophagusdivertikel *nt*.
esophageal dysrhythmia diffuser Ösophagusspasmus *m*.
esophageal erosion Speiseröhren-, Ösophaguserosion *f*.
esophageal fistula 1. → esophagotracheal fistula. 2. → esophagostoma.
esophageal foramen → esophageal hiatus.
esophageal glands Speiseröhrendrüsen *pl*, Gll. (o)esophageae.
esophageal hiatus Hiatus (o)esophageus.
esophageal impression of liver Speiseröhrenfurche *f* der Leber, Impressio (o)esophagea (hepatis).
esophageal injury Speiseröhrenverletzung *f*, -trauma *nt*, Ösophagusverletzung *f*, -trauma *nt*.
esophageal malignancy Speiseröhren-, Ösophagusmalignom *nt*, maligner Speiseröhrentumor *m*, maligne Speiseröhrengeschwulst *f*; Speiseröhrenkrebs *m*, -karzinom *nt*, Ösophaguskrebs *m*, -karzinom *nt*.

esophageal manometry Ösophagusmanometrie f, -druckmessung f.
esophageal motility Speiseröhren-, Ösophagusmotilität f.
esophageal mucosa Speiseröhren-, Ösophagusschleimhaut f, Tunica mucosa (o)esophagi.
esophageal necrosis Speiseröhren-, Ösophagusnekrose f.
esophageal obstruction Speiseröhren-, Ösophagusobstruktion f.
esophageal opening of diaphragm → esophageal hiatus.
esophageal operation Operation f an der Speiseröhre, Speiseröhren-, Ösophagusoperation f.
esophageal perforation Speiseröhren-, Ösophagusperforation f.
esophageal plexus vegetatives Speiseröhrengeflecht nt, Vagusgeflecht nt des Ösophagus, Plexus (o)esophagealis.
esophageal reflux Speiseröhren-, Ösophagusreflux m, gastroösophagealer Reflux m.
esophageal resection chir. Speiseröhren-, Ösophagusresektion f.
esophageal ring Schatzki-Ring m.
esophageal rupture Speiseröhrenriß m, -ruptur f, Ösophagusriß m, -ruptur f.
 postemetic/spontaneous e. Boerhaave-Syndrom nt, spontane/postemetische/emetogene Ösophagusruptur.
esophageal sound Ösophagussonde f.
esophageal spasm Speiseröhrenkrampf m, Ösophagusspasmus m, Ösophagospasmus m.
 symptomatic idiopathic diffuse e. abbr. SIDES idiopathischer diffuser Ösogusspasmus, symptomatic idiopathic diffuse esophageal spasm abbr. SIDES.
esophageal speech Ösophagusstimme f, -sprache f, -ersatzstimme f.
esophageal sphincter Speiseröhren-, Ösophagussphinkter m abbr. ÖS.
 lower e. abbr. LES unterer Ösopahagussphinkter abbr. uÖS.
 upper e. abbr. UES oberer Ösophagussphinkter abbr. oÖS, Ösophagusmund m.
esophageal stenosis Speiseröhrenverengerung f, Ösophagusstenose f.
esophageal stricture Speiseröhren-, Ösophagusstriktur f.
 peptic e. peptische Ösophagusstriktur.
esophageal surgery Speiseröhren-, Ösophaguschirurgie f.
esophageal temperature Ösophagustemperatur f.
esophageal trauma Speiseröhrenverletzung f, -trauma nt, Ösophagusverletzung f, -trauma nt.
esophageal ulcer Speiseröhren-, Ösophagusulkus nt.
esophageal variceal bleeding Ösophagusvarizenblutung f.
esophageal varices Ösophagusvarizen pl.
esophageal veins Speiseröhren-/Ösophagusvenen pl, Vv. (o)esophageales.
esophageal web → esophageal ring.
e·soph·a·gec·ta·sia [ɪˌsafədʒek'teɪʒ(ɪ)ə] n patho. Speiseröhrendehnung f, -dilatation f, -ektasie f, Ösophagusdehnung f, -dilatation f, -ektasie f.
e·soph·a·gec·ta·sis [ɪˌsafə'dʒektəsɪs] n → esophagectasia.
e·soph·a·gec·to·my [ˌ-'dʒektəmɪ] n chir. Speiseröhren-, Ösophagusresektion f, Ösophagektomie f.
e·soph·a·gism [ɪ'safədʒɪzəm] n → esophagospasm.
e·soph·a·gis·mus [ɪˌsafə'dʒɪzməs] n → esophagospasm.

e·soph·a·gi·tis [ɪˌsafə'dʒaɪtɪs] n Speiseröhrenentzündung f, Ösophagitis f, Oesophagitis f.
esophago- pref. Speiseröhren-, Ösophag(o)-, Oesophag(o)-, Ösophagus-.
e·soph·a·go·an·tros·to·my [ɪˌsafəgəʊænˈtrastəmɪ] n chir. Ösophagoantrostomie f.
e·soph·a·go·bron·chi·al [ˌ-'brɑŋkɪəl] adj Speiseröhre/Ösophagus u. Bronchus betr. od. verbindend, ösophagobronchial.
e·soph·a·go·car·di·o·my·ot·o·my [ˌ-ˌkɑːrdɪəʊmaɪˈatəmɪ] n chir. Speiseröhren-Kardia-Schnitt m, Ösophagokardiomyotomie f, Kardiotomie f.
e·soph·a·go·car·di·o·plas·ty [ˌ-'kɑːrdɪəplæstɪ] n chir. Speiseröhren-Kardia-Plastik f, Ösophagokardioplastik f.
e·soph·a·go·cele ['siːl] n Speiseröhrenbruch m, Ösophagozele f.
e·soph·a·go·co·lo·gas·tros·to·my [ˌ-ˌkəʊləgæs'trastəmɪ] n chir. Ösophagokologastrostomie f.
e·soph·a·go·co·lo·plas·ty [ˌ-'kəʊləplæstɪ] n chir. Ösophagusplastik f mit Koloninterposition, Ösophagokoloplastik f.
e·soph·a·go·du·o·de·nos·to·my [ˌ-ˌd(j)uːdɪ'nastəmɪ] n chir. Ösophagus-Duodenum-Anastomose f, Ösophagus-Duodenum-Fistel f, Ösophagoduodenostomie f.
e·soph·a·go·dyn·ia [ˌ-'diːnɪə] n Speiseröhren-, Ösophagusschmerz m, Ösophagodynie f.
e·soph·a·go·en·te·ros·to·my [ˌ-ˌentə'rastəmɪ] n chir. Ösophagus-Darm-Anastomose f, Ösophagus-Darm-Fistel f, Ösophagoenterostomie f.
e·soph·a·go·e·soph·a·gos·to·my [ˌ-ɪˌsafə'gastəmɪ] n chir. Ösophagoösophagostomie f.
e·soph·a·go·fun·do·pex·y [ˌ-'fʌndə'peksɪ] n chir. Ösophagofundopexie f.
e·soph·a·go·gas·trec·to·my [ˌ-gæs'trektəmɪ] n chir. Ösophagogastrektomie f.
e·soph·a·go·gas·tric [ˌ-'gæstrɪk] adj Speiseröhre/Ösophagus u. Magen/Gaster betr. od. verbindend, ösophagogastral, gastroösophageal.
esophagogastric junction ösophagogastrale/gastroösophageale Übergangszone f.
esophagogastric orifice Speiseröhren-, Ösophagus(ein)mündung f, Ostium cardiacum, Cardia f.
esophagogastric sphincter → esophageal sphincter, lower.
e·soph·a·go·gas·tro·a·nas·to·mo·sis [ˌ-ˌgæstrəʊˌnæstəˈməʊsɪs] n → esophagogastrostomy.
e·soph·a·go·gas·tro·my·ot·o·my [ˌ-ˌgæstrəmaɪˈatəmɪ] n → esophagocardiomyotomy.
e·soph·a·go·gas·tro·plas·ty [ˌ-'gæstrəplæstɪ] n chir. Speiseröhren-Magen-Plastik f, Ösophagogastroplastik f, Kardiaplastik f.
e·soph·a·go·gas·tros·co·py [ˌ-gæs'traskəpɪ] n Speiseröhren-Magen-Spiegelung f, Ösophagogastroskopie f.
e·soph·a·go·gas·tros·to·my [ˌ-gæs'trastəmɪ] n chir. Speiseröhren-Magen-Anastomose f, Speiseröhren-Magen-Fistel f, Ösophagogastrostomie f.
e·soph·a·go·gram [ɪ'safəgəgræm] n radiol. Ösophagogramm nt.
e·soph·a·gog·ra·phy [ɪˌsafə'gagrəfɪ] n radiol. Kontrastdarstellung f der Speiseröhre, Ösophagographie f.
e·soph·a·go·il·e·o·co·lo·plas·ty [ˌsafəgəʊˌɪlɪəʊ'kəʊləplæstɪ] n chir. Ösophagoileokoloplastik f.

e·soph·a·go·je·ju·no·gas·tros·to·mo·sis [ˌ-dʒɪˌdʒuːnəʊgæsˌtrastə'məʊsɪs] n → esophagojejunogastrostomy.
e·soph·a·go·je·ju·no·gas·tros·to·my [ˌ-dʒɪˌdʒuːnəʊgæs'trastəmɪ] n chir. Ösophagus-Jejunum-Anastomose f, -Fistel f, Ösophagojejunogastrostomie f.
e·soph·a·go·je·ju·no·plas·ty [ˌ-dʒɪ'dʒuːnəplæstɪ] n chir. Ösophagus-Jejunum-Plastik f, Ösophagojejunoplastik f.
e·soph·a·go·je·ju·nos·to·my [ˌ-dʒɪdʒuːˈnastəmɪ] n chir. Ösophagus-Jejunum-Anastomose f, Ösophagus-Jejunum-Fistel f, Ösophagojejunostomie f.
e·soph·a·go·lar·yn·gec·to·my [ˌ-ˌlærɪn'dʒektəmɪ] n chir. Ösophagolaryngektomie f.
e·soph·a·go·ma·la·cia [ˌ-mə'leɪʃ(ɪ)ə] n patho. Speiseröhrenerweichung f, Ösophagomalazie f.
e·soph·a·go·my·co·sis [ˌ-maɪ'kəʊsɪs] n Pilzbefall m od. -erkrankung f der Speiseröhre, Speiseröhren-, Ösophagusmykose f.
e·soph·a·go·my·ot·o·my [ˌ-maɪ'atəmɪ] n chir. 1. Ösophagomyotomie f. 2. → esophagocardiomyotomy.
e·soph·a·go·plas·ty ['plæstɪ] n chir. Speiseröhren-, Ösophagusplastik f.
e·soph·a·go·pli·ca·tion [ˌ-plaɪ'keɪʃn] n chir. Speiseröhrenplikatur f, -plikation f, Ösophagusplikatur f, -plikation f, Ösophagoplicatio f.
e·soph·a·gop·to·sia [ɪˌsafəgap'təʊsɪə] n → esophagoptosis.
e·soph·a·gop·to·sis [ɪˌsafəgap'təʊsɪs] n Speiseröhren-, Ösophagussenkung f, Ösophagoptose f.
e·soph·a·go·sal·i·var·y reflex [ˌ-'sælə,veriː, -vərɪ] Roger-Reflex m.
e·soph·a·go·scope [ɪ'safəgəʊskəʊp] n Ösophagoskop nt.
e·soph·a·gos·co·py [ɪˌsafə'gaskəpɪ] n Speiseröhrenspiegelung f, Ösophagoskopie f.
e·soph·a·go·spasm [ɪ'safəgəʊˌspæzəm] n Speiseröhrenkrampf m, Ösophagospasmus m.
e·soph·a·go·ste·no·sis [ˌ-stɪ'nəʊsɪs] n Speiseröhrenverengerung f, Ösophagus-, Ösophagostenose f.
e·soph·a·go·sto·ma [ɪˌsafə'gastəmə] n chir. Ösophagostoma nt.
e·soph·a·go·sto·mi·a·sis [ɪˌsafəgəʊstəʊ'maɪəsɪs] n Ösophagostomum-Infektion f, -Befall m, Oesophagostomiasis f.
e·soph·a·gos·to·my [ɪˌsafə'gastəmɪ] n chir. Speiseröhrenschnitt m, operative Eröffnung f der Speiseröhre, Ösophagotomie f, Oesophagotomia f.
e·soph·a·go·tra·che·al [ɪˌsafəgəʊ'treɪkɪəl] adj Speiseröhre/Ösophagus u. Luftröhre/Trachea betr. od. verbindend, ösophagotracheal, tracheoösophageal, Ösophago-tracheal-.
esophagotracheal fistula Ösophagotracheal-, Tracheoösophagealfistel f.
 distal e. untere Ösophagotrachealfistel.
 H-type e. (ösophagotracheale) H-Fistel.
 proximal e. obere Ösophagotrachealfistel.
esophagotracheal groove ösophagotracheale Grube/Rinne f.
esophagotracheal septum embryo. ösophagotracheale Scheidewand f, Septum (o)esophagotracheale.
e·soph·a·gram [ɪ'safəgræm] n → esophagogram.
e·soph·a·gus [ɪ'safəgəs] n, pl **-gi** [-dʒaɪ, -gaɪ] Speiseröhre f, Ösophagus m, Oesophagus m.

esophagus agenesis Speiseröhren-, Ösophagusagenesie f.
esophagus aplasia Speiseröhren-, Ösophagusaplasie f.
esophagus atresia Speiseröhren-, Ösophagusatresie f.
esophagus malformation Speiseröhren-, Ösophagusmißbildung f.
esophagus stenosis Speiseröhrenverengerung f, Ösophagus-, Ösophagostenose f.
es·o·pho·ria [esəˈfɔʊrɪə] n ophthal. latentes Einwärtsschielen nt, Esophorie f, Endophorie f, Strabismus convergens latens.
e·so·phor·ic [esəˈfɔːrɪk] adj Esophorie betr., von ihr betroffen, Esophorie-.
es·o·phy·lax·is [esəfɪˈlæksɪs] n Esophylaxie f.
es·o·sphe·noi·di·tis [esəˌsfiːnɔɪˈdaɪtɪs] n HNO Osteomyelitis f des Os sphenoidale.
es·o·tro·pia [ˌesəˈtroʊpɪə] n ophthal. Einwärtsschielen nt, Esotropie f, Strabismus convergens/internus.
es·o·trop·ic [ˌ-ˈtrɒpɪk, -ˈtroʊp-] adj Esotropie betr., von ihr gekennzeichnet, nach innen schielend, esotrop.
ESP abbr. → extrasensory perception.
es·pun·dia [eˈspuːndɪə] n Espundia f, südamerikanische Haut-Schleimhautleishmaniase f, mukokutane Leishmaniase Südamerikas f.
ESR abbr. 1. → electron spin resonance. 2. → erythrocyte sedimentation rate.
ESRD abbr. → end-stage renal disease.
ESR spectroscopy → electron spin resonance spectroscopy.
es·sence [ˈesəns] n 1. Essenz f, das Wesen, das Wesentliche, Kern m. 2. konzentrierte Zubereitung f, Essenz f, Essentia f.
es·sen·tia [əˈsentʃ(ɪ)ə] n → essence 2.
es·sen·tial [əˈsenʃl] I n Hauptsache f, das Wesentliche; (wesentliche) Voraussetzung f (to für). II adj 1. essentiell, wesentlich, grundlegend, fundamental, (unbedingt) erforderlich (to für); Haupt-, Grund-. 2. patho. essentiell; idiopathisch; primär. 3. ätherisch, Essenz(en) enthaltend.
essential albuminuria essentielle Albuminurie/Proteinurie f.
essential anosmia essentielle/idiopathische Anosmie f.
essential asthma essentielles/primäres Asthma nt.
essential atrophy of iris ophthal. essentielle Irisatrophie f.
essential blepharospasm ophthal. essentieller/idiopathischer Lidkrampf/Blepharospasmus m.
essential bradycardia essentielle Bradykardie f.
essential convulsion neuro. zentralbedingte Konvulsion f.
essential dysmenorrhea gyn. primäre/essentielle Dysmenorrhö f.
essential fever idiopathisches Fieber nt.
essential hematuria primäre Hämaturie f.
essential hypertension essentielle/idiopathische/primäre Hypertonie f.
essential hypotension essentielle/primäre/konstitutionelle Hypotonie f.
essential oil chem. ätherisches Öl nt.
essential pentosuria benigne essentielle Pentosurie f, Xylosurie f.
essential phthisis (of eye) ophthal. Augapfel-, Bulbuserweichung f, Ophthalmomalazie f.
essential proteinuria → essential albuminuria.
essential telangiectasia Angioma serpiginosum f.

essential thrombocythemia hämorrhagische/essentielle Thrombozythämie f, Megakaryozytenleukämie f, megakaryozytäre Myelose f.
essential thrombocytopenia idiopathische thrombozytopenische Purpura f abbr. ITP, essentielle/idiopathische Thrombozytopenie f, Morbus Werlhof m.
essential tremor hereditärer/essentieller Tremor m.
essential vertigo idiopathischer Schwindel m.
Esser [ˈesər]: **E.'s operation** HNO Esser-Plastik f.
EST abbr. → electroshock therapy.
es·ter [ˈestər] n Ester m.
es·ter·ase [ˈestəreɪz] n Esterase f.
esterase inhibitor Esterasehemmer m, -hemmstoff m, -inhibitor m.
esterase-negative adj histol. esterasenegativ.
esterase-positive adj histol. esterasepositiv.
ester bond chem. Esterbindung f.
es·ter·i·fi·ca·tion [eˌsterəfɪˈkeɪʃn] n chem. Veresterung f.
es·ter·i·fy [eˈsterəfaɪ] vt chem. verestern.
es·ter·ize [ˈestəraɪz] chem. I vt in einen Ester verwandeln. II vi in einen Ester umgewandelt werden.
es·te·rol·y·sis [estəˈrɒləsɪs] n chem. Esterhydrolyse f, -spaltung f.
es·ter·o·lyt·ic [ˌestəroʊˈlɪtɪk] adj esterspaltend, -hydrolisierend.
es·te·trol [ˈestətrɒl] n abbr. **E₄** Östetrol nt, Estetrol nt.
es·the·sia [esˈθiːʒ(ɪ)ə] n Sinneseindruck m, Gefühl nt, Empfindung f, Sensibilität f, Perzeption f, Ästhesie f.
esthesio- pref. Sinnes-, Sensibilitäts-, Gefühls-, Empfindungs-, Ästhesio-.
es·the·si·o·blast [esˈθiːz(ɪ)əblæst] n Ganglioblast m, embryonale Spinalganglienzelle f, Ästhesioblast m.
es·the·si·ol·o·gy [esˌθiːzɪˈɒlədʒɪ] n Ästhesiologie f.
es·the·si·om·e·ter [esˌθiːzɪˈɒmɪtər] n Ästhesiometer nt.
es·the·si·o·neu·ro·blas·to·ma [esˌθiːzɪəˌnjʊərəˈblæstəʊmə] n patho. Ästhesioneuroblastom nt.
es·the·si·o·neu·ro·sis [ˌ-ˌnjʊəˈrəʊsɪs] n Erkrankung f sensibler Nerven, Ästhesioneurose f.
es·the·si·on·o·sus [esˌθiːzɪˈɒnəsəs] n → esthesioneurosis.
es·thet·ic surgery [esˈθetɪk] kosmetische Chirurgie f, Schönheitschirurgie f.
es·ti·mate [n ˈestəmɪt, -meɪt; v -meɪt] I n 1. Schätzung f, Veranschlagung f. 2. Bewertung f, Beurteilung f. II vt 3. (ab-, ein-)schätzen, taxieren, veranschlagen (at auf). 4. (etw.) beurteilen, bewerten, s. eine Meinung bilden über. III vi schätzen.
es·ti·ma·tion [ˌestəˈmeɪʃn] n 1. → estimate 1. 2. Meinung f, Ansicht f, Urteil nt.
es·ti·val [ˈestɪvəl, eˈstaɪvəl] adj Sommer betr., im Sommer auftretend, sommerlich, Sommer-, Ästivo-.
es·ti·vo·au·tum·nal [ˌestɪvəʊˈtʌmnəl, eˌstaɪ-] adj Sommer u. Herbst betr., im Sommer u. Herbst auftretend, Ästivoautumnal-, Sommer-Herbst-.
Estlander [ˈestlændər]: **E. flap** Estlander-Plastik f.
E.'s operation 1. HNO Estlander-Plastik f. **2.** Estlander-Létievant-Operation f.
es·ton [ˈestən] n Aluminiumacetat nt.
es·tra·di·ol [ˌestrəˈdaɪɒl, -əl] n abbr. **E₂** Estradiol nt, Östradiol nt.

estradiol benzoate Estradiol-, Östradiolbenzoat nt.
estradiol dipropionate Estradiol-, Östradioldipropionat nt.
estradiol-6β-hydroxylase n → estradiol-6β-monooxygenase.
estradiol-6β-monooxygenase n Estradiol-6β-monooxygenase f, Östradiol-6β-monooxygenase f.
estradiol ondecylate Estradiol-, Östradiolondecylat nt.
estradiol valerate Estradiol-, Östradiolvalerat nt.
es·tra·mus·tine [ˌestrəˈmʌstiːn] n pharm. Estramustin nt.
es·trane [ˈestreɪn] n Östran nt, Estran nt.
es·tra·pen·ta·ene [ˌestrəˈpentəwiːn] n biochem. Estrapentaen(-Ring m) nt.
es·tra·tet·ra·ene [ˌ-ˈtetrəwiːn] n biochem. Estratetraen(-Ring m) nt.
es·tra·tri·ene [ˌ-ˈtraɪiːn] n biochem. Estratrien(-Ring m) nt.
es·trin [ˈestrɪn] n → estrogen.
estrin phase → estrogenic phase.
es·tri·ol [ˈestrɪɒl, -əl, -traɪ-] n abbr. **E₃** Estriol nt, Östriol nt.
es·tro·gen [ˈestrədʒən] n Estrogen nt, Östrogen nt.
es·tro·gen·ic [ˌestrəˈdʒenɪk] adj 1. Östrogen betr., östrogenartig (wirkend), östrogen. 2. Östrus auslösend.
estrogenic hormones östrogene Hormone pl.
estrogenic phase gyn. östrogene/proliferative Phase f, Proliferations-, Follikelreifungsphase f.
es·trog·e·nous [esˈtrɒdʒənəs] adj → estrogenic 1.
estrogen receptor Östrogen-, Estrogenrezeptor m.
estrogen-receptor activity Östrogen-, Estrogenrezeptorbindungskapazität f.
estrogen-receptor analysis Östrogen-, Estrogenrezeptoranalyse f, -bestimmung f, Östrogenrezeptoranalyse f, -bestimmung f.
estrogen-receptor protein Östrogenrezeptorprotein nt.
estrogen replacement therapy abbr. **ERT** Östrogen-, Estrogen(ersatz)therapie f.
estrogen therapy → estrogen replacement therapy.
es·trone [ˈestroʊn] n abbr. **E₁** Estron nt, Östron nt, Follikulin nt, Folliculin nt.
es·tro·stil·ben [ˌestrəˈstɪlbən] n pharm. Diäthylstilböstrol nt, Diethylstilbestrol nt abbr. **DES**.
es·trous [ˈestrəs] adj bio. Östrus betr., Östral-, Brunst-.
es·tru·al [ˈestrəwəl] adj → estrous.
es·tru·a·tion [estrəˈweɪʃn] n → estrus.
es·trum [ˈestrəm] n → estrus.
es·trus [ˈestrəs] n bio. Brunst f, Östrus m.
ESWL abbr. → extracorporeal shock wave lithotripsy.
es·y·late [ˈesɪleɪt] n Äthan-, Ethansulfonat nt.
et·a·fed·rine [etəˈfedriːn, -rɪn] n pharm. Etafedrin nt.
e·taf·e·none [ɪˈtæfənoʊn] n pharm. Etafenon nt.
e·tam·i·van [ɪˈtæmɪvæn] n → ethamivan.
e·tam·sy·late [ɪˈtæmsɪleɪt] n → ethamsylate.
ETEC abbr. → Escherichia coli, enterotoxicogenic.
eth·a·cryn·ate [ˌeθəˈkriːneɪt] n Etacrynat nt, Ethacrinat nt.
eth·a·cryn·ic acid [ˌeθəˈkrɪnɪk] Etacrynsäure f.
eth·al [ˈeθæl, ˈiːθ-] n Cetylalkohol m.
eth·al·de·hyde [ɪˈældəhaɪd] n Azet-, Acetaldehyd m, Äthanal nt, Ethanal nt.

e·tham·bu·tol [ɪ'θæmbjuːtɑl] *n pharm.* Ethambutol *nt.*
e·tham·i·van [ɪ'θæmɪvæn] *n pharm.* Etamivan *nt.*
e·tham·sy·late [ɪ'θæmsɪleɪt] *n pharm.* Etamsylat *nt.*
eth·a·nal ['eθənæl, -nl] *n* → ethaldehyde.
ethanal acid Glyoxalsäure *f*, Glyoxylsäure *f*.
eth·ane ['eθeɪn] *n* Äthan *nt*, Ethan *nt*.
eth·ane·di·al [ˌeθeɪn'daɪæl] *n* Glyoxal *nt*, Oxalaldehyd *m*.
eth·ane·di·a·mine [ˌ-'daɪəmiːn] *n* Äthylen-, Ethylendiamin *nt.*
eth·ane·di·o·ic acid [ˌ-daɪ'əʊɪk] Oxal-, Kleesäure *f*.
1,2-eth·ane·di·sul·fo·nate [ˌ-daɪsʌlfəneɪt] *n* Äthandisulfonat *nt.*
eth·a·no·ic acid [eθə'nəʊɪk] Essigsäure *f*, Äthan-, Ethansäure *f*.
eth·a·nol ['eθənɒl, -nɑl] *n* Äthanol *nt*, Ethanol *nt*, Äthylalkohol *m*; *inf.* Alkohol *m*.
eth·a·nol·a·mine [ˌeθə'nɑləmiːn, -'nəʊlə-, -nə'læmɪn] *n* Äthanol-, Ethanolamin *nt*, Colamin *nt*, Monoethanolamin *nt*.
ethanolamine kinase Ethanol-, Äthanolaminkinase *f*.
ethanolamine phosphoglyceride Ethanol-, Äthanolaminphosphoglycerid *nt*, Phosphatidyläthanolamin *nt*, -ethanolamin *nt.*
eth·a·nol·a·mine·sul·fon·ic acid [ˌeθə'nɑləmiːnsʌl'fɑnɪk] Ethanol-, Äthanolaminsulfonsäure *f*, Taurin *nt.*
eth·a·ver·ine [ˌeθə'veriːn] *n pharm.* Ethaverin *nt.*
eth·ene ['eθiːn] *n* → ethylene.
eth·e·nyl ['eθənɪl] *n* Vinyl-(Radikal *nt*).
eth·e·nyl·ben·zene [eθənɪl'benziːn] *n* Styrol *nt*, Vinylbenzol *nt.*
e·ther ['eθər] *n* **1.** Äther *m*, Ether *m.* **2.** Diäthyläther *m*, Diethylether *m*; *inf.* Äther *m.*
e·the·re·al [ɪ'θɪərɪəl] *adj* ätherisch, ätherhaltig, flüchtig, Äther-.
e·the·re·al·ize [ɪ'θɪərɪəlaɪz] *vt chem.* mit Äther behandeln, ätherisieren, äthern.
ethereal oil *chem.* ätherisches Öl *nt.*
e·the·re·ous [ɪ'θɪərɪəs] *adj* → ethereal.
ether bond *chem.* Äther-, Etherbindung *f.*
e·the·ri·al *adj* → ethereal.
e·ther·ic [ɪ'θerɪk, 'iːθərɪk] *adj* → ethereal.
e·ther·i·fi·ca·tion [ˌɪˌθerɪfɪ'keɪʃn, ˌiːθər-] *n chem.* Verätherung *f*, Veretherung *f.*
e·ther·i·fy [ɪ'θerəfaɪ, 'iːθər-] *vt* in einen Äther verwandeln.
e·ther·ism ['iːθərɪzəm] *n* Äthervergiftung *f.*
ether spirit Hoffmann-Tropfen *pl*, Ätherweingeist *m*, Spiritus aetherus.
eth·i·cal ['eθɪkl] *adj* **1.** Ethik betr., ethisch; moralisch, sittlich. **2.** dem Berufsethos entsprechend. **3.** moralisch einwandfrei, von ethischen Grundsätzen geleitet. **4.** *pharm.* rezeptpflichtig.
eth·ics ['eθɪks] *pl* Ethik *f.*
e·thid·i·um bromide [ɪ'θɪdɪəm] Äthidiumbromid *nt.*
e·thi·nyl *n* → ethynyl.
ethinyl estradiol *pharm.* Ethinylestradiol *nt*, Äthinylöstradiol *nt.*
eth·i·on·a·mide [ˌeθɪ'ɑnəmaɪd] *n pharm.* Ethionamid *nt.*
e·thi·o·nine [ɪ'θaɪəniːn, -nɪn] *n* Äthionin *nt*, Ethionin *nt.*
e·this·ter·one [ɪ'θɪstərəʊn] *n pharm.* Ethisteron *nt.*
eth·mo·ceph·a·lus [ˌeθmə'sefələs] *n embryo.* Ethmozephalus *m*, -kephalus *m.*
eth·mo·fron·tal [ˌ-'frʌntl] *adj* Siebbein u. Stirnbein betr., ethmofrontal.
eth·moid ['eθmɔɪd] **I** *n* Siebbein *nt*, Ethmoid *nt*, Os ethmoidale. **II** *adj* **1.** → ethmoidal. **2.** siebartig, kribriform.
eth·moi·dal [eθ'mɔɪdl] *adj* Siebbein/Os ethmoidale betr., ethmoidal, Siebbein-.
ethmoidal aircells Siebbeinzellen *pl*, Cellulae ethmoidales.
ethmoidal artery: anterior e. vordere Siebbeinarterie *f*, Ethmoidalis *f* anterior, A. ethmoidalis anterior.
posterior e. hintere Siebbeinarterie *f*, Ethmoidalis *f* posterior, A. ethmoidalis posterior.
ethmoidal bulla Bulla ethmoidalis.
ethmoidal cells → ethmoidal aircells.
ethmoidal concha: inferior e. mittlere Nasenmuschel *f*, Concha nasalis media.
superior e. obere Nasenmuschel *f*, Concha nasalis superior.
supreme e. oberste Nasenmuschel *f*, Concha nasalis suprema.
ethmoidal crest: e. of maxilla Crista ethmoidalis maxillae.
e. of palatine bone Crista ethmoidalis ossis palatinii.
ethmoidal foramen: anterior e. For. ethmoidale anterius.
posterior e. For. ethmoidale posterius.
ethmoidal forceps *HNO* Siebbeinzange *f.*
ethmoidal groove → ethmoidal sulcus (of nasal bone).
ethmoidal incisure of frontal bone Inc. ethmoidalis (ossis frontalis).
ethmoidal infundibulum Infundibulum ethmoidale.
e. of nasal cavity Infudibulum ethmoidale cavi nasi.
ethmoidal labyrinth Siebbeinlabyrinth *nt*, Labyrinthus ethmoidalis.
ethmoidal nerve: anterior e. N. ethmoidalis anterior.
posterior e. N. ethmoidalis posterior.
ethmoidal notch of frontal bone Inc. ethmoidalis (ossis frontalis).
ethmoidal process (of inferior nasal concha) Proc. ethmoidalis (conchae nasalis inferioris).
ethmoidal sinuses Sinus ethmoidales.
ethmoidal sinusitis → ethmoiditis 1.
ethmoidal spine of Macalister Crista sphenoidalis.
ethmoidal sulcus (of nasal bone) Sulcus ethmoidalis (ossis nasalis).
ethmoidal veins Siebbein-, Ethmoidalvenen *pl*, Vv. ethmoidales.
ethmoid antrum → ethmoidal bulla.
ethmoid bone → ethmoid I.
ethmoid cornu mittlere Nasenmuschel *f*, Concha nasalis media.
eth·moi·dec·to·my [eθmɔɪ'dektəmɪ] *n HNO, neurochir.* Siebbeinausräumung *f*, Ethmoidektomie *f.*
eth·moi·di·tis [ˌ-'daɪtɪs] *n* **1.** Entzündung *f* der Siebbeinzellen, Ethmoiditis *f*, Sinusitis ethmoidalis. **2.** Siebbeinentzündung *f*, Entzündung *f* des Os ethmoidale, Ethmoiditis *f.*
eth·moi·do·lac·ri·mal [eθˌmɔɪdəʊ'lækrɪml] *adj* → ethmolacrimal.
eth·moi·do·max·il·lar·y [ˌ-'mæksəˌleriː, -mækˌsɪlərɪ] *adj* → ethmomaxillary.
eth·moi·do·na·sal [ˌ-'neɪzl] *adj* → ethmonasal.
eth·moi·do·pal·a·tal [ˌ-'pælətl] *adj* → ethmopalatal.
eth·moi·do·sphe·noid [ˌ-'sfiːnɔɪd] *adj* → ethmosphenoid.
eth·moi·dot·o·my [ˌeθmɔɪ'dɑtəmɪ] *n HNO, neurochir.* operative Eröffnung *f* der Siebbeinzellen, Ethmoidotomie *f.*
eth·mo·lac·ri·mal [ˌeθməʊ'lækrɪml] *adj* Siebbein/Os ethmoidale u. Tränenbein/Os lacrimale betr.

ethmolacrimal suture Sutura ethmoidolacrimalis.
eth·mo·max·il·lar·y [ˌ-'mæksəˌleriː, -mækˌsɪlərɪ] *adj* Siebbein/Os ethmoidale u. Oberkiefer/Maxilla betr.
ethmomaxillary suture Sutura ethmoidomaxillaris.
eth·mo·na·sal [ˌ-'neɪzl] *adj* Siebbein/Os ethmoidale u. Nasenbein/Os nasale betr.
eth·mo·pal·a·tal [ˌ-'pælətl] *adj* Siebbein/Os ethmoidale u. Gaumenbein/Os palatinum betr.
eth·mo·sphe·noid [ˌ-'sfiːnɔɪd] *adj* Siebbein/Os ethmoidale u. Keilbein/Os sphenoidale betr.
eth·mo·vo·mer·ine [ˌ-'vəʊmərɪn] *adj* Siebbein/Os ethmoidale u. Vomer betr.
eth·nic ['eθnɪk] *adj* Volk(sgruppe) betr., ethnisch, Volks-, Völker-, Ethno-.
eth·nics ['eθnɪks] *pl* → ethnology.
eth·no·bi·ol·o·gy [ˌeθnəʊbaɪ'ɑlədʒɪ] *n* Ethnobiologie *f.*
eth·nog·ra·phy [eθ'nɑgrəfɪ] *n* Ethnographie *f.*
eth·nol·o·gy [eθ'nɑlədʒɪ] *n* Völkerkunde *f*, Ethnologie *f.*
eth·o·brom ['eθəʊbrəʊm] *n* Tribromethanol *nt*, -äthanol *nt.*
eth·o·caine ['eθəʊkeɪn] *n pharm.* Procain--Hydrochlorid *nt.*
eth·o·log·i·cal [ˌeθə'lɑdʒɪkl] *adj* Ethologie betr., ethologisch.
e·thol·o·gist [ɪ'θɑlədʒɪst] *n* Ethologe *m*, -login *f.*
e·thol·o·gy [ɪ'θɑlədʒɪ] *n* **1.** (vergleichende) Verhaltensforschung *f*, Ethologie *f.* **2.** Persönlichkeitsforschung *f*, Ethologie *f.*
eth·o·sux·i·mide [ˌeθəʊ'sʌksəmaɪd] *n pharm.* Ethosuximid *nt.*
eth·ox·zol·a·mide [ˌeθɑks'zəʊləmaɪd] *n pharm.* Ethoxzolamid *nt.*
eth·yl ['eθɪl] *n* Äthyl-, Ethyl-(Radikal *nt*).
ethyl acetate Äthyl-, Ethylacetat *nt.*
ethyl alcohol → ethanol.
eth·yl·al·de·hyde [ˌeθl'ældəhaɪd] *n* → ethaldehyde.
eth·yl·a·mine [ˌ-'æmiːn, -mɪn] *n* Äthyl-, Ethylamin *nt.*
ethyl aminobenzoate *pharm.* Benzocain *nt.*
eth·yl·ate ['eθəleɪt] *n* Äthylat *nt*, Ethylat *nt.*
eth·yl·a·tion [ˌeθə'leɪʃn] *n* Äthylieren *nt*, Äthylierung *f.*
ethyl carbamate Urethan *nt*, Carbaminsäureäthylester *nt.*
ethyl cellulose Äthyl-, Ethylcellulose *f.*
ethyl chloride Äthyl-, Ethylchlorid *nt*, Monochloräthan *nt*, -ethan *nt.*
ethyl cyanide Äthylzyanid *nt*, -cyanid *nt*, Ethylzyanid *nt*, -cyanid *nt*, Propionitril *nt.*
eth·yl·ene ['eθəliːn] *n* Äthylen *nt*, Ethylen *nt*, Äthen *nt*, Ethen *nt.*
eth·yl·ene·di·a·mine·tet·ra·ac·e·tate [ˌeθəliːnˌdaɪəmiːnˌtetrə'æsɪteɪt] *n* Äthylen-, Ethylendiamintetraacetat *nt*, Edetat *nt.*
eth·yl·ene·di·a·mine·tet·ra·ce·tic acid [ˌ-ˌdaɪəmiːnˌtetrəə'sɪtɪk, -əˈsetɪk] *abbr.*
EDTA Äthylendiamintetraessigsäure *f*, Ethylendiamintetraessigsäure *f* abbr. EDTA, AeDTE, Edetinsäure *f.*
ethylene dichloride Äthylen-, Ethylendichlorid *nt.*
eth·yl·en·i·mine [eθl'enəmiːn] *n* Äthylen-, Ethylenimin *nt.*
ethyl ether → ether 2.
ethyl green Brillantgrün *nt.*
eth·yl·ism ['eθəlɪzəm] *n* Äthylalkoholvergiftung *f*, -intoxikation *f*, Äthanolvergiftung *f*, -intoxikation *f*, Äthylismus *m.*
eth·yl·ma·lo·nic-adipic aciduria *abbr.*

EMA [ˌeθɪlməˈləʊnɪk, -ˈlɑn-] Äthylmalonyladipinazidurie *f*, Glutarsäure-Azidurie II B *f*.
eth·yl·mor·phine [ˌ-ˈmɔːrfiːn] *n pharm.* Äthyl-, Ethylmorphin *nt.*
ethylmorphine hydrochloride *pharm.* Ethylmorphinhydrochlorid *nt*, Aethylmorphinum hydrochloricum.
ethyl nitrite Äthyl-, Ethylnitrit *nt.*
ethyl urethan *pharm.* Äthyl-, Ethylurethan *nt.*
e·thy·no·di·ol [ɪˈθaɪnəʊˌdaɪəʊl, -ɔl] *n pharm.* Etynodiol *nt.*
e·thy·nyl [ɪˈθaɪnl] *n* Äthinyl-, Ethinyl-(Radikal *nt*).
e·ti·do·caine [ɪˈtaɪdəʊkeɪn] *n pharm., anes.* Etidocain *nt.*
e·ti·dro·nate [ɪtaɪˈdrəʊnaɪt] *n pharm.* Etidronat *nt.*
e·ti·dron·ic acid [ɪtaɪˈdrɒnɪk] *pharm.* Etidronsäure *f.*
et·il·ef·rine [etɪlˈefriːn] *n pharm.* Etilefrin *nt.*
e·ti·o·cho·lan·o·lone [ˌɪtɪəʊkəʊˈlænəloʊn] *n biochem.* Ätiocholanolon *nt.*
etiocholanolone fever Ätiocholanolon-Fieber *nt.*
e·ti·o·gen·ic [ˌ-ˈdʒenɪk] *adj* (*Ursache*) auslösend, verursachend, kausal.
e·ti·o·log·ic [ˌ-ˈlɑdʒɪk] *adj* → etiological.
e·ti·o·log·i·cal [ˌ-ˈlɑdʒɪkl] *adj* Ätiologie betr., ätiologisch.
e·ti·ol·o·gy [ɪtɪˈɑlədʒɪ] *n* 1. Lehre *f* von den Krankheitsursachen, Ätiologie *f.* 2. (Gesamtheit der) Krankheitsursachen *pl*, Ätiologie *f.*
e·ti·o·pa·thol·o·gy [ˌɪtɪəʊpəˈθɑlədʒɪ] *n* Krankheitsentstehung *f*, -entwicklung *f*, Pathogenese *f.*
e·ti·o·por·phy·rin [ˌ-ˈpɔːrfərɪn] *n* Ätioporphyrin *nt.*
e·ti·o·trop·ic [ˌ-ˈtrɑpɪk, -ˈtrəʊp-] *adj* auf die (Kranheits-)Ursache gerichtet, ätiotrop, kausal, Kausal-.
e·to·fen·a·mate [ˌɪtəʊˈfenəmeɪt] *n pharm.* Etofenamat *nt.*
e·to·fi·brate [ˌ-ˈfaɪbreɪt] *n pharm.* Etofibrat *nt.*
e·tom·i·date [ɪˈtɑmɪdeɪt] *n pharm., anes.* Etomidat *nt.*
e·to·po·side [ˌɪtəʊˈpəʊsaɪd] *n pharm.* Etoposid *nt.*
et·o·zo·lin [ˌ-ˈzəʊlɪn] *n pharm.* Etozolin *nt.*
Eu *abbr.* → europium.
eu- *pref.* Normal-, Eu-.
Eu·bac·te·ri·a·les [juːbækˌtɪərɪˈeɪliːz] *pl micro.* Eubacteriales *pl.*
Eu·bac·te·ri·um [juːbækˈtɪərɪəm] *n micro.* Eubacterium *nt.*
eu·bac·te·ri·um [juːbækˈtɪərɪəm] *n, pl* -**ria** [-rɪə] 1. echtes Bakterium *nt*, Eubakterium *nt*, Eubacterium *nt.* 2. Bakterium *nt* der Ordnung Eubacteriales. 3. Bakterium *nt* der Ordnung Eubacterium.
eu·bi·ot·ics [juːbaɪˈɑtɪks] *pl* Eubiotik *f.*
eu·caine [ˈjuːkeɪn] *n pharm.* Eukain *nt*, Eucain *m.*
eu·ca·lyp·tol [juːkəˈlɪptɑl] *n pharm.* Cineol *nt*, Eukalyptol *nt.*
eu·ca·lyp·tus oil [juːkəˈlɪptəs] Eukalyptusöl *nt.*
eu·cap·nia [juːˈkæpnɪə] *n physiol.* normale Kohlendioxidspannung *f* des Blutes, Eukapnie *f.*
eu·car·y·on *n* 1. → eukaryon. 2. → eukaryote.
eu·car·y·o·sis *n* → eukaryosis.
eu·car·y·ote *n* → eukaryote.
eu·car·y·ot·ic *adj* → eukaryotic.
Eu·ces·to·da [juːseˈstəʊdə] *pl micro.* Bandwürmer *pl*, Zestoden *pl*, Cestoda *pl*, Cestodes *pl.*

eu·chlor·hy·dria [juːklɔːrˈhaɪdrɪə, -klɔːr-] *n physiol.* Euchlorhydrie *f.*
eu·cho·lia [juːˈkəʊlɪə] *n physiol.* Eucholie *f.*
eu·chro·mat·ic [ˌjukrəˈmætɪk] *adj* Euchromatin betr., aus Euchromatin bestehend, euchromatisch, achromatisch.
eu·chro·ma·tin [juːˈkrəʊmətɪn] *n* Achromatin *nt*, Euchromatin *nt.*
eu·chro·ma·top·sy [juːˈkrəʊmətɑpsɪ] *n physiol. ophthal.* normales Farbensehen *nt*, Euchromatop(s)ie *f.*
eu·chro·mo·some [juːˈkrəʊməsəʊm] *n genet.* Autosom *nt.*
eu·chy·lia [juːˈkaɪlɪə] *n physiol.* Euchylie *f.*
eu·chy·mia [juːˈkaɪmɪə] *n physiol.* Euchymie *f.*
eu·coe·lom [juːˈsiːləm] *n embryo.* Zölom *nt*, Zölomhöhle *f*, Coeloma *nt.*
eu·col·loid [juːˈkɑlɔɪd] *n* Eukolloid *nt.*
eu·cra·sia [juːˈkreɪʒɪə] *n physiol.* Eukrasie *f.*
eu·di·e·mor·rhy·sis [juːdaɪəˈmɑrəsɪs] *n* normaler Kapillarfluß *m*, normale Kapillarzirkulation *f.*
eu·di·om·e·ter [juːdɪˈɑmɪtər] *n* Gasmeßröhre *f*, Eudiometer *nt.*
eu·dip·sia [juːˈdɪpsɪə] *n physiol.* Eudipsie *f.*
eu·es·the·sia [juːesˈθiːʒ(ɪ)ə] *n physiol.* normale Funktion *f* der Sinne, Euästhesie *f.*
Eu·flag·el·la·ta [juːˌflædʒəˈleɪtə] *pl old* → Mastigophora.
eu·ga·my [ˈjuːgəmɪ] *n* Eugamie *f.*
eu·gen·ic [juːˈdʒenɪk] *adj* Eugenik betr., eugenisch.
eugenic acid → eugenol.
eu·gen·i·cist [juːˈdʒenəsɪst] *n* Eugeniker(in *f*) *m.*
eu·gen·ics [juːˈdʒenɪks] *pl* Erbhygiene *f*, Eugenik *f*, Eugenetik *f.*
eu·gen·ist [juːˈdʒenɪst] *n* → eugenicist.
eu·gen·ol [juːˈdʒenɑl, -nəʊl] *n pharm.* Eugeninsäure *f*, Eugenol *nt.*
eu·glob·u·lin [juːˈglɑbjəlɪn] *n* Euglobulin *nt.*
eu·gly·ce·mia [juːglaɪˈsiːmɪə] *n physiol.* normaler Blutzuckerspiegel *m*, Euglykämie *f.*
eu·gly·ce·mic [juːglaɪˈsiːmɪk] *adj* Euglykämie *f* betr., euglykämisch.
eu·gna·thia [juːˈneɪθɪə] *n dent.* Eugnathie *f.*
eu·gno·sia [juːˈnəʊʒ(ɪ)ə] *n neuro., physiol.* Eugnosie *f.*
eu·gnos·tic [juːˈnɑstɪk] *adj* Eugnosie betr., eugnostisch.
eu·go·na·do·trop·ic hypogonadism [juːgəʊˌnædəˈtrɑpɪk, -ˈtrəʊ-, -ˌgɑnədəʊ-] eugonadotroper Hypogonadismus *m.*
eu·gon·ic [juːˈgɑnɪk] *adj micro.* üppig wachsend, mit üppigem Wachstum, eugonisch.
eu·hy·dra·tion [juːhaɪˈdreɪʃn] *n physiol.* Euhydra(ta)tion *f.*
eu·kar·y·on [juːˈkærɪɑn] *n* 1. Eukaryon *nt.* 2. → eukaryote.
eu·kar·y·o·sis [juːkærɪˈəʊsɪs] *n* Eukaryose *f.*
eu·kar·y·ote [juːˈkærɪɒt, -əʊt] *n bio.* Eukaryont *m*, Eukaryot *m.*
eu·kar·y·ot·ic [juːˌkærɪˈɑtɪk] *adj* Eukaryon od. Eukaryo(n)t betr., eukaryot, eukaryont(isch).
eukaryotic cell eukaryontische Zelle *f.*
eukaryotic protist *micro.* höherer Protist *m*, Eukaryo(n)t *m.*
eu·ker·a·tin [juːˈkerətɪn] *n* Eukeratin *nt.*
eu·ki·ne·sia [juːkɪˈniːʒ(ɪ)ə, -kaɪ-] *n* normale Beweglichkeit *f*, Normalität *f* der Bewegungsabläufe, Eukinesie *f.*
eu·ki·ne·sis [juːkɪˈniːsɪs, -kaɪ-] *n* → eukinesia.
eu·ki·net·ic [juːkɪˈnetɪk] *adj* Eukinesie betr., mit normalem Bewegungsablauf, eukinetisch.

Eulenburg [ˈɔɪlənbɜrg; ˈɔʏlənbʊrg]: **E.'s disease** Eulenburg-Krankheit *f*, -Syndrom *nt*, Paramyotonia congenita.
Euler-Liljestrand [ˈɔɪlər ˈlɪljəstrænd]: **E.-L. mechanism** (von) Euler-Liljestrand-Mechanismus *m.*
E.-L. reflex (von) Euler-Liljestrand-Reflex *m.*
eu·mel·a·nin [juːˈmelənɪn] *n* Eumelanin *nt.*
eu·men·or·rhea [juːˌmenəˈrɪə] *n gyn.* normale/regelrechte Monatsblutung/Menstruationsblutung *f*, Eumenorrhoe *f.*
eu·me·tria [juːˈmiːtrɪə] *n neuro.* Eumetrie *f.*
eu·mor·phism [juːˈmɔːrfɪzəm] *n histol.* Eumorphismus *m.*
Eu·my·ce·tes [juːmaɪˈsiːtiːz] *pl micro.* echte Pilze *pl*, Eumyzeten *pl*, Eumycetes *pl*, Eumycophyta *pl.*
eu·my·ce·to·ma [juːˌmaɪsəˈtəʊmə] *n* Eumyzetom *nt.*
Eu·my·co·phy·ta [juːˌmaɪkəʊˈfaɪtə] *pl* → Eumycetes.
eu·my·cot·ic mycetoma [juːmaɪˈkɑtɪk] Eumyzetom *nt.*
eu·nuch [ˈjuːnək] *n* Eunuch *m*, Eunuche *m.*
eu·nuch·ism [ˈjuːnəkɪzəm] *n* Eunuchismus *m.*
eu·nuch·oid [ˈjuːnəkɔɪd] I *n* Eunuchoid *m.* II *adj* einem Eunuchen ähnlich, eunuchoid.
eunuchoid gigantism eunuchoider Riesenwuchs *m.*
eu·nuch·oid·ism [ˈjuːnəkɔɪdɪzəm] *n* Eunuchoidismus *m.*
eu·os·mia [juːˈɑzmɪə] *n* 1. *physiol.* normaler Geruchssinn *m*, Euosmie *f.* 2. angenehmer Geruch *m*, Wohlgeruch *m.*
EUP *abbr.* → extrauterine pregnancy.
eu·pan·cre·a·tism [juːˈpæŋkrɪətɪzəm] *n physiol.* normale Pankreasfunktion *f*, Eupankreatismus *m.*
eu·pep·sia [juːˈpepsɪə] *n physiol.* normale Verdauung *f*, Eupepsie *f.*
eu·pep·sy [ˈjuːpepsɪ] *n* → eupepsia.
eu·pep·tic [juːˈpeptɪk] *adj* Eupepsie betr. *od.* fördernd, eupeptisch.
eu·per·i·stal·sis [juːˌperɪˈstælsɪs] *n physiol.* normale Peristaltik *f*, Euperistaltik *f.*
eu·pho·ret·ic [juːfəˈretɪk] *n, adj* → euphoriant.
eu·pho·ria [juːˈfɔːrɪə, -ˈfəʊr-] *n* 1. Hochgefühl *nt*, -stimmung *f*, Glücksgefühl *nt*, Euphorie *f.* 2. *psychia.* krankhaft gehobene Stimmung *f*, motivlose Heiterkeit *f*, motivloses Glücksgefühl *nt*, Euphorie *f.*
eu·pho·ri·ant [juːˈfɔːrɪənt, -ˈfəʊ-] I *n* euphorieauslösende Substanz *f*, Euphorikum *nt.* II *adj* euphorieauslösend, in Euphorie versetzend, euphorisierend.
eu·phor·ic [juːˈfɔːrɪk, -ˈfɑr-] *adj* Euphorie betr., euphorisch.
eu·pho·ri·gen·ic [juːˌfɔːrɪˈdʒenɪk] *adj* euphorieauslösend.
eu·pho·ris·tic [juːfəˈrɪstɪk] *adj* euphorieauslösend, euphorisierend.
eu·pho·ry [ˈjuːfərɪ] *n* → euphoria.
eu·pla·sia [juːˈpleɪʒ(ɪ)ə, -zɪə] *n histol.* Euplasie *f.*
eu·plas·tic [juːˈplæstɪk] *adj histol., patho.* euplastisch.
eu·ploid [ˈjuːplɔɪd] I *n* euploider Organismus *m.* II *adj* euploid.
eu·ploi·dy [ˈjuːplɔɪdɪ] *n genet.* euploide Beschaffenheit *f*, Euploidie *f.*
eup·nea [juːpˈniːə, juːpˈnɪə] *n* normale/freie/ungestörte Atmung *f*, normale Ruheatmung *f*, Eupnoe *f.*
eup·ne·ic [juːpˈniːɪk] *adj* Eupnoe betr., von Eupnoe gekennzeichnet, eupnoisch.
eup·noe·a *n* → eupnea.
eu·prax·ia [juːˈpræksɪə, -ʃə] *n physiol., neuro.* Eupraxie *f.*

eu·pro·tein·e·mia [juːˌprəʊtɪˈniːmɪə] *n* Euproteinämie *f*.
eu·rhyth·mia [juːˈrɪðmɪə] *n* **1.** *physiol*. Eurhythmie *f*. **2.** *card*. regelmäßiger Puls/Herzschlag *m*, Eurhythmie *f*.
Eu·ro·pe·an [ˌjʊərəˈpiːən]: **E. blastomycosis** europäische Blastomykose *f*, Kryptokokkose *f*, Cryptococcose *f*, Cryptococcus-Mykose *f*, Torulose *f*, Busse-Buschke-Krankheit *f*.
E. hookworm (europäischer) Hakenwurm *m*, Grubenwurm *m*, Ancylostoma duodenale.
E. relapsing fever epidemisches (europäisches) Rückfallfieber *nt*, Läuserückfallfieber *nt*.
E. typhus epidemisches/klassisches Fleckfieber *nt*, Läusefleckfieber *nt*, Fleck-, Hunger-, Kriegstyphus *m*, Typhus exanthematicus.
eu·ro·pi·um [jʊəˈrəʊpɪəm, jə-] *n abbr*. **Eu** Europium *nt abbr*. Eu.
eury- *pref*. Weit-, Breit-, Eury-.
eu·ry·ce·phal·ic [ˌjʊərəsɪˈfælɪk] *adj* Brachyzephalie betr., von Brachyzephalie betroffen, kurz-, rundköpfig, brachyzephal, -zephal.
eu·ry·cra·ni·al [ˌ-ˈkreɪnɪəl] *adj* kurzköpfig.
eu·ryg·nath·ic [ˌ-(g)ˈnæθɪk] *adj* Eurygnathismus betr., eurygnath.
eu·ryg·na·thism [jʊəˈrɪgnəθɪzəm] *n* Eurygnathismus *m*.
eu·ry·o·pia [ˌjʊərɪˈəʊpɪə] *n ophthal*. Euryopie *f*.
eu·ry·so·mat·ic [ˌ-səʊˈmætɪk] *adj* (*Konstitution*) breitwüchsig, eurysom.
eu·ry·ther·mal [ˌ-ˈθɜːml] *adj micro*. eurytherm.
eu·ry·ther·mic [ˌ-ˈθɜːmɪk] *adj* → eurythermal.
eu·sit·ia [juːˈsɪtɪə] *n* normaler Appetit *m*.
eu·splanch·nia [juːˈsplæŋknɪə] *n* normale Funktion *f* der inneren Organe, Eusplanchnie *f*.
eu·sple·nia [juːˈspliːnɪə] *n* normale Milzfunktion *f*, Eusplenie *f*.
eu·sta·chi·an [juːˈsteɪʃɪən, -kɪən]: **e. canal** Ohrtrompete *f*, Eustach'-Tube *f*, -Röhre *f*, Tuba auditiva/auditoria.
e. canal, osseous (Semi-)Canalis musculotubarius.
e. cartilage Tuben-, Ohrtrompetenknorpel *m*, Cartilago tubae auditoriae.
e. catheter *HNO* Tubenkatheter *m*.
e. muscle M. tensor tympani.
e. salpingitis → eustachitis.
e. tonsil Tubenmandel *f*, Tonsilla tubaria.
e. tube → e. canal.
e. valve *embryo*. Eustachio'-Klappe *f*, Sylvius'-Klappe *f*, Heister'-Klappe *f*, Valvula Eustachii, Valvula v. cavae inferioris.
eu·sta·chi·tis [juːstəˈkaɪtɪs] *n* Entzündung *f* der Tuba auditiva/auditoria, Tubenentzündung *f*, Syringitis *f*.
eu·sta·chi·um [juːˈsteɪkɪəm] *n* → eustachian canal.
eus·then·ia [juːsˈθiːnɪə] *n physiol*. Eusthenie *f*.
eus·then·u·ria [juːsθəˈn(j)ʊərɪə] *n physiol*. Eusthenurie *f*.
Eu·stron·gy·lus gigas [juːˈstrɒndʒɪləs] *micro*. Nierenwurm *m*, Riesenpalisadenwurm *m*, Eustrongylus gigas, Dioctophyma renale.
eu·sys·to·le [juːˈsɪstəlɪ] *n card*. Eusystole *f*.
eu·sys·tol·ic [juːsɪsˈtɒlɪk] *adj* Eusystole betr., eusystolisch.
eu·tec·tic [juːˈtektɪk] **I** *n chem*. Eutektikum *nt*. **II** *adj* eutektisch.
eutectic point *chem*. eutektischer Punkt *m*.
eu·tha·na·sia [ˌjuːθəˈneɪz(ɪ)ə, -zɪə] *n* **1.** leichter/schmerzloser Tod *m*, Euthanasie *f*. **2.** Sterbehilfe *f*, Euthanasie *f*.

eu·ther·mic [juːˈθɜːmɪk] *adj* eutherm.
eu·thy·mia [juːˈθaɪmɪə] *n* Euthymie *f*.
eu·thy·roid [juːˈθaɪrɔɪd] *adj* mit normaler Schilddrüsenfunktion, euthyreot.
euthyroid goiter euthyreote Struma *f*.
eu·thy·roid·ism [juːˈθaɪrɔɪdɪzəm] *n endo*. normale Schilddrüsenfunktion *f*, Euthyreose *f*.
eu·thy·scope [ˈjuːθaɪskəʊp] *n ophthal*. Euthyskop *nt*.
eu·thys·co·py [juːˈθɪskəpɪ] *n ophthal*. Euthyskopie *f*.
eu·to·cia [juːˈtəʊsɪə] *n gyn*. normale Entbindung *f*, Eutokie *f*.
eu·to·nia [juːˈtəʊnɪə] *n physiol*. (*Muskel*) normaler Tonus *m*, Eutonie *f*, Normotonie *f*.
eu·ton·ic [juːˈtɒnɪk] *adj physiol*. euton, normoton.
eu·to·pia [juːˈtəʊpɪə] *n* (*Organ*) normale/regelrechte Lage *f*, Eutopie *f*.
eu·top·ic [juːˈtɒpɪk] *adj* an normaler Stelle liegend, eutop(isch).
eutopic pregnancy *gyn*. eutopische/intrauterine Schwangerschaft/Gravidität *f*.
eu·tro·phia [juːˈtrəʊfɪə] *n* → eutrophy.
eu·troph·ic [juːˈtrɒfɪk, -ˈtrəʊ-] *adj* nährstoffreich, eutroph.
eu·troph·i·ca·tion [juːˌtrɒfɪˈkeɪʃn] *n bio*. Eutrophierung *f*.
eu·tro·phy [ˈjuːtrəfɪ] *n physiol.*, *ped*. guter Ernährungszustand *m*; gute/ausreichende Ernährung *f*, Eutrophie *f*.
eV *abbr*. → electron volt.
ev *abbr*. → electron volt.
e·vac·u·ant [ɪˈvækjəwənt] **I** *n* **1.** entleerendes/abführendes Mittel *nt*. **2.** Abführmittel *nt*, Evacantium *nt*, Kathartikum *nt*. **3.** Brechmittel *nt*, Emetikum *nt*. **4.** harntreibendes Mittel *nt*, Diuretikum *nt*. **II** *adj* **5.** die Entleerung fördernd, evakuierend. **6.** den Stuhlgang fördernd, abführend.
e·vac·u·ate [ɪˈvækjʊweɪt] **I** *vt* **1.** aus-, entleeren. **2.** (*Flüssigkeit, Luft*) absaugen, abziehen, abpumpen, evakuieren. **3.** (*Blase*) entleeren; (*Darm*) abführen. **to ~ the bowls** abführen. **4.** *gyn*. eine (Vakuum-)Kürettage durchführen. **II** *vi* (*Darm*) entleeren, Stuhlgang haben; (*Blase*) entleeren, urinieren, Wasser lassen.
e·vac·u·a·tion [ɪˌvækjəˈweɪʃn] *n* **1.** Aus-, Entleerung *f*, Evakuation *f*. **2.** (*Darm*) Entleerung *f*, Abführen *nt*; Stuhlgang *m*; (*Blase*) Entleerung *f*, Miktion *f*. **3.** Stuhl *m*, Fäzes *pl*, Faeces *pl*. **4.** *gyn*. (Vakuum-)-Kürettage *f*, Gebärmutterräumung *f*, Evakuation *f*, Evacuatio uteri.
evacuation reflex Entleerungsreflex *m*.
bladder e. Blasenentleerungsreflex.
colonic e. Darmentleerungsreflex.
e·vag·i·nate [ɪˈvædʒɪneɪt] *vt* ausstülpen.
e·vag·i·na·tion [ɪˌvædʒɪˈneɪʃn] *n* Ausstülpung *f*, Evagination *f*.
e·val·u·ate [ɪˈvæljueɪt] *vt* **1.** abschätzen, bewerten, beurteilen, evaluieren. **2.** berechnen, bestimmen. **3.** auswerten.
e·val·u·a·tion [ɪˌvæljuˈeɪʃn] *n* **1.** Schätzung *f*, Festsetzung *f*. **2.** Bewertung *f*, Beurteilung *f*. **3.** Berechnung *f*, Bestimmung *f*. **4.** Auswertung *f*.
ev·a·nes·cent [ˌevəˈnesnt] *adj* **1.** s. auflösend, s. verflüchtigend. **2.** flüchtig, vergänglich, von kurzer Dauer; instabil.
Evans [ˈevənz]: **E. blue** *histol*. Evansblau *nt*.
E.'s syndrome *hema*. Evans-Syndrom *nt*, Evans-Fisher-Syndrom *nt*.
e·vap·o·ra·ble [ɪˈvæpərəbl] *adj* verdunstbar.
e·vap·o·rate [ɪˈvæpəreɪt] **I** *vt* evaporieren, verdampfen *od*. verdunsten (lassen), zur Verdampfung bringen; eindampfen. **II** *vi* evaporieren, verdampfen, verdunsten; s. verflüchtigen.
e·vap·o·rat·ed milk [ɪˈvæpəreɪtɪd] Kondensmilch *f*, evaporierte Milch *f*.
e·vap·o·ra·tion [ɪˌvæpəˈreɪʃn] *n* Evaporation *f*, Verdampfung *f*, Verdunstung *f*; Verdampfen *nt*; Eindampfen.
evaporation heat transfer coefficient *abbr*. h_e Wärmeübergangszahl *f* für Evaporation *abbr*. h_e.
e·vap·o·ra·tive [ɪˈvæpəreɪtɪv] *adj* Verdunstungs-, Verdampfungs-.
e·vap·o·ra·tor [ɪˈvæpəreɪtər] *n* Evaporator *m*, Verdampfer *m*.
e·vap·o·rim·e·ter [ɪˌvæpəˈrɪmɪtər] *n* Evapori-, Evaporometer *nt*, Verdunstungsmesser *m*.
e·vap·o·rom·e·ter [ɪˌvæpəˈrɒmɪtər] *n* → evaporimeter.
e·va·sion [ɪˈveɪʒn] *n* **1.** Ausrede *f*, Ausflucht *f*, ausweichende Antwort *f*. **2.** *psychia*. Evasion *f*.
e·va·sive [ɪˈveɪsɪv] *adj* **1.** (*Verhalten*) ausweichend. **2.** schwer feststellbar *od*. faßbar.
e·vent [ɪˈvent] *n* **1.** Fall *m*. **at all ~s** auf alle Fälle, jedenfalls. **in the ~ of death** im Todesfall. **2.** Ereignis *nt*, Vorkommnis *nt*.
e·ven·tra·tion [ˌɪvenˈtreɪʃn] *n* **1.** *patho*. (Bauch-)Eingeweidevorfall *m*, Eventratio *f*, Eventratio (viscerum) *f*. **2.** → evisceration 1., 2.
event-related potential *abbr*. **ERP** ereigniskorreliertes Potential *nt abbr*. EKP, event-related potential *abbr*. ERP.
e·ver·sion [ɪˈvɜːʒn, -ʃn] *n* Auswärtsdrehung *f*, -kehrung *f*, -wendung *f*; Ausstülpung *f*, Verlagerung *f* nach außen, Eversion *f*.
e·vert [ɪˈvɜːt] *vt* auswärtsdrehen, -wenden, -kehren, ausstülpen.
e·ver·tor (**muscle**) [ɪˈvɜːtər] *anat*. Auswärtsdreher *m*, -wender *m*.
E.v.G. *abbr*. → elastica-van-Gieson stain.
e·vide·ment [evidˈmɑ̃] *n chir*. Ausräumung *f*, Ausschabung *f*, Auskratzung *f*, Kürettage *f*, Exkochleation *f*.
ev·i·dence [ˈevɪdəns] **I** *n* **1.** Klarheit *f*, Offenkundigkeit *f*, Augenscheinlichkeit *f*; Beweis *m*, Beweismittel *nt*, -stück *nt*, -material *nt*. **to give ~** aussagen. **2.** (An-)Zeichen *nt*, Spur *f*. **II** *vt* be-, nachweisen, zeigen.
ev·i·dent [ˈevɪdənt] *adj* offensichtlich, offenkundig, klar, augenscheinlich, evident.
e·vil [ˈiːvəl] **I** *n* **1.** Unheil *nt*, Unglück *nt*, Übel *nt*. **2.** Krankheit *f*. **II** *adj* übel, böse, schlecht, schlimm.
ev·i·ra·tion [ˌɪvaɪˈreɪʃn, ˌevə-] *n* **1.** Entmannung *f*, Kastration *f*. **2.** *patho*. Verweiblichung *f*, Feminisierung *f*. **3.** *psychia*. Verweiblichung *f*, Effemination *f*.
e·vis·cer·a·tion [ɪˌvɪsəˈreɪʃn] *n* **1.** *patho*. Eingeweidevorfall *m*, Evisceration *f*. **2.** *chir*. Eingeweideentfernung *f*, Evisceration *f*, Exenteration *f*. **3.** *ophthal*. Ausweidung *f* des Augapfels, Evisceration *f*.
ev·o·ca·tion [ˌevəˈkeɪʃn, ˌiːvəʊ-] *n embryo*. Evokation *f*.
ev·o·ca·tor [ˈevəkeɪtər, ˈiːvə-] *n embryo*. Evokator *m*.
e·voked potential [ɪˈvəʊkd] *abbr*. **EP** evoziertes Potential *nt abbr*. EP.
auditory e. *abbr*. **AEP** akustisch evoziertes Potential *abbr*. AEP.
somatic e. *abbr*. **SEP** somatisch/somatosensorisch evoziertes Potential *abbr*. SEP.
visual e. *abbr*. **VEP** visuell evoziertes Potential *abbr*. VEP.

evoked response audiometry *HNO* Electric-Response-Audiometrie *f abbr.* ERA, Evoked-Response-Audiometrie *f.*
evoked response olfactometry *abbr.* ERO evoked response olfactometry *abbr.* ERO, objective Olfaktometrie *f.*
ev·o·lute ['evəluːt] **I** *vt* entwickeln (*into* zu). **II** *vi* s. entwickeln (*into* zu).
ev·o·lu·tion [,evə'luːʃn] *n* **1.** Entfaltung *f*, Entwicklung *f*. **2.** *bio.* Entwicklung *f*, Evolution *f*. **3.** *phys.* Entwicklung *f*; *techn.* Umdrehung *f*, Bewegung *f*. **4.** *gyn.* Entwicklung *f*, Evolution *f*, Evolutio *f*.
ev·o·lu·tion·al [,evə'luːʃənl] *adj* Entwicklung betr., Entwicklungs-.
ev·o·lu·tion·ar·y [,evə'luːʃəˌneriː] *adj* **1.** Entwicklung betr., Entwicklungs-. **2.** *bio.* Evolution betr., Evolutions-. **3.** *phys.*, *techn.* Entwicklungs-, Bewegungs-.
e·volve [ɪ'vɑlv] **I** *vt* **1.** entwickeln, entfalten. **2.** *phys.* verströmen. **II** *vi* **3.** s. entwickeln, s. entfalten (*into* zu). **4.** entstehen (*from* aus).
e·volve·ment [ɪ'vɑlvmənt] *n* Entwicklung *f*, Entfaltung *f*.
e·vul·sion [ɪ'vʌlʃn] *n ortho.* (gewaltsames) Herausreißen *nt*, Herausziehen *nt*.
Ewald ['juːəld; 'evalt]: **E.'s node** Klavikulardrüse *f*, Virchow'-Knötchen *nt*, -Knoten *m*, -Drüse *f*.
Ewart ['juːərt]: **E.'s sign** Ewart-Zeichen *nt*, Pins-Zeichen *nt*.
Ewing ['juːɪŋ]: **E.'s sarcoma/tumor** Ewing'-(Knochen-)Sarkom *nt*, endotheliales Myelom *nt*.
Ew·ing·el·la [juːɪŋ'elə] *n micro.* Ewingella *f.*
ex- *pref.* Aus-, Ent-, Ver-, Ex-.
ex·ac·er·bate [ɪg'zæsərbeɪt] *vt* (*Krankheit, Schmerzen*) verschlimmern, verschärfen, exazerbieren; wiederaufbrechen.
ex·ac·er·ba·tion [ɪgˌzæsər'beɪʃn] *n* (*Krankheit, Schmerzen*) Verschlimmerung *f*, Verschärfung *f*, Steigerung *f*, Exazerbation *f*, Exacerbatio *f*; Wiederaufbrechen *nt*.
ex·ag·ger·ate [ɪg'zædʒəreɪt] **I** *vt* **1.** übertreiben, übertrieben darstellen. **2.** überbetonen. **II** *vi* übertreiben.
ex·ag·ger·a·tion [ɪgˌzædʒə'reɪʃn] *n* **1.** Übertreibung *f*, Übersteigerung *f*, Exaggeratio *f*. **2.** Überbetonung *f.*
ex·air·e·sis *n* → exeresis.
ex·alt [ɪg'zɔːlt] *vt* s. überschwenglich begeistern, s. verzückt gebärden; s. hysterisch erregen, exaltieren.
ex·al·ta·tion [,egzɔːl'teɪʃn] *n psychia.* hysterische Aufregung *f*, übertriebene Begeisterung *f*, Überspanntheit *f*, Exaltation *f.*
ex·alt·ed [ɪg'zɔːltɪd] *adj psychia.* hysterisch aufgeregt, überschwenglich begeistert, überspannt, exaltiert.
ex·am·i·na·tion [ɪgˌzæmə'neɪʃn] *n* **1.** Untersuchung *f*. **2.** Untersuchung *f*, Prüfung *f* (*of, into sth.* einer Sache). **3.** Prüfung *f*, Examen *nt.*
ex·am·i·na·tion·al [ɪg'zæmə'neɪʃənl] *adj* Prüfung *od.* Untersuchung betr., Prüfungs-, Untersuchungs-.
ex·am·ine [ɪg'zæmɪn] **I** *vt* **1.** untersuchen. **2.** untersuchen, prüfen (*for* auf). **3.** (*wissenschaftlich*) untersuchen, erforschen. **II** *vi* **to ~ into sth.** etw. prüfen *od.* untersuchen.
ex·am·i·nee [ɪgˌzæmə'niː] *n* Prüfling *m*, Prüfungs-, Examenskandidat(in *f*) *m.*
ex·am·in·er [ɪg'zæmɪnər] *n* Prüfer(in *f*) *m.*
ex·am·in·ing hook [ɪg'zæmɪnɪŋ] *chir.* Tasthaken *m.*
ex·am·ple [ɪg'zæmpl] *n* **1.** Muster *nt*, Probe *f*. **2.** Beispiel *nt* (*of* für). **for ~** zum Beispiel. **beyond/without ~** beispiellos. **3.** Vorbild *nt*, Beispiel *nt* (*to* für).

ex·a·nia [eg'zæniə] *n* Mastdarmvorfall *m*, Rektumprolaps *m*, Exanie *f.*
ex·an·i·mate [eg'zænəmɪt, -meɪt] *adj* **1.** entseelt, leblos. **2.** bewußtlos, komatös.
ex·an·i·ma·tion [egˌzænə'meɪʃn] *n* **1.** Leblosigkeit *f*. **2.** Bewußtlosigkeit *f*, Koma *nt.*
ex·an·them [eg'zænθəm] *n* **1.** Hautausschlag *m*, Exanthem *nt*, Exanthema *nt*. **2.** Erkrankung *f* mit Exanthem als Hauptsymptom, Exanthem *nt*, Exanthema.
ex·an·the·ma [,egzæn'θiːmə] *n*, *pl* **-mas, -the·ma·ta** [-'θemətə] → exanthem.
exanthema subitum Dreitagefieber *nt*, -exanthem *nt*, sechste Krankheit *f*, Exanthema subitum, Roseola infantum.
ex·an·them·a·tous [,egzæn'θemətəs] *adj* Exanthem betr., durch ein Exanthem gekennzeichnet, exanthemartig, exanthematisch, exanthematös.
exanthematous fever mit Exanthem einhergehendes Fieber *nt*, Febris exanthematica.
exanthematous typhus epidemisches/klassisches Fleckfieber *nt*, Läuseflieckfieber *nt*, Fleck-, Hunger-, Kriegstyphus *m*, Typhus exanthematicum.
e. of Sao Paulo Felsengebirgsfleckfieber *nt*, amerikanisches Zeckenbißfieber *nt*, Rocky Mountain spotted fever (*nt*) *abbr.* RMSF.
ex·an·thrope ['ekzænθrəʊp] *n* äußere/externe Krankheitsursache/Infektionsquelle *f.*
ex·an·throp·ic [,egzæn'θrɑpɪk] *adj* (*Krankheit, Infektion*) von außen kommend, nicht im Körper entstanden; exogen.
ex·ar·te·ri·tis [eksˌɑːrtə'raɪtɪs] *n* Periarteriitis *f.*
ex·ar·tic·u·la·tion [eksɑːrˌtɪkjə'leɪʃn] *n ortho.* Amputation *f od.* Absetzen *nt* einer Gliedmaße im Gelenk, Exartikulation *f.*
ex·ca·vate ['ekskəveɪt] *vt* aushöhlen, ausbuchten; *chir., dent.* exkavieren.
ex·ca·va·tio [,ekskə'veɪʃɪəʊ] *n* → excavation.
ex·ca·va·tion [,ekskə'veɪʃn] *n* **1.** Aushöhlung *f*, Ausbuchtung *f*, Höhle *f*, Vertiefung *f*; *anat.* Exkavation *f*, Excavatio *f*. **2.** Aushöhlen *nt*. **3.** *dent.* Exkavation *f.*
ex·ca·va·tor ['ekskəveɪtər] *n chir., dent.* Exkavator *m.*
ex·cen·tric [ɪk'sentrɪk] *n, adj* → eccentric.
ex·cer·e·bra·tion [,eksərə'breɪʃn] *n gyn., patho.* Gehirnentfernung *f*, Exzerebration *f.*
ex·cer·nent [ek'sɜːrnənt] *adj* Entleerung *od.* Ausfluß verursachend *od.* fördernd.
ex·cess [n ɪk'ses; *adj* 'ekses] **I** *n* **1.** Übermaß *nt*, -fluß *m* (*of* an). **2.** Überschuß *m*. **3.** Exzeß *m*. **II** *adj* überschüssig, Über-.
e. in birth rate Geburtenüberschuß.
ex·ces·sive length [ɪk'sesɪv] Überlänge *f.*
ex·change [ɪks'tʃeɪndʒ] **I** *n* (Aus-)Tausch *m*, Auswechs(e)lung *f*. **in ~** anstatt, als Ersatz. **II** *vt* (aus-)tauschen, (aus-)wechseln (*for* gegen).
exchange area Austauschfläche *f.*
exchange diffusion Austauschdiffusion *f.*
exchange process Austauschvorgang *m.*
ex·chang·er [ɪks'tʃeɪndʒər] *n phys., chem.* Austauscher *m.*
exchange reaction Austauschreaktion *f.*
exchange surface Austauschfläche *f.*
exchange transfusion (Blut-)Austauschtransfusion *f*, Blutaustausch *m.*
exchange transport Austausch-, Gegen-, Countertransport *m*, Antiport *m.*
ex·cip·i·ent [ɪk'sɪpɪənt] *n pharm.* Träger-(substanz *f*) *m*, Vehikel *nt.*
ex·cise [ɪk'saɪz] *vt chir.* (her-)ausschneiden, entfernen, exzidieren (*from* aus).
ex·ci·sion [ek'sɪʒn, ɪk-] *n chir.* **1.** (Her-)

Ausschneiden *nt*, Exzidieren *nt*. **2.** (Her-)Ausschneidung *f*, Entfernung *f*, Exzision *f* (*from* aus).
e. of the radial heat *ortho.* Radiusköpfchenresektion *f.*
ex·ci·sion·al [ek'sɪʒnl] *adj* Exzision *od.* Exzidieren betr., Exzisions-.
excisional biopsy Exzisionsbiopsie *f*, Probeexzision *f abbr.* PE.
excision repair *biochem.* Exzisionsreparatur *f.*
ex·cit·a·bil·i·ty [ɪkˌsaɪtə'bɪlətɪ] *n* **1.** *physiol.* Erregbarkeit *f*, Reizbarkeit *f*, Exzitabilität *f*. **2.** Nervosität *f*; Reiz-, Erregbarkeit *f.*
ex·cit·a·ble [ɪk'saɪtəbl] *adj* **1.** erregbar, reizbar, exzitabel. **2.** anregbar; nervös, reizbar, erregbar.
excitable area motorischer Kortex/Cortex *m*, motorische Rinde(nregion *f*) *f*, Motokortex *m*, -cortex *m.*
excitable cell *physiol.* erregbare Zelle *f.*
ex·cit·a·ble·ness [ɪk'saɪtəblnɪs] *n* → excitability.
ex·cit·ant [ɪk'saɪtnt, 'eksɪtənt] **I** *n pharm.* Reizmittel *nt*, Stimulans *nt*, Exzitans *nt*, Exzitantium *nt*, Analeptikum *nt*. **II** *adj* er-, anregend, belebend, stimulierend.
excitant drug → excitant I.
ex·ci·ta·tion [,eksaɪ'teɪʃn, -sɪ-] *n* **1.** *physiol.* Anregung *f*, Reizung *f*; Reiz *m*, Exzitation *f*. **2.** *psycho.* Erregung *f*, Exzitation *f*. **3.** *chem., electr.* An-, Erregung *f.*
excitation-contraction coupling *physiol.* Erregung-Kontraktionskopplung *f*, Kopplung *f* von Erregung und Kontraktion, elektromechanische Kopplung *f.*
excitation-contraction uncoupling *physiol.* elektromechanische Entkopplung *f.*
excitation energy *phys.* Anregung(senergie *f*) *f.*
excitation impulse Erregungsimpuls *m.*
excitation pattern Erregungsmuster *nt.*
excitation phase Erregungsphase *f.*
excitation voltage *electr.* Erregerspannung *f.*
excitation wave Erregungswelle *f.*
ex·ci·ta·tive [ɪk'saɪtətɪv] *adj* → excitatory.
excitative phase/stage *anes.* (*Narkose*) Exzitationsstadium *nt.*
ex·ci·ta·to·ry [ɪk'saɪtətɔːriː, -təʊ-] *adj* anod. erregend (wirkend), exzitativ, exzitatorisch.
excitatory nerve-terminal potential *abbr.* ENTP erregendes Nervenendpotential *nt*, excitatory nerve-terminal potential *abbr.* ENTP.
excitatory postsynaptic current *abbr.* EPSC erregender postsynaptischer Strom *m*, excitatory postsynaptic current *abbr.* EPSC.
excitatory postsynaptic potential *abbr.* EPSP erregendes postsynaptisches Potential *nt abbr.* EPSP, excitatory postsynaptic potential *abbr.* EPSP.
excitatory receptive field *abbr.* ERF exzitatorisches rezeptives Feld *nt abbr.* ERF.
excitatory synapse erregende/exzitatorische Synapse *f.*
excitatory transmitter erregender/exzitatorischer Transmitter *m.*
ex·cite [ɪk'saɪt] *vt* **1.** auf-, erregen. **to ~ o.s.** s. aufregen (*over* über). **2.** (*Nerv*) reizen, anregen; (*Appetit*) anregen; (*sexuell*) erregen. **3.** *phys.* erregen, anregen.
ex·cit·ed [ɪk'saɪtɪd] *adj* aufgeregt, (*a. sexuell*) erregt; *phys.* angeregt.
excited atom *phys.* angeregtes Atom *nt.*
excited state *phys.* angeregter Zustand *m.*
ex·cite·ment [ɪk'saɪtmənt] *n* **1.** Er-, Aufregung *f* (*over* über). **2.** *physiol.* Reizung *f*; (sexuelle) Erregung *f.*

ex·cit·ing [ɪk'saɪtɪŋ] adj anregend; erregend; aufregend.
exciting electrode aktive/differente Elektrode f.
ex·ci·to·an·a·bol·ic [ɪk͵saɪtəænə'bɑlɪk] adj den Aufbaustoffwechsel/Anabolismus anregend od. fördernd.
ex·ci·to·cat·a·bol·ic [͵-kætə'bɑlɪk] adj den Abbaustoffwechsel/Katabolismus fördernd od. anregend.
ex·ci·to·glan·du·lar [͵-'glændʒələr] adj die Drüsensekretion anregend od. fördernd.
ex·ci·to·met·a·bol·ic [͵-metə'bɑlɪk] adj den Stoffwechsel/Metabolismus fördernd od. anregend.
ex·ci·to·mo·tor [͵ᴵ-'moʊtər] adj die Bewegung od. Motorik anregend, exzitomotorisch.
excitomotor area motorischer Kortex/Cortex m, motorische Rinde(nregion f) f, Motokortex m, -cortex m.
ex·ci·to·mo·tor·y [͵-'moʊtərɪ] adj → excitomotor.
ex·ci·to·mus·cu·lar [͵-'mʌskjələr] adj die Muskelaktivität stimulierend od. anregend.
ex·ci·ton [ɪk'saɪtan, 'eksɪtan] n phys. Exziton nt, Exciton nt.
ex·ci·tor [ɪk'saɪtər, -tɔːr] n 1. pharm. anregendes (Heil-)Mittel nt, Stimulans nt. 2. motorischer/efferenter Nerv nt.
ex·ci·to·se·cre·to·ry [ɪk͵saɪtəsɪ'kriːtərɪ] adj die Sekretion anregend od. fördernd.
ex·ci·to·vas·cu·lar [͵-'væskjəlɑr] adj die Vasomotorik anregend.
ex·cla·ma·tion point hair [͵ekskləʹmeɪʃn] Ausrufungszeichenhaar nt.
ex·clave ['eksklɛɪv] n anat. vom Hauptorgan getrennt liegendes Organ(teil), ektop(isch)es/akzessorisches Organ(teil nt) nt.
ex·clude [ɪk'skluːd] vt ausschließen (from von).
ex·clud·ed volume [ɪk'skluːdɪd] phys. Ausschlußvolumen nt.
ex·clu·sion [ɪk'skluːʒn] n Ausschluß m, Ausschließung f (from von); Exklusion f. **to the ~ of** unter Ausschluß von.
exclusion chromatography Ausschlußchromatographie f, Gelfiltration f.
exclusion principle 1. mathe. Prinzip nt der Ausschließung. **2.** phys. Äquivalenzprinzip nt.
ex·coch·le·a·tion [eks͵kɑklɪ'eɪʃn] n chir. Auslöffeln nt, Auskratzen nt, Exkochleation f, Excochleatio f.
ex·con·ju·gant [eks'kɑndʒəgənt] n bio. Exkonjugant m.
ex·co·ri·ate [ɪk'skɔːrɪeɪt, -'skoʊr-] vt 1. (Haut) ritzen, abschürfen, wund reiben. 2. die Haut abziehen von.
ex·co·ri·at·ed acne [ɪk'skɔːrɪeɪtɪd, -'skoʊr-] derm. Akne/Acne excoriée des jeunes filles.
ex·co·ri·a·tion [ɪk͵skɔːrɪ'eɪʃn, -͵skoʊr-] n (Haut-)Abschürfung f, Exkoriation f, Excoriatio f.
ex·cre·ment ['ekskrəmənt] n 1. Ausscheidung f, Exkrement nt, Excrementum nt. 2. Stuhl m, Kot m, Exkremente pl, Fäzes pl, Faeces pl.
ex·cre·men·tal [ekskrə'mentl] adj → excrementitious.
ex·cre·men·ti·tious [͵ekskrəmən'tɪʃəs] adj Exkrement od. Fäzes betr., fäkal, kotig, Kot-, Fäkal-.
ex·cres·cence [ɪk'skresəns] n patho. Auswuchs m, Exkreszenz f, Excrescentia f.
ex·cre·ta [ɪk'skriːtə] pl Ausscheidungen pl, Exkrete pl Excreta pl.
ex·crete [ɪk'skriːt] vt ausscheiden; absondern; sezernieren.

ex·cre·tion [ɪk'skriːʃn] n 1. Ausscheidung f, Absonderung f, Exkretion f; Ausscheiden nt. 2. Ausscheidung f, Exkret nt, Excretum nt.
excretion pyelography Ausscheidungspyelographie f, intravenöse Pyelographie f.
excretion test Ausscheidungs-, Exkretionstest m.
excretion urography urol., radiol. Ausscheidungsurographie f.
ex·cre·to·ry ['ekskrə͵tɔːrɪ, -͵toʊ-, ek'skriːtərɪ] adj Exkretion betr., exkretorisch, sezernierend, ausscheidend, absondernd, Exkretions-, Ausscheidungs-.
excretory duct histol. Ausführungsgang m.
e. of gallbladder Gallenblasengang, Zystikus m, Cysticus m, Ductus cysticus.
primitive e. embryo. primitiver Ausführungsgang.
e. of seminal vesicle Ausführungsgang des Samenbläschens, Ductus excretorius (glandulae/vesiculae seminalis).
e. of testis Samenleiter m, Ductus/Vas deferens.
excretory ductules of lacrimal gland Ausführungsgänge pl der Tränendrüse, Ductuli excretorii (gl. lacrimalis).
excretory gland exkretorische Drüse f.
excretory organ exkretorisches Organ nt, Ausscheidungsorgan nt.
excretory product Exkretionsprodukt nt.
excretory urography → excretion urography.
ex·cru·ci·at·ing [ɪk'skruːʃɪ͵eɪtɪŋ] adj (Schmerz) unerträglich, qualvoll, peinigend (to für).
excruciating pain unerträglich starker Schmerz m, Schmerz m mit Vernichtungsgefühl.
ex·cur·rent [ɪk'skʌrənt] adj 1. → excretory. 2. zentrifugal, efferent; weg-, herausführend, heraus-, ableitend.
ex·cur·sion [ɪk'skɜrʒn, -ʃn] n 1. physiol. (Bewegungs-)Ausschlag m (aus einer Mittelstellung), Exkursion f. 2. phys. Ausschlag m, Exkursion f. 3. (wissenschaftliche) Exkursion f.
ex·cur·sive movements [ɪk'skɜrsɪv] → excursion 1.
ex·cy·clo·pho·ria [͵eksaɪkloʊ'fɔːrɪə] n ophthal. Exzyklophorie f.
ex·cy·clo·tro·pia [͵-'troʊpɪə] n ophthal. Exzyklotropie f.
ex·cys·ta·tion [͵eksɪs'teɪʃn] n micro. Exzystierung f.
ex·e·cute ['eksɪkjuːt] vt (Aufgabe) aus-, durchführen; erfüllen, wahrnehmen.
ex·e·cu·tion [͵eksɪ'kjuːʃn] n Aus-, Durchführung f; Erfüllung f, Wahrnehmung f. **to put sth. into ~** etw. ausführen.
execution phase Ausführungsphase f.
ex·e·mia [ek'siːmɪə] n akute Hämokonzentration f.
ex·en·ce·pha·lia [͵eksənsɪ'feɪljə] n → exencephaly.
ex·en·ceph·a·lon [͵ᴵ-'sefəlɑn] n → exencephaly.
ex·en·ceph·a·lous [͵-'sefələs] adj embryo. Exenzephalie betr., exenzephal, exenkephal.
ex·en·ceph·a·lus [͵-'sefələs] n embryo. Exenzephalus m, Exenkephalus m.
ex·en·ceph·a·ly [͵-'sefəlɪ] n embryo. Exenzephalie f, Exenkephalie f.
ex·en·ter·a·tion [ek͵sentəʹreɪʃn] n chir. Ausweidung f, Eingeweide-, Organentfernung f, Exenteration f, Exenteratio f.
ex·en·ter·i·tis [ek͵sentəʹraɪtɪs] n Entzündung/Peritonitis f des Peritoneum viscerale.

ex·er·cise ['eksərsaɪz] I n (körperliche od. geistige) Übung f, (körperliche) Bewegung f. II vt (Körper, Geist) üben, trainieren; (Körper) bewegen. III vi üben, trainieren.
exercise tests card. Belastungstests pl.
exercise therapy Bewegungstherapie f.
ex·er·e·sis [eks'erəsɪs] n, pl **-ses** [-siːz] chir. 1. (Teil-)Entfernung f, Resektion f, Exhärese f, Exhairese f. 2. Herausziehen nt, Exhärese f, Exhairese f.
ex·er·gon·ic [͵eksər'gɑnɪk] adj chem. energiefreisetzend, exergonisch.
exergonic reaction chem. exergonische Reaktion f.
ex·er·tion [ɪg'zɜrʃn] n Anstrengung f, Belastung f; Strapaze f.
ex·er·tion·al dyspnea [ɪg'zɜrʃnl] Belastungsdyspnoe f.
ex·fe·ta·tion [eksfɪ'teɪʃn] n gyn. ektopische od. extrauterine Schwangerschaft/Gravidität f.
ex·fo·li·ate [eks'foʊlɪeɪt] I vt (Haut) abschälen, ablegen. II vi abblättern, s. schälen.
ex·fo·li·a·tio [eks͵foʊlɪ'eɪʃɪoʊ] n → exfoliation.
ex·fo·li·a·tion [eks͵foʊlɪ'eɪʃn] n derm., patho. Abblättern nt, Abschälen nt; Abblätterung f, Abschälung f, Abstoßung f, Exfoliation f, Exfoliatio f.
ex·fo·li·a·tive [eks'foʊlɪətɪv] adj s. schuppend, abblätternd, exfoliativ, Exfoliativ-.
exfoliative cytodiagnosis/cytology Exfoliativzytologie f, exfoliative Zytodiagnostik f.
exfoliative dermatitis Wilson-Krankheit f, Dermatitis exfoliativa, Pityriasis rubra Hebra(-Jadassohn).
exfoliative gastritis erosive Gastritis f, Gastritis erosiva.
exfoliative psoriasis → erythrodermic psoriasis.
exfoliative toxin Exfoliativtoxin nt.
ex·ha·la·tion [͵eks(h)ə'leɪʃn] n 1. Ausatmen nt; Ausatmung f, Exhalation f. 2. Verströmen nt; Ausdünsten nt, Ausdünstung f, Geruch m.
ex·hale [eks'heɪl, ek'seɪl] I vt 1. ausatmen, exhalieren. 2. verströmen, ausdünsten, exhalieren. II vi 3. ausatmen, exhalieren. 4. ausströmen (from aus).
ex·haust [ɪg'zɔːst] I vt 1. erschöpfen, auf-, verbrauchen; jdn. erschöpfen, ermüden, entkräften. 2. (ent-)leeren, (her-)auspumpen; absaugen. II vi s. entleeren; (Dampf) entweichen, ausströmen.
ex·haust·ed [ɪg'zɔːstɪd] adj 1. (körperlich, geistig) erschöpft, entkräftet, ermüdet, ermattet. 2. verbraucht, erschöpft, aufgebraucht.
ex·haust·ing [ɪg'zɔːstɪŋ] adj anstrengend, strapaziös, ermüdend, erschöpfend.
ex·haus·tion [ɪg'zɔːstʃn] n 1. (extreme) Ermüdung f, Entkräftung f, Erschöpfung(szustand m) f, Exhaustio f. 2. (Ent-)Leerung f, (Her-)Auspumpen nt; Absaugung f. 3. (Gas) Herausströmen nt.
exhaustion atrophy Erschöpfungsatrophie f.
exhaustion psychosis Erschöpfungspsychose f.
ex·haus·tive [ɪg'zɔːstɪv] adj 1. erschöpfend, vollständig, exhaustiv. 2. old → exhausting.
exhaustive methylation chem. erschöpfende Methylierung f.
ex·hi·bi·tion [͵eksə'bɪʃn] n pharm. Medikamentenverabreichung f, -gabe f.
ex·hi·bi·tion·ism [͵eksə'bɪʃənɪzəm] n psychia. Exhibitionismus m.

exhibitionist

ex·hi·bi·tion·ist [ˌeksə'bɪʃənɪst] *n psychia.* Exhibitionist(in *f*) *m*.
ex·hil·a·rant [ɪg'zɪlərənt] *adj* (den Geist) belebend, erfrischend, aufheiternd.
ex·hu·ma·tion [ˌekshju:'meɪʃn] *n forens.* Exhumierung *f*, Exhumieren *nt*.
ex·hume [ɪg'z(j)u:m, eks'hju:m] *vt forens.* exhumieren.
ex·is·ten·tial psychiatry [egzɪ'stenʃl] existentielle Psychotherapie *f*.
ex·it dose ['egzɪt, 'eksɪt] *radiol.* Exit-, Austrittsdosis *f*.
ex·i·tus ['eksɪtəs] *n, pl* **exitus** 1. Tod *m*, Exitus (letalis) *m*. 2. Ausgang *m*.
exo- *pref.* Außen-, Ex(o)-, Ekto-.
exo-amylase *n* β-Amylase *f*, Exoamylase *f*.
ex·o·an·ti·gen [ˌeksəʊ'æntɪdʒən] *n* → ectoantigen.
ex·o·bi·ol·o·gy [ˌ-baɪ'ɑlədʒɪ] *n* Exo-, Ektobiologie *f*, extraterrestrische Biologie *f*.
ex·o·car·dia [ˌ-'kɑ:rdɪə] *n* → ectocardia.
ex·o·car·di·al [ˌ-'kɑ:rdɪəl] *adj* → extracardial.
ex·o·cat·a·pho·ria [ˌ-kætə'fɔ:rɪə] *n ophthal.* Exokataphorie *f*.
ex·o·cele ['-si:l] *n* → exocoelom.
ex·o·cel·lu·lar [ˌ-'seljələr] *adj* exozellulär.
ex·o·cer·vi·cal carcinoma [ˌ-'sɜrvɪkəl] *gyn.* Portiokarzinom *nt*.
ex·o·cer·vix [ˌ-'sɜrvɪks] *n gyn.* Ektozervix *f*, Portio vaginalis cervicis.
ex·o·coel ['-si:l] *n* → exocoelom.
ex·o·coele ['-si:l] *n* → exocoelom.
ex·o·coe·lom [ˌ-'si:ləm] *n* extraembryonales Zölom *nt*, Chorionhöhle *f*, Exozölom *nt*.
ex·o·coe·lo·ma [ˌ-sɪ'ləʊmə] *n* → exocoelom.
ex·o·coe·lom·ic cavity [ˌ-sɪ'lɑmɪk, -'ləʊm-] primärer Dottersack *m*.
exocoelomic cyst Exozölomzyste *f*.
exocoelomic membrane *embryo.* Heuser'-Membran *f*.
ex·o·crine ['eksəkrɪn, -kraɪn] **I** *n* 1. → exocrine gland. 2. exokrin sezernierte Substanz *f*. **II** *adj* nach außen absondernd *od.* ausscheidend, exokrin.
exocrine gland Drüse *f* mit äußerer Sekretion, exokrine Drüse *f*.
exocrine part of pancreas exokrines Pankreas(teil *m*), Pars exocrina pancreatica.
ex·o·cy·clic [ˌeksəʊ'saɪklɪk, -'sɪk-] *adj chem.* exozyklisch.
ex·o·cy·to·sis [ˌ-saɪ'təʊsɪs] *n* Exozytose *f*.
ex·o·cy·tot·ic [ˌ-saɪ'tɑtɪk] *adj* Exozytose betr., mittels Exozytose, exozytotisch, Exozytosen-.
ex·o·de·oxy·ri·bo·nu·cle·ase [ˌ-dɪˌɑksɪˌraɪbəʊ'n(j)u:klɪeɪz] *n* Exodesoxyribonuklease *f*.
ex·o·de·vi·a·tion [ˌ-dɪvɪ'eɪʃn] *n* 1. → exophoria. 2. → exotropia.
ex·o·en·zyme [ˌ-'enzaɪm] *n* 1. Exoenzym *nt*. 2. extrazelluläres Enzym *nt*, Ektoenzym *nt*.
ex·o·ep·i·the·li·al gland [ˌ-epɪ'θɪlɪəl] exoepitheliale Drüse *f*.
ex·o·er·gic [ˌ-'ɜrdʒɪk] *adj chem.* Energie freisetzend, exoerg(isch).
ex·o·e·ryth·ro·cyt·ic [ˌ-ɪˌrɪθrə'sɪtɪk] *adj micro.* exoerythrozytär.
exoerythrocytic cycle/phase *micro.* exoerythrozytärer Zyklus *m*, exoerythrozytäre Phase *f*.
ex·og·a·my [ek'sɑgəmɪ] *n bio.* Exogamie *f*.
ex·o·gas·tru·la [ˌeksəʊ'gæstrʊlə] *n embryo.* Exogastrula *f*.
ex·o·gas·tru·la·tion [ˌ-gæstrʊ'leɪʃn] *n embryo.* Exogastrulation *f*.
ex·o·ge·net·ic [ˌ-dʒə'netɪk] *adj* → exogenous.

ex·o·gen·ic [ˌ-'dʒenɪk] *adj* → exogenous.
ex·og·e·nous [ek'sɑdʒənəs] *adj* 1. von außen zugeführt *od.* stammend *od.* wirkend, durch äußere Ursachen entstehend, exogen. 2. an der Außenfläche ablaufend, exogen.
exogenous cycle *micro.* exogener Zyklus *m*.
exogenous disease exogene Krankheit *f*, Exopathie *f*.
exogenous infection exogene Infektion *f*.
exogenous pigment exogenes Pigment *nt*, Exopigment *nt*.
exogenous pyrogen exogenes Pyrogen *nt*.
exogenous reinfection exogene Reinfektion *f*, exogener Reinfekt *m*.
exogenous retrovirus *micro.* exogenes Retrovirus *n*.
exogenous syndactyly *embryo.* exogene Syndaktylie *f*.
ex·og·na·thia [ˌeksəg'næθɪə, -'neɪ-] *n* Prognathie *f*, Progenie *f*.
ex·om·pha·los [eks'ɑmfələs, -ləs] *n* 1. Nabelbruch *m*, Exomphalos *m*, Exomphalozele *f*, Hernia umbilicalis. 2. Nabelschnurbruch *m*, Exomphalos *m*, Exomphalozele *f*, Hernia funiculi umbilicalis.
exomphalos-macroglossia-gigantism syndrome Exomphalos-Makroglossie--Gigantismus-Syndrom *nt*, EMG-Syndrom *nt*, Beckwith-Wiedemann-Syndrom *nt*.
ex·o·mys·i·um [ˌeksəʊ'mɪsɪəm] *n* Muskelhüllgewebe *nt*, Perimysium *nt*.
ex·on ['eksən] *n genet.* Exon *nt*.
ex·o·nu·cle·ase [ˌeksəʊ'n(j)u:klɪeɪz] *n* Exonuklease *f*, -nuclease *f*.
ex·op·a·thy [eks'ɑpəθɪ] *n* durch äußere Ursachen hervorgerufene Krankheit *f*, exogene Krankheit *f*, Exopathie *f*.
ex·o·pep·ti·dase [ˌeksəʊ'peptɪdeɪz] *n* Exopeptidase *f*.
ex·o·pho·ria [ˌ-'fəʊrɪə] *n ophthal.* Exophorie *f*.
ex·o·phor·ic [ˌ-'fɔ:rɪk] *adj* Exophorie betr., von ihr gekennzeichnet, Exophorie-.
ex·oph·thal·mic [eksəf'θælmɪk] *adj* Exophthalmus betr., durch Exophthalmus gekennzeichnet, exophthalmisch, Exophthalmus-, Exophthalmo-.
exophthalmic goiter Basedow'-Krankheit *f*, Morbus Basedow *m*.
exophthalmic ophthalmoplegia exophthalmische Ophthalmoplegie *f*.
ex·oph·thal·mo·gen·ic [eksəfˌθælməʊ'dʒenɪk] *adj* Exophthalmus verursachend *od.* auslösend, exophthalmogen.
ex·oph·thal·mom·e·ter [eksəfˌθæl'mɑmɪtər] *n* Exophthalmometer *nt*.
ex·oph·thal·mom·e·try [ˌ-'mɑmətrɪ] *n* Exophthalmusmessung *f*, -bestimmung *f*, Exophthalmometrie *f*.
ex·oph·thal·mos [ˌeksəf'θælməs] *n* old Glotzauge *nt*, Exophthalmos *m*, Exophthalmus *m*, Exophthalmie *f*, Ophthalmoptose *f*, Protrusio/Protopsis bulbi.
exophthalmos-producing substance *abbr.* EPS Exophthalmus-produzierender Faktor *m abbr.* EPF, Exophthalmus--produzierende Substanz *abbr.* EPS.
ex·oph·thal·mus [ˌeksəf'θælməs] *n* → exophthalmos.
ex·o·phyt·ic [ˌeksəʊ'fɪtɪk] *adj patho.* nach außen wachsend, exophytisch.
exophytic carcinoma exophytisch-wachsendes/exophytisches Karzinom *nt*.
exophytic tumor exophytisch-wachsender/exophytischer Tumor *m*.
ex·o·plasm ['-plæzəm] *n* Ekto-, Exoplasma *nt*.
ex·or·bi·tism [ek'sɔ:rbətɪzəm] *n* → exophthalmos.

ex·o·ri·bo·nu·cle·ase [ˌeksəʊraɪbəʊ'n(j)u:klɪeɪz] *n* Exoribonuklease *f*, -nuclease *f*.
ex·o·sep·sis [ˌeksəʊ'sepsɪs] *n patho.* exogene Sepsis *f*, Exosepsis *f*.
ex·o·se·ro·sis [ˌ-sɪ'rəʊsɪs] *n patho., derm.* Exsudation *f* auf die äußere Körperoberfläche.
ex·o·skel·e·ton [ˌ-'skelɪtn] *n bio.* Außen-, Ekto-, Exoskelett *nt*.
ex·os·mose ['eksazməʊs] *vt* von innen nach außen diffundieren.
ex·os·mo·sis [ˌeksaz'məʊsɪs] *n* Exosmose *f*.
ex·o·spore [ˌeksəʊ'spɔər, -'spɔ:r] *n micro.* Ekto-, Exospore *f*.
ex·o·spo·ri·um [ˌ-'spəʊrɪəm, -'spɔ:r-] *n micro.* Exospor *nt*, Exosporium *nt*.
ex·os·tec·to·my [eksas'tektəmɪ] *n* → exostosectomy.
ex·os·to·sec·to·my [ekˌsastəʊ'sektəmɪ] *n ortho.* Exostosenentfernung *f*, -resektion *f*.
ex·os·to·sis [ˌeksas'təʊsɪs] *n, pl* **-ses** [-si:z] *ortho.*, *patho.* Exostose *f*, Exostosis *f*.
ex·os·tot·ic [ˌeksas'tɑtɪk] *adj* Exostose(n) betr., exostosenartig, -ähnlich, exostotisch.
ex·o·ter·ic [ˌeksəʊ'terɪk] *adj* → exogenous 1.
ex·o·the·li·o·ma [ˌ-ˌθi:lɪ'əʊmə] *n* Meningiom(a) *nt*, Meningeom(a) *nt*.
ex·o·ther·mal [ˌ-'θɜrml] *adj* → exothermic.
exothermal reaction *chem.* exotherme Reaktion *f*.
ex·o·ther·mic [ˌ-'θɜrmɪk] *adj chem.* Wärme abgebend, exotherm.
exothermic reaction → exothermal reaction.
ex·o·tox·ic [ˌ-'tɑksɪk] *adj* Exotoxin betr., durch Exotoxin(e) verursacht, exotoxinbildend, Exotoxin-.
exotoxic bacterium exotoxinbildendes Bakterium *nt*.
ex·o·tox·in [ˌ-'tɑksɪn] *n* Exo-, Ektotoxin *nt*.
ex·o·tro·pia [ˌ-'trəʊpɪə] *n ophthal.* Auswärtsschielen *nt*, Exotropie *f*, Strabismus divergens.
ex·o·trop·ic [ˌ-'trɑpɪk, -'trəʊ-] *adj ophthal.* Exotropie betr., nach außen schielend, exotrop.
ex·pand [ɪk'spænd] **I** *vt* ausbreiten, ausspannen, ausdehnen, ausweiten, erweitern, entfalten. **II** *vi* s. ausdehnen, s. erweitern, s. ausspannen, s. entfalten.
ex·panse [ɪk'spæns] *n* weite Fläche *f*, ausgedehnter Raum *m*, Ausdehnung *f*, Weite *f*.
ex·pan·si·ble [ɪk'spænsɪbl] *adj* (aus-)dehnbar.
ex·pan·sile [ɪk'spænsɪl, -saɪl] *adj* (aus-)dehnbar, Ausdehnungs-.
ex·pan·sion [ɪk'spænʃn] *n* 1. *phys.* Ausdehnen *nt*, Ausdehnung *f*, Ausweitung *f*. 2. → expanse. 3. *patho.* Ausbreitung *f*, Expansion *f*.
expansion chamber *phys.* Nebelkammer *f*.
ex·pan·sive [ɪk'spænsɪv] *adj* 1. (s.) ausdehnend, expansiv, Ausdehnungs-, Expansions-. 2. ausdehnungsfähig. 3. *patho.* (*Wachstum*) verdrängend, expansiv. 4. weit, umfassend, ausgedehnt, breit. 5. *psychia.* größenwahnsinnig.
expansive delusion expansiver Wahn *m*, Größenwahn *m*, Megalomanie *f*.
expansive growth *patho.* expansives/verdrängendes Wachstum *nt*.
ex·pan·sive·ness [ɪk'spænsɪvnɪs] *n* 1. Ausdehnung *f*. 2. Ausdehnungsvermögen *nt*. 3. → expansive delusion.
ex·pect·an·cy [ɪk'spektənsɪ] *n* Erwartung *f*; Hoffnung *f*, Aussicht *f*.
e. of life Lebenserwartung *f*.

expectancy potential Erwartungspotential *nt*.
ex·pect·ant [ɪkˈspektənt] *adj* 1. (*Behandlung*) er-, abwartend, exspektativ. to be ~ of sth. etw. erwarten. 2. schwanger.
ex·pec·to·rant [ɪkˈspektərənt] I *n* schleimlösendes/auswurfförderndes Mittel *nt*, Expektorans *nt*. II *adj* schleimlösend, auswurffördernd.
ex·pec·to·rate [ɪkˈspektəreɪt] *vt* (*Schleim*) auswerfen, aus-, abhusten, expektorieren; (*Blut*) spucken.
ex·pec·to·ra·tion [ɪkˌspektəˈreɪʃn] *n* 1. Aus-, Abhusten *nt*, Auswerfen *nt*, Expektoration *f*, Expektorieren *nt*. 2. (Aus-)Spucken *nt*. 3. Auswurf *m*, Expektorat *nt*, Sputum *nt*.
ex·pe·ri·ence [ɪkˈspɪərɪəns] I *n* 1. Erfahrung *f*; Erfahrenheit *f*; (praktische) Erfahrung *f*, Fach-, Sachkenntnis *f*. 2. Erlebnis *nt*. II *vt* erfahren, kennenlernen, erleben.
ex·pe·ri·en·tial [ɪkˌspɪərɪˈenʃl] *adj* auf Erfahrung beruhend, Erfahrungs-.
ex·per·i·ment [*n* ɪkˈsperəmənt; *v* ekˈsperəmənt] I *n* Versuch *m*, Experiment *nt*. II *vi* experimentieren, Versuche durchführen *od.* anstellen (*on* an; *with* mit).
ex·per·i·men·tal [ɪkˌsperəˈmentl] *adj* 1. experimentell, Versuchs-, Experimental-. 2. → experiential.
experimental allergic encephalitis → experimental allergic encephalomyelitis.
experimental allergic encephalomyelitis *abbr.* **EAE** experimentelle allergische Enzephal(omyel)itis *f abbr.* EAE.
experimental animal Versuchstier *nt*.
ex·per·i·men·tal·ist [ɪkˌsperəˈmentəlɪst] *n* → experimenter.
ex·per·i·men·tal·ize [ˌ-ˈmentəlaɪz] *vi* experimentieren (*on* an; *with* mit).
ex·per·i·men·tal·ly [ˌ-ˈmentəlɪ] *adv* experimentell, auf experimentellem Wege; versuchsweise.
experimental medicine experimentelle Medizin *f*, Experimentalmedizin *f*.
experimental pathology experimentelle Pathologie *f*.
experimental psychology experimentelle Psychologie *f*.
ex·per·i·men·ta·tion [ˌ-menˈteɪʃn] *n* Experimentieren *nt*.
ex·per·i·ment·er [ɪkˈsperɪmentər] *n* Experimentator *m*.
ex·per·i·men·tor *n* → experimenter.
ex·pert [ˈekspɜrt] I *n* Fachmann *m*, Experte *m*, Expertin *f*; Sachverständige(r *m*) *f*, Gutachter(in *f*) *m* (*at, in* in; *on* auf dem Gebiet). II *adj* 1. erfahren, Erfahrung haben in. 2. fachmännisch, fach-, sachkundig, sachverständig. 3. Sachverständigen-, Experten-. 4. geschickt, gewandt (*at, in* in).
ex·per·tise [ˌeksparˈtiːz] *n* 1. Expertise *f*. 2. Fach-, Sachkenntnis *f*.
ex·per·tize [ˈekspartaɪz] I *vt* begutachten. II *vi* ein Gutachten abgeben *od.* (er-)stellen (*on* über).
ex·pi·rate [ˈekspɪreɪt] *n* ausgeatmete/abgeatmete Luft *f*, Exspirat *nt*.
ex·pi·ra·tion [ˌekspɪˈreɪʃn] *n* 1. Ausatmen *nt*, Ausatmung *f*, Exspiration *f*, Exspiratio *f*, Exspirium *nt*. 2. *old* letzter Atemzug *m*, Tod *m*. 3. *fig.* Ende *nt*, Ablauf *m* (*einer Frist*).
expiration center Exspirationszentrum *nt*.
ex·pir·a·to·ry [ɪkˈspaɪərətɔːrɪː, -təʊ-] *adj* Exspiration betr., exspiratorisch, Ausatmungs-, Exspirations-.
expiratory dyspnea exspiratorische Dyspnoe *f*.
expiratory exchange ratio *physiol.* respiratorischer Austauschquotient *m*; respiratorischer Quotient *m abbr.* RQ.
expiratory neuron exspiratorisches Neuron *nt*.
expiratory reserve volume *abbr.* **ERV** exspiratorisches Reservevolumen *nt abbr.* ERV.
expiratory resistance exspiratorische Resistance *f*.
expiratory stridor exspiratorischer Stridor *m*.
ex·pire [ɪkˈspaɪər] I *vt* (*Luft*) ausatmen, exspirieren. II *vi* 1. ausatmen, exspirieren. 2. (*Frist*) ablaufen, enden; verfallen. 3. sterben.
ex·pi·ri·um [ɪkˈspɪərɪəm] *n old* → expiration 1.
ex·pi·ry [ɪkˈspaɪərɪ, ˈekspərɪ] *n*, *pl* -ries → expiration 3.
ex·plant [*n* ˈeksplænt; *v* eksˈplænt] I *n* Explantat *nt*. II *vt* explantieren.
ex·plan·ta·tion [ˌeksplænˈteɪʃn] *n* Explantation *f*.
ex·plode [ɪkˈspləʊd] I *vt* zur Explosion bringen, explodieren lassen. II *vi* 1. explodieren. 2. *s.* explosionsartig verbreiten *od.* vermehren, sprunghaft ansteigen.
ex·plo·ra·tion [ˌekspləˈreɪʃn] *n* 1. Untersuchung *f*, Erkundung *f*, Ausforschung *f*, Exploration *f*. 2. Anamneseerhebung *f*, Exploration *f*.
ex·plor·a·tive [ɪkˈsplɔːrətɪv] *adj* 1. untersuchend, exploratix, Explorativ-, Probe-. 2. (er-)forschend, Forschungs-.
exploratory laparotomy explorative Laparotomie *f*, Probelaparotomie *f*.
ex·plor·a·to·ry [ɪkˈsplɔːrətɔːrɪː, -təʊ-] *adj* → explorative.
exploratory operation operative Exploration *f*.
exploratory thoracotomy explorative Thorakotomie *f*, Probethorakotomie *f*.
ex·plore [ɪkˈsplɔːr, -ˈsplɔʊər] I *vt* untersuchen, erforschen, erkunden, explorieren, sondieren. II *vi* forschen.
ex·plo·sion [ɪkˈspləʊʒn] *n* 1. Explosion *f*, Explodieren *nt*. 2. plötzlicher/heftiger/explosionsartiger Ausbruch *m od.* Anstieg *m*, explosionsartige Vermehrung *f*, Explosion *f*.
explosion injury/trauma Explosionstrauma *nt*.
ex·plo·sive [ɪkˈspləʊsɪv] I *n* Explosiv-, Verschlußlaut *m*. II *adj* 1. leicht explodierend, explosiv, explosibel. 2. explosionsartig, heftig, sprunghaft (ansteigend), s. explosionsartig vermehrend. 3. *fig.* leicht erregbar, leicht aufbrausend.
explosive decompression explosive/rapide Dekompression *f*.
explosive speech *neuro.* explosive Sprache *f*.
ex·po·nent [ɪkˈspəʊnənt, ˈekspə-] *n mathe.* Hochzahl *f*, Exponent *m*.
ex·po·nen·tial [ˌekspəʊˈnenʃl, -spə-] *mathe.* I *n* Exponentialgröße *f*. II *adj* exponentiell, Exponential-.
exponential curve Exponentialkurve *f*.
exponential equation Exponentialgleichung *f*.
exponential function Exponentialfunktion *f*.
exponential growth exponentielles Wachstum *nt*.
exponential period/phase *micro.* (*Wachstum*) exponentielle Phase *f*, log-Phase *f*.
exponential series Exponentialreihe *f*.
ex·pose [ɪkˈspəʊz] *vt* 1. (*Kind*) aussetzen. 2. aussetzen, preisgeben (*to*). 3. *fig.* bloßstellen; ~ o.s. *s.* bloßstellen. 4. *chir.* bloß-, freilegen, darstellen. 5. entblößen, enthüllen, zeigen. 6. *phys.*, *radiol.* (*einer Einwirkung*) aussetzen; *photo.* belichten.
ex·posed [ɪkˈspəʊzd] *adj* 1. ausgesetzt (*to*). 2. offenliegend, unbedeckt, unverdeckt. 3. (*Lage, Stellung*) ungeschützt, exponiert.
ex·po·sure [ɪkˈspəʊʒər] *n* 1. (Kindes-)Aussetzung *f*. 2. Aussetzen *nt*, Preisgabe *f*, Exponieren *nt*, Exposition *f*. 3. Ausgesetztsein *nt*, Gefährdung *f*, Exposition *f* (*to* durch). 4. *chir.* Frei-, Bloßlegung *f*, Darstellung *f*. 5. ungeschützte *od.* exponierte Lage *f*. 6. *phys.* Belichtung(szeit *f*) *f*.
e. **to radiation** *radiol.* Strahlenbelastung *f*, -exposition.
exposure dose *radiol.* Ionendosis *f*.
exposure keratitis Keratitis/Keratopathia e lagophthalmo.
exposure meter *photo.* Belichtungsmesser *m*.
exposure time Expositionszeit *f*.
ex·press [ɪkˈspres] *vt* 1. (her-)ausdrücken, (her-)auspressen (*from, out of* aus). 2. ausdrücken, zum Ausdruck bringen, äußern; (*Gefühl*) zeigen. 3. *genet.* exprimieren.
ex·press·i·ble [ɪkˈspresɪbl] *adj* ausdrückbar.
ex·pres·sion [ɪkˈspreʃn] *n* 1. (Her-)Ausdrücken *nt*, (Her-)Auspressen *nt*; *gyn.* Expression *f*, Exprimieren *nt*. 2. *fig.* Ausdruck *m*, Äußerung *f*. 3. Gesichtsausdruck *m*, Mimik *f*. 4. Ausdruck *m*.
ex·pres·sion·less [ɪkˈspreʃnlɪs] *adj* ausdruckslos.
ex·pres·sive [ɪkˈspresɪv] *adj* ausdrucksvoll, -stark, expressiv; ausdrucksfähig, Ausdrucks-.
expressive aphasia *neuro.* motorische Aphasie *f*, Broca-Aphasie *f*.
ex·pres·sive·ness [ɪkˈspresɪvnɪs] *n* Ausdruckskraft *f* -fähigkeit *f*.
expressive-receptive aphasia *neuro.* Total-, Globalaphasie *f*.
ex·pres·siv·i·ty [ˌeksprəˈsɪvətɪ] *n genet.* Expressivität *f*.
ex·pul·sion [ɪkˈspʌlʃn] *n chir., gyn.* Austreibung *f*, Expulsion *f*.
ex·pul·sive [ɪkˈspʌlsɪv] *adj* austreibend, expulsiv, Austreibungs-, Expulsions-, Expulsiv-.
expulsive pains *gyn.* Austreibungsschmerz *m*.
expulsive stage *gyn.* Austreibungsphase *f*.
ex·san·gui·nate [eksˈsæŋgwəneɪt] I *adj* exsanguine. II *vt* 1. aus-, verbluten. 2. Blut abziehen; blutleer machen.
ex·san·gui·na·tion [eksˌsæŋgwəˈneɪʃn] *n* massiver Blutverlust *m*, Ausblutung *f*, Aus-, Verbluten *nt*, Exsanguination *f*.
exsanguination transfusion (Blut-)Austauschtransfusion *f*, Blutaustausch *m*, Exsanguinationstransfusion *f*.
ex·san·guine [eksˈsæŋgwɪn] *adj* blutleer, blutarm, anämisch.
ex·san·gui·no·trans·fu·sion [eksˌsæŋgwɪnəʊtrænsˈfjuːʒn] *n* (Blut-)Austauschtransfusion *f*, Blutaustausch *m*, Exsanguinationstransfusion *f*.
ex·scind [ekˈsɪnd] *vt* → exsect.
ex·sect [ekˈsekt] *vt chir.* (her-)ausschneiden, entfernen, exzidieren.
ex·sec·tion [ekˈsekʃn] *n* → excision.
ex·sic·cant [ekˈsɪkənt] *n* austrocknendes Mittel *nt*, (Aus-)Trockenmittel *nt*, Exsikkans *nt*.
ex·sic·cate [ˈeksɪkeɪt] *vt*, *vi* austrocknen.
ex·sic·ca·tion [ˌeksɪˈkeɪʃn] *n* (Aus-)Trocknen *nt*, Austrocknung *f*, Exsikkation *f*, Exsikkose *f*.
exsiccation fever *ped.* Durstfieber *nt*.

exsiccative

ex·sic·ca·tive ['eksɪkətɪv] **I** *n* → exsiccant. **II** *adj* austrocknend.
ex·sic·ca·tor ['eksɪkeɪtər] *n* Trockenapparat *m*, Exsikkator *m*.
ex·sorp·tion [ek'sɔːrpʃn] *n physiol*. Exsorption *f*.
ex·stro·phy ['ekstrəfɪ] *n patho., urol.* Ekstrophie *f*, Ekstrophia *f*, Exstrophie *f*, Extrophie *f*, Extrophia *f*.
  e. of bladder Spaltblase *f*, Blasenekstrophie, -exstrophie.
  e. of cloaca Kloakenekstrophie, -exstrophie.
ex·tend [ɪk'stend] **I** *vt* (*Hände*) ausstrecken; (aus-)dehnen; erweitern, vergrößern; (*a. zeitl.*) verlängern. **II** *vi* (*a. zeitl.*) s. erstrecken; s. ausdehnen, s. ausstrecken lassen.
ex·tend·ed [ɪk'stendɪd] *adj* ausgestreckt; (aus-)gedehnt; erweitert, vergrößert; verlängert.
extended form *chem.* offene/gestreckte Form *f*.
extended pyeolotomy *urol*. Gil-Vernet-Operation *f*.
ex·ten·si·bil·i·ty [ɪkˌstensə'bɪlɪtɪ] *n* (Aus-)Dehnbarkeit *f*.
ex·ten·si·ble [ɪk'stensəbl] *adj* (aus-)dehnbar; ausstreckbar.
ex·ten·sim·e·ter [ˌeksten'sɪmətər] *n phys.* Dehnungsmesser *m*.
ex·ten·sion [ɪk'stenʃn] *n* **1.** (*a. fig.*) Ausdehnung *f* (*to* auf); Erweiterung *f*, Vergrößerung *f*; (*a. zeitl.*) Verlängerung *f*. **2.** *chir., ortho.* Extension *f*, Zug *m*, Streckung *f*. **3.** (*Gliedmaße*) Strecken *nt*, Durchstrecken *nt*.
extension bandage *ortho.* Streck-, Extensionsverband *nt*.
extension splint *ortho.* Extensionsschiene *f*.
ex·ten·sive [ɪk'stensɪv] *adj* umfassend, umfangreich, ausgedehnt, beträchtlich.
ex·ten·sive·ness [ɪk'stensɪvnɪs] *n* Umfang *m*, Ausdehnung *f*, Größe *f*.
ex·ten·som·e·ter [ˌeksten'sɑmɪtər] *n* → extensimeter.
ex·ten·sor [ɪk'stensər, -sɔːr] *n* Strecker *m*, Streckmuskel *m*, Extensor *m*, M. extensor.
extensor carpi radialis accessorius (muscle) Extensor *m* carpi radialis accessorius, M. extensor carpi radialis accessorius.
extensor carpi radialis brevis (muscle) Extensor *m* carpi radialis brevis, M. extensor carpi radialis brevis.
extensor carpi radialis intermedius (muscle) Extensor *m* carpi radialis intermedius, M. extensor carpi radialis intermedius.
extensor carpi radialis longus (muscle) Extensor *m* carpi radialis longus, M. extensor carpi radialis longus.
extensor carpi radialis (muscle) radialer Handstrecker *m*, Extensor *m* carpi radialis, M. extensor carpi radialis.
extensor carpi ulnaris (muscle) ulnarer Handstrecker *m*, Extensor *m* carpi ulnaris, M. extensor carpi ulnaris.
extensor digiti minimi (muscle) Kleinfingerstrecker *m*, Extensor *m* digiti minimi, M. extensor digiti minimi.
extensor digitorum brevis (muscle) kurzer Zehenstrecker *m*, Extensor *m* digitorum brevis, M. extensor digitorum brevis.
extensor digitorum longus (muscle) langer Zehenstrecker *m*, Extensor *m* digitorum longus, M. extensor digitorum longus.
extensor digitorum (manus) (muscle) Fingerstrecker *m*, Extensor *m* digitorum (manus), M. extensor digitorum (manus).
extensor hallucis brevis (muscle) Extensor *m* hallucis brevis, M. extensor hallucis brevis.
extensor hallucis longus (muscle) *abbr.* **EHL** Extensor *m* hallucis longus, M. extensor hallucis longus.
extensor hallucis (muscle) Großzehenstrecker *m*, Extensor *m* hallucis, M. extensor hallucis.
extensor indicis (muscle) Zeigefingerstrecker *m*, Extensor *m* indicis, M. extensor indicis.
extensor muscle → extensor.
  deep e.s tiefe Streckmuskeln *pl*, -muskulatur *f*.
  e. of fingers → extensor digitorum (manus) (muscle).
  e. of great toe → extensor hallucis (muscle).
  e. of index (finger) → extensor indicis (muscle).
  e. of little finger → extensor digiti minimi (muscle).
  radial e. of wrist → extensor carpi radialis (muscle).
  superficial e.s oberflächliche Streckmuskeln *pl*, -muskulatur *f*.
  e. of thumb → extensor pollicis (muscle).
  e. of toes Zehenstrecker *m*, Extensor *m* digitorum pedis, M. extensor digitorum pedis.
  ulnar e. of wrist → extensor carpi ulnaris (muscle).
extensor pollicis brevis (muscle) Extensor *m* pollicis brevis, M. extensor pollicis brevis.
extensor pollicis longus (muscle) Extensor *m* pollicis longus, M. extensor pollicis longus.
extensor pollicis (muscle) Daumenstrecker *m*, Extensor *m* pollicis, M. extensor pollicis.
extensor reflex Streck-, Extensorreflex *m*.
  crossed e. gekreuzter Streckreflex.
extensor retinaculum: e. of foot Strecksehnenband *nt* des Fußes, Retinaculum mm. extensorum pedis.
  e. of hand Strecksehnenband *nt* der Hand, Retinaculum extensorum (manus), Lig. carpi dorsale.
  inferior e. of foot Y-Band *nt*, Retinaculum mm. extensorum (pedis) inferius.
  superior e. of foot oberes Strecksehnenband/Retinakulum *nt*, Retinaculum mm. extensorum (pedis) superius.
extensor side of wrist Rück-/Streckseite *f* der Handwurzel, Regio carpalis posterior.
extensor spasm *neuro*. Extensorenkrampf *m*, Extensorspasmus *m*.
extensor tendon Extensor-, Extensorensehne *f*, Streckersehne *f*.
ex·tent [ɪk'stent] *n* **1.** Ausdehnung *f*, Größe *f*, Länge *f*, Breite *f*. **2.** *fig.* (Aus-)Maß *nt*, Umfang *m*; Grad *m*.
ex·te·ri·or [ɪk'stɪərɪər] **I** *n* Äußere(s) *nt*; Außenseite *f*; äußere Erscheinung *f*. **II** *adj* **1.** äußerlich, äußere(r, s), Außen-. **2.** von außen (kommend *od.* einwirkend).
ex·te·ri·or·i·za·tion [ɪkˌstɪərɪɑːɪ'zeɪʃn] *n* **1.** *chir.* (*Organ*) Verlagerung *f* nach außen, Exteriorisation *f*. **2.** *psychia*. Externalisieren *nt*, Externalisierung *f*. **3.** *physiol*. Objektivierung *f*.
ex·te·ri·or·ize [ɪk'stɪərɪəraɪz] *vt* **1.** *chir.* (*Organ*) nach außen verlagern *od.* verlegen. **2.** *psychia*. (Konflikte, Schuldgefühle) nach außen verlagern, nach außen wenden, externalisieren. **3.** *physiol*. (Wahr-nehmung) objektivieren.
ex·ter·mi·nate [ɪk'stɜrməneɪt] *vt* ausrotten, vernichten, vertilgen.
ex·ter·mi·na·tion [ɪkˌstɜrmə'neɪʃn] *n* Ausrottung *f*, Vernichtung *f*, Vertilgung *f*.
ex·tern [*n* 'ekstɜrn; *adj* ɪk'stɜrn] **I** *n* Externe(r *m*) *f*; *nicht im Krankenhaus wohnender Arzt od. Student*. **II** *adj old* → external.
ex·ter·nal [ek'stɜrnl] *adj* **1.** außen befindlich *od*. gelegen, äußere(r, s), äußerlich, extern, Außen-. **2.** von außen kommend *od*. (ein-)wirkend. **for → use** äußerlich, zum äußeren Gebrauch.
external angle Außenwinkel *m*.
  e. of border of tibia *anat*. Margo interosseus tibiae.
  e. of scapula *anat*. Angulus lateralis (scapulae).
external aperture: e. of aqueduct of cochlea äußere Öffnung *f* des Aquaeductus cochleae, Apertura externa aqu(a)eductus cochleae.
  e. of aqueduct of vestibule äußere Öffnung *f* des Aquaeductus vestibuli, Apertura externa aqu(a)eductus vestibuli.
  e. of canaliculus of cochlea äußere Öffnung *f* des Canaliculus cochleae, Apertura externa canaliculi cochleae.
  e. of tympanic canaliculus äußere Öffnung *f* des Canaliculus tympanicus, Apertura inferior canaliculi tympanici.
external auditory meatus reflex *neuro*. Kehrer-Zeichen *nt*.
external axis of bulb/eye äußere/anatomische Augenachse *f*, Axis bulbi externus.
external band of Baillarger äußere Baillarger-Schicht *f*, äußerer Baillarger-Streifen *m*, Stria laminae granularis interna (corticis cerebri).
external base of cranium äußere Schädelbasis *f*, Basis cranii externa.
external border of scapula äußerer Skapularand *m*, Margo lateralis scapulae.
external branch: e. of accessory nerve Ramus externus n. accessorii.
  e. of superior laryngeal nerve äußerer Ast *m* des N. laryngeus superior, Ramus externus n. laryngei superioris.
external callus *ortho.* äußerer Kallus *m*.
external capsule äußere Kapsel *f*, Capsula externa.
external carotid steal syndrome Karotissyndrom *nt*, Karotis-Anzapfsyndrom *nt*, Karotis-Steal-Syndrom *nt*.
external coat: e. of capsule of graafian follicle Theka/Theca *f* externa, Tunica externa thecae folliculi.
  e. of esophagus Tunica adventitia (o)esophagi.
  e. of ureter Tunica adventitia ureteris.
external conjugate Conjugata externa, Diameter Baudelocque.
external criterion Außenkriterium *nt*.
external crus of superficial inguinal ring Crus laterale anuli inguinalis superficialis.
external ear äußeres Ohr *nt*, Auris externa.
external extremity of clavicle Extremitas acromialis.
external exudative retinopathy Coats-Syndrom *nt*, Morbus Coats *m*, Retinitis exsudativa externa.
external fistula *patho*. äußere Fistel *f*, Fistula externa.
external genitalia äußere Geschlechtsorgane/Genitalien *pl*, Organa genitalia externa.
external genu of facial nerve äußeres Fazialisknie *f*, Geniculum n. facialis.

external glomerulus *embryo.* äußerer Glomerulus *m*.
external hemorrhage äußere Blutung *f*.
external hemorrhoids äußere Hämorrhoiden *pl*.
external hernia *chir.* **1.** äußerer/indirekter/seitlicher/schräger Leistenbruch *m*, Hernia inguinalis externa/indirecta/lateralis/obliqua. **2.** äußere Hernie *f*, Hernia externa.
external hordeolum *ophthal.* Hordeolum externum.
external hydrocephalus *neuro., patho.* Hydrocephalus externus.
ex·ter·na·lia [ˌɛkstɜrˈneɪlɪə] *pl* → external genitalia.
ex·ter·nal·i·za·tion [ɪkˌstɜrnələˈzeɪʃn] *n* → exteriorization.
ex·ter·nal·ize [ɪkˈstɜrnlaɪz] *vt* → exteriorize.
external lamina: e. of peritoneum äußeres Blatt *nt* des Bauchfells, Peritoneum parietale.
e. of pterygoid process Lamina lateralis proc. pterygoidei.
e. of skull äußeres Blatt *nt* des knöchernen Schädeldachs, Lamina externa (cranii).
external layer: e. of myometrium supravaskuläre Schicht *f* des Myometriums, Stratum supravasculare (myometrii).
e. of skull → external lamina of skull.
e. of theca folliculi Theka/Theca *f* externa, Tunica externa thecae folliculi.
external line of Baillarger → external band of Baillarger.
external lip of iliac crest Labium externum cristae iliacae.
external malleolar sign Chaddock-Zeichen *nt*, -Reflex *m*.
external margin: e. of scapula → external border of scapula.
e. of testis konvexer/vorderer Hodenrand *m*, Margo anterior testis.
external medium → external phase.
external meningitis epidurale Pachymeningitis *f*, Pachymeningitis externa.
external mouth of uterus äußerer Muttermund *m*, Ostium uteri.
external nose äußere Nase *f*, Nasus externus.
external ophthalmopathy Ophthalmopathia externa.
external ophthalmoplegia *ophthal.* Ophthalmoplegia externa.
external orifice of aqueduct of vestibule Apertura externa aqu(a)eductus vestibuli.
external pacemaker *card.* externer Herzschrittmacher *m*.
external parasite Außenparasit *m*.
external perimysium Muskelhüllgewebe *nt* des Sekundärbündels, Perimysium externum.
external phase *phys.* äußere/dispergierende Phase *f*, Dispergens *nt*, Dispersionsmedium *nt*, -mittel *nt*.
external piles → external hemorrhoids.
external pneumatic compression pump. EPC (externe) pneumatische Kompression *f*.
external respiration äußere Atmung/Respiration *f*, Lungenatmung *f*.
external rotation Außenrotation *f*.
external segment of globus pallidus äußeres Pallidumglied/-segment *nt*.
external sheath of optic nerve äußere Durahülle *f* des N. opticus, Vagina externa n. optici.
external sphincter (muscle) of anus (*After*) äußerer Schließmuskel *m*, Sphinkter/Sphincter *m* ani externus, M. sphincter ani externus.

external squint → external strabismus.
external strabismus *ophthal.* Auswärtsschielen *nt*, Exotropie *f*, Strabismus divergens.
external stria/stripe of Baillarger → external band of Baillarger.
external substance of suprarenal gland Nebennierenrinde *f* *abbr.* NNR, Cortex (gl. suprarenalis).
external surface of eyelid äußere/vordere Lidfläche *f*, Facies anterior palpebrarum.
external tubercle of humerus Tuberculum majus humeri.
external tuber of Henle Tuberculum mentale.
external tuberosity of femur Epicondylus lateralis femoris.
external tunnel (*Ohr*) äußerer Tunnel *m*.
external urethrotomy *urol.* Urethrotomia externa.
external version *gyn.* äußere Wendung *f*.
external wall of cochlear duct äußere Ductus cochlearis-Wand *f*, Paries externus ductus cochlearis.
external work *physiol.* äußere Arbeit *f*.
ex·terne [ˈɛkstɜrn] *n, adj* → extern.
ex·ter·o·cep·tion [ˌɛkstərəˈsɛpʃn] *n* Extero(re)zeption *f*.
ex·ter·o·cep·tive [ˌ-ˈsɛptɪv] *adj* äußere Reize aufnehmend, extero(re)zeptiv.
exteroceptive nervous system extero(re)zeptives System *nt*.
exteroceptive sensibility extero(re)zeptive Sensibilität *f*.
ex·ter·o·cep·tor [ˌ-ˈsɛptər] *n* Extero(re)zeptor *m*.
ex·ter·o·fec·tion [ˌ-ˈfɛkʃn] *n* *patho., neuro.* Exterofektion *f*.
ex·ter·o·fec·tive [ˌ-ˈfɛktɪv] *adj* *patho., neuro.* auf äußere Reize reagierend, exterofektiv.
ex·ti·ma [ˈɛkstɪmə] *n, pl* **-mas, -mae** [-miː] **1.** (*Gefäß*) Adventitia *f*, Tunica adventitia. **2.** (*Organ*) Adventitia *f*, Tunica externa.
ex·tinct [ɪkˈstɪŋkt] *adj* erloschen; ausgestorben. **to become ~** aussterben.
ex·tinc·tion [ɪkˈstɪŋkʃn] *n* **1.** Ex(s)tinktion *f*, (Aus-, Er-)Löschen *nt*; Auslöschung *f*, Vernichtung *f*. **2.** *phys.* Abschwächung *f*, Extinktion *f*. **3.** *bio.* Aussterben *nt*. **4.** Abschaffung *f*, Aufhebung *f*. **5.** *psycho.* Extinktion *f*.
extinction coefficient *abbr.* ϵ Extinktionskoeffizient *m* *abbr.* ε.
molar e. *abbr.* **E** molarer Extinktionskoeffizient.
specific e. *abbr.* **a** spezifischer Extinktionskoeffizient.
ex·tin·guish [ɪkˈstɪŋgwɪʃ] *vt* **1.** (*Feuer, Licht*) (aus-)löschen; auslöschen, vernichten, zerstören. **2.** auslöschen, ersticken, (ab-)töten.
ex·tir·pate [ˈɛkstərpeɪt, ɪkˈstɜrpeɪt] *vt* **1.** *chir.* (völlig) entfernen, exstirpieren. **2.** (mit der Wurzel) ausreißen; ausmerzen, ausrotten.
ex·tir·pa·tion [ˌɛkstərˈpeɪʃn] *n* **1.** *chir.* (vollständige) Entfernung *f*, Exstirpation *f*. **2.** Ausrottung *f*, Ausmerzung *f*.
ex·tor·sion [ɪkˈstɔːrʃn] *n* **1.** Außenrotation *f*. **2.** *ophthal.* Extorsion *f*; (positive) Disklination *f*.
extra- *pref.* Außer-, Extra-.
extra-abdominal fibromatosis extraabdominelle/extraabdominale Fibromatose *f*.
extra-adrenal *adj* außerhalb der Nebenniere(n) (liegend), extraadrenal.
ex·tra·am·ni·ot·ic pregnancy [ˌɛkstrəˌæmnɪˈɑtɪk] Graviditas examnialis.

extra-anatomic reconstruction *chir.* extraanatomische Rekonstruktion *f*.
extra-anthropic *adj* → exanthropic.
extra-articular *adj* außerhalb eines Gelenks (liegend), extraartikulär.
extra-articular arthrodesis *ortho.* extraartikuläre Gelenkversteifung/Arthrodese *f*.
extra-articular fracture *ortho.* extraartikuläre Fraktur *f*.
ex·tra·au·ral [ˌɛkstrəˈɔːrəl] *adj* außerhalb des Ohres (liegend), extraaural.
ex·tra·bron·chi·al [ˌ-ˈbrɑŋkɪəl] *adj* außerhalb der Bronchien (liegend), extrabronchial.
ex·tra·bul·bar [ˌ-ˈbʌlbər] *adj* außerhalb eines Bulbus (liegend), extrabulbär.
ex·tra·ca·pil·lar·y glomerulonephritis [ˌ-kəˈpɪlərɪ] intra-extrakapilläre proliferative Glomerulonephritis *f*.
ex·tra·cap·su·lar [ˌ-ˈkæpsələr, -sjʊ-] *adj* außerhalb der Kapsel (liegend), extrakapsulär.
extracapsular ankylosis *ortho.* extrakapsuläre Ankylose *f*.
extracapsular fracture extrakapsuläre Fraktur *f*.
extracapsular ligaments extrakapsuläre Bänder *pl*, Ligg. extracapsularia.
ex·tra·car·di·al [ˌ-ˈkɑːrpəl] *adj* außerhalb des Herzens (liegend), extrakardial.
ex·tra·cel·lu·lar [ˌ-ˈsɛljələr] *adj* außerhalb der Zelle (liegend), extrazellulär, Extrazellular-.
extracellular cholesterolosis/cholesterosis Erythema elevatum diutinum.
extracellular enzyme → exoenzyme.
extracellular fluid *abbr.* **ECF** Extrazellularflüssigkeit *f* *abbr.* EZF, ECF.
extracellular space ES, ECS extrazellulärer Raum *m*, Extrazellularraum *m* *abbr.* EZ, EZR.
extracellular toxin Ekto-, Exotoxin *nt*.
extracellular water *abbr.* **ECW** extrazelluläres Wasser *nt* *abbr.* EZW.
ex·tra·cer·e·bel·lar [ˌ-sɛrəˈbɛlər] *adj* außerhalb des Kleinhirns (liegend), extrazerebellar, extrazerebellär.
ex·tra·cer·e·bral [ˌ-ˈsɛrəbrəl] *adj* außerhalb des Großhirns (liegend), extrazerebral.
extracerebral hematoma extrazerebrales Hämatom *nt*.
ex·tra·cho·ri·al pregnancy [ˌ-ˈkɔːrɪəl] Graviditas exochorialis.
ex·tra·chro·mo·so·mal [ˌ-ˌkroʊməˈsoʊml] *adj* außerhalb eines Chromosoms/der Chromosomen (liegend), extrachromosomal.
extrachromosomal inheritance extrachromosomale Vererbung *f*.
extrachromosomal resistance *micro.* extrachromosomale Resistenz *f*.
ex·tra·cor·po·ral [ˌ-ˈkɔːrpərəl] *adj* → extracorporeal.
ex·tra·cor·po·re·al [ˌ-kɔːrˈpɔːrɪəl] *adj* außerhalb des Körpers (liegend), extrakorporal.
extracorporeal circulation extrakorporaler Kreislauf *m*, extrakorporale Zirkulation *f*.
extracorporeal dialysis extrakorporale Dialyse *f*; Hämodialyse *f*.
extracorporeal membrane oxygenation *abbr.* **ECMO** extrakorporale Membranoxygenation *f* *abbr.* ECMO.
extracorporeal shock wave lithotripsy *abbr.* **ESWL** extrakorporale Stoßwellenlithotripsie *f* *abbr.* ESWL.
ex·tra·cor·pus·cu·lar [ˌ-kɔːrˈpʌskjələr] *adj* extrakorpuskulär.
ex·tra·cor·ti·co·spi·nal system [ˌ-ˌkɔːrtɪkoʊˈspaɪnl] → extrapyramidal system.

extracorticospinal tract → extrapyramidal system.

ex·tra·cra·ni·al [ˌekstrəˈkreɪnɪəl] *adj* außerhalb des (knöchernen) Schädels (liegend), extrakraniell, extrakranial.

extracranial bypass extrakranialer/extrakranieller Bypass/Shunt *m*.

extracranial-intracranial bypass *chir.*, *neurochir.* extrakranial-intrakranialer Bypass/Shunt *m*.

ex·tract [*n* ˈekstrækt; *v* ɪkˈstrækt] **I** *n* Extrakt *m*, Auszug *m* (*from* aus). **II** *vt* **1.** herausnehmen, -ziehen, -holen (*from* aus); (*Fremdkörper*) entfernen; (*Mineral*) gewinnen (*from* aus). **2.** (*Zahn*) ziehen, extrahieren. **3.** *mathe.* die Wurzel ziehen, extrahieren. **4.** *chem.* auszieheh, -scheiden, herauslösen, extrahieren.

ex·tract·a·ble [ɪkˈstræktəbl] *adj* (her-)ausziehbar, extrahierbar.

extractable nuclear antigens *abbr.* **ENA** *immun.* extrahierbare nukleäre Antigene *pl abbr.* ENA, extrahierbare Kernantigene *pl*.

ex·tract·i·ble *adj* → extractable.

ex·trac·tion [ɪkˈstrækʃn] *n* **1.** Herausziehen *nt*, -nehmen *nt*, -holen *nt*; (*Mineral*) Gewinnung *f*. **2.** (*Zahn*) Ziehen *nt*, Extraktion *f*, Extrahieren *nt*. **3.** *chir.* Herausziehen *nt*, Entfernen *nt*, Extrahieren *nt*, Extraktion *f*. **4.** *gyn.* Herausziehen *nt* des Kindes, Extraktion *f*. **5.** *mathe.* (Wurzel-)Ziehen *nt*, Extraktion *f*, Extrahieren *nt*. **6.** *chem.*, *phys.* Ausziehen *nt*, -scheiden *nt*, Extraktion *f*, Extrahieren *nt*. **7.** → extract I.

ex·trac·tive [ɪkˈstræktɪv] **I** *n* → extract I. **II** *adj* durch Extraktion (erfolgend), (her-)ausziehend, auslaugend, löslich, extraktiv, Extraktiv-.

ex·trac·tor [ɪkˈstræktər] *n* Extraktionszange *f*, Extraktor *m*; *gyn.* (Geburts-)Zange *f*.

ex·tra·cys·tic [ˌekstrəˈsɪstɪk] *adj* **1.** außerhalb der Gallenblase (liegend), extrabiliär. **2.** außerhalb der (Harn-)Blase (liegend), extravesikal. **3.** außerhalb einer Zyste (liegend).

ex·tra·du·ral [ˌ-ˈdʊərəl, -ˈdjʊər-] *adj* außerhalb der Dura mater (liegend), extradural; epidural.

extradural abscess epiduraler/extraduraler Abszeß *m*, Epiduralabszeß *m*.

extradural anesthesia extradurale Anästhesie *f*.

extradural bleeding Epiduralblutung *f*, epidurale/extradurale Blutung *f*.

extradural hematoma Epiduralhämatom *nt*, epidurales/extradurales Hämatom *nt*.

extradural hematorrhachis extradurale/subdurale Hämatorrhachis *f*, Haematorrhachis externa.

extradural hemorrhage → extradural bleeding.

extradural space → epidural space.

ex·tra·em·bry·on·ic [ˌ-ˌembrɪˈɒnɪk] *adj* außerhalb des Embryos (liegend), extraembryonal.

extraembryonic celom/coelom → exocoelom.

extraembryonic membranes *embryo.* Eihäute *pl*.

extraembryonic mesoderm extraembryonales Mesoderm *nt*.

ex·tra·ep·i·phys·e·al [ˌ-ˌepɪˈfɪzɪəl] *adj* außerhalb der Epiphyse (liegend), nicht mit der Epiphyse verbunden, extraepiphysär, extraepiphyseal.

ex·tra·fu·sal [ˌ-ˈfjuːzl] *adj* außerhalb einer Muskelspindel (liegend), extrafusal.

extrafusal fibers extrafusale Fasern *pl*.

ex·tra·gem·mal [ˌ-ˈdʒeməl] *adj* extragemmal.

extragemmal fibers extragemmale (Nerven-)Fasern *pl*.

ex·tra·gen·i·tal [ˌ-ˈdʒenɪtl] *adj* außerhalb der Geschlechtsorgane (liegend), nicht von den Geschlechtsorganen stammend, extragenital.

ex·tra·glan·du·lar perspiration [ˌ-ˈglændʒələr] extraglanduläre Wasserabgabe *f*, extraglandulärer Wasserverlust *m*, Perspiratio insensibilis.

extraglandular water loss → extraglandular perspiration.

ex·tra·he·pat·ic [ˌ-hɪˈpætɪk] *adj* nicht in der Leber (liegend), extrahepatisch.

extrahepatic cholestasis extrahepatische Gallestauung/Cholestase *f*.

extrahepatic jaundice extrahepatischer Ikterus *m*.

ex·tra·hy·po·tha·lam·ic [ˌ-ˌhaɪpəʊθəˈlæmɪk, -ˌhɪp-] *adj* außerhalb des Hypothalamus (liegend), extrahypothalamisch.

ex·tra·in·tes·ti·nal [ˌ-ɪnˈtestɪnl] *adj* außerhalb des Darm(trakt)s (liegend), extraintestinal.

extraintestinal air *radiol.* freie Luft *f* im Bauchraum.

extraintestinal amebiasis extraintestinale Amöbiasis *f*.

ex·tra·lem·mal [ˌ-ˈleməl] *adj* extralemmal.

ex·tra·lig·a·men·tous [ˌ-ˌlɪgəˈmentəs] *adj* außerhalb eines Bandes (liegend), nicht mit einem Band verbunden, extraligamentär.

ex·tra·ly·so·so·mal [ˌ-ˌlaɪsəˈsəʊml] *adj* extralysosomal.

ex·tra·mal·le·o·lus [ˌ-məˈlɪələs] *n anat.* Außenknöchel *m*, Malleolus lateralis.

ex·tra·med·ul·lar·y [ˌ-ˈmedəˌlerɪ, -ˈmedʒ-, -meˈdʌləri] *adj* außerhalb der (Knochen-, Rücken-)Marks (liegend), extramedullär.

extramedullary hemopoiesis extramedulläre Blutbildung *f*.

ex·tra·me·nin·ge·al [ˌ-mɪˈnɪndʒɪəl] *adj* außerhalb der Hirnhäute (liegend), extrameningeal.

ex·tra·mi·to·chon·dri·al [ˌ-maɪtəˈkɒndrɪəl] *adj* außerhalb der Mitochondrien (liegend), extramitochondrial.

ex·tra·mu·ral [ˌ-ˈmjʊərəl] *adj* außerhalb der (Organ-)Wand (liegend), extramural.

extramural ganglion extramurales Ganglion *nt*.

ex·tra·ne·ous [ɪkˈstreɪnɪəs] *adj* **1.** außerhalb des Organismus liegend *od.* ablaufend. **2.** äußere(r, s), Außen-. **3.** fremd (*to*).

ex·tra·nu·cle·ar [ˌekstrəˈn(j)uːklɪər] *adj* außerhalb des (Zell-)Kerns (liegend), extranukleär.

extranuclear inheritance extranukleäre/zytoplasmatische Vererbung *f*.

ex·tra·oc·u·lar muscles [ˌ-ˈɒkjələr] (äußere) Augenmuskeln *pl*, Mm. bulbi.

ex·tra·o·ral [ˌ-ˈɔːrəl] *adj* außerhalb der Mundhöhle (liegend), extraoral.

ex·tra·os·se·ous [ˌ-ˈɒsɪəs] *adj* außerhalb des Knochens (liegend), extraossär.

ex·tra·par·en·chy·mal [ˌekstrəpəˈreŋkɪməl] *adj* außerhalb des Parenchyms liegend *od.* ablaufend, extraparenchymal.

ex·tra·pel·vic [ˌ-ˈpelvɪk] *adj* außerhalb des Beckens (liegend), extrapelvin.

ex·tra·per·i·car·di·al [ˌ-ˌperɪˈkɑːrdɪəl] *adj* außerhalb des Herzbeutels/Pericardium (liegend), extraperikardial.

ex·tra·per·i·ne·al [ˌ-ˌperɪˈniːəl] *adj* nicht im Damm (liegend), extraperineal.

ex·tra·per·i·os·te·al [ˌ-ˌperɪˈɒstɪəl] *adj* außerhalb des Periosts (liegend), extraperiostal.

ex·tra·per·i·to·ne·al [ˌ-ˌperɪtəˈniːəl] *adj* außerhalb *od.* an der Außenfläche des Peritoneums (liegend), außerhalb der Bauchhöhle (liegend), extraperitoneal, Extraperitoneal-.

extraperitoneal fascia Fascia extraperitonealis.

extraperitoneal organ extraperitoneal liegendes Organ *nt*, Organum extraperitoneale.

extraperitoneal space Extraperitonealraum *m*, Spatium extraperitoneale.

extraperitoneal tissue Fascia extraperitonealis.

ex·tra·pla·cen·tal [ˌ-pləˈsentl] *adj* außerhalb der Plazenta (liegend), nicht mit der Plazenta verbunden, extraplazentar.

ex·tra·plan·tar [ˌ-ˈplæntər] *adj* an *od.* auf der Außenseite der Fußsohle (liegend), extraplantar.

ex·tra·pleu·ral [ˌ-ˈplʊərəl] *adj* außerhalb der Pleura *od.* Pleurahöhle (liegend), extrapleural.

extrapleural pneumothorax extrapleuraler Pneu(mothorax *m*) *m*.

ex·trap·o·late [ɪkˈstræpəleɪt] *vt*, *vi mathe.* extrapolieren.

ex·trap·o·la·tion [ɪkˌstræpəˈleɪʃn] *n mathe.*, *phys.* Extrapolation *f*.

ex·tra·pro·fes·sion·al [ˌekstrəprəˈfeʃənl] *adj* nicht zum Beruf gehörig, außerberuflich.

ex·tra·pros·tat·ic [ˌ-prəˈstætɪk] *adj* außerhalb der Prostata (liegend), nicht mit der Prostata verbunden, extraprostatisch.

ex·tra·pros·ta·ti·tis [ˌ-ˌprɒstəˈtaɪtɪs] *n urol.* Paraprostatitis *f*.

ex·tra·psy·chic conflict [ˌ-ˈsaɪkɪk] *psycho.* extrapsychischer Konflikt *m*.

ex·tra·pul·mo·nar·y [ˌ-ˈpʌlməˌnerɪː, -ˌnɔrɪ, ˌpʊl-] *adj* außerhalb der Lunge(n) (liegend), nicht mit der Lunge verbunden, extrapulmonal.

ex·tra·py·ram·i·dal [ˌ-pɪˈræmɪdl] *adj* außerhalb der Pyramidenbahn, extrapyramidal.

extrapyramidal disease extrapyramidales Syndrom *nt*, extrapyramidaler Symptomenkomplex *m*.

extrapyramidal motor system → extrapyramidal system.

extrapyramidal part of medial longitudinal fasciculus extrapyramidaler Anteil *m* des Fasciculus longitudinalis medialis.

extrapyramidal syndrome → extrapyramidal disease.

extrapyramidal system extrapyramidal-motorisches System *nt*.

extrapyramidal tract → extrapyramidal system.

ex·tra·rec·tus [ˌ-ˈrektəs] *n anat.* Rektus *m* lateralis, M. rectus lateralis.

ex·tra·re·nal [ˌ-ˈriːnl] *adj* außerhalb der Niere (liegend), nicht von der Niere ausgehend, extrarenal.

extrarenal azotemia extrarenale Azot(h)ämie *f*.

ex·tra·sac·cu·lar hernia [ˌ-ˈsækjələr] Gleithernie *f*, -bruch *m*.

ex·tra·sen·so·ry [ˌ-ˈsensərɪ] *adj* außer-, übersinnlich.

extrasensory perception *abbr.* **ESP** außersinnliche/übersinnliche Wahrnehmung *f*, extrasensory perception *abbr.* ESP.

ex·tra·so·mat·ic [ˌ-səʊˈmætɪk, -sə-] *adj* außerhalb des Körpers liegend *od.* ablaufend, nicht mit dem Körper verbunden, extrasomatisch, extrakorporal.

ex·tra·su·pra·re·nal [ˌ-ˌsuːprəˈriːnl] *adj* → extra-adrenal.

extra systole → extrasystole.

ex·tra·sys·to·le [ˌ-ˈsɪstəlɪ] *n card.* vorzeitige

Herz(muskel)kontraktion f, Extraschlag m, Extrasystole f abbr. ES.
ex·tra·ter·res·tri·al [ˌ-tə'restrɪəl] **I** n außerirdisches Wesen nt. **II** adj außerirdisch, extraterrestrisch.
ex·tra·tho·rac·ic [ˌ-θɔː'ræsɪk, -θə-] adj außerhalb des Thorax (liegend), extrathorakal.
ex·tra·tra·che·al [ˌ-'treɪkɪəl, -trə'kiːəl] adj außerhalb der Trachea (liegend), extratracheal.
ex·tra·tu·bal [ˌ-'t(j)uːbl] adj **1.** außerhalb einer Tube (liegend), extratubal. **2.** gyn. außerhalb der Eileiter (liegend), extratubal. **3.** HNO außerhalb der Ohrtrompete (liegend), extratubal.
ex·tra·tym·pan·ic [ˌ-tɪm'pænɪk] adj außerhalb der Paukenhöhle (liegend), extratympanal, extratympanisch.
ex·tra·u·ter·ine [ˌ-'juːtərɪn, -raɪn] adj außerhalb der Gebärmutter/des Uterus (liegend), extrauterin.
extrauterine pregnancy abbr. EUP Extrauterinschwangerschaft f, -gravidität f abbr. EU, EUG, ektopische Schwangerschaft f, Graviditas extrauterina.
ex·tra·vag·i·nal [ˌ-'vædʒənl] adj außerhalb der Scheide/Vagina (liegend), extravaginal.
ex·trav·a·sate [ɪk'strævəseɪt] **I** n Extravasat nt. **II** vt (Blut) (aus einem Gefäß) austreten lassen. **III** vi (Blut) (aus einem Gefäß) austreten.
ex·trav·a·sa·tion [ɪkˌstrævə'seɪʃn] n **1.** Flüssigkeitsaustritt m aus einem Gefäß, Extravasation f. **2.** Extravasat nt.
ex·tra·vas·cu·lar [ˌekstrə'væskjələr] adj außerhalb eines Gefäßes (liegend), extravasal.
ex·tra·ven·tric·u·lar [ˌ-ven'trɪkjələr] adj außerhalb eines Ventrikels (liegend), extraventrikulär.
ex·tra·ver·sion [ˌ-'vɜrʒn] n → extroversion.
ex·tra·vert ['-vɜrt] n, adj, vt → extrovert.
ex·treme [ɪk'striːm] **I** n das Äußerste, Extrem nt; äußerstes Ende nt. **II** adj äußerste(r, s), weiteste(r, s), höchste(r, s), extrem, maßlos, End-, Extrem-.
extreme capsule Capsula extrema.
extreme unction letzte Ölung f, Heilige Ölung f.
ex·trem·i·tal [ɪk'stremɪtl] adj Extremität betr., Extremitäten-, Gliedmaßen-.
ex·trem·i·ty [ɪk'stremətɪ] n, pl **-ties 1.** äußeres Ende nt, Endstück nt, das Äußerste, Spitze f; anat. Extremitas f. **2.** Extremität f, Gliedmaße f, Glied nt.
e. of kidney Nierenpol m, Extremitas renis.
e. of ovary Eierstockpol m, Extremitas ovarii.
e. of testis Hodenpol m, Extremitas testis.
extremity fracture Extremitätenfraktur f.
extremity injury Extremitätenverletzung f.
extremity paralysis neuro. Gliedmaßenlähmung f, -parese f, Extremitätenlähmung f, -parese f.
ex·trin·sic [ɪk'strɪnsɪk, -zɪk] adj von außen (kommend od. wirkend), äußerlich, äußere(r, s), exogen, extrinsisch, extrinsic.
extrinsic allergic alveolitis → extrinsic alveolitis.
extrinsic alveolitis exogen-allergische Alveolitis f, Hypersensitivitätspneumonitis f.
extrinsic asthma Extrinsic-Asthma nt, exogen-allergisches Asthma (bronchiale) nt.
extrinsic factor (Cyano-)Cobalamin nt, Vitamin B_{12} nt.

extrinsic muscles von außen einstrahlende Muskeln pl/Muskulatur f.
e. of larynx äußere/extrinsische Kehlkopfmuskeln/-muskulatur.
extrinsic pathway → extrinsic system.
extrinsic protein äußeres/peripheres (Membran-)Protein nt.
extrinsic reflex Fremdreflex m.
extrinsic system hema. Extrinsic-System nt.
ex·tro·gas·tru·la·tion [ˌekstrəʊˌgæstruː'leɪʃn] n embryo. Extrogastrulation f.
ex·tro·phia [ɪk'strəʊfɪə] n → exstrophy.
ex·tro·ver·sion [ˌekstrəʊ'vɜrʒn] n **1.** ortho. Auswärtsdrehung f, -wendung f, Extroversion f, Extraversion f. **2.** psychia. Extraversion f, Extravertiertheit f, Extroversion f.
ex·tro·vert ['-vɜrt] **I** n extravertierter Mensch m, Extravertierte(r m) f. **II** adj **1.** ortho. nach außen gedreht, extra-, extrovertiert. **2.** psychia. nach außen gewandt, (welt-)offen, extra-, extrovertiert. **III** vt **3.** ortho. nach außen drehen od. wenden, extra-, extrovertieren. **4.** psychia. nach außen wenden, s. der äußeren Welt zuwenden, extra-, extrovertieren.
ex·trude [ɪk'struːd] **I** vt ausstoßen, (her-)auspressen. **II** vi (her-)vorstehen (from aus).
ex·tru·sion [ɪk'struːʒn] n **1.** (a. fig.) (Her-)Ausstoßung f, (Her-)Ausstoßen nt. **2.** dent. Expulsion f, Extrusion f. **3.** physiol. (Sekret) Ausschleusung f, Extrusion f; Expulsion f.
ex·tu·bate [ek'st(j)uːbeɪt] vt einen Tubus entfernen, extubieren.
ex·tu·ba·tion [ˌekst(j)uː'beɪʃn] n Tubusentfernung f, Extubieren nt, Extubation f.
ex·u·ber·ant [ɪg'zuːbərənt] adj **1.** üppig, (über-)reichlich. **2.** patho. (Wachstum) übermäßig, stark wuchernd.
ex·u·date ['eksjʊdeɪt] n patho. Exsudat nt, Ausschwitzung f.
ex·u·da·tion [ˌeksjʊ'deɪʃn] n **1.** → exudate. **2.** patho. Ausschwitzung f, Ausschwitzen nt, Exsudation f.
ex·u·da·tive [ɪg'zuːdətɪv] adj Exsudat od. Exsudation betr., exsudativ.
exudative angina Croup m, Krupp m.
exudative arthritis exsudative Arthritis f, Arthritis exsudativa.
exudative ascites exsudativer Aszites m, Aszites m durch Exsudat.
exudative bronchitis kruppöse/membranöse/pseudomembranöse Bronchitis f, Bronchitis crouposa/fibrinosa/plastica/pseudomembranacea.
exudative calcifying fasciitis Kalzinose f, Calcinosis f.
exudative choroiditis ophthal. exsudative Chorioiditis f.
exudative diathesis exsudative Diathese f.
exudative discoid and lichenoid dermatitis derm. exsudative diskoide lichenoide Dermatitis f, oid-oid-disease (nt).
exudative enteropathy exsudative Enteropathie f.
exudative glomerulonephritis exsudative Glomerulonephritis f.
exudative inflammation exsudative Entzündung f.
exudative nephritis exsudative Nephritis f.
exudative neurodermatitis nummuläres/mikrobielles/nummulär-mikrobielles/parasitäres/diskoides Ekzem nt, bakterielles Ekzematoid nt, Dermatitis nummularis, Eccema nummularis.
exudative pleurisy/pleuritis exsudative Rippenfellentzündung/Pleuritis f, Pleuri-

tis exsudativa.
exudative retinitis/retinopathy ophthal. Coats-Syndrom nt, Retinitis exsudativa.
exudative tuberculosis exsudative Form/Phase f der Lungentuberkulose.
ex·um·bil·i·ca·tion [eksəmˌbɪlə'keɪʃn] n → exomphalos.
ex·u·vi·ate [ɪg'zuːvɪeɪt] (Haut) **I** vt abstreifen, (ab-)schälen. **II** vi s. schälen, s. häuten.
eye [aɪ] n **1.** Auge nt; anat. Oculus nt. **2.** (Nadel-)Öhr nt, Öse f. **3.** bot. Auge nt, Knospe f.
eye·ball ['aɪbɔːl] n Augapfel m, Bulbus m (oculi).
eyeball compression reflex → eyeball-heart reflex.
eyeball-heart reflex okulokardialer Reflex m, Bulbusdruckreflex m, Aschner--Dagnigni-Bulbusdruckversuch m.
eye bank Augenbank f.
eye bath ophthal. Augenbad nt.
eye·brow ['aɪbraʊ] n **1.** (Augen-)Braue f, Supercilium nt. **2.** Augenbrauenhaare pl, Supercilia pl.
eye center, occipital okzipitales Blickzentrum nt.
eye chart ophthal. Seh(proben)tafel f.
eye·cup ['aɪkʌp] n **1.** Augenschale f, -schälchen nt. **2.** embryo. Augenbecher m, Caliculus ophthalmicus.
eyed [aɪd] adj **1.** -äugig. **2.** mit Öse(n) (versehen).
eye doctor 1. Augenarzt m, -ärztin f, Ophthalmologe f, -login f. **2.** Optometrist(in f) m.
eye douche ophthal. **1.** Augenbad nt. **2.** Augendusche f.
eye drops Augentropfen pl.
eye·fold ['aɪfəʊld] n → epicanthus.
eye forceps ophthal. Augenpinzette f.
eye·glass ['aɪglæs, -glɑːs] n **1.** Monokel nt. **2. pair of ~es** Brille f. **3.** → eyepiece.
eye gnats micro. Hippelates pl.
eye·ground ['aɪgraʊnd] n Augenhintergrund m, Fundus m (oculi).
eye·hole ['aɪhəʊl] n **1.** Guckloch nt. **2.** anat. Augenhöhle f, Orbita f, Cavitas orbitale.
eye·lash ['aɪlæʃ] n (Augen-)Wimper f, Cilium nt.
eye lens Okular(linse f) nt.
eye·less ['aɪlɪs] adj **1.** blind. **2.** augenlos, ohne Augen.
eye level Augenhöhe f. **on ~** auf Augenhöhe.
eye·lid ['aɪlɪd] n (Augen-)Lid nt, Palpebra f.
eyelid closure reflex Korneal-, Blinzel-, Lidreflex m.
eyelid swelling Lidschwellung f.
eye lotion → eyewash.
eye memory visuelles/ikonisches Gedächtnis nt.
eye-minded adj mit visueller Erinnerung begabt, (Typ) visuell.
eye movement Augenbewegung f.
conjugated e. konjugierte Augenbewegung.
reflex e. reflektorische Augenbewegung.
eye muscle 1. Augenmuskel m. **2. ~s** pl (äußere) Augenmuskeln pl, Mm. bulbi.
eye-muscle nuclei (ZNS) Augenmuskelkerne pl.
eye-muscle paralysis Augenmuskellähmung f, -parese f.
eye patch Augenklappe f.
eye·piece ['aɪpiːs] n Okular nt.
eye·pit ['aɪpɪt] n anat. Augenhöhle f, Orbita f, Cavitas orbitale.
eye protector Augenklappe f, -schützer m.
eye reflex Fundusreflex m.

eye·shot ['aɪʃɒt] *n* Seh-, Sichtweite *f*. **(with-)in ~/out of ~** in/außer Sichtweite.
eye·sight ['aɪsaɪt] *n* Sehkraft *f*, -leistung *f*, -vermögen *nt*, Visus naturalis; Sehen *nt*. **to have good/poor ~** gute/schwache Augen haben. **to loose one's ~** das Augenlicht verlieren, erblinden.
eyesight test Sehtest *m*, Seh(schärfen)prüfung *f*; Augenuntersuchung *f*.
eye socket → eyepit.
eye speculum *ophthal.* Lidhalter *m*, Blepharostat *m*.
eye·strain ['aɪstreɪn] *n* Ermüdung *od.* Überanstrengung *f* der Augen, Asthenopie *f*.
eye·tooth ['aɪtuːθ] *n* Eck-, Reißzahn *m*, Dens caninus.
eye·wash ['aɪwɒʃ, -wɔʃ] *n pharm.* Augenwasser *nt*, Kollyrium *nt*, Collyrium *nt*.
eye worm *micro.* Augenwurm *m*, Wander-, Taglarvenfilarie *f*, Loa loa *f*.

F

F *abbr.* 1. → Fahrenheit. 2. → farad. 3. → Faraday's constant. 4. → fluorine.
f *abbr.* 1. → femto-. 2. → foot 4.
F₀ *abbr.* → oligomycin-sensitivity-conferring factor.
F₁ *abbr.* → filial generation 1.
F₂ *abbr.* → filial generation 2.
F I *abbr.* → factor I 1.
F II *abbr.* → factor II.
F III *abbr.* → factor III.
F IV *abbr.* → factor IV.
F V *abbr.* → factor V 1.
F VI *abbr.* → factor VI.
F VII *abbr.* → factor VII.
F VIII *abbr.* → factor VIII.
F IX *abbr.* → factor IX.
F X *abbr.* → factor X 1.
F XI *abbr.* → factor XI.
F XII *abbr.* → factor XII.
F XIII *abbr.* → factor XIII.
FA *abbr.* → fatty acid.
Fab *abbr.* → Fab fragment.
F(ab')₂ *abbr.* → F(ab')₂ fragment.
fa·bel·la [fə'belə] *n, pl* **-lae** [-li:] *anat.* Fabella *f.*
Faber ['fɑːbər]: **F.'s anemia/syndrome** Faber'-Anämie *f*, Chloranämie *f.*
Fab fragment *abbr.* **Fab** antigenbindendes Fragment *nt*, Fab-Fragment *nt abbr.* Fab.
F(ab')₂ fragment *abbr.* **F(ab')₂** F(ab')₂-Fragment *nt abbr.* F(ab')₂.
fa·bism ['feɪbɪzəm] *n* → favism.
FABP *abbr.* → fatty-acid binding protein.
fab·ri·ca·tion [ˌfæbrɪ'keɪʃn] *n* → fabulation.
Fabricius [fə'brɪʃ(ɪ)əs]: **bursa of F.** Bursa Fabricii.
Fabry ['fæbrɪ, 'fɑː-]: **F.'s disease** Fabry-Syndrom *nt*, Morbus Fabry *m*, hereditäre Thesaurismose *f* Ruiter-Pompen-Weyers, Ruiter-Pompen-Weyers-Syndrom *nt*, Thesaurismosis hereditaria lipoidica, Angiokeratoma corporis diffusum (Fabry), Angiokeratoma universale.
fab·u·la·tion [ˌfæbjə'leɪʃn] *n psychia.* Fabulieren *nt.*
face [feɪs] *n* **1.** Gesicht *nt*; *anat.* Facies *f.* **2.** Gesichtsausdruck *m*, Miene *f.* Grimasse *f.* **3.** Außenfläche *f*, Vorderseite *f*; *anat.* Facies *f.* **4.** *mathe.* (geometrische) Fläche *f.*
face·ache ['feɪseɪk] *n* Gesichtsschmerz *m*; Trigeminusneuralgie *f.*
face-centred *adj chem., phys.* flächenzentriert.
face-lift I *n* Gesichts(haut)straffung *f*, Facelifting *nt.* **to have a ~** s. das Gesicht liften lassen. II *vt* ein Facelifting durchführen, liften.
face lifting → face-lift I.
face mask *chir.* Mundschutz *m.*
face mite *micro.* Haarbalgmilbe *f*, Demodex folliculorum.
face pack (kosmetische) Gesichtspackung *f*, -maske *f.*

face phenomenon *neuro.* Chvostek-Zeichen *nt.*
face powder Gesichtspuder *m.*
face presentation *gyn.* Gesichtslage *f.*
fac·et ['fæsɪt] *n* **1.** (kleine) Fläche *f*, Facette *f.* **2.** Gelenkfacette *f.* **3.** *fig.* Seite *f*, Aspekt *m.*
facet articulation (of vertebrae) Zwischenwirbelgelenk *nt*, Intervertebralgelenk *nt*, Artic. intervertebralis.
fac·e·tec·to·my [ˌfæsɪ'tektəmɪ] *n ortho.*, *neurochir.* Facettektomie *f.*
fac·et·ed ['fæsətɪd] *adj* facettiert, Facetten-.
facet joint (of vertebrae) → facet articulation (of vertebrae).
fa·cette [fɑː'set] *n* → facet.
faci- *pref.* → facio-.
fa·cial ['feɪʃl] I *n* (kosmetische) Gesichtsbehandlung *f.* II *adj* Gesicht betr., zum Gesicht gehörend, fazial, facial, Gesichts-.
facial and masticatory muscles Gesichts- u. Kaumuskeln *pl*, Gesichts- u. Kaumuskulatur *f*, Mm. faciales et masticatorii.
facial anesthesia *neuro.* Sensibilitätsstörung *f* bei Fazialisparese.
facial artery 1. Gesichtsschlagader *f*, Facialis *f*, A. facialis. **2.** *old* → carotid artery, external.
   deep f. *old* → maxillary artery.
   transverse f. quere Gesichtsschlagader, Transversa *f* faciei, A. transversa faciei/ facialis.
facial atrophy *neuro.* Romberg(-Parry)-Syndrom *nt*, Romberg-Trophoneurose *f*, progressive halbseitige Gesichtsatrophie *f*, Hemiatrophia faciei/facialis progressiva, Atrophia (hemi-)facialis.
   progressive unilateral f. → facial atrophy.
facial bones Gesichtsknochen *pl*, Ossa faciei/facialia.
facial burn Gesichtsverbrennung *f*, Verbrennung im Gesicht.
facial canal Fazialiskanal *m*, Canalis facialis.
facial cleft *embryo.* Gesichtsspalte *f*, Fissura facialis, Prosoposchisis *f.*
   lateral f. laterale Gesichtsspalte.
   median f. mediane Gesichtsspalte.
   oblique f. schräge Gesichtsspalte/Wangenspalte, Meloschisis *f.*
   transverse f. → lateral f.
facial colliculus Fazialishügel *m*, Colliculus facialis.
facial deformity Gesichtsdeformität *f.*
facial diplegia *neuro.* Lähmung *f* beider Gesichtshälften, Diplegia facialis.
facial edema Gesichtsödem *nt.*
facial eminence → facial colliculus.
facial expression Gesichtsausdruck *m*, Mimik *f.*
facial fracture *ortho.* Fraktur *f* des Gesichtsschädels.
facial hairs Gesichtshaare *pl.*
facial hemiatrophy → facial atrophy.
facial hemiplegia Halbseitenlähmung *f* des Gesichts, faziale Hemiplegie *f.*

facial hillock → facial colliculus.
facial injury Gesichtsverletzung *f.*
fa·ci·a·lis phenomenon [feɪʃɪ'eɪlɪs] *neuro.* Chvostek-Zeichen *nt.*
facial massage Gesichtsmassage *f.*
facial muscles Gesichtsmuskulatur *f*, mimische Muskulatur *f*, Mm. faciales.
facial nerve Fazialis *m*, VII. Hirnnerv *m*, N. facialis [VII]; N. intermediofacialis.
facial nerve neuroma Fazialisneurinom *nt.*
facial nerve palsy → facial paralysis.
facial nerve paralysis → facial paralysis.
facial neuralgia Trigeminusneuralgie *f*, Neuralgia trigeminalis.
facial neuroma → facial nerve neuroma.
facial pack → face pack.
facial pain Gesichtsschmerz *m.*
   mandibular f. mandibulärer Gesichtsschmerz.
   odontogenous f. dentogener Gesichtsschmerz.
facial palsy → facial paralysis.
facial paralysis Fazialislähmung *f*, -parese *f*, Gesichtslähmung *f*, Fazioplegie *f*, Prosopoplegie *f.*
   central f. zentrale Fazialislähmung.
   otogenic f. otogene Fazialislähmung.
   peripheral f. periphere Fazialislähmung.
   traumatic f. traumatische Fazialislähmung.
   unilateral f. Bell-Lähmung, einseitige Fazialislähmung.
facial plexus vegetativer Plexus *m* der A. facialis.
facial prominences *embryo.* Gesichtswülste *pl.*
facial reflex bulbomimischer Reflex *m*, Mondonesi-Reflex *m.*
facial regions Gesichtsregionen *pl*, Regiones faciales.
facial root Fazialiswurzel *f*, Radix n. facialis.
facial sign *neuro.* Chvostek-Zeichen *nt.*
facial spasm Bell-Spasmus *m*, Fazialiskrampf *m*, Fazialis-Tic *m*, Gesichtszucken *nt*, mimischer Gesichtskrampf *m*, Tic convulsif/facial.
facial tic → facial spasm.
facial trauma Gesichtsverletzung *f.*
facial trophoneurosis → facial hemiatrophy.
facial vein Gesichtsvene *f*, V. facialis.
   anterior/common f. → facial vein.
   deep f. tiefe Gesichtsvene, V. profunda facialis/faciei.
   posterior f. V. retromandibularis.
   transverse f. quere Gesichtsvene, Begleitvene der A. transversa faciei, V. transversa facialis/faciei.
fa·ci·es ['feɪʃiːz, 'fæʃ-] *n, pl* **facies 1.** *anat.* Gesicht *nt*, Facies *f.* **2.** *anat.* Außenfläche *f*, Vorderseite *f*, Facies *f.* **3.** Gesichtsausdruck *m*, Miene *f.*
fa·cil·i·tate [fə'sɪlɪteɪt] *vt* erleichtern, fördern, ermöglichen.

facilitated diffusion 282

fa·cil·i·tat·ed diffusion [fə'sılıteıtıd] erleichterte/katalysierte/vermittelte Diffusion *f*.
facilitated transport vermittelter/erleichterter Transport *m*.
fa·cil·i·ta·tion [fə,sılı'teıʃn] *n* **1.** *physiol.* Bahnung *f*, Facilitation *f*. **2.** Förderung *f*, Erleichterung *f*.
fa·cil·i·ties [fə'sılıti:s] *pl* Einrichtung(en *pl*) *f*, Anlage(n *pl*) *f*.
fa·cil·i·tor·y [fı'sılətɔ:riː, -təʊ-] *adj* erleichternd, fördernd.
facio- *pref.* Gesichts-, Fazi(o)-.
fa·ci·o·bra·chi·al [,feıʃıəʊ'breıkıəl] *adj* Gesicht u. Arm betr., faziobrachial.
fa·ci·o·ceph·a·lal·gia [,-,sefə'læld3(ı)ə] *n neuro.* Gesichtsneuralgie *f*, Neuralgie *f* der Gesichtsnerven.
fa·ci·o·cer·vi·cal [,-'sɜːvɪkl] *adj* Gesicht u. Hals betr., faziozervikal.
fa·ci·o·dig·i·to·gen·i·tal dysplasia/syndrome [,-,dıdʒıtə'dʒenıtl] Aarskog-Syndrom *nt*.
fa·ci·o·fa·cial anastomosis [,-'feıʃl] *neurochir.* faziofaziale Anastomose *f*.
fa·ci·o·gen·i·tal dysplasia [,-'dʒenıtl] Arskog-Syndrom *nt*.
fa·ci·o·lin·gual [,-'lıŋɡwəl] *adj* Gesicht u. Zunge betr., faziolingual.
fa·ci·o·plas·ty [,-'plæstı] *n chir.* Gesichtsplastik *f*.
fa·ci·o·ple·gia [,-'pliːdʒ(ı)ə] *n* → facial paralysis.
fa·ci·o·scap·u·lo·hu·mer·al [,-,skæpjələʊ'h(j)uːmərəl] *adj* Gesicht, Schulterblatt u. Arm betr., fazio-skapulo-humeral.
facioscapulohumeral (muscular) atrophy/dystrophy Landouzy-Déjérine-Krankheit *f*, -Syndrom *nt*, -Typ *m*, fazio-skapulo-humerale Muskeldystrophie *f*.
fa·ci·o·ste·no·sis [,-stı'nəʊsıs] *n embryo.* Faziostenose *f*.
F-actin *n* fibrilläres Aktin *nt*, F-Aktin *nt*.
fac·ti·tial [fæk'tıʃl] *adj* künstlich herbeigeführt *od.* erzeugt.
factitial dermatitis Dermatitis artefacta.
factitial proctitis/rectitis *radiol.* Strahlenproktitis *f*.
fac·ti·tious [fæk'tıʃəs] *adj* künstlich (erzeugt), artifiziell, nicht natürlich.
factitious disorder factitious disorder/disease (*nt*).
factitious melanin Melanoid *nt*.
factitious urticaria *derm.* **1.** Hautschrift *f*, Dermographie *f*, -graphia *f*, -graphismus *m*. **2.** dermographische Urtikaria *f*, Urticaria factitia.
fac·tor ['fæktər] *n* **1.** *hema.*, *immun.* Faktor *m*. **2.** Erbfaktor *m*. **3.** Faktor *m*, (maßgebender) Umstand *m*, bestimmendes Element *nt*.
factor I 1. *abbr.* **F I** Fibrogen *nt*, Faktor I *m abbr.* F I. **2.** *immun.* C3b-Inaktivator *m abbr.* C3b-INA, Faktor I *m*.
factor I deficiency Fibrinogenmangel *m*, Hypofibrinogenämie *f*; Afibrinogenämie *f*.
factor II *abbr.* **F II** Prothrombin *nt*, Faktor II *m abbr.* F II.
factor II deficiency Faktor II-Mangel *m*, Hypoprothrombinämie *f*.
factor III *abbr.* **F III** Gewebsthromboplastin *nt*, Faktor III *m abbr.* F III.
factor IV *abbr.* **F IV** Kalcium *nt*, Calzium *nt*, Faktor IV *m abbr.* F IV.
factor V 1. *abbr.* **F V** Proakzelerin *nt*, Proaccelerin *nt*, Acceleratorglobulin *nt*, labiler Faktor *m*, Faktor V *m abbr.* F V. **2.** *micro.* (Wachstums-)Faktor V *m*.
factor V deficiency Parahämophilie (A) *f*,

Owren-Syndrom *nt*, Faktor V-Mangel-(krankheit *f*) *m*, Hypoproakzelerinämie *f*, Hypoproaccelerinämie *f*.
factor VI *abbr.* **F VI** Accelerin *nt*, Akzelerin *nt*, Faktor VI *m abbr.* F VI.
factor VII *abbr.* **F VII** Prokonvertin *nt*, -convertin *nt*, Faktor VII *m abbr.* F V II, Autothrombin I *nt*, Serum-Prothrombin-Conversion-Accelerator *m abbr.* SPCA, stabiler Faktor *m*.
factor VII deficiency Faktor VII-Mangel, Hypoproconvertinämie *f*, Hypoprokonvertinämie *f*, Parahämophilie B *f*.
factor VIII *abbr.* **F VIII** antihämophiles Globulin *nt abbr.* AHG, Antihämophiliefaktor *m abbr.* AHF, Faktor VIII *m abbr.* F VIII.
factor VIII-associated antigen Faktor VIII-assoziiertes-Antigen *nt*, von Willebrand-Faktor *m abbr.* vWF.
factor VIII: vWF → factor VIII-associated antigen.
factor IX *abbr.* **F IX** Faktor IX *m abbr.* F IX, Christmas-Faktor *m*, Autothrombin II *nt*.
factor IX complex Faktor IX-Komplex *m*.
factor IX deficiency Hämophilie B *f*, Christmas-Krankheit *f*, Faktor IX-Mangel(krankheit *f*) *m*.
factor X 1. *abbr.* **F X** Faktor X *m abbr.* F X, Stuart-Prower-Faktor *m*, Autothrombin III *nt*. **2.** *micro.* (Wachstums-)Faktor X *m*.
factor X deficiency Faktor X-Mangel *m*.
factor XI *abbr.* **F XI** Faktor XI *m abbr.* F XI, Plasmathromboplastinantecedent *m abbr.* PTA, antihämophiler Faktor C *m*, Rosenthal-Faktor *m*.
factor XI deficiency Faktor XI-Mangel, PTA-Mangel *m*.
factor XII *abbr.* **F XII** Faktor XII *m abbr.* F XII, Hageman-Faktor *m*.
factor XII deficiency Hageman-Syndrom *nt*, Faktor XII-Mangel(krankheit *f*) *m*.
factor XIII *abbr.* **F XIII** Faktor XIII *m abbr.* F XIII, fibrinstabilisierender Faktor *m abbr.* FSF, Laki-Lorand-Faktor F *m abbr.* LLF.
factor analysis *stat.* Faktoranalyse *f*.
factor B *immun.* C3-Proaktivator *m*, Faktor B *m*, glycinreiches Beta-Globulin *nt abbr.* GBG.
factor D *immun.* C3-Proaktivatorkonvertase *f*, Faktor D *m*.
factor h 1. *immun.* Faktor H *m*. **2.** Biotin *nt*, Vitamin H *nt*.
fac·to·ri·al [fæk'tɔːrɪəl, -'təʊr-] **I** *n mathe.* Fakultät *f*. **II** *adj* faktoriell, in Faktoren zerlegt, nach Faktoren aufgeschlüsselt.
factor P Properdin *nt*.
factor S Biotin *nt*, Vitamin H *nt*.
fac·ul·ta·tive ['fækəltətıv] *adj* **1.** *bio.* fakultativ. **2.** freigestellt, wahlweise, fakultativ.
facultative aerobe *bio.* fakultativer Aerobier *m*.
facultative anaerobe *bio.* fakultativer Anaerobier *m*.
facultative parasite fakultativer Parasit *m*.
fac·ul·ty ['fækəltı] *n*, *pl* **-ties 1.** Fähigkeit *f*, Vermögen *nt*, Kraft *f*. **2.** Begabung *f*, Talent *nt*, Gabe *f*. **3.** (*Universität*) Fakultät *f*.
  f. of hearing Hörvermögen.
  the medical f. die medizinische Fakultät.
  f. of smell Sehvermögen.
  f. of speech Sprech-, Sprachvermögen.
  f. of thought Denkvermögen.
FAD *abbr.* → flavin adenine dinucleotide.
fae·cal *adj Brit.* → fecal.
fae·ces *pl Brit.* → feces.

fag·o·py·rism [,fæɡəʊ'paırızəm] *n* Buchweizenkrankheit *f*, -ausschlag *m*, Fagopyrismus *m*.
fag·o·py·ris·mus [,-paı'rızməs] *n* → fagopyrism.
Fahr [fær; faːr]: **F.'s disease/syndrome** Fahr-Krankheit *f*, -Syndrom *nt*.
Fahraeus-Lindqvist [fɑː'reıəs, 'lındkwıst]: **F.-L. effect** Sigma-Effekt *m*, Fahraeus--Lindqvist-Effekt *m*.
Fahrenheit ['færənhaıt] *abbr.* **F** Fahrenheit *nt abbr.* F.
  F. scale Fahrenheit-Skala *f*.
  F. thermometer Fahrenheit-Thermometer *nt*.
Fahr-Volhard ['fɑːlhɑːrt; 'fɔlhaːrt]: **F.-V. disease** Fahr-Volhard-Nephrosklerose *f*, maligne Nephrosklerose *f*.
fail [feıl] **I** *vt* **1.** jdm. fehlen. **2.** (*Prüfung*) jdn. durchfallen lassen; durchfallen. **II** *vi* **3.** (*Funktion*) abnehmen, schwächer werden; versagen. **4.** fehlschlagen, scheitern, mißlingen. **5.** verfehlen, versäumen, unterlassen. **6.** fehlgehen, irren. **7.** (*Prüfung*) durchfallen.
fail·ing ['feılıŋ] **I** *n* Fehler *m*, Schwäche *f*. **II** *adj* (*Funktion*) nachlassend.
fail·ure ['feıljər] *n* **1.** *patho.* Versagen *nt*, Störung *f*, Insuffizienz. **2.** Fehlen *nt*, Nichtvorhandensein *nt*. **3.** Versiegen *nt*; Ausbleiben *nt*, Nichteintreten *nt*. **4.** Unterlassung *f*, Versäumnis *nt*. **5.** *techn.* Störung *f*, Defekt *m*. **6.** Fehlschlag *m*, Mißerfolg *m*; Scheitern *nt*, Mißlingen *nt*. **7.** (*Prüfung*) Durchfallen *nt*.
  f. of speech Sprachversagen, Aphasie *f*.
  f. to thrive *ped.* Gedeihstörung.
faint [feınt] **I** *n* Ohnmacht *f*, Ohnmachtsanfall *m*, Synkope *f*. **II** *adj* **1.** schwach, matt, kraftlos (*with* vor). **2.** (*Ton, Farbe*) schwach, matt. **III** *vi* ohnmächtig werden, in Ohnmacht fallen (*with, from* vor).
fair-skinned *adj* hellhäutig.
fal·cate ['fælkeıt] *adj* → falciform.
fal·cial ['fælʃl, -tʃl] *adj anat.* Falx betr., Falx-.
fal·ci·form ['fælsıfɔːrm] *adj anat.* sichelförmig, falciform, Sichel-.
falciform cartilage (*Kniegelenk*) Innenmeniskus *m*, Meniscus medialis artic. genus.
falciform hymen *gyn.* sichelförmiges Hymen *nt*, Hymen falciformis.
falciform ligament (of liver) sichelförmiges Leberband *nt*, Lig. falciforme (hepatis).
falciform margin: f. of fascia lata → f. of hiatus saphenous.
  f. of hiatus saphenous sichelförmiger Rand *m* der Fascia lata, Margo falciformis fasciae latae, Margo falciformis (hiatus saphenus).
  f. of white line of pelvic fascia Arcus tendineus fasciae pelvis.
falciform process Proc. falciformis.
  f. of cerebellum Kleinhirnsichel *f*, Falx cerebelli.
  f. of cerebrum (Groß-)Hirnsichel *f*, Falx cerebri.
fal·cine ['fælsıːn] *adj* → falcial.
fal·cip·a·rum fever/malaria [fæl'sıpərəm] Falciparum-Malaria *f*, Tropen-, Aestivoautumnalfieber *nt*, Malaria tropica.
fal·cu·la ['fælkjələ] *n* → falx cerebri.
fal·cu·lar ['fælkjələr] *adj* **1.** → falcial. **2.** → falciform.
fall [fɔːl] (*v* fell; fallen) **I** *n* **1.** Fall *m*, Sturz *m*; Fallen *nt*. **2.** (*Temperatur*) Sinken *nt*, Abnehmen *nt*, Abfallen *nt*. **3.** Abfall *m*, Gefälle *nt*, Neigung *f*. **4.** Herbst *m*. **5.** Zusammenbrechen, Einsturz *m*. **6.** *fig.* Nieder-, Untergang *m*, Verfall *m*. **II** *vi* **7.** (ab-)fallen; (um-, hin-, nieder-, herun-

ter-)fallen; (ab-, um-)stürzen. 8. *(Temperatur)* (ab-)fallen, abnehmen, sinken. 9. *(zeitlich)* eintreten.
fall behind *vi* zurückbleiben *od.* -fallen hinter.
fall down *vi* hin(unter)fallen, herunterfallen; umfallen; einstürzen.
fall in *vi* einfallen, einstürzen.
fall off *vi* abfallen.
fall out *vi* 1. herausfallen. 2. *fig.* ausfallen, ausgehen, s. erweisen als. 3. s. ereignen, geschehen.
fall over *vi* hin-, umfallen, stürzen; umkippen.
fall through *vi (a. fig.)* durchfallen.
fall·ing of the womb ['fɔ:lɪŋ] *gyn.* Gebärmuttersenkung *f*, Descensus uteri.
falling sickness Epilepsie *f*, Epilepsia *f*.
fal·lo·pi·an [fə'ləʊpɪən]: **f. aqueduct/arch** → f. canal.
f. artery Gebärmutter-, Uterusschlagader *f*, Uterina *f*, A. uterina.
f. canal Fazialiskanal *m*, Canalis facialis.
f. hiatus Hiatus canalis n. petrosi majoris.
f. ligament Leistenband *nt*, Arcus/Lig. inguinale.
f. neuritis Fazialislähmung *f*, -parese *f*, Gesichtslähmung *f*, Fazioplegie *f*, Prosopoplegie *f*.
f. pregnancy Eileiter-, Tuben-, Tubarschwangerschaft *f*, Tubargravidität *f*, Graviditas tubaria.
f. tube Eileiter *m*, Tube *f*, Oviduct *m*, Salpinx *f*, Tuba uterina.
f. valve Bauhin'-Klappe *f*, Ileozäkal-, Ileozökalklappe *f*, Valva ileocaecalis/ ilealis.
Fallopio [fə'ləʊpɪəʊ]: **foramen of F.** Hiatus canalis n. petrosi majoris.
Fallopius [fə'ləʊpɪəs]: **aqueduct of F.** Fazialiskanal *m*, Canalis facialis.
ligament of F. Leistenband *nt*, Arcus/Lig. inguinale.
Fallot [fæ'lo]: **F.'s disease** Fallot'-Tetralogie *f*, -Tetrade *f*, Fallot IV *m*.
pentalogy of F. Fallot'-Pentalogie *f*, Fallot V *m*.
F.'s syndrome/tetrad → F.'s disease.
tetralogy of F. → F.'s disease.
trilogy of F. Fallot'-Trilogie *f*, -Triade *f*, Fallot III *m*.
fall-out ['fɔ:laʊt] *n* 1. *phys.* Fallout *m*, radioaktiver Niederschlag *m*. 2. *fig.* Neben-, Abfallprodukt *nt*. 3. *fig.* (negative) Auswirkungen *pl*.
false [fɔ:ls] *adj* falsch; unwahr; fehlerhaft; unecht, Pseudo-, Schein-.
false albuminuria akzidentelle Albuminurie/Proteinurie *f*.
false aneurysm falsches Aneurysma *nt*, Aneurysma spurium.
f. of heart Herzwand-, Kammerwand-, Ventrikelaneurysma, Aneurysma cordis.
false angina Angina (pectoris) vasomotoria.
false ankylosis fibröse Ankylose *f*, Ankylosis fibrosa.
false anuria falsche Anurie *f*.
false articulation Pseudo-, Falsch-, Scheingelenk *nt*, Pseudarthrose *f*.
false cast *(Harn)* Pseudozylinder *m*, Zylindroid *m*.
false crepitus *ortho.* Gelenkreiben *nt*.
false crisis *(Fieber)* Pseudokrise *f*.
false croup falscher Krupp *m*, Pseudokrupp *m*, subglottische Laryngitis *f*, Laryngitis subglottica.
false cyanosis Pseudozyanose *f*, falsche Zyanose *f*.
false cyst Pseudozyste *f*, falsche Zyste *f*.
false denticle falscher/unechter Dentikel *m*.

false diverticulum falsches Divertikel *nt*, Diverticulum spurium.
false glottis Rima vestibuli.
false hematuria Pseudohämaturie *f*, falsche Hämaturie *f*.
false hermaphroditism falscher Hermaphroditismus *m*, Hermaphroditismus spurius, Pseudohermaphroditismus *m*.
false hypertrophy Pseudohypertrophie *f*.
false joint → false articulation.
false knot 1. *chir.* falscher Knoten *m*, Weiberknoten *m*. 2. *gyn.* falscher Nabelschnurknoten *m*.
false labor *gyn.* Senkwehen *pl*.
false membrane Pseudomembran *f*.
false neck of humerus chirurgischer Humerushals *m*, Collum chirurgicum humeri.
false-negative I *n* falschnegativer Test *m*, falschnegative Reaktion *f*. II *adj* falschnegativ.
false-negative reaction falsch-negative Reaktion *f*.
false neuroma 1. Amputationsneurom *nt*. 2. Neuroma spurium.
false nucleolus Karyosom *nt*.
false pains *gyn.* Senkwehen *pl*.
false paracusis *HNO* Paracusis Willisii.
false paralysis Pseudoparalyse *f*, -paralysis *f*.
false pelvis großes Becken *nt*, Pelvis major.
false-positive I *n* falschpositiver Test *m*, falschpositive Reaktion *f*. II *adj* falschpositiv.
false-positive reaction falsch-positive Reaktion *f*.
false pregnancy *gyn.* Scheinschwangerschaft *f*, Pseudokyesis *f*, Pseudogravidität *f*.
false proteinuria → false albuminuria.
false rib falsche/unechte Rippe *f*, Costa spuria.
false teeth (künstliches) Gebiß *nt*.
false tumor Pseudotumor *m*.
false twins binovuläre/dissimilare/dizygote/erbungleiche/heteroovuläre/zweieiige Zwillinge *pl*.
false vertebrae Vertebrae spuriae.
fal·si·fi·ca·tion [ˌfɔ:lsɪfɪ'keɪʃn] *n (Erinnerung)* (Ver-)Fälschung *f*.
fal·si·fy ['fɔ:lsɪfaɪ] *vt* 1. (ver-)fälschen, falsch *od.* irreführend darlegen. 2. widerlegen.
falx [fælks, fɔ:lks] *n*, *pl* **fal·ces** ['fælsi:z, 'fɔ:l] *anat.* Sichel *f*, sichelförmige Struktur *f*, Falx *f*.
f. of cerebellum Kleinhirnsichel, Falx cerebelli.
f. of cerebrum → falx cerebri.
falx cerebri *anat.* (Groß-)Hirnsichel *f*, Falx cerebri.
fa·mil·ial [fə'mɪljəl] *adj* familiär, Familien-.
familial acholuric jaundice hereditäre Sphärozytose *f*, Kugelzell(en)anämie *f*, Kugelzell(en)ikterus *m*, familiärer hämolytischer Ikterus *m*, Morbus Minkowski-Chauffard *m*.
familial aggregation *epidem.* familiäre Häufung *f*.
familial amyloidosis familiäre/hereditäre Amyloidose *f*.
familial apolipoprotein C-II deficiency → familial hyperlipoproteinemia, type I.
familial ataxia Friedreich-Ataxie *f*, spinale/spinozerebellare Heredoataxie *f*, Heredoataxia spinalis.
familial autonomic dysfunction Riley-Day-Syndrom *nt*, Dysautonomie *f*.
familial benign chronic pemphigus Hailey-Hailey-Syndrom *nt*, -Krankheit *f*, Morbus Hailey-Hailey *m*, familiärer gut-

artiger Pemphigus *m*, Pemphigus chronicus benignus familiaris (Hailey-Hailey), Gougerot-Hailey-Hailey-Krankheit *f*, Pemphigus Gougerot-Hailey-Hailey *m*, Dyskeratosis bullosa (hereditaria).
familial bilateral giant cell tumor Cherubismus *m*, Cherubinismus *m*.
familial broad-beta hyperlipoproteinemia → familial hyperlipoproteinemia, type III.
familial cancer/carcinoma familiär gehäuft auftretendes Karzinom *nt*, familiär gehäuft auftretender Krebs *m*.
familial centrolobar sclerosis Pelizaeus-Merzbacher-Krankheit *f*, -Syndrom *nt*, orthochromatische Leukodystrophie *f*, sudanophile Leukodystrophie *f* Typ Pelizaeus-Merzbacher.
familial chloride diarrhea → familial chloridorrhea.
familial chloridorrhea *ped.* familiäre Chlorverlustdiarrhö *f*, Chlorid-Diarrhö-Syndrom *nt*.
familial cholemia → familial nonhemolytic jaundice.
familial clustering *epidem.* familiäre Häufung *f*.
familial colloid degeneration *ophthal.* Altersdrusen *pl*, Chorioiditis guttata senilis.
familial combined hyperlipidemia 1. → familial hyperlipoproteinemia, type II. 2. → familial hyperlipoproteinemia, type IIb. 3. → familial hyperlipoproteinemia, type IV.
familial combined hyperlipoproteinemia 1. → familial hyperlipoproteinemia, type II. 2. → familial hyperlipoproteinemia, type IIb.
familial dysautonomia Riley-Day-Syndrom *nt*, Dysautonomie *f*.
familial dysbetalipoproteinemia → familial hyperlipoproteinemia, type III.
familial fat-induced hyperlipemia → familial hyperlipoproteinemia, type I.
familial fibrous dysplasia of jaw Cherubismus *m*, Cherubinismus *m*.
familial HDL deficiency Tangier-Krankheit *f*, Analphalipoproteinämie *f*, Hypo-Alpha-Lipoproteinämie *f*.
familial hemophagocytic reticulosis maligne Histiozytose *f*, maligne Retikulohistiozytose *f*, histiozytäre medulläre Retikulose *f*.
familial hepatitis Wilson-Krankheit *f*, -Syndrom *nt*, Morbus Wilson *m*, hepatolentikuläre/hepatozerebrale Degeneration *f*.
familial high density lipoprotein deficiency → familial HDL deficiency.
familial histiocytic reticulosis → familial hemophagocytic reticulosis.
familial hyperbetalipoproteinemia → familial hyperlipoproteinemia, type IIa.
f. and hyperprebetalipoproteinemia → familial hyperlipoproteinemia, type III.
familial hypercholesterolemia → familial hyperlipoproteinemia, type IIa.
f. and hyperlipemia → familial hyperlipoproteinemia, type III.
familial hypercholesteremic xanthomatosis → familial hyperlipoproteinemia, type IIa.
familial hyperchylomicronemia → familial hyperlipoproteinemia, type I.
f. and hyperprebetalipoproteinemia → familial hyperlipoproteinemia, type I.
familial hyperlipoproteinemia primäre/essentielle Hyperlipoproteinämie *f*.
type I f. Bürger-Grütz-Syndrom *nt*, (primäre/essentielle) Hyperlipoproteinämie Typ I, fettinduzierte/exogene Hypertri-

familial hyperparathyroidism

glyzeridämie f, fettinduzierte/exogene Hyperlipämie f, Hyperchylomikronämie f, familiärer C-II-Apoproteinmangel m.
type II f. (primäre/essentielle) Hyperlipoproteinämie Typ II, kombinierte Hyperlipoproteinämie f.
type IIa f. (primäre/essentielle) Hyperlipoproteinämie Typ IIa, essentielle/familiäre Hypercholesterinämie f, primäre Hyperbetalipoproteinämie f, familiäre idiopathische hypercholesterinämische Xanthomatose f, LDL-Rezeptordefekt m.
type IIb f. (primäre/essentielle) Hyperlipoproteinämie Typ IIb, (familiäre) kombinierte Hyperlipidämie f.
type III f. (primäre/essentielle) Hyperlipoproteinämie Typ III, Hypercholesterinämie f mit Hypertriglyzeridämie, Broad-Beta-Disease (nt), Hyperlipoproteinämie mit breiter Betabande.
type IV f. (primäre/essentielle) Hyperlipoproteinämie Typ IV, endogene/kohlenhydratinduzierte Hyperlipidämie/Triglyzeridämie f, familiäre Hypertriglyzeridämie f.
type V f. (primäre/essentielle) Hyperlipoproteinämie Typ V, fett- u. kohlenhydratinduzierte Hyperlipidämie/Hyperlipoproteinämie f, exogen-endogene Hyperlipoproteinämie, kalorisch-induzierte Hyperlipoproteinämie u. Hyperchylomikronämie u. Hyperpräbetalipoproteinämie.
familial hyperparathyroidism familiärer Hyperparathyroidismus m.
familial hypertriglyceridemia 1. → familial hyperlipoproteinemia, type I. **2.** → familial hyperlipoproteinemia, type IV.
familial hypophosphatemia familiäre Hypophosphatämie f, Vitamin D-resistente Rachitis f, (Vitamin D-)refraktäre Rachitis f.
familial immunity angeborene Immunität f.
familial intestinal polyposis → familial polyposis.
familial juvenile nephronophthisis/nephrophthisis familiäre juvenile Nephronophthisis f, hereditäre idiopathische Nephronophthisis f.
familial LCAT deficiency → familial lecithin-cholesterol acyltransferase deficiency.
familial lecithin-cholesterol acyltransferase deficiency Norum-Krankheit f, familiärer primärer LCAT-Mangel m.
familial lipoprotein lipase deficiency 1. → familial hyperlipoproteinemia, type I. **2.** → familial hyperlipoproteinemia, type V.
familial LPL deficiency 1. → familial hyperlipoproteinemia, type I. **2.** → familial hyperlipoproteinemia, type V.
familial Mediterranean fever familiäres Mittelmeerfieber nt, familiäre rekurrente Polyserositis f.
familial metaphyseal dysplasia Pyle'-Krankheit f, familiäre metaphysäre Dysplasie f.
familial myoglobinuria idiopathische/familiäre Myoglobinurie f.
familial nonhemolytic jaundice Meulengracht(-Gilbert)-Krankheit f, -Syndrom nt, intermittierende Hyperbilirubinämie Meulengracht f, Icterus juvenilis intermittens Meulengracht.
familial osseous dystrophy spondyloepiphysäre Dysplasie f, Morquio(-Ullrich)-Syndrom nt, Morquio-Brailsford-Syndrom nt, Mukopolysaccharidose f Typ IV abbr. MPS IV.

familial osteoarthropathy of fingers Thiemann'-Krankheit f.
familial osteochondrodystrophy → familial osseous dystrophy.
familial osteoectasia ortho. juveniler Morbus Paget m, Hyperostosis corticalis deformans juvenilis.
familial paroxysmal polyserositis familiäres Mittelmeerfieber nt, familiäre rekurrente Polyserositis f.
familial periodic paralysis familiäre paroxysmale hypokaliämische Lähmung f.
familial polyposis familiäre Polypose/Polyposis f, Polyposis familiaris, Adenomatosis coli.
familial polyposis syndrome → familial polyposis.
familial recurrent polyserositis → familial Mediterranean fever.
familial splenic anemia Gaucher'-Erkrankung f, -Krankheit f, Gaucher f, Morbus Gaucher m, Glukozerebrosidose f, Zerebrosidlipidose f, Lipoidhistiozytose f vom Kerasintyp, Glykosylzeramidlipidose f.
familial tremor hereditärer/essentieller Tremor m.
familial white folded (mucosal) dysplasia derm. weißer Schleimhautnävus m, Naevus spongiosus albus mucosae.
fam·i·ly ['fæməlɪ] **I** n **1.** Familie f. **2.** bio. Familie f. **II** adj Familien-.
family ataxia → familial ataxia.
family planning Familienplanung f, Geburtenregelung f.
family therapy Familientherapie f.
fam·ine dropsy ['fæmɪn] → famine edema.
famine edema Hungerödem nt.
famine fever Rückfallfieber nt, Febris recurrens.
fa·mo·ti·dine [fə'məʊtɪdiːn] n pharm. Famotidin nt.
Fañanas [fan'janas]: **F. cells/glia** Fañanas-Zellen m.
Fanconi [fæn'kəʊnɪ]: **F.'s anemia** Fanconi-Anämie f, -Syndrom nt, konstitutionelle infantile Panmyelopathie f.
F.'s disease 1. → F.'s anemia. **2.** → F.'s syndrome 2.
F.'s pancytopenia → F.'s anemia.
F.'s syndrome 1. → F.'s anemia. **2.** renal-glykosurische Rachitis f, Fanconi-Syndrom nt. **3.** Debré-de Toni-Fanconi-Syndrom nt.
fan·go ['fæŋgəʊ] n Fango m.
fan·go·ther·a·py [,fæŋgəʊ'θerəpɪ] n Fangobehandlung f, -therapie f.
fan·ta·size ['fæntəsaɪz] **I** vt s. jdn. od. etw. vorstellen. **II** vi **1.** phantasieren (about von). **2.** (tag-)träumen.
fan·tasm ['fæntæzəm] n Wahn-, Trugbild nt, Hirngespinst nt, Sinnestäuschung f, Phantasma f.
fan·tast ['fæntæst] n Träumer m, Phantast m.
fan·ta·sy ['fæntəsɪ] **I** n, pl **-sies 1.** Einbildung(skraft f) f, Vorstellungsvermögen nt, Phantasie f. **2.** Phantasie f, Phantasievorstellung f, -gebilde nt; Hirngespinst nt, Trugbild nt. **3.** Tag-, Wachtraum m. **4.** Phantasieren m. **II** vt, vi → fantasize.
F antigen → Forssman antigen.
Farabeuf [fara'bœf]: **F.'s amputation/operation** ortho. Beinamputation f nach Farabeuf.
far·ad ['færəd] n abbr. **F** Farad nt abbr. F.
far·a·da·ic [færə'deɪɪk] adj → faradic.
Faraday ['færədɪ, -daɪ]: **F.'s cage** Faraday'-Käfig m.
F.'s constant abbr. F Faraday'-Konstante f abbr. F.
F.'s law Faraday'-Gesetz nt.

fa·rad·ic [fə'rædɪk] adj phys. faradisch.
faradic current faradischer Strom m.
far·a·dism ['færədɪzəm] n **1.** → faradic current. **2.** → faradization.
far·a·di·za·tion [,færədɪ'zeɪʃn, -daɪ-] n Behandlung f mit faradischem Strom, Faradisation f, Faradotherapie f.
far·a·do·con·trac·til·i·ty [,færədəʊˌkɒntrækˈtɪlətɪ] n Muskelkontraktion f durch faradischen Strom.
far·a·do·ther·a·py [,-'θerəpɪ] n → faradization.
Farber ['fɑːrbər]: **F.'s disease/lipogranulomatosis** → F.'s syndrome.
F.'s syndrome Farber'-Krankheit f, disseminierte Lipogranulomatose f.
F.'s test ped. Farber-Test m.
Farber-Uzman ['ʊzmən, 'ʌz-]: **F.-U. syndrome** → Farber's syndrome.
far·cy ['fɑːrsɪ] n, pl **-cies** derm. Hautrotz m, Malleus farciminosus.
FA reaction → fluorescent antibody reaction.
Far Eastern hemorrhagic fever [fɑːr] epidemisches hämorrhagisches Fieber nt mit renalem Syndrom abbr. HFRS, koreanisches hämorrhagisches Fieber, hämorrhagische Nephrosonephritis f, Nephropathia epidemica.
Far East Russian encephalitis zentraleuropäische Zeckenenzephalitis f, Frühsommer-Enzephalitis f abbr. FSE, Frühsommer-Meningo-Enzephalitis f abbr. FSME, Central European encephalitis abbr. CEE.
far·i·na·ceous [,færɪ'neɪʃəs] adj **1.** mehlartig, mehlig, Mehl-. **2.** stärkehaltig, Stärke-.
farm·er's lung ['fɑːrmər] Farmerlunge f, Drescherkrankheit f, Dreschfieber nt.
farmer's skin Farmer-, Landmanns-, Seemannshaut f.
far·ne·sene alcohol ['fɑːrnəsiːn] → farnesol.
far·ne·sol ['fɑːrnəsɒl] n Farnesol nt.
far·ne·syl·py·ro·phos·phor·ic acid [,fɑːrnəsɪl,paɪrəfɒs'fɒrɪk] Farnesylpyrophosphorsäure f.
far·no·quin·one [,fɑːrnəʊ'kwɪnəʊn] n Menachinon nt, Vitamin K_2 nt.
far point ophthal. Fernpunkt m, Punctum remotum.
f. of convergence ophthal. Konvergenzfernpunkt.
Farre [feər]: **F.'s white line** Farre-Linie f.
far sight → farsightedness 1.
far·sight·ed [fɑːr'saɪtɪd] adj **1.** weitsichtig, hyperop. **2.** fig. weitblickend, umsichtig.
far·sight·ed·ness ['-nɪs] n **1.** Weitsichtigkeit f, Hyperopie f, Hypermetropie f. **2.** fig. Weitblick m, Umsicht f.
far vision Fernsehen nt, Fern-, Weitsicht f.
fas·ci·a ['fæʃ(ɪ)ə] n, pl **-ci·ae** [-ʃɪˌiː] **1.** anat. Faszie f, Fascia f. **2.** Binde f, Band nt.
f. of arm Oberarmfaszie, Fascia brachii/brachialis.
f. of clitoris Klitoris-, Clitorisfaszie, Fascia clitoridis.
f. of forearm Unterarmfaszie, Fascia antebrachii.
f. of leg oberflächliche Unterschenkelfaszie, Fascia cruris.
f. of nape Fascia nuchae/nuchalis.
f. of neck Halsfaszie, Fascia cervicalis.
f.e of Tenon Fasciae musculares (bulbi).
f. of thigh → fascia lata.
f. of urogenital trigone Urogenitaldiaphragma nt, Diaphragma urogenitale.
fas·ci·al ['fæʃ(ɪ)əl] adj Faszie betr., Faszien-, Faszio-.

fascia lata Oberschenkelfaszie *f*, Fascia lata (femoris).
fascial closure *chir.* Faszienverschluß *m*, -naht *f*.
fascial hernia Faszienbruch *m*, -hernie *f*.
fas·ci·a·plas·ty ['fæʃiəplæsti] *n chir.* Faszienplastik *f*.
fas·ci·cle ['fæsɪkl] *n* (Faser-)Bündel *nt*, Strang *m*, Faszikel *m*, *anat.* Fasciculus *m*.
fas·cic·u·lar [fə'sɪkjələr] *adj* **1.** *anat.* Faszikel betr., faszikulär. **2.** büschelförmig, faszikulär.
fascicular degeneration (*Muskel*) Faszikeldegeneration *f*, -atrophie *f*.
fascicular keratitis *ophthal.* Gefäßbändchen *nt*, Keratitis fascicularis, Wanderphlyktäne *f*.
fascicular repair *neurochir.* perineuriale Nervennaht *f*, Perineuralnaht *f*.
group f. interfaszikuläre Nervennaht.
fascicular sarcoma spindelzelliges Sarkom *nt*, Spindelzellsarkom *nt*.
fascicular zone *histol.* Bündelschicht *f*, Zona fasciculata.
fas·cic·u·late [fə'sɪkjəleɪt, -lɪt] *adj* → fascicular 2.
fas·cic·u·lat·ed ['-leɪtɪd] *adj* → fascicular 2.
fasciculated bladder Balkenblase *f*.
fas·cic·u·la·tion [fə,sɪkjə'leɪʃn] *n* **1.** Faszikelbildung *f*. **2.** faszikuläre Zuckungen *pl*, Faszikulation *f*.
fas·cic·u·lus [fə'sɪkjələs] *n, pl* **-li** [-laɪ] *anat.* kleines Bündel *nt*, Faserbündel *nt*, Muskel-, Nervenfaserbündel *nt*, -faserstrang *m*, Faszikel *m*, Fasciculus *m*.
f. of Burdach Burdach'-Strang, Fasciculus cuneatus (medullae spinalis).
f. of Goll Goll'-Strang, Fasciculus gracilis (medullae spinalis).
f. of Türck Türck'-Bündel *nt*, Tractus temporopontinus.
f. of Vicq d'Azyr Vicq d'Azyr'-Bündel, Fasciculus mamillothalamicus.
fasciculus gracilis: f. of medulla oblongata Fasciculus gracilis medullae oblongatae.
f. of spinal cord Goll'-Strang, Fasciculus gracilis (medullae spinalis).
fas·ci·ec·to·my [,fæʃi'ektəmɪ, ,fæsɪ-] *n ortho.* Faszienexzision *f*, -resektion *f*, Fasziektomie *f*.
fas·ci·i·tis [-'aɪtɪs] *n* Faszienentzündung *f*, Fasziitis *f*.
fas·ci·od·e·sis [,-'ɒdəsɪs] *n ortho.* Fasziodese *f*.
fas·ci·o·gen·ic [,fæsiə'dʒenɪk] *adj* von einer Faszie ausgehend, durch eine Faszie bedingt, fasziogen.
fasciogenic contracture *ortho.* fasziogene Kontraktur *f*.
Fas·ci·o·la [fə'sɪələ, -'saɪ-] *n micro.* Fasciola *f*.
F. gigantica Fasciola gigantica.
F. hepatica großer Leberegel *m*, Fasciola hepatica.
fas·ci·o·la [fə'sɪələ, -'saɪ-] *n, pl* **-las, -lae** [-liː] **1.** *anat.* Bändchen *nt*, Fasciola *f*. **2.** *ortho.* kleiner *od.* schmaler Verband *m*.
fas·ci·o·lar gyrus [fə'sɪələr] Gyrus fasciolaris.
fas·ci·o·li·a·sis [,fæsiəʊ'laɪəsɪs] *n* Leberegelkrankheit *f*, Fasciola-hepatica-Infektion *f*, Fasciola-gigantica-Infektion *f*, Fasziolose *f*, Fasziolosis *f*, Fascioliasis *f*.
fas·ci·o·lid [fə'sɪəlɪd, -'saɪ-] *n micro.* Fasziolid *m*, Fasciolid *m*.
fas·ci·o·lop·si·a·sis [,fæsɪəlɒp'saɪəsɪs] *n* Darmegelkrankheit *f*, Fasziolopsiasis *f*, Fasciolopsiasis *f*.
Fas·ci·o·lop·sis [,-'lɒpsɪs] *n micro.* Fasciolopsis *f*.

F. buski großer Darmegel *m*, Fasciolopsis buski.
fas·ci·o·plas·ty ['fæʃɪəplæstɪ] *n ortho.* Faszienplastik *f*.
fas·ci·or·rha·phy [fæʃɪ'ɔrəfɪ] *n ortho.* Fasziennaht *f*, Fasziorrhaphie *f*.
fas·ci·ot·o·my [fæʃɪ'ɒtəmɪ] *n ortho.* Faszienspaltung *f*, -schnitt *m*, Fasziotomie *f*.
fas·ci·tis [fæ'saɪtɪs] *n* → fasciitis.
fast [fæst, faːst] **I** *n* Fasten *nt*. **II** *adj* **1.** schnell, rasch. **2.** (*Film*) hochempfindlich; (*Linse*) lichtstark. **3.** fest, beständig. **4.** fest; befestigt, festgemacht, sicher. **to make** ~ festmachen, befestigen. **a ~ grip** ein fester Griff. **5.** widerstandsfähig, beständig (*to* gegen). **III** *adv* **6.** schnell, rasch. **7.** fest. **IV** *vi* fasten.
f. to light lichtecht.
fast asleep fest *od.* tief schlafen.
fas·ten [fæsn, faːsn] **I** *vt* **1.** festmachen, befestigen, festbinden (*to* an). **2.** (ver-, ab-)schließen, zumachen. **II** *vi s.* schließen lassen.
fas·ten·er ['fæsənər, 'faː-] *n* Verschluß(vorrichtung *f*) *m*.
fas·ten·ing ['fæsənɪŋ, 'faː-] **I** *n* **1.** Festmachen *nt*, Befestigen *nt*. **2.** → fastener. **II** *adj* Schließ-, Verschluß-, Befestigungs-.
fas·tid·i·ous [fæs'tɪdɪəs, fə-] *adj micro.* anspruchsvoll.
fas·tid·i·um [fæs'tɪdɪəm, fə-] *n* Ekel *m*, Abscheu *m*, Fastidium *n*.
fas·ti·ga·tum [fæstɪ'geɪtəm] *n anat.* Nc. fastigii.
fas·tig·i·al nucleus [fæs'tɪdʒɪəl] *anat.* Nc. fastigii.
fas·tig·i·um [fæs'tɪdʒɪəm] *n, pl* **-i·ums, -gia** [-dʒɪə] *n* **1.** (*ZNS*) Giebelkante *f*, Fastigium *nt*. **2.** (*Fieber, Krankheitsverlauf*) Gipfel *m*, Höhepunkt *m*, Fastigium *nt*.
fast·ing ['fæstɪŋ, 'faːst-] **I** *n* Fasten *nt*. **II** *adj* fastend, Fast-.
fasting cure Fasten-, Hungerkur *f*.
fasting hypoglycemia Fastenhypoglykämie *f*.
fast·ness ['fæstnɪs, 'faːst-] *n* Widerstandsfähigkeit *f*, -kraft *f*, Beständigkeit *f* (*to* gegen); Farb-, Lichtechtheit *f*.
fast sleep fester *od.* tiefer Schlaf *m*.
fast wave sleep REM-Schlaf *m*, Traumschlaf *m*, paradoxer/desynchronisierter Schlaf *m*.
fat [fæt] **I** *n* **1.** Fett *nt*, Lipid *nt*. **2.** Fettgewebe *nt*. **3.** → fatness. **II** *adj* **4.** dick, beleibt, fett(leibig), korpulent, adipös. **5.** fett, fettig, fetthaltig. **6.** *fig.* produktiv, einträglich. **III** *vt* fett(leibig)/dick machen; *biochem.* Fett(e) einbauen. **IV** *vi* fett(leibig)/dick werden.
fat out/up *vt* mästen.
fa·tal ['feɪtl] **I** *n* tödlicher (Verkehrs-)Unfall *m*. **II** *adj* **1.** tödlich, mit tödlichem Ausgang, fatal, letal. **2.** fatal, unheilvoll, verhängnisvoll (*to* für). **3.** unvermeidlich.
fatal disease tödlich verlaufende Erkrankung *f*.
fatal dose tödliche/letale Dosis *f abbr.* LD, ld, Dosis letalis *abbr.* DL, d.l.
fa·tal·i·ty [feɪ'tælɪtɪ] *n* **1.** Verhängnis *nt*; Geschick *nt*; Unglück *nt*, Schicksalsschlag *m*. **2.** (*Krankheit*) tödlicher Verlauf *m*; tödlicher Unfall *m*. **3.** (Todes-)Opfer *nt*.
fatality rate Sterbe-, Sterblichkeitsziffer *f*, -rate *f*, Mortalität *f*, Zahl *f* der Todesfälle.
fat body *anat.* Fettkörper *m*, Corpus adiposum.
f. of cheek Wangenfettpfropf *m*, Bichat'-Fettpfropf *m*, Corpus adiposum buccae.

infrapatellar f. Hoffa'-Fettkörper, Corpus adiposum infrapatellare.
f. of ischiorectal fossa Corpus adiposum fossae ischio-analis.
f. of orbit Corpus adiposum orbitae.
paranephric f. pararenales Fettpolster *m*, pararenaler Fettkörper, Corpus adiposum pararenale.
pararenal f. → paranephric f.
fat breakdown Fettabbau *m*.
fat cell Fettzelle *f*, Adipo-, Lipozyt *m*.
fat cell lipoma *patho.* braunes Lipom *nt*, Hibernom(a) *nt*, Lipoma feto-cellulare.
fat deposition Fetteinlagerung *f*.
fat digestion Fettverdauung *f*, -digestion *f*.
fat embolism Fettembolie *f*.
FA test → fluorescent antibody test.
fat heart 1. Fettherz *nt*, Cor adiposum. **2.** Herzmuskelverfettung *f*.
fa·ther ['fɑːðər] **I** *n* Vater *m*; Vorfahr *m*, Ahn *m*; *bio.* Vatertier *nt*. **II** *adj* Vater-. **III** *vt* **1.** ein Kind zeugen. **2.** die Vaterschaft anerkennen.
father complex *psychia.* Elektra-Komplex *m*.
father-in-law Schwiegervater *m*.
fat hernia → fatty hernia.
fat·i·ga·bil·i·ty [,fætɪgə'bɪlɪtɪ] *n patho.* leichte/schnelle Ermüdbarkeit *f*.
fat·i·ga·ble ['fætɪgəbl] *adj* leicht/schnell ermüdend.
fa·tigue [fə'tiːg] **I** *n* **1.** (*a. techn.*) Ermüdung *f*; Ermattung *f*, Erschöpfung *f*. **2.** Überanstrengung *f*, -müdung *f*. **II** *vt* (*a. techn.*) ermüden; erschöpfen. **III** *vi* (*a. techn.*) ermüden.
fatigue behavior Ermüdungsverhalten *nt*.
fa·tigued [fə'tiːgd] *adj* (*a. techn.*) ermüdet; erschöpft.
fatigue fever Fieber *nt* bei/durch Übermüdung.
fatigue fracture Ermüdungsfraktur *f*, -bruch *m*, Streßfraktur *f*, -bruch *m*.
fatigue neurosis 1. Beard-Syndrom *nt*, Nervenschwäche *f*, nervöse Übererregbarkeit *f*, Neurasthenie *f*, Neurasthenia *f*. **2.** Psychasthenie *f*.
fatigue nystagmus Ermüdungsnystagmus *m*.
fatigue rise *physiol.* Ermüdungsanstieg *m*.
fatigue test Ermüdungsprobe *f*, Dauerprüfung *f*.
fa·ti·guing [fə'tiːgɪŋ] *adj* ermüdend, erschöpfend; anstrengend, strapaziös, mühsam.
fat·less ['fætlɪs] *adj* fettfrei, ohne Fett, mager.
fat·like ['fætlaɪk] *adj* fettartig, -ähnlich, wie Fett.
fat malabsorption Fettmalabsorption *f*.
fat marrow gelbes fetthaltiges Knochenmark *nt*, Fettmark *nt*, Medulla ossium flava.
fat metabolism Fettstoffwechsel *m*, -metabolismus *m*.
fat-mobilizing hormone lipolytisches Hormon *nt*.
fat necrosis Fett(gewebs)nekrose *f*.
subcutaneous f. of the newborn Underwood'-Krankheit *f*, Fettdarre *f*, Sklerem(a) *nt*, Fettsklerem *nt* der Neugeborenen, Sclerema adiposum neonatorum.
fat·ness ['fætnɪs] *n* **1.** Fettleibigkeit *f*, Fettsucht *f*, Obesität *f*, Adipositas *f*, Obesitas *f*. **to run to** ~ Fett ansetzen. **2.** Fettigkeit *f*, Fett-, Ölhaltigkeit *f*.
fat pad Fettpolster *nt*, -pfropf *m*.
buccal f. Wangenfettpfropf, Bichat'-Fettpfropf, Corpus adiposum buccae.
ischiorectal f. Corpus adiposum fossae ischio-analis.

paranephric f. pararenales Fettpolster, pararenaler Fettkörper *m*, Corpus adiposum pararenale.
pararenal f. → paranephric f.
F_1-ATPase *n* Kopplungsfaktor F_1 *m*, F_1-ATPase *f*.
fat phanerosis Lipo-, Fettphanerose *f*.
fat-soluble *adj chem.* fettlöslich.
fat-soluble vitamin fettlösliches Vitamin *nt*.
fat-splitting enzyme Lipase *f*.
fat stain *histol.* Fettfärbung *f*.
fat-storing cell (*Leber*) Fettspeicherzelle *f*.
fat·ten ['fætn] **I** *vt* dick *od.* fett(leibig) machen; mästen. **II** *vi* dick *od.* fett(leibig) werden; s. mästen.
fatten up *vt* → fatten I.
fat·ten·ing ['fætnɪŋ] *adj* (*Essen*) dick machend.
fat tissue Fettgewebe *nt*.
fat tissue necrosis Fettgewebsnekrose *f*.
fat·ty ['fætɪ] *adj* **1.** fett, fettig, fetthaltig, adipös, Fett-. **2.** fett, fettleibig, adipös, Fett-.
fatty acid *abbr.* **FA** Fettsäure *f abbr.* **FS**.
 essential f. *abbr.* **EFA** essentielle Fettsäure.
 even-carbon f. Fettsäure mit gerader Anzahl von C-Atomen.
 free f. *abbr.* **FFA** freie Fettsäure *abbr.* **FFS**, nichtveresterte Fettsäure *abbr.* **NFS**, unveresterte Fettsäure *abbr.* **UFS**.
 α-hydroxy f. α-Hydroxyfettsäure.
 long-chain f. langkettige Fettsäure.
 medium-chain f. mittelkettige Fettsäure.
 monoenoic f. einfach ungesättigte Fettsäure, Monoen(fett)säure.
 monounsaturated f. → monoenoic f.
 nonesterified f. *abbr.* **NEFA** freie Fettsäure *abbr.* **FFS**, nichtveresterte Fettsäure *abbr.* **NFS**, unveresterte Fettsäure *abbr.* **UFS**.
 odd-carbon f. Fettsäure mit ungerader Anzahl von C-Atomen.
 polyenoic f. mehrfach ungesättigte Fettsäure, Polyen(fett)säure.
 polyunsaturated f. → polyenoic f.
 saturated f. gesättigte Fettsäure.
 short-chain f. kurzkettige Fettsäure.
 unesterified f. *abbr.* **UFA** → free f.
 unsaturated f. ungesättigte Fettsäure.
fatty acid activation *biochem.* Fettsäureaktivierung *f*.
fatty-acid binding protein *abbr.* **FABP** Fettsäure-bindendes Protein *nt*.
fatty acid catabolism Fettsäureabbau *m*, -katabolismus *m*.
fatty acid chain Fettsäurekette *f*.
fatty-acid cyclooxygenase Fettsäurezyklooxygenase *f*.
fatty acid ester Fettsäureester *m*.
fatty acid oxidation Fettsäureoxidation *f*.
fatty acid oxidation cycle Zyklus *m* der Fettsäureoxidation, Fettsäurezyklus *m*.
fatty acid peroxidase Fettsäureperoxidase *f*.
fatty acid shuttle Fettsäureshuttle *m*.
fatty acid synthase (**complex**) Fettsäuresynthase(komplex *m*) *f*.
fatty acid synthesis Fettsäuresynthese *f*.
fatty alcohol Fettalkohol *m*.
fatty ascites fettiger/adipöser Aszites *m*.
fatty atrophy fettige Atrophie *f*, Fettinfiltration *f* bei Atrophie.
fatty ball of Bichat → fat body of cheek.
fatty body → fat body.
fatty bone marrow → fat marrow.
fatty capsule of kidney Nierenfettkapsel *f*, perirenale Fettkapsel *f*, Capsula adiposa renis.
fatty cardiopathy *patho.* fettige/verfettende Kardiopathie *f*.
fatty cast (*Harn*) Fettkörnchenzylinder *m*.

fatty change → fatty metamorphosis.
fatty cirrhosis *patho.* Fettzirrhose *f*.
fatty compound *chem.* offene Kette(nverbindung *f*) *f*.
fatty degeneration *patho.* degenerative Verfettung *f*, fettige Degeneration *f*, Degeneratio adiposa.
 f. of liver Leber(epithel)verfettung, fettige Metamorphose/Degeneration der Leber.
 f. of myocardium fettige Herzmuskeldegeneration.
 f. of renal cortex Nierenrindenverfettung.
 renal cortical f. → f. of renal cortex.
fatty diarrhea Fettdurchfall *m*, Steatorrhö *f*, Steatorrhoea *f*.
fatty heart → fat heart.
fatty hepatitis *patho.* Fettleberhepatitis *f*.
fatty granular cell Fettkörnchenzelle *f*.
fatty granule cell → fatty granular cell.
fatty infiltration Fettzelldurchwachsung *f*.
fatty kidney Fettniere *f*.
fatty liver Fettleber *m*, Hepar adiposum.
fatty liver hepatitis Fettleberhepatitis *f*.
fatty marrow → fat marrow.
fatty metamorphosis fettige Metamorphose/Degeneration *f*.
 f. of liver Leber(epithel)verfettung *f*, fettige Metamorphose/Degeneration der Leber.
 central f. of liver zentrale Leberverfettung.
 diffuse f. of liver diffuse Leberverfettung.
 peripheral f. of liver periphere Leberverfettung.
fatty nevus Nävolipom *nt*, Naevus lipomatosus.
fatty stool Fettstuhl *m*.
fatty tissue → fat tissue.
fatty tumor Fettgeschwulst *f*, Lipom *nt*.
fau·ces ['fɔːsiːz] *n, pl* **fau·ces** *anat.* **1.** Schlund *m*, Schlundenge *f*, Fauces *f*. **2.** Rachen *m*, Pharynx *m*.
Fauchard [foʊ'ʃɑːr]: **F.'s disease** Alveolarpyorrhoe *f*, Parodontitis marginalis.
fau·cial ['fɔːʃl] *adj* Schlundengen *od.* Rachen betr., Rachen-, pharyngeal.
faucial cavity Schlund-, Rachenhöhle *f*, Cavitas pharyngis.
faucial diphtheria Rachendiphtherie *f*.
faucial paralysis *HNO* Schlundlähmung *f*, Isthmoplegie *f*.
faucial reflex Würg(e)reflex *m*.
faucial tonsil Gaumenmandel *f*, Tonsilla palatina.
fau·ci·tis [fɔː'saɪtɪs] *n HNO* Faucitis *f*.
fau·na ['fɔːnə] *n, pl* **-nas, -nae** [-niː] *bio.* Fauna *f*.
fa·va ['fɑːvə] *n* Saubohne *f*, Favabohne *f*, Vicia faba.
fa·ve·o·lar [fə'vɪələr] *adj* → foveolar.
fa·ve·o·late [fə'vɪəleɪt, -lɪt] *adj* wabenförmig; alveolär.
fa·ve·o·lus [fə'vɪələs] *n, pl* **-li** [-laɪ] → foveola.
fa·vic chan·de·liers ['fævɪk ˌʃændɪ'lɪər] *micro.* favic chandeliers *pl*.
fa·vid ['fævɪd] *n derm.* Favid *nt*.
fa·vism ['fɑːvɪzəm] *n* Bohnenkrankheit *f*, Favismus *m*, Fabismus *m*.
Favre-Durand-Nicolas ['fɑːvrə dyˈrɑ̃ nikɔ'lɑ]: **F.-D.-N. disease** Morbus Durand-Nicolas-Favre *m*, klimatischer Bubo *m*, vierte Geschlechtskrankheit *f*, Lymphogranuloma inguinale/venereum *abbr.* **LGV**, Lymphopathia venerea, Poradenitis inguinalis.
Favre-Nicolas-Durand: F.-N.-D. disease → Favre-Durand-Nicolas disease.
Favre-Racouchot [rakuˈʃo]: **nodular elastosis of F.-R.** → F.-R. syndrome.
F.-R. syndrome Favre-Racouchot-Krankheit *f*, Elastoidosis cutanea nodularis et cystica.

fa·vus ['feɪvəs] *n derm.* Erb-, Flechten-, Kopf-, Pilzgrind *m*, Favus *m*, Tinea (capitis) favosa, Dermatomycosis favosa.
Fazio-Londe ['fɑːtsɪəʊ, lɔ̃ːnd; 'fazjo]: **F.-L. atrophy** familiär progressive Bulbärparalyse *f*, Fazio-Londe-Syndrom *nt*.
FBC *abbr.* → full blood count.
Fc *abbr.* → Fc fragment.
F cells 1. (*Pankreas*) F-Zellen *pl*. **2.** *bact.* F-Zellen *pl*.
Fc fragment *immun.* kristallisierbares Fragment *nt*, Fc-Fragment *nt abbr.* **Fc**.
Fc receptors Fc-Rezeptoren *pl*.
Fd *abbr.* → Fd fragment.
Fd fragment *abbr.* **Fd** *immun.* Fd-Fragment *nt*.
FDP *abbr.* **1.** [fibrin/fibrinogen degradation products] → fibrinolytic split products. **2.** → flexor digitorum profundus (muscle). **3.** → fructose-1,6-diphosphate.
FDS *abbr.* → flexor digitorum superficialis (muscle).
F-duction *n micro.* Sexduktion *f*, F-Duktion *f*.
Fe *abbr.* [ferrum] → ferrum.
fear [fɪər] **I** *n* **1.** Furcht *f*, Angst *f* (*of* vor; *that* daß). **2.** Befürchtung *f*, Besorgnis *f*, Sorge *f*, Bedenken *pl*. **3.** Gefahr *f*, Risiko *nt*. **II** *vt* (s.) fürchten vor, Angst haben vor. **III** *vi* **4.** s. fürchten, Furcht *od.* Angst haben. **5.** bangen (*for* um).
feb·ri·cant ['febrɪkənt] *n, adj* → febrifacient.
feb·ri·cide ['febrɪsaɪd] **I** *n* fiebersenkendes Mittel *nt*, Antipyretikum *nt*. **II** *adj* fiebersenkend, antipyretisch.
fe·bric·i·ty [fɪ'brɪsətɪ] *n* Fieberhaftigkeit *f*, Fieberzustand *m*, febriler Zustand *m*.
fe·bric·u·la [fɪ'brɪkjələ] *n* leichtes Fieber *nt*, leichte fieberhafte Erkrankung *f*, Febricula *f*.
feb·ri·fa·cient [ˌfebrɪ'feɪʃənt] **I** *n* fiebererzeugendes Mittel *nt*, Pyretikum *nt*, Pyrogen *nt*. **II** *adj* fiebererzeugend, -verursachend, -erregend, pyrogen, pyretisch.
fe·brif·ic [fɪ'brɪfɪk] *adj* → febrifacient II.
fe·brif·u·gal [fɪ'brɪf(j)əgl] *adj* fiebersenkend, -mildernd, -reduzierend, antipyretisch.
feb·ri·fuge ['febrɪfjuːdʒ] **I** *n* fiebersenkendes Mittel *nt*, Antipyretikum *nt*. **II** *adj* → febrifugal.
feb·rile ['febrɪl, 'fiːb-] *adj* Fieber betr., mit Fieber, fieberhaft, febril, Fieber-.
febrile albuminuria Fieberalbuminurie *f*, Fieberproteinurie *f*, febrile Albuminurie/Proteinurie *f*.
febrile convulsion Fieberkrampf *m*.
febrile crisis Fieberkrise *f*.
febrile delirium Fieberdelir *nt*.
febrile pharyngitis akute febrile Pharyngitis *f*.
febrile proteinuria → febrile albuminuria.
febrile urine Fieberurin *m*.
fe·bris ['febrɪs, 'feɪ-] *n* → fever.
fe·cal ['fiːkl] *adj* Kot/Fäzes betr., kotig, fäkal, Fäkal-, Kot-, Stuhl-.
fecal abscess Kot-, Fäkalabszeß *m*.
fecal contamination fäkale Kontamination *f*, Kontamination *f* durch Faeces.
fecal continence Darm-, Stuhlkontinenz *f*.
fecal fistula Kotfistel *f*, Fistula stercoralis.
fecal flora Stuhlflora *f*.
fecal impaction Koteinklemmung *f*.
fecal incontinence Stuhl-, Darminkontinenz *f*, Incontinentia alvi.
fe·ca·lith ['fiːkəlɪθ] *n* Kotstein *m*, Koprolith *m*.
fecal matter → feces.
fe·cal·oid ['fiːkəlɔɪd] *adj* stuhlähnlich, kotartig, kotig, fäkulent.

fe·ca·lo·ma [fiːkəˈləʊmə] *n* Kotgeschwulst *f*, Fäkalom *nt*, Koprom *nt*, Sterkorom *nt*.
fecal peritonitis kotige/fäkulente Peritonitis *f*.
fecal softener Stuhlerweichungsmittel *nt*, Laxans *nt*.
fecal sterol fäkales Sterin *nt*.
fecal tumor → fecaloma.
fe·ca·lu·ri·a [fiːkəˈl(j)ʊərɪə] *n* Kotausscheidung *f* im Harn, Fäkalurie *f*.
fecal vomiting Koterbrechen *nt*, Kopremesis *f*.
fe·ces [ˈfiːsiːz] *pl* Stuhl *m*, Kot *m*, Fäzes *pl*, Faeces *pl*, Fäkalien *pl*.
Fechner [ˈfɛknər; ˈfɛç-]: **F.'s psychophysical law** Fechner psychophysisches Gesetz *nt*.
F.'s psychophysics Fechner'-Psychophysik *f*.
fec·u·la [ˈfɛkjələ] *n, pl* **-lae** [-liː] *chem.* Stärke *f*, Stärkemehl *nt*.
fec·u·lence [ˈfɛkjələns] *n* 1. Schlammigkeit *f*, Trübheit *f*. 2. Bodensatz *m*. 3. Kotartigkeit *f*, Fäkulenz *f*.
fec·u·lent [ˈfɛkjələnt] *adj* 1. kotig, kotartig, fäkulent. 2. schlammig, schmutzig, trübe, getrübt.
feculent vomiting fäkulentes Erbrechen *nt*; Koterbrechen *nt*, Kopremesis *f*..
fe·cun·date [ˈfiːkəndeɪt, ˈfɛ-] *vt* befruchten.
fe·cun·da·tion [ˌfiːkənˈdeɪʃn, ˌfɛ-] *n* Befruchtung *f*, Fertilisation *f*.
fe·cun·da·tive [fɪˈkʌndətɪv] *adj* befruchtend.
fe·cun·di·ty [fɪˈkʌndətɪ] *n* (erhöhte) Fruchtbarkeit *f*, Fertilität *f*.
fee·ble [ˈfiːbl] *adj* schwach, matt.
feeble-brained *adj* schwachköpfig.
feeble-mindedness *n old* Schwachsinn *m*, geistige Minderentwicklung *f*.
feed [fiːd] (*v* **fed; fed**) **I** *n* 1. (*Säugling*) Füttern *nt*, Mahlzeit *f*; *inf.* Essen *nt*. 2. *techn.* Versorgung *f*; (*Computer*) Eingabe *f* (*into* in). **II** *vt* 3. (*Kinder, Kranke*) füttern (*on, with* mit). **to ~ o.s.** (*Kind, Patient*) alleine *od.* ohne Hilfe essen (können). **to ~ at the breast** stillen. **to ~ by force** zwangsernähren. 4. (*Familie*) ernähren, unterhalten. 5. *techn.* (*Maschine*) versorgen beschicken (*with* mit); (*Computer*) füttern. **III** *vi* 6. Nahrung zu s. nehmen; (*Säugling*) gefüttert werden (*on, upon* mit). 7. s. (er-)nähren, leben (*on, upon* von).
feed back *vt electr.* rückkoppeln; (*Informationen*) zurückleiten (*to* an).
feed up *vt* jdn. auf-, hochpäppeln.
feed·back [ˈfiːdbæk] *n* Rückkopplung *f*, Feedback *m*.
feedback circuit *techn.* Feedback-, Rückkopplungskreis *m*.
feedback inhibition Rückkopplungs-, Rückwärts-, Feedbackhemmung *f*.
feedback inhibitor Feedbackinhibitor *m*.
feedback mechanism → feedback inhibition.
feedback system Rückkopplungs-, Feedbacksystem *nt*.
feed·er [ˈfiːdər] *n* 1. (Säuglings-, Saug-)Flasche *f*. 2. *Brit.* Lätzchen *nt*.
feeder pathway zuführender Stoffwechselweg *m*, Nachschubweg *m*.
feed-forward inhibition Vorwärts-, Feedforwardhemmung *f*.
feed·ing [ˈfiːdɪŋ] **I** *n* Füttern *nt*, (Er-)Nähren *nt*, Ernährung *f*, Mahlzeit *f*. **II** *adj techn.* versorgend, speisend, Zufuhr-.
feeding bottle → feeder 1.
feeding catheter Ernährungs-, Nahrungskatheter *m*.
feeding cup Schnabeltasse *f*.
feeding time (*Säugling*) Zeit *f* für die Mahlzeit.

feel [fiːl] (*v* **felt; felt**) **I** *n* 1. Gefühl *nt*. 2. Gefühl *nt*, Empfindung *f*, Eindruck *m*; Stimmung *f*. **II** *vt* 3. anfassen, (be-, an-)fühlen. 4. fühlen, (ver-)spüren, wahrnehmen. **III** *vi* 5. fühlen. 6. fühlen, durch Fühlen *od.* Tasten feststellen. 7. s. fühlen, s. befinden, sein. 8. finden, glauben (*that* daß). 9. s. anfühlen.
Feeley-Gorman [ˈfiːliː ˈgɔːrmən]: **F.-G. agar** Feeley-Gorman-Agar *m*/*nt*.
feel·ing [ˈfiːlɪŋ] *n* 1. Gefühl *nt*, Gefühlssinn *m*. 2. Stimmung *f*, Gefühlszustand *m*. 3. (Gefühls-)Eindruck *m*. 4. Empfindung *f*, Einstellung *f*, Ansicht *f*.
Feer [feːr]: **F.'s disease** Feer'-Krankheit *f*, Rosakrankheit *f*, vegetative Neurose *f* der Kleinkinder, Swift-Syndrom *nt*, Selter-Swift-Feer'-Krankheit *f*, Feer-Selter-Swift-Krankheit *f*, Akrodynie *f*, Acrodynia *f*.
feet [fiːt] *pl* → foot.
FEF *abbr.* → frontal eye field.
Fehling [ˈfeːlɪŋ]: **F.'s solution** Fehling'-Lösung *f*.
F.'s test Fehling'-Probe *f*.
feigned eruption [feɪnd] *derm.* Dermatitis artefacta.
Feitis [ˈfeɪtɪs]: **flecked spleen of F.** *patho.* Fleckenmilz *f*.
fel [fel] *n* Galle *f*, Fel *nt*.
Fel·der·struk·tur [ˈfɛltərʃtrʊkˈtuːr] *n histol.* Felderstruktur *f*.
Feldmann [ˈfɛldmən]: **F.'s dichotic speech test** *HNO* dichotischer Sprachtest *m* nach Feldmann.
F element → F factor.
fe·line [ˈfiːlaɪn] *adj* Katzen-.
feline leukemia virus *abbr.* **FeLV** Katzen-Leukämie-Virus *nt*, feline leukemia virus *abbr.* FeLV.
feline sarcoma virus *abbr.* **FeSV** Katzen-Sarkom-Virus *nt*, feline sarcoma virus *abbr.* FeSV.
Felix-Weil [ˈfiːlɪks waɪl]: **F.-W. reaction** Weil-Felix-Reaktion *f*, -Test *m*.
fel·late [fəˈleɪt] *vt* fellationieren, fellieren.
fel·la·tio [fəˈleɪʃɪəʊ] *n* Fellatio *f*, Coitus oralis.
fel·la·tion [fəˈleɪʃn] *n* → fellatio.
fel·la·to·rism [ˈfelətəːrɪzəm] *n* → fellatio.
fel·on [ˈfelən] *n* eitrige Fingerspitzenerkrankung *f*; tiefes Fingerpanaritium *nt*.
felt·work [ˈfeltwɜːrk] *n histol.* filzartiges Geflecht *nt*.
Felty [ˈfeltɪ]: **F.'s syndrome** Felty-Syndrom *nt*, Erwachsenenform *f* des Still-Syndroms.
FeLV *abbr.* → feline leukemia virus.
fe·male [ˈfiːmeɪl] **I** *n* 1. Frau *f*; Mädchen *nt*. 2. *bio.* Weibchen *nt*; weibl. Pflanze *f*. **II** *adj* 3. das weibliche Geschlecht betr., weiblich. 4. Frau(en) betr., von Frauen, weiblich, Frauen-.
female anisogamete Makrogamet *m*, Gynogamet *m*.
female castration beidseitige Eierstockentfernung/Oophorektomie/Ovariektomie *f*.
female circumscision 1. weibliche Beschneidung *f*, Klitoridektomie *f*, Klitorisektomie *f*. 2. Infibulation *f*.
female genitalia: external f. äußere weibliche Geschlechtsorgane/Genitalien *pl*, Organa genitalia feminina externa.
internal f. innere weibliche Geschlechtsorgane/Genitalien *pl*, Organa genitalia feminina interna.
female gonad weibliche Geschlechts-/Keimdrüse *f*, Eierstock *m*, Ovarium *nt*, Ovar *nt*, Oophoron *nt*.
female homosexuality weibliche Homosexualität *f*, Lesbianismus *m*, Sapphismus *m*.
female hypospadias Hypospadie *f* der weiblichen Harnröhre.
female pattern hair loss *derm.* weiblicher Typ *m* der Alopecia androgenetica.
female pronucleus → feminonucleus.
female pseudohermaphroditism Pseudohermaphroditismus feminius.
female pudendum (weibliche) Scham(gegend *f*) *f*, Vulva *f*, äußere weibliche Geschlechtsorgane/Genitalien *pl*, Pudendum *nt*.
female sterility weibliche Sterilität *f*.
fem·i·nal·i·ty [feməˈnælətɪ] *n* → femininity.
fem·i·ne·i·ty [feməˈniːətɪ] *n* → femininity.
fem·i·nine [ˈfemənɪn] *adj* 1. weiblich, Frauen-. 2. weibisch, feminin.
fem·i·nin·i·ty [feməˈnɪnətɪ] *n* 1. Weiblichkeit *f*. 2. Fraulichkeit *f*.
fem·i·nism [ˈfemənɪzəm] *n* 1. Verweiblichung *f*, Feminismus *m*. 2. Frauenrechtsbewegung *f*, Feminismus *m*.
fe·min·i·ty [fɪˈmɪnətɪ] *n* → femininity.
fem·i·ni·za·tion [ˌfemənaɪˈzeɪʃn] *n patho.* Verweiblichung *f*, Feminisierung *f*, Feminisation *f*.
fem·i·niz·ing testis syndrome [ˈfemənaɪzɪŋ] Goldberg-Maxwell-Morris-Syndrom *nt*, testikuläre Feminisierung *f*.
fem·i·no·nu·cle·us [ˌfemənəʊˈn(j)uːklɪəs] *n embryo.* weiblicher Vorkern/Pronukleus *m*.
fem·o·ral [ˈfemərəl] *adj* Oberschenkel(knochen) betr., femoral, Femur-, Oberschenkel(knochen)-.
femoral arch, superficial Leistenband *nt*, Lig. inguinale, Arcus inguinale.
femoral artery Oberschenkelschlagader *f*, -arterie *f*, Femoralis *f*, A. femoralis.
deep f. tiefe Oberschenkelarterie, Profunda *f* femoris, A. profunda femoris.
lateral circumflex f. äußere Oberschenkel-/Femurkranzarterie, Circumflexa *f* femoris lateralis, A. circumflexa femoris lateralis.
medial circumflex f. innere Oberschenkel-/Femurkranzarterie, Circumflexa *f* femoris medialis, A. circumflexa femoris medialis.
femoral artery injury Femoralisverletzung *f*, Femoralarterienverletzung *f*.
femoral articulation Hüftgelenk *nt*, Artic. coxae/iliofemoralis.
femoral aponeurosis Oberschenkelfaszie *f*, Fascia lata (femoris).
femoral bone → femur 1.
femoral branch of genitofemoral nerve Femoralast *m* des N. genitofemoralis, N. lumboinguinalis, Ramus femoralis (n. genitofemoralis).
femoral calcar *anat.* Schenkelsporn *m*, Calcar femorale/femoris.
femoral canal Canalis femoralis.
femoral crest Linea aspera.
femoral epiphysis Femurepiphyse *f*.
slipped capital/upper f. *abbr.* **SUFE** Lösung *f* der Femorepiphyse, Epiphyseolysis/Epiphysiolysis capitis femoris, Coxa vara adolescentium.
femoral fascia Oberschenkelfaszie *f*, Fascia lata (femoris).
femoral fracture Oberschenkelbruch *m*, -fraktur *f*, Femurfraktur *f*, Fractura femoris.
distal f. distale Oberschenkel-/Femurfraktur.
intercondylar f. interkondyläre Oberschenkel-/Femurfraktur.
intertrochanteric f. intertrochantäre Oberschenkel-/Femurfraktur.

femoral head 288

intracondylar f. intrakondyläre Oberschenkel-/Femurfraktur.
percondylar f. perkondyläre Oberschenkel-/Femurfraktur.
pertrochanteric f. pertrochantäre Oberschenkel-/Femurfraktur.
proximal f. proximale/hüftgelenksnahe Oberschenkel-/Femurfraktur.
subtrochanteric f. subtrochantäre Oberschenkel-/Fremurfraktur.
supracondylar f. suprakondyläre Oberschenkel-/Femurfraktur.
unicondylar f. monokondyläre Oberschenkel-/Femurfraktur.
femoral head Femur-, Oberschenkelkopf *m*, Caput femoris.
femoral head extractor *ortho*. (Hüft-, Femur-)Kopfextraktor *m*.
femoral head fracture Hüftkopf-, Femurkopffraktur *f*.
femoral head prosthesis *ortho*. Hüftkopfprothese *f*.
femoral hernia *chir*. Schenkelbruch *m*, -hernie *f*, Merozele *f*, Hernia femoralis/curalis.
  bilocular h. *chir*. Hey-Hernie *f*, Hernia encystica.
femoral joint → femoral articulation.
femoral muscle Vastus *m* intermedius, M. vastus intermedius.
femoral neck (Ober-)Schenkelhals *m*, Collum femoris.
  anteverted f. Coxa antetorta.
femoral neck fracture Schenkelhals-, Femurhalsfraktur *f*.
  lateral f. laterale Schenkelhalsfraktur.
  medial f. mediale/subkapitale Schenkelhalsfraktur.
  midcervical f. intermediäre Schenkelhalsfraktur.
  subcapital f. → mediale f.
  transcervical f. → lateral f.
femoral neck reamer *ortho*. (Femur-)Halsraspel *f*.
femoral nerve Femoralis *m*, N. femoralis.
  quadrate f. N. musculi quadrati femoris, N. quadratus femoris.
femoral nerve stretch test *neuro*. Femoralisdehnungstest *m*.
femoral plexus vegetativer Plexus *m* der A. femoralis, Plexus femoralis.
femoral pulse Femoralispuls *m*.
femoral reflex Femoralisreflex *m*, Remak--Zeichen *m*.
femoral region Oberschenkelregion *f*, Regio/Facies femoralis.
  anterior f. Oberschenkelvorderfläche *f*, Regio/Facies femoralis anterior.
  posterior f. Oberschenkelrückseite *f*, Regio/Facies femoralis posterior.
femoral ring Eingang *m* des Canalis femoralis, A(n)nulus femoralis.
femoral septum Cloquet-Septum *nt*, Septum femorale.
femoral shaft (Ober-)Schenkel-, Femurschaft *m*.
femoral shaft fracture Oberschenkelschaft-, Femurschaftfraktur *f*.
femoral shaft rasp *ortho*. Femurraspel *f*.
femoral surface → femoral region.
femoral trigone Schenkeldreieck *nt*, Scarpa'-Dreieck *nt*, Trigonum femorale.
femoral vein Oberschenkelvene *f*, V. femoralis.
  deep f. tiefe Oberschenkelvene, V. profunda femoris.
  lateral circumflex f.s Begleitvenen *pl* der A. circumflexa femoris lateralis, Vv. circumflexae laterales femorales.
  medial circumflex f.s Begleitvenen *pl* der A. circumflexa femoris medialis, Vv. circumflexae mediales femorales.

femoral vein thrombosis Thrombose *f* der V. femoralis.
femoro- *pref*. Femoral-, Oberschenkel-, Femur-.
fem·o·ro·ab·dom·i·nal reflex [ˌfeməræb-'dɑmɪnl] *neuro*. femoroabdominaler Reflex *m*.
fem·o·ro·cele ['-siːl] *n* → femoral hernia.
fem·o·ro·il·i·ac [ˌ-'ɪliæk] *adj* Femur u. Ilium betr., femoroiliakal.
fem·o·ro·pa·tel·lar dysplasia [ˌ-pə'telər] femoropatellare Dysplasie *f*.
fem·o·ro·pop·lit·e·al bypass [ˌ-pɑp'lɪtɪəl] *HTG* femoropoplitealer Bypass *m*.
fem·o·ro·tib·i·al [ˌ-'tɪbɪəl] *adj* Femur u. Tibia betr., femorotibial.
femto- *pref. abbr*. f Femto- *abbr*. f.
fe·mur ['fiːmər] *n, pl* **fe·mo·ra** [ˈfemərə], **-murs** 1. Oberschenkelknochen *m*, Femur *nt*, Os femoris. 2. Oberschenkel *m*.
fen·bu·fen [fen'bjuːfen] *n pharm*. Fenbufen *nt*.
fen·di·line ['fendɪlaɪn] *n pharm*. Fendilin *nt*.
fe·nes·tra [fɪ'nestrə] *n, pl* **-trae** [-triː] *anat., chir*. Fenster *nt*, fensterähnliche Öffnung *f*, Fenestra *f*.
  f. of cochlea rundes Fenster, Schneckenfenster, Fenestra cochleae.
fe·nes·tral [fɪ'nestrəl] *adj anat*. Fenster betr., fensterartig, fenestral.
fe·nes·trate ['fenəstreit] *chir., histol*. I *adj* mit Fenster(n)/Löchern (versehen), gefenstert, fenestriert. II *vt* fenstern.
fe·nes·trat·ed ['fenəstreɪtɪd] *adj* → fenestrate I.
fenestrated capillary gefensterte/fenestrierte Kapillare *f*, Typ 2-Kapillare *f*.
fenestrated hymen *gyn*. Hymen cribriformis.
fenestrated membrane gefensterte/fenestrierte Membran *f*.
fenestrated placenta Placenta fenestrata.
fen·es·tra·tion [ˌfenəˈstreɪʃn] *n* 1. *chir*. Fensterung(soperation) *f*, Fenestration *f*. 2. *patho*. Fenster *nt*; Defekt *m*.
fenestration operation → fenestration 1.
fen·eth·yl·line [fen'eθəliːn] *n pharm*. Fenetyllin *nt*.
fen·flur·a·mine [fen'fluərəmiːn] *n pharm*. Fenfluramin *nt*.
Fenn [fen]: **F. effect** Fenn-Effekt *m*.
fen·o·pro·fen [ˌfenəˈproufen] *n pharm*. Fenoprofen *nt*.
fen·o·ter·ol [ˌfenəˈterɒl] *n pharm*. Fenoterol *nt*.
fen·pip·ra·mide [fenˈpɪprəmaɪd] *n pharm*. Fenpipramid *nt*.
fen·ta·nyl ['fentənɪl] *n pharm., anes*. Fentanyl *nt*.
fen·ti·clor ['fentəklɔːr] *n pharm*. Fenticlor *nt*.
Fenwick ['fenwɪk]: **F.'s disease** (chronisch-)atrophische Gastritis *f*.
Fenwick-Hunner ['hʌnər]: **F.-H. ulcer** Fenwick-Ulkus *nt*, Hunner-Ulkus *nt*, Hunner-Fenwick-Ulkus *nt*, Fenwick--Hunner-Ulkus *m*.
Féréol-Graux [fereˈɔl gro]: **F.-G. palsy/paralysis** *ophthal*. Féréol-Lähmung *f*.
Ferguson [ˈfɜːrɡəsn]: **F.'s method** *ortho*. (Skoliose) Ferguson-Methode *f*.
  F.'s operation *urol*. Ferguson-Operation *f*.
  F.'s reflex Ferguson'-Reflex *m*.
Fergusson [ˈfɜːrɡəsn]: **F.'s incision** *HNO* Fergusson-Schnitt *m*, -Operation *f*.
  F.'s speculum *gyn*. Scheidenspekulum *nt* nach Fergusson.
fer·ment [*n* ˈfɜːrment; *v* fərˈment] I *n old* → enzyme. II *vt chem*. zum Gären bringen, vergären. III *vi chem*. gären, in Gärung sein.

fer·ment·a·bil·i·ty [ˌfɜːrməntəˈbɪlətɪ] *n* Gärungsfähigkeit *f*, gährungsfähige Beschaffenheit *f*.
fer·ment·a·ble [fərˈmentəbl] *adj* → fermentative 2.
fer·men·ta·tion [ˌfɜːrmenˈteɪʃn] *n chem*. Gärung *f*, Gärungsprozeß *m*, Fermentation *f*, Fermentierung *f*.
fermentation product Gärungsprodukt *nt*.
fermentation tube Gärungsröhrchen *nt*.
fer·ment·a·tive [fərˈmentətɪv] *adj chem*. 1. Gärung betr. *od*. bewirkend, gärend, fermentativ, enzymatisch, Gär(ungs)-. 2. gär(ungs)fähig, fermentierbar.
fermentative pathway glykolytischer/fermentativer Stoffwechselweg *m*.
fer·men·tive [fərˈmentɪv] *adj* → fermentative.
fer·men·tum [fərˈmentəm] *n* Hefe *f*.
fer·mi·um [ˈfɜːrmɪəm] *n chem. abbr*. **Fm** Fermium *nt abbr*. Fm.
Fernandez [ferˈnændez; ferˈnandeθ]: **F. reaction** Fernandez-Reaktion *f*.
fern·ing [ˈfɜːrnɪŋ] *n gyn*. Farnkrautphänomen *nt*, Arborisationsphänomen *nt*.
fern phenomenon [ˈfɜːrn] → ferning.
fern test *gyn*. Farnkrautphänomen *nt*, Farntest *m*.
Ferrata [feˈrɑːtə; feˈrɑːtə]: **F.'s cell** Ferrata--Zelle *f*, Hämohistioplast *m*.
fer·rat·ed [ˈfereɪtɪd] *adj chem*. eisenbeladen.
fer·re·dox·in [ˌferəˈdɑksɪn] *n* Ferredoxin *nt*.
ferredoxin-NADP oxidoreductase Ferredoxin-NADP-oxidoreduktase *f*.
ferredoxin-reducing substance *abbr*. **FRS** ferredoxin-reduzierende Substanz *f abbr*. FRS.
Ferrein [fəˈrɛ̃; feˈrɛ̃]: **F.'s canal** Tränenkanal *m*, Rivus lacrimalis.
  F.'s cords Stimmfalten *pl*, Plicae vocalis.
  F.'s foramen Hiatus canalis n. petrosi majoris.
  pyramids of F. (*Niere*) Markstrahlen *pl*, Radii medullares.
fer·ric [ˈferɪk] *adj chem*. dreiwertiges Eisen enthaltend, Ferri-, Eisen-III-.
ferric chloride Eisen-III-chlorid *nt*.
ferric chloride test *lab*. Eisenchloridprobe *f*, Fölling-Probe *f*.
ferric ferrocyanide Berliner-Blau *nt*, Ferriferrocyanid *nt*.
ferric hydroxide Eisen-III-hydroxid *nt*.
fer·ri·cy·a·nide [ˌferɪˈsaɪənaɪd, ˌferaɪ-] *n* Hexacyanoferrat (III) *nt*.
fer·ri·heme chloride [ˈ-hiːm] Teichmann--Kristalle *pl*, saures Hämin *m*, Hämin(kristalle *pl*) *nt*, Chlorhämin(kristalle *pl*) *nt*, Chlorhämatin *nt*.
fer·ri·he·mo·glo·bin [ˌ-ˈhiːməɡloubɪn] *n* Methämoglobin *nt abbr*. Met-Hb, Hämiglobin *nt*.
fer·ri·por·phy·rin chloride [ˌ-ˈpɔːrfərɪn] → ferriprotoporhyrin.
fer·ri·pro·to·por·phy·rin [ˌ-ˌproutouˈpɔːrfərɪn] *n* Teichmann-Kristalle *pl*, salzsaures Hämin *m*, Hämin(kristalle *pl*) *nt*, Chlorhämin(kristalle *pl*) *nt*, Chlorhämatin *nt*.
fer·ri·tin [ˈferɪtɪn] *n* Ferritin *nt*.
fer·ro·che·la·tase [ˌferouˈkiːləteɪz] *n* Ferrochelatase *f*, Goldberg'-Enzym *nt*.
fer·ro·cy·to·chrome c-oxygen oxyreductase [ˌ-ˈsaɪtəkroum] Cytochrom a₃ *nt*, Cytochrom(c)oxidase *f*, *old* Warburg'-Atmungsferment *nt*, Ferrocytochromc-Sauerstoff-Oxidoreduktase *f*.
fer·ro·ki·net·ic [ˌ-kɪˈnetɪk, -kaɪ-] *adj* Ferrokinetik betr., ferrokinetisch.
fer·ro·ki·net·ics [ˌ-kɪˈnetɪks] *pl* Ferrokinetik *f*.

fer·ro·pro·tein [ˌ-'prəʊtiːn, -tiːɪn] *n* Ferroprotein *nt*.
fer·ro·pro·to·por·phy·rin [ˌ-ˌprəʊtəʊ'pɔːrfərɪn] *n* Häm *nt*, Protohäm *nt*.
fer·ro·ther·a·py [ˌ-'θerəpɪ] *n* Eisentherapie *f*.
fer·rous ['ferəs] *adj chem* zweiwertiges Eisen enthaltend, Ferro-, Eisen-II-.
ferrous fumarate *pharm.* Ferrofumarat *nt*, Eisen-II-fumarat *nt*.
ferrous gluconate *pharm.* Ferrogluconat *nt*, Eisen-II-gluconat *nt*.
ferrous lactate *pharm.* Ferrolactat *nt*, Eisen-II-laktat *nt*.
ferrous succinate Ferrosuccinat *nt*, Eisen-II-succinat *nt*.
ferrous sulfate Ferrosulfat *nt*, Eisen-II-sulfat *nt*.
ferrous wheel hypothesis *biochem.* Ferrous-wheel-Hypothese *f*.
fer·rox·i·dase [fer'ɑksɪdeɪz] *n* Zörulo-, Zärulo-, Coerulo-, Caeruloplasmin *nt*, Ferroxidase I *f*.
fer·ru·gi·na·tion [fəˌruːdʒə'neɪʃn] *n patho.* Eiseneinlagerung *f*, -ablagerung *f*.
fer·ru·gi·nous [fə'ruːdʒɪnəs] *adj* 1. eisenhaltig, Eisen-. 2. rostfarben.
fer·rum ['ferəm] *n abbr.* **Fe** *chem.* Eisen *nt*, Ferrum *nt abbr.* Fe.
Ferry-Porter ['ferɪ 'pɔːrtər]: **F.-P. law** Ferry-Porter-Regel *f*.
fer·tile ['fɜːrtl; *Brit.* -taɪl] *adj* fruchtbar, zeugungs-, fortpflanzungsfähig, fertil.
fertile eunuch syndrome fertiler Eunuchoidismus *m*, Pasqualini-Syndrom *nt*.
fer·til·i·ty [fɜːr'tɪlətɪ] *n* Fruchtbarkeit *f*, Fertilität *f*; (männliche) Befruchtungs-/Zeugungsfähigkeit *f*.
fertility factor Fertilitätsfaktor *m*, F-Faktor *m*.
fer·ti·li·za·tion [ˌfɜːrtlə'zeɪʃn] *n* Befruchtung *f*, Fertilisation *f*.
fer·ti·lize ['fɜːrtlaɪz] *vt* befruchten, fruchtbar machen.
fer·ves·cence [fər'vesəns] *n* Temperaturanstieg *m*.
fes·ter ['festər] **I** *n* 1. Geschwür *nt*, Ulkus *nt*. 2. eiternde Wunde *f*. **II** *vt* zum Eitern bringen. **III** *vi* 3. eitern. 4. verwesen, verfaulen.
fes·ti·nant ['festɪnənt] *adj* beschleunigend.
fes·ti·na·tion [ˌfestə'neɪʃn] *n neuro.* Festination *f*.
FeSV *abbr.* → feline sarcoma virus.
fe·tal ['fiːtl] *adj* Fötus *od.* Fetalperiode betr., fötal, fetal, Feto-, Fetus-.
fetal adenoma fetales (Schilddrüsen-)Adenom *nt*.
fetal alcohol syndrome Alkoholembryopathie(syndrom *nt*) *f*.
fetal asphyxia fetale Asphyxie *f*.
fetal atelectasis (*Lunge*) fetale Atelektase *f*.
fetal bradycardia fetale Bradykardie *f*.
fetal cartilage embryonaler/fetaler Knorpel *m*.
fetal cell lipoma braunes Lipom *nt*, Hibernom(a) *nt*, Lipoma feto-cellulare.
fetal chondrodysplasia → fetal chondrodystrophia.
fetal chondrodystrophia Achondroplasie *f*, Chondrodystrophie *f*, Chondrodysplasia/Chondrodystrophia fetalis (Kaufmann).
hypoplastic f. Conradi-Syndrom *nt*, Conradi-Hünermann-(Raap)-Syndrom *nt*, Chondrodysplasia/Chondrodystrophia calcificans congenita.
fetal circulation kindlicher/fetaler Kreislauf *m*.
fetal component of placenta → fetal placenta.

fetal death intrauteriner Fruchttod *m*; Todgeburt *f*.
fetal distress fetaler Gefahrenzustand *m*, fetale Notsituation *f*, fetal distress.
fetal erythroblastosis fetale Erythroblastose *f*, Erythroblastosis fetalis, Morbus haemolyticus neonatorum *abbr.* MHN.
fetal face syndrome Robinow-Syndrom *nt*.
fetal fat braunes Fettgewebe *nt*.
fetal fracture kongenitale Fraktur *f*, intrauterin erworbene Fraktur *f*.
fetal hemoglobin *abbr.* **HbF** fetales Hämoglobin *nt abbr.* HbF.
fetal hydantoin syndrome embryopathisches Hydantoin-Syndrom *nt*.
fetal hydrops Hydrops fetalis, Hydrops congenitus/fetus universalis.
fe·tal·ism ['fiːtəlɪzəm] *n* → fetalization.
fe·tal·i·za·tion [ˌfiːtəlaɪ'zeɪʃn] *n patho.* Fetalisation *f*, Fötalisation *f*, Fetalismus *m*.
fetal life Fötal-, Fetalperiode *f*.
fetal lipoma → fetal cell lipoma.
fetal membranes *embryo.* Eihäute *pl*.
fetal movements *gyn.* Kindsbewegungen *pl*.
fetal period Fötal-, Fetalperiode *f*.
fetal placenta fötale Plazenta *f*, kindlicher Teil *m* der Plazenta, Placenta f(o)etalis, Pars f(o)etalis placentae.
fetal rhythm *card.* Pendel-Rhythmus *m*, Tick-Tack-Rhythmus *m*, Embryokardie *f*.
fetal rickets → fetal chondrodystrophia.
fetal tachycardia fetale Tachykardie *f*.
fe·ta·tion [fiː'teɪʃn] *n* 1. Schwangerschaft *f*, Gravidität *f*. 2. Fetusentwicklung *f*, -wachstum *nt*.
fe·ti·cide ['fiːtɪsaɪd] **I** *n* Fetusschädigung *f*, -abtötung *f*, Foetizid *m*, Fetizid *m*. **II** *adj* fetusschädigend, -abtötend, fetizid.
fet·id ['fetɪd, 'fiː-] *adj* übelriechend, stinkend, fetid, fötid.
fet·ish ['fetɪʃ, 'fiː-] *n psychia.* Fetisch *m*.
fet·ish·ism ['fetəʃɪzəm] *n psychia.* Fetischismus *m*.
fet·ish·ist ['fetəʃɪst] *n psychia.* Fetischist(in *f*) *m*.
fe·to·cel·lu·lar lipoma [ˌfiːtəʊ'seljələr] → fetal cell lipoma.
fe·to·gen·e·sis [ˌ-'dʒenəsɪs] *n* Föto-, Fetogenese *f*.
fe·tog·ra·phy [fiː'tɑgrəfɪ] *n* Fetographie *f*.
fe·tol·o·gy [fiː'tɑlədʒɪ] *n* Foetologie *f*, Fetologie *f*.
fe·to·ma·ter·nal hemorrhage [ˌfiːtəʊmə'tɜːrnl] → fetomaternal transfusion.
fetomaternal transfusion *gyn.* fetomaternale Transfusion *f*.
fe·tom·e·try [fiː'tɑmətrɪ] *n gyn.* Fetometrie *f*.
fe·top·a·thy [fiː'tɑpəθɪ] *n* 1. Embryopathie *f*, Embryopathia *f*. 2. Fetopathie *f*, Fetopathia *f*.
fe·to·pla·cen·tal [ˌfiːtəʊplə'sentl] *adj* Fetus u. Plazenta betr. *od.* verbindend, fetoplazentar.
α-fe·to·pro·tein [ˌ-'prəʊtiːn, -tiːɪn] *n* α₁-Fetoprotein *nt*, alpha₁-Fetoprotein *nt abbr.* AFP.
fe·tor ['fiːtər] *n* übler Geruch *m*, Fötor *m*, Foetor *m*.
fe·to·scope ['fiːtəskəʊp] *n* Fetoskop *nt*.
fe·to·scop·ic [ˌ-'skɑpɪk] *adj* Fetoskopie betr., mittels Fetoskopie, fetoskopisch.
fe·tos·co·py [fiː'tɑskəpɪ] *n* Fetoskopie *f*.
fe·tu·in ['fiːtjuːɪn] *n* Fetuin *nt*.
fe·tus ['fiːtəs] *n, pl* **-tus·es** Foetus *m*, Fetus *m*, Fötus *m*.
Feulgen ['fɔɪlgən; 'fɔʏl]: **F. (nuclear) reaction** *histol.* Feulgen'-Nuklearreaktion *f*.
F. stain/test → F. (nuclear) reaction.

FEV₁ *abbr.* → forced expiratory volume.
fe·ver ['fiːvər] *n* 1. Fieber *nt*, Febris *f*, Pyrexie *f*. 2. fieberhafte Erkrankung *f*, Fieber *nt*.
fever blister(s) Fieberbläschen *nt*, Herpes simplex der Lippen, Herpes febrilis/labialis.
fe·ver·ish ['fiːvərɪʃ] *adj* 1. fieb(e)rig, febril, Fieber-. 2. fiebererzeugend. 3. (*fig.*) fieberhaft, fiebrig.
fe·ver·ish·ness ['-nɪs] *n* → febricity.
feverish urine Fieberurin *m*.
Fèvre-Languepin ['fɛːvrə lɑ̃ɡ'pɛ̃]: **F.-L. syndrome** Fèvre-Languepin-Syndrom *nt*.
FF *abbr.* → filtration fraction.
FFA *abbr.* → fatty acid, free.
F factor Fertilitätsfaktor *m*, F-Faktor *m*.
FFP *abbr.* → fresh frozen plasma.
FFR *abbr.* → frequency-following responses.
F-G agar → Feeley-Gorman agar.
FH₄ *abbr.* → tetrahydrofolic acid.
FIA *abbr.* → fluoroimmunoassay.
fi·ber ['faɪbər] *n* 1. *techn., bio.* Faser *f*, Fiber *f*. 2. *anat.* Faser *f*, faserähnliche Struktur *f*, Fibra *f*. 3. Ballaststoffe *pl*.
f.s of stria terminalis Fibrae striae terminalis.
fiber bundle Faserbündel *nt*.
pallidosubthalamic f. pallidosubthalamisches Faserbündel.
pallidotegmental f. pallidotegmentales Faserbündel.
fiber cable Faserbündel *nt*.
fiber felt *histol.* Faserfilz *m*.
fi·ber·gas·tro·scope [ˌfaɪbər'ɡæstrəskəʊp] *n* Glasfaser-, Fibergastroskop *nt*.
fi·ber·glass ['-ɡlæs, -ɡlɑːs] *n* Fiberglas *nt*.
fiberglass cast *ortho.* Fiberglasverband *m*, Kunststoffgips *m*.
fi·ber·less ['-lɪs] *adj* faserlos, ohne Fasern.
fi·ber·op·tic bronchoscope [ˌ-'ɑptɪk] Glasfaser-, Fiberbronchoskop *nt*.
fiberoptic endoscope → fiberscope.
fi·ber·op·tics [ˌ-'ɑptɪks] *pl* (Glas-)Faser-, Fiberoptik *f*.
fi·ber·scope ['-skəʊp] *n* Fibroskop *nt*, Faser-, Fiberendoskop *nt*.
fiber tension Faserspannung *f*.
myocardial f. Myokardfaserspannung *f*.
fiber tract Faserbahn *f*.
fibr- *pref.* → fibro-.
fi·bra ['faɪbrə] *n, pl* **-brae** [-briː] → fiber 2.
fi·bre *n Brit.* → fiber.
fi·bre·mia [faɪ'briːmɪə] *n* → fibrinemia.
fi·bril ['faɪbrəl] *n* kleine *od.* dünne Faser *f*, Fibrille *f*, Filament *nt*, Filamentbündel *nt*.
fi·bril·la [faɪ'brɪlə] *n, pl* **-lae** [-liː] → fibril.
fi·bril·lar [faɪ'brɪlər] *adj* Fibrille betr., aus Fibrillen bestehend, (fein-)faserig, fibrillär, Fibrillen-.
fibrillar protein Faser-, Skleroprotein *nt*.
fi·bril·lary [faɪ'brɪleriː, 'fɪb-] *adj* → fibrillar.
fibrillary astrocytoma faserreiches/fibrilläres Astrozytom *nt*, Astrocyma fibrillare.
fibrillary contraction fibrilläre/faszikuläre Kontraktion *f*.
fi·bril·late [faɪ'brɪlert, 'fɪb-] **I** *adj* → fibrillar. **II** *vi* 1. zer-, auffasern, fibrillieren. 2. *patho.* zucken, flimmern, fibrillieren.
fi·bril·lat·ed ['faɪbrɪlertəd] *adj* → fibrillar.
fi·bril·la·tion [ˌ-'leɪʃn] *n* 1. *patho.* Faserbildung *f*, Auffaserung *f*. 2. *patho.* Fibrillieren *nt*, Fibrillation *f*. 3. *card.* Flimmern *nt*, Fibrillation *f*.
fibrillation potential Fibrillationspotential *nt*.
fi·brilled ['faɪbrɪld] *adj* → fibrillar.
Fi·bril·len·struk·tur [fɪˌbrɪlənʃtrʊk'uːr] *n histol.* Fibrillenstruktur *f*.

fibrilliform

fi·bril·li·form [faɪˈbrɪləfɔːrm, ˈfaɪbrɪ-] *adj* fibrillen-, faserähnlich, -artig, faserig.
fi·bril·lo·blast [ˈ-blæst] *n* Odontoblast *m*, Dentinoblast *m*.
fi·bril·lo·gen·e·sis [ˌ-ˈdʒenəsɪs] *n* Fibrillenbildung *f*, -formation *f*.
fi·bril·lol·y·sis [ˌfaɪbrɪˈlɒləsɪs] *n* Fibrillenauflösung *f*, -zerstörung *f*, Fibrillolyse *f*.
fi·bril·lo·lyt·ic [ˌfaɪbrɪləˈlɪtɪk, faɪˌbrɪlə-] *adj* fibrillenzerstörend, -auflösend, fibrillolytisch.
fi·brin [ˈfaɪbrɪn] *n* Fibrin *nt*.
fi·brin·ase [ˈfaɪbrɪneɪz] *n* **1.** Faktor XIII *m abbr*. F XIII, fibrinstabilisierender Faktor *m abbr*. FSF, Laki-Lorand-Faktor *m abbr*. LLF. **2.** → fibrinolysin.
fi·bri·na·tion [ˌfaɪbrəˈneɪʃn] *n* Fibrinbildung *f*.
fibrin calculus Fibrinstein *m*.
fibrin coagulum Fibringerinnsel *nt*.
fibrin degradation products *abbr*. **FDP** → fibrinolytic split products.
fi·bri·ne·mia [ˌfaɪbrəˈniːmɪə] *n* Fibrinämie *f*.
fibrin monomer Fibrinmonomer *nt*.
fibrino- *pref*. Fibrin-, Fibrino-.
fi·bri·no·cel·lu·lar [ˌfaɪbrɪnəʊˈseljələr] *adj* aus Fibrin u. Zellen bestehend, fibrinozellulär.
fi·brin·o·gen [faɪˈbrɪnədʒən] *n* Fibrinogen *nt*, Faktor I *m abbr*. F I.
fi·bri·nog·e·nase [ˌfaɪbrɪˈnɒdʒəneɪz] *n* Thrombin *nt*, Faktor IIa *m*.
fibrinogen deficiency Fibrinogenmangel *m*, Hypofibrinogenämie *f*.
fibrinogen degradation products *abbr*. **FDP** → fibrinolytic split products.
fi·bri·no·ge·ne·mia [faɪˌbrɪnədʒəˈniːmɪə] *n* Fibrinogenämie *f*, Hyperfibrinogenämie *f*.
fi·bri·no·gen·e·sis [ˌfaɪbrɪnəˈdʒenəsɪs] *n* Fibrinbildung *f*, Fibrinogenese *f*.
fi·bri·no·gen·ic [ˌ-ˈdʒenɪk] *adj* fibrinbildend, fibrinogen.
fi·bri·no·ge·nol·y·sis [ˌ-dʒɪˈnɒləsɪs] *n* Fibrinogenauflösung *f*, -spaltung *f*, -inaktivierung *f*, Fibrinogenolyse *f*.
fi·bri·no·gen·o·lyt·ic [ˌ-ˌdʒenəˈlɪtɪk] *adj* Fibrinogenolyse betr., fibrinogenauflösend, -spaltend, -inaktivierend, fibrinogenolytisch.
fi·bri·no·gen·o·pe·nia [ˌ-ˌdʒenəˈpiːnɪə] *n* Fibrinogenmangel *m*, Fibrinogenopenie *f*, Hypofibrinogenämie *f*, Fibrinopenie *f*.
fi·bri·nog·e·nous [faɪbrɪˈnɒdʒənəs] *adj* → fibrinogenic.
fi·bri·noid [ˈfaɪbrɪnɔɪd] **I** *n* Fibrinoid *nt*. **II** *adj* fibrinähnlich, -artig, fibrinoid.
fibrinoid degeneration fibrinoide Degeneration *f*.
fibrinoid swelling *patho*. fibrinoide Verquellung *f*.
fi·bri·no·ki·nase [faɪˌbrɪnəˈkaɪneɪz, -ˈkɪn-] *n* Fibrinokinase *f*.
fi·bri·nol·y·sin [ˌfaɪbrəˈnɒləsɪn] *n* Fibrinolysin *nt*, Plasmin *nt*.
fi·bri·nol·y·sis [ˌ-ˈnɒləsɪs] *n* Fibrinspaltung *f*, Fibrinolyse *f*.
fi·brin·o·ly·so·ki·nase [faɪˌbrɪnəˌlaɪsəˈkaɪneɪz, -ˈkɪn-] *n* Fibrinolysokinase *f*.
fi·bri·no·lyt·ic [ˌfaɪbrɪnəˈlɪtɪk] *adj* Fibrinolyse betr. *od*. verursachend, fibrinspaltend, fibrinolytisch.
fibrinolytic agent Fibrinolytikum *nt*.
fibrinolytic split products *abbr*. **FSP** Fibrinogen-, Fibrinspaltprodukte *pl abbr*. FSP, Fibrin-, Fibrinogendegradationsprodukte *pl abbr*. FDP.
fi·bri·no·pe·nia [ˌ-ˈpiːnɪə] *n* → fibrinogenopenia.
fi·bri·no·pep·tide [ˌ-ˈpeptaɪd] *n* Fibrinopeptid *nt*.
fi·bri·no·plate·let [ˌ-ˈpleɪtlɪt] *adj* aus Fibrin u. Thrombozyten bestehend.
fi·bri·no·pu·ru·lent [ˌ-ˈpjʊər(j)ələnt] *adj* fibrinös-eitrig.
ffibrinopurulent inflammation fibrinös-eitrige Entzündung *f*.
fi·brin·ous [ˈfaɪbrɪnəs] *adj* Fibrin betr. *od*. enthaltend, fibrinartig, -haltig, fibrinreich, fibrinös, Fibrin-.
fibrinous bronchitis kruppöse/membranöse/pseudomembranöse Bronchitis *f*, Bronchitis crouposa/fibrinosa/plastica/pseudomembranacea.
fibrinous cast (*Harn*) fibrinöser Zylinder *m*.
fibrinous cystitis fibrinöse (Harn-)Blasenentzündung/Zystitis *f*, Cystitis fibrinosa.
fibrinous degeneration fibrinöse Degeneration *f*.
fibrinous inflammation fibrinöse Entzündung *f*.
fibrinous iritis *ophthal*. fibrinöse Iritis *f*.
fibrinous pericarditis fibrinöse Perikardentzündung/Perikarditis *f*, Pericarditis fibrinosa.
fibrinous peritonitis fibrinöse Peritonitis *f*.
fibrinous pharyngitis fibrinöse Pharyngitis *f*.
fibrinous pleurisy/pleuritis fibrinöse Rippenfellentzündung/Pleuritis *f*, Pleuritis fibrinosa.
fibrinous pneumonia fibrinöse Pneumonie *f*.
fibrinous polyp *gyn*. fibrinöser Polyp *m*.
fibrinous rhinitis pseudomembranöse/fibrinöse Rhinitis *f*, Rhinitis pseudomembranacea.
fibrinous stomatitis fibrinöse Stomatitis *f*.
fibrin-platelet thrombus Fibrin-Plättchenthrombus *m*.
fibrin stabilizing factor *abbr*. **FSF** Faktor XIII *m abbr*. F XIII, fibrinstabilisierender Faktor *m abbr*. FSF, Laki-Lorand--Faktor *m abbr*. LLF.
fibrin stain *histol*. Fibrinfärbung *f*.
fibrin thrombus Fibrinthrombus *m*.
fi·brin·u·ria [ˌfaɪbrɪˈn(j)ʊərɪə] *n* Fibrinausscheidung *f* im Harn, Fibrinurie *f*.
fibro- *pref*. Faser-, Fibro-.
fi·bro·a·de·nia [ˌfaɪbrəʊəˈdiːnɪə] *n* *patho*. Fibroadenie *f*.
fi·bro·ad·e·no·ma [ˌ-ˌædəˈnəʊmə] *n* *patho*. Fibroadenom *nt*, -adenoma *nt*, Adenofibrom *nt*, Adenoma fibrosum.
f. of breast Fibroadenom der Brust.
fi·bro·ad·e·no·sis [ˌ-ˌædəˈnəʊsɪs] *n* *patho*. Fibroadenose *f*, Fibroadenomatosis.
fi·bro·ad·i·pose [ˌ-ˈædɪpəʊs] *adj* fibrös-fettig, fettig-fibrös.
fi·bro·an·gi·o·ma [ˌ-ˌændʒɪˈəʊmə] *n* *patho*. Fibroangiom *nt*.
fi·bro·a·re·o·lar [ˌ-əˈrɪələr] *adj* *histol*. fibroareolär.
fi·bro·blast [ˈ-blæst] *n* juvenile Bindegewebszelle *f*, Fibroblast *m*.
fi·bro·blas·tic [ˌ-ˈblæstɪk] *adj* **1.** fibroblastisch, Fibroblasten-. **2.** → fibroplastic.
fibroblastic osteosarcoma fibroblastisches Osteosarkom *m*.
fibroblastic sarcoma → fibrosarcoma.
fibroblast interferon β-Interferon *nt abbr*. IFN-β.
fi·bro·blas·to·ma [ˌ-blæsˈtəʊmə] *n* **1.** → fibroma. **2.** → fibrosarcoma.
fi·bro·bron·chi·tis [ˌ-brɒŋˈkaɪtɪs] *n* → fibrinous bronchitis.
fi·bro·car·ci·no·ma [ˌ-kɑːrsɪˈnəʊmə] *n* szirrhöses Karzinom *nt*, Faserkrebs *m*, Szirrhus *m*, Skirrhus *m*, Ca. scirrhosum.
fi·bro·car·ti·lage [ˌ-ˈkɑːrtɪldʒ] *n* fibröser Knorpel *m*, Faserknorpel *m*, Bindegewebsknorpel *m*, Cartilago fibrosa/collagenosa.
fi·bro·car·ti·lag·i·nous [ˌ-ˌkɑːrtɪˈlædʒənəs] *adj* Faserknorpel betr., aus Faserknorpel bestehend, fibrokartilaginär, -chondral, faserknorpelig.
fibrocartilaginous articulation Symphyse *f*, Synchondrose *f*.
fibrocartilaginous lip of acetabulum Pfannenlippe *f*, Labrum acetabulare.
fibrocartilaginous ring of tympanic membrane fibrokartilaginärer Trommelfellring *m*, A(n)nulus fibrocartilagineus (membranae tympani).
fi·bro·ca·se·ous [ˌ-ˈkeɪsɪəs] *adj* *patho*. fibrös-käsig, käsig-fibrös.
fi·bro·cel·lu·lar [ˌ-ˈseljələr] *adj* fibrozellulär.
fibrocellular tumor → fibroma.
fi·bro·ce·men·to·ma [ˌ-ˌsɪmenˈtəʊmə] *n* Zementfibrom *nt*, Zementoblastom *nt*.
fi·bro·chon·dri·tis [ˌ-kɒnˈdraɪtɪs] *n* *patho*. Faserknorpelentzündung *f*, Fibrochondritis *f*.
fi·bro·chon·dro·ma [ˌ-kɒnˈdrəʊmə] *n* *patho*. Fibrochondrom(a) *nt*.
fi·bro·cyst [ˈ-sɪst] *n* *patho*. zystisches Fibrom *nt*, Fibrozystom *nt*.
fi·bro·cys·tic [ˌ-ˈsɪstɪk] *adj patho*. fibrös-zystisch, zystisch-fibrös.
fibrocystic disease: f. of the breast *gyn*. zystische/fibrös-zystische Mastopathie *f*, Mammadysplasie *f*, Zystenmamma *f*, Mastopathia chronica cystica.
f. of the pancreas Mukoviszidose *f*, zystische (Pankreas-)Fibrose *f*, Fibrosis pancreatica cystica.
proliferative f. (of the breast) Schimmelbusch-Krankheit *f*, proliferierende Mastopathie *f*.
fi·bro·cys·to·ma [ˌ-sɪsˈtəʊmə] *n* → fibrocyst.
fi·bro·cyte [ˈfaɪbrəʊsaɪt] *n* Bindegewebszelle *f*, Fibrozyt *m*.
fi·bro·dys·pla·sia [ˌ-dɪsˈpleɪʒ(ɪ)ə, -zɪə] *n* *patho*. fibröse Dysplasie *f*, Fibrodysplasia *f*, Dysplasia fibrosa.
fi·bro·e·las·tic [ˌ-ɪˈlæstɪk] *adj* fibroelastisch.
fibroelastic membrane of larynx (fibroelastische) Kehlkopfmembran *f*, Membrana fibro-elastica laryngis.
fi·bro·e·las·to·ma [ˌ-ɪlæsˈtəʊmə] *n* *patho*. Fibroelastom *nt*.
fi·bro·e·las·to·sis [ˌ-ɪlæsˈtəʊsɪs] *n* *patho*. Fibroelastose *f*, Fibroelastosis *f*.
fi·bro·en·chon·dro·ma [ˌ-enkɒnˈdrəʊmə] *n* *patho*. Fibroenchondrom(a) *nt*.
fi·bro·ep·i·the·li·al [ˌ-epɪˈθɪlɪəl] *adj* fibroepithelial.
fibroepithelial interferon → fibroblast interferon.
fibroepithelial papilloma → fibropapilloma.
fi·bro·ep·i·the·li·o·ma [ˌ-epɪˌθɪlɪˈəʊmə] *n* *patho*. Fibroepitheliom(a) *nt*.
fi·bro·fas·ci·tis [ˌ-fəˈsaɪtɪs] *n* → fibrositis.
fi·bro·fat·ty [ˌ-ˈfætɪ] *adj patho*. fibrös-fettig, fettig-fibrös.
fi·bro·fi·brous [ˌ-ˈfaɪbrəs] *adj patho*. fibrofibrös.
fi·bro·gen·e·sis [ˌ-ˈdʒenəsɪs] *n* Fasersynthese *f*, -bildung *f*, Fibrogenese *f*.
fi·bro·gen·ic [ˌ-ˈdʒenɪk] *adj* Faserbildung induzierend, fibrogen.
fi·brog·li·a [faɪˈbrɒɡlɪə] *n histol*. Fibroglia *f*.
fi·bro·gli·o·ma [ˌfaɪbrəɡlaɪˈəʊmə] *n patho*. Faser-, Fibrogliom(a) *nt*.
fi·bro·gli·o·sis [ˌ-ɡlaɪˈəʊsɪs] *n patho*. Fibrogliose *f*.

fi·bro·his·ti·o·cyt·ic [ˌ-ˌhɪstɪəˈsɪtɪk] *adj* fibrohistiozytär.
fi·broid [ˈfaɪbrɔɪd] **I** *n* **1.** → fibroleiomyoma. **2.** → fibroma. **II** *adj* aus Fasern od. fibrösem Bindegewebe bestehend, fibroid.
fibroid adenoma → fibroadenoma.
fibroid degeneration fibröse Degeneration *f*, Fibrose *f*.
fi·broid·ec·to·my [ˌfaɪbrɔɪˈdektəmɪ] *n chir., gyn.* Fibroidektomie *f*, Fibromektomie *f*.
fibroid heart Cor fibrosum.
fibroid induration Zirrhose *f*, Cirrhosis *f*.
fibroid inflammation atrophische/fibroide Entzündung *f*.
fibroid tumor → fibroma.
fi·bro·in [ˈfaɪbrəwɪn] *n* Fibroin *nt*.
fi·bro·ker·a·to·ma [ˌfaɪbrəkerəˈtəʊmə] *n patho.* Fibrokeratom(a) *nt*.
fi·bro·lei·o·my·o·ma [ˌ-laɪəmaɪˈəʊmə] *n patho.* Fibroleiomyom(a) *nt*, Leiomyofibrom(a) *nt*.
fi·bro·li·po·ma [ˌ-lɪˈpəʊmə] *n patho.* Fibrolipom(a) *nt*, Lipoma fibrosum.
fi·bro·li·pom·a·tous [ˌ-lɪˈpɑmətəs] *adj* fibrolipomatös.
fi·bro·ma [faɪˈbrəʊmə] *n patho.* Bindegewebsgeschwulst *f*, Fibrom(a) *nt*.
fi·bro·ma·toid [faɪˈbrəʊmətɔɪd] *adj* fibromähnlich, -artig, fibromatös.
fi·bro·ma·to·sis [faɪˌbrəʊməˈtəʊsɪs] *n patho.* Fibromatose *f*, Fibromatosis *f*.
fi·bro·ma·tous [faɪˈbrəʊmətəs] *adj* Fibrom betr., fibromartig, fibromatös.
fi·brom·ec·to·my [ˌfaɪbrəʊˈmektəmɪ] *n chir.* Fibromentfernung *f*, -exzision *f*, Fibromektomie *f*.
fi·bro·mem·bra·nous [ˌ-ˈmembrənəs] *adj* fibromembranös, fibromembranartig.
fi·bro·mus·cu·lar [ˌ-ˈmʌskjələr] *adj* fibromuskulär.
fibromuscular dysplasia fibromuskuläre Dysplasie *f*.
fi·bro·my·ec·to·my [ˌ-maɪˈektəmɪ] *n* → fibromyomectomy.
fi·bro·my·o·ma [ˌ-maɪˈəʊmə] *n patho.* Fibromyom(a) *nt*.
fi·bro·my·o·mec·to·my [ˌ-maɪəˈmektəmɪ] *n chir.* Fibromyomexzision *f*, Fibromyomektomie *f*.
fi·bro·my·o·si·tis [ˌ-maɪəˈsaɪtɪs] *n patho.* Fibromyositis *f*.
fi·bro·myx·o·ma [ˌ-mɪkˈsəʊmə] *n patho.* Fibromyxom(a) *nt*.
fi·bro·myx·o·sar·co·ma [ˌ-ˌmɪksəsɑːˈkəʊmə] *n patho.* Fibromyxosarkom *nt*, -myxosarcoma *nt*.
fi·bro·nec·tin [ˌ-ˈnektɪn] *n* Fibronektin *nt*, -nectin *nt*.
fi·bro·neu·ro·ma [ˌ-njʊəˈrəʊmə] *n patho.* Neurofibrom *nt*, Fibroneurom *nt*.
fi·bro·nu·cle·ar [ˌ-ˈn(j)uːklɪər] *adj* fibronukleär.
fibro-osseous *adj* fibroossär.
fibro-osteoclastic *adj* fibroosteoklastisch.
fibro-osteoma *n patho.* verknöcherndes/ossifizierendes Fibrom *nt*, Fibroosteom *nt*.
fi·bro·pap·il·lo·ma [ˌ-ˌpæpəˈləʊmə] *n patho.* fibroepitheliales Papillom *nt*, Fibropapillom *nt*.
fi·bro·pla·sia [ˌ-ˈpleɪʒ(ɪ)ə, -zɪə] *n patho.* Fibroplasie *f*, Fibroplasia *f*.
fi·bro·plas·tic [ˌ-ˈplæstɪk] *adj* fibroplastisch.
fibroplastic tumor 1. → fibroma. **2.** → fibrosarcoma.
fi·bro·plate [ˈ-pleɪt] *n* Gelenk(zwischen)scheibe *f*, Discus articularis.
fi·bro·pol·y·pus [ˌ-ˈpɑlɪpəs] *n patho.* fibröser Polyp *m*.
fi·bro·pu·ru·lent [ˌ-ˈpjʊər(j)ələnt] *adj* fibrös-eitrig, eitrig-fibrös.
fi·bro·re·tic·u·late [ˌ-rɪˈtɪkjəlɪt, -leɪt] *adj histol.* fibroretikulär.
fi·bro·sar·co·ma [ˌ-sɑːˈkəʊmə] *n patho.* Fibrosarkom *nt*, -sarcoma *nt*.
fi·bro·sar·co·ma·tous [ˌ-sɑːˈkɑmətəs] *adj* fibrosarkomatös.
fi·brose [ˈfaɪbrəʊs] **I** *adj* → fibrous. **II** *vt* fibrosieren.
fi·bro·se·rous [ˌfaɪbrəʊˈsɪərəs] *adj* fibroserös, fibrös-serös, serofibrös.
fi·bros·ing alveolitis [ˈfaɪbrəʊsɪŋ] idiopathische Lungenfibrose *f*, fibrosierende Alveolitis *f*.
fibrosing osteochondroma Osteochondrofibrom(a) *nt*.
fi·bro·sis [faɪˈbrəʊsɪs] *n, pl* **-ses** [-siːz] *patho.* Fibrose *f*, Fibrosis *f*.
fi·bro·si·tis [ˌfaɪbrəˈsaɪtɪs] *n* Weichteil-, Muskelrheumatismus *m*, Fibrositis-Syndrom *nt*.
fi·bro·tho·rax [ˌ-ˈθɔːræks] *n patho.* Fibrothorax *m*.
fi·brot·ic [faɪˈbrɑtɪk] *adj* Fibrose betr., fibrotisch.
fi·brous [ˈfaɪbrəs] *adj* faserig, fibrös, Faser-.
fibrous actin → F-actin.
fibrous ankylosis fibröse Gelenkversteifung/Ankylose *f*, Ankylosis fibrosa.
fibrous annulus Faserring *m*, A(n)ulus fibrosus (disci intervertebralis).
fibrous appendage of liver → fibrous appendix of liver.
fibrous appendix of liver Leberzipfel *m*, Appendix fibrosa hepatis.
fibrous arch of soleus muscle Arcus tendineus m. solei.
fibrous astrocyte Spinnenzelle *f*, faseriger/fibrillärer Astrozyt *m*.
fibrous bone Bindegewebsknochen *m*.
fibrous capsule fibröse Kapsel *f*.
f. of graafian follicle Tunica externa thecae folliculi.
f. of kidney (fibröse) Nierenkapsel, Capsula fibrosa renis.
f. of liver → perivascular f.
perivascular f. Glisson'-Kapsel, Capsula fibrosa perivascularis.
f. of spleen fibröse Milzkapsel, Tunica fibrosa (lienis).
f. of thyroid (gland) Schilddrüsenkapsel, Capsula fibrosa gl. thyroideae.
fibrous cartilage → fibrocartilage.
fibrous cavernitis Peyronie-Krankheit *f*, Penisfibromatose *f*, Induratio penis plastica, Sclerosis fibrosa penis.
fibrous coat → fibrous tunic.
f. of corpus cavernosum Tunica albuginea corporum cavernosum.
f. of eyeball → fibrous tunic of eyeball.
f. of liver → fibrous tunic of liver.
f. of ovary Theca folliculi.
f. of testis Tunica albuginea testis.
fibrous cortical defect → fibroxanthoma of bone.
fibrous degeneration fibröse Degeneration *f*, Fibrose *f*.
fibrous dysplasia fibröse Dysplasie *f*, Fibrodysplasie *f*, -dysplasia *f*, Dysplasia fibrosa.
f. of bone Jaffé-Lichtenstein-Krankheit *f*, Jaffé-Lichtenstein-Uehlinger-Syndrom *nt*, fibröse (Knochen-)Dysplasie, nicht-ossifizierendes juveniles Osteofibrom *nt*, halbseitige von Recklinghausen-Krankheit *f*, Osteodystrophia fibrosa unilateralis.
f. of jaw Cherubismus *m*, Cherubinismus *m*.
polyostotic f. Albright-Syndrom *nt*, Albright-McCune-Syndrom *nt*, McCune-Albright-Syndrom *nt*, polyostotische fibröse Dysplasie.
fibrous giant cell tumor of bone nicht-osteogenes/nicht-ossifizierendes Knochenfibrom *nt*, xanthomatöser/fibröser Riesenzelltumor *m* des Knochens, Xanthogranuloma *nt* des Knochens.
fibrous glass → fiberglass.
fibrous goiter fibröse Struma *f*, Struma fibrosa.
fibrous histiocytoma *patho.* Fibrohistiozytom *nt*, fibröses Histiozytom *nt*, Dermatofibrom *nt*.
malignant f. malignes fibröses Histiozytom.
fibrous joint Bandverbindung *f*, Artic. fibrosa.
fibrous layer of articular capsule → fibrous membrane of articular capsule.
fibrous ligament: anterior f. Lig. sternoclaviculare anterius.
posterior f. Lig. sternoclaviculare posterius.
fibrous long-spacing collagen *abbr.* **FLSC** fibrous long-spacing collagen *abbr.* FLSC.
fibrous membrane of articular capsule Fibrosa *f*, Membrana fibrosa (capsulae articularis), Stratum fibrosum.
fibrous nephritis interstitielle Nephritis *f*.
fibrous pericarditis fibrinöse Perikardzündung/Perikarditis *f*, Pericarditis fibrinosa.
fibrous pericardium äußeres fibröses Perikard *nt*.
fibrous pneumonia fibrös-organisierte Pneumonie *f*.
chronic f. interstitielle Lungenfibrose *f*.
fibrous polyp fibröser Polyp *m*.
fibrous protein → fibrillar protein.
fibrous ring → fibrous annulus.
f.s of heart Faserringe *pl* der Herzostien, A(n)uli fibrosi cordis.
fibrous scarring Narbenfibromatose *f*.
fibrous septum of nose bindegewebiger Abschnitt *m* der Nasenscheidewand, Pars fibrosa septi nasi.
fibrous sheath of optic nerve äußere Durahülle *f* des N. opticus, Vagina externa (n. optici).
fibrous skeleton of heart Herzskelett *nt*.
fibrous tendon sheath fibröse Sehnenscheide *f*, Vagina fibrosa tendinis.
f.s of foot Vaginae fibrosae tendinum digitorum pedis.
f.s of toes Vaginae fibrosae digitorum pedis.
fibrous tissue fibröses Bindegewebe *nt*.
fibrous trigones of heart fibröse Bindegewebszwickel *pl* des Herzens, Trigona fibrosa cordis.
fibrous tunic faserig-bindegewebige Organhüllschicht/-kapsel *f*, Tunica fibrosa.
f. of eyeball äußere Augenhaut *f*, Tunica fibrosa bulbi.
f. of kidney → fibrous capsule of kidney.
f. of liver Bindegewebskapsel der Leber, Tunica fibrosa hepatis.
fi·bro·vas·cu·lar [ˌfaɪbrəʊˈvæskjələr] *adj* fibrovaskulär.
fi·bro·xan·tho·ma [ˌ-zænˈθəʊmə] *n patho.* Fibroxanthom(a) *nt*.
f. of bone nicht-ossifizierendes Fibrom *nt*, fibröser Kortikalisdefekt *m*, fibröser metaphysärer Defekt *m*, benignes fibröses Histiozytom *nt* des Knochens.
fib·u·la [ˈfɪbjələ] *n, pl* **-las, -lae** [-liː] Wadenbein *nt*, Fibula *f*.
fib·u·lar [ˈfɪbjələr] *adj* Wadenbein betr., fibular, Wadenbein-, Fibula-.
fibular artery Wadenbeinschlagader *f*, -arterie *f*, Fibularis *f*, A. fibularis.

fibular bone

fibular bone → fibula.
fibular border of foot Fußaußenrand m, Margo lateralis/fibularis pedis.
fibular bursa Bursa subtendinea m. bicipitis femoris inferior.
fibula fracture ortho. Wadenbeinbruch m, -fraktur f, Fibulafraktur f.
fibular hemimelia fibulare Hemimelie f.
fibular incisure (of tibia) Inc. fibularis (tibiae).
fib·u·la·ris (muscle) [ˌfɪbjəˈlεərɪs]: **long f.** old → peroneus longus (muscle).
  short f. old → peroneus brevis (muscle).
  third f. old → peroneus tertius (muscle).
fibular malleolus Außenknöchel m, Malleolus lateralis.
fibular margin of foot → fibular border of foot.
fibular muscle: long f. old → peroneus longus (muscle).
  short f. old → peroneus brevis (muscle).
  third f. old → peroneus tertius (muscle).
fibular nerve: common f. Fibularis/Peronäus m communis, N. fibularis/peron(a)eus communis.
  deep f. Fibularis/Peronäus m profundus, N. fibularis/peron(a)eus profundus.
  superficial f. Fibularis/Peronäus m superficialis, N. fibularis/peron(a)eus superficialis.
fibular node Lymphknoten m an der A. fibularis, Nodus fibularis.
fibular notch (of tibia) → fibular incisure (of tibia).
fibular trochlea (of calcaneus) Trochlea peron(a)ealis/fibularis (calcanei).
fibular veins Wadenbeinvenen pl, Vv. fibulares.
fib·u·lo·cal·ca·ne·al [ˌfɪbjələʊkælˈkeɪnɪəl] adj Fibula u. Kalkaneus betr. od. verbindend, fibulokalkaneal.
fi·cin [ˈfaɪsn] n Ficin nt.
Fick [ˈfɪk]: **F.'s first law of diffusion** Fick'-Diffusionsgesetz nt.
  F.'s formula Fick'-Gleichung f, -Formel f.
  F.'s law of diffusion → F.'s first law of diffusion.
  F.'s method → F.'s principle.
  F.'s principle Fick'-Prinzip nt.
fi·co·sis [faɪˈkəʊsɪs] n derm. Sykose f, Sycosis f.
fi·del·i·ty [fɪˈdelɪtɪ, faɪ-] n, pl **-ties** Genauigkeit f; genaue Übereinstimmung f.
Fiedler [ˈfiːdlər]: **F.'s disease** Weil'-Krankheit f, Leptospirosis icterohaemorrhagica.
  F.'s myocarditis idiopathische Myokarditis f, Fiedler'-Myokarditis f.
field [fiːld] n 1. (a. anat., fig.) Feld nt, Gebiet nt, Bezirk m, Bereich m. 2. electr., mathe., phys. Feld nt. 3. psycho. (Um-)Feld nt.
  f. of activity Arbeitsgebiet, Tätigkeitsbereich.
  f. of application Anwendungsbereich.
  f. of force phys. Kraftfeld.
  f. of gaze Blickfeld.
  f. of vision physiol. Augenfeld; Blick-, Gesichtsfeld.
field block Feldblock m.
field block anesthesia anes. Feldblock m.
field blocking → field block.
field fever 1. Zuckerrohrfieber nt, Zuckerplantagenleptospirose f, cane-field fever (nt). 2. Batavia-, Reisfeldfieber nt, Leptospirosis bataviae. 3. Feld-, Ernte-, Schlamm-, Sumpffieber nt, Erbsenpflückerkrankheit f, Leptospirosis grippotyphosa.
field H (of Forel) Forel'-H-Feld nt.
field H₁ (of Forel) Forel'-H₁-Feld nt.
field H₂ (of Forel) Forel'-H₂-Feld nt.

field hospital Feldlazarett nt.
Fielding [ˈfiːldɪŋ]: **F.'s membrane** Tapetum nt.
field intensity phys. Feldstärke f.
field-ion microscope phys. Feldionenmikroskop nt.
field lens Feldlinse f.
field strength phys. Feldstärke f.
field study stat. Feldstudie f.
Fiessinger-Leroy-Reiter [ˈfiːsəndʒər ləˈrwa ˈraɪtər]: **F.-L.-R. syndrome** Reiter'-Krankheit f, -Syndrom nt, Fiessinger-Leroy-Reiter-Syndrom nt, venerische Arthritis f, Okulourethrosynovitis f, urethro-okulo-synoviales Syndrom nt.
fièvre boutonneuse [ˈfjεːvrə butɔˈnœs] Boutonneuse-Fieber nt, Fièvre boutonneuse.
fifth disease [fɪfθ, fɪθ] Ringelröteln pl, Sticker-Krankheit f, fünfte Krankheit f, Morbus quintus, Erythema infectiosum, Megalerythem nt, Megalerythema epidemicum/infectiosum.
fifth finger Kleinfinger m, Digitus minimus/quintus.
fifth nerve Trigeminus m, V. Hirnnerv m, N. trigeminus.
fifth venereal disease Morbus Durand-Nicolas-Favre m, klimatischer Bubo m, vierte Geschlechtskrankheit f, Lymphogranuloma inguinale/venereum abbr. LGV, Lymphopathia venerea, Poradenitis inguinalis.
fifth ventricle Cavum septi pellucidi.
fight-or-flight reaction [faɪt] Alarmreaktion f.
FIGLU abbr. → formiminoglutamic acid.
fig·u·rate erythema [ˈfɪgjərɪt] derm. Erythema gyratum/figuratum.
figurate psoriasis derm. Psoriasis figurata.
fig·ure [ˈfɪgjər] I n 1. Zahl f, Ziffer f. 2. Betrag m, Summe f; Preis m. 3. Figur f, Form f, Gestalt f, Aussehen nt. 4. Figur f, Diagramm nt, Zeichnung f; Illustration f. II vt 5. formen, gestalten. 6. abbilden, bildlich darstellen. III vi 7. rechnen. 8. erscheinen, auftauchen, vorkommen.
fig·ured [ˈfɪgjərd] adj geformt, gestaltet, figuriert.
figure-of-eight bandage ortho. Achter(gang)verband m, Fächerverband m, Schildkrötenverband m.
figure-of-eight suture chir. 8er-Naht f, Achternaht f.
  Bunnell f. Achternaht ohne Ausziehdraht.
fig wart [fɪg] Feig-, Feuchtwarze f, spitzes Kondylom nt, Condyloma acuminatum, Papilloma acuminatum/venereum.
fi·la·ceous [fɪˈleɪʃəs] adj filamentös.
fil·a·ment [ˈfɪləmənt] n 1. Faser f; (a. electr., techn.) (dünner) Faden m, feiner Draht m. 2. anat. fadenförmiger Fortsatz m, Filament nt, Filamentum nt.
  f. of meninges Filum terminale/spinale.
fil·a·men·tous [fɪləˈmentəs] adj 1. fadenförmig, faserig, faserartig, Fasern-; anat. filiform. 2. filamentös.
filamentous colony micro. filamentöse/myzeliale Kolonie f.
fil·a·men·tum [fɪləˈmentəm] n, pl **-ta** [-tə] → filament 2.
fi·lar [ˈfaɪlər] adj 1. → fibrillar. 2. → filamentous.
Fi·la·ria [fɪˈlεərɪə] n micro. Filaria f.
  F. bancrofti Bancroft-Filarie f, Wuchereria bancrofti.
  F. diurna 1. Wanderfilarie f, Taglarvenfilarie f, Augenwurm m, Loa loa. 2. Microfilaria diurna.
  F. dracunculus Medina-, Guineawurm m, Dracunculus/Filaria medinensis.

F. immitis Herzwurm m, Dirofilaria immitis.
F. loa → F. diurna 1.
F. medinensis → F. dracunculus.
F. nocturna → F. bancrofti.
F. sanguinis-hominis → F. bancrofti.
F. volvulus Knäuelfilarie f, Onchocerca volvulus.
fi·lar·i·a [fɪˈlεərɪə] n, pl **-lar·i·ae** [-ˈlεərɪˌiː] micro. Filarie f, Filaria f.
fi·lar·i·al [fɪˈlεərɪəl] adj Filarie(n) betr., Filarien-.
filarial arthritis Filarienarthritis f.
filarial worm → filaria.
fil·a·ri·a·sis [ˌfɪləˈraɪəsɪs] n Filarieninfektion f, Filariose f, Filariasis f.
fi·lar·i·ci·dal [fɪˌlεərɪˈsaɪdl] adj filarien(ab)tötend, filarizid.
fi·lar·i·cide [fɪˈlεərɪsaɪd] n Filarienmittel nt, Filarizid nt.
fi·lar·i·form [fɪˈlεərɪfɔːrm] adj 1. filarienähnlich, -artig, filariform. 2. → filiform.
Fi·lar·i·i·cae [fɪˈlεərɪsiː] pl → Filarioidea.
fi·lar·i·id worm [fɪˈlεərɪɪd] → filaria.
Fi·la·ri·oi·dea [fɪˌlεərɪˈɔɪdɪə] pl micro. Filarioidea pl.
Filatov [fɪˈlætɔf]: **F.'s disease** Pfeiffer'-Drüsenfieber nt, infektiöse Mononukleose f, Monozytenangina f, Mononucleosis infectiosa.
  F. flap Rundstiellappen m.
  F.'s spots Koplik-Flecken pl.
Filatov-Dukes [d(j)uːks]: **F.-D. disease** Dukes'-Krankheit f, Dukes-Filatoff'-Krankheit f, Filatow-Dukes-Krankheit f, vierte Krankheit f, Parascarlatina f, Rubeola scarlatinosa.
Filatov-Gillies [ˈgɪliːz]: **F.-G. flap** Rundstiellappen m.
file¹ [faɪl] I n 1. Akte f, Ordner m, Aktenstück nt. 2. (Computer) Datei f. 3. Reihe f. II vt (ein-)ordnen, ab-, einheften.
file² [faɪl] I n ortho., techn. Feile f. II vt (zu-)feilen.
fil·i·al [ˈfɪlɪəl] adj genet. Filial-.
filial generation genet. Filialgeneration f.
  first f. → filial generation 1.
  second f. → filial generation 2.
filial generation 1 abbr. F₁ Tochtergeneration f, F₁-Generation f abbr. F₁.
filial generation 2 abbr. F₂ Enkelgeneration f, F₂-Generation f abbr. F₂.
fil·i·cin [ˈfɪləsɪn] n Filicin nt.
fil·i·form [ˈfɪlɪfɔːrm, ˈfaɪl-] adj fadenförmig, faserig, faserartig, Fasern-; anat. filiform.
filiform bougie Filiformbougie m, Gleitsonde f.
filiform papillae fadenförmige Papillen pl, Papillae filiformis.
filiform pulse fadenförmiger/dünner Puls m, Pulsus filiformis.
fil·i·o·pa·ren·tal [ˌfɪlɪəʊpəˈrεntl] adj Eltern-Kind-.
fill [fɪl] I n Füllung f. II vt 1. (voll-, an-, aus-)füllen; (Flüssigkeit) ein-, abfüllen. 2. (Essen) sättigen. 3. dent. füllen, plombieren. III vi s. füllen.
  fill in vt (Loch) auf-, ausfüllen, ergänzen.
  fill out vt (Formular) ausfüllen.
  fill up vt ausfüllen.
fill·er [ˈfɪlər] n 1. Abfüllmaschine f; Trichter m. 2. Füllstoff m, -masse f, -paste f.
fil·let [ˈfɪlɪt] n 1. Band nt, Streifen m, Strang m. 2. anat. Schleife f, Lemniskus m, Lemniscus m.
fill·ing [ˈfɪlɪŋ] I n 1. Füllung f, Füllmasse f, -material nt. 2. dent. (Zahn-)Füllung f, (-)Plombe f. 3. (Voll-, An-, Aus-)Füllen nt; dent. Plombieren nt. II adj (Essen) sättigend.
filling defect radiol. Füllungsdefekt m.

filling period *physiol.* Füllungsphase *f.*
filling pressure Füllungsdruck *m.*
  mean f. mittlerer Füllungsdruck, statischer Blutdruck.
fill-in test *psycho.* Lückentest *m.*
film [fɪlm] **I** *n* **1.** Film *m*, Membran(e) *f*, (dünnes) Häutchen *nt.* **2.** Schleier *m*; (*Auge*) Trübung *f.* **3.** Film *m*, Überzug *m*, (dünne) Schicht *f*, Haut *f*, Häutchen *nt*, Belag *m.* **4.** *photo.* Film *m.* **5.** feines Gewebe *nt*, Faser *f.* **II** *vt* überziehen (*with* mit); ein Häutchen bilden. **III** *vi* s. mit einem Häutchen überziehen; (*Glas*) anlaufen.
  film over *vi* → film III.
film badge *radiol.* Strahlenschutzplakette *f.*
film contrast *radiol.* Filmkontrast *m.*
film·i·ness ['fɪlmɪnɪs] *n* (hauch-)dünne Beschaffenheit *f.*
film oxygenator Filmoxygenator *m.*
film·y ['fɪlmɪ] *adj* **1.** (*Auge*) trüb, verschleiert. **2.** mit einem Häutchen bedeckt; häutchenartig. **3.** (hauch-)dünn, zart.
fi·lo·po·di·um [ˌfɪləˈpəʊdɪəm, ˌfaɪ-] *n*, *pl* **-dia** [-dɪə] *bio.* Fadenfüßchen *nt*, Filopodium *nt.*
fi·lo·var·i·co·sis [ˌværəˈkəʊsɪs] *n* *patho.* Filovarikose *f.*
Fi·lo·vir·i·dae [ˌ-ˈvɪrədiː] *pl micro.* Filoviridae *pl.*
fil·ter ['fɪltər] **I** *n chem.*, *phys.*, *photo.*, *electr.* Filter *m*/*nt.* **II** *vt* filtern, filtrieren. **III** *vi* durchsickern (*through* durch); (*Licht*) durchscheinen, -schimmern (*through* durch).
  filter off *vt* abfiltern.
fil·ter·a·bil·i·ty [ˌfɪltərəˈbɪlətɪ] *n* Filtrierbarkeit *f.*
fil·ter·a·ble ['fɪlt(ə)rəbl] *adj* filtrierbar.
filter bag Filtertüte *f.*
fil·ter·ing ['fɪlt(ə)rɪŋ] **I** *n* Filtern *nt*, Filtrieren *nt.* **II** *adj* Filtrier-, Filter-.
filtering paper → filter paper.
filter paper Filter-, Filtrierpapier *nt.*
filter-paper chromatography Papierchromatographie *f.*
fil·tra·ble ['fɪltrəbl] *adj* → filterable.
fil·trate ['fɪltreɪt] **I** *n* Filtrat *nt.* **II** *vt* (ab-)filtern, filtrieren.
filtrate factor *old* → pantothenic acid.
fil·tra·tion [fɪl'treɪʃn] *n* Filtration *f*, Filtrierung *f*, Filtrieren *nt.*
filtration angle Iridokorneal-, Kammerwinkel *m*, Angulus iridocornealis.
filtration coefficient *abbr.* **kF** Filtrationskoeffizient *m abbr.* k$_F$.
filtration equilibrium Filtrationsgleichgewicht *nt.*
filtration fraction *abbr.* **FF** (*Niere*) Filtrationsfraktion *f abbr.* FF.
filtration pressure Filtrationsdruck *m.*
filtration rate Filtrationsrate *f*, -geschwindigkeit *f.*
filtration reabsorption equilibrium Filtrations-Reabsorptionsgleichgewicht *nt.*
filtration slit *histol.* Schlitz-, Filtrationspore *f.*
fi·lum ['faɪləm] *n*, *pl* **-la** [-lə] *anat.* Faden *m*, fadenförmige Struktur *f*, Filum *nt.*
fim·bria ['fɪmbrɪə] *n*, *pl* **-bri·ae** [-briː] **1.** *anat.* Franse *f*, fransenartige Struktur *f*, Fimbrie *f*, Fimbria *f.* **2.** *-æ pl* Pili *pl*, Fimbrien *f.*
  f. of hippocampus Markbündel *nt* des Hippocampus, Fimbria hippocampi.
  f.e of uterine tube Tubenfimbrien *pl*, Fimbriae tubae.
fim·bri·ate ['fɪmbrɪɪt, -eɪt] *adj* mit Fransen/Fimbrien besetzt, befranst.
fim·bri·at·ed ['-eɪtɪd] *adj* → fimbriate.
fimbriated crest → fimbriated fold.
fimbriated fold Plica fimbriata.

fim·bri·ec·to·my [ˌfɪmbrɪˈektəmɪ] *n gyn.* Fimbrienentfernung *f*, Fimbriektomie *f.*
fim·bri·o·cele ['fɪmbrɪəsiːl] *n* Fimbriozele *f.*
fim·bri·o·den·tate sulcus [ˌ-ˈdenteɪt] Sulcus fimbriodentatus.
fim·bri·ol·y·sis [fɪmbrɪˈɒləsɪs] *n gyn.* Fimbrienlösung *f*, Fimbriolyse *f.*
fim·bri·o·plas·ty ['fɪmbrɪəplæstɪ] *n gyn.* Fimbrienplastik *f.*
fi·nal host ['faɪnl] *bio.*, *micro.* Endwirt *m.*
final phase Endphase *f*, -stadium *nt.*
find·ing ['faɪndɪŋ] *n* (*a. -s pl*) Befund *m*; Beobachtung *f*; Feststellung(en *pl*) *f.*
fine [faɪn] *adj* fein; dünn, zart, zierlich; rein, pur.
fine-needle aspiration biopsy Feinnadelaspiration(sbiopsie *f*) *f*, Feinnadel(punktions)biopsie *f.*
fine-needle biopsy Feinnadelbiopsie *f.*
fine-needle transhepatic cholangiography *abbr.* **FNTC** transhepatische Feinnadelcholangiographie *f.*
fine structure Feinbau *m*, Ultrastruktur *f.*
fine tremor feinschlägiger Tremor *m.*
fin·ger ['fɪŋɡər] **I** *n* **1.** Finger *m*; *anat.* Digitus *m.* **2.** Fingerbreit *m.* **3.** (Uhr-)Zeiger *m.* **4.** *techn.* Greifer *m.* **5.** (*Handschuh*) Fingerling *m.* **II** *vt* befühlen, betasten, (be-)fingern, anfassen, herumfingern (an).
fin·ger·ag·no·sia [ˌfɪŋɡəræɡˈnəʊʒ(ɪ)ə] *n neuro.* Fingeragnosie *f.*
finger amputation Fingeramputation *f.*
finger cellulitis → felon.
fingered ['fɪŋɡəd] *adj* mit Fingern.
finger fracture technique *chir.* (*Leber*) Fingerdissektion *f.*
fin·ger·ing ['fɪŋɡərɪŋ] *n* Betasten *nt*, Befühlen *nt*, (Be-)Fingern *nt.*
fin·ger·nail ['fɪŋɡərneɪl] *n* (Finger-)Nagel *m*; *anat.* Unguis *m.*
finger-nose test *neuro.* Finger-Nase-Versuch *m.*
finger percussion Finger-Finger-Perkussion *f.*
finger phenomenon Gordon-Fingerspreizreflex *m*, -Reflex *m.*
fin·ger·print ['fɪŋɡərprɪnt] *n* **1.** Fingerabdruck *m*, Daktylogramm *nt.* **2.** (unverwechselbares) Kennzeichen *nt.*
fingerprint degeneration *patho.* Fingerprintdegeneration *f.*
finger pulp Fingerkuppe *f*, -beere *f.*
finger ray Fingerstrahl *m.*
finger-thumb reflex Mayer-Reflex *m*, Daumenmitbewegungsphänomen *nt.*
fin·ger·tip ['fɪŋɡətɪp] *n* Fingerspitze *f.*
finger-to-finger test *neuro.* Finger-Finger-Versuch *m.*
Finkler and Prior ['fɪŋklər 'praɪər]: **spirillum of F.a.P.** Vibrio metschnikovii, Vibrio cholerae biovar proteus.
Finkelstein ['fɪŋkəlstaɪn, -ʃtaɪn]: **F.'s sign/test** Finkelstein-Zeichen *nt.*
Finney ['fɪnɪ]: **F.'s operation/pyloroplasty** *chir.* Pyloroplastik *f* nach Finney.
Finsen ['fɪnzn]: **F.'s apparatus/lamp** Finsen-Lampe *f.*
  F. light/rays Finsen-Licht *nt.*
Finsen-Reya ['reɪə]: **F.-R. lamp** Finsen-Reya-Lampe *f.*
fire ['faɪər] *n* **1.** Feuer *nt*, Flamme *f.* **2.** → fever. **3.** *patho.* Entzündung *f*, Inflammation *f*, Inflammatio *f.* **4.** *anat.* Wundrose *f*, Rose *f*, Erysipel *nt*, Erysipelas *nt*, Streptodermia cutanea lymphatica.
firm [fɜːm] *n* Ärzteteam *nt.*
fir·pene ['fɜːpiːn] *n* Pinen *nt.*
first aid [fɜːst] Erste Hilfe *f.*
first degree burn Verbrennung *f* 1. Grades.
first division of trigeminal nerve erster Trigeminusast *m*, N. ophthalmicus.

first finger Daumen *m*, Pollex *m.*
first head of triceps brachii muscle langer Trizepskopf *m*, Caput longum m. tricipitis brachii.
first law of thermodynamics erster Hauptsatz *m* der Thermodynamik.
first nerves Riechfäden *pl*, Fila olfactoria, Nn. olfactorii.
first-order reaction *chem.* Reaktion *f* erster Ordnung.
  apparent/pseudo f. pseudomonomolekulare Reaktion.
first rank symptoms *abbr.* **FRS** *psychia.* Symptome *pl* ersten Ranges.
first sound erster Herzton *m*, I. Herzton *m.*
first stage (of labor) *gyn.* Eröffnungsphase *f*, -periode *f.*
first substrate *biochem.* erstes/führendes Substrat *nt.*
Fischer ['fɪʃər]: **F. projection** *chem.* Fischer-Projektion *f.*
  F.'s projection formulas *chem.* Fischer-Projektionsformeln *pl.*
Fisher ['fɪʃər]: **F.'s syndrome** Fisher-Syndrom *nt.*
fish skin [fɪʃ] **1.** Fischschuppenkrankheit *f*, Ichthyosis vulgaris. **2.** Saurier-, Krokodil-, Alligatorhaut *f*, Sauriasis *f.*
fish-mouth mitral stenosis [fɪʃmaʊθ] *card.* (*Mitralis*) Knopflochstenose *f*, Fischmaulstenose *f.*
fish tapeworm *micro.* (breiter) Fischbandwurm *m*, Grubenkopfbandwurm *m*, Diphyllobothrium latum, Bothriocephalus latus.
fish tapeworm anemia Anämie *f* bei Fischbandwurmbefall.
fis·sile ['fɪsɪl] *adj* → fissionable.
fissile material *phys.* Spaltmaterial *nt*, spaltbares Material *nt.*
fis·sil·i·ty [fɪˈsɪlətɪ] *n* → fissionability.
fis·sion ['fɪʃn] **I** *n* **1.** Spaltung *f*, Spalten *nt.* **2.** *bio.* (Zell-)Teilung *f.* **3.** *phys.* Kernspaltung *f.* **II** *vt phys.* spalten. **III** *vi phys.* s. spalten.
fis·sion·a·bil·i·ty [ˌfɪʃənəˈbɪlətɪ] *n* Spaltbarkeit *f.*
fis·sion·a·ble ['fɪʃənəbl] *adj* spaltbar.
fission bomb Atombombe *f.*
fission fungi *micro.* Spaltpilze *pl*, Schizomyzeten *pl*, Schizomycetes *pl.*
fission product *phys.* Spaltungsprodukt *nt*, Spaltprodukt *nt.*
fis·sip·a·rous [fɪˈsɪpərəs] *adj bio.* s. durch Teilung vermehrend, fissipar.
fis·su·ral ['fɪʃərəl] *adj* Fissur betr., Fissuren-.
fis·sure ['fɪʃər] **I** *n* **1.** Spalt(e *f*) *m*, Ritze *f*, Riß *m.* **2.** *anat.* Spalt(e *f*) *m*, Furche *f*, Rinne *f*, Fissur *f*, Fissura *f.* **3.** Fissur *f* (Knochen-)Riß *m*; (*Haut*) Schrunde *f*, Rhagade *f.* **4.** Spaltung *f.* **II** *vt* spalten. **III** *vi* s. spalten, rissig werden, aufspringen, (*Haut*) schrundig werden.
  f. of Bichat Fissura transversa cerebralis.
  f. of glottis Stimmritze, Rima glottidis.
  f. of hippocampus Fissura hippocampi, Sulcus hippocampi/hippocampalis.
  f. of laryngeal vestibule Vorhofspalte, -ritze, Rima vestibuli laryngis.
  f. for ligamentum teres Fissura lig. teretis.
  f. for ligamentum venosum Fissura lig. venosi.
  f. of Monro Sulcus hypothalamicus.
  f. of Rolando Rolando'-Fissur *f*, Zentralfurche *f* des Großhirns, Sulcus centralis (cerebri).
  f. of round ligament (Leber-)Furche für Lig. teres hepatis, Fissura lig. teretis hepatis.
  f. of Sylvius Sylvius'-Furche *f*, Sulcus lateralis.

fissurectomy

f. of venous ligament Fissura lig. venosi.
f. of vestibule → f. of laryngeal vestibule.
fis·su·rec·to·my [fɪʃəˈrektəmɪ] *n chir.* Fissurektomie *f.*
fis·sured [ˈfɪʃərd] *adj* **1.** gespalten, eingerissen, rissig. **2.** (*Haut*) (auf-)gesprungen, schrundig, rissig.
fissured fracture Haarbruch *m*, Knochenfissur *f.*
fissured tongue Faltenzunge *f*, Lingua plicata/scrotalis.
fissure fracture → fissured fracture.
fist [fɪst] **I** *n* Faust *f.* **II** *vt* eine Faust machen, die Hand zur Faust ballen.
fist·ed [fɪstɪd] *adj* geballt.
fis·tu·la [ˈfɪstʃələ] *n, pl* **-las, -lae** [-liː] **1.** *patho.* Fistel *f*, Fistula *f.* **2.** *chir.* Fistel *f*; Shunt *m.*
fistula knife *chir.* Fistelmesser *nt*, Syringotom *nt.*
fis·tu·lar [ˈfɪstʃələr] *adj* → fistulous.
fistula symptom *HNO* Fistelsymptom *nt.*
fis·tu·lat·ed [ˈfɪstʃəleɪtɪd] *adj* → fistulous.
fistula test *HNO* Fistelprobe *f*, Fistelsymptomtest *m.*
fis·tu·la·tion [ˌfɪstʃəˈleɪʃn] *n* → fistulization.
fis·tu·la·tome [ˈfɪstʃələtəʊm] *n chir.* Fistelmesser *nt*, Syringotom *nt.*
fis·tu·lec·to·my [ˌfɪstʃəˈlektəmɪ] *n chir.* Fistelgangsexzision *f*, Fistulektomie *f*, Syringektomie *f.*
fis·tu·li·za·tion [ˌfɪstʃəlɪˈzeɪʃn] *n* **1.** *patho.* Fistelbildung *f.* **2.** *chir.* Anlegen *nt* einer Fistel *od.* eines Shunts, Fistelung *f.*
fis·tu·lize [ˈfɪstʃəlaɪz] *vt chir.* eine Fistel *od.* einen Shunt anlegen.
fis·tu·lo·en·ter·os·to·my [ˌfɪstʃələʊentəˈrɒstəmɪ] *n chir.* Ableitung *f* einer Fistel in den Darm, Fistuloenterostomie *f.*
fis·tu·lose [ˈfɪstʃələʊs] *adj* → fistulous.
fis·tu·lot·o·my [ˌfɪstʃəˈlɒtəmɪ] *n chir.* Fistelspaltung *f*, Fistulotomie *f*, Syringotomie *f.*
fis·tu·lous [ˈfɪstʃələs] *adj* Fistel betr., fistelartig, -ähnlich, Fistel-.
fistulous tract Fistelgang *m.*
fit¹ [fɪt] **I** *n* **1.** Sitz *m*, Paßform *f.* **a good/bad ~** es paßt gut/nicht gut. **a tight ~** stramm sitzen. **2.** Übereinstimmung *f*; Zusammenpassen *nt* **II** *adj* **3.** passend, geeignet; (*Zeitpunkt*) günstig. **4.** tauglich; verwendbar, brauchbar (*for* für). **5.** angemessen, angebracht (*to do zu tun*). **6.** *sport.* fit, (gut) in Form; gesund. **to keep ~ s.** fit halten. **to look ~** gesund aussehen. **III** *vt* **7.** anpassen (*to an*); passend machen (*for* für); einpassen, -setzen, -bauen (*into* in). **8.** an jdm. Maß nehmen; anprobieren (*on s.o.* jdm.). **9.** ausrüsten, ausstatten, einrichten (*with* mit). **10.** jdn. befähigen (*for* für, *to do* zu tun); jdn. ausbilden (*for* für). IV *vi* **11.** (*Prothese, Verband*) passen, sitzen. **12.** s. eignen. **13.** passen (*into* in); s. einfügen (*into* in); zusammenpassen. **fit in I** *vt* **1.** einfügen, -schieben, -setzen, -bauen, -pressen. **2.** jdm. einen Termin geben; einschieben. **II** *vi* übereinstimmen (*with* mit).
fit on I *vt* **1.** (*Kleidung*) anprobieren. **2.** anbringen, anpassen, (an-)montieren (*to* an). **II** *vi* passen.
fit out ausrüsten, ausstatten, einrichten (*with* mit).
f. to drink trinkbar.
f. to drive fahrtauglich, -tüchtig.
f. to eat eß-, genießbar.
f. for service (*Militär*) diensttauglich.
f. for transport transportfähig.
f. for work arbeitsfähig.
fit² [fɪt] *n* Anfall *m*, Ausbruch *m*, Episode *f.* **to have a ~** einen Anfall bekommen.

f. of anger → f. of temper.
f. of coughing Hustenanfall.
f. of nerves Nervenkrise *f.*
f. of temper Wutanfall, Zornesausbruch.
f. of perspiration Schweißausbruch.
FITC *abbr.* → fluorescein isothiocyanate.
fit·ful [ˈfɪtfəl] *adj* **1.** (*Schlaf*) unruhig. **2.** unregelmäßig, sporadisch; in Anfällen. **3.** unstet, unbeständig, sprunghaft, launenhaft.
fit·ful·ness [ˈ-nɪs] *n* Launen-, Sprunghaftigkeit *f.*
fit·ness [ˈfɪtnɪs] *n* **1.** Gesundheit *f*; Fitness *f*, Fitneß *f*, Kondition *f.* **2.** Geeignetsein *nt*, Eignung *f*, Tauglichkeit *f.* **3.** Angemessenheit *f.*
fitness training Fitneßtraining *nt.*
fitness room Fitneßraum *m.*
fitness test Fitneßtest *m.*
fit·ted [ˈfɪtɪd] *adj* **1.** befähigt (*for* für). **2.** passend, geeignet. **3.** nach Maß (zugeschnitten).
fit·ting [ˈfɪtɪŋ] **I** *n* **1.** (*Prothese*) Anprobe *f*, Anpassen *nt*, Einsetzen *nt.* **2.** *techn.* Montieren *nt*, Montage *f*; Einbauen *nt*, Einpassen *nt.* **3.** *techn.* Paßstück *nt*, -teil *nt/m.* **II** *adj* passend, geeignet; angebracht.
fit·tings [ˈfɪtɪŋz] *pl* Ausstattung *f*, Einrichtung *f.*
Fitz-Hugh and Curtis [fɪts hjuː ˈkɜːtɪs]: **F.-H. and C. syndrome** Fitz-Hugh-Curtis-Syndrom *nt*, Perihepatitis acuta gonorrhoica.
five-day fever [faɪv] Fünftagefieber *nt*, Wolhyn'-Fieber *m*, Wolhynienfieber *nt*, Febris quintana.
five-year survival rate Fünfjahresüberlebensrate *f.*
fix [fɪks] **I** *n sl.* Fix *m*, Drogeninjektion *f.* **to give o.s. a ~** *sl.* fixen. **II** *vt* **1.** festmachen, befestigen, anbringen, -heften (*to* an, auf). **2.** festsetzen, -legen (*at* auf); bestimmen, anberaumen; arrangieren, organisieren. **3.** *chem.* (*Flüssigkeit*) fest werden lassen; *histol., photo.* fixieren. **4.** reparieren, instand setzen. **5.** (*Augen*) (fest) richten *od.* heften (*on, upon* auf). **6.** (*Glied*) ruhigstellen. **III** *vi* **7.** *chem.* fest werden, erstarren. **8.** *sl.* fixen, s. Rauschgift einspritzen.
fix·ate [fɪkˈseɪt] *vt* **1.** → fix **1. 2.** *psycho.* fixiert sein (*on an*, auf).
fix·a·tion [fɪkˈseɪʃn] *n* **1.** Befestigung *f*, Fixierung *f.* **2.** Festsetzung *f*, -legung *f*, Bestimmung *f.* **3.** *chir.* Befestigung *f*, Fixierung *f*, Fixation *f.* **4.** *ophthal.* Einstellung *f*, Fixierung *f.* **5.** *chem., histol., photo.* Fixierung *f*, Fixieren *nt.* **6.** *psycho.* → fixed idea. **7.** *psycho.* Bindung *f*, Fixierung *f.* **8.** (*Glied*) Ruhigstellung *f*, Fixation *f.*
fixation forceps *chir.* Fixierpinzette *f.*
fixation nystagmus Fixationsnystagmus *m*, kongenitaler/hereditärer Pendelnystagmus *m.*
fixation period *physiol.* Fixationsperiode *f.*
fixation reaction Komplementbindung *f.*
fix·a·tive [ˈfɪksətɪv] **I** *n* Fixativ *nt*, Fixiermittel *nt.* **II** *adj* Fixier-.
fixed [fɪkst] *adj* **1.** befestigt, angebracht; (fest) eingebaut. **2.** festgesetzt, -gelegt, bestimmt. **3.** *chem.* gebunden, nicht flüssig; *histol., photo.* fixiert. **4.** (*Blick*) starr, starrend. **5.** (*Muskel, Sehne*) ansetzen (*to* an). **6.** (*Idee*) fix.
fixed idea fixe Idee *f*, Zwangsvorstellung *f*, Komplex *m.*
fixed point *mathe.* Fest-, Fixpunkt *m.*
fixed pupil starre/fixierte Pupille *f*, Pupillenstarre *f.*
fixed-rate pacemaker *card.* frequenzsta-

biler/festfrequenter/starrfrequenter Herzschrittmacher *m.*
fixed torticollis/wryneck *ortho.* fixierter Schiefhals *m.*
fix·er [ˈfɪksər] *n* **1.** → fixative **I. 2.** *sl.* Dealer *m*, Drogenhändler *m.*
fix·ing [ˈfɪksɪŋ] *n* **1.** Befestigen *nt*, Anbringen *nt*; (*Glied*) Ruhigstellen *nt.* **2.** Reparatur *f.* **3.** *photo., histol.* Fixieren *nt.*
fixing agent → fixative **I.**
fixing bath Fixierbad *nt.*
fix·i·ty [ˈfɪksətɪ] *n* Festigkeit *f*, Beständigkeit *f*, Stabilität *f.*
flab·by [ˈflæbɪ] *adj* schlaff, weich.
flac·cid [ˈflæksɪd] *adj* weich, schlaff.
flac·cid·a [ˈflæksɪdə] *n anat.* Flaccida *f*, Pars flaccida (membranae tympani).
flaccida cholesteatoma *HNO* Flaccidacholesteatom *nt*, primäres Kuppelraumcholesteatom *nt.*
flaccid areflexia *neuro.* schlaffe Areflexie *f.*
flaccid ectropion *ophthal.* Ektropium paralyticum.
flaccid hemiplegia schlaffe Hemiplegie *f*, Hemiplegia flaccida.
flaccid paralysis *neuro.* schlaffe Lähmung *f.*
flaccid paraplegia schlaffe Paraplegie *f.*
Flack [flæk]: **F.'s node** Sinus-Knoten *m*, Sinoatrial-Knoten *m*, SA-Knoten *m*, Keith-Flack'-Knoten *m*, Nodus sinuatrialis.
flag·el·lan·tism [ˈflædʒəlæntɪzəm] *n psychia.* Flagellantismus *m*, Flagellomanie *f.*
fla·gel·lar [fləˈdʒelər, ˈflædʒə-] *adj* Geißel/Flagellum betr., Geißel-.
flagellar agglutinin H-Agglutinin *nt*, Geißelagglutinin *nt.*
flagellar antigen *micro.* Geißelantigen *nt*, H-Antigen *nt.*
flagellar rootlet Rhizoplast *nt.*
flagellar stain *histol.* Geißelfärbung *f.*
Flag·el·la·ta [ˌflædʒəˈleɪtə] *pl micro.* Geißeltierchen *pl*, -infusorien *pl*, Flagellaten *pl*, Flagellata *pl*, Mastigophoren *pl*, Mastigophora *pl.*
flag·el·late [n ˈflædʒəlɪt, -leɪt; *adj* -lɪt; *v* -leɪt] **I** *n* **1.** Geißeltierchen *nt*, Flagellat *m*, Flagellatum *nt.* **2.** geißeltragender Mikroorganismus *m.* **II** *adj* Flagellat betr., geißeltragend, geißelförmig, begeißelt, mit Geißeln besetzt, Geißel-. **III** *vt* (*a. fig.*) geißeln.
flag·el·lat·ed [ˈflædʒəleɪtɪd] *adj* → flagellate **II.**
flagellated bodies (*Malaria*) Sichelkeime *pl.*
flag·el·la·tion [ˌflædʒəˈleɪʃn] *n* (*a. fig.*) Geißelung *f*; *psychia.* Flagellation *f.*
fla·gel·li·form [fləˈdʒelɪfɔːrm] *adj zoo.* geißel-, peitschenförmig.
flag·el·lin [ˈflædʒəlɪn] *n* Flagellin *nt.*
fla·gel·lo·spore [fləˈdʒeləspɔː, -spəʊr] *n bio.* Zoospore *f.*
fla·gel·lu·la [fləˈdʒeljələ] *n bio.* Zoospore *f.*
fla·gel·lum [fləˈdʒeləm] *n, pl* **-lums, -la** [-lə] Geißel *f*, Flimmer *m*, Flagelle *f*, Flagellum *nt.*
flail [fleɪl] *adj* übermäßig beweglich, schlotternd.
flail chest Brustwand-, Thoraxwandflattern *nt*, flail chest (*f*).
flail joint *ortho.* Schlottergelenk *nt.*
Flajani [fləˈdʒɑːnɪ]: **F.'s disease** Basedow'-Krankheit *f*, Morbus Basedow *m.*
flake fracture [fleɪk] *ortho.* Abschälungsfraktur *f*, flake fracture (*f*).
flame [fleɪm] **I** *n* Flamme *f.* **to be in ~s in** Flammen stehen. **II** *vt techn.* flammen. **III** *vi* flammen, lodern.

flame up vi auflodern, in Flammen aufgehen.
flame burn Verbrennung f durch (offene) Flamme(n).
flame-ionization detector Flammenionisationsdetektor m.
flame-less ['fleimlis] adj flammenlos.
flame-let ['fleimlit] n Flämmchen nt.
flame photometer Flamm(en)photometer nt.
flam·ma·ble ['flæməbl] I n Brennstoff m, -material nt; feuergefährlicher Stoff m. II adj brennbar, entflammbar, (leicht) entzündlich; feuergefährlich.
flam·me·ous nevus ['flæmiəs] derm. Feuer-, Gefäßmal nt, Portwein-, Weinfleck m, Naevus flammeus.
flank [flæŋk] n Flanke f, Weiche f; Lende f; Seite f.
flank bone Darmbein nt, Ilium nt, Os ilii/iliacum.
flank incision chir. Flanken-, Lenden-, Lumbalschnitt m.
flank pain Flankenschmerz m.
flap [flæp] n 1. chir. (Haut-, Gewebe-)Lappen m. 2. neuro. (grob-)schägiges Zittern nt, Flattern nt. 3. techn. (Verschluß-)Klappe f, Lasche f.
f. of the ear Ohrläppchen nt.
flap amputation chir. geschlossene Amputation f, Amputation f mit Lappendeckung.
flap-eared adj schlappohrig.
flap extraction ophthal. Lappenextraktion f.
flap·less amputation ['flæplis] ortho. offene Amputation f, Amputation f ohne Stumpfdeckung.
flap·ping tremor ['flæpiŋ] neuro. Flattertremor m, Flapping-tremor m, Asterixis f.
flap valves anat. Taschenklappen pl.
flare ['fleər] I n 1. derm. flächenhafte fortschreitende Hautrötung f, flammende Röte f. 2. → flare-up. II vi → flare up.
flare up vi aufflammen, aufflackern, auflodern.
flare-up n Aufflackern nt, Auflodern nt, Aufflammen nt; Ausbruch m.
flash keratoconjunctivitis [flæʃ] ophthal. Conjunctivitis actinica/photoelectrica, Keratoconjunctivitis/Ophthalmia photoelectrica.
flash ophthalmia → flash keratoconjunctivitis.
flask [flæsk, flɑːsk] n Flasche f, Kolben m, Gefäß nt.
flat [flæt] I n flache Seite f; Fläche f, Ebene f. II adj 1. flach, eben, Flach-. 2. (Nase) platt; (Stimme) ausdruckslos; (Foto) kontrastarm, matt; (Gesicht) flach; (Geräusch) dumpf, gedämpft. 3. flach liegend. **to lay ~** flach hinlegen. **to lie ~** flach liegen.
Flatau [flaˈtau]: **F.'s law** Flautau-Regel f.
Flatau-Schilder [ˈʃildər]: **F.-S. disease** Schilder'-Krankheit f, Encephalitis periaxialis diffusa.
flat back Flachrücken m.
flat bone platter Knochen m, Os planum.
flat chest flacher langer Thorax m.
flat condyloma breites Kondylom nt, Condyloma latum/syphiliticum.
flat EEG → flat electroencephalogram.
flat electroencephalogram neuro. Null-Linien-EEG nt, isoelektrisches Elektroenzephalogramm nt.
flat·foot ['flætfʊt] n, pl **-feet** [-fiːt] Plattfuß m, Pes planus.
flat-footed adj plattfüßig.
flat hand Platthand f.
flat-nosed adj plattnasig.

flat papular syphilid lentikuläres Syphilid nt.
flat pelvis flaches/plattes Becken nt, Pelvis plana.
flat suture Sutura plana.
flat·ten ['flætn] I vt flach od. eben od. glatt machen, abflachen. II vi flach od. eben od. glatt werden.
flat·tened ['flætnd] adj abgeflacht, abgeplattet, flach, platt.
flattened epithelium histol. abgeflachtes Epithel nt.
flat·u·lence ['flætʃələns] n Geblähtsein nt, Blähung(en pl) f, Flatulenz f. **to cause/produce ~** blähen, Blähungen verursachen.
flat·u·len·cy ['flætʃələnsi] n → flatulence.
flat·u·lent ['flætʃələnt] adj Blähungen verursachend, blähend, (auf-)gebläht.
flatulent colic Tympanie f, Tympania f.
fla·tus ['fleitəs] n 1. Wind m, Blähung f, Flatus m. 2. Darmluft f, -gas nt, Flatus m.
flat verruca derm. Flachwarze f, Verruca plana (juvenilis).
flat vertebra ortho. Plattwirbel m.
flat wart → flat verruca.
flat worm micro. Plattwurm m, Plathelminth f.
fla·val ligaments ['fleivl] gelbe Bänder pl, Ligg. flava.
fla·va·noid ['flævənɔid, 'flei-] n → flavonoid.
flav·a·none ['flævənəʊn, 'flei-] n Flavanon nt.
fla·vec·to·my [fləˈvektəmi] n ortho., neurochir. Teilentfernung f des Lig. flavum, Flavektomie f.
fla·ve·do [fləˈviːdəʊ] n derm. Flavedo f, Xanthodermie f.
fla·ves·cent [fləˈvesnt] adj gelb, gelblich.
fla·vin ['fleivin] n Flavin nt.
flavin adenine dinucleotide abbr. **FAD** Flavinadenindinukleotid nt abbr. FAD.
flavin-containing adj flavinhaltig, -enthaltend.
flavin-linked dehydrogenase flavingebundene/flavinabhängige Dehydrogenase f.
flavin-linked oxidase flavinabhängige Oxidase f.
flavin mononucleotide abbr. **FMN** Flavinmononukleotid nt abbr. FMN, Riboflavin(-5'-)phosphat nt.
flavin monooxygenase Aryl-4-hydroxylase f, unspezifische Monooxygenase f.
flavin nucleotide Flavinnukleotid nt.
flavin pigment Flavinpigment nt.
Fla·vi·vir·i·dae [ˌfleiviˈvirədiː, -ˈvair-] pl micro. Flaviviridae pl.
fla·vi·vi·rus [ˌ-ˈvairəs] n micro. Flavivirus nt.
Fla·vo·bac·te·ri·um [fleivəʊbækˈtiəriəm] n micro. Flavobakterium nt.
fla·vo·dox·in [ˌ-ˈdɒksin] n Flavodoxin nt.
fla·vo·en·zyme [ˌ-ˈenzaim] n Flavoenzym nt.
fla·vone ['fleivəʊn] n Flavon nt.
fla·vo·noid ['fleivənɔid] n Flavonoid nt.
fla·vo·pro·tein [ˌfleivəʊˈprəʊtiːn, -tiːin] n Flavoprotein nt.
fla·vor ['fleivər] n 1. Geschmack m, Aroma nt. 2. pharm. Geschmacksverbesserer m, -korrigens nt.
fla·vo·xan·thin [ˌfleivəʊˈzænθin] n Flavoxanthin nt.
fla·vox·ate [fləˈvɒkseit] n pharm. Flavoxat nt.
flax·seed [ˈflæksˌsiːd] n Flachs-, Leinsamen m.
fld. abbr. → fluid I.
flea [fliː] n micro. Floh m.
flea-bitten kidney patho. Fleck-, Flohstichniere f.

flea-borne typhus endemisches/murines Fleckfieber nt, Ratten-, Flohfleckfieber nt.
fle·cai·nide [fliˈkeinaid] n pharm. Flecainid nt.
Flechsig ['fleksiɡ]: **F.'s bundles** → F.'s fasciculi.
F.'s fasciculi Binnen-, Elementar-, Grundbündel pl des Rückenmarks, Intersegmentalfaszikel pl, F. proprii (medullae spinalis).
F.'s oval field Flechsig' ovales Feld nt.
F.'s tract Flechsig'-Bündel nt, Tractus spinocerebellaris dorsalis/posterior.
fleck [flek] I n 1. Fleck m, Flecken m, Tupfen m. 2. Hautfleck m; Sommersprosse f. II vt sprenkeln, tüpfeln.
flecked spleen of Feitis [flekt] patho. Fleckenmilz f.
fleck·fie·ber [flekˈfiːbər] n epidemisches/klassisches Fleckfieber nt, Läusefleckfieber nt, Hunger-, Kriegs-, Flecktyphus m, Typhus exanthematicus.
flec·tion n → flexion.
flec·tion·al adj → flexional.
Flegel ['fleːɡəl]: **F.'s disease** Morbus Flegel m, Hyperkeratosis lenticularis perstans (Flegel).
Fleischer ['flaiʃər]: **F. ring** ophthal. Fleischer-Ring m.
F.'s vortex Cornea verticillata.
Fleischer-Strümpell ['ʃtrimpəl; 'ʃtrym-]: **F.-S. ring** Kayser-Fleischer-Ring m.
Flemming ['flemiŋ]: **F. center** Keim-, Reaktionszentrum nt.
interfibrillar substance of F. Hyaloplasma nt, Grundzytoplasma nt, zytoplasmatische Matrix f.
flesh [fleʃ] n 1. Muskelgewebe nt; Fleisch nt. 2. (Frucht-, Tier-)Fleisch nt.
flesh·y columns of heart ['fleʃi] → fleshy trabeculae of heart.
fleshy mole gyn., patho. 1. Fleischmole f, Mola carnosa. 2. Blutmole f, Mola sanguinolenta.
fleshy trabeculae of heart Herztrabekel pl, Muskelbälkchen pl, Trabeculae carneae (cordis).
Fletcher ['fletʃər]: **F.'s factor** Präkallikrein nt, Fletcher-Faktor m.
flex [fleks] I n Biegen nt, Beugen nt. II vt 1. beugen, biegen. **to ~ one's arm.** 2. (Muskeln) anspannen. **to ~ one's muscles.** III vi s. biegen (lassen).
flex·i·bil·i·ty [ˌfleksəˈbilɪti] n Flexibilität f; (Material) Biegsamkeit f, Elastizität f; (Person) Beweglichkeit f; Anpassungsfähigkeit f; (Stimme) Modulationsfähigkeit f.
flex·i·ble ['fleksibl] adj flexibel; (Material) biegsam, elastisch; (Person) beweglich, anpassungsfähig; (Stimme) modulationsfähig.
flex·i·ble·ness ['-nis] n → flexibility.
flex·ile ['fleksil, -sail] adj → flexible.
flex·ion ['flekʃn] n 1. Beugung f, Biegung f, Krümmung f. 2. Flexion f, Beugen nt. 3. gyn. Flexio uteri. 4. gyn. Flexionslage f, -haltung f, Beugung f des Kindskopfes auf die Brust.
flex·ion·al ['flekʃnəl] adj flektiert, Beugungs-, Flexions-.
flexion contracture ortho. Flexions-, Beugekontraktur f.
flexion crease Querfurche f der Handflächen.
flexion deformity ortho. (Gelenk) Beugefehlstellung f.
Flexner ['fleksnər]: **F.'s bacillus** Flexner'-Bacillus m, Shigella flexneri.
F.'s dysentery Bakterienruhr f, bakterielle Ruhr f, Dysenterie f.

flexor 296

flex·or ['flɛksər] n Beuger m, Beugemuskel m, Flexor m, M. flexor.
flexor canal Handwurzelkanal m, -tunnel m, Karpalkanal m, -tunnel m, Canalis carpi/carpalis.
flexor carpi radialis (muscle) radialer Handbeuger m, Flexor m carpi radialis, M. flexor carpi radialis.
flexor carpi ulnaris (muscle) ulnarer Handbeuger m, Flexor m carpi ulnaris, M. flexor carpi ulnaris.
flexor digiti minimi brevis manus (muscle) kurzer Kleinfingerbeuger m, Flexor m digiti minimi brevis manus, M. flexor digiti minimi brevis manus.
flexor digiti minimi brevis pedis (muscle) kurzer Kleinzehenbeuger m, Flexor m digiti minimi brevis pedis, M. flexor digiti minimi brevis pedis.
flexor digitorum brevis (muscle) kurzer Zehenbeuger m, Flexor m digitorum brevis, M. flexor digitorum brevis.
flexor digitorum longus (muscle) langer Zehenbeuger m, Flexor m digitorum longus, M. flexor digitorum longus.
flexor digitorum manus (muscle) Fingerbeuger m, Flexor m digitorum manus, M. flexor digitorum manus.
flexor digitorum pedis (muscle) Zehenbeuger m, Flexor m digitorum pedis, M. flexor digitorum pedis.
flexor digitorum profundus (muscle) abbr. **FDP** tiefer Fingerbeuger m, Flexor m digitorum profundus, M. flexor digitorum profundus.
flexor digitorum superficialis (muscle) abbr. **FDS** oberflächlicher Fingerbeuger m, Flexor m digitorum superficialis, M. flexor digitorum superficialis.
flexor hallucis brevis (muscle) Flexor m hallucis brevis, M. flexor hallucis brevis.
flexor hallucis longus (muscle) Flexor m hallucis longus, M. flexor hallucis longus.
flexor hallucis (muscle) Großzehenbeuger m, Flexor m hallucis, M. flexor hallucis.
flexor muscle → flexor.
f. of fingers → flexor digitorum manus (muscle).
f. of great toe → flexor hallucis (muscle).
radial f. of wrist → flexor carpi radialis (muscle).
short f. of little finger → flexor digiti minimi brevis manus (muscle).
short f. of little toe → flexor digiti minimi brevis pedis (muscle).
f. of thumb → flexor pollicis (muscle).
f. of toes → flexor digitorum pedis (muscle).
ulnar f. of wrist → flexor carpi ulnaris (muscle).
flex·or·plas·ty ['flɛksərplæsti] n ortho. Flexorplastik f.
flexor pollicis brevis (muscle) kurzer Daumenbeuger m, Flexor m pollicis brevis, M. flexor pollicis brevis.
flexor pollicis longus (muscle) abbr. **FPL** langer Daumenbeuger m, Flexor m pollicis longus, M. flexor pollicis longus.
flexor pollicis (muscle) Daumenbeuger m, Flexor m pollicis, M. flexor pollicis.
flexor pulley ortho., anat. (Finger) Ringband nt der Beugeseite.
flexor reflex Flexorreflex m.
flexor retinaculum: f. of foot Halteband nt der Plantarflexoren, Retinaculum mm. flexorum (pedis).
f. of hand Retinaculum flexorum (manus), Lig. carpi transversum.
flexor side of wrist Vorder-/Beugeseite f der Handwurzel, Regio carpalis anterior.

flexor tendon Beugersehne f.
flexor tunnel Karpalkanal m, Canalis carpi.
flex·u·ose ['flɛkʃəwəʊs] adj s. schlängelnd, s. windend, geschlängelt.
flex·u·ous ['flɛkʃəwəs] adj → flexuose.
flex·u·ra [flɛkʃ'(j)ʊərə] n, pl -rae [-riː] → flexure 1.
flex·ur·al ['flɛkʃərəl] adj Biegung/Flexur betr., Biege-, Flexions-.
flexural psoriasis derm. Psoriasis inversa.
flexural stress phys. Biegespannung f.
flex·ure ['flɛkʃər] n **1.** Biegung f, Beugung f, Krümmung f, Flexur f; anat. Flexura f. **2.** Biegen nt, Beugen nt.
f. of duodenum Zwölffingerdarmkrümmung, Duodenalflexur, Flexura duodeni.
flick·er ['flɪkər] n **1.** Flackern nt. **2.** (Auge) Flimmern nt. **3.** Zucken nt. **4.** Flattern nt.
flicker-fusion frequency/threshold physiol. Flimmerfusionsfrequenz f, kritische Flimmerfrequenz f, critical flicker frequency abbr. **CFF**.
flight [flaɪt] n **1.** Flucht f. **2.** Flug m, Fliegen nt.
f. of ideas psychia. Ideenflucht.
flight behavior Fluchtverhalten nt.
flight blindness ophthal. Amaurosis fugax der Flieger.
fling·ing movement [flɪŋɪŋ] Schleuderbewegung f.
Flint [flɪnt] **F.'s murmur** card. Austin Flint-Geräusch nt, Flint-Geräusch nt.
flint [flɪnt] n **1.** Feuerstein m, Flint m. **2.** Zünd-, Feuerstein m.
flint disease Kalkstaublunge f, Chalikose f, Chalicosis (pulmonum) f.
flint·y liver ['flɪnti] patho. Feuersteinleber f.
flit·ter·ing scotoma ['flɪtərɪŋ] ophthal. Flimmerskotom nt, Scotoma scintillans.
float [fləʊt] **I** vt schwimmen od. treiben lassen. **II** vi **1.** (in einer Flüssigkeit) schweben, ziehen, flottieren. **2.** (auf dem Wasser) schwimmen, (im Wasser) treiben.
float·a·tion n → flotation.
float·ers ['fləʊtərz] pl ophthal. Mückensehen nt, Myiodesonsia f, Mouches volantes.
float·ing [ˌfləʊtɪŋ] adj **1.** schwimmend, treibend, Schwimm-, Schweb-. **2.** anat., patho. Wander-; fluktuierend, flottierend.
floating-beta disease (primäre/essentielle) Hyperlipoproteinämie Typ III f, Hypercholesterinämie f mit Hypertriglyzeridämie, Broad-Beta-Disease (nt), Hyperlipoproteinämie f mit breiter Betabande.
floating-beta proteinemia → floating-beta disease.
floating gallbladder flottierende Gallenblase f.
floating kidney patho. Wanderniere f, Ren mobilis/migrans.
floating liver patho. Lebersenkung f, -tiefstand m, Wanderleber f, Hepatoptose f, Hepar migrans/mobile.
floating patella ortho. tanzende Patella f.
floating ribs Costae fluitantes.
floating spleen patho. Wandermilz f, Lien migrans/mobilis.
floc·cil·la·tion [ˌflɑksə'lɪdʒɪəm] n → floccillation.
floc·ci·la·tion [ˌ-'leɪʃn] n neuro. Flockenlesen f, Floccilatio f, Floccilegium f, Karphologie f, Krozidismus m.
floc·cose ['flɑkəʊs] adj micro. flockig.
floc·cu·la·ble ['flɑkjəbl] adj chem. ausflockbar.
floc·cu·lant ['flɑkjələnt] n (Aus-)Flockungsmittel nt.

floc·cu·lar ['flɑkjələr] adj flockig.
floccular degeneration patho. albuminöse/albuminoide/albuminoid-körnige Degeneration f, trübe Schwellung f.
floccular fossa Fossa subarcuata.
floc·cu·late ['flɑkjəleɪt] vt, vi chem. (aus-)flocken.
floc·cu·la·tion [ˌflɑkjə'leɪʃn] n (Aus-)Flockung f, Ausflocken nt, Flockenbildung f.
flocculation test Flockungstest m.
floc·cule ['flɑkjuːl] n **1.** Flöckchen nt, flöckchenähnliche Substanz od. Masse f. **2.** (ZNS) old Flöckchen nt, Flocculus m.
floc·cu·lence ['flɑkjələns] n **1.** flockige Beschaffenheit f. **2.** → flocculation.
floc·cu·len·cy ['flɑkjələnsi] n → flocculence.
floc·cu·lent ['flɑkjələnt] adj **1.** chem. flockig, flockenartig. **2.** micro. flockig.
floc·cu·lo·nod·u·lar lobe [ˌflɑkjələʊ'nɑdʒələr] Lobus flocculonodularis.
floc·cu·lus ['flɑkjələs] n, pl -li [-laɪ] → floccule.
flood fever [flʌd] Tsutsugamushi-Fieber nt, japanisches Fleckfieber nt, Milbenfleckfieber nt, Scrub-Typhus m.
flood·ing ['flʌdɪŋ] n **1.** gyn. starke Uterusblutung f; Menorrhagie f. **2.** psychia. Reizüberflutung f.
floor [flɔːr, fləʊər] n Boden m; (Ulkus) Grund m.
f. of tympanic cavity Boden m der Paukenhöhle, Paries jugularis (cavitatis tympanicae).
floor plate embryo. Bodenplatte f.
flop·py ['flɑpi] adj schlaff (herabhängend), schlapp, schlotterig.
floppy infant floppy infant (nt).
floppy infant syndrome Floppy-infant-Syndrom nt.
floppy mitral valve syndrome card. Barlow-Syndrom nt, Mitralklappenprolaps-Syndrom m.
flo·ra ['flɔːrə, 'flɔː-] n, pl -ras, -rae [-riː] **1.** bot. Flora f, Pflanzenwelt f. **2.** (Bakterien-)Flora f.
flo·ral ['flɔːrəl, 'flɔː-] adj floral, Blumen-, Blüten-; (Geruch) blumig.
Florence ['flɔːrəns, 'flɑr-]: **F.'s crystals** Florence-Kristalle pl.
flo·res ['flɔːriːz, 'flɔː-] pl **1.** Blumen pl, Blüten pl, Flores pl. **2.** pharm. Blüte(n pl) f, Flores pl.
flor·id ['flɔːrɪd, 'flɔː-] adj **1.** patho. blühend, stark entwickelt od. ausgeprägt, florid(e). **2.** (leuchtend) rot.
flo·ri·form cataract ['flɔːrɪfɔːrm] ophthal. Blütenstar m, Cataracta floriformis.
floss silk [flɔs, flɑs] Zahnseide f.
flo·ta·tion [fləʊ'teɪʃn] n **1.** lab. Schaumschwimmaufbereitung f, Flotation f. **2.** Schwimmen nt, Treiben nt; Schweben nt.
flotation rate phys. Flotationsrate f, Flotation f.
flour mite ['flaʊər] micro. Tyrophagus farinae.
flour·y cornea ['flaʊəri] ophthal. Cornea farinata.
flow [fləʊ] **I** n **1.** Fließen nt, Rinnen nt, Strömen nt. **2.** (a. fig.) Fluß m, Strom m; phys. Flow m; Ab-, Zufluß m. **3.** Monatsblutung f, Periode f, Regel f, Menses pl, Menstruation f. **4.** electr. Strom(fluß m) m. **II** vi **5.** fließen, rinnen, strömen (from aus); zirkulieren. **6.** die Menstruation haben, menstruieren.
flow in vi hinein-, hereinströmen.
flow out of vi (her-)ausströmen.
flow birefringence phys. Strömungsdoppelbrechung f.

flow chart → flow sheet.
flow cytometry *urol.* Durchflußzytometrie *f.*
flow-directed catheter Einschwemmkatheter *m.*
flow·er ['flaʊər] *n* **1.** Blume *f*; Blüte *f.* **2.** ~s *pl chem., pharm.* Blüte(n *pl*) *f*, Flores *pl.*
f.s of sulfur Schwefelblume *f*, -blüte *f.*
flower-spray ending Flower-Spray-Endigung *f.*
flower spray of Bochdalek *anat.* Bochdalek'-Blumenkörbchen *nt.*
flow·ing ['fləʊɪŋ] *adj* fließend, strömend, zirkulierend, Fließ-.
flowing hyperostosis *ortho.* Melorheostose *f.*
flowing phase *phys.* Fließphase *f*, bewegliche Phase *f.*
flow·me·ter ['fləʊmɪtər] *n* (Durch-)Fluß-, (Durch-)Strömungsmesser *m*, Flowmeter *nt.*
flow pattern *phys.* Stromlinienbild *nt.*
flow potential Strömungspotential *nt.*
flow pulse Strom-, Strömungspuls *m.*
flow sheet Fließschema *nt.*
flox·ur·i·dine [flɑks'jʊərədiːn] *n* → 5-fluorodeoxyuridine.
fl. oz *abbr.* → fluid ounce.
FLSC *abbr.* → fibrous long-spacing collagen.
flu [fluː] *n inf.* Grippe *f*, Influenza *f.* **to have (the)** ~ (die) Grippe haben.
flu·an·i·sone [fluː'ænɪsəʊn] *n pharm.* Fluanison *nt.*
flu·clox·a·cil·lin [ˌfluːklɑksə'sɪlɪn] *n pharm.* Flucloxacillin *nt.*
fluc·tu·ant ['flʌktʃəwənt] *adj* schwankend, fluktuierend.
fluc·tu·ate ['flʌktʃəweɪt] *vi* schwanken, s. ändern, fluktuieren.
fluc·tu·a·tion [ˌflʌktʃə'weɪʃn] *n* Schwankung *f*, Fluktuation *f*; Schwanken *nt*, Fluktuieren *nt.*
fluctuation deafness *HNO* fluktuierende Schwerhörigkeit *f.*
flu·cy·to·sine [fluː'saɪtəsiːn, -sɪn] *n pharm.* Flucytosin *nt.*
flu·dro·cor·ti·sone [fluːdrə'kɔːrtɪzəʊn] *n pharm.* Fludrocortison *nt.*
flu·ent aphasia [fluːənt] *neuro.* Aphasie *f* mit flüssiger Spontansprache.
flu·fen·am·ic acid [fluː'fən'æmɪk] *pharm.* Flufenaminsäure *f.*
flu·id ['fluːɪd] **I** *n abbr.* **fld.** Flüssigkeit *f*; *chem.* nicht-festes Mittel *nt*, Fluid *nt.* **II** *adj* flüssig, fließend, fluid.
flu·id·al ['fluːɪdl] *adj* Flüssigkeits-.
fluid balance Flüssigkeitsbilanz *f*, -haushalt *m.*
fluid bed *chem.* Fließbett *nt*, Wirbelschicht *f.*
fluid cleft *histol.* Saftspalte *f.*
fluid compartment *physiol.* Flüssigkeitsraum *m*, -kompartiment *nt.*
fluid consumption Flüssigkeitsverbrauch *m.*
fluid content (*Gewebe*) Flüssigkeitsgehalt *m.*
fluid deficit Flüssigkeitsmangel *m*, -defizit *nt.*
fluid drachm 1. *US* 3,69 ccm. **2.** *Brit.* 3,55 ccm.
fluid dram → fluid drachm.
fluid elimination Flüssigkeitsausscheidung *f.*
fluid equilibrium → fluid balance.
flu·id·ex·tract [fluːɪd'ekstrækt] *n pharm.* flüssiger Extrakt *m*, Fluidextrakt *m*, Extractum fluidum/liquidum.
flu·id·ex·trac·tum [ˌfluːɪdeks'træktəm] *n* → fluidextract.

flu·id·i·fy [fluː'ɪdəfaɪ] **I** *vt* verflüssigen. **II** *vi* s. verflüssigen.
fluid intake Flüssigkeitszufuhr *f*, -aufnahme *f.*
flu·id·ism ['fluːɪdɪzəm] *n* Humoralpathologie *f.*
flu·id·i·ty [fluː'ɪdɪti] *n* Flüssigkeit *f*; *chem.* Fluidität *f.*
flu·id·i·za·tion [ˌfluːɪdə'zeɪʃn, -daɪ'z-] *n* Verflüssigung *f*; *chem.* Fluidisation *f.*
flu·id·ize ['fluːɪdaɪz] *vt* verflüssigen; *chem.* fluidisieren.
fluid loss Flüssigkeitsverlust *m.*
fluid lung 1. Flüssigkeitslunge *f*, Wasserlunge *f*, fluid lung (*f*). **2.** urämische Wasserlunge *f.*
fluid manometer Flüssigkeitsmanometer *nt.*
fluid medium *micro.* Flüssignährboden *m*, -medium *nt.*
fluid-mosaic model *biochem.* fluid-mosaic-Modell *nt.*
flu·id·ness ['fluːɪdnɪs] *n* → fluidity.
fluid output Flüssigkeitsausscheidung *f*, Flüssigkeitsabgabe *f.*
fluid ounce *abbr.* **fl. oz 1.** *US* 29,573 ccm. **2.** *Brit.* 28,413 ccm.
flu·id·ounce [fluːɪd'aʊns] *n* → fluid ounce.
fluid overload Flüssigkeitsüberladung *f*, -überbelastung *f.*
fluid pressure hydraulischer Druck *m.*
flu·id·rachm [fluːɪd'ræm] *n* → fluid drachm.
flu·id·ram [fluːɪd'ræm] *n* → fluid drachm.
fluid replacement Flüssigkeitsersatz *m.*
fluid requirement Flüssigkeitsbedarf *m.*
fluid restriction Flüssigkeitsbeschränkung *f.*
fluid retention Flüssigkeitsretention *f.*
fluid status Flüssigkeitsstatus *m.*
fluid supply Flüssigkeitszufuhr *f.*
fluid therapy Flüssigkeitstherapie *f.*
fluid uptake Flüssigkeitsaufnahme *f.*
fluke [fluːk] *n micro.* Saugwurm *m*, Egel *m*, Trematode *f.*
flu-like ['fluːlaɪk] *adj* grippeähnlich.
flu·meth·a·sone [fluː'meθəsəʊn] *n pharm.* Flumetason *nt.*
flu·nar·i·zine [fluː'nærəziːn] *n pharm.* Flunarizin *nt.*
flu·nis·o·lide [fluː'nɪsəʊlaɪd] *n pharm.* Flunisolid *nt.*
flu·ni·traz·e·pam [ˌfluːnɪ'treɪzəpæm] *n pharm.* Flunitrazepam *nt.*
flu·o·cin·o·lone acetonide [ˌfluːəʊ'sɪnələʊn] *n pharm.* Fluocinolonacetonid *nt.*
flu·o·cin·o·nide [ˌ-'sɪnənaɪd] *n pharm.* Fluocinonid *nt.*
flu·o·cor·tin butyl [ˌ-'kɔːrtɪn] *pharm.* Fluocortinbutyl *nt.*
flu·o·cor·to·lone [ˌ-'kɔːrtələʊn] *n pharm.* Fluocortolon *nt.*
flu·or ['fluːɔːr] *n patho.* Ausfluß *m*, Fluor *m.*
flu·o·resce [flʊə'res] *vi* fluoreszieren.
flu·o·res·ce·in [flʊə'resɪn, flɔː-] *n* Fluorescein *nt*, -zein *nt*, Resorcinphthalein *nt.*
fluorescein installation test *ophthal.* Fluoresceinversuch *m*, -augenprobe *f.*
fluorescein isothiocyanate *abbr.* **FITC** Fluoresceinisothiocyanat *nt abbr.* FITC.
flu·o·res·ce·in·u·ria [flʊəˌresɪn'(j)ʊərɪə] *n* Fluoresceinausscheidung *f* im Harn, Fluoresceinurie *f.*
flu·o·res·cence [flʊə'resəns] *n* Fluoreszenz *f.*
fluorescence microscope Fluoreszenzmikroskop *nt.*
fluorescence microscopy Fluoreszenzmikroskopie *f.*
fluorescence polarization *phys.* Fluoreszenzpolarisation *f.*

flu·o·res·cent [flʊə'resənt] *adj* fluoreszierend.
fluorescent antibody fluoreszierender Antikörper *m.*
fluorescent antibody reaction → fluorescent antibody test.
fluorescent antibody technique Immun(o)fluoreszenz(-Technik *f*) *f.*
fluorescent antibody test *immun.* Immunfluoreszenz(test *m*) *f*, Fluoreszenz-Antikörper-Reaktion *f.*
indirect f. *abbr.* **IFAR** indirekte Fluoreszenz *f*, indirekte Fluoreszenz-Antikörper-Reaktion *abbr.* IFAR, indirekter Fluoreszenztest, Sandwich-Technik *f.*
fluorescent dye → fluorochrome.
fluorescent microscope → fluorescence microscope.
fluorescent screen *radiol.* Leuchtschirm *m.*
fluorescent treponemal antibody *abbr.* **FTA** *immun.* Fluoreszenz-Treponemen--Antikörper *m abbr.* FTA.
fluorescent treponemal antibody absorption test *abbr.* **FTA-Abs** Fluoreszenz-Treponemen-Antikörper-Absorptionstest *m*, FTA-Abs-Test *m abbr.* FTA-Abs.
flu·o·res·cin [flʊə'resɪn] *n* Fluorescin *nt*, -reszin *nt.*
flu·o·ri·da·tion [ˌflʊərɪ'deɪʃn] *n* Fluoridierung *f*, Fluorierung *f.*
flu·o·ride ['flʊəraɪd, -ɪd] *n* Fluorid *nt.*
fluoride poisoning Fluorvergiftung *f.*
chronic f. → fluorosis.
flu·o·rim·e·ter [flʊə'rɪmɪtər] *n* → fluorometer.
flu·o·rim·e·try [flʊə'rɪmɪtri] *n* → fluorometry.
flu·o·rine ['flʊərɪn, -riːn] *n abbr.* **F** Fluor *nt abbr.* F.
fluorine poisoning Fluorvergiftung *f.*
chronic f. → fluorosis.
flu·o·ro·ac·e·tate [ˌflʊərəʊ'æsɪteɪt] *n* Fluoracetat *nt*, -acetat *nt.*
flu·o·ro·chrome ['-krəʊm] *n* fluoreszierender Farbstoff *m*, fluoreszierendes Färbemittel *nt*, Fluorochrom *nt.*
fluorochrome staining Fluoreszenzfärbung *f*, Fluorochromisierung *f.*
vital f. Vitalfluoreszenzfärbung, Vitalfluorochromisierung *f.*
flu·o·ro·cit·rate [ˌ-'sɪtreɪt, -'saɪ-] *n* Fluorzitrat *nt*, -citrat *nt.*
flu·o·ro·cyte ['-saɪt] *n* Fluorozyt *m*, Fluoreszyt *m.*
5-flu·o·ro·de·ox·y·u·ri·dine [ˌ-dɪˌɑksɪ'jʊərədiːn] *n abbr.* **FUDR, FUdr** (5-)Fluorodesoxyuridin *nt abbr.* FUDR.
flu·o·rog·ra·phy [flʊə'rɑgrəfi] *n radiol.* Röntgendurchleuchtung *f*, (Röntgen-)Schirmbildverfahren *nt.*
flu·o·ro·im·mu·no·as·say ['flʊərəʊˌɪmjənəʊˌæseɪ] *n abbr.* **FIA** Fluoreszenzimmunoassay *m abbr.* FIA.
flu·o·rom·e·ter [flʊə'rɑmɪtər] *n* Fluorometer *nt.*
flu·o·ro·meth·o·lone [ˌflʊərəʊ'meθələʊn] *n pharm.* Fluorometholon *nt.*
flu·o·ro·met·ric [ˌ-'metrɪk] *adj* Fluorometer *od.* Fluorometrie betr., fluorometrisch.
flu·o·rom·e·try [flʊə'rɑmətri] *n* Fluorometrie *f*, Fluoreszenzphotometrie *f.*
flu·o·ro·neph·e·lom·e·ter [ˌflʊərəˌnefɪ'lɑmɪtər] *n* Fluoronephelometer *nt.*
p-flu·o·ro·phen·yl·al·a·nine [ˌ-ˌfenl'ælənaɪn] *n p*-Fluorphenylalanin *nt.*
flu·o·ro·pho·tom·e·try [ˌ-fəʊ'tɑmɪtri] *n* Fluorophotometrie *f.*
flu·o·ro·roent·ge·nog·ra·phy [ˌ-rentgə'nɑgrəfi] *n radiol.* Röntgendurchleuch-

fluoroscope

tung f, (Röntgen-)Schirmbildverfahren nt.
flu·o·ro·scope ['-skəup] n radiol. Fluoroskop nt.
flu·o·ro·scop·i·cal [,-'skɒpɪkl] adj Fluoroskopie betr., fluoroskopisch.
flu·o·ros·co·py [fluə'rɒskəpɪ] n radiol. (Röntgen-)Durchleuchtung f, Fluoroskopie f.
flu·o·ro·sis [fluə'rəusɪs] n chronische Fluorvergiftung f, Fluorose f.
5-flu·o·ro·u·ra·cil [,fluərə'juərəsɪl] n abbr. **5-FU** pharm. 5-Fluorouracil nt abbr. 5-FU.
flu·ox·e·tine [flu:'ɒksəti:n] n pharm. Fluoxetin nt.
flu·pen·tix·ol [flu:'pen'tɪksɒl] n pharm. Flupentixol nt.
flu·phen·a·zine [flu:'fenəzi:n] n pharm. Fluphenazin nt.
flu·pred·nis·o·lone [flu:pred'nɪsələun] n pharm. Fluprednisolon nt.
flur·az·e·pam [fluə'ræzɪpæm] n pharm. Flurazepam nt.
flur·bi·pro·fen [fluə'baɪprəufen] n pharm. Flurbiprofen nt.
flush [flʌʃ] I n 1. Erröten nt; Röte f. 2. Wallung f, Hitze f, Flush m, Flushing nt. II vt erröten lassen. III vi → flush up.
flush out vt (aus-)spülen, (aus-)waschen.
flush up vi erröten, rot werden.
flu·spir·i·lene [flu:'spɪrəli:n] n pharm. Fluspirilen nt.
flu·ta·mide ['flu:təmaɪd] n pharm. Flutamid nt.
flut·ter ['flʌtər] I n card., neuro. Flattern nt. II vi flattern.
flutter-fibrillation n card. Flimmerflattern nt, Flatterflimmern nt.
flutter waves card. Flatterwellen pl.
flux [flʌks] I n 1. (a. phys., electr.) Fließen nt, Fluß m. 2. (a. patho., physiol.) Ausfluß m. 3. → flux density. 4. techn. Fluß-, Schmelzmittel nt. II vi (aus-)fließen.
flux density 1. phys. (magnetische) Flußdichte f. 2. electr. Stromdichte f.
flux·ion·ar·y hyperemia ['flʌkʃənerɪ] fluxionäre Hyperämie f.
flux map phys. Fließschema nt.
flux·me·ter ['flʌksmi:tər] n phys. Flußmesser m; electr. Strommesser m.
fly¹ [flaɪ] v (flew, flown) I n Fliegen nt, Flug m. II vt, vi fliegen.
fly² [flaɪ] n bio. Fliege f.
fly agaric bio. Fliegenpilz m, Amanita muscaria.
Fm abbr. → fermium.
FMN abbr. → flavin mononucleotide.
FMN adenylyltransferase FMN-Adenyltransferase f.
FNTC abbr. → fine-needle transhepatic cholangiography.
F₀ abbr. → oligomycin-sensitivity-conferring factor.
foam [fəum] I n Schaum m. II vt, vi schäumen.
foam cell 1. Schaum-, Xanthomzelle f. 2. Mikulicz-Zellen pl.
fo·cal ['fəukl] adj 1. mathe., phys. Brennpunkt/Fokus betr., im Brennpunkt (stehend), fokal, focal, Brennpunkt-, Fokal-. 2. patho. von einem Fokus verursacht od. ausgehend, fokal, Fokal-, Herd-.
focal appendicitis fokale Appendizitis f.
focal choroiditis pharm. herdförmige/fokale/lokalisierte Chorioiditis f.
focal depth phys. Schärfentiefe f, Tiefenschärfe f.
focal dermal hypoplasia (syndrome) fokale dermale Hypoplasie f, FDH-Syndrom nt, kongenitale ektodermale u. mesodermale Dysplasie f, Goltz-Gorlin-Syndrom II nt, Goltz-Peterson-Gorlin-Ravits-Syndrom nt, Jessner-Cole-Syndrom nt, Liebermann-Cole-Syndrom nt.
focal distance phys. Brennweite f.
focal dose oncol. Herddosis f.
focal embolic glomerulonephritis Löhlein'-Herdnephritis f.
focal epilepsy fokale Epilepsie f.
chronic f. Kojewnikow-, Koshewnikoff-, Koževnikov-Syndrom nt, -Epilepsie f, Epilepsia partialis continua.
focal glomerular sclerosis fokal-segmentale Glomerulosklerose f.
focal glomerulonephritis Berger-Krankheit f, -Nephropathie f, mesangiale IgA-Glomerulonephritis f, fokale/fokalbetonte Glomerulonephritis f.
focal infection Fokal-, Herdinfektion f.
fo·cal·i·za·tion [,fəukəlaɪ'zeɪʃn] n 1. Vereinigung f in einem Brennpunkt. 2. (Optik) Scharfeinstellung f.
fo·cal·ize ['fəukəlaɪz] I vt 1. fokussieren, (scharf) einstellen (on auf). 2. phys. im Brennpunkt vereinigen; (Strahlen) bündeln. 3. auf einen bestimmten Teil des Körpers beschränken. II vi 4. s. in einem Brennpunkt vereinigen, s. bündeln. 5. s. scharf einstellen. 6. s. auf einen bestimmten Teil des Körpers beschränken.
focal length phys. Brennweite f.
focal necrosis Fokalnekrose f.
focal nephritis → focal glomerulonephritis.
focal plane phys. Brennebene f.
focal pneumonia Herd-, Fokalpneumonie f, Bronchopneumonie f.
peribronchial f. peribronchiale Herdpneumonie.
focal point 1. phys. Brennpunkt m. 2. fig. → focus m.
focal reaction Lokalreaktion f, lokale/örtliche Reaktion f.
focal sclerosis patho. multiple Sklerose f, abbr. MS, Polysklerose f, Sclerosis multiplex, Encephalomyelitis disseminata.
focal segmental glomerulosclerosis fokal-segmentale Glomerulosklerose f.
fo·cim·e·ter [fəu'sɪmɪtər] n → focometer.
fo·com·e·ter [fəu'kɒmɪtər] n ophthal., phys. Fokometer nt.
fo·cus ['fəukəs] I n, pl **-cus·es**, **-ci** [-saɪ, -kaɪ] 1. mathe., phys. Brennpunkt m, Fokus m. 2. fig. Brenn-, Mittelpunkt m. 3. patho. Herd m, Fokus m. 4. (Optik) Scharfeinstellung f. **in ~/out of ~** scharf od. richtig eingestellt/falsch od. unscharf eingestellt. II radiol. Brennfleck m, Fokus m. II vt 6. fokussieren, (scharf) einstellen (on auf). 7. phys. im Brennpunkt vereinigen; (Strahlen) bündeln. 8. fig. konzentrieren (on auf). III vi 9. s. in einem Brennpunkt vereinigen, s. bündeln. 10. s. scharf einstellen. 11. fig. s. konzentrieren (on auf).
fo·cused grid ['fəukəst] radiol. Fokussierraster nt.
fo·cus·ing lens ['fəukəsɪŋ] Sammellinse f.
foetal adj → fetal.
foe·ta·tion n → fetation.
foe·tus n → fetus.
fog [fɒg, fɔg] n Nebel m.
Fogarty ['fəugɑrtɪ]: **F. catheter** Fogarty-Katheter m.
foil [fɔɪl] n (Metall-, Kunststoff-)Folie f.
Foix [fwa]: **F.'s syndrome** ophthal. Foix-Syndrom nt.
Foix-Alajouanine [,alaʒwa'nin]: **F.-M. myelitis** Foix-Alajouanine-Syndrom nt, subakute nekrotisierende Myelitis f, Myelitis necroticans.
fol·a·cin ['fɒləsɪn] n → folic acid.
fo·late ['fəuleɪt] n Folat nt.
folate deficiency Folsäuremangel m.
fold [fəuld] I n 1. anat. Falte f, Plica f. 2. Falz m, Kniff m; Falte f. II vt 3. falten. **to ~ one's arms** die Arme verschränken. 4. zusammenlegen, -falten, -klappen; kniffen, falzen. 5. etw. einschlagen od. -hüllen (in in).
f. of armpit Achselhöhlenfalte, Plica axillaris.
f. of chorda tympani Chordafalte, Plica chordae tympani.
f. of laryngeal nerve Plica nervi laryngei.
f. of left vena cava Plica v. cavae sinistrae.
f.s of uterine tube Tubenfalten pl, Plicae tubariae/tubales.
fold·ed fundus gallbladder ['fəuldɪd] phrygische Mütze f.
fold·ing fracture ['fəuldɪŋ] Wulstbruch m.
Foley ['fəulɪ]: **F. catheter** Foley-Katheter m.
F. operation urol. Foley-Plastik f.
F. Y-plasty pyeloplasty → F. operation.
fo·li·a·ceous [,fəulɪ'eɪʃəs] adj → foliate.
fo·li·an process ['fəulɪən] vorderer Hammerfortsatz m, Proc. anterior (mallei).
fo·li·ar ['fəulɪər] adj → foliate.
fo·li·ate ['fəulɪət, -eɪt] adj blattartig, -förmig, blätt(e)rig, Blatt-, Blätter-.
foliate papillae (Zunge) blattförmige Papillen pl, Papillae foliatae.
fo·lic acid ['fəulɪk,-fə-] Fol(in)säure f, Folacin nt, Pteroylglutaminsäure f, Vitamin B_c nt.
folic acid antagonist Folsäureantagonist m.
folic acid deficiency Folsäuremangel m.
folic acid deficiency anemia Folsäuremangelanämie f.
fo·lie [fɒ'li] n 1. psychische Erkrankung f, Psychose f, Folie f. 2. → folly.
folie à deux [fɒ'li ə du:; a də] psychia. induziertes Irresein nt, Folie à deux.
fo·lin·ic acid [fəu'lɪnɪk] Folinsäure f, N^{10}-Formyl-Tetrahydrofolsäure f, Leukovorin nt, Leucovorin nt, Citrovorum-Faktor m abbr. CF.
fo·li·um ['fəulɪəm] n, pl **-lia** [-lɪə] 1. bio. Blatt nt, blattartiges Gebilde nt, Folium nt. 2. anat. blattartige Struktur f, Folium nt.
Folius ['fəulɪəs]: **process of F.** → folian process.
folk medicine [fəuk] Laien-, Haus-, Volksmedizin f.
fol·li·cle ['fɒlɪkl] n anat. bläschenförmiges Gebilde nt, Follikel m, Folliculus m.
f.s of thyroid gland Schilddrüsenfollikel pl, Speicherfollikel pl, Folliculi gl. thyroideae.
follicle cell → follicular cell.
follicle maturation Follikelreifung f.
follicle-maturation phase → follicular phase.
follicle mite micro. Haarbalgmilbe f, Demodex folliculorum.
follicle stimulating hormone abbr. **FSH** follikelstimulierendes Hormon nt abbr. FSH, Follitropin nt, Follikelreifungshormon nt.
follicle stimulating hormone releasing factor **FRF, FSH-RF** Gonadotropin-releasing-Faktor m abbr. Gn-RF, Gonadotropin-releasing-Hormon nt abbr. Gn-RH.
follicle stimulating hormone releasing hormone abbr. **FSH-RH** → follicle stimulating hormone releasing factor.
follicle-stimulating principle → follicle-stimulating hormone.
fol·li·clis ['fɒlɪklɪs] n derm. Folliklis f, Folliclis f.
fol·lic·u·lar [fə'lɪkjələr] adj Follikel betr., von einem Follikel (ab-)stammend od. ausgehend, aus Follikeln bestehend, fol-

likelähnlich, follikular, follikulär, Follikel-.
follicular abscess Follikelabszeß *m*.
follicular adenocarcinoma follikuläres Adenokarzinom *nt*.
follicular adenoma follikuläres (Schilddrüsen-)Adenom *nt*.
follicular amyloidosis (*Milz*) Follikelamyloidose *f*.
follicular arteries of spleen (*Milz*) Zentralarterien *pl*.
follicular atresia Follikeluntergang *m*, -atresie *f*.
follicular blepharitis ophthal. Blepharitis follicularis.
follicular bronchiectasis follikuläre Bronchiektas(i)e *f*, Bronchiektas(i)e *f* mit Traubenbildung.
follicular cancer of thyroid → follicular carcinoma of thyroid.
follicular carcinoma follikuläres Karzinom *nt*.
f. of thyroid follikuläres Schilddrüsenkarzinom *nt*, metastasierendes Schilddrüsenadenom *nt*.
follicular cell 1. Follikelzelle *f*. **2.** ~s *pl* Follikelepithel *nt*, Granulosazellen *pl*.
follicular conjunctivitis ophthal. follikuläre Konjunktivitis *f*, Follikularkatarrh *m*, Conjunctivitis follicularis.
follicular cyst Follikelzyste *f*.
follicular cystitis Cystitis follicularis/nodularis.
follicular degeneration → follicular atresia.
follicular epithelial cell → follicular cell.
follicular epithelium Follikelepithel *nt*, Granulosazellen *pl*.
follicular fluid Follikelflüssigkeit *f*, Liquor folliculi.
follicular gastritis follikuläre Gastritis *f*.
follicular goiter parenchymatöse Struma *f*, Struma parenchymatosa.
follicular hyperkeratosis derm. Krötenhaut *f*, Phrynoderm *nt*, Hyperkeratosis follicularis (metabolica).
follicular impetigo Ostiofollikulitis/Ostiofolliculitis/Impetigo Bockhart, Staphyloderma follicularis, Impetigo follicularis Bockhart, Folliculitis staphylogenes superficialis, Folliculitis pustolosa, Staphylodermia Bockhart.
follicular iritis ophthal. follikuläre Iritis *f*.
follicular lymphoma Brill-Symmers-Syndrom *nt*, Morbus Brill-Symmers *m*, zentroblastisch-zentrozytisches (malignes) Lymphom *nt*, großfollikuläres Lymphoblastom/Lymphom *nt*.
follicular maturation Follikelreifung *f*.
follicular mucinosis Pinkus Alopezie *f*, Mucinosis follicularis, Alopecia mucinosa, Mucophanerosis intrafollicularis et seboglandularis.
follicular pharyngitis follikuläre Pharyngitis *f*.
follicular phase Proliferations-, Follikel- (reifungs)phase *f*, östrogene Phase *f*.
follicular rupture Ei-, Follikelsprung *m*, Ovulation *f*.
follicular salpingitis follikuläre Salpingitis *f*, Salpingitis follicularis.
follicular stage → follicular phase.
follicular stigma gyn. Stigma *nt*, Macula pellucida.
follicular syphilid kleinpapulöses/miliares/lichenoides Syphilid *nt*, Lichen syphiliticus.
follicular tonsillitis Kryptentonsillitis *f*, Angina follicularis.
follicular ureteritis follikuläre Harnleiterentzündung/Ureteritis *f*, Ureteritis follicularis.

fol·lic·u·late [fə'lɪkjəlɪt, -leɪt] *adj* → follicular.
fol·lic·u·lat·ed ['-leɪtɪd] *adj* → follicular.
fol·lic·u·lin [fə'lɪkjəlɪn] *n old* → estrone.
fol·lic·u·li·tis [fə͵lɪkjə'laɪtɪs] *n* **1.** Follikelentzündung *f*, Follikulitis *f*, Folliculitis *f*. **2.** *derm*. Haarfollikelentzündung *f*, Follikulitis *f*, Folliculitis *f*.
fol·lic·u·lo·ma [͵-'ləʊmə] *n patho*. Granulosa(zell)tumor *m*, Folliculoma *nt*, Ca. granulosocellulare.
fol·lic·u·lo·sis [͵-'ləʊsɪs] *n patho*. Follikulose *f*, Folliculosis *f*.
fol·lic·u·lus [fə'lɪkjələs] *n*, *pl* -**li** [-laɪ, -liː] → follicle.
Folling ['fɑlɪŋ]: **F.'s disease** Fölling-Krankheit *f*, -Syndrom *nt*, Morbus Fölling *m*, Phenylketonurie *f abbr.* PKU, Brenztraubensäureschwachsinn *m*, Oligophrenia phenylpyruvica.
fol·li·tro·pin [fɑlɪ'trəʊpɪn] *n* → follicle stimulating hormone.
fol·low·ing substrate ['fɑləʊɪŋ] *biochem*. zweites Substrat *nt*, Folgesubstrat *nt*.
follow-up *n* Nachbetreuung *f*, -behandlung *f*, -sorge *f*.
fol·ly ['fɑlɪ] *n*, *pl* -**lies** Verrücktheit *f*, Narrheit *f*, Torheit *f*.
fo·ment [fəʊ'ment] *vt* mit feucht-warmen Umschlägen behandeln, bähen.
fo·men·ta·tion [͵fəʊmen'teɪʃn] *n* **1.** feucht-warmer Umschlag *m*, Foment *nt*, Fomentation *f*. **2.** Behandlung *f* mit feucht-warmen Umschlägen, Fomentation *f*.
fo·mes ['fəʊmiːz] *n*, *pl* **fo·mi·tes** ['fɑmɪtiːz, 'fəʊ-] *n* fomite.
fo·mite ['fəʊmaɪt] *n epidem*. Ansteckungs-(über)träger *m*, infizierter Gegenstand *m*.
Fon·se·caea [fɑnsɪ'siːɪ] *n micro*. Fonsecaea *f*.
Fontana [fɑn'tænɑ]: **F.'s canal** Fontana-Kanal *m*, Sinus venosus sclerae.
spaces of F. (*Auge*) Fontana'-Räume *pl*, Spatia anguli iridocornealis.
fon·ta·nel *n* → fontanelle.
fon·ta·nelle [͵fɑntə'nel] *n anat*. Fontanelle *f*, Fonticulus *m*.
fon·tic·u·lus [fɑn'tɪkjələs] *n*, *pl* -**li** [-laɪ, -liː] → fontanelle.
food [fuːd] *n* **1.** Essen *nt*, Nahrung *f*, Kost *f*. **2.** → foodstuff.
food additive Nahrungsmittelzusatz *m*, -additiv *nt*, Lebensmittelzusatz *m*, -additiv *nt*.
food allergy Nahrungsmittelallergie *f*.
food asthma Extrinsic-Asthma *nt* durch Nahrungsmittelallergie.
food ball Phytobezoar *m*.
food-borne *adj* durch Nahrung(smittel) übertragen.
food chain bio. Nahrungskette *f*.
food coloring Lebensmittelfarbstoff *m*.
food conditions Ernährungslage *f*.
food consumption Nahrungsaufnahme *m*, -verbrauch *m*.
food ingestion Nahrungsaufnahme *f*.
food intake Nahrungsaufnahme *f*.
food mite Haus-, Wohnungs-, Polstermilbe *f*, Glycyphagus domesticus.
food poisoning Lebensmittelvergiftung *f*.
bacterial f. bakterielle Lebensmittelvergiftung.
food-sensitive *adj* ernährungsbewußt.
food·stuff ['fuːdstʌf] *n* Nahrungs-, Lebensmittel *nt*; Nährstoffe *pl*.
foot [fʊt] *n*, *pl* **1.-3. feet** [fiːt]; **4. foot, feet** [fiːt] **1.** Fuß *m*; *anat*. Pes *m*. **2.** Gang *m*, Schritt *m*. **3.** (*Strumpf*) Fuß *m*. (*Bett*) Fußende *nt*. **4.** *abbr*. **ft, f** Fuß *m* (= 30,48 cm).
foot-and-mouth disease (echte) Maul- u. Klauenseuche *f abbr*. MKS, Febris aphthosa, Stomatitis epidemica, Aphthosis epizootica.
foot-bath ['fʊtbæθ, -bɑːθ] *n* Fußbad *nt*; Fußbadewanne *f*.
foot cells 1. Sertoli'-Zellen *pl*, Stütz-, Ammen-, Fußzellen *pl*. **2.** (*Nase*) Basal-, Ersatzzellen *pl*.
foot clonus neuro. Fußklonus *m*.
foot deformity Fußdeformität *f*.
foot-drop *n* Spitzfußstellung *f* bei Fibularisfähmung.
foot-gear ['fʊtgɪər] *n* Fußbekleidung *f*, Schuhe *pl*, Schuhwerk *nt*.
foot gutter Rec. piriformis.
foot·less ['fʊtlɪs] *adj* ohne Füße.
foot·ling presentation ['fʊtlɪŋ] *gyn*. Fußlage *f*.
complete f. vollkommene Steiß-Fuß-Lage.
double f. vollkommene Fußlage.
incomplete f. unvollkommene Steiß-Fuß-Lage.
single f. unvollkommene Fußlage.
foot·pace ['fʊtpeɪs] *n* Schrittempo *nt*. **at a ~** im Schritt.
foot plate embryo. Fußplatte *f*.
foot presentation → footling presentation.
foot·print ['fʊtprɪnt] *n* Fußabdruck *m*.
foot process histol. (*Podozyt*) Füßchen *nt*.
foot·rest ['fʊtrest] *n* Fußstütze *f*.
foot skeleton Fußskelett *nt*.
foot·sore ['fʊtsɔːr, -sʊər] *adj* (*Füße*) wundgelaufen, wund.
foot-spray ['fʊtspreɪ] *n* Fußspray *m/nt*.
foot·stool ['fʊtstuːl] *n* Schemel *m*, Fußbank *f*.
foot·wear ['fʊtweər] *n* → footgear.
for·age [fə'rɑːʒ] *n chir*. Forage *f*.
fo·ra·men [fəʊ'reɪmən] *n*, *pl* -**ram·i·na** [-'ræmɪnə], -**mens** *anat*. Öffnung *f*, Loch *nt*, Foramen *nt*.
f. of Bochdalek Bochdalek'-Foramen *nt*, Hiatus pleuroperitonealis.
f. of Fallopio Hiatus canalis n. petrosi majoris.
f. of Key and Retzius → f. of Luschka.
f. of Luschka Luschka-Foramen, Apertura lateralis ventriculi quarti.
f. of saphenous vein Hiatus saphenus.
f. of Winslow Winslow'-Foramen, -Loch, For. epiploicum/omentale.
foramen cecum (of tongue) For. c(a)ecum linguae, For. Morgagni.
foramen magnum großes Hinterhauptsloch *nt*, For. magnum.
foramen ovale anat. For. ovale cordis.
patent/persistent f. offenes/persistierendes Foramen ovale, For. ovale persistens.
fo·ram·i·nal herniation [fə'ræmɪnl] Hernia tonsillaris.
foraminal node Lymphknoten *m* am For. epiploicum, Nodus foraminalis.
fo·ra·mi·not·o·my [fə͵ræmɪ'nɑtəmɪ] *n ortho*., *neurochir*. Foraminotomie *f*.
Forbes [fɔːrbz]: **F.' disease** Cori-Krankheit *f*, Forbes-Syndrom *nt*, hepatomuskuläre benigne Glykogenose *f*, Glykogenose *f* Typ III.
Forbes-Albright ['ɔːlbraɪt]: **F.-A. syndrome** Forbes-Albright-Syndrom *nt*.
force [fɔərs, fɔːrs] **I** *n* **1.** Kraft *f*, Wucht *f*, Stärke *f*. **by ~ of** durch, mittels. **2.** Gewalt-(anwendung) *f*, Zwang *m*, Druck *m*. **by ~** gewaltsam, mit Gewalt; zwangsweise. **to resort to ~** Gewalt anwenden. **3.** Überzeugungskraft *f*. **II** *vt* **4.** s./jdn. zwingen *od*. nötigen (*to do* zu tun). **5.** etw. erzwingen; etw. aufzwingen. **6.** zwängen, drängen, (unter-, heraus-)drücken, pressen.
force back *vt* (*Tränen*) unterdrücken, zurückdrängen.

forced

force down vt (*Essen*) hinunterzwingen; (*Lachen*) unterdrücken.
force out vt herausdrücken.
force together vt zusammenpressen.
forced [fɔːrst, fɔːrst] *adj* 1. erzwungen, Zwangs-. 2. gezwungen, gequält.
forced alimentation Zwangsernährung *f*.
forced attitude Zwangshaltung *f*, -stellung *f*, -lage *f*.
force development Kraftentwicklung *f*.
forced expiratory volume *abbr.* **FEV₁** (Ein-)Sekundenkapazität *f* *abbr.* ESK, Atemstoßtest *m*, Tiffeneau-Test *m*.
forced feeding Zwangsernährung *f*.
forced respiration forcierte Atmung *f*, willkürliche Hyperventilation *f*.
force-feed vt zwangsernähren.
force-ful ['fɔərsfəl, 'fɔːrs-] *adj* 1. (*Person*) energisch, kraftvoll. 2. eindrucks-, wirkungsvoll; überzeugend.
force parallelogram Kräfteparallelogramm *m*.
for·ceps ['fɔːrsəps, -seps] *n*, *pl* -**ceps**, -**ci·pes** [-səˈpiːz] 1. (*a.* **a pair of ~**) *chir.* Zange *f*, Klemme *f*; Pinzette *f*; Forzeps *m*, Forceps *m*. 2. *anat.* zwingenförmiges Organ *nt*, Forceps *m*. 3. *bio.* Schere *f*, Zange *f*.
forceps baby Zangengeburt *f*.
forceps delivery *gyn.* Zangengeburt *f*, -entbindung *f*, -extraktion *f*.
high f. hohe Zangengeburt.
low/outlet f. tiefe Zangengeburt.
forceps frontalis vordere Balkenzwinge *f*, Forceps frontalis/minor.
forceps major → forceps occipitalis.
forceps minor → forceps frontalis.
forceps occipitalis hintere Balkenzwinge *f*, Forceps occipitalis/major.
for·ci·ble ['fɔərsɪbl, 'fɔːr-] *adj* 1. gewaltsam; zwangsweise, Zwangs-. 2. → forceful.
forcible alimentation Zwangsernährung *f*.
forcible feeding Zwangsernährung *f*.
for·ci·pate ['fɔːrsɪpeɪt, 'fəʊr-] *adj* *bio.* zangen-, scherenähnlich.
for·ci·pat·ed [-peɪtɪd] *adj* → forcipate.
Fordyce ['fɔːrdaɪs]: **angiokeratoma of F.** Fordyce-Krankheit *f*, Angiokeratoma scroti Fordyce.
F.'s disease 1. Fordyce-Krankheit *f*, -Drüsen *pl*, -Zustand *m*, freie/ektopische Talgdrüsen *pl*. 2. Fox-Fordyce-Krankheit, apokrine Miliaria *f*, Hidradenoma eruptivum, Apocrinitis sudoripara pruriens, Akanthosis circumporalis pruriens.
F.'s granules/spots → F.'s disease 1.
fore [fɔːr, 'fəʊr] *adj* vordere(r, s), Vor-, Vorder-, Unter-.
fore·arm ['fɔːrɑːrm, 'fəʊr-] *n* Unter-, Vorderarm *m*; *anat.* Antebrachium *nt*.
forearm fracture *ortho.* Unterarmschaftfraktur *f*.
forearm sign *neuro.* Léri-Zeichen *nt*.
forearm stub *embryo.* Unterarmstumpf *m*.
fore·brain ['-breɪn] *n* *embryo.* Vorderhirn *nt*, Prosenzephalon *nt*, Prosencephalon *nt*.
forebrain bundle, medial mediales Vorderhirnbündel *nt*, Fasciculus prosencephalicus medialis.
forebrain vesicle *embryo.* Vorderhirnbläschen *nt*.
fore·fin·ger ['-fɪŋɡər] *n* Zeigefinger *m*; *anat.* Index *m*.
fore·foot ['-fʊt] *n* Vorfuß *m*.
forefoot amputation *ortho.* Vorfußamputation *f*.
fore·gut ['-ɡʌt] *n* *embryo.* Kopf-, Vorderdarm *m*.
fore·head ['fɔːrɪd, 'fɑːr-, 'fɔːrhed] *n* 1. Stirn *f*; *anat.* Frons *f*. 2. Front *f*, Stirnteil *nt*.

for·eign ['fɒrɪn] *adj* fremd (*to*); seltsam, unbekannt; nicht passend (*to* zu).
foreign antigen Fremdantigen *nt*.
foreign body Fremdkörper *m* *abbr.* FK, Corpus alienum.
foreign-body appendicitis Fremdkörperappendizitis *f*.
foreign-body aspiration Fremdkörperaspiration *f*.
foreign body giant cells Fremdkörperriesenzellen *pl*.
foreign-body granuloma Fremdkörpergranulom *nt*.
foreign-body reaction Fremdkörperreaktion *f*.
foreign matter → foreign body.
foreign protein Fremdeiweiß *nt*, -protein *nt*.
foreign serum Fremdserum *nt*.
foreign substance körperfremde Substanz *f*, Fremdsubstanz *f*; Fremdkörper *m*.
foreign tissue Fremdgewebe *nt*.
fore·kid·ney [ˌfɔːrˈkɪdnɪ, ˌfəʊr-] *n* Vorniere *f*, Pronephros *m*.
Forel [fɔˈrel]: **area H of F.** → field H of F.
area H₁ of F. → field H₁ of F.
area H₂ of F. → field H₂ of F.
F.'s areas Forel'-Felder *pl*.
F.'s axis Forel'-(Hirn-)Achse *f*.
F.'s decussation → F.'s tegmental decussation.
field H of F. Forel'-H-Feld *nt*.
field H₁ of F. Forel'-H₁-Feld *nt*.
field H₂ of F. Forel'-H₂-Feld *nt*.
F.'s fields → F.'s areas.
F.'s tegmental decussation Forel'-Haubenkreuzung *f*, vordere Haubenkreuzung *f*.
fore·limb ['fɔːrlɪm, 'fəʊr-] *n* *embryo.* obere Gliedmaße *f*, Arm *m*.
forelimb bud *embryo.* Armknospe *f*, -anlage *f*.
fore·milk ['-mɪlk] *n* Vormilch *f*, Kolostralmilch *f*, Kolostrum *nt*.
fore·name ['-neɪm] *n* Vorname *m*.
fo·ren·sic [fəˈrensɪk] *adj* forensisch, gerichtlich, Gerichts-.
forensic chemistry forensische/gerichtliche Chemie *f*, Gerichtschemie *f*.
forensic medicine forensische/gerichtliche Medizin *f*, Gerichtsmedizin *f*, Rechtsmedizin *f*.
forensic psychiatry forensische/gerichtliche Psychiatrie *f*.
forensic psychology forensische Psychologie *f*, Kriminalpsychologie *f*.
fore·part ['fɔːrpɑːrt, 'fəʊr-] *n* Vorderteil *m*/*nt*.
fore·play ['-pleɪ] *n* (sexuelles) Vorspiel *nt*.
fore·quar·ter amputation ['-kwɔːrtər] *ortho.* interskapulothorakale (Schulter-)-Amputation *f*.
fore·run·ner ['-rʌnər] *n* *fig.* Vorbote *m*, (erstes) Anzeichen *nt*.
fore·skin ['-skɪn] *n* Vorhaut *f*, Präputium *nt*, Pr(a)eputium penis.
Forestier [fɔrɛsˈtjeː]: **F.'s disease** Forestier'--Krankheit *f*, -Syndrom *nt*, Morbus Forestier *m*, Hyperostosis vertebralis senilis ankylosans.
fore·stomach ['fɔːrstʌmək, 'fəʊr-] *n* *anat.* Antrum cardiacum.
for·est-spring encephalitis ['fɔːrɪst, 'fɑːr-] russische Früh(jahr)-Sommer-Enzephalitis *f* *abbr.* RSSE, russische Zeckenenzephalitis *f*.
forest yaws südamerikanische Hautleishmaniase *f*, kutane Leishmaniase *f* Südamerikas, Chiclero-Ulkus *m*.
fore·tooth ['fɔːrtuːθ, 'fəʊr-] *n*, *pl* -**teeth** [-tiːθ] Schneidezahn *m*, Incisivus *m*, Dens incisivus.

fore·wat·ers ['-wɔːtərz] *pl* *gyn.* Vorwasser *nt*.
fork [fɔːrk] *n* 1. Gabel *f*. 2. Gabel *f*, Gabelung *f*, Abzweigung *f*.
forked uvula [fɔːrkt, 'fɔːrkɪd] Zäpfchen-, Uvulaspalte *f*, Uvula bifida.
form [fɔːrm] I *n* 1. Form *f*, Gestalt *f*. **to take ~ Form** *od.* Gestalt annehmen. **in the ~ of** in Form von. **in tablet ~** in Tablettenform. 2. (körperliche *od.* geistige) Verfassung *f*, Form *f*. **in one's ~** in Form. **out of one's ~** nicht in Form. **to be in good ~** gut in Form sein, in guter Verfassung sein. **at the top of one's ~** in Hochform. 3. *mathe.* Formel *f*. 4. *chem.* Form *f*, Konfiguration *f*. 5. Erscheinungsform *f*, -weise *f*. 6. Form *f*, Art (*u.* Weise) *f*; System *nt*. 7. Formular *nt*, Formblatt *nt*. 8. *techn.* Form *f*, Schablone *f*. II *v* 9. Form *f*, bilden, gestalten (*into* zu). 10. (*Charakter*) formen. 11. (an-)ordnen, zusammenstellen. 12. (*Plan*) entwerfen; (*Ideen*) entwickeln. 13. *techn.* (ver-)formen, s. bilden, s. gestalten, entstehen. **form·al·de·hyde** [fɔːrˈmældəˌhaɪd] *n* Formaldehyd *m*, Ameisensäurealdehyd *m*, Methanal *nt*.
formaldehyde dehydrogenase Formaldehyddehydrogenase *f*.
form·al·de·hy·do·gen·ic [fɔːrˌmældəˌhaɪdəʊˈdʒenɪk] *adj* formaldehydbildend.
for·ma·lin ['fɔːrməlɪn] *n* Formalin *nt*.
for·ma·lin·ize ['fɔːrməlɪnaɪz] *vt* mit Formalin *od.* Formaldehyd behandeln.
formalin pigment Formalinpigment *nt*.
form·am·i·dase [fɔːrˈæmɪdeɪz] *n* 1. Formamidase *f*. 2. → formylkynurenine hydrolase.
for·mant ['fɔːrmənt] *n* Formant *m*.
for·mate ['fɔːrmeɪt] *n* Formiat *nt*.
formate dehydrogenase Formiatdehydrogenase *f*.
formate hydrogenolyase → formate dehydrogenase.
for·ma·tio [fɔːrˈmeɪʃɪəʊ] *n*, *pl* -**nes** [-niːz] → formation 1.
for·ma·tion [fɔːrˈmeɪʃn] *n* 1. Bildung *f*, Gebilde *nt*, Formation *f*; *anat.* Formatio *f*. 2. Formung *f*, Gestaltung *f*; Bildung *f*, Entwicklung *f*, Entstehung *f*, Formation *f*. 3. Anordnung *f*, Struktur *f*, Zusammensetzung *f*.
form·a·tive ['fɔːrmətɪv] *adj* 1. gestaltend, bildend, formend, formativ; Entwicklungs-. 2. *bio.* morphogenetisch.
formative osteitis Ostitis condensans.
forme fruste [fɔːrm frʌst] abortive *od.* blande Verlaufsform *f*, forme fruste (*f*).
for·mic acid ['fɔːrmɪk] Ameisensäure *f*, Formylsäure *f*.
for·mi·ca·tion [ˌfɔːrmɪˈkeɪʃn] *n* *neuro, psychia.* Ameisenlaufen *nt*, Formicatio *f*.
for·mi·ci·a·sis [ˌfɔːrmɪˈsaɪəsɪs] *n* *derm.* Formiciasis *f*.
for·mim·i·no [fɔːrˈmɪmɪnəʊ] *n* Formimino-(Gruppe *f*).
for·mim·i·no·glu·ta·mate [fɔːrˌmɪmɪnəʊˈɡluːtəmeɪt] *n* Formiminoglutamat *nt*.
for·mim·i·no·glu·tam·ic acid [ˌ-ɡluːˈtæmɪk] *abbr.* **FIGLU** Formiminoglutaminsäure *f* *abbr.* FIGLU, FIGS.
for·mim·i·no·trans·fer·ase [ˌ-ˈtrænsfəreɪz] *n* Glutamatforminotransferase *f*.
form·less ['fɔːrmlɪs] *adj* formlos.
form·less·ness ['-nɪs] *n* Formlosigkeit *f*.
for·mo·cor·tal [ˌfəʊbəʊˈkɔːrtl] *n* *pharm.* Formocortal.
for·mol ['fɔːrmɒl, -məʊl] *n* wässrige Formaldehydlösung *f*, Formol *nt*.
formol titration *chem.* Formoltitration *f*.
form perception *physiol.* Gestaltwahrnehmung *f*.

form recognition *physiol.* Formerkennung *f.*
for·mu·la ['fɔːrmjəlɒ] *n, pl* **-las, -lae** [-liː] **1.** *chem., mathe.* Formel *f.* **2.** *pharm.* Rezeptur *f.* **3.** Zusammensetzung *f,* Formel *f.* **4.** *ped.* künstliche Säuglingsnahrung *f.*
for·mu·lar·y ['fɔːrmjəleriː, -ləri] *n pharm.* Vorschriftensammlung *f,* -buch *nt,* Formelsammlung *f,* -buch *nt.*
for·mu·late ['fɔːrmjəleɪt] *vt* **1.** formulieren, in einer Formel ausdrücken. **2.** *(Programm)* aufstellen.
for·mu·lize ['fɔːrmjəlaɪz] *vt* → formulate.
for·myl ['fɔːrmɪl] *n* Formyl-(Radikal *nt*).
for·myl·ase ['fɔːrmɪleɪz] *n* → formylkynurenine hydrolase.
for·myl·ate ['fɔːrmɪleɪt] *vt* formylieren.
for·myl·ky·nur·e·nine [,fɔːrmɪlkaɪˈnʊərəniːn] *n* Formylkynurenin *nt.*
formylkynurenine hydrolase Arylformamidase *f,* Formylkynureninhydrolase *f.*
for·myl·trans·fer·ase [,-'trænsfəreɪz] *n* Formyltransferase *f.*
Forney ['fɔːrni]: **F.'s syndrome** Forney--Robinson-Pascoe-Syndrom *nt.*
for·ni·cate ['fɔːrnɪkeɪt] **I** *adj* bogenförmig. **II** *vi* außerehelichen Geschlechtsverkehr haben; Unzucht treiben.
for·ni·ca·tion [fɔːrnɪˈkeɪʃn] *n* außerehelicher Geschlechtsverkehr *m*; Unzucht *f.*
fornication sign Tinel-Hoffmann'-Klopfzeichen *nt.*
for·nix ['fɔːrnɪks] *n, pl* **-ni·ces** [-nəsiːs] *anat.* **1.** Gewölbe *nt,* Kuppel *f,* Dach *nt,* Bogen *m,* Fornix *m.* **2.** Hirngewölbe *nt,* Fornix cerebri.
f. of cerebrum Hirngewölbe, Fornix cerebri.
f. of lacrimal sac Tränensackkuppel, Fornix sacci lacrimalis.
f. of pharynx Pharynxkuppel, Fornix pharyngis.
f. of stomach Magenkuppel, Fornix gastricus/ventricularis.
f. of vagina Scheidengewölbe, Fornix vaginae.
fornix column Gewölbsäule *f,* -pfeiler *m,* Fornixsäule *f,* -pfeiler *m,* Columna fornicis.
Forrester ['fɔrɪstər]: **F. splint** *ortho.* Forrester-Brown-Schiene *f.*
Forrester-Brown [braʊn]: **F.-B. splint** *ortho.* Forrester-Brown-Schiene *f.*
Forsius-Eriksson ['fɔːrsɪɒs ˈerɪksɒn]: **F.-E. type ocular albinism** → F.-E. syndrome.
F.-E. syndrome okulärer Albinismus (Forsius-Eriksson) *m.*
Forssman ['fɔːrsmən; 'fɔrsman]: **F. antibody** Forssman-Antikörper *m,* F-Antikörper *m.*
F. antigen Forssmanantigen *nt,* F-Antigen *nt.*
F. antigen-antibody reaction → F. reaction.
F. reaction Forssman-Antikörper-Reaktion *f.*
Förster ['ferstər; 'fœr-]: **F.'s choroiditis/disease** Förster-Chorioiditis *f,* Areolarchorioiditis *f,* Chorioiditis areolaris.
Fort Bragg fever [fɔːrt, faʊrt bræɡ] Fort-Bragg-Fieber *nt.*
for·ti·fi·ca·tion spectrum [,fɔːrtɪfɪˈkeɪʃn] *ophthal.* Teichopsie *f,* Teichoskopie *f,* Zackensehen *nt.*
for·tu·i·tous [fɔːrˈt(j)uːɪtəs] *adj* zufällig.
for·ward conduction ['fɔːrwərd] *card.* anterograde Erregunsleitung *f.*
forward failure Vorwärtsversagen *nt,* forward failure (*nt*).
fos·fo·my·cin [,fɒsfəˈmaɪsɪn] *n pharm.* Fosfomycin *nt.*
Foshay ['fɔːʃeɪ]: **F. test** Foshay-Reaktion *f.*

fos·sa ['fɒsə] *n, pl* **-sae** [-siː] *anat.* Grube *f,* Höhle *f,* Mulde *f,* Nische *f,* Fossa *f.*
f. of antihelix Fossa anthelicis.
f. of capitulum of radius Fovea capituli radii.
f. of coronoid process Fossa coronoidea.
f. of gall bladder Gallenblasengrube, -bett *nt,* Leberbett *nt,* Fossa vesicae felleae/biliaris.
f. of gasserian ganglion Impressio trigeminalis.
f. of head of femur Fossa capitis femoris.
f. of incus Fossa incudis.
f. of lacrimal gland Fossa gl. lacrimalis.
f. of lacrimal sac Fossa sacci lacrimalis.
f. of lateral malleolus Fossa malleoli lateralis.
f. of Morgagni Fossa navicularis urethrae.
f. of oval window Fossula fenestrae vestibuli.
f. of Sylvius 1. Sylvius'-Furche *f,* Sulcus lateralis. **2.** Fossa lateralis cerebralis.
f. of vestibule of vagina Fossa vestibuli vaginae.
fossa ovalis of thigh Hiatus saphenus.
fos·sette [fɒˈset] *n* **1.** *anat.* kleine Grube *f,* Grübchen *nt.* **2.** *ophthal.* kleines tiefes Hornhautgeschwür *nt.*
fos·su·la ['fɒsjələ] *n, pl* **-lae** [-liː] *anat.* kleine Grube *od.* Nische *f,* Grübchen *nt,* Fossula *f.*
f. of cochlear window Fossula fenestrae cochleae.
f. of oval window → f. of vestibular window.
f. of petrous ganglion Fossula petrosa.
f. of round window → f. of cochlear window.
f. of vestibular window Fossula fenestrae vestibuli.
Foster Kennedy ['fɒstər, 'fas-, 'kenɪdiː]: **F. K. syndrome** Foster-Kennedy-Syndrom *nt,* Kennedy-Syndrom *nt.*
Fothergill ['fɒðərɡɪl]: **F.'s disease 1.** Scarlatina anginosa. **2.** Trigeminusneuralgie *f,* Neuralgia trigeminalis..
F.'s neuralgia → F.'s disease 2.
F.'s operation *gyn.* Fothergill-Operation *f,* Manchester-Operation *f.*
F.'s sign Fothergill-Phänomen *nt.*
F.'s sore throat → F.'s disease 1.
fou·droy·ant [fuːˈdrɔɪənt] *adj* schlagartig einsetzend, foudroyant, fulminant.
found·ry·man's fever ['faʊndrɪmən] Metalldampffieber.
fou·chette [fʊərˈʃet] *n anat.* Frenulum labiorum pudendi.
Fournier [fʊrˈnjeɪ]: **F.'s disease** Fournier'--Gangrän *f,* -Krankheit *f,* Skrotalgangrän *f.*
F.'s gangrene → F.'s disease.
syphiloma of F. → F.'s disease.
fourth concha [faʊrθ, fɔːrθ] oberste Nasenmuschel *f,* Concha nasalis suprema.
fourth disease Dukes'-Krankheit *f,* Dukes-Filatoff-Krankheit *f,* Filatow--Dukes-Krankheit *f,* vierte Krankheit *f,* Parascarlatina *f,* Rubeola scarlatinosa.
fourth finger Ringfinger *m,* Digitus anularis/quartus.
fourth nerve Trochlearis *m,* IV. Hirnnerv *m,* N. trochlearis.
fourth sound *card.* IV. Herzton *m*; Vorhofton *m.*
fourth ventricle (of brain/cerebrum) vierter (Hirn-)Ventrikel *m,* Ventriculus quartus (cerebri).
four-vessel angiography [fəʊr, fɔːr] *radiol.* Viergefäßangiographie *f.*
fo·vea ['fəʊvɪə] *n, pl* **-ve·ae** [-viː] *anat.* kleine Grube *od.* Vertiefung *f,* Fovea *f.*

f. of capitulum of radius Fovea capituli radii.
f. of condyloid process Fovea pterygoidea.
f. of head of femur Fovea capitis femoris.
f. of Morgagni Fossa navicularis urethrae.
fo·ve·al vision ['fəʊvɪəl] direktes/zentrales Sehen *nt.*
fo·ve·ate ['fəʊvɪeɪt, -ɪt] *adj* eingedellt, eingedrückt; foveolär.
fo·ve·at·ed ['fəʊvɪeɪtɪd] *adj* → foveate.
foveated chest *ortho.* Trichterbrust *f,* Pectus excavatum/infundibulum/recurvatum.
fo·ve·o·la [fəʊˈvɪələ] *n, pl* **-las, -lae** [-liː] *anat.* Grübchen *nt,* winzige Vertiefung *f,* Foveaola *f.*
f. of retina Foveola retinae.
fo·ve·o·lar [fəʊˈvɪələr] *adj* → foveate.
foveolar hyperplasia *patho.* foveoläre Hyperplasie *f.*
fo·ve·o·late [fəʊˈvɪələt, -lɪt] *adj* → foveate.
fo·ve·o·lat·ed [fəʊˈvɪəleɪtɪd] *adj* → foveate.
Foville [fɔˈvɪl]: **F.'s syndrome** Foville-Syndrom *nt.*
fowl [faʊl] *n* Geflügel *nt,* Hühner *pl.*
Fowler ['faʊlər]: **F.'s loudness balance test** *HNO* Fowler-Test *m,* Lautheitsvergleich *m* nach Fowler.
F.'s position Fowler-Lagerung *f.*
fowl mite *micro.* Vogelmilbe *f,* Dermanyssus avium.
fowl pest/plague *micro.* Hühner-, Geflügelpest *f.*
fowl tick *micro.* Argas persicus.
Fox [fɒks]: **F.'s disease** → Fox-Fordyce disease.
Fox-Fordyce ['fɔːrdaɪs]: **F.-F. disease** Fox--Fordyce-Krankheit *f,* apokrine Miliaria *f,* Hidradenoma eruptivum, Apocrinitis sudoripara pruriens, Akanthosis circumporalis pruriens.
fox·glove ['fɒksɡlʌv] *n bio.* Fingerhut *m,* Digitalis *f.*
FP *abbr.* → freezing point.
f.p. *abbr.* → freezing point.
F1P *abbr.* → fructose-1-phosphate.
F6P *abbr.* → fructose-6-phosphate.
FPL *abbr.* → flexor pollicis longus (muscle).
F plasmid → F factor.
F protein F-Protein *nt,* Fusionsprotein *nt.*
Fr *abbr.* → francium.
frac·tion ['frækʃn] *n* **1.** *mathe.* Bruch *m.* **2.** *(a. fig.)* Bruchteil *m*; sehr geringer Teil, eine Spur. **3.** *chem.* Fraktion *f.*
frac·tion·al ['frækʃənəl] *adj* **1.** *mathe.* Bruch-. **2.** *fig.* geringfügig, minimal. **3.** *chem.* fraktioniert.
fractional distillation *chem.* fraktionierte Destillation *f.*
fractional dose fraktionierte Dosis *f,* Dosis refracta.
frac·tion·al·ize ['frækʃənlaɪz] *vt* in Bruchteile zerlegen.
fractional precipitation *phys., chem.* fraktionierte Ausfällung/Präzipitation *f.*
frac·tion·ate ['frækʃneɪt] *vt chem.* fraktionieren, auftrennen.
frac·tion·a·tion [,frækʃəˈneɪʃn] *n chem.* Fraktionierung *f,* Fraktionieren *nt.*
frac·tion·ize ['frækʃənaɪz] **I** *vt* teilen. **II** *vi s.* teilen.
frac·ture ['fræktʃər] **I** *n* **1.** Bruch *m,* Riß *m.* **2.** Knochenbruch, -fraktur *m,* Fractura *f,* *inf.* Bruch, Fraktur. **II** *vt, vi* brechen, frakturieren; zerbrechen.
f. of the anatomic neck of humerus Humerusfraktur durch das Collum anatomicum, Humeruskopffraktur.
f. of the anterior column (*Hüfte*) Bruch/Fraktur des vorderen Pfeilers, vordere Beckenpfeilerfraktur.

fracture blister

f. of C₁ Atlasfraktur.
f. of C₂ Axisfraktur.
f. of the capitellum Fraktur des Capitulum humeri.
f. of the clavicle Schlüsselbeinbruch, -fraktur, Klavikulafraktur.
f. of the coccyx Steißbeinbruch, -fraktur.
f. by contrecoup (*Schädel*) Contre-coup-Fraktur.
f. of the humerus Oberarmbruch, Humerusfraktur.
f. of the inferior pubic ramus untere Schambein(ast)fraktur.
f. of the ischial ramus Sitzbein(ast)fraktur.
f. of the olecranon Olekranonfraktur.
f. of the patella Kniescheibenbruch, Patellafraktur.
f. of the pelvic ring Beckenringfraktur.
f. of the posterior column (*Hüfte*) Bruch/Fraktur des hinteren Pfeilers, hintere Beckenpfeilerfraktur.
f. of the proximal humerus proximale Humerusfraktur.
f. of the pubic arch Schambogenfraktur.
f. of the radial styloid (Abriß-)Fraktur des Proc. styloideus radii.
f. of the sacrum Kreuzbeinbruch, -fraktur.
f. of the spinal column Wirbelsäulenfraktur.
f. of the superior pubic ramus obere Schambein(ast)fraktur.
f. of the tibial plateau Schienbeinkopffraktur, Tibiakopffraktur.
f. of the ulnar styloid Fraktur des Proc. styloideus ulnae.
fracture blister Spannungsblase *f*.
fracture callus (Fraktur-, Bruch-)Kallus *m*.
frac·tured ['fræktʃərd] *adj* gebrochen, frakturiert.
fractured acetabulum Hüftpfannenbruch *m*, Acetabulumfraktur *f*.
fractured capitellum Fraktur *f* des Capitulum humeri.
fractured clavicle Schlüsselbeinbruch *m*, -fraktur *f*, Klavikulafraktur *f*.
fractured coccyx Steißbeinbruch *m*, -fraktur *f*.
fractured dislocation → fracture-dislocation.
fractured femur Oberschenkelbruch *m*, -fraktur *f*, Femurfraktur *f*.
fractured fibula Wadenbeinbruch *m*, -fraktur *f*, Fibulafraktur *f*.
fractured heel bone Fersenbeinbruch *m*, -fraktur *f*, Kalkaneusfraktur *f*.
fractured humerus Oberarmbruch *m*, -fraktur *f*, Humerusfraktur *f*.
fracture-dislocation *n* Luxationsfraktur *f*, Verrenkungsbruch *m*.
fractured neck of femur Schenkelhalsbruch *m*, -fraktur *f*, Femurhalsfraktur *f*.
fractured olecranon Olekranonbruch *m*.
fractured patella Kniescheibenbruch *m*, -fraktur *f*, Patellafraktur *f*.
fractured radius Speichenbruch *m*, Radiusfraktur *f*.
fractured rib Rippenbruch *m*, -fraktur *f*.
fractured sacrum Kreuzbeinbruch *m*, -fraktur *f*.
fractured skull Schädel(dach)bruch *m*, -fraktur *f*.
fractured spine Wirbelsäulenbruch *m*, -fraktur *f*.
fractured sternum Brustbein-, Sternumfraktur *f*.
fractured talus Sprungbein-, Talusfraktur *f*.
fractured tibia Schienbeinbruch *m*, -fraktur *f*, Tibiafraktur *f*.
fractured ulna Ellenbruch *m*, Ulnafraktur *f*.

fractured wrist Handgelenksbruch *m*, -fraktur *f*.
fracture fragment Bruchstück *nt*, -fragment *nt*; Knochenfragment *nt*.
fracture healing Frakturheilung *f*.
fracture non-union Pseudarthrose(nbildung *f*) *f*.
fracture site Bruchstelle *f*.
fracture slipping Abrutschen *nt* der Frakturenden.
fracture treatment Frakturbehandlung *f*.
frag·ile ['frædʒəl; *Brit*. 'frædʒaɪl] *adj* zerbrechlich, brüchig, gebrechlich, fragil.
frag·ile·ness ['-nɪs] *n* → fragility.
fragile X syndrome fragile-X-Syndrom *nt*, Marker-X-Syndrom *nt*, Martin-Bell-Syndrom *nt*.
fra·gil·i·tas [frə'dʒɪlətæs] *n* → fragility.
fra·gil·i·ty [frə'dʒɪləti] *n* Zerbrechlichkeit *f*, Brüchigkeit *f*, Sprödigkeit *f*, Fragilität *f*.
f. of blood *physiol.* Erythrozytenresistenz *f*.
fragility test Erythrozytenresistenztest *m*.
fra·gil·o·cyte [frə'dʒɪlosaɪt] *n hema.* Fragilozyt *m*.
fra·gil·o·cy·to·sis [ˌ-saɪ'toʊsɪs] *n hema.* Fragilozytose *f*.
frag·ment ['frægmənt] **I** *n* Fragment *nt*, Bruchstück *nt*, -teil *m*. **II** *vi* (zer-)brechen, in Stücke brechen.
frag·men·tal [fræg'mentl] *adj* → fragmentary.
frag·men·tar·y ['frægməntəri] *adj* bruchstückhaft, unvollendet, lückenhaft, fragmentarisch, fragmentär.
frag·men·ta·tion [ˌfrægmən'teɪʃn] *n* **1.** Zersplitterung *f*, Zerkleinerung *f*, Zertrümmerung *f*, Zerfall *m*, Fragmentierung *f*, Fragmentation *f*. **2.** *bio.* Fortpflanzung *f* durch Abknospung, Fragmentation *f*. **3.** *biochem.* Fragmentation *f*, Fragmentierung *f*.
fraise [freɪz] **I** *n* (Bohr-)Fräse *f*. **II** *vt* fräsen.
Fraley ['freɪlɪ]: **F.'s syndrome** Fraley-Syndrom *nt*.
fram·be·sia [fræm'biːʒə] *n* Frambösie *f*, Pian *f*, Parangi *f*, Yaws *f*, Framboesia tropica.
fram·be·si·form syphilid [fræm'biːzɪfɔːrm] frambösiformes Syphilid *nt*.
fram·be·si·o·ma [fræmˌbiːzɪ'oʊmə] *n* Frambösiom *nt*, Mutterefloreszenz *f*, Primärläsion *f*.
fram·boe·sia *n* → frambesia.
fram·boe·si·o·ma *n* → frambesioma.
frame [freɪm] *n* **1.** Rahmen *m*, Gestell *nt*; *anat.* Gestell *nt*; Gerippe *nt*, Skelett *nt*. **2.** (Brillen-)Gestell *nt*. **3.** *fig.* Rahmen *m*, Struktur *f*, System *nt*. **within the ~ of** im Rahmen. **4.** (Gemüts-)Verfassung *f*, Gemütszustand *m*. **5.** (Körper-)Bau *m*, Gestalt *f*, Figur *f*.
f. of mind (Gemüts-)Verfassung *f*, Gemütszustand.
f. of reference *mathe.* Bezugs-, Koordinatensystem.
frame-shift mutation *genet.* Rasterverschiebung *f*, frame-shift-Mutation *f*.
frame·work ['freɪmwɜrk] *n* **1.** (*a. techn., histol., bio.*) (Grund-)Gerüst *nt*, Stützwerk *nt*; Gerippe *nt*. **2.** Gestell *nt*. **3.** *fig.* Rahmen *m*, Struktur *f*, System *nt*. **4.** *anat.* (Stütz-)Gerüst *nt* eines Organs, Stroma *nt*.
framework fiber *bio.* Gerüstfaser *f*.
Franceschetti [ˌfrantʃəˈskeɪti]: **F. syndrome** Franceschetti-Syndrom *nt*, Treacher-Collins-Syndrom *nt*, Dysostosis mandibulo-facialis.
Franceschetti-Jadassohn ['jaːdazoːn]: **F.-J. syndrome** Franceschetti-Jadassohn-Syndrom *nt*, Naegeli-Syndrom *nt*,

Naegeli-Bloch-Sulzberger-Syndrom *nt*, retikuläre Pigmentdermatose *f*, Melanophorennaevus *m*, familiärer Chromatophorennaevus *m*, Incontinentia pigmenti Typ Franceschetti-Jadassohn.
Francis ['frænsɪs]: **F. disease** Francis-Krankheit *f*, Ohara-Krankheit *f*, Hasen-, Nagerpest *f*, Lemming-Fieber *nt*, Tularämie *f*.
Fran·ci·sel·la [frænsɪ'selə] *n micro.* Francisella *f*.
fran·ci·um ['frænsɪəm] *n abbr.* **Fr** Francium *nt abbr.* Fr.
Franco ['fræŋkoʊ; frɑ'koː]: **F.'s operation** suprapubische Zystotomie *f*.
François [frɑ'swɑ]: **F.' syndrome** Dyskephaliesyndrom *nt* von François, Hallermann-Streiff(-François)-Syndrom *nt*, Dysmorphia mandibulo-oculo-facialis.
Fränkel ['frɛŋkəl; 'frɛŋ-]: **F.'s sign** Fränkel-Zeichen *nt*.
Frankenhäuser ['fraŋkənhɔʏsər]: **F.'s ganglion** Frankenhäuser'-Ganglion *nt*.
Frank·fort ['fræŋkfərt]: **F. horizontal** → F. plane.
F. horizontal plane → F. plane.
F. plane *radiol.* Deutsche Horizontale *f*, Frankfurter Horizontale *f*, Ohr-Augen-Ebene *f*.
Frankl-Hochwart ['fræŋkl 'hoʊkwɑrt; 'fraŋ- 'hoːxvaːrt]: **F.-H.'s disease** Frankl-Hochwart-Syndrom *nt*, Frankl-Hochwart-Pellizzi-Marburg-Syndrom *nt*.
Franklin ['fræŋklɪn]: **F.'s disease** Franklin-Syndrom *nt*, Schwerekettenkrankheit *f*, H-Krankheit *f*.
Frank-Starling [fræŋk 'stɑːrlɪŋ]: **F.-S.'s curve** Frank-Starling-Kurve *f*, Druck-Volumendiagramm *nt*.
F.-S. mechanism Frank-Starling-Mechanismus *m*, Starling'-Gesetz *nt*.
fra·ter·nal [frə'tɜrnl] *adj* brüderlich, Brüder-, Bruder-; *bio.* zweieiig.
fraternal twins binovuläre/dissimilare/dizygote/erbungleiche/zweieiige/heteroovuläre Zwillinge *pl*.
Fraunhofer ['frɔ(ə)nhoʊfər, -hɑf-]: **F.'s lines** *phys.* Fraunhofer'-Linien *pl*.
Frazier-Spiller ['freɪzər 'spɪlər]: **F.-S. operation** *neurochir.* Frazier-Spiller-Operation *f*, Neurotomia retrogasserina.
FRC *abbr.* → functional residual capacity.
freck·le ['frekl] **I** *n* **1.** Sommersprosse *f*, Ephelide *f*. **2.** (Haut-)Fleck *m*, Fleckchen *nt*. **II** *vt* tüpfeln, sprenkeln. **III** *vi* Sommersprossen bekommen.
freck·led ['frekld] *adj* sommersprossig.
freck·ly ['freklɪ] *adj* → freckled.
Fredet-Ramstedt [frɑ'dɛ 'ræmstet]: **F.-R. operation** *chir.* Weber-Ramstedt-Operation *f*, Ramstedt-Operation *f*, Pyloro(myo)tomie *f*.
free [friː] **I** *adj* **1.** frei, befreit (*from, of* von); ohne. **~ from infection** frei von ansteckenden Krankheiten. **~ from pain** schmerzfrei. **2.** *chem.* frei, ungebunden. **3.** frei, unabhängig, ungebunden, selbständig. **4.** kostenlos, gratis, frei-, Gratis-. **~ of charge** gebührenfrei. **II** *vt* befreien (*from* aus, von); (auf-)lösen.
free area *psycho.* Freiraum *m*.
free association *psycho.* freie Assoziation *f*.
free band of colon → free taenia.
free bilirubin freies/indirektes/unkonjugiertes Bilirubin *nt*.
free border of ovary → free margin of ovary.
free cells of connective tissue freie Bindegewebszellen *pl*.
free denticle freier Dentikel *m*.

free diffusion freie Diffusion f.
free edge of nail → free margin of nail.
free electron freies Elektron nt.
free energy phys., chem. freie od. ungebundene Energie f.
 standard f. of formation freie Bindungsenergie unter Standardbedingungen.
 standard f. of hydrolyse Standardwert der freien Energie der Hydrolyse, freie Energie der Hydrolyse unter Standardbedingungen.
free-energy change chem. Änderung f der freien Energie.
 standard f. Änderung der freien Energie unter Standardbedingungen.
free flap chir. freier (Haut-, Gewebe-)Lappen m.
free gingiva Periodontium insertionis.
free graft chir. freies Transplantat nt.
free gum → free gingiva.
free-ing of the arms [fri:'ɪŋ] gyn. Armlösung f.
free-ly movable joint ['fri:lɪ] echtes Gelenk nt, Diarthrose f, Artic./Junctura synovialis.
Freeman-Sheldon [·fri:mən 'ʃeld(ə)n]: **F.-S. syndrome** Freeman-Sheldon-Syndrom nt, kranio-karpo-tarsales Dysplasie-Syndrom nt, Dysplasia cranio-carpo-tarsalis.
free margin: f. of nail vorderer/freier Nagelrand m, Schnitt-, Abnutzungskante f, Margo liber unguis.
 f. of ovary freier/konvexer Eierstock-/Ovarialrand m, Margo liber ovarii.
free perforation chir. freie Perforation f.
free radical chem., radiol. freies Radikal nt.
free taenia freie Tänie f, Taenia libera.
 f. of colon freie Kolontänie, T(a)enia libera coli.
free villi freie (End-)Zotten pl.
free water freies Wasser nt.
freeze [fri:z] (v froze; frozen) I n (Ge-)Frieren nt; gefrorener Zustand m; Frost m, Kälte f. II vt **1.** gefrieren, einfrieren, tiefkühlen **2.** med. vereisen. **3.** fig. erstarren lassen. III vi **4.** frieren; gefrieren, zu Eis werden; hart od. fest werden, erstarren. **5.** fest-, anfrieren (to an); haften (to an). **6.** fig. (Lächeln) erstarren, eisig werden; (Blut) gerinnen, gefrieren.
freeze-cleaving n → freeze-etching.
freeze-dry vt gefriertrocknen.
freeze-dryer n Gefriertrockner m.
freeze-drying n Gefriertrocknung f, lyophile Trocknung f, Lyophilisation f.
freeze-etching n histol., patho. Gefrierätzung f, -ätzmethode f.
freeze-etch method → freeze-etching.
freez·er ['fri:zər] n Gefrierschrank m, -truhe f, Tiefkühlschrank m, -truhe f.
freez·ing ['fri:zɪŋ] I n **1.** Einfrieren nt. **2.** med. Vereisung f. **3.** Erstarrung f. **4.** Gefrierung f, Kongelation f, Congelatio f. **5.** Gefrieren nt, Gerinnen, Erstarren nt. II adj eiskalt; Gefrier-, Kälte-.
freezing point abbr. **Fp, f.p.** Gefrierpunkt m. **below ~** unter dem Gefrierpunkt, unter Null.
freezing-point depression phys. Gefrierpunktserniedrigung f.
freezing process Tiefkühlverfahren nt.
Frei [fraɪ]: **F.'s antigen** Frei-Antigen nt.
 F.'s disease Morbus Durand-Nicolas-Favre f, klimatischer Bubo m, vierte Geschlechtskrankheit f, Lymphogranuloma inguinale/venereum abbr. **LGV**, Lymphopathia venerea, Poradenitis inguinalis.
 F.'s reaction → F.'s skin reaction.

 F.'s skin reaction Frei-Hauttest m, -Intrakutantest m.
 F.'s (skin) test → F.'s skin reaction.
Freiberg ['fraɪbərg]: **F.'s disease/infarction** ortho. Freiberg-Köhler-Krankheit f, Morbus Köhler II m.
Frei-Hoffman ['hɑfmən]: **F.-H. reaction** → Frei's skin reaction.
Frejka ['freɪkɑ]: **F. pillow (splint)** ortho. Frejka-Spreizkissen nt.
trem·i·tus ['fremɪtəs] n tastbares od. hörbares Vibrieren nt, Vibration f, Schwirren nt, Fremitus m.
French [frentʃ]: **F. chalk** Talkum nt, Talcum m.
 F. flap Verschiebelappen m, -plastik f, Vorschiebelappen m, -plastik f.
 F. proof agar Sabouraud-Agar m/nt, Sabouraud-Glucose-Agar m/nt.
 F. scale Charrière-Scheibe f, -Skala f.
fre·nec·to·my [frɪ'nektəmɪ] n HNO Frenektomie f, Frenulektomie f.
Frenkel ['freŋkl]: **F.'s intracutaneous test** Frenkel'-Intrakutantest m.
fre·no·plas·ty [ˌfri:nə'plæstɪ] n HNO Zungenbändchenplastik f, Fren(ul)oplastik f.
fre·not·o·my [frɪ'nɑtəmɪ] n **1.** Frenulumdurchtrennung f, Fren(ul)otomie f. **2.** HNO Zungenbändchendurchtrennung f, Fren(ul)otomie f, Ankylotomie f.
fren·u·lum ['frenjələm] n, pl **-la** [-lə] anat. Bändchen nt, Frenulum nt.
 f. of clitoris Klitorisbändchen, Frenulum clitoridis.
 f. of cranial medullary velum Frenulum veli medullaris cranialis/rostralis/superioris.
 f. of ileocecal valve Bändchen der Bauhin'-Klappe, Frenulum valvae ilealis.
 f. of lower lip Unterlippenbändchen, Frenulum labii inferioris.
 f. of Morgagni → f. of ileocecal valve.
 f. of prepuce of penis Frenulum pr(a)eputii.
 f. of pudendal labia Frenulum labiorum pudendi.
 f. of rostral medullary velum → f. of cranial medullary velum.
 f. of superior medullary velum → f. of cranial medullary velum.
 f. of tongue Zungenbändchen, Frenulum linguae.
 f. of upper lip Oberlippenbändchen, Frenulum labii superioris.
fre·num ['fri:nəm] n, pl **-na** [-nə] anat. (Schleimhaut) Band nt, Falte f, Frenum nt.
 f. of labia Frenulum labiorum pudendi.
 f. of tongue Zungenbändchen nt, Frenulum linguae.
Frenzel ['frenzl]: **F's diagram** Frenzel-Schema nt.
 F.'s glasses/spectacles physiol. Frenzel-Brille f.
fren·zy ['frenzɪ] I n Ekstase f, Verzückung f; Besessenheit f, Manie f. II vt rasend machen, zur Raserei bringen.
fre·quen·cy ['fri:kwənsɪ] n **1.** electr., phys., stat. Frequenz f. **2.** Häufigkeit f.
frequency analysis Frequenzanalyse f.
frequency curve 1. bio., mathe. Häufigkeitskurve f. **2.** bio. Variationskurve f.
frequency-difference threshold Frequenzunterschiedsschwelle f.
frequency dispersion physiol. Frequenzdispersion f.
frequency distribution Häufigkeitsverteilung f.
frequency filter Frequenzfilter nt.
frequency-following responses abbr. **FFR** Frequency-Following-Responses pl abbr. **FFR**.

frequency inotropism Frequenzinotropie f.
frequency meter electr. Frequenzmesser m.
frequency modulation phys. Frequenzmodulation f.
frequency range electr. Frequenzbereich m.
frequency-selective adj frequenzselektiv.
fre·quent ['fri:kwənt] adj **1.** häufig (vorkommend), oft wiederkehrend, frequent; regelmäßig. **2.** (Puls) frequent, beschleunigt.
frequent pulse schneller/frequenter Puls m, Pulsus frequens.
fresh blood [freʃ] Frischblut nt.
fresh frozen plasma abbr. **FFP** Fresh-frozen-Plasma nt abbr. **FFP**.
fresh·wa·ter ['freʃwɔːtər] n Süßwasser nt.
fress·re·flex ['fresrɪfleks] n Freßreflex m.
Freud [frɔɪd; frɔʏt]: **F.'s theory** Freud'-Lehre f.
Freund [frɔɪnd; frɔʏnt]: **F. adjuvant** Freund-Adjuvans nt.
 F. complete adjuvant komplettes Freund-Adjuvans nt.
Frey [fraɪ]: **F.'s (irritation) hairs** Frey-Reizhaare pl.
 F.'s syndrome aurikulotemporales Syndrom nt, Frey-Baillarger-Syndrom nt, Geschmacksschwitzen nt.
FRF abbr. → follicle stimulating hormone releasing factor.
fri·a·bil·i·ty [fraɪə'bɪlətɪ] n Zerreibbarkeit f; Bröckligkeit f; (leichte) Zerreißbarkeit f.
fri·a·ble ['fraɪəbl] adj (leicht) zerreibbar; bröck(e)lig, krümelig, mürbe.
fri·a·ble·ness ['-nɪs] n → friability.
fric·a·tive ['frɪkətɪv] I n Reibelaut m, Frikativlaut m, Frikativ m. II adj reibend, frikativ, Reibe-.
fric·tion ['frɪkʃn] n **1.** phys. Reibung f, Friktion f. **2.** Ab-, Einreibung f, Frottieren nt.
 to apply ~ frottieren, ein-, abreiben.
fric·tion·al ['frɪkʃnəl, -ʃənl] adj Reibung betr., Reibungs-, Friktions-.
frictional electricity Reibungselektrizität f.
frictional force phys. Reibungskraft f, -widerstand m.
frictional resistance phys. Reibungswiderstand m.
friction burn Verbrennung f durch Reibung(shitze).
friction knot doppelter Knoten m.
fric·tion·less ['frɪkʃnlɪs] adj techn. reibungsfrei, -arm.
friction murmur → friction sound.
friction rub → friction sound.
friction sound card. Reibegeräusch nt, Reiben nt.
Friderichsen-Waterhouse [ˌfrɪdə'rɪksən 'wɔːtərhaʊs]: **F.-W. syndrome** Waterhouse-Friderichsen-Syndrom nt.
Friedländer ['fri:dlendər; -'lendər]: **F.'s bacillus** Friedländer-Bakterium nt, -Bacillus m, Bact. pneumoniae Friedländer, Klebsiella pneumoniae.
 F.'s bacillus pneumonia → F.'s pneumonia.
 F.'s disease Arteritis/Endarteritis obliterans.
 F.'s pneumobacillus → F.'s bacillus.
 F.'s pneumonia Friedländer-Pneumonie f, Klebsiellenpneumonie f.
Friedman ['fri:dmən]: **F.'s test** → Friedman-Lapham test.
Friedman-Lapham ['læfəm]: **F.-L. test** Friedman(-Lapham)-Reaktion f.
Friedmann ['fri:dmən]: **F.'s disease** Narkolepsie f.
 F.'s vasomotor syndrome Friedmann-Syndrom nt.

Friedreich

Friedreich ['fri:draɪk; -raɪç]: **F.'s ataxia** Friedreich-Ataxie *f*, spinale/spinozerebellare Heredoataxie *f*, Heredoataxia spinalis.
F.'s change of note → F.'s sign 2.
F.'s disease 1. → F.'s ataxia. **2.** Friedreich-Syndrom *nt*, Paramyoclonus multiplex.
F.'s foot Friedreich-Fuß *m*.
F.'s heredoataxia → F.'s ataxia.
F.'s phenomenon *pulmo*. Friedreich-Zeichen *nt*, -Kavernenzeichen *nt*.
F.'s sign 1. Friedreich-Zeichen *nt*, Halsvenenkollaps *m*. **2.** Friedreich-Zeichen *nt*, -Kavernenzeichen *nt*.
F.'s taxia → F.'s ataxia.
frig·id ['frɪdʒɪd] *adj* **1.** kalt, frostig, eisig, kühl. **2.** *psychia*. gefühlskalt; frigid, frigide.
fri·gid·i·ty [frɪ'dʒɪdətɪ] *n* **1.** Kälte *f*, Kühle *f*, Frostigkeit *f*, Frigidität *f*. **2.** *psychia*. Gefühlskälte *f*, Frigidität *f*.
frig·id·ness ['frɪdʒɪdnɪs] *n* → frigidity.
frig·o·la·bile [,frɪgə'leɪbəl, -baɪl] *adj* kältelabil, -instabil.
frig·o·rif·ic [,-'rɪfɪk] *adj* kälteerzeugend.
frig·o·sta·bile *adj* → frigostable.
frig·o·sta·ble [,-'steɪbl] *adj* kältestabil, -beständig.
frig·o·ther·a·py [,-'θerəpɪ] *n* Kältetherapie *f*, Kryotherapie *f*.
fringe [frɪndʒ] *n* **1.** Franse *f*. **2.** Rand *m*, Saum *m*, Einfassung *f*, Umrandung *f*.
fringe joint *ortho*. chronisch villöse Arthritis *f*, Arthritis chronica villosa.
frit [frɪt] **I** *n* Fritt-, Weich-, Knochenporzellanmasse *f*. **II** *vt* fritten, schmelzen.
Fritsch [frɪtʃ]: **F.'s catheter** Bozeman--Fritsch-Katheter *m*.
frog [frɒg, frɔg] *n zoo*. Frosch *m*.
frog-like position ['frɒglaɪk, 'frɔg-] Frosch(schenkel)stellung *f*.
Fröhlich ['frø:lɪk; 'frø:lɪç]: **F.'s afterimage** Fröhlich'-Nachbild *nt*.
F.'s syndrome Babinski-Fröhlich-Syndrom *nt*, Morbus Fröhlich *m*, Dystrophia adiposogenitalis (Fröhlich).
Froin [frwɛ̃]: **F.'s syndrome** Froin-Symptom *nt*, -Syndrom *nt*.
Froment [fro'mã]: **F.'s (paper) sign** *neuro*. Froment-Zeichen *nt*.
Frommel ['frɒməl]: **F.'s disease** → Frommel-Chiari syndrome.
Frommel-Chiari [kɪ'ɑ:rɪ]: **F.-C. syndrome** Chiari-Frommel-Syndrom *nt*, Laktationsatrophie *f* des Genitals.
frons [frɒnz] *n* Stirn *f*, Frons *f*.
front [frʌnt] **I** *n* **1.** Vorder-, Stirnseite *f*, Front *f*. **at the ~** vorn, auf der Vorderseite. **2.** Vorderteil *nt*. **3.** Vordergrund *m*. **in ~ of** vor. **II** *adj* Vorder-, Front-.
fron·tal ['frʌntl] **I** *n* → frontal bone. **II** *adj* **1.** stirnwärts, -seitig, frontal. **2.** Stirn *od*. Stirnbein/Os frontale betr., Stirn-, Vorder-.
frontal angle of parietal bone *anat*. Angulus frontalis (ossis parietalis).
frontal antrum Stirnhöhle *f*, Sinus frontalis.
frontal area → frontal cortex.
frontal artery innere Stirnarterie *f*, Supratrochlearis *f*, A. frontalis (medialis), A. supratrochlearis.
frontal bone Stirnbein *nt*, Os frontale.
frontal brain Frontal-, Stirnhirn *nt*.
frontal branch: anteromedial f. of callosomarginal artery Ramus frontalis anteromedialis a. callosomarginalis.
f.es of callosomarginal artery Stirnlappenäste *pl* der A. callosomarginalis, Rami frontales a. callosomarginalis.
f. of frontal nerve Stirnast *m* des N. frontalis, Ramus frontalis n. frontalis.

mediomedial f. of callosomarginal artery Ramus frontalis mediomedialis a. callosomarginalis.
f. of middle meningeal artery Stirnast *od*. vorderer Endast *m* der A. meningea media, Ramus frontalis a. meningeae mediae.
posteromedial f. of callosomarginal artery Ramus frontalis posteromedialis a. callosomarginalis.
f. of superficial temporal artery Stirnast *m* der A. temporalis superficialis, Ramus frontalis a. temporalis superficialis.
frontal convolution: ascending f. → frontal gyrus, ascending.
inferior f. → frontal gyrus, inferior.
middle f. → frontal gyrus, middle.
superior f. → frontal gyrus, superior.
frontal cortex frontaler Kortex *m*, Stirnlappenrinde *f*, -kortex *m*.
frontal crest Crista frontalis.
frontal eminence → frontal tuber.
frontal eye field *abbr*. **FEF** frontales Augenfeld *nt*.
frontal fontanelle vordere/große Fontanelle *f*, Stirnfontanelle *f*, Fonticulus anterior.
frontal foramen For. frontale, Inc. frontalis.
frontal gyrus: ascending f. *old* vordere Zentralwindung *f*, Gyrus pr(a)ecentralis.
inferior f. untere Stirnhirnwindung *f*, Gyrus frontalis inferior.
medial f. Gyrus frontalis medialis.
middle f. mittlere Stirnhirnwindung *f*, Gyrus frontalis medius.
superior f. obere Stirnhirnwindung *f*, Gyrus frontalis superior.
frontal hamulus Ala cristae galli.
frontal horn of lateral ventricle Vorderhorn *nt* des Seitenventrikels, Cornu anterius/frontale ventriculi lateralis.
frontal incisure Inc. frontalis, For. frontale.
fron·ta·lis (muscle) [,frʌn'tælɪs, ,frɑn-, -'teɪl-] Frontalis *m*, M. frontalis, Venter frontalis (m. occipitofrontalis).
frontal lobe Frontal-, Stirnlappen *m*, Lobus frontalis.
frontal-lobe abscess Stirnhirn-, Frontallappenabszeß *m*.
frontal-lobe lesion Stirnhirnläsion *f*.
frontal-lobe tumor Stirnhirn-, Frontallappentumor *m*.
frontal margin of parietal bone Scheitelbeinvorderrand *m*, Margo frontalis ossis parietalis.
frontal mirror Stirnspiegel *m*.
frontal muscle → frontalis (muscle).
frontal nerve Frontalis *m*, N. frontalis.
frontal notch → frontal incisure.
frontal operculum Operculum frontale, Pars opercularis (gyri frontalis inferioris).
frontal plane *anat*. Frontalebene *f*.
frontal pole of cerebral hemisphere Frontalpol *m*, Vorderende *nt* einer Großhirnhemisphäre, Polus frontalis (hemisph(a)erii cerebri).
frontal process: f. of maxilla Stirnfortsatz *m* des Oberkiefers, Proc. frontalis maxillae.
f. of zygomatic bone Stirnfortsatz *m* des Jochbeins, Proc. frontalis ossis zygomatici.
frontal prominence → frontal tuber.
frontal region *anat*. Stirngegend *f*, Frontalregion *f*, Regio frontalis.
frontal sinus Stirnhöhle *f*, Sinus frontalis.
bony/osseous f. knöcherne Stirnhöhle, Sinus frontalis osseus.
frontal sinusitis Stirnhöhlenentzündung *f*, Sinusitis frontalis.

frontal sinus lavage Stirnhöhlenspülung *f*.
frontal speech area motorisches Sprachzentrum *nt*, motorische/frontale Broca'--(Sprach-)Region *f*, Broca'-Feld *nt*.
frontal speech field/region → frontal speech area.
frontal sulcus: inferior f. Sulcus frontalis inferior.
superior f. Sulcus frontalis superior.
frontal suture Sutura frontalis/metopica.
frontal tuber Stirnhöcker *m*, Tuber frontale, Eminentia frontalis.
frontal veins 1. Stirn-, Frontallappenvenen *pl*, Vv. frontales. **2.** mediale Stirnvenen *pl*, Supratrochlearvenen *pl*, Vv. frontales.
fronto- *pref*. Stirn(bein)-, Fronto-.
fron·to·ba·sal artery [,frʌntəʊ'beɪzl]: **lateral f.** A. frontobasalis lateralis, Ramus orbitofrontalis lateralis (a. cerebri mediae).
medial f. A. frontobasalis medialis, Ramus orbitofrontalis medialis (a. cerebri anterioris).
fron·to·cor·ti·cal aphasia [,-'kɔ:rtɪkl] *neuro*. motorische Aphasie *f*, Broca-Aphasie *f*.
fron·to·eth·moi·dal suture [,-'eθmɔɪdl] Sutura fronto-ethmoidalis.
fron·to·lac·ri·mal suture [,-'lækrɪml] Sutura frontolacrimalis.
fron·to·ma·lar suture [,-'meɪlər] → frontozygomatic suture.
fron·to·max·il·lar·y [,-'mæksə,lerɪ:, -mæk'sɪlərɪ] *adj* Stirn *od*. Stirnbein u. Oberkiefer/Maxilla betr., frontomaxillär, frontomaxillar.
frontomaxillary suture Sutura frontomaxillaris.
fron·to·na·sal [,-'neɪzl] *adj* Stirn *od*. Stirnbein u. Nase betr., frontonasal.
frontonasal prominence *embryo*. Frontonasalhöcker *m*, -wulst *m*.
frontonasal suture Sutura frontonasalis.
fron·to·oc·cip·i·tal diameter [,-ɑk'sɪpɪtl] *gyn*., *ped*. frontookzipitaler/okzipitofrontaler Durchmesser *m*, Diameter frontooccipitalis/occipitofrontalis.
frontooccipital fasciculus, inferior Fasciculus fronto-occipitalis inferior.
fronto-orbital area orbitofrontale Rinde *f*, orbitofrontaler Kortex *m*.
fron·to·pa·ri·e·tal operculum [,-pə'raɪɪtl] Operculum frontoparietale.
fron·to·pon·tine fibers [,-'pɑntaɪn, -ti:n] frontopontine Fasern *pl*, Fibrae frontopontinae.
frontopontine tract Arnold'-Bündel *nt*, Tractus frontopontinus.
fron·to·tem·po·ral [,-'temp(ə)rəl] *adj* Stirnbein u. Schläfenbein betr., frontotemporal.
fron·to·zy·go·mat·ic suture [,-,zaɪgə'mætɪk, -,zɪgə-] Sutura frontozygomatica.
frost·bite ['frɒstbaɪt, 'frɔst-] *n* Erfrierung *f*, Kongelation *f*, Congelatio *f*.
frost·ed liver ['frɒstɪd, 'frɔst-] *patho*. Zuckergußleber *f*, Perihepatitis chronica hyperplastica.
frot·tage [frɔ'tɑ:ʒ] *n* **1.** Frottieren *nt*, Abreiben *nt*. **2.** *psychia*. Frottage *f*.
frot·teur [frɔ'tɜr, -'tœːr] *n psychia*. Frotteur *m*.
fro·zen ['frəʊzən] *adj* (ein-, zu-)gefroren, erfroren, Gefrier-.
frozen section *patho*., *histol*. Gefrierschnitt *m*.
frozen-section microtome Gefrier-(schnitt)mikrotom *nt*.
frozen shoulder schmerzhafte Schultersteife *f*, Periarthritis/Periarthropathia humeroscapularis *abbr*. PHS.

FRS abbr. 1. → ferredoxin-reducing substance. 2. → first rank symptoms.
fruc·tan ['frʌktæn] n Fruktan nt, Levan nt.
fruc·to·fu·ra·nose [ˌfrʌktə'fjʊrənəʊz] n Fruktofuranose f.
β-fruc·to·fur·a·no·sid·ase [ˌ-ˌfjʊrənəʊ'saɪdeɪz] n Saccharase f, β-Fructofuranosidase f, Invertase f.
fruc·to·ki·nase [ˌ-'kaɪneɪz, -'kɪn-] n Frukto-, Fructokinase f.
fruc·to·py·ra·nose [ˌ-'paɪrənəʊz] n → fructose.
fruc·to·sa·mine [ˌ-'sæmɪn] n Fructosamin nt.
fruc·to·san ['-sæn] n Fruktosan nt, Fructosan nt, L(a)evulan nt.
fruc·tose ['frʌktəʊs] n Fruchtzucker m, (D-)Fruktose f, (D-)Fructose f, L(a)evulose f.
fructose-1,6-bisphosphatase n → fructose-1,6-diphosphatase.
fructose-2,6-bisphosphatase n → fructose-2,6-diphosphatase.
fructose-1,6-bisphosphate n → fructose-1,6-diphosphate.
fructose-2,6-bisphosphate n → fructose-2,6-diphosphate.
fructose bisphosphate aldolase → fructose diphosphate aldolase.
fructose-1,6-diphosphatase n Fructose-1,6-diphosphatase f, Hexosediphosphatase f.
fructose-2,6-diphosphatase n Fructose-2,6-diphosphatase f.
fructose-1,6-diphosphate n abbr. **FDP** Fructose-1,6-diphosphat nt abbr. F-1,6-P, Harden-Young-Ester m.
fructose-2,6-diphosphate n Fructose-2,6-diphosphat nt abbr. F-2,6-P.
fructose diphosphate aldolase Fructosediphosphataldolase f, Fructosebisphosphataldolase f, Aldolase f abbr. ALD.
fructose intolerance (erbliche) Fruktoseintoleranz f, Fruktoseintoleranzsyndrom nt.
fruc·to·se·mia [ˌfrʌktəʊ'siːmɪə] n Fruktoseausscheidung f im Harn, Fruktosämie f, Fructosämie f.
fructose-1-phosphate n abbr. **F1P** Fructose-1-phosphat nt abbr. F-1-P.
fructose-6-phosphate n abbr. **F6P** Fructose-6-phosphat nt abbr. F-6-P, Neuberg-Ester m.
fructose-1-phosphate aldolase Isozym B nt der Fructosediphosphataldolase.
fruc·to·si·dase [ˌfrʌktə'saɪdeɪz] n → β-fructofuranosidase.
fruc·to·su·ria [ˌ-'s(j)ʊərɪə] n Fruktosurie f, Fructosurie f.
fruc·to·syl·trans·fer·ase [ˌ-ˌsɪl'trænsfəreɪz] n Fructosyltransferase f.
fruit [fruːt] n bot. Frucht f; Obst nt, Früchte pl.
fruit·ar·i·an [fruː'teərɪən] I n Rohköstler(in f) m. II adj Obst-, Frucht-.
fruit-body n → fruiting body.
fruit·ing body ['fruːtɪŋ] micro. Fruchtkörper m.
fruit juice Frucht-, Obstsaft m.
fruit pulp bot. Fruchtfleisch nt.
fruit sugar → fructose.
fruit·y ['fruːtɪ] adj (Geruch, Geschmack) frucht-, obstartig; Obst-, Frucht-.
frus·e·mide ['fruːsɪmaɪd] n → furosemide.
frus·tra·tion tolerance [frʌ'streɪʃn] Frustrationstoleranz f.
FSF abbr. → fibrin stabilizing factor.
FSH abbr. → follicle stimulating hormone.
FSH-RF abbr. → follicle stimulating hormone releasing factor.
FSH-RH abbr. [follicle stimulating hormone releasing hormone] → follicle stimulating hormone releasing factor.
FSP abbr. → fibrinolytic split products.
ft abbr. → foot 4.
FTA abbr. → fluorescent treponemal antibody.
FTA-Abs abbr. → fluorescent treponemal antibody absorption test.
FTA-Abs test → fluorescent treponemal antibody absorption test.
5-FU abbr. → 5-fluorouracil.
Fuchs [f(j)uːks; fʊks]: **F.' adenoma** ophthal. Fuchs-Adenom nt.
F.'s coloboma ophthal. Fuchs'-Kolobom nt.
crypts of F. Iriskrypten pl.
F.' dystrophy → F.' epithelial dystrophy.
F.' epithelial dystrophy ophthal. Fuchs'-Hornhautdystrophie f, Dystrophia epithelialis corneae.
F.'s syndrome ophthal. Fuchs-Syndrom nt, -Heterochromie f.
fuch·sin ['f(j)uːksɪn] n Fuchsin nt.
fuchsin agar Endo-Fuchsinagar m/nt.
fuchsin bodies Russell'-Körperchen pl.
fuch·sin·o·phil [f(j)uː'ksɪnəfɪl] histol. I n fuchsinophile Zelle od. Struktur f. II adj fuchsinophil.
fuch·sin·o·phil·ia [ˌf(j)uːksɪnə'fɪlɪə] n histol. Fuchsinophilie f.
fuch·sin·o·phil·ic [ˌ-'fɪlɪk] adj → fuchsinophil II.
fuch·si·noph·i·lous [ˌfjuːksə'nɑfɪləs] adj → fuchsinophil II.
fuchsin stain histol. Fuchsinfärbung f.
fu·cose ['fjuːkəʊs] n Fucose f.
α-L-fu·co·si·dase [fjuː'kaʊsɪdeɪz] n α-L-Fucosidase f.
fu·co·si·do·sis [ˌfjuːkəsɑˈdəʊsɪs] n Fucosidose(-Syndrom nt) f.
FUDR abbr. → 5-fluorodeoxyuridine.
FUdr abbr. → 5-fluorodeoxyuridine.
fu·el ['fjʊəl] n (a. physiol.) Brennstoff m; Heiz-, Brennmaterial nt, Treibstoff m; (a. fig.) Nahrung f.
fuel molecule Brennstoffmolekül nt.
fuel value physiol. Brennwert m.
fu·gac·i·ty [fjuː'gæsətɪ] n chem. Flüchtigkeit f, Fugazität f.
fu·gi·tive ['fjuːdʒɪtɪv] adj flüchtig, vergänglich, kurzlebig, vorübergehend; unbeständig, unecht.
fugitive wart/verruca derm. Flachwarze f, Verruca plana (juvenilis).
fu·gu·ism ['fjuːgəwɪzəm] n → fuguism.
fu·gu·is·mus [fjuːgə'wɪzməs] n Tetrodotoxinvergiftung f, Tetrodotoxismus m.
fu·gu toxin ['fjuːgəʊ] → fugutoxin.
fu·gu·tox·in [fjuːgə'tɑksɪn] n Tetrodotoxin nt abbr. TTX.
ful·crum ['fʊlkrəm, 'fʌl-] n, pl **-crums, -cra** [-krə] phys. Dreh-, Hebel-, Gelenk-, Stützpunkt m.
ful·gu·rant ['fʌlgjərənt] adj (auf-)blitzend, blitzartig.
fulgurant pain schießender Schmerz m.
ful·gu·rate ['fʌlgjəreɪt] vt 1. (auf-)blitzen. 2. durch Blitzeinschlag od. Funkenschlag zerstören.
ful·gu·ra·tion [ˌfʌlgjə'reɪʃn] n 1. patho. Blitzeinschlag m, -einwirkung f, Fulguration f. 2. chir. Elektrodesikkation f, Fulguration f.
fu·lig·i·nous [fjuː'lɪdʒənəs] adj rußig, (ruß-)schwarz, Ruß-.
full [fʊl] I n (das) Ganze. **in ~** vollständig, ganz. II adj 1. voll, angefüllt mit. 2. voll, ganz. 3. vollständig, ausführlich, genau. 4. (Gesicht) voll, rund; (Figur) vollschlank; (Stimme) voll, kräftig.
full bath Vollbad nt.
full blood count abbr. **FBC** großes Blutbild nt.
full diet Voll-, Normalkost f.
full·ness ['fʊlnɪs] n 1. Fülle f, Überfülle f. 2. Körperfülle f. 3. Völle(gefühl nt) f.
full pack Ganzpackung f.
full recovery vollständige/komplette Wiederherstellung od. Heilung od. Erholung f; chir. Restitutio ad integrum.
full-term adj gyn. (Geburt) termingerecht.
full-thickness burn Verbrennung f dritten Grades.
full thickness flap chir. Vollhautlappen m, Vollhauttransplantat nt.
full-thickness graft → full thickness flap.
ful·ly developed ['fʊlɪ] ausgebildet, ausgewachsen.
ful·mi·nant ['fʌlmɪnənt] adj plötzlich od. schlagartig (auftretend), fulminant, foudroyant; perakut.
fulminant hepatitis fulminante Hepatitis f, akute virusbedingte Lebernekrose f.
fulminant hyperpyrexia maligne Hyperthermie/Hyperpyrexie f.
ful·mi·nate ['fʌlmɪneɪt] vi plötzlich auftreten od. ausbrechen.
ful·mi·nat·ing anoxia ['fʌlmɪneɪtɪŋ] fulminante Anoxie f.
fulminating apoplexy fulminante Apoplexie f.
fulminating appendicitis fulminante/perakute Appendizitis f.
fulminating hypoxia fulminante Hypoxie f.
fu·ma·rase ['fjuːməreɪz] n → fumarate hydratase.
fu·ma·rate ['fjuːməreɪt] n Fumarat nt.
fumarate hydratase Fumarase f, Fumarathydratase f.
fumarate pathway biochem. Fumaratweg m.
fu·mar·ic acid [fjuː'mærɪk] Fumarsäure f.
fu·mar·o·yl·a·ce·to·ac·e·tate hydrolase [fjuːˌmærəwɪləˌsiːtəʊ'æsɪteɪt] → fumarylacetoacetase.
fu·ma·ryl·ac·e·to·ac·e·tase [ˌfjuːməriːləˌsiːtəʊ'æsɪteɪz] n Fumarylacetoacetase f.
4-fu·ma·ryl·ac·e·to·ac·e·tate [ˌ-əˌsiːtəʊ'æsɪteɪt] n 4-Fumarylacetoacetat nt, 4-Fumarylacetoazetat nt.
4-fu·ma·ryl·ac·e·to·ac·e·tic acid [ˌ-əˌsiːtəə'setɪk] 4-Fumarylacetessigsäure f, 4-Fumarylacetoessigsäure f.
fume [fjuːm] I n Dampf m, Dunst m, Rauch m, Nebel m. II vt 1. (Dämpfe) von s. geben, ausstoßen. 2. räuchern, beizen. (aus-)räuchern. III vi rauchen, dampfen.
fu·mi·gant ['fjuːmɪgənt] n Ausräucherungsmittel nt.
fu·mi·gate ['fjuːmɪgeɪt] vt ausräuchern.
fu·mi·ga·tion [fjuːmɪ'geɪʃn] n (Aus-)Räucherung f, Fumigation f.
func·tio ['fʌŋkʃɪəʊ] n → function 1.
func·tion ['fʌŋkʃn] I n 1. physiol. Funktion f, Tätigkeit f, Wirksamkeit f. 2. (Person) Pflicht f, Aufgabe f, Amt n. 3. mathe. Funktion f. 4. (Werkzeug) Funktion f, Zweck m. II vi fungieren od. tätig sein (as als); dienen (as als); physiol. funktionieren, arbeiten.
func·tion·al ['fʌŋkʃnəl] adj (a. mathe.) funktionell, Funktions-; physiol. funktionsfähig. **to be ~** funktionieren, arbeiten.
functional albuminuria funktionelle/physiologische/intermittierende Proteinurie/Albuminurie f.
functional amblyopia ophthal. funktionelle Amblyopie f.
functional analysis Funktionsanalyse f.
functional anatomy funktionelle Anatomie f.
functional anemia funktionelle Anämie f.
functional anosmia funktionelle Anosmie f.

functional aphasia

functional aphasia funktionelle Aphasie f.
functional asplenia/asplenism funktionelle Asplenie f.
functional blindness psychogene Blindheit f.
functional cardiovascular disease neurozirkulatorische Asthenie f, Effort-Syndrom nt, DaCosta-Syndrom nt, Soldatenherz nt, Phrenikokardie f.
functional circuit physiol. Funktionskreis nt.
functional congestion funktionelle Hyperämie f.
functional control Funktionskontrolle f.
functional deafness psychogene Schwerhörigkeit/Taubheit f.
functional disease funktionelle Erkrankung/Krankheit/Störung f, Funktionsstörung f.
functional disorder → functional disease.
functional diverticulum radiol. funktionelles Divertikel nt.
functional dysmenorrhea gyn. funktionelle Dysmenorrhö f.
functional dyspepsia funktionelle Dyspepsie f.
functional dyspnea funktionelle Dyspnoe f.
funtional group chem. funktionelle Gruppe f.
functional headache funktioneller/psychogener Kopfschmerz m.
functional histology funktionelle Histologie f.
functional hypertrophy funktionelle Hypertrophie f.
functional impairment Funktionsbeeinträchtigung f, -einschränkung f.
func·ti·o·na·lis [,fʌŋkʃɪəʊˈneɪlɪs] n Funktionalis f, Lamina/Pars functionalis, Stratum functionale endometrii.
functional layer of endometrium → functionalis.
functional limit physiol. Lähmungszeit f.
functional loop physiol. Funktionsschleife f.
functional metabolism physiol. Funktions-, Betriebsstoffwechsel m.
functional murmur card. funktionelles Herzgeräusch nt.
functional mydriasis ophthal. funktionelle Mydriasis f.
functional obstruction funktionelle Obstruktion f.
functional paralysis funktionelle Lähmung f.
functional pathology funktionelle Pathologie f.
functional proteinuria funktionelle/physiologische/intermittierende Proteinurie/Albuminurie f.
functional psychology Funktionspsychologie f.
functional reserve funktionelle Reserve f.
functional residual capacity abbr. FRC funktionelle Residualkapazität f abbr. FRK.
functional spasm funktioneller Krampf m.
functional stricture funktionelle/spastische Striktur f.
functional syncytium funktionelles Synzytium nt.
functional treatment funktionelle Behandlung f.
fun·dal [ˈfʌndl] adj Fundus betr., Fundus-, Fundo-.
fundal placenta Placenta fundalis.
fun·da·ment [ˈfʌndəmənt] n 1. Fundament nt, Grundlage f. 2. Gesäß nt. 3. Anus m, After m.
fun·da·men·tal [,fʌndəˈmentl] I n 1. Fundament nt, Grundlage f. 2. phys. Basis-, Fundamentaleinheit f. II adj fundamental, grundlegend, wesentlich (to für); grundsätzlich, elementar, Grund(lagen)-, Fundamental-.
fundamental bundles of spinal cord Binnen-, Elementar-, Grundbündel pl des Rückenmarks, Intersegmentalfaszikel pl, Fasciculi proprii (medullae spinalis).
fundamental columns Grundbündel pl, Fasciculi proprii.
fundamental frequency phys., physiol. Grundfrequenz f.
fundamental law mathe., phys. Hauptsatz m.
fundamental particle phys. Elementarteilchen nt.
fundamental research Grundlagenforschung f.
fun·dec·to·my [fʌnˈdektəmɪ] n → fundusectomy.
fun·dic [ˈfʌndɪk] adj → fundal.
fundic glands → fundus glands.
fun·di·form [ˈfʌndəfɔːrm] adj schleifen-, schlingenförmig, -artig.
fundiform ligament of penis Lig. fundiforme penis.
fun·do·pex·y [ˈfʌndəpeksɪ] n chir. Fundopexie f.
fun·do·pli·ca·tion [,-plɪˈkeɪʃn] n chir. Fundoplikation f nach Nissen, Fundoplicatio f.
fun·dus [ˈfʌndəs] n, pl -di [-daɪ] 1. anat. (Hinter-)Grund m, Boden m, Bodenteil nt, Fundus m. 2. → f. of eye. 3. → f. of stomach.
f. of bladder → f. of urinary bladder.
f. of eye Augenhintergrund, Fundus m, Fundus oculi.
f. of gallbladder Gallenblasenkuppel f, Fundus vesicae felleae/biliaris.
f. of internal acoustic meatus Boden des inneren Gehörganges, Fundus meatus acustici interni.
f. of stomach Magenfundus, Fundus gastricus/ventricularis.
f. of urinary bladder 1. (Harn-)Blasengrund, Fundus vesicae (urinariae). 2. (Harn-)Blasenspitze f, Apex vesicae/vesicalis (urinariae).
f. of uterus Gebärmutter-, Uterusfundus/-kuppe f, Fundus uteri.
f. of vagina Scheidengewölbe, Fornix vaginae.
fun·du·scope [ˈfʌndəskəʊp] n ophthal. Augenspiegel m, Funduskop nt, Ophthalmoskop nt.
fun·dus·co·py [fʌnˈdʌskəpɪ] n Augenspiegeln nt, Augenspiegelung f, Funduskopie f, Ophthalmoskopie f.
fundus-corpus region (Magen) Fundus-Corpus-Region f.
fun·do·sec·to·my [,fʌndəˈsektəmɪ] n chir. Fundusresektion f, Fundektomie f.
fundus glands Corpus- u. Fundusdrüsen pl, Gll. gastricae propriae.
fundus reflex Fundusreflex m.
fun·gal [ˈfʌŋgəl] adj Pilz/Fungus betr., fungal, Pilz-, Fungus-.
fungal arthritis Gelenkfungus m, Arthritis fungosa.
fungal endocarditis Pilzendokarditis f, Endocarditis mycotica.
fungal filament Pilzfaden m, Hyphe f.
fungal infection Pilzerkrankung f, -infektion f, Mykose f, Mycosis f.
fungal meningitis Pilzmeningitis f.
fungal pneumonia Pilzpneumonie f.
fun·gate [ˈfʌŋgeɪt] vi pilzartig od. schwammartig wachsen.
fun·ge·mia [fʌŋˈgiːmɪə] n patho. Pilzsepsis f, Fungämie f, Mykämie f.

Fun·gi [ˈfʌndʒaɪ, ˈfʌŋgaɪ] pl micro. Pilze pl, Fungi pl, Myzeten pl, Mycetes pl, Mycophyta pl, Mycota pl.
fun·gi pl of fungus.
fun·gi·cid·al [,fʌndʒəˈsaɪdl, ,fʌŋgə-] adj pilz(ab)tötend, fungizid.
fun·gi·cide [ˈ-saɪd] n pharm. fungizides Mittel nt, Fungizid nt.
fun·gi·ci·din [,-ˈsaɪdɪn] n pharm. Nystatin nt.
fun·gi·form [ˈ-fɔːrm] adj pilz-, schwammförmig, pilziform.
fungiform papillae pilzförmige Papillen pl, Papillae fungiformes.
fun·gi·sta·sis [,-ˈsteɪsɪs] n Fungistase f.
fun·gi·stat [ˈ-stæt] n pharm. fungistatisches Mittel nt, Fungistatikum nt.
fun·gi·stat·ic [,-ˈstætɪk] adj das Pilzwachstum hemmend, fungistatisch.
fun·gi·tox·ic [ˈ-ˈtɒksɪk] adj pilz-, fungitoxisch.
fun·gi·tox·ic·i·ty [,-tɒkˈsɪsətɪ] n Toxizität f für Pilze/Fungi.
fun·goid [ˈfʌŋgɔɪd] adj pilz-, schwammartig, fungoid, fungös.
fun·gos·i·ty [fʌŋˈgɒsətɪ] n pilzartiges/fungoides Wachstum nt, Fungosität f.
fun·gous [ˈfʌŋgəs] adj 1. → fungoid. 2. → fungal.
fungous foot Madurafuß m.
fungous gonitis primär synoviale Gonitis f.
fungous synovitis → fungal arthritis.
fun·gus [ˈfʌŋgəs] n, pl fun·gi [ˈfʌndʒaɪ, ˈfʌŋgaɪ] 1. → Fungi. 2. bio. Pilz m, Schwamm m. 3. patho. pilzartige/schwammartige Geschwulst f, schwammartiges Gebilde nt.
fungus ball Aspergillom nt.
fu·nic [ˈfjuːnɪk] adj 1. → funicular. 2. Nabelschnur betr., Nabelschnur-.
fu·ni·cle [ˈfjuːnɪkl] n → funicular.
fu·nic·u·lar [fjuːˈnɪkjələr, fə-] adj anat. band-, strangartig, funikulär, Band-, Strang-.
funicular artery Hodenarterie f, Testikularis f, A. testicularis.
funicular hydrocele Hydrocele funicularis.
funicular myelitis Dana-Lichtheim-Krankheit f, Lichtheim-Syndrom nt, Dana-Syndrom nt, Dana-Lichtheim-Putman-Syndrom nt, funikuläre Myelose f.
funicular myelopathy funikuläre Myelopathie f.
funicular myelosis → funicular myelitis.
fu·nic·u·li·tis [fjuːˌnɪkjəˈlaɪtɪs] n 1. Funiculusentzündung f, Funikulitis f, Funiculitis f. 2. urol. Samenstrangentzündung f, Funikulitis f, Funiculitis f. 3. neuro. Entzündung f der Spinalnervenwurzel, Funikulitis f, Funiculitis vertebralis.
fu·nic·u·lo·ep·i·did·y·mi·tis [fjuːˌnɪkjəlɒʊˌepɪˌdɪdəˈmaɪtɪs] n urol. Entzündung f von Samenstrang u. Epididymis, Funikuloepididymitis f.
fu·nic·u·lo·pex·y [ˈ-peksɪ] n urol. Funikulopexie f.
fu·nic·u·lus [fjuːˈnɪkjələs, fə-] n, pl -li [-laɪ] anat. kleiner (Gewebe-)Strang m, strangartiges Gebilde nt, Funiculus m.
f.li of spinal cord Markstänge pl des Rückenmarks, Funiculi medullae spinalis.
fu·ni·form [ˈfjuːnəfɔːrm] adj band-, seilartig.
fu·nis [ˈfjuːnɪs] n 1. anat. bandartige/seilartige Struktur f. 2. Nabelschnur f, Funiculus umbilicalis.
funis presentation gyn. Nabelschnurvorfall m.

fun·nel ['fʌnl] *n* Trichter *m*.
funnel breast Trichterbrust *f*, Pectus excavatum/infundibulum/recurvatum.
funnel chest → funnel breast.
funnel-shaped pelvis Trichterbecken *nt*.
fu·ran ['fjʊərǣn] *n* Furan *nt*, Furfuran *nt*.
fu·rane ['fjʊəreɪn] *n* → furan.
fu·ra·nose ['fjʊərənəʊs] *n* Furanose *f*.
furanose form *chem*. Furanoseform *f*.
furanose ring *chem*. Furanosering *m*.
furan ring *chem*. Furanring *m*.
fur·cal ['fɜrkl] *adj* gabelförmig; gegabelt, gespalten.
fur·cate [*adj* 'fɜrkeɪt, -kɪt; *v* 'fɜrkeɪt] **I** *adj* → furcal. **II** *vi* s. gabeln *od*. teilen.
furcate placenta gelappte Plazenta *f*, Lappenplazenta *f*, Placenta lobata.
fur·ca·tion [fɜr'keɪʃn] *n anat*. Gabelung *f*.
fur·fur ['fɜrfər] *n*, *pl* **fur·fur·es** ['fɜrfjə‚riːz] Hautschuppe *f*.
fur·fu·ra·ceous [‚fɜrf(j)ə'reɪʃəs] *adj* kleieförmig (schuppend).
fur·fu·ral ['fɜrf(j)ərǣl] *n* → furfurol.
fur·fur·an ['fɜrf(j)ərǣn] *n* → furan.
fur·fu·rol ['fɜrf(j)ərɒl] *n* Furfural *nt*, Furfurol *nt*.
fu·ri·bund ['fjʊərəbənd] *adj* wütend, rasend, tobsüchtig.
fu·ri·ous ['fjʊərəs] *adj* erregt, wütend, zornig, rasend.
fur·nace·men's cataract ['fɜrnɪsmen] Feuer-, Glasbläserstar *m*, Infrarotkatarakt *f*, Cataracta calorica.
fu·ro·cou·ma·rin [‚fjʊərəʊ'kumərɪn] *n pharm*. Fur(an)ocumarin *nt*.
fu·ror ['fjʊərɔːr, -rər] *n* 1. Wut *f*, Raserei *f*, Tobsucht *f*, Furor *m*. 2. Ekstase *f*, Begeisterungstaumel *m*.
fur·o·sem·ide [‚fjʊərəʊ'semɪd, -maɪd] *n pharm*. Furosemid *nt*.
fur·row ['fɜrəʊ, 'fʌr-] **I** *n* 1. (schmale) Rinne *od*. Furche *f*; *techn*. Rille *f*. 2. *anat*. Runzel *f*, Furche *f*; *bio*. Falz *m*. **II** *vt* (durch-)furchen; (*Gesicht*) runzeln. **III** *vi* s. furchen.
fur·rowed ['fɜrəʊd, 'fʌr-] *adj* ge-, zer-, durchfurcht, runz(e)lig, furchig.
furrowed tongue Faltenzunge *f*, Lingua plicata/scrotalis.
furrow keratitis Keratitis dendrica, Herpes-simplex-Keratitis *f*.
fur·row·y ['fɜrəwɪ, 'fʌr-] *adj* → furrowed.
fu·run·cle ['fjʊərʌŋkl] *n* Eiterbeule *f*, Furunkel *m/nt*, Furunculus *m*.
fu·run·cu·lar [fjʊə'rʌŋkjələr] *adj* Furunkel betr., furunkulös, Furunkel-.
furuncular otitis *HNO* Ohr-, Gehörgangsfurunkel *m*, Otitis externa furunculosa/circumscripta.
fu·run·cu·loid [fjʊə'rʌŋkjələɪd] *adj* furunkelähnlich, -artig.
fu·run·cu·lo·sis [fjʊə‚rʌŋkjə'ləʊsɪs] *n* Furunkulose *f*, Furunculosis *f*.
fu·run·cu·lus [fjʊə'rʌŋkjələs] *n*, *pl* **-li** [-laɪ] → furuncle.
fu·sar·i·o·tox·i·co·sis [fjuː‚zeərɪəʊtɑksɪ'kəʊsɪs] *n* Fusarium-Mykotoxikose *f*.
Fu·sar·i·um [fjuː'zeərɪəm] *n micro*. Fusarium *nt*.
fus·cin ['fjuːsɪn] *n* Fuszin *nt*, Fuscin *nt*.
fuse [fjuːz] **I** *n phys*., *techn*. (Schmelz-)Sicherung *f*. **II** *vt* 1. *phys*., *techn*. schmelzen. 2. *fig*. verschmelzen, vereinigen. **III** *vi* 3. *Brit. electr*. durchbrennen. 4. *techn*. schmelzen. 5. *fig*. s. vereinigen, s. verbinden, verschmelzen.
fused kidney [fjuːzd] Verschmelzungsniere *f*.
fused vertebrae *ortho*. Blockwirbel(bildung *f*) *pl*.
fu·sel oil ['fjuːzl] *chem*. Fuselöl *nt*.
fu·si·bil·i·ty [‚fjuːzə'bɪlətɪ] *n phys*. Schmelzbarkeit *f*.
fu·si·ble ['fjuːzɪbl] *adj* schmelzbar, Schmelz-.
fu·si·cel·lu·lar [‚fjuːzɪ'seljələr] *adj* → fusocellular.
fu·si·date ['-deɪt] *n* Fusidinat *nt*.
fu·sid·ic acid [fjuː'sɪdɪk] *pharm*. Fusidinsäure *f*.
fu·si·form ['fjuːzəfɔːrm] *adj* spindelförmig; *anat*. fusiform.
fusiform aneurysm fusiformes Aneurysma *nt*, Aneurysma fusiforme.
fusiform bacillus → fusobacterium.
fusiform bronchiectasis spindelförmige/fusiforme Bronchiektas(i)e *f*.
fusiform cataract *ophthal*. Spindelstar *m*, Cataracta fusiformis.
fusiform cell spindelförmige Zelle *f*.
fusiform-cell layer Spindelzellschicht *f*, Lamina multiformis.
fusiform gyrus Gyrus fusiformis.
fusiform layer of cerebral cortex multiforme Schicht *f*, Lamina multiformis corticis cerebri.
fusiform muscle spindelförmiger Muskel *m*, M. fusiformis.
fu·si·mo·tor [‚fjuːzɪ'məʊtər] *adj* fusimotorisch, Fusimoto(r)-.
fu·sion ['fjuːʒn] *n* 1. *phys*., *techn*. Schmelzen *nt*, Verschmelzen *nt*. 2. *bio*. (Zell-, Chromosomen-)Verschmelzung *f*, Fusion *f*. 3. *ophthal*., *physiol*. Fusion *f*. 4. *phys*. (Kern-)Fusion *f*. 5. *fig*. Verschmelzung *f*, Vereinigung *f*.
fu·sion·al ['fjuːʒnəl] *adj* Fusions-.
fusion beat *card*. Kombinationssystole *f*.
fusion bomb Wasserstoffbombe *f*.
fusion electrolysis *electr*. Schmelzflußelektrolyse *f*.
fusion frequency *physiol*. Fusionsfrequenz *f*.
fusion nucleus *bio*., *phys*. Verschmelzungskern *m*.
fusion point *phys*. Schmelzpunkt *m*.
fusion protein Fusionsprotein *nt*, F-Protein *nt*.
fusion reactor Fusionsreaktor *m*.
Fu·so·bac·te·ri·um [‚fjuːzəʊbæk'tɪərɪəm] *micro*. Fusobacterium *nt*.
fu·so·bac·te·ri·um [‚fjuːzəʊbæk'tɪərɪəm] *n*, *pl* **-ria** [-rɪə] *micro*. Fusobakterium *nt*.
fu·so·cel·lu·lar [‚-'seljələr] *adj* spindelzellig.
fu·so·spi·ril·lar·y [‚-'spaɪrə‚lerɪ] *adj* fusospirillär.
fusospirillary gingivitis Plaut-Vincent-Angina *f*, Vincent-Angina *f*, Fusospirillose *f*, Fusospirochätose *f*, Angina ulcerosa/ulceromembranacea.
fusospirillary stomatitis → fusospirillary gingivitis.
fu·so·spi·ril·lo·sis [‚-‚spaɪrɪ'ləʊsɪs] *n* → fusospirillary gingivitis.
fu·so·spi·ro·che·tal disease [‚-‚spaɪrəʊ'kiːtl] → fusospirochetosis.
fusospirochetal gingivitis/stomatitis → fusospirillary gingivitis.
fu·so·spi·ro·che·to·sis [‚-‚spaɪrəkɪ'təʊsɪs] *n* Fusospirochätose *f*, Fusoborreliose *f*.
fus·ti·ga·tion [‚fʌstə'geɪʃn] *n psychia*. Geißelung *f*, Fustigation *f*.
fu·tile ['fjuːtaɪl, -tl] *adj* 1. sinn-, zwecklos, nutzlos, wirkungslos, futil. 2. unbedeutend, nichtig, futil.
futile cycle *biochem*. sinnloser/futiler Zyklus *m*.
fuzz·y ['fʌzɪ] *adj* 1. *histol*. faserig, fusselig. 2. flockig, flaumig. 3. unscharf, verschwommen.
FW sleep → fast wave sleep.

G

G *abbr.* 1. → gauss. 2. → giga-. 3. → (D-)glucose. 4. → gravitational constant. 5. → guanine. 6. → guanosine.
g *abbr.* 1. → gram. 2. → gravity.
Γ *abbr.* → gamma.
γ *abbr.* → gamma.
GA *abbr.* → glutaric aciduria.
Ga *abbr.* → gallium.
GA II B *abbr.* → glutaric aciduria II B.
GABA *abbr.* → gamma-aminobutyric acid.
GABA·er·gic [gæbə'ɜːrdʒɪk] *adj* GABAerg.
GABAergic synapse GABAerge Synapse *f.*
G-actin *n* globuläres Aktin *nt*, G-Aktin *nt.*
gad·fly ['gædflaɪ] *n micro.* Pferdebremse *f*, Tabanus *m.*
gad·get ['gædʒɪt] *n* Apparat *m*, Gerät *nt*, Vorrichtung *f.*
gad·o·lin·i·um [gædə'lɪnɪəm] *n abbr.* **Gd** Gadolinium *nt*, -Atom *nt* abbr. Gd.
Gaenslen ['genzlən]: **G.'s sign/test** *ortho.* Gaenslen-Zeichen *nt*, -Handgriff *m.*
Gaffky ['gæfkɪ]: **G.'s scale** Gaffky-Skala *f.*
GAG *abbr.* → glycosaminoglycan.
gag [gæg] **I** *n* 1. Knebel *m.* 2. *chir., HNO* Mundsperrer *m*, -spreizer *m.* **II** *vt* 3. zum Würgen reizen. 4. den Mund zuhalten, knebeln. 5. *chir., HNO* jdm. den Mund mit einem Sperrer offenhalten. 6. verstopfen. **III** *vi* würgen.
gage [geɪdʒ] *n*, *vt* → gauge.
gag·ging ['gægɪŋ] *n* Würgen *nt.*
gag reflex Würg(e)reflex *m.*
gain [geɪn] **I** *n* 1. Gewinn *m*, Vorteil *m*, Nutzen *m (to für).* 2. Zunahme *f*, Steigerung *f.* 3. *phys.* Verstärkung *f.* **II** *vt* 4. *(Lebensunterhalt)* verdienen. 5. gewinnen. 6. erreichen; erlangen, erhalten, erringen. **III** *vi* 7. näherkommen, aufholen (gegenüber). 8. besser *od.* kräftiger werden; zunehmen *(in* an). 9. übergreifen *(on, upon* auf); s. ausbreiten *(on, upon* über).
Gaisböck ['gaɪsbek, -bœk]: **G.'s disease/syndrome** Gaisböck-Syndrom *nt*, Polycythaemia (rubra) hypertonica.
gait [geɪt] *n* Gang *m*, Gangart *f.*
gait ataxia Gangataxie *f*, lokomotorische Ataxie *f.*
gait pattern Gangbild *nt*, -muster *nt.*
galact- *pref.* → galacto-.
ga·lac·ta·cra·sia [gəˌlæktə'kreɪsɪə] *n gyn.* unphysiologische Zusammensetzung *f* der Muttermilch.
ga·lac·ta·gog·in [ˌ-'gɑgɪn] *n* humanes Plazenta-Laktogen *nt abbr.* HPL, Chorionsomatotropin *nt.*
ga·lac·ta·gogue [-'gɑg, -gɔg] **I** *n pharm.* Galaktagogum *nt*, Laktagogum *nt.* **II** *adj pharm., gyn.* den Milchfluß fördernd.
ga·lac·tan [gə'læktən] *n* Galaktan *nt.*
gal·ac·te·mia [ˌgælæk'tiːmɪə] *n* Galaktämie *f.*
ga·lac·tic [gə'læktɪk] **I** *n* → galactagogue I. **II** *adj* 1. Milch betr., Milch-, Galakt-, Lakt(o)-. 2. → galactagogue II.

ga·lac·ti·dro·sis [gəˌlæktɪ'drəʊsɪs] *n patho.* Milchschwitzen *nt*, Galakthidrose *f.*
ga·lac·tin [gə'læktɪn] *n old* → galactopoietic hormone.
gal·ac·tis·chia [ˌgælæk'tɪskɪə] *n gyn.* Unterdrückung *f* der Milchsekretion.
ga·lac·ti·tol [gə'læktɪtɑl] *n* Galaktit *nt*, Dulcit *nt.*
galacto- *pref.* Milch-, Milchzucker-, Galakt(o)-, Lakt(o)-.
ga·lac·to·blast [gə'læktəblæst] *n* Kolostrumkörperchen *nt*, Donné-Körperchen *nt.*
ga·lac·to·bol·ic [ˌ-'bɑlɪk] *adj* die Milchsekretion fördernd, galaktobol.
ga·lac·to·cele [-'siːl] *n* 1. Milchzyste *f*, Galaktozele *f.* 2. Hydrozele *f* mit milchigem Inhalt, Galaktozele *f.*
ga·lac·to·cer·e·bro·side [ˌ-'serəbrəʊsaɪd] *n* Galaktocerebrosid *nt.*
galactocerebroside β-galactosidase → galactosylceramidase.
ga·lac·to·gen [gə'læktədʒən] *n* Galaktogen *nt.*
gal·ac·tog·e·nous [gælæk'tɑdʒənəs] *adj* die Milchbildung fördernd, milchbildend, galaktogen.
ga·lac·to·gogue [gə'læktəgɑg, -gɔg] *n, adj* → galactagogue.
gal·ac·tog·ra·phy [gælæk'tɑgrəfɪ] *n radiol., gyn.* Galaktographie *f.*
ga·lac·to·ki·nase [gə'læktə'kaɪneɪz, -'kɪ-] *n* Galakto-, Galactokinase *f.*
galactokinase deficiency Galaktokinasemangel *m.*
ga·lac·to·lip·id [ˌ-'lɪpɪd, -'laɪp-] *n* Galaktolipid *nt.*
ga·lac·to·lip·in [ˌ-'lɪpɪn] *n* → galactolipid.
ga·lac·to·lip·ine [ˌ-'lɪpɪn] *n* → galactolipid.
gal·ac·to·ma [ˌgælæk'təʊmə] *n* → galactocele.
gal·ac·tom·e·ter [ˌgælæk'tɑmɪtər] *n lab., gyn.* Milchspindel *f*, Galakto-, Laktometer *nt*, Laktodensimeter *nt.*
ga·lac·to·pex·ic [gə'læktə'peksɪk] *adj biochem.* Galaktose bindend *od.* fixierend.
ga·lac·to·pex·y ['-peksɪ] *n biochem.* Galaktosebindung *f*, -fixierung *f.*
gal·ac·toph·a·gous [ˌgælæk'tɑfəgəs] *adj* von Milch lebend, galaktophag.
ga·lac·to·phle·bi·tis [gəˌlæktəflɪ'baɪtɪs] *n* Phlegmasia alba dolens.
ga·lac·to·phore ['-fəʊər] **I** *n* Milchgang *m*, Ductus lactiferus. **II** *adj* → galactophorous.
ga·lac·to·pho·ri·tis [ˌ-fə'raɪtɪs] *n gyn.* Milchgangentzündung *f*, Galaktophoritis *f.*
gal·ac·toph·o·rous [gælæk'tɑfərəs] *adj anat.* milchführend.
galactophorous canals → galactophorous ducts.
galactophorous ducts Milchgänge *pl*, Ductus lactiferi.

galactophorous tubules → galactophorous ducts.
ga·lac·to·poi·e·sis [gəˌlæktəpɔɪ'iːsɪs] *n* Milchbildung *f*, Galaktopoese *f.*
ga·lac·to·poi·et·ic [ˌ-pɔɪ'etɪk] **I** *n* galaktopoetische Substanz *f.* **II** *adj* Milchbildung betr. *od.* anregend, galaktopoetisch.
galactopoietic factor → galactopoietic hormone.
galactopoietic hormone Prolaktin *nt abbr.* PRL, Prolactin *nt*, laktogenes Hormon *nt.*
ga·lac·to·py·ra [ˌ-'paɪrə] *n gyn.* Milchfieber *nt*, Laktationsfieber *nt*, Galaktopyra *f.*
ga·lac·to·py·ra·nose [ˌ-'paɪrənəʊz] *n* Galaktopyranose *f.*
ga·lac·tor·rhea [ˌ-'rɪə] *n gyn.* Milchfluß *m*, Galaktorrhö *f*, Galaktorrhoe *f.*
galactorrhea-amenorrhea syndrome Galaktorrhö-Amenorrhö-Syndrom *nt*, Amenorrhö-Galaktorrhö-Syndrom *nt.*
ga·lac·tos·a·mine [gəˌlæk'təʊsəmiːn, -təʊs'æmɪn] *n* Galaktosamin *nt*, Chondrosamin *nt.*
galactosamine-6-sulfate sulfatase N-Acetylgalaktosamin-6-Sulfatsulfatase *f*, Chondroitinsulfatsulfatase *f.*
ga·lac·to·san [gə'læktəsæn, -sən] *n* Galaktosan *nt.*
gal·ac·tos·che·sis [ˌgælæk'tɑskəsɪs] *n* → galactischia.
ga·lac·to·scope [gə'læktəskəʊp] *n lab., gyn.* Galaktoskop *nt*, Laktoskop *nt.*
ga·lac·tose [gə'læktəʊs] *n* Galaktose *f*, Galactose.
galactose cataract Katarakt *f* bei Galaktosämie.
galactose diabetes 1. → galactosemia. 2. Galaktosediabetes *m*, Galaktokinasemangel *m.*
galactose elimination test Galaktosetoleranztest *m*, Bauer-Probe *f.*
galactose epimerase → galactowaldenase.
galactose epimerase deficiency Galaktowaldenase-Mangel *m*, benigne Galaktosämie *f.*
ga·lac·tos·e·mia [gəˌlæktə'siːmɪə] *n* (hereditäre/kongenitale) Galaktosämie *f*, Galaktoseintoleranz *f*, -unverträglichkeit *f.*
ga·lac·tos·e·mic cataract [ˌ-'iːmɪk] → galactose cataract.
galactose-1-phosphate *n* Galaktose-1-phosphat *nt.*
galactose-1-phosphate uridyltransferase UDPglukose-hexose-1-phosphaturidyltransferase *f*, UDPglukose-galaktose-1-phosphaturidyltransferase *f*, Galaktose-1-phosphaturidyltransferase *f.*
galactose tolerance test Galaktosetoleranztest *m*, Bauer-Probe *f.*
α-D-ga·lac·to·sid·ase [gəˌlæktə'saɪdeɪz] *n* α-D-Galaktosidase *f.*
α-D-galactosidase A α-D-Glaktosidase A *f*, Ceramidtrihexosidase *f.*

α-(D)-galactosidase A deficiency Fabry-
-Syndrom *nt*, Morbus Fabry *m*, hereditäre Thesaurismose *f* Ruiter-Pompen-
-Weyers, Ruiter-Pompen-Weyers-Syndrom *nt*, Thesaurismosis hereditaria lipoidica, Angiokeratoma corporis diffusum (Fabry), Angiokeratoma universale.
α-D-galactosidase B α-D-Galaktosidase
B *f*, α-*N*-Acetylgalaktosaminidase *f*.
β-galactosidase *n* β-Galaktosidase *f*,
Laktase *f*.
β-galactosidase deficiency Morquio-
-Syndrom Typ B *nt*.
ga·lac·to·side [gə'læktəsaɪd, -sɪd] *n* Galak-
tosid *nt*, Galactosid *nt*.
galactoside permease Galaktosidper-
mease *f*.
gal·ac·to·sis [ˌgælæk'təʊsɪs] *n, pl* **-ses**
[-siːz] (*Milchdrüsen*) Milchbildung *f*.
ga·lac·to·sta·sia [gəˌlæktə'steɪʒ(ɪ)ə, -ʃɪə] *n*
→ galactostasis.
gal·ac·tos·ta·sis [ˌgælæk'tɒstəsɪs] *n gyn*.
Milchstauung *f*, Galaktostase *f*.
ga·lac·to·su·ria [gəˌlæktə's(j)ʊərɪə] *n* Ga-
laktoseausscheidung *f* im Harn, Galak-
tosurie *f*.
ga·lac·to·syl·ce·ram·i·dase [gəˌlæktəsɪlsə-
'ræmɪdeɪz] *n* Galaktosylceramidase *f*,
Galaktocerebrosid-β-galaktosidase *f*.
ga·lac·to·syl·cer·a·mide [-sɪl'serəmaɪd] *n*
→ galactocerebroside.
galactosylceramide β-galactosidase →
galactosylceramidase.
**galactosylceramide β-galactosidase de-
ficiency** → galactosylceramide lipidosis.
**galactosylceramide β-galactosyl-hydro-
lase** → galactosylceramidase.
galactosylceramide lipidosis Krabbe-
-Syndrom *nt*, Globoidzellen-Leukodystrophie *f*, Galaktozerebrosidlipidose
f, Galaktozerebrosidose *f*, Angiomatosis
encephalo-cutanea, Leukodystrophia cerebri progressiva hereditaria.
ga·lac·to·syl·glu·cose [ˌ-sɪl'gluːkəʊz] *n*
Milchzucker *m*, Laktose *f*, Lactose *f*,
Laktobiose *f*.
ga·lac·to·ther·a·py [ˌ-'θerəpɪ] *n* **1.** Galakto-
therapie *f*, Laktotherapie *f*. **2.** Milchdiät
f, -kur *f*.
ga·lac·to·tox·in [ˌ-'tɒksɪn] *n* Galaktotoxin
nt.
ga·lac·to·tox·ism [ˌ-'tɒksɪzəm] *n* Milchver-
giftung *f*, Vergiftung *f* durch Milch.
gal·ac·tot·ro·phy [ˌgælæk'tɒtrəfɪ] *n ped*.
Milchfütterung *f*.
ga·lac·to·wal·den·ase [gəˌlæktə'wældən-
eɪz] *n* Galaktowaldenase *f*, UDP-Gluco-
se-4-Epimerase *f*, UDP-Galaktose-4-
-Epimerase *f*.
gal·ac·tox·ism [ˌgælæk'tɒksɪzəm] *n* →
galactotoxism.
gal·ac·tox·is·mus [ˌ-'tɒksɪzməs] *n* → galactotoxism.
gal·ac·tu·ria [ˌgælæk't(j)ʊərɪə] *n* Galakturie *f*, Chylurie *f*, Chylolipurie *f*.
ga·lac·tu·ron·ic acid [gəˌlæktjə'rɒnɪk] Ga-
lakturon-, Galacturonsäure *f*.
Galant [gə'lænt]: **G.'s reflex** Galant-Reflex
m.
Galassi [gə'læsɪ, -'lasɪ]: **G.'s pupillary phenomenon** Westphal-Piltz-Phänomen *nt*, Orbikularisphänomen *nt*, Lid-Pupillen-Reflex *m*.
ga·lea [ˈgeɪlɪə, ˈgæ-] *n, pl* **le·ae** [-liːɪ] *anat*.
1. Helm *m*, Haube *f*, haubenartiges
Gebilde *nt*, Galea *f*. **2.** Kopfschwarte *f*,
Galea aponeurotica, Aponeurosis epicranialis.
galea aponeurotica → galea 2.
Galeati [ˌgælɪ'ætiː]: **G.'s glands** Brunner'-
-Drüsen *pl*, Duodenaldrüsen *pl*, Gll. duodenales.

Galeazzi [ˌgælɪ'ætziː]: **G.'s fracture** *ortho*.
Galeazzi-Fraktur *f*.
G.'s fracture-dislocation/injury → G.'s frac-
ture.
G.'s sign *ortho*. Galeazzi-Zeichen *nt*, relative Beinverkürzung *f*.
Galen ['geɪlən]: **G.'s pore** Leistenkanal *m*,
Canalis inguinalis.
G.'s vein Galen-Vene *f*, Cerebri *f* magna,
V. magna cerebri.
ventricle of G. Kehlkopfventrikel *m*, Morgagni'-Ventrikel *m*, Galen'-Ventrikel *m*,
Ventriculus laryngis.
ga·len·ic [gə'liːnɪk, -'lenɪk] *adj* galenisch,
Galen-.
ga·len·i·ca [gə'lenɪkə] *pl* → galenicals.
ga·len·i·cals [gə'lenɪkəls] *pl pharm*. galeni-
sche Mittel *pl*, Galenika *pl*, Galenica *pl*.
ga·len·ics [gə'lenɪks] *pl* → galenicals.
gal·e·ro·pia [ˌgælə'rəʊpɪə] *n* → galeropsia.
gal·e·rop·sia [ˌ-'rɒpsɪə] *n ophthal*. Ga-
lerop(s)ie *f*.
gall [gɔːl] **I** *n* **1.** Galle *f*, Gallenflüssigkeit *f*,
Fel *nt*. **2.** Gallapfel *m*. **3.** → gallbladder. **4.**
wund geriebene Stelle *f*. **II** *vt* wund reiben
od. scheuern. **III** *vi* (s. wund) reiben *od.*
scheuern.
gal·la·mine ['gæləmiːn] *n pharm*. Gallamin
nt.
gal·late ['gæleɪt] *n* Gallat *nt*.
Gallavardin [galavar'dɛ̃]: **G.'s phenomenon**
Gallavardin-Phänomen *nt*.
gall·blad·der ['gɔːlblædər] *n* Gallenblase *f*,
inf. Galle *f*, Vesica fellea/biliaris.
gallbladder aplasia Gallenblasenaplasie
f.
gallbladder atresia Gallenblasenatresie *f*.
gallbladder bed → gallbladder fossa.
gallbladder bile (Gallen-)Blasengalle *f*.
gallbladder carcinoma Gallenblasenkar-
zinom *nt*.
gallbladder cholesteatosis Stippchengal-
lenblase *f*, Gallenblasencholesteatose *f*,
Cholesteatosis vesicae/vesicularis.
gallbladder cholesterolosis → gallbladder cholesteatosis.
gallbladder diseases Gallenblasener-
krankungen *pl*.
gallbladder empyema Gallenblasen-
empyem *nt*.
gallbladder fossa Gallenblasengrube *f*,
-bett *nt*, Leberbett *nt*, Fossa vesicae bili-
aris/felleae.
gallbladder hypoplasia Gallenblasenhy-
poplasie *f*.
gallbladder injury Gallenblasenverlet-
zung *f*.
gallbladder lipoidosis → gallbladder cholesteatosis.
gallbladder papilloma Gallenblasenpa-
pillom *nt*.
gallbladder perforation *chir*. Gallenbla-
senperforation *f*, -durchbruch *m*.
gallbladder rupture Gallenblasenruptur *f*,
-riß *m*.
gall duct Gallengang *m*.
gall duct probe *chir*. Gallengangssonde *f*.
gal·lic acid ['gælɪk, 'gɒl-] Gall-, Gallussäu-
re *f*.
gal·li·um ['gælɪəm] *n abbr*. **Ga** Gallium *nt*
abbr. Ga.
gall·nut ['gɔːlnʌt] *n* Gallapfel *m*.
gal·lon ['gælən] *n* Gallone *f*, Gallon *m/nt*.
gal·lop ['gæləp] *n card*. Galopp *m*, Galopprhythmus *m*.
gal·lop·ing consumption ['gæləpɪŋ] galop-
pierende (Lungen-)Schwindsucht *f*.
gallop rhythm *card*. Galopp *m*, Galopprhythmus *m*.
systolic g. systolischer Galopp.
gal·lo·tan·nic acid [ˌgælə'tænɪk] Tannin
nt, Gerbsäure *f*.

gal·lows traction ['gæləʊz, -əz] *ortho*.
Bryant-Extension *f*, vertikale Überkopfextension *f*, Overheadtraction *f*.
gall·stone ['gɔːlstəʊn] *n* Gallenstein *nt*,
Galle(n)konkrement *nt*, Cholelith *m*,
Calculus biliaris/felleus.
gallstone colic Gallenkolik *f*, Colica hepatica.
gallstone disease Gallensteinleiden *nt*,
Cholelithiasis *f*.
gallstone ileus Gallensteinileus *m*.
gallstone pancreatitis Gallensteinpan-
kreatitis *f*.
gallstone probe *chir*. Gallensteinsonde
f.
GALT *abbr*. → gut-associated lymphoid
tissue.
Galton ['gɔːltn]: **G.'s law** *genet*. Galton-Ge-
setz *nt*, -Regel *f*.
G.'s law of regression Galton'-Regres-
sionsregel *f*.
gal·van·ic [gæl'vænɪk] *adj* galvanisch.
galvanic bath galvanisches Bad *nt*.
galvanic cautery → galvanocautery.
galvanic current/electricity galvanischer
Strom *m*, konstanter Gleichstrom *m*.
galvanic nystagmus elektrischer Nystagmus *m*.
galvanic skin reaction → galvanic skin
response.
galvanic skin response *abbr*. **GSR** psychogalvanischer (Haut-)Reflex *m*.
galvanic threshold *phys*., *physiol*. Rheobase *f*.
gal·va·nism ['gælvənɪzəm] *n* **1.** → galvanic
current. **2.** → galvanization. **3.** Galvanismus *m*, Berührungselektrizität *f*.
gal·va·ni·za·tion [ˌgælvənɪ'zeɪʃn] *n* **1.** Gal-
vanisierung *f*, Galvanisieren *nt*. **2.** Behandlung *f* mit galvanischem Strom,
Galvanotherapie *f*.
gal·va·no·cau·ter·y [ˌgælvənəʊ'kɔːtərɪ] *n* **1.**
Galvanokaustik *f*, Elektrokaustik *f*,
Elektrokauterisation *f*. **2.** Galvanokauter
m, Elektrokauter *m*, Elektrokaustiknadel *f*.
gal·va·no·chem·i·cal [ˌ-'kemɪkl] *adj* elek-
tro-, galvanochemisch.
gal·va·no·con·trac·til·i·ty [ˌ-ˌkɒntræk'tɪlə-
tɪ] *n physiol*. Galvanokontraktilität *f*.
gal·va·no·far·a·di·za·tion [ˌ-ˌfærədɪ'zeɪʃn]
n Galvanofaradisation *f*.
gal·va·no·i·on·i·za·tion [ˌ-ˌaɪənɪ'zeɪʃn] *n*
old Iontophorese *f*.
gal·va·nol·y·sis [gælvə'nɒləsɪs] *n* Elektrolyse *f*.
gal·va·nom·e·ter [gælvə'nɒmɪtər] *n* Galvanometer *nt*.
gal·va·no·met·ric [ˌgælvənəʊ'metrɪk] *adj*
galvanometrisch.
gal·va·no·mus·cu·lar [ˌ-'mʌskjələr] *adj*
galvanomuskulär.
gal·va·no·sur·ger·y [ˌ-'sɜːdʒərɪ] *n chir*.
Galvanochirurgie *f*.
gal·va·no·tax·is [ˌ-'tæksɪs] *n* Galvanotaxis
f; Elektrotaxis *f*.
gal·va·no·ther·a·peu·tics [ˌ-ˌθerə'pjuːtɪks]
pl → galvanotherapy.
gal·va·no·ther·a·py [ˌ-'θerəpɪ] *n* Behand-
lung/Therapie *f* mit galvanischem Strom,
Galvanotherapie *f*.
gal·va·not·o·nus [gælvə'nɒtənəs] *n* **1.** Gal-
vanotonus *m*. **2.** Elektrotonus *m*.
gal·va·not·ro·pism [gælvə'nɒtrəpɪzəm] *n*
Galvanotropismus *m*; Elektrotropismus
m.
gam·a·sid ['gæməsɪd] *n micro*. Gamaside
f.
Ga·mas·i·dae [gə'mæsɪdiː] *pl micro*. Ga-
masidae *pl*.
Ga·mas·i·des [gə'mæsɪdiːz] *pl micro*. Ga-
masides *pl*.

gamasoidosis

gam·a·soi·do·sis [ˌgæməsɔɪ'dəʊsɪs] *n derm.* Vogelmilbenkrätze *f*, Gamasidiosis *f*.
Gam·bi·an ['gæmbɪən]: **G. fever** Gambian-(Rückfall-)Fieber *nt*.
G. sleeping sickness → G. trypanosomiasis.
G. trypanosomiasis westafrikanische Schlafkrankheit/Trypano(so)miasis *f*.
game·keep·er's thumb ['geɪmkiːpər] *ortho.* Skidaumen *m*.
gamet- *pref.* → gameto-.
gam·e·tan·gi·um [ˌgæmɪ'tændʒɪəm] *n, pl* **-gia** [-dʒɪə] Gametangium *nt*.
gam·ete ['gæmiːt, gə'miːt] *n* 1. reife Keimzelle *f*, Geschlechtszelle *f*, Gamet *m*, Gamozyt *m*. 2. *parasit.* (*Plasmodium*) Gametozyt *m*, Gamont *m*.
ga·met·ic [gə'metɪk] *adj* Gameten-.
gameto- *pref.* Gamet(o)-.
ga·me·to·ci·dal [gəˌmiːtə'saɪdl, ˌgæmɪtəʊ-] *adj* gametozid.
ga·me·to·cide ['-saɪd] *n* Gametozid *nt*.
ga·me·to·cyst ['-sɪst] *n* Gametozyst *m*.
ga·me·to·cyte ['-saɪt] *n* 1. Gametozyt *m*. 2. *micro.* Gamont *m*.
ga·me·to·cy·te·mia [ˌ-saɪ'tiːmɪə] *n micro.* Gametozytämie *f*.
ga·me·to·gen·e·sis [ˌ-'dʒenəsɪs] *n* Gametenbildung *f*, -entwicklung *f*, Gametogenese *f*.
ga·me·to·gen·ic [ˌ-'dʒenɪk] *adj* gametogen.
ga·me·tog·e·nous [gæmɪ'tɑdʒənəs] *adj* → gametogenic.
ga·me·tog·e·ny [gæmɪ'tɑdʒənɪ] *n* → gametogenesis.
ga·me·to·go·nia [gəˌmiːtə'gəʊnɪə, ˌgæmɪtəʊ-] *n* → gametogony.
gam·e·tog·o·ny [gæmɪ'tɑgənɪ] *n* 1. *micro.* Gamogonie *f*, Gametogonie *f*. 2. *bio.* geschlechtliche Fortpflanzung *f*, Gametogonie *f*, Gamogonie *f*, Gamogenese *f*.
gam·e·toid ['gæmɪtɔɪd] *adj* gametoid.
ga·me·top·a·thy [gæmɪ'tɑpəθɪ] *n genet.* Gametopathie *f*.
ga·me·to·pha·gia [gəˌmiːtə'fædʒɪə, ˌgæmɪtəʊ-] *n* → gamophagia.
ga·me·to·phore ['-fəʊər] *n* Gametophor *m*.
ga·me·to·phyte ['-faɪt] *n* Gametophyt *m*.
gam·ma ['gæmə] *n abbr.* Γ, γ Gamma *f abbr.* Γ, γ.
gamma alcoholism γ-Alkoholismus *m*.
gamma-aminobutyric acid *abbr.* **GABA** γ-Amino-n-Buttersäure *f*, Gammaaminobuttersäure *f abbr.* GABA.
gamma angle *ophthal.* Gamma-Winkel *m*.
gamma-benzene hexachloride Benzolhexachlorid *nt*, Hexachlorcyclohexan *nt abbr.* HCH; Lindan *nt*.
gamma camera *radiol.* Gammakamera *f*.
gamma cells: **g. of hypophysis** (*Hypophyse*) chromophobe Zellen *pl*, γ-Zellen *pl*.
g. of pancreas (*Pankreas*) C-Zellen *pl*, γ-Zellen *pl*.
gamma chain disease Gamma-Typ *m* der Schwerekettenkrankheit, γ-Typ *m*, γ-H-Kettenkrankheit *f*.
gam·ma·cism ['gæməsɪzəm] *n* Gammazismus *m*.
gamma fibers γ-Fasern *pl*, Aγ-Fasern *pl*.
gamma function *mathe.* Gammafunktion *f*.
gamma globulin 1. Gammaglobulin *nt*, γ-Globulin *nt*. 2. *old* Immunglobulin *nt*.
gam·ma·glob·u·lin·op·a·thy [ˌgæməˌglɑbjəlɪ'nɑpəθɪ] *n immun.* Gammopathie *f*.
gam·ma·gram ['gæməgræm] *n radiol.* Szintigramm *nt*.
gamma granules γ-Granula *pl*.
gamma hemolysis γ-Hämolyse *f*, Gammahämolyse *f*.

gamma-hemolytic *adj* gamma-hämolytisch, γ-hämolytisch, nicht-hämolytisch, nicht-hämolysierend.
gamma-hemolytic streptococci → gamma streptococci.
Gam·ma·her·pes·vir·i·nae [ˌgæməˌhɜrpiːz'vɪrəniː] *pl micro.* Gammaherpesviren *pl*, Gammaherpesvirinae *pl*.
gam·ma·her·pes·vi·rus·es [ˌ-ˌhɜrpiːz'vaɪrəsəs] *pl* → Gammaherpesvirinae.
gamma loop Gammaschleife *f*.
gamma motoneuron γ-Motoneuron *nt*.
gamma motor system → gamma loop.
gamma neuron γ-Neuron *nt*.
gamma radiation *phys.* Gammastrahlung *f*, γ-Strahlung *f*.
gamma rays Gammastrahlen *pl*, γ-Strahlen *pl*.
gamma rhythm γ-Rhythmus *m*, Gammarhythmus *m*.
gamma-scintigraphy *n radiol.* Gammaszintigraphie *f*.
gamma staphylolysin γ-Staphylolysin *nt*.
gamma streptococci *micro.* gamma-hämolysierende/nicht-hämolysierende Streptokokken *pl*.
gam·mop·a·thy [gæ'mɑpəθɪ] *n immun.* Gammopathie *f*.
Gamna ['gæmnə]: **G.'s disease** Gamna-Krankheit *f*.
G.'s nodules → Gamna-Gandy bodies.
Gamna-Favre ['faːvrə]: **G-F. bodies** Favre-Gamna-Körperchen *pl*.
Gamna-Gandy ['gændɪ, gɑ'diː]: **G.-G. bodies/nodules** Gamna-Gandy-Körperchen *pl*, -Knötchen *pl*.
ga·mo·bi·um [gə'məʊbɪəm, gæ-] *n, pl* **-bia** [-bɪə] Gamobium *nt*.
gam·o·gen·e·sis [ˌgæmə'dʒenəsɪs] *n* geschlechtliche Fortpflanzung *f*, Gamogenese *f*, Gamogenesis *f*, Gamogonie *f*.
gam·og·o·ny [gə'mɑgənɪ] *n* → gametogony.
gam·one ['gæməʊn] *n bio.* Gamon *n*.
gam·ont ['gæmɑnt] *n* Gamont *m*, Gametozyt *m*.
gam·o·pha·gia [ˌgæmə'feɪdʒ(ɪ)ə] *n* Gamophagie *f*, Gametophagie *f*.
gam·o·pho·bia [ˌ-'fəʊbɪə] *n psychia.* Gamophobie *f*; Misgamie *f*.
gamp·so·dac·ty·ly [ˌgæmpsə'dæktəlɪ] *n ortho.* Klauenfuß *m*.
Gamstorp ['gæmstɔːrp]: **G.'s disease** Gamstorp-Syndrom *nt*, Adynamia episodica hereditaria.
gan·ci·clo·vir [gæn'saɪkləvɪər] *n pharm.* Ganciclovir, Dihydroxypropoxymethylguanin *nt abbr.* DHPG.
Gandy-Gamna ['gændɪ 'gæmnə, gɑ'diː]: **G.-G. bodies/nodules** → Gamna-Gandy bodies.
G.-G. spleen siderotische Splenomegalie *f*.
Gandy-Nanta ['næntə]: **G.-N. disease** siderotische Splenomegalie *f*.
gangli- *pref.* → ganglio-.
gan·glia *pl* → ganglion.
gan·gli·al ['gæŋglɪəl] *adj* Ganglion betr., Ganglien-, Ganglio-.
gan·gli·ate ['gæŋglɪeɪt, -ɪt] *adj* → ganglionated.
gan·gli·at·ed ['gæŋglɪeɪtɪd] *adj* → ganglionated.
gangliated cord Grenzstrang *m*, Truncus sympatheticus/sympathicus.
gan·gli·ec·to·my [ˌgæŋglɪ'ektəmɪ] *n* → ganglionectomy.
gan·gli·form ['-fɔːrm] *adj* ganglionartig, -förmig.
gan·gli·it·is [ˌ-'aɪtɪs] *n* → ganglionitis.
ganglio- *pref.* Ganglien-, Ganglio-.
gan·gli·o·blast ['gæŋglɪəblæst] *n* Ganglioblast *m*.

gan·gli·o·cyte ['-saɪt] *n* → ganglion cell 1.
gan·gli·o·cy·to·ma [ˌ-saɪ'təʊmə] *n* → ganglioneuroma.
gan·gli·o·form ['-fɔːrm] *adj* → gangliform.
gan·gli·o·gli·o·ma [ˌ-glaɪ'əʊmə] *n* zentrales Ganglioneurom *nt*, Gangliogliom(a) *nt*.
gan·gli·o·gli·o·neu·ro·ma [ˌ-ˌglaɪənjʊə'rəʊmə] *n* → ganglioneuroma.
gan·gli·ol·y·sis [gæŋglɪ'ɑləsɪs] *n patho.* Gangliolyse *f*.
gan·gli·o·lyt·ic [ˌgæŋglɪə'lɪtɪk] *n, adj* ganglioplegic.
gan·gli·o·ma [gæŋglɪ'əʊmə] *n* → ganglioneuroma.
gan·gli·on ['gæŋglɪən] *n, pl* **-gli·ons**, **-glia** [-glɪə] 1. *anat.* (Nerven-)Knoten *m*, Ganglion *nt*. 2. *chir.* Überbein *nt*, Ganglion *nt*. 3. *fig.* Mittel-, Knotenpunkt *m*.
g. of autonomic plexuses Ganglien(zellgruppen *pl*) *pl* der vegetativen Plexus, Ggll. plexuum autonomicorum/visceralium.
g. of Müller oberes Glossopharyngeusganglion, Ehrenritter'-Ganglion, Müller'-Ganglion, Ggl. rostralis/superius n. glossopharyngei.
g.lia of sympathetic plexuses → g.lia of autonomic plexuses.
g.lia of sympathetic trunk Grenzstrangganglien *pl*, Ggll. trunci sympathetici.
g. of trigeminal nerve Gasser'-Ganglion, Ggl. trigeminale/semilunare/Gasseri.
g.lia of visceral plexuses → g.lia of autonomic plexuses.
gan·gli·o·nat·ed ['gæŋglɪəneɪtɪd] *adj* ganglienbesitzend.
ganglionated cord → gangliated cord.
ganglion-blocking agent *pharm.* Ganglienblocker *m*, Ganglioplegikum *nt*.
ganglion cell 1. Ganglienzelle *f*, Gangliozyt *m*. 2. (*Auge*) retinale Ganglienzelle *f*.
off-center g. Off-Zentrum-Ganglienzelle.
on-center g. On-Zentrum-Ganglienzelle.
on-off g. On-Off-Ganglienzelle.
pseudounipolar g. pseudounipolare Nerven- *od.* Ganglienzelle, pseudounipolarer Neurozyt/Gangliozyt *m*.
retinal g. retinale Ganglienzelle.
spinal g.s Spinalganglienzellen *pl*.
ganglion cell layer (*Auge*) Optikus-Ganglienzellschicht *f*.
gan·gli·on·ec·to·my [ˌgæŋglɪə'nektəmɪ] *n* 1. *ortho.* Ganglionexzision *f*, Gangliektomie *f*, Ganglionektomie *f*. 2. *neurochir.* Ganglionektomie *f*, Gangliektomie *f*.
gan·gli·o·neu·ro·blas·to·ma [ˌ-ˌnjʊərəblæs'təʊmə] *n* Ganglioneuroblastom(a) *nt*.
gan·gli·o·neu·ro·fi·bro·ma [ˌ-ˌnjʊərəfaɪ'brəʊmə] *n* → ganglioneuroma.
gan·gli·o·neu·ro·ma [ˌ-njʊə'rəʊmə] *n* Ganglioneurom *nt*, -neuroma *nt*, -zytom *nt*.
gan·gli·on·ic [gæŋglɪ'ɑnɪk] *adj* Ganglion betr., ganglionär, Ganglien-, Ganglio-.
ganglionic blockade Ganglienblockade *f*.
ganglionic blocking agent *pharm.* Ganglienblocker *m*, Ganglioplegikum *nt*.
ganglionic branches: **g. of maxillary nerve** Rami ganglionares n. maxillaris.
g. of sublingual nerve Äste *pl* des N. lingualis zum Ggl. submandibulare, Rami ganglionares/ganglionici n. lingualis.
ganglionic canal Rosenthal'-Kanal *m*, Schneckenspindelkanal *m*, Canalis ganglionaris, Canalis spiralis modioli.
ganglionic crest *embryo.* Neuralleiste *f*.
ganglionic cyst (*Knochen*) Geröll-, Trümmerzyste *f*.
intraosseous g. → ganglionic cystic defect of bone.

ganglionic cystic defect of bone intraossäres Ganglion *nt*, juxtaartikuläre Knochenzyste *f*.
ganglionic layer: g. of cerebellum Purkinje'-Zellschicht *f*, Stratum ganglionare/ganglionsum cerebelli.
g. of optic nerve → ganglionic stratum of optic nerve.
g. of retina → ganglionic stratum of retina.
ganglionic stratum: g. of optic nerve Stratum ganglionare n. optici.
g. of retina Stratum ganglionare retinae.
gan·gli·on·it·is [ˌgæŋglɪəˈnaɪtɪs] *n* Ganglion-, Ganglienentzündung *f*, Ganglionitis *f*, Gangliitis *f*.
gan·gli·on·o·ple·gic [ˌgæŋglɪˌɑnəˈpliːdʒɪk] *n, adj* → ganglioplegic.
gan·gli·o·ple·gic [ˌgæŋglɪəˈpliːdʒɪk] **I** *n pharm*. Ganglienblocker *m*, Ganglioplegikum *nt*. **II** *adj* ganglienblockend, ganglioplegisch.
gan·gli·o·side [-ˈsaɪd] *n* Gangliosid *nt*.
ganglioside lipidosis → gangliosidosis.
gan·gli·o·si·do·sis [ˌ-saɪˈdəʊsɪs] *n, pl* **-ses** [-siːz] Gangliosidose *f*.
gan·gli·o·sym·pa·thec·to·my [ˌ-ˌsɪmpəˈθɛktəmɪ] *n neurochir*. Gangliosympathektomie *f*.
gan·go·sa [gæŋˈgəʊsə] *n HNO* Gangosa *f*, Rhinopharyngitis mutilans.
gan·grene [ˈgæŋgriːn, gæŋˈgriːn] *n* Gangrän *f*, Brand *m*, gangräne Nekrose *f*, Gangraena *f*.
gan·gre·nous [ˈgæŋgrɪnəs] *adj* Gangrän betr., mit *od.* in Form einer Gangrän, gangränös.
gangrenous appendicitis gangränöse Appendizitis *f*, Appendicitis gangraenosa.
gangrenous balanitis Corbus-Krankheit *f*, gangränöse Balanitis *f*, Balanitis gangraenosa.
gangrenous bowel *chir*. gangrenöser Darm(abschnitt *m*) *m*.
gangrenous cellulitis Erysipelas gangraenosum.
gangrenous cholecystitis gangränöse Gallenblasenentzündung/Cholezystitis *f*, Cholecystitis gangraenosa.
gangrenous cystitis gangränöse (Harn-)Blasenentzündung/Zystitis *f*, Cystitis gangraenosa.
gangrenous emphysema Gasbrand *m*, -gangrän *f*, -ödem *nt*, -ödemerkrankung *f*, malignes Ödem *nt*, Gasphlegmone *f*, Gangraena emphysematosa.
gangrenous erysipelas Erysipelas gangraenosum.
gangrenous necrosis gangränöse Nekrose *f*.
gangrenous pharyngitis gangränöse Pharyngitis *f*.
gangrenous pneumonia gangränöse Pneumonie *f*.
gangrenous stomatitis Noma *f*, Wangenbrand *m*, Wasserkrebs *m*, infektiöse Gangrän *f* des Mundes, Cancer aquaticus, Chancrum oris, Stomatitis gangraenosa.
gan·o·blast [ˈgænəʊblæst] *n* Adamanto-, Amelo-, Ganoblast *m*.
Ganser [ˈgænzər; ˈgans-]: **G.'s commissure** jGanser'-Kommissur *f*, Commissura supraoptica dorsalis.
G.'s diverticula Ganser-Divertikel *pl*.
G.'s ganglion Nc. interpeduncularis.
G.'s syndrome Ganser-Syndrom *nt*, Pseudodemenz *f*, Scheinblödsinn *m*, Zweckpsychose *f*.
GAP *abbr*. → glyceraldehyde-3-phosphate.
gap [gæp] *n* 1. Lücke *f*. **to fill/close a ~** eine Lücke (aus-)füllen/schließen. 2. Spalt(e *f*) *m*, Öffnung *f*, Loch *nt*, Riß *m*.
GAPD *abbr*. → glyceraldehyde-3-phosphate dehydrogenase.
gap·ing [ˈgeɪpɪŋ, ˈgæp-] *adj* (*Wunde*) klaffend, weit geöffnet.
gap junction offener Zellkontakt *m*, Nexus *m*.
gap·less [ˈgæplɪs] *adj* lückenlos.
Gap₁ period *bio*. G₁-Phase *f*.
Gap₂ period *bio*. G₂-Phase *f*.
gap-toothed *adj* 1. mit Zahnlücken. 2. mit weiter Zahnstellung, mit auseinanderstehenden Zähnen.
Gardner [ˈgɑːrdnər]: **G.'s syndrome** Gardner-Syndrom *nt*.
Gardner-Diamond [ˈdaɪ(ə)mənd]: **G.-D. syndrome** Erythrozytenautosensibilisierung *f*, schmerzhafte Ekchymosen-Syndrom *nt*, painful bruising syndrome (*nt*).
Gard·ner·el·la [gɑːrdnəˈrelə] *n micro*. Gardnerella *f*.
Garel [gaˈrel]: **G.'s sign** Burger-Zeichen *nt*, Heryng-Zeichen *nt*.
gar·gal·es·the·sia [ˌgɑːrglˌænəsˈθiːʒə] *n* Gargalanästhesie *f*.
gar·gal·es·the·sia [ˌ-esˈθiː(ɪ)ə] *n* Gargalästhesie *f*, Gargaläsie *f*.
gar·gle [ˈgɑːrgl] **I** *n* 1. Gurgeln *nt*. 2. Gurgelmittel *nt*, -wasser *nt*; Mundwasser *nt*. **II** *vt, vi* gurgeln.
gar·goyl·ism [ˈgɑːrgɔɪlɪzəm] *n* 1. Wasserspeiergesicht *nt*, Fratzengesichtigkeit *f*, Gargoylfratze *f*, Gargoylismus *m*. 2. (**autosomal recessive type**) Hurler-Krankheit *f*, -Syndrom *nt*, (von) Pfaundler-Hurler-Krankheit *f*, -Syndrom *nt*, Mukopolysaccharidose I-H *f abbr*. MPS I-H, Lipochondrodystrophie *f*, Dysostosis multiplex.
Garland [ˈgɑːrlənd]: **G.'s curve** Ellis-Damoiseau'-Linie *f*.
G.'s triangle Garland-Dreieck *nt*.
gar·ment [ˈgɑːrmənt] *n* 1. Kleidung *f*, Kleidungsstück *nt*. 2. Hülle *f*, Gewand *nt*.
Garré [gaˈre]: **G.'s disease** sklerosierende/nicht-eitrige Osteomyelitis *f*, Garré'-Osteomyelitis *f*, -Krankheit *f*, Osteomyelitis sicca Garré.
G.'s osteitis/osteomyelitis → G.'s disease.
Garrod [ˈgærəd]: **G.'s nodes** Garrod'-Knötchen *pl*, (echte) Fingerknöchelpolster *pl*.
gar·rot(t)e tourniquet [gəˈrəʊt, -ˈrat] *ortho*. Abbindung *f*.
Garter [ˈgɑːrtər]: **G. strapping** *ortho*. redressierender Verband *m* mit Fixierung der Nachbarphalanx.
Gartner [ˈgɑːrtnər]: **G.'s canal** Gartner'-Gang *m*, Längsgang *m* des Epoophorons, Ductus epoophorontis longitudinalis.
G.'s cyst Gartner-Zyste *f*.
G.'s duct → G.'s canal.
Gärtner [ˈgɛrtnər]: **G.'s bacillus** Gärtner-Bazillus *m*, Salmonella enteritidis.
G.'s (vein) phenomenon *card*. Gärtner-Zeichen *nt*.
gart·ne·ri·an cyst [gɑːrˈtnɪərɪən] Gartner-Zyste *f*.
gas [gæs] **I** *n, pl* **-es, -ses** 1. *chem*. Gas *nt*. 2. (Gift-)Gas *nt*, Kampfstoff *m*. 3. Lachgas *nt*, Distickstoffoxid *nt*, Stickoxidul *nt*. **to have ~** Lachgas bekommen. 4. Blähung *f*, Wind *m*, Flatus *m*. **II** *vt* 5. mit Gas füllen. 6. mit Gas verseuchen *od.* vergiften, vergasen. 7. *techn*. mit Gas behandeln, begasen.
gas abscess Gasabszeß *m*.
gas-absorbing *adj* gasabsorbierend.
gas bacillus Welch-Fränkel-(Gasbrand-)Bazillus *m*, Clostridium perfringens.
gas bottle Gasflasche *f*.
gas burner Gasbrenner *m*.

gas cell *chem., phys*. Gaszelle *f*.
gas chromatography *abbr*. **GC** Gaschromatographie *f abbr*. GC.
gas coal Gaskohle *f*.
gas constant *abbr*. **R** Gaskonstante *f abbr*. R.
gas cyst Gaszyste *f*, gashaltige Zyste *f*.
gas-discharge tube *electr*. Gasentladungs-, Ionenröhre *f*.
gas dynamics *phys*. Gasdynamik *f*.
gas embolism Luft-, Gasembolie *f*.
gas endarterectomy *chir*. Gasendarterektomie *f*.
gas·e·ous [ˈgæsɪəs, ˈgæfəs] *adj chem*. gasförmig, -artig, gasig, Gas-.
gaseous anesthetic gasförmiges Anästhetikum *nt*, Narkosegas *nt*.
gaseous cholecystitis emphysematöse Gallenblasenentzündung/Cholezystitis *f*, Cholecystitis emphysematosa.
gaseous diffusion Gasdiffusion *f*.
gaseous edema Gasödem *nt*.
gaseous gangrene → gas gangrene.
gaseous hydrogen gasförmiger Wasserstoff *m*.
gas·e·ous·ness [ˈgæsɪəsnɪs, ˈgæfəs-] *n* Gasförmigkeit *f*, Gaszustand *m*.
gaseous pericholecystitis emphysematöse Gallenblasenentzündung/Cholezystitis *f*, Cholecystitis emphysematosa.
gaseous state gasförmiger (Aggregat-)Zustand *m*.
gas exchange Gasaustausch *m*.
gas-filled *adj* gasgefüllt.
gas gangrene *patho*. Gasbrand *m*, -gangrän *f*, -ödem *nt*, -ödemerkrankung *f*, malignes Ödem *nt*, Gasphlegmone *f*, Gangraena emphysematosa.
gas·i·fi·ca·tion [ˌgæsəfɪˈkeɪʃn] *n techn*. Vergasung *f*.
gas·i·form [ˈgæsɪfɔːrm] *adj* → gaseous.
gas·i·fy [ˈgæsɪfaɪ] **I** *vt* vergasen, in Gas verwandeln. **II** *vi zu* Gas werden.
gas jet 1. Gasflamme *f*. 2. Gasbrenner *m*.
Gaskell [ˈgæskəl]: **G.'s bridge** His'-Bündel, Fasciculus atrioventricularis.
gas laser *phys*. Gaslaser *m*.
gas law *phys*. Gasgesetz *nt*.
gas-light [ˈgæslaɪt] *n* 1. Gaslicht *nt*. 2. Gasbrenner *m*.
gas-liquid chromatography *abbr*. **GLC** Gas-Flüssigkeitschromatographie *f*.
gas liquor *chem*. konzentrierter Salmiakgeist *m*.
gas mask Gasmaske *f*.
gas mixture Gasgemisch *nt*.
alveolar g. alveoläres Gasgemisch, *old* Alveolarluft *f*.
gas·o·gen·ic [gæsəˈdʒɛnɪk] *adj* gasbildend, -produzierend.
gas·o·line [ˈgæsəliːn, ˈgæsəliːn] *n chem*. Gasolin *nt*.
gas·om·e·ter [gæˈsɑmɪtər] *n* Gasometer *m*.
gas·o·met·ric [ˌgæsəˈmɛtrɪk] *adj* gasometrisch.
gas·om·e·try [gæˈsɑmɪtrɪ] *n* Gasometrie *f*.
gasp [gæsp, gɑːsp] **I** *n* Keuchen *nt*, Schnaufen *nt*, schweres Atmen *nt*, Schnappatmung *f*. **II** *vi* keuchen, schnaufen, schwer atmen. **to ~ for breath** nach Luft schnappen *od.* ringen.
gas phase *phys*. Gasphase *f*.
gasp·ing [ˈgæspɪŋ, ˈgɑːsp-] **I** *n* → gasp **I**. **II** *adj* keuchend, schnaufend, schwer atmend.
gas-proof [ˈgæspruːf] *adj* gasdicht.
Gasser [ˈgæsər]: **G.'s ganglion** Gasser'-Ganglion *nt*, Ganglion trigeminale/semilunare/Gasseri.
G.'s syndrome Gasser-Syndrom *nt*, hämolytisch-urämisches Syndrom *nt abbr*. HUS.

gasserian

gas·se·ri·an [gæˈsɪərɪən]: **g. duct** Müller'-Gang *m*, Ductus paramesonephricus.
g. ganglion → Gasser's ganglion.
g. ganglionitis Herpes zoster ophthalmicus, Zoster ophthalmicus.
gas-solid chromatography *abbr.* **GSC** Gas-Adsorptionschromatographie *f*.
gas·sy [ˈgæsɪ] *adj* **1.** gashaltig, -artig, voll Gas. **2.** kohlensäurehaltig.
gas tank Gasbehälter *m*.
gas·ter [ˈgæstər] *n anat.* Magen *m*, Gaster *f*, Ventriculus *m*.
gas·ter·al·gia [ˌgæstərˈældʒ(ɪ)ə] *n* → gastralgia.
Gas·ter·o·phil·i·dae [ˌgæstərəʊˈfɪlədiː] *pl micro.* Gasterophilidae *pl*.
Gas·ter·oph·i·lus [gæstəˈrɒfɪləs] *n micro.* Gastrophilus *m*.
gas thermometer Gasthermometer *nt*.
gas·tight [ˈgæstaɪt] *adj* gasdicht.
gastr- *pref.* → gastro-.
gas·trad·e·ni·tis [ˌgæstrædɪˈnaɪtɪs] *n* Magendrüsenentzündung *f*, Gastr(o)adenitis *f*.
gas·tral·gia [gæˈstrældʒ(ɪ)ə] *n* **1.** Magenschmerz(en *pl*) *m*, Gastrodynie *f*, Gastralgie *f*. **2.** Magenkrampf *m*, -kolik *f*, Gastrospasmus *m*.
gas·tra·mine [ˈgæstrəmiːn, -mɪn] *n* Betazol *nt*.
gastramine hydrochloride Betazolhydrochlorid *nt*.
gas·tra·tro·phia [ˌgæstrəˈtrəʊfɪə] *n* chronisch-atrophische Gastritis *f*.
gas·trec·ta·sia [gæstrekˈteɪʒ(ɪ)ə] *n* Magenerweiterung *f*, Gastrektasie *f*.
gas·trec·ta·sis [gæsˈtrektəsɪs] *n* → gastrectasia.
gas·trec·to·my [gæsˈtrektəmɪ] *n chir.* Magenentfernung *f*, totale Magenresektion *f*, Gastrektomie *f*.
gas·tric [ˈgæstrɪk] *adj* Magen betr., gastrisch, gastral, Magen-, Gastro-.
gastric achylia Magensaftmangel *m*, Achylie *f*, Achylia gastrica.
gastric acid Magensäure *f*.
gastric adenocarcinoma Adenokarzinom *nt* des Magens.
gastric anacidity Magenanazidität *f*, Magensäuremangel *m*, Achlorhydrie *f*.
gastric anti-pernicious anemia factor Intrinsic-Faktor *m*, intrinsic factor (*m*).
gastric antrum präpylorischer Magenabschnitt *m*, Antrum *nt* (pyloricum).
gastric areas Magenschleimhautfelder *pl*, Areae gastricae.
gastric artery Magenschlagader *f*, -arterie *f*, A. gastrica.
  inferior left g. → gastroepiploic artery, left.
  inferior right g. → gastroepiploic artery, right.
  left g. linke Magen(kranz)arterie, Gastrica *f* sinistra, A. gastrica sinistra.
  posterior g., A. gastrica posterior.
  right g. rechte Magen(kranz)arterie, Gastrica *f* dextra, A. gastrica dextra.
  short g.s kurze Magenarterien *pl*, Aa. gastrici breves.
gastric atonia → gastroatonia.
gastric atrophy Magen(schleimhaut)atrophie *f*.
  idiopathic g. chronisch-atrophische Gastritis *f*.
gastric biopsy Magen-, Gastrobiopsie *f*.
gastric bleeding Magenblutung *f*.
gastric body Magenkörper *m*, Corpus gastricum/ventriculare.
gastric branches: anterior g. of vagus nerve vordere Magenäste *pl* des N. vagus, Rami gastrici anteriores (n. vagi).
  g. of left gastroepiploic artery Magenäste *pl* der A. gastroepiploica sinistra, Rami gastrici a. gastroepiploicae/gastro-omentalis sinistrae.
  g. of left gastroomental artery → g. of left gastroepiploic artery.
  posterior g. of vagus nerve hintere Magenäste *pl* des N. vagus, Rami gastrici posteriores (n. vagi).
  g. of right gastroepiploic artery Magenäste *pl* der A. gastroepiploica dextra, Rami gastrici a. gastroepiploicae/gastro-omentalis dextrae.
  g. of right gastroomental artery → g. of right gastroepiploic artery.
gastric bubble Magenblase *f*.
gastric calculus → gastrolith.
gastric canal Magenstraße *f*, Canalis gastricus/ventricularis.
gastric cancer/carcinoma Magenkrebs, -karzinom *nt*.
  early g. Frühkarzinom des Magens, Magenfrühkarzinom.
gastric cirrhosis entzündlicher Schrumpfmagen *m*, Magenszirrhus *m*, Brinton--Krankheit *f*, Linitis plastica.
gastric colic Magenkrampf *m*, -kolik *f*, Gastrospasmus *m*, Colica gastrica.
gastric crisis *neuro.* gastrische Krise *f*.
gastric curvature Magenkrümmung *f*, -kurvatur *f*, Curvatura gastrica/ventricularis.
  greater g. große (Magen-)Kurvatur, Curvatura gastrica/ventricularis major.
  lesser g. kleine (Magen-)Kurvatur, Curvatura gastrica/ventricularis minor.
gastric cycle Magenzyklus *m*.
gastric digestion Magenverdauung *f*, peptische Verdauung *f*.
gastric dilatation Magen(über)dehnung *f*, -dilatation *f*.
gastric emptying Magenentleerung *f*.
gastric fibers, oblique schräge Muskel(faser)züge *pl* der Magenwand, Fibrae obliquae.
gastric fields → gastric areas.
gastric fistula 1. *patho.* Magenfistel *f*, Fistula gastrica. **2.** *chir.* Magenfistel *f*, Gastrotomie *f*.
gastric folds Magenschleimhautfalten *pl*, Plicae gastricae.
gastric follicles 1. → gastric glands. **2.** Folliculi lymphatici gastrici.
gastric fornix Magenkuppel *f*, Fornix gastricus/ventricularis.
gastric foveolae Magengrübchen *pl*, Foveolae gastricae.
gastric fundic flap *chir.* (gestielter) Magenfunduslappen *m*.
gastric fundic patch → gastric fundic flap.
gastric fundus Magenfundus *m*, Fundus gastricus/ventricularis.
gastric glands Magendrüsen *f*, Fundus- u. Korpusdrüsen *pl*, Gll. gastricae propriae.
gastric hemorrhage Magenblutung *f*.
gastric herniation Magenvorfall *m*, -herniation *f*.
gastric hyperacidity Hyperazidität *f* des Magensaftes, Hyperchlorhydrie *f*.
gastric impression of liver Magenabdruck *m* auf der Leberoberfläche, Impressio gastrica (hepatis).
gastric indigestion *patho.* Dyspepsie *f*, Dyspepsia *f*.
gastric inhibitory polypeptide *abbr.* **GIP** → glucose dependent insulinotropic peptide.
gastric interposition *chir.* **1.** Mageninterposition *f*. **2.** Mageninterponat *nt*.
gastric intrinsic factor Intrinsic-Faktor *m*, intrinsic factor (*m*).
gastric juice Magensaft *m*, -speichel *m*, Sucus gastricus.
gastric lymph nodes: left g. linke Lymphknotengruppe *f* der kleinen Magenkurvatur, Nodi lymphatici viscerales gastrici sinistri.
  right g. rechte Lymphknotengruppe *f* der kleinen Magenkurvatur, Nodi lymphatici viscerales gastrici dextri.
gastric lymphoma Lymphom/Lymphogranulom *nt* des Magens.
gastric metaplasia gastrale Metaplasie *f*, Metaplasie *f* der Magenschleimhaut.
gastric motility Magenmotilität *f*.
gastric mucosal barrier Magenschleimhautbarriere *f*.
gastric mucosal bleeding Magenschleimhautblutung *f*.
gastric mucosal hemorrhage → gastric mucosal bleeding.
gastric mucosal ulcer Magenschleimhautgeschwür *nt*, Ulcus ventriculi simplex.
gastric mucosal ulceration → gastric mucosal ulcer.
gastric neoplasm Magengeschwulst *f*, -tumor *m*.
gastric nerves Trunci vagales anterior et posterior.
gastric notch Magenknieeinschnitt *m*, Inc. angularis (ventriculi/gastris).
gastric outlet obstruction Magenausgangsstenose *f*.
gastric outlet stenosis → gastric outlet obstruction.
gastric pH Magensaft-pH *m*.
gastric phase (*Verdauung*) gastrale Phase *f*.
gastric pits → gastric foveolae.
gastric plexus: g.es *pl* Magenplexus *pl*, Plexus gastrici.
  anterior g. → gastric branches of vagus nerve, anterior.
  posterior g. → gastric branches of vagus nerve, posterior.
gastric plicae → gastric folds.
gastric polyp Magenpolyp *m*.
gastric polyposis Magenpolypose *f*, Polyposis gastrici/ventriculi.
gastric resection Magen(teil)resektion *f*, partielle Gastrektomie *f*.
gastric sclerosis → gastric cirrhosis.
gastric secrete Magensekret *nt*.
gastric secretion 1. Magensekretion *nt*. **2.** Magensekret *nt*.
gas·tric·sin [ˈgæstrɪksɪn] *n* Pepsin C *nt*, Gastrizin *nt*.
gastric spasm → gastrospasm.
gastric stump cancer *chir.* Magenstumpfkarzinom *nt*.
gastric surgery Magenchirurgie *f*.
gastric tumor Magengeschwulst *f*, -tumor *m*.
gastric ulcer Magengeschwür *nt*, -ulkus *nt*, Ulcus ventriculi.
gastric varices Magen(fundus)varizen *pl*.
gastric vein: left g. linke Magenkranzvene *f*, V. gastrica sinistra.
  right g. rechte Magenkranzvene *f*, V. gastrica dextra.
  short g.s kurze Magenvenen *pl*, Vv. gastricae breves.
gastric vertigo Magenschwindel *m*, Vertigo gastrica.
gastric volvulus *chir.* Magenvolvulus *m*, -torsion *f*, Volvulus ventriculi.
gas·trin [ˈgæstrɪn] *n physiol.* Gastrin *nt*.
gas·trin·o·ma [ˌgæstrɪˈnəʊmə] *n* Gastrinom *nt*.
gas·trit·ic [gæsˈtrɪtɪk] *adj* Gastritis betr., gastritisch.
gas·tri·tis [gæsˈtraɪtɪs] *n* Magenkatarrh *m*, Magen(schleimhaut)entzündung *f*, Gastritis *f*.

gastro- *pref.* Magen-, Gastro-.
gas·tro·a·ceph·a·lus [ˌgæstrəʊɛrˈsefələs] *n embryo.* Gastroazephalus *m.*
gas·tro·ad·e·ni·tis [ˌ-ædəˈnaɪtɪs] *n* → gastradenitis.
gas·tro·a·mor·phus [ˌ-əˈmɔːrfəs] *n embryo.* Gastroamorphus *m.*
gas·tro·a·nas·to·mo·sis [ˌ-əˌnæstəˈməʊsɪs] *n* → gastrogastrostomy.
gas·tro·a·to·nia [ˌ-əˈtəʊnɪə, -eɪ-] *n* Magenatonie *f*, Gastroatonie *f.*
gas·tro·cam·er·a [ˌ-ˈkæm(ə)rə] *n* Gastrokamera *f.*
gas·tro·car·di·ac [ˌ-ˈkɑːrdɪæk] *adj* Magen u. Herz betr., gastrokardial.
gastrocardiac syndrome gastrokardialer Symptomenkomplex *m*, Roemheld-Symptomenkomplex *m*, -Syndrom *nt.*
gas·tro·cele [ˈ-siːl] *n* 1. Magenhernie *f*, Gastrozele *f.* 2. Magendivertikel *nt*, Gastrozele *f.*
gas·troc·ne·mio·sem·i·mem·bra·nous bursa [ˌ-,(k)niːmɪəʊˌsemɪˈmembrənəs] Bursa *m.* semimembranosi.
gas·troc·ne·mi·us (muscle) [ˌgæstrakˈniːmɪəs, ˌgæstrəˈniː-] Gastroknemius *m*, Gastrocnemius *m*, M. gastrocnemius.
gas·tro·coel(e) [ˈgæstrəʊsiːl] *n* Urdarm *m*, Archenteron *nt.*
gas·tro·col·ic [ˌ-ˈkɔlɪk] *adj* Magen/Gaster u. Kolon betr., gastrokolisch.
gastrocolic fistula Magen-Kolon-Fistel *f*, gastrokolische Fistel *f*, Fistula gastrocolica.
gastrocolic ligament Lig. gastrocolicum.
gastrocolic omentum großes Netz *nt*, Omentum majus.
gastrocolic reflex gastrokolischer Reflex *m.*
gas·tro·co·li·tis [ˌ-kəˈlaɪtɪs] *n* Entzündung *f* von Magen u. Kolon, Gastrokolitis *f.*
gas·tro·co·lop·to·sis [ˌ-kəʊləpˈtəʊsɪs] *n patho.* Senkung *f* von Magen u. Kolon, Gastrokoloptose *f.*
gas·tro·co·los·to·my [ˌ-kəˈlɒstəmɪ] *n chir.* Magen-Kolon-Anastomose *f*, Gastrokolostomie *f.*
gas·tro·co·lot·o·my [ˌ-kəˈlɒtəmɪ] *n chir.* Gastrokolotomie *f.*
gas·tro·cu·ta·ne·ous fistula [ˌ-kjuːˈteɪnɪəs] äußere Magenfistel *f*, gastrokutane Fistel *f.*
gas·tro·di·aph·a·nos·co·py [ˌ-daɪˌæfəˈnɑskəpɪ] *n* → gastrodiaphany.
gas·tro·di·aph·a·ny [-daɪˈæfənɪ] *n* Gastrodiaphanie *f.*
gas·tro·did·y·mus [ˌ-ˈdɪdəməs] *n embryo.* Gastrodidymus *m.*
gas·tro·dis·ci·a·sis [ˌ-dɪsˈkaɪəsɪs] *n* Gastrodisciasis *f*, Gastrodiscoidiasis *f.*
Gas·tro·dis·coi·des [ˌ-dɪˈskɔɪdiːz] *n micro.* Gastrodiscoides *f.*
G. hominis Gastrodiscoides hominis.
Gas·tro·dis·cus [ˌ-ˈdɪskəs] *n* → Gastrodiscoides.
gas·tro·du·o·de·nal [ˌ-,(d)juːəʊˈdiːnl, -d(j)uːˈædnəl] *adj* Magen/Gaster u. Zwölffingerdarm/Duodenum betr. *od.* verbindend, gastroduodenal.
gastroduodenal artery Magen-Duodenum-Arterie *f*, Gastroduodenalis *f*, A. gastroduodenalis.
gastroduodenal fistula Magen-Duodenum-Fistel *f*, gastroduodenale Fistel *f.*
gastroduodenal orifice Ostium pyloricum.
gas·tro·du·o·de·nec·to·my [ˌ-,(d)juːədɪˈnektəmɪ] *n chir.* (Teil-)Entfernung *f* von Magen u. Duodenum, Gastroduodenektomie *f.*
gas·tro·du·o·de·ni·tis [ˌ-,(d)juːədɪˈnaɪtɪs] *n* Entzündung *f* von Magen u. Duodenum,

Gastroduodenitis *f.*
gas·tro·du·o·de·nos·co·py [ˌ-,(d)juːədɪˈnɒskəpɪ] *n* Gastroduodenoskopie *f.*
gas·tro·du·o·de·nos·to·my [ˌ-,(d)juːədɪˈnɒstəmɪ] *n chir.* gastroduodenale Anastomose *f*, Gastroduodenostomie *f.*
gas·tro·dyn·ia [ˌgæstrəˈdiːnɪə] *n* Magenschmerz(en *pl*) *m*, Gastrodynie *f*, Gastralgie *f.*
gas·tro·en·ter·al·gia [ˌ-ˌentəˈrældʒ(ɪ)ə] *n* Schmerzen *pl* in Magen u. Darm, Magen--Darm-Schmerz *m.*
gas·tro·en·ter·ic [ˌ-enˈterɪk] *adj* → gastrointestinal.
gastroenteric anastomosis → gastroenterostomy.
gastroenteric influenza (Magen-)Darmgrippe *f.*
gas·tro·en·ter·i·tis [ˌ-entəˈraɪtɪs] *n* Magen--Darm-Entzündung *f*, -Katarrh *m*, Gastroenteritis *f.*
gas·tro·en·ter·o·a·nas·to·mo·sis [ˌ-ˌentərəʊəˌnæstəˈməʊsɪs] *n chir.* → gastroenterostomy.
gas·tro·en·ter·o·co·li·tis [ˌ-ˌentərəʊkəˈlaɪtɪs] *n* Magen-Darm-Kolon-Entzündung *f*, -Katarrh *m*, Gastroenterokolitis *f.*
gas·tro·en·ter·o·co·los·to·my [ˌ-ˌentərəʊkəˈlɒstəmɪ] *n chir.* Gastroenterokolostomie *f.*
gas·tro·en·ter·ol·o·gist [ˌ-ˌentəˈrɒlədʒɪst] *n* Gastroenterologe *m*, -login *f.*
gas·tro·en·ter·ol·o·gy [ˌ-ˌentəˈrɒlədʒɪ] *n* Gastroenterologie *f.*
gas·tro·en·ter·op·a·thy [ˌ-ˌentəˈrɑpəθɪ] *n* Magen-Darm-Erkrankung *f*, Gastroenteropathie *f.*
gas·tro·en·ter·o·plas·ty [ˌ-ˈentərəʊplæstɪ] *n chir.* Magen-Darm-Plastik *f*, Gastroenteroplastik *f.*
gas·tro·en·ter·op·to·sis [ˌ-ˌentərɑpˈtəʊsɪs] *n* Magen-Darm-Senkung *f*, -Tiefstand *m*, Gastroenteroptose *f.*
gas·tro·en·ter·os·to·my [ˌ-ˌentəˈrɒstəmɪ] *n chir.* Magen-Darm-Anastomose *f*, Gastroenteroanastomose *f*, gastrointestinale Anastomose *f*, Gastroenterostomie *f abbr.* G.E.
gas·tro·en·ter·ot·o·my [ˌ-ˌentəˈrɒtəmɪ] *n chir.* Gastroenterotomie *f.*
gas·tro·ep·i·plo·ic [ˌgæstrəʊˌepɪˈpləʊɪk] *adj* Magen/Gaster u. Netz/Epiploon betr. *od.* verbindend, gastroomental, gastroepiploisch.
gastroepiploic artery: left g. linke Magen--Netz-Arterie *f*, Gastroepiploica *f* sinistra, A. gastroepiploica/gastro-omentalis sinistra.
right g. rechte Magen-Netz-Arterie *f*, Gastroepiploica *f* dextra, A. gastroepiploica/gastro-omentalis dextra.
gastroepiploic lymph nodes: left g. → gastroomental lymph nodes, left.
right g. → gastroomental lymph nodes, right.
gastroepiploic vein: left g. Begleitvene *f* der A. gastroepiploica sinistra, V. gastroepiploica/gastro-omentalis sinistra.
right g. Begleitvene *f* der A. gastroepiploica dextra, V. gastroepiploica/gastro--omentalis dextra.
gas·tro·e·soph·a·ge·al [ˌ-ˌɪˌsɒfəˈdʒiːəl, -ɪsəˈfædʒɪəl] *adj* Magen/Gaster u. Speiseröhre/Ösophagus betr. *od.* verbindend, gastroösophageal, ösophagogastral.
gastroesophageal hernia paraösophageale (Hiatus-)Hernie *f.*
gastroesophageal junction ösophagogastrale/gastroösophageale Übergangszone *f.*
gastroesophageal reflux *abbr.* **GER** gastroösophagealer Reflux *m.*

gastroesophageal varices gastroösophageale Varizen *pl.*
gas·tro·e·soph·a·gi·tis [ˌ-ɪˌsɒfəˈdʒaɪtɪs] *n* Entzündung *f* von Magen u. Speiseröhre, Gastroösophagitis *f.*
gas·tro·fi·bro·scope [ˌ-ˈfaɪbrəskəʊp] *n* Gastrofibroskop *nt.*
gas·tro·gas·tros·to·my [ˌ-gæsˈtrɒstəmɪ] *n chir.* Gastroanastomose *f*, Gastrogastrostomie *f.*
gas·tro·ga·vage [ˌ-gəˈvɑːʒ] *n* Ernährung *f* mittels Magensonde.
gas·tro·gen·ic [ˌ-ˈdʒenɪk] *adj* vom Magen ausgehend, aus dem Magen stammend, gastrogen.
gastrogenic diarrhea gastrogene Diarrhö *f*, Magendiarrhö *f.*
gas·trog·e·nous diarrhea [gæsˈtrɒdʒənəs] → gastrogenic diarrhea.
gas·tro·graph [ˈgæstrəgræf] *n radiol.* Gastrokinetograph *m.*
gas·tro·he·pat·ic [ˌ-hɪˈpætɪk] *adj* Magen/Gaster u. Leber/Hepar betr. *od.* verbindend, gastrohepatisch.
gastrohepatic ligament Lig. hepatogastricum.
gastrohepatic omentum kleines Netz *nt*, Omentum minus.
gas·tro·il·e·al [ˌ-ˈɪlɪæl] *adj* Magen/Gaster u. Ileum betr., gastroileal.
gastroileal reflex Gastroilealreflex *m.*
gas·tro·il·e·i·tis [ˌ-ɪlɪˈaɪtɪs] *n* Entzündung *f* von Magen u. Ileum, Gastroileitis *f.*
gas·tro·il·e·os·to·my [ˌ-ɪlɪˈɑstəmɪ] *n chir.* Magen-Ileum-Anastomose *f*, Gastroileostomie *f.*
gas·tro·in·tes·ti·nal [ˌ-ɪnˈtestənl; *Brit.* -ɪnˈtestaɪnl] *adj abbr.* **GI** Magen/Gaster u. Darm/Intestinum betr., gastrointestinal, gastroenteral, Magen-Darm-, Gastroentero-, Gastrointestino-.
gastrointestinal allergy Nahrungsmittelallergie *f.*
gastrointestinal anastomosis → gastroenterostomy.
gastrointestinal anthrax Darmmilzbrand *m*, Anthrax intestinalis.
gastrointestinal bleeding Magen-Darm--Blutung *f*, gastrointestinale Blutung *f.*
upper g. obere Magen-Darm-Blutung, obere gastrointestinale Blutung.
gastrointestinal bypass *chir.* Magen--Darm-Bypass *m*, gastrointestinaler Bypass *m.*
gastrointestinal canal → gastrointestinal tract.
gastrointestinal digestion gastrointestinale/primäre Verdauung *f*, Verdauung *f* im Magen-Darm-Trakt.
gastrointestinal duplications Duplikaturen *pl* des Magen-Darm-Traktes.
gastrointestinal fistula *patho.* Magen--Darm-Fistel *f*, gastrointestinale Fistel *f.*
gastrointestinal hemorrhage → gastrointestinal bleeding.
gastrointestinal hormone gastrointestinales Hormon *nt.*
gastrointestinal influenza (Magen-)-Darmgrippe *f.*
gastrointestinal peptide gastrointestinales Peptid *nt.*
gastrointestinal tract Magen-Darm--Trakt *m*, -Kanal *m*, Gastrointestinaltrakt *m.*
gastrointestinal tract tumor Tumor *m* des Gastrointestinaltraktes.
gas·tro·je·ju·nal anastomosis [ˌ-dʒɪˈdʒuːnl] → gastrojejunostomy.
gastrojejunal loop obstruction syndrome *chir.* Syndrom *nt* der zuführenden Schlinge, Afferent-loop-Syndrom *nt.*

gastrojejunocollic fistula

gas·tro·je·ju·no·col·ic fistula [ˌ-dʒɪˌdʒuːnəˈkɑlɪk] *patho.* Magen-Jejunum-Kolon-Fistel *f.*
gas·tro·je·ju·no·e·soph·a·gos·to·my [ˌ-dʒɪˌdʒuːnəɪˌsafəˈgastəmɪ] *n chir.* Ösophagojejunogastrostomie *f.*
gas·tro·je·ju·nos·to·my [ˌ-dʒɪˌdʒuːˈnastəmɪ] *n chir.* Magen-Jejunum-Anastomose *f*, Gastrojejunostomie *f.*
gas·tro·ki·ne·to·graph [ˌ-kɪˈniːtəgræf, -ˈnetə-] *n radiol.* Gastrokinetograph *m.*
gas·tro·la·vage [ˌ-ləˈvɑːʒ] *n* Magenspülung *f*, Gastrolavage *f.*
gas·tro·li·e·nal [ˌ-laɪˈiːnl, -ˈlaɪənl] *adj* Magen/Gaster u. Milz/Lien betr., gastrolienal.
gastrolienal ligament Magen-Milz-Band *nt*, Lig. gastrolienale/gastrosplenicum.
gas·tro·lith [ˈ-lɪθ] *n* Magenstein *m*, Gastrolith *m.*
gas·tro·li·thi·a·sis [ˌ-lɪˈθaɪəsɪs] *n* Gastrolithiasis *f.*
gas·trol·o·gist [gæˈstrɑlədʒɪst] *n* Gastrologe *m*, -login *f.*
gas·trol·o·gy [gæˈstrɑlədʒɪ] *n* Gastrologie *f.*
gas·trol·y·sis [gæˈstrɑləsɪs] *n chir.* Magenlösung *f*, -mobilisierung *f*, Gastrolyse *f.*
gas·tro·ma·la·cia [ˌgæstrəməˈleɪʃ(ɪ)ə] *n patho.* (saure) Magenerweichung *f*, Gastromalazie *f*, Gastromalacia (acida) *f.*
gas·tro·meg·a·ly [ˌ-ˈmegəlɪ] *n* Magenvergrößerung *f*, Gastromegalie *f.*
gas·trom·e·lus [gæˈstramələs] *n embryo.* Gastromelus *m.*
gas·tro·my·co·sis [ˌgæstrəmaɪˈkəʊsɪs] *n* Pilzerkrankung/Mykose *f* des Magens, Gastromykose *f.*
gas·tro·my·ot·o·my [ˌ-maɪˈɑtəmɪ] *n chir.* Gastromyotomie *f.*
gas·tro·myx·or·rhea [ˌ-ˌmɪksəˈrɪə] *n* übermäßige Schleimabsonderung *f* des Magens, Myxorrhoea gastrica.
gas·trone [ˈgæstrəʊn] *n* Gastron *nt.*
gas·tro·ne·ste·os·to·my [ˌgæstrənestɪˈastəmɪ] *n* → gastrojejunostomy.
gas·tro·o·men·tal [ˌ-əʊˈmentl] *adj* → gastroepiploic.
gastroomental artery: left g. → gastroepiploic artery, left.
right g. → gastroepiploic artery, right.
gastroomental lymph nodes: left g. linke Lymphknotengruppe *f* der großen Magenkurvatur, Nodi lymphatici viscerales gastro-omentales sinistri.
right g. rechte Lymphknotengruppe *f* der großen Magenkurvatur, Nodi lymphatici viscerales gastro-omentales dextri.
gastroomental vein: left g. → gastroepiploic vein, left.
right g. → gastroepiploic vein, right.
gas·tro·pa·gus [gæˈstrapəgəs] *n embryo.* Gastropagus *m.*
gas·tro·pan·cre·at·ic [ˌgæstrəˌpænkrɪˈætɪk, -ˌpæn-] *adj* Magen/Gaster u. Bauchspeicheldrüse/Pancreas betr. *od.* verbindend.
gastropancreatic fold Plica gastropancreatica.
gastropancreatic ligament of Huschke → gastropancreatic fold.
gas·tro·pan·cre·a·ti·tis [ˌ-ˌpænkrɪəˈtaɪtɪs] *n* Entzündung *f* von Magen u. Pankreas, Gastropankreatitis *f.*
gas·tro·pa·ral·y·sis [ˌ-pəˈrælɪsɪs] *n* 1. → gastroparesis. 2. → gastroatonia.
gas·tro·pa·re·sis [ˌ-pəˈriːsɪs, -ˈpærə-] *n* Magenlähmung *f*, Gastroparese *f*, -paralyse *f*, -plegie *f.*
gas·tro·path·ic [ˌ-ˈpæθɪk] *adj* Gastropathie betr.
gas·tropa·thy [gæˈstrapəθɪ] *n* Magenerkrankung *f*, -leiden *nt*, Gastropathie *f*, -pathia *f.*
gas·tro·per·i·o·dyn·ia [ˌgæstrəperɪəˈdiːnɪə] *n* periodischer Magenschmerz *m.*
gas·tro·per·i·to·ni·tis [ˌ-perɪtəˈnaɪtɪs] *n* Entzündung *f* von Magen u. Peritoneum, Gastroperitonitis *f.*
gas·tro·pex·y [ˈ-peksɪ] *n chir.* Magenanheftung *f*, Gastropexie *f.*
Gas·tro·phil·i·dae [ˌ-ˈfɪlədiː] *pl* → Gasterophilidae.
Gas·troph·i·lus [gæˈstrafɪləs] *n* → Gasterophilus.
gas·tro·phren·ic [ˌgæstrəˈfrenɪk] *adj* Magen/Gaster u. Zwerchfell betr., gastrophrenisch.
gastrophrenic ligament Lig. gastrophrenicum.
gas·tro·plas·ty [ˈgæstrəplæstɪ] *n chir.* Magenplastik *f*, Gastroplastik *f.*
gas·tro·ple·gia [ˌ-ˈpliːdʒ(ɪ)ə] *n* → gastroparesis.
gas·tro·pli·ca·tion [ˌ-plaɪˈkeɪʃn] *n chir.* Gastroplikation *f*, Gastroplicatio *f.*
gas·tro·pneu·mon·ic [ˌ-n(j)uːˈmɑnɪk] *adj* Magen/Gaster u. Lunge(n) betr., gastropulmonal.
gas·tro·pod [ˈ-pɑd] *n bio.* Schnecke *f*, Gastropode *m.*
Gas·trop·o·da [gæˈstrapədə] *pl bio.* Schnecken *pl*, Gastropoden *pl*, Gastropoda *pl.*
gas·trop·to·sis [ˌgæstrapˈtəʊsɪs] *n patho.* Magensenkung *f*, -tiefstand *m*, Gastroptose *f.*
gas·trop·tyx·is [ˌgæstrapˈtɪksɪs] *n* → gastroplication.
gas·tro·pul·mo·nar·y [ˌ-ˈpʌlməˌnerɪː, -nərɪ] *adj* Magen/Gaster u. Lunge(n) betr., gastropulmonal.
gas·tro·py·lo·rec·to·my [ˌ-ˌpaɪləˈrektəmɪ] *n chir.* Gastropylorektomie *f.*
gas·tro·py·lor·ic [ˌ-paɪˈlɔːrɪk, -pɪ-] *adj* gastropylorisch.
gas·tror·rha·gia [ˌ-ˈrædʒ(ɪ)ə] *n* Magenblutung *f*, Gastrorrhagie *f.*
gas·tror·rha·phy [gæˈstrɔrəfɪ] *n chir.* 1. Magennaht *f*, Naht *f* der Magenwand, Gastrorrhaphie *f.* 2. → gastroplication.
gas·tror·rhea [ˌgæstrəˈrɪə] *n patho.* Magenfluß *m*, Hypersekretion *f* des Magens, Gastrorrhoe *f.*
gas·tror·rhex·is [ˌ-ˈreksɪs] *n patho.* Magenruptur *f*, Gastrorrhexis *f.*
gas·tros·chi·sis [gæˈstraskəsɪs] *n embryo.* Bauchspalte *f*, Gastroschisis *f.*
gas·tro·scope [ˈgæstrəskəʊp] *n* Gastroskop *nt.*
gas·tro·scop·ic [ˌ-ˈskɑpɪk] *adj* Gastroskop *od.* Gastroskopie betr., mittels Gastroskop *od.* Gastroskopie, gastroskopisch.
gas·tros·co·py [gæˈstraskəpɪ] *n* Magenspiegelung *f*, Gastroskopie *f.*
gas·tro·se·lec·tive [ˌgæstrəsɪˈlektɪv] *adj* magenselektiv, gastroselektiv.
gas·tro·spasm [ˈ-spæzəm] *n* Magenkrampf *m*, -kolik *f*, Gastrospasmus *m*; Colica gastrica.
gas·tro·splen·ic [ˌ-ˈspliːnɪk, -ˈsplenɪk] *adj* → gastrolienal.
gastrosplenic ligament → gastrolienal ligament.
gastrosplenic omentum → gastrolienal ligament.
gas·tro·stax·is [ˌ-ˈstæksɪs] *n patho.* 1. Sickerblutung *f* aus der Magenschleimhaut, Gastrostaxis *f.* 2. hämorrhagische Gastritis *f.*
gas·tro·ste·no·sis [ˌ-stɪˈnəʊsɪs] *n* Magenverengung *f*, -stenose *f*, Gastrostenose *f.*
gas·tros·to·ga·vage [gæˌstrastəgəˈvɑːʒ] *n* Ernährung *f* mittels Magensonde.
gas·tros·to·ma [gæˈstrastəmə] *n chir.* äußere Magenfistel *f*, Gastrostoma *nt.*
gas·tros·to·my [gæˈstrastəmɪ] *n chir.* Gastrostomie *f.*
gas·tro·suc·cor·rhe·a [ˌgæstrəsʌkəˈrɪə] *n* Reichmann-Syndrom *nt*, Gastrosukorrhoe *f.*
gas·tro·tho·ra·cop·a·gus [ˌ-ˌθɔːrəˈkapəgəs, -ˌθɔː-] *n embryo.* Gastrothorakopagus *m.*
gas·tro·tome [ˈ-təʊm] *n chir.* Gastrotomiemesser *nt*, Gastrotom *nt.*
gas·trot·o·my [gæsˈtratəmɪ] *n chir.* Magenerößnung *f*, -schnitt *m*, Gastrotomie *f.*
gas·tro·to·nom·e·ter [ˌgæstrətəˈnamɪtər] *n* Gastrotonometer *nt.*
gas·tro·to·nom·e·try [ˌgæstrətəˈnamətrɪ] *n* Gastrotonometrie *f.*
gas·tro·trop·ic [ˌgæstrəˈtrapɪk, -ˈtrəʊp-] *adj* gastrotrop.
gas·tro·tym·pa·ni·tis [ˌ-tɪmpəˈnaɪtɪs] *n* Magenüberblähung *f.*
gas·tro·vas·cu·lar cavity [ˌ-ˈvæskjələr] *embryo.* Gastrovaskularraum *m*, -system *nt.*
gas·tru·la [ˈgæstrələ] *n, pl* **-las, -lae** [-liː] *embryo.* Gastrula *f.*
gas·tru·la·tion [ˌgæstrʊˈleɪʃn] *n embryo.* Gastrulation *f.*
gate [geɪt] *n* 1. Tor *nt*, Pforte *f*, (enger) Durchgang *m*, Schranke *f.* 2. *fig.* Zugang *m*, Weg *m* (*to* zu); Schranke *f.*
gate-control hypothesis Gate-Control-Theorie *f*, Kontrollschrankentheorie *f.*
gate-control theory → gate-control hypothesis.
gate hypothesis → gate-control hypothesis.
gate theory → gate-control hypothesis.
gate·way [ˈgeɪtweɪ] *n* (*a. fig.*) Ein-, Zugang *m*, Tor *nt*, Weg *m* (*to* zu).
gat·ing current [ˈgeɪtɪŋ] *physiol.* Torstrom *m.*
Gaucher [ɡoˈʃeɪ]: **G.'s cell** Gaucher-Zelle *f.*
G.'s disease Gaucher'-Erkrankung *f*, -Krankheit *f*, -Syndrom *nt*, Morbus Gaucher *m*, Glukozerebrosidose *f*, Zerebrosidlipidose *f*, Lipoidhistiozytose *f* vom Kerasintyp, Glykosylzeramidlipidose *f.*
G.'s disease, acute neuronopathic type → G.'s disease, type 2.
G.'s disease, adult type → G.'s disease, type 1.
G.'s disease, chronic non-neuronopathic type → G.'s disease, type 1.
G.'s disease, infantile type → G.'s disease, type 2.
G.'s disease, juvenile type → G.'s disease, type 3.
G.'s disease, subacute neuronopathic type → G.'s disease, type 3.
G.'s disease, type 1 Gaucher-Krankheit Typ I *f*, chronische nicht-neuronopathische Form *f*, adulte Form *f.*
G.'s disease, type 2 Gaucher-Krankheit Typ II *f*, akute neuronopathische Form *f*, infantile Form *f.*
G.'s disease, type 3 Gaucher-Krankheit Typ III *f*, subakute neuronopathische Form *f*, juvenile Form *f.*
G.'s splenomegaly → G.'s disease.
Gauer-Henry [ˈɡaʊər ˈhenrɪ]: **G.-H. reflex** Gauer-Henry-Reflex *m.*
gauge [ɡeɪdʒ] **I** *n* 1. Meßgerät *nt*, Messer *m*, Anzeiger *m.* 2. Maß-, Zollstab *m.* 3. Normal-, Eichmaß *nt.* 4. Umfang *m*, Inhalt *m.* **II** *vt* 5. (ab-, aus-)messen, prüfen. 6. eichen, justieren, kalibrieren.
Gault [ɡɔːlt]: **G.'s cochleopalpebral reflex** Gault-Reflex *m.*

gaunt·let anesthesia ['gɔːntlɪt, 'gɑnt-] *neuro.* Handschuhanästhesie *f.*
gauntlet bandage *ortho.* Handschuhverband *m.*
gauntlet flap Stiellappen *m*, gestielter (Haut-)Lappen *m.*
gauss [gaʊs] *n abbr.* **G** Gauß *nt abbr.* G.
gauss·i·an ['gaʊsɪən]: **g. curve** *stat.* Glockenkurve *f*, Gauss-Kurve *f.* **g. distribution** *stat.* Gauss'-Normalverteilung *f.*
gauze [gɔːz] *n* Gaze *f*, Verband(s)mull *m.*
gauze bandage Mullbinde *f.*
gauze dressing Gazeverband *m.*
gauze wick Gazestreifen *m.*
ga·vage [gəˈvɑːʒ] *n* 1. Zwangsernährung *f* (mittels Magensonde). 2. therapeutische Hyperalimentation *f.*
Gay [geɪ]: **G.'s glands** zirkumanale Drüsen *pl*, Gll. anales/circumanales.
Gay-Lussac [lyˈsak]: **G.-L.'s law** *phys.* Gay--Lussac'-Gesetz *nt.*
gaze [geɪz] **I** *n* (starrer) Blick *m*, Starren *nt.* **II** *vi* anstarren, starren (*at* auf).
gaze center Blickzentrum *nt.*
gaze-evoked nystagmus → gaze nystagmus.
gaze hyperkinesia Blickhyperkinesie *f.*
gaze nystagmus Blickrichtungs-, Blicklähmungsnystagmus *m.*
gaze-paretic nystagmus → gaze nystagmus.
gaze saccade Blicksakkade *f.*
G band (*Chromosom*) G-Bande *f.*
G-banding *genet.* G-Banding *nt*, Giemsa--Banding *nt.*
GBG *abbr.* → glycine-rich β-glycoprotein.
GBM *abbr.* → glomerular basement membrane.
GBS *abbr.* → Guillain-Barré syndrome.
GC *abbr.* → gas chromatography.
g-cal *abbr.* → gram calorie.
G cell 1. (*Pankreas*) G-Zelle *f*, Gastrinzelle *f.* 2. (*Hypophyse*) G-Zelle *f*, Gammazelle *f.*
G cell tumor (*Pankreas*) G-Zell(en)-Tumor *m.*
γ chain γ-Kette *f.*
Gd *abbr.* → gadolinium.
GDP *abbr.* → guanosine(-5'-)diphosphate.
Ge *abbr.* → germanium.
ge- *pref.* → geo-.
gear [gɪər] *n* Ausrüstung *f*, Gerät *nt*, Werkzeug(e *pl*) *nt*, Zubehör *nt*, Vorrichtung *f.*
Gee [giː]: **G.'s disease** → Gee-Herter-Heubner disease.
Gee-Herter ['hɜrtər]: **G.-H. disease** → Gee-Herter-Heubner disease.
Gee-Herter-Heubner ['hɔybnər]: **G.-H.-H. disease/syndrome** Herter-Heubner-Syndrom *nt*, Gee-Herter-Heubner-Syndrom *nt*, Heubner-Herter-Krankheit *f*, (infantile Form der) Zöliakie *f*, glutenbedingte Enteropathie *f.*
Gee-Thaysen ['θaɪsn]: **G.-T. disease** Erwachsenenform *f* der Zöliakie, einheimische Sprue *f.*
Gegenbaur ['geɪgnbaʊər; 'geːgən-]: **G.'s cell** Osteoblast *m*, -plast *m.*
ge·gen·hal·ten [ˌgeɪgənˈhæltn; 'geːgənhaltn] *n neuro.* Gegenhalten *nt.*
Geigel ['gaɪgəl]: **G.'s reflex** Geigel-Reflex *m*, Leistenreflex *m*, Femoroabdominalreflex *m.*
Geiger ['gaɪgər]: **G. counter** Geiger-Zählrohr *m*, -Zähler *m*, Geiger-Müller-Zählrohr *nt*, -Zähler *m.*
Geiger-Müller ['mɪlər; 'mʏlər]: **G.-M. counter/tube** → Geiger counter.
gel [dʒel] **I** *n* Gel *nt.* **II** *vi* gelieren, ein Gel bilden.

ge·las·mus [dʒɪˈlæzməs] *n psychia.* zwanghaftes/hysterisches Lachen *nt*, Lachkrampf *m*, Gelasma *nt.*
ge·las·tic [dʒɪˈlæstɪk] *adj* lachend, Lach-.
gel·ate ['dʒeleɪt] *vi* → gel II.
gel·at·i·fi·ca·tion [dʒəˌlætɪfɪˈkeɪʃn] *n* Gelatinieren *nt*, Gelatinierung *f.*
gel·a·tin ['dʒelətɪn; *Brit.* -tiːn] *n* Gelatine *f*, Gelatina *f*, Gallerte *f*, Gelee *m/nt.*
gel·a·tin·ase [dʒəˈlætɪneɪz, 'dʒelətɪneɪz] *n* Gelatinase *f.*
gel·at·i·nate [dʒəˈlætɪneɪt] *vt, vi* → gelatinize.
gelatin culture medium Gelatinenährboden *m*, -medium *nt.*
gel·a·tine *n* → gelatin.
gelatine sugar Aminoessigsäure *f*, Glyzin *nt*, Glycin *nt*, Glykokoll *nt abbr.* Gly.
gel·a·tin·if·er·ous [ˌdʒelətɪˈnɪfərəs] *adj* gelatinbildend.
gelatin form cancer/carcinoma [dʒeləˈtɪnəfɔːrm] → gelatinous carcinoma.
gelatiniform degeneration gallertige Degeneration *f.*
ge·lat·i·nize [dʒəˈlætɪnaɪz, 'dʒelətn-] **I** *vt* gelatinieren lassen. **II** *vi* gelatinieren.
gelatin medium → gelatin culture medium.
ge·lat·i·noid [dʒəˈlætɪnɔɪd] **I** *n* gallertartige Substanz *f.* **II** *adj* → gelatinous 1.
ge·lat·i·nous [dʒəˈlætɪnəs] *adj* 1. gel-, gallert-, gelatineartig, gelatinös, Gallert-. 2. Gel enthaltend.
gelatinous ascites Gallertbauch *m*, Pseudomyxoma peritonei.
gelatinous cancer → gelatinous carcinoma.
gelatinous carcinoma Gallert-, Schleim-, Kolloidkrebs *m*, -karzinom *nt*, Ca. colloides/gelatinosum/mucoides/mucosum.
gelatinous infiltration (*Lunge*) graue Infiltration *f.*
gelatinous nucleus Gallertkern *m*, Nc. pulposus.
gelatinous pneumonia gelatinöse Pneumonie *f.*
gelatinous polyp Myxom(a) *nt.*
gelatinous substance: **central g.** Substantia gelatinosa centralis. **g. of spinal cord** Substantia gelatinosa.
gelatinous tissue gallertartiges/gallertiges Bindegewebe.
gelatinous tumor Myxom(a) *nt.*
ge·la·tion [dʒəˈleɪʃn] *n* 1. Einfrieren *nt.* 2. Gelierung *f.*
geld [geld] (**gelded**; **geld**) *vt bio.* kastrieren, verschneiden.
gel diffusion test Geldiffusionstest *m*, Agardiffusionstest *m.*
geld·ing ['geldɪŋ] *n bio.* Kastrieren *nt*, Verschneiden *nt.*
gel electrophoresis *lab.* Gelelektrophorese *f.*
gel filtration Gelfiltration *f*, Molekularsiebfiltration *f*, molekulare Ausschlußchromatographie *f.*
gel-filtration chromatography Gel(filtrations)chromatographie *f.*
Gélineau [ʒeliˈno]: **G.'s syndrome** Narkolepsie *f.*
Gell and Coombs [gel kuːms]: **G.a.C. classification** *immun.* Gell-Coombs-Klassifikation *f.*
Gellé [ʒəˈle]: **G.'s test** *HNO* Gellé-Versuch *m.*
gel·ose ['dʒeləʊs] *n* Agar *m/nt.*
ge·lo·sis [dʒɪˈləʊsɪs] *n*, *pl* **-ses** [-siːz] *patho.* knotenförmige Gewebsverhärtung *f*, Gelose *f*; Myogelose *f.*
gel·o·trip·sy ['dʒelətrɪpsi] *n* Gelotripsie *f.*
gel-permeation chromatography Gel(filtrations)chromatographie *f.*

gem·el·lar·y ['dʒemɪleriː] *adj* Zwillinge betr., Zwillings-.
gemellary pregnancy Zwillingsschwangerschaft *f.*
gem·el·lip·a·ra [ˌdʒeməˈlɪpərə] *n gyn.* Patientin *f* mit Zwillingsgeburt, Gemellipara *f.*
gem·el·lol·o·gy [ˌdʒeməˈlɑlədʒɪ] *n* Zwillingsforschung *f*, Geminologie *f.*
ge·mel·lus inferior (**muscle**) [dʒɪˈmeləs] Gemellus *m* inferior/tuberalis, M. gemellus inferior.
gemellus (**muscle**) Gemellus *m*, M. gemellus.
gemellus superior (**muscle**) Gemellus *m* superior/spinalis, M. gemellus superior.
gem·i·nate [*adj* 'dʒemənɪt, -neɪt; *v* -neɪt] *adj* paarweise (auftretend), gepaart, Doppel-. **II** *vt* verdoppeln. **III** *vi* s. verdoppeln.
gem·i·ni *pl* → geminus.
gem·i·nous ['dʒemɪnəs] *adj, vt, vi* → geminate.
gem·i·nus ['dʒemɪnəs] *n*, *pl* **-ni** [-niː, -naɪ] Zwilling *m*, Geminus *m.*
gem·is·to·cyte [dʒəˈmɪstəsaɪt] *n* gemistozytischer Astrozyt *m*, Gemistozyt *m.*
gem·is·to·cyt·ic astrocyte [ˌ-ˈsɪtɪk] → gemistocyte.
gemistocytic astrocytoma gemistozytisches Astrozytom *nt.*
gemistocytic cell → gemistocyte.
gem·ma ['dʒemə] *n* 1. *anat.* Knospe *f*, knospenähnliche Struktur *f*, Gemma *f.* 2. Geschmacksknospe *f*, Gemma gustatoria, Caliculus gustatorius. 3. *bio.* Brutkörper *m*, Gemme *f.*
gem·man·gi·o·ma [ˌdʒemændʒɪˈəʊmə] *n* Hämangioendotheliom(a) *nt.*
gem·ma·tion [dʒəˈmeɪʃn] *n bio.* Knospung *f*; Knospenbildung *f.*
gem·mif·e·rous [dʒəˈmɪfərəs] *adj bio.* knospentragend.
gem·mule ['dʒem(j)uːl] *n bio.* Keim-, Dauerknospe *f*, Gemmula *f.*
ge·nal ['dʒiːnl, 'gen-] *adj* Wange betr., bukkal, Wangen-, Backen-.
gen·der ['dʒendər] *n* (anatomisches) Geschlecht *nt.*
gene [dʒiːn] *n* Gen *nt*, Erbfaktor *m*, -einheit *f*, -anlage *f.*
gene action Genwirkung *f.*
gene activation Genaktivierung *f.*
gene activity Gentätigkeit *f*, -aktivität *f.*
gene balance genetische Balance *f*, Genbalance *f.*
gene combination Genkombination *f.*
gene complex Genkomplex *m.*
gene conversion Genkonversion *f.*
gene duplication Genverdopplung *f*, -duplikation *f.*
gene exchange Genaustausch *m.*
gene expression Genausprägung *f*, -manifestierung *f*, -manifestation *f*, -expression *f.*
gene flow Genfluß *m*, Gen-flow *m.*
gene frequency Genhäufigkeit *f*, -frequenz *f.*
gene function Genfunktion *f.*
gene interaction Genwechselwirkung *f.*
gene linkage Genkopplung *f*, Faktorenkopplung *f.*
gene map Genkarte *f.*
gene mapping Genkartierung *f.*
gene mutation Genmutation *f.*
gene pool Genpool *m.*
gen·e·ra *pl* → genus.
gen·er·al ['dʒenərəl] *adj* allgemein, generell, Allgemein-; allgemeingültig, üblich. **the ~ practice** das übliche Verfahren. **as a ~ rule** meistens. **for ~ use** für den allgemeinen *od.* normalen Gebrauch.

general-adaptation reaction → general-adaptation syndrome.
general-adaptation syndrome Adaptationssyndrom *nt*, allgemeines Anpassungssyndrom *nt abbr.* AAS.
general anatomy allgemeine Anatomie *f*.
general anesthesia Voll-, Allgemeinnarkose *f*, -anästhesie *f*, *inf.* Narkose *f*.
general anesthetic (Allgemein-)Narkotikum *nt*, Narkosemittel *nt*.
general condition Allgemeinzustand *m*, -befinden *nt*.
general donor *immun.* Universalspender *m*.
general gas equation allgemeine Gasgleichung *f*.
general health Allgemeinzustand *m*.
general hospital allgemeines Krankenhaus *nt*.
gen·er·al·i·za·tion [ˌdʒenərəliˈzeɪʃn] *n* 1. Verallgemeinerung *f*, Generalisation *f*. 2. *patho.* Generalisierung *f*, Generalisation *f*, Ausbreitung *f* auf dem gesamten Körper; Metastasierung *f*. 3. *psycho.* Generalisierung *f*.
gen·er·al·ize [ˈdʒenərəlaɪz] I *vt* verallgemeinern, generalisieren. II *vi* 1. verallgemeinern, allgemeine Schlüsse ziehen (*from* aus). 2. (*Krankheit*) *s.* generalisieren.
gen·er·al·ized amnesis [ˈdʒenərəlaɪzd] generalisierte Amnesie *f*, Totalamnesie *f*.
generalized anaphylaxis anaphylaktischer Schock *m*, Anaphylaxie *f*.
generalized anxiety disorder generalisierte Angst(neurose) *f*.
generalized chondromalacia (von) Meyenburg-Altherr-Uehlinger-Syndrom *nt*, rezidivierende Polychondritis *f*, systematisierte Chondromalazie *f*.
generalized cortical hyperostosis van Buchem-Syndrom *nt*, Hyperostosis corticalis generalisata.
generalized elastolysis generalisierte Elastolyse *f*, Fall-, Schlaffhaut *f*, Dermatochalasis *f*, Dermatomegalie *f*, Chalodermie *f*, Chalazodermie *f*, Cutis laxa (-Syndrom *nt*).
generalized emphysema panazinäres/panlobuläres/diffuses Lungenemphysem *nt*.
generalized epilepsy generalisierte Epilepsie *f*.
generalized essential telangiectasia generalisierte essentielle Teleangiektasie *f*.
generalized flexion epilepsy *neuro.* Hypsarrhythmie *f*.
generalized gangliosidosis → GM₁-gangliosidosis.
generalized glycogenosis → glycogen storage disease, type II.
generalized lipodystrophy Lawrence-Syndrom *nt*, lipatrophischer Diabetes *m*.
generalized morphea *derm.* Morphea generalisata.
generalized psoriasis *derm.* Psoriasis generalisata/universalis.
generalized pustular psoriasis of Zumbusch *derm.* Psoriasis pustulosa vom Typ Zumbusch, Psoriasis pustulosa generalisata, Psoriasis pustulosa gravis Zumbusch.
generalized scleroderma progressive/diffuse/systemische Sklerodermie *f*, systemische Sklerose *f*, Systemsklerose *f*, Sclerodermia diffusa/progressiva.
generalized transduction generalisierte/allgemeine Transduktion *f*.
general knowledge Allgemeinwissen *nt*, Allgemeinbildung *f*.
gen·er·al·ly contracted pelvis [ˈdʒenərəli]

allgemein verengtes Becken *nt*.
general medicine Allgemeinmedizin *f*.
general paralysis → general paralysis of the insane.
 g. of the insane *abbr.* **GPI** progressive Paralyse *f abbr.* PP, Paralysis progressiva.
general paresis → general paralysis of the insane.
general pathology allgemeine Pathologie *f*.
general peritonitis generalisierte Bauchfellentzündung *f*, Peritonitis diffusa.
general practitioner *abbr.* **GP** praktischer Arzt *m*, praktische Ärztin *f*, Arzt *m*/Ärztin *f* für Allgemeinmedizin, Allgemeinmediziner(in *f*) *m*.
general recipient *immun.* Universalempfänger(in *f*) *m*.
general sensation *physiol.* Allgemeinempfindung *f*.
general surgery Allgemeinchirurgie *f*.
general surgical disease allgemeinchirurgische Erkrankung *f*.
general term Allgemeinbegriff *m*.
general transduction → generalized transduction.
general tuberculosis Miliartuberkulose *f*, miliare Tuberkulose *f*, Tuberculosis miliaris.
gen·er·ate [ˈdʒenəreɪt] *vt* 1. *electr.* erzeugen (*from* aus); (*Wärme, Rauch*) entwickeln. 2. *fig.* verursachen, hervorbringen, bewirken. 3. *bio.* zeugen.
gen·er·at·ing [ˈdʒenəreɪtɪŋ] *adj* erzeugend.
gen·er·a·tion [ˌdʒenəˈreɪʃn] *n* 1. Generation *f*; Menschenalter *nt*. 2. *chem., phys., electr.* Erzeugung *f*; Entwicklung *f*. 3. Zeugung *f*, Fortpflanzung *f*. 4. Entstehung *f*.
 g. of force Krafterzeugung, -entwicklung.
gen·er·a·tion·al [ˌdʒenəˈreɪʃnəl] *adj* Generations-.
generational conflict Generationskonflikt *m*, -unterschied *m*.
generation index *bio.* Generationsindex *m*.
generation interval Generationsintervall *nt*.
generation time Generationszeit *f*, -dauer *f*.
gen·er·a·tive [ˈdʒenərətɪv, -reɪtɪv] *adj* 1. Zeugung *od.* Fortpflanzung betr., generativ, geschlechtlich, Zeugungs-, Fortpflanzungs-. 2. fortpflanzungsfähig, fruchtbar.
generative cell reife Keimzelle *f*, Geschlechtszelle *f*, Gamet *m*, Gamozyt *m*.
gen·er·a·tive·ness [ˈdʒenəreɪtɪvnɪs] *n* Fortpflanzungsfähigkeit *f*, Generativität *f*.
generative organs → genitalia.
generative power Zeugungskraft *f*.
gen·er·a·tor [ˈdʒenəreɪtər] *n* 1. *electr.* Generator *m*, Stromerzeuger *m* Dynamomaschine *f*. 2. *chem.* Entwickler *m*. 3. *bio.* (Er-)Zeuger *m*.
generator potential Generatorpotential *nt*.
gene recombination Genrekombination *f*.
gene reduplication Genverdoppelung *f*, -reduplikation *f*.
gene regulation Genregulation *f*.
gene repression *genet.* Genrepression *f*.
gene repressor Genrepressor *m*.
ge·ner·ic [dʒəˈnerɪk] I *n* (*meist ~s pl*) → generic drugs. II *adj* 1. *bio.* Geschlecht *nt*. Gattung betr., generisch, Gattungs-. 2. → general.
ge·ner·i·cal [dʒəˈnerɪkl] *adj* → generic II.
generic drugs *pharm.* Fertigarzneimittel *pl*, Generika *pl*, Generica *pl*.

316

generic name 1. *pharm.* Freiname *m*, generic name (*m*). 2. *bio.* Gattungsname *m*, -bezeichnung *f*.
ge·ne·si·al [dʒəˈniːʒ(ɪ)əl] *adj* → generic 1.
ge·nes·ic [dʒəˈnesɪk, -niː-] *adj* → generic 1.
gen·e·sis [ˈdʒenəsɪs] *n* Entstehung *f*, Erzeugung *f*, Entwicklung *f*, Genese *f*, Genesis *f*.
ge·net·ic [dʒəˈnetɪk] *adj* Genetik *od.* Gene betr., durch Gene bedingt, genetisch, erbbiologisch, Vererbungs-, Erb-, Entwicklungs-.
ge·net·i·cal [dʒəˈnetɪkl] *adj* → genetic.
genetic analysis Erbanalyse *f*.
genetic assimilation genetische Assimilation *f*.
genetic code genetischer Kode/Code *m*.
genetic complement Genbestand *m*.
genetic continuity genetische Kontinuität *f*.
genetic counseling genetische Beratung *f*.
genetic coupling Genkopplung *f*, Faktorenkopplung *f*.
genetic damage Genschaden *m*, -schädigung *f*, genetische Schädigung *f*.
genetic disease genetische/genetisch-bedingte Erkrankung/Krankheit *f*.
genetic disorder → genetic disease.
genetic drift genetische Drift *f*, Gendrift *f*.
genetic engineering Genmanipulation *f*, genetische Manipulation *f*, Genetic engineering *n*.
genetic exchange Genaustausch *m*.
genetic immunity angeborene Immunität *f*.
genetic information Erbinformation *f*, -substanz *f*.
genetic interactions *micro.* (*Virus*) genetische Wechselwirkungen *pl*.
ge·net·i·cist [dʒəˈnetəsɪst] *n* Genetiker(in *f*) *m*.
genetic map Genkarte *f*.
genetic material genetisches Material *nt*, Genmaterial *nt*.
genetic memory genetisches Gedächtnis *nt*.
genetic mutant genetische Mutante *f*.
genetic polymorphism genetischer Polymorphismus *m*.
genetic rearrangement genetischer Umbau *m*.
genetic reassortment genetisches Reassortment *nt*.
ge·net·ics [dʒəˈnetɪks] *pl* 1. Genetik *f*, Erb-, Vererbungslehre *f*. 2. Erbanlagen *pl*.
genetic sex chromosomales/genetisches Geschlecht *nt*.
ge·net·o·troph·ic [dʒəˌnetəˈtrɑfɪk, -ˈtroʊ-] *adj* genetotroph(isch).
gene transfer Genübertragung *f*, -transfer *m*.
Ge·ne·va Convention [dʒəˈniːvə] Genfer Konvention *f*.
Gengou [ʒɑ̃ˈɡu]: **G. phenomenon** Gengou-Phänomen *nt*, Komplementbindung *f*.
geni- *pref.* → genio-.
ge·ni·al [dʒəˈnaɪəl, ˈdʒiːnɪəl] *adj* Kinn betr., Kinn-, Geni(o)-, Mento-; Unterkiefer-.
genial apophysis Spina mentalis.
ge·ni·an [dʒəˈnaɪən, ˈdʒiːnɪən] *adj* → genial.
gen·ic [ˈdʒenɪk] *adj* Gen(e) betr., durch Gene bedingt, Gen-.
genic action Genwirkung *f*.
genic balance genetische Balance *f*, Genbalance *f*.
ge·nic·u·lar [dʒəˈnɪkjələr] *adj* Knie(gelenk) betr., Knie-, Kniegelenks-
genicular artery: descending g. absteigende Kniegelenksarterie *f*, A. descendens genicularis.

lateral inferior g. A. inferior lateralis genus.
lateral superior g. A. superior lateralis genus.
medial inferior g. A. inferior medialis genus.
medial superior g. A. superior medialis genus.
middle g. A. media genus.
genicular veins Knie(gelenks)venen *pl*, Vv. geniculares.
ge·nic·u·late [dʒə'nɪkjəlɪt, -leɪt] *adj anat.* knoten-, knieförmig.
geniculate body: lateral g. *abbr.* **LGB** lateraler Kniehöcker *m*, Corpus geniculatum laterale *abbr.* CGL.
medial g. *abbr.* **MGB** medialer Kniehöcker *m*, Corpus geniculatum mediale *abbr.* CGM.
geniculate cells Geniculatumzellen *pl*, Zellen *pl* des Kniehöckers.
ge·nic·u·lat·ed [dʒə'nɪkjəleɪtɪd] *adj* → geniculate.
geniculate ganglion (sensorisches) Fazialis(knie)ganglion *nt*, Ggl. geniculatum/ geniculi (n. facialis).
geniculate neuralgia *neuro.* Genikulatumneuralgie *f*, Ramsay Hunt-Syndrom *nt*, Neuralgia geniculata, Zoster oticus, Herpes zoster oticus.
geniculate nucleus: lateral g. Kern *m* des lateralen Kniehöckers, Nc. geniculatus lateralis.
medial g. Kern *m* des medialen Kniehöckers, Nc. geniculatus medialis.
geniculate otalgia → geniculate neuralgia.
ge·nic·u·lo·cal·car·ine radiation [dʒə,nɪkjələʊ'kælkəraɪn] → geniculocalcarine tract.
geniculocalcarine tract Gratiolet'-Sehstrahlung *f*, Radiatio optica.
ge·nic·u·lum [dʒə'nɪkjələm] *n, pl* **-la** [-lə] *anat.* kleines Knie *nt*, kleine knieähnliche Struktur *f*, Geniculum *nt*.
g. of facial canal Knie des Fazialiskanals, Geniculum canalis facialis.
g. of facial nerve äußeres Fazialisknie, Geniculum n.facialis.
genio- *pref.* Kinn-, Geni(o)-, Mento-; Unterkiefer-.
ge·ni·o·chei·lo·plas·ty [,dʒi:nɪəʊ'kaɪləplæsti] *n chir.* Lippen-Kinn-Plastik *f*.
ge·ni·o·glos·sus (muscle) [,-'glɑsəs, -'glɒs-] Genioglossus *m*, M. genioglossus.
ge·ni·o·hy·o·glos·sus [,-haɪə'glɑsəs] *n* → genioglossus (muscle).
ge·ni·o·hy·oi·de·us (muscle) [,-haɪ'ɔɪdɪəs] Geniohyoideus *m*, M. geniohyoideus.
ge·ni·o·hy·oid (muscle) [,-'haɪɔɪd] → geniohyoideus (muscle).
ge·ni·o·plas·ty ['-plæsti] *n chir.* Kinnplastik *f*, Genioplastik *f*.
genit- *pref.* → genito-.
gen·i·tal ['dʒenɪtl] *adj* 1. Zeugung *od.* Vermehrung betr., genital, Zeugungs-, Fortpflanzungs-. 2. Geschlechtsorgane/Genitalien betr., genital, Geschlechts-, Genital-.
genital branch of genitofemoral nerve Genitalast *m* des N. genitofemoralis, N. spermaticus externus, Ramus genitalis (n. genitofemoralis).
genital canal → genital duct.
genital center geniospinales Zentrum *nt*, Centrum genitospinale.
genital cleft *embryo.* Genitalspalte *f*.
genital corpuscles Nervenkörperchen *pl* der Corpitalregion, Corpuscula genitalia.
genital cycle Genital-, Monats-, Sexual-, Menstrual-, Menstruationszyklus *m*.

genital duct *embryo.* Genitalgang *m*, -kanal *m*.
genital eminence → genital tubercle.
genital fold *embryo.* Geschlechts-, Genitalfalte *f*, -leiste *f*.
genital gland 1. weibliche Geschlechts-/ Keimdrüse *f*, Eierstock *m*, Ovarium *nt*, Ovar *nt*, Oophoron *nt*. 2. männliche Geschlechts-/Keimdrüse *f*, Hode(n) *m*, Testikel *m*, Testis *m*, Orchis *m*.
genital herpes Herpes genitalis.
gen·i·ta·lia [,dʒenɪ'teɪlɪə, -'teɪljə] *pl* Geschlechts-, Genitalorgane *pl*, Genitalien *pl*, Genitale *pl*, Organa genitalia.
gen·i·tal·ic [dʒenɪ'tælɪk] *adj* → genital 2.
genital ligament: caudal g. *embryo.* kaudales Keimdrüsenband *nt*.
cranial g. *embryo.* kraniales Keimdrüsenband *nt*.
genital organs → genitalia.
genital phase *psycho.* genitale Phase *f*.
genital pruritus Pruritus genitalis.
genital reflex Genitalreflex *m*.
genital ridge → genital fold.
gen·i·tals ['dʒenɪtlz] *pl* → genitalia.
genital stage → genital phase.
genital swelling *embryo.* Geschlechts-, Genitalwulst *m*.
genital tubercle *embryo.* Genitalhöcker *m*.
genital tuberculosis Genitaltuberkulose *f*.
genital wart Feig-, Feuchtwarze *f*, spitzes Kondylom *nt*, Condyloma acuminatum, Papilloma acuminatum/venereum.
genito- *pref.* Genital-, Genito-.
gen·i·to·cru·ral [,dʒenɪtəʊ'krʊərəl] *adj* Genitale *od.* Inguinalregion u. Oberschenkel betr., genitokrural, genitofemoral.
gen·i·to·fem·o·ral nerve [,-'femərəl] Genitofemoralis *m*, N. genitofemoralis.
gen·i·to·in·gui·nal ligament [,-'ɪŋgwənl] *embryo.* Lig. genito-inguinale.
gen·i·to·spi·nal center [,-'spaɪnl] → genital center.
gen·i·to·u·ri·nar·y [,-'jʊərɪneri:] *adj abbr.* **GU** Harn- u. Geschlechtsorgane betr., urogenital, Urogenital-.
genitourinary apparatus Urogenitalsystem *nt*, -trakt *m*, Harn- u. Geschlechtsapparat *m*, Apparatus urogenitalis, Systema urogenitale.
genitourinary injury Verletzung *f* des Urogenitalapparates.
genitourinary region Urogenitalgegend *f*, -region *f*, Regio urogenitalis.
genitourinary schistosomiasis Urogenitalbilharziose *f*, (Harn-)Blasenbilharziose *f*, Schistosomiasis urogenitalis.
genitourinary system → genitourinary apparatus.
genitourinary tract → genitourinary apparatus.
genitourinary tract injury → genitourinary injury.
genitourinary tuberculosis Urogenitaltuberkulose *f*.
gen·ius ['dʒi:nɪəs] *n, pl* **gen·ius·es** 1. Genie *nt*, genialer Mensch *m*; Genialität *f*. 2. Geist *m*, eigener Charakter *m*, Genius *m*.
Gennari [dʒə'nɑ:ri:]: **band of G.** Gennari'- -Streifen *m*.
line of G. → band of G.
G.'s stain Gennari'-Versilberung *f*.
stria of G. → band of G.
stripe of G. → band of G.
gen·o·cop·y ['dʒenəkɒpi] *n genet.* Genokopie *f*.
gen·o·der·ma·tol·o·gy [,-,dɜːrmə'tɑlədʒi] *n* Genodermatologie *f*.
gen·o·der·ma·to·sis [,-,dɜːrmə'təʊsɪs] *n* Genodermatose *f*, Genodermie *f*.
ge·nom *n* → genome.

ge·nome ['dʒi:nəʊm] *n* Erbinformation *f*, Genom *nt*.
ge·no·mic [dʒɪ'nəʊmɪk, -'nɑm-] *adj* Genom betr., Genom-.
genomic mutation Genommutation *f*.
ge·no·tox·ic [,dʒi:nə'tɑksɪk] *adj* gen(om)schädigend.
gen·o·type ['dʒenətaɪp, 'dʒi:n-] *n* Genotyp(us *m*) *m*, Erbbild *nt*.
gen·o·typ·ic [dʒenə'tɪpɪk, dʒi:n-] *adj* Genotyp(us) betr., auf ihm beruhend, durch ihn bestimmt, genotypisch.
genotypic reversion *genet.* genotypische Reversion *f*.
gen·ta·mi·cin [,dʒentə'maɪsɪn] *n pharm.* Gentamicin *nt*.
gen·ta·my·cin *n* → gentamicin.
gen·ti·an·ic acid [dʒentʃɪ'ænɪk] → gentisin.
gen·ti·an·in ['dʒentʃənɪn] *n* → gentisin.
gen·tian·o·phil ['dʒentʃənəfɪl] *histol.* **I** *n* gentianophile Struktur *od.* Zelle *f*. **II** *adj* leicht mit Gentianaviolett färbend, gentianophil.
gen·tian·o·phil·ic [,-'fɪlɪk] *adj* → gentianophil **II**.
gen·tia·noph·i·lous [,dʒentʃə'nɑfɪləs] *adj* → gentianophil **II**.
gen·tian·o·pho·bic [,dʒentʃənə'fəʊbɪk] *adj histol.* nicht mit Gentianaviolett färbend, gentianophob.
gen·tian·ose ['dʒentʃənəʊs] *n* Gentianose *f*.
gen·tian violet ['dʒenʃn] Gentianaviolett *nt*.
gen·tia·vern ['dʒenʃɪəvɜrn] *n* → gentian violet.
gen·ti·sate ['dʒentɪseɪt] *n* Genti(ni)sat *nt*.
gen·tis·ic acid [dʒen'tɪsɪk] Gentisinsäure *f*, Dihydroxybenzoesäure *f*.
gen·ti·sin ['dʒentɪsɪn] *n* Gentisin *nt*, Gentianin *nt*, Gentiin *nt*.
ge·nu ['dʒi:njʊ], dʒe-] *n, pl* **ge·nua** ['dʒenjʊə] *anat.* 1. Knie *nt*, Genu *nt*. 2. Knick *m*, Abknickung *f*.
g. of corpus callosum Balkenknie, Genu corporis callosi.
g. of facial canal Geniculum canalis facialis.
g. of internal capsule Kapselknie, Knie der inneren Kapsel, Genu capsulae internae.
gen·u·al [dʒenjəwəl] *adj* Knie betr., knieartig, -ähnlich, Knie-.
genual bursa: anterior g. Bursa anserina.
external inferior g. Bursa subtendinea m. bicipitis femoris inferior.
internal superior g.e Bursae subtendineae m. sartorii.
posterior g. Bursa m. semimembranosi.
gen·u·cu·bi·tal position [,dʒenjə'kju:bɪtl] *chir.* Knie-Ellenbogen-Lage *f*.
gen·u·pec·to·ral position [,-'pektərəl] *chir.* Knie-Brust-Lage *f*.
genu recurvatum überstreckbares Knie *nt*, Hohlknie *nt*, Genu recurvatum.
congenital g. angeborenes Genu recurvatum.
constitutional g. konstitutionelles Genu recurvatum.
ge·nus ['dʒi:nəs] *n, pl* **gen·e·ra** ['dʒenərə] *bio.* Gattung *f*, Genus *nt*.
genus name Gattungsname *m*.
genu valgum X-Bein *nt*, Genu valgum.
genu varum O-Bein *nt*, Genu varum.
geo- *pref.* Erde-, Geo-.
ge·o·bi·ol·o·gy [,dʒi:əʊbaɪ'ɑlədʒi] *n* Geobiologie *f*.
ge·o·chem·i·cal [,-'kemɪkl] *adj* geochemisch.
ge·o·chem·is·try [,-'kemɪstri] *n* Geochemie *f*.
ge·o·graph·i·cal pathology [,-'græfɪkl] Geopathologie *f*.

ge·o·graph·ic tongue [ˌ-'græfɪk] Landkartenzunge *f*, Wanderplaques *pl*, Lingua geographica, Exfoliatio areata linguae/dolorosa, Glossitis exfoliativa marginata, Glossitis areata exsudativa.
ge·o·mag·net·ic [ˌ-mæg'netɪk] *adj* geo-, erdmagnetisch.
ge·o·mag·net·ism [ˌ-'mægnɪtɪzəm] *n phys.* Erd-, Geomagnetismus *m*.
ge·o·med·i·cine [ˌ-'medəsən, -'medsɪn] *n* Geomedizin *f*.
ge·o·met·ric [ˌ-'metrɪk] *adj* geometrisch.
ge·o·met·ri·cal [ˌ-'metrɪkl] *adj* → geometric.
geometrical isomerism cis-trans Isomerie *f*, geometrische Isomerie *f*.
geometric mean *mathe.* geometrisches Mittel *n*.
ge·o·path·o·log·i·cal [ˌ-pæθə'lɑdʒɪkl] *adj* geopathologisch.
ge·o·pa·thol·o·gy [ˌ-pə'θɑlədʒɪ] *n* Geopathologie *f*.
ge·o·pha·gia [ˌ-'feɪdʒ(ɪ)ə] *n psychia.* Erdeessen *nt*, Geophagie *f*.
ge·oph·a·gism [dʒɪ'ɑfədʒɪzəm] *n* → geophagia.
ge·oph·a·gy [dʒɪ'ɑfədʒɪ] *n* → geophagia.
ge·o·phil·ic [ˌdʒiːə'fɪlɪk] *adj bio.* geophil.
ge·oph·i·lous [dʒɪ'ɑfɪləs] *adj* → geophilic.
ge·o·sphere ['dʒiːəʊsfɪər] *n* Geosphäre *f*.
ge·o·tac·tic [ˌ-'tæktɪk] *adj* Geotaxis betr., geotaktisch.
ge·o·tax·is [ˌ-'tæksɪs] *n* Geotaxis *f*.
ge·ot·ri·cho·sis [dʒɪˌɑtrɪ'kəʊsɪs] *n* Geotrichiuminfektion *f*, Geotrichose *f*.
Ge·ot·ri·chum [dʒɪ'ɑtrɪkəm] *n micro.* Geotrichum *nt*.
G. candidum Milchschimmel *m*, Geotrichum candidum.
ge·o·trop·ic [ˌdʒiːə'trɑpɪk, -'trəʊ-] *adj* geotrop(isch).
ge·ot·ro·pism [dʒɪ'ɑtrəpɪzəm] *n bio.* Geotropismus *m*.
ge·phy·ro·pho·bia [dʒɪˌfaɪrə'fəʊbɪə] *n psychia.* Brückenangst *f*, Gephyrophobie *f*.
GER *abbr.* → gastroesophageal reflux.
ger- *pref.* → geronto-.
ge·ra·ni·ol [dʒə'reɪnɪɒl] *n* Geraniol *nt*.
ge·ra·nyl·py·ro·phos·phor·ic acid [dʒəˌreɪnlˌpaɪrəʊfɑs'fɒrɪk, ˌdʒerənɪl-] Geranylpyrophosphorsäure *f*.
ge·rat·ic [dʒə'rætɪk] *adj* → gerontal.
ger·a·tol·o·gy [ˌdʒerə'tɑlədʒɪ] *n* → gerontology.
Gerdy [ʒer'di]: **G.'s fibers** Lig. metacarpale transversum superficiale.
G.'s hyoid fossa Karotisdreieck *nt*, Trigonum caroticum.
Gerhardt ['gerhɑːrt]: **G.'s disease** Gerhardt-Syndrom *nt*, Mitchell-Gerhardt-Syndrom *nt*, Weir-Mitchell-Krankheit *f*, Erythromelalgie *f*, Erythralgie *f*, Erythermalgie *f*, Akromelalgie *f*.
G.'s phenomenon → G.'s sign.
G.'s reaction → G.'s test.
G.'s sign Biermer-Schallwechsel *m*, Gerhardt-Schallwechsel *m*.
G.'s test Gerhardt'-Probe *f*.
Gerhardt-Semon [sə'mɔ̃]: **G.-S. law** HNO Gerhardt-Simon-Regel *f*, -Gesetz *nt*.
ger·i·at·ric [ˌdʒerɪ'ætrɪk, ˌdʒiər-] *adj* Alter *od.* Geriatrie betr., geriatrisch, Alters-.
geriatric agent *pharm.* Geriatrikum *nt*.
ger·i·a·tri·cian [ˌdʒerɪə'trɪʃn] *n* Geriater *m*.
geriatric medicine → geriatrics.
ger·i·at·rics [ˌdʒerɪ'ætrɪks, ˌdʒiər-] *pl* Alters-, Greisenheilkunde *f*, Geriatrie *f*, Presbyatrie *f*.
geriatric therapy → gerontotherapeutics.
Gerlach ['gerlæk]: **G.'s tonsil** Tubenmandel *f*, Tonsilla tubaria.

G.'s valve Gerlach-Klappe *f*, Valvula proc. vermiformis.
Gerlier [ʒer'lje]: **G.'s disease/syndrome** Vertigo epidemica.
germ [dʒɜrm] **I** *n* **1.** Keim *m*, Anlage *f*. **2.** Keim *m*, Bazillus *m*, Bakterium *nt*, (Krankheits-)Erreger *m*. **II** *vt* keimen lassen. **III** *vi* keimen.
Ger·man measles ['dʒɜrmən] Röteln *pl*, Rubella *f*, Rubeola *f*.
German measles virus Rötelnvirus *nt*.
ger·ma·nin ['dʒɜrmənɪn] *n* Germanin *f*, Suramin-Natrium *f*.
ger·ma·ni·um [dʒɜr'meɪnɪəm] *n abbr.* **Ge** Germanium *nt abbr.* Ge.
germ-bearing hillock Eihügel *m*, Discus proligerus/oophorus, Cumulus oophorus.
germ carrier Bazillen-, Keimträger *m*.
germ cell Germinal-, Keimzelle *f*.
mature g. reife Keimzelle *f*, Geschlechtszelle *f*, Gamet *m*, Gamozyt *m*.
primordial g.s *embryo.* Urkeimzellen *pl*.
germ cell tumor → germinoma.
germ disk Keimscheibe *f*, -schild *m*, Blastodiskus *m*.
bilaminar g. zweiblättrige Keimscheibe.
trilaminar g. dreiblättrige Keimscheibe.
germ hillock → germ-bearing hillock.
ger·mi·cid·al [ˌdʒɜrmɪ'saɪdl] *adj* keim(ab)-tötend, germizid.
ger·mi·cide ['dʒɜrmɪsaɪd] *n* keim(ab)tötendes Mittel *nt*, Germizid *nt*.
ger·mi·nal ['dʒɜrmɪnl] *adj* **1.** Keim *od.* Keim(bahn)zellen betr., germinal, germinativ, Keim(zellen)-, Germinal-. **2.** bakteriell, Keim-, Bakterien-.
germinal center Keim-, Reaktionszentrum *nt*.
germinal disk → germ disk.
germinal epithelium 1. Peritoneal-/Keimepithel *nt* des Ovars, Epithelium germinale. **2.** Keim-/Seminalepithel *nt* des Hodens.
germinal layer Keimzone *f*, -schicht *f*.
germinal membrane Keimhaut *f*, Blastoderm *nt*.
germinal mutation gametische Mutation *f*.
germinal streak *embryo.* Keimstreifen *m*.
germinal tumor → germinoma.
germinal vesicle Keimbläschen *nt*.
ger·mi·nant ['dʒɜrmɪnənt] *adj* keimend, sprossend.
ger·mi·nate ['dʒɜrmɪneɪt] **I** *vt* zum Keimen bringen, keimen lassen. **II** *vi* keimen, sprießen.
ger·mi·na·tion [ˌdʒɜrmɪ'neɪʃn] *n* Keimen *nt*, Keimung *f*, Germination *f*.
ger·mi·na·tive ['dʒɜrmɪnətɪv, -nətɪv] *adj* **1.** → germinal. **2.** Keimung bewirkend *od.* auslösend.
germinative area *embryo.* Keimfleck *m*, Macula germinativa.
germinative layer Regenerationsschicht *f*, Stratum germinativum epidermidis.
g. of epidermis Regenerationsschicht *f*, Stratum germinativum epidermidis.
g. of nail Wachstumsschicht *f* des Nagels, Stratum germinativum unguis.
germinative streak → germinal streak.
ger·mi·no·blast [ˈdʒɜrmɪnəblæst] *n* **1.** Germinoblast *m*. **2.** *hema.* Germinoblast *m*, Zentroblast *m*.
ger·mi·no·cyte ['-saɪt] *n* **1.** Keimzelle *f*, Germinozyt *m*. **2.** *hema.* Germinozyt *m*, Zentrozyt *m*.
ger·mi·no·ma [ˌdʒɜrmɪ'nəʊmə] *n* Keimzelltumor *m*, Germinom *nt*.
Ger·mis·ton virus ['dʒɜrməstən] Germiston-Virus *nt*.
germ killer Desinfektionsmittel *nt*.

germ layer *embryo.* Keimblatt *nt*.
ectodermal g. äußeres Keimblatt *nt*, Ektoblast *nt*, Ektoderm *nt*.
entodermal g. inneres Keimblatt *nt*, Entoderm *nt*.
mesodermal g. mittleres/drittes Keimblatt *nt*, Mesoderm *nt*.
germ-line ['dʒɜrmlaɪn] *n* Keimbahn *f*, Germen *nt*.
germ membrane → germinal membrane.
germ plasma Keimplasma *nt*, Erb-, Idioplasma *nt*.
germ-proof ['dʒɜrmpruːf] *adj* keimsicher, -frei.
germ ridge → genital fold.
germ tissue Keimgewebe *nt*.
germ warfare biologische Kriegsführung *f*.
gero- *pref.* → geronto-.
ger·o·co·mia [ˌdʒerə'kəʊmɪə] *n* **1.** Pflege u. Betreuung alter Patienten, Gerontokomie *f*. **2.** Altershygiene *f*, Gerontokomie *f*, Gerohygiene *f*.
ger·o·co·my ['-kəʊmɪ] *n* → gerocomia.
ger·o·der·ma ['-dɜrmə] *n* → gerodermia.
ger·o·der·mia [ˌ-'dɜrmɪə] *n* **1.** Gerodermie *f*, Geroderma *nt*. **2.** atrophische Altershaut *f*, Greisenhaut *f*, Geroderma *nt*.
ger·ok·o·my [dʒɜr'ɑkəmɪ] *n* → gerocomia.
ger·o·ma·ras·mus [ˌdʒerəmə'ræzməs] *n* senile Atrophie *f*.
ger·o·mor·phism [ˌ-'mɔːrfɪzəm] *n* vorzeitige Senilität *f*.
geront- *pref.* → geronto-.
ge·ron·tal [dʒɪ'rɑntl] *adj* Alter betr., Alters-, Geronto-, Gero-.
ger·on·tin [dʒɜr'ɑntɪn, dʒɜrən-] *n* Spermin *nt*.
ger·on·tine ['-tiːn] *n* → gerontin.
geronto- *pref.* Alters-, Geronto-, Gero-.
ger·on·tol·o·gist [ˌdʒɜrən'tɑlədʒɪst] *n* Gerontologe *m*, -login *f*.
ger·on·tol·o·gy [ˌ-'tɑlədʒɪ] *n* Altersforschung *f*, Lehre *f* vom Altern, Gerontologie *f*, Gerontologie *f*, Geratologie *f*.
ge·ron·to·phil·ia [dʒəˌrɑntə'fɪlɪə] *n psychia.* Gerontophilie *f*.
ge·ron·to·ther·a·peu·tics [ˌ-ˌθerə'pjuːtɪks] *pl* Behandlung *f* alter Patienten, Gero-, Gerontotherapie *f*.
ge·ron·to·ther·a·py [ˌ-'θerəpɪ] *n* → gerontotherapeutics.
ge·ron·to·tox·on [ˌ-'tɑksən] *n* → gerontoxon.
ger·on·tox·on [ˌdʒerən'tɑksən] *n ophthal.* Gerontoxon *nt*, Arcus senilis (corneae).
ger·o·psy·chi·a·try [ˌdʒerəʊsaɪ'kaɪətrɪ] *n* Geronto-, Geropsychiatrie *f*.
Gerota [ɡe'rəʊtə]: **G.'s capsule/fascia** Gerota'-Fazie *f*, -Kapsel *f*, Fascia renalis.
Gerstmann ['ɡerstman]: **G.'s syndrome** Gerstmann-Syndrom *nt*.
ges·ta·gen ['dʒestədʒən] *n* Gestagen *nt*, gestagenes Hormon *nt*.
ges·ta·gen·ic [ˌdʒestə'dʒenɪk] *adj* Gestagen betr., gestagen.
gestagenic hormone → gestagen.
gestagenic phase *gyn.* gestagene Phase *f*, Sekretions-, Lutealphase *f*.
ge·stal·tism [ɡə'ʃtaltɪzəm, -'ʃtalt-] *n psychia., psycho.* Gestalttheorie *f*.
ge·stalt theory [ɡə'ʃalt, -'ʃtalt; ɡeː'ʃtalt] → gestaltism.
gestalt therapy Gestalttherapie *f*.
ges·ta·tion [dʒe'steɪʃn] *n* **1.** Schwangerschaft *f*, Gravidität *f*. **2.** *bio.* Trächtigkeit *f*, Gestation *f*.
ges·ta·tion·al diabetes [dʒe'steɪʃnl] Gestationsdiabetes *m*.
gestational edema Schwangerschaftsödem *nt*.

gestational proteinuria Schwangerschaftsproteinurie f, -albuminurie f.
gestational psychosis Schwangerschaftspsychose f.
gestational toxicosis → gestosis.
gestation period Schwangerschaftsdauer f; bio. Tragzeit f.
gestation time → gestation period.
ges·to·sis [dʒesˈtəʊsɪs] n, pl **-ses** [-siːz] gyn. Gestations-, Schwangerschaftstoxikose f, Gestose f.
get [get] (got; gotten) I vt 1. bekommen, kriegen, erhalten; (Wunde) s. zuziehen; (Erkältung) s. holen. 2. erwerben, erzielen; s. besorgen, s. beschaffen; (Hilfe) holen. II vi werden. to ~ dressed s. anziehen. to ~ drunk betrunken werden. to ~ married heiraten. to ~ old alt werden. to ~ tired müde werden. to ~ o.s. pregnant schwanger werden.
get about vi (nach einer Krankheit) s. bewegen können, auf den Beinen sein.
get across I vt klar od. verständlich machen (to sb. jdm.). II vi s. verständlich machen (to); verständlich werden (to).
get along vi 1. voran-, vorwärts-, weiterkommen. 2. s. vertragen (with mit).
get around vi 1. (Person) vermeiden. 2. jdn. überreden, herumkriegen.
get at vi 1. erreichen, herankommen an. 2. etw. herausfinden, -bekommen, einer Sache auf den Grund kommen.
get away vi entkommen, entwischen (from aus; jdm.).
get back vi zurückbekommen, -erhalten, -gewinnen.
get by vi zurecht-, aus-, durchkommen.
get down I vt 1. (Essen) hinunterbringen, -schlucken. 2. deprimieren, fertigmachen. 3. (Fieber) herunterbringen. 4. (Kleidung) abnehmen. II vi s. bücken.
get into vi 1. hineinpassen od. -kommen in. 2. s. angewöhnen. to ~ a habit s. eine Gewohnheit annehmen, s. angewöhnen (of doing sth. etw. zu tun). 3. in Wut od. Panik geraten.
get off I vt ~ into sleep jdn. zum (Ein-)Schlafen bringen. II vi (a. ~ to sleep) einschlafen.
get on vi 1. voran-, vorwärtskommen; a. ~ well Fortschritte machen. 2. s. vertragen (with mit). 3. ~ one's nerves jdm. auf die Nerven gehen.
get out I vt (Splitter) herausmachen, -ziehen. II vi ~ of bed aufstehen.
get over vi s. erholen von, überstehen; (Problem) überwinden.
get round vi ~ get around.
get through I vt 1. durchbringen, durch(be)kommen (durch). 2. etw. klarmachen (to s.o. jdm.). II vi durchkommen.
get up vi aufstehen; s. (vom Stuhl) erheben.
GeV abbr. → giga electron volt.
Gev abbr. → giga electron volt.
GFR abbr. → glomerular filtration rate.
GGT abbr. → γ-glutamyltransferase.
GH abbr. 1. → growth hormone. 2. → growth hormone inhibiting hormone.
GH-IF abbr. [growth hormone inhibiting factor] → growth hormone inhibiting hormone.
GH-IH abbr. → growth hormone inhibiting hormone.
GHK equation → Goldmann equation.
Ghon [ɡɑːn]: **G. complex** → G. focus.
G. focus pulmo. Ghon'-Primärkomplex m, -Herd m.
G. primary lesion/tubercle → G. focus.
Ghon-Sachs [sæks; zaks]: **G.-S. bacillus** Pararauschbrandbazillus m, Clostridium septicum.

ghost [ɡəʊst] n 1. → ghost cell. 2. micro. Ghost m.
ghost cell histol. Erythrozytenghost m, Schattenzelle f, Blutkörperchenschatten m, Ghost m.
GH-RF abbr. [growth hormone releasing factor] → growth hormone releasing hormone.
GH-RH abbr. → growth hormone releasing hormone.
GH-RIF abbr. [growth hormone release inhibiting factor] → growth hormone inhibiting hormone.
GH-RIH abbr. [growth hormone release inhibiting hormone] → growth hormone inhibiting hormone.
GI abbr. → gastrointestinal.
Giacomini [ˌdʒakəˈmiːni]: **G.'s band** Giacomini'-Bändchen nt.
Gianelli [dʒaˈneli]: **G.'s sign** ophthal. Tournay-Zeichen nt.
Giannuzzi [dʒaˈnutsi]: **G.'s body** (von) Ebner'-Halbmond, Giannuzzi'-Halbmond, Heidenhain'-Halbmond, seröser Halbmond.
G.'s cell → G.'s body.
crescent of G. → G.'s body.
G.'s demilune → G.'s body.
Gianotti-Crosti [dʒaːˈnati ˈkrɔːsti]: **G.-C. syndrome** Gianotti-Crosti-Syndrom nt, infantile papulöse Akrodermatitis f, Acrodermatitis papulosa eruptiva infantilis.
gi·ant [ˈdʒaɪənt] I n Riese m; riesiges Exemplar nt. II adj riesenhaft, riesig, Riesen-.
giant axon Riesenaxon nt.
giant cell Riesenzelle f.
bone marrow g. Knochenmarksriesenzelle, Megakaryozyt m.
foreign body g. Fremdkörperriesenzelle.
Langhans' g.s Langhans'-Riesenzellen pl.
muscle g. Muskelriesenzelle.
placental g. Plazentariesenzelle.
Sternberg's g.s Sternberg'-Riesenzellen pl.
Touton's g.s Touton'-Riesenzellen pl.
trophoblast g. Trophoblastriesenzelle.
tumor g. Tumorriesenzelle.
giant cell aortitis Riesenzellaortitis f.
giant-cell arteritis (senile) Riesenzellarteriitis f, Horton'-Riesenzellarteriitis f, Horton-Syndrom nt, Horton-Magath-Brown-Syndrom nt, Arteriitis cranialis/gigantocellularis/temporalis.
giant cell carcinoma Riesenzellkarzinom nt, Ca. gigantocellulare.
giant cell epulis Riesenzellepulis f, Epulis gigantocellularis.
giant cell formation Riesenzellbildung f.
giant cell granuloma → giant cell epulis.
giant cell hepatitis (neonatale) Riesenzellhepatitis f.
giant cell myeloma → giant cell tumor of bone.
giant cell myocarditis Riesenzellmyokarditis f.
giant cell pneumonia Masernpneumonie f, Riesenzellpneumonie f.
giant-cell reparative granuloma: central g. (Knochen) reparatives Riesenzellgranulom nt.
peripheral g. → giant cell epulis.
giant cell sarcoma Riesenzellsarkom nt, Sarcoma gigantocellulare.
giant cell thyroiditis de Quervain-Thyr(e)oiditis f, subakute nicht-eitrige Thyr(e)oiditis f, granulomatöse Schilddrüsenentzündung/Thyr(e)oiditis f, Riesenzellthyr(e)oiditis f.
giant cell tumor Riesenzelltumor m.
aneurysmal g. aneurysmatische/hämorrhagische/hämangiomatöse Knochenzyste f, aneurysmatischer Riesenzelltumor.

benignes Knochenaneurysma nt.
g. of bone Riesenzelltumor des Knochens, Osteoklastom nt.
brown g. (Knochen) brauner Riesenzelltumor.
familial bilateral g. Cherubismus m, Cherubinismus m.
fibrous g. of bone → xanthomatous g. of bone.
subperiosteal g. subperiostaler Riesenzelltumor, ossifizierendes periostales Hämangiom nt.
g. of tendon sheath Riesenzelltumor der Sehnenscheide, pigmentierte villonoduläre Synovitis f abbr. PVNS, benignes Synovialom nt, Tendosynovitis nodosa.
xanthomatous g. xanthomatöser Riesenzelltumor.
xanthomatous g. of bone nicht-osteogenes/nicht-ossifizierendes (Knochen-)Fibrom nt, xanthomatöser/fibröser Riesenzelltumor des Knochens, Xanthogranulom(a) nt des Knochens.
giant chromosome 1. Riesenchromosom nt. 2. Lampenbürstenchromosom nt.
giant colon Megakolon nt, -colon nt.
giant condyloma (**acuminatum**) derm. Buschke-Löwenstein-Tumor m, -Kondylom nt, Condylomata gigantea.
giant congenital pigmented nevus kongenitaler Riesenpigmentnävus m.
giant edema Quincke-Ödem nt, angioneurotisches Ödem nt.
giant fibroadenoma of breast Riesenfibroadenom nt der Brust.
giant follicle lymphoma → giant follicular lymphoma.
giant follicular lymphoma Brill-Symmers-Syndrom nt, Morbus Brill-Symmers m, großfollikuläres Lymphoblastom/Lymphom nt, zentroblastisch-zentrozytisches (malignes) Lymphom nt.
giant follicular thyroiditis → giant cell thyroiditis.
giant hairy nevus 1. → giant congenital pigmented nevus. 2. Badehosennävus m, Schwimmhosennävus m.
giant hypertrophic gastritis Riesenfaltengastritis f, Ménétrier-Syndrom nt, Morbus Ménétrier m, Gastropathia hypertrophica gigantea.
giant hypertrophy of gastric mucosa → giant hypertrophic gastritis.
giant intestinal fluke micro. großer Darmegel m, Fasciolopsis buski.
giant intracanalicular myxoma gyn. Riesenfibroadenom nt der Brust.
gi·ant·ism [ˈdʒaɪəntɪzəm] n 1. → gigantism. 2. übermäßige Größe f.
giant pelvis allgemein vergrößertes Becken nt.
giant pigmented nevus 1. → giant congenital pigmented nevus. 2. Badehosennävus m, Schwimmhosennävus m.
giant platelet disease/syndrome Bernard-Soulier-Syndrom nt.
giant pyramidal cells Betz'-Riesen(pyramiden)zellen pl.
giant pyramids → giant pyramidal cells.
giant urticaria Quincke-Ödem nt, angioneurotisches Ödem nt.
Gi·ar·dia [dʒɪˈɑːrdɪə, ˈdʒɑːr-] n micro. Giardia f.
gi·ar·di·a·sis [ˌdʒɪɑːrˈdaɪəsɪs] n Giardia-Infektion f, Lamblia-Infektion f, Giardiasis f, Lambliasis f.
gib·ber·ish aphasia [ˈdʒɪbərɪʃ, ˈgɪb-] Jargonaphasie f.
gib·bos·i·ty [ɡɪˈbɒsəti] n 1. Buckligkeit f. 2. Buckel m, Höcker m. 3. Kyphose f.
gib·bous [ˈgɪbəs] adj 1. gewölbt, konvex. 2. buck(e)lig, höckerig. 3. kyphotisch.

Gibbs-Donnan

Gibbs-Donnan [gɪbz 'dɑnən]: **G.-D. equilibrium** (Gibbs-)Donnan-Gleichgewicht nt.
gib·bus ['gɪbəs] n ortho. Spitzbuckel m, Buckel m, anguläre Kyphose f, Gibbus m.
Gibson ['gɪbsən]: **G.'s murmur** card. Gibson-Geräusch nt.
gid·di·ness ['gɪdnɪs] n 1. (subjektiver) Schwindel m, Schwind(e)ligkeit f. 2. Schwindelanfall m. 3. Benommenheit f.
gid·dy ['gɪdɪ] adj 1. schwind(e)lig. 2. verwirrt, benommen. 3. wirr, konfus.
Giemsa ['gi:mzə]: **G. banding** (Chromosom) Giemsa-G-Banding nt.
G.'s stain Giemsa-Färbung f.
Gierke ['gɪərkə]: **G.'s cells** Gierke-Zellen pl.
G.'s disease → glycogen storage disease, type I.
Gieson → van Gieson.
GIF abbr. [growth hormone inhibiting factor] → growth hormone inhibiting hormone.
Gifford ['gɪfərd, -fɔːrd]: **G.'s reflex** Westphal-Piltz-Phänomen nt, Orbikularisphänomen nt, Lid-Pupillen-Reflex m.
G.'s sign ophthal. Gifford-Zeichen nt.
Gifford-Galassi [gə'læsɪ, -'lɑsɪ]: **G.-G. reflex** Westphal-Piltz-Phänomen nt, Orbikularisphänomen nt, Lid-Pupillen-Reflex m.
giga- pref. abbr. **G** Giga- abbr. G.
gi·ga electron volt ['gɪgə] abbr. **GeV**, **Gev** Gigaelektronenvolt nt abbr. GeV.
gigant- pref. → giganto-.
gi·gan·tism [dʒaɪ'gæntɪzəm, dʒɪ-] n Riesenwuchs m, Gigantismus m, Gigantosomie f.
giganto- pref. Riesen-, Gigant(o)-.
gi·gan·to·blast [dʒaɪ'gæntəʊblæst] n hema. Gigantoblast m.
gi·gan·to·mas·tia [,-'mæstɪə] n gyn. Gigantomastie f; Makromastie f.
gi·gan·to·me·lia [,-'miːlɪə, -jə] n patho. Gigantomelie f.
Gi·gan·to·rhyn·chus cestodiformis [,-'rɪŋkəs] micro. Moniliformis moniliformis.
gi·gan·to·so·ma [,-'səʊmə] n → gigantism.
Gigli ['dʒɪljiː]: **G.'s operation** gyn. Gigli-Operation f.
GIH abbr. → growth hormone inhibiting hormone.
gi·ki·yam·i [gɪkɪ'jæmɪ] n Nanukayami(-Krankheit f) nt, (japanisches) Siebentagefieber nt, japanisches Herbstfieber nt.
GIK solution → glucose-insulin-kalium solution.
Gilbert [ʒɪl'bɛr]: **G.'s cholemia** intermittierende Hyperbilirubinämie Meulengracht f, Meulengracht-Krankheit f, -Syndrom nt, Meulengracht-Gilbert-Krankheit f, -Syndrom nt, Icterus juvenilis intermittens Meulengracht.
G.'s disease → G.'s cholemia.
G.'s sign Gilbert-Zeichen nt.
G.'s syndrome → G.'s cholemia.
Gilchrist ['gɪlkrɪst]: **G. bandage** Gilchrist--Verband m.
G.'s disease/mycosis Gilchrist-Krankheit f, nordamerikanische Blastomykose f.
gill [gɪl] n 1. zoo. Kieme f, Branchie f. 2. bot. (Pilz) Lamelle f.
gill cleft embryo. Schlundfurche f, Kiemenspalte f.
Gilles de la Tourette [dʒil də la tu'ret]: **G.'s disease/syndrome** Gilles-de-la-Tourette--Syndrom nt, Tourette-Syndrom nt, Maladie des tics, Tic impulsif.
Gilliam ['gɪljəm, -ɪəm]: **G.'s operation** gyn. Gilliam-Operation f.
Gillies ['gɪliːz]: **G.' flap** Rundstiellappen m.
G.' operation 1. ophthal. Gillies-Operation f. 2. HNO Gillies-Technik f.

Gil-Vernet [gɪl vɜr'net; hɪl]: **G.-V. operation** urol. Gil-Vernet-Operation f.
Gimbernat [gɪmbər'næt; hɪmbər'nɑːt]: **G.'s hernia** Gimbernat-Hernie f, Laugier-Hernie f.
G.'s ligament Gimbernat-Band nt, Lig. lacunare.
reflex ligament of G. Lig. reflexum.
gin·ger ['dʒɪndʒər] n Ingwer m.
ginger paralysis Ingwerlähmung f.
gingiv- pref. → gingivo-.
gin·gi·va [dʒɪn'dʒaɪvə, 'dʒɪndʒə-] n, pl **-vae** [-viː] Zahnfleisch nt, Gingiva f, Periodontium protectoris.
gin·gi·val [dʒɪn'dʒaɪvl, 'dʒɪndʒə-] adj Zahnfleisch betr., gingival, Zahnfleisch-, Gingiva(l)-.
gingival abscess Zahnfleischabszeß m.
gingival branches: **inferior g. of inferior dental plexus** Zahnfleischäste pl des Plexus dentalis inferior, Rami gingivales inferiores (plexus dentalis inferioris).
superior g. of superior dental plexus Zahnfleischäste pl des Plexus dentalis superior, Rami gingivales superiores (plexus dentalis superioris).
gingival cyst Zahnfleischzyste f.
gingival fibromatosis Fibromatosis gingivae, Elephantiasis gingivae.
gingival hyperplasia Zahnfleischhyperplasie f.
gingival line 1. Zahnfleischrand m, Margo gingivalis. 2. Zahnfleischsaum m.
gingival margin → gingival line 1.
gingival papilla Interdentalpapille f, Papilla gingivalis/interdentalis.
gingival sulcus Zahnfleischtasche f, Sulcus gingivalis.
gin·gi·vec·to·my [,dʒɪndʒə'vektəmɪ] n HNO Zahnfleischabtragung f, Gingivektomie f, Gingivoektomie f.
gin·gi·vi·tis [,-'vaɪtɪs] n Zahnfleischentzündung f, Gingivitis f.
gingivo- pref. Zahnfleisch-, Gingiv(o)-.
gin·gi·vo·den·tal ligament [,dʒɪndʒəvəʊ-'dentl] Wurzelhaut f, Desmodont nt, Periodontium nt.
gin·gi·vo·glos·si·tis [,-glɑ'saɪtɪs] n Entzündung f von Zahnfleisch u. Zunge, Gingivoglossitis f.
gin·gi·vo·la·bi·al [,-'leɪbɪəl] adj Zahnfleisch u. Lippe(n) betr., gingivolabial.
gin·gi·vo·per·i·o·don·ti·tis [,-perɪəʊ,dɑn-'taɪtɪs] n Entzündung f von Zahnfleisch u. Wurzelhaut, Gingivoperiodontitis f.
gin·gi·vo·plas·ty ['-plæstɪ] n Zahnfleischplastik f, Gingivoplastik f.
gin·gi·vo·sis [,dʒɪndʒɪ'vəʊsɪs] n chronisch desquamative Gingivitis f.
gin·gi·vo·sto·ma·ti·tis [,dʒɪndʒɪvəʊ,stəʊ-mə'taɪtɪs] n Entzündung f von Zahnfleisch u. Mundschleimhaut, Gingovostomatitis f.
gin·gly·form ['dʒɪŋglɪfɔːrm, 'gɪŋ-] adj → ginglymoid.
gin·gly·moid ['-mɔɪd] adj Scharniergelenk/Ginglymus betr., ginglymusähnlich.
ginglymoid articulation/joint → ginglymus.
gin·gly·mus ['-məs] n Scharniergelenk nt, Ginglymus m.
gin·seng ['dʒɪnsæŋ] n Ginseng m, Panax ginseng.
Giordano [dʒɔr'dɑːnəʊ]: **G.'s sphincter** M. sphincter ductus choledochi.
GIP abbr. [gastric inhibitory polypeptide] → glucose dependent insulinotropic peptide.
Giraldés [hɪrɑl'deɪz]: **G.' organ** Paradidymis f.
Girard [ʒɪ'rɑr]: **G.'s method/operation** chir. Girard'-Hernienoperation f.

gir·dle ['gɜrdl] n (a. anat.) Gürtel m, gürtelförmige Struktur od. Zone f, Cingulum nt.
g. of inferior member Beckengürtel, Cingulum membri inferioris, Cingulum pelvicum.
g. of superior member Schultergürtel, Cingulum membri superioris, Cingulum pectorale.
girdle anesthesia neuro. gürtelförmige Anästhesie(zone f) f.
girdle pain gürtelförmiger Schmerz m.
girdle sensation neuro. Gürtelgefühl nt, Zonästhesie f.
Girdlestone ['gɜrdlstəʊn]: **G. procedure** ortho. Girdlestone-Operation f.
git·a·lin ['dʒɪtəlɪn, dʒɪ'taɪl-, -'tæl-] n Gitalin nt.
git·a·lox·in [,dʒɪtə'lɑksɪn] n Gitaloxin nt.
gith·a·gism ['gɪθədʒɪzəm] n Githaginvergiftung f, Githagismus m.
git·og·e·nin [dʒɪ'tɑdʒənɪn, -niːn] n Gitogenin nt.
gi·to·nin [dʒɪ'təʊnɪn, 'dʒɪtənɪn] n Gitonin nt.
gi·tox·i·gen·in [dʒɪ'tɑksɪdʒenɪn] n Gitoxigenin nt.
gi·tox·in [dʒɪ'tɑksɪn] n Gitoxin nt.
git·ter cell ['gɪtər] Gitterzelle f.
git·ter·zel·le ['gɪtərzelɪ; -'tselə] n Gitterzelle f.
give [gɪv] (v **gave**; **given**) **I** n Elastizität f; Federung f; fig. Flexibilität f, Nachgiebigkeit f.
II vt 1. geben; übergeben, -reichen; (Rat, Befehl) erteilen; (Zimmer) zuteilen, -weisen. 2. etw. zugestehen; (Zeit) geben, gewähren; (Hilfe) gewähren; (Medikament) verabreichen; (Spritze) geben. **to ~ relief** Linderung verschaffen. 3. äußern, von s. geben. **to ~ a cry** einen Schrei ausstoßen. 4. verursachen. **to ~ sb. pain** jdm. weh tun, jdm. Schmerzen bereiten. 5. (er-)geben. **to ~ no result** ohne Ergebnis bleiben.
III vi 6. geben; (Geld) spenden (to). 7. (Beine) nachgeben; (Nerven) versagen 8. (Material) s. dehnen od. weiten, s. anpassen (to an); nachgeben; federn.
give in vi nach-, aufgeben; s. jdm. geschlagen geben (to sb.).
give off vt (Geruch) verbreiten, von s. geben, ausströmen; (Gas) aus-, verströmen. 2. (Gefäße) abgehen, abzweigen.
give out I vt → give off. **II** vi (Kräfte) zu Ende gehen; (Stimme, Nieren) versagen.
give up I vt aufgeben, aufhören mit. **to ~ smoking** das Rauchen aufgeben; (Hoffnung, einen Kranken) aufgeben. **II** vi s. geschlagen geben, aufgeben; resignieren.
gia·bel·la [glə'belə] n, pl **-lae** [-liː, -laɪ] anat. Glabella f.
gla·bel·lum [glə'beləm] n → glabella.
gla·brate ['glæbreɪt] adj → glabrous.
gla·brose ['gleɪbrəʊs] n oberflächliche Trichophytie f des Körpers, Tinea/Trichophytia/Epidermophytia corporis.
gla·brous ['gleɪbrəs] adj bio. kahl, haarlos.
glabrous skin glatte haarlose Haut f.
glad·i·ate ['glædɪt, -eɪt] adj schwertförmig.
glad·i·o·lus [,glædɪ'əʊləs] n, pl **-li** [-laɪ] Corpus sterni.
gland [glænd] n anat. Drüse f, drüsenförmiges Gebilde nt, Glandula f.
g.s of biliary mucosa Schleimdrüsen pl der Gallengänge, Gll. biliares.
g.s of Haller präputiale (Talg-)Drüsen pl, Tyson-Drüsen pl, Vorhaut-, Präputialdrüsen pl, Gll. pr(a)eputiales.
g.s of mouth Gll. oris.
g.s of mucous membranes Schleimhautdrüsen pl.

g.s of tongue Zungen(speichel)drüsen *pl*, Gll. linguales.
g.s of Tyson präputiale (Talg-)Drüsen *pl*, Tyson-Drüsen *pl*, Vorhaut-, Präputialdrüsen *pl*, Gll. pr(a)eputiales.
g.s of Zeis Zeis'-Drüsen *pl*, Gll. sebaceae conjunctivales.
gland cell Drüsenzelle *f*.
glan·der·ous ['glændərəs] *adj* Rotz/Malleus betr., von Malleus betroffen, Malleus-.
glan·ders ['glændərz] *n* Rotz *m*, Malleus *m*, Maliasmus *m*.
glanders bacillus *micro.* Pseudomonas/Malleomyces/Actinobacillus mallei.
glan·des *pl* → glans.
glan·di·lem·ma [,glændı'lemə] *n* Drüsenkapsel *f*, Glandilemm(a) *nt*.
glan·do·trop·ic [,glændoʊ'trɑpɪk, 'troʊ-] *adj* auf Drüsen einwirkend, glandotrop.
glandotropic hormone glandotropes Hormon *nt*.
gland primordium *embryo.* Drüsenanlage *f*.
glan·du·la ['glændʒələ] *n*, *pl* **-lae** [-liː, -laɪ] → gland.
glan·du·lar ['glændʒələr] *adj* **1.** Drüse/Glandula betr., glandulär, Drüsen-. **2.** Glans clitoridis/penis betr., Glans-.
glandular branches: g. of facial artery A. facialis-Äste *pl* zur Gl. submandibularis, Rami glandulares a. facialis.
g. of inferior thyroid artery A. thyroidea inferior-Äste *pl* zu Schilddrüse u. Nebenschilddrüse, Rami glandulares a. thyroideae inferiores.
g. of submandibular ganglion Ggl. submandibularis-Äste *pl* zur Gl. submandibularis, Rami glandulares ggl. submandibularis.
g.es of superior thyroid artery Drüsenäste *pl* der A. thyroidea superior, Rami glandulares a. thyroideae superioris.
glandular cancer → glandular carcinoma.
glandular carcinoma Adenokarzinom *nt*, Adenocarcinom *nt*, Ca. adenomatosum.
glandular crest of larynx Lig. vestibulare.
glandular-cystic hyperplasia *gyn.* glandulär-zystische Hyperplasie *f*.
glandular cystoma *patho.* glanduläres Kystom/Zystom *nt*.
glandular duct Drüsenausführungsgang *m*.
glandular epispadias *urol.* glanduläre Epispadie *f*.
glandular epithelium Drüsenepithel *nt*.
glandular fever infektiöse Mononukleose *f*, Pfeiffer'-Drüsenfieber *nt*, Monozytenangina *f*, Mononucleosis infectiosa.
glandular foramen: g.mina of Littre Lacunae urethralis.
g. of Morgagni For. caecum linguae.
g. of tongue For. caecum linguae.
glandular fossa of frontal bone Fossa gl. lacrimalis.
glandular hyperplasia glanduläre Hyperplasie *f*.
glandular hypospadias *urol.* glanduläre Hypospadie *f*.
glandular lobe of pituitary (gland) Adenohypophyse *f*, Hypophysenvorderlappen *m abbr.* HVL, Adenohypophysis *f*, Lobus anterior hypophyseus.
glandular mastitis parenchymatöse Mastitis *f*.
glandular parenchyma of prostate Drüsenparenchym *nt* der Prostata, Parenchyma (gl.) prostatae.
glandular part of hypophysis → glandular lobe of pituitary (gland).
glandular perspiration glandulärer Wasserverlust *m*, Wasserverlust *m od.* -abga-

be *f* durch Schwitzen, Perspiratio sensibilis.
glandular pharyngitis follikuläre Pharyngitis *f*.
glandular plague Beulen-, Bubonenpest *f*, Pestis bubonica/fulminans/major.
glandular substance of prostate Drüsensubstanz *f* der Prostata, Substantia (gl.) prostatae.
glandular tissue Drüsengewebe *nt*, drüsenbildendes Gewebe *nt*.
glandular tularemia glanduläre Tularämie *f*.
glandular ureteritis glanduläre Harnleiterentzündung/Ureteritis *f*, Ureteritis glandularis.
glandular water loss → glandular perspiration.
glan·dule ['glændjuːl] *n* kleine Drüse *f*.
glan·du·lo·pap·il·lar·y [,glændʒəloʊpə-'pılərı] *adj* glandulär-papillär, glandulopapillär.
glan·du·lous ['glændʒələs] *adj* → glandular 1.
glans [glænz] *n*, *pl* **glan·des** ['glændiːz] *anat.* Eichel *f*, Glans *f* (penis), Balanos *f*.
g. of clitoris Klitoris-, Clitorisspitze *f*, Glans clitoridis.
g. of penis → glans.
glan·u·lar ['glænjələr] *adj* Glans clitoridis/penis betr., Glans-/Eichel-.
Glanzmann ['glænzmən; 'glantsman]: **G.'s disease/thrombasthenia** Glanzmann-Naegeli-Syndrom *nt*, Thrombasthenie *f*.
glare [gleər] *n ophthal.* Blendung *f*.
gla·rom·e·ter [gleə'rɑmıtər] *n ophthal.* Glarometer *nt*.
gla·se·ri·an fissure [gleɪ'zɪərıən] Glaser'--Spalte *f*, Fissura petrotympanica.
Glasgow ['glæsgoʊ, -koʊ]: **G.'s sign** *card.* Glasgow-Zeichen *nt*.
glass [glæs, glɑːs] **I** *n* **1.** Glas *nt*; Glasscheibe *f*; Spiegel *m*; Trinkglas *nt*. **2.** (*a.* **a pair of ~es**) *pl* Brille *f*. **3.** Vergrößerungsglas *nt*, Linse *f*, Augenglas *nt*. **II** *vt* verglasen.
glass·blow·er's cataract ['glæsbloʊər] *ophthal.* Feuer-, Glasbläserstar *m*, Infrarotkatarakt *f*, Cataracta calorica.
glass capillary Glaskapillare *f*.
glass-capillary electrode Glaskapillarelektrode *f*.
glass electrode Glaselektrode *f*.
glass eye Glasauge *nt*, künstliches Auge *nt*.
glass factor Faktor XII *m abbr.* F XII, Hageman-Faktor *m*.
glass fiber Glasfaser *f*, -fiber *f*.
glass·i·ness ['glæsɪnɪs, -'glɑːs-] *n* **1.** (*Augen*) Glasigkeit *f*. **2.** glasiges Aussehen *nt*.
glass·like cartilage ['glæslaɪk] hyaliner Knorpel *m*, Hyalinknorpel *m*, Cartilago hyalina.
glass pox weiße Pocken *pl*, Alastrim *nt*, Variola minor.
glass·work·er's cataract ['glæswɜrkər] → glassblower's cataract.
glass·y ['glæsɪ, 'glɑː-] *adj* **1.** glasähnlich, -artig, gläsern, glasig; *anat.* hyalin. **2.** (*Augen*) glasig, starr.
glassy degeneration hyaline Degeneration *f*, Hyalinose *f*, Hyalinisierung *f*, Hyalinisation *f*.
glassy membrane 1. Slavjansky'-Membran *f*, (Follikel-)Glashaut *f*. **2.** Lamina basalis.
Glauber ['glaʊbər]: **G.'s salt** Glaubersalz *nt*, Natriumsulfat *nt*.
glau·co·ma [glɔː'koʊmə, gloʊ-] *n* grüner Star *m*, Glaukom *nt*, Glaucoma *nt*.
glau·co·ma·to·cy·clit·ic crisis [glɔː,koʊ-mətoʊsaɪ'klıtık] zyklitisches Glaukom *nt*,

Posner-Schlossmann-Syndrom *nt*, glaukomatozyklitische Krise *f*.
glau·co·ma·tous [glɔː'koʊmətəs, gloʊ-] *adj* Glaukom betr., glaukomatös, Glaukom-.
glaucomatous cataract Glaukomflecken *pl*, Cataracta glaucomatosa.
glaucomatous cup → glaucomatous excavation.
glaucomatous excavation *ophthal.* Glaukomexkavation *f*.
glaucomatous halo *ophthal.* Halo glaucomatosus.
glaucomatous ring → glaucomatous halo.
glau·co·sis [glɔː'koʊsɪs] *n* Blindheit *f* als Glaukomfolge, Glaukose *f*.
glau·co·su·ria [,glɔːkə's(j)ʊərıə] *n old* → indicanuria.
glau·kom·fleck·en ['glaʊkɒm'flekn; -'flɛkən] *pl* → glaucomatous cataract.
glaze [gleɪz] **I** *n* **1.** Glasur *f*, Glasurmasse *f*. **2.** Glasigkeit *f*. **II** *vt* **3.** glasieren, mit Glasur überziehen. **4.** (*Augen*) glasig machen.
GLC *abbr.* → gas-liquid chromatography.
gleet [gliːt] *n* **1.** chronisch gonorrhoische Urethritis *f*. **2.** Harnröhrenausfluß *m*.
Glenn [glen]: **G.'s operation** Glenn-Operation *f*, Kava-Pulmonalis-Anastomose *f*.
gle·no·hu·mer·al [,glenoʊ'(h)juːmərəl, ,gliːnoʊ-] *adj* Humerus u. Cavitas glenoidalis betr., glenohumeral.
glenohumeral articulation Schultergelenk *nt*, Artic. humeri/glenohumeralis.
glenohumeral ligaments Ligg. glenohumeralia.
gle·noid ['gliːnɔɪd, 'gle-] *adj anat.* höhlenartig, -förmig, glenoidal.
glenoid cavity Gelenkpfanne *f* der Skapula, Cavitas glenoidalis.
glenoid fossa 1. → glenoid cavity. **2.** → g. of temporal bone.
g. of temporal bone Fossa mandibularis.
g. of scapula → glenoid cavity.
glenoid labrum Labrum glenoidale.
glenoid ligament: g.s of Cruveilhier Ligg. plantaria articc. metatarsophalangearum.
g. of humerus Labrum glenoidale.
g. of Macalister Labrum glenoidale.
glenoid lip → glenoid labrum.
Gley [gleɪ]: **G.'s cells** Gley'-Zellen *pl*, Interstitialzellen *pl* des Hodens.
G.'s gland Nebenschilddrüse *f*, Epithelkörperchen *nt*, Parathyr(e)oidea *f*, Gl. parathyroidea.
gli·a ['glaɪə, 'gliːə] *n anat.* Glia *f*, Neuroglia *f*.
gli·a·blast ['glaɪəblæst, 'gliː-] *n* → glioblast.
glia cell → gliacyte.
gli·a·cyte ['-saɪt] *n* (Neuro-)Gliazelle *f*, Gliozyt *m*.
gli·a·din ['glaɪəd(ı)n] *n* Gliadin *nt*.
glia filament Gliafilament *nt*.
gli·al ['glaɪəl] *adj* (Neuro-)Glia betr., gliär, Glia-.
glial architectonics Gliaarchitektonik *f*.
glial boundary membrane → glial limiting membrane.
glial capsule Gliazellkapsel *f*.
glial cell → gliacyte.
glial fibril Gliafibrille *f*.
glial limiting membrane Gliagrenzmembran *f*, Membrana limitans gliae.
outer g. → superficial g.
perivascular g. perivaskuläre Gliamembran, Membrana limitans gliae perivascularis.
superficial g. oberflächliche Gliagrenzmembran, Membrana limitans gliae superficialis.

glial membrane

glial membrane → glial limiting membrane.
glial scar Glianarbe f.
gli·ben·cla·mide [glaɪ'benkləmaɪd] n pharm. Glibenclamid.
gli·born·ur·ide [glaɪ'bɔːrnjʊəraɪd] n pharm. Glibornurid nt.
gli·cen·tin [glaɪ'sentɪn] n Enteroglukagon nt, intestinales Glukagon nt.
glid·ing ['glaɪdɪŋ] I n Gleiten nt. II adj gleitend, Gleit-.
gliding articulation/joint Artic. plana.
gliding sheath Gleithülle f, -scheide f.
gli·o·blast ['glaɪəʊblæst] n Glioblast m, Spongioblast m.
gli·o·blas·to·ma [ˌ-blæs'təʊmə] n patho. Glioblastom(a) nt, Gliablastom nt.
glioblastoma multiforme buntes Glioblastom, Glioblastoma multiforme.
gli·o·cyte ['-saɪt] n (Neuro-)Gliazelle f, Gliozyt m.
gli·o·cy·to·ma [ˌ-saɪ'təʊmə] n → glioma.
gli·og·e·nous [glaɪ'ɑdʒənəs] adj von Gliazellen gebildet, gliogen.
gli·o·ma [glaɪ'əʊmə] n Gliageschwulst f, -tumor m, Gliom(a) nt.
glioma-polyposis syndrome Turcot-Syndrom m.
gli·o·ma·to·sis [ˌglaɪəmə'təʊsɪs] n patho. Gliomatose f.
gli·o·ma·tous [glaɪ'əmətəs] adj gliomartig, gliomatös.
gli·o·myx·o·ma [ˌglaɪəmɪk'səʊmə] n patho. Gliomyxom nt.
gli·o·neu·ro·ma [ˌ-njʊə'rəʊmə] n patho. Glioneurom nt, Glioneuroblastom nt.
gli·o·pha·gia [ˌ-'feɪdʒ(ɪ)ə] n Gliophagie f.
gli·o·pil ['-pɪl] n Gliafilz m, Gliopil nt.
gli·o·sar·co·ma [ˌ-sɑː'kəʊmə] n Gliosarkom nt, Glioma sarcomatosum.
gli·o·sis [glaɪ'əʊsɪs] n patho. Gliose f, Gliosis f.
glip·i·zide ['glɪpəzaɪd] n pharm. Glipizid nt.
gli·qui·done ['glaɪkwədəʊn] n pharm. Gliquidon nt.
Glisson ['glɪsn] G.'s capsule Glisson'-Kapsel f, Capsula fibrosa perivascularis.
G.'s cirrhosis Glisson'-Zirrhose f.
G.'s disease Rachitis f.
G.'s sling Glisson-Schlinge f.
G.'s sphincter M. sphincter ampullae hepatopancreaticae, Sphincter ampullae.
glis·so·ni·tis [glɪsə'naɪtɪs] n Entzündung f der Glisson'-Kapsel, Glissonitis f.
Gln abbr. → glutamine.
glob·al ['glǝʊbl] adj umfassend, global, Gesamt-, Global-, Total-.
global aphasia neuro. Total-, Globalaphasie f.
globe [glǝʊb] I n Kugel f; kugelförmiger Gegenstand m. II vt zusammenballen, kugelförmig machen. III vi s. zusammenballen.
g. of eye Augapfel m, Bulbus oculi.
globe cell anemia hereditäre Sphärozytose f, Kugelzell(en)anämie f, Kugelzell(en)ikterus m, familiärer hämolytischer Ikterus m, Morbus Minkowski-Chauffard m.
glo·bi ['glǝʊbaɪ] pl 1. → globus. 2. Lepraglobi pl.
glo·bin ['glǝʊbɪn] n Globin nt.
glo·boid ['glǝʊbɔɪd] I n bio. Globoid nt. II adj → globose.
globoid cell Globoidzelle f.
globoid cell leukodystrophy Krabbe-Syndrom nt, Globoidzellen-Leukodystrophie f, Galaktozerebrosidlipidose f, Galaktozerebrosidose f, Angiomatosis encephalo-cutanea, Leukodystrophia cerebri progressiva hereditaria.

globoid leukodystrophy → globoid cell leukodystrophy.
glo·bose ['glǝʊbǝʊs, glǝʊ'bǝʊs] adj kugelförmig, sphärisch, globulär, globoid, kugelig, Kugel-.
globose nucleus Kugelkern m, Nc. globosus.
glo·bo·side ['glǝʊbǝsaɪd] n Globosid nt.
glo·bos·i·ty [glǝʊ'bɒsǝtɪ] n Kugelform f, -gestalt f.
glo·bous ['glǝʊbǝs] adj → globose.
glob·u·lar ['glɑbjǝlǝr] adj 1. → globose. 2. aus Kügelchen od. Tröpfchen bestehend, globulär.
globular actin globuläres Aktin nt, G-Aktin nt.
glob·u·la·ri·a·cit·rin [ˌglɑbjǝˌleǝrɪǝ'sɪtrɪn] n Rutin nt, Rutosid nt.
globular model biochem. globuläres Modell nt, Untereinheitenmodell nt.
globular protein globuläres Eiweiß/Protein nt.
globular sputum Sputum globosum.
globular value Färbeindex m abbr. FI, Hämoglobinquotient m.
glob·ule ['glɑbjuːl] n 1. Kügelchen nt. 2. Tröpfchen nt.
glob·u·li·ci·dal [ˌglɑbjǝlɪ'saɪdl] adj Erythrozyten zerstörend, globulizid.
glob·u·li·cide ['glɑbjǝlɪsaɪd] n Globulizid nt.
glob·u·lin ['glɑbjǝlɪn] n Globulin nt.
glob·u·li·nu·ria [ˌglɑbjǝlɪ'n(j)ʊǝrɪǝ] n Globulinausscheidung f im Harn, Globulinurie f.
glob·u·lous ['glɑbjǝlǝs] adj → globular.
glob·u·lus ['glɑbjǝlǝs] n, pl -li [-laɪ] 1. → globose nucleus. 2. pharm. kugelförmige Arzneizubereitung f, Globulus m; Zäpfchen nt.
glo·bus ['glǝʊbǝs] n, pl -bi [-baɪ] (a. anat.) Kugel f, Klumpen m, Globus m.
globus pal·li·dus ['pælɪdǝs] medialer Teil m des Linsenkerns, Globus pallidus, Pallidum nt.
lateral g. lateraler Teil m des Globus pallidus, Globus pallidus lateralis.
medial g. medialer Teil m des Globus pallidus, Globus pallidus medialis.
glo·mal ['glǝʊmǝl] adj Glomus betr., Glomus-.
glo·man·gi·o·ma [glǝʊˌmændʒɪ'ǝʊmǝ] n → glomus tumor.
glo·mec·to·my [glǝʊ'mektǝmɪ] n chir. Glomus(-caroticum)-Entfernung f, Glomektomie f.
glom·er·ate ['glɑmǝrɪt, -reɪt] adj (zusammen-)geballt, gehäuft, geknäuelt, knäuelig.
glom·er·a·tion [ˌglɑmǝ'reɪʃn] n (Zusammen-)Ballung f, Anhäufung f; Knäuel nt/m.
glomerul- pref. → glomerulo-.
glo·mer·u·lar [glǝʊ'merjǝlǝr, glǝ-] adj 1. Glomerulus/Glomerulum betr., glomerulär, Glomerulo-. 2. → glomerate.
glomerular arteriole: afferent g. zuführende Glomerulusarterie/-arteriole f, Arteriola glomerularis afferens, Vas afferens (glomeruli).
efferent g. abführende Glomerulusarteriole/-arteriole f, Arteriola glomerularis efferens, Vas efferens (glomeruli).
glomerular basement membrane abbr. GBM (Glomerulum-)Basalmembran f.
glomerular capillary glomeruläre Kapillare f.
glomerular capsule Bowman'-Kapsel f, Capsula glomerularis.
glomerular cell Glomuszelle f.
glomerular filtrate Glomerulumfiltrat nt, glomeruläres Filtrat nt.

glomerular filtration glomeruläre Filtration f.
glomerular filtration rate abbr. GFR glomeruläre Filtrationsrate f abbr. GFR.
glomerular loop Glomerulumschlinge f.
glomerular membrane Glomerulum-, Glomerularmembram f.
glomerular nephritis → glomerulonephritis.
glomerular zone histol. Zona glomerulosa.
glo·mer·u·late [glǝʊ'merjǝleɪt, -lɪt] adj → glomerate.
glom·er·ule ['glɑmǝruːl] n → glomerulus.
glo·mer·u·li·tis [glǝʊˌmerjǝ'laɪtɪs] n patho. Glomerulumentzündung f, Glomerulitis f.
glomerulo- pref. Glomerulum-, Glomerulo-.
glo·mer·u·lo·cap·su·lar nephritis [glǝʊˌmerjǝlǝʊ'kæpsǝlǝr] Nephritis f mit Beteiligung der Glomeruluskapsel.
glo·mer·u·lo·ne·phri·tis [ˌ-nɪ'fraɪtɪs] n abbr. GN Glomerulonephritis f abbr. GN.
glo·mer·u·lo·ne·phrop·a·thy [ˌ-nɪ'frɑpǝθɪ] n Glomerulonephrose f, Glomerulonephropathie f.
glo·mer·u·lop·a·thy [glǝʊˌmerjǝ'lɑpǝθɪ] n Glomerulopathie f.
glo·mer·u·lo·sa [ˌ-'lǝʊsǝ] n Zona glomerulosa.
glomerulosa cell Zona-glomerulosa-Zelle f.
glo·mer·u·lo·scle·ro·sis [glǝʊˌmerjǝlǝʊ'sklɪǝrǝʊsɪs] n patho. Glomerulosklerose f.
glo·mer·u·lose [glǝʊ'merjǝlǝʊs] adj → glomerular.
glo·mer·u·lus [glǝʊ'merjǝlǝs, glǝ-] n, pl -li [-laɪ] 1. anat. Knäuel nt/m, Glomerulus m, Glomerulum nt. 2. (Nieren-)Glomerulus m, Glomerulus renalis.
glomerulus-type synapse glomerulusartige Synapse f.
glo·mic ['glǝʊmɪk] adj Glomus betr., Glomus-.
glo·mi·form body/gland ['glǝʊmɪfɔːrm] → glomus organ.
glo·moid ['glǝʊmɔɪd] adj glomusähnlich, -artig, glomoid.
glo·mus ['glǝʊmǝs] n, pl -mi [-maɪ], **glo·mer·a** ['glɑmǝrǝ] anat. 1. Gefäß-, Nervenknäuel nt/m, Glomus nt. 2. → glomus organ.
glomus body → glomus organ.
glomus cell Glomuszelle f.
glomus jugulare tumor Glomus-jugulare-Tumor m.
glomus organ Glomusorgan nt, Masson-Glomus nt, Hoyer-Grosser-Organ nt, Knäuelanastomose f, Glomus neuromyoarteriale, Anastomosis arteriovenosa glomeriformis.
glomus tumor Glomustumor m, Glomangiom(a) nt, Angiomyoneurom nt.
glomus tympanicum tumor Glomus-tympanicum-Tumor m.
gloss- pref. → glosso-.
glos·sa ['glɑsǝ, 'glɒs-] n, pl -sae [-siː] anat. Zunge f, Glossa f, Lingua f.
glos·sa·gra [glɑ'sægrǝ] n gichtbedingte Zungenschmerzen pl, Glossagra f.
glos·sal ['glɑsl, 'glɒs-] adj Zunge/Glossa betr., zungenförmig, lingual, Zungen-, Glosso-.
glossal-facial anastomosis anat. Hypoglossus-Fazialis-Anastomose f.
glos·sal·gia [glɑ'sældʒ(ɪ)ǝ] n Zungenbrennen nt, Zungenschmerz(en pl) m, Glossalgie f, Glossodynie f.
glos·san·thrax [glɑ'sænθræks] n Milz-

brandkarbunkel *m* der Zunge, Glossanthrax *m*.
glos·sec·to·my [glɑ'sektəmɪ] *n chir.* Zungen(teil)amputation *f*, Glossektomie *f*.
Glos·si·na [glɑ'saɪnə] *n micro.* Zungen-, Tsetsefliege *f*, Glossina *f*.
glos·si·tis [glɑ'saɪtɪs] *n* Zungen(schleimhaut)entzündung *f*, Glossitis *f*.
glosso- *pref.* Zunge/Glossa betr., Zungen-, Glosso-.
glos·so·cele ['glasəʊsiːl, 'glɒs-] *n* 1. Glossozele *f*. 2. zystische Zungengeschwulst *f*, Glossozele *f*.
glos·so·cin·es·thet·ic [ˌ-sɪnes'θetɪk] *adj* → glossokinesthetic.
glos·so·dy·na·mom·e·ter [ˌ-ˌdaɪnə'mamɪtər] *n* Glossodynamometer *f*.
glos·so·dyn·ia [ˌ-'diːnɪə] *n* → glossalgia.
glos·so·ep·i·glot·tic [ˌ-ˌepɪ'glatɪk] *adj* Zunge/Glossa u. Kehldeckel/Epiglottis betr., glossoepiglottisch.
glossoepiglottic fold: lateral g. Plica glosso-epiglottica lateralis.
median g. Plica glosso-epiglottica mediana.
glos·so·ep·i·glot·tid·e·an [ˌ-ˌepɪglɑ'tiːdɪən] *adj* → glossoepiglottic.
glos·so·fa·cial anastomosis [ˌ-'feɪʃl] → glossal-facial anastomosis.
glos·so·graph ['-græf] *n* Glossograph *m*.
glos·so·hy·al [ˌ-'haɪəl] *adj* Zunge/Glossa u. Zungenbein/Os hyoideum betr., glossohyal.
glos·so·kin·es·thet·ic [ˌ-kɪnes'θetɪk] *adj* glossokinästhetisch.
glos·so·la·bi·al paralysis [ˌ-'leɪbɪəl] Duchenne-Syndrom *nt*, (progressive) Bulbärparalyse *f*.
glos·so·la·lia [ˌ-'leɪlɪə] *n psychia.* Glossolalie *f*.
glos·sol·y·sis [glɑ'salɪsɪs] *n* → glossoplegia.
glos·son·cus [glɑ'saŋkəs] *n* Zungenschwellung *f*.
glos·so·pal·a·tine [ˌglasəʊ'pælətaɪn, -tɪn, ˌglɒs-] *adj* Zunge/Glossa u. Gaumen/Palatum betr.
glossopalatine arch vorderer Gaumenbogen *m*, Arcus palatoglossus.
glos·so·pal·a·ti·nus (muscle) [ˌ-ˌpælæ'taɪnəs] Palatoglossus *m*, M. palatoglossus.
glos·so·p·a·thy [glɑ'sapəθɪ] *n* Zungenerkrankung *f*, Glossopathie *f*.
glos·so·pha·ryn·ge·al [ˌglasəʊfə'rɪndʒ(ɪ)əl] rɪn'dʒiːəl, ˌglɒs-] *adj* Zunge/Glossa u. Rachen/Pharynx betr., glossopharyngeal.
glossopharyngeal muscle → glossopharyngeus (muscle).
glossopharyngeal nerve Glossopharyngeus *m*, IX. Hirnnerv *m*, N. glossopharyngeus [IX].
glossopharyngeal neuralgia Glossopharyngeusneuralgie *f*, Neuralgia glossopharyngealis.
glos·so·pha·ryn·ge·us (muscle) [ˌ-fə'rɪndʒ(ɪ)əs] *old* M. glossopharyngeus, Pars glossopharyngea (m. constrictoris pharyngis superioris).
glos·so·pha·ryn·go·la·bi·al paralysis [ˌ-fəˌrɪŋgəʊ'leɪbɪəl] → glossolabial paralysis.
glos·so·pho·bia [ˌ-'fəʊbɪə] *n psychia.* Glossophobie *f*, Lalophobie *f*.
glos·so·phyt·ia [ˌ-'fɪtɪə] *n* schwarze Haarzunge *f*, Glossophytie *f*, Melanoglossie *f*, Lingua pilosa/villosa nigra.
glos·so·plas·ty ['-plæstɪ] *n chir.* Zungenplastik *f*, Glossoplastik *f*.
glos·so·ple·gia [ˌ-'pliːdʒ(ɪ)ə] *n* Zungenlähmung *f*, Glossoplegie *f*.
glos·sop·to·sis [ˌglasap'təʊsɪs] *n* Zurück-

sinken *nt* der Zunge, Glossoptose *f*.
glos·so·py·ro·sis [ˌglasəpaɪ'rəʊsɪs, ˌglɒs-] *n* Zungenbrennen *nt*, Glossopyrie *f*, -pyrosis *f*.
glos·sor·rha·phy [glɑ'sɔrəfɪ] *n chir.* Zungennaht *f*, Glossorrhaphie *f*.
glos·sos·co·py [glɑ'saskəpɪ] *n* Zungenuntersuchung *f*, -inspektion *f*.
glos·so·spasm ['glasəspæzəm, 'glɒs-] *n* Zungenkrampf *m*, Glossospasmus *m*.
glos·so·ste·re·sis [ˌ-stə'riːsɪs] *n* → glossectomy.
glos·sot·o·my [glɑ'satəmɪ] *n chir.* Zungenschnitt *m*, -durchtrennung *f*, Glossotomie *f*.
glos·so·trich·ia [ˌglasə'trɪkɪə, ˌglɒs-] *n* Haarzunge *f*, Glossotrichie *f*, Trichoglossie *f*, Lingua villosa/pilosa.
gloss·y ['glasɪ, 'glɒsɪ] *adj* glänzend.
glossy skin Glanzhaut *f*, Atrophoderma neuriticum.
glot·tal ['glatl] *adj* Glottis betr., glottisch, Glottis.
glot·tic [glatɪk] *adj* 1. → glossal. 2. → glottal.
glottic spasm Stimmritzenkrampf *m*, Laryngospasmus *m*.
glot·tis ['glatɪs] *n, pl* **-tis·es**, **-ti·des** [-tɪdiːz] Stimmapparat *m* des Kehlkopfs, Glottis *f* (vocalis).
glot·ti·tis [glɑ'taɪtɪs, glɒ-] *n* Glottisentzündung *f*, Glottitis *f*.
glove [glʌv] *n* Handschuh *m*.
glove anesthesia *neuro.* Handschuhanästhesie *f*.
glow [gləʊ] **I** *n* 1. Glut *f*. 2. Glühen *nt*, Leuchten *nt*; Hitze *f*, Röte *f*. **II** *vt* 3. glühen. 4. glühen, leuchten, strahlen; (*Gesicht*) brennen.
glow·ing ['gləʊɪŋ] *adj* 1. glühend. 2. glühend, leuchtend, strahlend; brennend.
Glu *abbr.* → glutamic acid.
gluc- *pref.* → gluco-.
glu·ca·gon ['gluːkəgan] *n* Glukagon *nt*, Glucagon *nt*.
glu·ca·go·no·ma [gluːkəgɑ'nəʊmə] *n* Glukagonom *nt*, Glucagonom(a) *nt*, A--Zell(en)-Tumor *m*.
glucagonoma syndrome Glukagonom--Syndrom *nt*.
glu·can ['gluːkæn] *n* Glukan *nt*, Glucan *nt*, Glukosan *m*.
1,4-α-glucan branching enzyme Branchingenzym *nt*, Glucan-verzweigende Glykosyltransferase *f*, 1,4-α-Glucan--branching-Enzym *nt*.
α-glucan-branching glycosyltransferase → 1,4-α-glucan branching enzyme.
glucan chain Glucankette *f*.
glucan-1,4-α-glucosidase *n* Glukan-1,4--α-Glucosidase *f*, lysosomale α-Glukosidase *f*.
α-glucan glycosyl 4:6-transferase → 1,4--α-glucan branching enzyme.
α(1→4)glucan phosphorylase α(1→4)-Glukanphosphorylase *f*.
(D-)glu·car·ic acid [gluː'kærɪk] D-Glucarsäure *f*, D-Zuckersäure *f*.
glu·ce·mia [gluː'siːmɪə] *n old* → glycemia.
glu·ci·num [gluː'sɪnɪəm] *n old* → beryllium.
glu·ci·tol ['gluːsətɒl, -təʊl] *n* Sorbit *nt*, Sorbitol *nt*, Glucit *nt*, Glucitol *nt*.
gluco- *pref.* Glukose-, Gluko-, Gluco-.
glu·co·cer·e·bro·si·dase [ˌgluːkəʊˌserəˈbrəʊsɪdeɪz] *n* Glukozerebrosidase *f*, Gluko-, Glucocerebrosidase *f*.
glu·co·cer·e·bro·side [ˌ-'serəbrəʊsaɪd] *n* Glukozerebrosid *nt*, Gluko-, Glucocerebrosid *nt*.
glu·co·cor·ti·coid [ˌ-'kɔːrtɪkɔɪd] **I** *n* Glukokortikoid *nt*, Glucocorticoid *nt*, Gluko-

steroid *nt*. **II** *adj* Glukokortikoid(e) betr., glukokortikoidähnliche Wirkung besitzend, glukokortikoidähnlich.
glucocorticoid hormone → glucocorticoid I.
glu·co·fu·ra·nose [ˌ-'fjʊərənəʊz] *n* Gluko-, Glucofuranose *f*.
glu·co·gen·e·sis [ˌ-'dʒenəsɪs] *n* Glukosebildung *f*, Gluko-, Glyko-, Glucogenese *f*.
glu·co·gen·ic [ˌ-'dʒenɪk] *adj* glukogen, glucogen.
glu·co·he·mia [ˌ-'hiːmɪə] *n* → glycemia.
glu·co·ki·nase [ˌ-'kaɪneɪz, -'kɪn-] *n* 1. Gluko-, Glucokinase *f*. 2. glukosespezifische Hexokinase *f*.
glu·co·ki·net·ic [ˌ-kɪ'netɪk] *adj* Glukose aktivierend, glukokinetisch.
glu·co·lip·id [ˌ-'lɪpɪd] *n* Gluko-, Glucolipid *nt*.
glu·col·y·sis [gluː'kalɪsɪs] *n* → glycolysis.
glu·co·lyt·ic [ˌgluːkəʊ'lɪtɪk] *adj* → glycolytic.
glu·co·nate ['-neɪt] *n* Glukonat *nt*, Gluconat *nt*.
glu·co·ne·o·gen·e·sis [ˌ-ˌniːə'dʒenəsɪs] *n* Gluko-, Glyko-, Gluconeogenese *f*.
glu·co·ne·o·ge·net·ic [ˌ-ˌniːədʒə'netɪk] *adj* Glukoneogenese betr., glukoneogenetisch.
glu·con·ic acid [gluː'kanɪk] Glukon-, Gluconsäure *f*.
glu·co·pe·nia [ˌgluːkəʊ'piːnɪə] *n* → glycopenia.
glu·co·pro·tein [ˌ-'prəʊtiːn, -tiːn] *n* 1. Gluko-, Glucoprotein *nt*. 2. → glycoprotein.
glu·co·py·ra·nose [ˌ-'paɪrənəʊz] *n* Gluko-, Glucopyranose *f*.
glu·co·re·cep·tor [ˌ-rɪ'septər] *n* Gluko-, Glucorezeptor *m*.
glu·co·sac·char·ic acid [ˌ-sə'kærɪk] → (D-)glucaric acid.
glu·co·sa·mine [gluː'kəʊsəmiːn, -mɪn] *n* Glukosamin *nt*, Aminoglukose *f*.
(D-)glu·cose ['gluːkəʊz] *n abbr.* **G** (D-)-Glukose *f*, Traubenzucker *m*, Dextrose *f*, Glucose *f*, α-D-Glucopyranose *f*, Glykose *f*.
glucose-alanine cycle Glukose-Alanin--Zyklus *m*.
glucose carrier Glukosecarrier *m*.
glucose catabolism Glukosekatabolismus *m*.
glucose-cystine blood agar *micro.* Blut-Traubenzucker-Cystein-Agar *m/nt*.
glucose dependent insulinotropic peptide gastrisches inhibitorisches Polypeptid *nt abbr.* GIP.
glucose-1,6-diphosphate *n* Glukose-1,6-diphosphat *nt*.
glucose-insulin-kalium solution Glukose-Insulin-Kalium-Lösung *f*.
glucose-insulin-potassium solution Glukose-Insulin-Kalium-Lösung *f*.
glucose intolerance Glukoseintoleranz *f*.
glucose-lactate cycle Cori-Zyklus *m*.
glucose level (Blut-)Zuckerspiegel *m*, (Blut-)Zuckerwert *m*, Glukosespiegel *m*.
glucose metabolism Glukosestoffwechsel *m*.
glucose oxidase Glukoseoxidase *f abbr.* GOD.
glucose oxidase paper strip test Glukosurienachweis *m* mit Glukoseoxidaseteststreifen.
glucose-6-phosphatase *n* Glukose-6-phosphatase *f abbr.* G-6-Pase.
glucose-6-phosphatase deficiency → glycogen storage disease, type I.
glucose-1-phosphate *n abbr.* **G1P** Glukose-1-phosphat *nt abbr.* G-1-P, Cori-Ester *m*.

glucose-6-phosphate

glucose-6-phosphate *n abbr.* **G6P** Glukose-6-phosphat *nt abbr.* G-6-P, Robison--Ester *m*.
glucose-1-phosphate adenylyltransferase Glukose-1-phosphat-adenylyltransferase *f*.
glucose-6-phosphate dehydrogenase *abbr.* **G6PD** Glukose-6-phosphatdehydrogenase *f abbr.* G-6-PDH, GPP.
glucose-6-phosphate dehydrogenase deficiency → glucose-6-phosphate dehydrogenase disease.
glucose-6-phosphate dehydrogenase deficiency anemia Anämie *f* durch Glukose-6-phosphatdehydrogenasemangel.
glucose-6-phosphate dehydrogenase disease Glukose-6-Phosphatdehydrogenasemangel(krankheit *f*) *m*, G-6-PDH--Mangel(krankheit *f*) *m*.
glucose-6-phosphate isomerase Glukose(-6-)phosphatisomerase *f*, Phosphohexoseisomerase *f abbr.* PHI, Phosphoglucoseisomerase *f abbr.* PGI.
glucosephosphate isomerase deficiency Glucosephosphatisomerase-Mangel *m*, Glucosephosphatisomerase-Defekt *m*.
glucose-1-phosphate kinase Phosphoglukokinase *f*, -glucokinase *f*.
glucose-1-phosphate uridylyltransferase Glukose-1-phosphat-uridylyltransferase *f*.
glucose-repressed *adj biochem.* durch Glukose reprimiert.
glucose-repressible *adj biochem.* durch Glukose reprimierbar.
glucose threshold (*Niere*) Glukoseschwelle *f*.
glucose tolerance *abbr.* **GT** Glukosetoleranz *f*.
  impaired g. *abbr.* **IGT** pathologische Glukosetoleranz.
glucose tolerance test *abbr.* **GTT** Glukosetoleranztest *m abbr.* GTT.
  oral g. *abbr.* **oGTT** oraler Glukosetoleranztest *abbr.* oGTT.
glucose value → glucose level.
glu·co·si·dase [glu:'kəʊsɪdeɪz] *n* Gluko-, Glucosidase *f*.
α-1,4-glucosidase deficiency → glycogen storage disease, type II.
glu·co·side ['glu:kəsaɪd] *n* Glukosid *nt*, Glucosid *nt*.
glu·co·sum [glu:'kəʊsəm] *n* → (D-)glucose.
glu·cos·u·ria [glu:kə's(j)ʊərɪə] *n* (Trauben-)Zuckerausscheidung *f* im Harn, Glukosurie *f*, Glucosurie *f*, Glukurese *f*, Glucurese *f*, Glykosurie *f*, Glykurie *f*.
glu·co·syl ['glu:kəsɪl] *n* Glykosyl-(Radikal *nt*).
glu·co·syl·cer·am·i·dase [,glu:kəsɪlsə'ræmɪdeɪz] *n* → glucocerebrosidase.
glu·co·syl·cer·a·mide lipidosis [,-'serəmaɪd] Gaucher'-Erkrankung *f*, -Krankheit *f*, -Syndrom *nt*, Morbus Gaucher *m*, Glukozerebrosidose *f*, Zerebrosidlipidose *f*, Lipoidhistiozytose *f* vom Kerasintyp, Glykosylzeramidlipidose *f*.
glu·co·syl·trans·fer·ase [,-'trænsfəreɪz] *n* Glykosyltransferase *f*.
glu·cu·ro·lac·tone [glu:kjərəʊ'læktəʊn] *n* Glucuro(no)lacton *nt*.
glu·cu·ro·nate [glu:'kjʊərəneɪt] *n* Glukuronat *nt*, Glucuronat *nt*.
glucuronate reductase Glukuronatreduktase *f*.
glu·cu·ron·ic acid [,glu:kjə'rɒnɪk] Glukuron-, Glucuronsäure *f*.
β-glu·cu·ron·i·dase [,glu:kjʊərənɪdeɪz] *n* β-Glucuronidase *f abbr.* GRD, β-GU.
β-glucuronidase deficiency Sly-Syndrom *nt*, Mukopolysaccharidose VIII *f abbr.* MPS VIII.

glu·cu·ro·nide [glu:'kjʊərənaɪd] *n* → glucuronoside.
glucuronide transferase → glucuronosyltransferase.
glu·cu·ro·no·lac·tone [,glu:kə,rəʊnəʊ'læktəʊn] *n* → glucurolactone.
glu·cu·ron·o·side [,glu:kjə'rɒnəsaɪd] *n* Glukuronid *nt*, Glucuronid *nt*, Glukuronosid *nt*.
glu·cu·ron·o·syl·trans·fer·ase [,glu:kjə,rɒnəsɪl'trænsfəreɪz] *n* Glukuronyltransferase *f*.
glu·cu·ron·yl transferase [glu:'kjʊərənɪl] → glucuronosyltransferase.
glue [glu:] *n* Leim *m*, Kleber *m*, Klebstoff *m*.
glue ear *HNO* Seromukotympanon *nt*.
glue·y ['glu:ɪ] *adj* klebrig; zähflüssig.
glu·ta·mate ['glu:təmeɪt] *n* Glutamat *nt*.
glutamate acetyltransferase Glutamatacetyltransferase *f*.
glutamate decarboxylase Glutamatdecarboxylase *f*.
glutamate dehydrogenase Glutamatdehydrogenase *f abbr.* GLD, GLDH, Glutaminsäuredehydrogenase *f abbr.* GSDH.
glutamate formiminotransferase Glutamatformiminotransferase *f*.
glutamate kinase Glutamatkinase *f*.
glutamate synapse Glutamatsynapse *f*.
glutamate synthase Glutamatsynthase *f*.
glu·tam·ic acid [glu:'tæmɪk] *abbr.* **Glu** Glutaminsäure *f abbr.* Glu, α-Aminoglutarsäure *f*.
glutamic acid formiminotransferase → glutamate formiminotransferase.
glutamic acid semialdehyde Glutaminsäuresemialdehyd *m*.
glutamic-oxaloacetic transaminase *abbr.* **GOT** Glutamatoxalacettransaminase *f abbr.* GOT, Aspartataminotransferase *f abbr.* AST, Aspartattransaminase *f*.
glutamic-pyruvic transaminase *abbr.* **GPT** Glutamatpyruvattransaminase *f abbr.* GPT, Alaninaminotransferase *f abbr.* ALT, Alanintransaminase *f*.
glu·ta·min·ase [glu:'tæmɪneɪz] *n* Glutaminase *f*.
glu·ta·mine ['glu:təmi:n, -mɪn] *n abbr.* **Gln** Glutamin *nt abbr.* Gln.
glutamine amidotransferase Glutaminamidotransferase *f*.
glutamine synthetase Glutaminsynthetase *f*.
glu·tam·i·nyl [glu:'tæmɪnɪl] *n* Glutaminyl(-Radikal *nt*).
glutaminyl-peptide γ-glutamyltransferase Faktor XIIIa *m*.
glu·ta·myl ['glu:təmɪl, glu:'tæm-] *n* Glutamyl-(Radikal *nt*).
γ-glutamyl amino acid γ-Glutamylaminosäure *f*.
γ-glutamyl carboxylase γ-Glutamylcarboxylase *f*.
γ-glutamyl cycle γ-Glutaminsäurezyklus *m*.
γ-glu·ta·myl·cy·clo·trans·fer·ase [,glu:təmɪl,saɪkləʊ'trænsfəreɪz] *n* γ-Glutamylcyclotransferase *f*.
γ-glu·ta·myl·cys·te·ine [,-'sɪsti:n] *n* γ-Glutamylcystein *nt*.
γ-glutamylcysteine synthetase γ-Glutamylcysteinsynthetase *f*.
γ-glutamyl phosphate γ-Glutamylphosphat *nt*.
γ-glu·ta·myl·trans·fer·ase [,-'trænsfəreɪz] *n abbr.* **GGT** γ-Glutamyltransferase *f abbr.* γ-GT, γ-Glutamyltranspeptidase *f abbr.* GGTP.
(γ-)glutamyl transpeptidase → γ-glutamyltransferase.

γ-glutamyl transpeptidase deficiency γ-Glutamyltransferasemangel *m*, Glutathionurie *f*.
glu·ta·ral ['glu:tərəl] *n* → glutaraldehyde.
glu·tar·al·de·hyde [glu:tə'rældəhaɪd] *n* Glutar(säuredi)aldehyd *m*.
glu·tar·ic acid [glu:'tærɪk] Glutarsäure *f*.
glutaric aciduria *abbr.* **GA** vermehrte Glutarsäureausscheidung *f* im Harn, Glutarsäureazidurie *f*.
glutaric aciduria IIB *abbr.* **GA IIB** Äthylmalonyladipinazidurie *f*, Glutarsäureazidurie *f* IIB.
glu·ta·thi·one [glu:tə'θaɪəʊn] *n* Glutathion *nt*, γ-Glutamylcysteinglycin *nt*.
  oxidized g. *abbr.* **GSSG** oxidiertes Glutathion, Glutathiondisulfid *nt abbr.* GSSG.
  reduced g. *abbr.* **GSH** reduziertes Glutathion, Glutathionsulfhydryl *nt abbr.* GSH.
glu·ta·thi·o·ne·mia [glu:tə,θaɪəʊ'ni:mɪə] *n* Glutathionämie *f*.
glutathione peroxidase Glutathionperoxidase *f*.
glutathione reductase (NAD(P)H) Glutathionreductase (NAD(P)H) *f abbr.* GR.
glutathione synthethase Glutathionsynthetase *f*.
glutathione synthetase deficiency Glutathionsynthetasemangel *m*.
glu·ta·thi·o·nu·ria [glu:tə,θaɪə'n(j)ʊərɪə] *n* **1.** vermehrte Glutathionausscheidung *f* im Harn, Glutathionurie *f*. **2.** γ-Glutamyltransferasemangel *m*, Glutathionurie *f*.
glu·te·al ['glu:tɪəl, glu:'ti:əl] *adj* Gesäß-(muskulatur) betr., glutäal, gluteal, Gesäß-, Gesäßmuskel-.
gluteal artery: inferior g. untere Gesäßarterie *f*, Glutäa *f* inferior, A. glut(a)ealis inferior.
  superior g. obere Gesäßarterie *f*, Glutäa *f* superior, A. glut(a)ealis superior.
gluteal cleft Gesäßspalte *f*, Afterfurche *f*, Crena ani, Rima ani.
gluteal crest Tuberositas glut(a)ealis.
gluteal eminence (of femur) Tuberositas glut(a)ealis.
gluteal fold → gluteal groove.
gluteal furrow → gluteal groove.
gluteal groove Gesäßfurche *f*, -falte *f*, Sulcus glut(a)ealis.
gluteal hernia Beckenhernie *f*, Ischiozele *f*, Hernia ischiadica.
gluteal intermuscular bursae Bursae intermusculares mm. glut(a)eorum.
gluteal line: anterior g. Linea glut(a)ealis anterior.
  inferior g. Linea glut(a)ealis inferior.
  posterior g. Linea glut(a)ealis posterior.
gluteal lymph nodes: inferior g. Lymphknoten *pl* der A. gluteaa inferior, Nodi lymphatici glut(a)eales inferiores.
  superior g. Lymphknoten *pl* der A. gluteaa superior, Nodi lymphatici glut(a)eales superiores.
gluteal muscle → gluteus.
gluteal nerve: inferior g. 1. Glutäus *m* inferior, N. glut(a)eus inferior. **2. ~s** *pl* untere Clunialnerven *pl*, Rami clunium/glut(a)eales inferiores.
  middle g.s mittlere Clunialnerven *pl*, Rami clunium/glut(a)eales medii.
  superior g. Glutäus *m* superior, N. glut(a)eus superior.
gluteal reflex Glutäal-, Glutealreflex *m*.
gluteal region Gesäßgegend *f*, -region *f*, Regio glut(a)ealis.
gluteal sulcus → gluteal groove.
gluteal tuberosity of femur Tuberositas glut(a)ealis.
gluteal veins: inferior g. Begleitvenen *pl*

der A. glutaea inferior, Vv. glut(a)eales inferiores.
superior g. Begleitvenen *pl* der A. glutaea superior, Vv. glut(a)eales superiores.
glu·te·lin ['gluːtlɪn] *n* Glutelin *nt*.
glu·ten ['gluːt(ɪ)n] *n* Klebereiweiß *nt*, Gluten *nt*.
gluten enteropathy gluteninduzierte Enteropathie *f*, Zöliakie *f*.
gluten flour Gluten-, Klebermehl *nt*.
glu·te·nin ['gluːtnɪn] *n* Glutenin *nt*.
glu·te·o·fas·ci·al bursae [ˌgluːtɪəˈfæʃ(ɪ)əl] → gluteal intermuscular bursae.
glu·te·o·fem·o·ral bursae [ˌ-ˈfemərəl] → gluteal intermuscular bursae.
glu·te·o·in·gui·nal [ˌ-ˈɪŋgwɪnl] *adj* gluteoinguinal.
glu·te·o·tu·ber·o·sal bursa [ˌ-t(j)uːbəˈrəʊsl] Bursa ischiadica/sciatica m. glut(a)ei maximi.
glu·teth·i·mide [gluːˈteθəmaɪd] *n pharm.* Glutethimid *nt*.
glu·te·us ['gluːtɪəs, gluːˈtiːəs -] *n*, *pl* **-tei** [-tɪaɪ, -ˈtiːaɪ] Glutäus *m*, M. glut(a)eus.
gluteus maximus (muscle) Glutäus *m* maximus, M. glut(a)eus maximus.
gluteus medius (muscle) Glutäus *m* medius, M. glut(a)eus medius.
gluteus minimus (muscle) Glutäus *m* minimus, M. glut(a)eus minimus.
gluteus muscle → gluteus.
greatest g. → gluteus maximus (muscle).
least g. → gluteus minimus (muscle).
middle g. → gluteus medius (muscle).
glu·ti·nous ['gluːtnəs] *adj* klebrig; zähflüssig.
glu·ti·tis [gluːˈtaɪtɪs] *n* Gesäßentzündung *f*, Glutitis *f*.
Gly *abbr.* → glycine.
gly·bu·ride [glaɪˈbjʊəraɪd] *n* → glibenclamide.
glyc- *pref.* → glyco-.
gly·can [ˈglaɪkæn] *n* Polysaccharid *nt*, Glykan *nt*, Glycan *nt*.
gly·ce·mia [glaɪˈsiːmɪə] *n* Zuckergehalt *m* des Blutes, Glykämie *f*.
gly·ce·mic gangrene [glaɪˈsiːmɪk] diabetische Gangrän *f*.
gly·cen·tin [glaɪˈsentɪn] *n* Enteroglukagon *nt*, intestinales Glukagon *nt*.
glyc·er·al·de·hyde [ˌglɪsəˈrældəhaɪd] *n* Glycerin-, Glycerinaldehyd *m*, Glyceraldehyd *m*.
glyceraldehyde-3-phosphate *abbr.* **GAP** Glycerinaldehyd-3-phosphat *nt abbr.* GAP, 3-Phosphoglyzerinaldehyd *m*.
glyceraldehyde-3-phosphate dehydrogenase *abbr.* **GAPD** Glycerinaldehyd(-3)dehydrogenase *f abbr.* GAPD(H), 3--Phosphoglyzerinaldehyddehydrogenase *f*.
glyc·er·ate [ˈglɪsəreɪt] *n* Glyzerat *nt*, Glycerat *nt*.
gly·cer·ic acid [glɪˈserɪk] Glyzerin-, Glycerinsäure *f*.
glyceric aldehyde → glyceraldehyde.
glyc·er·i·dase [ˈglɪsərɪdeɪz] *n* Lipase *f*.
glyc·er·ide [ˈglɪsəraɪd, -ɪd] *n* Acylglycerin *nt*, Glyzerid *nt*, Glycerid *nt*.
glyc·er·in [ˈglɪsərɪn] *n* **1.** → glycerol **2.** glyzerinhaltige Zubereitung *f*.
glycerin aldehyde → glyceraldehyde.
glyc·er·in·at·ed [ˈglɪsərəneɪtɪd] *adj* mit Glyzerin behandelt *od.* versetzt, glyzerinhaltig.
glyc·er·i·num [ˌglɪsəˈraɪnəm] *n* → glycerol.
glyc·er·ol [ˈglɪsərɒl, -rɒl] *n* Glyzerin *nt*, Glycerin *nt*, Glycerol *nt*, Propan-1,2,3--triol *nt*.
glyc·er·o·lize [ˈglɪsərəlaɪz] *vt* mit Glyzerin behandeln, in Glyzerin konservieren.
glycerol kinase Glyzerinkinase *f*.

glycerol lipid Glyzerinfett *nt*, -lipid *nt*.
glycerol-3-phosphate *n* Glyzerin-3-phosphat *nt*.
glycerol phosphate acyltransferase Glyzerinphosphatacyltransferase *f*.
glycerol-3-phosphate dehydrogenase Glyzerin-3-phosphatdehydrogenase *f*.
cytosol g. → glycerol-3-phosphate dehydrogenase (NAD+).
glycerol-3-phosphate dehydrogenase (NAD+) zytoplasmatische Glyzerin-3--phosphatdehydrogenase *f*, Glyzerinphosphatdehydrogenase (NAD+) *f*.
glycerol phosphate shuttle Glyzerinphosphatshuttle *m*.
glycerol phosphatide Phosphoglyzerid *nt*, Glycerophosphatid *nt*, *inf.* Phospholipid *nt*, Phosphatid *nt*.
glycerol-3-phosphorylcholine *n* Glyzerin--3-phosphorylcholin *nt abbr.* GPC.
glycerol teichoic acid Glycerinteichonsäure *f*.
glycerol tripalmitate Palmitin *nt*.
glyc·er·one [ˈglɪsərəʊn] *n* Glyzeron *nt*, Glyceron *nt*, Dihydroxyaceton *nt*.
glycerone phosphate Dihydroxyacetonphosphat *nt*.
glyc·er·o·phil·ic [ˌglɪsərəˈfɪlɪk] *adj* glyzerophil.
glyc·er·o·phos·pha·tase [ˌ-ˈfɒsfəteɪz] *n* Glycerophosphatase *f*.
glyc·er·ose [ˈglɪsərəʊz] *n* Glycerose *f*, Glyzerose *f*.
glyc·er·o·tri·o·le·ate [ˌglɪsərəʊtraɪˈəʊleɪt] *n* Olein *nt*, Triolen *nt*.
glyc·er·yl [ˈglɪsərɪl] *n* Glyzeryl-, Glyceryl--(Radikal *nt*).
glyceryl guaiacolate *pharm.* Guaifenesin *nt*, Guajacolglyzerinäther *m*.
glyceryl triacetate *pharm.* Triacetin *nt*, Glycerintriacetat *nt*, Glyceroltriacetat *nt*.
glyceryl trinitrate *pharm.* Glyceroltrinitrat *nt*, Nitroglyzerin *nt*.
gly·ci·nate [ˈglaɪsɪneɪt] *n* Glyzinat *nt*, Glycinat *nt*.
gly·cine [ˈglaɪsiːn, -sɪn] *n abbr.* **Gly** Glyzin *nt*, Glycin *nt abbr.* Gly, Glykokoll *nt*, Aminoessigsäure *f*.
glycine amidinotransferase Glycinamidinotransferase *f*.
glycine aminotransferase Glycinaminotransferase *f*, Glutaminsäure-glycin--transaminase *f*.
glycine antagonist Glycinantagonist *m*.
gly·ci·ne·mia [ˌglaɪsəˈniːmɪə] *n* erhöhter Glycingehalt *m* des Blutes, Hyperglyzinämie *f*, Hyperglycinämie *f*, Glykollkrankheit *f*, Glyzinose *f*, Glycinosis *f*, Glyzinurie *f* mit Hyperglyzinämie.
gly·ci·ner·gic [ˌ-ˈnɜːdʒɪk] *adj* glycinerg.
glycinergic synapse glycinerge Synapse *f*.
glycine-rich β-glycoprotein *abbr.* **GBG** *immun.* C3-Proaktivator *m*, Faktor B *m*, glycinreiches Beta-Globulin *nt abbr.* GBG.
glycine synthase Glycinsynthase *f*.
gly·ci·nu·ria [ˌ-ˈn(j)ʊərɪə] *n* Glycinausscheidung *f* im Harn, Glyzinurie *f*, Glycinurie *f*.
Gly·ciph·a·gus [glaɪˈsɪfəgəs] *n* → Glycyphagus.
glyco- *pref.* Glykogen-, Glyk(o)-, Glyc(o)-, Zucker-, Glyzerin-.
gly·co·ca·lix [ˌglaɪkəˈkeɪlɪks] *n* Glyko-, Glycokalix *f*.
gly·co·ca·lyx *n* → glycocalix.
gly·co·che·no·de·ox·y·cho·late [ˌ-ˌkiːnəʊdɪˌɒksɪˈkəʊleɪt] *n* Glykochenodesoxycholat *nt*.
gly·co·che·no·de·ox·y·cho·lic acid [ˌ-ˌkiːnəʊdɪˌɒksɪˈkəʊlɪk, -ˈkɒl-] Glykochenodesoxycholsäure *f*.

glycohemoglobin

gly·co·cho·late [ˌ-ˈkəʊleɪt, -ˈkɒl-] *n* Glykocholat *nt*.
gly·co·cho·lic acid [ˌ-ˈkəʊlɪk, -ˈkɒl-] Glykocholsäure *f*.
gly·co·cine [ˈ-siːn, -sɪn] *n* → glycine.
gly·co·clas·tic [ˌ-ˈklæstɪk] *adj* → glycolytic.
gly·co·coll [ˈ-kɒl] *n* → glycine.
gly·co·cy·a·mine [ˌ-ˈsaɪəmiːn, -saɪˈæmɪn] *n* Guanidinoessigsäure *f*.
gly·co·gen [ˈglaɪkədʒən] *n* Glykogen *nt*, tierische Stärke *f*.
gly·co·ge·nase [ˈ-dʒɪneɪz] *n* Glykogenase *f*; α-Amylase *f*; β-Amylase *f*.
gly·co·gen·e·sis [ˌ-ˈdʒenəsɪs] *n* **1.** Glykogenbildung *f*, Glykogenese *f*. **2.** Zuckerbildung *f*.
gly·co·ge·net·ic [ˌ-dʒəˈnetɪk] *adj* → glycogenic.
gly·co·gen·ic [-ˈdʒenɪk] *adj* Glykogenese *od.* Glykogen betr., Glykogenese fördernd, glykogenetisch.
gly·co·ge·nol·y·sis [ˌ-dʒɪˈnɒləsɪs] *n* Glykogenabbau *m*, Glykogenolyse *f*.
gly·co·gen·o·lyt·ic [ˌ-dʒenəˈlɪtɪk] *adj* Glykogenolyse betr. *od.* fördernd, glykogenspaltend, -abbauend, glykogenolytisch.
gly·co·ge·no·sis [ˌ-dʒɪˈnəʊsɪs] *n* → glycogen storage disease.
gly·cog·e·nous [glaɪˈkɒdʒənəs] *adj* → glycogenic.
glycogen phosphorylase Glykogenphosphorylase *f*.
glycogen phosphorylase kinase Phosphorylasekinase *f*.
glycogen storage disease Glykogenspeicherkrankheit *f*, Glykogenthesaurismose *f*, Glykogenose *f*.
g., type I (von) Gierke-Krankheit, van Creveld-von Gierke-Krankheit, hepatorenale Glykogenose, Glykogenose Typ I.
g., type II Pompe-Krankheit, generalisierte maligne Glykogenose, Glykogenose Typ II.
g., type III Cori-Krankheit, Forbes-Syndrom *nt*, hepatomuskuläre benigne Glykogenose, Glykogenose Typ III.
g., type IV Andersen-Krankheit, Amylopektinose *f*, leberzirrhotische retikuloendotheliale Glykogenose, Glykogenose Typ IV.
g., type V McArdle-Krankheit, -Syndrom *nt*, muskuläre Glykogenose, Muskelphosphorylasemangel *m*, Myophosphorylaseinsuffizienz *f*, Glykogenose Typ V.
g., type VI Hers-Erkrankung, -Syndrom *nt*, -Glykogenose, Leberphosphorylaseinsuffizienz *f*, Glykogenose Typ VI.
g., type VII Tarui-Krankheit, Muskelphosphofruktokinaseinsuffizienz *f*, Glykogenose Typ VII.
g., type VIII hepatische Glykogenose, Phosphorylase-b-kinase-Insuffizienz *f*, Glykogenose Typ VIII.
glycogen storage myopathy Glykogenspeichermyopathie *f*.
glycogen synthase Glykogensynthase *f*, -synthetase *f*.
glycogen synthase a aktive Glykogensynthetase *f*, Glykogensynthetase a *f*.
glycogen synthase b inaktive Glykogensynthetase *f*, Glykogensynthetase b *f*.
glycogen synthase D *old* → glycogen synthase b.
glycogen synthase I *old* → glycogen synthase a.
glycogen synthetase → glycogen synthase.
gly·co·geu·sia [ˌglaɪkəˈgjuːʒ(ɪ)ə] *n* Glykogeusie *f*.
gly·co·he·mia [ˌ-ˈhiːmɪə] *n* → glycemia.
gly·co·he·mo·glo·bin [ˌ-ˈhiːməgləʊbɪn,

glycohistechia

-'hemə-] *n* glykosyliertes Hämoglobin *nt*, Glykohämoglobin *nt*.
gly·co·his·tech·ia [ˌ-hɪs'tekɪə] *n patho.* Glykohistechia *f*.
gly·col ['glaɪkɔl, -kəl] *n* Glykol *nt*.
gly·co·late ['glaɪkəleɪt] *n* Glykolat *nt*.
glycolate oxidase Glykolatoxidase *f*.
gly·col·ic acid [glaɪ'kɑlɪk] Glykolsäure *f*, Hydroxyessigsäure *f*.
gly·co·lip·id [ˌglaɪkə'lɪpɪd] *n* Glykolipid *nt*.
glycolipid lipidosis Fabry-Syndrom *nt*, Morbus Fabry *m*, hereditäre Thesaurismose *f* Ruiter-Pompen-Weyers, Ruiter-Pompen-Weyers-Syndrom *nt*, Thesaurismosis hereditaria lipoidica, Angiokeratoma corporis diffusum (Fabry), Angiokeratoma universale.
gly·co·lur·ic acid [ˌ-'lʊərɪk] Hydantoinsäure *f*, Uraminessigsäure *f*.
gly·col·y·sis [glaɪ'kɑləsɪs] *n* Glyko-, Glycolyse *f*, Embden-Meyerhof-Weg *m*.
gly·co·lyt·ic [ˌglaɪkə'lɪtɪk] *adj* Glykolyse betr. *od.* fördernd, glykolytisch.
glycolytic enzyme glykolytisches Enzym *nt*.
glycolytic pathway glykolytischer Stoffwechselweg *m*.
gly·co·met·a·bol·ic [ˌ-ˌmetə'bɑlɪk] *adj* Zuckerstoffwechsel betr.
gly·co·me·tab·o·lism [ˌ-mə'tæbəlɪzəm] *n* Zuckerstoffwechsel *m*, -metabolismus *m*.
gly·cone ['glaɪkəʊn] *n pharm.* Glyzerinzäpfchen *nt*, -suppositorium *nt*.
gly·co·ne·o·gen·e·sis [ˌglaɪkəˌniːəʊ'dʒenəsɪs] *n* → gluconeogenesis.
gly·co·nu·cle·o·pro·tein [ˌ-ˌn(j)uːklɪə'prəʊtiːn, -tɪːn] *n* Glykonukleoprotein *nt*.
gly·co·pe·nia [ˌ-'piːnɪə] *n patho.* Glykopenie *f*.
gly·co·pep·tide [ˌ-'peptaɪd] *n* Glykopeptid *nt*.
gly·co·pex·ic [ˌ-'peksɪs] *adj biochem.* die Zucker- *od.* Glykogenspeicherung fördernd, zucker-, glykogenspeichernd.
gly·co·pex·is [ˌ-'peksɪs] *n biochem.* Zuckerspeicherung *f*, -bindung *f*, Glykogenspeicherung *f*, -bindung *f*.
Gly·coph·a·gus [glaɪ'kɑfəgəs] *n* → Glycyphagus.
gly·co·phor·in [ˌglaɪkə'fɔːrɪn] *n* Glykophorin *nt*.
gly·co·phos·pho·glyc·er·ide [ˌ-ˌfɑsfəʊ-'glɪsəraɪd, -ɪd] *n* Glykophosphoglycerid *nt*.
gly·co·pri·val [ˌ-'praɪvəl] *adj* Glukosemangel betr., durch Glukosemangel hervorgerufen, glykopriv.
gly·co·pro·tein [ˌ-'prəʊtiːn, -tɪːn] *n* Glykoprotein *nt*, -proteid *nt*, Glycoprotein *nt*, -proteid *nt*.
gly·co·pty·a·lism [ˌ-'taɪəlɪzəm] *n* → glycosialia.
gly·co·pyr·ro·late [ˌ-'pɪrəleɪt] *n pharm.* Glycopyrroniumbromid *nt*.
gly·co·pyr·ro·ni·um bromide [ˌ-pɪ'rəʊnɪəm] → glycopyrrolate.
gly·co·reg·u·la·tion [ˌ-ˌregjə'leɪʃn] *n* Kontrolle *f* des Zuckerstoffwechsels.
gly·cor·rha·chia [ˌ-'reɪkɪə, -'rækɪ-] *n* Auftreten *nt* von Zucker im Liquor cerebrospinalis.
gly·co·sam·ine [ˌ-'sæmɪn, -sə'miːn] *n* Glykosamin *nt*, Aminozucker *m*.
gly·cos·a·mi·no·gly·can [ˌglaɪkəʊsəˌmiːnəʊ'glaɪkæn] *n abbr.* **GAG** Glykosaminoglykan *nt abbr.* GAG.
gly·cos·a·mi·no·lip·id [ˌglaɪkəʊsəˌmiːnəʊ-'lɪpɪd] *n* Glykosaminolipid *nt*.
gly·co·se·mia [ˌglaɪkəʊ'siːmɪə] *n* → glycemia.
gly·co·si·a·lia [ˌ-saɪ'eɪlɪə, -'ælɪə] *n* Glukoseausscheidung *f* im Speichel, Glykoptyalismus *m*, Glykosialie *f*.
gly·co·si·dase [glaɪ'kəʊsɪdeɪz] *n* Glykosidase *f*, Glykosidhydrolase *f*.
gly·co·side ['glaɪkəsaɪd] *n* Glykosid *nt*, Glycosid *nt*.
gly·co·sid·ic [ˌglaɪkə'sɪdɪk] *adj* glykosidisch.
glycosidic bond/linkage *chem.* glykosidische Bindung *f*.
gly·co·sphin·go·lip·id [ˌ-ˌsfɪŋgəʊ'lɪpɪd] *n* Glykosphingolipid *nt*, Sphingoglykolipid *nt*.
gly·co·sphin·go·lip·i·do·sis [ˌ-ˌsfɪŋgəʊlɪpə'dəʊsɪs] *n* Fabry-Syndrom *nt*, Morbus Fabry *m*, Ruiter-Pompen-Weyers-Syndrom *nt*, hereditäre Thesaurismose *f* Ruiter-Pompen-Weyers, Thesaurismosis hereditaria lipoidica, Angiokeratoma corporis diffusum (Fabry), Angiokeratoma universale.
gly·co·stat·ic [ˌ-'stætɪk] *adj* glykostatisch.
gly·co·su·ria [ˌ-'s(j)ʊərɪə] *n* (Trauben-)-Zuckerausscheidung *f* im Harn, Glukosurie *f*, Glucosurie *f*, Glykosurie *f*, Glykurie *f*, Glukurese *f*, Glucurese *f*.
gly·co·su·ric acid [ˌ-'sjʊərɪk] Homogentisinsäure *f*, 2,5-Dihydroxyphenylessigsäure *f*.
gly·co·syl ['-sɪl] *n* Glykosyl-(Radikal *nt*).
gly·co·syl·ac·yl·glyc·er·ol [ˌ-sɪlˌæsɪl-'glɪsərɔl, -rɑl] *n* Glykosylacylglycerin *nt*.
N-gly·co·syl·a·mine [ˌ-sɪlə'miːn, -'æmɪn] *n* N-Glycosylamin *nt*, N-Glykosid *nt*.
gly·co·syl·at·ed [glaɪ'kəʊsɪleɪtɪd] *adj* glykosyliert.
glycosylated hemoglobin glykosyliertes Hämoglobin *nt*.
glycosylated hemoglobin test HbA₁c-Bestimmung *f*.
gly·co·syl·a·tion [ˌglaɪkəsɪ'leɪʃn] *n* Glykosylierung *f*.
gly·co·syl·cer·am·i·dase [ˌglaɪkəsɪls-'ræmɪdeɪz] *n* Glukozerebrosidase *f*, Gluko-, Glucozerebrosidase *f*.
gly·co·syl·cer·a·mide lipidosis [ˌ-sɪl'serəmaɪd] Gaucher'-Erkrankung *f*, -Krankheit *f*, -Syndrom *nt*, Morbus Gaucher *m*, Glukozerebrosidose *f*, Zerebrosidlipidose *f*, Glykosylzeramidlipidose *f*, Lipoidhistiozytose *f* vom Kerasintyp.
glycosyl diacylglycerol Glykosyldiacylglycerin *nt*.
glycosyl-1-phosphate nucleotidyltransferase Glykosyl-1-phosphatnucleotidyltransferase *f*, Pyrophosphorylase *f*.
gly·co·syl·sphin·go·sine [ˌ-sɪl'sfɪŋgəsɪːn, -sɪn] *n* Glykosylsphingosin *nt*.
gly·co·syl·trans·fer·ase [ˌ-sɪl'trænsfəreɪz] *n* Glykosyltransferase *f*.
gly·co·troph·ic [ˌ-'trɑfɪk, -'trəʊ-] *adj* → glycotropic.
gly·co·trop·ic [ˌ-'trɑpɪk, -'trəʊ-] *adj* Hyperglykämie verursachend, glykotrop.
gly·cu·res·is [ˌglaɪkjʊ'riːsɪs] *n* → glycosuria.
gly·cu·ron·ic acid [ˌglaɪkjʊ'rɑnɪk] Glukuronsäure *f*.
gly·cu·ro·nide [ˌglaɪ'kjʊərənaɪd] *n* Glukuronid *nt*.
gly·cu·ro·nu·ria [glaɪˌkjʊərə'n(j)ʊərɪə] *n* Glykuronsäureausscheidung *f* im Harn, Glykuronurie *f*.
glyc·yl ['glaɪsɪl] *n* Glyzyl-, Glycyl-(Radikal *nt*).
glycyl chain (*Insulin*) A-Kette *f*.
glycyl-tRNA synthetase Glycyl-tRNA-synthetase *f*.
Gly·cyph·a·gus [glaɪ'sɪfəgəs] *n micro.* Glycyphagus *m*.
G. domesticus Haus-, Wohnungs-, Polstermilbe *f*, Glycyphagus domesticus.
glyc·yr·rhi·za [glɪsə'raɪzə] *n pharm.* Süßholz(wurzel *f*) *nt*, Radix liquiritiae.

glyc·yr·rhi·zic acid [glɪsə'raɪzɪk] → glycyrrhizin.
glyc·yr·rhi·zin [glɪsə'raɪzn] *n* Glycyrrhizin *nt*.
gly·ke·mia [glaɪ'kiːmɪə] *n* → glycemia.
glykemic gangrene → glycemic gangrene.
gly·ox·al [glaɪ'ɑksəl] *n* Glyoxal *nt*, Oxalaldehyd *m*.
gly·ox·a·lase [glaɪ'ɑksəleɪz] *n* Glyoxalase *f*.
glyoxalase I Glyoxalase I *f*, Lactoylglutathionlyase *f*.
glyoxalase II Glyoxalase II *f*, Hydroxyacylglutathionhydrolase *f*.
gly·ox·a·line [glaɪ'ɑksəliːn, -lɪn] *n* Imidazol *nt*, Glyoxalin *nt*.
gly·ox·i·some *n* → glyoxosome.
gly·ox·o·some [glaɪ'ɑksəsəʊm] *n* Glyoxysom *nt*.
gly·ox·y·late [glaɪ'ɑksəleɪt] *n* Glyoxylat *nt*, Glyoxalat *nt*.
glyoxylate cycle Glyoxalatzyklus *m*.
gly·ox·yl·ic acid [ˌglaɪɑk'sɪlɪk] Glyoxalsäure *f*, Glyoxylsäure *f*.
gm *abbr.* → gram.
Gm allotypes [gamma chain marker] Gm-Allotypen *pl*.
Gm antigens Gm-Antigene *pl*.
Gmelin ['meɪlɪn; 'gmeliːn]: **G.'s reaction/test** Gmelin-Probe *f*.
GM₁-gangliosidosis *n* generalisierte Gangliosidose *f*, GM₁-Gangliosidose *f* Typ I.
GM₂-gangliosidosis *n* Tay-Sachs-Erkrankung *f*, -Syndrom *nt*, infantile amaurotische Idiotie *f*, GM₂-Gangliosidose *f* Typ I.
GMP *abbr.* → guanosine monophosphate.
3',5' GMP *abbr.* → guanosine 3',5'-cyclic phosphate.
GMP synthetase GMP-Synthetase *f*, Guanylsäuresynthetase *f*.
GMW *abbr.* → gram-molecular weight.
GN *abbr.* → glomerulonephritis.
gnash [næʃ] *vt, vi* mit den Zähnen knirschen.
gnash·ing ['næʃɪŋ] *n* Zähneknirschen *nt*.
gnat [næt] *n* **1.** *US* Kriebelmücke *f*. **2.** *Brit.* (Stech-)Mücke *f*.
gnath- *pref.* → gnatho-.
gna·thal·gia [næ'θældʒ(ɪ)ə] *n* Kieferschmerz(en *pl*) *m*, Gnathalgie *f*, Gnathodynie *f*.
gnath·ic ['næθɪk, 'neɪ-] *adj* Kiefer betr., Kiefer-, Gnath(o)-.
gna·thi·on ['næθɪɑn, 'neɪ-] *n* Gnathion *nt*.
gna·thi·tis [næ'θaɪtɪs] *n* Kieferentzündung *f*, Gnathitis *f*.
gnatho- *pref.* Kiefer-, Gnath(o)-.
gnath·o·ceph·a·lus [ˌnæθə'sefələs] *n embryo.* Gnathozephalus *m*.
gnath·o·dyn·ia [ˌ-'dɪnɪə] *n* → gnathalgia.
gnath·o·pal·a·tos·chi·sis [ˌ-ˌpælə'tɑskəsɪs] *n embryo.* Kiefer-Gaumen-Spalte *f*, Gnathopalatoschisis *f*.
gnath·o·plas·ty ['-plæstɪ] *n chir., HNO* Kieferplastik *f*, Gnathoplastik *f*.
gna·thos·chi·sis [næ'θɑskəsɪs] *n embryo.* Kieferspalte *f*, Gnathoschisis *f*.
Gna·thos·to·ma [næ'θɑstəmə] *n micro.* Gnathostoma *nt*.
G. spinigerum Magenwurm *m* der Ratte, Gnathostoma spinigerum.
gnath·o·sto·mi·a·sis [ˌnæθə'staɪəsɪs] *n* Gnathostomainfektion *f*, Gnathostomiasis *f*.
Gna·thos·to·mum [næ'θɑstəmʊm] *n* → Gnasthostoma.
gno·to·bi·ol·o·gy [ˌnəʊtəʊbaɪ'ɑlədʒɪ] *n* gnotobiotics.
gno·to·bi·ote [ˌ-'baɪəʊt] *n* Gnotobio(n)t *m*.

gno·to·bi·ot·ic [ˌ-baɪˈɒtɪk] *adj* gnotobiotisch.
gno·to·bi·ot·ics [ˌ-baɪˈɒtɪks] *pl* Gnotobiologie *f*, Gnotobiose *f*.
GnRF *abbr.* → gonadotropin releasing factor.
GnRH *abbr.* [gonadotropin releasing hormone] → gonadotropin releasing factor.
go [gəʊ] (*v* went, gone) **I** *n, pl* **goes 1.** Gehen *nt*; Gang *m*; Verlauf *m*. **2.** Versuch *m*. **to have a ~ at** (doing) sth. etw. probieren *od.* versuchen. **at one ~** auf Anhieb. **in one ~** auf einmal. **3.** Anfall *m*.
II *adj techn. inf.* funktionstüchtig.
III *vi* **4.** gehen (*to* nach); s. (fort-)bewegen. **to ~ on foot** zu Fuß gehen. **5.** anfangen, losgehen. **6.** s. erstrecken, reichen, gehen (*to* bis). **7.** gehen, passen (*into*, in in). **8.** gehören (*in*, *into* in; *on* auf). **9.** *techn.* gehen, laufen, funktionieren, arbeiten. **10.** werden. **to ~ bad** verderben, schlecht werden. **to ~ blind** erblinden. **to ~ mad** verrückt *od.* wahnsinnig werden. **to ~ hungry** hungern. **to ~ sick** s. krankmelden. **to ~ to sleep** einschlafen. **to ~ with child** schwanger sein. **11.** verlaufen, s. entwickeln. **12.** (*Entscheidung*) ausfallen. **13.** s. vertragen, gehen, harmonisieren (*with* mit); passen (*with* zu). **14.** sterben. **15.** zusammenbrechen; (*Kräfte*) nachlassen; kaputtgehen, versagen.
go at *vi* losgehen auf, angreifen.
go back *vi* zurückgehen; *fig.* zu (alten Gewohnheiten) zurückkehren (*to*).
go down *vi* **1.** (*Essen*) hinunterrutschen. **2.** (*Fieber*) fallen, sinken, zurückgehen; nachlassen, s. beruhigen. **3.** (*beim Test*) durchfallen.
go for *vi* **1.** (*Arzt*) holen (gehen). **2.** losgehen auf, s. stürzen auf, angreifen.
go into *vi* **1.** (genau) untersuchen/prüfen, s. befassen mit. **2.** einen Anfall bekommen; ins Koma fallen. **3.** **to ~ mourning** trauern, Trauer tragen.
go off *vi* **1.** (*Schmerz*) nachlassen. **2.** s. verschlechtern; (*Nahrungsmittel*) verderben. **3.** ohnmächtig werden. **4.** einschlafen. **5.** geraten (*in, into* in). **to ~ in a fit** einen Anfall bekommen. **to ~ one's head** verrückt werden; sehr wütend werden. **6.** (*Bombe*) losgehen. **7.** ausgehen, nicht (mehr) funktionieren.
go on *vi* **1.** weitermachen, fortfahren (*with* mit, *doing* zu tun). **2.** passieren, vor s. gehen. **3.** weitergehen *od.* -fahren. **to ~ the pill** die Pille nehmen. **to ~ a diet** eine Schlankheitskur machen.
go out *vi* **1.** (*Licht, Feuer*) ausgehen, erlöschen. **2.** zu Ende gehen, enden. **3.** → go off 3, 4.
go round *vi* **1.** vorbeigehen (*to* bei). **2.** s. drehen.
go through *vi* **1.** durchgehen, -nehmen, -sprechen. **2.** durchmachen, erleiden. **3. ~ with** zu Ende führen, aus-, durchführen, durchziehen.
go under *vi* **1.** eine Narkose haben. **2.** einer Krankheit zum Opfer fallen.
go up *vi* (*Fieber*) steigen.
go with *vi* **1.** jdn./etw. begleiten. **2.** passen zu.
go without *vi* auskommen ohne, s. behelfen ohne, verzichten (müssen) auf.
goat louse [gəʊt] *micro.* Linognathus stenopsis.
goat's milk anemia Ziegenmilchanämie *f*.
gob·let [ˈgɒblət] *n* Becher *m*.
goblet cell Becherzelle *f*.
gog·gle [ˈgɒgl] *n* **1.** Augenschutz(schild *nt*) *m*. **2. ~s** *pl* Schutzbrille *f*.
goi·ter [ˈgɔɪtər] *n* Kropf *m*, Struma *f*.
goi·tre *n Brit.* → goiter.

goi·tro·gen [ˈgɔɪtrədʒən] *n* strumigene Substanz *f*.
goi·tro·gen·ic [ˌgɔɪtrəˈdʒenɪk] *adj* Kropf/ Struma verursachend *od.* auslösend, strumigen.
goitrogenic substance → goitrogen.
goi·trog·e·nous [gɔɪˈtrɒdʒənəs] *adj* → goitrogenic.
goi·trous [ˈgɔɪtrəs] *adj* Struma betr., kropfartig, strumaartig, Kropf-, Struma-.
gold [gəʊld] *n* Gold *nt*; *chem.* Aurum *nt abbr.* Au.
Goldberger [ˈgəʊldbɜːrgər]: **G.'s augmented limb leads** Goldberger-(Extremitäten-)- Ableitungen *pl*.
G.'s method → G.'s augmented limb leads.
Goldberg-Maxwell [ˈgəʊldbɜːrg ˈmækswel]: **G.-M. syndrome** testikuläre Feminisierung *f*, Goldberg-Maxwell-Morris- -Syndrom *nt*.
Goldblatt [ˈgəʊldblæt]: **G. hypertension** → G.'s mechanism.
G.'s kidney Goldblatt-Niere *f*, vaskuläre Schrumpfniere *f*.
G.'s mechanism Goldblatt-Mechanismus *m*, -Phänomen *nt*.
G.'s phenomenon → G.'s mechanism.
Goldenhar [ˈgəʊldənhɑːr]: **G.'s syndrome** Goldenhar-Syndrom *nt*, okuloaurikuläres/okulo-aurikulo-vertebrales Syndrom *nt*, okulo-aurikulo-vertebrale Dysplasia *f*, Dysplasia oculo-auricularis, Dysplasia oculo-auriculo-vertebralis.
Goldflam [ˈgɒltflæm]: **G.'s disease** → Goldflam-Erb disease.
Goldflam-Erb [ɜːrb]: **G.-E. disease** Erb- -Goldflam-Syndrom *nt*, -Krankheit *f*, Erb-Oppenheim-Goldflam-Syndrom *nt*, -Krankheit *f*, Hoppe-Goldflam-Syndrom *nt*, Myasthenia gravis pseudoparalytica.
Goldman [ˈgəʊldmən]: **G.'s applanation tonometer** *ophthal.* Goldmann-Applanationstonometer *nt*.
G. equation Goldman-Gleichung *f*, Goldman-Hodgkin-Katz-Gleichung *f*.
Goldman-Hodgkin-Katz [ˈhɒdʒkɪn kæts]: **G.-H.-K. equation** → Goldman equation.
gold orange Methylorange *nt*, Heliantin *nt*.
gold reaction Goldsolreaktion *f*. **colloidal g.** → gold reaction.
Goldscheider [ˈgəʊldʃaɪdər]: **G.'s disease** Goldscheider'-Krankheit *f*, Köbner'- -Krankheit *f*, Epidermolysis bullosa hereditaria simplex (Köbner), Epidermolysis bullosa simplex Köbner, Pemphigus héréditaire traumatique.
Goldstein [ˈgəʊldstaɪn]: **G.'s disease** hereditäre Teleangiektasie *f*, Morbus Osler *m*, Osler-Rendu-Weber-Krankheit *f*, -Syndrom *nt*, Rendu-Osler-Weber-Krankheit *f*, -Syndrom *nt*, Teleangiectasia hereditaria haemorrhagica.
G.'s sign Goldstein-Zehenzeichen *nt*.
golf arm [gɑːlf, gɒlf] *ortho.* Golfschulter *f*, -spielerarm *m*.
Golgi [ˈgɒldʒi]: **G.'s apparatus** Golgi-Apparat *m*, -Komplex *m*.
G.'s body → G. apparatus.
G.'s cell 1. Golgi-Zelle *f*. **2.** → G. type I neuron. **3.** → G. type II neuron.
G.'s complex → G. apparatus.
G.'s corpuscle → G.'s organ.
G. impregnation Golgi-Imprägnation *f*.
G. interneuron Golgi-Interneuron *n*.
G. material *embryo.* Golgi-Material *nt*.
G.'s method → G.'s stain.
G.'s organ Golgi-Sehnenorgan *nt*, -Sehnenspindel *f*.
G.'s stain Golgi-Färbung *f*.
G.'s staining method → G.'s stain.

G.'s tendon organ → G.'s organ.
G. type I neuron Neuron vom Deiters-Typ.
G. type II neuron Neuron vom Golgi-Typ.
Golgi-Mazzoni [mædˈzəʊni]: **G.-M. corpuscle** Golgi-Mazzoni'-Körperchen *nt*.
gol·gi·o·ki·ne·sis [ˌgɒldʒɪəʊkɪˈniːsɪs, -kaɪ-] *n bio.* Golgiokinese *f*, Diktyokinese *f*.
gol·gi·o·some [ˈ-səʊm] *n* Diktyosom *nt*.
Goll [gɑl, gɒl]: **G.'s column** → G.'s fasciculus.
G.'s fasciculus Goll-Strang *m*, Fasciculus gracilis (medullae spinalis).
G.'s fibers Goll'-Fasern *pl*.
G.'s nucleus Nc. gracilis.
G.'s tract → G.'s fasciculus.
Goltz [gəʊlts, gɒlts]: **G.' syndrome** fokale dermale Hypoplasie *f*, FDH-Syndrom *nt*, kongenitale ektodermale u. mesodermale Dysplasie *f*, Goltz-Gorlin-Syndrom II *nt*, Goltz-Peterson-Gorlin-Ravits- -Syndrom *nt*, Jessner-Cole-Syndrom *nt*, Liebermann-Cole-Syndrom *nt*.
Goltz-Gorlin [ˈgɔːrlɪn]: **G.-G. syndrome** → Goltz's syndrome.
Gombault [gɡ̃ˈbo]: **G.'s degeneration/neuritis** Déjérine-Sottas-Krankheit *f*, -Syndrom *nt*, hypertrophische Neuropathie (Déjérine-Sottas) *f*, hereditäre motorische u. sensible Neuropathie Typ III *f abbr.* HMSN.
Gombault-Philippe [fiˈlip]: **G.-P. triangle** Gombault-Philippe'-Triangel *f*, Philippe-Gombault'-Triangel *f*.
Gomori [gəˈmɔːri]: **G.'s silver impregnation stain** Gomori-Silberimprägnation *f*.
gom·phol·ic joint [gɑmˈfɑlɪk] → gomphosis.
gom·pho·sis [gɑmˈfəʊsɪs] *n* **1.** Einkeilung *f*, Einzapfung *f*, Gomphosis *f*. **2.** Artic. dentoalveolaris, Gomphosis *f*.
gon- *pref.* **1.** → gono-. **2.** Knie-, Gon-.
gon·a·cra·tia [ˌgɑnəˈkreɪʒ(ɪ)ə] *n* Samenfluß *m*, Spermatorrhoe *f*.
gonad- *pref.* → gonado-.
go·nad [ˈgəʊnæd, ˈgɑ-] *n* Keim-, Geschlechtsdrüse *f*, Gonade *f*.
go·nad·al [gəʊˈnædl, gɑ-] *adj* Gonade(n) betr., gonadal, Gonad(o)-, Gonaden-.
gonadal agenesia Gonadenagenesie *f*.
gonadal dysgenesis Gonadendysgenesie *f*.
  mixed g. gemischte Gonadendysgenesie.
  pure g. reine Gonadendysgenesie, Swyer- -Syndrom *nt*.
gonadal insufficiency Gonadeninsuffizienz *f*.
gonadal mesenchyma Gonadenmesenchym *nt*.
gonadal ridge *embryo.* Genitalleiste *f*, -falte *f*, Geschlechtsleiste *f*, -falte *f*.
gonadal sex *genet.* Gonadengeschlecht *nt*.
gonadal shield *radiol.* Gonadenschutz *m*.
go·nad·ec·to·mize [gəʊnæˈdektəmaɪz] *vt chir., urol., gyn.* die Gonaden entfernen, eine Gonadektomie durchführen.
go·nad·ec·to·my [gəʊnæˈdektəmɪ] *n chir., urol., gyn.* Gonadenentfernung *f*, Gonadektomie *f*.
go·na·di·al [gəʊˈneɪdɪəl] *adj* → gonadal.
gonado- *pref.* Gonaden-, Gonad(o)-.
go·na·do·blas·to·ma [gəʊˌnædəblæsˈtəʊmə, ˌgɑnədəʊ-] *n patho.* Gonadoblastom *nt*.
go·na·do·gen·e·sis [ˌ-ˈdʒenəsɪs] *n embryo.* Gonadenentwicklung *f*, Gonadogenese *f*.
go·na·do·in·hib·i·to·ry [ˌ-ɪnˈhɪbətɔːriː, -təʊ-] *adj* die Gonadenaktivität hemmend.
go·na·do·ki·net·ic [ˌ-kɪˈnetɪk] *adj* die Gonadenaktivität stimulierend.
go·na·do·lib·er·in [ˌ-ˈlɪbərɪn] *n* → gonadotropin releasing factor.

gonadopathy

go·na·dop·a·thy [gɒnæ'dɑpəθɪ] *n* Gonadenerkrankung *f*, Gonadopathie *f*.
go·nad·o·pause [gəʊ'næɾəpɔːz, 'ɡɑnədəʊ-] *n* Gonadopause *f*.
go·nad·o·rel·in [,-'relɪn] *n* synthetisches Gonadotropin-releasing-Hormon *nt*.
go·nad·o·trope ['-trəʊp] *n* → gonadotroph.
go·nad·o·troph ['-trəʊf] *n* **1.** gonadotrope Substanz *f*. **2.** (*HVL*) gonadotrope Zelle *f*; β-Zelle *f*, Beta-Zelle *f*; D-Zelle *f*, Delta-Zelle *f*.
gonadotroph cell (*HVL*) gonadotrope Zelle *f*; β-Zelle *f*, Beta-Zelle *f*; D-Zelle *f*, Delta-Zelle *f*.
go·na·do·troph·ic [,-'trafɪk, -'trəʊ-] *adj* → gonadotropic.
go·na·do·tro·phin [,-'trəʊfɪn] *n* → gonadotropin.
go·na·do·trop·ic [,-'trapɪk, -'trəʊ-] *adj* auf die Gonaden wirkend, gonadotrop.
gonadotropic hormone → gonadotropin.
go·na·do·tro·pin [,-'trəʊpɪn] *n* gonadotropes Hormon *nt*, Gonadotropin *nt*.
gonadotropin releasing factor *abbr.* **GnRF** Gonadotropin-releasing-Faktor *m abbr.* GnRF, Gonadotropin-releasing-Hormon *nt abbr.* GnRH, Gonadoliberin *nt*.
gonadotropin releasing hormone *abbr.* **GnRH** → gonadotropin releasing factor.
gon·a·duct ['gɒnədʌkt] *n* **1.** abführender/ableitender Samengang *m*. **2.** Eileiter *m*, Tuba uterina.
go·nag·ra [ɡɑ'nægrə, -neɪ-] *n* Kniegicht *f*, Gonagra *f*.
go·nal·gia [ɡəʊ'næld3(ɪ)ə] *n* Knieschmerz *m*, Gonalgie *f*.
gon·an·gi·ec·to·my [,ɡanænd3ɪ'ektəmɪ] *n urol.* Vasektomie *f*, Vasoresektion *f*.
gon·ar·thri·tis [ɡɑnɑː'θraɪtɪs] *n* Knie(gelenk)entzündung *f*, Gonitis *f*, Gonarthritis *f*.
gon·ar·throc·a·ce [,ɡɑnɑː'θrɑkəsɪ:] *n old* tuberkulöse Knie(gelenk)entzündung/ Gonitis *f*, Gonitis tuberculosa.
gon·ar·thro·men·in·gi·tis [ɡɑn,ɑːrθrə,menɪn'dʒaɪtɪs] *n* Kniegelenk(s)synovitis *f*.
gon·ar·thro·sis [,ɡɑnɑː'θrəʊsɪs] *n* Kniegelenkarthrose *f*, Gonarthrose *f*.
gon·ar·throt·o·my [,ɡɑnɑː'θrɑtəmɪ] *n ortho.* Gonarthrotomie *f*.
go·nat·o·cele [ɡəʊ'nætəsɪ:l] *n* Knie(gelenk)geschwulst *f*.
gon·e·cyst ['ɡɑnəsɪst] *n* Bläschendrüse *f*, Samenblase *f*, -bläschen *nt*, Gonezystis *f*, Spermatozystis *f*, Vesicula seminalis.
gon·e·cys·tis [,-'sɪstɪs] *n* → gonecyst.
gon·e·cys·ti·tis [,-sɪs'taɪtɪs] *n* Samenblasenentzündung *f*, Vesikulitis *f*, Vesiculitis *f*, Spermatozystitis *f*.
gon·e·cys·to·lith [,-'sɪstəlɪθ] *n* Samenblasenstein *m*, Spermatozystolith *m*.
gon·e·i·tis [ɡɑnɪ'aɪtɪs] *n* → gonitis.
Gon·gy·lo·ne·ma [,ɡɑndʒɪləʊ'niːmə] *f micro.* Gongylonema *nt*.
gon·gy·lo·ne·mi·a·sis [,-nɪ'maɪəsɪs] *n* Gongylonemainfektion *f*, Gongylonemiasis *f*.
goni- *pref.* → gonio-.
go·ni·al angle ['ɡəʊnɪəl] Angulus mandibulae.
gon·id·an·gi·um [,ɡɑnə'dændʒɪəm] *n micro.* Gonidangium *nt*.
go·nid·i·o·spore [ɡəʊ'nɪdɪəspəʊər] *n micro.* Gonidiospore *f*.
go·nid·i·um [ɡə'nɪdɪəm] *n, pl* **-dia** [-dɪə] *micro.* Gonidie *f*, Gonidium *nt*.
Gonin [ɡɔ'nɛ̃]: **G.'s operation** *ophthal.* Gonin-Operation *f*.
gonio- *pref.* Winkel-, Goni(o)-.
gon·i·o·ma [,ɡɑnɪ'əʊmə] *n patho.* Goniom(a) *nt*.

go·ni·om·e·ter [,ɡəʊnɪ'ɑmɪtər] *n* Goniometer *nt*.
go·ni·om·e·try [,ɡəʊnɪ'ɑmətrɪ] *n* Goniometrie *f*.
go·ni·on ['ɡəʊnɪɑn] *n, pl* **-nia** [-nɪə] Gonion *nt*, äußerster Punkt des Unterkieferwinkels.
go·ni·o·punc·ture [,ɡəʊnɪə'pʌŋ(k)tʃər] *n ophthal.* Kammerwinkelpunktion *f*, Goniopunktion *f*.
go·ni·o·scope ['-skəʊp] *n ophthal.* Gonioskop *nt*.
go·ni·os·co·py [,ɡəʊnɪ'ɑskəpɪ] *n ophthal.* Gonioskopie *f*.
go·ni·o·syn·ech·ia [,ɡəʊnɪəsɪ'nekɪə, -'niː-] *n ophthal.* Goniosynechie *f*.
go·ni·o·tome [-'təʊm] *n ophthal.* Goniotomiemesser *nt*, Goniotom *nt*.
go·ni·ot·o·my [ɡəʊnɪ'ɑtəmɪ] *n ophthal.* Goniotomie *f*, Trabekulotomie *f*.
go·ni·tis [ɡəʊ'naɪtɪs] *n* Knie(gelenk)entzündung *f*, Gonitis *f*, Gonarthritis *f*.
gono- *pref.* Gon(o)-.
gon·o·blen·nor·rhea [,ɡɑnəʊ,blenə'rɪə] *n* gonorrhoische Bindehautentzündung *f*, Gonoblennorrhoe *f*, Conjunctivitis gonorrhoica.
gon·o·cele ['-siːl] *n* Gonozele *f*, Spermatozele *f*.
gon·o·cho·rism [,-'kɔːrɪzəm] *n* Gonochorismus *m*.
gon·o·cho·ris·mus [,-kɔː'rɪzməs] *n* → gonochorism.
gon·o·cide ['-saɪd] *n, adj* → gonococcide.
gon·o·coc·cal [,-'kɑkəl] *adj* Gonokokken betr., Gonokokken-.
gonococcal arthritis Gonokokkenarthritis *f*, gonorrhoische Arthritis *f*, Arthritis gonorrhoica.
gonococcal cervicitis Gonokokkenzervizitis *f*.
gonococcal conjunctivitis → gonoblennorrhea.
gonococcal endocarditis Gonokokkenendokarditis *f*.
gonococcal endometritis gonorrhoische Endometritis *f*, Endometritis gonorrhoica.
gonococcal perihepatitis gonorrhoische Perihepatitis *f*.
gonococcal proctitis Gonokokkenproktitis *f*.
gonococcal salpingitis Gonokokkensalpingitis *f*.
gonococcal stomatitis Gonokokkenstomatitis *f*.
gonococcal urethritis gonorrhoische Urethritis *f*, Urethritis gonorrhoica.
gon·o·coc·ce·mia [,-kɑk'siːmɪə] *n* Gonokokkämie *f*, Gonokokkensepsis *f*.
gon·o·coc·ci *pl* → gonococcus.
gon·o·coc·cic [,-'kɑksɪk] *adj* → gonococcal.
gon·o·coc·cide [,-'kɑksaɪd] **I** *n* gonokokken(ab)tötendes Mittel *nt*. **II** *adj* gonokokken(ab)tötend.
gon·o·coc·cide [,-'kɑksaɪd] *n, adj* → gonococcide.
gon·o·coc·cus [,-'kɑkəs] *n, pl* **-coc·ci** [-'kɑksaɪ, -siː] Gonokokkus *m*, Gonococcus *m*, Neisseria gonorrhoeae.
gon·o·cyte ['-saɪt] *n* Gonozyt *m*.
gon·o·mer·y [ɡəʊ'nɑmərɪ] *n genet.* Gonomerie *f*.
gon·o·phage ['ɡɑnəfeɪdʒ] *n* Gonophage *m*.
gon·o·phore ['-fɔʊər, -fɔːr] *n* Gonophore *f*.
gon·or·rhea [,-'rɪə] *n* Tripper *m*, Gonorrhö *f*, Gonorrhoe(a) *f abbr.* GO.
gon·or·rhe·al [,-'rɪəl] *adj* Gonorrhö betr., gonorrhoisch, Gonorrhö-.
gonorrheal arthritis → gonococcal arthritis.

gonorrheal conjunctivitis → gonoblennorrhea.
gonorrheal coxitis gonorrhoische Koxitis *f*, Coxitis gonorrhoica.
gonorrheal gonitis Tripperrheumatismus *m*, Gonitis gonorrhoica.
gonorrheal ophthalmia gonorrhoische Ophthalmie *f*, Ophthalmia gonorrhoica.
gonorrheal stomatitis → gonococcal stomatitis.
gonorrheal urethritis → gonococcal urethritis.
gon·o·some ['-səʊm] *n genet.* Sex-, Hetero-, Geschlechtschromosom *nt*, Gonosom *nt*, Heterosom *nt*, Allosom *nt*.
gony- *pref.* Knie-, Gon-.
gon·y·camp·sis [,ɡɑnɪ'kæmpsɪs] *n* Kniegelenkdeformität *f*; Kniegelenkversteifung *f*, -ankylose *f*.
gon·y·cro·te·sis [,-krəʊ'tiːsɪs] *n* X-Bein *nt*, Genu valgum.
gon·y·ec·ty·po·sis [,-,ektɪ'pəʊsɪs] *n* O-Bein *nt*, Genu varum.
gon·y·o·cele ['ɡɑnɪəsɪːl] *n* **1.** Kniegelenksynovitis *f*. **2.** tuberkulöse Gonitis *f*, Gonitis tuberculosa.
gon·y·on·cus [ɡɑnɪ'ɑŋkəs] *n* Knie(gelenk)schwellung *f*.
Good [ɡʊd]: **G.'s syndrome** Good-Syndrom *nt*, Thymom *nt* mit Agammaglobulinämie.
Goodman ['ɡʊdmən]: **G.' syndrome** Goodman-Syndrom *nt*.
good-natured *adj* gutartig.
Goodpasture [ɡʊd'pæstʃər]: **G.'s stain** Peroxidasefärbung *f* nach Goodpasture.
G.'s syndrome Goodpasture-Syndrom *nt*.
Goormaghtigh ['ɡɔːrmətaɪ]: **apparatus of G.** juxtaglomerulärer Apparat *m*.
G. cell Goormaghtigh'-Zelle *f*.
goose flesh [ɡuːs] Gänsehaut *f*, Cutis anserina.
go-over *n* gründliche Untersuchung *f*.
Gopalan [ɡəʊ'pɑlən]: **G.'s syndrome 1.** Gopalan-Syndrom *nt*. **2.** Gopalan-Syndrom *nt*, Syndrom *nt* der brennenden Füße, heiße Greisenfüße *pl*, Burning-feet-Syndrom *nt*.
Gordon ['ɡɔːrdn]: **G.'s reflex** Gordon-Reflex *m*, Gordon-Scharfer-Reflex *m*, Gordon-Zehenzeichen *nt*.
G.'s sign Gordon-Fingerspreizzeichen *nt*.
G.'s test Gordon-Test *m*.
Gorham ['ɡɔːr(h)əm]: **G.'s disease** Gorham(-Staut)-Erkrankung *f*.
Gorlin ['ɡɔːrlɪn]: **G.'s syndrome 1.** → Gorlin-Chaudhry-Moss syndrome. **2.** → Gorlin-Goltz syndrome.
Gorlin-Chaudhry-Moss ['tʃɔːdrɪ mɔs]: **G.-C.-M. syndrome** Gorlin-Chaudhry-Moss-Syndrom *nt*.
Gorlin-Goltz [ɡəʊlts; ɡɒlts]: **G.-G. syndrome** Gorlin-Goltz-Syndrom *nt*, Basalzellnävus-Syndrom *nt*, nävoides Basalzell(en)karzinom-Syndrom *nt*, nävoide Basaliome *pl*, Naevobasaliome *pl*, Naevobasaliomatose *f*.
go·ron·dou [ɡəʊ'rɑnduː] *n* → goundou.
Gosselin [ɡɒs'lɛ̃]: **G.'s fracture** *ortho.* Gosselin-Fraktur *f*.
gos·sy·pol ['ɡɑsəpɑl, -pɒl] *n* Gossypol *nt*.
GOT *abbr.* → glutamic-oxaloacetic transaminase.
Gottron ['ɡɒtron]: **G.'s papule 1.** Acrogeria Gottron, Gottron-Syndrom I *nt*. **2.** Gottron-Syndrom II *nt*, Erythrokeratodermia progressiva symmetrica Gottron, Erythrokeratodermia verrucosa progressiva, Erythrodermia congenitalis progressiva symmetrica.
G.'s sign → **G.'s papule 2.**

gouge [gaʊdʒ] *n ortho., chir.* Hohlbeitel *m*, -meißel *m*.
Gougerot-Blum [guːʒeˈro blʌm; blym]: **G.-B. disease/syndrome** *derm.* Gougerot--Blum-Syndrom *nt*, Blum-Syndrom *nt*, Gougerot-Dermatitis *f*, lichenoide Purpura *f*, Dermatite lichénoide purpurique et pigmentée, Dermatitis lichenoides purpurica et pigmentosa.
Gougerot-Carteaud [karˈto]: **G.-C. syndrome** Gougerot-Carteaud-Syndrom *nt*, Papillomatosis confluens et reticularis.
Gougerot-Nulock-Houwer [ˈnʊlɑk ˈhaʊər; nyˈlok]: **G.-N.-H. syndrome** Sjögren-Syndrom *nt*.
Gougerot-Sjögren [ˈsjœgrən]: **G.-S. disease** Sjögren-Syndrom *nt*.
Gould [guːld]: **G.'s suture** *chir.* Gould-Naht *f*.
goun·dou [ˈgundu:] *n* Gundu-, Goundou--Syndrom *nt*.
gout [gaʊt] *n* Gicht *f*.
gout kidney Urat-, Gichtniere *f*.
gout nephropathy Urat-, Gichtnephropathie *f*.
gout·y [ˈgaʊti] *adj* Gicht betr., von ihr betroffen, gichtartig, Gicht-.
gouty arthritis Gichtarthritis *f*, Arthritis urica.
  acute g. akute Gichtarthritis, akuter Gichtanfall *m*.
gouty crystals Gichtkristalle *pl*.
gouty diathesis Gichtdiathese *f*, harnsaure/uratische Diathese *f*, Diathesis urica.
gouty iritis *ophthal.* Iritis uratica.
gouty kidney Gicht-, Uratniere *f*.
gouty nephropathy Urat-, Uratnephropathie *f*.
gouty synovitis Gichtsynovitis *f*.
gouty ulcer Gichtgeschwür *nt*.
gouty urethritis Gichturethritis *f*.
gouty urine Gichtharn *m*.
Gowers [ˈgaʊərs]: **G.' column** Gowers'--Bündel *nt*, Tractus spinocerebellaris anterior/ventralis.
  G.' fasciculus → G.' column.
  G.' phenomenon *neuro.* Gowers-Zeichen *nt*, An-sich-selbst-Hochklettern *nt*.
  G.' sign → G.' phenomenon.
  G.' syndrome vasovagale Synkope *f*.
  G.' tract → G.' column.
Goyon [ˈgɔɪən]: **G.'s canal** Goyon-Loge *f*, Ulnartunnel *m*.
Goyrand [gwaˈrɑ̃]: **G.'s injury** *ortho.* Chassaignac-Lähmung *f*, Subluxation *f* des Radiusköpfchens, Pronatio dolorosa, Subluxatio radii peranularis.
G1P *abbr.* → glucose-1-phosphate.
G6P *abbr.* → glucose-6-phosphate.
G6PD *abbr.* → glucose-6-phosphate dehydrogenase.
G6PD disease → glucose-6-phosphate dehydrogenase disease.
G_1 period → G_1 phase.
G_2 period → G_2 phase.
G_1 phase *bio.* G_1-Phase *f*.
G_2 phase *bio.* G_2-Phase *f*.
GPI *abbr.* → general paralysis of the insane.
GPT *abbr.* → glutamic-pyruvic transaminase.
gr *abbr.* → grain 2.
graaf·ian follicles/vesicles [ˈgrɑːfiən, ˈgræ-] Graaf'-Follikel *pl*, Tertiärfollikel *pl*, reife Follikel *pl*, Folliculi ovarici vesiculosi.
grac·ile lobe of cerebellum [ˈgræsaɪl, -sɪl] Lobulus gracilis/paramedianus (cerebelli).
gracile tubercle Tuberculum gracile.
grac·i·lis (muscle) [ˈgræsəlɪs] Grazilis *m*, M. gracilis.

grad. *abbr.* → gradient I.
gra·date [ˈgreɪdeɪt] **I** *vt* **1.** (*Farben*) abstufen, abtönen, gegeneinander absetzen, ineinander übergehen lassen. **2.** abstufen. **II** *vi* **3. s.** abstufen, stufenweise ineinander übergehen. **4.** stufenweise übergehen (*into in*).
gra·da·tion [greɪˈdeɪʃn] *n* **1.** (*Farben*) Abstufung *f*, Abtönung *f*; stufenweise Anordnung *f*, Staffelung *f*. **2.** Stufengang *m*, -folge *f*, -leiter *f*. **3.** *radiol.* Gradation *f*.
gra·da·tion·al [greɪˈdeɪʃənl] *adj* **1.** stufenweise, abgestuft. **2.** stufenweise fortschreitend.
grade [greɪd] **I** *n* **1.** Grad *m*, Stufe *f*, Rang *m*, Klasse *f*. **2.** Art *f*, Gattung *f*, Sorte *f*. **3.** Phase *f*, Stufe *f*. **4.** *bio.* Kreuzung *f*, Mischling *m*. **II** *vt* **5.** sortieren, einteilen, klassieren, einstufen. **6.** *bio.* kreuzen.
Gradenigo [ɡrɑːdəˈnɪɡəʊ]: **G.'s syndrome/triad** Gradenigo-Syndrom *nt*.
gra·di·ent [ˈɡreɪdɪənt] **I** *n abbr.* **grad.** Neigung *f*, Steigerung *f*, Gefälle *nt*; *mathe., phys.* Gradient *m*. **II** *adj* (stufenweise) steigend *od.* fallend.
gradient elution *phys.* Gradientenelution *f*.
grad·ing [ˈɡreɪdɪŋ] *n patho.* Grading *nt*.
grad·u·ate [*n, adj* ˈɡrædʒʊɪt, -weɪt; *v* -weɪt] **I** *n* Hochschulabsolvent(in *f*) *m*, Akademiker(in *f*) *m*; Graduierte(r *m*) *f*; Schulabgänger(in *f*) *m*. **II** *adj* Akademiker-. **III** *vt* **1.** graduieren, jdm. einen akademischen Grad verleihen. **2.** *phys., techn.* mit einer Maßeinteilung versehen, in Grade einteilen, graduieren. **3.** abstufen, staffeln. **4.** *chem.* gradieren. **IV** *vi* **5.** graduieren, einen akademischen Grad erwerben; die Abschlußprüfung bestehen. **6. s.** entwickeln, aufsteigen (*into* zu). **7. s.** staffeln, **s.** abstufen. **8.** allmählich übergehen (*into* in).
grad·u·at·ed [ˈɡrædʒəweɪtɪd] *adj* **1.** abgestuft, gestaffelt. **2.** graduiert, mit einer Gradeinteilung versehen.
graduated pipette Meßpipette *f*.
graduate nurse diplomierte/geprüfte Schwester *f*.
grad·u·a·tion [ɡrædʒəˈweɪʃn] *n* **1.** Abstufung *f*, Staffelung *f*. **2.** *phys., techn.* Grad-, Teilstrich *m*; Gradeinteilung *f*, Graduierung *f*. **3.** *chem.* Gradierung *f*. **4.** Erteilung *f* od. Erlangung *f* eines akademischen Grades, Graduierung *f*.
Graefe [ˈɡreɪfɪ; ˈɡreːfə]: **G.'s disease** (von) Graefe-Syndrom *nt*, obere Bulbärparalyse *f*, Ophthalmoplegia chronica progressiva.
  G.'s operation *ophthal.* **1.** von Graefe-Operation *f*, -Schielkorrektur *f*. **2.** von Graefe-Operation *f*, -Linsenextraktion *f*.
  G.'s sign von Graefe-Zeichen *nt*.
  G.'s spot von Graefe-Fleck *m*.
  G.'s test *ophthal.* von Graefe-Versuch *m*.
graft [ɡræft, ɡrɑːft] **I** *n* **1.** Transplantat *nt*, transplantiertes Gewebe *nt*. **2.** Transplantation *f*. **II** *vt* transplantieren, eine Transplantation durchführen.
graft destruction *immun.* Transplantatzerstörung *f*.
graft·ing [ˈɡræftɪŋ, ˈɡrɑːftɪŋ] *n* Transplantation *f*, Implantation *f*.
graft rejection *immun.* Transplantatabstoßung *f*.
graft-versus-host disease → graft--versus-host reaction.
graft-versus-host reaction Transplantat--Wirt-Reaktion *f*, Graft-versus-Host--Reaktion *f*, GvH-Reaktion *f abbr.* GvHR.

granular-cell myoblastoma

Graham [ˈɡreɪəm, ɡræm]: **G.'s law** Graham-Regel *f*.
  G.'s peroxidase stain Peroxidasefärbung *f* nach Graham.
  G.'s sclerosing goiter Graham-Tumor *m*, sklerosierende Struma Graham *f*.
Graham Little [ˈlɪtl]: **G. L. syndrome** Graham Little-Syndrom *nt*, Little-Syndrom *nt*.
Graham Steell [stiːl]: **G. S.'s murmur** Graham Steell-Geräusch *nt*, Steell-Geräusch *nt*.
grain [ɡreɪn] *n* **1.** Korn *nt*. **2.** *abbr.* **gr** *pharm.* Gran *nt*.
grain itch *derm.* Gersten-, Getreidekrätze *f*, Akarodermatitis urticaroides.
grain itch mite *micro.* Gersten-, Getreidemilbe *f*, Pediculoides ventricosus, Acarus tritici.
Gram [ɡræm]: **G.'s method/stain** Gram-Färbung *f*.
gram [ɡræm] *n abbr.* **g, gm** Gramm *nt abbr.* **g**.
gram atom *phys.* Grammatom(gewicht *nt*) *nt*, Atomgramm *nr*.
gram-atomic weight *phys.* → gram atom.
gram calorie *abbr.* **g-cal** *phys.* (Gramm-, Standard-)Kalorie *f abbr.* **cal**, kleine Kalorie *f*.
gram-equivalent *n chem.* Grammäquivalent *nt*.
gram·i·ci·din [ˌɡræməˈsaɪdn] *n pharm.* Gramizidin *nt*.
gram ion → gram-ion.
gram-ion *n chem.* Grammion *nt*.
gramme *n Brit.* → gram.
gram-mole [ˈɡræmˌməʊl] *n* → gram-molecular weight.
gram-molecular weight *abbr.* **GMW** Grammolekül *nt*, Mol *nt*, Grammol *nt*, Grammolekulargewicht *nt*.
gram molecule → gram-molecular weight.
gram-negative *adj* Gram-negativ, gramnegativ.
gram-negative bacteria gram-negative Bakterien *pl*.
gram-positive *adj* Gram-positiv, grampositiv.
gram-positive bacteria gram-positive Bakterien *pl*.
gra·na [ˈɡreɪnə] *pl bio.* Grana *pl*.
grand·daugh·ter cyst [ˈɡrænˌdɔːtər] Enkelzyste *f*, tertiäre Zyste *f*.
gran·di·ose delusion [ˈɡrændɪəʊs] expansiver Wahn *m*, Größenwahn *m*, Megalomanie *f*.
grand mal [ɡræn mal, mæl; ɡrɑ̃ mal] → grand mal epilepsy.
grand mal epilepsy Grand-mal(-Epilepsie *f*) *nt abbr.* **GM**.
Grandry [ˈɡrɑːndri]: **G.'s corpuscles** Merkel-Tastzellen *pl*, -Tastscheibe *f*, Meniscus tactus.
Grandry-Merkel [ˈmɜːrkl; ˈmɛrkəl]: **G.-M. corpuscles** Merkel-Tastzellen *pl*, -Tastscheibe *f*, Meniscus tactus.
Granit [ˈɡrɑːnɪt]: **G.'s loop** Gammaschleife *f*.
gran·ny knot [ˈɡræni] *chir.* falscher Knoten *m*, Weiberknoten *m*.
gran·u·lar [ˈɡrænjələr] *adj* körnig, gekörnt, granulär, granular, granulös, granulär.
granular atrophy, red (*Niere*) rote Granularatrophie *f*.
granular cast *urol.* granulierter Zylinder *m*.
granular cell Körnerzelle *f*.
  basal g.s basalgekörnte Zellen *pl*.
granular-cell myoblastoma *patho.* Abrikossoff-Geschwulst *f*, -Tumor *m*, Myoblastenmyom *nt*, Myoblastom *nt*, Granularzelltumor *m*.

granular-cell myoblastomyoma/schwannoma/tumor → granular-cell myoblastoma.
granular conjunctivitis Trachom(a) nt, ägyptische Körnerkrankheit f, trachomatöse Einschlußkonjunktivitis f, Conjunctivitis (granulosa) trachomatosa.
granular cortex (*ZNS*) granuläre Rinde f, Koniokortex m.
granular degeneration *patho.* albuminöse/albuminoide/albuminoid-körnige Degeneration f, trübe Schwellung f.
granular foveolae Foveolae granulares.
granular induration Zirrhose f, Cirrhosis f.
granular isocortex → granular cortex.
granular layer: g. of cerebellum innere Körnerschicht f der Kleinhirnrinde, Stratum granulare/granulosum.
g. of epidermis Stratum granulosum epidermidis.
external g. of cerebral cortex äußere Körnerschicht f (der Großhirnrinde), Lamina granularis externa.
g. of follicle Granulärschicht f des Follikels, Stratum granulosum folliculi ovarici.
internal g. of cerebral cortex innere Körnerschicht f (der Großhirnrinde), Lamina granularis interna (corticis cerebri/cerebralis).
g. of olfactory bulb Lamina granularis bulbi olfactorii.
g. of Tomes → Tomes' g.
Tomes' g. Tomes'-Körnerschicht f.
granular leukoblast Promyelozyt m.
granular leukocyte → granulocyte.
granular lids → granular conjunctivitis.
granular ophthalmia → granular conjunctivitis.
granular pharyngitis granuläre Pharyngitis f.
granular pits Foveolae granulares.
granular pneumocyte Nischenzelle f, Alveolarzelle f Typ II, Pneumozyt m Typ II.
granular pneumonocyte → granular pneumocyte.
granular powder *pharm.* Granulat nt.
gran·u·late ['grænjəleɪt] **I** vt körnen, granulieren. **II** vi körnig werden, granulieren.
gran·u·lat·ed ['grænjəleɪtɪd] adj granuliert, gekörnt, körnig.
gran·u·la·tio [grænjə'leɪʃɪəʊ] n, pl **-la·ti·o·nes** [-leɪʃɪ'əʊniːz] → granulation 1.
gran·u·la·tion [ˌgrænjʊ'leɪʃn] n **1.** *anat.* körnchenähnliche Struktur f, Granulation f, Granulatio f. **2.** Körnchenbildung f, Körnen nt, Granulieren. **3.** *patho.* Granulation f; Granulierung f. **4.** → granulation tissue. **5.** *techn.*, *chem.* Granulieren nt, Granulierung f.
granulation tissue *patho.* Granulationsgewebe nt, Granulatio f.
granulation tumor → granuloma.
gran·ule ['grænjuːl] n **1.** Körnchen nt; *histol.* Zell-, Speicherkörnchen nt, Granulum nt.
granule cell Körnerzelle f.
granule layer → granular layer of cerebellum.
gran·u·lo·blast ['grænjələʊblæst] n Myeloblast m.
gran·u·lo·cyte ['-saɪt] n Granulozyt m, granulärer Leukozyt m.
granulocyte count 1. Granulozytenzahl f. **2.** Granulozytenzählung f, Bestimmung f der Granulozytenzahl.
granulocyte series *hema.* granulozytäre Reihe f.
gran·u·lo·cyt·ic [ˌ-'sɪtɪk] adj Granulozyt(en) betr., granulozytär, Granulozyten-, Granulozyto-.

granulocytic leukemia myeloische/granulozytäre Leukämie f.
granulocytic sarcoma *patho.* Chlorosarkom nt, Chlorom nt, Chloroleukämie f.
granulocytic series → granulocyte series.
gran·u·lo·cy·top·a·thy [ˌ-saɪ'tɒpəθɪ] n Granulozytopathie f.
gran·u·lo·cy·to·pe·nia [ˌ-ˌsaɪtə'piːnɪə] n **1.** Granulo(zyto)penie f; Neutropenie f; Leukopenie f. **2.** Agranulozytose f, maligne/perniziöse Neutropenie f.
gran·u·lo·cy·to·poi·e·sis [ˌ-ˌsaɪtəpɔɪ'iːsɪs] n → granulopoiesis.
gran·u·lo·cy·to·poi·et·ic [ˌ-ˌsaɪtəpɔɪ'etɪk] adj → granulopoietic.
gran·u·lo·cy·to·sis [ˌ-saɪ'təʊsɪs] n *hema.* Granulozytose f.
gran·u·lo·ma [grænjə'ləʊmə] n, pl **-mas, -ma·ta** [-mətə] Granulationsgeschwulst f, Granulom nt, Granuloma n.
gran·u·lo·ma·to·sis [grænjəˌləʊmə'təʊsɪs] n Granulomatose f, Granulomatosis f.
gran·u·lom·a·tous [grænjə'ləʊmətəs] adj granulomatös.
granulomatous arteritis (senile) Riesenzellarteriitis f, Horton'-Riesenzellarteriitis f, Horton-Syndrom nt, Horton-Magath-Brown-Syndrom nt, Arteriitis cranialis/gigantocellularis/temporalis.
granulomatous carcinoma granulomatöses Karzinom nt, Ca. granulomatosum.
granulomatous colitis granulomatöse Kolitis f, Colitis granulomatosa.
granulomatous disease (progressive) septische Granulomatose f, kongenitale Dysphagozytose f.
granulomatous enteritis Crohn'-Krankheit f, Morbus Crohn m, Enteritis regionalis, Ileocolitis regionalis/terminalis, Ileitis regionalis/terminalis.
granulomatous epulis granulomatöse Epulis f, Epulis granulomatosa.
granulomatous ileocolitis → granulomatous enteritis.
granulomatous infection granulomatöse Infektion f.
granulomatous inflammation granulomatöse Entzündung f.
granulomatous inflammatory disease of the colon Enteritis regionalis Crohn des Dickdarms, Colitis regionalis.
granulomatous lymphoma Hodgkin-Krankheit f, -Lymphom nt, Morbus Hodgkin m, (Hodgkin-)Paltauf-Steinberg-Krankheit f, (maligne) Lymphogranulomatose f, Lymphogranulomatosis maligna.
granulomatous myocarditis granulomatöse Myokarditis f.
granulomatous orchitis granulomatöse Hodenentzündung/Orchitis f, Orchitis granulomatosa.
granulomatous rosacea *derm.* lupoide Rosazea f, Rosacea granulomatosa.
granulomatous thyroiditis de Quervain-Thyr(e)oiditis f, subakute nicht-eitrige Thyr(e)oiditis f, granulomatöse Schilddrüsenentzündung/Thyr(e)oiditis f, Riesenzellthyr(e)oiditis f.
granulomatous uveitis *ophthal.* granulomatöse Uveitis f, Uveitis granulomatosa.
granuloma tropicum Framboesie f, Pian f, Parangi f, Yaws f, Framboesia tropica.
gran·u·lo·mere ['grænjələʊmɪər] n Granulomer nt.
gran·u·lo·pe·nia [ˌ-'pɪnɪə] n → granulocytopenia.
gran·u·lo·plasm ['-plæzəm] n Granuloplasma nt.
gran·u·lo·plas·tic [ˌ-'plæstɪk] adj körnchen-, granulabildend.
gran·u·lo·poi·e·sis [ˌ-pɔɪ'iːsɪs] n Granulo-

zytenbildung f, Granulozytopo(i)ese f, Granulopoese f.
gran·u·lo·poi·et·ic [ˌ-pɔɪ'etɪk] adj Granulopoese betr. *od.* stimulierend, granulo(zyto)poetisch.
gran·u·lo·sa [grænjə'ləʊzə] n *histol.* Granulosa f, Stratum granulosum ovarii.
granulosa carcinoma → granulosa cell carcinoma.
granulosa cell carcinoma Granulosa(zell)tumor m, Folliculoma nt, Ca. granulosocellulare.
granulosa cells Follikelepithel nt, Granulosazellen pl.
primitive g. präfollikuläre Zellen pl, primitive Granulosazellen pl.
granulosa-lutein cells Granulosaluteinzellen pl.
granulosa-theca cell tumor Granulosa-Thekazelltumor m, Theka-Granulosazelltumor m.
granulosa tumor → granulosa cell carcinoma.
gran·u·lose ['grænjələʊs] adj → granular.
gran·u·lo·sis [grænjə'ləʊsɪs] n Körnerkrankheit f, Granulose f, Granulosis f.
granulosis viruses *micro.* Baculoviren pl, Baculoviridae pl.
gran·u·los·i·ty [grænjə'lɒsətɪ] n → granulosis.
gran·u·lo·vac·u·o·lar [ˌgrænjələˌvækjə'wəʊlər, -'vækjələr] adj granulär-vakulär, granulovakulär.
gra·num ['greɪnəm] n, pl **-na** [-nə] → grain 1.
grape [greɪp] n Weintraube f, -beere f.
grape cell *hema.* Morula-, Traubenzelle f.
grape mole Traubenmole f, Mola bothryoides.
grape sugar → (D-)glucose.
graph- *pref.* → grapho-.
graph [græf, grɑːf] n **1.** graphische Darstellung f, Diagramm nt, Schaubild nt, Kurvenblatt nt, -bild nt; *mathe.* Kurve f, Graph m.
graph·es·thia [ˌgræfes'θiːʒ(ɪ)ə] n Graphästhesie f.
graph·ic ['græfɪk] adj **1.** graphisch, zeichnerisch. **2.** anschaulich, plastisch.
graph·i·cal ['græfɪkl] adj → graphic.
graphic aphasia *neuro.* zerebrale Agraphie f.
graphic formula *chem.* Strukturformel f.
graphic representation graphische Darstellung f.
graph·ite ['græfaɪt] n Graphit m.
graph·i·to·sis [græfɪ'təʊsɪs] n *patho.* Graphitlunge f.
grapho- *pref.* Schreib-, Schreiben-, Graph(o)-.
gra·phol·o·gy [græ'fɒlədʒɪ] n Graphologie f, Handschrift(en)deutung f.
graph·o·ma·ni·a [græfə'meɪnɪə, -jə] n *psychia.* Schreibwut f, Graphomanie f.
graph·o·mo·tor aphasia [ˌ-'məʊtər] *neuro.* zerebrale Agraphie f.
graph·or·rhea [ˌ-'rɪə] n *psychia.* Kritzelsucht f, Graphorrhoe f.
graph·o·spasm ['-spæzəm] n Schreibkrampf m, Graphospasmus m, Mogigraphie f.
graph paper Millimeterpapier nt.
Graser ['græsər; 'grɑːzər]: **G.'s diverticulum** Graser-Divertikel nt.
Grashey ['græʃɪ]: **G.'s aphasia** Grashey'-Aphasie f.
grasp [græsp, grɑːsp] **I** n **1.** (fester) Griff m. **2.** Auffassungskraft f, Fassungskraft f, Verständnis nt. **II** vt **3.** packen, (er-)greifen. **4.** verstehen, begreifen, erfassen. **III** vi (fest) zugreifen *od.* zupacken.

grasp·ing reflex ['græspɪŋ, 'grɑːsp-] → grasp reflex.
grasp reflex Greifreflex *m.*
grass bacillus [græs, grɑːs] *micro.* Heubazillus, Bacillus subtilis.
grass dermatitis Wiesengräserdermatitis *f*, Wiesengrasdermatitis *f*, Pflanzendermatitis *f*, Phyto-, Photodermatitis *f*, Dermatitis (bullosa) pratensis, Photodermatitis phytogenica.
Grasset [grɑ'seː]: **G.'s law** Landouzy--Grasset-Gesetz *nt.*
G.'s phenomenon 1. → G.'s sign. **2.** → Grasset-Gaussel-Hoover sign.
G.'s sign Grasset-Zeichen *nt*, Bychowski--Zeichen *nt.*
Grasset-Bychowski [baɪ'tʃəʊskɪ]: **G.-B. sign** → Grasset's sign.
Grasset-Gaussel [goˈsel]: **G.-G. phenomenon** → Grasset-Gaussel-Hoover sign.
Grasset-Gaussel-Hoover ['huːvər]: **G.-G.-H. sign** Grasset-Zeichen *nt*, Hoover-Zeichen *nt*, Phänomen *nt* der komplementären Opposition.
grate [greɪt] **I** *n* Gitter *nt.* **II** *vt* **1.** knirschen *od.* kratzen (mit). **to ~ one's teeth** mit den Zähnen knirschen. **2.** zerreiben. **III** *vi* knirschen, kratzen, knarren.
grat·ing ['greɪtɪŋ] **I** *n* **1.** Kratzen *nt*, Knirschen *nt*, Knarren *nt.* **2.** Gitter(werk *nt*) *nt*, Vergitterung *f.* **3.** *phys.* (Beugungs-)Gitter *nt.* **II** *adj* knirschend, kratzend, reibend.
grating spectrum *phys.* Gitterspektrum *nt.*
Gratiolet [grɑˌtioˈleː]: **G.'s fibers** Gratiolet--Sehstrahlung *f*, Radiatio optica.
radiation of G. → G.'s fibers.
G.'s radiating fibers → G.'s fibers.
grat·tage [græˈtɑːʒ, grɑ-; grɑˈtɑːʒ] *n chir.* Aufreiben *nt*, Aufrauhen *nt*, Aufraspeln *nt.*
grave¹ [greɪv] *n* Grab *nt.*
grave² [greɪv] **(graven; graved)** *vt* (ein-)schnitzen, (ein-)schneiden, (ein-)meißeln.
grave³ [greɪv] *adj* ernst, bedenklich, bedrohlich.
grave fat → grave-wax.
grav·el ['grævəl] *n urol.* Harngrieß *m.*
Graves ['greɪvz]: **G.' disease** Basedow'--Krankheit *f*, Morbus Basedow *m.*
G.' eye signs Augensymptome *pl* bei Morbus Basedow.
grave-wax *n* Fett-, Leichenwachs *nt*, Adipocire *f.*
grav·id ['grævɪd] *adj* schwanger, gravid.
grav·i·da ['grævɪdə] *n*, *pl* **-das, -dae** [-diː] Schwangere *f*, Gravida *f.*
grav·i·da·tion abscess [grævɪ'deɪʃn] Senkungsabszeß *m.*
gra·vid·ic [græˈvɪdɪk] *adj* Schwangerschaft *od.* Schwangere betr., während der Schwangerschaft auftretend, Schwangeren-, Schwangerschafts-, Graviditäts-.
gravidic retinitis → gravidic retinopathy.
gravidic retinopathy Retinopathia eclamptica gravidarum.
grav·id·ism ['grævɪdɪzəm] *n* → gravidity.
gra·vid·i·tas [grəˈvɪdətəs] *n* → gravidity.
gra·vid·i·ty [grəˈvɪdətɪ] *n* Schwangerschaft *f*, Gravidität *f*, Graviditas *f.*
grav·i·do·pu·er·per·al [ˌgrævɪdəʊpjuːˈɜːp(ə)rəl] *adj* Schwangerschaft u. Wochenbett betr.
gravid uterus Schwangerschaftsuterus *m.*
gra·vim·e·ter [grəˈvɪmɪtər] *n* Gravimeter *nt.*
grav·i·met·ric [ˌgrævɪˈmetrɪk] *adj* Gravimetrie betr., mittels Gravimetrie, gravimetrisch.
grav·i·met·ri·cal [ˌ-ˈmetrɪkl] *adj* → gravimetric.

gravimetric analysis → gravimetry 1.
gra·vim·e·try [grəˈvɪmətrɪ] *n* **1.** Gewichtsanalyse *f*, gravimetrische Analyse *f*, Gravimetrie *f.* **2.** *phys.* Gravimetrie *f.*
grav·i·tate ['grævɪteɪt] *vi s.* (durch Schwerkraft) fortbewegen.
grav·i·ta·tion [ˌgrævɪˈteɪʃn] *n phys.* Massenanziehung *f*, Gravitation *f.*
grav·i·ta·tion·al [ˌgrævɪˈteɪʃnl] *adj* Gravitations-, Schwer(e)-.
gravitational acceleration Erdbeschleunigung *f*, Gravitationsbeschleunigung *f.*
gravitational constant *abbr.* **G** Gravitationskonstante *f.*
gravitational field Schwere-, Gravitationsfeld *nt.*
gravitational force Gravitations-, Schwerkraft *f.*
gravitational pull Anziehungskraft *f.*
gravitational ulcer Stauungsulkus *nt*, Ulcus (cruris) venosum.
grav·i·ta·tive ['grævɪteɪtɪv] *adj* → gravitational.
grav·i·ty ['grævɪtɪ] *n*, *pl* **-ties** *abbr.* **g** Schwerkraft *f*, Gravitation(skraft *f*) *f.*
gravity abscess Senkungsabszeß *m.*
Grawitz ['grɑːvɪts; 'grɑ-]: **G.' tumor** Grawitz-Tumor *m*, Hypernephrom *nt*, hypernephroides Karzinom *nt*, klarzelliges Nierenkarzinom *nt.*
gray¹ [greɪ] *n abbr.* **Gy** *radiol.* Gray *nt abbr.* Gy.
gray² [greɪ] **I** *n* **1.** Grau *nt*, graue Farbe *f.* **2.** → gray matter. **II** *adj* **3.** grau. **4.** trübe, grau. **5.** *techn.* neutral, farblos, naturfarben. **6.** grau(haarig), ergraut. **III** *vi* grau werden, ergrauen.
gray atrophy *ophthal.* graue/sekundäre Optikusatrophie *f.*
gray body *phys.* Graustrahler *m.*
gray column: g.s Säulen *pl* der grauen (Rückenmarks-)Substanz, Columnae griseae.
anterior g. of spinal cord Vordersäule *f* (des Rückenmarks), Columna anterior/ventralis medullae spinalis.
lateral g. of spinal cord Seitensäule *f* (des Rückenmarks), Columna lateralis medullae spinalis.
posterior g. of spinal cord Hintersäule *f* (des Rückenmarks), Columna dorsalis/posterior (medullae spinalis).
gray degeneration graue Degeneration *f.*
gray fibers marklose (Nerven-)Fasern *pl*, Remak-Fasern *pl.*
gray-headed *adj* grauhaarig.
gray hepatisation *patho.* graue Hepatisation *f.*
gray induration *patho.* graue Induration *f.*
gray infiltration (*Lunge*) graue Infiltration *f.*
gray·ing ['greɪɪŋ] *n* (*Haar*) Ergrauen *nt.*
gray·ish ['greɪɪʃ] *adj* graulich, gräulich.
gray matter graue Gehirn- u. Rückenmarksubstanz *f*, graue Substanz *f*, Substantia grisea.
    central intermediate g. of spinal cord Substantia (grisea) intermedia centralis (medullae spinalis).
    lateral intermediate g. of spinal cord Substantia (grisea) intermedia lateralis (medullae spinalis).
    g. of spinal cord graue Rückenmarkssubstanz *f*, Substantia grisea medullae spinalis.
gray·ness ['greɪnɪs] *n* Grau *nt*, graue Farbe *f*; *fig.* Trübheit *f.*
gray ramus, communicans Ramus communicans griseus.
gray scale *phys.* Grauskala *f.*
gray substance → gray matter.

central g. of cerebrum zentrales Höhlengrau *nt*, Substantia grisea centralis.
g. of spinal cord → gray matter of spinal cord.
gray syndrome Gray-Syndrom *nt.*
gray tuber Tuber cinereum.
gray tubercle 1. Tuber cinerum. **2.** Tuberculum trigeminale.
great [greɪt] *adj* groß; (*Anzahl*) sehr viele; (*zeitlich*) lang; (*Alter*) hoch; bedeutend, wichtigste(r, s), Groß-, Haupt-.
great cistern Cisterna magna/cerebellomedullaris.
great·er circle of iris ['greɪtər] Ziliarabschnitt *m* der Iris, A(n)nulus iridis major.
greater circulation großer (Körper-)Kreislauf *m.*
greater cul-de-sac Magenfundus *m*, Fundus gastricus/ventricularis.
greater curvature of stomach große Magenkurvatur *f*, Curvatura gastrica/ventricularis major.
greater fossa of Scarpa Scarpa'-Dreieck *nt*, Trigonum femorale.
greater horn of hyoid bone Cornu majus (ossis hyoidei).
greater lip of pudendum große Schamlippe *f*, Labium majus pudendi.
greater muscle of helix M. helicis major.
greater omentectomy *chir.* (Teil-)Resektion *f* des Omentum majus.
greater omentum großes Netz *nt*, Omentum majus.
greater pelvis großes Becken *nt*, Pelvis major.
greater ring of iris → greater circle of iris.
greater tubercle of humerus Tuberculum majus (humeri).
greater tuberosity fracture (Abriß-)Fraktur *f* des Tuberculum majus (humeri).
greater tuberosity of humerus Tuberculum majus (humeri).
greater wing of sphenoid bone großer Keilbeinflügel *m*, Ala major (ossis sphenoidalis).
great foramen großes Hinterhauptsloch *nt*, For. magnum.
great head: g. of adductor hallucis muscle Caput obliquum m. adductoris hallucis.
g. of triceps brachii muscle lateraler/äußerer Trizepskopf *m*, Caput laterale m. tricipitis brachii.
g. of triceps femoris muscle M. adductor magnus.
great lacuna of urethra Fossa navicularis urethrae.
great-toe reflex Babinski-Zeichen *nt*, -Reflex *m*, (Groß-)Zehenreflex *m.*
great vessel injury Verletzung *f* der großen Gefäße.
great wing of sphenoid bone → greater wing of sphenoid bone.
green [griːn] *n* Grün *nt*, grüne Farbe *f*, grüner Farbstoff *m.* **II** *adj* **1.** grün. **2.** (*Wunde*) frisch, neu. **3.** *fig.* grün, unerfahren, unreif, naiv; jugendlich, rüstig.
green blindness *ophthal.* Grünblindheit *f*, -schwäche *f*, Deuteranop(s)ie *f.*
green cancer *patho.* Chlorom *nt*, Chloroleukämie *f*, Chlorosarkom *nt.*
Greenfield ['griːnfiːld]: **G.'s disease** Greenfield-Syndrom *nt*, spätinfantile Form *f* der metachromatischen Leukodystrophie.
green hemoglobin Choleglobin *nt*, Verdohämoglobin *nt.*
Greenhow ['griːnhəʊ]: **G.'s disease** *derm.* Vaganten-, Vagabundenhaut *f*, Cutis vagantium.
green monkey virus Marburg-Virus *nt.*
green sickness *hema.* Chlorose *f*, Chlorosis *f.*

green soap Kali(schmier)seife f, Sapo kalinus/mollis.
green-stick fracture ['gri:nstɪk] ortho. Grünholzbruch m, -fraktur f.
green vision Grünsehen nt, Chlorop(s)ie f.
Greig [gri:g]: **G.'s syndrome** Greig-Syndrom nt, okulärer Hypertelorismus m.
grenz rays [grenz] radiol. Bucky-Strahlen pl, Grenzstrahlen pl.
grey n, adj, v Brit. → gray.
Grey Turner [greɪ 'tɜrnər]: **G. T.'s sign** Turner'-Zeichen nt.
GRF abbr. [growth hormone releasing factor] → growth hormone releasing hormone.
GRH abbr. → growth hormone releasing hormone.
Grice [graɪs]: **G. arthrodesis of subtalar joint** ortho. extraartikuläre Arthrodese f nach Grice.
  G. operation → G. arthrodesis of subtalar joint.
  G. procedure (for talipes valgus) → G. arthrodesis of subtalar joint.
Grice-Green [gri:n]: **G.-G. arthrodesis/operation/procedure** → Grice arthrodesis of subtalar joint.
grid [grɪd] n 1. Gitter(netz nt) nt. 2. radiol. Streustrahlenblende f; Gitterblende f, Rasterblende f.
grid·i·ron incision ['grɪdaɪərn] chir. Schräginzision f nach McBurney.
grief [gri:f] n Gram m, Kummer m, Leid nt, Schmerz m.
Griesinger ['gri:sɪŋər]: **G.'s sign/symptom** Griesinger'-Zeichen nt.
grif·fin claw ['grɪfɪn] Krallen-, Klauenhand m.
Griffith ['grɪfɪθ]: **G.'s operation** Griffith'--Hernienoperation f.
  G.'s sign Griffith-Zeichen nt.
grind [graɪnd] (v ground) I n Knirschen nt. II vt 1. (zer-)mahlen, zerreiben, -stoßen, -kleinern. 2. (Messer) schleifen nt. 3. (Zähne) knirschen. **to ~ one's teeth** mit den Zähnen knirschen. III vi mahlen, knirschen.
grind down vt → grind 1.
grind·er ['graɪndər] n 1. Backen-, Mahlzahn m, Molar m. 2. Schleifmaschine f.
grinder's disease Quarz-, Kiesel-, Steinstaublunge f, Silikose f, Silicosis f.
grind·ing ['graɪndɪŋ] n 1. Mahlen nt; Knirschen nt. 2. Schleifen nt, Schärfen nt. II adj knirschen; (zer-)mahlend, Mahl-, Schleif-.
grinding surface (of tooth) (Zahn) Mahl-, Kaufläche f.
grip¹ [grɪp] (v gripped) I n 1. (Grob-, Breit-)-Griff m. 2. fig. Griff m, Halt m; Herrschaft f, Gewalt f, Zugriff m; Verständnis f. II vt 3. ergreifen, packen. 4. fig. begreifen, verstehen. III vi ortho. (Schraube) greifen, Halt finden.
grip² [grɪp] n Grippe f, Influenza f.
gripe [graɪp] I n (meist ~s pl) Bauchschmerzen pl, Krämpfe pl, Kolik f. II vt Bauchschmerzen/eine Kolik verursachen. **to be ~d** Bauchschmerzen/eine Kolik haben. III vi Bauchschmerzen/eine Kolik auslösen od. haben.
gripp·al ['grɪpl] adj Grippe betr., grippal, Grippe-.
grippe [grɪp] n old Grippe f, Influenza f.
gris·e·o·ful·vin [ˌgrɪsɪəʊ'fʌlvɪn] n pharm. Griseofulvin f.
Gritti ['grɪti]: **G.'s amputation/operation** ortho. Beinamputation f nach Gritti.
Gritti-Stokes ['stəʊks]: **G.-S. amputation** ortho. Beinamputation f nach Gritti--Stokes.

Grocco ['grɔkəʊ]: **G.'s sign 1.** Grocco-Leberzeichen nt. **2.** Grocco-Rauchfuß-Dreieck nt.
  G.'s triangle → G.'s sign 2.
  G.'s triangular dullness → G.'s sign 2.
groin [grɔɪn] n anat. Leiste f, Leistengegend f, -region f, Regio inguinalis.
groin ulcer Granuloma inguinale/venereum, Granuloma pudendum chronicum, Donovaniosis f.
grommet ['grɑmɪt] n HNO Paukenröhrchen nt.
grommet (drain) tube → grommet.
Grönblad-Strandberg ['grenblæd 'strændbɑrg]: **G.-S. syndrome** derm. (Darier-)-Grönblad-Strandberg-Syndrom nt, systematische Elastorrhexis f, Pseudoxanthoma elasticum.
groove [gru:v] n Furche f, Rinne f; techn. Nut f, Rille f.
  g. for eustachian tube Sulcus tubae auditivae/auditoriae.
  g. of great superficial petrosal nerve Sulcus n. petrosi majoris.
  g. for inferior v. cava Vena-cava-Rinne, Sulcus v. cavae (hepatis).
  g. of lacrimal bone Sulcus lacrimalis ossis lacrimalis.
  g. for medial meningeal artery Sulcus a. meningeae mediae.
  g. for nasal nerve Sulcus ethmoidalis (ossis nasalis).
  g. for occipital artery Sulcus a. occipitalis.
  g. for radial nerve Radialisrinne, Sulcus (n.) radialis.
  g. for sigmoid sinus Sulcus sinus sigmoidei.
  g. for subclavian artery Sulcus a. subclaviae.
  g. for subclavian muscle Sulcus m. subclavii.
  g. of ulnar nerve Sulcus n. ulnaris.
grooved [gru:vd] adj gefurcht, furchig, rinnig; gerillt.
grooved tongue Faltenzunge f, Lingua plicata/scrotalis.
gross [grəʊs] adj 1. grob(körnig). 2. mit bloßem Auge sichtbar, makroskopisch, Makro-. 3. (Fehler) schwer, grob. 4. (Wachstum) dicht, stark, üppig. 5. brutto, gesamt, Brutto-, Gesamt-, Roh-.
gross anatomy makroskopische Anatomie f.
gross hematuria makroskopische Hämaturie f, Makrohämaturie f.
gross lesion makroskopische Läsion f.
ground [graʊnd] I n 1. Grund m, Boden m. 2. Grundlage f, Basis f. 3. fig. Ursache f, (Beweg-)Grund m. **on health/medical ~s** aus gesundheitlichen/medizinischen Gründen. **on ~s of age** aus Altersgründen. **on the ~s of** auf Grund von. 4. ~s pl (Boden-)Satz m. 5. Hinter-, Untergrund m. II adj gegründet. III vt fig. gründen, basieren, aufbauen (on, in auf).
ground bundles of spinal cord Binnen-, Elementar-, Grundbündel pl des Rückenmarks, Interfaszikel pl, Fasciculi proprii (medullae spinalis).
ground-glass hepatocyte patho. Milchglashepatozyt m.
ground itch anemia Anämie f bei Hakenwurmbefall.
ground lamellae (Knochen) Schaltlamellen pl.
ground state phys. Grundzustand m.
ground substance Grund-, Kitt-, Interzellular-, Zwischenzellsubstanz f.
  amorphous g. amorphe Grund-, Kitt-, Interzellularsubstanz.
  bone g. Knochengrundsubstanz.
  cartilage g. Knorpelgrundsubstanz, Chondroid nt.

ground line mathe. Grundlinie f.
ground plane Horizontalebene f.
ground water Grundwasser nt.
group [gru:p] I n 1. Gruppe f; (Patienten-)-Kollektiv nt. 2. chem. Gruppe f, Radikal nt. II vt gruppieren, in Gruppen einteilen od. anordnen; klassifizieren. III vi s. gruppieren.
group agglutination Gruppenagglutination(sreaktion f) f.
group agglutinin Gruppenagglutinin nt.
group analysis psycho., psychia. Gruppenanalyse f.
group antigen Gruppenantigen nt.
  erythrocyte g. Erythrozytengruppenantigen nt.
group-conscious adj socio. gruppenbewußt.
group consciousness socio. Gruppenbewußtsein nt.
group-dynamic adj socio. gruppendynamisch.
group dynamics socio. Gruppendynamik f.
group·ing ['gru:pɪŋ] n Gruppierung f, Anod. Einordnung f (in Gruppen); Gruppenbestimmung f.
group JK corynebacterium micro. Corynebacterium nt der Gruppe JK.
group medicine → group practice.
group practice Gemeinschaftspraxis f.
group reaction Gruppenagglutination f.
group-reactive adj immun. gruppenreaktiv.
group-reactive antigen gruppenreaktives Antigen nt, gruppenspezifisches kreuzreagierendes Antigen nt.
group-specific adj gruppenspezifisch.
group therapy psycho., psychia. Gruppentherapie f.
group-transfer n chem. Gruppenübertragung f, -transfer m.
group-transferring adj chem. gruppenübertragend.
group-transferring reaction chem. gruppenübertragende Reaktion f.
group translocation genet. Gruppentranslokation f.
group treatment psycho., psychia. Gruppentherapie f.
Grover ['grəʊvər]: **G.'s disease** Morbus Grover m, Grover-Krankheit f, transitorische akantholytische Dermatose f.
grow [grəʊ] (grew; grown) I vt züchten. II vi 1. wachsen; (Person) größer werden, wachsen. **to ~ together** zusammenwachsen. 2. fig. zunehmen, s. vergrößern (in an). 3. werden, s. entwickeln, s. bilden. **to ~ warm** s. erwärmen, warm werden.
grow up vi auf-, heranwachsen; erwachsen werden.
grow·ing ['grəʊɪŋ] I n Wachsen nt, Wachstum nt. II adj wachsend, Wachstums-; (Kind) heranwachsend; fig. zunehmend, ansteigend.
growing pains Wachstumsschmerzen pl.
growth [grəʊθ] n 1. a. fig. Wachsen nt, Wachstum m; Wuchs m, Größe f. 2. Entwicklung f. 3. fig. Zuwachs m, Zunahme f, Anwachsen nt. 4. patho. Gewächs nt, Wucherung f, Auswuchs m, Geschwulst f, Neoplasma nt. 5. Kultivierung f, Züchtung f.
growth curve Wachstumskurve f.
growth cycle Wachstumszyklus m.
growth disk epiphysäre Wachstumszone f, Epiphysenfuge f.
growth factor Wachstumsfaktor m.
growth factor V micro. (Wachstums-)Faktor V m.
growth factor X micro. (Wachstums-)Faktor X m.

growth hormone *abbr.* **GH** Wachstumshormon *nt*, somatotropes Hormon *nt abbr.* STH, Somatotropin *nt*.
 placental g. humanes Plazenta-Laktogen *nt abbr.* HPL, Choriosomatotropin *nt*.
growth hormone inhibiting factor *abbr.* **GIF, GH-IF** → growth hormone inhibiting hormone.
growth hormone inhibiting hormone *abbr.* **GH, GIH** Somatostatin *nt*, growth hormone release inhibiting hormone *abbr.* GH-RIH, somatotropin (release) inhibiting hormone/factor *abbr.* SH-IF, SR-IF, growth hormone inhibiting factor *abbr.* GH-IF.
growth hormone release inhibiting factor *abbr.* **GH-RIF** → growth hormone inhibiting hormone.
growth hormone release inhibiting hormone *abbr.* **GH-RIH** → growth hormone inhibiting hormone.
growth hormone releasing factor *abbr.* **GH-RF, GRF** → growth hormone releasing hormone
growth hormone releasing hormone *abbr.* **GH-RH, GRH** Somatoliberin *nt*, Somatotropin-releasing-Faktor *m abbr.* SRF, growth hormone releasing factor *abbr.* GRF, GH-RF, growth hormone releasing hormone *abbr.* GRH, GH-RH.
growth-onset diabetes (mellitus) insulinabhängiger Diabetes (mellitus) *m*, Typ 1 Diabetes (mellitus).
growth parameter Wachstumsparameter *m*, wachstumsbeeinflußender Parameter *m*.
growth phase Wachstumsphase *f*, -periode *f*.
growth plate → growth disk.
growth rate Wachstumsrate *f*, -geschwindigkeit *f*.
growth retardation Wachstumsverzögerung *f*.
Gruber ['gruːbər]: **G.'s reaction** Gruber-Widal-Reaktion *f*, -Test *m*, Widal-Reaktion *f*, -Test *m*.
 G.'s syndrome Meckel-Syndrom *nt*, Dysencephalia splanchnocystica.
 G.'s test → G.'s reaction.
Gruber-Landzert ['lændzərt]: **G.-L. fossa** Rec. duodenalis inferior.
Gruber-Widal [viˈdal]: **G.-W. reaction/test** → Gruber's reaction.
grum·bling appendix ['grʌmblɪŋ] *inf.* Blinddarmreizung *f*.
gru·mose ['gruːməʊs] *adj* → grumous.
gru·mous ['gruːməs] *adj* (*Blut*) geronnen, dick, klumpig.
Grünbaum-Widal ['griːnbaʊm viˈdal; 'gryːn-]: **G.-W. test** → Gruber's reaction.
Grynfeltt ['grɪnfelt; 'gryːn-]: **G.'s hernia** *chir.* Grynfeltt-Hernie *f*.
 triangle of G. and Lesgaft → G.'s triangle.
 G.'s triangle Grynfeltt-Dreieck *nt*, Trigonum lumbale superior.
gry·pho·sis [grɪˈfəʊsɪs] *n* → gryposis.
gry·po·sis [grɪˈpəʊsɪs] *n patho.* abnorme Krümmung *f*, Gryposis *f*.
GSC *abbr.* → gas-solid chromatography.
GSH *abbr.* → glutathione, reduced.
GSR *abbr.* → galvanic skin response.
GSSG *abbr.* → glutathione, oxidized.
G-strophantin *n* g-Strophanthin *nt*, Ouabain *nt*.
G syndrome G-Syndrom *nt*.
GT *abbr.* → glucose tolerance.
GTP *abbr.* → guanosine(-5'-)triphosphate.
GTP cyclohydrolase GTP-cyclohydrolase *f*.
GTT *abbr.* → glucose tolerance test.
GU *abbr.* → genitourinary.

guai·ac (gum) ['gwaɪæk] Guajak(harz *nt*) *nt*.
guai·a·col ['gwaɪəkɒl, -kɔl] *n pharm.* Guajacol *nt*, Guajacolum *nt*.
guaiac test Guajaktest *m*, -probe *f*.
guai·fen·e·sin [gwaɪˈfenəsɪn] *n pharm.* Guaifenesin *nt*, Guajacolglyzerinäther *m*.
guai·phen·e·sin *n* → guaifenesin.
Gua·ma virus ['gwɑːmə] *micro.* Guama-Virus *nt*.
gua·na·benz ['gwɑːnəbenz] *n pharm.* Guanabenz *nt*.
gua·nase ['gwɑːneɪz] *n* → guanine deaminase.
guan·eth·i·dine [gwɑːˈnɛθɪdiːn] *n pharm.* Guanethidin *nt*.
guan·i·dase ['gwænɪdeɪz] *n* Guanidase *f*.
guan·i·dine ['gwænɪdiːn, -dɪn] *n* Guanidin *nt*, Iminoharnstoff *m*.
guanidine-acetic acid → guanidinoacetic acid.
gua·ni·di·ne·mia [ˌgwɑːnədɪˈniːmɪə] *n* Guanidinämie *f*.
guanidine phosphate Phosphoguanidin *nt*, Guanidinphosphat *nt*.
gua·ni·di·no·a·ce·tic acid [gwɑːnəˌdiːnəʊ-əˈsiːtɪk] Guanidinoessigsäure *f*.
guanido-acetic acid → guanidinoacetic acid.
gua·ni·do·u·rea [ˌgwɑːnɪdəʊˈjʊərɪə] *n* Guanidoharnstoff *m*.
guan·i·dyl·ate [ˌgwænɪˈdɪleɪt] *n* Guanidylat *nt*.
guanidylate cyclase Guanidylatcyclase *f*.
guanidylate kinase Guanidylatkinase *f*.
Guanieri [gwɑˈnɪərɪ]: **G.'s gelatin agar** Guanieri-Gelatineagar *m/nt*.
gua·nine ['gwɑːniːn] *n abbr.* **G** Guanin *nt abbr.* G.
guanine aminase → guanine deaminase.
guanine cell Zelle *f* mit Guaninkristallen.
guanine deaminase Guanindeaminase *f*, Guanase *f*.
guanine nucleotide → guanosine monophosphate.
guanine ribonucleotide → guanosine monophosphate.
gua·no·sine ['gwɑːnəsiːn, -sɪn] *n abbr.* **G** Guanosin *nt abbr.* G.
guanosine 3',5'-cyclic phosphate *abbr.* **3',5'GMP, cGMP, cyclic GMP** zyklisches Guanosin-3',5'-Phosphat *nt abbr.* 3',5'GMP, , zyklisches GMP, Zyklo-GMP *nt*, Cyclo-GMP *nt abbr.* cGMP.
guanosine(-5'-)diphosphate *n abbr.* **GDP** Guanosin(-5'-)diphosphat *nt abbr.* GDP.
guanosine monophosphate *abbr.* **GMP** Guanosin(-5')monophosphat *nt abbr.* GMP, Guanylsäure *f*.
 cyclic g. → guanosine 3',5'-cyclic phosphate.
guanosine(-5'-)triphosphate *n abbr.* **GTP** Guanosin(-5')triphosphat *nt abbr.* GTP.
gua·nyl·ic acid [gwɑːˈnɪlɪk] *n* → guanosine monophosphate.
guanylic acid synthetase → GMP synthetase.
gua·ra·nine [ˈgwærənɪn, gwəˈrɑː-, -nɪn] *n* Koffein *nt*, Coffein *nt*, Methyltheobromin *nt*, 1,3,7-Trimethylxanthin *nt*.
guard [gɑːrd] **I** *n* **1.** Schutz *m*, Schutzvorrichtung *f*, -gitter *nt*. **2.** Vorsichtsmaßnahme *f*, Sicherung *f*. **II** *vt* (be-)hüten, (be-)schützen, bewachen, wachen über; bewahren, sichern (*against, from* gegen, vor).
guard·ing ['gɑːrdɪŋ] *n chir.* (*Bauchdecke*) Abwehrspannung *f*.
Guarnieri [gwarˈnɪerɪ]: **G.'s bodies** Guanieri-Einschlußkörperchen *pl*.
 G.'s corpuscles/inclusions → G.'s bodies.

Guarua [gwɑˈrɔːə]: **G. virus** Guarua-Virus *nt*.
gu·ber·nac·u·lum [ˌg(j)uːbərˈnækjələm] *n, pl* **-la** [-lə] *anat.* Leit-, Führungsband *nt*, Gubernaculum *nt*.
Gubler ['guːblər]: **G.'s hemiplegia** → G.'s syndrome.
 G.'s line Gubler-Linie *f*.
 G.'s paralysis → G.'s syndrome.
 G.'s sign Gubler-Tumor *m*, -Zeichen *nt*.
 G.'s syndrome Gubler-Lähmung *f*, Millard-Gubler-Syndrom *nt*, Brücken--Mittelhirn-Syndrom *nt*, Hemiplegia alternans inferior.
 G.'s tumor → G.'s sign.
Gudden ['gʊdn]: **G.'s commissure** Gudden'-Kommissur *f*, Commissura supraoptica ventralis.
 G.'s ganglion Nc. interpeduncularis.
Guérin [geˈrɛ̃]: **G.'s fold** Valvula fossae navicularis.
 G.'s fracture Guérin-Fraktur *f*, LeFort I-Fraktur *f*.
guid·ance ['gaɪdns] *n* **1.** Leitung *f*, Führung *f*. **2.** Anleitung *f*, Unterweisung *f*, Belehrung *f*. **3.** Beratung *f*, Führung *f*, Betreuung *f*.
guide [gaɪd] **I** *n* **1.** Führer(in *f*) *m*, Leiter(in *f*) *m*. **2.** Leitfaden *m*, Einführung *f* (*to* in); Handbuch *nt*. **3.** Berater(in *f*) *m*. **4.** Richtschnur *f*, Anhaltspunkt *m*, Hinweis *m*. **II** *vt* steuern, lenken, führen, leiten.
guide dog Blindenhund *m*.
guide-line ['gaɪdlaɪn] *n* Leit-, Richtlinie *f*, Richtschnur *f*.
guide plane Führungsebene *f*.
guide wire *ortho., techn.* Bohr-, Führungsdraht *m*.
Guidi ['gwiːdɪ]: **G.'s canal** Canalis pterygoideus.
guid·ing plane ['gaɪdɪŋ] Führungsebene *f*.
guiding symptom charakteristisches Zeichen *nt*.
Guillain-Barré [giˈjɛ̃ baˈre]: **G.-B. polyneuritis** → G.-B. syndrome.
 G.-B. reflex Weingrow-Reflex *m*.
 G.-B. syndrome *abbr.* **GBS** Guillain-Barre--Syndrom *nt*, (Poly-)Radikuloneuritis *f*, Neuronitis *f*.
Guillen ['gwɪlən]: **G.'s view** *radiol.*, *HNO* Aufnahme *f* nach Guillen.
guil·lo·tine ['gɪlətiːn, 'gɪə-] *n chir.*, *HNO* Guillotine *f*.
guillotine amputation *ortho.* offene Amputation *f*, Amputation *f* ohne Stumpfdeckung.
guin·ea pig ['gɪnɪ] **1.** Meerschweinchen *nt*. **2.** *fig.* Versuchskaninchen *nt*.
Guin·ea worm ['gɪnɪ] *micro.* Medina-, Guineawurm *m*, Dracunculus medinensis, Filaria medinensis.
Guinea worm disease Medinawurmbefall *m*, -infektion *f*, Guineawurmbefall *m*, -infektion *f*, Drakunkulose *f*, Drakontiase *f*, Dracunculosis *f*, Dracontiasis *f*.
Guinon [giˈnõ]: **G.'s disease** Gilles-de-la--Tourette-Syndrom *nt*, Tourette-Syndrom *nt*, Maladie des tics, Tic impulsif.
Guldberg and Waage ['gʊldbərg vɑːgə; 'vɑːgə]: **G. and W.'s law** Massenwirkungsgesetz *nt*.
Gulf Coast tick [gʌlf] *micro.* Amblyomma maculatum.
Gull [gʌl]: **G.'s disease** *old* → myxedema.
gul·let ['gʌlɪt] *n* **1.** Schlund *m*, Kehle *f*, Gurgel *f*. **2.** Speiseröhre *f*, Ösophagus *m*, Oesophagus *m*.
Gullstrand ['gʌlstrænd]: **G.'s formula** Gullstrand-Formel *f*.
 G.'s slit lamp Gullstrand-Lampe *f*.
gu·lon·ic acid [gjuːˈlɒnɪk] Gulonsäure *f*.

L-gulonolactone 334

L-gu·lo·no·lac·tone [,gju:lənəʊ'læktəʊn] *n* L-Gulonolacton *nt*.
gu·lose ['g(j)u:ləʊz] *n* Gulose *f*.
gum [gʌm] *n* 1. *anat*. Zahnfleisch *nt*, Gingiva *f*. 2. Gummi *m/nt*; Klebstoff *m*. 3. Gummi *m/nt*, Gummiharz *nt*, Kautschuk *m*.
gum acid *chem*. Harzsäure *f*.
gum ammoniac *chem*. Ammoniakgummi *nt*.
gum arabic Gummi arabicum.
gum-boil ['gʌmbɔɪl] *n* Zahnfleischabszeß *m*; Parulis *f*.
gum elastic Naturgummi *nt*, Kautschuk *m*.
gum hypertrophy Zahnfleischhypertrophie *f*.
gum line Zahnfleischrand *m*, Margo gingivalis.
gum·ma ['gʌmə] *n*, *pl* **-mas, -ma·ta** [-mətə] *patho*. 1. Gummiknoten *m*, -geschwulst *f*, Gumma *nt*. 2. Syphilom *nt*, Gumma (syphiliticum) *nt*. 3. benigne Spätsyphilis *f*.
gum·ma·tous ['gʌmətəs] *adj* Gumma betr., gummaartig, gummatös, gummös.
gummatous abscess syphilitischer Abszeß *m*.
gummatous osteitis gummatöse Osteitis *f*.
gummatous syphilid → gumma 2.
gummatous ulcer gummöses/hypodermitisches Ulkus *nt*.
gum·my ['gʌmɪ] *adj* 1. gummiartig, gummiabsondernd, klebrig, zäh(flüssig). 2. aus Gummi, Gummi-; gummihaltig. 3. → gummatous.
gummy tumor → gumma.
Gumprecht ['gʌmpreçt]: **G.'s shadows** *hema*. Gumprecht'-Kernschatten *pl*, -Schatten *pl*.
gum sugar L-Arabinose *f*.
gum tragacanth Tragant *m*.
gun·cot·ton ['gʌnkɑtn] *n* Schießbaumwolle *f*, Nitrozellulose *f*.
Gunn [gʌn]: **G.'s crossing sign** → G.'s sign 1. **G.'s phenomenon** → G.'s sign 2. **G.'s sign** 1. Gunn-Zeichen *nt*, Kreuzungsphänomen *nt*. 2. Gunn-Zeichen *nt*, Kiefer-Lid-Phänomen *nt*. **G.'s syndrome** → G.'s sign 2.
gun·shot ['gʌnʃɑt] *n* Schußwunde *f*, -verletzung *f*.
gunshot injury *HNO* (*Ohr*) Knalltrauma *nt*.
gunshot wound Schußwunde *f*, -verletzung *f*.
gun·stock deformity ['gʌnstɑk] *ortho*. Cubitus varus.
Günther ['gɪntər; 'gyn-]: **G.'s disease** Günther'-Krankheit *f*, Morbus Günther *m*, kongenitale erythropoetische Porphyrie *f* *abbr*. CEP, Porphyria erythropo(i)etica congenita, Porphyria congenita Günther.
Günzburg ['gɪntsbɜrg; 'gyntsbʊrk]: **G.'s test** Günzburg-Probe *f*.
gur·gling rales ['gɜrglɪŋ] großblasige Rasselgeräusche *pl*.
Gussenbauer ['gʊsnbaʊər]: **G.'s suture** *chir*. Gussenbauer-Naht *f*.
gus·ta·tion [gʌ'steɪʃn] *n* 1. Geschmackssinn *m*, -vermögen *nt*. 2. Schmecken *nt*.
gus·ta·tive ['gʌstətɪv] *adj* → gustatory.
gus·ta·to·ry [gʌstə,tɔːriː, -təʊ-] *adj* Geschmackssinn betr., gustatorisch, gustativ, Geschmacks-.
gustatory anesthesia Verlust *m* des Geschmackssinnes, Hypo-, Ageusie *f*.
gustatory anosmia gustatorische Anosmie *f*.
gustatory audition Auditio gustatoria.
gustatory bud Geschmacksknospe *f*, Caliculus gustatorius, Gemma gustatoria.

gustatory bulb → gustatory bud.
gustatory cells Geschmackssinneszellen *pl*, Schmeckzellen *pl*.
gustatory center Geschmackszentrum *nt*.
gustatory fibers Geschmacksfasern *pl*.
gustatory glands (von) Ebner'-Drüsen *pl*, (von) Ebner'-Spüldrüsen *pl*.
gustatory hallucination *psychia*. gustatorische Halluzination *f*, Geschmackshalluzination *f*.
gustatory hyperesthesia *neuro*. gustatorische Hyperästhesie *f*, Hypergeusie *f*.
gustatory hyp(o)esthesia verminderte Geschmacksempfindung *f*, gustatorische Hypästhesie *f*, Hypogeusie *f*.
gustatory nucleus Nc. (tractus) solitarius.
gustatory olfaction gustatorisches Riechen *nt*.
gustatory organ Geschmacksorgan *nt*, Organum gustatorium/gustus.
gustatory papillae Zungenpapillen *pl*, Papillae linguales.
gustatory pore Geschmackspore *f*, Porus gustatorius.
gustatory receptor Geschmacksrezeptor *m*.
gustatory sweating syndrome aurikulotemporales Syndrom *nt*, Frey-Baillarger- -Syndrom *nt*, Geschmacksschwitzen *nt*.
gus·tom·e·ter [gʌs'tɑmɪtər] *n* Gustometer *nt*.
gus·tom·e·try [gʌs'tɑmətrɪ] *n* Gustometrie *f*.
gut [gʌt] *n* 1. Darm(kanal *m*) *m*; Gedärme *pl*, Eingeweide *pl*; *anat*. Intestinum *nt*. 2. *chir*. Catgut *nt*. 3. *inf*. Bauch *m*.
gut-associated lymphoid tissue *abbr*. **GALT** darmassoziiertes lymphatisches System *nt*, gut-associated lymphoid tissue *nt*, GALT.
gut glucagon Enteroglukagon *nt*, intestinales Glukagon *nt*.
Guthrie ['gʌθrɪ]: **G.'s muscle** M. sphincter urethrae. **G. test** Guthrie-Hemmtest *m*.
gut·ta ['gʌtə] *n*, *pl* **gut·tae** ['gʌtɪ] Tropfen *m*; *pharm*. Gutta *f*.
gutta-per·cha ['pɜrtʃə] *n* Guttapercha *f*.
gut·tate ['gʌteɪt] *adj* *histol*. (tropfenförmig) gesprenkelt.
guttate choroidopathy *ophthal*. Altersdrusen *pl*, Chorioiditis guttata senilis.
guttate morphea *derm*. Morphea guttata.
guttate parapsoriasis *derm*. Parapsoriasis guttata, Pityriasis lichenoides.
guttate psoriasis *derm*. Psoriasis guttata.
gut·ta·tion [gʌ'teɪʃn] *n* *bio*. Guttation *f*.
gut·ti·form ['gʌtəfɔːrm] *adj* tropfenförmig.
gut·tur ['gʌtər] *n* *anat*. Kehle *f*, vorderer Teil *m* des Halses.
gut·tur·al ['gʌtərəl] *adj* 1. Kehle/Guttur betr., guttural, kehlig, Kehl-. 2. (*Stimme*) rauh, heiser, kehlig, guttural.
guttural cartilage Stell-, Gießbecken-, Aryknorpel *m*, Cartilago aryt(a)enoidea.
guttural duct Ohrtrompete *f*, Eustach'Kanal *m*, -Röhre *f*, Tuba auditiva/auditoria.
Guyon [gwi'jɑ̃]: **G.'s amputation** *ortho*. (tiefe) Unterschenkelamputation *f* nach Guyon. **G.'s canal** Guyon'-Loge *f*. **G.'s operation** → G.'s amputation.
GVH disease/reaction → graft-versus- -host reaction.
Gy *abbr*. → gray[1].
gym·nas·tics [dʒɪm'næstɪks] *pl* Gymnastik *f*, Übung(en *pl*) *f*; Turnen *nt*.
Gym·no·as·ca·ce·ae [,dʒɪmnəʊæs'keɪsɪiː] *pl* *micro*. Gymnoascaceae *pl*.
gym·no·car·pic [,-'kɑːrpɪk] *adj* → gymnocarpus.

gym·no·car·pous [,-'kɑːrpəs] *adj* *micro*. nacktfrüchtig, gymnokarp.
gym·no·pho·bia [,-'fəʊbɪə] *n* *psychia*. Angst *f* vorm Nacktsein *od*. vor Nackten, Gymnophobie *f*.
gym·no·spore ['-spəʊər, -spɔːr] *n* Gymnospore *f*.
gyn- *pref*. → gyneco-.
gynaeco- *pref*. *Brit*. → gyneco-.
gyn·an·der [dʒɪ'nændər] *n* echter Zwitter *m*, Gynander *m*, Hermaphrodit *m*.
gyn·an·dria [dʒɪ'nændrɪə] *n* → gynandrism.
gyn·an·drism [dʒɪ'nændrɪzəm] *n* 1. Zwittrigkeit *f*, Zwittertum *nt*, Hermaphroditismus *m*, Hermaphrodismus *m*. 2. Gynandrie *f*, Gynandrismus *m*, Pseudohermaphroditismus femininus. 3. → gynandromorphism.
gyn·an·dro·blas·to·ma [dʒɪ,nændrəʊblæs-'təʊmə] *n* *gyn*., *patho*. Gynandroblastom *nt*.
gyn·an·droid [dʒɪ'nændrɔɪd] **I** *n* 1. → gynander. 2. weiblicher Scheinzwitter/Pseudohermaphrodit *m*, Gynandroid *m*. **II** *adj* gynandroid.
gyn·an·dro·morph [dʒɪ'nændrəmɔːrf] *n* *bio*. Gynandromorpher *m*.
gyn·an·dro·mor·phism [dʒɪ,nændrə'mɔːrfɪzəm] *n* *bio*. Scheinzwittertum *nt*, Gynandromorphismus *m*, Gynandromorphie *f*.
gyn·an·dro·mor·phous [dʒɪ,nændrə'mɔːrfəs] *adj* *bio*. gynandromorph.
gyn·an·dry [dʒɪ'nændrɪ] *n* → gynandrism.
gyn·a·tre·sia [,dʒɪnə'triːʒ(ɪ)ə] *n* *patho*., *gyn*. Gynatresie *f*.
gyne- *pref*. → gyneco-.
gynec- *pref*. → gyneco-.
gy·ne·cic [dʒɪ'niːsɪk] *adj* Frau(en) betr., Frau(en)-, Gyn-, Gynäko-, Gyno-.
gy·ne·ci·um [dʒɪ'niːsɪən, -ʃɪ-] *n* *bio*. Gynäzium *nt*.
gyneco- *pref*. Frau(en)-, Gynäko-, Gyn-, Gyno-.
gy·ne·cog·ra·phy [,dʒɪnɪ'kɑgrəfɪ, ,gaɪnɪ-] *n* *gyn*., *radiol*. Kontrastdarstellung *f* von Gebärmutter u. Eileiter, Utero-, Metro-, Hysterosalpingographie *f* *abbr*. HSG, Utero-, Metro-, Hysterotubographie *f*.
gy·ne·coid ['dʒɪnɪkɔɪd, 'gaɪnɪ-] *adj* frauenähnlich, -artig, gynäkoid, gynoid.
gynecoid pelvis gynäkoides Becken *nt*.
gy·ne·co·log·ic [,dʒɪnɪkə'lɑdʒɪk, ,gaɪnɪ-] *adj* Gynäkologie betr., gynäkologisch.
gy·ne·co·log·i·cal [,-'lɑdʒɪkl] *adj* → gynecologic.
gynecological forceps Geburtszange *f*.
gynecological perineum Sehnenplatte *f* des Damms, Centrum tendineum perinei.
gynecologic disease gynäkologische Erkrankung *f*.
gy·ne·col·o·gist [,dʒɪnɪ'kɑlədʒɪst, ,gaɪnɪ-] *n* Frauenarzt *m*, -ärztin *f*, Gynäkologe *m*, -login *f*.
gy·ne·col·o·gy [,-'kɑlədʒɪ] *n* Frauenheilkunde *f*, Gynäkologie *f*.
gy·ne·co·ma·nia [,dʒɪnɪkə'meɪnɪə, ,gaɪnɪkəʊ-] *n* *psychia*. Satyriasis *f*, Satyrismus *m*.
gy·ne·co·mas·tia [,-'mæstɪə] *n* Vergrößerung *f* der männlichen Brust(drüse), Gynäkomastie *f*.
gy·ne·co·mas·tism [,-'mæstɪzəm] *n* → gynecomastia.
gy·ne·co·mas·ty ['-mæstɪ] *n* → gynecomastia.
gy·ne·co·ma·zia [,-'meɪzɪə] *n* → gynecomastia.
gy·ne·cop·a·thy [,dʒɪnɪ'kɑpəθɪ, ,gaɪnɪ-] *n* Gynäkopathie *f*.
gy·ne·coph·o·ral canal [,-'kɑfərəl] *micro*. Canalis gynaecophorus.

gyn·e·coph·o·rous canal [ˌ-'kɑfərəs] *micro.* Canalis gynaecophorus.
gy·ne·pho·bia [ˌ-'fəʊbɪə] *n psychia.* krankhafte Angst *f* vor *od.* Abneigung *f* gegen Frauen, Gynäkophobie *f*.
gyn·e·plas·ty ['-plæstɪ] *n* → gynoplasty.
gy·ni·at·rics [ˌdʒɪnɪ'ætrɪks, ˌdʒaɪ-, ˌgaɪ-] *pl* Behandlung *f* von Frauenkrankheiten.
gy·ni·at·ry [ˌ-'ætrɪ] *n* → gyniatrics.
gyno- *pref.* → gyneco-.
gyn·o·gam·on [ˌdʒɪnə'gæməʊn] *n* Gynogamon *nt*.
gyn·o·gen·e·sis [ˌ-'dʒenəsɪs] *n bio.* Gynogenese *f*.
gyn·o·me·rog·o·ny [ˌ-mə'rɑgənɪ] *n bio.* Gynomerogonie *f*.
gyn·op·a·thy [dʒɪ'nɑpəθɪ] *n* Frauenkrankheit *f*, Gynopathie *f*.
gy·no·pho·bia [ˌdʒɪnə'fəʊbɪə, ˌdʒaɪ-, ˌgaɪ-] *n* → gynephobia.
gy·no·plas·tic [ˌ-'plæstɪk] *adj* Gynoplastik betr., gynoplastisch.
gy·no·plas·tics [ˌ-'plæstɪks] *pl* → gynoplasty.
gy·no·plas·ty ['-plæstɪ] *n chir., gyn.* Chirurgie *f* der weiblichen Geschlechtsorgane, Gynoplastik *f*.
gyp·sum ['dʒɪpsəm] *n* Gips *m*.
gy·rase ['dʒaɪreɪz] *n micro.* Gyrase *f*.
gyrase inhibitor Gyrasehemmer *m*.
gy·rate ['dʒaɪreɪt] *adj* gewunden, geschlängelt.
gyrate atrophy of choroid and retina *ophthal.* Atrophia gyrata choroideae et retinae.
gyrate erythema Erythema gyratum/figuratum.
gyrate impressions Impressiones digitatae/gyrorum.
gyrate psoriasis *derm.* Psoriasis gyrata.
gyrate scalp *derm.* faltenartige Pachydermie *f*, Cutis/Pachydermia verticis gyrata, Naevus cerebriformis.
gy·ra·tion [dʒaɪ'reɪʃn] *n* Kreis-, Drehbewegung *f*, Drehung *f*.

gyre [dʒaɪər] *n* → gyrus.
gy·rec·to·my [dʒaɪ'rektəmɪ] *n neurochir.* Gyrektomie *f*.
gyr·en·ce·phal·ic [ˌdʒaɪənsɪ'fælɪk, ˌdʒaɪ-] *adj* (*Gehirn*) mit vielen Windungen versehen, gyrenzephal.
gy·ro·sa [dʒaɪ'rəʊsə] *n* Magenschwindel *m*, Gyrosa *f*, Vertigo gyrosa.
gy·rose ['dʒaɪrəʊs] *adj histol., bio.* gewunden, gewellt.
gy·ro·spasm ['dʒaɪrəspæzəm] *n* Drehkrampf *m* des Kopfes, Gyrospasmus *m*.
gy·rous ['dʒaɪrəs] *adj* → gyrose.
gy·rus ['dʒaɪrəs] *n, pl* **-ri** [-raɪ] *anat.* Kreis *m*, Windung *f*, Hirnwindung *f*, Gyrus *m*.
g.i of cerebellum Kleinhirnwindungen *pl*, Gyri/Folia cerebelli.
g.i of cerebrum (Groß-)Hirnwindungen *pl*, Gyri cerebrales.
g.i of frontal lobe Stirnhirnwindungen *pl*.
g.i of insula Windungen/Gyri *pl* der Insel, Gyri insulae.

H

H abbr. 1. → heat content. 2. → henry. 3. → histamine. 4. → histidine. 5. → hydrogen. 6. → hyperopia.
h abbr. 1. → hecto-. 2. [hora] → hour. 3. → Planck's constant.
H⁺ abbr. → hydrogen ion.
[H⁺] abbr. → hydrogen ion concentration.
H₀ abbr. → null hypothesis.
H₁ abbr. → alternative hypothesis.
²H abbr. 1. → deuterium. 2. → heavy hydrogen.
³H abbr. → tritium.
HA abbr. 1. → hemagglutinin 2. 2. → hepatitis A. 3. → hyaluronic acid.
Ha abbr. → hahnium.
HAA abbr. [hepatitis-associated antigen] → hepatitis B surface antigen.
Haab [ha:b]: **H.'s reflex** Haab-Reflex m, Rindenreflex m der Pupille.
Haase ['ha:sǝ]: **H.'s rule** Haase'-Regel f.
ha·be·na [hǝ'bi:nǝ] n, pl **-nae** [-ni:] → habenula.
ha·be·nal [hǝ'bi:nl] adj Habena betr.
ha·be·nar [hǝ'bi:nǝr] adj → habenal.
ha·ben·u·la [hǝ'benjǝlǝ] n, pl **-lae** [-li:] anat. 1. Zügel m, Habenula f. 2. Zirbeldrüsen-, Epiphysenstiel m, Habenula f.
ha·ben·u·lar commissure [hǝ'benjǝlǝr] Commissura habenularis/habenularum.
habenular nuclei Ncc. habenulae medialis et lateralis.
habenular sulcus Sulcus habenulae/habenularis.
habenular trigone Trigonum habenulae/habenulare.
ha·ben·u·lo·in·ter·pe·dun·cu·lar tract [hǝ‚benjǝlǝʊ‚ɪntǝrpɪ'dʌnkjǝlǝr] Meynert'--Bündel nt, Fasciculus reflexus, Tractus habenulointerpeduncularis.
ha·ben·u·lo·pe·dun·cu·lar tract [‚-pɪ'dʌŋkjǝlǝr] habenulopeduncular tract.
ha·ben·u·lo·tec·tal fibers [‚-'tektl] habenulotektale Fasern pl.
habenulotectal tract habenulotektale Bahn f, Tractus habenulotectalis.
ha·ben·u·lo·teg·men·tal tract [‚-teg'mentl] habenulotegmentale Bahn f, Tractus habenulotegmentalis.
Habermann ['hæbǝrmǝn; 'ha:bǝrman]: **H.'s disease** Mucha-Habermann-Syndrom nt, Pityriasis lichenoides et varioliformis acuta (Mucha-Habermann).
hab·it ['hæbɪt] n 1. (An-)Gewohnheit f. out of ~/by ~ gewohnheitsmäßig, aus Gewohnheit. 2. (Drogen) Sucht f, Süchtigkeit f. 3. psycho. Habit nt/m. 4. Konstitution f, Verfassung f.
h.s of life Lebensgewohnheiten pl.
hab·i·tat ['hæbɪtæt] n bio. Habitat nt, Lebensraum m, -bezirk m.
habit-forming adj Sucht od. Gewöhnung erzeugend, suchterzeugend.
habit spasm Tic m, Tick m, (nervöses) Zucken nt.
ha·bit·u·al [hǝ'bɪtʃʊǝl] adj 1. gewohnheitsmäßig, habitual, habituell, wiederholt auftretend, Gewohnheits-. 2. üblich, ständig, gewohnt.
habitual abortion gyn. habitueller Abort m.
habitual dislocation ortho. habituelle Luxation f.
ha·bit·u·al·ness [hǝ'bɪtʃǝwǝlnɪs] n Gewohnheitsmäßigkeit f.
ha·bit·u·ate [hǝ'bɪtʃǝweɪt] I vt ~ o.s. s. gewöhnen (to an). II vi 1. süchtig machen. 2. zur Gewohnheit werden.
ha·bit·u·a·tion [hǝ‚bɪtʃǝ'weɪʃn] n 1. Gewöhnung f (to an). 2. physiol., psycho. Gewöhnung f, Habituation f. 3. pharm. Gewöhnung f, Habituation f.
habituation dependence psychische Abhängigkeit f.
hab·i·tude ['hæbɪt(j)u:d] n 1. (An-)Gewohnheit f. 2. Neigung f, Veranlagung f.
hab·i·tus ['hæbɪtǝs] n, pl **-tus** 1. Körperbau(typus m) m, Konstitution f, Habitus m. 2. Körperhaltung f, -stellung f, Habitus m. 3. gyn. Fruchthaltung f, Habitus m.
Hab·ro·ne·ma [‚hæbrǝʊ'ni:mǝ] n micro. Habronema nt.
hab·ro·ne·mi·a·sis [‚-nɪ'maɪǝsɪs] n Habronemainfektion f, Habronematosis f, Habronemosis f.
hack·ing cough ['hækɪŋ] abgehackter Husten m.
Hadfield-Clarke ['hædfi:ld 'klɑ:rk]: **H.-C. syndrome** zystische (Pankreas-)Fibrose f, Mukoviszidose f.
HAE abbr. → hereditary angioedema.
haem [hi:m] n → heme.
haem- pref. Brit. → hemo-.
haema- pref. Brit. → hemo-.
Hae·ma·dip·sa [‚hi:mǝ'dɪpsǝ, ‚hem-] n micro. Haemadipsa nt.
Hae·ma·phy·sa·lis [‚-'faɪsǝlɪs] n micro. Haemaphysalis f.
haemat(o)- pref. Brit. → hemato-.
Hae·ma·to·bia [‚-'tǝʊbɪǝ] n micro. Haematobia f.
Hae·ma·to·si·phon [‚hi:mǝtǝʊ'saɪfǝn, ‚hem-] n micro. Haematosiphon nt.
H. indorus mexikanische Geflügelwanze f, Haematosiphon indorus.
Haem·en·te·ria [hi:mǝn'tɪǝrɪǝ] n micro. Haementeria f.
H. officinalis Haementeria officinalis, Placobdella officinalis.
haemo- pref. Brit. → hemo-.
Hae·mo·bar·ton·el·la [‚hi:mǝ‚bɑ:rtǝ'nelǝ, ‚hem-] n micro. Haemobartonella f.
Hae·mo·dip·sus [‚-'dɪpsǝs] n micro. Haemodipsus m.
Hae·mo·greg·a·ri·na [‚-‚gregǝ'raɪnǝ] n micro. Haemogregarina f.
Hae·mon·chus [hi:'mɒŋkǝs] n micro. Haemonchus m.
Hae·moph·i·lus [hi:'mɒfɪlǝs] n micro. Haemophilus m.
H. aegyptius Koch-Weeks-Bazillus m, Haemophilus aegypti(c)us/conjunctivitidis.
H. ducreyi Streptobacillus m des weichen Schankers, Haemophilus ducreyi, Coccobacillus ducreyi.
H. duplex Diplobakterium Morax-Axenfeld nt, Moraxella (Moraxella) lacunata.
H. influenzae Pfeiffer'-(Influenza-)Bazillus m, Haemophilus influenzae, Bact. influenzae.
H. pertussis Keuchhustenbakterium nt, Bordet-Gengou-Bakterium nt, Bordetella/Haemophilus pertussis.
Haemophilus influenzae meningitis Influenzabazillenmeningitis f, Haemophilus-influenzae-Meningitis f.
haem·or·rha·gia [‚hemǝ'reɪdʒɪǝ] n → hemorrhage I.
Hae·mo·spo·rid·ia [‚hi:mǝspǝ'rɪdɪǝ, ‚hem-] pl micro. Haemosporidien pl, Haemosporidia pl.
hae·mo·zo·in [‚-'zǝʊɪn] n → hemozoin.
Haff disease [hæf] Haffkrankheit f.
haf·ni·um ['hæfnɪǝm] n abbr. **Hf** Hafnium nt abbr. Hf.
Haf·nia ['hæfnɪǝ] n micro. Hafnia f.
Hageman ['hægǝmǝn]: **H. factor** abbr. **HF** Faktor XII m abbr. F XII, Hageman--Faktor m.
H. factor deficiency Hageman-Syndrom nt, Faktor XII-Mangel(krankheit f) m.
H. syndrome → H. factor deficiency.
Hagen-Poiseuille ['heɪgǝn, pwa:'sœj; 'ha:gǝn]: **H.-P. law** Hagen-Poiseuille'-Gesetz nt.
H agglutination micro., immun. H-Agglutination f.
Haglund ['ha:glʊnd]: **H.'s disease** 1. Haglund-Krankheit f, Apophysitis calcanei. 2. Haglund-Ferse f, -Exostose f.
H.'s deformity → H.'s disease 2.
hahn·e·mann·ism ['hɑ:nǝmǝnɪzǝm] n → homeopathy.
hahn·i·um ['hɑ:nɪǝm] n abbr. **Ha** Hahnium nt abbr. Ha.
HAI abbr. 1. → hemagglutination inhibition. 2. → hemagglutination inhibition test.
Hailey-Hailey ['heɪlɪ]: **H.-H. disease** Hailey-Hailey-Krankheit f, -Syndrom nt, Morbus Hailey-Hailey m, familiärer gutartiger Pemphigus m, Gougerot-Hailey-Hailey-Krankheit f, Pemphigus chronicus benignus familiaris (Hailey-Hailey), Pemphigus Gougerot-Hailey-Hailey, Dyskeratosis bullosa (hereditaria).
hair [heǝr] n 1. Haar nt; anat. Pilus m. 2. Haar nt, Haare pl; (Körper-)Haare pl, Behaarung f. to lose one's ~ die Haare verlieren, kahl werden. 3. Faser f, Härchen nt.
h.s of axilla Achsel(höhlen)haare pl, Hirci pl.
h.s of external acoustic meatus Haare des äußeren Gehörganges, Tragi pl.
h.s of eyebrow Augenbrauenhaare pl, Supercilia pl.
h.s of head Kopfhaare pl, Capilli pl.

h.s of nose Nasenhaare *pl*, Haare *pl* des Naseneingangs, Vibrissae *pl*.
h.s of vestibule of nose → h.s of nose.
hair-ball ['heərbɔːl] *n* Haarball *m*, Trichobezoar *m*.
hair-brush ['heərbrʌʃ] *n* 1. Haarbürste *f*. 2. Haarpinsel *m*.
hair bulb Haarzwiebel *f*, Bulbus pili.
hair canal Haarkanal *m*.
hair cells: acoustic/auditory h. akustische Haarzellen *pl*.
 cochlear h. Corti'-Haarzellen *pl*.
 inner h. (*Ohr*) innere Haarzellen *pl*.
 outer h. (*Ohr*) äußere Haarzellen *pl*.
 vestibular h. vestibuläre Haarzellen *pl*.
hair crosses Cruces pilorum.
hair cuticle Haarkutikula *f*.
hair cycle Haarzyklus *m*.
haired [heəd] *adj* behaart; -haarig.
hair follicle Haarfollikel *m*, -balg *m*, Folliculus pili.
hair-follicle cyst piläre Hautzyste *f*.
hair follicle infection Haarbalginfektion *f*.
hair follicle mite Haarbalgmilbe *f*, Demodex folliculorum.
hair-follicle sensor Haarfollikelsensor *m*.
hair growth Haarwachstum *nt*.
hair·i·ness ['heərɪnɪs] *n* Behaartheit *f*, Haarigkeit *f*.
hair·less ['heəlɪs] *adj* ohne Haar(e), haarlos, unbehaart, kahl.
hair·less·ness ['heəlɪsnɪs] *n* Haarlosigkeit *f*; Kahlheit *f*.
hair·like ['heəlaɪk] *adj* haarähnlich, -artig.
hair·line ['heəlaɪn] I *n* Haaransatz *m*. II *adj* haarfein, sehr fein *od.* dünn.
hair-line fracture *ortho.* Haarbruch *m*, Knochenfissur *f*.
hair loss Haarausfall *m*; Alopezie *f*.
hair-matrix carcinoma Basalzell(en)karzinom *m*, Ca. basocellulare.
hair medulla Haarmark *nt*.
hair-on-end appearance/configuration *radiol.* Bürstenschädel *m*.
hair papilla Haarpapille *f*, Papilla pili.
hair receptor Haarrezeptor *m*.
hair restorer Haarwuchsmittel *nt*.
hair root Haarwurzel *f*, Radix pili.
hair root epithelium Haarwurzelepithel *nt*.
hair shaft Haarschaft *m*, Scapus pili.
hair sheath (Haar-)Wurzelscheide *f*.
hair streams Streichrichtungen *pl* der Haare, Flumina pilorum.
hair teeth Dentes acustici.
hair transplant Haartransplantation *f*, -verpflanzung *f*.
hair vortices Haarwirbel *pl*, Vortices pilorum.
hair·y ['heərɪ] *adj* haarig, behaart, Haar-; haarartig.
hairy cell *hema.* Haarzelle *f*.
hairy cell leukemia *hema.* Haarzellenleukämie *f*, leukämische Retikuloendotheliose *f*.
hairy heart Zottenherz *nt*, Cor villosum.
hairy mole → hairy nevus.
hairy nevus Haarnävus *m*, -mal *nt*, Naevus pilosus.
hairy tongue Haarzunge *f*, Glossotrichie *f*, Trichoglossie *f*, Lingua pilosa/villosa.
 black h. schwarze Haarzunge, Glossophytie *f*, Melanoglossie *f*, Lingua pilosa/villosa nigra.
hal- *pref.* → halo-.
hal·a·zone ['hæləzəʊn] *n pharm.* Halazon *nt*.
Halberstaedter-Prowazek ['halbərstetər pro'vatsek]: **H.-P. bodies** Halberstädter-Prowazek-(Einschluß-)Körperchen *pl*, Prowazek-(Einschluß-)Körperchen *pl*.

hal·cin·o·nide [hæl'sɪnənaɪd] *n pharm.* Halcinonid *nt*.
Haldane ['hɔːldeɪn]: **H.'s apparatus** Haldane-Apparat *m*.
 H. chamber → H.'s apparatus.
 H. effect (Christiansen-Douglas-)-Haldane-Effekt *m*.
half [hæf, hɑːf] I *n*, *pl* **halves** [hævz, hɑːvz] Hälfte *f*. II *adj* halb. III *adv* halb, zur Hälfte; fast, nahezu; (*zeitlich*) halb.
half-antigen *n* Halbantigen *nt*, Hapten *nt*.
half bath Halbbad *nt*.
half-blood *n* 1. → half-breed. 2. Halbbruder *m od.* -schwester *f*.
half-blooded *adj* von Eltern verschiedener Rassen abstammend.
half-breed *n* Mischling *m*; *bio.* Bastard *m*, Hybride *f*.
half brother Halbbruder *m*.
half-caste *n* → half-breed.
half desmosome Hemi-, Halbdesmosom *nt*.
half face Profil *nt*.
half-hour I *n* halbe Stunde *f*. II *adj* halbstündig, halbstündlich.
half-hourly *adj* → half-hour II.
half lamella Halblamelle *f*.
half-live *n abbr.* T ½, t ½ *pharm., chem., phys.* Halbwert(s)zeit *f abbr.* HWZ, T ½, t ½.
 biological h. biologische Halbwertzeit.
 effective h. effektive Halbwertzeit.
half-live period → half-live.
half-saturation pressure Halbsättigungsdruck *m*.
half sister Halbschwester *f*.
half-time *n* → half-live.
half-value layer *abbr.* **HVL** *radiol.* Halbwert(schicht)dicke *f abbr.* HWD, d ½.
 second l. *radiol.* Halbwertschichtdicke der zweiten Schicht.
half-value thickness → half-value layer.
half-way house ['hɑːfweɪ, 'hæf-] 1. Rehabilitationszentrum *nt*. 2. *fig.* Zwischenstufe *f*, -station *f*.
hal·ide ['hælaɪd, 'heɪ-] *chem.* I *n* Halogenid *nt*, Halid *nt*, Haloid *nt*. II *adj* salzähnlich, haloid.
hal·i·pha·gia [ˌhælɪ'feɪdʒ(ɪ)ə] *n* Salzessen *nt*, Haliphagie *f*.
hal·i·ste·re·sis [ˌ-stɪ'riːsɪs] *n patho.* Halisterese *f*, Halisteresis *f*.
hal·i·ste·ret·ic [ˌ-stə'retɪk] *adj* Halisterese betr., salz-, kalkarm.
hal·i·to·sis [ˌhælɪ'təʊsɪs] *n* (über) Mund-, Atemgeruch *m*, Halitose *f*, Halitosis *f*, Kakostomie *f*, Foetor ex ore.
hal·i·tus ['hælɪtəs] *n* Atem *m*, Ausdünstung *f*, Geruch *m*, Halitus *m*.
Haller ['halər]: **H.'s arch** 1. äußerer Haller'-Bogen *m*, Quadratusarkade *f*, Lig. arcuatum laterale, Arcus lumbocostalis lateralis. 2. innerer Haller'-Bogen *m*, Psoasarkade *f*, Lig. arcuatum mediale, Arcus lumbocostalis medialis.
 circle of H. Haller'-, Zinn'-Gefäßkranz *m*, Circulus vasculosus n. optici.
 H.'s cones Lobuli/Coni epididymidis.
 crypts of H. → glands of H.
 glands of H. präputiale (Talg-)Drüsen *pl*, Präputialdrüsen *pl*, Gll. pr(a)eputiales.
 H.'s line vordere Mittelfurche *f*, Fissura mediana anterior/ventralis medullae oblongatae.
 H.'s membrane Haller'-Membran *f*, Lamina vasculosa (choroidea).
 rete of H. Haller'-Netz *nt*, Rete testis.
 H.'s tripod Truncus c(o)eliacus.
 H.'s unguis Calcar avis.
 H.'s vascular tissue → H.'s membrane.
Hallermann-Streiff ['hælərmən straɪf]:

H.-S. syndrome → Hallermann-Streiff-François syndrome.
Hallermann-Streiff-François [frɑ̃'swa]: **H.-S.-F. syndrome** Hallermann-Streiff-(-François)-Syndrom *nt*, Dyskephaliesyndrom *nt* von François, Dysmorphia mandibulo-oculo-facialis.
Hallervorden ['halərfɔrdən]: **H. syndrome** → Hallervorden-Spatz disease.
Hallervorden-Spatz [ʃpats]: **H.-S. disease/syndrome** Hallervorden-Spatz-Erkrankung *f*, -Syndrom *nt*.
hal·lex ['hælɪks] *n*, *pl* **-li·ces** ['hælɪsiːz] → hallux.
Hallgren ['hɔlgrən]: **H.'s syndrome** Hallgren-Syndrom *nt*.
Hallopeau [alo'po]: **H.'s acrodermatitis/disease** Hallopeau'-Krankheit *f*, -Eiterflechte *f*, Akrodermatitis suppurativa continua.
hal·lu·cal ['hæljəkl] *adj* Hallux betr., Hallux-, Großzeh(en)-.
hal·lu·ces *pl* → hallux.
hal·lu·ci·nate [hə'luːsɪneɪt] I *vt* halluzinieren, Halluzination(en) auslösen. II *vi* halluzinieren, Halluzination(en) haben, unter Halluzinationen leiden.
hal·lu·ci·na·tion [həˌluːsɪ'neɪʃn] *n* Halluzination *f*, Sinnestäuschung *f*.
 h. of smell olfaktorische Halluzination, Geruchshalluzination.
 h. of taste gustatorische Halluzination, Geschmackshalluzination.
hal·lu·ci·na·tive [hə'luːsɪneɪtɪv] *adj* auf Halluzinationen beruhend, halluzinativ.
hal·lu·ci·na·to·ry [hə'luːsɪnəˌtɔːriː, -təʊ-] *adj* mit Halluzinationen einhergehend, halluzinatorisch.
hal·lu·ci·no·gen [hə'luːsɪnədʒən] *n* Halluzinogen *nt*.
hal·lu·ci·no·gen·e·sis [həˌluːsɪnəʊ'dʒenəsɪs] *n* Halluzinationsbildung *f*, Halluzinogenese *f*.
hal·lu·ci·no·ge·net·ic [ˌ-dʒə'netɪk] *adj* → hallucinogenic II.
hal·lu·ci·no·gen·ic [ˌ-'dʒenɪk] I *n* → hallucinogen. II *adj* Halluzination(en) bewirkend *od.* auslösend, halluzinogen.
hal·lu·ci·no·sis [həˌluːsɪ'nəʊsɪs] *n psychia.* Halluzinose *f*.
hal·lu·ci·not·ic [ˌ-'nɒtɪk] *adj* Halluzinose betr., Halluzinosen-.
hal·lux ['hæləks] *n*, *pl* **hal·lu·ces** ['hæljəsiːz] Großzehe *f*, Hallux *m*, Digitus primus pedis.
hallux valgus Ballengroßzehe *f*, X-Großzehe *f*, Hallux valgus.
Hallwachs ['halvaks]: **H. effect** photo-/lichtelektrischer Effekt *m*, Photoeffekt *m*.
hal·ma·to·gen·e·sis [ˌhælmətəʊ'dʒenəsɪs] *n genet.* sprunghafte Variation *f*, Halmatogenese *f*, -genesis *f*.
halo- *pref.* Salz-, Hal(o)-.
ha·lo ['heɪləʊ] *n*, *pl* **-los, loes** 1. Ring *m*, Kreis *m*, Hof *m*, Saum *m*, Halo *m*. 2. *phys.* Lichthof *m*, Farbenkreis *m*, Halo *m*. 3. Ring *m* um die Augen, Halo *m*. 4. Warzenvorhof *m*, Areola mammae. 5. *patho., derm.* Halo *m*. 6. *ortho.* Halo *m*.
hal·o·der·mia [ˌhælə'dɜːmɪə] *n derm.* Halodermie *f*.
halo-femoral traction *ortho.* halo-femorale Extension *f*.
hal·o·gen [ˈ-dʒən] *n* Salzbildner *m*, Halogen *nt*.
halogen acne *derm.* Halogenakne *f*.
hal·o·gen·at·ed hydrocarbon [ˈ-dʒeneɪtɪd] *chem.* halogenierter Kohlenwasserstoff *m*.
hal·o·gen·a·tion [ˌ-dʒə'neɪʃn] *n* Halogenierung *f*, Halogenation *f*.

haloid

hal·oid ['hæloɪd, 'heɪ-] *adj* → halide II.
haloid acid Halogenwasserstoff(säure *f*) *m*.
halo immobilization → halo traction.
ha·lom·e·ter [heɪ'lɑmɪtər] *n* **1.** *hema*. Halometer *nt*. **2.** *ophthal*. Halometer *nt*.
ha·lom·e·try [heɪ'lɑmətrɪ] *n* **1.** *hema*. Halometrie *f*. **2.** *ophthal*. Halometrie *f*.
halo nevus Halo-Nävus *m*, Sutton-Nävus *m*, perinaevische Vitiligo *f*, Leucoderma centrifugum acquisitum, Vitiligo circumnaevalis.
halo-pelvic apparatus *ortho*. Halo-Becken-Apparat *m*, Halo-Pelvis-Apparat *m*.
halo-pelvic traction *ortho*. Halo-Becken-Extension *f*.
hal·o·per·i·dol [ˌhælə'perɪdɔl, -dɑl] *n pharm*. Haloperidol *nt*.
hal·o·phil ['-fɪl] *adj* → halophilic.
hal·o·phile ['-faɪl] *bio*. **I** *n* halophiler Mikroorganismus *m*. **II** *adj* → halophilic.
hal·o·phil·ic [ˌ-'fɪlɪk] *adj bio*. salzliebend, halophil.
ha·loph·i·lous [hæ'lɑfələs] *adj* → halophilic.
hal·o·pro·gin [ˌhælə'proʊdʒɪn] *n pharm*. Haloprogin *nt*.
halo sign *radiol*. Halozeichen *nt*, Deuel--Halozeichen *nt*.
hal·o·ste·re·sis [ˌ-stə'riːsɪs] *n* → halisteresis.
halo symptom *ophthal*. Halo glaucomatosus.
hal·o·thane ['-θeɪn] *n anes*. Halothan *nt*, Fluothan *nt*.
halothane hepatitis Halothanhepatitis *f*.
halo traction *ortho*. Halo-Extension *f*.
halo-vest brace *ortho*. Halo-Fixateur externe *m*.
halo vision Halosehen *nt*.
Halsted ['hɔːlstɪd, -stɪd]: **H.'s ligament** Lig. costoclaviculare.
H.'s mastectomy Halsted-Operation *f*, radikale Mastektomie *f*, Mammaamputation *f*, Ablatio mammae.
H.'s operation 1. → H.'s mastectomy. **2.** → Halsted-Ferguson operation.
H.'s suture *chir*. Halsted-Naht *f*.
Halsted-Ferguson ['fɜrɡəsən]: **H.-F. operation** *chir*. Herniotomie *f* nach Halsted(-Ferguson).
ham·am·e·lose [hə'mæmələʊs] *n* Hamamelose *f*.
ha·mar·tia [hɑ'mɑːrʃɪə] *n embryo*. Hamartie *f*.
ha·mar·to·blas·to·ma [həˌmɑːrtəʊblæs-'təʊmə] *n patho*. Hamartoblastom *nt*, malignes Hamartom *nt*.
ham·ar·to·ma [ˌhæmər'təʊmə] *n, pl* **-mas, -ma·ta** [-mətə] *patho*. Hamartom *nt*.
ham·ar·to·ma·to·sis [ˌhæmɑːrtəʊmə'təʊ-sɪs] *n* Hamartomatose *f*, Hamartomatosis *f*, Hamartosis *f*, Hamartosis *f*.
ham·ar·to·pho·bia [ˌ-'fəʊbɪə] *n psychia*. krankhafte Angst *f* vor Fehlhandlungen, Hamartophobie *f*.
ha·mate ['heɪmeɪt] *adj anat*. hakenförmig, krumm, Haken-.
hamate bone Hakenbein *nt*, Hamatum *nt*, Os hamatum.
ha·ma·tum [hə'meɪtəm] *n, pl* **-tums, -ta** [-tə] → hamate bone.
Hamburger ['hæmbɜrɡər]: **H.'s interchange** → H. phenomenon.
H.'s law Hamburger-Gesetz *nt*.
H. phenomenon Hamburger-Phänomen *nt*, -Gesetz *nt*, Chloridverschiebung *f*.
H.'s shift → H. phenomenon.
Hamilton ['hæmɪltən]: **H.'s method** *gyn*. Hamilton-Methode *f*.
Hamilton Russell ['rʌsl]: **H. R. traction**

ortho. Extension(s)behandlung *f* nach Hamilton-Russell.
Hamman ['hæmæn]: **H.'s disease/syndrome** Hamman-Syndrom *nt*, (spontanes) Mediastinalemphysem *nt*, Pneumomediastinum *nt*.
Hamman-Rich [rɪtʃ]: **H.-R. syndrome** Hamman-Rich-Syndrom *nt*, diffuse progressive interstitielle Lungenfibrose *f*.
ham·mer ['hæmər] *n* **1.** *anat*. Hammer *m*, Malleus *m*. **2.** Hammer *m*.
hammer finger *ortho*. Hammerfinger *m*.
hammer nose Kartoffel-, Säufer-, Pfund-, Knollennase *f*, Rhinophym *nt*, Rhinophyma *nt*.
Hammerschlag ['hæmərʃlɑːɡ; 'hɑmərʃlɑːk]: **H.'s method** *hema*. Hammerschlag-Methode *f*.
hammer toe *ortho*. Hammerzehe *f*, Digitus malleus.
Hammond ['hæmənd]: **H.'s disease** Hammond-Syndrom *nt*, Athetosis duplex.
Hampton ['hæmptən]: **H. line** *radiol*. Hampton-Linie *f*.
ham·string ['hæmstrɪŋ] *n* Kniesehne *f*, Sehne *f* der ischiokruralen Muskeln.
hamstring muscles ischiokrurale Muskeln *pl*/Muskulatur *f*.
ham·strings ['hæmstrɪŋz] *pl* → hamstring muscles.
ham·u·lar ['hæmjələr] *adj* → hamate.
hamular groove Sulcus hamuli pterygoidei.
ham·u·lus ['hæmjələs] *n, pl* **-li** [-laɪ] *anat*., *bio*. kleiner Haken *m*, hakenförmiger Fortsatz *m*, Hamulus *m*.
h. of bony spiral lamina Hamulus laminae spiralis.
h. of ethmoid bone Proc. uncinatus ossis ethmoidalis.
h. of hamate (bone) Hamulus ossis hamati.
Hancock ['hænkɑk]: **H.'s amputation/operation** *ortho*. Hancock-Amputation *f*, supramalleoläre Unterschenkelamputation *f* nach Hancock.
H. valve *HTG* Hancock-Prothese *f*.
Hand [hænd]: **H.'s disease/syndrome** → Hand-Schüller-Christian disease.
hand [hænd] *n* **1.** Hand *f*; *anat*. Manus *f*. **2.** *zoo*. Hand *f*, Fuß *m*. **3.** (Uhr-)Zeiger *m*. **4.** (Hand-)Schrift *f*.
hand-and-foot syndrome Hand-Fuß-Syndrom *nt*, Sichelzellendaktylitis *f*.
hand·ba·sin ['hændbeɪsn] *n* (Hand-)Waschbecken *nt*.
hand·book ['hændbʊk] *n* Handbuch *nt*.
hand·breadth ['hændbredθ] *n* Handbreit *f*.
hand·cream ['hændkriːm] *n* Handcreme *f*.
hand eczema Handekzem *nt*.
hand·ed·ness ['hændɪdnɪs] *n* Händigkeit *f*.
hand-foot-and-mouth disease/syndrome falsche Maul- u. Klauenseuche *f*, Hand--Fuß-Mund-Exanthem *nt*, Hand-Fuß--Mund-Krankheit *f*.
hand glass 1. → hand lens. **2.** Handspiegel *m*.
hand·grip ['hændɡrɪp] *n* Händedruck *m*, (Hand-)Griff *m*.
hand·i·cap ['hændɪkæp] *n* Handikap *nt*; Nachteil *m*, Hindernis *nt* (*to* für); Behinderung *f*.
hand·i·capped ['hændɪkæpt] **I** the ~ *pl* die Behinderten. **II** *adj* gehandikapt, benachteiligt, behindert (*with* durch).
han·dle ['hændl] **I** *n* Griff *m*, Stiel *m*, Henkel *m*. **II** *vt* **1.** anfassen, berühren. **2.** handhaben, gebrauchen, umgehen *od*. fertig werden mit, anfassen, anpacken.
h. of malleus Hammerstiel *m*, Manubrium mallei.
hand lens Vergrößerungsglas *nt*, Lupe *f*.

han·dling ['hændlɪŋ] *n* **1.** Berührung *f*, Berühren *nt*. **2.** Handhabung *f*, Gebrauch *m*; Ver-, Bearbeitung *f*. **3.** (*Patient*) Umgang *m* (*of* mit).
hand plate *embryo*. Handplatte *f*.
Hand-Schüller-Christian ['ʃɪlər 'krɪstʃən]: **H.-S.-C. disease** Hand-Schüller-Christian-Krankheit *f*, Schüller-Hand-Christian-Krankheit *f*, Schüller-Krankheit *f*.
H.-S.-C. syndrome → H.-S.-C. disease.
hand·shake ['hændʃeɪk] *n* Händedruck *m*.
hand-shoulder syndrome Schulter-Arm--Syndrom *nt*.
hand surgeon Handchirurg(in *f*) *m*.
hand surgery Handchirurgie *f*.
hand·writ·ing ['hændraɪtɪŋ] *n* (Hand-)Schrift *f*.
HANE *abbr*. [hereditary angioneurotic edema] → hereditary angioedema.
Hanger ['hæŋər]: **H.'s test** Hanger--Flockungstest *m*, Kephalin-Cholesterin-Test *m*.
hang·ing arm cast ['hæŋɪŋ] *ortho*. Hänge-, Pendelgips(verband *m*) *m*, hanging cast (*m*).
hanging-block culture *micro*. Kultur *f* im hängenden Block.
hanging cast → hanging arm cast.
hanging drop *micro*. hängender Tropfen *m*.
hanging-drop culture *micro*. Kultur *f* im hängenden Tropfen.
hanging drop technique *micro*. hängender Tropfen *m*.
hang·man's fracture ['hæŋmən] *ortho*. Axisfraktur *f* mit beidseitigem Bruch der Bogenwurzel, Hangman's fracture (*f*).
Hanhart ['hænhɑːrt]: **H.'s syndrome** Hanhart-Syndrom *nt*.
Hankow fever ['hæŋkaʊ; hɑn'kəʊ] japanische Schistosomiasis/Bilharziose *f*, Schistosomiasis japonica.
Hannover ['hænəʊvər]: **H.'s canal** *ophthal*. Hannover-Kanal *m*.
Hanot [a'noʊ]: **H.'s cirrhosis 1.** biliäre (Leber-)Zirrhose *f*, Hanot-Zirrhose *f*, Cirrhosis biliaris. **2.** primär biliäre (Leber-)Zirrhose *f*.
H.'s disease/syndrome → H.'s cirrhosis.
Hanot-Chauffard [ʃoʊ'fɑːr]: **H.-C. syndrome** Hanot-Chauffard-Syndrom *nt*.
Hansen ['hɑnsən]: **H.'s bacillus** Hansen-Bazillus *m*, Mycobacterium leprae, Leprabazillus *m*, -bakterium *nt*.
H.'s disease Hansen-Krankheit *f*, Morbus Hansen *m*, Aussatz *m*, Lepra *f*, Hansenosis *f*.
Hantaan ['hæntæn]: **H. virus** Ha(n)taan-Virus *nt*.
H antigen *micro*. Geißelantigen *nt*, H-Antigen *nt*.
haph·al·ge·sia [ˌhæfæl'dʒɪzɪə, -dʒiːʒə] *n psychia*. Berührungsüberempfindlichkeit *f* der Haut, Haphalgesie *f*.
haph·e·pho·bia [ˌhæfɪ'foʊbɪə] *n psychia*. krankhafte Angst *f* vor dem Berührtwerden, Haphephobie *f*, Haptophobie *f*.
hapl(o)- *pref*. Einzel-, Einfach-, Hapl(o)-.
hap·lo·dont ['hæplədɑnt] *adj dent*. haplodont.
hap·loid ['hæplɔɪd] *genet*. **I** *n* Zelle *f* od. Individuum *nt* mit haploidem Chromosomensatz *m*. **II** *adj* haploid.
haploid phase → haplophase.
hap·loi·dy ['hæplɔɪdɪ] *n genet*. Haploidie *f*.
hap·lo·my·co·sis [ˌhæpləmaɪ'kəʊsɪs] *n* (Lungen-)Adiaspiromykose *f*.
hap·lont ['hæplɑnt] *n genet*. Haplont *m*.
hap·lop·a·thy [hæp'lɑpəθɪ] *n patho*. einfache/unkomplizierte Erkrankung *f*.

hap·lo·phase ['hæpləfeɪz] *n* Haplophase *f*.
hap·lo·pia [hæp'loʊpɪə] *n ophthal.* Einfachsehen *nt*, Haplopie *f*.
hap·lo·scope ['hæpləskoʊp] *n ophthal.* Haploskop *nt*.
hap·lo·scop·ic [ˌ-'skɑpɪk] *adj* haploskopisch.
hap·lo·spo·ran·gin [ˌ-spə'rændʒɪn] *n* Haplosporangin *nt*.
Hap·lo·spo·ran·gi·um [ˌ-spə'rændʒɪəm] *n micro.* Emmonsia *f*.
hap·lo·type ['-taɪp] *n* Haplotyp *m*.
Hapsburg lip ['hæpsbɜrɡ] Habsburger-Lippe *f*.
hap·ten ['hæptən] *n* Halbantigen *nt*, Hapten *nt*.
hapten carrier complex Hapten-Carrier-Komplex *m*.
hap·tene ['-tiːn] *n* → hapten.
hap·ten·ic [hæp'tenɪk] *adj* Hapten betr., durch Haptene bedingt, Hapten-.
hap·te·pho·bia [ˌhæptə'foʊbɪə] *n* → haphephobia.
hap·tic ['hæptɪk] *adj* Tastsinn betr., haptisch, taktil.
haptic hallucination *psychia.* haptische/taktile Halluzination *f*.
hap·tics ['hæptɪks] *pl physiol.* Lehre *f* vom Tastsinn, Haptik *f*.
hap·to·glo·bin [ˌhæptoʊ'ɡloʊbɪn] *n* Haptoglobin *nt*.
hap·tom·e·ter [hæp'tɑmɪtər] *n physiol.* Haptometer *nt*.
Harada [hə'rædə]: **H.'s disease/syndrome** Harada-Syndrom *nt*.
ha·rar·a [hə'reərə] *n derm.* Urticaria multiformis endemica.
hard [hɑːrd] *adj* 1. hart; fest. 2. schwierig, schwer. 3. widerstandsfähig, zäh. 4. hart, gefühllos; schroff. 5. (*Getränk*) sauer, herb; (*Droge*) hart; (*Laut*) stimmlos; (*Wasser*) hart.
   h. of hearing schwerhörig.
hard-bodied ticks → hard ticks.
hard cancer szirrhöses Karzinom *nt*, Faserkrebs *m*, Szirrhus *m*, Skirrhus *m*, Ca. scirrhosum.
hard cataract harte Katarakt *f*, Cataracta dura.
hard cerumen *HNO* angetrockneter/verkeilter Zeruminalpfropf *m*.
hard chancre harter Schanker *m*, Hunter-Schanker *m*, syphilitischer Primäraffekt *m*, Ulcus durum.
hard·en ['hɑːrdn] **I** *vt* 1. härten, hart *od.* härter machen. 2. *fig.* ab-, verhärten, abstumpfen (*to* gegen). **II** *vi* 3. erhärten, hart werden. 4. *fig.* s. ab- *od.* verhärten, abstumpfen (*to* gegen).
hard·en·er ['hɑːrdnər] *n* Härtemittel *nt*, Härter *m*.
hard·en·ing ['hɑːrdnɪŋ] *n* Härten *nt*, (Ver-, Ab-)Härtung *f*.
   h. of the arteries *inf.* Arterienverkalkung *f*, Arteriosklerose *f*, -sclerosis *f*.
Harden-Young ['hɑːrdn jʌŋ]: **H.-Y. ester** Harden-Young-Ester *m*, Fructose-1,6-diphosphat *nt abbr.* F-1,6-P.
hard fibroma hartes Fibrom *nt*, Fibroma durum.
hard·ness ['hɑːrdnɪs] *n* 1. Härte *f*, Festigkeit *f*. 2. (Wasser-)Härte *f*. 3. Schwere *f*, Schwierigkeit *f*. 4. Widerstandsfähigkeit *f*. 5. *fig.* Härte *f*, Schroffheit *f*.
hardness number Härte *f*.
hard palate harter Gaumen *m*, Palatum durum.
   bony h. knöcherner Gaumen, Palatum osseum.
hard pulse harter/gespannter Puls *m*, Pulsus durus.

hard rays harte/energiereiche Röntgenstrahlung *f*.
hard sore → hard chancre.
hard stuff *inf.* Hard stuff, harte Droge(n *pl*) *f*.
hard ticks *micro.* Schild-, Haftzecken *pl*, Holzböcke *pl*, Ixodidae *pl*.
hard ulcer → hard chancre.
hard water hartes Wasser *nt*.
hard work Schwerarbeit *f*.
hard x-rays → hard rays.
Hardy-Weinberg ['hɑːrdɪ 'waɪnbɜrɡ]: **H.-W. equilibrium/law/rule** Hardy-Weinberg-Gesetz *nt*.
Hare [heər]: **H.'s syndrome** Pancoast-Syndrom *nt*.
hare·lip ['heərlɪp] *n* Hasenscharte *f*, Lippenspalte *f*, Cheiloschisis *f*.
har·le·quin color change syndrome ['hɑːrləkwɪn, -kɪn] → harlequin reaction.
harlequin fetus 1. *ped.*, *derm.* Harlekinfetus *m*, Ichthyosis congenita (gravis/universalis), Keratosis diffusa maligna, Hyperkeratosis universalis congenita. 2. → harlequin reaction.
harlequin reaction *ped.* Harlekinfetus *m*, Harlekin-Farbwechsel *m*.
harlequin sign → harlequin reaction.
Harley ['hɑːrlɪ]: **H.'s disease** intermittierende Hämoglobinurie *f*, Harley-Krankheit *f*.
har·mo·ni·a [hɑːr'moʊnɪə] *n anat.* falsche Naht *f*, Harmonia *f*, Sutura plana.
har·mon·ic [hɑːr'mɑnɪk] *n phys.* Harmonische *f*, Oberlaut *m*, -ton *m*, Oberwelle *f*.
harmonic suture → harmonia.
har·mo·ni·za·tion [ˌhɑːrmənaɪ'zeɪʃn] *n* Harmonisierung *f*, Angleichung *f*.
har·mo·nize [hɑːr'mənaɪz] **I** *vt* in Einklang bringen, angleichen, harmonisieren, (*with* an). **II** *vi* in Einklang stehen, übereinstimmen, harmonieren (*with* mit).
har·ness ['hɑːrnɪs] *n* 1. *ped.* Laufgeschirr *nt*. 2. *ortho.* Gurt *m*, Zügel *m*, Bandage *f*. 3. *inf.* Uniform *f*, Tracht *f*.
har·poon [hɑːr'puːn] *n chir.* Harpune *f*.
Harrington ['hærɪŋtən]: **H. instrumentation** → H. operation.
H. operation Skoliosekorrektur *f* nach Harrington.
H. rod Harrington-Stab *m*.
H. technique → H. operation.
Harris ['hærɪs]: **H.'** lines *radiol.* Harris-Linien *pl*.
H.' migrainous neuralgia Bing-Horton-Syndrom *nt*, -Neuralgie *f*, Horton-Syndrom *nt*, -Neuralgie *f*, Erythroprosopschmerz *m*, -kephalgie *f*, Erythroprosopalgie *f*, Cephalaea histaminica, cluster headache (*nt*).
H.'s syndrome Harris-Syndrom *nt*.
H. tube Harris-Sonde *f*.
Harrison ['hærɪsən]: **H.'s curve** Harrison-Furche *f*.
H.'s groove → H.'s curve.
H. spot test Harrison-Test *m*.
H.'s sulcus → H.'s curve.
harsh respiration [hɑːrʃ] bronchovesikuläres/vesikobronchiales Atmen/Atmungsgeräusch *nt*.
Hartmann ['hɑːrtmən]: **H.'s colostomy** → H.'s operation.
H.'s critical point Sudeck-Punkt *m*.
H.'s operation *chir.* Hartmann-Operation *f*.
H.'s point → H.'s critical point.
H.'s pouch Hartmann-Sack *m*.
H.'s procedure → H.'s operation.
H.'s speculum *HNO* Ohrtrichter *m* nach Hartmann.
Hart·ma·nel·la [ˌhɑːrtmə'nelə] *n micro.* Hartmanella *f*.

hart·ma·nel·li·a·sis [ˌhɑːrtmənə'laɪəsɪs] *f* Hartmanellainfektion *f*, Hartmanellose *f*, Hartmanelliasis *f*.
Hartnup ['hɑːrtnəp]: **H. disease/syndrome** Hartnup-Krankheit *f*, -Syndrom *nt*.
har·vest ['hɑːrvɪst] *chir.* (*Transplantat*) **I** *n* Ernte *f*, Entnahme *f*. **II** *vt* entnehmen.
harvest bug *micro.* Chigger *m*, Trombicula-Larve *f*.
har·ves·ter's lung ['hɑːrvəstər] Farmerlunge *f*, Drescherkrankheit *f*, Dreschfieber *nt*.
harvest mite → harvest bug.
Hasami [hə'sɑːmɪ]: **H. fever** Hasami-Fieber *nt*.
has·a·mi·ya·mi [ˌhæsəmɪ'jæmɪ] *n* Sakushu-, Akiyami-, Hasamiyami-Fieber *nt*.
hash·eesh ['hɑːʃiːʃ, hɑː'ʃiːʃ] *n* → hashish.
Hashimoto [hæʃɪ'moʊtoʊ]: **H. disease/struma/thyroiditis** Hashimoto-Thyreoiditis *f*, Struma lymphomatosa.
hash·ish ['hæʃiːʃ, -ɪʃ, hæ'ʃiːʃ] *n* Haschisch *nt*.
Hasner ['hæsnər]: **H.'s fold/valve** Hasner'-Klappe *f*, Plica lacrimalis.
Hassall ['hæsəl]: **H.'s bodies/corpuscles** Hassall'-Körperchen *pl*.
hasty eating ['heɪstɪ] hastiges/überstürztes Essen *nt*, Tachyphagie *f*.
Hataan [hə'tɑːn]: **H. virus** *micro.* Ha(n)taan-Virus *nt*.
Hatchcock ['hætʃkɑk]: **H.'s sign** *HNO* Hatchcock-Zeichen *nt*.
Hatch-Slack [hætʃ slæk]: **H.-S. cycle/pathway** Hatch-Slack-Zyklus *m*, C_4-Zyklus *m*.
HAT medium [hypoxanthine, aminopterin, thymidine] HAT-Medium *nt*.
Haudek ['hɔːdek; 'haʊ-]: **H.'s niche/sign** *radiol.* Haudek-Nische *f*.
haus·tel·lum [hɔː'stɛləm] *n*, *pl* -la [-lə] *micro.* Saugrüssel *m*.
haus·to·ri·um [hɔː'stɔːrɪəm] *n*, *pl* -ri·a [-rɪə] *micro.* Saugfortsatz *m*, Saugwarze *f*, Haustorium *nt*.
haus·tral ['hɔːstrəl] *adj* Haustren *od.* Haustrierung betr., haustrenartig.
haus·trat·ed ['hɔːstreɪtɪd] *adj* → haustral.
haus·tra·tion [hɔː'streɪʃn] *n* 1. Haustrenbildung *f*, Haustrierung *f*. 2. Haustrum *nt*.
haus·trum ['hɔːstrəm] *n*, *pl* -tra [-trə] *anat.* segmentale Aussackung *f*, Haustrum *nt*.
   h.a of colon Dickdarm-, Kolonhaustren *pl*, Haustra/Sacculations coli.
haut mal [oʊ; oʊ mɑl] → haut mal epilepsy.
haut mal epilepsy Grand-mal-(Epilepsie *f*) *nt abbr.* GM.
HAV *abbr.* → hepatitis A virus.
Haverhill ['heɪvərhɪl]: **H. fever** Rattenbißkrankheit II *f*, Haverhill-Fieber *nt*, atypisches Rattenbißfieber *nt*, Haverhill-Fieber *nt*, Bakterien-Rattenbißfieber *nt*, Streptobazillen-Rattenbißfieber *nt*, Erythema arthriticum epidemicum.
Ha·ver·hil·lia multiformis [heɪvər'hɪlɪə] *micro.* Haverhillia multiformis, Streptobacillus moniliformis.
ha·ver·sian [hə'vɜrʒn, heɪ-]: **h. canal** Havers'-Kanal *m*, Canalis nutriens.
h. glands Synovialzotten *pl*, Villi synoviales.
h. lamella Havers'-(Knochen-)Lamelle *f*.
h. space → h. canal.
h. system Havers'-System *nt*, Havers'-Ringlamellensystem *nt*.
h. vessel Zentralgefäß *nt* des Osteons, Havers'-Gefäß *nt*.
HA-1 virus → hemadsorption type 1 virus.
HA-2 virus → hemadsorption type 2 virus.

Haworth

Haworth ['hɑwərθ, 'hɔ-]: **H. formula** Haworth-Projektionsformel *f*.
H. projection Haworth-Projektion *f*.
Hay [heɪ]: **H.'s test** Hay-Schwefelblumenprobe *f*.
hay bacillus [heɪ] Heubazillus, Bacillus subtilis.
Hayem [ɛ'jem]: **H.'s solution** Hayem'-Lösung *f*.
Hayem-Widal [vi'dal]: **H.-W. syndrome** Widal-Abrami-Anämie *f*, -Ikterus *m*, Widal-Anämie *f*, -Ikterus *m*.
hay fever Heufieber *nt*, -schnupfen *m*. **nonseasonal/perennial h.** perenniale (allergische) Rhinitis.
Haygarth ['heɪgɑːrθ]: **H.'s nodes/nodosities** Haygarth-Knoten *pl*.
HB *abbr*. → hepatitis B.
Hb *abbr*. → hemoglobin.
HbA *abbr*. → hemoglobin A.
HbA$_{1c}$ *abbr*. → hemoglobin A$_{1c}$.
HbA$_2$ *abbr*. → hemoglobin A$_2$.
H band H-Bande *f*, H-Streifen *m*, H-Zone *f*, helle Zone *f*, Hensen'-Zone *f*.
HBB *abbr*. → 2-(α-hydroxybenzyl)-benzimidazole.
HbC *abbr*. → hemoglobin C.
HB$_c$Ag *abbr*. → hepatitis B core antigen
HbCN *abbr*. → cyanmethemoglobin.
HbD *abbr*. → hemoglobin D.
HBDH *abbr*. → α-hydroxybutyrate dehydrogenase.
HBDNAP *abbr*. → hepatitis B DNA polymerase.
HBE *abbr*. → His bundle electrogram.
HbE *abbr*. → hemoglobin E.
HB$_e$Ag *abbr*. → hepatitis B e antigen.
HbF *abbr*. → hemoglobin F.
HbH *abbr*. → hemoglobin H.
HbI *abbr*. → hemoglobin I.
HBIG *abbr*. → hepatitis B immune globulin.
HBLV *abbr*. → human B-lymphotropic virus.
HbM *abbr*. → hemoglobin M.
HbO$_2$ *abbr*. → oxyhemoglobin.
H$_2$ breath test H$_2$-Atemtest *m*, Wasserstoffatemtest *m*.
HbS *abbr*. → hemoglobin S.
HB$_s$Ag *abbr*. → hepatitis B surface antigen.
HB$_s$ antigen → hepatitis B surface antigen.
HB surface antigen → hepatitis B surface antigen.
HBV *abbr*. → hepatitis B virus.
HB vaccine Hepatitis B-Vakzine *f*.
HBV carrier HBV-Träger *m*.
h$_c$ *abbr*. → convective heat transfer coefficient.
HCG *abbr*. → human chorionic gonadotropin.
hCG *abbr*. → human chorionic gonadotropin.
H chain *biochem*. H-Kette *f*, schwere Kette *f*.
HCl *abbr*. → hydrogen chloride.
HCM *abbr*. → hypertrophic cardiomyopathy.
HCN *abbr*. → hydrogen cyanide.
H colony *micro*. H-Form *f*, Hauchform *f*.
HCT *abbr*. → hematocrit 1.
HCV *abbr*. → human coronavirus.
HDAg *abbr*. → hepatitis delta antigen.
HDCC *abbr*. → human diploid cell culture.
HDCV *abbr*. → human diploid cell vaccine.
H disease → Hartnup disease.
H disk → H band.
HDL *abbr*. → high-density lipoprotein.
HDN *abbr*. → hemolytic disease of the newborn.

HDV *abbr*. → hepatitis delta virus.
HE *abbr*. → hematoxylin-eosin.
He *abbr*. → helium.
h$_e$ *abbr*. → evaporation heat transfer coefficient.
Head [hed]: **H.'s areas/lines/zones** Head'-Zonen *pl*.
head [hed] **I** *n* **1.** Kopf *m*, Haupt *nt*. **2.** *anat*. Kopf *m*, Caput *m*. **3.** Kopf *m*, vorderes *od*. oberes Ende *nt*, Spitze *f*, Vorderteil *nt*. **4.** Kopf *m*, Verstand *m*. **5.** Höhepunkt *m*, Krise *f*. **6.** Leiter(in *f*) *m*, Chef(in *f*) *m*, Direktor(in *f*) *m*. **7.** (*Abszeß*) Durchbruchstelle *f*. **to come to a ~** eitern, durch-, aufbrechen. **8.** *phys*. (Dampf-, Wasser-, Gas-)Druck *m*. **II** *adj* führend, oberste(r, s), vorderste(r, s), erste(r, s), Kopf-, Spitzen-, Vorder-.
h. of biceps brachii muscle Bizepskopf, Caput m. bicipitis brachii.
h. of caudate nucleus Caudatuskopf, Kopf des Nc. caudatus, Caput nc. caudati.
h. of condyloid process of mandible → h. of mandible.
h. of dorsal horn of spinal cord Kopf des Hinterhorns, Caput cornus dorsalis/posterioris medullae spinalis.
h. of epididymis Nebenhodenkopf, Caput epididymidis.
h. of femur Femur-, Oberschenkelkopf, Caput femoris.
h. of fibula Wadenbein-, Fibulaköpfchen *nt*, Caput fibulae/fibulare.
h. of humerus Humerus-, Oberarmkopf, Caput humeri/humerale.
h. of malleus Hammerkopf, Caput mallei.
h. of mandible Gelenkkopf des Unterkiefers, Caput mandibulae.
h. of metacarpal bone Metakarpalköpfchen *nt*, Caput metacarpale.
h. of metatarsal bone Metatarsalköpfchen *nt*, Caput metatarsale.
h. of muscle Muskelkopf, Caput musculi.
h. of pancreas Pankreaskopf, Caput pancreatis.
h. of penis Eichel *f*, Glans penis.
h. of phalanx Caput/Trochlea phalangis.
h. of posterior horn of spinal cord → h. of dorsal horn of spinal cord.
h. of radius Speichen-, Radiuskopf, Caput radii/radiale.
h. of rib Rippenköpfchen *nt*, Caput costae.
h. of spermatozoon Spermienkopf.
h. of spleen oberer Milzpol *m*, Extremitas posterior (lienis/splenis).
h. of stapes Steigbügelkopf, Caput stapedis.
h. of talus Taluskopf, Caput tali/talare.
h. of testis oberer Hodenpol *m*, Extremitas superior testis.
h. of triceps brachii muscle Trizepskopf, Caput m. tricipitis brachii.
h. of ulna Ellen-, Unlaköpfchen *nt*, Caput ulnae.
head·ache ['hedeɪk] *n* Kopfschmerz(en *pl*) *m*, Kopfweh *nt*, Kephalgie *f*, Kephalalgie *f*, Kephal(a)ea *f*, Cephalgia *f*, Cephalalgia *f*, Cephal(a)ea *f*, Cephalodynie *f*, Zephalgie *f*, Zephalalgie *f*. **to have a ~** Kopfschmerzen haben.
head·ach·y ['hedeɪkɪ] *adj* Kopfschmerzen verursachend, an Kopfschmerzen leidend, Kopfschmerz-.
head·band ['hedbænd] *n* Stirn-, Kopfband *nt*.
head bend → head fold.
head cap (*Spermium*) Kopfkappe *f*, Akrosom *nt*.
head fold *embryo*. Kopffalte *f*.
head·gut ['hedgʌt] *n embryo*., *bio*. Kopfdarm *m*.

head injury 1. Kopfverletzung *f*, -trauma *nt*. **2.** Schädelverletzung *f*, -trauma *nt*. **open h.** offene Schädelverletzung, offenes Schädeltrauma.
head kidney Vorniere *f*, Pronephros *m*.
head·less ['hedlɪs] *adj* kopflos, ohne Kopf.
head louse Kopflaus *f*, Pediculus humanus capitis.
head mirror Stirnspiegel *m*.
head·most ['hedməʊst] *adj* vorderste(r, s).
head·phone ['hedfəʊn] *n* Kopfhörer *m*.
head presentation *gyn*. Kopf-, Schädellage *f*.
head process *embryo*. Chordafortsatz *m*.
head regions *anat*. Kopfregionen *pl*, Regiones capitis.
head·rest ['hedrest] *n* Kopfstütze *f*, -lehne *f*.
head restraint → head rest.
head shaking nystagmus Kopfschüttelnystagmus *m*.
head trauma → head injury.
Heaf [hiːf]: **H. test** Heaf-Test *m*.
HE agar → Hektoen enteric agar.
heal [hiːl] **I** *vt* heilen (*sb. of sth.* jdn. von einer Krankheit), gesund machen. **II** *vi* (ver-, zu-)heilen; (aus-)heilen; gesund werden, genesen.
heal up/over → heal II.
healed tuberculosis [hiːld] inaktive/vernarbte/verheilte Tuberkulose *f*.
healed ulcer verheiltes Ulkus *nt*.
healed yellow atrophy (of liver) postnekrotische Leberzirrhose *f*.
heal·er ['hiːlər] *n* Heiler(in *f*) *m*; Heilmittel *nt*.
heal·ing ['hiːlɪŋ] **I** *n* **1.** Heilung *f*, (Aus-, Zu-, Ver-)Heilen *nt*. **2.** Gesundung *f*, Genesung *f*. **II** *adj* heilend, heilsam, Heil-, Heilungs-.
healing by first intention primäre Wundheilung *f*, Primärheilung *f*, Heilung *f* per primam intentionem, p.p.-Heilung *f*.
healing by granulation → healing by second intention.
healing by second intention sekundäre Wundheilung *f*, Sekundärheilung *f*, Heilung *f* per secundam intentionem, p.s.-Heilung *f*.
health [helθ] *n* **1.** Gesundheit *f*. **2.** Gesundheitszustand *m*. **in good ~** gesund. **in poor ~** kränklich.
health care medizinische Versorgung *f*, Gesundheitsfürsorge *f*.
health center Ärzte-, Gesundheitszentrum *nt*.
health certificate ärztliches Attest *nt*, Gesundheitszeugnis *f*.
health education Gesundheitserziehung *f*.
health food Reformkost *f*; Biokost *f*.
health food store Reformhaus *nt*; Bioladen *m*.
health·ful ['helθfʊl] *adj* → healthy.
health hazard Gesundheitsrisiko *nt*.
health·i·ness ['helθɪnɪs] *n* Gesundheit *f*.
health insurance Krankenversicherung *f*.
health resort Kurort *m*.
health spa Kurbad *nt*, Heilbad *nt*.
health worker Gesundheitsfürsorger(in *f*) *m*.
health·y ['helθɪ] *adj* gesund; gesundheitsfördernd, bekömmlich, heilsam.
healthy coloring gesunde Hautfarbe *f*.
heap [hiːp] **I** *n* Haufen *m*. **II** *vt* häufen. **a ~ed spoonful** ein gehäufter Löffel (voll).
hear [hɪər] (**heard**; **heard**) *vt*, *vi* hören.
hear·a·ble ['hɪərəbl] *adj* hörbar.
hear·ing ['hɪərɪŋ] *n* **1.** Gehör(sinn *m*) *nt*, Hörvermögen *f*. **2.** Hören *nt*. **within ~/out of ~** in Hörweite/außer Hörweite.
h. of pure tones Reintongehör.
hearing aid Hörgerät *nt*, -apparat *m*, -hilfe *f*.

hearing center Hörzentrum *nt*.
hearing difficulty → hearing loss.
hearing disorders Hörstörungen *pl*.
hearing distance Hörweite *f*.
hearing education Hörerziehung *f*.
hearing impairment Einschränkung *f* des Hörvermögens.
hearing loss *abbr*. **HL** (Ge-)Hörverlust *m*, Hörstörung *f*, Schwerhörigkeit *f*.
 acoustic trauma h. → noise-induced h.
 acquired h. erworbene Schwerhörigkeit.
 bilateral h. beidseitige Schwerhörigkeit.
 central h. zentrale Hörstörung/Schwerhörigkeit.
 cochleoneural h. kochleoneurale Schwerhörigkeit.
 conduction/conductive h. Schalleitungsstörung, -schwerhörigkeit, Mittelohrschwerhörigkeit, -taubheit *f*.
 congenital h. kongenitale Schwerhörigkeit.
 fluctuation h. fluktuierende Schwerhörigkeit.
 functional h. psychogene Schwerhörigkeit/Taubheit *f*.
 high-frequency h. Hörverlust für hohe Frequenzen.
 hysterical h. → functional h.
 industrial h. → noise-induced h.
 inner ear h. Innenohrtaubheit *f*.
 labyrinthine h. → inner ear h.
 low-tone h. Gehörverlust für niedrige Frequenzen.
 middle ear h. → conduction h.
 moderate h. mittelgradiger Hörverlust.
 nerve/neural h. → retrocochlear h.
 noise-induced h. chronische Lärmschwerhörigkeit.
 occupational h. → noise-induced h.
 pancochlear h. pankochleärer Gehörverlust, pankochleäre Taubheit *f*.
 perceptive h. → sensorineural h.
 psychic/psychogenic h. → functional h.
 retrocochlear h. retrokochleäre Schwerhörigkeit.
 sensorineural h. Schallempfindungsstörung, Schallempfindungsschwerhörigkeit *f*.
 sensory h. → sensorineural h.
 severe h. hochgradige Schwerhörigkeit.
 slight h. geringgradiger Gehörverlust.
 h. for speech Hörverlust für Sprache.
 h. for speech comprehension Hörverlust für Sprachverständnis.
 transmission h. → conduction h.
 unilateral h. einseitige Schwerhörigkeit.
hearing range Hörbereich *m*, -dynamik *f*.
hearing test Hörprüfung *f*.
hearing threshold Hörschwelle *f*.
hearing training Hörtraining *nt*.
heart [hɑːrt] *n* **1.** Herz *nt*; *anat*. Cor *nt*, Cardia *f*. **2.** *fig*. Herz *nt*, Seele *f*. **3.** das Innere, Kern *m*, Mitte *f*; das Wesentliche.
heart arrest Herzstillstand *m*.
heart atrophy Herzatrophie *f*.
heart attack Herzanfall *m*, -attacke *f*; Herzinfarkt *m*.
heart-beat ['hɑːrtbiːt] *n* Puls-, Herzschlag *m*, -aktion *f*, -zyklus *m*.
heart block *card*. Herzblock *m*, kardialer Block *m*.
 aborization h. Aborisations-, Ast-, Verzweigungsblock.
 atrioventricular h. atrioventrikulärer Block, AV-Block.
 bundle-branch h. *abbr*. **BBB** Schenkelblock.
 complete h. → third degree h.
 first degree h. AV-Block I. Grades.
 incomplete h. → second degree h.
 interventricular h. → bundle-branch h.
 intraventricular h. intraventrikulärer Block.
 left bundle-branch h. *abbr*. **LBBB** Linksschenkelblock *abbr*. LSB.
 Mobitz h. Mobitz-Typ *m*, -Block, AV-Block II. Grades Typ II.
 partial h. → second degree h.
 right bundle-branch h. *abbr*. **RBBB** Rechtsschenkelblock *abbr*. RSB.
 second degree h. partieller AV-Block, AV-Block II. Grades.
 sinoatrial/sinoauricular/sinus h. sinuatrialer/sinuaurikulärer Block, SA-Block.
 third degree h. kompletter/totaler AV-Block, AV-Block III. Grades.
 Wenckebach h. Wenckebach-Periode *f*, AV-Block II. Grades Typ I.
heart bulge *embryo*. Herzvorwölbung *f*.
heart-burn ['hɑːrtbɜrn] *n* Sodbrennen *nt*, Pyrosis *f*.
heart defect Herzfehler *m*, (Herz-)Vitium *nt*, Vitium cordis.
 congenital h. angeborener/kongenitaler Herzfehler.
 organic h. → heart defect.
heart disease Herzerkrankung *f*, -krankheit *f*, -leiden *nt*.
 coronary h. *abbr*. **CHD** koronare Herzkrankheit *abbr*. KHK, koronare Herzerkrankung *abbr*. KHE, stenosierende Koronarklerose *f*, degenerative Koronarerkrankung.
 thyrotoxic h. Thyreokardiopathie *f*.
 valvular h. Herzklappenerkrankung.
heart-disease cell → heart-failure cell.
heart failure *abbr*. **HF** Herzinsuffizienz *f*, -versagen *nt*, Myokardinsuffizienz *f*, Herzmuskelschwäche *f*, Insufficientia cordis.
 acute h. akute Herzinsuffizienz.
 backward h. Rückwärtsversagen, backward failure (*nt*).
 chronic h. chronische Herzinsuffizienz.
 congestive h. *abbr*. **CHF** dekompensierte Herzinsuffizienz.
 forward h. Vorwärtsversagen, forward failure (*nt*).
 high-output h. high-output failure (*nt*).
 left-sided h. Links(herz)insuffizienz, Linksversagen.
 left-ventricular h. → left-sided h.
 low-output h. low-output failure (*nt*).
 right-sided h. Rechts(herz)insuffizienz.
 right-ventricular h. → right-sided h.
heart-failure cell Herzfehlerzelle *f*.
heart-hand syndrome Holt-Oram-Syndrom *nt*.
heart hypertrophy Herz(muskel)hypertrophie *f*.
 left h. Linksherzhypertrophie, linksventrikuläre Hypertrophie.
 right h. Rechtsherzhypertrophie, rechtsventrikuläre Hypertrophie.
heart insufficiency → heart failure.
heart-lesion cell → heart-failure cell.
heart-like ['hɑːrtlaɪk] *adj* herzähnlich, -förmig.
heart loop *embryo*. Herzschleife *f*.
heart-lung machine Herz-Lungen-Maschine *f*.
heart-lung transplantation Herz-Lungen-Transplantation *f*.
heart malformation Herzmißbildung *f*, -fehlentwicklung *f*, -malformation *f*.
heart murmur *card*. Herzgeräusch *nt*.
heart rate Herzfrequenz *f*.
heart reflex Abrams'-Herzreflex *m*.
heart sac Herzbeutel *m*, Perikard *nt*, Pericardium *nt*.
heart shadow *radiol*. Herzschatten *m*.
heart-shaped *adj* herzförmig.
heart-shaped pelvis Kartenherzbecken *nt*.
heart-shaped uterus herzförmiger Uterus *m*, Uterus cordiformis.
heart sound Herzton *m*.
 abnormal h. Herzgeräusch *nt*.
 first h. erster Herzton, I. Herzton.
 fourth h. vierter Herzton, IV. Herzton, Vorhofton.
 second h. zweiter Herzton, II. Herzton.
 third h. dritter Herzton, III. Herzton.
heart stroke **1.** Herzschlag *m*. **2.** Herzbräune *f*, Stenokardie *f*, Angina pectoris.
heart sugar Inosit *nt*, Inositol *nt*.
heart surgery Herzchirurgie *f*.
 open h. offene Herzchirurgie, Chirurgie am offenen Herzen.
heart throb Herzschlag *m*.
heart tones Herztöne *pl*.
heart transplant Herztransplantat *nt*.
heart transplantation Herztransplantation *f*, -verpflanzung *f*.
 heterotopic h. heterotope Herztransplantation.
 orthotopic h. orthotope Herztransplantation.
heart tube *embryo*. Herzschlauch *m*.
heart valve Herzklappe *f*.
 prosthetic h. künstliche Herzklappe, Herzklappenersatz *m*, -prothese *f*.
heart-worm ['hɑːrtwɜrm] *n micro*. Dirofilaria immitis.
heat [hiːt] **I** *n* **1.** Hitze *f*, (große) Wärme *f*; (*Körper*) Erhitztheit *f*. **2.** *zoo*. Brunst *f*, Brunft *f*; Läufigkeit *f*. **3.** *fig*. Hitze *f*, Erregtheit *f*, Leidenschaft(lichkeit *f*) *f*.) **II** *vt* erwärmen, erhitzen, heiß *od*. warm machen. **III** *vi* s. erwärmen, s. erhitzen, heiß *od*. warm werden.
heat up I *vt* → heat II. **II** *vi* → heat III.
 h. of combustion *phys*. Verbrennungswärme.
 h. of evaporation *phys*. Verdampfungswärme.
 h. of fusion *phys*. Fusionswärme.
 h. of reaction *phys*. Reaktionswärme.
 h. of solution *phys*. Lösungswärme.
 h. of sublimation *phys*. Sublimierungswärme.
 h. of vaporization → h. of evaporation.
heat-a-ble ['hiːtəbl] *adj* erhitzbar; heizbar.
heat adaptation Hitzeadaptation *f*.
heat apoplexy Hitzschlag *m*, Thermoplegie *f*.
heat balance Wärmehaushalt *m*, -bilanz *f*.
heat blood agar Kochblutagar *m/nt*, Schokoladenagar *m/nt*.
heat capacity *abbr*. **C** Wärmekapazität *f*.
 specific h. *abbr*. **c** spezifische Wärmekapazität.
heat cataract *ophthal*. Feuer-, Glasbläserstar *m*, Infrarotkatarakt *f*, Cataracta calorica.
heat collapse → heat exhaustion.
heat conduction Wärmeleitung *f*, Konduktion *f*.
heat conductivity Wärmeleitfähigkeit *f*.
heat content *abbr*. **H** Enthalpie *f* *abbr*. H.
heat cramp Hitzekrampf *m*, -tetanie *f*.
heat dissipation Wärmeabgabe *f*.
heat-ed ['hiːtɪd] *adj* **1.** *fig*. erregt (*with* von). **2.** ge-, beheizt; heiß geworden.
heat-er ['hiːtər] *n* Heizgerät *nt*, -körper *m*.
heat exhaustion Hitzeerschöpfung *f*, -kollaps *m*.
heat hyperpyrexia → heatstroke.
heat-ing ['hiːtɪŋ] **I** *n* **1.** Heizung *f*. **2.** (Be-)Heizen *nt*, Erwärmen *nt*, Erhitzen *nt*. **II** *adj* heizend, erwärmend, Heiz-.
heating pad Heizkissen *nt*.
heat-labile *adj* hitzelabil.
heat lamp Infrarotlicht *nt*, -lampe *f*, -strahler *m*.
heat loss Wärmeabgabe *f*, -verlust *m*.
 dry h. trockene Wärmeabgabe.

heat production

evaporative h. evaporative Wärmeabgabe, Wärmeabgabe durch Verdampfung.
heat production Wärmebildung f, -produktion f.
heat-proof ['hi:tpru:f] adj hitze-, wärmebeständig, thermostabil.
heat prostration → heat exhaustion.
heat radiation Wärmestrahlung f.
heat rash derm. Roter Hund m, tropische Flechte f, Miliaria rubra.
heat rays Infrarotstrahlen pl.
heat-regulatory center thermoregulatorisches Zentrum nt.
heat resistance Hitzebeständigkeit f.
heat-resistant adj → heatproof.
heat-resisting adj → heatproof.
heat sensation Wärme-, Hitzeempfindung f.
heat-sensitive adj wärme-, hitzeempfindlich.
heat shock Hitzeschock m.
heat-shock proteins Hitzeschockproteine pl.
heat-shock response Hitzeschockreaktion f.
heat spots Schweißfrieseln pl, -bläschen pl, Hitzepickel pl, -blattern pl, Schwitzbläschen pl, Miliaria pl, Dermatitis hidrotica.
heat-stable adj wärme-, hitzebeständig, thermostabil.
heat sterilization Hitzesterilisation f. **moist h.** Dampfsterilisation.
heat stress Wärme-, Hitzebelastung f.
heat stroke → heatstroke.
heat-stroke ['hi:tstrəʊk] n Hitzschlag m, Thermoplegie f.
heat syncope Hitzekollaps m.
heat transfer phys. Wärmeübertragung f, -transfer m.
heat-treat vt wärmebehandeln.
heat treatment Wärmebehandlung f.
heat unit phys. Wärmeeinheit f.
heat urticaria Wärmeurtikaria f, Urticaria e calore.
heave [hi:v] (v heaved; heaved) I n (Hoch-)Heben nt. II vt 1. (hoch-)heben, (-)stemmen, (-)hieven. 2. schwer atmen, (Seufzer) ausstoßen. 3. inf. erbrechen. III vi 4. s. heben u. senken, wogen. 5. keuchen. 6. inf. s. übergeben.
heav-i-ness ['hevɪnɪs] n 1. Schwere f; Stärke f. 2. Schwerfälligkeit f. 3. Druck m, Last f. 4. Schläfrigkeit f.
heav-y ['hevɪ] adj 1. schwer. 2. groß, beträchtlich; (Schlaf) tief; (Raucher, Trinker) stark, übermäßig; (Essen) schwer, schwerverdaulich; (Alkohol) stark. 3. bedrückt, niedergeschlagen; ernst; (be-)drückend. 4. plump, schwerfällig. 5. schläfrig, benommen (with von). 6. folgenschwer. **of ~ consequences** mit weitreichenden Folgen.
heavy chain biochem. schwere Kette f, H-Kette f.
heavy-chain disease Franklin-Syndrom nt, Schwerekettenkrankheit f, H-Krankheit f.
heavy current Starkstrom m.
heavy-footed adj mit schwerem Gang.
heavy-handed adj unbeholfen, plump.
heavy-hearted adj niedergeschlagen.
heavy hydrogen abbr. ²H schwerer Wasserstoff m, Deuterium nt abbr. D, ²H.
heavy meromyosin schweres Meromyosin nt, H-Meromyosin nt.
heavy metal Schwermetall nt.
heavy metal poisoning Schwermetallvergiftung f.
heavy metal stain histol. Schwermetallfärbung f.

heavy water schweres Wasser nt, Deuteriumoxid nt abbr. D₂O.
heavy work Schwerarbeit f.
he·be·phre·nia [,hi:bə'fri:nɪə, ,heb-] n psychia. Hebephrenie f, hebephrene Schizophrenie f.
he·be·phren·ic [,-'frenɪk, 'fri:n-] I n Patient(in f) m mit Hebephrenie. II adj hebephren betr., hepephren.
hebephrenic dementia hebephrene Demenz f.
hebephrenic schizophrenia → hebephrenia.
Heberden ['hebərdən]: **H.'s angina** → H.'s asthma.
H.'s asthma Herzbräune f, Stenokardie f, Angina pectoris.
H.'s disease 1. → H.'s rheumatism. **2.** → H.'s asthma.
H.'s nodes Heberden-Knoten pl.
H.'s nodosities → H.'s nodes.
H.'s rheumatism Heberden'-Polyarthrose f.
H.'s signs → H.'s nodes.
he·bet·ic [hɪ'betɪk] adj Pubertät betr., pubertär, Pubertäts-.
heb·e·tude ['hebɪt(j)u:d] n (Sinne) Stumpfheit f, Abstumpfung f, Hebetudo f.
Hebra ['hi:brə]: **H.'s disease/prurigo** Hebra'-Krankheit f, Kokardenerythem nt, Erythema (exsudativum) multiforme, Hidroa vesiculosa.
hec·a·ter·o·mer·ic [,hekətərə'merɪk] adj → hecatomeral.
hec·a·tom·er·al [,-'tɒmərəl] adj hekatomer(al).
hec·a·to·mer·ic [,-tə'merɪk] adj → hecatomeral.
Hecht [hekt; heçt]: **H. phenomenon** Rumpel-Leede-Phänomen nt.
H.'s pneumonia Masernpneumonie f, Riesenzellpneumonie f.
heck·le cell ['hekl] (Haut) Stachelzelle f.
hect- pref. → hecto-.
hec·tic ['hektɪk] adj anhaltend unruhig, auszehrend, schwindsüchtig, hektisch.
hectic fever Febris hectica.
hectic flush hektische Röte f.
hecto- pref. abbr. **h** hekt(o)-, Hekt(o)- abbr. **h**.
hec·to·gram ['hektəgræm] n abbr. **hg** Hektogramm nt abbr. hg.
hec·to·li·ter ['-lɪtər] n abbr. **hl** Hektoliter m/nt abbr. hl.
hec·to·me·ter ['-mɪtər] n abbr. **hm** Hektometer m/nt abbr. hm.
HECV abbr. → human enteric coronavirus.
he·don·ic [hi:'dɒnɪk] adj hedonistisch.
he·do·nism ['hi:dnɪzəm] n Hedonismus m, Hedonik f.
he·do·no·pho·bia [,hi:dənəʊ'fəʊbɪə] n psychia. Hedonophobie f.
hed·ro·cele ['hedrəsi:l] n chir. Hedrozele f.
heel [hi:l] n 1. anat. Ferse f, Fersenregion f, Calx f, Regio calcanea. 2. (Schuh) Absatz m; (Strumpf) Ferse f.
heel bone Fersenbein nt, Kalkaneus m, Calcaneus m.
heel bone fracture → heel fracture.
heel fracture ortho. Fersenbeinbruch m, -fraktur f, Kalkaneusfraktur f.
heel-knee test Knie-Hacken-Versuch m.
heel tendon Achillessehne f, Tendo calcaneus.
heel-toe walking ortho. (Fuß) Abrollen nt.
Heerfordt ['heərfɔ:rt]: **H.'s disease/syndrome** Heerfordt-Syndrom nt, Febris uveoparotidea.
Hegar ['heɪga:r]: **H.'s bougie** Hegarstift m.
H.'s dilatator/dilator → H.'s bougie.
H.'s sign gyn. Hegar-Zeichen nt.
H.'s uterine dilatator/dilator → H.'s bougie.

342

Hegglin ['heglɪn]: **H.'s anomaly** hema. May-Hegglin-Anomalie f, Hegglin-Syndrom nt.
H.'s change in neutrophils and platelets → H.'s anomaly.
H.'s syndrome → H.'s anomaly.
Hegouménakis [hɪ'gju:menækɪs]: **H.'s sign** Hegouménakis-Zeichen nt.
Heiberg-Esmarch ['haɪbɜrg 'esma:rk]: **H.-E. maneuver** Esmarch(-Heiberg)-Handgriff m, Heiberg-Handgriff m.
Heidenhain ['haɪdnhaɪn]: **H.'s azan stain** Heidenhain'-Azanfärbung f.
H.'s cell (Magen) Beleg-, Parietalzelle f.
H.'s iron hematoxylin stain Heidenhain'-Hämatoxylinfärbung f.
H.'s myelin stain Markscheidenfärbung f nach Heidenhain.
H. pouch Heidenhain-Magentasche f.
H.'s syndrome Heidenhaim-Syndrom nt.
height [haɪt] n 1. Höhe f, Größe f; Körpergröße f. 2. Höhepunkt m, Gipfel m.
height vertigo Höhenschwindel m.
Heim-Kreysig [haɪm 'kraɪsɪg]: **H.-K. sign** radiol. Heim-Kreysig-Zeichen nt.
Heimlich ['haɪmlɪk]: **H. maneuver** Heimlich-Handgriff m.
Heineke-Mikulicz ['haɪnɪkɪ 'mɪkjəlɪtʃ]: **H.-M. operation/pyloroplasty** chir. Heineke-Mikulicz-Operation f, -Pyloroplastik f.
Heine-Medin ['haɪnə 'meɪdɪn]: **H.-M. disease** (epidemische/spinale) Kinderlähmung f, Heine-Medin-Krankheit f, Poliomyelitis (epidemica) anterior acuta.
Heinz [haɪnts]: **H. bodies** → Heinz-Ehrlich bodies.
H. body anemia Anämie f mit Heinz'-Innenkörperchen.
H. granules → H. bodies.
Heinz-Ehrlich ['eərlɪk, e:rlɪç]: **H.-E. bodies** Heinz'-Innenkörperchen pl, Heinz-Ehrlich-Körperchen pl.
Heister ['haɪstər]: **H.'s diverticulum** Bulbus superius v. jugularis.
H.'s fold Heister'-Klappe f, Plica spiralis.
H.'s valve → H.'s fold.
Hektoen ['hektəʊn]: **H. enteric agar** Hektoen-Agar m/nt.
HeLa cells HeLa-Zellen pl.
hel·coid ['helkɔɪd] adj geschwürartig, ulkusähnlich.
hel·co·ma [hel'kəʊmə] n ophthal. Hornhautgeschwür nt, -ulkus nt, Ulcus corneae.
hel·co·me·nia [,helkəʊ'mi:nɪə] n gyn. Geschwürbildung f während der Menstruation.
hel·co·plas·ty ['-plæstɪ] n chir. Geschwürplastik f, -versorgung f, Ulkusplastik f, -versorgung f, Helkoplastik f.
hel·co·sis [hel'kəʊsɪs] n Geschwür(s)leiden nt, Helkosis f.
Held [held]: **H.'s bundle** Held'-Bündel nt, Tractus vestibulospinalis.
H.'s limiting membrane Blut-Hirn-Schranke f.
hel·e·nine ['helənɪ:n] n pharm. Helenin nt.
heli- pref. → helio-.
he·li·an·thin [,hi:lɪ'ænθɪn] n → helianthine.
he·li·an·thine [,-'ænθɪ:n] n Methylorange nt, Helianthin nt.
he·li·a·tion [,-'eɪʃn] n derm. → heliotherapy.
hel·i·cal ['helɪkəl] adj schrauben-, spiral-, schnecken-, helixförmig, helikal.
helical fracture Torsionsbruch m, -fraktur f, Drehbruch m, -fraktur f, Spiralbruch m, -fraktur f.
helical symmetry helikale Symmetrie f.
Hel·i·cel·la [,hɪlɪ'selə] n micro. Helicella f.
Hel·i·cel·li·dae [,-'selɪdiː] pl micro. Helicellidae pl.

hel·i·cine ['helisi:n, -sɪn] *adj* 1. spiral-, schneckenförmig. 2. Helix betr., helikal.
helicine arteries Rankenarterien *pl.*
h. of penis Rankenarterien (des Penis), Aa. helicinae (penis).
helicine branches of uterine artery Rami helicini (a. uterinae).
hel·i·cis major (muscle) ['helɪsɪs] M. helicis major.
helicis minor (muscle) M. helicis minor.
hel·i·coid ['helɪkɔɪd] *adj* spiral- *od.* schneckenförmig, spiralig.
hel·i·co·tre·ma [‚helɪkə'tri:mə] *n* Breschet-Hiatus *m*, Schneckenloch *nt*, Helicotrema *nt.*
he·li·en·ceph·a·li·tis [‚hi:lɪen‚sefə'laɪtɪs] *n* Helioenzephalitis *f.*
helio- *pref.* Sonnen-, Heli(o)-.
he·li·o·aer·o·ther·a·py [‚hi:lɪəʊ‚eərəʊ'θerəpɪ] *n* Helioaerotherapie *f.*
he·li·on ['hi:lɪən] *n* → helium.
he·li·op·a·thy [hi:lɪ'ɑpəθɪ] *n* durch Sonnenlicht hervorgerufene Erkrankung *f*, Heliopathie *f.*
he·li·o·pho·bia [‚hi:lɪə'fəʊbɪə] *n psychia.* krankhafte Angst *f* vor Sonnenlicht, Heliophobie *f.*
he·li·o·sis [hi:lɪ'əʊsɪs] *n* Sonnenstich *m*, Heliosis *f.*
he·li·o·tax·is [‚hi:lɪə'tæksɪs] *n bio.* Heliotaxis *f.*
he·li·o·ther·a·py [‚-'θerəpɪ] *n* Behandlung *f* mit Sonnenlicht, Heliotherapie *f.*
he·li·ot·ro·pism [‚hi:lɪ'ɑtrəpɪzəm] *n bio.* Heliotropismus *m.*
he·li·um ['hi:lɪəm] *n abbr.* **He** Helium *nt abbr.* He.
helium dilution method Heliumeinwaschmethode *f*, Heliumverdünnungsmethode *f.*
he·lix ['hi:lɪks] *n, pl* **-lix·es, hel·i·ces** ['helɪ‚sɪz, 'hi:-] 1. *anat.* äußerer Ohrmuschelrand *m*, Helix *f.* 2. *biochem.* Helix *f.* 3. *allg.* schneckenförmige Struktur *f*, Spirale *f*, Helix *f.*
α-helix *n biochem.* α-Helix *f.*
hel·le·bore ['heləbɔ:r, -bəʊr] *n pharm.* Nieswurz *f*, Helleborus *f.*
hel·le·bor·ism ['-bəʊrɪzəm] *n* Nieswurzvergiftung *f*, Helleborismus *m.*
Hellendall ['heləndæl]: **H.'s sign** Cullen-Zeichen *nt*, -Syndrom *nt*, Cullen-Hellendall-Zeichen *nt*, -Syndrom *nt.*
Heller ['helər]: **H.'s operation** Heller-Kardiomyotonie *f.*
H.'s plexus Heller-Plexus *m.*
H.'s test 1. Heller-Probe *f*, -Eiweißnachweis *m.* 2. Heller-Blutnachweiß *m*, -Probe *f.*
Heller-Döhle ['di:lɪ]: **H.-D. disease** Aortensyphilis *f*, Mesaortitis luetica, Aortitis syphilitica.
Hellin ['helɪn]: **H.'s law** *gyn.* Hellin'-Regel *f.*
Hellin-Zeleny [zə'li:nɪ]: **H.-Z. law** → Hellin's law.
hel·met cell ['helmɪt] *hema.* Schistozyt *m.*
Helmholtz ['helmhəʊlts]: **H. theory** → H. theory of hearing.
H. theory of accommodation von Helmholtz-Akkomodationstheorie *f.*
H. theory of color vision Dreifarbentheorie *f*, Young-Helmholtz-Theorie *f.*
H. theory of hearing Helmholtz-Hörtheorie *f*, Resonanzhypothese *f.*
hel·minth ['helmɪnθ] *n micro.* parasitischer Wurm *m*, Helminthe *f.*
hel·min·tha·gogue [hel'mɪnθəgɔg, -gag] **I** *n* Wurmmittel *nt*, Anthelmintikum *nt.* **II** *adj* gegen Würmer wirkend, wurm(ab)tötend, anthelmintisch.
hel·min·them·e·sis [‚helmɪn'θeməsɪs] *n*

Wurm-, Würmererbrechen *nt*, Helminthemesis *f.*
hel·min·thi·a·sis [‚-'θaɪəsɪs] *n* Wurmerkrankung *f*, Helminthiasis *f*, Helminthose *f.*
hel·min·thic [hel'mɪnθɪk] **I** *n* → helminthagogue I. **II** *adj* 1. Helminthen betr., durch Helminthen verursacht, Helminthen-, Wurm-. 2. → helminthagogue II.
helminthic abscess Helminthen-, Wurmabszeß *m.*
helminthic appendicitis Appendizitis *f* durch Wurmbefall, Appendicitis helminthica/vermicularis.
helminthic disease → helminthiasis.
hel·min·thi·cide [hel'mɪnθəsaɪd] *n* Vermizid *nt*, Vermicidum *nt.*
hel·min·thism ['helmɪnθɪzəm] *n* Helminthen-, Wurmbefall *m*; Helminthiasis *f.*
hel·min·thoid [hel'mɪnθɔɪd] *adj* wurmähnlich, helminthoid.
hel·min·thol·o·gy [‚helmɪn'θɑlədʒɪ] *n* Helminthologie *f.*
hel·min·tho·ma [‚-'θəʊmə] *n* Wurmknoten *m*, Helminthom(a) *nt.*
hel·min·tho·pho·bia [hel‚mɪnθə'fəʊbɪə] *n psychia.* Helminthophobie *f.*
hel·min·thous [hel'mɪnθəs] *adj* Helminthen betr., mit Helminthen infiziert, Helminthen-, Wurm-.
he·lo·ma [hɪ'ləʊmə] *n, pl* **-mas, -ma·ta** [-mətə] Hautschwiele *f*, Heloma *nt.*
he·lo·sis [hɪ'ləʊsɪs] *n* Hühneraugen(bildung *f*) *pl*, Helose *f.*
he·lot·o·my [hɪ'lɑtəmɪ] *n chir., derm.* Helotomie *f.*
help·er cell ['helpər] T-Helferzelle *f.*
helper virus *micro.* Helfer-, Helpervirus *nt.*
Hel·vel·la [hel'velə] *n micro.* Helvella *f.*
Hel·vel·la·ce·ae [‚helvə'leɪsi:] *pl micro.* Helvellaceae *f.*
hel·vel·lic acid [hel'velɪk] Helvellasäure *f.*
Helweg ['helveg]: **H.'s bundle/tract** Helweg'-Dreikantenbahn *f*, Tractus olivospinalis.
hem- *pref.* → hemo-.
hema- *pref.* → hemo-.
he·ma·chro·ma·to·sis [‚hi:mə‚krəʊmə'təʊsɪs, ‚hem-] *n* → hemochromatosis.
hem·a·chrome ['-krəʊm] *n* 1. Blutfarbstoff *m.* 2. sauerstofftransportierendes Blutpigment *nt.*
hem·a·cyte ['-saɪt] *n* → hemocyte.
hem·a·cy·tom·e·ter [‚-saɪ'tɑmɪtər] *n* → hemocytometer.
hem·a·cy·tom·e·try [‚-saɪ'tɑmətrɪ] *n* → hemocytometry.
hem·a·cy·to·zo·on [‚-‚saɪtə'zəʊɑn] *n* → hemocytozoon.
hem·ad·os·te·no·sis [‚hemædəʊstɪ'nəʊsɪs] *n* Blutgefäß-, Arterienstenose *f.*
he·ma·drom·e·ter [‚hi:mə'drɑmɪtər, ‚hemə-] *n* → hemodrometer.
he·ma·dro·mo·graph [‚-'drəʊməgræf] *n* → hemodromograph.
he·ma·dro·mom·e·ter [‚-drəʊ'mɑmɪtər] *n* → hemodromometer.
hem·ad·sor·bent [‚hemæd'sɔ:rbənt] *adj* hämadsorbierend, hämadsorptiv.
hem·ad·sorp·tion [‚hemæd'sɔ:rpʃn] *n* Hämadsorption *nt abbr.* HAD.
hemadsorption agent 1 → hemadsorption type 1 virus.
hemadsorption agent 2 → hemadsorption type 2 virus.
hemadsorption test Hämadsorptionstest *m.*
hemadsorption type 1 virus *micro.* Parainfluenza-3-Virus *nt*, Parainfluenzavirus Typ 3 *nt.*

hemadsorption type 2 virus *micro.* Parainfluenza-1-Virus *nt*, Parainfluenzavirus Typ 1 *nt.*
hemadsorption virus test → hemadsorption test.
he·ma·dy·na·mom·e·ter [‚hi:mə‚daɪnə'mɑmɪtər, ‚hem-] *n* → hemodynamometer.
hem·a·dy·na·mom·e·try [‚-‚daɪnə'mɑmətrɪ] *n* → hemodynamometry.
hem·a·fa·cient [‚-'feɪʃnt] *n, adj* → hemopoietic.
hem·a·fe·cia [‚-'fi:sɪə] *n* blutiger/bluthaltiger Stuhl *m*, Blutstuhl *m.*
he·mag·glu·ti·na·tion [‚-‚glu:tə'neɪʃn] *n* Hämagglutination *f.*
hemagglutination inhibition *abbr.* **HI, HAI** Hämagglutinationshemmung *f.*
hemagglutination-inhibition assay → hemagglutination inhibition test.
hemagglutination-inhibition reaction → hemagglutination inhibition test.
hemagglutination inhibition test *abbr.* **HI, HAI** Hämagglutinationshemmtest *m abbr.* HAH, HHT, Hämagglutinationshemmungsreaktion *f.*
hem·ag·glu·ti·na·tive [‚-'glu:tneɪtɪv] *adj* Hämagglutination betr. *od.* verusachend, hämagglutinativ, hämagglutinierend.
he·mag·glu·ti·nin [‚-'glu:tənɪn] *n* 1. Hämagglutinin *nt.* 2. *abbr.* **HA** *micro.* Hämagglutinin *nt abbr.* HA.
hemagglutinin neuraminidase protein *micro.* Hämagglutinin-Neuraminidaseprotein *nt*, HN-Protein *nt.*
hem·ag·glu·tin·o·gen [‚-'glu:tɪnədʒən] *n* Hämagglutinogen *nt.*
he·ma·gog·ic [‚-'gɑdʒɪk] *adj* den Blutfluß fördernd.
he·ma·gogue ['-gɔg, -gag] *n* 1. blutungsförderndes Mittel *nt*, Haemagogum *nt.* 2. Emmagogum *n.*
he·mal ['hi:məl] *adj* 1. Blut *od.* Blutgefäße betr., Blut-, Häma-, Häm(o)-, Blutgefäß-. 2. *embryo.* hämal.
hemal arch *embryo.* Hämalbogen *m.*
he·ma·lum [hɪ'mæləm] *n* Hämalaun *nt.*
hemalum-eosin stain Hämalaun-Eosin-Färbung *f.*
hemalum stain Hämalaunfärbung *f.*
he·ma·nal·y·sis [‚hi:mə'nɑləsɪs, ‚hem-] *n* Blutuntersuchung *f*, -analyse *f*, Häm(o)analyse *f.*
he·man·gi·ec·ta·sia [hɪ‚mændʒɪek'teɪʒ(ɪ)ə] *n* → hemangiectasis.
he·man·gi·ec·ta·sis [‚-'ektəsɪs] *n* Blutgefäßerweiterung *f*, Hämangiektasie *f*, Haemangiectasia *f.*
he·man·gi·o·am·el·o·blas·to·ma [hɪ‚mændʒɪəʊəmələʊblæs'təʊmə] *n patho.* Hämangioameloblastom(a) *nt.*
he·man·gi·o·blast [hɪ'mændʒɪəʊblæst] *n* Hämangioblast *m.*
he·man·gi·o·blas·to·ma [‚-blæs'təʊmə] *n* Lindau-Tumor *m*, Hämangioblastom *nt*, Angioblastom *nt.*
he·man·gi·o·en·do·the·li·o·blas·to·ma [‚-‚endəʊ‚θi:lɪəblæs'təʊmə] *n patho.* Hämangioendothelioblastom(a) *nt.*
he·man·gi·o·en·do·the·li·o·ma [‚-‚endəʊθi:lɪ'əʊmə] *n* Hämangioendotheliom(a) *nt.*
he·man·gi·o·en·do·the·li·o·sar·co·ma [‚-‚endəʊ‚θi:lɪəsɑ:r'kəʊmə] *n* → hemangiosarcoma.
he·man·gi·o·fi·bro·ma [‚-faɪ'brəʊmə] *n patho.* Hämangiofibrom(a) *nt.*
he·man·gi·o·ma [hɪ‚mændʒɪ'əʊmə] *n patho., derm.* Hämangiom *nt*, Haemangioma *nt.*
hemangioma-thrombocytopenia syndrome Kasabach-Merritt-Syndrom *nt*,

hemangiomatosis 344

Thrombo(zyto)penie-Hämangiom-Syndrom *nt*.
he·man·gi·o·ma·to·sis [hɪˌmændʒɪəʊmə'təʊsɪs] *n patho*., *derm*. Hämangiomatose *f*, Haemangiomatosis *f*.
he·man·gi·o·ma·tous epulis [hɪˌmændʒɪə'mətəs] teleangiektatisches Granulom *nt*, Granuloma pediculatum/pyogenicum/teleangiectaticum.
he·man·gi·o·per·i·cyte [ˌ-'perɪsaɪt] *n* Adventitiazelle *f*, Perizyt *m*.
he·man·gi·o·per·i·cy·to·ma [ˌ-ˌperɪsaɪ'təʊmə] *n patho*. Hämangioperizytom *nt*.
he·man·gi·o·sar·co·ma [ˌ-sɑːr'kəʊmə] *n patho*. malignes/sarkomatöses Hämangioendotheliom *nt*, Hämangiosarkom *nt*.
hem·a·phe·re·sis [ˌheməfə'riːsɪs] *n* Hämapherese *f*.
hem·a·poi·e·sis [ˌ-pɔɪ'iːsɪs] *n* → hemopoiesis.
hem·a·poi·et·ic [ˌ-pɔɪ'etɪk] *n, adj* → hemopoietic.
he·mar·thron [hɪ'mɑːrθrɒn] *n* → hemarthrosis.
he·mar·thros [hɪ'mɑːrθrəʊs] *n* → hemarthrosis.
he·mar·thro·sis [hɪmɑːr'θrəʊsɪs] *n* blutiger Gelenkerguß *m*, Hämarthros *m*, Hämarthrose *f*.
hem·ar·to·ma [ˌ-'təʊmə] *n* → hemangioma.
hemat- *pref*. → hemato-.
he·ma·ta·chom·e·ter [ˌhiːmətə'kɒmɪtər] *n* → hemotachometer.
he·ma·tal ['hiːmətəl, 'hem-] *adj* → hemal 1.
he·mat·a·pos·te·ma [ˌ-pɒs'tiːmə] *n patho*. Abszeß *m* mit Einblutung.
he·ma·te·in [ˌhiːmə'tiːɪn, 'hiːmətiːɪn, 'hem-] *n* Hämatein *nt*.
he·ma·tem·e·sis [hiːmə'teməsɪs, hem-] *n* Bluterbrechen *nt*, Hämatemesis *f*, Vomitus cruentus.
he·mat·en·ceph·a·lon [ˌhiːmæten'sefələn] *n* Großhirn(ein)blutung *f*, Hirn(ein)blutung *f*, zerebrale Blutung *f*.
he·ma·ther·a·py [ˌhiːmə'θerəpɪ, ˌhemə-] *n* → hemotherapy.
he·ma·therm ['-θɜːrm] *n* → homeotherm.
he·ma·ther·mal [ˌ-'θɜːrml] *adj* → homeothermic.
he·ma·ther·mous [ˌ-'θɜːrməs] *adj* → homeothermic.
he·mat·hi·dro·is [ˌhiːmæθaɪ'drəʊsɪs, ˌhem-] *n* → hematidrosis.
he·ma·tho·rax [hiːmə'θɔːræks, hem-] *n* → hemothorax.
he·mat·ic [hɪ'mætɪk] **I** *n* → hematinic I. **II** *adj* 1. Blut betr., im Blut enthalten, Blut-, Häma-, Häm(o)-. 2. → hematinic II.
he·ma·ti·dro·sis [ˌhiːmətɪ'drəʊsɪs, ˌhem-] *n* Blutschwitzen *nt*, Blutschwitzen *nt*, Hämat(h)idrosis *f*, Hämhidrose *f*, Häm(h)idrosis *f*.
hem·a·tim·e·ter [ˌhemə'tɪmətər, ˌhemə-] *n* → hemocytometer.
hem·a·tim·e·try [ˌ-'tɪmətrɪ] *n* → hemocytometry.
he·ma·tin ['hiːmətɪn, 'hem-] *n* Hämatin *nt*, Hydroxyhämin *nt*.
hematin chloride Teichmann-Kristalle *pl*, salzsaures Hämin *nt*, Hämin(kristalle *pl*) *nt*, Chlorhämin(kristalle *pl*) *nt*, Chlorhämatin *nt*.
he·ma·ti·ne·mia [ˌhiːmətɪ'niːmɪə; ˌhiːmə-] *n* Hämatinämie *f*.
he·ma·tin·ic [ˌ-'tɪnɪk] **I** *n pharm*. Hämatikum *nt*. **II** *adj* Hämatin betr., Hämatin-.
hem·a·tin·om·e·ter [ˌ-tɪ'nɒmɪtər] *n* → hemoglobinometer.
hem·a·tin·u·ri·a [ˌ-tɪ'n(j)ʊərɪə] *n* Hämatinausscheidung *f* im Harn, Hämatinurie *f*.

hemato- *pref*. Blut-, Häma-, Häm(o)-, Hämat(o)-.
hem·a·to·bil·ia [ˌhemətəʊ'bɪlɪə, ˌhiːmə-] *n* → hemobilia.
hem·a·to·blast ['-blæst] *n* → hemocytoblast.
hem·a·to·cele ['-siːl] *n* 1. Blutbruch *m*, Hämatozele *f*, Haematocele *f*. 2. *urol*. Hämatozele *f*, Haematocele testis. 3. Einblutung *f* in eine Körperhöhle, Hämatozele *f*.
hem·a·to·ce·lia [ˌ-'siːlɪə] *n* → hematocele 3.
hem·a·to·ceph·a·lus [ˌ-'sefələs] *n* Hämatozephalus *m*, -kephalus *m*, Haem(at)ocephalus *m*.
hem·a·to·che·zia [ˌ-'kiːzɪə] *n* 1. Blutstuhl *m*, Hämatochezie *f*, Haematochezia *f*. 2. Abgang *m* von Blutstuhl, Hämatochezie *f*.
hem·a·to·chlo·rin [ˌ-'klɔːrɪn, -'klɒː-] *n* Hämatochlorin *nt*.
hem·a·to·chro·ma·to·sis [ˌ-ˌkrəʊmə'təʊsɪs] *n* 1. Gewebefärbung *f* durch Blutpigmente. 2. → hemochromatosis.
hem·a·to·chy·lu·ria [ˌ-kaɪ'l(j)ʊərɪə] *n* Hämatochylurie *f*.
hem·a·to·coe·lia [ˌ-'siːlɪə] *n* → hematocele 3.
hem·a·to·col·pom·e·tra [ˌ-kɒlpə'miːtrə] *n gyn*. Hämatokolpometra *f*.
hem·a·to·col·pos [ˌ-'kɒlpəs] *n gyn*. Hämatokolpos *m*, Hämokolpos *m*.
he·mat·o·crit ['-krɪt] *n* 1. *abbr*. **HCT** Hämatokrit *m abbr*. Hk, Hkt. 2. Hämatokritröhrchen *nt*.
hem·a·toc·ry·al [ˌhemə'tɒkrɪəl] *adj bio*. wechselwarm, poikilotherm.
hem·a·to·crys·tal·lin [ˌhemətəʊ'krɪstəlɪn, ˌhiːm-] *n* → hemoglobin.
hem·a·to·cy·a·nin [ˌ-'saɪənɪn] *n* → hemocyanin.
hem·a·to·cyst ['-sɪst] *n* 1. hämorrhagische/blutgefüllte Zyste *f*, Blutzyste *f*, Haem(at)ocystis *f*. 2. → hematocystis.
hem·a·to·cys·tis [ˌ-'sɪstɪs] *n* Blutansammlung *f* in Harn- *od*. Gallenblase, Haem(at)ocystis *f*.
hem·a·to·cyte ['-saɪt] *n* → hemocyte.
hem·a·to·cy·to·blast [ˌ-'saɪtəblæst] *n* → hemocytoblast.
hem·a·to·cy·tol·y·sis [ˌ-saɪ'tɒləsɪs] *n* → hemolysis.
hem·a·to·cy·tom·e·ter [ˌ-saɪ'tɒmɪtər] *n* → hemocytometer.
hem·a·to·cy·to·pe·nia [ˌ-ˌsaɪtə'piːnɪə] *n* → hema. Panzytopenie *f*.
hem·a·to·cy·to·zo·on [ˌ-ˌsaɪtə'zəʊɒn] *n* → hemocytozoon.
hem·a·to·cy·tu·ria [ˌ-saɪ'tʊərɪə] *n* (echte) Hämaturie *f*, Erythrozyturie *f*, Hämazyturie *f*.
hem·a·to·di·al·y·sis [ˌ-daɪ'æləsɪs] *n* → hemodialysis.
hem·a·to·dys·cra·sia [ˌ-dɪs'kreɪʒ(ɪ)ə] *n* → hemodyscrasia.
hem·a·to·dys·tro·phy [ˌ-'dɪstrəfɪ] *n* → hemodystrophy.
he·ma·to·en·ceph·al·ic barrier [ˌhemətəʊˌensə'fælɪk, ˌhiːmə-] Blut-Hirn-Schranke *f*.
he·ma·to·gen·e·sis [ˌ-'dʒenəsɪs] *n* → hemopoiesis.
hem·a·to·gen·ic [ˌ-'dʒenɪk] **I** *n* → hemopoietic I. **II** *adj* 1. → hemopoietic II. 2. → hematogenous.
hematogenic shock Volumenmangelschock *m*, hypovolämischer Schock *m*.
he·ma·tog·e·nous [ˌhiːmə'tɒdʒənəs, ˌhemə-] *adj* 1. im Blut entstanden, aus dem Blut stammend, hämatogen. 2. durch Blut übertragen, über den Blutweg, hämatogen.

hematogenous abscess hämatogener Abszeß *m*.
hematogenous hyalin → hematohyaloid.
hematogenous jaundice → hemolytic icterus.
hematogenous metastasis hämatogene Metatase *f*.
hematogenous osteitis hämatogene Ostitis *f*.
hematogenous pigment hämoglobinogenes Pigment *nt*.
hematogenous spread hämatogene Aussaat *f*.
hematogenous tuberculosis hämatogene postprimäre Tuberkulose *f*.
he·mat·o·glo·bin [ˌhemətəʊ'gləʊbɪn, ˌhiːmətəʊ-] *n* → hemoglobin.
he·ma·to·glo·bin·u·ria [ˌ-gləʊbɪ'n(j)ʊərɪə] *n* → hemoglobinuria.
he·ma·to·glob·u·lin [ˌ-'glɒbjəlɪn] *n* → hemoglobin.
he·ma·to·hi·dro·sis [ˌ-haɪ'drəʊsɪs, -hɪ-] *n* → hematidrosis.
he·ma·to·his·ti·o·blast [ˌ-'hɪstɪəblæst] *n* → hemohistioblast.
he·ma·to·his·ton [ˌ-'hɪstən] *n* Globin *nt*.
he·ma·to·hy·a·loid [ˌ-'haɪəlɔɪd] *n* Hämatohyaloid *nt*, hämatogenes Hyalin *nt*.
he·ma·toid ['hiːmətɔɪd, 'hem-] *adj* blutähnlich, -artig, hämatoid.
he·ma·toi·din (**crystals**) [ˌhiːmə'tɔɪdɪn, ˌhem-] Hämatoidin(kristalle *pl*) *nt*.
he·ma·to·kol·pos [ˌ-'kɒlpəs] *n* → hematocolpos.
he·ma·to·lith ['hemətəʊlɪθ, 'hiːm-] *n old* → hemolith.
he·ma·tol·o·gist [ˌhiːmə'tɒlədʒɪst, ˌhem-] *n* Hämatologe *m*, -login *f*.
he·ma·tol·o·gy [ˌ-'tɒlədʒɪ] *n* Hämatologie *f*, Hämologie *f*.
he·ma·to·lymph·an·gi·o·ma [ˌhemətəʊlɪmfænʒɪ'əʊmə, ˌhiːm-] *n* Hämato-, Hämolymphangiom *nt*.
he·ma·tol·y·sis [ˌhemə'tələsɪs, ˌhiːm-] *n* → hemolysis.
he·ma·to·lyt·ic [ˌhemətəʊ'lɪtɪk, ˌhiːm-] *adj* → hemolytic.
he·ma·to·ma [ˌhemə'təʊmə, ˌhiːm-] *n, pl* **-mas**, **-ma·ta** [-mətə] Bluterguß *m*, Hämatom *nt*, Haematoma *nt*.
he·ma·to·ma·nom·e·ter [ˌhemətəʊmə'nɒmɪtər, ˌhiːm-] *n* Blutdruckmeßgerät *nt*, -apparat *m*, Sphygmomanometer *nt*.
he·ma·to·me·di·as·ti·num [ˌ-ˌmɪdɪə'staɪnəm] *n* → hemomediastinum.
hem·a·to·me·tra [ˌ-'miːtrə] *n gyn*. Hämato-, Hämometra *f*.
hem·a·to·me·tro·col·pos [ˌ-ˌmiːtrə'kɒlpəs] *n gyn*. Hämatometrokolpos *m*.
he·ma·tom·e·try [ˌhiːmə'tɒmɪtrɪ, ˌhem-] *n* 1. Hämoglobin- *od*. Hämatokritbestimmung *f*, Hämatometrie *f*. 2. Blutdruckmessung *f*, Hämometra *f*.
he·ma·to·mole [hɪ'mætəməʊl] *n gyn*. Breus'-Mole *f*.
hem·a·tom·phal·o·cele [ˌhiːmətɒm'fæləsiːl, ˌhem-] *n* Nabelhernie *f* mit Einblutung, Hämatomphalozele *f*.
he·ma·to·my·e·lia [ˌhemətəʊmaɪˈiːlɪə, ˌhiːm-] *n* Rückenmarks(ein)blutung *f*, Hämatomyelie *f*.
he·ma·to·my·e·li·tis [ˌ-maɪə'laɪtɪs] *n* akute hämorrhagische Myelitis *f*, Hämatomyelitis *f*.
he·ma·to·ne·phro·sis [ˌ-nɪ'frəʊsɪs, -ne-] *n* Blutansammlung *f* im Nierenbecken, Hämatonephrose *f*, Hämatopelvis *f*.
he·ma·ton·ic [hiːmə'tɒnɪk, ˌhem-] *n* → hematinic I.
hem·a·to·pa·thol·o·gy [ˌhemətəʊpə'θɒlədʒɪ, ˌhiːm-] *n* → hemopathology.
he·ma·top·a·thy [hiːmə'tɒpəθɪ, ˌhem-] *n* → hemopathy.

hem·a·to·pe·nia [ˌhemətoʊ'piːnɪə, ˌhiːm-] *n* Blutmangel *m*, Hämatopenie *f*.
hem·a·to·per·i·car·di·um [ˌ-ˌperɪ'kɑːrdɪəm] *n* → hemopericardium.
hem·a·to·per·i·to·ne·um [ˌ-ˌperɪtə'niːəm] *n* → hemoperitoneum.
hem·a·to·phage ['-feɪdʒ] *n* → hemophagocyte.
hem·a·to·pha·gia [ˌ-'feɪdʒɪə] *n* 1. bio. Hämato-, Hämophagie *f*. 2. psychia. Hämato-, Hämophagie *f*. 3. → hemocytophagia.
hem·a·to·phag·o·cyte [ˌ-'fægəsaɪt] *n* → hemophagocyte.
he·ma·toph·a·gous [ˌhiːmə'tafəgəs] *adj* bio., micro. blutsaugend, hämatophag.
he·ma·toph·a·gy [ˌ-'tafədʒɪ] *n* → hematophagia.
hem·a·to·phil·ia [ˌhemətoʊ'fɪlɪə, ˌhiːm-] *n* → hemophilia.
hem·a·to·pho·bia [ˌ-'foʊbɪə] *n* → hemophobia.
hem·a·to·pi·e·sis [ˌ-'paɪəsɪs] *n* Blutdruck *m*.
hem·a·to·plas·tic [ˌ-'plæstɪk] *adj* blutbildend, hämatoplastisch.
he·mat·o·poi·e·sis [ˌ-pɔɪ'iːsɪs] *n* → hemopoiesis.
hem·a·to·poi·et·ic [ˌ-pɔɪ'etɪk] *n*, *adj* → hemopoietic.
hematopoetic system hämopoetisches System *nt*.
hematopoietic tissue hämopoetisches/ blutbildendes Gewebe *nt*.
hem·a·to·poi·e·tin [ˌ-'pɔɪətɪn] *n* → hemopoietin.
hem·a·to·por·phyr·ia [ˌ-pɔːrfɪ'ərɪə, -faɪr-] *n* 1. Porphyrie *f*, Porphyria *f*. 2. erythropoetische Porphyrie *f*, Günther-Krankheit *f*, -Syndrom *nt*, Hämatoporphyrie *f*, Porphyria erythropoetica congenita Günther.
hem·a·to·por·phy·rin [ˌ-'pɔːrfərɪn] *n* Hämatoporphyrin *nt*.
hem·a·to·por·phy·rin·e·mia [ˌ-pɔːrfərɪ'niːmɪə] *n* Hämatoporphyrinämie *f*.
hem·a·to·por·phy·rin·u·ria [ˌ-pɔːrfərɪ'nʊərɪə] *n* Hämatoporphyrinausscheidung *f* im Harn, Hämatoporphyrinurie *f*.
hem·a·tor·rha·chis [ˌhemə'tɔːrəkɪs] *n* 1. spinale Meningealapoplexie *f*, Hämatorrhachis *f*, Apoplexia spinalis. 2. → hematomyelia.
hem·a·tor·rhe·a [ˌhemətoʊ'rɪə, ˌhiːm-] *n* 1. massive Blutung *f*, Massenblutung *f*, Blutsturz *m*, Hämatorrhö *f*. 2. → hemoptysis.
hem·a·to·sal·pinx [ˌ-'sælpɪŋks] *n gyn*. Blutansammlung *f* im Eileiter, Hämatosalpinx *f*.
hem·a·tos·che·o·cele [ˌhemə'taskɪəsɪːl] *n* Blutansammlung *f* im Skrotum, Hämatoscheozele *f*.
hem·a·to·sep·sis [ˌhemətoʊ'sepsɪs, ˌhiːm-] *n* (Hämato-)Sepsis *f*, Septikämie *f*.
he·ma·to·sin [ˌhiːmə'toʊsɪn] *n* → hematin.
hem·a·to·sis [ˌ-'toʊsɪs] *n* 1. → hemopoiesis. 2. *physiol*. Arterialisation *f*.
hem·a·to·spec·tro·pho·tom·e·ter [ˌheməˌtoʊˌspektrəfoʊ'tamɪtər, ˌhiːm-] *n lab*. Hämato-, Hämospektrophotometer *nt*.
hem·a·to·spec·tro·scope [ˌ-'spektrəskoʊp] *n lab*. Hämato-, Hämospektroskop *nt*.
hem·a·to·spec·tros·co·py [ˌ-spek'traskəpɪ] *n lab*. Hämato-, Hämospektroskopie *f*.
hem·a·to·sper·mat·o·cele [ˌ-spɜr'mætəsiːl] *n urol*. Hämatospermatozele *f*.
hem·a·to·sper·mia [ˌ-'spɜrmɪə] *n* → hemospermia.
hem·a·to·spher·i·ne·mia [ˌ-ˌsfɪərə'niːmɪə] *n* → hemoglobinemia.

hem·a·to·stat·ic [ˌ-'stætɪk] **I** *n* → hemostatic I. **II** *adj* 1. → hemostatic II. 2. Blutstauung/Hämostase betr., hämatostatisch.
hem·a·tos·te·on [ˌhemə'tastɪən] *n* (Knochen) Markhöhlen(ein)blutung *f*, Haematosteon *nt*.
hem·a·to·ther·a·py [ˌhemətoʊ'θerəpɪ, ˌhiːm-] *n* → hemotherapy.
hem·a·to·ther·mal [ˌ-'θɜrml] *adj* → homeothermic.
hem·a·to·tho·rax [ˌ-'θɔːræks] *n* → hemothorax.
hem·a·to·tox·ic [ˌ-'taksɪk] *adj* → hemotoxic.
hem·a·to·tox·i·co·sis [ˌ-taksɪ'koʊsɪs] *n* Hämatotoxikose *f*.
hem·a·to·tox·in [ˌ-'taksɪn] *n* → hemotoxin.
hem·a·to·trop·ic [ˌ-'trapɪk, -'troʊp-] *adj* → hemotropic.
hem·a·to·tym·pa·num [ˌ-'tɪmpənəm] *n* → hemotympanum.
hem·a·tox·ic [ˌhemə'taksɪk, ˌhiːm-] *adj* → hemotoxic.
hem·a·tox·in [ˌ-'taksɪn] *n* → hemotoxin.
he·ma·tox·y·lin [ˌ-'taksəlɪn] *n* Hämatoxylin *nt*.
hematoxylin-eosin *n abbr*. **HE** *histol*. Hämatoxylin-Eosin *abbr*. HE.
hematoxylin-eosin stain Hämatoxylin-Eosin-Färbung *f*, HE-Färbung *f*.
he·ma·to·zo·al [ˌhemətoʊ'zoʊəl, ˌhiːm-] *adj* → hemozoic.
he·ma·to·zo·an [ˌ-'zoʊən] **I** *n* → hemozoon. **II** *adj* → hemozoic.
he·ma·to·zo·ic [ˌ-'zoʊɪk] *adj* → hemozoic.
he·ma·to·zo·on [ˌ-'zoʊən] *n* → hemozoon.
hem·a·tu·re·sis [ˌhemətjə'riːsɪs] *n* → hematuria.
hem·a·tu·ria [ˌhiːmə't(j)ʊərɪə, ˌhem-] *n* Blutharnen *nt*, Blutausscheidung *f* im Harn, Hämaturie *f*, Haematuria *f*.
hem·a·tur·ic bilious fever [ˌ-'t(j)ʊərɪk] Schwarzwasserfieber *nt*, Febris biliosa et haemoglobinurica.
heme [hiːm] *n* 1. Häm *nt*, Protohäm *nt*. 2. Protohäm IX *nt*.
heme enzyme Hämenzym *nt*.
hem·en·do·the·li·o·ma [ˌhemendoʊˌθiːlɪ'oʊmə] *n* → hemangioendothelioma.
He·men·te·ria [ˌhiːmən'tɪərɪə] *n* → Haementeria.
heme protein hämhaltiges Protein *nt*, Hämoprotein *nt*.
hem·er·a·lope ['hemərəloʊp] *n* Patient(in *f*) *m* mit Hemeralopie, Hemeralope(r *m*) *f*.
hem·er·a·lo·pia [ˌ-'loʊpɪə] *n ophthal*. Tagblindheit *f*, Nykteralopie *f*, Nyktalopie *f*.
hem·er·a·no·pia [ˌ-'noʊpɪə] *n* → hemeralopia.
heme synthetase Hämsynthetase *f*, Goldberg-Enzym *nt*, Ferrochelatase *f*.
hemi- *pref*. Halb-, Hemi-.
hem·i·a·car·di·us [ˌhemɪa'kɑːrdɪəs] *n embryo*. Hemicardius *m*, Hemicardiacus *m*.
hem·i·ac·e·tal [ˌ-'æsɪtæl] *n* Halb-, Hemiacetal *nt*.
hem·i·a·chro·ma·top·si·a [ˌ-ˌəkroʊmə'tapsɪə] *n ophthal*. Farbenhemianopsie *f*, Hemiachromatopsie *f*, Hemichromatopsie *f*.
hem·i·a·geu·si·a [ˌ-ə'gjuːzɪə] *n neuro*. Hemiageusie *f*.
hem·i·a·geus·tia [ˌ-ə'gjuːstɪə] *n* → hemiageusia.
hem·i·al·bu·min [ˌ-æl'bjuːmɪn] *n* → hemialbumose.
hem·i·al·bu·mose [ˌ-'ælbjəmoʊs] *n patho*. Hemialbumin *nt*, Hemialbumose *f*.

hem·i·al·bu·mo·su·ria [ˌ-ˌælbjuːmə's(j)ʊərɪə] *n patho*. Hemialbumosurie *f*.
hem·i·al·gia [ˌ-'ældʒ(ɪ)ə] *n neuro*. Halbseitenschmerz *m*, Hemialgie *f*.
hem·i·am·bly·o·pia [ˌ-ˌæmblɪ'oʊpɪə] *n* → hemianopia.
hem·i·a·my·os·the·nia [ˌ-eɪˌmaɪəs'θiːnɪə] *n* → hemiparesis.
hem·i·an·a·cu·sia [ˌ-ænə'kjuːzɪə] *n HNO* einseitige Taubheit *f*, Hemianakusis *f*.
hem·i·an·al·ge·si·a [ˌ-ænl'dʒiːzɪə] *n neuro*. halbseitige Analgesie *f*, Hemianalgesie *f*.
hem·i·an·en·ceph·a·ly [ˌ-ˌænən'sefəlɪ] *n embryo*. halbseitiger Hirnmangel *m*, Hemianenzephalie *f*.
hem·i·an·es·the·sia [ˌ-ænəs'θiːʒə] *n neuro*. Hemianästhesie *f*, Hemianaesthesia *f*.
hem·i·an·gi·ec·ta·tic hypertrophy [ˌ-ˌændʒɪek'tætɪk] Klippel-Feil-Syndrom *nt*.
hem·i·a·no·pia [ˌ-ə'noʊpɪə] *n ophthal*., *neuro*. Halbseitenblindheit *f*, Hemianopsie *f*, -anopie *f*.
hem·i·a·no·pic [ˌ-ə'napɪk] *adj* Hemianop(s)ie betr., hemianopisch, hemianoptisch.
hemianopic scotoma *ophthal*. hemianopes Skotom *nt*.
hem·i·a·nop·sia [ˌ-ə'napsɪə] *n* → hemianopia.
hem·i·a·nop·tic [ˌ-ə'naptɪk] *adj* → hemianopic.
hem·i·an·os·mia [ˌ-ə'nazmɪə] *n neuro*. halbseitige/einseitige Anosmie *f*, Hemianosmie *f*.
hem·i·a·pla·sia [ˌ-ə'pleɪʒ(ɪ)ə] *n patho*. halbseitige/einseitige Aplasie *f*, Hemiaplasie *f*.
hem·i·a·prax·ia [ˌ-ə'præksɪə] *n neuro*. einseitige/halbseitige Apraxie *f*, Hemiapraxie *f*.
hem·i·ar·thro·plas·ty [ˌ-'ɑːrθroʊplæstɪ] *n ortho*. Hemiarthroplastik *f*, Hemiprothese *f*.
hem·i·a·syn·er·gia [ˌ-eɪsɪ'nɜrdʒ(ɪ)ə] *n neuro*. halbseitige/einseitige Asynergie *f*, Hemiasynergie *f*.
hem·i·a·tax·ia [ˌ-ə'tæksɪə] *n neuro*. einseitige/halbseitige Ataxie *f*, Hemiataxie *f*.
hem·i·a·tax·y [ˌ-ə'tæksɪ] *n* → hemiataxia.
hem·i·ath·e·to·sis [ˌ-æθə'toʊsɪs] *n neuro*. halbseitige/einseitige Athetose *f*, Hemiathetose *f*.
hem·i·at·ro·phy [ˌ-'ætrəfɪ] *n* halbseitige/einseitige Atrophie *f*, Hemiatrophie *f*, Hemiatrophia *f*.
hem·i·az·y·gous vein [ˌ-'æzɪgəs, -ə'zaɪ-] Hemiazygos *f*, V. hemiazygos.
accessory h. Hemiazygos *f* accessoria, V. hemiazygos accessoria.
hem·i·az·y·gos vein [ˌ-'æzɪgəs, -ə'zaɪ-] *n* → hemiazygous vein.
hem·i·bal·lism [ˌ-'bælɪzəm] *n* → hemiballismus.
hem·i·bal·lis·mus [ˌ-bə'lɪzməs] *n neuro*. Hemiballismus *m*.
hem·i·block ['-blak] *n card*. Hemiblock *m*.
he·mic ['hiːmɪk, 'hem-] *adj* Blut betr., Blut-, Häma-, Hämat(o)-, Häm(o)-.
hem·i·car·dia [ˌhemɪ'kɑːrdɪə] *n embryo*. Hemikardie *f*, Hemicardia *f*.
hem·i·car·di·us [ˌ-'kɑːrdɪəs] *n embryo*. Hemikardius *m*, Hemicardius *m*.
hemic calculus → hemolith.
hem·i·cel·lu·lose [ˌ-'seljəloʊs] *n* Hemicellulose *f*.
hemic distomiasis Schistosomiasis *f*, Bilharziose *f*.
hem·i·ceph·a·lal·gia [ˌ-ˌsefə'lældʒ(ɪ)ə] *n* → hemicrania 1.
hem·i·ce·pha·lia [ˌ-sɪ'feɪlɪə] *n embryo*. partielle Anenzephalie *f*, Hemizephalie *f*, -kephalie *f*, Hemicephalia *f*.

hem·i·ceph·a·lus [ˌ-'sefələs] *n embryo*. Hemizephalus *m*, -kephalus *m*.

hem·i·ce·re·brum [ˌ-sə'riːbrəm, -'serə-] *n* (Groß-)Hirnhemisphäre *f*, Hemisph(a)erium cerebralis.

hem·i·cho·rea [ˌ-kə'rɪə, -'kɔː-, -'kəʊ-] *n neuro*. halbseitige/einseitige Chorea *f*, Hemichorea *f*.

hem·i·chro·ma·top·sia [ˌ-krəʊmə'tɒpsɪə] *n* → hemiachromatopsia.

hem·i·co·lec·to·my [ˌ-kə'lektəmɪ] *n chir*. Hemikolektomie *f*.

hem·i·cor·ti·cec·to·my [ˌ-ˌkɔːrtɪ'sektəmɪ] *n neurochir*. Hemikortikektomie *f*.

hem·i·cra·nia [ˌ-'kreɪnɪə] *n* 1. Halbseitenkopfschmerz *m*, halbseitiger/einseitiger Kopfschmerz *m*, Hemikranie *f*, Hemicrania *f*. 2. → hemicephalia.

hem·i·cra·ni·ec·to·my [ˌ-ˌkreɪnɪ'ektəmɪ] *n neurochir*. Hemikraniektomie *f*, Hemikraniotomie *f*.

hem·i·cra·ni·o·sis [-ˌkreɪnɪ'əʊsɪs] *n* Hemikraniose *f*.

hem·i·de·cor·ti·ca·tion [ˌ-dɪˌkɔːrtɪ'keɪʃn] *n neurochir*. Hemidekortikation *f*.

hem·i·de·per·son·al·i·za·tion [ˌ-dɪˌpərsnəlɪ'zeɪʃn, -laɪ-] *n psychia*. Hemidepersonalisation *f*.

hem·i·des·mo·some [ˌhemɪ'dezməsəʊm] *n* → half desmosome.

hem·i·di·a·pho·re·sis [-ˌdaɪəfə'riːsɪs] *n* 1. → hemihidrosis. 2. → hemihyperhidrosis.

hem·i·dro·sis [ˌ-'drəʊsɪs] *n* 1. → hematidrosis. 2. → hemihidrosis.

hem·i·dys·es·the·sia [ˌ-dɪses'θiːʒ(ɪ)ə] *n neuro*. halbseitige/einseitige Dysästhesie *f*, Hemidysästhesie *f*.

hem·i·dys·tro·phy [ˌ-'dɪstrəfɪ] *n patho*. halbseitige/einseitige Dystrophie *f*, Hemidystrophie *f*.

hem·i·ec·tro·me·lia [ˌ-ˌektrəʊ'miːlɪə] *n embryo*. halbseitige/einseitige Ektromelie *f*, Hemiektromelie *f*.

hem·i·en·ceph·a·lus [ˌ-en'sefələs] *n* → hemicephalus.

hem·i·ep·i·lep·sy [ˌ-'epɪlepsɪ] *n neuro*. halbseitige/einseitige Epilepsie *f*, Hemiepilepsie *f*.

hem·i·fac·e·tec·to·my [ˌ-ˌfæsɪ'tektəmɪ] *n ortho*. Hemifacettektomie *f*.

hem·i·fa·cial [ˌ-'feɪʃl] *adj* eine Gesichtshälfte betr., hemifazial.

hemifacial atrophy halbseitige Gesichtsatrophie *f*, Atrophia hemifacialis.

hem·i·gas·trec·to·my [ˌ-gæs'trektəmɪ] *n chir*. Hemigastrektomie *f*.

hem·i·geu·sia [ˌ-'gjuːzɪə] *n* → hemiageusia.

hem·i·gi·gan·tism [ˌ-'dʒaɪgæntɪzəm, -dʒɪ-] *n* Halbseitenriesenwuchs *m*, Hemigigantismus *m*.

hem·i·glos·sal [ˌ-'glɒsl] *adj* eine Zungenhälfte betr., hemiglossal, hemilingual.

hem·i·glos·sec·to·my [ˌ-glɒ'sektəmɪ] *n chir*., *HNO* Hemiglossektomie *f*.

hem·i·glos·si·tis [ˌ-glɒ'saɪtɪs] *n* Hemiglossitis *f*.

hem·i·gnath·ia [ˌ-'næθɪə] *n embryo*. Hemignathie *f*.

hem·i·hep·a·tec·to·my [ˌ-ˌhepə'tektəmɪ] *n chir*. Hemihepatektomie *f*.

hem·i·hi·dro·sis [ˌ-haɪ'drəʊsɪs] *n* Hemihidrose *f*, Hemihidrosis *f*, Hemidrosis *f*.

hem·i·hyp·al·ge·sia [ˌ-hɪpæl'dʒiːzɪə] *n neuro*. halbseitige/einseitige Hypalgesie *f*, Hemihypalgesie *f*, -hypalgie *f*.

hem·i·hy·per·es·the·sia [ˌ-ˌhaɪpəres-'θiːʒ(ɪ)ə] *n neuro*. halbseitige/einseitige Hyperästhesie *f*, Hemihyperästhesie *f*.

hem·i·hy·per·hi·dro·sis [ˌ-ˌhaɪpərhaɪ'drəʊsɪs] *n* halbseitige/einseitige Hyperhidrose *f*, Hemihyperhidrose *f*, -hidrosis *f*.

hem·i·hy·per·pla·sia [ˌ-ˌhaɪpər'pleɪʒ(ɪ)ə, -zɪə] *n patho*. halbseitige/einseitige Hyperplasie *f*, Hemihyperplasie *f*.

hem·i·hy·per·to·nia [ˌ-ˌhaɪpər'təʊnɪə] *n neuro*. halbseitige/einseitige Hypertonie *f*, Hemitonie *f*.

hem·i·hy·per·tro·phy [ˌ-haɪ'pərtrəfɪ] *n* halbseitige/einseitige Hypertrophie *f*, Hemihypertrophie *f*, Curtius-Syndrom *nt*.

hem·i·hyp·es·the·sia [ˌ-ˌhaɪpes'θiːʒ(ɪ)ə] *n* einseitige/halbseitige Hyp(o)ästhesie *f*, Hemihypästhesie *f*.

hem·i·hy·po·es·the·sia [ˌ-ˌhaɪpəes'θiːʒ(ɪ)ə] *n* → hemihypesthesia.

hem·i·hy·po·pla·sia [ˌ-ˌhaɪpə'pleɪʒ(ɪ)ə, -zɪə] *n patho*. einseitige/halbseitige Hypoplasie *f*, Hemihypoplasie *f*.

hem·i·hy·po·to·nia [ˌ-ˌhaɪpə'təʊnɪə] *n neuro*. halbseitige/einseitige Hypotonie *f*, Hemihypotonie *f*.

hem·i·kar·y·on [ˌ-'kærɪɒn] *n bio*., *histol*. Hemikaryon *nt*.

hem·i·ke·tal [ˌ-'kiːtæl] *n* Halb-, Hemiketal *nt*.

hem·i·lam·i·nec·to·my [ˌ-ˌlæmɪ'nektəmɪ] *n chir*., *neurochir*. Hemilaminektomie *f*.

hem·i·lar·yn·gec·to·my [ˌ-ˌlærɪn'dʒektəmɪ] *n HNO* Hemilaryngektomie *f*.

hem·i·lat·er·al [ˌ-'lætərəl] *adj* halb-, einseitig, hemilateral.

hemilateral chorea → hemichorea.

hem·i·le·sion [ˌ-'liːʒn] *n neuro*. Halbseitenläsion *f*.

hem·i·lin·gual [ˌ-'lɪŋgwəl] *adj* → hemiglossal.

hem·i·mac·ro·glos·sia [ˌ-ˌmækrə'glɒsɪə] *n patho*., *HNO* Hemimakroglossie *f*.

hem·i·man·dib·u·lec·to·my [ˌ-ˌmændɪbjə'lektəmɪ] *n HNO* Hemimandibulektomie *f*.

hem·i·max·il·lec·to·my [ˌ-ˌmaksɪ'lektəmɪ] *n HNO* Hemimaxillektomie *f*.

hem·i·me·lia [ˌ-'miːlɪə, -jə] *n embryo*. Hemimelie *f*.

hem·i·me·lus [ˌ-'miːləs] *n embryo*. Hemimelus *m*.

he·min ['hiːmɪn] *n* 1. Hämin *nt*. 2. Teichmann-Kristalle *pl*, salzsaures Hämin *nt*, Hämin(kristalle *pl*) *nt*, Chlorhämin(kristalle *pl*) *nt*, Chlorhämatin *nt*.

hemin chloride → hemin 2.

hemin crystals → hemin 2.

hem·i·ne·phrec·to·my [ˌhemɪnɪ'frektəmɪ] *n chir*., *urol*. Heminephrektomie *f*.

hem·i·neph·ro·u·re·ter·ec·to·my [ˌ-ˌnefrəʊəˌriːtə'rektəmɪ] *n urol*. Heminephroureterektomie *f*.

hemin form *chem*. Häminform *f*.

hemin test Teichmann-Probe *m*.

hem·i·o·pia [ˌhemɪ'əʊpɪə] *n* → hemianopia.

hem·i·op·ic [ˌ-'ɒpɪk] *adj* → hemianopic.

hemiopic reaction Wernicke-Phänomen *nt*.

hem·ip·a·gus [he'mɪpəgəs] *n embryo*. Hemipagus *m*.

hem·i·par·al·y·sis [ˌhemɪpə'ræləsɪs] *n* → hemiplegia.

hem·i·par·an·es·the·sia [ˌ-ˌpærænes'θiːʒə] *n neuro*. Hemiparanästhesie *f*.

hem·i·par·a·ple·gia [ˌ-ˌpærə'pliːdʒ(ɪ)ə] *n neuro*. Hemiparaplegie *f*.

hem·i·par·a·site [ˌ-'pærəsaɪt] *n bio*., *micro*. Halbschmarotzer *m*, Halbparasit *m*, Hemiparasit *m*.

hem·i·pa·re·sis [ˌ-pə'riːsɪs, -'pærə-] *n neuro*. Halbseitenschwäche *f*, leichte/unvollständige Halbseitenlähmung *f*, Hemiparese *f*.

hem·i·par·es·the·sia [ˌ-ˌpæres'θiːʒə] *n neuro*. halbseitige/einseitige Parästhesie *f*, Hemiparästhesie *f*.

hem·i·pa·ret·ic [ˌ-pə'retɪk] I *n* Hemiparetiker(in *f*) *m*. II *adj* Hemiparese betr., von ihr betroffen, hemiparetisch.

hem·i·par·kin·son·ism [ˌ-'pɑːrkɪnsənɪzəm] *n neuro*. Hemiparkinsonismus *m*.

hem·i·pel·vec·to·my [ˌ-pel'vektəmɪ] *n ortho*. Hemipelvektomie *f*.

hem·i·phal·an·gec·to·my [ˌ-ˌfælən'dʒektəmɪ] *n ortho*. Hemiphalangektomie *f*.

hem·i·ple·gia [ˌ-'pliːdʒ(ɪ)ə] *n neuro*. (vollständige) Halbseitenlähmung *f*, Hemiplegie *f*, Hemiplegia *f*.

hem·i·ple·gic [ˌ-'pliːdʒɪk] I *n* Hemiplegiker(in *f*) *m*. II *adj* Hemiplegie betr., durch sie bedingt, hemiplegisch.

He·mip·ter·a [he'mɪptərə] *pl micro*. Halbflügler *pl*, Hemipteren *pl*, Hemiptera *pl*.

hem·i·py·lor·ec·to·my [ˌhemɪpaɪlɔː'rektəmɪ] *n chir*. Hemipylorektomie *f*.

hem·i·py·o·ne·phro·sis [ˌ-ˌpaɪənɪ'frəʊsɪs] *n urol*. Hemipyonephrose *f*.

hem·i·rha·chis·chi·sis [ˌ-rə'kɪskəsɪs] *n embryo*. Hemirhachischisis *f*.

hem·i·sa·cral·i·za·tion [ˌ-sækrəlɪ'zeɪʃn, -seɪ-, -laɪ-] *n embryo*., *ortho*. Hemisakralisation *f*.

hem·i·sco·to·sis [ˌ-skə'təʊsɪs] *n* → hemianopia.

hem·i·so·ton·ic [ˌ-sə'tɒnɪk] *adj* (*Blut*) isoton, isotonisch.

hem·i·spasm ['-spæzəm] *n neuro*. Halbseitenkrampf *m*, Hemispasmus *m*.

hem·i·sphere ['-sfɪər] *n* Hemisphäre *f*, Halbkugel *f*; *anat*. Hemisph(a)erium *nt*.

hem·i·spher·ec·tomy [ˌ-sfɪər'ektəmɪ] *n neurochir*. Hemisphärektomie *f*.

hem·i·spher·ic [ˌ-'sferɪk] *adj* halbkug(e)lig, hemisphärisch.

hem·i·spher·i·cal [ˌ-'sferɪkl] *adj* → hemispheric.

hemispheric dominance *neuro*. Hemisphärendominanz *f*.

hemispheric gliosis unilaterale/hemisphärische Gliose *f*.

hemispheric vesicles of brain vesicle *embryo*. Hemisphärenbläschen *pl*.

hem·i·sphe·ri·um [ˌ-'sfɪərɪəm] *n*, *pl* -ria [-rɪə] 1. Hemisphäre *f*, Halbkugel *f*; *anat*. Hemisph(a)erium *nt*. 2. Kleinhirnhälfte *f*, -hemisphäre, Hemisph(a)erium cerebelli. 3. Groß-, Endhirnhälfte *f*, Groß-, Endhirnhemisphäre, Hemisph(a)erium cerebralis.

He·mis·po·ra stel·la·ta [he'mɪspərə] *n micro*. Hemispora stellata.

hem·i·spo·ro·sis [ˌhemɪspə'rəʊsɪs] *n* Hemisporose *f*.

hem·i·stru·mec·to·my [ˌ-struː'mektəmɪ] *n chir*. Hemistrumektomie *f*.

hem·i·syn·drome [ˌ-'sɪndrəʊm] *n* Halbseitensyndrom *nt*, Hemisyndrom *nt*.

hem·i·sys·to·le [ˌ-'sɪstəlɪ] *n card*. Halbseitenkontraktion *f*, Hemisystolie *f*.

hem·i·tet·a·ny [ˌ-'tetənɪ] *n neuro*. halbseitige/einseitige Tetanie *f*, Hemitetanie *f*.

hem·i·ther·mo·an·es·the·sia [ˌ-ˌθɜːrməˌænəs'θiːʒə] *n neuro*. halbseitige/einseitige Thermoanästhesie *f*, Hemithermoanästhesie *f*.

hem·i·tho·rax [ˌ-'θɔːræks, -'θəʊə-] *n* Brustkorb-, Thoraxhälfte *f*, Hemithorax *f*.

hem·i·thy·roid·ec·to·my [ˌ-ˌθaɪrɔɪ'dektəmɪ] *n chir*. Hemithyreoidektomie *f*.

hem·i·to·nia [ˌ-'təʊnɪə] *n* → hemihypertonia.

hem·i·trem·or [ˌ-'tremər] *n neuro*. Halbseitentremor *m*, Hemitremor *m*.

hem·i·va·go·to·my [ˌ-veɪ'gɒtəmɪ] *n neuro*. Hemivagotomie *f*.

hem·i·ver·te·bra [ˌ-'vɜːrtəbrə] *n embryo*., *ortho*. Halbwirbel *m*.

hem·i·zy·gos·i·ty [ˌ-zaɪˈɡɒsətɪ] *n genet.* Hemizygotie *f.*
hem·i·zy·gote [ˌ-ˈzaɪɡəʊt] *n* hemizygote Zelle *f,* hemizygotes Individuum *nt.*
hem·i·zy·gous [ˌ-ˈzaɪɡəəs] *adj* hemizygot.
hemo- *pref.* Blut-, Häma-, Hämato-, Häm(o)-.
he·mo·ag·glu·ti·na·tion [ˌhiːməʊˌɡluːtəˈneɪʃn, ˌhem-] *n* → hemagglutination.
he·mo·ag·glu·ti·nin [ˌ-əˈɡluːtənɪn] *n* → hemagglutinin.
he·mo·bil·ia [ˌ-ˈbɪlɪə] *n* Hämobilie *f,* Hämatobilie *f.*
he·mo·blast [ˈ-blæst] *n* → hemocytoblast.
he·mo·blas·tic leukemia [ˌ-ˈblæstɪk] *hema.* Stammzellenleukämie *f,* akute undifferenzierte Leukämie *f abbr.* AUL.
he·mo·blas·to·sis [ˌ-blæsˈtəʊsɪs] *n hema.* Hämoblastose *f.*
he·mo·ca·thar·sis [ˌ-kəˈθɑːrsɪs] *n* Blutreinigung *f,* Hämato-, Hämokatharsis *f.*
he·mo·ca·ther·e·sis [ˌ-kəˈθerəsɪs] *n* Blutzellenzerstörung *f.*
he·mo·cath·e·ret·ic [ˌ-ˌkæθəˈretɪk] *adj* Blutzellen zerstörend.
he·mo·cho·le·cyst [ˌ-ˈkəʊləsɪst, -ˈkɒlə-] *n* 1. atraumatische Gallenblasenblutung *f.* 2. Blutansammlung *f* in der Gallenblase, Hämato-, Hämocholecystis *f.*
he·mo·cho·le·cys·ti·tis [ˌ-ˌkəʊləsɪsˈtaɪtɪs, -ˌkɒlə-] *n* hämorrhagische Gallenblasenentzündung/Cholezystitis *f,* Cholecystitis haemorrhagica.
he·mo·cho·ri·al [ˌ-ˈkɔːrɪəl, -ˈkəʊr-] *adj* hämochorial.
hemochorial placenta hämochoriale Plazenta *f,* Placenta h(a)emochorialis.
he·mo·chro·ma·to·sis [ˌ-ˌkrəʊməˈtəʊsɪs] *n* Eisenspeicherkrankheit *f,* Hämochromatose *f,* Siderophilie *f,* Bronzediabetes *m.*
he·mo·chro·ma·tot·ic [ˌ-ˌkrəʊməˈtɒtɪk] *adj* Hämochromatose betr.
he·mo·chrome [ˈ-krəʊm] *n* Hämochrom *nt,* Hämochromogen *nt.*
he·mo·chro·mo·gen [ˌ-ˈkrəʊmədʒən] *n* → hemochrome.
he·mo·cla·sia [ˌ-ˈkleɪʒ(ɪ)ə] *n* 1. Hämoklasie *f.* 2. Erythroklasie *f.*
he·moc·la·sis [hɪˈmɒkləsɪs] *n* → hemoclasia.
he·mo·clas·tic crisis [ˌhiːməˈklæstɪk, ˌhem-] hämoklastische Krise *f.*
hemoclastic reaction hämoklastische Reaktion *f.*
he·mo·con·cen·tra·tion [ˌ-ˌkɒnsənˈtreɪʃn] *n hema.* Bluteindickung *f,* Hämokonzentration *f.*
he·mo·con·ges·tion [ˌ-kənˈdʒestʃn] *n* Blutstauung *f.*
he·mo·co·nia [ˌ-ˈkəʊnɪə] *pl* Blutstäubchen *pl,* Hämokonien *pl,* -konia *pl.*
he·mo·co·ni·o·sis [ˌ-ˌkəʊnɪˈəʊsɪs] *n* Hämokoniose *f.*
he·mo·cry·os·co·py [ˌ-kraɪˈɒskəpɪ] *n lab.* Gefrierpunktsbestimmung *f* des Blutes, Hämokryoskopie *f.*
he·mo·cul·ture [ˈ-kʌltʃər] *n micro.* Blutkultur *f.*
he·mo·cu·pre·in [ˌ-ˈkjuːprɪˌɪn] *n* Hämocuprein *nt,* Erythrocuprein *nt,* Superoxiddismutase *f abbr.* SOD.
he·mo·cy·a·nin [ˌ-ˈsaɪənɪn] *n* Hämocyanin *nt.*
he·mo·cyte [ˈ-saɪt] *n* Blutzelle *f,* Hämozyt *m.*
he·mo·cy·to·blast [ˌ-ˈsaɪtəblæst] *n* (Blut-)Stammzelle *f,* Hämozytoblast *m.*
he·mo·cy·to·blas·tic leukemia [ˌ-ˌsaɪtəˈblæstɪk] → hemoblastic leukemia.
he·mo·cy·to·blas·to·ma [ˌ-ˌsaɪtəblæsˈtəʊmə] *n hema.* Stammzelltumor *m,* Hämozytoblastom *nt.*

he·mo·cy·to·ca·ther·e·sis [ˌ-ˌsaɪtəkəˈθerəsɪs] *n* Blutzellenzerstörung *f.*
he·mo·cy·tol·y·sis [ˌ-saɪˈtɒləsɪs] *n* → hemolysis.
he·mo·cy·tom·e·ter [ˌ-saɪˈtɒmɪtər] *n lab.* Zählkammer *f,* Hämozytometer *nt.*
he·mo·cy·tom·e·try [ˌ-saɪˈtɒmətrɪ] *n* Hämozytometrie *f.*
he·mo·cy·to·pha·gia [ˌ-ˌsaɪtəˈfeɪdʒ(ɪ)ə] *n* Hämozytophagie *f,* Hämophagozytose *f.*
he·mo·cy·to·poi·e·sis [ˌ-ˌsaɪtəpɔɪˈiːsɪs] *n* → hemopoiesis.
he·mo·cy·to·trip·sis [ˌ-saɪtəˈtrɪpsɪs] *n* druckbedingte/traumatische Hämolyse *f.*
he·mo·cy·to·zo·on [ˌ-ˌsaɪtəˈzəʊɒn] *n, pl* **-zoa** [-ˈzəʊə] einzelliger Blutparasit *m,* Hämozytozoon *nt.*
he·mo·di·ag·no·sis [ˌhiːmədaɪəɡˈnəʊsɪs, ˌhem-] *n* Hämodiagnostik *f.*
he·mo·di·al·y·sis [ˌ-daɪˈæləsɪs] *n* Blutwäsche *f,* Hämodialyse *f;* extrakorporale Dialyse *f.*
he·mo·di·a·lyz·er [ˌ-ˈdaɪəlaɪzər] *n* Hämodialysator *m,* künstliche Niere *f.*
he·mo·di·a·stase [ˌ-ˈdaɪəsteɪz] *n* Blutamylase *f.*
he·mo·di·lu·tion [ˌ-daɪˈl(j)uːʃn, -dɪ-] *n* Blutverdünnung *f,* Hämodilution *f.*
he·mo·drom·o·graph [ˌ-ˈdrɒməɡræf] *n* Hämodromograph *m.*
he·mo·dro·mom·e·ter [ˌ-drəˈmɒmɪtər] *n* Hämodromometer *nt.*
he·mo·dy·nam·ic [ˌ-daɪˈnæmɪk] *adj* hämodynamisch.
he·mo·dy·nam·ics [ˌ-daɪˈnæmɪks] *pl* Hämodynamik *f.*
he·mo·dy·na·mom·e·ter [ˌ-daɪnəˈmɒmɪtər] *n* Blutdruckmeßgerät *nt,* -apparat *m;* Sphygmomanometer *nt.*
he·mo·dy·na·mom·e·try [ˌ-daɪnəˈmɒmɪtrɪ] *n* Blutdruckmessung *f.*
he·mo·dys·cra·sia [ˌ-dɪsˈkreɪʒ(ɪ)ə] *n* Hämato-, Hämodyskrasie *f.*
he·mo·dys·tro·phy [ˌ-ˈdɪstrəfɪ] *n* Hämodystrophie *f.*
he·mo·en·do·the·li·al placenta [ˌ-ˌendəˈθiːlɪəl] Placenta haemo-endothelialis.
he·mo·fer·rum [ˌ-ˈferəm] *n* Hämoglobineisen *nt.*
he·mo·fil·ter [ˈ-fɪltər] *n* Hämofilter *m/nt.*
he·mo·fil·tra·tion [ˌ-fɪlˈtreɪʃn] *n* Hämofiltration *f.*
he·mo·flag·el·late [ˌ-ˈflædʒəlɪt, -leɪt] *n micro.* Blutflagellat *m.*
he·mo·fus·cin [ˌ-ˈfjuːsɪn] *n* Hämofuscin *nt,* -fuszin *nt.*
he·mo·gen·e·sis [ˌ-ˈdʒenəsɪs] *n* → hemopoiesis.
he·mo·gen·ic [ˌ-ˈdʒenɪk] *adj* 1. → hematogenous. 2. → hemopoietic II.
he·mo·glo·bin [ˌ-ˈɡləʊbɪn] *n abbr.* **Hb** Blutfarbstoff *m,* Hämoglobin *nt abbr.* Hb.
hemoglobin A *abbr.* **HbA** Erwachsenenhämoglobin *nt,* Hämoglobin A *nt abbr.* HbA.
hemoglobin A$_{1c}$ *abbr.* **HbA$_{1c}$** Hämoglobin A$_{1c}$ *nt abbr.* HbA$_{1c}$.
hemoglobin A$_2$ *abbr.* **HbA$_2$** Hämoglobin A$_2$ *nt abbr.* HbA$_2$.
he·mo·glo·bin·at·ed [ˌ-ˈɡləʊbɪneɪtɪd] *adj* hämoglobinhaltig.
hemoglobin Bart's Hämoglobin Bart's *nt.*
hemoglobin C *abbr.* **HbC** Hämoglobin C *nt abbr.* HbC.
hemoglobin cast *urol.* Hämoglobinpräzipitat *nt,* -zylinder *m.*
hemoglobin C disease Hämoglobin-C-Krankheit *f.*
hemoglobin Chesapeake Hämoglobin Chesapeake *nt.*
hemoglobin C-thalassemia (disease)

Hämoglobin-C-Thalassämie *f,* HbC-Thalassämie *f.*
hemoglobin D *abbr.* **HbD** Hämoglobin D *nt abbr.* HbD.
hemoglobin disease Hämoglobinopathie *f.*
hemoglobin E *abbr.* **HbE** Hämoglobin E *nt abbr.* HbE.
he·mo·glo·bi·ne·mia [ˌ-ˌɡləʊbɪˈniːmɪə] *n* Hämoglobinämie *f.*
hemoglobin E-thalassemia (disease) Hämoglobin-E-Thalassämie *f,* HbE-Thalassämie *f.*
hemoglobin F *abbr.* **HbF** fetales Hämoglobin *nt,* Hämoglobin F *nt abbr.* HbF.
hemoglobin Gower Hämoglobin Gower *nt.*
hemoglobin H *abbr.* **HbH** Hämoglobin H *nt abbr.* HbH.
hemoglobin H disease Hämoglobin-H-Krankheit, HbH-Krankheit *f,* α-Thalassämie *f.*
hemoglobin I *abbr.* **HbI** Hämoglobin I *nt abbr.* HbI.
hemoglobin Kansas Hämoglobin Kansas *nt.*
hemoglobin Lepore Hämoglobin Lepore *nt.*
hemoglobin M *abbr.* **HbM** Hämoglobin M *abbr.* HbM.
he·mo·glo·bi·no·cho·lia [ˌ-ˌɡləʊbɪnəˈkəʊlɪə] *n* Hämoglobinocholie *f.*
he·mo·glo·bi·nol·y·sis [ˌ-ˌɡləʊbɪˈnɒləsɪs] *n* Hämoglobinabbau *m,* -spaltung *f,* Hämoglobinolyse *f.*
he·mo·glo·bi·nom·e·ter [ˌ-ˌɡləʊbɪˈnɒmɪtər] *n lab.* Hämoglobinometer *nt.*
he·mo·glo·bi·nom·e·try [ˌ-ˌɡləʊbɪˈnɒmətrɪ] *n lab.* Hämoglobinometrie *f.*
he·mo·glo·bi·nop·a·thy [ˌ-ˌɡləʊbɪˈnɒpəθɪ] *n* Hämoglobinopathie *f.*
he·mo·glo·bi·no·pep·sia [ˌ-ˌɡləʊbɪnəˈpepsɪə] *n* → hemoglobinolysis.
he·mo·glo·bi·nous [ˌ-ˈɡləʊbɪnəs] *adj* hämoglobinhaltig.
hemoglobin precipitate → hemoglobin cast.
hemoglobin precipitation Hämoglobinpräzipitation *f,* -ausfällung *f.*
hemoglobin Rainier Hämoglobin Rainier *nt.*
hemoglobin S *abbr.* **HbS** Sichelzellhämoglobin *nt,* Hämoglobin S *nt abbr.* HbS.
hemoglobin Seattle Hämoglobin Seattle *nt.*
he·mo·glo·bi·nu·ria [ˌhiːməˌɡləʊbɪˈn(j)ʊərɪə, ˌhem-] *n* Hämoglobinausscheidung *f* im Harn, Hämoglobinurie *f,* Haemoglobinuria *f.*
he·mo·glo·bi·nu·ric [ˌ-ˌɡləʊbɪˈn(j)ʊərɪk] *adj* Hämoglobinurie betr., durch Hämoglobinurie gekennzeichnet, hämoglobinurisch.
hemoglobinuric fever Schwarzwasserfieber *nt,* Febris biliosa et haemoglobinurica.
hemoglobinuric nephrosis hämoglobinurische Nephrose *f.*
hemoglobin Yakima Hämoglobin Yakima *nt.*
he·mo·gram [ˈ-ɡræm] *n hema.* Hämogramm *nt;* Differentialblutbild *nt.*
he·mo·his·ti·o·blast [ˌ-ˈhɪstɪəblæst] *n* Ferrata-Zelle *f,* Hämohistioblast *m.*
he·mo·his·ti·o·blas·tic syndrome [ˌ-ˌhɪstɪəˈblæstɪk] Retikuloendotheliose *f.*
he·mo·ki·ne·sis [ˌ-kɪˈniːsɪs, -kaɪ-] *n* Blutfluß *m,* -zirkulation *f,* Hämokinese *f.*
he·mo·ki·net·ic [ˌ-kɪˈnetɪk] *adj* den Blutfluß betr. *od.* fördernd, hämokinetisch.
he·mo·lith [ˈ-lɪθ] *n* Gefäßstein *m,* Angiolith *m,* Hämolith *m.*

hemology 348

he·mol·o·gy [hɪˈmalədʒɪ] n → hematology.
he·mo·lymph [ˈhiːməlɪmf, ˈhem-] n Hämolymphe f.
he·mo·lymph·an·gi·o·ma [ˌ-lɪmˌfændʒɪˈəʊmə] n hematolymphangioma.
he·mol·y·sate [hɪˈmaləseɪt] n Hämolysat nt.
he·mol·y·sin [hɪˈmaləsɪn, ˌhiːməˈlaɪsɪn, ˌhem-] n **1.** hämolyseverursachendes Toxin nt, Hämolysegift nt, Hämolysin nt. **2.** hämolyseauslösender Antikörper m, Hämolysin nt.
hemolysin unit Hämolysineinheit f.
he·mol·y·sis [hɪˈmaləsɪs] n Erythrozytenauflösung f, -zerstörung f, -abbau m, Hämolyse f, Hämatozytolyse f.
α-hemolysis n α-Hämolyse f, Alphahämolyse f.
β-hemolysis n β-Hämolyse f, Betahämolyse f.
γ-hemolysis n γ-Hämolyse f, Gammahämolyse f.
he·mo·lyt·ic [ˌhiːməˈlɪtɪk, ˌhem-] adj Hämolyse betr. od. auslösend, hämolytisch.
α-hemolytic adj alphahämolytisch, α-hämolytisch.
β-hemolytic adj betahämolytisch, β-hämolytisch.
γ-hemolytic adj γ-hämolytisch, gamma-hämolytisch, nicht-hämolytisch, nicht-hämolysierend.
hemolytic anemia hämolytische Anämie f.
  angiopathic h. angiopathische hämolytische Anämie.
  aquired h. erworbene hämolytische Anämie.
  autoimmune h. abbr. **AIHA** autoimmunhämolytische Anämie.
  autoimmune h., cold-antibody type autoimmunhämolytische Anämie mit Kälteantikörpern.
  autoimmune h., warm-antibody type autoimmunhämolytische Anämie mit Wärmeantikörpern.
  congenital h. kongenitale hämolytische Anämie.
  constitutional h. hereditäre Sphärozytose f, Kugelzell(en)anämie, Kugelzell(en)ikterus nt, familiärer hämolytischer Ikterus m, Morbus Minkowski-Chauffard m.
  immune h. immunhämolytische Anämie, serogene hämolytische Anämie, immunotoxisch-bedingte hämolytische Anämie.
  immune h., drug-induced medikamentös-induzierte immunhämolytische Anämie, medikamentös-induzierte immunologische hämolytische Anämie.
  infectious h. infektiöse/infektiös-bedingte hämolytische Anämie.
  microangiopathic h. Moschcowitz-Syndrom nt, Moschcowitz-Singer-Symmers-Syndrom nt, thrombotisch-thrombozytopenische Purpura f, thrombotische Mikroangiopathie f, Purpura Moschcowitz, Purpura thrombotica (thrombocytopenica).
  h. of the newborn → hemolytic disease of the newborn.
  nonspherocytic h. hämolytische Anämie ohne Sphärozyten.
  toxic h. toxische hämolytische Anämie.
hemolytic crisis hämolytische Krise f.
hemolytic disease of the newborn abbr. **HDN** fetale Erythroblastose f, Erythroblastosis fetalis, Morbus haemolyticus neonatorum abbr. MHN.
hemolytic icteroanemia Widal-Anämie f, -Ikterus m, Widal-Abrami-Anämie f, -Ikterus.
hemolytic icterus hämolytische Gelbsucht f, hämolytischer Ikterus m.

aquired h. Widal-Anämie f, -Ikterus, Widal-Abrami-Anämie f, -Ikterus.
congenital h. → hemolytic anemia, constitutional.
hemolytic jaundice → hemolytic icterus.
hemolytic malaria Schwarzwasserfieber nt, Febris biliosa et haemoglobinurica.
hemolytic plaque assay micro. Jerne--Technik f, (Hämolyse-)Plaquetechnik f.
hemolytic splenomegaly hämolytische Splenomegalie f.
hemolytic streptococci hämolytische Streptokokken pl.
β-hemolytic streptococci β-hämolytische Streptokokken pl.
hemolytic unit 1. Hämolysineinheit f. **2.** Komplementeinheit f.
hemolytic-uremic syndrome abbr. **HUS** Gasser-Syndrom nt, hämolytisch-urämisches Syndrom nt abbr. HUS.
he·mo·lyz·a·ble [ˌhiːməˈlaɪzəbl, ˌhem-] adj hämolysierbar.
he·mo·ly·za·tion [ˌ-laɪˈzeɪʃn] n Hämolyseauslösung f, -verursachung f.
he·mo·lyze [ˈ-laɪz] vt, vi hämolysieren.
he·mo·ma·nom·e·ter [ˌ-məˈnamɪtər] n Blutdruckmeßgerät nt, -apparat m; Sphygmomanometer nt.
he·mo·me·di·as·ti·num [ˌ-ˌmɪdɪəˈstaɪnəm] n Hämomediastinum nt.
he·mom·e·ter [hɪˈmamɪtər] n → hemoglobinometer.
he·mo·me·tra [ˌhiːməˈmiːtrə, ˌhem-] n → hematometra.
he·mom·e·try [hɪˈmamətrɪ] n → hematometry.
he·mo·ne·phro·sis [ˌhiːmənɪˈfrəʊsɪs, ˌhem-] n → hematonephrosis.
he·mo·nor·mo·blast [ˌ-ˈnɔːrməblæst] n Erythroblast m.
he·mo·pa·thol·o·gy [ˌ-pəˈθalədʒɪ] n Hämopathologie f.
he·mop·a·thy [hɪˈmapəθɪ] n Erkrankung f des Blutes od. der blutbildenden Gewebe, Hämopathie f.
he·mo·per·i·car·di·um [-ˈhiːməˌperɪˈkaːrdɪəm, ˌhemə-] n Blutansammlung f im Herzbeutel, Hämo-, Hämatoperikard nt.
he·mo·per·i·to·ne·um [ˌ-ˌperɪtəˈniːəm] n Blutansammlung f in der Bauchhöhle, Hämo-, Hämatoperitoneum nt.
he·mo·pex·in [ˌ-ˈpeksɪn] n Hämopexin f abbr. Hx.
he·mo·phage [ˈ-feɪdʒ] n → hemophagocyte.
he·mo·phag·o·cyte [ˌ-ˈfægəsaɪt] n Hämophagozyt m, Hämophage m.
he·mo·phag·o·cy·to·sis [ˌ-ˌfægəsaɪˈtəʊsɪs] n Hämophagozytose f, Hämozytophagie f.
he·mo·phil [ˈ-fɪl] **I** n hämophiler Mikroorganismus m. **II** adj micro. blutliebend, hämophil.
he·mo·phile [ˈ-faɪl] adj → hemophil II.
he·mo·phil·ia [ˌ-ˈfɪlɪə] n Bluterkrankheit f, Hämophilie f, Haemophilia f.
hemophilia A klassische Hämophilie f, Hämophilie A f, Faktor-VIII-Mangel m, Haemophilia vera.
hemophilia B Hämophilie B f, Faktor-IX--Mangel(krankheit f) m, Christmas--Krankheit f.
hemophilia C Faktor XI-Mangel, PTA--Mangel m.
he·mo·phil·i·ac [ˌ-ˈfɪlɪæk] n Bluter m, Hämophiler m.
he·mo·phil·ic [ˌ-ˈfɪlɪk] adj **1.** → hemophil II. **2.** Hämophilie betr., von Hämophilie betroffen, hämophil, Bluter-.
hemophilic arthritis/arthropathy Blutergelenk nt, hämophile Arthritis f, Arthropathia haemophilica.

hemophilic bacterium hämophiles Bakterium nt.
hemophilic joint → hemophilic arthritis.
he·mo·phil·i·oid [ˌ-ˈfɪlɪɔɪd] n Hämophilioid nt, Pseudohämophilie f.
He·moph·i·lus [hɪˈmafɪləs] n → Haemophilus.
he·mo·pho·bia [ˌhiːməˈfəʊbɪə, ˌhem-] n psychia. krankhafte Angst f vor Blut, Hämo-, Hämatophobie f.
he·moph·thal·mia [ˌhɪmafˈθælmɪə] n → hemophthalmus.
he·moph·thal·mos n → hemophthalmus.
he·moph·thal·mus [ˌ-ˈθælməs] n Bluterguß m ins Auge, Hämophthalmus m.
he·mo·pi·e·zom·e·ter [ˌhiːməˌpaɪəˈzamɪtər, ˌhem-] n Blutdruckmeßgerät nt, -apparat m.
he·mo·plas·tic [ˌ-ˈplæstɪk] adj → hematoplastic.
he·mo·pleu·ra [ˌ-ˈplʊərə] n → hemothorax.
he·mo·pneu·mo·per·i·car·di·um [ˌ-ˌn(j)uːməˌperɪˈkaːrdɪəm] n Hämopneumoperikard nt.
he·mo·pneu·mo·tho·rax [ˌ-ˌn(j)uːməˈθɔːræks] n Hämopneumothorax m.
he·mo·poi·e·sic [ˌ-pɔɪˈiːsɪk] n, adj → hemopoietic.
he·mo·poi·e·sis [ˌ-pɔɪˈiːsɪs] n Blutbildung f, Hämatopo(i)ese f, Hämopo(i)ese f.
he·mo·poi·et·ic [ˌ-pɔɪˈetɪk] **I** n hämopoesefördernes Mittel nt. **II** adj die Blut(zell)bildung betr. od. anregend, hämopoetisch.
hemopoietic tissue → hematopoietic tissue.
he·mo·poi·e·tin [ˌ-ˈpɔɪətɪn] n erythropoetischer Faktor m, Erythropo(i)etin nt, Hämato-, Hämopo(i)etin nt.
he·mo·por·phy·rin [ˌ-ˈpɔːrfərɪn] n → hematoporphyrin.
he·mo·pre·cip·i·tin [ˌ-prɪˈsɪpətɪn] n Hämopräzipitin nt.
he·mo·proc·tia [ˌ-ˈprakʃə] n Rektum-, Mastdarmblutung f, rektale Blutung f.
he·mo·pro·tein [ˌ-ˈprəʊtiːn, -tiːn] n Hämoprotein nt.
he·mop·so·nin [ˌhɪmapˈsəʊnɪn] n Hämopsonin nt.
he·mop·tic [hɪˈmaptɪk] adj → hemoptysic.
he·mop·to·ic [hɪmapˈtəʊɪk] adj → hemoptysic.
he·mop·ty·sic [ˌhɪmapˈtaɪsɪk] adj Bluthusten/Hämoptyse betr., durch Bluthusten gekennzeichnet.
he·mop·ty·sis [hɪˈmaptəsɪs] n Bluthusten nt, -spucken nt, Hämoptoe f, Hämoptyse f, Haemoptysis f.
he·mo·py·e·lec·ta·sia [ˌhiːməpaɪəlekˈteɪʒ(ɪ)ə, ˌhem-] n urol. Hämopyelektasie f.
he·mo·py·el·ec·ta·sis [ˌ-paɪəˈlektəsɪs] n → hemopyelectasia.
hem·o·rhe·ol·o·gy [ˌ-rɪˈalədʒɪ] n → hemorheology.
he·mor·rha·chis [hɪˈmarəkɪs] n **1.** → hematomyelia. **2.** → hematorrhachis.
hem·or·rhage [ˈhemərɪdʒ, ˈhemrɪdʒ] **I** n Blutung f, Einblutung f, Hämorrhagie f, Haemorrhagia f. **II** vi (schwach), bluten, sickern.
hem·or·rha·gen·ic [ˌhemərəˈdʒenɪk] adj Blutung/Hämorrhagie auslösend od. verursachend.
hem·or·rhag·ic [ˌheməˈrædʒɪk] adj Blutung betr., durch Blutung gekennzeichnet, hämorrhagisch, Blutungs-.
hemorrhagic anemia (akute) Blutungsanämie f, akute (post-)hämorrhagische Anämie f.
hemorrhagic ascites hämorrhagischer/blutiger Aszites m, Hämaskos m.
hemorrhagic bronchitis hämorrhagische

Bronchitis *f*, Bronchitis haemorrhagica, Bronchospirochaetosis Castellani.
hemorrhagic cyst hämorrhagische Zyste *f*.
hemorrhagic cystitis hämorrhagische (Harn-)Blasenentzündung/Zystitis *f*, Cystitis haemorrhagica.
hemorrhagic dengue Dengue-hämorrhagisches Fieber *nt*.
hemorrhagic diathesis Blutungsneigung *f*, hämorrhagische Diathese *f*.
hemorrhagic disease of the newborn hämorrhagische Diathese *f* der Neugeborenen, Morbus haemorrhagicus neonatorum, Melaena neonatorum vera.
hemorrhagic encephalitis hämorrhagische Enzephalitis *f*, Encephalitis haemorrhagica.
hemorrhagic enteropathy hämorrhagische Enteropathie *f*.
hemorrhagic exudative erythema Schoenlein-Henoch-Syndrom *nt*, (anaphylaktoide) Purpura Schoenlein-Henoch *f*, rheumatoide Purpura *f*, Immunkomplexpurpura *f*, -vaskulitis *f*, Purpura anaphylactoides/rheumatica (Schoenlein-Henoch), athrombopenische Purpura *f*.
hemorrhagic fever *abbr.* **HF** hämorrhagisches Fieber *nt abbr.* HF.
African h. afrikanisches hämorrhagisches Fieber.
Argentine/Argentinean h. argentinisches hämorrhagisches Fieber, Juninfieber.
Bolivian h. *abbr.* **BHF** bolivianisches hämorrhagisches Fieber *abbr.* BHF, Madungofieber.
Congo-Crimean h. → Crimean h.
Crimean h. Kongo-Krim-Fieber, hämorrhagisches Krim-Fieber.
Crimean-Congo h. → Crimean h.
dengue h. Dengue-hämorrhagisches Fieber.
Ebola h. Ebola-Fieber, Ebola hämorrhagisches Fieber.
epidemic h. → h. with renal syndrome.
Far Eastern h. → h. with renal syndrome.
Korean h. → h. with renal syndrome.
Lassa h. Lassafieber.
Manchurian h. → h. with renal syndrome.
Omsk h. *abbr.* **OHF** Omsk hämorrhagisches Fieber *abbr.* OHF.
Philippine h. → dengue h.
h. with renal syndrome *abbr.* **HFRS** hämorrhagisches Fieber mit renalem Syndrom *abbr.* HFRS, koreanisches hämorrhagisches Fieber, akute hämorrhagische Nephrosonephritis *f*, Nephropathia epidemica.
Thai h. → dengue h.
viral h. 1. → hemorrhagic fever. 2. → Ebola h.
hemorrhagic gastritis hämorrhagische Gastritis *f*, Gastritis haemorrhagica.
hemorrhagic gingivitis hämorrhagische Gingivitis *f*.
hemorrhagic glaucoma hämorrhagisches Glaukom *nt*, Glaucoma haemorrhagicum/apoplecticum.
hemorrhagic infarct hämorrhagischer/roter Infarkt *m*.
hemorrhagic infarction hämorrhagische Infarzierung *f*.
h. of small intestine hämorrhagische Dünndarminfarzierung *f*.
hemorrhagic inflammation hämorrhagische Entzündung *f*.
hemorrhagic iritis *ophthal.* hämorrhagische Iritis *f*.
hemorrhagic measles hämorrhagische Masern *pl*.
hemorrhagic metropathy hämorrhagische Metropathie *f*, Metropathia haemorrhagica.
hemorrhagic myelitis hämorrhagische Myelitis/Myelopathie *f*.
hemorrhagic myelopathy hämorrhagische Myelopathie *f*.
hemorrhagic necrotizing bronchopneumonia hämorrhagisch-nekrotisierende Bronchopneumomie *f*.
hemorrhagic necrotizing pancreatitis hämorrhagisch-nekrotisierende Pankreatitis *f*.
hemorrhagic necrotizing pneumonia → hemorrhagic necrotizing bronchopneumonia.
hemorrhagic necrotizing tracheitis hämorrhagisch-nekrotisierende Tracheitis *f*.
hemorrhagic nephritis hämorrhagische Nephritis *f*, Nephritis haemorrhagica.
hemorrhagic oozing Sickerblutung *f*.
hemorrhagic pachymeningitis Pachymeningitis/Pachymeningiosis *f* haemorrhagica interna.
hemorrhagic pericarditis hämorrhagische Perikarditis *f*, Pericarditis haemorrhagica.
hemorrhagic peritonitis hämorrhagische Bauchfellentzündung/Peritonitis *f*.
hemorrhagic pian Peruwarze *f*, Verruga peruana.
hemorrhagic plague hämorrhagische Beulenpest/Bubonenpest *f*.
hemorrhagic pleurisy hämorrhagische Brustfellentzündung/Pleuritis *f*, Pleuritis haemorrhagica.
hemorrhagic pneumonia hämorrhagische Pneumonie *f*.
hemorrhagic polioencephalitis, superior Wernicke'-Enzephalopathie *f*, -Syndrom *nt*, Polioencephalitis haemorrhagica superior (Wernicke).
hemorrhagic pulmonary infarction hämorrhagischer Lungeninfarkt *m*.
hemorrhagic retinopathy hämorrhagische Retinopathie/Retinitis *f*, Retinitis/Retinopathia haemorrhagica.
hemorrhagic rickets rachitischer Säuglingskorbut *m*, Möller-Barlow-Krankheit *f*.
hemorrhagic scurvy → hemorrhagic rickets.
hemorrhagic shock hämorrhagischer Schock *m*, Blutungsschock *m*.
hemorrhagic thrombocythemia hämorrhagische/essentielle Thrombozythämie *f*, Megakaryozytenleukämie *f*, megakaryozytäre Myelose *f*.
hem·or·rhag·in [ˌheməˈrædʒɪn, -ˈreɪdʒ-] *n* Hämorrhagin *nt*.
hem·or·rha·gip·a·rous [ˌheməˌrɪˈdʒɪpərəs] *adj* → hemorrhagic.
hem·or·rhea [ˌheməˈriə] *n* 1. → hematorrhea 1. 2. → hemoptysis.
he·or·rhe·ol·o·gy [ˌ-rɪˈɑlədʒɪ] *n* Hämo(r)rheologie *f*.
hem·or·rhoid [ˈhemərɔɪd] *sing* → hemorrhoids.
hem·or·rhoi·dal [ˌ-ˈrɔɪdl] *adj* Hämorrhoiden betr., hämorrhoidal, hämorrhoidenähnlich, Hämorrhoidal-.
hemorrhoidal artery: inferior h. untere Mastdarm-/Rektumarterie *f*, Rektalis *f* inferior, A. rectalis inferior.
middle h. mittlere Mastdarm-/Rektumarterie *f*, Rektalis *f* media, A. rectalis media.
superior h. obere Mastdarm-/Rektumarterie *f*, Rektalis *f* superior, A. rectalis superior.
hemorrhoidal nerves, inferior untere Rektal-/Analnerven *pl*, Nn. rectales inferiores, Nn. anales/h(a)emorrhoidales inferiores.
hemorrhoidal plexus rektaler Venenplexus *m*, Hämorrhoidalplexus *m*, Plexus h(a)emorrhoidalis, Plexus venosus rectalis.
middle h. Plexus h(a)emorrhoidalis medius, Plexus rectalis medius.
superior h. Plexus h(a)emorrhoidalis superior, Plexus rectalis superior.
hemorrhoidal thrombosis Hämorrhoidenthrombose *f*, -thrombosierung *f*.
hemorrhoidal vein: inferior h.s untere Mastdarm-/Rektumvenen *pl*, Vv. rectales inferiores.
middle h.s mittlere Mastdarm-/Rektumvenen *pl*, Vv. rectales mediae.
superior h. obere Rektumvene *f*, V. rectalis superior.
hemorrhoidal zone Hämorrhoidalzone *f*, -ring *m*, Zona h(a)emorrhoidalis.
hem·or·rhoid·ec·to·my [ˌheməɹɔɪˈdektəmɪ] *n chir.* Hämorrhoidenexzision *f*, Hämorrhoidektomie *f*.
hem·or·rhoids [ˈhemərɔɪds] *pl* Hämorrhoiden *pl*.
he·mo·sal·pinx [ˌhiːməˈsælpɪŋks, ˌhem-] *n* → hematosalpinx.
he·mo·sid·er·in [ˌ-ˈsɪdərɪn] *n* Hämosiderin *nt*.
he·mo·sid·er·in·u·ria [ˌ-ˌsɪdərɪnˈ(j)ʊərɪə] *n* Hämosiderinausscheidung *f* im Harn, Hämosiderinurie *f*.
he·mo·sid·er·o·sis [ˌ-sɪdəˈrəʊsɪs] *n* Hämosiderose *f*.
he·mo·site [ˈheməʊsaɪt] *n old* Blutparasit *m*.
he·mo·sper·mia [ˌhiːməˈspɜrmɪə, ˌhem-] *n urol.* Hämato-, Hämospermie *f*.
he·mo·spo·ri·an [ˌ-ˈspɔːriæn, -ˈspəʊr-] I *n* Hämosporidie *f*. II *adj* Hämosporidien betr.
hem·o·spo·rid·i·an [ˌ-spəˈrɪdiæn] *n*, *adj* → hemosporian.
he·mo·sta·sia [ˌ-ˈsteɪʒ(ɪ)ə, -ziə] *n* → hemostasis.
he·mos·ta·sis [hɪˈmɑstəsɪs, ˌhiːməˈsteɪsɪs, ˌhem-] *n* 1. Blut(ungs)stillung *f*, Hämostase *f*. 2. Blutstauung *f*, -stockung *f*, (Hämo-)Stase *f*.
he·mo·stat [ˈhiːməstæt, ˈhem-] *n* 1. (Blut-)Gefäßklemme *f*, -klammer *f*, Arterienklemme *f*, -klammer *f*. 2. topisches Hämostatikum *nt*.
he·mo·stat·ic [ˌ-ˈstætɪk] I *n* Blutstillungsmittel *nt*, blutstillendes Mittel *nt*, Hämostatikum *nt*, Hämostyptikum *nt*. II *adj* Hämostase betr., blut(ungs)stillend, hämostatisch, hämostyptisch.
he·mo·styp·tic [ˌ-ˈstɪptɪk] *n*, *adj* → hemostatic.
he·mo·ta·chom·e·ter [ˌ-tæˈkɑmɪtər] *n* Hämato-, Hämatochometer *nt*.
he·mo·ther·a·peu·tics [ˌ-θerəˈpjuːtɪks] *pl* → hemotherapy.
he·mo·ther·a·py [ˌ-ˈθerəpɪ] *n* Bluttherapie *f*, Hämato-, Hämotherapie *f*; Transfusionstherapie *f*.
he·mo·tho·rax [ˌ-ˈθɔːræks] *n* Blutbrust *f*, Hämo-, Hämatothorax *m*.
he·mo·tox·ic [ˌ-ˈtɑksɪk] *adj* hämotoxisch.
hemotoxic anemia (hämo-)toxische Anämie *f*.
he·mo·tox·in [ˌ-ˈtɑksɪn] *n* Hämotoxin *nt*.
he·mo·troph [ˈ-trɑf, -trəʊf] *n gyn.* Gesamtheit *f* der mütterlichen Nährstoffe.
he·mo·trophe *n* → hemotroph.
he·mo·trop·ic [ˌ-ˈtrɑpɪk, -ˈtrəʊp-] *adj* hämato-, hämotrop.
he·mo·tym·pa·num [ˌ-ˈtɪmpənəm] *n HNO* Bluterguß *m* in die Paukenhöhle, Hämo-, Hämatotympanon *nt*.
he·mo·zo·ic [ˌ-ˈzəʊɪk] *adj* Blutparasiten betr., Blutparasiten-.

hemozoin

he·mo·zo·in [ˌ-'zəʊɪn] *n* Hämozoin *nt*.
he·mo·zo·on [ˌ-'zəʊɒn] *n*, *pl* **-zo·a** [-'zəʊə] *micro.* (ein- *od.* vielzelliger) Blutparasit *m*, Hämozoon *nt*.
HEMPAS antigen HEMPAS-Antigen *nt*.
HEMPAS cell HEMPAS-Zelle *f*.
hen·bane ['henbeɪn] *n* → hyoscyamus.
Henderson-Hasselbalch ['hendərsən 'hæslbælk]: **H.-H. equation** Henderson--Hasselbalch-Gleichung *f*.
Henderson-Jones ['dʒəʊnz]: **H.-J. disease/syndrome** Henderson-Jones-Syndrom *nt*, Reichel-Syndrom, polytope Gelenkchondromatose *f*.
Henle ['henli:, -lə] : **H.'s ampulla** Samenleiterampulle *f*, Ampulla ductus deferentis.
  H.'s canal → H.'s loop.
  crural canal of H. Schenkel-, Adduktorenkanal *m*, Canalis adductorius.
  external tuber of H. Tuberculum mentale.
  H.'s fenestrated (elastic) membrane Membrana elastica interna.
  H.'s fiber Henle'-Fortsatz *m*.
  H.'s layer (*Haar*) Henle'-Schicht *f*, -Membran *f*.
  H.'s ligament Leistensichel *f*, Falx inguinalis, Tendo conjunctivus.
  H.'s loop Henle'-Schleife *f*.
  H.'s membrane Lamina basalis.
  palatine incisure of H. Inc. sphenopalatina (ossis palatini).
  restiform process of H. unterer Kleinhirnstiel *m*, Pedunculus cerebellaris caudalis/inferior.
  scapular tuberosity of H. Proc. coracoideus.
  H.'s sheath Endoneurium *nt*.
  H.'s sphincter Henle-Sphinkter *m*.
  spine of H. Spina suprameatica/suprameatalis.
hen·na ['henə] *n pharm.* Henna *f/nt*.
Hennebert [en'bɛr]: **H.'s (fistula) sign/test** Hennebert'-Fistelsymptom *nt*.
Henoch ['henəʊk; 'henɔx]: **H.'s disease** → Henoch-Schönlein purpura.
  H.'s purpura 1. → Henoch-Schönlein purpura. **2.** Purpura Henoch, Purpura fulminans.
Henoch-Schönlein ['ʃeɪnlaɪn; 'ʃøːn-]: **H.-S. purpura/syndrome** Schoenlein--Henoch-Syndrom *nt*, (anaphylaktoide) Purpura Schoenlein-Henoch *f*, rheumatoide/athrombopenische Purpura *f*, Immunkomplexpurpura *f*, Immunkomplexvaskulitis *f*, Purpura anaphylactoides (Schoenlein-Henoch), Purpura rheumatica (Schoenlein-Henoch).
hen·o·gen·e·sis [ˌhenəʊ'dʒenəsɪs] *n* Ontogenese *f*.
hen·pu·ye [hen'pjuːjɪ] *n* Gundu-, Goundou-Syndrom *nt*.
Henry ['henrɪ] : **H.'s law** Henry'-Absorptionsgesetz *nt*.
hen·ry ['henrɪ] *n abbr.* **H** Henry *nt abbr.* **H**.
Henry-Gauer [gaʊər]: **H.-G. reflex** Henry--Gauer-Reflex *m*.
Hensen ['hensn]: **H.'s canal** → H.'s duct.
  H.'s cells → supporting cells of H.
  H.'s disk H-Bande *f*, H-Streifen *m*, H-Zone *f*, helle Zone *f*, Hensen'-Zone *f*.
  H.'s duct Hensen'-Gang *m*, -Kanal *m*, Ductus reuniens.
  H.'s knot → H.'s node.
  H.'s line → H.'s disk.
  H.'s node *embryo.* Primitivknoten *m*.
  supporting cells of H. Hensen'-(Stütz-)Zellen *pl*.
he·pad·na·vi·rus·es [həˌpædnə'vaɪrəsəs] *pl micro.* Hepadnaviren *pl*, Hepadnaviridae *pl*.
he·par ['hiːpær] *n anat.* Leber *f*, Hepar *nt*.
hep·a·ran-α-glucosaminide acetyltransferase ['hepəræn] Acetyl-CoA:α-Glukosamid-*N*-Acetyltransferase *f*.
heparan *N*-sulfatase Heparan-*N*-sulfatase *f*.
heparan sulfate Heparansulfat *nt*.
heparan sulfate sulfamidase → heparan--*N*-sulfatase.
heparan sulfate sulfatase → heparan--*N*-sulfatase.
hep·a·rin ['hepərɪn] *n* Heparin *nt*.
hep·a·rin·ase ['hepəreɪz] *n* Heparinase *f*, Heparinlyase *f*.
hep·a·rin·ate ['hepəreɪt] *n* Heparinat *nt*.
heparin eliminase → heparinase.
hep·a·rin·e·mia [ˌhepərɪ'niːmɪə] *n* Heparinämie *f*.
hep·a·rin·ic acid [hepə'rɪnɪk] → heparin.
hep·a·rin·i·za·tion [ˌhepərɪnə'zeɪʃn] *n* Heparinisieren *nt*, Heparinisierung *f*.
hep·a·rin·ize ['hepərɪnaɪz] *vt* mit Heparin behandeln *od.* versetzen, heparinisieren.
heparin lyase → heparinase.
hep·a·rin·oid ['hepərɪnɔɪd] *n* Heparinoid *nt*.
hep·a·ri·tin sulfate ['hepərɪtɪn] → heparan sulfate.
hepat- *pref.* → hepato-.
hep·a·tal·gi·a [hepə'tældʒ(ɪ)ə] *n* Leberschmerz *m*, Hepatalgie *f*, Hepatodynie *f*.
hep·a·ta·tro·phia [hepətə'trəʊfɪə] *n* Leberatrophie *f*.
hep·a·tat·ro·phy [hepə'tætrəfɪ] *n* → hepatatrophia.
hep·a·tec·to·mize [ˌhepə'tektəmaɪz] *vt chir.* eine Hepatektomie durchführen, hepatektomieren.
hep·a·tec·to·my [hepə'tektəmɪ] *n chir.* Leberentfernung *f*, -resektion *f*, Hepatektomie *f*.
hepatic- *pref.* → hepatico-.
he·pat·ic [hɪ'pætɪk] *adj* **1.** Leber/Hepar betr., zur Leber gehörig, hepatisch, Leber-, Hepat(o)-. **2.** rotbraun.
hepatic abscess Leberabszeß *m*.
  amebic h. Amöbenabszeß.
  bacterial h. bakterieller Leberabszeß.
  candidal h. Candidaabszeß.
  cryptogenic h. kryptogener Leberabszeß.
  pyelophlebitic h. pyelophlebitischer Leberabszeß.
  pyogenic h. pyogener/metastatisch-pyämischer Leberabszeß.
  traumatic h. posttraumatischer Leberabszeß.
hepatic amebiasis/amebiosis Amöbenhepatitis *f*, Leberamöbiasis *f*.
hepatic arteriography *radiol.* Arteriographie *f* der A. hepatica propria.
hepatic artery Leberarterie *f*, Hepatika *f*, Hepatica *f* propria, A. hepatica propria.
  common h. Hepatica *f* communis, A. hepatica communis.
  proper h. → hepatic artery.
hepatic artery aneurysm Aneurysma *nt* der A. hepatica propria.
hepatic artery ligation *chir.* Ligatur *f* der A. hepatica propria.
hepatic artery-portal venous fistula *patho.* Fistel *f* zwischen A. hepatica u. V. portae, A. hepatica-V. portae-Fistel *f*, Hepatica-Porta-Fistel *f*.
hepatic bed of gallbladder Gallenblasengrube *f*, -bett *nt*, Leberbett *nt*, Fossa vesicae felleae/biliaris.
hepatic branches of vagus nerve Leberäste *pl* des N. vagus, Rami hepatici (n. vagi).
hepatic capsulitis *n* Entzündung *f* der Leberkapsel, Perihepatitis *f*.
hepatic cell, (parenchymal) Leber(epithel)zelle *f*, Hepatozyt *m*, Leberparenchymzelle *f*.

hepatic cell adenoma Leberzelladenom *nt*.
hepatic circulation Leberkreislauf *m*.
hepatic cirrhosis Leberzirrhose *f*, Cirrhosis hepatis.
  hypertrophic h. primär biliäre Zirrhose *abbr.* **PBZ**, nicht-eitrige destruierende Cholangitis *f*.
hepatic colic Gallenkolik *f*, Colica hepatica.
hepatic coma Leberkoma *nt*, hepatisches Koma *nt*, Coma hepaticum.
  endogenous h. Leberzerfallskoma, endogenes Leberkoma.
  exogenous h. Leberausfallskoma, exogenes Leberkoma.
hepatic cords Leber(zell)bälkchen *pl*.
hepatic crisis *neuro.* hepatische Krise *f*, Leberkrise *f*.
hepatic cyst Leberzyste *f*.
hepatic diverticulum *embryo.* Leberdivertikel *nt*.
hepatic duct: common h. gemeinsamer Gallengang *m* der Leberlappen, Hepatikus *m*, Hepaticus *m*, Ductus hepaticus communis.
  left h. linker (Leber-)Gallengang *m*, Ductus hepaticus sinister.
  right h. rechter (Leber-)Gallengang *m*, Ductus hepaticus dexter.
hepatic duct bifurcation *chir.*, *radiol.* Hepaticusbifurkation *f*, -gabel *f*.
hepatic dystrophy *patho.* Leberdystrophie *f*.
  acute h. akute Leberdystrophie.
  acute yellow h. akute gelbe Leberdystrophie.
  subacute h. subakute Leberdystrophie.
  subacute red h. subakute rote Leberdystrophie.
hepatic edema hepatogenes Ödem *nt*.
hepatic encephalopathy hepatische/portosystemische Enzephalopathie *f*, hepatozerebrales Syndrom *nt*, Encephalopathia hepatica *f*.
hepatic failure Leberinsuffizienz *f*, -versagen *nt*.
  fulminant h. perakute Leberinsuffizienz.
hepatic fibrosis Leberfibrose *f*.
  periportal h. periportale Leberfibrose.
hepatic flexure of colon rechte Kolonflexur *f*, Flexura hepatica coli, Flexura coli dextra.
hepatic function test Leberfunktionstest *m*.
hepatic funiculus → hepatocystic duct.
h. of Rauber *old* → hepatic artery.
hepatic glands Schleimdrüsen *pl* der Gallengänge, Gll. biliares.
hepatic graft Lebertransplantat *nt*.
hepatic infantilism hepatischer Infantilismus *m*.
hepatic injury Leberverletzung *f*, -trauma *nt*.
hepatic insufficiency Leberinsuffizienz *f*, -versagen *nt*.
hepatic laceration *chir.* Leber(ein)riß *m*.
hepatic ligaments Leberbänder *pl*, Ligg. hepatis.
hepatic lobe Leberlappen *m*, Lobus hepatis.
  left h. linker Leberlappen, Lobus hepatis sinister.
  right h. rechter Leberlappen, Lobus hepatis dexter.
hepatic lobectomy *chir.* Leberlappenresektion *f*, Leberlobektomie *f*.
hepatic lobules Leberläppchen *pl*, Lobuli hepatis.
hepatic metastasis Lebermetastase *f*.
hepatic necrosis *patho.* Leber(zell)nekrose *f*.

hepatico- *pref.* Hepatikus-, Hepaticus-, Hepatiko-.
he·pat·i·co·cho·lan·gi·o·en·te·ros·to·my [hɪˌpætɪkəʊkəʊˌlændʒɪəentə'rɒstəmɪ] *n chir.* Hepatikocholangioenterostomie *f.*
he·pat·i·co·cho·lan·gi·o·je·ju·nos·to·my [ˌ-kəʊˌlændʒɪədʒɪdʒuː'nɒstəmɪ] *n chir.* Hepatikocholangiojejunostomie *f.*
he·pat·i·co·cho·led·o·chos·to·my [-kəˌledə'kɒstəmɪ] *n chir.* Hepatikocholedochostomie *f.*
he·pat·i·co·do·chot·o·my [ˌ-də'kɒtəmɪ] *n chir.* Hepatikodochotomie *f.*
he·pat·i·co·du·o·de·nos·to·my [ˌ-d(j)uːədɪ'nɒstəmɪ] *n chir.* Hepatikoduodenostomie *f.*
he·pat·i·co·en·ter·os·to·my [ˌ-entə'rɒstəmɪ] *n chir.* Hepatikoenterostomie *f.*
he·pat·i·co·gas·tros·to·my [ˌ-gæs'trɒstəmɪ] *n chir.* Hepatikogastrostomie *f.*
he·pat·i·co·je·ju·nos·to·my [ˌ-dʒɪdʒuː'nɒstəmɪ] *n chir.* Hepatikojejunostomie *f.*
Hep·a·tic·o·la [hepə'tɪkjələ] *n micro.* Capillaria *f.*
he·pat·i·co·li·a·sis [hɪˌpætɪkəʊ'laɪəsɪs] *n* **1.** Capillaria-Infektion *f,* Capillariasis *f.* **2.** intestinale Capillariasis *f,* Capillariasis philippinensis.
he·pat·i·co·li·thot·o·my [ˌ-lɪ'θɒtəmɪ] *n chir.* Hepatikolithotomie *f.*
he·pat·i·co·lith·o·trip·sy [ˌ-'lɪθətrɪpsɪ] *n chir.* Hepatikolithotripsie *f.*
he·pat·i·co·pan·cre·at·ic duct [ˌ-ˌpæŋkrɪ'ætɪk] → hepatopancreatic duct.
hepatic ophthalmia Ophthalmia hepatica.
he·pat·i·co·pul·mo·nar·y [ˌ-'pʌlmə‚nerɪː, -nərɪ] *adj* → hepatopneumonic.
he·pat·i·cos·to·my [hɪˌpætɪ'kɒstəmɪ] *n chir.* Hepatikostomie *f.*
he·pat·i·cot·o·my [hɪˌpætɪ'kɒtəmɪ] *n chir.* Hepatikotomie *f.*
hepatic phosphorylase deficiency Hers-Erkrankung, -Syndrom *nt,* Glykogenose *f,* Leberphosphorylaseinsuffizienz *f,* Glykogenose Typ VI *f.*
hepatic phosphorylase kinase deficiency hepatische Glykogenose *f,* Glykogenose Typ VIII *f,* Phosphorylase-b-kinase-Insuffizienz *f.*
hepatic plexus Plexus hepaticus.
hepatic porphyria hepatische Porphyrie *f,* Porphyria hepatica.
hepatic portal Leberpforte *f,* Porta hepatis.
hepatic portoenterostomy *chir.* intrahepatische Cholangiojejunostomie *f,* Hepato(porto)enterostomie *f.*
hepatic pulse Leberpuls *m.*
hepatic resection Leberresektion *f,* -teilentfernung *f.*
   major h. subtotale Leberresektion.
   radical h. radikale Leberresektion, Dreiviertelresektion.
hepatic schistosomiasis hepatolienale Schistosomiasis *f.*
hepatic segments Lebersegmente *pl,* Segmenta hepatis.
hepatic siderosis *patho.* Lebersiderose *f,* Siderose *f* der Leber.
hepatic toxicity → hepatotoxicity.
hepatic transplant Lebertransplantat *nt.*
hepatic transplantation Lebertransplantation *f.*
hepatic trauma Leberverletzung *f,* -trauma *nt.*
hepatic triad Glisson'-Trias *f.*
hepatic tumor Lebertumor *m,* -geschwulst *f.*
   mixed h. → hepatoblastoma.
hepatic veins Leber(binnen)venen *pl,* Vv. hepaticae.
   intermediate h. Venen aus dem Lobus cau-

datus, Vv. hepaticae intermediae.
   left h. Venen aus dem linken Leberlappen, Vv. hepaticae sinistrae.
   middle h. → intermediate h.
   right h. Venen aus dem rechten Leberlappen, Vv. hepaticae dextrae.
hepatic vessels Lebergefäße *pl.*
hep·a·tin ['hepətɪn] *n* Glykogen *nt,* tierische Stärke *f.*
hep·a·tism ['hepətɪzəm] *n* Gesundheitsverschlechterung *f* durch Leberleiden, Hepatismus *m.*
hep·a·tit·ic [hepə'tɪtɪk] *adj* Hepatitis betr., hepatitisch, Hepatitis-.
hep·a·ti·tis [hepə'taɪtɪs] *n* Leberentzündung *f,* Hepatitis *f.*
hepatitis A *abbr.* **HA** (Virus-)Hepatitis A *f abbr.* HA, epidemische Hepatitis *f,* Hepatitis epidemica.
hepatitis antigen → hepatitis B surface antigen.
hepatitis-associated antigen *abbr.* **HAA** → hepatitis B surface antigen.
hepatitis A virus *abbr.* **HAV** Hepatitis-A-Virus *nt abbr.* HAV.
hepatitis B *abbr.* **HB** (Virus-)Hepatitis B *f abbr.* HB, Serumhepatitis *f.*
hepatitis B core antigen *abbr.* **HB$_c$Ag** Hepatitis-B-Kernantigen *nt,* Hepatitis B core-Antigen *nt abbr.* HB$_c$Ag.
hepatitis B DNA polymerase *abbr.* **HBDNAP** Hepatitis-B-DNA-polymerase *f abbr.* HBDNAP.
hepatitis B e antigen *abbr.* **HB$_e$Ag** Hepatitis-B$_e$-Antigen *nt,* Hepatitis B e-Antigen *nt abbr.* HB$_e$Ag.
hepatitis B immune globulin *abbr.* **HBIG** Hepatitis-B-Immunglobulin *nt abbr.* HBIG.
hepatitis B surface antigen *abbr.* **HB$_s$Ag** Australiaantigen *nt,* Hepatitis B surface--Antigen *nt abbr.* HB$_s$Ag, HB$_s$-Antigen *nt,* Hepatits B-Oberflächenantigen *nt.*
hepatitis B vaccine Hepatitis-B-Vakzine *f,* HB-Vakzine *f.*
hepatitis B virus *abbr.* **HBV** Hepatitis-B--Virus *nt abbr.* HBV.
hepatitis C virus Hepatitis-C-Virus *nt,* Non-A-Non-B-Hepatitis-Virus *nt,* NANB-Hepatitisvirus *nt.*
hepatitis D Deltahepatitis *f,* Hepatitis D *f.*
hepatitis delta antigen *abbr.* **HDAg** (Hepatitis-)Deltaantigen *nt abbr.* HDAg.
hepatitis delta virus *abbr.* **HDV** Deltaagens *nt,* Hepatitis-Delta-Virus *nt abbr.* HDV.
hepatitis virus Hepatitisvirus *nt.*
   non-A,non-B h. → hepatitis C virus.
hep·a·ti·za·tion [ˌhepətɪ'zeɪʃn, -taɪ-] *n patho.* Hepatisation *f.*
hepato- *pref.* Leber-, Hepat(o)-.
hep·a·to·bil·i·ar·y [ˌhepətəʊ'bɪliˌerɪ, -'bɪljərɪ] *adj* Leber/Hepar u. Galle *od.* Gallenblase betr., hepatobiliär.
hepatobiliary capsule Glisson'-Kapsel *f,* Capsula fibrosa perivascularis.
hep·a·to·blas·to·ma [ˌ-blæs'təʊmə] *n patho.* Lebermischtumor *nt,* Hepatoblastom *nt.*
hep·a·to·bron·chi·al [ˌ-'brɒŋkɪəl] *adj* Leber/Hepar u. Bronchus betr. *od.* verbindend, hepatobronchial.
hepatobronchial fistula *patho.* Leber--Bronchus-Fistel *f,* hepatobronchiale Fistel *f.*
hep·a·to·car·cin·o·gen·ic [ˌ-ˌkɑːrsɪnə'dʒenɪk] *adj patho.* Leberkrebs verursachend.
hep·a·to·car·ci·no·ma [ˌ-ˌkɑːrsɪ'nəʊmə] *n* → hepatocellular carcinoma.
hep·a·to·car·di·ac channel [ˌ-'kɑːrdɪæk] *embryo.* Leber-Herz-Kanal *m.*

he·pat·o·cele [hɪ'pætəsiːl] *n patho.* Leberbruch *m,* Hepatozele *f.*
hep·a·to·cel·lu·lar [ˌhepətəʊ'seljələr] *adj* Leberzelle(n) betr., hepatozellulär, Leberzell(en)-.
hepatocellular adenoma Leberzelladenom *nt.*
hepatocellular carcinoma (primäres) Leberzellkarzinom *nt,* hepatozelluläres Karzinom *nt,* malignes Hepatom *nt,* Ca. hepatocellulare.
hepatocellular cholestasis hepatozelluläre/intrahepatische Gallestauung/Cholestase *f.*
hepatocellular jaundice hepatozellulärer Ikterus *m,* Parenchymikterus *m.*
hepatocellular necrosis Leber(zell)nekrose *f.*
hep·a·to·ce·re·bral [ˌ-'serebrəl, -sə'riːb-] *adj* Leber/Hepar u. Großhirn/Cerebrum betr., hepatozerebral.
hep·a·to·cho·lan·ge·i·tis [ˌ-kəʊlændʒɪ'aɪtɪs] *n patho.* Entzündung *f* von Leber u. Gallengängen, Hepatocholangitis *f.*
hep·a·to·cho·lan·gi·o·car·ci·no·ma [ˌ-kəʊˌlændʒɪəʊˌkɑːrsɪ'nəʊmə] *n patho.* Cholangiohepatom(a) *nt,* Hepatocholangiokarzinom *nt.*
hep·a·to·cho·lan·gi·o·du·o·de·nos·to·my [ˌ-kəʊˌlændʒɪəʊˌd(j)uːədɪ'nɒstəmɪ] *n chir.* Hepatocholangioduodenostomie *f.*
hep·a·to·cho·lan·gi·o·en·ter·os·to·my [ˌ-kəʊˌlændʒɪəʊˌentə'rɒstəmɪ] *n chir.* Hepatocholangioenterostomie *f.*
hep·a·to·cho·lan·gi·o·gas·tros·to·my [ˌ-kəʊˌlændʒɪəʊgæs'trɒstəmɪ] *n chir.* Hepatocholangiogastrostomie *f.*
hep·a·to·cho·lan·gi·o·je·ju·nos·to·my [ˌ-kəʊˌlændʒɪəʊdʒɪdʒuː'nɒstəmɪ] *n chir.* Hepatocholangiojejunostomie *f.*
hep·a·to·cho·lan·gi·os·to·my [ˌ-kəʊˌlændʒɪ'ɒstəmɪ] *n chir.* Hepatocholangiostomie *f.*
hep·a·to·cho·lan·gi·tis [ˌ-kəʊlæn'dʒaɪtɪs] *n* → hepatocholangeitis.
hep·a·to·cir·rho·sis [ˌ-sɪ'rəʊsɪs] *n* Leberzirrhose *f,* Cirrhosis hepatis.
hep·a·to·col·ic [ˌ-'kɒlɪk, -'kəʊ-] *adj* Leber/Hepar u. Kolon betr., hepatokolisch.
hepatocolic ligament Lig. hepatocolicum.
hep·a·to·cu·pre·in [ˌ-'kjuːpriːɪn] *n* **1.** Hämatocuprein *nt.* **2.** → hemocuprein.
hep·a·to·cys·tic [ˌ-'sɪstɪk] *adj* Leber/Hepar u. Gallenblase betr., hepatobiliär.
hepatocystic duct Choledochus *m,* Ductus choledochus/biliaris.
hep·a·to·cyte ['hepətəsaɪt] *n* Leber(epithel)zelle *f,* Leberparenchymzelle *f,* Hepatozyt *m.*
hep·a·to·du·o·de·nal [ˌ-ˌd(j)uə'diːnl, -ˌd(j)uː'ɒdnəl] *adj* Leber/Hepar u. Zwölffingerdarm/Duodenum betr., hepatoduodenal.
hepatoduodenal ligament Lig. hepatoduodenale.
hep·a·to·du·o·de·nos·to·my [ˌ-ˌd(j)uːədɪ'nɒstəmɪ] *n* **1.** → hepaticoduodenostomy. **2.** → hepatocholangioduodenostomy.
hep·a·to·dyn·i·a [ˌ-'diːnɪə] *n* → hepatalgia.
hep·a·to·dys·tro·phy [ˌ-'dɪstrəfɪ] *n patho.* akute gelbe Leberdystrophie *f.*
hep·a·to·en·ter·ic [ˌ-en'terɪk] *adj* Leber u. Darm betr., hepatointestinal, hepatoenteral, hepatointestinal.
hep·a·to·en·ter·os·to·my [ˌ-entə'rɒstəmɪ] *n* **1.** → hepaticoenterostomy. **2.** → hepatocholangioenterostomy.
hep·a·tof·u·gal [hepə'tæfjəgəl] *adj* von der Leber weg(fließend *od.* gerichtet), hepatofugal.
hep·a·to·gas·tric [ˌhepətəʊ'gæstrɪk] *adj* Leber/Hepar u. Magen/Gaster betr., hepatogastral, -ventrikulär.

hepatogastric ligament

hepatogastric ligament Lig. hepatogastricum.
hep·a·to·gen·ic [ˌ-'dʒenɪk] *adj* **1.** *embryo.* Lebergewebe bildend, hepatogen. **2.** von der Leber ausgehend, in der Leber entstanden, hepatogen.
hepatogenic jaundice hepatogener/hepatischer Ikterus *m*.
hep·a·tog·e·nous [hepə'tadʒənəs] *adj* → hepatogenic.
hepatogenous jaundice → hepatogenic jaundice.
hepatogenous pigment hepatogenes Pigment *nt*.
hep·a·to·gram ['hepətəgræm] *n* **1.** *radiol.* Hepatogramm *nt*, Kontrastaufnahme *f* der Leber. **2.** Lebersphygmogramm *nt*.
hep·a·tog·ra·phy [hepə'tagrəfɪ] *n* **1.** *radiol.* Kontrastdarstellung *f* der Leber, Hepatographie *f*. **2.** Lebersphygmographie *f*.
hep·a·to·he·mia [ˌhepətə'hi:mɪə] *n* Leberstauung *f*.
hep·a·toid ['hepətɔɪd] *adj* leberähnlich, -artig, hepatoid.
hep·a·to·jug·u·lar reflex/reflux [ˌhepətəʊ-'dʒʌgjələr] *card.* hepatojugulärer Reflux *m*.
hep·a·to·len·tic·u·lar degeneration/disease [ˌ-len'tɪkjələr] Wilson-Krankheit *f*, -Syndrom *nt*, Morbus Wilson *m*, hepatolentikuläre/hepatozerebrale Degeneration *f*.
hep·a·to·li·e·nal [ˌ-laɪ'i:nl, -'laɪənl] *adj* Leber/Hepar u. Milz/Lien betr., hepatolienal.
hepatolienal fibrosis Banti-Krankheit *f*, -Syndrom *nt*.
hepatolienal hemopoiesis hepatolienale Blutbildung/Hämopo(i)ese *f*.
hepatolienal phase *hema.* Phase *f* der hepatolienalen Blutbildung.
hep·a·to·li·e·nog·ra·phy [ˌ-ˌlaɪə'nagrəfɪ] *n* radiol. Hepatolienographie *f*, Hepatosplenographie *f*; Splenoportographie *f*.
hep·a·to·li·e·no·meg·a·ly [ˌ-ˌlaɪənə'megəlɪ] *n* → hepatosplenomegaly.
hep·a·to·lith ['-lɪθ] *n* Leberstein *m*, intrahepatischer Gallenstein *m*, Hepatolith *m*.
hep·a·to·li·thec·to·my [ˌ-lɪ'θektəmɪ] *n* chir. Hepatolithentfernung *f*, Hepatolithektomie *f*.
hep·a·to·li·thi·a·sis [ˌ-lɪ'θaɪəsɪs] *n* patho. Hepatolithiasis *f*.
hep·a·tol·o·gist [hepə'talədʒɪst] *n* Hepatologe *m*, -login *f*.
hep·a·tol·o·gy [hepə'talədʒɪ] *n* Hepatologie *f*.
hep·a·tol·y·sin [hepə'talɪsɪn] *n* patho. Leberzellen-zerstörendes Zytolysin *nt*, Hepatolysin *m*.
hep·a·tol·y·sis [hepə'taləsɪs] *n* patho. Leberzellzerstörung *f*, Hepatolyse *f*.
hep·a·to·lyt·ic [hepə'lɪtɪk] *adj* Hepatolyse betr. *od.* auslösend, hepatolytisch.
hep·a·to·ma [hepə'təʊmə] *n* (primärer) Lebertumor *m*, Hepatom(a) *nt*.
hep·a·to·ma·la·cia [ˌhepətəmə'leɪʃ(ɪ)ə] *n* patho. Lebererweichung *f*, Hepatomalazie *f*, -malacia *f*.
hep·a·to·me·ga·lia [ˌ-mɪ'geɪlɪə] *n* → hepatomegaly.
hep·a·to·meg·a·ly [ˌ-'megəlɪ] *n* Lebervergrößerung *f*, -schwellung *f*, Hepatomegalie *f*.
hep·a·to·mel·a·no·sis [ˌ-melə'nəʊsɪs] *n* patho. Hepatomelanose *f*, -melanosis *f*.
hep·a·tom·e·try [hepə'tamətrɪ] *n* Bestimmung *f* der Lebergröße, Hepatometrie *f*.
hep·a·tom·pha·lo·cele [hepə'tamfələsi:l] *n* chir. Hepatomphalozele *f*.
hep·a·tom·pha·los [hepə'tamfələs] *n* embryo., patho. Hepatomphalos *m*.

hep·a·to·ne·cro·sis [ˌhepətənɪ'krəʊsɪs] *n* Leber(zell)nekrose *f*.
hep·a·to·neph·ric [ˌ-'nefrɪk] *adj* → hepatorenal.
hepatonephric syndrome → hepatorenal syndrome.
hep·a·to·ne·phrit·ic [ˌ-nɪ'frɪtɪk] *adj* Hepatonephritis betr., hepatonephritisch.
hep·a·to·ne·phri·tis [ˌ-nɪ'fraɪtɪs] *n* patho. Hepatonephritis *f*.
hep·a·to·neph·ro·meg·a·ly [ˌ-ˌnefrə'megəlɪ] *n* patho. Vergrößerung/Schwellung *f* von Leber u. Niere(n), Hepatonephromegalie *f*.
hep·a·to·pan·cre·at·ic [ˌ-ˌpænkrɪ'ætɪk, -ˌpæŋ-] *adj* Leber/Hepar u. Bauchspeicheldrüse/Pancreas betr., hepatopankreatisch.
hepatopancreatic ampulla Vater'-Ampulle *f*, Ampulla hepatopancreatica.
hepatopancreatic duct Wirsung'-Gang *m*, -kanal *m*, Pankreasgang *m*, Ductus pancreaticus.
accessory h. Ductus pancreaticus accessorius.
hepatopancreatic fold Plica hepaticopancreatica.
hep·a·to·path ['-pæθ] *n* Patient(in *f*) *m* mit Lebererkrankung, Leberkranke(r *m*) *f*.
hep·a·to·path·ic [ˌ-'pæθɪk] *adj* leberschädigend, hepatopathisch.
hep·a·top·a·thy [hepə'tapəθɪ] *n* Lebererkrankung *f*, -leiden *nt*, Hepatopathie *f*, Hepatopathia *f*.
hep·a·to·per·i·to·ni·tis [ˌhepətəˌperɪtə'naɪtɪs] *n* Entzündung *f* der Leberkapsel, Perihepatitis *f*.
hep·a·top·e·tal [hepə'tapətəl] *adj* zur Leber hin(fließend *od.* gerichtet), hepatopetal.
hep·a·to·pex·y ['hepətəpeksɪ] *n* chir. Leberfixierung *f*, -anheftung *f*, Hepatopexie *f*.
hep·a·to·phle·bi·tis [ˌ-flɪ'baɪtɪs] *n* Lebervenenentzündung *f*, Hepatophlebitis *f*.
hep·a·to·phle·bog·ra·phy [ˌ-flɪ'bagrəfɪ] *n* radiol. Leber-, Hepatophlebographie *f*.
hep·a·to·phos·pho·ryl·ase deficiency glycogenosis [ˌ-fas'fɔrəleɪz, -'farə-] Hers'-Erkrankung *f*, -Syndrom *nt*, -Glykogenose *f*, Leberphosphorylaseinsuffizienz *f*, Glykogenose Typ VI *f*.
hep·a·to·pleu·ral [ˌ-'plʊərəl] *adj* Leber/Hepar u. Pleura *od.* Pleurahöhle betr. *od.* verbindend, hepatopleural.
hepatopleural fistula Leber-Pleurahöhlen-Fistel *f*, hepatopleurale Fistel *f*.
hep·a·to·pneu·mon·ic [ˌ-n(j)u:'manɪk] *adj* Leber/Hepar und Lunge(n) betr. *od.* verbindend, hepatopulmonal.
hep·a·to·por·tal [ˌ-'pɔ:rtl, -'pəʊr-] *adj* Leberpforte *od.* Pfortader(system) betr., hepatoportal.
hep·a·to·por·to·en·ter·os·to·my [ˌ-ˌpɔ:rtəˌentə'rastəmɪ] *n* → hepatic portoenterostomy.
hep·a·top·to·sis [ˌhepətap'təʊsɪs] *n* **1.** Lebersenkung *f*, -tiefstand *m*, Wanderleber *f*, Hepar migrans/mobile, Hepatoptose *f*. **2.** Chilaiditi-Syndrom *nt*, Interpositio coli/hepatodiaphragmatica.
hep·a·to·pul·mo·nar·y [ˌhepətə'pʌlmə-ˌneri:, -nərɪ] *adj* → hepatopneumonic.
hep·a·to·re·nal [ˌ-'ri:nl] *adj* Leber/Hepar u. Niere/Ren betr., hepatorenal.
hepatorenal glycogenosis (von) Gierke'-Krankheit *f*, van Creveld-von Gierke'-Krankheit *f*, hepatorenale Glykogenose *f*, Glykogenose Typ I.
hepatorenal glycogen storage disease → hepatorenal glycogenosis.
hepatorenal ligament Lig. hepatorenale.

hepatorenal pouch → hepatorenal recess.
hepatorenal recess hepatorenale Peritonealgrube *f*, Rec. hepatorenalis.
hepatorenal syndrome hepatorenales Syndrom *nt*.
hepatorenal tyrosinemia hereditäre/hepatorenale Tyrosinämie *f*, Tyrosinose *f*.
hep·a·tor·rha·gia [ˌ-'reɪdʒ(ɪ)ə] *n* Leberblutung *f*, Lebereinblutung *f*, Hepatorrhagie *f*.
hep·a·tor·rha·phy [hepə'tɔrəfɪ] *n* chir. Lebernaht *f*, Hepatorrhaphie *f*.
hep·a·tor·rhea [ˌhepətə'rɪə] *n* übermäßiger Galle(n)fluß *m*, übermäßige Galle(n)ausscheidung *f*, Cholorrhoe *f*.
hep·a·tor·rhex·is [ˌ-'reksɪs] *n* Leberriß *m*, -ruptur *f*, Hepatorrhexis *f*.
hep·a·tos·co·py [hepə'taskəpɪ] *n* (direkte) Leberuntersuchung *f*, Hepatoskopie *f*.
hep·a·to·sis [hepə'təʊsɪs] *n* funktionelle Lebererkrankung/Leberschädigung *f*, Hepatose *f*.
hep·a·to·sple·ni·tis [ˌhepətəsplɪ'naɪtɪs] *n* Entzündung *f* von Leber u. Milz, Hepatosplenitis *f*.
hep·a·to·sple·nog·ra·phy [ˌ-splɪ'nagrəfɪ] *n* → hepatolienography.
hep·a·to·sple·no·meg·a·ly [ˌ-ˌsplɪnə'megəlɪ] *n* Vergrößerung/Schwellung *f* von Leber u. Milz, Hepatosplenomegalie *f*.
hep·a·to·sple·nop·a·thy [ˌ-splɪ'napəθɪ] *n* kombinierte Erkrankung *f* von Leber u. Milz, Hepatosplenopathie *f*.
hep·a·tos·to·my [hepə'tastəmɪ] *n* chir. Hepatostomie *f*.
hep·a·to·ther·a·py [ˌhepətə'θerəpɪ] *n* **1.** Behandlung *f* von Lebererkrankheiten, Hepatotherapie *f*. **2.** Behandlung *f* mit Leberpräparaten, Hepatotherapie *f*.
hep·a·tot·o·my [hepə'tatəmɪ] *n* chir. Leberschnitt *m*, Hepatotomie *f*.
hep·a·to·tox·e·mia [ˌhepətətak'si:mɪə] *n* Autotoxämie *f* bei Leberversagen, Hepatotoxämie *f*.
hep·a·to·tox·ic [ˌ-'taksɪk] *adj* leber(zell)-schädigend, hepatotoxisch.
hep·a·to·tox·ic·i·ty [ˌ-tak'sɪsətɪ] *n* Lebergiftigkeit *f*, -schädlichkeit *f*, Hepatotoxizität *f*.
hep·a·to·tox·in [ˌ-'taksɪn] *n* Lebergift *nt*, hepatotoxische Substanz *f*, Hepatotoxin *nt*.
hep·a·to·trop·ic [ˌ-'trapɪk, -'trəʊp-] *adj* Lebergewebe bevorzugend, hepatotrop.
hep·a·to·um·bil·i·cal ligament [ˌ-ʌm'bɪlɪkl] Lig. teres hepatis.
hep·a·tox·ic [hepə'taksɪk] *adj* → hepatotoxic.
hept(a)- *pref.* sieben-, hept(a)-.
hep·tad ['heptæd] *n chem.* siebenwertiges Element *nt*.
hep·ta·dac·tyl·ia [ˌheptədæk'tɪlɪə] *n* → heptadactyly.
hep·ta·dac·ty·lism [ˌ-'dæktəlɪzəm] *n* → heptadactyly.
hep·ta·dac·ty·ly [ˌ-'dæktəlɪ] *n* embryo. Polydaktylie *f* mit sieben Fingern *od.* Zehen, Heptadaktylie *f*.
hep·ta·ene ['heptəwi:n] *n chem.* Heptaen *nt*.
hep·tam·i·nol [hep'tæmɪnɒl] *n pharm.* Heptaminol *nt*.
hep·tane ['heptein] *n chem.* Heptan *nt*.
hep·ta·pep·tide [ˌheptə'peptaɪd] *n* Heptapeptid *nt*.
hep·ta·tom·ic [ˌ-'tamɪk] *adj* → heptavalent.
hep·ta·va·lent [ˌ-'veɪlənt] *adj chem.* siebenwertig, heptavalent.
hep·tose ['heptəʊs] *n* Heptose *f*.
hep·to·su·ria [ˌheptə's(j)ʊərɪə] *n* Heptoseausscheidung *f* im Harn, Heptosurie *f*.

hep·tu·lose ['heptəlʊs, 'heptʃə-] n Ketoheptose f, Heptulose f.
hep·tyl·pen·i·cil·lin [ˌheptɪlˌpenəˈsɪlɪn] n pharm. Heptylpenicillin nt, Penicillin K nt, Penicillin IV nt.
herb [(h)ɜrb] n 1. bio. Kraut nt. 2. pharm. (Heil-)Kraut nt.
her·ba·ceous [(h)ɜrˈbeɪʃəs] adj krautartig, krautig, Kraut-, Kräuter-.
her·bal [(h)ɜrbl] I n Kräuter-, Pflanzenbuch nt. II adj Kräuter od. Pflanzen betr., Kräuter-, Pflanzen-.
her·bi·cide ['(h)ɜrbəsaɪd] n Pflanzen-, Unkrautvernichtungsmittel nt, Herbizid nt.
her·bi·vore ['hɜrbəvɔːr, -vʊr] n bio. Pflanzen-, Krautfresser m, Herbivore f.
her·biv·o·rous [(h)ɜrˈbɪvərəs] adj bio. pflanzen-, krautfressend.
herd instinct [hɜrd] psycho. Herdentrieb m.
he·red·i·ta·bil·i·ty [həˌredɪtəˈbɪlətɪ] n Erblichkeit f, Vererbbarkeit f.
he·red·i·ta·ble [həˈredɪtəbl] adj → heritable.
he·red·i·tar·y [həˈredɪterɪ] adj ererbt, vererbt, erblich, erbbedingt, Erb-; angeboren.
hereditary allergy atopische Allergie f.
hereditary amyloidosis familiäre/hereditäre Amyloidose f.
hereditary angioedema abbr. HAE hereditäres Angioödem nt, hereditäres Quincke-Ödem nt.
hereditary angioneurotic edema abbr. HANE → hereditary angioedema.
hereditary areflexic dysstasia/dystasia Roussy-Lévy-Syndrom nt, erbliche areflektorische Dysstasie f.
hereditary ataxia Heredoataxie f.
hereditary ataxic dysstasia/dystasia → hereditary areflexic dysstasia.
hereditary benign intraepithelial dyskeratosis (syndrome) derm. hereditäre benigne intraepitheliale Dyskeratose f.
hereditary cerebral leukodystrophy Pelizaeus-Merzbacher-Krankheit f, -Syndrom nt, sudanophile Leukodystrophie f Typ Pelizaeus-Merzbacher, orthochromatische Leukodystrophie f.
hereditary chorea Erbchorea f, Chorea Huntington, Chorea chronica progressiva hereditaria.
hereditary deforming chondrodysplasia Ollier'-Erkrankung f, -Syndrom nt, Enchondromatose f, multiple kongenitale Enchondrome pl, Hemichondrostrophie f.
hereditary deforming chondrodystrophy → hereditary multiple exostoses.
hereditary disease/disorder hereditäre/ erbliche Erkrankung f, Erbkrankheit f, -leiden nt.
hereditary dystopic lipidosis Fabry-Syndrom nt, Morbus Fabry m, hereditäre Thesaurismose Ruiter-Pompen-Weyers f, Ruiter-Pompen-Weyers-Syndrom nt, Thesaurismosis hereditaria lipoidica, Angiokeratoma corporis diffusum (Fabry), Angiokeratoma universale.
hereditary ectodermal polydysplasia derm. anhidrotisch ektodermale Dysplasie f, ektodermale (kongenitale) Dysplasie f, Christ-Siemens-Syndrom nt, Guilford-Syndrom nt, Jacquet'-Syndrom nt, Anhidrosis hypotrichotica/congenita.
hereditary elliptocytosis hereditäre Elliptozytose f, Ovalo-, Kamelozytose f, Elliptozytenanämie f.
hereditary essential tremor hereditärer/ essentieller Tremor m.
hereditary familial/family ataxia spinale/ spinozerebellare Heredoataxie f, Heredoataxia spinalis, Friedreich-Ataxie f.
hereditary fragility of bone Osteogenesis imperfecta, Osteopsathyrosis f.
hereditary hemiplegia angeborene/hereditäre Hemiplegie f.
hereditary hemorrhagic telangiectasia hereditäre Teleangiektasie f, Morbus Osler m, Rendu-Osler-Weber-Krankheit f, -Syndrom nt, Osler-Rendu-Weber-Krankheit f, -Syndrom nt, Teleangiectasia hereditaria haemorrhagica.
hereditary hemorrhagic thrombasthenia Glanzmann-Naegeli-Syndrom nt, Thrombasthenie f.
hereditary hypersegmentation of neutrophils hema. Hereditär-Anomalie f.
hereditary hypertrophic neuropathy Déjérine-Sottas-Krankheit f, -Syndrom nt, hereditäre motorische u. sensible Neuropathie Typ III f abbr. HMSN, hypertrophische Neuropathie (Déjérine-Sottas) f.
hereditary lymphedema hereditäres/kongenitales Lymphödem/Trophödem nt.
hereditary methemoglobinemic cyanosis enzymopathische/hereditäre Methämoglobinämie f.
hereditary multiple exostoses multiple kartilaginäre Exostosen pl, hereditäre multiple Exostosen pl, multiple Osteochondrome pl, Ecchondrosis ossificans.
hereditary multiple trichoepithelioma Trichoepitheliom f, Brooke'-Krankheit f, multiple Trichoepitheliome pl, Trichoepithelioma papulosum multiplex, Epithelioma adenoides cysticum.
hereditary opalescent dentin dent. Capdepont-Zahndysplasie f, -Syndrom nt, Stainton-Syndrom nt, Glaszähne pl, Dentinogenesis imperfecta hereditaria.
hereditary progressive arthro-ophthalmopathy erbliche progressive Arthro-Ophthalmopathie f, Stickler-Syndrom nt.
hereditary pseudohemophilia (von) Willebrand-Jürgens-Syndrom nt, konstitutionelle Thrombopathie f, hereditäre/ vaskuläre Pseudohämophilie f, Angiohämophilie f.
hereditary spherocytosis Minkowski--Chauffard(-Gänsslen)-Syndrom nt, hereditäre Sphärozytose f, konstitutionelle hämolytische Kugelzellanämie f, familiärer hämolytischer Ikterus m, Morbus Minkowski-Chauffard m.
hereditary trait erbliche Belastung f.
hereditary transmission 1. Vererbung f, Erbgang m. **2.** Erblichkeit f, Heredität f.
hereditary trophedema → hereditary lymphedema.
hereditary tyrosinemia hereditäre/hepatorenale Tyrosinämie f, Tyrosinose f.
hereditary vitelliform dystrophy ophthal. kongenitale Makuladegeneration f.
he·red·i·ty [həˈredətɪ] n, pl **-ties** 1. Heredität f, Erblichkeit f, Vererbbarkeit f. 2. Vererbung f, Erbgang m. 3. Erbmasse f, ererbte Anlagen pl, Erbanlagen pl.
her·e·do·a·tax·ia [ˌherədoʊəˈtæksɪə] n neuro. Heredoataxie f.
her·e·do·de·gen·er·a·tion [ˌ-dɪˌdʒenəˈreɪʃn] n 1. Heredodegeneration f. 2. Nonne-Marie-Krankheit f, (Pierre) Marie-Krankheit f, zerebellare Heredoataxie f, Heredoataxia cerebellaris.
her·e·do·di·ath·e·sis [ˌ-daɪˈæθəsɪs] n patho. erblich-bedingte/hereditäre Veranlagung f, erblich-bedingte/hereditäre Prädisposition f.
her·e·do·fa·mil·ial [ˌ-fəˈmɪljəl] adj heredofamiliär.

heredofamilial amyloidosis → hereditary amyloidosis.
heredofamilial tremor hereditärer/essentieller Tremor m.
her·e·do·lu·es [ˌ-ˈluːˌiːz] n angeborene/ kongenitale Syphilis f, Lues connata/ congenita, Syphilis connata/congenita.
her·e·do·mac·u·lar degeneration [ˌ-ˈmækjələr] hereditäre Makuladegeneration f.
her·e·do·path·ia [ˌ-ˈpæθɪə] n Erbkrankheit f, -leiden nt, Heredopathie f, -pathia f.
her·e·do·syph·i·lis [ˌ-ˈsɪfəlɪs] n → heredolues.
Hérelle → d'Hérelle.
He·rel·lea vaginicola [hɪˈrelɪə] → Acinetobacter calcoaceticus.
Hering ['heɪrɪŋ, 'heː-]: **H.'s afterimage** ophthal., physiol. Hering'-Nachbild nt.
canals of H. Hering'-Kanälchen pl.
H.'s nerve Hering'-Blutdruckzügler m, Karotissinusnerv m, Ramus sinus carotici n. glossopharyngei.
H.'s sinus nerve → H.'s nerve.
H.'s test ophthal. Hering-Test m.
H.'s theory Hering'-Farbentheorie f, Gegenfarbentheorie f.
Hering-Breuer ['brɔyər]: **H.-B. reflex** Hering-Breuer-Reflex m.
her·it·a·bil·i·ty [ˌherɪtəˈbɪlətɪ] n 1. Erblichkeit f, Heritabilität f. 2. Erblichkeitsgrad m, Heritabilität f.
her·it·a·ble ['herɪtəbl] adj vererbbar, erblich, hereditär, Erb-.
Herlitz ['hɜrlɪts]: **H.'s disease** Herlitz-Syndrom nt, kongenitaler nicht-syphilitischer Pemphigus m, Epidermolysis bullosa (hereditaria) letalis, Epidermolysis bullosa atrophicans generalisata gravis Herlitz.
Hermansky-Pudlak ['hɜrmænskɪ 'pudlæk]: **H.-P. syndrome** abbr. HPS Hermansky-Pudlak-Syndrom nt.
her·maph·ro·dism [hɜrˈmæfrədɪzəm] n → hermaphroditism.
her·maph·ro·dite [hɜrˈmæfrədaɪt] I n Hermaphrodit m, Zwitter m. II adj → hermaphroditic.
her·maph·ro·dit·ic [hɜrˌmæfrəˈdɪtɪk] adj zwittrig, hermaphroditisch, zwitterhaft, Zwitter-.
her·maph·ro·di·tism [hɜrˈmæfrədaɪtɪzəm] n Zwittrigkeit f, Zwittertum nt, Hermaphroditismus m, Hermaphrodismus m.
her·maph·ro·di·tis·mus [hɜrˌmæfrədaɪˈtɪzməs] n → hermaphroditism.
her·met·ic [hɜrˈmetɪk] adj hermetisch, dicht(verschlossen); luftdicht.
her·nia ['hɜrnɪə] n, pl **-nias**, **-niae** [-nɪiː] patho., chir. (Eingeweide-)Bruch m, Hernie f, Hernia f.
h. of bladder Blasenhernie, -bruch, -vorfall m, Zystozele f, Cystocele f.
h. of liver Leberbruch, Hepatozele f.
hernia knife → herniotome.
her·ni·al ['hɜrnɪəl] adj Hernie betr., Hernien-, Hernio-, Bruch-.
hernial canal Bruchkanal m, -pforte f.
hernial hydrocele Hydrocele hernialis.
hernial sac Bruchsack m.
hernia sac Bruchsack m.
her·ni·at·ed disk ['hɜrnɪeɪtɪd] → herniation of intervertebral disk.
her·ni·a·tion [ˌhɜrnɪˈeɪʃn] n 1. Bruch-, Hernienbildung f, Herniation f. 2. Einklemmung f, Herniation f.
h. of intervertebral disk Bandscheibenvorfall m, -prolaps m, -hernie f, Hernia disci intervertebralis.
h. of nucleus pulposus Nucleus-pulposus--Vorfall m.
hernio- pref. Bruch-, Hernien-, Hernio-

her·ni·o·ap·pen·dec·to·my [ˌhɜrnɪəˌæpən-'dektəmɪ] *n chir.* kombinierte Appendektomie *f* u. Herniotomie.
her·ni·o·en·te·rot·o·my [ˌ-ˌentə'rɑtəmɪ] *n chir.* kombinierte Herniotomie *f* u. Enterotomie.
her·ni·og·ra·phy [hɜrnɪ'ɑgrəfɪ] *n radiol.* Herniographie *f.*
her·ni·oid ['hɜrnɪɔɪd] *adj* hernienähnlich, -artig.
her·ni·o·lap·a·rot·o·my [ˌhɜrnɪəˌlæpə'rɑtəmɪ] *n chir.* Herniolaparotomie *f.*
her·ni·o·plas·ty ['-plæstɪ] *n chir.* Hernien-, Hernioplastik *f.*
her·ni·o·punc·ture [ˌ-'pʌŋkʃər] *n chir.* Hernienpunktion *f.*
her·ni·or·rha·phy [ˌhɜrnɪ'ɔrəfɪ] *n chir.* Hernienoperation *f*, Herniorrhaphie *f.*
her·ni·o·tome ['hɜrnɪətəʊm] *n chir.* Bruchmesser *nt*, Herniotom *nt.*
her·ni·ot·o·my [ˌhɜrnɪ'ɑtəmɪ] *n chir.* Hernien-, Bruchoperation *f*, Herniotomie *f.*
her·o·in ['herəʊɪn] *n pharm.* Heroin *nt*, Dia(cetyl)morphin *nt.*
herp·an·gi·na [hɜrpæn'dʒaɪnə] *n* Herpangina *f*, Zahorsky-Syndrom *nt*, Angina herpetica.
herpangina viruses Herpanginaviren *pl.*
her·pes ['hɜrpi:z] *n* 1. Herpes *m*. 2. → herpes genitalis. 3. → herpes simplex.
herpes B virus Herpes-B-Virus *nt*, Herpesvirus simiae.
herpes encephalitis Herpesenzephalitis *f*, Herpes-simplex-Enzephalitis *f*, HSV-Enzephalitis *f.*
herpes febrilis Fieberbläschen *nt*, Herpes simplex der Lippen, Herpes febrilis/labialis.
herpes genitalis Herpes genitalis.
herpes infection Herpesinfektion *f.*
herpes labialis → herpes febrilis.
herpes ophthalmicus → herpes zoster ophthalmicus.
herpes progenitalis → herpes genitalis.
herpes sepsis/septicemia Herpessepsis *f.*
herpes simplex Herpes simplex.
herpes simplex encephalitis → herpes encephalitis.
herpes simplex virus *abbr.* **HSV** Herpes-simplex-Virus *nt abbr.* HSV, Herpesvirus huminis *abbr.* HVH.
herpes simplex virus encephalitis → herpes encephalitis.
herpes simplex virus type I Herpes-simplex-Virus Typ I *abbr.* HSV-I, HSV-Typ I *m.*
herpes simplex virus type II Herpes-simplex-Virus Typ II *abbr.* HSV-II, HSV-Typ II *m.*
Her·pes·vir·i·dae [ˌhɜrpi:s'vɪrɪdi:, -'vaɪr-] *pl* Herpesviren *pl*, Herpesviridae *pl.*
Her·pes·vi·rus [ˌ-vaɪrəs] *n micro.* Herpesvirus *nt.*
her·pes·vi·rus [ˌ-'vaɪrəs] *n micro.* Herpesvirus *nt.*
herpesvirus simiae → herpes B virus.
herpes zoster Gürtelrose *f*, Zoster *m*, Zona *f*, Herpes zoster.
herpes zoster auricularis Genikulatumneuralgie *f*, Ramsay Hunt-Syndrom *nt*, Zoster oticus, Herpes zoster oticus, Neuralgia geniculata.
herpes zoster ophthalmicus Zoster ophthalmicus, Herpes zoster ophthalmicus.
herpes zoster oticus → herpes zoster auricularis.
her·pet·ic [hɜr'petɪk] *adj* 1. Herpes betr., mit Herpes einhergehend, herpetisch, Herpes-. 2. Herpesviren betr., durch sie verursacht, herpetisch, Herpes-.
herpetic encephalitis → herpes encephalitis.

herpetic fever Febris herpetica.
herpetic gingivitis Herpesgingivitis *f.*
herpetic gingivostomatitis aphthöse Stomatitis *f*, Gingivostomatitis/Stomatitis herpetica.
herpetic keratitis Herpes-Keratitis *f*, Herpes corneae (simplex).
herpetic keratoconjunctivitis herpetische Keratokonjunktivitis *f*, Herpes-Keratokonjunktivitis *f*, Keratoconjunctivitis herpetica.
herpetic meningoencephalitis Herpesmeningoenzephalitis *f*, Meningoencephalitis herpetica.
herpetic paronychia/perionychia → herpetic whitlow.
herpetic stomatitis → herpetic gingivostomatitis.
herpetic ulcer Herpesgeschwür *nt*, -ulkus *nt.*
herpetic whitlow Herpesparonychie *f.*
her·pet·i·form [hɜr'petɪfɔ:rm] *adj* herpesähnlich, -artig, herpetiform.
her·pe·to·pho·bia [ˌhɜrpətəʊ'fəʊbɪə] *n psychia.* Herpetophobie *f.*
Her·pe·to·vir·i·dae [ˌ-'vɪrədi:, -'vaɪr-] *pl micro.* Herpetoviridae *pl.*
her·pe·to·vi·rus [ˌ-'vaɪrəs] *n micro.* Herpetovirus *nt.*
Herrick ['herɪk] *n:* **H.'s anemia** Sichelzell(en)anämie *f*, Herrick-Syndrom *nt.*
Herring ['herɪŋ] *n:* **H.'s bodies** Herring'-Körper *pl.*
her·ring·bone pattern ['herɪŋbəʊn] *patho.*, *histol.* fischzugartiges Muster *nt.*
herring-worm disease Heringswurmkrankheit *f*, Anisakiasis *f.*
Hers [hɜrz] *n:* **H.' disease** Hers-Erkrankung *f*, -Syndrom *nt*, -Glykogenose *f*, Leberphosphorylaseinsuffizienz *f*, Glykogenose *f* Typ VI.
her·sage [ɛr'sɑ:ʒ] *n neurochir.* interfaszikuläre Neurolyse *f*, Endoneurolyse *f.*
Herter ['hɜrtər] *n:* **H.'s disease/infantilism** → Herter-Heubner disease.
Herter-Heubner ['hɜʊbnər] *n:* **H.-H. disease** (Gee-)Herter-Heubner-Syndrom *nt*, Heubner-Herter-Krankheit *f*, (infantile Form der) Zöliakie *f*, glutenbedingte Enteropathie *f.*
Hertwig-Magendie ['hɜrtvɪg mɑʒɑ:'di; 'hɜrtvɪk] *n:* **H.-M. phenomenon/syndrome** *ophthal.* Hertwig-Magendie-Phänomen *nt*, -Syndrom *nt*, Magendie-Hertwig-Schielstellung *f*, Magendie-Schielstellung *f*, -Zeichen *nt.*
hertz ['hɜrts] *n abbr.* **Hz** Hertz *nt abbr.* Hz.
hertz·ian rays ['hɜrtsɪən, 'hɜrts-] Radiowellen *pl.*
hertzian waves → hertzian rays.
Herxheimer ['hɜrkshaɪmər; 'hɜrks-] *n:* **H.'s reaction** Jarisch-Herxheimer-Reaktion *f.*
Heryng ['herɪŋ] *n:* **H.'s sign** Burger-Zeichen *nt*, Heryng-Zeichen *nt.*
HES *abbr.* → hydroxyethyl starch.
Heschl [heʃl; he-] *n:* **H.'s convolution** Heschl'-Querwindung *f*, Gyrus temporalis transversus anterior.
H.'s gyri Heschl'-Querwindungen *pl*, Gyri temporales transversi.
hes·per·i·din [hes'perədɪn] *n pharm.* Hesperidin *nt.*
Hess [hes; 'hes] *n:* **H.' afterimage** *physiol.*, *ophthal.* Hess'-Nachbild *nt.*
H.' test Rumpel-Leede-Test *m.*
Hesselbach ['heslbax] *n:* **H.'s hernia** Hesselbach-Hernie *f*, Cooper-Hernie *f.*
H.'s ligament Hesselbach-Band *nt*, Lig. interfoveolare.
H.'s triangle Trigonum inguinale.
HE stain → hematoxylin-eosin stain.

het·a·cil·lin [ˌhetə'sɪlɪn] *n pharm.* Hetacillin *nt.*
HETE *abbr.* → hydroxyeicosatetraenoic acid.
het·er·a·del·phus [ˌhetərə'delfəs] *n embryo.* Heteradelphus *m.*
het·er·e·cious [hetər'eʃəs] *adj micro.* wirtswechselnd, heterözisch, heteroezisch.
het·er·e·cism [hetər'esɪzəm] *n micro.* Heterözie *f.*
het·er·es·the·sia [hetəres'θi:ʒ(ɪ)ə] *n neuro.* Heterästhesie *f.*
hetero- *pref.* Fremd-, Heter(o)-.
het·er·o·ag·glu·ti·na·tion [ˌhetərəˌglu:tə-'neɪʃn] *n* Heteroagglutination *f.*
het·er·o·ag·glu·ti·nin [ˌ-ə'glu:tənɪn] *n* Heteroagglutinin *nt.*
het·er·o·al·bu·mose [ˌ-'ælbjəməʊs] *n* Heteroalbumin *nt*, -albumose *f.*
het·er·o·al·bu·mo·su·ria [ˌ-ˌælbjəməʊ-'s(j)ʊərɪə] *n* Heteroalbumosurie *f.*
het·er·o·an·ti·bod·y [ˌ-'æntɪbɑdɪ] *n* Hetero-, Xenoantikörper *m*, heterogener/xenogener Antikörper *m.*
het·er·o·an·ti·gen [ˌ-'æntɪdʒən] *n* Heteroantigen *nt*, heterogenes/xenogenes Antigen *nt.*
het·er·o·at·om [ˌ-'ætəm] *n chem.* Heteroatom *nt.*
het·er·o·aux·in [ˌ-'ɔ:ksɪn] *n* Heteroauxin *nt*, Indol-3-essigsäure *f abbr.* IES.
Het·er·o·bil·har·zi·a [ˌ-bɪl'hɑ:rzɪə] *n micro.* Heterobilharzia *f.*
het·er·o·blas·tic [ˌ-'blæstɪk] *adj embryo.* von mehreren Geweben abstammend, heteroblastisch.
het·er·o·cel·lu·lar [ˌ-'seljələr] *adj* aus verschiedenen Zellen bestehend, heterozellulär.
het·er·o·cen·tric [ˌ-'sentrɪk] *adj* heterozentrisch.
heterocentric chromosome heterozentrisches Chromosom *nt.*
het·er·o·ceph·a·lus [ˌ-'sefələs] *n embryo.* Heterokephalus *m*, -zephalus *m.*
het·er·o·chei·ral [ˌ-'kaɪrəl] *adj* heterochiral.
het·er·o·chi·ral [ˌ-'kaɪrəl] *adj* heterochiral.
het·er·o·chro·mat·ic [ˌ-krəʊ'mætɪk] *adj* heterochromatisch.
het·er·o·chro·ma·tin [ˌ-'krəʊmətɪn] *n* Heterochromatin *nt.*
het·er·o·chro·ma·tin·i·za·tion [ˌ-ˌkrəʊmətɪnə'zeɪʃn] *n* 1. Heterochromatinbildung *f.* 2. *genet.* Lyonisierung *f.*
het·er·o·chro·ma·ti·za·tion [ˌ-ˌkrəʊmətaɪ-'zeɪʃn] *n* 1. Heterochromatinbildung *f.* 2. *genet.* Lyonisierung *f.*
het·er·o·chro·ma·to·sis [ˌ-ˌkrəʊmə'təʊsɪs] *n* → heterochromia.
het·er·o·chro·mia [ˌ-'krəʊmɪə] *n* Heterochromie *f*, Heterochromatose *f.*
het·er·o·chro·mic cyclitis [ˌ-'krəʊmɪk] *ophthal.* Heterochromiezyklitis Fuchs *f.*
het·er·o·chro·mo·some [ˌ-'krəʊməsəʊm] *n* Sex-, Geschlechts-, Heterochromosom *nt*, Genosom *nt*, Allosom *nt*, Heterosom *nt.*
het·er·o·chro·mous [ˌ-'krəʊməs] *adj bio.* verschiedenfarbig, heterochrom, -chromatisch.
het·er·o·chron ['hetərəkrɑn] *n physiol.* Heterochron *m.*
het·er·o·chro·nia [ˌ-'krəʊnɪə] *n* 1. *embryo.* Heterochronie *f.* 2. *physiol.* Heterochronie *f.*
het·er·o·chron·ic [ˌ-'krɑnɪk] *adj* → heterochronous.
het·er·och·ro·nous [ˌhetə'rɑkrənəs] *adj* zeitlich versetzt *od.* verschoben, heterochron.
het·er·och·tho·nous [hetə'rɑktənəs] *adj* heterochthon.

het·er·o·chy·lia [ˌhetərə'kaılıə] *n patho.* (*Magen*) Heterochylie *f.*
het·er·o·clad·ic anastomosis [ˌ-'klædık] *anat.* heterokladische Anastomose *f.*
het·er·o·crine ['-krın, -kraın, -kri:n] *adj* heterokrin.
heterocrine gland seromuköse Mischdrüse *f*, gemischte Drüse *f*, Gl. seromucosa.
het·er·oc·ri·sis [ˌhetə'rakrısəs] *n patho.* Heterokrise *f.*
het·er·o·cy·clic [ˌhetərə'saıklık, -'sık-] *adj chem.* heterozyklisch.
heterocyclic base *chem.* heterozyklische Base *f.*
heterocyclic compound *chem.* heterozyklische Verbindung *f.*
heterocyclic ring *chem.* heterozyklischer Ring *m*, heterozyklische Ringstruktur *f.*
het·er·o·cy·to·tro·pic antibody [ˌ-ˌsaıtə'troʊpık, -'trap-] heterozytotroper Antikörper *m.*
het·er·o·der·mic graft [ˌ-'dɜrmık] *chir.* heterologes Hauttransplantat *nt.*
het·er·o·did·y·mus [ˌ-'dıdəməs] *n* → heterodymus.
het·er·o·di·mer [ˌ-'daımər] *n* Heterodimer *nt.*
het·er·o·dis·perse [ˌ-'dıspɜrs] *adj* (*Tropfen*) von unterschiedlicher Größe, heterodispers.
het·er·o·dont ['-dant] *adj dent.* heterodont, anisodont.
het·er·od·ro·mous [hetə'radrəməs] *adj* in entgegengesetzter Richtung (ablaufend), heterodrom.
het·er·od·y·mus [hetə'radıməs] *n embryo.* Hetero(di)dymus *m.*
het·er·o·e·cious [ˌhetərə'i:ʃəs] *adj bio., micro.* 1. wirtswechselnd, heterözisch, heteroezisch. 2. getrennt geschlechtig, heterözisch, heteroezisch.
het·er·o·e·rot·i·cism [ˌ-ı'ratəsızəm] *n* Alloerotismus *m.*
het·er·o·er·o·tism [ˌ-'erətızəm] *n* Alloerotismus *m.*
het·er·o·fer·men·ta·tion [ˌ-ˌfɜrmən'teıʃn] *n* → heterolactic fermentation.
het·er·o·gam·ete [ˌ-'gæmi:t, -gə'mi:t] *n* Hetero-, Anisogamet *m.*
het·er·o·ga·met·ic [ˌ-gæ'metık] *adj genet.* hetero-, digametisch.
het·er·og·a·me·ty [ˌ-'gæməti] *n genet.* Hetero-, Digametie *f.*
het·er·og·a·mous [hetə'ragəməs] *adj* Heterogamie betr., hetero-, anisogam.
het·er·og·a·my [hetə'ragəmı] *n* Hetero-, Anisogamie *f.*
het·er·o·gan·gli·on·ic [ˌhetərəˌgæŋglı'anık] *adj* heteroganglionär.
het·er·o·ge·ne·ic [ˌ-dʒə'ni:ık] *adj* → heterogenous 2.
heterogeneic antigen → heteroantigen.
het·er·o·ge·ne·i·ty [ˌ-dʒə'ni:əti] *n* Verschiedenartigkeit *f*, Ungleichartigkeit *f*, Heterogenität *f.*
het·er·o·ge·ne·ous [ˌ-'dʒi:nıəs, -jəs] *adj* uneinheitlich, ungleich-, verschiedenartig, heterogen.
heterogeneous catalysis heterogene Katalyse *f*, Kontaktkatalyse *f.*
heterogeneous fluid heterogene/nicht-Newtonsche Flüssigkeit *f.*
heterogeneous nuclear ribonucleic acid → heterogeneous nuclear RNA.
heterogeneous nuclear RNA *abbr.* hnRNA heterogene Kern-RNS *f abbr.* hnRNS, heterogene Kern-RNA *f abbr.* hnRNA.
het·er·o·gen·e·sis [ˌ-'dʒenəsıs] *n* 1. *genet.* Heterogenese *f*, Heterogonie *f.* 2. *bio.* asexuelle Entstehung/Bildung *f*, Heterogenese *f*, Heterogonie *f.* 3. *bio.* Spontanentstehung *f*, -bildung *f*, Heterogenese *f*, Heterogonie *f.*
het·er·o·ge·net·ic [ˌ-dʒə'netık] *adj* 1. Heterogenese betr., heterogenetisch. 2. von verschiedener Herkunft, von einer anderen Art stammend, heterogenetisch.
heterogenetic antibody → heterologous antibody.
heterogenetic antigen heterophiles Antigen *nt.*
het·er·o·gen·ic [ˌ-'dʒenık] *adj* → heterogenous 2.
het·er·o·ge·nic·i·ty [ˌ-dʒə'nısəti] *n* → heterogeneity.
het·er·o·ge·note [ˌ-'dʒınoʊt] *n genet.* Heterogenote *f.*
het·er·og·e·nous [ˌhetə'radʒənəs] *adj* 1. → heterogeneous. 2. von verschiedener Herkunft, von einer anderen Art (stammend), heterogenetisch, heterogen, xenogen, xenogenetisch.
heterogenous graft → heterograft.
heterogenous system heterogenes System *nt.*
heterogenous vaccine heterogener Impfstoff *m.*
het·er·og·e·ny [hetə'radʒənı] *n genet.* Heterogenie *f.*
het·er·o·gly·can [ˌhetərə'glaıkæn] *n* Heteroglykan *nt.*
het·er·og·o·ny [ˌhetə'ragənı] *n* → heterogenesis.
het·er·o·graft ['hetərəgræft] *n* heterogenes/heterologes/xenogenes/xenogenetisches Transplantat *nt*, Xeno-, Heterotransplantat *nt.*
het·er·o·hem·ag·glu·ti·na·tion [ˌ-ˌheməˌgluːtə'neıʃn] *n* Heterohämagglutination *f.*
het·er·o·hem·ag·glu·ti·nin [ˌ-ˌhemə'gluːtənın] *n* Heterhämagglutinin *nt*, heterophiles Hämagglutinin *nt.*
het·er·o·he·mol·y·sin [ˌ-ˌhı'maləsın] *n* Heterohämolysin *nt.*
het·er·o·hex·o·san [ˌ-'heksəsæn] *n* Heterohexosan *nt.*
het·er·o·hyp·no·sis [ˌ-hıp'noʊsıs] *n* Heterohypnose *f.*
het·er·o·im·mune [ˌ-ı'mjuːn] *adj* Heteroimmunität betr., heteroimmun.
het·er·o·im·mu·ni·ty [ˌ-ı'mjuːnəti] *n* Heteroimmunität *f.*
het·er·o·in·fec·tion [ˌ-ın'fekʃn] *n* Heteroinfektion *f.*
het·er·o·in·tox·i·ca·tion [ˌ-ınˌtaksə'keıʃn] *n* Heterointoxikation *f*, Vergiftung *f* von außen.
het·er·o·kar·y·on [ˌ-'kærıan] *n* Heterokaryon *nt.*
het·er·o·kar·y·o·sis [ˌ-ˌkærı'oʊsıs] *n* Heterokaryose *f.*
het·er·o·ker·a·to·plas·ty [ˌ-'kerətəplæsti] *n ophthal.* heterologe Hornhautplastik *f*, Heterokeratoplastik *f.*
het·er·o·ki·ne·sia [ˌ-kı'niːʒ(ı)ə, -kaı-] *n neuro.* Heterokinesie *f*, -kinese *f.*
het·er·o·ki·ne·sis [ˌ-kı'niːsıs, -kaı-] *n* 1. *genet.* Heterokinese *f.* 2. → heterokinesia.
het·er·o·lac·tic fermentation [ˌ-'læktık] heterolaktische/heterofermentative/gemischte Milchsäuregärung *f.*
het·er·o·la·lia [ˌ-'leılıə] *n* → heterophasia.
het·er·o·lat·er·al [ˌ-'lætərəl] *adj* auf der anderen Seite (liegend), die andere (Körper-)Seite betr., hetero-, kontralateral.
het·er·o·lip·id [ˌ-'lıpıd] *n chem.* Heterolipid *nt.*
het·er·ol·o·gous [ˌhetə'raləgəs] *adj* 1. abweichend, nicht übereinstimmend, heterolog. 2. artfremd, heterolog, xenogen.
heterologous antibody → heteroantibody.
heterologous chromosome → heterochromosome.
heterologous graft → heterograft.
heterologous insemination heterologe Insemination *f*, künstliche Befruchtung *f* mit Spendersperma.
heterologous interference *micro., immun.* heterologe Interferenz *f.*
heterologous protein Fremdeiweiß *nt.*
heterologous serum heterologes Serum *nt.*
heterologous stimulus heterologer Reiz *m.*
heterologous tissue heterologes Gewebe *nt.*
heterologous transplantation → heterotransplantation.
heterologous tumor heterologer Tumor *m.*
heterologous twins binovuläre/dissimiläre/dizygote/erbungleiche/heteroovuläre/zweieiige Zwillinge *pl.*
heterologous vaccine heterologer Impfstoff *m*, heterologe Vakzine *f.*
het·er·ol·o·gy [hetə'ralədʒı] *n* Abweichung *f* in Art *od.* Form *od.* Funktion, Heterologie *f.*
het·er·ol·y·sin [hetə'ralısın] *n* 1. Hetero(zyto)lysin *nt.* 2. Heterolysin *nt.*
het·er·ol·y·sis [hetə'raləsıs] *n* Heterolyse *f.*
het·er·o·ly·so·some [ˌhetəroʊ'laısəsoʊm] *n* Heterolysosom *nt.*
het·er·o·lyt·ic [ˌ-'lıtık] *adj* heterolytisch.
het·er·o·mas·ti·gote [ˌ-'mæstıgoʊt] *n micro.* Heteromastigote *f.*
het·er·om·er·al [ˌhetə'ramərəl] *adj* → heteromerous.
heteromeral cell Kommissurenzelle *f.*
het·er·o·mer·ic [ˌhetəroʊ'merık] *adj* → heteromerous.
heteromeric cell → heteromeral cell.
het·er·om·er·ous [ˌhetə'ramərəs] *adj* heteromer.
het·er·o·met·a·pla·sia [ˌhetərəˌmetə'pleıʒ(ı)ə, -zıə] *n patho.* Heterometaplasie *f.*
het·er·o·me·tro·pia [ˌ-mı'troʊpıə] *n ophthal.* Heterometropie *f.*
het·er·o·mor·phic [ˌ-'mɔrfık] *adj* verschiedengestaltig, heteromorph.
het·er·o·mor·phism [ˌ-'mɔrfızəm] *n* → heteromorphy.
het·er·o·mor·pho·sis [ˌ-mɔːr'foʊsıs] *n* Heteromorphose *f.*
het·er·o·mor·phous [ˌ-'mɔrfəs] *adj* → heteromorphous.
het·er·o·mor·phy ['-mɔrfı] *n* Heteromorphie *f*, -morphismus *m.*
het·er·on·o·mous [ˌhetə'ranəməs] *adj* 1. *bio.* ungleichartig, -wertig, heteronom. 2. unselbständig, von fremden Gesetzen abhängig, heteronom.
het·er·on·o·my [ˌhetə'ranəmı] *n* 1. *bio.* Heteronomie *f*, Ungleichartigkeit *f*, -wertigkeit *f.* 2. Unselbständigkeit *f.*
het·er·on·y·mous [hetə'ranıməs] *adj* ungleichnamig, heteronym.
heteronymous diplopia *ophthal.* gekreuzte/heteronyme/temporale Diplopie *f.*
heteronymous hemianopia/hemianopsia *ophthal.* heteronyme/gekreuzte Hemianop(s)ie *f.*
heteronymous image *ophthal.* heteronymes Bild *nt.*
hetero-osteoplasty *n ortho.* heterologe Knochentransplantation *f.*
hetero-ovular *adj embryo.* heteroovulär; dizygot.
hetero-ovular twins → heterologous twins.
het·er·op·a·gus [hetə'rapəgəs] *n embryo.* Heteropagus *m.*
het·er·op·a·thy [hetə'rapəθı] *n* 1. *neuro.* ab-

heteropentosan

norme/abnormale Reizempfindlichkeit f, Heteropathie f. 2. Hetero-, Allopathie f.
het·er·o·pen·to·san [ˌhetərə'pentəsæn] n Heteropentosan nt.
het·er·o·phag·ic [ˌ-'fædʒɪk] adj Heterophagie betr., heterophagisch.
heterophagic vacuole/vesicle → heterophagosome.
het·er·o·phag·o·some [ˌ-'fægəsəʊm] n heterophagische Vakuole f, Heterophagosom nt.
het·er·oph·a·gy [hetər'ɒfədʒɪ] n Heterophagie f.
het·er·o·pha·sia [ˌhetərə'feɪʒ(ɪ)ə] n neuro. Vorbeireden nt, Heterolalie f, Heterophasie f.
het·er·o·pha·sis [ˌ-'feɪsɪs] n → heterophasia.
het·er·o·phe·mia [ˌ-'fiːmɪə] n → heterophasia.
het·er·oph·e·my [hetə'rɒfəmɪ] n → heterophasia.
het·er·o·phil ['hetərəfɪl] I n 1. bio. heterophiler Leukozyt m. 2. → heterophilic antigen. II adj heterophil.
heterophil agglutination test 1. Paul-Bunnel-Test m. 2. modifizierter Paul-Bunnel-Test m mit Pferdeerythrozyten.
heterophil antibody heterologer/heterophiler Antikörper m.
heterophil antibody test → heterophil agglutination test.
heterophil antigen → heterophilic antigen.
het·er·o·phile ['-faɪl] I n 1. bio. heterophiler Leukozyt m. 2. → heterophilic antigen. II adj heterophil.
heterophile antibody → heterophil antibody.
heterophile antigen → heterophilic antigen.
heterophile hemolysin heterophiles Hämolysin m.
het·e·ro·phil·ic [ˌ-'fɪlɪk] adj → heterophile II.
heterophilic antigen heterophiles Antigen nt.
het·er·o·pho·nia [ˌ-'fəʊnɪə] n 1. Stimmbruch m, Mutation f, Mutatio f. 2. Stimmveränderung f, Heterophonie f.
het·er·o·pho·ral·gia [ˌ-fə'rældʒ(ɪ)ə] n ophthal. Heterophoralgie f.
het·er·o·pho·ria [ˌ-'fəʊrɪə] n ophthal. Neigung f zum Schielen, Heterophorie f.
het·er·o·phor·ic [ˌ-'fəʊrɪk, -'fɒr-] adj ophthal. zum Schielen neigend, heterophor(isch).
het·er·oph·thal·mia [ˌhetərɒf'θælmɪə] n ophthal. Heterophthalmus m.
het·er·oph·thal·mos [ˌhetərɒf'θælməs] n → heterophthalmia.
het·er·oph·thal·mus [ˌhetərɒf'θælməs] n → heterophthalmia.
het·er·oph·thon·gia [ˌhetərɒf'θɒndʒɪə] n → heterophonia.
het·er·o·phy·di·a·sis [ˌhetərəfə'daɪəsɪs] n → heterophyiasis.
Het·er·oph·y·es [ˌhetə'rɒfɪˌiːz] n micro. Heterophyes f.
H. heterophyes Zwergdarmegel m, Heterophyes heterophyes.
het·er·o·phy·i·a·sis [ˌhetərəfaɪ'aɪəsɪs] n: Heterophyes-Infektion f, Heterophyiasis f, Heterophydiasis f, Heterophyose f.
het·er·o·pla·sia [ˌ-'pleɪʒ(ɪ)ə] n Heteroplasie f, Alloplasie f.
het·er·o·plas·tic [ˌ-'plæstɪk] adj 1. Heteroplasie od. Heteroplastik betr., heteroplastisch. 2. → heterologous.
heteroplastic graft → heterograft.
heteroplastic transplantation → heterotransplantation.

het·er·o·plas·tid [ˌ-'plæstɪd] n → heterograft.
het·er·o·plas·ty ['-plæstɪ] n, pl -ties 1. → heterotransplantation. 2. → heteroplasia.
het·er·o·ploid ['-plɔɪd] I n heteroploide Zelle f; heteroploider Organismus m. II adj heteroploid.
het·er·o·ploi·dy ['-plɔɪdɪ] n Heteroploidie f.
het·er·o·pol·y·mer [ˌ-'pɒlɪmər] n Heteropolymer nt.
het·er·o·pol·y·mer·ic [ˌ-pɒlɪ'merɪk] adj heteropolymer.
het·er·o·pol·y·sac·cha·ride [ˌ-pɒlɪ'sækəraɪd, -rɪd] n Heteropolysaccharid nt.
het·er·o·pro·so·pus [ˌ-'prəʊsəpəs] n embryo. Januskopf m, Janiceps m.
het·er·o·pro·tein [ˌ-'prəʊtiːn, -tiːɪn] n Heteroprotein nt.
het·er·o·pro·tein·e·mia [ˌ-ˌprəʊtɪ'niːmɪə] n Heteroproteinämie f.
het·er·op·sia [hetə'rɒpsɪə] n ophthal. Heteropie f, Heteropsie f, Heteroskopie f.
Het·er·op·ter·a [hetə'rɒptərə] pl micro. Wanzen pl, Heteropteren pl, Heteroptera pl.
het·er·o·pyk·no·sis [ˌhetərəpɪk'nəʊsɪs] n Heteropyknose f.
het·er·o·pyk·not·ic [ˌ-pɪk'nɒtɪk] adj heteropyknotisch.
het·er·o·sac·cha·ride [ˌ-'sækəraɪd, -rɪd] n Heterosaccharid nt.
het·er·o·scope ['-skəʊp] n ophthal. Heteroskop nt.
het·er·o·sco·py [hetə'rɒskəpɪ] n ophthal. 1. → heteropsia. 2. Heteroskopie f.
het·er·o·sex·u·al [ˌhetərə'sekʃəwəl; Brit. -'sekʃʊəl] I n Heterosexuelle(r m) f. II adj heterosexuell.
het·er·o·sex·u·al·i·ty [ˌ-ˌsekʃə'wælətɪ; Brit. -sjʊ'ælətɪ] n Heterosexualität f.
het·er·o·sis [hetə'rəʊsɪs] n genet. Heterosis f.
het·er·os·mia [hetə'rɒsmɪə] n neuro. Heterosmie f.
het·er·o·some ['hetərəsəʊm] n → heterochromosome.
het·er·o·spe·cif·ic graft [ˌ-spə'sɪfɪk] → heterograft.
het·er·o·spore ['-spəʊər, -spɔːr] n bio., micro. heterosporer Organismus m.
het·er·os·po·rous [hetə'rɒspərəs] adj bio., micro. verschiedensporig, heterospor.
het·er·os·po·ry [hetə'rɒspərɪ] n bio., micro. Heterosporie f.
het·er·o·sug·ges·tion [ˌhetərəsə'dʒestʃn] n Heterosuggestion f.
het·er·o·syn·ap·sis [ˌ-sɪ'næpsɪs] n Heterosynapsis f.
het·er·o·syn·ap·tic facilitation [ˌ-sɪ'næptɪk] heterosynaptische Bahnung f.
het·er·o·tax·ia [ˌ-'tæksɪə] n embryo., patho. Eingeweide-, Organverlagerung f, Heterotaxie f; Situs inversus.
het·er·o·tax·ic [ˌ-'tæksɪk] adj Heterotaxie betr., von ihr betroffen.
het·er·o·tax·is [ˌ-'tæksɪs] n → heterotaxia.
het·er·o·tax·y [ˌ-'tæksɪ] n → heterotaxia.
het·er·o·thal·lic [ˌ-'θælɪk] adj bio., micro. heterothallisch.
het·er·o·thal·lism [ˌ-'θælɪzəm] n bio., micro. Heterothallie f.
het·er·o·thal·ly [ˌ-'θælɪ] n → heterothallism.
het·er·o·therm [ˌ-'θɜːrm] n bio. heterothermer Organismus m.
het·er·o·ther·mic [ˌ-'θɜːrmɪk] adj bio. heterotherm.
het·er·o·ther·my ['-θɜːrmɪ] n bio. Heterothermie f.
het·er·o·to·nia [ˌ-'təʊnɪə] n card. Heterotonie f.
het·er·o·ton·ic [ˌ-'tɒnɪk] adj heteroton, -tonisch.

het·er·o·to·pia [ˌ-'təʊpɪə] n 1. embryo. Heterotopie f, Dystopie f, Ektopie f. 2. Wortentstellung f.
het·er·o·top·ic [ˌ-'tɒpɪk] adj an atypischer Stelle liegend od. entstehend, heterotop(isch), dystop, ektop.
heterotopic pancreas heterotopes/ektopes Pankreas(gewebe nt) nt, Pankreasektopie f, -heteropie f.
heterotopic pregnancy 1. Extrauterinschwangerschaft f, -gravidität f abbr. EU, EUG. 2. kombinierte uterine u. extrauterine Schwangerschaft f.
heterotopic stimulus heterotoper Reiz m.
heterotopic transplantation heterotope Transplantation f.
het·er·ot·o·py [ˌhetə'rɒtəpɪ] n → heterotopia.
het·er·o·trans·plant [ˌhetərə'trænzplænt] n heterogenes/heterologes/xenogenes/xenogenetisches Transplantat nt, Xeno-, Heterotransplantat nt.
het·er·o·trans·plan·ta·tion [ˌ-ˌtrænzplæn'teɪʃn] n heterogene/heterologe/xenogene/xenogenetische Transplantation f, Xeno-, Heterotransplantation f, Xeno-, Heteroplastik f.
het·er·o·tri·cho·sis [ˌ-trɪ'kəʊsɪs] n derm. Heterotrichosis f; Heterochromie f.
het·er·o·troph ['-trɒf, -trəʊf] n heterotropher Organismus m.
het·er·o·tro·phia [ˌ-'trəʊfɪə] n → heterotrophy.
het·er·o·troph·ic [ˌ-'trɒfɪk, -'trəʊ-] adj Heterotrophie betr., heterotroph.
heterotrophic bacteria heterotrophe Bakterien pl.
heterotrophic cell heterotrophe Zelle f.
het·er·ot·ro·phy [ˌhetə'rɒtrəfɪ] n Heterotrophie f.
het·er·o·tro·pia [ˌhetərə'trəʊpɪə] n ophthal. Schielen nt, Strabismus m.
het·er·o·trop·ic enzyme [ˌ-'trɒpɪk, -'trəʊ-] heterotropes Enzym nt.
het·er·ot·ro·py [hetə'rɒtrəpɪ] n → heterotropia.
het·er·o·type mitosis ['hetərətaɪp] → heterotypic mitosis.
het·er·o·typ·ic [ˌ-'tɪpɪk] adj heterotyp, heterotypisch.
het·er·o·typ·i·cal [ˌ-'tɪpɪkl] adj → heterotypic.
heterotypical cortex Archicortex m, Archipallium nt, Cortex medialis pallii, Arch(a)eocortex m.
heterotypic isocortex → heterotypical cortex.
heterotypic mitosis heterotypische Mitose f.
heterotypic tumor → heterologous tumor.
heterotypic vaccine → heterologous vaccine.
het·er·o·vac·cine [ˌ-'væksiːn] n Heterovakzine f.
het·er·ox·e·nous [hetə'rɒksənəs] adj micro. mehrwirtig, heteroxen.
het·er·o·zy·go·sis [ˌhetərəzaɪ'gəʊsɪs] n → heterozygosity.
het·er·o·zy·gos·i·ty [ˌ-zaɪ'gɒsətɪ] n genet. Ungleich-, Mischerbigkeit f, Heterozygotie f.
het·er·o·zy·gote [ˌ-'zaɪgəʊt] n heterozygote Zelle f, Heterozygot m, Heterozygote f.
het·er·o·zy·gous [ˌ-'zaɪgəs] adj Heterozygotie betr., ungleicherbig, heterozygot.
heterozygous form of β-thalassemia heterozygote β-Thalassämie f, Thalassaemia minor.
heterozygous β-thalassemia → heterozygous form of β-thalassemia.

Heubner ['hɔybnər]: **H.'s disease** Heubner'-Krankheit f, -Endarteriitis f. **H.'s (specific) endarteritis** → H.'s disease.
Heubner-Herter ['hɜrtər]: **H.-H. disease** → Herter-Heubner disease.
Heuser ['hɔɪzər]: **H.'s membrane** embryo. Heuser'-Membran f.
hex(a)- pref. sechsfach, sechs-, Hex(a)-.
hex·a·ba·sic [,heksə'beɪsɪk] adj sechsbasisch.
hex·a·bi·ose [,-'baɪəʊs] n old → disaccharide.
hex·a·car·ba·cho·line bromide [,-,kɑːrbə-'kəʊliːn] pharm., anes. Hexacarbacholinbromid nt.
hex·a·chlo·ro·ben·zene [,-,klɔːrəʊ'benziːn] n Hexachlorbenzol nt, Perchlorbenzol nt.
hex·a·chlo·ro·cy·clo·hex·ane [,-,klɔːrəʊ-,saɪkləʊ'heksein] n Benzolhexachlorid nt, Hexachlorcyclohexan nt abbr. HCH; Lindan nt.
hex·a·chlo·ro·phene [,-'klɔːrəfiːn] n pharm. Hexachlorophen nt.
hex·a·co·sane [,-'kəʊseɪn] n Hexacosan nt.
hex·ad ['heksæd] n 1. chem. sechswertiges Element nt. 2. Sechsergruppe f, Hexade f.
hex·a·dac·tyl·ia [,heksədæk'tiːlɪə] n → hexadactyly.
hex·a·dac·ty·lism [,-'dæktəlɪzəm] n → hexadactyly.
hex·a·dac·ty·ly [,-'dæktəlɪ] n embryo. Polydaktylie f mit sechs Fingern od. Zehen, Hexadaktylie f.
hex·a·dec·a·no·ate [,-,dekə'nəʊeɪt] n Hexadecanoat nt, Palmitat nt.
hex·a·dec·a·no·ic acid [,-,dekə'nəʊɪk] Palmitinsäure f, n-Hexadecansäure f.
2,4-hex·a·di·e·no·ic acid [,-,daɪə'nəʊɪk] 2,4-Hexadiensäure f, Sorbinsäure f.
hex·a·ene ['heksəwiːn] n chem. Hexaen nt.
hex·a·gon ['heksəgən, -gən] n Sechseck nt, Hexagon nt.
hex·ag·o·nal [hek'sægənl] adj sechseckig, hexagonal.
hex·a·mer ['heksəmər] n Hexamer nt.
hex·a·me·tho·ni·um [,heksəmɪ'θəʊnɪəm] n pharm. Hexamethonium nt.
hexamethonium bromide pharm. Hexamethoniumbromid nt.
hex·a·meth·y·lat·ed [,-'meθəleɪtɪd] adj chem. sechsfach methyliert, hexamethyliert.
hex·a·meth·yl·en·am·ine [,-,meθəlɪn'æmɪn] n → hexamine.
hex·a·meth·yl·ene·di·am·ine [,-,meθəliːn-'daɪəmiːn] n Hexamethylendiamin nt.
hex·a·meth·yl·en·tet·ra·mine [,-,meθəlɪn-'tetræmiːn] n → hexamine.
hex·a·meth·yl violet ['-meθɪl] Gentianaviolett nt.
hex·am·i·dine [heks'æmədiːn] n pharm. Hexamidin nt.
hex·a·mine ['heksəmiːn] n Hexamin nt, Methenamin nt, Hexamethylentetramin nt.
hex·ane ['hekseɪn] n Hexan nt.
hex·ane·di·o·ic acid [,heksemdaɪ'əʊɪk] Pimelinsäure f.
hex·a·no·ic acid [,heksə'nəʊɪk] Kapronsäure f, Capronsäure f, Butylessigsäure f, Hexansäure f.
hex·a·ploid ['-plɔɪd] adj genet. hexaploid.
hex·a·ploi·dy ['-plɔɪdɪ] n genet. Hexaploidie f.
Hex·ap·o·da [hek'sæpədə] pl 1. bio. Sechsfüßler pl, Hexapoden pl. 2. bio., micro. Kerbtiere pl, Kerfe pl, Insekten pl, Insecta pl, Hexapoden pl, Hexapoda pl.
hex·a·tom·ic [,heksə'tɑmɪk] adj chem. sechsatomig.

hex·a·va·lent [,-'veɪlənt] adj chem. sechswertig, hexavalent.
hex·en·milch ['heksənmɪlx] n ped. Hexenmilch nt, Lac neonatorum.
hex·es·trol [hek'sestrɒl, -rəʊl] n Hexöstrol nt, Hex(o)estrol nt.
hex·et·i·dine [hek'setədiːn] n pharm. Hexetidin nt.
hex·i·tol ['heksɪtɒl] n Hexitol nt, Hexit nt.
hex·o·bar·bi·tal [,heksə'bɑːrbɪtɒl, -tæl] n pharm. Hexobarbital nt.
hex·o·bar·bi·tone [,-'bɑːrbɪtəʊn] n → hexobarbital.
hex·o·ben·dine [,-'bendiːn] n pharm. Hexobendin nt.
hex·o·cy·cli·um methylsulfate [-'saɪklɪəm] pharm. Hexocyciummetilsulfat nt.
hex·o·ki·nase [,-'kaɪneɪz] n Hexokinase f abbr. HK.
hex·on ['heksɒn] n micro. (Virus) Hexon nt.
hex·one bases ['heksəʊn] Hexonbasen pl.
hex·on·ic acid [hek'sɒnɪk] Hexonsäure f.
hex·os·a·mine [hek'sɒsəmiːn] n Hexosamin nt.
hex·os·a·min·i·dase [hek,sɒsə'mɪnɪdeɪz] n 1. Hexosaminidase f. 2. β-N-Acetylgalaktosaminidase f, N-Acetyl-β-Hexosaminidase A f.
hex·o·san ['heksəsæn] n Hexosan nt.
hex·ose ['heksəʊs] n Hexose f.
hexose diphosphatase Hexosediphosphatase f, Fructose-1,6-diphosphatase f.
hexose diphosphate Hexosediphosphat nt.
hexose monophosphate Hexosemonophosphat nt abbr. HMP.
hexose monophosphate shunt Pentosephosphatzyklus m, Phosphogluconatweg m.
hex·ose·phos·pha·tase [,heksəʊs'fɒsfəteɪz] n Hexosephosphatase f.
hex·ose·phos·phate [,-'fɒsfeɪt] n Hexosephosphat nt, Hexosephosphorsäure f.
hexosephosphate isomerase Glukose-(-6-)phosphatisomerase f, Phosphohexoseisomerase f abbr. PHI, Phosphoglucoseisomerase f abbr. PGI.
hexose-1-phosphate uridylyltransferase UDPglukose-hexose-1-phosphaturidylyltransferase f, UDPglukose-galaktose-1-phosphaturidylyltransferase f, Galaktose-1-phosphat-uridylyltransferase f.
hex·o·syl·trans·fer·ase [,heksəsɪl'trænsfəreɪz] n Hexosyltransferase f.
hex·u·lose ['heksjələʊs] n Ketohexose f, Hexulose f.
hex·u·ron·ic acid [,heksjə'rɒnɪk] Hexuronsäure f.
hex·yl ['heksɪl] n Hexyl-(Radikal nt).
n-hex·yl·a·mine [,heksɪl'æmɪn, -ə'miːn] n n-Hexylamin nt.
Hey [heɪ]: **H.'s amputation** Hey-Amputation f, Vorfußamputation f nach Hey. **H.'s hernia** chir. Hey-Hernie f, Hernia encystica. **H.'s ligament** 1. Margo falciformis (hiatus saphenus). 2. Cornu superius hiatus saphenus. **H.'s operation** → H.'s amputation.
Heyer-Pudenz ['heɪər 'pjuːdənz]: **H.-P. valve** neurochir. Heyer-Pudenz-Ventil nt.
HF abbr. 1. → Hageman factor. 2. → heart failure. 3. → hemorrhagic fever.
Hf abbr. → hafnium.
Hfr abbr. → high-frequency of recombination.
Hfr cell genet. Hfr-Zelle f.
HFR deficiency Dihydrofolatreduktasemangel m, DHFR-Mangel m.
HFRS abbr. → hemorrhagic fever with renal syndrome.

Hg abbr. → hydrargyrum.
hg abbr. → hectogram.
H gene → histocompatibility gene.
HGF abbr. → hyperglycemic-glycogenolytic factor.
HG factor → hyperglycemic-glycogenolytic factor.
HGH abbr. → human growth hormone.
hGH abbr. → human growth hormone.
HGPRT abbr. → hypoxanthine guanine phosphoribosyltransferase.
HGPRT deficiency Lesch-Nyhan-Syndrom nt, Automutilationssyndrom nt.
H graft chir. portokavaler Interpositionsshunt m.
HHT abbr. → hydroxyheptadecatrienoic acid.
HI abbr. 1. → hemagglutination inhibition. 2. → hemagglutination inhibition test.
5-HIAA abbr. → 5-hydroxyindoleacetic acid.
hi·a·tal [haɪ'eɪtl] adj Hiatus betr., hiatal, Hiatus-.
hiatal hernia Hiatushernie f.
axial h. gleitende Hiatushernie, Gleitbruch m, -hernie.
paraesophageal/parahiatal h. paraösophageale (Hiatus-)Hernie.
sliding h. gleitende Hiatushernie, Gleitbruch m, -hernie.
type I h. → sliding h.
type II h. → paraesophageal h.
hi·a·tus [haɪ'eɪtəs] n, pl **-tus**, **-tus·es** anat. Spalt(e f) m, Ritze f, schmale Öffnung f, Hiatus m.
h. of Winslow Winslow'-Foramen nt, -Loch nt, For. epiploicum/omentale.
hiatus hernia → hiatal hernia.
Hibbs [hɪbs]: **H.' instrumentation/operation/technique** ortho. Skoliosekorrektur f nach Hibbs, Hibbs-Operation f.
hi·ber·na·tion [,haɪbər'neɪʃn] n bio. Winterschlaf m, Hibernation f.
hi·ber·no·ma [,-'nəʊmə] n patho. braunes Lipom nt, Hibernom(a) nt, Lipoma fetocellulare.
hic·cough n, vi → hiccup.
hic·cup ['hɪkəp, -əp] **I** n Schluckauf m, Singultus m. **II** vi Schluckauf haben.
Hickey-Hare ['hɪkɪ heər]: **H.-H. test** Hickey-Hare-Test m.
hick·o·ry-stick fracture ['hɪkərɪ] ortho. Grünholzbruch m, -fraktur f.
Hicks [hɪks]: **H. version** gyn. Braxton--Hicks-Version f, Hicks-Version f.
hidden margin of nail ['hɪdn] hinterer Nagelrand m, Margo occultus (unguis).
hidr- pref. → hidro-.
hi·drad·e·ni·tis [,haɪdrædɪ'naɪtɪs] n Schweißdrüsenentzündung f, Hidradenitis f, Hidrosadenitis f.
hi·drad·e·no·ma [,haɪdrædɪ'nəʊmə] n Schweißdrüsenadenom nt, Hidradenom(a) nt, Syringom(a) nt, Adenoma sudoriparum.
hidro- pref. Schweiß-, Schweißdrüsen-, Hidr(o)-.
hid·roa → hydroa.
hid·ro·ad·e·no·ma [,haɪdrəædə'nəʊmə] n → hidradenoma.
hid·ro·cys·to·ma [,-,sɪs'təʊmə] n Schweißdrüsenzyste f, Hidrokystom nt, -zystom nt.
hid·ro·poi·e·sis [,-pɔɪ'iːsɪs] n Schweißbildung f, Hidropoese f.
hid·ro·poi·et·ic [,-pɔɪ'etɪk] adj Schweißbildung betr. od. fördernd, hidropoetisch.
hi·dros·ad·e·ni·tis [,haɪdrəsædɪ'naɪtɪs] n → hidradenitis.
hid·ros·che·sis [haɪ'drɒskəsɪs] n verminderte od. fehlende Schweißbildung f, Anhidrose f, Anidrose f, Anhidrosis f.

hi·dro·sis [hɪˈdrəʊsɪs, haɪ-] *n* Schweißabsonderung *f*, Hidrose *f*, Hidrosis *f*.
hi·drot·ic [hɪˈdrɒtɪk, haɪ-] **I** *n* schweißtreibendes Mittel *nt*, Hidrotikum *nt*, Hidroticum *nt*, Diaphoretikum *nt*, Diaphoreticum *nt*. **II** *adj* Schweißabsonderung betr. *od.* fördernd, schweißtreibend, hidrotisch, diaphoretisch.
hidrotic ectodermal dysplasia Clouston-Syndrom *nt*, hidrotische ektodermale Dysplasie *f*.
hi·er·ar·chic [ˌhaɪəˈrɑːrkɪk] *adj* hierarchisch.
hi·er·ar·chi·cal [ˌhaɪərəˈrɑːrkɪkl] *adj* → hierarchic.
hi·er·ar·chy [ˈhaɪərɑːrkɪ] *n*, *pl* **-chies** Rangordnung *f*, -folge *f*, Hierarchie *f*.
high [haɪ] *adj* **1.** hoch, hochgelegen; Hoch-, Ober-, Haupt-. **2.** (*Temperatur, Druck, Fieber*) hoch; (*Leistung*) gut, erstklassig; (*Stimme*) hoch, schrill. **3.** *sl.* **to be ~ on drugs/drinks** 'high' sein/'blau' *od.* betrunken sein.
high-altitude chamber Höhenkammer *f*.
high-altitude climate Höhenklima *nt*.
high-altitude illness → high-altitude sickness.
high-altitude intoxication Höhenrausch *m*.
high-altitude nausea → high-altitude sickness.
high-altitude sickness (akute) Höhenkrankheit *f*.
high-assimilation pelvis hohes Assimilationsbecken *nt*.
high-blood pressure Bluthochdruck *m*, (arterielle) Hypertonie *f*, Hypertension *f*, Hypertonus *m*, Hochdruckkrankheit *f*.
high-ceiling diuretic *pharm.* Schleifendiuretikum *nt*.
high-chair [ˈhaɪˌtʃeər] *n* (Kinder-)Hochstuhl *m*.
high-density lipoprotein *abbr.* **HDL** Lipoprotein *nt* mit hoher Dichte, high density lipoprotein *abbr.* HDL, α-Lipoprotein *nt*.
high-dose tolerance high-dose-Immunotoleranz *f*.
high-duty *adj* Hochleistungs-.
high enema Dünndarmeinlauf *m*, hoher Einlauf *m*, Enteroklysma *nt*.
high-energy bond *chem.* energiereiche Bindung *f*.
high-energy compound *chem.* energiereiche Verbindung *f*.
high-energy linkage → high-energy bond.
high-energy phosphate bond energiereiche Phosphatbindung *f*.
high-energy physics Hochenergie-, Elementarteilchenphysik *f*.
high·er protist [ˈhaɪər] *bio.* höherer Protist *m*, Eukaryo(n)t *m*.
high·est concha [ˈhaɪəst] oberste Nasenmuschel *f*, Concha nasalis suprema.
high-fiber diet ballaststoffreiche Diät/Kost *f*.
high frequency Hochfrequenz *f*.
   h. of recombination *abbr.* **Hfr** *genet., micro.* high-frequency of recombination *abbr.* Hfr.
high-frequency *adj* hochfrequent, Hochfrequenz-.
high-frequency current Hochfrequenzstrom *m*, Tesla-Strom *m*.
high-frequency deafness Schwerhörigkeit *f* für hohe Frequenzen.
high-frequency transduction *genet.* hochfrequente Transduktion *f*.
high-frequency treatment Diathermie *f*.
high lithotomy hoher Blasenschnitt *m*, Sectio alta.
high·ly selective vagotomy [ˈhaɪlɪ] *chir.* supraselektive Vagotomie *f*.
high-melting *adj* bei hoher Temperatur schmelzend.
high-molecular-weight *adj abbr.* **HMW** *chem.* hochmolekular.
high-molecular-weight kininogen *abbr.* **HMWK** hochmolekulares Kininogen *nt*, HMW-Kininogen *nt abbr.* HMWK.
high-molecular-weight neutrophil chemotactic factor *abbr.* **HMW-NCF** Neutrophilen-chemotaktischer Faktor *m abbr.* NCF.
Highmore [ˈhaɪmɔːr, -məʊr]: **antrum of H.** Kieferhöhle *f*, Sinus maxillaris.
high-performance liquid chromatography → high-pressure liquid chromatography.
high-pitched *adj* (*Ton*) hoch.
high-pitched bowel sounds *chir.* hochgestellte Darmgeräusche *pl*, klingendes Preßstrahlgeräusch *nt*.
high-powered *adj* stark, Hochleistungs-.
high-pressure *adj* Hochdruck-.
high-pressure liquid chromatography *abbr.* **HPLC** (Hoch-)Druckflüssigkeitschromatographie *f*.
high-pressure oxygen Sauerstoffüberdrucktherapie *f*, hyperbare Sauerstofftherapie/Oxygenation *f*.
high-pressure system *physiol.* Hochdrucksystem *nt*.
   arterial h. arterielles (Hochdruck-)System.
high-proof *adj chem.* (*Alkohol*) hochprozentig.
high-resolution banding *genet.* hochauflösendes Banding *nt*.
high-risk patient Risikopatient(in *f*) *m*, Patient(in *f*) *m* mit erhöhtem Risiko.
high steppage gait *neuro.* Steppergang *m*.
high-temperature *adj* Hochtemperatur-.
high-tension *adj electr.* Hochspannungs-.
high-voltage *adj electr.* Hochspannungs-.
high-zone tolerance high-dose-Immunotoleranz *f*.
hi·lar [ˈhaɪlər] *adj* Hilum betr., hilär, Hilum-, Hilus-.
hilar carcinoma hilusnahes Lungenkarzinom *nt*.
hilar cells (*Ovar*) Berger-, Hiluszellen *pl*.
hilar cell tumor Hiluszelltumor *m*, Berger-Zell(en)tumor *m*.
hilar dissection *chir.* (*Leber*) Hiluspräparation *f*.
hilar region Hilumregion *f*, -gegend *f*.
hi·li·tis [haɪˈlaɪtɪs] *n* **1.** Hilusentzündung *f*, Entzündung *f* im Bereich eines Hilus, Hilitis *f*. **2.** Lungenhilusentzündung *f*, Hilitis *f*.
Hill [hɪl]: **H. force-velocity relation** Hill'-Kraft-Geschwindigkeitsbeziehung *f*.
   H.'s operation *chir.* posteriore Gastropexie *f* nach Hill.
   H.'s posterior gastropexy → H.'s operation.
   H. reaction Hill'-Reaktion *f*.
   H. reagent Hill'-Reagenz *nt*.
   H.'s sign card. Hill-Zeichen *nt*.
hill·ock [ˈhɪlək] *n* Höcker *m*, (kleiner) Hügel *m*.
Hill-Sachs [zaks]: **H.-S. lesion** Hill-Sachs--Impression *f*.
Hilton [ˈhɪltn]: **H.'s law** Hilton-Regel *f*.
   H.'s muscle M. aryepiglotticus.
   H.'s sac Kehlkopfblindsack *m*, Sacculus laryngis, Appendix ventriculi laryngis.
   H.'s white line Hilton-Linie *f*.
   white line of H. Hilton'-Linie *f*.
hi·lum [ˈhaɪləm] *n*, *pl* **-la** [-lə] *anat.* Hilus *m*, Hilum *nt*.
   h. of caudal olivary nucleus Hilum nc. olivaris caudalis/inferioris.
   h. of dentate nucleus Hilum nc. dentati.
   h. of kidney Nierenhilus, *old* Hilus renalis, Hilum renale.
   h. of inferior olivary nucleus → h. of caudal olivary nucleus.
   h. of lung Lungenhilus, Hilum pulmonis.
   h. of lymph node Lymphknotenhilus, Hilum nodi lymphatici.
   h. of ovary Eierstockhilus, Hilum ovarii.
   h. of spleen Milzhilus, Hilum lienalis/splenicum.
   h. of suprarenal gland Nebennierenhilus, Hilum gl. suprarenalis.
hi·lus [ˈhaɪləs] *n*, *pl* **-li** [-laɪ] *old* → hilum.
   h. of kidney → hilum of kidney.
   h. of lung → hilum of lung.
   h. of lymph node → hilum of lymph node.
   h. of ovary → hilum of ovary.
hilus cells (*Ovar*) Berger-, Hiluszellen *pl*.
hilus cell tumor → hilar cell tumor.
hi·man·to·sis [ˌhaɪmænˈtəʊsɪs] *n patho., HNO* (übermäßig) langes Zäpfchen *nt*.
hinch·a·zon [ˌhɪntʃəˈzan] *n* Beriberi *f*, Vitamin B_1-Mangel(krankheit *f*) *m*, Thiaminmangel(krankheit *f* *m*.
hind·brain [ˈhaɪndbreɪn] *n* Rautenhirn *nt*, Rhombenzephalon *nt*, Rhomencephalon *nt*.
hindbrain vesicle Rautenhirnbläschen *nt*.
hind·foot [ˈhaɪndfʊt] *n* Rückfuß *m*.
hind·gut [ˈhaɪndɡʌt] *n embryo.* Hinterdarm *m*; Enddarm *m*.
hind-kidney *n embryo.* Nachniere *f*, Metanephros *nt*.
hind-limb [ˈhaɪndlɪm] *n embryo.* untere Gliedmaße *f*, Bein *nt*.
hindlimb bud *embryo.* Beinknospe *f*, -anlage *f*.
hind-quar·ter amputation [ˈhaɪndkwɔːrtər] *ortho.* interiliabdominale Amputation *f*; Hemipelvektomie *f*.
Hines and Brown [haɪnz braʊn]: **H.a.B. test** Hines-Brown-Test *m*, Cold-pressure-Test *m*, CP-Test *m*.
hinge [hɪndʒ] **I** *n* Scharnier *nt*, Angel *f*, Gelenk *nt*. **II** *vi* mit einem Scharnier verbinden *od.* versehen.
hinge articulation Scharniergelenk *nt*, Ginglymus *m*.
hinge joint → hinge articulation.
hinge region *immun.* Gelenk-, Scharnierregion *f*.
hip [hɪp] *n* **1.** Hüfte *f*, Coxa *f*. **2.** → hip joint.
hip arthroplasty *ortho.* **1.** Hüftgelenk(s)plastik *f*, Hüftarthroplastik *f*. **2.** → hip prosthesis.
hip bath Sitzbad *nt*.
hip·bone [ˈhɪpbəʊn] *n* Hüftbein *nt*, -knochen *m*, Os coxae/pelvicum.
hip fracture proximale/hüftgelenksnahe Oberschenkel-/Femurfraktur *f*.
hip hemiarthroplasty *ortho.* Hüftkopfprothese *f*.
hip joint Hüftgelenk *nt*, Artic. coxae/iliofemoralis.
hip-joint disease 1. Hüftgelenkserkrankung *f*, Koxarthropathie *f*. **2.** Hüftgelenkstuberkulose *f*, Coxitis tuberculosa.
hip pain Hüft(gelenk)schmerz *m*, Koxalgie *f*, Coxalgie *f*, Coxalgia *f*.
Hippel [ˈhɪpl]: **H.'s disease** → Hippel-Lindau disease.
Hip·pe·la·tes [hɪpəˈleɪtiːz] *n micro.* Hippelates *f*.
Hippel-Lindau [ˈlɪndaʊ]: **H.-L. disease** (von) Hippel-Lindau-Syndrom *nt*, Netzhautangiomatose *f*, Angiomatosis retinae cystica, Angiomatosis cerebelli et retinae.
Hip·po·bos·ca [hɪpəˈbɒskə] *n micro.* Hippobosca *f*.

Hip·po·bos·ci·dae [ˌhɪpəˈbɒskədiː] pl micro. Lausfliegen pl, Hippoboscidae pl.
hip·po·cam·pal [ˌhɪpəˈkæmpl] adj Hippokampus betr., hippokampal, Hippokampus-.
hippocampal commissure Fornix-, Hippocampuskommissur, Commissura hippocampi/fornicis.
hippocampal convolution Gyrus hippocampi/parahippocampalis.
hippocampal cortex Hippokampusrinde f.
hippocampal fissure Fissura hippocampi, Sulcus hippocampalis/hippocampi.
hippocampal formation Hippokampusformation f.
hippocampal gyrus → hippocampal convolution.
hippocampal sulcus → hippocampal fissure.
hip·po·cam·pus [ˌhɪpəˈkæmpəs] n, pl **-pi** [-paɪ, -piː] Ammonshorn nt, Hippokampus m, Hippocampus m.
Hippocrates [hɪˈpɒkrətiːz]: **H. manipulation** ortho. Schulter(gelenk)reposition f nach Hippokrates.
hip·po·crat·ic angina [ˌhɪpəˈkrætɪk] Retropharyngealabszeß m.
hippocratic face/facies Hippokrates-Gesicht nt, Facies hippocratica.
hippocratic fingers Trommelschlegelfinger pl, Digiti hippocratici.
Hippocratic Oath hippokratischer Eid m, Eid m des Hippokrates.
hip prosthesis ortho. Hüftgelenkprothese f, inf. künstliche Hüfte f, Hüftendoprothese f.
total h. Hüfttotalendoprothese, Hüft--TEP f.
hip·pu·rate [ˈhɪpjəreɪt, hɪˈpjʊər-] n Hippurat nt.
hip·pu·ria [hɪˈp(j)ʊərɪə] n übermäßige Hippursäureausscheidung f im Harn, Hippurie f.
hip·pu·ric acid [hɪˈpjʊərɪk] Hippursäure f, Benzoylaminoessigsäure f, Benzolglykokoll nt.
hip·pu·ri·case [hɪˈpjʊərɪkeɪz] n Aminoacylase f, Hippurikase f.
hip·pus [ˈhɪpəs] n neuro. Pupillenzittern nt, Irisblinzeln nt, Hippus m (pupillae), Atetosis pupillaris.
hip replacement → hip prosthesis.
total h. abbr. **THR** → hip prosthesis, total.
hip-shot [ˈhɪpʃɒt] adj mit verrenkter Hüfte.
hip spica ortho. Becken-Bein-Verband m, Spica coxae.
hip spica cast ortho. Becken-Bein-Gips(verband m) m.
hir·ci [ˈhɜːsaɪ, ˈhɪər-] pl, sing **-cus** [-kəs] Achselhaare pl, Hirci pl.
hir·cis·mus [hɜːˈsɪzməs, hɪər-] n derm. Achselgeruch m.
hir·cus sing → hirci.
Hirschsprung [ˈhɪrʃsprʊŋ; -ʃprʊŋ]: **H.'s disease** aganglionäres/kongenitales Megakolon nt, Hirschsprung-Krankheit f, Morbus Hirschsprung m, Megacolon congenitum.
hir·sute [ˈhɜːsuːt, hɜːˈsuːt] adj **1.** haarig. **2.** mit zottigem od. struppigem Haar.
hir·su·ties [hɜːˈsuːʃɪˌiːz] n → hirsutism.
hir·sut·ism [ˈhɜːsətɪzəm] n Hirsutismus m, Hirsuties f.
hi·ru·di·ci·dal [hɪˌruːdəˈsaɪdl] adj pharm. Blutegel(ab-)tötend.
hi·ru·di·cide [hɪˈruːdəsaɪd] n pharm. Blutegelmittel nt, Blutegel-abtötendes Mittel nt.
hir·u·din [ˈhɪr(j)ədɪn, hɪˈruːdɪn] n Hirudin nt.
Hir·u·di·na·ri·a [ˌhɪrədɪˈneərɪə] n micro. Hirudinaria f.

Hir·u·din·ea [ˌhɪrʊˈdɪnɪə] n Blutegel m, Hirudinea f.
hir·u·di·ni·a·sis [ˌhɪrʊdɪˈnaɪəsɪs] n Befall m durch Blutegel, Hirudiniasis f.
hi·ru·di·ni·za·tion [hɪˌruːdɪnaɪˈzeɪʃn] n **1.** Behandlung f mit Hirudin. **2.** Blutegeltherapie f.
Hi·ru·do [hɪˈruːdəʊ] n micro. Hirudo f.
H. medicinalis medizinischer Blutegel m, Hirudo medicinalis.
His abbr. → histidine.
His [hɪz]: **H.' band** → bundle of H.
bundle of H. His'-Bündel nt, Fasciculus atrioventricularis.
H. bundle electrocardiography His-Bündelableitung f.
H. bundle electrogram abbr. **HBE** His-Bündel-Elektrogramm nt abbr. HBE.
H.' disease Wolhyn'-Fieber nt, Fünftagefieber nt, Wolhynienfieber nt, Febris quintana.
duct of H. → H.' canal.
isthmus of H. embryo. Isthmus rhombencephali.
H.' perivascular space His'-Raum m.
H.' space → H.' perivascular space.
H.' spindle Aortenspindel f.
hiss [hɪs] **I** n Zischen nt; Zischlaut m. **II** vi zischen.
hiss·ing [ˈhɪsɪŋ] n Zischen nt.
his·tam·i·nase [hɪˈstæmɪneɪz] n Histaminase f, Diaminoxidase f.
his·ta·mine [ˈhɪstəmiːn, -mɪn] n abbr. **H** Histamin nt abbr. **H**.
histamine blocker Histaminblocker m, Histaminrezeptoren-Antagonist m, -Blocker m, Antihistaminikum nt.
histamine cephalalgia → histamine headache.
histamine flush Histaminflush m.
histamine headache Histaminkopfschmerz m, -kephalgie f, (Bing-)Horton--Syndrom nt, -Neuralgie f, Cephalaea histaminica, Erythroprosopalgie f, cluster headache m.
his·ta·mi·ne·mia [hɪsˌtæmɪˈniːmɪə] n Histaminämie f.
histamine receptor Histaminrezeptor m, H-Rezeptor m.
histamine 1 receptor Histamin 1-Rezeptor m, H_1-Rezeptor m.
histamine 2 receptor Histamin 2-Rezeptor m, H_2-Rezeptor m.
histamine receptor-blocking agent → histamine blocker.
histamine releasing factor Histamin--Releasing-Faktor m.
his·ta·mi·ner·gic [hɪstəmɪˈnɜːdʒɪk] adj histaminerg.
histamine-sensitizing factor abbr. **HSF** old Pertussistoxin nt abbr. PT.
histamine shock Histaminschock m.
histamine test Histamintest m.
his·ta·mi·nu·ria [ˌhɪstəmɪˈn(j)ʊərɪə] n Histaminausscheidung f im Harn, Histaminurie f.
his·tan·ox·ia [ˌhɪstəˈnɒksɪə] n Gewebeanoxie f.
histi- pref. → histio-.
his·tic [ˈhɪstɪk] adj Gewebe betr., Gewebe-, Histo-.
his·ti·dase [ˈhɪstədeɪz] n → histidine ammonia-lyase.
his·ti·di·nase [ˈhɪstədɪneɪz] n → histidine ammonia-lyase.
his·ti·dine [ˈhɪstədiːn, -diːn] n abbr. **H, His** Histidin nt abbr. H, His.
histidine ammonia-lyase Histidinammoniaklyase f, Histid(in)ase f.
histidine decarboxylase Histidindecarboxylase f.

histidine enzyme Histidinenzym nt.
histidine loading test Histidinbelastungstest m, FIGLU-Test m.
his·ti·di·ne·mia [hɪstədɪˈniːmɪə] n (Hyper-)Histidinämie f.
his·ti·di·nol [ˈhɪstədɪnɒl] n Histidinol nt.
histidinol dehydrogenase Histidinoldehydrogenase f.
histidinol phosphatase Histidinolphosphatase f.
histidinol phosphate Histidinolphosphat nt.
histidinol phosphate transaminase Histidinolphosphattransaminase f, Histidinolphosphataminotransferase f.
his·ti·di·nu·ria [ˌhɪstədɪˈn(j)ʊərɪə] n erhöhte Histidinausscheidung f im Harn, Histidinurie f.
histio- pref. Gewebe-, Histio-, Histo-.
his·ti·o·blast [ˈhɪstɪəblæst] n Histo-, Histioblast m.
his·ti·o·cyte [ˈ-saɪt] n Gewebsmakrophag m, Histiozyt m.
his·ti·o·cyt·ic [ˌ-ˈsɪtɪk] adj Histiozyte(n) betr., histiozytisch, histiozytär.
histiocytic granuloma histiozytäres Granulom nt.
histiocytic leukemia (akute) Monozytenleukämie f abbr. AMOL.
histiocytic lymphoma immunoblastisches (malignes) Lymphom nt, Retikulumzellensarkom nt.
histiocytic medullary reticulosis maligne Histiozytose f, maligne Retikulohistiozytose f, histiozytäre medulläre Retikulose f.
his·ti·o·cy·to·ma [ˌ-saɪˈtəʊmə] n Histiozytom nt, Histiocytoma nt.
his·ti·o·cy·to·ma·to·sis [ˌ-saɪtəməˈtəʊsɪs] n Histiozytomatose f, Histiocytomatosis f.
his·ti·o·cy·to·sis [ˌ-saɪˈtəʊsɪs] n Histiozytose f, Histiocytosis f.
histiocytosis X Histiozytose/Histiocytosis X f.
his·ti·o·gen·ic [ˌ-ˈdʒenɪk] adj → histogenous.
his·ti·oid [ˈhɪstɪɔɪd] adj → histoid.
histioid tumor Bindegewebstumor m.
his·ti·o·ma [hɪstɪˈəʊmə] n → histoma.
his·ti·on·ic [hɪstɪˈɒnɪk] adj Gewebe betr., von einem Gewebe abstammend, Gewebe-, Histio-, Histo-.
histo- pref. → histio-.
his·to·blast [ˈhɪstəblæst] n → histioblast.
his·to·chem·i·cal [ˌ-ˈkemɪkl] adj Histochemie betr., histochemisch.
his·to·chem·is·try [ˌ-ˈkemɪstrɪ] n Histochemie f.
his·to·clas·tic [ˌ-ˈklæstɪk] adj gewebeabbauend, histoklastisch.
his·to·clin·i·cal [ˌ-ˈklɪnɪkl] adj klinisch-histologisch.
his·to·com·pat·i·bil·i·ty [ˌ-kəmˌpætəˈbɪlətɪ] n Gewebeverträglichkeit f, Histokompatibilität f.
histocompatibility antigens/complex Histokompatibilitätsantigene pl, HLA-Antigene pl.
histocompatibility gene Histokompatibilitätsgen nt, HLA-Gen nt.
histocompatibility locus → histocompatibility gene.
his·to·com·pat·i·ble [ˌ-kəmˈpætɪbl] adj gewebsverträglich, histokompatibel.
his·to·cyte [ˈ-saɪt] n → histiocyte.
his·to·cy·to·sis [ˌ-saɪˈtəʊsɪs] n → histiocytosis.
his·to·di·ag·no·sis [ˌ-daɪəgˈnəʊsɪs] n Gewebe-, Histodiagnose f.
his·to·di·al·y·sis [ˌ-daɪˈæləsɪs] n Gewebeauflösung f, -desintegration f.

histodifferentiation 360

his·to·dif·fer·en·ti·a·tion [ˌ-ˌdɪfəˌrenʃɪˈeɪʃn] n embryo. Gewebedifferenzierung f.
his·to·flu·o·res·cence [ˌ-ˌfluəˈresns] n Gewebe-, Histofluoreszenz f.
histofluorescence microscopy Histofluoreszenzmikroskopie f.
his·to·gen·e·sis [ˌ-ˈdʒenəsɪs] n Gewebeentstehung f, Histogenese f, Histogenie f, Histiogenese f.
his·to·ge·net·ic [ˌ-dʒəˈnetɪk] adj Histogenese betr., gewebebildend, histogenetisch.
his·tog·e·nous [hɪsˈtadʒənəs] adj vom Gewebe gebildet, aus dem Gewebe stammend, histogen.
his·tog·e·ny [hɪsˈtadʒənɪ] n → histogenesis.
his·to·gram [ˈhɪstəgræm] n stat. Histogramm nt.
his·to·hem·a·tog·e·nous [ˌ-hiːməˈtadʒənəs] adj von Gewebe u. Blut gebildet, histohämatogen.
his·to·hy·pox·ia [ˌ-haɪˈpaksɪə] n Gewebehypoxie f.
his·toid [ˈhɪstɔɪd] adj 1. gewebsartig, -ähnlich, histoid. 2. patho. histoid.
his·to·in·com·pat·i·bil·i·ty [ˌhɪstɔɪnkəmˌpætɪˈbɪlətɪ] n Gewebeunverträglichkeit f, Histoinkompatibilität f.
histoincompatibility gene Histoinkompatibilitätsgen nt.
his·to·in·com·pat·i·ble [ˌ-ɪnkəmˈpætɪbl] adj gewebsunverträglich, histoinkompatibel.
his·to·log·ic [ˌ-ˈladʒɪk] adj → histological.
histologic accommodation histologische Anpassung f, Pseudometaplasie f.
his·to·log·i·cal [ˌ-ˈladʒɪkl] adj Histologie betr., histologisch.
histologic anatomy Gewebelehre f, Histologie f; mikroskopische Anatomie f, Mikroanatomie f.
histologic lesion mikroskopische Schädigung/Läsion f.
his·tol·o·gist [hɪsˈtalədʒɪst] n Histologe m, Histologin f.
his·tol·o·gy [hɪsˈtalədʒɪ] n 1. Gewebelehre f, Histologie f. 2. (mikroskopische) (Gewebs-, Organ-)Struktur f.
his·tol·y·sis [hɪsˈtaləsɪs] n patho. Gewebeauflösung f, Histolyse f.
his·to·lyt·ic [ˈhɪstəˈlɪtɪk] adj Histolyse betr. od. auslösend, histolytisch.
his·to·ma [hɪsˈtəʊmə] n Gewebetumor m, -geschwulst f, Histom(a) nt, Histiom(a) nt.
his·to·met·a·plas·tic [ˌhɪstəˌmetəˈplæstɪk] adj Gewebsmetaplasie auslösend, histometaplastisch.
his·to·mor·phol·o·gy [ˌ-mɔːrˈfalədʒɪ] n Histomorphologie f.
his·tone [ˈhɪstəʊn] n Histon nt.
histone bases Hexonbasen pl.
his·to·neu·rol·o·gy [ˌhɪstənjʊəˈralədʒɪ] n Neurohistologie f.
his·to·nu·ria [ˌ-ˈn(j)ʊərɪə] n patho. Histonurie f.
his·to·path·o·gen·e·sis [ˌ-ˌpæθəˈdʒenəsɪs] n Histopathogenese f.
his·to·path·o·log·ic [ˌ-ˌpæθəˈladʒɪk] adj Histopathologie betr., histopathologisch.
his·to·pa·thol·o·gy [ˌ-pəˈθalədʒɪ] n Gewebe-, Histopathologie f.
his·toph·a·gous [hɪsˈtafəgəs] adj micro. gewebefressend, histophag.
his·to·phys·i·ol·o·gy [ˌhɪstəˌfɪzɪˈalədʒɪ] n Gewebe-, Histophysiologie f.
His·to·plas·ma [ˌ-ˈplæzmə] n micro. Histoplasma f.
his·to·plas·min [ˌ-ˈplæzmɪn] n micro., derm. Histoplasmin nt.
histoplasmin-latex test Histoplasmin-Latextest m.

histoplasmin skin test → histoplasmin test.
histoplasmin test Histoplasmin-(Haut-)-Test m.
his·to·plas·mo·ma [ˌ-plæzˈməʊmə] n Histoplasmom nt.
his·to·plas·mo·sis [ˌ-plæzˈməʊsɪs] n Darling'-Krankheit f, Histoplasmose f, retikuloendotheliale Zytomykose f.
his·to·ra·di·og·ra·phy [ˌ-ˌreɪdɪˈagrəfɪ] n histol. Historadiographie f.
his·to·re·ten·tion [ˌ-rɪˈtenʃn] n Gewebespeicherung f, Speicherung f im Gewebe.
his·tor·rhex·is [ˌ-ˈreksɪs] n patho. nicht-infektiöse Gewebeauflösung f, Historrhexis f.
his·to·ry [ˈhɪstərɪ, ˈhɪstrɪ] n 1. Vor-, Krankengeschichte f; Anamnese f. 2. (Entwicklungs-)Geschichte f, Werdegang m. 3. Lebensbeschreibung f, -lauf m. 4. zusammenhängende od. zusammenfassende Darstellung/Beschreibung f, Geschichte f.
his·to·ther·a·py [ˌhɪstəˈθerəpɪ] n Gewebe-, Histotherapie f.
his·to·tome [ˈ-təʊm] n histol. Mikrotom nt.
his·tot·o·my [hɪsˈtatəmɪ] n histol. Anfertigung f von Gewebe(e)schnitten.
his·to·tox·ic [ˌhɪstəˈtaksɪk] adj gewebeschädigend, histotoxisch.
histotoxic anoxia histotoxische/zytotoxische Anoxie f.
histotoxic hypoxia histotoxische/zytotoxische Hypoxie f.
his·to·trop·ic [ˌ-ˈtrapɪk, -ˈtrəʊp-] adj mit besonderer Affinität zu Gewebe od. Gewebezellen, histotrop.
his·to·zo·ic [ˌ-ˈzəʊɪk] adj micro. im Gewebe lebend, histozoisch.
his·tri·on·ic [hɪstrɪˈanɪk] adj physiol., psychia. (Verhalten) theatralisch.
histrionic personality → hysterical personality.
histrionic spasm mimischer Gesichtskrampf m, Bell-Spasmus m, Fazialiskrampf m, Gesichtszucken nt, Fazialis--Tic m, Tic convulsif/facial.
his·tri·o·nism [ˈhɪstrɪənɪzəm] n physiol., psychia. Histrionismus m.
His-Werner [hɪz ˈwɜrnər]: **H.-W. disease** → His' disease.
Hitzelberger [ˈhɪtsəlbɜrgər]: **H.'s sign** Hitzelberger'-Zeichen nt.
Hitzig [ˈhɪtsɪɡ]: **H.'s girdle** Hitzig-Zone f.
HIV abbr. → human immunodeficiency virus.
hive [haɪv] n derm. Quaddel f, Urtica f.
hives [haɪvz] pl derm. Nesselsucht f, -ausschlag m, Urtikaria f, Urticaria f.
HIV infection HIV-Infektion f.
HL abbr. → hearing loss.
Hl abbr. → latent hyperopia.
hl abbr. → hectoliter.
HLA abbr. → human leukocyte antigens.
HLA complex → human leucocyte antigens.
HLA gene → histocompatibility gene.
HLA-identical adj HLA-identisch.
HLA system HLA-System nt.
HLA typing HLA-Typing nt, -Typisierung f.
Hm abbr. → manifest hyperopia.
hm abbr. → hectometer.
H meromyosin schweres Meromyosin nt, H-Meromyosin f.
HMG abbr. → human menopausal gonadotropin.
hMG abbr. → human menopausal gonadotropin.
HMG-CoA abbr. → β-hydroxy-β-methylglutaryl-CoA.
HMW abbr. → high-molecular-weight.

HMWK abbr. → high-molecular-weight kininogen.
HMW kininogen → high-molecular-weight kininogen.
HMW-NCF abbr. → high-molecular-weight neutrophil chemotactic factor.
HN2 abbr. → nitrogen mustard.
HNCM abbr. → hypertrophic non-obstructive cardiomyopathy.
HN protein → hemagglutinin neuraminidase protein.
hnRNA abbr. → heterogeneous nuclear RNA.
Ho abbr. → holmium.
H₀ abbr. → null hypothesis.
hoarse [hɔːrs, həʊrs] adj (Stimme) heiser, rauh.
hoarse·ness [ˈhɔːrsnɪs, ˈhəʊrs-] n (Stimme) Heiserkeit f.
hob·nail liver [ˈhabneɪl] patho. 1. Schuhzweckenleber f. 2. Kartoffelleber f.
HOCM abbr. → hypertrophic obstructive cardiomyopathy.
Hodge [hadʒ]: **H.'s planes** Hodge-Ebenen pl.
Hodgen [ˈhadʒən]: **H. splint** ortho. Hodgen-Schiene f.
Hodgkin [ˈhadʒkɪn]: **H. cell** Hodgkin-Zelle f.
  H. cycle Hodgkin-Zyklus m.
  H.'s disease Hodgkin-Krankheit f, -Lymphom nt, Morbus Hodgkin m, (Hodgkin-)Paltauf-Steinberg-Krankheit f, (maligne) Lymphogranulomatose f, Lymphogranulomatosis maligna.
  H.'s granuloma/lymphoma → H.'s disease.
  non-H.'s lymphoma non-Hodgkin-Lymphom nt abbr. NHL.
  H.'s sarcoma Hodgkin-Sarkom nt.
Hodgkin-Key [kiː]: **H.-K. murmur** Hodgkin-Key-Geräusch nt.
Hofbauer [ˈhafbaʊər]: **H. cell** Hofbauer'-Zelle f.
Hoff → van't Hoff.
Hoffa [ˈhafə]: **H.'s disease** Hoffa'-Erkrankung f.
Hoffmann [ˈhafmən]: **H.'s atrophy** Werdnig-Hoffmann-Krankheit f, infantile Form f der spinalen Muskelatrophie.
  H.'s drops Hoffmann-Tropfen pl, Ätherweingeist m, Spiritus aethereus.
  H.'s phenomenon neuro. Hoffmann-Phänomen f.
  H.'s reflex → H.'s sign 2.
  H.'s sign 1. Hoffmann'-Trigeminuszeichen nt. 2. neuro. Fingerbeugereflex m, Trömner-Reflex m, -Fingerzeichen nt, Knipsreflex m.
Hoffmann-Werdnig [ˈverdnɪɡ]: **H.-W. syndrome** → Hoffmann's atrophy.
Hofmann [ˈhafmən]: **H.'s bacillus** Löffler'-Pseudodiphtheriebazillus m, Corynebacterium hofmannii/pseudodiphtheriticum.
Hofmeister [ˈhəʊfmaɪstər]: **H.'s modification/operation** chir. Hofmeister-Operation f, nach Hofmeister modifizierte Billroth II-Magenresektion.
  H.'s series/tests Hofmeister-Reihen pl, lyotrope Reihen pl.
hog's bean [haɡ] pharm. Bilsenkraut nt, Hyoscyamus niger.
Hohmann [ˈhəʊmən]: **H.'s operation/osteotomy** ortho. Hohmann-Operation f, -Keilosteotomie f.
  H.'s retractor Hohmann-Knochenhebel m.
hol·an·dric [haˈlændrɪk, həʊ-] adj genet. holandrisch.
holandric gene Y-gebundenes Gen nt, holandrisches Gen nt.
holandric inheritance holandrische Vererbung f.

hol·ar·thrit·ic [ˌhɑlɑːrˈθrɪtɪk, ˌhɔʊl-] *adj* Holarthritis betr., holarthritisch; polyarthritisch.
hol·ar·thri·tis [ˌhɑlɑːrˈθraɪtɪs, ˌhɔʊl-] *n patho., ortho.* Holarthritis *f*; Polyarthritis *f*.
hold·fast (organ/organelle) [ˈhɔʊldfæst, -fɑːst] *bio., histol.* Haftorgan *nt*, Haftscheibe *f*.
ho·lism [ˈhɔʊlɪzəm] *n psycho., psychia.* Holismus *m*.
ho·lis·tic [hɔʊˈlɪstɪk] *adj* holistisch, Ganzheits-.
holistic medicine holistische Medizin *f*.
holistic psychology holistische Psychologie *f*, Ganzheitspsychologie *f*.
Hollander [ˈhɑləndər]: **H.'s test** Hollander-Hypoglykämietest *m*.
hol·low [ˈhɑlɔʊ] **I** *n* **1.** Vertiefung *f*, Mulde *f*, Senke *f*. **2.** Höhle *f*, (Aus-)Höhlung *f*, Hohlraum *m*. **II** *adj* **3.** hohl, Hohl-; (*Ton*) hohl; (*Stimme*) dumpf; (*Wangen*) eingefallen, hohl; (*Augen*) tiefliegend. **4.** hungrig, leer. **III** *vt* aushöhlen. **IV** *vi* hohl werden.
hollow out I *vt* → hollow III. **II** *vi* → hollow IV.
hollow back Hohl(rund)rücken *m*, Hohlkreuz *nt*.
hollow-cheeked *adj* hohlwangig.
hollow chisel *ortho.* Hohlmeißel *m*.
hollow-eyed *adj* hohläugig.
hollow viscus Hohlorgan *nt*.
Holmes [hɔʊmz]: **H.'s degeneration** *neuro.* zerebellooliväre Atrophie Typ Holmes *f*. **H.' phenomenon** → H.'s sign.
H.'s sign *neuro.* Holmes-Phänomen *nt*, Holmes-Stewart-Phänomen *nt*, Rückstoß-, Rückschlag-, Reboundphänomen *nt*.
Holmes-Adie [ˈædɪ]: **H.-A. syndrome** Adie-Syndrom *nt*.
Holmes-Stewart [ˈst(j)uːərt]: **H.-S. phenomenon** → Holmes' sign.
Holmgren [ˈhɔʊ(l)mgrən]: **H. method/test** *ophthal.* Holmgren-Test *m*.
Holmgren-Golgi [ˈgɔldʒɪ]: **H.-G. canals** Holmgren-Golgi-Kanälchen *pl*, (intra-)zytoplasmatische Kanälchen *pl*.
hol·mi·um [ˈhɔʊlmɪəm] *n abbr.* **Ho** Holmium *nt abbr.* Ho.
holo- *pref.* Holo-, Pan-, Voll-.
hol·o·a·car·di·us [ˌhɑlɔeɪˈkɑːrdɪəs, ˌhɔʊl-] *n embryo.* Holoakardius *m*, -acardius *m*.
hol·o·a·cra·nia [ˌ-eɪˈkreɪnɪə] *n embryo.* Hol(o)akranie *f*, Hol(o)acrania *f*.
hol·o·an·en·ceph·a·ly [ˌ-ænənˈsefəlɪ] *n embryo.* Holoanenzephalie *f*.
hol·o·an·ti·gen [ˌ-ˈæntɪdʒən] *n* Voll-, Holoantigen *nt*.
hol·o·blas·tic [ˌ-ˈblæstɪk] *adj embryo.* holoblastisch.
holoblastic cleavage holoblastische Furchung(steilung *f*) *f*.
holoblastic ovum *bio.* holoblastisches Ei *nt*.
hol·o·crine [ˈ-krɪn, -kraɪn] *adj* holokrin.
holocrine extrusion holokrine Extrusion *f*.
holocrine gland holokrine Drüse *f*.
hol·o·di·as·tol·ic [ˌ-daɪəˈstɑlɪk] *adj card.* während der ganzen Diastole, holo-, pandiastolisch.
hol·o·en·dem·ic [ˌ-enˈdemɪk] *adj epidem.* holoendemisch.
hol·o·en·zyme [ˌ-ˈenzaɪm] *n* Holoenzym *nt*.
hol·o·gam·ete [ˌ-ˈgæmiːt, gəˈmiːt] *n* Hologamet(e *f*) *m*.
hol·o·ga·mous [hɔˈlɑgəməs] *adj* hologam.
hol·o·gram [ˈ-græm] *n* Hologramm *nt*.
ho·log·ra·phy [həˈlɑgrəfɪ] *n* Holographie *f*.
hol·o·gyn·ic [ˌhɑləˈdʒɪnɪk, -ˈgaɪnɪk, ˌhɔʊl-] *adj genet.* hologyn.
hol·o·mas·ti·gote [ˌ-ˈmæstɪgɔʊt] *n micro.* Holomastigote *f*.
hol·o·par·a·site [ˌ-ˈpærəsaɪt] *n bio.* Vollschmarotzer *m*, -parasit *m*, Holoparasit *m*.
hol·o·phyt·ic [ˌ-ˈfɪtɪk] *adj micro.* holophytisch.
hol·o·pros·en·ceph·a·ly [ˌ-prɑsənˈsefəlɪ] *n embryo.* Holoprosenzephalie(-Syndrom *nt*) *f*, Arhinenzephalie-Syndrom *nt*.
hol·o·pro·tein [ˌ-ˈprɔʊtiːɪn, -tiːn] *n* Holoprotein *nt*.
hol·o·ra·chis·chi·sis [ˌ-rəˈkɪskəsɪs] *n* totale/vollständige Wirbelsäulenspalte *f*, Holor(h)achischisis *f*.
hol·o·sac·cha·ride [ˌ-ˈsækəraɪd, -rɪd] *n* Holosaccharid *nt*.
hol·o·schi·sis [ˌ-ˈskaɪsɪs] *n* direkte Zellteilung *f*, Amitose *f*.
hol·o·sys·tol·ic [ˌ-sɪsˈtɑlɪk] *adj card.* während der ganzen Systole, holosystolisch, pansystolisch.
holosystolic murmur *card.* pansystolisches/holosystolisches Geräusch *nt*.
ho·lot·o·py [həˈlɑtəpɪ] *n anat.* Holotopie *f*.
ho·lot·ri·chous [həˈlɑtrɪkəs] *n micro.* holotrich.
hol·o·type [ˈ-taɪp] *n micro.* Holostandard *m*, -typ *m*, Standardtyp *m*.
hol·o·zo·ic [ˌ-ˈzɔʊɪk] *adj bio.* holozoisch, phagotroph.
Holth [hɔʊlθ]: **H.'s operation** *ophthal.* Iriseinklemmung *f*, Iridenkleisis *f*, Iridenklisis *f*.
Holthouse [ˈhɔlthaʊs]: **H.'s hernia** Holthouse-Hernie *f*.
Holt-Oram [hɔʊlt ˈɔːræm]: **H.-O. syndrome** Holt-Oram-Syndrom *nt*.
Holzknecht [ˈhɔltsknɛçt]: **H.'s movement** Holzknecht'-Massenbewegung *f*. **H.'s space** Holzknecht-Raum *m*, Retrokardialraum *m*.
hom- *pref.* → homo-.
hom·a·log·ra·phy [ˌhɑməˈlɑgrəfɪ] *n* Schichtanatomie *f*, Homalographie *f*.
Homans [ˈhɔʊmənz]: **H.'s sign** *chir.* Homans-Zeichen *nt*.
ho·mat·ro·pine [hɔʊˈmætrəpiːn, -pɪn] *n pharm.* Homatropin *n*.
homatropine hydrobromide Homatropinhydrobromid *nt*.
hom·ax·i·al [hɔʊˈmæksɪəl, hɑˈm-] *adj* mit gleichlangen Achsen, hom(o)axial.
home(o)- *pref.* Homöo(o)-, Homoio-.
ho·me·o·ki·ne·sis [ˌhɔʊmɪɔʊkɪˈniːʒ(ɪ)ə, -kaɪ-] *n bio., histol.* Homöokinese *f*.
ho·me·o·mor·phous [ˌ-ˈmɔːrfəs] *adj* von gleicher Form u. Struktur, homöomorph.
homeo-osteoplasty *n ortho.* homologe Knochentransplantation *f*.
ho·me·o·path [ˈ-pæθ] *n* → homeopathist.
ho·me·o·path·ic [ˌ-ˈpæθɪk] *adj* Homöopathie betr., homöopathisch.
ho·me·op·a·thist [ˌhɔʊmɪˈɑpəθɪst] *n* Homöopath(in *f*) *m*.
ho·me·op·a·thy [hɔʊmɪˈɑpəθɪ] *n* Homöopathie *f*.
ho·me·o·pla·sia [ˌhɔʊmɪəˈpleɪʒ(ɪ)ə, -zɪə] *n* Homöoplasie *f*.
ho·me·o·plas·tic [ˌ-ˈplæstɪk] *adj* Homöoplasie betr., homöoplastisch.
ho·me·o·sis [ˌhɔʊmɪˈɔʊsɪs] *n* Homöosis *f*.
ho·me·o·sta·sis [ˌhɔʊmɪəˈsteɪsɪs] *n* Homöo-, Homoiostase *f*, Homöostasie *f*, Homöostasis *f*.
ho·me·o·stat·ic [ˌ-ˈstætɪk] *adj* Homöostase betr., zu ihr beruhend, homöostatisch.
homeostatic drives homöostatische Triebe *pl*.
ho·me·o·ther·a·peu·tic [ˌ-ˌθerəˈpjuːtɪk] *adj* **1.** → homeopathic. **2.** Homöotherapie betr., homöotherapeutisch.
ho·me·o·ther·a·py [ˌ-ˈθerəpɪ] *n* Homöotherapie *f*.
ho·me·o·therm [ˈ-θɜrm] *n* warmblütiges/homöothermes Lebewesen *nt*, Warmblüter *m*.
ho·me·o·ther·mal [ˌ-ˈθɜrml] *adj* → homeothermic.
ho·me·o·ther·mic [ˌ-ˈθɜrmɪk] *adj bio.* dauerwarm, warmblütig, homöo-, homoiotherm.
ho·me·o·ther·mism [ˌ-ˈθɜrmɪzəm] *n bio.* → homeothermy.
ho·me·o·ther·my [ˈ-θɜrmɪ] *n bio.* Warmblütigkeit *f*, Homöo-, Homoiothermie *f*.
ho·me·o·typ·ic [ˌ-ˈtɪpɪk] *adj* → homeotypical.
ho·me·o·typ·i·cal [ˌ-ˈtɪpɪkl] *adj histol.* homöotypisch, homotypisch.
home·sick·ness [ˈhɔʊmsɪknɪs] *n psycho., psychia.* Heimweh *nt*, Nostalgie *f*.
hom·i·cid·al [ˌhɑməˈsaɪdl, ˌhɔʊm-] *adj* **1.** *psychia.* mörderisch, mordlustig. **2.** Mord-, Totschlags-.
hom·i·cide [ˈ-saɪd] *n* Mord *m*, Tötung *f*, Totschlag *m*.
hom·i·nal [ˈhɑmɪnəl] *adj* Mensch betr., Menschen-, Human-.
hom·i·nid [ˈhɑmɪnɪd] **I** *n* menschenartiges Wesen *nt*, Hominid(e) *m*. **II** *adj* menschenartig, -ähnlich, hominid.
Ho·min·i·dae [hɔʊˈmɪnədiː] *pl* Menschenartige *pl*, Hominiden *pl*, Hominidae *pl*.
hom·in·i·nox·ious [ˌhɑmənɪˈnɑkʃəs] *adj* für den Menschen schädlich, den Menschen schädigend.
hom·i·ni·za·tion [ˌ-ˈzeɪʃn] *n bio.* Menschwerdung *f*, Hominisation *f*.
hom·i·noid [ˈhɑmənɔɪd] *n* menschenähnliches Wesen *nt*, Hominoid(e) *m*.
Hom·i·noi·dea [ˌhɑmɪˈnɔɪdɪə] *pl* Menschenähnliche *pl*, Hominoiden *pl*, Hominoidea *pl*.
Ho·mo [ˈhɔʊmɔʊ] *n* Mensch *m*, Homo *m*.
homo- *pref.* **1.** gleich-, hom(o)-. **2.** *chem.* Homo-.
ho·mo [ˈhɔʊmɔʊ] *n* Mensch *m*, Homo *m*.
ho·mo·bi·o·tin [ˌhɔʊmɔʊˈbaɪətɪn, ˌhɑm-] *n* Homobiotin *nt*.
ho·mo·car·no·si·nase [ˌ-ˈkɑːrnəsɪneɪz] *n* Homokarnosinase *f*, -carnosinase *f*.
ho·mo·car·no·sine [ˌ-ˈkɑːrnəsiːn] *n* Homokarnosin *nt*, -carnosin *nt*.
ho·mo·car·no·sin·o·sis [ˌ-kɑːrˌnɔʊsɪˈnɔʊsɪs] *n patho.* Homokarnosinose *f*, -carnosinose *f*.
ho·mo·cel·lu·lar [ˌ-ˈseljələr] *adj* homozellulär.
homocellular transport homozellulärer Transport *m*.
ho·mo·cen·tric [ˌ-ˈsentrɪk] *adj* einen gemeinsamen Mittelpunkt habend, homozentrisch.
ho·mo·chro·mat·ic [ˌ-krɔʊˈmætɪk] *adj phys.* einfarbig, monochromatisch.
ho·mo·chrome [ˈ-krɔʊm] *adj* → homochromatic.
ho·moch·ro·nous [hɔʊˈmɑkrənəs] *adj* **1.** gleichzeitig, gleichlaufend, synchron (*with* mit). **2.** *genet.* in derselben Generation auftretend, homochron.
ho·mo·cit·rate [ˌhɔʊmɔʊˈsɪtreɪt, ˌhɑm-] *n* Homozitrat *nt*, -citrat *nt*.
homocitrate synthase Homocitratsynthase *f*.

ho·mo·cit·ric acid [ˌ-'sɪtrɪk] Homozitronensäure f, -citronensäure f.
ho·mo·clad·ic anastomosis [ˌ-'klædɪk] anat. homokladische Anastomose f.
ho·mo·cy·clic [ˌ-'saɪklɪk, -'sɪk-] adj chem. homozyklisch.
homocyclic compound chem. isozyklische Verbindung f.
homocyclic ring chem. homozyklischer Ring m, homozyklische Ringstruktur f.
ho·mo·cys·te·ine [ˌ-'sɪsti:in] n Homozystein nt, -cystein nt.
homocysteine methyltransferase Homocystein-methyltransferase f.
homocysteine:tetrahydrofolate methyltransferase Homocystein-tetrahydrofolat-methyltransferase f, 5-Methyltetrahydrofolat-homocystein-methyltransferase f.
ho·mo·cys·tine [ˌ-'sɪsti:n, -tɪn] n Homozystin nt, -cystin nt.
ho·mo·cys·ti·ne·mia [ˌ-ˌsɪstəˈniːmɪə] n Homozystinämie f, -cystinämie f.
ho·mo·cys·ti·nu·ria [ˌ-ˌsɪstəˈn(j)ʊərɪə] n Homocystinurie f, -zystinurie f.
ho·mo·cy·to·tro·pic antibody [ˌhəʊməˌsaɪtəˈtrɒpɪk, ˌhæmə-] homozytotroper Antikörper m.
ho·mo·dont ['-['həʊmədɒnt] adj dent. homodont.
ho·mo·dro·mous [həʊˈmædrəməs] adj physiol. in die gleiche Richtung (ablaufend), homodrom.
homoe(o)- pref. → home(o)-.
ho·moe·o·sis [ˌhəʊmɪˈəʊsɪs] n → homeosis.
ho·mo·e·rot·ic [ˌhəʊməʊˈrɒtɪk] adj homoerotisch.
ho·mo·e·rot·i·cism [ˌ-ɪˈrɒtəsɪzəm] n Homoerotik f, Homoerotismus m.
ho·mo·er·o·tism [ˌ-ˈerətɪzəm] n → homoeroticism.
ho·mo·gam·ete [ˌ-ˈgæmiːt, -gəˈmiːt] n genet. Homogamet m.
ho·mo·ga·met·ic [ˌ-gəˈmetɪk] adj genet. homogametisch.
ho·mog·a·mous [həʊˈmægəməs] adj genet. homogam.
ho·mog·a·my [həʊˈmægəmɪ] n 1. genet. Homogamie f. 2. socio. Homogamie f.
ho·mo·ge·ne·i·ty [ˌhəʊmədʒəˈniːɪtɪ, ˌhæm-] n Gleichartigkeit f, Einheitlichkeit f, Homogenität f.
homogeneity coefficient radiol. Homogenitätsgrad m.
ho·mo·ge·ni·za·tion [ˌ-ˌdʒɪnɪəˈzeɪʃn] n → homogenization.
ho·mo·ge·ne·ous [ˌ-ˈdʒiːnɪəs, -jəs] adj gleichartig, einheitlich, übereinstimmend, homogen.
homogeneous fluid homogene Flüssigkeit f, Newtonsche Flüssigkeit f.
ho·mo·ge·ne·ous·ness [ˌ-ˈdʒiːnɪəsnɪs] n → homogeneity.
ho·mo·gen·e·sis [ˌ-ˈdʒenəsɪs] pl bio. Homogenese f.
ho·mo·ge·net·ic [ˌ-dʒəˈnetɪk] adj Homogenese betr., homogenetisch.
ho·mo·ge·net·ical [ˌ-dʒəˈnetɪkl] adj → homogenetic.
homogenetic cortex Neokortex m, Neocortex m.
ho·mo·gen·ic [ˌ-ˈdʒenɪk] adj → homozygous.
ho·mo·ge·nic·i·ty [ˌ-dʒəˈnɪsətɪ] n → homogeneity.
ho·mo·ge·ni·za·tion [həˌmædʒənɪˈzeɪʃn, həʊ-] n Homogenisierung f, Homogenisation f.
ho·mog·e·nize [həˈmædʒənaɪz, həʊ-] vt homogen od. gleichartig od. einheitlich machen, homogenisieren.
ho·mog·e·nized milk [həˈmædʒənaɪzd, həʊ-] homogenisierte Milch f.
ho·mog·e·nous [həˈmædʒənəs, həʊ-] adj 1. → homogeneous. 2. → homoplastic. 3. → homologous.
homogenous system homogenes System nt.
ho·mo·gen·ti·sate [ˌhəʊməʊˈdʒentɪseɪt] n Homogentisat nt.
homogentisate 1,2-dioxygenase → homogentisic acid 1,2-dioxygenase.
homogentisate oxidase → homogentisic acid 1,2-dioxygenase.
ho·mo·gen·tis·ic acid [ˌ-dʒenˈtɪsɪk] Homogentisinsäure f, 2,5-Dihydroxyphenylessigsäure f.
homogentisic acid 1,2-dioxygenase Homogentisinsäure(-1,2-)dioxygenase f, Homogentisinatoxidase f, Homogentisin(säure)oxygenase f.
homogentisic acid oxidase → homogentisic acid 1,2-dioxygenase.
homogentisic acid oxidase deficiency Homogentisinsäureoxigenasemangel m, Alkaptonurie f.
ho·mo·gen·tis·i·case [ˌ-dʒenˈtɪsɪkeɪz] n → homogentisic acid 1,2-dioxygenase.
ho·mo·gen·ti·su·ria [ˌ-ˌdʒentɪˈs(j)ʊərɪə] n Homogentisinsäureausscheidung f im Harn, Homogentisinurie f.
ho·mog·e·ny [həˈmædʒənɪ, həʊ-] n → homogenesis.
ho·mo·gly·can [ˌ-ˈglaɪkæn] n → homopolysaccharide.
ho·mo·graft ['-ɡræft] n homologes/allogenes/allogenetisches Transplantat nt, Homo-, Allotransplantat nt.
homograft reaction Allotransplantatabstoßung(sreaktion f) f.
homoi(o)- pref. → home(o)-.
ho·moi·o·pla·sia [həʊˌmɔɪəˈpleɪʒ(ɪ)ə, -zɪə] n → homeoplasia.
ho·moi·os·ta·sis [ˌhəʊmɔɪˈæstəsɪs] n → homeostasis.
ho·moi·o·ther·mal [həʊˌmɔɪəˈθɜːrml] adj → homeothermic.
ho·moi·so·cit·ric acid [ˌhəʊməʊˌaɪsəˈsɪtrɪk, ˌhæm-] Homoisozitronensäure f.
ho·mo·ker·a·to·plas·ty [ˌ-ˈkerətəplæstɪ] n ophthal. homologe Hornhautplastik f, Homokeratoplastik f.
ho·mo·lac·tic [ˌ-ˈlæktɪk] adj biochem. homolaktisch, homofermentativ.
homolactic fermentation homolaktische/homofermentative Milchsäuregärung f.
ho·mo·lat·er·al [ˌ-ˈlætərəl] adj dieselbe (Körper-)Seite betr., auf derselben Seite (liegend), homo-, ipsilateral.
ho·mo·lip·id ['-lɪpɪd] n Homolipid nt.
ho·mo·lo·gen [həʊˈmælədʒən] n → homologue 2.
ho·mo·log·i·cal [ˌhəʊməˈlɒdʒɪkl, ˌhæm-] adj → homologous.
ho·mol·o·gous [həˈmæləgəs, həʊ-] adj 1. entsprechend, übereinstimmend, ähnlich, artgleich, homolog. 2. immun. homolog, allogen, allogenetisch. 3. chem. gleichliegend, -laufend, homolog.
homologous antigen 1. homologes Antigen nt. 2. Isoantigen nt.
homologous chromosome Autosom nt.
homologous graft → homograft.
homologous hepatitis → hepatitis B.
homologous insemination homologe Insemination f, künstliche Befruchtung f mit Sperma des Ehemannes.
homologous interference immun., micro. homologe Interferenz f.
homologous recombination genet. homologe/legitime Rekombination f.
homologous series chem. homologe Reihe f.
homologous serum homologes Serum nt.
homologous serum hepatitis → hepatitis B.
homologous serum jaundice → hepatitis B.
homologous stimulus homologer Reiz m.
homologous tissue homologes Gewebe nt.
homologous transplant → homograft.
homologous transplantation homologe/allogene/allogenetische Transplantation f, Homo-, Allotransplantation f.
homologous tumor homologer Tumor m.
ho·mo·logue ['həʊməlɒɡ, -lɑːɡ, 'həʊ-] n 1. bio. homologes Organ nt. 2. chem. homologe Verbindung f.
ho·mol·o·gy [həˈmælədʒɪ, həʊ-] n, pl -gies Übereinstimmung f, Entsprechung f, homologe Beschaffenheit f, Homologie f.
ho·mol·y·sin [həʊˈmælɪsɪn] n immun. homologes Lysin nt, Homolysin nt.
ho·mol·y·sis [həʊˈmælɪsɪs] n immun. Homolyse f.
ho·mo·mor·phic [ˌhəʊməʊˈmɔːrfɪk, ˌhæm-] adj gleichgestaltig, homomorph.
ho·mo·mor·phous [ˌ-ˈmɔːrfəs] adj → homomorphic.
ho·mon·o·mous [həʊˈmænəməs] adj gleichartig, gleichwertig, von gleicher Funktion, homonom.
ho·mon·y·mous [həˈmænɪməs, həʊ-] adj gleichnamig, homonym(isch).
homonymous diplopia ophthal. direkte/gleichseitige/ungekreuzte/homonyme Diplopie f, Diplopia simplex.
homonymous hemianopia/hemianopsia ophthal. homonyme/gleichseitige Hemianop(s)ie f.
homonymous image ophthal. homonymes Bild nt.
ho·mo·phile ['həʊməfaɪl] n, adj → homosexual.
ho·mo·plas·ty ['həʊməplæstɪ] n 1. chir. Homo-, Homöo-, Homoioplastik f. 2. → homoplasy.
ho·mo·plas·tic [ˌ-ˈplæstɪk] adj 1. chir. Homoplastik betr., homoplastisch. 2. homoplastisch, homolog, allogen. 3. bio. homoplastisch.
homoplastic graft → homograft.
ho·mop·la·sy [həʊˈmæplɪsɪ, 'həʊməplæsɪ, -pleɪsɪ] n bio. Homoplasie f.
ho·mo·pol·y·mer [ˌhəʊməˈpɒlɪmər, ˌhæm-] n Homopolymer nt.
ho·mo·pol·y·pep·tide [ˌ-ˌpɒlɪˈpeptaɪd] n Homopolypeptid nt.
ho·mo·pol·y·sac·cha·ride [ˌ-ˌpɒlɪˈsækəraɪd, -rɪd] n Homopolysaccharid nt, Homoglykan nt.
ho·mo·pro·line [ˌ-ˈprəʊlɪn, -liːn] n Pipecolinsäure f, Homoprolin nt.
ho·mo·ser·ine [ˌ-ˈserɪn, -riːn] n Homoserin nt.
homoserine acyltransferase Homoserin-acyltransferase f.
homoserine deaminase Cystathionin-γ-lyase f.
homoserine dehydratase → homoserine deaminase.
homoserine dehydrogenase Homoserin-dehydrogenase f.
homoserine kinase Homoserinkinase f.
homoserine phosphate Homoserinphosphat nt.
homoserine phosphoric acid Homoserinphosphorsäure f.
ho·mo·sex·u·al [ˌ-ˈsekʃəwəl, -ˈseksjʊəl] I n Homosexuelle(r m) f. II adj homosexuell, -phil, -erotisch.
ho·mo·sex·u·al·i·ty [ˌ-ˌsekʃəˈwælətɪ, -ˌsek-

sju'æləti] n Homosexualität f, -erotik f, -philie f.
ho·mos·po·rous [həʊ'mɒspərəs] adj bio., micro. gleichsporig, iso-, homospor.
ho·mos·po·ry [həʊ'mɒspəri] n bio., micro. Homosporie f, Isosporie f.
ho·mo·stim·u·lant [ˌhəʊməʊ'stɪmjələnt, ˌham-] n Homostimulans nt.
hom·o·thal·lic [ˌ-'θælɪk] adj micro. homothallisch.
hom·o·thal·lism [ˌ-'θælɪzəm] n micro. Homothallie f.
ho·mo·therm ['-θɜrm] n → homeotherm.
ho·mo·ther·mal [ˌ-'θɜrml] adj → homeothermic.
ho·mo·ther·mic [ˌ-'θɜrmɪk] adj → homeothermic.
ho·mo·top·ic [ˌ-'tɒpɪk] adj homotop; orthotop.
homotopic transplantation orthotope Transplantation f.
ho·mo·trans·plant [ˌ-'trænzplænt] n → homograft.
ho·mo·trans·plan·ta·tion [ˌ-ˌtrænzplæn'teɪʃn] n → homologous transplantation.
ho·mo·trop·ic [ˌ-'trɒpɪk, -'trəʊ-] adj homotrop.
homotropic enzyme homotropes Enzym nt.
ho·mo·typ·al [ˌ-'taɪpl] adj → homotypic.
ho·mo·type ['-taɪp] n homotypes Organ nt, Homotyp m.
ho·mo·typ·ic [ˌ-'tɪpɪk] adj homöotyp, -typisch, homotyp(isch).
ho·mo·typ·i·cal [ˌ-'tɪpɪkl] adj → homotypic.
homotypical cortex → homotypic isocortex.
homotypic isocortex hom(ö)otyper/hom(ö)otypischer Isocortex m.
homotypic tumor → homologous tumor.
ho·mo·va·nil·lic acid [ˌ-və'nɪlɪk] abbr. HVA Homovanillinsäure f.
ho·mo·zo·ic [ˌ-'zəʊɪk] adj bio. homozoisch.
ho·mo·zy·go·sis [ˌ-zaɪ'gəʊsɪs] n Gleich-, Reinerbigkeit f, Erbgleichheit f, Homozygotie f.
ho·mo·zy·gos·i·ty [ˌ-zaɪ'gɒsəti] n → homozygosis.
ho·mo·zy·gote [ˌ-'zaɪgəʊt] n homozygote Zelle f, homozygoter Organismus m, Homozygot m, Homozygote f.
ho·mo·zy·got·ic [ˌ-zaɪ'gɒtɪk] adj → homozygous.
ho·mo·zy·gous [ˌ-'zaɪgəs] adj gleich-, reinerbig, homozygot.
homozygous form of β-thalassemia → homozygous β-thalassemia.
homozygous β-thalassemia Cooley-Anämie f, homozygote β-Thalassämie f, Thalassaemia major.
ho·mun·cu·lus [hə'mʌŋkjələs, həʊ-] n, pl -li [-laɪ] Homunkulus m, Homunculus m.
hon·ey·comb appearance/configuration ['hʌnɪkəʊm] histol., radiol. Bienenwaben-, Honigwabenstruktur f.
honeycomb lung Wabenlunge f.
honeycomb ringworm Favus m, Erb-, Flechten-, Kopf-, Pilzgrind m, Tinea (capitis) favosa, Dermatomycosis favosa.
Hong Kong influenza ['hɒŋ 'kɒŋ] Hongkonggrippe f.
Hong Kong toe Athleten-, Sportlerfuß m, Fußpilz m, Fußpilzerkrankung f, Fußmykose f, Tinea f der Füße, Tinea pedis/pedum f, Epidermophytia pedis/pedum.
hoof-and-mouth disease [huːf] (echte) Maul- u. Klauenseuche f abbr. MKS, Febris aphthosa, Stomatitis epidemica, Aphthosis epizootica.
hook [hʊk] n chir. Haken m.

hook forceps chir. Hakenzange f.
hook·less tapeworm ['hʊklɪs] micro. Rinder(finnen)bandwurm m, Taenia saginata, Taeniarhynchus saginatus.
hook-up n 1. phys., physiol. System nt, Schaltung f, Schaltbild nt, -schema nt. 2. Zusammenschluß m, Zusammenschaltung f.
hook·worm ['hʊkwɜrm] n micro. 1. Hakenwurm m. 2. (europäischer) Hakenwurm m, Grubenwurm m, Ancylostoma duodenale.
h. of the dog Ancylostoma caninum.
hookworm anemia Anämie f bei Hakenwurmbefall.
hookworm disease Hakenwurmbefall m, -infektion f, Ankylostomiasis f, Ankylostomatosis f, Ankylostomatidose f.
Hoppe-Goldflam ['hɒpə 'gəʊltflam]: H.-G. disease Erb-Goldflam-Syndrom nt, -Krankheit f, Erb-Oppenheim-Goldflam-Syndrom nt, -Krankheit f, Hoppe-Goldflam-Syndrom nt, Myasthenia gravis pseudoparalytica.
hor·de·in ['hɔːrdɪɪn] n Hordein nt.
hor·de·o·lum [hɔːr'dɪələm] n ophthal. Gerstenkorn nt, Zilienabszeß m, Hordeolum nt.
ho·ri·zo·car·dia [həˌraɪzə'kɑːrdɪə] n card. Horizontallage/Querlage f des Herzens, Horizokardie f.
hor·i·zon·tal [ˌhɔːrɪ'zɒntl, ˌhɑrə-] I n Horizontale f, Waag(e)rechte f. II adj horizontal, waag(e)recht.
horizontal cells (Retina) Horizontalzellen pl.
h.s of Cajal Cajal-Zellen pl.
horizontal disparity Querdisparation f, horizontale Paration f.
horizontal fissure: h. of cerebellum Fissura horizontalis cerebelli.
great h. → h. of cerebellum.
h. of right lung horizontaler Interlobärspalt m, Fissura horizontalis (pulmonis dextris).
horizontal folds of rectum Plicae transversae recti.
horizontal heart 1. physiol. Horizontaltyp m. 2. → horizocardia.
horizontal lamina of palatine bone → horizontal plate of palatine bone.
horizontal maxillary fracture Guérin-Fraktur f, LeFort I-Fraktur f.
horizontal nystagmus horizontaler Nystagmus m.
horizontal part of duodenum unterer/horizontaler Duodenumabschnitt m, Pars horizontalis/inferior duodeni.
horizontal plane Horizontalebene f, Horizontale f.
horizontal plate of palatine bone horizontale Platte f des Gaumenbeins, Lamina horizontalis (ossis palatini).
horizontal transmission horizontale Infektionsübertragung/Transmission f.
horizontal vertigo horizontaler Schwindel m.
hor·mic psychology ['hɔːrmɪk] hormische Psychologie f, Antriebspsychologie f, Hormismus m.
hor·mism ['hɔːrmɪzəm] n → hormic psychology.
Hor·mo·den·drum [ˌhɔːrmə'dendrəm] n micro. Hormodendron nt.
hor·mon·a·gogue [ˌhɔːrˈmɒnəgɒg, -gag] n pharm. Hormonbildung-anregendes Mittel nt, Hormonagogum nt.
hor·mo·nal ['hɔːrməʊnl, 'hɔːrməʊn] adj hormonal, hormonell, Hormon-.
hor·mo·nal·ly-dependent ['hɔːrmənəlɪ] adj hormonabhängig.
hormonal response hormonelle/hormon-

gesteuerte Reizantwort/Reaktion/Anpassung f.
hormonal therapy Hormontherapie f.
hor·mone ['hɔːrməʊn] n Hormon nt.
hormone blocker Hormonblocker m, -antagonist m, Antihormon nt.
hormone breakdown Hormonabbau m.
hormone chemistry Chemie f der Hormone.
hormone-dependent adj hormonabhängig.
hormone-like adj hormonähnlich.
hormone preprotein → hormonogen.
hormone receptor Hormonrezeptor m.
hormone-receptor complex Hormonrezeptorkomplex m.
hormone release Hormonausschüttung f, -ausscheidung f, -abgabe f.
hormone replacement therapy abbr. HRT Hormon(ersatz)therapie f.
hormone-sensitive adj hormonsensitiv.
hormone-sensitive lipase hormonsensitive Lipase f.
hormone therapie Hormontherapie f.
hormone-withdrawal bleeding Hormonentzugsblutung f.
hor·mon·ic [hɔːr'mɒnɪk, -'məʊn-] adj → hormonal.
hor·mon·o·gen ['hɔːrmənədʒən] n Prohormon nt, Hormonogen nt, Hormogen nt.
hor·mo·no·gen·e·sis [ˌhɔːrmənəʊ'dʒenəsɪs] n Hormonbildung f, Hormonogenese f.
hor·mo·no·gen·ic [ˌ-'dʒenɪk] adj Hormonbildung betr. od. stimulierend, hormonbildend, homonogen.
hor·mo·no·poi·e·sis [ˌ-pɔɪ'iːsɪs] n → hormonogenesis.
hor·mo·no·poi·et·ic [ˌ-pɔɪ'etɪk] adj → hormonogenic.
hor·mo·no·priv·ia [ˌ-'prɪvɪə] n old Hormonmangel m.
hor·mo·no·ther·a·py [ˌ-'θerəpɪ] n Hormontherapie f.
Horn [hɒːrn]: H.'s sign chir. (ten) Horn-Zeichen nt.
horn [hɔːrn] n 1. Horn nt, hornförmige Struktur f; anat. Cornu nt. 2. zoo. Horn nt; (Insekt) Fühler m. 3. chem. Horn nt, Keratin nt.
h. of Ammon 1. Ammonshorn, Hippokampus m, Hippocampus m. 2. (eigentliches) Ammonshorn, Cornu Ammonis, Pes hippocampi.
h. of hyoid bone Zungenbeinhorn, Cornu ossis hyoidei.
h. of sacrum Cornu sacrale.
h. of thyroid cartilage Schildknorpelhorn, Cornu cartilaginis thyroideae.
h. of uterus Gebärmutterzipfel m, Cornu uteri.
horn cell 1. (Epidermis) Hornzelle f. 2. (ZNS) Vorder- od. Hinterhornzelle f.
horned [hɔːrnd] adj gehörnt, Horn-.
Horner ['hɔːrnər]: H.'s law Horner-Gesetz nt, -Regel f.
H.'s muscle Horner-Muskel m, Pars lacrimalis m. orbicularis oculi.
H.'s ptosis → H.'s syndrome.
H.'s sign gyn. Spalding-Zeichen nt.
H.'s syndrome Horner-Syndrom nt, -Trias f, -Symptomenkomplex m.
Horner-Bernard [bɛr'nar]: H.-B. syndrome → Horner's syndrome.
hor·ni·fi·ca·tion [ˌhɔːrnɪfɪ'keɪʃn] n Verhornung f, Verhornen nt, Keratinisation f.
horn·less ['hɔːrnlɪs] adj ohne Horn/Hörner, hornlos.
horn·y ['hɔːrnɪ] adj 1. → horned. 2. hornig, schwielig. 3. aus Horn, Horn-.
horny layer: h. of epidermis epidermale

horny scale

Hornschicht f, Stratum corneum epidermidis.
h. of nail verhornter Nagelteil m, Stratum corneum unguis.
horny scale (*Haut*) Hornschuppe f.
ho·rop·ter [hə'rɑptər, hɔ-] n Sehgrenze f, Horopter m.
horopter circle Horopterkreis m.
hor·op·ter·ic [ˌhɔrɑp'tɛrɪk] adj Horopter betr-, Horopter-.
hor·rip·i·la·tion [hɔˌrɪpə'leɪʃn] n derm. Horripilatio f.
horse cell test [hɔːrs] immun. modifizierter Paul-Bunnell-Test m mit Pferdeerythrozyten.
horse chestnut pharm. Roßkastanie f, Aesculus hippocastanum.
horse-fly ['hɔːrsflaɪ] n micro. Pferdebremse f, Tabanus m.
horse louse micro. Trichodectis pilosus.
horse·pow·er ['hɔːrspaʊər] n abbr. **h.p.**, **HP** phys. Pferdestärke f abbr. PS.
horse-pox ['hɔːrspɑks] n Pferdepocken pl, Variola equina.
horse-rad·ish peroxidase ['hɔːrsrædɪʃ] Meerrettichperoxidase f.
horse·shoe abscess ['hɔːrsʃuː, 'hɔːrʃ-] Hufeisenabszeß m.
horseshoe fistula Hufeisenfistel f.
horseshoe kidney Hufeisenniere f, Ren arcuatus.
horseshoe placenta Hufeisenplazenta f.
horse tick micro. Dermacentor albipictus.
Hortega [hɔːr'teɪgə]: **H. cell** Hortega-Zelle f, H-Zelle f, Mikrogliazelle f.
H. glia Mesoglia f, Hortega-Glia f, -Zellen pl.
H. method Hortega-Silberimprägnierung f, -Versilberung f.
H.'s neuroglia stain → H. method.
hor·to·be·zoar [ˌhɔːrtə'biːzɔːr, -zəʊr] n Phytobezoar m.
Horton ['hɔːrtn]: **H.'s arteritis** → H.'s disease 1.
H.'s cephalgia → H.'s disease 2.
H.'s disease 1. Horton'-Riesenzellarteriitis f, -Syndrom nt, senile Riesenzellarteriitis f, Horton-Magath-Brown-Syndrom nt, Arteriitis cranialis/gigantocellularis/temporalis. **2.** (Bing-)Horton-Syndrom nt, -Neuralgie f, Histaminkopfschmerz m, Kephalgie f, Erythroprosopalgie f, Cephalaea histaminica, cluster headache (nt).
H.'s headache → H.'s disease 2.
H.'s syndrome → H.'s disease.
hos·pice ['hɑspɪs] n Sterbeklinik f.
hos·pi·tal ['hɑspɪtl] n **1.** Krankenhaus nt, Klinik f. **2.** Lazaret nt. **3.** Pflegeheim nt, Hospital m.
hospital-acquired infection nosokomiale Infektion f, nosokomialer Infekt m, Nosokomialinfektion f.
hospital fever epidemisches/klassisches Fleckfieber nt, Läusefleckfieber nt, Fleck-, Hunger-, Kriegstyphus m, Typhus exanthematicus.
hospital gangrene Wundliegen nt, Dekubitalulkus nt, -geschwür nt, Dekubitus m, Decubitus m.
hos·pi·tal·ism ['hɑspɪtlɪzəm] n **1.** psycho., psychia. Hospitalismus m. **2.** patho. Hospitalismus m.
hos·pi·tal·i·za·tion [ˌhɑspɪtlə'zeɪʃn] n **1.** Aufnahme/Einweisung/Einlieferung f ins Krankenhaus, Hospitalisierung f. **2.** Krankenhausaufenthalt m.
hos·pi·tal·ize ['hɑspɪtlaɪz] vt ins Krankenhaus einweisen od. einliefern, hospitalisieren, (stationär) aufnehmen.
hospital nurse Krankenhausschwester f.
host [həʊst] n bio., micro. Wirt m, Wirtstier

nt, -pflanze f, -zelle f. **to act as a ~** als Wirt dienen.
host alternation Wirtswechsel m.
host bacterium Wirtsbakterium nt.
host cell micro. Wirtszelle f.
host-parasite interaction/relationship micro. Wirt-Parasit-Wechselwirkung f.
host range Wirtsspektrum nt.
host reservoir Parasitenreservoir nt.
host resistance Wirtsresistenz f.
host selection Wirtswahl f.
host-specific adj wirtsspezifisch.
host specificity Wirtsspezifität f.
host-versus-graft reaction Wirt-anti--Transplantat-Reaktion f, Host-versus--Graft-Reaktion f abbr. HvG, HvGR.
HOT abbr. → hyperbaric oxygen therapy.
hot [hɑt] adj **1.** warm, heiß. **2.** fig. erhitzt, heiß. **3.** phys. heiß, stark radioaktiv. **4.** phys. stromführend.
hot abscess heißer Abszeß m.
hot-air bath Heißluftbad nt.
hot-cold hemolysin Kalt-Warm-Hämolysin m.
hot flushes gyn. fliegende Hitze f, Hitzewallungen pl.
hot nodule (*Schilddrüse*) heißer Knoten m.
hot pack heiße Packung f.
Hounsfield ['haʊnzfiːld]: **H. unit** radiol. Hounsfield-Einheit f.
hour ['aʊər] n abbr. **h** Stunde f abbr. h.
hour·glass gallbladder ['aʊərglæs, -glɑːs] patho. Sanduhrgallenblase f.
hourglass stomach patho. Sanduhrmagen m.
house dust mite ['haʊs] micro. Hausstaubmilbe f, Dermatophagoides pteronyssius.
house·maid's knee ['haʊsmeɪd] ortho. Bursitis praepatellaris.
Houssay [uː'saɪ]: **H. phenomenon** Houssay--Phänomen nt, -Effekt m.
H. syndrome Houssay-Syndrom nt.
Houston ['hjuːstn]: **H.'s folds/valves** zirkuläre Mastdarmfalten pl, Plicae transversae recti.
Howel-Evans ['haʊəl 'ɛvənz]: **H.-E.' syndrome** Howel-Evans-Syndrom nt.
Howell ['haʊəl]: **H.'s bodies** → Howell-Jolly bodies.
H.'s test urol., lab. Howard-Test m.
Howell-Jolly [ʒɔ'liː]: **H.-J. bodies** (Howell-)-Jolly-Körperchen pl.
H.'s symptom Howship-von Romberg--Zeichen nt.
Howship-Romberg ['rɑmbərg]: **H.-R. sign** Romberg-Zeichen nt, -Phänomen nt, Howship-von Romberg-Zeichen nt, -Phänomen nt.
Hoyer ['hɔɪər]: **H.'s canals** Sucquet-Hoyer--Kanäle pl.
HP abbr. → horsepower.
h.p. abbr. → horsepower.
HPETE abbr. → hydroperoxyeicosatetraenoic acid.
HPL abbr. → human placental lactogen.
hPL abbr. → human placental lactogen.
HPLC abbr. → high-pressure liquid chromatography.
HPRT abbr. [hypoxanthine guanine phosphoribosyltransferase] → hypoxanthine phosphoribosyltransferase.
HPRT deficiency Lesch-Nyhan-Syndrom nt, Automutilationssyndrom nt.
HPS abbr. → Hermansky-Pudlak syndrome.
HPV abbr. → human papillomavirus.
h$_r$ abbr. → radiation heat transfer coefficient.
H-R conduction time card. HR-Intervall nt.

H receptor Histaminrezeptor m, H-Rezeptor m.
H$_1$ receptor Histamin 1-Rezeptor m, H$_1$--Rezeptor m.
H$_2$ receptor Histamin 2-Rezeptor m, H$_2$--Rezeptor m.
H-reflex n Hoffmann-Reflex m, H-Reflex m.
HRT abbr. → hormone replacement therapy.
HSF abbr. → histamine-sensitizing factor.
H space → Holzknecht's space.
HSV abbr. → herpes simplex virus.
HSV encephalitis → herpes encephalitis.
Ht abbr. → total hyperopia.
5-HT abbr. → 5-hydroxytryptamine.
HTACS abbr. → human thyroid adenylate cyclase stimulator.
HTLV abbr. → human T-cell lymphotropic virus.
HTLV III abbr. [human T-cell lymphotropic virus, type III] → human immunodeficiency virus.
H-type fistula (ösophagotracheale) H-Fistel f.
Hübener-Thomsen-Friedenreich ['(h)juːbənər 'tɑmsən 'friːdnraɪx]: **H.-T.-F. phenomenon** Thomsen-Phänomen nt, Hübener--Thomsen-Friedenreich-Phänomen nt, T-Agglutinationsphänomen nt.
Hubrecht ['huːprɛçt]: **H.'s protochordal knot** embryo. Primitivknoten m.
Huchard [yʃɑːr]: **H.'s disease** Huchard'--Krankheit f, Präsklerose f.
H.'s symptom Huchard-Syndrom nt.
Hudson ['hʌdsən]: **H.'s line** ophthal. Stähli'-Linie f.
Hudson-Stähli ['ʃtɛːli]: **H.-S. line** ophthal. Stähli'-Linie f.
hue [(h)juː] n **1.** (Farb-)Ton m, Tönung f, Schattierung f. **2.** Farbe f.
Hueck [hɛk; hyk]: **H.'s ligament** Hueck'-, Stenon'-Band nt, iridokorneales Balkenwerk nt, Reticulum trabeculare (anguli iridocornealis), Lig. pectinatum (anguli iridocornealis).
Hueter [hjuːtər; 'hyːtər]: **H.'s line** Hueter--Linie f.
H.'s maneuver Hueter-Methode f.
H.'s sign ortho. Hueter-Zeichen nt.
Hueter-Mayo ['meɪoʊ]: **H.-M. operation** chir. Operation f nach Hueter-Mayo.
Hüfner ['hyːfnər]: **H.'s number** Hüfner'--Zahl f.
Huggins ['hʌgɪnz]: **H.' operation** Huggins--Operation f.
Huguier [ygi'je]: **H.'s sinus** Fossula fenestrae vestibuli.
Huhner ['hjuːnər]: **H. test** gyn. Huhner--Test m, Huhner-Sims-Test m, postkoitaler Spermakompatibilitätstest m.
hum [hʌm] **I** n Summen nt; Brummen nt. **II** vi summen; brummen.
hu·man [(h)juːmən] **I** n Mensch m. **II** adj **1.** den Menschen betr-, im Menschen vorkommend, vom Menschen stammend, human, Human-. **2.** menschlich, menschenfreundlich, menschenwürdig, human, Menschen-.
human being Mensch m.
human B-lymphotropic virus abbr. **HBLV** humanes B-lymphotropes-Virus nt abbr. HBLV, humanes Herpesvirus C nt.
human botfly micro. Dasselfliege f, Dermatobia hominis.
human chorionic gonadotropin abbr. **HCG, hCG** humanes Choriongonadotropin nt abbr. HCG.
human coronavirus abbr. **HCV** humanes Coronavirus nt abbr. HCV.
human dignity Menschenwürde f.

human diploid cell culture *abbr.* **HDCC** humane diploide Zell(en)kultur *f*, human diploid cell culture *abbr.* HDCC.
human diploid cell vaccine *abbr.* **HDCV** Human-Diploid-Zell-Vakzine *f*, human diploid cell vaccine *abbr.* HDCV.
hu·mane [(h)juːˈmeɪn] *adj* → human 2.
human enteric coronavirus *abbr.* **HECV** humanes enterisches Coronavirus *nt abbr.* HECV, human enteric coronavirus (*nt*).
human fibrinogen Humanfibrinogen *nt*.
human flea *micro.* Menschenfloh *m*, Pulex irritans.
human follicle-stimulating hormone Menotropin *nt*, Menopausengonadotropin *nt*, humanes Menopausengonadotropin *nt abbr.* HMG.
human growth hormone *abbr.* **HGH, hGH** Wachstumshormon *nt*, Somatotropin *nt*, somatotropes Hormon *nt abbr.* STH.
human herpesvirus 1 → herpes simplex virus type I.
human herpesvirus 2 → herpes simplex virus type II.
human herpesvirus 3 *micro.* Varicella--Zoster-Virus *nt abbr.* VZV.
human herpesvirus 4 *micro.* Epstein--Barr-Virus *nt abbr.* EBV, EB-Virus *nt*.
human herpesvirus 5 *micro.* Zyto-, Cytomegalievirus *nt abbr.* CMV.
human herpesvirus C → human B-lymphotropic virus.
human immunodeficiency virus *abbr.* **HIV** human immunodeficiency virus (*nt*) *abbr.* HIV, humanes T-Zell-Leukämie--Virus III *abbr.* HTLV III, Lymphadenopathie-assoziiertes Virus *nt abbr.* LAV, Aids-Virus *nt*.
human leukocyte antigens *abbr.* **HLA** Histokompatibilitätsantigene *pl*, Transplantationsantigene *pl*, HLA-Antigene *pl*, human leukocyte antigens *abbr.* HLA, humane Leukozytenantigene *pl abbr.* HLA.
human louse *micro.* Menschenlaus *f*, Pediculus humanus.
human medicine Humanmedizin *f*.
human menopausal gonadotropin *abbr.* **HMG, hMG** Menotropin *nt*, Menopausengonadotropin *nt*, humanes Menopausengonadotropin *nt abbr.* HMG.
human nature menschliche Natur *f*.
human papillomavirus *abbr.* **HPV** humanes Papillomavirus *nt abbr.* HPV.
human parasite *micro.* Humanparasit *m*, Parasit *m* des Menschen.
human physiology Physiologie *f* des Menschen, Humanphysiologie *f*.
human placental lactogen *abbr.* **HPL, hPL** humanes Plazenta-Laktogen *nt abbr.* HPL, Choriosomatotropin *nt*.
human race Menschengeschlecht *nt*.
human serum Humanserum *nt*.
human serum jaundice → hepatitis B.
human T-cell leukemia/lymphoma virus → human T-cell lymphotropic virus.
human T-cell lymphotropic virus *abbr.* **HTLV** *micro.* humanes T-Zell-lymphotropes-Virus *nt abbr.* HTLV, humanes T-Zell-Leukämievirus *nt abbr.* HTLV.
human T-cell lymphotropic virus type III *abbr.* **HTLV III** → human immunodeficiency virus.
human thyroid adenylate cyclase stimulator *abbr.* **HTACS** Thyroidea-stimulierendes Immunglobulin *nt abbr.* TSI, thyroid-stimulating immunoglobulin *abbr.* TSI, long-acting thyroid stimulator *abbr.* LATS.
hu·mec·tant [(h)juːˈmektənt] **I** *n chem.* Feuchthaltemittel *nt*, Feuchthalter *m*. **II** *adj* **1.** feucht. **2.** an-, befeuchtend, benetzend.
hu·mec·ta·tion [ˌ(h)juːmekˈteɪʃn] *n* **1.** *patho.* seröse Gewebeinfiltration *f*. **2.** An-, Befeuchten *nt*. **3.** Einweichen *nt*.
hu·mer·al [ˈ(h)juːmərəl] *adj* **1.** Oberarm *od.* Oberarmknochen/Humerus betr., humeral, Humerus-. **2.** Schulter betr., Schulter-.
humeral bone *old* → humerus.
humeral epicondyle Humerusepikondyle *f*, Epicondylus humeri.
lateral h. Epicondylus lateralis humeri.
medial h. Epicondylus medialis humeri.
humeral head: h. of flexor carpi ulnaris muscle Caput humerale m. flexoris carpi ulnaris.
h. of flexor digitorum superficialis muscle Caput humero-ulnare m. flexoris digitorum superficialis.
h. of pronator teres muscle Caput humerale m. pronatoris teretis.
humeral incisure of ulna Inc. trochlearis (ulnae).
humeral shaft Oberarm-, Humerusschaft *m*.
humeral shaft fracture Oberarmschaftbruch *m*, Humerusschaftfraktur *f*.
humero- *pref.* Oberarm-, Humerus-, humeral; Schulter-.
hu·mer·o·ra·di·al [ˌ(h)juːməroʊˈreɪdiəl] *adj* Humerus u. Radius betr., humeroradial, Humeroradial-.
humeroradial articulation Humeroradialgelenk *nt*, Artic. humeroradialis.
humeroradial joint → humeroradial articulation.
hu·mer·o·scap·u·lar [ˌ-ˈskæpjələr] *adj* Humerus u. Skapula betr., humeroskapular, skapulohumeral.
hu·mer·o·ul·nar [ˌ-ˈʌlnər] *adj* Humerus u. Ulna betr., humeroulnar, Humeroulnar-.
humeroulnar articulation Humeroulnargelenk *nt*, Artic. humeroulnaris.
humeroulnar head of flexor digitorum superficialis muscle → humeral head of flexor digitorum superficialis muscle.
humeroulnar joint → humeroulnar articulation.
hu·mer·us [ˈ(h)juːmərəs] *n*, *pl* **-ri** [-raɪ] Oberarmknochen *m*, Humerus *m*.
hu·mid [ˈ(h)juːmɪd] *adj* feucht.
humid gangrene *patho.* feuchte Gangrän *f*.
hu·mid·i·fi·er [(h)juːˈmɪdəfaɪər] *n* (Luft-)Befeuchter *m*.
hu·mid·i·fy [(h)juːˈmɪdəfaɪ] *vt* befeuchten.
hu·mid·i·ty [(h)juːˈmɪdətɪ] *n* (Luft-)Feuchtigkeit *f*; Feuchtigkeitsgehalt *m*.
hum·ming [ˈhʌmɪŋ] *adj* summend; brummend.
humming-top murmur *card.* Nonnensausen *nt*, -geräusch *nt*, Kreiselgeräusch *nt*, Bruit de diable.
hum nose [hʌm] Kartoffel-, Säuferpfund-, Knollennase *f*, Rhinophym *nt*, Rhinophyma *nt*.
hu·mor [ˈ(h)juːmər] *n* **1.** *physiol.* (Körper-)Flüssigkeit *f*, Humor *m*. **2.** (Gemüts-)Verfassung *f*, Stimmung *f*, Laune *f*. **in a good/ bad ~** *fig.* guter/schlechter Laune. **out of ~** schlecht gelaunt.
hu·mor·al [ˈ(h)juːmərəl] *adj* (Körper-)Flüssigkeit(en) betr., humoral, Humoral-.
humoral antibody humoraler Antikörper *m*.
humoral doctrine Humoralpathologie *f*.
humoral immunity humorale Immunität *f*.
hu·mor·al·ism [ˈ(h)juːmərəlɪzəm] *n* → humoral doctrine.
hu·mor·ism [ˈ(h)juːmərɪzəm] *n* → humoral doctrine.

hump [hʌmp] *n* Buckel *m*, Höcker *m*.
hump back Kyphose *f*.
hump nose Höckernase *f*.
hu·mus [ˈ(h)juːməs] *n bio.* Humus *m*.
hunch·back [ˈhʌntʃbæk] *n* Kyphose *f*.
hun·ger [ˈhʌŋɡər] **I** *n* **1.** Hunger *m*, Hungergefühl *nt*. **2.** *fig.* Hunger *m*, Verlangen *nt* (*for* nach). **II** *vi* **1.** Hunger haben, hungern. **2.** *fig.* hungern (*for* nach).
hunger edema Hungerödem *nt*.
hunger osteopathy alimentäre/nutritive Osteopathie *f*, Hungerosteopathie *f*.
hunger osteoporosis Hungerosteoporose *f*.
hunger strike Hungerstreik *m*. **to go on (a) ~** in (den) Hungerstreik treten.
hun·gry [ˈhʌŋɡrɪ] *adj* **1.** hungrig. **to be/feel ~** Hunger haben, hungrig sein. **to get ~** Hunger bekommen. **to go ~** hungern. **2.** *fig.* hungrig (*for* nach).
Hunner [ˈhʌnər]: **H.'s stricture** *urol.* Hunner-Striktur *f*.
H.'s ulcer Fenwick-Ulkus *nt*, Hunner-Ulkus *nt*, Hunner-Fenwick-Ulkus *nt*, Fenwick-Hunner-Ulkus *nt*.
Hunt [hʌnt]: **H.'s atrophy** Hunt-(Handmuskel-)Atrophie *f*.
H.'s disease 1. → H.'s syndrome 1. **2.** → H.'s syndrome 3.
juvenile paralysis agitans of H. → H.'s syndrome 2.
H.'s neuralgia → H.'s syndrome 1.
H.'s syndrome 1. Genikulatumneuralgie *f*, Ramsay Hunt-Syndrom *nt*, Zoster oticus, Herpes zoster oticus, Neuralgia geniculata. **2.** Pallidumsyndrom *nt*, progressive Pallidumatrophie Hunt *f*, Paralysis agitans juveniles. **3.** Hunt-Syndrom *nt*, Dyssynergia cerebellaris myoclonica.
Hunter [ˈhʌntər]: **H.'s canal** Adduktorenkanal *m*, Canalis adductorius.
H.'s glossitis atrophische Glossitis *f*, Hunter'-Glossitis *f*, Möller-Hunter'-Glossitis *f*.
H.'s gubernaculum Hunter'-Band *nt*, Gubernaculum testis.
H.'s ligament rundes Mutterband *nt*, Lig. teres uteri.
H.'s line Linea alba.
H.'s syndrome → Hunter-Hurler syndrome.
Hunter-Hurler [ˈhɜrlər; ˈhuːr-]: **H.-H. syndrome** Morbus Hunter *m*, Hunter-Syndrom *nt*, Mukopolysaccharidose II *f abbr.* MPS II.
hun·te·ri·an chancre [hʌnˈtɪərɪən] harter Schanker *m*, Hunter-Schanker *m*, syphilitischer Primäraffekt *m*, Ulcus durum.
Hunter-Schreger [ˈʃreɪɡər; ˈʃreːɡ-]: **bands of H.-S.** → H.-S. lines.
H.-S. lines *dent.* Schreger-Hunter'-Linien *pl*.
Huntington [ˈhʌntɪŋtən]: **H.'s chorea/disease** Erbchorea *f*, Chorea Huntington, Chorea chronica progressiva hereditaria.
Hurler [ˈhɜrlər; ˈhuːr-]: **H.'s disease** Hurler--Krankheit *f*, -Syndrom *nt*, Lipochondrodystrophie *f*, von Pfaundler-Hurler--Krankheit *f*, -Syndrom *nt*, Dysostosis multiplex, Mukopolysaccharidose I-H *f abbr.* MPS I-H.
pseudo-H. polydystrophy Mukolipidose III *f*, Pseudo-Hurler-Dystrophie *f*.
H.'s syndrome/type → H.'s disease.
Hurler-Scheie [ˈʃaɪə]: **H.-S. compound/syndrome/type** Hurler-Scheie-Variante *f*, Mukopolysaccharidose I-H/S *f abbr.* MPS I-H/S.
hur·loid facies [ˈhɜrlɔɪd] Wasserspeiergesicht *nt*, Gargoylfratze *f*.
Hurst [hɜrst]: **H. bougies** *chir.* Hurst-Sonden *pl*.

Hürthle

Hürthle ['hɜrtl; 'hyrtlə]: **H. cell adenoma** Hürthle-Tumor m, -Zelladenom nt, -Struma f, oxyphiles Schilddrüsenadenom nt.
H. cell carcinoma Hürthle-Zell-Karzinom nt, malignes Onkozytom nt.
H. cells Hürthle-Zellen pl.
H. cell tumor → H. cell adenoma.
H. cell tumor, malignant → H. cell carcinoma.
HUS abbr. → hemolytic-uremic syndrome.
Huschke ['hʊʃkə]: **auditory teeth of H.** Dentes acustici.
gastropancreatic ligament of H. → H.'s ligament.
H.'s ligament Plica gastropancreatica.
H.'s valve → Hasner's fold.
husk·y ['hʌskɪ] adj (Stimme) heiser, rauh.
Hutchinson ['hʌtʃɪnsən]: **H.'s disease 1.** polymorphe Lichtdermatose (Haxthausen) f, polymorpher Lichtausschlag m, Lichtekzem nt, Sommerprurigo f, Lupus erythematodes-artige Lichtdermatose f, Prurigo aestevalis, Eccema solare, Dermatopathia photoelectrica. **2.** Angioma serpiginosum. **3.** Chorioiditis gutta senilis, Altersdrusen pl.
H.'s facies Hutchinson-Gesicht nt, Facies Hutchinson.
H.'s freckle prämaligne Melanose f, melanotische Präkanzerose f, Dubreuilh--Krankheit f, -Erkrankung f, Dubreuilh--Hutchinson-Krankheit f, -Erkrankung f, Lentigo maligna, Melanosis circumscripta praeblastomatosa/praecancerosa Dubreuilh.
H.'s incisors → H.'s teeth.
melanotic freckle of H. → H.'s freckle.
H.'s neuroblastoma Hutchinson-Sympathoblastom nt.
H.'s patch ophthal. Hornhautfleck(en pl) m bei konnataler Lues.
H.'s pupil Hutchinson-Pupille f.
summer prurigo of H. 1. → H.'s disease 1. **2.** Sommerprurigo Hutchinson f, Hidroa vacciniformia/aestivalia/vacciniformis, Hydroa aestivale/vacciniforme, Dermatopathia photogenica.
H.'s syndrome → H.'s disease.
H.'s teeth Hutchinson-Zähne pl.
H.'s triad Hutchinson'-Trias f.
H.'s type Hutchinson-Sympathoblastom nt.
Hutchinson-Gilford ['ɡɪlfɔːrd, -fəʊrd]: **H.-G. disease/syndrome** Hutchinson--Gilford-Syndrom nt, Gilford-Syndrom nt, Progerie f, greisenhafter Zwergwuchs m, Progeria Hutchinson-Gilford, Progeria infantilis.
Hutchison ['hʌtʃɪsən]: **H. syndrome/type** Hutchison-Syndrom nt.
Hutinel [ytɪ'nel]: **H.'s disease** Hutinel'--Krankheit f, -Zirrhose f.
Huxley ['hʌkslɪ]: **H.'s layer/membrane/sheath** Huxley-Schicht f, -Membran f.
HVA abbr. → homovanillic acid.
H-V conduction time card. HV-Intervall nt.
HVG reaction → host-versus-graft reaction.
HV interval card. HV-Intervall nt.
HVL abbr. → half-value layer.
hyal- pref. → hyalo-.
hy·al ['haɪəl] adj → hyoid II.
hy·a·lin ['haɪəlɪn] n → hyaline I.
hy·a·line [n 'haɪəliːn, -lɪn; adj -lɪn, -laɪn] **I** n **1.** biochem. Hyalin nt. **2.** glasartig transparente Substanz f. **II** adj **3.** Hyalin betr., Hyalin-. **4.** transparent, durchscheinend; glasartig, glasig, hyalin. **5.** amorph, nicht kristallin.
hyaline arteriolar nephrosclerosis benigne Nephrosklerose f.
hyaline arteriosclerosis patho. hyaline Arteriosklerose f.
hyaline bodies Councilman-Körperchen pl.
hyaline cartilage hyaliner Knorpel m, Hyalinknorpel m, Cartilago hyalina.
hyaline casts urol. Hyalinzylinder pl, hyaline (Nieren-)Zylinder pl.
hyaline degeneration hyaline Degeneration f, Hyalinose f; Hyalinisierung f, Hyalinisation f.
hyaline leukocyte old → monocyte.
hyaline membrane hyaline Membran f.
hyaline membrane disease (of the newborn) hyaline Membrankrankheit f der Lungen, Membransyndrom nt (der Früh- u. Neugeborenen).
hyaline membrane syndrome → hyaline membrane disease (of the newborn).
hyaline thrombus hyaliner Thrombus m.
hy·a·lin·i·za·tion [ˌhaɪəlɪnɪ'zeɪʃn] n patho. Hyalinisierung f, Hyalinisation f.
hy·a·li·no·sis [haɪəlɪ'nəʊsɪs] n patho. hyaline Degeneration f, Hyalinose f.
hy·a·li·nu·ria [ˌ-'n(j)ʊərɪə] n Ausscheidung f von Hyalin od. Hyalinzylindern im Harn, Hyalinurie f.
hy·a·li·tis [haɪə'laɪtɪs] n ophthal. Glaskörperentzündung f, Hyalitis f, Hyaloiditis f.
hyalo- pref. **1.** Hyalin-. **2.** Glaskörper-. **3.** Glas-.
hy·a·lo·bi·u·ron·ic acid [ˌhaɪələʊbaɪə'rɑnɪk] Hyalobiuronsäure f.
hy·a·lo·cyte ['-saɪt] n Hyalozyt m.
hy·al·o·gen [haɪ'ælədʒən] n Hyalogen nt.
hy·a·loid ['haɪəlɔɪd] adj anat. transparent, glasig, glasartig, hyaloid.
hyaloid artery embryo. Glaskörperschlagader f.
hyaloid body Glaskörper m, Corpus vitreum.
hyaloid canal Cloquet'-Kanal m, Canalis hyaloideus.
hyaloid degeneration patho. amyloide Degeneration f, Amylodose f.
hy·a·loi·de·o·ret·i·nal degeneration [haɪəˌlɔɪdɪə'retɪnl] Wagner'-Krankheit f, hereditäre vitreoretinale Degeneration f.
hyaloid fossa Glaskörpermulde f, Fossa hyaloidea.
hy·a·loid·in [haɪə'lɔɪdɪn] n Hyaloidin nt.
hy·a·loid·i·tis [haɪəlɔɪ'daɪtɪs] n → hyalitis.
hyaloid membrane Glaskörpermembran f, Membrana vitrea/hyaloidea.
hy·a·lo·mere ['haɪələmɪər] n Hyalomer m.
hy·a·lo·mit·ome [ˌ-'mɪtəʊm] n old → hyaloplasm.
Hy·a·lom·ma [haɪə'lɑmə] n micro. Hyalomma f.
hy·a·lo·mu·coid [ˌhaɪələ'mjuːkɔɪd] adj hyalomukoid.
hy·a·lo·nyx·is [ˌ-'nɪksɪs] n ophthal. Glaskörperpunktion f.
hy·a·lo·pha·gia [ˌ-'feɪdʒ(ɪ)ə] n psychia. Glasessen nt, Hyalophagie f.
hy·a·loph·a·gy [haɪə'lɑfədʒɪ] n → hyalophagia.
hy·al·o·plasm ['haɪələplæzəm] n Grundzytoplasma nt, zytoplasmatische Matrix f, Hyaloplasma nt.
hy·a·lo·plas·ma [ˌ-'plæzmə] n → hyaloplasm.
hy·a·lo·plas·mat·ic [ˌ-plæz'mætɪk] adj Hyaloplasma betr., im Hyaloplasma liegend, hyaloplasmatisch.
hy·a·lo·plas·mic [ˌ-'plæzmɪk] adj → hyaloplasmatic.
hy·a·lo·se·ro·si·tis [ˌ-sɪrəʊ'saɪtɪs] n patho. Hyaloserositis f.
hy·a·lo·sis [haɪə'ləʊsɪs] n ophthal. degenerative Veränderung f des Humor vitreus.

hy·al·o·tome [haɪ'ælətəʊm] n → hyaloplasm.
hy·a·lu·rate [haɪə'lʊəreɪt] n → hyaluronate.
hy·a·lu·ro·nate [ˌhaɪə'lʊrəneɪt] n Hyaluronsäureester m, -salz nt, Hyaluronat nt.
hyaluronate lyase Hyaluronatlyase f.
hy·al·u·ron·ic acid [ˌhaɪəlʊ'rɑnɪk] abbr. **HA** Hyaluronsäure f.
hyaluronic lyase → hyaluronate lyase.
hy·a·lu·ron·i·dase [ˌ-'rɑnɪdaɪz] n hyaluronsäure-spaltendes Enzym nt, Hyaluronidase f.
hy·a·lu·ron·o·glu·co·sa·min·i·dase [haɪəlʊˌrɑnəˌɡluːkəʊsə'mɪnədeɪz] n Hyaluron(o)glukosaminidase f.
hy·a·lu·ron·o·glu·cu·ron·i·dase [ˌ-,ɡluːkə'rɑnɪdeɪz] n Hyaluron(o)glucuronidase f.
H-Y antigen H-Y-Antigen nt.
hy·bar·ox·ia [ˌhaɪbə'rɑksɪə] n Sauerstoffüberdrucktherapie f, hyperbare (Sauerstoff-)Therapie/Oxygenation f.
hy·brid ['haɪbrɪd] **I** n Bastard m, Kreuzung f, Mischling m, Hybride f. **II** adj hybrid, Bastard-, Misch-.
hybrid antibody hybrider Antikörper m.
hybrid chromosome hybrides Chromosom nt.
hy·brid·ism ['haɪbrədɪzəm] n **1.** Hybridisierung f, Hybridität f. **2.** Hybridität f.
hy·brid·i·ty [haɪ'brɪdətɪ] n → hybridism 2.
hy·brid·i·za·tion [ˌhaɪbrɪdɪ'zeɪʃn] n **1.** Hybridisierung f, Hybridisation f. **2.** Hybridisation, Bastardisierung f. **3.** chem. Hybridisierung f, Hybridisierungstechnik f.
hy·brid·ize ['haɪbrɪdaɪz] v **I** vt hybridisieren, bastadieren, kreuzen. **II** vi s. kreuzen.
hy·brid·o·ma [haɪbrɪ'dəʊmə] n Hybridom nt.
hybridoma growth factor Humaninterferon β2 nt abbr. Human-IFN-β2.
hybrid vigor genet. Heterosis f.
hy·dan·to·ic acid [ˌhaɪdæn'təʊɪk] Hydantoinsäure f, Uraminessigsäure f.
hy·dan·to·in [haɪdæn'təʊɪn] n Hydantoin nt, Glykolylharnstoff m.
hy·dan·to·in·ate [haɪdæn'təʊɪneɪt] n Hydantoinat nt.
hy·da·tid ['haɪdətɪd] n **1.** anat. zystenähnliche Struktur f, Hydatide f. **2.** parasit. Echinokokkenblase f, -zyste f, Hydatide f.
h.s of Morgagni Morgagni'-Hydatiden pl, Appendices vesiculosae (epoophorontis).
hydatid cyst parasit. Echinokokkenblase f, -zyste f, Hydatide f.
alveolar h. → multilocular h.
multilocular h. multilokuläre Echinokokkuszyste/Hydatidenzyste.
multiloculate h. → multilocular h.
osseous h. verkalkte Echinokokkuszyste/Hydatidenzyste.
hydatid disease Hydatidose f, Echinokokkenkrankheit f, -infektion f, Echinokokkose f.
alveolar/multilocular h. alveoläre Echinokokkose f.
unilocular h. zystische Echinokokkose f.
hydatid fremitus Hydatidenschwirren nt.
hy·da·tid·i·form [haɪdə'tɪdəfɔːrm] adj hydatidenartig, -förmig, -ähnlich, hydatidiform.
hydatidiform mole → hydatid mole.
hydatid mole gyn. Blasenmole f, Mola hydatidosa.
hy·da·tid·o·cele [haɪdə'tɪdəsiːl] n patho., chir. Hydatidozele f.
hy·da·ti·do·ma [haɪdətɪ'dəʊmə] n Hydatidom nt.
hy·da·ti·do·sis [ˌ-'dəʊsɪs] n → hydatid disease.

hy·da·ti·dos·to·my [,-'dɒstəmɪ] *n chir., urol.* Hydatideneröffnung *f*, -drainage *f*.
hydatid polyp zystischer Polyp *m*; gestielte Zyste *f*.
hydatid resonance Hydatidenschwirren *nt*.
hydatid tapeworm *micro.* Blasenbandwurm *m*, Hundebandwurm *m*, Echinococcus granulosus, Taenia echinococcus.
hydatid thrill *card.* Hydatidenschwirren *nt*.
Hy·da·tig·en·a [haɪdə'tɪdʒənə] *n micro.* Taenia *f*.
hy·da·toid ['haɪdətɔɪd] **I** *n* 1. Kammerwasser *nt*, Humor aquosus. 2. → hyaloid membrane. **II** *adj* Kammerwasser betr., Kammerwasser-.
Hyde [haɪd]: **H.'s disease** nodulöse Prurigo *f*, Prurigo nodularis Hyde.
hydr- *pref.* → hydro-.
hy·drad·e·ni·tis *n* → hidradenitis.
hy·drad·e·no·ma *n* → hidradenoma.
hy·draer·o·per·i·to·ne·um [haɪ,dreərəʊ-,perɪtə'niːəm] *n* Hydropneumoperitoneum *nt*.
hy·dra·gogue ['haɪdrəgɒg, -gag] **I** *n* Wasserausscheidung-förderndes Mittel *nt*, Hydragogum *nt*. **II** *adj* die Wasserausscheidung fördernd.
hy·dral·a·zine [haɪ'drælǝziːn] *n pharm.* Hydralazin *nt*, 1-Hydrazinophthalazin *nt*.
hy·dra·mine ['haɪdrəmiːn] *n chem.* Hydramin *nt*.
hy·dram·ni·on [haɪ'dræmnɪɒn] *n gyn.* Hydramnion *nt*.
hy·dram·ni·os [haɪ'dræmnɪɒs] *n* → hydramnion.
hy·dran·en·ceph·a·ly [,haɪdrænən'sefəlɪ] *n embryo.* Blasenhirn *nt*, Hydranzephalie *f*.
hy·drar·gyr·ia [,haɪdrɑːr'dʒɪərɪə] *n* Quecksilbervergiftung *f*, Hydrargyrie *f*, Hydrargyrose *f*, Merkurialismus *m*.
hy·drar·gy·rism [haɪ'drɑːrdʒərɪzəm] *n* → hydrargyria.
hy·drar·gy·ro·ma·nia [haɪ'drɑːrdʒaɪrəʊ-'meɪnɪə, -jə] *n patho., psychia.* Hydrargyromanie *f*.
hy·drar·gy·ro·sis [,-dʒɪ'rəʊsɪs] *n* → hydrargyria.
hy·drar·gy·rum [haɪ'drɑːrdʒərəm] *n abbr.* **Hg** Quecksilber *nt*; *chem.* Hydragyrum *nt abbr.* Hg.
hy·drar·thro·di·al [,haɪdrɑː'rəʊdɪəl] *adj* Hydarthrose betr.
hy·drar·thron [haɪ'drɑːrθrɒn] *n* → hydrarthrosis.
hy·drar·thro·sis [haɪdrɑː'rəʊsɪs] *n ortho.* seröser Gelenkerguß *m*, Hydarthros(e) *f*) *m*, Hydrarthros(e) *f*) *m*, Hydrops articularis.
hy·drar·thrus [haɪ'drɑːrθrəs] *n* → hydrarthrosis.
hy·drase ['haɪdreɪz] *n* → hydratase.
hy·dra·tase ['haɪdrəteɪz] *n* Hydratase *f*.
hy·drate ['haɪdreɪt] **I** *n* Hydrat *nt*. **II** *vt* hydratisieren.
hy·drat·ed ['haɪdreɪtɪd] *adj* hydratisiert.
hy·dra·tion [haɪ'dreɪʃn] *n* 1. Wasseranlagerung *f*, Hydratbildung *f*, Hydration *f*, Hydratation *f*. 2. Wasseraufnahme *f*, Hydratation *f*, Hydration *f*.
hy·dra·tion·al shell [haɪ'dreɪʃənl] *chem.* Wasserhülle *f*, Hydra(ta)tionshülle *f*.
hy·drau·lics [haɪ'drɒlɪks, -'drɑːlɪks] *pl* Hydraulik *f*.
hy·dra·zide ['haɪdrəzaɪd, -zɪd] *n* Hydrazid *nt*.
hy·dra·zine ['-ziːn] *n* Hydrazin *nt*, Diamid *nt*.
hy·dra·zin·ol·y·sis [,haɪdrəzɪ'nɒləsɪs] *n* Hydrazinolyse *f*.
hy·dra·zone ['haɪdrəzəʊn] *n* Hydrazon *nt*.

hy·dre·mia [haɪ'driːmɪə] *n* Hydrämie *f*, Hydroplasmie *f*; Verdünnungsanämie *f*.
hy·dre·mic edema [haɪ'driːmɪk] hydrämisches Ödem *nt*.
hydremic nephritis nephrotisches Syndrom *nt*; Nephrose *f*.
hy·dren·ceph·a·lo·cele [,haɪdrən'sefələ-siːl] *n* Enzephalozystozele *f*, Hydroenzephalozele *f*.
hy·dren·ceph·a·lo·me·nin·go·cele [,-,sefə-ləmɪ'nɪŋgəsiːl] *n* Enzephalozystomeningozele *f*, Enzephalomeningozele *f*, Meningoenzephalozele *f*.
hy·dren·ceph·a·lus [,-'sefələs] *n* → hydrocephalus.
hy·dren·ceph·a·ly [,-'sefəlɪ] *n* → hydrocephalus.
hy·dri·at·ic [,haɪdrɪ'ætɪk] *adj* → hydriatric.
hy·dri·at·ric [,-'ætrɪk] *adj* Hydrotherapie betr., hydrotherapeutisch, hydriatrisch.
hy·dri·at·rics [,-'ætrɪks] *pl* Wasserheilkunde *f*, Hydrotherapie *f*, Hydriatrie *f*.
hy·dric ['haɪdrɪk] *adj* Wasserstoff betr. *od.* enthaltend, Wasserstoff-, Hydro-.
hy·dride ['haɪdraɪd, -drɪd] *n* Hydrid *nt*.
hy·dri·on ['haɪdrɪɒn] *n* → hydrogen ion.
hydro- *pref.* 1. Wasser-, Hydr(o)-. 2. *chem.* Wasserstoff-, Hydro-.
hy·droa [haɪ'drəʊə] *n derm.* Hidroa *f*, Hydroa *f*.
hy·dro·a·dip·sia [,haɪdrəʊə'dɪpsɪə] *n* Hydroadipsie *f*.
hy·dro·ap·pen·dix [,haɪdrəʊə'pendɪks] *n* Hydroappendix *f*, Hydrops appendices.
hy·dro·ar·o·mat·ic acid [,-,ærə'mætɪk] hydroaromatische Säure *f*.
hy·dro·bil·i·ru·bin [,-'bɪlərʊbɪn] *n* Hydrobilirubin *nt*.
hy·dro·bleph·a·ron [,-'blefərən] *n* Lidödem *nt*, Hydroblepharon *nt*.
hy·dro·bro·mate [,-'brəʊmeɪt] *n* Hydrobromat *nt*.
hy·dro·bro·mic acid [,-'brəʊmɪk] Bromwasserstoffsäure *f*.
hy·dro·bro·mide [,-'brəʊmaɪd, -mɪd] *n* Hydrobromid *nt*.
hy·dro·cal·y·co·sis [,-kælɪ'kəʊsɪs] *n urol.* Hydrokalykose *f*, Hydrocalycosis *f*.
hy·dro·ca·lyx [,-'keɪlɪks] *n urol.* Hydrokalix *m*.
hy·dro·car·ba·rism [,-'kɑːrbərɪzəm] *n* → hydrocarbonism.
hy·dro·car·bon [,-'kɑːrbən] *n* Kohlenwasserstoff *m*.
hydrocarbon chain Kohlenwasserstoffkette *f*.
hy·dro·car·bo·nism [,-'kɑːrbənɪzəm] *n* Vergiftung/Intoxikation *f* durch Kohlenwasserstoffe.
hydrocarbon phase *biochem.* Kohlenwasserstoffphase *f*.
hydrocarbon tail → hydrocarbon chain.
hy·dro·car·dia [,-'kɑːrdɪə] *n* → hydropericardium.
hy·dro·cele ['-siːl] *n* 1. Wasserbruch *m*, Hydrozele *f*, Hydrocele *f*. 2. Hydrocele testis.
hy·dro·ce·phal·ic [,haɪdrəsɪ'fælɪk] *adj* Hydrozephalus betr., hydrozephal, Hydrozephalus-.
hy·dro·ceph·a·lo·cele [,-'sefələsiːl] *n* → hydrencephalocele.
hy·dro·ceph·a·loid [,-'sefələɪd] **I** *n* → hydrocephaloid disease *nt adj* hydrozephaloidähnlich, hydrozephaloid.
hydrocephaloid disease Hydrozephaloid *nt*, Encephalomeningitis acuta.
hy·dro·ceph·a·lus [,-'sefələs] *n* Wasserkopf *m*, Hydrozephalus *m*, Hydrocephalus *m*.
hy·dro·ceph·a·ly [,-'sefəlɪ] *n* → hydrocephalus.

hy·dro·chlor·ic acid [,-'klɔːrɪk, -'klɔʊr-] Salzsäure *f*.
hy·dro·chlo·ride [,-'klɔːraɪd, -rɪd, -'klɔʊ-] *n* Hydrochlorid *nt*.
hy·dro·chlo·ro·thi·a·zide [,-,klɔːrə'θaɪə-zaɪd, -,klɔʊ-] *n pharm.* Hydrochlorothiazid *nt*.
hy·dro·cho·le·cys·tis [,-,kɒʊlə'sɪstɪs, -,kɒlə-] *n patho.* Gallenblasenhydrops *m*, Hydrops vesicae felleae.
hy·dro·chol·e·re·sis [,-,kɒʊlɪ'riːsɪs, -,kɒl-] *n* Hydrocholerese *f*.
hy·dro·chol·e·ret·ic [,-,kɒʊlə'retɪk, ,kɒl-] *adj* Hydrocholerese betr. *od.* verursachend, hydrocholeretisch.
hy·dro·cho·les·ter·ol [,-kə'lestərɒʊl, -rɒl] *n* Hydrocholesterin *nt*, -cholesterol *nt*.
hy·dro·cir·so·cele [,-'sɜːrsəsiːl] *n* kombinierte Hydrozele *f* u. Varikozele.
hy·dro·co·done [,-'kəʊdəʊn] *n pharm.* Hydrocodon *nt*.
hy·dro·col·loid [,-'kɒlɔɪd] *n* Hydrokolloid *nt*.
hy·dro·col·po·cele [,-'kɒlpəsiːl] *n* → hydrocolpos.
hy·dro·col·pos [,-'kɒlpəs] *n gyn.* Scheidenretentionszyste *f*, Hydrokolpos *m*.
hy·dro·cor·ti·sone [,-'kɔːrtɪzəʊn] *n* Kortisol *nt*, Cortisol *nt*, Hydrocortison *nt*.
hy·dro·cy·an·ic acid [,-saɪ'ænɪk] → hydrogen cyanide.
hy·dro·cy·an·ism [,-'saɪənɪzəm] *n* Blausäurevergiftung *f*.
hy·dro·cyst ['-sɪst] *n* seröse (Retentions-)-Zyste *f*, Hydrozyste *f*.
hy·dro·cyst·ad·e·no·ma [,-sɪstædə'nəʊmə] *n* papilläres Hidradenom *nt*, Hydrokystadenom *nt*, Hidrozystadenom *nt*.
hy·dro·cys·to·ma [,-sɪs'təʊmə] *n* Hydrozystom *nt*, Hydrokystom *nt*.
hy·dro·dif·fu·sion [,-dɪ'fjuːʒn] *n* Hydrodiffusion *f*.
hy·dro·dip·sia [,-'dɪpsɪə] *n* Wasserdurst *m*, Hydrodipsie *f*.
hy·dro·dip·so·ma·nia [,-dɪpsə'meɪnɪə, -jə] *n psychia.* Hydrodipsomanie *f*.
hy·dro·di·u·re·sis [,-daɪə'riːsɪs] *n* Wasser-, Hydrodiurese *f*.
hy·dro·dy·nam·ic [,-daɪ'næmɪk] *adj* Hydrodynamik betr., hydrodynamisch.
hy·dro·dy·nam·ics [,-daɪ'næmɪks] *pl* Hydrodynamik *f*.
hy·dro·e·lec·tric [,-ɪ'lektrɪk] *adj* hydroelektrisch.
hydroelectric bath hydroelektrisches Bad *nt*.
hy·dro·en·ceph·a·lo·cele [,-en'sefələsiːl] *n* → hydrencephalocele.
hy·dro·flu·or·ic acid [,-'flɔːrɪk] Flußsäure *f*.
hy·dro·gel ['-dʒel] *n chem.* Hydrogel *nt*.
hy·dro·gen ['-dʒən] *n abbr.* **H** Wasserstoff *m*; *chem.* Hydrogenium *nt abbr.* H.
hydrogen acceptor Wasserstoffakzeptor *m*.
hy·dro·gen·ase ['haɪdrədʒəneɪz, haɪ'drɑː-dʒəneɪz] *n* Hydrogenase *f*.
hy·dro·gen·ate [,-dʒəneɪt, haɪ'drɑːdʒəneɪt] *vt* 1. Wasserstoff anlagern, hydrieren. 2. (*Öl, Fett*) härten.
hy·dro·gen·a·tion [,-dʒə'neɪʃn] *n chem.* Hydrierung *f*.
hydrogen atom Wasserstoffatom *nt*.
hydrogen bacteria *micro.* Wasserstoffbakterien *pl*, -bildner *pl*.
hydrogen-binding capacity Wasserstoffbindungskapazität *f*.
hydrogen bomb Wasserstoffbombe *f*.
hydrogen bond Wasserstoffbrückenbindung *f*.
hydrogen-bonding capacity Wasserstoffbindungskapazität *f*.

hydrogen breath test

hydrogen breath test Wasserstoffatemtest m, H_2-Atemtest m.
hydrogen bromide Bromwasserstoff m.
hydrogen chloride abbr. **HCl** Chlorwasserstoff m abbr. HCl.
hydrogen cyanide abbr. **HCN** Cyanwasserstoff m abbr. HCN; Blausäure f.
hydrogen dioxide → hydrogen peroxide.
hydrogen electrode Wasserstoffelektrode f.
hydrogen ion abbr. **H+** Wasserstoffion nt abbr. H+.
hydrogen ion concentration abbr. **[H+]** Wasserstoffionenkonzentration f abbr. [H+].
hy·dro·gen·ize ['-dʒənaɪz, haɪ'drɑdʒə-] vt → hydrogenate.
hy·dro·gen·ly·ase [ˌhaɪdrədʒən'laɪeɪz] n 1. Hydrogenlyase f. 2. Hydrogenase f.
hydrogen nucleus Wasserstoffkern m.
hydrogen peroxide Wasserstoff(su)peroxid nt.
hydrogen sulfide Schwefelwasserstoff m.
hy·dro·gym·nas·tics [ˌhaɪdrədʒɪm'næstɪks] pl Unterwassergymnastik f, Hydrogymnastik f.
hy·dro·hal·o·gen acid [ˌ-'hælədʒən] Halogenwasserstoff(säure f) m.
hy·dro·hem·a·to·ne·phro·sis [ˌ-ˌhemətəʊnɪ'frəʊsɪs] n urol. Hydrohäm(at)onephrose f.
hy·dro·hem·a·to·tho·rax [ˌ-ˌhemətə'θɔːræks] n Hydrohäm(at)othorax m.
hy·dro·ki·net·ic [ˌ-kɪ'netɪk] adj Hydrokinetik betr., hydrokinetisch.
hy·dro·ki·net·ics [ˌ-kɪ'netɪks] pl Hydrokinetik f.
hy·dro·la·bile [ˌ-'leɪbɪl] adj hydrolabil.
hy·dro·la·bil·i·ty [ˌ-lə'bɪlətɪ] n Hydrolabilität f.
hy·dro·lab·y·rinth [ˌ-'læbərɪn(t)θ] n HNO Hydrolabyrinth nt, Hydrops labyrinthi.
hy·dro·lase ['-leɪz] n Hydrolase f.
hydro-lyase Hydrolyase f, Hydratase f, Dehydratase f.
hy·drol·y·sate [haɪ'drəlɪseɪt] n Hydrolysat nt.
hy·drol·y·sis [haɪ'drɒləsɪs] n, pl **-ses** [-siːz] Hydrolyse f.
hy·dro·lyst ['haɪdrəlɪst] n hydrolyseförderndes Agens nt, Hydrolysator m.
hy·dro·lyte ['-laɪt] n Hydrolyt m.
hy·dro·lyt·ic [ˌ-'lɪtɪk] adj Hydrolyse betr. od. fördernd, hydrolytisch.
hydrolytic enzyme → hydrolase.
hy·dro·lyz·a·ble ['-laɪzəbl] adj hydrolysierbar.
hy·dro·ly·zate n → hydrolysate.
hy·dro·lyze ['haɪdrəlaɪz] vt, vi hydrolisieren.
hy·dro·ma [haɪ'drəʊmə] n → hygroma.
hy·dro·mas·sage [ˌhaɪdrəʊmə'sɑːʒ] n Unterwassermassage f.
hy·dro·men·in·gi·tis [ˌ-menɪn'dʒaɪtɪs] n seröse Meningitis f, Hydromeningitis f.
hy·dro·me·nin·go·cele [ˌ-mɪ'nɪŋgəsiːl] n Hydromeningozele f, Meningozele f.
hy·drom·e·ter [haɪ'drɒmɪtər] n Wassermesser m, Hydrometer nt.
hy·dro·me·tra [ˌhaɪdrə'miːtrə] n gyn. Hydrometra f.
hy·dro·met·ric [ˌ-'metrɪk] adj Hydrometrie betr., hydrometrisch.
hy·dro·me·tro·col·pos [ˌ-ˌmiːtrə'kɒlpəs] n gyn. Hydrometrokolpos m.
hy·drom·e·try [haɪ'drɒmətrɪ] n Hydrometrie f.
hy·dro·mi·cro·ceph·a·ly [ˌhaɪdrəˌmaɪkrə'sefəlɪ] n patho. Hydromikrozephalie f.
hy·dro·mor·phone [ˌ-'mɔːrfəʊn] n pharm. Hydromorphon nt.
hy·drom·pha·lus [haɪ'drɒmfələs] n Hydromphalus m.
hy·dro·my·e·lia [ˌhaɪdrə'maɪ'iːlɪə] n embryo. Hydromyelie f, Hydrorrhachis interna.
hy·dro·my·e·lo·cele [ˌ-'maɪələʊsiːl] n Hydromyelozele f.
hy·dro·my·e·lo·me·nin·go·cele [ˌ-ˌmaɪələʊmɪ'nɪŋgəsiːl] n Hydromyelomeningozele f, Meningomyelozele f.
hy·dro·my·o·ma [ˌ-maɪ'əʊmə] n zystisches Leiomyom nt, Hydromyom nt.
hy·dro·ne·phro·sis [ˌ-nɪ'frəʊsɪs] n urol. Harnstauungs-, Wassersackniere f, Hydronephrose f, Uronephrose f.
hy·dro·ne·phrot·ic [ˌ-nɪ'frɒtɪk] adj Hydronephrose betr., hydronephrotisch.
hy·dro·ni·um [haɪ'drəʊnɪəm] n Hydroniumion nt, Hydroxoniumion nt.
hydronium ion → hydronium.
hy·dro·path·ic [ˌhaɪdrə'pæθɪk] adj 1. Hydropathie betr., hydropathisch. 2. → hydrotherapeutic.
hy·drop·a·thy [haɪ'drɒpəθɪ] n Hydropathie f.
hy·dro·pe·nia [ˌhaɪdrə'piːnɪə] n Wassermangel m.
hy·dro·per·i·car·di·tis [ˌ-ˌperɪkɑː'daɪtɪs] n seröse Perikarditis f, Hydroperikarditis f.
hy·dro·per·i·car·di·um [ˌ-ˌperɪ'kɑːrdɪəm] n Herzbeutelwassersucht f, Hydroperikard nt, -perikardium nt, Hydrokardie f, Hydrops pericardii.
hy·dro·per·i·to·ne·um [ˌ-ˌperɪtə'niːəm] n Bauchwassersucht f, Aszites m.
hy·dro·per·i·to·nia [ˌ-ˌperɪ'təʊnɪə] n → hydroperitoneum.
hy·dro·per·ox·ide [ˌ-pə'rɒksaɪd] n → hydrogen peroxide.
hy·dro·per·ox·y·ei·co·sa·tet·rae·no·ic acid [ˌ-pəˌrɒksaɪˌkəʊsəˌtetrəɪ'nəʊɪk] abbr. **HPETE** Hydroperoxyeicosatetraensäure f abbr. HPETE.
hy·dro·pex·ia [ˌ-'peksɪə] n → hydropexis.
hy·dro·pex·ic [ˌ-'peksɪk] adj wasserbindend, -fixierend, hydropektisch.
hy·dro·pex·is [ˌ-'peksɪs] n Wasserbindung f, -einlagerung f, -fixierung f, Hydropexie f.
hy·dro·phil ['-fɪl] adj → hydrophilic.
hy·dro·phile ['-fɪl, -faɪl] adj → hydrophilic.
hy·dro·phil·ia [ˌ-'fiːlɪə, -jə] n Hydrophilie f.
hy·dro·phil·ic [ˌ-'fɪlɪk] adj wasserliebend, Wasser/Feuchtigkeit aufnehmend, Wasser anziehend, hydrophil.
hydrophilic colloid hydrophiles Kolloid nt.
hy·droph·i·lism [haɪ'drɒfəlɪzəm] n → hydrophilia.
hy·droph·i·lous [haɪ'drɒfɪləs] adj → hydrophilic.
hy·dro·pho·bia [ˌhaɪdrə'fəʊbɪə] n 1. Wasserscheu f, Hydrophobie f. 2. old → rabies.
hy·dro·pho·bic [ˌ-'fəʊbɪk] adj 1. wasserscheu; wasserabstoßend, hydrophob. 2. Tollwut/Rabies betr., tollwütig.
hydrophobic bond chem. hydrophobe Wechselwirkung/Bindung f.
hydrophobic colloid hydrophobes Kolloid nt.
hydrophobic interaction chem. hydrophobe Wechselwirkung f.
hy·dro·pho·bic·i·ty [ˌ-fəʊ'bɪsətɪ] n → hydrophobism.
hydrophobic phase phys. hydrophobe Phase f.
hy·dro·pho·bism ['-fəʊbɪzəm] n chem. Hydrophobie f.
hy·dro·pho·bous [ˌ-'fəʊbəs] adj → hydrophobic.
hy·droph·thal·mia [ˌhaɪdrəf'θælmɪə] n → hydrophthalmos.

hy·droph·thal·mos [ˌ-'θælməs] n ophthal. Ochsenauge nt, Glaukom nt der Kinder, angeborenes Glaukom nt, Hydrophthalmus m, Buphthalmus m.
hy·droph·thal·mus n → hydrophthalmos.
hy·dro·phy·so·me·tra [ˌhaɪdrəˌfaɪzə'miːtrə] n gyn. Physohydrometra f.
hy·drop·ic [haɪ'drɒpɪk] adj Hydrops betr., mit Hydrops einhergehend, hydropisch.
hydropic degeneration hydropische Degeneration f.
hydropic nephrosis hypokaliämische Nephropathie f.
hy·dro·pig·e·nous nephritis [ˌhaɪdrəʊ'pɪdʒənəs] nephrotisches Syndrom nt; Nephrose f.
hy·dro·pneu·ma·to·sis [ˌ-n(j)uːmə'təʊsɪs] n patho. kombiniertes Emphysem nt u. Ödem, Hydropneumatosis f.
hy·dro·pneu·mo·g·o·ny [ˌ-n(j)uːmə'mɒgənɪ] n ortho., radiol. Arthropneumographie f zur Ergußdiagnostik.
hy·dro·pneu·mo·per·i·car·di·um [ˌ-ˌn(j)uːməˌperɪ'kɑːrdɪəm] n Hydropneumoperikard nt, Pneumohydroperikard nt.
hy·dro·pneu·mo·per·i·to·ne·um [ˌ-ˌn(j)uːməˌperɪ'niːəm] n Hydropneumoperitoneum nt, Pneumohydroperitoneum nt.
hy·dro·pneu·mo·tho·rax [ˌ-ˌn(j)uːmə'θɔːræks] n Hydropneumothorax m, Pneumohydrothorax m.
hy·dro·pon·ics [ˌ-'pɒnɪks] pl bio. Hydrokultur f, Hydroponik f.
hy·drops ['haɪdrɒps] n Wassersucht f, Hydrops m.
h. of gallbladder Gallenblasenhydrops, Hydrops vesicae felleae.
hy·dro·py·o·ne·phro·sis [ˌhaɪdrəˌpaɪənɪ'frəʊsɪs] n urol. Hydropyonephrose f.
hy·dro·qui·none [ˌ-kwɪ'nəʊn] n Hydrochinon nt, Parahydroxybenzol nt.
hy·dror·a·chis [haɪ'drɒrəkɪs] n Hydrorrhachis f.
hy·dror·rhea [ˌhaɪdrə'rɪə] n seröser Ausfluß m, Hydrorrhoe f, Hydrorrhoea f.
hy·dro·sal·pinx [ˌ-'sælpɪŋks] n gyn. Hydrosalpinx f, Hydrops tubae, Sactosalpinx serosa.
hy·dro·sar·ca [ˌ-'sɑːrkə] n Anasarka f.
hy·dro·sar·co·cele [ˌ-'sɑːrkəsiːl] n kombinierte Hydrozele f u. Sarkozele, Hydrosarkozele f.
hy·dro·sol ['-sɒl, -sal] n Hydrosol nt.
hy·dro·sol·u·ble [ˌ-'sæljəbəl] adj wasserlöslich.
hy·dro·sphyg·mo·graph [ˌ-'sfɪgməgræf] n physiol. Hydrosphygmograph m.
hy·dro·spi·rom·e·ter [ˌ-spaɪ'rɒmɪtər] n physiol. Hydrospirometer nt.
hy·dro·sta·bile [ˌ-'steɪbɪl] adj hydrostabil.
hy·dro·stat ['-stæt] n Hydrostat m.
hy·dro·stat·ic [ˌ-'stætɪk] adj Hydrostatik betr., hydrostatisch.
hydrostatic indifference level physiol. hydrostatische Indifferenzebene f.
hydrostatic pressure hydrostatischer Druck m.
hy·dro·stat·ics [ˌ-'stætɪks] pl Hydrostatik f.
hy·dro·sul·fu·ric acid [ˌ-sʌl'fjʊərɪk] → hydrogen sulfide.
hy·dro·sy·rin·go·my·e·lia [ˌ-sɪˌrɪŋgəʊmaɪ'iːlɪə] n Hydrosyringomyelie f, Syringomyelie f.
hy·dro·tax·is [ˌ-'tæksɪs] n Hydrotaxis f.
hy·dro·ther·a·peu·tic [ˌ-θerə'pjuːtɪk] adj Hydrotherapie betr., hydrotherapeutisch, hydriatrisch.
hy·dro·ther·a·peu·tics [ˌ-ˌθerə'pjuːtɪks] pl → hydrotherapy.
hy·dro·ther·a·py [ˌ-'θerəpɪ] n Wasserkur f; Wasserheilkunde f, -verfahren nt, Hydriatrie f, Hydrotherapie f.

hy·dro·thi·o·ne·mia [ˌ-θaɪəˈniːmɪə] *n patho*. Auftreten *nt* von Schwefelwasserstoff im Blut, Hydrothionämie *f*.
hy·dro·tho·rax [ˌ-ˈθɔːræks] *n* Brustwassersucht *f*, Hydrothorax *m*.
hy·drot·o·my [haɪˈdrɒtəmɪ] *n chir., histol*. Hydrotomie *f*.
hy·drot·ro·pism [haɪˈdrɒtrəpɪzəm] *n* **1.** *bio*. Hydrotropismus *m*. **2.** *chem*. Hydrotropie *f*.
hy·dro·tu·ba·tion [ˌhaɪdrətjuːˈbeɪʃn] *n gyn*. Hydrotubation *f*, Hydropertubation *f*.
hy·dro·u·re·ter [ˌ-ˈjʊərətər] *n urol*. Hydroureter *m*, Hydrureter *m*.
hy·dro·u·re·ter·o·ne·phro·sis [ˌ-jʊəˌriːtərəʊnɪˈfrəʊsɪs] *n urol*. Hydroureteronephrose *f*.
hy·dro·u·re·ter·o·sis [ˌ-jʊəˌriːtəˈrəʊsɪs] *n* → hydroureter.
hy·dro·u·ria [ˌ-ˈ(j)ʊərɪə] *n* → hydruria.
hy·drous [ˈhaɪdrəs] *adj* wasserhaltig.
hy·dro·va·ri·um [ˌhaɪdrəˈveərɪəm] *n gyn*. Hydrovarium *nt*, Hydrops ovarii.
hy·drox·ide [haɪˈdrɒksaɪd, -sɪd] *n* Hydroxid *nt*.
hydroxide ion Hydroxidion *nt*.
hy·drox·o·co·bal·a·min [haɪˌdrɒksəʊkəʊˈbæləmɪn] *n* Hydroxocobalamin *nt*, Aquocobalamin *nt*, Vitamin B_{12b} *nt*.
hy·drox·o·co·be·mine [haɪˈdrɒksəkəʊbəmiːn] *n* → hydroxocobalamin.
hydroxy- *pref*. Hydroxy-.
hy·drox·y·a·ce·tic acid [haɪˌdrɒksɪəˈsiːtɪk, -əˈset-] Hydroxyessigsäure *f*, Glykolsäure *f*.
hy·drox·y acid [haɪˈdrɒksɪ] Hydroxysäure *f*.
3-hy·drox·y·ac·yl-CoA [haɪˌdrɒksɪˈæsɪl, -iːl] *n* 3-Hydroxyacyl-CoA *nt*.
3-hydroxyacyl-CoA dehydrogenase 3-Hydroxyacyl-CoA-dehydrogenase *f*.
3-hydroxyacyl-CoA epimerase 3-Hydroxyacyl-CoA-epimerase *f*.
hy·drox·y·ac·yl·glu·ta·thi·one hydrolase [ˌ-ˌæsɪlˌgluːtəˈθaɪəʊn] Hydroxyacylglutathionhydrolase *f*, Glyoxalase II *f*.
3-hy·drox·y·an·thra·nil·ic acid [ˌ-ˌænθrəˈnɪlɪk] 3-Hydroxyanthranilsäure *f*.
3-hydroxyanthranilic acid 3,4-dioxygenase 3-Hydroxyanthranilsäure-3,4-dioxygenase *f*.
hy·drox·y·ap·a·tite [ˌ-ˈæpətaɪt] *n* Hydroxi-, Hydroxyl)apatit *f/nt*.
hydroxyapatite crystal Hydroxyapatitkristall *m*.
2-(α-hydroxybencyl)-benzimidazole *n abbr*. **HBB** 2-(α-Hydroxybenzyl)-Benzimidazol *nt abbr*. HBB.
2-hy·drox·y·ben·za·mide [ˌ-ˈbenzəmaɪd] *n pharm*. Salizylamid *nt*, Salicylamid *nt*, Salicylsäureamid *nt*, *o*-Hydroxybenzamid *nt*.
hy·drox·y·ben·zene [ˌ-ˈbenziːn] *n* Phenol *nt*, Karbolsäure *f*, Monohydroxybenzol *nt*.
2-hy·drox·y·ben·zo·ic acid [ˌ-benˈzəʊɪk] Salizylsäure *f*, Salicylsäure *f*, *o*-Hydroxybenzoesäure *f*.
***p*-hy·drox·y·ben·zyl·pen·i·cil·lin** [ˌ-ˌbenzɪlpenəˈsɪlɪn] *n pharm*. Penicillin X *nt*, Penicillin III *nt*, Hydroxybenzylpenicillinsäure *f*.
β-hy·drox·y·bu·tyr·ate [ˌ-ˈbjuːtəreɪt] *n* β-Hydroxybutyrat *nt*.
α-hydroxybutyrate dehydrogenase *abbr*. **HBDH** α-Hydroxybutyratdehydrogenase *f abbr*. HBDH.
β-hydroxybutyrate dehydrogenase β-Hydroxybutyratdehydrogenase *f*, 3-Hydroxybutyratdehydrogenase *f*.
hy·drox·y·bu·tyr·ic acid [ˌ-bjuːˈtɪrɪk] Hydroxybuttersäure *f*.

β-hydroxybutyric acid β-Hydroxybuttersäure *f*.
β-hydroxybutyric dehydrogenase → β-hydroxybutyrate dehydrogenase.
hy·drox·y·car·ba·mide [ˌ-ˈkɑːrbəmaɪd] *n* → hydroxyurea.
hy·drox·y·chlo·ro·quine [ˌ-ˈklɔːrəkwɪn] *n pharm*. Hydroxychloroquin *nt*.
25-hy·drox·y·cho·le·cal·cif·e·rol [ˌ-ˌkəʊləkælˈsɪfərɒl, -ˌkalə-] *n* 25-Hydroxycholecalciferol *nt*, Calcidiol *nt*.
17-hy·drox·y·cor·ti·co·ster·oid [ˌ-ˌkɔːrtɪkəʊˈsterɔɪd, -ˈstɪər-] *n abbr*. **17-OH-CS** 17-Hydroxikortikosteroid *nt*, 17-Hydroxicorticosteroid *nt abbr*. 17-OH-CS.
17-hydroxycorticosteroid test Porter--Silber-Methode *f*.
17-hy·drox·y·cor·ti·cos·ter·one [ˌ-ˌkɔːrtɪˈkɒstərəʊn] *n* Kortisol *nt*, Cortisol *nt*, Hydrocortison *nt*.
18-hydroxycorticosterone *n* 18-Hydroxicorticosteron *nt*.
hy·drox·y·ei·co·sa·tet·ra·e·no·ic acid [ˌ-ˌaɪkəʊsəˌtetrəˈnəʊɪk] *abbr*. **HETE** Hydroxyeicosatetraensäure *f abbr*. HET.
25-hy·drox·y·er·go·cal·cif·e·rol [ˌ-ˌɜːrgəkælˈsɪfərɒl] *n* 25-Hydroxyergocalciferol *nt*.
hy·drox·y·es·trin benzoate [ˌ-ˈestrɪn] *pharm*. Estradiolbenzoat *nt*.
hy·drox·y·eth·yl starch [ˌ-ˈeθəl] *abbr*. **HES** Hydroxyäthylstärke *f abbr*. HES.
γ-hy·drox·y·glu·tam·ic acid [ˌ-ˈgluːˈtæmɪk] γ-Hydroxyglutaminsäure *f*.
hy·drox·y·he·min [ˌ-ˈhiːmɪn] *n* → hematin.
hy·drox·y·hep·ta·dec·a·tri·e·no·ic acid [ˌ-ˌheptəˌdekəˌtraɪˈnəʊɪk] *abbr*. **HHT** Hydroxyheptadecatriensäure *f abbr*. HHT.
5-hy·drox·y·in·dole·a·ce·tic acid [ˌ-ɪndəʊləˈsiːtɪk, -ˈset-] *abbr*. **5-HIAA** 5-Hydroxyindolessigsäure *f abbr*. 5-HIE.
β-hy·drox·y·i·so·bu·tyr·ic acid [ˌ-ˌaɪsəbjuːˈtɪrɪk] β-Hydroxyisobuttersäure *f*.
β-hydroxyisobutyric acid dehydrogenase β-Hydroxyisobuttersäuredehydrogenase *f*.
β-hy·drox·y·i·so·bu·tyr·yl-CoA hydrolase [ˌ-ˌaɪsəˈbjuːtərɪl] β-Hydroxyisobutyryl--CoA-hydrolase *f*.
hy·drox·yl [haɪˈdrɒksɪl] *n* Hydroxyl-(Radikal *nt*).
hy·drox·yl·ap·a·tite [haɪˌdrɒksɪlˈæpətaɪt] *n* → hydroxyapatite.
hy·drox·y·lase [haɪˈdrɒksɪleɪz] *n* Hydroxylase *f*.
11β-hydroxylase *n* 11β-Hydroxylase *f*, Steroid-11β-monooxygenase *f*.
17α-hydroxylase *n* 17α-Hydroxylase *f*, Steroid-17α-monooxygenase *f*.
17-hydroxylase deficiency syndrome 17-Hydroxylasemangel-Syndrom *nt*.
21-hydroxylase *n* 21-Hydroxylase *f*, Steroid-21-monooxygenase *f*.
hy·drox·y·ly·sine [ˌhaɪdrɒksɪˈlaɪsiːn] *n* Hydroxylysin *nt*.
5-hy·drox·y·meth·yl·cy·to·sine [ˌ-ˌmeθlˈsaɪtəsiːn, -sɪn] *n* 5-Hydroxymethylcytosin *nt*.
5-hy·drox·y·meth·yl·fur·fur·al [ˌ-ˌmeθlˈfɜːrf(j)ərəl] *n* 5-Hydroxymethylfurfural *nt*.
3-hydroxy-3-methylglutaric acid 3-Hydroxy-3-methylglutarsäure *f*.
β-hydroxy-β-methylglutaryl-CoA *n abbr*. **HMG-CoA** β-Hydroxy-β-methylglutaryl--CoA *nt abbr*. HMG-CoA.
β-hydroxy-β-methylglutaryl-CoA lyase β-Hydroxy-β-methylglutaryl-CoA-lyase *f*, HMG-CoA-lyase *f*.
β-hydroxy-β-methylglutaryl-CoA reductase β-Hydroxy-β-methylglutaryl-CoA--reduktase *f*, HMG-CoA-reduktase *f*.
β-hydroxy-β-methylglutaryl-CoA synthase β-Hydroxy-β-methylglutaryl-CoA-synthase *f*, HMG-CoA-synthase *f*.
hy·drox·y·meth·yl·trans·fer·ase [ˌ-ˌmeθlˈtrænsfəreɪz] *n* Hydroxymethyltransferase *f*.
5-hy·drox·y·meth·yl·u·ra·cil [ˌ-ˌmeθlˈjʊərəsɪl] *n* 5-Hydroxymethyluracil *nt*.
hy·drox·y·ner·vone [ˌ-ˈnɜːrvəʊn] *n* Hydroxynervon *nt*.
hy·drox·y·phen·yl·al·a·nine [ˌ-fenlˈæləniːn] *n* Tyrosin *nt abbr*. Tyr.
hy·drox·y·phen·yl·eth·yl·a·mine [ˌ-fenlˌeθɪləˈmiːn, -ˈæmɪn] *n* Tyramin *nt*, Tyrosamin *nt*.
4-hy·drox·y·phen·yl·pyr·u·vate [ˌ-ˌfenlˈpaɪruːveɪt] *n* 4-Hydroxyphenylpyruvat *nt*, *p*-Hydroxyphenylpyruvat *nt*.
4-hydroxyphenylpyruvate dioxygenase 4-Hydroxyphenylpyruvatdioxygenase *f*, 4-Hydroxyphenylpyruvatoxidase *f*.
***p*-hydroxyphenylpyruvate oxidase** → 4-hydroxyphenylpyruvate dioxygenase.
4-hy·drox·y·phen·yl·py·ru·vic acid [ˌ-fenlpaɪˈruːvɪk] 4-Hydroxyphenylbrenztraubensäure *f*.
hy·drox·y·phen·yl·u·ria [ˌ-fenlˈ(j)ʊərɪə] *n* Hydroxyphenylurie *f*.
17α-hy·drox·y·preg·nen·o·lone [ˌ-pregˈniːnələʊn] *n* 17α-Hydroxypregnenolon *nt*.
17α-hy·drox·y·pro·ges·ter·one [ˌ-prəʊˈdʒestərəʊn] *n* 17α-Hydroxyprogesteron *nt*.
hydroxyprogesterone caproate *pharm*. Hydroxyprogesteroncaproat *nt*.
hy·drox·y·pro·line [ˌ-ˈprəʊliːn, -lɪn] *n* Hydroxyprolin *nt*.
hy·drox·y·pro·li·ne·mia [ˌ-ˌprəʊlɪˈniːmɪə] *n* Hydroxyprolinämie *f*.
hydroxyproline oxidase Hydroxyprolinoxidase *f*.
4-hydroxy-L-proline oxidase deficiency → hydroxyprolinemia.
hy·drox·y·pro·li·nu·ria [ˌ-ˌprəʊlɪˈn(j)ʊərɪə] *n* Hydroxyprolinausscheidung *f* im Harn, Hydroxyprolinurie *f*.
6-hy·drox·y·pu·rine [ˌ-ˈpjʊəriːn, -rɪn] *n* → hypoxanthine.
hy·drox·y·pyr·u·vate [ˌ-ˈpaɪruːveɪt] *n* Hydroxypyruvat *nt*.
(17-)hy·drox·y·ste·roid [ˌ-ˈstɪərɔɪd, -ˈster-] *n* (17-)Hydroxysteroid *nt*.
hydroxysteroid dehydrogenase Hydroxysteroiddehydrogenase *f*.
5-hy·drox·y·tryp·ta·mine [ˌ-ˈtrɪptəmiːn] *n abbr*. **5-HT** 5-Hydroxytryptamin *nt abbr*. 5-HT, Serotonin *nt*.
5-hy·drox·y·tryp·to·phan [ˌ-ˈtrɪptəfæn] *n* 5-Hydroxytryptophan *nt*.
hy·drox·y·ty·ra·mine [ˌ-ˈtaɪrəmiːn] *n* Dopamin *nt*, Hydroxytyramin *nt*.
hy·drox·y·u·rea [ˌ-jʊəˈrɪə, -ˈjʊərɪə] *n* Hydroxyharnstoff *nt*, Hydroxyurea *nt*.
hy·drox·y·val·ine [ˌ-ˈvæliːn, -ɪn, ˈveɪ-] *n* Hydroxyvalin *nt*.
hy·drox·y·zine [haɪˈdrɒksəziːn] *n pharm*. Hydroxyzin *nt*.
hy·dru·ria [haɪˈdr(j)ʊərɪə] *n* Hydrurie *f*; Polyurie *f*.
hy·dru·ric [haɪˈd(j)ʊərɪk] *adj* Hydrurie *od*. Polyurie betr., hydrurisch, polyurisch.
hy·gi·eist [ˈhaɪdʒɪɪst] *n* → hygienist.
hy·giene [ˈhaɪdʒiːn] *n* Hygiene *f*.
hy·gi·en·ic [haɪˈdʒiːnɪk, haɪˈdʒɪ-] **I** *sl pl* Hygiene *f*. **II** *adj* **1.** Hygiene betr., auf Hygiene beruhend, der Gesundheit dienend, hygienisch. **2.** Hygiene betr., sauber, frei von Verschmutzung, hygienisch.
hy·gien·ist [haɪˈdʒiːnɪst, -ˈdʒen-, ˈhaɪdʒɪ-] *n* Hygieniker(in *f*) *m*.
hygr- *pref*. → hygro-.

hygric

hy·gric ['haɪgrɪk] *adj* Feuchtigkeit betr., Feuchtigkeits-, Hygro-.
hygro- *pref.* Feuchtigkeits-, Hygro-.
hy·gro·ma [haɪ'grəʊmə] *n*, *pl* **-mas, -ma·ta** [-mətə] Wassergeschwulst *f*, Hygrom(a) *nt*.
hy·gro·ma·tous [haɪ'grəʊmətəs] *adj* Hygrom betr., hygromartig, hygromatös.
hy·gro·me·ter [haɪ'grɒmɪtər] *n* Luftfeuchtigkeitsmesser *m*, Hygrometer *nt*.
hy·gro·met·ric [ˌhaɪgrə'metrɪk] *adj* Hygrometrie betr., hygrometrisch.
hy·grom·e·try [haɪ'grɒmətrɪ] *n* Luftfeuchtigkeitsmessung *f*, Hygrometrie *f*.
hy·gro·pho·bia [ˌhaɪgrə'fəʊbɪə] *n psychia.* krankhafte Angst *f* vor Feuchtigkeit, Hygrophobie *f*.
hy·gro·scop·ic [ˌ-'skɒpɪk] *adj* Wasser *od.* (Luft-)Feuchtigkeit anziehend *od.* aufnehmend, hygroskopisch.
hy·gro·sto·mia [ˌ-'stəʊmɪə] *n* (übermäßiger) Speichelfluß *m*, Sialorrhoe *f*, Ptyalismus *m*, Hypersalivation *f*.
hy·lic ['haɪlɪk] *adj embryo.* hylisch.
hy·me·cro·mone [ˌhaɪmɪ'krəʊməʊn] *n pharm.* Hymecromon *nt*.
hy·men ['haɪmən] *n* Jungfernhäutchen *nt*, Hymen *m/nt*.
hy·men·al ['haɪmənl] *adj* Jungfernhäutchen/Hymen betr., hymenal, Hymenal-.
hymenal atresia Hymenalatresie *f*, Atresia hymenalis.
hymenal caruncles Fleischwärzchen *pl* (der Scheide), Hymenalkarunkeln *pl*, Carunculae hymenales (myrtiformes).
hymenal membrane → hymen.
hy·men·ec·to·my [ˌhaɪmə'nektəmɪ] *n gyn.* Hymenexzision *f*, Hymenektomie *f*.
hy·men·i·tis [haɪmə'naɪtɪs] *n gyn.* Hymenentzündung *f*, Hymenitis *f*.
hy·me·ni·um [haɪ'mɪnɪəm] *n, pl* **-nia** [-nɪə] *micro.* Sporen-, Fruchtlager *nt*, Hymenium *nt*.
hy·me·noid ['haɪmənɔɪd] *adj* 1. hymenartig, -ähnlich, hymenoid. 2. Membran betr., häutig, membranartig, membranös, Membran-.
hy·me·no·le·pi·a·sis [ˌhaɪmənəʊlə'paɪəsɪs] *n* Zwergbandwurminfektion *f*, Hymenolepiasis *f*, Hymenolepidose *f*.
Hy·men·o·le·pid·i·dae [-lə'pɪdɪdiː] *pl micro.* Hymenolepididae *pl*.
Hy·me·nol·e·pis [haɪmɪ'nɑləpsɪs] *n micro.* Hymenolepis *f*.
H. **diminuta** Ratten-, Mäusebandwurm *m*, Hymenolepis diminuta.
H. **nana** Zwergbandwurm *m*, Hymenolepis nana.
Hy·me·nop·tera [haɪmɪ'nɒptərə] *pl bio.* Hautflügler *pl*, Hymenopteren *pl*, Hymenoptera *pl*.
hy·men·op·ter·ism [ˌhaɪmə'nɒptərɪzəm] *n* Hymenopterismus *m*.
hy·men·or·rha·phy [ˌhaɪmə'nɔrəfɪ] *n gyn.* Hymennaht *f*, Hymenorrhaphie *f*.
hy·men·ot·o·my [haɪmɪ'nɒtəmɪ] *n gyn.* Hymendurchtrennung *f*, -durchschneidung *f*, -spaltung *f*, Hymenotomie *f*.
hy·o·bran·chi·al cleft [ˌhaɪəʊ'brænkɪəl] *embryo.* Hyobranchialspalt *m*, -furche *f*.
hy·o·ep·i·glot·tic [ˌ-epɪ'glɒtɪk] *adj* Zungenbein/Os hyoideum u. Kehldeckel/Epiglottis betr., hyoepiglottisch.
hyoepiglottic ligament Lig. hyoepiglotticum.
hy·o·ep·i·glot·tid·e·an [ˌ-ˌepɪglə'tiːdɪən] *adj* → hyoepiglottic.
hy·o·glos·sal muscle [ˌ-'glɒsl, -'gləʊ-] *n* hyoglossus (muscle).
hy·o·glos·sus (muscle) [ˌ-'glɒsəs, -'gləʊ-] *old* Zungenbeinzungenmuskel *m*, Hyoglossus *m*, M. hyoglossus.

hy·oid ['haɪɔɪd] I *n* Zungenbein *nt*, Os hyoideum. II *adj* Zungenbein betr., Zungenbein-.
hy·oi·dal [haɪ'ɔɪdl] *adj* → hyoid II.
hyoid arch *embryo.* Hyoidbogen *m*, II. Schlundbogen *m*.
hyoid artery Ramus suprahyoideus a. lingualis.
hyoid bone → hyoid I.
hyoid bursa Bursa subcutanea prominentiae laryngealis.
hyoid cleft → hyomandibular cleft.
hy·oi·de·an [haɪ'ɔɪdɪən] *adj* → hyoid II.
hy·o·man·dib·u·lar cleft [ˌhaɪəʊmæn'dɪbjələr] *embryo.* Hyomandibularspalt *m*, -furche *f*.
hy·os·cine ['siːn, -sɪn] *n* Scopolamin *nt*.
hy·os·cy·a·mine [ˌ-'saɪəmiːn, -mɪn] *n* Hyoscyamin *nt*, Hyoszyamin *nt*.
d/l-hyoscyamine *n* Atropin *nt*.
Hy·os·cy·a·mus [ˌ-'saɪəməs] *n pharm.* Bilsenkraut *nt*, Hyoscyamus niger.
hy·o·thy·roid [ˌ-'θaɪrɔɪd] *adj* Zungenbein/Os hyoideum u. Schildknorpel betr. *od.* verbindend, thyr(e)ohyoid.
hyothyroid membrane Membrana thyrohyoidea.
hyp- *pref.* → hypo-.
hyp·a·cu·sia [ˌhɪpə'k(j)uːzɪə, -ʒɪə, ˌhaɪ-] *n* → hypacusis.
hyp·a·cu·sis [ˌ-'k(j)uːsɪs] *n HNO* Hörschwäche *f*, Hyp(o)akusis *f*.
hyp·al·bu·min·e·mia [ˌ-æl,bjuːmɪ'niːmɪə] *n* verminderter Albumingehalt *m* des Blutes, Hyp(o)albuminämie *f*.
hyp·al·bu·mi·no·sis [ˌ-æl,bjuːmɪ'nəʊsɪs] *n* Hypalbuminose *f*.
hyp·al·ge·sia [ˌhɪpæl'dʒiːzɪə, -dʒiːʒə, ˌhaɪp-] *n* verminderte Schmerzempfindung *f*, Hypalgesie *f*, Hypalgie *f*.
hyp·al·ge·sic [ˌæl'dʒiːzɪk] *adj* Hypalgesie betr. *od.* verursachend, hypalgetisch, hypalgisch.
hyp·al·get·ic [ˌæl'dʒetɪk] *adj* → hypalgesic.
hyp·al·gia [ˌ-'ældʒ(ɪ)ə] *n* → hypalgesia.
hyp·am·ni·on [ˌ-'æmnɪən] *n gyn.* Fruchtwassermangel *m*, Hypamnion *nt*.
hyp·am·ni·os [ˌ-'æmnɪɒs] *n* → hypamnion.
hyp·an·a·ci·ne·sia [ˌ-ænəsɪ'niːʒ(ɪ)ə] *n* → hypokinesia.
hyp·an·a·ci·ne·sis [ˌ-sɪ'niːsɪs] *n* → hypokinesia.
hyp·an·a·ki·ne·sia [ˌ-kɪ'niːʒ(ɪ)ə, -kaɪ-] *n* → hypokinesia.
hyp·an·a·ki·ne·sis [ˌ-kɪ'niːsɪs, -kaɪ-] *n* → hypokinesia.
hyp·ar·te·ri·al [ˌhɪpɑːr'tɪərɪəl, ˌhaɪp-] *adj* unterhalb einer Arterie liegend.
hyparterial bronchi Bronchus lobaris medius/inferius dexter, Bronchus lobaris superior/inferior sinister, Rami bronchiales hyparteriales.
hyp·ax·i·al [ˌ-'æksɪəl] *adj* hypaxial.
hyp·az·o·tu·ria [ˌ-æzə'tj(ʊ)ərɪə] *n* verminderte Stickstoffausscheidung *f* im Harn, Hypazoturie *f*.
hyper- *pref.* Über-, Hyper-.
hy·per·ab·duc·tion syndrome [ˌhaɪpər·æb'dʌkʃn] Hyperabduktionssyndrom *nt*, Hyperelevationssyndrom *nt*.
hy·per·ab·sorp·tion [ˌ-æb'sɔːrpʃn] *n* übermäßige/gesteigerte Absorption *f*, Hyperabsorption *f*.
hy·per·ac·an·tho·sis [ˌ-ˌækən'təʊsɪs] *n derm.* Akanthose *f*, Acanthosis *f*.
hy·per·ac·id [ˌ-'æsɪd] *adj* übermäßig sauer, hyperazid, superazid.
hy·per·ac·id·am·in·u·ria [ˌ-ˌæsɪdˌæmɪ'n(j)ʊərɪə] *n* vermehrte Aminosäureausscheidung *f* im Harn, Hyperaminoazidurie *f*.

hy·per·a·cid·i·ty [ˌ-ə'sɪdətɪ] *n* Übersäuerung *f*, Hyperazidität *f*.
hy·per·a·cou·sia [ˌ-ə'k(j)uːzɪə, -ʒɪə] *n* → hyperacusis.
hy·per·ac·tive [ˌ-'æktɪv] *adj* 1. *patho.* übermäßig aktiv, hyperaktiv; hyperkinetisch. 2. *psychia., ped.* hyperaktiv.
hyperactive child syndrome hyperkinetisches Syndrom *nt* des Kindesalters.
hy·per·ac·tiv·i·ty [ˌ-æk'tɪvətɪ] *n* 1. *patho.* Hyperaktivität *f*, Hyperkinese *f*, -kinesie *f*. 2. *psychia., ped.* Hyperaktivität *f*.
hy·per·a·cu·sia [ˌ-ə'k(j)uːzɪə, -ʒɪə] *n* → hyperacusis.
hy·per·a·cu·sis [ˌ-ə'k(j)uːsɪs] *n HNO, psychia.* Hyperakusis *f*.
hy·per·a·cute [ˌ-ə'kjuːt] *adj* (*Verlauf, Reaktion*) hyperakut, perakut.
hyperacute rejection *chir.* (*Transplantat*) hyperakute/perakute Abstoßung *f*.
hy·per·ad·e·no·sis [ˌ-ædɪ'nəʊsɪs] *n* Drüsenvergrößerung *f*; gesteigerte Drüsentätigkeit *f*, Hyperadenosis *f*, Hyperadenie *f*.
hy·per·ad·i·po·sis [ˌ-ædɪ'pəʊsɪs] *n* extreme Fettleibigkeit *f*.
hy·per·ad·i·pos·i·ty [ˌ-ædɪ'pɒsətɪ] *n* → hyperadiposis.
hy·per·ad·re·nal·cor·ti·cal·ism [ˌ-əˌdriːnl'kɔːrtɪkəlɪzm] *n* → hyperadrenocorticism.
hy·per·ad·re·nal·ism [ˌ-ə'driːnəlɪzəm] *n* gesteigerte Hormonausschüttung *f* der Nebenniere, Hyperadrenalismus *m*, Hyperadrenie *f*.
hy·per·ad·re·no·cor·ti·cal·ism [ˌ-əˌdriːnəʊ'kɔːrtɪkəlɪzəm] *n* → hyperadrenocorticism.
hy·per·ad·re·no·cor·ti·cism [ˌ-ə'driːnəʊ'kɔːrtəsɪzəm] *n* Überfunktion *f* der Nebennierenrinde, Hyperkortizismus *m*.
hy·per·a·ku·sis [ˌ-ə'k(j)uːsɪs] *n* → hyperacusis.
hy·per·al·bu·min·e·mia [ˌ-ˌæl,bjuːmɪ'niːmɪə] *n* Hyperalbuminämie *f*.
hy·per·al·bu·mi·no·sis [ˌ-æl,bjuːmɪ'nəʊsɪs] *n* Hyperalbuminose *f*.
hy·per·al·do·ste·ro·ne·mia [ˌ-ˌældəʊˌstɪərə'niːmɪə] *n* Hyperaldosteronämie *f*.
hy·per·al·do·ste·ro·nism [ˌ-ˌældəʊ'sterənɪzm] *n* Hyperaldosteronismus *m*, Aldosteronismus *m*.
hy·per·al·do·ster·on·u·ria [ˌ-ˌældəʊˌstɪərə'n(j)ʊərɪə] *n* Hyperaldosteronurie *f*.
hy·per·al·ge·sia [ˌ-æl'dʒiːzɪə, -dʒiːʒə] *n* Schmerzüberempfindsamkeit *f*, gesteigerte Schmerzempfindlichkeit *f*, Hyperalgesie *f*, Hyperalgie *f*.
hy·per·al·ge·sic [ˌ-æl'dʒiːzɪk] *adj* Hyperalgesie betr., hyperalgetisch.
hy·per·al·get·ic [ˌ-æl'dʒetɪk] *adj* → hyperalgesic.
hy·per·al·gia [ˌ-'ældʒ(ɪ)ə] *n* → hyperalgesia.
hy·per·al·i·men·ta·tion [ˌ-ˌælɪmen'teɪʃn] *n* 1. Überernährung *f*, Hyperalimentation *f*. 2. hochkalorische Ernährung *f*, Hyperalimentation *f*.
hy·per·al·i·men·to·sis [ˌ-ˌælɪmen'təʊsɪs] *n* Hyperalimentationssyndrom *nt*.
hy·per·al·ka·les·cence [ˌ-ˌælkə'lesns] *n* → hyperalkalinity.
hy·per·al·ka·lin·i·ty [ˌ-ˌælkə'lɪnətɪ] *n* übermäßige Alkalität *f*, Hyperalkalität *f*.
hy·per·al·lan·to·in·u·ria [ˌ-ˌælæntəʊɪ'n(j)ʊərɪə] *n* gesteigerte Allantoinausscheidung *f* im Harn, Hyperallantoinurie *f*.
hy·per·al·pha·li·po·pro·tein·e·mia [ˌ-ˌælfəˌlɪpəˌprəʊtiː'niːmɪə] *n* Hyperalphalipoproteinämie *f*.
hy·per·am·i·no·ac·i·de·mia [ˌ-əˌmiːnəʊˌæsɪ'diːmɪə] *n* erhöhter Aminosäuregehalt *m* des Blutes, Hyperaminoazidämie *f*.

hy·per·am·i·no·ac·id·u·ria [ˌ-əˌmiːnəʊˌæsɪ-'d(j)ʊərɪə] *n* gesteigerte Aminosäureausscheidung *f* im Harn, Hyperaminoazidurie *f*.
hy·per·am·mo·ne·mia [ˌ-ˌæməˈniːmɪə] *n* erhöhter Ammoniakgehalt *m* des Blutes, Hyperammon(i)ämie *f*, Ammon(i)ämie *f*.
hy·per·am·mo·ni·e·mia [ˌ-ˌməʊnɪˈiːmɪə] *n* → hyperammonemia.
hy·per·am·mo·nu·ria [ˌ-ˌæməˈn(j)ʊərɪə] *n* erhöhte Ammoniakausscheidung *f* im Harn, Hyperammonurie *f*.
hy·per·am·y·las·e·mia [ˌ-ˌæməleɪsˈiːmɪə] *n patho.* erhöhter Amylasegehalt *m* des Blutes, Hyperamylasämie *f*.
hy·per·an·a·ci·ne·sia [ˌ-ænəsɪˈniːʒ(ɪ)ə] *n* → hyperkinesia.
hy·per·an·a·ci·ne·sis [ˌ-ænəsɪˈniːsɪs, -saɪ-] *n* → hyperkinesia.
hy·per·an·a·ki·ne·sia [ˌ-ænəkɪˈniːʒ(ɪ)ə, -kaɪ-] *n* → hyperkinesia.
hy·per·an·a·ki·ne·sis [ˌ-ænəkɪˈniːsɪs, -kaɪ-] *n* → hyperkinesia.
hy·per·an·dro·gen·ism [ˌ-ˈændrədʒenɪzəm] *n* Hyperandrogenismus *m*.
hy·per·a·phia [ˌ-ˈeɪfɪə, -ˈæf-] *n neuro.* taktile Hyperästhesie *f*, Hyper(h)aphie *f*.
hy·per·ar·gi·nin·e·mia [ˌ-ˌɑːrdʒənɪˈniːmɪə] *n* Arginasemangel *m*, Hyperargininämie *f*, Argininämie *f*.
hy·per·az·o·te·mia [ˌ-æzəˈtiːmɪə] *n* Hyperazotämie *f*.
hy·per·az·o·tu·ria [ˌ-æzəˈt(j)ʊərɪə] *n* übermäßige Stickstoffausscheidung *f* im Harn, Hyperazoturie *f*.
hy·per·bar·ic [ˌ-ˈbærɪk] *adj* hyperbar, Überdruck-.
hyperbaric anesthesia *anes.* hyperbare Anästhesie *f*, Überdruckanästhesie *f*, -narkose *f*.
hyperbaric chamber Überdruck-, Dekompressionskammer *f*.
hyperbaric oxygen → hyperbaric oxygen therapy.
hyperbaric oxygen therapy *abbr.* **HOT** Sauerstoffüberdrucktherapie *f*, hyperbare (Sauerstoff-)Therapie/Oxygenation *f*.
hyperbaric pressure Überdruck *m*.
hy·per·bas·o·phil·ic [ˌ-ˌbeɪsəˈfɪlɪk] *adj histol.* hyperbasophil.
hy·per·be·ta·l·a·nin·e·mia [ˌ-ˌbeɪtəˌæləˈniːmɪə] *n* Hyperbetaalaninämie *f*, β-Alaninämie *f*.
hyper-beta carnosinemia Karnosinämie-, Carnosinämie-Syndrom *nt*.
hy·per·be·ta·lip·o·pro·tein·e·mia [ˌ-ˌbeɪtəˌlɪpəprəʊtiːnˈiːmɪə] *n* Hyperbetalipoproteinämie *f*.
hy·per·bi·car·bo·nat·e·mia [ˌ-baɪˌkɑːrbəneɪˈtiːmɪə] *n* Hyperbicarbonatämie *f*, Bicarbonatämie *f*.
hy·per·bil·i·ru·bi·ne·mia [ˌ-ˌbɪləˌruːbɪˈniːmɪə] *n* vermehrter Bilirubingehalt *m* des Blutes, Hyperbilirubinämie *f*.
hy·per·bil·i·ru·bi·nu·ria [ˌ-ˌbɪləˌruːbɪˈn(j)ʊərɪə] *n* erhöhte Bilirubinausscheidung *f* im Harn, Hyperbilirubinurie *f*.
hy·per·blas·to·sis [ˌ-blæsˈtəʊsɪs] *n* Hyperblastose *f*, Hyperblastosis *f*.
hy·per·bo·la [haɪˈpɜːrbələ] *n, pl* **-las, -lae** [-liː, -laɪ] *mathe.* Hyperbel *f*.
hy·per·bol·ic [ˌhaɪpərˈbɒlɪk] *adj mathe.* Hyperbel betr., in Form einer Hyperbel, hyperbolisch.
hy·per·bol·i·cal [ˌ-ˈbɒlɪkl] *adj* → hyperbolic.
hy·per·brach·y·ceph·a·ly [ˌ-ˌbrækɪˈsefəlɪ] *n* extreme Brachyzephalie *f*, Hyperbrachyzephalie *f*, -kephalie *f*.
hy·per·brad·y·ki·nin·e·mia [ˌ-ˌbrædɪˌkaɪnɪˈniːmɪə] *n* Hyperbradykininämie *f*.
hy·per·cal·ce·mia [ˌ-kælˈsiːmɪə] *n* erhöhter Kalziumgehalt *m* des Blutes, Hyperkalz(i)ämie *f*.
hypercalcemia syndrome 1. Hyperkalzämiesyndrom *nt*. 2. alimentäre Hyperkalzämie *f*, Milch-Alkali-Syndrom *nt*, Burnett-Syndrom *nt*.
hy·per·cal·ce·mic crisis [ˌ-kælˈsiːmɪk] hyperkalzämische/hyperparathyreoide Krise *f*, akuter Hyperparathyr(e)oidismus *m*.
hy·per·cal·ci·ne·mia [ˌ-ˌkælsɪˈniːmɪə] *n* → hypercalcemia.
hy·per·cal·ci·nu·ria [ˌ-ˌkælsɪˈn(j)ʊərɪə] *n* → hypercalciuria.
hy·per·cal·ci·pex·y [ˌ-ˈkælsɪpeksɪ] *n* übermäßige Kalziumeinlagerung/-fixierung *f* im Gewebe, Hyperkalzipexie *f*.
hy·per·cal·ci·to·ni·ne·mia [ˌ-ˌkælsɪˌtəʊnɪˈniːmɪə] *n* erhöhter Kalzitoningehalt *m* des Blutes, Hyperkalzitoninämie *f*, Kalzitoninämie *f*, Hyperkalcitoninämie *f*, Calcitoninämie *f*.
hy·per·cal·ci·u·ria [ˌ-kælsɪˈ(j)ʊərɪə] *n* vermehrte Kalziumausscheidung *f* im Harn, Hyperkalzurie *f*, Hyperkalziurie *f*.
hy·per·cal·ci·u·ric [ˌ-kælsɪˈ(j)ʊərɪk] *adj* Hyperkalziurie betr., hyperkalz(i)urisch.
hy·per·cap·nia [ˌ-ˈkæpnɪə] *n* Erhöhung *f* der arteriellen Kohlendioxidspannung, Hyperkapnie *f*, Hyperkarbie *f*.
hy·per·cap·nic [ˌ-ˈkæpnɪk] *adj* Hyperkapnie betr., durch sie gekennzeichnet.
hypercapnic acidosis respiratorische/atmungsbedingte Azidose *f*.
hy·per·car·bia [ˌ-ˈkɑːrbɪə] *n* → hypercapnia.
hy·per·car·dia [ˌ-ˈkɑːrdɪə] *n* Herzhypertrophie *f*.
hy·per·car·o·te·ne·mia *n* → hypercarotinemia.
hy·per·car·o·ti·ne·mia [ˌ-ˌkærətɪˈniːmɪə] *n* Hyperkarotinämie *f*.
hy·per·cel·lu·lar [ˌ-ˈseljələr] *adj* Hyperzellularität betr., von ihr gekennzeichnet, hyperzellulär.
hy·per·cel·lu·lar·i·ty [ˌ-ˌseljəˈleərətɪ] *n* Hyperzellularität *f*.
hy·per·ce·men·to·sis [ˌ-ˌsɪmenˈtəʊsɪs] *n dent.* Hypercementose *f*, Zementhyperplasie *f*.
hy·per·chlo·re·mia [ˌhaɪpərkləʊˈriːmɪə] *n* erhöhter Chloridgehalt *m* des Blutes, Hyperchlorämie *f*.
hy·per·chlo·re·mic [ˌ-kləʊˈriːmɪk] *adj* Hyperchlorämie betr., durch sie gekennzeichnet, hyperchlorämisch.
hyperchloremic acidosis hyperchlorämische Azidose *f*.
hy·per·chlor·hy·dria [ˌ-kləʊrˈhaɪdrɪə] *n (Magen)* erhöhte Salzsäureproduktion *f*, Hyperazidität *f*, Hyperchlorhydrie *f*.
hy·per·chlor·u·ria [ˌ-kləʊˈr(j)ʊərɪə] *n* erhöhte Chloridausscheidung *f* im Harn, Hyperchlorurie *f*.
hy·per·cho·les·ter·e·mia [ˌ-kəˌlestəˈriːmɪə] *n* → hypercholesterolemia.
hy·per·cho·les·ter·e·mic [ˌ-kəˌlestəˈriːmɪk] *adj* → hypercholesterolemic.
hy·per·cho·les·ter·in·e·mia [ˌ-kəˌlestərɪˈniːmɪə] *n* → hypercholesterolemia.
hy·per·cho·les·ter·ol·e·mia [ˌ-kəˌlestərəˈliːmɪə] *n* erhöhter Cholesteringehalt *m* des Blutes, Hypercholesterinämie *f*.
hy·per·cho·les·ter·ol·e·mic [ˌ-kəˌlestərəˈliːmɪk] *adj* Hypercholesterinämie betr. *od.* verursachend, durch Hypercholesterinämie gekennzeichnet.
hy·per·cho·les·ter·ol·ia [ˌ-kəˌlestəˈrəʊlɪə] *n* erhöhter Cholesteringehalt *m* der Galle.
hy·per·cho·lia [ˌ-ˈkəʊlɪə] *n* übermäßige Galleproduktion *od.* -sekretion *f*, Hypercholie *f*.

hy·per·chon·dro·pla·sia [ˌ-ˌkɒndrəˈpleɪʒ(ɪ)ə, -zɪə] *n ortho.* Hyperchondroplasie *f*.
hy·per·chro·ma·sia [ˌ-krəʊˈmeɪʒ(ɪ)ə] *n* → hyperchromatism.
hy·per·chro·mat·ic [ˌ-krəʊˈmætɪk] *adj* hyperchromatisch.
hyperchromatic anemia → hyperchromic anemia.
hyperchromatic cell hyperchromatische/hyperchrome Zelle *f*.
hy·per·chro·ma·tin [ˌ-ˈkrəʊmətɪn] *n* Hyperchromatin *nt*.
hyperchromatin granules azurophile Granula *pl*.
hy·per·chro·ma·tism [ˌ-ˈkrəʊmətɪzəm] *n* Hyperchromatose *f*.
hy·per·chro·ma·to·sis [ˌ-ˌkrəʊməˈtəʊsɪs] *n* 1. Hyperchromasie *f*. 2. Hyperchromatose *f*.
hy·per·chro·me·mia [ˌ-krəʊˈmiːmɪə] *n hema.* Hyperchromie *f*, Hyperchromasie *f*.
hy·per·chro·mia [ˌ-ˈkrəʊmɪə] *n* → hyperchromatism.
hy·per·chro·mic [ˌ-ˈkrəʊmɪk] *adj* 1. hyperchromatisch. 2. hyperchrom.
hyperchromic anemia hyperchrome Anämie *f*.
hyperchromic effect *biochem.* hyperchromer Effekt *m*.
hy·per·chy·lia [ˌ-ˈkaɪlɪə] *n* übermäßige Magensaftsekretion *f*, Hyperchylie *f*.
hy·per·chy·lo·mi·cro·ne·mia [ˌ-ˌkaɪləˌmaɪkrəˈniːmɪə] *n* Hyperchylomikronämie *f*, Chylomikronämie *f*.
hy·per·ci·ne·sia [ˌ-sɪˈniːʒ(ɪ)ə] *n* → hyperkinesia.
hy·per·ci·ne·sis [ˌ-sɪˈniːsɪs, -saɪ-] *n* → hyperkinesia.
hy·per·co·ag·u·la·bil·i·ty [ˌ-kəʊˌægjələˈbɪlətɪ] *n hema.* erhöhte Gerinnbarkeit *f* des Blutes, Hyperkoagulabilität *f*.
hy·per·co·ag·u·la·ble [ˌ-kəʊˈægjələbl] *adj hema.* leicht gerinnbar, mit erhöhter Gerinnbarkeit.
hy·per·cor·ti·cal·ism [ˌ-ˈkɔːrtɪkəlɪzəm] *n* → hyperadrenocorticism.
hy·per·cor·ti·coid·ism [ˌ-ˈkɔːrtɪkɔɪdɪzəm] *n* Hyperkortikoidismus *m*.
hy·per·cor·ti·so·lism [ˌ-ˈkɔːrtɪsəʊlɪzəm] *n* Hyperkortisolämie *f*.
hy·per·cor·ti·sol·ism [ˌ-ˈkɔːrtɪsəʊlɪzəm] *n* 1. Hyperkortisolismus *m*, -cortisolismus *m*. 2. → hyperadrenocorticism.
hy·per·cre·a·tin·e·mia [ˌ-krɪətɪˈniːmɪə] *n* erhöhter Kreatingehalt *m* des Blutes, Hyperkreatinämie *f*.
hy·per·cri·nia [ˌ-ˈkrɪnɪə] *n* Hyperkrinie *f*.
hy·per·crin·ism [ˈ-krɪnɪzəm] *n* → hypercrinia.
hy·per·cry·al·ge·sia [ˌ-kraɪælˈdʒiːzɪə, -dʒiːʒə] *n* → hypercryesthesia.
hy·per·cry·es·the·sia [ˌ-kraɪesˈθiːʒ(ɪ)ə] *n neuro.* erhöhte Kälteempfindlichkeit *f*, Hyperkryästhesie *f*.
hy·per·cu·pre·mia [ˌ-k(j)uˈpriːmɪə] *n* erhöhter Kupfergehalt *m* des Blutes, Kuprämie *f*.
hy·per·cu·pri·u·ria [ˌ-ˌk(j)uprɪˈ(j)ʊərɪə] *n* erhöhte Kupferausscheidung *f* im Harn, Kuprurese *f*.
hy·per·cy·a·not·ic [ˌ-saɪəˈnɒtɪk] *adj* extrem zyanotisch, hyperzyanotisch.
hy·per·cy·e·sia [ˌ-saɪˈiːzɪə] *n* → hypercyesis.
hy·per·cy·e·sis [ˌ-saɪˈiːsɪs] *n embryo.* Überbefruchtung *f*, Superfetatio *f*.
hy·per·cy·the·mia [ˌ-saɪˈθiːmɪə] *n hema.* pathologische Erhöhung *f* der Erythrozytenzahl, Erythrozythämie *f*, Erythrozytose *f*, Hypererythrozythämie *f*, Hyperzythämie *f*.

hypercytochromia

hy·per·cy·to·chro·mia [ˌ-saɪtə'krəʊmɪə] n Hyperzytochromie f.
hy·per·cy·to·sis [ˌ-saɪ'təʊsɪs] n 1. pathologische Erhöhung f der Zellzahl, Hyperzytose f. 2. Erhöhung f der Leukozytenzahl, Leukozytose f.
hy·per·dac·tyl·ia [ˌ-dæk'tiːlɪə] n → hyperdactyly.
hy·per·dac·tyl·ism [ˌ-'dæktəlɪzəm] n → hyperdactyly.
hy·per·dac·ty·ly [ˌ-'dæktəlɪ] n embryo. Hyperdaktylie f, Polydaktylie f.
hy·per·den·se ['haɪpərdens] adj radiol. hyperdens.
hy·per·di·as·to·lic hypotension [ˌ-daɪə-'stɑlɪk] hyperdiastolische Hypotonie f.
hy·per·di·crot·ic [ˌ-daɪ'krɑtɪk] adj card. hyperdikrot.
hy·per·dip·loid [ˌ-'dɪplɔɪd] adj genet. hyperdiploid.
hy·per·dip·sia [ˌ-'dɪpsɪə] n übermäßiger Durst m, Hyperdipsie f.
hy·per·dis·ten·tion [ˌʌ-dɪ'stenʃn] n Überdehnung f, -blähung f.
hy·per·dy·nam·ia [ˌ-daɪ'næmɪə] n übermäßige Muskelaktivität f, Hyperdynamie f.
hy·per·dy·nam·ic [ˌ-daɪ'næmɪk] adj Hyperdynamie betr., hyperdynamisch.
hyperdynamic ileus chir. spastischer Ileus m.
hyperdynamic phase hyperdynamische Phase f, hyperdynamisches Stadium nt.
hy·per·e·lec·tro·ly·te·mia [ˌ-ɪˌlektrəlaɪ'tiːmɪə] n Erhöhung f der Elektrolytkonzentration im Blut, Hyperelektrolytämie f.
hy·per·em·e·sis [ˌ-'eməsɪs] n übermäßiges Erbrechen nt, Hyperemesis f.
hy·per·e·met·ic [ˌ-ə'metɪk] adj Hyperemesis betr., durch Hyperemesis gekennzeichnet, hyperemetisch.
hy·per·e·mia [ˌ-'iːmɪə] n vermehrte Blutfülle f, Hyperämie f.
hy·per·e·mic [ˌ-'iːmɪk] adj durch Hyperämie gekennzeichnet, hyperämisch.
hyperemic headache Stauungskopfschmerz m.
hy·per·e·mi·za·tion [ˌ-ˌemɪ'zeɪʃn] n Hyperämisierung f, Hyperämisieren nt.
hy·per·en·dem·ic [ˌ-en'demɪk] adj epidem. hyperendemisch.
hy·per·en·zym·e·mia [ˌ-enzaɪ'miːmɪə] n erhöhte Enzymaktivität f im Blut, Hyperenzymämie f, Hyperenzymie f.
hy·per·e·o·sin·o·phil·ia [ˌ-ɪəˌsɪnə'fɪlɪə, -lJə] n hema. übermäßige Eosinophilie f, Hypereosinophilie f.
hy·per·eph·i·dro·sis [ˌ-efɪ'drəʊsɪs] n → hyperhidrosis.
hy·per·ep·i·neph·ri·ne·mia [ˌ-epɪˌnefrɪ'niːmɪə] n Hyperadrenalinämie f.
hy·per·er·e·thism [ˌ-'erəθɪzəm] n extreme Reizbarkeit/Irritabilität f.
hy·per·er·ga·sia [ˌ-ɜr'geɪʒ(ɪ)ə] n pathologisch erhöhte funktionelle Aktivität f, Hyperergasie f.
hy·per·er·gia [ˌ-'ɜrdʒɪə] n 1. → hyperergasia. 2. → hyperergy.
hy·per·er·gic [ˌ-'ɜrdʒɪk] adj Hyperergie betr., hypererg(isch).
hyperergic encephalitis hyperergische Enzephalitis f.
hy·per·er·gy ['-ɜrdʒɪ] n immun. gesteigerte Empfindlichkeit f, verstärkte Reaktion(sbereitschaft f) f, Hyperergie f; Allergie f.
hy·per·e·ryth·ro·cy·the·mia [ˌ-ˌrɪθrə-saɪ'θiːmɪə] n → hypercythemia.
hy·per·es·o·pho·ria [ˌ-esə'fɔːrɪə] n ophthal. Hyperesophorie f, Esohyperphorie f.
hy·per·es·the·sia [ˌ-es'θiːʒ(ɪ)ə] n neuro.

Überempfindlichkeit f, Hyperästhesie f, Hyperaesthesia f.
hy·per·es·thet·ic [ˌ-es'θetɪk] adj neuro. Hyperästhesie betr., durch sie gekennzeichnet, überempfindlich, hyperästhetisch.
hy·per·es·tri·ne·mia [ˌ-estrɪ'niːmɪə] n → hyperestrogenemia.
hy·per·es·trin·ism [ˌ-'estrənɪzəm] n → hyperestrogenism.
hy·per·es·tro·ge·ne·mia [ˌ-ˌestrədʒɪ'niː-mɪə] n pathologisch erhöhter Östrogengehalt m des Blutes, Hyperöstrogenämie f.
hy·per·es·tro·gen·ism [ˌ-'estrədʒenɪzəm] n Hyperöstrogenismus m.
hy·per·eu·ry·o·pia [ˌ-jʊərɪ'əʊpɪə] n ophthal. Euryopie f.
hy·per·ex·cit·a·bil·i·ty [ˌ-ɪkˌsaɪtə'bɪlətɪ] n neuro. Übererregbarkeit f, Hyperexzitabilität f.
hy·per·ex·cit·a·ble [ˌ-ɪk'saɪtəbl] adj neuro. übererregbar, hyperexzitabel.
hy·per·ex·cre·to·ry [ˌ-'ekskrətɔːrɪ, -ˌtəʊ-] adj durch Übersekretion gekennzeichnet, hyperexkretorisch.
hy·per·ex·o·pho·ria [ˌ-eksəʊ'fɔʊrɪə] n ophthal. Hyperexophorie f, Exohyperphorie f.
hy·per·ex·tend [ˌ-ɪk'stend] (Gelenk) I vt überstrecken, hyperextendieren. II vi überstreckt werden.
hy·per·ex·tend·a·bil·i·ty n → hyperextendibility.
hy·per·ex·tend·a·ble adj → hyperextendible.
hy·per·ex·tend·i·bil·i·ty [ˌ-ˌɪkstendə'bɪlətɪ] n (Gelenk) Überstreckbarkeit f, Hyperextendibilität f.
hy·per·ex·tend·i·ble [ˌ-ɪk'stendɪbl] adj (Gelenk) überstreckbar, hyperextendierbar.
hy·per·ex·ten·sion [ˌ-ɪk'stenʃn] n f. 1. Überstreckung f, Hyperextension f. 2. Überstrecken nt, Hyperextendieren nt.
hyperextension deformity ortho. (Gelenk) Hyperextensionsfehlstellung f.
hy·per·fer·re·mia [ˌ-fə'riːmɪə] n pathologisch erhöhter Eisengehalt m des Blutes.
hy·per·fer·ri·ce·mia [ˌ-ferɪ'siːmɪə] n → hyperferremia.
hy·per·fi·brin·o·ge·ne·mia [ˌ-fɪ'brɪnədʒə-'niːmɪə] n vermehrter Fibrinogengehalt m des Blutes, Hyperfibrinogenämie f.
hy·per·flex·ion [ˌ-'flekʃn] n ortho. (Gelenk) übermäßige Beugung f, Hyperflexion f.
hy·per·func·tion [ˌ-'fʌŋkʃn] n Über-, Hyperfunktion f.
hy·per·func·tion·ing [ˌ-'fʌŋkʃənɪŋ] n → hyperfunction.
hy·per·ga·lac·tia [ˌ-gə'lækʃɪə, -tɪə] n gyn. übermäßige/überschießende Milchsekretion f, Hypergalaktie f.
hy·per·gal·ac·to·sis [ˌ-gælək'təʊsɪs] n → hypergalactia.
hy·per·ga·lac·tous [ˌ-gə'læktəs] adj Hypergalaktie betr. od. verursachend, mit überschießender Milchbildung einhergehend.
hy·per·gam·ma·glob·u·li·ne·mia [ˌ-gæmə-ˌglɑbjəlɪ'niːmɪə] f immun. Hypergammaglobulinämie f.
hyp·er·ga·sia [ˌ-'geɪzɪə] n → hypoergasia.
hy·per·gas·tri·ne·mia [ˌ-gæs'traɪniːmɪə] n erhöhter Gastringehalt m des Blutes, Hypergastrinämie f.
hy·per·gen·e·sis [ˌ-'dʒenəsɪs] n embryo. Überentwicklung f, Hypergenese f.
hy·per·ge·net·ic [ˌ-dʒə'netɪk] adj embryo. Hypergenese betr., hypergenetisch, überentwickelt.
hy·per·gen·i·tal·ism [ˌ-'dʒenɪtəlɪzəm] n Hypergenitalismus m.
hy·per·geus·es·the·sia [ˌ-ˌgjuːzes'θiːʒ(ɪ)ə] n → hypergeusia.

hy·per·geu·sia [ˌ-'gjuːʒ(ɪ)ə] n neuro. gustatorische Hyperästhesie f, Hypergeusie f.
hy·per·gia [haɪ'pɜrdʒɪə] n 1. immun. verminderte Reaktivität f, Hypergie f. 2. → hypoergasia.
hy·per·gic [haɪ'pɜrdʒɪk] adj 1. Hypergie betr., hyperg. 2. → hyperergic.
hy·per·glob·u·lia [ˌ-haɪpərɡlə'bjuːlɪə] n hema. Hyperglobulie f, Polyglobulie f.
hy·per·glob·u·lin·e·mia [ˌ-ˌglɑbjəlɪ'niːmɪə] n Hyperglobulinämie f.
hyp·er·glob·u·lin·e·mic purpura [ˌ-ˌglɑb-jəlɪ'niːmɪk] Purpura hyperglobulinaemica (Waldenström).
hy·per·glob·u·lism [ˌ-'glɑbjəlɪzəm] n → hyperglobulia.
hy·per·glu·ca·go·ne·mia [ˌ-gluːkəɡə'niː-mɪə] n pathologisch erhöhter Glukagongehalt m des Blutes, Hyperglukagonämie f.
hy·per·gly·ce·mia [ˌ-glaɪ'siːmɪə] n pathologische Blutzuckererhöhung f, Hyperglykämie f, Hyperglyzämie f.
h. of injury streßbedingte Hyperglykämie f, Streßdiabetes m.
hy·per·gly·ce·mic [ˌ-glaɪ'siːmɪk] adj Hyperglykämie betr. od. verursachend, hyperglykämisch.
hyperglycemic-glycogenolytic factor abbr. HGF Glukagon nt, Glucagon nt.
hyperglycemic glycosuria hyperglykämische Glukosurie f, Glykosurie f.
hy·per·glyc·er·i·de·mia [ˌ-glɪsərɪ'diːmɪə] n erhöhter Glyceridgehalt m des Blutes, Hyperglyceridämie f.
hy·per·gly·ci·ne·mia [ˌ-glaɪsə'niːmɪə] n erhöhter Glycingehalt m des Blutes, Hyperglycinämie f, Hyperglycinämie f, Glykokollkrankheit f, Glyzinose f, Glycinosis f, Glyzinurie f mit Hyperglyzinämie f.
hy·per·gly·ci·nu·ria [ˌ-glaɪsə'n(j)ʊərɪə] n vermehrte Glycinausscheidung f im Harn, Hyperglyzinurie f, Hyperglycinurie f.
h. with hyperglycinemia → hyperglycinemia.
hy·per·gly·co·ge·nol·y·sis [ˌ-glaɪkədʒɪ-'nɑləsɪs] n übermäßige Glykogenolyse f, Hyperglykogenolyse f.
hy·per·gly·cor·rha·chia [ˌ-glaɪkə'reɪkɪə, -'ræk-] n erhöhter Zuckergehalt m des Liquor cerebrospinalis.
hy·per·gly·co·se·mia [ˌ-glaɪkə'siːmɪə] n → hyperglycemia.
hy·per·gly·co·su·ria [ˌ-ˌglaɪkə's(j)ʊərɪə] n stark erhöhte Zuckerausscheidung f im Harn, Hyperglykosurie f.
hy·per·gly·ke·mia [ˌ-glaɪ'kiːmɪə] n → hyperglycemia.
hy·per·go·nad·ism [ˌ-'gəʊnædɪzəm, -'gɑ-] n Gonadenüberfunktion f, Hypergonadismus m.
hy·per·go·na·do·troph·ic [ˌ-ˌgəʊnədəʊ-'trɑfɪk, -'trəʊ-] adj hypergonadotroph(isch), hypergonadotrop.
hy·per·go·na·do·trop·ic [ˌ-ˌgəʊnədəʊ-'trɑpɪk, -'trəʊ-] adj → hypergonadotrophic.
hypergonadotropic hypogonadism primärer/hypergonadotroper Hypogonadismus m.
hy·per·gua·ni·di·ne·mia [ˌ-ˌgwɑnədɪ'niː-mɪə] n erhöhter Guanidingehalt m des Blutes, Hyperguanidinämie f.
hy·per·he·do·nia [ˌ-hɪ'dəʊnɪə] n psychia. übersteigertes Lustgefühl nt, Hyperhedonie f.
hy·per·he·don·ism [ˌ-'hiːdnɪzəm] n → hyperhedonia.
hy·per·he·mo·glo·bi·ne·mia [ˌ-ˌhiːməglə-bɪ'niːmɪə, ˌhem-] n hema. extreme Hämoglobinämie f, Hyperhämoglobinämie f.

hy·per·hep·a·rin·e·mia [ˌ-ˌhepərɪn'iːmɪə] n Hyperheparinämie f.
hy·per·he·pat·ia [ˌ-hɪ'pætɪə] n Überfunktion f der Leber.
hy·per·hi·dro·sis [ˌ-haɪ'drəʊsɪs, -hɪ-] n übermäßiges Schwitzen nt, Hyperhidrose f, Hyper(h)idrosis f, Polyhidrose f, Poly(h)idrosis f.
hy·per·hy·dra·tion [ˌ-haɪ'dreɪʃn] n Überwässerung f, übermäßiger Wassergehalt m des Körpers, Hyperhydratation f.
hy·per·hy·dro·chlo·ria [ˌ-ˌhaɪdrə'klɔːrɪə] n → hyperchlorhydria.
hy·per·hy·dro·chlo·rid·ia [ˌ-ˌhaɪdrəklɔː'rɪdɪə] n → hyperchlorhydria.
hy·per·hy·dro·pex·is [ˌ-ˌhaɪdrə'peksɪs] n übermäßige Wassereinlagerung f im Gewebe, Hyperhydropexie f.
hy·per·hy·dro·pex·y [ˌ-'haɪdrəpeksɪ] n → hyperhydropexis.
hy·per·hy·drox·y·pro·lin·e·mia [ˌ-haɪˌdrɑksɪprəʊlɪ'niːmɪə] n Hyperhydroxyprolinämie f, Hydroxyprolinämie f.
hy·per·i·dro·sis [ˌ-ɪ'drəʊsɪs] n → hyperhidrosis.
hy·per·im·i·do·di·pep·ti·du·ria [ˌ-ˌɪmɪdəʊdaɪpeptɪ'd(j)ʊərɪə] n Prolidasemangel m.
hy·per·im·mune [ˌ-ɪ'mjuːn] adj hyperimmun.
hyperimmune serum Hyperimmunserum nt.
hy·per·im·mu·ni·ty [ˌ-ɪ'mjuːnətɪ] n Hyperimmunität f.
hy·per·im·mu·ni·za·tion [ˌ-ˌɪmjənɪ'zeɪʃn] n Hyperimmunisierung f.
hy·per·im·mu·no·glob·u·li·ne·mia [ˌ-ˌɪmjənəʊˌglɑbjəlɪ'niːmɪə] n Hyperimmunglobulinämie f.
hyperimmunoglobulinemia E syndrome Buckley-Syndrom nt, Hyperimmunglobulinämie E f.
hy·per·in·fla·tion [ˌ-ɪn'fleɪʃn] n (Lunge) Überblähung f.
hy·per·in·o·se·mia [ˌhaɪpərɪnə'siːmɪə, -aɪnəʊ-] n → hyperinosis.
hy·per·i·no·sis [ˌ-aɪ'nəʊsɪs] n Hyperinose f.
hy·per·in·su·lin·e·mia [ˌ-ˌɪn(t)sjəlɪ'niːmɪə] n erhöhter Insulingehalt m des Blutes, Hyperinsulinämie f.
hy·per·in·su·lin·ism [ˌ-'ɪn(t)sjəlɪnɪzəm] n 1. vermehrte Insulinsekretion f, Hyperinsulinismus m. 2. Insulinschock m. 3. → hyperinsulinemia.
hy·per·in·vo·lu·tion [ˌ-ɪnvə'luːʃn] n übermäßige Organrückbildung/Involution f, Hyper-, Superinvolution f, Superinvolutio f.
hy·per·i·o·de·mia [ˌ-aɪə'diːmɪə] n erhöhter Jodgehalt m des Blutes, Hyperjodämie f, Hyperiodämie f.
hy·per·i·so·ton·ic [ˌ-aɪsə'tɑnɪk] adj → hypertonic.
hy·per·ka·le·mia [ˌ-kə'liːmɪə] n erhöhter Kaliumgehalt m des Blutes, Hyperkal(i)ämie f.
hy·per·ka·le·mic [ˌ-kə'liːmɪk] adj Hyperkal(i)ämie betr., von ihr gekennzeichnet, hyperkal(i)ämisch.
hyperkalemic acidosis hyperkaliämische Azidose f.
hyperkalemic periodic paralysis Gamstorp-Syndrom nt, Adynamia episodica hereditaria.
hy·per·ka·li·e·mia [ˌ-ˌkælɪ'iːmɪə] n → hyperkalemia.
hy·per·ker·a·tin·i·za·tion [ˌ-ˌkerətɪnə'zeɪʃn] n → hyperkeratosis 1.
hy·per·ker·a·to·sis [ˌ-kerə'təʊsɪs] n 1. derm. Hyperkeratose f, Hyperkeratosis f. 2. ophthal. Kornea-, Hornhauthypertrophie f.
h. of palms and soles Palmoplantarkeratose f, Keratodermia/Keratosis palmoplantaris.
hyperkeratosis lenticularis perstans Morbus Flegel m, Hyperkeratosis lenticularis perstans (Flegel).
hy·per·ke·to·ne·mia [ˌ-ˌkiːtə'niːmɪə] n erhöhte Ketonkörperkonzentration f des Blutes, Hyperketonämie f, Ketonämie f.
hy·per·ke·to·nu·ria [ˌ-ˌkiːtə'n(j)ʊərɪə] n übermäßige Ketonkörperausscheidung f im Harn, Hyperketonurie f.
hy·per·ke·to·sis [ˌ-kɪ'təʊsɪs] n übermäßige Ketonkörperbildung f, Hyperketose f.
hy·per·ki·ne·mia [ˌ-kaɪ'niːmɪə] n card. pathologisch erhöhtes Herzzeitvolumen nt.
hy·per·ki·ne·sia [ˌ-kɪ'niːʒ(ɪ)ə, -kaɪ-] n 1. neuro. übermäßige Bewegungsaktivität f, gesteigerte Spontanmotorik f, Hyperkinese f, -kinesie f, -kinesis f, Hypermotilität f. 2. psychia. Bewegungsunruhe f, Hyperkinese f, -kinesie f, -kinesis f, -aktivität f.
hy·per·ki·ne·sis [ˌ-kɪ'niːsɪs, -kaɪ-] n → hyperkinesia.
hyperkinesis sign Claude'-(Hyperkinese-)Zeichen nt.
hy·per·ki·net·ic [ˌ-kɪ'netɪk] adj Hyperkinese betr., hyperkinetisch.
hyperkinetic heart syndrome hyperkinetisches Herzsyndrom nt.
hyperkinetic reaction/syndrome hyperkinetisches Syndrom nt des Kindesalters.
hy·per·lact·ac·i·de·mia [ˌ-ˌlæktæsɪ'diːmɪə] n pathologisch erhöhte Laktatkonzentration f des Blutes, Hyperlaktazidämie f, -lactazidämie f.
hy·per·lac·ta·tion [ˌ-læk'teɪʃn] n gyn. verstärkte u. verlängerte Milchsekretion f, Hyper-, Superlaktation f.
hy·per·lec·i·thi·ne·mia [ˌ-ˌlesɪθɪ'niːmɪə] n erhöhter Lezithingehalt m des Blutes, Hyperlezithinämie f, -lecithinämie f.
hy·per·leu·ko·cy·to·sis [ˌ-ˌluːkəsaɪ'təʊsɪs] n hema. extreme Leukozytose f, Hyperleukozytose f, leukämoide Reaktion f, Pseudoleukämie f.
hy·per·ley·dig·ism [ˌ-'laɪdɪgɪzəm] n Überaktivität f der Leydig-Zellen.
hy·per·li·pe·mia [ˌ-laɪ'piːmɪə] n vermehrter Neutralfettgehalt m des Blutes, Hyperlipämie f, Lipämie f.
hy·per·li·pe·mic [ˌ-laɪ'piːmɪk] adj Hyperlipämie betr., durch sie gekennzeichnet, hyperlipämisch.
hyperlipemic hyponatremia Hyponatr(i)ämie f bei Hyperlipämie.
hy·per·lip·i·de·mia [ˌ-lɪpə'diːmɪə] n vermehrter Gesamtlipidgehalt m des Blutes, Erhöhung f der Serumlipide, Hyperlipidämie f, Lipidämie f.
hy·per·li·poi·de·mia [ˌ-laɪpɔɪ'diːmɪə] n → hyperlipidemia.
hy·per·lip·o·pro·tein·e·mia [ˌ-ˌlɪpəprəʊtɪ'niːmɪə] n vermehrter Lipoproteingehalt m des Blutes, Hyperlipoproteinämie f.
hy·per·li·the·mia [ˌ-lɪ'θiːmɪə] n erhöhter Lithiumgehalt m des Blutes, Hyperlithämie f.
hy·per·li·thu·ria [ˌ-lɪ'θ(j)ʊərɪə] n vermehrte Harnsäureausscheidung f, Hyperlithurie f.
hy·per·lor·do·sis [ˌ-lɔːr'dəʊsɪs] n ortho. extreme Lordose f, Hyperlordose f.
hy·per·lu·cen·cy [ˌ-'luːsnsɪ] n radiol. erhöhte Strahlendurchlässigkeit f.
hy·per·lu·te·in·i·za·tion [ˌ-ˌluːtɪənɪ'zeɪʃn, -naɪ-] n gyn. Hyperluteinisation f.
hy·per·ly·sin·e·mia [ˌ-ˌlaɪsə'niːmɪə] n erhöhter Lysingehalt m des Blutes, Hyperlysinämie f, Lysinintoleranz f.
hy·per·ly·sin·u·ria [ˌ-ˌlaɪsə'n(j)ʊərɪə] n erhöhte Lysinausscheidung f im Harn, Hyperlysinurie f.
hy·per·mag·ne·se·mia [ˌ-ˌmægnɪ'siːmɪə] n erhöhter Magnesiumgehalt m des Blutes, Hypermagnesiämie f.
hy·per·mas·tia [ˌ-'mæstɪə] n gyn. 1. Hypermastie f, Polymastie f. 2. Brust(drüsen)hypertrophie f, Hypermastie f, Makromastie f.
hy·per·ma·ture [ˌ-mə't(j)ʊər, -'tʃʊər] adj überreif.
hypermature cataract ophthal. überreifer Star m, Cataracta hypermatura.
hy·per·mel·a·not·ic [ˌ-melə'nɑtɪk] adj hypermelanotisch.
hy·per·men·or·rhea [ˌ-menə'rɪə] n gyn. übermäßig starke Menstruation(sblutung f) f, Hypermenorrhoe f.
hy·per·met·a·bol·ic [ˌ-metə'bɑlɪk] adj hypermetabolisch.
hypermetabolic state hypermetabolischer Zustand m.
hy·per·me·tab·o·lism [ˌ-mɪ'tæbəlɪzəm] n gesteigerter Stoffwechsel m, Hypermetabolismus m.
hy·per·met·a·mor·pho·sis [ˌ-ˌmetəmɔːr'fəʊsɪs] n psychia. Hypermetamorphose f.
hy·per·met·a·pla·sia [ˌ-metə'pleɪʒ(ɪ)ə, -zɪə] n pathologisch erhöhte Metaplasie f, Hypermetaplasie f.
hy·per·me·thi·o·nin·e·mia [-mɪˌθaɪənɪ'niːmɪə] n hereditäre/hepatorenale (Hyper-)-Tyrosinämie f, Tyrosinose f.
hy·per·me·tria [ˌ-'miːtrɪə] n neuro. Hypermetrie f.
hy·per·me·trope [ˌ-'metrəʊp] n → hyperope.
hy·per·me·tro·pia [ˌ-mɪ'trəʊpɪə] n → hyperopia.
hy·per·me·trop·ic [ˌ-mɪ'trɑpɪk, -'trəʊp-] adj → hyperopic.
hypermetropic astigmatism ophthal. kombinierte Hyperopie f u. Astigmatismus.
hy·per·mim·ia [ˌ-'mɪmɪə] n übermäßige/übertriebene Gestik f, Hypermimie f.
hy·per·min·er·al·i·za·tion [ˌ-ˌmɪnərələ'zeɪʃn, -laɪ-] n radiol. Hypermineralisation f.
hy·perm·ne·sia [ˌhaɪpərm'niːʒə] n übersteigertes Erinnerungsvermögen nt, abnorme Gedächtnisstärke f, Hypermnesie f.
hyp·er·mo·bile kidney [ˌ-'məʊbəl, -biːl] patho. Wanderniere f, Ren mobilis/migrans.
hy·per·mo·bil·i·ty [ˌ-məʊ'bɪlətɪ] n ortho. (Gelenk) übermäßige Beweglichkeit f, Überstreckbarkeit f, Hypermobilität f.
hy·per·morph ['-mɔːrf] n 1. Stehriese m. 2. genet. hypermorphes Gen nt.
hy·per·mor·phic [ˌ-'mɔːrfɪk] adj genet. hypermorph.
hy·per·mo·til·i·ty [ˌ-məʊ'tɪlətɪ] n gesteigerte Motilität f, Hypermotilität f; (Darm) Hyperperistaltik f.
hy·per·my·es·the·sia [ˌ-maɪes'θiːʒ(ɪ)ə] n neuro. Muskelhyperästhesie f, Hypermyästhesie f.
hy·per·my·o·to·nia [ˌ-maɪə'təʊnɪə] n neuro. gesteigerter Muskeltonus m, Hypermyotonie f.
hy·per·my·ot·ro·phy [ˌ-maɪ'ɑtrəfɪ] n Muskelhypertrophie f.
hy·per·na·tre·mia [ˌ-nə'triːmɪə] n erhöhter Natriumgehalt m des Blutes, Hypernatriämie f.
hy·per·na·tre·mic [ˌ-nə'triːmɪk] adj Hypernatriämie betr. od. verursachend, hypernatriämisch.
hypernatremic encephalopathy hypernatriämische/hypernatriämisch-bedingte Enzephalopathie f.

hy·per·na·tro·ne·mia [ˌ-nætrə'niːmɪə] *n* → hypernatremia.
hy·per·ne·o·cy·to·sis [ˌ-ˌnɪəsaɪ'təʊsɪs] *n hema.* Hyperleukozytose *f* mit starker Linksverschiebung.
hy·per·neph·roid [ˌ-'nefrɔɪd] *adj* der Nebennierenrinde ähnlich, hypernephroid.
hypernephroid (renal) carcinoma hypernephroides (Nieren-)Karzinom *nt*, klarzelliges Nierenkarzinom *nt*, (maligner) Grawitz-Tumor *m*, Hypernephrom *nt*.
hy·per·ne·phro·ma [ˌ-nə'frəʊmə] *n* **1.** → hypernephroid (renal) carcinoma. **2.** benigner Grawitz-Tumor *m*, Hypernephrom *nt*.
hy·per·noi·a [ˌ-'nɔɪə] *n* übermäßige geistige *od.* seelische Aktivität *f*, Hypernoia *f*.
hy·per·nom·ic [ˌ-'nɑmɪk] *adj* extrem, exzessiv, ungehemmt.
hy·per·nor·mal [ˌ-'nɔːrml] *adj* übermäßig, über-, hypernormal; pathologisch.
hy·per·nu·tri·tion [ˌ-n(j)uː'trɪʃn] *n* Überernährung *f*.
hy·per·o·don·tia [ˌ-ə'dɑntʃ(ɪ)ə] *n* angeborene Überzahl *f* von Zähnen, Hyperodontie *f*.
hy·per·on ['haɪpərən] *n phys.* Hyperon *nt*.
hy·per·on·cot·ic [ˌhaɪpərɑn'kɑtɪk] *adj physiol.* (*Druck*) hyperonkotisch.
hy·per·o·nych·ia [ˌ-əʊ'nɪkɪə] *n* Nagelhypertrophie *f*, Hyperonychie *f*.
hy·per·ope ['-əʊp] *n* Weitsichtige(r *m*) *f*, Hyperope(r *m*) *f*.
hy·per·o·pia [ˌ-'əʊpɪə] *n abbr.* **H** Über-, Weitsichtigkeit *f*, Hyperopie *f*, Hypermetropie *f*.
hy·per·op·ic [ˌ-'əʊpɪk] *adj* Weitsichtigkeit betr., weitsichtig, hypermetropisch, hyperop.
hyperopic astigmatism *abbr.* **ah** *opthal.* kombinierte Hyperopie *f* u. Astigmatismus.
hy·per·or·chi·dism [ˌ-'ɔːrkədɪzəm] *n* Hyperorchidismus *m*.
hy·per·o·rex·ia [ˌ-əʊ'reksɪə] *n* **1.** Heißhunger *m*, Eß-, Freßsucht *f*, Hyperorexie *f*, Bulimie *f*. **2.** Bulimia nervosa *f*, Bulimarexie *f*, Freß-Kotzsucht *f*, Eß-Brechsucht *f*.
hy·per·or·tho·cy·to·sis [ˌ-ˌɔːrθəsaɪ'təʊsɪs] *n hema.* Hyperleukozytose *f* ohne Linksverschiebung.
hy·per·os·mia [ˌ-'ɑzmɪə] *n neuro.* pathologisch gesteigertes Geruchsvermögen *nt*, olfaktorische Hyperästhesie *f*, Hyperosmie *f*.
hy·per·os·mo·lal·i·ty [ˌ-ɑzmə'læləti] *n* Hyperosmolalität *f*.
hy·per·os·mo·lar [ˌ-az'məʊlər] *adj* hyperosmolar.
hy·per·os·mo·lar·i·ty [ˌ-ɑzmə'leərəti] *n* Hyperosmolarität *f*.
hyperosmolar nonketotic coma hyperosmolares Koma *nt*.
hy·per·os·mot·ic [ˌ-ɑz'mɑtɪk] *adj* hyperosmotisch.
hyperosmotic thirst hyperosmotischer Durst *m*.
hy·per·os·phre·sia [ˌ-ɑz'friːʒ(ɪ)ə] *n* → hyperosmia.
hy·per·os·phre·sis [ˌ-zs'friːsɪs] *n* → hyperosmia.
hy·per·os·te·og·e·ny [ˌ-ɑstɪ'ɑdʒəni] *n* übermäßige/überschießende Knochenentwicklung/Knochenbildung *f*.
hy·per·os·to·sis [ˌ-ɑs'təʊsɪs] *n* **1.** Knochenhypertrophie *f*, -hyperplasie *f*, Hyperostose *f*, Exostosis *f*. **2.** *ortho., patho.* Exostose *f*, Exostosis *f*.
hy·per·os·tot·ic [ˌ-ɑs'tɑtɪk] *adj* Hyperostose betr., hyperostotisch.
hy·per·o·var·ia [ˌ-əʊ'veərɪə] *n* → hyperovarianism.

hy·per·o·var·i·an·ism [ˌ-əʊ'veərɪənɪzəm] *n gyn., ped.* Pseudopubertas praecox durch vorzeitige Ovarialfunktion.
hy·per·o·va·rism [ˌ-'əʊvərɪzəm] *n* → hyperovarianism.
hy·per·ox·al·e·mia [ˌ-ɑksə'liːmɪə] *n* erhöhter Oxalsäuregehalt *m* des Blutes, Hyperoxalämie *f*.
hy·per·ox·al·u·ria [ˌ-ˌɑksə'l(j)ʊərɪə] *n* erhöhte Oxalsäureausscheidung *f* im Harn, Hyperoxalurie *f*, Oxalurie *f*.
hy·per·ox·e·mia [ˌ-ɑk'siːmɪə] *n* erhöhter Säuregehalt *m* des Blutes, Hyperoxämie *f*.
hy·per·ox·ia [ˌ-'ɑksɪə] *n* **1.** erhöhter Sauerstoffgehalt *m* im Gewebe, Hyperoxie *f*. **2.** erhöhte Sauerstoffspannung *f*, Hyperoxie *f*.
hy·per·ox·ic [ˌ-'ɑksɪk] *adj* Hyperoxie betr., hyperoxisch.
hy·per·ox·i·da·tion [ˌ-ˌɑksɪ'deɪʃn] *n chem.* Hyperoxidation *f*.
hy·per·ox·ide [ˌ-'ɑksaɪd] *n* Hyperoxid *nt*, Superoxid *nt*, Peroxid *nt*.
hy·per·pal·les·the·sia [ˌ-ˌpælɪs'θiːʒə] *n* pathologisch erhöhte Vibrationsempfindlichkeit *f*, Hyperpallästhesie *f*.
hy·per·pan·cre·a·tism [ˌ-'pæŋkrɪətɪzəm] *n patho.* übermäßige Pankreasaktivität *f*, Hyperpankreatismus *m*.
hy·per·pan·cre·or·rhea [ˌ-ˌpæŋkrɪə'rɪə] *n* übermäßige Pankreassekretion *f*.
hy·per·par·a·site [ˌ-'pærəsaɪt] *n micro.* Über-, Sekundär-, Hyperparasit *m*.
hy·per·par·a·sit·ic [ˌ-ˌpærə'sɪtɪk] *adj micro.* hyperparasitisch.
hy·per·par·a·thy·roid crisis [ˌ-ˌpærə'θaɪrɔɪd] → hypercalcemic crisis.
hy·per·par·a·thy·roid·ism [ˌ-ˌpærə'θaɪrɔɪdɪzəm] *n* Nebenschilddrüsenüberfunktion *f*, Hyperparathyreoidismus *m abbr.* HPT, Hyperparathyroidismus *m*, Hyperparathyreose *f*.
hy·per·pa·rot·i·dism [ˌ-pə'rɑtədɪzəm] *n* erhöhte Aktivität *f* der Gl. parotidia.
hy·per·path·ia [ˌ-'pæθɪə] *n neuro.* Hyperpathie *f*.
hy·per·pep·sia [ˌ-'pepsɪə, -ʃə] *n* **1.** pathologisch gesteigerte Verdauung *f*, Hyperpepsie *f*. **2.** Verdauungsstörung *f* bei Hyperchlorhydrie, Hyperpepsie *f*.
hy·per·pep·sin·e·mia [ˌ-ˌpepsɪ'niːmɪə] *n* pathologisch erhöhter Pepsingehalt *m* des Blutes, Hyperpepsinämie *f*.
hy·per·pep·sin·ia [ˌ-'pep'sɪnɪə] *n* übermäßige Pepsinsekretion *f*, Hyperpepsinie *f*.
hy·per·pep·sin·u·ria [ˌ-ˌpepsɪ'n(j)ʊərɪə] *n* pathologisch erhöhte Pepsinausscheidung *f* im Harn, Hyperpepsinurie *f*.
hy·per·per·i·stal·sis [ˌ-ˌperɪ'stɔːlsɪs, -stæl-] *n* übermäßige Peristaltik *f*, Hyperperistaltik *f*.
hy·per·per·me·a·bil·i·ty [ˌ-ˌpɜrmɪə'bɪləti] *n* übermäßige Durchlässigkeit *f*, Hyperpermeabilität *f*.
hy·per·pha·gia [ˌ-'feɪdʒ(ɪ)ə] *n* Eß-, Freßsucht *f*, Gefräßigkeit *f*, Hyperphagie *f*, Polyphagie *f*.
hy·per·pha·lan·gia [ˌ-fə'lændʒ(ɪ)ə, -feɪ-] *n embryo.* überzählige Phalangen *pl*, Hyperphalangie *f*, Polyphalangie *f*.
hy·per·pha·lan·gism [ˌ-fə'lændʒɪzəm] *n* → hyperphalangia.
hy·per·phen·yl·al·a·nin·e·mia [ˌ-ˌfenlˌælə'niːmɪə] *n* erhöhter Phenylalaningehalt *m* des Blutes, Hyperphenylalaninämie *f*, Phenylalaninämie *f*.
type I h. Fölling-Krankheit *f*, Morbus Fölling *m*, Phenylketonurie *f abbr.* PKU, Brenztraubensäureschwachsinn *m*, Oligophrenia phenylpyruvica.
type II h. Hyperphenylalaninämie Typ II, persistierende Hyperphenylalaninämie.

type III h. Hyperphenylalaninämie Typ III, transitorische Hyperphenylalaninämie.
type IV h. Hyperphenylalaninämie Typ IV, maligne Hyperphenylalaninämie, Dihydropteridinreduktasemangel *m*, DHPR-Mangel *m*.
type V h. Hyperphenylalaninämie Typ V, atypische Phenylketonurie *f*, Dihydrobiopterinreduktasemangel *m*.
type VI h. Hyperphenylalaninämie Typ VI, persistierende Hyperphenylalaninämie mit Tyrosinämie.
type VII h. transitorische Tyrosinämie *f* des Neugeborenen.
type VIII h. hereditäre/hepatorenale Tyrosinämie *f*, Tyrosinose *f*.
hy·per·pho·ria [ˌ-'fɔːrɪə] *n ophthal.* latentes Höhenschielen *nt*, Hyperphorie *f*.
hy·per·phos·pha·ta·se·mia [ˌ-ˌfɑsfəteɪ'siːmɪə] *n* pathologische Erhöhung *f* der alkalischen Phosphatase im Blut, Hyperphosphatasämie *f*, Hyperphosphatasemia *f*.
hy·per·phos·pha·ta·sia [ˌ-ˌfɑsfə'teɪzɪə] *n* → hyperphosphatasemia.
hy·per·phos·pha·te·mia [ˌ-ˌfɑsfə'tiːmɪə] *n* Vermehrung *f* des anorganischen Phosphats im Blut, Hyperphosphatämie *f*.
hy·per·phos·pha·tu·ria [ˌ-ˌfɑsfə't(j)ʊərɪə] *n* erhöhte Phosphatausscheidung *f* im Harn, Hyperphosphaturie *f*.
hy·per·phos·pho·re·mia [ˌ-ˌfɑsfə'riːmɪə] *n* erhöhter Gehalt *m* an Phosphorverbindungen im Blut, Hyperphosphorämie *f*.
hy·per·phre·nia [ˌ-'friːnɪə] *n* **1.** pathologisch gesteigerte geistige Aktivität *f*, Hyperphrenie *f*. **2.** überdurchschnittlich hohe Intelligenz *f*.
hy·per·pi·e·sia [ˌ-paɪ'iːzɪə] *n* → hyperpiesis.
hy·per·pi·e·sis [ˌ-paɪ'iːsɪs] *n* essentielle/idiopathische/primäre Hypertonie *f*.
hy·per·pig·men·ta·tion [ˌ-ˌpɪgmən'teɪʃn] *n* vermehrte Pigmentierung *f*, Hyperpigmentierung *f*.
hy·per·pin·e·al·ism [ˌ-'pɪnɪəlɪzəm] *n* gesteigerte Funktion *f* der Epiphyse, Hyperpinealismus *m*.
hy·per·pi·tu·i·tar·ism [ˌ-pɪ't(j)uːətərɪzəm] *n* Hypophysenüberfunktion *f*, Hyperpituitarismus *m*.
hy·per·pi·tu·i·tar·y gigantism [ˌ-pɪ't(j)uːəˌteriː] *n* hypophysärer Riesenwuchs *m*.
hy·per·pla·sia [ˌ-'pleɪʒ(ɪ)ə, -zɪə] *n* Hyperplasie *f*, -plasia *f*, numerische Hypertrophie *f*.
hy·per·plas·mia [ˌ-'plæzmɪə] *n* **1.** vermehrtes Blutplasmavolumen *nt*, Hyperplasmie *f*. **2.** *hema.* Erythrozytenschwellung *f*, -vergrößerung *f*.
hy·per·plas·tic [ˌ-'plæstɪk] *adj* Hyperplasie betr., von ihr gekennzeichnet, hyperplastisch.
hyperplastic arteriolar nephrosclerosis maligne Nephrosklerose *f*.
hyperplastic arteriosclerosis hyperplastische Arteriosklerose *f*.
hyperplastic chondrodystrophy hyperplastische Chondrodystrophie *f*.
hyperplastic gingivitis hyperplastische/hypertrophische Gingivitis *f*, Gingivitis hyperplastica/hypertrophicans.
hyperplastic inflammation proliferative/produktive Entzündung *f*.
hyperplastic osteoarthritis → hypertrophic pulmonary osteoarthropathy.
hyperplastic periostosis Caffey-de Toni-Syndrom *nt*, Caffey-Silverman-Syndrom *nt*, Caffey-Smith-Syndrom *nt*, Hyperostosis corticalis infantilis.
hyperplastic polyp hyperplastischer Polyp *m*.

hyperplastic pulmonary osteoarthritis → hypertrophic pulmonary osteoarthropathy.

hyperplastic rhinitis chronisch-hyperplastische Rhinitis/Rhinopathie *f*, Rhinitis hyperplastica/hypertrophicans, Rhinopathia chronica hyperplastica.

hyperplastic tissue hyperplastisches Gewebe *nt*.

hy·per·ploid ['-plɔɪd] *genet*. **I** *n* hyperploide Zelle *f*, hyperploider Organismus *m*. **II** *adj* hyperploid.

hy·per·ploi·dy [‚-'plɔɪdɪ] *n genet*. Hyperploidie *f*.

hy·perp·nea [‚haɪpərp'nɪə, ‚haɪpər'nɪə] *n* vertiefte Atmung *f*, Hyperpnoe *f*.

hy·per·pne·ic [‚haɪpər'niːɪk] *adj* Hyperpnoe betr., hyperpno(e)isch.

hy·per·po·lar·i·za·tion [‚-‚pəʊləraɪ'zeɪʃn] *n* Hyperpolarisation *f*.

hy·per·po·lar·iz·ing afterpotential [‚-'pəʊləraɪzɪŋ] hyperpolarisierendes Nachpotential *nt*.

hy·per·pol·y·pep·ti·de·mia [‚-‚palɪ‚peptɪ'diːmɪə] *n* erhöhter Polypeptidgehalt *m* des Blutes, Hyperpolypeptidämie *f*.

hy·per·pot·as·se·mia [‚-‚pɑtə'siːmɪə] *n* → hyperkalemia.

hy·per·pra·gia [‚-'preɪdʒɪə] *n psychia*. übersteigerte geistige Aktivität *f*.

hy·per·prax·ia [‚-'præksɪə] *n neuro*. übersteigerte Aktivität *f*, Hyperpraxie *f*.

hy·per·pre·be·ta·lip·o·pro·tein·e·mia [‚-‚priː‚beɪtə‚lɪpəprəʊtɪ'niːmɪə] *n* Erhöhung *f* der Präbetalipoproteine im Blut, Hyperpräbetalipoproteinämie *f*.

hy·per·pres·by·o·pia [‚-‚prezbɪ'əʊpɪə] *n ophthal*. übermäßige Presbyopie *f*, Hyperpresbyopie *f*.

hy·per·pro·cho·re·sis [‚-‚prəʊkə'riːsɪs] *n* → hyperperistalsis.

hy·per·pro·lac·tin·e·mia [‚-‚prəʊ‚læktɪ'niːmɪə] *n* erhöhter Prolaktingehalt *m* des Blutes, Hyperprolaktinämie *f*, -prolactinämie *f*.

hy·per·pro·lac·tin·e·mic amenorrhea [‚-‚prəʊ‚læktɪ'niːmɪk] *gyn*. hyperprolaktinämische Amenorrhoe *f*.

hy·per·pro·li·ne·mia [‚-‚prəʊlɪ'niːmɪə] *n* erhöhter Prolingehalt *m* des Blutes, Hyperprolinämie *f*.
  type I h. Hyperprolinämie Typ I, Prolinoxidasemangel *m*.
  type II h. Hyperprolinämie Typ II, Pyrrolin-5-carboxylat-Dehydrogenasemangel *m*.

hy·per·pro·sex·ia [‚-‚prəʊ'seksɪə] *n psychia*. pathologisch gesteigerte Aufmerksamkeit *f*, Hyperprosexie *f*.

hy·per·pro·tein·e·mia [‚-‚prəʊtɪ'niːmɪə] *n* Erhöhung *f* der Plasmaproteine, Hyperproteinämie *f*.

hy·per·pro·te·o·sis [‚-‚prəʊtɪ'əʊsɪs] *n* Erkrankung *f* durch übermäßige Proteinzufuhr.

hy·perp·sel·a·phe·sia [‚haɪpərp‚selə'fiːzɪə] *n neuro*. taktile Hyperästhesie *f*, Hyperpselaphesie *f*.

hy·per·pty·a·lism [‚haɪpər'taɪəlɪzəm] *n* Speichelfluß *m*, pathologisch gesteigerte Speichelabsonderung *f*, Ptyalismus *m*, Sialorrhoe *f*, Hypersalivation *f*, Salivatio *f*.

hy·per·py·ret·ic [‚-paɪ'retɪk] *adj* Hyperpyrexie betr. *od*. verursachend, hyperpyretisch, Hyperpyrexie-.

hy·per·py·rex·ia [‚-paɪ'reksɪə] *n* hohes Fieber *nt*, Hyperpyrexie *f*.
  h. of anesthesia maligne Hyperpyrexie/Hyperthermie *f*.

hy·per·py·rex·i·al [‚-paɪ'reksɪəl] *adj* → hyperpyretic.

hy·per·re·ac·tive [‚-rɪ'æktɪv] *adj* übermäßig stark reagierend, hyperreaktiv.

hy·per·re·flex·ia [‚-rɪ'fleksɪə] *n neuro*. Reflexsteigerung *f*, Hyperreflexie *f*.

hy·per·re·nin·e·mia [‚-‚riːnɪn'iːmɪə] *n* erhöhter Reningehalt *m* des Blutes, Hyperreninismus *m*, Hyperreninämie *f*.

hy·per·res·o·nance [‚-'rezənən(t)s] *n* **1.** Hyperresonanz *f*. **2.** (*Perkussion*) hypersonorer Klopfschall *m*.

hy·per·sal·e·mia [‚-‚sæl'iːmɪə] *n* erhöhter Salzgehalt *m* des Blutes, Hypersal(i)ämie *f*, Hypersalie *f*.

hy·per·sa·line [‚-'seɪlaɪn] *adj* übermäßig salzhaltig, hypersalin.

hy·per·sal·i·va·tion [‚-‚sælɪ'veɪʃn] *n* → hyperptyalism.

hy·per·sar·co·sin·e·mia [‚-‚sɑːrkəsɪ'niːmɪə] *n* erhöhter Sarkosingehalt *m* des Blutes, Hypersarkosinämie *f*, Sarkosinämie *f*.

hy·per·se·cre·tion [‚-sɪ'kriːʃn] *n* übermäßige Absonderung/Sekretion *f*, Hypersekretion *f*, Supersekretion *f*.

hy·per·seg·men·ta·tion [‚-‚segmən'teɪʃn] *n* Hypersegmentierung *f*.

hy·per·sen·si·bil·i·ty [‚-‚sensə'bɪlətɪ] *n* **1.** → hyperesthesia. **2.** Reizüberempfindlichkeit *f*, Hypersensibilität *f*.

hy·per·sen·si·tive [‚-'sensətɪv] *adj* **1.** überempfindlich, hypersensibel. **2.** *immun*. überempfindlich, allergisch (*to* gegen).

hy·per·sen·si·tive·ness [‚-'sensətɪvnɪs] *n* → hypersensitivity.

hy·per·sen·si·tiv·i·ty [‚-‚sensə'tɪvətɪ] *n* **1.** Reizüberempfindlichkeit *f*, Hypersensitivität *f*, -sensitation *f*, -sensibilität *f*. **2.** *immun*. Überempfindlichkeit *f*, Allergie *f*.
  type I h. anaphylaktische Überempfindlichkeit/Allergie, anaphylaktischer Typ *m* der Überempfindlichkeitsreaktion, Überempfindlichkeitsreaktion *f* vom Soforttyp, Typ I der Überempfindlichkeitsreaktion.
  type II h. Überempfindlichkeitsreaktion *f* vom zytotoxischen Typ, Typ II der Überempfindlichkeitsreaktion.
  type III h. Immunkomplex-vermittelte Überempfindlichkeitsreaktion *f*, Arthus-Typ *m* der Überempfindlichkeitsreaktion, Typ III der Überempfindlichkeitsreaktion.
  type IV h. T-zellvermittelte Überempfindlichkeitsreaktion *f*, Tuberkulin-Typ/Spät-Typ/Typ IV der Überempfindlichkeitsreaktion.

hypersensitivity pneumonitis exogen allergische Alveolitis *f*, Hypersensitivitätspneumonitis *f*.

hypersensitivity reaction Überempfindlichkeitsreaktion *f*.
  delayed h. T-zellvermittelte Überempfindlichkeitsreaktion *f*, Tuberkulin-Typ/Spät-Typ/Typ IV der Überempfindlichkeitsreaktion.
  immediate h. anaphylaktische Überempfindlichkeit/Allergie, anaphylaktischer Typ *m* der Überempfindlichkeitsreaktion, Überempfindlichkeitsreaktion *f* vom Soforttyp, Typ I der Überempfindlichkeitsreaktion.

hypersensitivity vasculitis Immunkomplexvaskulitis *f*, leukozytoklastische Vaskulitis *f*, Vasculitis allergica, Arteriitis allergica cutis.

hy·per·sen·si·ti·za·tion [‚-‚sensətɪ'zeɪʃn] *immun*. Erzeugung *f* einer Überempfindlichkeit(sreaktion), Allergisierung *f*.

hy·per·sen·si·tize [‚-'sensɪtaɪz] *vt* eine Überempfindlichkeit hervorrufen, allergisieren.

hy·per·ser·o·to·ne·mia [‚-‚sɪərətəʊ'niːmɪə, -‚serə-] *n* erhöhter Serotoningehalt *m* des Blutes, Hyperseroton(in)ämie *f*, Hyperserotoni(ni)smus *m*.

hy·per·sex·u·al·i·ty [‚-‚seksʃə'wælətɪ] *n psychia*. übermäßiges sexuelles Verlangen *nt*, Hypersexualität *f*.

hy·per·ske·o·cy·to·sis [‚-‚skɪəsaɪ'təʊsɪs] *n* → hyperneocytosis.

hy·per·so·ma·to·trop·ism [‚-‚səʊmətə'trəʊpɪzəm] *n* erhöhter Somatotropingehalt *m* des Blutes, Hypersomatotropismus *m*.

hy·per·so·mia [‚-'səʊmɪə] *n* Riesenwuchs *m*, Hypersomie *f*, Gigantismus *m*.

hy·per·so·mic [‚-'səʊmɪk] *adj* Hypersomie betr., an Hypersomie leidend, riesenwüchsig, hypersom.

hy·per·som·nia [‚haɪpər'sɑmnɪə] *n neuro*., *psychia*. Schlafsucht *f*, Hypersomnie *f*.

hypersomnia-bulimia syndrome Kleine-Levin-Syndrom *nt*.

hy·per·son·ic [‚-'sɑnɪk] *adj* Hyperschall betr., hypersonisch, Hyperschall-, Überschall-.

hy·per·sper·mia [‚-'spɜrmɪə] *n* Hyper(zoo)spermie *f*.

hy·per·sper·mic [‚-'spɜrmɪk] *adj* Hyper(zoo)spermie betr., hyper(zoo)sperm.

hy·per·sple·nia [‚-'spliːnɪə] *n* → hypersplenism.

hy·per·sple·nic neutropenia [‚-'spliːnɪk] Hypersplenie-bedingte Neutropenie *f*.

hypersplenic pancytopenia Hypersplenie-bedingte Panzytopenie *f*.

hy·per·sple·nism [‚-'spliːnɪzəm] *n* Milzüberfunktion *f*, Hypersplenie *f*, Hyperspleniesyndrom *nt*, Hyperplenismus *m*.

hy·per·ste·a·to·sis [‚-stɪə'təʊsɪs] *n derm*. vermehrte Talgabsonderung *f* der Haut, Hypersteatose *f*.

hy·per·ster·e·o·roent·gen·og·ra·phy [‚-‚sterɪərəntɡə'nɑɡrəfɪ, -‚stɪərɪə-] *n radiol*. Hyperröntgenstereographie *f*.

hy·per·ster·e·o·ski·ag·ra·phy [‚-‚sterɪə‚skaɪ'æɡrəfɪ, -‚stɪərɪə-] *n* → hyperstereoroentgenography.

hy·per·sthen·u·ria [‚-sθɪn(j)ʊərɪə] *n* Ausscheidung *f* eines hochgestellten Harns, Hypersthenurie *f*.

hy·per·su·pra·re·nal·ism [‚-‚suːprə'riːnəlɪzəm] *n* → hyperadrenalism.

hy·per·sus·cep·ti·bil·i·ty [‚-sə‚septə'bɪlətɪ] *n* Überempfindlichkeit *f*.

hy·per·sym·path·i·co·to·nus [‚-‚sɪm‚pæθɪkəʊ'təʊnəs] *n* erhöhter Sympathikotonus *m*, Hypersympathikotonus *m*, Hypersympathikotonie *f*.

hy·per·sys·to·le [‚-'sɪstəlɪ] *n card*. Hypersystole *f*.

hy·per·sys·tol·ic [‚-sɪs'tɑlɪk] *adj* Hypersystole betr., hypersystolisch.

hy·per·ta·rach·ia [‚-tə'rækɪə] *n* extreme Reizempfindlichkeit *f* des Nervensystems.

hy·per·te·lia [‚-'tiːlɪə] *n* → hypertely.

hy·per·tel·or·ism [‚-'telərɪzəm] *n* **1.** Hypertelorismus *m*. **2.** Greig-Syndrom *nt*, okulärer Hypertelorismus *m*.

hypertelorism-hypospadias syndrome Hypertelorismus-Hypospadie-Syndrom *nt*, BBB-Syndrom *nt*.

hy·per·te·ly [‚-'tiːlɪ] *n embryo*. Überentwicklung *f*, Hypertelie *f*.

hy·per·ten·sin [‚-'tensɪn] *n old* → angiotensin.

hy·per·ten·sin·ase [‚-'tensɪneɪz] *n old* → angiotensinase.

hy·per·ten·sin·o·gen [‚-ten'sɪnədʒən] *n old* → angiotensinogen.

hy·per·ten·sion [‚-'tenʃn] *n* Bluthochdruck *m*, (arterielle) Hypertonie *f*, Hyperten-

hypertensive

sion f, Hypertonus m, Hochdruckkrankheit f.
hy·per·ten·sive [,-'tensɪv] **I** n Hochdruckpatient(in f) m, Hypertoniker(in f) m. **II** adj Hypertonie/Hypertension betr., hypertensiv.
hypertensive arteriopathy hypertensive Arteriopathie f.
hypertensive arteriosclerosis hypertensive Arteriosklerose f.
hypertensive cardiopathy hypertensive Kardiopathie f.
hypertensive encephalopathy Hypertensionsenzephalopathie f, Encephalopathia hypertensiva.
hypertensive ischemic ulcer ischämisches Ulkus nt, Infarktulkus nt, Ulcus hypertonicum.
hypertensive patient → hypertensive I.
hypertensive retinitis → hypertensive retinopathy.
hypertensive retinopathy Retinopathia hypertensiva (maligna).
hy·per·ten·sor [,-'tensər] n blutdrucksteigerndes Mittel nt.
hy·per·tes·toid·ism [,-'testɔɪdɪzəm] n männl. Hypergonadismus m.
hy·per·the·co·sis [,haɪpərθɪ'kəʊsɪs] n gyn. Thekazellenhyperplasie f, Hyperthekose f.
hy·per·the·lia [,-'θi:lɪə] n überzählige Brustwarzen pl, Hyperthelie f, Polythelie f.
hy·per·ther·mal [,-'θɜrml] adj hypertherm.
hy·per·ther·mal·ge·sia [,-,θɜrmæl'dʒi:zɪə, -dʒi:ʒə] n neuro. pathologisch erhöhte Wärmeempfindlichkeit f, Hyperthermalgesie f.
hy·per·ther·mes·the·sia [,-,θɜrmes'θi:-ʒ(ɪ)ə] n neuro. erhöhte Wärmeempfindlichkeit f, Hyperthermästhesie f.
hy·per·ther·mia [,-'θɜrmɪə] n Überwärmung f, -hitzung f, pathologische Erhöhung f der Körpertemperatur, Hyperthermie f.
h. of anesthesia maligne Hyperthermie/Hyperpyrexie f.
hy·per·ther·mo·es·the·sia [,-,θɜrməʊes-'θi:ʒ(ɪ)ə] n → hyperthermesthesia.
hy·per·ther·my [,-'θɜrmɪ] n → hyperthermia.
hy·per·throm·bin·e·mia [,-,θrɒmbɪ'ni:mɪə] n pathologisch erhöhter Thrombingehalt m des Blutes, Hyperthrombinämie f.
hy·per·thy·mia [,-'θaɪmɪə] n psychia. Hyperthymie f.
hy·per·thy·mic [,-'θaɪmɪk] adj 1. Hyperthymie betr., hyperthym. 2. Hyperthymismus betr.
hy·per·thy·mism [,-'θaɪmɪzəm] n Hyperthymismus m.
hy·per·thy·mi·za·tion [,-,θaɪmə'zeɪʃn] n → hyperthymism.
hy·per·thy·rea [,-'θaɪrɪə] n → hyperthyroidism.
hy·per·thy·re·o·sis [,-θaɪrɪ'əʊsɪs] n → hyperthyroidism.
hy·per·thy·roid [,-'θaɪrɔɪd] adj hyperthyreot.
hy·per·thy·roid·ism [,-'θaɪrɔɪdɪzəm] n Schilddrüsenüberfunktion f, Hyperthyreose f, Hyperthyreoidismus m, Hyperthyreoidie f.
hy·per·thy·roi·do·sis [,-θaɪrɔɪ'dəʊsɪs] n → hyperthyroidism.
hy·per·thy·rox·i·ne·mia [,-θaɪ,rɒksɪ'ni:-mɪə] n erhöhter Thyroxingehalt m des Blutes, Hyperthyroxinämie f.
hy·per·to·nia [,-'təʊnɪə] n erhöhte Spannung f, erhöhter Tonus m, Hypertonie f, Hypertonus m.
hy·per·ton·ic [,-'tɒnɪk] adj physiol. hypertonisch, hyperton.

hypertonic dehydratation hypertone Dehydratation f.
hypertonic hyperhydration hypertone Hyperhydratation f.
hy·per·to·nic·i·ty [,-təʊ'nɪsətɪ] n Hypertonie f.
hypertonic solution hypertone Lösung f.
hy·per·to·nus [,-'təʊnəs] n → hypertonia.
hy·per·tri·chi·a·sis [,-trɪ'kaɪəsɪs] n → hypertrichosis.
hy·per·tri·cho·sis [,-trɪ'kəʊsɪs] n derm. verstärkte Behaarung f, Hypertrichose f, Hypertrichie f, Hypertrichosis f.
hy·per·tri·glyc·er·id·e·mia [,-traɪ,ɡlɪsəraɪ-'di:mɪə] n erhöhter Triglyzeridgehalt m des Blutes, Hypertriglyzeridämie f, -triglyceridämie f.
hy·per·tro·phia [,-'trəʊfɪə] n → hypertrophy.
hy·per·troph·ic [,-'trɒfɪk, -'trəʊfɪk] adj Hypertrophie betr., hypertroph(isch).
hypertrophic angioma Hämangioendotheliom(a) nt.
hypertrophic arthritis degenerative Gelenkentzündung f, Osteo-, Gelenkarthrose f, Arthrosis deformans.
hypertrophic cardiomyopathy abbr. **HCM** hypertrophische Kardiomyopathie/Cardiomyopathie f abbr. HCM.
hypertrophic cirrhosis primär biliäre Zirrhose abbr. PBZ, nicht-eitrige destruierende Cholangitis f.
hypertrophic gastritis 1. hypertrophische Gastritis f. 2. Ménétrier-Syndrom nt, Morbus Ménétrier m, Riesenfaltengastritis f, Gastropathia hypertrophica gigantea.
hypertrophic nodular gliosis hypertrophisch-noduläre Gliose f.
hypertrophic non-obstructive cardiomyopathy abbr. **HNCM** hypertrophische nichtobstruktive Kardiomyopathie/Cardiomyopathie f abbr. HNCM.
hypertrophic obstructive cardiomyopathy abbr. **HOCM** hypertrophische obstruktive Kardiomyopathie/Cardiomyopathie f abbr. HOCM.
hypertrophic pharyngitis Pharyngitis hypertrophicans.
hypertrophic pneumonic osteoarthropathy → hypertrophic pulmonary osteoarthropathy.
hypertrophic pulmonary osteoarthropathy hypertrophische pulmonale Osteoarthropathie f, Marie-Bamberger-Syndrom nt, Bamberger-Marie-Syndrom nt, Akropachie f.
hypertrophic pyloristenosis/pylorostenosis hypertrophe Pylorusstenose f.
hypertrophic rhinitis → hyperplastic rhinitis.
hypertrophic scar hypertrophe Narbe f.
hypertrophic tonsillitis hypertrophische Tonsillitis f.
hy·per·tro·phy [haɪ'pɜrtrəfɪ] **I** n übermäßige Volumenzunahme f, Hypertrophie f. **II** vt hypertrophieren lassen, zu Hypertrophie führen. **III** vi hypertrophieren, sich (übermäßig) vergrößern.
hy·per·tro·pia [,haɪpər'trəʊpɪə] n ophthal. Höhenschielen nt, Hypertropie f, Strabismus verticalis.
hy·per·ty·ro·sin·e·mia [,-taɪrəsɪ'ni:mɪə] n (Hyper)Tyrosinämie f.
hy·per·u·re·sis [,-jə'ri:sɪs] n old → polyuria.
hy·per·u·ric·ac·id·e·mia [,-juərɪk,æsɪ'di:-mɪə] n → hyperuricemia.
hy·per·u·ric·ac·id·u·ria [,-juərɪk,æsɪ-'d(j)uərɪə] n → hyperuricuria.
hy·per·u·ri·ce·mia [,-juərɪ'si:mɪə] n erhöh-

ter Harnsäuregehalt m des Blutes, Hyperurikämie f, Hyperurikosämie f.
hy·per·u·ri·ce·mic [,-juərɪ'si:mɪk] adj Hyperurikämie betr., Hyperurikämie-.
hy·per·u·ri·cu·ria [,-juərɪ'k(j)uərɪə] n erhöhte Harnsäureausscheidung f, Hyperurikurie f, Hyperurikosurie f.
hy·per·vac·ci·na·tion [,-,væksə'neɪʃn] n immun. 1. Auffrischungsimpfung f, Hypervakzination f. 2. Hyperimmunisierung f, Hypervakzination f.
hy·per·val·i·ne·mia [,-vælɪ'ni:mɪə] n erhöhter Valingehalt m des Blutes, Hypervalinämie f, Valinämie f.
hy·per·var·i·a·ble region [,-'veərɪəbl] hypervariable Region f.
hy·per·vas·cu·lar [,-'væskjələr] adj stark vaskularisiert, hypervaskularisiert.
hy·per·vas·cu·lar·i·ty [,-,væskjə'lærətɪ] n übermäßiger Gefäßreichtum m, Hypervaskularisation f.
hy·per·ven·ti·la·tion [,-,ventɪ'leɪʃn] n Überventilation f, Hyperventilation f.
hyperventilation syndrome Hyperventilationssyndrom nt.
hyperventilation tetany Hyperventilationstetanie f.
hy·per·vis·cos·i·ty [,-vɪs'kɒsətɪ] n übermäßig hohe Viskosität f, Hyperviskosität f.
hyperviscosity syndrome Hyperviskositätssyndrom nt.
hy·per·vi·ta·min·o·sis [,-,vaɪtəmɪ'nəʊsɪs] n Hypervitaminose f.
hy·per·vo·le·mia [,-vəʊ'li:mɪə] n vermehrtes Plasmavolumen nt, Hypervolämie f.
hy·per·vo·le·mic [,-vəʊ'li:mɪk] adj Hypervolämie betr., hypervolämisch.
hyp·es·the·sia [haɪpes'θi:ʒ(ɪ)ə] n → hypoesthesia.
hy·pha ['haɪfə] n, pl **-phae** [-faɪ, -fi:] micro. Pilzfaden m, Hyphe f.
hy·phal ['haɪfl] adj micro. Hyphe(n) betr., Hyphen-.
hyphal fungi → Hyphomycetes.
hyp·he·do·nia [haɪfə'dəʊnɪə] n psychia. Hyphedonie f.
hy·phe·ma [haɪ'fi:mə] n ophthal. Bluterguß m in die vordere Augenkammer, Hyphäma nt, Hyphaema nt.
hy·phe·mia [haɪ'fi:mɪə] n 1. → hyphema. 2. old → oligemia.
hyp·hi·dro·sis [,haɪphɪ'drəʊsɪs, -haɪ-] n → hypohidrosis.
hy·pho·my·cete [,haɪfəʊ'maɪsi:t] n micro. Fadenpilz m, Hyphomyzet m.
Hy·pho·my·ce·tes [,-maɪ'si:ti:z] pl micro. Fadenpilze pl, Hyphomyzeten pl, Hyphomycetes pl.
hy·pho·my·ce·tic [,-maɪ'si:tɪk] adj Hyphomyzeten betr., durch sie verursacht, Fadenpilz-, Hyphomyzeten-.
hyp·i·so·ton·ic [,hɪp,aɪsə'tɒnɪk, -,ɪsə-] adj → hypotonic.
hypn- pref. → hypno-.
hyp·na·gog·ic [hɪpnə'ɡɒdʒɪk] adj 1. schlaferzeugend, einschläfernd, hypnagog. 2. beim Einschlafen od. im Halbschlaf auftretend, hypnagog.
hypnagogic hallucination psychia. hypnagoge Halluzination f.
hyp·na·gogue ['hɪpnəɡɒɡ, -ɡæɡ] **I** n Schlafmittel nt, Hypnagogum nt, Hypnotikum nt, Hypnoticum nt. **II** adj schlaferzeugend, einschläfernd, hypnagog.
hyp·nal·gia [hɪp'nældʒ(ɪ)ə] n Schlafschmerz m, Hypnalgie f.
hyp·nic ['hɪpnɪk] adj Schlaf betr., Schlaf erzeugend, Schlaf-, Hypno-.
hypno- pref. Schlaf-, Hypno-, Hypnose-.
hyp·no·a·nal·y·sis [,hɪpnəʊə'næləsɪs] n psychia. Psychoanalyse f unter Anwendung von Hypnose, Hypnoanalyse f.

hyp·no·an·es·the·sia [ˌ-ˌænəsˈθiːʒə] *n anes.* Hypnonarkose *f*, -anästhesie *f*.
hyp·no·ca·thar·sis [ˌ-kəˈθɑːrsɪs] *n psychia.* Hypnokatharsis *f*.
hyp·no·cin·e·mat·o·graph [ˌ-sɪnəˈmætəɡræf] *n* Hypno-, Somnokinematograph *m*.
hyp·no·cyst [ˈ-sɪst] *n micro.* Ruhezyste *f*.
hyp·no·gen·e·sis [ˌ-ˈdʒenəsɪs] *n* Herbeiführen *nt* von Schlaf *od.* Hypnose, Hypnogenese *f*.
hyp·no·ge·net·ic [ˌ-dʒəˈnetɪk] *adj* → hypnogenic.
hyp·no·gen·ic [ˌ-ˈdʒenɪk] *adj* schlaf-, hypnoseerzeugend, hypnogen.
hyp·nog·e·nous [hɪpˈnɑdʒənəs] *adj* → hypnogenic.
hyp·noid [ˈhɪpnɔɪd] *adj* hypnoseähnlich, schlafähnlich, hypnoid.
hyp·noi·dal [hɪpˈnɔɪdl] *adj* → hypnoid.
hyp·no·lep·sy [ˈhɪpnəlepsɪ] *n neuro.* Narkolepsie *f*.
hyp·nol·o·gist [hɪpˈnɑlədʒɪst] *n* → hypnotist.
hyp·no·po·dia [ˌhɪpnəˈpəʊdɪə] *n* Lernen *nt* im Schlaf, Hypnopädie *f*.
hyp·no·pho·bia [ˌ-ˈfəʊbɪə] *n psychia.* krankhafte Angst *f* vor dem Einschlafen, Hypnophobie *f*.
hyp·no·pom·pic [ˌ-ˈpɑmpɪk] *adj* im Halbschlaf *od.* während der Aufwachphase auftretend, hypnopomp.
hypnopompic hallucination *psychia.* hypnopompe Halluzination *f*.
hyp·no·sis [hɪpˈnəʊsɪs] *n, pl* **-ses** [-siːz] Hypnose *f*.
hypnosis anesthesia → hypnoanesthesia.
hyp·no·ther·a·py [ˌhɪpnəˈθerəpɪ] *n* 1. Schlaftherapie *f*, Hypnotherapie *f*. 2. *psychia.* Behandlung *f* durch/unter Hypnose, Hypnotherapie *f*.
hyp·not·ic [hɪpˈnɑtɪk] **I** *n* 1. Schlafmittel *nt*, Hypnagogum *nt*, Hypnotikum *nt*, Hypnoticum *nt*. 2. hypnotisierte Person *f*. **II** *adj* 3. schlaferzeugend, einschläfernd, hypnagog. 4. Hypnose betr., hypnotisch, Hypnose-.
hyp·no·tism [ˈhɪpnətɪzəm] *n* 1. Hypnotismus *m*. 2. → hypnosis.
hyp·no·tist [ˈhɪpnətɪst] *n* Hypnotiseur *m*.
hyp·no·ti·za·tion [ˌhɪpnətɪˈzeɪʃn] *n* Hypnotisieren *nt*.
hyp·no·tize [ˈhɪpnətaɪz] *vt* hypnotisieren, in Hypnose versetzen.
hyp·no·tiz·er [ˈhɪpnətaɪzər] *n* → hypnotist.
hyp·no·toid [ˈhɪpnətɔɪd] *adj* hypnoseähnlich, hypnotoid.
hyp·no·zo·ite [ˌhɪpnəˈzəʊaɪt] *n micro.* Hypnozoit *m*.
hypo- *pref.* Unter-, Hyp(o)-.
hy·po [ˈhaɪpəʊ] *n inf.* 1. → hypodermic inoculation. 2. → hypodermic syringe.
hy·po·a·cid·i·ty [ˌhaɪpəʊəˈsɪdətɪ] *n* Säuremangel *m*, Hyp(o)azidität *f*, Subazidität *f*.
hy·po·ac·tive [ˌ-ˈæktɪv] *adj* Hypoaktivität betr. *od.* zeigend, hypoaktiv.
hy·po·ac·tiv·i·ty [ˌ-ækˈtɪvətɪ] *n* verminderte Aktivität *f*, Hypoaktivität *f*.
hy·po·a·cu·sis [ˌ-əˈk(j)uːsɪs] *n HNO* Hörschwäche *f*, Hyp(o)akusis *f*.
hy·po·a·dre·nal·ism [ˌ-əˈdriːnəlɪzəm] *n* 1. Nebenniereninsuffizienz *f*, Hyp(o)adrenalismus *m*. 2. → hypoadrenocorticism.
hy·po·a·dre·no·cor·ti·cism [ˌ-əˈdriːnəʊˌkɔːrtɪsɪzəm] *n* Nebennierenrindeninsuffizienz *f*, NNR-Insuffizienz *f*, Hypoadrenokortizismus *m*, Hypokortikalismus *m*, Hypokortizismus *m*.
hy·po·al·bu·min·e·mia [ˌ-ælˌbjuːmɪˈniːmɪə] *n* verminderter Albumingehalt *m* des Blutes, Hyp(o)albuminämie *f*.

hy·po·al·bu·mi·no·sis [ˌ-ælˌbjuːmɪˈnəʊsɪs] *n* Hyp(o)albuminose *f*.
hy·po·al·do·ste·ro·ne·mia [ˌ-ˌældəʊˌstɪərəˈniːmɪə] *n* verminderter Aldosterongehalt *m* des Blutes, Hypoaldosteronämie *f*.
hy·po·al·do·ste·ro·nism [ˌ-ˌældəʊˈsterənɪzəm] *n* Aldosteronmangel *m*, Hypoaldosteronismus *m*.
hy·po·al·do·ste·ro·nu·ria [ˌ-ˌældəʊˌstɪərəˈn(j)ʊərɪə] *n* verminderte Aldosteronausscheidung *f* im Harn, Hypoaldosteronurie *f*.
hy·po·al·ge·sia [ˌ-ælˈdʒiːzɪə, -dʒɪˈʒə] *n* verminderte Schmerzempfindung *f*, Hypalgesie *f*, Hypalgie *f*.
hy·po·al·i·men·ta·tion [ˌ-ˌælɪmenˈteɪʃn] *n* Unterernährung *f*, Hyp(o)alimentation *f*.
hy·po·al·ka·line [ˌ-ˈælkəlaɪn, -lɪn] *adj* Hypoalkalität betr. *od.* zeigend, hyp(o)alkalisch.
hy·po·al·ka·lin·i·ty [ˌ-ˌælkəˈlɪnətɪ] *n* verminderte Alkalität *f*, Hyp(o)alkalität *f*.
hy·po·am·i·no·ac·i·de·mia [ˌ-əˌmiːnəʊˌæsɪˈdiːmɪə] *n* verminderter Aminosäuregehalt *m* des Blutes, Hypoaminoazidämie *f*.
hy·po·an·dro·gen·ism [ˌ-ˈændrədʒenɪzəm] *n* Hyp(o)androgenismus *m*.
hy·po·az·o·tu·ria [ˌ-æzəˈt(j)ʊərɪə] *n* verminderte Stickstoffausscheidung *f* im Harn, Hypazoturie *f*.
hy·po·bar·ia [ˌ-ˈbeərɪə] *n* → hypobarism.
hy·po·bar·ic [ˌ-ˈbærɪk] *adj* 1. hypobar, Unterdruck-. 2. *(Flüssigkeit)* von geringerer Dichte, hypobar.
hy·po·bar·ism [ˌ-ˈbærɪzəm] *n* Hypobarismus *m*.
hy·po·ba·rop·a·thy [ˌ-bəˈrɑpəθɪ] *n* Erkrankung *f* durch Unterdruck, Hypobaropathie *f*.
hy·po·be·ta·lip·o·pro·tein·e·mia [ˌ-ˌbeɪtəˌlɪpəprəʊtɪːnˈiːmɪə] *n* verminderter Betalipoproteingehalt *m* des Blutes, Hypobetalipoproteinämie *f*.
hy·po·bil·i·ru·bi·ne·mia [ˌ-ˌbɪləˌruːbɪˈniːmɪə] *n* verminderter Bilirubingehalt *m* des Blutes, Hypobilirubinämie *f*.
hy·po·blast [ˈ-blæst] *n embryo.* inneres Keimblatt *nt*, Entoderm *nt*.
hy·po·blas·tic [ˌ-ˈblæstɪk] *adj* Entoderm betr., vom Entoderm abstammend, entodermal.
hy·po·bran·chi·al eminence [ˌ-ˈbræŋkɪəl] *embryo.* Hypobranchialhöcker *m*, Copula *f* (linguae).
hy·po·bro·mite [ˌ-ˈbrəʊmaɪt] *n* Hypobromit *nt*.
hy·po·bro·mous acid [ˌ-ˈbrəʊməs] unterbromige Säure *f*.
hy·po·cal·ce·mia [ˌ-kælˈsiːmɪə] *n* verminderter Kalziumgehalt *m* des Blutes, Hypokalz(i)ämie *f*.
hy·po·cal·ce·mic tetany [ˌ-kælˈsiːmɪk] hypokalz(i)ämische Tetanie *f*.
hy·po·cal·cia [ˌ-ˈkælsɪə] *n* Kalziummangel *m*, Hypokalzie *f*.
hy·po·cal·ci·fi·ca·tion [ˌ-ˌkælsəfɪˈkeɪʃn] *n* verminderte/mangelhafte Kalzifizierung *f*, Hypokalzifizierung *f*, Hypokalzifikation *f*.
hy·po·cal·ci·pex·y [ˌ-ˈkælsɪpeksɪ] *n* verminderte/mangelhafte Kalziumeinlagerung *f*, Hypokalzipexie *f*.
hy·po·cal·ci·u·ria [ˌ-ˌkælsɪˈ(j)ʊərɪə] *n* pathologisch verminderte Kalziumausscheidung *f* im Harn, Hypokalziurie *f*.
hy·po·cap·nia [ˌ-ˈkæpnɪə] *n* verminderte Kohlendioxidspannung *f* des Blutes, Hypokapnie *f*, Hypokarbie *f*.
hy·po·cap·nic [ˌ-ˈkæpnɪk] *adj* Hypokapnie betr. *od.* zeigend, hypokapnisch.
hy·po·car·bia [ˌ-ˈkɑːrbɪə] *n* → hypocapnia.
hy·po·cel·lu·lar [ˌ-ˈseljələr] *adj* mit verminderter Zellzahl, hypozellulär, zellarm.

hy·po·cel·lu·lar·i·ty [ˌ-ˌseljəˈleərətɪ] *n* Zellarmut *f*, Hypozellularität *f*.
hy·po·chlo·re·mia [ˌ-kləʊˈriːmɪə] *n* verminderter Chloridgehalt *m* des Blutes, Hypochlorämie *f*.
hy·po·chlo·re·mic [ˌ-kləʊˈriːmɪk] *adj* Hypochlorämie betr., hypochlorämisch.
hypochloremic alkalosis hypochlorämische Alkalose *f*.
hypochloremic azotemia hypochlorämische/chloroprive Azotämie *f*.
hy·po·chlor·hy·dria [ˌ-kləʊrˈhaɪdrɪə] *n* verminderte Salzsäuresekretion *f* des Magens, Hypochlorhydrie *f*.
hy·po·chlo·ri·da·tion [ˌ-ˌklɔːrɪˈdeɪʃn] *n* Chloridmangel *m*.
hy·po·chlo·ri·de·mia [ˌ-kləʊrɪˈdiːmɪə] *n* → hypochloremia.
hy·po·chlo·rite [ˌ-ˈklɔːraɪt] *n* Hypochlorit *nt*.
hy·po·chlo·ri·za·tion [ˌ-ˌklɔːrɪˈzeɪʃn] *n* Reduktion *f* des Kochsalzgehaltes in der Nahrung.
hy·po·chlo·rous acid [ˌ-ˈklɔːrəs] hypochlorige Säure *f*.
hy·po·chlor·u·ria [ˌ-kləʊˈr(j)ʊərɪə] *n* verminderte Chloridausscheidung *f* im Harn, Hypochlorurie *f*.
hy·po·cho·les·ter·e·mia [ˌ-kəˌlestəˈriːmɪə] *n* → hypocholesterolemia.
hy·po·cho·les·ter·e·mic [ˌ-kəˌlestəˈriːmɪk] *adj* → hypocholesterolemic.
hy·po·cho·les·ter·in·e·mia [ˌ-kəˌlestərɪˈniːmɪə] *n* → hypocholesterolemia.
hy·po·cho·les·ter·ol·e·mia [ˌ-kəˌlestərɒlˈiːmɪə] *n* verminderter Cholesteringehalt *m* des Blutes, Hypocholesterinämie *f*.
hy·po·cho·les·ter·ol·e·mic [ˌ-kəˌlestərɒlˈiːmɪk] *adj* Hypocholesterinämie betr. *od.* verursachend, hypocholesterinämisch.
hy·po·cho·lia [ˌ-ˈkəʊlɪə] *n* verminderte/mangelhafte Galle(n)sekretion *f*, Hypocholie *f*, Oligocholie *f*.
hy·po·chol·u·ria [ˌ-kəʊlˈ(j)ʊərɪə] *n* verminderte Galle(n)ausscheidung *f* im Harn, Hypocholurie *f*.
hy·po·chon·dria [ˌ-ˈkɑndrɪə] *n* 1. Hypochondrie *f*, -chondria *f*, Krankheitswahn *m*. 2. *pl* → hypochondrium.
hy·po·chon·dri·ac [ˌ-ˈkɑndrɪæk] **I** *n psycho.* Hypochonder *m*. **II** *adj* 1. *anat.* Hypochondrium betr. 2. *psycho.* Hypochondrie/Hypochonder betr., von Hypochondrie betroffen, an Hypochondrie leidend, hypochondrisch.
hy·po·chon·dri·a·cal [ˌ-kənˈdraɪəkl] *adj* → hypochondriac 2.
hypochondriacal neurosis → hypochondria 1.
hypochondriac region → hypochondrium.
hy·po·chon·dri·al [ˌ-ˈkɑndrɪəl] *adj* → hypochondriac 2.
hy·po·chon·dri·a·sis [ˌ-kənˈdraɪəsɪs] *n* → hypochondria 1.
hy·po·chon·dri·um [ˌ-ˈkɑndrɪəm] *n, pl* **-dria** [-drɪə] *anat.* Hypochondrium *nt*, Regio hypochondriaca.
hy·po·chon·dro·pla·sia [ˌ-ˌkɑndrəˈpleɪʒ(ɪ)ə, -zɪə] *n ortho.* Hypochondroplasie *f*.
hy·po·chro·ma·sia [ˌ-ˌkrəʊˈmeɪʒ(ɪ)ə] *n* 1. Hypochromasie *f*. 2. Hypochromie *f*.
hy·po·chro·mat·ic [ˌ-krəʊˈmætɪk] *adj* hypochromatisch.
hy·po·chro·ma·tism [ˌ-ˈkrəʊmətɪzəm] *n* Hypochromie *f*.
hy·po·chro·ma·to·sis [ˌ-ˌkrəʊməˈtəʊsɪs] *n* Hypochromatose *f*.
hy·po·chrome [ˈhaɪpəkrəʊm] *n* hypochrome Substanz *f*.

hypochromemia

hy·po·chro·me·mia [ˌ-krəˈmiːmɪə] *n* hypochrome Anämie *f*.
hy·po·chro·mia [ˌ-ˈkroʊmɪə] *n* 1. Hypochromie *f*. 2. Hypochromatose *f*.
hy·po·chro·mic [ˌ-ˈkroʊmɪk] *adj* 1. hypochrom. 2. hypochromatisch.
hypochromic anemia hypochrome Anämie *f*.
 idiopathic h. idiopathische hypochrome Anämie.
hy·po·chrom·ism [ˌ-ˈkroʊmɪzəm] *n* Hypochromizität *f*.
hy·po·chro·mo·trich·ia [ˌ-ˌkroʊmoʊˈtrɪkɪə] *n* verminderte Haarpigmentierung *f*, Haarpigmentmangel *m*, Hypochromotrichie *f*.
hy·po·chro·my [ˌ-ˈkroʊmɪ] *n* Hypochromie *f*.
hy·po·chro·sis [ˌ-ˈkroʊsɪs] *n hema*. Hypochromie *f*.
hy·po·chy·lia [ˌ-ˈkaɪlɪə] *n* verminderte Magensaftbildung *f*, Hypochylie *f*, Oligochylie *f*.
hy·po·ci·ne·sia [ˌ-sɪˈniːʒ(ɪ)ə] *n* → hypokinesia.
hy·po·ci·ne·sis [ˌ-sɪˈniːsɪs, -saɪ-] *n* → hypokinesia.
hy·po·ci·tra·te·mia [ˌ-sɪtrəˈtiːmɪə] *n* verminderter Zitratgehalt *m* des Blutes, Hypozitratämie *f*.
hy·po·ci·tra·tu·ria [ˌ-sɪtrəˈt(j)ʊərɪə] *n* verminderte Zitratausscheidung *f* im Harn, Hypozitraturie *f*.
hy·po·ci·tre·mia [ˌ-sɪˈtriːmɪə] *n* → hypocitratemia.
hy·po·ci·tru·ria [ˌ-sɪˈtrʊərɪə] *n* → hypocitraturia.
hy·po·co·ag·u·la·bil·i·ty [ˌ-koʊˌægjələˈbɪlətɪ] *n* verminderte Gerinnbarkeit *f*, Hypokoagulabilität *f*.
hy·po·co·ag·u·la·ble [ˌ-koʊˈægjələbl] *adj* mit verminderter Gerinnbarkeit, hypokoagulabel.
hy·po·com·ple·ment·e·mia [ˌ-ˌkɑmpləmenˈtiːmɪə] *n* verminderter Komplementgehalt *m* des Blutes, Hypokomplementämie *f*.
hy·po·con·dy·lar [ˌ-ˈkɑndɪlər] *adj* unterhalb einer Kondyle (liegend), hypokondylär.
hy·po·cor·ti·cal·ism [ˌ-ˈkɔːrtɪkəlɪzəm] *n* hypoadrenocorticism.
hy·po·cor·ti·cism [ˌ-ˈkɔːrtəsɪzəm] *n* → hypoadrenocorticism.
hy·po·cu·pre·mia [ˌ-k(j)uˈpriːmɪə] *n* verminderter Kupfergehalt *m* des Blutes, Hypokrupämie *f*.
hy·po·cy·clo·sis [ˌ-saɪˈkloʊsɪs] *n ophthal*. Akkommodationsschwäche *f*.
hy·po·cy·the·mia [ˌ-saɪˈθiːmɪə] *n* Verminderung *f* der Erythrozytenzahl, Hypozythämie *f*.
hy·po·cy·to·sis [ˌ-saɪˈtoʊsɪs] *n* Verminderung *f* der Blutzellzahl, Hypozytose *f*.
hy·po·dac·tyl·ia [ˌ-dækˈtɪlɪə] *n* → hypodactyly.
hy·po·dac·tyl·ism [ˌ-ˈdæktəlɪzəm] *n* → hypodactyly.
hy·po·dac·ty·ly [ˌ-ˈdæktəlɪ] *n embryo*. angeborenes Fehlen *nt* von Fingern *od*. Zehen, Hypodaktylie *f*.
hy·po·dense [ˈhaɪpədens] *adj radiol*. hypodens.
hy·po·derm [ˈ-dɜrm] *n* Unterhautzellgewebe *nt*, Subkutis *f*, Hypodermis *f*, Tela subcutanea.
Hy·po·der·ma [ˌ-ˈdɜrmə] *n micro*. Hypoderma *f*.
hy·po·der·ma [ˌ-ˈdɜrmə] *n* → hypoderm.
hy·po·der·mal [ˌ-ˈdɜrməl] *adj* unter der Haut (liegend), in der Subkutis (liegend), subkutan, hypodermal.

hy·po·der·mat·ic [ˌ-dərˈmætɪk] *adj* → hypodermic II.
hy·po·der·ma·toc·ly·sis [ˌ-dərməˈtɑkləsɪs] *n* → hypodermoclysis.
hy·po·der·mat·o·my [ˌ-dərˈmætəmɪ] *n chir*. Durchtrennung *f* der Subkutis.
hy·po·der·mi·a·sis [ˌ-dərˈmaɪəsɪs] *n* Infektion *f* durch Hypodermalarven, Hypodermosis *f*.
hy·po·der·mic [ˌ-ˈdɜrmɪk] **I** *n* 1. → hypodermic injection. 2. → hypodermic syringe. **II** *adj* 3. unter der Haut (liegend), in der Subkutis (liegend), subkutan, hypodermal. 4. subkutan verabreicht *od*. appliziert.
hypodermic injection subkutane Injektion *f*.
hypodermic inoculation subkutane Injektion *f*.
hypodermic needle Nadel *f* zur subkutanen Injektion.
hypodermic syringe Spritze *f* zur subkutanen Injektion.
hy·po·der·mis [ˌ-ˈdɜrmɪs] *n* → hypoderm.
hy·po·der·moc·ly·sis [ˌ-dərˈmɑkləsɪs] *n* subkutane Infusion *f*.
hy·po·der·mo·li·thi·a·sis [ˌ-ˌdərməlɪˈθaɪəsɪs] *n* subkutane Kalkablagerung *f*.
hy·po·di·a·phrag·mat·ic [ˌ-ˌdaɪəfrægˈmætɪk] *adj* unterhalb des Zwerchfells (liegend), hypo-, subphrenisch.
hy·po·dip·loid [ˌ-ˈdɪplɔɪd] *genet*. **I** *n* hypodiploide Zelle *f*, hypodiploider Organismus *m*. **II** *adj* hypodiploid.
hy·po·dip·loi·dy [ˌ-ˈdɪplɔɪdɪ] *n genet*. Hypodiploidie *f*.
hy·po·dip·sia [ˌ-ˈdɪpsɪə] *n* pathologisch verminderter Durst *m*, Hypodipsie *f*.
hy·po·don·tia [ˌ-ˈdɑnʃɪə] *n dent*. Hypodontie *f*, Hypodontia *f*.
hy·po·dy·nam·ia [ˌ-daɪˈnæmɪə] *n* Hypodynamie *f*.
hy·po·dy·nam·ic [ˌ-daɪˈnæmɪk] *adj* hypodynam, hypodynamisch; kraftlos, schwach, geschwächt.
hypodynamic phase hypodynamische Phase *f*, hypodynamisches Stadium *nt*.
hy·po·dys·fi·brin·o·ge·ne·mia [ˌ-ˌdɪsfəˌbrɪnədʒəˈniːmɪə] *n* Hypodysfibrinogenämie *f*.
hy·po·ec·cri·sia [ˌ-ɪˈkrɪsɪə] *n* verminderte Ausscheidung/Exkretion *f*.
hy·po·ec·cri·sis [ˌ-ˈɛkrəsɪs] *n* → hypoeccrisia.
hy·po·e·cho·ic [ˌ-ɪˈkoʊɪk] *adj* schallarm.
hy·po·e·lec·tro·ly·te·mia [ˌ-ɪˌlɛktrəlaɪˈtiːmɪə] *n* verminderter Elektrolytgehalt *m* des Blutes, Hyp(o)elektrolytämie *f*.
hy·po·e·mia [ˌ-ˈiːmɪə] *n* Ischämie *f*.
hy·po·e·o·sin·o·phil·ia [ˌ-ɪəˌsɪnəˈfɪlɪə, -ljə] *n hema*. Eosinopenie *f*.
hy·po·ep·i·neph·ri·ne·mia [ˌ-ɛpɪˌnɛfrɪˈniːmɪə] *n* verminderter Adrenalingehalt *m* des Blutes, Hyp(o)adrenalinämie *f*.
hy·po·er·ga·sia [ˌ-ɜrˈgeɪʒ(ɪ)ə] *n* pathologisch verminderte funktionelle Aktivität *f*, Hyp(o)ergasie *f*.
hy·po·er·gia [ˌ-ˈɜrdʒɪə] *n* 1. → hypoergasia. 2. verminderte Reaktion(sfähigkeit *f*) *f*, abgeschwächte Reizempfindlichkeit *f*, Hypergie *f*.
hy·po·er·gic [ˌ-ˈɜrdʒɪk] *adj* 1. mit verminderter Aktivität/Energie, hypergisch. 2. Hypergie betr. *od*. zeigend, hyperg(isch).
hy·po·er·gy [ˌ-ˈɜrdʒɪ] *n* → hypoergia 2.
hy·po·es·o·pho·ria [ˌ-esəˈfɔːrɪə] *n ophthal*. Esohypophorie *f*, Hypoesophorie *f*.
hy·po·es·the·sia [ˌ-esˈθiːʒ(ɪ)ə] *n neuro*. verminderte Reizempfindlichkeit *f*, Hyp(o)ästhesie *f*, Hypästhesie *f*.
hy·po·es·thet·ic [ˌ-esˈθɛtɪk] *adj* Hypoästhesie betr., hyp(o)ästhetisch.

hy·po·es·tri·ne·mia [ˌ-estrɪˈniːmɪə] *n* → hypoestrogenemia.
hy·po·es·tro·ge·ne·mia [ˌ-ˌestroʊdʒɪˈniːmɪə] *n* verminderter Östrogengehalt *m* des Blutes, Hypöstrogenämie *f*.
hy·po·ex·o·pho·ria [ˌ-ˌeksoʊˈfɔːrɪə] *n ophthal*. Exohypophorie *f*, Hypoexophorie *f*.
hy·po·fer·re·mia [ˌ-fəˈriːmɪə] *n* verminderter Eisengehalt *m* des Blutes, Hypoferrämie *f*.
hy·po·fer·ric anemia [ˌ-ˈfɛrɪk] Eisenmangelanämie *f*, sideropenische Anämie *f*.
hy·po·fer·rism [ˌ-ˈfɛrɪzəm] *n* Eisenmangel *m*.
hy·po·fer·tile [ˌ-ˈfɜrtl, -taɪl] *adj* hypofertil.
hy·po·fer·til·i·ty [ˌ-fɜrˈtɪlətɪ] *n* verminderte Fruchtbarkeit *f*, Hypofertilität *f*.
hy·po·fi·brin·o·ge·ne·mia [ˌ-fɪˈbrɪnədʒəˈniːmɪə] *n* verminderter Fibrinogengehalt *m* des Blutes, Fibrinogenmangel *m*, Hypofibrinogenämie *f*.
hy·po·func·tion [ˌ-ˈfʌŋkʃn] *n* Unter-, Hypofunktion *f*.
hy·po·ga·lac·tia [ˌ-gəˈlækʃɪə, -tɪə] *n gyn*. verminderte/ungenügende Milchsekretion *f*, Hypogalaktie *f*.
hy·po·ga·lac·tous [ˌ-gəˈlæktəs] *adj* zu wenig Milch bildend *od*. sezernierend.
hy·po·gam·ma·glo·bin·e·mia [ˌ-ˌgæməˌgloʊbəˈniːmɪə] *n* → hypogammaglobulinemia.
hy·po·gam·ma·glob·u·li·ne·mia [ˌ-ˌgæməˌglɑbjəlɪˈniːmɪə] *n* Gammaglobulinmangel *m*, Hypogammaglobulinämie *f*.
hy·po·gas·tric [ˌ-ˈgæstrɪk] *adj* 1. unterhalb des Magens (liegend). 2. Unterbauch/Hypogastrium betr., hypogastrisch, Unterbauch-. 3. A. iliaca interna betr.
hypogastric artery innere Hüftarterie *f*, Hypogastrika *f*, Iliaka *f* interna, *old* A. hypogastrica, A. iliaca interna.
hypogastric fascia Beckenfaszie *f*, Fascia pelvis.
hypogastric fossa innere/mittlere Leistengrube *f*, Fossa inguinalis medialis.
hypogastric nerve: left h. N. hypogastricus sinister. **right h.** N. hypogastricus dexter.
hypogastric plexus: inferior h. Beckengeflecht *nt*, -plexus *m*, Plexus pelvicus, Plexus hypogastricus inferior.
superior h. N. pr(a)esacralis, Plexus hypogastricus superior.
hypogastric reflex *neuro*. femoroabdominaler Reflex *m*.
hypogastric region → hypogastrium.
hypogastric vein innere Hüftvene *f*, *old* V. hypogastrica, V. iliaca interna.
hypogastric zone → hypogastrium.
hy·po·gas·tri·um [ˌ-ˈgæstrɪəm] *n* Unterbauch(gegend *f*) *m*, Scham(inbegriff *f*) *f*, Hypogastrium *nt*, Regio pubica.
hy·po·gas·tro·cele [ˌ-ˈgæstrəsiːl] *n* Hypogastrozele *f*.
hy·po·gas·trop·a·gus [ˌ-gæsˈtrɑpəgəs] *n embryo*. Hypogastropagus *m*.
hy·po·gas·tros·chi·sis [ˌ-gæsˈtrɑskəsɪs] *n embryo*. Bauchspalte *f* in der Unterbauchgegend, Hypogastroschisis *f*.
hy·po·gen·e·sis [ˌˌhaɪpoʊˈdʒɛnəsɪs] *n embryo*. Unterentwicklung *f*, defekte Embryonalentwicklung *f*, Hypogenesie *f*, Hypogenese *f*.
hy·po·ge·net·ic [ˌ-dʒəˈnɛtɪk] *adj* Hypogenese betr., unterentwickelt, fehlentwickelt, hypogenetisch.
hy·po·gen·i·tal·ism [ˌ-ˈdʒɛnɪtəlɪzəm] *n* Unterentwicklung *f* der Geschlechtsorgane, Hypogenitalismus *m*.
hy·po·geu·es·the·si·a [ˌ-gjuːzesˈθiːʒ(ɪ)ə] *n* → hypogeusia.

hy·po·geu·sia [ˌ-ˈgjuːʒ(ɪ)ə] *n* verminderte Geschmacksempfindung *f*, gustatorische Hypästhesie *f*, Hypogeusie *f*.
hy·po·glob·u·lia [ˌ-glaˈbjuːlɪə] *n* Verminderung *f* der Erythrozytenzahl, Hypoglobulie *f*.
hy·po·glos·sal [ˌ-ˈglɑsl, -ˈglɔsl] **I** *n* → hypoglossal nerve. **II** *adj* unter der Zunge (liegend), sublingual, Unterzungen-; N. hypoglossus betr., Hypoglossus-.
hypoglossal canal Canalis hypoglossi.
hypoglossal nerve Hypoglossus *m*, XII. Hirnnerv *m*, N. hypoglossus [XII].
hypoglossal nucleus Ursprungskern *m* des XII. Hirnnerven, Hypoglossuskern *m*, Nc. n. hypoglossi, Nc. hypoglossalis.
hypoglossal trigone Trigonum hypoglossale, Trigonum n. hypoglossi.
hy·po·glos·sia-hypodactyly syndrome [ˌ-ˈglɑsɪə] Hypoglossie-Hypodaktylie-Syndrom *nt*, Aglossie-Adaktylie-Syndrom *nt*.
hy·po·glos·sis [ˌ-ˈglɑsɪs] *n* → hypoglottis.
hy·po·glos·so·hy·oid triangle [ˌ-ˌglɑsəʊ-ˈhaɪɔɪd] Pirogoff'-Dreieck *nt*.
hy·po·glos·sus [ˌ-ˈglɑsəs] *n*, *pl* **-si** [-saɪ] → hypoglossal nerve.
hy·po·glot·tis [ˌ-ˈglɑtɪs] *n* Zungenunterseite *f*.
hy·po·glu·ca·gon·e·mia [ˌ-ˌgluːkəgəˈniːmɪə] *n* verminderter Glukagongehalt *m* des Blutes, Hypoglukagonämie *f*, -glucagonämie *f*.
hy·po·gly·ce·mia [ˌ-glaɪˈsiːmɪə] *n* pathologische Verminderung *f* des Blutzuckers, Hypoglykämie *f*, Glukopenie *f*.
hy·po·gly·ce·mic [ˌ-glaɪˈsiːmɪk] **I** *n* blutzuckersenkendes Mittel *nt*, Hypoglykämikum *nt*. **II** *adj* Hypoglykämie betr. *od.* verursachend, durch Hypoglykämie bedingt, hypoglykämisch.
hypoglycemic coma hypoglykämisches Koma *nt*, hypoglykämischer Schock *m*, Coma hypoglycaemicum.
hypoglycemic encephalopathy hypoglykämische Enzephalopathie *f*.
hypoglycemic shock hypoglykämischer Schock *m*, hypoglykämisches Koma *nt*, Coma hypoglycaemicum.
hy·po·gly·co·ge·nol·y·sis [ˌ-glaɪkədʒɪˈnɑləsɪs] *n* verminderter Glykogenabbau *m*, Hypoglykogenolyse *f*.
hy·po·gly·cor·rha·chia [ˌ-glaɪkəˈreɪkɪə, -ˈræk-] *n* verminderter Zuckergehalt *m* des Liquor cerebrospinalis.
hy·po·gnath·ia [ˌ-ˈnæθɪə] *n* Unterentwicklung *f* des Unterkiefers, Hypognathie *f*.
hy·pog·na·thous [haɪˈpɑgnəθəs] *adj embryo.* hypognath.
hy·pog·na·thus [haɪˈpɑgnəθəs] *n embryo.* Hypognathus *m*.
hy·po·go·nad·ism [ˌ-ˈgəʊnædɪzəm, -ˈgɑ-] *n* Unterfunktion *f* der Keimdrüsen/Gonaden, Hypogonadismus *m*.
h. with anosmia → hypogonadotropic eunuchoidism.
hy·po·gon·a·do·troph·ic [ˌ-ˌgɑnədəʊˈtrɑfɪk, -ˈtrəʊ-] *adj* → hypogonadotropic.
hy·po·gon·a·do·trop·ic [ˌˌgɑnədəʊˈtrɑpɪk, -ˈtrəʊ-] *adj* Gonadotropinmangel betr., durch Gonadotropinmangel verursacht, hypogonadotrop.
hypogonadotropic eunuchoidism (Gauthier-)Kallmann-Syndrom *nt*, olfakto-genitales Syndrom *nt*.
hypogonadotropic hypogonadism sekundärer/hypogonadotroper Hypogonadismus *m*.
hy·po·gran·u·lo·cy·to·sis [ˌ-ˌgrænjələʊsaɪˈtəʊsɪs] *n hema.* Granulozytenverminderung *f*, Granulozytopenie *f*.

hy·po·he·pat·ia [ˌ-hɪˈpætɪə] *n* Unterfunktion *f* der Leber.
hy·po·hi·dro·sis [ˌ-hɪˈdrəʊsɪs] *n* verminderte Schweißsekretion *f*, Hypo(h)idrose *f*, Hypo(h)idrosis *f*.
hy·po·hi·drot·ic [ˌ-hɪˈdrɑtɪk] *adj* Hypohidrosis betr. *od.* verursachend, hypohidrotisch.
hy·po·hy·dra·tion [ˌ-haɪˈdreɪʃn] *n* 1. Wassermangel *m*, Dehydration *f*, Dehydratation *f*. 2. Entwässerung *f*, Dehydratation *f*.
hy·po·hy·dre·mia [ˌ-haɪˈdriːmɪə] *n* Blutplasmamangel *m*.
hy·po·hy·dro·chlo·ria [ˌ-ˌhaɪdrəˈklɔʊrɪə] *n* → hypochlorhydria.
hy·po·hyp·not·ic [ˌ-hɪpˈnɑtɪk] *adj* (*Schlaf*) leicht.
hy·po·i·dro·sis [ˌ-ɪˈdrəʊsɪs] *n* → hypohidrosis.
hy·po·in·su·lin·e·mia [ˌ-ɪn(t)sjəlɪˈniːmɪə] *n* verminderter Insulingehalt *m* des Blutes, Insulinmangel *m*, Hypoinsulinämie *f*, Insulinämie *f*.
hy·po·in·su·lin·ism [ˌ-ˈɪn(t)sjəlɪnɪzəm] *n* verminderte/mangelhafte Insulinsekretion *f* des Pankreas, Hypoinsulinismus *m*.
hy·po·i·o·de·mia [ˌ-aɪəˈdiːmɪə] *n* verminderter Jodgehalt *m* des Blutes, Hypojodämie *f*.
hy·po·i·o·di·dism [ˌ-aɪˈəʊdədɪzəm] *n* Jodidmangel *m*, Hypojodidismus *f*.
hy·po·i·so·ton·ic [ˌ-aɪsəˈtɑnɪk, -ˌɪsə-] *adj* → hypotonic.
hy·po·ka·le·mia [ˌ-kəˈliːmɪə] *n* verminderter Kaliumgehalt *m* des Blutes, Hypokal(i)ämie *f*.
hy·po·ka·le·mic [ˌ-kəˈliːmɪk] *adj* Hypokaliämie betr., durch sie gekennzeichnet, hypokal(i)ämisch.
hypokalemic alkalosis hypokaliämische Alkalose *f*.
hypokalemic nephropathy hypokaliämische Nephropathie *f*.
hypokalemic nephrosis hypokaliämische Nephropathie *f*.
hypokalemic periodic paralysis familiäre paroxysmale hypokaliämische Lähmung *f*.
hypokalemic tubulopathy (*Niere*) hypokaliämische Tubulopathie *f*.
hy·po·ka·li·e·mia [ˌˌkælɪˈiːmɪə] *n* → hypokalemia.
hy·po·ki·ne·mia [ˌ-kɪˈniːmɪə] *n radiol.* verminderte Herzleistung *f*, vermindertes Herzminutenvolumen *nt*.
hy·po·ki·ne·sia [ˌ-kɪˈniːʒ(ɪ)ə, -kaɪ-] *n* Bewegungsarmut *f*, verminderte Spontanmotorik *f*, Hypokinese *f*, Hypokinesie *f*, Hypomotilität *f*.
hy·po·ki·ne·sis [ˌ-kɪˈniːsɪs, -kaɪ-] *n* → hypokinesia.
hy·po·ki·net·ic [ˌ-kɪˈnetɪk] *adj* Hypokines(i)e betr., durch sie gekennzeichnet, hypokinetisch.
hy·po·lem·mal [ˌ-ˈleməl] *adj* hypolemmal.
hy·po·leu·ke·mia [ˌ-luːˈkiːmɪə] *n* subleukämische Leukämie *f*.
hy·po·ley·dig·ism [ˌ-ˈlɪdɪgɪzəm] *n* Unterfunktion *f* der Leydig'-Zellen.
hy·po·li·pe·mia [ˌ-lɪˈpiːmɪə] *n* verminderter Lipidgehalt *m* des Blutes, Hypolipämie *f*, Hypolipidämie *f*.
hy·po·lip·i·de·mic [ˌ-lɪpəˈdiːmɪk] *adj* Hypolip(id)ämie betr., hypolipämisch, hypolipidämisch.
hy·po·lip·o·pro·tein·e·mia [ˌ-ˌlɪpəˌprəʊtiˈniːmɪə] *n* verminderter Lipoproteingehalt *m* des Blutes, Hypolipoproteinämie *f*.
hy·po·li·po·sis [ˌ-lɪˈpəʊsɪs] *n* Lipidmangel *m* der Gewebe.

hy·po·li·quor·rhea [ˌ-lɪkwɔːˈrɪə] *n* Liquormangel *m*, Hypoliquorrhoe *f*.
hy·po·lym·phe·mia [ˌ-lɪmˈfiːmɪə] *n hema.* Lymphozytenmangel *m*, Lympho(zyto)penie *f*.
hy·po·mag·ne·se·mia [ˌ-ˌmægnɪˈsiːmɪə] *n* verminderter Magnesiumgehalt *m* des Blutes, Hypomagnesiämie *f*.
hy·po·ma·nia [ˌ-meɪnɪə] *n psychia.* leichte Manie *f*, Hypomanie *f*.
hy·po·man·ic [ˌ-ˈmænɪk] *adj* Hypomanie betr., hypomanisch.
hy·po·mas·tia [ˌhaɪpəʊˈmæstɪə] *n* Unterentwicklung *f* der Brustdrüsen, Hypomastie *f*.
hy·po·ma·zia [ˌ-ˈmeɪzɪə] *n* → hypomastia.
hy·po·mel·an·cho·lia [ˌ-ˌmelənˈkəʊlɪə, -lɪə] *n psychia.* leichte Melancholie *f*, Hypomelancholie *f*.
hy·po·mel·a·no·sis [ˌ-meləˈnəʊsɪs] *n hema.* Pigmentmangel *m* der Haut, Hypomelanose *f*, Hypomelanosis *f*; Leukoderm *nt*, Leucoderma *nt*, Leukodermie *f*.
h. of Ito Incontinentia pigmenti achromians (Ito).
hy·po·men·or·rhea [ˌ-menəˈrɪə] *n gyn.* (zu) schwache Menstruationsblutung *f*, Hypomenorrhoe *f*.
hy·po·mere [ˈ-mɪər] *n embryo.* Hypomer *nt*.
hy·po·met·a·bol·ic [ˌ-metəˈbɑlɪk] *adj* Hypometabolismus betr., hypometabol(isch).
hy·po·me·tab·o·lism [ˌ-mɪˈtæbəlɪzəm] *n* verminderter Stoffwechsel *m*, Hypometabolismus *m*.
hy·po·me·tria [ˌ-ˈmiːtrɪə] *n neuro.* Hypometrie *f*.
hy·po·min·er·al·i·za·tion [ˌ-ˌmɪnrələˈzeɪʃn, -lai-] *n radiol.* Hypomineralisation *f*.
hy·pom·ne·sia [ˌhaɪpəʊmˈniːʒə] *n* Gedächtnisstörung *f*, Hypomnesie *f*.
hy·po·morph [ˈhaɪpəmɔːrf] *adj genet.* hypomorph.
hy·po·mor·phic [ˌ-ˈmɔːrfɪk] *adj* → hypomorph.
hy·po·mo·til·i·ty [ˌ-məʊˈtɪlətɪ] *n* 1. verringerte Motilität *f*, Hypomotilität *f*. 2. → hypokinesia.
hy·po·my·o·to·nia [ˌ-maɪəˈtəʊnɪə] *n* verringerter Muskeltonus *m*, Hypomyotonie *f*.
hy·po·myx·ia [ˌ-ˈmɪksɪə] *n* verringerte Schleimsekretion *f*.
hy·po·na·tre·mia [ˌ-nəˈtriːmɪə] *n* verminderter Natriumgehalt *m* des Blutes, Hyponatriämie *f*.
hy·po·na·tru·ria [ˌ-nəˈtr(j)ʊərɪə] *n* verminderte Natriumausscheidung *f* im Harn, Hyponatriurie *f*.
hy·po·ne·o·cy·to·sis [ˌ-nɪəsaɪˈtəʊsɪs] *n hema.* Leukopenie *f* mit Linksverschiebung.
hy·po·ni·tre·mia [ˌ-nɪˈtriːmɪə] *n* verminderter Stickstoffgehalt *m* des Blutes.
hy·po·noi·a [ˌ-ˈnɔɪə] *n psychia.* eingeengte/abgeflachte Bewußtseinslage *f*, Hyponoia *f*.
hy·po·nych·i·al [ˌ-ˈnɪkɪəl] *adj* 1. unter dem Nagel (liegend), hyponychal, subungual. 2. Hyponychium betr., Nagelbett-.
hy·po·nych·i·um [ˌ-ˈniːkɪəm] *n* Nagelbettepithel *nt*, Hyponychium *nt*.
hy·pon·y·chon [haɪˈpænɪkɑn] *n* (Ein-)Blutung *f* unter dem Nagel.
hypo-oncotic *adj* (*Druck*) hypoonkotisch, hypoonkotisch.
hypo-orchidism *n* endokrine Hodeninsuffizienz *f*, Hyporchidie *f*.
hypo-orthocytosis *n hema.* Leukopenie *f* ohne Linksverschiebung.
hypo-osmolality *n* Hypo(o)smolalität *f*.

hypo-osmolar

hypo-osmolar *adj* hyp(o)osmolar.
hypo-ovarianism *n* endokrine Eierstockinsuffizienz *f*, Hypovarismus *m*.
hy·po·pal·les·the·sia *n* [ˌhaɪpəˌpæles'θiːʒ(ɪ)ə] *neuro.* verminderte Vibrationsempfindlichkeit *f*, Hypopallästhesie *f*.
hy·po·pan·cre·a·tism [ˌ-'pæŋkrɪətɪzəm] *n* herabgesetzte/verminderte Pankreasfunktion *f*.
hy·po·pan·cre·or·rhea [ˌ-pæŋkrɪə'rɪə] *n* verminderte Pankreassekretion *f*.
hy·po·par·a·thy·roid·ism [ˌ-ˌpærə'θaɪrɔɪdɪzəm] *n* Nebenschilddrüseninsuffizienz *f*, Unterfunktion *f* der Nebenschilddrüsen, Hypoparathyr(e)oidismus *m*, Hypoparathyreose *f*.
hy·po·par·a·thy·roid tetany [ˌ-pærə'θaɪrɔɪd] parathyreoprive Tetanie *f*, Tetania parathyreopriva.
hy·po·pep·sia [ˌ-'pepsɪə, -ʃə] *n* mangelhafte Verdauung *f*, Hypopepsie *f*, Oligopepsie *f*.
hy·po·pep·sin·ia [ˌ-pep'sɪnɪə] *n* (*Magen*) mangelhafte Pepsinsekretion *f*.
hy·po·per·fused [ˌ-pər'fjuːzd] *adj* minderdurchblutet, hypoperfundiert.
hy·po·per·fu·sion [ˌ-pər'fjuːʒn] *n* Minder-, Mangeldurchblutung *f*, Hypoperfusion *f*.
hy·po·per·i·stal·sis [ˌ-perɪ'stɔːlsɪs, -stæl-] *n* verminderte Peristaltik *f*, Hypoperistaltik *f*.
hy·po·per·i·stal·tic [ˌ-perɪ'stɔːltɪk, -stæl-] *adj* Hypoperistaltik betr., hypoperistaltisch.
hy·po·pha·lan·gism [ˌ-fə'lændʒɪzəm] *n embryo.* angeborenes Fehlen *nt* von Finger-/od. Zehengliedern, Hypophalangie *f*.
α-hy·poph·a·mine [haɪ'pɑfəmiːn] *n* Oxytozin *nt*, Oxytocin *nt*.
β-hypophamine *n* Vasopressin *nt*, Antidiuretin *nt*, antidiuretisches Hormon *nt abbr.* ADH.
hy·po·pha·ryn·ge·al [ˌhaɪpəfə'rɪndʒɪəl] *adj* Hypopharynx betr., hypopharyngeal, Hypopharyngo-, Hypopharynx-.
hypopharyngeal diverticulum Zenker'-Divertikel *nt*, pharyngoösophageales Divertikel *nt*.
hy·po·phar·yn·go·scope [ˌ-fə'rɪŋgəskoʊp] *n HNO* Hypopharyngoskop *nt*.
hy·po·phar·yn·gos·co·py [ˌ-ˌfærɪŋ'gɑskəpɪ] *n HNO* Hypopharynxuntersuchung *f*, Hypopharyngoskopie *f*.
hy·po·phar·ynx [ˌ-'færɪŋks] *n* Hypo-, Laryngopharynx *m*, Pars laryngea pharyngis.
hy·po·pho·ne·sis [ˌ-foʊ'niːsɪs] *n* Schalldämpfung *f*, abgeschwächtes Atemgeräusch *nt*, gedämpfter Klopfschall *m*, Hypophonie *f*, Hypophonesie *f*.
hy·po·pho·nia [ˌ-'foʊnɪə] *n HNO* Stimmschwäche *f*, Hypophonie *f*, Hypophonesie *f*, Phonasthenie *f*.
hy·po·pho·ria [ˌ-'foʊrɪə] *n ophthal.* Hypophorie *f*.
hy·po·phos·pha·ta·se·mia [ˌ-ˌfɑsfətər'siːmɪə] *n* → hypophosphatasia.
hy·po·phos·pha·ta·sia [ˌ-fɑsfə'teɪzɪə] *n* Hypophosphatasie *f*.
hy·po·phos·pha·te·mia [ˌ-fɑsfə'tiːmɪə] *n* verminderter Phosphatgehalt *m* des Blutes, Hypophosphatämie *f*.
hy·po·phos·pha·te·mic [ˌ-fɑsfə'tiːmɪk] *adj* Hypophosphatämie betr., von ihr gekennzeichnet, hypophosphatämisch.
hy·po·phos·pha·tu·ria [ˌ-fɑsfə't(j)ʊərɪə] *n* verminderte Phosphatausscheidung *f* im Harn, Hypophosphaturie *f*.
hy·po·phos·pho·re·mia [ˌ-fɑsfə'riːmɪə] *n* → hypophasphatemia.
hy·po·phra·sia [ˌ-'freɪʒ(ɪ)ə, -zɪə] *n psychia.* Hypophrasie *f*.

hy·po·phre·nia [ˌ-'friːnɪə] *n psychia.* geistige Behinderung *f*, *inf.* Schwachsinn *m*, Hypophrenie *f*, Oligophrenie *f*.
hy·po·phren·ic [ˌ-'frenɪk] *adj* 1. unterhalb des Zwerchfells (liegend), subphrenisch, hypophrenisch. 2. geistig behindert, *inf.* schwachsinnig, oligophren.
hy·poph·y·se·al *adj* → hypophysial.
hypophyseal fossa → hypophysial fossa.
hypophyseal stalk → hypophysial stalk.
hy·poph·y·sec·to·mize [haɪˌpɑfə'sektəmaɪz] *vt neurochir.* eine Hypophysektomie durchführen, die Hypophyse entfernen, hypophysektomieren.
hy·poph·y·sec·to·my [haɪˌpɑfə'sektəmɪ] *n neurochir.* Hypophysenentfernung *f*, Hypophysektomie *f*.
hy·po·phys·e·o·por·tal circulation [ˌhaɪpəˌfɪzɪə'pɔːrtl] hypophysärer Pfortader-/Portalkreislauf *m*, hypophysäres Pfortader-/Portalsystem *nt*.
hypophyseoportal system → hypophyseoportal circulation.
hy·po·phys·e·o·priv·ic *adj* → hypophysioprivic.
hy·po·phys·e·o·trop·ic *adj* → hypophysiotropic.
hy·poph·y·si·al [haɪˌpɑfə'zɪəl, ˌhaɪpə'fiːz-] *adj* Hypophyse betr., aus der Hypophyse stammend, hypophysär, pituitär, Hypophysen-.
hypophysial artery: inferior h. untere Hypophysenarterie *f*, A. hypophysialis inferior.
superior h. obere Hypophysenarterie *f*, A. hypophysialis superior.
hypophysial atrophy Hypophysenatrophie *f*.
hypophysial cachexia Simmonds'-Kachexie *f*.
hypophysial cartilage *embryo.* Hypophysenknorpel *m*.
hypophysial cavity Hypophysenhöhle *f*.
hypophysial dwarf hypophysärer Zwerg *m*.
hypophysial dwarfism Lorain-Syndrom *nt*, hypophysärer Zwergwuchs/Minderwuchs *m*.
hypophysial fossa Hypophysengrube *f*, Fossa hypophysialis.
hypophysial infantilism → hypophysial dwarfism.
hypophysial infarct Hypopyhseninfarkt *m*, -infarzierung *f*.
hypophysial necrosis Hypophysennekrose *f*.
hypophysial stalk Hypophysenstiel *m*, Infundibulum hypothalami.
hy·po·phys·i·o·por·tal circulation/system [ˌhaɪpɪˌfɪzɪə'pɔːrtl] → hypophyseoportal circulation.
hy·po·phys·i·o·priv·ic [ˌ-ˌfɪzɪə'prɪvɪk] *adj* hypophysiopriv, hypophysiopriv.
hy·po·phys·i·o·trop·ic [ˌ-ˌfɪzɪoʊ'trɑpɪk] *adj* hypophysiotrop, hypophyseotrop.
hypophysiotropic hormone hypophysiotropes Hormon *nt*.
hypophysiotropic zone hypophysiotrope Zone *f*.
hy·poph·y·sis [haɪ'pɑfəsɪs] *n, pl* -**ses** [-sɪːz] Hirnanhangsdrüse *f*, Hypophyse *f*, Hypophysis cerebri, Gl. pituitaria.
hy·poph·y·si·tis [haɪˌpɑfə'saɪtɪs] *n* Hypophysenentzündung *f*, Hypophysitis *f*.
hy·po·pi·e·sia [ˌhaɪpəpaɪ'iːzɪə] *n* → hypotension 1.
hy·po·pi·e·sis [ˌ-paɪ'iːsɪs] *n* → hypotension 1.
hy·po·pig·men·ta·tion [ˌ-ˌpɪgmən'teɪʃn] *n* mangelnde *od.* fehlende Pigmentierung *f*, Hypopigmentierung *f*.
hy·po·pin·e·al·ism [ˌ-'pɪnɪəlɪzəm] *n* Unter-

funktion *f* der Zirbeldrüse, Hypopinealismus *m*.
hy·po·pi·tu·i·tar·ism [ˌ-pɪ't(j)uːətərɪzəm] *n* Hypophysenvorderlappeninsuffizienz *f*, HVL-Insuffizienz *f*, Simmonds-Syndrom *nt*, Hypopituitarismus *m*.
hy·po·pla·sia [ˌ-'pleɪʒ(ɪ)ə, -zɪə] *n* (Organ-)Unterentwicklung *f*, Hypoplasie *f*, -plasia *f*.
hy·po·plas·tic [ˌ-'plæstɪk] *adj* Hypoplasie betr., von ihr gekennzeichnet, hypoplastisch.
hypoplastic anemia hypoplastische Anämie *f*.
congenital h. 1. Blackfan-Diamond-Anämie, -Syndrom *nt*, chronische kongenitale aregenerative Anämie. **2.** Fanconi-Anämie *f*, -Syndrom *nt*, konstitutionelle infantile Panmyelopathie *f*.
hypoplastic chondrodystrophy hypoplastische Chondrodystrophie *f*.
hypoplastic fetal chondrodystrophy Chondrodysplasia/Chondrodystrophia calcificans congenita, Conradi-Syndrom *nt*, Conradi-Hünermann(-Raap)-Syndrom *nt*.
hypoplastic heart hypoplastisches Herz *nt*.
hypoplastic left-heart syndrome Linkshypoplasie-Syndrom *nt*.
hy·po·plas·ty ['-plæstɪ] *n* → hypoplasia.
hy·po·ploid ['-plɔɪd] *adj genet.* hypoploid.
hy·po·ploi·dy [ˌ-'plɔɪdɪ] *n genet.* Hypoploidie *f*.
hy·po·pnea [ˌhaɪpoʊ'niːə] *n* flache langsame Atmung *f*, Hypopnoe *f*.
hy·po·pne·ic [ˌ-'niːɪk] *adj* Hypopnoe betr., von ihr gekennzeichnet, hypopnoisch.
hy·po·pneu·ma·ti·za·tion [ˌ-n(j)uːmətɪ'zeɪʃn] *n HNO* Pneumatisationshemmung *f*, Hypopneumatisation *f*.
hy·po·po·ro·sis [ˌ-pə'roʊsɪs] *n ortho.* mangelhafte (Fraktur-)Kallusbildung *f*.
hy·po·po·tas·se·mia [ˌ-pətə'siːmɪə] *n* → hypokalemia.
hy·po·po·tas·se·mic [ˌ-pətə'siːmɪk] *adj* → hypokalemic.
hy·po·prax·ia [ˌ-'præksɪə] *n* pathologisch verminderte Aktivität *f*, Hypopraxie *f*.
hy·po·pro·ac·cel·er·in·e·mia [ˌ-proʊækˌselərɪ'niːmɪə] *n* Owen-Syndrom *nt*, Faktor-V-Mangel *m*, Parahämophilie (A) *f*, Hypoproakzelerinämie *f*, Hypoproaccelerinämie *f*.
hy·po·pro·con·ver·tin·e·mia [ˌ-proʊkənˌvɜrtə'niːmɪə] *n* Faktor-VII-Mangel *m*, Parahämophilie B *f*, Hypoprokonvertinämie *f*, Hypoproconvertinämie *f*.
hy·po·pro·tein·e·mia [ˌ-proʊti(ɪ)n'iːmɪə] *n* verminderter Proteingehalt *m* des Blutes, Hypoproteinämie *f*.
hy·po·pro·tein·ia [ˌ-proʊ'tiːnɪə] *n* allgemeiner Proteinmangel *m*.
hy·po·pro·tein·o·sis [ˌ-proʊti(ɪ)n'oʊsɪs] *n* Proteinmangelerkrankung *f*, Hypoproteinose *f*.
hy·po·pro·throm·bi·ne·mia [ˌ-proʊˌθrɑmbɪ'niːmɪə] *n* Faktor-II-Mangel *m*, Hypoprothrombinämie *f*.
hy·pop·sel·a·phe·sia [ˌhaɪpɑpˌselə'fiːzɪə] *n* taktile Hypästhesie *f*, Hypopselaphesie *f*.
hy·po·pty·a·lism [ˌ-'taɪəlɪzəm] *n* verminderte Speichelsekretion *f*, Hypoptyalismus *m*, Hyposalivation *f*.
hy·po·py·on [haɪ'poʊpɪən] *n micro.* Eiteransammlung *f* in der vorderen Augenkammer, Hypopyon *nt*.
hypopyon keratitis Hypopyonkeratitis *f*, Ulcus corneae serpens.
hypopyon keratoiritis → hypopyon keratitis.
hy·po·re·flex·ia [ˌhaɪpoʊrɪ'fleksɪə] *n neuro.* Reflexabschwächung *f*, Hyporeflexie *f*.

hy·po·re·nin·e·mia [ˌ-riːnɪnˈiːmɪə] *n* verminderter Reningehalt *m* des Blutes, Hyporeninämie *f*.
hy·po·ri·bo·fla·vi·no·sis [ˌ-ˌraɪbəʊˈfleɪvɪˈnəʊsɪs] *n* Riboflavinmangel *m*, Ariboflavinose *f*.
hy·por·rhea [ˌ-ˈrɪə] *n* leichte Blutung *f*, Sickerblutung *f*.
hy·po·sal·e·mia [ˌ-səˈliːmɪə] *n* verminderter Salzgehalt *m* des Blutes, Hyposaliämie *f*.
hy·po·sal·i·va·tion [ˌ-sælɪˈveɪʃn] *n* → hypoptyalism.
hy·po·sar·ca [ˌ-ˈsɑːkə] *n* Anasarka *f*.
hy·po·scle·ral [ˌ-ˈsklɪərəl, -ˈskle-] *adj* unter der Sklera (liegend), hypo-, subskleral.
hy·po·se·cre·tion [ˌ-sɪˈkriːʃn] *n* verminderte Sekretion *f*, Hyposekretion *f*.
hy·po·sen·si·tive [ˌ-ˈsensətɪv] *adj* **1.** vermindert reizempfindlich, hyposensibel. **2.** *immun.* vermindert reaktionsfähig, hyperg, hypergisch.
hy·po·sen·si·tiv·i·ty [ˌ-sensəˈtɪvətɪ] *n immun.* verminderte Reaktion(sfähigkeit *f*) *f*, Hypergie *f*.
hy·po·sen·si·ti·za·tion [ˌ-ˌsensətɪˈzeɪʃn] *n immun.* Hyposensibilisierung *f*, Desensibilisierung *f*.
hy·po·sex·u·al·i·ty [ˌ-seksʃʊˈwælətɪ] *n* pathologische Verminderung *f* des Sexualtriebs, Hyposexualität *f*.
hy·po·si·al·ad·e·ni·tis [ˌ-ˌsaɪælˌædəˈnaɪtɪs] *n* HNO Entzündung *f* der submaxillären Speicheldrüsen, Hyposialadenitis *f*.
hy·po·si·a·lo·sis [ˌ-saɪəˈləʊsɪs] *n* → hypoptyalism.
hy·po·ske·o·cy·to·sis [ˌ-ˌskɪəsaɪˈtəʊsɪs] *n* → hyponeocytosis.
hys·po·mia [haɪˈpɑzmɪə] *n neuro.* vermindertes Geruchsvermögen *nt*, olfaktorische Hypästhesie *f*, Hyposmie *f*.
hy·po·mo·lar·i·ty [haɪˌpɑsməˈlærətɪ] *n* verminderte Osmolarität *f*, Hyposmolarität *f*.
hy·pos·mo·sis [ˌhaɪpɑzˈməʊsɪs] *n* verlangsamte Osmose *f*, Hyposmose *f*.
hy·po·so·ma·to·trop·ism [ˌhaɪpəʊˌsəʊmətəˈtrəʊpɪzəm] *n* verminderte Somatotropinsekretion *f*, Somatotropinmangel *m*, Hyposomatotropismus *m*.
hy·po·so·mia [ˌ-ˈsəʊmɪə] *n* pathologischer Kleinwuchs *m*, Kümmerwuchs *m*, Hyposomie *f*.
hy·po·som·nia [ˌ-ˈsɑmnɪə] *n* leichte Schlaflosigkeit *f*, Schlafstörung *f*, Hyposomnie *f*.
hy·po·spa·dia [ˌ-ˈspeɪdɪə] *n* → hypospadias.
hy·po·spa·di·ac [ˌ-ˈspeɪdɪæk] **I** *n* Patient *m* mit Hypospadie. **II** *adj* Hypospadie betr., hypospadisch, Hypospadie-.
hy·po·spa·di·as [ˌ-ˈspeɪdɪəs] *n* untere Harnröhrenspalte *f*, Hypospadie *f*, Fissura urethrae inferior.
hy·po·sper·mia [ˌ-ˈspɜːmɪə] *n* Hypo(zoo)spermie *f*.
hy·po·sper·mic [ˌ-ˈspɜːmɪk] *adj* Hypo(zoo)spermie betr., hypo(zoo)sperm.
hy·po·phre·sia [ˌhaɪpɑsˈfriːzɪə] *n* → hyposmia.
hy·po·splen·ism [ˌhaɪpəʊˈsplenɪzəm] *n* Milzunterfunktion *f*, Hyposplenismus *m*.
hy·pos·ta·sis [haɪˈpɑstəsɪs] *n, pl* **-ses** [-siːz] **1.** Senkung *f*, Hypostase *f*. **2.** *patho.* passive Blutfülle *f*, Senkungsblutfülle *f*, Hypostase *f*, Hypostasis *f*. **3.** *genet.* Überdeckung *f*, Hypostase *f*, Hypostasie *f*.
hy·po·stat·ic [ˌhaɪpəˈstætɪk] *adj* **1.** Hypostase betr., hypostatisch. **2.** *s.* senkend, *s.* absetzend, hypostatisch.
hypostatic abscess Senkungsabszeß *m*.

hypostatic congestion hypostatische Blutstauung/Hyperämie *f*.
hypostatic pneumonia hypostatische Pneumonie *f*.
hy·po·ste·a·tol·y·sis [ˌ-stɪəˈtɑləsɪs] *n biochem.* unzureichende Fettspaltung *f*.
hy·pos·the·nia [ˌhaɪpɑsˈθiːnɪə] *n* allgemeine (Körper-, Muskel-)Schwäche *f*, Hyposthenie *f*.
hy·pos·the·ni·ant [ˌhaɪpɑsˈθiːnɪənt] *adj* schwächend.
hy·pos·then·ic [ˌhaɪpɑsˈθenɪk] *adj* Hyposthenie betr., von ihr gekennzeichnet, schwach, geschwächt, hyposthenisch.
hy·pos·then·u·ria [ˌhaɪpɑsθɪˈn(j)ʊərɪə] *n* verminderte Harnkonzentration *f*, verminderte Konzentrationsleistung *f* der Nieren, Hyposthenurie *f*.
hy·po·sto·mia [ˌhaɪpəˈstəʊmɪə] *n embryo.* Hypostomie *f*.
hy·pos·to·sis [ˌhaɪpɑsˈtəʊsɪs] *n ortho.* mangelhafte Knochenentwicklung *f*, Hypostose *f*.
hy·po·sul·fite [ˌhaɪpəˈsʌlfaɪt] *n* Thiosulfat *nt*.
hy·po·su·pra·re·nal·ism [ˌ-ˌsuːprəˈriːnəlɪzəm] *n* → hypoadrenalism.
hy·po·sym·path·i·co·to·nus [ˌ-sɪmˌpæθɪkəʊˈtəʊnəs] *n* verminderter Sympathikotonus *m*, Hyposympath(ik)otonus *m*.
hy·po·sys·to·le [ˌ-ˈsɪstəlɪ] *n card.* unvollständige *od.* abgeschwäche Systole *f*, Hyposystole *f*.
hy·po·tax·ia [ˌ-ˈtæksɪə] *n* **1.** *psychia.* mittlerer Grad *m* der Hypnose, Hypotaxe *f*, Hypotaxie *f*, Hypotaxis *f*. **2.** *neuro.* leichte Ataxie *f*, Hypotaxie *f*, Hypotaxis *f*.
hy·po·tel·or·ism [ˌhaɪpəˈtelərɪzəm] *n* Hypotelorismus *m*.
hy·po·ten·sion [ˌ-ˈtenʃn] *n* **1.** niedriger Blutdruck *m*, Hypotonie *f*, Hypotonus *m*, Hypotonia *f*, Hypotension *f*. **2.** → hypotonia *2*.
hy·po·ten·sive [ˌ-ˈtensɪv] **I** *n* Patient(in *f*) *m* mit Hypotonie, Hypotoniker(in *f*) *m*. **II** *adj* Hypotonie betr. *od.* verursachend, hypotensiv.
hypotensive agent blutdrucksenkendes Mittel *nt*, Blutdrucksenker *m*.
hypotensive anesthesia *anes.* Hypotensionsanästhesie *f*, Vollnarkose *f* mit Hypotonie.
hy·po·ten·sor [ˌ-ˈtensər] *n* blutdrucksenkendes Mittel *nt*, Blutdrucksenker *m*.
hy·po·tha·lam·ic [ˌ-θəˈlæmɪk] *adj* Hypothalamus betr., vom Hypothalamus stammend, unterhalb des Thalamus liegend, hypothalamisch, Hypothalamus-.
hypothalamic amenorrhea *gyn.* hypothalamische Amenorrhoe *f*.
hypothalamic area: anterior h. vordere Hypothalamusregion *f*, Area/Regio hypothalamica anterior.
 dorsal h. dorsale Hypothalamusregion *f*, Area/Regio hypothalamica dorsalis.
 lateral h. seitliche Hypothalamusregion *f*, Area/Regio hypothalamica lateralis.
 posterior h. hintere Hypothalamusregion *f*, Regio hypothalamica posterior.
hypothalamic branch of posterior communicating artery Hypothalamusast *m* der A. communicans posterior, Ramus hypothalamicus a. communicantis posterioris.
hypothalamic centers hypothalamische Zentren *pl*.
hypothalamic nucleus: h.i *pl* Hypothalamuskerne *pl*, Ncc. hypothalamici.
 anterior h. vorderer Hypothalamuskern *m*, Nc. hypothalamicus anterior.
 dorsal h. dorsaler Hypothalamuskern *m*, Nc. hypothalamicus dorsalis.

dorsomedial h. dorsomedialer Hypothalamuskern *m*, Nc. hypothalamicus dorsomedialis.
 posterior h. hinterer Hypothalamuskern *m*, Nc. hypothalamicus posterior.
 ventrolateral h. ventrolateraler Hypothalamuskern *m*, Nc. hypothalamicus ventrolateralis.
hy·po·tha·lam·i·co·hy·poph·y·si·al tract [ˌ-θəˈlæmɪkəʊhaɪˌpɑfəˈsiːəl] → hypothalamohypophysial tract.
hypothalamic pathways Hypothalamusbahnen *pl*.
hypothalamic-pituitary system Hypothalamus-Hypophysen-System *nt*, Hypophysenzwischenhirnsystem *nt*.
hypothalamic-posterior pituitary system Hypothalamus-Neurohypophysen-System *nt*, hypothalamisch-neurohypophysäres System *nt*.
hypothalamic region: anterior h. → hypothalamic area, anterior.
 dorsal h. → hypothalamic area, dorsal.
 intermediate h. intermediäre Hypothalamusregion *f*, Regio hypothalamica intermediae.
 lateral h. → hypothalamic area, lateral.
 posterior h. → hypothalamic area, posterior.
hypothalamic sulcus Hypothalamusrinne *f*, Sulcus hypothalamicus.
hy·po·thal·a·mo·hy·poph·y·si·al tract [ˌ-ˌθæləməʊhaɪˌpɑfəˈsiːəl] hypothalamo--hypophysäres System *nt*, Tractus hypothalamohypophysialis.
hy·po·thal·a·mo·tha·lam·ic fibers [ˌ-ˌθæləməʊθəˈlæmɪk] hypothalamo-thalamische Fasern *pl*, Fibrae hypothalamothalamicae.
hy·po·thal·a·mot·o·my [ˌ-θæləˈmɑtəmɪ] *n neurochir.* Hypothalamotomie *f*.
hy·po·thal·a·mus [ˌ-ˈθæləməs] *n, pl* **-mi** [-maɪ] Hypothalamus *m abbr.* HT.
hy·po·the·nal [ˌ-ˈθiːnl] *adj* → hypothenar II.
hy·po·the·nar [haɪˈpɑθənər, -ˌnɑːr, ˌhaɪpəˈθiː-] **I** *n* Kleinfingerballen *m*, Hypothenar *nt*, Eminentia hypothenaris. **II** *adj* Hypothenar betr., Hypothenar-.
hypothenar eminence → hypothenar I.
hy·po·ther·mal [ˌhaɪpəˈθɜːml] *adj* **1.** (*Körper*) unterkühlt, hypothermal. **2.** lau, lauwarm.
hy·po·ther·mia [ˌ-ˈθɜːmɪə] *n* **1.** Unterkühlung *f*, Hypothermie *f*. **2.** *anes., chir.* künstliche/kontrollierte Hypothermie *f*.
hy·po·ther·mic [ˌ-ˈθɜːmɪk] *adj* Hypothermie betr. *od.* zeigend, unterkühlt, hypothermal.
hypothermic anesthesia Vollnarkose *f* mit Hypothermie.
hy·po·ther·my [ˌ-ˈθɜːmɪ] *n* → hypothermia.
hy·poth·e·sis [haɪˈpɑθəsɪs, hɪ-] *n, pl* **-ses** [-siːz] Hypothese *f*, Annahme *f*, Vermutung *f*, Voraussetzung *f*.
hy·poth·e·size [haɪˈpɑθəsaɪz, hɪ-] *vt* annehmen, voraussetzen. **II** *vi* eine Hypothese aufstellen.
hy·po·thet·ic [ˌhaɪpəˈθetɪk] *adj* → hypothetical.
hy·po·thet·i·cal [ˌ-ˈθetɪkl] *adj* hypothetisch.
hy·po·threp·sia [ˌ-ˈθrepsɪə] *n* Mangelernährung *f*, Hypot(h)repsie *f*.
hy·po·throm·bin·e·mia [ˌ-ˌθrɑmbəˈniːmɪə] *n* verminderter Thrombingehalt *m* des Blutes, Thrombinmangel *m*, Hypothrombinämie *f*.
hy·po·thy·mia [ˌ-ˈθaɪmɪə] *n psychia.* Verstimmung *f*, Unlustgefühl *nt*, Hypothymie *f*.

hypothymic

hy·po·thy·mic [,-'θaɪmɪk] *adj psychia.* unlustig, verstimmt, hypothym.
hy·po·thy·rea [,-'θaɪrɪə] *n* → hypothyroidism.
hy·po·thy·re·o·sis [,-θaɪrɪ'əʊsɪs] *n* → hypothyroidism.
hy·po·thy·roid [,-'θaɪrɔɪd] *adj* Hypothyr(e)oidismus betr., durch Hypothyr(e)oidismus gekennzeichnet *od.* bedingt, hypothyreot.
hypothyroid dwarf hypothyreotischer Zwerg *m.*
hypothyroid dwarfism Kretinismus *m.*
hy·po·thy·roi·dea [,-θaɪ'rɔɪdɪə] *n* → hypothyroidism.
hy·po·thy·roid·ism [,-'θaɪrɔɪdɪzəm] *n* Schilddrüsenunterfunktion *f*, Hypothyreose *f*, Hypothyr(e)oidismus *m.*
hy·po·thy·ro·sis [,-θaɪ'rəʊsɪs] *n* → hypothyroidism.
hy·po·thy·rox·in·e·mia [,-θaɪˌrɒksɪ'ni:mɪə] *n* verminderter Thyroxingehalt *m* des Blutes, Hypothyroxinämie *f.*
hy·po·to·nia [,-'təʊnɪə] *n* 1. Druck-, Spannungs-, Tonuserniedrigung *f*, -verminderung *f*, Hypotonie *f*, Hypotonus *m*, Hypotonia *f.* 2. verminderter/reduzierter Muskeltonus *m*, Muskelhypotonie *f.*
hy·po·ton·ic [,-'tɒnɪk] *adj* 1. mit *od.* bei niedrigem Tonus *od.* Druck, hypoton(isch). 2. mit geringerem osmotischem Druck, hypoton(isch).
hypotonic dehydration hypotone Dehydra(ta)tion/Hypohydratation *f.*
hypotonic hyperhydration hypotone Hyperhydratation *f.*
hypotonic hypohydration → hypotonic dehydration.
hy·po·to·nic·i·ty [,-təʊ'nɪsətɪ] *n* 1. → hypotonia. 2. Hypotonizität *f.*
hypotonic solution hypotone Lösung *f.*
hy·po·to·nus [,-'təʊnəs] *n* → hypotonia.
hy·pot·o·ny [haɪ'pɒtənɪ] *n* → hypotonia.
hy·po·tri·chi·a·sis [ˌhaɪpəʊtrɪ'kaɪəsɪs] *n* 1. angeborener Haarmangel *m*, kongenitale Alopezie *f*, Alopecia/Atrichia congenita. 2. → hypotrichosis.
hy·po·tri·cho·sis [,-trɪ'kəʊsɪs] *n* spärliche Behaarung *f*, Haarmangel *m*, Hypotrichose *f*, -trichosis *f*, -trichia *f.*
hy·pot·ri·chous [haɪ'pɒtrɪkəs] *adj micro.* hypotrich.
hy·pot·ro·phy [haɪ'pɒtrəfɪ] *n patho.* Unterentwicklung *f*, Hypotrophie *f.*
hy·po·tro·pia [ˌhaɪpə'trəʊpɪə] *n ophthal.* Hypotropie *f*, Strabismus deorsum vergens.
hy·po·tym·pa·not·o·my [,-ˌtɪmpə'nɒtəmɪ] *n HNO* Hypotympanoneröffnung *f*, Hypotympanotomie *f.*
hy·po·tym·pa·num [,-'tɪmpənəm] *n anat.* unterster Teil *m* der Paukenhöhle, Hypotympanon *nt*, Hypotympanum *nt*, Hypotympanicum *nt.*
hy·po·u·re·mia [,-jə'ri:mɪə] *n* verminderter Harnstoffgehalt *m* des Blutes, Hypourämie *f.*
hy·po·u·re·sis [,-jə'ri:sɪs] *n* verminderte Harnausscheidung *f*, Oligurie *f.*
hy·po·u·ri·ce·mia [,-jʊərɪ'si:mɪə] *n* verminderter Harnsäuregehalt *m* des Blutes, Hypourikämie *f*, -urikosämie *f.*
hy·po·u·ri·cu·ria [,-jʊərɪ'k(j)ʊərɪə] *n* verminderte Harnsäureausscheidung *f*, Hypourikurie *f*, -urikosurie *f.*
hy·po·va·ria [,-'veərɪə] *n* → hypo-ovarianism.
hy·po·va·ri·an·ism [,-'veərɪənɪzəm] *n* → hypo-ovarianism.
hy·po·ven·ti·la·tion [,-ventə'leɪʃn] *n* alveoläre Minderbelüftung *f*, Mangel-, Minderventilation *f*, Hypoventilation *f.*

hy·po·vi·ta·min·o·sis [,-vaɪtəmɪ'nəʊsɪs] *n* Vitaminmangelkrankheit *f*, Hypovitaminose *f.*
hy·po·vo·le·mia [,-vəʊ'li:mɪə] *n* Verminderung *f* der zirkulierenden Blutmenge, Hypovolämie *f.*
hy·po·vo·le·mic [,-vəʊ'li:mɪk] *adj* Hypovolämie betr., durch Hypovolämie gekennzeichnet *od.* verursacht, hypovolämisch.
hypovolemic shock Volumenmangelschock *m*, hypovolämischer Schock *m.*
  endogenous h. endogener Volumenmangelschock.
  exogenous h. exogener Volumenmangelschock.
hypovolemic thirst hypovolämischer Durst *m.*
hy·po·xan·thine [,-'zænθi:n, -θɪn] *n* Hypoxanthin *nt*, 6-Hydroxypurin *nt.*
hypoxanthine guanine phosphoribosyltransferase *abbr.* **HGPRT** Hypoxanthin(-Guanin)-phosphoribosyltransferase *f abbr* HGPRT.
hypoxanthine guanine phosphoribosyltransferase deficiency Lesch-Nyhan-Syndrom *nt*, Automutilationssyndrom *nt.*
hypoxanthine oxidase Xanthinoxidase *f abbr.* XO, Schardinger'-Enzym *nt.*
hypoxanthine phosphoribosyltransferase *abbr.* **HPRT** → hypoxanthine guanine phosphoribosyltransferase.
hypoxanthine phosphoribosyltransferase deficiency → hypoxanthine guanine phosphoribosyltransferase deficiency.
hy·pox·e·mia [haɪˌpɒk'si:mɪə] *n* verminderter Sauerstoffgehalt *m* des arteriellen Blutes, arterielle Hypoxie *f*, Hypoxämie *f.* 2. → hypoxia.
hy·pox·e·mic [haɪˌpɒk'si:mɪk] *adj* Hypoxämie betr., durch Hypoxämie gekennzeichnet *od.* bedingt, hypoxämisch.
hy·pox·ia [haɪ'pɒksɪə] *n* Sauerstoffmangel *m*, Sauerstoffnot *f*, Hypoxie *f.*
hy·pox·ic [haɪ'pɒksɪk] *adj* Hypoxie betr., durch Hypoxie gekennzeichnet *od.* bedingt, hypoxisch.
hypoxic hypoxia hypoxische/anoxische Hypoxie/Anoxie *f.*
hy·pox·i·do·sis [haɪˌpɒksɪ'dəʊsɪs] *n* Hypoxidose *f*, Hypoxydose *f.*
hyps- *pref.* → hypsi-.
hyp·sa·rhyth·mia *n* → hypsarrhythmia.
hyp·sar·rhyth·mia [ˌhɪpsə'rɪθmɪə] *n neuro.* Hypsarrhythmie *f.*
hypsi- *pref.* Hoch-, Hypsi-, Hyps(o)-.
hyp·si·ce·phal·ic [ˌhɪpsəsə'fælɪk] *adj* Akrozephalie/Oxyzephalie betr., von Akrozephalie gekennzeichnet, spitz-, turmschädelig, akro-, oxy-, hypsi-, turrizephal.
hyp·si·ceph·a·ly [,-'sefəlɪ] *n* Turm-, Spitzschädel *m*, Akrozephalie *f*, -cephalie *f*, Oxyzephalie *f*, -cephalie *f*, Hypsizephalie *f*, -cephalie *f*, Turrizephalie *f*, -cephalie *f.*
hyp·si·ceph·a·lous [,-'sefələs] *adj* → hypsicephalic.
hyp·si·loid ['hɪpsɪlɔɪd] *adj* Y-förmig.
hypsiloid cartilage Y-Fuge *f*, Y-Knorpel *m.*
hypso- *pref.* → hypsi-.
hyp·so·ceph·a·lous [ˌhɪpsə'sefələs] *adj* → hypsicephalic.
hyp·so·ceph·a·ly [,-'sefəlɪ] *n* → hypsicephaly.
hyp·so·chrome ['-krəʊm] *n chem.* hypsochrome Gruppe *f.*
hyp·so·chro·mic [,-'krəʊmɪk] *adj phys.* farbaufhellend, hypsochrom.
hyp·so·no·sus [hɪp'səʊnəsəs] *n* Höhenkrankheit *f.*

Hyrtl ['hɪərtl; 'hɜrtl]: **H.'s anastomosis/loop** *anat.* Hyrtl'-Anastomose *f.*
  H.'s recess Kuppelraum *m*, Attikus *m*, Epitympanum *nt*, Epitympanon *nt*, Rec. epitympanicus.
  H.'s sphincter Hyrtl-Sphinkter *m.*
hyster- *pref.* → hystero-.
hys·ter·al·gia [ˌhɪstər'ældʒ(ɪ)ə] *n gyn.* Gebärmutterschmerz(en *pl*) *m*, Hysteralgie *f*, Hysterodynie *f*, Metralgie *f*, Metrodynie *f.*
hys·ter·a·tre·sia [,-ə'tri:ʒ(ɪ)ə] *n gyn.* Gebärmutter-, Uterusatresie *f.*
hys·ter·ec·to·mize [hɪstə'rektəmaɪz] *vt gyn.* die Gebärmutter entfernen, eine Hysterektomie durchführen, hysterektomieren.
hys·ter·ec·to·my [hɪstə'rektəmɪ] *n gyn.* Gebärmutterentfernung *f*, Hysterektomie *f*, Hysterectomia *f*, Uterusexstirpation *f.*
hys·ter·e·sis [hɪstə'ri:sɪs] *n* 1. verzögerter Wirkungseintritt *m*, verzögerte Reaktion *f*, Hysterese *f*, Hysteresis *f.* 2. *phys.* magnetische Hysterese *f.* 3. *card.* Hysterese *f*, Hysteresis *f.* 4. *chem.* sekundäre Verfestigung *f* von Kolloiden, Hysterese *f*, Hysteresis *f.*
hys·ter·eu·ry·sis [ˌhɪstər'jʊərəsɪs] *n gyn.* Muttermundaufdehnung *f*, -dilatation *f.*
hys·te·ria [hɪ'stɪərɪə, -'stɪər-] *n psychia.* 1. klassische Hysterie *f*, klassisches Konversionssyndrom *nt.* 2. hysterische Reaktion/Neurose *f*, Konversionsreaktion *f*, -neurose *f*, -hysterie *f.* 3. hysterische Angst *m*; Angstneurose *f.* 4. hysterische/histrionische Persönlichkeit(sstörung *f*) *f.* 5. übertriebene Erregbarkeit *f*, Erregtheit *f*, grundlose Erregung *f*, Hysterie *f.*
hys·ter·ic [hɪ'sterɪk] **I** *n* Hysteriker(in *f*) *m.* **II** *adj* → hysterical.
hys·ter·i·cal [hɪ'sterɪkl] *adj* 1. Hysterie betr., auf Hysterie beruhend, an Hysterie leidend, hysterisch. 2. leicht erregbar, übertrieben erregt, übernervös, hysterisch.
hysterical anesthesia *neuro.* hysterische/psychogene Anästhesie *f.*
hysterical aphonia → hysteric aphonia.
hysterical arthralgia hysterische/psychogene Arthralgie *f.*
hysterical asthenopia hysterische Asthenopie *f.*
hysterical ataxia hysterische Ataxie *f.*
hysterical blindness psychogene Blindheit *f.*
hysterical contracture hysterische/psychogene Kontraktur *f.*
hysterical convulsion hysterische/psychogene Konvulsion *f.*
hysterical deafness psychogene Schwerhörigkeit/Taubheit *f.*
hysterical glossolabial hemispasm Brissaud-Syndrom *nt.*
hysterical neurosis hysterische Reaktion/Neurose *f*, Konversionsreaktion *f*, -neurose *f*, -hysterie *f.*
hysterical nystagmus hysterischer Nystagmus *m.*
hysterical paralysis hysterische/psychogene Lähmung *f.*
hysterical personality hysterische/histrionische Persönlichkeit(sstörung *f*) *f.*
hysterical polydipsia *psychia.* psychogene Polydipsie *f.*
hysterical pseudodementia psychogene Pseudodemenz *f.*
hysterical scoliosis hysterische/psychogene Skoliose *f.*
hysterical torticollis hysterischer/psychogener Schiefhals *m.*
hysterical vertigo psychogener Schwindel *m.*

hysterical vomiting psychogenes/hysterisches Erbrechen *nt*.
hysterical wryneck → hysterical torticollis.
hysteric amnesia hysterische/psychogene Amnesie *f*.
hysteric aphonia hysterische/psychogene Aphonie *f*.
hysteric contracture → hysterical contracture.
hysteric pregnancy psychogene Scheinschwangerschaft *f*.
hys·ter·i·form [hɪ'sterɪfɔːrm] *adj* hysterieähnlich, -förmig, hysteriform.
hystero- *pref*. 1. Gebärmutter-, Uterus-, Hyster(o)-. 2. Hysterie-.
hys·ter·o·car·ci·no·ma [ˌhɪstərəʊˌkɑːrsɪ'nəʊmə] *n* Endometriumkarzinom *nt*, Ca. endometriale.
hys·ter·o·cele ['-siːl] *n chir., gyn*. Hysterozele *f*, Hernia uterina.
hys·ter·o·cer·vi·cot·o·my [ˌ-ˌsɜrvɪ'kɑtəmɪ] *n* → hysterotrachelotomy.
hys·ter·o·clei·sis [ˌ-'klaɪsɪs] *n gyn*. operativer Gebärmutterverschluß *m*, Hysterokleisis *f*.
hys·ter·o·col·pec·to·my [ˌ-kɑl'pektəmɪ] *n gyn*. Hysterokolpektomie *f*.
hys·ter·o·col·po·scope [ˌ-'kɑlpəskəʊp] *n gyn*. Hysterokolposkop *nt*.
hys·ter·o·col·pos·co·py [ˌ-kɑl'pɑskəpɪ] *n* Endoskopie *f* von Scheide u. Gebärmutter, Hysterokolposkopie *f*.
hys·ter·o·cys·tic [ˌ-'sɪstɪk] *adj* Gebärmutter u. Harnblase betr., uterovesikal.
hys·ter·o·cys·to·clei·sis [ˌ-ˌsɪstə'klaɪsɪs] *n gyn*. Bozeman-Operation *f*, Hysterozystokleisis *f*.
hys·ter·o·cys·to·pex·y [ˌ-'sɪstəpeksɪ] *n gyn*. Hysterozystopexie *f*.
hys·ter·o·dyn·ia [ˌ-'diːnɪə] *n* → hysteralgia.
hys·ter·o·ep·i·lep·sy [ˌ-'epɪlepsɪ] *n* → hysterical convulsion.
hys·ter·o·gram ['-græm] *n radiol*. Hysterogramm *nt*.
hys·ter·o·graph ['-græf] *n gyn*. Hysterograph *m*.

hys·te·rog·ra·phy [hɪstə'rɑgrəfɪ] *n* 1. *radiol*. Kontrastdarstellung *f* der Gebärmutterhöhle, Hysterographie *f*, Uterographie *f*. 2. *gyn*. Hysterographie *f*.
hys·ter·oid ['hɪstərɔɪd] *adj* hysterieähnlich, -förmig, hysteriform, hysteroid.
hysteroid convulsion → hysterical convulsion.
hys·ter·o·lith ['hɪstərəlɪθ] *n* Gebärmutter-, Uterusstein *m*, Hysterolith *m*, Uterolith *m*.
hys·te·rol·y·sis [hɪstə'rɑləsɪs] *n gyn*. Gebärmutterlösung *f*, Hysterolyse *f*.
hys·ter·om·e·ter [hɪstə'rɑmɪtər] *n gyn*. Hysterometer *nt*.
hys·ter·om·e·try [hɪstə'rɑmətrɪ] *n gyn*. Hysterometrie *f*.
hys·ter·o·my·o·ma [ˌhɪstərəʊmaɪ'əʊmə] *n* Gebärmutter-, Uterusmyom *nt*.
hys·ter·o·my·o·mec·to·my [ˌ-ˌmaɪə'mektəmɪ] *n gyn*. operative Entfernung *f* eines Uterusmyoms, Hysteromyomektomie *f*.
hys·ter·o·my·ot·o·my [ˌ-maɪ'ɑtəmɪ] *n gyn*. Hysteromyotomie *f*.
hystero-oophorectomy *n gyn*. Entfernung *f* von Gebärmutter u. Eierstöcken, Hystero-oophorektomie *f*, Hysteroovariektomie *f*.
hys·te·rop·a·thy [hɪstə'rɑpəθɪ] *n* Gebärmutter-, Uteruserkrankung *f*, Hystero-, Metro-, Uteropathie *f*.
hys·ter·o·pex·y ['hɪstərəʊpeksɪ] *n gyn*. Gebärmutterfixierung *f*, -anheftung *f*, Hysteropexie *f*, Uteropexie *f*.
hys·ter·op·to·sia [ˌhɪstərɑp'təʊzɪə] *n* → hysteroptosis.
hys·ter·op·to·sis [ˌ-ɑp'təʊsɪs] *n gyn*. Gebärmuttersenkung *f*, Metroptose *f*, Hysteroptose *f*, Descensus uteri.
hys·ter·or·rha·phy [hɪstə'rɔrəfɪ] *n gyn*. 1. Gebärmutter-, Uterusnaht *f*, Hysterorrhaphie *f*. 2. → hysteropexy.
hys·ter·or·rhex·is [ˌhɪstərəʊ'reksɪs] *n gyn*. Gebärmutter-, Uterusruptur *f*, -riß *m*, Hystero-, Metrorrhexis *f*.
hys·ter·o·sal·pin·gec·to·my [ˌ-sælpɪn'dʒektəmɪ] *n gyn*. Entfernung *f* von Gebärmutter u. Eileiter(n), Hysterosalpingektomie *f*.
hys·ter·o·sal·pin·gog·ra·phy [ˌ-sælpɪŋ'gɑgrəfɪ] *n radiol*. Kontrastdarstellung *f* von Gebärmutter u. Eileitern, Utero-, Metro-, Hysterotubographie *f*, Utero-, Metro-, Hysterosalpingographie *f abbr*. HSG.
hysterosalpingo-oophorectomy *n gyn*. Entfernung *f* von Gebärmutter, Eileitern u. Eierstöcken, Hysterosalpingo-oophorektomie *f*, Hysterosalpingoovariektomie *f*.
hys·ter·o·sal·pin·gos·to·my [ˌhɪstərəˌsælpɪŋ'gɑstəmɪ] *n gyn*. Hysterosalpingostomie *f*.
hys·ter·o·scope ['hɪstərəskəʊp] *n gyn*. Hysteroskop *nt*.
hys·te·ros·co·py [hɪstə'rɑskəpɪ] *n gyn*. Gebärmutterspiegelung *f*, Hysteroskopie *f*.
hys·ter·o·spasm ['hɪstərəspæzəm] *n gyn*. Gebärmutter-; Uteruskrampf *m*, Hystero-, Uterospasmus *m*.
hys·ter·o·ther·mom·e·try [ˌ-θɜr'mɑmətrɪ] *n gyn*. Messung *f* der Gebärmuttertemperatur.
hys·te·rot·o·my [hɪstə'rɑtəmɪ] *n gyn*. Gebärmutterschnitt *m*, -eröffnung *f*, Hysterotomie *f*, Hysterotomia *f*.
hys·ter·o·trach·e·lec·ta·sia [ˌhɪstərəˌtrækəlek'teɪʒ(ɪ)ə, -treɪk-] *n gyn*. Zervixdehnung *f*, -dilatation *f*.
hys·ter·o·trach·e·lec·to·my [ˌ-ˌtrækəl'ektəmɪ, -treɪk-] *n gyn*. Gebärmutterhalsentfernung *f*, Zervixresektion *f*.
hys·ter·o·trach·e·lo·plas·ty [ˌ-'trækələʊplæstɪ, -treɪk-] *n gyn*. Gebärmutterhals-, Zervixplastik *f*.
hys·ter·o·trach·e·lor·rha·phy [ˌ-ˌtrækə'lɔrəfɪ, -treɪk-] *n gyn*. Zervixnaht *f*.
hys·ter·o·trach·e·lot·o·my [ˌ-ˌtrækə'lɑtəmɪ, -treɪk-] *n gyn*. Zervixschnitt *m*.
hys·ter·o·tu·bog·ra·phy [ˌ-t(j)uː'bɑgrəfɪ] *n* → hysterosalpingography.
Hz *abbr*. → hertz.
H zone H-Bande *f*, H-Streifen *m*, H-Zone *f*, helle Zone *f*, Hensen'-Zone *f*.

I

I *abbr.* 1. → inosine. 2. → iodine. 3. → isoleucine.
IAHA *abbr.* → immune adherence hemagglutination assay.
iatr- *pref.* → iatro-.
i·at·ric [aɪ'ætrɪk] *adj* Medizin *od.* Arzt betr., ärztlich, medizinisch, Arzt-, Iatro-.
i·at·ri·cal [aɪ'ætrɪkl] *adj* → iatric.
iatro- *pref.* Medizin-, Arzt-, Iatr(o)-.
i·at·ro·chem·is·try [aɪˌætrə'keməstrɪ] *n histor.* Iatrochemie *f*, Chemiatrie *f*.
i·at·ro·gen·ic [ˌ-'dʒenɪk] *adj* durch den Arzt hervorgerufen, durch ärztliche Einwirkung entstanden, iatrogen.
iatrogenic infection iatrogene Infektion *f*.
iatrogenic injury iatrogene Verletzung/ Schädigung *f*.
i·at·ro·phys·ics [ˌ-'fɪsɪks] *pl* 1. *histor.* Iatrophysik *f*, Iatromechanik *f*. 2. medizinische/klinische Physik *f*. 3. physikalische Therapie *f*, Physiotherapie *f*.
I.B. *abbr.* → inclusion body.
I band I-Bande *f*, I-Streifen *m*, I-Zone *f*, isotrope Bande *f*.
IBC *abbr.* → iron-binding capacity.
I$_{BS}$ neuron I$_{BS}$-Neuron *nt*, bulbospinal inspiratorisches Neuron *nt*.
i·bu·pro·fen [aɪ'bjuːprəʊfən] *n pharm.* Ibuprofen *n*.
IC *abbr.* 1. → immune complex. 2. → inspiratory capacity.
ice [aɪs] **I** *n* Eis *nt*. **II** *vt* 1. mit Eis bedecken *od.* überziehen. 2. in Eis verwandeln, gefrieren lassen. **III** *vi* 3. gefrieren. 4. zufrieren; vereisen (*up, over*).
ice bag Eisbeutel *m*.
Ice·land disease ['aɪslænd] epidemische Neuromyasthenie *f*, Encephalomyelitis benigna myalgica.
Ice·lan·dic disease [aɪs'lændɪk] → Iceland disease.
I-cell disease I-Zellen-Krankheit *f*, Mukolipidose II *f*.
I cells I-Zellen *pl*, Inklusionszellen *pl*.
ice pack Eispackung *f*.
ICF *abbr.* → intracellular fluid.
ICH *abbr.* → infantile cortical hyperostosis.
ich·no·gram ['ɪknəgræm] *n* Fußsohlenabdruck *m*, Ichnogramm *nt*.
i·chor ['aɪkɔːr, 'aɪkər] *n* (eitrig-seröses) Wundsekret *n*.
i·chor·e·mia [ˌaɪkə'riːmɪə] *n* Septikämie *f*, Septikhämie *f*, Blutvergiftung *f*; Sepsis *f*.
i·chor·oid ['-rɔɪd] *adj* eitrig-serös.
i·chor·ous ['-rəs] *adj* eitrig-serös, purulent.
i·chor·rhea [ˌ-'rɪə] *n* eitrig-seröser Ausfluß *m*.
i·chor·rhe·mia [ˌ-'riːmɪə] *n* → ichoremia.
ich·tham·mol ['ɪkθəmɒl, -məʊl] *n pharm., derm.* Ichthammol *nt*, Ammonium bituminosulfonicum/sulfoichthyolicum.
ichthy- *pref.* → ichthyo-.
ich·thy·ism ['ɪkθɪɪzəm] *n* → ichthyotoxism.
ich·thy·is·mus [ɪkθɪ'ɪzməs] *n* → ichthyotoxism.
Ichthyo- *pref.* Fisch-, Ichthy(o)-.

ich·thy·o·a·can·tho·tox·in [ˌɪkθɪəʊəˌkæn-θə'taksɪn] *n* Ichthyoakanthotoxin *nt*.
ich·thy·o·a·can·tho·tox·ism [ˌ-əˌkænθə-'taksɪzəm] *n* Ichthyoakanthotoxismus *m*.
ich·thy·o·he·mo·tox·in [ˌ-ˌhiːmə'taksɪn, -ˌhemə-] *n* Ichthyohämotoxin *nt*.
ich·thy·o·he·mo·tox·ism [ˌ-ˌhiːmə'taksɪzəm, -ˌhemə-] *n* Ichthyohämotoxismus *m*.
ich·thy·oid ['ɪkθɪɔɪd] *adj* fischähnlich, -artig, -förmig, ichthyoid.
ich·thy·ol·sul·fo·nate [ɪkθɪɒl'sʌlfəneɪt] *n* Ichthyolsulfonat *nt*.
ich·thy·ol·sul·fon·ic acid [ˌ-sʌl'fɒnɪk] Ichthyolsulfonsäure *f*.
ich·thy·o·o·tox·in [ˌɪkθɪəʊə'taksɪn] *n* Ichthyootoxin *nt*.
ich·thy·o·o·tox·ism [ˌ-'taksɪzəm] *n* Ichthyootoxismus *m*.
ich·thy·oph·a·gous [ɪkθɪ'afəgəs] *adj bio.* fischfressend, s. von Fisch ernährend, ichthyophag.
ich·thy·o·pho·bia [ˌɪkθɪəʊ'fəʊbɪə] *n psychia.* krankhafte Angst *f* vor Fischen, Ichthyophobie *f*.
ich·thy·o·sar·co·tox·in [ˌ-saːrkə'taksɪn] *n* Ichthyosarkotoxin *nt*.
ich·thy·o·sar·co·tox·ism [ˌ-ˌsaːrkə'taksɪzəm] *n* Ichthyosarkotoxismus *m*.
ich·thy·o·si·form [ɪkθɪ'əʊsɪfɔːrm] *adj derm.* einer Ichthyosis ähnlich, ichthyosiform.
ichthyosiform erythroderma Erythrodermia congenitalis ichthyosiformis bullosa.
ich·thy·o·sis [ˌ-'əʊsɪs] *n, pl* -ses [-siːz] *derm.* 1. Ichthyose *f*, Ichthyosis *f*. 2. Fischschuppenkrankheit *f*, Ichthyosis simplex/vulgaris.
ich·thy·ot·ic [ˌ-'atɪk] *adj* Ichthyosis betr., von Ichthyosis gekennzeichnet.
ich·thy·o·tox·ic [ˌ-'taksɪk] *adj* durch Fischtoxin(e) hervorgerufen.
ich·thy·o·tox·i·con [ˌ-'taksɪkan] *n* → ichthyotoxin.
ich·thy·o·tox·in [ˌ-'taksɪn] *n* Fischgift *nt*, -toxin *nt*, Ichthyotoxin *nt*.
ich·thy·o·tox·ism [ˌ-'taksɪzəm] *n* Fischvergiftung *f*, Ichthyismus *m*, Ichthysmus *m*, Ichthyotoxismus *m*.
ic·ing liver ['aɪsɪŋ] *patho.* Zuckergußleber *f*, Perihepatitis chronica hyperplastica.
i·con·ic memory [aɪ'kɒnɪk] visuelles/ikonisches Gedächtnis *nt*.
i·co·sa·he·dral symmetry [aɪˌkəʊsə'hiː-drəl] *micro.* Ikosaeder-Symmetrie *f*.
icosahedral viruses *micro.* Ikosaeder-Viren *pl*.
i·co·sa·he·dron [ˌ-'hiːdrən] *n, pl* **-drons, -dra** [-drə] *mathe.* Ikosaeder *nt*.
i·co·sa·no·ic acid [ˌ-'nəʊɪk] Arachinsäure *f*, n-Eicosansäure *f*.
ICP *abbr.* → infantile cerebral palsy.
ICS *abbr.* 1. → intercostal space. 2. → intracellular space.
ICSH *abbr.* → interstitial cell stimulating hormone.
ICT *abbr.* [insulin coma therapy] → insulin shock therapy.

ic·tal ['ɪktəl] *adj* Anfall/Iktus betr., durch einen Anfall gekennzeichnet *od.* bedingt, Anfalls-.
icter- *pref.* → ictero-.
ic·ter·ep·a·ti·tis [ɪktərˌepə'taɪtɪs] *n* → icterohepatitis.
ic·ter·ic [ɪk'terɪk] *adj* Gelbsucht/Ikterus betr., von Gelbsucht betroffen, gelbsüchtig, ikterisch, Ikterus-.
ic·ter·i·tious [ɪktə'rɪʃəs] *adj* → icteric.
ictero- *pref.* Ikterus-, Ictero-.
ic·ter·o·a·ne·mia [ˌɪktərəʊə'niːmɪə] *n* Widal-Anämie *f*, -Ikterus *m*, Widal--Abrami-Anämie *f*, -Ikterus *m*.
ic·ter·o·gen·ic [ˌ-'dʒenɪk] *adj* Gelbsucht/ Ikterus verursachend, ikterogen.
icterogenic spirochetosis Weil'-Krankheit *f*, Leptospirosis icterohaemorrhagica.
ic·ter·o·hem·a·tu·ria [ˌ-ˌhemə't(j)ʊərɪə] *n* Ikterus *m* mit Hämaturie.
ic·ter·o·he·mo·glo·bi·nu·ria [ˌ-ˌhiːməgləʊ-bɪ'n(j)ʊərɪə] *n* Ikterus *m* mit Hämoglobinurie.
ic·ter·o·he·mo·lyt·ic anemia [ˌ-ˌhiːmə'lɪt-ɪk, -ˌhem-] hämolytische Anämie *f* mit Ikterus.
ic·ter·o·he·mor·rha·gia [ˌ-ˌhemə'rædʒ(ɪ)ə] *n* Ikterus *m* mit Hämorrhagie.
ic·ter·o·hep·a·ti·tis [ˌ-ˌhepə'taɪtɪs] *n* ikterische Hepatitis *f*, Hepatitis *f* mit Ikterus.
ic·ter·oid ['ɪktərɔɪd] *adj* gelbsüchtig, ikterisch.
ic·ter·us ['ɪktərəs] *n* Gelbsucht *f*, Ikterus *m*, Icterus *m*.
ic·tus ['ɪktəs] *n* 1. plötzlicher Anfall *m*, Attacke *f*, Synkope *f*, plötzlich auftretendes Symptom *nt*, Iktus *m*, Ictus *m*. 2. Schlag *m*, Stoß *m*, Ictus *m*.
ICU *abbr.* → intensive care unit.
ICW *abbr.* → intracellular water.
I.D. *abbr.* → infective dose.
id [ɪd] *n* 1. *psychia.* Id *nt*, Es *nt*. 2. *immun.* → id reaction.
I.D.$_{50}$ *abbr.* → infective dose, median.
IDA *abbr.* → iminodiacetic acid.
IDD *abbr.* → insulin-dependent diabetes.
IDDM *abbr.* [insulin-dependent diabetes mellitus] → insulin-dependent diabetes.
i·de·a [aɪ'dɪə, -'diːl] **I** *n* 1. Idee *f*, Vorstellung *f*; Gedanke *m*. 2. Meinung *f*, Ansicht *f*; Absicht *f*, Plan *m*.
i·de·al [aɪ'dɪəl, -'diːl] **I** *n* 1. Ideal *nt*, Idealvorstellung *f*; das Ideelle. 2. *mathe.* Ideal *nt*. **II** *adj* 3. ideell, Ideen-, nur gedacht. 4. ideal, vollkommen, Ideal-. 5. *mathe.* ideell.
i·de·al·ist [aɪ'dɪəlɪst] *n* Idealist(in *f*) *m*.
i·de·al·is·tic [aɪˌdɪə'lɪstɪk, ˌaɪdɪə-] *adj* idealistisch.
i·de·al·i·za·tion [aɪˌdɪələ'zeɪʃn] *n psychia.* Idealisierung *f*.
i·de·al·ize [aɪ'dɪəlaɪz] *vt, vi psychia.* idealisieren.
ideal weight Idealgewicht *nt*.
i·de·a·tion [ˌaɪdɪ'eɪʃn] *n* 1. *physiol.* Ideen-, Begriffsbildung *f*, Ideation *f*, Ideierung *f*. 2. *neuro.* Ideation *f*.

i·de·a·tion·al agnosia [ˌ-'eɪʃənl] *neuro.* ideatorische Agnosie *f*.
ideational apraxia ideatorische Apraxie *f*.
i·de·a·to·ry apraxia [aɪ'dɪətɔːriː, 'aɪdɪə-, -təʊ-] → ideational apraxia.
i·dée fixe [i'de fiks] *psychia.* fixe Idee *f*.
i·den·ti·cal [aɪ'dentɪkl, ɪ'den-] *adj* identisch, gleich (*with* mit); *bio.* artgleich.
identical points *opthal.* korrespondierende Netzhautpunkte *pl*.
identical reduplication identische Reduplikation *f*, Autoreduplikation *f*.
identical twins eineiige/erbgleiche/identische/monovuläre/monozygote Zwillinge *pl*.
i·den·ti·fi·a·ble [aɪ'dentɪfaɪəbl, ɪ'den-] *adj* identifizierbar, feststellbar; nachweisbar, diagnostizierbar.
i·den·ti·fi·ca·tion [aɪˌdentəfɪ'keɪʃn, ɪˌden-] *n* Identifizierung *f*, Feststellung *f*.
i·den·ti·fy [aɪ'dentɪfaɪ, ɪ'den-] **I** *vt* identifizieren, (Identität) feststellen, nachweisen, bestimmen, erkennen. **II** *vi* s. identifizieren (*with* mit).
i·den·ti·ty [aɪ'dentɪtɪ, ɪ'den-] *n, pl* **-ties 1.** Identität *f*, Persönlichkeit *f*. **to establish s.o.'s ~** jds. Identität feststellen, jdn. identifizieren. **2.** Nachweis *m*. **3.** *bio.* Artgleichheit *f*; Gleichheit *f*, Identität *f*, Übereinstimmung *f*.
identity crisis *psychia.* Identitätskrise *f*.
identity disorder Identitätsstörung *f*, -krise *f*.
i·de·o·ki·net·ic [ˌaɪdɪəkɪ'netɪk, ˌɪd-] *adj* → ideomotor.
ideokinetic apraxia ideokinetische/ideomotorische Apraxie *f*.
i·de·o·mo·tion [ˌ-'məʊʃn] *n* Ideo-, Psychomotorik *f*.
i·de·o·mo·tor [ˌ-'məʊtər] *adj* psycho-, ideomotorisch, ideokinetisch.
ideomotor apraxia ideokinetische/ideomotorische Apraxie *f*.
i·de·o·mus·cu·lar [ˌ-'mʌskjələr] *adj* → ideomotor.
id·e·o·pho·bia [ˌ-'fəʊbɪə] *n psychia.* krankhafte Angst *f* vor Ideen, Ideophobie *f*.
i·de·o·plas·tia [ˌ-'plæstɪə] *n psychia.* Ideoplastie *f*, -plasie *f*.
i·de·o·vas·cu·lar [ˌ-'væskjələr] *adj* ideovaskulär.
idi(o)- *pref.* Selbst-, Eigen-, Idi(o)-.
id·i·o·ag·glu·ti·nin [ˌɪdɪəə'gluːtənɪn] *n* Idioagglutinin *nt*.
id·i·o·blast ['-blæst] *n bio.* Idioblast *m*.
id·i·o·chro·ma·tin [ˌ-'krəʊmətɪn] *n* Idiochromatin *nt*.
id·i·o·chro·mo·some [ˌ-'krəʊməsəʊm] *n* Geschlechts-, Sexchromosom *nt*, Gonosom *nt*, Heterosom *nt*.
id·i·o·cy ['ɪdɪəsɪ] *n, pl* **-cies 1.** *psychia.* hochgradiger Schwachsinn *m*, Idiotie *f*; Idiotismus *m*. **2.** *fig.* Blödheit *f*, Dummheit *f*, Schwachsinn *m*.
id·i·o·dy·nam·ic [ˌɪdɪədaɪ'næmɪk] *adj* unabhängig aktiv, idiodynamisch.
id·i·o·gen·e·sis [ˌ-'dʒenəsɪs] *n* idiopathische Krankheitsentstehung *f*, Idiogenese *f*.
id·i·o·glos·sia [ˌ-'glɒsɪə] *n ped.* Idioglossie *f*.
id·i·o·glot·tic [ˌ-'glɒtɪk] *adj* Idioglossie betr., von Idioglossie betroffen.
id·i·o·gram ['-græm] *n genet.* Idio-, Karyogramm *nt*.
id·i·o·graph·ic [ˌ-'græfɪk] *adj psycho.* idiographisch.
id·i·o·het·er·o·ag·glu·ti·nin [ˌ-ˌhetərəə'gluːtənɪn] *n* Idioheteroagglutinin *nt*.
id·i·o·het·er·ol·y·sin [ˌ-hetə'rɒləsɪn] *n* Idioheterolysin *nt*.
id·i·o·hyp·no·tism [ˌ-'hɪpnətɪzəm] *n* Selbst-, Idio-, Autohypnose *f*.
id·i·o·i·so·ag·glu·ti·nin [ˌ-ˌaɪsəə'gluːtənɪn] *n* Idioisoagglutinin *nt*.
id·i·o·i·sol·y·sin [ˌ-aɪ'sɒləsɪn] *n* Idioisolysin *nt*.
id·i·o·la·lia [ˌ-'leɪlɪə] *n ped., psychia.* Idiolalie *f*.
id·i·o·lect ['-lekt] *n* Individualsprache *f*, Idiolekt *m*.
id·i·o·lec·tal [ˌ-'lektl] *adj* Idiolekt betr., auf ihm beruhend, idiolektal.
id·i·o·lec·tic [ˌ-'lektɪk] *adj* → idiolectal.
id·i·ol·y·sin [ɪdɪ'ɒləsɪn] *n* Idiolysin *nt*.
id·i·om ['ɪdɪəm] *n* Idiom *nt*.
id·i·o·mat·ic [ˌɪdɪə'mætɪk] *adj* idiomatisch.
id·i·o·mat·i·cal [ˌ-'mætɪkl] *adj* → idiomatic.
id·i·o·mere ['-mɪər] *n* Idiomer *nt*, Chromomer *nt*.
id·i·o·mus·cu·lar [ˌ-'mʌskjələr] *adj* idiomuskulär.
idiomuscular contraction idiomuskuläre Kontraktion *f*.
i·di·o·neu·ro·sis [ˌ-n(j)ʊə'rəʊsɪs] *n* Idioneurose *f*, -neurosis *f*.
id·i·o·no·dal [ˌ-'nəʊdl] *adj* im AV-Knoten entstehend *od.* entstanden, idionodal.
id·i·o·pa·thet·ic [ˌ-pə'θetɪk] *adj* → idiopathic.
id·i·o·path·ic [ˌ-'pæθɪk] *adj* ohne erkennbare Ursache (entstanden), unabhängig von anderen Krankheiten, selbständig, idiopathisch; essentiell, primär, genuin.
idiopathic abortion *gyn.* idiopathischer Abort *m*.
idiopathic amyloidosis primäre/idiopathische (System-)Amyloidose *f*, Paramyloidose *f*.
idiopathic anemia idiopathische/essentielle/primäre Anämie *f*.
idiopathic atrophic gastritis (chronisch-)atrophische Gastritis *f*.
idiopathic atrophoderma/atrophodermia of Pasini and Pierini *derm.* Atrophodermia idiopathica Pasini-Pierini.
idiopathic avascular necrosis of the femoral head *ortho.* idiopathische Hüftkopfnekrose *f* des Erwachsenen, avaskuläre/ischämische Femurkopfnekrose *f*.
idiopathic benign hypertrophy of pylorus idiopathische benigne Pylorushypertrophie *f*, Billroth-Syndrom *nt*.
idiopathic bradycardia idiopathische/essentielle Bradykardie *f*.
idiopathic cardiomyopathy primäre/idiopathische Kardiomyopathie *f*.
idiopathic disease idiopathische Erkrankung *f*.
idiopathic edema idiopathisches Ödem *nt*.
idiopathic epilepsy idiopathische/essentielle/endogene/kryptogenetische/genuine Epilepsie *f*.
idiopathic fibrous mediastinitis Mediastinalfibrose *f*.
idiopathic gastric atrophy → idiopathic atrophic gastritis.
idiopathic guttate hypomelanosis idiopathische fleckförmige Hypomelanose *f*, Hypomelanosis guttata idiopathica, Leucoderma lenticulare disseminatum.
idiopathic hypercalcemia idiopathische Hyperkalzämie *f*.
idiopathic hyperlipemia Bürger-Grütz--Syndrom *nt*, (primäre/essentielle) Hyperlipoproteinämie *f* Typ I, fettinduzierte/exogene Hypertriglyzeridämie *f*, fettinduzierte/exogene Hyperlipämie *f*, Hyperchylomikronämie *f*, familiärer C-II--Apoproteinmangel *m*.
idiopathic hypertension essentielle/idiopathische/primäre Hypertonie *f*.

idiopathic hypertrophic osteoarthropathy Pachydermoperiostose *f*, Touraine--Solente-Golé-Syndrom *nt*, familiäre Pachydermoperiostose *f*, idiopathische hypertrophische Osteoarthropathie *f*, Akropachydermie *f* mit Pachydermoperiostose, Hyperostosis generalisata mit Pachydermie.
idiopathic hypertrophic subaortic stenosis *abbr.* **IHSS** idiopathische hypertrophische subaortale Stenose *f abbr.* IHSS, Subaortenstenose *f*.
idiopathic hypoparathyroidism idiopathischer Hypoparathyreoidismus *m*.
idiopathic infantilism proportionierter Zwergwuchs/Minderwuchs *m*.
idiopathic megacolon idiopathisches Megakolon *nt*, Megacolon idiopathicum.
idiopathic multiple pigmented hemorrhagic sarcoma Kaposi-Sarkom *nt*, Morbus Kaposi *m*, Retikuloangiomatose *f*, Angioretikulomatose *f*, idiopathisches multiples Pigmentsarkom Kaposi *nt*, Sarcoma idiopathicum multiplex haemorrhagicum.
idiopathic myocarditis idiopathische Myokarditis *f*, Fiedler-Myokarditis *f*.
idiopathic myoglobinuria idiopathische/familiäre Myoglobinurie *f*.
idiopathic neuralgia idiopathische Neuralgie *f*.
idiopathic neutropenia Agranulozytose *f*, maligne Neutropenie *f*.
idiopathic osteoporosis idiopathische Osteoporose *f*.
idiopathic pericarditis idiopathische Herzbeutelentzündung/Perikarditis *f*.
idiopathic polyneuritis Guillain-Barre--Syndrom *nt*, (Poly-)Radikuloneuritis *f*, Neuronitis *f*.
idiopathic pulmonary fibrosis idiopathische Lungenfibrose *f*, fibrosierende Alveolitis *f*.
idiopathic respiratory distress of the newborn Atemnotsyndrom *nt* des Neugeborenen *abbr.* ANS, Respiratory-distress-Syndrom *nt* des Neugeborenen *abbr.* RDS.
idiopathic scoliosis *ortho.* idiopathische Skoliose *f*.
idiopathic thrombocythemia hämorrhagische/essentielle Thrombozythämie *f*, Megakaryozytenleukämie *f*, megakaryozytäre Myelose *f*.
idiopathic thrombocytopenic purpura *abbr.* **ITP** idiopathische thrombozytopenische Purpura *f abbr.* ITP, essentielle/idiopathische Thrombozytopenie *f*, Morbus Werlhof *m*.
id·i·op·a·thy [ɪdɪ'ɒpəθɪ] *n patho.* idiopathische Erkrankung *f*.
id·i·o·plasm ['ɪdɪəplæzəm] *n* Erbsubstanz *f*, Erb-, Keimplasma *nt*, Idioplasma *nt*.
id·i·o·re·flex [ˌ-'rɪfleks] *n neuro.* Eigen-, Idioreflex *m*.
id·i·o·some ['-səʊm] *n* → idiozome.
id·i·o·spasm ['ɪdɪəspæzəm] *n* lokalisierter Krampf/Spasmus *m*.
id·i·o·syn·cra·sy [ˌ-'sɪnkrəsɪ] *n* **1.** Eigenart *f*, Idiosynkrasie *f*. **2.** Veranlagung *f*, Natur *f*, Idio(syn)krasie *f*. **3.** *immun.* (angeborene) Überempfindlichkeit *f*, Hypersensibilität *f*, Idio(syn)krasie *f*. **4.** *psychia.* heftige Abneigung *f*, starker Widerwillen *m*, Idiosynkrasie *f*.
id·i·o·syn·crat·ic [ˌ-sɪn'krætɪk] *adj* **1.** *immun.* Idiosynkrasie betr., überempfindlich, allergisch, idiosynkratisch. **2.** *psychia.* Idiosynkrasie betr., auf ihr beruhend, idiosynkratisch.
idiosyncratic neutropenia Agranulozytose *f*, maligne/perniziöse Neutropenie *f*.

idiot

id·i·ot ['ɪdɪət] *n* **1.** hochgradig Schwachsinnige(r *m*) *f*, Idiot *m*, Idiotin *f*. **2.** *fig.* Trottel *m*, Dummkopf *m*, Idiot *m*.
id·i·ot·ic [ɪdɪ'ɑtɪk] *adj* **1.** hochgradig schwachsinnig, idiotisch. **2.** *fig.* blöd, vertrottelt, schwachsinnig, idiotisch.
id·i·ot·ism ['ɪdɪətɪzəm] *n old* → idiocy.
id·i·o·tope ['-təʊp] *n genet.* Idiotop *nt*, Idiotypendeterminante *f*.
id·i·o·top·y ['-təpɪ] *n anat.* Idiotopie *f*.
id·i·o·troph·ic [,-'trafɪk, -'trəʊ-] *adj bio.* idiotroph.
id·i·o·trop·ic [,-'trɑpɪk, -'trəʊ-] *adj psychia.* idiotrop; introvertiert; egozentrisch.
id·i·o·type ['-taɪp] *n genet.* Idiotyp *m*, Idiotypus *m*, Genotyp *m*, -typus *m*.
id·i·o·typ·ic [,-'tɪpɪk] *adj* Idiotyp(en) betr., idiotypisch, Idiotypen-.
idiotypic antibody anti-idiotypischer Antikörper *m*.
idiotypic antigenic determinant → idiotope.
idiotypic determinant → idiotope.
idiotypic variation idiotypische Variation *f*.
id·i·o·ty·py ['-taɪpɪ] *n genet.* Idiotypie *f*.
id·i·o·var·i·a·tion [,-,veərɪ'eɪʃn, -,verɪ-] *n genet.* **1.** Idiovariation *f*. **2.** Mutation *f*.
id·i·o·ven·tric·u·lar [,-ven'trɪkjələr] *adj card.* nur den Ventrikel betr., idioventrikulär.
idioventricular rhythm idioventrikuläre Erregungsbildung *f*, Kammerautomatie *f*, -automatismus *m*.
id·i·o·zome ['-zəʊm] *n histol.* Idiozom *nt*.
I disk → I band.
id·i·tol ['ɪdɪtɔl, -təʊl] *n* Iditol *nt*.
L-iditol dehydrogenase L-Iditoldehydrogenase *f*, Iditdehydrogenase *f*, Sorbitdehydrogenase *f abbr.* SHD.
IDL *abbr.* → intermediate-density lipoprotein.
i·dose ['aɪdəʊs, 'ɪd-] *n* Idose *f*.
i·dox·ur·i·dine [,aɪdɑks'jʊərɪdi:n] *n abbr.*
IDU Idoxuridin *nt abbr.* IDU, IDUR, Jododesoxyuridin *nt*.
id reaction Id-Typ *m*, -Reaktion *f*.
IDU *abbr.* → idoxuridine.
id·u·ron·ate-2-sulfatase [,aɪdjə'rɑneɪt] *n* Iduronat-2-sulfatase *f*, Iduronatsulfat-sulfatase *f*.
id·u·ron·ic acid [,-'rɑnɪk] Iduronsäure *f*.
iduronic sulfatase → iduronate-2-sulfatase.
α-L-id·u·ron·i·dase [,-'rɑnɪdeɪz] *n* α-L-Iduronidase *f*.
α-L-iduronidase deficiency Hurler-Krankheit *f*, -Syndrom *nt*, von Pfaundler-Hurler-Krankheit *f*, -Syndrom *nt*, Lipochondrodystrophie *f*, Dysostosis multiplex, Mukopolysaccharidose I-H *f abbr.* MPS I-H.
IEP *abbr.* → immunoelectrophoresis.
IF *abbr.* **1.** → inhibiting factor. **2.** → initiation factor.
IFAR *abbr.* [indirect fluorescent antibody reaction] → indirect fluorescent antibody test.
IFA test → indirect fluorescent antibody test.
IFN *abbr.* → interferon.
IFN-α *abbr.* → interferon-α.
IFN-β *abbr.* → interferon-β.
IFN-γ *abbr.* → interferon-γ.
I form *biochem.* I-Form *f*.
i·fos·fa·mide [aɪ'fɑsfəmaɪd] *n pharm.* Ifosfamid *nt*.
Ig *abbr.* → immunoglobulin.
IgA *abbr.* → immunoglobulin A.
IgA deficiency, isolated/selective *immun.* selektiver IgA-Mangel *m*.
IgA glomerulonephritis Berger-Krankheit *f*, -Nephropathie *f*, mesangiale/fokale/fokalbetonte Glomerulonephritis *f*.
IgA nephropathy → IgA glomerulonephritis.
IgA$_1$ protease IgA$_1$-Protease *f*.
Ig class switch *immun.* Ig-Klassen-Switch *m*.
IgD *abbr.* → immunoglobulin D.
IgE *abbr.* → immunoglobulin E.
IGF *abbr.* → insulin-like growth factors.
IGF I *abbr.* → insulin-like growth factor I.
IgG *abbr.* → immunoglobulin G.
IgM *abbr.* → immunoglobulin M.
IgM anti-HAV → IgM class antibody to HAV.
IgM anti-HB$_C$ → IgM class antibody to HB$_C$Ag.
IgM class antibody to HAV Anti-HAV-IgM *nt*, Antikörper *m* gegen HAV der IgM-Klasse.
IgM class antibody to HB$_C$Ag Anti-HB$_C$-IgM *nt*, Antikörper *m* gegen HB$_C$Ag der IgM-Klasse.
ig·ni·punc·ture ['ɪgnəpʌŋ(k)tʃər] *n* Ignipunktur *f*.
ig·no·tine ['ɪgnətɪn] *n* Karnosin *nt*, Carnosin *nt*, β-Alanin-L-Histidin *nt*.
IGT *abbr.* → glucose tolerance, impaired.
IH *abbr.* → inhibiting hormone.
IHA test → indirect hemagglutination antibody test.
IL *abbr.* **1.** → interleukin. **2.** → intermediate lobe (of hypophysis).
IL-1 *abbr.* → interleukin 1.
IL-2 *abbr.* → interleukin-2.
IL-3 *abbr.* → interleukin-3.
ILA *abbr.* [insulin-like activity] → insulin-like growth factors.
Ile *abbr.* → isoleucine.
ile- *pref.* → ileo-.
il·e·ac ['ɪliæk] *adj* **1.** Ileum betr., ileal, Ileo-, Ileum-. **2.** ileusartig.
il·e·a·del·phus [ɪlɪə'delfəs] *n* → iliopagus.
il·e·al ['ɪliəl] *adj* → ileac 1.
ileal arteries Ileumarterien *pl*, Ileumäste *pl* der A. mesenterica superior, Aa. ileales.
ileal atresia Ileumatresie *f*.
ileal branch of ileocolic artery Ileumast *m* der A. ileocolica, Ramus ilealis a. ileocolicae.
ileal bypass *chir.* Ileumausschaltung *f*, ilealer/jejunaler Bypass/Shunt *m*.
ileal carcinoid Ileumkarzinoid *nt*.
ileal conduit *chir.* Ileumblase *f*, -conduit *nt*/*m*.
ileal diverticulum Meckel'-Divertikel *nt*.
ileal loop Ileumschlinge *f*.
ileal mucosa Ileumschleimhaut *f*.
ileal papilla → ileocecal papilla.
ileal secretion Ileumsekret *nt*.
ileal shunt → ileal bypass.
ileal stoma *chir.* Ileostoma *nt*.
ileal veins Ileumvenen *pl*, Vv. ileales.
il·e·ec·to·my [ɪlɪ'ektəmɪ] *n chir.* Ileumresektion *f*, Ileektomie *f*.
il·e·i·tis [ɪlɪ'aɪtɪs] *n* Ileumentzündung *f*, Ileitis *f*.
ileo- *pref.* **1.** Ileum betr., Ileo-, Ileum-. **2.** Ilium betr., Ilio-. **3.** Ilias betr., Ilio-, Ilia-.
il·e·o·ce·cal [ɪlɪəʊ'si:kl] *adj* Ileum u. Zäkum betr. *od.* verbindend, ileozäkal, -zökal.
ileocecal fistula *patho.* ileozäkale Fistel *f*, Ileozäkalfistel *f*.
ileocecal fold Plica ileoc(a)ecalis.
ileocecal fossa: inferior i. → ileocecal recess, inferior.
superior i. → ileocecal recess, superior.
ileocecal opening Ileumeinmündung *f* ins Zäkum, Ostium valvae ilealis.
ileocecal papilla Papilla ilealis.

ileocecal recess ileozäkale Bauchfelltasche *f*, Rec. ileoc(a)ecalis.
inferior i. Rec. ileoc(a)ecalis inferior.
superior i. Rec. ileoc(a)ecalis superior.
ileocecal valve Bauhin'-Klappe *f*, Ileozäkal-, Ileozökalklappe *f*, Valva ileoc(a)ecalis/ilealis.
il·e·o·ce·cos·to·my [,-sɪ'kɑstəmɪ] *n chir.* Ileum-Zäkum-Fistel *f*, Ileozäkostomie *f*, Zäkoileostomie *f*.
il·e·o·ce·cum [,-'si:kəm] *n* Ileozäkum *nt*.
il·e·o·col·ic [,-'kɑlɪk] *adj* Ileum u. Kolon betr. *od.* verbindend, ileokolisch.
ileocolic artery A. ileocolica.
ascending i. A. ascendens ileocolica, Ramus colicus a. ileocolicae.
ileocolic fossa → ileocecal recess, superior.
ileocolic intussusception *chir.* ileokolische Invagination *f*.
ileocolic plexus vegetativer Plexus *m* der A. ileocolica.
ileocolic valve → ileocecal valve.
ileocolic vein Ileozäkalvene *f*, V. ileocolica.
il·e·o·co·li·tis [,-kə'laɪtɪs] *n* Entzündung *f* von Ileum u. Kolon, Ileokolitis *f*, Ileocolitis *f*.
il·e·o·co·lon·ic [,-kəʊ'lɑnɪk] *adj* → ileocolic.
il·e·o·co·los·to·my [,-kə'lɑstəmɪ] *n chir.* Ileum-Kolon-Fistel *f*, Ileokolostomie *f*.
il·e·o·co·lot·o·my [,-kə'lɑtəmɪ] *n chir.* Ileokolotomie *f*.
il·e·o·cys·to·plas·ty [,-'sɪstəplæstɪ] *n urol.* Ileozystoplastik *f*.
il·e·o·cys·tos·to·my [,-sɪs'tɑstəmɪ] *n chir.* Ileum-Blasen-Fistel *f*, Ileozystostomie *f*.
il·e·o·il·e·al fistula [,-'ɪlɪəl] ileoileale Fistel *f*.
ileoileal intussusception *chir.* ileoileale Invagination *f*.
il·e·o·il·e·os·to·my [,-ɪlɪ'ɑstəmɪ] *n chir.* Ileoileostomie *f*, -anastomose *f*.
il·e·o·je·ju·ni·tis [,-dʒɪdʒu:'naɪtɪs] *n* Entzündung *f* von Ileum u. Jejunum, Ileojejunitis *f*.
il·e·o·je·ju·nos·to·my [,-,dʒɪdʒu:'nɑstəmɪ] *n chir.* Ileum-Jejunum-Fistel *f*, Ileojejunostomie *f*, Jejunoileostomie *f*.
il·e·o·pex·y ['-peksɪ] *n chir.* Ileumfixierung *f*, -anheftung *f*, Ileopexie *f*.
il·e·o·proc·tos·to·my [,-prɑ'tɑstəmɪ] *n* → ileorectostomy.
il·e·o·rec·tal [,-'rektəl] *adj* Ileum u. Rektum betr. *od.* verbindend, ileorektal.
ileorectal anastomosis ileorektale Anastomose *f*.
ileorectal fistula *patho.* Ileum-Rektum-Fistel *f*, ileorektale Fistel *f*.
il·e·o·rec·tos·to·my [,-rek'tɑstəmɪ] *n chir.* Ileum-Rektum-Fistel *f*, Ileoproktostomie *f*, Ileorektostomie *f*.
il·e·or·rha·phy [ɪlɪ'ɔrəfɪ] *n chir.* Ileumnaht *f*, Ileorrhaphie *f*.
il·e·o·sig·moid fistula [,ɪlɪəʊ'sɪgmɔɪd] *patho.* Ileum-Sigma-Fistel *f*, Ileosigmoidalfistel *f*.
il·e·o·sig·moi·dos·to·my [,-,sɪgmɔɪ'dɑstəmɪ] *n chir.* Ileum-Sigma-Fistel *f*, Ileosigmoidostomie *f*.
il·e·os·to·my [ɪlɪ'ɑstəmɪ] *n* **1.** *chir.* Ileumfistelung *f*, Ileostomie *f*. **2.** ileal stoma.
ileostomy bag Ileostomabeutel *m*.
il·e·ot·o·my [ɪlɪ'ɑtəmɪ] *n chir.* Ileumeröffnung *m*, -schnitt *m*, Ileotomie *f*.
il·e·o·trans·verse colostomy [,ɪlɪəʊtræns'vɜrs] → ileotransversostomy.
il·e·o·trans·ver·sos·to·my [,-trænsvɜrs'ɑstəmɪ] *n chir.* Ileotransversostomie *f*.
il·e·o·ty·phus [,-'taɪfəs] *n old* → typhoid fever.

il·e·o·u·re·thros·to·my [ˌ-jʊərɪ'θrɑstəmɪ] n → ileal conduit.
il·e·um ['ɪlɪəm] n Ileum nt, Intestinum ileum.
il·e·us ['ɪlɪəs] n chir. Darmverschluß m, Ileus m.
Ilfeld ['ɪlfəld]: **I. splint** ortho. Ilfeld-Schiene f.
Ilhéus [ɪ'ljeu:s]: **I. encephalitis** Ilhéus-Enzephalitis f.
  I. fever Ilhéus-Fieber nt.
  I. virus micro. Ilhéus-Virus nt.
ili- pref. → ilio-.
il·i·ac ['ɪlɪæk] adj Darmbein/Os ilium betr., iliakal, Darmbein-.
iliac artery: anterior i. → external i.
  circumflex i., deep tiefe Hüftkranzarterie f, Zirkumflexa f iliaka profunda, A. circumflexa iliaca profunda.
  circumflex i., superficial oberflächliche Hüftkranzarterie f, Zirkumflexa f iliaka superficialis, A. circumflexa iliaca superficialis.
  common i. gemeinsame Hüftschlagader/-arterie f, Iliaka f communis, A. iliaca communis.
  external i. äußere Hüftarterie f, Iliaka f externa, A. iliaca externa.
  internal i. innere Hüftarterie f, Hypogastrika f, Iliaka f interna, old A. hypogastrica, A. iliaca interna.
  small i. → iliolumbar artery.
iliac artery aneurysm Aneurysma nt der A. iliaca communis.
iliac bone Darmbein nt, Ilium nt, Os ilii/iliacum.
iliac branch of iliolumbar artery Beckenkammast m der A. iliolumbalis, Ramus iliacus a. iliolumbalis.
iliac bursa, subtendinous Bursa subtendinea iliaca.
iliac canal Lacuna musculorum.
iliac colon absteigendes Kolon nt, Colon descendens.
iliac crest Becken-, Darmbeinkamm m, Crista iliaca.
iliac crest puncture Beckenkammpunktion f.
iliac fascia Fascia iliaca.
iliac fossa Fossa iliaca.
iliac lymph nodes: common i. Lymphknoten pl der A. iliaca communis, Nodi lymphatici parietales iliaci communes.
  common intermediate i. Nodi lymphatici parietales iliaci communes intermedii.
  common lateral i. Nodi lymphatici parietales iliaci communes laterales.
  common medial i. Nodi lymphatici parietales iliaci communes mediales.
  common promontory i. Nodi lymphatici parietales iliaci communes promontorii.
  common subaortic i. Lymphknoten pl der Aortengabel, Nodi lymphatici parietales iliaci communes subaortici.
  external i. Lymphknoten pl der A. iliaca externa, Nodi lymphatici parietales iliaci externi.
  external interiliac i. zwischen A. iliaca interna u. A. iliaca externa liegende Lymphknoten, Nodi lymphatici parietales (iliaci externi) interiliaci.
  external intermediate i. Nodi lymphatici parietales iliaci externi intermedii.
  external lateral i. Nodi lymphatici parietales iliaci externi laterales.
  external medial i. Nodi lymphatici parietales iliaci externi mediales.
  internal i. Lymphknoten pl der A. iliaca interna, Nodi lymphatici parietales iliaci interni.
iliac mesocolon Mesokolon nt des Sigmas, Mesosigma nt, Mesocolon sigmoideum.
iliac muscle → iliacus (muscle).
il·i·a·co·sub·fas·ci·al fossa [ˌɪlaɪəkəʊsʌb-'fæʃ(ɪ)əl, -'feɪ-] Fossa iliacosubfascialis.
iliac plexuses vegetative Plexus pl der Aa. iliacae, Plexus iliaci.
iliac spine Spina iliaca.
  anterior inferior i. Spina iliaca anterior inferior.
  anterior superior i. Spina iliaca anterior superior.
  posterior inferior i. Spina iliaca posterior inferior.
  posterior superior i. Spina iliaca posterior superior.
iliac tubercle Tuberculum iliacum.
iliac tuberosity Tuberositas iliaca.
il·i·a·cus (muscle) [ɪ'laɪəkəs] Iliakus m, M. iliacus.
iliac vein: common i. gemeinsame Hüftvene f, V. iliaca communis.
  deep circumflex i. Begleitvene f der A. circumflexa iliaca profunda, V. circumflexa iliaca profunda.
  external i. äußere Hüftvene f, V. iliaca externa.
  internal i. innere Hüftvene f, old V. hypogastrica, V. iliaca interna.
  superficial circumflex i. Begleitvene f der A. circumflexa ilium superficialis, V. circumflexa iliaca superficialis.
iliac vein thrombosis Thrombose f der V. iliaca interna.
il·i·a·del·phus [ˌɪlɪə'delfəs] n → iliopagus.
ilio- pref. Ilio-, Darmbein-.
il·i·o·coc·cyg·e·al [ˌɪlɪəʊkak'sɪdʒɪəl] adj Darmbein/Os ilium u. Steißbein/Os coccygis betr., iliokokzygeal.
iliococcygeal muscle → iliococcygeus (muscle).
il·i·o·coc·cyg·e·us (muscle) [ˌ-kak'sɪdʒɪəs] Iliokokzygeus m, M. iliococcygeus.
il·i·o·cos·tal [ˌ-'kɑstl] adj Darmbein/Os ilium u. Rippen/Costae betr., iliokostal.
il·i·o·cos·ta·lis [ˌ-kɑs'tælɪs, -'teɪl-] n Iliokostalis m, M. iliocostalis.
iliocostalis cervicis (muscle) Iliokostalis m cervicis, M. iliocostalis cervicis.
iliocostalis lumborum (muscle) Iliokostalis m lumborum, M. iliocostalis lumborum.
iliocostalis muscle → iliocostalis.
iliocostalis thoracis (muscle) Iliokostalis m thoracis, M. iliocostalis thoracis.
iliocostal ligament Lig. lumbocostale.
iliocostal muscle → iliocostalis.
  i. of back → iliocostalis thoracis (muscle).
  i. of neck → iliocostalis cervicis (muscle).
il·i·o·fem·or·al [ˌ-'femərəl] adj Darmbein/Os ilium u. Oberschenkel/Femur betr., iliofemoral.
iliofemoral ligament Bigelow'-Band nt, Lig. iliofemorale.
iliofemoral triangle ortho. Bryant'-Dreieck nt, Iliofemoraldreieck f.
il·i·o·hy·po·gas·tric nerve [ˌ-ˌhaɪpə'gæstrɪk] Iliohypogastrikus m, N. iliohypogastricus.
il·i·o·in·gui·nal nerve [ˌ-'ɪŋgwənl] Ilioinguinalis m, N. ilioinguinalis.
il·i·o·lum·bar [ˌ-'lʌmbər, -bɑr] adj Darmbein/Os ilium u. Lumbalregion betr., iliolumbal.
iliolumbar artery Iliolumbalis f, A. iliolumbalis.
iliolumbar ligament Lig. iliolumbale.
iliolumbar vein Begleitvene f der A. iliolumbalis, V. iliolumbalis.
il·i·op·a·gus [ɪlɪ'apəgəs] n embryo. Iliopagus m.
il·i·o·pec·tin·e·al [ˌɪlɪəʊpek'tɪnɪəl] adj Darmbein/Os ilium u. Schambein/Os pubis betr., iliopektineal, iliopubisch.
iliopectineal arch Arcus iliopectineus.
iliopectineal bursa Bursa iliopectinea.
iliopectineal crest: i. of iliac bone Linea arcuata ossis ilii.
  i. of pelvis Linea terminalis (pelvis).
  i. of pubis Eminentia iliopubica.
iliopectineal eminence → iliopubic eminence.
iliopectineal fascia → iliopectineal arch.
iliopectineal fossa Fossa iliopectinealis.
iliopectineal line Linea arcuata ossis ilii.
iliopectineal tubercle → iliopubic eminence.
il·i·o·pel·vic [ˌ-'pelvɪk] adj Darmbein/Os ilium u. Becken/Pelvis betr., iliopelvin.
il·i·o·pso·as (muscle) [ˌ-'səʊəs] Iliopsoas m, M. iliopsoas.
iliopsoas sign chir. Cope-Zeichen nt, Psoaszeichen nt.
iliopsoas test → iliopsoas sign.
il·i·o·pu·bic [ˌ-'pju:bɪk] adj → iliopectineal.
iliopubic eminence Eminentia iliopubica/iliopectinea.
iliopubic tract Tractus iliopubicus.
iliopubic tuber → iliopubic eminence.
iliopubic tubercle → iliopubic eminence.
iliopubic vesicular bursa Bursa iliopectinea.
il·i·o·sa·cral [ˌ-'seɪkrəl, '-sæ-] adj Darmbein/Os ilium u. Kreuzbein/Os sacrum betr., iliosakral.
iliosacral articulation Kreuzbein-Darmbein-Gelenk nt, Iliosakralgelenk nt abbr. ISG, Artic. sacroiliaca.
iliosacral joint → iliosacral articulation.
iliosacral ligaments Ligg. sacroiliaca.
  anterior i. Ligg. sacroiliaca ventralia/anteriora.
  interosseous i. Ligg. sacroiliaca interossea.
  long i. Ligg. sacroiliaca dorsalia/posteriora.
il·i·o·spi·nal [ˌ-'spaɪnl] adj Darmbein/Os ilium u. Rückenmark betr., iliospinal.
il·i·o·tho·ra·cop·a·gus [ˌ-ˌθɔrə'kɑpəgəs, -ˌθɔ:-] n embryo. Iliothorakopagus m.
il·i·o·tib·i·al [ˌ-'tɪbɪəl] adj Darmbein/Os ilium u. Schienbein/Tibia betr. od. verbindend, iliotibial.
iliotibial band → iliotibial tract.
iliotibial ligament of Maissiat → iliotibial tract.
iliotibial tract Maissiat'-Streifen m, -Band nt, Tractus iliotibialis.
il·i·o·xi·phop·a·gus [ˌ-zɪ'fɑpəgəs] n embryo. Ilioxiphopagus m.
il·i·um ['ɪlɪəm] pl **il·ia** ['ɪlɪə] Darmbein nt, Ilium nt, Os ilii/iliacum.
ill [ɪl] **I** n **1.** Übel nt, Unglück nt, Mißgeschick nt; Mißstand m. **2.** → illness. **II** adj **3.** krank, erkrankt. **to be taken ~/to fall ~** krank werden, erkranken (with an). **4.** ungünstig, nachteilig; schlecht, übel, schlimm, schädlich.
il·lac·ri·ma·tion [ˌɪlækrə'meɪʃn] n ophthal. Tränenträufeln nt, Dakryorrhoe f, Epiphora f.
il·laq·ue·a·tion [əˌlækwɪ'eɪʃn] n ophthal. Illaqueation f.
il·le·git·i·mate recombination [ˌɪlɪ'dʒɪtəmɪt] genet. illegitime/nichthomologe Rekombination f.
il·li·ni·tion [ɪlə'nɪʃn] n (Salbe) Einreiben nt, Einreibung f.
ill·ness ['ɪlnɪs] n Krankheit f, Erkrankung f, Leiden nt.
il·lu·mi·nate [ɪ'lu:məneɪt] vt be-, ausleuchten.
il·lu·mi·na·tion [ɪˌlu:mə'neɪʃn] n Be-, Ausleuchtung f.

il·lu·mi·na·tor [ɪ'lu:məneɪtər] *n phys., histol.* Beleuchtungsgerät *nt*, -quelle *f*, Illuminator *m*.
il·lu·sion [ɪ'lu:ʒn] *n* **1.** Sinnestäuschung *f*, Illusion *f*. **2.** *psychia.* Trugwahrnehmung *f*, Einbildung *f*, Selbsttäuschung *f*, Wahn *m*, Illusion *f*.
i. of doubles Capgras-Syndrom *nt*.
il·lu·sion·al [ɪ'lu:ʒnəl] *adj* Illusion betr., durch Illusionen gekennzeichnet, Illusions-.
il·lu·sion·ar·y [ɪ'lu:ʒənerɪ] *adj* → illusional.
I.M., i.m. *abbr.* → intramuscular.
im·age ['ɪmɪdʒ] **I** *n* **1.** *phys., mathe., opt.* Bild *nt*. **2.** Erscheinungsform *f*, Gestalt *f*. **3.** *psycho.* Wiedererleben *nt*. **4.** Vorstellung *f*, Bild *nt*. **II** *vt* **5.** bildlich darstellen. **6.** s. etw. vorstellen.
image formation *physiol.* Bildentstehung *f*.
image intensifyer *radiol.* Bildverstärker *m*.
im·ag·i·nar·y [ɪ'mædʒəˌnerɪ] *adj* eingebildet, imaginär; erfunden, frei ersonnen.
im·ag·i·na·tion [ɪˌmædʒɪ'neɪʃn] *n* Vorstellen *nt*; Vorstellung *f*, Einbildung *f*; Phantasie *f*, Vorstellungs-, Einbildungskraft *f*, Imagination *f*. **in ~** in der Vorstellung, im Geiste. **to have (a vivid) ~** (eine rege) Phantasie haben.
im·ag·i·na·tive [ɪ'mædʒənətɪv, -ˌneɪt-] *adj* phantasievoll, -reich, einfallsreich.
im·ag·i·na·tiveness ['-neɪtɪvnɪs] *n* Phantasie *f*, Ideen-, Einfallsreichtum *m*.
im·ag·ine [ɪ'mædʒɪn] *vt* s. (aus-)denken, s. vorstellen, ersinnen.
im·ag·ing method/procedure ['ɪmədʒɪŋ] *radiol.* bildgebendes Verfahren *nt*.
i·ma·go [ɪ'meɪgəʊ] *n, pl* **-goes, i·mag·i·nes** [ɪ'mædʒɪniːz] **1.** *psycho.* Imago *f*. **2.** *zoo.* ausgewachsenes *od.* geschlechtsreifes Insekt *nt*, Vollinsekt *nt*, Imago *f*.
im·bal·ance [ɪm'bæləns] *n* **1.** Ungleichgewicht *nt*, Gleichgewichtsstörung *f*, Unausgewogenheit *f*. **2.** *fig.* Unausgeglichenheit *f*.
im·be·cile ['ɪmbəsɪl] **I** *n* **1.** mittelgradig Schwachsinnige(r *m*) *f*, Imbezi(l)le(r *m*) *f*. **2.** *inf.* Idiot *m*, Trottel *m*. **II** *adj* **3.** mittelgradig schwachsinnig, imbezil(l). **4.** *inf.* idiotisch, vertrottelt, schwachsinnig.
im·be·cil·i·ty [ɪmbə'sɪlətɪ] *n* mittelgradiger Schwachsinn *m*, Imbezil(l)ität *f*.
im·bed [ɪm'bed] *vt* **1.** (*a. histol.*) (ein-)betten; (ein-)lagern. **2.** (fest) umschließen, um-, einhüllen.
im·bibe [ɪm'baɪb] *vt* **1.** trinken. **2.** (*Feuchtigkeit*) aufsaugen.
im·bi·bi·tion [ˌɪmbə'bɪʃn] *n* **1.** (*Flüssigkeit*) Absorption *f*. **2.** Durchtränkung *f*, Durchtränken *nt*, Imbibition *f*.
im·bri·cate ['ɪmbrəkt, -keɪt] *adj histol.* dachziegelartig *od.* schuppenartig angeordnet, geschuppt.
im·bri·cat·ed ['-keɪtɪd] *adj* → imbricate.
Imerslund ['ɪmərslənd]: **I. syndrome** → Imerslund-Graesbeck syndrome.
Imerslund-Graesbeck ['greɪsbek]: **I.-G. syndrome** Imerslund-Gräsbeck-Syndrom *nt*.
im·id·am·ine [ˌɪmɪd'æmɪn] *n pharm.* Antazolin *nt*.
im·id·az·ole [ˌɪ-'æzəʊl] *n* Imidazol *nt*, Glyoxalin *nt*.
imidazole acetol phosphate Imidazolacetolphosphat *nt*.
imidazole glycerol phosphate Imidazolglyzerinphosphat *nt*.
imidazole glycerol phosphate dehydratase Imidazolglyzerinphosphat-dehydratase *f*.
im·id·az·o·lyl·eth·yl·a·mine [ˌɪmɪdˌæzəʊ-

lɪlˌeθəl'æmɪn] *n* Histamin *nt abbr.* H.
im·ide ['ɪmaɪd] *n* Imid *nt*.
imido- *pref.* Imido-.
im·i·do·di·pep·ti·dase [ˌɪmɪdəʊdaɪ'peptɪˌdeɪz] *n* Prolidase *f*, Prolindipeptidase *f*.
im·in·az·ole [ˌɪmɪn'æzəʊl, ɪmɪnə'zəʊl] *n* → imidazole.
imino- *pref.* Imino-.
im·i·no acid ['ɪmɪnəʊ] Iminosäure *f*.
im·i·no·di·a·ce·tic acid [ˌɪmɪnəʊdaɪə'si:tɪk, -'set-, ˌɪˌmi:n-] *abbr.* **IDA** Iminodiessigsäure *f*.
α-im·i·no·glu·ta·rate [ˌ-'glu:təreɪt] *n* α-Iminoglutarat *nt*.
α-im·i·no·glu·tar·ic acid [ˌ-glu:'tærɪk] α-Iminoglutarsäure *f*.
im·i·no·gly·ci·nu·ria [ˌ-glaɪsə'n(j)ʊərɪə] *n* (*renale*) Iminoglycinurie *f*, Iminoazidurie *f*.
im·i·no·u·rea [ˌ-'jʊərɪə] *n* Guanidin *nt*, Iminoharnstoff *m*.
im·ip·ra·mine [ɪ'mɪprəmi:n] *n pharm.* Imipramin *nt*.
im·ma·ture ['ɪmətʃʊər, -'t(j)ʊər] *adj* unreif, unausgereift.
immature cataract beginnender Star *m*, Cataracta incipiens.
immature infant Frühgeborenes *nt*.
immature labor vorzeitige Geburt *f*, Frühgeburt *f*.
immature teratoma unreifes/malignes Teratom *nt*, Teratoma inguinale.
im·ma·tu·ri·ty [ˌɪmə'tʃʊərɪtɪ, -'t(j)ʊər-] *n* **1.** Unreife *f*. **2.** *ped., gyn.* Unreife *f* des Frühgeborenen, Immaturität *f*.
im·me·di·ate [ɪ'mi:dɪɪt] *adj* **1.** unmittelbar, direkt. **2.** (*zeitlich*) unmittelbar (bevorstehend), unverzüglich, sofort, nächste(r, s), Sofort-, Immediat-; (*räumlich*) nächst(gelegen), in unmittelbarer Nähe, Immediat-. **3.** direkt betreffend, unmittelbar berührend.
immediate allergy → immediate hypersensitivity.
immediate auscultation direkte Auskultation *f*.
immediate hypersensitivity anaphylaktische Überempfindlichkeit/Allergie *f*, anaphylaktischer Typ *m* der Überempfindlichkeitsreaktion *f*, Überempfindlichkeitsreaktion *f* vom Soforttyp, Typ I der Überempfindlichkeitsreaktion.
immediate hypersensitivity reaction → immediate hypersensitivity.
immediate percussion direkte Perkussion *f*.
immediate postsurgical prosthesis prosthetische Sofortversorgung *f*.
immediate transfusion direkte Transfusion *f*.
im·med·i·ca·ble [ɪ'medɪkəbl] *adj* (*Krankheit*) unheilbar, inkurabel.
im·merse [ɪ'mɜrs] *vt* (ein-)tauchen (*in* in).
im·mer·sion [ɪ'mɜrʒn, -ʃn] *n* (Ein-, Unter-)Tauchen *nt*; *phys.* Immersion *f*.
immersion lens → immersion objective.
immersion objective Immersionsobjektiv *nt*.
im·mi·nent ['ɪmənənt] *adj* nahe bevorstehend, drohend, imminent.
imminent abortion *gyn.* drohender Abort *m*, Abortus imminens.
im·mis·ci·bil·i·ty [ˌɪmɪsə'bɪlətɪ] *n* Unvermischbarkeit *f*.
im·mis·ci·ble [ɪ'mɪsəbl] *adj phys.* nicht-mischbar.
im·mo·bile [ɪ'məʊbl, -bi:l] *adj* unbeweglich, immobil; bewegungslos; starr, fest.
im·mo·bil·i·ty [ˌɪməʊ'bɪlətɪ] *n* Unbeweglichkeit *f*; Bewegungslosigkeit *f*.
im·mo·bi·li·za·tion [ɪˌməʊbəlaɪ'zeɪʃn] *n* **1.** *ortho.* Ruhigstellung *f*, Immobilisierung

f, Immobilisation *f*. **2.** Feststellen *nt*, Immobilisieren *nt*.
immobilization osteoporosis *ortho.* Immobilisationsosteoporose *f*.
im·mo·bi·lize [ɪ'məʊbəlaɪz] *vt* **1.** *ortho.* ruhigstellen, immobilisieren. **2.** unbeweglich machen, feststellen, immobilisieren.
im·mo·bi·liz·ing antibody [ɪ'məʊbəlaɪzɪŋ] *immun.* Treponema-immobilisierender Antikörper *m*.
immobilizing bandage *ortho.* Immobilisationsverband *m*.
im·mo·tile [ɪ'məʊtl] *adj* feststehend, unbeweglich.
immotile-cilia syndrome immotile-Cilia--Syndrom *nt*.
im·mov·a·ble joint [ɪ'mu:vəbl] Bandverbindung *f*, Artic. fibrosa.
immun- *pref.* → immuno-.
im·mune [ɪ'mju:n] **I** *n* immune Person *f*. **II** *adj* **1.** *fig.* immun, geschützt (*against*, *to* gegen); gefeit (*against*, *to* gegen); unempfänglich. **2.** Immunsystem *od.* Immunantwort betr., immun (*against*, *to* gegen); Immun(o)-.
immune adherence Immunadhärenz *f*.
immune adherence factor Immunadhärenzfaktor *m*.
immune adherence hemagglutination assay *abbr.* **IAHA** Immunadhärenz--Hämagglutinationstest *m*.
immune adsorption Immunadsorption *f*.
immune agglutinin Immunagglutinin *nt*.
immune antibody Immunantikörper *m*.
immune assay → immunoassay.
immune body Antikörper *m abbr.* AK, Ak.
immune complex *abbr.* **IC** Immunkomplex *m abbr.* IK, IC, Antigen-Antikörper-Komplex *m abbr.* AAK.
immune-complex disease/disorder Immunkomplexkrankheit *f*.
immune complex glomerulonephritis Immunkomplexglomerulonephritis *f*.
immune complex hypersensitivity Immunkomplex-vermittelte Überempfindlichkeitsreaktion *f*, Arthus-Typ *m* der Überempfindlichkeitsreaktion, Typ III *m* der Überempfindlichkeitsreaktion.
immune complex nephritis Immunkomplexnephritis *f*.
immune conglutinin → immunoconglutinin.
immune deficiency → immunodeficiency.
immune deviation Immundeviation *f*.
immune globulin Immunglobulin *n*.
cytomegalovirus i. *abbr.* **CMVIG** Zytomegalievirusimmunoglobulin.
hepatitis B i. *abbr.* **HBIG** Hepatitis B-Immunglobulin *abbr.* HBIG.
rabies i., human *abbr.* **RIG** humanes Rabiesimmunglobulin *abbr.* RIG.
tetanus i. *abbr.* **TIG** Tetanusimmunglobulin.
varicella-zoster i. *abbr.* **VZIG** Varicella--Zoster-Immunglobulin *abbr.* VZIG.
immune globulin chain Immunglobulinkette *f*.
immune hemolysin Immunhämolysin *nt*.
immune hemolysis Immunhämolyse *f*.
immune interferon γ-Interferon *nt abbr.* IFN-γ.
immune mechanism Immunmechanismus *m*.
immune opsonin opsonisierender Antikörper *m*.
immune paralysis Immunparalyse *f*.
immune protein → immune body.
immune reaction → immune response.
immune response Immunantwort *f*, -reaktion *f*, immunologische Reaktion *f*.
cellular i. zelluläre Immunantwort.

delayed i. Immunreaktion vom verzögerten Typ.
humoral i. humorale Immunantwort.
immediate i. Immunreaktion vom Soforttyp.
primary i. Primärantwort, -reaktion.
secondary i. Sekundärantwort, -reaktion.
immune response genes Immunantwort-Gene *pl*, Immune-response-Gene *pl*, Ir-Gene *pl*.
immune serum Immun-, Antiserum *nt*.
immune suppressor genes Immunsuppressionsgene *pl*, Is-Gene *pl*.
immune surveillance → immunosurveillance.
immune system Immunsystem *nt*.
immune system suppression → immunosuppression.
immune thrombocytopenia Immunthrombocytopenie *f*.
immune thyroiditis Hashimoto-Thyreoiditis *f*, Struma lymphomatosa.
immune tolerance 1. Immuntoleranz *f abbr.* IT. **2.** Immunparalyse *f*.
im·mu·ni·fa·cient [ɪˌmjuːnəˈfeɪʃənt] *adj* Immunität hervorrufend, immunisierend.
im·mu·ni·ty [ɪˈmjuːnətɪ] *n* Immunität *f*, Unempfänglichkeit *f (from, against* gegen*)*.
immunity deficiency → immunodeficiency.
im·mu·ni·za·tion [ˌɪmjənəˈzeɪʃn, ˌmjuː-] *n* Immunisierung *f*, Immunisation *f*.
im·mu·nize [ˈɪmjənaɪz, ˈmjuː-] *vt* immunisieren, immun machen *(against* gegen*)*.
immuno- *pref.* Immun-, Immuno-.
im·mu·no·ad·ju·vant [ˌɪmjənəʊˈædʒəvənt ˌmjuː-] *n* Immun(o)adjuvans *nt*.
im·mu·no·ad·sor·bent [ˌ-ædˈsɔːrbənt] *n* Immunadsorbens *nt*, Immunosorbens *nt*.
im·mu·no·ad·sorp·tion [ˌ-ædˈsɔːrpʃn] *n* Immunadsorption *f*.
im·mu·no·ag·glu·ti·na·tion [ˌ-əˌɡluːtəˈneɪʃn] *n* Immunagglutination *f*.
im·mu·no·as·say [ˌ-əˈseɪ, -ˈæseɪ] *n* Immunoassay *m*.
im·mu·no·bi·ol·o·gy [ˌ-baɪˈɒlədʒɪ] *n* Immunbiologie *f*.
im·mu·no·blast [ˈ-blæst] *n* Immunoblast *m*.
im·mu·no·blas·tic lymphadenopathy [ˌ-ˈblæstɪk] angioimmunoblastische/immunoblastische Lymphadenopathie *f*, Lymphogranulomatosis X *f*.
immunoblastic (malignant) lymphoma immunoblastisches (malignes) Lymphom *nt*, Retikulumzellensarkom *nt*.
immunoblastic sarcoma → immunoblastic (malignant) lymphoma.
B-cell i. B-Zellen-immunoblastisches Sarkom *nt*.
T-cell i. T-Zellen-immunoblastisches Sarkom *nt*.
im·mu·no·chem·i·cal [ˌ-ˈkemɪkl] *adj* Immun(o)chemie betr., immunochemisch.
im·mu·no·chem·is·try [ˌ-ˈkeməstrɪ] *n* Immun(o)chemie *f*.
im·mu·no·che·mo·ther·a·py [ˌ-ˌkiːməʊˈθerəpɪ, -ˌkem-] *n* kombinierte Immun- u. Chemotherapie *f*, Immun(o)chemotherapie *f*.
im·mu·no·com·pe·tence [ˌ-ˈkɒmpətəns] *n* Immunkompetenz *f*.
im·mu·no·com·pe·tent [ˌ-ˈkɒmpətənt] *adj* immunologisch kompetent, immunkompetent.
immunocompetent cell Immunozyt *m*, immunkompetente Zelle *f*.
im·mu·no·com·plex [ˌ-ˈkɒmpleks] *n* → immune complex.
im·mu·no·com·pro·mised [ˌ-ˈkɒmprəmaɪzd] *adj* mit geschwächter (Immun-)Abwehr, abwehrgeschwächt.
im·mu·no·con·glu·ti·nin [ˌ-kɒnˈɡluːtɪnɪn, -kən-] *n* Immunkonglutinin *nt*.
im·mu·no·cyte [ˌ-ˈsaɪt] *n* immunkompetente Zelle *f*, Immunozyt *m*.
im·mu·no·cy·to·ad·her·ence [ˌ-ˌsaɪtəædˈhɪərəns] *n* Immunozytoadhärenz *f*.
im·mu·no·cy·to·chem·is·try [ˌ-ˌsaɪtəˈkeməstrɪ] *n* Immunozytochemie *f*.
im·mu·no·cy·to·ma [ˌ-saɪˈtəʊmə] *n* Immunozytom *nt*, lymphoplastozytisches/lympho-plasmozytoides Lymphom *nt*.
im·mu·no·de·fi·cien·cy [ˌ-dɪˈfɪʃənsɪ] *n*, *pl* **-cies** Immundefekt *m*, Immunmangelkrankheit *f*, Defektimmunopathie *f*.
i. with elevated IGM Immundefektsyndrom *nt* mit IGM-Überproduktion.
i. with hyper-IGM → i. with elevated IGM.
i. with increased IGM → i. with elevated IGM.
i. with short-limbed dwarfism Immunmangel mit disproportioniertem Zwergwuchs.
i. with thrombocytopenia and eczema Wiskott-Aldrich-Syndrom *n*.
i. with thymoma Immundefekt mit Thymom.
immunodeficiency disease/disorder/syndrome → immunodeficiency.
im·mu·no·de·pres·sant [ˌ-dɪˈpresənt] *n* → immunosuppressive agent.
im·mu·no·de·pres·sion [ˌ-dɪˈpreʃn] *n* → immunosuppression.
im·mu·no·de·pres·sive [ˌ-dɪˈpresɪv] **I** *n* → immunosuppressive agent. **II** *adj* → immunosuppressive II.
im·mu·no·de·pres·sor [ˌ-dɪˈpresər] *n* → immunosuppressive agent.
im·mu·no·der·ma·tol·o·gy [ˌ-ˌdɜːrməˈtɒlədʒɪ] *n* Immundermatologie *f*.
im·mu·no·de·vi·a·tion [ˌ-dɪvɪˈeɪʃn] *n* Immundeviation *f*.
im·mu·no·di·ag·no·sis [ˌ-daɪəɡˈnəʊsɪs] *n* Sero-, Serumdiagnostik *f*.
im·mu·no·dif·fu·sion [ˌ-dɪˈfjuːʒn] *n* Immun(o)diffusion *f*.
im·mu·no·dom·i·nance [ˌ-ˈdɒmɪnəns] *n* Immun(o)dominanz *f*.
im·mu·no·dom·i·nant [ˌ-ˈdɒmɪnənt] *adj* immun(o)dominant.
im·mu·no·e·lec·tro·pho·re·sis [ˌ-ɪˌlektrəʊfəˈriːsɪs] *n*, IEP Immun(o)elektrophorese *f*.
im·mu·no·fer·ri·tin [ˌ-ˈferɪtɪn] *n* Antikörper-Ferritin-Konjugat *nt*.
im·mu·no·fil·tra·tion [ˌ-fɪlˈtreɪʃn] *n* Immunofiltration *f*.
im·mu·no·flu·o·res·cence [ˌ-flʊəˈresəns, -flɔː-, -fləʊ-] *n* Immun(o)fluoreszenz *f*.
immunofluorescence microscopy Immun(o)fluoreszenzmikroskopie *f*.
im·mu·no·flu·o·res·cent stain [ˌ-flʊəˈresnət] Immun(o)fluoreszenzfärbung *f*.
im·mu·no·gen [ˈɪmjuːnədʒən] *n* Immunogen *nt*.
im·mu·no·ge·net·ic [ˌɪmjənəʊdʒəˈnetɪk, ˌmjuː-] *adj* Immungenetik betr., immungenetisch.
im·mu·no·ge·net·ics [ˌ-dʒəˈnetɪks] *pl* Immungenetik *f*.
im·mu·no·gen·ic [ˌ-ˈdʒenɪk] *adj* Immunität hervorrufend, eine Immunantwort auslösend, immunogen.
im·mu·no·ge·nic·i·ty [ˌ-dʒəˈnɪsətɪ] *n* Immunogenität *f*.
im·mu·no·glob·u·lin [ˌ-ˈɡlɒbjəlɪn] *n abbr.* **Ig** Immunglobulin *nt abbr.* Ig.
immunoglobulin A *abbr.* **IgA** Immunglobulin A *nt abbr.* IgA.
immunoglobulin class switch Ig-Klassen-Switch *m*.
immunoglobulin D *abbr.* **IgD** Immunglobulin D *nt abbr.* IgD.
immunoglobulin E *abbr.* **IgE** Immunglobulin E *nt abbr.* IgE.
immunoglobulin G *abbr.* **IgG** Immunglobulin G *nt abbr.* IgG.
immunoglobulin genes Immunoglobulingene *pl*.
immunoglobulin M *abbr.* **IgM** Immunglobulin M *nt abbr.* IgM.
im·mu·no·glob·u·li·nop·a·thy [ˌ-ˌɡlɒbjəlɪˈnɒpəθɪ] *n* Gammapathie *f*.
im·mu·no·he·ma·tol·o·gy [ˌ-hiːməˈtɒlədʒɪ, -hem-] *n* Immunhämatologie *f*.
im·mu·no·he·mol·y·sis [ˌ-hɪˈmɒləsɪs] *n* Immun(o)hämolyse *f*.
im·mu·no·his·to·chem·i·cal [ˌ-hɪstəˈkemɪkl] *adj* Immunhistochemie betr., immunhistochemisch.
im·mu·no·his·to·che·mis·try [ˌ-hɪstəˈkeməstrɪ] *n* Immunhistochemie *f*.
im·mu·no·his·to·flu·o·res·cence [ˌ-ˌhɪstəflʊəˈresəns] *n* Immunhistofluoreszenz *f*.
im·mu·no·in·com·pe·tence [ˌ-ɪnˈkɒmpətəns] *n* Immuninkompetenz *f*.
im·mu·no·in·com·pe·tent [ˌ-ɪnˈkɒmpətənt] *adj* immunologisch inkompetent, immuninkompetent.
im·mu·no·log·ic [ˌɪmjənəˈlɒdʒɪk, ˌmjuː-] *adj* → immunological.
im·mu·no·log·i·cal [ˌ-ˈlɒdʒɪkl] *adj* Immunologie betr., immunologisch, Immun(o)-.
immunological deficiency → immunodeficiency.
immunological deficiency syndrome → immunodeficiency.
im·mu·no·log·i·cal·ly competent [ˌ-ˈlɒdʒɪklɪ] → immunocompetent.
immunologically competent cell → immunocyte.
immunologically incompetent → immunoincompetent.
immunological memory immunologisches Gedächtnis *nt*.
immunological reaction → immune response.
immunological response → immune response.
immunological surveillance → immunosurveillance.
immunological tolerance → immunologic tolerance.
immunologic competence → immunocompetence.
immunologic enhancement immunologische Verstärkung *f*.
immunologic incompetence → immunoincompetence.
immunologic paralysis Immunparalyse *f*.
immunologic resistance Immunresistenz *f*.
immunologic tolerance 1. Immuntoleranz *f abbr.* IT. **2.** Immunparalyse *f*.
acquired i. erworbene Immuntoleranz.
high-dose i. high-dose-Immuntoleranz.
high-zone i. → high-dose i.
low-dose i. low-dose-Immuntoleranz.
low-zone i. → low-dose i.
im·mu·nol·o·gist [ˌɪmjəˈnɒlədʒɪst] *n* Immunologe *m*, -login *f*.
im·mu·nol·o·gy [ˌɪmjəˈnɒlədʒɪ] *n* Immunologie *f*, Immunitätsforschung *f*, -lehre *f*.
im·mu·no·mod·u·la·tion [ˌɪmjənəʊmɒdʒəˈleɪʃn, ˌmjuː-] *n* Immunmodulation *f*.
im·mu·no·mod·u·la·tor [ˌ-ˈmɒdʒəleɪtər] *n* Immunmodulator *m*.
im·mu·no·par·a·si·tol·o·gy [ˌ-ˌpærəsaɪˈtɒlədʒɪ] *n* Immunparasitologie *f*.
im·mu·no·path·o·gen·e·sis [ˌ-ˌpæθəˈdʒenəsɪs] *n* Immunpathogenese *f*.
im·mu·no·path·o·log·ic [ˌ-ˌpæθəˈlɒdʒɪk] *adj* Immunpathologie betr., immun(o)pathologisch.

immunopathology

im·mu·no·pa·thol·o·gy [,-pə'θalədʒɪ] n Immun(o)pathologie f.
im·mu·no·phys·i·ol·o·gy [,-fɪzɪ'alədʒɪ] n Immunphysiologie f.
im·mu·no·po·ten·ti·a·tion [,-pə,tentʃɪ'eɪʃn] n Verstärkung f der Immunantwort.
im·mu·no·po·ten·ti·a·tor [,-pə'tentʃɪeɪtər] n die Immunantwort verstärkendes Mittel nt.
im·mu·no·pre·cip·i·ta·tion [,-prɪ,sɪpə'teɪʃn] n Immunpräzipitation f.
im·mu·no·pro·lif·er·a·tive [,-prə'lɪfəreɪtɪv] adj immunproliferativ.
immunoproliferative disorder immunproliferative Erkrankung f.
im·mu·no·pro·phy·lax·is [,-prəʊfə'læksɪs] n Immunprophylaxe f.
im·mu·no·ra·di·o·met·ric assay [,-,reɪdɪə-'metrɪk] immunradiometrische Bestimmung/Analyse f.
im·mu·no·ra·di·om·e·try [,-reɪdɪ'amətrɪ] n Immun(o)radiometrie f.
im·mu·no·re·ac·tion [,-rɪ'ækʃn] n → immune response.
im·mu·no·re·ac·tive [,-rɪ'æktɪv] adj eine Immunreaktion zeigend od. gebend, immun(o)reaktiv.
im·mu·no·re·ac·tiv·i·ty [,-rɪæk'tɪvətɪ] n Immunreaktivität f.
im·mu·no·reg·u·la·tion [,-regjə'leɪʃn] n Steuerung f der Immunantwort, Immunregulation f.
im·mu·no·scin·tig·ra·phy [,-sɪn'tɪgrəfɪ] n radiol. Immunszintigraphie f.
im·mu·no·se·lec·tion [,-sɪ'lekʃn] n Immunselektion f.
im·mu·no·sor·bent [,-'sɔːrbənt] n Immunadsorbens nt, Immunosorbens nt.
im·mu·no·stim·u·lant [,-'stɪmjələnt] n immun(system)stimulierende Substanz f, Immunstimulans nt.
im·mu·no·stim·u·la·tion [,-stɪmjə'leɪʃn] n Immunstimulation f.
im·mu·no·stim·u·la·to·ry agent [,-'stɪmjə-lə,tɔːrɪ, -təʊ-] → immunostimulant.
im·mu·no·sup·pres·sant [,-sə'presənt] n → immunosuppressive agent.
im·mu·no·sup·pressed [,-sə'prest] adj immunsupprimiert.
im·mu·no·sup·pres·sion [,-sə'preʃn] n Unterdrückung od. Abschwächung f der Immunreaktion, Immun(o)suppression f, Immun(o)depression f.
im·mu·no·sup·pres·sive [,-sə'presɪv] I n → immunosuppressive agent. II adj die Immunreaktion unterdrückend od. abschwächend, immun(o)suppressiv, immun(o)depressiv.
immunosuppressive agent Immun(o)-suppressivum nt, Immun(o)depressivum nt, immun(o)suppressive/immun(o)depressive Substanz f.
immunosuppressive drug → immunosuppressive agent.
immunosuppressive therapy Immunsuppression f.
im·mu·no·sur·veil·lance [,-sɜːr'veɪl(j)əns] n Immunüberwachung f, -surveillance f.
im·mu·no·ther·a·py [,-'θerəpɪ] n Immuntherapie f.
im·mu·no·tol·er·ance [,-'talərən(t)s] n → immunologic tolerance.
im·mu·no·tox·in [,-'taksɪn] n Immun(o)toxin nt.
im·mu·no·trans·fu·sion [,-trænz'fjuːʃn] n Immun(o)transfusion f.
im·mu·no·type [ɪ'mjuːnətaɪp] n Serotyp m, Serovar m.
immunotype-specific antigen (immuno-)-typenspezifisches Antigen nt.
i·mol·a·mine [aɪ'maləmɪn] n pharm. Imolamin nt.

IMP abbr. → inosine monophosphate.
im·pact¹ ['ɪmpækt] n 1. Zusammenprall m, Anprall m; Auftreffen nt, Aufprall m. 2. phys. Stoß m, Schlag m; Wucht f. 3. fig. (Ein-)Wirkung f, Auswirkungen pl, (starker) Einfluß m (on auf).
im·pact² [ɪm'pækt] vt 1. einkeilen, ein-, festklemmen. 2. zusammenpressen, -drücken. 3. ver-, vollstopfen.
im·pact·ed [ɪm'pæktɪd] adj eingekeilt, verkeilt, impaktiert.
impacted cerumen Ohrschmalz-, Zeruminalpfropf m, Cerumen obturans.
impacted earwax → impacted cerumen.
impacted fracture eingestauchte Fraktur f.
im·pac·tion [ɪm'pækʃn] n ortho. Einkeilung f, Verkeilung f, Impaktion f.
im·pair [ɪm'peər] vt beeinträchtigen; (ab-)-schwächen; (Gesundheit) schädigen.
im·pair·ment [ɪm'peərmənt] n Beeinträchtigung f, (Ab-)Schwächung f; (Gesundheit) Schädigung f.
im·pal·pa·ble [ɪm'pælpəbl] adj 1. (Pulver) sehr fein. 2. (Puls) nicht palpierbar. 3. unfühlbar, ungreifbar; kaum (er-)faßbar.
im·par ['ɪmpaːr] adj anat. ungleich, ungerade, impar; ungepaart.
im·pa·tent [ɪm'peɪtənt] adj (Gang) verschlossen, nicht durchgängig.
im·pa·tience [ɪm'peɪʃns] n Ungeduld f, ungeduldiges Verlangen nt (for nach).
im·pa·tient [ɪm'peɪʃənt] adj 1. ungeduldig. 2. unduldsam, intolerant (gegenüber).
IMP cyclohydrolase IMP-Cyclohydrolase f, Inosinsäurecyclohydrolase f.
IMP dehydrogenase IMP-Dehydrogenase f, Inosinsäuredehydrogenase f.
im·ped·ance [ɪm'piːdns] n 1. abbr. **Z** electr. Scheinwiderstand m, Impedanz f abbr. Z. 2. akustischer Widerstand m, akustische Impedanz f, (Schall-)Impedanz f.
impedance adaptation physiol. Impedanzanpassung f, -adaptation f.
impedance audiometry HNO Impedanzaudiometrie f.
impedance matching phys. Impedanzanpassung f.
im·pen·e·tra·bil·i·ty [ɪm,penɪtrə'bɪlətɪ] n phys. Undurchdringlichkeit f.
im·pen·e·tra·ble [ɪm'penɪtrəbl] adj phys. undurchdringlich (by für).
im·per·cep·ti·ble [,ɪmpər'septɪbl] adj 1. nicht wahrnehmbar, unmerklich, imperzeptibel. 2. verschwindend klein.
im·per·cep·tion [,-'sepʃn] n eingeschränkte/verminderte Wahrnehmungsfähigkeit f.
im·per·cep·tive [,-'septɪv] adj → impercipient.
im·per·cip·i·ent [,-'sɪpɪənt] adj 1. ohne Wahrnehmung, nicht wahrnehmend. 2. fig. begriffsstutzig, beschränkt.
im·per·fect [ɪm'pɜːrfɪkt] adj unvollkommen, unvollständig, unvollendet, imperfekt; mangelhaft, fehlerhaft, schwach.
imperfect fungi micro. unvollständige Pilze pl, Fungi imperfecti, Deuteromyzeten pl, Deuteromycetes pl, Deuteromycotina pl.
imperfect stage micro. ungeschlechtliche/vegetative Phase f.
imperfect yeast micro. unechte/imperfekte Hefe f.
im·per·fo·rate [ɪm'pɜːrfərɪt, -reɪt] adj patho. ohne Öffnung, verschlossen, nicht-perforiert, atretisch.
imperforate anus embryo. Analatresie f, Atresia ani.
imperforate hymen nicht-perforiertes Hymen nt, Hymen imperforatus.

im·per·fo·ra·tion [ɪm,pɜːrfə'reɪʃn] n patho. angeborener Verschluß m, angeborene Atresie f, Imperforatio f.
im·per·me·a·bil·i·ty [ɪm,pɜːrmɪə'bɪlətɪ] n Undurchdringbarkeit f, Undurchlässigkeit f, Impermeabilität f.
im·per·me·a·ble [ɪm'pɜːrmɪəbl] adj undurchdringbar, undurchlässig, impermeabel (to für).
im·per·vi·ous [ɪm'pɜːrvɪəs] adj 1. → impermeable. 2. unempfindlich (to gegen).
im·per·vi·ous·ness ['-nɪs] n 1. → impermeability. 2. Unempfindlichkeit f (to gegen).
im·pe·tig·i·ni·za·tion [,ɪmpe,tɪdʒənaɪ'zeɪʃn] n derm. Impetiginisierung f, Impetiginisation f.
im·pe·tig·i·nous [,-'tɪdʒənəs] adj derm. Impetigo betr., impetigoartig, borkig, impetiginös.
impetiginous cheilitis Lippenimpetigo f.
impetiginous syphilid impetiginöses Syphilid nt.
im·pe·ti·go [,ɪmpə'tiːgəʊ, -taɪ-] n derm. 1. Eiter-, Grind-, Krusten-, Pustelflechte f, feuchter Grind m, Impetigo contagiosa/vulgaris. 2. Schälblasenausschlag m, Pemphigoid nt der Neugeborenen, Impetigo bullosa, Pemphigus (acutus) neonatorum f.
impetigo-like adj derm. impetigoähnlich, impetiginoid.
im·pe·tus ['ɪmpətəs] n 1. phys. Stoß-, Triebkraft f, Antrieb m, Schwung m, Impetus m. 2. fig., psycho. Antrieb m, Anstoß m, Impuls m, Schwung m, Impetus m.
im·pi·la·tion [,ɪmpaɪ'leɪʃn] n hema. Geldrollenbildung f, -agglutination f, Rouleau-Bildung f.
im·plant [n 'ɪmplænt; v ɪm'plænt] chir., ortho. I n Implantat nt. II vt ein-, ver-, überpflanzen (in, into); implantieren.
im·plan·ta·tion [,ɪmplæn'teɪʃn] n 1. gyn., embryo. Einnistung f, Implantation f, Nidation f. 2. chir., ortho. Ein-, Ver-, Überpflanzung f, Implantation f. 3. dent. Implantation f.
implantation cone Axonhügel m, Ursprungskegel m.
implantation cyst Implantationszyste f.
implantation dermoid Epidermal-, Epidermoid-, Epidermiszyste f, epidermale Zyste f.
implantation metastasis Implantationsmetastase f.
im·plant·ed pacemaker [ɪm'plæntɪd] card. interner/implantierter Herzschrittmacher m.
implant forceps chir. Implantationspinzette f.
im·ple·ment ['ɪmplɪmənt] I n Werkzeug nt, (Arbeits-)Gerät nt, Utensilien pl, Zubehör nt; Hilfsmittel nt. II vt aus-, durchführen.
im·plic·it [ɪm'plɪsɪt] adj 1. → implied. 2. mathe. implizit. 3. verborgen, hintergründig. 4. absolut, vorbehaltlos, bedingungslos.
im·plied [ɪm'plaɪd] adj inbegriffen, mitverstanden, mitenthalten, einbezogen.
im·plode [ɪm'pləʊd] vi phys. implodieren.
im·plo·sion [ɪm'pləʊʒn] n phys. Implosion f; implodieren nt.
im·po·tence ['ɪmpətəns] n 1. Unvermögen nt, Unfähigkeit f, Impotenz f; Schwäche f, Kraftlosigkeit f. 2. andro. männliche Unfähigkeit f zum Geschlechtsverkehr, Impotentia coeundi. 3. andro. Zeugungsunfähigkeit f, Unvermögen nt, Sterilität f des Mannes, Impotentia generandi.
im·po·ten·cy ['ɪmpətənsɪ] n → impotence.

390

im·po·tent ['ɪmpətənt] *adj* **1.** unfähig (*in doing, to do* zu tun); hilflos, ohnmächtig; schwach, kraftlos. **2.** *andro.* impotent; zeugungsunfähig.

im·po·ten·tia [,ɪmpə'tenʃɪə] *n* → impotence.

im·preg·na·ble [ɪm'pregnəbl] *adj* imprägnierbar.

im·preg·nate [*adj* ɪm'pregnɪt, -neɪt; *v* -neɪt, 'ɪmpregneɪt] **I** *adj* befruchtet; schwanger. **II** *vt* **1.** befruchten; schwängern. **2.** *chem.* sättigen, durchdringen; *phys.* imprägnieren, (durch-)tränken (*with* mit).

im·preg·na·tion [,ɪmpreg'neɪʃn] *n* **1.** *bio.* Befruchtung *f*, Imprägnation *f*; Schwängerung *f*. **2.** *phys., chem.* Sättigen *nt*, Sättigung *f*, Imprägnierung *f*; gesättigter Zustand *m*; Durchtränkung *f*.

im·press·i·bil·i·ty [ɪm,presə'bɪlətɪ] *n* Empfänglichkeit *f*.

im·press·i·ble [ɪm'presɪbl] *adj* empfänglich (*to* für); leicht zu beeindrucken (*to* durch).

im·pres·sio [ɪm'presɪəʊ] *n* → impression 1.

im·pres·sion [ɪm'preʃn] *n* **1.** *anat.* Eindruck *m*, Abdruck *m*, Impressio *f*. **2.** Eindruck *m* (*of* von); Vermutung *f*, Gefühl *nt*; *psycho.* (Sinnes-)Eindruck *m*, sinnlicher Reiz *m*. **3.** Einwirkung *f* (*on* auf). **4.** Eindrücken *nt* (*in, into* in).
i. for/of costoclavicular ligament Impressio lig. costoclavicularis.

im·pres·sion·a·ble [ɪm'preʃənəbl] *adj* **1.** → impressible. **2.** leicht zu beeindrucken, für Eindrücke empfänglich.

impression preparation *histol.* Abklatschpräparat *nt*.

impression tonometer *ophthal.* Impressionstonometer *nt*.

impression tonometry *ophthal.* Impressionstonometrie *f*.

impressive aphasia [ɪm'presɪv] sensorische Aphasie *f*, Wernicke-Aphasie *f*.

im·print·ing [ɪm'prɪntɪŋ] *n physiol.* Prägung *f*.

im·prob·a·bil·i·ty [ɪm,prɒbə'bɪlətɪ] *n* Unwahrscheinlichkeit *f*.

im·prob·a·ble [ɪm'prɒbəbl] *adj* unwahrscheinlich.

im·prove [ɪm'pruːv] **I** *vt* verbessern; (*Methode*) verfeinern. **II** *vi* s. (ver-)bessern, besser werden, Fortschritte machen, s. erholen.

im·prove·ment [ɪm'pruːvmənt] *n* **1.** (Ver-)Besserung *f*; Erholung *f*; (*Methode*) Verfeinerung *f*. **2.** Vermehrung *f*, Erhöhung *f*, Steigerung *f*.

im·pulse ['ɪmpʌls] *n* **1.** Stoß *m*, Antrieb *m*. **2.** *fig.* Anreiz *m*, Anregung *f*, Impuls *m*. **(to act) on ~** impulsiv *od.* aus einem Impuls heraus (handeln). **3.** *phys.* Impuls *m*; *electr.* (Strom-, Spannungs-)Stoß *m*. **4.** *physiol.* (Nerven-)Impuls *m*, (An-)Reiz *m*. **5.** *psycho.* Impuls *m*.

impulse-conducting fibers Purkinje-Fasern *pl*.

impulse volley Impulsserie *f*.

im·pul·sion [ɪm'pʌlʃn] *n* **1.** *psycho.* Trieb *m*, Drang *m*, Zwang *m*. **2.** Antrieb(skraft *f*) *m*, Triebkraft *f*.

im·pul·sive [ɪm'pʌlsɪv] *adj* **1.** impulsiv, spontan. **2.** (an-)treibend, Trieb-.

im·pul·sive·ness [-nɪs] *n* → impulsivity.

im·pul·siv·i·ty [,ɪmpʌl'sɪvətɪ] *n* impulsives Wesen *od.* Verhalten *nt*, Spontaneität *f*, Impulsivität *f*.

im·pure [ɪm'pjʊər] *adj* unrein, schmutzig, verunreinigt, unsauber; verfälscht; gemischt.

im·pure·ness ['-nɪs] *n* → impurity.

im·pu·ri·ty [ɪm'pjʊərətɪ] *n* Schmutz *m*, Verunreinigung *f*, Unreinheit *f*.

IMV *abbr.* → intermittent mandatory ventilation.

IMViC character [indole production, methyl red test, Voges-Proskauer reaction, citrate utilisation] *micro.* IMViC-Eigenschaften *pl*.

IMViC reactions/test *micro.* IMViC-Testkombination *f*.

In *abbr.* → indium.

in·a·bil·i·ty [ɪnə'bɪlətɪ] *n* Unfähigkeit *f*, Unvermögen *nt*.

in·ac·cu·ra·cy [ɪn'ækjərəsɪ] *n* **1.** Ungenauigkeit *f*. **2.** Fehler *m*, Irrtum *m*.

in·ac·cu·rate [ɪn'ækjərɪt] *adj* **1.** ungenau. **2.** unrichtig, falsch.

in·ac·cu·rate·ness ['-nɪs] *n* Ungenauigkeit *f*.

in·a·cid·i·ty [ɪnə'sɪdətɪ] *n* Anazidität *f*.

in·ac·tion [ɪn'ækʃn] *n* **1.** Untätigkeit *f*. **2.** Trägheit *f*, Faulheit *f*. **3.** Ruhe *f*.

in·ac·ti·vate [ɪn'æktɪveɪt] *vt* **1.** *immun.* unwirksam machen, inaktivieren. **2.** *micro.* inaktivieren.

in·ac·ti·vat·ed vaccine [ɪn'æktɪveɪtɪd] Totimpfstoff *m*, -vakzine *f*, inaktivierter Impfstoff *m*.

in·ac·ti·va·tion [ɪn,æktɪ'veɪʃn] *n* Inaktivieren *nt*, Inaktivierung *f*.

in·ac·ti·va·tor [ɪn'æktɪveɪtər] *n* inaktivierende Substanz *f*, Inaktivator *m*.

in·ac·tive [ɪn'æktɪv] *adj* **1.** untätig, nicht aktiv. **2.** träge, faul; lustlos. **3.** *chem., phys.* unwirksam, inaktiv; ohne optische Aktivität; nicht radioaktiv. **4.** *patho.* ruhend, inaktiv, Inaktivitäts-.

inactive tuberculosis inaktive/vernarbte/ verheilte Tuberkulose *f*.

in·ac·tiv·i·ty [ɪnæk'tɪvətɪ] *n* **1.** → inaction 1, 2. **2.** *chem., phys.* Unwirksamkeit *f*, Inaktivität *f*. **3.** *patho.* Untätigkeit *f*, Ruhen *nt*, Inaktivität *f*.

in·a·dapt·a·bil·i·ty [ɪnə,dæptə'bɪlətɪ] *n* **1.** Mangel *m* an Anpassungsfähigkeit. **2.** Unverwendbarkeit *f*.

in·a·dapt·a·ble [ɪnə'dæptəbl] *adj* **1.** nicht anpassungsfähig (*to* an). **2.** unverwendbar (*to* für).

in·ad·e·qua·cy [ɪn'ædɪkwəsɪ] *n* **1.** Unangemessenheit *f*, Inadäquatheit *f*. **2.** Unzulänglichkeit *f*.

in·ad·e·quate [ɪn'ædɪkwɪt] *adj* **1.** nicht passend, nicht entsprechend, unangemessen (*to*); inadäquat. **2.** unzulänglich, ungenügend, inadäquat.

inadequate stimulus unterschwelliger Reiz *m*.

in·a·li·men·tal [ɪnælə'mentl] *adj* nicht nahrhaft, nicht als Nahrungsmittel geeignet.

in·an·i·mate [ɪn'ænɪmɪt] *adj bio.* unbelebt, leblos.

in·an·i·mate·ness [-'ænɪmətnɪs] *n* Unbelebtheit *f*, Leblosigkeit *f*.

in·an·i·ma·tion [ɪn,ænɪ'meɪʃn] *n* → inanimateness.

in·a·ni·tion [ɪnə'nɪʃn] *n patho.* Inanition *f*.

inanition fever *pat.* Durstfieber *nt*.

in·ap·pa·rent [ɪnə'pærənt] *adj* symptomlos, symptomarm, klinisch nicht in Erscheinung tretend, inapparent, nicht sichtbar, nicht wahrnehmbar.

inapparent infection inapparente Infektion *f*.

in·ap·pe·tence [ɪn'æpɪtəns] *n* **1.** fehlendes Verlangen *nt* nach Nahrung, Appetitlosigkeit *f*, Inappetenz *f*. **2.** *psychia.* Fehlen *nt* der sexuellen Appetenz, Inappetenz *f*. **3.** Unlust *f*, Lustlosigkeit *f*.

in·ap·pe·ten·cy [ɪn'æpətənsɪ] *n* → inappetence.

in·ap·pe·tent [ɪn'æpətənt] *adj* **1.** appetitlos. **2.** lustlos, unlustig.

in·ar·tic·u·late [,ɪnɑː'tɪkjəlɪt] *adj* **1.** (*Sprache*) undeutlich (ausgesprochen), unverständlich, unartikuliert. **2.** unfähig s. klar auszudrücken. **3.** unaussprechlich. **4.** *bio.* ungegliedert, ohne Gelenke.

in·ar·tic·u·lat·ed [,-'tɪkjəleɪtɪd] *adj* **1.** inarticulate 1. **2.** *bio.* ungegliedert, ohne Gelenke.

in·ar·tic·u·late·ness [,-'tɪkjəlɪtnɪs] *n* **1.** (*Sprache*) Undeutlichkeit *f*, Unverständlichkeit *f*. **2.** Unfähigkeit *f* (deutlich) zu sprechen.

in·as·sim·i·la·ble [ɪnə'sɪmələbl] *adj biochem.* nicht assimilierbar.

in·at·ten·tion [ɪnə'tenʃn] *n* Unaufmerksamkeit *f*.

in·at·ten·tive [ɪnə'tentɪv] *adj* unachtsam, unaufmerksam (*to* gegen).

in·at·ten·tive·ness ['-nɪs] *n* Unaufmerksamkeit *f*.

in·au·di·bil·i·ty [ɪn,ɔːdə'bɪlətɪ] *n* Unhörbarkeit *f*.

in·au·di·ble [ɪn'ɔːdɪbl] *adj* unhörbar.

in·au·di·ble·ness ['-nɪs] *n* Unhörbarkeit *f*.

in·born ['ɪnbɔːrn] *adj* angeboren, bei der Geburt vorhanden.

inborn reflex angeborener Reflex *m*.

in·bred ['ɪnbred] *adj* **1.** angeboren; tief eingewurzelt. **2.** durch Inzucht erzeugt.

in·breed ['ɪnbriːd] *vt bio.* durch Inzucht züchten.

in·breed·ing ['ɪnbriːdɪŋ] *n bio., genet.* Inzucht *f*.

in·can·des·cent [,ɪnkæn'desənt] *adj* (weiß-)glühend.

in·ca·pa·bil·i·ty [ɪn,keɪpə'bɪlətɪ] *n* **1.** Unfähigkeit *f*. **2.** Untauglichkeit *f*. **3.** Hilflosigkeit *f*.

in·ca·pa·ble [ɪn'keɪpəbl] *adj* **1.** unfähig (*of* zu); nicht im Stande (*of doing* zu tun). **2.** hilflos. **3.** ungeeignet, untauglich (*for* für).

in·ca·pac·i·tate [ɪnkə'pæsɪteɪt] *vt* **1.** unfähig *od.* untauglich machen (*for sth.* für etw.). **2.** behindern, arbeits- *od.* erwerbsunfähig machen.

in·ca·pac·i·tat·ed [,ɪnkə'pæsɪteɪtɪd] *adj* **1.** behindert. **2.** arbeits-, erwerbsunfähig.

in·ca·pac·i·ta·tion [,ɪnkə,pæsɪ'teɪʃn] *n* **1.** Unfähigmachen *nt*. **2.** → incapacity.

in·ca·pac·i·ty [ɪnkə'pæsətɪ] *n* Unfähigkeit *f*, Untauglichkeit *f*.
i. for work Arbeitsunfähigkeit; Erwerbsunfähigkeit.

in·cap·su·late [ɪn'kæpsəleɪt, -sjʊ-] *vt* einverkapseln.

in·car·cer·ate [ɪn'kɑːrsəreɪt] *vt patho., chir.* einklemmen, inkarzerieren.

in·car·cer·at·ed [ɪn'kɑːrsəreɪtɪd] *adj chir., patho.* eingeklemmt, inkarzeriert.

incarcerated hernia inkarzerierte/eingeklemmte Hernie *f*, Hernia incarcerata.

incarcerated placenta eingeklemmte Plazenta *f*, Placenta incarcerata.

in·car·cer·a·tion [ɪn,kɑːrsə'reɪʃn] *n chir., patho.* Einklemmung *f*, Inkarzeration *f*, Incarceratio *f*.

incarceration syndrome Dietl-Krise *f*, -Syndrom *nt*.

in·ca·ri·al bone [ɪŋ'keərɪəl] Inkabein *nt*, Os interparietale.

in·car·nant [ɪn'kɑːrənt] *adj patho.* die Granulationsbildung fördernd.

in·car·na·tio [ɪnkɑːr'neɪʃɪəʊ] *n patho.* Einwachsen *nt*, Inkarnation *f*, Incarnatio *f*.

in·car·na·tive [ɪn'kɑːrnətɪv] **I** *n* die Granulationsbildung förderndes Mittel *nt*. **II** *adj* → incarnant.

in·cen·di·a·rism [ɪn'sendɪərɪzəm] *n* **1.** Brandstiftung *f*. **2.** *psychia.* Pyromanie *f*.

in·cen·tive [ɪn'sentɪv] **I** *n* Ansporn *m*, Antrieb *m*, Anreiz *m* (*to* zu). **II** *adj* anspornend, antreibend, anreizend (*to* zu).

incentive spirometer

incentive spirometer Atemrohr *nt*.
in·cest ['ɪnsest] *n* Blutschande *f*, Inzest *m*.
in·cest·u·ous [ɪn'sestʃəwəs] *adj* in der Art eines Inzests, als Inzest, inzestuös.
inch [ɪntʃ] *n* Inch *m*, Zoll *nt*.
in·cha·cao [ɪntʃə'kɑːəʊ] *n* Beriberi *f*, Vitamin B₁-Mangel(krankheit *f*) *m*, Thiaminmangel(krankheit *f*) *m*.
in·ci·dence ['ɪnsɪdəns] *n* **1.** Auftreten *nt*, Vorkommen *nt*, Häufigkeit *f*, Verbreitung *f*, Inzidenz *f*. **2.** Auftreffen *nt* (*on, upon* auf); *phys*. Einfall(en *nt*) *m*.
incidence rate Inzidenzrate *f*.
in·ci·dent ['ɪnsɪdənt] **I** *n* Vorfall *m*, Ereignis *nt*, Vorkommnis *nt*, Episode *f*. **II** *adj* **1.** auftreffend; (*Licht*) einfallend, -strahlend. **2.** verbunden (*to* mit); gehörend (*to* zu).
in·ci·den·tal [ˌɪnsɪ'dentl] **I** *n* Nebenumstand *m*, Nebensächlichkeit *f*. **II** *adj* **1.** nebensächlich, Neben-. **2.** beiläufig; gelegentlich; zufällig. **3.** folgend (*on, upon* auf), nachher (auftretend).
incidental finding Zufallsbefund *m*.
incidental murmur *card*. akzidentelles (Herz-)Geräusch *nt*.
incidental parasite *micro*. Zufallsparasit *m*.
incident angle *phys*. Inzidenz-, Einfallswinkel *m*.
incident ray *phys*. einfallender Strahl *m*.
in·cin·er·ate [ɪn'sɪnəreɪt] *vt* verbrennen.
in·cin·er·a·tion [ɪnˌsɪnə'reɪʃn] *n* **1.** Verbrennung *f*. **2.** Feuerbestattung *f*, Kremation *f*, Veraschung *f*.
in·cin·er·a·tor [ɪn'sɪnəreɪtər] *n* Verbrennungsofen *m*; Verbrennungsanlage *f*.
in·cip·i·ence [ɪn'sɪpɪəns] *n* Beginn *m*, Anfang *m*; Anfangsstadium *nt*.
in·cip·i·ent [ɪn'sɪpɪənt] *adj* beginnend, anfangend, anfänglich, inzipient, Anfangs-.
incipient abortion *gyn*. beginnender Abort *m*, Abortus incipiens.
incipient cataract beginnender Star *m*, Cataracta incipiens.
in·ci·sal [ɪn'saɪzl] *adj* schneidend, Schneide-.
incisal edge → incisal margin (of tooth).
incisal margin (of tooth) Schneidekante *f*, Margo incisalis.
in·cise [ɪn'saɪz] *vt* ein-, aufschneiden, durch Inzision eröffnen, inzidieren.
in·cised [ɪn'saɪzd] *adj* eingeschnitten, Schnitt-.
incise drape *chir*. Inzisionsfolie *f*.
incised wound Schnittwunde *f*, Schnitt *m*.
in·ci·sion [ɪn'sɪʒn] *n* **1.** Schnittwunde *f*, Schnitt *m*. **2.** (Ein-)Schnitt *m*, Eröffnung *f*, Inzision *f*, Incisio *f*. **3.** Einschneiden *nt*, Inzidieren *nt*.
 i. of fascia Faszienspaltung *f*, -schnitt, Fasziotomie *f*.
in·ci·sion·al biopsy [ɪn'sɪʒnəl] Inzisionsbiopsie *f*, Probeinzision *f*.
incisional hernia Narbenbruch *m*, -hernie *f*.
incisional pain schneidender Schmerz *m*.
in·ci·sive [ɪn'saɪzɪv] *adj* **1.** (ein-)schneidend. **2.** Schneidezahn betr., Schneide- **3.** *fig*. scharf.
incisive bone Zwischenkieferknochen *m*, Os incisivum.
incisive canal Canalis incisivus.
incisive duct → incisor duct.
incisive foramen For. incisivum.
incisive fossa Fossa incisiva.
incisive margin → incisal margin (of tooth).
in·ci·sive·ness [ɪn'saɪzɪvnɪs] *n fig*. Schärfe *f*.
incisive papilla Papilla incisiva.
incisive suture Sutura incisiva.

incisive tooth → incisor.
in·ci·sor [ɪn'saɪzər] *n* Schneidezahn *m*, Incisivus *m*, Dens incisivus.
incisor canaliculus → incisor duct.
incisor duct Ductus incisivus.
incisor tooth → incisor.
in·ci·su·ra [ˌɪnsaɪ'zʊərə, ˌɪn(t)sɪ-] *n, pl* **-rae** [-riː] **1.** → incisure. **2.** *physiol*. Inzisur *f*.
incisurae helicis (muscle) M. incisurae helicis.
in·cis·ure [ɪn'sɪʒər, -'saɪ-] *n anat*. Einschnitt *m*, Einbuchtung *f*, Inzisur *f*, Incisura *f*.
 i. of acetabulum Inc. acetabuli/acetabularis.
 i. of apex of heart Herzspitzeneinschnitt, -inzisur, Inc. apicis cordis.
 i. of mandible Inc. mandibulae.
 i. of Rivinus Inc. tympanica.
 i. of scapula Inc. scapulae/scapularis.
 i. of tentorium of cerebellum Inc. tentorii.
in·clin·a·ble [ɪn'klaɪnəbl] *adj* tendierend, neigend (*to* zu).
in·cli·na·tio [ˌɪnklɪ'neɪʃɪəʊ] *n anat*. → inclination 1.
in·cli·na·tion [ˌ-'neɪʃn] *n* **1.** Neigung *f*; Gefälle *nt*; Schräge *f*, geneigte Fläche *f*; Neigungswinkel *m*; *anat*. Inklination *f*, Inclinatio *f*. **2.** (*Person*) Neigung *f*, Tendenz *f*, Hang *m*, Anlage *f* (*for, to* zu). **3.** Neigen *nt*, Beugen *nt*.
 i. of pelvis Beckenneigung, Inclinatio pelvis.
in·cline [*n* 'ɪnklaɪn, ɪn'klaɪn; *v* ɪn'klaɪn] **I** *n* Gefälle *nt*, (Ab-)Hang *m*, Neigung *f*; *mathe*., *phys*. schiefe Ebene *f*. **II** *vt* neigen, beugen, schräg stellen; (*Kopf*) senken. **III** *vi* **1.** *fig*. neigen, eine Anlage/Neigung haben (*to* zu). **2.** s. neigen, (*to, towards* nach); abfallen; geneigt sein (*to, toward* zu).
in·clined [ɪn'klaɪnd] *adj* **1.** schräg, geneigt. **2.** *fig*. neigend (*to* zu). **to be ~ to do sth.** dazu neigen, etw. zu tun.
inclined plane *phys*. schiefe Ebene *f*.
in·cli·nom·e·ter [ˌɪnklə'nɑmɪtər] *n* **1.** Neigungsmesser *m*. **2.** *ophthal*. Inklinometer *nt*.
in·clu·sion [ɪn'kluːʒn] *n* Einschluß *m*, Einschließen *nt* (*in* in); Inklusion *f*.
inclusion body *abbr*. **I.B.** Einschluß-, Elementarkörperchen *nt*.
inclusion body disease Zytomegalie(-Syndrom *nt*) *f*, Zytomegalievirusinfektion *f*, zytomegale Einschlußkörperkrankheit *f*.
inclusion body encephalitis subakute sklerosierende Panenzephalitis *f abbr*. SSPE, subakute sklerosierende Leukenzephalitis van Bogaert *f*, Einschlußkörperenzephalitis Dawson *f*.
inclusion cell disease I-Zellen-Krankheit *f*, Mukolipidose II *f*.
inclusion cells Inklusionszellen *pl*, I-Zellen *pl*.
inclusion conjunctivitis *ophthal*. Einschluß-, Schwimmbadkonjunktivitis *f*.
inclusion conjunctivitis virus *old* → Chlamydia trachomatis.
inclusion cyst Einschlußzyste *f*.
 epidermal/epidermoid i. epidermale Einschlußzyste.
inclusion disease Einschluß(körperchen)krankheit *f*.
in·co·ag·u·la·bil·i·ty [ˌɪnkəʊˌægjələ'bɪlətɪ] *n* Ungerinnbarkeit *f*.
in·co·ag·u·la·ble [ˌ-'ægjələbl] *adj* nicht gerinnbar, ungerinnbar.
in·co·er·ci·ble [ˌ-'ɜrsɪbl] *adj* **1.** unerzwingbar, nicht zu erzwingen(d). **2.** *phys*. nicht komprimierbar.
in·co·her·ence [ˌ-'hɪərəns, -'her-] *n* Zusam-

menhangslosigkeit *f*, Unverbundenheit *f*, Inkohärenz *f*.
in·co·her·en·cy [ˌ-'hɪərənsɪ] *n* → incoherence.
in·co·her·ent [ˌ-'hɪərənt] *adj* unzusammenhängend, unverbunden, zusammenhangslos, inkohärent.
incoherent speech *psychia*. inkohärente/unzusammenhängende Sprache *f*.
in·com·i·tant strabismus [ɪn'kɑmɪtənt] *ophthal*. Lähmungsschielen *nt*, Strabismus paralyticus.
in·com·pat·i·bil·i·ty [ˌɪnkəmˌpætə'bɪlətɪ] *n* Unvereinbarkeit *f*, Unverträglichkeit *f*, Gegensätzlichkeit *f*, Inkompatibilität *f*.
incompatibility reaction Unverträglichkeitsreaktion *f*.
in·com·pat·i·ble [ˌ-'pætɪbl] *adj* unvereinbar, unverträglich, nicht zusammenpassend, inkompatibel (*with* mit).
incompatible blood transfusion reaction Transfusionszwischenfall *m*.
in·com·pat·i·ble·ness [ˌ-'pætɪblnɪs] *n* → incompatibility.
in·com·pe·tence [ɪn'kɑmpɪtəns] *n* **1.** Unfähigkeit *f*, Untüchtigkeit *f*, Inkompetenz *f*. **2.** Unzulänglichkeit *f*, Insuffizienz *f*.
 i. of the cardiac valves (Herz-)Klappeninsuffizienz.
in·com·pe·ten·cy [ɪn'kɑmpɪtənsɪ] *n* → incompetence.
in·com·pe·tent [ɪn'kɑmpɪtənt] *adj* **1.** unfähig (*to do* zu tun); untüchtig. **2.** unqualifiziert, nicht sach- *od*. fachkundig, inkompetent. **3.** nicht ausreichend (*for* für); unzulänglich, mangelhaft, insuffizient.
in·com·plete [ˌɪnkəm'pliːt] *adj* **1.** unvollständig, unvollkommen, unvollzählig, inkomplett. **2.** unfertig.
incomplete abortion *gyn*. inkompletter/unvollständiger Abort *m*, Abortus incompletus.
incomplete achromatopsy *ophthal*. atypische/inkomplette Farbenblindheit *f*.
incomplete agglutinin → incomplete antibody.
incomplete antibody nicht-agglutinierender/inkompletter/blockierender Antikörper *m*.
incomplete cleavage *embryo*. partielle/meroblastische Furchung(steilung *f*) *f*.
incomplete dislocation *ortho*. unvollständige Verrenkung *f*, Ausrenkung *f*, Subluxation *f*.
incomplete dominance *genet*. unvollständige Dominanz *f*, Semidominanz *f*.
incomplete duplication of spinal cord *embryo*. Diastematomyelie *f*.
incomplete fistula inkomplette/blinde Fistel *f*, Fistula incompleta.
incomplete fracture unvollständiger Bruch *m*, unvollständige Fraktur *f*, Fractura imperfecta.
incomplete hemianopia/hemianopsia *ophthal*. inkomplette Hemianop(s)ie *f*.
incomplete hernia inkomplette Hernie *f*, Hernia incompleta.
incomplete monochromasy → incomplete achromatopsy.
in·com·plete·ness [ˌ-nɪs] *n* Unvollständigkeit *f*, Unvollkommenheit *f*.
incomplete ophthalmoplegia Ophthalmoplegia partialis.
incomplete paralysis leichte *od*. unvollständige Paralyse/Lähmung *f*, motorische Schwäche *f*, Parese *f*.
in·com·ple·tion [ˌɪnkəm'pliːʃn] *n* → incompleteness.
in·com·press·i·bil·i·ty [ˌ-ˌpresə'bɪlətɪ] *n* Inkompressibilität *f*.
in·com·press·i·ble [ˌ-'presɪbl] *adj* nicht-komprimierbar, inkompressibel.

in·con·gru·ence [ɪnˈkɑŋgruəns] *n* Nichtübereinstimmung *f; mathe.* Inkongruenz *f.*
in·con·gru·ent [ɪnˈkɑŋgruənt] *adj* **1.** nicht übereinstimmen *(to, with* mit*).* **2.** nicht passend, unvereinbar *(to, with* mit*).* **3.** *mathe.* inkongruent.
incongruent nystagmus dissoziierter Nystagmus *m.*
in·con·gru·i·ty [ɪnkənˈgruːətɪ] *n, pl* **-ties 1.** Nichtübereinstimmung *f;* Unvereinbarkeit *f.* **2.** *mathe.* Inkongruenz *f.* **3.** Ungereimtheit *f,* Widersinnigkeit *f.*
in·con·gru·ous [ɪnˈkɑŋgrəwəs] *adj* → incongruent.
in·con·gru·ous·ness [ˈ-nɪs] *n* → incongruity.
in·con·stan·cy [ɪnˈkɑnstənsɪ] *n* Unbeständigkeit *f,* Veränderlichkeit *f,* Inkonstanz *f.*
in·con·stant [ɪnˈkɑnstənt] *adj* unbeständig, veränderlich, inkonstant; variabel.
in·con·ti·nence [ɪnˈkɑntnəns] *n* **1.** Unmäßigkeit *f,* Zügellosigkeit *f.* **2.** *patho.* Inkontinenz *f,* Incontinentia *f.*
i. of feces Stuhl-, Darminkontinenz, Incontinentia alvi.
i. of urine Harninkontinenz, Incontinentia urinae.
in·con·ti·nen·cy [ɪnˈkɑntnənsɪ] *n* → incontinence.
in·con·ti·nent [ɪnˈkɑntnənt] *adj* **1.** unmäßig, zügellos. **2.** *patho.* inkontinent.
in·con·ti·nen·tia [ɪnˌkɑntəˈnenʃɪə] *n* → incontinence.
in·co·or·di·na·tion [ɪnkəʊˌɔːrdəˈneɪʃn] *n neuro.* mangelhafte *od.* fehlende Koordination *f,* Inkoordination *f.*
in·cor·po·rate [ɪnˈkɔːrpəreɪt] **I** *vt* **1.** vereinigen, verbinden, zusammenschließen *(with, into,* in mit*).* **2.** einverleiben, aufnehmen *(in, into* in*);* eingliedern, einbauen, inkorporieren. **3.** *chem., techn.* vermischen *(into* zu*).* **4.** *techn., biochem.* einbauen *(into* in*).* **5.** *fig.* verkörpern. **II** *vi* s. verbinden *od.* vereinigen *od.* zusammenschließen *(with* mit*).*
in·cor·po·ra·tion [ɪnˌkɔːrpəˈreɪʃn] *n* **1.** Vereinigung *f,* Verbindung *f,* Zusammenschluß *m.* **2.** Einverleibung *f,* Eingliederung *f,* Inkorporation *f.*
in·crease [*n* ˈɪnkriːs; *v* ɪnˈkriːs] **I** *n* **1.** Vergrößerung *f,* Vermehrung *f,* Verstärkung *f,* Zunahme *f,* Zuwachs *m,* Wachstum *nt.* **2.** Anwachsen *nt,* Wachsen *nt,* Steigen *nt,* Steigerung *f,* Erhöhung *f.* **II** *vt* vergrößern, verstärken, vermehren, erhöhen, steigern. **III** *vi* **3.** zunehmen, größer werden, wachsen, anwachsen, steigen, ansteigen, s. vergrößern, s. vermehren, s. erhöhen, s. verstärken, s. steigern. **4.** s. *(durch Fortpflanzung)* vermehren.
in·creased metabolism [ɪnˈkriːst] erhöhter/gesteigerter Stoffwechsel *m,* Hypermetabolismus *m.*
in·cre·ment [ˈɪnkrəmənt, ˈɪŋ-] *n (a. mathe., phys.)* Zuwachs *m,* Zunahme *f,* Inkrement *nt.*
in·cre·men·tal [ˌ-ˈmentl] *adj* Inkrement betr., inkremental, Zuwachs-.
incremental lines Retzius'-Streifung *f.*
in·cre·tion [ɪnˈkriːʃn] *n physiol.* **1.** innere Sekretion *f,* Inkretion *f.* **2.** Inkret *nt.*
in·cre·to·ry [ˈ-təʊrɪ, -tərɪ] *adj* innere Sekretion betr., inkretorisch, innersekretorisch; endokrin.
incretory gland Drüse *f* mit innerer Sekretion, endokrine Drüse *f,* Gl. endocrina, Gl. sine ductibus.
in·crust [ɪnˈkrʌst] **I** *vt* mit einer Kruste überziehen, ver-, überkrusten. **II** *vi* **1.** s. verkrusten, s. überkrusten. **2.** eine Kruste bilden.

in·crus·ta·tion [ˌɪnkrʌˈsteɪʃn] *n* **1.** Kruste *f,* Grind *m,* Schorf *m.* **2.** *patho.* Verkrustung *f,* Inkrustation *f.*
in·cu·bate [ˈɪnkjəbət, ˈɪŋ-] **I** *n* Inkubat *nt.* **II** *vt* **1.** *micro.* inkubieren, im Inkubator züchten. **2.** (be-, aus-)brüten. **III** *vi* **3.** ausgebrütet werden. **4.** s. im Inkubator entwickeln. **5.** *fig.* s. entwickeln, reifen.
in·cu·ba·tion [ˌ-ˈbeɪʃn] *n* **1.** *micro.* (Be-, Aus-)Brüten *nt,* Inkubation *f.* **2.** *ped.* Aufzucht *f* im Inkubator, Inkubation *f.* **3.** → incubation period 1.
incubation period 1. *patho.* Inkubationszeit *f.* **2.** *micro.* Inkubationszeit *f,* Latenzperiode *f.* **3.** → extrinsic i.
extrinsic i. *micro.* äußere Inkubationszeit, Inkubationszeit im Vektor.
in·cu·ba·tive stage [ˈ-beɪtɪv] → incubation period.
in·cu·ba·tor [ˈ-beɪtər] *n* **1.** *micro.* Brutschrank *m,* Inkubator *m.* **2.** *ped.* Brutkasten *m,* Inkubator *m.*
in·cu·bus [ˈɪnkjəbəs, ˈɪŋ-] *n, pl* **-bi** [-baɪ], **-bus·es** Alptraum *m,* Alpdrücken *nt,* Inkubus *m,* Incubus *m.*
in·cu·dal [ˈɪnkjədl, ˈɪŋ-] *adj* Amboß/Incus betr., Amboß-, Incus-.
incudal fold Plica incudialis.
incudal fossa Fossa incudis.
in·cu·date [ˈɪnkjədeɪt, -dɪt, ˈɪŋ-] *adj* → incudal.
in·cu·dec·to·my [ˌ-ˈdektəmɪ] *n* HNO Amboßentfernung *f,* -exstirpation *f,* Inkudektomie *f.*
in·cu·di·form [ɪnˈkjuːdəfɔːrm] *adj anat.* amboßförmig.
in·cu·do·mal·le·al [ˌɪŋkədəʊˈmælɪəl] *adj anat.* Incus u. Malleus betr.
in·cu·do·mal·le·o·lar articulation [ˌ-məˈlɪələr] Hammer-Amboß-Gelenk *nt,* Inkudomalleolargelenk *nt,* Artic. incudomallearis.
incudomalleolar joint → incudomalleolar articulation.
in·cu·do·sta·pe·di·al articulation [ˌ-stəˈpɪdɪəl] Amboß-Steigbügel-Gelenk *nt,* Inkudostapedialgelenk *nt,* Artic. incudostapedialis.
incudostapedial joint → incudostapedial articulation.
in·cur·a·bil·i·ty [ɪnˌkjʊərəˈbɪlətɪ] *n (Krankheit)* Unheilbarkeit *f,* Inkurabilität *f.*
in·cur·a·ble [ɪnˈkjʊərəbl] *adj (Krankheit)* unheilbar, nicht heilbar, inkurabel.
in·cur·vate [*adj* ɪnˈkɜːrvət, ɪnˈkɜːrvɪt; *v* ˈɪnkɜːrveɪt, ɪnˈkɜːrveɪt] **I** *adj* (nach innen) gekrümmt, (ein-)gebogen; verkrümmt. **II** *vt* (nach innen) krümmen, (ein-)biegen.
in·cur·va·tion [ˌɪnkɜːrˈveɪʃn] *n* **1.** (Einwärts-)Krümmung *f,* Verkrümmung *f.* **2.** Krümmen *nt.*
in·curve [ɪnˈkɜːrv] **I** *n* → incurvation. **II** *adj* → incurvate **I**. **III** *vt* → incurvate **II**.
in·cus [ˈɪŋkəs, ˈɪn-] *n, pl* **-cu·des** [-ˈkjuːdiːz] *anat.* Amboß *m,* Incus *m.*
in·cy·clo·duc·tion [ɪnˌsaɪkləˈdʌkʃn] *n ophthal.* Inzyklovergenz *f,* Konklination *f.*
in·cy·clo·pho·ria [ˌ-ˈfəʊrɪə] *n ophthal.* Inzyklophorie *f.*
in·cy·clo·tro·pia [ˌ-ˈtrəʊpɪə] *n ophthal.* Inzyklotropie *f.*
in·dane·di·one [ˌɪndeɪnˈdaɪəʊn] *n* Indandion *nt.*
in·dem·ni·fi·ca·tion [ɪnˌdemnɪfɪˈkeɪʃn] *n* **1.** *forens.* Entschädigung *f,* Ersatzleistung *f.* **2.** Entschädigung(ssumme *f) f,* Vergütung *f,* Abfindung(sbetrag *m) f.*
in·dem·ni·fy [ɪnˈdemnəfaɪ] *vt* jdn. entschädigen, jdm. Schadensersatz leisten *(for* für*).*
in·dem·ni·tee [ɪnˌdemnəˈtiː] *n forens.* Entschädigungsberechtigte(r *m) f.*

in·dem·ni·ty [ɪnˈdemnɪtɪ] *n* Entschädigung(ssumme *f) f,* Vergütung *f,* Abfindung(sbetrag *m) f.*
in·den·i·za·tion [ɪnˌdenɪˈzeɪʃn] *n* → innidiation.
in·dent [*n* ˈɪndent, ɪnˈdent; *v* ɪnˈdent] **I** *n* Einbeulung *f,* Vertiefung *f,* Delle *f.* **II** *vt* eindrücken, einbeulen.
in·den·ta·tion tonometer [ˌɪndenˈteɪʃn] *ophthal.* Impressionstonometer *nt.*
in·de·pend·ence [ˌɪndəˈpendəns] *n* Unabhängigkeit *f (of* von*);* Selbständigkeit *f.*
in·de·pend·en·cy [ˌ-ˈpendənsɪ] *n* → independence.
in·de·pend·ent [ˌ-ˈpendənt] *adj* unabhängig *(of* von*);* selbständig; unbeeinflußt.
independent form *biochem.* I-Form *f.*
in·de·ter·mi·nate [ˌɪndɪˈtɜːrmənɪt] *adj* nicht-determiniert.
indeterminate cleavage *embryo.* nicht-determinierte Furchung *f.*
indeterminate leprosy indeterminierte Lepra *f abbr.* IL, Lepra indeterminata.
in·dex [ˈɪndeks] *n, pl* **-dex·es, -di·ces** [-dɪsiːz] **1.** Zeigefinger *m,* Index *m,* Digitus secundus. **2.** Register *nt,* Verzeichnis *nt,* Katalog *m,* Index *m.* **3.** Kartei *f.* **4.** *fig.* Hinweis *m (of, to* auf*);* Anhaltspunkt *m,* (An-)Zeichen *nt (of, to* von, für*).* **5.** Index *m,* Meßziffer *f,* Meß-, Vergleichszahl *f.* **6.** (Uhr-)Zeiger *m;* (*Waage*) Zunge *f.*
i. of refraction Brechungs-, Refraktionsindex.
index ametropia *ophthal.* Indexametropie *f.*
index card Karteikarte *f.*
index file Kartei *f.*
index finger Zeigefinger *m,* Index *m,* Digitus secundus.
index myopia *ophthal.* Brechungsmyopie *f.*
In·di·an [ˈɪndɪən] **I.** flap Schwenklappen(plastik *f) m.*
I. operation HNO Indische Methode/Rhinoplastik *f.*
I. relapsing fever indisches Rückfallfieber *nt.*
I. rhinoplasty → I. operation.
I. tick typhus Boutonneuse-Fieber *nt,* Fièvre boutonneuse.
In·dia rubber [ˈɪndɪə] Naturgummi *nt,* Kautschuk *m.*
India rubber skin Ehlers-Danlos-Syndrom *nt.*
in·di·can [ˈɪndɪkən] *n* **1.** (Pflanzen-)Indikan *nt.* **2.** Harnindikan *nt,* Kaliumindoxylsulfat *nt.*
in·di·can·e·mia [ˌɪndɪkæˈniːmɪə] *n* erhöhter Indikangehalt *m* des Blutes, Indikanämie *f.*
in·di·can·i·dro·sis [ˌɪndɪkænɪˈdrəʊsɪs] *n* Indikanausscheidung *f* im Schweiß.
in·di·can·o·ra·chia [ˌɪndɪkænəˈrækɪə] *n* Vorkommen *nt* von Indikan im Liquor cerebrospinalis.
in·di·cant [ˈɪndɪkənt] **I** *n* → indication. **II** *adj* → indicative.
in·di·can·u·ria [ˌɪndɪkæˈn(j)ʊərɪə] *n* vermehrte Indikanausscheidung *f* im Harn, Indikanurie *f.*
in·di·car·mine [ˌɪndɪˈkɑːrmɪn, -miːn] *n* Indigokarmin *nt.*
in·di·cate [ˈɪndəkeɪt] *vt* **1.** hinweisen, -deuten auf, schließen lassen auf; *techn.* (an-)zeigen. **2.** *(Therapie)* erfordern, angezeigt erscheinen lassen, indizieren.
in·di·cat·ed [ˈ-keɪtɪd] *adj* angezeigt, angebracht, indiziert.
in·di·ca·tio [ˌ-ˈkeɪʃɪəʊ] *n* → indication.
in·di·ca·tion [ˌ-ˈkeɪʃn] *n* **1.** (An-)Zeichen *nt (of* für*);* Hinweis *m (of* auf*).* **2.** *med.* Heilanzeige *f,* Indikation *f,* Indicatio *f.* **3.** Deuten *nt,* (An-)Zeigen *nt.*

indicative

in·dic·a·tive [ɪnˈdɪkətɪv] *adj* aufzeigend, andeutend (*of*). **to be ~ of** schließen lassen auf, hindeuten auf.
in·di·ca·tor [ˈɪndəkeɪtər] *n* **1.** Zeigefinger *m*, Index *m*, Digitus secundus. **2.** *anat.* M. extensor indicis. **3.** *chem.* Indikator *m*. **4.** *stat.* Indikator *m*. **5.** *techn.* (An-)Zeiger *m*, Zähler *m*, Messer *m*, Meß-, Anzeigegerät *nt*.
indicator-dilution curve Indikator-, Farbstoffverdünnungskurve *f*.
indicator-dilution method Farbstoff-, Indikatorverdünnungsmethode *f*, -technik *f*.
indicator-dilution technique → indicator-dilution method.
indicator dye Farbindikator *m*.
in·dif·fer·ence [ɪnˈdɪf(ə)rəns] *n* **1.** Teilnahmslosigkeit *f*, Gleichgültigkeit *f*, Desinteresse *nt*, Indifferenz *f* (*to, towards* gegenüber). **2.** Bedeutungslosigkeit *f*.
in·dif·fer·ent [ɪnˈdɪf(ə)rənt] *adj* **1.** teilnahmslos, gleichgültig, indifferent (*to, towards* gegenüber). **2.** *chem., phys.* neutral, unbestimmt, indifferent. **3.** *bio.* (*Zelle, Gewebe*) nicht differenziert *od.* spezialisiert.
indifferent electrode inaktive/indifferente/passive Elektrode *f*.
indifferent gonad *embryo.* indifferente Gonadenanlage *f*.
indifferent stage *embryo.* indifferentes Stadium *nt*.
indifferent streptococci *micro.* nicht-hämolysierende/gamma-hämolytische Streptokokken *pl*.
in·di·gene [ˈɪndɪdʒiːn] *n* **1.** Eingeborene(r *m*) *f*. **2.** *bio.* einheimisches Tier *nt*; einheimische Pflanze *f*.
in·dig·e·nous [ɪnˈdɪdʒənəs] *adj* eingeboren; einheimisch.
in·di·gest·i·bil·i·ty [ˌɪndɪˌdʒestəˈbɪlɪtɪ, -daɪ-] *n* Unverdaulichkeit *f*, Unverdaubarkeit *f*.
in·di·gest·i·ble [ˌ-ˈdʒestəbl] *adj* un-, schwerverdaulich.
in·di·ges·tion [ˌ-ˈdʒestʃn] *n* **1.** Verdauungsstörung *f*, Indigestion *f*. **2.** Magenverstimmung *f*, verdorbener Magen *m*.
in·di·ges·tive [ˌ-ˈdʒestɪv] *adj* mit Indigestion verbunden; an Indigestion leidend.
in·di·gi·ta·tion [ɪnˌdɪdʒəˈteɪʃn] *n* → intussusception.
in·di·go [ˈɪndɪɡəʊ] *n, pl* **-gos, -goes 1.** Indigo *m*. **2.** → indigo blue.
indigo blue Indigoblau *n*.
indigo-blue *adj* indigoblau.
indigo calculus *urol.* Indigostein *m*.
in·di·go·car·mine [ˌɪndɪɡəʊˈkɑːrmɪn, -maɪn] *n* Indigokarmin *nt*.
in·di·go·tin [ɪnˈdɪɡətɪn, ˌɪndɪˈɡəʊtn] *n* → indigo blue.
in·di·go·tin·di·sul·fo·nate sodium [ˌ-daɪˈsʌlfəneɪt] → indigocarmine.
in·di·go·u·ria [ˌɪndɪɡəʊˈ(j)ʊərɪə] *n* → indiguria.
in·di·gu·ria [ɪndɪˈɡ(j)ʊərɪə] *n* Indigoausscheidung *f* im Harn, Indigurie *f*.
in·di·rect [ˌɪndəˈrekt, -daɪ-] *adj* mittelbar, auf Umwegen, nicht gerade *od.* direkt, indirekt.
indirect ballottement *gyn.* Ballottement *nt* des kindlichen Kopfes.
indirect bilirubin freies/indirektes/unkonjugiertes Bilirubin *nt*.
indirect calorimetry indirekte Kalorimetrie *f*.
indirect emetic *pharm.* zentrales Emetikum *nt*.
indirect fluorescent antibody reaction *abbr.* **IFAR** → indirect fluorescent antibody test.
indirect fluorescent antibody test indirekte Fluoreszenz-Antikörper-Reaktion *f* *abbr.* **IFAR**, indirekte Fluoreszenz *f*, indirekter Fluoreszenztest *m*, Sandwich--Technik *f*.
indirect fracture indirekte Fraktur *f*.
indirect hemagglutination indirekte/passive Hämagglutination *f*.
indirect hemagglutination antibody test indirekter Hämagglutinations-Antikörper-Test *m*, IHA-Test *m*.
indirect hernia äußerer/seitlicher/indirekter/schräger Leistenbruch *m*, Hernia inguinalis externa/indirecta/lateralis/obliqua.
indirect laryngoscopy *HNO* indirekte Kehlkopfspiegelung/Laryngoskopie *f*.
indirect metaplasia indirekte Metaplasie *f*.
indirect ophthalmoscopy indirekte Ophthalmoskopie *f*.
indirect oxidase Peroxidase *f*.
indirect reflex gekreuzter/diagonaler/konsensueller Reflex *m*.
indirect transfusion indirekte Transfusion *f*.
indirect vision indirektes/peripheres Sehen *nt*.
in·di·ru·bin [ˌɪndɪˈruːbɪn] *n* Indirubin *nt*.
in·di·ru·bin·u·ria [ˌ-ˌruːbɪˈn(j)ʊərɪə] *n* Indirubinausscheidung *f* im Harn, Indirubinurie *f*.
in·dis·crete [ˌɪndɪˈskriːt, ɪnˈdɪskriːt] *adj* zusammenhängend, kompakt, homogen.
in·dis·pen·sa·bil·i·ty [ˌ-ˌspensəˈbɪlɪtɪ] *n* Unentbehrlichkeit *f*, Unerläßlichkeit *f*.
in·dis·pen·sa·ble [ˌ-ˈspensəbl] *adj* unentbehrlich, unbedingt notwendig, unerläßlich (*to life*). **~ to life** unentbehrlich.
in·dis·pen·sa·ble·ness [ˌ-ˈspensəblnɪs] *n* → indispensability.
in·dis·po·si·tion [ˌɪndɪspəˈzɪʃn] *n* Unpäßlichkeit *f*, Unwohlsein *nt*, Indisposition *f*, Indisponiertheit *f*.
in·dis·sol·u·bil·i·ty [ˌɪndɪˌsɑljəˈbɪlɪtɪ] *n* **1.** *phys.* Unlöslichkeit *f*. **2.** *fig.* Unauflösbarkeit *f*.
in·dis·sol·u·ble [ɪndɪˈsɑljəbl] *adj* **1.** *phys.* unlöslich. **2.** *fig.* unauflösbar.
in·dis·sol·u·ble·ness [ˈ-nɪs] *n* → indissolubility.
in·dis·tinct [ɪndɪˈstɪŋkt] *adj* **1.** undeutlich, unscharf. **2.** unklar, verworren, dunkel, verschwommen.
in·dis·tinct·ness [ˈ-nɪs] *n* **1.** Undeutlichkeit *f*; Unschärfe *f*. **2.** Unklarheit *f*, Verschwommenheit *f*.
in·di·um [ˈɪndɪəm] *n abbr.* **In** Indium *n abbr.* **In**.
in·di·vid·u·al [ˌɪndəˈvɪdʒuːəl] I *n* **1.** Einzelmensch *m*, -wesen *nt*, -person *f*, Individuum *nt*, Einzelne(r *m*) *f*. **2.** *bio.* Einzelorganismus *m*, -wesen *nt*. II *adj* **3.** einzeln, individuell, Einzel-, Individual-. **4.** persönlich, eigentümlich, eigenwillig, charakteristisch, individuell.
in·di·vid·u·al·ism [ˌ-ˈvɪdʒuːəlɪzəm] *n* **1.** Individualismus *m*. **2.** → individuality 1.
in·di·vid·u·al·i·ty [ˌ-ˌvɪdʒuːˈælɪtɪ] *n* **1.** (persönliche) Eigenart *od.* Note *f*, Besonderheit *f*, Individualität *f*. **2.** Einzelwesen *nt*, -mensch *m*. **3.** individuelle Existenz *f*, Individualität *f*.
in·di·vid·u·al·i·za·tion [ˌ-ˌvɪdʒuːəlaɪˈzeɪʃn] *n* Betrachtung *f od.* Behandlung *f* des Einzelnen, individuelle Behandlung *od.* Betrachtung *f*, Individualisierung *f*, Individualisation *f*.
in·di·vid·u·al·ize [ˌ-ˈvɪdʒuːəlaɪz] *vt* jdn. als Einzelwesen betrachten *od.* behandeln, individuell behandeln, einzeln betrachten, individualisieren. **2.** individuell gestalten.
in·di·vid·u·al·ly [ˌ-ˈvɪdʒəlɪ] *adv* **1.** einzeln, jede(r, s) für sich. **2.** einzeln betrachtet, für s. genommen. **3.** persönlich.
individual psychology Individualpsychologie *f*.
individual therapy/treatment *psychia.* Individualtherapie *f*.
in·di·vid·u·ate [ˌ-ˈvɪdʒuːeɪt] *vt* **1.** unterscheiden (*from* von). **2.** → individualize 2.
in·di·vid·u·a·tion [ˌ-ˌvɪdʒuːˈeɪʃn] *n* **1.** *psycho.* Ausbildung *f* der Individualität, Individuation *f*, individuelle Selbstfindung *f*. **2.** individuelle/persönliche Gestaltung *f*.
in·do·lac·e·tu·ria [ˌɪndəʊˌlæsɪˈt(j)ʊərɪə] *n* Indolessigsäureausscheidung *f* im Harn, Indolazeturie *f*, -aceturie *f*.
in·dol·a·mine [ɪnˈdɑləmiːn] *n* Indolamin *nt*.
in·dole [ˈɪndəʊl] *n* Indol *nt*, 2,3-Benzopyrrol *nt*.
in·dole·a·ce·tic acid [ˌɪndəʊləˈsiːtɪk, -ˈsetɪk] Indolyl-, Indolessigsäure *f*.
in·do·lence [ˈɪndəlns] *n* **1.** Trägheit *f*, Indolenz *f*. **2.** (*Schmerz*) Unempfindlichkeit *f*, Schmerzlosigkeit *f*, Indolenz *f*. **3.** *patho.* langsamer Verlauf *m*, langsamer Heilungsprozeß *m*.
in·do·lent [ˈɪndəlnt] *adj* **1.** gleichgültig, träge. **2.** (schmerz-)unempfindlich, indolent. **3.** schmerzlos, indolent. **4.** langsam voranschreitend, langsam heilend, indolent.
indolent bubo schmerzloser/indolenter Bubo *m*, Bubo indolens.
in·do·log·e·nous [ˌɪndəˈlɑdʒənəs] *adj* indolproduzierend.
in·dol·u·ria [ɪndəˈl(j)ʊərɪə] *n* Indolausscheidung *f* im Harn, Indolurie *f*.
in·do·meth·a·cin [ˌɪndəʊˈmeθəsɪn] *n pharm.* Indometacin *nt*.
in·do·phe·nol [ˌ-ˈfiːnɔl, -nɑl] *n* Indophenol *nt*.
in·do·phe·no·lase [ˌ-ˈfiːnəleɪz] *n* Indophenoloxidase *f*, Zytochromoxidase *f*, Cytochromoxidase *f*.
indophenol blue Indophenolblau *nt*.
indophenol oxidase → indophenolase.
in·do·pro·fen [ˌ-ˈprəʊfən] *n pharm.* Indoprofen *nt*.
in·dor·a·min [ɪnˈdɔːrəmɪn] *n pharm.* Indoramin *nt*.
in·dox·yl [ɪnˈdɑksɪl] *n* Indoxyl *nt*, 3-Hydroxyindol *nt*.
in·dox·yl·e·mia [ɪnˌdɑksɪˈliːmɪə] *n* Auftreten *nt* von Indoxyl im Blut, Indoxylämie *f*.
indoxyl-sulfate *n* Indoxylsulfat *n*.
in·dox·yl·u·ria [ɪnˌdɑksɪˈl(j)ʊərɪə] *n* Indoxylausscheidung *f* im Harn, Indoxylurie *f*.
in·duce [ɪnˈd(j)uːs] *vt* **1.** jdn. veranlassen *od.* bewegen (*to do* zu tun). **2.** (*Narkose, Schlaf*) bewirken, auslösen, herbeiführen, induzieren; (*Geburt*) einleiten. **3.** *electr.* erzeugen, induzieren. **4.** *genet.* induzieren.
in·duced [ɪnˈd(j)uːst] *adj* **1.** auf Induktion beruhend, induziert. **2.** (künstlich) herbeigeführt, induziert. **3.** *phys.* sekundär, induziert, Induktions-.
induced abortion *gyn.* **1.** artifizieller/induzierter Abort *m*, Schwangerschaftsabbruch *m*, Abortus artificialis. **2.** indizierter Abort *m*.
induced current *electr.* Induktionsstrom *m*, faradischer Strom *m*.
induced draft Saugzug *m*, künstlicher Zug *m*.
induced enzyme induzierbares Enzym *nt*.

induced-fit hypothesis Induced-fit-Hypothese f.
induced glomerulonephritis Serumnephritis f.
induced insanity psychia. induziertes Irresein nt, Folie à deux.
induced labor induzierte Geburt f.
induced mutation induzierte Mutation f.
induced pneumothorax künstlicher Pneu(mothorax m) m.
induced psychotic disorder → induced insanity.
induced radioactivity künstliche Radioaktivität f.
induced sleep künstlich erzeugter Schlaf m.
in·duce·ment [ɪn'd(j)u:smənt] n Anlaß m, Beweggrund m; Anreiz m.
in·duc·er [ɪn'd(j)u:sər] n genet. Induktor m, Inducer m.
in·duc·i·ble [ɪn'd(j)u:sɪbl] adj induzierbar.
inducible enzyme → induced enzyme.
in·duc·ing [ɪn'd(j)u:sɪŋ] adj induzierend.
inducing agent induzierendes Agens nt, induzierende Substanz f.
in·duct·ance [ɪn'dʌktəns] n electr. 1. Induktion f, Induktivität f. 2. Induktanz f, induktiver Widerstand m.
in·duc·tion [ɪn'dʌkʃn] n 1. Herbeiführung f, Auslösung f, Einleitung f, Induktion f. 2. genet., biochem. Induktion f. 3. anes. Einleitung(sphase f) f, Induktionsphase f. 4. phys. Induktion f. 5. biochem. (Enzym-)Induktion f.
i. of labor Geburtseinleitung.
induction period bio. Induktionsphase f.
in·duc·tive [ɪn'dʌktɪv] adj Induktion betr., durch Induktion entstehend, induktiv, Induktions-.
inductive phase anes. Einleitung(sphase f) f, Induktionsphase f.
inductive resistance phys. Blindwiderstand m, Reaktanz f.
in·duc·tor [ɪn'dʌktər] n 1. bio. Induktor m. 2. biochem. Induktor m, Reaktionsbeschleuniger m.
in·du·lin ['ɪndjəlɪn] n histol. Indulin nt.
in·du·lin·o·phil [-'lɪnəfɪl] I n indulinophile Struktur f. II adj mit Indulin anfärbbar, indulin(o)phil.
in·du·lin·o·phile [-,lɪnəfaɪl] adj → indulinophil II.
in·du·lin·o·phil·ic [-,lɪnə'fɪlɪk] adj → indulinophil II.
in·du·rate [adj 'ɪnd(j)uərɪt, ɪn'd(j)uə-; v 'ɪnd(j)uəreɪt] I adj verhärtet, induriert. II vt 1. härten, hart machen, indurieren. 2. fig. ab-, verhärten, abstumpfen (against, to gegen). III vi 3. s. verhärten, hart werden. 4. fig. abstumpfen, abgehärtet werden.
in·du·rat·ed ['ɪnd(j)uəreɪtɪd] adj → indurate I.
in·du·ra·tion [,-'reɪʃn] n 1. patho. (Gewebs-)Verhärtung f, Induration f, Induratio f. 2. fig. Ab-, Verhärtung f, Abstumpfung f.
in·du·ra·tive ['-reɪtɪv] adj Induration betr., von Induration betroffen, durch Induration gekennzeichnet, indurativ.
indurative pleurisy indurative Brustfellentzündung/Pleuritis f.
indurative pneumonia indurative Pneumonie f, chronische Indurativpneumonie f.
in·du·si·um gris·e·um [ɪn'd(j)u:zɪəm, -ʒɪəm 'grɪsɪəm] Gyrus supracallosus, Indusium griseum.
in·dus·tri·al [ɪn'dʌstrɪəl] adj industriell, gewerblich, Industrie-, Betriebs-, Arbeits-; industrialisiert.

industrial accident Arbeits-, Betriebsunfall m.
industrial chemistry angewandte Chemie f.
industrial deafness chronische Lärmschwerhörigkeit f.
industrial dermatitis berufsbedingte Kontaktdermatitis f.
industrial dermatosis → industrial dermatitis.
industrial disease Berufskrankheit f.
industrial hygiene Gesundheitsschutz m am Arbeitsplatz.
industrial injury Betriebsunfall m.
industrial medicine Arbeitsmedizin f.
industrial psychology Arbeits-, Betriebspsychologie f.
industrial spectacles Schutzbrille f.
in·dwell·ing catheter [ɪn'dwelɪŋ] Verweil-, Dauerkatheter m.
in·e·bri·ant [ɪn'i:brɪənt] I n berauschendes Mittel nt. II adj berauschend, betäubend.
in·e·bri·ate [n ɪn'i:brɪɪt; v -eɪt] I n 1. Betrunkene(r m) f. 2. (Gewohnheits-)Trinker(in f) m. II vt 3. berauschen, betrunken machen. 4. fig. betäuben.
in·e·bri·a·tion [ɪn,i:brɪ'eɪʃn] n (Be-)Trunkenheit f.
in·e·bri·e·ty [,ɪnɪ'braɪətɪ] n → inebriation.
in·ed·i·ble [ɪn'edəbl] adj ungenießbar, nicht eßbar.
in·ert [ɪ'nɜːt] adj 1. phys., chem. untätig, (reaktions-)träge, inert. 2. träg(e), lust-, kraftlos, schwerfällig.
inert gas Edelgas nt.
in·er·tia [ɪ'nɜːʃ(j)ə] n 1. Trägheit f, Langsamkeit f, Schwäche f, Inertia f, Inertie f. 2. phys. (Massen-)Trägheit f; chem. Reaktionsträgheit f.
inertial force Trägheitskraft f.
in·er·tial [ɪ'nɜːʃ(j)əl] adj Trägheits-, Inertial-.
inertial resistance phys. Trägheitswiderstand m.
inertial system Inertialsystem nt.
inertia theory HNO, physiol. Massenträgheitstheorie f.
inertia uteri gyn. Wehenschwäche f, Inertia uteri.
in·fan·cy ['ɪnfənsɪ] n, pl -cies 1. frühe Kindheit f, frühes Kindesalter nt, Säuglingsalter nt. 2. forens. Minderjährigkeit f. 3. fig. Anfangsstadium nt, Anfang m.
in·fant ['ɪnfənt] I n 1. Säugling m; (kleines) Kind nt. 2. forens. Minderjährige(r m) f. II adj 3. Säuglings-. 4. (noch) klein, im Kindesalter; Kinder-, Kindes-. 5. forens. minderjährig. 6. fig. in den Anfängen steckend, im Anfangsstadium, jung.
infant botulism Säuglingsbotulismus m.
infant death Säuglingstod m, Tod m im ersten Lebensjahr.
in·fan·ti·cide [ɪn'fæntɪsaɪd] n 1. Kind(es)tötung f. 2. Kind(es)-, Kindermörder(in f) m.
in·fan·tile ['ɪnfəntaɪl, -tɪl] adj 1. Kind od. Kindheit betr., kindlich, im Kindesalter, infantil. 2. psychia. kindisch, zurückgeblieben, unterentwickelt, infantil.
infantile acrodermatitis derm. Gianotti-Crosti-Syndrom nt, infantile papulöse Akrodermatitis f, Acrodermatitis papulosa eruptiva infantilis.
infantile amaurotic (familial) idiocy Tay-Sachs-Erkrankung f, -Syndrom nt, infantile amaurotische Idiotie f, GM_2-Gangliosidose Typ I f.
infantile arteriosclerosis infantile Arteriosklerose f.
infantile arteritis infantile Arteriitis f.
infantile atrophy Säuglingsdystrophie f, Marasmus m.

infantile autism frühkindlicher Autismus m, Kanner-Syndrom nt.
infantile beriberi akute Säuglingsberiberi f.
infantile cerebral palsy abbr. ICP neuro. zerebrale Kinderlähmung f, infantile Zerebralparese f.
infantile cortical hyperostosis abbr. ICH Caffey-Silverman-Syndrom nt, Caffey--de Toni-Syndrom nt, Caffey-Smith-Syndrom nt, Hyperostosis corticalis infantilis.
infantile coxitis Säuglingskoxitis f.
infantile diarrhea Sommerdiarrhö f.
infantile digital fibromatosis infantile digitale Fibromatose f, juvenile Fibromatose f.
infantile diplegia neuro., ped. Geburtslähmung f, infantile Diplegie f.
infantile form of celiac disease Zöliakie f, Herter-Heubner-Syndrom nt, Heubner--Herter-Krankheit f, Gee-Herter-Heubner-Syndrom nt.
infantile genetic agranulocytosis infantile hereditäre Agranulozytose f, Kostmann-Syndrom nt.
infantile glaucoma Ochsenauge nt, Glaukom nt der Kinder, angeborenes Glaukom nt, Hydrophthalmus m (congenitus), Buphthalmus m (congenitus), Glaucoma infantile.
infantile GM_1-gangliosidosis generalisierte Gangliosidose f, GM_1-Gangliosidose (Typ I) f.
infantile hemiplegia geburtstraumatische Hemiplegie f.
infantile hypothyroidism Kretinismus m.
infantile leishmaniasis mediterrane Kinder-Kala-Azar f.
infantile myxedema infantiles Myxödem nt.
infantile papular acrodermatitis → infantile acrodermatitis.
infantile paralysis (epidemische/spinale) Kinderlähmung f, Heine-Medin-Krankheit f, Poliomyelitis (epidemica) anterior acuta.
infantile pelvis infantiles/juveniles Becken nt.
infantile pressure alopecia Säuglingsglatze f, Dekubitalalopezie f, Alopecia decubitalis.
infantile purulent conjunctivitis ophthal. bakterielle Konjunktivitis f der Neugeborenen.
infantile scoliosis ortho., ped. Säuglingsskoliose f.
infantile scurvy rachitischer Säuglingsskorbut m, Möller-Barlow-Krankheit f.
infantile spastic paralysis → infantile cerebral palsy.
infantile type of Gaucher's disease Gaucher-Krankheit Typ II f, infantile Form f, akute neuronopathische Form f.
in·fan·ti·lism ['ɪnfntɪlɪzəm] n 1. körperlicher/physischer/somatischer Infantilismus m. 2. psychischer Infantilismus m.
in·fan·til·i·ty [,ɪnfən'tɪlətɪ] n 1. psychia. infantiler Zustand m, Kindlichkeit f, kindisches Wesen nt, Infantilität f. 2. Kindlichkeit f.
infant mortality Säuglingssterblichkeit f, Erstjahressterblichkeit f.
in·farct ['ɪnfɑːrkt, ɪn'fɑːrkt] n Infarkt m, infarzierter Areal m.
in·farc·tion [ɪn'fɑːrkʃn] n 1. Infarzierung f, Infarktbildung f. 2. Infarkt m.
i. of small intestine Dünndarminfarzierung.
in·faust [ɪn'faʊst] adj ungünstig, aussichtslos, infaust.
in·fect [ɪn'fekt] vt 1. patho. jdn. od. etw.

infected

infizieren, jdn. anstecken (with mit; by durch). **to become ~ed** s. infizieren od. anstecken. **2.** bio. befallen. **3.** (Luft) verpesten; fig. vergiften.
in·fect·ed [ɪnˈfektɪd] adj infiziert (with mit).
infected abortion gyn. infektiöser Abort m.
infected bile infizierte Galle f.
in·fect·i·ble [ɪnˈfektɪbl] adj infizierbar.
in·fec·tion [ɪnˈfekʃn] n **1.** Ansteckung f, Infektion f. **to catch/take an ~** s. infizieren od. anstecken. **2.** Infekt m, Infektion f, Infektionskrankheit f. **3.** bio. Befall m. **4.** (Luft-)Verpestung f; fig. Vergiftung f.
infection-immunity n Infektions-, Infektimmunität f.
in·fec·ti·os·i·ty [ɪnˌfekʃɪˈɑsətɪ] n Ansteckungsfähigkeit f, Infektiosität f.
in·fec·tious [ɪnˈfekʃəs] adj ansteckungsfähig, ansteckend, infektiös; übertragbar.
infectious agent micro. infektiöses Agens nt, infektiöse Einheit f.
infectious-allergic myocarditis infektiös--allergische/infektallergische Myokarditis f.
infectious aneurysm infektiöses Aneurysma nt.
infectious arthritis Infektarthritis f.
infectious bulbar paralysis Aujeszky'--Krankheit f, Pseudowut f, -lyssa f, -rabies f.
infectious disease Infekt m, Infektion f, Infektionskrankheit f.
infectious eczematoid dermatitis Engman-Krankheit f, infektiöse ekzematoide Dermatitis f.
infectious endocarditis infektiöse Endokarditis f.
infectious hepatitis (Virus-)Hepatitis A f abbr. HA, epidemische Hepatitis f, Hepatitis epidemica.
infectious icterus Weil'-Krankheit f, Leptospirosis icterohaemorrhagica.
infectious jaundice 1. → infectious hepatitis. **2.** → infectious icterus.
infectious mononucleosis Pfeiffer'-Drüsenfieber nt, infektiöse Mononukleose f, Monozytenangina f, Mononucleosis infectiosa.
in·fec·tious·ness [ɪnˈfekʃəsnɪs] n → infectiosity.
infectious purpura infektiöse Purpura f.
infectious rhinitis infektiöse Rhinitis f.
infectious spirochetal jaundice → infectious icterus.
infectious spondylitis infektiöse Spondylitis f, Spondylitis infectiosa.
infectious unit → infectious agent.
infectious wart derm. gemeine/gewöhnliche Warze f, Stachelwarze f, Verruca vulgaris.
in·fec·tive [ɪnˈfektɪv] adj → infectious.
infective asthma infektallergisches Asthma nt.
infective disease → infectious disease.
infective dose abbr. **I.D.** micro. infektiöse Dosis f, Infektionsdosis f abbr. ID, Dosis infectiosa abbr. DI.
median d. abbr. **I.D.$_{50}$** mittlere Infektionsdosis abbr. ID$_{50}$, Dosis infectiosa media abbr. DIM.
infective embolism infektiöse/septische Embolie f.
infective endocarditis infektiöse Endokarditis f.
infective jaundice 1. → infectious hepatitis. **2.** → infectious icterus.
in·fec·tive·ness [ɪnˈfektɪvnɪs] n → infectiosity.
infective polyneuritis Guillain-Barre--Syndrom nt, (Poly-)Radikuloneuritis f, Neuronitis f.

infective silicosis Silikotuberkulose f.
infective thrombus infektiöser Thrombus m.
in·fec·tiv·i·ty [ɪnfekˈtɪvətɪ] n → infectiosity.
in·fe·cund [ɪnˈfiːkənd, -ˈfekənd] adj unfruchtbar, infertil; steril.
in·fe·cun·di·ty [ˌɪnfɪˈkʌndətɪ] n (weibliche) Unfruchtbarkeit f, Infertilität f; Sterilität f.
in·fe·ri·or [ɪnˈfɪərɪər] adj **1.** tiefer od. weiter unten liegend, untere(r, s), inferior, Unter-. **2.** (Qualität) minderwertig, minder. **3.** untergeordnet, niedriger, geringer.
inferior angle: anterior i. of parietal bone Angulus sphenoidalis (ossis parietalis).
posterior i. of parietal bone Angulus mastoideus (ossis parietalis).
i. of scapula Angulus inferior (scapulae).
inferior aperture: i. of minor pelvis untere Öffnung f des kleinen Beckens, Beckenausgang m, Apertura pelvis/pelvica inferior.
i. of thorax Brustkorbausgang m, untere Thoraxapertur f, Apertura thoracis inferior.
i. of tympanic canaliculus äußere Öffnung f des Canaliculus tympanicus, Apertura inferior canaliculi tympanici.
inferior border of spleen unterer Milzrand m, Margo inferior lienis/splenis.
inferior branch: i. of oculomotor nerve unterer Okulomotoriusast m, Ramus inferior n. oculomotorii.
posterior i.es of greater palatine nerve Rami nasales posteriores inferiores n. palatini majoris.
i. of superior gluteal artery unterer Ast m der A. glut(a)ea superior, Ramus inferior a. glut(a)eae superioris.
i.es of transverse cervical nerve untere Äste pl des N. transversus colli, Rami inferiores n. transversi colli.
i. of vestibular nerve unterer Teil des N. vestibularis, Pars caudalis/inferior n. vestibularis.
inferior bulb of jugular vein Bulbus inferior v. jugularis.
inferior bursa of biceps femoris muscle Bursa subtendinea m. bicipitis femoris inferior.
inferior cartilage of nose Cartilago alaris major.
inferior colliculus unterer/hinterer Hügel m der Vierhügelplatte, Colliculus caudalis/inferior.
inferior concha untere Nasenmuschel f, Concha nasalis inferior.
inferior extremity: i. of kidney unterer Nierenpol m, Extremitas inferior renis.
i. of testis unterer Hodenpol m, Extremitas inferior testis.
inferior fascia of urogenital diaphragm Fascia diaphragmatis urogenitalis inferior.
inferior fossa of omental sac Rec. inferior omentalis.
inferior fovea Fovea inferior.
inferior ganglion: i. of glossopharyngeal nerve unteres Glossopharyngeusganglion nt, Ggl. caudalis/inferius n. glossopharyngei.
i. of vagus nerve unteres Vagusganglion nt, Ggl. caudalis/inferius n. vagi.
inferior horn: i. of lateral ventriculus Unterhorn nt des Seitenventrikels, Cornu inferius/temporale ventriculi lateralis.
i. of saphenous opening Cornu inferius hiatus saphenus.
in·fe·ri·or·i·ty [ɪnˌfɪərɪˈɔrətɪ] n Unterlegenheit f (to gegenüber); Minderwertigkeit f.
inferiority complex psycho. Minderwertigkeitskomplex m.

inferiority feeling psycho. Minderwertigkeitsgefühl nt.
inferior lamina of sphenoid bone Proc. pterygoideus (ossis sphenoidalis).
inferior lip Unterlippe f, Labium inferius.
i. of ileocecal valve Labium inferius valvulae coli.
inferior margin: i. of lung unterer/vorderer Lungenrand m, Margo anterior/inferior pulmonis.
i. of spleen → inferior border of spleen.
inferior mediastinum unterer Mediastinalraum m, unteres Mediastinum nt, Mediastinum inferius, Cavum mediastinale inferius.
inferior myocardial infarction diaphragmaler/inferiorer (Myokard-)Infarkt m.
inferior nucleus of trigeminal nerve spinaler/unterer Trigeminuskern m, Nc. inferior/spinalis n. trigeminalis.
inferior opening of pelvis Beckenausgang m, Apertura pelvis/pelvica inferior.
inferior part of duodenum unterer/horizontaler Duodenumabschnitt m, Pars horizontalis/inferior duodeni.
inferior polioencephalitis Polioencephalitis inferior.
inferior ramus of pubis unterer Schambeinast m, Ramus inferior ossis pubis.
inferior root: i. of ansa cervicalis untere/vordere Wurzel f der Ansa cervicalis, Radix inferior/anterior ansae cervicalis.
i. of cervical loop → i. of ansa cervicalis.
i. of vestibulocochlear nerve unterer/kochleärer Anteil m des N. vestibulocochlearis, Radix cochlearis/inferior n. vestibulocochlearis.
inferior segment of kidney Segmentum inferius.
inferior strait Beckenausgang m, Apertura pelvis inferior.
inferior syndrome of red nucleus neuro. Claude-Syndrom nt, unteres Ruber-Syndrom nt, unteres Syndrom nt des Nc. ruber.
inferior tarsus Lidplatte f des Unterlids, Tarsus inferior (palpebrae).
inferior tracheotomy unterer Luftröhrenschnitt m, untere Tracheotomie f.
inferior trunk of brachial plexus unterer Primärfaszikel m des Plexus brachialis, Truncus inferior (plexus brachialis).
inferior vein: i.s of cerebellar hemisphere Vv. hemisphaerii (cerebelli) inferiores, Vv. inferiores cerebelli.
i. of vermis untere Kleinhirnwurm-/Vermisvene f, V. vermis inferior, V. inferior vermis.
in·fe·ro·fron·tal fissure [ˌɪnfərəʊˈfrʌntl] Sulcus frontalis inferior.
in·fe·ro·lat·er·al [ˌ-ˈlætərəl] adj anat. unten u. außen (liegend), inferolateral.
inferolateral myocardial infarction inferolateraler (Myokard-)Infarkt m.
in·fe·ro·me·di·an [ˌ-ˈmiːdɪən] adj anat. unten u. in der Mittellinie (liegend), inferomedian.
in·fe·ro·na·sal [ˌ-ˈneɪzl] adj ophthal. inferonasal.
in·fe·ro·pos·te·ri·or [ˌ-pɒˈstɪərɪər, -pəʊ-] adj anat. unten u. hinten (liegend), inferoposterior.
in·fe·ro·tem·po·ral [ˌ-ˈtemp(ə)rəl] adj ophthal. inferotemporal.
in·fer·tile [ɪnˈfɜːtl; Brit. -taɪl] adj **1.** unfruchtbar, infertil. **2.** bio. unfruchtbar, steril.
in·fer·til·i·tas [ˌɪnfərˈtɪlətæs] n → infertility.
in·fer·til·i·ty [ˌ-ˈtɪlətɪ] n **1.** gyn. (weibliche) Unfruchtbarkeit f, Infertilität f, Impotentia generandi. **2.** andro. (männliche) Unfruchtbarkeit f, Sterilität f, Infertilität

f, Impotentia generandi. **3.** *bio.* Unfruchtbarkeit *f*, Sterilität *f*.
in·fest [ɪn'fest] *vt micro.* (*Parasit*) verseuchen, befallen.
in·fes·ta·tion [ɪnfes'teɪʃn] *n* Parasitenbefall *m*, -infektion *f*, Infestation *f*.
in·fest·ed [ɪn'festɪd] *adj* (*Parasit*) verseucht, befallen, infiziert.
infested abortion *gyn.* infektiöser Abort *m*.
in·fib·u·la·tion [ɪnˌfɪbjə'leɪʃn] *n gyn., histor.* Infibulation *f*.
in·fil·trate [ɪn'fɪltreɪt, 'ɪnfɪltreɪt] **I** *n patho.* Infiltrat *nt*. **II** *vt* **1.** *patho.* einsickern (in), eindringen, infiltrieren. **2.** durchsetzen, -dringen, -tränken (*with* mit). **III** *vi* einsickern, eindringen (*into* in).
in·fil·trat·ing ['ɪnfɪltreɪtɪŋ] *adj* einsickernd, eindringend, infiltrierend.
infiltrating ductal carcinoma with productive fibrosis szirrhöses Brust(drüsen)karzinom *nt*, Szirrhus *m*, Ca. solidum simplex der Brust.
infiltrating lipoma Liposarkom *nt*, Liposarcoma *nt*.
infiltrating tumor infiltrativ-wachsender Tumor *m*.
in·fil·tra·tion [ˌɪnfɪl'treɪʃn] *n* **1.** *patho.* Infiltration *f*, Infiltrierung *f*. **2.** *patho.* Infiltrat *nt*. **3.** Einsickern *nt*, Infiltration *f*. **4.** Durchsetzen *nt*, -dringen *nt*, -tränken *nt*.
infiltration analgesia/anesthesia *anes.* Infiltrationsanästhesie *f*.
in·fil·tra·tive dermopathia ['ɪnfɪltreɪtɪv, ɪn'fɪl-] prätibiales Myxödem *nt*, Myxoedema circumscriptum tuberosum, Myxoedema praetibiale symmetricum.
infiltrative tumor infiltrierender/infiltrativ-wachsender Tumor *m*.
in·firm [ɪn'fɜrm] *adj* schwach, gebrechlich.
in·fir·ma·ry [ɪn'fɜrməri] *n, pl* **-ries 1.** Krankenhaus *nt*. **2.** Krankenzimmer *nt*, -stube *f*, -revier *nt*; Sanitätsstation *f*.
in·fir·mi·ty [ɪn'fɜrməti] *n, pl* **-ties 1.** Schwäche *f*, Gebrechlichkeit *f*; Gebrechen *nt*. **2.** Geistesschwäche *f*.
in·firm·ness [ɪn'fɜrmnɪs] *n* → infirmity.
in·flame [ɪn'fleɪm] **I** *vt* entzünden. **to become** ~*d* s. entzünden. **II** *vi* **1.** s. entzünden. **2.** Feuer fangen, s. entzünden. **3.** *fig.* s. erhitzen, wütend werden.
in·flamed [ɪn'fleɪmd] *adj* **1.** entzündet. **2.** brennend.
inflamed ulcer entzündetes Ulkus *nt*.
in·flam·ma·bil·i·ty [ɪnˌflæmə'bɪləti] *n* **1.** Entflammbarkeit *f*, Brennbarkeit *f*, Entzündlichkeit *f*. **2.** Feuergefährlichkeit *f*. **3.** *fig.* Erregbarkeit *f*.
in·flam·ma·ble [ɪn'flæməbl] **I** *n* Brennstoff *m*, -material *nt*, leicht entzündliche *od.* feuergefährliche Substanz *f*. **II** *adj* **1.** entflammbar, brennbar, (leicht) entzündlich; feuergefährlich. **2.** *fig.* reizbar, leicht erregbar, jähzornig.
in·flam·ma·tion [ˌɪnflə'meɪʃn] *n* **1.** *patho.* Entzündung *f*, Inflammation *f*, Inflammatio *f*. **2.** *fig.* Erregung *f*, Entflammung *f*.
inflammation theory of ulcer formation Entzündungstheorie *f* der Ulkusentstehung.
in·flam·ma·to·ry [ɪn'flæmətɔːri, -təʊ-] *adj* Entzündung betr., durch eine Entzündung gekennzeichnet, entzündlich, Entzündungs-.
inflammatory arthritis, chronic rheumatoide Arthritis *f*, progrediente/primär chronische Polyarthritis *f abbr.* PCP, PcP.
inflammatory arthropathy entzündliche Gelenkerkrankung *f*.
inflammatory atrophy entzündliche Atrophie *f*.

inflammatory bowel disease entzündliche Darmerkrankung *f*.
inflammatory cells *patho.* Entzündungszellen *pl*.
inflammatory dysmenorrhea *gyn.* entzündlich-bedingte Dysmenorrhö *f*.
inflammatory edema entzündliches Ödem *nt*.
inflammatory exudate entzündliches Exsudat *nt*.
inflammatory gangrene entzündliche Gangrän *f*.
inflammatory glaucoma entzündlich-bedingtes Glaukom *nt*, Glaucoma inflammatorium *nt*.
inflammatory hyperplasia entzündliche Hyperplasie *f*.
inflammatory infiltrate/infiltration entzündliches Infiltrat *nt*.
inflammatory joint disease entzündliche Gelenkerkrankung/Gelenkaffektion *f*.
inflammatory osteoarthritis entzündliche/rapid-progressive Arthrose *f*.
inflammatory polyp entzündlicher Polyp *m*.
inflammatory response Entzündungsreaktion *f*.
inflammatory rheumatism rheumatisches Fieber *nt abbr.* RF, Febris rheumatica, akuter Gelenkrheumatismus *m*, Polyarthritis rheumatica acuta.
inflammatory scoliosis *ortho.* infektiös-bedingte Skoliose *f*.
inflammatory vasculitis entzündliche Vaskulitis *f*.
in·flat·a·ble [ɪn'fleɪtəbl] *adj* aufblasbar.
in·flate [ɪn'fleɪt] **I** *vt* **1.** *patho.* aufblähen, auftreiben. **2.** aufblasen, mit Luft *od.* Gas füllen, aufpumpen. **II** *vi* aufgeblasen *od.* aufgepumpt werden, s. mit Luft *od.* Gas füllen.
in·flat·ed [ɪn'fleɪtɪd] *adj* **1.** *patho.* aufgebläht, aufgetrieben. **2.** aufgeblasen.
in·fla·tion [ɪn'fleɪʃn] *n* **1.** *patho.* Aufblähen *nt*, Auftreiben *nt*. **2.** Aufblasen *nt*, Aufpumpen *nt*.
in·flect [ɪn'flekt] *vt* (einwärts-)biegen, (-)beugen, nach innen beugen.
in·flec·tion [ɪn'flekʃn] *n* (Einwärts-)Biegung *f*, (-)Beugung *f*, (-)Krümmung *f*, Inflektion *f*.
inflection point *mathe.* Umkehrpunkt *m*.
in·flex·ion *n Brit.* → inflection.
in·flict [ɪn'flɪkt] *vt* (*Schaden*) zufügen, (*Wunde*) beibringen (*on, upon*).
in·flow ['ɪnfləʊ] *n* Zustrom *m*, -fluß *m*, Einströmen *nt*.
in·flu·en·za [ˌɪnflu'enzə] *n* Grippe *f*, Influenza *f*.
influenza A A-Grippe *f*, Influenza A *f*.
influenza A virus → influenza type A virus.
influenza B B-Grippe *f*, Influenza B *f*.
influenza bacillus Pfeiffer'-(Influenza-)-Bazillus *m*, Haemophilus influenzae, Bact. influenzae.
influenza B virus → influenza type B virus.
influenza C C-Grippe *f*, Influenza C *f*.
influenza C virus → influenza type C virus.
in·flu·en·zal [ˌɪnflu'enzl] *adj* Grippe betr., grippal, Influenza-, Grippe-.
influenzal encephalitis Grippe-, Influenzaenzephalitis *f*.
influenza-like *adj* grippe-, influenzaähnlich, grippal.
influenzal otitis Grippeotitis *f*.
influenzal pneumonia 1. Grippe-, Influenzapneumonie *f*. **2.** Haemophilus-influenza-Pneumonie *f*.
influenzal virus → influenza virus.

influenza pneumonia → influenzal pneumonia.
influenza type A virus Influenza A-Virus *nt*.
influenza type B virus Influenza B-Virus *nt*.
influenza type C virus Influenza C-Virus *nt*.
In·flu·en·za·vi·rus [ˌɪnfluːˌenzə'vaɪrəs] *n micro.* Influenzavirus *nt*.
influenza virus Grippe-, Influenzavirus *nt*.
i. A → influenza virus type A.
i. B → influenza virus type B.
i. C → influenza virus type C.
influenza virus pneumonia → influenzal pneumonia 1.
influenza virus type A Influenza A-Virus *nt*.
influenza virus type B Influenza B-Virus *nt*.
influenza virus type C Influenza C-Virus *nt*.
influenza virus vaccine Grippe-, Influenzaimpfstoff *m*, -vakzine *f*.
in·flux ['ɪnflʌks] *n* → inflow.
in·fold [ɪn'fəʊld] *vt* **1.** einhüllen (*in* in); umhüllen (*with* mit). **2.** falten.
in·fold·ing [ɪn'fəʊldɪŋ] *n* **1.** Um-, Einhüllen *nt*. **2.** Falten *nt*, Faltung *f*.
in·form [ɪn'fɔːrm] *vt* unterrichten, benachrichtigen, in Kenntnis setzen, informieren (*of, about* über). **to** ~ **sb. of sth.** jdn. über etw. informieren, jdn. von etw. unterrichten.
in·for·ma·tion [ˌɪnfər'meɪʃn] *n* **1.** Benachrichtigung *f*, Unterrichtung *f*. **2.** (wissenschaftliche) Tatsachen *pl*. **3.** Auskunft *f*, Information(en *pl*) *f* (*on* über). **to give** ~ Auskunft geben. **a piece of** ~ eine Auskunft/Information.
in·for·ma·tion·al [ˌɪnfər'meɪʃnl] *adj* informatorisch, Informations-.
informational macromolecule *biochem.* informatives/informationstragendes Makromolekül *nt*.
information flow Informationsfluß *m*.
information storage Informationsspeicherung *f*.
information theory Informationstheorie *f*.
information transfer Informationsvermittlung *f*, -übertragung *f*.
information-transmitting system informationsübertragendes System *nt*.
in·form·a·tive [ɪn'fɔːrmətɪv] *adj* aufschlußreich, lehrreich, informativ.
in·form·a·to·ry [ɪn'fɔːrmətɔːri, -təʊr-] *adj* **1.** → informational. **2.** → informative.
in·formed [ɪn'fɔːrmd] *adj* informiert, unterrichtet. **to keep sb./o.s.** ~ jdn./s. auf dem Laufenden halten (*of* über).
informed consent informierte Einwilligung *f*, informed consent.
in·form·o·some [ɪn'fɔːrməsəʊm] *n genet.* Informosom *nt*.
infra- *pref.* Infra-, Sub-
infra-axillary *adj* unterhalb der Axilla (liegend), infra-, subaxillär, subaxillar.
in·fra·cal·ca·rine gyrus [ˌɪnfrə'kælkəraɪn] Gyrus lingualis.
in·fra·car·di·ac [ˌɪnfrə'kɑːrdɪæk] *adj* unterhalb des Herzens/d. der Herzebene (liegend), infra-, subkardial.
in·fra·cer·e·bral [ˌɪnfrə'serəbrəl] *adj* unterhalb des Großhirns (liegend), subzerebral.
in·fra·cla·vic·u·lar [ˌɪnfrəklə'vɪkjələr] *adj* unterhalb des Schlüsselbeins/der Clavicula (liegend), infra-, subklavikulär.
infraclavicular fossa Mohrenheim'-Grube *f*, Trigonum deltoideopectorale, Fossa infraclavicularis.
infraclavicular infiltrate *patho.* infraklavikuläres Infiltrat *nt*.

infraclavicular part of brachial plexus

infraclavicular part of brachial plexus infraklavikulärer Teil *m* des Plexus brachialis, Pars infraclavicularis (plexus brachialis).
infraclavicular region → infraclavicular fossa.
infraclavicular triangle → infraclavicular fossa.
in·fra·cli·noid aneurysm [,-'klaɪnɔɪd] infraclinoidales Aneurysma *nt*.
in·fra·cor·ti·cal [,-'kɔːrtɪkl] *adj* unterhalb der Rinde (liegend), infra-, subkortikal.
in·fra·cos·tal [,-'kɑstl] *adj* unterhalb einer Rippe *od.* der Rippen (liegend), infra-, subkostal.
infracostal artery Ramus costalis lateralis a. thoracicae internae.
infracostal line Planum subcostale.
in·fra·cot·y·loid [,-'kɑtlɔɪd] *adj* unterhalb des Azetabulums (liegend), subazetabulär.
in·frac·tion [ɪn'frækʃn] *n ortho.* Haarbruch *m*, (Knochen-)Fissur *f*, Infraktur *f*, Infraktion *f*.
in·frac·ture [ɪn'fræktʃər] *n* → infraction.
in·fra·di·a·phrag·mat·ic [,ɪnfrədaɪə'frægmætɪk] *adj* unterhalb des Zwerchfells (liegend), infradiaphragmal, -diaphragmatisch, subdiaphragmatisch, -phrenisch.
in·fra·duc·tion [,-'dʌkʃn] *n ophthal.* Abwärtswendung *f* eines Auges, Infraduktion *f*.
in·fra·du·o·de·nal fossa [,-,d(j)uːəʊ'diːnl] Rec. retroduodenalis.
in·fra·gle·noid [,-'gliːnɔɪd] *adj* unterhalb der Cavitas glenoidalis (liegend), infra-, subglenoidal.
infraglenoid tubercle Tuberculum infraglenoidale.
infraglenoid tuberosity → infraglenoid tubercle.
in·fra·glot·tic [,-'glɑtɪk] *adj* unterhalb der Glottis (liegend), infra-, subglottisch.
infraglottic cavity infraglottischer Raum *m*, Cavitas infraglottica.
infraglottic space → infraglottic cavity.
in·fra·he·pat·ic [,-hɪ'pætɪk] *adj* unterhalb der Leber (liegend), subhepatisch.
in·fra·hy·oid [,-'haɪɔɪd] *adj* unterhalb des Zungenbeins (liegend), infrahyoidal, subhyoid(al).
infrahyoid branch of superior thyroid artery Ramus infrahyoideus a. thyroideae superioris.
infrahyoid bursa Bursa infrahyoidea.
infrahyoid muscles infrahyoidale Muskulatur *f*, Mm. infrahyoidei.
in·fra·ma·mil·lary [,-'mæməlɛrɪ, 'mæmɪlərɪ] *adj* unterhalb der Brustwarze (liegend), infra-, submamillär.
in·fra·mam·ma·ry [,-'mæmərɪ] *adj* unterhalb der Brust(drüse) (liegend), infra-, submammär.
inframammary region Regio inframammaria.
in·fra·man·dib·u·lar [,-mæn'dɪbjələr] *adj* unterhalb des Unterkiefers (liegend), inframandibulär, -mandibular, submandibulär, -mandibular.
in·fra·mar·gin·al [,-'mɑːrdʒɪnl] *adj* unterhalb einer Grenze (liegend), infra-, submarginal.
in·fra·max·il·lary [,-'mæksəlɛrɪ, -mæk'sɪlərɪ] *adj* unterhalb des Oberkiefers (liegend), inframaxillär, -maxillar, submaxillär, -maxillar.
in·fra·nod·al extrasystole [,-'nəʊdl] *card.* ventrikuläre Extrasystole *f*.
in·fra·nu·cle·ar [,-'n(j)uːklɪər] *adj* unterhalb eines Kerns (liegend), infranukleär, -nuklear, subnukleär, -nuklear.

in·fra·oc·cip·i·tal nerve [,-ɑk'sɪpɪtl] N. suboccipitalis.
in·fra·or·bit·al [,-'ɔːrbɪtl] *adj* unterhalb der Orbita/Augenhöhle (liegend), auf dem Orbitaboden liegend, infra-, suborbital.
infraorbital artery *old* Augenhöhlenbodenschlagader *f*, Infraorbitalis *f*, A. infraorbitalis.
infraorbital canal Infraorbitalkanal *m*, Canalis infraorbitalis.
infraorbital foramen For. infraorbitale.
infraorbital groove of maxilla → infraorbital sulcus of maxillae.
infraorbital margin: i. of maxilla Margo infraorbitalis maxillae.
 i. of orbita unterer Augenhöhlenrand *m*, Margo infraorbitalis orbitae.
infraorbital nerve Infraorbitalis *m*, N. infraorbitalis.
infraorbital region Infraorbitalregion *f*, Regio infraorbitalis.
infraorbital sulcus of maxilla Infraorbitalfurche *f*, Sulcus infraorbitalis (maxillae).
infraorbital suture Sutura infra-orbitalis.
in·fra·pal·pe·bral sulcus [,-'pælpəbrəl, -pæl'piːbrəl] Unterlidfurche *f*, Sulcus infrapalpebralis.
in·fra·pa·tel·lar [,-pə'tɛlər] *adj* unterhalb der Kniescheibe/Patella (liegend), infrapatellar, -patellär, subpatellar.
infrapatellar branch of saphenous nerve infrapatellärer Ast *m* des N. saphenus, Ramus infrapatellaris n. spheni.
infrapatellar bursa: deep i. Bursa infrapatellaris profunda.
 inferior i., superficial Bursa subcutanea tuberositatis tibiae.
 subcutaneous i. Bursa subcutanea infrapatellaris.
infrapatellar fold Plica synovialis infrapatellaris.
infrapatellar synovial fold Plica synovialis infrapatellaris.
in·fra·pir·i·form foramen [,-'pɪrəfɔːrm] For. infrapiriforme.
in·fra·psy·chic [,-'saɪkɪk] *adj* unterhalb der Bewußtseinsebene, unbewußt; automatisch.
in·fra·red [,-'rɛd] **I** *n* **1.** *abbr.* **IR** Ultrarot *nt abbr.* IR. **2.** Infrarot-, Ultrarotlicht *nt*, IR-Licht *nt*, UR-Licht *nt*. **II** *adj* ultra-, infrarot.
infrared cataract Feuer-, Glasbläserstar *m*, Infrarotkatarakt *f*, Cataracta calorica.
infrared lamp Infrarotlicht, -lampe *f*, -strahler *m*.
infrared light Infrarot-, Ultrarotlicht *nt*, IR-Licht *nt*, UR-Licht *nt*.
infrared rays Infrarotstrahlen *pl*.
infrared waves Infrarotwellen *pl*.
in·fra·scap·u·lar [,-'skæpjələr] *adj* unterhalb des Schulterblattes/der Scapula (liegend), infraskapular, -skapulär, subskapulär, -skapular.
infrascapular region Unterschulterblattregion *f*, Regio infrascapularis.
in·fra·son·ic [,-'sɑnɪk] *adj* infrasonar, Infraschall-.
in·fra·son·ics [,-'sɑnɪks] *pl* Lehre *f* vom Infraschall.
infrasonic sound Infraschall *m*.
infrasonic waves → infrasonic sound.
in·fra·spi·nal [,-'spaɪnl] *adj* → infraspinous.
in·fra·spi·na·tus [,-spaɪ'neɪtəs] *n* Infraspinatus *m*, M. infraspinatus.
infraspinatus muscle → infraspinatus.
infraspinatus reflex Infraspinatusreflex *m*.
in·fra·spi·nous [,-'spaɪnəs] *adj* unterhalb der Spina scapulae (liegend), infraspinal.
infraspinous fossa Fossa infraspinata/infraspinosa.
infraspinous muscle → infraspinatus (muscle).
in·fra·splen·ic [,-'spliːnɪk, -'splɛn-] *adj* unterhalb der Milz (liegend), subsplenisch.
in·fra·ster·nal [,-'stɜrnl] *adj* unterhalb des Brustbeins/Sternums (liegend), infra-, substernal.
infrasternal angle epigastrischer Winkel *m*, Rippenbogenwinkel *m*, Angulus infrasternalis.
in·fra·struc·ture ['-strʌktʃər] *n* **1.** *histol., bio.* Feinstruktur *f*, Infrastruktur *f*. **2.** Infrastruktur *f*.
in·fra·tem·po·ral [,-'tɛmp(ə)rəl] *adj* unterhalb der Schläfe *od.* Schläfengrube (liegend), infratemporal.
infratemporal crest Crista infratemporalis.
infratemporal fossa Unterschläfengrube *f*, Fossa infratemporalis.
infratemporal region → infratemporal fossa.
in·fra·ten·to·ri·al [,-tɛn'tɔːrɪəl, -'təʊr-] *adj* unterhalb des Tentorium cerebelli (liegend), infra-, subtentorial.
infratentorial tumor infratentorieller Tumor *m*.
in·fra·tho·rac·ic [,-θɔː'ræsɪk, -θə-] *adj* unterhalb des Brustkorbs (liegend), subthorakal.
in·fra·ton·sil·lar [,-'tɑnsɪlər] *adj* unterhalb der Gaumenmandel (liegend), infra-, subtonsillär.
in·fra·tra·che·al [,-'treɪkɪəl] *adj* unterhalb der Luftröhre/Trachea (liegend), infra-, subtracheal.
in·fra·troch·le·ar nerve [,-'trɑklɪər] Infratrochlearis *m*, N. infratrochlearis.
in·fra·um·bil·i·cal [,-ʌm'bɪlɪkl] *adj* unterhalb des Nabels (liegend), infra-, subumbilikal.
in·fra·ver·gence [,-'vɜrdʒəns] *n ophthal.* Infravergenz *f*.
in·fra·ver·sion [,-'vɜrʒn] *n* **1.** *ophthal.* Abwärtswendung *f* beider Augen, Infraversion *f*. **2.** Drehung *f* nach unten.
in·fre·quence [ɪn'friːkwəns] *n* **1.** Seltenheit *f*. **2.** Spärlichkeit *f*.
in·fre·quen·cy [ɪn'friːkwənsɪ] *n* → infrequence.
in·fre·quent [ɪn'friːkwənt] *adj* selten; spärlich.
infrequent menstruation Oligomenorrhoe *f*.
infrequent pulse langsamer Puls *m*, Pulsus rarus.
in·fric·tion [ɪn'frɪkʃn] *n* (*Salbe, Öl*) Einreiben *nt*, Einreibung *f*.
in·fun·dib·u·lar [,ɪnfən'dɪbjələr] *adj* **1.** *anat.* trichterförmig, infundibulär. **2.** Infundibulum betr., -infundibulär.
infundibular body Neurohypophyse *f*, Hypophysenhinterlappen *m abbr.* HHL, Neurohypophysis *f*, Lobus posterior hypophyseos.
infundibular nucleus of hypothalamus Nc. arcuatus/infundibularis (hypothalami).
infundibular part of adenohypophysis Trichterlappen *m*, Pars infundibularis/tuberalis adenohypophyseos.
infundibular process Neurallappen *m* der Neurohypophyse, Lobus nervosus neurohypophyseos.
infundibular pulmonary stenosis *card.* Infundibulumstenose *f*, subvalvuläre/infundibuläre Pulmonalstenose *f*.
infundibular recess Rec. infundibularis/infundibuli.

infundibular stalk Hypophysenstiel *m*, Infundibulum hypothalami.
infundibular stem → infundibular stalk.
infundibular stenosis → infundibular pulmonary stenosis.
in·fun·dib·u·lec·to·my [ˌɪnfəndɪbjəˈlektəmɪ] *n HTG* Infundibulektomie *f*, Infundibulumresektion *f*.
in·fun·dib·u·li·form [ˌ-ˈdɪbjəlɪfɔːrm] *adj anat.* trichterförmig.
infundibuliform recess Rosenmüller'-Grube *f*, Rec. pharyngeus.
in·fun·dib·u·lo·ma [ˌ-ˌdɪbjəˈləʊmə] *n patho.* (*Hypophyse*) Tumor *m* der Pars tuberalis.
in·fun·dib·u·lo·pel·vic ligament [ˌ-ˌdɪbjələʊˈpelvɪk] Lig. suspensorium ovarii.
in·fun·dib·u·lo·ven·tric·u·lar crest [ˌ-ˌdɪbjələʊvenˈtrɪkjələr] (*Herz*) supraventrikuläre Muskelleiste *f*, Crista supraventricularis.
in·fun·dib·u·lum [ˌɪnfənˈdɪbjələm] *n*, *pl* **-la** [-lə] **1.** *anat.* Trichter *m*, trichterförmige Struktur *f*, Infundibulum *nt*. **2.** Conus arteriosus, Infundibulum *nt*.
i. of heart → infundibulum 2.
i.la of kidney Nierenkelche *pl*, Calices renales.
i. of urinary bladder (Harn-)Blasengrund *m*, (Harn-)Blasenfundus *m*, Fundus vesicae (urinariae).
i. of uterine tube Tubentrichter, -infundibulum, Infundibulum tubae uterinae.
in·fuse [ɪnˈfjuːz] *vt* mittels Infusion einführen, infundieren.
in·fu·si·ble [ɪnˈfjuːzɪbl] *adj* unschmelzbar.
in·fu·sion [ɪnˈfjuːʒn] *n* **1.** Infusion *f*. **2.** *pharm.* Aufgießen *nt*; Ziehenlassen *nt*; Aufguß *m*, Infus *nt*, Infusum *nt*; Tee *m*.
infusion apparatus Infusionsgerät *nt*.
infusion bottle Infusionsflasche *f*.
infusion cannula Infusionskanüle *f*.
infusion chemotherapy Infusionschemotherapie *f*.
infusion cholangiography *radiol.* Infusioncholangiographie *f*.
infusion fluid Infusionsflüssigkeit *f*.
infusion solution Infusionslösung *f*.
infusion therapy Infusionstherapie *f*.
infusion urography *radiol.* Infusionsurographie *f*.
In·fu·so·ri·a [ˌɪnfjʊˈsɔːrɪə, -ˈsəʊr-] *pl micro.* Aufguß-, Wimpertierchen *pl*, Infusorien *pl*, Ciliata *pl*.
in·fu·so·ri·al [ˌ-ˈsɔːrɪəl] *adj* infusorienartig, Infusorien-.
infusorial earth Kieselgur *nt*, Infusorienerde *f*.
in·fu·so·ri·an [ˌ-ˈsɔːrɪən] **I** *n* → Infusoria. **II** *adj* → infusorial.
in·fu·so·ri·um [ˌ-ˈsɔːrɪəm] *sing* → Infusoria.
in·fu·sum [ɪnˈfjuːsəm] *n pharm.* Aufguß *m*, Infus *nt*, Infusum *nt*.
in·gest [ɪnˈdʒest] *vt* (*Nahrung*) aufnehmen *od.* zu s. nehmen.
in·ges·ta [ɪnˈdʒestə] *pl* Ingesta *pl*, aufgenommene Nahrung *f*.
in·ges·tion [ɪnˈdʒestʃn] *n* (Nähr-)Stoffaufnahme *f*, Nahrungsaufnahme *f*, Ingestion *f*.
in·ges·tive [ɪnˈdʒestɪv] *adj* Nahrungsaufnahme betr., zur Nahrungsaufnahme dienend, Ingestions-.
Ingrassia [ɪnˈɡræsɪə]: **I.'s apophysis/process** kleiner Keilbeinflügel *m*, Ala minor (ossis sphenoidalis).
I.'s wing 1. → I.'s apophysis. **2.** ~s *pl* Keilbeinflügel *pl*.
in·gra·ves·cence [ˌɪnɡrəˈvesn(t)s] *n* (langsam-progrediente) Verschlimmerung *f*.
in·gra·ves·cent [ˌ-ˈvesnt] *adj* s. (allmählich) verschlimmernd, langsam-progredient.

ingravescent apoplexy langsam-progrediente Apoplexie *f*.
in·grow·ing [ˈɪnɡrəʊɪŋ] *adj* einwärtswachsend, einwachsend; eingewachsen.
in·grown [ˈɪnɡrəʊn] *adj* eingewachsen.
ingrown hairs Pili incarnati/recurvati; Pseudofolliculitis barbae.
in·growth [ˈɪnɡrəʊθ] *n* **1.** Einwachsen *nt*. **2.** Einwachs *m*.
in·guen [ˈɪŋɡwen] *n anat.* Leiste *f*, Leistengegend *f*, Inguen *nt*.
in·gui·nal [ˈɪŋɡwɪnl] *adj* Leiste(ngegend) betr., inguinal, Inguinal-, Leisten-.
inguinal arch → inguinal ligament.
inguinal arteries → inguinal branches of femoral artery.
inguinal branches of femoral artery A. femoralis-Äste *pl* zur Leistenregion, Rami inguinales a. femoralis.
inguinal bubo Leistenbubo *m*.
inguinal canal Leistenkanal *m*, Canalis inguinalis.
inguinal falx Leistensichel *f*, Falx inguinalis, Tendo conjunctivus.
inguinal fold *embryo.* untere Gonadenfalte *f*.
inguinal fossa Leistengrube *f*, Fossa inguinalis.
external i. äußere/seitliche Leistengrube, Fossa inguinalis lateralis.
internal i. innere/mittlere Leistengrube, Fossa inguinalis medialis.
lateral i. → external i.
medial i. → internal i.
middle i. → internal i.
inguinal fovea → inguinal fossa.
inguinal hernia Leistenbruch *m*, -hernie *f*, Hernia inguinalis.
acquired h. erworbener Leistenbruch, Hernia inguinalis acquisita.
congenital h. angeborener Leistenbruch, Hernia inguinalis congenita.
direct h. direkter/innerer/gerader Leistenbruch, Hernia inguinalis interna/medialis/directa.
external h. äußerer/seitlicher/indirekter/schräger Leistenbruch, Hernia inguinalis externa/indirecta/lateralis/obliqua.
indirect h. → external h.
internal h. → direct h.
medial h. → direct h.
oblique h. → external h.
inguinal ligament Leistenband *nt*, Lig. inguinale, Arcus inguinale.
i. of Cooper Lig. pectineale.
reflex i. Lig. inguinale reflexum.
inguinal lymph nodes Leisten-, Inguinallymphknoten *pl*, Nodi lymphatici inguinales.
deep i. tiefe Leistenlymphknoten, Nodi lymphatici inguinales profundi.
inferior i. untere Leistenlymphknoten, Nodi lymphatici inguinales inferiores.
inferior superficial i. untere oberflächliche Leistenlymphknoten, Nodi lymphatici inguinales (superficiales) inferiores.
superficial i. oberflächliche Leistenlymphknoten, Nodi lymphatici inguinales superficiales.
superolateral i. obere seitliche Leistenlymphknoten, Nodi lymphatici inguinales superolaterales.
superolateral superficial i. laterale Gruppe *f* der oberflächlichen Leistenlymphknoten, Nodi lymphatici inguinales (superficiales) superolaterales.
superomedial i. obere mediale Leistenlymphknoten, Nodi lymphatici inguinales superomediales.
superomedial superficial i. mediale Gruppe *f* der oberflächlichen Leistenlymph-

knoten, Nodi lymphatici inguinales (superficiales) superomediales.
inguinal plexus lymphatischer Leistenplexus *m*.
inguinal reflex Geigel-Reflex *m*, Leistenreflex *m*, Femoroabdominalreflex *m*.
inguinal region Leiste *f*, Leistengegend *f*, -region *f*, Regio inguinalis.
inguinal ring Leistenring *m*, A(n)nulus inguinalis.
abdominal i. → deep i.
deep i. innerer Leistenring, A(n)nulus inguinalis profundus.
external i. → superficial i.
internal i. → abdominal i.
subcutaneous i. → superficial i.
superficial i. äußerer Leistenring, A(n)nulus inguinalis superficialis.
inguinal testis Leisten-, Inguinalhoden *m*.
in·gui·no·ab·dom·i·nal [ˌɪŋɡwɪnəʊæbˈdɑmɪnl] *adj* Leiste(ngegend) u. Abdomen betr., inguinoabdominal.
in·gui·no·cru·ral [ˌ-ˈkruːrəl] *adj* Leiste(ngegend) u. Oberschenkel betr., inguinokrural, -femoral.
inguinocrural hernia kombinierte Leisten- u. Schenkelhernie *f*.
in·gui·no·dyn·ia [ˌ-ˈdiːnɪə] *n* Leistenschmerz *m*.
in·gui·no·fem·o·ral hernia [ˌ-ˈfemərəl] → inguinocrural hernia.
in·gui·no·la·bi·al [ˌ-ˈleɪbɪəl] *adj* Leiste(ngegend) u. Schamlippe(n) betr., inguinolabial.
in·gui·no·pro·per·i·to·ne·al hernia [ˌ-prəʊˌperɪtəˈnɪəl] Krönlein-, Bruggiser-Hernie *f*.
in·gui·no·scro·tal [ˌ-ˈskrəʊtl] *adj* Leiste(ngegend) u. Skrotum betr., inguinoskrotal.
INH *abbr.* [isonicotinic acid hydrazide] → isoniazid.
in·hal·ant [ɪnˈheɪlənt] **I** *n* **1.** Inhalat *nt*. **2.** Inhalationsmittel *nt*, -präparat *nt*. **II** *adj* einatmend, Inhalations-.
in·ha·la·tion [ˌɪnhəˈleɪʃn] *n* **1.** Einatmung *f*, Einatmen *nt*, Inhalation. **2.** → inhalant 2.
in·ha·la·tion·al [ˌ-ˈleɪʃnəl] *adj* inhalativ, Inhalations-.
inhalational anthrax Lungenmilzbrand *m*, Wollsortierer-, Lumpensortierer-, Hadernkrankheit *f*.
inhalation allergy Inhalationsallergie *f*.
inhalation anesthesia Inhalationsnarkose *f*.
inhalation anesthetic Inhalationsnarkotikum *nt*.
inhalation injury inhalative Atemwegsverletzung *f*, Inhalationsverletzung *f*.
inhalation pneumonia 1. Aspirationspneumonie *f*. **2.** Bronchopneumonie *f* durch Gasinhalation.
inhalation therapy Inhalationstherapie *f*.
inhalation tuberculosis Inhalationstuberkulose *f*.
in·ha·la·tor [ˈɪnhəleɪtər] *n* Inhalationsapparat *m*, Inhalator *m*.
in·hale [ɪnˈheɪl] *vt*, *vi* einatmen, inhalieren; (*Zigarette*) auf die Lunge rauchen.
in·hal·er [ɪnˈheɪlər] *n* Inhalator *m*.
in·her·ent [ɪnˈhɪərənt, -ˈher-] *adj* innewohnend, eigen (*in*); intrinsisch; angeboren.
inherent immunity angeborene Immunität *f*.
in·her·it [ɪnˈherɪt] **I** *vt* (er-)erben (*from* von). **II** *vi* erben.
in·her·it·a·ble [ɪnˈherɪtəbl] *adj* vererbbar, erblich, Erb-.
in·her·it·ance [ɪnˈherɪtəns] *n* **1.** Vererbung *f*. **by** ~ erblich, durch Vererbung. **2.** Erbgut *nt*.
in·her·it·ed [ɪnˈherɪtɪd] *adj* ver-, ererbt, Erb-.

inherited immunity angeborene Immunität *f*.
in·hib·in [ɪn'hɪbɪn] *n* Inhibin *nt*.
in·hib·it [ɪn'hɪbɪt] *vt* **1.** *biochem. physiol.* hemmen, (ver-)hindern, inhibieren. **2.** jdn. zurückhalten (*from* von); jdn. hindern (*from* an).
in·hib·it·ing antibody [ɪn'hɪbɪtɪŋ] univalenter/hemmender Antikörper *m*.
inhibiting factor *abbr.* **IF** Inhibiting-Faktor *m abbr.* IF.
inhibiting hormone *abbr.* **IH** Inhibiting--Hormon *nt abbr.* IH.
in·hi·bi·tion [ˌɪn(h)ɪ'bɪʃn] *n biochem. physiol.* Hemmung *f*, Inhibition *f*.
inhibition zone *micro.* Hemmhof *m*, -zone *f*.
in·hib·i·tive [ɪn'hɪbɪtɪv] *adj* → inhibitory.
in·hib·i·tor [ɪn'hɪbɪtər] *n chem., biochem.* Hemmstoff *m*, Hemmer *m*, Inhibitor *m*.
inhibitor constant Inhibitorkonstante *f*.
in·hib·i·to·ry [ɪn'hɪbətɔːriː, -təʊ-] *adj* hemmend, hindernd, inhibitorisch, Hemmungs-.
inhibitory center (*ZNS*) hemmendes/inhibierendes/inhibitorisches Zentrum *n*.
inhibitory modulator hemmender/negativer Modulator *m*.
inhibitory nerve-terminal potential *abbr.* **INTP** inhibitorisches Nervenendpotential *nt*, inhibitory nerve-terminal potential *abbr.* INTP.
inhibitory postsynaptic current *abbr.* **IPSC** inhibitorischer postsynaptischer Strom *m*, inhibitory postsynaptic current *abbr.* IPSC.
inhibitory postsynaptic potential *abbr.* **IPSP** inhibitorisches postsynaptisches Potential *nt abbr.* IPSP, inhibitory postsynaptic potential *abbr.* IPSP.
inhibitory receptive field *abbr.* **IRF** inhibitorisches rezeptives Feld *nt abbr.* IRF.
inhibitory reflex hemmender/inhibitorischer Reflex *m*, Hemmreflex *m*. **intestino-intestinal i.** intestino-intestinaler Hemmreflex.
inhibitory synapse inhibitorische/hemmende Synapse *f*.
inhibitory transmitter hemmender/inhibitorischer Transmitter *m*.
in·ho·mo·ge·ne·i·ty [ˌɪnˌhəʊmədʒə'nɪətɪ, -ˌhæm-] *n* inhomogene Beschaffenheit *f*, Inhomogenität *f*.
in·ho·mo·ge·ne·ous [ˌɪnˌhəʊmə'dʒiːnɪəs, -ˌhæm-] *adj* nichthomogen, ungleichmäßig, inhomogen.
in·i·ac ['ɪnɪæk] *adj anat.* Inion betr.
in·i·ad ['ɪnɪæd] *adj* in Richtung auf das Inion.
in·i·al ['ɪnɪəl] *adj anat.* Inion betr.
in·i·en·ceph·a·lus [ˌɪnɪen'sefələs] *n embryo.* Inienzephalus *m*.
in·i·en·ceph·a·ly [-'sefəlɪ] *n embryo.* Inienzephalie *f*, -encephalia *f*.
in·i·od·y·mus [ɪnɪ'ɑdɪməs] *n* → iniopagus.
in·i·on ['ɪnɪən] *n anat.* Inion *nt*.
in·i·op·a·gus [ɪnɪ'ɑpəgəs] *n embryo.* Iniopagus *m*, Iniodymus *m*, Craniopagus occipitalis.
in·i·ops ['ɪnɪɑps] *n embryo.* Iniops *m*.
in·i·tial [ɪ'nɪʃl] *adj* anfänglich, erste(r, s), initial, Anfangs-, Ausgangs-, Initial-.
initial atelectasis (*Lunge*) primäre Atelektase *f*.
initial body Retikular-, Initialkörperchen *nt*.
initial cell Germinal-, Keimzelle *f*.
initial dose *pharm.* Initial-, Aufsättigungsdosis *f*.
initial focus *patho.* Initialherd *m*.
initial heat initiale Wärme *f*, Initialwärme *f*.

initial hematuria initiale Hämaturie *f*.
initial injury initiale Verletzung *f*, Ausgangs-, Erstverletzung *f*.
initial pain erster Schmerz *m*, Initialschmerz *m*.
initial temperature Ausgangstemperatur *f*.
initial velocity Ausgangs-, Initialgeschwindigkeit *f*.
in·i·ti·ate [ɪ'nɪʃɪeɪt] *vt* anfangen, beginnen, einleiten, in die Wege leiten, initiieren.
in·i·ti·a·tion [ɪˌnɪʃɪ'eɪʃn] *n* Einleitung *f*; Anfang *m*, Beginn *m*, Initiierung *f*, Initiation *f*. **i. of contraction** Kontraktionsinitiation.
initiation codon Initial-, Initiations-, Starterkodon *nt*.
initiation complex Initial-, Initiations-, Starterkomplex *m*.
initiation factor *abbr.* **IF** Initial-, Initiationsfaktor *m abbr.* IF.
initiation phase Initiations-, Einleitungsphase *f*.
initiation point Start-, Initiationspunkt *m*.
in·i·ti·a·tive [ɪ'nɪʃətɪv, -ʃɪətɪv] **I** *n* Initiative *f*. **II** *adj* anfänglich, beginnend, einführend, einleitend, Einführungs-.
in·i·ti·a·tor [ɪ'nɪʃɪeɪtər] *n* **1.** Initiator *m*, Urheber *m*. **2.** *chem.* Initiator *m*.
initiator protein Initiator-, Starterprotein *nt*.
initiator tRNA Initiator-tRNA *f*, Starter-tRNA *f*.
in·i·ti·a·to·ry [ɪ'nɪʃɪətɔːrɪ, -təʊ-] *adj* einleitend, initiatorisch.
in·i·tis [ɪn'aɪtɪs] *n* Muskelentzündung *f*, Myositis *f*.
in·ject [ɪn'dʒekt] *vt* (ein-)spritzen, injizieren.
in·ject·a·ble [ɪn'dʒektəbl] **I** *n* Injektionsmittel *nt*. **II** *adj* injizierbar.
in·ject·ed [ɪn'dʒektɪd] *adj* **1.** eingespritzt, injiziert. **2.** *patho.* blutüberfüllt, injiziert.
in·jec·tio [ɪn'dʒekʃɪəʊ] *n* → injection.
in·jec·tion [ɪn'dʒekʃn] *n* **1.** Injektion *f*, Einspritzung *f*, Spritze *f*. **2.** *pharm.* Injektion *f*, Injektionslösung *f*, -präparat *nt*. **3.** *patho.* Gefäßinjektion *f*. **4.** *patho.* Blutüberfüllung *f*, Kongestion *f*; Hyperämie *f*. **5.** *techn.* Einspritzung *f*.
injection equipment (*Drogenszene*) Besteck *nt*.
injection syringe (Injektions-)Spritze *f*.
in·jure ['ɪndʒər] *vt* **1.** verletzen, verwunden; traumatisieren. **2.** (*etw.*) beschädigen, verletzen. **3.** *fig.* schaden, schädigen. **4.** *fig.* (*Gefühle*) kränken, verletzen, jdm. wehtun.
in·jured ['ɪndʒərd] **I** *n* Verletzte *m/f*. **II** *adj* **1.** verletzt. **2.** schadhaft, beschädigt. **3.** *fig.* geschädigt. **4.** *fig.* gekränkt, verletzt.
in·ju·ri·ous [ɪn'dʒʊərɪəs] *adj* **1.** schädlich (*to* für); abträglich. **2.** kränkend, verletzend. **i. to health** gesundheitsschädlich.
in·ju·ry ['ɪndʒərɪ] *n, pl* -**ries 1.** Verletzung *f* (*to* an; *from* durch, von); Wunde *f*, Schaden *m*, Schädigung *f*, Trauma *nt*. **2.** (Be-)Schädigung *f*, Schaden *m* (*to* an). **i. from ischemia** ischämie-bedingte Schädigung, Schädigung durch Ischämie.
injury potential Demarkationspotential *nt*.
in knee X-Bein *nt*, Genu valgum.
in·lay [*n* 'ɪnleɪ; *v* 'ɪnleɪ, ɪn'leɪ] **I** *n* **1.** *chir., ortho.* Inlay *nt*, Implantat *nt*, Einlagespan *m*, Knochenspan *m*. **2.** *dent.* Einlagefüllung *f*, Inlay *nt*. **II** *vt* einlegen.
in·lay·er ['ɪnleɪər] *n* innere Schicht *f*.
in·let ['ɪnlet] *n* Eingang *m*, Zugang *m*; Einlaß *m*.
in·mate ['ɪnmeɪt] *n* (*Anstalt*) Insasse *m*, Insassin *f*.

in·most ['ɪnməʊst; *Brit.* -məst] *adj* → innermost.
I.N.N. *abbr.* → International Nonproprietary Names.
in·nate [ɪ'neɪt, 'ɪneɪt] *adj* **1.** angeboren (*in*); bei der Geburt vorhanden; kongenital; hereditär. **2.** innewohnend, eigen (*in*).
innate immunity angeborene Immunität *f*.
innate reflex angeborener Reflex *m*.
in·ner ['ɪnər] *adj* **1.** innere(r, s), inwendig, Innen-, Endo-. **2.** *fig.* innere(r, s), engere(r, s), vertraut; geistig, innerlich. **3.** *chem.* intramolekular.
inner angle of humerus Margo medialis humeri.
inner band of Baillarger innere Baillarger-Schicht *f*, innerer Baillarger--Streifen *m*, Stria laminae pyramidalis ganglionaris/interna (corticis cerebri).
inner callus *ortho.* innerer/zentraler Kallus *m*.
inner conflict (innerer/seelischer) Konflikt *m*.
inner ear Innenohr *nt*, Auris interna.
inner ear deafness Innenohrtaubheit *f*.
inner ear injury Innenohrverletzung *f*.
inner ear lesion Innenohrschädigung *f*.
inner ear trauma Innenohrverletzung *f*.
inner life Innen-, Seelenleben *nt*.
inner line of Baillarger → inner band of Baillarger.
inner margin Innenrand *m*. **i. of iris** innerer Rand *od.* Pupillenrand der Iris, Margo pupillaris (iridis).
inner mesaxon inneres Mesaxon *nt*.
in·ner·most ['ɪnərməʊst; *Brit.* -məst] *adj* **1.** innerste(r, s). **2.** *fig.* tiefste(r, s), geheimste(r, s).
inner periosteum innere Knochenhaut *f*, Endost(eum) *nt*, Periosteum internum.
inner plate of cranial bone innere Blatt *nt* des knöchernen Schädeldaches, Lamina interna (ossis cranii).
inner ridge *embryo.* (*Ohr*) innere Leiste *f*.
inner sheath of optic nerve innere Meningealscheide *f* des N. opticus, Vagina interna (n. optici).
inner stria of Baillarger → inner band of Baillarger.
inner stripe of Baillarger → inner band of Baillarger.
inner surface Innenfläche *f*, -seite *f*. **i. of eyelid** innere/hintere Lidfläche, Facies posterior palpebraris.
inner table of skull Lamina interna.
inner tunnel (*Ohr*) innerer Tunnel *m*.
in·ner·vate ['ɪnərveɪt] *vt physiol.* **1.** mit (Nerven-)Reizen versorgen, innervieren. **2.** (durch) Nervenreize anregen, stimulieren, innervieren.
in·ner·va·tion [ˌɪnər'veɪʃn] *n* nervale Versorgung *f*, Versorgung *f* mit Nerven(reizen), Innervation *f*.
innervation apraxia motorische Apraxie *f*.
innervation density Innervationsdichte *f*.
inner wall Innenwand *f*.
in·nid·i·a·tion [ɪˌnɪdɪ'eɪʃn] *n patho.* Einnisten *nt*, Innidation *f*.
in·no·cent murmur ['ɪnəsent] *card.* funktionelles (Herz-)Geräusch *nt*.
innocent tumor gutartiger/benigner Tumor *m*.
in·no·cu·i·ty [ˌɪnə'kjuːətɪ] *n* Unschädlichkeit *f*, Harmlosigkeit *f*.
in·noc·u·ous [ɪ'nɑkjəwəs] *adj* unschädlich, harmlos.
in·nom·i·nate [ɪ'nɑmənɪt] *adj* **1.** namenlos, unbenannt. **2.** anonym.
innominate aneurysm Aneurysma *nt* des Truncus brachiocephalicus.
innominate artery Truncus brachiocephalicus.

innominate bone Hüftbein *nt*, -knochen *m*, Os coxae.
innominate cartilage Ring-, Krikoidknorpel *m*, Cartilago cricoidea.
innominate fossa of auricle Cavum/Cavitas conchalis.
innominate osteotomy *ortho.* Beckenosteotomie *f.*
innominate veins Vv. brachiocephalicae (dextra et sinistra).
in·nox·ious [ɪˈnɒkʃəs] *adj* unschädlich, harmlos.
in·nu·tri·tion [ˌɪn(j)uːˈtrɪʃn] *n* Nahrungsmangel *m.*
ino *abbr.* → inosine.
in·o·chon·dri·tis [ˌɪnəʊkənˈdraɪtɪs] *n patho.* Faserknorpelentzündung *f.*
in·oc·u·la·ble [ɪˈnɒkjələbl] *adj* **1.** inokulierbar, durch Inokulation/Impfung übertragbar, impfbar. **2.** durch Inokulation/Impfung infizierbar.
in·oc·u·late [ɪˈnɒkjəleɪt] *vt* **1.** durch Inokulation übertragen, inokulieren. **2.** *micro.* (be-, über-)impfen, inokulieren.
in·oc·u·la·tion [ɪˌnɒkjəˈleɪʃn] *n* Beimpfung *f*, Überimpfung *f*, Impfung *f*, Inokulation *f.*
inoculation hepatitis (Virus-)Hepatitis B *f abbr.* HB, Serumhepatitis *f.*
in·oc·u·lum [ɪˈnɒkjələm] *n, pl* **-la** [-lə] Inokulum *nt.*
in·og·lia [ɪnˈɒɡlɪə] *n* Fibroglia *f.*
in·o·my·o·si·tis [ˌɪnəmaɪəˈsaɪtɪs] *n patho.* Fibromyositis *f.*
in·op·er·a·ble [ɪnˈɒpərəbl] *adj* **1.** *chir.*, *patho.* inoperabel, nicht operierbar. **2.** undurchführbar.
in·op·er·a·tive [ɪnˈɒp(ə)rətɪv] *adj* **1.** unwirksam, wirkungslos. **2.** *techn.* außer Betrieb, nicht einsatzfähig.
in·or·gan·ic [ˌɪnɔːˈɡænɪk] *adj* **1.** *chem.* anorganisch. **2.** unorganisch.
inorganic acid anorganische Säure *f*, Mineralsäure *f.*
inorganic chemistry anorganische Chemie *f.*
inorganic compound anorganische Verbindung *f.*
inorganic murmur *card.* funktionelles (Herz-)Geräusch *nt.*
inorganic phosphate anorganisches Phosphat *nt.*
inorganic pyrophosphatase anorganische Pyrophosphatase *f.*
in·os·co·py [ɪnˈɒskəpɪ] *n histol.*, *patho.* Inoskopie *f.*
in·os·cu·late [ɪnˈɒskjəleɪt] *vt* eine Anastomose bilden, anastomosieren.
in·os·cu·la·tion [ɪnˌɒksjəˈleɪʃn] *n* **1.** *anat.* Anastomose *f*, Anastomosis *f.* **2.** *chir.* Anastomose *f*; Shunt *m*; Fistel *f.*
in·ose [ˈɪnəʊs] *n* → inositol.
in·o·se·mia [ˌɪnəˈsiːmɪə] *n* **1.** erhöhter Inositgehalt *m* des Blutes, Inositämie *f.* **2.** erhöhter Fibringehalt *m* des Blutes, Hyperfibrinämie *f.*
in·o·si·nate [ɪˈnəʊsɪneɪt] *n* Inosinat *nt.*
in·o·sine [ˈɪnəsiːn, -sɪn, -sɪn] *n abbr.* **I, Ino** Inosin *nt abbr.* I, Ino.
inosine monophosphate *abbr.* **IMP** Inosinmonophosphat *nt abbr.* IMP, Inosinsäure *f.*
inosine phosphorylase Purinnukleosidphosphorylase *f.*
inosine triphosphate *abbr.* **ITP** Inosintriphosphat *nt abbr.* ITP.
in·o·sin·ic acid [ɪnəˈsɪnɪk] → inosine monophosphate.
inosinic acid cyclohydrolase → IMP cyclohydrolase.
inosinic acid dehydrogenase → IMP dehydrogenase.

in·o·site [ˈɪnəsaɪt] *n* → inositol.
in·o·si·tol [ɪˈnəʊsɪtɒl, -təʊl] *n* **1.** Inosit *nt*, Inositol *nt.* **2.** meso-Inosit *m*, meso--Inositol *nt*, myo-Inosit *m*, myo-Inositol *nt.*
inositol niacinate *pharm.* Inositolnicotinat *nt.*
inositol triphosphate *abbr.* **IP₃** Inosittriphosphat *nt abbr.* IP₃, Phosphoinositol *nt.*
in·o·si·tol·u·ria [ˌɪnəʊˌsaɪtəˈl(j)ʊərɪə] *n* → inosituria.
in·o·si·tu·ria [ˌɪnəsɪˈt(j)ʊərɪə] *n* Inositausscheidung *f* im Harn, Inositurie *f*, Inositolurie *f.*
in·o·su·ria [ɪnəˈs(j)ʊərɪə] *n* **1.** → inosituria. **2.** vermehrte Fibrinausscheidung *f* im Harn, (Hyper-)Fibrinurie *f.*
i·no·trop·ic [ˌɪnəˈtrɒpɪk, -ˈtrəʊp-] *adj* inotrop.
i·not·ro·pism [ɪˈnɒtrəpɪzəm] *n* inotrope Wirkung *f*, Inotropie *f.*
in·quest [ˈɪnkwɛst] *n forens.* (gerichtliche) Untersuchung *f.*
in·qui·line [ˈɪnkwəlaɪn, -lɪn] *n bio.*, *micro.* Einmieter *m*, Raumparasit *m*, Inquilin *m.*
in·quire [ɪnˈkwaɪər] **I** *vt* **1.** erkundigen nach, erfragen (*of s.o.* bei jdm.). **II** *vi* **1.** (nach-)fragen (*after, for* nach; *about* wegen); sich erkundigen (*after, for* nach; *about* wegen); Erkundigungen einziehen (*about* über, wegen). **2.** Untersuchungen anstellen, (nach-, er-)forschen, prüfen (*into sth.*).
in·quir·er [ɪnˈkwaɪərər] *n* **1.** Untersuchende(r *m*) *f.* **2.** (An-)Fragende(r *m*) *f*, Fragesteller(in *f*) *m.*
in·quir·ing [ɪnˈkwaɪrɪŋ] *adj* **1.** forschend, fragend. **2.** wißbegierig.
in·quir·y [ɪnˈkwaɪrɪ] *n, pl* **-quir·ies 1.** Untersuchung *f*, Prüfung *f* (*of, into*); Nachforschung *f*, Ermittlung *f.* **2.** Erkundigung *f*, An-, Nachfrage *f.*
in·sal·i·vate [ɪnˈsælɪveɪt] *vt* (*Nahrung*) einspeicheln, mit Speichel versetzen *od.* vermischen.
in·sal·i·va·tion [ɪnˌsælɪˈveɪʃn] *n* (*Nahrung*) Durchmischung *f* mit Speichel, Insalivation *f.*
in·sa·lu·bri·ous [ˌɪnsəˈluːbrɪəs] *adj* ungesund, unzuträglich, unbekömmlich.
in·sa·lu·bri·ty [ˌɪnsəˈluːbrətɪ] *n* Unbekömmlichkeit *f*, Unzuträglichkeit *f.*
in·sane [ɪnˈseɪn] *adj* geisteskrank, wahnsinnig, irrsinnig.
insane root *pharm.* Bilsenkraut *nt*, Hyoscyamus niger.
in·san·i·tar·y [ɪnˈsænɪtərɪ] *adj* unhygienisch, gesundheitsschädlich.
in·san·i·ta·tion [ɪnˌsænɪˈteɪʃn] *n* unhygienischer Zustand *m.*
in·san·i·ty [ɪnˈsænətɪ] *n, pl* **-ties 1.** *psychia.* Geisteskrankheit *f*, Irresein *nt*, Irrsinn *m*, Wahnsinn *m*, Insania *f.* **2.** *fig.* Verrücktheit *f*, Tollheit *f*, Wahnsinn *m.*
in·sa·tia·bil·i·ty [ɪnˌseɪʃ(ɪ)əˈbɪlətɪ] *n* (*Durst, Hunger*) Unstillbarkeit *f*; *fig.* Unersättlichkeit *f.*
in·sa·tia·ble [ɪnˈseɪʃ(ɪ)əbl] *adj* (*Durst, Hunger*) unstillbar; *fig.* unersättlich.
in·sa·tia·ble·ness ['-nɪs] *n* → insatiability.
in·sa·ti·ate [ɪnˈseɪʃɪɪt] *adj* → insatiable.
in·scrip·tio [ɪnˈskrɪpʃɪəʊ] *n* **1.** → inscription. **2.** → intersection.
in·scrip·tion [ɪnˈskrɪpʃn] *n* **1.** *pharm.* Inscriptio *f.* **2.** Inschrift *m*, Eintrag *m*; Eintragung *f.* **3.** *mathe.* Einbeschreibung *f.*
in·sect [ˈɪnsɛkt] *n bio.*, *micro.* Kerbtier *nt*, Insekt *nt.*
in·sec·ta [ɪnˈsɛktə] *pl bio.*, *micro.* Kerbtiere *pl*, Kerfe *pl*, Insekten *pl*, Insecta *pl*, Hexapoden *pl*, Hexapoda *pl.*

insect bite Insektenstich *m.*
insect dermatitis Insektendermatitis *f.*
insect host *micro.* Wirtsinsekt *nt.*
in·sec·ti·cid·al [ɪnˌsɛktɪˈsaɪdl] *adj* Insekten (ab-)tötend, insektizid.
in·sec·ti·cide [ɪnˈsɛktɪsaɪd] *n* Insektenbekämpfungs-, Insektenvertilgungsmittel *nt*, Insektizid *nt.*
in·sec·ti·fuge [ɪnˈsɛktɪfjuːdʒ] *n* Insektenvertreibungsmittel *nt*, Insektenschutzmittel *nt*, Repellent *nt.*
in·sec·tion [ɪnˈsɛkʃn] *n* Einschnitt *m.*
in·sec·tiv·o·ra [ˌɪnsɛkˈtɪvərə] *pl bio.* Insektenfresser *pl*, Insektivoren *pl*, Insectivora *pl.*
in·sec·ti·vore [ɪnˈsɛktəvɔːr, -vəʊr] *n bio.* Insektenfresser *m*, Insektivore *m.*
in·sec·tiv·o·rous [ˌɪnsɛkˈtɪvərəs] *adj bio.* insektenfressend, insektivor, entomophag.
in·sec·tol·o·gy [ˌɪnsɛkˈtɒlədʒɪ] *n bio.* Insektenkunde *f*, Entomologie *f.*
insect pest Insektenplage *f.*
insect-repellent I *n* → insectifuge. **II** *adj* insektenvertreibend.
insect vector *micro.* Vektorinsekt *nt.*
in·se·cure [ˌɪnsɪˈkjʊər] *adj* **1.** ungesichert, nicht fest. **2.** *fig.* unsicher; ungewiß, riskant.
in·se·cu·ri·ty [ˌɪnsɪˈkjʊərətɪ] *n, pl* **-ties** Unsicherheit *f.*
in·sem·i·nate [ɪnˈsɛmɪneɪt] *vt* **1.** befruchten. **2.** *bio.* befruchten, besamen. **3.** (ein-)pflanzen.
in·sem·i·na·tion [ɪnˌsɛmɪˈneɪʃn] *n* **1.** Befruchtung *f*, Insemination *f.* **2.** *bio.* Befruchtung *f*, Besamung *f*, Insemination *f.* **3.** (Ein-)Pflanzen *nt.*
in·se·nes·cence [ˌɪnsəˈnɛsəns] *n* Altern *nt*, Altwerden *nt.*
in·sen·sate [ɪnˈsɛnseɪt, -sɪt] *adj* **1.** gefühllos; empfindungslos, leblos. **2.** unsinnig, unvernünftig. **3.** *fig.* unempfänglich (*of, to* für); gleichgültig (*of, to* gegen).
in·sen·sate·ness ['-nɪs] *n* **1.** Gefühllosigkeit *f*; Empfindungs-, Leblosigkeit *f.* **2.** Unsinnigkeit *f*, Unvernunft *f.* **3.** *fig.* Unempfänglichkeit *f* (*of, to* für); Gleichgültigkeit *f* (*of, to* gegen).
in·sen·si·bil·i·ty [ɪnˌsɛnsɪˈbɪlətɪ] *n* **1.** Empfindungs-, Gefühllosigkeit *f* (*to* gegen). **2.** Bewußtlosigkeit *f.* **3.** *fig.* Gleichgültigkeit *f* (*of, to* gegenüber); Unempfänglichkeit *f* (*of, to* für).
i. to pain Schmerzunempfindlichkeit.
insensible perspiration extralgradualte Wasserabgabe *f*, Perspiratio insensibilis.
insensible thirst (pathologisch) verminderter Durst *m*, Hypodipsie *f.*
insensible water loss → insensible perspiration.
in·sen·si·tive [ɪnˈsɛnsɪtɪv] *adj* **1.** *chem.*, *phys.* unempfindlich (*to* gegen). **2.** → insensible 1, 3.
i. to light lichtunempfindlich.
i. to radiation strahlenunempfindlich.
in·sen·si·tive·ness ['-nɪs] *n* **1.** Unempfindlichkeit *f* (*to* gegen). **2.** → insensibility 1, 3.
in·sen·si·tiv·i·ty [ɪnˌsɛnsəˈtɪvətɪ] *n* → insensitiveness.
in·sen·ti·ent [ɪnˈsɛnʃ(ɪ)ənt] *adj* gefühl-, empfindungslos, unempfindlich.
in·sert [ɪnˈsɜːt] *vt* **1.** (*Muskel*) inserieren, ansetzen. **2.** einsetzen, einfügen; (*Kanüle*) einführen, einstechen; (*Sonde*) einschieben.
in·ser·tio [ɪnˈsɜːrʃɪəʊ] *n* → insertion.
in·ser·tion [ɪnˈsɜːʃn] *n* **1.** (*Muskel*) Ansatz

insertion sequence

m, Insertion *f*. **2.** (*Instrument*) Einführung *f*, Einfügen *nt*, Einbringen *nt*; Einstich *m*. **3.** *genet.* Einfügung *f*, Insertion *f*.
insertion sequence *genet.* Insertionssequenz *f abbr.* IS.
in·sheathed [ɪn'ʃiːðt] *adj* von einer Scheide *od.* Kapsel umgeben.
in·sid·i·ous [ɪn'sɪdɪəs] *adj* **1.** *patho.* schleichend, langsam-progredient. **2.** *fig.* heimtückisch, hinterhältig, hinterlistig.
in·sight ['ɪnsaɪt] *n psychia.* Einsicht *f*, (Selbst-)Verständnis *nt*, (Selbst-)Erkennung *f*.
in si·tu [ɪn 'saɪt(j)uː] am Ort, in natürlicher Lage, in situ.
in·so·late ['ɪnsəʊleɪt] *vt* den Sonnenstrahlen aussetzen.
in·so·la·tion [ˌɪnsəʊ'leɪʃn] *n* **1.** Sonnenbestrahlung *f*, Insolation *f*, Insolatio *f*. **2.** Sonnenstich *m*, Insolation *f*, Insolatio *f*.
in·sole ['ɪnsəʊl] *n ortho.* Einlage *f*, Einlegesohle *f*.
in·sol·u·bil·i·ty [ɪnˌsɒljə'bɪlɪtɪ] *n* Un(auf)löslichkeit *f*.
in·sol·u·ble [ɪn'sɒljəbl] **I** *n chem.* unlösliche Substanz *f*. **II** *adj* un(auf)löslich.
i. in water wasserunlöslich, unlöslich in Wasser.
in·som·nia [ɪn'sɒmnɪə] *n* Schlaflosigkeit *f*, (pathologische) Wachheit *f*, Insomnie *f*, Insomnia *f*.
in·som·ni·ac [ɪn'sɒmnɪæk] **I** *n* an Schlaflosigkeit Leidende(r *m*) *f*. **II** *adj* **1.** an Schlaflosigkeit leidend. **2.** zu Schlaflosigkeit führend, Schlaflosigkeit verursachend.
in·som·nic [ɪn'sɒmnɪk] *adj* → insomniac 1.
in·sorp·tion [ɪn'sɔːrpʃn] *n* Aufnahme *f* ins Blut.
in·spec·tion [ɪn'spekʃn] *n* äußerliche Untersuchung *f*, Inspektion *f*.
in·spi·rate ['ɪnspɪreɪt] *n* eingeatmetes Gas *nt*, eingeatmete Luft *f*, Inspirat *nt*; Inhalat *nt*.
in·spi·ra·tion [ˌɪnspə'reɪʃn] *n* **1.** Einatmung *f*, Inspiration *f*. **2.** *psycho.* Eingebung *f*, Inspiration *f*.
in·spi·ra·tor ['ɪnspəreɪtər] *n* Inhalationsapparat *m*, Inhalator *m*.
in·spi·ra·to·ry [ɪn'spaɪərətɔːrɪ, -təʊr-, -tərɪ] *n* Inspirations betr., inspiratorisch, Einatem-, Einatmungs-, Inspirations-.
inspiratory capacity *abbr.* **IC** Inspirationskapazität *f abbr.* IK, IC.
inspiratory center Einatem-, Inspirationszentrum *nt*.
inspiratory dyspnea inspiratorische Dyspnoe *f*.
inspiratory muscle Einatem-, Inspirationsmuskel *m*.
inspiratory neuron inspiratorisches Neuron *nt*.
inspiratory reserve volume *abbr.* **IRV** inspiratorisches Reservevolumen *nt abbr.* IRV.
inspiratory resistance inspiratorische Resistance *f*.
inspiratory stridor inspiratorischer Stridor *m*.
inspiratory work inspiratorische Arbeit *f*.
in·spire [ɪn'spaɪər] *vt*, *vi* einatmen; inhalieren.
in·spired [ɪn'spaɪərd] *adj* eingeatmet; inspiriert.
inspired air → inspirate.
in·spis·sat·ed ['ɪnspɪseɪtɪd] *adj* eingedickt, eingetrocknet.
inspissated bile syndrome Syndrom *nt* der eingedickten Galle, Gallenpfropf-Syndrom *nt*.
inspissated cerumen angetrockneter/eingetrockneter/verhärteter Zeruminalpfropf *m*.
in·spis·sa·tion [ˌɪnspɪ'seɪʃn] *n* Eintrocknen *nt*, Eindicken *nt*.
in·sta·bil·i·ty [ˌɪnstə'bɪlɪtɪ] *n* **1.** mangelnde Festigkeit *f*. Stabilität *f*, Instabilität *f*. **2.** *fig.* Unbeständigkeit *f*, Labilität *f*.
in·sta·ble [ɪn'steɪbl] *adj* **1.** instabil. **2.** *fig.* unbeständig; labil.
in·step ['ɪnstep] *n anat.* (*Fuß*) Rist *m*, Spann *m*.
in·stil *vt* → instill.
in·still [ɪn'stɪl] *vt* **1.** einträufeln, instillieren (*into*). **2.** *fig.* einflößen, einimpfen, beibringen.
in·stil·la·tion [ˌɪnstə'leɪʃn] *n* **1.** Einträufelung *f*, Instillation *f*; Tropfinfusion *f*. **2.** *fig.* Einflößung *f*, Einimpfung *f*.
in·stil·la·tor [ˌɪnstə'leɪtər] *n* Tropfapparat *m*, Tropfer *m*, Instillator *m*.
in·stil·la·ment [ɪn'stɪlmənt] *n* instillation.
in·still·ment [ɪn'stɪlmənt] *n* → instillation.
in·stinct ['ɪnstɪŋkt] *n* **1.** angeborener Trieb *m*, Naturtrieb *m*, Instinkt *m*. **by/from** ~ instinktiv. **2.** (sicherer) Instinkt *m*, natürliche Begabung *f* (*for* für); instiktives Gefühl *nt* (*for* für).
in·stinc·tive [ɪn'stɪŋktɪv] *adj* instinktiv, instinktmäßig, triebmäßig; unwillkürlich; angeboren.
in·sti·tute ['ɪnstɪt(j)uːt] **I** *n* **1.** Institut *nt*, Anstalt *f*, Akademie *f*, Gesellschaft *f*. **2.** Institut(sgebäude *nt*) *nt*; Anstalt(sgebäude *nt*) *f*. **3.** höhere technische Schule *f*; Universitätsinstitut *nt*. **II** *vt* einrichten, errichten, gründen, ins Leben rufen.
in·sti·tu·tion [ˌɪnstə't(j)uːʃn] *n* **1.** Institution *f*, Einrichtung *f*; Institut *nt*; Anstalt *f*; Heim *nt*; Stiftung *f*; Gesellschaft *f*. **2.** Institut(sgebäude *nt*) *nt*; Anstalt(sgebäude *nt*) *f*; Heim *nt*. **3.** *socio.* Institution *f*, Einrichtung *f*. **4.** Errichtung *f*, Einrichtung *f*, Gründung *f*. **5.** Ingangsetzung *f*, Initiierung *f*.
in·sti·tu·tion·al·ize [-'t(j)uːʃənlaɪz] *vt* **1.** in ein Heim *od.* eine Anstalt einweisen. **2.** zu einer Institution machen, institutionalisieren.
in·struct [ɪn'strʌkt] *vt* **1.** unterrichten (*in* in); ausbilden, schulen (*in* in). **2.** informieren, unterrichten. **3.** instruieren, anweisen, beauftragen (*to* zu *inf*).
in·struc·tion [ɪn'strʌkʃn] *n* **1.** Unterricht *m*; Ausbildung *f*, Schulung *f*. **2.** Informierung *f*, Unterrichtung *f*. **3.** Anweisung *f*, Auftrag *m*, Instruktion *f*.
in·struc·tion·al [ɪn'strʌkʃnəl] *adj* **1.** Unterrichts-, Lehr-, Ausbildungs-, Schulungs-. **2.** → instructive.
in·struc·tive [ɪn'strʌktɪv] *adj* instruktiv, lehrreich, eindringlich, einprägsam, aufschlußreich.
in·struc·tor [ɪn'strʌktər] *n* Lehrer *m*, Ausbilder *m*.
in·struc·tress [ɪn'strʌktrɪs] *n* Lehrerin *f*, Ausbilderin *f*.
in·stru·ment ['ɪnstrəmənt] **I** *n* **1.** Instrument *nt*, (feines) Werkzeug *nt*, (Meß-)Gerät *nt*. **2.** *fig.* Instrument *nt*, (Hilfs-)Mittel *nt*. **3.** Instrumente *pl*, Apparate-, Geräte-. **III** *vt* instrumentieren, mit Instrumenten ausrüsten.
in·stru·men·tal [ˌɪnstrə'mentl] *adj* **1.** instrumentell, mit Hilfe von Instrumenten, Instrumenten-. **2.** förderlich, dienlich, behilflich (*in* bei).
instrumental conditioning operante/instrumentelle Konditionierung *f*.
instrumental percussion instrumentelle Perkussion *f*.
in·stru·men·tar·i·um [ˌɪnstrəmen'teərɪəm] *n*, *pl* **-ria** [-rɪə] *chir.*, *ortho.* Instrumentarium *nt*.
in·stru·men·ta·tion [ˌɪnstrəmen'teɪʃn] *n* Anwendung von *od.* Ausstattung mit Instrumenten, Instrumentierung *f*.
in·su·da·tion [ˌɪnsjə'deɪʃn] *n* **1.** Insudation *f*. **2.** Insudat *nt*.
in·suf·fi·cien·cy [ˌɪnsə'fɪʃənsɪ] *n*, *pl* **-cies 1.** *patho.* Funktionsschwäche *f*, Insuffizienz *f*, Insufficientia *f*. **2.** Unzulänglichkeit *f*; Untauglichkeit *f*, Unfähigkeit *f*.
insufficiency disease Mangelkrankheit *f*.
in·suf·fi·cient [ˌɪnsə'fɪʃənt] *adj* **1.** unzulänglich, ungenügend, nicht ausreichend, insuffizient. **2.** untauglich, unfähig (*to do* zu *tun*).
in·suf·flate [ɪn'sʌfleɪt, 'ɪnsəfleɪt] *vt* **1.** einblasen, insufflieren. **2.** hineinblasen in; ausblasen.
in·suf·fla·tion [ˌɪnsə'fleɪʃn] *n* **1.** Einblasen *nt*, Insufflation *f*. **2.** *techn.* Einblasung *f*; Ausblasung *f*.
insufflation anesthesia *anes.* Insufflationsnarkose *f*, -anästhesie *f*.
in·suf·fla·tor ['ɪnsəfleɪtər] *n* Insufflationsapparat *m*.
in·su·la ['ɪns(j)ələ] *n*, *pl* **-lae** [-liː] *anat.* → insular lobe.
i.e of Peyer Peyer'-Plaques *pl*, Folliculi lymphatici aggregati.
i. of Reil → insular lobe.
in·su·lant ['ɪns(j)ələnt] *n phys.*, *electr.* Isolierstoff *m*, -material *nt*.
in·su·lar ['ɪns(j)ələr] *adj* **1.** Lobus insularis *od.* Langerhans'-Inseln betr., Insel-. **2.** inselartig, -förmig, insular(isch), Insel-.
insular area → insular lobe.
insular arteries Inselarterien *pl*, Aa. insulares.
insular cortex → insular lobe.
insular lobe Insel *f*, Inselrinde *f*, Insula *f*, Lobus insularis.
insular part of middle cerebral artery Inselabschnitt *m* der A. cerebri media, Pars insularis (a. cerebri mediae).
insular region Inselregion *f*.
insular sclerosis *patho.* multiple Sklerose *f abbr.* MS, Polysklerose *f*, Sclerosis multiplex, Encephalomyelitis disseminata.
insular veins Inselvenen *pl*, Anfangsäste *pl* der V. cerebri media profunda, Vv. insulares.
in·su·late ['ɪns(j)əleɪt] *vt* **1.** *phys.*, *electr.* isolieren. **2.** (*Schall*, *Wärme*) dämmen, abisolieren. **3.** *fig.* absondern, isolieren (*from* von); schützen (*from* vor); abschirmen (*from* gegen).
in·su·lat·ing ['-leɪtɪŋ] *adj* isolierend, Isolier-.
insulating layer Isolierschicht *f*, Isolator *m*.
in·su·la·tion [ˌ-'leɪʃn] *n* **1.** *phys.*, *electr.* Isolierung *f*, Isolation *f*. **2.** Isoliermaterial *nt*, -stoff *m*.
insulation resistance Isolationswiderstand *m*.
in·su·la·tor ['-leɪtər] *n electr.* Isolator *m*; Nichtleiter *m*, Isolierstoff *m*.
in·su·lin ['ɪnsələn, 'ɪns(j)ʊ-] *n* Insulin *nt*; *old* Inselhormon *nt*.
insulin antagonist Insulinantagonist *m*.
insulin-antagonistic *adj* insulinantagonistisch.
insulin antibody Insulinantikörper *m*.
in·su·lin·ase ['ɪnsəlɪneɪz] *n* Insulinase *f*.
insulin coma therapy *abbr.* **ICT** → insulin shock therapy.
insulin coma treatment → insulin shock therapy.
insulin-dependent diabetes *abbr.* **IDD** insulinabhängiger Diabetes (mellitus) *m*, Typ 1 Diabetes *m* (mellitus), Insulinmangeldiabetes *m*.

insulin edema Insulinödem *nt*.
in·su·lin·e·mia [ˌɪns(j)əlɪ'niːmɪə] *n* erhöhter Insulingehalt *m* des Blutes, (Hyper-)Insulinämie *f*.
insulin-glucagon system Insulin-Glukagon-System *nt*.
insulin hypoglycemia test Hollander-Hypoglykämietest *m*.
insulin-induced *adj* insulininduziert, -bedingt.
in·su·lin·ize ['ɪns(j)əlɪnaɪz] *vt* mit Insulin behandeln.
insulin-like *adj* insulinähnlich.
insulin-like activity *abbr*. **ILA** → insulin-like growth factors.
insulin-like growth factors *abbr*. **IGF** insulinähnliche Wachstumsfaktoren *pl*, insulin-like growth factors *abbr*. IGF, insulinähnliche Aktivität *f*.
insulin-like growth factor I *abbr*. **IGF I** Somatomedin C *nt*.
in·su·lin·lip·o·dys·tro·phy [ˌɪns(j)əlɪnˌlɪpə'dɪstrəfɪ, -ˌlaɪpə-] *n* Insulinlipodystrophie *f*.
in·su·lin·o·gen·e·sis [ˌɪns(j)əlɪnə'dʒenəsɪs] *n* Insulinbildung *f*.
in·su·lin·o·gen·ic [ˌ-'dʒenɪk] *adj* Insulinbildung betr. *od*. fördernd, insulinbildend.
in·su·lin·oid ['ɪns(j)əlɪnɔɪd] *adj* insulinartig (wirkend).
in·su·li·no·ma [ˌɪns(j)əlɪ'nəʊmə] *n*, *pl* **-mas**, **-ma·ta** [-mətə] Insulinom *nt*, B-Zell(en)-Tumor *m*.
in·su·lin·o·pe·nic [ˌɪns(j)əlɪnə'piːnɪk] *adj* den Insulinspiegel senkend, mit einem erniedrigten Insulinspiegel einhergehend.
insulinopenic diabetes Insulinmangeldiabetes *m*.
insulin receptor Insulinrezeptor *m*.
insulin resistance Insulinresistenz *f*.
insulin shock Insulinschock *m*.
insulin shock therapy *abbr*. **IST** Insulinschocktherapie *f*.
insulin shock treatment → insulin shock therapy.
insulin unit Insulineinheit *f*.
in·su·lism ['ɪnsjəlɪzəm] *n* Hyperinsulinismus *m*.
in·su·li·tis [ɪnsjə'laɪtɪs] *n* Entzündung *f* der Langerhans'-Inseln, Insulitis *f*.
in·su·lo·gen·ic [ˌɪns(j)əlǝʊ'dʒenɪk] *adj* → insulinogenic.
in·su·lo·ma [ɪns(j)ə'ləʊmə] *n* → insulinoma.
in·sult [*n* 'ɪnsʌlt; *v* ɪn'sʌlt] **I** *n* **1**. Verletzung *f*, Wunde *f*, Trauma *nt*. **2**. Beleidigung (*to* für). **II** *vt* beleidigen (*by* durch, mit).
in·sus·cep·ti·bil·i·ty [ˌɪnsəˌseptə'bɪlətɪ] *n* Unempfindlichkeit *f* (*to* gegen); Unempfänglichkeit *f* (*to* für); Immunität *f*.
in·sus·cep·ti·ble [ˌɪnsə'septɪbl] *adj* nicht anfällig (*to* für); unempfindlich (*to* gegen); unempfänglich (*to* für); immun.
in·take ['ɪnteɪk] *n* **1**. Aufnahme *f*; aufgenommene Menge *f*, Zufuhr *f*. **2**. (*Patienten*) (Neu-)Aufnahme(n *pl*) *f*, (Neu-)Zugänge *pl*. **3**. Ein-, Ansaugen *nt*.
inte·gral ['ɪntɪgrəl, ɪn'tegrəl] **I** *n mathe*. Integral *nt*. **II** *adj* **1**. *mathe*. ganz(zahlig), Integral-. **2**. integral, wesentlich, unabdingbar. **3**. vollständig, vollkommen.
integral absorbed dose → integral dose.
integral dose *radiol*. Integraldosis *f*.
integral protein integrales (Membran-)Protein *m*.
integral vector Integralvektor *m*.
in·te·grate ['ɪntəgreɪt] **I** *vt* **1**. integrieren, einfügen, -gliedern, -bauen, -beziehen, aufnehmen (*into* in). **2**. *mathe*. integrieren, das Integral berechnen. **II** *vi* s. integrieren, s. eingliedern (lassen), s. einbeziehen lassen (*into* in).

in·te·grat·ed ['-greɪtɪd] *adj* integriert.
integrated circuit integrierter Schaltkreis *m*.
in·te·grat·ing ['-greɪtɪŋ] *adj* integrierend.
in·te·gra·tion [ˌ-'greɪʃn] *n* **1**. Integration *f*, Integrierung *f*, Eingliederung *f*, Einfügung *f*, Aufnahme *f*, Einbeziehung *f* (*into* in); Zusammenschluß *m* (*into* zu). **2**. *mathe*. Berechnung *f* des Integrals, Integration *f*. **3**. *psycho*. Integration *f*. **4**. *genet*. Coadaptation *f*, Integration *f*.
in·te·gra·tion·al nucleus [ˌ-'greɪʃnəl] Integrationskern *m*.
integration center *physiol*. Integrationsorgan *nt*, -zentrum *nt*.
in·te·gra·tive [ˌ-'greɪtɪv] *adj* Integrations-.
integrative organ Integrationsorgan *nt*.
in·te·gra·tor cell ['-greɪtər] → interneuron.
in·teg·ri·ty [ɪn'tegrətɪ] *n* Unversehrtheit *f*, Integrität *f*.
in·teg·u·ment [ɪn'tegjəmənt] *n* **1**. Bedeckung *f*, Hülle *f*, Integument *nt*. **2**. äußere Haut *f*, Integumentum commune.
in·teg·u·men·tal [ɪnˌtegjə'mentl] *adj* Integument betr., Haut-.
in·teg·u·men·ta·ry [ˌ-'ment(ə)rɪ] *adj* → integumental.
in·teg·u·men·tum [ˌ-'mentəm] *n* → integument.
in·tel·lect ['ɪntlekt] *n* Verstand *m*, Denk-, Erkenntnisvermögen *nt*, Urteilskraft *f*.
in·tel·lec·tion [ɪntə'lekʃn] *n* **1**. Denken *nt*, Verstandes-, Denktätigkeit *f*. **2**. Gedanke *m*, Idee *f*.
in·tel·lec·tive [ɪntə'lektɪv] *adj* **1**. denkend. **2**. intelligent. **3**. Verstand betr., Verstandes-.
in·tel·lec·tu·al [ɪntə'lektʃ(əw)əl] **I** *n* Intellektuelle(r *m*) *f*, Verstandesmensch *m*, Geistesarbeiter(in *f*) *m*. **II** *adj* **1**. verstandesmäßig, geistig, intellektuell, Verstandes-, Geistes-. **2**. klug, vernünftig, intelligent. **3**. (geistig) anspruchsvoll, intellektuell.
intellectual aphasia echte/organisch-bedingte Aphasie *f*.
in·tel·lec·tu·al·i·za·tion [ɪntəˌlektʃə(wə)lɪ'zeɪʃn, -laɪ-] *n* intellektuelle Behandlung *f*, Intellektualisierung *f*.
in·tel·lec·tu·al·ize [ɪntə'lektʃə(wə)laɪz] *vt* intellektuell behandeln, intellektualisieren.
in·tel·li·gence [ɪn'telɪdʒəns] *n* **1**. Intelligenz *f*. **2**. schnelle Auffassungsgabe *f*, Klugheit *f*, Intelligenz *f*.
intelligence quotient *abbr*. **IQ** Intelligenzquotient *m abbr*. IQ.
intelligence test Intelligenztest *m*.
in·tel·li·gent [ɪn'telɪdʒənt] *adj* **1**. klug, geistig begabt, intelligent. **2**. vernünftig, verständig; verstehend.
in·tem·per·ance [ɪn'temp(ə)rəns] *n* **1**. Unmäßigkeit *f*. **2**. Unbeherrschtheit *f*. **3**. Trunksucht *f*. **4**. (*Klima*) Rauhheit *f*.
in·tem·per·ate [ɪn'temp(ə)rɪt] *adj* **1**. unmäßig, ausschweifend, zügellos; maßlos. **2**. unbeherrscht. **3**. trunksüchtig. **4**. (*Klima*) rauh.
intemperate bacteriophage nichttemperenter/lytischer/virulenter Bakteriophage *m*.
in·tend·ed [ɪn'tendɪd] *adj* (*Motorik*) beabsichtigt, geplant, absichtlich, intendiert.
in·tense [ɪn'tens] *adj* intensiv; (*Fieber*, *Schmerz*, *Verlangen*) heftig, stark; (*Farbe*) tief, satt; (*Licht*) grell, hell; (*Geräusch*) durchdringend; *photo*. (*Negativ*) dicht.
intense homesickness *psycho*., *psychia*. pathologisches Heimweh *nt*, Nostomanie *f*.

in·tense·ness ['-nɪs] *n* → intensity.
in·ten·si·fi·ca·tion [ɪnˌtensəfɪ'keɪʃn] *n* Intensivierung *f*, Verstärkung *f*; Erhöhung *f*, Steigerung *f*.
in·ten·si·fi·er [ɪn'tensɪfaɪər] *n* Verstärker *m*.
in·ten·si·fy [ɪn'tensɪfaɪ] **I** *vt* intensivieren, verstärken; erhöhen, steigern. **II** *vi* s. verstärken, s. erhöhen, s. steigern.
in·ten·si·ty [ɪn'tensɪtɪ] *n* Intensität *f*; (*Schmerz*) Stärke *f*, Heftigkeit *f*; (*Farbe*) Tiefe *f*, Sattheit *f*; (*Licht*) Grelle *f*, Grellheit *f*; *photo*. (*Negativ*) Dichte *f*; *phys*., *electr*. (Strom-, Licht-)Stärke *f*, Stärkegrad *m*.
i. of radiation Strahlungsintensität.
intensity-difference threshold Intensitätsunterschiedsschwelle *f*.
intensity sensor Intensitätssensor *m*.
in·ten·sive [ɪn'tensɪv] *adj* **1**. intensiv, heftig, stark; stark wirkend. **2**. Intensiv-.
intensive care Intensivpflege *f*. **to be in ~** auf der Intensivstation sein.
intensive care unit *abbr*. **ICU** Intensiv-, Wachstation *f*.
in·ten·tion [ɪn'tenʃn] *n* **1**. Absicht *f*, Vorhaben *nt*, Vorsatz *m*, Planung *f*, Intention *f*. **2**. Heilprozeß *m*, Wundheilung *f*, Intention *f*. **3**. *chir*., *ortho*. Verfahren *nt*, Technik *f*, Operation *f*.
intention spasm Intensionsspasmus *m*, -krampf *m*.
intention tremor *neuro*. Intentionstremor *m*.
inter- *pref*. Zwischen-, Inter-; Gegen-, Wechsel-.
in·ter·ac·i·nar [ˌɪntər'æsɪnər, -nɑː] *adj histol*. zwischen Azini (liegend), interazinär.
in·ter·ac·i·nous [ˌ-'æsɪnəs] *adj* → interacinar.
in·ter·act [ˌ-'ækt] *vi* s. gegenseitig beeinflussen; *psycho*. interagieren; *phys*. wechselwirken.
in·ter·ac·tion [ˌ-'ækʃn] *n* gegenseitige Einwirkung *f*, (*a. phys*.) Wechselwirkung *f*; *psycho*. Interaktion *f*.
in·ter·ac·tive [ˌ-'æktɪv] *adj* aufeinander (ein-)wirkend, s. gegenseitig beeinflussend; *psycho*. interagierend; *phys*. wechselwirkend.
in·ter·al·ve·o·lar [ˌ-æl'vɪələr] *adj* zwischen Alveolen (liegend), interalveolär, -alveolar, Interalveolar-.
interalveolar pores Kohn'-Poren *pl*, (Inter-)Alveolarporen *pl*.
interalveolar septa 1. interalveolare Trennwände *pl*, Septa interalveolaria. **2.** (*Lunge*) (Inter-)Alveolarsepten *pl*.
in·ter·an·gu·lar [ˌ-'æŋgjələr] *adj* zwischen zwei *od*. mehreren Winkeln liegend *od*. auftretend.
in·ter·an·nu·lar [ˌ-'ænjələr] *adj* interanulär.
interannular segment → internodal segment.
in·ter·ar·tic·u·lar [ˌ-ɑː'tɪkjələr] *adj* zwischen Gelenkflächen (liegend), interartikulär.
interarticular cartilage Gelenkzwischenscheibe *f*, Discus articularis.
interarticular disk → interarticular cartilage.
interarticular fibrocartilage → interarticular cartilage.
interarticular ligament intraartikuläres Band/Ligament *nt*.
i. of head of rib Lig. capitis costae intraarticulare.
i. of hip joint Lig. capitis femoris.
interarticular sulcus of talus Sulcus tali.
in·ter·ar·y·te·noid [ˌ-ærɪ'tiːnɔɪd, -ə'rɪtnɔɪd] *adj* zwischen den Aryknorpeln (liegend), interarytänoid.

interarytenoid fold interarytänoide Schleimhautfalte *f*, Plica interaryt(a)enoidea.
interarytenoid incisure (of larynx) Inc. interaryt(a)enoidea.
interarytenoid notch → interarytenoid incisure (of larynx).
in·ter·a·tom·ic [ˌ-ə'tɑmɪk] *adj* zwischen Atomen (liegend), interatomar.
in·ter·a·tri·al [ˌ-'eɪtrɪəl] *adj* zwischen den Vorhöfen (liegend), die Vorhöfe verbindend, interatrial.
interatrial septum (of heart) Vorhofseptum *nt*, Septum interatriale (cordis).
in·ter·au·ric·u·lar [ˌ-ɔː'rɪkjələr] *adj* → interatrial.
interauricular septum → interatrial septum (of heart).
in·ter·brain ['-breɪn] *n* Zwischenhirn *nt*, Dienzephalon *nt*, Diencephalon *nt*.
interbrain vesicle *embryo*. Zwischenhirnbläschen *nt*.
in·ter·breed [ˌ-'briːd] **I** *vt* kreuzen, durch Kreuzung züchten. **II** *vi* **1.** s. kreuzen. **2.** s. untereinander vermehren.
in·ter·ca·lar·y [ɪn'tɜrkəˌlerɪː, ˌɪntər'kælərɪ] *adj* eingeschaltet, eingeschoben, eingekeilt, interkaliert, interkalar.
intercalary neuron → interneuron.
in·ter·ca·late [ɪn'tɜrkəleɪt] *vt* einschieben, einschalten, dazwischenschieben.
in·ter·ca·lat·ed [ɪn'tɜrkəleɪtɪd] *adj* → intercalary.
intercalated disk Glanzstreifen *m*, Discus intercalaris.
intercalated nucleus Nc. intercalatus.
in·ter·can·a·lic·u·lar [ˌɪntərˌkænə'lɪkjələr] *adj* interkanalikulär.
in·ter·cap·il·lar·y [ˌ-'kæpəlerɪː, -kəˈpɪlərɪ] *adj* zwischen Kapillaren (liegend), Kapillaren verbindend, interkapillär.
intercapillary cell Mesangial-, Mesangiumzelle *f*.
intercapillary glomerulosclerosis Kimmelstiel-Wilson-Syndrom *nt*, diabetische Glomerulosklerosis *f*.
intercapillary nephrosclerosis interkapilläre Nephrosklerose *f*, Glomerulosklerose *f*.
in·ter·ca·pit·u·lar veins [ˌ-kəˈpɪtʃələr]: **i. of foot** Vv. intercapitulares pedis.
i. of hand Vv. intercapitulares manus.
in·ter·ca·rot·ic [ˌ-'rɑtɪk] *adj* zwischen der A. carotis externa u. der A. carotis interna (liegend).
in·ter·ca·rot·id [ˌ-kəˈrɑtɪd] *adj* → intercarotic.
intercarotid body Karotisdrüse *f*, Paraganglion *nt* der Karotisgabel, Glomus/Paraganglion caroticum.
in·ter·car·pal [ˌ-'kɑːrpl] *adj* zwischen Handwurzel-/Karpalknochen (liegend), interkarpal.
intercarpal articulations Interkarpalgelenke *pl*, Articc. intercarpales.
intercarpal joints → intercarpal articulations.
intercarpal ligaments Ligg. intercarpalia.
dorsal i. Ligg. intercarpalia dorsalia.
interosseous i. Ligg. intercarpalia interossea.
palmar i. Ligg. intercarpalia palmaria.
volar i. → palmar i.
in·ter·car·ti·lag·i·nous [ˌ-ˌkɑːrtə'lædʒɪnəs] *adj* → interchondral.
in·ter·cav·ern·ous [ˌ-'kævərnəs] *adj* zwischen Hohlräumen (liegend), Hohlräume verbindend, interkavernös.
intercavernous plexus Sinus cavernosi--verbindender Venenplexus.
intercavernous sinuses Sinus intercavernosi.

in·ter·cel·lu·lar [ˌ-'seljələr] *adj* zwischen Zellen (liegend), im Interzellularraum (liegend), Zellen verbindend, interzellulär, -zellular, Interzellular-.
intercellular cleft Interzellulärspalt *m*.
intercellular space Interzellularraum *m*.
intercellular substance Zwischenzell-, Interzellular-, Grund-, Kittsubstanz *f*.
in·ter·cen·tral [ˌ-'sentrəl] *adj (ZNS)* zwischen mehreren Zentren (liegend), mehrere Zentren verbindend, interzentral.
in·ter·cept [ˌ-'sept] *vt* auffangen, unterbrechen.
in·ter·cep·tion [ˌ-'sepʃn] *n (Strahl)* Auffangen *nt*; Unterbrechung *f*.
in·ter·cer·e·bral [ˌ-'serəbrəl] *adj* zwischen den Großhirnhemisphären (liegend), interzerebral.
in·ter·change [*n* '-tʃeɪndʒ; *v* ˌ-'tʃeɪndʒ] **I** *n* **1.** *genet*. Translokation *f*. **2.** Auswechslung *f*, Austausch *m*. **II** *vt* auswechseln, (aus-)tauschen, gegeneinander austauschen.
in·ter·change·a·ble [ˌ-'tʃeɪndʒəbl] *adj* austausch-, auswechselbar.
in·ter·change·a·bil·i·ty [ˌ-ˌtʃeɪndʒə'bɪlətɪ] *n* Austauschbar-, Auswechselbarkeit *f*.
in·ter·chang·er [ˌ-'tʃeɪndʒər] *n techn.* *(Wärme etc.)* Austauscher *m*.
in·ter·chon·dral [ˌ-'kɑndrəl] *adj* zwischen Knorpeln (liegend), knorpelverbindend, interchondral.
interchondral articulations Articc. interchondrales.
interchondral joints → interchondral articulations.
in·ter·cil·i·um [ˌ-'sɪlɪəm] *n anat*. Glabella *f*.
in·ter·cis·tron·ic [ˌ-sɪs'trɑnɪk] *adj* intercistronisch.
in·ter·cla·vic·u·lar [ˌ-klə'vɪkjələr] *adj* die Schlüsselbeine verbindend, interklavikular.
interclavicular incisure Inc. jugularis sterni.
interclavicular ligament Lig. interclaviculare.
interclavicular notch → interclavicular incisure.
in·ter·coc·cyg·e·al [ˌ-kɑk'sɪdʒɪəl] *adj* zwischen den Steißbeinsegmenten (liegend), interkokzygeal.
in·ter·co·lum·nar [ˌ-kə'lʌmnər] *adj* zwischen Kolumnen *od*. Pfeilern (liegend), interkolumnar.
intercolumnar fibers Fibrae intercrurales.
intercolumnar tubercle Subfornikalorgan *nt*, Organum subfornicale.
in·ter·con·dy·lar [ˌ-'kɑndɪlər] *adj* zwischen Kondylen (liegend), interkondylär.
intercondylar area of tibia Area intercondylaris (tibiae).
anterior i. Area intercondylaris anterior (tibiae).
posterior i. Area intercondylaris posterior (tibiae).
intercondylar eminence → intercondylar tubercle.
intercondylar fossa: anterior i. of tibia → intercondylar area of tibia, anterior.
i. of femur Fossa intercondylaris (femoris).
posterior i. of tibia → intercondylar area of tibia, posterior.
intercondylar fracture of the femur *ortho.* interkondyläre Oberschenkelfraktur/Femurfraktur *f*.
intercondylar line Linea intercondylaris (femoris).
intercondylar notch of femur → intercondylar fossa of femur.
intercondylar process of tibia → intercondylar tubercle.
intercondylar tubercle Eminentia intercondylaris (tibiae).
lateral i. Tuberculum intercondylare laterale.
medial i. Tuberculum intercondylare mediale.
in·ter·con·dy·loid [ˌ-'kɑndlɔɪd] *adj* → intercondylar.
intercondyloid line → intercondylar line.
in·ter·con·dy·lous [ˌ-'kɑndɪləs] *adj* → intercondylar.
in·ter·con·nect [ˌ-kə'nekt] *vt* miteinander verbinden, zusammenschalten.
in·ter·con·nec·tion [ˌ-kə'nekʃn] *n* (gegenseitige) Verbindung *od*. Beziehung *f*, Wechselbeziehung *f*, Zusammenschaltung *f*, -schluß *m*.
in·ter·cos·tal [ˌ-'kɑstl] *adj* zwischen Rippen (liegend), Zwischenrippenraum betr., interkostal.
intercostal anesthesia → intercostal nerve block.
intercostal aponeurosis: external i. → intercostal membrane, anterior.
internal i. → intercostal membrane, posterior.
intercostal artery: anterior i.ies Rami intercostales anteriores a. thoracicae internae.
highest i. oberste Interkostalarterie *f*, Interkostalis *f* suprema, A. intercostalis suprema.
posterior i.ies hintere Interkostalarterien *pl*, Aa. intercostales posteriores.
superior → highest i.
intercostal articulations Articc. interchondrales.
intercostal block → intercostal nerve block.
intercostal branches of internal thoracic artery, anterior → intercostal arteries, anterior.
in·ter·cos·ta·lis [ˌ-'kɑsteɪlɪs] *n* → intercostal muscles.
intercostalis externus (muscle) → intercostal muscles, external.
intercostalis internus (muscle) → intercostal muscles, internal.
intercostalis intimus (muscle) → intercostal muscles, innermost.
intercostalis muscle → intercostal muscles.
intercostal joints → intercostal articulations.
intercostal lymph nodes paravertebrale Interkostallymphknoten *pl*, Nodi lymphatici intercostales.
intercostal membrane Zwischenrippen-, Interkostalmembran *f*, Membrana intercostalis.
anterior i. äußere Zwischenrippen-/Interkostalmembran, Membrana intercostalis externa.
posterior i. innere Zwischenrippen-/Interkostalmembran, Membrana intercostalis interna.
intercostal muscles Zwischenrippen-, Interkostalmuskeln *pl*, -muskulatur *f*, Mm. intercostales.
external i. äußere Interkostalmuskeln, Mm. intercostales externi.
innermost i. innerste Interkostalmuskeln, Mm. intercostales intimi.
internal i. innere Interkostalmuskeln, Mm. intercostales interni.
intercostal nerve block Interkostalanästhesie *f*.
intercostal nerves Zwischenrippen-, Interkostalnerven *pl*, Rami anteriores/ventrales nn. thoracicorum, Nn. intercostales.

intercostal neuralgia Interkostalneuralgie f.
intercostal space abbr. **ICS** Zwischenrippen-, Interkostalraum m, Spatium intercostale.
intercostal vein Zwischenrippen-, Interkostalvene f.
 anterior i.s vordere Interkostalvenen pl, Vv. intercostales anteriores.
 highest i. oberste Interkostalvene, V. intercostalis suprema.
 posterior i.s hintere Interkostalvenen pl, Vv. intercostales.
 superior i., left V. intercostalis superior sinistra.
 superior i., right V. intercostalis superior dextra.
in·ter·cos·to·bra·chi·al nerve [ˌ-ˌkɑstəʊ-ˈbreɪkɪəl, -ˈbræk-] N. intercostobrachialis.
in·ter·course [ˈkɔːrs, -kəʊrs] n 1. Umgang m, Verkehr m, Beziehung(en pl) f (with mit). 2. (Geschlechts-)Verkehr m, Koitus m.
in·ter·cri·co·thy·rot·o·my [ˌ-ˌkraɪkəθaɪˈrɑtəmɪ] n Interkrikothyrotomie f, Krikothyreotomie f.
in·ter·cris·tal diameter [ˌ-ˈkrɪstl] gyn. Distantia cristarum/intercristalis.
in·ter·crit·i·cal [ˌ-ˈkrɪtɪkəl] adj patho. zwischen zwei Krankheitsschüben, interkritisch.
intercritical gout symptomfreie Gicht f, Intermediärphase f.
in·ter·cross [n ˈ-krɔs, -krɑs; v ˌ-ˈkrɔs, -ˈkrɑs] (a. bio.) I n Kreuzung(sprodukt nt) f; Kreuzen nt. II vt kreuzen. III vi s. kreuzen.
in·ter·cru·ral [ˌ-ˈkrʊərəl] adj zwischen Schenkeln (liegend), interkrural.
intercrural fibers Fibrae intercrurales.
in·ter·cu·ne·i·form [ˌ-ˈkjuːn(ɪ)ɪfɔːrm, -kjəˈniːə-] adj die Keilbeine verbindend, zwischen den Keilbeinen (liegend), intercuneiform.
intercuneiform articulations/joints Articc. intercuneiformes.
intercuneiform ligaments: dorsal i. Ligg. intercuneiformia dorsalia.
 interosseous i. Ligg. intercuneiformia interossea.
 plantar i. Ligg. intercuneiformia plantaria.
in·ter·cur·rent [ˌ-ˈkɜrənt, -ˈkʌr-] adj hinzukommend, dazwischentretend, zwischenzeitlich (auftretend), interkurrent, interkurrierend.
intercurrent disease interkurrente Erkrankung/Krankheit f.
in·ter·den·tal [ˌ-ˈdentl] adj zwischen Zähnen (liegend), Zähne verbindend, interdental, Interdental-.
interdental papilla Interdentalpapille f, Papilla gingivalis/interdentalis.
interdental septa → interalveolar septa 1.
in·ter·den·ti·um [ˌ-ˈdenʃɪəm] n anat., dent. Interdentalraum m, Interdentium nt.
in·ter·de·pend [ˌ-dɪˈpend] vi voneinander abhängen.
in·ter·de·pend·ence [ˌ-dɪˈpendəns] n gegenseitige Abhängigkeit f.
in·ter·de·pend·en·cy [-dɪˈpendənsɪ] n → interdependence.
in·ter·de·pend·ent [ˌ-dɪˈpendənt] adj voneinander abhängig.
in·ter·di·ges·tive myoelectric motor complex [ˌ-daɪˈdʒestɪv, -daɪ-] interdigestiver myoelektrischer Motorkomplex m.
in·ter·dig·it [ˌ-ˈdɪdʒɪt] n Finger- od. Zehenzwischenraum m, Interdigitalraum m.
in·ter·dig·i·tal [ˌ-ˈdɪdʒɪtl] adj zwischen Fingern od. Zehen (liegend), Finger- od. Zehen verbindend, Interdigitalraum betr., interdigital.

in·ter·dig·i·tate [ˌ-ˈdɪdʒɪteɪt] I vt miteinander verflechten. II vi 1. verflochten sein (with mit). 2. ineinandergreifen.
in·ter·dig·i·tat·ing (reticular) cells [ˌ-ˌdɪdʒɪˈteɪtɪŋ] interdigitierende Retikulumzellen pl.
in·ter·face [ˈ-feɪs] n 1. chem., phys. Grenz-, Trennungsfläche f. 2. electr. Schnittstelle f; (Computer) Nahtstelle f.
in·ter·fas·ci·al space [ˌ-ˈfæʃɪəl] Tenon'-Raum m, Spatium episclerale.
in·ter·fas·cic·u·lar [ˌ-fəˈsɪkjələr] adj zwischen Faszikeln (liegend), interfaszikulär.
interfascicular fasciculus Schultze'-Komma nt, Fasciculus interfascicularis/semilunaris.
interfascicular glia interfaszikuläre Glia f.
in·ter·fem·o·ral [ˌ-ˈfemərəl] adj zwischen den Oberschenkeln (liegend).
in·ter·fere [ˌ-ˈfɪər] vi 1. stören, behindern, hemmen (with); etw. beeinträchtigen (with). 2. s. einmischen (in in). 3. phys. s. überlagern, interferieren.
in·ter·fer·ence [ˌ-ˈfɪərəns] n 1. Störung f, Behinderung f, Hemmung f (with); Beeinträchtigung f (with). 2. Einmischung f, Einschaltung f (in in). 3. psycho., card., bio. Interferenz f. 4. phys. Überlagerung f, Interferenz f. 5. micro. Virusinterferenz f.
interference microscope Interferenzmikroskop nt.
interference pattern phys. Interferenzmuster nt.
in·ter·fe·ren·tial [ˌ-fəˈrenʃəl] adj Interferenz-.
in·ter·fer·ing [ˌ-ˈfɪərɪŋ] adj störend, behindernd; s. einmischend; phys. s. überlagernd, interferierend.
in·ter·fer·om·e·ter [ˌ-fəˈrɑmɪtər] n Interferometer nt.
in·ter·fer·om·e·try [ˌ-fəˈrɑmətrɪ] n Interferometrie f.
in·ter·fer·on [ˌ-ˈfɪərɑn] n abbr. **IFN** Interferon nt abbr. IFN.
interferon-α n abbr. **IFN-α** Leukozyteninterferon nt, α-Interferon nt abbr. IFN-α.
interferon-β n abbr. **IFN-β** Fibroblastininterferon nt, β-Interferon nt abbr. IFN-β.
interferon-γ n abbr. **IFN-γ** Immuninterferon nt, γ-Interferon nt abbr. IFN-γ.
in·ter·fi·bril·lar [ˌ-ˈfaɪbrɪlər] adj zwischen Fibrillen (liegend), interfibrillär.
interfibrillar substance of Flemming Hyaloplasma nt, Grundzytoplasma nt, zytoplasmatische Matrix f.
in·ter·fi·bril·lar·y [ˌ-ˈfaɪbrəˌleriː] adj → interfibrillar.
in·ter·fi·brous [ˌ-ˈfaɪbrəs] adj zwischen Fasern (liegend), interfibrös.
in·ter·fi·la·men·tous [ˌɪntərfɪləˈmentəs] adj zwischen Filamenten (liegend), interfilamentär.
in·ter·fi·lar mass/substance [ˌ-ˈfaɪlər] → interfibrillar substance of Flemming.
in·ter·fol·lic·u·lar cells [ˌ-fəˈlɪkjələr] Hürthle-Zellen pl.
in·ter·fo·ve·o·lar ligament [ˌ-foʊˈvɪələr] Lig. interfoveolare.
in·ter·fron·tal [ˌ-ˈfrʌntl] adj zwischen Stirnbeinhälften (liegend), interfrontal.
in·ter·gan·gli·on·ic [ˌ-gæŋglɪˈɑnɪk] adj zwischen Ganglien (liegend), Ganglien verbindend, interganglionär.
interganglionic branches Verbindungsäste pl der Grenzstrangganglien, Rami interganglionares.
in·ter·gem·mal [ˌ-ˈdʒeml] adj intergemmal.

in·ter·glob·u·lar [ˌ-ˈglɑbjələr] adj interglobulär, -globular.
interglobular spaces of Owen Czermak-Räume pl, Interglobulärräume pl, Spatia interglobularia.
in·ter·glu·te·al [ˌ-ˈgluːtɪəl] adj zwischen den Gesäßbacken (liegend), interglutäal, intergluteal, internatal.
in·ter·gra·da·tion [ˌ-greɪˈdeɪʃn] n 1. allmähliches Ineinanderübergehen nt. 2. bio., genet. Intergradation f.
in·ter·grade [n ˈ-greɪd; v ˌ-ˈgreɪd] I n Zwischenstufe f, -form f, -stadium nt. II vi allmählich ineinander übergehen.
in·ter·gran·u·lar [ˌ-ˈgrænjələr] adj intergranulär.
in·ter·gy·ral [ˌ-ˈdʒaɪrəl] adj zwischen Gyri (liegend), intergyral.
in·ter·hem·i·cer·e·bral [ˌ-ˌhemɪˈserəbrəl] adj → interhemispheric.
in·ter·hem·i·spher·ic [ˌ-ˌhemɪˈsferɪk] adj zwischen Hemisphären (liegend), Hemisphären verbindend, interhemisphärisch.
interhemispheric fibers (ZNS) interhemisphärische Fasern pl.
in·ter·ic·tal [ˌ-ˈɪktl] adj zwischen zwei Anfällen (auftretend).
in·ter·il·i·ac lymph nodes [ˌ-ˈɪlɪæk] → iliac lymph nodes, external interiliac.
in·ter·il·i·o·ab·dom·i·nal amputation [ˌ-ˌɪlɪoʊæbˈdɑmɪnl] ortho. interilioabdominale Amputation f; Hemipelvektomie f.
in·ter·in·nom·i·no·ab·dom·i·nal amputation [ˌ-ˌɪnɑmɪnoʊæbˈdɑmɪnl] → interilioabdominal amputation.
in·ter·i·on·ic [ˌ-aɪˈɑnɪk] adj zwischen Ionen (liegend), interionisch.
in·te·ri·or [ɪnˈtɪərɪər] I n das Innere; Innenraum m, -seite f. II adj 1. innere(r, s), innen, Innen-. 2. privat, intern.
interior angle mathe. Innenwinkel m.
in·ter·ja·cent [ˌɪntərˈdʒeɪsənt] adj dazwischenliegend.
in·ter·ki·ne·sis [ˌ-kɪˈniːsɪs, -kaɪ-] n bio. Interkinese f.
in·ter·la·bi·al [ˌ-ˈleɪbɪəl] adj zwischen den Lippen (liegend), interlabial.
in·ter·lace [ˌ-ˈleɪs, -ˈleɪs] I vt (miteinander) verflechten, verknüpfen, vernetzen, verweben. II vi s. verflechten, s. verweben, s. (über-)kreuzen.
in·ter·la·mel·lar [ˌ-ləˈmelər, -ˈlæmə-] adj zwischen Lamellen (liegend), interlamellär.
in·ter·leu·kin [ˈ-luːkɪn] n abbr. **IL** Interleukin nt abbr. IL.
interleukin-1 n abbr. **IL-1** Interleukin-1 nt abbr. IL-1.
interleukin-2 n abbr. **IL-2** Interleukin-2 nt abbr. IL-2.
interleukin-3 n abbr. **IL-3** Interleukin-3 nt abbr. IL-3.
in·ter·lig·a·men·ta·ry [ˌ-ˈlɪgəməntərɪ] adj zwischen Ligamenten (liegend), interligamentär.
in·ter·lig·a·men·tous [ˌ-ˌlɪgəˈmentəs] adj → interligamentary.
in·ter·link [n ˈ-lɪŋk; v ˌ-ˈlɪŋk] I n Bindeglied, Zwischenglied nt. II vt (miteinander) verbinden od. verketten od. verknüpfen, ineinanderhängen.
in·ter·lo·bar [ˌ-ˈloʊbər, -bɑr] adj zwischen Organlappen (liegend), Organlappen verbindend, interlobär.
interlobar arteries of kidney renale Zwischenlappen-/Interlobarterien pl, Aa. interlobares renis.
interlobar empyema interlobäres Empyem nt.
interlobar grooves → interlobar sulci of cerebrum.

interlobar sulci of cerebrum Interlobarfurchen *pl* des Großhirns, Sulci interlobares (cerebri).
interlobar veins of kidney Zwischenlappen-, Interlobarvenen *pl*, Vv. interlobares renis.
in·ter·lo·bi·tis [ˌ-ləʊˈbaɪtɪs] *n* Interlobärpleuritis *f*, Pleuritis interlobaris.
in·ter·lob·u·lar [ˌ-ˈlɒbjələr] *adj* zwischen Organläppchen (liegend), interlobulär.
interlobular arteries: i. of kidney Interlobular-, Radialarterien *pl*, Aa. interlobulares renis.
  i. of liver Interlobulararterien *pl*, Aa. interlobulares hepatis.
interlobular bile canals interlobuläre Gallengänge *pl*, Ductuli interlobulares hepatis.
interlobular bile ducts → interlobular bile canals.
interlobular duct *histol.* interlobulärer (Ausführungs-)Gang *m*.
interlobular ductules of liver → interlobular bile canals.
interlobular emphysema interlobuläres Lungenemphysem *nt*.
interlobular pleurisy → interlobitis.
interlobular septa (of lung) (*Lunge*) Läppchengrenzmembranen *pl*, Septa interlobularia.
interlobular veins: i. of kidney Interlobularvenen *pl*, Vv. interlobulares renis.
  i. of liver Interlobularvenen *pl*, Vv. interlobulares hepatis.
in·ter·lock·ing screw [ˌ-ˈlɒkɪŋ] *ortho.* Verriegelungsschraube *f*.
in·ter·loop abscess [ˌ-ˈluːp] Darmschlingenabszeß *m*, zwischen Darmschlingen liegender Abszeß *m*.
in·ter·lude [ˈ-luːd] *n* (kurze) Zeit *f*, Periode *f*; Unterbrechung *f* (*in*).
in·ter·mal·le·o·lar [ˌ-məˈlɪələr] *adj* zwischen den Knöcheln/Malleoli (liegend), intermalleolär.
in·ter·ma·mil·lar·y [ˌ-ˈmæmələrɪ] *adj* zwischen den Brustwarzen (liegend), intermamillär.
in·ter·mam·ma·ry [ˌ-ˈmæmərɪ] *adj* zwischen den Brüsten (liegend), intermammär.
in·ter·mar·riage [ˌ-ˈmærɪdʒ, ˈ-mærɪdʒ] *n* 1. Heirat *f* zwischen (Bluts-)Verwandten. 2. Heirat *f* zwischen Angehörigen verschiedener Rassen, Mischehe *f*.
in·ter·mar·ry [ˌɪntərˈmærɪ] *vi* 1. untereinander heiraten. 2. eine Mischehe eingehen.
in·ter·max·il·lar·y [ˌ-ˈmæksəˌlerɪ, -ˈmæksɪlərɪ] *adj* intermaxillär, -maxillar.
intermaxillary segment *embryo.* Zwischenkiefer-, Intermaxillarsegment *nt*.
intermaxillary suture Sutura intermaxillaris.
in·ter·me·di·ar·y [ˌ-ˈmiːdɪərɪ] *I n* 1. Vermittler(in *f*) *m*. 2. Zwischenform *f*, -stadium *nt*. **II** *adj* → intermediate II.
intermediary filament intermediäres Filament *nt*, Intermediärfilament *nt*.
intermediary metabolism Zwischenstoffwechsel *m*, Intermediärstoffwechsel *m*, -metabolismus *m*.
intermediary nerve → intermediate nerve.
in·ter·me·di·ate [ˌ-ˈmiːdjət, -dɪət; *v* -dɪeɪt] **I** *n* 1. Zwischenglied *nt*, Zwischenprodukt *nt*, Intermediärsubstanz *f*. 2. Vermittler(in *f*) *m*. **II** *adj* 3. dazwischenliegend, zwischen-, -form *f*; *chem.* Zwischen-, Mittel-, Intermediär-. 4. verbindend, vermittelnd, Verbindungs-, Zwischen-. **III** *vi* intervenieren, einschreiten; vermitteln.
intermediate bone Mondbein *nt*, Os lunatum.
intermediate callus *ortho.* Intermediärkallus *m*.
intermediate carcinoma basosquamöses/intermediäres Karzinom *nt*.
intermediate cell (*ZNS*) Binnenzelle *f*.
intermediate-density lipoprotein *abbr.* **IDL** Lipoprotein *nt* mit mittlerer Dichte, intermediate-density lipoprotein *abbr.* IDL.
intermediate disk Z-Linie *f*, Z-Streifen *m*, Zwischenscheibe *f*, Telophragma *nt*.
intermediate eminence Eminentia intercondylaris.
intermediate erythroblast polychromatischer Normoblast *m*.
intermediate ganglia Ggll. intermedia.
intermediate gray substance: central i. of spinal cord Substantia (grisea) intermedia centralis medullae spinalis.
  lateral i. of spinal cord Substantia (grisea) intermedia lateralis medullae spinalis.
intermediate groove: dorsal i. of spinal cord Sulcus intermedius dorsalis/posterior (medullae spinalis).
  posterior i. of spinal cord → dorsal i. of spinal cord.
intermediate heart *physiol.* Normal-, Indifferenztyp *m*.
intermediate host *micro.* Zwischenwirt *m*.
intermediate junction Zonula adherens.
intermediate lamellae (*Knochen*) Schaltlamellen *pl*.
intermediate line of iliac crest Linea intermedia (cristae iliacae).
intermediate lobe → intermediate lobe of hypophysis.
intermediate lobe inhibiting factor Melanotropin-inhibiting-Faktor *m* *abbr.* MIF, MSH-inhibiting-Faktor *m*.
intermediate lobe of hypophysis *abbr.* **IL** Hypophysenzwischenlappen *m* *abbr.* HZL, Pars intermedia adenohypophyseos.
intermediate mass (of thalamus) Massa intermedia, Adh(a)esio interthalamica.
intermediate mesoderm intermediäres Mesoderm *nt*.
intermediate nerve Intermedius *m*, N. intermedius.
intermediate neuron → interneuron.
intermediate normoblast polychromatischer Normoblast *m*.
intermediate nuclei of auditory tract Zwischenkerne *pl* der Hörbahn.
intermediate part: i. of adenohypophysis Hypophysenmittellappen *m* *abbr.* HML, Pars intermedia adenohypophyseos.
  i. of bulbus of vestibule Pars intermedia bulborum.
intermediate product Zwischenprodukt *nt*.
intermediate sinuses Intermediärsinus *m*.
intermediate sleep mittlerer Schlaf *m*.
intermediate stage Zwischen-, Intermediärphase *f*.
intermediate substance: central i. of spinal cord Substantia (grisea) intermedia centralis medullae spinalis.
  lateral i. of spinal cord Substantia (grisea) intermedia lateralis medullae spinalis.
intermediate sulcus of spinal cord: dorsal i. → intermediate groove of spinal cord, dorsal.
  posterior i. → intermediate groove of spinal cord, dorsal.
intermediate vein mittlere Kolonvene *f*, V. colica intermedia/media.
intermediate zone (of hypophysis) Zona intermedia hypophyseos.
in·ter·me·din [ˌ-ˈmiːdɪn] *n* Melanotropin *nt*, melanotropes Hormon *nt*, melanozytenstimulierendes Hormon *nt* *abbr.* MSH.
in·ter·me·di·o·fa·cial nerve [ˌ-ˌmiːdɪəʊˈfeɪʃl] Fazialis *m*, VII. Hirnnerv *m*, N. facialis [VII]; N. intermediofaciālis.
in·ter·me·di·o·lat·er·al [ˌ-ˌmiːdɪəʊˈlætərəl] *adj* intermediolateral.
intermediolateral column of spinal cord intermediolaterale (Rückenmarks-)Säule *f*, Columna autonomica/intermediolateralis medullae spinalis.
intermediolateral nucleus Nc. intermediolateralis.
intermediolateral substance of spinal cord Substantia intermediolateralis, Substantia intermedia lateralis medullae spinalis.
intermediolateral tract Seitensäule *f* (des Rückenmarks), Columna lateralis medullae spinalis.
in·ter·me·di·o·me·di·al nucleus [ˌ-ˌmiːdɪəʊˈmiːdɪəl] Nc. intermediomedialis.
in·ter·mem·bra·nous [ˌ-ˈmembrənəs] *adj* zwischen Membranen (liegend *od.* auftretend), intermembranös.
in·ter·me·nin·ge·al [ˌ-mɪˈnɪndʒɪəl] *adj* zwischen den Meningen (liegend), intermeningeal.
in·ter·men·stru·al [ˌ-ˈmenstrʊəl, -strəwəl, -strəl] *adj* zwischen zwei Menstruationen (liegend), intermenstrual, -menstruell, Intermenstrual-.
intermenstrual pain *gyn.* Mittelschmerz *m*, Intermenstrualschmerz *m*.
intermenstrual stage → intermenstruum.
in·ter·men·stru·um [ˌ-ˈmenstr(ʊ)əm, -strəwəm] *n*, *pl* **-stru·ums, -strua** [-str(ʊ)ə, -strəwə] Intermenstrualphase *f*, -stadium *nt*, -interval *nt*, Intermenstruum *nt*.
in·ter·mes·en·ter·ic plexus [ˌ-ˌmesənˈterɪk] Plexus intermesentericus.
in·ter·met·a·car·pal [ˌ-ˌmetəˈkɑːpəl] *adj* zwischen Metakarpalknochen (liegend), Metakarpalknochen verbindend, intermetakarpal.
intermetacarpal arteries, palmar palmare Mittelhandarterien *pl*, Aa. metacarpales palmares.
intermetacarpal articulations/joints Intermetakarpalgelenke *pl*, Articc. intermetacarpales.
intermetacarpal ligament Lig. metacarpale.
in·ter·met·a·mer·ic [ˌ-ˌmetəˈmerɪk] *adj* *embryo.* zwischen zwei Metameren (liegend), intermetamer(isch).
in·ter·met·a·tar·sal [ˌ-ˌmetəˈtɑːrsl] *adj* zwischen Metatarsalknochen (liegend), Metatarsalknochen verbindend, intermetatarsal.
intermetatarsal articulations/joints Intermetatarsalgelenke *pl*, Articc. intermetatarsales.
intermetatarsal ligament Lig. metatarsale.
in·ter·mis·sion [ˌ-ˈmɪʃn] *n* 1. Pause *f*, Unterbrechung *f*. 2. *med.* symptomfreie Phase *f* im Krankheitsverlauf, Intermission *f*.
in·ter·mit [ˌ-ˈmɪt] *I vt* unterbrechen, aussetzen mit. **II** *vi* aussetzen, vorübergehend aufhören.
in·ter·mi·tot·ic [ˌ-maɪˈtɒtɪk] *adj* *bio.* zwischen zwei Mitosen liegend *od.* auftretend, intermitotisch, Intermitose-.
in·ter·mit·tence [ˌ-ˈmɪtns] *n* 1. Unterbrechung *f*, Aussetzen *nt*. 2. → intermission 2.
in·ter·mit·ten·cy [ˌ-ˈmɪtnsɪ] *n* → intermittence.
in·ter·mit·tent [ˌ-ˈmɪtnt] *adj* (zeitweilig) aussetzend, mit Unterbrechungen, periodisch (auftretend), intermittierend.

intermittent albuminuria funktionelle/physiologische/intermittierende Proteinurie/Albuminurie *f*.
intermittent claudication → i. of the leg.
i. of the cauda equina → i. of the spinal cord.
i. of the leg intermittierendes Hinken *nt*, Charcot-Syndrom *nt*, Claudicatio intermittens, Angina cruris, Dysbasia intermittens/angiospastica.
i. of the spinal cord Claudicatio intermittens des Rückenmarks/der Cauda equina.
intermittent cramp 1. Tetanus *m*, Tetanie *f*. **2.** neuromuskuläre Übererregbarkeit *f*, Tetanie *f*.
intermittent fever (*Malaria*) Wechselfieber *nt*, Febris intermittens.
intermittent hemoglobinuria intermittierende Hämoglobinurie *f*, Harley-Krankheit *f*.
intermittent hepatic fever intermittierendes Fieber *nt* bei Cholelithiasis.
intermittent hydrosalpinx *gyn.* Hydrops tubae profluens, Hydrorrhoea tubae intermittens.
intermittent incontinence intermittierende Harninkontinenz *f*.
intermittent malaria → intermittent fever.
intermittent malarial fever → intermittent fever.
intermittent mandatory ventilation *abbr.* **IMV** intermittierende mandatorische Beatmung *f*, intermittent mandatory ventilation *abbr.* IMV.
intermittent pain intermittierender Schmerz *m*.
intermittent parasite *micro.* vorübergehender Parasit *m*.
intermittent positive pressure breathing *abbr.* **IPPB** intermittierende positive Druck(be)atmung *f*, intermittierende Überdruckbeatmung *f*.
intermittent positive pressure respiration *abbr.* **IPPR** → intermittend positive pressure breathing.
intermittent positive pressure ventilation *abbr.* **IPPV** → intermittend positive pressure breathing.
intermittent proteinuria funktionelle/physiologische/intermittierende Proteinurie/Albuminurie *f*.
intermittent pulse intermittierender Puls *m*, Pulsus intermittens.
intermittent strabismus *ophthal.* intermittierendes Schielen *nt*.
intermittent torticollis *ortho.* intermittierender Schiefhals/Torticollis *m*.
intermittent tremor intermittierender Tremor *m*.
in·ter·mix [,-'mɪks] **I** *vt* vermischen. **II** *vi s.* vermischen.
in·ter·mix·ture [,-'mɪkstʃər] *n* **1.** Gemisch *nt*, Mischung *f*. **2.** Beimischung *f*, Zusatz *m*. **3.** Vermischen *nt*.
in·ter·mo·lec·u·lar [,-məˈlekjələr, -məʊ-] *adj chem., phys.* zwischen Molekülen (liegend *od.* wirkend), intermolekular.
in·ter·mus·cu·lar [,ɪntərˈmʌskjələr] *adj* zwischen Muskeln (liegend), Muskeln verbindend, intermuskulär.
intermuscular hernia intermuskuläre/interparietale Hernie *f*, Hernia intermuscularis/interparietalis.
intermuscular ligament Septum intermusculare.
external i. of arm Septum intermusculare brachii laterale.
external i. of thigh Septum intermusculare femoris laterale.
fibular i. Septum intermusculare curis anterius.
internal i. of arm Septum intermusculare brachii mediale.
lateral i. of arm Septum intermusculare brachii laterale.
lateral i. of thigh Septum intermusculare femoris laterale.
medial i. of arm Septum intermusculare brachii mediale.
medial i. of thigh Septum intermusculare femoris mediale.
intermuscular septum Septum intermusculare.
anterior i. of (lower) leg Septum intermusculare cruris anterius.
i. of arm Septum intermusculare brachii.
crural i. → i. of (lower) leg.
crural i., anterior → anterior i. of (lower) leg.
crural i., posterior → posterior i. of (lower) leg.
external i. of thigh Septum intermusculare femoris laterale.
lateral i. of arm Septum intermusculare brachii laterale.
lateral i. of thigh → external i. of thigh.
i. of (lower) leg Septum intermusculare cruris.
medial i. of arm Septum intermusculare brachii mediale.
medial i. of thigh Septum intermusculare femoris mediale.
posterior i. of (lower) leg Septum intermusculare cruris posterius.
i. of thigh Septum intermusculare femoris.
in·ter·nal [ɪnˈtɜrnl] **I** ~s *pl* innere Organe *pl*. **II** *adj* **1.** innere(r, s), intern, Innen-. **2.** *pharm.* innerlich (anzuwenden). **for ~ application/use** zum inneren Gebrauch, zur inneren Anwendung.
internal angle of tibia Margo medialis tibiae.
internal aperture of tympanic canaliculus innere Öffnung *f* des Canaliculus tympanicus, Apertura superior canaliculi tympanici.
internal axis of bulb/eye innere Augenachse *f*, Axis bulbi internus.
internal band of Baillarger → inner band of Baillarger.
internal base of cranium innere Schädelbasis *f*, Basis cranii interna.
internal branch: i. of accessory nerve Ramus internus n. accessorii.
i. of superior laryngeal nerve innerer Ast *m* des N. laryngeal superior, Ramus internus n. laryngei superioris.
internal callus *ortho.* innerer/zentraler Kallus *m*.
internal capsule innere Kapsel *f*, Capsula interna.
internal clock *physiol.* biologische Uhr *f*, innere Uhr *f*.
internal coat: i. of capsule of graafian follicle Tunica interna thecae folliculi.
i. of pharynx of Luschka Tela submucosa pharyngis.
internal conjugate Conjugata anatomica.
internal crus: i. of greater alar cartilage Crus mediale cartilago alaris majoris.
i. of superficial inguinal ring Crus mediale anuli inguinalis superficialis.
internal ear Innenohr *nt*, Auris interna.
internal endometriosis *gyn.* Endometriosis uteri interna, *old* Adenomyosis interna.
internal extremity of clavicle Extremitas sternalis.
internal fistula innere Fistel *f*, Fistula interna.
internal fixation *ortho.* operative Frakturbehandlung *f*, -stabilisierung *f*, Osteosynthese *f*.
internal genu of facial nerve inneres Fazialisknie *nt*, Genu n. facialis.
internal glomerulus *embryo.* innerer Glomerulus *m*.
internal growth interstitielles Wachstum *nt*.
internal hemorrhagic pachymeningitis Pachymeningitis/Pachymeningiosis haemorrhagica interna.
internal hemorrhoids innere Hämorrhoiden *pl*.
internal hernia direkter/innerer/gerader Leistenbruch *m*, Hernia inguinalis interna/medialis/directa.
internal hordeolum *ophthal.* Hordeolum internum.
internal hydrocephalus Hydrocephalus internus.
internal injury innere Verletzung *f*.
in·ter·nal·i·za·tion [ɪn,tɜrnlaɪˈzeɪʃn] *n psycho.* Verinnerlichung *f*, Internalisierung *f*.
in·ter·nal·ize [ɪnˈtɜrnlaɪz] *vt psycho.* verinnerlichen, internalisieren.
internal lamina: i. of pterygoid process Lamina medialis proc. pterygoidei.
i. of skull inneres Blatt *nt* des knöchernen Schädeldaches, Lamina interna (cranii).
internal layer: i. of myometrium subvaskuläre Schicht *f* des Myometriums, Stratum subvasculare/submucosum (myometrii).
i. of skull → internal lamina of skull.
i. of theca folliculi Theka/Theca *f* interna, Tunica interna thecae folliculi.
internal limb of greater alar cartilage Crus mediale cartilago alaris majoris.
internal line of Baillarger → inner band of Baillarger.
internal lip of iliac crest Labium internum cristae iliacae.
in·ter·nal·ly compensated isomer [ɪnˈtɜrnlɪ] *chem.* intern kompensiertes Isomer *nt*, meso-Form *f*.
internal margin of testis hinterer Hodenrand *m*, Margo posterior testis.
internal medicine innere Medizin *f*; *inf.* Innere *f*.
internal meningitis subdurale Pachymeningitis *f*, Pachymeningitis interna.
internal ophthalmopathy Ophthalmopathia interna.
internal ophthalmoplegia Ophthalmoplegia interna.
internal organs innere Organe *pl*.
internal pacemaker *card.* interner/implantierter Herzschrittmacher *m*.
internal parasite *micro.* Binnen-, Innenschmarotzer *m*, Endo-, Entoparasit *m*, Endosit *m*.
internal pathology medizinische Pathologie *f*.
internal perimysium Muskelhüllgewebe *nt* des Primärbündels, Perimysium internum.
internal phase *phys.* disperse/innere Phase *f*, Dispersum *nt*.
internal respiration innere Atmung *f*, Zell-, Gewebeatmung *f*.
internal rotation Innenrotation *f*.
internal segment of globus pallidus inneres Pallidumsegment *nt*.
internal sheath of optic nerve → inner sheath of optic nerve.
internal sphincter (muscle) innerer Schließmuskel *m*.
internal sphincterotomy *chir.* Sphinkterotomie *f* des Sphincter ani internus.
internal strabismus *ophthal.* Einwärtsschielen *nt*, Esotropie *f*, Strabismus convergens/internus.

internal stria of Baillarger

internal stria of Baillarger → inner band of Baillarger.
internal stripe of Baillarger → inner band of Baillarger.
internal surface of eyelid innere/hintere Lidfläche *f*, Facies posterior palpebraris.
internal tubercle of humerus Tuberculum minus humeri.
internal tuberosity of femur Epicondylus medialis femoris.
internal urethrotomy *urol.* endourethrale Urethrotomie *f*, Urethrotomia interna.
internal version *gyn.* innere Wendung *f*.
in·ter·na·sal [ˌɪntərˈneɪzl] *adj* internasal.
internasal suture Sutura internasalis.
in·ter·na·tal [ˌ-ˈneɪtl] *adj* zwischen den Gesäßbacken (liegend), internatal, interglutäal, intergluteal.
in·ter·na·tion·al [ˌ-ˈnæʃənl] *adj* zwischen-, überstaatlich, international, weltweit, Welt-.
International Nonproprietary Names *abbr.* **I.N.N.** *pharm.* internationale Freinamen *pl* pharmazeutischer Grundstoffe, International Nonproprietary Names *abbr.* INN.
International System of Units internationales Einheitensystem *nt*, Système international d'Unites, SI-System *nt*.
international unit *abbr.* **I.U.** internationale Einheit *f abbr.* I.E., international unit *abbr.* I.U.
i. of enzyme activity internationale Einheit der Enzymaktivität, Enzymeinheit.
in·ter·neu·ral synapse [ˌ-ˈnjʊərəl, -ˈnʊrəl] interneurale Synapse *f*.
in·ter·neu·ron [ˌ-ˈn(j)ʊərɑn] *n* Zwischen-, Schalt-, Interneuron *nt*.
in·tern·ist [ˈɪntɜrnɪst, ɪnˈtɜrn-] *n* Internist(in *f*) *m*, (Fach-)Arzt/Ärztin für innere Krankheiten.
in·ter·nod·al [ˌɪntərˈnoʊdl] *adj* zwischen zwei Knoten (liegend), internodal.
internodal segment internodales/interanuläres Segment *nt*, Internodium *nt*.
internodal zone internodale Zone *f*.
in·ter·node (of Ranvier) [ˈ-noʊd] *n* → internodal segment.
in·ter·nu·cle·ar [ˌ-ˈn(j)uːkliər] *adj bio.* zwischen (Zell-)Kernen (liegend), internukleär, -nuklear.
internuclear ophthalmoplegia *ophthal.* internukleäre Ophthalmoplegie *f*.
in·ter·nun·cial cells [ˌ-ˈnʌnʃl] (*ZNS*) Schaltzellen *pl*.
internuncial fibers (*ZNS*) Verbindungsfasern *pl*.
internuncial neuron → interneuron.
in·ter·o·cep·tion [ˌɪntəroʊˈsepʃn] *n* Intero(re)zeption *f*, Entero(re)zeption *f*.
in·ter·o·cep·tive [ˌ-ˈseptɪv] *adj* innere körpereigene Reize aufnehmend, intero(re)zeptiv, entero(re)zeptiv.
interoceptive nervous system intero(re)zeptives System *nt*.
interoceptive sensibility interozeptive Sensibilität *f*.
in·ter·o·cep·tor [ˌ-ˈseptər] *n* Intero(re)zeptor *m*, Entero(re)zeptor *m*.
in·ter·oc·u·lar [ˌɪntərˈɑkjələr] *adj* zwischen den Augen (liegend), interokular.
in·ter·or·bit·al [ˌ-ˈɔːrbɪtl] *adj* zwischen den Augenhöhlen (liegend), interorbital.
in·ter·os·se·al [ˌ-ˈɑsɪəl] *adj* 1. → interosseous. 2. Mm. interossei betr.
in·ter·os·sei (muscles) [ˌ-ˈɑsɪaɪ] *old* Zwischenknochenmuskeln *pl*, Interossärmuskeln *pl*, Mm. interossei.
dorsal i. of foot dorsale Interossärmuskeln des Fußes, Interossei *pl* dorsales pedis, Mm. interossei dorsales pedis.
dorsal i. of hand dorsale Interossärmuskeln der Hand, Interossei *pl* dorsales manus, Mm. interossei dorsales manus.
palmar i. palmare Interossärmuskeln, Interossei *pl* palmares, Mm. interossei palmares.
plantar i. plantare Interossärmuskeln, Interossei *pl* plantares, Mm. interossei plantares.
in·ter·os·se·ous [ˌ-ˈɑsɪəs] *adj* zwischen Knochen (liegend), Knochen verbindend, interossär.
interosseous artery: anterior i. Interossea *f* anterior, A. interossea anterior.
common i. Interossea *f* communis, A. interossea communis.
dorsal i. of forearm → posterior i.
posterior i. Interossea *f* posterior, A. interossea posterior.
posterior i. of forearm → posterior i.
recurrent i. Interossea *f* recurrens, A. interossea recurrens.
volar i. → anterior i.
interosseous border: i. of fibula Margo interosseus fibulae.
i. of radius Margo interosseus radii.
i. of tibia Margo interosseus tibiae.
i. of ulna Margo interosseus ulnae.
interosseous cartilage Zwischenknorpel *m* von fibrösen Verbindungen *od.* Symphysen.
interosseous crest: i. of fibula Margo interosseus fibulae.
i. of radius Margo interosseus radii.
i. of tibia Margo interosseus tibiae.
i. of ulna Margo interosseus ulnae.
interosseous groove of calcaneus Sulcus calcanei.
interosseous ligaments of knee Kreuzbänder *pl*, Ligg. cruciata genus/genualia.
interosseous margin Margo interosseus.
i. of fibula Margo interosseus fibulae.
i. of radius Margo interosseus radii.
i. of tibia Margo interosseus tibiae.
i. of ulna Margo interosseus ulnae.
interosseous membrane Membrana interossea.
i. of forearm Membrana interossea antebrachii.
i. of leg Membrana interossea cruris.
interosseous muscles → interossei (muscles).
dorsal i. of foot → interossei (muscles) of foot, dorsal.
dorsal i. of hand → interossei (muscles) of hand, dorsal.
palmar i. → interossei (muscles), palmar.
plantar i. → interossei (muscles), plantar.
interosseous nerve: anterior i. of forearm N. interosseus (antebrachii) anterior.
i. of leg N. interosseus cruris.
posterior i. of forearm N. interosseus (antebrachii) posterior.
interosseous ridge: i. of fibula Margo interosseus fibulae.
i. of radius Margo interosseus radii.
i. of tibia Margo interosseus tibiae.
i. of ulna Margo interosseus ulnae.
interosseous veins: anterior i. Vv. interosseae anteriores.
dorsal i. of foot dorsale Mittelfußvenen *pl*, Vv. metatarsales dorsales.
posterior i. Vv. interosseae posteriores.
in·ter·pal·pe·bral [ˌɪntərˈpælpəbrəl] *adj* zwischen den Augenlidern (liegend), interpalpebral.
in·ter·pa·ri·e·tal [ˌ-pəˈraɪɪtl] *adj* 1. interparietal. 2. intermural.
interparietal bone Inkabein *nt*, Os interparietale.
interparietal fissure Sulcus intraparietalis.
interparietal hernia intermuskuläre/interparietale Hernie *f*, Hernia intermuscularis/interparietalis.
interparietal plane of occipital bone Planum occipitale.
interparietal sulcus → intraparietal sulcus.
in·ter·par·ox·ys·mal [ˌ-pærəkˈsɪzml] *adj* zwischen zwei Anfällen/Paroxysmen auftretend, interparoxysmal.
in·ter·pec·to·ral lymph node [ˌ-ˈpektərəl] Brustwand-, Pektoralislymphknoten *m*, Nodus lymphaticus (axillaris) interpectoralis.
in·ter·pe·dic·u·late distance [ˌ-pɪˈdɪkjəlɪt, -lɪt] *radiol.* Interpedikulärabstand *m*.
in·ter·pe·dun·cu·lar cistern [ˌ-pɪˈdʌŋkjələr] Cisterna basalis/interpeduncularis.
interpeduncular fossa Fossa interpeduncularis.
interpeduncular nucleus Nc. interpeduncularis.
in·ter·pel·vi·ab·dom·i·nal amputation [ˌ-ˌpelvɪæbˈdɑmɪnl] *ortho.* Jaboulay-Amputation *f*, -Operation *f*, -Hemipelvektomie *f*.
in·ter·per·son·al [ˌ-ˈpɜrsnl] *adj* 1. zwischen mehreren Personen ablaufend, mehrere Personen betr., interpersonal, -personell. 2. zwischenmenschlich.
in·ter·pha·lan·ge·al [ˌ-fəˈlændʒɪəl] *adj* zwischen Finger- *od.* Zehengliedern (liegend), Finger- *od.* Zehenglieder verbindend, interphalangeal.
interphalangeal articulations → interphalangeal joints.
interphalangeal joint: i.s *pl* Mittel- *od.* Endgelenke *pl* von Finger *od.* Zehe, Interphalangealgelenke *pl*, IP-Gelenke *pl*, Articc. interphalangeales.
distal i. *abbr.* **DIPJ** Endgelenk von Finger *od.* Zehe, distales Interphalangealgelenk *nt*, DIP-Gelenk *nt*, Artic. interphalangealis distalis.
proximal i. *abbr.* **PIPJ** Mittelgelenk von Finger *od.* Zehe, proximales Interphalangealgelenk *nt*, PIP-Gelenk *nt*, Artic. interphalangealis proximalis.
in·ter·phase [ˈ-feɪz] *n bio.* Interphase *f*.
interphase cell Interphasenzelle *f*.
interphase nucleus *histol.* Interphase-, Ruhe-, Arbeitskern *m*.
in·ter·pi·al [ˌ-ˈpaɪəl] *adj* zwischen zwei Schichten der Pia mater (liegend), interpial.
in·ter·plant [ˈ-plænt] *n embryo.* Interplantat *nt*.
in·ter·plant·ing [ˌ-ˈplæntɪŋ] *n embryo.* Interplantation *f*.
in·ter·pleu·ral [ˌ-ˈplʊərəl] *adj* zwischen zwei Pleuraschichten (liegend), interpleural.
in·ter·plex·i·form cells [ˌ-ˈpleksəfɔːrm] interplexiforme Zellen *pl*.
in·ter·po·lar [ˌ-ˈpoʊlər] *adj* zwischen den Polen (liegend), die Pole verbindend, interpolar.
in·ter·po·late [ɪnˈtɜrpəleɪt] *vt* 1. einschalten, einfügen, interpolieren. 2. *mathe.* interpolieren.
in·ter·po·lat·ed [ɪnˈtɜrpəleɪtɪd] *adj* eingefügt, eingeschoben, interpoliert; interpoliert.
interpolated extrasystole *card.* interpolierte Extrasystole *f*.
interpolated flap Schwenklappen(plastik *f*) *m*.
in·ter·po·la·tion [ɪnˌtɜrpəˈleɪʃn] *n* 1. Einschaltung *f*, Einfügung *f*, Interpolation *f*. 2. Einschalten *nt*, Einfügen *nt*, Interpolieren *nt*. 3. *mathe.* Interpolation *f*.
in·ter·pose [ˌɪntərˈpoʊz] **I** *vt* dazwischenstellen, -legen, -bringen; zwischen-, ein-

schalten, interponieren. **II** *vi* dazwischenkommen, -treten.
in·ter·posed [ˌ-'pəʊzd] *adj* eingeschoben, zwischengeschaltet, zwischengesetzt, interponiert.
in·ter·po·si·tion [ˌ-pə'zɪʃn] *n* **1.** Dazwischentreten *nt*, -legen *nt*, -bringen *nt*. **2.** Zwischen-, Einschaltung *f*. **3.** *chir.* (Transplantat-)Zwischenschaltung *f*, Zwischenlagerung *f*, Interposition *f*; Interponat *nt*.
interposition graft Interpositionstransplantat *nt*, Interponat *nt*.
interposition H graft *chir.* portokavaler Interpositionsshunt *m*.
in·ter·pret [ɪn'tɜrprɪt] *vt* interpretieren, deuten, auslegen (*as* als); (*Daten*) auswerten.
in·ter·pre·ta·tion [ɪnˌtɜrprɪ'teɪʃn] *n* Interpretierung *f*, Interpretation *f*, Deutung *f*, Auslegung *f*; (*Daten*) Auswertung *f*.
in·ter·pre·ta·tive [ɪn'tɜrprɪteɪtɪv] *adj* interpretierend.
in·ter·pre·tive [ɪn'tɜrprɪtɪv] *adj* → interpretative.
in·ter·prox·i·mal papilla [ˌ-'prɑksɪməl] → interdental papilla.
in·ter·pu·bic [ˌ-'pjuːbɪk] *adj* zwischen den Schambeinen (liegend), interpubisch.
interpubic lamina, fibrocartilaginous *old* Lamina fibrocartilaginea interpubica, Discus interpubicus.
interpubic ligament → interpubic lamina, fibrocartilaginous.
in·ter·pu·pil·lar·y [ˌ-'pjuːpəˌleriː] *adj* zwischen den Pupillen (liegend), interpupillar.
interpupillary distance *ophthal.* Interpupillar-, Pupillardistanz *f*.
in·ter·re·act [ˌ-rɪ'ækt] *vi* aufeinander *od.* wechselseitig reagieren, s. gegenseitig beeinflussen.
in·ter·re·ac·tion [ˌ-rɪ'ækʃn] *n* gegenseitige Beeinflussung *f*, wechselseitige Reaktion *f*.
in·ter·re·nal [ˌ-'riːnl] *adj* zwischen den Nieren (liegend), interrenal.
interrenal organ *embryo.* Interrenalorgan *nt*.
interrenal system Nebennierenrinde *f* *abbr.* NNR, Cortex (gl. suprarenales).
in·ter·rupt [*n* 'ɪntərʌpt; *v* ˌɪntə'rʌpt] **I** *n* Unterbrechung *f*. **II** *vt* **1.** ab-, unterbrechen. **to ~ a pregnancy** eine Schwangerschaft abbrechen. **2.** stören, hindern, aufhalten; versperren. **III** *vi* unterbrechen.
in·ter·rupt·ed suture [ˌɪntə'rʌptɪd] *chir.* Einzelnaht *f*.
in·ter·rup·tion [ˌɪntə'rʌpʃn] *n* **1.** Unterbrechung *f*. **without ~** ohne Unterbrechung, ununterbrochen. **2.** Störung *f*, Behinderung *f*; Versperrung *f*.
i. of pregnancy Schwangerschaftsabbruch *m*, -unterbrechung.
in·ter·sa·cral canals [ˌɪntər'seɪkrəl, '-sæ-] Forr. intervertebralia ossis sacri.
in·ter·scap·u·lar [ˌ-'skæpjələr] *adj* zwischen den Schulterblättern (liegend), interskapulär.
in·ter·scap·u·lo·tho·rac·ic amputation [ˌ-ˌskæpjələʊθəˈræsɪk] *ortho.* interskapulothorakale (Schulter-)Amputation *f*.
in·ter·sect [ˌ-'sekt] *vt* **1** *vt* (durch-)kreuzen, (-)schneiden. **II** *vi* s. (durch-, über-)schneiden, s. kreuzen.
in·ter·sec·tio [ˌ-'sekʃɪəʊ] *n* → intersection 1.
in·ter·sec·tion [ˌ-'sekʃn] *n* **1.** Kreuzung *f*, Schnitt-, Kreuzungspunkt *m*; *anat.* Intersectio *f*. **2.** Kreuzen *nt*, Durchschneiden *nt*.

in·ter·sec·tion·al [ˌ-'sekʃənl] *adj* Kreuzungs-, Schnitt(punkt)-.
in·ter·seg·ment [ˌ-'segmənt] *n* Zwischen-, Intersegment *nt*.
in·ter·seg·men·tal [ˌ-seg'mentl] *adj* zwischen Segmenten (liegend), Segmente verbindend, intersegmental, intersegmentär.
intersegmental fasciculi of spinal cord: anterior i. Fasciculi proprii anteriores/ventrales medullae spinalis.
dorsal i. Fasciculi proprii dorsales/posteriores medullae spinalis.
lateral i. Fasciculi proprii laterales medullae spinalis.
posterior i. → dorsal i.
ventral i. → anterior i.
intersegmental tracts of spinal cord: anterior i. Fasciculi proprii anteriores/ventrales medullae spinalis.
dorsal i. Fasciculi proprii dorsales/posteriores medullae spinalis.
lateral i. Fasciculi proprii laterales medullae spinalis.
posterior i. → dorsal i.
ventral i. → anterior i.
in·ter·sep·tal [ˌɪntər'septl] *adj* zwischen Septen (liegend), interseptal.
in·ter·sep·tum [ˌ-'septəm] *n anat.* Zwerchfell *nt*, Diaphragma *nt*.
in·ter·sex ['-seks] *n bio.* **1.** Intersex *nt*. **2.** Zwitter *m*, Hermaphrodit *m*, Intersex *nt*. **3.** → intersexualism.
in·ter·sex·u·al [ˌ-'sekʃəwəl, -sjʊəl] *adj bio.* intersexuell.
in·ter·sex·u·al·ism [ˌ-'sekʃəwəlɪzəm, -sjʊəl-] *n bio.* Zwischengeschlechtlichkeit *f*, Intersexualität *f*.
in·ter·sex·u·al·i·ty [ˌ-sekʃə'wælətɪ, -sjʊ-'ælə-] *n* → intersexualism.
in·ter·sig·moi·dal recess [ˌ-sɪg'mɔɪdl] Rec. intersigmoideus.
in·ter·sig·moid fossa [ˌ-'sɪgmɔɪd] Rec. intersigmoideus.
in·ter·space [*n* '-speɪs; *v* ˌ-'speɪs] **I** *n* Zwischenraum *m*. **II** *vt* (Zwischen-)Raum lassen zwischen.
in·ter·spa·tial [ˌ-'speɪʃl] *adj* Zwischenraum-.
in·ter·spi·nal [ˌ-'spaɪnl] *adj* zwischen Dornfortsätzen (liegend), Dornfortsätze verbindend, interspinal.
in·ter·spi·na·les [ˌ-ˌspaɪ'neɪliːz] *pl* → interspinales muscles.
interspinales cervicis (muscle) zervikale Interspinalmuskeln *pl*, Interspinales *pl* cervices, Mm. interspinales cervicis.
interspinales lumborum (muscles) lumbale Interspinalmuskeln *pl*, Interspinales *pl* lumborum, Mm. interspinales lumborum.
interspinales muscles Interspinalmuskeln *pl*, Mm. interspinales.
interspinales thoracis (muscles) thorakale Interspinalmuskeln *pl*, Interspinales *pl* thoracis, Mm. interspinales thoracis.
interspinal ligaments Ligg. interspinalia.
interspinal line Planum interspinale.
interspinal muscles → interspinales muscles.
lumbar i. → interspinales lumborum (muscles).
i. of neck → interspinales cervicis (muscles).
i. of thorax → interspinales thoracis (muscles).
interspinal plane *anat.* Planum interspinale.
in·ter·spi·nous [ɪntər'spaɪnəs] *adj* → interspinal.
interspinous ligaments → interspinal ligaments.

interstitial tissue

in·ter·stice [ɪn'tɜrstɪs] *n*, *pl* **-stic·es** [-stəsɪz] **1.** (schmale) Lücke *od.* Spalte *f*; Zwischenraum *m*. **2.** *histol.* (Gewebs-)Zwischenraum *m*, Interstitium *nt*.
in·ter·sti·tial [ˌɪntər'stɪʃl] *adj* im Interstitium (liegend), interstitiell, Interstitial-.
interstitial atrophy interstitielle Knochenatrophie *f*.
interstitial cells 1. Leydig-(Zwischen-)Zellen *pl*, Interstitialzellen *pl*, interstitielle Drüsen *pl*. **2.** (*Leber*) interstitielle Fettspeicherzellen *pl*. **3.** Interstitialzellen *pl* des Corpus pineale. **4.** interstitielle Eierstockzellen *pl*, -drüsen *pl*.
i. of testis Gley-Zellen *pl*, Interstitialzellen *pl* des Hodens.
interstitial cell stimulating hormone *abbr.* ICSH luteinisierendes Hormon *nt* *abbr.* LH, Luteinisierungshormon *nt*, Interstitialzellen-stimulierendes Hormon *nt*, interstitial cell stimulating hormone *abbr.* ICSH.
interstitial denticle interstitieller Dentikel *m*.
interstitial disease interstitielle Erkrankung *f*.
interstitial edema interstitielles Ödem *nt*.
interstitial emphysema 1. Darmemphysem *nt*, Emphysema intestini. **2.** Darmwandemphysem *nt*, Pneumatosis cystoides intestini.
interstitial fluid *abbr.* **ISF** interstitielle Flüssigkeit *f* *abbr.* IF.
interstitial glands 1. → interstitial cells 1. **2.** → interstitial cells 4.
interstitial growth interstitielles Wachstum *nt*.
interstitial hernia Hernia interstitialis.
interstitial hypertrophic neuritis Déjérine-Sottas-Syndrom *nt*, -Krankheit *f*, hereditäre motorische u. sensible Neuropathie Typ III *f*, hypertrophische Neuropathie (Déjérine-Sottas) *f*.
interstitial implantation *gyn.*, *embryo.* interstitielle Einnistung/Implantation *f*.
interstitial inflammation interstitielle Entzündung *f*.
interstitial keratitis interstitielle/parenchymatöse Keratitis *f*, Keratitis interstitialis/parenchymatosa.
interstitial lamellae (*Knochen*) Schaltlamellen *pl*.
interstitial mastitis interstitielle Mastitis *f*.
interstitial myocarditis interstitielle Myokarditis *f*.
interstitial myositis interstitielle Myositis *f*, Myositis fibrosa.
interstitial nephritis interstitielle Nephritis *f*.
acute i. akute interstitielle Nephritis.
chronic i. chronische interstitielle Nephritis.
interstitial neuritis interstitielle Neuritis *f*.
interstitial nucleus (of Cajal) Cajal'-Kern *m*, -Zellen *pl*, Nc. interstitialis.
interstitial plasma cell pneumonia Pneumocystis-Pneumonie *f*, interstitielle Plasmazellpneumonie *f*, Pneumocystose *f*.
interstitial pneumonia interstitielle Pneumonie *f*, Pneumonitis *f*.
interstitial pregnancy intramurale/interstitielle Schwangerschaft *f*, Graviditas interstitialis.
interstitial space *histol.* (Gewebs-)Zwischenraum *m*, Interstitium *nt*.
interstitial substance Kitt-, Interzellular-, Zwischenzellsubstanz *f*.
interstitial system (*Knochen*) Schaltlamellen *pl*.
interstitial tissue Zwischenzell-, Interstitialgewebe *nt*.

in·ter·sti·ti·o·spi·nal fasciculus [ˌ-ˌstɪʃɪəʊ-spaɪnl] Fasciculus interstitiospinalis.
in·ter·sti·tium [ˌ-'stɪʃɪəm] n 1. histol. (Gewebs-)Zwischenraum m, Interstitium nt. 2. → interstitial tissue.
in·ter·tar·sal [ˌɪntər'tɑːrsl] adj zwischen Tarsalknochen (liegend), Tarsalknochen verbindend, intertarsal.
intertarsal articulation Intertarsalgelenk nt, Artic. intertarsalis.
intertarsal joint → intertarsal articulation.
intertarsal ligaments Ligg. tarsi.
 dorsal i. Ligg. tarsi dorsalia.
 interosseous i. Ligg. tarsi interossea.
 plantar i. Ligg. tarsi plantaria.
in·ter·ten·di·nous connection [ˌ-'tendɪnəs] anat. Con(n)exus intertendineus.
in·ter·tha·lam·ic adhesion [ˌ-θə'læmɪk] interthalamische Adhäsion f, Adh(a)esio interthalamica, Massa intermedia.
interthalamic commissure → interthalamic adhesion.
interthalamic connexus → interthalamic adhesion.
in·ter·trag·ic incisure [ˌ-'trædʒɪk] Inc. intertragica.
in·ter·trans·ver·sa·rii muscles [ˌ-trænsvər'særiaɪ] → intertransverse muscles.
in·ter·trans·verse [ˌ-ɪntər'vɜrs] adj (Wirbelsäule) zwischen Querfortsätzen (liegend), Querfortsätze verbindend, intertransversal.
intertransverse ligaments Ligg. intertransversaria.
intertransverse muscles Intertransversalmuskeln pl, Mm. intertransversarii.
 cervical i. zervikale Intertransversalmuskeln, Mm. intertransversarii cervicis.
 lumbar i. lumbale Intertransversalmuskeln, Mm. intertransversarii lumborum.
 i. of lumbar spine → lumbar i.
 i. of neck → cervical i.
 thoracic i. thorakale Intertransversalmuskeln, Mm. intertransversarii thoracis.
 i. of thorax → thoracic i.
in·ter·trig·i·nous [ˌ-'trɪdʒənəs] adj derm. von Intertrigo betroffen, in Form einer Intertrigo, intertriginös.
in·ter·tri·go [ˌ-'traɪgəʊ] n derm. Wundsein nt, (Haut-)Wolf m, Intertrigo f, Dermatitis intertriginosa.
in·ter·tro·chan·ter·ic [ˌ-trəʊkən'terɪk] adj zwischen den Trochanteren (liegend), intertrochantär.
intertrochanteric crest Crista intertrochanterica.
intertrochanteric fracture intertrochantäre Oberschenkel-/Femurfraktur f.
intertrochanteric line Linea intertrochanterica.
intertrochanteric ridge → intertrochanteric crest.
in·ter·trop·i·cal anemia [ˌ-'trɒpɪkl] Anämie f bei Hakenwurmbefall.
intertropical hyphemia Hakenwurmbefall m, -infektion f, Ankylostomiasis f, Ankylostomatosis f, Ankylostomatidose f.
in·ter·tu·ber·cu·lar [ˌ-t(j)uː'bɜrkjələr] adj zwischen Tuberkuli (liegend), intertuberkulär.
intertubercular groove Bizepsrinne f des Humerus, Sulcus intertubercularis (humeri).
intertubercular line Planum intertuberculare.
intertubercular plane anat. Planum intertuberculare.
intertubercular sulcus → intertubercular groove.
in·ter·tu·bu·lar [ˌ-'t(j)uːbjələr] adj zwischen Tubuli (liegend), intertubulär.

in·ter·u·re·ter·al [ˌ-jʊə'riːtərəl] adj → interureteric.
in·ter·u·re·ter·ic [ˌ-jʊərə'terɪk] adj zwischen den Harnleitern/Ureteren (liegend), interureterisch, interuretär.
interureteric fold interureterische Schleimhautfalte f, Plica interureterica.
interureteric ridge → interureteric fold.
in·ter·vag·i·nal space [ˌ-'vædʒənl, -və'dʒaɪn] Tenon'-Raum m, Spatium episclerale.
 i. of optic nerve Spatium intervaginale (n. optici).
in·ter·val ['ɪntərvəl] n 1. (zeitlicher u. räumlicher) Abstand m, Intervall nt. **at ~s** in Abständen, ab u. zu. **at regular ~s** in regelmäßigen Abständen. **at five-minute ~s** in Abständen von fünf Minuten, alle fünf Minuten. **at four-hourly ~s** alle vier Stunden, vierstündlich. 2. mathe. Intervall nt.
interval appendectomy chir. Appendektomie f im Intervallstadium.
in·ter·val·ic adj → intervallic.
in·ter·val·lic [ˌɪntər'vælɪk] adj Intervall betr., Intervall-.
interval scale Intervallskala f.
interval training Intervalltraining nt.
in·ter·val·vu·lar [ˌ-'vælvjələr] adj zwischen Klappen/Valvae (liegend), intervalvulär.
in·ter·vas·cu·lar [ˌ-'væskjələr] adj zwischen (Blut-)Gefäßen (liegend), intervaskulär, -vaskular.
in·ter·vene [ˌ-'viːn] vi 1. eingreifen, einschreiten, intervenieren. 2. vermitteln (in, between in, zwischen). 3. (plötzlich) eintreten, (unerwartet) dazwischenkommen.
in·ter·ven·ing sequence [ˌ-'viːnɪŋ] genet. Intron nt.
in·ter·ve·nous tubercle [ˌ-'viːnəs] Tuberculum intervenosum.
in·ter·ven·tion [ˌ-'venʃn] n Eingriff m, Einschreiten nt, Eingreifen nt, (therapeutische od. prophylaktische) Maßnahme f, Intervention f.
in·ter·ven·tric·u·lar [-ven'trɪkjələr] adj zwischen Kammern/Ventrikeln (liegend), Ventrikel verbindend, interventrikulär, Interventrikular-.
interventricular artery, anterior vordere Interventrikulararterie f, Ramus interventricularis anterior (a. coronariae sinistrae) abbr. RIVA.
interventricular block card. Schenkelblock m.
interventricular branch: anterior i. of left coronary artery → interventricular artery, anterior.
 posterior i. of right coronary artery Endast m der A. coronaria dextra, hintere Interventrikulararterie f, Ramus interventricularis posterior (a. coronariae dextrae).
interventricular cistern Cisterna interventricularis.
interventricular foramen Monro'-Foramen nt, For. Monroi, For. interventriculare.
 i. of heart embryo. interventrikuläres Foramen, For. interventriculare cordis.
interventricular groove: anterior i. → interventricular sulcus, anterior.
 inferior i. → interventricular sulcus, inferior.
interventricular septum Kammer-, Interventrikular-, Ventrikelseptum nt, Septum interventriculare (cordis).
interventricular sulcus Interventrikularfurche f, Sulcus interventricularis.
 anterior i. vordere Interventrikularfurche, Sulcus interventricularis anterior.
 inferior i. hintere Interventrikularfurche, Sulcus interventricularis inferior/posterior.
 posterior i. → inferior i.
interventricular vein: anterior i. V. interventricularis anterior.
 posterior i. V. interventricularis posterior.
in·ter·ver·te·bral [ˌ-'vɜrtəbrəl] adj zwischen Wirbeln (liegend), intervertebral, Zwischenwirbel-, Intervertebral-.
intervertebral ankylosis ortho. Intervertebralankylose f, Ankylosis intervertebralis.
intervertebral body Wirbelkörper, Corpus vertebrae/vertebrale.
intervertebral cartilage → intervertebral disk.
intervertebral chondrosis ortho. Chondrosis intervertebralis.
intervertebral disk Intervertebral-, Zwischenwirbelscheibe f, Bandscheibe f, Discus intervertebralis.
intervertebral disk degeneration ortho. Bandscheibendegeneration f.
intervertebral disk disease Bandscheibenschaden m.
intervertebral fibrocartilage → intervertebral disk.
intervertebral foramen Zwischenwirbelloch nt, For. intervertebrale.
intervertebral ligament 1. Längsband nt, Lig. longitudinale. 2. → intervertebral disk.
intervertebral osteochondrosis ortho. Osteochondrosis intervertebralis.
intervertebral spondylosis ortho. Unkovertebralarthrose f, Spondylosis intervertebralis/uncovertebralis.
intervertebral symphysis Intervertebralverbindung f, Symphysis intervertebralis.
intervertebral vein Intervertebralvene f, V. intervertebralis.
in·ter·vil·lous [ˌ-'vɪləs] adj zwischen Zotten/Villi (liegend), intervillös.
intervillous space intervillöser Raum/Spalt m.
in·ter·zon·al [ˌ-'zəʊnl] adj interzonal, Interzonen-.
in·tes·ti·nal [ɪn'testənl; Brit. ˌɪntes'taɪnl] adj Darm/Intestinum betr., intestinal, Darm-, Eingeweide-, Intestinal-.
intestinal amebiasis Amöbenruhr f, -dysenterie f, intestinale Amöbiasis f.
intestinal anastomosis chir. Darmanastomose f, Enteroanastomose f.
intestinal angina Morbus Ortner m, Ortner-Syndrom II m, Angina abdominalis/intestinalis, Claudicatio intermittens abdominalis.
intestinal anthrax Darmmilzbrand m.
intestinal arteries Darmarterien pl, Aa. intestinales.
intestinal atresia Darmatresie f.
intestinal bacteria Entero-, Darmbakterien pl.
intestinal bilharziasis Manson'-Krankheit f, -Bilharziose f, Schistosomiasis mansoni/intestinalis.
intestinal bleeding Darmblutung f.
 upper i. Magen-Darm-Blutung, gastrointestinale Blutung.
intestinal bypass → intestinal anastomosis.
intestinal calculus Darmstein m, Enterolith m.
intestinal canal Darmrohr nt, Canalis intestinalis.
intestinal candidiasis Intestinalcandidose f.
intestinal clamp chir. Darmklemme f.

intestinal colic Darmkolik *f*, Colica intestinalis.
intestinal complaints Darmbeschwerden *pl*.
intestinal crisis *neuro.* intestinale Krise *f*.
intestinal digestion Darmverdauung *f*, intestinale Verdauung *f*.
intestinal disaccharidase deficiency Disaccharidintoleranz *f*.
intestinal diverticulum Darmdivertikel *nt*.
intestinal dyspepsia intestinale Dyspepsie *f*.
intestinal emphysema → intestinal pneumatosis.
intestinal fistula *patho.* Darmfistel *f*.
intestinal flora Darmflora *f*.
intestinal fluke *micro.* Darmegel *m*.
  giant i. großer Darmegel, Fasciolopsis buski.
intestinal follicles → intestinal glands.
intestinal gangrene Darmgangrän *f*.
intestinal glands Lieberkühn'-Drüsen *pl*, -Krypten *pl*, Darmdrüsen *pl*, Gll. intestinales.
intestinal glucagon Enteroglukagon *nt*, intestinales Glukagon *nt*.
intestinal hemorrhage Darmblutung *f*.
  upper i. Magen-Darm-Blutung, gastrointestinale Blutung.
intestinal infantilism intestinaler Infantilismus *m*.
intestinal infarct Darminfarzierung *f*.
intestinal infarction Darminfarkt *m*.
intestinal influenza Darmgrippe *f*.
intestinal intoxication Selbstvergiftung *f*, Autointoxikation *f*.
intestinal lipodystrophy intestinale Lipodystrophie *f*, Whipple'-Krankheit *f*, Morbus Whipple *m*, lipophage Intestinalgranulomatose *f*, Lipodystrophia intestinalis.
intestinal loop Darmschleife *f*.
  primitive i. *embryo.* Nabelschleife.
intestinal malrotation *embryo., chir.* Malrotation *f* des Darmes.
intestinal metaplasia intestinale Metaplasie *f*, Metaplasie *f* der Darmschleimhaut.
intestinal motility Darmmotilität *f*.
intestinal mucosa Darmschleimhaut *f*.
intestinal neoplasm → intestinal tumor.
intestinal obstruction Darmverlegung *f*, -obstruktion *f*, -verschluß *m*, Ileus *m*.
intestinal parasite *micro.* Darmparasit *m*.
intestinal peritoneum Peritoneum *nt* der Baucheingeweide, viszerales Peritoneum *nt*, Peritoneum viscerale.
intestinal phase *physiol.* (*Verdauung*) intestinale Phase *f*.
intestinal plexus, submucous Meissner'-Plexus *m*, Plexus submucosus.
intestinal pneumatosis Darm(wand)emphysem *nt*, Pneumatosis cystoides intestini.
intestinal polyposis gastrointestinale Polypose *f*, Polyposis intestinalis.
intestinal resection *chir.* Darmresektion *f*.
intestinal schistosomiasis → intestinal bilharziasis.
intestinal stasis Enterostase *f*.
intestinal stenosis Darmstenose *f*.
intestinal stone → intestinal calculus.
intestinal surface of uterus (*Uterus*) Darmfläche *f*, Facies intestinalis (uteri).
intestinal tonsil Peyer'-Plaques *pl*, Folliculi lymphatici aggregati.
intestinal trunks intestinale Lymphstämme *pl*, Trunci intestinales.
intestinal tube Darmrohr *nt*, -sonde *f*.
intestinal tuberculosis Darm-, Intestinaltuberkulose *f*.
intestinal tumor Darmgeschwulst *f*, -tumor *m*, -neoplasma *nt*.

intestinal villi Darmzotten *pl*, Villi intestinales.
intestinal volvulus *chir., ped.* Darmverschlingung *f*, Volvulus intestini.
intestinal wall Darmwand *f*.
in·tes·tine [ɪn'testɪn] *n* Darm *m*; *anat.* Intestinum *nt*; **~s** *pl* Eingeweide *pl*, Gedärme *pl*.
intestino-intestinal *adj* intestino-intestinal.
intestino-intestinal reflex intestino-intestinaler Reflex *m*.
in·tes·ti·no·tox·in [ɪn,testɪnəʊ'tɒksɪn] *n* Enterotoxin *nt*.
in·tes·ti·num [ˌɪntes'taɪnəm] *n*, *pl* **-na** [-nə] → intestine.
in·ti·ma ['ɪntɪmə] *n*, *pl* **-mae** [-miː] *anat.* Intima *f*, Tunica intima (vasorum).
in·ti·ma·cy ['ɪntɪməsɪ] *n* Vertrautheit *f*, Intimität *f*; intime *od.* sexuelle Beziehung *f*.
in·ti·mal ['ɪntɪməl] *adj anat.* Intima betr., Intima-.
intimal arteriosclerosis Intimasklerose *f*.
intimal damage Intimaschaden *m*, -schädigung *f*.
intimal edema Intimaödem *nt*.
intimal scar Intimanarbe *f*.
intimal tear Intima(ein)riß *m*.
in·ti·mate ['ɪntəmɪt] **I** *n* Vertraute(r *m*) *f*, Intimus *m*. **II** *adj* **1.** vertraut, eng verbunden, intim. **2.** (*sexuell*) intim. **3.** innerste(r, s). **4.** (*Kenntnisse*) gründlich, genau.
in·ti·mate·ness ['ɪntəmeɪtnɪs] *n* → intimacy.
in·ti·mi·tis [ɪntə'maɪtɪs] *n* Intimaentzündung *f*, Intimitis *f*.
in·tol·er·ance [ɪn'tɒlərəns] *n* **1.** Unduldsamkeit *f*, Intoleranz *f* (*to* gegen). **2.** *bio., patho.* Überempfindlichkeit *f* (*to* gegen); Unverträglichkeit *f*, Intoleranz *f*.
in·tol·er·ant [ɪn'tɒlərənt] *adj* **1.** unduldsam, intolerant (*of* gegenüber). **2.** *patho., bio.* überempfindlich, nicht widerstandsfähig, intolerant (*of* gegen).
in·tor·sion [ɪn'tɔːrʃn] *n ophthal.* Intorsion *f*.
in to·to [ɪn 'təʊtəʊ] im ganzen, vollständig, in toto.
in·tox·i·cant [ɪn'tɒksɪkənt] **I** *n* Rauschmittel *nt*, berauschendes Getränk *nt*. **II** *adj* berauschend; vergiftend.
in·tox·i·cate [ɪn'tɒksɪkeɪt] **I** *vt* **1.** berauschen, in einen Rauschzustand versetzen. **2.** vergiften. **II** *vi* berauschen, berauschend wirken.
in·tox·i·ca·tion [ɪn,tɒksɪ'keɪʃn] *n* **1.** Rausch *m*. **2.** *patho.* Vergiftung *f*, Intoxikation *f*; Toxikose *f*. **3.** Alkoholintoxikation *f*, akuter Alkoholrausch *m*, Trunkenheit *f*.
intoxication amaurosis *ophthal.* toxische Amblyopie *f*.
INTP *abbr.* → inhibitory nerve-terminal potential.
intra- *pref.* inner-, intra-.
intra-abdominal *adj* in(nerhalb) der Bauchhöhle (liegend), intraabdominal, -abdominell.
intra-abdominal abscess intraabdominaler/intraabdomineller Abszeß *m*.
intra-abdominal bleeding intraabdominelle Blutung *f*.
intra-abdominal hemorrhage intraabdominelle Blutung *f*.
intra-abdominal infection intraabdominelle Infektion *f*.
intra-abdominal pressure intraabdomineller Druck *m*.
intra-abdominal sepsis intraabdominale Sepsis *f*.
intra-acinous *adj* innerhalb eines Azinus (liegend), intraazinös, intraazinär.
intra-alveolar edema intraalveoläres (Lungen-)Ödem *nt*.

intra-alveolar pressure intraalveolärer/intrapulmonaler Druck *m*.
intra-appendicular *adj* innerhalb einer Appendix (liegend), intraappendikular.
intra-arterial *adj* in einer Arterie (liegend), in eine Arterie, intraarteriell.
intra-arterial chemotherapy transarterielle lokale Chemotherapie *f*.
intra-arterial line intraarterieller Zugang/Katheter *m*.
intra-articular *adj* innerhalb eines Gelenks (liegend), intrartikulär.
intra-articular arthrodesis *ortho.* intraartikuläre Arthrodese *f*.
intra-articular bleeding Gelenk(ein)blutung *f*, intraartikuläre Blutung *f*.
intra-articular disk Gelenkzwischenscheibe *f*, Discus articularis.
intra-articular fracture intraartikuläre Fraktur *f*.
  i. of distal tibia Pilon-Fraktur, Pilon tibial.
intra-articular hemorrhage → intra-articular bleeding.
intra-articular ligament of head of rib Lig. capitis costae intraarticulare.
intra-articular tuberculosis intraartikuläre Tuberkulose *f*.
intra-atomic *adj* innerhalb eines Atoms (liegend), intraatomar.
intra-atrial *adj* in einem Vorhof (liegend), intraatrial.
intra-atrial block *card.* intraatrialer Block *m*.
intra-atrial conduction *card.* intraatriale Erregungsleitung/Erregungsausbreitung *f*.
intra-aural *adj* im Ohr (liegend), im Inneren des Ohres, intraaural.
intra-auricular *adj* → intra-atrial.
intra-axonal *adj* innerhalb eines Axons (liegend), intraaxonal.
in·tra·bron·chi·al [ˌɪntrə'brɒŋkɪəl] *adj* in einem Bronchus (liegend), intra-, endobronchial.
in·tra·buc·cal [ˌ-'bʌkəl] *adj* im Mund *od.* in der Wange, intrabukkal.
in·tra·ca·nic·u·lar fibroadenoma [ˌ,-ˌkænə'lɪkjələr] *gyn.* intrakanalikuläres/intrakanalikulär-wachsendes Fibroadenom *nt* der Brust, Fibroadenoma intracanaliculare.
intracanalicular fibroma → intracanalicular fibroadenoma.
intracanalicular papilloma intrakanalikuläres Papillom *n*.
intracanalicular part of optic nerve Canalis-opticus-Abschnitt *m* des N. opticus, Pars intracanalicularis n. optici.
intracanalicular spread *patho.* intrakanalikuläre Aussaat *f*.
in·tra·cap·il·lar·y glomerulonephritis [ˌ-kə'pɪlərɪ] mesangioproliferative Glomerulonephritis *f*.
in·tra·cap·su·lar [ˌ-'kæps(j)ələr] *adj* innerhalb einer Kapsel (liegend), intrakapsulär.
intracapsular ankylosis *ortho.* intrakapsuläre Ankylose *f*.
intracapsular fracture intrakapsuläre Fraktur *f*.
intracapsular ligament intrakapsuläres Band/Ligament *nt*, Lig. intracapsularia.
in·tra·car·di·ac [ˌ-'kɑːrdɪæk] *adj* innerhalb des Herzens (liegend), ins Herz hinein, intrakardial, endokardial.
intracardiac catheter Herzkatheter *m*.
in·tra·car·pal [ˌ-'kɑːrpl] *adj* im Handgelenk (liegend), zwischen den Karpalknochen (liegend), intrakarpal.
in·tra·car·ti·lag·i·nous [ˌ,-ˌkɑːrtə'lædʒɪnəs] *adj* im Knorpel (liegend), endochondral, intrakartilaginär.

intracavitary

in·tra·cav·i·ta·ry [ˌɪ-ˈkævɪteri:] *adj* in einer Höhle (liegend), intrakavitär.
in·tra·ce·li·al [ˌɪ-ˈsiːliəl] *adj* in einer Körperhöhle (liegend).
in·tra·cel·lu·lar [ˌɪ-ˈseljələr] *adj* innerhalb einer Zelle (liegend *od.* ablaufend), intrazellulär, intrazellular.
intracellular compartmentation intrazelluläre Kompartimentierung *f.*
intracellular enzyme Endoenzym *nt,* intrazelluläres Enzym *nt.*
intracellular fluid *abbr.* **ICF** intrazelluläre Flüssigkeit *f,* Intrazellularflüssigkeit *f abbr.* IZF, ICF.
intracellular messenger intrazelluläre Botensubstanz *f,* intrazellulärer Bote *m.*
intracellular space *abbr.* **ICS, IS** intrazellulärer Raum *m,* Intrazellularraum *m abbr.* IZR, IZ.
intracellular toxin Endotoxin *nt.*
intracellular transport intrazellulärer Transport *m.*
intracellular water *abbr.* **ICW** intrazelluläres Wasser *nt abbr.* IZW.
in·tra·cer·e·bel·lar [ˌɪ-serəˈbelər] *adj* innerhalb des Kleinhirns (liegend), intrazerebellär.
intracerebellar nuclei Kleinhirnkerne *pl,* Ncc. cerebelli.
in·tra·cer·e·bral bleeding [ˌɪ-ˈserəbrəl, -səˈriːbrəl] intrazerebrale Blutung *f.*
intracerebral calcification intrazerebrale Kalzifikation *f.*
intracerebral hematoma intrazerebrales Hämatom *nt.*
intracerebral hemorrhage → intracerebral bleeding.
in·tra·cer·vi·cal [ˌɪ-ˈsɜrvɪkl, -sərˈvaɪkl] *adj gyn.* in der Zervix (liegend), im Halskanal, intra-, endozervikal.
in·tra·chon·dral [ˌɪ-ˈkɑndrəl] *adj* → intracartilaginous.
in·tra·chon·dri·al [ˌɪ-ˈkɑndriəl] *adj* → intracartilaginous.
in·tra·chord·al [ˌɪ-ˈkɔːrdl] *adj* intrachordal.
in·tra·cis·ter·nal [ˌɪ-sɪsˈtɜrnl] *adj* in einer Zisterne/Cisterna (liegend).
intracisternal puncture Subokzipital-, Zisternen-, Hirnzisternenpunktion *f.*
in·tra·col·ic [ˌɪ-ˈkɑlɪk] *adj* im Kolon (liegend), intrakolisch.
in·tra·con·dy·lar fracture of femur [ˌɪ-ˈkɑndɪlər] intrakondyläre Oberschenkel-/Femurfraktur.
in·tra·cor·dal [ˌɪ-ˈkɔːrdl] *adj* → intracardiac.
in·tra·cor·di·al [ˌɪ-ˈkɔːrdiəl, -dʒəl] *adj* → intracardiac.
in·tra·cor·po·ral [ˌɪ-ˈkɔːrp(ə)rəl] *adj* → intracorporeal.
in·tra·cor·po·re·al [ˌɪ-kɔːrˈpɔːriəl, -ˈpəʊr-] *adj* im Körper (liegend), intrakorporal.
in·tra·cor·pus·cu·lar [ˌɪ-kɔːrˈpʌskjələr] *adj* intrakorpuskulär.
in·tra·cos·tal [ˌɪ-ˈkɑstl, -ˈkɔstl] *adj* auf der Innenseite der Rippen (liegend), intrakostal.
in·tra·cra·ni·al [ˌɪ-ˈkreɪniəl] *adj* in(nerhalb) der Schädelhöhle (liegend), intrakranial, intrakraniell.
intracranial abscess intrakranieller Abszeß *m.*
intracranial aerocele traumatischer Pneum(at)ozephalus *m.*
intracranial aneurysm intrakranielles Aneurysma *nt.*
intracranial bleeding intrakranielle Blutung *f.*
intracranial cavity Schädelhöhle *f,* Cavitas cranii.
intracranial hematoma intrakranielles Hämatom *nt.*

intracranial hemorrhage → intracranial bleeding.
intracranial part: i. of optic nerve intrakranieller Abschnitt *m* des N. opticus, Pars intracranialis n. optici.
i. of vertebral artery intrakranieller Abschnitt *m* der A. vertebralis, Pars intracranialis a. vertebralis.
intracranial pneumatocele Pneum(at)ozephalus *m.*
intracranial pressure intrakranialer Druck *m,* Hirndruck *m.*
in·trac·ta·ble [ɪnˈtræktəbl] *adj* **1.** (*Krankheit*) hartnäckig, therapierefraktär. **2.** unlenkbar, eigensinnig.
in·tra·cu·ta·ne·ous [ˌɪntrəkjuˈteɪniəs] *adj* in der Haut (liegend), in die Haut, intrakutan, intradermal.
intracutaneous reaction Intrakutanreaktion *f.*
intracutaneous test *derm.* Intrakutantest *m,* -probe *f,* Intradermaltest *m.*
in·tra·cu·ti reaction [ˌɪntrəˈkjuːtaɪ] Frei--Hauttest *m,* -Intrakutantest *m.*
in·tra·cys·tic [ˌɪ-ˈsɪstɪk] *adj* in einer Zyste (liegend), intrazystisch.
in·tra·cy·to·plas·mic [ˌɪ-saɪtəˈplæzmɪk] *adj* innerhalb des Zytoplasmas (liegend), intrazytoplasmatisch.
intracytoplasmic canals Holmgren--Golgi-Kanälchen *pl,* (intra-)zytoplasmatische Kanälchen *pl.*
in·tra·de·cid·u·al implanation [ˌɪ-dɪˈsɪdʒʊəl, -dʒuəl] intradeziduale Einnistung/Implantation/Nidation *f.*
in·tra·der·mal [ˌɪ-ˈdɜrməl] *adj* → intracutaneous.
intradermal nevus intradermaler/dermaler/korialer Nävus *m.*
intradermal reaction → intracutaneous reaction.
intradermal test → intracutaneous test.
in·tra·der·mic [ˌɪ-ˈdɜrmɪk] *adj* → intracutaneous.
in·tra·duc·tal [ˌɪ-ˈdʌktl] *adj* in einem Gang/Ductus (liegend), intraductal.
intraductal carcinoma intraduktales/intrakanalikuläres Karzinom *nt,* Ca. intraductale.
intraductal papilloma (*Brustdrüse*) intraduktales Papillom *nt.*
in·tra·du·o·de·nal [ˌɪ-d(j)uːəʊˈdiːnl] *adj* im Duodenum (liegend), intraduodenal.
in·tra·du·ral [ˌɪ-ˈd(j)ʊərəl] *adj* in der Dura (liegend), innerhalb der Durahöhle, intradural.
intradural abscess intraduraler Abszeß *m.*
in·tra·em·bry·on·ic [ˌɪ-ˌembrɪˈɑnɪk] *adj* innerhalb des Embryos (liegend), intraembryonal.
intraembryonic circulation intraembryonaler Kreislauf *m.*
intraembryonic coelom intraembryonale Zölomhöhle *f.*
intraembryonic ectoderm intraembryonales Ektoderm *nt.*
intraembryonic mesoderm intraembryonales Mesoderm *nt.*
in·tra·ep·i·der·mal [ˌɪ-epɪˈdɜrml] *adj* in der Epidermis (liegend), in die Epidermis, intraepidermal.
intraepidermal carcinoma intraepidermales Karzinom *nt,* Ca. in situ der Haut.
intraepidermal epithelioma Borst--Jadassohn intraepidermales Epitheliom *nt* Borst-Jadassohn.
in·tra·ep·i·phys·e·al [ˌɪ-epɪˈfiːziəl] *adj* innerhalb einer Epiphyse (liegend), intraepiphysär.
in·tra·ep·i·phys·i·al *adj* → intraepiphyseal.

in·tra·ep·i·the·li·al [ˌɪ-epɪˈθiːliəl] *adj* innerhalb des Epithels (liegend), intraepithelial.
intraepithelial carcinoma Oberflächenkarzinom *nt,* präinvasives/intraepitheliales Karzinom *nt,* Carcinoma in situ *abbr.* CIA.
intraepithelial cyst intraepitheliale Zyste *f.*
intraepithelial gland endoepitheliale/intraepitheliale Drüse *f.*
in·tra·e·ryth·ro·cyt·ic [ˌɪ-ˌɪrɪθrəˈsɪtɪk] *adj* innerhalb eines Erythrozyten (liegend), intraerythrozytär.
in·tra·fas·cic·u·lar [ˌɪ-fəˈsɪkjələr] *adj* innerhalb eines Faszikels (liegend), intrafaszikulär.
in·tra·feb·rile [ˌɪ-ˈfebrɪl, -ˈfiːb-] *adj* während des Fieberstadiums.
in·tra·fe·ta·tion [ˌɪ-fɪˈteɪʃn] *n embryo.* Intrafetation *f.*
in·tra·fis·su·ral [ˌɪ-ˈfɪʃərəl] *adj* innerhalb einer Fissura (liegend), intrafissural.
in·tra·fis·tu·lar [ˌɪ-ˈfɪstʃələr] *adj* in einer Fistel (liegend), intrafistulär.
in·tra·fol·lic·u·lar [ˌɪ-fəˈlɪkjələr] *adj* innerhalb eines Follikels (liegend), intrafollikulär.
in·tra·fu·sal [ˌɪ-ˈfjuːzl] *adj* innerhalb einer Muskelspindel (liegend), intrafusal.
intrafusal fibers intrafusale Fasern *pl.*
in·tra·gas·tric [ˌɪ-ˈgæstrɪk] *adj* im Magen (liegend), in den Magen, intragastral.
in·tra·gem·mal [ˌɪ-ˈdʒeml] *adj* intragemmal.
intragemmal fibers intragemmale Nervenfasern *pl.*
in·tra·gen·ic [ˌɪ-ˈdʒenɪk] *adj genet.* in einem Gen.
in·tra·glan·du·lar [ˌɪ-ˈglændʒələr] *adj* innerhalb einer Drüse (liegend), intraglandulär.
intraglandular lymph nodes in der Parotis liegende Lymphknoten *pl,* Nodi lymphatici intraglandulares.
in·tra·glob·u·lar [ˌɪ-ˈglɑbjələr] *adj* intraglobulär, intraglobular.
in·tra·gy·ral [ˌɪ-ˈdʒaɪrəl] *adj* in einem Gyrus (liegend), intragyral.
in·tra·he·pat·ic [ˌɪ-hɪˈpætɪk] *adj* innerhalb der Leber liegend *od.* ablaufend, intrahepatisch.
intrahepatic abscess intrahepatischer Abszeß *m.*
intrahepatic cholangiojejunostomy *chir.* Hepato(porto)enterostomie *f,* intrahepatische Cholangiojejunostomie *f.*
intrahepatic cholestasis intrahepatische Gallestauung/Cholestase *f.*
intrahepatic jaundice intrahepatischer Ikterus *m.*
in·tra·hy·po·tha·lam·ic [ˌɪ-ˌhaɪpəʊθəˈlæmɪk, -ˌhɪp-] *adj* intrahypothalamisch.
in·tra·ic·tal [ˌɪ-ˈɪktəl] *adj* während eines Anfalls.
in·tra·in·tes·ti·nal [ˌɪ-ɪnˈtestɪnl] *adj* im Darm (liegend), intraintestinal.
in·tra·jug·u·lar [ˌɪ-ˈdʒʌgjələr] *adj* intrajugular.
intrajugular process Proc. intrajugularis.
i. of occipital bone Proc. intrajugularis ossis occipitalis.
i. of temporal bone Proc. intrajugularis ossis temporalis.
in·tra·la·mel·lar [ˌɪ-ləˈmelər] *adj* intralamellär.
in·tra·lam·i·nar [ˌɪ-ˈlæmɪnər] *adj* intralaminar, intralaminär.
intralaminar nuclei of thalamus intralaminäre Thalamuskerne *pl,* Ncc. reticulares (intralaminares thalami).
intralaminar part of optic nerve Lamina-

-cribrosa-Abschnitt *m* des N. opticus, Pars intralaminaris n. optici.
in·tra·la·ryn·ge·al [ˌ-lə'rɪndʒ(ɪ)əl] *adj* im Larynx (liegend), intra-, endolaryngeal.
in·tra·leu·ko·cy·tic [ˌ-ˌluːkə'sɪtɪk] *adj* innerhalb eines Leukozyten (liegend), intraleukozytär.
in·tra·lig·a·men·ta·ry pregnancy [ˌ-lɪgə-'mentərɪ] ektopische Schwangerschaft *f* im Lig. latum uteri.
in·tra·lig·a·men·tous [ˌ-lɪgə'mentəs] *adj* in einem Band/Ligament (liegend), intraligamentär.
intraligamentous pregnancy → intraligamentary pregnancy.
in·tra·lin·gual [ˌ-'lɪŋgwəl] *adj* innerhalb der Zunge (liegend), intralingual, intraglossal.
in·tra·lo·bar [ˌ-'loʊbər] *adj* in einem Lappen/Lobus (liegend), intralobär.
in·tra·lob·u·lar [ˌ-'labjələr] *adj* in einem Läppchen/Lobulus (liegend), intralobulär.
in·tra·lum·bar [ˌ-'lʌmbər] *adj* im Lumbalkanal (liegend), in den Lumbalkanal, intralumbal.
in·tra·lu·mi·nal cyst [ˌ-'luːmɪnəl] intraluminale Zyste *f*.
intraluminal manometry intraluminale Manometrie *f*.
intraluminal pressure intraluminaler Druck *m*.
in·tra·mam·ma·ry [ˌ-'mæmərɪ] *adj* in der Brust (liegend), intramammär.
in·tra·mas·toid abscess [ˌ-'mæstɔɪd] Abszeß *m* des Proc. mastoideus.
in·tra·mat·ri·cal [ˌ-'meɪtrɪkəl, -'mæ-] *adj* innerhalb der Matrix (liegend).
in·tra·me·a·tal [ˌ-mɪ'eɪtl] *adj* im Gehörgang (liegend), intrameatal.
in·tra·med·ul·lar·y [ˌ-'medʒələrɪː] *adj* **1.** im Rückenmark (liegend), in das Rückenmark, intramedullär. **2.** in der Medulla oblongata (liegend), intramedullär. **3.** im Knochenmark (liegend), in das Knochenmark, intramedullär.
intramedullary anesthesia *anes.* intramedulläre/intraossäre Anästhesie *f*.
intramedullary hematoma intramedulläres Hämatom *nt*.
intramedullary hemorrhage Rückenmarks(ein)blutung *f*, Hämatomyelie *f*.
intramedullary nail *ortho.* Marknagel *m*.
triflange i. Dreikantlamellenmarknagel.
intramedullary nailing *ortho.* Marknagelung *f*.
blind i. gedeckte Marknagelung.
open i. offene Marknagelung.
in·tra·mem·bra·nous [ˌ-'membrənəs] *adj* innerhalb einer Membran (liegend *od.* auftretend), intramembranös.
intramembranous ossification direkte/ desmale Knochenbildung *od.* Verknöcherung *f*, Osteogenesis membranacea.
in·tra·me·nin·ge·al [ˌ-mɪ'nɪndʒəl] *adj* innerhalb der Meningen (liegend), von den Meningen umschlossen, intrameningeal.
in·tra·mi·to·chon·dri·al [ˌ-ˌmaɪtə'kandrɪəl] *adj* intramitochondrial.
in·tra·mo·lec·u·lar [ˌ-mə'lekjələr] *adj chem.* innerhalb eines Moleküls, inner-, intramolekular.
in·tra·mu·ral [ˌ-'mjʊərəl] *adj* innerhalb einer Organwand liegend *od.* auftretend, intramural.
intramural abscess intramuraler Abszeß *m*.
intramural ganglion intramurales Ganglion *nt*.
intramural hematoma intramurales Hämatom *nt*.
intramural part of uterine tube intramuraler Tubenabschnitt *m*, Pars intramuralis tubae uterinae.
intramural perforation *chir.* intramurale Perforation *f*.
intramural plexus intramuraler Plexus *m*.
intramural pregnancy → interstitial pregnancy.
intramural reflex intramuraler Reflex *m*.
in·tra·mus·cu·lar [ˌ-'mʌskjələr] *adj abbr.* **I.M., i.m.** innerhalb des Muskels (liegend), in den Muskel, intramuskulär *abbr.* i.m.
in·tra·my·o·car·di·al [ˌ-ˌmaɪə'kɑːrdɪəl] *adj* innerhalb des Myokards (liegend), intramyokardial.
in·tra·my·o·me·tri·al [ˌ-ˌmaɪə'miːtrɪəl] *adj* innerhalb des Myometriums (liegend), intramyometrial.
in·tra·na·sal [ˌ-'neɪzl] *adj* in der Nase (liegend), in die Nase, intranasal.
intranasal anesthesia 1. Intranasalanästhesie *f*, intranasale Lokalanästhesie *f*. **2.** pernasale Anästhesie *f*.
intranasal block Intranasalanästhesie *f*, intranasale Lokalanästhesie *f*.
in·tra·neu·ral [ˌ-'nj(ʊ)ərəl, -'nu-] *adj* in einem Nerven (liegend), in einen Nerv, intra-, endoneural.
in-transit metastasis *patho.* In-transit-Metastase *f*.
in·tra·nu·cle·ar [ˌ-'n(j)uːklɪər] *adj* im (Zell-)Kern (liegend), intranukleär.
intranuclear inclusions Einschlußkörperchen *pl*.
in·tra·oc·cip·i·tal synchondrosis [ˌ-ɑk'sɪpɪtl] Synchondrosis intra-occipitalis.
anterior i. Synchondrosis intra-occipitalis anterior.
posterior i. Synchondrosis intra-occipitalis posterior.
in·tra·oc·u·lar [ˌ-'ɑkjələr] *adj* im Auge *od.* Augapfel (liegend), intraokular, intraokulär.
intraocular fluid Kammerwasser *nt*, Humor aquosus.
intraocular neuritis intraokuläre Entzündung *f* des N. opticus.
intraocular part of optic nerve Augapfelabschnitt *m* des N. opticus, Pars intraocularis n. optici.
intraocular pressure/tension intraokulärer Druck *m*.
in·tra·op·er·a·tive [ˌ-'ɑp(ə)rətɪv, -'ɑpərei-] *adj* während einer Operation, intraoperativ.
intraoperative hemolysis intraoperative Hämolyse *f*.
intraoperative monitoring intraoperative Überwachung *f*.
intraoperative pancreatography *chir.* intraoperative Pankreat(ik)ographie *f*.
in·tra·o·ral [ˌ-'ɔːrəl, -'ɔːr-] *adj* im Mund *od.* in der Mundhöhle (liegend), intraoral.
intraoral anesthesia 1. intraorale Lokalanästhesie *f*. **2.** perorale Anästhesie *f*.
in·tra·or·bit·al [ˌ-'ɔːrbɪtl] *adj* in der Augenhöhle (liegend), intraorbital.
in·tra·os·se·ous [ˌ-'ɑsɪəs] *adj* im Knochen (liegend), in den Knochen, intraossär, intraossal, endostal.
intraosseous anesthesia intraossäre Lokalanästhesie *f*.
intraosseous bleeding Knochen(ein)blutung *f*, intraossäre Blutung *f*.
intraosseous fixation *ortho.* operative Frakturbehandlung *f*, -stabilisierung *f*, Osteosynthese *f*.
intraosseous hemorrhage → intraosseous bleeding.
in·tra·os·te·al [ˌ-'ɑstɪəl] *adj* → intraosseous.
in·tra·o·var·i·an [ˌ-oʊ'veərɪən] *adj* innerhalb des Eierstocks (liegend), intraovarial.
in·tra·ov·u·lar [ˌ-'ɑvjələr, -'oʊv-] *adj* im Ei/ Ovum (liegend), intraovulär.
in·tra·par·en·chym·a·tous [ˌ-ˌpærəŋ'kɪmətəs] *adj* innerhalb des Parenchyms (liegend), intraparenchymal, intraparenchymatös.
in·tra·pa·ri·e·tal sulcus [ˌ-pə'raɪɪtl] Sulcus intraparietalis.
in·tra·par·tum [ˌ-'pɑːrtəm] *adj* während/ unter der Geburt, intra partum, intrapartal.
intrapartum hemorrhage intrapartale Blutung *f*, Blutung *f* unter der Geburt.
in·tra·pel·vic [ˌ-'pelvɪk] *adj* innerhalb des Beckens (liegend), intrapelvin.
intrapelvic protrusion *ortho.* Protrusio acetabuli.
in·tra·per·i·car·di·ac [ˌ-ˌperɪ'kɑːrdɪæk] *adj* → intrapericardial.
in·tra·per·i·car·di·al [ˌ-ˌperɪ'kɑːrdɪəl] *adj* innerhalb des Perikards (liegend), intraperikardial.
in·tra·per·i·ne·al [ˌ-ˌperɪ'niːəl] *adj* im Perineum (liegend), intraperineal.
in·tra·per·i·os·te·al fracture [ˌ-ˌperɪ'ɑstɪəl] Fraktur *f* ohne Periostverletzung.
in·tra·per·i·to·ne·al [ˌ-ˌperɪtə'niːəl] *adj* in der Bauchfellhöhle (liegend), von Bauchfell/Peritoneum umgeben, intraperitoneal.
intraperitoneal abscess intraperitonealer Abszeß *m*.
intraperitoneal pregnancy Bauchhöhlenschwangerschaft *f*, Abdominalschwangerschaft *f*, abdominale Schwangerschaft *f*, Graviditas abdominalis.
intraperitoneal transfusion intraperitoneale Transfusion *f*.
in·tra·per·son·al [ˌ-'pɜːrsnəl] *adj* → intrapsychic.
intrapersonal conflict *psychia.* intrapsychischer Konflikt *m*.
in·tra·pi·al [ˌ-'paɪəl] *adj* innerhalb der Pia mater (liegend), intrapial.
in·tra·pi·tu·i·tar·y cyst [ˌ-pɪ't(j)uːəterɪː] Rathke'-Zyste *f*.
in·tra·pla·cen·tal [ˌ-plə'sentl] *adj* innerhalb der Plazenta (liegend), intraplazentar.
in·tra·pleu·ral [ˌ-'plʊərəl] *adj* in der Pleurahöhle (liegend), intrapleural.
intrapleural pressure intrapleuraler Druck *m*.
in·tra·pon·tine [ˌ-'pɑntaɪn, -tiːn] *adj* in der Pons cerebri (liegend), intrapontin.
in·tra·pros·tat·ic [ˌ-prɑs'tætɪk] *adj* innerhalb der Prostata (liegend), intraprostatisch.
in·tra·pro·to·plas·mic [ˌ-ˌproʊtoʊ'plæzmɪk] *adj* innerhalb des Protoplasmas (liegend), intraprotoplasmatisch.
in·tra·psy·chic [ˌ-'saɪkɪk] *adj* intrapsychisch.
intrapsychic conflict *psychia.* intrapsychischer Konflikt *m*.
in·tra·pul·mo·nar·y [ˌ-'pʌlmənerɪ, -'pʊl-] *adj* innerhalb der Lunge (liegend), im Lungenparenchym (liegend), intrapulmonal.
intrapulmonary pressure → intraalveolar pressure.
intrapulmonary shunt *physiol., patho.* intrapulmonaler Shunt *m*.
in·tra·py·ret·ic [ˌ-paɪ'retɪk] *adj* während des Fieberstadiums.
in·tra·ra·chid·i·an [ˌ-rə'kɪdɪən] *adj* → intraspinal.
in·tra·rec·tal [ˌ-'rektl] *adj* im Rektum (liegend), in das Rektum, intrarektal.
in·tra·re·nal [ˌ-'riːnl] *adj* in der Niere (liegend), intrarenal.

intrarenal abscess intrarenaler Abszeß m, Nierenabszeß m.
intrarenal reflux intrarenaler Reflux m.
in·tra·ret·i·nal [ˌ-'retnəl] adj innerhalb der Netzhaut/Retina (liegend), intraretinal.
intraretinal space embryo. Sehventrikel m.
in·tra·rha·chid·i·an [ˌ-rə'kɪdɪən] adj → intraspinal.
in·tra·scle·ral [ˌ-'sklɪərəl] adj innerhalb der Lederhaut/Sklera (liegend), intraskleral.
intrascleral plexus intraskleraler Venenplexus m.
in·tra·scro·tal [ˌ-'skrəʊtl] adj im Hodensack/Skrotum (liegend), intraskrotal.
in·tra·seg·men·tal [ˌ-seg'mentl] adj innerhalb eines Segments (liegend), intrasegmental.
in·tra·sel·lar [ˌ-'selər] adj in der Sella turcica (liegend), intrasellär.
in·tra·spi·nal [ˌ-'spaɪnl] adj in der Wirbelsäule od. im Wirbelkanal (liegend), in den Wirbelkanal, intraspinal.
intraspinal anesthesia → intraspinal block.
intraspinal block Spinalanästhesie f; inf. Spinale f.
intraspinal neurons intraspinale Binnenzellen pl, Binnenzellen pl des Eigenapparates.
in·tra·splen·ic [ˌ-'splenɪk, -'spliː-] adj innerhalb der Milz (liegend).
in·tra·ster·nal [ˌ-'stɜrnl] adj im Sternum (liegend), ins Sternum, intrasternal.
in·tra·stro·mal [ˌ-'strəʊml] adj im Stroma (liegend).
in·tra·syn·o·vi·al [ˌ-sɪ'nəʊvɪəl] adj innerhalb des Synovialis (liegend), intrasynovial.
in·tra·tar·sal [ˌ-'tɑrsl] adj in der Fußwurzel, zwischen Tarsalknochen (liegend), intratarsal.
in·tra·ten·di·nous bursa of olecranon [ˌ-'tendɪnəs] Bursa intratendinea olecrani.
in·tra·tes·tic·u·lar [ˌ-tes'tɪkjələr] adj innerhalb des Hodens (liegend), in den Hoden, intratestikulär.
in·tra·tha·lam·ic fibers [ˌ-θə'læmɪk] intrathalamische (Verbindungs-)Fasern pl, Fibrae intrathalamicae.
in·tra·the·cal [ˌ-'θiːkl] adj 1. innerhalb des Liquorraumes (liegend), intrathekal. 2. innerhalb einer Scheide (liegend); von einer Scheide umgeben.
intrathecal pressure intrathekaler Druck m.
in·tra·tho·rac·ic [ˌ-θɔ'ræsɪk, -θəʊ-] adj im Brustkorb (liegend), intra-, endothorakal.
intrathoracic goiter intrathorakale Struma f, Struma endothoracica; Tauchkropf m.
intrathoracic infection intrathorakale Infektion f.
intrathoracic pressure intrathorakaler Druck m.
in·tra·ton·sil·lar [ˌ-'tɒnsɪlər] adj in einer Mandel/Tonsilla (liegend), intratonsillär, intratonsillar.
in·tra·tra·bec·u·lar [ˌ-trə'bekjələr] adj intratrabekulär.
in·tra·tra·che·al [ˌ-'treɪkɪəl] adj in der Luftröhre/Trachea (liegend), in die Luftröhre, intra-, endotracheal.
in·tra·tu·bal [ˌ-'t(j)uːbl] adj 1. in der Ohrtrompete/Tuba auditiva (liegend), intratubar. 2. im Eileiter/in der Tuba uterina (liegend), intratubar.
in·tra·tu·bu·lar [ˌ-'t(j)uːbjələr] adj in einem Tubulus (liegend), intratubulär.
in·tra·tym·pan·ic [ˌ-tɪm'pænɪk] adj in der Paukenhöhle (liegend), intratympanisch, intratympanal.
in·tra·u·re·ter·al [ˌ-jʊə'riːtərəl, -jə-] adj in einem Harnleiter/Ureter (liegend), intraurethär, intraureterisch.
in·tra·u·re·thral [ˌ-jʊə'riːθrəl] adj in der Harnröhre (liegend), in die Harnröhre, intraurethral.
in·tra·u·ter·ine [ˌ-'juːtərɪn, -raɪn] adj in der Gebärmutter(höhle), in die Gebärmutter, intrauterin.
intrauterine amputation embryo. kongenitale/intrauterine Amputation f.
intrauterine contraceptive device abbr. IUCD gyn. Intrauterinpessar nt abbr. IUP.
intrauterine device abbr. IUD gyn. Intrauterinpessar nt abbr. IUP.
intrauterine dislocation ortho. intrauterine Luxation f.
intrauterine fracture kongenitale Fraktur f, intrauterin-erworbene Fraktur f.
intrauterine immunity intrauterin-erworbene Immunität f.
intrauterine infection intrauterine Infektion f.
intrauterine life Intrauterinperiode f.
intrauterine parabiotic syndrome fetofetale Transfusion f.
intrauterine pneumonia intrauterine Pneumonie f.
intrauterine pregnancy gyn. eutopische/intrauterine Schwangerschaft/Gravidität f.
intrauterine transfusion gyn. intrauterine Transfusion f.
in·tra·vag·i·nal [ˌ-'vædʒənl; -və'dʒaɪnl] adj gyn. innerhalb der Scheide/Vagina (liegend), in die Scheide, intravaginal.
in·tra·vas·cu·lar [ˌ-'væskjələr] adj innerhalb eines Gefäßes (liegend), in ein Gefäß, intravasal, intravaskulär.
intravascular agglutination intravaskuläre (Erythrozyten-)Aggregation f.
intravascular hemolysis intravaskuläre Hämolyse f.
in·tra·ve·nous [ˌ-'viːnəs] 1 n 1. intravenöse Injektion f. 2. intravenöse Infusion f. II adj abbr. I.V., i.v. innerhalb der Vene (liegend), in eine Vene hinein, intravenös abbr. i.v.
intravenous anesthesia intravenöse Anästhesie f.
intravenous anesthetic (agent) intravenöses Injektionsanästhetikum nt.
intravenous cholecystogram intravenöses Cholezystogramm nt, inf. i.v.-Galle f.
intravenous drip intravenöse Tropfinfusion f.
intravenous feeding intravenöse Ernährung f.
intravenous glucose tolerance test abbr. IVGTT intravenöser Glukosetoleranztest m abbr. IVGTT.
intravenous infusion intravenöse Infusion f, i.v.-Infusion f.
intravenous instillation intravenöse Tropfinfusion f.
intravenous pyelogram abbr. IVP intravenöses Pyelogramm nt, i.v.-Pyelogramm nt.
intravenous pyelography Ausscheidungspyelographie f, intravenöse Pyelographie f.
intravenous regional anesthesia intravenöse Regionalanästhesie f abbr. IVRA.
intravenous tension venöser Blutdruck m.
intravenous therapy intravenöse Therapie f.
intravenous urography urol., radiol. Ausscheidungsurographie f.
in·tra·ven·tric·u·lar [ˌ-ven'trɪkjələr] adj in einem Ventrikel (liegend), intraventrikulär, intraventrikular.
intraventricular block intraventrikulärer Block m.
intraventricular bleeding Ventrikel(ein)blutung f, intraventrikuläre Blutung f.
intraventricular conduction card. intraventrikuläre Erregungsleitung/Erregungsausbreitung f.
intraventricular hemorrhage → intraventricular bleeding.
intraventricular pressure intraventrikulärer Druck m, Ventrikel-, Kammerdruck m.
in·tra·ver·te·bral [ˌ-'vɜrtəbrəl] adj → intraspinal.
intravertebral body Wirbelkörper m, Corpus vertebrae/vertebrale.
in·tra·ves·i·cal [ˌ-'vesɪkəl] adj in der Harnblase (liegend), intravesikal.
intravesical pressure intravesikaler Druck m.
in·tra·vil·lous [ˌ-'vɪləs] adj intravillös.
in·tra·vi·tal [ˌ-'vaɪtl] adj während des Lebens, in lebendem Zustand, intravital, Intravital-.
intravital stain/staining Intravital-, Vitalfärbung f.
intra vi·tam ['ɪntrə 'vaɪtəm] während des Lebens, intra vitam, intravital.
in·tra·vit·re·ous [ˌ-'vɪtrɪəs] adj innerhalb des Glaskörpers (liegend), intravitreal.
in·trin·sic [ɪn'trɪnsɪk] adj (a. psycho.) innere(r, s), von innen kommend od. wirkend, innewohnend, innerhalb, endogen, intrinsisch.
in·trin·si·cal [ɪn'trɪnsɪkl] adj → intrinsic.
intrinsic albuminuria intrinsische Albuminurie/Proteinurie f.
intrinsic asthma Intrinsic-Asthma nt.
intrinsic cells: intraspinal i. intraspinale Binnenzellen pl, Binnenzellen pl des Eigenapparates.
i. of spinal cord → intraspinal i.
intrinsic dysmenorrhea gyn. primäre/essentielle Dysmenorrhö f.
intrinsic factor Intrinsic-Faktor m, intrinsic factor (m).
intrinsic light physiol. Eigengrau nt.
intrinsic protein integrales (Membran-)Protein nt.
intrinsic muscles Binnenmuskel pl, -muskulatur f.
intrinsic musculature of larynx innere Kehlkopf-, Larynxmuskulatur f.
intrinsic pathway hema. intrinsic-System nt.
intrinsic proteinuria → intrinsic albuminuria.
intrinsic reflex Eigenreflex m.
intrinsic system → intrinsic pathway.
intro- pref. Intro-.
in·tro·duce [ˌɪntrə'd(j)uːs] vt 1. einführen. 2. (Narkose) einleiten. 3. (Krankheit) einschleppen (into in).
in·tro·duc·er [ˌ-'d(j)uːsər] n anes. Intubator m.
in·tro·duc·tion [ˌ-'dʌkʃn] n 1. Einführung f. 2. (Narkose) Einleitung f. 3. (Krankheit) Einschleppung f. 4. Einleitung f, Vorrede f, Vorwort nt.
in·tro·flec·tion [ˌ-'flekʃn] n Biegung/Beugung f nach innen, Introflexion f.
in·tro·flex·ion [ˌ-'flekʃn] → introflection.
in·tro·gres·sion [ˌ-'greʃn] n genet. Introgression f.
in·tro·i·tus [ɪn'trəʊətəs, -trɔɪ-] n, pl **in·tro·i·tus** anat. Eingang m, Introitus m.
in·tro·jec·tion [ˌɪntrə'dʒekʃn] n psychia. Introjektion f.
in·tro·mis·sion [ˌ-'mɪʃn] n Einführen nt, Hineinstecken nt, Intromission f.

in·tron ['ɪntrɑn] n genet. Intron nt.
in·tro·spect [ˌɪntrə'spekt] vi psycho., psychia. s. selbst beobachten.
in·tro·spec·tion [ˌ-'spekʃn] n psycho., psychia. Selbstbeobachtung f, Introspektion f.
in·tro·spec·tive [ˌ-'spektɪv] adj psycho., psychia. nach innen gewendet, s. selbst beobachtend, auf Selbstbeobachtung beruhend, introspektiv.
in·tro·sus·cep·tion [ˌ-sə'sepʃn] n → intussusception.
in·tro·ver·sion [ˌ-'vɜrʒn, -ʃn] n psycho. Introversion f, Introvertiertheit f.
in·tro·vert [n, adj '-vɜrt; v ˌ-'vɜrt] **I** n psycho. introvertierter Mensch m. **II** adj psycho. nach innen gekehrt, introvertiert. **III** vt 1. (Gedanken) nach innen richten. 2. histol., bio. einstülpen.
in·tu·bate ['ɪnt(j)u:beɪt] vt anes. intubieren, eine Intubation vornehmen (an).
in·tu·ba·tion [ˌɪnt(j)u:'beɪʃn] n Intubation f, Intubieren nt.
in·tu·ba·tor ['ɪnt(j)u:beɪtər] n anes. Intubator m.
in·tu·i·tion [ˌɪnt(j)u:'ɪʃn] n 1. unmittelbares Erkennen od. Wahrnehmen nt, (plötzliche) Eingebung od. Erkenntnis f, Intuition f. 2. intuitives Wissen nt.
in·tu·i·tive [ɪn't(j)u:ɪtɪv] adj intuitiv, Intuitions-.
in·tu·mesce [ˌɪnt(j)u:'mes] vi anschwellen.
in·tu·mes·cence [ˌ-'mesəns] n 1. Anschwellung f, Intumeszenz f, Intumescentia f. 2. Anschwellen nt.
in·tu·mes·cent [ˌ-'mesənt] adj s. aufblähend, anschwellend, intumeszent.
intumescent cataract Cataracta intumescentia.
in·tu·mes·cen·tia [ˌ-mə'senʃɪə] n → intumescence 1.
in·tus·sus·cep·tion [ˌɪntəsə'sepʃn] n patho., chir. Invagination f, Indigitation f, Intussuszeption f.
in·tus·sus·cep·tion·al [ˌ-'sepʃnəl] adj intussuszeptionell.
in·tus·sus·cep·tum [ˌ-'septəm] n, pl **-ta** [-tə] patho., chir. Invaginat nt, Intussuszeptum nt, Intussusceptum nt.
in·tus·sus·cip·i·ens [ˌ-'sɪpɪənz] n, pl **-cip·i·en·tes** [-sɪpɪ'entɪːz] patho., chir. Invaginans nt, Intussuszipiens nt, Intussuscipiens nt.
in·u·lase ['ɪnjəleɪz] n Inulase f, Inulinase f.
in·u·lin ['ɪnjəlɪn] n → inulase.
in·u·lin·ase ['ɪnjəleɪnz] n → inulase.
inulin clearance Inulinclearance f.
in·unc·tion [ɪ'nʌŋ(k)ʃn] n Einreibung f, Einsalbung f, Inunktion f, Inunctio f.
in·un·da·tion fever [ˌɪnən'deɪʃn] → island fever.
in u·ter·o [ɪn 'ju:tərəʊ] im Uterus (liegend od. befindlich), in utero, intauterin.
in·vac·ci·na·tion [ɪnˌvæksə'neɪʃn] n Invakzination f.
in va·cu·o [ɪn 'wɑːkʊəʊ; 'vækju:əʊ] im luftleeren Raum, in vacuo.
in·vade [ɪn'veɪd] vt eindringen in, s. ausbreiten über/in, s. eindrängen in.
in·vag·i·nate [adj ɪn'vædʒənɪt, -neɪt; v -neɪt] **I** adj eingestülpt, nach innen gefaltet, invaginiert. **II** vt einstülpen, nach innen falten. **III** vi s. einstülpen, nach innen falten.
invaginate planula embryo. Gastrula f.
in·vag·i·nat·ed synapse [ɪn'vædʒəneɪtɪd] invaginierte Synapse f.
in·vag·i·na·tion [ɪnˌvædʒə'neɪʃn] n 1. Einstülpen nt, Einstülpung f, Invagination f. 2. embryo. Invagination f. 3. → intussusception.
in·va·lid ['ɪnvəlɪd; -liːd] **I** n Kranke(r m) f,

Gebrechliche(r m) f, Invalide m, Arbeits-, Erwerbsunfähige(r m) f. **II** adj kränklich, krank, gebrechlich, invalid(e), arbeits-, erwerbsunfähig, Kranken-. **III** vt 1. zum Invaliden machen. 2. jdn. als invalid anerkennen, invalidisieren.
in·va·lid·ism ['ɪnvəlɪdɪzəm] n 1. (körperliches) Gebrechen nt. 2. → invalidity. 3. Gesundheitsfanatismus m.
in·va·lid·i·ty [ɪnvə'lɪdətɪ] n Arbeits-, Erwerbs-, Dienstunfähigkeit f, Invalidität f.
InV allotypes genet. KM-Allotypen pl, InV-Allotypen pl.
in·va·sin [ɪn'veɪsɪn] n Hyaluronidase f.
in·va·sion [ɪn'veɪʒn] n 1. patho. (Erreger) Eindringen nt, Invasion f. 2. micro. Invasion f. 3. pharm. Invasion f. 4. patho. (Tumor) Invasion f; Infiltration f.
invasion factor Hyaluronidase f.
in·va·sive [ɪn'veɪzɪv] adj 1. patho. eindringend, invasiv. 2. chir. invasiv.
invasive carcinoma invasives/infiltrierendes Karzinom nt.
invasive mole gyn. destruierende Blasenmole f, destruierendes Chorionadenom nt.
in·va·sive·ness [ɪn'veɪsɪvnɪs] n 1. Fähigkeit f zur Invasion, Invasivität f. 2. patho. Fähigkeit f zur Invasion/Infiltration.
invasive thyroiditis eisenharte Struma f, Riedel-Struma f, chronische hypertrophische Thyreoiditis f.
in·vent [ɪn'vent] vt erfinden; ersinnen; erfinden, erdichten.
in·ven·tion [ɪn'venʃn] n 1. Erfindung f; Erfinden nt. 2. Erfindungsgabe f, Fantasie f, Einfallsreichtum m. 3. Erfindung f, Märchen nt.
in·ven·tive [ɪn'ventɪv] adj 1. erfinderisch, Erfindungs-. 2. originell, einfallsreich.
in·ven·tive·ness [ɪn'ventɪvnɪs] n → invention 2.
in·ven·tor [ɪn'ventər] n Erfinder(in f) m.
in·ven·to·ry ['ɪnvəntɔːriː, -təʊ-] n, pl **-ries** psycho., psychia. Inventar nt, Inventarium nt, Inventory nt.
in·verse [ɪn'vɜrs, 'ɪnvɜrs] **I** n 1. Umkehrung f, Gegenteil nt. 2. mathe. Inverse(s) nt, Reziproke(s) nt. **II** adj 3. umgekehrt, entgegengesetzt. 4. verkehrt. 5. mathe. invers, reziprok, umgekehrt, entgegengesetzt.
inverse astigmatism ophthal. inverser Astigmatismus m, Astigmatismus m gegen die Regel, Astigmatismus inversus.
inverse psoriasis derm. Psoriasis inversa.
in·ver·sion [ɪn'vɜrʒn, -ʃn] n 1. phys., chem. Umkehrung f, Inversion f. 2. genet. (Chromosomen-)Inversion f. 3. psycho. Homosexualität f, (sexuelle) Inversion f. 4. patho. Umstülpung f eines Hohlorgans, Inversion f, Inversio f. 5. mathe. Inversion f.
i. of chromosome genet. Chromosomeninversion f.
i. of uterus gyn. Inversio uteri.
in·vert [n, adj 'ɪnvɜrt; v ɪn'vɜrt] **I** n 1. das Umgekehrte, das Nachaußen-Gekehrte. 2. psycho. Invertierte(r m) f, Homosexuelle(r m) f. **II** adj chem. einer Inversion unterliegend. **III** vt 3. einwärtsdrehen, -kehren, umstülpen, umkehren, -wenden. 4. chem. invertieren.
in·ver·tase [ɪn'vɜrteɪz, 'ɪnv-] n Invertase f, β-Fruktofuranosidase f.
In·ver·te·bra·ta [ɪnˌvɜrtə'breɪtə] pl bio. Wirbellose pl, Invertebraten pl.
in·ver·te·brate [ɪn'vɜrtəbrɪt, -breɪt] **I** n bio. wirbelloses Tier nt, Wirbelloser m, Invertebrat m. **II** adj wirbellos.
in·vert·ed [ɪn'vɜrtɪd] adj 1. umgekehrt, in-

vertiert. 2. psycho. invertiert, homosexuell.
inverted follicular keratosis Akrotrichom nt, follikuläres Porom nt, invertierte follikuläre Keratose f, Keratosis follicularis inversa.
inverted image phys. wirkliches/reelles Bild nt.
inverted nipple gyn. Hohl-, Schlupfwarze f.
inverted reflex paradoxer Reflex m.
inverted repetition genet. inverse Repetition f.
inverted Y field radiol. umgekehrtes Ypsilon-Feld nt.
inverted Y (field) technique radiol. umgekehrte Ypsilon-Bestrahlung f.
in·vert·ose [ɪn'vɜrtəʊz, 'ɪnv-] n Invertzucker m.
invert sugar → invertose.
in·vest [ɪn'vest] vt 1. (a. anat.) umgeben, um-, einhüllen, bekleiden. 2. allg. investieren, anlegen (in in).
in·ves·ti·gate [ɪn'vestɪgeɪt] **I** vt untersuchen, erforschen, recherchieren. **II** vi Untersuchungen/Nachforschungen anstellen (into über); recherchieren.
in·ves·ti·ga·tion [ɪnˌvestɪ'geɪʃn] n (Er-)Forschung f, Untersuchung f (into, of); Nachforschung f, Recherche f, Überprüfung f.
i. of behavior Verhaltensforschung.
in·ves·ti·ga·tive [ɪn'vestɪgeɪtɪv] adj Forschungs-, Forscher-.
in·ves·ti·ga·to·ry [ɪn'vestɪgətɔːriː, -təʊ-] adj → investigative.
investigatory reflex Orientierungsreaktion f.
in·vest·ing [ɪn'vestɪŋ] n Um-, Einhüllen nt.
investing cartilage Gelenkknorpel m, Cartilago articularis.
in·vest·ment [ɪn'vestmənt] n Um-, Einhüllung f.
in·vet·er·a·cy [ɪn'vetərəsɪ] n patho. (Krankheit) Hartnäckigkeit f.
in·vet·er·ate [ɪn'vetərɪt] adj patho. (Krankheit) lange bestehend, hartnäckig, verschleppt, inveteriert.
inveterate edema inveteriertes Lungenödem nt.
in·vig·or·ant [ɪn'vɪgərənt] n pharm. Stärkungs-, Kräftigungsmittel nt.
in·vig·or·ate [ɪn'vɪgəreɪt] vt stärken, kräftigen; beleben, anregen.
in·vig·or·a·tion [ɪnˌvɪgə'reɪʃn] n Stärkung f, Kräftigung f; Belebung f, Anregung f; Er-, Aufmunterung f.
in·vig·or·a·tive [ɪn'vɪgəreɪtɪv] adj stärkend, kräftigend; belebend, anregend; er-, aufmunternd.
in·vis·i·bil·i·ty [ɪnˌvɪzə'bɪlətɪ] n Unsichtbarkeit f.
in·vis·i·ble [ɪn'vɪzəbl] **I** n das Unsichtbare. **II** adj unsichtbar, invisibel.
invisible differentiation embryo. Chemodifferenzierung f.
in vi·tro [ɪn 'viːtrəʊ] im (Reagenz-)Glas, außerhalb des Organismus, in vitro.
in vitro fertilization In-vitro-Fertilisation f, abbr. IVF.
in vi·vo [ɪn 'viːvəʊ] im lebendigen Organismus, in vivo, intravital.
in·vo·lu·cre ['ɪnvəluːkər] n → involucrum.
in·vo·lu·crum [ˌɪnvə'luːkrəm] n, pl **-cra** [-krə] Hülle f, Scheide f, Involucrum nt.
in·vol·un·tar·y [ɪnˌvɒlən'terɪ, -tərɪ] adj 1. unwillkürlich. 2. unfreiwilig. 3. unabsichtlich, unbeabsichtigt, ungewollt.
involuntary guarding chir. reflektorische Abwehrspannung f.
involuntary muscles unwillkürliche Muskulatur f.

involuntary nervous system autonomes/ vegetatives Nervensystem *nt abbr.* ANS, Pars autonomica systematis nervosi, Systema nervosum autonomicum.

in·vo·lute [*n, adj* 'ɪnvəluːt; *v* ˌɪnvə'luːt] **I** *n mathe.* Involute *f*, Evolvente *f*. **II** *adj* **1.** kompliziert, verwickelt. **2.** nach innen gerollt, eingerollt. **III** *vi* **3.** s. einrollen. **4.** s. (zu-)rückbilden, s. (zu-)rückentwickeln.

in·vo·lu·tion [ˌ-'luːʃn] *n* **1.** Rückbildung *f*, Rückentwicklung *f*, Involution *f*. **2.** *mathe.* Involution *f*. **3.** *psychia.* Involution *f*.
i. of uterus *gyn.* postpartale Uterusinvolution, Involutio uteri.

in·vo·lu·tion·al [ˌ-'luːʃənl] *adj* Involutions-.
involutional melancholia → involutional psychosis.
involutional osteoporosis *ortho.* Involutionsosteoporose *f*.
involutional psychosis Involutionspsychose *f*.
involution cyst *gyn.* Involutionszyste *f*.
Io *abbr.* → ionium.
io·ben·zam·ic acid [ˌaɪəben'zæmɪk] Iobenzaminsäure *f*.
io·car·mic acid [ˌ-'kɑːrmɪk] Iocarminsäure *f*.
io·ce·tam·ic acid [ˌ-sɪ'tæmɪk] Iocetaminsäure *f*.
io·da·mide [aɪ'əʊdəmaɪd] *n* Iodamid *nt*.
Iod·a·moe·ba [aɪˌəʊdə'miːbə, aɪɑd-] *n micro.* Iodamoeba *f*, Jodamoeba *f*.
io·date [aɪədeɪt] *n* Iodat *nt*, Jodat *nt*.
iod-Basedow *n* Jodbasedow *m*, jodinduzierte Hyperthyreose *f*.
i·od·ic [aɪ'ɑdɪk] *adj* jodhaltig, Jod-, Iod-.
iodic acid Iod-, Jodsäure *f*.
io·dide [aɪədaɪd, -dɪd] *n* Iodid *nt*, Jodid *nt*.
iodide acne Jodakne *f*.
iodide goiter Jodstruma *f*.
iodide peroxidase Iodid-, Jodidperoxidase *f*, Jodinase *f*.
io·dim·e·try [aɪə'dɪmətrɪ] *n* Jodimetrie *f*.
io·din·ase ['aɪədneɪz] *n* → iodide peroxidase.
io·din·ate ['aɪədneɪt] *vt chem.* mit Jod behandeln, jodieren, jodieren.
io·din·a·tion [ˌaɪədɪ'neɪʃn] *n* Iodierung *f*, Jodierung *f*, Jodination *f*.
io·dine [aɪədiːn, -dɪn] *n abbr.* **I** Jod *nt abbr.* **J**, Iod *nt abbr.* **I**.
iodine deficiency Jodmangel *m*.
iodine number *chem.* Jodzahl *f*.
iodine value → iodine number.
io·din·o·phil [aɪə'dɪnəfɪl] **I** *n* jodophile Zelle *od.* Struktur *f*. **II** *adj* → iodinophilous.
io·din·o·phile ['-faɪl] **I** *n* → iodinophil **I**. **II** *adj* → iodinophilous.
io·di·noph·i·lous [aɪdɪ'nɑfɪləs] *adj histol.* leicht mit Jod anfärbbar, jodophil.
io·dism ['aɪədɪzəm] *n* chronische Jodvergiftung/Jodintoxikation *f*, Jodismus *m*.
io·di·za·tion [ˌaɪədaɪ'zeɪʃn] *n* → iodination.
io·dize ['aɪədaɪz] *vt* → iodinate.
io·do·ac·e·tate [aɪˌəʊdə'æsɪteɪt, aɪˌədə-] *n* Jod-, Iodacetat *nt*.
io·do·a·ce·tic acid [ˌ-ə'siːtɪk, -ə'set-] Jod-, Iodessigsäure *f*.
io·do·chlor·hy·drox·y·quin [ˌ-ˌklɔːrhaɪ'drɑksɪkwɪn] *n pharm.* Clioquinol *nt*.
5-io·do·de·ox·y·ur·i·dine [ˌ-dɪˌɑksɪ'jʊərɪdiːn] *n* → idoxuridine.
io·do·der·ma [ˌ-'dɜːrmə] *n* Jodausschlag *m*, Jododerma *nt*.
io·do·form ['-fɔːrm] *n* Jodoform *nt*.
io·do·form·ism ['-fɔːrmɪzəm] *n* Jodoformvergiftung *f*.
io·do·for·mum [ˌ-'fɔːrməm] *n* → iodoform.
io·do·gor·go·ic acid [ˌ-gɔːr'gəʊɪk] (3,5-)-Dijodtyrosin *nt*.

io·do·met·ric [ˌ-'metrɪk] *adj* Jodometrie betr., jodometrisch.
io·dom·e·try [aɪə'dɑmətrɪ] *n* Jodo-, Iodometrie *f*.
io·do·pa·no·ic acid [aɪˌəʊdəpə'nəʊɪk, aɪˌədə-] → iopanoic acid.
io·do·phe·nol [ˌ-'fiːnɔl, -nɑl] *n* (Mono-)-Jodphenol *nt*.
io·do·phil ['-fɪl] **I** *n* → iodinophil **I**. **II** *adj* → iodinophilous.
iodophil granules jodophile Granula *pl*.
io·do·phil·ia [ˌ-'fɪlɪə] *n histol.* Jodophilie *f*.
io·do·phthal·ein [ˌ-'θælɪɪn, -liːn] *n* Jodophthalein *nt*.
io·dop·sin [aɪə'dɑpsɪn] *n* Jodopsin *nt*, Iodopsin *nt*, Tagessehstoff *m*.
io·do·ther·a·py [aɪˌəʊdə'θerəpɪ] *n* Behandlung *f* mit Jod *od.* Jodiden.
io·do·thy·ro·glob·u·lin [ˌ-ˌθaɪrə'glɑbjəlɪn] *n* Thyreoglobulin *nt*.
io·do·thy·ro·nine [ˌ-'θaɪrəniːn, -nɪn] *n* Jodthyronin *nt*.
io·do·ty·ro·sine [ˌ-'taɪrəsiːn, -sɪn] *n* Jodtyrosin *nt*.
iodotyrosine dehalogenase → iodotyrosine deiododinase.
iodotyrosine deiododinase Jodtyrosindejododinase *f*.
io·dous [aɪ'əʊdəs, aɪ'ɑdəs] *adj chem.* jodhaltig, jodähnlich, Jod-.
io·dox·am·ic acid [ˌaɪədɑk'sæmɪk] Iodoxaminsäure *f*.
io·dum [aɪ'əʊdəm] *n* → iodine.
io·du·ria [aɪə'd(j)ʊərɪə] *n* Jod- *od.* Jodidausscheidung *f* im Harn.
io·glic·ic acid [aɪə'glɪsɪk] Ioglicinsäure *f*.
io·gly·cam·ic acid [ˌaɪəglaɪ'kæmɪk] Ioglycaminsäure *f*.
ion ['aɪən, 'aɪɑn] *n* Ion *nt*.
ion channel Ionenkanal *m*.
ion concentration Ionenkonzentration *f*.
Ionescu [jə'neskəʊ, ɪə-]: **I. valve** *HTG* Ionescu-Klappe *f*.
ion exchange Ionenaustausch *m*.
ion-exchange chromatography Ionenaustausch(er)chromatographie *f*.
ion-exchange resin Ionenaustauscherharz *nt*, Resin *nt*.
ion flow Ionenstrom *m*, -fluß *m*.
ion gradient Ionengradient *m*, -gefälle *nt*.
i·on·ic [aɪ'ɑnɪk] *adj* Ion(en) betr., ionisch, Ionen-.
ionic bond *chem.* Ionenbindung *f*, elektrovalente/heteropolare/ionogene Bindung *f*.
ionic compound ionische Verbindung *f*.
ionic concentration → ion concentration.
ionic conductivity Ionenleitfähigkeit *f*.
ionic interaction ionische Wechselwirkung *f*.
ionic lattice Ionengitter *nt*.
ionic linkage → ionic bond.
ionic migration *chem., phys.* Ionenwanderung *f*.
ionic rays α-Strahlen *pl*, Alphastrahlen *pl*, -Strahlung *f*.
ionic solution ionische Lösung *f*.
ionic strength Ionenstärke *f*.
ionic theory of excitation *physiol.* Ionentheorie *f* der Erregung.
io·ni·um [aɪ'əʊnɪəm] *n abbr.* **Io** Ionium *nt abbr.* Io.
ion·iz·a·ble ['aɪənaɪzəbl] *adj* ionisierbar.
ion·i·za·tion [ˌaɪənaɪ'zeɪʃn] *n* **1.** Ionisation *f*, Ionisierung *f*. **2.** → ionophoresis.
ionization chamber *phys.* Ionisationskammer *f*.
ionization product *chem.* Ionisationsprodukt *nt*.
ionization state Ionisierungs-, Ionisationszustand *m*.
ion·ize ['aɪənaɪz] **I** *vt* ionisieren, eine Ioni-

sation erzeugen. **II** *vi* in Ionen zerfallen.
ion·ized atom ['aɪənaɪzd] ionisiertes Atom *nt*, Ion *nt*.
ion·iz·er ['aɪənaɪzər] *n phys.* Ionisator *m*.
ion·iz·ing radiation ['-aɪzɪŋ] ionisierende Strahlung *f*.
ion·o·gen·ic [aɪˌənə'dʒenɪk] *adj* **1.** Ionen bildend *od.* liefernd. **2.** durch Ionen entstanden, auf Ionen beruhend, ionogen.
io·no·gram ['aɪənəgræm] *n* Elektropherogramm *nt*.
ion·om·e·ter [aɪə'nɑmɪtər] *n* Ionometer *nt*.
ion·om·e·try [aɪə'nɑmətrɪ] *n* Ionometrie *f*.
ion·o·phore [aɪ'ɑnəfɔːr, -fəʊr] *n* Ionophor *nt*.
ion·o·pho·re·sis [aɪˌɑnəfə'riːsɪs] *n* Ionophorese *f*, Elektrophorese *f*.
ion·o·pho·ret·ic [aɪˌɑnəfə'retɪk] *adj* Elektrophorese betr., mittels Elektrophorese, elektrophoretisch.
io·no·ther·a·py [ˌaɪənə'θerəpɪ] *n* **1.** Behandlung *f* mit Ionenstrahlen. **2.** → iontophoresis.
ion product *chem.* Ionenprodukt *nt*.
ion selectivity Ionenselektivität *f*.
ion·ther·a·py [aɪən'θerəpɪ] *n* → iontophoresis.
ion·to·pho·re·sis [aɪˌɑntəfə'riːsɪs] *n* Ionentherapie *f*, Kataphorese *f*, Iontophorese *f*.
ion·to·pho·ret·ic [ˌ-fə'retɪk] *adj* Iontophorese betr., iontophoretisch.
ion·to·quan·tim·e·ter [ˌ-kwæn'tɪmətər] *n* → ionometer.
ion·to·ra·di·om·e·ter [ˌ-reɪdɪ'ɑmɪtər] *n* → ionometer.
ion·to·ther·a·py [ˌ-'θerəpɪ] *n* → iontophoresis.
io·pam·i·dol [ˌaɪə'pæmɪdɔl, -əʊl] *n radiol.* Iopamidol *nt*.
io·pa·no·ic acid [aɪəpæ'nəʊɪk] Iopansäure *f*.
io·py·dol [aɪə'paɪdɔl, -əʊl] *n radiol.* Iopydol *nt*.
io·py·done [aɪə'paɪdəʊn] *n radiol.* Iopydon *nt*.
io·ta·cism [aɪ'əʊtəsɪzəm] *n* Jotazismus *m*, Itazismus *m*.
io·thal·a·mate [aɪə'θæləmeɪt] *n radiol.* Iotalamat, Iotalamint *nt*.
io·tha·lam·ic acid [aɪəθə'læmɪk] *radiol.* Iotalaminsäure *f*.
io·trox·ic acid [aɪə'trɑksɪk] *radiol.* Iotroxinsäure *f*.
IP *abbr.* → isoelectric point.
IP₃ *abbr.* → inositol triphosphate.
I-para *n* Erstgebärende *f*, Primipara *f*.
ip·e·cac ['ɪpəkæk] *n* → ipecacuanha.
ip·e·cac·u·an·ha [ˌɪpəˌkækjuː'ænə] *n pharm.* Brechwurzel *f*, Ipekakuanha *f*, Ipecacuanha *f*, Radix ipecacuanhae.
IPPB *abbr.* → intermittent positive pressure breathing.
IPPR *abbr.* [intermittent positive pressure respiration] → intermittent positive pressure breathing.
IPPV *abbr.* [intermittent positive pressure ventilation] → intermittent positive pressure breathing.
i·pra·tro·pi·um bromide [ɪprə'trəʊpɪəm] *pharm.* Ipratropiumbromid *nt*.
IPSC *abbr.* → inhibitory postsynaptic current.
ip·si·lat·er·al [ˌɪpsɪ'lætərəl] *adj* auf gleicher Seite (liegend), ipsilateral, kollateral.
ipsilateral reflex homolateraler/homonymer Reflex *m*.
IPSP *abbr.* → inhibitory postsynaptic potential.
IPTG *abbr.* → isopropyl thiogalactoside.
IPV *abbr.* → poliovirus vaccine inactivated.

IQ *abbr.* → intelligence quotient.
IR *abbr.* → infrared 1.
Ir *abbr.* → iridium.
IRF *abbr.* → inhibitory receptive field.
Ir genes → immune response genes.
irid- *pref.* → irido-.
ir·i·dal ['ɪrədl, 'aɪr-] *adj* Regenbogenhaut/Iris betr., Iris-, Irido-.
iridal angle → iridocorneal angle.
ir·i·dal·gia [ɪrə'dældʒ(ɪ)ə, ˌaɪrə-] *n ophthal.* Irisschmerz *m*, Iridalgie *f*.
ir·id·aux·e·sis [ˌɪrɪdɔːg'ziːsɪs, ˌaɪrə-] *n ophthal.* Irisverdickung *f*.
ir·i·dec·tome [ˌɪrɪ'dektəʊm, ˌaɪrə-] *n ophthal.* Iridektom *nt*, Iridektomiemesser *nt*.
ir·i·dec·to·mize [ˌ-'dektəmaɪz] *vt* eine Iridektomie durchführen, iridektomieren.
ir·i·dec·to·my [ˌ-'dektəmɪ] *n ophthal.* Irisresektion *f*, -ausschneidung *f*, -entfernung *f*, Iridektomie *f*.
iridectomy scissors *ophthal.* Iridektomieschere *f*.
ir·i·dec·tro·pi·um [ˌ-dek'trəʊpɪəm] *n ophthal.* Iridektropium *nt*, Ektropium uveae.
ir·i·de·mia [ˌ-'diːmɪə] *n ophthal.* Irisblutung *f*.
ir·i·den·clei·sis [ˌ-den'klaɪsɪs] *n ophthal.* Iriseinklemmung *f*, Iridenkleisis *f*, Iridenklisis *f*.
ir·i·den·tro·pi·um [ˌ-den'trəʊpɪəm] *n ophthal.* Iridentropium *nt*, Entropium uveae.
ir·i·de·re·mia [ˌ-də'riːmɪə] *n ophthal.* angeborenes Fehlen *nt* der Regenbogenhaut, Irisaplasie *f*, Irideremie *f*; Aniridie *f*.
ir·i·des·cence [ˌɪrɪ'desns] *n* Schillern *nt*, Irisieren *nt*.
ir·i·des·cent [ɪrɪ'desnt] *adj* schillernd, irisierend.
ir·i·de·sis [ɪ'rɪdəsɪs] *n ophthal.* Iridesis *f*, Iridodesia *f*.
ir·i·di·ag·no·sis [ˌɪrɪdaɪəg'nəʊsɪs] *n* → iridodiagnosis.
irid·i·al [aɪ'rɪdɪəl, ɪ'-] *adj* → iridal.
iridial folds Irisfalten *pl*, Plicae iridis.
iridial part of retina Irisabschnitt *m* der Retina, Pars iridica retinae.
irid·i·an [-'rɪdɪən] *adj* → iridal.
irid·ic [-'rɪdɪk] *adj* → iridal.
irid·i·um [ɪ'rɪdɪəm aɪ'r-] *n abbr.* **Ir** Iridium *nt abbr.* Ir.
irido- *pref.* Regenbogenhaut-, Iris-, Irid(o)-.
ir·i·do·a·vul·sion [ˌɪrɪdəʊə'vʌlʃn, ˌaɪrɪ-] *n ophthal.* Irisabriß *m*.
ir·i·do·cap·su·li·tis [ˌ-kæpsə'laɪtɪs, -ˌkæpsjʊ-] *n ophthal.* Entzündung *f* von Iris u. Linsenkapsel, Iridokapsulitis *f*.
ir·i·do·cele ['-siːl] *n ophthal.* Irisprolaps *m*, -hernie *f*, Iridozele *f*, -cele *f*.
ir·i·do·cho·roid·i·tis [ˌ-ˌkɔːrɔɪ'daɪtɪs] *n ophthal.* Entzündung *f* von Iris u. Aderhaut, Iridochorioiditis *f*.
ir·i·do·col·o·bo·ma [ˌ-ˌkɑlə'bəʊmə] *n ophthal.* angeborener Regenbogenhautdefekt *m*, Iriskolobom *nt*.
ir·i·do·cor·ne·al angle [ˌ-'kɔːrnɪəl] Iridokorneal-, Kammerwinkel *m*, Angulus iridocornealis.
iridocorneal mesodermal dysgenesis *ophthal.* Rieger-Anomalie *f*.
ir·i·do·cor·ne·o·scle·rec·to·my [ˌ-ˌkɔːrnɪəʊsklɪ'rektəmɪ] *n ophthal.* Iridokorneosklerektomie *f*.
ir·i·do·cy·clec·to·my [ˌ-sɪk'lektəmɪ, -saɪ-] *n ophthal.* Iridozyklektomie *f*.
ir·i·do·cy·cli·tis [ˌ-sɪk'laɪtɪs, -saɪ-] *n ophthal.* Entzündung *f* von Iris u. Ziliarkörper, Iridozyklitis *f*, -cyclitis *f*.

ir·i·do·cy·clo·cho·roid·i·tis [ˌ-ˌsaɪkləˌkɔːrɔɪ'daɪtɪs] *n ophthal.* Entzündung *f* von Iris, Aderhaut u. Ziliarkörper, Iridozyklochorioiditis *f*.
ir·i·do·cys·tec·to·my [ˌ-sɪs'tektəmɪ] *n ophthal.* Iridozystektomie *f*.
ir·i·dod·e·sis [ɪrɪ'dɑdəsɪs] *n* → iridesis.
ir·i·do·di·ag·no·sis [ˌɪrɪdəʊdaɪəg'nəʊsɪs, ˌaɪrɪ-] *n* Augendiagnose *f*, Iridodiagnose *f*.
ir·i·do·di·al·y·sis [ˌ-daɪ'æləsɪs] *n ophthal.* Irisablösung *f* vom Ziliarrand, Iridodialyse *f*, -dialysis *f*.
ir·i·do·di·as·ta·sis [ˌ-daɪ'æstəsɪs] *n ophthal.* Iridodiastase *f*.
ir·i·do·di·la·tor [ˌ-daɪ'leɪtər, -dɪ-] *I n* 1. M. dilator pupillae. 2. pupillenerweiterndes Mittel *nt*. **II** *adj* pupillenerweiternd.
ir·i·do·do·ne·sis [ˌ-də'niːsɪs] *n ophthal.* Irisschlottern *nt*, Iridodonesis *f*.
ir·i·do·ker·a·ti·tis [ˌ-kerə'taɪtɪs] *n ophthal.* Entzündung *f* von Iris u. Kornea, Iridokeratitis *f*.
ir·i·do·ki·ne·sia [ˌ-kɪ'niːʒ(ɪ)ə, -kaɪ-] *n* → iridokinesis.
ir·i·do·ki·ne·sis [ˌ-kɪ'niːsɪs, -kaɪ-] *n ophthal.* Irisbewegungen *pl*, Iridokinese *f*.
ir·i·do·ki·net·ic [ˌ-kɪ'netɪk] *adj* Iridokinese betr., iridokinetisch, iridomotorisch.
ir·i·do·lep·tyn·sis [ˌ-lep'tɪnsɪs] *n ophthal.* Irisausdünnung *f*, -atrophie *f*.
ir·i·do·ma·la·cia [ˌ-mə'leɪʃ(ɪ)ə] *n ophthal.* Iriserweichung *f*, Iridomalazie *f*, -malacia *f*.
ir·i·do·mes·o·di·al·y·sis [ˌ-ˌmezədaɪ'æləsɪs] *n ophthal.* Iridomesodialysis *f*.
ir·i·do·mo·tor [ˌ-'məʊtər] *adj* → iridokinetic.
ir·i·don·co·sis [ˌɪrɪdɑŋ'kəʊsɪs, ˌaɪrɪ-] *ophthal.* Irisverdickung *f*.
ir·i·don·cus [ˌ-'dɑŋkəs] *n ophthal.* Irisschwellung *f*.
ir·i·do·pa·ral·y·sis [ˌɪrɪdəʊpə'ræləsɪs, ˌaɪrɪ-] *n* → iridoplegia.
ir·i·dop·a·thy [ɪrɪ'dɑpəθɪ, ˌaɪrɪ-] *n ophthal.* pathologische Veränderung *f* der Regenbogenhaut, Iridopathie *f*, -pathia *f*.
ir·i·do·per·i·pha·ki·tis [ˌɪrɪdəʊˌperɪfə'kaɪtɪs, ˌaɪrɪ-] *n ophthal.* Iridoperiphakitis *f*.
ir·i·do·ple·gia [ˌ-'pliːdʒ(ɪ)ə] *n* Lähmung *f* des M. sphincter pupillae, Iridoplegie *f*, Iridoparalysis *f*, Iridoparese *f*.
ir·i·dop·to·sis [ˌɪrɪdɑp'təʊsɪs, ˌaɪrɪ-] *n* Irisprolaps *m*, Iridoptose *f*, Iridoptosis *f*.
ir·i·do·pu·pil·lar·y [ˌɪrɪdəʊ'pjuːpələrɪ, -ˌleri, ˌaɪrɪ-] *adj* Regenbogenhaut/Iris u. Pupille betr. *od.* verbindend, iridopupillär.
iridopupillary membrane Iridopupillarmembran *f*, Membrana iridopupillaris.
ir·i·dor·rhex·is [ˌ-'reksɪs] *n ophthal.* 1. Irisriß *m*, Iridorrhexis *f*. 2. Irisabriß *m*.
ir·i·dos·chi·sis [ɪrɪ'dɑskəsɪs, ˌaɪrɪ-] *n ophthal.* Iridoschisis *f*.
ir·i·do·scle·rot·o·my [ˌɪrɪdəʊsklɪ'rɑtəmɪ, ˌaɪrɪ-] *n ophthal.* Iridosklerotomie *f*.
ir·i·do·ste·re·sis [ˌ-stə'riːsɪs] *n ophthal.* Verlust *m od.* Fehlen *nt* der Regenbogenhaut.
ir·i·dot·o·my [ˌɪrɪ'dɑtəmɪ, ˌaɪrɪ-] *n ophthal.* Irisschnitt *m*, -durchtrennung *f*, -einschnitt *m*, Iridotomie *f*, Iritomie *f*.
ir·i·do·vir·i·dae [ˌɪrɪdəʊ'vɪrədiː, -'vaɪr-, ˌaɪrɪ-] *pl micro.* Iridoviridae *pl*.
ir·i·do·vi·rus [ˌ-'vaɪrəs] *n micro.* Iridovirus *nt*.
iris ['aɪərɪs] *n, pl* **iris·es** [-sɪz], **iri·des** ['ɪrɪˌdiːz, 'aɪrɪ-] Regenbogenhaut *f*, Iris *f*.
iris bombé *ophthal.* Napfkucheniris *f*, Iris bombans/bombata.
iris contraction reflex 1. Pupillenreflex *m*, -reaktion *f*. 2. (*Pupille*) Lichtreaktion *f*, -reflex *m*.

iris hook *ophthal.* Irishäkchen *nt*.
iris-op·sia [aɪrɪs'ɑpsɪə] *n ophthal.* Regenbogenfarbensehen *nt*, Iridopsie *f*.
irit·ic [aɪ'rɪtɪk, ɪ'r-] *adj* Iritis betr., iritisch.
iri·tis [aɪ'raɪtɪs, ɪ'r-] *n* Regenbogenhautentzündung *f*, Iritis *f*.
irit·o·my [aɪ'rɪtəmɪ, ɪ'r-] *n* → iridotomy.
I_R-neuron *n physiol.* I_R-Neuron *nt*, ramp--inspiratorisches Neuron *nt*.
i·ron ['aɪərn] **I** *n* 1. *chem.* Eisen *nt*, Ferrum *nt abbr.* Fe. 2. *pharm.* Eisen(präparat *nt*) *nt*, eisenhaltiges Arzneimittel *nt*. **to take ~** Eisen nehmen. **II** *adj* eisern, Eisen-; eisenfarbig.
iron-binding capacity *abbr.* **IBC** Eisenbindungskapazität *f abbr.* EBK.
iron-calcium deposits *patho.* Eisen-Kalziumkrustation *f*.
iron clearance (Plasma-)Eisenclearance *f*.
iron compound eisenhaltige Verbindung *f*, Eisenverbindung *f*.
iron deficiency Eisenmangel *m*.
iron deficiency anemia Eisenmangelanämie *f*, sideropenische Anämie *f*.
iron fumarate Eisen-II-fumarat *nt*, Ferrofumarat *nt*.
iron-hard thyroiditis eisenharte Struma *f*, Riedel-Struma *f*, chronische hypertrophische Thyreoiditis *f*.
iron hematoxylin Eisen-Hämatoxylin *nt*.
iron hematoxylin stain Eisen-Hämatoxylin-Färbung *f*.
iron hydroxide Eisen-III-hydroxid *nt*.
iron lung eiserne Lunge *f*, Tankrespirator *m*.
iron protein Eisen-, Ferroprotein *nt*, eisenhaltiges Protein *nt*.
iron salt Eisensalz *nt*.
iron storage disease Eisenspeicherkrankheit *f*, Hämochromatose *f*.
iron sulfate Eisen-II-sulfat *nt*, Ferrosulfat *nt*.
iron-sulfur center *biochem.* Eisen-Schwefel-Zentrum *nt*.
iron-sulfur protein Eisen-Schwefel-Protein *nt*.
i·rot·o·my [aɪ'rɑtəmɪ] *n* → iridotomy.
ir·ra·di·ance [ɪ'reɪdɪəns] *n phys.* Strahlungsintensität *f*; spezifische Strahlungsenergie *f*.
ir·ra·di·an·cy [ɪ'reɪdɪənsɪ] *n* → irradiance.
ir·ra·di·ant [ɪ'reɪdɪənt] *adj* strahlend (*with* vor).
ir·ra·di·ate [ɪ'reɪdɪeɪt] *vt* 1. *radiol.* bestrahlen, mit Strahlen behandeln. 2. erleuchten, aus-, anstrahlen; (*Schmerz*) ausstrahlen. 3. (*Licht*) ausstrahlen, verbreiten; (*Strahlen*) aussenden.
ir·ra·di·at·ed ergosterol [ɪ'reɪdɪeɪtɪd] Ergocalciferol *nt*, Vitamin D_2 *nt*.
ir·ra·di·a·tion [ɪˌreɪdɪ'eɪʃn] *n* 1. *radiol.* Bestrahlung *f*, Strahlentherapie *f*. 2. Erleuchtung *f*, Anstrahlung *f*, Ausleuchtung *f*. 3. (*Schmerz*) Ausstrahlung *f*, Irradiation *f*. 4. *physiol.* Ausbreitung *f*, Irradiation *f*. 5. (*Licht*) Ausstrahlung *f*, Aussendung *f*. 6. *phys.* Strahlungsintensität *f*; spezifische Strahlungsenergie *f*. 7. *psycho.* Irradiation *f*.
ir·ra·tion·al [ɪ'ræʃənl] **I** *n mathe.* irrationale Zahl *f*. **II** *adj* irrational, unvernünftig; vernunftlos; vernunftwidrig, unlogisch.
ir·re·duc·i·ble [ɪrɪ'd(j)uːsəbl] *adj* 1. *chir.* nicht-reponierbar, irreponibel. 2. *chem.* nicht-reduzierbar. 3. *ortho.* nicht-einrenkbar, irreponibel.
irreducibel hernia inkarzerierte/eingeklemmte Hernie *f*, Hernia incarcerata.
ir·reg·u·lar [ɪ'regjələr] *adj* 1. unregelmäßig, ungleichmäßig; uneben; irregulär. 2. ungesetzlich, nicht statthaft, ungültig, regelwidrig. 3. ungeregelt, ungeordnet.

irregular astigmatism ophthal. irregulärer Astigmatismus m.
irregular bone komplizierter Knochen m, Os irregulare.
irregular emphysema irreguläres/unregelmäßiges Emphysem nt.
irregular gout extraartikuläre/viszerale Gicht f.
ir·reg·u·lar·i·ty [ɪˌregjəˈlærətɪ] n, pl **-ties 1.** Unregelmäßigkeit f, Ungleichmäßigkeit f, Uneinheitlichkeit f, Unebenheit f. **2.** Ungesetzlichkeit f, Ungültigkeit f, Regelwidrigkeit f. **3.** Regellosigkeit f, Unordentlichkeit f.
i. of pulse Herzrhythmusstörung f, Arrhythmie f, Arrhythmia f.
irregular pulse unregelmäßiger Puls m, Pulsus irregularis.
ir·rep·a·ra·ble [ɪˈrepərəbl] adj **1.** nicht wiederherstellbar, nicht heilbar, irreparabel. **2.** unersetzlich, unersetzbar.
ir·res·pi·ra·ble [ɪˈrespɪrəbl] adj nicht einatembar, nicht respirabel.
ir·re·spon·sive [ɪrɪˈspɑnsɪv] adj nicht ansprechend od. reagierend (to auf); nicht empfänglich (to für).
ir·re·vers·i·bil·i·ty [ɪrɪˌvɜrsəˈbɪlətɪ] n **1.** irreversible Beschaffenheit f, Irreversibilität f. **2.** Unwiderruflichkeit f, Unabänderlichkeit f.
ir·re·vers·i·ble [ɪrɪˈvɜrsəbl] adj **1.** chem., phys., mathe. nicht umkehrbar, nur in einer Richtung verlaufend, irreversibel. **2.** unwiderruflich, unabänderlich, nicht rückgängig zu machen.
irreversible colloid instabiles/irreversibles Kolloid n.
irreversible coma Hirntod m, biologischer Tod m.
irreversible inhibition irreversible Hemmung f.
irreversible shock irreversibler/paralytischer/refraktärer Schock m.
irreversible thermodynamics Thermodynamik f offener Systeme, Thermodynamik f irreversibler Prozesse.
ir·ri·gate [ˈɪrɪgeɪt] vt (aus-)spülen, auswaschen.
ir·ri·ga·tion [ɪrɪˈgeɪʃn] n **1.** (Aus-, Durch-)Spülung f, Spülen nt, Irrigation f. **2.** (Spül-)Lösung f, Irrigans nt.
irrigation syringe Spülspritze f.
ir·ri·ga·tor [ˈɪrɪgeɪtər] n Spülkanne m, Irrigator m.
ir·ri·ta·bil·i·ty [ɪrətəˈbɪlətɪ] n **1.** physiol. Reiz-, Erregbarkeit f, Irritabilität f. **2.** psycho. irritierbares Wesen nt, Irritierbarkeit f.
ir·ri·ta·ble [ˈɪrɪtəbl] adj **1.** physiol. reiz-, erregbar, irritabel. **2.** patho., psycho. (leicht) reizbar, (über-)empfindlich; gereizt; nervös.
irritable bladder Reizblase f.
irritable bowel Reizkolon nt, irritables/spastisches Kolon nt, Kolonneurose f, Colon irritabile/spasticum.
irritable bowel syndrome → irritable bowel.
irritable colon → irritable bowel.
irritable colon syndrome → irritable bowel.
irritable heart Soldatenherz nt, neurozirkulatorische Asthenie f, Effort-Syndrom nt, Da Costa-Syndrom nt, Phrenikokardie f.
ir·ri·tant [ˈɪrɪtnt] **I** n Reizstoff m, -mittel nt, Irritans nt. **II** adj einen Reiz auslösend, reizend, Reiz-.
irritant agent → irritant I.
irritant dermatitis nicht-allergische Kontaktdermatitis f, toxische Kontaktdermatitis f, toxisches Kontaktekzem nt.

ir·ri·tate [ˈɪrɪteɪt] vt **1.** reizen, irritieren. **2.** reizen, (ver-)ärgern, irritieren.
ir·ri·ta·tion [ɪrɪˈteɪʃn] n **1.** physiol. Reiz m, Reizung f, Reizen nt. **2.** patho. Reizzustand m, Reizung f. **3.** Verärgerung f, Reizung f, Irritation f.
irritation cells Türk'-Reizformen pl.
irritation fibroma Irritationsfibrom nt, Lappenfibrom nt.
irritation therapy Reiztherapie f.
ir·ri·ta·tive [ˈɪrɪteɪtɪv] adj **1.** als Reiz wirkend, erregend, irritativ. **2.** reizbar; gereizt.
irritative diarrhea irritative Diarrhö f.
IRV abbr. → inspiratory reserve volume.
IS abbr. → intracellular space.
is- pref. → iso-.
is·chae·mia n → ischemia.
is·che·mia [ɪˈskiːmɪə, -mjə] n Ischämie f.
is·che·mic [ɪˈskiːmɪk, -ˈskemɪk] adj Ischämie betr., von Ischämie betroffen, durch Ischämie bedingt, blutleer, ischämisch, Ischämie-.
ischemic colitis ischämische Kolitis f.
ischemic contracture ortho. ischämische/ischämie-bedingte Kontraktur f.
ischemic hypoxia ischämische Anoxie/Hypoxie f, Stagnationsanoxie f, -hypoxie f.
ischemic infarct ischämischer/anämischer/weißer/blasser Infarkt m.
ischemic injury ischämie-bedingte Schädigung f, Schädigung f durch Ischämie.
ischemic necrosis ischämische Nekrose f.
  epiphyseal i. aseptische Epiphysennekrose, Osteochondrose f, -chondrosis f.
ischemic neuropathy ischämische Neuropathie f.
ischemic palsy ischämische Lähmung/Paralyse f.
ischemic paralysis → ischemic palsy.
ischemic phase of endometrium (Endometrium) ischämische Phase f.
ischemic proctitis ischämische Proktitis f.
ischemic reflex Ischämiereflex m, -reaktion f.
ischemic tolerance patho. Ischämietoleranz f.
is·che·sis [ɪsˈkiːsɪs] n patho. Unterdrückung f der (normalen) Sekretion.
ischi- pref. → ischio-.
is·chi·a·del·phus [ɪskɪəˈdelfəs] n → ischiodidymus.
is·chi·ad·ic [ɪskɪˈædɪk] adj → ischial.
ischiadic bursa Bursa ischiadica/sciatica m. obturatoris interni.
ischiadic foramen: greater i. For. ischiadicum/sciaticum majus.
  lesser i. For. ischiadicum/sciaticum minus.
ischiadic nerve Ischiasnerv m, N. ischiadicus/sciaticus.
ischiadic plexus 1. Kreuzbein-, Sakralplexus m, Plexus sacralis. **2.** Plexus venosus sacralis.
is·chi·al [ˈɪskɪəl] adj Sitzbein betr., zum Sitzbein gehörend, Ischias-, Sitzbein-.
ischial bone → ischium.
ischial bursa: i. of gluteus maximus muscle Bursa ischiadica/sciatica m. glut(a)ei maximi.
  i. of internal obturator muscle → ischiadic bursa.
is·chi·al·gia [ɪskɪˈældʒ(ɪ)ə] n **1.** Hüftschmerz m, Ischialgie f. **2.** Ischias m/nt/f, Ischiassyndrom nt.
ischial incisure Inc. ischiadica/ischialis.
  greater i. Inc. ischiadica/ischialis major.
  lesser i. Inc. ischiadica/ischialis minor.
ischial notch → ischial incisure.
  greater i. → ischial incisure, greater.
  lesser i. → ischial incisure, lesser.

ischial ramus Sitzbeinast m, Ramus ossis ischii.
ischial spine Spina ischiadica/ischialis.
ischial tuberosity Sitzbeinhöcker m, Tuber ischiadicum/ischiale.
is·chi·at·ic [ɪskɪˈætɪk] adj → ischial.
ischiatic hernia Beckenhernie f, Ischiozele f, Hernia ischiadica.
is·chi·a·ti·tis [ɪskɪəˈtaɪtɪs] n Entzündung f des N. ischiadicus.
ischio- pref. Sitzbein-, Ischias-, Hüft(e)-, Ischio-.
is·chi·o·a·nal [ɪskɪəʊˈeɪnl] adj Sitzbein/Ischium u. Anus betr., ischioanal.
is·chi·o·bul·bar [-ˈbʌlbər, -bɑːr] adj Sitzbein/Ischium u. Bulbus penis betr., ischiobulbär.
is·chi·o·cap·su·lar ligament [-ˈkæps(j)ələr] Lig. ischiofemorale.
is·chi·o·ca·ver·no·sus (muscle) [-ˌkævərˈnəʊsəs] Ischiokavernosus m, -cavernosus m, M. ischiocavernosus.
is·chi·o·cav·ern·ous muscle [-ˈkævərnəs] → ischiocavernosus (muscle).
is·chi·o·cele [-ˈsiːl] n → ischiatic hernia.
is·chi·o·coc·cyg·e·al [-kɑkˈsɪdʒɪəl] adj Sitzbein/Ischium u. Steißbein/Coccyx betr., ischiokokzygeal.
is·chi·o·coc·cy·ge·us [-kɑkˈsɪdʒɪəs] n M. coccygeus.
is·chi·o·did·y·mus [-ˈdɪdəməs] n embryo. Ischiodidymus m.
is·chi·o·dyn·ia [-ˈdiːnɪə] n → ischialgia.
is·chi·o·fem·o·ral [-ˈfemərəl] adj Sitzbein/Ischium u. Femur betr., ischiofemoral.
ischiofemoral ligament Lig. ischiofemorale.
is·chi·o·fib·u·lar [-ˈfɪbjələr] adj Sitzbein/Ischium u. Wadenbein/Fibula betr., ischiofibulär.
is·chi·o·glu·te·al bursitis [-ˈgluːtɪəl] Entzündung f der Bursa ischiadica m. glut(a)ei maximi.
is·chi·om·e·lus [ɪskɪˈɑmələs] n embryo. Ischiomelus m.
is·chi·o·ni·tis [ɪskɪəˈnaɪtɪs] n Sitzbeinentzündung f.
is·chi·o·pa·gia [-ˈpædʒɪə] n embryo. Ischiopagie f.
is·chi·op·a·gus [ɪskɪˈɑpəgəs] n embryo. Ischiopagus m.
is·chi·op·a·gy [ɪskɪˈɑpədʒɪ] n embryo. Ischiopagie f.
is·chi·o·per·i·ne·al [ɪskɪəʊˌperəˈniːəl] adj Sitzbein/Ischium u. Damm/Perineum betr., ischioperineal.
is·chi·o·pu·bic foramen [-ˈpjuːbɪk] For. obturatorium.
is·chi·o·rec·tal [-ˈrektl] adj Sitzbein/Ischium u. Rektum betr. od. verbindend, ischiorektal.
ischiorectal abscess ischiorektaler Abszeß m.
ischiorectal aponeurosis Fascia diaphragmatis pelvis inferior.
ischiorectal cavity → ischiorectal fossa.
ischiorectal fascia → ischiorectal aponeurosis.
ischiorectal fat pad Corpus adiposum fossae ischiorectalis.
ischiorectal fossa Fossa ischio-analis.
ischiorectal hernia Dammbruch m, Perineozele f, Hernia perinealis/ischiorectalis.
is·chi·o·sa·cral [-ˈsækrəl, -ˈseɪ-] adj Sitzbein/Ischium u. Kreuzbein/Os sacrale betr., ischiosakral.
is·chi·o·tho·ra·cop·a·gus [-ˌθɔːrəˈkɑpəgəs, -ˈθɔː-] n → iliothoracopagus.
is·chi·o·vag·i·nal [-ˈvædʒɪnl, -vəˈdʒaɪnl] adj Sitzbein/Ischium u. Scheide/Vagina betr., ischiovaginal.

is·chi·o·ver·te·bral [ˌ-ˈvɜrtəbrəl] *adj* Sitzbein/Ischium u. Wirbelsäule betr., ischiovertebral.
is·chi·um [ˈɪskɪəm] *n*, *pl* **-chia** [-kɪə] Sitzbein *nt*, Ischium *nt*, Os ischii.
is·cho·chy·mia [ˌɪskoʊˈkaɪmɪə] *n* (*Magen*) Ischochymie *f*.
is·chu·ret·ic [ˌɪskjəˈretɪk] *adj* Ischurie betr., ischurisch.
is·chu·ria [ɪsˈk(j)ʊərɪə] *n urol.* Harnverhalt *m*, -verhaltung *f*, -sperre *f*, Ischurie *f*, Ischuria *f*.
is·ei·co·nia [ˌaɪsaɪˈkoʊnɪə] *n* → isoiconia.
is·ei·con·ic [ˌ-ˈkɑnɪk] *adj* → isoiconic.
is·ei·ko·nia [ˌ-ˈkoʊnɪə] *n* → isoiconia.
is·ei·kon·ic lens [ˌ-ˈkɑnɪk] Aniseikoniglas *nt*.
ISF *abbr.* → interstitial fluid.
Is genes → immune suppressor genes.
Ishihara [ɪʃɪˈhɑːrə]: **I.'s test** *ophthal.* Ishihara-Test *m*.
is·land [ˈaɪlənd] *n* **1.** Insel *f*. **2.** *anat.* Insel *f*, isolierter Zellhaufen *od.* Gewebeverband *m*.
i.s of Langerhans Langerhans'-Inseln *pl*, endokrines Pankreas *nt*, Inselorgan *nt*, Pankreasinseln *pl*, Pars endocrina pancreatis.
i. of Reil Insel *f*, Inselrinde *f*, Insula *f*, Lobus insularis.
island disease → island fever.
island fever Tsutsugamushi-Fieber *m*, japanisches Fleckfieber *nt*, Milbenfleckfieber *nt*, Scrub-Typhus *m*.
island flap Insellappen *m*.
is·let [ˈaɪlɪt] *n* **1.** Inselchen *nt*. **2.** → island *1*.
i.s of Langerhans → islands of Langerhans.
islet-activating protein *old* → pertussis toxin.
islet adenoma → islet cell adenoma.
islet carcinoma → islet cell carcinoma.
islet cell adenoma Inselzelladenom *nt*, Adenoma insulocellulare, Nesidioblastom *nt*, Nesidiom *nt*.
islet cell carcinoma Inselzellkarzinom *nt*, Ca. insulocellulare.
islet cell hyperplasia Insel(zell)hyperplasie *f*.
islet cells Inselzellen *pl*, Zellen *pl* der Langerhans'-Inseln.
islet cell tumor Inselzelltumor *m*.
non-beta i. nicht-beta-Inselzelltumor.
islet hyperplasia → islet cell hyperplasia.
islet tissue → islands of Langerhans.
iso- *pref.* **1.** is(o)-, Is(o)-. **2.** *chem.* iso-.
i·so·ag·glu·ti·na·tion [ˌaɪsəəˌɡluːtəˈneɪʃn] *n* Isoagglutination *f*.
i·so·ag·glu·ti·nin [ˌ-əˈɡluːtənɪn] *n* Isoagglutinin *nt*.
i·so·al·lele [ˌ-əˈliːl] *n genet.* Isoallel *nt*.
i·so·al·lox·a·zine [ˌ-əˈlɑksəziːn] *n* Isoalloxazin *nt*.
i·so·am·yl·am·ine [ˌ-emɪlˈæmɪn] *n* Isoamylamin *nt*.
i·so·am·yl·eth·yl·bar·bi·tu·ric acid [ˌ-ˌæmɪlˌeθəlˌbɑːrbɪˈt(j)ʊərɪk] *pharm.* Amobarbital *nt*.
i·so·am·yl nitrite [ˌ-ˈæmɪl] Amylnitrit *nt*.
i·so·an·dros·ter·one [ˌ-ænˈdrɑstərən] *n* Iso-, Epiandrosteron *nt*.
i·so·an·ti·bod·y [ˌ-ˈæntɪbɑdɪ] *n* Allo-, Isoantikörper *m*.
i·so·an·ti·gen [ˌ-ˈæntɪdʒən] *n* Allo-, Isoantigen *nt*.
i·so·bam·ate [ˌ-ˈbæmeɪt] *n pharm.* Carisoprodol *m*.
i·so·bar [ˈ-bɑːr] *n* **1.** *chem.* Isobar *nt*. **2.** *phys.* Isobare *f*.
i·so·bar·ic [ˌ-ˈbærɪk] *adj* isobar.
i·so·bu·ta·nol [ˌ-ˈbjuːtnɒl, -əl] *n* Isobutanol *m*, Isobutylalkohol *m*.

i·so·bu·tyl alcohol [ˌ-ˈbjuːtɪl] → isobutanol.
i·so·bu·tyl·ene [ˌ-ˈbjuːtliːn] *n* Isobutylen *nt*.
i·so·bu·tyr·ic acid [ˌ-bjuːˈtɪrɪk] Isobuttersäure *f*.
i·so·ca·lor·ic [ˌ-kəˈlɔːrɪk] *adj* mit der selben Kalorienmenge, isokalorisch.
i·so·cel·lu·lar [ˌ-ˈseljələr] *adj* aus gleichartigen Zellen bestehend, isozellulär.
i·so·cho·les·ter·in [ˌ-kəˈlestərɪn] *n* Lanosterin *nt*.
i·so·cho·les·ter·ol [ˌ-kəˈlestərəʊl, -ɒl] *n* Lanosterin *nt*.
i·so·cho·ria [ˌ-ˈkoʊrɪə, -ˈkɔː-] *n ophthal.* gleiche Pupillenweite *f* beider Augen, Isokorie *f*.
i·so·chor·ic [ˌ-ˈkɔːrɪk, -ˈkəʊr-] *adj* → isovolumic.
i·so·chro·mat·ic [ˌ-krəʊˈmætɪk] *adj* isochrom, isochromatisch, farbtonrichtig, gleichfarbig; gleichmäßig gefärbt.
i·so·chro·mat·o·phil [ˌ-krəˈmætəfɪl, -ˈkrəʊmətə-] *adj histol.* isochromatophil.
i·so·chro·mic anemia [ˌ-ˈkrəʊmɪk] normochrome Anämie *f*.
i·so·chro·mo·some [ˌ-ˈkrəʊməsəʊm] *n* Isochromosom *nt*.
i·soch·ro·nal [aɪˈsɑkrənl] *adj* → isochronous.
i·so·chro·nia [ˌaɪsəˈkrəʊnɪə] *n* **1.** *physiol.* Isochronaxie *f*. **2.** *phys.* Isochronismus *m*.
i·so·chron·ic [ˌ-ˈkrɑnɪk] *adj* → isochronous.
i·soch·ro·nism [aɪˈsɑkrənɪzəm] *n* → isochronia.
i·soch·ro·nous [aɪˈsɑkrənəs] *adj* gleich lang dauernd, von gleicher Dauer, isochron.
i·soch·ro·ous [aɪˈsɑkrəʊəs] *adj* isochromatic.
i·so·ci·trase [ˌaɪsəˈsɪtreɪz] *n* → isocitrate lyase.
i·so·cit·ra·tase [ˌ-ˈsɪtrəteɪz] *n* → isocitrate lyase.
i·so·cit·rate [ˌ-ˈsaɪtreɪt, -ˈsɪt-] *n* Isocitrat *nt*, Isozitrat *nt*.
isocitrate dehydrogenase Isozitrat-, Isocitratdehydrogenase *f abbr.* ICD, IDH.
NADP-specific i. → isocitrate dehydrogenase (NADP+).
NAD-specific i. → isocitrate dehydrogenase (NAD+).
isocitrate dehydrogenase (NAD+) NAD-spezifische Isocitratdehydrogenase *f*.
isocitrate dehydrogenase (NADP+) NADP-spezifische Isocitratdehydrogenase *f*.
isocitrate lyase Isozitrat-, Isocitratlyase *f*.
i·so·cit·ric acid [ˌ-ˈsɪtrɪk] Isocitronen-, Isozitronensäure *f*.
isocitric acid dehydrogenase → isocitrate dehydrogenase.
i·so·cit·ri·tase [ˌ-ˈsɪtrəteɪz] *n* → isocitrate lyase.
i·so·col·loid [ˌ-ˈkɑlɔɪd] *n* Isokolloid *nt*.
i·so·co·na·zole [ˌ-ˈkɑnəzəʊl] *n pharm.* Isoconazol *nt*.
i·so·cor·tex [ˌ-ˈkɔːrteks] *n* **1.** Isokortex *m*, -cortex *m*. **2.** Neokortex *m*, Neocortex *m*.
i·so·cy·a·nate asthma [ˌ-ˈsaɪəneɪt, -nɪt] Isozyanatasthma *nt*.
i·so·cy·an·ic acid [ˌ-saɪˈænɪk] Isocyansäure *f*.
i·so·cy·a·nide [ˌ-ˈsaɪənaɪd, -nɪd] *n* Isocyanid *nt*, Isonitril *nt*.
i·so·cy·clic [ˌ-ˈsaɪklɪk, -ˈsɪk-] *adj chem.* iso-, homozyklisch.
isocyclic compound *chem.* isozyklische Verbindung *f*.
isocyclic ring isozyklische/homozyklische Ringstruktur *f*.

i·so·cy·tol·y·sin [ˌ-saɪˈtɑləsɪn] *n* Isozytolysin *nt*.
i·so·cy·to·sis [ˌ-saɪˈtəʊsɪs] *n hema.* Isozytose *f*.
i·so·dac·ty·lism [ˌ-ˈdæktəlɪzəm] *n ortho.* Isodaktylie *f*.
i·so·des·mo·sine [ˌ-ˈdezməsiːn] *n* Isodesmosin *nt*.
i·so·dis·per·soid [ˌ-dɪsˈpɜrsɔɪd] *n* → isocolloid.
i·so·don·tic [ˌ-ˈdɑntɪk] *adj dent.* isodont(isch).
i·so·dose [ˈ-dəʊs] *n radiol.* Isodose *f*.
isodose curve Isodose(nkurve *f*) *f*.
i·so·dul·cite [ˌ-ˈdʌlsaɪt] *n* Isodulcit *nt*, Rhamnose *f*.
i·so·dy·nam·ic [ˌ-daɪˈnæmɪk] *adj* isodynamisch.
isodynamic effect isodynamischer Effekt *m*, Isodynamie *f*.
i·so·dy·na·mo·gen·ic [ˌ-ˌdaɪnəməʊˈdʒenɪk] *adj* isodynamogen.
i·so·e·lec·tric [ˌ-ɪˈlektrɪk] *adj* isoelektrisch.
isoelectric EEG → isoelectric electroencephalogram.
isoelectric electroencephalogram *neuro.* Null-Linien-EEG *nt*, isoelektrisches Elektroenzephalogramm *nt*.
isoelectric focusing *immun.*, *lab.* Elektrofokussierung *f*, isoelektrische Fokussierung *f*.
isoelectric line isoelektrische Linie *f*.
isoelectric period *card.* (*EKG*) isoelektrische Periode *f*.
isoelectric point *abbr.* **IP** isoelektrischer Punkt *m abbr.* IP.
isoelectric precipitation isoelektrische Ausfällung/Präzipitation *f*.
isoelectric zone isoelektrische Zone *f*.
i·so·e·lec·tro·en·ceph·a·lo·gram [ˌ-ɪˌlektrəʊenˈsefələɡræm] *n neuro.* Null-Linien--EEG *nt*, isoelektrisches Elektroenzephalogramm *nt*.
i·so·en·er·get·ic [ˌ-ˌenərˈdʒetɪk] *adj* mit gleicher Energie, isoenergetisch.
i·so·en·zyme [ˌ-ˈenzaɪm] *n* Iso(en)zym *nt*.
i·so·eth·a·rine [ˌ-ˈeθəriːn] *n pharm.* Isoetarin *nt*.
i·so·flu·rane [ˌ-ˈflʊəreɪn] *n anes.* Isoflu(o)ran *nt*.
i·so·flur·o·phate [ˌ-ˈflʊərəfeɪt] *n* Diisopropylfluorphosphat *nt abbr.* DFP, Fluostigmin *nt*.
i·sog·a·me [aɪˈsɑɡəmɪ] *n* → isogamy.
i·so·gam·ete [ˌaɪsəˈɡæmiːt] *n* Isogamet *m*.
i·so·ga·met·ic [ˌ-ɡəˈmetɪk] *adj* isogametisch, Isogameten-.
i·sog·a·mous [aɪˈsɑɡəməs] *adj* Isogamie betr., isogam.
i·sog·a·my [aɪˈsɑɡəmɪ] *n* Isogamie *f*.
i·so·ge·ne·ic [ˌaɪsədʒəˈniːɪk] *adj genet.* isogen(etisch), syngen(etisch).
isogeneic antigen → isoantigen.
isogeneic graft → isograft.
isogeneic homograft → isograft.
isogeneic transplantation → isotransplantation.
i·so·gen·e·sis [ˌ-ˈdʒenəsɪs] *n embryo.* Übereinstimmung *f* der Entwicklung, Isogenese *f*.
i·so·gen·ic [ˌ-ˈdʒenɪk] *adj* → isogeneic.
i·so·gen·o·mat·ic [ˌ-dʒenəˈmætɪk] *adj* → isogenomatisch.
i·so·ge·nom·ic [ˌ-dʒɪˈnɑmɪk] *adj* → isogenomatic.
i·so·glu·tam·ic acid [ˌ-ɡluːˈtæmɪk] Isoglutaminsäure *f*.
i·so·glu·ta·mine [ˌ-ˈɡluːtəmiːn, -mɪn] *n* Isoglutamin *nt*.
i·so·graft [ˈ-ɡræft] *n* isologes/isogenes/syngenes/syngenetisches/isogenetisches Transplantat *nt*, Isotransplantat *nt*.

isohemagglutination

i·so·hem·ag·glu·ti·na·tion [ˌ-hiːməˌgluːtɪn-'eɪʃn, -ˌheməʔ-] n Iso(häm)agglutination f.
i·so·hem·ag·glu·ti·nin [ˌ-hiːməˈgluːtɪnɪn, -ˌheməʔ-] n Iso(häm)agglutinin nt.
i·so·he·mol·y·sin [ˌ-hɪˈmæləsɪn] n Isohämolysin nt.
i·so·he·mol·y·sis [ˌ-hɪˈmæləsɪs] n Isohämolyse f.
i·so·he·mo·lyt·ic [ˌ-hiːməˈlɪtɪk, -ˌhem-] adj Isohämolyse betr., durch Isohämolyse gekennzeichnet, isohämolytisch.
i·so·hy·dria [ˌ-ˈhaɪdrɪə] n physiol. Isohydrie f.
i·so·hy·dric [ˌ-ˈhaɪdrɪk] adj physiol. isohydrisch.
isohydric cycle isohydrischer Zyklus m.
i·so·i·co·nia [ˌ-aɪˈkəʊnɪə] n ophthal. Isoikonie f.
i·so·i·con·ic [ˌ-aɪˈkɑnɪk] adj ophthal. Isoikonie betr., isoikon(isch).
i·so·im·mu·ni·za·tion [ˌ-ˌɪmjənɪˈzeɪʃn] n Iso-, Alloimmunisierung f.
i·so·i·on·ic [ˌ-aɪˈɑnɪk] adj isoionisch.
isoionic point isoionischer Punkt m.
i·so·late [n ˈaɪsəlɪt, -leɪt; v -leɪt] I n bio., micro. Isolat nt. II vt 1. (a. chem., phys.) absondern, isolieren (from von). 2. fig. isoliert od. getrennt betrachten; trennen (from von).
i·so·lat·ed [ˈ-leɪtɪd] adj 1. abgesondert, abgetrennt, isoliert. 2. einzeln, vereinzelt, Einzel-. 3. chem., phys. isoliert.
isolated hypoaldosteronism isolierter/selektiver Hypoaldosteronismus m.
i·so·la·tion [ˌ-ˈleɪʃn] n 1. Abtrennen nt, Isolieren nt; Abtrennung f, Isolation f. 2. Absonderung f, Getrennthaltung f, Isolierung f, Isolation f. 3. psychia. (Affekt-)Isolierung f.
isolation ward Isolierabteilung f, -station f.
i·so·la·tor [ˈ-leɪtər] n Isoliermaterial nt; Isolator m.
i·so·lec·i·thal [ˌ-ˈlesɪθəl] adj embryo., bio. isolezithal.
isolecithal ovum bio. isolezithales Ei nt.
i·so·leu·cine [ˌ-ˈluːsiːn, -sɪn] n abbr. I, Ile Isoleucin nt abbr. I, Ile.
i·so·leu·ko·ag·glu·ti·nin [ˌ-ˌluːkəəˈgluːtənɪn] n (natürliches) Leukozytenagglutinin nt.
i·sol·o·gous [aɪˈsɑləgəs] adj genetisch-identisch, artgleich, isolog, homolog; syngen(etisch), isogen(etisch).
isologous graft → isograft.
isologous transplantation → isotransplantation.
i·sol·y·sin [aɪˈsɑləsɪn] n Isolysin nt.
i·sol·y·sis [aɪˈsɑləsɪs] n Isolyse f.
i·so·lyt·ic [ˌaɪsəˈlɪtɪk] adj Isolyse betr., isolytisch.
i·so·malt·ase [ˌ-ˈmɔːlteɪz] n α-Dextrinase f, Oligo-1,6-α-glukosidase f.
i·so·malt·ose [ˌ-ˈmɔːltəʊs] n Isomaltose f, Dextrinose f.
i·so·mas·ti·gote [ˌ-ˈmæstɪgəʊt] n Isomastigote f.
i·so·mer [ˈ-mər] n Isomer(e) nt.
i·som·er·ase [aɪˈsɑmərеɪz] n Isomerase f.
i·so·mer·ic [ˌ-ˈmerɪk] adj Isomerie betr. od. zeigend, isomer.
i·som·er·ide [aɪˈsɑməraɪd] n → isomer.
i·som·er·ism [aɪˈsɑmərɪzəm] n Isomerie f.
i·som·er·i·za·tion [aɪˌsɑməraɪˈzeɪʃn] n Isomerenbildung f, Isomerisation f.
i·som·er·ize [aɪˈsɑməraɪz] vt isomerisieren.
i·som·er·ous [aɪˈsɑmərəs] adj → isomeric.
i·so·meth·ep·tene [ˌaɪsəˈmeθeptiːn] n pharm. Isomethepten nt.
i·so·met·ric [ˌ-ˈmetrɪk] adj physiol. bei konstanter Länge, isometrisch.
isometric contraction isometrische Kontraktion f.
isometric period card. isometrische Kontraktionsphase f, Phase f der isometrischen Anspannung.
i·so·me·tro·pia [ˌ-mɪˈtrəʊpɪə] n ophthal. Gleichsichtigkeit/Refraktionsgleichheit f beider Augen, Isometropie f.
i·som·e·try [aɪˈsɑmətrɪ] n Längenkonstanz f, Isometrie f.
i·so·mor·phic [ˌaɪsəˈmɔːrfɪk] adj → isomorphous.
isomorphic effect Koebner-Phänomen nt, isomorpher Reizeffekt m.
isomorphic gliosis isomorphe Gliose f.
isomorphic response → isomorphic effect.
i·so·mor·phism [ˌ-ˈmɔːrfɪzəm] n histol. Gleichgestaltigkeit f, Isomorphie f, Isomorphismus m.
i·so·mor·phous [ˌ-ˈmɔːrfəs] adj gleichgestaltig, von gleicher Form u. Gestalt, isomorph.
i·so·naph·thol [ˌ-ˈnæfθɒl, -θɑl] n Betanaphthol nt, β-Naphthol nt.
i·so·ni·a·zid [ˌaɪsəˈnaɪəzɪd] n pharm. Isoniazid nt, Isonicotinsäurehydrazid nt abbr. INH, Pyridin-4-carbonsäurehydrazid nt.
isoniazid neuropathy Isoniazidneuropathie f, INH-Polyneuropathie f.
i·so·nic·o·tin·ic acid [ˌ-ˌnɪkəˈtɪnɪk] Isonicotinsäure f, Isonicotinsäure f.
isonicotinic acid hydrazide abbr. **INH** → isoniazid.
i·so·nic·o·ti·no·yl·hy·dra·zine [ˌ-ˌnɪkəˈtiːnəwɪlˈhaɪdrəziːn] n → isoniazid.
i·so·nic·o·ti·nyl·hy·dra·zine [ˌ-ˌnɪkəˈtiːnɪlˈhaɪdrəziːn] n → isoniazid.
i·so·ni·tril [ˌ-ˈnaɪtrɪl] n → isocyanide.
iso-oncotic adj physiol. iso(o)nkotisch.
iso-osmotic adj iso(o)smotisch.
i·so·par·or·chis [ˌaɪsəpɑːrˈɔːrkɪs] n micro. Isoparorchis m.
i·sop·a·thy [aɪˈsɑpəθɪ] n Isopathie f.
i·so·pen·te·nyl-diphosphate δ-isomerase [ˌaɪsəˈpentənɪl] → isopentenyl pyrophosphate isomerase.
isopentenyl pyrophosphate Isopentenylpyrophosphat nt, aktives Isopren nt.
isopentenyl pyrophosphate isomerase Isopentenylpyrophosphatisomerase f.
3-isopentenyl pyrophosphoric acid 3-Isopentenylpyrophosphorsäure f.
i·so·per·i·stal·tic anastomosis [ˌ-ˌperɪˈstɒltɪk, -ˈstæl-, -ˈstɑːl-] chir. isoperistaltische (Entero-)Anastomose/Enterostomie f.
i·soph·a·gy [aɪˈsɑfədʒɪ] n Selbstauflösung f, Autolyse f; Selbstverdauung f, Autodigestion f.
i·so·phil antibody [ˈaɪsəfɪl] isophiler Antikörper m.
i·so·phile antigen [ˈ-faɪl] Allo-, Isoantigen nt.
i·so·phone [ˈ-fəʊn] n Isophone f.
i·so·pho·ria [ˌ-ˈfəʊrɪə] n ophthal. Isophorie f.
i·so·pia [aɪˈsəʊpɪə] n ophthal. gleiche Sehschärfe f beider Augen, Isopie f.
i·so·plas·tic graft [ˌaɪsəˈplæstɪk] → isograft.
i·so·pleth [ˈ-pleθ] n phys. Isoplethe f.
i·so·po·ten·tial line [ˌ-pəˈtenʃl] Isopotentiallinie f.
i·so·pre·cip·i·tin [ˌ-prɪˈsɪpətɪn] n Isopräzipitin nt.
i·so·pren·a·line [ˌ-ˈprenəliːn] n pharm. Isoprenalin nt, Isoproterenol nt, Isopropylnoradrenalin nt.
i·so·prene [ˈ-priːn] n Isopren nt, 2-Methyl-1,3-butadien nt.
isoprene unit Isopreneinheit f.
i·so·pren·oid [ˌ-ˈpriːnɔɪd] n Isoprenoid nt.
isoprenoid alcohol → isoprenol.
i·so·pre·nol [ˌ-ˈprenɒl, -əʊl] n Isoprenol nt, Isoprenoidalkohol m.
i·so·pro·pa·mide iodide [ˌ-ˈprəʊpəmaɪd] pharm. Isopropamidjodid nt.
i·so·pro·pa·nol [ˌ-ˈprəʊpənɒl, -nɑl] n Isopropanol nt, Isopropylalkohol m.
i·so·pro·pyl alcohol [ˌ-ˈprəʊpɪl] → isopropanol.
isopropyl-aminacetic acid Valin nt abbr. Val, α-Aminoisovaleriansäure f.
i·so·pro·pyl·ar·ter·e·nol [ˌ-ˌprəʊpɪlˌɑːrˈterənɒl, -nɑːl] n → isoprenaline.
i·so·pro·pyl·car·bi·nol [ˌ-ˌprəʊpɪlˈkɑːrbɪnɒl, -nɑːl] n → isopropanol.
isopropyl malate Isopropylmalat nt.
α-isopropyl malate dehydratase α-Isopropylmalatdehydratase f.
α-isopropyl malate dehydrogenase α-Isopropylmalatdehydrogenase f.
α-isopropyl malate synthase α-Isopropylmalatsynthase f.
isopropyl malic acid Isopropyläpfelsäure f.
isopropyl meprobamate pharm. Carisoprodol nt.
isopropyl thiogalactoside abbr. **IPTG** Isopropylthiogalaktosid nt abbr. IPTG.
i·so·pro·ter·e·nol [ˌ-ˌprəʊˈterənɒl, -nɑːl] → isoprenaline.
i·sop·ter [aɪˈsɑptər] n ophthal. Isoptere f.
i·so·pyk·nic [ˌ-ˈpɪknɪk] adj von gleicher Dichte od. Dicke.
i·so·quin·o·line [ˌ-ˈkwɪnəliːn, -lɪn] n Isochinolin nt.
i·sor·rhea [ˌ-ˈrɪə] n physiol. Flüssigkeitshomöostase f, Isorrhoe f.
i·so·sen·si·ti·za·tion [ˌ-ˌsensətɪˈzeɪʃn, -taɪ-] n Allo-, Isosensitivierung f.
i·so·ser·ine [ˌ-ˈseriːn, -ˌsɪər-, -ɪn] n Isoserin nt.
i·so·se·rum treatment [ˌ-ˈsɪərəm] Iso(immun)serumbehandlung f.
i·so·sex·u·al [ˌ-ˈsekʃəwəl] adj gleichgeschlechtlich, isosexuell.
is·os·mot·ic [aɪsɑzˈmɒtɪk] adj → iso-osmotic.
is·os·mot·ic·i·ty [aɪsɑzməˈtɪsətɪ] n Iso(o)smie f.
isosmotic swelling patho. albuminöse/albuminoide/albuminoid-körnige Degeneration f, trübe Schwellung f.
i·so·sor·bide dinitrate [ˌaɪsəˈsɔːrbaɪd] pharm. Isosorbiddinitrat nt abbr. ISDN.
Isos·po·ra [aɪˈsɑspərə] pl micro. Isospora pl.
i·so·spore [ˈaɪsəspʊər, -spɔːr] n micro. Isospore f.
isos·po·ri·a·sis [aɪˌsɑspəˈraɪəsɪs] n Isosporainfektion f, Isoporiasis f, Isosporose f.
i·so·spo·ro·sis [ˌaɪsəspəˈrəʊsɪs] n → isosporiasis.
i·so·spo·rous [aɪˈsɑspərəs] adj iso-, homospor.
i·sos·po·ry [aɪˈsɑspərɪ, ˈaɪsəspʊrɪ] n Gleichsporigkeit f, Iso-, Homosporie f.
i·so·stere [ˈaɪsəstɪər] n Isoster(es) nt.
i·sos·the·nu·ria [aɪsəsθɪˈn(j)ʊərɪə] n Harnstarre f, Isosthenurie f.
i·so·ther·a·py [ˌaɪsəˈθerəpɪ] n → isopathy.
i·so·therm [ˈ-θɜːrm] n Isotherme f.
i·so·ther·mal [ˈ-θɜːrml] adj bei konstanter Temperatur verlaufend, gleichwarm, isotherm.
isothermal line Isotherme f.
i·so·ther·mic [ˌ-ˈθɜːrmɪk] adj → isothermal.
i·so·thi·o·cy·a·nate [ˌ-ˌθaɪəʊˈsaɪəneɪt] n Isothiocyanat nt.
i·so·thi·o·cy·an·ic acid [ˌ-ˌθaɪəsaɪˈænɪk] Isothiozyansäure f.

i·so·thi·pen·dyl [ˌ-θaɪˈpendɪl] *n pharm.* Isothipendyl *nt*.
i·so·tone [ˈ-təʊn] *n phys.* Isoton *nt*.
i·so·to·nia [ˌ-ˈtəʊnɪə] *n* Isotonie *f*.
i·so·ton·ic [ˌ-ˈtɒnɪk] *adj* isoton(isch).
isotonic contraction isotonische Kontraktion *f*.
isotonic dehydration isotone Dehydra(ta)tion *f*.
isotonic hyperhydration isotone Hyperhydratation *f*.
i·so·to·nic·i·ty [ˌ-təˈnɪsətɪ] *n* Isotonie *f*, Isotonizität *f*.
isotonic saline isotone (Koch-)Salzlösung *f*.
i·so·tope [ˈ-təʊp] *n phys.* Isotop *nt*.
isotope clearance Radioisotopenclearance *f*.
i·so·top·ic [ˌ-ˈtɒpɪk] *adj phys.* Isotop betr., isotop, Isotopen-.
isotopic labeling Isotopenmarkierung *f*.
isotopic number *phys., chem.* Isotopenzahl *f*.
isotopic scan Radionuklid-Scan *m*.
i·sot·o·py [aɪˈsɒtəpɪ] *n phys.* Isotopie *f*.
i·so·trans·plant [ˌaɪsəˈtrænzplænt] *n* → isograft.
i·so·trans·plan·ta·tion [ˌ-ˌtrænzplænˈteɪʃn] *n* isologe/isogene/isogenetische/syngene/syngenetische Transplantation *f*, Isotransplantation *f*.
i·so·tron [ˈ-trɒn] *n phys.* Isotron *nt*.
i·so·trop·ic [ˌ-ˈtrɒpɪk, -ˈtrəʊ-] *adj* **1.** *phys.* einfachbrechend, isotrop. **2.** *chem., phys.* Isotropie betr., isotrop.
isotropic band I-Bande *f*, I-Streifen *m*, I-Zone *f*, isotrope Bande *f*.
isotropic disk → isotropic band.
i·sot·ro·pous [aɪˈsɒtrəpəs] *adj* → isotropic.
i·sot·ro·py [aɪˈsɒtrəpɪ] *n phys.* Isotropie *f*.
i·so·type [ˈ-taɪp] *n immun.* Isotyp *m*.
i·so·typ·ic [ˌ-ˈtɪpɪk] *adj* Isotypie *od.* Isotypen betr., isotypisch.
isotypic variation isotypische Variation *f*.
i·sot·y·py [aɪˈsɒtɪpɪ] *n immun.* Isotypie *f*.
i·so·va·ler·ic acid [ˌaɪsəvəˈlerɪk, -ˈlɪər-] Isovaleriansäure *f*.
isovaleric acid-CoA dehydrogenase → isovaleryl-CoA dehydrogenase.
isovaleric acid-CoA dehydrogenase deficiency → isovalericacidemia.
i·so·va·ler·ic·ac·i·de·mia [ˌ-vəˌlerɪkˌæsəˈdiːmɪə] *n* Isovalerianazidämie *f*.
i·so·val·er·yl-CoA dehydrogenase [ˌ-ˈvæl-ərɪl] Isovaleryl-CoA-dehydrogenase *f*.
i·so·vol·u·met·ric [ˌ-ˌvaljəˈmetrɪk] *adj* → isovolumic.
isovolumetric contraction isovolumetrische Kontraktion *f*.
i·so·vol·u·mia [ˌ-vɒlˈjuːmɪə] *n physiol.* Volumenkonstanz *f*, Isovolämie *f*.
i·so·vol·u·mic [ˌ-vɒlˈjuːmɪk] *adj* bei *od.* mit konstantem Volumen, isovolumetrisch, isochor.
i·sox·a·zo·lyl penicillins [aɪˌsɒksəˈzəʊlɪl] *pharm.* Isoxazolyl-Penicilline *pl*.
i·sox·i·cam [aɪˈsɒksɪkæm] *n pharm.* Isoxicam *nt*.
i·sox·su·prine [aɪˈsɒksəpriːn] *n pharm.* Isoxsuprin *nt*.
i·so·zyme [ˈaɪsəzaɪm] *n* Iso(en)zym *nt*.
is·sue [ˈɪʃuː, *Brit.* ˈɪsjuː] *n* **1.** *patho.*

(Eiter-, Blut-, Serum-)Ausfluß *m*. **2.** *patho.* eiterndes Geschwür *nt*. **3.** Ausgang *m*, Ergebnis *nt*, Resultat *nt*, Schluß *m*. **4.** (*Buch, Zeitschrift*) (Her-)Ausgabe *f*, Veröffentlichung *f*, Auflage *f*; Ausgabe *f*, Nummer *f*. **5.** Streitfrage *f*, -punkt *m*. **II** *vt* (*Buch, Zeitung*) herausgeben, veröffentlichen, auflegen, publizieren. **III** *vi* **6.** herausstrüren, -brechen. **7.** herausfließen, -strömen. **8.** (*Buch*) herauskommen, herausgegeben werden.
IST *abbr.* → insulin shock therapy.
isth·mec·to·my [ɪs(θ)ˈmektəmɪ] *n chir.* Isthmusresektion *f*, Isthmektomie *f*.
isth·mi·an [ˈɪs(θ)mɪən] *adj* → isthmic.
isth·mic [ˈɪs(θ)mɪk] *adj* Isthmus betr., Isthmus-, Isthmo-.
isth·mi·tis [ɪs(θ)ˈmaɪtɪs] *n HNO* Entzündung *f* der Schlundenge, Isthmitis *f*.
isth·mo·pa·ral·y·sis [ˌɪs(θ)məpəˈræləsɪs] *n* → isthmoplegia.
isth·mo·ple·gia [ˌ-ˈpliːdʒ(ɪ)ə] *n HNO* Schlundlähmung *f*, Isthmoplegie *f*.
isth·mo·spasm [ˈ-spæzəm] *n* Isthmospasmus *m*.
isth·mus [ˈɪs(θ)məs] *n, pl* **-mus·es, -mi** [-maɪ] schmale enge Verbindung *f*, Verengung *f*, Enge *f*, Isthmus *m*.
i. of aorta Aortenisthmus, Isthmus aortae.
i. of auditory tube Tubenenge, -isthmus, Isthmus tubae auditoriae.
i. of auricular cartilage Isthmus cartilaginis auricularis.
i. of cingulate gyrus Isthmus gyri cinguli, Isthmus cingulatus.
i. of eustachian tube → i. of auditory tube.
i. of fallopian tube → i. of uterine tube.
i. of fauces Schlund-, Rachenenge, Isthmus faucium.
i. of His *embryo.* Isthmus rhombencephali.
i. of limbic lobe → i. of cingulate gyrus.
i. of prostate (gland) Prostataisthmus, Isthmus prostatae.
i. of rhombencephalon *embryo.* Isthmus rhombencephali.
i. of thyroid (gland) Schilddrüsenisthmus, Isthmus gl. thyroideae.
i. of urethra Harnröhrenenge, -isthmus, Isthmus urethrae.
i. of uterine tube Tubenisthmus, -enge, Isthmus tubae uterinae.
i. of uterus Gebärmutter-, Uterusisthmus, Isthmus uteri.
isthmus stenosis *card.* Aortenisthmusstenose *f*, Coarctatio aortae.
i·su·ria [aɪˈs(j)ʊərɪə] *n urol., neuro.* Isurie *f*.
I-tai-Itai disease [ˈaɪtaɪ] Itai-Itai-Krankheit *f*.
I·tal·ian [ɪˈtæljən]: **I. flap** Fernplastik *f*.
I. operation *HNO* italienische Methode/Rhinoplastik *f*.
I. rhinoplasty → I. operation.
itch [ɪtʃ] **I** *n* **1.** Jucken *nt*, Juckreiz *m*; Pruritus *m*. **2.** *med.* Krätze *f*, Scabies *f*. **II** *vt* jdn. jucken, kratzen. **III** *vi* jucken.
itch·i·ness [ˈɪtʃɪnɪs] *n* → itch 1.
itch·ing [ˈɪtʃɪŋ] **I** *n* → itch 1. **II** *adj* juckend, Juck-.
itching powder Juckpulver *nt*.

itching purpura ekzematidartige Purpura *f*, epidemische purpurisch-lichenoide Dermatitis *f*, disseminierte pruriginöse Angiodermatitis *f*.
itch mite *micro.* Krätzmilbe *f*, Sarcoptes/Acarus scabiei.
itch point *physiol.* Juckpunkt *m*.
itch·y [ˈɪtʃɪ] *adj* **1.** → itching II. **2.** krätzig.
it·er [ˈɪtɪər, ˈaɪtɪər] *n anat.* (Verbindungs-)-Gang *m*.
it·er·ance [ˈɪtərəns] *n* → iteration.
it·er·ant [ˈɪtərənt] *adj* s. wiederholend.
it·er·ate [ˈɪtəreɪt] *vt* wiederholen.
it·er·a·tion [ɪtəˈreɪʃn] *n* **1.** Wiederholung *f*. **2.** *psychia.* Iteration *f*. **3.** *mathe.* Iteration *f*.
it·er·a·tive [ˈɪtəreɪtɪv, ˈɪtərətɪv] *adj* **1.** (s.) wiederholend, verdoppelnd, iterativ. **2.** *mathe.* iterativ.
ith·y·cy·phos [ˌɪθəˈsaɪfəʊs] *n* → ithyokyphosis.
ith·y·lor·do·sis [ˌ-lɔːrˈdəʊsɪs] *n ortho.* Ithy(o)lordose *f*, -lordosis *f*.
ith·y·ky·pho·sis [ɪθɪkaɪˈfəʊsɪs] *n ortho.* Ithyokyphose *f*, -kyphosis *f*.
Ito [ˈiːtəʊ]: **I. cells** Ito-Zellen *pl*.
hypomelanosis of I. Incontinentia pigmenti achromians (Ito).
I.'s nevus deltoido-akromiale Melanozytose *f*, Nävus Ito *m*, Naevus fuscocoeruleus/acromiodeltoideus/deltoideoacromialis.
Ito-Reenstierna [riːnˈstɪərnə]: **I.-R. reaction/test** Ito-Reenstierna-Reaktion *f*.
ITP *abbr.* → idiopathic thrombocytopenic purpura. **2.** inosine triphosphate.
I-transferase *n* Jodtransferase *f*.
I.U. *abbr.* → international unit.
IUCD *abbr.* → intrauterine contraceptive device.
IUD *abbr.* → intrauterine device.
131I uptake test Radiojodtest *m*.
I.V., i.v. *abbr.* → intravenous II.
i.v. drug abuser Fixer *m*.
Ivemark [ˈaɪvmɑːrk]: **I.'s syndrome** Ivemark-Syndrom *nt*.
IVGTT *abbr.* → intravenous glucose tolerance test.
i·vo·ry bones [ˈaɪvərɪ, ˈaɪvrɪ] Marmorknochenkrankheit *f*, Albers-Schönberg-Krankheit *f*, Osteopetrosis *f*.
ivory vertebra *radiol., ortho.* Elfenbeinwirbel *m*.
IVP *abbr.* → intravenous pyelogram.
Iwanoff [ˈɪwænɒf]: **I.'s cysts** *ophthal.* Blessig-Zysten *pl*.
Ix·o·des [ɪkˈsəʊdiːz] *n micro.* Ixodes *m*.
ix·o·di·a·sis [ˌɪksəʊˈdaɪəsɪs] *n* **1.** Ixodiasis *f*. **2.** Zeckenbefall *m*. **3.** durch Zecken übertragene Krankheit *f*.
ix·od·ic [ɪkˈsɒdɪk, -ˈsəʊd-] *adj* durch Zecken übertragen *od.* verursacht, Zecken-.
Ix·od·i·dae [ɪkˈsɒdədiː] *pl micro.* Schild-, Holzzecken *pl*, Holzböcke *pl*, Ixodidae *pl*.
ix·od·i·des [ɪkˈsɒdədiːz] *pl micro.* Zecken *pl*, Ixodides *pl*.
ix·o·diph·a·gus [ˌɪksəˈdɪfəɡəs] *n micro.* Ixodiphagus *m*.
ix·o·dism [ˈɪksədɪzəm] *n* → ixodiasis.
Ix·o·doi·dea [ˌɪksəˈdɔɪdɪə] *pl micro.* Ixodoidea *pl*.

J

J abbr. → joule.
jab [dʒæb] **I** n **1.** Stich m, Stoß m. **2.** inf. Spritze f, Injektion f; Impfung f. **II** vt (hinein-)stechen, (hinein-)stoßen (into in). **III** vi stechen, stoßen (at nach; with mit).
Jaboulay [ʒabu'lɛ]: **J.'s amputation** Jaboulay-Amputation f, -Operation f, -Hemipelvektomie f.
J.'s method HTG Jaboulay-Methode f, Jaboulay-Brian-Methode f.
J.'s operation → J.'s amputation.
J.'s pyloroplasty Pyloroplastik f nach Jaboulay.
Jaccoud [ʒa'ku]: **J.'s sign/syndrome** Jaccoud-Zeichen nt.
jack-et ['dʒækɪt] **I** n **1.** Jacke f, Jacket nt. **2.** techn. Mantel m, Ummantelung f, Umhüllung f, Umwicklung f, Hülle f, Verkleidung f. **3.** phys. Hülle f, Hülse f. **II** vt **4.** (mit einer Jacke) bekleiden. **5.** techn. ummanteln, verkleiden.
jacket cancer Panzerkrebs m, Cancer en cuirasse.
jacket crown dent. Jacketkrone f.
jack-knife position ['dʒæknaɪf] chir. Klappmesserposition f, Jackknife-Lagerung f.
Jackson ['dʒæksən]: **J.'s law** Jackson-Gesetz nt.
J.'s syndrome Jackson-Syndrom nt, -Lähmung f.
jack-so-ni-an epilepsy [dʒæk'səʊnɪən] Jackson-Epilepsie f.
Jacob ['dʒeɪkəb]: **J.'s membrane** Schicht f der Stäbchen u. Zapfen, Stratum neuroepitheliale retinae.
Jacob-Monod [ʒa'kɔ mɔ'nɔ]: **J.-M. hypothesis/model** Jacob-Monod-Hypothese f, -Modell nt.
Jacobson [dʒeɪkəbsən]: **J.'s canal** Canaliculus tympanicus.
J.'s cartilage Jacobson'-Knorpel m, Cartilago vomeronasalis.
J.'s nerve N. tympanicus.
J.'s organ Jacobson'-Organ nt, Vomeronasalorgan nt, Organum vomeronasale.
J.'s plexus Jacobson'-Plexus m, Plexus tympanicus.
J.'s retinitis Retinitis syphilitica.
J.'s sulcus 1. Sulcus promontorii. **2.** Sulcus tympanicus.
Jacod [ʒa'kɔ]: **J.'s syndrome** Jacod-Syndrom nt, -Trias f, Jacod-Negri-Syndrom nt, petrosphenoidales Syndrom f.
Jacquet [ʒa'kɛ]: **J.'s dermatitis/erythema** Windeldermatitis f, posterosives Syphiloid nt, Dermatitis ammoniacalis, Dermatitis glutaealis infantum, Erythema glutaeale, Erythema papulosum posterosivum.
jac-ta-tio [dʒæk'teɪʃɪəʊ] n → jactitation.
jac-ta-tion [dʒæk'teɪʃn] n → jactitation.
jac-ti-ta-tion [ˌdʒæktɪ'teɪʃn] n neuro. Jaktation f, Jactatio f.
Jadassohn ['ja:dazo:n]: **nevus sebaceus of J.** Talgdrüsennävus Jadassohn m, Nävo-

lipom nt, Naevus sebaceus/lipomatosus.
Jadassohn-Lewandowsky [levən'davski]: **J.-L. syndrome** Jadassohn-Lewandowsky-Syndrom nt, Pachyonychie-Syndrom nt, Pachyonychia congenita.
Jadassohn-Tièche [tjɛʃ]: **J.-T. nevus** derm. blauer Nävus m, Jadassohn-Tièche-Nävus m, Naevus caeruleus/coeruleus.
Jaffé [ʒa'fe]: **J.'s reaction/test** Jaffé-Probe f.
Jaffé-Lichtenstein ['lɪktənstiːn; 'lɪçtənʃtaɪn]: **J.-L. disease/syndrome** Jaffé-Lichtenstein-Krankheit f, Jaffé-Lichtenstein-Uehlinger-Syndrom nt, fibröse (Knochen-)Dysplasie f, nicht-ossifizierendes juveniles Osteofibrom nt, halbseitige von Recklinghausen-Krankheit f, Osteodystrophia fibrosa unilateralis.
Jahnke ['ja:nkə]: **J.'s syndrome** Jahnke-Syndrom nt.
jake paralysis [dʒeɪk] Ingwerlähmung f.
Jakob ['jakɔp]: **J.'s disease** → Jakob-Creutzfeld disease.
Jakob-Creutzfeldt ['krɔytsfɛlt]: **J.-C. disease** abbr. JCD Creutzfeldt-Jakob-Erkrankung f abbr. CJE, -Syndrom nt, Jakob-Creutzfeldt-Erkrankung f, -Syndrom nt.
J.-C. virus Jakob-Creutzfeldt-Virus nt, JC-Virus nt.
Jaksch [jakʃ]: **J.'s anemia/disease** von Jaksch-Hayem-Anämie f, -Syndrom nt, Anaemia pseudoleucaemica infantum.
jail fever [dʒeɪl] epidemisches/klassisches Fleckfieber nt, Läusefleckfieber nt, Fleck-, Hunger-, Kriegstyphus m, Typhus exanthematicus.
Ja·mai·ca ginger paralysis/polyneuritis [dʒə'meɪkə] Ingwerlähmung f.
ja-mais vu [ʒa'mɛ vy] neuro. Jamais-vu-Erlebnis nt.
James [dʒeɪmz]: **J. fibers** James'-Fasern pl, -Bündel nt.
Janet [ʒa'nɛ]: **J.'s disease** Psychasthenie f.
jan·i·ceps ['dʒænɪseps] n embryo. Januskopf m, Janiceps m.
Jansen ['janzən]: **J.'s disease** Jansen-Syndrom nt, Dysostosis enchondralis metaphysaria.
J.'s operation HNO Jansen-Operation f.
Jansky ['dʒænskɪ; janskɪ]: **J.'s classification** hema. Jansky-Klassifikation f.
Jansky-Bielschowsky [ˌbiːl'ʃɔvski, ˌbɛl-]: **J.-B. disease** Jansky-Bielschowsky-Krankheit f, Bielschowsky-Syndrom nt, spätinfantile Form f der amaurotischen Idiotie.
Ja·nus green B stain ['dʒeɪnəs] Janusgrünfärbung f.
Jap·a·nese [ˌdʒæpə'niːz]: **J. B encephalitis** abbr. JBE japanische B-Enzephalitis f abbr. JBE, Encephalitis japonica B.
J. B encephalitis virus japanische B-Enzephalitis-Virus nt, JBE-Virus nt.
J. blood fluke japanischer Pärchenegel m, Schistosoma japonicum.
J. dysentery Bakterienruhr f, bakterielle

Ruhr f, Dysenterie f.
J. flood fever Tsutsugamushi-Fieber nt, japanisches Fleckfieber nt, Milbenfleckfieber nt, Scrub-Typhus m.
J. river fever → J. flood fever.
J. schistosomiasis japanische Schistosomiasis/Bilharziose f, Schistosomiasis japonica.
jar¹ [dʒɑːr] n Gefäß nt, Krug m, Topf m.
jar² [dʒɑːr] **I** n **1.** Erschütterung f; Stoß m. **2.** Kratzen nt, Quietschen nt. **II** vt **3.** erschüttern; durchrütteln. **4.** kratzen od. quietschen (mit). **III** vi zittern, beben.
jar·gon aphasia ['dʒɑːrgən] Jargonaphasie f.
jar·gon·a·pha·sia [ˌdʒɑːrgənə'feɪʒə] n → jargon aphasia.
Jarisch-Herxheimer ['jarɪʃ 'hɛrkshaɪmər]: **J.-H. reaction** Jarisch-Herxheimer-Reaktion f, Herxheimer-Jarisch-Reaktion f.
jaun·dice ['dʒɔːndɪs, 'dʒɑːn-] **I** n **1.** patho. Gelbsucht f, Ikterus m, Icterus m. **2.** Voreingenommenheit f; Neid m, Eifersucht f; Feindseligkeit f. **II** vt voreingenommen machen; neidisch od. eifersüchtig machen; feindselig machen.
j. of the newborn Neugeborenenikterus, Icterus neonatorum.
jaun·diced ['dʒɔːndɪst, 'dʒɑːn-] adj **1.** patho. gelbsüchtig, ikterisch. **2.** voreingenommen; neidisch, eifersüchtig; feindselig.
jaundiced patient ikterischer Patient m, ikterische Patientin f, Patient(in f) m mit Gelbsucht/Ikterus.
jaundice infectious hepatitis (Virus-)Hepatitis A f abbr. HA, epidemische Hepatitis f, Hepatitis epidemica.
jaw [dʒɔː] n **1.** anat. Kiefer m, Kinnlade f. **2.** → jawbone. **3.** ~s pl zoo. Maul nt, Rachen m; Mundöffnung f. **4.** techn. Klaue f.
jaw·bone ['dʒɔːbəʊn] n anat. Kiefer(knochen m) m.
jaw jerk → jaw reflex.
Jaworski [ja'wɔrski]: **J.'s bodies/corpuscles** Jaworski-Körperchen pl.
jaw reflex Masseter-, Unterkieferreflex m.
jaw-winking phenomenon Gunn-Zeichen nt, Kiefer-Lid-Phänomen nt.
jaw-winking syndrome → jaw-winking phenomenon.
jaw-working reflex → jaw-winking phenomenon.
JBE abbr. → Japanese B encephalitis.
JBE virus → Japanese B encephalitis virus.
JCD abbr. → Jakob-Creutzfeldt disease.
J chain immun. J-Kette f.
JC virus → Jakob-Creutzfeldt virus.
J disk I-Bande f, I-Streifen m, I-Zone f, isotrope Bande f.
Jefferson ['dʒefərsən]: **J. fracture** Atlasfraktur f.
Jeghers-Peutz ['jeɪgərz pɔyts]: **J.-P. syndrome** Peutz-Jeghers-Syndrom nt, Polyposis intestini Peutz-Jeghers.

jejun- *pref.* → jejuno-.
je·ju·nal [dʒɪˈdʒuːnl] *adj* Jejunum betr., jejunal, Jejunal-, Jejuno-.
jejunal arteries Jejunal-, Jejunumarterien *pl*, Aa. jejunales.
jejunal atresia Jejunumatresie *f*.
jejunal bypass *chir.* Ileumausschaltung *f*, ilealer/jejunaler Bypass/Shunt *m*.
jejunal interposition *chir.* 1. Jejunuminterposition *f.* 2. Jejunuminterponat *nt*.
jejunal secretion Jejunal-, Jejunumsekret *nt*.
jejunal shunt → jejunal bypass.
jejunal syndrome *chir.* Dumpingsyndrom *nt*.
jejunal ulcer Jejunal-, Jejunumulkus *nt*, Ulcus jejuni.
jejunal veins Jejunumvenen *pl*, Vv. jejunales.
je·ju·nec·to·my [ˌdʒɪdʒuːˈnektəmɪ] *n chir.* Jejunumexzision *f*, -resektion *f*, Jejunektomie *f*.
je·ju·ni·tis [ˌ-ˈnaɪtɪs] *n* Jejunumentzündung *f*, Jejunitis *f*.
jejuno- *pref.* Jejunal-, Jejuno-, Jejunum-.
je·ju·no·ce·cos·to·my [dʒɪˌdʒuːnəʊsɪˈkɑstəmɪ] *n chir.* Jejunum-Zäkum-Fistel *f*, Jejunozäkostomie *f*.
je·ju·no·co·los·to·my [ˌ-kəˈlɑstəmɪ] *n chir.* Jejunum-Kolon-Fistel *f*, Jejunokolostomie *f*.
je·ju·no·il·e·al [ˌ-ˈɪlɪəl] *adj* Jejunum u. Ileum betr. *od.* verbindend, jejunoileal, ileojejunal.
jejunoileal bypass *chir.* 1. jejunoilealer Bypass/Shunt *m*. 2. Ileumausschaltung *f*, ilealer/jejunaler Bypass/Shunt *m*.
jejunoilileal shunt → jejunoileal bypass.
je·ju·no·il·e·i·tis [ˌ-ɪlɪˈaɪtɪs] *n* Entzündung *f* von Jejunum u. Ileum, Jejunoileitis *f*.
je·ju·no·il·e·os·to·my [ˌ-ɪləˈɑstəmɪ] *n chir.* Jejunum-Ileum-Fistel *f*, Jejunoileostomie *f*.
je·ju·no·je·ju·nos·to·my [ˌ-ˌdʒɪdʒuːˈnɑstəmɪ] *n chir.* Jejunojejunostomie *f*.
je·ju·no·plas·ty [ˈ-plæstɪ] *n chir.* Jejunumplastik *f*.
je·ju·nor·rha·phy [ˌdʒɪdʒuːˈnɔrəfɪ] *n chir.* Jejunumnaht *f*, Jejunorrhaphie *f*.
je·ju·nos·to·my [ˌ-ˈnɑstəmɪ] *n chir.* Jejunal-, Jejunumfistel *f*, Jejunostomie *f*.
je·ju·not·o·my [ˌ-ˈnɑtəmɪ] *n chir.* Jejunumeröffnung *f*, -schnitt *m*, Jejunotomie *f*.
je·ju·num [dʒɪˈdʒuːnəm] *n old* Leerdarm *m*, Jejunum *nt*, Intestinum jejunum.
jell [dʒel] I *vt* → jelly II. II *vi* → jelly III.
Jellinek [ˈjelinek]: **J.'s sign/symptom** Jellinek-Zeichen *nt*.
jel·ly [ˈdʒelɪ] I *n*, *pl* **-lies** Gallert(e *f*) *nt*, Gelee *m*, Sülze *f*, Aspik *m*; geleeartige *od.* gallertartige Masse *f*. II *vt* zum Gelieren bringen, gelieren lassen. III *vi* gelieren.
Jendrassik [jenˈdrasɪk]: **J.'s maneuver** Jendrassik'-Handgriff *m*.
J.'s sign Jendrassik-Zeichen *nt*.
Jensen [ˈjenzən]: **J.'s disease/retinitis/retinochorioiditis** *ophthal.* Retinochorioiditis juxtapapillaris Jensen.
J.'s sarcoma Jensen-Sarkom *nt*.
Jer·i·cho boil [ˈdʒerɪkəʊ] kutane Leishmaniose/Leishmaniase *f*, Hautleishmaniose *f*, Orientbeule *f*, Leishmaniasis cutis.
jerk [dʒɜrk] I *n* 1. (plötzlicher) Reflex *m*, unwillkürliche *od.* ruckartige Bewegung *f*; Zuckung *f*, Zucken *nt*; Ruck *m*. at one ∼ auf einmal. by ∼s ruckweise. to give a ∼ (zusammen-)zucken. with a ∼ plötzlich, mit einem Ruck. 2. ∼s *pl Brit. inf.* gymnastische Übungen *pl*. II *vi* (zusammen-)zucken; *s.* ruckartig bewegen.
jerk nystagmus Rucknystagmus *m*.

jerk·y [ˈdʒɜrkɪ] *adj* ruckartig, ruck- *od.* stoßweise.
jerky nystagmus → jerk nystagmus.
Jerne [ˈjernə]: **J. plaque assay/technique** *immun.* Jerne-Technik *f*, (Hämolyse-)-Plaquetechnik *f*.
Jervell and Lange-Nielsen [ˈdʒɜrvel ˈlæŋə ˈniːlzən]: **J.a.L. syndrome** Jervell--Lange-Nielsen-Syndrom *nt*.
Jes·u·it bark [ˈdʒeʒuːɪt, ˈdʒez(j)uː-] *pharm.* Chinarinde *f*.
jet [dʒet] I *n* 1. Strahl *m*. 2. *techn.* Düse *f*, Strahlrohr *nt*. II *vt* 3. ausstrahlen, ausstoßen, -spritzen. 4. an-, bespritzen (*with* mit). III *vi* (heraus-, hervor-)schießen (*from* aus).
jet atomisation Düsenvernebelung *f*.
jet fatigue → jet lag.
jet lag Jet-lag *m*.
jet lag syndrome → jet lag.
jet nebulisation Düsenvernebelung *f*.
jet syndrome → jet lag.
Jeune [ʒœn]: **J.'s syndrome** Jeune'-Krankheit *f*, asphyxierende Thoraxdysplasie *f*.
j-g complex → juxtaglomerular apparatus.
JH virus Echovirus Typ 28 *nt*.
jig·ger [ˈdʒɪɡər] *n micro.* Sandfloh *m*, Tunga/Dermatophilus penetrans.
Job syndrome [dʒəʊb] Hiob-Syndrom *nt*.
Jo·cas·ta complex [dʒəˈkæstə] *psychia.* Jokaste-Komplex *m*.
jock itch [dʒɑk] Tinea inguinalis, Epidermophytia inguinalis, Eccema marginatum, Ekzema marginatum Hebra.
JODA *abbr.* → juvenile-onset diabetes of adult.
jod·bas·e·dow [ˌaɪəʊdˈbɑːzədəʊ] *n* Jodbasedow *m*, jodinduzierte Hyperthyreose *f*.
Johne [ˈjoːnə]: **J.'s bacillus** Johne-Bazillus *m*, Mycobacterium paratuberculosis.
Johnson-Stevens [ˈdʒɑnsən ˈstiːvənz]: **J.-S. disease** Stevens-Johnson-Syndrom *nt*, Stevens-Johnson-Fuchs-Syndrom *nt*, Fissinger-Rendu-Syndrom *nt*, Dermatostomatitis Baader *f*, Ectodermose érosive pluriorificielle, Erythema exsudativum multiforme majus.
join·ing [ˈdʒɔɪnɪŋ] *immun.* J-Kette *f*.
joint [dʒɔɪnt] I *n* 1. *anat.* Gelenk *nt*, Articulatio *f*. 2. Verbindung(sstelle *f*) *f*, Fuge *f*, Naht(stelle *f*) *f*; *techn.* Gelenk *nt*, Verbindung(sstück *nt*) *f*, Bindeglied *nt*. 3. *sl.* 'Joint'. II *adj* gemeinsam, gemeinschaftlich, Gemeinschafts-; vereint. III *vt* verbinden, zusammenfügen.
j.s of foot Fußgelenke *pl*, Articc. pedis.
j.s of free inferior limb Articc. membri inferioris liberi.
j.s of free superior limb Articc. membri superioris liberi.
j.s of hands Handgelenke *pl*, Articc. manus.
j. of head of rib Rippenkopfgelenk *f*, Artic. capitis costae/costalis.
j.s of inferior limb Articc. membri inferioris.
j.s of inferior limb girdle Articc. cinguli pelvici.
j.s of the pelvic girdle → j.s of inferior limb girdle.
j.s of the shoulder girdle Articc. cinguli pectoralis.
j.s of superior limb Articc. membri superioris.
j.s of superior limb girdle Articc. cinguli pectoralis.
joint afferent Gelenkafferenz *f*.
joint body *ortho.* Gelenk(fremd)körper *m*, Enarthrum *nt*, Enarthron *nt*.
joint calculus *ortho.* Gelenkstein *m*, -konkrement *nt*.

jugal suture

joint capsule Gelenkkapsel *f*, Capsula articularis.
joint cartilage Gelenk(flächen)knorpel *m*, Cartilago articularis.
joint cavity Gelenkhöhle *f*, -raum *m*, -spalt *m*, Cavitas articularis.
joint chondromatosis *ortho.* Gelenkchondromatose *f*.
joint crepitus *ortho.* Gelenkreiben *nt*.
joint disease Gelenkerkrankung *f*, -affektion *f*, Arthropathie *f*.
  degenerative j. degenerative Gelenkerkrankung, Osteoarthrose *f*, Gelenkarthrose *f*, Arthrosis deformans.
  inflammatory j. entzündliche Gelenkerkrankung/Gelenkaffektion *f*.
joint·ed [ˈdʒɔɪntɪd] *adj* mit Gelenken versehen, gegliedert.
joint effusion Gelenkerguß *m*.
  purulent j. eitriger Gelenkerguß.
  sanguineous j. blutiger Gelenkerguß.
  serofibrinous j. serofibrinöser Gelenkerguß.
  serous j. seröser Gelenkerguß.
joint fracture Fraktur *f* gelenkbildender Knochen.
joint infection Gelenkinfektion *f*.
joint meniscus sichel- *od.* halbmondförmige Gelenk(zwischen)scheibe *f*, Meniskus *m*, Meniscus articularis.
joint mouse Gelenkmaus *f*, freier Gelenkkörper *m*, Corpus liberum.
  cartilaginous j. knorpeliger/chondraler freier Gelenkkörper.
  osseous j. knöcherner/ossärer freier Gelenkkörper.
joint pain Gelenkschmerz *m*, Arthralgie *f*, Arthrodynie *f*.
joint replacement *ortho.* Gelenkersatz *m*, künstliches Gelenk *nt*.
  total j. Totalendoprothese *f abbr.* TEP.
joint resection *ortho.* Gelenkresektion *f*.
joint sensation → joint sensibility.
joint sensibility Gelenkempfindung *f*, -sensibilität *f*, Arthrästhesie *f*.
joint sensor Gelenksensor *m*.
joint space → joint cavity.
joint space narrowing *radiol., ortho.* Gelenkspaltverschmälerung *f*.
joint space widening *radiol., ortho.* Gelenkspalterweiterung *f*.
joint stability Gelenkstabilität *f*.
joint stiffness *ortho.* Gelenksteife *f*, -versteifung *f*.
joint synovectomy Gelenk(s)synovektomie *f*.
joint tuberculosis Gelenktuberkulose *f*.
Jolly [ˈʒɔˈliː]: **J.'s bodies** (Howell-)Jolly--Körperchen *pl*.
Jolly [ˈdʒɔlɪ]: **J.'s reaction** Jolly-Reaktion *f*, myasthenische Reaktion *f*.
Jones [dʒəʊnz]: **J.' cylinder** Sekretkörnchen *nt* der Samenbläschen.
  J. fracture Jones-Fraktur *f*.
Jonnesco [jɔˈnesko]: **J.'s fossa** Rec. duodenalis superior.
Jonston [ˈdʒɑnstən; ˈjɔn-]: **J.'s alopecia/arc/area** *derm.* kreisrunder Haarausfall *m*, Pelade *f*, Alopecia areata, Area Celsi.
Joseph [ˈjoːsef]: **J. disease** Machado--Joseph-Syndrom *nt*, Azorenkrankheit *f*.
joule [dʒuːl, dʒaʊl] *n abbr.* **J** Joule *nt abbr.* **J**.
J point *card.* J-Punkt *m*.
juc·cu·ya [juːˈkjuːjə] *n* kutane Leishmaniose/Leishmaniase *f*, Hautleishmaniose *f*, Orientbeule *f*, Leishmaniasis cutis.
Judkins [ˈdʒʌdkɪnz]: **J. technique** *radiol.* Judkins-Technik.
ju·gal bone [ˈdʒuːɡl] *old* → cheekbone.
jugal suture Pfeilnaht *f*, Sutura sagittalis.

ju·gate ['dʒuːgeɪt, -gɪt] *adj bio.* paarig, gepaart.
jug·u·lar ['dʒʌgjələr, 'dʒuːgjə-] **I** *n* → jugular vein. **II** *adj* Hals betr; Jugularvene betr., jugular, Jugular-.
jugular bruit *card.* Nonnensausen *nt*, -geräusch *nt*, Kreiselgeräusch *nt*, Bruit de diable.
jugular eminence Tuberculum jugulare.
jugular foramen For. jugulare.
jugular foramen syndrome Vernet-Syndrom *nt*.
jugular fossa 1. Drosselgrube *f*, Fossa jugularis. **2.** Fossa jugularis ossis temporalis.
j. of temporal bone → jugular fossa 2.
jugular ganglion: j. of glossopharyngeal nerve Müller'-Ganglion *nt*, Ehrenritter'- -Ganglion *nt*, oberes Glossopharyngeusganglion *nt*, Ggl. rostralis/superius n. glossopharyngei.
j. of vagus nerve oberes Vagusganglion *nt*, Ggl. rostralis/superius n. vagi.
jugular glomus Glomus jugulare/tympanicum.
jugular incisure: j. of occipital bone Inc. jugularis ossis occipitalis.
j. of sternum Inc. jugularis sterni.
j. of temporal bone Inc. jugularis ossis temporalis.
jugular lymph nodes: anterior j. vordere jugulare Lymphknoten *pl*, Nodi lymphatici jugulares anteriores.
lateral j. laterale jugulare Lymphknoten *pl*, Nodi lymphatici jugulares laterales.
jugular nerve N. jugularis.
jugular notch: j. of occipital bone Inc. jugularis ossis occipitalis.
j. of sternum Inc. jugularis sterni.
j. of temporal bone Inc. jugularis ossis temporalis.
jugular plexus lymphatischer Plexus *m* der V. jugularis interna.
jugular process Proc. jugularis.
jugular pulse Jugularispuls *m*.
jugular sign Queckenstedt-Zeichen *nt*.
jugular trunk: left j. Truncus jugularis sinister.
right j. Truncus jugularis dexter.
jugular tubercle of occipital bone Tuberculum jugulare (ossis occipitalis).
jugular vein Drosselvene *f*, Jugularvene *f*, Jugularis *f*, V. jugularis.
anterior j. Jugularis anterior, V. jugularis anterior.
external j. äußere Jugularvene, Jugularis externa, V. jugularis externa.
internal j. innere Jugularvene, Jugularis interna, V. jugularis interna.
jugular venous distension *abbr.* **JVD** Jugularvenenerweiterung *f*, -stauung *f*.
jugular wall of tympanic cavity Boden *m* der Paukenhöhle, Paries jugularis (cavitatis tympanicae).
ju·gu·late ['dʒuːgjələt, 'dʒʌgjə-] *vt* **1.** (*Krankheitsverlauf*) kupieren. **2.** *forens.* die Kehle durchschneiden.
jug·u·lo·di·gas·tric lymph node [,dʒʌgjələʊdaɪ'gæstrɪk, ,dʒʌgjə-] oberster tiefer Halslymphknoten *m*, Nodus (lymphaticus) jugulodigastricus.
jugulo-omohyoid lymph node Nodus (lymphaticus) jugulo-omohyoideus.
jug·u·lo·tym·pan·ic body [,tɪm'pænɪk] → jugular glomus.
ju·gum ['dʒuːgəm] *n, pl* **-gums, -ga** [-gə] *anat.* Joch *nt*, jochartige Struktur *f*, Erhebung *f*, Jugum *nt*.
ju·gu·max·il·lar·y [,dʒuːgə'mæksələri, -mæk'sɪlərɪ] *adj* Jochbein u. Maxilla betr.
juice [dʒuːs] *n* **1.** Saft *m*; **~s** *pl* (Körper-)Säfte *pl*. **2.** *fig.* das Wesentliche.

jump flap [dʒʌmp] Wanderlappen *m*, Wanderlappen-Fernplastik *f*.
jump·ing disease ['dʒʌmpɪŋ] Gilles-de-la- -Tourette-Syndrom *nt*, Tourette-Syndrom *nt*, Maladie des tics, Tic impulsif.
junc·tion ['dʒʌŋkʃn] **I** *n* **1.** Verbinden *nt*, Vereinigen *nt*; Verbindung *f*, Vereinigung *f*. **2.** Verbindungsstelle *f*, -punkt *m*, Anschluß *f*, Vereinigungsstelle *f*, Junktion *f*. **3.** Zusammenfluß *m*; Kreuzung *f*. **II** *adj* Verbindungs-, Anschluß-.
junc·tion·al complex ['dʒʌŋkʃənl] Haftkomplex *m*, junctional complex (*m*).
junctional cyst Junktionszyste *f*.
junctional epidermolysis bullosa Herlitz-Syndrom *nt*, kongenitaler nicht-syphilitischer Pemphigus *m*, Epidermolysis bullosa (hereditaria) letalis, Epidermolysis bullosa atrophicans generalisata gravis Herlitz.
junctional nevus *derm.* Grenz-, Übergangs-, Abtropfungs-, Junktionsnävus *m*, junktionaler Nävus *m*.
junction folds, subneural subneuraler Faltenapparat *m*, subneurales Faltenfeld *nt*.
junction nevus → junctional nevus.
junc·tu·ra [dʒʌn'tʃʊərə] *n, pl* **-rae** [-riː] *anat.* Verbindung *f*, Junctura *f*.
junc·ture ['dʒʌŋktʃər] *n* **1.** Vereinigung(s- stelle *f*) *f*, Verbindungsstelle *od.* -stück *f*, Gelenk *nt*; Naht *f*; Fuge *f*. **2.** Verbinden *nt*, Vereinigen *nt*. **3.** kritischer Augenblick *od.* Zeitpunkt *m*.
June cold [dʒuːn] Heuschnupfen *m*, -fieber *nt*.
Jung [jʊŋ] **J.'s muscle** M. pyramidalis auricularis.
jung·i·an psychoanalysis ['jʊŋɪən] analytische Psychologie *f*.
jun·gle fever ['dʒʌŋgəl] Sumpf-, Wechselfieber *nt*, Malaria *f*.
Jüngling ['jyŋlɪŋ] **J.'s disease** Jüngling- -Krankheit *f*, Perthes-Jüngling-Krankheit *f*, Ostitis multiplex cystoides.
Junin fever ['dʒuːnɪn] Juninfieber *nt*, argentinisches hämorrhagisches Fieber *nt*.
Junin fever virus Juninfiebervirus *nt*.
Juster [ʒysˈte]: **J. reflex** Juster-Reflex *m*.
jus·ti·fi·a·ble abortion ['dʒʌstɪfaɪəbl] *gyn.* indizierter Abort *m*.
ju·van·tia [dʒuːˈvænʃɪə] *pl* Heilmittel *pl*, therapeutische Maßnahmen *pl*, Juvantia *pl*.
ju·ve·nile ['dʒuːvənl, -naɪl] **I** *n* Jugendliche(r *m*) *f*. **II** *adj* **1.** jugendlich, jung, juvenil, Jugend-, Juvenil-. **2.** unreif, Entwicklungs-; kindisch.
juvenile angiofibroma (juveniles) Nasenrachenfibrom *nt*, Schädelbasisfibrom *nt*, Basalfibroid *nt*, -fibrom *nt*.
juvenile arrhythmia *card.* Sinusarrhythmie *f* des Jugendlichen.
juvenile cataract juvenile Katarakt *f*, Cataracta juvenilis.
juvenile cell jugendlicher Granulozyt *m*, Metamyelozyt *m*; *inf.* Jugendlicher *m*.
juvenile chorea Sydenham-Chorea *f*, Chorea minor (Sydenham), Chorea juvenilis/rheumatica/infectiosa/simplex.
juvenile cirrhosis chronisch-aktive/chronisch-aggressive Hepatitis *f abbr.* CAH.
juvenile deforming metatarsophalangeal osteochondritis Freiberg-Köhler- -Krankheit *f*, Morbus Köhler II *m*.
juvenile diabetes → juvenile-onset diabetes.
juvenile elastoma juveniles Elastom *nt*, Elastoma juvenilis.
juvenile form → juvenile cell.
j. of metachromatic leukodystrophy Scholz-Bielschowsky-Henneberg-Skle-

rosetyp *m*, Scholz-Syndrom *nt*.
juvenile glaucoma juveniles Glaukom *nt*, Glaucoma juvenile.
juvenile GM₁-gangliosidosis juvenile/ spätinfantile GM₁-Gangliosidose *f*, GM₁-Gangliosidose *f* Typ II.
juvenile GM₂-gangliosidosis juvenile (Form *f* der) GM₂-Gangliosidose *f*.
juvenile goiter Adoleszentenstruma *f*, Struma adolescentium/juvenilis.
juvenile involution Pubertätsinvolution *f*.
juvenile kyphosis Scheuermann'-Krankheit *f*, Morbus Scheuermann *m*, Adoleszentenkyphose *f*, Osteochondritis/Osteochondrosis deformans juvenilis.
juvenile melanoma Spindelzellnävus *m*, Spitz-Tumor *m*, Allen-Spitz-Nävus *m*, Spitz-Nävus *m*, Nävus Spitz *m*, Epitheloidzellnävus *m*, benignes juveniles Melanom *nt*.
juvenile nasopharyngeal fibroma (juveniles) Nasenrachenfibrom *nt*, Schädelbasisfibrom *nt*, Basalfibroid *nt*, -fibrom *nt*.
juvenile-onset diabetes insulinabhängiger Diabetes (mellitus) *m*, Typ 1 Diabetes *m* (mellitus), Insulinmangeldiabetes *m*.
j. of adult *abbr.* **JODA** Typ-I-Diabetes mellitus *m* des Erwachsenen, juvenile-onset diabetes of adult *abbr.* JODA.
juvenile Paget's disease juveniler Morbus Paget *m*, Hyperostosis corticalis deformans juvenilis.
juvenile paradentitis Parodontitis *f*, Periodontitis *f*.
juvenile paralysis agitans of Hunt progressive Pallidumatrophie Hunt *f*, Pallidumsyndrom *nt*, Paralysis agitans juvenilis.
juvenile pelvis infantiles/juveniles Becken *nt*.
juvenile periodontitis → juvenile paradentitis.
juvenile polyposis juvenile Polypose *f*.
juvenile rheumatoid arthritis juvenile Form *f* der chronischen Polyarthritis, Morbus Still *m*, Still-Syndrom *nt*, Chauffard-Ramon-Still-Krankheit *f*.
juvenile stage Entwicklungsstadium *nt*.
juvenile type: j. of amaurotic idiocy juvenile Form *f* der amaurotischen Idiotie, Stock-Vogt-Spielmeyer-Syndrom *nt*, Batten-Spielmeyer-Vogt-Syndrom *nt*, neuronale/juvenile Zeroidlipofuszinose/ Ceroidlipofuscinose *f*.
j. of Gaucher's disease juvenile Form *f*, subakute neuronopathische Form *f*, Gaucher-Krankheit *f* Typ III.
juvenile verruca Flachwarze *f*, Verruca plana (juvenilis).
juvenile wart → juvenile verruca.
juvenile xanthogranuloma juveniles Xanthogranulom/Riesenzellgranulom *nt*, Naevoxanthoendotheliom *nt*, Xanthogranuloma juvenile, Naevoxanthom *nt*.
ju·ve·nil·i·ty [dʒuːvə'nɪlətɪ] *n* Jugendlichkeit *f*, Juvenilität *f*.
juxta- *pref.* nahe bei, in der Nähe von, juxta-.
juxta-articular *adj* in Gelenknähe (liegend), gelenknah, juxt(a)artikulär.
jux·ta·cor·ti·cal chondroma [,dʒʌksta- 'kɔːrtɪkl] *ortho.* juxtakortikales/periostales/perossales Chondrom *nt*.
juxtacortical ossifying sarcoma *ortho.* periostales Osteosarkom *nt*, perossales Sarkom *nt*, periostales (osteogenes) Sarkom *nt*.
juxtacortical sarcoma *ortho.* parostales/ juxtakortikales Sarkom *nt*.
jux·ta·ep·i·phys·e·al [,-ˌepɪˈfiːzɪəl] *adj* in Epiphysennähe (liegend), epiphysennah, juxtaepiphysär.

jux·ta·glo·mer·u·lar [ˌ-gloʊˈmerjələr] *adj* in Glomerulusnähe liegend, juxtaglomerulär.
juxtaglomerular apparatus juxtaglomerulärer Apparat *m*.
juxtaglomerular cell Goormaghtigh'-Zelle *f*.
juxtaglomerular cell hyperplasia Bartter-Syndrom *nt*, Hyperplasie *f* des juxtaglomerulären Apparates.
juxtaglomerular complex → juxtaglomerular apparatus.
juxta-intestinal (lymph) nodes juxtaintestinale Lymphknoten *pl*, Nodi lymphatici mesenterici juxta-intestinales.
jux·ta·med·ul·lar·y [ˌ-ˈmedələrɪ, -ˈmedʒə-, -məˈdʌləri] *adj* in Marknähe liegend, marknah, juxtamedullär.
jux·ta·pap·il·lar·y choroiditis [ˌ-pəˈpɪləri, -ˈpæpəˌleriː] *ophthal*. juxtapapilläre Chorioiditis *f*, Chorioiditis juxtapapillaris.
jux·ta·po·si·tion [ˌ-pəˈzɪʃn] *n* Anlagerung *f* von außen, Apposition *f*, Juxtaposition *f*.
jux·ta·py·lor·ic [ˌ-paɪˈlɔrɪk, -ˈlɑr-, -pɪ-] *adj* in Pylorusnähe (liegend), pylorusnah, juxtapylorisch.
jux·ta·spi·nal [ˌ-ˈspaɪnl] *adj* in Wirbelsäulennähe (liegend), wirbelsäulennah, juxtaspinal.
jux·ta·ves·i·cal [ˌ-ˈvesɪkl] *adj* in Harnblasennähe (liegend), (harn-)blasennah, juxtavesikal.
JVD *abbr*. → jugular venous distension.

K

K *abbr.* **1.** → bulk modulus of elasticity. **2.** → dissociation constant. **3.** → encephalization factor. **4.** → kalium. **5.** → kelvin.
K' *abbr.* → dissociation constant, apparent.
k *abbr.* → kilo-.
K *abbr.* → kappa.
κ *abbr.* → kappa.
ka·bu·re [kə'bʊərɪ] *n* japanische Schistosomiasis/Bilharziose *f*, Schistosomiasis japonica.
Kahler ['ka:lər]: **K.'s disease** Kahler-Krankheit *f*, Huppert-Krankheit *f*, Morbus Kahler *m*, Plasmozytom *nt*, multiples Myelom *nt*, plasmozytisches Immunozytom *nt*, plasmozytisches Lymphom *nt*) *m*.
Kahn [ka:n]: **K.'s albumin A reaction** Kahn-Flockungsreaktion *f*.
kak·ke ['kækə] *n* Beriberi *f*, Vitamin B₁-Mangel(krankheit *f*) *m*, Thiaminmangel(krankheit *f*) *m*.
kak·o·dyl ['kækədɪl] *n* Kakodyl *nt*, Tetramethyldiarsin *nt*.
kak·os·mia [kæk'ɑzmɪə] *n neuro.* Kakosmie *f*.
ka·la·a·zar [,kɑ:lə'zɑ:r] *n* viszerale Leishmaniose *f*, Kala-Azar *f*, Splenomegalia tropica.
ka·le·mia [kə'li:mɪə] *n* (vermehrter) Kaliumgehalt *m* des Blutes, (Hyper-)Kaliämie *f*.
ka·li ['keɪlɪ] *n* Pottasche *f*, Kaliumkarbonat *nt*.
ka·li·e·mia [kælɪ'i:mɪə, keɪ-] *n* → kalemia.
ka·lim·e·ter [kə'lɪmətər] *n* Alkalimeter *nt*.
ka·li·o·pe·nia [,kælɪo'pɪnɪə, keɪ-] *n* Kaliummangel *nt*, Kaliopenie *f*; Hypokaliämie *f*.
ka·li·o·pe·nic [-'pɪnɪk] *adj* Kaliopenie betr. *od.* verursachend, durch sie gekennzeichnet *od.* verursacht, kaliopenisch.
ka·li·um ['keɪlɪəm] *n abbr.* **K** Kalium *nt abbr.* K.
ka·li·u·re·sis [,kælɪjə'ri:sɪs, ,keɪ-] *n* Kaliumausscheidung *f* im Harn, Kaliurese *f*.
ka·li·u·ret·ic [,-je'retɪk] **I** *n* kaliuretisches Mittel *nt*. **II** *adj* Kaliurese betr. *od.* fördernd, kaliuretisch.
kal·li·din ['kælədɪn] *n* Kallidin *nt*, Lysyl-Bradykinin *nt*.
kallidin I Bradykinin *nt*.
kallidin II → kallidin.
kallidin 9 Bradykinin *nt*.
kallidin 10 → kallidin.
kal·li·kre·in [,kælɪ'kri:ɪn] *n* Kallikrein *nt*.
kallikrein-kinin system Kallikrein-Kinin-System *nt*.
kal·li·krei·no·gen [,kælə'kraɪnədʒən] *n* Kallikreinogen *nt*, Präkallikrein *nt*, Fletscher-Faktor *m*.
kallikrein system → kallikrein-kinin system.
Kallmann ['kælmən]: **K.'s syndrome** (Gauthier-)Kallmann-Syndrom *nt*, olfakto-genitales Syndrom *nt*.
Kal·muck type ['kælmʌk, kæl'mʌk] Down-

-Syndrom *nt*, Trisomie 21(-Syndrom *nt*) *f*, Mongolismus *m*, Mongoloidismus *m*.
Kalmuk → Kalmuck.
kal·u·re·sis [,kæljə'ri:sɪs] *n* → kaliuresis.
kal·u·ret·ic [,-'retɪk] *n, adj* → kaliuretic.
Ka·me·run swelling [kamə'ru:n] Calabar-Beule *f*, -Schwellung *f*, Kamerun-Schwellung *f*, Loiasis *f*, Loiase *f*.
Kammerer-Battle ['kæmərər 'bætl]: **K.-B. incision** Battle-Schnitt *m*.
kan·a·my·cin [,kænə'maɪsɪn] *n pharm.* Kanamycin *nt*.
kanamycin-vancomycin blood agar *abbr.* **KVBA** *micro.* Kanamycin-Vancomycin-Blutagar *m/nt*.
kanamycin-vancomycin laked blood agar *micro.* Kanamycin-Vancomycin-Hämin-Agar *m/nt*.
Kanavel [kə'nævəl]: **K.'s sign** Kanavel'-Zeichen *nt*.
K.'s triangle Kanavel-Dreieck *nt*.
Kan·da·har sore [,kændə'hɑ:r] kutane Leishmaniose/Leishmaniase *f*, Hautleishmaniose *f*, Orientbeule *f*, Leishmaniasis cutis.
kang cancer [kaŋ] → kangri cancer.
kan·gri burn carcinoma ['kæŋgrɪ] → kangri cancer.
kangri cancer Kangri-Krebs *m*.
Kanner ['kænər]: **K.'s syndrome** Kanner-Syndrom *nt*, frühkindlicher Autismus *m*.
K antigen Kapselantigen *nt*, K-Antigen *nt*.
Kantor ['kæntər]: **K.'s sign** *radiol.* Kantor'-Zeichen *nt*, String sign (*nt*).
ka·o·lin [ˈkeɪəlɪn] *n* → kaoline.
ka·o·line [ˈkeɪəlɪn] *n* Kaolin *nt*.
ka·o·lin·o·sis [keɪəlɪ'nəʊsɪs] *n* Kaolin(staub)lunge *f*, Kaolinose *f*.
Kaposi ['kæpəsɪ, 'kæpəsi]: **K.'s sarcoma** Kaposi-Sarkom *nt*, Morbus Kaposi *m*, Retikuloangiomatose *f*, Angioretikulomatose *f*, idiopathisches multiples Pigmentsarkom Kaposi *nt*, Sarcoma idiopathicum multiplex haemorrhagicum.
K.'s varicelliform eruption Kaposi-Dermatitis *f*, Ekzema/Eccema herpeticatum/herpetiformis, varizelliforme Eruption Kaposi *f*, Pustulosis acuta varicelliformis.
kap·pa ['kæpə] *n abbr.* **K, κ** Kappa *nt abbr.* K, κ.
kappa angle *ophthal.* Kappa-Winkel *m*.
kappa chain *biochem.* kappa-Kette *f*, κ-Kette *f*.
kap·pa·cism ['kæpəsɪzəm] *n* Kappazismus *m*, Kappatismus *m*.
kappa granules azurophile Granula *pl*.
Kappeler ['kapələr]: **K.'s maneuver** Kappeler-Handgriff *m*.
ka·ra·ya (gum) [kə'raɪə] Karaya-Gummi *nt*, -Harz *nt*.
Karnofsky [kɑ:r'nɑfskɪ]: **K. performance index/scale** Karnofsky-Index *m*, -Skala *f*.
Kartagener [kɑ:r'tægɪnər]: **K.'s syndrome/triad** Kartagener-Syndrom *nt*.
kary- *pref.* → karyo-.

kar·y·en·chy·ma [,kærɪ'eŋkɪmə] *n* → karyolymph.
karyo- *pref.* Kern-, Zellkern-, Kary(o)-, Nukle(o)-, Nucle(o)-.
kar·y·o·chy·le·ma [,kærɪəʊkaɪ'li:mə] *n* → karyolymph.
kar·y·o·chrome cell ['-krəʊm] karyochrome (Nerven-)Zelle *f*.
kar·y·oc·la·sis *n* → karyoklasis.
kar·y·o·clas·tic *adj* → karyoklastic.
kar·y·o·cyte ['-saɪt] *n* **1.** kernhaltige Zelle *f*, Karyozyt *m*. **2.** *hema.* Normoblast *m*.
kar·y·o·gam·ic [,-'gæmɪk] *adj* Karyogamie betr., karyogam.
kar·y·og·a·my [,kærɪ'ɑgəmɪ] *n* Karyogamie *f*.
kar·y·o·gen·e·sis [,kærɪəʊ'dʒenəsɪs] *n* Zellkernentwicklung *f*, Karyogenese *f*.
kar·y·o·gen·ic [,-'dʒenɪk] *adj* Karyogenese betr., den Zellkern bildend, karyogen.
kar·y·o·gram ['-græm] *n* Karyogramm *nt*, Idiogramm *nt*.
kar·y·o·ki·ne·sis [,-kɪ'ni:sɪs, -kaɪ-] *n* **1.** mitotische Kernteilung *f*, Karyokinese *f*. **2.** Mitose *f*.
kar·y·o·ki·net·ic [,-kɪ'netɪk] *adj* Karyokinese betr., karyokinetisch; mitotisch.
kar·y·o·kla·sis [,kærɪ'akləsɪs] *n* Kernzerbrechlichkeit *f*, Kernauflösung *f*, Karyoklasie *f*.
kar·y·o·klas·tic [,kærɪəʊ'klæstɪk] *adj* **1.** Karyoklasie betr., karyoklastisch. **2.** mitosehemmend.
kar·y·o·lymph ['-lɪmf] *n* Kernsaft *m*, Karyolymphe *f*.
kar·y·ol·y·sis [,kærɪ'ɑləsɪs] *n* (Zell-)Kernauflösung *f*, Karyolyse *f*.
kar·y·o·lyt·ic [,kærɪəʊ'lɪtɪk] *adj* Karyolyse betr. *od.* auslösend, von ihr gekennzeichnet, karyolytisch.
kar·y·o·meg·a·ly [,-'megəlɪ] *n* Kernvergrößerung *f*, Karyomegalie *f*.
kar·y·o·mere ['-mɪər] *n* Karyomer *nt*, Karyomerit *m*.
kar·y·om·er·ite [,kærɪ'amərait] *n* → karyomere.
kar·y·om·e·try [,kærɪ'amətrɪ] *n* Zellkernmessung *f*, Karyometrie *f*.
kar·y·o·mi·to·sis [,kærɪəʊmai'təʊsɪs] *n* mitotische Kernteilung *f*, Karyomitose *f*.
kar·y·o·mi·tot·ic [,-mai'tatɪk] *adj* Karyomitose betr., karyomitotisch.
kar·y·on ['kærɪan] *n* Zellkern *m*, Nukleus *m*, Nucleus *m*, Karyon *nt*.
kar·y·o·phage ['kærɪəfeɪdʒ] *n micro.* Karyophage *m*.
kar·y·o·plasm ['-plæzəm] *n* (Zell-)Kernprotoplasma *nt*, Karyoplasma *nt*, Nukleoplasma *nt*.
kar·y·o·plas·mat·ic [,-plæz'mætɪk] *adj* → karyoplasmic.
kar·y·o·plas·mic [,-'plæzmɪk] *adj* Karyoplasma betr., nukleoplasmatisch.
karyoplasmic ratio Kern-Zytoplasma-Relation *f*.
kar·y·o·plast ['-plæst] *n* → karyon.

kar·y·o·pyk·no·sis [ˌ-pɪk'nəʊsɪs] *n* Kernschrumpfung *f*, -verdichtung *f*, (Kern-)Pyknose *f*, Karyopyknose *f*.
kar·y·o·pyk·not·ic [ˌ-pɪk'nɑtɪk] *adj* Karyopyknose betr. *od.* auslösend, von Karyopyknose gekennzeichnet, karyopyknotisch.
kar·y·or·rhec·tic [ˌ-'rektɪk] *adj* Karyorrhexis betr. *od.* verursachend, karyorrhektisch.
kar·y·or·rhex·is [ˌ-'reksɪs] *n, pl* **-rhex·es** [-'reksiːz] (Zell-)Kernzerfall *m*, Karyo(r)rhexis *f*.
kar·y·o·some ['-səʊm] *n* Karyosom *nt*.
kar·y·os·ta·sis [ˌkærɪ'ɑstəsɪs] *n* Kernruhe *f*; Interphase *f*.
kar·y·o·the·ca [ˌkærɪəʊ'θiːkə] *n* Kernmembran *f*, Karyothek *f*.
kar·y·o·tin ['kærɪətɪn] *n* Chromatin *nt*.
kar·y·o·type ['-taɪp] *n* Karyotyp *m*.
kar·y·o·typ·ic [ˌ-'tɪpɪk] *adj* Karyotyp(en) betr., Karyotypen-.
kar·y·o·typ·ing [ˌ-'taɪpɪŋ] *n* Chromosomenanalyse *f*.
kar·y·o·zo·ic [ˌ-'zəʊɪk] *adj micro.* karyozoisch.
Kasabach-Merritt ['kæsəbak 'merɪt]: **K.-M. syndrome** Kasabach-Merritt-Syndrom *nt*, Thrombo(zyto)penie-Hämangiom-Syndrom *nt*.
Kasai [kə'saɪ]: **K. operation/portoenterostomy** *chir.* Hepatojejunostomie *f* nach Kasai.
Kaschin-Beck → Kashin-Beck.
Kashin-Beck ['kæʃɪn bek]: **K.-B. disease** Kaschin-Beck-Krankheit *f*, -Syndrom *nt*.
Kast [kæst, kɑːst]: **K.'s syndrome** Maffucci-Kast-Syndrom *nt*.
kat *abbr.* → katal.
kat·a·did·y·mus [ˌkætə'dɪdəməs] *n embryo.* Katadidymus *m*.
kat·al ['kætæl] *n abbr.* **kat** Katal *nt abbr.* kat.
kat·a·ther·mom·e·ter [ˌkætəθɜr'mɑmɪtər] *n phys., physiol.* Katathermometer *nt*.
Katayama [kætə'jɑːmə]: **K. disease/fever/syndrome** Katayama-Krankheit *f*, -Fieber *nt*, -Syndrom *nt*.
kath·i·so·pho·bia [ˌkæθɪsəʊ'fəʊbɪə] *n psychia.* krankhafte Angst *f* vorm Hinsetzen, Kathisophobie *f*.
kat·i·on ['kæt,aɪən, -ən] *n* Kation *nt*.
kat·o·pho·ria [ˌkætə'fəʊrɪə] *n ophthal.* Kataphorie *f*.
kat·o·tro·pia [ˌ-'trəʊpɪə] *n* → katophoria.
Kauffmann-White ['kaʊfmən (h)waɪt]: **K.-W. classification** Kauffmann-White-Schema *nt*.
Kawasaki [kɑːwɑ'sɑːkɪ]: **K. disease/syndrome** Kawasaki-Syndrom *nt*, Morbus Kawasaki *m*, mukokutanes Lymphknotensyndrom *nt abbr.* MCLS, akutes febriles mukokutanes Lymphadenopathiesyndrom *nt*.
Kayser ['kaɪzər]: **K.'s disease** Wilson-Krankheit *f*, -Syndrom *nt*, Morbus Wilson *m*, hepatolentikuläre/hepatozerebrale Degeneration *f*.
Kayser-Fleischer ['flaɪʃər]: **K.-F. ring** Kayser-Fleischer-Ring *m*.
Kb *abbr.* → kilobase.
Kbp *abbr.* → kilobase pairs.
kcal *abbr.* → kilocalorie.
K cells 1. K-Zellen *pl*, Killerzellen *pl*. **2.** zytotoxische T-Lymphozyten *od.* T-Zellen *pl*.
K channel Kaliumkanal *m*, K⁺-Kanal *m*.
kCi *abbr.* → kilocurie.
KCl *abbr.* → potassium chloride.
K complex *neuro.* K-Komplex *m*.
KDO *abbr.* → 2-keto-3-deoxy-octanic acid.
Kearns [kɜrnz]: **K.' syndrome** Kearns-Sayre-Syndrom *nt*.
Kearns-Sayre [seər]: **K.-S. syndrome** Kearns-Sayre-Syndrom *nt*.
keb·o·ceph·a·ly [ˌkebəʊ'sefəlɪ] *n embryo.* Affenkopf *m*, Kebo-, Zebo-, Cebozephalie *f*.
keb·u·zone ['kebəzəʊn] *n pharm.* Kebuzon *nt*.
Ke·da·ni fever [kə'dɑːnɪ] Tsutsugamushi-Fieber *nt*, japanisches Fleckfieber *nt*, Milbenfleckfieber *nt*, Scrub-Typhus *m*.
Kedani mite *micro.* Trombicula akamushi.
keeled chest ['kiːld] Kiel-, Hühnerbrust *f*, Pectus gallinatum/carinatum.
Keen [kiːn]: **K.'s sign** *ortho.* Keen-Zeichen *nt*.
keep [kiːp] (*v* kept; kept) **I** *n* **1.** (Lebens-)Unterhalt *m*. **2.** Unterkunft u. Verpflegung *f*. **3.** Unterhaltskosten *pl*. **4.** Obhut *f*. **II** *vt* **5.** (be-)halten, haben. **6.** *fig.* (er-)halten, (be-)wahren. **to ~ one's temper** s. beherrschen. **7.** aufheben, (auf-)bewahren. **to ~ cool** kühl aufbewahren. **to ~ dry/to ~ in a dry place** trocken aufbewahren. **to ~ a note of** s. etw. notieren. **to ~ warm** warm halten. **8.** (*Beziehung*) pflegen. **to ~ alive** am Leben erhalten. **to ~ clean** sauber *od.* rein halten. **to ~ in good repair** in gutem Zustand erhalten, instand halten. **10.** (*Bett*) hüten. **11.** (*Regel*) einhalten, befolgen; (*Versprechen*) halten. **12.** ernähren, er-, unterhalten, versorgen. **13.** behüten, aufpassen auf. **III** *vi* bleiben. **to ~ in bed** im Bett bleiben. **to ~ in good health** gesund bleiben.
keep at *vi* weitermachen mit, dranbleiben an.
keep away I *vt* jdn./etw. fernhalten (*from* von). **II** *vi* s. fernhalten (*from* von); wegbleiben (*from* von).
keep back *vt* **1.** (*Tränen*) unterdrücken. **2.** (*Informationen*) verschweigen (*from sb.* jdm.). **3.** etw. verzögern, aufhalten; (*Urin*) verhalten, (*Wasser*) stauen.
keep down *vt* **1.** (*Kosten*) niedrig halten. **2.** (*Gefühle*) unter Kontrolle halten; (*Wut*) unterdrücken. **3.** (*Nahrung*) bei s. behalten.
keep in *vt* (*Atem*) anhalten; (*Bauch*) einziehen; (*Gefühle*) unterdrücken, unter Kontrolle halten.
keep off I *vt* jdn./etw. fernhalten von. **II** *vi* s. fernhalten von, wegbleiben, vermeiden.
keep on *vi* **1.** weitermachen, nicht aufhören. **2.** leben *od.* s. ernähren von.
keep out I *vt* nicht hereinlassen (*of* in); fernhalten (*of* von). **II** *vi fig.* s. heraushalten (*of* aus).
keep to I *vi* festhalten an, bleiben bei. **II** *vt* **to keep sth. to a minimum** etw. auf ein Minimum beschränken.
keep under *vt* **1.** (*Gefühle*) unterdrücken. **2.** jdn. unter Narkose behandeln. **3.** unter Kontrolle halten. **to ~ observation** jdn. beobachten (lassen).
keep up *vt* **1.** (*Beziehung*) weiterpflegen. **2.** etw. in Ordnung halten.
keep up with *vi* Schritt halten mit.
ke·fir [kə'fɪər] *n* Kefir *m*.
Kehr [keːr]: **K.'s sign** *chir.* Kehr-Zeichen *nt*.
Kehrer ['keːrər]: **K.'s sign** *neuro.* Kehrer-Zeichen *nt*.
Keith [kiːθ]: **K.'s bundle** → Keith-Flack's bundle.
K.'s node → Keith-Flack node.
Keith-Flack [flæk]: **K.-F.'s bundle** Keith-Flack-Bündel *nt*, Sinuatrialbündel *nt*.

K.-F.'s node Sinus-Knoten *m*, Sinoatrial-Knoten *m*, SA-Knoten *m*, Keith-Flack'-Knoten *m*, Nodus sinuatrialis.
Kell [kel]: **K. blood group (system)** Kell-Blutgruppe *f*, -Blutgruppensystem *nt*, Kell-Cellano-System *nt*.
Keller-Blake ['kelər bleɪk]: **K.-B. splint** *ortho.* Keller-Blake-Schiene *f*.
Kelly ['kelɪ]: **K.'s operation 1.** *gyn.* Kelly-Operation *f*. **2.** *HNO* Kelly-Operation *f*, Kelly-Arytänoidopexie *f*.
ke·loid ['kiːlɔɪd] *n* Wulstnarbe *f*, Keloid *nt*.
k. of gums Fibromatosis gingivae, Elephantiasis gingivae.
ke·loid·al blastomycosis [kɪ'lɔɪdl] Lobo-Krankheit *f*, Lobomykose *f*, Keloidblastomykose *f*, Blastomycosis queloidana.
ke·loi·do·sis [kiːlɔɪ'dəʊsɪs] *n* Keloidose *f*.
ke·lo·plas·ty ['kiːləplæstɪ] *n chir.* operative Narben- *od.* Keloidentfernung *f*.
ke·lo·so·mia [ˌ-'səʊmɪə] *n embryo.* Zelosomie *f*.
ke·lot·o·my [kɪ'lɑtəmɪ] *n chir.* Hernien-, Bruchoperation *f*, Herniotomie *f*.
Kelvin ['kelvɪn]: **K. scale** Kelvin-Skala *f*.
K. thermometer Kelvin-Thermometer *nt*.
kel·vin ['kelvɪn] *n abbr.* **K** Kelvin *nt abbr.* K.
Ke·me·ro·vo virus ['kemərəʊvə] Kemerova-Virus *nt*.
Kendall ['kendl]: **K.'s compound A** 11-Dehydrocorticosteron *nt*, Kendall-Substanz A *f*.
K.'s compound B Kortiko-, Corticosteron *nt*, Compound B Kendall.
K.'s compound E Kortison *nt*, Cortison *nt*.
K.'s compound F Kortisol *nt*, Cortisol *nt*, Hydrocortison *nt*.
Kennedy ['kenɪdɪː]: **K.'s syndrome** Foster Kennedy-Syndrom *nt*, Kennedy-Syndrom *nt*.
Kent [kent]: **K.'s bundle** Kent'-Bündel *nt*.
Kent-His [hɪz]: **K.-H. bundle** His'-Bündel *nt*, Fasciculus atrioventricularis.
Ken·yan tick typhus ['kenjən, 'kiːn-] Boutonneuse-Fieber *nt*, Fièvre boutonneuse.
Ken·ya tick ['kenjə, 'kiːn-] *micro.* Rhipicephalus appendiculatus.
K enzyme K-Enzym *nt*.
keph·a·lin ['kefəlɪn] *n* Kephalin *nt*, Cephalin *nt*.
ker·a·sin ['kerəsɪn] *n* Kerasin *nt*.
kerasin histiocytosis Gaucher'-Erkrankung *f*, -Krankheit *f*, -Syndrom *nt*, Morbus Gaucher *m*, Glukozerebrosidose *f*, Zerebrosidlipidose *f*, Lipoidhistiozytose *f* vom Kerasintyp, Glykosylzeramidlipidose *f*.
kerat- *pref.* → kerato-.
ker·a·tal·gia [kerə'tældʒ(ɪ)ə] *n ophthal.* Hornhautschmerz *m*, Keratalgie *f*, Keratalgia *f*.
ker·a·tan sulfate ['kerətæn] Keratansulfat *nt*.
ker·a·tan·sul·fa·tu·ria [ˌkerətæn,sʌlfə'tj(ʊ)ərɪə] *n* Morquio-Syndrom *nt*, Morquio-Ullrich-Syndrom *nt*, Morquio-Brailsford-Syndrom *nt*, spondylepiphysäre Dysplasie *f*, Mukopolysaccharidose *f* Typ IV *abbr.* MPS IV.
ker·a·tec·ta·sia [kerətek'teɪʒ(ɪ)ə] *n ophthal.* Hornhautvorwölbung *f*, -staphylom *nt*, Keratektasie *f*, Kerektasie *f*.
ker·a·tec·to·my [ˌ-'tektəmɪ] *n ophthal.* Hornhautentfernung *f*, -exzision *f*, Keratektomie *f*.
ker·a·ti·a·sis [ˌ-'taɪəsɪs] *n* → keratosis.
ke·rat·ic [kə'rætɪk] *adj* **1.** Keratin betr., Keratin-. **2.** Hornhaut/Kornea betr., Hornhaut-, Kerato-. **3.** hornartig, Horn-.

keratin

ker·a·tin ['kerətɪn] *n* Hornstoff *m*, Keratin *nt*.
ker·a·tin·ase ['-tɪneɪz] *n* Keratinase *f*.
ker·a·tin·i·za·tion [,-tɪnə'zeɪʃn] *n* Verhornung *f*, Keratinisation *f*.
ker·a·tin·ize ['-tɪnaɪz, kə'rætnaɪz] *vi* verhornen, hornig werden.
ker·a·tin·iz·ing layer of epidermis ['kerətɪnaɪzɪŋ, kə'rætn-] Hornbildungsschicht *f*, Stratum granulosum u. Stratum lucidum.
ke·rat·i·no·cyte [kɪ'rætnəʊsaɪt] *n* Keratinozyt *m*, Hornzelle *f*, Malpighi-Zelle *f*.
ke·rat·i·nous [kɪ'rætnəs] *adj* hornig, verhornt, aus Horn, Horn-.
ker·a·ti·tis [kerə'taɪtɪs] *n ophthal*. Hornhautentzündung *f*, Keratitis *f*.
kerato- *pref*. Hornhaut-, Kerato-, Korneal-.
ker·a·to·ac·an·tho·ma [,kerətəʊæ,kæn'θəʊmə] *n derm*. Keratoakanthom *nt*, selbstheilendes Stachelzellkarzinom *nt*, selbstheilender Stachelzell(en)krebs *m*, Molluscum sebaceum/pseudocarcinomatosum.
ker·a·to·an·gi·o·ma [,-ændʒɪ'əʊmə] *n* Angiokeratom(a) *nt*.
ker·a·to·at·ro·pho·der·ma [,-ætrəfəʊ'dɜːmə] *n derm*. 1. Porokeratosis, Keratoatrophodermie *f*, Keratoatrophodermie *f*, Parakeratosis anularis. 2. Mibelli'-Krankheit *f*, Porokeratosis/Parakeratosis Mibelli *f*, Keratoatrophodermie *f*, Hyperkeratosis concentrica, Hyperkeratosis figurata centrifuga atrophicans, Keratodermia excentrica.
ker·a·to·cele ['-siːl] *n ophthal*. Vorfall *m* der Descemet'-Membran, Keratozele *f*, Descemetozele *f*.
ker·a·to·con·junc·ti·vi·tis [,-kən,dʒʌŋktə'vaɪtɪs] *n ophthal*. Entzündung *f* von Horn- u. Bindehaut, Keratokonjunktivitis *f*, Keratoconjunctivitis *f*.
ker·a·to·co·nus [,-'kəʊnəs] *n ophthal*. Hornhautkegel *m*, Keratokonus *m*.
ker·a·to·cyte ['-saɪt] *n* Keratozyt *m*.
ker·a·to·der·ma [,-'dɜːmə] *n derma*. 1. Hautverhornung *f*, Hornhautbildung *f*, Keratoderma *nt*. 2. übermäßige Verhornung *f*, Keratoderma *nt*, -dermatose *f*, -dermia *f*.
k. of eye *anat*. (Augen-)Hornhaut *f*, Kornea *f*, Cornea *f*.
ker·a·to·der·ma·ti·tis [,-,dɜːrmə'taɪtɪs] *n derm*. Keratodermatitis *f*.
ker·a·to·der·ma·to·cele [,-dɜːr'mætəsiːl] *n* → keratocele.
ker·a·to·der·mia [,-'dɜːrmɪə] *n* → keratoderma.
ker·a·to·ec·ta·sia [,-ek'teɪʒ(ɪ)ə] *n* → keratectasia.
ker·a·to·gen·e·sis [,-'dʒenəsɪs] *n* Hornbildung *f*, Keratogenese *f*, Keratinisation *f*.
ker·a·to·gen·et·ic [,-dʒə'netɪk] *adj* Keratogenese betr., keratogenetisch.
ker·a·tog·e·nous [kerə'tɑdʒənəs] *adj* Hornbildung *nt*. Verhornung fördernd, keratogen.
keratogenous membrane Matrix unguis.
ker·a·to·glo·bus [,kerətə'gləʊbəs] *n ophthal*. Keratoglobus *m*.
ker·a·to·glos·sus [,-'glɑsəs] *n anat*. M. chondroglossus.
ker·a·to·hel·co·sis [,-hel'kəʊsɪs] *n ophthal*. Ulzeration/Geschwürsbildung *f* der Hornhaut, Keratohelkose *f*.
ker·a·to·hy·a·lin [,-'haɪəlɪn] *n* Keratohyalin *nt*, Keratohyalin *f*.
ker·a·to·hy·a·line [,-'haɪəliːn, -laɪn] I *n* → keratohyalin. II *adj* keratohyalin.
keratohyalin granules → keratohyalin.
ker·a·toid ['kerətɔɪd] *adj* 1. hornartig, keratoid. 2. Hornhaut(gewebe) ähnlich, keratoid.
ker·a·toi·di·tis [,kerətɔɪ'daɪtɪs] *n* → keratitis.
ker·a·to·ir·i·do·cyc·li·tis [,kerətəʊ,ɪrɪdəʊsɪk'laɪtɪs] *n ophthal*. Entzündung *f* von Kornea, Iris u. Ziliarkörper, Keratoiridozyklitis *f*.
ker·a·to·i·ri·tis [,-aɪ'raɪtɪs] *n* Entzündung *f* von Kornea u. Iris, Keratoiritis *f*, Iridokeratitis *f*.
ker·a·tol·y·sis [kerə'tɑləsɪs] *n derm*. 1. Ablösung *f* der Hornschicht, Keratolyse *f*, Keratolysis *f*. 2. Auflösung/Erweichung *f* der Hornsubstanz der Haut, Keratolyse *f*. 3. Auflösung *f* der Keratolysis *f*.
ker·a·to·lyt·ic [,kerətəʊ'lɪtɪk] I *n* Keratolytikum *nt*. II *adj* Keratolyse betr. od. auslösend, keratolytisch.
ker·a·to·ma [kerə'təʊmə] *n, pl* -mas, -mata [-mətə] 1. Hornschwiele *f*, Kallus *m*, Callus *m*, Callositas *f*. 2. Keratom *nt*, Keratoma *nt*.
ker·a·to·ma·la·cia [,kerətəʊmə'leɪʃɪə, -sɪə] *n ophthal*. Hornhauterweichung *f*, Keratomalazie *f*.
ker·a·tome ['kerətəʊm] *n* → keratotome.
ker·a·tom·e·ter [kerə'tɑmɪtər] *n ophthal*. Keratometer *nt*, Ophthalmometer *nt*.
ker·a·to·met·ric [,kerətə'metrɪk] *adj* Keratometrie betr., keratometrisch, ophthalmometrisch.
ker·a·tom·e·try [kerə'tɑmətrɪ] *n ophthal*. Keratometrie *f*, Ophthalmometrie *f*.
ker·a·to·mi·leu·sis [,kerətəʊmɪ'luːsɪs] *n ophthal*. Keratomileusis *f*.
ker·a·to·my·co·sis [,-maɪ'kəʊsɪs] *n ophthal*. Pilzinfektion *f* der Hornhaut, Hornhaut-, Keratomykose *f*, Keratitis mycotica.
ker·a·ton·o·sus [kerə'tɑnəsəs] *n ophthal*. degenerative Hornhauterkrankung *f*, Keratonose *f*.
ker·a·to·nyx·is [,kerətə'nɪksɪs] *n ophthal*. Hornhautstich *m*, Keratonyxis *f*; Vorderkammerpunktion *f*.
ker·a·top·a·thy [kerə'tɑpəθɪ] *n ophthal*. nichtentzündliche Hornhauterkrankung *f*, Keratopathie *f*.
ker·a·to·plas·ty ['kerətəplæstɪ] *n ophthal*. Hornhaut-, Keratoplastik *f*, Hornhauttransplantation *f*.
ker·a·to·pros·the·sis [,-prɑs'θiːsɪs] *n ophthal*. Keratoprothese *f*.
ker·a·tor·rhex·is *n* → keratorrhexis.
ker·a·tor·rhex·is [,-'reksɪs] *n ophthal*. Hornhautriß *m*, -ruptur *f*, Keratorrhexis *f*.
ker·a·to·scle·ri·tis [-sklɪ'raɪtɪs] *n ophthal*. Entzündung *f* von Hornhaut u. Sklera, Keratoskleritis *f*, -scleritis *f*.
ker·a·to·scope ['-skəʊp] *n ophthal*. Placido-Scheibe *f*, Keratoskop *nt*.
ker·a·tos·co·py [kerə'tɑskəpɪ] *n ophthal*. Hornhautuntersuchung *f*, Keratoskopie *f*.
ker·a·to·sis [kerə'təʊsɪs] *n derm*. Verhornungsstörung *f*, Keratose *f*, Keratosis *f*.
ker·a·to·sul·fate [,kerətəʊ'sʌlfeɪt] *n* → keratan sulfate.
ker·a·tot·ic [kerə'tɑtɪk] *adj derm*. Keratose betr. od. auslösend, keratotisch, Keratose-.
ke·rat·o·tome [kə'rætətəʊm, 'kerətə-] *n ophthal*. Hornhautmesser *nt*, Keratotom *nt*.
ker·a·tot·o·my [kerə'tɑtəmɪ] *n ophthal*. Hornhautschnitt *m*, -durchtrennung *f*, Keratotomie *f*, Korneotomie *f*.
ke·rau·no·neu·ro·sis [kə,rɔːnənjʊə'rəʊsɪs, -nʊ-] *n psycho., psychia*. Keraunoneurose *f*.
ke·rau·no·pho·bia [-'fəʊbɪə] *n psychia*. krankhafte Angst *f* vor Gewittern, Keraunophobie *f*.
Kerckring ['kɜrkrɪŋ]: **K.'s center** Kerckring-Knochenkern *m*.
K.'s (circular) folds Kerckring'-Falten *pl*, Plicae circulares (Kerckringi).
K.'s ossicle → K.'s center.
K.'s valve → K.'s (circular) folds.
ke·rec·ta·sis [kə'rektəsɪs] *n* → keratectasia.
ke·rec·to·my [kə'rektəmɪ] *n* → keratectomy.
ke·ri·on ['kɪrɪɑn] *n derm*. Kerion *nt*.
Kerkring → Kerckring.
Kerley ['kɜrlɪ]: **K. (B) lines** Kerley-B-Linien *pl*.
ker·ma [kɜrmə] *abbr*. [kinetic energy released in material] Kerma *f*.
Kern plasma relation theory [kɜrn] Kern-Plasma-Relationstheorie *f*.
ker·nic·ter·us [kɜr'nɪktərəs] *n ped*. Kernikterus *m*, Bilirubinenzephalopathie *f*.
Kernig ['kernɪg]: **K.'s sign** *neuro*. Kernig'-Zeichen *nt*.
ker·oid ['kerɔɪd] *adj* → keratoid.
ker·o·sene ['kerəsiːn] *n* → kerosine.
ker·o·ther·a·py [,kerə'θerəpɪ] *n* Behandlung *f* mit Wachs- od. Paraffinpräparaten.
Kessler ['keslər]: **K. grasping suture** *ortho*. Kessler-Naht *f*.
ke·tal [kiːtæl] *n* Ketal *nt*.
ketal bond/linkage Ketalbindung *f*.
ke·ta·mine [kiːtəmiːn, -mɪn] *n pharm., anes*. Ketamin *nt*.
ke·ta·zo·lam ['ketəzəʊlæm] *n pharm*. Ketazolam *nt*.
ke·ti·mine ['ketɪmiːn, -mɪn] *n* Ketimin *nt*.
keto- *pref*. Keto(n)-.
ke·to ac·id [kiːtəʊ] Keto(n)säure *f*.
3-keto acid-CoA transferase 3-Ketosäure-CoA-transferasae *f*.
keto acid decarboxylase → α-keto acid dehydrogenase, branched-chain.
keto acid decarboxylase deficiency Ahornsirup-Krankheit *f*, -Syndrom *nt*, Valin-Leucin-Isoleucinurie *f*, Verzweigtkettendecarboxylase-Mangel *m*.
α-keto acid dehydrogenase α-Ketosäuredehydrogenase *f*.
branched-chain k. verzweigtkettige (α-)Ketosäuredehydrogenase/Ketosäuredecarboxylase *f*.
ke·to·ac·i·de·mia [,kiːtəʊæsɪ'diːmɪə] *n* Ketoazidämie *f*.
ke·to·ac·i·do·sis [,-,æsɪ'dəʊsɪs] *n* Ketoazidose *f*, -acidose *f*.
ke·to·ac·i·dot·ic [,-,æsɪ'dɑtɪk] *adj* Ketoazidose betr. od. verursachend, ketoazidotisch.
ke·to·ac·i·du·ria [,-,æsɪ'd(j)ʊərɪə] *n* Ketosäureausscheidung *f* im Harn, Ketoazidurie *f*.
ke·to·a·mi·no·ac·i·de·mia [,-ə,miːnəʊæsə'diːmɪə] *n* → keto acid decarboxylase deficiency.
β-ke·to·ac·yl-ACP reductase [,kiːtəʊ'æsɪl] β-Ketoacyl-ACP-reduktase *f*.
β-ketoacyl-ACP synthase β-Ketoacyl-ACP-synthase *f*.
3-ketoacyl-CoA thiolase Acetyl-CoA-acyltransferase *f*.
α-ke·to·a·dip·ic acid [-ə'dɪpɪk] α-Ketoadipinsäure *f*.
α-keto-ε-amino caproic acid α-Keto-ε-aminocapronsäure *f*.
α-ke·to·bu·tyr·ic acid [-bjuː'tɪrɪk] α-Ketobuttersäure *f*.
β-ketobutyric acid Azetessigsäure *f*, β-Ketobuttersäure *f*.

ke·to·co·na·zole [ˌ-'kəʊnəzəʊl, -zɒl] *n pharm.* Ketoconazol *nt.*
2-keto-3-deoxy-octanic acid *abbr.* KDO 2-Keto-3-desoxyoctansäure *f abbr.* KDO.
keto-enol tautomerism Keto-Enol-Tautomerie *f.*
keto form *chem.* Ketoform *f.*
ke·to·gen·e·sis [kiːtəʊ'dʒenəsɪs] *n* Keto(n)körperbildung *f*, Ketogenese *f.*
ke·to·ge·net·ic [ˌ-dʒə'netɪk] *adj* → ketogenic.
ke·to·gen·ic [ˌ-'dʒenɪk] *adj* Keton(körper)bildend, ketogen, ketoplastisch.
ketogenic hormone lipolytisches Hormon *nt.*
α-ke·to·glu·ta·rate [ˌ-'gluːtəreɪt] *n* α-Ketoglutarat *nt.*
α-ketoglutarate dehydrogenase α-Ketoglutaratdehydrogenase *f.*
α-ketoglutarate-malate carrier α-Ketoglutarat-Malat-Carrier *m.*
α-ketoglutarate pathway *biochem.* α-Ketoglutaratweg *m.*
ketoglutarate reductase (lysine) Saccharopindehydrogenase (NADP+, L-Lysin-bildend) *f.*
α-ke·to·glu·tar·ic acid [ˌ-gluː'tærɪk] α-Ketoglutarsäure *f.*
ke·to·hep·tose [ˌ-'heptəʊs] *n* Ketoheptose *f.*
ke·to·hex·o·ki·nase [ˌ-ˌheksə'kaɪneɪz] *n* Keto(hexo)kinase *f*, Fructokinase *f.*
ke·to·hex·ose [ˌ-'heksəʊs] *n* Ketohexose *f.*
ke·to·hy·drox·y·es·trin [ˌ-haɪˌdrɒksɪ'estrɪn] *n* Estron *nt*, Östron *nt*, Follikulin *nt*, Folliculin *nt.*
α-ke·to·i·so·cap·ro·ate [ˌ-ˌaɪsə'kæprəweɪt] *n* α-Ketoisocaproat *nt.*
α-ke·to·i·so·ca·pro·ic acid [ˌ-ˌaɪsəkə'prəʊɪk] α-Ketoisocapronsäure *f.*
α-ketoisocaproic acid dehydrogenase α-Ketoisocapronsäuredehydrogenase *f.*
α-ke·to·i·so·val·er·ate [ˌ-ˌaɪsə'væləreɪt] *n* α-Ketoisovalerat *nt.*
α-ketoisovalerate dehydrogenase α-Ketoisovaleratdehydrogenase *f.*
α-ke·to·i·so·va·ler·ic acid [ˌ-ˌaɪsəvə'lerɪk, -'lɪər-] α-Ketoisovaleriansäure *f.*
α-ketoisovaleric acid dehydrogenase α-Ketoisovaleriansäuredehydrogenase *f.*
ke·tol ['kiːtɒl, -təʊl] *n* Ketol *nt.*
ketol-isomerase *n* Ketolisomerase *f.*
ke·tol·y·sis [kɪ'tɒləsɪs] *n* Ketolyse *f.*
ke·to·lyt·ic [ˌkiːtə'lɪtɪk] *adj* Ketolyse betr. *od.* fördernd, ketolytisch.
α-keto-β-methylvalerate *n* α-Keto-β-methylvalerat *nt.*
α-keto-β-methylvaleric acid α-Keto-β-methylvaleriansäure *f.*
ke·tone ['kiːtəʊn] *n chem.* Keton *nt.*
ketone bodies Keto(n)körper *pl.*
ke·to·ne·mia [ˌkiːtəʊ'niːmɪə] *n* erhöhter Keton(körper)gehalt *m* des Blutes, Ketonämie *f.*
ke·ton·ic [kiː'tɒnɪk] *adj* Keton(e) betr., Keton-, Keto-.
ke·to·ni·za·tion [ˌkiːtəʊnaɪ'zeɪʃn] *n chem.* Umwandlung *f* in ein Keton.
ke·to·nu·ria [ˌ-'n(j)ʊərɪə] *n* Ketonkörperausscheidung *f* im Harn, Ketonurie *f.*
keto-octose *n* Ketooctose *f.*
ke·to·pen·tose [ˌ-'pentəʊs] *n* Ketopentose *f.*
ke·to·phen·yl·bu·ta·zone [ˌ-ˌfenl'bjuːtəzəʊn, -ˌfiːnl] *n* → kebuzone.
ke·to·pla·sia [ˌ-'pleɪʒ(ɪ)ə, -zɪə] *n* Keto(n)körperbildung *f.*
ke·to·plas·tic [ˌ-'plæstɪk] *adj* → ketogenic.
ke·to·pro·fen [ˌ-'prəʊfen] *n pharm.* Ketoprofen *nt.*
α-ke·to·pro·pi·on·ic acid [ˌ-ˌprəʊpɪ'ɒnɪk,

-'əʊnɪk] Brenztraubensäure *f*, Acetylameisensäure *f*, α-Ketopropionsäure *f.*
β-keto-reductase *n* 3-Hydroxyacyl-CoA-dehydrogenase *f.*
ke·tose ['kiːtəʊs] *n* Keto(n)zucker *m*, Ketose *f.*
ke·to·sis [kɪ'taʊsɪs] *n patho.* Azeton-, Ketonämie *f*, Ketoazidose *f*, Ketose *f*, Ketosis *f.*
ketosis-prone diabetes insulinabhängiger Diabetes (mellitus) *m*, Typ 1 Diabetes (mellitus), Insulinmangeldiabetes *m.*
ketosis-resistant diabetes nicht-insulinabhängiger Diabetes mellitus *m*, Typ-II--Diabetes mellitus *m*, non-insulin-dependent diabetes (mellitus) *abbr.* NIDD(M).
17-ke·tos·ter·oid [kɪ'tɒstərɔɪd] *n abbr.* 17-KS.
17-KS 17-Ketosteroid *nt abbr.* 17-KS, 17-Oxosteroid *nt.*
ke·to·suc·cin·ic acid [ˌkiːtəʊ'sʌksɪnɪk] Oxalessigsäure *f.*
keto sugar acid Ketozuckersäure *f.*
ke·to·su·ria [ˌ-'s(j)ʊərɪə] *n* Ketoseausscheidung *f* im Harn, Ketosurie *f.*
ke·to·tet·rose [ˌ-'tetrəʊz] *n* Ketotetrose *f.*
3-ke·to·thi·o·lase [ˌ-'θaɪəleɪz] *n* Acetyl--CoA-acyltransferase *f.*
ke·tot·ic hyperglycinemia [kɪ'tɒtɪk] ketotische Hyperglycinämie *f.*
ke·to·trans·fer·ase [ˌkiːtəʊ'trænsfəreɪz] *n* Transketolase *f abbr.* TK.
ke·to·tri·ose [ˌ-'traɪəʊs] *n* Ketotriose *f.*
ke·tox·ime [kɪ'tɒksiːm] *n* Ketoxim *nt.*
keV, kev *abbr.* → kilo electron volt.
Kew Gardens (spotted) fever [kjuː] Rickettsienpocken *pl*, Pockenfleckfieber *nt.*
key [kiː] I *n* 1. Schlüssel *m.* 2. *fig.* Schlüssel *m (to* zu); Erklärung *f (to* für); Lösung *f.* 3. Taste *f*, Druckknopf *m*; Taster *m*, Tastkontakt *m*, Tastschalter *m.* II Schlüssel-. III *vt* 4. ver-, festkeilen. 5. (*Computer*) eintippen, eingeben.
key in *vt* → key 4, 5.
key on *vt* → key 4.
Key and Retzius [kiː 'retzɪəs]: **(connective tissue) sheath of K.a.R.** Endoneurium *nt.*
key·hole pupil ['kiːhəʊl] *ophthal.* Schlüssellochpupille *f.*
key-in-lock maneuver *gyn.* (de) Lee--Spiegelhandgriff *m.*
k_F *abbr.* → filtration coefficient.
KFD *abbr.* → Kyasanur Forest disease.
kg *abbr.* → kilogram.
khel·lin ['kelɪn] *n pharm.* Khellin *nt.*
KHN *abbr.* → Knoop hardness number.
kHz *abbr.* → kilohertz.
kick [kɪk] *n* 1. (Fuß-)Tritt *m*, Stoß *m.* 2. *electr.* (Strom-)Stoß *m*, Impuls *m.* 3. (*Zeiger*) Ausschlag *m.*
Kidd [kɪd]: **K. blood group (system)** Kidd--Blutgruppe *f*, -Blutgruppensystem *nt.*
kid·ney ['kɪdnɪ] *n* Niere *f*; *anat.* Ren *m*, Nephros *m.*
kidney abscess Nierenabszeß *m.*
kidney biopsy Nierenbiopsie *f*, -punktion *f.*
kidney carbuncle Nierenkarbunkel *m.*
kidney clamp *chir.* Nierenfaßzange *f.*
kidney condition Nierenleiden *nt.*
kidney disease Nierenerkrankung *f*, -leiden *nt*, Nephropathie *f.*
  polycystic k. polyzystische Nieren *pl.*
  acute k. akutes Nierenversagen *nt.*
  high-output k. polyurisches Nierenversagen.
  non-oliguric k. nicht-oligurisches Nierenversagen.
  oliguric k. oligurisches Nierenversagen.
  polyuric k. polyurisches Nierenversagen.
kidney function Nierenfunktion *f.*

kidney function test Nierenfunktionsprüfung *f.*
kidney graft → kidney transplant.
kidney insufficiency Niereninsuffizienz *f.*
kidney machine künstliche Niere *f.*
kidney pedicle Nierenstiel *m.*
kidney pedicle clamp *chir.* Nierenstielklemme *f.*
kidney-shaped *adj* nierenförmig.
kidney-shaped placenta nierenförmige Plazenta *f*, Placenta reniformis.
kidney stone Nierenstein *m*, Nephrolith *m*, Calculus renalis.
kidney transplant Nierentransplantat *nt.*
  cadaveric k. Kadaver-, Leichenniere(ntransplantat *nt*) *f.*
  related k. Verwandtenniere(ntransplantat *nt*) *f.*
kidney transplantation Nierentransplantation *f*, -verpflanzung *f.*
kidney worm *micro.* Nieren-, Riesenpalisadenwurm *m*, Dioctophyma renale, Eustrongylus gigas.
Kienböck ['kiːnbek]: **K.'s disease 1.** Kienböck'-Krankheit *f*, Morbus Kienböck *m*, Lunatummalazie *f.* **2.** (post-)traumatische Syringomyelie *f.*
K.'s disease of the lunate → K.'s disease 1.
K.'s dislocation *ortho.* Luxation *f* des Os lunatum, Lunatumluxation *f.*
K.'s phenomenon *radiol.* Kienböck-Zeichen *nt.*
Kiesselbach ['kiːzəlbax]: **K.'s area** Kiesselbach'-Ort *m*, Locus Kiesselbachi.
kill [kɪl] **I** *vt* **1.** töten, umbringen, ermorden; **to ~ o.s.** s. umbringen. **2.** arg zu schaffen machen. **my back is ~ing me** mein Rücken bringt mich (noch) um. **3.** (*Wirkung*) neutralisieren, unwirksam machen, aufheben; (*Maschine*) ab-, ausschalten; (*Keime*) abtöten; (*Schmerz*) stillen; (*Hoffnung*) vernichten; (*Gefühle*) töten. **II** *vi* töten, den Tod verursachen.
killed vaccine [kɪld] Todimpfstoff *m*, -vakzine *f*, inaktivierter Impfstoff *m.*
kill·er ['kɪlər] **I** *n* **1.** Mörder *m*, Killer *m.* **2.** Vernichtungs-, Vertilungsmittel *nt.* **3.** tödlich verlaufende Krankheit *f.* **II** *adj* tödlich, Killer-.
killer cells 1. Killer-Zellen *pl*, K-Zellen *pl.* **2.** zytotoxische T-Zellen *pl*, zytotoxische T-Lymphozyten *pl.*
killer T cells → killer cells 2.
Killian ['kɪlɪən]: **K.'s nasal speculum** *HNO* Killian-Nasenspekulum *nt.*
kill·ing ['kɪlɪŋ] **I** *n* Töten *m*, Tötung *f.* **II** *adj* tödlich; (*a. fig.*) vernichtend, mörderisch.
kilo- *pref. abbr.* k Kilo- *abbr.* k.
kil·o·base ['kɪləbeɪs] *n abbr.* **Kb** Kilobase *f.*
kilobase pairs *abbr.* **Kbp** Kilobasenpaare *pl abbr.* Kbp.
kil·o·cal·o·rie ['-kælərɪ] *n abbr.* **kcal, C, Cal** (große) Kalorie *f*, Kilokalorie *f abbr.* Kcal, Cal.
kil·o·cu·rie ['-kjʊərɪ, -kjʊəˌrɪ] *n abbr.* **kCi** Kilocurie *nt abbr.* kCi.
kilo electron volt *abbr.* **keV, kev** Kiloelektronenvolt *nt abbr.* keV.
kil·o·gram ['-græm] *n abbr.* **kg** Kilogramm *nt abbr.* kg.
kil·o·hertz ['-hɜːts] *n abbr.* **kHz** Kilohertz *nt abbr.* kHz.
kil·o·li·ter ['-liːtər] *n abbr.* **kl** Kiloliter *m/nt abbr.* kl.
kil·o·me·ter [kɪ'lɒmɪtər, 'kɪləmɪtər] *n abbr.* **km** Kilometer *m abbr.* km.
kil·o·met·ric [ˌkɪlə'metrɪk] *adj* kilometrisch.
kil·o·volt ['-vəʊlt] *n abbr.* **kV, kv** Kilovolt *nt abbr.* kV.
kil·o·watt ['-wɒt] *n abbr.* **kW, kw** Kilowatt *nt abbr.* kW.

kilowatt-hour

kilowatt-hour *n abbr.* **kWh, kwhr** Kilowattstunde *f abbr.* kWh.
Kimmelstiel-Wilson ['kɪməlstiːl 'wɪlsən]: **K.-W. disease/syndrome** Kimmelstiel-Wilson-Syndrom *nt*, diabetische Glomerulosklerose *f*.
Kimura [kɪ'mʊərə]: **K.'s disease** Kimura-Krankheit *f*, -Syndrom *nt*, Morbus Kimura *m*, papulöse Angioplasie *f*, angiolymphoide Hyperplasie *f* mit Eosinophilie (Kimura).
kin- *pref.* → kino-.
kin·an·es·the·sia [kɪnˌænəs'θiːʒə] *n neuro.* Verlust *f* der Bewegungsempfindung, Kinanästhesie *f*.
ki·nase ['kaɪneɪz, 'kɪ-] *n* Kinase *f*.
kine- *pref.* → kino-.
kin·e·mat·ic [ˌkɪnə'mætɪk] *adj* Kinematik betr., auf ihr beruhend, kinematisch.
kin·e·mat·ics [ˌ-'mætɪks] *pl* Bewegungslehre *f*, Kinematik *f*.
kinematic viscosity *abbr.* **v** *phys.* kinematische Viskosität *f abbr.* v.
ki·ne·mia [kaɪ'niːmɪə] *n card.* Herzzeitvolumen *nt abbr.* HZV.
kin·e·plas·tic amputation [ˌkɪnə'plæstɪk] → kineplasty.
kin·e·plas·tics [ˌ-'plæstɪks] *pl* → kineplasty.
kin·e·plas·ty ['-plæstɪ] *n chir., ortho.* plastische Amputation *f*, Kineplastik *f*. (*Muskel*) Bewegungsschmerz *m*, Kines(i)algie *f*.
kin·e·scope ['-skəʊp] *n ophthal.* Kineskop *nt*.
kinesi- *pref.* → kinesio-.
ki·ne·sia [kɪ'niːʒ(ɪ)ə, kaɪ-] *n* → kinetosis.
ki·ne·si·al·gia [kɪˌniːsɪ'ældʒ(ɪ)ə] *n* → kinesalgia.
ki·ne·si·at·rics [ˌ-'ætrɪks] *pl* → kinesitherapy.
ki·ne·sics [kɪ'niːsɪks] *pl* Kinesik *f*.
kinesi-esthesiometer *n neuro., physiol.* Kinesiästhesiometer *nt*.
kin·e·sim·e·ter [kɪnə'sɪmətər, kaɪ-] *n* Bewegungsmesser *m*, Kinesi(o)meter *nt*.
kinesio- *pref.* Bewegungs-, Kinesi(o)-.
ki·ne·si·ol·o·gy [kɪˌniːsɪ'ɒlədʒɪ] *n* Bewegungslehre *f*, Kinesiologie *f*.
ki·ne·si·om·e·ter [ˌ-'ɒmɪtər] *n* → kinesimeter.
ki·ne·si·o·neu·ro·sis [kɪˌniːzɪəʊnjʊə'rəʊsɪs, kaɪ-, -nʊ-] *n* Bewegungs-, Motilitäts-, Kinesioneurose *f*.
ki·ne·si·o·ther·a·py [ˌ-'θerəpɪ] *n* → kinesitherapy.
ki·ne·sip·a·thy [kɪnə'sɪpəθɪ] *n* → kinesitherapy.
ki·ne·sis [kɪ'niːsɪs, kaɪ-] *n* Bewegung *f*, Kinesie *f*, Kinesis *f*.
ki·ne·si·ther·a·py [kɪˌniːsɪ'θerəpɪ] *n* Bewegungstherapie *f*, Kinesio-, Kinesitherapie *f*.
kin·es·the·sia [ˌkɪnəs'θiːʒ(ɪ)ə, -zɪə] *n* Bewegungs- u. Lagesinn *m*, Muskelsinn *m*, Bewegungsempfindung *f*, Kinästhesie *f*.
kin·es·the·si·om·e·ter [ˌ-ˌθiːʒɪ'ɒmɪtər] *n neuro., physiol.* Kinästhesiometer *nt*.
kin·es·the·sis [ˌ-'θiːsɪs] *n* → kinesthesia.
kin·es·thet·ic [ˌ-'θetɪk] *adj* Kinästhesie betr., kinästhetisch.
kinesthetic aura *neuro.* kinästhetische Aura *f*.
kinesthetic hallucination *psychia.* kinästhetische Halluzination *f*.
kinesthetic sense Muskelsensibilität *f*, -sinn *m*, Myästhesie *f*.
kinesthetic sensibility Proprio(re)zeption *f*, Tiefensensibilität *f*, kinästhetische Sensibilität *f*.
kinet- *pref.* → kineto-.

ki·net·ic [kɪ'netɪk, kaɪ-] *adj* Kinetik od. Bewegung betr. od. fördernd od. verursachend, kinetisch, Bewegungs-.
kinetic ataxia *neuro.* motorische Ataxie *f*.
kinetic emphysema kinetisches (Lungen-)Emphysem *nt*.
kinetic energy Bewegungsenergie *f*, kinetische Energie *f*.
kinetic labyrinth *physiol.* kinetisches Labyrinth *nt*, Bogengangsapparat *m*.
kinetic perimetry *ophthal.* kinetische/dynamische Perimetrie *f*.
ki·net·ics [kɪ'netɪks, kaɪ-] *pl* Kinetik *f*.
kinetic tremor Bewegungstremor *m*.
ki·ne·tin [kaɪ'niːtɪn] *n bio.* Kinetin *nt*.
kineto- *pref.* Bewegungs-, Kinet(o)-.
ki·ne·to·chore [kɪ'niːtəkɔːr, -'netə-, kaɪ-] *n* Kinetochor *nt*, Zentromer *nt*.
ki·ne·to·gen·ic [ˌ-'dʒenɪk] *adj* Bewegung auslösend, kinetogen.
ki·ne·to·nu·cle·us [ˌ-'n(j)uːklɪəs] *n* → kinetoplast.
ki·ne·to·plasm ['-plæzəm] *n* Kinetoplasma *nt*.
ki·ne·to·plast ['-plæst] *n micro.* Kinetoplast *m*, Kinetonukleus *m*, Blepharoplast *m*.
Ki·ne·to·plas·ti·da [ˌ-'plæstɪdə] *pl micro.* Kinetoplastida *pl*.
ki·ne·to·scope [ˌ-'skəʊp] *n physiol., neuro.* Kinetoskop *nt*.
ki·ne·tos·co·py [ˌkaɪnɪ'tɒskəpɪ] *n physiol., neuro.* Kinetoskopie *f*.
kin·e·to·sis [ˌkɪnə'təʊsɪs] *n, pl* **-ses** [-siːz] Bewegungs-, Reisekrankheit *f*, Kinetose *f*.
ki·ne·to·some [kɪ'niːtəsəʊm, -'netə-, kaɪ-] *n* Basalkörperchen *nt*, -körnchen *nt*, Kinetosom *nt*.
ki·ne·to·ther·a·py [ˌ-'θerəpɪ] *n* → kinesitherapy.
King [kɪŋ]: **K.'s operation** *HNO* Kelly-Operation *f*, Kelly-Arytänoidopexie *f*.
King·el·la [kɪŋ'elə] *n micro.* Kingella *f*.
ki·nin ['kaɪnɪn, 'kɪ-] *n* Kinin *nt*.
kininase I Carboxypeptidase N *f*.
kininase II (Angiotensin-)Converting-Enzym *nt abbr.* ACE.
ki·nin·o·gen [ˌˌ'kaɪnɪnədʒən] *n* Kininogen *nt*.
kinin system → kallikrein-kinin system.
kink [kɪŋk] **I** *n* Knick *m*, Abknickung *f*. **II** *vt, vi* (ab-)knicken.
kinked aorta [kɪŋkt] Knick- *od.* Buckelbildung *f* der Aorta, Pseudocoarctatio aortae.
Kinkiang fever [kɪŋkɪ'æn] japanische Schistosomiasis/Bilharziose *f*, Schistosomiasis japonica.
kink·y-hair disease ['kɪŋkɪ] Menkes-Syndrom *nt*, -Stahlhaarkrankheit *f*, Kraushaarsyndrom *nt*, Trichopoliodystrophie *f*, kinky-hair disease (*nt*), Pili torti mit Kupfermangel.
kinky-hair syndrome → kinky-hair disease.
kino- *pref.* Bewegungs-, Kine-, Kinet(o)-, Kin(o)-.
ki·no·cen·trum [ˌkɪnə'sentrəm, ˌkaɪ-] *n* Kinozentrum *nt*, Zentrosom *nt*.
ki·no·cil·i·um [ˌ-'sɪlɪəm] *n, pl* **-cil·ia** [-'sɪlɪə] (Kino-)Zilie *f*, Flimmerhaar *nt*.
ki·nol·o·gy [kaɪ'nɒlədʒɪ] *n* → kinesiology.
kin·o·mere ['kɪnəmɪər, 'kaɪ-] *n* Zentromer *nt*.
kin·o·plasm ['-plæzəm] *n* → kinetoplasm.
kin·o·plas·mic [ˌ-'plæzmɪk] *adj* Kinetoplasma betr., kinetoplasmatisch.
ki·no·sphere ['-sfɪər] *n bio., histol.* Aster *f*, Astrosphäre *f*.
Kinsbourne ['kɪnzbɔːrn, -bəʊrn]: **K. syndrome** Kinsbourne-Syndrom *nt*, myoklonisch infantile Enzephalopathie *f*.
Kirchner ['kɪərknər; 'kɪrçnər] **K.'s diverticulum** Kirchner-Divertikel *nt*.
Kirk [kɜrk]: **K.'s amputation/technique** *ortho.* suprakondyläre Oberschenkelamputation *f* nach Kirk, Kirk-Amputation *f*.
Kirschner ['kɪrʃnər]: **K.'s apparatus** → K.'s wire.
K.'s wire Kirschner-Draht *m*.
K.'s wire splint → K.'s wire.
kiss·ing bugs ['kɪsɪŋ] *micro.* Raubwanzen *pl*, Reduviiden *pl*, Reduviidae *pl*.
kissing disease Pfeiffer'-Drüsenfieber *nt*, infektiöse Mononukleose *f*, Monozytenangina *f*, Mononucleosis infectiosa.
kissing spine *ortho.* Baastrup'-Zeichen *nt*, -Syndrom *nt*, -Krankheit *f*, Arthrosis interspinosa.
kissing ulcer Abklatschgeschwür *nt*.
kit·a·sa·my·cin [ˌkɪtəsə'maɪsɪn] *n pharm.* Leucomycin *nt*, Kitasamycin *nt*.
Kitasato [kiːtə'sɑːtəʊ]: **K.'s bacillus** Pestbakterium *nt*, Yersinia/Pasteurella pestis.
Kite [kaɪt]: **K. (corrective) cast** *ortho.* Umstellungsgipsverband *m* nach Kite.
k.j. *abbr.* → knee jerk.
Kjeldahl ['keldɑːl]: **K.'s method** Kjeldahl-Verfahren *nt*, Kjdahlometrie *f*.
kl *abbr.* → kiloliter.
Klapp [klap]: **K.'s method** *ortho.* Klapp-Kriechübungen *pl*.
Klatskin ['klætskɪn]: **K. tumor** *patho.* Gallengangskarzinom *nt* an der Hepatikusgabelung.
Klebs [klɛbs]: **K.'** **disease** Glomerulonephritis *f abbr.* GN.
Kleb·si·el·la [ˌklɛbzɪ'elə] *n micro.* Klebsiella *f*.
K. friedländeri → K. pneumoniae.
K. ozaenae → K. pneumoniae ozaenae.
K. pneumoniae Friedländer-Bakterium *nt*, -Bazillus *m*, Klebsiella pneumoniae, Bact. pneumoniae Friedländer.
K. pneumoniae ozaenae Ozäna-Bakterium *nt*, Klebsiella (pneumoniae) ozaenae, Bact. ozaenae.
K. pneumoniae rhinoscleromatis Rhinosklerom-Bakterium *nt*, Klebsiella (pneumoniae) rhinoscleromatis, Bact. rhinoscleromatis.
K. rhinoscleromatis → K. pneumoniae rhinoscleromatis.
Klebsiella pneumonia Klebsiellenpneumonie *f*, Friedländer-Pneumonie *f*.
Klebs-Löffler ['leflər; 'lœf-]: **K.-L. bacillus** Diphtheriebazillus *m*, -bakterium *nt*, (Klebs-)Löffler-Bazillus *m*, Corynebacterium/Bact. diphtheriae.
Kleine-Levin ['klaɪnə 'levɪn]: **K.-L. syndrome** Kleine-Levin-Syndrom *nt*.
Klein-Waardenburg [klaɪn 'vɑːrdnbɜrg]: **K.-W. syndrome** Waardenburg-Syndrom *nt*, Klein-Waardenburg-Syndrom *nt*.
Klemperer ['klɛmpərər]: **K.'s disease** Banti-Krankheit *f*, -Syndrom *nt*.
klep·to·ma·nia [ˌklɛptə'meɪnɪə, -njə] *n psychia.* krankhafter Stehltrieb *m*, Kleptomanie *f*.
klep·to·ma·ni·ac [ˌ-'meɪnɪæk] *psychia.* **I** *n* Kleptomane *m*, -manin *f*. **II** *adj* an Kleptomanie leidend, kleptomanisch.
klep·to·pho·bia [ˌ-'fəʊbɪə] *n psychia.* Kleptophobie *f*.
Klinefelter ['klaɪnfɛltər]: **K.'s syndrome** Klinefelter-Syndrom *nt*.
Klippel-Feil ['klɪp'el faɪl]: **K.-F. syndrome** Klippel-Feil-Syndrom *nt*.
Klippel-Trénaunay [treno'nɛ]: **K.-T. syndrome** Klippel-Trénaunay-Syndrom *nt*,

Klippel-Trénaunay-Weber-Syndrom *nt*, Osteoangiohypertrophie-Syndrom *nt*, angio-osteo-hypertrophisches Syndrom *nt*, Haemangiectasia hypertrophicans.
Klippel-Trénaunay-Weber ['webər, 'veɪ-]: **K.-T.-W. syndrome** → Klippel--Trénaunay syndrome.
klis·e·om·e·ter [klɪsɪ'ɑmɪtər] *n* Klisiometer *nt*.
Klumpke ['klʊmpkə]: **K.'s palsy/paralysis** *neuro*. Klumpke-Déjérine-Lähmung *f*, Klumpke'-Lähmung *f*, untere Armplexuslähmung *f*.
Klumpke-Déjérine [deʒe'rin]: **K.-D. paralysis/syndrome** → Klumpke's palsy.
Klüver-Bucy ['kluːvər 'bjuːsɪ]: **K.-B. syndrome** *neuro*. Klüver-Bucy-Syndrom *nt*.
K_m *abbr*. → Michaelis constant.
km *abbr*. → kilometer.
Km allotypes [kappa chain marker] Km--Allotypen *pl*, InV-Allotypen *pl*.
Km antigens Km-Antigene *pl*.
Knapp [knæp]: **K.'s operation** *ophthal*. Knapp-Operation *f*.
knead [niːd] *vt* (*Muskel*) (durch-)kneten, massieren.
knead·ing ['niːdɪŋ] *n* (*Muskel*) (Durch-)Kneten *nt*, Massieren *nt*.
knee [niː] *n* 1. Knie *nt*; *anat*. Genu *nt*. **on one's ~s** kniend. 2. Kniegelenk *nt*, Artic. genus/genualis. 3. (*a. techn.*) knieförmige Struktur *f*, Knie(stück *nt*) *nt*.
k. of internal capsule Kapselknee, Knie der inneren Kapsel, Genu capsulae internae.
knee bend Kniebeuge *f*.
knee cap 1. Kniescheibe *f*, Patella *f*. 2. Knieschützer *m*.
knee-chest position *chir*. Knie-Brust-Lage *f*.
knee-elbow position *chir*. Knie-Ellenbogen-Lage *f*.
knee injury Knieverletzung *f*, -trauma *nt*.
knee jerk *abbr*. **k.j.** Patellarsehnenreflex *m* *abbr*. PSR, Quadrizepssehnenreflex *m* *abbr*. QSR.
knee-jerk reflex → knee jerk.
knee joint Kniegelenk *nt*, Artic. genus/genualis.
kneel [niːl] (**knelt; kneeled**) *vi* 1. knien, auf den Knien. 2. (*s.*) hinknien, niederknien.
kneel down *vi* → kneel 2.
knee pad Knieschützer *m*.
knee pan → knee cap 1.
knee phenomenon → knee jerk.
knee presentation *gyn*. Knielage *f*.
knee reflex → knee jerk.
knee region Kniegegend *f*, -region *f*, Regio genus/genualis.
anterior k. Knievorderseite *f*, Regio genus/genualis anterior.
posterior k. Knierückseite *f*, Regio genus/genualis posterior.
knee trauma Knieverletzung *f*, -trauma *nt*.
kneipp·ism ['naɪpɪzəm] *n* Kneipp-Kur *f*.
Kne·mi·do·kop·tes [ˌniːmɪdəʊ'kɑptiːz] *n* *micro*. Knemidokoptes *pl*.
knife [naɪf] I *n*, *pl* **knives** [naɪvz] 1. Messer *nt*. 2. *chir*., *patho*. Messer *nt*, Skalpell *nt*. II *vt* 3. schneiden, mit einem Messer bearbeiten. 4. mit einem Messer stechen (*o.* verletzen).
knife blade Messerklinge *f*.
knife edge Messerschneide *f*.
knife handle Messergriff *m*.
knife point Messerspitze *f*.
knif·er ['naɪfər] *n forens*. Messerstecher *m*.
knif·ing ['naɪfɪŋ] *n forens*. Messerstecherei *f*.
knife rest crystals *urol*. Sargdeckelkristalle *pl*.

knock [nɑk] I *n* 1. Schlag *m*, Stoß *m*. 2. Klopfen *nt*, Pochen *nt*. II *vt* 3. schlagen, stoßen. 4. schlagen, klopfen. III *vi* 5. schlagen, pochen, klopfen. 6. schlagen, prallen, stoßen (*against*, *into* gegen; *on* auf). 7. *techn*. rattern, rütteln; klopfen.
knob [nɑb] *n* 1. *anat*. Vorsprung *m*, Höcker *m*, Verdickung *f*, Beule *f*; *inf*. Knubbel *m*. 2. Knopf *m*, Knauf *m*.
knobbed [nɑbd] *adj* → knobby.
knob·ble ['nɑbl] *n* Knötchen *nt*.
knob·bly ['nɑblɪ] *adj* → knobby.
knob·by ['nɑbɪ] *adj* knotig; uneben, höckerig; *inf*. knubbelig.
knock-knee *n* X-Bein *nt*, Genu valgum.
knock-kneed *adj* X-beinig.
Knoop [nuːp; knoːp]: **K. hardness number** *abbr*. KHN Knoop-Härte *f abbr*. HK.
K.'s theory Knoop-Regel *f*.
knot [nɑt] *n* 1. *anat*. knotenförmige Struktur *f*, Knoten *m*, Nodus *m*. 2. *patho*. knotenartige Struktur *f*, Knoten *m*. 3. (*a. chir*.) Knoten *m*, Schleife *f*, Schlinge *f*. **to make/tie a ~** einen Knoten machen. II *vt* einen Knoten machen in; (ver-)knoten, (ver-)knüpfen. III *vi* 4. (einen) Knoten bilden, s. verknoten. 5. s. verwickeln.
knot together *vt* verknoten.
knot·ted ['nɑtɪd] *adj* 1. ge-, verknotet, geknüpft. 2. → knotty.
knotted hair 1. Trichonodose *f*, Trichonodosis *f*. 2. Haarknötchenkrankheit *f*, Trichorrhexis nodosa, Nodositas crinium.
knot·ty ['nɑtɪ] *adj* knotig, voller Knoten.
know [noʊ] (**knew; known**) I *vt* wissen; kennen; können; *s*. auskennen in. II *vi* wissen (*of* von, um); Bescheid wissen (*about* über).
knowl·edge ['nɑlɪdʒ] *n* 1. Kenntnis *f*. **to have ~ of** Kenntnis haben von. **to my ~** soviel ich weiß; meines Wissens. 2. Wissen *nt*, Kenntnisse *pl* (*of*, *in* in).
knowl·edge·a·ble ['nɑlɪdʒəbl] *adj* kenntnisreich; klug, gescheit.
knowledge memory Wissensgedächtnis *nt*.
Knowles [noʊlz]: **K. pin** *ortho*. Knowles--Nagel *m*.
known [noʊn] I *adj* bekannt (*as* als; *to s.o.* jdm.); anerkannt. II *ptp* → know.
knuck·le ['nʌkl] *n* 1. (Finger-)Knöchel *m*. 2. Fingergrundgelenk *nt*. 3. (*a. techn*.) Gelenköse *f*.
knuck·le·bone ['nʌklbəʊn] *n anat*. Mittelhand-, Metakarpalknochen *m*.
knuckle joint 1. Fingergrundgelenk *nt*, MP-Gelenk *nt*, Artic. metacarpophalangealis. 2. *techn*. einachsiges Gelenk *nt*, (Kreuz-, Gabel-)Gelenk *nt*.
knuckle pads Fingerknöchelpolster *pl*.
dorsal k. Garrod'-Knötchen *pl*, (echte) Fingerknöchelpolster *pl*.
Koch [kɑk, kɔx]: **K.'s bacillus** 1. Tuberkelbazillus *m*, -bakterium *nt*, Tuberkulosebazillus *m*, -bakterium *nt*, TB-Bazillus *m*, TB-Erreger *m*, Mycobacterium tuberculosis, Mycobacterium tuberculosis var. hominis. 2. Komma-Bazillus *m*, Vibrio cholerae/comma.
K.'s law → K.'s postulates.
K.'s node Atrioventrikularknoten *m*, AV-Knoten *m*, Aschoff-Tawara'-Knoten *m*, Nodus atrioventricularis.
K.'s phenomenon Koch-Phänomen *nt*.
K.'s postulates Koch'-Regeln *pl*, -Postulate *pl*.
K.'s tuberculin Alttuberkulin *nt* *abbr*. AT, Tuberkulin-Original-Alt *nt* *abbr*. TOA.
Kocher ['kɑkər, 'kɔxər]: **K.'s clamp** Kocher-Klemme *f*.
K.'s forceps Kocher-Klemme *f*.

K.'s incision Kocher-(Rippenbogenrand-)Schnitt *m*.
K.'s maneuver *chir*. Kocher'-Duodenalmobilisierung *f*.
K.'s operation 1. *ortho*. Kocher-Reposition *f*. 2. Kocher-Strumaoperation *f*. 3. Kocher-Duodenalmobilisierung *f*.
Kocher-Debré-Sémélaigne [dəˈbre seməˈlɛːn]: **K.-D.-S. syndrome** Debré-Sémélaigne-Syndrom *nt*.
koch·er·i·za·tion [ˌkoʊkəraɪˈzeɪʃn] *n* → Kocher's maneuver.
Koch-Weeks [wiːks]: **K.-W. bacillus** Koch--Weeks-Bazillus *m*, Haemophilus aegypti(c)us/conjunctividis.
K.-W. conjunctivitis *ophthal*. Koch--Weeks-Konjunktivitis *f*, akute kontagiöse Konjunktivitis *f*, Konjunktivitis *f* durch Haemophilus aegyptius.
Koebner ['kebnər; 'kœb-]: **K.'s phenomenon** Koebner-Phänomen *nt*, isomorpher Reizeffekt *m*.
Koerber-Salus-Elschnig ['kœrbər 'seɪləs 'elʃnɪɡ]: **K.-S.-E. syndrome** Retraktionsnystagmus *m*, Nystagmus retractorius.
Koettstorfer ['kɛtstɔːrfər]: **K. number** Verseifungszahl *f*.
Kohler ['koʊlər]: **K.'s principle** Kohler'--Prinzip *nt*.
Köhler ['køːlər]: **K.'s (bone) disease** 1. Köhler-Krankheit *f*, Köhler-Müller--Weiss-Syndrom *nt*, Morbus Köhler I. 2. → Köhler's second disease.
K.'s principle Kohler'-Prinzip *nt*.
K.'s second disease Freiberg-Köhler--Krankheit *f*, Morbus Köhler II.
Köhler-Pellegrini-Stieda [pelə'griːnɪ 'stiːdə]: **K.-P.-S. disease** *ortho*. Stieda--Pellegrini-Schatten *m*, Pellegrini-Schatten *m*.
Köhlmeier-Degos ['køːlmaɪər deˈɡɔ]: **K.-D. disease** Köhlmeier-Degos-Syndrom *nt*, Degos-Delort-Tricot-Syndrom *nt*, tödliches kutaneointestinales Syndrom *nt*, Papulosis maligna atrophicans (Degos), Papulosis atrophicans maligna, Thrombangitis cutaneaintestinalis disseminata.
Kohlrausch ['koːlraʊʃ]: **K.'s fold** Kohlrausch'-Falte *f*, Plica transversalis recti.
K.'s valve → K.'s fold.
K. veins Kohlrausch'-Venen *pl*.
Kohn [koːn]: **K.'s pores** Kohn-Poren *pl*, (Inter-)Alveolarporen *pl*.
koil(o)- *pref*. Hohl-, Koil(o)-.
koi·lo·nych·ia [ˌkɔɪləˈnɪkɪə] *n derm*. Löffel-, Hohlnagel *m*, Koilonychie *f*.
koi·lo·ster·nia [ˌ-ˈstɜːrnɪə] *n* Trichterbrust *f*, Pectus excavatum/infundibulum/recurvatum.
Kojewnikoff → Koschewnikow.
ko·jic acid [ˈkoʊdʒɪk] Kojisäure *f*.
Kölliker ['kɛlɪkər; 'kœl-]: **K.'s dental crest** Os incisivum.
K.'s membrane Membrana reticularis (ductus cochlearis).
K.'s nucleus Kölliker'-Kernsubstanz *f*, Substantia intermedia centralis.
Kolmer ['koʊlmər]: **K. test** *immun*. Kolmer-Test *m*, Cardiolipin-Komplementbindungsreaktion *f* nach Kolmer.
ko·ly·pep·tic [ˌkɑlɪˈpɛptɪk] *adj* verdauungshemmend, kolypeptisch.
ko·lyt·ic [kəˈlɪtɪk] *adj* 1. hemmend, inhibitorisch. 2. (*Person*) gehemmt, zurückgezogen.
König ['keɪnɪɡ; 'køːnɪɡ]: **K. syndrome** König-Syndrom *nt*.
ko·nim·e·ter [kəʊˈnɪmətər] *n* → konometer.
ko·ni·o·cor·tex [ˌkəʊnɪəʊˈkɔːrteks] *n* granulärer Kortex *m*, Koniocortex *m*.

ko·nom·e·ter [kəʊˈnɑmɪtər] *n* Koni(o)meter *nt*.
Koon-gol virus [ˈkuːŋgɒl] Koongol-Virus *nt*.
ko·phe·mia [kəˈfiːmɪə] *n* Worttaubheit *f*, akustische Aphasie *f*.
Koplik [ˈkɑplɪk]: **K.'s sign/spots** Koplik-Flecken *pl*.
Kopp [kɑp]: **K.'s asthma** Stimmritzenkrampf *m*, Laryngismus stridulus.
kop·ro·ste·rin [kɑprəˈsterɪn] *n* Koprosterin *nt*.
Korányi-Grocco [kəʊˈrænji: ˈgrɑkəʊ]: **K.-G. triangle** Grocco-Rauchfuß-Dreieck *nt*.
Ko·re·an [kəˈrɪən, kəʊ-]: **K. hemorrhagic fever** hämorrhagisches Fieber *nt* mit renalem Syndrom *abbr*. HFRS, koreanisches hämorrhagisches Fieber *nt*, akute hämorrhagische Nephrosonephritis *f*, Nephropathia epidemica.
K. hemorrhagic fever virus Ha(n)taan-Virus *nt*.
K. hemorrhagic nephrosonephritis → K. hemorrhagic fever.
Ko·rin fever [ˈkəʊrɪn] → Korean hemorrhagic fever.
ko·ro [ˈkɔːrəʊ, ˈkəʊrəʊ] *n psychia*. Koro *nt*, Shook jang *nt*.
ko·ros·co·py [kəˈrɑskəpɪ] *n ophthal*. Koroskopie *f*, Retinoskopie *f*, Skiaskopie *f*.
Korotkoff [kəˈrɑtkɒf]: **K.'s method** auskultatorische Blutdruckmessung *f* nach Korotkow.
K.'s sounds Korotkov-Geräusche *pl*.
K.'s test Korotkow-Test *m*.
Korsakoff [ˈkɔːrsəkɒf]: **K.'s psychosis/syndrome** Korsakow-Psychose *f*, -Syndrom *nt*.
Korsakov → Korsakoff.
Koschewnikow [kəʊˈʃevnɪkɒf]: **K.'s disease/epilepsy** Kojewnikow-, Koshewnikoff-, Koževnikov-Syndrom *nt*, -Epilepsie *f*, Epilepsia partialis continua.
Koshevnikoff → Koschewnikow.
Kostmann [ˈkəʊstmən]: **K.'s syndrome** infantile hereditäre Agranulozytose *f*, Kostmann-Syndrom *nt*.
Kovalevsky [kəʊvəˈlefskɪ]: **K.'s canal** *embryo*. Canalis neurentericus.
Koyter [ˈkɔɪtər]: **K.'s muscle** M. corrugator supercilii.
Kozhevnikov → Koschewnikow.
Kr *abbr*. → krypton.
Krabbe [ˈkræbi; ˈkrɑbə]: **K.'s disease** Krabbe-Syndrom *nt*, Globoidzellen-Leukodystrophie *f*, Galaktozerebrosidlipidose *f*, Galaktozerebrosidose *f*, okuloenzephalische/enzephalookuläre Angiomatose *f*, Angiomatosis encephalocutanea, Leukodystrophia cerebri progressiva hereditaria.
K.'s leukodystrophy/syndrome → K.'s disease.
Kraske [ˈkræski; ˈkrɑskə]: **K.'s operation** *chir*. Kraske-Operation *f*.
K. position *chir*. Klappmesserposition *f*, Jackknife-Lagerung *f*.
kra·tom·e·ter [kræˈtɑmɪtər] *n ophthal*. Kratometer *nt*.
krau·o·ma·nia [ˌkrɔːwəˈmeɪnɪə, -jə] *n neuro*. Krauomanie *f*.
krau·ro·sis [krɔːˈrəʊsɪs] *n derm., patho*. Kraurose *f*, Kraurosis *f*, Craurosis *f*.
kraurosis vulvae Breisky-Krankheit *f*, Kraurosis/Craurosis vulvae.
Krause [ˈkraʊzə]: **bulbs of K.** → K.'s corpuscles.
K.'s corpuscles Krause'-Endkolben *pl*, Corpuscula bulboidea.
K.'s end bulbs → K.'s corpuscles.
end bulbs of K. → K.'s corpuscles.

K.'s glands Krause-Drüsen *pl*, Konjunktivaldrüsen *pl*, Gll. conjunctivales.
K.'s ligament Lig. transversum perinei.
K.'s line Z-Linie *f*, Z-Streifen *m*, Zwischenscheibe *f*, Telophragma *nt*.
K.'s membrane → K.'s line.
nympha of K. Kitzler *m*, Klitoris *f*, Clitoris *f*.
K.'s syndrome Krause-Reese-Syndrom *nt*, Reese-Syndrom *nt*, Dysplasia encephalo-ophthalmica.
K.'s valve Krause'-Klappe *f*, Valvula sacci lacrimalis inferior.
Krause-Wolfe [wʊlf]: **K.-W. graft** Krause-Wolfe-Lappen *m*, Wolfe-Krause-Lappen *m*.
kre·a·tin [ˈkrɪatɪn] *n* Kreatin *nt*, Creatin *nt*, α-Methylguanidinoessigsäure *f*.
Krebs [kreːps]: **K. cycle 1.** Krebs-Zyklus *m*, Zitronensäure-, Citratzyklus *m*, Tricarbonsäurezyklus *m*. **2.** → Krebs-Henseleit cycle.
K. ornithine cycle → Krebs-Henseleit cycle.
K. urea cycle → Krebs-Henseleit cycle.
Krebs-Henseleit [ˈhɛnsəlaɪt]: **K.-H. cycle** Harnstoff-, Ornithinzyklus *m*, Krebs-Henseleit-Zyklus *m*.
kres·ol [ˈkresɔl, -sɑl] *n* Kresol *nt*.
Kretschmer [ˈkrɛtʃmər]: **K. types** Kretschmer-Typen *pl*.
Kreysig [ˈkraɪzɪg]: **K.'s sign** *radiol*. Heim-Kreysig-Zeichen *nt*.
Kristeller [ˈkrɪstələr]: **K.'s expression/method/technique** *gyn*. Kristeller-Handgriff *m*, Kristellern *nt*.
Krogh [krəʊg; krɒx]: **K.'s diffusion coefficient** Krogh'-Diffusionskoeffizient *m*.
Kromayer [ˈkrɒmaɪər]: **K.'s lamp** Kromayer-Lampe *f*.
Krompecher [ˈkrɒmpekər]: **K.'s carcinoma/tumor** *old* Ulcus rodens.
Krönig [ˈkreɪnɪg; ˈkrøːn-]: **K. fields** Krönig-Schallfelder *pl*.
Krönlein [ˈkreɪnlɪn; ˈkrøːnlaɪn]: **K.'s hernia** Krönlein-Hernie *f*, Bruggiser-Hernie *f*.
Krukenberg [ˈkrʊkənbɜːrg]: **K.'s tumor** Krukenberg-Tumor *m*.
K.'s veins Zentralvenen *pl*, Vv. centrales (hepatis).
kry·os·co·py [kraɪˈɑskəpɪ] *n lab*. Kryoskopie *f*.
kryp·ton [ˈkrɪptɑn] *n abbr*. **Kr** Krypton *nt abbr*. Kr.
K$_S$ *abbr*. → substrate constant.
17-KS *abbr*. → 17-ketosteroid.
k-stro·phan·thin [strəˈfænθɪn] *n pharm*. k-Strophanthin *nt*.
k-strophanthin-α *n pharm*. k-Strophanthin-α *nt*, Cymarin *nt*.
ku·bis·a·ga·ri [kjuːˌbɪsəˈgɑːrɪ] *n* Vertigo epidemica.
ku·bis·ga·ri [ˌkjuːbɪsˈgɑːrɪ] *n* → kubisagari.
Kufs [kuːfz]: **K.' disease** Kufs-Syndrom *nt*, Kufs-Hallervorden-Krankheit *f*, Erwachsenenform *f* der amaurotischen Idiotie.
Kugelberg-Welander [ˈkuːgəlbɜːrg ˈwelændər]: **K.-W. disease** Kugelberg-Welander-Krankheit *f*, -Syndrom *nt*, Atrophia musculorum spinalis pseudomyopathica (Kugelberg-Welander), juvenile Form *f* der spinalen Muskelatrophie.
Kuhn [kuːn]: **K.'s tube** Kuhn-Tubus *m*.
Kühne [ˈkiːnə; ˈkyːn-]: **K.'s spindle** Muskelspindel *f*.
Kuhnt-Junius [kuːnt ˈdʒuːnɪəs]: **K.-J. degeneration/disease** Kuhnt-Junius-Krankheit *f*, scheibenförmige/disziforme senile feuchte Makuladegeneration *f*.

Kulchitsky [kuːlˈtʃɪtskɪ]: **K.-cell carcinoma** Kultschitzky-Tumor *m*.
K.'s cells enterochromaffine/gelbe/argentaffine/enterendokrine Zellen *pl*, Kultschitzky-Zellen *pl*..
Kulenkampff [ˈkuːlənkæmpf]: **K.'s anesthesia** *anes*. Kulenkampff-Plexusanästhesie *f*.
Külz [kɪlts; kylts]: **K.'s cast/cylinder** (*Harn*) Komazylinder *m*.
Kümmell [ˈkɪməl; ˈkyməl]: **K.'s disease/spondylitis** → Kümmell-Verneuil disease.
Kümmell-Verneuil [vɛrˈnœj]: **K.-V. disease** Kümmell-Verneuil-Krankheit *f*, -Syndrom *nt*, traumatische Kyphose *f*, Spondylopathia traumatica.
Kunkel [ˈkʌŋkl]: **K.'s syndrome** lupoide Hepatitis *f*, Bearn-Kunkel(-Slater)-Syndrom *nt*.
Küntscher [ˈkɪntʃər; ˈkyn-]: **K. nail** *ortho*. Küntscher-Nagel *m*.
K. nailing *ortho*. Küntscher-Marknagelung *f*.
Kupffer [ˈkʊpfər]: **K.'s cells** (von) Kupffer'-(Stern-)Zellen *pl*.
Kupressoff [kjuːˈpresɒf]: **K.'s center** spinales Blasenzentrum *nt*.
Kurloff [ˈkuːrlɒf]: **K.'s bodies** Kurloff-Körper *pl*.
Kurlov → Kurloff.
Kur·thia [ˈkɜːrθɪə] *n micro*. Kurthia *f*, Proteus zenkeri.
ku·ru [ˈkuːru] *n* Lach-, Schüttelkrankheit *f*, Kuru *nt*, Kuru-Kuru *nt*.
Kurzrok-Miller [ˈkɜːrtsrɑk ˈmɪlər]: **K.-M. test** *gyn*. Kurzrok-Miller-Test *m*, Invasionstest *m*.
Kus·kok·wim syndrome [kʌsˈkɑkwɪm] Kuskokwim-Krankheit *f*.
Kussmaul [ˈkɒsmaʊl]: **K.'s aphasia** Kussmaul-Aphasie *f*.
K. breathing Lufthunger *m*, Kussmaul-Atmung *f*, Kussmaul-Kien-Atmung *f*.
K.'s coma Kussmaul-Koma *nt*, diabetisches/hyperglykämisches Koma *nt*, Coma diabeticum/hyperglycaemicum.
K.'s disease → Kussmaul-Meier disease.
K.'s (paradoxical) pulse paradoxer Puls *m*, Pulsus paradoxus.
K. respiration → K. breathing.
Kussmaul-Kien [kiːn]: **K.-K. breathing/respiration** → Kussmaul breathing.
Kussmaul-Meier [ˈmaɪər]: **K.-M. disease** Kussmaul-Meier-Krankheit *f*, Panarteriitis/Periarteriitis/Polyarteriitis nodosa.
Küstner [ˈkɪstnər; ˈkystnər]: **K.'s sign** Küstner-Zeichen *nt*.
Küttner [ˈkɪtnər; ˈkytnər]: **K.'s ganglion** oberster tiefer Halslymphknoten *m*, Nodus (lymphaticus) jugulodigastricus.
K.'s tumor Küttner-Tumor *m*.
kV, kv *abbr*. → kilovolt.
KVBA *abbr*. → kanamycin-vancomycin blood agar.
Kveim [k(ə)ˈveɪm]: **K. antigen** Kveim-Antigen *nt*.
K. test Kveim-Hauttest *m*, Kveim-Nickerson-Test *m*.
KVLB agar → kanamycin-vancomycin laked blood agar.
kW, kw *abbr*. → kilowatt.
kwa·shi·or·kor [ˌkwɑːʃɪˈɔːrkər] *n ped*. Kwashiorkor *nt*.
kWh *abbr*. → kilowatt-hour.
kwhr *abbr*. → kilowatt-hour.
Ky·a·sa·nur Forest disease [ˈkaɪəsənʊər] *abbr*. **KFD** Kyasanur-Waldfieber *nt*, Kyasanurwald-Fieber *nt*.
Kyasanur Forest disease virus KFD-Virus *nt*, Kyasanur-Waldfieber-Virus *nt*.

ky·ma·tism ['kaɪmətɪzəm] *n neuro.* Myokymie *f*.
ky·mo·gram ['-græm] *n* Kymogramm *nt*.
ky·mo·graph ['-græf] *n* Kymograph *m*.
ky·mog·ra·phy [kaɪ'mɑgrəfɪ] *n* Kymographie *f*.
ky·mo·scope ['kaɪməskəʊp] *n* Kymoskop *nt*.
kyn·u·ren·ic acid [ˌkɪnjə'renɪk, -'riː-, ˌkaɪn-] Kynurensäure *f*.
kyn·u·ren·in *n* → kynurenine.

kyn·u·ren·i·nase [ˌkɪnjə'renɪneɪz, ˌkaɪn-] *n* Kynureninase *f*.
kyn·u·ren·ine [kaɪ'njʊərəniːn, ˌkɪnjə'riːnɪn] *n* Kynurenin *nt*.
kynurenine-3-hydroxylase *n* → kynurenine-3-monooxygenase.
kynurenine-3-monooxygenase *n* Kynurenin-3-monooxygenase *f*.
ky·phos ['kaɪfɑs] *n ortho.* Buckel *m*.
ky·pho·sco·li·o·sis [ˌkaɪfəˌskəʊlɪ'əʊsɪs, -ˌskɑl-] *n ortho.* Kyphoskoliose *f*.
ky·pho·sco·li·ot·ic pelvis [ˌ-ˌskəʊlɪ'ɑtɪk] Kyphoskoliosebecken *nt*.
ky·pho·sis [kaɪ'fəʊsɪs] *n, pl* **-ses** [-siːz] *ortho.* Kyphose *f*.
ky·phot·ic [kaɪ'fɑtɪk] *adj* Kyphose betr., von ihr betroffen, kyphotisch, Kyphose-.
kyphotic angle *ortho.* Kyphosewinkel *m*.
kyphotic pelvis Kyphosebecken *nt*.
Kyrle ['kɪərlə; 'kyrlə]: **K.'s disease** Kyrle--Krankheit *f*, Morbus Kyrle *m*, Hyperkeratosis follicularis et parafollicularis in cutem penetrans (Kyrle).
kyt(o)- *pref.* Zell-, Zyt(o)-, Cyt(o)-.

L

L *abbr.* → 1. → leucine. 2. → solubility product.
l *abbr.* → liter.
Λ *abbr.* → lambda.
λ *abbr.* → lambda.
La *abbr.* → lanthanum.
lab [læb] *n* 1. *old* → rennin. 2. *inf.* → laboratory.
Labbé [la'be]: **L.'s triangle** Labbé'-Dreieck *nt*.
 L.'s vein Labbé'-Vene *f*, V. anastomotica inferior.
la·bel ['leɪbəl] **I** *n* Etikett *nt*, Aufkleber *m*, Label *nt*; Aufschrift *f*, Beschriftung *f*; Schild *nt*, Anhänger *m*. **II** *vt* etikettieren, mit einem Aufkleber/Anhänger/Etikett versehen, beschriften.
la·beled atom ['leɪbəld] *phys.* radioaktiv- -markiertes Atom *nt*, radioaktives Atom *nt*, radioaktives Markeratom *nt*.
labeled phosphorus radioaktiver Phosphor *m*, Radiophosphor *m*.
la·bel·ing ['leɪbəlɪŋ] *n* Markieren *nt*, Markierung *f*, Kennzeichnung *f*.
labeling machine Etikettiermaschine *f*.
labeling reagent Markierungsreagenz *nt*.
la·bel·ling → labeling.
la·bet·a·lol [lə'betələl, -lɒl] *n pharm.* Labetalol *nt*.
la·bi·al ['leɪbɪəl] *adj* Lippe/Labium betr., labial, Lippen-, Labial-.
labial artery: inferior l. Unterlippenschlagader *f*, -arterie *f*, Labialis *f* inferior, A. labialis inferior.
 posterior l.ies of vulva → labial branches of internal pudendal artery, posterior.
 superior l. Oberlippenschlagader *f*, -arterie *f*, Labialis *f* superior, A. labialis superior.
labial branches: anterior l. of femoral artery Schamlippenäste *pl* der A. femoralis, Rami labiales anteriores a. femoralis.
 inferior l. of mental nerve Unterlippenäste *pl* des N. mentalis, Rami labiales inferiores n. mentalis.
 posterior l. of internal pudendal artery Schamlippenäste *pl* der A. pudenda interna, Rami labiales posteriores a. pudendae internae.
 superior l. of infraorbital nerve Oberlippenäste *pl* des N. infraorbitalis, Rami labiales superiores n. infraorbitalis.
labial component of intermaxillary segment *embryo.* Lippenanteil *m* des Zwischenkiefersegmentes.
labial edema *gyn.* Schamlippenödem *nt*.
labial frenulum Lippenbändchen *nt*, Frenulum labii.
 inferior l. Unterlippenbändchen *nt*, Frenulum labii inferius.
 superior l. Oberlippenbändchen *nt*, Frenulum labii superius.
labial glands Lippen(speichel)drüsen *pl*, Gll. labiales.
labial hernia Hernia labialis.
 posterior l. Hernia vaginolabialis, Hernia labialis posterior.

la·bi·al·ism ['leɪbɪəlɪzəm] *n neuro.* Labialismus *m*.
labial nerves: anterior l. vordere Schamlippennerven *pl*, Nn. labiales anteriores.
 posterior l. hintere Schamlippennerven *pl*, Nn. labiales posteriores.
labial paralysis *neuro.* Duchenne-Syndrom *nt*, progressive Bulbärparalyse *f*.
labial region: inferior l. Unterlippenregion *f*, Regio labialis inferior.
 superior l. Oberlippenregion *f*, Regio labialis superior.
labial sound Labial-, Lippenlaut *m*.
labial vein Lippenvene *f*, V. labialis.
 anterior l.s vordere Schamlippenvenen *pl*, Vv. labiales anteriores.
 inferior l.s Unterlippenvenen *pl*, Vv. labiales inferiores.
 posterior l.s hintere Schamlippenvenen *pl*, Vv. labiales posteriores.
 superior l. Oberlippenvene *f*, V. labialis superior.
la·bi·cho·rea [ˌleɪbɪkə'rɪə, -koʊ-] *n* → labiochorea.
la·bile ['leɪbəl, -baɪl] *adj* 1. *phys.* labil, schwankend, unbeständig; *chem.* zersetzlich. 2. *psycho.* labil, unsicher; *med.* nicht widerstandfähig.
labile factor Proakzelerin *nt*, Proaccelerin *nt*, Acceleratorglobulin *nt*, labiler Faktor *m*, Faktor V *m abbr.* F V.
labile hypertension labile Hypertonie *f*.
labile pulse labiler Puls *m*.
la·bil·i·ty [leɪ'bɪlətɪ] *n* Labilität *f*.
labio- *pref.* Lippen-, Schamlippen-, Labio-.
la·bi·o·al·ve·o·lar [ˌleɪbɪoʊæl'vɪələr] *adj* Lippen u. Zahnalveolen betr., labioalveolär.
la·bi·o·cho·rea [ˌ-kə'rɪə, -koʊ-] *n neuro.* chronischer Lippenkrampf *m*.
la·bi·o·den·tal [ˌ-'dentl] **I** *n* Labiodental-(laut *m*) *m*, Lippenzahnlaut *m*. **II** *adj* Lippe(n) u. Zähne betr., labiodental.
la·bi·o·glos·so·la·ryn·ge·al [ˌˌglɒsoʊlə- 'rɪndʒ(ɪ)əl] *adj* Lippen, Zunge u. Larynx betr., labioglossolaryngeal.
labioglossolaryngeal paralysis → labial paralysis.
la·bi·o·glos·so·pha·ryn·ge·al [ˌ-ˌglɒsəfə- 'rɪndʒ(ɪ)əl] *adj* Lippen, Zunge u. Pharynx betr., labioglossopharyngeal.
labioglossopharyngeal paralysis → labial paralysis.
la·bi·o·graph ['-græf] *n* Labiograph *m*.
la·bi·o·lin·gual [ˌ-'lɪŋgwəl] *adj* Lippe(n) u. Zunge betr., labiolingual, labioglossal.
la·bi·o·men·tal [ˌ-'mentl] *adj* Lippe u. Kinn betr., labiomental.
la·bi·o·my·co·sis [ˌ-maɪ'koʊsɪs] *n* Lippenmykose *f*.
la·bi·o·na·sal [ˌ-'neɪzl] **I** *n* Labionasal(laut *m*) *m*, Lippennasenlaut *m*. **II** *adj* Lippe(n) u. Nase betr., labionasal.
la·bi·o·pal·a·tine [ˌ-'pælətaɪn, -tɪn] *adj* → labiovelar II.
la·bi·o·plas·ty ['-plæstɪ] *n* Lippen-, Labio-, Cheiloplastik *f*.

la·bi·o·scro·tal swelling [ˌ-'skroʊtl] *embryo.* Geschlechts-, Genitalwulst *m*.
la·bi·o·ve·lar [ˌ-'viːlər] **I** *n* Labiovelar(laut *m*) *m*, Lippengaumenlaut *m*. **II** *adj* Lippe(n) u. Gaumen betr., labiovelar.
la·bi·um ['leɪbɪəm] *n*, *pl* **-bia** [-bɪə] *anat.* 1. Lippe *f*, Labium *nt*. 2. Schamlippe *f*, Labium pudendi.
la·bor ['leɪbər] **I** *n* 1. Wehen *pl*, Labores (parturientinum). **to be in ~** in Wehen liegen, kreißen. **to go into ~/enter ~** Wehen bekommen. 2. (schwere) Arbeit *f*. 3. Anstrengung *f*, Mühe *f*. **II** *vi* 4. in den Wehen liegen, kreißen. 5. (schwer) arbeiten (*at* an); s. abmühen (*at, with* mit); s. quälen.
lab·o·ra·to·ry ['læbrətɔːrɪ, -toʊ-; *Brit.* lə- 'bɒrət(ə)rɪ] *n* Laboratorium *nt*, Labor *nt*.
laboratory animal Laboratoriumstier *nt*.
laboratory assistant Laborant(in *f*) *m*.
laboratory culture Laboratoriums-, Laborkultur *f*.
laboratory experiment Laborversuch *m*, -test *m*.
laboratory medium *micro.* Labornährboden *m*, -medium *nt*.
laboratory population Laborpopulation *f*.
laboratory test Laborversuch *m*, -test *m*.
laboratory value Laborwert *m*.
la·bored ['leɪbərd] *adj* mühsam, schwer; schwerfällig.
labored breathing/respiration erschwerte Atmung *f*, Atemnot *f*, Dyspnoe *f*.
labor-intensive *adj* arbeitsintensiv.
la·bo·ri·ous [lə'bɔːrɪəs] *adj* mühsam, mühselig, schwierig; schwerfällig, fleißig.
labor pains *gyn.* Geburtsschmerzen *pl*, Schmerzen *pl* unter der Geburt.
la·bour, *vi Brit.* → labor.
lab·ro·cyte ['læbrəsaɪt] *n* Mastzelle *f*, Mastozyt *m*.
la·brum ['leɪbrəm, 'læ-] *n*, *pl* **-bra** [-brə] 1. *anat.* Lippe *f*, Rand *m*, Labrum *nt*. 2. *zoo.* (*Insekt*) Oberlippe *f*, Labrum *nt*.
la·bu·ri·nine [læ'bjʊərənɪːn] *n* Zytisin *nt*, Cytisin *nt*.
lab·y·rinth ['læbərɪnθ] *n* 1. Labyrinth *nt*, irrgangähnliches Gebilde *nt*; *anat.* Labyrinthus *m*. 2. Innenohr(labyrinth *nt*) *nt*, Labyrinth *nt*.
 l. of cochlea Schneckenlabyrinth, Labyrinthus cochlearis.
lab·y·rin·thec·to·my [ˌlæbərɪn'θektəmɪ] *n* HNO, *neurochir.* Labyrinthexzision *f*, Labyrinthektomie *f*.
lab·y·rin·thi·an [ˌlæbə'rɪnθɪən] *adj* → labyrinthine.
lab·y·rin·thic [ˌ-'rɪnθɪk] *adj* → labyrinthine.
lab·y·rin·thine [ˌ-'rɪnθɪn, -θiːn] *adj* Labyrinth betr., labyrinthisch, labyrinthär, Labyrinth-.
labyrinthine artery 1. A. labyrinthi, Ramus meatus acustici interni a. basilaris. 2. A. labyrinthina.
labyrinthine ataxia labyrinthäre/vestibuläre Ataxie *f*.

labyrinthine branch of basilar artery → labyrinthine artery 1.
labyrinthine deafness *HNO* Innenohrtaubheit *f*.
labyrinthine dysplasia *HNO* Labyrinthdysplasie *f*.
labyrinthine fluid Cotunnius'-Flüssigkeit *f*, Perilymphe *f*, Perilympha *f*, Liquor cotunnii.
labyrinthine hydrops Ménière'-Krankheit *f*, Morbus Ménière *m*.
labyrinthine hypoplasia *HNO* Labyrinthhypoplasie *f*.
labyrinthine nystagmus vestibulärer Nystagmus *m*, Labyrinthnystagmus *m*.
labyrinthine placenta Placenta labyrinthina.
labyrinthine reaction *HNO* Labyrinthreaktion *f*.
  thermal l. thermale/kalorische Labyrinthreaktion.
labyrinthine reflexes Labyrinthreflexe *pl*.
labyrinthine righting reflex Labyrinthstellreflex *m*.
labyrinthine segment of facial nerve labyrinthäres Segment *nt* des N. facialis.
labyrinthine sense Gleichgewichtssinn *m*.
labyrinthine testing *HNO* Labyrinthprüfung *f*.
  caloric l. thermische/kalorische Labyrinthprüfung.
labyrinthine veins 1. Labyrinthvenen *pl*, Vv. labyrinthi. **2.** Vv. labyrinthinae.
labyrinthine vertigo Ménière'-Krankheit *f*, Morbus Ménière *m*.
labyrinthine wall of tympanic cavity mediale Wand *f* der Paukenhöhle, Paries labyrinthicus (cavitatis tympanicae).
lab·y·rin·thi·tis [ˌlæbərɪnˈθaɪtɪs] *n* **1.** Labyrinthentzündung *f*, Labyrinthitis *f*. **2.** Innenohrentzündung *f*, Otitis interna.
lab·y·rin·thot·o·my [ˌ-ˈθɑtəmɪ] *n HNO* Labyrintheröffnung *f*, Labyrinthotomie *f*.
lab·y·rin·thus [ˌlæbəˈrɪnθəs] *n, pl* **-thi** [-θaɪ] → labyrinth.
lac [læk] *n, pl* **lac·ta** [ˈlæktə] **1.** Milch *f*, Lac *nt*. **2.** milchartige Flüssigkeit *f*, Milch *f*. **3.** Gummilack *m*, Lackharz *nt*.
lac·er·a·ble [ˈlæsərəbl] *adj* zerreißbar.
lac·er·ate [*adj* ˈlæsəreɪt, -ɪt; *v* -eɪt] **I** *adj* → lacerated. **II** *vt* verletzen, zerschneiden, ein-, aufreißen, lazerieren, zerfetzen.
lac·er·at·ed [ˈlæsəreɪtɪd] *adj* (aus-)gefranst; zerfetzt, ein-, aufgerissen, lazeriert; verletzt.
lacerate foramen: anterior l. Augenhöhlendachspalte *f*, obere Orbitaspalte *f*, Fissura orbitalis superior.
  middle l. For. lacerum.
  posterior l. For. jugulare.
lac·er·a·tion [ˌlæsəˈreɪʃn] *n* **1.** Zerreißen *nt*, Lazerieren *nt*. **2.** Riß-, Kratz-, Platz-, Schnittwunde *f*, Riß-, Kratz-, Platz-, Schnittverletzung *f*, Lazeration *f*.
la·cer·tus [ləˈsɜrtəs] *n anat.* Lacertus *m*.
lach·ry·mal *adj* → lacrimal.
la·cin·i·ate [ləˈsɪnɪeɪt, -ɪt] *adj bot.*, *zoo.* (aus-)gezackt, zackig, gefranst.
laciniate ligament Retinaculum mm. flexorum (pedis).
lack [læk] **I** *n* Mangel *m*, Knappheit *f* (*of* an). **for/through ~ of (time)** aus Mangel an (Zeit). **II** *vt* Mangel haben *od.* leiden an, nicht haben.
  l. of appetite Appetitlosigkeit *f*.
  l. of exercise Bewegungsmangel.
  l. of interest Interesselosigkeit *f*, Desinteresse *nt*.
  l. of oxygen Sauerstoffmangel.
  l. of tone Tonusmangel *m*.

lac·mus [ˈlækməs] *n* Lackmus *nt*.
lac·ri·ma [ˈlækrɪmə] *n, pl* **-mae** [-miː] Träne *f*, Lacrima *f*.
lac·ri·mal [ˈlækrɪml] *adj* Tränen *od.* Tränendrüse *od.* Tränenkanal betr., lakrimal, Tränen-.
lacrimal abscess Tränensackabszeß *m*.
lacrimal apparatus Tränenapparat *m*, Apparatus lacrimalis.
lacrimal artery Tränendrüsenarterie *f*, A. lacrimalis, A. lacrimalis.
lacrimal bay → lacus lacrimalis.
lacrimal bone Tränenbein *nt*, Os lacrimale.
lacrimal border of maxilla Margo lacrimalis maxillae.
lacrimal calculus Tränenstein *m*, Dakryolith *m*.
lacrimal canal Kanal *m* des Ductus nasolacrimalis, Canalis nasolacrimalis.
lacrimal canaliculus Tränengang *m*, -kanal *m*, Ductus/Canaliculus lacrimalis.
lacrimal caruncle Tränenwärzchen *nt*, Karunkel *f*, Caruncula lacrimalis.
lacrimal crest: anterior l. Crista lacrimalis anterior.
  posterior l. Crista lacrimalis posterior.
lacrimal duct → lacrimal canaliculus.
lacrimal fissure Sulcus lacrimalis ossis lacrimalis.
lacrimal fistula Tränengangs-, Tränensackfistel *f*.
lacrimal fluid Tränenflüssigkeit *f*.
lacrimal fold Hasner'-Klappe *f*, Plica lacrimalis.
lacrimal fossa 1. Tränendrüsengrube *f*, Fossa glandulae lacrimalis. **2.** Sulcus lacrimalis ossis lacrimalis.
  l. of lacrimal gland → lacrimal fossa 1.
lacrimal gland Tränendrüse *f*, Gl. lacrimalis.
  accessory l.s Nebentränendrüsen *pl*, Gll. lacrimales accessoriae.
lacrimal hamulus Hamulus lacrimalis.
lacrimal incisure of maxilla Inc. lacrimalis.
lacrimal lake → lacus lacrimalis.
lacrimal margin of maxilla → lacrimal border of maxilla.
lacrimal nerve N. lacrimalis.
lacrimal notch of maxilla → lacrimal incisure of maxilla.
lacrimal nucleus Nc. lacrimalis.
lacrimal papilla Tränenpapille *f*, Papilla lacrimalis.
lacrimal point Tränenpünktchen *nt*, Punctum lacrimale.
lacrimal process (of inferior nasal concha) Proc. lacrimalis (conchae nasalis inferior).
lacrimal reflex Tränenreflex *m*.
lacrimal sac Tränensack *m*, Saccus lacrimalis.
lacrimal secretion Tränenflüssigkeit *f*.
lacrimal sound Tränengangssonde *f*.
lacrimal sulcus: l. of lacrimal bone Tränenfurche *f* des Tränenbeins, Sulcus lacrimalis ossis lacrimalis.
  l. of maxilla Tränenkanalfurche *f* der Maxilla, Sulcus lacrimalis maxillae.
lacrimal vein Tränendrüsenvene *f*, V. lacrimalis.
lac·ri·ma·tion [ˌlækrɪˈmeɪʃn] *n* Tränenkretion *f*, Lakrimation *f*.
lac·ri·ma·tor [ˈlækrɪmeɪtər] *n* tränentreibende/lakrimogene Substanz *f*.
lacrimator gas Tränengas *nt*.
lac·ri·ma·to·ry [ˈlækrɪməˌtɔːrɪ, -təʊ-] *adj* die Tränensekretion fördernd, lakrimogen.
lac·ri·mo·con·chal suture [ˌlækrɪməʊˈkɒŋkəl] Sutura lacrimoconchalis.

lacrimo-gustatory reflex gustatorisches Weinen *nt*.
lac·ri·mo·max·il·lar·y suture [ˌ-mækˈsɪlərɪ, -ˈmæksələrɪ] Sutura lacrimomaxillaris.
lac·ri·mo·na·sal [ˌ-ˈneɪzl] *adj* Tränensack u. Nase betr. *od.* verbindend, nasolakrimal.
lacrimonasal duct Tränen-Nasen-Gang *m*, Ductus nasolacrimalis.
lac·ri·mot·o·my [ˌlækrɪˈmɒtəmɪ] *n HNO* Tränensackeröffnung *f*, Tränengangseröffnung *f*, Lakrimotomie *f*.
La Crosse encephalitis [ləˈkrɒs] La Crosse-Enzephalitis *f*.
La Crosse virus La Crosse-Virus *nt*.
lact- *pref.* → lacto-.
lac·tac·i·de·mia [lækˌtæsɪˈdiːmɪə] *n* erhöhter Milchsäuregehalt *m* des Blutes, Laktazidämie *f*, Lactazidämie *f*, Hyperlaktazidämie *f*.
lac·tac·i·du·ria [lækˌtæsɪˈd(j)ʊərɪə] *n* Milchsäureausscheidung *f* im Harn, Lakt-, Lactazidurie *f*, Laktatazidurie *f*.
lac·ta·gogue [ˈlæktəgɒg, -gɑg] *gyn.* **I** *n* milchtreibendes Mittel *nt*, Laktagogum *nt*, Galaktogogum *nt*. **II** *adj* milchtreibend.
(α-)lac·tal·bu·min [ˌlæktælˈbjuːmɪn] *n* (α-)Lakt-, Lactalbumin *nt*.
lac·tam [ˈlæktæm] *n* Laktam *nt*, Lactam *nt*, Laktonamin *nt*.
β-lactam antibiotic β-Lactam-Antibiotikum *nt*.
β-lac·tam·ase [ˈlæktəmeɪz] *n* β-Laktamase *f*, β-Lactamase *f*, beta-Laktamase *f*, beta-Lactamase *f*.
β-lactamase-resistant *adj* β-Lactamase-fest, β-Lactamase-resistent.
β-lactamase-resistant penicillin β-Lactamase-festes Penicillin *nt*.
β-lactam drug → β-lactam antibiotic.
lactam form *chem.* Lactamform *f*.
lac·tam·ide [lækˈtæmɪd] *n* Laktamid *nt*, Lactamid *nt*.
β-lactam ring β-Lactamring *m*.
lac·tar·i·an [lækˈtɛərɪən] *n* → lactovegetarian.
lac·tase [ˈlækteɪz] *n* Laktase *f*, Lactase *f*, β-Galaktosidase *f*.
lactase deficiency Laktasemangel *m*.
lac·tate [ˈlækteɪt] **I** *n* Laktat *nt*, Lactat *nt*. **II** *vi* Milch absondern, laktieren.
lactate dehydrogenase *abbr.* **LDH** Laktatdehydrogenase *f* abbr. LDH.
lac·ta·tion [lækˈteɪʃn] *n* **1.** Milchsekretion *f*, Laktation *f*. **2.** Laktationsperiode *f*, Laktation *f*.
lac·ta·tion·al [lækˈteɪʃnl] *adj* Laktation betr., Laktations-.
lactation amenorrhea *gyn.* Laktationsamenorrhoe *f*.
lactation-amenorrhea syndrome Laktations-Amenorrhoe-Syndrom *nt*.
lactation hormone Prolaktin *nt* *abbr.* PRL, Prolactin *nt*, laktogenes Hormon *nt*.
lac·te·al [ˈlæktɪəl] **I** *n* (*Darm*) Lymphkapillare *f*. **II** *adj* Milch betr. *od.* produzierend, milchig, Lakt(o)-, Lact(o)-, Milch-.
lacteal calculus *gyn.* (*Brust*) Milchgangstein *m*.
lacteal cyst *gyn.* Laktations-, Milchzyste *f*.
lacteal fistula Milch(gangs)fistel *f*.
lacteal sinuses Milchsäckchen *pl*, Sinus lactiferi.
lacteal tumor 1. Brust(drüsen)abszeß *m*. **2.** Milchzyste *f*, Galaktozele *f*.
lacteal vessel (*Darm*) Lymphkapillare *f*.
lac·te·ous [ˈlæktɪəs] *adj* → lacteal II.
lac·tes·cent [lækˈtesənt] *adj* **1.** milchartig, milchig. **2.** laktierend, Milch absondernd.

lactic 436

lac·tic ['læktɪk] *adj chem.*, *physiol.* Milch betr., Milch-, Lakt(o)-, Lact(o)-, Galakt(o)-, Galact(o)-.
lactic acid Milchsäure *f*, α-Hydroxypropionsäure *f*.
lactic acid bacteria milchsäurebildende Bakterien *pl*.
lactic acid dehydrogenase → lactate dehydrogenase.
lac·tic·ac·i·de·mia [ˌlæktɪkˌæsɪ'diːmɪə] *n* → lactacidemia.
lactic acid fermentation Milchsäuregärung *f*.
lactic acid-forming bacteria → lactic acid bacteria.
lactic acidosis Laktazidose *f*, Laktatazidose *f*, Lactazidose *f*.
lactic aciduria → lactaciduria.
lactic streptococci *micro.* N-Streptokokken *pl*, Streptokokken *pl* der Gruppe N.
lac·tif·er·ous [læk'tɪfərəs] *adj* Milch produzierend *od.* (ab-)leitend *od.* führend.
lactiferous ducts Milchgänge *pl*, Ductus lactiferi.
lactiferous gland Brustdrüse *f*, Gl. mammaria.
lactiferous sinuses → lacteal sinuses.
lactiferous tubules → lactiferous ducts.
lac·tif·u·gal [læk'tɪfjəgəl] *adj* → lactifuge II.
lac·ti·fuge ['læktɪfjuːdʒ] *gyn.* **I** *n* Milchsekretion-hemmendes Mittel *nt*, Lakti-, Lactifugum *nt*. **II** *adj* die Milchsekretion hemmend, milchvermindernd, milchhemmend.
lac·tig·e·nous [læk'tɪdʒənəs] *adj* milchbildend, milchsezernierend.
lac·tig·er·ous [læk'tɪdʒərəs] *adj* → lactiferous.
lac·tim ['læktɪm] *n* Laktim *nt*, Lactim *nt*, Laktonimin *nt*.
lac·tin ['læktɪn] *n* → lactose.
lac·ti·nat·ed ['læktɪneɪtɪd] *adj* Milchzucker/Laktose enthaltend, mit Laktose zubereitet.
lacto- *pref.* Milch-, Lakt(o)-, Lact(o)-. Galakt(o)-, Galact(o)-.
Lac·to·bac·il·la·ce·ae [ˌlæktəʊˌbæsə'leɪsɪˌiː] *pl micro.* Milchsäurebakterien *pl*, Lactobacillaceae *pl*.
Lac·to·ba·cil·lus [ˌ-bə'sɪləs] *n, pl* **-cil·li** [-'sɪlaɪ] *micro.* Milchsäurestäbchen *pl*, Lakto-, Lactobacillus *m*.
L. bifidus Bifidus-Bakterium *nt*, Lactobacillus bifidus, Bifidobacterium bifidum.
Lactobacillus casei factor Fol(in)säure *f*, Folacin *nt*, Pteroylglutaminsäure *f*, Vitamin B₉ *nt*.
lac·to·bu·ty·rom·e·ter [ˌ-ˌbjuːtə'rɒmɪtər] *n lab.* Milchfettmesser *m*, Laktobutyrometer *nt*.
lac·to·cele ['-siːl] *n* Milchzyste *f*, Galaktozele *f*.
lac·to·chrome ['-krəʊm] *n* Ribo-, Laktoflavin *nt*, Vitamin B₂ *nt*.
lac·to·crit ['-krɪt] *n lab.* Milchfettmesser *m*, Laktokrit *m*.
lac·to·den·sim·e·ter [ˌ-den'sɪmɪtər] *n* → lactometer.
lac·to·fer·rin [ˌ-'ferɪn] *n* Lakto-, Lactoferrin *nt*, -transferin *nt*.
lac·to·fla·vin [ˌ-'fleɪvɪn] *n* Ribo-, Laktoflavin *nt*, Vitamin B₂ *nt*.
lac·to·gen ['-dʒən] *n* 1. laktationsfördernde Substanz *f*. 2. Prolaktin *nt abbr.* PRL, Prolactin *nt*, laktogenes Hormon *nt*.
lac·to·gen·e·sis [ˌ-'dʒenəsɪs] *n* Milchbildung *f*, Laktogenese *f*.
lac·to·gen·ic [ˌ-'dʒenɪk] *adj* Laktogenese betr. *od.* fördernd, laktogen.

lactogenic factor/hormone Prolaktin *nt abbr.* PRL, Prolactin *nt*, laktogenes Hormon *nt*.
lac·to·glob·u·lin [ˌ-'glɒbjəlɪn] *n* Lakto-, Lactoglobulin *nt*.
lac·tom·e·ter [lɒk'tɒmɪtər] *n* Milchwaage *f*, Lakto-, Galaktometer *nt*, Laktodensimeter *nt*.
lac·to·nase ['læktəneɪz] *n* Laktonase *f*, Lactonase *f*.
lac·tone ['læktəʊn] *n* Lakton *nt*, Lacton *nt*.
lac·to·pro·tein [ˌlæktəʊ'prəʊtiːn, -tiːɪn] *n* Milcheiweiß *nt*, Lakto-, Lactoprotein *nt*.
lac·tor·rhea [ˌ-'rɪə] *n gyn.* Milchfluß *m*, Galaktorrhö *f*, Galaktorrhoe *f*.
lac·to·sa·zone [ˌ-'seɪzəʊn] *n* Lactosazon *nt*.
lac·to·scope ['-skəʊp] *n* Laktoskop *nt*, Galaktoskop *nt*.
lac·tose ['læktəʊs] *n* Milchzucker *m*, Laktose *f*, Lactose *f*, Laktobiose *f*.
lactose intolerance Laktoseintoleranz *f*, -malabsorption *f*.
lactose-litmus agar *bio.* Laktose-Lackmus-Agar *m/nt*.
lactose synthase Laktosesynthase *f*, -synthetase *f*.
lac·to·side ['læktəsaɪd] *n* Laktosid *nt*, Lactosid *nt*.
lac·to·si·do·sis [ˌ-saɪ'dəʊsɪs] *n, pl* **-ses** [-siːz] Laktosidspeicherkrankheit *f*, Laktosidose *f*.
lac·to·sum [læk'təʊsəm] *n* → lactose.
lac·to·su·ria [ˌlæktə's(j)ʊərɪə] *n* Laktoseausscheidung *f* im Harn, Laktosurie *f*.
lac·to·syl-N-acylsphingosine [ˌ-sɪl] Lactosyl-N-acylsphingosin *nt*, Lactosylceramid *nt*.
lactosyl ceramidase Lactosylceramidase *f*.
lactosyl ceramidase I Galaktosylceramidase *f*, Galaktocerebrosid-β-galaktosidase *f*.
lactosyl ceramidase II β-Galaktosidase *f*, Laktase *f*.
lac·to·syl·cer·a·mide [læk,təʊsɪl'serəmaɪd] *n* → lactosyl-N-acylsphingosine.
lactosylceramide galactosyl hydrolase → lactosyl ceramidase.
lac·to·syl·cer·a·mi·do·sis [ˌlæktəsɪlˌserəmaɪ'dəʊsɪs] *n* Lactosylceramidose *f*, neutrale β-Galaktosidase-Defekt *m*.
lactosyl cerebrosidase Lactosylcerebrosidase *f*.
lac·to·ther·a·py [ˌlæktə'θerəpɪ] *n* 1. Galakto-, Laktotherapie *f*. 2. Milchdiät *f*, -kur *f*.
lac·to·trope ['-trəʊp] *n* → lactotroph.
lac·to·troph ['-trɒf, -trəʊf] *n* Prolaktin-Zelle *f*, mammotrope Zelle *f*.
lactotroph cell → lactotroph.
lac·to·tro·phin [ˌ-'trəʊfɪn] *n* Prolaktin *nt abbr.* PRL, Prolactin *nt*, laktogenes Hormon *nt*.
lac·to·trop·ic [ˌ-'trɒpɪk, -trəʊ-] *adj* laktotrop.
lactotropic cell → lactotroph.
lac·to·tro·pin [ˌ-'trəʊpɪn, ˌ-'trɒp-] *n* → lactotrophin.
lac·to·veg·e·tar·i·an [ˌ-ˌvedʒɪ'terɪən, -'teər-] **I** *n* Laktovegetarier(in *f*) *m*. **II** *adj* Laktovegetarismus betr., laktovegetarisch.
lac·to·yl·glu·ta·thi·one lyase [ˌlæktəwɪlˌgluːtə'θaɪəʊn] Lactoylglutathionlyase *f*, Glyoxalase I *f*.
lac·tu·lose ['læktjələʊs] *n pharm.* Lactulose *f*.
la·cu·na [lə'k(j)uːnə] *n, pl* **-nae** [-niː] *anat.* Hohlraum *m*, Spalt(e *f*) *m*, Lücke *f*, Lakune *f*, Lacuna *f*. 2. Lücke *f*, Spalt(e *f*) *m*; Grube *f*.

l. of muscles *old* Lacuna musculorum.
l.e of urethra Urethrallakunen *pl*, -buchten *pl*, Morgagni'-Lakunen *pl*, Lacunae urethrales.
l. of vessels *old* Lacuna vasorum.
la·cu·nal [lə'kjuːnl] *adj* → lacunar.
la·cu·nar [lə'k(j)uːnər] *adj* Lakune(n) betr. *od.* enthaltend, lückenhaft, lakunar, lakunär, Lakunen-.
lacunar angina Angina/Tonsillitis lacunaris.
lacunar cells *hema.* Lakunenzellen *pl*.
lacunar ligament Lig. lacunare.
lacunar node: intermediate l. mittlerer Lymphknoten *m* der Lacuna vasorum, Nodus lacunaris intermedius.
lateral l. lateraler Lymphknoten *m* der Lacuna vasorum, Nodus lacunaris lateralis.
medial l. medialer Lymphknoten *m* der Lacuna vasorum, Nodus lacunaris medialis.
lacunar space intervillöser Raum/Spalt *m*.
lacunar stage *embryo.* lakunäres Stadium *nt*.
lacunar tonsillitis *HNO* Angina/Tonsillitis lacunaris.
lac·u·nar·y ['lækjuːˌnerɪ, lə'kjuːnərɪ] *adj* → lacunar.
la·cune [lə'k(j)uːn] *n* → lacuna.
la·cu·nule [lə'k(j)uːnjuːl] *n* 1. *anat.* kleine schmale Bucht *od.* Ausbuchtung *f*, kleine Lakune/Lacuna *f*. 2. kleine Lücke/Spalte/Grube *f*.
la·cus lacrimalis ['leɪkəs, 'læk-] Tränensee *m*, Lacus lacrimalis.
Ladd [læd] **L.'s band** *embryo.*, *chir.* Ladd'-Band *nt*.
L.'s operation/procedure *chir.* Ladd-Operation *f*.
L.'s syndrome Ladd-Syndrom *nt*.
Ladd-Franklin ['fræŋklɪn] **L.-F. theory** Ladd-Franklin-Theorie *f*.
Ladewig ['leɪdwɪg] **L. stain** *histol.* Ladewig-Färbung *f*.
Laennec [leɪ'nek] **L.'s cirrhosis** mikronoduläre/kleinknotige/organisierte Leberzirrhose *f*.
L.'s disease 1. dissezierendes Aneurysma *nt*, Aneurysma dissecans. 2. → L.'s cirrhosis.
laev(o)- *pref.* → levo-.
laev·u·lose ['levjələʊz] *n* Fruchtzucker *m*, (D-)Fruktose *f*, (D-)Fructose *f*, L(a)evulose *f*.
LAF *abbr.* [lymphocyte-activating factor] *old* → interleukin-1.
Lafora [lə'fɔːrə] **L.'s bodies** Lafora-Körperchen *pl*.
L.'s disease Lafora-Syndrom *nt*, Unverricht-Syndrom *nt*, Myoklonusepilepsie *f*, myoklonische Epilepsie *f*.
lag [læg] (*v* **lagged**) **I** *n* 1. Zurückbleiben *nt*, Nachhinken *nt*. 2. *phys.* negative Phasenverschiebung *f*. **II** *vi* → lag behind.
lag behind *vi* 1. zurückbleiben, nicht mitkommen, nachhinken. 2. *s.* verzögern; nacheilen.
la·gen·i·form [lə'dʒenɪfɔːrm] *adj* flaschenförmig.
Lag·o·chi·las·ca·ris minor [ˌlægəʊkaɪ'læskərɪs] *micro.* Lagochilascaris minor.
lag·oph·thal·mia [ˌlægɒf'θælmɪə] *n* → lagophthalmos.
lag·oph·thal·mic keratitis [ˌ-'θelmɪk] Keratitis/Keratopathia e lagophthalmo.
lag·oph·thal·mos [ˌ-'θelməs] *n ophthal.* Hasenauge *nt*, Lagophthalmus *m*.
lag·oph·thal·mus *n* → lagophthalmos.
lag period/phase *micro.* lag-Phase *f*, Lagphase *f*, Latenzphase *f*.

Lagrange [lə'greɪndʒ; la'grɑ̃:ʒ]: **L.'s operation** *ophthal.* Lagrange-Operation *f*, Sklerektoiridektomie *f*.
Lahore sore [lə'hʊər, -'hɔː(ə)r] kutane Leishmaniose/Leishmaniase *f*, Hautleishmaniose *f*, Orientbeule *f*, Leishmaniasis cutis.
Laimer ['leɪmər]: **L.'s area** Laimer'-Dreieck *nt*.
LAK cell lymphokin-aktivierte Killerzelle *f*, LAK-Zelle *f*.
laked blood agar [leɪkt] *micro.* Hämin--Agar *m/nt*.
Laki-Lorand ['lækɪ lə'rænd]: **L.-L. factor** *abbr.* **LLF** Faktor XIII *m abbr.* F XIII, fibrinstabilisierender Faktor *m abbr.* FSF, Laki-Lorand-Faktor *m abbr.* LLF.
laky blood ['leɪkɪ] hämolysiertes Blut *nt*.
lallation [læ'leɪʃn] *n* Lallen *nt*, Lallatio *f*.
Lallemand [lal'mɑ̃]: **L.'s bodies** Sekretkörnchen *pl* der Samenbläschen.
Lallemand-Trousseau [tru'so]: **L.-T. bodies** → Lallemand's bodies.
lalo- *pref.* Sprach-, Sprech-, Lalo-.
lalognosis [ˌlælɒg'nəʊsɪs] *n* Sprachverständnis *nt*.
laloneurosis [ˌlælənjʊə'rəʊsɪs, -nʊ-] *n* Laloneurose *f*.
lalopathy [læ'lɒpəθɪ] *n* Sprach-, Sprechstörung *f*, Lalopathie *f*.
lalophobia [ˌlælə'fəʊbɪə] *n* Sprechangst *f*, -scheu *f*, Lalophobie *f*.
laloplegia [ˌ-'pliːdʒ(ɪ)ə] *n* Sprachlähmung *f*, Laloplegie *f*.
lalorrhea [ˌ-'rɪə] *n* → logorrhea.
Lalouette [lalu'et]: **L.'s pyramid** Lobus pyramidalis.
lambda ['læmdə] *n abbr.* **Λ, λ** Lambda *nt abbr.* Λ, λ.
lambda chain lambda-Kette *f*, λ-Kette *f*.
lambdacism ['læmdəsɪzəm] *n* Lambdazismus *m*.
lambdacismus ['-sɪzməs] *n* Lambdazismus *m*.
lambdoid ['læmdɔɪd] *adj* λ-förmig, λ-, Lambda-.
lambdoidal [læm'dɔɪdl] *adj* → lambdoid.
lambdoid margin Margo lambdoideus.
lambdoid suture Lambdanaht *f*, Sutura lambdoidea.
Lambert-Beer ['læmbərt bɪər]: **L.-B.'s law** Lambert-Beer'-Gesetz *nt*.
Lambert-Eaton ['iːtn]: **L.-E. syndrome** Lambert-Eaton-Rooke-Syndrom *nt*, pseudomyasthenisches Syndrom *nt*.
Lamblia ['læmblɪə] *n micro.* Lamblia *f*, Giardia *f*.
lambliasis [læm'blaɪəsɪs] *n* Giardia-Infektion *f*, Lamblia-Infektion *f*, Giardiasis *f*, Lambliasis *f*.
lambliosis [ˌlæmblɪ'əʊsɪs] *n* → lambliasis.
Lambrinudi [læmbrɪ'nuːdɪ]: **L.'s operation** *ortho.* Lambrinudi-Operation *f*.
lame [leɪm] **I** *adj* lahm; gelähmt. **II** *vt* lähmen.
lamella [lə'melə] *n, pl* **-las, -lae** [-liː, -laɪ] dünnes Plättchen *nt*, dünne Membran *f*, Lamelle *f*.
lamellar [lə'melər] *adj* → lamellate.
lamellar bone lamellärer Knochen *m*, Lamellenknochen *m*.
lamellar cataract Schichtstar *m*, Cataracta zonularis.
lamellar corpuscles Vater-Pacini'-(Lamellen-)Körperchen *pl*, Corpuscula lamellosa.
lamellar ichthyosis lamelläre Ichthyosis *f*, lamelläre Desquamation *f* bei Neugeborenen, Ichthyosis lamellosa.
lamellar layer, outer *histol.* äußere Lamellenschicht *f*.

lamellate ['læməleɪt, lə'meleɪt, -lɪt] *adj* aus Lamellen aufgebaut *od.* bestehend, plättchenähnlich, -artig, lamellenähnlich, -artig, geschichtet, lamellär, lamellar, Lamellen-.
lamellated ['læməleɪtɪd] *adj* → lamellate.
lamellated bone → lamellar bone.
lamellated corpuscles → lamellar corpuscles.
lamelliform [lə'melɪfɔːrm] *adj* lamellenförmig.
lamellose [lə'meləʊs, 'læmələʊs] *adj* → lamellate.
lamina ['læmɪnə] *n, pl* **-nas, -nae** [-niː] 1. *anat. bio.* dünne Platte *od.* Schicht *f*, Überzug *m*, Blättchen *nt*, Lamina *f*. 2. *anat.* → l. of vertebra.
l. of cricoid cartilage Ringknorpelplatte, Lamina cartilaginis cricoideae.
l. of modiolus Endplatte der Lamina spiralis ossea, Lamina modioli.
l. of septum pellucidum Lamina septi pellucidi.
l. of tectum of mesencephalon Vierhügelplatte, Lamina quadrigemina, Lamina tecti/tectalis (mesencephali).
l. of tubal cartilage laterale Knorpelplatte des Tubenknorpels, Lamina cartilaginis lateralis (tubae auditivae).
l. of vertebra Wirbel(bogen)platte, Lamina arcus vertebrae/vertebralis.
l. of vertebral arch → l. of vertebra.
lamina affixa Lamina affixa.
lamina fusca Lamina fusca sclerae.
laminagram ['læmɪnəgræm] *n radiol.* Schichtaufnahme *f*, Tomogramm *nt*.
laminagraphy [læmɪ'nɑgrəfɪ] *n radiol.* Schichtröntgen *nt*, Tomographie *f*.
laminal ['læmɪnl] *adj* → laminar.
lamina muscularis mucosae *histol.* Muskularis/Muscularis *f* mucosae, Lamina muscularis mucosae.
lamina propria *histol.* Lamina *f* propria, Propria *f* mucosae, Lamina propria mucosae.
laminar ['læmɪnər] *adj* aus Schichten bestehend, blätterig, lamellenförmig, -artig, laminar, laminal.
laminar flow 1. *phys.* laminare Strömung *f*, Laminar-, Schichtenströmung *f*. 2. *chir.* Laminar-flow *m*.
laminary [læmɪ'neːrɪ] *adj* → laminar.
laminate ['læmɪneɪt, -nɪt] *adj* 1. → laminated. 2. → laminar.
laminated ['-neɪtɪd] *adj* aus Lamellen bestehend, in Schichten, lamellös, lamellär, lamellar.
laminated epithelium mehrschichtiges Epithel *nt*.
laminated thrombus *patho.* Abscheidungsthrombus *m*.
laminate induration *patho.* schiefrige Induration *f*.
lamina tragi Lamina tragi.
laminectomy [læmɪ'nektəmɪ] *n ortho., neurochir.* Wirbelbogenresektion *f*, Laminektomie *f*.
laminogram ['læmɪnəgræm] *n* → laminagram.
laminography [læmɪ'nɒgrəfɪ] *n* → laminagraphy.
laminotomy [læmɪ'nɒtəmɪ] *n ortho., neurochir.* Wirbelbogendurchtrennung *f*, Laminotomie *f*.
laminous ['læmɪnəs] *adj* 1. → laminated. 2. → laminar.
lamp [læmp] *n* Lampe *f*; Leuchte *f*, Beleuchtungskörper *m*; Glühbirne *f*.
lamp-brush chromosome ['læmpbrʌʃ] *genet.* Lampenbürstenchromosom *nt*.
lana ['lænə] *n* Wolle *f*, Lana *f*.

lanatoside [lə'nætəsaɪd] *n pharm.* Lanatosid *nt*.
lanatoside C Lanatosid C *nt*.
lance [læns, lɑːns] **I** *n* → lancet. **II** *vt chir., ortho.* mit einer Lanzette eröffnen *od.* aufschneiden *od.* aufstechen.
Lancefield ['lænsfiːld]: **L. classification** *micro.* Lancefield-Einteilung *f*, -Klassifikation *f*.
L. groups Lancefield-Gruppen *pl*.
L. precipitation test *micro.* Lancefield-Präzipitationstest *m*.
lanceolate ['lænsɪəleɪt, -lɪt] *adj* lanzenförmig.
Lancereaux-Mathieu [lɑ̃səˈro maˈtjø]: **L.-M. disease** Weil'-Krankheit *f*, Leptospirosis icterohaemorrhagica.
lancet ['lænsɪt, 'lɑːn-] *n chir., ortho.* Lanzette *f*.
lancet fluke *micro.* kleiner Leberegel *m*, Lanzettegel *m*, Dicrocoelium dendriticum/lanceolatum.
lancinating ['lænsɪneɪtɪŋ] *adj* bohrend, stechend, blitzartig, lanzinierend.
lancinating pain stechender/lanzinierender Schmerz *m*.
Lancisi [læn'tʃiːsɪ]: **lateral L.'s stria** lateraler Längsstreifen *m* des Balkens, Stria longitudinalis lateralis (corporis callosi).
medial L.'s stria medialer Längsstreifen *m* des Balkens, Stria longitudinalis medialis (corporis callosi).
L.'s sign *card.* Lancisi-Zeichen *nt*.
Landau ['landaʊ]: **L.'s reflex** *ped.* Landau-Reflex *m*.
Landolt [lɑ̃'dɔlt]: **L.'s ring** Landolt'-Ring *m*.
Landouzy [læn'duːzɪ; lɑ̃du'zi]: **L. atrophy** → Landouzy-Déjérine atrophy
L.'s disease Weil'-Krankheit *f*, Leptospirosis icterohaemorrhagica.
L.'s dystrophy/type → Landouzy--Déjérine atrophy
Landouzy-Déjérine [deʒe'riːn]: **L.-D. atrophy** fazio-skapulo-humerale Muskeldystrophie *f*, Landouzy-Déjérine-Krankheit *f*, -Syndrom *nt*, -Typ *m*.
L.-D. dystrophy/type → L.-D. atrophy.
Landouzy-Grasset [grɑ'se]: **L.-G. law** Landouzy-Grasset-Gesetz *nt*.
Landry [lɑ̃'dri]: **L.'s disease/palsy** → L.'s paralysis.
L.'s paralysis Landry-Lähmung *f*, -Paralyse *f*, -Typ *m*, Paralysis spinalis ascendens acuta.
L.'s syndrome → L.'s paralysis.
land scurvy [lænd] idiopathische thrombozytopenische Purpura *f abbr.* ITP, essentielle idiopathische Thrombozytopenie *f*, Morbus Werlhof *m*.
Landsteiner-Donath ['lændstaɪnər; 'lantʃtaɪnər]: **L.-D. test** Donath-Landsteiner--Reaktion *f*, Landsteiner-Reaktion *f*.
Landzert ['lændsərt]: **L.'s fossa** Rec. paraduodenalis.
Lane [leɪn]: **L.'s plates** *ortho.* Lane-Platten *pl*.
Langat ['læŋgət]: **L. virus** Langat-Virus *nt*.
Lange ['læŋə]: **L.'s reaction** Goldsolreaktion *f*.
Langenbeck ['laŋənbek]: **L.'s amputation** *ortho.* Langenbeck-Amputation *f*.
L.'s needle holder Langenbeck-Nadelhalter *m*.
L.'s operation *chir.* Langenbeck-Hämorrhoidenentfernung *f*, -Operation *f*.
L.'s retractor Langenbeck-Haken *m*.
Langer ['læŋər]: **L.'s arch** → L.'s axillary arch.
L.'s axillary arch Langer'-Achselbogen *m*.

Langerhans

L.'s lines Langer'-Linien *pl*, Hautspalt-, Hautspannungslinien *pl*.
L.'s muscle → L.'s axillary arch.
Langerhans ['læŋərhænz; 'laŋərhans]: **L.' cell** Langerhans'-Zelle *f*.
L.' cell granulomatosis eosinophiles (Knochen-)Granulom *nt*.
L.' granules Birbeck-Granula *pl*.
islands/islets of L. Langerhans'-Inseln *pl*, endokrines Pankreas *nt*, Inselorgan *nt*, Pankreasinseln *pl*, Pars endocrina pancreatis.
lang·er·han·si·an adenoma [ˌlæŋər'hænʃɪən] Inselzelladenom *nt*, Adenoma insulocellulare, Nesidioblastom *nt*, Nesidiom *nt*.
Langhans ['læŋhænz; 'laŋhans]: **L.' cell 1.** Zytotrophoblast *m*, Langhans'-Zelle *f*, -Zellschicht *f*. **2.** *patho.* Langhans'-Riesenzelle *f*.
L.' giant cells Langhans'-Riesenzellen *pl*.
L.' layer Zytotrophoblastenschicht *f*, Langhans'-Zellschicht *f*.
L.' proliferating goiter → L.' struma.
L.' stria → L.' layer.
L.' struma organoide Struma *f*, wuchernde Struma *f* Langhans, Langhans-Struma *f*.
lan·guage ['læŋgwɪdʒ] *n* **1.** Sprache *f*. **2.** Rede-, Ausdrucksweise *f*. **3.** (Fach-)Sprache *f*, Terminologie *f*. **4.** Sprachwissenschaft *f*.
language-dominant *adj physiol.* sprachdominant.
lan·o·lin ['lænlɪn] *n* Wollwachs *nt*, Lanolin *nt*.
la·nos·ter·ol [lə'nɒstərɒl] *n* Lanosterin *nt*.
Lan·sing virus ['lænsɪŋ] *micro.* Lansing-Stamm *m*, -Virus *nt*, Poliovirus Typ II *nt*.
Lanterman ['læntərmæn]: **L.'s clefts/incisures** Schmidt-Lanterman'-Einkerbungen *pl*, -Inzisuren *pl*.
Lanterman-Schmidt [ʃmɪt]: **L.-S.'s clefts/incisures** → Lanterman's clefts.
lan·tha·nic ['lænθənɪk] *adj (Krankheit)* symptomlos.
lan·tha·nides ['lænθənaɪds, -nɪds] *pl chem.* seltene Erden *pl*, Lanthaniden *pl*.
lan·tha·num ['lænθənəm] *n abbr.* **La** Lanthan *nt abbr.* La.
la·nu·gi·nous [lə'n(j)u:dʒɪnəs] *adj* von Lanugohaaren bedeckt, lanugoartig, lanuginös.
la·nu·go [lə'n(j)u:gəʊ] *n, pl* **-gos** *ped.*, *embryo.* Flaum *m*, Wollhaar(kleid *nt*) *nt*, Lanugo *f*.
lanugo hair Lanugo-, Wollhaar *nt*.
la·num ['leɪnəm] *n* Lanum *nt*.
Lanz [lænz]: **L.'s line** Planum interspinale.
L.'s point *chir.* Lanz'-Punkt *m*.
LAP *abbr.* **1.** → leucine aminopeptidase. **2.** → leukocyte alkaline phosphatase.
lapar- *pref.* → laparo-.
lap·a·rec·to·my [læpə'rektəmɪ] *n chir.* Bauchwandexzision *f*, Bauchdeckenplastik *f*, Laparektomie *f*.
laparo- *pref.* Bauch-, Bauchdecken-, Bauchwand-, Bauchhöhlen-, Lapar(o)-.
lap·a·ro·cele ['læpərəsi:l] *n chir.* Bauch(wand)hernie *f*, Bauch(wand)bruch *m*, Laparozele *f*, Hernia abdominalis/ventralis.
lap·a·ro·cho·le·cys·tot·o·my [ˌlæpərəʊˌkəʊləsɪs'tɒtəmɪ] *n chir.* Gallenblaseneröffnung *f*, Cholezystotomie *f*.
lap·a·ro·co·lec·to·my [ˌlæpərəʊkə'lektəmɪ, -kəʊ-] *n chir.* Dickdarmentfernung *f*, -exstirpation *f*, Kolonentfernung *f*, -exstirpation *f*, Kolektomie *f*.
lap·a·ro·co·los·to·my [ˌlæpərəʊkə'lɒstəmɪ] *n chir.*

lap·a·ro·co·lot·o·my [ˌlæpərəʊkə'lɒtəmɪ] *n chir.* Dickdarmeröffnung *f*, -durchtrennung *f*, Koloneröffnung *f*, -durchtrennung *f*, Kolotomie *f*.
lap·a·ro·cys·tec·to·my [ˌlæpərəʊsɪs'tektəmɪ] *n chir.* transabdominelle Zystektomie *f*, Laparozystektomie *f*.
lap·a·ro·cys·ti·dot·o·my [ˌlæpərəʊsɪstə'dɒtəmɪ] *n* **1.** *chir.*, *gyn.* transabdominelle Zystotomie *f*, Laparozystotomie *f*. **2.** *chir.*, *urol.* suprabubischer Blasenschnitt *m*, Laparozystotomie *f*.
lap·a·ro·cys·tot·o·my [ˌlæpərəʊsɪs'tɒtəmɪ] *n* → laparocystidotomy.
lap·a·ro·en·te·ros·to·my [ˌlæpərəʊentə'rɒstəmɪ] *n chir.* Laparoenterostomie *f*.
lap·a·ro·en·te·rot·o·my [ˌlæpərəʊentə'rɒtəmɪ] *n chir.* kombinierte Laparotomie *f* u. Enterotomie, Laparoenterotomie *f*.
lap·a·ro·gas·tros·co·py [ˌlæpərəʊgæs'trɒskəpɪ] *n chir.* Laparogastroskopie *f*.
lap·a·ro·gas·tros·to·my [ˌlæpərəʊgæs'trɒstəmɪ] *n chir.* Laparo-, Zöliogastrostomie *f*.
lap·a·ro·gas·trot·o·my [ˌlæpərəʊgæs'trɒtəmɪ] *n chir.* kombinierte Laparotomie *f* u. Gastrotomie, Laparo-, Zöliogastrotomie *f*.
lap·a·ro·hep·a·tot·o·my [ˌlæpərəʊhepə'tɒtəmɪ] *n chir.* Laparohepatotomie *f*.
lap·a·ro·hys·ter·ec·to·my [ˌlæpərəʊhɪstə'rektəmɪ] *n gyn.* transabdominelle Hysterektomie *f*, Laparohysterektomie *f*, Hysterectomia abdominalis.
laparohystero-oophorectomy *n gyn.* Laparotomie *f* mit Entfernung von Gebärmutter u. Eierstöcken, Laparohystero-oophorektomie *f*, Laparohystero-ovariektomie *f*.
lap·a·ro·hys·ter·o·pex·y [ˌlæpərəʊ'hɪstərəpeksɪ] *n gyn.* transabdominelle Hysteropexie *f*, Laparohysteropexie *f*.
laparohysterosalpingo-oophorectomy *n gyn.* Laparohysterosalpingo-oophorektomie *f*, Laparohysterosalpingo-ovariektomie *f*.
lap·a·ro·hys·te·rot·o·my [ˌlæpərəʊhɪstə'rɒtəmɪ] *n gyn.* transabdominelle Hysterotomie *f*, Abdomino-, Laparo-, Zöliohysterotomie *f*.
lap·a·ro·il·e·ot·o·my [ˌlæpərəʊɪlɪ'ɒtəmɪ] *n chir.* kombinierte Laparotomie *f* u. Ileotomie, Laparoileotomie *f*.
lap·a·ro·my·i·tis [ˌlæpərəʊmaɪ'aɪtɪs] *n* → laparomyositis.
lap·a·ro·my·o·mec·to·my [ˌlæpərəʊmaɪə'mektəmɪ] *n chir.*, *gyn.* transabdominelle Myomektomie *f*, Laparomyomektomie *f*.
lap·a·ro·my·o·mot·o·my [ˌlæpərəʊmaɪə'mɒtəmɪ] *n chir.*, *gyn.* transabdominelle Myomotomie *f*, Laparomyomotomie *f*.
lap·a·ro·my·o·si·tis [ˌlæpərəʊmaɪə'saɪtɪs] *n* Entzündung *f* der seitlichen Bauchwandmuskeln, Laparomyositis *f*.
lap·a·ro·ne·phrec·to·my [ˌlæpərəʊnɪ'frektəmɪ] *n chir.*, *urol.* transperitoneale Nierenentfernung/Nephrektomie *f*.
lap·a·ror·rha·phy [læpə'rɒrəfɪ] *n chir.* Bauchwandnaht *f*, Zölio-, Laparorrhaphie *f*.
lap·a·ro·sal·pin·gec·to·my [ˌlæpərəˌsælpɪn'dʒektəmɪ] *n gyn.* transabdominelle Salpingektomie *f*, Zölio-, Laparosalpingektomie *f*.
laparosalpingo-oophorectomy *n gyn.* transabdominelle Salpingo-oophorektomie *f*, Laparosalpingo-oophorektomie *f*, Laparosalpingo-ovariektomie *f*.
lap·a·ro·sal·pin·got·o·my [ˌlæpərəˌsælpɪn'dʒɒtəmɪ] *n gyn.* transabdominelle Salpingotomie *f*, Zölio-, Laparosalpingotomie *f*.
lap·a·ro·scope ['læpərəskəʊp] *n* Laparoskop *nt*.

lap·a·ros·co·py [ˌlæpə'rɒskəpɪ] *n* Bauchspiegelung *f*, Laparoskopie *f*.
lap·a·ro·sple·nec·to·my [ˌlæpərəsplɪ'nektəmɪ] *n chir.* kombinierte Laparotomie *f* u. Splenektomie, Laparosplenektomie *f*.
lap·a·ro·sple·not·o·my [ˌlæpərəsplɪ'nɒtəmɪ] *n chir.* Laparosplenotomie *f*.
lap·a·rot·o·my [læpə'rɒtəmɪ] *n chir.* (operative) Bauchhöhleneröffnung *f*, Laparotomie *f*.
lap·a·ro·u·te·rot·o·my [ˌlæpərəju:tə'rɒtəmɪ] *n* → laparohysterotomy.
Lapidus ['læpɪdəs]: **L.' operation** *ortho.* Lapidus-Operation *f*.
lap·i·ni·za·tion [ˌlæpɪnɪ'zeɪʃn] *n micro.*, *immun.* Lapinisation *f*.
lap·in·ize ['læpɪnaɪz] *vt micro.*, *immun.* lapinisieren.
lap·in·ized ['læpɪnaɪzd] *adj micro.*, *immun.* lapinisiert.
lap·is ['læpɪs, 'leɪpɪs] *n* Stein *m*, Lapis *m*.
Laplace [lə'plɑ:s]: **L.'s law/relation** Laplace'-Gesetz *nt*, -Beziehung *f*.
lap pad [læp] *chir.* Bauchtuch *nt*.
lapse [læps] **I** *n* **1.** Versehen *nt*, Fehler *m*, Lapsus *m*. **2.** *patho.* Fall *m*, Absinken *nt*, Lapsus *m*; Ptose *f*. **3.** *(Zeit)* Ab-, Verlauf *m*; Zeitspanne *f*. **4.** Verfall *m*, Absinken *nt*, Niedergang *m*. **5.** Verschwinden *nt*, Aussterben *nt*; Aufhören *nt*. **II vi 6.** *(Zeit)* verstreichen; *(Frist)* ablaufen. **7.** verfallen, versinken *(into* in*)*. **8.** absinken, abgleiten, verfallen *(into* in*)*. **9.** verschwinden, aussterben.
lap·sus ['læpsəs] *n* → lapse 1, 2.
lard [lɑ:rd] *n* (Schweine-)Fett *nt*, Adeps suillus.
lar·da·ceous [lɑ:r'deɪʃəs] *adj* fettartig, -ähnlich.
lardaceous degeneration *patho.* amyloide Degeneration *f*; Amyloidose *f*.
lardaceous kidney *o* → amyloid kidney.
lardaceous liver Amyloidleber *f*.
lardaceous spleen Wachsmilz *f*.
large ['lɑ:(r)dʒ] **I** *n* **at ~** im großen u. ganzen, im allgemeinen; ausführlich, detailliert. **II** *adj* **1.** groß, Groß-; *(Person)* stark, korpulent. **2.** ausgedehnt, umfassend, bedeutend. **III** *adv* (sehr) groß.
large-bore catheter großlumiger Katheter *m*.
large bowel Dickdarm *m*, Intestinum crassum.
large bowel cancer/carcinoma Dickdarmkrebs *m*, -karzinom *nt*.
large bowel diverticulum Dickdarmdivertikel *nt*.
large bowel obstruction Dickdarmverschluß *m*.
large calorie *abbr.* **C, Cal** große Kalorie *f*, Kilokalorie *f abbr.* kcal, Cal.
large-cell anaplastic carcinoma → large cell carcinoma.
large-cell auditory nucleus Deiters'-Kern *m*, Nc. vestibularis lateralis.
large-cell carcinoma großzelliges/großzellig-anaplastisches Bronchialkarzinom *nt*, *inf.* Großzeller *m*.
large granule cells *histol.* L-Zellen *pl*.
large intestine → large bowel.
large·ness ['lɑ:(r)dʒnɪs] *n* **1.** Größe *f*. **2.** Umfang *m*, Bedeutung *f*; Ausgedehntheit *f*.
large pelvis großes Becken *nt*, Pelvis major.
large plaque parapsoriasis *derm.* großherdig-entzündliche Form *f* der Parapsoriasis en plaques, prämaligne Form *f* der Parapsoriasis en plaques, Parapsoriasis en plaques simples.
large red kidney Stauungsniere *f*.
large-scale structure Grobstruktur *f*.

la·rith·mics [ləˈrɪðmɪks] *pl* Bevölkerungsstatistik *f*.
Larrey [laˈrɛj]: **L.'s amputation/operation** *ortho*. Larrey-Amputation *f*, Schultergelenkexartikulation *f* nach Larrey.
L.'s spaces Larrey'-Spalten *pl*.
Larrey-Weil [vaɪl]: **L.-W. disease** Weil'-Krankheit *f*, Leptospirosis icterohaemorrhagica.
Larsen [ˈlɑːrzn]: **L.'s disease** → Larsen-Johansson disease.
L.'s syndrome Larsen-Syndrom *nt*.
Larsen-Johansson [jəʊˈhænsən]: **L.-J. disease** Larsen-Johansson-Krankheit *f*, Osteopathia patellae juvenilis.
lar·va [ˈlɑːrvə] *n, pl* **-vae** [-viː] *bio., micro*. Larve *f*, Larva *f*.
lar·va·ceous [lɑːrˈveɪʃəs] *adj* → larvate.
lar·val [ˈlɑːrvəl] *adj* **1.** Larve(n) betr., Larven-. **2.** → larvate.
larval conjunctivitis *ophthal*. Myiasis *f* der Bindehaut.
larval epilepsy latente/larvierte Epilepsie *f*.
larval form *micro., bio*. Larvenform *f*.
larval nephrosis larvierte Nephrose *f*.
larval parasitism *micro., bio*. Larvenparasitismus *m*.
larval plague abortive Pest *f*, Pestis minor.
larval stage *micro., bio*. Larvenstadium *nt*.
larva migrans *derm*. Hautmaulwurf *m*, Larva migrans, Myiasis linearis migrans, creeping disease (*nt*).
cutaneous l. Larva migrans cutanea.
visceral l. Larva migrans visceralis.
lar·vate [ˈlɑːrveɪt] *adj* (*Krankheit, Symptom*) versteckt, verkappt, maskiert, larviert.
lar·vat·ed [ˈlɑːrveɪtɪd] *adj* → larvate.
lar·vi·cid·al [ˌlɑːrvəˈsaɪdl] *adj* larven(ab)tötend, larvizid.
lar·vi·cide [ˈlɑːrvəsaɪd] *n* Larvenvertilgungsmittel *nt*, Larvizid *nt*.
lar·vi·form [ˈlɑːrvəfɔːrm] *adj* larvenförmig.
lar·vip·a·rous [lɑːrˈvɪpərəs] *adj* larvenübertragend.
lar·vi·phag·ic [ˌlɑːrvɪˈfædʒɪk] *adj* → larvivorous.
lar·viv·o·rous [lɑːrˈvɪvərəs] *adj bio., micro*. larvenfressend.
laryng- *pref*. → laryngo-.
lar·yn·gal·gia [lærɪnˈgældʒ(ɪ)ə] *n* Larynx-, Kehlkopfschmerz *m*, Laryngalgie *f*.
la·ryn·ge·al [ləˈrɪndʒ(ɪ)əl, ˌlærɪnˈdʒiːəl] *adj* Kehlkopf/Larynx betr., laryngeal, Kehlkopf-, Laryng(o)-, Larynx-.
laryngeal anomaly Larynxfehlbildung *f*, -mißbildung *f*, Kehlkopffehlbildung *f*, -mißbildung *f*.
laryngeal artery: inferior l. untere Kehlkopfschlagader/-arterie *f*, Laryngea *f* inferior, A. laryngealis inferior.
superior l. obere Kehlkopfschlagader/-arterie *f*, Laryngea *f* superior, A. laryngea superior.
laryngeal atresia Larynx-, Kehlkopfatresie *f*.
laryngeal carcinoma Kehlkopfkrebs *m*, Larynxkarzinom *nt*.
laryngeal cartilage: l.s *pl* Kehlkopfknorpel *pl*, Cartilagines laryngeales.
l. of Luschka Sesamknorpel *m* des Stimmbandes, Cartilago sesamoidea (lig. vocalis).
laryngeal cavity Kehlkopfinnenraum *m*, Cavitas laryngis.
laryngeal crisis *neuro*. (tabische) Larynxkrise *f*.
laryngeal diphtheria Kehlkopf-, Larynxdiphtherie *f*.

laryngeal diverticulum Kehlkopfdivertikel *nt*.
laryngeal edema Larynx-, Kehlkopfödem *nt*.
laryngeal epilepsy Kehlkopfschlag *m*, Epilepsia laryngealis.
laryngeal fracture Kehlkopffraktur *f*, Larynx(knorpel)fraktur *f*.
laryngeal glands Kehlkopf-, Larynxdrüsen *pl*, Gll. laryngeales.
laryngeal lymphatic follicles (*Kehlkopf*) Lymphfollikel *nt*, Noduli/Folliculi lymphatici laryngis.
laryngeal mirror *HNO* Kehlkopfspiegel *m*.
laryngeal musculature Kehlkopf-, Larynxmuskulatur *f*, Mm. laryngis.
laryngeal nerve: inferior l. N. laryngealis inferior.
recurrent l. Rekurrens *m*, N. laryngealis recurrens.
superior l. N. laryngealis superior.
superior l., internal Ramus internus n. laryngei superioris.
laryngeal obstruction Larynx-, Kehlkopfobstruktion *f*.
laryngeal papillomatosis Larynx-, Kehlkopfpapillomatose *f*.
laryngeal polyp Larynx-, Kehlkopfpolyp *m*.
laryngeal pouch → laryngeal sacculus.
laryngeal prominence Adamsapfel *m*, Prominentia laryngea.
laryngeal protuberance → laryngeal prominence.
laryngeal sacculus Kehlkopfblindsack *m*, Sacculus laryngis, Appendix ventriculi laryngis.
laryngeal sinus → laryngeal ventricle.
laryngeal skeleton Kehlkopfskelett *nt*.
laryngeal spasm → laryngospasm.
laryngeal stridor Stridor laryngealis.
congenital l. Stridor congenitus/connatus, Stridulus *m*.
laryngeal syncope 1. Larynx-, Kehlkopfschwindel *m*, Vertigo laryngica. **2.** Hustenschlag *m*, -synkope *f*.
laryngeal tuberculosis Larynx-, Kehlkopftuberkulose *f*, Laryngophthise *f*.
laryngeal vein: inferior l. untere Kehlkopfvene *f*, V. laryngea inferior.
superior l. obere Kehlkopfvene *f*, Begleitvene *f* der A. laryngea superior, V. laryngealis superior.
laryngeal ventricle Morgagni-Ventrikel *m*, -Tasche *f*, Galen'-Ventrikel *m*, -Tasche *f*, Kehlkopftasche *f*, Ventriculus laryngis.
laryngeal vertigo → laryngeal syncope 1.
laryngeal vestibule Kehlkopfvorhof *m*, oberer Kehlkopfinnenraum *m*, Vestibulum laryngis.
laryngeal web *embryo., HNO* partielle Larynxatresie *f*.
lar·yn·gec·to·mee [ˌlærɪnˈdʒektəmiː] *n HNO* Patient(in *f*) *m* nach Laryngektomie, laryngektomierter Patient *m*.
lar·yn·gec·to·mize [ˌlærɪnˈdʒektəmaɪz] *vt HNO* eine Laryngektomie durchführen *od*. vornehmen, laryngektomieren.
lar·yn·gec·to·my [ˌlærɪnˈdʒektəmɪ] *n HNO* Larynxentfernung *f*, -exstirpation *f*, Kehlkopfentfernung *f*, -exstirpation *f*, Laryngektomie *f*.
lar·yn·gis·mus [ˌləˈdʒɪzməs] *n, pl* **-mi** [-maɪ] Larynx-, Kehlkopfkrampf *m*.
laryngismus stridulus 1. → laryngospasm. **2.** falscher Krupp *m*, Pseudokrupp *m*, subglottische Laryngitis *f*, Laryngitis subglottica.
lar·yn·git·ic [ˌlærɪnˈdʒɪtɪk] *adj* Laryngitis betr., von ihr gekennzeichnet, laryngitisch.

lar·yn·gi·tis [ˌlærɪnˈdʒaɪtɪs] *n, pl* **-git·i·des** [-ˈdʒɪtədiːz] Larynx-, Kehlkopfentzündung *f*, Laryngitis *f*.
laryngo- *pref*. Kehlkopf-, Laryng(o)-, Larynx-.
la·ryn·go·cele [ləˈrɪŋgəʊsiːl] *n HNO* Luftsack *m*, -geschwulst *f*, Laryngozele *f*, -cele *f*.
la·ryn·go·cen·te·sis [ˌ-senˈtiːsɪs] *n HNO* Kehlkopfpunktion *f*, Laryngozentese *f*.
la·ryn·go·fis·sure [ˌ-ˈfɪʃər] *n HNO* mediane Kehlkopfspaltung/Laryngotomie *f*, Laryngofissur *f*.
la·ryn·go·gram [ˈ-græm] *n radiol*. Laryngogramm *nt*.
la·ryn·go·graph [ˈ-græf] *n HNO* Laryngograph *m*.
la·ryn·gog·ra·phy [ˌlærɪnˈgɑgrəfɪ] *n radiol., HNO* Laryngographie *f*.
la·ryn·go·hy·po·phar·ynx [ləˌrɪŋgəʊhaɪpəˈfærɪŋks] *n* Laryngohypopharynx *m*.
la·ryn·gol·o·gy [ˌlærɪnˈgɑlədʒɪ] *n* Laryngologie *f*.
la·ryn·go·ma·la·cia [ləˌrɪŋgəʊməˈleɪʃ(ɪ)ə] *n* Kehlkopferweichung *f*, Laryngomalazie *f*.
lar·yn·gom·e·try [ˌlærɪnˈgɑmətrɪ] *n HNO* Laryngometrie *f*.
la·ryn·go·pa·ral·y·sis [ləˌrɪŋgəʊpəˈrælʌsɪs] *n* Larynx-, Kehlkopflähmung *f*, Laryngoparalyse *f*, Laryngoplegie *f*.
lar·yn·gop·a·thy [ˌlærɪnˈgɑpəθɪ] *n HNO* Kehlkopferkrankung *f*, Laryngopathie *f*.
la·ryn·go·pha·ryn·ge·al [ləˌrɪŋgəʊfəˈrɪndʒ(ɪ)əl] *adj* Kehlkopf/Larynx u. Rachen/Pharynx betr. *od*. verbindend, laryngopharyngeal, Laryngopharyng(o)-.
laryngopharyngeal branches of superior cervical ganglion Äste *pl* des Ggl. cervicalis superior zu Larynx u. Pharynx, Rami laryngopharyngeales ggl. cervicalis superioris.
laryngopharyngeal cavity → laryngopharynx.
laryngopharyngeal recess Rec. piriformis.
la·ryn·go·phar·yn·gec·to·my [ˌ-ˌfærɪnˈdʒektəmɪ] *n HNO* kombinierte Laryngektomie *f* u. Pharyngektomie, Laryngopharyngektomie *f*.
la·ryn·go·pha·ryn·ge·us [ˌ-fəˈrɪndʒɪəs] *n* M. constrictor pharyngis inferior.
la·ryn·go·phar·yn·gi·tis [ˌ-ˌfærɪnˈdʒaɪtɪs] *n* Entzündung *f* von Larynx u. Pharynx, Laryngopharyngitis *f*.
la·ryn·go·phar·ynx [ˌ-ˈfærɪŋks] *n* Hypo-, Laryngopharynx *m*, Pars laryngea pharyngis.
lar·yn·goph·o·ny [ˌlærɪnˈgɑfənɪ] *n* Laryngophonie *f*.
lar·yn·goph·thi·sis [ˌ-ˈgɑfθəsɪs] *n* Larynx-, Kehlkopftuberkulose *f*, Laryngophthise *f*.
la·ryn·go·plas·ty [ləˈrɪŋgəʊplæstɪ] *n HNO* Larynx-, Kehlkopfplastik *f*.
la·ryn·go·ple·gia [ˌ-ˈpliːdʒ(ɪ)ə] *n* → laryngoparalysis.
la·ryn·gop·to·sis [ˌ-ˈtəʊsɪs] *n HNO* Kehlkopfsenkung *f*, Laryngoptosis *f*.
la·ryn·go·py·o·cele [ˌ-ˈpaɪəsiːl] *n HNO* mit Eiter gefüllte Laryngozele *f*, Laryngopyozele *f*.
la·ryn·go·rhi·nol·o·gy [ˌ-ˌraɪˈnɑlədʒɪ] *n* Laryngorhinologie *f*.
lar·yn·gor·rha·gia [ˌ-ˈrædʒ(ɪ)ə] *n* Larynx-, Kehlkopfblutung *f*, Laryngorrhagie *f*.
lar·yn·gor·rha·phy [ˌ-ˈgɑrəfɪ] *n HNO* Kehlkopfnaht *f*, Laryngorrhaphie *f*.
lar·yn·gor·rhea [ləˌrɪŋgəˈrɪə] *n HNO* Laryngorrhoe *f*.
lar·yn·go·scope [ˈ-skəʊp] *n HNO* Laryngoskop *nt*.

laryngoscopic

la·ryn·go·scop·ic [ˌ-'skɒpɪk] *adj* Laryngoskopie betr., laryngoskopisch.
lar·yn·gos·co·py [ˌlærɪŋ'gɒskəpɪ] *n HNO* Kehlkopfspiegelung *f*, -untersuchung *f*, Laryngoskopie *f*.
la·ryn·go·spasm [lə'rɪŋgəspæzəm] *n* Stimmritzenkrampf *m*, Laryngospasmus *m*.
la·ryn·go·spas·tic reflex [ˌ-'spæstɪk] → larngospasm.
la·ryn·gos·ta·sis [ˌlærɪn'gɒstəsɪs] *n* Croup *m*, Krupp *m*.
la·ryn·go·ste·no·sis [lə,rɪŋgəʊstɪ'nəʊsɪs] *n* Larynxverengung *f*, -stenose *f*, Kehlkopfverengung *f*, -stenose *f*, Laryngostenose *f*.
la·ryn·gos·to·my [ˌlærɪn'gɒstəmɪ] *n HNO* **1.** Laryngostomie *f*. **2.** Kehlkopffistel *f*, Laryngostoma *nt*.
lar·yn·go·strob·o·scope [ˌlærɪŋgə'strəʊbəskəʊp] *n HNO* Laryngostroboskop *nt*.
lar·yn·go·stro·bos·co·py [ˌ-strəʊ'bɒskəpɪ] *n HNO* Laryngostroboskopie *f*.
la·ryn·go·tome ['-təʊm] *n HNO* Laryngotom *nt*.
la·ryn·got·o·my [ˌlærɪn'gɒtəmɪ] *n HNO* Kehlkopferöffnung *f*, -spaltung *f*, Laryngotomie *f*.
la·ryn·go·tra·che·al [lə,rɪŋgəʊ'treɪkɪəl] *adj* Larynx u. Trachea betr., laryngotracheal.
laryngotracheal bronchitis laryngotracheale Bronchitis *f*.
laryngotracheal diphtheria → laryngeal diphtheria.
laryngotracheal separation *HNO, ortho.* laryngotrachealer Abriß *m*.
la·ryn·go·tra·che·i·tis [ˌ-treɪkɪ'aɪtɪs] *n HNO* Entzündung *f* von Kehlkopf/Larynx u. Luftröhre/Trachea, Laryngotracheitis *f*.
la·ryn·go·tra·che·o·bron·chi·tis [ˌ-,treɪkɪəʊbrɒŋ'kaɪtɪs] *n* Entzündung *f* von Larynx, Trachea u. Bronchien, Laryngotracheobronchitis *f*.
la·ryn·go·tra·che·o·bron·chos·co·py [ˌ-,treɪkɪəʊbrɒn'kɒskəpɪ] *n HNO* Laryngotracheobronchoskopie *f*.
la·ryn·go·tra·che·o·e·soph·a·ge·al cleft [ˌ-,treɪkɪəʊɪ,safə'dʒɪəl, -ɪsə'fædʒɪəl] Larynx-Trachea-Ösophagus-Spalte *f*.
la·ryn·go·tra·che·os·co·py [ˌ-,treɪkɪ'ɒskəpɪ] *n* Laryngotracheoskopie *f*.
la·ryn·go·tra·che·ot·o·my [ˌ-,treɪkɪ'ɒtəmɪ] *n HNO* Eröffnung *f* von Kehlkopf u. Luftröhre, Laryngotracheotomie *f*.
la·ryn·go·ves·ti·bu·li·tis [ˌ-,vestɪbjə'laɪtɪs] *n HNO* Laryngovestibulitis *f*.
la·ryn·go·xe·ro·sis [ˌ-zɪ'rəʊsɪs] *n HNO* pathologische Trockenheit *f* der Kehlkopfschleimhaut, Laryngoxerose *f*, -xerosis *f*.
lar·ynx ['lærɪŋks] *n, pl* **lar·ynx·es, la·ryn·ges** [lə'rɪndʒiːz] Kehlkopf *m*, Larynx *m*.
LAS *abbr.* → lymphadenopathy syndrome.
lase [leɪz] **I** *vt* mit Laser bestrahlen. **II** *vi* Laserlicht ausstrahlen, lasen.
Lasègue [la'seg]: **L.'s sign** *neuro., ortho.* Lasègue-Zeichen *nt*.
la·ser ['leɪzər] *abbr.* [lightwave amplification by stimulated emission of radiation] Laser *m*.
laser beam Laserstrahl *m*.
laser fusion Laserfusion *f*.
laser microscope Laser-Scan-Mikroskop *nt*.
laser surgery Laserchirurgie *f*.
Las·sa (hemorrhagic) fever ['lɒsə] Lassafieber *nt*.
Lassa virus *micro.* Lassavirus *nt*.
las·si·tude ['læsɪt(j)uːd] *n* Schwäche *f*, Erschöpfung *f*, Mattigkeit *f*, Abgespanntheit *f*.
Latarget [latar'ʒɛt]: **L.'s nerve** Plexus hypogastricus superior, N. pr(a)esacralis.
late [leɪt] *adj* spät, Spät-; verspätet, zu spät; letzter(r, s), frühere(r, s), ehemalig; verstorben.
late abortion *gyn.* Spätabort *m*, später Abort *m*.
late-appearing factor *old* Pertussistoxin *nt abbr.* PT.
late complication Spätkomplikation *f*.
late cortical potentials späte kortikale Gleichspannungspotentiale *pl*, contingent negative variation *abbr.* CNV.
late deceleration *gyn.* Spätdezeleration *f*, Spättief *nt*, späte Dezeleration *f*, Dip II *m*.
late developer *ped.* Spätentwickler *m*.
late diastolic murmur *card.* präsystolisches/spät-diastolytisches (Herz-)Geräusch *m*.
late erythroblast azidophiler/orthochromatischer/oxaphiler Normoblast *m*.
late-expiratory neuron spätexspiratorisches Neuron *nt*, E-Neuron *nt*.
late infantile type of amaurotic idiocy *ped., neuro.* spätinfantile Form *f* der amaurotischen Idiotie, Bielschowsky--Syndrom *nt*, Jansky-Bielschowsky--Krankheit *f*.
late injury Spätschaden *m*, -schädigung *f*.
late-inspiratory neuron spätinspiratorisches Neuron *nt*, L-I-Neuron *nt*.
late juvenile type of cerebral sphingolipidosis *neuro., ped.* juvenile Form *f* der amaurotischen Idiotie, neuronale/juvenile Ceroidlipofuscinose *f*, Batten--Spielmeyer-Vogt-Syndrom *nt*, Stock--Vogt-Spielmeyer-Syndrom *nt*, neuronale/juvenile Zeroidlipofuszinose *f*.
late latent syphilis Spätlatenz *f*, Syphilis/Lues latens seronegativa.
late morbidity Spätmorbidität *f*.
la·ten·cy ['leɪtnsɪ] *n* **1.** Verborgenheit *f*, latente Beschaffenheit *od.* Phase *f*, Latenz *f*. **2.** *physiol.* Latenz *f*, Latenzzeit *f*. **3.** *patho.* Symptomlosigkeit *f*, Latenz *f*.
latency period → latency phase.
latency phase 1. *psycho.* Latenzphase *f*. **2.** *micro.* Latenzzeit *f*, Inkubationszeit *f*.
latency stage Latenzperiode *f*.
late normoblast azidophiler/orthochromatischer/oxaphiler Normoblast *m*.
la·tent ['leɪtnt] *adj* verborgen, inapparent, unsichtbar, versteckt, latent; *phys., patho., psycho.* latent.
latent allergy latente Überempfindlichkeit/Allergie *f*.
latent cancer → latent carcinoma.
latent carcinoma latentes Karzinom *nt*.
latent deviation *ophthal.* latentes Schielen *nt*, Heterophorie *f*, Strabismus latens.
latent diabetes *old* pathologische Glukosetoleranz *f*.
latent epilepsy latente/larvierte Epilepsie *f*.
latent gout latente Gicht *f*.
latent heat *phys.* latente Wärme *f*.
l. of evaporation Verdampfungswärme.
l. of fusion Fusionswärme.
l. of sublimation Sublimierungswärme.
l. of vaporization → l. of evaporation.
latent hyperopia *abbr.* Hl *ophthal.* latente Weitsichtigkeit/Hyperopie *f*.
latent infection latente Infektion *f*.
latent jaundice okkulter/latenter Ikterus *m*.
latent mydriasis *ophthal.* latente Mydriasis *f*.
latent neuritis latente Neuritis *f*.
latent nystagmus latenter Nystagmus *m*.
latent period 1. *micro.* Latenzzeit *f*, Inkubationszeit *f*. **2.** *physiol.* Latenz *f*, Latenzzeit *f*.
latent reflex latenter Reflex *m*.
latent schizophrenia latente Schizophrenie *f*, Borderline-Psychose *f*, Borderline--Schizophrenie *f*.
latent sinusitis *HNO* okkulte/latente Nebenhöhlenentzündung/Sinusitis *f*.
latent strabismus *ophthal.* latentes Schielen *nt*, Heterophorie *f*, Strabismus latens.
latent syphilis seropositives Stadium *nt*, Latenzstadium *nt*, Syphilis/Lues latens.
early l. Frühlatenz *f*, Syphilis/Lues latens seropositiva.
late l. Spätlatenz *f*, Syphilis/Lues latens seronegativa.
latent tetany latente Tetanie *f*.
latent typhoid Typhus ambulatorius/levissimus.
latent typhus (fever) Brill-Krankheit *f*, Brill-Zinsser-Krankheit *f*.
late postprandial dumping (syndrome) *chir.* postalimentäres Spätsyndrom *nt*, Spät-Dumping *nt*, reaktive Hypoglykämie *f*.
late post-traumatic epilepsy späte (post-)traumatische Epilepsie *f*.
late protein *micro.* (*Virus*) Spätprotein *nt*.
lat·er·al ['lætərəl] *adj* an *od.* auf der Seite, zur Körperseite hin liegend, seitlich, seitwärts, lateral, Seiten-, Lateral-.
lateral and medial nuclei of mamillary body Ncc. corporis mamillaris medialis et lateralis.
lateral aneurysm laterales/seitliches Aneurysma *nt*.
lateral angle: l. of border of tibia Margo interosseus tibiae.
l. of eye seitlicher/äußerer Augenwinkel *m*, Angulus oculi lateralis.
l. of humerus Margo lateralis humeri.
lateral aperture of fourth ventricle Luschka-Foramen *nt*, Apertura lateralis ventriculi quarti.
lateral basal segment of lung seitliches Basalsegment *nt*, Segmentum basale laterale [S. IX].
lateral border: l. of foot Fußaußenrand *m*, Margo lateralis/fibularis pedis.
l. of forearm Außenrand *m* des Unterarms, Margo lateralis/radialis antebrachii.
l. of humerus Humerusaußenkante *f*, Margo lateralis humeri.
l. of scapula Schulterblattaußenrand *m*, Margo lateralis scapulae.
lateral branch: l. of anterior interventricular branch of left coronary artery Ramus lateralis interventricularis anterioris a. coronariae sinistrae.
l.es of anterolateral central arteries Rami laterales aa. centralium anterolateralium.
l. of left hepatic duct Ramus lateralis ductus hepatici sinistri.
l. of right pulmonary artery Ramus lateralis a. pulmonalis dextrae.
l. of superior thyroid artery Ramus glandularis lateralis a. thyroideae superioris.
l. of supraorbital nerve lateraler Ast *m* des N. supraorbitalis, Ramus lateralis n. supraorbitalis.
lateral bursa of gastrocnemius muscle Bursa subtendinea m. gastrocnemii lateralis.
lateral chain *chem.* Seitenkette *f*.
lateral column of spinal cord Seitensäule *f* (des Rückenmarks), Columna lateralis (medullae spinalis).
lateral commissure of eye lid seitliche/

äußere Augenlidkommissur *f*, Commissura palpebralis lateralis.
lateral condylar fracture → lateral epicondylar fracture.
lateral condyle: **l. of femur** äußere/laterale/fibulare Femurkondyle *f*, äußere/laterale/fibulare Oberschenkelkondyle *f*, Condylus lateralis femoris.
l. of tibia äußere/laterale Tibiakondyle *f*, Condylus lateralis tibiae.
lateral cord of brachial plexus laterales Bündel *nt* des Plexus brachialis, Fasciculus lateralis (plexus brachialis).
lateral crest of fibula Seiten- *od.* Hinterkante *f* des Wadenbeins, Margo posterior fibulae.
lateral crus: **l. of greater alar cartilage** Crus laterale cartilago alaris majoris.
l. of superficial inguinal ring Crus laterale anuli inguinalis superficialis.
lateral curvature ortho. Skoliose *f*.
lateral decubitus Seitenlage *f*.
lateral dominance physiol. Seitendominanz *f*.
lateral epicondylar fracture Fraktur *f* des Epicondylus lateralis humeri.
lateral fissure of cerebrum Sulcus lateralis.
lateral folding embryo. laterale Abfaltung *f*.
lateral fornix → lateral part of fornix of vagina.
lateral fossa of brain Fossa lateralis cerebralis.
lateral fracture of neck of femur ortho. laterale Schenkelhalsfraktur *f*.
lateral funiculus: **l. of medulla oblongata** Seitenstrang *m* des Markhirns, Funiculus lateralis medullae oblongatae.
l. of spinal cord Seitenstrang *m* (des Rückenmarks), Funiculus lateralis (medullae spinalis).
lateral head: **l. of abductor hallucis muscle** Caput laterale m. abductoris hallucis.
l. of gastrocnemius muscle Caput laterale m. gastrocnemii.
l. of triceps brachii muscle lateraler/äußerer Trizepskopf *m*, Caput laterale m. tricipitis brachii.
lateral hemianopia/hemianopsia neuro. homonyme/gleichseitige Hemianop(s)ie *f*.
lateral hermaphroditism Hermaphroditismus (verus) dimidiatus/lateralis.
lateral horn of spinal cord Seitenhorn *nt* (des Rückenmarks), Cornu laterale (medullae spinalis).
lateral hypothalamus lateraler Hypothalamus *m*.
lateral incisure of sternum Inc. clavicularis (sterni).
lateral inhibition physiol. laterale Hemmung *f*.
lat·er·al·i·ty [ˌlætəˈræləti] *n* physiol., psycho. Lateralität *f*.
lat·er·al·iza·tion [ˌlætərəlɪˈzeɪʃn] *n* neuro. Lateralisation *f*.
lat·er·al·ize [ˈlætərəlaɪz] *vt* neuro. lateralisieren.
lateral lacunae (of superior sagittal sinus) Seitennischen *pl* des Sinus sagittalis superior, Lacunae laterales.
lateral lamina: **l. of cartilage of auditory tube** → l. of tubal cartilage.
l. of pterygoid process Lamina lateralis proc. pterygoidei.
l. of tubal cartilage laterale Knorpelplatte *f* des Tubenknorpels, Lamina cartilaginis lateralis (tubae auditivae).
lateral lemniscus Lemniscus lateralis.
lateral ligament Außen-, Lateralband *nt*, laterales Ligament *nt*, Lig. laterale/collaterale.

l. of ankle (joint) Außenknöchelband.
l. of colon Taenia omentalis.
l of knee äußeres Seitenband, Außenband, Lig. collaterale fibulare.
l. of malleus seitliches Malleusband, Lig. mallei laterale.
radial l. of carpus Lig. collaterale carpi radiale.
ulnar l. of carpus Lig. collaterale carpi ulnare.
lateral limb of greater alar cartilage Crus laterale cartilago alaris majoris.
lateral lobe hyperplasia (of the prostate) urol. (*Prostata*) Seitenlappenhyperplasie *f*.
lateral lobe of prostate (*Prostata*) Seitenlappen *m*, Lobus prostatae.
left l. linker (Seiten-)Lappen, Lobus sinister prostatae.
right l. rechter (Seiten-)Lappen, Lobus dexter prostatae.
lateral malleolar fracture Außenknöchelbruch *m*, -fraktur *f*.
lateral malleolus Außenknöchel *m*, Malleolus lateralis.
lateral margin: **l. of foot** → lateral border of foot.
l. of forearm → lateral border of forearm.
l. of humerus → lateral border of humerus.
l. of kidney seitlicher/konvexer Nierenrand *m*, Margo lateralis renis.
l. of nail Seitenrand *m* des Nagels, Margo lateralis unguis.
l. of orbit seitlicher Orbitarand *m*, Margo lateralis orbitae.
l. of scapula → lateral border of scapula.
l. of tongue Margo linguae.
lateral mass: **l. of atlas** Massa lateralis atlantis.
l. of ethmoid bone Labyrinthus ethmoidalis.
l. of sacrum Pars/Massa lateralis ossis sacri.
lateral medullary syndrome Wallenberg-Syndrom *nt*, dorsolaterales Oblongata-Syndrom *nt*.
lateral meniscus of knee Außenmeniskus *m*, Meniscus lateralis (artic. genus).
lateral mesoderm Seitenplattenmesoderm *nt*.
lateral nucleus: **l. of amygdaloid body** Nc. lateralis corporis amygdaloidei.
dorsal l. of thalamus Nc. lateralis dorsalis thalami.
posterior l. of thalamus Nc. lateralis posterior thalami.
lateral nystagmus horizontaler Nystagmus *m*.
lateral part: **l. of fornix of vagina** Seitengewölbe *nt*, Pars lateralis fornicis vaginae.
l. of globus pallidus lateraler Teil *m* des Globus pallidus, Globus pallidus lateralis.
lateral plate embryo. Seitenplatte *f*.
lateral plate mesoderm → lateral mesoderm.
lateral process: **l. of cartilage of nasal septum** Proc. lateralis.
l. of malleus seitlicher Hammerfortsatz, Proc. lateralis mallei.
l. of mammary gland Achselfortsatz *m* der Brustdrüse, Proc. axillaris/lateralis gl. mammariae.
l. of talus Proc. lateralis tali.
lateral recess: **l. of fourth ventricle** seitliche Ausstülpung *f* des IV. Ventrikels, Rec. lateralis (ventriculi quarti).
l. of nasopharynx Rosenmüller'-Grube *f*, Rec. pharyngeus (Rosenmülleri).
lateral recumbent position gyn. Sims-Lage *f*.

lateral region: **left l.** linke Seiten-/Lateralregion *f*, Regio lateralis sinistra.
l. of neck hinteres Halsdreieck *nt*, Regio cervicalis lateralis, Trigonum cervicale posterius.
right l. rechte Seiten-/Lateralregion *f*, Regio lateralis dextra.
lateral root: **l. of median nerve** laterale Medianuswurzel *f*, Radix lateralis n. mediani.
l. of optic tract lateraler Zweig/Ast *m* des Tractus opticus, Radix lateralis tractus optici.
lateral sclerosis Lateralsklerose *f*.
lateral segment: **l. of left lobe of liver** Segmentum laterale.
l. of right lung Lateralsegment *nt* des Mittellappens, Segmentum laterale [S. IV].
lateral spinal sclerosis → lateral sclerosis.
lateral spondylosis of the vertebral body ortho. Unkovertebralarthrose *f*, Spondylosis intervertebralis/uncovertebralis.
lateral sulcus: **anterior l. of medulla oblongata** Vorderseitenfurche *f* der Medulla oblongata, Sulcus anterolateralis/ventrolateralis medullae oblongatae.
anterior l. of spinal cord Vorderseitenfurche *f* des Rückenmarks, Sulcus anterolateralis/ventrolateralis medullae spinalis.
posterior l. of medulla oblongata Hinterseitenfurche *f* der Medulla oblongata, Sulcus posterolateralis medullae oblongatae.
posterior l. of spinal cord Hinterseitenfurche *f* des Rückenmarks, Sulcus posterolateralis medullae spinalis.
lateral tubercle of posterior process of talus Tuberculum laterale.
lateral tuberosity of femur Epicondylus lateralis femoris.
lateral ventricle of brain/cerebrum Seitenventrikel *m*, Ventriculus lateralis (cerebri).
lateral view radiol. Seitenaufnahme *f*; Seitenansicht *f*.
lateral wing of sphenoid bone großer Keilbeinflügel *m*, Ala major (ossis sphenoidalis).
late reaction Spätreaktion *f*.
late receptor potential abbr. **LRP** spätes/sekundäres Rezeptorpotential *nt*, late receptor potential abbr. LRP.
lat·er·i·ceous [ˌlætəˈrɪʃəs] *adj* → lateritious.
lat·er·i·flec·tion [ˌlætərɪˈflekʃn] *n* → lateroflexion.
lat·er·i·flex·ion [ˌ-ˈflekʃn] *n* → lateroflexion.
lat·er·i·tious [ˌlætəˈrɪʃəs] *adj* histol. ziegelrot.
latero- pref. Seiten-, Latero-, Lateral-.
lat·er·o·ab·dom·i·nal [ˌlætərəʊæbˈdɑmɪnl] *adj* lateroabdominal.
lat·er·o·de·vi·a·tion [ˌ-dɪviˈeɪʃn] *n* (geringe) Seitwärtsverlagerung *f*, -beugung *f*, -biegung *f*.
lat·er·o·duc·tion [ˌ-ˈdʌkʃn] *n* Bewegung *f* zur Seite, Lateroduktion *f*.
lat·er·o·flec·tion *n* → lateroflexion.
lat·er·o·flex·ion [ˌ-ˈflekʃn] *n* Beugung *f* zur Seite, Lateroflexion *f*, Lateroflexio *f*.
lat·er·o·lat·er·al anastomosis [ˌ-ˈlætərəl] Seit-zu-Seit-Anastomose *f*, laterolaterale Anastomose *f*.
laterolateral pancreaticojejunostomy chir. Puestow-Mercadier I-Operation *f*, longitudinale laterolaterale Pankreatikojejunostomie *f*.
lat·er·o·pha·ryn·ge·al space [ˌ-fəˈrɪndʒ(i)əl] Lateropharyngealraum *m*, Spatium lateropharyngeum.
lat·er·o·po·si·tion [ˌ-pəˈzɪʃn] *n* Seitwärts-

lateropulsion

verlagerung *f*, Lateroposition *f*, Lateropositio *f*.
lat·er·o·pul·sion [ˌ-'pʌlʃn] *n neuro.* (unwillkürliche) Seitwärtsneigung *f*, -bewegung *f*, Lateropulsion *f*.
lat·er·o·ter·mi·nal anastomosis [ˌ-'tɜːmnəl] Seit-zu-End-Anastomose *f*, lateroterminale Anastomose *f*.
lateroterminal pancreaticojejunostomy *chir.* Puestow-Mercadier II-Operation *f*, longitudinale lateroterminale Pankreatikojejunostomie *f*.
lat·er·o·tor·sion [ˌ-'tɔːrʃn] *n* seitliches Verdrehen *nt*, Laterotorsion *f*.
lat·er·o·ver·sion [ˌ-'vɜrʒn] *n* Drehung *od.* Wendung *f* zur Seite, Lateroversion *f*, Lateroversio *f*.
late syphilis Spätsyphilis *f*, Tertiärstadium *nt*, Lues III *f*.
late systole Prädiastole *f*.
la·tex ['leɪteks] *n, pl* **la·tex·es, lat·i·ces** ['lætəsiːz] Latex *m*.
latex agglutination assay/test Latex(agglutinations)test *m*.
latex fixation assay/test → latex agglutination assay.
lath·y·rism ['læθərɪzəm] *n* Kichererbsenvergiftung *f*, Lathyrismus *m*, Lathyrismus-Syndrom *nt*.
la·tis·si·mus dor·si (muscle) [lə'tɪsəməs 'dɔːrsaɪ] Latissimus *m* dorsi, M. latissimus dorsi.
lat·ro·dec·tism [ˌlætrə'dektɪzəm] *n* Latrodektismus *m*.
Lat·ro·dec·tus [ˌ-'dektəs] *n bio.* Latrodectus *f*.
LATS *abbr.* → long-acting thyroid stimulator.
lat·tice ['lætɪs] *n* 1. Gitter *nt*; *phys.* Kristallgitter *nt*. 2. Gittermuster *nt*, -anordnung *f*.
lattice constant *phys.* Gitterkonstante *f*.
lattice dystrophy (of cornea) *ophthal.* Haab-Dimmer-Dystrophie *f*.
lattice fiber Retikulum-, Retikulinfaser *f*, Gitterfaser *f*, argyrophile Faser *f*.
lattice hypothesis *immun.* Gittertheorie *f*.
lattice work Gitterwerk *n*, -gerüst *nt*.
la·tus ['lætəs, 'leɪ-] *n anat.* Seite *f*, Latus *nt*.
lau·da·num ['lɔːdnəm] *n* 1. Opium *nt*, Laudanum *nt*. 2. Opiumtinktur *f*, Tinktura opii, Laudanum liquidum.
Lauenstein ['lauənstaɪn]: **L. technique** *radiol.* Lauenstein-Technik *f*.
laugh [læf, lɑːf] I *n* Lachen *nt*, Gelächter *nt*. II *vi*, *vi* lachen.
laugh·ing ['læfɪŋ, 'lɑːfɪŋ] I *n* Lachen *nt*, Gelächter *nt*. II *adj* lachend, Lach-.
laughing disease Lach-, Schüttelkrankheit *f*, Kuru, Kuru-Kuru *nt*.
laughing gas Lachgas *nt*, Distickstoffoxid *nt*.
laughing sickness Pseudobulbärparalyse *f*.
laugh·ter ['læftər, 'lɑːf-] *n* Lachen *nt*, Gelächter *nt*.
laughter reflex Lachreflex *m*.
Laugier [loʒi'je]: **L.'s hernia** Gimbernat-Hernie *f*, Laugier-Hernie *f*.
L.'s sign *ortho.* Laugier-Zeichen *nt*.
Laumonier [lomɔ̃'nje]: **L.'s ganglion** 1. Ganglion *nt* des Plexus caroticus internus. 2. Schmiedel'-Ganglion *nt*.
Launois [lo'nwa]: **L.'s syndrome** Launois-Syndrom *nt*, hypophysärer Riesenwuchs *m*.
Launois-Cléret [kleˈrɛ]: **L.-C. syndrome** Babinski-Fröhlich-Syndrom *nt*, Morbus Fröhlich *m*, Dystrophia adiposogenitalis (Fröhlich).
Laurell ['lɔrəl, 'lɑ-]: **L.'s (rocket) immunoelectrophoresis** → L. technique.

L. technique Laurell'-Immunoelektrophorese *f*..
Laurence-Biedl ['lɔːrəns 'biːdəl]: **L.-B. syndrome** → Laurence-Moon-Bardet-Biedl syndrome.
Laurence-Moon [muːn]: **L.-M. syndrome** Laurence-Moon-Syndrom *nt*.
Laurence-Moon-Bardet-Biedl [barˈde]: **L.-M.-B.-B. syndrome** Laurence-Moon-Bardet-Biedl-Syndrom *nt*, Laurence-Moon-Biedl-Syndrom *nt*, Laurence-Moon-Biedl-Bardet-Syndrom *nt*, dienzephalo-retinale Degeneration *f*.
Laurence-Moon-Biedl: **L.-M.-B. syndrome** → Laurence-Moon-Bardet-Biedl syndrome.
lau·ric acid ['lɔːrɪk, 'lɑ-] Laurinsäure *f*, n-Dodecansäure *f*.
lau·ro·yl ['lɔːrəwɪl, 'lɑ-] *n* Lauroyl-(Radikal *nt*).
Lauth [lɔːθ]: **L.'s canal** Schlemm'-Kanal *m*, Sinus venosus sclerae.
L.'s ligament Lig. transversum atlantis.
L.'s sinus → L.'s canal.
L.'s violet Thionin *nt*, Lauth'-Violett *nt*.
LAV *abbr.* (lymphadenopathy-associated virus) *old* → human immunodeficiency virus.
la·vage [ləˈvɑːʒ, ˈlævɪdʒ] I *n* (Aus-)Waschen *nt*, (Aus-)Spülen *nt*, Spülung *f*, Lavage *f*, Lavement *nt*. II *vt* (aus-)waschen, (aus-)spülen.
l. of the maxillary sinus Kieferhöhlenspülung, -lavage.
l. of the sinuses Nebenhöhlenspülung, -lavage.
lavage cannula Spülkanüle *f*.
law [lɔː] *n* 1. Gesetz *nt*, Recht *nt*, Gesetze *pl*; einzelnes Gesetz *nt*. **according to ∼** nach dem Gesetz. **by ∼** gesetzlich. **contrary to ∼** gesetz(es)widrig. **in ∼** vor dem Gesetz. 2. Gesetz *nt*, Gesetzmäßigkeit *f*, Prinzip *nt*, (Grund-, Lehr-)Satz *m*, Regel *f*. 3. Rechtswissenschaft *f*, Jura.
l. of conservation of energy Gesetz/Satz von der Erhaltung der Energie.
l. of conservation of matter Gesetz/Satz von der Erhaltung der Materie.
l. of contrary innervation Meltzer-Regel, -Gesetz.
l. of definite proportions Gesetz der konstanten Proportionen, Proust-Gesetz.
l. of excitation 1. Erregungsgesetz. 2. DuBois-Reymond-Gesetz.
l. of gravitation Newton'-Gravitationsgesetz.
l. of the heart Starling'-Kontraktionsgesetz.
l. of independent assortment *genet.* Rekombinations-, Unabhängigkeitsgesetz.
l. of inertia Trägheitsgesetz.
l. of mass action Massenwirkungsgesetz.
l. of multiple proportions Gesetz der multiplen Proportionen.
l. of nature Naturgesetz.
l. of reciprocal proportions Gesetz der multiplen Proportionen.
l. of refraction Brechungsgesetz.
l. of regression Galton-Regressionsgesetz.
l. of segregation *genet.* Spaltungsgesetz.
l. of sines Descartes'-Brechungsgesetz.
l. of specific irritability Müller-Gesetz (der spezifischen Reizbarkeit).
Lawford ['lɔːfɔːrd, -fərd]: **L.'s syndrome** Lawford-Syndrom *nt*.'l
law·ful ['lɔːfəl] *adj* gesetz-, rechtmäßig, legal; legitim; anerkannt, rechtsgültig.
lawn tennis arm [lɔːn] Tennisellenbogen *m*, Epicondylitis radialis humeri.
Lawrence-Seip ['lɔːrəns, 'lɑr-]: **L.-S. syndrome** Lawrence-Syndrom *nt*, lipatrophischer Diabetes *m*.
law·ren·ci·um [lɔːˈrensəm] *n abbr.* **Lw, Lr** Lawrencium *nt abbr.* Lw, Lr.
lax [læks] *adj* 1. (*Gelenk*, *Band*) locker, schlaff, lose, lax. 2. *physiol.* gut/normal arbeitend. 3. an Durchfall leidend.
lax·a·tion [lækˈseɪʃn] *n* Darmentleerung *f*, Stuhlgang *m*, Defäkation *f*.
lax·a·tive ['læksətɪv] I *n* Abführmittel *nt*, Laxans *nt*, Laxativ(um) *nt*. II *adj* abführend, laxativ, laxierend, Abführ-.
laxative abuse Abführmittelabusus *m*, -mißbrauch *m*, Laxanzienabusus *m*, -mißbrauch *m*.
lax·i·ty ['læksətɪ] *n* 1. (*Gelenk*, *Band*) Schlaffheit *f*, Laxheit *f*, Lockerheit *f*. 2. Unklarheit *f*, Verschwommenheit *f*.
lax·ness ['læksnɪs] *n* → laxity.
lax skin *derm.* Schlaff-, Fallhaut *f*, Dermatochalasis *f*, Dermatolysis *f*, Dermatomegalie *f*, Chalodermie *f*, Chalazodermie *f*, Cutis laxa-Syndrom *nt*, Zuviel-Haut-Syndrom *nt*.
lay·er ['leɪər] I *n* Schicht *f*, Lage *f*, Blatt *nt*; *anat.* Lamina *f*, Stratum *nt*. **in ∼s** schicht-, lagenweise. II *vt* schichtweise legen, schichten.
l. of fat Fettschicht.
l. of rods and cones Schicht der Stäbchen u. Zapfen, Stratum neuroepitheliale retinae.
l.s of rostral colliculus Strata (grisea et alba) colliculi superioris.
l.s of superior colliculus → l.s of rostral colliculus.
laz·a·ret [læzə'ret] *n* 1. Leprastation *f*, -hospital *nt*. 2. Krankenhaus *nt* für ansteckende Krankheiten. 3. Quarantäne-, Isolierstation *f*.
laz·a·ret·to [læzə'retəʊ] *n* → lazaret.
laz·a·rine leprosy ['læzəriːn, -raɪn] Lucio-Phänomen *nt*.
la·zy leukocyte syndrome ['leɪzɪ] Lazy-Leukocyte-Syndrom *nt*.
lb. *abbr.* [libra] → pound² 1.
LB agar *micro.* Luria-Bertani-Agar *m/nt*.
LBBB *abbr.* → bundle-branch block, left.
LCAT *abbr.* → lecithin-cholesterol acyltransferase.
LCAT deficiency, familial Norum-Krankheit *f*, familiärer primärer LCAT-Mangel *m*.
L cells 1. *histol.* L-Zellen *pl*. 2. *micro.* L-Zellen *pl*.
L-chain *biochem.* L-Kette *f*, leichte Kette *f*.
L-chain disease/myeloma Bence-Jones-Plasmozytom *nt*, -Krankheit *f*, L-Kettenkrankheit *f*, Leichte-Kettenkrankheit *f*.
L.C.L. bodies → Levinthal-Coles-Lillie bodies.
LCM *abbr.* → lymphocytic choriomeningitis.
LCM virus LCM-Virus *nt*.
L.D. *abbr.* → lethal dose.
L.D.$_{50}$ *abbr.* → lethal dose, median.
ld *abbr.* → dual logarithm.
LD agar *micro.* Natriumdesoxycholatagar *m/nt* nach Leifson, Leifson-Agar *m/nt*.
LD antigens Lymphozyten-definierte Antigene *pl*, LD-Antigene *pl*.
L.D. body → Leishman-Donovan body.
LDC agar *micro.* Desoxycholat-Zitrat-Agar *m/nt* nach Leifson.
LDH *abbr.* 1. → lactate dehydrogenase. 2. → low-dose heparin.
LDL *abbr.* → low-density lipoprotein.
LDL receptor LDL-Rezeptor *m*.
LDL-receptor disorder (primäre/essentielle) Hyperlipoproteinämie *f* Typ IIa, essentielle/familiäre Hypercholesterin-

ämie f, primäre Hyperbetalipoproteinämie f, familiäre idiopathische hypercholesterinämische Xanthomatose f, LDL--Rezeptordefekt m.
LE abbr. → lupus erythematosus.
leach·ing [liːtʃɪŋ] n chem. Auslaugen nt, Auslaugung f.
lead¹ [led] I n Blei nt; chem. Plumbum nt abbr. Pb. II vt verbleien, mit Blei überziehen; mit Blei beschweren od. füllen.
lead² [liːd] I n 1. physiol. (EKG) Ableitung f. 2. Führung f, Leitung f, Spitze f. 3. Hinweis m, Indiz nt, Anhaltspunkt m. 4. electr. Leitung(skabel nt) f; Zuleitung f. II adj Führungs-, Leit-, Haupt-.
lead acetate Bleiazetat nt.
lead anemia Bleianämie f.
lead-chamber process chem. Bleikammerverfahren nt.
lead chloride Bleichlorid nt.
lead chromate Bleichromat nt, Chromgelb nt.
lead colic Bleikolik f, Colica saturnina.
lead content chem. Bleigehalt m.
lead·en [ˈledn] adj 1. bleiern, bleiartig, -haltig, Blei-. 2. fig. bleiern, bleischwer; bleifarben.
lead encephalitis → lead encephalopathy.
lead encephalopathy Bleienzephalopathie f, Encephalopathia saturnina.
lead hand ortho. Bleihand f.
lead·ing [ˈliːdɪŋ] I n Führung f, Leitung f. II adj leitend, führend, erste(r, s), Haupt-, Leit-, Führungs-.
leading strand biochem. Hauptstrang m, leading strand.
leading substrate biochem. erstes/führendes Substrat n.
lead line patho. Bleisaum m.
lead neuritis Bleineuropathie f, Neuritis saturnina.
lead nephropathy → lead neuritis.
lead palsy Bleilähmung f.
lead paralysis Bleilähmung f.
lead pipe colon radiol. (Colitis ulcerosa) glattes Kolon nt, Fahrradschlauch m.
lead-pipe rigidity plastischer Rigor m.
lead poisoning Bleivergiftung f, Saturnismus m, Saturnialismus m.
lead soap chem. Bleiseife f.
lead stomatitis Stomatitis saturnina.
lead tetroxide Bleitetroxid nt, Bleimennige f, rotes Bleioxid nt.
lead·y [ˈledɪ] adj → leaden 1.
leaf [liːf] I n, pl **leaves** [liːvz] 1. bot. Blatt nt. 2. (Buch) Blatt nt, Seite f. 3. Blatt nt, (dünne) Folie f, Lamelle f. II vt durchblättern.
leaf through vi durchblättern.
leaf·let [ˈliːflɪt] n 1. bot. Blättchen nt. 2. Hand-, Reklamezettel m, Flugblatt nt; Merkblatt nt; Prospekt m.
leak [liːk] I n 1. Leck nt, undichte Stelle f; Loch nt. 2. Auslaufen nt; Durchsickern nt. II vi durchlassen. III vi lecken, leck sein.
leak in vi eindringen, -strömen.
leak out vi auslaufen, -strömen, -treten, entweichen.
leak·ing capillary syndrome [ˈliːkɪŋ] Syndrom nt der blutenden Kapillaren.
leak point (Niere) Glukoseschwelle f.
leap·ing mydriasis [ˈliːpɪŋ] ophthal. alternierende/springende Mydriasis f, Mydriasis alternans.
Lear [lɪər]: **L. complex** psychia. Lear-Komplex m.
learn [lɜrn] (**learned; learnt**) I vt 1. (er-)lernen. 2. erfahren (from). **to ~ the truth** die Wahrheit erfahren. II vi 1. lernen. 2. erfahren, hören (about, of von).
learned [lɜrnd] adj 1. erlernt. 2. gelehrt; wissenschaftlich; akademisch. 3. erfahren (in in).
learned reflex erlernter Reflex m.
learn·ing [ˈlɜrnɪŋ] n (Er-)Lernen nt.
learning disability Lernbehinderung f.
learning-disabled adj lernbehindert.
learning process Lernprozess m.
learning theory Lerntheorie f.
leath·er bottle stomach [ˈleðər] entzündlicher Schrumpfmagen m, Brinton-Krankheit f, Magenszirrhus m, Linitis plastica.
Leber [ˈleɪbər; ˈleːbər]: **L.'s congenital amaurosis** → L.'s disease 2.
L.'s corpuscles Hassall'-Körperchen pl.
L.'s disease 1. Leber'-Optikusatrophie f. 2. kongenitale Amaurose (Leber) f.
L.'s optic atrophy → L.'s disease 1.
L.'s plexus Leber-Plexus m.
LE bodies L.e.-Körper pl, L.E.-Körper pl, Lupus erythematodes-Körper pl.
Lecat [liˈka]: **L.'s gulf** Lecat-Bucht f.
LE cell phenomenon L.e.-Zellphänomen nt, L.E.-Zellphänomen nt.
LE cells L.e.-Zellen pl, L.E.-Zellen pl, Lupus erythematodes-Zellen pl.
lech·o·py·ra [lekəˈpaɪrə] n Wochenbett-, Kindbettfieber nt, Puerperalfieber nt, -sepsis f, Febris puerperalis.
lec·i·thal [ˈlesɪθəl] adj lezithal.
lec·ith·al·bu·min [lesɪθˈælbjəmɪn] n Lezith-, Lecithalbumin n.
lec·i·thin [ˈlesɪθɪn] n Lezithin nt, Lecithin nt, Phosphatidylcholin nt abbr. PC.
lecithin acyltransferase → lecithin--cholesterol acyltransferase.
lec·i·thi·nase [ˈlesɪθɪneɪz] n Lezithinase f, Lecithinase f.
lecithinase A Phospholipase A_1 f, Phospholipase A_2 f, Lecithinase A f.
lecithinase B Lysophospholipase f, Lecithinase B f, Phospholipase B f.
lecithinase C Phospholipase C f, Lecithinase C f, Lysophosphodiesterase I f.
lecithinase D Phospholipase D f, Lecithinase D f.
lecithin-cholesterol acyltransferase abbr. LCAT Lecithin-Cholesterin-Acyltransferase f abbr. LCAT.
lec·i·thi·ne·mia [lesəθɪˈniːmɪə] n (erhöhter) Lezithingehalt m des Blutes, Lezithinämie f, Lecithinämie f.
lecithin-sphingomyelin ratio Lezithin--Sphingomyelin-Quotient m, L/S-Quotient m.
lec·i·tho·pro·tein [lesɪθoʊˈproʊtiːn, -tiːɪn] n Lecithoprotein nt.
lec·tin [ˈlektɪn] n Lektin nt, Lectin nt.
lec·ture [ˈlektʃər] I n Vortrag f, Vorlesung m (on über; to vor). **to give/read a ~** einen Vortrag od. eine Vorlesung halten. II vt einen Vortrag od. eine Vorlesung halten vor. III vi einen Vortrag od. eine Vorlesung halten, lesen (on über; to vor).
lec·tur·er [ˈlektʃərər] n Vortragende(r m) f, Dozent(in f) m.
Ledderhose [ˈlɛdərhoːzə]: **L.'s disease** Ledderhose-Syndrom nt, Dupuytren'--Kontraktur f der Plantarfaszie, plantare Fibromatose f, Morbus Ledderhose m, Plantaraponeurosenkontraktur f, Fibromatosis plantae.
Lederer [ˈlɛdərər]: **L.'s anemia/disease** hema. Lederer-Anämie f.
Lee [liː]: **L.'s ganglion** Frankenhäuser'--Ganglion nt.
L.'s speech delay test HNO Sprachverzögerungstest m nach Lee.
leech [liːtʃ] n Blutegel m.
leech·es [ˈliːtʃəs] pl Blutegel pl, Hirudinea pl.
Leede-Rumpel [ˈliːdɪ ˈrʌmpl]: **L.-R. phenomenon** Rumpel-Leede-Phänomen nt.
Leeuwenhoek [ˈleɪvənhuːk]: **L.'s canal** Havers'-Kanal m, Canalis nutriens.
Lee-White [liː (h)waɪt]: **L.-W. method** Lee--White-Probe f, -Test m.
LE factors antinukleäre Antikörper pl abbr. ANA.
LeFort [ləˈfɔːr]: **L.'s amputation** ortho. LeFort-Amputation f, Fußamputation f nach LeFort.
L. I fracture Guérin-Fraktur f, LeFort I-Fraktur f.
L. II fracture LeFort II-Fraktur f.
L. III fracture LeFort III-Fraktur f.
L.'s operation → L.'s amputation.
L. sound LeFort-Sonde f.
Le Fort-Neugebauer [ˈnɔɪɡəbaʊər]: **L.-N. operation** Le Fort-Neugebauer-Operation f.
left [left] I n die Linke, Linke(r, s), linke Seite f. **on/at/to the ~** links (of von); auf der linken Seite (of von). II adj linke(r, s), Links-. III adv links (of von); auf der linken Seite.
left anterior hemiblock card. linksanteriorer Hemiblock m.
left atrium linker (Herz-)Vorhof m, Atrium cordis sinistrum.
left auricle (of heart) linkes Herzohr nt, Auricula sinistra.
left auricula of heart → left auricle (of heart).
left branch: l. of av-bundle linker Tawara--Schenkel m, linker Schenkel m des His'-Bündels, Crus sinistrum fasciculi atrioventricularis.
l. of portal vein Ramus sinister v. portae hepatis.
l. of proper hepatic artery A. hepatica propria-Ast m zum linken Leberlappen, Ramus sinister a. hepaticae propriae.
left crus of diaphragm linker Zwerchfellschenkel m, Crus sinistrum diaphragmatis.
left duct of caudate lobe Ductus lobi caudati sinister.
left flexure of colon linke Kolonflexur f, Flexura lienalis coli, Flexura coli sinistra.
left-handed adj 1. linkshändig. 2. phys. linksdrehend, lävorotatorisch.
left-handedness n Linkshändigkeit f.
left-handed person Linkshänder(in f) m.
left-hander n Linkshänder(in f) m.
left-hand side linke Seite f.
left heart Linksherz nt.
left heart bypass HTG Linksbypass m.
left heart dilatation card. Linksherzdilatation f, Dilatation f des linken Ventrikels.
left heart hypertrophy card. Linksherzhypertrophie f, linksventrikuläre Hypertrophie f.
left hemicolectomy chir. linksseitige Hemikolektomie f.
left leg of av-bundle → left branch of av-bundle.
left lobe of liver linker Leberlappen m, Lobus hepatis sinister.
left lung linke Lunge f, linker Lungenflügel m, Pulmo sinister.
left margin of uterus Margo uteri sinister.
left mesocolon Mesokolon nt des Colon descendens, Mesocolon descendens.
left posterior hemiblock card. linksposteriorer Hemiblock m.
left-sided appendicitis 1. linksseitige Appendizitis f bei Situs inversus. 2. Linksappendizitis f, Divertikulitis f.
left-to-right shunt Links-Rechts-Shunt m.
left ventricle of heart linke Herzkammer f, linker Ventrikel m, Ventriculus sinister cordis.
left-ventricular adj (Herz) linksventrikulär.

left-ventricular dilatation → left heart dilatation.
left-ventricular failure Links(herz)insuffizienz f, Linksversagen nt.
left-ventricular hypertrophy → left heart hypertrophy.
left·ward ['leftwərd] adj nach links (gerichtet), Links-.
leftward shift physiol., hema. Linksverschiebung f.
leg [leg] n **1.** (Unter-)Schenkel m; anat. Crus nt. **2.** Bein nt. **3.** (Hosen-)Bein nt; (Tisch-, Stuhl-)Bein nt; (Zirkel) Schenkel m; mathe. Kathete f.
Legal [le'ga:l]: **L.'s disease** Cephal(al)gia pharyngotympanica.
L.'s test Legal'-Probe f.
le·gal medicine ['li:gəl] forensische/gerichtliche Medizin f, Gerichtsmedizin f, Rechtsmedizin f.
legal procedure gerichtliches Verfahren nt.
legal psychiatry forensische/gerichtliche Psychiatrie f.
leg edema Beinödem nt.
Legg [leg]: **L.'s disease** → Legg-Calvé-Perthes disease.
Legg-Calvé [kal've]: **L.-C. disease** → Legg-Calvé-Perthes disease.
Legg-Calvé-Perthes ['pertez]: **L.-C.-P. disease** Perthes-Krankheit f, Morbus Perthes m, Legg-Calvé-Perthes-Krankheit f, Legg-Calvé-Perthes-Krankheit f, Legg-Calvé-Perthes-Waldenström--Krankheit f, Osteochondropathia deformans coxae juvenilis, Coxa plana (idiopathica).
L.-C.-P. syndrome → L.-C.-P. disease.
Legg-Calvé-Waldenström ['valdənstre:m]: **L.-C.-W. disease** → Legg-Calve-Perthes disease.
Le·gion·el·la [li:dʒə'nelə] n micro. Legionella f.
L. micdadei Legionella micdadei, Pittsburgh pneumonia agent abbr. PPA.
L. pittsburgensis → L. micdadei.
le·gion·el·la [li:dʒə'nelə] n, pl -lae [-li:] micro. Legionelle f, Legionella f.
Le·gion·el·la·ce·ae [li:dʒənə'leɪsi,i:] pl micro. Legionellaceae f.
le·gion·el·lo·sis [,-'ləʊsɪs] n **1.** Legionelleninfektion f, Legionellose f. **2.** → legionnaire's disease.
le·gion·naire's bacillus [ledʒə'neər] Legionella pneumophila.
legionnaire's disease Legionärs-, Veteranenkrankheit f.
le·git·i·mate recombination [lɪ'dʒɪtəmɪt] genet. legitime/homologe Rekombination f.
leg·less ['leglɪs] adj beinlos, ohne Beine.
leg phenomenon Pool-Beinphänomen nt, Pool-Schlesinger-Phänomen nt.
leg·ume ['legju:m, lɪ'gju:m] n bot. **1.** Hülse f, Legumen nt. **2.** Hülsenfrucht f, Leguminose f.
le·gu·me·lin [lɪ'gju:məlɪn] n Legumelin nt.
le·gu·min [lɪ'gju:mən, 'legjəmɪn] n Legumin nt.
le·gu·mi·nous [lɪ'gju:mənəs] adj erbsen-, bohnen-, hülsenartig, hülsentragend, Hülsen-.
leguminous plants Hülsenfrüchte pl, Leguminosen pl.
Leichtenstern ['laɪktənstərn; 'laɪçtənʃtern]: **L.'s encephalitis** hämorrhagische Enzephalitis f, Encephalitis haemorrhagica.
L.'s phenomenon Leichtenstern-Phänomen nt.
L.'s sign → L.'s phenomenon.
L.'s type → L.'s encephalitis.

Leifson ['li:fsən]: **L. deoxycholate agar** micro. Natriumdesoxycholatagar m/nt nach Leifson, Leifson-Agar m/nt.
L. deoxycholate citrate agar micro. Desoxycholat-Zitrat-Agar m/nt nach Leifson.
L.'s selenite broth Selenitbouillon f nach Leifson.
Leigh [li:]: **L.'s disease/syndrome** Leigh--Syndrom nt, -Enzephalomyelopathie f, nekrotisierende Enzephalomyelopathie f.
Leiner ['laɪnər]: **L.'s disease** Leiner'-Dermatitis f, -Erythrodermie f, Erythrodermia desquamativa Leiner.
leio- pref. Glatt-, Leio-.
lei·o·der·mia [,laɪə'dɜrmɪə] n Glanzhaut f, Lioderma nt, Leioderma nt, Leiodermie f.
lei·o·my·o·blas·to·ma [,-,maɪəblæ'stəʊmə] n epitheliales Leiomyom nt, Leiomyoblastom nt.
lei·o·my·o·fi·bro·ma [,-,maɪfaɪ'brəʊmə] n Leiomyofibrom nt, Fibroleiomyom nt.
lei·o·my·o·ma [,-maɪ'əʊmə] n, pl -mas, -mata [-mətə] Leiomyom(a) nt.
lei·o·my·o·ma·to·sis [,-,maɪəmə'təʊsɪs] n Leiomyomatose f, Leiomyomatosis f.
lei·o·my·om·a·tous [,-maɪ'mætəs] adj Leiomyom betr., leiomyomatös.
lei·o·my·o·sar·co·ma [,-,maɪəsɑr'kəʊmə] n Leiomyosarkom nt, Leiomyosarcoma f.
leip(o)- pref. lipo-.
Leishman ['li:ʃmæn]: **L.'s chrome cells** patho. Leishman-Zellen pl.
L.'s stain Leishman-Färbung f.
Leishman-Donovan ['dɒnəvən]: **L.-D. body** amastigote Form f, Leishman--Donovan-Körperchen nt, Leishmania--Form f.
Leish·ma·nia [li:ʃ'mænɪə, -'meɪn-] n micro. Leishmania f.
leish·ma·nia [li:ʃ'mænɪə, -'meɪn-] n micro. Leishmanie f, Leishmania f.
leish·ma·ni·al [li:ʃ'mænɪəl, -'meɪn-] adj Leishmanien betr., durch sie verursacht, Leishmanien-.
leish·ma·ni·a·sis [,li:ʃmə'naɪəsɪs] n Leishmanieninfektion f, Leishmaniase f, Leishmaniasis f, Leishmaniose f, Leishmaniosis f.
leish·man·i·cal [li:ʃ'mænɪ'saɪdl] adj leishmanien(ab)tötend, leishmanizid.
leish·man·i·cide [li:ʃ'mænɪsaɪd] n Leishmanizid nt.
leish·man·id ['li:ʃmænɪd] n Hautleishman(o)id nt, Leishmanid nt.
leish·man·in ['li:ʃmənɪn, li:ʃ'mænɪn] n Leishmanin nt.
leishmanin test Leishmanin-Test m, Montenegro-Test m.
leish·man·i·o·sis [li:ʃ,mænɪ'əʊsɪs] n → leishmaniasis.
leish·ma·noid ['li:ʃmənɔɪd] n Leishmanoid nt.
le·ma ['li:mə] n Augenlidtalg m, Sebum palpebrale.
Lembert [lɑ̃'bɛːr]: **L.'s suture** chir. Lembert-Naht f.
lem·o·blast ['lemablæst] n → lemnoblast.
lem·o·cyte ['leməsaɪt] n → lemnocyte.
lem·nis·cal fibers [lem'nɪskl] Lemniskusfasern pl.
lemniscal system Hinterstrang-, Lemniskussystem nt.
lem·nis·cus [lem'nɪskəs] n, pl -nis·ci [-'nɪsaɪ, -'nɪski:] anat. Schleife f, Lemniskus m, Lemniscus m.
lem·no·blast ['lemnəblæst] n Lemnoblast m.

lem·no·cyte ['-saɪt] n Lemnozyt m, Mantelzelle f.
lem·on ['lemən] I n **1.** Zitrone f. **2.** Limone f. **3.** Zitronengelb nt. II adj zitronengelb; Zitronen-.
lemon oil Zitronenöl nt.
le·mo·pa·ral·y·sis [,li:məpə'ræləsɪs] n Speiseröhrenlähmung f, Ösophagusparalyse f.
le·mo·ste·no·sis [,-stɪ'nəʊsɪs] n Speiseröhrenverengung f, -stenose f, Ösophagusstenose f.
Lenègre [lə'nɛ:grə]: **L.'s disease** Lenègre-Krankheit f.
length [leŋkθ, leŋθ, leŋθ] n **1.** Länge f. **2.** (zeitliche) Länge f, Dauer f. **of some ~** ziemlich lange, von einiger Dauer.
length-control system Längenkontrollsystem nt.
length·en ['leŋkθən, 'leŋ-, 'len-] I vt **1.** verlängern, länger machen. **2.** ausdehnen. **3.** strecken, verdünnen. II vi länger werden.
length-tension diagram Längenspannungsdiagramm nt.
length unit Längeneinheit f.
length·ways ['leŋkθweɪz, 'leŋθ-, 'lenθ-] adj Längs-. II adv längs, der Länge nach, in der Länge.
lengthways cut Längsschnitt m.
length·wise ['-waɪz] adj, adv → lengthways.
len·i·tive ['lenɪtɪv] I n Linderungsmittel nt, Lenientium nt. II adj lindernd, mildernd.
Lennert ['lenərt]: **L.'s lesion** → L.'s lymphoma.
L.'s lymphoma lymphoepithelioides Lymphom nt, Lennert'-Lymphom nt.
Lennox ['lenəks]: **L. syndrome** Lennox--Syndrom nt.
lens [lenz] n **1.** photo., phys. Linse f, Objektiv nt. **2.** anat. (Augen-)Linse f, Lens f (cristallina). **3.** (Brillen-)Glas nt. **4.** Vergrößerungsglas nt, Lupe f.
lens capsule Linsenkapsel f, Capsula lentis.
lens diopter Linsendioptrie f.
lens fibers Linsenfasern pl, Fibrae lentis.
lens-induced uveitis ophthal. phakogene Uveitis f.
lens pit embryo. Linsengrübchen nt.
lens placode embryo. Linsenplatte f, -plakode f.
lens sac → lens vesicle.
lens system Linsensystem nt.
lens vesicle embryo. Linsenbläschen nt.
lens zonule Zinn'-(Strahlen-)Zone f, Zonula ciliaris.
len·ti·co·nus [,lentɪ'kəʊnəs] n ophthal. Lentikonus m.
len·tic·u·la [len'tɪkjələ] n, pl -las, -lae [-li:] → lenticular nucleus.
len·tic·u·lar [len'tɪkjələr] adj **1.** linsenförmig, lentikular, lentikulär; phys. bikonvex. **2.** anat. (Auge) Linse betr., lental, Linsen-. **3.** Linsenkern/Nc. lenticularis betr.
lenticular apophysis → lenticular process of incus.
lenticular astigmatism ophthal. Linsenastigmatismus m.
lenticular bone old → pisiform I.
lenticular capsule Linsenkapsel f, Capsula lentis.
lenticular carcinoma Ca. lenticulare.
lenticular cataract Linsenstar m.
lenticular fasciculus Linsenkernbündel nt, Fasciculus lenticularis.
lenticular fossa (of vitreous body) Glaskörpermulde f, Fossa hyaloidea.
lenticular loop Linsenkernschlinge f, Ansa lenticularis.
lenticular loop and bundle Linsenkern-

schleife *f* u. -bündel *nt*, Ansa et fasciculus lenticulares.
lenticular nucleus Linsenkern *m*, Nc. lenticularis/lentiformis.
lenticular process of incus Proc. lenticularis (incudis).
lenticular progressive degeneration hepatolentikuläre/hepatozerebrale Degeneration *f*, Wilson-Krankheit *f*, -Syndrom *nt*, Morbus Wilson *m*.
lenticular syphilid lentikuläres Syphilid *nt*.
lenticular vesicle → lens vesicle.
lenticulo-optic *adj* Linsenkern u. Sehbahn betr.
len·tic·u·lo·stri·ate [lenˌtɪkjələʊˈstraɪɪt, -eɪt] *adj* Linsenkern u. Corpus striatum betr.
len·tic·u·lo·tha·lam·ic part of internal capsule [ˌ-θəˈlæmɪk] Pars thalamolenticularis capsulae internae.
len·tic·u·lus [lenˈtɪkjələs] *n, pl* **-li** [-laɪ] **1.** *derm.* Lenticula *f*, Lenticulus *m*. **2.** *ophthal.* Linsenprothese *f*, intraokulare (Kunststoff-)Linse *f abbr.* IOL.
len·ti·form [ˈlentɪfɔːrm] *adj* linsenförmig; *anat.* lentiform.
lentiform bone *old* → pisiform I.
lentiform nucleus → lenticular nucleus.
lentiform papillae linsenförmige Papillen *pl*, kurze pilzförmige Papillen *pl*, Papillae lentiformis.
len·tig·i·no·sis [lenˌtɪdʒəˈnəʊsɪs] *n derm.* Lentiginose *f*, Lentiginosis *f*.
len·tig·i·nous [lenˈtɪdʒɪnəs] *adj* Lentigo betr., nach Art einer Lentigo, lentiginös.
len·ti·glo·bus [lentɪˈɡləʊbəs] *n ophthal.* Lentiglobus *m*.
len·ti·go [lenˈtaɪɡəʊ, -ˈtɪ-] *n, pl* **len·tig·i·nes** [lenˈtɪdʒəniːz] *derm.* Linsenmal *nt*, Linsen-, Leberfleck *m*, Lentigo *f* (benigna/juvenilis/simplex).
lentigo maligna Dubreuilh-Krankheit *f*, -Erkrankung *f*, Dubreuilh-Hutchinson--Krankheit *f*, -Erkrankung *f*, prämaligne Melanose *f*, melanotische Präkanzerose *f*, Lentigo maligna, Melanosis circumscripta praeblastomatosa/praecancerosa (Dubreuilh).
lentigo-maligna melanoma *abbr.* **LMM** Lentigo-maligna-Melanom *nt abbr.* LMM.
Len·ti·vir·i·nae [lentɪˈvɪərəniː] *pl micro.* Lentiviren *pl*, Lentivirinae *pl*.
len·ti·vi·rus [lentɪˈvaɪrəs] *n micro.* Lentivirus *nt*.
len·to·chol reaction [ˈlentəkəl] Lentochol--Reaktion *f*, Sachs-Georgi-Reaktion *f*.
lentochol test Lichtheim-Prüfung *f*.
Lenz [lents]: **L.'s syndrome** Lenz-Syndrom *nt*.
Leon [ˈlɪən]: **L. virus** *micro.* Leon-Stamm *m*, -Virus *nt*, Poliovirus Typ III *nt*.
Leonard [ˈlenərd; ˈlɒnɑːrd]: **L. tube** Kathodenstrahlröhre *f*.
le·on·ti·a·sis [lɪənˈtaɪəsɪs] *n patho.* Leontiasis *f*, Facies leontina, Löwengesicht *nt*.
le·on·tine facies [ˈlɪəntaɪn] → leontiasis.
leop·ard's bane [ˈlepərd] *pharm.* Bergwohlverleih *m*, Arnika *f*, Arnica montana.
leopard fundus *ophthal.* Fundus tabulatus.
leopard retina *ophthal.* Fundus tabulatus.
leopard syndrome Lentiginosis-Syndrom *nt*, LEOPARD-Syndrom *nt*.
Leopold [ˈlɪəpəʊlt; ˈleəpɒlt]: **L.'s law** *gyn.* Leopold'-Regel *f*.
L.'s maneuvers *gyn.* Leopold'-Handgriffe *pl*.
LE panniculitis Lupus erythematodes profundus.

lep·er [ˈlepər] *n* Leprakranke(r *m*) *f*, Aussätzige(r *m*) *f*.
leper hospital Leprastation *f*, -krankenhaus *nt*, Leprosorium *nt*.
LE phenomenon LE-Phänomen *nt*, Lupus-erythematodes-Phänomen *nt*.
L.E. phenomenon → LE phenomenon.
lepid- *pref.* → lepido-.
le·pid·ic [ləˈpɪdɪk] *adj* Schuppen *od.* Schuppung betr., schuppig, Schuppen-, Lepido-.
lepido- *pref.* Schuppen-, Lepid(o)-.
lep·i·do·sis [lepəˈdəʊsɪs] *n, pl* **-ses** [-siːz] *derm.* Schuppenbildung *f*, Lepidosis *f*.
lep·o·thrix [ˈlepəθrɪks] *n, pl* **-thrixes** [-θrɪksɪz] *derm.* Trichobacteriosis/Trichomycosis axillaris, Trichonocardiosis *f*.
lep·ra [ˈleprə] *n* → leprosy.
lepra bacillus *micro.* Hansen-Bazillus *m*, Mycobacterium leprae.
lepra cell (Virchow'-)Leprazelle *f*.
lepra reaction Leprareaktion *f*.
lep·re·chaun·ism [ˈleprəkɒnɪzəm] *n* Leprechaunismus(-Syndrom *nt*) *m*.
lep·rid [ˈleprɪd] *n* Leprid *nt*.
lep·ride [ˈlepraɪd, -rɪd] *n* Leprid *nt*.
lep·ro·ma [lepˈrəʊmə] *n, pl* **-mas**, **-mata** [-mətə] Lepraknoten *m*, Leprom *nt*.
lep·rom·a·tous [lepˈrɒmətəs] *adj* Leprom betr., lepromatös.
lepromatous leprosy lepromatöse Lepra *f abbr.* LL, Lepra lepromatosa.
lep·ro·min [ˈleprəmɪn] *n* Lepromin *nt*, Mitsuda-Antigen *nt*.
lepromin reaction Leprominreaktion *f*, Mitsuda-Reaktion *f*.
lepromin test Lepromintest *m*.
lep·ro·sar·i·um [leprəˈseərɪəm] *n, pl* **-riums**, **-ria** [-rɪə] Leprastation *f*, -krankenhaus *nt*, -kolonie *f*, Leprosorium *nt*.
lep·ro·sar·y [ˈleprəsərɪ] *n* → leprosarium.
lep·rose [ˈleprəʊs] *adj* → leprous.
lep·ro·ser·y [ˈleprəsərɪ] *n* → leprosarium.
lep·ro·stat·ic [leprəˈstætɪk] **I** *n* Leprostatikum *nt*. **II** *adj* leprostatisch.
lep·ro·sy [ˈleprəsɪ] *n* Lepra *f*, Aussatz *m*, Hansen-Krankheit *f*, Morbus Hansen *m*, Hansenosis *f*.
leprosy bacillus → lepra bacillus.
lep·rot·ic [lepˈrɒtɪk] *adj* → leprous.
lep·rous [ˈleprəs] *adj* Lepra betr., von ihr betroffen, leprös, Lepra-.
lept(o)- *pref.* Lept(o)-.
lep·to·ce·phal·ic [leptəsɪˈfælɪk] *adj* schmalköpfig, schäd(e)lig, leptozephal, -kephal.
lep·to·ceph·a·lous [-ˈsefələs] *adj* → leptocephalic.
lep·to·ceph·a·lus [ˌ-ˈsefələs] *n* Leptozephalus *m*, -kephalus *m*.
lep·to·ceph·a·ly [ˌ-ˈsefəlɪ] *n* Schmalköpfigkeit *f*, -schäd(e)ligkeit *f*, Leptozephalie *f*, -kephalie *f*.
lep·to·cyte [ˈ-saɪt] *n hema.* Leptozyt *m*, Planozyt *m*.
lep·to·cy·to·sis [ˌ-saɪˈtəʊsɪs] *n hema.* Leptozytose *f*.
lep·to·dac·ty·lous [ˌ-ˈdæktɪləs] *adj* schmalfingrig, leptodaktyl.
lep·to·dac·ty·ly [ˌ-ˈdæktəlɪ] *n* Schmalfingrigkeit *f*, Leptodaktylie *f*.
lep·to·me·nin·ge·al [ˌ-mɪˈnɪndʒɪəl] *adj* Leptomeninx betr., leptomeningeal.
leptomeningeal cyst Arachnoidalzyste *f*.
lep·to·me·nin·gi·o·ma [ˌ-mɪˌnɪndʒɪˈəʊmə] *n* Meningiom *nt* der weichen Hirnhäute, Leptomeningiom(a) *nt*.
lep·to·men·in·gi·tis [ˌ-menɪnˈdʒaɪtɪs] *n* Entzündung *f* der weichen Hirnhäute, Leptomeningitis *f*.
lep·to·men·in·gop·a·thy [ˌ-menɪnˈɡɒpəθɪ]

n Erkrankung *f* der weichen Hirnhäute, Leptomeningopathie *f*.
lep·to·me·ninx [ˌ-ˈmiːnɪŋks] *n, pl* **-me·nin·ges** [-mɪˈnɪndʒiːz] weiche Hirn- u. Rückenmarkshaut *f*, Leptomeninx *f*.
lep·tom·o·nad [lepˈtɒmənæd, ˌleptəˈməʊnæd] **I** *n* → leptomonas. **II** *adj micro.* Leptomonas betr., Leptomonaden-, Leptomonas-.
Lep·tom·o·nas [lepˈtæmənəs, ˌleptəˈməʊnæs] *n micro.* Leptomonas *f*.
lep·tom·o·nas [lepˈtæmənəs, ˌleptəˈməʊnæs] *n micro.* **1.** Leptomonade *f*, Leptomonas *f*. **2.** Leptomonas-Form *f*.
lep·to·ne·ma [ˌleptəˈniːmə] *n histol.* Leptonem(a) *nt*.
lep·to·pro·so·pia [ˌleptəprəˈsəʊpɪə] *n* Schmalgesichtigkeit *f*, Leptoprosopie *f*.
lep·to·pro·sop·ic [ˌ-prəˈsəʊpɪk, -ˈsɒp-] *adj* schmalgesichtig, leptoprosop.
lep·tor·rhine [ˈ-raɪn] *adj* schmalnasig, leptorrhin.
lep·to·scope [ˈ-skəʊp] *n* Leptoskop *nt*.
lep·to·so·mat·ic [ˌ-səʊˈmætɪk] *adj* schmalwüchsig, leptosom.
lep·to·some [ˈ-səʊm] *n* Leptosome *f*/*m*, Leptosomatiker(in *f*) *m*; Astheniker(in *f*) *m*.
lep·to·so·mic [ˌ-ˈsəʊmɪk] *adj* → leptosomatic.
Lep·to·spi·ra [ˌ-ˈspaɪrə] *n micro.* Leptospira *f*.
L. biflexa apathogene Leptospiren *pl*, Wasserleptospiren *pl*, Leptospira biflexa.
L. icterohaemorrhagiae Weil'-Leptospire *f*, -Spirochaete *f*, Leptospira (interrogans serovar) icterohaemorrhagiae.
lep·to·spi·ra [ˌ-ˈspaɪrə] *n, pl* **-rae** [-riː] *micro.* Leptospire *f*, Leptospira *f*.
Lep·to·spi·ra·ce·ae [ˌ-spaɪˈreɪsɪˌiː] *n micro.* Leptospiraceae *pl*.
lep·to·spi·ral [ˌ-ˈspaɪrəl] *adj* Leptospire(n) betr., durch sie verursacht, Leptospiren-.
leptospiral disease → leptospirosis.
leptospiral jaundice Weil'-Krankheit *f*, Leptospirosis icterohaemorrhagica.
lep·to·spire [ˈ-spaɪər] *n* → leptospira.
lep·to·spi·ro·sis [ˌ-spaɪˈrəʊsɪs] *n* Leptospirenerkrankung *f*, Leptospirose *f*, Leptospirosis *f*.
lep·to·spi·ru·ria [ˌ-spaɪˈr(j)ʊərɪə] *n patho.* Leptospirenausscheidung *f* im Harn, Leptospirurie *f*.
lep·to·tene [ˈ-tiːn] *n* Leptotän *nt*.
lep·to·thri·co·sis [ˌ-θraɪˈkəʊsɪs] *n* → leptotrichosis.
Lep·to·thrix [ˈ-θrɪks] *n micro.* Leptothrix *f*.
lep·to·thrix [ˈ-θrɪks] *n micro.* Leptothrix *f*.
Lep·to·trich·ia [ˌ-ˈtrɪkɪə] *n micro.* Leptotrichia *f*.
lep·to·tri·cho·sis [ˌ-trɪˈkəʊsɪs] *n* Leptothrix-Infektion *f*, Leptotrichose *f*, Leptotrichosis *f*.
Lep·to·trom·bid·i·um [ˌ-trɒmˈbɪdɪəm] *n micro.* Leptotrombidium *f*.
Léri [ˈlerɪ; leˈriː]: **L.'s pleonosteosis** Léri--Layani-Weill-Syndrom *nt*.
L.'s sign Léri-Zeichen *nt*.
Leriche [ləˈriːʃ]: **L.: 's disease** Sudeck'-Dystrophie *f*, Sudeck-Syndrom *nt*, Morbus Sudeck *m*.
L.'s operation Leriche-Operation *f*, periarterielle Sympatektomie *f*.
L.'s syndrome Leriche-Syndrom *nt*, Aortenbifurkationssyndrom *nt*.
Léri-Weill [weɪl]: **L.-W. disease/syndrome** Léri-Layani-Weill-Syndrom *nt*.
Lermoyez [lɛrmwaˈjeː]: **L.'s syndrome** Lermoyez-Anfall *m*.
LES *abbr.* = esophageal sphincter, lower.
les·bi·an [ˈlezbɪən] **I** *n* Lesbierin *f*. **II** *adj* lesbisch.

les·bi·an·ism [ˈlezbɪənɪzəm] *n* weibliche Homosexualität *f*, Lesbianismus *m*, Sapphismus *m*.
Lesch-Nyhan [leʃ ˈnaɪən]: **L.-N. syndrome** Lesch-Nyhan-Syndrom *nt*, Automutilationssyndrom *nt*.
Lesgaft [ˈlesgæft]: **L.'s space** Grynfeltt-Dreieck *nt*, Trigonum lumbale superior.
L.'s triangle → L.'s space.
triangle of Grynfeltt and L. → L.'s space.
le·sion [ˈliːʒn] *n* **1.** Verletzung *f*, Wunde *f*, Schädigung *f*, Läsion *f*, Läsio *f*. **2.** Funktionsstörung *f*, -ausfall *m*, Läsion *f*, Läsio *f*.
Lesser [ˈlesər]: **L.'s triangle** Lesser-Dreieck *nt*.
less·er [ˈlesər] *adj* **1.** kleiner, geringer. **2.** weniger bedeutend.
lesser circle of iris Pupillarabschnitt *m* der Iris, A(n)nulus iridis minor.
lesser circulation kleiner Kreislauf *m*, Lungenkreislauf *m*.
lesser cul-de-sac (*Magen*) Antrum *nt*, Antrum pyloricum.
lesser curvature of stomach kleine Magenkurvatur *f*, Curvatura gastrica/ventricularis minor.
lesser ganglion of Meckel Faesebeck'-Ganglion *nt*, Blandin'-Ganglion *nt*, Ggl. submandibulare.
lesser horn of hyoid bone Cornu minus (ossis hyoidei).
lesser incisure of ischium Inc. ischiadica/ischialis minor.
lesser lip of pudendum kleine Schamlippe *f*, Labium minus pudendi.
lesser muscle of helix M. helicis minor.
lesser omentectomy *chir.* (partielle) Resektion *f* des Omentum minus.
lesser omentum kleines Netz *nt*, Omentum minus.
lesser pancreas Proc. uncinatus (pancreatis).
lesser pelvis kleines/echtes Becken *nt*, Pelvis minor.
lesser ring of iris → lesser circle of iris.
lesser sac of peritoneal cavity Netzbeutel *m*, Bauchfelltasche *f*, Bursa omentalis.
lesser tubercle of humerus Tuberculum minus humeri.
lesser tuberosity → lesser tubercle of humerus.
lesser tuberosity fracture Fraktur *f* des Tuberculum minus humeri.
lesser wing of sphenoid bone kleiner Keilbeinflügel *m*, Ala minor (ossis sphenoidalis).
let [let] (**let; let**) *vt* lassen; jdm. erlauben. **to ~ sb./sth. alone** jdn./etw. in Ruhe lassen. **to ~ go** loslassen. **to ~ o.s. go 1.** lockerlassen, s. gehenlassen, aus s. herausgehen, s. entspannen. **2.** s. gehenlassen, s. vernachlässigen. **to ~ s.o. know** jdn. wissen lassen, jdm. Bescheid geben.
let down *vt* jdn. im Stich lassen (*over* mit); jdn. enttäuschen.
let in *vt* (*her-, hin-*)einlassen; (*Flüssigkeitkeit*) durchlassen. **II** *vi* undicht sein; (*Flüssigkeit*) durchlassen.
let out *vt* heraus-, hinauslassen (*of* aus); (*Schrei*) ausstoßen.
let through *vt* durchlassen.
let-down reflex *gyn.* Milchejektionsreflex *m*.
le·thal [ˈliːθəl] **I** *n* **1.** → lethal gene. **2.** letale Substanz *f*. **II** *adj* tödlich, letal, Todes-, Letal-.
lethal dose *abbr.* **L.D.** tödliche/letale Dosis *f abbr.* LD, ld, Letaldosis *f abbr.* LD, Dosis letalis *abbr.* DL, d.l.
median l. *abbr.* **L.D.₅₀** mittlere letale Dosis *abbr.* LD₅₀, Dosis letalis media.
minimal l. *abbr.* **M.L.D.** minimale letale Dosis, Dosis letalis minima *abbr.* Dlm.
lethal factor → lethal gene.
lethal gene *genet.* Letalfaktor *m*, Letalgen *nt*.
lethal infection tödlich verlaufende Infektion *f*.
le·thal·i·ty [lɪˈθælətɪ] *n* Letalität *f*.
lethal midline granuloma letales Mittelliniengranulom *nt*, Granuloma gangraenescens nasi.
lethal mutant letale Mutante *f*, Letalmutante *f*.
lethal mutation → lethal gene.
lethal synthesis *biochem.* Letalsynthese *f*.
le·thar·gic [ləˈθɑːrdʒɪk] *adj* → lethargical.
le·thar·gi·cal [ləˈθɑːrdʒɪkl] *adj* **1.** teilnahmslos, träge, stumpf, lethargisch. **2.** *patho.* schlafsüchtig, lethargisch.
lethargic encephalitis (von) Economo-Krankheit *f*, -Enzephalitis *f*, europäische Schlafkrankheit *f*, Encephalitis epidemica/lethargica.
leth·ar·gy [ˈleθərdʒɪ] *n*, *pl* **-gies 1.** Teilnahmslosigkeit *f*, Trägheit *f*, Stumpfheit *f*, Lethargie *f*. **2.** *patho.* Schlafsucht *f*, Lethargie, Lethargia *f*.
LETS *abbr.* [large external transformation-sensitive factor] Fibronektin *nt*.
Letterer-Siwe [ˈletərər ˈsaɪwiː; ˈziːwə]: **L.-S. disease** Letterer-Siwe-Krankheit *f*, Abt-Letterer-Siwe-Krankheit *f*, maligne/akute Säuglingsretikulose *f*, maligne generalisierte Histiozytose *f*.
let-up *n inf.* **1.** Nachlassen *nt*; Pause *f*. **2.** Aufhören *nt*.
Leu *abbr.* → leucine.
leuc- *pref.* → leuko-.
leu·ce·mia [luːˈsiːmɪə] *n* → leukemia.
leu·cine [ˈluːsiːn, -sɪn] *n abbr.* **L, Leu** Leuzin *nt*, α-Aminoisocapronsäure *f*, Leucin *nt abbr.* L, Leu.
leucine aminopeptidase *abbr.* **LAP** Leucinaminopeptidase *f abbr.* LAP, Leucinarylamidase *f*.
leucine aminotransferase Leucinaminotransferase *f*, Leucintransaminase *f*.
leucine arylamidase → leucine aminopeptidase.
leucine enkephalin Leu-Enkephalin *nt*, Leucin-Enkephalin *nt*.
leucine hypoglycemia → leucine-induced hypoglycemia.
leucine-induced hypoglycemia Leucin-empfindliche Hypoglykämie *f*.
leucine transaminase → leucine aminotransferase.
leu·ci·no·sis [luːsɪˈnəʊsɪs] *n patho.* Leuzinose *f*, Leucinose *f*.
leu·ci·nu·ria [luːsɪˈn(j)ʊərɪə] *n* Leuzinausscheidung *f* im Harn, Leuzinurie *f*, Leucinurie *f*.
leu·cism [ˈluːsɪzəm] *n derm.* Leuzismus *m*; Albinismus partialis.
leu·ci·tis [luːˈsaɪtɪs] *n ophthal.* Lederhaut-, Skleraentzündung *f*, Skleritis *f*, Scleritis *f*.
leuco- *pref.* → leuko-.
leu·co·cyte → leukocyte.
leu·co·cy·to·sis *n* → leukocytosis.
leu·co·my·cin [luːkəˈmaɪsɪn] *n pharm.* Leucomycin *nt*.
leu·cop·ter·in [luːˈkɑptərɪn] *n* Leukopterin *nt*.
Leu·co·thrix [ˈluːkəθrɪks] *n micro.* Leucothrix *f*.
leu·cot·o·my *n* → leukotomy.
Leu·co·tri·cha·ce·ae [ˌluːkətrɪˈkeɪsɪiː] *pl micro.* Leucotrichaceae *pl*.
leu·co·vo·rin [luːˈkɑvərɪn] *n* Folinsäure *f*, N¹⁰-Formyl-Tetrahydrofolsäure *f*, Leukovorin *nt*, Leucovorin *nt*, Citrovorum-Faktor *m abbr.* CF.

leu-enkephalin *n* → leucine enkephalin.
leuk- *pref.* → leuko-.
leu·ka·phe·re·sis [ˌluːkəfɪˈriːsɪs] *n hema., lab.* Leukapherese *f*.
leu·ke·mia [luːˈkiːmɪə] *n* Leukämie *f*, Leukose *f*.
leu·ke·mic [luːˈkiːmɪk] *adj* Leukämie betr., von ihr betroffen, leukämisch.
leukemic erythrocytosis Morbus Vaquez-Osler *m*, Vaquez-Osler-Syndrom *nt*, Osler-Krankheit *f*, Vaquez-Osler-Krankheit *f*, Polycythaemia (rubra) vera, Erythrämie *f*.
leukemic hiatus Hiatus leucaemicus.
leukemic infiltration leukämisches Infiltrat *nt*, leukämische Infiltration *f*.
leukemic leukemia leukämische Leukämie *f*.
leukemic meningitis leukämische Hirnhautinfiltration *f*, Meningitis/Meningiosis leucaemica.
leukemic reaction → leukemoid reaction.
leukemic reticuloendotheliosis Haarzellenleukämie *f*, leukämische Retikuloendotheliose *f*.
leukemic reticulosis (akute) Monozytenleukämie *f abbr.* AMOL.
leukemic retinitis → leukemic retinopathy.
leukemic retinopathy leukämische Netzhautinfiltration *f*.
leu·ke·mid [luːˈkiːmɪd] *n* Leukämid *nt*.
leu·ke·mo·gen [luːˈkiːmədʒən] *n* leukämieauslösende Substanz *f*, Leukämogen *nt*.
leu·ke·mo·gen·e·sis [luːˌkiːməˈdʒenəsɪs] *n* Leukämogenese *f*.
leu·ke·mo·gen·ic [luːˌkiːməˈdʒenɪk] *adj* leukämieauslösend, -verursachend, leukämogen.
leu·ke·moid [luːˈkiːmɔɪd] **I** *n* → leukemoid reaction. **II** *adj* leukämieartig, -ähnlich, leukämoid.
leukemoid reaction leukämoide/leukämische Reaktion *f*, Leukämoid *nt*.
leuk·en·ceph·a·li·tis [ˌluːkənˌsefəˈlaɪtɪs] *n* → leukoencephalitis.
leu·kin [ˈluːkɪn] *n* Leukin *nt*.
leuko- *pref.* Leuk(o)-, Leuc(o)-.
leu·ko·ag·glu·tin·in [ˌluːkəəˈɡluːtənɪn] *n* Leukozytenagglutinin *nt*, Leukoagglutinin *nt*.
leukoagglutinin reaction (*Transfusion*) Leukoagglutininreaktion *f*.
leu·ko·blast [ˈ-blæst] *n* Leukoblast *m*.
leu·ko·blas·to·sis [ˌ-blæsˈtəʊsɪs] *n* Leukoblastose *f*.
leu·ko·ci·din [ˌ-ˈsaɪdɪn] *n* Leukozidin *nt*, Leukocidin *nt*.
leu·ko·co·ria *n* → leukokoria.
leu·ko·crit [ˈ-krɪt] *n* Leukokrit *m*.
leu·ko·cy·tac·tic [ˌ-saɪˈtæktɪk] *adj* → leukotactic.
leu·ko·cy·tal [ˌ-ˈsaɪtæl] *adj* → leukocytic.
leu·ko·cy·tax·ia [ˌ-saɪˈtæksɪə] *n* → leukotaxis.
leu·ko·cy·tax·is [ˌ-saɪˈtæksɪs] *n* → leukotaxis.
leu·ko·cyte [ˈ-saɪt] *n* weiße Blutzelle *f*, weißes Blutkörperchen *nt*, Leukozyt *m*.
leukocyte agglutinin → leukoagglutinin.
leukocyte alkaline phosphatase *abbr.* **LAP** alkalische Leukozytenphosphatase *f abbr.* ALP, aLP.
leukocyte antigens Leukozytenantigene *pl*.
human l. *abbr.* **HLA** Histokompatibilitätsantigene *pl*, Transplantationsantigene *pl*, humane Leukozytenantigene *pl abbr.* HLA, HLA-Antigene *pl*, human leukocyte antigens *abbr.* HLA.
leukocyte cast *urol.* Leukozytenzylinder *m*.

leukocyte count 1. Leukozytenzahl *f.* **2.** Leukozytenzählung *f.*
leukocyte cream Leukozytenmanschette *f*, buffy coat.
leukocyte diapedesis Leukozytendiapedese *f.*
leukocyte inclusions Döhle'-(Einschluß-)-Körperchen *pl.*
leukocyte inhibitory factor *abbr.* **LIF** Leukozytenmigration-inhibierender Faktor *m abbr.* LIF.
leukocyte interferon α-Interferon *nt abbr.* IFN-α.
leukocyte number Leukozytenzahl *f.*
leukocyte progenitor Leukozytenvorläufer(zelle *f*) *m.*
leu·ko·cy·the·mia [ˌ-saɪˈθiːmɪə] *n* → leukemia.
leu·ko·cyt·ic [ˌ-ˈsɪtɪk] *adj* Leukozyten betr., leukozytär, Leukozyten-, Leukozyto-.
leukocytic crystals Asthmakristalle *pl*, Charcot-Leyden-Kristalle *pl.*
leukocytic diapedesis Leukopedese *f*, Leukozyten-, Leukodiapedese *f.*
leukocytic pyrogen endogenes Pyrogen *nt abbr.* EP.
leukocytic sarcoma 1. → leukosarcoma. **2.** → leukemia.
leukocyte series *hema.* granulozytäre Reihe *f.*
leu·ko·cy·to·blast [ˌ-ˈsaɪtəblæst] *n* Leukoblast *m.*
leu·ko·cy·to·clas·tic angiitis [ˌ-ˌsaɪtəˈklæstɪk] → leukocytoclastic vasculitis.
leukocytoclastic vasculitis Immunkomplexvaskulitis *f*, leukozytoklastische Vaskulitis *f*, Vasculitis allergica, Vasculitis hyperergica cutis, Arteriitis allergica cutis.
leu·ko·cy·to·gen·e·sis [ˌ-saɪtəˈdʒenəsɪs] *n* Leukozytenbildung *f*, Leukozytogenese *f.*
leu·ko·cy·toid [ˈ-saɪtɔɪd] *adj* leukozytenartig, -ähnlich, -förmig, leukozytoid.
leu·ko·cy·tol·y·sin [ˌ-saɪˈtɑləsɪn] *n* Leukolysin *nt*, Leukozytolysin *f.*
leu·ko·cy·tol·y·sis [ˌ-saɪˈtɑləsɪs] *n* Leukozytenauflösung *f*, Leukolyse *f*, Leukozytolyse *f.*
leu·ko·cy·to·lyt·ic [ˌ-saɪtəˈlɪtɪk] **I** *n* leukolytische Substanz *f.* **II** *adj* Leuko(zyto)lyse betr. *od.* auslösend, leuko(zyto)lytisch.
leu·ko·cy·to·ma [ˌ-saɪˈtoʊmə] *n* Leukozytom *nt*, Leukocytoma *nt.*
leu·ko·cy·to·pe·nia [ˌ-ˌsaɪtəˈpiːnɪə] *n* → leukopenia.
leu·ko·cy·toph·a·gy [ˌ-saɪˈtɑfədʒɪ] *n* Leukozytophagie *f*, Leukophagozytose *f.*
leu·ko·cy·to·poi·e·sis [ˌ-ˌsaɪtəpɔɪˈiːsɪs] *n* → leukopoiesis.
leu·ko·cy·to·sis [ˌ-saɪˈtoʊsɪs] *n* Erhöhung *f* der Leukozytenzahl, Leukozytose *f.*
leu·ko·cy·to·tac·tic [ˌ-ˌsaɪtəˈtæktɪk] *adj* → leukotactic.
leu·ko·cy·to·tax·ia [ˌ-ˌsaɪtəˈtæksɪə] *n* → leukotaxis.
leu·ko·cy·to·tax·is [ˌ-ˌsaɪtəˈtæksɪs] *n* → leukotaxis.
leu·ko·cy·to·ther·a·py [ˌ-ˌsaɪtəˈθerəpɪ] *n* Leukozytotherapie *f.*
leu·ko·cy·to·tox·ic·i·ty [ˌ-ˌsaɪtətɑkˈsɪsətɪ] *n* Leukozytentoxizität *f.*
leu·ko·cy·to·tox·in [ˌ-ˌsaɪtəˈtɑksɪn] *n* Leuko(zyto)toxin *nt.*
leu·ko·cy·to·trop·ic [ˌ-ˌsaɪtəˈtrɑpɪk] *adj* mit besonderer Affinität für Leukozyten, leukozytotrop.
leu·ko·cy·tu·ria [ˌ-saɪˈt(j)ʊərɪə] *n* Leukozytenausscheidung *f* im Harn, Leukozyturie *f.*
leu·ko·der·ma [ˌ-ˈdɜrmə] *n derm.* Leukoderm *nt*, -derma *nt*, Leucoderma *nt*, Leukopathie *f*, -pathia *f.*
leu·ko·der·ma·tous [ˌ-ˈdɜrmətəs] *adj* Leukoderm(a) betr.
leu·ko·der·mia [ˌ-ˈdɜrmɪə] *n* → leukoderma.
leu·ko·der·mic [ˌ-ˈdɜrmɪk] *adj* → leukodermatous.
leu·ko·dys·tro·phy [ˌ-ˈdɪstrəfɪ] *n patho.* Leukodystrophie *f*, -dystrophia *f.*
leu·ko·e·de·ma [ˌ-ɪˈdiːmə] *n derm.* Leuködem *nt.*
leu·ko·en·ceph·a·li·tis [ˌ-enˌsefəˈlaɪtɪs] *n* Entzündung *f* der weißen Hirnsubstanz, Leukoenzephalitis *f*, Leukenzephalitis *f*, Leucoencephalitis *f.*
leu·ko·en·ceph·a·lop·a·thy [ˌ-enˌsefəˈlɑpəθɪ] *n patho.* krankhafte Veränderung *f* der weißen Hirnsubstanz, Leukoenzephalopathie *f.*
leu·ko·en·ceph·a·ly [ˌ-enˈsefəlɪ] *n* → leukoencephalopathy.
leu·ko·e·ryth·ro·blas·tic anemia [ˌ-ɪˌrɪθrəˈblæstɪk] leukoerythroblastische Anämie *f*, idiopathische/primäre myeloische Metaplasie *f*, Leukoerythroblastose *f.*
leu·ko·e·ryth·ro·blas·to·sis [ˌ-ɪˌrɪθrəblæsˈtoʊsɪs] *n* → leukoerythroblastic anemia.
leu·ko·gram [ˈ-græm] *n hem.* Leukogramm *nt.*
leu·ko·ker·a·to·sis [ˌ-kerəˈtoʊsɪs] *n* → leukoplakia *f.*
leu·ko·ki·ne·sis [ˌ-kɪˈniːsɪs, -kaɪ-] *n* Leukokinese *f.*
leu·ko·ki·net·ic [ˌ-kɪˈnetɪk] *adj* Leukokinese betr., leukokinetisch.
leu·ko·ki·nin [ˌ-ˈkaɪnɪn, -ˈkɪn-] *n* Leukokinin *nt.*
leu·ko·ko·ria [ˌ-ˈkoʊrɪə] *n ophthal.* Leukokorie *f.*
leu·ko·krau·ro·sis [ˌ-krɔːˈroʊsɪs] *n derm., gyn.* Breisky'-Krankheit *f*, Kraurosis/Craurosis vulvae.
leu·ko·lym·pho·sar·co·ma [ˌ-ˌlɪmfəsɑːrˈkoʊmə] *n* **1.** Lymphosarkomzellenleukämie *f.* **2.** → leukosarcoma.
leu·kol·y·sin [luːˈkɑləsɪn] *n* → leukocytolysin.
leu·kol·y·sis [luːˈkɑləsɪs] *n* → leukocytolysis.
leu·ko·lyt·ic [ˌluːkəˈlɪtɪk] *n, adj* → leukocytolytic.
leu·ko·ma [luːˈkoʊmə] *n ophthal.* weißer Hornhautfleck *m*, Leukom(a) *nt*, Leucoma *nt*, Albugo *f.*
leu·ko·maine [ˈluːkəmeɪn] *n* Leukomain *nt.*
leu·ko·main·e·mia [ˌ-meɪˈniːmɪə] *n* erhöhter Leukomaingehalt *m* des Blutes, Leukomainämie *f.*
leu·kom·a·tous [luːˈkɑmətəs] *adj ophthal.* Leukom betr., leukomatös.
leu·ko·my·e·li·tis [ˌluːkəmaɪəˈlaɪtɪs] *n patho.* Entzündung *f* der weißen Rückenmark(s)substanz, Leukomyelitis *f.*
leu·ko·my·e·lop·a·thy [ˌ-maɪəˈlɑpəθɪ] *n patho.* krankhafte Veränderung *f* der weißen Rückenmark(s)substanz, Leukomyelopathie *f.*
leu·ko·my·o·ma [ˌ-maɪˈoʊmə] *n* → lipomyoma.
leu·kon [ˈluːkɑn] *n hema.* Leukon *nt.*
leu·ko·nych·ia [luːkəˈnɪkɪə] *n derm.* Weißfärbung *f* der Nägel, Leukonychie *f*, Leukonychia *f*, Leuconychia *f.*
leu·kop·a·thia [luːˈpæθɪə] *n derm.* Pigmentverlust *m* der Haut, Leukopathie *f*, -pathia *f*, Leukoderm *nt*, -derma *nt*, Leucoderma *nt.*
leu·kop·a·thy [luːˈkɑpəθɪ] *n* → leukopathia.
leu·ko·pe·de·sis [ˌluːkəpɪˈdiːsɪs] *n* Leukopedese *f*, Leukozyten-, Leukodiapedese *f.*
leu·ko·pe·nia [ˌ-ˈpiːnɪə] *n* verminderter Leukozytengehalt *m* des Blutes, Leukopenie *f*, Leukozytopenie *f.*
leu·ko·pe·nic [ˌ-ˈpiːnɪk] *adj* Leukopenie betr. *od.* verursachend, leukopenisch.
leukopenic agammaglobulinemia Schweizer-Typ *m* der Agammaglobulinämie, schwerer kombinierter Immundefekt *m.*
leukopenic leukemia 1. aleukämische Leukämie *f.* **2.** subleukämische Leukämie *f.*
leu·ko·phag·o·cy·to·sis [ˌ-ˌfæɡəsaɪˈtoʊsɪs] *n* → leukocytophagy.
leu·ko·phe·re·sis [ˌ-fəˈriːsɪs] *n* Leukopherese *f.*
leu·ko·phleg·ma·sia [ˌ-flegˈmeɪʒ(ɪ)ə, -ʒɪə] *n derm.* Milchbein *nt*, Leukophlegmasie *f*, Phlegmasia alba dolens.
leu·ko·phyl(l) [ˈ-fɪl] *n bio.* Leukophyl *nt.*
leu·ko·pla·kia [ˌ-ˈpleɪkɪə] *n* **1.** Weißschwielenkrankheit *f*, Leukoplakie *f*, -plakia *f*, Leucoplacia *f.* **2.** orale Leukoplakie *f*, Leukoplakie *f* der Mundschleimhaut, Leukoplakia oris.
leu·ko·pla·kic [ˌ-ˈpleɪkɪk] *adj* Leukoplakie betr., von ihr gekennzeichnet, leukoplakisch.
leukoplakic thickening leukoplakische Verdickung *f.*
leukoplakic vulvitis leukoplakische Vulvitis *f.*
leu·ko·plast [ˈ-plæst] *n bio.* Leukoplast *m.*
leu·ko·plas·tid [ˌ-ˈplæstɪd] *n* → leukoplast.
leu·ko·poi·e·sis [ˌ-pɔɪˈiːsɪs] *n* Leukozytenbildung *f*, Leukopoese *f*, Leukozytopoese *f.*
leu·ko·poi·et·ic [ˌ-pɔɪˈetɪk] *adj* Leukopoese betr., leukopoetisch, leukozytopoetisch.
leu·ko·pre·cip·i·tin [ˌ-prɪˈsɪpətɪn] *n* Leukozytenpräzipitin *nt.*
leu·ko·pro·te·ase [ˌ-ˈproʊteɪz] *n* Leukoprotease *f.*
leu·kop·sin [luːˈkæpsɪn] *n* Sehweiß *nt*, Leukopsin *nt.*
leu·kor·rha·gia [ˌluːkəˈrædʒ(ɪ)ə] *n gyn.* starke Leukorrhoe *f*, Leukorrhagie *f.*
leu·kor·rhea [ˌ-ˈrɪə] *n gyn.* Weißfluß *m*, Leukorrhoe *f.*
leu·kor·rhe·al [ˌ-ˈrɪəl] *adj* Leukorrhoe betr.
leu·ko·sar·co·ma [ˌ-sɑːrˈkoʊmə] *n hema.* Leukosarkom *nt*, Leukolymphosarkom *nt.*
leu·ko·sar·co·ma·to·sis [ˌ-sɑːrˌkoʊməˈtoʊsɪs] *n hema.* Leukosarkomatose *f.*
leu·ko·sis [luːˈkoʊsɪs] *n*, *pl* **-ses** [-siːz] **1.** Leukose *f.* **2.** → leukemia.
leu·ko·tac·tic [ˌluːkəˈtæktɪk] *adj* Leukotaxis betr., leukotaktisch.
leu·ko·tax·ia [ˌ-ˈtæksɪə] *n* → leukotaxine.
leu·ko·tax·in [ˌ-ˈtæksɪn] *n* → leukotaxine.
leu·ko·tax·ine [ˌ-ˈtæksɪn] *n* Leukotaxin *nt*, Leukozytotaxis *f.*
leu·ko·thrix [ˈ-θrɪks] *n* → Leucothrix.
leu·ko·tome [ˈ-toʊm] *n neurochir.* Leukotom *nt.*
leu·kot·o·my [luːˈkɑtəmɪ] *n neurochir.* Leukotomie *f.*
leu·ko·tox·ic [ˌluːkəˈtɑksɪk] *adj* leukozytenzerstörend, -schädigend, leukotoxisch, leukozytotoxisch.
leu·ko·tox·ic·i·ty [ˌ-tɑkˈsɪsətɪ] *n* Leuko(zyto)toxizität *f.*
leu·ko·tox·in [ˌ-ˈtɑksɪn] *n* Leuko(zyto)toxin *nt.*
Leu·ko·tri·cha·ce·ae *pl* → Leucotrichaceae.
leu·ko·trich·ia [ˌ-ˈtrɪkɪə] *n derm.* Weißhaarigkeit *f*, Leukotrichosis *f*, Leukotrichia *f.*

leukotriene

leu·ko·tri·ene [ˌ-'traɪiːn] *n abbr.* **LT** Leukotrien *nt abbr.* LT.
leu·ko·u·ro·bi·lin [ˌ-jʊərə'baɪlɪn] *n* Leukourobilin *nt.*
Lev [lef]: **L.'s disease** Lev'-Krankheit *f.*
lev- *pref.* → levo-.
Levaditi [levə'diːtɪ]: **L.'s stain** *histol.* Levaditi-Färbung *f*, -Versilberung *f.*
lev·al·lor·phan [levə'lɔːrfən] *n pharm.* Levallorphan *nt.*
lev·an ['levæn] *n* Fructan *nt*, Levan *nt*, Poly-D-Fruktose *f.*
lev·ar·ter·e·nol [levɑːr'tɪərɪnɒl, -nəʊl] *n* Noradrenalin *nt*, Norepinephrin *nt*, Arterenol *nt*, Levarterenol *nt.*
le·va·tor [lɪ'veɪtər, -tər] *n, pl* **-to·res** [levə'tɔːriːz, -'tə℧r-] **1.** *anat.* Hebemuskel *m*, Levator *m*, M. levator. **2.** *chir.* Elevatorium *nt.*
levator anguli oris (muscle) Levator *m* anguli oris, M. levator anguli oris, *old* M. caninus.
levator ani (muscle) Levator *m* ani, M. levator ani.
levator costae (muscle) Levator *m* costae, M. levator costae.
levator glandulae thyroideae (muscle) Levator *m* gl. thyroideae, M. levator glandulae thyroideae.
levator hernia Levatorhernie *f.*
levator labii superioris alaeque nasi (muscle) Levator *m* labii superioris alaeque nasi, M. levator labii superioris alaeque nasi.
levator labii superioris (muscle) Levator *m* labii superioris, M. levator labii superioris.
levator loop Levatorschlinge *f.*
levator muscle → levator l.
l. of angle of mouth → levator anguli oris (muscle).
l. of palatine velum → levator veli palatini (muscle).
l. of prostate → levator prostatae (muscle).
l. of ribs → levator costae (muscle).
l. of scapula → levator scapulae (muscle).
l. of thyroid gland → levator glandulae thyroideae (muscle).
l. of upper lid → levator palpebrae superioris (muscle).
l. of upper lip → levator labii superioris (muscle).
l. of upper lip and nasal wing → levator labii superioris alaeque nasi (muscle).
levator palpebrae superioris (muscle) Oberlidheber *m*, Levator *m* palpebrae superioris, M. levator palpebrae superioris.
levator prostatae (muscle) Levator *m* prostatae, M. levator prostatae, M. pubovaginalis.
levator scapulae (muscle) Levator *m* scapulae, M. levator scapulae.
levator syndrome Levator-ani-Syndrom *nt.*
levator veli palatini (muscle) Levator *m* veli palatini, M. levator veli palatini.
LeVeen [lə'viːn]: **L. (peritoneovenous) shunt** LeVeen-Shunt *m.*
lev·el ['levəl] **I** *n* **1.** ebene Fläche *f*, Ebene *f*; Horizontale *f*, Waag(e)rechte *f*. **2.** (*Alkohol etc.*) Spiegel *m*, Stand *m*, Pegel *m*, Gehalt *m*, Konzentration *f*, Anteil *m*. **3.** *fig.* Niveau *nt*, Stand *m*, Grad *m*. **a high ~ of intelligence** ein hoher Intelligenzgrad. **4.** *techn.* Wasserwaage *f*. **II** *adj* **5.** eben; waag(e)recht, horizontal; *fig.* gleich, auf gleichem Niveau (*with* mit). **a ~ teaspoon** ein gestrichener Teelöffel (voll). **6.** gleichmäßig, ausgeglichen, gleichbleibend; (*Person*) vernünftig, ruhig.
level down *vt* nach unten ausgleichen, auf

ein tieferes Niveau bringen, herabsetzen.
level off I *vt* ausgleichen; gleichmachen, nivellieren. **II** *vi* s. ausgleichen, s. einpendeln.
level out *vt, vi* → level off.
level up *vt* nach oben ausgleichen, auf ein höheres Niveau bringen, erhöhen.
l. of amputation *ortho.* Amputationshöhe *f.*
l. of metabolic activity Stoffwechselumsatz *m.*
l. of metabolism → l. of metabolic activity.
l. of sound Geräuschpegel, Tonstärke *f.*
lev·er ['levər, 'liː-] **I** *n phys., techn.* Hebel *m*; Brechstange *f.* **II** *vt* hebeln, (hoch-)stemmen.
lever out *vt* herausstemmen (*of* aus).
lev·er·age ['levərɪdʒ, 'liː-] *n* Hebelkraft *f*, -wirkung *f.*
lever arm *phys.* Hebelarm *m.*
lev·i·cel·lu·lar [levɪ'seljələr] *adj histol.* glattzellig.
lev·i·gate [*adj* 'levɪgɪt, -geɪt; *v* -geɪt] **I** *adj bio.* glatt. **II** *vt* **1.** pulverisieren, (*zu einer Paste*) verreiben. **2.** *chem.* homogenisieren.
lev·i·ga·tion [levɪ'geɪʃn] *n* Pulverisieren *nt*, Verreiben *nt.*
Lévi-Lorain [le'vi lɔ'rɛ̃]: **L.-L. dwarf** hypophysärer Zwerg *m.*
L.-L. dwarfism/infantilism Lorain-Syndrom *nt*, hypophysärer Zwergwuchs/ Minderwuchs *m.*
Levin ['levɪn]: **L.'s tube** Levin-Sonde *f.*
Levinthal-Coles-Lillie ['levɪnθəl 'kəʊlz 'lɪlɪ; 'levɪntəl]: **L.-C.-L. bodies** Levinthal-Coles-Lillie-Körperchen *pl.*
lev·i·tate ['levɪteɪt] **I** *vt* **1.** IC (*einen Patienten*) auf Luftkissen betten *od.* lagern. **2.** *psycho., psychia.* frei schweben lassen, levitieren. **II** *vi psycho., psychia.* frei schweben, levitieren.
lev·i·ta·tion [levɪ'teɪʃn] *n* **1.** IC (*Verbrennung*) Luftkissenlagerung *f*. **2.** *psycho., psychia.* Levitation *f.*
levo- *pref.* Links-, Läv(o)-, Lev(o)-.
le·vo·car·dia [ˌliːvə'kɑːrdɪə] *n* Lävokardie *f.*
le·vo·car·di·o·gram [ˌ-'kɑːrdɪəgræm] *n* Lävokardiogramm *nt.*
le·vo·cli·na·tion [ˌklaɪ'neɪʃn] *n ophthal.* Lävoklination *f.*
le·vo·cy·clo·duc·tion [ˌ-ˌsaɪklə'dʌkʃn] *n* → levoduction.
le·vo·do·pa [ˌ-'dəʊpə] *n pharm.* Levodopa *nt.*
le·vo·duc·tion [ˌ-'dʌkʃn] *n ophthal.* Lävoduktion *f.*
lev·o·gram ['-græm] *n card.* Lävogramm *nt.*
le·vo·gy·ral [ˌ-'dʒaɪrəl] *adj* → levorotatory.
le·vo·gy·ra·tion [ˌ-dʒaɪ'reɪʃn] *n* → levorotation.
le·vo·gy·rous [ˌ-'dʒaɪrəs] *adj* → levorotatory.
le·vo·me·pro·ma·zine [ˌ-mɪ'prəʊməziːn] *n pharm.* Levomepromazin *nt.*
le·vo·pro·pox·y·phene [ˌ-prəʊ'pɑksɪfiːn] *n pharm.* Levopropoxyphen *nt.*
le·vo·ro·ta·ry [ˌ-'rəʊtərɪ] *adj* → levorotatory.
le·vo·ro·ta·tion [ˌ-rəʊ'teɪʃn] *n chem., phys.* Linksdrehung *f*, Lävorotation *f.*
le·vo·ro·ta·to·ry [ˌ-'rəʊtətɔːrɪ, -təʊ-] *adj chem., phys.* linksdrehend, lävorotatorisch.
le·vo·thy·rox·ine sodium [ˌ-θaɪ'rɑksiːn] *pharm.* Levothyroxin-Natrium *nt.*
le·vo·tor·sion [ˌ-'tɔːrʃn] *n* → levoclination.
le·vo·ver·sion [ˌ-'vɜːrʒn] *n ophthal.* Lävoversion *f.*

lev·u·lan ['levjələn] *n* Fruktosan *nt*, Fructosan *nt*, L(a)evulan *nt.*
lev·u·lo·san [levjə'ləʊsæn] *n* → levulan.
lev·u·lose ['levjələʊz] *n* Fruchtzucker *m*, Fruktose *f*, Fructose *f*, Lävulose *f.*
lev·u·lo·se·mia [ˌlevjələʊ'siːmɪə] *n* Fruktoseausscheidung *f* im Harn, Fruktosämie *f*, Fruktosämie *f.*
lev·u·lo·su·ria [ˌ-'s(j)ʊərɪə] *n* Fruktosurie *f*, Fructosurie *f.*
Lévy-Roussy [le'vi ru'si]: **L.-R. syndrome** Roussy-Lévy-Syndrom *nt*, erbliche areflektorische Dysstasie *f.*
Lewandowsky ['lewændɒwskɪ]: **nevus elasticus of L.** Naevus elasticus Lewandowsky.
Lewandowsky-Lutz [lʊts]: **L.-L. disease** Lewandowsky-Lutz-Krankheit *f*, -Syndrom *nt*, Epidermodysplasia verruciformis, Verrucosis generalisata (Lewandowsky-Lutz).
Lewis ['luːɪs]: **L. acid** Lewis-Säure *f.*
L. base Lewis-Base *f.*
L. blood group (system) Lewis-Blutgruppe *f*, -Blutgruppensystem *nt.*
lew·is·ite ['luːəsaɪt] *n* Lewisit *nt.*
Lewy ['luːɪ]: **L. bodies** Lewy-Korpuskel *pl.*
Leyden ['laɪdn]: **L.'s ataxia** Pseudotabes *f.*
L.'s crystals Charcot-Leyden-Kristalle *pl.*
Leyden-Möbius ['mɪbɪəs]: **L.-M. muscular dystrophy** → L.-M. syndrome.
L.-M. syndrome Leyden-Möbius-Krankheit *f*, -Syndrom *nt*, Gliedgürtelform *f* der progressiven Muskeldystrophie.
L.-M. type → L.-M. syndrome.
Leydig ['laɪdɪg]: **L.'s cells** Leydig'-Zellen *pl*, Leydig'-Zwischenzellen *pl*, Interstitialzellen *pl*, interstitielle Drüsen *pl.*
L. cell tumor Leydig-Zell(en)tumor *m.*
L.'s cylinders Leydig-Zylinder *pl.*
L.'s duct *embryo.* Wolff'-Gang *m*, Urnierengang *m*, Ductus mesonephricus.
L-form *micro.* L-Form *f*, L-Phase *f*, L-Organismus *m.*
LGB *abbr.* → geniculate body, lateral.
LGV *abbr.* → lymphogranuloma venereum.
LH *abbr.* → luteinizing hormone.
Lhermitte ['lɛrmɪt]: **L.'s sign** Lhermitte-Zeichen *nt.*
Lhermitte-McAlpine [mə'kælpaɪn]: **L.-M. syndrome** Lhermitte-McAlpine-Syndrom *nt.*
LH-RF *abbr.* [luteinizing hormone releasing factor] → luteinizing hormone releasing hormone.
LH-RH *abbr.* → luteinizing hormone releasing hormone.
Li *abbr.* → lithium.
LIA *abbr.* → lysine-iron agar.
li·bid·i·nal [lɪ'bɪdnəl] *adj* → libidinous.
li·bid·i·nous [lɪ'bɪdnəs] *adj* Libido betr., durch Libido bestimmt, libidinös, triebhaft.
li·bi·do [lɪ'biːdəʊ, -'baɪ-] *n* **1.** Geschlechts-, Sexualtrieb *m*, Libido *f*. **2.** *psychia.* Libido *f*, Lebenswille *m*, Lebenskraft *f.*
Libman-Sacks ['lɪbmən 'zæks]: **L.-S. disease** → L.-S. endocarditis.
L.-S. endocarditis Libman-Sacks-Syndrom *nt*, Endokarditis Libman-Sacks *f*, atypische verruköse Endokarditis *f*, Endocarditis thrombotica.
L.-S. syndrome → L.-S. endocarditis.
li·bra ['laɪbrə] *n, pl* **-brae** [-briː] *abbr.* **lb.** → pound² 1.
lice *pl* → louse.
li·chen ['laɪkən] *n* **1.** *derm.* Lichen *m*. **2.** *bio.* Flechte *f.*
lichen amyloidosus *derm.* Lichen amyloidosus.

li·chen·i·fi·ca·tion [laɪˌkenəfɪ'keɪʃn] *n derm.* Lichenifikation *f*, Lichenisation *f*.
li·chen·in ['laɪkənɪn] *n* Lichenin *nt*, Lichen-, Moosstärke *f*.
li·chen·i·za·tion [ˌlaɪkənɪ'zeɪʃn] *n* → lichenification.
li·chen·oid ['laɪkənɔɪd] **I** *n derm.* Lichenoid *nt*. **II** *adj* lichenartig, flechtenähnlich, lichenoid.
lichenoid dermatosis lichenoide Dermatose *f*.
lichenoid eczema lichenifiziertes Ekzem *nt*.
Lichtheim ['lɪkthaɪm; 'lɪçt-]: **L.'s disease** Dana-Lichtheim-Krankheit *f*, Dana--Syndrom *nt*, Lichtheim-Syndrom *nt*, Dana-Lichtheim-Putnam-Syndrom *nt*, funikuläre Myelose *f*.
L.'s plaques Lichtheim-Flecken *pl*.
L.'s sign Déjérine-Phänomen *nt*, Déjérine-Lichtheim-Phänomen *nt*.
L.'s syndrome → L.'s disease.
lick [lɪk] **I** *n* Lecken *nt*. **II** *vt* (ab-, be-)lecken. **III** *vi* lecken.
lick·ing ['lɪkɪŋ] *n* Lecken *nt*.
lic·o·rice ['lɪkərɪʃ, 'lɪkrɪʃ] *n* **1.** Lakritzen-, Süßholzsaft *m*. **2.** licorice root.
licorice root Süßholz(wurzel *f*) *nt*.
lid [lɪd] *n* **1.** (Augen-)Lid *nt*, Palpebra *f*. **2.** Deckel *m*.
Liddel and Sherrington ['lɪdl 'ʃerɪŋtən]: **L.a.S. reflex** Muskeldehnungsreflex *m*.
lid edema Lidödem *nt*.
lid hook *ophthal.* Lidhaken *m*.
li·do·caine ['laɪdəkeɪn] *n pharm.* Lidocain *nt*.
li·do·fla·zine [ˌ-'fleɪziːn] *n pharm.* Lidoflazin *nt*.
lid reflex Korneal-, Blinzel-, Lidreflex *m*.
lid retractor *ophthal.* Lidsperrer *m*.
lid swelling Lidschwellung *f*.
lie¹ [laɪ] (*v* lied) **I** *n* Lüge *f*. **II** *vi* lügen, trügen, täuschen.
lie² [laɪ] (*v* lay; lain) **I** *n* Lage *f*. **II** *vi* liegen.
lie back *vi* s. zurücklegen *od.* -lehnen.
lie down *vi* s. hin- *od.* niederlegen.
lie up *vi* das Bett *od.* das Zimmer hüten (müssen).
Lieberkühn ['liːbə(r)k(j)uːn; -kyːn]: **L.'s crypts** Lieberkühn'-Drüsen *pl*, -Krypten *pl*, Darmdrüsen *pl*, Gll. intestinales.
L.'s follicles/glands → L.'s crypts.
Liebermann-Burchard ['bɑːrkhɑːd; 'bʊrxaːrd]: **L.-B. reaction** *lab.* Liebermann--Burchard-Reaktion *f*.
L.-B. test → L.-B. reaction.
lie detector Lügendetektor *m*.
lien- *pref.* → lieno-.
li·en ['laɪən] *n* Milz *f*; *anat.* Splen *m*, Lien *m*.
li·e·nal [laɪ'iːnl, 'laɪənl] *adj* Milz/Splen betr., von der Milz ausgehend, lienal, splenisch, Milz-, Lienal-, Splen(o)-.
lienal artery Milzarterie *f*, Lienalis *f*, A. lienalis/splenica.
lienal plexus Plexus lienalis/splenicus.
lienal vein Milzvene *f*, Lienalis *f*, V. lienalis/splenica.
li·en·cu·lus [laɪ'eŋkjələs] *n, pl* -**li** [-laɪ] *anat.* Nebenmilz *f*, Lienculus *m*, Lien accessorius.
li·en·ec·to·my [laɪə'nektəmɪ] *n chir.* Milzentfernung *f*, -exstirpation *f*, Splenektomie *f*.
li·en·i·tis [laɪə'naɪtɪs] *n* Milzentzündung *f*, Splenitis *f*, Lienitis *f*.
lieno- *pref.* Milz-, Lienal-, Splen(o)-.
li·e·no·cele [laɪ'iːnəsiːl, 'laɪənəʊ-] *n* **1.** Splenozele *f*. **2.** Milztumor *m*, Splenom(a) *nt*.
li·e·nog·ra·phy [laɪə'nɒgrəfɪ] *n radiol.* Kontrastdarstellung *f* der Milz, Splenographie *f*.

li·e·no·ma·la·cia [ˌlaɪənəʊmə'leɪʃ(ɪ)ə, laɪˌiːnə-] *n* Milzerweichung *f*, Splenomalazie *f*.
li·e·no·med·ul·la·ry [-'medəˌlerɪː] *adj* Milz/Splen u. Knochenmark betr., splenomedullär.
li·e·no·my·e·log·e·nous [ˌ-maɪə'lɑdʒənəs] *adj* → lienomedullary.
li·e·no·my·e·lo·ma·la·cia [ˌ-ˌmaɪələʊmə'leɪʃ(ɪ)ə] *n* Splenomyelomalazie *f*.
li·e·no·pan·cre·at·ic [ˌ-ˌpæŋkrɪ'ætɪk] *adj* Milz/Splen u. Bauchspeicheldrüse/Pankreas betr., lieno-, splenopankreatisch.
li·e·nop·a·thy [laɪə'nɑpəθɪ] *n* Milzerkrankung *f*, Splenopathie *f*.
li·e·no·phren·ic ligament [ˌlaɪənəʊ'frenɪk, laɪˌiːnəʊ-] Lig. splenorenale/lienorenale/phrenicosplenicum.
li·e·no·re·nal [ˌ-'riːnl] *adj* Milz/Splen u. Niere/Ren betr., splenorenal, lienorenal.
li·en·ter·ic [laɪən'terɪk] *adj* Lienterie betr., lienterisch.
lienteric diarrhea Diarrhoea lienterica.
li·en·ter·y ['laɪəntəriː] *n patho.* Lienterie *f*.
li·en·un·cu·lus [ˌlaɪən'ʌŋkjələs] *n* → lienculus.
Lieutaud [ljø'tɔː]: **L.'s body/triangle/trigone** Lieutaud'-Dreieck *nt*, Blasendreieck *nt*, Trigonum vesicae.
L.'s uvula Blasenzäpfchen *nt*, Uvula vesicae.
LIF *abbr.* → leukocyte inhibitory factor.
life [laɪf] *n*, *pl* **lives** **1.** Leben *nt*. **to bring s.b. back to ~** jdn. wiederbeleben. **to come back to ~** wieder zu s. kommen, wieder zu Bewußtsein kommen. **early in ~** in jungen Jahren. **later in ~** in späteren Jahren, in vorgerücktem Alter. **for ~** fürs (ganze) Leben. **2.** (Menschen-)Leben *nt*. **to take s.b.'s ~** jdn. umbringen. **to take one's own ~** s. das Leben nehmen. **3.** Lebensdauer *f*, -zeit *f*, Leben *nt*. **4.** Lebensweise *f*, -wandel *m*, -art *f*. **5.** Leben *nt*, Schwung *m*. **full of ~** voller Leben, lebhaft, lebendig.
life-belt cataract *ophthal.* ringförmige/scheibenförmige Katarakt *f*.
life cycle Lebenszyklus *m*, Lebens-, Entwicklungsphase *f*.
life expectancy Lebenserwartung *f*.
life experience Lebenserfahrung *f*.
life force Lebenskraft *f*.
life·ful ['laɪfəl] *adj* lebhaft, lebendig, voller Leben.
life-giving *adj* lebenspendend.
life history Lebensgeschichte *f*; *bio.* Entwicklungsgeschichte *f*.
life instinct *psycho.* Geschlechts-, Sexualtrieb *m*.
life insurance Lebensversicherung *f*.
life island keimfreies Milieu *nt*, Life-island *nt*.
life·less ['laɪflɪs] *adj* **1.** leblos, tot. **2.** unbelebt. **3.** *fig.* matt, teilnahmslos.
life·line ['-laɪn] *n* (Hand) Lebenslinie *f*.
life-long ['-lɔːŋ, -lɑŋ] *adj* lebenslang.
life-saving **I** *n* Lebensrettung *f*. **II** *adj* lebensrettend, (Lebens-)Rettungs-.
life science Biowissenschaft *f*.
life space *psycho.* Lebensraum *m*.
life span ~ lifetime.
life style Lebensstil *m*, -wandel *m*.
life-sustaining measures lebenserhaltende Maßnahmen *pl*.
life table Sterblichkeitstabelle *f*.
life-threatening *adj* lebensbedrohlich, -gefährdend, -gefährlich.
life·time ['laɪftaɪm] *n* Leben *nt*, Lebenszeit *f*; (*a. techn.*) Lebensdauer *f*.
lig·a·ment ['lɪgəmənt] *n anat.* Band *nt*, Ligament *nt*, Ligamentum *nt*; Chorda *f*, Plica *f*.

l. of ankle (joint) Innenknöchelband, Außenknöchelband.
l.s of auditory ossicles Bänder *pl* der Gehörknöchelchen, Ligg. ossiculorum auditoriorum.
l.s of auricle Ohrmuschelbänder *pl*, Ligg. auricularia.
l. of Botallo Lig. arteriosum.
l.s of colon Kolontänien *pl*, Taeniae coli.
l. of Fallopius Leistenband, Lig. inguinale, Arcus inguinalis.
l. of head of femur Lig. capitis femoris.
l. of knee Knie(gelenks)band.
l.s of liver Leberbänder *pl*, Ligg. hepatis.
l. of Maissiat Maissiat-Band, Tractus iliotibialis.
l. of nape Nackenband, Lig. nuchae.
l.s of tarsus Lig. tarsi.
l.s of Valsalva → l.s of auricle.
l. of Vesalius Leistenband, Lig. inguinale, Arcus inguinalis.
lig·a·men·to·pex·is [lɪgə'mentəpeksɪs] *n* → ligamentopexy.
lig·a·men·to·pex·y [lɪgə'mentəpeksɪ] *n chir.*, *gyn.* Ligamentopexie *f*.
lig·a·men·tous ['lɪgəmentəs] *adj* Ligament betr., ligamentär, Band-.
ligamentous articulation Syndesmose *f*, Junctura fibrosa.
ligamentous joint → ligamentous articulation.
ligamentous membrane Membrana tectoria.
lig·a·men·tum [ˌlɪgə'mentəm] *n, pl* -**ta** [-tə] → ligament.
ligamentum arteriosum *embryo.* Lig. arteriosum.
ligamentum venosum *embryo.* Lig. venosum (Arantii).
li·gand ['laɪgənd, 'lɪ-] *n chem.*, *biochem.* Ligand *m*.
ligand specificity *chem.* Ligandenspezifität *f*.
li·gase ['laɪgeɪz] *n* Ligase *f*, Synthetase *f*.
li·gate ['laɪgeɪt] *vt chir.* ligieren, unterbinden.
li·ga·tion [laɪ'geɪʃn] *n chir.* Ligatur *f*, Unterbindung *f*.
lig·a·ture ['lɪgətʃər, -tʃʊər] *chir.* **I** *n* Ligatur *f*. **II** *vt* → ligate.
ligature groove *embryo.*, *gyn.* Schnürfurche *f*.
light¹ [laɪt] (*v* lighted; lit) **I** *n* Licht *nt*, Helligkeit *f*; Beleuchtung *f*, Licht(quelle *f*) *nt*; (Tages-)Licht *nt*. **II** *adj* hell, licht. **~ hair** helles Haar. **III** *vt* → light up.
light up *vt* anzünden; (*Licht*) anmachen; be-, erleuchten, erhellen.
light² [laɪt] *adj* (*a.* Nicht schwer); (*Schlaf*) leicht; (*Krankheit*) leicht, unbedeutend; (*Essen*) leicht (verdaulich); (*Aufgabe*) leicht, nicht schwierig. **a ~ eater** kein großer Esser.
light-absorbing *adj* lichtabsorbierend.
light-absorbing pigment lichtabsorbierendes Pigment *nt*.
light absorption Lichtabsorption *f*.
light-absorption spectrum (Licht-)Absorptionsspektrum *nt*.
light adaptation *ophthal.* Helladaptation *f*, -anpassung *f*.
light-adapted *adj ophthal.* helladaptiert.
light bath Lichtbad *nt*.
light cells (*Schilddrüse*) parafollikuläre Zellen *pl*, C-Zellen *pl*.
light chain *biochem.* leichte Kette *f*, Leichtkette *f*, L-Kette *f*.
light corpuscle *phys.* Lichtkorpuskel *nt*.
light-dark adaptation Hell-Dunkel-Adaptation *f*.
light-dark contrast Hell-Dunkel-Kontrast *m*.

light-dependent *adj* lichtabhängig.
light diaphragm (*Mikroskop*) Leuchtfeldblende *f*.
light emission *phys.* Lichtemission *f*.
light energy Lichtenergie *f*.
light-fast ['laɪtfæst, -fɑːst] *adj* lichtecht.
light-fast-ness ['-nɪs] *n* Lichtechtheit *f*.
light guide Glasfaser *f*, -fiber *f*.
light-headed *adj* (leicht) benommen.
light-headedness *n* (leichte) Benommenheit *f*.
light hydrogen leichter Wasserstoff *m*, Protium *nt*.
light-independent *adj* lichtunabhängig.
light-independent phosphorylation lichtunabhängige Phosphorylierung *f*.
light-induced *adj* lichtinduziert.
light-insensitive *adj* lichtunempfindlich.
light intensity Lichtintensität *f*.
light meromyosin *biochem.* leichtes Meromyosin *nt*, L-Meromyosin *nt*.
light metal Leichtmetall *nt*.
light meter *photo.* Belichtungsmesser *m*.
light microscope Lichtmikroskop *nt*.
light-ness ['laɪtnɪs] *n* Leichtheit *f*; Leichtigkeit *f*, geringes Gewicht *nt*; Leichtverdaulichkeit *f*.
light-ning ['laɪtnɪŋ] *n* Blitz *m*. **struck by ~** vom Blitz erschlagen.
lightning pain schießender Schmerz *m*.
lightning stroke Blitzschlag *m*.
light-proof ['laɪtpruːf] *adj* lichtundurchlässig, -dicht.
light quantum *phys.* Licht-, Strahlungsquant *nt*; Photon *nt*, Quant *nt*.
light reaction: l.s *pl biochem.* Lichtreaktionen *pl*, -phase *f*.
consensual l. *ophthal.* konsensuelle Lichtreaktion.
light receptor Lichtrezeptor *m*.
light-red *n* Hellrot *nt*.
light reflex 1. *HNO* Trommelfellreflex *m*, Lichtreflex *m*. **2.** *ophthal.* Lichtreflex *m*, -reaktion *f*.
direct l. direkter Lichtreflex *m*.
light response *physiol.* (*Auge*) Lichtreaktion *f*.
consensual l. konsensuelle Lichtreaktion.
direct l. direkte Lichtreaktion.
light scattering Lichtstreuung *f*.
light-sensitive *adj* lichtempfindlich.
light sensitive eruption *derm.* polymorphe Lichtdermatose (Haxthausen) *f*, polymorpher Lichtausschlag *m*, Sommerprurigo *f*, Prurigo aestivalis, Lupus-erythematodes-artige Lichtdermatose *f*, Lichtekzem *nt*, Eccema solare, Dermatopathia photoelectrica.
light sensitivity Lichtempfindlichkeit *f*.
light-skinned *adj* hellhäutig.
light sleep leichter Schlaf *m*.
light source Lichtquelle *f*.
light therapy Licht-, Phototherapie *f*.
light-tight ['laɪttaɪt] *adj Brit.* → lightproof.
light treatment → light therapy.
light urticaria Sonnen-, Sommer-, Lichturtikaria *f*, photoallergische Urtikaria *f*, Urticaria solaris/photogenica.
light waves Lichtwellen *pl*.
Lightwood ['laɪtwʊd]: **L.'s syndrome** Lightwood-Syndrom *nt*.
Lightwood-Albright ['ɔːlbraɪt]: **L.-A. syndrome** Lightwood-Albright-Syndrom *nt*.
Lignac ['lɪgnæk]: **L.'s disease/syndrome** → Lignac-Fanconi disease.
Lignac-Fanconi [fæn'kəʊnɪ]: **L.-F. disease** Lignac-Fanconi-Erkrankung *f*, -Krankheit *f*, Lignac-Syndrom *nt*, Aberhalden--Fanconi(-Lignac)-Syndrom *nt*, Zystinspeicherkrankheit *f*, Zystinose *f*, Cystinose *f*.
L.-F. syndrome → L.-F. disease.

lig-ne-ous ['lɪgnɪəs] *adj* holzartig, holzig, Holz-.
ligneous struma → ligneous thyroiditis.
ligneous thyroiditis eisenharte Struma *f*, Riedel-Struma *f*, chronisch hypertrophische Thyreoiditis *f*.
lig-nin ['lɪgnɪn] *n* Lignin *nt*.
lig-no-caine ['lɪgnəkeɪn] *n* → lidocaine.
lig-no-cer-ic acid [ˌlɪgnə'serɪk, -'sɪər-] Lignocerinsäure *f*, n-Tetracosansäure *f*.
lig-num ['lɪgnəm] *n* Holz *nt*, Lignum *nt*.
lig-ro-in ['lɪgrəwɪn] *n* Ligroin *nt*, Lackbenzin *nt*.
lig-ro-ine ['lɪgrəwiːn] *n* → ligroin.
lil-li-pu-tian [ˌlɪlɪ'pjuːʃn] **I** *n* Liliputaner(in *f*) *m*. **II** *adj* winzig, zwergenhaft.
lilliputian hallucination Liliput-Halluzination *f*.
limb [lɪm] *n* Glied *nt*, Gliedmaße *f*, Extremität *f*; *fig.* Arm *m*, Bein *m*; Ast *m*.
l.s of anthelix Anthelixschenkel *pl*, Crura anthelicis.
l.s of bony semicircular canales Crura ossea.
l. of helix Crus helicis.
lim-bal ['lɪmbl] *adj* → limbic.
limb amputation *ortho.* Gliedmaßenamputation *f*.
limb anomaly Gliedmaßenanomalie *f*, -fehlbildung *f*, Extremitätenanomalie *f*, -fehlbildung *f*.
limb bud *embryo.* Extremitätenknospe *f*, -anlage *f*, Gliedmaßenknospe *f*, -anlage *f*.
lower l. Beinknospe, -anlage.
upper l. Armknospe, -anlage.
lim-bic ['lɪmbɪk] *adj* Limbus betr., randständig, marginal, limbisch, Rand-.
limbic cortex limbische Rinde *f*, limbischer Cortex *m*.
limbic gyrus Gyrus cinguli/cingulatus.
limbic system limbisches System *nt*.
limb-kinetic apraxia gliedkinetische Apraxie *f*.
limb lead *physiol.* (*EKG*) Extremitätenableitung *f*.
Goldberger's augmented l.s Ableitungen *pl* nach Goldberger.
limb recording → limb lead.
lim-bus ['lɪmbəs] *n*, *pl* **-bi** [-baɪ] *anat.* **1.** Saum *m*, Rand *m*, Kante *f*, Limbus *m*. **2.** → l. of cornea.
l. of cornea Perikornealring *m*, Limbus corneae.
l. of spiral lamina Limbus laminae spiralis osseae.
lime [laɪm] *n* **1.** Kalziumoxid *nt*, Calciumoxid *nt*, gebrannter Kalk *m*. **2.** *bot.* Limone *f*, Limonelle *f*.
li-men ['laɪmən] *n*, *pl* **li-mens**, **lim-i-na** ['lɪmənə] *anat.*, *physiol.*, *psycho.* Grenze *f*, Schwelle *f*, Limen *nt*.
l. of insula Inselschwelle, Limen insulae.
limen nasi Limen nasi.
lime-stone ['laɪmstəʊn] *n* Kalkstein *m*.
lime-wa-ter ['-wɔːtər] *n* **1.** kalkhaltiges Wasser *nt*. **2.** Kalkmilch *f*, -lösung *f*.
lim-i-nal ['lɪmənl] *adj* Grenz-, Schwellen-, Limen-.
liminal stimulus Grenz-, Schwellenreiz *m*.
lim-it ['lɪmɪt] **I** *n* **1.** Grenze *f*; Begrenzung *f*, Beschränkung *f*, Limit *nt*. **off ~** Zutritt verboten (*to* für). **over the ~** zuviel; (*zeitlich*) zu lange. **to the ~** bis zum Letzten. **within ~s** bis zu einem gewissen Grade, in (gewissen) Grenzen. **without ~(s)** grenzenlos, unbeschränkt, unbegrenzt. **2.** Grenzlinie *f*, Grenze *f*. **3.** *mathe.* Grenzwert *m*. **II** *vt* begrenzen, ein-, beschränken (*to* auf); limittieren.
lim-i-ta-tion [ˌlɪmɪ'teɪʃn] *n* Ein-, Beschränkung *f*, Begrenzung *f*, Limitierung *f*, Limitation *f*.

lim-i-ta-tive ['lɪmɪteɪtɪv] *adj* begrenzend, ein-, beschränkend, limitativ.
limit dextrin Grenzdextrin *nt*.
limit dextrinase α-Dextrinase *f*, Oligo-1,6-α-Glukosidase *f*.
limit dextrinosis Cori-Krankheit *f*, Forbes-Syndrom *nt*, hepatomuskuläre benigne Glykogenose *f*, Glykogenose Typ III *f*.
lim-it-ed ['lɪmɪtɪd] *adj* begrenzt, beschränkt (*to* auf); lokalisiert, umschrieben. **~ in time** befristet.
lim-it-ing ['lɪmɪtɪŋ] *adj* ein-, beschränkend, Grenz-.
limiting angle *phys.* kritischer Einfallswinkel *m*, Grenzwinkel *m*.
limiting factor *physiol.* Begrenzungsfaktor *m*, limitierender Faktor *m*.
limiting lamina: anterior l. → limiting membrane, anterior.
posterior l. Descemet'-Membran *f*, hintere Basalmembran *f*, Lamina elastica posterior Descemeti, Lamina limitans posterior (corneae).
limiting membrane Grenzmembran *f*, -schicht *f*.
anterior l. Bowman'-Membran *f*, vordere Basalmembran *f*, Lamina elastica anterior (Bowmani), Lamina limitans anterior (corneae).
external l. äußere Grenzmembran *f*, Membrana limitans externa.
glial l., outer Membrana limitans gliae superficialis.
glial l., perivascular Membrana limitans gliae perivascularis.
glial l., superficial → glial l., outer.
Held's l. Blut-Hirn-Schranke *f*.
inner l. → internal l.
internal l. innere Grenzmembran *f*, Membrana limitans interna.
outer l. → external l.
posterior l. Descemet'-Membran *f*, hintere Basalmembran *f*, Lamina elastica posterior Descemeti, Lamina limitans posterior (corneae).
limiting ring: anterior l. vorderer Schwalbe'-Grenzring *m*.
posterior l. hinterer Schwalbe'-Grenzring *m*.
limiting sulcus: l. of brain Seitenfurche *f* des Großhirns, Sulcus limitans.
l. of Reil Sulcus circularis insulae.
l. of rhomboid fossa Seitenfurche *f* der Rautengrube, Sulcus limitans fossae rhomboideae.
limit-less ['lɪmɪtlɪs] *adj* grenzenlos.
Lim-na-tis ['lɪm'nætɪs] *n micro.* Limnatis *f*.
lim-ne-mia [lɪm'niːmɪə] *n* chronische Malaria *f*.
lim-o-nene ['lɪmənɪːn] *n chem.* Limonen *nt*.
li-mo-sis [laɪ'məʊsɪs] *n* abnormer/krankhafter Hunger *m*.
limp[1] [lɪmp] **I** *n* Hinken *nt*. **II** *vi* hinken, humpeln.
limp[2] [lɪmp] *adj* **1.** schlaff, schlapp. **2.** biegsam, weich.
limp chorea *neuro.* Chorea mollis.
lim-pid ['lɪmpɪd] *adj* durchsichtig, klar.
lim-pid-i-ty [lɪm'pɪdətɪ] *n* Durchsichtigkeit *f*, Klarheit *f*.
lim-pid-ness ['lɪmpɪdnɪs] *n* → limpidity.
limp-ness ['lɪmpnɪs] *n* Schlaff-, Schlappheit *f*.
lim-u-lus test ['lɪmjələs] Limulustest *m*.
lim-y ['laɪmɪ] *adj* kalkig, kalkartig, kalkhaltig, Kalk-.
limy bile *patho.* Kalk-, Kalkmilchgalle *f*.
lin-co-my-cin [ˌlɪŋkəʊ'maɪsɪn] *n pharm.* Lincomycin *nt*.
linc-ture ['lɪŋktʃər] *n pharm.* Linctus *m*.
linc-tus ['lɪŋktəs] *n pharm.* Linctus *m*.

lin·dane ['lɪndeɪn] n Benzolhexachlorid nt, Hexachlorcyclohexan nt abbr. HCH; Lindan nt.
Lindau ['lɪndaʊ]: **L.'s disease** (von) Hippel--Lindau-Syndrom nt, Netzhautangiomatose f, Angiomatosis retinae cystica, Angiomatosis cerebelli et retinae.
L.'s tumor Lindau-Tumor m, Hämangioblastom nt, Angioblastom nt.
Lindau-von Hippel [vɒn 'hɪpəl]: **L.-v. H. disease** → Lindau's disease.
line¹ [laɪn] I n 1. anat. Linie f, Grenzlinie f, Linea f. 2. (Hand-)Linie f; (Gesichts-)Falte f, Runzel f; (Gesichts-)Zug m. 3. Linie f, Strich m. 4. Linie f, Richtung f; fig. Taktik f; ~s pl Richtlinien pl. 5. Methode f, Verfahren nt. 6. Grenze f, Grenzlinie f. 7. Leine f, Schnur f. 8. Reihe f, Linie f. **in ~** in Übereinstimmung (with mit). **to be in ~** übereinstimmen (with mit). **to be out of ~** nicht übereinstimmen (with mit). 9. (Abstammungs-)Linie f, Geschlecht nt. **the male ~** die männl. Linie. **in direct ~** in direkter Linie. II vt 10. (Gesicht) (zer-)furchen, zeichnen. 11. (ein-)säumen.
line off vt abgrenzen.
l. of Amici Z-Linie f, Z-Streifen m, Zwischenscheibe f, Telophragma f.
l. of attachment Ansatz-, Befestigungsstelle f, -linie f.
l. of demarcation Grenz-, Demarkationslinie f.
l. of Gennari Gennari'-Streifen m.
l. of intersection Schnittlinie f.
l.s of orientation anat. Orientierungslinien pl.
l. of origin Ursprung m, Ursprungsstelle f, -linie f.
l.s of Owen dent. Owen'-Linien pl.
l. of reasoning Denkweise f.
l.s of Retzius dent. Retzius'-Streifung f.
l.s of Schreger Schreger-Hunter'-Linien pl.
l.s of tension Spannungslinien pl.
l. of thought Auffassung f, Denkrichtung f, -weise f.
l. of vision ophthal. optische Augenachse f, Sehachse f, Axis opticus.
line² [laɪn] vt auskleiden, (aus-)füttern, überziehen. **~d with** ausgekleidet mit.
lin·ea ['lɪnɪə] n, pl **lin·e·ae** [-niː] anat. Linie f, Linea f.
linea alba Linea alba (abdominis).
linea aspera Linea aspera (femoris).
lin·e·age ['lɪnɪɪdʒ] n Geschlecht nt, Abstammung f.
lin·e·al measure ['lɪnɪəl] Längenmaß nt.
lin·e·a·ments ['lɪnɪəmənts] pl (Gesichts-)Züge pl, Konturen pl.
lin·e·ar ['lɪnɪər] adj 1. geradlinig, linear, Linear-; Längen-. 2. linienförmig, Strich-, Linien-.
linear acceleration phys. Linearbeschleunigung f.
linear fracture längsverlaufende Fraktur f.
linear measure → lineal measure.
linear morphea derm. lineare Sklerodermie f, bandförmige zirkumskripte Sklerodermie f, Morphea linearis.
linear movement phys. Linearbewegung f.
linear nucleus: intermediate l. Nc. linearis intermedius.
superior l. Nc. linearis superior.
linear osteotomy ortho. lineare Osteotomie f.
linear scleroderma → linear morphea.
linear vection Linearvektion f.
line-breed vi reinzüchten.
line-breed·ing ['laɪnbriːdɪŋ] n Reinzucht f, Linienzucht f.

lined [laɪnd] adj (Gesicht) faltig, gezeichnet.
lin·en ['lɪnən] I n Leinen nt, Leinwand f; (Bett-)Wäsche f. II adj leinen, Leinen-.
line spectrum phys. Linienspektrum nt.
L-I neuron → late-inspiratory neuron.
Lineweaver-Burk ['laɪnwiːvər bɜrk]: **L.-B. equation** Lineweaver-Burk-Gleichung f.
L.-B. plot Lineweaver-Burk-Darstellung f.
lingu- pref. → linguo-.
lin·gua ['lɪŋgwə] n, pl **-guae** [-gwiː] Zunge f; anat. Lingua f, Glossa f.
lin·gual ['lɪŋgwəl] adj lingual, Zungen-, Lingual-.
lingual aponeurosis Zungenaponeurose f, Aponeurosis lingualis.
lingual artery Zungenschlagader f, -arterie f, Lingualis f, A. lingualis.
deep l. tiefe Zungenschlagader/-arterie, A. profunda linguae.
lingual bone Zungenbein nt, Os hyoideum.
lingual branch: dorsal l.es of lingual artery Rami dorsales linguae a. lingualis.
l. of facial nerve Zungenast m des N. facialis, Ramus lingualis n. facialis.
l.es of glossopharyngeal nerve Zungenäste pl des N. glossopharyngeus, Rami linguales n. glossopharyngei.
l.es of hypoglossal nerve Zungenäste pl des N. hypoglossus, Rami linguales n. hypoglossi.
l.es of lingual nerve Zungenäste pl des N. lingualis, Rami linguales n. lingualis.
lingual follicle Zungenbalg m, Folliculus lingualis.
lingual frenotomy HNO Zungenbändchendurchtrennung f, Frenulotomie f, Frenotomie f, Ankylotomie f.
lingual frenulum/frenum Zungenbändchen nt, Frenulum linguae.
lingual gland: l.s pl Zungen(speichel)drüsen pl, Gll. linguales.
anterior l. (Blandin-)Nuhn'-Drüse f, Gl. lingualis anterior, Gl. apicis linguae.
lingual goiter Zungengrundstruma f, Struma baseos linguae.
lingual gyrus Gyrus lingualis.
lingual mucosa Zungenschleimhaut f, Tunica mucosa linguae.
lingual muscles Zungenmuskeln pl, -muskulatur f, Mm. linguae.
lingual nerve Lingualis m, N. lingualis.
lingual papillae Zungenpapillen pl, Papillae linguales.
lingual paralysis Zungenlähmung f.
lingual plexus vegetativer Plexus m der A. lingualis.
lingual septum Zungenseptum nt, Septum linguale.
lingual spatula Zungenspatel m.
lingual swellings embryo. Zungenwülste pl.
lingual thyroid Zungengrundschilddrüse f.
lingual titubation Stammeln nt; Stottern nt.
lingual tonsil Zungen(grund)mandel f, Tonsilla lingualis.
lingual trophoneurosis halbseitiger Zungenschwund m, Hemiatrophia linguae.
lingual vein Zungenvene f, V. lingualis.
deep l. tiefe Zungenvene, V. profunda linguae.
dorsal l.s Zungenrückenvenen pl, Vv. dorsales linguae.
lingual villi fadenförmige Papillen pl, Papillae filiformis.
Lin·guat·u·la [lɪŋ'gwætʃələ] n micro. Zungenwurm m, Linguatula f.
L. rhinaria/serrata Nasenwurm m, Linguatula serrata.

lin·guat·u·li·a·sis [lɪŋˌgwætʃə'laɪəsɪs] n Linguatula-Infektion f, Linguatuliasis f.
Lin·gua·tu·li·dae [ˌlɪŋgwə't(j)uːlədɪ] pl micro. Linguatulidae pl.
lin·guat·u·lo·sis [lɪŋˌgwætʃə'ləʊsɪs] n → linguatuliasis.
lin·gui·form ['lɪŋgwəfɔːrm] adj zungenförmig.
linguiform lobe (Leber) Riedel'-Lappen m.
lin·gu·la ['lɪŋgjələ] n, pl **-lae** [-liː] anat. Zünglein nt, zungenförmiges Gebilde nt, Lingula f.
l. of cerebellum Lingula, Lingula cerebelli.
l. of (left) lung Lungenzipfel m, Lingula pulmonis (sinistri).
l. of mandible Lingula mandibulae.
l. of sphenoid bone Lingula sphenoidalis.
lin·gu·lar ['lɪŋgjələr] adj Lingula betr., zungenförmig, Lingular-.
lingular branch of left pulmonary artery: inferior l. Ramus lingularis inferior a. pulmonalis sinistrae.
superior l. Ramus lingularis superior a. pulmonalis sinistrae.
lingular bronchus: inferior l. Bronchus lingularis inferior.
superior l. Bronchus lingularis superior.
lingular segment of (left) lung: inferior l. (Lunge) unteres Lingularsegment nt, Segmentum lingulare inferius [S. V].
superior l. (Lunge) oberes Lingularsegment nt, Segmentum lingulare superius [S. IV].
lin·gu·late ['lɪŋgjəlɪt, -leɪt] adj zungenförmig.
lin·gu·lat·ed ['lɪŋgjəleɪtɪd] adj → lingulate.
lin·gu·lec·to·my [lɪŋgjə'lektəmɪ] n HTG Lingulektomie f, Resektion f der Lingula pulmonis.
linguo- pref. Zungen-, Linguo(-).
lin·guo·cer·vi·cal ridge [ˌlɪŋgwə'sɜrvɪkəl] dent. Cingulum nt.
lin·guo·den·tal [ˌ-'dentl] adj Zunge und Zähne betr., linguodental.
lin·guo·fa·cial trunk [ˌ-'feɪʃl] Truncus linguofacialis.
lin·guo·gin·gi·val ridge [ˌ-dʒɪn'dʒaɪvl, -'dʒɪndʒə-] dent. Cingulum nt.
lin·guo·pap·il·li·tis [ˌ-pæpɪ'laɪtɪs] n Entzündung f der Zungenrandpapillen, Linguopapillitis f.
lin·i·ment ['lɪnəmənt] n pharm. Liniment nt, Linimentum nt.
lin·i·men·tum [lɪnə'mentəm] n → liniment.
li·nin ['laɪnɪn] n Linin nt.
lin·ing ['laɪnɪŋ] n Belag m, Überzug m; Auskleidung f; Deckschicht f; (Aus-)Fütterung f.
lining cell 1. → lining cell of alveoli. 2. wandständiger Makrophage m von Blut- u. Lymphsinus.
l. of alveoli Deckzelle f, Alveolarzelle f Typ I, Pneumozyt m Typ I.
li·ni·tis [lɪ'naɪtɪs, laɪ-] n patho. Linitis f.
link [lɪŋk] I n (Binde-, Ketten-, Befestigungs-)Glied nt, Verbindung(stück nt) f, Bindung f. II vt verbinden, verknüpfen (to, with mit). III vi s. verbinden, s. verknüpfen (to with mit).
link up I vt → link II. II vi → link III.
link·age ['lɪŋkɪdʒ] n 1. chem. Bindung f (to an). 2. Verkettung f, Verbindung f, Verknüpfung f. 3. bio. Kopplung f.
link-up ['lɪŋkʌp] n → linkage 2.
Li·nog·na·thus [lɪ'nɒgnəθəs] n micro. Linognathus m.
li·no·le·ate [lɪ'nəʊlɪeɪt] n Linoleat nt.
lin·o·le·ic acid [lɪnə'liːɪk, lɪ'nəʊ-] Linolsäure f, Leinölsäure f.
lin·o·le·nic acid [lɪnə'liːnɪk, -'len-] Linolensäure f.

linolic acid

li·no·lic acid [lɪˈnəʊlɪk] → linoleic acid.
lin·seed [ˈlɪnsiːd] n bot. Leinsamen m.
linseed oil Leinöl nt.
Lin·sto·wi·i·dae [lɪnstəˈwaɪədiː] pl micro. Linstowiidae pl.
Linton-Nachlas [ˈlɪntn ˈnæxlæs]: L.-N. tube Linton-Nachlas-Sonde f.
li·num [ˈlaɪnəm] n linseed.
li·o·thy·ro·nine [laɪəʊˈθaɪrəniːn] n pharm. Liothyronin nt.
lip- pref. → lipo-.
lip [lɪp] I n 1. Lippe f; anat. Labium oris. 2. anat. lippenähnliche Struktur f, Labium nt, Labrum nt. 3. Rand m; Wundrand m. 4. (Gefäß) Schnabel m, Tülle f. 5. techn. Schneide f. II adj Lippen-.
lip·ac·i·de·mia [lɪpæsəˈdiːmɪə] n Lipazidämie f, Hyperlipazidämie f.
lip·ac·i·du·ri·a [lɪpæsəˈd(j)ʊərɪə] n Lipazidurie f.
lip·ar·o·cele [ˈlɪpˈærəsiːl] n 1. Fettbruch m, Liparozele f, Lipozele f, Adipozele f. 2. urol. Liparozele f, Lipozele f.
lip·a·roid [ˈlɪpərɔɪd] adj fettig, fettartig, lipoid.
li·pase [ˈlaɪpeɪz, ˈlɪ-] n 1. Lipase f. 2. Triacylglycerinlipase f, Triglyceridlipase f.
li·pa·sic [laɪˈpeɪsɪk] adj 1. Lipase betr., Lipase-. 2. → lipolytic.
lip·as·u·ria [ˌlɪpeɪˈs(j)ʊərɪə, laɪ-] n Lipaseausscheidung f im Harn, Lipasurie f.
lip·ec·to·my [lɪˈpektəmɪ] n chir. Fett(gewebs)entfernung f, Lipektomie f.
lip·e·de·ma [lɪpɪˈdiːmə] n Lipödem nt.
li·pe·mia [lɪˈpiːmɪə, laɪ-] n Lipämie f, Lipaemia f, Hyperlipämie f.
lip·id [ˈlɪpɪd, ˈlaɪ-] n Lipid nt.
lipid A Lipid A nt.
lip·i·dase [ˈlɪpɪdeɪz] n → lipase 1.
lipid-containing viruses lipidhaltige Viren pl.
lipid dermatoarthritis multiple Retikulohistiozytome pl, multizentrische Retikulohistiozytose f, Lipoiddermatoarthritis f, Reticulohistiocytosis disseminata.
lipid digestion Fettverdauung f, -digestion f.
lip·ide [ˈlɪpaɪd, ˈlaɪ-, -ɪd] n → lipid.
lip·i·de·mia [lɪpɪˈdiːmɪə] n Lipidämie f, Hyperlipidämie f.
lipid granulomatosis Xanthomatose f.
lipid hormone Lipidhormon nt.
li·pid·ic [lɪˈpɪdɪk] adj Lipid(e) betr. od. enthaltend, Lipid-, Lipo-.
lipid membrane Lipidmembran nt.
lipid metabolism Lipidstoffwechsel m, -metabolismus m.
lipid nephrosis → lipoid nephrosis.
lip·i·dol [ˈlɪpɪdɑl] n Fett-, Lipidalkohol m.
lip·i·dol·y·sis [lɪpɪˈdɑləsɪs] n Lipidspaltung f, Lipidolyse f.
lip·i·do·lyt·ic [ˌlɪpɪdəˈlɪtɪk] adj Lipidolyse betr. od. verursachend, lipidolytisch.
lip·i·do·sis [lɪpɪˈdəʊsɪs] n → lipid storage disease.
lipid pneumonia Lipidpneumonie f, Öl-, Fettaspirationspneumonie f.
lipid proteinosis → lipoproteinosis.
lipid-soluble adj lipidlöslich.
lipid storage disease Lipidspeicherkrankheit f, Lipidose f, Lipoidose f.
lipid storage myopathy Lipidspeichermyopathie f.
lip·id·u·ria [lɪpɪˈd(j)ʊərɪə] n Lipidausscheidung f im Harn, Lipidurie f, Lipurie f.
lip-in [ˈlɪpɪn, ˈlaɪ-] n lipid.
lipo- pref. Fett-, Lip(o)-.
lip·o·ad·e·no·ma [ˌlɪpəˌædəˈnəʊmə] n Lipoadenom nt.
lip·o·am·ide [ˌ-ˈæmaɪd, -mɪd] n Lip(o)amid nt.

lipoamide dehydrogenase Lip(o)amiddehydrogenase f, Dihydrolipoyldehydrogenase f.
lip·o·a·mi·no acid [ˌ-əˈmiːnəʊ] Lipoaminsäure f, O-Aminoacylphosphatidylglycin nt.
lip·o·ar·thri·tis [ˌ-ɑːrˈθraɪtɪs] n ortho. Entzündung f des periartikulären Fettgewebes, Lipoarthritis f.
lip·o·ate acetyltransferase [ˈlɪpəʊeɪt] Lipoatacetyltransferase f, Dihydrolipoyltransacetylase f.
lip·o·a·tro·phia [ˌlɪpəəˈtrəʊfɪə] n → lipoatrophy.
lip·o·a·troph·ic diabetes [ˌ-ˈtrəʊfɪk, -ˈtrɑf-] 1. Lawrence-Syndrom nt, lipatrophischer Diabetes m. 2. → lipoatrophy 1.
lip·o·at·ro·phy [ˌ-ˈætrəfɪ] n 1. Fettgewebsschwund m, Atrophie f, Lipoatrophie f, Lipatrophie f, Lipoatrophia f, Lipatrophia f. 2. → lipodystrophy.
lip·o·blast [ˈ-blæst] n Lipoblast m.
lip·o·blas·tic lipoma [ˌ-ˈblæstɪk] → liposarcoma.
lip·o·blas·to·ma [ˌ-blæsˈtəʊmə] n 1. Lipoblastom(a) nt. 2. → liposarcoma.
lip·o·cal·ci·gran·u·lo·ma·to·sis [ˌ-ˌkælsɪˌgrænjəˌləʊməˈtəʊsɪs] n Lipokalzinogranulomatose f, Calcinosis universalis interstitialis.
lip·o·cat·a·bol·ic [ˌ-ˌkætəˈbɑlɪk] adj Fettabbau betr. od. fördernd, lipokatabol(isch).
lip·o·cele [ˈ-siːl] n → liparocele 1.
lip·o·cere [ˈ-sɪər] n Fettwachs nt, Leichenwachs nt, Adipocire f.
lip·o·chon·dro·dys·tro·phy [ˌ-ˌkɑndrəˈdɪstrəfɪ] n Hurler-Krankheit f, -Syndrom nt, von Pfaundler-Hurler-Krankheit f, -Syndrom nt, Lipochondrodystrophie f, Dysostosis multiplex, Mukopolysaccharidose I-H f abbr. MPS I-H.
lip·o·chon·dro·ma [ˌ-kɑnˈdrəʊmə] n Lipochondrom(a) nt, benignes Mesenchymom nt.
lip·o·chrome [ˈ-krəʊm] n Lipochrom nt, Lipoidpigment nt.
lip·o·chro·me·mia [ˌ-krəʊˈmiːmɪə] n Lipochromämie f.
lipochrome pigment → lipochrome.
lip·o·chro·mo·gen [ˌ-ˈkrəʊmədʒən] n Lipochromogen nt.
li·poc·la·sis [lɪˈpɑkləsɪs] n → lipolysis.
lip·o·clas·tic [ˌlɪpəˈklæstɪk] adj → lipolytic.
lip·o·cyte [ˈ-saɪt] n 1. Fett(gewebs)zelle f, Lipozyt m, Adipozyt m. 2. (Leber) Fettspeicherzelle f.
lip·o·di·er·e·sis [ˌ-daɪˈerəsɪs] n → lipolysis.
lip·o·di·e·ret·ic [ˌ-daɪəˈretɪk] adj → lipolytic.
lip·o·dys·tro·phia [ˌ-dɪˈstrəʊfɪə] n → lipodystrophy.
lip·o·dys·tro·phy [ˌ-ˈdɪstrəfɪ] n Lipodystrophie f, Lipodystrophia f.
li·pof·er·ous [lɪˈpɑfərəs] adj fettleitend, -transportierend.
lip·o·fi·bro·ma [ˌlɪpəfaɪˈbrəʊmə] n Lipofibrom(a) nt.
lip·o·fus·cin [ˌ-ˈfʌsɪn, -ˈfjuːsɪn] n 1. Abnutzungspigment nt, Lipofuszin nt. 2. → lipochrome.
lip·o·fus·ci·no·sis [ˌ-ˌfjuːsəˈnəʊsɪs] n Lipofuszinose f.
lip·o·gen·e·sis [ˌ-ˈdʒenəsɪs] n Fett(bio)synthese f, Lipogenese f.
lip·o·ge·net·ic [ˌ-dʒəˈnetɪk] adj → lipogenic.
lip·o·gen·ic [ˌ-ˈdʒenɪk] adj fettbildend od. -produzierend, lipogen.
lip·og·e·nous [lɪˈpɑdʒənəs] adj Fettleibigkeit verursachend.
lip·o·gran·u·lo·ma [ˌ-ˌgrænjəˈləʊmə] n Lipogranulom nt, Oleogranulom nt.

lip·o·gran·u·lo·ma·to·sis [ˌ-ˌgrænjəˌləʊməˈtəʊsɪs] n Lipogranulomatose f.
lip·o·he·mar·thro·sis [ˌ-ˌhiːmɑːrˈθrəʊsɪs] n ortho. Lipohämarthros m, Lipohämarthrose f.
lip·o·he·mia [ˌ-ˈhiːmɪə] n → lipemia.
lip·o·hy·a·lin [ˌ-ˈhaɪəlɪn] n Lipohyalin nt.
li·po·ic acid [lɪˈpəʊɪk] Liponsäure f, Thiooctansäure f.
lip·oid [ˈlɪpɔɪd, ˈlaɪ-] I n 1. biochem. Lipoid nt. 2. → lipid. II adj fettartig, -ähnlich, lipoid.
lip·oi·dal [lɪˈpɔɪdl, laɪ-] adj → lipoid II.
lipoidal degeneration lipoide Degeneration f.
lipoid dermatoarthritis multiple Retikulohistiozytome pl, multizentrische Retikulohistiozytose f, Lipoiddermatoarthritis f, Reticulohistiocytosis disseminata.
lip·oi·de·mia [ˌ-ˈdiːmɪə] n → lipemia.
lipoid granuloma Lipoidgranulom nt.
lipoid granulomatosis Xanthomatose f.
lipoid histiocytoma Fibroxanthom(a) nt.
li·poid·ic [lɪˈpɔɪdɪk] adj → lipoid II.
lipoid nephrosis Lipoidnephrose f, Lipidnephrose f, Minimal-change-Glomerulonephritis f.
li·poi·do·lyt·ic [lɪˌpɔɪdəˈlɪtɪk] adj → lipidolytic.
li·poi·do·sis [lɪpɔɪˈdəʊsɪs] n 1. → lipid storage disease. 2. Lipoidose f.
lipoid pneumonia → lipoid pneumonia.
lipoid proteinosis → lipoproteinosis.
lip·oid·pro·tein·o·sis [ˌlɪpɔɪdˌprəʊtiːˈnəʊsɪs] n → lipoproteinosis.
lip·oid·sid·er·o·sis [ˌ-sɪdəˈrəʊsɪs] n Lip(o)idsiderose f.
lipoid thesaurismosis → lipid storage disease.
lip·oi·du·ria [lɪpɔɪˈd(j)ʊərɪə] n → lipiduria.
lip·o·lip·oi·do·sis [ˌlɪpəˌlɪpɔɪˈdəʊsɪs] n Lipolipoidose f.
li·pol·y·sis [lɪˈpɑləsɪs] n Fettspaltung f, -abbau m, Lipolyse f.
lip·o·lyt·ic [lɪpəˈlɪtɪk] adj Lipolyse betr. od. verursachend, lipolytisch.
li·po·ma [lɪˈpəʊmə] n, pl -mas, -ma·ta [-mətə] Fett(gewebs)geschwulst f, -tumor m, Lipom(a) nt.
li·pom·a·toid [lɪˈpɑmətɔɪd] adj lipomartig, -ähnlich, lipomatös.
li·pom·a·to·sis [lɪˌpəʊməˈtəʊsɪs] n Lipomatose f, Lipomatosis f.
li·pom·a·tous [lɪˈpɑmətəs] adj → lipomatoid.
lipomatous myxoma Myxoma lipomatodes.
lipomatous nevus Nävolipom nt, Naevus lipomatosus.
lip·o·mel·a·not·ic reticulosis [ˌlɪpəʊmeləˈnɑtɪk] derm. Pautrier-Woringer-Syndrom nt, dermatopathische Lymphopathie/Lymphadenitis f, lipomelanotische Retikulose f.
lip·o·me·nin·go·cele [ˌ-mɪˈnɪŋgəsiːl] n Lipomeningozele f.
lip·o·me·tab·o·lic [ˌ-metəˈbɑlɪk] adj Fettstoffwechsel betr., lipometabolisch.
lip·o·me·tab·o·lism [ˌ-məˈtæbəlɪzəm] n Fettstoffwechsel m, -metabolismus m.
lip·o·mi·cron [ˌ-ˈmaɪkrɑn] n Lipomikron nt, Chylomikron nt.
lip·o·mu·co·pol·y·sac·cha·ri·do·sis [ˌ-ˌmjuːkəʊˌpɑlɪsækərɪˈdəʊsɪs] n Mukolipidose I f, Lipomukopolysaccharidose f.
lip·o·my·o·he·man·gi·o·ma [ˌ-ˌmaɪəʊhɪˌmændʒɪˈəʊmə] n Lipomyohämangiom nt.
lip·o·my·o·ma [ˌ-maɪˈəʊmə] n Lipomyom(a) nt.
lip·o·myx·o·ma [ˌ-mɪksˈəʊmə] n Lipomyxom(a) nt.

lip·o·ne·phro·sis [ˌ-nɪˈfrəʊsɪs] *n* → lipoid nephrosis.
lip·o·nu·cle·o·pro·tein [ˌ-ˌn(j)uːklɪəʊˈprəʊtiːn, -tiːɪn] *n* Liponukleoprotein *nt*.
li·pop·a·thy [lɪˈpəpəθɪ] *n* Fettstoffwechselstörung *f*, Lipopathie *f*.
lip·o·pec·tic [ˌlɪpəˈpektɪk] *adj* Lipopexie betr., lipopektisch.
lip·o·pe·nia [ˌ-ˈpiːnɪə] *n* Lipidmangel *m*, Lipopenie *f*.
lip·o·pe·nic [ˌ-ˈpiːnɪk] *adj* Lipopenie betr., von Lipopenie betroffen, durch Lipopenie gekennzeichnet, lipopenisch.
lip·o·pep·tid [ˌ-ˈpeptɪd] *n* Lipopeptid *nt*.
lip·o·pex·ia [ˌ-ˈpeksɪə] *n* Fettspeicherung *f*, -einlagerung *f*, Lipopexie *f*.
lip·o·pex·ic [ˌ-ˈpeksɪk] *adj* → lipopectic.
lip·o·phage [ˈ-feɪdʒ] *n* Lipophage *m*.
lip·o·pha·gia [ˌ-ˈfeɪdʒɪə] *n* → lipophagy.
lip·o·phag·ic [ˌ-ˈfædʒɪk] *adj* Lipophagie betr., lipophagisch.
lipophagic granuloma lipophages Granulom *nt*, Lipogranulom *nt*.
lipophagic intestinal granulomatosis Whipple'-Krankheit *f*, Morbus Whipple *m*, intestinale Lipodystrophie *f*, lipophage Intestinalgranulomatose *f*, Lipodystrophia intestinalis.
li·poph·a·gy [lɪˈpəfədʒɪ] *n* Lipophagie *f*.
lip·o·phan·er·o·sis [ˌlɪpəˌfænəˈrəʊsɪs, ˌlaɪpə-] *n* Fett-, Lipophanerose *f*.
lip·o·phil [ˈ-fɪl] *n* lipophile Substanz *f*.
lip·o·phile [ˈ-faɪl] *adj* → lipophilic.
lip·o·phil·ia [ˌ-ˈfiːlɪə] *n* 1. *chem.* Fettlöslichkeit *f*, Lipophilie *f*. 2. Neigung *f* zu Fettleibigkeit, Lipophilie *f*.
lip·o·phil·ic [ˌ-ˈfɪlɪk] *adj* Lipohilie betr., lipophil.
lip·o·pol·y·sac·cha·ride [ˌ-ˌpəlɪˈsækəraɪd, -rɪd] *n abbr.* **LPS** Lipopolysaccharid *nt abbr.* LPS.
lip·o·pro·tein [ˌ-ˈprəʊtiːn, -tiːɪn] *n* Lipoprotein *nt*.
α-lipoprotein *n* Lipoprotein *nt* mit hoher Dichte, α-Lipoprotein *nt*, high-density lipoprotein *abbr.* HDL, α-Lipoprotein *nt*.
β-lipoprotein *n* Lipoprotein *nt* mit geringer Dichte, β-Lipoprotein *nt*, low-density lipoprotein *abbr.* LDL.
lipoprotein electrophoresis *lab.* Lipoproteinelektrophorese *f*.
lipoprotein lipase *abbr.* **LPL** Lipoproteinlipase *f abbr.* LPL.
lipoprotein-X *n* Lipoprotein X *nt abbr.* LP-X.
lip·o·pro·tein·e·mia [ˌ-ˌprəʊtɪˈniːmɪə] *n* Lipoproteinämie *f*.
α-lipoproteinemia *n* Tangier-Krankheit *f*, Analphalipoproteinämie *f*, Hypo-Alpha--Lipoproteinämie *f*.
β-lipoproteinemia *n* Abetalipoproteinämie *f*, A-Beta-Lipoproteinämie *f*, Bassen-Kornzweig-Syndrom *nt*.
lip·o·pro·tein·o·sis [ˌ-ˌprəʊtɪˈnəʊsɪs] *n* Urbach-Wiethe-Syndrom *nt*, Lipoidproteinose (Urbach-Wiethe) *f*, Hyalinosis cutis et mucosae.
lip·o·sar·co·ma [ˌ-saːrˈkəʊmə] *n* Liposarkom *nt*, Liposarcoma *nt*.
li·po·sis [lɪˈpəʊsɪs] *n* → lipomatosis.
lip·o·si·tol [lɪˈpəʊsɪtəl, -təʊl] *n* Inosit *nt*, Inositol *nt*.
lip·o·sol·u·ble [ˌlɪpəˈsɒljəbl] *adj* fettlöslich.
lip·o·some [ˈ-səʊm] *n* Liposom *nt*.
lip·o·tei·cho·ic acid [ˌ-taɪˈkəʊɪk] *n* Lipoteichonsäure *f*.
lip·o·troph·ic [ˌ-ˈtrɒfɪk, -ˈtrəʊ-] *adj* Lipotrophie betr., lipotroph(isch).
li·pot·ro·phy [lɪˈpətrəfɪ] *n* Lipotrophie *f*.
lip·o·trop·ic [ˌlɪpəˈtrəpɪk, -ˈtrəʊ-] *adj* mit besonderer Affinität zu Fett, lipotrop.

β-lip·o·tro·pin [ˌ-ˈtrəʊpɪn] *n* β-Lipotropin *f*.
li·pot·ro·pism [lɪˈpətrəpɪzəm] *n* Lipotropie *f*.
li·pot·ro·py [lɪˈpətrəpɪ] *n* → lipotropism.
li·pox·i·dase [lɪˈpɒksɪdeɪz] *n* → lipoxygenase.
li·pox·y·ge·nase [lɪˈpɒksɪdʒɪneɪz] *n* Lipoxygenase *f*.
lipoxygenase pathway *biochem.* Lipoxygenaseweg *m*.
lip·o·yl transacetylase [ˈlɪpəwɪl] → lipoate acetyltransferase.
lip·pa [ˈlɪpə] *n* → lippitude.
lipped [lɪpt] *adj* 1. eine Lippe *od.* Lippen habend, -lippig; lippenförmig. 2. mit einem Schnabel *od.* Tülle versehen, gerandet.
lip·pi·tude [ˈlɪpət(j)uːd] *n ophthal.* Triefauge *nt*, Lidrandentzündung *f*, Lippitudo *f*, Blepharitis ciliaris/marginalis.
lip·pi·tu·do [lɪpəˈt(j)uːdəʊ] *n* → lippitude.
lip-read [ˈlɪpriːd] *vt*, *vi* von den Lippen ablesen.
lip-read·ing [ˈ-riːdɪŋ] *n* Lippenlesen *nt*.
lip reflex *ped.* Lippenreflex *m*.
Lipschütz [ˈlɪpʃɪts; -ʃʏts]: **L. bodies** Lipschütz'-Körperchen *pl*.
L.'s cell Zentrozyt *m*.
L.'s disease/ulcer Ulcus vulvae acutum (Lipschütz).
lip-smacking automatisms *neuro.* Schmatzautomatismen *pl*.
li·pu·ria [lɪˈp(j)ʊərɪə] *n* Lipidausscheidung *f* im Harn, Lipurie *f*, Lipidurie *f*.
li·pu·ric [lɪˈp(j)ʊərɪk] *adj* Lipidurie betr., lipurisch, lipidurisch.
liq·ue·fa·cient [ˌlɪkwəˈfeɪʃənt] **I** *n* Verflüssigungsmittel *nt*. **II** *adj* verflüssigend.
liq·ue·fac·tion [ˌ-ˈfækʃn] *n* Verflüssigung *f*, Liquefaktion *f*; Schmelzung *f*.
liquefaction degeneration → liquefaction necrosis.
liquefaction necrosis Kolliquationsnekrose *f*.
liq·ue·fac·tive [ˌ-ˈfæktɪv] *adj* verflüssigend.
liq·ue·fi·a·ble [ˌ-ˈfaɪəbl] *adj* verflüssigbar; schmelzbar.
liq·ue·fi·er [ˈ-faɪər] *n* Verflüssiger *m*, Verflüssigungsapparat *m*.
liq·ue·fy [ˈ-faɪ] **I** *vt* verflüssigen, liqueszieren; schmelzen. **II** *vi* verflüssigen, liqueszieren; schmelzen.
li·quesce [lɪˈkwes] *vt*, *vi* → liquefy.
li·ques·cent [lɪˈkwesnt] *adj s.* verflüssigend; schmelzend.
liq·uid [ˈlɪkwɪd] **I** *n* 1. Flüssigkeit *f*. 2. Schwing-, Schmelz-, Fließlaut *m*, Liquida (laut *m*), Liquida *f*. **II** *adj* 3. flüssig, liquid(e), Flüssigkeits-. 4. klar, wässrig, durchsichtig, transparent. 5. Liquid(laut) darstellend, liquid.
liquid air flüssige Luft *f*.
liquid body flüssiger Körper *m*.
liquid chromatography Flüssigkeitschromatographie *f*.
high-performance l. (Hoch-)Druckflüssigkeitschromatographie *f*.
high-pressure l. *abbr.* **HPLC** → high-performance l.
liquid crystal Flüssigkristall *m*, flüssiger Kristall *m*.
liquid extract flüssiger Extrakt *m*, Extractum fluidum/liquidum.
liquid-in-glass thermometer Flüssigkeitsthermometer *nt*.
li·quid·i·ty [lɪˈkwɪdətɪ] *n* 1. flüssiger Zustand *m*. 2. Klarheit *f*, Transparenz *f*.
liquid-liquid chromatography Flüssigkeits-Flüssigkeitschromatographie *f*, Verteilungschromatographie *f*.

liquid oxygen flüssiger Sauerstoff *m*, Flüssigsauerstoff *m*.
liquid phase flüssige Phase *f*.
liquid water flüssiges Wasser *nt*, Wasser *nt* in flüssigem Zustand.
liq·ui·fy [ˈlɪkwɪfaɪ] *vt*, *vi* → liquefy.
liq·uor [ˈlɪkər; ˈlɪkwɔːr] *n* 1. Flüssigkeit *f*. 2. *anat.* seröse Körperflüssigkeit *f*, Liquor *m*. 3. *pharm.* Arzneilösung *f*, Liquor *m*.
l. of Scarpa Endolymphe *f*, Endolympha *f*.
liq·uo·rice [ˈlɪkərɪʃ, ˈlɪkrɪʃ] *n* 1. Lakritzensaft *m*, Süßholzsaft *m*. 2. Süßholz(wurzel *f*) *nt*.
liquorice root Süßholz(wurzel *f*) *nt*.
Lisfranc [lɪsˈfraːŋk; lɪsˈfrɑ̃]: **L.'s amputation** → L.'s operation.
L.'s articulation Lisfranc'-Gelenklinie *f*, Articc. tarsometatarsales.
L.'s dislocation *ortho.* Lisfranc-Luxation *f*, Vorfußluxation *f* im Lisfranc'-Gelenk.
L.'s joint → L.'s articulation.
L.'s operation 1. Lisfranc'-(Vorfuß-)Amputation *f*, Amputation *f* durch die Lisfranc'-Gelenklinie. 2. *ortho.* Schultergelenk(s)exartikulation *f* nach Dupuytren.
L.'s tubercle Tuberculum *m.* scaleni anterioris.
lisp [lɪsp] **I** *n* Lispeln *nt*, Sigmatismus *m*; Parasigmatismus *m*. **II** *vi* 1. lispeln, mit der Zunge anstoßen. 2. stammeln.
lisp·ing [ˈlɪspɪŋ] *n* → lisp I.
Lissauer [ˈlɪsaʊər]: **L.'s bundle** → L.'s fasciculus.
column of L. → L.'s fasciculus.
L.'s fasciculus Lissauer'-Randbündel *nt*, Tractus dorsolateralis.
L.'s marginal tract → L.'s fasciculus.
L.'s marginal zone → L.'s fasciculus.
L.'s paralysis Lissauer-Paralyse *f*.
Lis·sen·ceph·a·la [ˌlɪsenˈsefələ] *pl bio.* Lissencephala *pl*.
lis·sen·ce·pha·lia [ˌ-sɪˈfeɪljə] *n* 1. Lissenzephalie *f*. 2. Agyrie *f*.
lis·sen·ce·phal·ic [ˌ-ˈfælɪk] *adj* 1. *bio.* Lissencephala betr. 2. lissenzephal. 3. agyral.
lis·sen·ceph·a·ly [ˌ-ˈsefəlɪ] *n* → lissencephalia.
lis·so·sphinc·ter [ˌlɪsəʊˈsfɪŋktər] *n anat.* unwillkürlicher Schließmuskel *m*, Lissosphinkter *m*.
Lister [ˈlɪstər]: **L.'s antiseptic** Quecksilber--Zink-Zyanid *nt*.
L.'s tubercle Tuberculum dorsale (radii).
Lis·ter·el·la [ˌlɪstəˈrelə] *n* → Listeria.
lis·ter·el·lo·sis [ˌlɪstərəˈləʊsɪs] *n* → listeriosis.
Lis·te·ria [lɪˈstɪərɪə] *n micro.* Listeria *f*.
lis·te·ri·al [lɪˈstɪərɪəl] *adj* Listeria betr., durch Listeria verursacht, Listerien-, Listeria-.
Listeria meningitis Listerienmeningitis *f*.
Listeria meningoencephalitis Listerienmeningoenzephalitis *f*.
lis·te·ri·o·sis [lɪˌstɪərɪˈəʊsɪs] *n, pl* **-ses** [-siːz] Listerieninfektion *f*, Listeriose *f*.
Liston [ˈlɪstn]: **L.'s splint** *ortho.* Liston-Schiene *f*.
li·ter [ˈliːtər] *n abbr.* **l** Liter *nt/m abbr.* l.
lit·er·al agraphia [ˈlɪtərəl] *neuro.* literale Agraphie *f*.
lith- *pref.* → litho-.
lith·a·gogue [ˈlɪθəgɒg, -gag] *n pharm.* Lithagogum *nt*.
lith·arge [ˈlɪθɑːdʒ, lɪˈθɑːdʒ] *n* Bleiglätte *f*, Bleioxid *nt*, Lithargyrum *nt*.
li·thec·bo·le [lɪˈθekbəlɪ] *n patho.* Steinaustoßung *f*, -expulsion *f*.
li·thec·ta·sy [lɪˈθektəsɪ] *n urol.* transurethrale Steinextraktion *f*, Lithektasie *f*.
li·thec·to·my [lɪˈθektəmɪ] *n* → lithotomy.

lithiasic

li·thi·a·sic [lɪ'θaɪəsɪk] *adj* Lithiasis betr.
li·thi·a·sis [lɪ'θaɪəsɪs] *n* Steinleiden *nt*, Lithiasis *f*.
lithiasis conjunctivitis *ophthal.* Conjunctivitis petrificans.
lith·ic ['lɪθɪk] *adj* 1. *patho.* Stein betr., Stein-. 2. *chem.* Lithium betr.
lithic acid Harnsäure *f*.
lith·i·um ['lɪθɪəm] *n abbr.* **Li** Lithium *nt abbr.* Li.
lithium borohydride Lithiumborhydrid *nt*.
litho- *pref.* Stein-, Lith(o)-.
lith·o·ce·no·sis [ˌlɪθəsɪ'nəʊsɪs] *n* → litholapaxy.
lith·o·clast ['-klæst] *n* → lithotriptor.
lith·o·cho·late [ˌ-'kəʊleɪt] *n* Lithocholat *nt*.
lith·o·cho·lic acid [ˌ-'kəʊlɪk, -'kɑ-] Lithocholsäure *f*.
lith·o·cho·lyl·gly·cine [ˌ-ˌkəʊlɪl'glaɪsiːn] *n* Glycinlithocholat *nt*.
lith·o·cho·lyl·tau·rine [ˌ-ˌkəʊlɪl'tɔːriːn, -rɪn] *n* Taurinlithocholat *nt*.
lith·o·cys·tot·o·my [ˌ-sɪs'tɒtəmɪ] *n urol.* Blasensteinschnitt *m*, Lithozystotomie *f*.
lith·o·di·al·y·sis [ˌ-daɪ'æləsɪs] *n* Steinauflösung *f*, Lithodialyse *f*.
lith·o·gen·e·sis [ˌ-'dʒenəsɪs] *n* Stein-, Konkrementbildung *f*, Lithogenese *f*.
lith·o·gen·ic [ˌ-'dʒenɪk] *adj* die Steinbildung fördernd, steinbildend, lithogen.
lithogenic bile lithogene Galle *f*.
li·thog·e·nous [lɪ'θɒdʒənəs] *adj* → lithogenic.
lith·o·kel·y·pho·pe·di·on [ˌlɪθəˌkelɪfəʊ'pɪdɪən] *n embryo.* Lithokelyphopädion *nt*.
lith·o·kel·y·phos [ˌ-'kelɪfəs] *n embryo.* Steinmole *f*, Lithokelyphos *m*.
li·thol·a·pax·y [lɪ'θæləpæksɪ] *n urol.* Litholapaxie *f*.
li·thol·y·sis [lɪ'θɒləsɪs] *n* Steinauflösung *f*, Litholyse *f*.
lith·o·lyt·ic [ˌlɪθə'lɪtɪk] I *n* litholytische Substanz *f*, Litholytikum *nt*. II *adj* steinauflösend, litholytisch.
li·thom·e·ter [lɪ'θɒmɪtər] *n* Lithometer *nt*.
lith·o·ne·phrot·o·my [ˌlɪθənɪ'frɒtəmɪ, -ne-] *n chir.* operative Nierensteinentfernung *f*, Nephrolithotomie *f*.
lith·o·pe·di·on [ˌ-'pɪdɪən] *n embryo.* Steinkind *nt*, Lithopädion *nt*.
lith·o·pe·di·um [ˌ-'pɪdɪəm] *n* → lithopedion.
lith·o·tome ['-təʊm] *n chir.* Steinmesser *nt*, Lithotom *nt*.
li·thot·o·my [lɪ'θɒtəmɪ] *n chir., urol.* 1. Steinschnitt *m*, Lithotomie *f*. 2. Blasensteinschnitt *m*; Blasenschnitt *m*.
lithotomy position Steinschnittlage *f*.
lith·o·trip·sy [ˈlɪθə'trɪpsɪ] *n, pl* -sies *urol.* Steinzertrümmerung *f*, Lithotripsie *f*, Lithoklasie *f*.
lith·o·trip·ter *n* → lithotriptor.
lith·o·trip·tic [ˌ-'trɪptɪk] *adj* Lithotripsie betr.
lith·o·trip·tor ['-trɪptər] *n urol.* Lithotripter *m*, -triptor *m*, -konion *nt*, -klast *m*, -fraktor *m*.
lith·o·trip·to·scope [ˌ-'trɪptəskəʊp] *n* Lithotriptoskop *nt*.
lith·o·trip·tos·co·py [ˌ-trɪp'tɒskəpɪ] *n* Lithotriptoskopie *f*.
lith·o·trite ['-traɪt] *n* → lithotriptor.
li·thot·ri·ty [lɪ'θɒtrətɪ] *n* → lithotripsy.
lith·o·troph ['lɪθətrɒf, -trəʊf] *n bio.* lithotroph.
lith·ous ['lɪθəs] *adj* steinartig, kalkulös, Stein-.
lith·ox·i·du·ria [lɪθˌɒksɪ'd(j)ʊərɪə] *n* Xanthinausscheidung *f* im Harn, Xanthinurie *f*.

lith·u·re·sis [ˌlɪθjə'riːsɪs] *n* Blasengrießabgang *m*, Lithurese *f*.
lith·u·re·te·ria [ˌlɪθərɪ'tɪərɪə] *n* Ureterolithiasis *f*.
lith·u·ri·a [lɪθ'j(ʊ)ərɪə] *n* übermäßige Harnsäureausscheidung *f*, Lithurie *f*.
lit·mus ['lɪtməs] *n* Lackmus *nt*.
litmus-milk (culture) medium *micro.* Lackmus-Milchbouillon *f*, -Milchmedium *nt*.
litmus paper Lackmuspapier *nt*.
Litten ['lɪtn]: **L.'s (diaphragm) phenomenon** Litten-Phänomen *nt*.
L.'s sign Litten-Phänomen *nt*.
lit·ter ['lɪtər] *n* 1. Trage *f*, Bahre *f*. 2. *zoo.* Wurf *m*.
Little ['lɪtl]: **L.'s area** Kiesselbach'-Ort *m*, Locus Kiesselbachi.
L.'s disease Little'-Krankheit *f*, Diplegia spastica infantilis.
lit·tle ['lɪtl] I *n* **a** ~ **(better)** etwas, ein wenig (besser). **after a** ~ nach einer Weile. **for a** ~ für ein Weilchen. ~ **by** ~ nach und nach, allmählich. II *adj* klein, Klein-; wenig; kurz; gering(fügig), unbedeutend. III *adv* wenig, kaum.
little finger Kleinfinger *m*, Digitus minimus/quintus manus.
little fossa: l. of cochlear window Fossula fenestrae cochleae.
l. of vestibular window Fossula fenestrae vestibuli.
little head of humerus Capitulum humeri.
little head of mandible Proc. condylaris.
Littman ['lɪtmən]: **L. agar** Littman-Agar *m*/*nt*.
lit·to·ral cell ['lɪtərəl] wandständiger Makrophage *m* von Blut- u. Lymphsinus.
Littre ['liːtrə]: **crypts of L.** Präputialdrüsen *pl*, Gll. pr(a)eputiales.
L.'s glands Littre'-Drüsen *pl*, Urethraldrüsen *pl*, Gll. urethrales urethrae masculinae.
glandular foramina of L. Lacunae urethrales.
L.'s hernia 1. Littre'-Hernie *f*, Darmwandbruch *m*. 2. Hernie *f* mit Meckel'--Divertikel im Bruchsack.
lit·tri·tis [lɪ'traɪtɪs] *n* Entzündung *f* der Littre'-Drüsen, Littre'-Abszeß *m*, Littritis *f*, Littreitis *f*.
live[1] [laɪv] *adj* 1. lebend, lebendig, Lebend-. 2. glühend, brennend; aktiv; *phys.* spannungs-, stromführend, unter Spannung/Strom stehend.
live[2] [lɪv] *vt* leben. II *vi* 1. leben, am Leben bleiben. **she is going to** ~ sie wird am Leben bleiben, sie wird durchkommen. 2. leben (*on*, *upon* von); s. ernähren (*on*, *upon* von; *by* durch, von). 3. leben, wohnen (*with* bei).
live birth Lebendgeburt *f*.
li·ve·do [lɪ'viːdəʊ] *n patho., derm.* Livedo *f*.
liv·e·doid ['lɪvɪdɔɪd] *adj* Livedo betr., livedoartig.
livedoid dermatitis livedoartige Dermatitis *f*, Dermatitis livedoides.
liv·er ['lɪvər] I *n* 1. Leber *f*; *anat.* Hepar *nt*. 2. Rotbraun *nt*. II *adj* rotbraun.
liver abscess Leberabszeß *m*.
  amebic l. Amöbenabszeß *m*.
  bacterial l. bakterieller Leberabszeß *m*.
  candidal l. Candidaabszeß *m*.
  cryptogenic l. kryptogener Leberabszeß *m*.
  pyelophlebitic l. pyelophlebitischer Leberabszeß *m*.
  pyogenic l. pyogener/metastatisch-pyämischer Leberabszeß *m*.
  traumatic l. (post-)traumatischer Leberabszeß *m*.
liver atrophy Leberatrophie *f*.

  acute yellow l. akute gelbe Leberdystrophie/-atrophie *f*.
  brown l. braune Leberatrophie.
  healed yellow l. postnekrotische Leberzirrhose *f*.
  subacute red l. subakute rote Leberdystrophie/-atrophie *f*.
liver bile Lebergalle *f*.
liver biopsy Leberbiopsie *f*, -punktion *f*.
  percutaneous l. perkutane Leberpunktion.
liver breath Foetor hepaticus.
liver bud *embryo.* Leberknospe *f*, -anlage *f*.
liver cell, (parenchymal) Leber(epithel)zelle *f*, (Leber-)Parenchymzelle *f*, Hepatozyt *m*.
liver cell adenoma Leberzelladenom *nt*.
liver cell carcinoma (primäres) Leberzellkarzinom *nt*, hepatozelluläres Karzinom *nt*, malignes Hepatom *nt*, Ca. hepatocellulare.
liver cirrhosis Leberzirrhose *f*, Cirrhosis hepatis.
liver complaint → liver disease.
liver cyst Leberzyste *f*.
liver disease Lebererkrankung *f*, -leiden *nt*, Hepatopathie *f*.
  end-stage l. terminale Leberinsuffizienz *f*.
  parenchymal l. Leberparenchymerkrankung *f*.
liver failure → liver insufficiency.
liver filtrate factor *old* → pantothenic acid.
liver flap *neuro.* Asterixis *f*, Flattertremor *m*, Flapping-tremor *m*.
liver fluke *micro.* Leberegel *m*.
  Asian l. hinterindischer Leberegel, Opisthorchis viverrini.
  cat l. Katzenleberegel, Opisthorchis felineus.
  Chinese l. chinesischer Leberegel, Clonorchis/Opisthorchis sinensis.
  civet l. hinterindischer Leberegel, Opisthorchis viverrini.
  sheep l. großer Leberegel, Fasciola hepatica.
  Sibirian l. → cat l.
liver function Leberfunktion *f*.
liver function test Leberfunktionstest *m*.
liver graft Lebertransplantat *nt*.
liver injury Leberverletzung *f*, -trauma *nt*.
liver insufficiency Leberinsuffizienz *f*, -versagen *nt*.
liv·er·ish ['lɪvərɪʃ] *adj* 1. leberleidend. **to be** ~ es mit der Leber zu tun haben. 2. leberähnlich, -artig, Leber-; rotbraun, rötlichbraun. 3. mürrisch.
liver-kidney syndrome hepatorenales Syndrom *nt*.
liver Lactobacillus casei factor Fol(in)säure *f*, Folacin *nt*, Pteroylglutaminsäure *f*, Vitamin B$_c$ *nt*.
liver metastasis Lebermetastase *f*.
liver necrosis Lebernekrose *f*.
  hypoxic l. hypoxämische Lebernekrose.
liver parenchyma Leberparenchym *nt*.
liver primordium *embryo.* Leberanlage *f*.
liver resection *chir.* Leber(teil)entfernung *f*, Leberresektion *f*.
  major l. subtotale Leberresektion.
  radical l. radikale Leberresektion, Dreiviertelresektion.
liver retractor *chir.* Leberhaken *m*.
liver rupture Leberruptur *f*, -riß *m*.
liver scan *radiol.* 1. Leberszintigraphie *f*. 2. Leberszintigramm *nt*.
liver sinusoid Lebersinusoid *nt*, sinusoide (Leber-)Kapillare *f*.
liver spot *patho.* Leberfleck *m*.
liver surgery Leberchirurgie *f*.
liver transplant Lebertransplantat *nt*.
liver transplantation Leberverpflanzung *f*, -transplantation *f*.

liver trauma Leberverletzung f, -trauma nt.
liver tumor Lebergeschwulst f, -tumor m, Hepatom nt.
  metastatic l. Lebermetastasen pl, sekundärer Lebertumor.
  primary l. primärer Lebertumor.
liv·er·y ['lɪvərɪ] adj → liverish.
live vaccine Lebendimpfstoff m, -vakzine f.
liv·id ['lɪvɪd] adj blaßbläulich, fahl, livid, livide, bläulich verfärbt.
li·vid·i·ty [lɪ'vɪdətɪ] n bläuliche (Haut-)Verfärbung f, Lividität f.
Livierato [,lɪvɪə'rætəʊ]: **L.'s reflex** Abrams'-Herzreflex m.
liv·ing conditions ['lɪvɪŋ] Wohnverhältnisse pl.
Livingston ['lɪvɪŋstən]: **L.'s triangle** Livingston-Dreieck nt.
li·vor ['laɪvɔːr, -vər] n **1.** → lividity. **2.** → livor mortis.
livor mortis Totenflecke pl, Livor mortis, Livores pl.
lix·iv·i·ate [lɪk'sɪvɪət] vt chem. auslaugen.
lix·iv·i·a·tion [lɪk,sɪvɪ'eɪʃn] n chem. Auslaugen nt, Auslaugung f.
lix·iv·i·um [lɪk'sɪvɪəm] n chem. Lauge f.
LLD factor Zyano-, Cyanocobalamin nt, Vitamin B₁₂ nt.
LLF abbr. → Laki-Lorand factor.
Lloyd-Hunter [lɔɪd 'hʌntər]: **L.-H. classification** Lloyd-Hunter-Einteilung f, -Klassifikation f.
L-meromyosin n leichtes Meromyosin nt, L-Meromyosin nt.
LMF abbr. → lymphocyte mitogenic factor.
LMM abbr. → lentigo maligna melanoma.
LMW abbr. → low-molecular-weight.
LMWK abbr. → low-molecular-weight kininogen.
LMW kininogen → low-molecular-weight kininogen.
LNPF abbr. → lymph node permeability factor.
Loa ['ləʊə] n micro. Loa f.
  L. loa Wanderfilarie f, Taglarvenfilarie f, Augenwurm m, Loa loa.
load [ləʊd] **I** n physiol. Belastung f; (a. techn., phys.) Last f. **II** vt **1.** (be-)laden, belasten (with mit); (Magen) überladen. **2.** beschweren. **III** vi (auf-, ein-)laden; beladen werden.
load up vi load III.
load-bearing capacity ortho. (Gelenk) mechanische Belastbarkeit f.
load capacity Belastbarkeit f, Leistungsaufnahme f.
load·ed ['ləʊdɪd] adj **1.** be-, geladen; beschwert. **2.** inf. betrunken.
load·ing dose ['ləʊdɪŋ] pharm. Initial-, Aufsättigungsdosis f.
load resistance electr. Belastungs-, Arbeitswiderstand m.
load test Belastungsprobe f.
load-tolerance limit physiol. Belastbarkeitsgrenze f.
lo·a·i·a·sis [laɪə'aɪəsɪs] n → loiasis.
lo·bar ['ləʊbər] adj (Organ-)Lappen/Lobus betr., lobär, Lappen-, Lobär-, Lobar-.
lobar atelectasis (Lunge) Lappenatelektase f.
lobar atrophy Pick'-Krankheit f, Pick'-Syndrom nt, Pick'-(Hirn-)Atrophie f.
lobar bronchus (Lunge) Lappen-, Lobärbronchus m, Bronchus lobaris.
  left inferior l. Bronchus lobaris inferior sinister.
  left superior l. Bronchus lobaris superior sinister.
  right inferior l. Bronchus lobaris inferior dexter.
  right middle l. Bronchus lobaris medius dexter.
  right superior l. Bronchus lobaris superior dexter.
lobar collaps (Lunge) kollabierter Lappen m; Lappenatelektase f.
lobar emphysema lobäres Lungenemphysem nt.
lobar gliosis lobäre Gliose f.
lobar pneumonia (Lunge) Lobär-, Lappenpneumonie f.
lo·bate ['ləʊbeɪt] adj gelappt, lappig.
lobe [ləʊb] n anat. (Organ-)Lappen m, Lobus m.
  l.s of cerebrum Hirnlappen pl, Lobi cerebrales.
  l.s of liver Leberlappen pl, Lobi hepatis.
  l. of lung Lungenlappen m, Lobus pulmonis.
  l.s of mammary gland Brustdrüsenlappen pl, Lobi gl. mammariae.
  l. of thyroid (gland) Schilddrüsenlappen, Lobus gl. thyroideae.
lo·bec·to·my [ləʊ'bektəmɪ] n chir. **1.** (Organ-)Lappenresektion f, Lobektomie f. **2.** (Lunge) Lobektomie f.
lobed [ləʊbd] adj gelappt, lappig.
lobed placenta gelappte Plazenta f, Lappenplazenta f, Placenta lobata.
lob·e·line ['ləʊbəliːn, -lɪn] n pharm. Lobelin nt.
lo·bi·tis [ləʊ'baɪtɪs] n patho. Lappenentzündung f, Lobitis f.
Lobo ['ləʊbəʊ]: **L.'s disease** Lobo-Krankheit f, Lobomykose f, Keloidblastomykose f, Blastomycosis queloidana.
Lo·bo·a lo·boi [ləʊ'bəʊə, 'ləʊbɔɪ] micro. Loboa loboi f.
lo·bo·my·co·sis [,ləʊbəʊmaɪ'kəʊsɪs] n → Lobo's disease.
lo·bo·po·di·um [,-'pəʊdɪəm] n, pl -**dia** [-dɪə] bio. Lappenfüßchen nt, Lobopodium nt.
lo·bose ['ləʊbəʊs] adj → lobate.
lo·bot·o·my [ləʊ'bɒtəmɪ] n **1.** chir. Lobotomie f. **2.** neurochir. Lobotomie f, Leukotomie f.
  prefrontal l. neurochir. Leukotomie, Lobotomie.
  transorbital l. transorbitale Leukotomie/Lobotomie.
lo·bous ['ləʊbəs] adj → lobate.
Lobstein ['ləʊbstaɪn; 'loːpʃtaɪn]: **L.'s disease/syndrome** Lobstein-Krankheit f, -Syndrom nt, Lobstein-Typ m der Osteogenesis imperfecta, Osteogenesis imperfecta tarda, Osteogenesis imperfecta Typ Lobstein.
lob·ster-claw ['lɒbstər] n ortho. Spalthand f.
lob·u·lar ['lɒbjələr] adj Läppchen/Lobulus betr., läppchenförmig, lobulär, Läppchen-, Lobulus-.
lobular atelectasis (Lunge) Fleckenatelektase f.
lobular bronchioles Terminalbronchiolen pl, Bronchioli terminales.
lobular carcinoma lobuläres Karzinom nt, Ca. lobulare.
lobular carcinoma in situ (Brust) Ca. lobulare in situ abbr. CLIS.
lobular fibroma Irritationsfibrom nt, Lappenfibrom nt.
lobular glomerulonephritis membranoproliferative Glomerulonephritis f.
lobular liver Lappenleber f, Hepar lobatum.
lobular pneumonia Bronchpneumonie f, lobuläre Pneumonie f, Herd-, Fokalpneumonie f.
lob·u·lat·ed ['lɒbjəleɪtɪd] adj gelappt, lappig.
lobulated tongue Lappenzunge f, Lingua lobata.
lob·u·la·tion [,lɒbjə'leɪʃn] n Lappung f.
lob·ule ['lɒbjuːl] n **1.** anat. (Organ-, Drüsen-)Läppchen nt, Lobulus m. **2.** → l. of auricle.
  l. of auricle Ohrläppchen, Lobulus auricularis.
  l.s of epididymis Läppchen pl des Nebenhodenkopfes, Lobuli/Coni epididymidis.
  l.s of liver Leberläppchen pl, Lobuli hepatis.
  l.s of lung Lungenläppchen pl, Segmenta bronchopulmonalia.
  l.s of mammary glands Brustdrüsenläppchen pl, Lobuli gl. mammariae.
  l.s of testis Hodenläppchen pl, Lobuli testis.
  l.s of thymus Thymusläppchen pl, Lobuli thymi.
  l.s of thyroid (gland) Schilddrüsenläppchen pl, Lobuli gl. thyroideae.
lob·u·lo·nod·u·lar glomerulonephritis [,lɒbjələʊ'nɒdʒələr] → lobular glomerulonephritis.
lob·u·lose ['lɒbjələʊs] adj → lobulated.
lob·u·lous ['lɒbjələs] adj → lobulated.
lob·u·lus ['lɒbjələs] n, pl **-li** [-laɪ] anat. → lobule.
lobulus simplex cerebelli unterer Teil m des Lobulus quadrangularis cerebelli, Lobulus simplex cerebelli, Pars inferoposterior lobuli quadrangularis.
lo·bus ['ləʊbəs] n, pl **-bi** [-baɪ] anat. → lobe.
lo·cal ['ləʊkəl] adj lokal, örtlich (begrenzt), Orts-, Lokal-.
local adaptation Lokaladaptation f.
local anesthesia Lokal-, Regionalanästhesie f.
  Bier's l. intravenöse Regionalanästhesie abbr. IVRA.
  vein l. → Bier's l.
local anesthetic Lokalanästhetikum nt.
local glomerulonephritis segmentale Glomerulonephritis f.
local infiltration lokale Injektion/Infiltration f.
local inflammation örtliche od. lokale Entzündung f.
lo·cal·iz·a·ble ['ləʊkəlaɪzəbl] adj lokalisierbar.
lo·cal·i·za·tion [,ləʊkəlɪ'zeɪʃn] n **1.** Ortsbestimmung f, örtliche Lage f, Lokalisierung f, Lokalisation f. **2.** patho. (Tumor etc.) Lokalisation f, Lokalisierung f. **3.** (Wachstum) Beschränkung f.
lo·cal·ize ['ləʊkəlaɪz] **I** vt lokalisieren, örtlich festlegen od. bestimmen; begrenzen (to auf). **II** v/s. festsetzen (in in); s. konzentrieren (on auf).
lo·cal·ized ['ləʊkəlaɪzd] adj lokalisiert, umschrieben, örtlich beschränkt.
localized albinism partieller/umschriebener Albinismus m, Albinismus circumscriptus, Piebaldismus m.
localized chronic pemphigoid lokalisiertes bullöses Pemphigoid nt.
localized epilepsy fokale Epilepsie f.
localized myeloma solitäres/lokalisiertes Myelom/Plasmozytom nt.
localized neurodermatitis Vidal-Krankheit f, Lichen Vidal m, Lichen simplex chronicus (Vidal), Neurodermitis circumscriptus.
localized osteoporosis Sudeck'-Dystrophie f, -Syndrom nt, Morbus Sudeck m.
localized pericarditis chronische lokalisierte Perikarditis f.
localized peritonitis örtlich umschriebene

localized scleroderma

Bauchfellentzündung *f*, Peritonitis circumscripta.
localized scleroderma zirkumskripte Sklerodermie *f*, lokalisierte Sklerodermie *f*, Sclerodermia circumscripta, Morphoea *f*, Morphaea *f*.
localized transient osteoporosis → localized osteoporosis.
lo·cal·iz·er ['ləʊkəlaɪzər] *n radiol.* Lokalisator *m*.
lo·cal·iz·ing electrode ['ləʊkəlaɪzɪŋ] aktive/differente Elektrode *f*.
local malignancy *patho.* örtliche Malignität *f*.
local nerve block Regionalanästhesie *f*.
local reaction Lokalreaktion *f*, lokale/örtliche Reaktion *f*.
local recurrence Lokalrezediv *nt*.
local relapse → local recurrence.
local symptom Lokalsymptom *nt*.
local treatment Lokalbehandlung *f*.
lo·cate ['ləʊkeɪt, ləʊ'keɪt] *vt* 1. ausfindig machen, auffinden, feststellen, aufspüren, lokalisieren. 2. örtlich bestimmen *od.* festlegen, lokalisieren.
lo·ca·tion [ləʊ'keɪʃn] *n* 1. Platz *m*, Stelle *f*; Lage *f*. 2. Lokalisierung *f*; Auffinden *nt*.
lo·chia ['ləʊkɪə, 'lɑkɪə] *n gyn.* Wochenfluß *m*, Lochia *f*, Lochien *pl*.
lo·chi·al ['ləʊkɪəl, 'lɑkɪəl] *adj* Lochien betr., Lochial-, Lochien-, Lochio-.
lo·chi·o·col·pos [,ləʊkɪ'kɑlpəs, ,lɑk-] *n gyn.* Lochiokolpos *m*.
lo·chi·o·me·tra [,-'miːtrə] *n* Lochiometra *f*.
lo·chi·o·me·tri·tis [,-mɪ'traɪtɪs] *n gyn.* Metritis puerperalis.
lo·chi·o·py·ra [,-'paɪrə] *n* Puerperalfieber *nt*, -sepsis *f*, Wochenbett-, Kindbettfieber *nt*, Febris puerperalis.
lo·chi·or·rha·gia [,-'rædʒ(ɪ)ə] *n* → lochiorrhea.
lo·chi·or·rhea [,-'rɪə] *n gyn.* Lochiorrhoe *f*, Lochiorrhagie *f*.
lo·chi·os·che·sis [,ləʊkɪ'askəsɪs, ,lɑk-] *n* → lochiostasis.
lo·chi·os·ta·sis [,-'astəsɪs] *n gyn.* Lochienstauung *f*, Lochiostase *f*, Lochiostasis *f*.
lo·cho·me·tri·tis [,ləʊkəʊmɪ'traɪtɪs] *n* → lochiometritis.
lo·ci *pl* → locus.
lock [lɑk] *n* Schloß *nt*, Verschluß *m*.
lock-and-key model *biochem.* Schlüssel-Schloß-Modell *nt*.
lock-and-key relationship *biochem.* Schlüssel-Schloß-Beziehung *f*.
locked-in syndrome Locked-in-Syndrom *nt*.
lock finger schnellender/schnappender/federnder Finger *m*, Trigger finger *f*.
lock·jaw ['lɑkdʒɔː] *n* Kiefersperre *f*, -klemme *f*, Trismus *m*.
lo·co·mo·tion [,ləʊkə'məʊʃn] *n* Bewegung *f*, Fortbewegung(sfähigkeit *f*) *f*, Ortsveränderung *f*, Lokomotion *f*.
lo·co·mo·tive [,-'məʊtɪv] *adj* fortbewegungsfähig, lokomotorisch, Fortbewegungs-.
lo·co·mo·tor [,-'məʊtər] *adj* Bewegung/Fortbewegung betr., (fort-)bewegend, lokomotorisch.
locomotor apparatus Bewegungsapparat *m*.
locomotor ataxia lokomotorische Ataxie *f*, Gangataxie *f*.
lo·co·mo·to·ri·um [ləʊkə[,-məʊ'tɔːrɪəm, -'tɔːr-] *n* Bewegungsapparat *m*.
lo·co·mo·to·ry [,-'məʊtərɪ] *adj* → locomotor.
loc·u·lar ['lɑkjələr] *adj histol.* gekammert.
loc·u·late [lɑkjəleɪt, -lɪt] *adj histol.* gekammert.
loc·u·la·tion syndrome [,lɑkjə'leɪʃn]

Froin-Symptom *nt*, -Syndrom *nt*.
lo·cum (tenens) ['ləʊkəm] Stellvertreter(in *f*) *m*.
lo·cus ['ləʊkəs] *n*, *pl* **-ca** [-kə], **-ci** [-saɪ, -kaɪ] 1. Ort *m*, Platz *m*, Stelle *f*; *anat.* Lokus *m*, Locus *m*. 2. *genet.* Genlocus *m*, -ort *m*.
locus caeruleus/ceruleus/coeruleus Locus c(a)eruleus/coeruleus.
loem·pe ['lempɪ] *n* Beriberi *f*, Vitamin B_1-Mangel(krankheit *f*) *m*, Thiaminmangel(krankheit *f*) *m*.
Loevit ['liːfɪt; 'lœːvɪt]: **L.'s cell** *old* → erythroblast.
Löffler ['lɛflər; 'lœflər]: **L.'s agar** Löffler--Serum(nährboden *m*) *nt*.
L.'s alkaline methylene blue Löffler-Methylenblau *nt*.
L.'s alkaline methylene blue stain (alkalische) Löffler'-Methylenblaufärbung *f*.
L.'s bacillus Löffler'-Bazillus *m*, Corynebacterium diphtheriae.
L.'s blood culture medium → L.'s agar.
L.'s coagulated serum medium → L.'s agar.
L.'s disease → L.'s endocarditis.
L.'s endocarditis Löffler-Endokarditis *f*, -Syndrom *nt*, Endocarditis parietalis fibroplastica.
L.'s eosinophilia Löffler-Syndrom *nt*, eosinophiles Lungeninfiltrat *nt*.
L.'s (parietal) fibroplastic endocarditis → L.'s endocarditis.
L.'s pneumonia → L.'s eosinophilia.
L.'s serum → L.'s agar.
L.'s syndrome 1. → L.'s endocarditis. 2. → L.'s eosinophilia.
log- *pref.* → logo-.
log·ag·no·sia [,lɑgæg'nəʊʒ(ɪ)ə, -ʒɪə] *n neuro.* Logagnosie *f*.
log·a·graph·ia [,-eɪ'græfɪə] *n neuro.* Logagraphie *f*.
log·am·ne·sia [,-æm'niːʒə] *n neuro.* sensorische Aphasie *f*.
log·a·pha·sia [,-ə'feɪʒə] *n neuro.* expressive Aphasie *f*.
log·a·rith·mic period/phase [,lɔgə'rɪðmɪk, ,lɑgə-, -rɪθ-] *micro.* log-Phase *f*, exponentielle Phase *f*.
log·as·the·ni·a [lɑgæs'θiːnɪə] *n neuro.* Logasthenie *f*.
logo- *pref.* Wort-, Sprach-, Log(o)-.
log·o·clon·ia [lɑgə'kləʊnɪə, lɔg-] *n neuro.* Logoklonie *f*.
log·o·gram ['-græm] *n* Logogramm *nt*.
log·o·klon·y ['-klɑnɪ] *n* → logoclonia.
log·o·ko·pho·sis [,-kəʊ'fəʊsɪs] *n neuro.* Worttaubheit *f*, akustische Aphasie *f*.
log·o·ma·nia [,-'meɪnɪə, -jə] *n neuro.* Logo(mono)manie *f*.
lo·gop·a·thy [ləʊ'gɑpəθɪ] *n* Sprachstörung *f*, Logopathie *f*.
log·o·pe·dia [,lɑgə'piːdɪə, ,lɔg-] *n* → logopedics.
log·o·pe·dics [,-'piːdɪks] *pl* Stimm- u. Sprachheilkunde *f*, Stimm- u. Sprachtherapie *f*, Logopädie *f*.
log·o·pe·dist [,-'piːdɪst] *n* Logopäde *m*, -pädin *f*.
log·o·ple·gia [,-'pliːdʒ(ɪ)ə] *n neuro.* Logoplegie *f*.
log·or·rhea [,-'rɪə] *n neuro., psychia.* Redesucht *f*, Polyphrasie *f*, Zungendelirium *nt*, Logorrhö *f*.
log period/phase *micro.* log-Phase *f*, exponentielle Phase *f*.
Löhlein ['løːlaɪn]: **L.'s focal embolic glomerulonephritis/nephritis** Löhlein'-Herdnephritis *f*.
Löhlein-Baehr [beːr]: **L.-B. lesion** Löhlein'-Herdnephritis *f*.
Lohmann ['ləʊmən]: **L. reaction** Lohmann-Reaktion *f*.

lo·i·a·sis [ləʊ'aɪəsɪs] *n* Loa-loa-Infektion *f*, -Filariose *f*, Filaria-loa-Infektion *f*, Loiasis *f*, Loaose *f*.
loin [lɔɪn] *n anat.* Lende *f*, Lumbus *m*.
Lombard [lɔ̃'baːr]: **L.'s (voice-reflex) test** *HNO* Lombard-Leseversuch *m*.
lo·mus·tine [ləʊ'mʌstiːn] *n* Lomustine *nt*.
Lone-Star fever [ləʊn stɑːr] Bullis-Fieber *nt*, Lone-Star-Fieber *nt*.
Lone-Star tick *micro.* Amblyomma americanum.
long [lɔŋ, lɑŋ] **I** *adj* lang, länglich, groß; hoch; weit; lang(wierig); langfristig. **II** *adv* lang(e).
long-acting *adj* langwirkend, langanhaltend.
long-acting thyroid stimulator *abbr.* **LATS** Thyroidea-stimulierendes Immunglobulin *nt abbr.* TSI, thyroid-stimulating immunoglobulin *abbr.* TSI, long-acting thyroid stimulator *abbr.* LATS.
long arm cast Oberarmgips(verband *m*) *m*.
long axis Längsachse *f*.
l. of body Körperlängsachse *f*.
long bone langer Knochen *m*, Os longum.
long branch of ciliary ganglion sensorischer Ast *m* des Ziliarganglions, Radix/Ramus nasociliaris ggl. ciliaris.
long-chain *adj chem.* langkettig.
long crus of incus langer Amboßfortsatz/-schenkel *m*, Crus longum (incudis).
long-eared *adj* langohrig.
lon·gev·i·ty [lɑn'dʒɛvətɪ, lɔn-] *n* Langlebigkeit *f*.
lon·ge·vous [-'dʒiːvəs] *adj* langlebig.
long gyrus of insula lange Inselwindung *f*, Gyrus longus insulae.
long-haired *adj* langhaarig, mit langen Haaren.
long head: **l. of adductor hallucis muscle** Caput obliquum m. adductoris hallucis.
l. of biceps brachii muscle langer Bizepskopf *m*, Caput longum m. bicipitis brachii.
l. of biceps femoris muscle langer Kopf *m* des M. biceps femoris, Caput longum m. bicipitis femoris.
l. of biceps flexor cruris muscle → l. of biceps femoris muscle.
l. of triceps brachii muscle langer Trizepskopf *m*, Caput longum m. tricipitis brachii.
l. of triceps femoris muscle M. adduktor longus.
long-headed *adj* langköpfig, -schädelig; dolichozephal, -kephal.
long-headedness *n embryo.* Langköpfigkeit *f*, Langschädel *m*, Dolichokephalie *f*, -zephalie *f*.
long incubation hepatitis (Virus-)Hepatitis B *f abbr.* HB, Serumhepatitis *f*.
long·ish ['lɔŋɪʃ, 'lɑŋ-] *adj* länglich, ziemlich lang.
lon·gis·si·mus [lɑn'dʒɪsəməs] *n* Longissimus *m*, M. longissimus.
longissimus capitis (muscle) Longissimus *m* capitis, M. longissimus capitis.
longissimus cervicis (muscle) Longissimus *m* cervicis, M. longissimus cervicis.
longissimus muscle → longissimus.
l. of back → longissimus thoracis (muscle).
l. of head → longissimus capitis (muscle).
l. of neck → longissimus cervicis (muscle).
longissimus thoracis (muscle) Longissimus *m* thoracis, M. longissimus thoracis.
lon·gi·tu·di·nal [,lɑndʒə't(j)uːdɪnl] *adj* in Längsrichtung verlaufend, längs verlaufend, longitudinal, Längen-, Längs-, Longitudinal-.

longitudinal arch of foot Fußlängsgewölbe *nt*.
longitudinal bands of colon Kolontänien *pl*, Taeniae coli.
longitudinal canals of modiolus longitudinale Spindel-/Modioluskanälchen *pl*, Canales longitudinales modioli.
longitudinal duct of epoophoron Gartner'-Gang *m*, Längsgang *m* des Epoophorons, Ductus epoophori/epoophorontis longitudinalis.
longitudinal fasciculus: dorsal l. Schütz'-(Längs-)Bündel *nt*, dorsales Längsbündel *nt*, Fasciculus longitudinalis dorsalis.
inferior l. of cerebrum unteres Längsbündel *nt*, Fasciculus longitudinalis inferior cerebri.
medial l. mediales Längsbündel *nt*, Fasciculus longitudinalis medialis.
superior l. of cerebrum oberes Längsbündel *nt*, Fasciculus longitudinalis superior cerebri.
longitudinal fibers: l. of ciliary muscle Brücke'-Fasern *pl*, -Muskel *m*, Fibrae longitudinales/meridionales m. ciliaris.
l. of pons longitudinale Brückenfasern *pl*, Fibrae pontis longitudinalis.
longitudinal fissure of cerebrum mediale Längsspalte *f* des Großhirns, Fissura longitudinalis cerebralis.
longitudinal fracture Längsbruch *m*, -fraktur *f*.
longitudinal growth Längenwachstum *nt*.
lon·gi·tu·di·na·lis inferior linguae (muscle) [ˌlɒndʒəˌt(j)uːdɪˈneɪlɪs] Longitudinalis *m* inferior/profundus linguae, M. longitudinalis inferior (linguae).
longitudinalis superior linguae (muscle) Longitudinalis *m* superior/superficialis linguae, M. longitudinalis superior (linguae).
longitudinal laterolateral pancreaticojejunostomy *chir.* longitudinale laterolaterale Pankreatikojejunostomie *f*, Puestow-Mercadier I-Operation *f*.
longitudinal lateroterminal pancreaticojejunostomy *chir.* longitudinale lateroterminale Pankreatikojejunostomie *f*, Puestow-Mercadier II-Operation *f*.
longitudinal layer: l. of muscular tunic of colon Stratum longitudinale tunicae muscularis coli.
l. of muscular tunic of rectum Stratum longitudinale tunicae muscularis recti.
l. of muscular tunic of small intestine Stratum longitudinale tunicae muscularis intestini tenuis.
l. of muscular tunic of stomach Stratum longitudinale tunicae muscularis gastris.
longitudinal ligament Längsband *nt* der Wirbelsäule, Lig. longitudinale.
anterior l. vorderes Längsband, Lig. longitudinale anterius.
posterior l. hinteres Längsband, Lig. longitudinale posterius.
longitudinal muscle of tongue: inferior l. → longitudinalis inferior linguae (muscle).
superior l. → longitudinalis superior linguae (muscle).
longitudinal oval pelvis longitudinal-ovales Becken *nt*.
longitudinal pyramidal fracture Pyramidenlängsfraktur *f*.
longitudinal raphe: (median) l. of tongue Sulcus medianus linguae.
longitudinal resistance *phys.* Längswiderstand *m*.
longitudinal section Längsschnitt *m*.
longitudinal sinus: inferior l. Sinus sagittalis inferior.
superior l. Sinus sagittalis superior.

longitudinal stria of corpus callosum: lateral l. lateraler Längsstreifen *m* des Balkens, Stria longitudinalis lateralis (corporis callosi).
medial l. medialer Längsstreifen *m* des Balkens, Stria longitudinalis medialis (corporis callosi).
longitudinal sulcus of heart Interventrikularfurche *f*, Sulcus interventricularis.
longitudinal suture Pfeilnaht *f*, Sutura sagittalis.
longitudinal system (*Muskel*) Longitudinalsystem *nt*, L-System *nt*.
longitudinal traction Längszug *m*.
longitudinal wave Longitudinalwelle *f*.
long-lasting *adj* langwierig; langdauernd, langanhaltend; strapazierfähig.
long leg cast Oberschenkelgips(verband *m*) *m*.
long-legged *adj* langbeinig.
long-life milk H-Milch *f*, haltbare Milch *f*.
long limb of incus → long crus of incus.
long-lived *adj* langlebig.
long measure → lineal measure.
Longmire [ˈlɒŋmaɪər, ˈlɑŋ-]: **L.'s operation** *chir.* Longmire-Operation *f*.
long muscle: l. of head → longus capitis (muscle).
l. of neck → longus colli (muscle).
long pulse schleichender Puls *m*, Pulsus tardus.
long root of ciliary ganglion → long branch of ciliary ganglion.
long-run *adj* langfristig.
long sight → long-sightedness.
long-sighted *adj* Weitsichtigkeit betr., weitsichtig, hypermetropisch, hyperop.
long-sightedness *n* Über-, Weitsichtigkeit *f*, Hyperopie *f*, Hypermetropie *f*.
long-standing *adj* seit langer Zeit bestehend, alt, langjährig.
long-term *adj* langfristig, Dauer-, Langzeit-.
long-term drain *chir.* Dauerdrain *m*.
long terminal repeat *abbr.* **LTR** *biochem.* LTR-Sequenz *f*.
long-term memory *abbr.* **LTM** Langzeitgedächtnis *nt*.
declarative l. deklaratives Langzeitgedächtnis.
episodic l. episodisches Langzeitgedächtnis.
procedural l. prozedurales Langzeitgedächtnis.
semantic l. semantisches Langzeitgedächtnis.
long-term performance Langzeit-, Ausdauerleistung *f*.
long-term prescription Dauerverordnung *f*.
long-time *adj* → long-standing.
long tract cells (*ZNS*) Strangzellen *pl*.
lon·gus capitis (muscle) [ˈlæŋgəs, ˈlɒŋ-] Longus *m* capitis, M. longus capitis.
longus colli (muscle) Longus *m* colli, M. longus colli.
long wave *phys.* Langwelle *f*.
long-wave *adj phys.* langwellig, Langwellen-.
long-wearing *adj* strapazierfähig.
long-winded *adj* (*Person*) ausdauernd.
long-windedness *n* Ausdauer *f*.
look [lʊk] **I** *n* **1.** Blick *m* (*at* auf). **to cast/throw ~ at** einen Blick werfen auf. **to give sth. a second ~** etw. nochmals *od.* genauer ansehen. **to have/take a (good) ~ at** (s.) etw. (genau) ansehen. **2.** Miene *f*, (Gesichts-)Ausdruck *m*. **3. ~s** *pl* Aussehen *nt*. **by/from the ~s of it** (so) wie es aussieht. **good ~s** gutes Aussehen. **to have the ~s of** aussehen wie. **II** *vt* jdm. in die Augen schauen *od.* blicken *od.* sehen. **III** *vi* **4.**

schauen, gucken, sehen. **5.** nachschauen, -sehen, suchen. **6.** aussehen, -sehen. **to ~ ill** krank aussehen.
look after *vi* aufpassen auf; s. kümmern um, sorgen für.
look around *vi* s. umschauen *od.* -sehen (in; *for* nach).
look at *vi* **1.** ansehen, -blicken, -schauen, -gucken, betrachten. **2.** s. etw. anschauen, etw. prüfen.
look back *vi* **1.** *a. fig.* zurückblicken, -schauen (*upon*, *to* auf). **2. she never looked back** sie machte ständig Fortschritte, es ging ständig mit ihr bergauf.
look for *vi* **1.** suchen (nach). **2.** erwarten; hoffen auf.
look in *vi* einen kurzen Besuch machen (*on* bei); kurz vorbeischauen.
look into *vi* untersuchen, prüfen.
look out for *vi* **1.** Ausschau halten *od.*, s. vorsehen vor. **look out! Paß auf! Vorsicht!**. **2.** Ausschau halten nach, s. umsehen nach.
look over *vi* einen Blick werfen in, etw. (über-)prüfen, etw. durchgehen.
look round *vi* → look around.
look through *vt*, *vi* etw. durchsehen *od.* -schauen.
look to *vi* **1.** achten *od.* aufpassen auf; s. kümmern um. **2.** s. verlassen auf.
look up I *vt* (*in einem Buch*) nachschlagen. **II** *vi* herauf-, hinauf-, aufblicken, -sehen, -schauen.
look·out [ˈlʊkaʊt] *n* **1.** Ausschau *f*. **to be on the ~** Ausschau halten (*for* nach). **to keep a good ~ for** auf der Hut sein. **2.** Aussichten *pl*.
look-over *n* **to give sth. a ~** s. etw. ansehen, etw. (über-)prüfen.
look-through *n* Durchsicht *f*. **to give sth. a ~** etw. durchsehen *od.* -schauen.
loop [luːp] **I** *n* **1.** Schlinge *f*, Schleife *f*, Schlaufe *f*, Öse *f*; *anat.* Ansa *f*. **2.** *techn.* geschlossener Stromkreis *m*, geschlossenes magnetisches Feld *nt*. **3.** *gyn.* Intrauterinpessar *m*, Spirale *f*. **II** *vt* schlingen (*round* um). **III** *vi* s. schlingen (*round* um); eine Schleife machen, eine Schlinge bilden.
l. of hypoglossal nerve Hypoglossusschlinge, Ansa cervicalis.
l. of Vieussens Ansa subclavia.
loop colostomy *chir.* doppelläufiges Kolostoma *nt*.
loop diuretic *pharm.* Schleifendiuretikum *nt*.
loop obstruction *patho.* (Darm-)Schlingenobstruktion *f*.
loose [luːs] **I** *adj* **1.** los(e), locker, frei. **to come/get ~** s. lockern, s. ablösen, abblättern. **2.** (*Gewebe*) locker. **3.** (*Gedanken*) unlogisch, wirr. **II** *vt* **4.** los-, freilassen. **5.** lösen, befreien (*from* von).
loose body freier Gelenkkörper *m*, Gelenkmaus *f*, Corpus liberum.
Looser [ˈluːzər; ˈloːzər]: **L.'s transformation zone** Looser-Umbauzone *f*.
Looser-Milkman [ˈmɪlkmən] **L.-M. syndrome** Looser-Syndrom *nt*, Milkman-Syndrom *nt*, Looser-Milkman-Syndrom *nt*.
loose skin Fall-, Schlaffhaut *f*, Cutis laxa--Syndrom *m*, Zuviel-Haut-Syndrom *nt*, Dermatochalasis *f*, Dermatolysis *f*, Dermatomegalie *f*, Chalazodermie *f*, Chalodermie *f*.
lop ear [lɒp] abstehende Ohrmuschel *f*, abstehendes Ohr *nt*.
lo·per·a·mide [loʊˈpɛrəmaɪd] *n* Loperamid *nt*.
lo·phot·ri·chate [ləˈfɑtrəkɪt] *adj* → lophotrichous.

lophotrichous 458

lo·phot·ri·chous [ləˈfɑtrɪkəs] *adj micro.* lophotrich.
Lorain [lɔˈrɛ̃]: **L.'s disease/infantilism** → L.'s syndrome.
L.'s syndrome Lorain-Syndrom *nt*, hypophysärer Zwergwuchs *m*, hypophysärer Minderwuchs *m*.
Lorain-Lévi [lˈvɪ]: **L.-L. dwarfism/infantilism/syndrome** → Lorain's syndrome.
lor·a·ze·pam [lɔːrˈæzəpæm] *n pharm.* Lorazepam *nt*.
lor·cai·nide [lɔːrˈkeɪnaɪd] *n pharm.* Lorcainid *nt*.
lor·do·sco·li·o·sis [ˌlɔːrdəʊskəʊlɪˈəʊsɪs, -skal-] *n ortho.* kombinierte Lordose *f* u. Skoliose, Lordoskoliose *f*.
lor·do·sis [lɔːrˈdəʊsɪs] *n, pl* **-ses** [-siːz] ventralkonvexe Biegung *f* (der Wirbelsäule), Lordose *f*, Lordosis *f*.
lor·dot·ic [lɔːrˈdɑtɪk] *adj* Lordose betr., lordotisch.
lordotic albuminuria orthostatische/lordotische Albuminurie/Proteinurie *f*.
lordotic pelvis Lordosebecken *nt*.
lordotic proteinuria → lordotic albuminuria.
Lorenz [ˈlɔrənz, ˈləʊr-; ˈloːrənz]: **L.'s brace** Lorenz-Gips *m*.
L.'s operation/osteotomy Lorenz'-Umstellungsosteotomie *f*.
L.'s position Lorenz-Stellung *f*, Froschstellung *f*.
Loschmidt [ˈləʊʃmɪt]: **L.'s number** Lohschmidt'-Zahl *f*.
loss [lɔːs, lɑs] *n* Verlust *m*, Schaden *m*, Einbuße *f*.
l. of appetite Appetitverlust; Anorexie *f*.
l. of function Funktionsverlust, -einschränkung *f*, Functio laesa.
l. of identity Identitätsverlust.
l. of libido Libidoverlust.
l. of motion *ortho.* Bewegungseinschränkung *f*, Verlust der Beweglichkeit.
Lostorfer [ˈlɔstə(r)fər]: **L.'s corpuscles** Lostorfer-Körperchen *pl*.
lo·tio [ˈləʊʃɪəʊ] *n* → lotion.
lo·tion [ˈləʊʃn] *n pharm.* Lotion *f*, Lotio *f*.
loud [laʊd] *adj* **1.** laut. **2.** *fig.* grell, schreiend; aufdringlich.
loud·ness [ˈ-nɪs] *n* **1.** *phys., physiol.* Lautstärke *f*. **2.** Lautheit *f*, das Laute. **3.** Lärm *m*.
loudness level Lautstärkepegel *m*.
loud noise Lärm *m*.
loud noise deafness Lärmschwerhörigkeit *f*.
loud·speak·er [ˈlaʊdspiːkər] *n* Lautsprecher *m*, Schall-, Tonverstärker *m*.
Louis [ˈluːɪz]: **L.'s angle** Angulus Ludovici/sterni/sternalis.
Louis-Bar [lwi baːr]: **L.-B. syndrome** *neuro.* Louis-Bar-Syndrom *nt*, Ataxia--Teleangiectasia *f*, Teleangiektasie--Ataxie-Syndrom *nt*, Ataxia teleangiectatica, progressive zerebelläre Ataxie *f*.
loupe [luːp] *n* Vergrößerungsglas *nt*, Lupe *f*.
loup·ing ill [ˈlaʊpɪŋ, ˈluː-] (*Schafe*) louping ill, Spring-, Drehkrankheit *f*.
louping ill virus *micro.* louping-ill-Virus *nt*.
louse [laʊs] *n*, *pl* **lice** [laɪs] *micro.* Laus *f*.
louse-borne *adj* durch Läuse übertragen, Läuse-.
louse-borne relapsing fever endemisches Rückfallfieber *nt*, Zeckenrückfallfieber *nt*.
louse-borne typhus epidemisches/klassisches Fleckfieber *nt*, Läusefleckfieber *nt*, Fleck-, Hunger-, Kriegstyphus *m*, Typhus exanthematicus.
louse flies *micro.* Hippoboscidae *pl*.

louse mite *micro.* Pyemotes *pl*.
lous·i·cide [ˈlaʊsəsaɪd] **I** *n* Pedikulizid *nt*. **II** *adj* läuse(ab)tötend, pedikulizid.
lou·si·ness [ˈlaʊzɪnɪs] *n* Läusebefall *m*, Verlausung *f*, Pedikulose *f*, Pediculosis *f*.
lou·sy [ˈlaʊzɪ] *adj* mit Läusen infestiert, von Läusen befallen.
Lovén [lɔˈven, -ˈviːn]: **L.'s reflex** Lovén--Reflex *m*.
low [ləʊ] **I** *n fig.* Tief *nt*, Tiefpunkt *m*, -stand *m*. **to reach a (new)** ~ einen (neuen) Tiefpunkt erreichen. **II** *adj* **1.** (*a. fig.*) tief, niedrig, tief gelegen; (*Qualität*) minderwertig, gering; (*Licht*) gedämpft; (*Vorräte*) fast leer, knapp. **to run/get** ~ zur Neige gehen. **2.** (*Stirn, Temperatur*) tief; (*Puls*) schwach, niedrig; (*Nahrung*) wenig nahrhaft; einfach; (*Herztöne, Stimme*) leise. **in a** ~ **voice** leise. **3.** (*Stimmung*) deprimiert, gedrückt, niedergeschlagen. **to feel** ~ niedergeschlagen sein. **to be** ~ **in health** bei schlechter Gesundheit sein. **4.** *socio.* nieder, niedrig; *bio.* primitiv, nieder. ~ **forms of life** niedere Lebensformen.
low-assimilation pelvis niedriges Assimilationsbecken *nt*.
low-caloric diet → low-calorie diet.
low-calorie *adj* kalorienarm.
low-calorie diet energiearme/kalorienarme Diät/Kost *f*, Magerkost *f*.
low-density lipoprotein *abbr.* **LDL** Lipoprotein *nt* mit geringer Dichte, β-Lipoprotein *nt*, low-density lipoprotein *abbr.* LDL.
low-density lipoprotein receptor LDL--Rezeptor *m*.
low diet → low-energy diet.
low-dose heparin *abbr.* **LDH** low-dose--Heparin *nt*, LD-Heparin *nt abbr.* LDH.
low-dose immunologic tolerance *immun.* Low-dose-Immuntoleranz *f*.
low-dose tolerance → low-dose immunologic tolerance.
Lowe [ləʊ]: **L.'s disease/syndrome** Lowe--Syndrom *nt*, Lowe-Terrey-Mac-Lachlan-Syndrom *nt*, okulo-zerebro-renales Syndrom *nt*.
Löwenberg [ˈleɪvənbɜrg, ˈløːvənberk]: **scala of L.** (häutiger) Schneckengang *m*, Ductus cochlearis.
Löwenstein-Jensen [ˈleɪvənstaɪn ˈjɛnzən, ˈløːvənstaɪn]: **L.-J.** (**culture**) **medium** Löwenstein-Jensen-Nährboden *nt*, -Medium *nt*.
low-energy compound *chem.* energiearme Verbindung *f*.
low-energy diet energiearme/kalorienarme Diät/Kost *f*, Magerkost *f*.
Löwenthal [ˈleɪvəntæl, ˈløːvəntaːl]: **L.'s tract** Löwenthal'-Bahn *f*, Tractus tectospinalis.
Lower [ˈləʊər]: **L.'s ring** Anulus fibrosus.
L.'s tubercle Tuberculum intervenosum.
low·er [ˈləʊər] **I** *adj* tiefer, niedriger, Nieder-; untere(r, s), Unter-. **II** *vt* **1.** (*Augen, Stimme, Temperatur*) senken, niedriger machen; herunterlassen. **2.** verringern, senken, herabsetzen, (ab-)schwächen. **III** *vi fig.* sinken, fallen; niedriger werden.
lower arm type of brachial palsy/paralysis Klumpke'-Lähmung *f*, Klumpke--Déjérine-Lähmung *f*, untere Armplexuslähmung *f*.
low·ered [ˈləʊərd] *adj* herabgesetzt, vermindert, abgeschwächt.
lower extremity Bein *nt*, untere Extremität *f*, Membrum inferius.
l. of kidney unterer Nierenpol *m*, Extremitas inferior renis.
lower ganglion: l. of glossopharyngeal nerve unteres Glossopharyngeusgangli-

on *nt*, Ggl. caudalis/inferius n. glossopharyngei.
l. of vagus nerve unteres Vagusganglion *nt*, Ggl. caudalis/inferius n. vagi.
low·er·ing [ˈləʊərɪŋ] *n* Herabsetzung *f*, Senkung *f*.
lower jaw (**bone**) Unterkiefer(knochen *m*) *m*, Mandibula *f*.
lower leg Unterschenkel *m*.
lower lid Unterlid *nt*, Palpebra inferior.
lower limbs untere Gliedmaßen/Extremitäten *pl*, Beine *pl*.
lower lip Unterlippe *f*, Labium inferius oris.
low·er·most [ˈləʊərməʊst] *adj* niedrigste(r, s); unterste(r, s).
lower motoneuron spinales Motoneuron *nt*.
lower nephron nephrosis akute Tubulusnekrose *f*, Crush-Niere *f*, Chromoproteinniere *f*, chromoproteinurische Niere *f*.
lower palpebra Unterlid *nt*, Palpebra inferior.
lower protist *bio.* niederer Protist *m*, Prokaryo(n)t *m*.
lower radicular syndrome → lower arm type of brachial palsy.
lower ramus of pubis unterer Schambeinast *m*, Ramus inferior ossis pubis.
lower teeth Zähne *pl od.* Zahnreihe *f* des Unterkiefers.
Lowe-Terrey-MacLachlan [ləʊ ˈtɛri mækˈlæklən]: **L.-T.-M. syndrome** Lowe-Syndrom *nt*, Lowe-Terrey-MacLachlan--Syndrom *nt*, okulo-zerebro-renales Syndrom *nt*.
low-fat *adj* fettarm.
low frequency *phys.* Niederfrequenz *f*.
low-grade *adj* **1.** minderwertig. **2.** (*Fieber*) leicht, geringgradig.
low-grade fever leichtes Fieber *nt*, (mäßig) erhöhte Temperatur *f*.
low-income *adj* einkommensschwach.
low-level *adj* niedrig.
low-lying *adj* tiefgelegen, tiefliegend.
low-molecular-weight *adj abbr.* **LMW** *chem.* niedermolekular.
low-molecular-weight dextran niedermolekulares Dextran *nt*.
low-molecular-weight heparin niedermolekulares Heparin *nt*.
low-molecular-weight kininogen *abbr.* **LMWK** niedermolekulares Kininogen *nt*, low-molecular-weight kininogen *abbr.* LMWK.
low·ness [ˈləʊnɪs] *n* Niedrigkeit *f*; Minderwertigkeit *f*; Knappheit *f*; Schwäche *f*; (*Ton*) Tiefe *f*; Niedergeschlagenheit *f*, Deprimiertheit *f*.
Lown-Ganong-Levine [laʊn ˈgænɔŋ lɪˈvaɪn]: **L.-G.-L. syndrome** Lown--Ganong-Levine-Syndrom *nt*, LGL-Syndrom *nt*.
low-noise *adj* rauscharm.
low-octane *adj chem.* mit niedriger Oktanzahl.
low-output failure *card.* low-output failure (*nt*).
low-pitched *adj* (*Ton*) tief; mit geringer Neigung.
low pressure Niederdruck *m*.
low-pressure system *physiol.* Niederdrucksystem *nt*.
low race primitive Rasse *f*.
low-salt *adj* salzarm.
low salt syndrome Salzmangelsyndrom *nt*.
low sodium syndrome Salzmangelsyndrom *nt*.
low-spirited *adj* niedergeschlagen, deprimiert, bedrückt, gedrückt.

low-spiritedness *n* Niedergeschlagenheit *f*, Deprimiertheit *f*, Be-, Gedrücktheit *f*.
low tension *electr.* Niederspannung *f*.
low-tension glaucoma Niederdruckglaukom *nt*.
low-tone deafness *HNO* Gehörverlust *m* für niedrige Frequenzen.
low voltage *electr.* Niederspannung *f*.
low-zone immunologic tolerance *immun.* Low-dose-Immuntoleranz *f*.
low-zone tolerance → low-zone immunologic tolerance.
lox·ia ['lɑksɪə] *n* Schiefhals *m*, Torticollis *m*, Loxia *f*, Caput obstipum.
lox·oph·thal·mus [lɑksɑf'θælməs] *n old* → strabismus.
loz·enge ['lɑzɪndʒ] *n pharm.* Tablette *f*, Pastille *f*, Trochiskus *m*.
LPF *abbr.* → lymphocytosis promoting factor.
L-phase variant *micro.* L-Form *f*, L-Phase *f*, L-Organismus *m*.
LPL *abbr.* → lipoprotein lipase.
LPS *abbr.* → lipopolysaccharide.
Lr *abbr.* → lawrencium.
LRF *abbr.* [luteinizing hormone releasing factor] → luteinizing hormone releasing hormone.
LRP *abbr.* → late receptor potential.
LSD *abbr.* → lysergic acid diethylamide.
L-S disease → Letterer-Siwe disease.
L-sided appendicitis 1. linkseitige Appendizitis *f* bei Situs inversus. 2. Linksappendizitis *f*, Divertikulitis *f*.
L/S ratio → lecithin-sphingomyelin ratio.
L system (*Muskel*) Longitudinalsystem *nt*, L-System *n*.
LT *abbr.* → leukotriene.
LTF *abbr.* [lymphocyte transforming factor] → lymphocyte mitogenic factor.
LTH *abbr.* [luteotropic hormone] → luteotropin.
LTM *abbr.* → long-term memory.
LTR *abbr.* → long terminal repeat.
Lu *abbr.* → lutetium.
Lubarsch ['lu:bɑ:rʃ]: **L.'s crystals** Lubarsch-Kristalle *pl*.
lu·bri·cant ['lu:brəkənt] **I** *n* Gleitmittel *nt*, Lubrikans *nt*; Schmiermittel *nt*. **II** *adj* gleitfähig machend, Gleit-; schmierend.
lu·bri·cate ['-keɪt] *vt* gleitfähig machen; einfetten, -schmieren.
lu·bri·cat·ing ['-keɪtɪŋ] *adj* Gleit-; Schmier-.
lubricating agent Gleitmittel *nt*, Lubrikans *nt*.
lubricating mucus Gleitschleim *m*.
lu·bri·ca·tion [,-'keɪʃn] *n* Schmieren *nt*, Ölen *nt*.
lu·bri·ca·tor ['-keɪtər] *n* → lubricant I.
lu·bri·cous ['lu:brɪkəs] *adj* schlüpfrig, glatt.
Luc [lʌk; lyk]: **L.'s operation** *HNO* Caldwell-Luc-Operation *f*.
lu·cen·cy ['lu:snsɪ] *n* 1. Durchsichtigkeit *f*, Klarheit *f*. 2. Glanz *m*.
lu·cent ['lu:snt] *adj* 1. durchsichtig, klar. 2. glänzend.
Lucey-Driscoll ['lu:sɪ 'drɪskəl]: **L.-D. syndrome** Lucey-Driscoll-Syndrom *nt*, Muttermilchikterus *m*.
Luciani [lu:tʃɪ'ɑ:nɪ, lu:'ʃɑ:nɪ]: **L.'s triad** Luciani-Syndrom *nt*.
lu·cid ['lu:sɪd] *adj* (*Gedanke etc.*) klar, hell.
lucid interval *psycho.* heller *od.* lichter Augenblick *m*.
lu·cid·i·ty [lu:'sɪdətɪ] *n* → lucidness.
lu·cid·ness ['lu:sɪdnɪs] *n* (*Gedanke etc.*) Klarheit *f*.
lu·cif·er·ase [lu:'sɪfəreɪz] *n* Luciferase *f*.
lu·cif·er·in [lu:'sɪfərɪn] *n* Luciferin *nt*.

Lu·cil·ia [lu:'sɪlɪə] *pl micro.* Schmeißfliegen *pl*, Lucilia *pl*.
Lucio ['lu:ʃəʊ]: **diffuse leprosy of L.** → L.'s leprosy.
L.'s leprosy Lucio-Phänomen *nt*.
L.'s phenomenon → L.'s leprosy.
Ludloff ['lʊdlɔf]: **L.'s sign** *ortho.* 1. Ludloff-Zeichen *nt*. 2. Ludloff-Hohmann-Zeichen *nt*.
Ludwig ['lʊdvɪg]: **L.'s angina** Ludwig-Angina *f*, tiefe Halsphlegmone *f*, Angina Ludovici.
L.'s angle Angulus Ludovici, Angulus sterni/sternalis.
L.'s theory Ludwig-Theorie *f*.
Luer ['lu:ər]: **L. bone rongeur** Luer-Knochenzange *f*.
L. forceps → L. bone rongeur.
L. rongeur → L. bone rongeur.
L. syringe Luer-Spritze *f*.
lu·es ['lu:i:z] *n* harter Schanker *m*, Morbus Schaudinn *m*, Schaudinn-Krankheit *f*, Syphilis *f*, Lues (venerea) *f*.
lu·et·ic [lu:'etɪk] *adj* Syphilis betr., von Syphilis betroffen, durch Syphilis verursacht, syphilitisch, luetisch, Syphilis-.
luetic aortitis → luetic mesaortitis.
luetic granuloma Syphilom *nt*, Gumma (syphiliticum) *nt*.
luetic mesaortitis Aortensyphilis *f*, Mesaortitis luetica, Aortitis syphilitica.
luetic osteochondritis kongenitale Knochensyphilis *f*, Osteochondritis syphilitica, Wegner'-Krankheit *f*.
Lugol [lu:'gɔl; ly'gɔl]: **L.'s solution** Lugol'-Lösung *f*.
lu·lib·er·in [lu:'lɪbərɪn] *n* → luteinizing hormone releasing hormone.
lu·lib·er·i·ner·gic [lu:,lɪbərɪ'nɜrdʒɪk] *adj* → lutiliberinergic.
lum·ba·go [lʌm'beɪgəʊ] *n* Hexenschuß *m*, Muskelrheumatismus *m* der Lendengegend, Lendenweh *nt*, Lumbalgie *f*, Lumbago *f*.
lum·bar ['lʌmbər] *adj* lumbal, Lumbal-, Lenden-, Lumbo-.
lumbar anesthesia Lumbalanästhesie *f*.
lumbar artery: l.ies *pl* Lenden-, Lumbalarterien *pl*, Aa. lumbales.
fifth l. → lowest l.
lowest l. unterste Lenden-/Lumbalarterie *f*, A. lumbalis ima.
lumbar branch of iliolumbar artery Lumbalast *m* der A. iliolumbalis, Ramus lumbalis a. iliolumbalis.
lumbar enlargement (of spinal cord) *anat.* Intumescentia lumbosacralis.
lumbar ganglia Lumbalganglien *pl*, Ggll. lumbalia/lumbaria.
lumbar hernia *chir.* Lendenbruch *m*, Hernia lumbalis.
lum·bar·i·za·tion [,lʌmbərɪ'zeɪʃn] *n ortho.*, *embryo.* Lumbalisation *f*.
lumbar lordosis Lendenlordose *f*.
lumbar lymph nodes: intermediate l. intermediäre Lumballymphknoten *pl*, Nodi lymphatici parietales lumbales/lumbares intermedii.
left l. lumbale Lymphknoten *pl* der Bauchaorta, Nodi lymphatici parietales lumbales/lumbares sinistri.
right l. lumbale Lymphknoten *pl* der V. cava inferior, Nodi lymphatici parietales lumbales/lumbares dextri.
lumbar nephrectomy *urol.* hintere Nierenentfernung/Nephrektomie *f*.
lumbar nerves lumbale Spinalnerven *pl*, Lendennerven *pl*, Nn. lumbales/lumbares.
lumbar pain → lumbago.
lumbar part: l. of autonomic nervous system Bauchabschnitt *m* des vegetativen Nervensystems, Pars abdominalis systematis autonomici, Pars abdominalis autonomica.
l. of spinal cord Lenden-, Lumbalsegmente *pl*, Lendenabschnitt *m* des Rückenmarks, Lumbaria *pl*, Pars lumbaris (medullae spinalis).
lumbar plexus 1. Lenden-, Lumbalplexus *m*, Plexus lumbalis/lumbaris. 2. lymphatischer Lendenplexus *m*, Plexus lumbalis.
lumbar puncture Lumbalpunktion *f*.
lumbar puncture headache Kopfschmerz *m* nach Lumbalpunktion.
lumbar region *anat.* Lende *f*, Lendengegend *f*, -region *f*, Regio lumbalis/lumbaris.
lumbar rheumatism → lumbago.
lumbar rib Lendenrippe *f*.
lumbar scoliosis *ortho.* Lendenskoliose *f*.
lumbar segments of spinal cord Lenden-, Lumbalsegmente *pl*, Lendenmark *nt*, Lendenabschnitt *m* des Rückenmarks, Lumbaria *pl*, Pars lumbaris (medullae spinalis).
lumbar spine Lendenwirbelsäule *f abbr.* LWS.
lumbar sympathectomy *neurochir.*, *anes.* lumbale Sympathektomie *f*.
lumbar triangle Lumbaldreieck *nt*, Petit'-Dreieck *nt*, Trigonum lumbale, Trigonum Petiti.
superior l. Grynfeltt-Dreieck *nt*, Trigonum lumbale superior.
lumbar trigone → lumbar triangle.
lumbar trunk: left l. Truncus lumbaris sinister.
right l. Truncus lumbaris dexter.
lumbar vein: l.s *pl* Lumbalvenen *pl*, Vv. lumbales.
ascending l. aufsteigende Lendenvene *f*, V. lumbalis ascendens.
lumbar vertebrae Lenden-, Lumbalwirbel *pl*, Vertebrae lumbales.
lumbo- *pref.* Lumbal-, Lenden-, Lumbo-.
lum·bo·ab·dom·i·nal [,lʌmbəʊæb'dɑmɪnl] *adj* Lende u. Abdomen betr., lumboabdominal.
lum·bo·co·los·to·my [-kə'lɑstəmɪ] *n chir.* Lumbarkolostomie *f*.
lum·bo·co·lot·o·my [-kə'lɑtəmɪ] *n chir.* Lumbarkolotomie *f*.
lum·bo·cos·tal [,-'kɑstl] *adj* Lumbalregion u. Rippen betr., lumbokostal.
lumbocostal arch: external l. Quadratusarkade *f*, Lig. arcuatum laterale, Arcus lumbocostalis lateralis (Halleri).
internal l. Psoarsarkade *f*, Lig. arcuatum mediale, Arcus lumbocostalis medialis (Halleri).
lumbocostal ligament Lig. lumbocostale.
lum·bo·dor·sal [,-'dɔrsl] *adj* lumbodorsal.
lumbodorsal fascia Fascia thoracolumbalis.
lum·bo·dyn·ia [,-'dɪnɪə] *n* → lumbago.
lum·bo·in·gui·nal nerve [,-'ɪŋgwənl] Femoralast *m* des N. genitofemoralis, N. lumboinguinalis, Ramus femoralis (n. genitofemoralis).
lum·bo·sa·cral [,-'seɪkrəl] *adj* Lumbalregion u. Sakrum betr., lumbosakral.
lumbosacral angle Lumbosakral-, Sakrovertebralwinkel *m*.
lumbosacral articulation Lumbosakralgelenk *nt*, Artic. lumbosacralis.
lumbosacral cord Truncus lumbosacralis.
lumbosacral enlargement (of spinal cord) *anat.* Intumescentia lumbosacralis.
lumbosacral joint → lumbosacral articulation.
lumbosacral plexus Plexus lumbosacralis.

lumbosacral trunk Truncus lumbosacralis.
lum·bri·cal ['lʌmbrɪkəl] *n* Lumbrikalmuskel *m*, M. lumbricalis.
lumbrical muscles: l. of foot Lumbrikalmuskeln *pl* des Fußes, Mm. lumbricales pedis.
  l. of hand Lumbrikalmuskeln *pl* der Hand, Mm. lumbricales manus.
lum·bri·ci·dal [ˌlʌmbrɪ'saɪdl] *adj* askarizid.
lum·bri·cide ['lʌmbrɪsaɪd] *n* Askarizid *nt*.
lum·bri·coid ['lʌmbrɪkɔɪd] **I** *n micro.* Spulwurm *m*, Ascaris lumbricoides. **II** *adj* wurmförmig, -artig.
lum·bri·co·sis [ˌlʌmbrɪ'kəʊsɪs] *n* Spulwurminfektion *f*, Askariasis *f*, Askari(d)ose *f*, Askaridiasis *f*.
Lum·bri·cus ['lʌmbrɪkəs] *n micro.* Lumbricus *m*.
lum·bus ['lʌmbəs] *n*, *pl* **-bi** [-baɪ] *anat.* Lende *f*, Lumbus *m*.
lu·men ['lu:mən] *n*, *pl* **-mi·na** [-mɪnə] **1.** *anat.* Lichtung *f*, Hohlraum *m*, Lumen *nt*. **2.** *phys.* Lumen *nt abbr.* lm.
lu·mi·nance ['lu:mɪnəns] *n physiol.* Leuchtdichte *f*.
lu·mi·nesce [ˌlu:mɪ'nes] *vi phys.* lumineszieren.
lu·mi·nes·cence [ˌ-'nesəns] *n* Lumineszenz *f*.
lu·mi·nes·cent [ˌ-'nesənt] *adj* lumineszierend.
lu·mi·nif·er·ous [ˌ-'nɪfərəs] *adj* lichterzeugend; leuchtend; lichtfortpflanzend.
lu·mi·no·phore ['lu:mɪnəfɔ:r, -fəʊr] *n* Luminophor *m*.
lu·mi·nos·i·ty [ˌlu:mɪ'nɒsɪtɪ] *n* Leuchten *nt*; Leuchtkraft *f*; *phys.* Lichtstärke *f*, Helligkeit *f*.
lu·mi·nous ['lu:mɪnəs] *adj* strahlend, leuchtend, Leucht-; *fig.* glänzend.
luminous energy Leuchtkraft *f*; Licht-, Strahlungsenergie *f*.
lu·mi·nous·ness ['-nɪs] *n* → luminosity.
lump [lʌmp] *n* **1.** Schwellung *f*, Beule *f*, Höcker *m*, Geschwulst *f*, Knoten *m*. **2.** Klumpen *m*, Brocken *m*.
lump·ec·to·my [lʌm'pektəmɪ] *n gyn.* (*Brust*) Segment-, Quadrantenresektion *f*, Lumpektomie *f*, Tylektomie *f*.
lump kidney *patho.* Kuchen-, Klumpenniere *f*.
lu·na·cy ['lu:nəsɪ] *n* Wahnsinn *m*, Geistesgestörtheit *f*, Geistesstörung *f*.
lu·nar ['lu:nɑ:r] *adj* **1.** Mond-, Lunar-. **2.** *chem.* Silber-.
lu·na·re [lu:'nærɪ] *n* → lunate I.
lu·nate ['lu:neɪt] **I** *n* Mondbein *nt*, Os lunatum. **II** *adj* (halb-)mondförmig.
lunate bone → lunate I.
lu·nat·ed ['lu:neɪtɪd] *adj* → lunate II.
lunate malacia → lunatomalacia.
lunate sulcus *old* Affenspalte *f*, Sulcus lunatus.
lunate surface (of acetabulum) Facies lunata (acetabuli).
lu·na·tic ['lu:nətɪk] **I** *n* Wahnsinnige(r *m*) *f*, Geistesgestörte(r *m*) *f*; Verrückte(r *m*) *f*. **II** *adj* wahnsinnig, geistesgestört; verrückt; irrsinnig, irre.
lu·na·tism ['lu:nətɪzəm] *n psychia.* Mondsüchtigkeit *f*, Lunatismus *m*.
lu·na·to·ma·la·cia [ˌlu:nətəʊmə'leɪʃ(ɪ)ə] *n ortho.* Lunatummalazie *f*, Kienbeck'-Krankheit *f*, Morbus Kienbeck *m*.
Lundh [lʌnd]: **L. test** Bestimmung *f* der Trypsinaktivität nach Lundh.
lung [lʌŋ] *n* Lunge *f*, Lungenflügel *m*; *anat.* Pulmo *m*.
lung abscess Lungenabszeß *m*.
lung biopsy Lungenbiopsie *f*, -punktion *f*.
lung buds *embryo.* Lungenknospen *pl*.

lung calculus Bronchialstein *m*, Broncholith *m*, Calculus bronchialis.
lung cancer → lung carcinoma.
lung carcinoma Lungenkrebs *m*, -karzinom *nt*.
lung contusion Kontusionslunge *f*, Lungenkontusion *f*, -quetschung *f*.
lung disease Lungenerkrankung *f*, -krankheit *f*, -leiden *nt*.
  chronic obstructive l. *abbr.* **COLD** chronisch-obstruktive Lungenerkrankung/ Atemwegserkrankung.
  obstructive l. obstruktive Lungenerkrankung.
  restrictive l. restriktive Lungenerkrankung.
lung fluke *micro.* Lungenegel *m*, Paragonimus ringeri/westermani.
lung fluke disease Lungenegelbefall *m*, Paragonimiasis *f*, Paragonimose *f*.
lung graft Lungentransplantat *nt*.
lung injury Lungenverletzung *f*, -trauma *nt*.
lung malformation *embryo.* Lungenfehlbildung *f*, -malformation *f*.
  adenomatoid l. kongenitale Zystenlunge *f*.
lung perfusion Lungendurchblutung *f*, -perfusion *f*.
lung plague Lungenpest *f*, Pestpneumonie *f*.
lung stone → lung calculus.
lung transplant Lungentransplantat *nt*.
lung transplantation Lungenverpflanzung *f*, -transplantation *f*.
lung trauma Lungenverletzung *f*, -trauma *nt*.
lung tumor Lungentumor *m*.
lung volumes *physiol.* Lungenvolumina *pl*.
lung-worms ['lʌŋwɜːmz] *pl* Lungenwürmer *pl*.
lu·nu·la ['lu:njələ] *n*, *pl* **-lae** [-liː] **1.** *anat.* halbmondförmige/sichelförmige Struktur *f*, Lunula *f*. **2.** Nagelhalbmond *m*, Lunula unguis.
  l.e of aortic semilunar valves halbmondförmiger Randstreifen *m* der Aortenklappe, Lunulae valvularum semilunarium aortae *pl*.
  l. of nail Nagelhalbmond *m*, Lunula unguis.
  l.e of pulmonary semilunar valves halbmondförmiger Randstreifen *m* der Pulmonal(is)klappe, Lunulae valvularum semilunarium trunci pulmonalis.
  l.e of semilunar valves halbmondförmige Randstreifen *m* der Semilunarklappen, Lunulae valvularum semilunarium.
lu·nu·lar ['lu:njələr] *adj* halbmondförmig, lunular.
lu·nu·late ['-leɪt] *adj* → lunular.
lu·nu·lat·ed ['-leɪtɪd] *adj* → lunular.
lu·nule ['lu:njuːl] *n* → lunula.
Lun·yo virus ['lʌnjəʊ] Lunyo-Virus *nt*.
lu·pi·form ['lu:pɪfɔ:rm] *adj* → lupoid.
lu·pi·no·sis [ˌ-'nəʊsɪs] *n* Lupinenvergiftung *f*, -krankheit *f*, Lupinose *f*.
lu·poid ['lu:pɔɪd] *adj derm.* Lupus betr., lupusähnlich, lupös, lupoid.
lupoid hepatitis lupoide Hepatitis *f*, Bearn-Kunkel(-Slater)-Syndrom *nt*.
lupoid rosacea *derm.* lupoide Rosazea *f*, Rosacea granulomatosa.
lu·po·ma [lu:'pəʊmə] *n* Lupusknötchen *nt*, Lupom *nt*.
lu·pous ['lu:pəs] *adj* → lupoid.
lu·pus ['lu:pəs] *n derm.* Lupus *m*.
lupus anticoagulant Lupusantikoagulans *nt*.
lupus erythematosus *abbr.* **LE** *derm.* Lupus erythematodes *abbr.* LE, L.e., L.E., Lupus erythematosus, Erythematodes *m*.

chilblain l. Lupus pernio.
chronic discoid l. → discoid l.
cutaneous l. Lupus erythematodes chronicus/integumentalis.
discoid l. *abbr.* **DLE** Discoid-Lupus erythematosus *abbr.* DLE, Lupus erythematodes chronicus discoides.
disseminated l. → systemic l.
hypertrophic l. Lupus erythematodes hypertrophicus.
systemic l. systemischer Lupus erythematodes *abbr.* SLE, Systemerythematodes *m*, Lupus erythematodes visceralis, Lupus erythematodes integumentalis et visceralis.
lupus erythematosus cells L.e.-Zellen *pl*, L.E.-Zellen *pl*, Lupus-erythematodes--Zellen *pl*.
lupus nephritis Lupusnephritis *f*, -nephropathie *f*.
lupus panniculitis Lupus erythematodes profundus.
Luque ['luːk]: **L.'s instrumentation/operation/technique** *ortho.* Skolioseoperation *f* nach Luque.
Lüscher ['lyʃər]: **L.'s test** HNO Lüscher--Test *m*, Tonintensitätsunterschiedsschwelle *f*.
Luschka ['lɒʃka]: **L.'s body** Glomus coccygeum.
L.'s bursa Bursa pharyngealis.
L.'s cartilage Luschka-Knorpel *m*, Sesamknorpel *m* des Stimmbandes, Cartilago sesamoidea (lig. vocalis).
ducts of L. Luschka'-Gänge *pl*.
foramen of L. Luschka-Foramen *nt*, Apertura lateralis ventriculi quarti.
L.'s fossa Rec. ileoc(a)ecalis superior.
L.'s ganglion → L.'s body.
L.'s gland → L.'s body.
internal coat of pharynx of L. Tela submucosa pharyngis.
laryngeal cartilage of L. → L.'s cartilage.
L.'s ligaments Ligg. sternopericardiaca.
L.'s nerve 1. N. ethmoidalis posterior. **2.** Ramus meningeus n. spinalium.
L.'s tonsil Rachenmandel *f*, Tonsilla pharyngealis/adenoidea.
L.'s tubercle Carina urethralis vaginae.
Lust [lʌst]: **L.'s phenomenon** Lust-Phänomen *nt*, Fibularisphänomen *nt*.
L.'s reflex/sign → L.'s phenomenon.
lu·te·al ['lu:tɪəl] *adj* Corpus luteum betr., luteal, Luteal-.
luteal cells Corpus-luteum-Zellen *pl*.
luteal phase *gyn.* gestagene Phase *f*, Sekretions-, Lutealphase *f*.
luteal phase defect/deficiency *gyn.* (dysfunktioneller) Lutealphasendefekt *m*, Lutealinsuffizienz *f*, Luteal(phase)defekt *m*.
lu·te·ci·um *n* → lutetium.
lu·te·in ['lu:ti:n, -tɪn] *n* Lutein *nt*.
lutein cells → luteal cells.
lutein cyst Luteinzyste *f*.
lu·te·in·ic [lu:tɪ'ɪnɪk] *adj* **1.** → luteal. **2.** Lutein betr., Lutein-. **3.** Luteinisation betr., luteinisierend.
lu·te·in·i·za·tion [ˌlu:tɪənɪ'zeɪʃn] *n* Luteinisation *f*, Luteinisierung *f*.
lu·te·in·ized granulosa-theca cell tumor ['lu:tɪənaɪzd] Luteom(a) *nt*, Luteinom(a) *nt*.
lu·te·in·iz·ing hormone ['lu:tɪənaɪzɪŋ] *abbr.* **LH** luteinisierendes Hormon *nt abbr.* LH, Luteinisierungshormon *nt*, Interstitialzellen-stimulierendes Hormon *nt*, interstitial cell stimulating hormone *abbr.* ICSH.
luteinizing hormone releasing factor *abbr.* **LH-RF, LRF** → luteinizing hormone releasing hormone.

luteinizing hormone releasing hormone abbr. **LH-RH** Luliberin nt, Lutiliberin nt, LH-releasing-Faktor m abbr. LH-RF, LH-releasing-Hormon nt abbr. LH-RH.
luteinizing principle → luteinizing hormone.
lu·te·i·no·ma [luːtɪəˈnəʊmə] n → luteoma 1.
Lutembacher [ˈluːtəmbaxər]: **L.'s complex/disease/syndrome** Lutembacher-Komplex m, -Syndrom nt.
lu·te·o·hor·mone [ˌluːtɪəˈhɔːrməʊn] n Gelbkörperhormon nt, Progesteron nt, Corpus-luteum-Hormon nt.
lu·te·ol·y·sis [luːtɪˈɒləsɪs] n Luteolyse f.
lu·te·o·ma [luːtɪˈəʊmə] n, pl -mas, -ma·ta [-mətə] **1.** Luteom(a) nt, Luteinom(a) nt. **2.** Luteoma gravidarum.
lu·te·o·troph·ic [ˌluːtɪəˈtrəʊfɪk, -ˈtrɑːf-] adj → luteotropic.
lu·te·o·troph·in [ˌ-ˈtrəʊfɪn, -ˈtrɑːf-] n → luteotropin.
lu·te·o·trop·ic [ˌ-ˈtrɒpɪk, -ˈtrəʊp-] adj luteotrop.
luteotropic hormone abbr. **LTH** → luteotropin.
luteotropic lactogenic hormone Prolaktin nt abbr. **PRL**, Prolactin nt, laktogenes Hormon nt.
lu·te·o·tro·pin [ˌ-ˈtrəʊpɪn] n bio. Luteotropin nt, luteotropes Hormon nt abbr. **LTH**.
lu·te·ti·um [luːˈtiːʃɪəm] n abbr. **Lu** Lutetium nt abbr. Lu.
Lu·ther·an blood group (system) [ˈluːθərən] Lutheran-Blutgruppe f, -Blutgruppensystem nt.
lu·ti·lib·er·in [ˌluːtɪˈlɪbərɪn] n → luteinizing hormone releasing hormone.
lu·ti·lib·er·i·ner·gic [ˌ-ˌlɪbərɪˈnɜrdʒɪk] adj lu(ti)liberinerg.
Lut·zo·myi·a [lʊtzəʊˈmaɪə] n micro. Lutzomyia f.
Lutz-Splendore-Almeida [lʌts splenˈdɔːrɪ alˈmeɪdə; lʊts]: **L.-S.-A. disease** Lutz-Splendore-Almeida-Krankheit f, brasilianische/südamerikanische Blastomykose f, Parakokzidioidomykose f, Granuloma paracoccidiales.
lux [lʌks] n, pl **lu·ces** [ˈluːsiːz] phys. Lux nt abbr. lx.
lux·a·tio [lʌkˈseɪʃɪəʊ] n → luxation.
lux·a·tion [lʌkˈseɪʃn] n ortho. Verrenkung f, Luxation f, Luxatio f; Dislokation f.
l. of lens (Auge) Linsenluxation f.
lux·ot·o·my [lʌksˈɒtəmɪ] n ortho. Amputation f mit Ovalärschnitt.
Luys [lyˈiːs]: **L.' body** → nucleus of L.
body of L. syndrome Hemiballismus m.
centromedian nucleus of L. Nc. centromedianus thalami.
nucleus of L. Luys'-Kern m, -Körper m, Corpus Luys, Nc. subthalamicus.
Lw abbr. → lawrencium.
ly·ase [ˈlaɪeɪz] n Lyase f, Synthase f.
ly·can·thro·py [laɪˈkænθrəpɪ] n psychia. Lykanthropie f.
ly·cine [ˈlaɪsiːn] n Betain nt, Trimethylglykokoll nt, Glykokollbetain nt.
ly·co·pene [ˈlaɪkəpiːn] n Lykopin nt.
ly·co·pe·ne·mia [ˌlaɪkəpiːˈniːmɪə] n Lykopinämie(-Syndrom nt) f.
LYDMA abbr. → lymphocyte-determined membrane antigen.
lye [laɪ] **I** n Lauge f. **II** vt mit Lauge behandeln, ablaugen.
Lyell [ˈlaɪəl]: **L.'s disease/syndrome** (medikamentöses) Lyell-Syndrom nt, Syndrom nt der verbrühten Haut, Epidermolysis acuta toxica, Epidermolysis necroticans combustiformis.
ly·ing-in [ˈlaɪɪŋ] **I** n **1.** Niederkunft f, Entbindung f. **2.** Kindbett nt, Wochenbett nt, Puerperium nt. **II** adj Wochenbett/Puerperium betr., puerperal, Puerperal-.
Lyme arthritis/disease [laɪm] Lyme-Krankheit f, -Borreliose f, -Disease nt, Erythema-migrans-Krankheit f abbr. **EMK**.
lymph [lɪmf] n **1.** Lymphe f, Lymphflüssigkeit f, Lympha f. **2.** lymphähnliche Flüssigkeit f.
lym·pha [ˈlɪmfə] n → lymph.
lym·pha·den [ˈlɪmfədən] n → lymph node.
lymph·ad·e·nec·ta·sis [lɪmˌfædəˈnektəsɪs] n Lymphknotenvergrößerung f, Lymphadenektasie f.
lymph·ad·e·nec·to·my [lɪmˌfædəˈnektəmɪ] n chir. Lymphknotenentfernung f, -exstirpation f, Lymphadenektomie f.
lymph·ad·en·hy·per·tro·phy [lɪmˌfædənhaɪˈpɜrtrəfɪ] n Lymphknotenhypertrophie f.
lymph·a·de·nia [lɪmfəˈdiːnɪə] n **1.** → lymphadenhypertrophy. **2.** → lymphadenopathy.
lymph·ad·e·ni·tis [lɪmˌfædəˈnaɪtɪs] n Lymphknotenentzündung f, Lymphadenitis f.
lymph·ad·e·no·cele [lɪmˈfædənəsiːl] n Lymphknotenzyste f, Lymphadenozele f.
lymph·ad·e·no·gram [lɪmˈfædənəgræm] n radiol. Lymphadenogramm nt.
lymph·ad·e·nog·ra·phy [lɪmˌfædɪˈnɒgrəfɪ] n radiol. Kontrastdarstellung f von Lymphknoten, Lymphadenographie f.
lymph·ad·e·noid [lɪmˈfædɪnɔɪd] adj histol. lymphadenoid.
lymphadenoid goiter Hashimoto-Thyreoiditis f, Struma lymphomatosa.
lymph·ad·e·no·ma [ˌlɪmfædɪˈnəʊmə] n **1.** Lymphadenom(a) nt. **2.** → lymphoma.
lymphadenoma cells Sternberg-(Reed)-Riesenzelle f.
lymph·ad·e·nop·a·thy [lɪmˌfædɪˈnɑpəθɪ] n Lymphknotenerkrankung f, Lymphadenopathie f.
lymphadenopathy-associated virus abbr. **LAV** old → human immunodeficiency virus.
lymphadenopathy syndrome abbr. **LAS** Lymphadenopathiesyndrom nt abbr. **LAS**.
lymph·ad·e·no·sis [lɪmˌfædɪˈnəʊsɪs] n Lymphknotenschwellung f, Lymphadenose f, Lymphadenosis f.
lymph·ad·e·not·o·my [lɪmˌfædɪˈnɑtəmɪ] n chir. Lymphadenotomie f.
lymph·an·ge·i·tis [ˌlɪmfændʒɪˈaɪtɪs] n → lymphangitis.
lymph·an·gi·ec·ta·sia [lɪmˌfændʒɪekˈteɪʒ(ɪ)ə] n → lymphangiectasis.
lymph·an·gi·ec·ta·sis [lɪmˌfændʒɪˈektəsɪs] n Lymphgefäßerweiterung f, Lymphangiektasie f.
l. of bone skelettale Lymphangiomatose/Hämangiomatose f, Angiomatose/Lymphangiektasie f des Knochens.
lymph·an·gi·ec·tat·ic [lɪmˌfændʒɪekˈtætɪk] adj Lymphangiektasie betr., lymphangiektatisch.
lymph·an·gi·ec·to·my [lɪmˌfændʒɪˈektəmɪ] n chir. Lymphgefäßresektion f, -exstirpation f, Lymphangiektomie f.
lymph·an·gi·i·tis [lɪmˌfændʒɪˈaɪtɪs] n → lymphangitis.
lymph·an·gi·o·ad·e·nog·ra·phy [lɪmˌfændʒɪəʊˌædəˈnɒgrəfɪ] n → lymphography.
lymph·an·gi·o·en·do·the·li·o·blas·to·ma [ˌ-ˌendəʊˌθiːlɪəˈblæstəʊmə] n → lymphangioendothelioma.
lymph·an·gi·o·en·do·the·li·o·ma [ˌ-ˌendəʊˌθiːlɪˈəʊmə] n Lymphangioendotheliom(a) nt, Lymphoendotheliom(a) nt.
lymph·an·gi·o·fi·bro·ma [ˌ-faɪˈbrəʊmə] n Lymphangiofibrom(a) nt.
lymph·an·gi·o·gram [ˈ-græm] n → lymphogram.
lymph·an·gi·og·ra·phy [lɪmˌfændʒɪˈɒgrəfɪ] n → lymphography.
lymph·an·gi·o·ma [lɪmˌfændʒɪˈəʊmə] n Lymphangiom(a) nt.
lymph·an·gi·om·a·tous [lɪmˌfændʒɪˈɑmətəs] adj Lymphangiom betr., lymphangiomatös.
lymph·an·gi·o·my·o·ma·to·sis [lɪmˌfændʒɪəʊˌmaɪəməˈtəʊsɪs] n gyn. Lymphangiomyomatosis(-Syndrom nt) f.
lymph·an·gi·on [lɪmˈfændʒɪən] n → lymphatic vessel.
lymph·an·gi·o·phle·bi·tis [lɪmˌfændʒɪəʊflɪˈbaɪtɪs] n Lymphangiophlebitis f.
lymph·an·gi·o·sar·co·ma [ˌ-sɑːrˈkəʊmə] n Lymphangiosarkom nt.
lymph·an·gi·o·sis [lɪmˌfændʒɪˈəʊsɪs] n Lymphangiosis f.
lym·phan·gi·tis [ˌlɪmfænˈdʒaɪtɪs] n Lymphgefäßentzündung f, Lymphangitis f, Lymphangiitis f.
lymphangitis carcinomatosa Lymphangiosis carcinomatosa.
lym·pha·phe·re·sis [ˌlɪmfəfəˈriːsɪs] n → lymphocytapheresis.
lym·phat·ic [lɪmˈfætɪk] **I** n **1.** Lymphgefäß nt, Vas lymphaticum. **2.** ~**s** pl Lymphgefäße pl, Lymphsystem nt. **II** adj Lymphe od. lymphatisches Organ betr., lymphatisch, Lymph(o)-.
lymphatic angina Monozytenangina f.
lymphatic capillary Lymphkapillare f, Vas lymphocapillare.
lymphatic drainage Lymphabfluß m, -drainage f.
lymphatic duct: l.s pl Hauptlymphgänge pl, Ductus lymphatici.
right l. rechter Hauptlymphgang m, Ductus lymphaticus/thoracicus dexter.
lymphatic edema → lymphedema.
lymphatic fistula Lymphfistel f, Fistula lymphatica.
lymphatic follicle Lymphfollikel m, -knötchen nt, Folliculus/Nodulus lymphaticus, Lymphonodulus m.
aggregated l.s Peyer'-Plaques pl, Folliculi lymphatici aggregati.
l.s of stomach Folliculi lymphatici gastrici.
l. of tongue Zungenbalg m, Folliculus lingualis.
lymphatic gland → lymph node.
lymphatic leukemia lymphatische/lymphozytische Leukämie f.
lym·phat·i·cos·to·my [lɪmˌfætɪˈkɑstəmɪ] n chir. Lymphatikostomie f.
lymphatic plexus Lymphgefäßnetz nt, Plexus lymphaticus.
axillary l. axillärer Lymph(gefäß)plexus m, Plexus lymphaticus axillaris.
lymphatic progenitor Lymphozytenvorläuferzelle f.
lymphatic pump Lymphpumpe f.
lymphatic ring, cardiac Lymphknotenring m um die Kardia, An(n)ulus lymphaticus cardiae.
lym·phat·ics pl → lymphatic 2.
lymphatic sarcoma → lymphosarcoma.
lymphatic sinus Lymph(knoten)sinus m.
lymphatic spread patho. lymphogene Aussaat/Streuung f.
lymphatic system lymphatisches System nt, Lymphsystem nt, Systema lymphaticum.
lymphatic tissue lymphatisches Gewebe nt.
lymphatic trunks Lymphstämme pl, Hauptlymphgefäße pl, Trunci lymphatici.

lymphatic valve Lymph(gefäß)klappe *f*, Valvula lymphatica.
lymphatic vessel Lymphgefäß *nt*, Vas lymphaticum.
 deep l. tiefes Lymphgefäß, Vas lymphaticum profundum.
 superficial l. oberflächliches Lymphgefäß, Vas lymphaticum superficiale.
lym·pha·tism ['lɪmfətɪzəm] *n* Lymphatismus *m*, lymphatische Diathese *f*, Status lymphaticus.
lym·pha·ti·tis [ˌlɪmfə'taɪtɪs] *n* → lymphangitis.
lym·pha·tol·y·sis [ˌ-'talǝsɪs] *n* Zerstörung *od.* Auflösung *f* des lymphatischen Gewebes, Lymphatolyse *f*.
lymph capillary → lymphatic capillary.
lymph cell → lymphocyte.
lymph circulation Lymphkreislauf *m*, -zirkulation *f*.
lymph cords (*Lymphknoten*) Markstränge *pl*.
lymph dialysis Lymphdialyse *f*.
lymph·e·de·ma [ˌlɪmfɪ'diːmǝ] *n* Lymphödem *nt*, Lymphoedema *nt*.
lymph·ep·i·the·li·o·ma [ˌlɪmfɛpɪˌθɪlɪ'əʊmǝ] *n* → lymphoepithelioma.
lymph follicle Lymphfollikel *m*, -knötchen *nt*, Folliculus/Nodulus lymphaticus, Lymphonodulus *m*.
 mucosal l. Lymphfollikel der Schleimhaut.
 primary l. Primärfollikel.
 secondary l. Sekundärfollikel.
lymph gland → lymph node.
lym·phi·za·tion [ˌlɪmfə'zeɪʃn] *n* Lymphbildung *f*.
lymph node Lymphknoten *m*, *old* Lymphdrüse *f*, Nodus lymphaticus, Lymphonodus *m*.
 abdominal l.s abdominelle Lymphknoten *pl*, Bauchlymphknoten *pl*, Nodi lymphatici abdominis.
 anorectal l.s → pararectal l.s.
 aortic l.s, lateral laterale Aortenlymphknoten *pl*, Nodi lymphatici aortici laterales.
 apical l.s apikale Achsellymphknoten *pl*, Nodi lymphatici axillares apicales.
 appendicular l.s Appendixlymphknoten *pl*, Nodi lymphatici appendiculares.
 l. of arch of azygos vein Lymphknoten am Azygosbogen, Nodus arcus v. azygos.
 axillary l.s Achsellymphknoten *pl*, Nodi lymphatici axillares.
 axillary l.s, apical → apical l.s.
 axillary l.s, brachial → brachial l.s.
 axillary l.s, deep tiefe Achsellymphknoten *pl*, Nodi lymphatici axillares profundi.
 axillary l., interpectoral → interpectoral l.
 axillary l.s, lateral → brachial l.s.
 axillary l., pectoral → interpectoral l.
 axillary l.s, subscapular → subscapular l.s.
 axillary l.s, superficial oberflächliche Achsellymphknoten *pl*, Nodi lymphatici axillares superficiales.
 brachial l.s Oberarmlymphknoten *pl*, Nodi lymphatici (axillares) brachiales.
 bronchopulmonary l.s Hiluslymphknoten *pl*, Nodi lymphatici bronchopulmonales/hilares.
 buccal l. Wangenlymphknoten *m*, Nodus (lymphaticus) buccinatorius.
 buccinator l. → buccal l.
 caval l.s, lateral laterale Cavalymphknoten *pl*, Nodi lymphatici cavales laterales.
 celiac l.s Lymphknoten *pl* des Truncus coeliacus, Nodi lymphatici viscerales coeliaci.
 cervical l.s Hals-, Zervikallymphknoten *pl*, Nodi lymphatici cervicales.
 cervical l.s, anterior vordere Halslymphknoten *pl*, Nodi lymphatici cervicales anteriores.
 cervical l.s, deep tiefe Halslymphknoten *pl*, Nodi lymphatici cervicales profundi.
 cervical l.s, deep anterior tiefe vordere Halslymphknoten *pl*, Nodi lymphatici cervicales anteriores profundi.
 cervical l.s, deep lateral tiefe seitliche Halslymphknoten *pl*, Nodi lymphatici cervicales laterales profundi.
 cervical l.s, lateral seitliche Halslymphknoten *pl*, Nodi lymphatici cervicales laterales.
 cervical l.s, prelaryngeal → prelaryngeal l.s.
 cervical l.s, superficial oberflächliche Halslymphknoten *pl*, Nodi lymphatici cervicales superficiales.
 cervical l.s, superficial anterior vordere oberflächliche Halslymphknoten *pl*, Nodi lymphatici cervicales anteriores superficiales.
 cervical l.s, superficial lateral seitliche oberflächliche Halslymphknoten *pl*, Nodi lymphatici cervicales laterales superficiales.
 colic l.s, left Lymphknoten *pl* der A. colica sinistra, Nodi lymphatici mesocolici colici sinistri.
 colic l.s, middle Lymphknoten *pl* der A. colica media, Nodi lymphatici mesocolici colici medii.
 colic l.s, right Lymphknoten *pl* der A. colica dextra, Nodi lymphatici mesocolici colici dextri.
 collecting l.s Sammellymphknoten *pl*.
 cubital l.s kubitale Lymphknoten *pl*, Nodi lymphatici cubitales.
 deep l.s of upper limb tiefe Armlymphknoten *pl*, Nodi lymphatici profundi (membri superioris).
 diaphragmatic l.s → phrenic l.s, superior.
 epigastric l.s, inferior Lymphknoten *pl* der A. epigastrica inferior, Nodi lymphatici parietales epigastrici inferiores.
 facial l.s Gesichtslymphknoten *pl*, Nodi lymphatici faciales.
 gastric l.s, left linke Lymphknotengruppe *f* der kleinen Magenkurvatur, Nodi lymphatici viscerales gastrici sinistri.
 gastric l.s, right rechte Lymphknotengruppe *f* der kleinen Magenkurvatur, Nodi lymphatici viscerales gastrici dextri.
 gastroepiploic l.s, left → gastroomental l.s, left.
 gastroepiploic l.s, right → gastroomental l.s., right.
 gastroomental l.s, left linke Lymphknotengruppe *f* der großen Magenkurvatur, Nodi lymphatici viscerales gastro-omentales sinistri.
 gastroomental l.s, right rechte Lymphknotengruppe *f* der großen Magenkurvatur, Nodi lymphatici viscerales gastro-omentales dextri.
 gluteal l.s, inferior Lymphknoten *pl* der A. glutaea inferior, Nodi lymphatici glut(a)eales inferiores.
 gluteal l.s, superior Lymphknoten *pl* der A. glutaea superior, Nodi lymphatici glut(a)eales superiores.
 hepatic l.s Leber(hilus)lymphknoten *pl*, Nodi lymphatici viscerales hepatici.
 hilar l.s → bronchopulmonary l.s.
 ileocolic l.s Lymphknoten *pl* der A. ileocolica, Nodi lymphatici ileocolici.
 iliac l.s, common Lymphknoten *pl* der A. iliaca communis, Nodi lymphatici parietales iliaci communes.
 iliac l.s, common intermediate Nodi lymphatici parietales iliaci communes intermedii.
 iliac l.s, common lateral Nodi lymphatici parietales iliaci communes laterales.
 iliac l.s, common medial Nodi lymphatici parietales iliaci communes mediales.
 iliac l.s, common promontory Nodi lymphatici parietales iliaci communes promontorii.
 iliac l.s, common subaortic Lymphknoten *pl* der Aortengabel, Nodi lymphatici parietales iliaci communes subaortici.
 iliac l.s, external Lymphknoten *pl* der A. iliaca externa, Nodi lymphatici parietales iliaci externi.
 iliac l.s, external interiliac zwischen A. iliaca interna u. A. iliaca externa liegende Lymphknoten, Nodi lymphatici parietales (iliaci externi) interiliaci.
 iliac l.s, external intermediate Nodi lymphatici parietales iliaci externi intermedii.
 iliac l.s, external lateral Nodi lymphatici parietales iliaci externi laterales.
 iliac l.s, external medial Nodi lymphatici parietales iliaci externi mediales.
 iliac l.s, internal Lymphknoten *pl* der A. iliaca interna, Nodi lymphatici parietales iliaci interni.
 infraauricular l.s infraaurikuläre Lymphknoten *pl*, Nodi lymphatici infraauriculares.
 inguinal l.s Leisten-, Inguinallymphknoten *pl*, Nodi lymphatici inguinales.
 inguinal l.s, deep tiefe Leisten-, Inguinallymphknoten *pl*, Nodi lymphatici inguinales profundi.
 inguinal l.s, inferior untere Leistenlymphknoten *pl*, Nodi lymphatici inguinales inferiores.
 inguinal l.s, inferior superficial untere oberflächliche Leistenlymphknoten *pl*, Nodi lymphatici inguinales (superficiales) inferiores.
 inguinal l.s, superficial oberflächliche Leistenlymphknoten *pl*, Nodi lymphatici inguinales superficiales.
 inguinal l.s, superolateral obere seitliche Leistenlymphknoten *pl*, Nodi lymphatici inguinales superolaterales.
 inguinal l.s, superolateral superficial laterale Gruppe der oberflächlichen Leistenlymphknoten, Nodi lymphatici inguinales (superficiales) superolaterales.
 inguinal l.s, superomedial obere mediale Leistenlymphknoten *pl*, Nodi lymphatici inguinales superomediales.
 inguinal l.s, superomedial superficial mediale Gruppe der oberflächlichen Leistenlymphknoten, Nodi lymphatici inguinales (superficiales) superomediales.
 intercostal l.s paravertebrale Interkostallymphknoten *pl*, Nodi lymphatici intercostales.
 interiliac l.s → iliac l.s, external interiliac.
 interpectoral l. Brustwand-, Pektoralislymphknoten, Nodus lymphaticus (axillaris) interpectoralis.
 intraglandular l.s in der Parotis liegende Lymphknoten, Nodi lymphatici intraglandulares.
 jugular l.s, anterior vordere jugulare Lymphknoten *pl*, Nodi lymphatici jugulares anteriores.
 jugular l.s, lateral laterale jugulare Lymphknoten *pl*, Nodi lymphatici jugulares laterales.
 jugulodigastric l. oberster tiefer Halslymphknoten, Nodus (lymphaticus) jugulodigastricus.

jugulo-omohyoid l. Nodus (lymphaticus) jugulo-omohyoideus.
juxta-esophageal l.s, pulmonary juxtaösophageale Lymphknoten *pl*, Nodi lymphatici juxta-oesophageales pulmonales.
juxta-intestinal l.s juxtaintestinale Lymphknoten *pl*, Nodi lymphatici mesenterici juxta-intestinales.
lienal l.s → splenic l.s.
lumbar l.s, intermediate intermediäre Lumballymphknoten *pl*, Nodi lymphatici parietales lumbales/lumbares intermedii.
lumbar l.s, left lumbale Lymphknoten *pl* der Bauchaorta, Nodi lymphatici parietales lumbales/lumbares sinistri.
lumbar l.s, right lumbale Lymphknoten *pl* der V. cava inferior, Nodi lymphatici parietales lumbales/lumbares dextri.
malar l. Wangenlymphknoten, Nodus lymphaticus malaris.
mandibular l. Unterkieferlymphknoten, Nodus (lymphaticus) mandibularis.
mastoid l.s retroauriculäre Lymphknoten *pl*, Nodi lymphatici mastoidei/retro--auriculares.
mediastinal l.s, anterior vordere Mediastinallymphknoten *pl*, Nodi lymphatici mediastinales anteriores.
mediastinal l.s, posterior hintere Mediastinallymphknoten *pl*, Nodi lymphatici mediastinales posteriores.
mesenteric l.s Mesenteriallymphknoten *pl*, Nodi lymphatici mesenterici.
mesenteric l.s, inferior untere Mesenteriallymphknoten *pl*, Nodi lymphatici mesenterici inferiores.
mesenteric l.s, superior obere Mesenteriallymphknoten *pl*, Nodi lymphatici mesenterici superiores, Nodi superiores centrales.
mesocolic l.s mesokolische Lymphknoten *pl*, Nodi lymphatici mesocolici.
nasolabial l. Lymphknoten der Nasolabialfalte, Nodus (lymphaticus) nasolabialis.
obturator l.s Lymphknoten *pl* der A. obturatoria, Nodi lymphatici parietales iliaci externi obturatorii.
occipital l.s okzipitale Lymphknoten *pl*, Nodi lymphatici occipitales.
pancreatic l.s, inferior untere Pankreaslymphknoten *pl*, Nodi lymphatici viscerales pancreatici inferiores.
pancreatic l.s, superior obere Pankreaslymphknoten *pl*, Nodi lymphatici viscerales pancreatici superiores.
pancreaticoduodenal l.s, inferior untere pankreatikoduodenale Lymphknoten *pl*, Nodi lymphatici viscerales pancreaticoduodenales inferiores.
pancreaticoduodenal l.s, superior obere pankreatikoduodenale Lymphknoten *pl*, Nodi lymphatici viscerales pancreaticoduodenales superiores.
paracolic l.s parakolische Lymphknoten *pl*, Nodi lymphatici mesocolici paracolici.
parammary l.s seitliche Brustdrüsen-, Mammalymphknoten *pl*, Nodi lymphatici parammarii.
pararectal l.s pararektale/anorektale Lymphknoten *pl*, Nodi lymphatici viscerales pararectales/anorectales.
parasternal l.s parasternale Lymphknoten *pl*, Nodi lymphatici parasternales.
paratracheal l.s paratracheale Lymphknoten *pl*, Nodi lymphatici paratracheales.
parauterine l.s parauterine Lymphknoten *pl*, Nodi lymphatici viscerales para-uterini.

paravaginal l.s paravaginale Lymphknoten *pl*, Nodi lymphatici viscerales paravaginales.
paravesicular l.s paravesikale Lymphknoten *pl*, Nodi lymphatici viscerales paravesiculares.
parotid l.s, deep tiefe Parotislymphknoten *pl*, Nodi lymphatici parotidei profundi.
parotid l.s, superficial oberflächliche Parotislymphknoten *pl*, Nodi lymphatici parotidei superficiales.
pectoral l. → interpectoral l.
pelvic l.s Beckenlymphknoten *pl*, Nodi lymphatici pelvis.
pericardial l.s perikardiale Lymphknoten *pl*, Nodi lymphatici pericardiales.
pericardial l.s, lateral laterale perikardiale Lymphknoten *pl*, Nodi lymphatici pericardiales laterales.
perivesicular l.s perivesikuläre Lymphknoten *pl*, Nodi lymphatici perivesiculares.
phrenic l.s, inferior untere Zwerchfellymphknoten *pl*, Nodi lymphatici parietales phrenici inferiores.
phrenic l.s, superior obere Zwerchfellymphknoten *pl*, Nodi lymphatici phrenici superiores.
popliteal l.s, deep tiefe Kniekehlen-, Popliteallymphknoten *pl*, Nodi lymphatici popliteales profundi.
popliteal l.s, superficial oberflächliche Kniekehlen-, Popliteallymphknoten *pl*, Nodi lymphatici popliteales superficiales.
postaortic l.s retroaortale Lymphknoten *pl*, Nodi lymphatici postaortici.
postcaval l.s retrokavale Lymphknoten *pl*, Nodi lymphatici postcavales.
postvesicular l.s postvesikale Lymphknoten *pl*, Nodi lymphatici postvesiculares.
preaortic l.s präaortale Lymphknoten *pl*, Nodi lymphatici pr(a)e-aortici.
preauricular l.s präauriculäre Lymphknoten *pl*, Nodi lymphatici pr(a)e-auriculares.
precaval l.s präkavale Lymphknoten *pl*, Nodi lymphatici pr(a)ecavales.
prececal l.s präzäkale Lymphknoten *pl*, Nodi lymphatici pr(a)ececales.
prelaryngeal l.s prälaryngeale Lymphknoten *pl*, Nodi lymphatici pr(a)elaryngeales.
prepericardial l.s präperikardiale Lymphknoten *pl*, Nodi lymphatici pr(a)epericardiales.
pretracheal l.s prätracheale Lymphknoten *pl*, Nodi lymphatici pr(a)etracheales.
prevertebral l.s prävertebrale Lymphknoten *pl*, Nodi lymphatici pr(a)evertebrales.
prevesicular l.s prävesikale Lymphknoten *pl*, Nodi lymphatici pr(a)evesiculares.
pulmonary l.s Lungenlymphknoten *pl*, Nodi lymphatici pulmonales.
pyloric l.s Pylorislymphknoten *pl*, Nodi lymphatici viscerales pylorici.
rectal l.s, superior Lymphknoten *pl* der A. rectalis superior, Nodi lymphatici rectales superiores.
regional l.s regionale Lymphknoten *pl*, Nodi (lymphatici) regionales.
retroaortic l.s → postaortic l.s.
retroauricular l.s → mastoid l.s.
retrocecal l.s retrozäkale Lymphknoten *pl*, Nodi lymphatici retroc(a)ecales.
retropharyngeal l.s retropharyngeale Lymphknoten *pl*, Nodi lymphatici retropharyngeales.

retropyloric l.s retropylorische Lymphknoten *pl*, Nodi (lymphatici) retropylorici.
Rosenmüller's l. 1. oberster tiefer Leistenlymphknoten. **2.** ~s *pl* → inguinal l.s, deep.
sacral l.s sakrale Lymphknoten *pl*, Nodi lymphatici sacrales.
sigmoid l.s Lymphknoten *pl* der A. sigmoidea, Nodi (lymphatici) sigmoidei.
splenic l.s Milzlymphknoten *pl*, Nodi lymphatici lienales/splenici.
submandibular l.s submandibuläre Lymphknoten *pl*, Nodi lymphatici submandibulares.
submental l.s Kinnlymphknoten *pl*, Nodi lymphatici submentales.
subpyloric l.s subpylorische Lymphknoten *pl*, Nodi lymphatici subpylorici.
subscapular l.s subskapuläre Lymphknoten *pl*, Nodi lymphatici (axillares) subscapulares.
superficial l.s of upper limb oberflächliche Lymphknoten *pl* des Arms, Nodi lymphatici membri superioris superficiales.
supraclavicular l.s supraklavikuläre Lymphknoten *pl*, Nodi lymphatici supraclaviculares.
suprapyloric l.s suprapylorische Lymphknoten *pl*, Nodi (lymphatici) suprapylorici.
supratrochlear l.s → cubital l.s.
thyroid l.s Schilddrüsenlymphknoten *pl*, Nodi lymphatici thyroidei.
tracheal l.s → paratracheal l.s.
tracheobronchial l.s, inferior untere tracheobronchiale Lymphknoten *pl*, Nodi lymphatici tracheobronchiales inferiores.
tracheobronchial l.s, superior obere tracheobronchiale Lymphknoten *pl*, Nodi lymphatici tracheobronchiales superiores.
vesicular l.s, lateral laterale paravesikale Lymphknoten *pl*, Nodi lymphatici vesiculares laterales.
lymph node disease (*Tumor*) Lymphknotenbefall *m*, Lymphknotenmetastase *f*, -metastasierung *f*.
lymph node dissection *chir.* Lymphknotenentfernung *f*, -dissektion *f*.
lymph node metastasis Lymphknotenmetastase *f*.
lymph node permeability factor *abbr.* **LNPF** Lymphknotenpermeabilitätsfaktor *m*, lymph node permeability factor *abbr.* LNPF.
lymph node tuberculosis Lymphknotentuberkulose *f*, Lymphadenitis tuberculosa.
lymph node tumor Lymphknotengeschwulst *f*, -tumor *m*.
lymph·no·di·tis [ˌlɪmfnəʊˈdaɪtɪs] *n* → lymphadenitis.
lymph nodule → lymph follicle.
lym·pho·blast [ˈlɪmfəblæst] *n* Lymphoblast *m*, Lymphozytoblast *m*.
lym·pho·blas·tic [ˌ-ˈblæstɪk] *adj* lymphoblastisch.
lymphoblastic leukemia akute lymphoblastische Leukämie *f*, Lymphoblastenleukämie *f*.
lymphoblastic lymphoma lymphoblastisches Lymphom *nt*.
lymphoblastic lymphosarcoma lymphoblastisches Lymphosarkom *nt*.
lym·pho·blas·to·ma [ˌ-blæsˈtəʊmə] *n* **1.** Lymphoblastom(a) *nt*. **2.** → lymphoblastic lymphoma.
lym·pho·blas·to·sis [ˌ-blæsˈtəʊsɪs] *n* Lymphoblastose *f*, -blastosis *f*.
lym·pho·cap·il·lar·y [ˌ-ˈkæpələrɪ, -kəˈpɪlə-

lymphocapillary network

rı] *adj* Lymphkapillare(n) betr., lymphokapillär.
lymphocapillary network Lymphkapillarennetz *nt*, Rete lymphocapillare.
lymphocapillary rete → lymphocapillary network.
lymphocapillary vessel Lymphkapillare *f*, Vas lymphocapillare.
lym·pho·cele ['-siːl] *n* Lymphozele *f*, -cele *f*.
lym·pho·ci·ne·sia [ˌ-sɪ'niːʒ(ı)ə] *n* → lymphokinesis.
lym·pho·cy·ta·phe·re·sis [ˌ-ˌsaɪtəfə'riːsɪs] *n lab.* Lymphozytenpherese *f*, Lympho(zyto)pherese *f*.
lym·pho·cyte ['-saɪt] *n* Lymphzelle *f*, Lymphozyt *m*, -cyt *m*.
lymphocyte-activating factor *abbr.* **LAF** *old* → interleukin-1.
lymphocyte blastogenic factor → lymphocyte mitogenic factor.
lymphocyte culture Lymphozytenkultur *f*.
lymphocyte-defined antigens Lymphozyten-definierte Antigene *pl*, LD-Antigene *pl*.
lymphocyte-detected membrane antigen → lymphocyte-determined membrane antigen.
lymphocyte-determined membrane antigen *abbr.* **LYDMA** lymphozyten-determiniertes Membranantigen *nt*, lymphocyte-determined membrane antigen *abbr.* LYDMA.
lymphocyte mitogenic factor *abbr.* **LMF** Lymphozytenmitogen *nt*, Lymphozytentransformationsfaktor *m abbr.* LTF.
lymphocyte proliferation assay/test gemischte Lymphozytenkultur *f*, Lymphozytenmischkultur *f*, mixed lymphocyte culture *abbr.* MLC, MLC-Assay *m*, MLC-Test *m*.
lymphocyte recirculation Lymphozytenrezirkulation *f*.
lymphocyte series *hema.* lymphozytäre Reihe *f*.
lymphocyte transformation *immun.* Lymphozytentransformation *f*.
lymphocyte transforming factor *abbr.* **LTF** → lymphocyte mitogenic factor.
lymphocyte wall Lymphozytenwall *m*, -mantel *m*.
lym·pho·cy·the·mia [ˌlɪmfəsaɪ'θiːmɪə] *n* → lymphocytosis.
lym·pho·cyt·ic [ˌ-'sɪtɪk] *adj* Lymphozyten betr., lymphozytär, Lymphozyten-.
lymphocytic choriomeningitis *abbr.* **LCM** Armstrong'-Krankheit *f*, lymphozytäre Choriomeningitis *f abbr.* LCM.
lymphocytic choriomeningitis virus LCM-Virus *nt*.
lymphocytic leukemia lymphatische/lymphozytische Leukämie *f*.
lymphocytic leukocytosis → lymphocytosis.
lymphocytic leukopenia Lymphopenie *f*.
lymphocytic lymphosarcoma lymphozytisches Lymphosarkom *nt*, zentrozytisches (malignes) Lymphom *nt*.
lymphocytic meningitis lymphozytäre Meningitis *f*.
lymphocytic series → lymphocyte series.
lymphocytic thyroiditis Hashimoto--Thyreoiditis *f*, Struma lymphomatosa.
lym·pho·cy·to·blast [ˌ-'saɪtəblæst] *n* → lymphoblast.
lym·pho·cy·to·ma [ˌ-saɪ'təʊmə] *n* Lymphozytom *nt*, Lymphocytoma *nt*; Pseudolymphom *nt*.
lym·pho·cy·to·pe·nia [ˌ-ˌsaɪtə'piːnɪə] *n* Lymphopenie *f*, Lymphozytopenie *f*.
lym·pho·cy·to·phe·re·sis [ˌ-ˌsaɪtəfə'riːsɪs] *n* → lymphocytapheresis.

lym·pho·cy·to·poi·e·sis [ˌ-ˌsaɪtəpɔɪ'iːsɪs] *n* → lymphopoiesis 2.
lym·pho·cy·to·poi·et·ic [ˌ-ˌsaɪtəpɔɪ'etɪk] *adj* → lymphopoietic.
lym·pho·cy·to·sis [ˌ-saɪ'təʊsɪs] *n* Lymphozytose *f*, Lymphocytosis *f*, Lymphozythämie *f*.
lymphocytosis promoting factor *abbr.* **LPF** *old* Pertussistoxin *nt abbr.* PT.
lym·pho·cy·to·tox·ic [ˌ-ˌsaɪtə'tɑksɪk] *adj* lymphozytenzerstörend, lymphozytotoxisch.
lymphocytotoxic antibody lymphozytotoxischer Antikörper *m*.
lymphocytotoxic cross-match *immun.* (*Transplantation*) Zytotoxizitätstest *m*.
lym·pho·cy·to·tox·ic·i·ty [ˌ-ˌsaɪtətɑk'sɪsətɪ] *n* Lymphozytotoxizität *f*.
lym·pho·di·a·pe·de·sis [ˌ-ˌdaɪəpɪ'diːsɪs] *n* Lympho(zyten)diapedese *f*.
lym·pho·duct ['-dʌkt] *n* → lymphatic vessel.
lym·pho·ep·i·the·li·al carcinoma [ˌ-epɪ-'θiːlɪəl, -jəl] → lymphoepithelioma.
lymphoepithelial tumor → lymphoepithelioma.
lym·pho·ep·i·the·li·o·ma [ˌ-epɪˌθɪlɪ'əʊmə] *n* Lymphoepitheliom *nt*, lymphoepitheliales Karzinom *nt*, Schmincke-Tumor *m*.
lym·pho·gen·e·sis [ˌ-'dʒenəsɪs] *n* Lymphbildung *f*, Lymphogenese *f*.
lym·pho·gen·ic [ˌ-'dʒenɪk] *adj* → lymphogenous 2.
lym·phog·e·nous [lɪm'fɑdʒənəs] *adj* 1. Lymphe produzierend. 2. aus Lymphe *od.* lymphatischen Gefäßen stammend, lymphogen.
lymphogenous leukemia → lymphocytic leukemia.
lym·pho·glan·du·la [ˌlɪmfə'glændʒələ] *n*, *pl* **-lae** [-liː, -laɪ] → lymph node.
lym·pho·gram ['-græm] *n radiol.* Lymphogramm *nt*, Lymphangiogramm *nt*.
lym·pho·gran·u·lo·ma [ˌ-ˌgrænjʊ'ləʊmə] *n* 1. Lymphogranulom(a) *nt*. 2. Hodgkin--Krankheit *f*, -Lymphom *nt*, (maligne) Lymphogranulomatose *f*, Morbus Hodgkin *m*, Lymphogranulomatosis maligna, (Hodgkin-)Paltauf-Steinberg--Krankheit *f*.
lymphogranuloma inguinale → lymphogranuloma venereum.
lym·pho·gran·u·lo·ma·to·sis [ˌ-ˌgrænjə-ˌləʊmə'təʊsɪs] *n* 1. Lymphogranulomatose *f*, -matosis *f*. 2. → lymphogranuloma.
lymphogranuloma venereum *abbr.* **LGV** Lymphogranuloma inguinale/venereum *nt abbr.* LGV, Lymphopathia venerea, Morbus Durand-Nicolas-Favre *m*, klimatischer Bubo *m*, vierte Geschlechtskrankheit *f*, Poradenitis inguinalis.
lymphogranuloma venereum antigen Frei-Antigen *nt*.
lymphogranuloma venereum virus *old* → Chlamydia trachomatis.
lym·phog·ra·phy [lɪm'fɑgrəfɪ] *n radiol.* Kontrastdarstellung *f* von Lymphgefäßen u. Lymphknoten, Lymphographie *f*, Lymphangiographie *f*.
lym·pho·he·ma·tog·e·nous [ˌlɪmfəˌhiːmə-'tɑdʒənəs] *adj* lymphohämatogen.
lymphohematogenous spread lymphohämatogene Aussaat *f*.
lym·pho·his·ti·o·cyt·ic [ˌ-ˌhɪstɪə'sɪtɪk] *adj* lympho-histiozytär.
lym·pho·his·ti·o·plas·ma·cyt·ic [ˌ-ˌhɪstɪə-ˌplæzmə'sɪtɪk] *adj* lympho-histio-plasmazytär.
lym·phoid ['lɪmfɔɪd] *adj* lymphartig, lymphatisch, lymphozytenähnlich, lymphoid, Lymph-.

lymphoid cell 1. Lymphoidzelle *f*. 2. Lymphozyt *m*.
lym·phoid·ec·to·my [ˌlɪmfɔɪ'dektəmɪ] *n chir.* Lymphoidektomie *f*.
lymphoid follicle → lymph follicle.
lymphoid hemoblast of Pappenheim Proerythroblast *m*.
lymphoid leukemia → lymphocytic leukemia.
lymphoid leukocyte agranulärer/lymphoider Leukozyt *m*, Agranulozyt *m*.
lym·phoi·do·cyte [lɪm'fɔɪdəsaɪt] *n* Lymphoidzelle *f*.
lymphoid organ lymphatisches Organ *nt*.
lymphoid ring Waldeyer'-Rachenring *m*, lymphatischer Rachenring *m*.
lymphoid sheath (*Milz*) periarterielle Lymphscheide *f*.
lymphoid thyroiditis → lymphocytic thyroiditis.
lymphoid tissue lymphatisches Gewebe *nt*.
gut-associated l. *abbr.* **GALT** darmassoziiertes lymphatisches System *nt*, gut-associated lymphoid tissue *abbr.* GALT.
lym·pho·kine ['lɪmfəkaɪn] *n* Lymphokin *nt*.
lymphokine-activated killer cell lymphokin-aktivierte Killerzelle *f*, LAK-Zelle *f*.
lym·pho·ki·ne·sis [ˌ-kɪ'niːsɪs] *n* 1. Lymphzirkulation *f*. 2. *HNO* Endolymphzirkulation *f*.
lym·phol·y·sis [lɪm'fɑləsɪs] *n* Lymphozytenauflösung *f*, Lympholyse *f*, -lysis *f*, Lymphozytolyse *f*.
lym·pho·lyt·ic [ˌlɪmfə'lɪtɪk] *adj* Lymphozyten auflösend *od.* zerstörend, lympho(zyto)lytisch.
lym·pho·ma [lɪm'fəʊmə] *n*, *pl* **-mas**, **-ma·ta** [-mətə] 1. Lymphknotenschwellung *f*, -tumor *m*, Lymphom(a) *nt*. 2. → lymphogranuloma. 3. non-Hodgkin-Lymphom *abbr.* NHL.
lym·pho·ma·toid [lɪm'fəʊmətɔɪd] *adj* lymphomartig, -ähnlich, lymphomatoid.
lymphomatoid papulosis *derm.* lymphomatoide Papulose *f*, T-Zell-Pseudolymphom *nt*.
lym·pho·ma·to·sis [lɪmˌfəʊmə'təʊsɪs] *n*, *pl* **-ses** [-siːz] Lymphomatose *f*, -matosis *f*.
lym·pho·ma·tous [lɪm'fəʊmətəs] *adj* Lymphom betr., lymphomartig, lymphomatös.
lym·pho·myx·o·ma [ˌlɪmfəmɪk'səʊmə] *n* Lymphomyxom(a) *nt*.
lym·pho·nod·u·lus [ˌ-'nɑdʒələs] *n*, *pl* **-li** [-laɪ] → lymph follicle.
lym·pho·no·dus [ˌ-'nəʊdəs] *n*, *pl* **-di** [-daɪ] → lymph node.
lym·pho·path·ia [ˌ-'pæθɪə] *n* → lymphopathy.
lymphopathia venereum → lymphogranuloma venereum.
lym·phop·a·thy [lɪm'fɑpəθɪ] *n* Erkrankung *f* des lymphatischen Systems, Lymphopathie *f*, Lymphopathia *f*.
lym·pho·pe·nia [ˌlɪmfə'piːnɪə] *n* Lymphopenie *f*, Lymphozytopenie *f*.
lym·pho·pe·nic agammaglobulinemia [ˌ-'piːnɪk] Schweizer-Typ *m* der Agammaglobulinämie, schwerer kombinierter Immundefekt *m*.
lym·pho·pla·sia [ˌ-'pleɪʒ(ı)ə, -zɪə] *n* Lymphoplasie *f*, -plasia *f*.
lym·pho·plas·ma·cel·lu·lar [ˌ-ˌplæzmə-'seljələr] *adj* lympho-plasmazellulär.
lym·pho·plas·ma·cyt·ic immunocytoma [ˌ-ˌplæzmə'sɪtɪk] Waldenström-Krankheit *f*, Morbus Waldenström *m*, Makroglobulinämie Waldenström *f*.
lym·pho·plas·ma·cy·toid immunocytoma [ˌ-ˌplæzmə'saɪtɔɪd] lymphoplasmozytoides Immunozytom *nt*.

lym·pho·poi·e·sis [ˌ-pɔɪˈiːsɪs] *n* **1.** Lymphbildung *f*. **2.** Lymphozytenbildung *f*, Lymphopo(i)ese *f*, Lymphozytopo(i)ese *f*.
lym·pho·poi·et·ic [ˌ-pɔɪˈetɪk] *adj* Lymphozytopo(i)ese betr. *od.* stimulierend, lympho(zyto)poetisch.
lym·pho·pro·lif·er·a·tive disease/disorder/syndrome [ˌ-prəˈlɪfəˌreɪtɪv] lymphoproliferative Erkrankung *f*.
lymphoproliferative system lymphoproliferatives System *nt*.
lymphoproliferative tumor Tumor *m* des lymphoproliferativen Systems.
lym·pho·re·tic·u·lar diseases/disorders/syndrome [ˌ-rɪˈtɪkjələr] lymphoretikuläre Erkrankungen *pl*, Erkrankungen *pl* des lymphoretikulären Systems.
lymphoreticular system lymphoretikuläres System *nt*.
lym·pho·re·tic·u·lo·sis [ˌ-rɪˌtɪkjəˈləʊsɪs] *n* Lymphoretikulose *f*.
lym·phor·rha·gia [ˌ-ˈrædʒ(ɪ)ə] *n* → lymphorrhea.
lym·phor·rhea [ˌ-ˈrɪə] *n* Lymphorrhagie *f*, Lymphorrhö *f*.
lym·pho·sar·co·ma [ˌ-sɑːrˈkəʊmə] *n* Lymphosarkom *nt*.
lymphosarcoma cell leukemia Lymphosarkomzellenleukämie *f*.
lym·pho·sar·co·ma·to·sis [ˌ-ˌsɑːrkəʊməˈtəʊsɪs] *n* Lymphosarkomatose *f*.
lym·phos·ta·sis [lɪmˈfæstəsɪs] *n* Lymphstauung *f*, Lymphostase *f*.
lym·pho·tax·is [ˌlɪmfəˈtæksɪs] *n* Lymphotaxis *f*.
lym·pho·tox·in [ˌ-ˈtɑksɪn] *n* Lymphotoxin *nt*, zytotoxisches Lymphokin *nt*.
lym·phous [ˈlɪmfəs] *adj* Lymphe betr., lymphhaltig, Lymph-.
lymph scrotum Elephantiasis scroti.
lymph sinus *n* lymphatic sinus.
lymph-vascular *adj* Lymphgefäße betr., lympho-vaskulär.
lymph-vascular system Lymphgefäßsystem *nt*.
lymph vessel Lymphgefäß *nt*, Vas lymphaticum.
  afferent l. zuführendes/afferentes Lymphgefäß, Vas afferens lymphaticum.
  deep l. tiefes Lymphgefäß, Vas lymphaticum profundum.
  efferent l. ableitendes/efferentes Lymphgefäß, Vas efferens lymphaticum.
  superficial l. oberflächliches Lymphgefäß, Vas lymphaticum superficiale.
lyn·es·tre·nol [lɪnˈestrənɒl, -nɑl] *n* Lynestrenol *nt*.
lyo- *pref.* Lyo-.
ly·o·chrome [ˈlaɪəkrəʊm] *n* Flavin *nt*.
ly·o·gel [ˈlaɪədʒel] *n* Lyogel *nt*.
Lyon [ˈlaɪən] : **L. hypothesis** *genet.* Lyon-Hypothese *f*.
ly·on·i·za·tion [ˌlaɪənaɪˈzeɪʃn] *n genet.* Lyonisierung *f*.
ly·on·ized [ˈlaɪənaɪzd] *adj genet.* lyonisiert.
ly·o·phil [ˈlaɪəfɪl] *n chem.* lyophile Substanz *f*.
ly·o·phile [ˈ-faɪl] **I** *n* → lyophil. **II** *adj* → lyophilic.
ly·o·phil·ic [ˌ-ˈfɪlɪk] *adj chem.* lyophil.
lyophilic colloid lyophiles Kolloid *nt*.
ly·oph·i·li·za·tion [laɪˌɑfəlɪˈzeɪʃn] *n* Gefriertrocknung *f*, Lyophilisation *f*, Lyophilisierung *f*.
ly·oph·i·lize [laɪˈɑfəlaɪz] *vt* gefriertrocknen, lyophilisieren.
ly·o·phobe [ˈlaɪəfəʊb] *n chem.* lyophobe Substanz *f*.
ly·o·pho·bic [ˌ-ˈfəʊbɪk] *adj chem.* lyophob.
ly·o·sol [ˈ-sɒl, -sɑl] *n chem.* Lyosol *nt*.
ly·o·sorp·tion [ˌ-ˈsɔːrpʃn] *n chem.* Lyosorption *f*.
ly·o·trop·ic [ˌ-ˈtrɑpɪk, -ˈtrəʊp-] *adj chem.* lyotrop.
lyotropic colloid lyotropes Kolloid *nt*.
lyotropic series Hofmeister-Reihen *pl*, lyotrope Reihen *pl*.
ly·pres·sin [laɪˈpresɪn] *n pharm.* Lypressin *nt*.
Lys *abbr.* → lysine.
lys- *pref.* → lyso-.
ly·sate [ˈlaɪseɪt] *n* **1.** *biochem.* Lyseprodukt *nt*, Lysat *nt*. **2.** *pharm.* Lysat *nt*.
lyse [laɪs] **I** *vt* etw. auflösen. **II** *vi* s. auflösen.
ly·ser·ga·mide [laɪˈsɜːrdʒəmaɪd] *n* → lysergic acid amide.
ly·ser·gic acid [laɪˈsɜːrdʒɪk] Lysergsäure *f*.
lysergic acid amide Lysergsäureamid *nt*, Lysergamid *f*.
lysergic acid diethylamide *abbr.* **LSD** Lysergsäurediäthylamid *nt abbr.* LSD, Lysergid *nt*.
ly·ser·gide [ˈlɪsərdʒaɪd] *n* → lysergic acid diethylamide.
ly·sim·e·ter [laɪˈsɪmɪtər] *n* Lysimeter *nt*.
ly·sin [ˈlaɪsɪn] *n immun.* Lysin *nt*.
ly·sine [ˈlaɪsiːn, -sɪn] *n abbr.* **Lys** Lysin *nt*.
lysine dehydrogenase Lysindehydrogenase *f*.
lysine dehydrogenase deficiency → lysine intolerance.
lysine enzyme Lysinenzym *nt*.
lysine intolerance erhöhter Lysingehalt *m* des Blutes, Hyperlysinämie *f*, Lysinintoleranz *f*.
lysine-iron agar *abbr.* **LIA** Lysin-Eisen-Agar *m/nt*.
lysine ketoglutarate reductase Saccharopindehydrogenase *f* (lysinbildend).
lysine-ketoglutarate reductase deficiency → lysine intolerance.
L-lysine:NAD oxidoreductase → lysine dehydrogenase.
L-lysine:NAD oxidoreductase deficiency → lysine intolerance.
ly·sin·o·gen [laɪˈsɪnədʒən] *n* Lysinogen *nt*.
ly·si·no·gen·ic [ˌlaɪsɪnəˈdʒenɪk] *adj* lysinogen.
ly·si·nu·ria [ˌlaɪsɪˈn(j)ʊərɪə] *n* Lysinausscheidung *f* im Harn, Lysinurie *f*.
ly·sis [ˈlaɪsɪs] *n, pl* **-ses** [-siːz] **1.** *patho.* Lyse *f*, Lysis *f*. **2.** (*Fieber*) Lyse *f*, Lysis *f*, lytische Defervszenz *f*, allmählicher Fieberabfall *m*. **3.** *bio., biochem.* Auflösung *f*, Lyse *f*. **4.** *chir.* Lösung *f*, Lyse *f*.
lyso- *pref.* Lys(o)-.
ly·so·ceph·a·lin [laɪsəˈsefəlɪn] *n* Lysokephalin *nt*, -cephalin *nt*.
ly·so·gen [ˈ-dʒən] *n* **1.** Lysinogen *nt*. **2.** lyseverursachendes/lytisches Agens *nt*. **3.** lysogeniertes Bakterium *nt*.
ly·so·gen·e·sis [ˌ-ˈdʒenəsɪs] *n immun.* Lysinbildung *f*.
ly·so·gen·ic [ˌ-ˈdʒenɪk] *adj* **1.** *immun.* lysinbildend, Lyse verursachend, lysogen. **2.** *micro.* Lysogenie betr., lysogen.
lysogenic bacterium *micro.* lysogenes Bakterium *nt*.
lysogenic conversion *micro.* lysogene Konversion *f*, Phagenkonversion *f*.
lysogenic factor Bakteriophage *m*, Phage *m*, bakterienpathogenes Virus *nt*.
ly·so·ge·nic·i·ty [ˌ-dʒəˈnɪsəti] *n* **1.** Fähigkeit *f* zur Lysinproduktion. **2.** Lysogenisation *f*. **3.** Lysogenie *f*.
ly·so·ge·ni·za·tion [ˌ-dʒenɪˈzeɪʃn] *n micro.* Lysogenisation *f*.
ly·sog·e·ny [laɪˈsɑdʒəni] *n micro.* Lysogenie *f*.
ly·so·ki·nase [ˌlaɪsəˈkaɪneɪz, ˈkɪ-] *n* Lysokinase *f*.
ly·so·lec·i·thin [ˌ-ˈlesɪθɪn] *n* Lysolezithin *nt*, Lysolecithin *nt*, Lysophosphatidylcholin *nt*.
ly·so·phos·pha·tide [ˌ-ˈfɑsfətaɪd] *n* Lysophosphatid *nt*.
ly·so·phos·pha·tid·ic acid [ˌ-fɑsfəˈtɪdɪk] Lysophosphatidsäure *f*.
ly·so·phos·pho·glyc·er·ide [ˌ-fɑsfəʊˈglɪsəraɪd, -rɪd] *n* Lysophosphoglyzerid *nt*.
ly·so·phos·pho·li·pase [ˌ-fɑsfəʊˈlaɪpeɪz, -lɪ-] *n* Lysophospholipase *f*, Lecithinase B *f*, Phospholipase B *f*.
ly·so·so·mal [ˌ-ˈsəʊml] *adj* Lysosom betr., lysosomal.
lysosomal enzymopathy → lysosomal storage disease.
lysosomal α-glucosidase Glukan-1,4-α-Glukosidase *f*, lysosomale α-Glukosidase *f*.
lysosomal storage disease lysosomale Speicherkrankheit *f*.
ly·so·some [ˈ-səʊm] *n* Lysosom *nt*.
lysosome membrane Lysosomenmembran *f*.
ly·so·type [ˈ-taɪp] *n* Lysotyp *m*, Phagovar *m*.
ly·so·zyme [ˈ-zaɪm] *n* Lysozym *nt*.
ly·so·zy·mu·ria [ˌ-zaɪˈm(j)ʊərɪə] *n* Lysozymausscheidung *f* im Harn, Lysozymurie *f*.
lyss- *pref.* → lysso-.
lys·sa [ˈlɪsə] *n* Tollwut *f*, Rabies *f*, Lyssa *f*, *old* Hydrophobie *f*.
Lys·sa·vi·rus [ˈlɪsəvaɪrəs] *n micro.* Lyssavirus *nt*.
lys·sic [ˈlɪsɪk] *adj* Tollwut betr., Tollwut-, Rabies-, Lyssa-.
lysso- *pref.* Tollwut-, Lyssa-, Rabies-.
lys·soid [ˈlɪsɔɪd] *adj* tollwutähnlich, -artig.
ly·syl [ˈlaɪsɪl] *n* Lysyl-(Radikal *nt*).
lysyl-bradykinin *n* Kallidin *nt*, Lysyl-Bradykinin *nt*.
lysyl oxidase Lysyloxidase *f*.
lyt·ic [ˈlɪtɪk] *adj* **1.** Lyse betr., Lyse-. **2.** Lysin betr., Lysin-. **3.** eine Lyse auslösend, lytisch. **4.** allmählich sinkend *od.* abfallend, zurückgehend, lytisch.
lytic bacteriophage nichttemperenter/lytischer/virulenter Bakteriophage *m*.
lytic cocktail lytischer Cocktail *m*, Cocktail lytique.
lytic virus lytisches Virus *nt*.
lyt·ta [ˈlɪtə] *n* → lyssa.
lyx·ose [ˈlɪksəʊz] *n* Lyxose *f*.
lyze *vt, vi* → lyse.

M

M *abbr.* 1. → meg(a)-. 2. → methionine. 3. → molar 3.
m *abbr.* 1. → meter 1. 2. → milli-. 3. → molal.
m- *pref.*, *abbr.* → meta- 2.
μ *abbr.* 1. → micro-. 2. [micron] → micrometer 1.
M.A. *abbr.* → mental age.
mA *abbr.* → milliampere.
μA *abbr.* → microampere.
MAA *abbr.* → macroaggregated albumin.
MAb *abbr.* → monoclonal antibody.
MAC *abbr.* 1. → maximal allowance concentration. 2. → membrane attack complex. 3. → minimal alveolar concentration.
Ma·ca·ca [məˈkɑːkə]: **M. mulatta** Rhesusaffe *m*, Macaca mulatta/rhesus.
Macalister [məˈkælɪstər]: **glenoid ligament of M.** Labrum glenoidale.
 xiphocostal ligaments of M. Ligg. costoxiphoidea.
Macchiavello [mɑkɪəˈveləʊ]: **M.'s stain** Macchiavello-Färbung *f*.
MacConkey [məˈkɒŋkiː]: **M. agar** MacConkey-Agar *m*/*nt*.
mac·er·ate [ˈmæsəreɪt] **I** *vt* 1. auf-, erweichen, aufquellen, mazerieren; *(Nahrung)* aufschließen. 2. ausmergeln, auszehren. **II** *vi* weich werden, aufweichen.
mac·er·a·tion [ˌmæsəˈreɪʃn] *n* 1. Auf-, Erweichen *nt*, Aufquellen *nt*, Mazeration *nt*; *(Nahrung)* Aufschließen *nt*. 2. Ausmergelung *f*, Auszehrung *f*.
Macewen [məˈkjuːən]: **M.'s sign/symptom** Macewen-Zeichen *nt*, Schädelschettern *nt*.
Mach [mæk; mɑx]: **M. band** Mach-Band *nt*.
 M.'s sound wastage theory Mach'-Schallabflußtheorie *f*.
Machado [məˈʃɑːdəʊ]: **M.'s test** Machado-Test *m*, Machado-Guerreiro-Reaktion *f*, Komplementbindungsreaktion *f* nach Machado.
Machado-Guerreiro [geˈreɪrəʊ]: **M.-G. test** → Machado's test.
Machado-Joseph [dʒəʊˈsef]: **M.-J. disease** Machado-Joseph-Syndrom *nt*, Azorenkrankheit *f*.
Mache [ˈmɑke; ˈmɑxə]: **M. unit** *abbr.* **M.U.** *phys.* Mache-Einheit *f abbr.* M.E.
ma·chine [məˈʃiːn] *n phys.*, *techn.* Maschine *f*, Apparat *m*, Vorrichtung *f*, Automat *m*.
ma·chin·er·y murmur [məˈʃiːnərɪ] *card.* Maschinengeräusch *nt*.
Ma·chu·po virus [mɑˈtʃuːpəʊ] *micro.* Machupo-Virus *nt*.
MAC INH *abbr.* → membrane attack complex inhibitor.
Mackay-Marg [məˈkeɪ mɑːrg]: **M.-M. tonometer** *ophthal.* MacKay-Marg-Tonometer *nt*.
Mackenrodt [ˈmɑknrəʊt]: **M.'s incision** Mackenrodt-Schnitt *m*.
 M.'s ligament Plica recto-uterina.

Mackenzie [məˈkenzɪ]: **M.'s amputation** *ortho.* Mackenzie-Amputation *f*, Fußamputation *f* nach Mackenzie.
Maclagan [məkˈlɑːgən]: **M.'s test** Maclagan-Reaktion *f*, Thymoltrübungstest *m*.
MacLean [məkˈliːn, -ˈleɪn]: **M. test** MacLean-Test *m*.
Macleod [məˈklaʊd]: **M.'s syndrome** Swyer-James-Syndrom *nt*.
macr- *pref.* → macro-.
Mac·ra·can·tho·rhyn·chus [ˌmækrəˌkænθəˈrɪŋkəs] *n micro.* Riesenkratzer *m*, Macracanthorhynchus *m*.
mac·ren·ce·pha·lia [ˌmækrənsɪˈfeɪljə, -lɪə] *n* → macrencephaly.
mac·ren·ceph·a·ly [ˌ-ˈsefəlɪ] *n* Makroenzephalie *f*, Makrenzephalie *f*.
macro- *pref.* Makr(o)-, Macr(o)-.
mac·ro·ad·e·no·ma [ˌmækrəʊædəˈnəʊmə] *n* Makroadenom *nt*.
mac·ro·ag·gre·gate [ˌ-ˈægrɪgɪt, -geɪt] *n* Makroaggregat *nt*.
mac·ro·ag·gre·gat·ed albumin [ˌ-ˈægrɪgeɪtɪd] *abbr.* **MAA** Makroalbuminaggregat *nt abbr.* MAA.
mac·ro·a·leu·ri·o·spore [ˌ-əˈlʊərɪəspəʊər, -spɔːr] *n micro.* Makroaleurospore *f*.
mac·ro·am·y·lase [ˌ-ˈæmɪleɪz] *n* Makroamylase *f*.
mac·ro·a·nal·y·sis [ˌ-əˈnæləsɪs] *n chem.* Makroanalyse *f*.
mac·ro·bac·te·ri·um [ˌ-bækˈtɪərɪəm] *n micro.* Makro-, Megabakterium *nt*.
mac·ro·bi·o·sis [ˌ-baɪˈəʊsɪs] *n* Langlebigkeit *f*, Makrobiose *f*.
mac·ro·bi·ot·ic [ˌ-baɪˈɒtɪk] *adj* makrobiotisch.
mac·ro·bi·ot·ics [ˌ-baɪˈɒtɪks] *pl* Makrobiotik *f*.
mac·ro·blast [ˈ-blæst] *n* Makroblast *m*.
mac·ro·ble·pha·ria [ˌ-bləˈfeərɪə] *n ophthal.* Makroblepharie *f*.
mac·ro·bra·chia [ˌ-ˈbreɪkɪə] *n embryo.* Makrobrachie *f*.
mac·ro·cel·lu·lar [ˌ-ˈseljələr] *adj* großzellig, makrozellulär.
mac·ro·ce·pha·lia [ˌ-sɪˈfeɪlɪə] *n* → macrocephaly.
mac·ro·ce·phal·ic [ˌ-sɪˈfælɪk] *adj* makrozephal, -kephal.
mac·ro·ceph·a·lous [ˌ-ˈsefələs] *adj* → macrocephalic.
mac·ro·ceph·a·lus [ˌ-ˈsefələs] *n* → macrocephaly.
mac·ro·ceph·a·ly [ˌ-ˈsefəlɪ] *n* Großköpfigkeit *f*, Makrozephalie *f*, -kephalie *f*.
mac·ro·chei·lia [ˌ-ˈkeɪlɪə] *n* Makroch(e)ilie *f*.
mac·ro·chei·ria [ˌ-ˈkeɪrɪə] *n* Makroch(e)irie *f*, Megaloch(e)irie *f*.
mac·ro·chem·i·cal [ˌ-ˈkemɪkl] *adj* Makrochemie betr., makrochemisch.
mac·ro·chem·is·try [ˌ-ˈkemɪstrɪ] *n* Makrochemie *f*.
mac·ro·chi·lia *n* → macrocheilia.
mac·ro·chi·ria *n* → macrocheiria.

mac·ro·chy·lo·mi·cron [ˌ-ˌkaɪləˈmaɪkrɒn] *n* Makrochylomikron *nt*.
mac·ro·clit·o·ris [ˌ-ˈklɪtərɪs] *n* Klitorishypertrophie *f*, Makroklitoris *f*.
mac·ro·co·lon [ˌ-ˈkəʊlən] *n* → megacolon.
mac·ro·co·nid·i·um [ˌ-kəˈnɪdɪəm] *n*, *pl* **-dia** [-dɪə] *micro.* Makrokonidie *f*, -konidium *nt*.
mac·ro·cor·nea [ˌ-ˈkɔːrnɪə] *n* → megalocornea.
mac·ro·cra·nia [ˌ-ˈkreɪnɪə] *n embryo.* Makrokranie *f*.
mac·ro·cyst [ˈ-sɪst] *n* 1. Makrozyste *f*. 2. *micro.* Makrozyste *f*.
mac·ro·cyte [ˈ-saɪt] *n* Makrozyt *m*.
mac·ro·cy·the·mia [ˌ-saɪˈθiːmɪə] *n* → macrocytosis.
mac·ro·cyt·ic [ˌ-ˈsɪtɪk] *adj* Makrozyt betr., makrozytisch, Makrozyten-.
macrocytic anemia makrozytäre Anämie *f*.
 nutritional m. Folsäuremangelanämie *f*.
 m. of pregnancy makrozytäre Schwangerschaftsanämie.
mac·ro·cy·to·sis [ˌ-saɪˈtəʊsɪs] *n* Makrozytose *f*.
mac·ro·dac·tyl·ia [ˌ-dækˈtɪlɪə, -ljə] *n* → macrodactyly.
mac·ro·dac·tyl·ism [ˌ-ˈdæktəlɪzəm] *n* → macrodactyly.
mac·ro·dac·ty·ly [ˌ-ˈdæktəlɪ] *n* Makrodaktylie *f*.
mac·ro·don·tia [ˌ-ˈdɒnʃɪə] *n dent.* übermäßige Größe *f* der Zähne, Makrodontie *f*, -dontie *f*.
mac·ro·don·tism [ˌ-ˈdɒntɪzəm] *n* → macrodontia.
mac·ro·e·lec·trode [ˌ-ɪˈlektrəʊd] *n* Makroelektrode *f*.
mac·ro·el·e·ment [ˌ-ˈeləmənt] *n chem.* Makroelement *nt*.
mac·ro·en·ceph·a·ly [ˌ-enˈsefəlɪ] *n* → macrencephaly.
mac·ro·e·ryth·ro·blast [ˌ-ɪˈrɪθrəblæst] *n* → macroblast.
mac·ro·e·ryth·ro·cyte [ˌ-ɪˈrɪθrəsaɪt] *n* → macrocyte.
mac·ro·es·the·sia [ˌ-esˈθiːʒə] *n* Makroästhesie *f*.
mac·ro·fau·na [ˌ-ˈfɔːnə] *n* Makrofauna *f*.
mac·ro·fi·bril [ˌ-ˈfaɪbrɪl, -fɪb-] *n* Makrofibrille *f*.
mac·ro·flo·ra [ˌ-ˈflɔːrə, -ˈfləʊ-] *n* Makroflora *f*.
mac·ro·fol·lic·u·lar adenoma [ˌ-fəˈlɪkjələr] (*Schilddrüse*) Kolloidadenom *nt*, makrofolliculäres Adenom *nt*.
mac·ro·gam·ete [ˌ-ˈgæmiːt] *n* Makrogamet(e) *f*) *m*, Gynogamet *m*.
mac·ro·ga·me·to·cyte [ˌ-gəˈmiːtəsaɪt] *n* Makrogametozyt *m*, Makrogamont *m*.
mac·ro·gam·ont [ˌ-ˈgæmɒnt] *n* → macrogametocyte.
mac·ro·gen·i·to·so·mia [ˌ-ˌdʒenɪtəʊˈsəʊmɪə] *n* Makrogenitosomie *f*, -genitalismus *f*.

mac·ro·gin·gi·vae [ˌ-dʒɪnˈdʒaɪviː] *pl* Fibromatosis gingivae, Elephantiasis gingivae.
mac·rog·lia [məˈkrɑɡlɪə] *n* Makroglia *f*, Astroglia *f*.
macroglia cell Makrogliazelle *f*, Astrozyt *m*.
(α₂-)mac·ro·glob·u·lin [ˌmækrəʊˈɡlɑbjəlɪn] *n* (α₂-)Makroglobulin *nt*.
mac·ro·glob·u·li·ne·mia [ˌ-ˌɡlɑbjəlɪˈniːmɪə] *n patho*. Makroglobulinämie *f*.
mac·ro·glos·sia [ˌ-ˈɡlɑsɪə] *n* Makroglossie *f*.
mac·ro·gna·thia [ˌ-ˈneɪθɪə, -ˈnæθ-] *n* Makrognathie *f*.
mac·ro·gra·phia [ˌ-ˈɡræfɪə] *n* → macrography.
mac·rog·ra·phy [məˈkrɑɡrəfɪ] *n neuro*. Makro-, Megalographie *f*.
mac·ro·gy·ria [ˌmækrəʊˈdʒaɪrɪə] *n* Makrogyrie *f*.
mac·ro·la·bia [ˌ-ˈleɪbɪə] *n* → macrocheilia.
mac·ro·lec·i·thal [ˌ-ˈlesɪθəl] *adj bio*. makrolezithal.
macrolecithal ovum *bio*. makrolezithales Ei *nt*.
mac·ro·leu·ko·blast [ˌ-ˈluːkəblæst] *n* Makroleukoblast *m*.
mac·ro·lide [ˈ-laɪd] *n* **1.** *chem*. Makrolid *nt*. **2.** Makrolid-Antibiotikum *nt*.
mac·ro·lym·pho·cyte [ˌ-ˈlɪmfəsaɪt] *n* Makrolymphozyt *m*.
mac·ro·lym·pho·cy·to·sis [ˌ-ˌlɪmfəsaɪˈtəʊsɪs] *n* Makrolymphozytose *f*.
mac·ro·ma·nia [ˌ-ˈmeɪnɪə, -jə] *n* **1.** *psychia*. expansiver Wahn *m*, Größenwahn *m*, Megalomanie *f*. **2.** *neuro*. Makromanie *f*.
mac·ro·mas·tia [ˌ-ˈmæstɪə] *n* Makromastie *f*.
mac·ro·ma·zia [ˌ-ˈmeɪzɪə] *n* → macromastia.
mac·ro·me·lia [ˌ-ˈmiːlɪə, -ljə] *n* Großgliedrigkeit *f*, Makromelie *f*.
ma·crom·e·lus [məˈkrɑmələs] *n embryo*. Makromelus *m*.
mac·ro·mere [ˈmækrəmɪər] *n* Makromere *f*.
mac·ro·meth·od [ˌ-ˈmeθəd] *n chem*. Makromethode *f*.
mac·ro·mo·lec·u·lar [ˌ-məˈlekjələr] *adj* hoch-, makromolekular.
mac·ro·mol·e·cule [ˌ-ˈmɑlɪkjuːl] *n* Riesen-, Makromolekül *nt*.
mac·ro·mon·o·cyte [ˌ-ˈmɑnəsaɪt] *n* Makromonozyt *m*.
mac·ro·my·e·lo·blast [ˌ-ˈmaɪələblæst] *n* Makromyeloblast *m*.
mac·ro·nod·u·lar [ˌ-ˈnɑdʒələr] *adj* großknotig, makronodulär.
mac·ro·nor·mo·blast [ˌ-ˈnɔːrməblæst] *n* **1.** Makronormoblast *m*. **2.** Makroblast *m*.
mac·ro·nu·cle·us [ˌ-ˈn(j)uːklɪəs] *n* Makro-, Megankleus *m*.
mac·ro·nych·ia [ˌ-ˈnɪkɪə] *n* Makronychie *f*, Megalonychie *f*.
macro-osmatic *adj* → macrosmatic II.
mac·ro·par·a·site [ˌ-ˈpærəsaɪt] *n* Makroparasit *m*.
mac·ro·pa·thol·o·gy [ˌ-pəˈθɑlədʒɪ] *n* Makropathologie *f*.
mac·ro·pe·nis [ˌ-ˈpiːnɪs] *n* → macrophallus.
mac·ro·per·fo·ra·tion [ˌ-ˌpɜːrfəˈreɪʃn] *n chir*. Makroperforation *f*.
mac·ro·phage [ˈ-feɪdʒ] *n* Makrophag(e) *m*.
macrophage-activating factor *abbr*. **MAF** Makrophagenaktivierungsfaktor *m abbr*. MAF.
macrophage chemotactic factor *abbr*. **MCF** Makrophagen-chemotaktischer Faktor *m abbr*. MCF.
macrophage cytotoxicity-inducing factor *abbr*. **MCIF** macrophage cytotoxicity--inducing factor *abbr*. MCIF.

macrophage deactivating factor *abbr*. **MDF** macrophage deactivating factor *abbr*. MDF.
macrophage disappearance factor *abbr*. **MDF** macrophage disappearance factor *abbr*. MDF.
macrophage growth factor *abbr*. **MGF** Makrophagenwachstumsfaktor *m*, macrophage growth factor *abbr*. MGF.
macrophage Ia recruiting factor *abbr*. **MIRF** macrophage Ia recruiting factor *abbr*. MIRF.
macrophage inhibitory factor → migration inhibiting factor.
macrophage migration inhibition test Makrophagen-Migrationshemmtest *m*.
macrophage slowing factor *abbr*. **MSF** macrophage slowing factor *abbr*. MSF.
macrophage spreading inhibitory factor *abbr*. **MSIF** macrophage spreading inhibitory factor *abbr*. MSIF.
macrophage system Makrophagensystem *nt*.
mac·ro·phag·o·cyte [ˌ-ˈfæɡəsaɪt] *n* → macrophage.
ma·croph·a·gus [məˈkrɑfəɡəs] *n* → macrophage.
mac·ro·phal·lus [ˌmækrəˈfæləs] *n* Makrophallus *m*.
ma·croph·thal·mia [məkrɑfˈθælmɪə] *n* Makrophthalmie *f*.
mac·ro·phys·ics [ˌmækrəʊˈfɪzɪks] *pl* Makrophysik *f*.
mac·ro·phyte [ˈ-faɪt] *n* Makrophyt *m*.
mac·ro·pla·sia [ˌ-ˈpleɪʒ(ɪ)ə] *n* Makroplasie *f*.
mac·ro·plas·tia [ˌ-ˈplæstɪə] *n* → macroplasia.
mac·ro·po·dia [ˌ-ˈpəʊdɪə] *n* Makropodie *f*.
mac·ro·pol·y·cyte [ˌ-ˈpɑlɪsaɪt] *n* Makropolyzyt *m*.
mac·ro·pro·lac·ti·no·ma [ˌ-prəʊˌlæktɪˈnəʊmə] *n* Makroprolaktinom *nt*.
mac·ro·pro·my·e·lo·cyte [ˌ-prəʊˈmaɪələsaɪt] *n* Makropromyelozyt *m*.
mac·ro·pro·so·pia [ˌ-prəʊˈsəʊpɪə] *n* Makroprosopie *f*.
mac·ro·pro·tein [ˌ-ˈprəʊtiːn, -tiːɪn] *n* Makroprotein *nt*.
ma·crop·sia [məˈkrɑpsɪə] *n* Makropsie *f*, Megalopsie *f*.
mac·ro·rhin·ia [ˌmækrəˈrɪnɪə] *n* Makrorhinie *f*.
mac·ro·sce·lia [ˌ-ˈsiːlɪə] *n* Makroskelie *f*.
mac·ro·scop·ic [ˌ-ˈskɑpɪk] *adj* mit bloßem Auge sichtbar, makroskopisch.
macroscopic agglutination Makroagglutination *f*.
mac·ro·scop·i·cal [ˌ-ˈskɑpɪkl] *adj* → macroscopic.
macroscopic(al) anatomy makroskopische Anatomie *f*.
macroscopic hematuria Makrohämaturie *f*, makroskopische Hämaturie *f*.
ma·cros·co·py [məˈkrɑskəpɪ] *n* Betrachtung/Untersuchung *f* mit bloßem Auge, Makroskopie *f*.
mac·ro·sig·moid [ˌmækrəʊˈsɪɡmɔɪd] *n* Megasigma *nt*.
ma·cros·mat·ic [ˌmækræzˈmætɪk] **I** *n* makrosmatisches Tier *od*. Lebewesen *nt*, Makrosmatiker *m*. **II** *adj* makrosmatisch.
mac·ro·so·ma·tia [ˌmækrəʊsəˈmeɪʒ(ɪ)ə, -ʃə] *n* Hoch-, Großwuchs *m*, Makrosomie *f*.
mac·ro·so·mia [ˌ-ˈsəʊmɪə] *n* → macrosomatia.
mac·ro·spo·ran·gi·um [ˌ-spəˈrændʒɪəm] *n micro*. Makro-, Megasporangium *nt*.
mac·ro·spore [ˈ-spəʊər, -spɔːr] *n micro*. Makro-, Megaspore *f*, Gynospore *f*.

mac·ro·ster·e·og·no·sia [ˌ-ˌsterɪəʊˈnəʊsɪə, -ˌstɪər-] *n* Makrostereognosie *f*.
mac·ro·ster·e·og·no·sis [ˌ-ˌsterɪɑɡˈnəʊsɪs] *n* → macrostereognosia.
mac·ro·sto·mia [ˌ-ˈstəʊmɪə] *n* Makrostomie *f*.
mac·ro·throm·bo·cyte [ˌ-ˈθrɑmbəsaɪt] *n* Riesen-, Makrothrombozyt *m*.
ma·cro·tia [mæˈkrəʊʃ(ɪ)ə] *n* Makrotie *f*.
mac·ro·tome [ˈmækrətəʊm] *n* Makrotom *nt*.
mac·u·la [ˈmækjələ], *pl* **-las**, **-lae** [-liː] **1.** Fleck *m*, Verdickung *f*; *anat*. Macula *f*. **2.** diskolorierte Hautstelle *f*, Macula *f*. **3.** → macula lutea.
m. of sacculus Macula sacculi.
m. of utricle Macula utriculi.
macula adherens Haftplatte *f*, Macula adhaerens, Desmosom *nt*.
macula densa Macula densa.
macula lutea gelber Fleck *m*, Makula *f*, Macula *f*, Macula lutea/retinae.
macula organ Makula-, Macula-, Statolithenorgan *nt*.
mac·u·lar [ˈmækjələr] *adj* **1.** gefleckt, fleckig, Flecken-. **2.** Makula betr., makulös, makulär.
macular arteriole: inferior m. untere Makulaarteriole *f*, Arteriola macularis inferior.
superior m. obere Makulaarteriole *f*, Arteriola macularis superior.
macular atrophy *derm*. Anetodermie *f*.
macular choroiditis *ophthal*. Chorioiditis macularis.
macular coloboma *ophthal*. Makulakolobom *nt*.
macular degeneration *ophthal*. Makuladegeneration *f*.
congenital m. Best'-Krankheit *f*.
disciform m. scheibenförmige/disziforme senile feuchte Makuladegeneration, Kuhnt-Junius-Krankheit *f*.
vitelliform/vitelline m. → congenital m.
macular disciform degeneration → macular degeneration, disciform.
macular edema Makulaödem *nt*.
macular erythema Roseola *f*.
macular evasion *ophthal*. Horror fusionis.
macular syphilid *derm*. makulöses Syphilid *nt*, Roseola syphilitica.
macular venule: inferior m. untere Makulavene *f*, Venula macularis inferior.
superior m. obere Makulavene *f*, Venula macularis superior.
mac·u·late [*adj* ˈmækjəlɪt; *v* -leɪt] **I** *adj* gefleckt, fleckig; beschmutzt. **II** *vt* beflecken.
mac·u·la·tion [ˌmækjəˈleɪʃn] *n* **1.** (Be-)Fleckung *f*, Fleckigsein *nt*, Geflecktsein *nt*. **2.** Fleck(en *m*) *m*, Makel *m*.
mac·ule [ˈmækjuːl] *n* **1.** Fleck *m*, Verdickung *f*; *anat*. Macula *f*. **2.** diskolorierte Hautstelle *f*, Macula *f*.
mac·u·lo·cer·e·bral [ˌmækjələʊˈserəbrəl, -səˈriːbr-] *adj ophthal*., *neuro*. Makula u. Zerebrum betr., makulozerebral.
maculo-ocular reflex makulookulärer Reflex *m*.
mac·u·lo·pap·u·lar [ˌ-ˈpæpjələr] *adj derm*. makulopapulös.
mac·u·lo·spi·nal reflex [ˌ-ˈspaɪnl] makulospinaler Reflex *m*.
mac·u·lo·ve·sic·u·lar [ˌ-vəˈsɪkjələr] *adj derm*. makulovesikulär.
mad [mæd] *adj* **1.** wahnsinnig; verrückt, toll, irr(e). **2.** tollwütig.
mad·a·ro·sis [ˌmædəˈrəʊsɪs] *n, pl* **-ses** [-siːz] *derm*. Madarosis *f*.
Madelung [ˈmɑdəlʊŋ]: **M.'s deformity** → M.'s disease 1.

mad itch

M.'s disease 1. Madelung'-Deformität *f*. **2.** Madelung'-Fetthals *m*.
M.'s neck → M.'s disease 2.
mad itch Pseudowut *f*, -lyssa *f*, -rabies *f*, Aujeszky'-Krankheit *f*.
Madlener ['madlənər]: **M.'s operation** *gyn*. Madlener-Operation *f*.
mad·man ['mædmæn, -mən] *n* Verrückte(r *m*) *f*, Wahnsinnige(r *m*) *f*, Irre(r *m*) *f*.
mad·ness ['mædnɪs] *n* Wahnsinn *m*; Tollheit *f*, Verrücktheit *f*.
Ma·don·na fingers [mə'dɑnə] Madonnenfinger *pl*.
Ma·dun·go fever [mə'dʌŋgəʊ] bolivianisches hämorrhagisches Fieber *nt abbr*. BHF, Madungofieber *nt*.
Madungo virus Madungo(fieber)virus *nt*.
Ma·du·ra foot [mə'dʊərə; 'mædʒərə] *derm*. Madurafuß *m*.
Mad·u·rel·la [,mædjʊə'relə] *n micro*. Madurella *f*.
mad·u·ro·my·co·sis [,mædjʊərəʊmaɪ'kəʊsɪs] *n* Madurymykose *f*, Myzetom *nt*, Mycetoma *nt*.
MAF *abbr*. → macrophage-activating factor.
ma·fe·nide ['meɪfɪnaɪd] *n pharm*. Mafenid *nt*.
Maffucci [mɑ'futʃi:]: **M.'s syndrome** Maffucci-Kast-Syndrom *nt*.
mag·al·drate ['mægældreɪt] *n pharm*. Magaldrat *nt*.
ma·gen·bla·se ['mɑːgənblɑːzə] *n radiol*. Magenblase *f*.
Magendie [maʒɑː'di]: **M.'s foramen** Magendie'-Foramen *nt*, For. Magendii, Apertura mediana ventriculi quarti.
M.'s law Bell(-Magendie)-Regel *f*.
M.'s sign Magendie-Hertwig sign.
M.'s spaces Magendie-Räume *pl*.
M.'s symptom → Magendie-Hertwig sign.
Magendie-Hertwig ['hɑrtvɪg; 'hɛrtvɪk]: **M.-H. sign** *ophthal*. Hertwig-Magendie--Phänomen *nt*, -Syndrom *nt*, Magendie--Hertwig-Schielstellung *f*, Magendie--Schielstellung *f*, -Zeichen *nt*.
M.-H. syndrome → M.-H. sign.
ma·gen·stras·se ['mɑːgənstræsə; -ʃtrɑːsə] *n* Magenstraße *f*.
ma·gen·ta [mə'dʒentə] *histol*. **I** *n* Magenta *nt*. **II** *adj* magenta(rot).
mag·got ['mægət] *n bio*. Made *f*, Larve *f*.
mag·is·tral ['mædʒɪstrəl] *adj pharm*. magistral.
mag·ma ['mægmə] *n*, *pl* **-mas**, **-ma·ta** [-mətə] dünnflüssiger Brei *m*, knetbare Masse *f*, Teig *m*, Magma *nt*.
Magnan ['mægnən]: **M.'s movement** Magnan-Zeichen *nt*.
M.'s sign → M.'s movement.
M.'s trombone movement → M.'s movement.
mag·ne·se·mia [mægnə'siːmɪə] *n* erhöhter Magnesiumgehalt *m* des Blutes, Magnesämie *f*.
mag·ne·sia [mæg'niːʒə, -ʃə] *n* Magnesia *nt*, Magnesiumoxid *nt*.
magnesia alba → magnesium carbonate.
magnesia calcinata → magnesia.
mag·ne·si·um [mæg'niːzɪəm, -ʒəm, -ʃɪəm] *n abbr*. **Mg** Magnesium *nt*, Mg.
magnesium ammonium phosphate Magnesium-Ammonium-phosphat *nt*, Tripelphosphat *nt*.
magnesium ammonium phosphate calculus Magnesium-Ammonium-phosphat-Stein *m*, Tripelphosphatstein *m*.
magnesium carbonate Magnesiumkarbonat *nt*.
magnesium chloride Magnesiumchlorid *nt*.

magnesium hydroxide Magnesiumhydroxid *nt*.
magnesium oxide → magnesia.
magnesium peroxide Magnesiumperoxid *nt*, -superoxid *nt*, -perhydrol *nt*.
magnesium phosphate Magnesiumphosphat *nt*.
magnesium sulfate Magnesiumsulfat *nt*, Bittersalz *nt*.
magnesium trisilicate Magnesiumtrisilikat *nt*.
mag·net ['mægnɪt] *n* Magnet *m*.
mag·net·ic [mæg'netɪk] *adj* Magnet *od*. Magnetismus betr., magnetisch, Magnet-.
magnetic attraction magnetische Anziehung(skraft *f*) *f*.
magnetic bottle *phys*. magnetische Flasche *f*.
magnetic core *phys*. Magnetkern *m*.
magnetic field magnetisches Feld *nt*, Magnetfeld *nt*.
magnetic field strength → magnetic field.
magnetic flux *phys*. Magnet-, Induktionsfluß *m*, magnetischer (Kraft-)Fluß *m*.
magnetic induction → magnetoinduction.
magnetic intensity → magnetic field.
magnetic needle *phys*. Magnetnadel *f*.
mag·net·ics [mæg'netɪks] *pl* Lehre vom Magnetismus, Magnetik *f*.
mag·net·ism ['mægnɪtɪzəm] *n* Magnetismus *m*.
mag·net·i·za·tion [,mægnɪtɪ'zeɪʃn] *n* Magnetisieren *nt*, Magnetisierung *f*.
mag·net·ize ['mægnɪtaɪz] *vt* magnetisieren.
mag·net·iz·ing field/force ['mægnɪtaɪzɪŋ] → magnetic field.
mag·ne·to·car·di·o·graph [,mægnətəʊ'kɑːdɪəgrɑːf] *n* Magnetokardiograph *m*.
mag·ne·to·e·lec·tric [,-ɪ'lektrɪk] *adj* magnetoelektrisch.
mag·ne·to·en·ceph·a·lo·graph [,-en'sefələgrɑːf] *n* Magnetoenzephalograph *m*.
mag·ne·to·en·ceph·a·log·ra·phy [,-en,sefə'lɑgrəfɪ] *n abbr*. **MEG** Magnetoenzephalographie *f abbr*. MEG.
mag·ne·to·in·duc·tion [,-ɪn'dʌkʃn] *n phys*. magnetische Induktion *f*.
mag·ne·tom·e·ter [,mægnɪ'tɑmɪtər] *n* Magnetometer *nt*.
mag·ne·ton ['mægnɪtɑn] *n phys*. Magneton *nt*.
mag·ne·to·ther·a·py [,mægnətəʊ'θerəpɪ] *n* Magnettherapie *f*.
magnet reaction Magnetreaktion *f*.
magnet reflex → magnet reaction.
magnet resonance imaging *abbr*. **MRI** *radiol*. Kernspinresonanztomographie *f*, NMR-Tomographie *f*, MR-Tomographie *f abbr*. MRT.
mag·ne·tron ['mægnɪtrɑn] *n* Magnetron *nt*.
mag·ni·cel·lu·lar [,mægnɪ'seljələr] *adj* magnozellular.
mag·ni·fi·ca·tion [,mægnəfɪ'keɪʃn] *n* Vergrößern *nt*; Vergrößerung *f*; *electr*. Verstärkung *f*; *phys*. Vergrößerung(sstärke *f*) *f*.
mag·ni·fi·er ['mægnɪfaɪər] *n* **1.** Vergrößerungsglas *nt*, Lupe *f*. **2.** *electr*. Verstärker *m*.
mag·ni·fy ['mægnɪfaɪ] *vt* **1.** vergrößern. **2.** *electr*. verstärken.
mag·ni·fy·ing glass/loupe ['mægnɪfaɪɪŋ] → magnifier 1.
mag·ni·tude ['mægnɪt(j)uːd] *n* Größe *f*, Größenordnung *f*.
mag·no·cel·lu·lar [,mægnəʊ'seljələr] *adj histol*. großzellig, magnozellular, -zellulär.
magnocellular part of nucleus ruber

großzelliger Abschnitt *m* des Nc. ruber, Pars magnocellularis (nc. rubri).
mag·num ['mægnəm] *n anat*. Os capitatum.
Mahaim [mɑ'(h)aɪm]: **M. fibers** Mahaim'-Fasern *pl*, -Bündel *nt*.
Maher [meɪər]: **M.'s disease** *gyn*. Parakolpitis *f*, -vaginitis *f*.
Mahler ['mɑːlər]: **M.'s sign** Mahler-Zeichen *nt*.
maid·en·head ['meɪdnhed] *n* **1.** *inf*. Jungfernhäutchen *nt*, Hymen *m/nt*. **2.** Jungfräulichkeit *f*.
mai·dism ['meɪdɪzəm] *n* Pellagra *f*, Vitamin-B₂-Mangelsyndrom *nt*, Niacinmangelsyndrom *nt*.
Maier ['maɪər]: **sinus of M.** Maier-Sinus *m*, Arlt'-Sinus *m*.
maim [meɪm] *vt* verstümmeln, zum Krüppel machen.
main [meɪn] *n* **1.** Hauptleitung *f*, -rohr *nt*, -kabel *nt*. **2. the ~s** *pl* (öffentliches) Versorgungsnetz *nt*; Stromnetz *nt*; Haupthahn *m*, -schalter *m*. **in the ~** *fig*. im großen u. ganzen. **II** *adj* größte(r, s), wichtigste(r, s), Haupt-.
main bronchus Primär-, Haupt-, Stammbronchus *m*, Bronchus principalis.
main-line ['meɪnlaɪn] **I** *n sl*. **1.** Hauptvene *f*. **2.** *(Heroin)* Schuß *m*. **II** *vi*, *sl*. fixen.
main-lin·er ['meɪnlaɪnər] *n sl*. Fixer(in *f*) *m*.
mains voltage Netzspannung *f*.
main·tain [meɪn'teɪn] *vt* **1.** *(Zustand)* (aufrecht-)erhalten, bewahren, beibehalten. **2.** *(Familie)* unterhalten. **3.** *techn*. instandhalten, warten, pflegen.
main·te·nance ['meɪntənəns] *n* **1.** (Aufrecht-)Erhaltung *f*, Beibehaltung *f*, Wahrung *f*. **2.** *(Familie)* Unterhalt *m*. **3.** *techn*. Instandhaltung *f*, Wartung *f*, Pflege *f*.
maintenance costs Unterhaltskosten *pl*.
maintenance dose *pharm*. Erhaltungsdosis *f*.
maintenance heat Erhaltungswärme *f*.
maintenance level (of metabolism) *physiol*. Erhaltungsumsatz *m*.
maintenance work Haltearbeit *f*.
Maissiat [mɛsi'ja]: **M.'s band** → ligament of M.
M.'s ligament → ligament of M.
ligament of M. Maissiat-Band *nt*, Tractus iliotibialis.
M.'s tract → ligament of M.
Maissoneuve [mɛsɔ'nœf]: **M.'s amputation** Maissoneuve-Amputation *f*.
M.'s sign *ortho*. Maisonneuve-Zeichen *nt*.
maize [meɪz] *n* **1.** Mais *m*. **2.** Maiskorn *nt*. **3.** Maisgelb *nt*.
Majocchi [ma'jɔki]: **M.'s disease** Purpura Majocchi, Majocchi'-Krankheit *f*, Purpura anularis teleangiectodes (atrophicans), Teleangiectasia follicularis anulata.
M.'s granuloma Granuloma trichophyticum.
M.'s purpura → M.'s disease.
ma·jor ['meɪdʒər] *adj* Haupt-; *(a. fig.)* größere(r, s); bedeutend, wichtig.
major agglutinin Haupt-, Majoragglutinin *nt*.
major caruncle of Santorini Papilla duodeni major.
major circulation großer Kreislauf *m*, Körperkreislauf *m*.
major component Hauptbestandteil *m*.
major curve *ortho*. *(Skoliose)* Hauptkrümmung *f*, Majorkurve *f*.
major epilepsy 1. generalisierte Epilepsie *f*. **2.** Grand-mal(-Epilepsie *f*) *nt abbr*. GM.
major gene Majorgen *nt*.

major histocompatibility antigens 1. Histokompatibilitätsantigene *pl*, Transplantationsantigene *pl*, HLA-Antigene *pl*, human leukocyte antigens *abbr.* HLA, humane Leukozytenantigene *pl abbr.* HLA. **2.** MHC-Antigene *pl*.
major histocompatibility complex *abbr.* MHC **1.** Haupthistokompatibilitätskomplex *m*, major Histokompatibilitätskomplex *m abbr.* MHC. **2.** Histokompatibilitätsantigene *pl*, Transplantationsantigene *pl*, HLA-Antigene *pl*, human leukocyte antigens *abbr.* HLA, humane Leukozytenantigene *pl abbr.* HLA.
major illness schwer(er)e Krankheit *f*.
major periodicity *biochem.* Hauptperiodizität *f*.
major test *immun.* Majortest *m*, -probe *f*.
major tranquilizer Antipsychotikum *nt*, Neuroleptikum *nt*.
major wing of sphenoid bone großer Keilbeinflügel *m*, Ala major (ossis sphenoidalis).
make [meɪk] (*v* made; made) **I** *n* **1.** Erzeugnis *nt*, Produkt *nt*, Fabrikat *nt*. **2.** Beschaffenheit *f*, Zustand *m*, Struktur *f*. **3.** Veranlagung *f*, Natur *f*. **4.** (Körper-)Bau *m*; Bau *m*, Gefüge *nt*. **5.** Anfertigung *f*, Herstellung *f*, Produktion *f*.
II *vt* **6.** machen; anfertigen, herstellen, erzeugen (*from, of, out of* von, aus); bauen; (*Termin, Versuch, Vorschlag, Fehler, Untersuchung*) machen; (*Tee, Aufguß*) kochen, zubereiten; (*Text*) verfassen, schreiben; (*Entscheidung*) treffen, fällen; (*Geld*) verdienen; (*Profit*) machen. **7.** verarbeiten, bilden, formen (*to, into* in, zu). **8.** schaffen, erlangen, erzielen; *mathe.* ergeben, s. belaufen auf, machen.
III *vi* den Versuch machen (*to do zu* tun).
make out *vt* **1.** (*Dokument*) anfertigen; (*Formular*) ausfüllen; (*Liste*) aufstellen. **2.** erkennen, ausmachen. **3.** entziffern.
make up I *vt* **1.** (*Bericht*) zusammenstellen; (*Liste*) anfertigen; (*Tabelle*) auf-, zusammenstellen; (*Rezept*) an-, ausfertigen; (*Bett*) zurechtmachen. **2.** jdn. zurechtmachen *od.* herrichten; jdn. schminken. **3. to ~ one's mind** s. entschließen en, zu tun, einen Entschluß fassen. **4.** vervollständigen, ergänzen, voll *od.* komplett machen. **5.** (*Geschichte*) erfinden, s. ausdenken. **6.** ausgleichen; nach-, auf-, einholen. **II** *vi* s. schminken, s. zurechtmachen.
make up for *vi* ausgleichen, aufholen, wiedergutmachen, wettmachen.
make·shift ['meɪkʃɪft] **I** *n* Übergangslösung *f*, Notbehelf *m*. **II** *adj* behelfsmäßig, provisorisch, Behelfs-, Not-.
make-up *n* **1.** Körperbau *m*, Konstitution *f*; Struktur *f*, Bau *m*, Zusammensetzung *f*. **2.** Veranlagung *f*, Natur *f*. **3.** Make-up *nt*, Schminke *f*; Make-up *nt*, Schminken *nt*.
mak·ing ['meɪkɪŋ] *n* **1.** Machen *nt*, Schaffen *nt*. **2.** Erzeugung *f*, Herstellung *f*, Zubereitung *f*. **3.** Produkt *nt*. **4.** Zusammensetzung *f*, Aufbau *m*, Bau(art *f*) *m*.
Ma·kon·de virus [məˈkəʊndeɪ] Makonde--Virus *nt*.
mal [mɑl, mæl] *n* Krankheit *f*, Übel *nt*.
 m. de Cayenne Elephantiasis tropica.
 m. de mer Seekrankheit *f*, Naupathie *f*, Nausea marina.
 m. del pinto Pinta *f*, Mal del Pinto, Carate *f*.
 m. de San Lazaro Elephantiasis tropica.
ma·la ['meɪlə] *n, pl* **-lae** [-liː] *anat.* **1.** Wange *f*, Mala *f*. **2.** Jochbein *nt*, Os zygomaticum.

Mal·a·bar leprosy ['mæləbɑːr] Elephantiasis tropica.
Malabar ulcer Tropen-, Wüstengeschwür *nt*, Ulcus tropicum.
mal·ab·sorp·tion [mæləbˈzɔːrpʃn] *n* Malabsorption *f*.
malabsorption syndrome Malabsorptionssyndrom *nt*.
Malacarne [ˌmæləˈkærneɪ]: **M.'s pyramid** oberer Teil *m* der Pyramis vermis.
 M.'s space Substantia perforata interpeduncularis/posterior.
mal·a·chite green ['mæləkaɪt] Malachitgrün *nt*.
ma·la·cia [məˈleɪʃ(ɪ)ə] *n patho.* (krankhafte) Erweichung *f*, Malazie *f*, Malacia *f*.
ma·la·ci·al [məˈleɪʃ(ɪ)əl] *adj* Malazie betr., von Malazie gekennzeichnet, Erweichungs-.
malacial focus *patho.* Erweichungsherd *m*.
ma·la·cic [məˈleɪsɪk] *adj* → malacial.
mal·a·co·pla·kia [ˌmæləkəʊˈpleɪkɪə] *n* **1.** *patho.* Malakoplakie *f*, Malacoplacia *f*. **2.** *urol.* Malacoplacia vesicae urinariae.
mal·a·co·sis [mæləˈkəʊsɪs] *n* → malacia.
mal·a·cos·te·on [ˌ-ˈkɒstɪən] *n* Knochenerweichung *f*, Osteomalazie *f*, -malacia *f*.
mal·a·cot·ic [ˌ-ˈkɒtɪk] *adj* → malacial.
ma·lac·tic [məˈlæktɪk] **I** *n* beruhigendes *od.* linderndes Mittel *nt*. **II** *adj* beruhigend, lindernd.
mal·a·die [mæləˈdɪ; malaˈdi] *n French* Krankheit *f*, Gebrechen *nt*.
 m. de Roger Roger-Syndrom *nt*, Morbus Roger *m*.
 m. du sommeil afrikanische Schlafkrankheit/Trypanosomiasis *f*.
 m. des tics Gilles-de-la-Tourette-Syndrom *nt*, Tourette-Syndrom *nt*, Maladie des tics, Tic impulsif.
mal·ad·just·ed [mæləˈdʒʌstɪd] *adj* **1.** *psychia.* nicht angepaßt, dissozial, milieugestört. **2.** schlecht angepaßt, schlecht angeglichen, unausgeglichen.
mal·ad·just·ment [mæləˈdʒʌstmənt] *n* **1.** *psychia.* mangelnde Anpassungsfähigkeit *f*, mangelnde Anpassung *f*, Milieustörung *f*. **2.** schlechte Anpassung *od.* Angleichung *f*.
mal·a·dy [ˈmælədɪ] *n, pl* **-dies** → maladie.
ma·laise [mæˈleɪz, mə-; maˈlɛːz] *n French* Unwohlsein *nt*, Unpäßlichkeit *f*, Kränklichkeit *f*.
mal·a·ko·pla·kia *n* → malacoplakia.
mal·a·lign·ment [mæləˈlaɪnmənt] *n ortho.* (*Fraktur*) fehlerhafte Ausrichtung *f* der Bruchstücke, Fehlstellung *f*.
mal·a·line·ment *n* → malalignment.
ma·lar [ˈmeɪlər] **I** *n old für* Jochbein *nt*, Os zygomaticum. **II** *adj* Wange *od.* Backe betr., Wangen-, Backen-; Jochbein betr.
malar arch Jochbeinbogen *m*, Arcus zygomaticus.
malar bone → malar I.
malar flush Wangenröte *f*.
ma·lar·ia [məˈleərɪə] *n* Sumpf-, Wechselfieber *nt*, Malaria *f*.
ma·lar·i·a·cid·al [məˌleərɪəˈsaɪdl] *adj* Malariaparasiten abtötend, plasmodizid.
malaria cycle *micro.* Malariazyklus *m*.
ma·lar·i·al [məˈleərɪəl] *adj* Malaria betr., durch Malaria bedingt, Malaria-.
malarial cachexia chronische Malaria *f*.
malarial crescents (*Malaria*) Sichelkeime *pl*.
malarial fever → malaria.
malarial hemoglobinuria Schwarzwasserfieber *nt*, Febris biliosa et haemoglobinurica.
malarial parasite → malaria parasite.
malarial pigment Malariapigment *nt*.

malaria melanin Malariamelanin *nt*.
malaria parasite Malariaerreger *m*, -plasmodium *nt*, Plasmodium *nt*.
ma·lar·i·a·ther·a·py [məˌleərɪəˈθerəpɪ] *n* Malariatherapie *f*.
ma·lar·i·o·ther·a·py [məˌleərɪəʊˈθerəpɪ] *n* Malariatherapie *f*.
ma·lar·i·ous [məˈleərɪəs] *adj* → malarial.
malar process Jochfortsatz *m* des Oberkiefers, Proc. zygomaticus maxillae.
Malassez [malaˈze]: **M.'s disease** Hodenzyste *f*.
 epithelial rests of M. Malassez'-Epithelreste *pl*.
Mal·as·se·zia [mæləˈsiːzɪə] *n micro.* Malassezia *f*; Pityrosporon *n*.
mal·as·sim·i·la·tion [mæləˌsɪməˈleɪʃn] *n* Malassimilation *f*.
mal·ate [ˈmæleɪt] *n* Malat *nt*.
malate-aspartate shuttle Malat-Aspartat-Shuttle *m*.
malate dehydrogenase *abbr.* **MDH** Malatdehydrogenase (NAD+) *f abbr.* MDH.
malate dehydrogenase (NADP+) Malatdehydrogenase (NADP+) *f*, Malatenzym *nt*.
malate-NAD dehydrogenase → malate dehydrogenase.
malate-NADPH dehydrogenase → malate dehydrogenase (NADP+).
Malatesta [mæləˈtestə]: **M.'s syndrome** Malatesta-Syndrom *nt*, Orbitaspitzensyndrom *nt*, Apex-orbitae-Syndrom *nt*.
malate synthase Malatsynthase *f*.
ma·la·thi·on [mæləˈθaɪɒn] *n pharm.* Malathion *nt*.
ma·lax·ate [ˈmæləkseɪt, məˈlæk-] *vt* (durch-)kneten.
ma·lax·a·tion [ˌmæləkˈseɪʃn, məˌlækˈs-] *n* (Durch-)Kneten *nt*.
Ma·lay·an filariasis [məˈleɪən] Brugia--malayi-Filariose *f*, Brugiose *f*, Filariasis malayi.
Ma·lay bugs [məˈleɪ] *micro.* Raubwanzen *pl*, Reduviiden *pl*, Reduviidae *pl*.
mal·de·vel·op·ment [mældɪˈveləpmənt] *n patho.* abnorme Entwicklung *f*, abnormes Wachstum *nt*.
mal·di·ges·tion [maldɪˈdʒestʃn] *n* ungenügende/unvollständige Verdauung *f*, Maldigestion *f*.
male [meɪl] **I** *n* Mann *m*; *zoo.* Männchen *nt*. **II** *adj* männlich, Männer-.
male animal männliches Tier *nt*, Männchen *nt*.
mal·e·ate [ˈmæleɪt, -ɪt] *n* Maleat *nt*, Maleinat *nt*.
male breast männliche Brust(drüse *f*) *f*, Mamma masculina.
male castration Kastration *f*, bilaterale Orchiektomie *f*.
male child Junge *m*.
Malecot [malˈko]: **M.'s catheter** Malecot--Katheter *m*.
male doctor Arzt *m*.
male genitalia: external m. äußere männliche Geschlechtsorgane/Genitalien *pl*, Organa genitalia masculina externa.
 internal m. innere männliche Geschlechtsorgane/Genitalien *pl*, Organa genitalia masculina interna.
male gonad männliche Geschlechts-/Keimdrüse *f*, Hode(n) *m*, Testikel *m*, Testis *m*, Orchis *m*.
male hypogonadism Eunuchoidismus *m*.
ma·le·ic acid [məˈliːɪk] Maleinsäure *f*.
male nurse Krankenpfleger *m*.
male pattern alopecia/baldness androgenetische Alopezie *f*, Haarausfall *m* vom männlichen Typ, männliche Glatzenbildung *f*, androgenetisches Effluvium *nt*,

male pronucleus

Alopecia androgenetica, Calvities hippocratica.
male pronucleus *embryo.* männlicher Vorkern/Pronukleus *m.*
male pseudohermaphroditism Pseudohermaphroditismus masculinus.
male sterility männliche Sterilität *f.*
male Turner syndrome Noonan-Syndrom *nt*, Pseudo-Ullrich-Turner-Syndrom *nt.*
mal·e·yl·a·ce·to·ac·e·tate [ˌmælɘwɪlɘˌsiːtɘʊˈæsteɪt] *n* Maleylacetoacetat *nt.*
maleylacetoacetate isomerase Maleylacetoacetatisomerase *f.*
4-mal·e·yl·a·ce·to·a·cet·ic acid [ˌ-ɘˌsiːtɘʊɘˈsiːtɪk, -ɘˈsetɪk] 4-Maleylacetessigsäure *f.*
maleylacetoacetic acid isomerase → maleylacetoacetate isomerase.
mal·for·ma·tion [mælfɔːrˈmeɪʃn] *n embryo.* Fehl-, Mißbildung *f*, Malformation *f.*
mal·func·tion [mælˈfʌŋkʃn] *n* Funktionsstörung *f*, Dysfunktion *f*, Dysfunctio *f.*
Malgaigne [mælˈgeɪn; malˈgɛɲə]: **M.'s amputation** *ortho.* Malgaigne-Amputation *f*, Fußamputation *f* nach Malgaigne.
M.'s fossa Karotisdreieck *nt*, Trigonum caroticum.
M.'s luxation Chassaignac-Lähmung *f*, Subluxation *f* des Radiusköpfchens, Pronatio dolorosa, Subluxatio radii peranularis.
M.'s triangle → M.'s fossa.
Malherbe [malˈɛrb]: **M.'s calcifying epithelioma** → M.'s disease.
M.'s disease verkalktes Epitheliom *nt*, Pilomatrixom *nt*, Pilomatricoma *nt*, Epithelioma calcificans (Malherbe).
mal·i·as·mus [mælɪˈæsmɘz] *n* Rotz *m*, Malleus *m*, Maliasmus *m.*
mal·ic acid [ˈmælɪk, ˈmeɪ-] Äpfel-, Apfelsäure *f.*
malic acid dehydrogenase → malate dehydrogenase.
malic enzyme → malate dehydrogenase (NADP+).
ma·lign [mɘˈlaɪn] *adj* → malignant.
ma·lig·nan·cy [mɘˈlɪɡnɘnsi] *n*, *pl* **-cies 1.** *patho.* Bösartigkeit *f*, Malignität *f.* **2.** bösartige Geschwulst *f*, Malignom *nt.* **3.** Schädlichkeit *f*, Verderblichkeit *f.*
malignancy-associated *adj* malignom-assoziiert.
ma·lig·nant [mɘˈlɪɡnɘnt] *adj* **1.** *patho.* bösartig, maligne. **2.** verderblich, schädlich. **3.** bösartig, böswillig, feindselig.
malignant adenoma Adenokarzinom *nt*, Adenocarcinom *nt*, Ca. adenomatosum.
malignant anemia perniziöse Anämie *f*, Biermer-Anämie *f*, Addison-Anämie *f*, Morbus Biermer *m*, Perniciosa *f*, Perniziosa *f*, Anaemia perniciosa, Vitamin B₁₂-Mangelanämie *f.*
malignant angina Angina gangraenosa.
malignant aphthae (echte) Maul- u. Klauenseuche *f abbr.* MKS, Febris aphthosa, Stomatitis epidemica, Aphthosis epizootica.
malignant ascites maligner Aszites *m.*
malignant atrophic papulosis Köhlmeier-Degos-Syndrom *nt*, Degos-Delort-Tricot-Syndrom *nt*, tödliches kutaneo-intestinales Syndrom *nt*, Papulosis maligna atrophicans (Degos), Papulosis atrophicans maligna, Thrombangitis cutaneaintestinalis disseminata.
malignant bubo maligner Bubo *m.*
malignant carbuncle Milzbrandkarbunkel *m.*
malignant carcinoid syndrome Flush-, Karzinoidsyndrom *nt*, Biörck-Thorson-Syndrom *nt.*

malignant cholangioma Gallengangskarzinom *nt*, malignes Cholangiom *nt*, cholangiozelluläres Karzinom *nt*, Ca. cholangiocellulare.
malignant diphtheria maligne Diphtherie *f.*
malignant disease bösartige/maligne Erkrankung *f*, Malignom *nt.*
malignant dysentery Dysenteria maligna.
malignant edema malignes Ödem *nt.*
malignant enchondroma Knorpel-, Chondrosarkom *nt*, Chondroma sarcomatosum, Enchondroma malignum.
malignant endocarditis septische Endokarditis *f.*
malignant epithelioma Karzinom *nt*, *inf.* Krebs *m*, Carcinoma *nt abbr.* Ca.
malignant exophthalmus hochgradiger Exophthalmus *m* bei Hyperthyreose.
malignant glaucoma malignes Glaukom *nt*, Ziliarblockglaukom *nt.*
malignant glioma Glioblastom(a) *nt*, Gliablastom *nt.*
malignant glomerulonephritis maligne Glomerulonephritis *f*, rasch progrediente Glomerulonephritis *f*, rapidly progressive glomerulonephritis.
malignant goiter Schilddrüsenkrebs *m*, -karzinom *nt.*
malignant granuloma letales Mittelliniengranulom *nt*, Granuloma gangraenescens nasi.
malignant granulomatosis → malignant lymphoma 1.
malignant hemangioendothelioma malignes/sarkomatöses Hämangioendotheliom *nt*, Hämangiosarkom *nt.*
malignant hepatoma (primäres) Leberzellkarzinom *nt*, hepatozelluläres Karzinom *nt*, malignes Hepatom *nt*, Ca. hepatocellulare.
malignant hyperphenylalaninemia Hyperphenylalaninämie *f* Typ IV, maligne Hyperphenylalaninämie *f*, Dihydropteridinreduktasemangel *m*, DHPR-Mangel *m.*
malignant hyperpyrexia maligne Hyperpyrexie/Hyperthermie *f.*
malignant hypertension maligne Hypertonie *f.*
malignant hyperthermia → malignant hyperpyrexia.
malignant lentigo Lentigo maligna, Dubreuilh-Krankheit *f*, -Erkrankung *f*, Dubreuilh-Hutchinson-Krankheit *f*, -Erkrankung *f*, prämaligne Melanose *f*, melanotische Präkanzerose *f*, Melanosis circumscripta praeblastomatosa/praecancerosa (Dubreuilh).
malignant lentigo melanoma *abbr.* **MLM** Lentigo-maligna-Melanom *nt abbr.* LMM.
malignant leukopenia Agranulozytose *f*, maligne/perniziöse Neutropenie *f.*
malignant lymphogranulomatosis → malignant lymphoma 1.
malignant lymphoma 1. Hodgkin-Krankheit *f*, -Lymphom *nt*, Morbus Hodgkin *m*, (Hodgkin-)Paltauf-Steinberg-Krankheit *f*, (maligne) Lymphogranulomatose *f*, Lymphogranulomatosis maligna. **2.** non-Hodgkin-Lymphom *nt abbr.* NHL.
m. of bone Retikulumzellsarkom/Retikulosarkom/Retothelsarkom *nt* des Knochens, malignes Lymphom des Knochens.
centroblastic m. zentroblastisches Lymphom.
centroblastic-centrocytic m. zentroblastisch-zentrozytischen (malignes) Lymphom *nt*, Brill-Symmers-Syndrom *nt*,

Morbus Brill-Symmers *m*, großfollikuläres Lymphom/Lymphoblastom *nt.*
centrocytic m. zentrozytisches (malignes) Lymphom, lymphozytisches Lymphosarkom *nt.*
immunoblastic m. Retikulumzellensarkom *nt*, immunoblastisches (malignes) Lymphom.
malignant malnutrition Kwashiorkor *nt.*
malignant melanoma *abbr.* **MM** malignes Melanom *nt abbr.* MM, Melano(zyto)blastom *nt*, Nävokarzinom *nt*, Melanokarzinom *nt*, Melanomalignom *nt*, malignes Nävoblastom *nt.*
amelanotic m. *abbr.* **AMM** amelanotisches (malignes) Melanom *abbr.* AMM.
malignant mesenchymoma malignes Mesenchymom *nt.*
malignant mole *gyn.* destruierende Blasenmole *f*, destruierendes Chorionadenom *nt.*
malignant myopia *ophthal.* bösartige/maligne Myopie *f.*
malignant neoplasm maligne Geschwulst *f*, malignes Neoplasma *nt*, Malignom *nt.*
malignant nephrosclerosis Fahr-Volhard-Nephrosklerose *f*, maligne Nephrosklerose *f.*
malignant neutropenia Agranulozytose *f*, maligne Neutropenie *f.*
malignant osteomyelitis *old* → multiple myeloma.
malignant purpura Meningokokkenmeningitis *f.*
malignant pustule Pustula maligna.
malignant pyoderma/pyodermia maligne Pyodermie *f.*
malignant synovialoma/synovioma malignes Synovialom/Synoviom *nt*, Synovialsarkom *nt.*
malignant teratoma malignes/embryonales/unreifes Teratom *nt*, Teratoma embryonale.
malignant tertian fever Tropen-, Aestivoautumnalfieber *nt*, Falciparum-Malaria *f*, Malaria tropica.
malignant tertian malaria → malignant tertian fever.
malignant trophoblastic teratoma *abbr.* **MTT** malignes trophoblastisches Teratom *nt.*
malignant tumor Krebs *m*, maligner Tumor *m*, Malignom *nt.*
ma·lig·ni·ty [mɘˈlɪɡnɘti] *n* → malignancy.
ma·lin·ger [mɘˈlɪŋɡɘr] *vt* s. krankstellen, simulieren.
ma·lin·ger·er [mɘˈlɪŋɡɘrɘr] *n* Simulant *m.*
ma·lin·ger·ing [mɘˈlɪŋɡɘrɪŋ] *n* Simulieren *nt.*
mal·le·a·bil·i·ty [ˌmælɪɘˈbɪlɘti] *n phys.*, *techn.* Dehn-, Streckbarkeit *f*; Verformbarkeit *f.*
mal·le·a·ble [ˈmælɪɘbl] *adj phys.*, *techn.* dehn-, streckbar; verformbar.
mal·le·al [ˈmælɪɘl] *adj* → mallear.
mal·le·ar [ˈmælɪɘr] *adj* Hammer/Malleus betr., mallear.
mallear fold: anterior m. Plica mallearis anterior.
posterior m. Plica mallearis posterior.
mallear prominence of tympanic membrane Prominentia mallearis (membranae tympanicae).
mallear stria of tympanic membrane Stria mallearis (membranae tympani).
mal·le·o·in·cu·dal [ˌmælɪɘˈɪŋkjɘdl, -ˈɪŋ-] *adj* Malleus u. Incus betr., malleoinkudal, inkudomalleolar.
mal·le·o·lar [mɘˈlɪɘlɘ(r)] *adj* **1.** (Fuß-)Knöchel *od.* Knöchelregion betr., malleolar, Knöchel-. **2.** (Ohr) Hammer/Malleus betr., malleolar.

malleolar artery: anterior m., lateral vordere äußere Knöchelarterie *f*, A. malleolaris anterior lateralis.
anterior m., medial vordere innere Knöchelarterie *f*, A. malleolaris anterior medialis.
posterior m.ies, lateral → malleolar branches of fibular artery, lateral.
posterior m.ies, medial → malleolar branches of posterior tibial artery, medial.
malleolar branches: lateral m. of fibular artery Außenknöcheläste *pl* der A. fibularis, Rami malleolares laterales a. peron(a)eae/fibularis.
medial m. of posterior tibial artery Innenknöcheläste *pl* der A. tibialis posterior, Rami malleolares mediales a. tibialis posterioris.
malleolar fracture Knöchelbruch *m*, Malleolarfraktur *f*, Fractura malleolaris.
lateral m. Außenknöchelbruch, -fraktur.
medial m. Innenknöchelbruch, -fraktur.
malleolar network: lateral m. Arteriengeflecht *nt* am Außenknöchel, Rete malleolare laterale.
medial m. Arteriengeflecht *nt* des Innenknöchels, Rete malleolare mediale.
malleolar region: anterior m. vordere Knöchelregion/-gegend *f*, Regio talocruralis anterior.
posterior m. hintere Knöchelregion/-gegend *f*, Regio talocruralis posterior.
malleolar rete: lateral m. → malleolar network, lateral.
medial m. → malleolar network, medial.
malleolar sulcus: m. of fibula Sulcus malleolaris fibulae.
m. of tibia Sulcus malleolaris tibiae.
mal·le·o·lus [mə'lɪələs] *n*, *pl* **-li** [-laɪ] (Fuß-)Knöchel *m*, Malleolus *m*.
Mal·le·o·my·ces [ˌmælɪə'maɪsi:z] *n micro.* Malleomyces *m*, Actinobacillus *m*.
mal·le·ot·o·my [mælɪ'ɒtəmɪ] *n* HNO Malleotomie *f*.
mal·let ['mælɪt] *n* Hammer *m*, Fäustel *m*.
mallet finger Hammerfinger *m*.
mallet toe Hammerzehe *f*, Digitus malleus.
mal·le·us ['mælɪəs] *n*, *pl* **mal·lei** [-lɪaɪ] 1. (Ohr) Hammer *m*, Malleus *m*. 2. *micro.* Maliasmus *m*, Rotz *m*, Malleus *m*.
Mal·loph·a·ga [mə'lɒfəgə] *pl micro.* Läuslinge *pl*, Kieferläuse *pl*, Mallophaga *f*.
Ma·llor·ca acne [mə'jɔ:rkə] Mallorca--Akne *f*, Akne/Acne aestivalis.
Mallory ['mælərɪ]: **M.'s bodies** Mallory--Körperchen *pl*.
Mallory-Weiss [vaɪs]: **M.-W. lesion** Schleimhautlazeration *f* bei Mallory--Weiss-Syndrom, Mallory-Weiss-Risse *pl*.
M.-W. syndrome Mallory-Weiss-Syndrom *nt*.
M.-W. tears → M.-W. lesion.
mal·nour·ished [mæl'nərɪʃt, -'nʌr-] *adj* fehl-, mangel-, unterernährt.
mal·nu·tri·tion [ˌmæln(j)u:'trɪʃn] *n* Fehl-, Mangel-, Unterernährung *f*, Malnutrition *f*.
mal·o·nate ['mælənɪt, -nɪt] *n* Malonat *nt*.
Maloney [mə'ləʊnɪ]: **M. bougie** Maloney--Bougie *f*.
ma·lo·nic acid [mə'ləʊnɪk, -'lɒn-] Malonsäure *f*.
mal·o·nyl ['mælənɪl, -ni:l] *n* Malonyl-(Radikal *nt*).
malonyl-CoA *n* → malonyl coenzyme A.
malonyl coenzyme A Malonyl-Coenzym A *nt*, Malonyl-CoA *nt*.
Malpighi [mæl'pi:gɪ; mal'pi:gi]: **pyramids of M.** Nierenpyramiden *pl*, Pyramides renales.

M.'s vesicles Lungenalveolen *pl*, -bläschen *pl*, Alveoli pulmonis.
mal·pigh·i·an [mæl'pi:gɪən]: **m. bodies (of spleen)** Malpighi-Körperchen *pl*, Milzknötchen *pl*, weiße Pulpa *f*, Folliculi lymphatici splenici, Lymphonoduli splenici.
m. body of kidney Nierenkörperchen *nt*, Malpighi'-Körperchen *nt*, Corpusculum renalis.
m. capsule Bowman'-Kapsel *f*, Capsula glomeruli.
m. cell Keratinozyt *m*, Hornzelle *f*, Malpighi-Zelle *f*.
m. corpuscle of kidney → m. body of kidney.
m. corpuscles (of spleen) → m. bodies (of spleen).
m. glomerulus (Nieren-)Glomerulus *m*, Glomerulus renalis.
m. layer Regenerationsschicht *f*, Stratum germinativum epidermidis.
m. rete → m. layer.
m. tuft → m. glomerulus.
mal·po·si·tion [mælpə'zɪʃn] *n* Stellungs-, Lageanomalie *f*, Fehlstellung *f*, Malposition *f*, Malpositio *f*.
mal·prac·tice [mæl'præktɪs] *n* (ärztlicher) Behandlungsfehler *m*, falsche Behandlung *f*, Kunstfehler *m*; Fahrlässigkeit *f*.
mal·prax·is [mæl'præksɪs] *n* → malpractice.
mal·pre·sen·ta·tion [mælˌpri:zen'teɪʃn, -ˌprezn-] *n gyn.* anomale Kindslage *f*.
mal·ro·ta·tion [mælrəʊ'teɪʃn] *n patho.* Malrotation *f*.
malt [mɔ:lt] *n* Malz *nt*.
Mal·ta fever ['mɔ:ltə] 1. Bruzellose *f*, Brucellose *f*, Brucellosis *f*. 2. Malta-, Mittelmeerfieber *nt*, Febris mediterranea/melitensis.
malt·ase ['mɔ:lteɪz] *n* Maltase *f*, α-D-Glucosidase *f*.
malt extract Malzextrakt *m*.
malt extract agar Malzextraktagar *m/nt*.
mal·to·bi·ose [ˌmɔ:ltəʊ'baɪəʊs] *n* → maltose.
mal·to·dex·trin [ˌ-'dekstrɪn] *n* Maltodextrin *nt*.
mal·tose ['mɔ:ltəʊz] *n* Malzzucker *m*, Maltose *f*.
maltose phosphorylase Maltosephosphorylase *f*.
mal·to·side ['mɔ:ltəʊsaɪd] *n* Maltosid *nt*.
mal·to·su·ria [ˌ-'s(j)ʊərɪə] *n* Maltoseausscheidung *f* im Harn, Maltosurie *f*.
mal·to·tri·ose [ˌ-'traɪəʊs] *n* Maltotriose *f*.
malt sugar → maltose.
malt-worker's lung Malzarbeiterlunge *f*.
ma·lum ['mɑ:ləm] *n*, *pl* **-la** [-lə] Leiden *nt*, Gebrechen *nt*, Krankheit *f*.
mal·un·ion [mæl'ju:njən] *n ortho.* (*Fraktur*) Verheilung *f* in Fehlstellung.
ma·mil·la [mə'mɪlə, mæ-] *n*, *pl* **-lae** [-li:] 1. *anat.* Brustwarze *f*, Mamille *f*, Papilla mammae. 2. warzenähnliche Struktur *f*, Mamille *f*, Mamilla *f*.
ma·mil·lar·y ['mæməˌlerɪ] *adj* Brustwarze betr., mamillär, mamillenförmig, Warzen-, Brustwarzen-.
mamillary body Corpus mamillare.
mamillary ducts Milchgänge *pl*, Ductus lactiferi.
mamillary eminence Mamillarhöcker *m*.
mamillary line Mamillarlinie *f*, Linea mamillaris.
mamillary process Proc. mamillaris.
m. of temporal bone Proc. mastoideus (ossis temporalis).
mamillary tubercle Proc. mamillaris.
m. of hypothalamus Corpus mamillare.
mam·il·late ['mæməleɪt] *adj* → mamillated.

mam·il·lat·ed ['mæməleɪtɪd] *adj* mit (Brust-)Warzen besetzt.
ma·mil·li·form [mə'mɪləfɔ:rm] *adj* (brust-)warzenförmig.
ma·mil·li·plas·ty [mə'mɪləplæstɪ] *n gyn.* Mamillenplastik *f*.
mam·il·li·tis [mæmə'laɪtɪs] *n* Brustwarzenentzündung *f*, Mamillitis *f*.
ma·mil·lo·teg·men·tal fasciculus/tract [məˌmɪləʊteg'mentl] Gudden'-Haubenbündel *nt*, Fasciculus mamillotegmentalis.
ma·mil·lo·tha·lam·ic fasciculus/tract [ˌ-θə'læmɪk] Vicq d'Azyr'-Bündel *nt*, Fasciculus mamillothalamicus.
mamm- *pref.* → mammo-.
mam·ma ['mæmə] *n*, *pl* **-mae** [-mi:] 1. *anat.* (weibliche) Brust *f*, Brustdrüse *f*, Mamma *f*. 2. *zoo.* Euter *m*, Zitze *f*.
mam·mal ['mæməl] *n zoo.* Säugetier *m*, Säuger *m*.
mam·mal·gia [mə'mældʒ(ɪ)ə] *n* → mastalgia.
Mam·ma·lia [mə'meɪlɪə, mæ-, -ljə] *pl zoo.* Säuger *pl*, Säugetiere *pl*, Mammalia *pl*.
mam·ma·li·an [mə'meɪlɪən, -ljən] **I** *n* Säugetier *nt*, Säuger *m*. **II** *adj* Säugetier-.
mammalian adenovirus *micro.* Mastadenovirus *nt*.
mam·ma·plas·ty ['mæməplæstɪ] *n gyn.* Brust(drüsen)plastik *f*, Mammaplastik *f*.
mam·ma·ry ['mæmərɪ] *adj* 1. Brust/Mamma betr. Milchdrüse betr., Mamma-, Brust(warzen)-, Milch(drüsen)-. 2. *zoo.* Euter-.
mammary abscess Brust(drüsen)abszeß *m*.
mammary artery: external m. seitliche Brustwandarterie *f*, Thoracica *f* lateralis, A. thoracica lateralis.
internal m. innere Brustwandarterie *f*, Mammaria/Thoracica *f* interna, A. thoracica interna.
mammary branches: m. of internal thoracic artery Brust(drüsen)-Äste *pl* der A. thoracica interna, Rami mammarii mediales a. thoracicae internae.
lateral m. of lateral thoracic artery Brust(drüsen)-Äste *pl* der A. thoracica lateralis, Rami mammarii laterales a. thoracicae lateralis.
medial m. of internal thoracic artery → m. of internal thoracic artery.
mammary calculus (*Brust*) Milchgangstein *m*.
mammary cancer → mammary carcinoma.
mammary cancer virus of mice → mammary tumor virus.
mammary carcinoma Brust(drüsen)krebs *m*, -karzinom *nt*, Mammakarzinom *nt*, *inf.* Mamma-Ca, Ca. mammae.
colloid m. verschleimendes/muzinöses Brust(drüsen)karzinom.
cribriform m. kribriformes Brust(drüsen)karzinom.
ductal m. Milchgangskarzinom.
ductal m. with productive fibrosis, infiltrating → scirrhous m.
familial m. familiäres/familiär-gehäuftes Brust(drüsen)karzinom.
inflammatory m. inflammatorisches Brust(drüsen)karzinom.
intraductal m. intraduktales/intraduktalwachsendes Brust(drüsen)karzinom.
lobular m. lobuläres Brust(drüsen)karzinom.
medullary m. medulläres Brust(drüsen)karzinom.
minimal m. Minimalkrebs, -karzinom, intraduktales *od.* lobuläres Carcinoma in situ.

mammary cycle

mucinous m. → colloid m.
papillary m. papilläres Brust(drüsen)karzinom.
scirrhous m. szirrhöses Brust(drüsen)karzinom, Szirrhus *m*, Carcinoma solidum simplex der Brust.
tubulary m. tubuläres Brust(drüsen)karzinom.
mammary cycle Brustzyklus *m*, zyklische Brustveränderungen *pl*.
mammary duct ectasia *gyn*. Plasmazell-, Komedomastitis *f*.
mammary ducts Milchgänge *pl*, Ductus lactiferi.
mammary dysplasia *gyn*. zystische/fibrös-zystische Mastopathie *f*, Mammadysplasie *f*, Zystenmamma *f*, Mastopathia chronica cystica.
mammary feminism Vergrößerung *f* der männl. Brust(drüse), Gynäkomastie *f*.
mammary fistula Milch(gangs)fistel *f*.
mammary gland Brustdrüse *f*, Gl. mammaria.
accessory m.s zusätzliche/akzessorische Brustdrüsen *pl*, Mammae aberrantes/accessoriae/erraticae, Polymastie *f*.
active m. laktierende/aktive Brustdrüse.
lactating m. → active m.
supernumerary m.s → accessory m.s.
mammary gland carcinoma → mammary carcinoma.
mammary line *embryo*. Milchleiste *f*.
mammary papilla Brustwarze *f*, Mamille *f*, Papilla mammaria.
mammary region Mammaregion *f*, Regio mammaria.
mammary ridge → mammary line.
mammary tumor Brust(drüsen)geschwulst *f*, -tumor *m*.
mammary tumor agent Mäuse-Mamma--Tumorvirus *nt* abbr. MMTV.
mammary tumor virus of mice → mammary tumor agent.
mam·ma·troph ['mæmətrɒf, -trəʊf] *n* → mammotroph.
mam·mec·to·my [mə'mektəmɪ] *n* gyn. Brust(drüsen)entfernung *f*, Mammaamputation *f*, Mastektomie *f*.
mam·mi·form ['mæmɪfɔːrm] *adj* brustförmig.
mam·mil·la *n* → mamilla.
mam·mil·la·plas·ty [mə'mɪləplæstɪ] *n* gyn. Mamillenplastik *f*.
mam·mil·lary *adj* → mamillary.
mam·mil·lat·ed *adj* → mamillated.
mam·mil·li·form *adj* → mamilliform.
mam·mil·li·tis *n* → mamillitis.
mam·mi·pla·sia [ˌmæmɪ'pleɪʒ(ɪ)ə, -zɪə] *n* → mammoplasia.
mam·mi·tis [mæ'maɪtɪs] *n* → mastitis.
mammo- *pref*. Brust-, Brustdrüsen-, Mamm(o)-, Mast(o)-.
mam·mo·gen·e·sis [ˌmæmə'dʒenəsɪs] *n* Brustdrüsenentwicklung *f*, Mammogenese *f*.
mam·mo·gen·ic hormone [ˌ-'dʒenɪk] mammogenes Hormon *nt*.
mam·mo·gram ['-græm] *n radiol*. Mammogramm *nt*.
mam·mog·ra·phy [mə'mɒgrəfɪ] *n radiol*. Mammographie *f*.
mam·mo·pla·sia [ˌmæmə'pleɪʒ(ɪ)ə, -zɪə] *n* Brustentwicklung *f*, Mammoplasie *f*, Mastoplasie *f*.
mam·mo·plas·ty ['-plæstɪ] *n* → mammaplasty.
mam·mose [mə'məʊs, 'mæm-] *adj* **1.** großbrüstig. **2.** → mamillated. **3.** → mammiform.
mam·mot·o·my [mæ'mɒtəmɪ] *n* → mastotomy.
mam·mo·troph ['mæmətrɒf, -trəʊf] *n* (*Adenohypophyse*) Prolaktin-Zelle *f*, mammotrope Zelle *f*.
mam·mo·troph·ic [ˌ-'trɒfɪk, -'trəʊ-] *adj* → mammotropic.
mam·mo·tro·phin [ˌ-'trəʊfɪn] *n old* → prolactin.
mam·mo·trop·ic [ˌ-'trɒpɪk, -'trəʊp-] *adj* auf die Brustdrüse wirkend, mammotrop.
mam·mot·ro·pin [mə'mɒtrəpɪn, ˌmæmə'trəʊpɪn] *n old* → prolactin.
man·age·ment ['mænɪdʒmənt] *n* Behandlung *f*, Pflege *f*.
Man·ches·ter brown ['mæntʃestər] Bismarckbraun *nt*.
Manchester operation Fothergill-Operation *f*, Manchester-Operation *f*.
Man·chu·ri·an hemorrhagic fever [mæn'tʃʊərɪən] hämorrhagisches Fieber *nt* mit renalem Syndrom abbr. HFRS, koreanisches hämorrhagisches Fieber *nt*, akute hämorrhagische Nephrosonephritis *f*, Nephropathia epidemica.
Manchurian typhus → murine typhus.
man·da·to·ry ['mændətɔːriː, -təʊ-] *adj* obligatorisch, verbindlich, zwingend, vorgeschrieben.
man·del·ate ['mændəleɪt] *n* Mandelat *nt*.
man·del·ic acid [mæn'delɪk, -'diːl-] Mandelsäure *f*.
man·de·lyt·ro·pine [mændə'lɪtrəpiːn] *n* Homatropin *nt*.
man·di·ble ['mændɪbl] *n* Unterkiefer(knochen *m*) *m*, Mandibel *f*, Mandibula *f*.
man·dib·u·la [mæn'dɪbjələ] *n, pl* -**lae** [-liː] → mandible.
man·dib·u·lar [mæn'dɪbjələr] *adj* Unterkiefer(knochen)/Mandibula betr., mandibular, Mandibular-, Unterkiefer-.
mandibular arch 1. *embryo*. Mandibularbogen *m*, erster Schlundbogen *m*. **2.** Unterkieferzahnreihe *f*, mandibuläre Zahnreihe *f*, Arcus dentalis inferior.
mandibular artery Unterkieferschlagader *f*, -arterie *f*, Alveolaris *f* inferior, A. alveolaris inferior.
mandibular articulation Kiefergelenk *nt*, Temporomandibulargelenk *nt*, Artic. temporomandibularis.
mandibular branch of facial nerve, marginal Unterkieferast *m* des N. facialis, Ramus marginalis mandibularis n. facialis.
mandibular canal Unterkieferkanal *m*, Canalis mandibulae.
mandibular cartilage → Meckel's cartilage.
mandibular condyle Proc. condylaris mandibulae.
mandibular division of trigeminal nerve → mandibular nerve.
mandibular foramen For. mandibulae.
mandibular fossa Fossa mandibularis.
mandibular gland Unterkieferdrüse *f*, Gl. submandibularis.
mandibular hypoplasia *embryo*. kongenitale Kleinheit *f* des Unterkiefers.
mandibular joint → mandibular articulation.
mandibular nerve dritter Trigeminusast *m*, Mandibularis *m*, N. mandibularis.
mandibular notch Inc. mandibulae.
mandibular prominences *embryo*. Unterkieferwülste *pl*.
mandibular reflex Masseter-, Unterkieferreflex *m*.
mandibular symphysis Symphysis mandibulae/mentalis.
mandibular teeth Zähne *pl od*. Zahnreihe *f* des Unterkiefers.
mandibular torus Torus mandibularis.
man·dib·u·lec·to·my [mænˌdɪbjə'lektəmɪ] *n* HNO, chir. Unterkieferentfernung *f*, -resektion *f*, Mandibulektomie *f*.
man·dib·u·lo·fa·cial dysostosis [mænˌdɪbjələʊ'feɪʃl] Treacher-Collins-Syndrom *nt*, Franceschetti-Syndrom *nt*, Dysostosis mandibulo-facialis.
m. with epibulbar dermoids Goldenhar--Syndrom *nt*, okuloaurikuläres/okulo--aurikulo-vertebrales Syndrom *nt*, okulo-aurikulo-vertebrale Dysplasie *f*, Dysplasia oculo-auricularis, Dysplasia oculo-auriculo-vertebralis.
mandibulofacial dysplasia → mandibulofacial dysostosis.
mandibulofacial syndrome → mandibulofacial dysostosis.
mandibulo-oculofacial dyscephaly → mandibulo-oculofacial syndrome.
mandibulo-oculofacial dysmorphia → mandibulo-oculofacial syndrome.
mandibulo-oculofacial syndrome Hallermann-Streiff(-Francois)-Syndrom *nt*, Dyskephaliesyndrom *nt* von Francois, Dysmorphia mandibulo-oculo-facialis.
man·dib·u·lo·pha·ryn·ge·al [mænˌdɪbjələʊfə'rɪndʒɪəl] *adj* Unterkiefer u. Pharynx betr., mandibulopharyngeal.
man·drin ['mændrɪn] *n* Mandrin *m*.
ma·neu·ver [mə'nuːvər] *n* Methode *f*, Technik *f*, Prozedur *f*, Manöver *nt*.
man·ga·nese ['mæŋgəniːz] *n abbr*. **Mn** Mangan *nt abbr*. Mn.
manganese poisoning → manganism.
man·gan·ic ['mæŋ'gænɪk] *adj* **1.** manganhaltig, Mangan-. **2.** dreiwertiges Mangan enthaltend, Mangan-III-.
manganic acid Mangansäure *f*.
man·ga·nism ['mæŋgənɪzəm] *n* (chronische) Manganvergiftung *f*, Manganismus *m*, Manganose *f*.
man·ga·nous ['mæŋgənəs, mæn'gænəs] *adj* zweiwertiges Mangan enthaltend, Mangan-II-.
man·ga·num ['mæŋgənəm] *n* → manganese.
mange [meɪndʒ] *n bio*. Räude *f*.
man·go fly ['mæŋgəʊ] *micro*. Mango-, Mangrovefliege *f*, Crysops dimidiata.
man·grove fly ['mæŋgrəʊv, 'mæn-] → mango fly.
ma·nia [ˈmeɪnɪə, -jə] *n psychia*. Manie *f*, Mania *f*.
ma·ni·ac ['meɪnɪæk] **I** *n* **1.** Maniker(in *f*) *m*. **2.** Wahnsinnige(r *m*) *f*, Rasende(r *m*) *f*, Verrückte(r *m*) *f*. **II** *adj* **3.** → maniacal. **4.** wahnsinnig, verrückt, irr(e).
ma·ni·a·cal [mə'naɪəkl] *adj* an einer Manie leidend, manisch.
ma·nic ['mænɪk] **I** *n* Maniker(in *f*) *m*. **II** *adj* Manie betr., an einer Manie leidend, manisch.
manic-depressive *adj psychia*. manisch--depressiv.
manic-depressive disorder manisch-depressive Psychose/Krankheit *f*.
manic-depressive illness/psychosis → manic-depressive disorder.
man·i·fest ['mænɪfest] **I** *adj* offenbar, offenkundig, augenscheinlich, deutlich (erkennbar), manifest. **II** *vt* be-, erweisen. **III** *vi* erscheinen, s. zeigen.
man·i·fes·ta·tion [ˌmænɪfə'steɪʃn] *n* **1.** *patho*. Offenbar-, Erkennbarwerden *nt*, Manifestation *f*. **2.** *genet*. Manifestation *f*. **3.** Äußerung *f*, Erscheinung *f*, Anzeichen *nt*, Symptom *nt*, Manifestation *f*.
manifest hyperopia *abbr*. **Hm** *ophthal*. manifeste Weitsichtigkeit/Hyperopie *f*.
manifest strabimus *ophthal*. manifestes Schielen *nt*, manifester Strabismus *m*, Heterotropie *f*.
manifest tetany manifeste Tetanie *f*.

man·i·kin ['mænɪkɪn] n Modell nt, Phantom nt, Gliederpuppe f.
ma·nil·o·quism [mə'nɪləkwɪzəm] n Daktylologie f (Finger- u. Gebärdensprache der Taubstummen).
ma·nip·u·la·tion [mə,nɪpjə'leɪʃn] n **1.** Handlung f, Tätigkeit f, Hantierung f, Manipulation f. **2.** (Hand-)Griff m, Verfahren nt, Manipulation f.
Mann [mæn]: **M.'s sign** Mann-Zeichen nt.
man·na ['mænə] n Manna nt.
man·nan ['mænæn, -nən] n Mannan nt.
man·nans ['mænæns] pl Mannane pl.
man·ner·ism ['mænərɪzəm] n psychia. Gespreiztheit f, Manieriertheit f, Manierismus m.
man·nite ['mænaɪt] n → mannitol.
man·ni·tol ['mænɪtɒl, -tɒl] n Mannit nt, Mannitol nt.
man·ni·tose ['mænɪtəʊs] n → mannose.
D-man·nos·a·mine ['mænəʊsəmi:n] n D-Mannosamin nt.
man·no·san ['mænəsæn] n → mannan.
man·nose ['mænəʊs] n Mannose f.
mannose-1-phosphate n Mannose-1-Phosphat nt.
mannose-6-phosphate n Mannose-6-Phosphat nt.
mannose-6-phosphate isomerase Mannose-6-phosphatisomerase f, Mannosephosphatisomerase f.
α-man·no·si·dase ['mænəʊsɪdeɪz] n α-Mannosidase f.
man·no·side ['mænəsaɪd] n Mannosid nt.
man·no·si·do·sis [,mænəsɪ'dəʊsɪs] n Mannosidasemangel(-Syndrom nt) m, Mannosidosis f.
D-man·nu·ron·ic acid [mænjə'rɒnɪk] D-Mannuronsäure f.
Mann-Whitney ['(h)wɪtnɪ]: **M.-W. test** stat. Rangsummentest m, Wilcoxon-Test m.
Mann-Whitney-Wilcoxon [wɪl'kɒksən]: **M.-W.-W. test** → Mann-Whitney test.
ma·nom·e·ter [mə'nɒmɪtər] n Druckmesser m, Manometer nt.
man·o·met·ric [,mænə'metrɪk] adj Manometer betr., manometrisch.
man·o·met·ri·cal [,-'metrɪkl] adj → manometric.
man·slaugh·ter ['mænslɔ:tər] n forens. Totschlag m, Körperverletzung f mit Todesfolge.
Manson ['mænsən]: **M.'s disease/schistosomiasis** Manson'-Krankheit f, -Bilharziose f, Schistosomiasis mansoni.
Man·son·el·la [,mænsə'nelə] n micro. Mansonella f.
man·so·nel·li·a·sis [,mænsəne'laɪəsɪs] n → mansonellosis.
man·so·nel·lo·sis [,mænsəne'ləʊsɪs] n Mansonellainfektion f, Mansonelliasis f, Mansonellose f.
Man·so·nia [mæn'səʊnɪə] n micro. Mansonia f.
Man·so·ni·oi·des [,mænsənɪ'ɔɪdi:z] pl micro. Mansonioides pl.
M antigen M-Antigen nt.
man·tle ['mæntl] n Mantel m, Hülle f, Umhüllung f.
mantle field radiol. Mantelfeld nt.
mantle field technique radiol. Mantelfeldbestrahlung f.
mantle layer embryo. Mantelschicht f.
mantle zone → mantle layer.
Mantoux [mæn'tu:, mɑ̃'tu]: **M. reaction/test** Mendel-Mantoux-Probe f, -Test nt.
man·u·al ['mænjuəl] **I** n Handbuch nt, Leitfaden m, Vorschrift f. **II** adj mit der Hand od. den Händen, manuell, Hand-, Manual-.
manual alphabet Fingeralphabet nt (der Taubstummen).

ma·nu·bri·o·ster·nal [mə,n(j)u:brɪəʊ'stɜrnl] adj Manubrium u. Corpus sterni betr., manubriosternal.
manubriosternal articulation → manubriosternal symphysis.
manubriosternal joint → manubriosternal symphysis.
manubriosternal symphysis Manubriosternalgelenk nt, Synchondrosis/Symphysis manubriosternalis.
manubriosternal synchondrosis → manubriosternal symphysis.
ma·nu·bri·um [mə'n(j)u:brɪəm] n, pl -bria [-brɪə], -bri·ums anat. Schwertgriff m, Manubrium nt, Manubrium sterni.
m. of malleus anat. Hammergriff m, Manubrium mallei.
m. of sternum → manubrium.
manubrium sterni → manubrium.
MAO abbr. **1.** → maximal acid output. **2.** → monoamine oxidase.
MAOI abbr. → monoamine oxidase inhibitor.
MAP abbr. → mean arterial pressure.
map [mæp] **I** n Karte f; Plan m. **II** vt kartographisch darstellen od. erfassen, auf einer Karte eintragen.
ma·ple bark disease ['meɪpl] Ahornrindenschälerkrankheit f.
maple sugar disease → maple syrup urine disease.
maple syrup disease → maple syrup urine disease.
maple syrup urine disease abbr. **MSUD** Ahornsirup-Krankheit f, -Syndrom nt, Valin-Leucin-Isoleucinurie f, Verzweigtkettendecarboxylase-Mangel m.
map-like skull radiol. Landkartenschädel m.
map·ping ['mæpɪŋ] n genet., card. Mapping nt.
map·py tongue ['mæpɪ] Landkartenzunge f, Wanderplaques pl, Lingua geographica, Exfoliatio areata linguae/dolorosa, Glossitis exfoliativa marginata, Glossitis areata exsudativa.
ma·pro·ti·line [mə'prɒtɪli:n] n Maprotilin nt.
ma·ran·tic [mə'ræntɪk] adj → marasmic.
marantic atrophy → marasmus f.
marantic edema marantisches Ödem nt.
marantic endocarditis atypische verruköse Endokarditis f, Libman-Sacks-Syndrom nt, Endokarditis Libman-Sacks, Endocarditis thrombotica.
mar·as·mat·ic [,mæræz'mætɪk] adj → marasmic.
ma·ras·mic [mə'ræzmɪk] adj Marasmus betr., durch Marasmus hervorgerufen, an Marasmus leidend, abgezehrt, verfallen, marantisch, marastisch.
ma·ras·moid [mə'ræzmɔɪd] adj marasmusähnlich, -artig.
ma·ras·mus [mə'ræzməs] n **1.** Verfall m, Kräfteschwund m, Marasmus m. **2.** Säuglingsdystrophie f, Marasmus m.
mar·ble ['mɑ:rbl] **I** n Marmor m. **II** vt sprenkeln, marmorieren.
marble bone disease → marble bones.
marble bones Marmorknochenkrankheit f, Albers-Schönberg-Krankheit f, Osteopetrosis f.
mar·ble·i·za·tion [,mɑ:rblaɪ'zeɪʃn] n Marmorierung f.
mar·ble·ize ['mɑ:rbəlaɪz] vt sprenkeln, marmorieren.
marble skin Cutis marmorata, Livedo reticularis.
marble state Vogt-Syndrom nt, -Erkrankung f, Status marmoratus.
mar·bo·ran [mɑ:rbə'ræn] n pharm. Methisazon nt, Marboran nt.

Mar·burg disease ['mɑ:rbɜrg; 'mɑrbʊrk] Marburg-Krankheit f, -Fieber nt.
Marburg virus Marburg-Virus nt.
Marburg virus disease → Marburg disease.
marc [mɑ:rk] n unlöslicher Rückstand m, Satz m.
mar·ces·cin [mɑ:r'sesɪn] n Marzeszin nt, Marcescin f.
March [mɑ:rtʃ]: **M.'s disease** Basedow'-Krankheit f, Morbus Basedow m.
Marchand ['mɑ:rʃænd]: **M.'s cells** Adventitialzellen pl, Makrophagen pl der Gefäßwand.
Marchesani [mɑrtʃə'sɑ:nɪ]: **M.'s syndrome** Marchesani-Syndrom nt, Weill-Marchesani-Syndrom nt.
march foot/fracture [mɑ:rtʃ] Marschfraktur f, Deutschländer-Fraktur f.
march hemoglobinuria Marschhämoglobinurie f.
Marchi ['mɑ:rkɪ]: **M.'s phase** Marchi-Phase f, -Stadium nt.
M.'s reaction Marchi'-Reaktion f.
M.'s tract Löwenthal'-Bahn f, Tractus tectospinalis.
Marchiafava-Bignami [mɑ:rkɪə'fɑ:və bɪn'jɑ:mɪ]: **M.-B. disease/syndrome** Marchiafava-Bignami-Syndrom nt.
Marchiafava-Micheli [mɪ'kelɪ]: **M.-M. anemia/disease/syndrome** Marchiafava-Micheli-Anämie f, paroxysmale nächtliche Hämoglobinurie f abbr. **PNH**.
Marcus Gunn ['mɑ:rkəs gʌn]: **M. G. phenomenon** → M. G.'s sign 2.
M. G.'s sign 1. Gunn-Zeichen nt, Kreuzungsphänomen nt. **2.** Gunn-Zeichen nt, Kiefer-Lid-Phänomen nt.
M. G. syndrome → M. G.'s sign 2.
Marek ['mærɪk, 'mɑ:r-]: **M.'s (disease)** virus Marek-Virus nt.
Marey [mɑ'rɛ]: **M.'s law** Marey-Regel f, -Gesetz nt.
Marfan [mɑ:r'fæn; mɑr'fɑ̃]: **M.'s disease** Marfan-Syndrom nt, Arachnodaktylie-Syndrom nt.
M.'s sign Marfan-Zeichen nt.
M.'s syndrome → M.'s disease.
mar·fan·oid ['mɑ:rfænɔɪd] adj marfanoid.
marfanoid appearance marfanoide Erscheinung/Gestalt f.
mar·ga·rine ['mɑ:rdʒərɪn, -ri:n, 'mɑ:rdʒrɪn] n Margarine f.
mar·gar·i·to·ma [,mɑ:rgərɪ'təʊmə] n HNO Perlgeschwulst f, Cholesteatom nt.
Mar·gar·o·pus [mɑ:r'gærəpəs] n micro. Margaropus f.
mar·gin ['mɑ:rdʒɪn] n **1.** Rand m, Saum m, Kante f, anat. Margo m. **2.** Spielraum m. **3.** Grenze f.
m. of acetabulum Azetabularand, Limbus acetabuli, Margo acetabularis.
m. of oval fossa of heart Rand der Fossa ovalis, Limbus fossae ovalis.
m. of tongue Margo linguae.
m. of uterus Uterusrand, Margo uteri.
mar·gin·al ['mɑ:rdʒɪnl] adj **1.** marginal, randständig, wandständig, am Rand(e), Rand-. **2.** unwesentlich, geringfügig, nebensächlich, Grenz-.
marginal artery: left m. Ramus marginalis sinister.
right m. Ramus marginalis dexter.
marginal blepharitis ophthal. Triefauge nt, Lidrandentzündung f, Lippitudo f, Blepharitis ciliaris/marginalis.
marginal cells (von) Ebner'-Halbmond m, Giannuzzi'-Halbmond m, seröser Halbmond m, Heidenhain'-Halbmond m.
marginal cistern marginale Zisterne f, Randzisterne f.

marginal crest of tooth

marginal crest of tooth Randleiste *f* von Schneide- u. Eckzähnen, Crista marginalis.
marginal cyst (*Gelenk*) Randzyste *f*.
marginal emphysema (*Lunge*) Randemphysem *nt*.
marginal follicle Rindenfollikel *m*.
marginal gingiva Zahnfleischsaum *m*, Gingiva marginalis.
marginal gingivitis Gingivitis marginalis.
marginal gyrus (of Turner) Gyrus frontalis medialis.
marginal keratitis Randkeratitis *f*, Keratitis marginalis.
marginal layer *embryo.* Randschleier *m*, Marginalzone *f*.
marginal periodontitis Parodontitis marginalis, Alveolarpyorrhoe *f*.
marginal ridge Crista marginalis.
m. of tooth → marginal crest of tooth.
marginal sinus 1. Rand-, Marginalsinus *m*. **2.** Sinus marginalis.
marginal tract: crossed m. → Spitzka's m. Spitzka's m. Lissauer'-Randbündel *nt*, Tractus dorsolateralis.
marginal tubercle of zygomatic bone Tuberculum marginale (ossis zygomatici).
marginal ulcer *chir.* Stoma-, Randulkus *nt*.
marginal vein: lateral m. V. marginalis lateralis.
medial m. V. marginalis medialis.
right m. V. marginalis dextra.
marginal zone 1. Randzone *f*. **2.** Grenzzone *f*, -schicht *f*.
Lissauer's m. Lissauer'-Randbündel *nt*, Tractus dorsolateralis.
Spitzka's m. → Lissauer's m.
mar·gin·a·tion [ˌmɑːrdʒəˈneɪʃn] *n patho.* Margination *f*.
mar·gin·o·plas·ty [ˌmɑːrˈdʒɪnəplæstɪ] *n ophthal.* Lidrandplastik *f*.
ma·ri·a·hua·na [mærɪəˈ(h)wɑːnə] *n* → marihuana.
ma·ri·a·jua·na *n* → marihuana.
Marie [maˈri]: **M.'s ataxia** → M.'s disease 3.
M.'s disease 1. Marie-Krankheit *f*, -Syndrom *nt*, Akromegalie *f*. **2.** → Marie--Bamberger disease. **3.** Nonne-Marie--Krankheit *f*, -Syndrom *nt*, (Pierre) Marie-Krankheit *f*, -Syndrom *nt*, zerebellare Heredoataxie *f*, Heredoataxia cerbellaris. **4.** Bechterew-Krankheit *f*, Morbus Bechterew *m*, Bechterew--Strümpell-Marie-Krankheit *f*, Marie--Strümpell-Krankheit *f*, Spondylarthritis/Spondylitis ankylopoetica/ankylosans.
M.'s sclerosis → M.'s disease 3.
M.'s syndrome → Marie-Bamberger disease.
Marie-Bamberger [ˈbæmbərgər]: **M.-B. disease/syndrome** Marie-Bamberger--Syndrom *nt*, Bamberger-Marie-Syndrom *nt*, hypertrophische pulmonale Osteoarthropathie *f*, Akropachie *f*.
Marie-Foix [fwa]: **M.-F. sign** Marie-Foix--Reflex *m*.
Marie-Robinson [ˈrɒbɪnsən]: **M.-R. syndrome** Marie-Robinson-Syndrom *nt*.
Marie-Strümpell [ˈstrɪmpəl; ˈʃtrympəl]: **M.-S. disease** → Marie's disease 4.
M.-S. spondylitis/syndrome → Marie's disease 4.
mar·i·gua·na *n* → marihuana.
mar·i·hua·na [ˌmærɪəˈ(h)wɑːnə] *n* Marihuana *m*.
mar·i·jua·na *n* → marihuana.
Marinesco [mærɪˈneskəʊ]: **M.'s sign** → M.'s succulent hand.

M.'s succulent hand Tatzenhand *f*; Safthand *f*.
Marinesco-Garland [ˈɡɑːrlənd]: **M.-G. syndrome** → Marinesco-Sjögren syndrome.
Marinesco-Sjögren [ˈʃəʊɡrən]: **M.-S. syndrome** Marinesco-Sjögren-Syndrom *nt*.
Marion [ˈmærɪən; marˈjɔ̃]: **M.'s disease** Marion-Syndrom *nt*.
Mariotte [ˌmærɪˈɒt; marˈjɔt]: **M.'s law** Boyle-Mariotte'-Gesetz *nt*.
M.'s spot (*Auge*) blinder Fleck *m*.
mar·i·tal [ˈmærɪtl] *adj* ehelich, Ehe-, Gatten-.
marital counseling Eheberatung *f*.
mar·i·time climate [ˈmærɪtaɪm] Seeklima *nt*, maritimes Klima *nt*.
Marjolin [marʒɔˈlɛ̃]: **M.'s ulcer** Marjolin--Ulkus *nt*.
mark [mɑːrk] **I** *n* **1.** Mal *nt*, Fleck *m*, Nävus *m*. **2.** Markierung *f*, Bezeichnung *f*, Mal *nt*, Marke *f*. **3.** Strieme *f*, Schwiele *f*, Furche *f*, Narbe *f*. **4.** Kerbe *f*, Einschnitt *m*. **5.** (Schul-)Note *f*, Zensur *f*. **II** *vt* **6.** markieren, kennzeichnen, (be-)zeichnen. **7.** kennzeichnen, kennzeichnend sein für. **III** *vi* markieren.
mark·er [ˈmɑːrkər] *n* **1.** Kennzeichen *nt*, Markierung *f*. **2.** Marker *m*, Markersubstanz *f*, Markierungsgen *nt*.
mark·ing [ˈmɑːrkɪŋ] *n* Markierung *f*, Kennzeichnung *f*.
mar·mo·rat·ed [ˈmɑːrmərentɪd] *adj* (*Haut*) marmoriert.
mar·mo·ra·tion [ˌmɑːrməˈreɪʃn] *n* Marmorierung *f*.
mar·mo·re·al [mɑːrˈməʊrɪəl] *adj* marmorartig, Marmor-.
mar·mo·set [ˈmɑːrməset] *n zoo.* Krallenaffe *m*.
Maroteaux-Lamy [maroˈtoʊ laˈmi]: **M.-L. syndrome** Maroteaux-Lamy-Syndrom *nt*, Morbus Maroteaux-Lamy *m*, Mukopolysaccharidose VI *f abbr.* MPS VI.
mar·riage [ˈmærɪdʒ] *n* **1.** Heirat *f*, Vermählung *f*, Hochzeit *f*. **2.** Ehe *f*.
mar·ried life [ˈmærɪd] Eheleben *nt*.
mar·row [ˈmærəʊ] *n* **1.** anat. Mark *nt*, Medulla *f*. **2.** anat. Knochenmark *nt*, Medulla ossium. **3.** *fig.* Mark *nt*, Kern *m*.
marrow abscess Knochenmark(s)abszeß *m*.
mar·row·brain [ˈmærəʊbreɪn] *n* → myelencephalon 1.
marrow canal 1. (Knochen-)Markhöhle *f*. **2.** Zahnwurzelkanal *m*, Canalis radicis dentis.
marrow cavity Markhöhle *f*, Cavitas medullaris.
primary m. *embryo.* primäre Markhöhle.
secondary m. *embryo.* sekundäre Markhöhle.
marrow cell (hämopoetische) Knochenmark(s)zelle *f*.
marrow nail *ortho.* Marknagel *m*.
marrow nailing *ortho.* Marknagelung *f*.
blind m. gedeckte Marknagelung.
marrow necrosis Knochenmark(s)nekrose *f*.
marrow space → marrow cavity.
Mar·seilles fever [marˈsɛj] Boutonneusefieber *nt*, Fièvre boutonneuse.
Marsh [mɑːrʃ]: **M.'s disease** Basedow'--Krankheit *f*, Morbus Basedow *m*.
Marshall [ˈmɑːrʃl]: **M.'s fold** → M.'s vestigial fold.
M.'s oblique vein Marshall'-Vene *f*, V. obliqua atrii sinistri.
vestigial fold of M. → M.'s vestigial fold.
M.'s vestigial fold Marshall-Falte *f*, Plica venae cavae sinistrae.
Marshall-Marchetti-Krantz [marˈketɪ

kræntz]: **M.-M.-K. operation** *gyn.* Marshall-Marchetti-Krantz-Operation *f*.
marsh fever [mɑːrʃ] **1.** Sumpf-, Wechselfieber *nt*, Malaria *f*. **2.** Feld-, Ernte-, Schlamm-, Sumpffieber *nt*, Erbsenpflückerkrankheit *f*, Leptospirosis grippotyphosa.
marsh gas → methane.
mar·su·pi·al [mɑːrˈsuːpɪəl] **I** *n zoo.* Beuteltier *nt*. **II** *adj* **1.** Beuteltier betr., Beuteltier-. **2.** beutelartig, Beutel-.
Mar·su·pi·a·lia [mɑːrˌsuːpɪˈeɪlɪə] *pl zoo.* Beuteltiere *pl*, Marsupialier *pl*, Didelphier *pl*.
mar·su·pi·al·i·za·tion [mɑːrˌsuːpɪəlaɪˈzeɪʃn] *n chir.* Marsupialisation *f*.
marsupial pouch → marsupium.
mar·su·pi·um [mɑːrˈsuːpɪəm] *n, pl -pia* [-pɪə] **1.** Hodensack *m*, Skrotum *nt*, Scrotum *nt*. **2.** *bio.* Brutbeutel *m*, Marsupium *nt*.
mar·tial [ˈmɑːrʃl] *adj* eisenhaltig, Eisen-.
Martin-Lester [ˈmɑːrtn ˈlestər]: **M.-L. agar/medium** Martin-Lester-Agar *m/nt*, -Medium *nt*.
Martin-Lewis [ˈluːɪs]: **M.-L. agar/medium** Martin-Lewis-Agar *m/nt*, -Medium *nt*.
Martinotti [martiˈnɔti]: **M.'s cells** Martinotti-Zellen *pl*.
Martorell [martɔˈrel]: **M.'s syndrome** Martorell-Krankheit *f*, -Syndrom *nt*, Takayasu-Krankheit *f*, -Syndrom *nt*, Pulslos-Krankheit *f*, pulseless disease (*nt*).
mas·cu·line [ˈmæskjʊlɪn] **I** *n* Mann *m*. **II** *adj* **1.** Mann betr., männlich, Männer-. **2.** männlich, mannhaft, maskulin; vital, robust; kräftig, stark.
masculine pelvis männliches/viriles Becken *nt*.
mas·cu·lin·i·ty [ˌmæskjəˈlɪnətɪ] *n* Männlichkeit *f*, Mannhaftigkeit *f*; Vitalität *f*, Robustheit *f*.
mas·cu·lin·i·za·tion [ˌmæskjəlɪnəɪˈzeɪʃn] *n* Vermännlichung *f*, Maskulinisierung *f*, Maskulinierung *f*, Virilisierung *f*.
mas·cu·lin·ize [ˈmæskjəlɪnaɪz] *vt* männlich machen, vermännlichen, maskulinisieren.
ma·ser [ˈmeɪzər] *abbr.* [microwave amplification by stimulated emission of radiation] Maser *m*.
mask [mæsk, mɑːsk] **I** *n* **1.** (Schutz-, Gesichts-)Maske *f*. **2.** Gasmaske *f*. **3.** Maske *f*, maskenhaftes Gesicht *nt*. **4.** *phys.* (Abdeck-)Blende *f*, Maske *f*. **II** *vt* **5.** jdn. maskieren, verkleiden. **6.** verschleiern, verhüllen, verdecken, verbergen, maskieren. **III** *vi* eine Maske tragen.
m. of pregnancy Melasma *nt*, Chloasma *nt*.
masked [mæskt, mɑːskt] *adj* **1.** verdeckt, verborgen, maskiert. **2.** verborgen, larviert.
masked gout latente Gicht *f*.
mask-like face [ˈmæsklaɪk, mɑːsk] *patho., neuro.* Maskengesicht *nt*.
mas·och·ism [ˈmæsəkɪzəm] *n psychia.* Masochismus *m*, Passivismus *m*.
mas·och·ist [ˈmæsəkɪst] *n psychia.* Masochist(in *f*) *m*.
mas·och·is·tic [ˌmæsəˈkɪstɪk] *adj* Masochismus betr., masochistisch.
mass [mæs] **I** *n* **1.** (a. *socio.*) Masse *f*, große Menge *f*, Anhäufung *f*, Ansammlung *f*. **2.** Stoff *m*, Substanz *f*; (Isolier-, Knet-)Masse *f*. **3.** *phys.* Masse *f*; *mathe.* Volumen *nt*, Inhalt *m*. **II** *adj* Massen-. **III** *vt* (an-)häufen, (an-)sammeln, zusammenballen, -ziehen. **IV** *vi s.* (an-)häufen, (an-)sammeln, s. zusammenballen.

mas·sa ['mæsə] *n, pl* **-sae** [-iː] Masse *f*, Massa *f*.
mass-action constant Massenwirkungskonstante *f*.
mas·sage [məˈsɑːʒ, -ˈsɑːdʒ] **I** *n* Massage *f*, Massieren *nt*. **II** *vt* massieren.
mas·sag·er [məˈsɑːʒər, -ˈsɑːdʒər] *n* → masseur.
mass concentration Massenkonzentration *f*.
mas·se·ter [mæˈsiːtər] *n* → masseter muscle.
mas·se·ter·ic [ˌmæsəˈterɪk] *adj* M. masseter betr., Masseter-.
masseteric artery A. masseterica.
masseteric fascia Fascia masseterica.
masseteric nerve N. massetericus.
masseteric tuberosity Tuberositas masseterica.
masseteric veins Vv. massetericae.
masseter muscle Kaumuskel *m*, Masseter *m*, M. masseter.
masseter reflex Masseter-, Unterkieferreflex *m*.
mas·seur [məˈsɜr; maˈsœːr] *n* **1.** Masseur *m*. **2.** Massagegerät *nt*.
mas·seuse [məˈsuːs, -ˈsɜrs; maˈsøːz] *n* Masseurin *f*, Masseuse *f*.
mass flexor reflex *neuro.* Flexormassenreflex *m*.
mass gradient Massengradient *m*.
Masshoff ['mæsʰɒf]: **M.'s lymphadenitis** Masshoff'-Lymphadenitis *f*, Lymphadenitis mesenterialis acuta.
mas·si·cot ['mæsɪkɒt] *n* Bleioxid *nt*.
mas·sive ['mæsɪf] *adj* **1.** massiv; massig; gewaltig, heftig. **2.** stark, anhaltend.
massive bleeding massive Blutung *f*, Massenblutung *f*.
massive coagulation Froin-Symptom *nt*.
massive hemorrhage → massive bleeding.
massive osteolysis Gorham-Erkrankung *f*, Gorham-Staut-Erkrankung *f*.
massive pneumonia massive Pneumonie *f*.
mass law Massenwirkungsgesetz *nt*.
mass movement Holzknecht'-Massenbewegung *f*.
mass number *abbr.* **A** *phys.* Massenzahl *f* *abbr.* A.
mass peristalsis Holzknecht'-Massenbewegung *f*.
Masson ['mæsən; maˈsɔ̃ː]: **M. stain** Masson-Färbung *f*.
Masson-Goldner [ˈɡoʊldnər]: **M.-G. stain** Masson-Goldner-Färbung *f*.
mass prolapse *ortho.* (*Bandscheiben*) Massenprolaps *m*.
mass reflex Massenreflex *m*.
mass spectrograph → mass spectrometer.
mass spectrometer Massenspektrometer *nt*.
mass unit Masseneinheit *f*.
 atomic m. *abbr.* **amu** Atommasseneinheit *f* *abbr.* AME.
mast- *pref.* → masto-.
mas·tad·e·ni·tis [ˌmæstædɪˈnaɪtɪs] *n* → mastitis.
mas·tad·e·no·ma [ˌmæstædɪˈnoʊmə] *n* Brust(drüsen)adenom *nt*.
Mast·ad·e·no·vi·rus [ˌmæstædnoʊˈvaɪrəs] *n* Mastadenovirus *nt*.
mas·tal·gia [mæsˈtældʒ(i)ə] *n* schmerzhafte Brustdrüse *f*, Mastalgie *f*, Mastodynie *f*.
mas·ta·tro·phia [mæstəˈtroʊfiə] *n* → mastatrophy.
mas·tat·ro·phy [mæsˈtætrəfi] *n* Brustdrüsenatrophie *f*, Mastatrophie *f*.

mas·tauxe [mæsˈtɔːksi] *n* Brustvergrößerung *f*, -hypertrophie *f*.
mast cell [mæst] Mastzelle *f*, Mastozyt *m*.
 blood m. Blutmastzelle, basophiler Granulozyt.
 tissue m. Gewebsmastzelle.
mast cell growth factor *abbr.* **MCGF** Interleukin-3 *nt abbr.* IL-3.
mast cell leukemia Basophilenleukämie *f*, Blutmastzell-Leukämie *f*.
mast cell tumor → mastocytoma.
mas·tec·to·my [mæsˈtektəmi] *n* Brust(drüsen)entfernung *f*, Mammaamputation *f*, Mastektomie *f*.
Master ['mæstər]: **M.'s (two-step exercise) test card.** Master-Test *m*, Zweistufentest *m*.
mas·ti·ca·ble ['mæstɪkəbl] *adj* kaubar.
mas·ti·cate ['mæstɪkeɪt] *vt* (zer-)kauen; zerkleinern.
mas·ti·ca·tion [ˌmæstɪˈkeɪʃn] *n* (Zer-)Kauen *nt*, Kauvorgang *m*, -funktion *f*, Mastikation *f*.
mas·ti·ca·to·ry ['mæstɪkətɔːri, -toʊ-, -təri] **I** *n pharm.* Kaumittel *nt*, Mastikatorium *nt*. **II** *adj* Kauen *a*. Kauapparat betr., mastikatorisch, Kau-.
masticatory apparatus Kauapparat *m*.
masticatory diplegia *neuro.* Diplegia masticatoria.
masticatory muscles Kaumuskeln *pl*, -muskulatur *f*, Mm. masticatorii.
masticatory paralysis Lähmung *f* der Kaumuskulatur.
masticatory spasm Kaumuskelkrampf *m*.
masticatory surface (*Zahn*) Kaufläche *f*, Facies occlusalis/masticatoria (dentis).
masticatory system → masticatory apparatus.
Mas·ti·goph·o·ra [ˌmæstɪˈɡɒf(ə)rə] *pl bio.* Geißelinfusorien *pl*, -tierchen *pl*, Flagellaten *pl*, Flagellata *pl*, Mastigophoren *pl*, Mastigophora *pl*.
mas·ti·goph·o·ran [ˌ-ˈɡɒf(ə)rən] *n bio.* Geißeltierchen *nt*, Flagellat *m*.
mas·ti·goph·o·rous [ˌ-ˈɡɒf(ə)rəs] *adj* Mastigophora betr.
mas·ti·gote ['-ɡoʊt] *n* → mastigophoran.
mas·ti·tis [mæsˈtaɪtɪs] *n gyn.* Brust(drüsen)entzündung *f*, Mastitis *f*, Mastadenitis *f*.
mastitis neonatorum Neugeborenenmastitis *f*, Mastitis neonatorum.
masto- *pref.* Brust-, Brustdrüsen-, Mast(o)-, Mamm(o)-.
mas·to·car·ci·no·ma [ˌmæstoʊˌkɑːrsəˈnoʊmə] *n* → mammary carcinoma.
mas·toc·cip·i·tal [mæstəkˈsɪpɪtl] *adj* → masto-occipital.
mas·to·chon·dro·ma [ˌmæstoʊkɒnˈdroʊmə] *n* Brust(drüsen)chondrom *nt*.
mas·to·cyte ['-saɪt] *n* → mast cell.
mas·to·cy·to·ma [ˌ-saɪˈtoʊmə] *n* Mastzelltumor *m*, Mastozytom *nt*.
mas·to·cy·to·sis [ˌ-saɪˈtoʊsɪs] *n* Mastozytose *f*.
mastocytosis syndrome Mastozytose-Syndrom *nt*.
mas·to·dyn·ia [ˌ-ˈdiːniə] *n* → mastalgia.
mas·to·gram ['-ɡræm] *n* → mammogram.
mas·tog·ra·phy [mæsˈtɒɡrəfi] *n* → mammography.
mas·toid ['mæstɔɪd] **I** *n* Warzenfortsatz *m*, Mastoid *nt*, Proc. mastoideus (ossis temporalis). **II** *adj* **1.** brust(warzen)förmig, warzenähnlich. **2.** Mastoid/Warzenfortsatz betr., mastoid.
mastoid abscess Mastoidabszeß *m*, Abszeß *m* der Warzenfortsatzzellen.
mastoid air cells Warzenfortsatzzellen *pl*, Cellulae mastoideae.
mas·toi·dal [mæsˈtɔɪdl] *adj* → mastoid 2.

mas·toid·al·gia [ˌmæstɔɪˈdældʒ(i)ə] *n* Schmerzen *pl* über dem Proc. mastoideus, Mastoidalgie *f*.
mastoid angle Angulus mastoideus.
mastoid antrum → mastoid cavity.
mastoid arteries Rami mastoidei a. auricularis posterioris.
mastoid bone → mastoid I.
mastoid branch: m. of occipital artery Ramus mastoideus a. occipitalis.
 m.es of posterior auricular artery → mastoid arteries.
mastoid canaliculus Canaliculus mastoideus.
mastoid cavity Warzenfortsatzhöhle *f*, Antrum mastoideum.
mastoid cells → mastoid air cells.
mas·toi·dea [mæsˈtɔɪdiə] *n* → mastoid I.
mas·toid·ec·to·my [ˌmæstɔɪˈdektəmi] *n* *HNO* Mastoidektomie *f*.
mastoid empyema → mastoiditis.
mas·toi·de·um [mæsˈtɔɪdiəm] *n* → mastoid I.
mastoid fontanelle hintere Seitenfontanelle *f*, Warzenfontanelle *f*, Fonticulus mastoideus/posterolateralis.
mastoid foramen For. mastoideum.
mastoid fossa Foveola suprameatica/suprameatalis.
mastoid incisure of temporal bone Inc. mastoidea (ossis temporalis).
mas·toid·i·tis [ˌmæstɔɪˈdaɪtɪs] *n* *HNO* Mastoiditis *f*.
mastoid margin of occipital bone Margo mastoideus (squamae occipitalis).
mastoid notch Inc. mastoidea (ossis temporalis).
mastoid operation → mastoidectomy.
mas·toid·ot·o·my [ˌmæstɔɪˈdɒtəmi] *n* *HNO* Mastoidotomie *f*.
mastoid process → mastoid I.
mastoid segment of facial nerve mastoidales Segment *nt* des N. facialis.
mastoid sinuses → mastoid air cells.
mastoid wall of tympanic cavity Hinterwand *f* der Paukenhöhle, Paries mastoideus (cavitatis tympanicae), Adnexa mastoidea.
mas·to·me·nia [ˌmæstəˈmiːniə] *n gyn.* Mastomenie *f*.
mas·ton·cus [mæsˈtɒŋkəs] *n gyn.* Brust(drüsen)schwellung *f*, -tumor *m*.
mas·to-oc·cip·i·tal *adj* masto-okzipital.
mas·to·pa·ri·e·tal [ˌmæstoʊpəˈraɪtl] *adj* mastoparietal.
mas·to·path·ia [ˌ-ˈpæθiə] *n* → mastopathy.
mas·top·a·thy [mæsˈtɒpəθi] *n gyn.* Brustdrüsenerkrankung *f*, Mastopathie *f*, -pathia *f*.
mas·to·pex·y ['mæstəpeksi] *n gyn.* Mastopexie *f*.
mas·to·plas·ia [ˌ-ˈpleɪʒ(i)ə, -ziə] *n* → mammoplasia.
mas·to·plas·ty ['-plæsti] *n* → mammaplasty.
mas·top·to·sis [ˌmæstə(p)ˈtoʊsɪs] *n* Hängebrust *f*, Mastoptose *f*, Mamma pendulans.
mas·tor·rha·gia [ˌmæstəˈrædʒ(i)ə] *n* blutende Mamma *f*, Mastorrhagie *f*.
mas·to·scir·rhus [ˌ-'s(k)ɪrəs] *n* → mammary carcinoma, scirrhous.
mas·to·squa·mous [ˌ-ˈskweɪməs] *adj* mastosquamös.
mas·tos·to·my [mæsˈtɒstəmi] *n gyn.* Mastostomie *f*.
mas·to·syr·inx [ˌmæstəˈsɪrɪŋks] *n* Brustdrüsenfistel *f*.
mas·tot·o·my [mæsˈtɒtəmi] *n gyn.* Brustdrüsenschnitt *m*, Mastotomie *f*.
mas·tur·bate [ˈmæstərbeɪt] *vt* masturbieren, onanieren.

mas·tur·ba·tion [mæstər'beɪʃn] n Masturbation f, Onanie f.
Masugi [mɑ'suːgɪ]: **M.'s nephritis** Masugi-Nephritis f, nephrotoxische Serumnephritis f.
Matas ['mætæs]: **M.' test** Matas-Moskowicz-Test m.
mat burn [mæt] Verbrennung f durch Reibung(shitze).
match¹ [mætʃ] **I** n **1.** Gegenstück nt, passende Sache od. Person f; (zusammenpassendes) Paar nt, Gespann nt. **2.** Heirat f. **II** vt **3.** bio. paaren. **4.** jdn. od. etw. vergleichen (with mit). **5.** passend machen, anpassen (to, with an). **6.** entsprechen, passen zu. **7.** phys. angleichen, anpassen. **III** vi zusammenpassen, übereinstimmen (with mit); entsprechen (to).
match² [mætʃ] n Zünd-, Streichholz m.
match·ing ['mætʃɪŋ] **I** n Anpassung f, Anpassen nt, Matching nt. **II** adj (dazu) passend.
mate [meɪt] **I** n **1.** Lebensgefährte m, -gefährtin f, Gatte m, Gattin f. **2.** zoo. Männchen nt, Weibchen nt, Geschlechts-, Paarungs-, Fortpflanzungspartner m. **II** vt zoo. paaren. **III** vi zoo. s. paaren.
ma·te·ri·al [mə'tɪərɪəl] **I** n **1.** Material nt, (Roh-, Grund-)Stoff m, (Roh-, Grund-)Substanz f; techn. Werkstoff m. **2.** fig. Material nt, Stoff m (for zu). **II** adj materiell, physisch, körperlich; stofflich, Material-.
material defect Materialfehler m.
material fatigue Materialermüdung f.
material test(ing) Materialprüfung f.
ma·te·ria med·i·ca [mə'tɪərɪə 'medɪkə] pharm. **1.** Arzneimittel pl. **2.** Pharmakologie f, Arzneimittellehre f, -forschung f.
ma·ter·nal [mə'tɜrnl] adj **1.** Mutter/Mater betr., mütterlich, maternal, Mutter-. **2.** mütterlicherseits.
maternal antibodies mütterliche/maternale Antikörper pl.
maternal circulation embryo. mütterlicher/maternaler Kreislauf m.
maternal component of placenta → maternal placenta.
maternal deprivation syndrome ped. Deprivationssyndrom nt.
maternal instinct psycho. Mutterinstinkt m.
maternal phenylketonuria maternale Phenylketonurie f.
maternal placenta maternale Plazenta f, mütterlicher Teil m der Plazenta, Pars uterina/materna placentae.
ma·ter·ni·ty [mə'tɜrnətɪ] **I** n **1.** Mutterschaft f, Maternität f; Mütterlichkeit f. **2.** Entbindungsstation f, -klinik f. **II** adj Schwangerschafts-, Umstands-, Wöchnerin(nen)-.
maternity allowance Mutterschaftsgeld nt, -beihilfe f.
maternity benefit → maternity allowance.
maternity care Schwangeren-, Schwangerschaftsbetreuung f.
maternity dress Umstandskleid nt.
maternity home → maternity hospital.
maternity hospital Entbindungsklinik f, -heim nt.
maternity leave Mutterschaftsurlaub m.
maternity ward Entbindungsstation f.
mat·ing ['meɪtɪŋ] n bio. Paarung f.
ma·tri·ar·chal [ˌmeɪtrɪ'ɑːrkl] adj Matriarchat betr., matriarchal, matriarchalisch.
ma·tri·ar·chal·ism [ˌ-'ɑːrkəlɪzəm] n matriarchalisches System nt.
ma·tri·ar·chate ['-ɑːrkɪt, -keɪt] n Matriarchat nt.
ma·tri·ar·chic [ˌ-'ɑːrkɪk] adj → matriarchal.

ma·tri·ar·chy ['-ɑːrkɪ] n → matriarchate.
mat·ri·cal ['mætrɪkəl] adj Matrix betr., Matrix-.
ma·tri·ci·al [mæ'trɪʃl] adj matrikal.
mat·ri·cli·nous [ˌmætrɪ'klaɪnəs, ˌmeɪ-] adj → matroclinous.
ma·tric·u·late [n mə'trɪkjəlɪt; v -leɪt] **I** n Immatrikulierte(r m) f. **II** vt immatrikulieren, einschreiben. **III** vi s. immatrikulieren, s. einschreiben.
ma·tric·u·la·tion [məˌtrɪkjə'leɪʃn] n Einschreibung f, Immatrikulation f.
mat·ri·lin·e·al [ˌmætrɪ'lɪnɪəl] adj genet. durch die mütterliche Linie vererbt.
mat·ri·mo·ni·al [ˌmætrɪ'məʊnɪəl] adj Ehe betr., ehelich, matrimoniell, Ehe-.
mat·ri·mo·ny ['mætrɪməʊnɪ] n Ehe(stand m) f.
ma·trix ['meɪtrɪks, 'mæ-] n, pl **ma·trix·es, ma·tri·ces** [-trɪsiːz] **1.** (a. anat., physiol.) Nähr-, Grundsubstanz f, Grundgewebe f, Matrix f; Mutterboden m; Grund-, Ausgangsgewebe nt, Matrix f. **2.** Vorlage f, Modell nt, Matrize f. **3.** bot. Nährboden m.
matrix calculus urol. Matrixstein m.
matrix cell Matrixzelle f.
matrix protein Matrixprotein nt.
mat·ro·cli·nous [ˌmætrə'klaɪnəs] adj matroklin.
mat·ro·cli·ny ['mætrəklaɪnɪ, 'meɪ-] n Matroklinie f.
mat·ter ['mætər] **I** n **1.** Material nt, Substanz f, Stoff m, Materie f. **2.** anat., physiol. Substanz f. **3.** patho. Eiter m. **4.** Angelegenheit f, Sache f. **II** vi patho. eitern.
mat·tress ['mætrɪs] n Matratze f.
mattress suture chir. Matratzennaht f.
horizontal m. horizontale Matratzennaht.
vertical m. vertikale Matratzennaht.
mat·u·rate ['mætʃəreɪt] vi **1.** (a. fig.) reifen. **2.** (Abszeß) reifen; zur Eiterung bringen.
mat·u·rate·ness ['-nɪs] n → maturity.
mat·u·ra·tion [ˌmætʃə'reɪʃn] n **1.** (Heran-)Reifen nt, Reifung f; micro. Maturation f; fig. Entwicklung f. **2.** bio. (Zell-)Reifung f. **3.** (Abszeß) (Aus-)Reifung f.
m. of follicle Follikelreifung.
m. of ovum Eireifung f, Oogenie f, Ovo-, Oogenese f.
maturation division **1.** Reifeteilung f. **2.** Reduktion(steilung f) f, Meiose f.
maturation factor Zyano-, Cyanocobalamin nt, Vitamin B₁₂ nt.
maturation phase embryo. Reifungsphase f, -periode f.
maturation process Reifungs-, Maturationsprozeß m.
ma·tur·a·tive [mə'tʃʊərətɪv, 'mætʃəreɪ-] **I** n Eiterung-förderndes Mittel m. **II** adj **1.** die Eiterung fördernd, zur Eiterung bringend. **2.** Reifung(sprozeß) fördernd, zur Reife bringen.
ma·ture [mə't(j)ʊər, -'tʃʊər] **I** adj **1.** reif, (aus-)gereift, vollentwickelt, ausgewachsen. **2.** (Person) reif, vernünftig. **II** vt (aus-)reifen lassen; reif werden lassen; reifer machen. **III** vi (aus-)reifen, reif werden; heranreifen.
mature bacteriophage reifer Phage m.
mature cataract reifer Star m, Cataracta matura.
mature cell leukemia chronische myeloische Leukämie f abbr. CML, chronische granulozytäre Leukämie f, chronische Myelose f.
ma·tured [mə't(j)ʊərd, -'tʃʊərd] adj (aus-)gereift, reif.
mature infant Reifgeborenes nt, reifer Säugling m.
mature phage reifer Phage m.

mature teratoma **1.** reifes/adultes Teratom nt, Dermoidzyste f. **2.** Dermoidzyste f des Ovars, zystisches Teratom nt, Teratoma coaetaneum.
ma·tu·ri·ty [mə't(j)ʊərətɪ, -'t(j)ʊər-] n (a. fig.) Reife f, Ausgereiftheit f, Maturität f.
maturity-onset diabetes nicht-insulinabhängiger Diabetes mellitus m, Typ-II--Diabetes mellitus m, non-insulin-dependent diabetes (mellitus) abbr. NIDD(M).
m. of youth abbr. **MODY** Typ-II-Diabetes mellitus bei Jugendlichen, maturity-onset diabetes of youth abbr. MODY.
ma·tu·ti·nal [mə't(j)uːtnl] adj morgendlich, Morgen-.
Mauchart ['maʊkɑːrt; -çɑrt]: **M.'s ligaments** Flügelbänder pl, Ligg. alaria.
Maunoir [moʊ'nwɑː]: **M.'s hydrocele** Hydrocele colli.
Maurer ['maʊrər]: **M.'s clefts** → **M.'s dots**.
M.'s dots hema. Maurer-Körnelung f, -Tüpfelung f.
M.'s spots/stippling → **M.'s dots**.
Mauriac [mɔːrɪ'ak]: **M. syndrome** Mauriac-Syndrom nt.
Mauthner ['maʊtnər]: **M.'s sheath** Axolemm nt.
M.'s test ophthal. Mauthner-Test m.
maw worm [mɔː] micro. Spulwurm m, Askaris f, Ascaris f.
max·il·la [mæk'sɪlə] n, pl **-lae** [-liː] Oberkiefer(knochen m) m, Maxilla f.
max·il·lar·y ['mæksəˌlerɪ; mæk'sɪlərɪ] **I** n → maxilla. **II** adj (Ober-)Kiefer/Maxilla betr., maxillär, maxillar, (Ober-)Kiefer-.
maxillary antrum Kieferhöhle f, Sinus maxillaris.
maxillary arch Oberkieferzahnreihe f, maxilläre Zahnreihe f, Arcus dentalis superior.
maxillary artery Oberkieferschlagader f, Maxillaris f, A. maxillaris.
internal m. → maxillary artery.
external m. old → facial artery 1.
maxillary articulation → mandibular articulation.
maxillary bone → maxilla.
inferior m. old → mandible.
superior m. old → maxilla.
maxillary division of trigeminal nerve → maxillary nerve.
maxillary hiatus Hiatus maxillaris.
maxillary hypoplasia embryo. kongenitale Kleinheit f des Oberkiefers.
maxillary joint → mandibular articulation.
maxillary ligament: lateral m. Lig. laterale (artic. temporomandibularis).
middle m. Lig. sphenomandibulare.
maxillary nerve zweiter Trigeminusast m, Maxillaris m, N. maxillaris.
maxillary process (of inferior nasal concha) Proc. maxillaris (conchae nasalis inferioris).
maxillary prominences embryo. Oberkieferwülste pl.
maxillary sinus (Ober-)Kieferhöhle f, Sinus maxillaris.
bony/osseous m. Sinus maxillaris osseus.
maxillary sinus cannula HNO Kieferhöhlenspülkanüle f.
maxillary sinusitis Kieferhöhlenentzündung f, Sinusitis maxillaris.
maxillary teeth Zähne pl od. Zahnreihe f des Oberkiefers.
maxillary tuber Tuber maxillare, Eminentia maxillaris.
maxillary veins Oberkiefervenen pl, Vv. maxillares.
max·il·lec·to·my [mæksɪ'lektəmɪ] n HNO Oberkieferresektion f, Maxillektomie f.

max·il·li·tis [mæksɪ'laɪtɪs] *n* Oberkieferentzündung *f*, Maxillitis *f*.
max·il·lo·fa·cial [mæk,sɪlǝʊ'feɪʃl] *adj* Kiefer u. Gesichtsknochen betr., die untere Gesichtshälfte betr., maxillofazial.
maxillofacial surgery Gesichts- u. Kieferchirurgie *f*.
max·il·lo·ju·gal [,-'dʒuːgl] *adj* Oberkiefer u. Wange betr., maxillojugal.
max·il·lo·la·bi·al [,-'leɪbɪǝl] *adj* Oberkiefer u. Lippe betr., maxillolabial.
max·il·lo·man·dib·u·lar [,-mæn'dɪbjǝlǝr] *adj* Oberkiefer u. Unterkiefer betr., maxillomandibulär.
max·il·lo·pal·a·tine [,-'pælǝtaɪn] *adj* Oberkiefer u. Gaumen betr., maxillopalatinal.
max·il·lo·pha·ryn·ge·al [,-fǝ'rɪndʒ(ɪ)ǝl] *adj* Oberkiefer u. Rachen betr., maxillopharyngeal.
max·il·lot·o·my [mæksɪ'lɑtǝmɪ] *n HNO* Maxillotomie *f*.
max·il·lo·tur·bi·nal bone [mæk,sɪlǝʊ'tɜrbɪnl] untere Nasenmuschel *f*, Concha nasalis inferior.
max·i·mal ['mæksɪmǝl] *adj* → maximum 1.
maximal acid output *abbr.* **MAO** *physiol.* (*Magen*) maximale Säuresekretion *f*, maximal acid output *abbr.* MAO.
maximal allowance concentration *abbr.* **MAC** maximal zulässige Konzentration *f abbr.* MZK.
maximal breathing capacity *abbr.* **MBC** *physiol.* Atemgrenzwert *m abbr.* AGW.
maximal discrimination *HNO* (*Gehör*) maximale Verständlichkeit/Diskrimination *f*.
maximal performance capacity Höchstleistungsfähigkeit *f*.
maximal permissible dose *abbr.* **M.P.D.** *radiol.* Maximaldosis *f*.
maximal possible rate of shortening *physiol.* maximale Verkürzungsgeschwindigkeit *f*.
maximal rate of pressure increase *physiol.* maximale Druckanstiegsgeschwindigkeit *f*.
maximal rate of shortening → maximal possible rate of shortening.
maximal work place concentration *abbr.* **MWC** *physiol.* maximale Arbeitsplatzkonzentration *f abbr.* MAK.
max·i·mize ['mæksɪmaɪz] *vt* den Höchstwert anstreben, bis zum Höchstmaß steigern, maximieren, maximalisieren.
max·i·mum ['mæksɪmǝm] **I** *n*, *pl* **-mums**, **-ma** [-mǝ] Maximalwert *m*, -grenze *f*, -maß *nt*, -stand *m*, Höchstwert *m*, -grenze *f*, -maß *nt*, -stand *m*, Maximum *nt*; *mathe.* oberer Grenzwert *m*. **II** *adj* 1. maximal, größte(r, s), Höchst-, Maximal-. 2. höchstzulässig, maximal.
maximum and minimum thermometer Maximum-Minimum-Thermometer *nt*.
maximum dose *pharm.* Maximaldosis *f abbr.* MD, Dosis maximalis.
maximum load Höchst-, Maximalbelastung *f*.
maximum performance Höchst-, Spitzenleistung *f*.
maximum thermometer Maximumthermometer *nt*.
maximum velocity Höchst-, Maximalgeschwindigkeit *f*.
maximum voltage *electr.* Maximalspannung *f*.
maximum voluntary ventilation *abbr.* **MVV** → maximal breathing capacity.
max·well [mækswel, -wǝl] *n* Maxwell *nt*.
Mayaro [meɪ'jɑːrǝʊ]: **M. virus** Mayaro-Virus *nt*.
Maydl ['meɪdl]: **M.'s operation** *urol.* Maydl-Operation *f*.

Mayer ['maɪǝr, 'meɪǝr]: **M.'s ligament** Lig. carpi radiatum.
radiate ligament of M. → M.'s ligament.
M.'s reflex Mayer-Reflex *m*, Daumenmitbewegungsphänomen *nt*.
M.'s view *radiol., HNO* Aufnahme *f* nach Mayer.
M.'s waves *physiol.* Mayer-Wellen *pl*, Blutdruckschwankungen III. Ordnung.
Mayer-Rokitansky-Küster-Hauser [rɑkɪ'tænskɪ 'kɪstǝr 'haʊsǝr; 'kystǝr]: **M.-R.-K.-H. syndrome** MRK-Syndrom *nt*, Mayer-Rokitansky-Küster-Syndrom *nt*, Rokitansky-Küster-Syndrom *nt*.
May-Grünwald [meɪ 'griːnvɑlt; 'gryːnvalt]: **M.-G.'s stain** May-Grünwald-Färbung *f*.
May-Grünwald-Giemsa ['giːmzǝ]: **M.-G.-G. stain** May-Grünwald-Giemsa-Färbung *f*.
May-Hegglin ['heglɪn]: **M.-H. anomaly** *hema.* May-Hegglin-Anomalie *f*, Hegglin-Syndrom *nt*.
Maylard ['meɪlɑːrd]: **M. incision** *gyn.* Maylard-Schnitt *m*.
Mayo ['meɪǝʊ]: **M.'s operation** 1. Mayo-Operation *f*, -Magenresektion *f*. 2. Mayo-Operation *f*, -Hernienoperation *f*. 3. Mayo-Operation *f*, -Venenexhärese *f*.
M.'s vein Pylorusvene *f*, V. pr(a)epylorica.
Mayo-Robson ['rǝʊbsǝn]: **M.-R. point** Mayo-Robson-Punkt *m*.
M.-R.'s position Mayo-Robson-Lagerung *f*.
maz- *pref.* → masto-.
maze [meɪz] *n* Irrgarten *m*, Labyrinth *nt*.
ma·zin·dol ['meɪzɪndǝʊl] *n pharm.* Mazindol *nt*.
mazo- *pref.* → masto-.
ma·zo·dyn·ia [,meɪzǝʊ'diːnɪǝ] *n* → mastalgia.
ma·zol·y·sis [meɪ'zɑlǝsɪs] *n gyn.* Plazentalösung *f*.
ma·zo·path·ia [,meɪzǝʊ'pæθɪǝ] *n* → mastopathy.
ma·zop·a·thy [meɪ'zɑpǝθɪ] *n* → mastopathy.
ma·zo·pex·y [meɪzǝʊpeksɪ] *n* → mastopexy.
Mazzoni [mæd'zǝʊnɪ]: **M.'s corpuscles** Mazzoni'-Lamellenkörperchen *pl*.
Mb *abbr.* → myoglobin.
mb *abbr.* → millibar.
M band M-Streifen *m*, M-Linie *f*, Mittelstreifen *m*, Mesophragma *nt*.
mbar *abbr.* → millibar.
MBC *abbr.* 1. → maximal breathing capacity. 2. → minimal bactericidal concentration.
MBq *abbr.* → megabecquerel.
MC *abbr.* → motor cortex.
mC *abbr.* → millicoulomb.
μC *abbr.* → microcoulomb.
MC agar → MacConkey agar.
McArdle [mǝ'kɑːrdl]: **M.'s disease/syndrome** McArdle-Krankheit *f*, -Syndrom *nt*, muskuläre Glykogenose *f*, Muskelphosphorylasemangel *m*, Myophosphorylaseinsuffizienz *f*, Glykogenose *f* Typ V.
McArdle-Schmid-Pearson [ʃmɪd 'pɪǝrsǝn]: **M.-S.-P. disease** → McArdle's disease.
McBride [mǝk'braɪd]: **M.'s operation** *chir.* Operation *f* nach McBride.
McBurney [mǝk'bɜrnɪ]: **M.'s incision** Schräginzision *f* nach McBurney.
M.'s operation McBurney-Operation *f*.
M.'s point McBurney'-Punkt *m*.
M.'s sign McBurney-Zeichen *nt*.
McCarthy [mǝ'kɑːrθɪ]: **M.'s reflex** Supra-

orbitalis-Reflex *m*.
McCune-Albright [mǝ'kjuːn 'ɔːlbraɪt]: **M.-A. syndrome** Albright-Syndrom *nt*, McCune-Albright-Syndrom *nt*, McCune-Syndrom *nt*, polyostotische fibröse Dysplasie *f*.
M cells M-Zellen *pl*.
MCF *abbr.* → macrophage chemotactic factor.
mcg *abbr.* → microgram.
MCGF *abbr.* → mast cell growth factor.
McGinn-White [mǝ'gɪn (h)waɪt]: **M.-W. sign** McGinn-White-Syndrom *nt*.
MCH *abbr.* → mean corpuscular hemoglobin.
MCHC *abbr.* → mean corpuscular hemoglobin concentration.
m-chromosome *n* → mitochondrial chromosome.
MCi *abbr.* → megacurie.
mCi *abbr.* → millicurie.
μCi *abbr.* → microcurie.
MCIF *abbr.* → macrophage cytotoxicity-inducing factor.
McLaughlin [mǝk'lʌflɪn]: **M. nail** *ortho.* McLaughlin-Nagel *m*.
McLean [mǝ'kliːn]: **M. tonometer** *ophthal.* Impressionstonometer *nt*.
McMurray [mǝk'mɜrɪ, -'mʌrɪ]: **M.'s sign/test** *ortho.* McMurray-Zeichen *nt*.
M colony *micro.* M-Kolonie *f*, M-Form *f*, mukoide Form *f*.
M component M-Gradient *m*, Myelomgradient *m*.
MCP *abbr.* 1. → metacarpophalangeal. 2. → myocardiopathy.
MCPJ *abbr.* → metacarpophalangeal joint.
MCP joint → metacarpophalangeal joint.
MCT *abbr.* → medium-chain triglyceride.
MCV *abbr.* → mean corpuscular volume.
Md *abbr.* → mendelevium.
MDF *abbr.* 1. → macrophage deactivating factor. 2. → macrophage disappearance factor. 3. → myocardial depressant factor.
MDH *abbr.* → malate dehydrogenase.
M disk → M band.
MEA *abbr.* [multiple endocrine adenomatosis] → multiple endocrine neoplasia.
mead·ow dermatitis ['medǝʊ] Wiesengräserdermatitis *f*, Wiesendermatitis *f*, Pflanzendermatitis *f*, Phyto-, Photodermatitis *f*, Dermatitis (bullosa) pratensis, Photodermatitis phytogenica.
meadow-grass dermatitis → meadow dermatitis.
meal[1] [miːl] *n* Mehl *nt*; Pulver *nt*.
meal[2] [miːl] *n* Mahl *nt*, Mahlzeit *f*, Essen *nt*.
meal mite *micro.* Tyrophagus.
meal·y ['miːlɪ] *adj* 1. mehlig; mehlhaltig. 2. (*Gesicht*) blaß.
mean [miːn] **I** *n* 1. ~ *pl* (Hilfs-)Mittel *nt/pl*, Werkzeug *nt*; (Geld-)Mittel *pl*. 2. Mitte *f*, Mittel *nt*, Durchschnitt *m*; *mathe.* Mittel(wert) *m*. **II** *adj* 3. mittel, durchschnittlich, mittlere(r, s), Durchschnitts-, Mittel-. 4. dazwischenliegend, Zwischen-.
mean arterial pressure *abbr.* **MAP** arterieller Mitteldruck *m*.
mean cell hemoglobin → mean corpuscular hemoglobin.
mean corpuscular hemoglobin *abbr.* **MCH** Färbekoeffizient *m abbr.* Hb_E, mean corpuscular hemoglobin *abbr.* MCH.
mean corpuscular hemoglobin concentration *abbr.* **MCHC** Sättigungsindex *m*, mittlere Hämoglobinkonzentration *f* der Erythrozyten, mean corpuscular hemoglobin concentration *abbr.* MCHC.

mean corpuscular volume *abbr.* **MCV** mittleres Erythrozyten(einzel)volumen *nt*, mean corpuscular volume *abbr.* MCV.
mean life *phys.* Halbwertszeit *f.*
mean luminance *physiol.* mittlere Leuchtdichte *f.*
mean pressure *physiol.* Mitteldruck *m*, mittlerer Druck *m.*
mean temperature Durchschnittstemperatur *f.*
mea·sles ['miːzəlz] *pl* Masern *pl*, Morbilli *pl.*
measles antigen Masernantigen *nt.*
measles encephalitis Masernenzephalitis *f.*
measles exanthema Masernexanthem *nt.*
measles, mumps, and rubella vaccine live MMR-Lebendvakzine *f*, Masern--Mumps-Röteln-Lebendvakzine *f.*
measles otitis Masernotitis *f.*
measles rash Masernexanthem *nt.*
measles vaccine → measles virus vaccine.
measles virus Masern-, Morbillivirus *nt.*
measles virus live vaccine Masern(virus)lebendvakzine *f*, -impfstoff *m.*
measles virus vaccine Masern-Vakzine *f.*
measles virus vaccine live Masern(virus)lebendvakzine *f*, -impfstoff *m.*
mea·sly ['miːzlɪ] *adj micro.* finnenhaltig, finnig.
measly tapeworm Schweine(finnen)bandwurm *m*, Taenia solium.
meas·ur·a·bil·i·ty [ˌmeʒərə'bɪlətɪ] *n* Meßbarkeit *f.*
meas·ur·a·ble ['meʒərəbl] *adj* meßbar.
meas·ur·a·ble·ness ['-nɪs] *n* → measurability.
meas·ure ['meʒər] **I** *n* **1.** (*a. phys., mathe.*) Maß(einheit *f*) *nt.* **2.** Maßnahme *f*, Vorkehrung *f.* **to take ~s** Maßnahmen ergreifen. **3.** *fig.* Ausmaß *nt.* **4.** Messen *nt*, Maß *nt.* **made to ~** nach Maß (gearbeitet). **5.** Meßgerät *nt*, Maß *nt*, Maßstab *m*, Meßbecher *m.* **II** *vt* **6.** (ab-, ver-, aus-)messen, Maß nehmen. **7.** *fig.* beurteilen, (ab-)schätzen.
measure off *vt* abmessen.
measure out *vt* abmessen; abwiegen.
measure up 1. ab-, vermessen. **2.** *fig.* ein-, abschätzen.
m. of capacity Hohlmaß.
m. of length Längenmaß.
meas·ured ['meʒərd] *adj* (ab-)gemessen.
measured value Meßwert *m.*
meas·ur·ement ['meʒərmənt] *n* **1.** Messen *nt*, (Ver-)Messung *f.* **2.** Maß *nt.* **to take s.o.'s ~s** an/bei jdm. Maß nehmen. **3.** ~s *pl* (Aus-)Maße *pl*, Größe *f.*
m. of stapedius reflex *HNO* Stapediusreflexmessung *f.*
measurement electrode Meßelektrode *f.*
measurement method Meßmethode *f*, -technik *f.*
measurement technique → measurement method.
meas·ur·ing ['meʒərɪŋ] **I** *n* Messen *nt*, (Ver-)Messung *f.* **II** *adj* Meß-.
measuring glass *lab.* Meßglas *nt*, -zylinder *m*, Mensur *f.*
measuring instrument Meßgerät *nt*, -instrument *nt.*
measuring range Meßbereich *m.*
measuring tape Maß-, Meßband *nt.*
measuring voltage *electr.* Meßspannung *f.*
me·a·tal [mɪ'eɪtəl] *adj* Meatus betr., meatal, Meatus-.
meatal atresia Gehörgangsatresie *f.*
meatal cartilage Gehörgangsknorpel *m*, Cartilago meatus acustici.

meatal cholesteatoma Gehörgangscholesteatom *nt.*
meatal furuncle Gehörgangsfurunkel *m*, Ohrfurunkel *m*, Otitis externa circumscripta/furunculosa.
meatal plug *embryo.* Gehörgangsplatte *f.*
meatal segment of facial nerve meatales Segment *nt* des N. facialis.
meatal toilet Gehörgangstoilette *f.*
meato- *pref.* Meatus-, Meato-; Gehörgangs-.
me·a·to·mas·toi·dec·to·my [mɪˌeɪtəʊˌmæstɔɪ'dektəmɪ] *n HNO* Meatomastoidektomie *f.*
me·a·tome ['mɪətəʊm] *n* → meatotome.
me·a·tom·e·ter [mɪə'tɑmɪtər] *n urol.* Meatometer *nt.*
me·a·tor·rha·phy [mɪə'tɔrəfɪ] *n urol.* Urethranaht *f*, Meatorrhaphie *f.*
me·at·o·scope [mɪ'eɪtəskəʊp] *n* Meatoskop *nt*; Urethroskop *nt.*
me·a·tos·co·py [ˌmɪə'tɑskəpɪ] *n* Meatoskopie *f*; Urethroskopie *f.*
me·at·o·tome [mɪ'eɪtətəʊm] *n HNO, urol.* Meatotom *nt.*
me·a·tot·o·my [mɪə'tɑtəmɪ] *n HNO, urol.* Meatotomie *f.*
meat poisoning [miːt] Fleischvergiftung *f.*
me·a·tus [mɪ'eɪtəs] *n, pl* **-tus, tus·es** *anat.* Gang *m*, Kanal *m*, Öffnung *f*, Foramen *nt*, Meatus *m.*
m. of nose Nasengang, Meatus nasi.
meatus temperature Gehörgangstemperatur *f.*
me·ben·da·zole [mɪ'bendəzəʊl] *n pharm.* Mebendazol *nt.*
me·bev·er·ine [mɪ'bevəriːn] *n pharm.* Mebeverin *nt.*
meb·hy·dro·line [meb'haɪdrəʊliːn] *n pharm.* Mebhydrolin *nt.*
me·chan·ic [mə'kænɪk] **I** *n* Mechaniker(in *f*) *m.* **II** *adj* → mechanical.
me·chan·i·cal [mə'kænɪkl] *adj* **1.** mechanisch, Bewegungs-; maschinell, Maschinen; mit einem Mechanismus versehen. **2.** *fig.* mechanisch, unbewußt, unwillkürlich, automatisch.
mechanical acne *derm.* Akne/Acne mechanica.
mechanical anosmia mechanische/respiratorische Anosmie *f.*
mechanical antidote mechanisches Antidot *nt.*
mechanical cleansing mechanische Reinigung *f.*
mechanical cystitis mechanische (Harn-)Blasenentzündung/Zystitis *f.*
mechanical diarrhea mechanische/mechanisch-bedingte Diarrhö *f.*
mechanical dysmenorrhea *gyn.* mechanische Dysmenorrhö *f.*
mechanical energy mechanische Energie *f.*
mechanical heart künstliches Herz *nt.*
mechanical ileus mechanischer Darmverschluß/Ileus *m.*
mechanical irritability *physiol.* mechanische Erregbarkeit *f.*
mechanical irritation mechanische Reizung *f.*
mechanical jaundice Verschlußikterus *m*, mechanischer Ikterus *m.*
mechanical obstruction mechanische Verlegung/Obstruktion *f.*
mechanical power *phys.* mechanische Leistung *f.*
mechanical stimulation *physiol.* mechanischer Reiz *m.*
mechanical stimulus mechanischer Reiz *m.*
mechanical stress mechanischer Stress *m*, mechanische Belastung *f.*

mechanical summation *physiol.* mechanische Summation *f.*
mechanical-traumatic *adj* mechanisch-traumatisch.
mechanical ventilation mechanische Beatmung *f.*
mechanical vertigo mechanischer Schwindel *m.*
mechanical work mechanische Arbeit *f.*
me·chan·i·co·re·cep·tor [məˌkænɪkəʊrɪ'septər] *n* → mechanoreceptor.
me·chan·i·co·ther·a·peu·tics [ˌ-ˌθerə'pjuːtɪks] *pl* → mechanotherapy.
me·chan·i·co·ther·a·py [ˌ-'θerəpɪ] *n* → mechanotherapy.
me·chan·ics [mə'kænɪks] *pl* **1.** Bewegungslehre *f*, Mechanik *f.* **2.** Mechanismus *m.*
mech·an·ism ['mekənɪzəm] *n techn., psycho.* Mechanismus *m.*
m. of defense 1. *psycho.* Abwehrmechanismus *m.* **2.** *physiol.* Abwehrapparat *m*, -mechanismus *m.*
mech·a·no·car·di·og·ra·phy [ˌmekənəʊˌkɑrdɪ'ɑgrəfɪ] *n card.* Mechanokardiographie *f abbr.* MKG.
mech·a·no·chem·i·cal [ˌ-'kemɪkl] *adj* mechanochemisch.
mech·a·no·chem·is·try [ˌ-'kemɪstrɪ] *n* Mechanochemie *f.*
mech·a·no·cyte ['-saɪt] *n* (in vitro) Fibroblast *m.*
mech·a·no·gen·ic [ˌ-'dʒenɪk] *adj physiol.* mechanogen.
mechanogenic autoregulation *physiol.* mechanogene/myogene Autoregulation *f.*
mech·a·no·gram ['-græm] *n physiol.* Mechanogramm *nt.*
mech·a·no·per·cep·tion [ˌ-pər'sepʃn] *n physiol.* Mechanoperzeption *f.*
mech·a·no·re·cep·tion [ˌ-rɪ'sepʃn] *n physiol.* Mechanorezeption *f.*
mech·a·no·re·cep·tor [ˌ-rɪ'septər] *n* Mechanorezeptor *m.*
mech·a·no·sen·si·tive [ˌ-'sensətɪv] *adj physiol.* mechanosensitiv.
mechanosensitive receptor → mechanosensor.
mech·a·no·sen·sor [ˌ-'sensər] *n physiol.* Mechanosensor *m*, mechanosensitiver Rezeptor *m.*
mech·a·no·ther·a·py [ˌ-'θerəpɪ] *n* Mechanotherapie *f.*
me·chlor·eth·a·mine [ˌmeklɔːr'eθəmiːn] *n* Stickstoff-Lost *nt*, N-Lost *nt*, Chlormethin *nt.*
Meckel ['mekəl]: **M.'s band** *HNO* Meckel'-Band *nt.*
M.'s cartilage *embryo.* Meckel'-Knorpel *m.*
M.'s cavity Meckel'-Raum *m*, Cavum trigeminale, Cavitas trigeminalis.
M.'s diverticulum Meckel'-Divertikel *nt.*
M.'s ganglion Meckel'-Ganglion *nt*, Ggl. pterygopalatinum.
lesser ganglion of M. Faesebeck'-Ganglion *nt*, Blandin'-Ganglion *nt*, Ggl. submandibulare.
M.'s ligament → M.'s band.
M.'s rod → M.'s cartilage.
M.'s space → M.'s cavity.
M.'s syndrome Meckel-Syndrom *nt*, Dysencephalia splanchnocystica.
tubercle of M. Tuberculum majus humeri.
meck·el·ec·to·my [mekə'lektəmɪ] *n chir., neurochir.* Exzision *f* des Meckel'-Ganglions.
Meckel-Gruber ['gruːbər]: **M.-G. syndrome** → Meckel's syndrome.
me·clas·tine [mɪ'klæstiːn] *n pharm.* Clemastin *nt.*

mec·li·zine ['meklɪziːn] *n pharm.* Meclozin *nt.*
mec·lo·cy·cline [ˌmekləʊ'saɪkliːn] *n pharm.* Meclocyclin *nt.*
me·clo·fen·ox·ate [ˌ-fen'ɒkseɪt] *n pharm.* Meclofenoxat *nt.*
mec·lo·zine ['-ziːn] *n pharm.* Meclozin *nt.*
mec·o·nate ['mekəneɪt] *n* Mekonat *nt.*
me·con·ic acid [mɪ'kɑnɪk, -'kəʊn-] Mekonsäure *f.*
me·co·ni·or·rhea [mɪˌkəʊnɪəʊ'rɪə] *n ped.* übermäßige Mekoniumausscheidung *f.*
me·co·nism ['miːkəʊnɪzəm] *n* Opiat-, Opiumvergiftung *f*, Mekonismus *m.*
me·co·ni·um [mɪ'kəʊnɪəm] *n* **1.** *gyn., ped.* Kindspech *nt*, Mekonium *nt*, Meconium *nt.* **2.** Opium *nt*, Laudanum *nt*, Meconium *nt.*
meconium aspiration Mekoniumaspiration *f.*
meconium blockage syndrome → meconium plug syndrome.
meconium corpuscles Mekoniumkörperchen *pl.*
meconium cyst Mekoniumzyste *f.*
meconium ileus Mekoniumileus *m.*
meconium peritonitis Mekoniumperitonitis *f.*
meconium plug syndrome *ped.* Mekoniumpfropfsyndrom *nt.*
me·daz·e·pam [mɪ'dæzɪpæm] *n pharm.* Medazepam *nt.*
me·dia ['miːdɪə] **1.** *n, pl* **-di·ae** [-dɪiː] *anat.* Media *f*, Tunica media. **2.** *pl* → medium.
me·di·al ['miːdɪəl] *adj* **1.** in der Mitte liegend, mittlere(r, s), medial, Mittel-. **2.** Media betr., Media-.
medial angle: m. of eye medialer/innerer Augenwinkel *m*, Angulus oculi medialis.
m. of humerus Margo medialis humeri.
m. of scapula Angulus superior (scapulae).
m. of tibia Margo medialis tibiae.
medial arteriole of retina mediale Netzhautarteriole *f*, Arteriola medialis retinae.
medial arteriosclerosis → medial calcification.
medial artery of foot, superficial Ramus superficialis a. plantaris medialis.
medial border: m. of foot Fußinnenrand *m*, Margo medialis/tibialis pedis.
m. of forearm Margo medialis/ulnaris antebrachii.
m. of humerus Humerusinnenrand *m*, Margo medialis humeri.
m. of scapula Innenrand *m* der Skapula, Margo medialis scapulae.
m. of tibia Schienbeininnenrand *m*, Margo medialis tibiae.
medial branch: m.es of anterolateral central arteries Rami mediales aa. centralium anterolateralium.
m. of left hepatic duct Ramus medialis ductus hepatici sinistri.
m. of right pulmonary artery Ramus medialis a. pulmonalis dextrae.
m. of supraorbital nerve medialer Ast *m* des N. supraorbitalis, Ramus medialis n. supraorbitalis.
medial bursa of gastrocnemius muscle Bursa subtendinea m. gastrocnemii medialis.
medial calcification Mediaverkalkung *f*, Mediasklerose *f.*
medial commissure of eye lid innere/mediale Augenlidkommissur *f*, Commissura palpebralis medialis.
medial condylar fracture → medial epicondylar fracture.
medial condyle of femur innere/mediale/ tibiale Femurkondyle/Oberschenkelkondyle *f*, Condylus medialis femoris.
medial cord of brachial plexus mittleres Bündel *nt* des Plexus brachialis, Fasciculus medialis (plexus brachialis).
medial crest of fibula Margo medialis fibulae.
medial crus: m. of greater alar cartilage Crus mediale cartilago alaris majoris.
m. of superficial inguinal ring Crus mediale anuli inguinalis superficialis.
medial eminence of rhomboid fossa medialer Längswulst *m* der Rautengrube, Eminentia medialis fossae rhomboideae.
medial epicondylar fracture Fraktur *f* des Epicondylus medialis humeri.
medial fracture of the neck of femur *ortho.* mediale/subkapitale Schenkelhals-/Femurhalsfraktur *f.*
medial head: m. of abductor hallucis muscle Caput mediale m. abductoris hallucis.
m. of gastrocnemius muscle Caput mediale m. gastrocnemii.
m. of triceps brachii muscle medialer/innerer Trizepskopf *m*, Caput mediale m. tricipitis brachii.
medial hernia direkter/innerer/gerader Leistenbruch *m*, Hernia inguinalis interna/medialis/directa.
medial hypothalamus medialer Hypothalamus *m.*
medial lamina: m. of cartilage of auditory tube → m. of tubal cartilage.
m. of pterygoid process Lamina medialis proc. pterygoidei.
m. of tubal cartilage mediale Knorpelplatte *f* des Tubenknorpels, Lamina cartilaginis medialis (tubae auditivae).
medial lemniscus Lemniscus medialis.
medial ligament Innenband *nt*, mediales Ligament *nt*, Lig. mediale.
m. of elbow joint Lig. collaterale ulnare.
m. of wrist Lig. collaterale carpi ulnare.
medial limb of greater alar cartilage Crus mediale cartilago alaris majoris.
medial malleolus Innenknöchel *m*, Malleolus medialis.
medial margin: m. of foot → medial border of foot.
m. of forearm → medial border of forearm.
m. of humerus → medial border of humerus.
m. of kidney medialer/konkaver Nierenrand *m*, Margo medialis renis.
m. of orbit Margo medialis orbitae.
m. of scapula → medial border of scapula.
m. of suprarenal gland Margo medialis gl. suprarenalis.
m. of tibia → medial border of tibia.
medial meniscus (of knee) Innenmeniskus *m*, Meniscus medialis (artic. genus).
**medial necrosis: m. of medionecrosis.
medial nucleus: m. of amygdaloid body Nc. medialis corporis amygdaloidei.
dorsal m. of thalamus Hauptkern *m* der medialen Kerngruppe, Nc. medialis dorsalis (thalami).
m.i of thalamus mediale Kerngruppe *f* des Thalamus, Ncc. mediales (thalami).
medial part of globus pallidus medialer Teil *m* des Globus pallidus, Globus pallidus medialis.
medial process of calcaneal tuberosity Proc. medialis tuberis calcanei.
medial root: m. of median nerve mediale Medianuswurzel *f*, Radix medialis n. mediani.
m. of optic tract medialer Zweig/Ast *m* des Tractus opticus, Radix medialis tractus optici.

medial segment: m. of left lobe of liver Segmentum mediale.
m. of right lung (*Lunge***)** mediales Segment *nt* des Mittellappens, Segmentum mediale [S. V].
medial sulcus of crus cerebri Sulcus n. oculomotorii, Sulcus oculomotorius.
medial tubercle of posterior process of talus Tuberculum mediale.
medial tuberosity of femur Epicondylus medialis femoris.
medial venule of retina mediale Netzhautvene *f*, Venula retinae medialis, Venula medialis retinae.
medial wall of tympanic cavity mediale Wand *f* der Paukenhöhle, Paries labyrinthicus cavitatis tympanicae.
me·di·an ['miːdɪən] *adj* in der Mitte liegend, die Mitte bildend, mittlere(r, s), median, Median-, Mittel-.
median aperture of fourth ventricle → Magendie's foramen.
median artery Begleitarterie *f* des N. medianus, A. comitans n. mediani.
median eminence (of tuber) Eminentia mediana tuberis.
median fissure: anterior m. of medulla oblongata vordere Mittelfurche *f*, Fissura mediana anterior/ventralis medullae oblongatae.
anterior m. of spinal cord vordere Rückenmarksfissur *f*, Fissura mediana anterior medullae spinalis.
dorsal m. of medulla oblongata hintere Mittelfurche *f*, Sulcus medianus dorsalis/ posterior medullae oblongatae.
dorsal m. of spinal cord hintere Rückenmarksfurche *f*, Sulcus medianus dorsalis/ posterior medullae spinalis.
posterior m. of medulla oblongata → dorsal m. of medulla oblongata.
posterior m. of spinal cord → dorsal m. of spinal cord.
ventral m. of medulla oblongata → anterior m. of medulla oblongata.
ventral m. of spinal cord → anterior m. of spinal cord.
median line: anterior m. (of trunk) vordere vertikale Rumpfmittellinie *f*, Linea mediana anterior.
posterior m. (of trunk) hintere vertikale Rumpfmittellinie *f*, Linea mediana posterior.
median lobe of prostate (*Prostata***)** Mittellappen *m*, Lobus medius prostatae.
median nerve Medianus *m*, N. medianus.
median nucleus: central m. of thalamus Nc. centromedianus thalami.
m.i of thalamus mediane Kerngruppe *f* des Thalamus, Ncc. mediani (thalami).
median plane *anat.* Medianebene *f*, Mediansagittale *f*, Mediansagittalebene *f.*
median raphe: m. of medulla oblongata Raphe (mediana) medullae oblongatae.
m. of pons Raphe (mediana) pontis.
median rhinoscopy *HNO* Rhinoscopia media.
median rhomboid glossitis Glossitis mediana rhombica, Glossitis rhombica mediana.
median septum: dorsal m. hinteres Rückenmarksseptum *nt*, Septum medianum dorsale/posterius.
posterior m. → dorsal m.
median sulcus: dorsal m. of medulla oblongata → median fissure of medulla oblongata, dorsal.
dorsal m. of spinal cord → median fissure of spinal cord, dorsal.
m. of fourth ventricle Medianfurche *f* des IV. Ventrikels, Sulcus medianus (ventriculi quarti).

median vein

posterior m. of medulla oblongata → median fissure of medulla oblongata, dorsal.
posterior m. of spinal cord → median fissure of spinal cord, dorsal.
m. of tongue mediane Zungenlängsfurche f, Sulcus medianus linguae.
median vein: m. of elbow Intermedia/Mediana f cubiti, V. mediana cubiti.
m. of forearm Intermedia/Mediana f antebrachii, V. intermedia/mediana antebrachii.
me·di·as·ti·nal [ˌmiːdiæˈstaɪnl] adj Mittelfell/Mediastinum betr., im Mediastinum liegend, mediastinal, Mediastinal-.
mediastinal arteries: anterior m. → mediastinal branches of internal thoracic artery.
posterior m. → mediastinal branches of thoracic aorta.
mediastinal branches: m. of internal thoracic artery Mediastinumäste pl der A. thoracica interna, vordere Mediastinalarterien pl, Rami mediastinales a. thoracicae internae.
m. of thoracic aorta Mediastinumäste pl der Aorta thoracica, Rami mediastinales aortae thoracicae.
mediastinal cavity → mediastinum 2.
mediastinal emphysema Hamman-Syndrom nt, (spontanes) Mediastinalemphysem nt, Pneumomediastinum nt.
mediastinal fibrosis Mediastinalfibrose f.
mediastinal flutter Mediastinalflattern nt.
mediastinal pleura Mediastinalpleura f, Pleura mediastinalis.
mediastinal shift Mediastinalverschiebung f, Verschiebung f des Mediastinums.
mediastinal space → mediastinum 2.
mediastinal tumor Mediastinaltumor m.
mediastinal veins Mediastinumvenen pl, Vv. mediastinales.
me·di·as·ti·ni·tis [ˌmɪdiˌæstɪˈnaɪtɪs] n Mediastinitis f.
me·di·as·ti·no·gram [ˌmɪdiæsˈtaɪnəgræm] n radiol. Mediastinogramm nt.
me·di·as·ti·nog·ra·phy [ˌmɪdiˌæstɪˈnɑgrəfi] n radiol. Kontrastdarstellung f des Mediastinums, Mediastinographie f.
me·di·as·ti·no·per·i·car·di·tis [ˌmɪdiˌæstɪnəʊˌperɪkɑːˈdaɪtɪs] n patho. Mediastinoperikarditis f.
me·di·as·ti·no·scope [ˌmɪdiəˈstɪnəskəʊp] n Mediastinoskop nt.
me·di·as·ti·no·scop·ic [ˌmɪdiˌæstɪnəʊˈskɑpɪk] adj Mediastinoskop od. Mediastinoskopie betr., mediastinoskopisch.
me·di·as·ti·nos·co·py [ˌmɪdiˌæstɪˈnɑskəpi] n Mediastinoskopie f.
me·di·as·ti·not·o·my [ˌmɪdiˌæstɪˈnɑtəmi] n chir. Mediastinumeröffnung f, Mediastinotomie f.
me·di·as·ti·num [ˌmɪdiæˈstaɪnəm] n, pl -na [-nə] 1. anat. in der Mitte liegende Scheidewand od. Abtrennung f, Mittelfell nt. 2. (Thorax) Mittelfell-, Mediastinalraum m, Mediastinum nt, Cavum mediastinale.
me·di·ate [adj ˈmiːdiət; v -dieɪt] I adj 1. indirekt, mittelbar. 2. in der Mitte (liegend), mittler(r, s), Mittel-. II vt vermitteln; (Wissen) weitergeben (to an). III vi vermitteln (between zwischen); ein Bindeglied darstellen (between zwischen).
mediate auscultation indirekte Auskultation f.
me·di·at·ed transport [ˈmiːdieɪtɪd] physiol. vermittelter/erleichterter Transport m.
mediate percussion indirekte Perkussion f.

mediate transfusion indirekte Transfusion f.
me·di·a·tion [ˌmiːdiˈeɪʃn] n Vermittlung f.
me·di·a·tor [ˈmiːdieɪtər] n 1. Vermittler m. 2. Mediator m, Mediatorsubstanz f.
me·di·a·to·ri·al [ˌmiːdiəˈtɔːriəl, -ˈtoʊr-] adj vermittelnd, (Ver-)Mittler-.
me·di·a·to·ry [ˈmiːdiətɔːri, -toʊr-] adj → mediatorial.
med·ic [ˈmedɪk] n 1. Mediziner(in f) m, Arzt m, Ärztin f. 2. Medizinstudent(in f) m. 3. (Militär) Sanitäter m.
med·i·ca·ble [ˈmedɪkəbl] adj heilbar.
med·i·cal [ˈmedɪkl] I n 1. (praktischer) Arzt m, (praktische) Ärztin f. 2. → medical examination. II adj 3. medizinisch, ärztlich, Kranken-. on ~ grounds aus gesundheitlichen Gründen. 4. heilend, Heil-. 5. internistisch. 6. behandlungsbedürftig.
medical adrenalectomy pharmakologische Adrenalektomie f.
medical association Ärzteverband m.
medical attendance ärztliche Behandlung f.
medical attendant Krankenpfleger(in f) m.
medical bacteriology medizinische Bakteriologie f.
medical board Gesundheitsbehörde f.
medical care ärztliche Behandlung od. Betreuung od. Versorgung f.
medical certificate ärztliches Attest nt.
medical chemistry medizinische Chemie f.
medical climatology medizinische Klimatologie f.
medical diathermy Thermopenetration f.
medical disease internistische/nicht-chirurgische Erkrankung f.
medical disorder → medical disease.
medical ethics ärztliche/medizinische Ethik f.
medical examination ärztliche Untersuchung f.
medical examiner 1. ärztlicher Leichen(be)schauer m. 2. Vertrauensarzt m, -ärztin f, Amtsarzt m, -ärztin f.
medical faculty, (the) die Medizinische Fakultät.
medical jurisprudence forensische/gerichtliche Medizin f, Gerichtsmedizin f, Rechtsmedizin f.
medical laboratory technician medizinisch-technischer Assistent m abbr. MTA, medizinisch-technische Assistentin f abbr. MTA.
medical language medizinische Fachsprache f.
medical microbiology medizinische Mikrobiologie f.
medical parasitology medizinische Parasitologie f.
medical pathology medizinische Pathologie f.
medical practicioner praktischer Arzt m, praktische Ärztin f.
medical profession Ärzteschaft f.
medical psychology medizinische Psychologie f.
medical record Krankenblatt nt, -akte f.
medical school medizinische Fakultät f.
medical science → medicine 1.
medical specialist Facharzt m, -ärztin f.
medical staff ärztliches Personal nt, Arztpersonal nt (eines Krankenhauses).
medical student Medizinstudent(in f) m.
medical treatment ärztliche Behandlung f.
medical vagotomy Vagusblock(ade f) m.
medical ward Innere Abteilung f.
me·dic·a·ment [məˈdɪkəmənt, ˈmedɪkə-] I

n Medikament nt, Arznei-, Heilmittel nt. II vt medikamentös behandeln.
med·i·ca·men·tous [məˌdɪkəˈmentəs] adj mit Hilfe von Medikamenten, medikamentös.
med·i·cant [ˈmedɪkənt] n → medicament I.
med·i·cate [ˈmedɪkeɪt] vt 1. (medizinisch od. medikamentös) behandeln. 2. mit Arzneistoff(en) imprägnieren od. versetzen.
med·i·cat·ed bath [ˈmedɪkeɪtɪd] Heilbad nt; medizinisches Bad nt.
medicated candles Räucherkerzen pl.
medicated cotton (wool) medizinische Watte f.
medicated wine Medizinalwein m.
med·i·ca·tion [ˌmedɪˈkeɪʃn] n 1. (Arzneimittel-)Anwendung f, (-)Verabreichung f, (-)Verordnung f, (-)Verschreibung f, Medikation f. 2. → medicament I. 3. Beimischung f von od. Imprägnierung f mit Arzneistoffen.
med·i·ca·tive [ˈmedɪkeɪtɪv] adj → medicinal 1.
med·i·ca·tor [ˈmedɪkeɪtər] n Applikator m.
me·dic·i·nal [mɪˈdɪsnl] adj 1. heilend, heilkräftig, medizinisch, medizinal, Heil-, Medizinal-, Medizin-. 2. → medical II.
medicinal chemistry pharmazeutische Chemie f.
medicinal eruption derm. Arzneimitteldermatitis f, -exanthem nt, Dermatitis medicamentosa.
medicinal herbs Heilkräuter pl.
medicinal soft soap Kali(schmier)seife f, Sapo kalinus/mollis.
medicinal spring Heilquelle f.
med·i·cine [ˈmedɪsən; Brit. ˈmedsɪn] I n 1. Medizin f, Heilkunst f, -kunde f, ärztliche Wissenschaft f. to practice ~ den Arztberuf ausüben. 2. Medikament nt, Medizin f, Heilmittel nt, Arznei(mittel nt) f. to take one's ~ seine Arznei (ein-)nehmen. 3. Innere Medizin f. II vt Arznei/Medizin verabreichen (to zu).
medicine chest Arzneischränkchen nt, Hausapotheke f.
medicine dropper Tropfenzähler m.
medicine glass Medizin-, Tropfenglas nt.
me·dic·i·ner [məˈdɪsnər, ˈmed(ə)sɪn-] n Mediziner(in f) m, Arzt m, Ärztin f.
medico- pref. medizinisch.
med·i·co [ˈmedɪkəʊ] n, pl -cos inf. 1. Mediziner(in f) m, Arzt m, Ärztin f. 2. Medizinstudent(in f) m.
med·i·co·chi·rur·gi·cal [ˌmedɪkəʊkaɪˈrɜːdʒɪkəl] adj medizinisch-chirurgisch, medikochirurgisch.
med·i·co·den·tal [ˌ-ˈdentl] adj Heilkunde u. Zahnheilkunde betr.
med·i·co·le·gal [ˌ-ˈliːgəl] adj gerichtsmedizinisch, rechtsmedizinisch, medikolegal.
med·i·co·phys·ics [ˌ-ˈfɪsɪks] pl medizinische Physik f.
med·i·co·psy·chol·o·gy [ˌ-saɪˈkɑlədʒi] n medizinische Psychologie f.
Me·di·na worm [mɪˈdiːnə] micro. Medina-, Guineawurm m, Dracunculus medinensis, Filaria medinensis.
me·di·o·car·pal articulation [ˌmiːdiəʊˈkɑːrpl] Artic. mediocarpalis.
mediocarpal joint → mediocarpal articulation.
me·di·oc·cip·i·tal [ˌmɪdiɑkˈsɪpɪtl] adj mediookzipital.
me·di·o·cla·vic·u·lar line [ˌmiːdiəʊkləˈvɪkjələr] Medioklavikularlinie f, Linea mediocalvicularis.
me·di·o·lat·er·al [ˌ-ˈlætərəl] adj in der Mitte u. auf der Seite (liegend), mediolateral.
me·di·o·ne·cro·sis [ˌ-nɪˈkrəʊsɪs] n Medianekrose f, Medionecrosis f.

m. of aorta Erdheim-Gsell-Syndrom *nt*, Gsell-Erdheim-Syndrom *nt*, Medionecrosis Erdheim-Gsell.
me·di·o·tar·sal amputation [,-'tɑːrsl] *ortho.* Chopart-Amputation *f*, -Exartikulation *f*.
me·di·sca·le·nus [,miːdɪskə'liːnəs] *n* M. scalenus medius.
me·di·sect ['miːdɪsekt] *vt* in der Mitte teilen.
med·i·tate ['medɪteɪt] **I** *vt* im Sinn haben, planen, vorhaben, erwägen. **II** *vi* nachsinnen, nachdenken, grübeln, meditieren (*on upon* über).
med·i·ta·tion [,medɪ'teɪʃn] *n* 1. Nachdenken *nt*, Sinnen *nt*. 2. Meditation *f*.
Med·i·ter·ra·ne·an anemia [,medɪtə'reɪnɪən] Cooley-Anämie *f*, homozygote β-Thalassämie *f*, Thalassaemia major.
Mediterranean fever 1. Malta-, Mittelmeerfieber *nt*, Febris mediterranea/melitensis. 2. Boutonneusefieber *nt*, Fièvre boutonneuse. 3. familiäres Mittelmeerfieber *nt*, familiäre rekurrente Polyserositis *f*.
me·di·um ['miːdɪəm] **I** *n*, *pl* **-di·ums, -dia** [-dɪə] 1. Medium *nt*, (Hilf-)Mittel *nt*, Werkzeug *nt*; *chem.*, *phys.* Medium *nt*, Träger *m*. 2. *bact.* Kultursubstrat *nt*, (künstlicher) Nährboden *m*. 3. Konservierungsstoff *m*, -mittel *nt*. 4. Durchschnitt *nt*, Mittel *nt*. 5. (*Hypnose*) Medium *nt*. 6. *fig.* Mittel *nt*, Mitte *f*, Mittelweg *m*. 7. Umgebung *f*, Umwelt *f*, Milieu *nt*. **II** *adj* mittelmäßig, mittlere(r, s), Mittel-, Durchschnitts-. **of ~ height** mittelgroß.
medium-cell histiocytosis → monocytic leukemia.
medium-chain triglyceride *abbr.* MCT mittelkettiges Triglycerid *nt*.
medium-sized *adj* mittelgroß.
medium-term *adj* mittelfristig.
medium-term performance *physiol.* Mittelzeitleistung *f*.
me·di·us ['miːdɪəs] *n*, *pl* **-di·i** [-dɪaɪ] *anat.* → middle finger.
med·or·rhea [medə'rɪə] *n* Harnröhrenausfluß *m*, Urethrorrhoe *f*.
med·ro·ges·tone [,medrəʊ'dʒestəʊn] *n pharm.* Medrogeston *nt*.
me·drox·y·pro·ges·ter·one [mɪ,drɒksɪprəʊ'dʒestərəʊn] *n pharm.* Medroxyprogesteron *nt*.
med·ryl·a·mine [med'rɪləmiːn] *n pharm.* Medrylamin *nt*.
med·ry·sone ['medrɪsəʊn] *n pharm.* Medryson *nt*.
me·dul·la [me'dʌlə, mɪ-] *n*, *pl* **-las, -lae** [-liː] *anat.* 1. Mark *nt*, markartige Substanz *f*, Medulla *f*. 2. → medulla oblongata. 3. Knochenmark *nt*, Medulla ossium.
m. of bone Knochenmark *nt*, Medulla ossium.
m. of kidney Nierenmark *nt*, Medulla renalis.
m. of ovary *embryo.* Ovarialmark, Medulla ovarii.
m. of suprarenal gland Nebennierenmark *abbr.* NNM, Medulla gl. suprarenalis.
m. of thymus Thymusmark, Medulla thymi.
medulla oblongata Markhirn *nt*, verlängertes Mark *nt*, Medulla oblongata, Bulbus *m* (medullae spinalis), Myelencephalon *nt*.
med·ul·lar·y ['medələrɪ, 'medjʊ-, me'dʌlərɪ] *adj anat.* 1. Mark/Medulla betr., markähnlich *od.* -haltig, markig, medullar, medullär, Mark-. 2. Medulla oblongata betr., medullär. 3. Knochenmark betr., medullär.
medullary artery A. nutricia/nutriens.

medullary body: m. of cerebellum Kleinhirnmark *nt*, Corpus medullare cerebelli.
m. of vermis (*Kleinhirn*) Markkörper *m*, Arbor vitae (cerebelli).
medullary branches of posterior inferior cerebellar artery, medial and lateral Medulla-Äste *pl* der A. inferior posterior cerebelli, Rami medullares mediales et lateralis a. inferioris posterioris cerebelli.
medullary callus *ortho.* zentraler/innerer Kallus *m*.
medullary canal 1. → medullary cavity. 2. Wirbel(säulen)-, Vertebralkanal *m*, Canalis vertebralis.
medullary canal reamer *ortho.* Markraumbohrer *m*, -raspel *f*.
medullary cancer → medullary carcinoma.
medullary carcinoma medulläres Karzinom *nt*, Ca. medullare.
medullary cavity Markraum *m*, -höhle *f*, Cavitas medullaris.
medullary center Centrum semiovale.
m. of cerebellum Corpus medullare.
medullary chromaffinoma Phäochromozytom *nt*.
medullary cone Conus medullaris.
medullary conus syndrome Konussyndrom *nt*, Conus-medullaris-Syndrom *nt*.
medullary cords 1. *embryo.* Hodenstränge *pl*. 2. (*Lymphknoten*) Markstränge *pl*.
medullary cystic disease familiäre juvenile Nephronophthisis *f*, hereditäre idiopathische Nephronophthisis *f*.
medullary fibrosarcoma medulläres Fibrosarkom *nt*.
medullary folds *embryo.* Neuralfalten *pl*.
medullary hemopoiesis medulläre/myelopoetische Blutbildung *f*.
medullary lamina: external m. of corpus striatum äußere Marklamelle *f* des Corpus striatum, Lamina medullaris lateralis corporis striati.
internal m. of corpus striatum innere Marklamelle *f* des Corpus striatum, Lamina medullaris medialis corporis striati.
lateral m. of corpus striatum → external m. of corpus striatum.
medial m. of corpus striatum → internal m. of corpus striatum.
m.e of thalamus Markstränge *pl* des Thalamus, Laminae medullares thalami interna et externa.
medullary layers of thalamus → medullary laminae of thalamus.
medullary membrane innere Knochenhaut *f*, Endost *nt*, Endosteum *nt*.
medullary nail *ortho.* Marknagel *m*.
medullary nailing *ortho.* Marknagelung *f*.
blind m. gedeckte Marknagelung.
medullary paraganglioma Phäochromozytom *nt*.
medullary phase *hema.* medulläre Periode/Phase *f*.
medullary plate *embryo.* Medullaplatte *f*.
medullary porencephaly Markporenzephalie *f*.
medullary rays of kidney (*Nierenrinde*) Markstrahlen *pl*, Radii medullares.
medullary segment Marksegment *nt*.
medullary sheath → myelin sheath.
medullary sinus Marksinus *m*.
medullary space → medullary cavity.
medullary sponge kidney Schwammniere *f*, Cacchi-Ricci-Syndrom *nt*.
medullary stria: external m. of corpus striatum → medullary lamina of corpus striatum, external.
m.e of fourth ventricle Striae medullares ventriculi quarti.
internal m. of corpus striatum → medullary lamina of corpus striatum, internal.

lateral m. of corpus striatum → medullary lamina of corpus striatum, external.
medial m. of corpus striatum → medullary lamina of corpus striatum, internal.
m.e of thalamus Markstreifen *pl* des Thalamus, Striae medullares thalami.
medullary substance: m. of bone Knochenmark *nt*, Medulla ossium.
m. of kidney Nierenmark *nt*, Medulla renalis.
m. of suprarenal gland Nebennierenmark *nt abbr* NNM, Medulla (gl. suprarenalis) *f*.
medullary taenia of thalamus T(a)enia thalami.
medullary tube *embryo.* Neuralrohr *nt*.
medullary velum Marksegel *nt*, Velum medullare.
anterior m. oberes Marksegel, Velum medullare anterius/cranialis/rostralis/superius.
caudal m. unteres Marksegel, Velum medullare caudale/inferius/posterius.
cranial m. → anterior m.
inferior m. → caudal m.
posterior m. → caudal m.
rostral m. → anterior m.
superior m. → anterior m.
medullary zone Markzone *f*.
med·ul·lat·ed ['medletɪd, 'medʒə-, mə'dʌleɪtɪd] *adj* 1. → myelinated. 2. markhaltig.
medullated nerve → myelinated nerve.
med·ul·la·tion [,medə'leɪʃn, ,-medjʊ-] *n* → myelogenesis 2.
med·ul·lec·to·my [,med(j)ə'lektəmɪ] *n chir.* Markexzision *f*, Medullektomie *f*.
med·ul·li·ad·re·nal [mɪ,dʌlɪə'driːnl] *adj* → medulloadrenal.
med·ul·li·tis [med(j)ə'laɪtɪs] *n* → myelitis.
medullo- *pref.* Mark-, Medullo-, Medullar-; Myel(o)-.
med·ul·lo·ad·re·nal [mɪ,dʌləʊə'driːnl, ,med(j)ələʊ-] *adj* Nebennierenmark betr., Nebennierenmark-, NNM-.
med·ul·lo·blast ['-blæst] *n* Medulloblast *m*, Neuroblast *m*.
med·ul·lo·blas·to·ma [,-blæs'təʊmə] *n* Medulloblastom(a) *nt*.
med·ul·lo·en·ce·phal·ic [,-,ensɪ'fælɪk] *adj* → myeloencephalic.
med·ul·lo·ep·i·the·li·o·ma [,-,epɪ,θɪlɪ'əʊmə] *n* Neuroepitheliom(a) *nt*.
med·ul·lo·my·o·blas·to·ma [,-,maɪəblæs'təʊmə] *n* Medullomyoblastom(a) *nt*.
med·ul·lo·su·pra·re·no·ma [,-,suːprəriː'nəʊmə] *n* Phäochromozytom *nt*.
Me·du·sa's head [mə'd(j)uːzə] Medusenhaupt *nt*, Caput Medusae, Cirsomphalus *m*.
Meeh [meː]: **M.'s formula** Meeh'-Formel *f*.
Meeh-Dubois [dy'bwɑ]: **M.-D. formula** → Meeh's formula.
Mees [miːz]: **M.' lines** *patho.* Mees'-Streifen *pl*.
M.' stripes → M.' lines.
mef·e·nam·ic acid [mefə'næmɪk] *pharm.* Mefenaminsäure *f*.
me·fen·o·rex [mɪ'fenəreks] *n pharm.* Mefenorex *nt*.
mef·ru·side ['mefruːsaɪd] *n pharm.* Mefrusid *nt*.
MEG *abbr.* → magnetoencephalography.
meg(a)- *pref. abbr.* **M** Groß-, Meg(a)- *abbr.* M.
meg·a·bac·te·ri·um [,megəbæk'tɪərɪəm] *n* Makro-, Megabakterium *nt*.
meg·a·bec·que·rel [,-bekɑ'rel] *n abbr.* **MBq** Megabecquerel *nt* MBq.
meg·a·blad·der [,-'blædər] *n urol.* hochgradige Erweiterung *f* der Harnblase, Megazystis *f*, Megavesica *f*.

meg·a·car·dia [ˌ-'kɑːrdɪə] n Herzvergrößerung f, Kardiomegalie f.
meg·a·car·y·o·blast n → megakaryoblast.
meg·a·car·y·o·cyte n → megakaryocyte.
meg·a·ce·cum [ˌ-'siːkəm] n Megazäkum nt.
meg·a·ce·phal·ic [ˌ-sɪ'fælɪk] adj → megalocephalic.
meg·a·ceph·a·lous [ˌ-'sefələs] adj → megalocephalic.
meg·a·ceph·a·ly [ˌ-'sefəlɪ] n → megalocephaly.
meg·a·cho·led·o·chus [ˌ-kə'ledəkəs] n Megacholedochus m.
meg·a·co·lon [ˌ-'kəʊlən] n Megakolon nt, -colon nt.
meg·a·cu·rie [ˌ-'kjʊərɪ, -kjʊə'rɪ] n abbr. **MCi** Megacurie nt abbr. MCi.
meg·a·cys·tis [ˌ-'sɪstɪs] n → megabladder.
megacystis-megaureter syndrome Megaureter-Megazystis-Syndrom nt.
meg·a·dac·tyl·ia [ˌ-dæk'tiːlɪə] n → megalodactyly.
meg·a·dac·tyl·ism [ˌ-'dæktəlɪzəm] n → megalodactyly.
meg·a·dac·ty·ly [ˌ-'dæktəlɪ] n → megalodactyly.
meg·a·dol·i·cho·co·lon [ˌ-ˌdalɪkəʊ'kəʊlən] n Megadolichokolon nt, -colon nt.
meg·a·du·o·de·num [ˌ-d(j)uːəʊ'diːnəm] n Megaduodenum nt.
meg·a·e·soph·a·gus [ˌ-ɪ'safəgəs] n Megaösophagus m.
meg·a·ga·mete [ˌ-'gæmiːt, -gæ'miːt] n → macrogamete.
meg·a·gna·thia [ˌ-'neɪθɪə, -'næθ-] n → macrognathia.
meg·a·hertz ['-hɑrts] n abbr. **MHz** Megahertz nt abbr. MHz.
meg·a·kar·y·o·blast [ˌ-'kærɪəblæst] n Megakaryoblast m.
meg·a·kar·y·o·cyte [ˌ-'kærɪəsaɪt] n Knochenmarksriesenzelle f, Megakaryozyt m.
meg·a·kar·y·o·cyt·ic leukemia [ˌ-ˌkærɪə-'sɪtɪk] Megakaryozytenleukämie f, megakaryozytäre Myelose f, hämorrhagische/essentielle Thrombozythämie f.
meg·a·kar·y·o·cy·to·poi·e·sis [ˌ-ˌkærɪəˌsaɪtəpɔɪ'iːsɪs] n Megakaryozytopo(i)ese f.
meg·a·kar·y·o·cy·to·sis [ˌ-ˌkærɪəsaɪ'təʊsɪs] n Megakaryozytose f.
megal- pref. → megalo-.
meg·a·lec·i·thal [ˌmegə'lesɪθəl] adj bio. makrolezithal.
megalecithal ovum → macrolecithal ovum.
meg·al·en·ceph·a·ly [ˌmegəlen'sefəlɪ] n Megalenzephalie f, Makroenzephalie f, Makrenzephalie f, Kephalonie f, Enzephalomegalie f.
meg·a·ler·y·the·ma [ˌmegələrə'θiːmə] n → megaloerythema.
me·gal·gia [meg'ældʒ(ɪ)ə] n starker Schmerz m.
megalo- pref. Groß-, Mega-, Megal(o)-; Makr(o)-.
meg·a·lo·blast ['megələʊblæst] n Megaloblast m.
meg·a·lo·blas·tic anemia [ˌ-'blæstɪk] megaloblastäre Anämie f.
familial m. Imerslund-Gräsbeck-Syndrom nt.
megaloblastic hemopoiesis megaloblastische Blutbildung/Hämopo(i)ese f.
megaloblastic phase (Blut) megaloblastische Periode/Phase f.
meg·a·lo·blas·toid [ˌ-'blæstɔɪd] adj megaloblastoid.
meg·a·lo·bul·bus [ˌ-'bʌlbəs] n radiol. Megabulbus m.
meg·a·lo·car·dia [ˌ-'kɑːrdɪə] n Herzvergrößerung f, Kardiomegalie f.

meg·a·lo·car·y·o·cyte [ˌ-'kærɪəsaɪt] n → megakaryocyte.
meg·a·lo·ce·pha·lia [ˌ-sɪ'feɪlɪə] n → megalocephaly.
meg·a·lo·ce·phal·ic [ˌ-sɪ'fælɪk] adj Megalozephalie betr., von Megalozephalie gekennzeichnet, megalozephal, -kephal.
meg·a·lo·ceph·a·ly [ˌ-'sefəlɪ] n Megalozephalie f, -kephalie f.
meg·a·lo·chei·ria [ˌ-'kaɪrɪə] n Megaloch(e)irie f, Makroch(e)irie f.
meg·al·o·chi·ria n → megalocheiria.
meg·a·lo·clit·o·ris [ˌ-'klɪtərɪs] n Klitorisvergrößerung f.
meg·al·o·cor·ne·a [ˌ-'kɔːrnɪə] n ophthal. Megakornea f, Megalokornea f.
meg·a·lo·cys·tis [ˌ-'sɪstɪs] n → megabladder.
meg·a·lo·cyte ['-saɪt] n Megalozyt m.
meg·a·lo·cy·the·mia [ˌ-saɪ'θiːmɪə] n → macrocytosis.
meg·a·lo·cyt·ic anemia [ˌ-'sɪtɪk] → macrocytic anemia.
meg·a·lo·cy·to·sis [ˌ-saɪ'təʊsɪs] n → macrocytosis.
meg·a·lo·dac·tyl·ia [ˌ-dæk'tiːlɪə] n → megalodactyly.
meg·a·lo·dac·tyl·ism [ˌ-'dæktəlɪzəm] n → megalodactyly.
meg·a·lo·dac·ty·ly [ˌ-'dæktəlɪ] n Megalo-, Makrodaktylie f, Makrodactylia f.
meg·a·lo·don·tia [ˌ-'dɑnʃɪə] n → macrodontia.
meg·a·lo·en·ceph·a·ly [ˌ-en'sefəlɪ] n → megalencephaly.
meg·a·lo·er·y·the·ma [ˌ-erə'θiːmə] n derm. Megalerythem(a) nt.
meg·a·lo·e·soph·a·gus [ˌ-ɪ'safəgəs] n Megaösophagus m.
meg·a·lo·gas·tria [ˌ-'gæstrɪə] n übermäßige Magenerweiterung f, Megalo-, Megagastrie f.
meg·a·lo·glos·sia [ˌ-'glɑsɪə] n → macroglossia.
meg·a·lo·gra·phia [ˌ-'græfɪə] n → macrography.
meg·a·log·ra·phy [megə'lɑgrəfɪ] n → macrography.
meg·a·lo·he·pat·ia [ˌmegələʊhɪ'pætɪə] n Lebervergrößerung f, -schwellung f, Hepatomegalie f.
meg·a·lo·kar·y·o·cyte [ˌ-'kærɪəsaɪt] n → megakaryocyte.
meg·a·lo·ma·nia [ˌ-'meɪnɪə, -jə] n psychia. expansiver Wahn m, Größenwahn m, Makro-, Megalomanie f.
meg·a·lo·ma·ni·ac [ˌ-'meɪnɪæk] **I** n Größenwahnsinne(r m) f. **II** adj größenwahnsinnig, megalomani(sch).
meg·a·lo·me·lia [ˌ-'miːlɪə] n → macromelia.
meg·a·lo·nych·ia [ˌ-'nɪkɪə] n Megalonychie f, Makronychie f.
meg·a·lo·pe·nis [ˌ-'piːnɪs] n → macrophallus.
meg·a·loph·thal·mos [megəlɑf'θælmɑs] n ophthal. Makrophthalmus m, Megalophthalmus m.
meg·a·loph·thal·mus n → megalophthalmos.
meg·a·lo·pia [ˌmegə'lɑpɪə] n → macropsia.
meg·a·lo·po·dia [ˌmegələʊ'pəʊdɪə] n → macropodia.
meg·a·lop·sia [ˌmegə'lɑpsɪə] n → macropsia.
meg·a·lo·sple·nia [ˌmegələʊ'spliːnɪə] n Milzvergrößerung f, -schwellung f, -tumor m, Splenomegalie f, -megalia f.
meg·a·lo·spore ['-spəʊər, -spɔːr] n → macrospore.
meg·a·lo·syn·dac·tyl·ia [ˌ-sɪndæk'tiːlɪə] n → megalosyndactyly.

meg·a·lo·syn·dac·ty·ly [ˌ-sɪn'dæktəlɪ] n Megalosyndaktylie f.
meg·a·lo·thy·mus [ˌ-'θaɪməs] n Thymusvergrößerung f.
meg·a·lo·u·re·ter [ˌ-'jʊərətər, -jʊə'riːtər] n Megaureter m.
meg·a·lo·u·re·thra [ˌ-jʊə'riːθrə] n Megaurethra f.
meg·a·nu·cle·us [ˌmegə'n(j)uːklɪəs] n → macronucleus.
meg·a·pro·so·pia [ˌ-prəʊ'səʊpɪə] n → macroprosopia.
meg·a·rec·tum [ˌ-'rektəm] n Megarektum nt.
meg·a·sig·moid [ˌ-'sɪgmɔɪd] n Megasigma nt.
meg·a·so·mia [ˌ-'səʊmɪə] n → macrosomatia.
meg·a·spo·ran·gi·um [ˌ-spə'ændʒɪəm, -spəʊ-] n → macrosporangium.
meg·a·spore ['-spəʊər, -spɔːr] n **1.** → macrospore. **2.** → macroconidium.
me·gas·tria [mɪ'gæstrɪə] n → megalogastria.
meg·a·throm·bo·cyte [ˌmegə'θrɑmbəsaɪt] n Megathrombozyt m.
meg·a·u·re·ter [ˌ-'jʊərətər, -jʊə'riːtər] n Megaureter m.
meg·a·u·re·thra [ˌ-jʊə'riːθrə] n Megaurethra f.
meg·a·volt ['-vəʊlt] n abbr. **MV** Megavolt nt abbr. MV.
meg·a·vol·tage radiation [ˌ-'vəʊltɪdʒ] radiol. Megavoltstrahlung f.
megavoltage therapy radiol. Megavolt-, Hochenergiestrahlentherapie f.
me·ges·trol acetate [mɪ'dʒestrəʊl] pharm. Megestrolacetat nt.
meg·ohm ['megəʊm] n phys. Megaohm nt, Megohm nt.
meg·oph·thal·mos [megɑf'θælməs] n → megalophthalmos.
me·grim ['miːgrɪm] n → migraine.
mehl·nähr·schad·en [ˌmeːlnɛːr'ʃaːdən] n Mehlnährschaden m.
Meibom ['maɪbəʊm]: **M.'s glands** → meibomian glands.
mei·bo·mi·an [maɪ'bəʊmɪən]: **m. conjunctivitis** Conjunctivitis meibomiana.
m. cyst Hagelkorn nt, Chalazion nt.
m. foramen For. c(a)ecum linguae, For. Morgagni.
m. glands Meibom'-Drüsen pl, Gll. tarsales.
m. sty/stye Hordeolum internum.
mei·bo·mi·a·ni·tis [maɪˌbəʊmɪə'naɪtɪs] n ophthal. Entzündung f der Meibom'-Drüsen, Meibomitis f.
mei·bo·mi·tis [ˌmaɪbəʊ'maɪtɪs] n → meibomianitis.
Meige [mɛːʒ]: **M.'s disease** Meige-Syndrom nt, Trophödem/Lymphödem nt Typ Meige.
Meigs [megz]: **M.' syndrome** Meigs-Syndrom nt.
Meinicke ['maɪnɪkɪ; -kə]: **M. reaction** Meinicke-Klärungsreaktion f.
mei·o·sis [maɪ'əʊsɪs] n Reduktion(s teilung f) f, Meiose f.
mei·ot·ic [maɪ'ɑtɪk] adj Meiose betr., meiotisch.
meiotic cell division → meiosis.
meiotic division → meiosis.
Meissner ['maɪsnər]: **M.'s ganglion** Ganglienzellgruppe f des Meissner'-Plexus.
M.'s oval corpuscles → M.'s tactile corpuscles.
M.'s plexus Meissner'-Plexus m, Plexus submucosus.
M.'s tactile corpuscles Meissner'-(Tast-)-Körperchen pl, Corpuscula tactus.

M.'s touch corpuscles → M.'s tactile corpuscles.
mel [mel] *n* Honig *m*, Mel *nt*.
me·lag·ra [mɪˈlægrə] *n* Melagra *f*.
me·lal·gia [mɪˈlældʒ(ɪ)ə] *n* Gliederschmerz(en *pl*) *m*, Melalgie *f*.
mel·a·mine [ˈmeləmiːn] *n* Melamin *nt*, Cyanursäureamid *nt*.
melamine resin Melaminharz *nt*.
melan- *pref.* → melano-.
mel·an·cho·lia [ˌmelənˈkəʊlɪə, -jə] *n* 1. *psychia.* endogene Depression *f*, Melancholie *f*. 2. Depression *f*, Gemütskrankheit *f*; Schwermut *f*, Trübsinn *m*, Melancholie *f*.
mel·an·cho·li·ac [ˌmelənˈkəʊlɪæk] *n* Melancholiker(in *f*) *m*.
mel·an·chol·ic [ˌmelənˈkɒlɪk] **I** *n* Melancholiker(in *f*) *m*. **II** *adj* 1. Melancholie betr., melancholisch, depressiv. 2. schwermütig, trübsinnig, melancholisch.
mel·an·chol·y [ˈmelənkəlɪ] *n* → melancholia.
mel·an·e·de·ma [ˌmelənɪˈdiːmə] *n* Kohlenstaublunge *f*, Anthrakose *f*, Anthracosis pulmonum.
mel·a·ne·mia [meləˈniːmɪə] *n* Melanämie *f*.
mel·an·i·dro·sis [ˌmelənɪˈdrəʊsɪs, mɪˌlænɪ-] *n* Melanidrosis *f*.
mel·a·nif·er·ous [meləˈnɪfərəs] *adj* melaninhaltig.
mel·a·nin [ˈmelənɪn] *n* Melanin *nt*.
mel·a·nism [ˈmelənɪzəm] *n* (angeborene) Melanose *f*.
melano- *pref.* Schwarz-, Melan(o)-.
mel·a·no·ac·an·tho·ma [ˌmelənəʊækænˈθəʊmə] *n* Melanoakanthom *nt*.
mel·a·no·am·el·o·blas·to·ma [ˌ-ˌæmələʊblæsˈtəʊmə] *n* Melanoameloblastom *nt*
me·lan·o·blast [ˈ-blæst] *n* Melanoblast *m*.
mel·a·no·blas·to·ma [ˌ-blæsˈtəʊmə] *n* → malignant melanoma.
mel·a·no·blas·to·sis [ˌ-blæsˈtəʊsɪs] *n* Melanoblastose *f*, Melanoblastosis *f*.
mel·a·no·car·ci·no·ma [ˌ-ˌkɑːrsɪˈnəʊmə] *n* → malignant melanoma.
me·lan·o·cyte [ˈ-saɪt] *n* Melanozyt *m*.
melanocyte stimulating hormone *abbr.* **MSH** Melanotropin *nt*, melanotropes Hormon *nt*, melanozytenstimulierendes Hormon *nt* *abbr.* MSH.
melanocyte stimulating hormone inhibiting factor *abbr.* **MIF** Melanotropin-inhibiting-Faktor *m* *abbr.* MIF, MSH-inhibiting-Faktor *m*.
melanocyte stimulating hormone releasing factor *abbr.* **MRF, MSH-RF** Melanoliberin *nt*, Melanotropin-releasing-Faktor *m* *abbr.* MRF, MSH-releasing-Faktor *m* *abbr.* MSH-RF.
mel·a·no·cyt·ic [ˌ-ˈsɪtɪk] *adj* Melanozyt(en) betr., melanozytär, -zytisch.
melanocytic nevus melanozytärer Nävus *m*, Melanozytennävus *m*.
mel·a·no·cy·to·ma [ˌ-saɪˈtəʊmə] *n* Melanozytom *nt*, -cytoma *nt*.
mel·a·no·cy·to·sis [ˌ-saɪˈtəʊsɪs] *n* Melanozytose *f*, -cytosis *f*.
mel·a·no·den·dro·cyte [ˌ-ˈdendrəsaɪt] *n* → melanocyte.
mel·a·no·der·ma [ˌ-ˈdɜːrmə] *n* Melanoderm *nt*, -derma *nt*, -dermie *f*, -dermia *f*.
mel·a·no·der·ma·ti·tis [ˌ-ˌdɜːrməˈtaɪtɪs] *n* Melanodermatitis *f*, -dermitis *f*.
me·lan·o·gen [məˈlænədʒən] *n* Melanogen *nt*.
mel·a·no·gen·e·sis [ˌmelənəʊˈdʒenəsɪs] *n* Melaninbildung *f*, Melanogenese *f*.
mel·a·no·gen·ic [ˌ-ˈdʒenɪk] *adj* melaninbildend.
mel·a·no·glos·sia [ˌ-ˈglɒsɪə] *n* schwarze Haarzunge *f*, Melanoglossie *f*, Glosso-phytie *f*, Lingua pilosa/villosa nigra.
mel·a·noid [ˈmelənɔɪd] **I** *n* Melanoid *nt*. **II** *adj* melaninartig, melanoid.
mel·a·no·leu·ko·der·ma [ˌmelənəʊˌluːkəˈdɜːrmə] *n* Melanoleukodermie *f*
mel·a·no·ma [meləˈnəʊmə] *n, pl* **-mas, -ma·ta** [-mətə] 1. Melanom *nt*. 2. malignes Melanom *nt* *abbr.* MM, Melano(zyto)blastom *nt*, Nävokarzinom *nt*, Melanokarzinom *nt*, Melanomalignom *nt*, malignes Nävoblastom *nt*.
mel·a·no·ma·to·sis [ˌmeləˌnəʊməˈtəʊsɪs] *n, pl* **-ses** [-siːz] Melanomatose *f*.
mel·a·no·ma·tous [meləˈnəʊmətəs] *adj* Melanom betr., melanomartig, melanomatös.
mel·a·no·nych·ia [ˌmelənəʊˈnɪkɪə] *n* Melanonychie *f*, Melanonychia *f*, Melonychie *f*.
mel·a·nop·a·thy [meləˈnɒpəθɪ] *n* Melanopathie *f*.
mel·a·no·phage [ˈmelənəʊfeɪdʒ] *n* Melanophage *m*.
mel·a·no·phore [məˈlænəfəʊər, -fɔːr, ˈmelənə-] *n* Melanophore *f*.
melanophore stimulating hormone → melanocyte stimulating hormone.
mel·a·no·pla·kia [ˌmelənəʊˈpleɪkɪə] *n* Melanoplakie *f*, -plakia *f*.
mel·a·nor·rha·gia [ˌ-ˈreɪdʒ(ɪ)ə] *n* → melena 1.
mel·a·nor·rhea [ˌ-ˈrɪə] *n* → melena 1.
mel·a·no·sis [meləˈnəʊsɪs] *n* Melanose *f*, Melanosis *f*.
mel·a·no·some [ˈmelənəʊsəʊm] *n* Melanosom *nt*.
mel·a·not·ic [meləˈnɒtɪk] *adj* Melanin betr., melaninhaltig, melanotisch.
melanotic ameloblastoma → melanoameloblastoma.
melanotic cancer/carcinoma → melanoma 2.
melanotic freckle (of Hutchinson) prämaligne Melanose *f*, melanotische Präkanzerose *f*, Dubreuilh-Krankheit *f*, -Erkrankung *f*, Dubreuilh-Hutchinson-Krankheit *f*, -Erkrankung *f*, Lentigo maligna, Melanosis circumscripta praeblastomatosa/praecancerosa Dubreuilh.
melanotic neuroectodermal tumor → melanoameloblastoma.
melanotic pigment → melanin.
melanotic progonoma → melanoameloblastoma.
melanotic prurigo *derm.* Prurigo melanotica.
melanotic sarcoma → melanoma 2.
mel·a·no·trich·ia [ˌmelənəʊˈtrɪkɪə] *n* Melanotrichie *f*, -trichia *f*.
mel·a·not·ri·chous [meləˈnɒtrɪkəs] *adj* dunkelhaarig, schwarzhaarig.
mel·a·no·troph [ˈmelənətrɒf, -trəʊf] *n* MSH-bildende Zelle *f*.
mel·a·no·trop·ic [ˌ-ˈtrɒpɪk, -ˈtrəʊp-] *adj* melanotrop.
mel·an·u·re·sis [ˌmelənjəˈriːsɪs] *n* → melanuria.
mel·a·nu·ria [meləˈn(j)ʊərɪə] *n* Melanurie *f*.
mel·a·nu·ric nephrosis [meləˈn(j)ʊərɪk] melanurische Nephrose *f*.
me·las·ma [məˈlæzmə] *n* Melasma *nt*, Chloasma *nt*.
mel·a·to·nin [meləˈtəʊnɪn] *n* Melatonin *nt*.
me·le·na [məˈliːnə] *n* 1. Teerstuhl *m*, Meläna *f*, Melaena *f*. 2. dunkelbraunes Erbrochenes *nt*.
Meleney [məˈliːnɪ]: **M.'s chronic undermining ulcer** → M.'s gangrene.
M.'s gangrene Meleney-Geschwür *nt*, Pyoderma gangraenosum, Dermatitis ulcerosa, Pyodermia ulcerosa serpiginosa.
M.'s synergistic gangrene → M.'s gangrene.
M.'s ulcer → M.'s gangrene.
me·lez·i·tose [məˈlezɪtəʊz] *n* Melezitose *f*.
mel·i·bi·ase [ˌmelɪˈbaɪeɪz] *n* α-D-Galaktosidase *f*.
mel·i·bi·ose [ˌ-ˈbaɪəʊs] *n* Melibiose *f*.
me·lic·i·tose [məˈlɪsɪtəʊz] *n* → melezitose.
mel·i·oi·do·sis [ˌmelɪɔɪˈdəʊsɪs] *n* Whitmore-Krankheit *f*, Pseudomalleus *m*, Pseudorotz *m*, Melioidose *f*, Melioidosis *f*, Malleoidose *f*.
me·li·tis [mɪˈlaɪtɪs] *n* Wangenentzündung *f*.
mel·i·tose [ˈmelɪtəʊs] *n* Raffinose *f*, Melitose *f*, Melitriose *f*.
mel·i·tra·cen [ˌ-ˈtreɪsən] *n* *pharm.* Melitracen *nt*.
mel·i·tri·ose [ˌ-ˈtraɪəʊs] *n* → melitose.
mel·i·tu·ria [ˌmelɪˈt(j)ʊərɪə] *n* 1. Zuckerausscheidung *f* im Harn, Melitiurie *f*, Mellitiurie *f*. 2. Ausscheidung *f* von Nicht-Glucosen im Harn, Melitiurie *f*, Mellitiurie *f*.
me·liz·i·tose [məˈlɪzɪtəʊs] *n* → melezitose.
Melkersson [ˈmelkərsən]: **M.'s syndrome** Melkersson-Rosenthal-Syndrom *nt*.
Melkersson-Rosenthal [ˈrəʊzənθæl; -tɑːl]: **M.-R. syndrome** Melkersson-Rosenthal-Syndrom *nt*.
mel·li·tu·ria [ˌmelɪˈt(j)ʊərɪə] *n* → melituria.
mel·o·cer·vi·co·plas·ty [ˌmeləˈsɜːrvɪkəʊplæstɪ] *n* *HNO* Wangen- u. Halsplastik *f*.
mel·o·did·y·mus [ˌ-ˈdɪdəməs] *n* *embryo.* Melodidymus *m*.
mel·o·ma·nia [ˌ-ˈmeɪnɪə, -jə] *n* *psychia.* Melomanie *f*.
mel·om·e·lus [mɪˈlɒmələs] *n* *embryo.* Melomelus *m*.
mel·on·cus [mɪˈlɒŋkəs] *n* Wangenschwellung *f*, -tumor *m*.
me·lo·no·plas·ty [mɪˈlɒnəplæstɪ] *n* → meloplasty.
mel·o·plas·ty [ˈmeləplæstɪ] *n* Wangenplastik *f*, Melo(no)plastik *f*.
mel·o·rhe·os·to·sis [ˌmelɪərɪəsˈtəʊsɪs] *n* *ortho.* Melorheostose *f*.
mel·o·sal·gia [meləˈsældʒ(ɪ)ə] *n* Beinschmerzen *pl*.
mel·os·chi·sis [mɪˈlɒskəsɪs] *n* Wangenspalte *f*, Meloschisis *f*.
mel·pha·lan [ˈmelfələn] *n* *pharm.* Melphalan *nt*.
melt [melt] (*v* **melted; molten**) **I** *n* 1. Schmelzen *nt*. 2. Schmelze *f*, geschmolzene Masse *f*, Schmelzmasse *f*. **II** *vt* (*a. techn.*) schmelzen, (zer-)schmelzen lassen (*into* in); zerlassen; auflösen. **III** *vi* (zer-)schmelzen, flüssig werden, zergehen, s. (auf-)lösen.
melt down *vt* nieder-, einschmelzen.
melt out *vt* ausschmelzen.
melt·age [ˈmeltɪdʒ] *n* Schmelzen *nt*, Schmelze *f*.
melt·ing [ˈmeltɪŋ] *adj* schmelzend, Schmelz-.
melting point *abbr.* T_m, **m.p.** *phys.* Schmelzpunkt *m*.
Meltzer [ˈmeltsər]: **M.'s law** Meltzer-Regel *f*, -Gesetz *nt*.
mem·ber [ˈmembər] *n* 1. Mitglied *nt*, Angehörige(r *m*) *f*. 2. *anat.* Glied(maße *f*) *nt*, Membrum *nt*. 3. Glied *nt*, Teil *nt*.
mem·bra·na [memˈbreɪnə, -brɑːnə] *n, pl* **-nae** [-niː, -naɪ] → membrane.
mem·bra·na·ceous [ˌmembrəˈneɪʃəs] *adj* → membranous.
membranaceous ampulla Bogengangsampulle *f*, Ampulla membranacea.
anterior m. Ampulle des vorderen Bogenganges, Ampulla membranacea anterior.
lateral m. Ampulle des seitlichen Bogenganges, Ampulla membranacea lateralis.

membranate 484

posterior m. Ampulle des hinteres Bogenganges, Ampulla membranacea posterior.
mem·bra·nate ['membrəneɪt] *adj* membranartig, membranös.
mem·brane ['membreɪn] *n* **1.** *anat.* (zarte) Haut *od.* Schicht *f*, Häutchen *nt*, Membran(e) *f*, Membrana *f*. **2.** *phys., chem.* Membran(e) *f*.
m. of perineum Membrana perinei.
m. of Slaviansky Slavjanski'-Membran, (Follikel-)Glashaut.
membrane attack complex *abbr.* **MAC** *immun.* (*Komplement*) terminaler Komplex *m*, C5b-9-Komplex *m*, Membranangriffskomplex *m abbr.* MAC.
membrane attack complex inhibitor *abbr.* **MAC INH** S-Protein *nt*, Vitronektin *nt*.
membrane bone Deckknochen *m*.
membrane-bound *adj* membrangebunden, -ständig.
membrane-bound antibody membrangebundener Antikörper *m*.
membrane-bound immunoglobulin membrangebundenes Immunglobulin *nt*.
membrane capacitance *physiol.* Membrankapazität *f*.
membrane channel *physiol.* Membrankanal *m*, -tunnel *m*.
membrane charge *physiol.* Membranladung *f*.
membrane component *biochem.* Membrankomponente *f*.
membrane conductance *physiol.* Membranleitfähigkeit *f*.
mem·bra·nec·to·my [membrə'nektəmɪ] *n chir.* Membranentfernung *f*, Membranektomie *f*.
membrane current *physiol.* Membranstrom *m*.
membrane depot *histol.* Membrandepot *nt*.
membrane ionic theory Ionentheorie *f* der Erregung.
membrane length constant *physiol.* Membranlängenkonstante *f*.
mem·bra·nelle [membrə'nel] *n* Membranelle *f*.
membrane manometer Membranmanometer *nt*.
mem·bra·ne·ous [mem'breɪnɪəs, -njəs] *adj* → membranous.
membrane oxygenator Membranoxygenator *m*.
membrane patch clamp *physiol.* Membranfleckklemme *f*, Patchclamp *f*.
membrane polarization *physiol.* Membranpolarisation *f*.
membrane potential *physiol.* Membranpotential *nt*.
membrane protein Membranprotein *nt*.
extrinsic m. äußeres/peripheres Membranprotein.
integral/intrinsic m. intrinsisches/integrales Membranprotein.
major outer m. *abbr.* **Momp** major outer membrane protein *abbr.* Momp.
outer m. *abbr.* **Omp** äußeres Membranprotein, outer membrane protein *abbr.* Omp.
peripheral m. → extrinsic m.
membrane pump *physiol.* Membranpumpe *f*.
membrane resistance *physiol.* Membranwiderstand *m*.
membrane system *histol.* Membransystem *nt*.
membrane teichoic acid Lipoteichonsäure *f*.
membrane transport system *histol.* Membrantransportsystem *nt*.
membrane vesiculation *histol.* Membranvesikulation *f*.

mem·bra·ni·form [mem'breɪnɪfɔːrm] *adj* membranartig, -förmig.
mem·bra·no·car·ti·lag·i·nous [membrənəʊˌkɑːrtɪ'lædʒɪnəs] *adj* membranokartilaginär.
mem·bra·noid ['membrənɔɪd] *adj* membranartig, membranoid.
mem·bra·nol·y·sis [membrə'nɒləsɪs] *n* Membranauflösung *f*, Membranolyse *f*.
mem·bra·no·pro·lif·er·a·tive glomerulonephritis [membrənəʊprə'lɪfəˌreɪtɪv] membranoproliferative Glomerulonephritis *f*.
mem·bra·nous ['membrənəs] *adj* Membran betr., häutig, membranartig, membranös, Membran-.
membranous bone Faserknochen *m*.
membranous bronchitis kruppöse/membranöse/pseudomembranöse Bronchitis *f*, Bronchitis crouposa/fibrinosa/plastica/pseudomembranacea.
membranous cataract Cataracta membranacea.
membranous cochlea (häutiger) Schneckengang *m*, Ductus cochlearis.
membranous conjunctivitis Conjunctivitis diphtherica.
membranous croup echter Krupp *m* bei Diphtherie, Kehlkopfdiphtherie.
membranous crus: m.ra Schenkel *pl* der Bogengänge, Crura membranacea.
ampullary m.ra of semicircular duct Ampullenteil der Bogengangsschenkel, Crura membranacea ampullaria.
common m. of semicircular duct gemeinsame Mündung des vorderen u. hinteren Bogenganges, Crus membranaceum commune.
simple m. of semicircular duct hinterer Schenkel *m* des seitlichen Bogenganges, Crus membranaceum simplex.
membranous dysmenorrhea *gyn.* Dysmenorrhoea membranacea.
membranous glomerulonephritis membranöse Glomerulonephritis *f*.
membranous labyrinth häutiges/membranöses Labyrinth *nt*, Labyrinthus membranaceus.
membranous lamina of auditory tube membranöser Wandanteil der Pars cartilagina, Lamina membranacea (tubae auditivae).
membranous laryngitis membranöse Laryngitis *f*.
membranous nephropathy → membranous glomerulonephritis.
membranous neurocranium *embryo.* Bindegewebsschädel *m*, Desmokranium *nt*, Desmocranium *nt*.
membranous part: m. of interventricular septum membranöser Teil *m* des Kammerseptums, Pars membranacea septi interventricularis cordis.
m. of male urethra membranöser/diaphragmaler Abschnitt *m* der (männlichen) Harnröhre, Pars membranacea urethrae masculinae.
m. of nasal septum membranöser Abschnitt der Nasenscheidewand, Pars membranacea septi nasi.
membranous pharyngitis kruppöse/pseudomembranöse Pharyngitis *f*.
membranous pneumocyte Deckzelle *f*, Alveolarzelle *f* Typ I, Pneumozyt *m* Typ I.
membranous pneumonocyte → membranous pneumocyte.
membranous rhinitis pseudomembranöse/fibrinöse Rhinitis *f*, Rhinitis pseudomembranacea.
membranous septum of nose → membranous part of nasal septum.

membranous stomatitis pseudomembranöse Stomatitis *f*.
membranous wall of trachea membranöse Tracherückwand *f*, Paries membranaceus tracheae.
mem·brum ['membrəm] *n, pl* **-bra** [-brə] *anat.* Glied(maße *f*) *nt*, Membrum *nt*, Extremitas *f*.
mem·o·rize ['meməraɪz] *vt s.* einprägen, auswendig lernen.
mem·o·ry ['memərɪ] *n, pl* **-ries 1.** Gedächtnis *nt*, Erinnerung(svermögen *nt*) *f*, Merkfähigkeit *f*. **from/by ~** aus dem Gedächtnis/Kopf. **to escape s.o.'s ~** jds. Gedächtnis entfallen. **to have a good ~ (for)** ein gutes Gedächtnis haben. **to have a weak ~ (for)** ein schwaches *od.* schlechtes Gedächtnis haben. **2.** Erinnerung *f* (*of an*). **3.** (*Computer*) Speicher *m*.
memory bank Daten-, Speicherbank *f*.
memory cell *immun.* Gedächtniszelle *f*, memory-cell.
memory defect Gedächtnisstörung *f*.
memory image *psycho.* Erinnerungsbild *nt*.
memory pattern → memory trace.
memory span *psycho.* Gedächtnisspanne *f*.
memory trace *physiol.* Gedächtnisspur *f*, Engramm *nt*; Erinnerungsbild *nt*.
MEN *abbr.* → multiple endocrine neoplasia.
men- *pref.* → meno-.
men·ac·me [mə'nækmɪ, mɪ-] *n gyn.* Menakme *f*.
men·a·di·ol [menə'daɪɒl] *n* Menadiol *nt*, Vitamin K_4 *nt*.
men·a·di·one [ˌmenə'daɪəʊn] *n* Menadion *nt*, Vitamin K_3 *nt*.
me·naph·thone [mə'næfθəʊn] *n* → menadione.
men·a·qui·none [menə'kwɪnəʊn] *n* Menachinon *nt*, Vitamin K_2 *nt*.
men·ar·chal [mə'nɑːrkl] *adj gyn.* Menarche betr.
men·ar·che ['menɑːrkɪ, me'nɑːrkɪ, mə-] *n gyn.* Menarche *f*.
men·ar·che·al [mə'nɑːrkɪəl] *adj* Menarche betr.
men·ar·chi·al *adj* → menarcheal.
Ménard-Shenton [me'nɑːr 'ʃentn]: **M.-S. line** *radiol.* Ménard-Shenton-Linie *f*.
Mendel ['mendl]: **M.'s dorsal reflex of foot** → M.'s reflex.
M.'s laws Mendel'-Gesetze *pl*, -Regeln *pl*.
M.'s reflex Mendel-Bechterew-Reflex *m*, -Zeichen *nt*.
M.'s test Mendel-Mantoux-Test *m*, -Probe *f*.
Mendel-Bechterew ['bektəˌref]: **M.-B. reflex/sign** → Mendel's reflex.
Mendel-Bekhterev ['bektəˌref]: **M.-B. reflex/sign** → Mendel's reflex.
Mendeléeff [ˌmendə'leɪef]: **M.'s law** Mendelejew-Regel *f*, Periodenregel *f*.
M.'s table Periodensystem *nt* der Elemente.
Mendeleev → Mendeléeff.
men·de·le·vi·um [ˌmendə'liːvɪəm] *n abbr.* **Md** Mendelevium *nt abbr.* Md.
men·de·li·an [men'diːlɪən, -ljən]: **m. laws** → Mendel's laws.
m. genetics Mendel'-Genetik *f*.
m. theory → Mendel's laws.
Mendelson ['mendlsən]: **M.'s syndrome** *gyn.* Mendelson-Syndrom *nt*.
Ménétrier [menetri'e]: **M.'s disease/syndrome** Ménétrier-Syndrom *nt*, Morbus Ménétrier *m*, Riesenfaltengastritis *f*, Gastropathia hypertrophica gigantea.
Mengert ['meŋgərt]: **M.'s shock syndrome** *gyn.* Kavakompressionssyndrom *nt*.

Menghini [meŋ'gɪnɪ]: **M.'s needle** Menghini-Nadel f.
men·hi·dro·sis [menhɪ'drəʊsɪs] n gyn. Menhidrosis f, Menidrosis f.
men·i·dro·sis [menɪ'drəʊsɪs] n → menhidrosis.
Ménière [me'njɛːr]: **M.'s attack** Ménière--Anfall m.
M.'s disease/syndrome Ménière'-Krankheit f, Morbus Ménière m.
M.'s triad Ménière'-Trias f.
mening- pref. → meningo-.
me·nin·ge·al [mɪ'nɪndʒɪəl] adj Hirnhäute/Meninges betr., meningeal, Hirnhaut-, Meningeal-.
meningeal anthrax zerebraler Milzbrand m.
meningeal artery A. meningea.
  accessory m. Ramus meningeus accessorius a. meningeae mediae.
  anterior m. vordere Hirnhautarterie f, Meningea f anterior, A. meningea anterior, Ramus meningeus anterior a. ethmoidalis anterioris.
  middle m. mittlere Hirnhautarterie f, Meningea f media, A. meningea media.
  posterior m. hintere Hirnhautarterie f, Meningea f posterior, A. meningea posterior.
meningeal bleeding Meningealblutung f, Blutung f in die Hirnhäute.
meningeal branch Hirnhaut-, Meningealast m, Ramus meningeus.
  accessory m. of middle meningeal artery Ramus meningeus accessorius a. meningeae mediae.
  anterior m. of anterior ethmoidal artery Ramus meningeus anterior a. ethmoidalis anterioris.
  m. of internal carotid artery Ramus meningeus a. carotidis internae.
  m. of mandibular nerve Hirnhaut-/Meningealast des N. mandibularis, Ramus meningeus n. mandibularis, N spinosus.
  middle m. of maxillary nerve Hirnhautast des N. maxillaris, Ramus meningeus (medius) n. maxillaris.
  m. of occipital artery Hirnhautast der A. occipitalis, Ramus meningeus a. occipitalis.
  recurrent m. of lacrimal artery Ramus meningeus recurrens a. lacrimalis.
  m. of spinal nerves Spinalnervenast zur Rückenmarkshaut, Ramus meningeus nn. spinalium.
  m. of vagus nerve Hirnhautast des N. vagus, Ramus meningeus n. vagi.
  m.es of vertebral artery Hirnhautäste pl der A. vertebralis, Rami meningei a. vertebralis.
meningeal filament Filum terminale/spinale.
meningeal granules Arachnoidalzotten pl, Pacchioni-Granulationen pl, Granulationes arachnoideae.
meningeal hemorrhage → meningeal bleeding.
meningeal injury Hirnhaut- od. Rückenmarkshautverletzung f.
meningeal irritation Hirnhautreizung f.
meningeal leukemia leukämische Hirnhautinfiltration f, Meningitis/Meningiosis leucaemica.
meningeal nerve → meningeal branch of maxillary nerve, middle.
meningeal plague Pestmeningitis f.
meningeal sulci Schädelwandfurchen pl für Meningealarterien, Sulci arteriales.
meningeal syndrome meningeales Syndrom nt.
meningeal thread, terminal Filum terminale/spinale.

meningeal veins Hirnhaut-, Duravenen pl, Vv. meningeae.
  middle m. mittlere Duravenen, Vv. meningeae mediae.
me·nin·gem·a·to·ma [mɪˌnɪndʒemə'təʊmə] n Durahämatom nt.
me·nin·ge·o·cor·ti·cal [mɪˌnɪndʒɪəʊ'kɔːrtɪkl] adj Hirnhaut u. Hirnrinde betr., meningeokortikal.
me·nin·ge·o·ma [mɪˌnɪndʒɪ'əʊmə] n → meningioma.
me·nin·ge·or·rha·phy [mɪˌnɪndʒɪ'ɔrəfɪ] n neurochir. Hirnhautnaht f.
me·ninges [mɪ'nɪndʒiːz], sing **me·ninx** ['miːnɪŋks] Hirn- u. Rückenmarkshäute pl, Meningen pl, Meninges pl.
me·nin·ghem·a·to·ma [mɪˌnɪndʒhemə'təʊmə] n Durahämatom nt.
men·in·gin·i·tis [ˌmenɪndʒɪ'naɪtɪs] n Entzündung f der weichen Hirnhaut, Leptomeningitis f.
me·nin·gi·o·ma [mɪˌnɪndʒɪ'əʊmə] n, pl **-mas, ma·ta** [-mətə] Meningiom(a) nt, Meningeom(a) nt.
me·nin·gi·o·ma·to·sis [mɪˌnɪndʒɪˌəʊmə'təʊsɪs] n Meningiomatose f.
me·nin·gism [mɪ'nɪndʒɪzəm, 'menɪn-] Meningismus m; Pseudomeningitis f.
men·in·git·ic [ˌmenɪn'dʒɪtɪk] adj Meningitis betr., von ihr betroffen, meningitisch, Meningitis-.
men·in·gi·tis [ˌ-'dʒaɪtɪs] n, pl **-git·i·des** [-'dʒɪtədiːz] Hirn- od. Rückenmarkshautentzündung f, Meningitis f.
meningo- pref. Hirnhaut-, Mening(o)-.
me·nin·go·ar·te·ri·tis [mɪˌnɪŋgəˌɑːrtə'raɪtɪs] n Entzündung f der Meningealarterien.
me·nin·go·blas·to·ma [ˌ-blæs'təʊmə] n malignes Melanom nt der Hirnhaut.
me·nin·go·cele ['-siːl] n Meningozele f, -cele f.
me·nin·go·ceph·a·li·tis [ˌ-ˌsefə'laɪtɪs] n → meningoencephalitis.
me·nin·go·cer·e·bri·tis [ˌ-serə'braɪtɪs] n → meningoencephalitis.
meningococcal meningitis [ˌ-'kɒkl] Meningokokkenmeningitis f, Meningitis cerebrospinalis epidemica.
me·nin·go·coc·ce·mia [ˌ-kɒk'siːmɪə] n Meningokokkensepsis f, Meningokokkämie f.
me·nin·go·coc·co·sis [ˌ-kɒ'kəʊsɪs] n Meningokokkeninfektion f, Meningokokkose f.
me·nin·go·coc·cus [ˌ-'kɒkəs] n Meningokokke m, Meningococcus m, Neisseria meningitidis.
meningococcus conjunctivitis Meningokokkenkonjunktivitis f.
me·nin·go·cor·ti·cal [ˌ-'kɔːrtɪkl] adj Hirnhaut u. Hirnrinde betr., meningokortikal.
me·nin·go·en·ceph·a·li·tis [ˌ-enˌsefə'laɪtɪs] n Meningoenzephalitis f, -encephalitis f, Enzephalo-, Encephalomeningitis f.
me·nin·go·en·ceph·a·lo·cele [ˌ-enˌsefələʊsiːl] n Meningoenzephalozele f, Enzephalomeningozele f.
me·nin·go·en·ceph·a·lo·my·e·li·tis [ˌ-enˌsefələʊmaɪə'laɪtɪs] n Meningoenzephalomyelitis f.
me·nin·go·en·ceph·a·lo·my·e·lop·a·thy [ˌ-enˌsefələʊmaɪə'lɒpəθɪ] n Meningoenzephalomyelopathie f.
me·nin·go·en·ceph·a·lop·a·thy [ˌ-enˌsefə'lɒpəθɪ] n Meningoenzephalopathie f, Enzephalomeningopathie f.
me·nin·go·fi·bro·blas·to·ma [ˌ-ˌfaɪbrəblæs'təʊmə] n → meningioma.
me·nin·go·gen·ic [ˌ-'dʒenɪk] adj von den Meningen ausgehend, meningogen.

men·in·go·ma [ˌmenɪn'gəʊmə] n → meningioma.
me·nin·go·ma·la·cia [mɪˌnɪŋgəʊmə'leɪʃ(ɪ)ə] n Meningomalazie f, -malacia f.
me·nin·go·my·e·li·tis [ˌ-maɪə'laɪtɪs] n Meningomyelitis f.
me·nin·go·my·e·lo·cele [ˌ-'maɪələʊsiːl] n Meningomyelozele f.
me·nin·go·my·e·lo·en·ceph·a·li·tis [ˌ-ˌmaɪələʊenˌsefə'laɪtɪs] n → meningoencephalomyelitis.
me·nin·go·my·e·lo·ra·dic·u·li·tis [ˌ-ˌmaɪələʊrəˌdɪkjə'laɪtɪs] n Meningomyeloradikulitis f.
men·in·gop·a·thy [ˌmenɪn'gɒpəθɪ] n Hirnhauterkrankung f, Meningopathie f.
me·nin·go·ra·dic·u·lar [mɪˌnɪŋgəʊrə'dɪkjələr] adj Hirnhäute u. Spinalnervenwurzeln betr., meningoradikulär.
me·nin·go·ra·dic·u·li·tis [ˌ-rəˌdɪkjə'laɪtɪs] n Meningoradikulitis f.
me·nin·gor·rha·gia [ˌ-'rædʒ(ɪ)ə] n Meningorrhagie f.
me·nin·gor·rhea [ˌ-'rɪə] n Meningorrhö f.
men·in·go·sis [ˌmenɪn'gəʊsɪs] n Meningose f.
me·nin·go·the·li·o·ma [mɪˌnɪŋgəˌθiːlɪ'əʊmə] n → meningioma.
me·nin·go·vas·cu·lar [ˌ-'væskjələr] adj Meningealgefäße betr., meningovaskulär.
meningovascular neurosyphilis → meningovascular syphilis.
meningovascular syphilis meningovaskuläre (Neuro-)Syphilis f.
men·in·gu·ria [ˌmenɪn'g(j)ʊərɪə] n patho. Meningurie f.
me·ninx → meninges.
me·nis·cal [mɪ'nɪskəl] adj Meniskus betr., Meniskus-, Menisko-.
meniscal clamp ortho. Meniskusfaßzange f.
meniscal retractor ortho. Meniskushaken m.
men·is·cec·to·my [ˌmenɪ'sektəmɪ] n chir., ortho. Meniskusentfernung f, -exzision f, Meniskektomie f.
men·i·che·sis [ˌmenɪ'skiːsɪs] n → menoschesis.
men·i·sci·tis [ˌmenɪ'saɪtɪs] n Meniskusentzündung f, Meniszitis f, Meniskitis f.
me·nis·co·cyte [mɪ'nɪskəsaɪt] n Sichelzelle f.
me·nis·co·cy·to·sis [mɪˌnɪskəʊsaɪ'təʊsɪs] n Sichelzell(en)anämie f, Herrick-Syndrom nt.
me·nis·co·fem·o·ral ligament [ˌ-'femərəl]
  anterior m. Lig. meniscofemorale anterius.
  posterior m. Lig. meniscofemorale posterius.
me·nis·coid [mɪ'nɪskɔɪd] adj meniskusähnlich, -förmig, meniskoid.
me·nis·co·syn·o·vi·al [mɪˌnɪskəsɪn'əʊvɪəl] adj meniskosynovial.
me·nis·co·tome [mɪ'nɪskətəʊm] n ortho. Meniskotom nt.
me·nis·cus [mɪ'nɪskəs] n, pl **-cus·es, -nis·ci** [-'nɪs(k)aɪ, -kiː] **1.** sichelförmige/halbmondförmige Gelenk(zwischen)scheibe f, Meniskus m, Meniscus articularis. **2.** sichelförmiger/halbmondförmiger Körper m. **3.** phys. (Flüssigkeit) Meniskus m. **4.** phys. konkav-konvexe Linse f, Meniskus m.
meniscus lens ophthal. Meniskus(glas nt) m.
  converging m. Konkavokonvexlinse f.
  diverging m. Konvexokonkavlinse f.
  negative m. → diverging m.
  positive m. → converging m.
meniscus sign radiol. Carman-Meniskus m.

Menkes

Menkes ['meŋkəs]: **M.' disease/syndrome** Menkes-Syndrom nt, -Stahlhaarkrankheit f, Kraushaarsyndrom nt, Trichopoliodystrophie f, kinky hair disease (nt), Pili torti mit Kupfermangel.
Mennell [mə'nel]: **M.'s sign** Mennell-Zeichen nt.
meno- pref. Men(o)-, Menstruations-.
men·o·met·ror·rha·gia [ˌmenəˌmiːtrə-'rædʒ(ɪ)ə, -ˌmetrə-] n gyn. Menometrorrhagie f.
men·o·paus·al [ˌ-'pɔːzl] adj Menopause betr., menopausal, Menopausen-.
menopausal arthritis klimakterische Arthropathie f, Arthropathia ovaripriva.
menopausal syndrome Menopausensyndrom nt.
men·o·pause ['-pɔːz] n Menopause f.
men·or·rha·gia [ˌ-'reɪdʒ(ɪ)ə] n gyn. Menorrhagie f.
men·or·rhal·gia [ˌ-'rældʒ(ɪ)ə] n Dysmenorrhoe f, Dysmenorrhoea f
men·or·rhea [ˌ-'rɪːə] n gyn. Menorrhoe f.
me·nos·che·sis [mə'nɑskəsɪs, ˌmenə'skiːsɪs] n gyn. Unterdrückung f der Menstruation, Menoschesis f.
men·o·sta·sia [ˌmenə'steɪzɪə] n gyn. Amenorrhoe f, Amenorrhoea f.
men·o·sta·sis [ˌ-'steɪsɪs] n → menostasia.
men·o·stax·is [ˌ-'stæksɪs] n übermäßig starke Menstruation(sblutung f) f, Hypermenorrhoe f.
men·o·tro·pin [ˌ-'trəʊpɪn] n Menotropin nt, Menopausengonadotropin nt, humanes Menopausengonadotropin nt abbr. HMG.
men·ses ['mensiːz] pl → menstruation.
men·stru·al ['menstrʊəl, -strəwəl, -strəl] adj Menstruation betr., menstrual, Menstruations-, Regel-.
menstrual bleeding Menstrual-, Monatsblutung f.
menstrual colic Dysmenorrhoe f, Dysmenorrhoea f.
menstrual cycle Genital-, Monats-, Sexual-, Menstrual-, Menstruationszyklus m.
menstrual decidua während der Menstruation abgestoßene Lamina functionalis.
menstrual flow → menstruation.
menstrual phase → menstruation.
menstrual stage → menstruation.
menstrual towel hyg. (Monats-, Damen-)Binde f.
men·stru·ate ['menstrəweɪt, -streɪt] vi die Menstruation haben, menstruieren.
men·stru·a·tion [ˌmenstrə'weɪʃn, -'streɪ-] n Monatsblutung f, Periode f, Regel f, Menses pl, Menstruation f.
men·stru·ous ['menstrəwəs, -strəs] adj Menstruations-.
men·stru·um ['menztr(əw)əm] n, pl **-struums, -strua** [-ztr(əw)ə] chem. Lösungsmittel nt.
men·su·al ['menʃəwəl] adj monatlich, mensual.
ment- pref. → mento-.
men·ta·gra [men'tægrə] n derm. Haarfollikelentzündung f, Sykose f, Sycosis f.
men·ta·graph·y·ton [ˌmentə'grɑfɪtən] n micro. Trichophyton mentagrophytes.
men·tal ['mentl] I n inf. Verrückte(r m) f. II adj 1. mental, geistig, innerlich, intellektuell, Geistes-. 2. geisteskrank, geistesgestört. 3. mental, seelisch, psychisch, Gemüts-. 4. Kinn betr., zum Kinn gehörend, mental, Kinn-.
mental activity geistige Aktivität f.
mental age abbr. **M.A.** psycho. Intelligenzalter nt, geistiger Entwicklungszustand m.
mental agraphia zerebrale Agraphie f.

mental alienation psychia. Entfremdungspsychose f, Alienation f.
mental arithmetic Kopfrechnen nt.
mental artery Kinnschlagader f, A. mentalis, Ramus mentalis a. alveolaris inferioris.
mental blackout Bewußtseinsstörung f.
mental block psycho. (mentale) Blockierung f, Sperre f.
mental branch: m. of inferior alveolar artery → mental artery.
m.es of mental nerve Kinnäste pl des N. mentalis, Rami mentales n. mentalis.
mental breakdown Nervenzusammenbruch m.
mental canal For. mentale.
mental capacity Zurechnungsfähigkeit f.
mental condition geistige/psychische Verfassung f, Geisteszustand m.
mental confusion geistige Verwirrung f.
mental defective Geistesgestörte(r m) f.
mental deficiency → mental retardation.
mental derangement → mental retardation.
mental disease Geisteskrankheit f.
mental disorder → mental disease.
mental fatigue psychische/zentrale Ermüdung f.
mental foramen For. mentale.
mental handicap geistige Behinderung f.
mental hospital psychiatrische Klinik f, (Nerven-)Heilanstalt f.
mental hygiene Psychohygiene f.
mental illness Geisteskrankheit f.
mental institution → mental hospital.
men·ta·lis (muscle) [men'tælɪs, -'teɪ-] Kinnmuskel m, Mentalis m, M. mentalis.
men·tal·i·ty [men'tælətɪ] n 1. Mentalität f, geistige Einstellung f, Haltung f, Gesinnung f. 2. geistige Fähigkeiten pl.
men·tal·ly ['mentlɪ] adv geistig, geistes-.
mentally-deficient adj geistesgestört.
mentally-handicapped adj geistig behindert.
mentally-ill adj geisteskrank.
mental nerve N. mentalis.
mental patient Geisteskranke(r m) f.
mental process 1. Denkprozeß f. 2. anat. Protuberantia mentalis.
mental protuberance Kinn nt, Kinnvorsprung m, Protuberantia mentalis.
mental ratio Intelligenzquotient m.
mental region Kinngegend f, -region f, Regio mentalis.
mental retardation Geistesschwäche f, -störung f.
mild m. leichte Debilität f.
moderate m. Debilität f.
profound m. Idiotie f.
severe m. Imbezillität f.
mental spine Spina mentalis.
mental state Geisteszustand m, geistige/mentale Verfassung f.
mental status → mental state.
mental subnormality → mental retardation.
mental symphysis Symphysis mandibulae/mentalis.
mental test psychologischer Test m.
mental tubercle Tuberculum mentale (mandibulae).
mental work geistige/mentale Arbeit f.
men·ta·tion [men'teɪʃn] n geistige Aktivität f.
Men·tha ['menθə] n bot., pharm. Minze f, Mentha f.
M. piperita Pfefferminze, Mentha piperita.
men·thol ['menθɒl, -θal] n Menthol nt, Mentholum nt, Pfefferminzkampfer m.
men·tho·lat·ed ['menθəleɪtɪd] adj Menthol enthaltend, mit Menthol behandelt.

men·thyl ['menθɪl] n Menthyl-(Radikal nt).
mento- pref. Kinn-, Ment(o)-, Geni(o)-.
men·to·an·te·ri·or [ˌmentəʊæn'tɪərɪər] adj gyn. mentoanterior.
mentoanterior position gyn. mentoanteriore (Gesichts-)Lage f.
men·to·la·bi·al [ˌ-'leɪbɪəl] adj Kinn u. Lippe betr. od. verbindend, mentolabial.
mentolabial furrow Lippenkinnfurche f, Sulcus mentolabialis.
mentolabial sulcus → mentolabial furrow.
mento-occipital diameter gyn., ped. okzipitomentaler/mentookzipitaler Durchmesser m, Diameter occipitomentalis/mentoocciptialis.
men·to·plas·ty ['-plæstɪ] n chir., HNO Kinnplastik f, Mentoplastik f.
men·to·pos·te·ri·or [ˌ-pɑ'stɪərɪər] adj gyn. mentoposterior.
mentoposterior position gyn. mentoposteriore (Gesichts-)Lage f.
men·to·trans·verse [ˌ-'trænz'vɜrs] adj gyn. mentotransvers.
mentotransverse position gyn. mentotransverse (Gesichts-)Lage f.
men·tum ['mentəm] n, pl **-ta** [-tə] anat. Kinn nt, Mentum nt.
M enzyme M-Enzym nt.
mep·a·crine ['mepəkrɪn, -kriːn] n pharm. Mepacrin nt.
me·per·i·dine [mə'perədiːn, -dɪn] n pharm., anes. Pethidin nt.
me·phen·a·mine [mə'fenəmiːn, -mɪn] n pharm. Orphenadrin nt.
me·phen·e·sin [mə'fenəsɪn] n pharm. Mephenesin nt.
me·phit·ic [mɪ'fɪtɪk] adj (Luft) verpestet, giftig, mephitisch.
mephitic gangrene Gasbrand m, -gangrän f, -ödem nt, -ödemerkrankung f, malignes Ödem nt, Gasphlegmone f, Gangraena emphysematosa.
me·phi·tis [mɪ'faɪtɪs] n faule Ausdünstung f.
me·piv·a·caine [mə'pɪvəkeɪn] n pharm., anes. Mepivacain nt.
me·pro·ba·mate [mə'prəʊbəmeɪt, ˌmeprəʊ'bæment] n pharm. Meprobamat nt.
me·pyr·a·mine [mə'pɪrəmiːn] n pharm. Mepyramin nt.
me·pyr·a·pone [mə'pɪrəpəʊn] n → metyrapone
mEq. abbr. → milliequivalent.
meq. abbr. → milliequivalent.
me·ral·gia [mə'rældʒ(ɪ)ə] n Oberschenkelschmerz(en pl) m, Schmerzen pl im Oberschenkel, Meralgia f.
mer·bro·min [mər'brəʊmɪn] n pharm. Merbromin nt.
mer·cap·tan [mər'kæptæn] n Merkaptan nt, -captan nt.
mer·cap·tide [mər'kæptaɪd] n Merkaptid nt, -captid nt.
mer·cap·to·eth·a·nol [mərˌkæptəʊ'eθɒnɒl, -nal] n Merkaptoäthanol nt, -ethanol nt.
mer·cap·tol [mər'kæptɒl] n Merkaptol nt.
6-mer·cap·to·pu·rine [mərˌkæptəʊ'pjʊəriːn] n abbr. **6-MP** 6-Mercaptopurin nt abbr. 6-MP.
3-mer·cap·to·py·ru·vate sulfur-transferase [ˌ-paɪ'ruːveɪt, -pɪ-] 3-Mercaptopyruvatsulfurtransferase f.
mer·cap·to·py·ru·vic acid [ˌ-paɪ'ruːvɪk, -pɪ-] Mercaptobrenztraubensäure f.
Mercier [mɛrsi'e]: **M.'s bar** Plica intereruterica.
M.'s sound Mercier-Katheter m.
M.'s valve → M.'s bar.
mer·cur·a·mide [mər'kjʊəramaɪd] n → mersalyl.

mer·cu·rate ['mɜrkjəreɪt] **I** *n* Quecksilbersalz *nt*. **II** *vt chem.* mit Quecksilber(salz) verbinden *od.* behandeln, merkurieren.
mer·cu·ri·al [mər'kjʊərɪəl] **I** *n pharm.* Quecksilberzubereitung *f*, -präparat *nt*. **II** *adj* Quecksilber betr., Quecksilber-; quecksilberhaltig, -artig.
mercurial cachexia chronische Quecksilbervergiftung *f*.
mer·cu·ri·al·ism [mər'kjʊərɪəlɪzəm] *n* Quecksilbervergiftung *f*, Merkurialismus *m*, Hydrargynie *f*, -gyrose *f*.
mer·cu·ri·al·ize [mər'kjʊərɪəlaɪz] *vt* mit Quecksilber behandeln.
mercurial line Quecksilberlinie *f*, -saum *m*.
mercurial poisoning → mercury poisoning.
mercurial stomatitis Stomatitis *f* bei Quecksilbervergiftung, Stomatitis mercurialis.
mercurial thermometer Quecksilberthermometer *nt*.
mer·cu·ri·ate [mər'kjʊərɪɪt, -eɪt] *n* → mercurate I.
mer·cu·ric [mər'kjʊərɪk] *adj* zweiwertiges Quecksilber betr. *od.* enthaltend, Merkuri-, Mercuri-, Quecksilber-II-.
mercuric chloride → mercury bichloride.
mer·cu·rize ['mɜrkjəraɪz] *vt* → mercurate II.
mer·cu·rous [mər'kjʊərəs, 'mɜrkjə-] *adj* einwertiges Quecksilber betr. *od.* enthaltend, Merkuro-, Mercuro-, Quecksilber-I-.
mercurous chloride Kalomel *nt*, Calomel *nt*, Quecksilber-I-Chlorid *nt*.
mer·cu·ry ['mɜrkjərɪ] *n* **1.** Quecksilber *nt*, *chem.* Hydrargyrum *nt abbr.* Hg. **2.** Quecksilber(säule *f*) *nt*. **3.** → mercurial I.
mercury arc *phys.* Quecksilberlichtbogen *m*.
mercury bichloride Sublimat *nt*, Quecksilber-II-chlorid *nt*.
mercury bichloride nephrosis Sublimatnephrose *f*.
mercury lamp Quecksilberdampflampe *f*.
mercury manometer Quecksilbermanometer *nt*.
mercury perchloride → mercury bichloride.
mercury poisoning Quecksilbervergiftung *f*, Merkurialismus *m*, Hydrargynie *f*, -gyrose *f*.
mercury pressure gauge Quecksilbermanometer *nt*.
mercury vapor lamp Quecksilberdampflampe *f*.
mer·cy killing ['mɜrsɪ] Sterbehilfe *f*, Euthanasie *f*.
Merendino [merən'di:nəʊ]: **M.'s technique** *HTG* Merendino-Operation *f*.
me·rid·i·an [mə'rɪdɪən] *n* Meridian *m*.
m.s of eye ball Meridiani bulbi oculi.
me·rid·i·o·nal [mə'rɪdɪənl] *adj* meridional, Meridian-.
meridional cleavage *bio.* meridionale Furchung(steilung *f*) *f*.
meridional fibers of ciliary muscle Brücke'-Fasern *pl*, -Muskel *m*, Fibrae longitudinales/meridionales m. ciliaris.
mer·i·stem ['merəstem] *n bio.* Meristem *nt*, Bildungsgewebe *nt*.
mer·i·ste·mat·ic tissue [ˌ-stə'mætɪk] → meristem.
mer·i·sto·ma [ˌ-'stəʊmə] *n* Meristom *nt*, Zytoblastom *nt*.
Merkel ['mɜrkl]: **M.'s cells 1.** Merkel'-Tastzellen *pl*, -Tastscheibe *f*, Meniscus tactus. **2.** Merkelzellen *pl*.
M.'s corpuscles → M.'s cells 1.
M.'s disks → M.'s cells 1.

M.'s muscle M. ceratocricoideus.
M.'s tactile cells → M.'s cells 1.
M.'s touch cells → M.'s cells 1.
Merkel-Ranvier [rɑ̃vi'e]: **M.-R. cells** → Merkel's cells.
mer·maid deformity ['mɜrmeɪd] *embryo.* Sirenbildung *f*, Sirene *f*, Sirenomelie *f*, Sympodie *f*.
mer·o·a·cra·nia [ˌmerəʊə'kreɪnɪə] *n embryo.* Mero(a)kranie *f*.
mer·o·blas·tic [ˌ-'blæstɪk] *adj bio.* meroblastisch.
meroblastic cleavage partielle/meroblastische Furchung(steilung *f*) *f*.
meroblastic ovum *bio.* meroblastisches Ei *nt*.
mer·o·cele ['-siːl] *n* Schenkelhernie *f*, Merozele *f*, Hernia femoralis/cruralis.
mer·o·cox·al·gia [ˌ-kɑk'sældʒ(ɪ)ə] *n* Schmerzen *pl* in Oberschenkel u. Hüfte, Merokoxalgie *f*.
mer·o·crine ['-kraɪn] *adj* merokrin.
merocrine gland merokrine Drüse *f*.
mer·o·cyst ['-sɪst] *n* Merozyst(e *f*) *m*.
mer·o·cyte ['-saɪt] *n embryo.* Merozyte *f*.
mer·o·di·as·tol·ic [ˌ-ˌdaɪə'stɑlɪk] *adj card.* merodiastolisch.
mer·o·dip·loid [ˌ-'dɪplɔɪd] *adj genet.* merodiploid.
mer·o·gam·ete [ˌ-'gæmiːt] *n* Merogamet *m*.
me·rog·a·my [mə'ragəmɪ] *n* Merogamie *f*.
mer·o·gas·tru·la [ˌmerə'gæstrʊlə] *n* Merogastrula *f*.
mer·o·gen·e·sis [ˌ-'dʒenəsɪs] *n bio.* Merogenese *f*.
mer·o·ge·net·ic [ˌ-dʒə'netɪk] *adj* Merogenese betr., merogenetisch, merogen.
mer·o·gen·ic [ˌ-'dʒenɪk] *adj* → merogenetic.
mer·o·gon·ic [ˌ-'gɑnɪk] *adj* Merogonie betr., merogon(isch).
me·rog·o·ny [mə'ragənɪ] *n* Merogonie *f*.
mer·o·me·lia [ˌmerə'miːlɪə] *n embryo.* Gliedmaßendefekt *m*, Meromelie *f*.
mer·o·mi·cro·so·mia [ˌ-ˌmaɪkrə'səʊmɪə] *n embryo.* Meromikrosomie *f*.
mer·o·my·o·sin [ˌ-'maɪəsɪn] *n* Meromyosin *nt*.
me·ro·nec·ro·bi·o·sis [ˌ-ˌnekrəbaɪ'əʊsɪs] *n patho.* Zellnekrose *f*.
me·ro·ne·cro·sis [ˌ-nə'krəʊsɪs] *n patho.* Zellnekrose *f*.
mer·ont ['merɑnt] *n micro.* Meront *m*.
mer·o·ra·chis·chi·sis [ˌmerərə'kɪskəsɪs] *n* Merorrhachischisis *f*, R(h)achischisis partialis.
mer·or·rha·chis·chi·sis *n* → merorachischisis.
me·ros·mia [mə'rɑsmɪə] *n* Merosmie *f*, partielle/elektive Anosmie *f*.
mer·o·sys·tol·ic [ˌmerəsɪs'tɑlɪk] *adj card.* merosystolisch.
me·rot·o·my [mə'rɑtəmɪ] *n* Merotomie *f*.
mer·o·zo·ite [ˌmerə'zəʊaɪt] *n micro.* Merozoit *m*.
mer·o·zy·gote [ˌ-'zaɪgəʊt, -'zɪ-] *n micro.* Merozygote *f*.
Merrifield ['merɪfiːld]: **M. technique** *biochem.* Merrifield-Technik *f*.
mer·sal·yl [mer'sælɪl, -liːl] *n pharm.* Mersalyl *nt*.
Mer·se·burg triad ['mɜrsəbʊrk] Merseburger Trias *f*.
Méry [me'ri]: **M.'s glands** Cowper'-Drüsen *pl*, Bulbourethraldrüsen *pl*, Gll. bulbourethrales.
Merzbacher-Pelizaeus ['mertsbækər pelɪ'zaɪəs; 'mɜrtsbaxər peːli'tsɛʊs]:
M.-P. disease Pelizaeus-Merzbacher--Krankheit *f*, -Syndrom *nt*, orthochromatische Leukodystrophie *f*, sudanophile Leukodystrophie *f* Typ Pelizaeus--Merzbacher.
mes- *pref.* Mes(o)-.
me·sal [mezl, 'miː-] *adj* → mesial.
mes·an·gi·al [mes'ændʒɪəl] *adj* Mesangium betr., mesangial, Mesangial-.
mesangial cell Mesangial-, Mesangiumzelle *f*.
mes·an·gi·o·cap·il·lar·y [mesˌændʒɪəʊ-'kæpə'lerɪː] *adj* mesangiokapillar, -kapillär.
mesangiocapillary glomerulonephritis membranoproliferative Glomerulonephritis *f*.
mes·an·gi·o·pro·lif·er·a·tive glomerulonephritis [ˌ-prə'lɪfəˌreɪtɪv] mesangioproliferative Glomerulonephritis *f*.
mes·an·gi·um [mes'ændʒɪəm] *n* Mesangium *nt*.
mes·a·or·ti·tis [ˌmesɪɔː'raɪtɪs] *n* Entzündung *f* der Aortenmedia, Mediaentzündung *f* der Aorta, Mesaortitis *f*.
mes·a·ra·ic [ˌmezə'reɪɪk] *adj* → mesenteric.
mes·a·re·ic [ˌmezə'reɪɪk] *adj* → mesenteric.
mes·ar·te·ri·tis [mesɑːrtɪ'raɪtɪs] *n* Mediaentzündung *f*, Mesarteritis *f*.
me·sat·i·ce·phal·ic [meˌsætɪsɪ'fælɪk, ˌmesətɪ-] *adj* mesozephal, mesokephal, normokephal, normozephal.
me·sat·i·pel·lic pelvis [ˌ-'pelɪk] rundes Becken *nt*.
mes·ax·on [mes'æksɑn] *n* Mesaxon *nt*.
mes·ca·line ['meskəliːn] *n* Meskalin *nt*, Mescalin *nt*.
mes·ca·lism ['meskəlɪzəm] *n* Mescalinintoxikation *f*, Mescalismus *m*, Mescalinismus *m*.
mes·ec·to·derm [mes'ektədərm] *n embryo.* Mesektoderm *nt*.
mes·en·ce·phal [mes'ensəfæl] *n* → mesencephalon.
mes·en·ce·phal·ic [mesˌensə'fælɪk, ˌmesən-] *adj* Mittelhirn/Mesencephalon betr., mesenzephalisch, Mesencephalon-, Mittelhirn-.
mesencephalic arteries Mittelhirnarterien *pl*, Aa. mesencephalicae.
mesencephalic flexure *embryo.* Scheitelbeuge *f*.
mesencephalic nucleus Nc. mesencephalicus.
trigeminal m. oberer Trigeminuskern *m*, Mittelhirnkern *m* des N. trigeminus, Nc. tractus mesencephalici n. trigeminalis, Nc. mesencephalicus trigeminalis, Nc. mesencephalicus n. trigeminalis.
m. of trigeminal nerve → trigeminal m.
mesencephalic tegmentum Mittelhirnhaube *f*, Tegmentum mesencephalicum.
mesencephalic tract of trigeminal nerve Mittelhirnabschnitt *m* des N. trigemini, Tractus mesencephalicus n. trigeminalis.
mesencephalic veins Mittelhirn-, Hirnstammvenen *pl*, Vv. mesencephalicae, Vv. trunci encephalici.
mes·en·ceph·a·li·tis [mesˌensefə'laɪtɪs, ˌmesən-] *n* Mittelhirnentzündung *f*, Mesencephalonentzündung *f*, Mesenzephalitis *f*, Mesencephalitis *f*.
mes·en·ceph·a·lon [ˌmesən'sefələn] *n* Mittelhirn *nt*, Mesenzephalon *nt*, Mesencephalon *nt*.
mesencephalon vesicle *embryo.* Mittelhirnbläschen *nt*.
mes·en·ceph·a·lot·o·my [ˌmesənˌsefə'lɑtəmɪ] *n neurochir.* Mesenzephalotomie *f*.
me·sen·chy·ma [mɪ'zeŋkɪmə] *n* Mesenchym *nt*, embryonales Bindegewebe *nt*.
mes·en·chy·mal [mes'eŋkɪməl] *adj* Mesenchym betr., aus Mesenchym enstehend, mesenchymal, Mesenchym-.

mesenchymal cell

mesenchymal cell Mesenchymzelle f.
mesenchymal chondrosarcoma mesenchymales Chondrosarkom nt.
mesenchymal tissue → mesenchyma.
mesenchymal tumor mesenchymaler Tumor m.
mes·en·chyme ['mes(ə)ŋkaɪm] n → mesenchyma.
mes·en·chy·mo·ma [ˌmesənkaɪ'məʊmə] n patho. Mesenchymom(o) nt.
mes·en·te·rec·to·my [ˌmesəntə'rektəmɪ] n chir. Mesenteriumresektion f, Mesenterektomie f.
mes·en·ter·ic [ˌmesən'terɪk] adj Mesenterium betr., zum Mesenterium gehörend, mesenterisch, mesenterial, Mesenterial-, Gekröse(n)-.
mesenteric adenitis → mesenteric lymphadenitis.
acute m. → mesenteric lymphadenititis, acute.
mesenteric arterial thrombosis Mesenterialarterienthrombose f.
mesenteric arteriogram radiol. Arteriogramm nt der Mesenterialarterien.
mesenteric arteriography radiol. Arteriographie f der Mesenterialarterien.
mesenteric artery: inferior m. Mesenterica f inferior, A. mesenterica inferior.
superior m. Mesenterica f superior, A. mesenterica superior.
mesenteric canal embryo. Canalis neurentericus.
mesenteric cyst Mesenterialzyste f.
mesenteric diverticulum mesenteriales Dünndarmdivertikel nt.
mesenteric ganglion: inferior m. Ggl. mesentericum inferius.
superior m. Ggl. mesentericum superius.
mesenteric hernia Hernia mesentericoparietalis.
mesenteric infarction Mesenterialinfarkt m.
mesenteric ischemia, acute → mesenteric infarction.
mesenteric lymphadenitis Mesenteriallymphadenitis f, Lymphadenitis mesenterica/mesenterialis, Entzündung f der Mesenteriallymphknoten.
acute m. Masshoff'-Lymphadenitis, Lymphadenitis mesenterialis acuta.
mesenteric lymph nodes Mesenteriallymphknoten pl, Nodi lymphatici mesenterici.
inferior m. untere Mesenteriallymphknoten pl, Nodi lymphatici mesenterici inferiores.
superior m. obere Mesenteriallymphknoten pl, Nodi lymphatici mesenterici superiores, Nodi superiores centrales.
mes·en·ter·i·co·pa·ri·e·tal fossa/recess [mesənˌterɪkəʊpə'raɪɪtl] Broesike'-Raum m, Fossa parajejunalis.
mesenteric plexus: inferior m. Plexus mesentericus inferior.
superior m. Plexus mesentericus superior.
mesenteric vascular embolus Mesenterialgefäßembolus m.
mesenteric vascular thrombosis Mesenterialgefäßthrombose f.
mesenteric vein: inferior m. untere Mesenterialvene f, V. mesenterica inferior.
superior m. obere Mesenterialvene f, V. mesenterica superior.
mesenteric vessels Mesenterialgefäße pl.
mes·en·ter·i·o·lum [ˌmesəntər'ɪəʊləm] n, pl -la [-lə] anat. Mesenteriolum nt.
mes·en·ter·i·o·pex·y [ˌmesən'terɪəʊpeksɪ] n chir. Mesenteriumfixation f, Mesenteriopexie f.
mes·en·ter·i·or·rha·phy [ˌmesənˌterɪ'ɔrəfɪ] n chir. Mesenteriumnaht f, Mesenteriorrhaphie f, Mesorrhaphie f.
mes·en·ter·i·pli·ca·tion [ˌmesənˌterɪplɪ'keɪʃn] n chir. Mesenteriplikation f.
mes·en·ter·i·tis [ˌmesəntə'raɪtɪs] n Mesenteriumentzündung f, Mesenteritis f.
mes·en·te·ri·um [ˌmes(ə)n'tɪərɪəm] n, pl -ria [-rɪə] → mesentery.
mes·en·ter·on [mes'entərən] n embryo. Mitteldarm m, Mesenteron nt.
mes·en·ter·y ['mesənˌterɪː] n, pl -ter·ies 1. (Dünndarm-)Gekröse nt, Mesenterium nt. 2. Bauchfellduplikatur f.
m. of ascending (part of) colon Meso(kolon) nt des aufsteigenden Kolons, Mesocolon ascendens.
m. of descending (part of) colon Meso(kolon) nt des Colon descendens, Mesocolon descendens.
m. of rectum Mesorektum nt.
m. of sigmoid colon Meso(kolon) nt des Sigmas, Mesosigma nt, Mesocolon sigmoideum.
m. of transverse (part of) colon Meso(kolon) nt des Colon transversum, Mesocolon transversum.
m. of vermiform appendix Mesoappendix nt.
mes·en·tor·rha·phy [ˌmesən'tɔrəfɪ] n → mesenteriorrhaphy.
mes·ep·i·the·li·um [mesepɪ'θiːlɪəm] n → mesothelium.
mesh graft [meʃ] Mesh-Graft f/nt, Mesh--Transplantat nt, Maschen-, Gittertransplantat nt.
mesh·work ['meʃwɜrk] n Netzwerk nt, Maschen pl.
me·si·al ['meziəl, 'miː-] adj anat., dent. mesial.
me·si·o·dens ['meziədenz, 'miːz-] n anat., dent. Mesiodont m, Mesiodens m.
me·sit·y·lene [mɪ'sɪtliːn] n Mesitylen nt.
meso- pref. Mes(o)-.
meso-aortitis n → mesaortitis.
mes·o·ap·pen·di·ci·tis [ˌmezəʊəˌpendə-'saɪtɪs] n Entzündung f der Mesoappendix, Mesoappendizitis f, -appendicitis f.
mes·o·ap·pen·dix [ˌ-ə'pendɪks] n, pl -dix·es, -di·ces [-dɪsiːz] Mesoappendix nt.
mes·o·ar·ri·al [ˌ-'eərɪəl] adj → mesoarterial.
mes·o·ar·i·um [ˌ-'eərɪəm] n → mesovarium.
mes·o·a·tri·al shunt [ˌ-'eɪtrɪəl] chir. mesoatriale Anastomose f, mesoatrialer Shunt m.
mes·o·bi·lin [ˌ-'baɪlɪn] n Mesobilin nt.
mes·o·bil·i·ru·bin [ˌ-'bɪlərʊbɪn] n Mesobilirubin nt.
mes·o·bil·i·ru·bin·o·gen [ˌ-ˌbɪləruː'bɪnədʒən] n Mesobilirubinogen nt.
mes·o·bil·i·vi·o·lin [ˌ-ˌbɪlə'vaɪəlɪn] n Mesobiliviolin nt.
mes·o·blast ['blæst] n embryo. mittleres Keimblatt nt, Mesoblast m, Mesoderm nt.
mes·o·blas·te·ma [ˌ-blæ'stiːmə] n Mesoblastem nt.
mes·o·blas·tic [ˌ-'blæstɪk] adj Mesoblast/Mesoderm betr., mesoblastisch, mesodermal.
mesoblastic segment Ursegment nt, Somit m.
mes·o·bron·chi·tis [ˌ-brɒŋ'kaɪtɪs] n patho. Mesobronchitis f.
mes·o·car·dia [ˌ-'kɑrdɪə] n patho. Mesokardie f.
mes·o·car·di·um [ˌ-'kɑrdɪəm] n embryo. Mesokard nt.
mes·o·ca·val shunt [ˌ-'keɪvəl, -'kɑ-] chir. mesokavale Anastomose f, mesokavaler Shunt m.
mes·o·ce·cal [ˌ-'siːkəl] adj Mesozäkum betr.
mes·o·ce·cum [ˌ-'siːkəm] n Mesozäkum nt, Mesoc(a)ecum nt.
mes·o·ce·phal·ic [ˌ-sɪ'fælɪk] adj 1. mesozephal, mesokephal, normokephal, normozephal. 2. Mittelhirn/Mesencephalon betr., mesenzephalisch, Mesencephalon-, Mittelhirn-.
mes·o·ceph·a·lon [ˌ-'sefələn] n → mesencephalon.
mes·o·ceph·a·lous [ˌ-'sefələs] adj → mesocephalic.
Mes·o·ces·toi·des [ˌ-ses'tɔɪdiːz] pl micro. Mesocestoides pl.
Mes·o·ces·toi·di·dae [ˌ-ses'tɔɪdɪdiː] pl micro. Mesocestoididae pl.
mes·o·chon·dri·um [ˌ-'kɑndrɪəm] n Mesochondrium nt.
mes·o·cho·roi·dea [ˌ-kə'rɔɪdɪə] n Mesochoroidea f.
mes·o·col·ic [ˌ-'kɑlɪk] adj Mesokolon betr., mesokolisch.
mesocolic band → mesocolic taenia.
mesocolic taenia mesokolische Tänie f, Taenia mesocolica.
mes·o·co·lon [ˌ-'kəʊlən] n, pl -lons, -la [-lə] Mesokolon nt, -colon nt.
mes·o·co·lo·pex·y [ˌ-'kəʊləpeksɪ] n chir. Mesokolonfixation f, Mesokolopexie f.
mes·o·co·lo·pli·ca·tion [ˌ-ˌkəʊləplaɪ'keɪʃn] n chir. Mesokoloplikation f.
mes·o·cor·nea [ˌ-'kɔrnɪə] n Mesokornea f, Substantia propria corneae.
mes·o·cor·tex [ˌ-'kɔrteks] n Übergangskortex m, Mesokortex m, -cortex m.
mes·o·cu·ne·i·form [ˌkjuːnɪəfɔːrm] n anat. Os cuneiforme intermedium.
mes·o·cy·to·ma [ˌ-saɪ'təʊmə] n Bindegewebstumor m.
mes·o·derm ['-dɜrm] n embryo. mittleres/drittes Keimblatt nt, Mesoderm nt; Mesoblast m.
mes·o·der·mal [ˌ-'dɜrml] adj Mesoderm betr., vom Mesoderm ausgehend, aus dem Mesoderm entstehend, mesodermal, Mesoderm(al)-.
mesodermal cell Mesodermzelle f.
mesodermal segment Ursegment nt, Somit m.
mes·o·der·mic [ˌ-'dɜrmɪk] adj → mesodermal.
mes·o·di·as·tol·ic [ˌmezəʊdaɪə'stɑlɪk] adj mesodiastolisch.
mes·o·du·o·de·nal [ˌ-ˌd(j)uːə'diːnl, -d(j)uː-'ɑdnəl] adj Mesoduodenum betr., mesoduodenal.
mes·o·du·o·de·num [ˌ-ˌd(j)uːə'diːnəm, -d(j)uː'ɑdnəm] n embryo. Mesoduodenum nt.
mes·o·en·ter·i·o·lum [ˌ-entə'rɪələm] n → mesenteriolum.
mes·o·ep·i·did·y·mis [ˌ-epɪ'dɪdɪmɪs] n Mesoepididymis f.
mes·o·e·soph·a·gus [ˌ-ɪ'sɑfəgəs] n Mesoösophagus m.
meso form meso-Form f.
mes·o·gas·ter [ˌ-'gæstər] n → mesogastrium.
mes·o·gas·tric [ˌ-'gæstrɪk] adj Mesogastrium betr., mesogastrisch.
mesogastric fossa Rec. duodenalis superior.
mes·o·gas·tri·um [ˌ-'gæstrɪəm] n embryo. Mesogastrium nt.
me·sog·lia [mɪ'sɑglɪə] n Mesoglia f, Hortega-Glia f, -Zellen pl.
mes·o·gli·al cells [ˌmezə'glɪəl] → mesoglia.
mes·o·glu·te·us [ˌ-'gluːtɪəs] n anat. M. glut(a)eus medius.
mes·o·hy·lo·ma [ˌ-haɪ'ləʊmə] n → mesothelioma.
mes·o·il·e·um [ˌ-'ɪlɪəm] n Mesoileum nt.

meso-inositol n Meso-, Myo-Inosit nt, Meso-, Myo-Inositol nt.
mes·o·je·ju·num [ˌ-dʒɪˈdʒuːnəm] n Mesojejunum nt.
mes·o·lec·i·thal [ˌ-ˈlesɪθəl] adj bio. mesolezithal.
mes·o·me·lia [ˌ-ˈmiːlɪə] n embryo. Mesomelie f.
mes·o·mel·ic [ˌ-ˈmelɪk, -ˈmiː-] adj embryo. Mesomelie betr., mesomel.
mes·o·mere [ˈ-mɪər] n Mesomere f.
mes·o·mer·ic [ˌ-ˈmerɪk] adj Mesomerie betr., mesomer.
me·som·er·ism [mɪˈzɑmərɪzəm] n Strukturresonanz f, Mesomerie f.
mes·o·me·tri·tis [ˌmezəʊmɪˈtraɪtɪs] n → myometritis.
mes·o·me·tri·um [ˌ-ˈmɪtrɪəm] n 1. Mesometrium nt. 2. → myometrium.
mes·o·mor·phic [ˌ-ˈmɔːrfɪk] adj Mesomorphie betr., mesomorph.
mes·o·mor·phy [ˈ-mɔːrfɪ] n Mesomorphie f.
me·som·u·la [mɪˈsɑmjələ] n bio., embryo. Mesomula f.
me·son [ˈmiːzɑn, ˈmez-] n Meson nt.
mes·o·neph·ric [ˌmezəˈnefrɪk] adj embryo. Urnieren/Mesonephros betr., mesonephrogen, Urnieren-, Mesonephros-.
mesonephric adenocarcinoma → mesonephroma.
mesonephric duct embryo. Wolff-Gang m, Urnierengang m, Ductus mesonephricus.
mesonephric ridge embryo. Urnierenleiste f.
mesonephric system embryo. Urnierensystem nt.
mesonephric tissue embryo. Urnierengewebe nt.
mesonephric tubules embryo. Urnierenkanälchen pl.
mes·o·ne·phro·ma [ˌ-nəˈfrəʊmə] n patho. Mesonephrom(a) nt.
mes·o·neph·ron [ˌ-ˈnefrən] n → mesonephros.
mes·o·neph·ros [ˌ-ˈnefrɑs] n, pl -roi [-rɔɪ] embryo. Urniere f, Wolff-Körper m, Mesonephron nt, Mesonephros m.
meso-omentum n Mesoomentum nt.
mes·o·pal·li·um [ˌ-ˈpælɪəm] n Paläopallium nt, Pal(a)eopallium nt.
mes·o·pex·y [ˈ-peksɪ] n → mesenteriopexy.
mes·o·phile [ˈ-faɪl, -fɪl] I n bio. mesophiler Organismus m. II adj → mesophilic.
mes·o·phil·ic [ˌ-ˈfɪlɪk] adj bio. mesophil.
mesophilic bacterium mesophiles Bakterium nt.
me·soph·i·lous [mɪˈzɑfələs] adj → mesophilic.
mes·o·phle·bi·tis [ˌmezəʊflɪˈbaɪtɪs] n patho. Mediaentzündung f einer Vene, Mesophlebitis f.
mes·o·phrag·ma [ˌ-ˈfrægmə] n → M band.
me·soph·ry·on [məˈzæfrɪən, -ɑn] n anat. Mesophryon nt.
mes·o·phyll [ˈmezəfɪl] n bio. Mesophyll nt.
mesophyll cells bio. Mesophyllzellen pl.
mes·o·pneu·mon [ˌ-ˈnjuːmɑn, -ˈnʊ-] n embryo. Mesopneumonium nt.
mes·o·pneu·mo·ni·um [ˌ-ˌnjuːˈməʊnɪəm, -ˈnʊ-] n → mesopneumon.
mes·o·por·phy·rin [ˌ-ˈpɔːrfɪrɪn] n Mesoporphyrin nt.
mes·o·ra·chis·chi·sis [ˌ-rəˈkɪskəsɪs] n → merorachischisis.
me·sor·chi·um [mɪˈsɔːrkɪəm] n, pl -chia [-kɪə] Mesorchium nt.
mes·o·rec·tum [ˌmezəʊˈrektəm] n Mesorektum nt.
mes·or·rha·chis·chi·sis [ˌ-rəˈkɪskəsɪs] n → merorachischisis.

mes·or·rha·phy [məˈsɔrəfɪ] n → mesenteriorrhaphy.
mes·o·sal·pinx [ˌmezəʊˈsælpɪŋks] n, pl -sal·pinges [-sælˈpɪndʒiːz] Mesosalpinx f.
mes·o·sig·moid [ˌ-ˈsɪgmɔɪd] n Meso(kolon nt) nt des Sigmas, Mesosigma nt, Mesocolon sigmoideum.
mes·o·sig·moi·di·tis [ˌ-ˌsɪgmɔɪˈdaɪtɪs] n Mesosigmaentzündung f.
mes·o·sig·moi·do·pex·y [ˌ-sɪgˈmɔɪdəpeksɪ] n chir. Mesosigmoidopexie f.
mes·o·some [ˈ-səʊm] n bio. Mesosom nt.
mes·o·ste·ni·um [ˌ-ˈstiːnɪəm] n → mesentery.
mes·o·ster·num [ˌ-ˈstɜrnəm] n anat. Corpus sterni.
mes·o·sys·tol·ic [ˌ-sɪsˈtɑlɪk] adj mesosystolisch.
mes·o·ten·di·ne·um [ˌ-tenˈdɪnɪəm] n Mesotendineum nt, Mesotenon m.
mes·o·ten·don [ˌ-ˈtendən] n → mesotendineum.
mes·o·ten·on [ˌ-ˈtenən] n → mesotendineum.
mes·o·the·li·al [ˌ-ˈθiːlɪəl] adj Mesothel betr., mesothelial, Mesothel-.
mesothelial cell Mesothelzelle f.
mesothelial tumor mesothelialer Tumor m.
mes·o·the·li·o·ma [ˌ-ˌθiːlɪˈəʊmə] n Mesotheliom(a) nt.
mes·o·the·li·um [ˌ-ˈθiːlɪəm] n Mesothel nt.
mes·oth·e·nar [mesˈæθɪnɑːr] n anat. M. adductor pollicis.
mes·o·tho·ri·um [ˌmezəˈθɔːrɪəm, -ˈθəʊr-, ˌmiːz-] n Mesothorium nt.
mes·o·tron [ˈ-trɑn] n → meson.
mes·o·trop·ic [ˌ-ˈtrɑpɪk, -ˈtrəʊp-] adj mesotrop.
mes·o·tym·pa·num [ˌ-ˈtɪmpənəm] n Mesotympanum nt, Mesotympanicum nt.
mes·o·var·i·al [ˌ-ˈveərɪəl] adj Mesovarium betr., mesovarial, Mesovarial-.
mesovarial margin of ovary Mesovarial-, Vorderrand f des Eierstocks/Ovars, Margo mesovaricus (ovarii).
mes·o·var·i·an [ˌ-ˈveərɪən] adj → mesovarial.
mes·o·var·i·um [ˌ-ˈveərɪəm] n, pl -var·ia [-ˈveərɪə] Mesovarium nt.
mes·sen·ger [ˈmesɪndʒər] I n Bote m. II adj genet. biochem. Boten-.
messenger RNA abbr. **mRNA** Boten-, Matrizen-, Messenger-RNA f abbr. mRNA, Boten-, Messenger-, Matrizen--RNS f abbr. mRNS.
messenger substance biochem. Botensubstanz f, -stoff m.
mes·ter·o·lone [mesˈterələʊn] n pharm. Mesterolon nt.
mes·tra·nol [ˈmestrənɔl, -nɑl] n pharm. Mestranol nt.
me·sul·phen [mɪˈsʌlfən] n pharm. Mesulfen nt.
mes·y·late [ˈmesɪleɪt] n Methansulfonat nt.
Met abbr. → methionine.
met(a)- pref. 1. Über-, Met(a)-. 2. abbr. **m-** chem. meta- abbr. m-.
me·tab·a·sis [məˈtæbəsɪs] n patho. Übergang m, Metabasis f.
met·a·bi·o·sis [ˌmetəbaɪˈəʊsɪs] n micro. Metabiose f.
met·a·bol·ic [ˌ-ˈbɑlɪk] adj 1. Stoffwechsel/ Metabolismus betr., stoffwechselbedingt, metabolisch, Stoffwechsel-. 2. bio. veränderlich, s. verwandelnd.
metabolic acidosis metabolische/stoffwechselbedingte Azidose f.
metabolic activity → metabolism.
metabolic adaptation metabolische Anpassung/Adaptation f.

metacarpal artery

metabolic alkalosis metabolische/stoffwechselbedingte Alkalose f.
metabolic antagonism metabolischer Antagonismus m.
metabolic antagonist metabolischer Antagonist m, Stoffwechselantagonist m.
metabolic autoregulation metabolische Autoregulation f.
metabolic block biochem. Stoffwechselblock m.
metabolic calculus Cholesterinstein m.
metabolic cataract metabolische/stoffwechselbedingte Katarakt f.
metabolic chemistry physiologische Chemie f, Biochemie f.
metabolic cirrhosis metabolische Leberzirrhose f, Leberzirrhose f bei Stoffwechseldefekt.
metabolic coma metabolisches Koma nt.
metabolic degradation Stoffwechseldegradation f, metabolische Degradation f.
metabolic disease Stoffwechselerkrankung f.
metabolic disorder Stoffwechselstörung f.
metabolic encephalopathy metabolische Enzephalopathie f.
metabolic energy Stoffwechselenergie f, metabolische Energie f.
metabolic hormone Stoffwechselhormon nt.
metabolic myopathy metabolische/stoffwechselbedingte Myopathie f.
metabolic pathway Stoffwechselweg m.
metabolic poison Stoffwechselgift nt.
metabolic product Stoffwechselprodukt nt.
metabolic rate physiol. Stoffwechselumsatz m.
 basal m. abbr. **BMR** Basal-, Grundumsatz abbr. GU, basal metabolic rate abbr. BMR.
 leisure m. Freizeitumsatz m.
 m. at rest Ruheumsatz m.
 working m. Arbeitsumsatz m.
metabolic regulation Stoffwechselkontrolle f, -regulation f.
metabolic response Stoffwechselreaktion f, metabolische Reizantwort/Reaktion f.
metabolic stone Cholesterinstein m.
metabolic turnover biochem. Stoffwechselsumsatz m.
metabolic water Verbrennungswasser nt.
met·a·bo·lim·e·ter [ˌ-bəˈlɪmɪtər] n physiol. Metabolimeter nt.
met·a·bo·lim·e·try [ˌ-bəˈlɪmɪtrɪ] n physiol. Stoffwechselmessung f, Metabolimetrie f.
me·tab·o·lism [məˈtæbəlɪzəm] n physiol. Stoffwechsel m, Metabolismus m.
me·tab·o·lite [məˈtæbəlaɪt] n Stoffwechsel-(zwischen)produkt nt, Metabolit m.
metabolite transport Metabolitentransport m.
me·tab·o·liz·a·ble [məˈtæbəlaɪzəbl] adj im Stoffwechsel abbaubar, metabolisierbar.
me·tab·o·lize [məˈtæbəlaɪz] vt, vi verstoffwechseln, umwandeln, metabolisieren.
met·a·car·pal [ˌmetəˈkɑːrpl] I ~ pl → metacarpal bones. II adj Mittelhand(knochen) betr., metakarpal, Mittelhand-, Metakarpal-.
metacarpal artery: dorsal m.ies dorsale Mittelhandarterien pl, Aa. metacarpales dorsales.
 palmar m.ies palmare Mittelhandarterien pl, Aa. metacarpales palmares.
 ulnar m.ies gemeinsame palmare Fingerarterien pl, Aa. digitales palmares communes.
 volar m., deep Ramus palmaris profundus a. ulnaris.

metacarpal bones

metacarpal bones Mittelhand-, Metakarpalknochen *pl*, Metacarpalia *pl*, Ossa metacarpi.
metacarpal fracture Mittelhandbruch *m*, Metakarpalfraktur *f*.
metacarpal head Metakarpalköpfchen *nt*, Caput metacarpale.
metacarpal ligament Lig. metacarpale.
   dorsal m.s Ligg. metacarpalia dorsalia.
   interosseous m.s Ligg. metacarpalia interossea.
   palmar m.s Ligg. metacarpalia palmaria.
   transverse m., deep Lig. metacarpale transversum profundum.
   transverse m., superficial Lig. metacarpale transversum superficiale.
metacarpal veins: dorsal (interosseous) m. dorsale Mittelhandvenen *pl*, Vv. metacarpales dorsales.
   palmar m. palmare Mittelhandvenen *pl*, Vv. metacarpales palmares.
met·a·car·pec·to·my [ˌ-kɑːr'pektəmi] *n ortho*. Metakarpalknochenexzision *f*, -resektion *f*.
metacarpo- *pref*. Mittelhand-, Metakarpo-.
met·a·car·po·car·pal [-ˌkɑːrpəʊ'kɑːrpl] *adj* Handwurzel(knochen) u. Mittelhand(knochen) betr., karpometakarpal, Karpometakarpal-.
metacarpocarpal articulation Karpometakarpalgelenk *nt*, Artic. carpometacarpale.
metacarpocarpal joint → metacarpocarpal articulation.
met·a·car·po·pha·lan·ge·al [ˌ-ˌkɑːrpəʊfə-'lændʒɪəl] *adj abbr*. **MCP** Mittelhand(knochen) u. Finger betr., metakarpophalangeal, Metakarpophalangeal-.
metacarpophalangeal articulation → metacarpophalangeal joint.
metacarpophalangeal joint *abbr*. **MCPJ** Fingergrundgelenk *nt*, Metakarpophalangealgelenk *nt*, MP-Gelenk *nt*, Artic. metacarpophalangeis.
metacarpophalangeal ligaments Ligg. palmaria.
met·a·car·po·the·nar reflex [ˌ-ˌkɑːrpəʊ-'θiːnɑːr] Daumenreflex *m*.
met·a·car·pus [ˌ-'kɑːrpəs] *n*, *pl* **-pi** [-paɪ] Mittelhand *f*, Metakarpus *m*.
met·a·cele *n* → metacoele.
met·a·cen·tric [ˌ-'sentrɪk] *adj* metazentrisch.
metacentric chromosome metazentrisches Chromosom *nt*.
met·a·cer·car·ia [ˌ-sɜːr'keəriə] *n*, *pl* **-riae** [-riˌiː] *micro*. Metazerkarie *f*.
met·a·chro·ma·sia [ˌ-krəʊ'meɪziə] *n histol*. Metachromasie *f*.
met·a·chro·mat·ic [ˌ-krəʊ'mætɪk, -krə-] *adj* metachromatisch.
metachromatic bodies Volutinkörnchen *pl*, metachromatische Granula *pl*, Babès-Ernst-Körperchen *pl*.
metachromatic dye metachromatischer Farbstoff *m*.
metachromatic granules → metachromatic bodies.
metachromatic leukodystrophy metachromatische Leukodystrophie/Leukoenzephalopathie *f*.
metachromatic leukoencephalopathy/leukoencephaly → metachromatic leukodystrophy.
met·a·chro·ma·tin [ˌ-'krəʊmətɪn] *n* Metachromatin *nt*.
met·a·chro·ma·tism [ˌ-'krəʊmətɪzəm] *n* → metachromasia.
met·a·chro·mia [ˌ-'krəʊmɪə] *n* → metachromasia.
met·a·chro·mic [ˌ-'krəʊmɪk] *adj* → metachromatic.

met·a·chro·mo·phil [ˌ-'krəʊməfɪl] *adj* → metachromatic.
met·a·chro·mo·phile [ˌ-'krəʊməfaɪl] *adj* → metachromatic.
met·a·chro·mo·some [ˌ-'krəʊməsəʊm] *n* Metachromosom *nt*.
me·tach·ro·nous [mə'tækrənəs] *adj* zu verschiedenen Zeiten auftretend, metachron.
me·tach·y·sis [mə'tækəsɪs] *n* Bluttransfusion *f*.
met·a·coele ['metəsiːl] *n* 1. Metazöl *nt*. 2. Metazölom *nt*.
met·a·coe·lo·ma [ˌ-sɪ'ləʊmə] *n* → metacoele 2.
met·a·cor·tan·dra·cin [ˌ-kɔːr'tændrəsɪn] *n pharm*. Prednison *nt*.
met·a·cor·tan·dra·lone [ˌ-kɔːr'tændrələʊn] *n pharm*. Prednisolon *nt*.
met·a·cre·sol [ˌ-'kriːsɔl, -sɑl] *n m*-Kresol *nt*, meta-Kresol *nt*.
met·a·cryp·to·zo·ite [ˌ-krɪptə'zəʊaɪt] *n micro*. Metakryptozoit *n*.
met·a·cy·e·sis [ˌ-saɪ'iːsɪs] *n* extrauterine/ektope Schwangerschaft *f*, Extrauteringravidität *f*.
met·a·cyst ['-sɪst] *n* Metazyste *f*.
met·a·du·o·de·num [ˌ-ˌd(j)uːəʊ'diːnəm] *n* Metaduodenum *nt*.
me·ta·fe·male [ˌ-'fiːmeɪl] *n genet*. 1. Metafemale *f*, Patientin *f* mit Drei-X-Syndrom *nt*. 2. Drei-X-Syndrom *nt*, Triplo-X-Syndrom *nt*, XXX-Syndrom *nt*.
met·a·gas·tru·la [ˌ-'gæstrʊlə] *n embryo*. Metagastrula *f*.
met·a·gen·e·sis [ˌ-'dʒenəsɪs] *n bio*. Ammenzeugung *f*, Metagenese *f*, -genesis *f*.
met·a·go·ni·mi·a·sis [ˌ-ˌgəʊnɪ'maɪəsɪs] *n* Metagonimus-Befall *m*, Metagonimiasis *f*, Metagonimose *f*.
Met·a·gon·i·mus [ˌ-'gɑnɪməs] *n micro*. Metagonimus *m*.
M. ovatus/yokogawai Metagonimus yokogawai.
met·a·he·mo·glo·bin [ˌ-'hiːməgləʊbɪn, -'hemə-] *n* → methemoglobin.
met·a·her·pet·ic keratitis [ˌ-hɜr'petɪk] Keratitis metaherpetica.
met·a·ic·ter·ic [ˌ-ɪk'terɪk] *adj patho*. metaikterisch.
met·a·in·fec·tive [ˌ-ɪn'fektɪv] *adj patho*. metainfektiös.
met·a·ki·ne·sis [ˌ-kɪ'niːsɪs, -kaɪ-] *n* 1. Metakinese *f*. 2. Prometaphase *f*.
met·al ['metl] **I** *n* Metall *nt*. **II** *adj* aus Metall, metallen, Metall-.
met·al·bu·min [metæl'bjuːmən] *n* Metalbumin *nt*, Pseudomuzin *nt*.
metal catalyst Metallkatalysator *m*.
metal complexing agent *chem*. Chelatbildner *m*.
metal cover Metallüberzug *m*.
met·al·de·hyde [mɪ'tældəhaɪd, me-] *n* Metaldehyd *m*.
metal fume fever Metalldampffieber *nt*.
me·tal·lic [mə'tælɪk] *adj* 1. Metall betr., aus Metall bestehend, Metall enthaltend, metallisch, metallen, Metall(o)-. 2. (*Klang*) metallisch.
metallic oxide *chem*. Metalloxyd *nt*.
metallic rales *pulmo*. metallische Rasselgeräusche *pl*, metallisches Rasseln *nt*.
metallic sound metallisches Geräusch *nt*.
metallic tinkles (*Auskultation*) Metallklang *m*, metallisches Klingen *nt*.
me·tal·lo·cy·a·nide [məˌtæləʊ'saɪənaɪd, -nɪd] *n* Metall(o)cyanid *nt*.
me·tal·lo·en·zyme [ˌ-'enzaɪm] *n* Metall(o)enzym *nt*.
me·tal·lo·fla·vo·pro·tein [ˌ-ˌfleɪvəʊ'prəʊtiːn, -tɪn] *n* Metall(o)flavoprotein *nt*.
met·al·loid ['metlɔɪd] **I** *n* Nicht-, Halbme-

tall *nt*, Metalloid *nt*. **II** *adj* metallähnlich, metalloid(isch).
met·al·loi·dal ['metlɔɪdl] *adj* → metalloid II.
me·tal·lo·phil·ic [məˌtæləʊ'fɪlɪk] *adj histol*. metallophil.
me·tal·lo·pho·bia [ˌ-'fəʊbɪə] *n psychia*. Metallophobie *f*.
me·tal·lo·por·phy·rin [ˌ-'pɔːrfərɪn] *n* Metall(o)porphyrin *nt*.
me·tal·lo·pro·tein [ˌ-'prəʊtiːn, -tiːɪn] *n* Metall(o)protein *nt*.
metal-on-metal prosthesis *ortho*. Metall-Metall-Prothese *f*.
metal prosthesis Metallprothese *f*.
met·a·lu·es ['metəluːˌiːz] *n* → metasyphilis.
met·a·lu·et·ic [ˌ-luː'etɪk] *adj* → metasyphilitic.
met·a·mere ['-mɪər] *n* Metamer *nt*.
met·a·mer·ic [ˌ-'merɪk] *adj* Metamerie betr., durch Metamerie gekennzeichnet, metamer(isch).
metameric innervation metamere Innervation *f*.
met·am·er·ism [mə'tæmərɪzəm] *n anat*., *chem*., *bio*. Metamerie *f*.
met·a·mor·phop·sia [ˌmetəmɔːr'fɑpsɪə] *n ophthal*. Metamorphopsie *f*.
met·a·mor·pho·sis [ˌ-mɔːr'fəʊsɪs, -'mɔːrfəsɪs] *n* Umgestaltung *f*, -formung *f*, -wandlung *f*, Metamorphose *f*.
met·a·mor·phot·ic [ˌ-mɔːr'fɑtɪk] *adj* Metamorphose betr., von Metamorphose gekennzeichnet, metamorph(isch).
met·a·my·e·lo·cyte [ˌ-'maɪələsaɪt] *n* jugendlicher Granulozyt *m*, Metamyelozyt *m*; *inf*. Jugendlicher *m*.
met·a·neph·ric [ˌ-'nefrɪk] *adj* Nachniere/Metanephros betr., metanephrogen, Nachnieren-.
metanephric blastema *embryo*. metanephrogenes Blastem *nt*.
metanephric bud *embryo*. Ureterknospe *f*, -anlage *f*.
metanephric duct Harnleiter *m*, Ureter *m*.
metanephric mesoderm *embryo*. metanephrogenes Mesoderm *nt*.
metanephric system *embryo*. Nachnierensystem *nt*.
met·a·neph·rine [ˌ-'nefrɪn] *n* Metanephrin *nt*.
met·a·neph·ron [ˌ-'nefrɑn] *n* → metanephros.
met·a·neph·ros [ˌ-'nefrɑs] *n*, *pl* **-roi** [-rɔɪ] *embryo*. Nachniere *f*, Metanephros *nt*.
met·a·neu·tro·phil [ˌ-'n(j)uːtrəfɪl] *adj histol*. metaneutrophil.
met·a·neu·tro·phile [ˌ-'n(j)uːtrəfaɪl] *adj* → metaneutrophil.
met·a·nu·cle·us [ˌ-'n(j)uːklɪəs] *n bio*. Metanukleus *m*.
met·a·phase ['-feɪz] *n* Metaphase *f*.
metaphase plate Äquatorialplatte *f*.
metaphase spindle Metaphasenspindel *f*.
met·a·phos·phor·ic acid [ˌ-fɑs'fɔːrɪk] Metaphosphorsäure *f*.
me·taph·y·se·al [mə'tæfəsəl, ˌmetə'fiːzɪəl] *adj* Metaphyse betr., metaphysär, Metaphysen-.
metaphyseal chondrodysplasia → metaphyseal dysostosis.
metaphyseal dysostosis *ortho*. Jansen-Syndrom *nt*, Dysostosis enchondralis metaphysaria.
metaphyseal dysplasia Pyle'-Krankheit *f*, familiäre metaphysäre Dysplasie *f*.
metaphyseal fibrous cortical defect nicht-ossifizierendes Fibrom *nt*, fibröser Kortikalisdefekt *m*, fibröser metaphysärer Defekt *m*, benignes fibröses Histiozytom *nt* des Knochens.

me·taph·y·si·al *adj* → metaphyseal.
me·taph·y·sis [mə'tæfəsɪs] *n*, *pl* **-ses** [-siːz] Zone *f* zwischen Epi- u. Diaphyse, Knochenwachstumszone *f*, Metaphyse *f*, Metaphysis *f*.
me·taph·y·si·tis [ˌmetəfɪ'saɪtɪs, məˌtæfɪ-] *n ortho*. Metaphysenentzündung *f*, Metaphysitis *f*.
met·a·pla·sia [ˌmetə'pleɪʒ(ɪ)ə] *n* Metaplasie *f*.
met·a·plasm ['plæzəm] *n* Metaplasma *nt*.
met·a·plas·tic [ˌ-'plæstɪk] *adj* **1.** Metaplasie betr., durch Metaplasie gekennzeichnet, metaplastisch. **2.** Metaplasma betr., aus Metaplasma bestehend, metaplasmatisch.
metaplastic ossification ektope/ektopische Knochenbildung/Verknöcherung *f*.
met·a·plex·us [ˌ-'pleksəs] *n* Plexus choroideus des IV. Ventrikels, Plexus choroideus ventriculi quarti.
met·a·pneu·mon·ic [ˌ-n(j)u:'mɑnɪk] *adj* nach einer Pneumonie, metapneumonisch, postpneumonisch.
metapneumonic pleurisy metapneumonische/postpneumonische Pleuritis *f*.
met·a·psy·chol·o·gy [ˌ-saɪ'kɑlədʒɪ] *n psycho*. Metapsychologie *f*.
met·a·py·rone [ˌ-'paɪrəʊn] *n* → metyrapone.
met·a·ram·i·nol [ˌ-'ræmɪnɒl] *n pharm*. Metaraminol *nt*.
met·a·rho·dop·sin [ˌ-rəʊ'dɑpsɪn] *n* Metarhodopsin *nt*.
met·ar·te·ri·ole [metˌɑ:r'tɪərɪəʊl] *n* Metarteriole *f*, Präkapillare *f*.
met·a·ru·bri·cyte [ˌ-'ru:brəsaɪt] *n* azidophiler/orthochromatischer/oxaphiler Normoblast *m*.
met·a·sta·ble [ˌ-'steɪbl] *adj chem., phys.* metastabil.
me·tas·ta·sis [mə'tæstəsɪs] *n*, *pl* **-ses** [-siːz] **1.** Absiedelung *f*, Tochtergeschwulst *f*, Metastase *f*, Metastasis *f*. **2.** Metastasierung *f*, Filialisierung *f*. **3.** Abszedierung *f*, Metastasierung *f*.
me·tas·ta·size [mə'tæstəsaɪz] *vt* Metastasen bilden *od*. setzen, metastasieren.
me·tas·ta·siz·ing mole [mə'tæstəsaɪzɪŋ] *gyn*. destruierendes Chorionadenom *nt*, destruierende Blasenmole *f*.
met·a·stat·ic [ˌmetə'stætɪk] *adj* Metastase(n) betr., metastasierend, metastatisch, Metastasen-.
metastatic abscess metastatischer Abszeß *m*.
metastatic calcification/calcinosis metastatische Verkalkung/Kalzinose *f*, Calcinosis metastatica.
metastatic cancer → metastatic carcinoma.
metastatic carcinoid syndrome Flush-, Karzinoidsyndrom *nt*, Biörck-Thorson--Syndrom *nt*.
metastatic carcinoma 1. Karzinommetastase *f*, -absiedlung *f*, sekundäres Karzinom *nt*. **2.** metastasierendes Karzinom *nt*.
metastatic choroiditis *ophthal*. metastatische Chorioiditis *f*, Chorioiditis metastatica.
metastatic disease 1. Metastasierung *f*, Filialisierung *f*. **2.** Krankheit(ssymptome *pl*) *f* durch Metastasierung.
metastatic echinococcosis metastasierende Hydatidose/Echinokokkose *f*.
metastatic hydatidosis → metastatic echinococcosis.
metastatic infection Pyämie *f*, Pyohämie *f*.
metastatic inflammation metastatische Entzündung *f*.

metastatic ophthalmia 1. sympathische Ophthalmie *f*, Ophthalmia sympathica. **2.** metastatische Ophthalmie *f*, Ophthalmia metastatica.
metastatic pattern Metastasierungsmuster *nt*.
metastatic pneumonia metastatische Pneumonie *f*.
metastatic retinitis septische Retinitis *f*.
metastatic tumor Tumormetastase *f*.
met·a·ster·num [ˌ-'stɜrnəm] *n anat*. Schwertfortsatz *m*, Proc. xiphoideus.
Met·a·stron·gyl·i·dae [ˌ-ˌstrɑn'dʒɪləˌdi:] *pl micro*. Metastrongylidae *pl*.
Met·a·stron·gy·lus [ˌ-'strɑndʒələs] *n micro*. Metastrongylus *m*.
met·a·syph·i·lis [ˌ-'sɪf(ə)lɪs] *n* Metasyphilis *f*, Metalues *f*.
met·a·syph·i·lit·ic [ˌ-sɪfə'lɪtɪk] *adj* Metasyphilis betr., metasyphilitisch, metaluetisch.
met·a·tar·sal [ˌ-'tɑ:rsl] **I ~s** *pl* Mittelfuß-, Metatarsalknochen *pl*, Ossa metatarsi, Metatarsalia *pl*. **II** *adj* Mittelfuß(knochen) betr., metatarsal, Mittelfuß-, Metatarsal-.
metatarsal arteries: dorsal m. dorsale Mittelfußarterien *pl*, Aa. metatarsales dorsales.
plantar m. plantare Mittelfußarterien *pl*, Aa. metatarsales plantares.
metatarsal bones → metatarsal I.
metatarsal fracture Mittelfußbruch *m*, Metatarsalfraktur *f*.
met·a·tar·sal·gia [ˌ-tɑːr'sældʒ(ɪ)ə] *n* Mittelfußschmerz *m*, Metatarsalgie *f*.
metatarsal head Metatarsalköpfchen *nt*, Caput metatarsale.
metatarsal ligament Lig. metatarsale.
dorsal m.s Ligg. metatarsalia dorsalia.
interosseous m.s Ligg. metatarsalia interossea.
plantar m.s Ligg. metatarsea/metatarsalia plantaria.
transverse m., deep Lig. metatarsale transversum profundum.
transverse m., superficial Lig. metatarsale transversum superficiale.
metatarsal reflex Mendl's reflex.
metatarsal veins: dorsal m. dorsale Mittelfußvenen *pl*, Vv. metatarsales dorsales.
plantar m. plantare Mittelfußvenen *pl*, Vv. metatarsales plantares.
met·a·tar·sec·to·my [ˌ-tɑːr'sektəmɪ] *n ortho*. Metatarsalknochenexzision *f*, -resektion *f*, Metatarsektomie *f*.
metatarso- *pref*. Mittelfuß-, Metatarsal-.
met·a·tar·so·pha·lan·ge·al [ˌ-ˌtɑːrsəʊfə-'lændʒɪəl] *adj abbr*. **MTP** Mittelfuß(knochen) u. Zehen betr., metatarsophalangeal, Metatarsophalangeal-.
metatarsophalangeal articulation → metatarsophalangeal joint.
metatarsophalangeal joint *abbr*. **MTPJ** Zehengrundgelenk *nt*, Metatarsophalangealgelenk *nt*, MT-Gelenk *nt*, Artic. metatarsophalangealis.
met·a·tar·sus [ˌ-'tɑːrsəs] *n*, *pl* **-si** [-saɪ] Mittelfuß *m*, Metatarsus *m*.
met·a·tha·lam·ic nuclei [ˌ-θə'læmɪk] Ncc. metathalami.
met·a·thal·a·mus [ˌ-'θæləməs] *n* Metathalamus *m*.
met·a·typ·ic [ˌ-'tɪpɪk] *adj* → metatypical.
met·a·typ·i·cal [ˌ-'tɪpɪkl] *adj patho*. metatypisch.
metatypical carcinoma basosquamöses/intermediäres Karzinom *nt*.
met·a·xe·nia [ˌ-'zi:nɪə, -jə] *n bio*. Metaxenie *f*, Ektogonie *f*.
me·tax·e·ny [mɪ'tæksənɪ] *n* → metaxenia.

Met·a·zoa [ˌmetə'zəʊə] *pl bio*. Mehr-, Vielzeller *pl*, Metazoen *pl*.
met·a·zoa *pl* → metazoon.
met·a·zo·al [ˌ-'zəʊəl] *adj* → metazoan II.
met·a·zo·an [ˌ-'zəʊən] *bio*. **I** *n* → metazoon. **II** *adj* vielzellig, metazoisch.
met·a·zo·ic [ˌ-'zəʊɪk] *adj* → metazoan II.
met·a·zo·on [ˌ-'zəʊən] *n*, *pl* **-zoa** [-'zəʊə] *bio*. Mehr-, Vielzeller *m*, Metazoon *nt*.
met·en·ce·phal [ˌmetən'sefələn] *n* → metencephalon.
met·en·ce·phal·ic [ˌmetˌensɪ'fælɪk, -ˌenkə-] *adj* Nachhirn/Metenzephalon betr., Metenzephalon-.
met·en·ceph·a·lon [ˌmetən'sefələn] *n* **1.** Brücke *f*, Pons *m* (cerebri). **2.** Nachhirn *nt*, Metenzephalon *nt*, Metencephalon *nt*.
met·enkephalin *n* Met-Enkephalin *nt*, Methionin-Enkephalin *nt*.
me·te·or·ism ['mi:tɪərɪzəm] *n* Blähsucht *f*, Meteorismus *m*, Tympania *f*.
me·te·or·o·pa·thol·o·gy [ˌmi:tɪˌɔːrəpə'θɑlədʒɪ] *n* Meteoropathologie *f*.
me·te·or·o·rop·a·thy [ˌmi:tɪə'rɑpəθɪ] *n* Meteoropathie *f*.
me·te·or·o·sen·si·tive [ˌmi:tɪˌɔːrə'sensətɪv] *adj* wetterfühlig.
me·te·or·o·trop·ic [ˌ-'trɑpɪk, -'trəʊp-] *adj* durch das Wetter/Klima bedingt, meteotrop.
me·te·or·o·trop·ism [mi:tɪə'rɑtrəpɪzəm] *n* Meteorotropismus *m*, -tropie *f*.
met·ep·en·ceph·a·lon [metepən'sefələn] *n* → myelencephalon.
me·ter ['mi:tər] **I** *n* **1.** *abbr*. **m** Meter *nt*/*m abbr*. **m**. **2.** Meter *nt*, Messer *m*, Zähler *m*, Meßinstrument *nt*. **II** *vt* messen.
meter-candle *n phys*. Lux *nt abbr*. lx.
met·er·ga·sia [metər'geɪʒ(ɪ)ə] *n* → metergasis.
met·er·ga·sis [ˌ-'geɪsɪs] *n* Funktionswechsel *m*, Metergie *f*.
met·es·trum [mə'testrəm] *n* → metestrus.
met·es·trus [mə'testrəs] *n bio*. Nachbrunst *f*, Metöstrus *m*.
met·for·min [met'fɔːrmɪn] *n pharm*. Metformin *nt*.
meth·ac·ry·late [meθ'ækrəleɪt] *n* Methacrylat *nt*.
meth·a·cryl·ic acid [ˌmeθə'krɪlɪk] Methacrylsäure *f*.
meth·a·done ['meθədəʊn] *n pharm*. Methadon *nt*.
meth·am·phet·a·mine [meθæm'fetəmi:n, -mɪn] *n pharm*. Methamphetamin *nt*.
meth·ane ['meθeɪn] *n* Sumpf-, Grubengas *nt*, Methan *nt*.
methane-producing bacteria → methanogenic bacteria.
meth·ane·sul·fo·nate [ˌmeθeɪn'sʌlfəneɪt] *n* Methansulfonat *nt*.
meth·ane·sul·fon·ic acid [ˌ-sʌl'fɑnɪk] Methansulfonsäure *f*.
meth·a·no·gen ['meθənəʊdʒən] *n* methanbildender Mikroorganismus *m*, Methanbildner *m*.
meth·a·no·gen·ic [ˌ-'dʒenɪk] *adj* methanbildend.
methanogenic bacteria methanbildende Bakterien *pl*, Methanbildner *pl*.
meth·a·nol ['meθənɒl, -nɑl] *n* Methanol *nt*, Methylkohol *m*.
meth·an·the·line [meθ'ænθəli:n] *n pharm*. Methanthelin *nt*.
meth·a·qua·lone [mə'θækwələʊn, ˌmeθə-'kweɪləʊn] *n pharm*. Methaqualon *nt*.
Met-Hb *abbr*. → methemoglobin.
met·hem·al·bu·min [ˌmethi:mæl'bju:mən] *n* Methämalbumin *nt*.
met·hem·al·bu·mi·ne·mia [ˌmethemælˌbju:mɪ'ni:mɪə] *n* Methämalbuminämie *f*.

met·heme ['methi:m] *n* Hämatin *nt*, Hydroxyhämin *nt*.
met·he·mo·glo·bin [met'hi:məgləʊbɪn, -'heməˌ-] *n abbr.* **Met-Hb** Methämoglobin *nt abbr.* Met.-Hb, Hämiglobin *nt*.
met·he·mo·glo·bi·ne·mia [metˌhi:məˌgləʊbɪ'ni:mɪə] *n* erhöhter Methämoglobingehalt *m* des Blutes, Methämoglobinämie *f*.
met·he·mo·glo·bi·ne·mic [metˌhi:məˌgləʊbɪ'ni:mɪk] *adj* Methämoglobinämie betr. *od.* verursachend, methämoglobinämisch.
methemoglobin reductase (NADPH) Methämoglobinreduktase (NADPH) *f*.
met·he·mo·glo·bi·nu·ri·a [metˌhi:məˌgləʊbɪ'n(j)ʊərɪə] *n* Methämoglobinausscheidung *f* im Harn, Methämoglobinurie *f*.
me·the·na·mine [meθ'i:nəmi:n, -mɪn] *n* Methenamin *nt*, Hexamin *nt*, Hexamethylentetramin *nt*.
meth·ene ['meθi:n] *n* → methylene.
methene bridge *chem.* Methinbrücke *f*.
meth·ex·e·nyl [meθ'eksənɪl] *n pharm.* Hexobarbital *nt*.
meth·i·cil·lin [ˌmeθə'sɪlɪn] *n pharm.* Methizillin *nt*, -cillin *nt*.
methicillin sodium *pharm.* Methicillin--Natrium *nt*.
meth·im·a·zole [meθ'ɪməzəʊl, -'θaɪmə-] *n pharm.* Methimazol *nt*, Thiamazol *nt*.
meth·ine ['meθi:n, -ɪn] *n* → methylidyne.
me·thi·o·late-formaline fixative [məˈθaɪəlert] Methiolat-Formalin-Fixierlösung *f*, MF-Fixierlösung *f*.
methiolate-iodine-formaline fixative Methiolat-Iod-Formalin-Fixierlösung *f*, MIF-Fixierlösung *f*.
me·thi·o·nine [mɪˈθaɪəni:n, -nɪn] *n abbr.* **M, Met** Methionin *nt abbr.* M, Met.
methionine adenosyltransferase Methioninadenosyltransferase *f*.
methionine aminopeptidase Methioninaminopeptidase *f*.
methionine enkephalin → met-enkephalin.
methionine malabsorption syndrome Methioninmalabsorptionssyndrom *nt*.
methionine synthase → 5-methyltetrahydrofolate-homocysteine methyltransferase.
me·thi·o·nyl [məˈθaɪənɪl] *n* Methionyl-(Radikal *nt*).
methionyl-tRNA synthetase Methionyl--tRNA-synthetase *f*.
meth·is·a·zone [meθ'ɪsəzəʊn] *n* Methisazon *nt*, Marboran *nt*.
meth·o·car·ba·mol [ˌmeθəˈkɑːrbəmɒl] *n pharm., anes.*, Methocarbamol *nt*.
meth·od ['meθəd] *n* Methode *f*, Verfahren *nt*; Vorgehens-, Verfahrensweise *f*; System *nt*.
m. of application Anwendungsweise.
m. of constant stimuli *physiol.* Konstanzverfahren, Methode der konstanten Reize.
m. of measuring Meßverfahren, -methode, -technik *f*.
m. of operation Verfahrensweise, Arbeitsmethode.
m. for thyroid activity Schilddrüsenfunktionstest *m*, -analyse *f*.
me·thod·ic [məˈθɒdɪk] *adj* methodisch, planmäßig, systematisch, durchdacht.
me·thod·i·cal [məˈθɒdɪkl] *adj* methodic.
meth·o·hex·i·tal [ˌmeθəʊˈheksɪtæl] *n pharm.* Methohexital *nt*.
meth·o·ma·nia [ˌ-'meɪnɪə, -jə] *n psychia.* Methomanie *f*.
meth·o·trex·ate [ˌ-'treksert] *n pharm.* Methotrexat *nt*.
meth·o·tri·mep·ra·zine [ˌ-traɪ'meprəzi:n] *n*

pharm. Levomepromazin *nt*.
me·thox·a·len [meˈθɒksələn] *n* → 8-methoxypsoralen.
me·thox·y·chlor [məˈθɒksɪklɔːr, -klʊər] *n chem.* Methoxychlor *nt*.
meth·ox·y·flu·rane [məˌθɒksɪˈflʊəreɪn] *n anes.* Methoxifluran *nt*, Methoxyfluran *nt*.
8-me·thox·y·psor·a·len [ˌ-'sɔːrələn] *n pharm., derm.* 8-Methoxypsoralen *nt*.
meth·phen·ox·y·di·ol [meθfenˌɒksɪ'daɪɒl] *n pharm.* Guaifenesin *nt*, Guajacolglyzerinäther *m*.
meth·sco·pol·a·mine bromide [meθskə-'pɒləmi:n, -mɪn] *pharm.* Scopolaminum hydrobromicum.
meth·yl ['meθəl] *n* Methyl-(Radikal *nt*).
methyl acetal Methylacetal *nt*.
α-meth·yl·a·ce·to·ac·e·tyl CoA-β-ketothiolase [ˌmeθələˌsiːtəʊˈæsətɪl] Acetyl--CoA-Acetyltransferase *f*, (Acetoacetyl-)Thiolase *f*.
methyl adenine Methyladenin *nt*.
methyl alcohol → methanol.
methyl aldehyde Formaldehyd *m*, Ameisensäurealdehyd *m*, Methanal *nt*.
meth·yl·a·mine [ˌmeθəlˈæmi:n, -'æmɪn] *n* Methylamin *nt*.
meth·yl·ate ['meθəleɪt] *chem.* **I** *n* Methylat *nt*. **II** *vt* **1.** methylieren. **2.** denaturieren.
meth·yl·at·ed ['meθəleɪtɪd] *adj* **1.** methyliert. **2.** denaturiert, vergällt.
methylated alcohol vergällter/denaturierter Alkohol *m*.
meth·yl·a·tion [meθə'leɪʃn] *n* Methylierung *f*.
methyl benzene Toluol *nt*, Methylbenzol *nt*.
meth·yl·ben·ze·tho·ni·um chloride [ˌmeθəlˌbenzəˈθəʊnɪəm] *pharm.* Methylbenzethoniumchlorid *nt*.
meth·yl·ben·zol [ˌ-'benzɒl, -zɒl] *n* → methyl benzene.
methyl blue Methylblau *nt*.
2-methyl-1,3-butadien *n* Isopren *nt*, 2-Methyl-1,3-butadien *nt*.
methyl cellulose Methylcellulose *f*.
methyl chloride Methylchlorid *nt*, (Mono-)Chlormethan *nt*.
meth·yl·co·bal·a·mine [ˌ-kəʊˈbæləmi:n] *n* Methylcobalamin *nt*.
β-meth·yl·cro·ton·o·yl-CoA carboxylase [ˌ-krəʊˈtænəwɪl] β-Methylcrotonyl--CoA-carboxylase *f*.
β-methylcrotonyl-CoA carboxylase deficiency → β-methylcrotonylglycinuria.
β-meth·yl·cro·to·nyl·gly·ci·nu·ria [ˌ-təʊnɪlˌglaɪsɪ'n(j)ʊərɪə] *n* β-Methylcrotonyl-CoA-carboxylase-Mangel *m*, β-Methylcrotonylglycinurie *f*, β-Methylcrotonylglycinurie *f*.
methyl cyanide Acetonitril *nt*.
meth·yl·cy·to·sine [ˌ-'saɪtəsi:n, -sɪn] *n* Methylcytosin *nt*.
meth·yl·do·pa [ˌ-'dəʊpə] *n pharm.* Methyldopa *nt*.
meth·yl·ene ['meθɪliːn] *n* Methylen *nt*, Methen *nt*.
methylene blue Methylenblau *nt*, Tetramethylthioninchlorid *nt*.
methylene blue stain *histol.* Methylenblaufärbung *f*.
Löffler's alkaline m. (alkalische) Löffler'-Methylenblaufärbung.
methylene (di)chloride Methylenchlorid *nt*, Dichlormethan *nt*.
5,10-meth·yl·ene·tet·ra·hy·dro·fo·late [ˈmeθəlˌi:nˌtetrəˌhaɪdrəˈfəʊleɪt] *n* 5,10-Methylentetrahydrofolat *nt*.
5,10-methylenetetrahydrofolate reductase (FADH$_2$) 5,10-Methylentetrahydrofolatreduktase (FADH$_2$) *f*.

methylenetetrahydrofolate reductase deficiency 5,10-Methylentetrahydrofolatreduktase-Defekt *m*.
5,10-meth·yl·ene·tet·ra·hy·dro·fo·lic acid [ˌ-ˌtetrəˌhaɪdrəˈfəʊlɪk, -'fɒl-] 5,10-Methylentetrahydrofolsäure *f*.
meth·y·len·o·phil [ˌmeθəˈlenəfɪl, -'li:nə-] *adj histol.* methylenophil, leicht mit Methylenblau anfärbbar *od.* färbend.
meth·y·len·o·phile [ˌ-'lenəfaɪl, -'li:nə-] *adj* → methylenophil.
meth·y·len·o·phil·ic [ˌ-lenəˈfɪlɪk, -'li:nə-] *adj* → methylenophil.
meth·yl·e·noph·i·lous [ˌmeθəlɪˈnɒfɪləs] *adj* → methylenophil.
meth·yl·er·go·met·rine [ˌmeθəlˌɜːrɡəʊˈmetriːn] *n* → methylergonovine.
meth·yl·er·go·no·vine [ˌ-ˌɜːrɡəʊˈnəʊviːn] *n pharm., gyn.* Methylergometrin *nt*, Methylergonovin *nt*.
methyl ether Methyläther *m*, -ether *m*.
meth·yl·gly·cine [ˌ-'ɡlaɪsiːn] *n* Sarkosin *nt*, Methylglykokoll *nt*, -glycin *nt*.
methyl glycoside Methylglykosid *nt*.
meth·yl·gly·ox·a·lase [ˌ-ɡlaɪˈɒksəleɪz] *n* Lactoylglutathionlyase *f*, Glyoxalase I *f*.
meth·yl·guan·i·dine [ˌ-'ɡwænɪdi:n, -dɪn] *n* Methylguanidin *nt*.
N-methyl-guanidinoacetic acid Kreatin *nt*, Creatin *nt*, α-Methylguanidinoessigsäure *f*.
meth·yl·gua·nine [ˌ-'ɡwɑːniːn] *n* Methylguanin *nt*.
meth·yl·hex·a·mine [ˌ-'heksəmi:n, -heksæmɪn] *n* → methylhexaneamine.
meth·yl·hex·ane·am·ine [ˌ-ˌheksem'æmɪn] *n* Methylhexanamin *nt*, 1,3-Dimethylamylamin *nt*.
meth·yl·his·ti·dine [ˌ-'hɪstɪdi:n] *n* Methylhistidin *nt*.
meth·yl·hy·dan·to·in [ˌ-haɪ'dæntəwɪn] *n* Methylhydantoin *nt*.
methyl hydride → methane.
me·thyl·ic [meˈθɪlɪk] *adj chem.* Methyl-.
me·thyl·i·dyne [meˈθɪlɪdaɪn] *n* Methin--(Radikal *nt*).
methyl iodide Methyliodid *nt*, -jodid *nt*.
meth·yl·ly·sine [ˌmeθəlˈlaɪsiːn] *n* Methyllysin *nt*.
meth·yl·ma·lon·ic acid [ˌ-məˈlɒnɪk, -'lɑn-] Methylmalonsäure *f*.
methylmalonic aciduria Methylmalonazidurie *f*.
meth·yl·ma·lo·nyl-CoA epimerase [ˌ-ˈmælənɪl, -ni:l] Methylmalonyl-CoA--epimerase *f*, Methylmalonyl-CoA-racemase *f*.
methylmalonyl-CoA mutase Methylmalonyl-CoA-mutase *f*.
methylmalonyl-CoA racemase → methylmalonyl-CoA epimerase.
meth·yl·mer·cap·tan [ˌ-mərˈkæptæn] *n* Methylmercaptan *nt*.
methyl methacrylate Methylmethacrylat *nt*.
meth·yl·meth·ane [ˌ-'meθeɪn] *n* Äthan *nt*, Ethan *nt*.
meth·yl·mor·phine [ˌ-'mɔːrfiːn] *n* Kodein *nt*, Codein *nt*, Methylmorphin *nt*.
methyl orange Methylorange *nt*, Helianthin *nt*.
meth·yl·phen·i·date [ˌ-'fenɪdeɪt] *n pharm.* Methylphenidat *nt*.
methyl phenol Kresol *nt*.
meth·yl·phen·yl·hy·dra·zine [ˌ-ˌfenlˈhaɪdrəzi:n] *n* Methylphenylhydrazin *nt*.
meth·yl·pred·nis·o·lone [ˌ-predˈnɪsələʊn] *n pharm.* Methylprednisolon *nt*.
6-meth·yl·pte·rin [ˌ-'terɪn] *n* 6-Methylpterin *nt*.
meth·yl·pu·rine [ˌ-'pjʊəri:n, -ɪn] *n* Methylpurin *nt*.

meth·yl·py·ra·pone [ˌ-'paɪrəpəʊn, -'pɪrə-] n → metyrapone.
methyl red Methylrot nt.
5-meth·yl·re·sor·cin·ol [ˌ-rɪ'sɔːrsɪnɒl] n Orcinol nt.
meth·yl·ros·an·i·line chloride [ˌ-rəʊ'zænəlɪn, -liːn] Kristallviolett nt, Methylrosaliniumchlorid nt.
meth·yl·tes·tos·ter·one [ˌ-tes'tɒstərəʊn] n pharm. Methyltestosteron nt.
meth·yl·tet·ra·hy·dro·fo·late [ˌ-ˌtetrəˌhaɪdrə'fəʊleɪt] n Methyltetrahydrofolat nt.
5-methyltetrahydrofolate-homocysteine methyltransferase 5-Methyltetrahydrofolat-homocystein-methyltransferase f, Homocystein-Tetrahydrofolatmethyltransferase f.
meth·yl·tet·ra·hy·dro·fo·lic acid [ˌ-ˌtetrəˌhaɪdrə'fəʊlɪk, -'fɒl-] Methyltetrahydrofolsäure f.
meth·yl·the·o·bro·mine [ˌ-θiːə'brəʊmiːn, -mɪn] n Koffein nt, Coffein nt, Methyltheobromin nt, 1,3,7-Trimethylxanthin nt.
meth·yl·thi·o·nine chloride [ˌ-'θaɪəniːn] → methylene blue.
meth·yl·thi·o·u·ra·cil [ˌ-ˌθaɪə'jʊərəsɪl] n abbr. MTU pharm. Methylthiouracil nt abbr. MTU.
meth·yl·trans·fer·ase [ˌ-'trænsfəreɪz] n Methyltransferase f, Transmethylase f.
meth·yl·u·ra·cil [ˌ-'jʊərəsɪl] n Methyluracil nt.
5-methyluracil n Thymin nt abbr. T, 5-Methyluracil nt.
meth·yl·u·ram·ine [ˌ-jʊə'ræmiːn] n → methylguanidine.
methyl violet Methylviolett nt.
methyl violet stain histol. Methylviolettfärbung f.
meth·yl·xan·thine [ˌ-'zænθiːn, -θɪn] n Methylxanthin nt.
meth·y·pry·lon [ˌmeθɪ'praɪlɒn] n pharm. Methyprylon nt.
meth·y·ser·gide [meθə'sɜːrdʒaɪd] n pharm. Methysergid nt.
me·thys·ti·cine [mə'θɪstəsiːn] n pharm. Kavain nt.
me·ti·a·mide [mɪ'taɪəmaɪd] n Metiamid nt.
met·my·o·glo·bin [metˌmaɪə'gləʊbɪn] n Metmyoglobin nt.
met·o·clo·pra·mide [ˌmetəʊklə'præmaɪd] n pharm. Metoclopramid nt.
met·oes·trum [met'estrəm] n → metestrus.
met·oes·trus n → metestrus.
me·to·la·zone [me'təʊləzəʊn] n pharm. Metolazon nt.
me·ton·y·my [mɪ'tɒnəmɪ] n psychia. Metonymie f.
metopo- pref. → metopo-.
me·top·a·gus [mɪ'tɒpəgəs] n → metopopagus.
me·top·ic [mɪ'tɒpɪk] adj Stirn betr., frontal, Stirn-.
metopic point → metopion.
metopic suture Sutura frontalis/metopica.
me·to·pi·on [mə'təʊpɪən] n anat. Metopion nt.
metopo- pref. Stirn-, Metop(o)-.
met·o·po·dyn·ia [ˌmetəpəʊ'diːnɪə] n frontale Kopfschmerzen pl, Metopodynie f.
met·o·pop·a·gus [ˌmetəʊ'pɒpəgəs] n embryo. Meto(po)pagus m.
me·to·pro·lol [mə'təʊprəlɒl] n pharm. Metoprolol nt.
me·tox·e·nous [mə'tɒksənəs] adj bio. wirtswechselnd, heterözisch.
me·tox·e·ny [mə'tɒksənɪ] n bio. Wirtswechsel m.
metr- pref. → metro-.

me·tra ['miːtrə] n, pl **-trae** [-triː] Gebärmutter f, Uterus m, Metra f.
me·tral·gia [mɪ'trældʒ(ɪ)ə] n gyn. Gebärmutterschmerz(en pl) m, Hysteralgie f, Hysterodynie f, Metralgie f, Metrodynie f.
me·tra·to·nia [ˌmiːtrə'təʊnɪə] n gyn. Gebärmutter-, Uterusatonie f.
me·tra·tro·phia [ˌ-'trəʊfɪə] n gyn. Gebärmutter-, Uterusatrophie f.
me·trec·to·my [mɪ'trektəmɪ] n gyn. Gebärmutterentfernung f, Hysterektomie f, Hysterectomia f, Uterusexstirpation f.
me·tria ['miːtrɪə] n gyn. Gebärmutterentzündung f während der Puerperalperiode; Metritis puerperalis.
met·ric ['metrɪk] adj metrisch, Maß-, Meter-.
met·ri·cal ['metrɪkl] adj → metric.
metric method of analysis chem. Maßanalyse f.
metric system metrisches System nt.
me·tri·tis [mɪ'traɪtɪs] n gyn. Gebärmutter-, Uterusentzündung f, Metritis f.
me·tri·za·mide [mɪ'trɪzəmaɪd] n radiol. Metrizamid nt.
metro- pref. Gebärmutter-, Metr(o)-, Hyster(o)-, Uter(o)-.
me·tro·car·ci·no·ma [ˌmiːtrəʊˌkɑːrsɪ'nəʊmə] n Endometriumkarzinom nt, Ca. endometriale.
me·tro·cele ['-siːl] n chir. Hysterozele f.
me·tro·col·po·cele [ˌ-'kɒlpəsiːl] n chir. Hysterokolpozele f.
me·tro·cyte ['-saɪt] n Mutterzelle f.
me·tro·dyn·ia [ˌ-'diːnɪə] n → metralgia.
me·tro·en·do·me·tri·tis [ˌ-ˌendəʊmɪ'traɪtɪs] n gyn. Metroendometritis f.
me·tro·fi·bro·ma [ˌ-faɪ'brəʊmə] n Uterusfibrom nt.
me·trog·ra·phy [mɪ'tɒgrəfɪ] n **1.** radiol. Kontrastdarstellung f der Gebärmutterhöhle, Hysterographie f, Uterographie f. **2.** gyn. Hysterographie f.
me·tro·lym·phan·gi·tis [ˌmiːtrəʊˌlɪmfæn'dʒaɪtɪs] n gyn. Entzündung f der Lymphgefäße des Uterus.
me·tro·ma·la·cia [ˌ-mə'leɪʃ(ɪ)ə] n patho. Metromalazie f.
me·tro·mal·a·co·ma [ˌ-ˌmælə'kəʊmə] n → metromalacia.
me·tro·mal·a·co·sis [ˌ-ˌmælə'kəʊsɪs] n → metromalacia.
met·ro·ma·nia [ˌ-'meɪnɪə, -jə] n patho. Metromanie f.
me·tro·men·or·rha·gia [ˌ-ˌmenə'reɪdʒ(ɪ)ə] n gyn. Metromenorrhagie f.
met·ro·ni·da·zole [ˌ-'maɪdəzəʊl, -'nɪdə-] n pharm. Metronidazol nt.
me·tro·par·al·y·sis [ˌmiːtrəʊpə'rælɪsɪs] n gyn. Gebärmutter-, Uteruslähmung f.
me·tro·path·ia [ˌ-'pæθɪə] n → metropathy.
me·tro·path·ic [ˌ-'pæθɪk] adj Metropathie betr.
me·trop·a·thy [mɪ'trɒpəθɪ] n Gebärmutter-, Uteruserkrankung f, Metropathie f.
me·tro·per·i·to·ne·al [ˌmiːtrəʊˌperɪtəʊ'niːəl] adj Uterus u. Peritoneum betr. od. verbindend, metroperitoneal.
metroperitoneal fistula uteroperitoneale/metroperitoneale Fistel f.
me·tro·per·i·to·ni·tis [ˌ-ˌperɪtəʊ'naɪtɪs] n gyn. Metroperitonitis f.
me·tro·phle·bi·tis [ˌ-flɪ'baɪtɪs] n gyn. Entzündung f der Gebärmuttervenen, Metrophlebitis f.
me·tro·plas·ty ['metrəʊplæstɪ, 'miː-] n gyn. Gebärmutter-, Uterusplastik f.
me·tro·pto·sis [ˌ-'təʊsɪs, -ptəʊ-, -trap-] n gyn. Gebärmuttersenkung f, Metroptose f, Hysteroptose f, Descensus uteri.
me·tror·rha·gia [ˌ-'reɪdʒ(ɪ)ə] n gyn. Gebär-

mutter-, Uterusblutung f, Metrorrhagie f.
me·tror·rhea [ˌ-'rɪə] n gyn. Metrorrhoe f.
me·tror·rhex·is [ˌ-'reksɪs] n gyn. Gebärmutter-, Uterusruptur f, Metrorrhexis f, Hysterorrhexis f.
me·tro·sal·pin·gi·tis [ˌ-ˌsælpɪn'dʒaɪtɪs] n gyn. Entzündung f von Uterus u. Eileiter, Hystero-, Metrosalpingitis f.
me·tro·sal·pin·gog·ra·phy [ˌ-ˌsælpɪn'gɒgrəfɪ] n radiol. Kontrastdarstellung f von Uterus u. Eileiter, Utero-, Metro-, Hysterosalpingographie f abbr. HSG, Utero-, Metro-, Hysterotubographie f.
met·ro·scope ['-skəʊp] n gyn. Hysteroskop nt.
me·tro·stax·is ['-ˌstæksɪs] n gyn. Metrostaxis f, Hysterostaxis f.
me·tro·ste·no·sis [ˌ-stɪ'nəʊsɪs] n gyn. Metrostenose f.
me·trot·o·my [mɪ'trɒtəmɪ] n gyn. Gebärmutterschnitt m, -eröffnung f, Hysterotomie f, Hysterotomia f.
me·tro·tu·bog·ra·phy [ˌmiːtrətjuː'bɒgrəfɪ] n → metrosalpingography.
me·tyr·a·pone [mə'tɪərəpəʊn] n Metyrapon nt.
metyrapone test Metyrapon-Test m.
Meuse fever [mjuːz; mɜːz] Wolhyn'-Fieber nt, Fünftagefieber nt, Wolhynienfieber nt, Febris quintana.
me·val·o·nate [me'væləneɪt] n Mevalonat nt.
mevalonate kinase Mevalonatkinase f.
mev·a·lon·ic acid [ˌmevə'lɒnɪk] Mevalonsäure f.
Mex·i·can ['meksɪkən]: **M. hat cell** hema. Targetzelle f.
M. hat erythrocyte hema. Targetzelle f.
M. spotted fever Felsengebirgsfleckfieber nt, amerikanisches Zeckenbißfieber nt, Rocky Mountain spotted fever (nt) abbr. RMSF.
M. typhus endemisches/murines Fleckfieber nt, Ratten-, Flohfleckfieber nt.
Meyenburg ['meɪənbɜːrg; 'maɪənbʊrk]:
M.'s complexes Meyenburg'-Komplexe pl.
M.'s disease (von) Meyenburg-Altherr-Uehlinger-Syndrom nt, rezidivierende Polychondritis f, systematisierte Chondromalazie f.
Meyenburg-Altherr-Uehlinger ['altheːr'yːlɪŋər]: **M.-A.-U. syndrome** → Meyenburg's disease.
Meyer ['maɪər]: **M.'s disease** Adenoide pl, adenoide Vegetationen pl.
M. mastectomy gyn. Halsted-Operation f, radikale Mastektomie f, Mammaamputation f, Ablatio mammae.
Meyer-Betz [bets]: **M.-B. disease** idiopathische/familiäre Myoglobinurie f.
M.-B. syndrome Myoglobinurie f.
Meyer-Schwickerath ['ʃvɪkəraːt]: **M.-S. and Weyers syndrome** okulodentodigitales Syndrom nt, Meyer-Schwickerath-Weyers-Syndrom nt.
Meynert ['maɪnərt]: **M.'s axis** Meynert'-(Hirn-)Achse f.
basal nucleus of M. Nc. basalis Meynert.
M.'s bundle Meynert'-Bündel nt, Fasciculus retroflexus, Tractus habenulointerpeduncularis.
M.'s cells Meynert'-Zellen pl, Riesensternzellen pl.
M.'s commissures Meynert'-Kommissuren pl, Commissurae supraopticae.
M.'s decussation Meynert'-Haubenkreuzung f, hintere Haubenkreuzung f.
M.'s fasciculus → M.'s bundle.
M.'s layer Meynert'-Schicht f, Pyramidenzellschicht f.
M.'s tract → M.'s bundle.

Meynet

Meynet [mɛ'nɛ]: **M.'s nodes** Meynet-Knötchen pl.
M.'s nodosities → M.'s nodes.
mez·lo·cil·lin [ˌmezlə'sɪlɪn] n pharm. Mezlocillin nt.
μF abbr. → microfarad.
MF fixative → methiolate-formaline fixative.
Mg abbr → magnesium.
mg abbr. → milligram.
μg abbr. → microgram.
MGB abbr. → geniculate body, medial.
MGF abbr. → macrophage growth factor.
MGG stain → May-Grünwald-Giemsa stain.
MHC abbr. → major histocompatibility complex.
MHC antigens MHC-Antigene pl.
MHC molecule MHC-Molekül nt.
MHC protein MHC-Protein nt.
MHC restriction MHC-Restriktion f.
mho abbr. → siemens.
MHz abbr. → megahertz.
MI abbr. → myocardial infarction.
mi·a·na bug/tick ['mɪəneɪ] micro. Argas persicus.
Mi·a·neh bug ['mɪəneɪ] micro. Argas persicus.
Mianeh disease/fever persisches Rückfallfieber nt.
mi·an·ser·in [mɪ'ænsərɪn] n pharm. Mianserin nt.
Mibelli [mɪ'belɪ]: **M.'s angiokeratoma** Angiokeratoma nt Mibelli.
M.'s disease derm. Mibelli'-Krankheit f, Porokeratosis/Parakeratosis Mibelli f, Keratoatrophodermie f, Hyperkeratosis concentrica, Hyperkeratosis figurata centrifugata atrophicans, Keratodermia excentrica.
porokeratosis of M. → M.'s disease.
MIC abbr. → minimal inhibitory concentration.
mi·cel·la [mɪ'selə, maɪ-] n, pl **-lae** [-liː] → micelle.
mi·cel·lar [mɪ'selər] adj mizellenartig, Mizellen-.
mi·cel·la·ri·za·tion [mɪˌselərɪ'zeɪʃn] n Mizellenbildung f.
mi·celle [mɪ'sel, maɪ-] n chem. Mizelle f, Micelle f.
Michaelis [mə'keɪlɪz]: **M. constant** abbr. K_m Michaelis-Konstante f abbr. K_m, Michaelis-Menten-Konstante f.
Michaelis-Gutmann ['guːtman]: **M.-G. bodies** Michaelis-Gutmann-Körperchen pl.
Michaelis-Menten ['mentən]: **M.-M. constant** → Michaelis constant.
M.-M. equation Michaelis-Menten-Gleichung f.
Michel ['mɪkəl, 'mɪxəl]: **M.'s deafness** HNO Michel-Schwerhörigkeit f, Michel-Typ m der angeborenen Taubheit.
mi·con·a·zole [mɪ'kanəzɒl] n pharm. Miconazol nt.
micr- pref. abbr. → micro-.
mi·cran·at·o·my [ˌmaɪkrən'ætəmɪ] n → microanatomy.
mi·cran·gi·op·a·thy [ˌmaɪkrændʒɪ'apəθɪ] n → microangiopathy.
mi·cren·ce·pha·lia [ˌmaɪkrənsɪ'feɪljə] n → microencephaly.
mi·cren·ceph·a·lon [ˌ-'sefələn] n → microencephaly.
mi·cren·ceph·a·ly [ˌ-'sefəlɪ] n → microencephaly.
micro- pref. abbr. μ Mikr(o)-, Micr(o)- abbr. μ.
mi·cro·ab·scess [ˌmaɪkroʊ'æbses] n Mikroabzeß m.

mi·cro·ad·e·no·ma [ˌ-ædə'noʊmə] n Mikroadenom nt.
mi·cro·aer·o·bi·on [ˌ-eə'roʊbɪˌan] n → microaerophile I.
mi·cro·aer·o·phil [ˌ-'eərəfɪl] adj → microaerophile II.
mi·cro·aer·o·phile [ˌ-'eərəfaɪl] bio. **I** n mikroaerophiler Organismus m. **II** adj mikroaerophil.
mi·cro·aer·o·phil·ic [ˌ-ˌeərə'fɪlɪk] adj → microaerophile II.
mi·cro·aer·oph·i·lous [ˌ-eə'rafɪləs] adj → microaerophile II.
mi·cro·ag·gre·gate [ˌ-'ægrɪgɪt, -geɪt] n Mikroaggregat nt.
mi·cro·am·me·ter [ˌ-'æmiːtər] n phys. Mikroamperemeter nt.
mi·cro·am·pere [ˌ-'æmpɪər, -æm'pɪər] n abbr. **μA** Mikroampere nt abbr. μA.
mi·cro·a·nal·y·sis [ˌ-ə'næləsɪs] n, pl **-ses** [-siːz] chem. Mikroanalyse f.
mi·cro·an·a·lyt·ic [ˌ-ænə'lɪtɪk] adj Mikroanalyse betr., mikroanalytisch.
mi·cro·a·nas·to·mo·sis [ˌ-əˌnæstə'moʊsɪs] n Mikroanastomose f.
mi·cro·a·nat·o·my [ˌ-ə'nætəmɪ] n → microanatomie f, Histologie f.
mi·cro·an·eu·rysm [ˌ-'ænjərɪzəm] n Mikroaneurysma nt.
mi·cro·an·gi·o·path·ic [ˌ-ˌændʒɪoʊ'pæθɪk] adj mikroangiopathisch.
microangiopathic hemolytic anemia → microangiopathic hemolytic anemia.
microangiopathic hemolytic anemia thrombotisch-thrombozytopenische Purpura f, Moschcowitz-Syndrom nt, Moschcowitz-Singer-Symmers-Syndrom nt, thrombotische Mikroangiopathie f, Purpura thrombotica (thrombocytopenica), Purpura Moschcowitz.
mi·cro·an·gi·op·a·thy [ˌ-ˌændʒɪ'apəθɪ] n Mikroangiopathie f.
mi·cro·an·gi·os·co·py [ˌ-ˌændʒɪ'askəpɪ] n Kapillarmikroskopie f, Kapillaroskopie f.
mi·cro·ar·chi·tec·ture [ˌ-'aːrkɪtektʃər] n Mikroarchitektur f.
Mi·cro·bac·te·ri·um [ˌ-bæk'tɪərɪəm] n micro. Microbacterium nt.
mi·cro·bac·te·ri·um [ˌ-bæk'tɪərɪəm] n, pl **-ri·a** [-rɪə] 1. Mikrobakterium nt, Microbacterium nt. 2. Mikroorganismus m.
mi·cro·bar ['-baːr] n Mikrobar nt.
mi·crobe ['maɪkroʊb] n bio. Mikrobe f, Mikroorganismus m, Mikrobion nt.
mi·cro·bi·al [maɪ'kroʊbɪəl] adj Mikrobe(n) betr., mikrobisch, mikrobiell, Mikroben-.
microbial concentration Mikrobenkonzentration f.
microbial eczema mikrobielles Ekzem nt.
microbial genetics Mikrobengenetik f.
microbial physiology Mikrobenphysiologie f.
mi·cro·bi·an [maɪ'kroʊbɪən] **I** n → microbe. **II** adj → microbial.
mi·cro·bic [maɪ'kroʊbɪk] adj → microbial.
microbic dissociation bakterielle Dissoziation f.
mi·cro·bi·cid·al [ˌmaɪkroʊbɪ'caɪdl] adj mikrobenabtötend, entkeimend, mikrobizid.
mi·cro·bi·cide ['-bɪsaɪd] n mikrobizides Mittel nt, Mikrobizid nt; Antibiotikum nt.
mic·ro·bid [maɪ'kroʊbɪd] n derm. Mikrobid nt.
mi·cro·bi·o·as·say [ˌmaɪkroʊˌbaɪoʊ'seɪ, -'æseɪ] n Mikrobioassay m.
mi·cro·bi·o·log·ic [ˌ-baɪə'ladʒɪk] adj → microbiologic.
mi·cro·bi·o·log·i·cal [ˌ-baɪə'ladʒɪk] adj → microbiologic.

mi·cro·bi·ol·o·gist [ˌ-baɪ'alədʒɪst] n Mikrobiologe m, -biologin f.
mi·cro·bi·ol·o·gy [ˌ-baɪ'alədʒɪ] n Mikrobiologie f.
mi·cro·bi·ot·ic [ˌ-baɪ'atɪk] adj 1. kurzlebig. 2. → microbial.
mi·cro·bism ['-bɪzəm] n Mikrobeninfektion f, Mikrobismus m.
mi·cro·blast ['-blæst] n Mikroblast m.
mi·cro·ble·pha·ria [ˌ-blə'færɪə] n ophthal. Mikroblepharie f, blepharon nt.
mi·cro·bleph·a·rism [ˌ-'blefərɪzəm] n → microblepharia.
mi·cro·bleph·a·ron [ˌ-'blefəran] n → microblepharia.
mi·cro·bleph·a·ry [ˌ-'blefərɪ] n → microblepharia.
mi·cro·bod·y ['-badɪ] n Peroxisom nt, Microbody m.
mi·cro·bra·chia [ˌ-'breɪkɪə] n embryo. Mikrobrachie f.
mi·cro·bra·chi·us [ˌ-'breɪkɪəs] n embryo. Mikrobrachius m.
mi·cro·bu·ret(te) [ˌ-bjʊə'ret] n Mikrobürette f.
mi·cro·cal·ci·fi·ca·tion [ˌ-ˌkælsɪfɪ'keɪʃn] n patho. Mikroverkalkung f, -kalzifikation f.
mi·cro·cal·ix [ˌ-'kælɪks] n patho. Mikrokalix m.
mi·cro·cal·lus [ˌ-'kæləs] n ortho. Mikrokallus m.
mi·cro·cal·yx n → microcalix.
mi·cro·car·ci·no·ma [ˌ-ˌkaːrsə'noʊmə] n patho. Mikrokarzinom nt.
mi·cro·car·dia [ˌ-'kaːrdɪə] n embryo. Mikrokardie f.
mi·cro·cen·trum [ˌ-'sentrəm] n Mikrozentrum nt, Zentrosphäre f.
mi·cro·ce·pha·lia [ˌ-sɪ'feɪljə] n → microcephaly.
mi·cro·ce·phal·ic [ˌ-sɪ'fælɪk] adj mikrozephal, -kephal.
mi·cro·ceph·a·lism [ˌ-'sefəlɪzəm] n → microcephaly.
mi·cro·ceph·a·lous [ˌ-'sefələs] adj → microcephaly.
mi·cro·ceph·a·lus [ˌ-'sefələs] n, pl **-li** [-laɪ] Mikrozephalus m.
mi·cro·ceph·a·ly [ˌ-'sefəlɪ] n embryo. Mikrozephalie f, -kephalie f, Mikrozephalus m.
mi·cro·chei·lia [ˌ-'keɪlɪə] n embryo. Mikroch(e)ilie f.
mi·cro·chei·ria [ˌ-'kaɪrɪə] n embryo. Mikroch(e)irie f.
mi·cro·chem·i·cal [ˌ-'kemɪkl] adj Mikrochemie betr., mikrochemisch.
mi·cro·chem·is·try [ˌ-'kemɪstrɪ] n Mikrochemie f.
mi·cro·chi·lia n → microcheilia.
mi·cro·chi·ria n → microcheiria.
mi·cro·cin·e·ma·tog·ra·phy [ˌ-ˌsɪnəmə'tagrəfɪ] n Mikrokinematographie f.
mi·cro·cir·cuit·ry [ˌ-'sɜːrkɪtrɪ] n phys., physiol. Mikroverschaltung f.
mi·cro·cir·cu·la·tion [ˌ-ˌsɜːrkjə'leɪʃn] n Mikrozirkulation f.
mi·cro·cli·mate [ˌ-'klaɪmɪt] n Mikroklima nt.
Mi·cro·coc·ca·ce·ae [ˌ-kə'keɪsɪˌiː] pl micro. Micrococcaceae pl.
mi·cro·coc·cal [ˌ-'kakəl] adj Mikrokokken-.
Mi·cro·coc·cus [ˌ-'kakəs] n micro. Micrococcus m.
mi·cro·coc·cus [ˌ-'kakəs] n, pl **-coc·ci** [-'kaksaɪ, -siː] bact. Mikrokokke f, Mikrokokkus m, Micrococcus m.
mi·cro·co·lon [ˌ-'koʊlən] n Mikrokolon nt.
mi·cro·col·o·ny [ˌ-'kalənɪ] n Mikrokolonie f.

mi·cro·con·cen·tra·tion [ˌ-ˌkɑnsən'treɪʃn] n Mikrokonzentration f.
mi·cro·co·nid·i·um [ˌ-kə'nɪdɪəm] n, pl **-dia** [-dɪə] micro. Mikrokonidium nt.
mi·cro·co·ria [ˌ-'kɔːrɪə] n ophthal. Mikrokorie f.
mi·cro·cor·nea [ˌ-'kɔːrnɪə] n ophthal. Mikrokornea f.
mi·cro·cos·mic [ˌ-'kɑzmɪk] adj mikrokosmisch.
mi·cro·cou·lomb [ˌ-'kuːlɑm, -kuː'lɑm, -ləʊm] n abbr. **µC** Mikrocoulomb nt abbr. µC.
mi·cro·cra·nia [ˌ-'kreɪnɪə] n embryo. Mikrokranie f.
mi·cro·crys·tal ['-krɪstl] n Mikrokristall m.
mi·cro·crys·tal·line [ˌ-'krɪstlɪn] adj mikrokristallin.
mi·cro·cul·ture ['-kʌltʃər] n Mikrokultur f.
mi·cro·cu·rie [ˌ-'kjʊərɪ, -kjʊə'rɪ] n abbr. **µCi** Mikrocurie nt abbr. µCi.
mi·cro·cyst ['-sɪst] n Mikrozyste f.
mi·cro·cyte ['-saɪt] n Mikrozyt m.
mi·cro·cy·the·mia [ˌ-saɪ'θiːmɪə] n → microcytosis.
mi·cro·cyt·ic anemia [ˌ-'sɪtɪk] mikrozytäre Anämie f.
hypochromic m. hypochrome mikrozytäre Anämie.
mi·cro·cy·to·sis [ˌ-saɪ'təʊsɪs] n Mikrozytose f.
mi·cro·dac·tyl·ia [ˌ-dæk'tɪːlɪə] n → microdactyly.
mi·cro·dac·ty·ly [ˌ-'dæktəlɪ] n Mikrodaktylie f.
mi·cro·den·si·tom·e·ter [ˌ-ˌdensɪ'tɑmɪtər] n Mikrodensitometer nt.
mi·cro·der·ma·tome [ˌ-'dɜːrmətəʊm] n chir. Mikrodermatom nt.
mi·cro·don·tia [ˌ-'dɑnʃɪə] n embryo., dent. Mikrodontie f.
mi·cro·don·tism [ˌ-'dɑntɪzəm] n → microdontia.
mi·cro·drep·a·no·cyt·ic anemia/disease [ˌ-ˌdrepənəʊ'sɪtɪk] → microdrepanocytosis.
mi·cro·drep·a·no·cy·to·sis [ˌ-ˌdrepənəʊsaɪ'təʊsɪs] n hema. Sichelzell(en)thalassämie f, Mikrodrepanozytenkrankheit f, HbS-Thalassämie f.
mi·cro·e·co·sys·tem [ˌ-'ekəʊsɪstəm, -'iːkəʊ-] n Mikroökosystem nt.
mi·cro·e·lec·tric waves [ˌ-ɪ'lektrɪk] → microwaves.
mi·cro·e·lec·trode [ˌ-ɪ'lektrəʊd] n Mikroelektrode f.
mi·cro·e·lec·tron·ics [ˌ-ɪlek'trɑnɪks] pl phys. Mikroelektronik f.
mi·cro·e·lec·tro·pho·re·sis [ˌ-ɪˌlektrəʊfə'riːsɪs] n Mikroelektrophorese f.
mi·cro·e·lec·tro·pho·ret·ic [ˌ-ɪˌlektrəʊfə'retɪk] adj Mikroelektrophorese betr., mittels Mikroelektrophorese, mikroelektrophoretisch.
mi·cro·em·bo·lus [ˌ-'embələs] n, pl **-li** [-laɪ] Mikroembolus m.
mi·cro·en·ceph·a·lon [ˌ-en'sefəlɑn] n → microencephaly.
mi·cro·en·ceph·a·ly [ˌ-en'sefəlɪ] n Mikr(o)enzephalie f.
mi·cro·en·vi·ron·ment [ˌ-en'vaɪ(r)ənmənt] n Mikromilieu nt, -umwelt f.
mi·cro·e·ryth·ro·blast [ˌ-ɪ'rɪθrəblæst] n Mikroblast m.
mi·cro·e·ryth·ro·cyte [ˌ-ɪ'rɪθrəsaɪt] n → microcrocyte.
mi·cro·e·vo·lu·tion [ˌ-evə'luːʃn] n Mikroevolution f.
mi·cro·far·ad [ˌ-'færəd, -æd] n abbr. **µF** Mikrofarad nt abbr. µF.
mi·cro·fau·na [ˌ-'fɔːnə] n Mikrofauna f.

mi·cro·fi·bril [ˌ-'faɪbrɪl, -'fɪb-] n Mikrofibrille f.
mi·cro·fil·a·ment [ˌ-'fɪləmənt] n Mikrofilament nt.
mi·cro·fil·a·re·mia [ˌ-ˌfɪlə'riːmɪə] n Mikrofilariensepsis f, Mikrofilarämie f.
mi·cro·fi·lar·ia [ˌ-fɪ'leərɪə] n, pl **-lar·i·ae** [-'leərɪˌiː] micro. Mikrofilarie f, Microfilaria f.
mi·cro·film ['-fɪlm] **I** n Mikrofilm m. **II** vt auf Mikrofilm aufnehmen.
mi·cro·flo·ra [ˌmaɪkrəʊ'flɔːrə, -'fləʊ-] n Mikroflora f.
mi·cro·fluo·rom·e·try [ˌ-fluə'rɑmətrɪ] n Mikrospektrophotometrie f, Zytophotometrie f.
mi·cro·fol·i·cu·lar [ˌ-fə'lɪkjələr] adj histol. mikrofollikulär.
microfollicular adenoma mikrofollikuläres (Schilddrüsen-)Adenom nt.
microfollicular goiter mikrofollikuläre Struma f.
mi·cro·frac·ture ['-fræktʃər] n ortho. Mikrofraktur f.
mi·cro·gam·ete [ˌ-'gæmiːt, -gæ'miːt] n micro. Mikrogamet m, Androgamet m.
mi·cro·ga·me·to·cyte [ˌ-gə'miːtəsaɪt] n → microgamont.
mi·cro·gam·ma [ˌ-'gæmə] n old → picogram.
mi·cro·gam·ont [ˌ-'gæmɑnt] n micro. Mikrogametozyt m, Mikrogamont m.
mi·crog·a·my [maɪ'krɑgəmɪ] n micro. Mikrogamie f.
mi·cro·gas·tria [ˌmaɪkrə'gæstrɪə] n embryo. Mikrogastrie f.
mi·cro·gen·e·sis [ˌ-'dʒenəsɪs] n Mikrogenese f.
mi·cro·ge·nia [ˌ-'dʒiːnɪə] n Mikrogenie f.
mi·crog·lia [maɪ'krɑglɪə] n **1.** Mesoglia f, Hortega-Glia f, -Zellen pl. **2.** Mikroglia f.
mi·crog·li·a·cyte [maɪ'krɑglɪəsaɪt] n → microglia 1.
mi·crog·li·al [maɪ'krɑglɪəl] adj Mikroglia betr., Mikroglia-.
microglial cells → microglia.
mi·cro·gli·o·cyte [maɪ'krɑglɪəʊsaɪt] n → microglia 1.
mi·cro·gli·o·ma [ˌmaɪkrəglaɪ'əʊmə] n patho. Mikrogliom nt.
β₂-mi·cro·glob·u·lin [ˌ-'glɑbjəlɪn] n β₂-Mikroglobulin nt, beta₂-Mikroglobulin nt.
mi·cro·glos·sia [ˌ-'glɑsɪə] n Mikroglossie f.
mi·cro·gna·thi·a [ˌ-'neɪθɪə, -'næθ-, maɪˌkræg-] n Mikrognathie f.
mi·cro·gram ['maɪkrəgræm] n abbr. **mcg, µg** Mikrogramm nt abbr. µg.
mi·cro·graph ['-græf] n **1.** Mikrograph m. **2.** mikrographische Darstellung f.
mi·crog·ra·phy [maɪ'krɑgrəfɪ] n **1.** neuro. Mikrographie f. **2.** Untersuchung f mit dem Mikroskop.
mi·cro·gy·ria [ˌmaɪkrəʊ'dʒaɪrɪə] n Mikrogyrie f.
mi·cro·gy·rus [ˌ-'dʒaɪrəs] n, pl **-gy·ri** [-'dʒaɪraɪ] Mikrogyrus m.
mi·cro·ham·ar·to·ma [ˌ-ˌhæm(r)'təʊmə] n patho. Mikrohamartom nt.
mi·cro·he·mat·o·crit [ˌ-hɪ'mætəkrɪt] n lab. Mikrohämatokrit m.
mi·cro·hem·or·rhage [ˌ-'hemərɪdʒ] n Mikroblutung f.
mi·cro·he·pa·tia [ˌ-hɪ'pætɪə] n embryo. Mikrohepatie f.
mi·cro·his·tol·o·gy [ˌ-hɪs'tɑlədʒɪ] n mikroskopische Histologie f, Mikrohistologie f.
mi·cro·in·farct [ˌ-'ɪnfɑːrkt] n patho. Mikroinfarkt m.
mi·cro·in·jec·tion [ˌ-ɪn'dʒekʃn] n Mikroinjektion f.

mi·cro·in·va·sion [ˌ-ɪn'veɪʒn] n patho. Mikroinvasion nt.
mi·cro·in·va·sive carcinoma [ˌ-ɪn'veɪsɪv] mikroinvasives Karzinom nt.
mi·cro·kin·e·ma·tog·ra·phy [ˌ-ˌkɪnəmæ'tɑgrəfɪ] n Mikrokinematographie f.
mi·cro·lar·yn·gos·co·py [ˌ-ˌlærɪn'gɑskəpɪ] n HNO Mikrolaryngoskopie f.
mi·cro·lec·i·thal [ˌ-'lesɪθəl] adj bio. mikrolezithal.
microlecithal ovum bio. mikrolezithales Ei nt.
mi·cro·le·sion [ˌ-'liːʒn] n patho. Mikroläsion nt.
mi·cro·leu·ko·blast [ˌ-'luːkəblæst] n → myeloblast.
mi·cro·li·ter ['-liːtər] n abbr. **µl** Mikroliter m abbr. µl.
mi·cro·lith [ˌ-'lɪθ] n patho. Mikrolith m.
mi·cro·li·thi·a·sis [ˌ-lɪ'θaɪəsɪs] n patho. Mikrolithiasis f.
mi·cro·man·di·ble [ˌ-'mændɪbl] n embryo. kongenitale Kleinheit f des Unterkiefers.
mi·cro·ma·nia [ˌ-'meɪnɪə, -jə] n psychia. Kleinheitswahn m, Mikromanie f.
mi·cro·ma·nip·u·la·tion [ˌ-məˌnɪpjə'leɪʃn] n chir. Mikromanipulation f.
mi·cro·ma·nip·u·la·tor [ˌ-mə'nɪpjəleɪtər] n chir. Mikromanipulator m.
mi·cro·ma·nom·e·ter [ˌ-mə'nɑmɪtər] n Mikromanometer nt.
mi·cro·ma·no·met·ric [ˌ-ˌmænə'metrɪk] adj mikromanometrisch.
mi·cro·mas·tia [ˌ-'mæstɪə] n Mikromastie f.
mi·cro·max·il·la [ˌ-mæk'sɪlə] n kongenitale Kleinheit f des Oberkiefers.
mi·cro·ma·zia [ˌ-'meɪzɪə] n → micromastia.
mi·cro·me·lia [ˌ-'miːlɪə] n Mikromelie f.
mi·cro·mel·ic dwarf [-'melɪk, -'miː-] mikromeler Zwerg m.
mi·crom·e·lus [maɪ'krɑmələs] n Patient(in f) m mit Mikromelie, Mikromelus m.
mi·cro·mere ['maɪkrəmɪər] n Mikromere f.
mi·cro·me·tab·o·lism [ˌ-mə'tæbəlɪzəm] n Mikrometabolismus m.
mi·cro·met·a·stat·ic disease [ˌ-ˌmetə'stætɪk] Mikrometastasierung f.
mi·cro·me·tas·ta·sis [ˌ-mɪ'tæstəsɪs] n Mikrometastase f.
mi·cro·me·ter [1 'maɪkrəʊmɪːtər; 2 maɪ'krɑmɪtər] n **1.** abbr. **µm** Mikrometer m/ nt abbr. µm. **2.** (Gerät) Mikrometer m.
mi·cro·meth·od ['maɪkrəmeθəd] n Mikromethode f.
mi·cro·met·ric [ˌ-'metrɪk] adj phys. mikrometrisch.
mi·cro·met·ri·cal [ˌ-'metrɪkl] adj → micrometric.
micromicro- pref. old → pico.
mi·cro·mi·lieu [ˌmaɪkrəʊmɪːl'jiː, -'jʊ] n → microenvironment.
mi·cro·mo·lar [ˌ-'məʊlər] adj abbr. **µM** mikromolar abbr. µM.
mi·cro·mo·lec·u·lar [ˌ-mə'lekjələr] adj mikromolekular.
Mi·cro·mo·nos·po·ra [ˌ-məʊ'nɑspərə] n micro. Micromonospora f.
Mi·cro·mo·nos·po·ra·ce·ae [ˌ-məʊˌnɑspə'reɪsˌiː] pl micro. Micromonosporaceae pl.
mi·cro·mor·phol·o·gy [ˌ-mɔːr'fɑlədʒɪ] n Mikromorphologie f.
mi·cro·my·e·lia [ˌ-maɪ'iːlɪə] n Mikromyelie f.
mi·cro·my·e·lo·blast [ˌ-'maɪələblæst] n Mikromyeloblast m.
mi·cro·my·e·lo·lym·pho·cyte [ˌ-ˌmaɪələ'lɪmfəsaɪt] n micromyeloblast.
mi·cron ['maɪkrən] n, pl **-crons, -cra** [-krə] abbr. **µ** old → micrometer 1.

microneurosurgery

mi·cro·neu·ro·sur·ger·y [ˌmaɪkrəʊˌnjʊərə-ˈsɜrdʒərɪ, -ˌnʊ-] n Mikroneurochirurgie f.
mi·cro·nod·u·lar [ˌ-ˈnɑdʒələr] adj patho. kleinknotig, mikronodulär.
micronodular cirrhosis mikronoduläre/kleinknotige/organisierte Leberzirrhose f.
micronodular tuberculid derm. lupoide Rosazea f, Rosacea granulomatosa.
mi·cro·nu·cle·us [ˌ-ˈn(j)uːklɪəs] n, pl **-cle·us·es, -cle·i** [-klɪaɪ] 1. histol. Kernkörperchen nt, Nukleolus m, Nucleolus m. 2. bio. Mikronukleus m, Kleinkern m der Ziliaten.
mi·cro·nych·ia [ˌ-ˈnɪkɪə] n Mikronychie f.
micro-orchidia n → micro-orchidism.
micro-orchidism n Mikrorchidie f, Mikrorchie f.
mi·cro·or·gan·ic [ˌ-ɔːrˈgænɪk] adj mikroorganisch.
mi·cro·or·gan·ism [ˌ-ˈɔːrgəˈnɪzəm] n Mikroorganismus m.
mi·cro·par·a·site [ˌ-ˈpærəsaɪt] n Mikroparasit m.
mi·cro·pa·thol·o·gy [ˌ-pəˈθɑlədʒɪ] n Mikropathologie f.
mi·cro·pe·nis [ˌ-ˈpiːnɪs] n → microphallus.
mi·cro·per·fo·ra·tion [ˌ-ˌpɜrfəˈreɪʃn] n chir. Mikroperforation f.
mi·cro·per·fu·sion [ˌ-ˈperˈfjuːʒn] n Mikroperfusion f.
mi·cro·phage [ˈ-feɪdʒ] n Mikrophage m.
microphage system Mikrophagensystem nt.
mi·cro·phag·o·cyte [ˌ-ˈfægəsaɪt] n → microphage.
mi·cro·pha·kia [ˌ-ˈfeɪkɪə] n ophthal. Mikrophakie f.
mi·cro·phal·lus [ˌ-ˈfæləs] n Mikrophallus m.
mi·cro·phone [ˈ-fəʊn] n Mikrophon nt, Mikrofon nt.
mi·cro·phon·ic [ˌ-ˈfɑnɪk] adj Mikrophon betr., Mikrophon-.
microphonic potentials physiol. (kochleäre) Mikrophonpotentiale pl.
mi·cro·phon·ics [ˌ-ˈfɑnɪks] pl → microphonic potenitals.
mi·cro·pho·to·graph [ˌ-ˈfəʊtəgræf] n 1. Mikrofoto nt, -photo nt. 2. Mikrofotografie f, -photographie f.
mi·croph·thal·mia [maɪkrɑfˈθælmɪə] n → microphthalmos.
mi·croph·thal·mos [maɪkrɑfˈθælməs] n ophthal. Mikrophthalmie f, Mikrophthalmus m.
mi·croph·thal·mus n → microphthalmos.
mi·cro·phys·ics [ˌmaɪkrəʊˈfɪzɪks] pl Mikrophysik f.
mi·cro·phys·i·ol·o·gy [ˌ-fɪzɪˈɑlədʒɪ] n Mikrophysiologie f.
mi·cro·pin·o·cy·to·sis [ˌ-ˌpɪnəsaɪˈtəʊsɪs, -ˌpaɪnə-] n Mikropinozytose f.
mi·cro·pi·pet [ˌ-paɪˈpet, -pɪ-] n Mikropipette f.
mi·cro·pla·sia [ˌ-ˈpleɪʒ(ɪ)ə, -zɪə] n Minderr-, Zwergwuchs m.
mi·cro·pleth·ys·mog·ra·phy [ˌ-ˌpleθɪzˈmɑgrəfɪ] n physiol. Mikroplethysmographie f.
mi·cro·po·dia [ˌ-ˈpəʊdɪə] n Mikropodie f.
mi·cro·pol·y·gy·ria [ˌ-ˌpɑlɪˈdʒaɪrɪə] n Mikropolygyrie f.
mi·cro·pore [ˈ-pəʊər, -pɔːr] n bio. Keimmund m, Mikropyle f.
mi·cro·pre·cip·i·ta·tion [ˌ-prɪˌsɪpəˈteɪʃn] n Mikropräzipitation f.
microprecipitation test Mikropräzipitationstest m.
mi·cro·probe [ˈ-prəʊb] n chir. Mikrosonde f.
mi·cro·pro·lac·ti·no·ma [ˌ-prəʊˌlæktɪˈnəʊmə] n Mikroprolaktinom nt.
mi·crop·sia [maɪˈkrɑpsɪə] n Mikropsie f, Mikropie f.
mi·cro·punc·ture [ˈmaɪkrəpʌŋktʃər] n Mikro-, Kapillarpunktion f.
mi·cro·pyle [ˈ-paɪl] n 1. embryo. Mikropyle f. 2. → micropore.
mi·cro·ra·di·o·gram [ˌ-ˈreɪdɪəgræm] n radiol., histol. Mikroradiogramm nt.
mi·cro·ra·di·og·ra·phy [ˌ-reɪdɪˈɑgrəfɪ] n radiol., histol. Mikroradiographie f.
mi·cror·chid·ia [ˌmaɪkrɔːrˈkɪdɪə] n → micro-orchidism.
mi·cro·re·frac·tom·e·ter [ˌmaɪkrərɪˌfrækˈtɑmɪtər] n Mikrorefraktometer nt.
mi·cro·res·pi·rom·e·ter [ˌ-ˌrespɪˈrɑmɪtər] n physiol. Mikrorespirometer nt.
mi·cro·rhin·ia [ˌ-ˈrɪnɪə] n Mikrorhinie f.
mi·cro·sac·cade [ˌ-sæˈkɑːd, -sə-] n Mikrosakkade f.
mi·cro·sce·lous [ˌ-ˈskeləs, maɪˈkræskələs] adj kurzbeinig.
microscope stage Objektivtisch m.
mi·cro·scop·ic [ˌ-ˈskɑpɪk] adj 1. winzig klein, mit bloßem Auge nicht sichtbar, mikroskopisch. 2. Mikroskop(ie) betr., mittels Mikroskop(ie), mikroskopisch, Mikroskop-.
microscopic agglutination Mikroagglutination f.
mi·cro·scop·i·cal [ˌ-ˈskɑpɪkl] adj → microscopic.
microscopical anatomy Gewebelehre f, Histologie f; mikroskopische Anatomie f, Mikroanatomie f.
microscopic examination mikroskopische Untersuchung f.
microscopic anatomy → microscopical anatomy.
microscopic hematuria Mikrohämaturie f, mikroskopische Hämaturie f.
microscopic slide → microslide.
microscopic structure Feinstruktur f, -aufbau m, -anatomie f.
mi·cros·co·py [maɪˈkrɑskəpɪ, ˈmaɪkrəˌskəʊpɪ] n Mikroskopie f, Untersuchung f mittels Mikroskop.
mi·cro·sec·ond [ˌmaɪkrəʊˈsekənd] n abbr. µs Mikrosekunde f abbr. µs.
mi·cro·slide [ˈ-slaɪd] n Objektträger m.
mi·cros·mat·ic [maɪkrɑzˈmætɪk] adj mikrosmatisch.
mi·cro·so·ma [ˌmaɪkrəˈsəʊmə] n Kleinwuchs m, Mikrosomie f.
mi·cro·so·mal [ˌ-ˈsəʊməl] adj Mikrosome(n) betr., von Mikrosomen stammend, mikrosomal.
mi·cro·so·mat·ic [ˌ-səʊˈmætɪk] I n Mikrosomatiker m. II adj mikrosomatisch.
mi·cro·some [ˈ-səʊm] n Mikrosom nt.
mi·cro·so·mia [ˌ-ˈsəʊmɪə] n Kleinwuchs m, Mikrosomie f.
mi·cro·spec·tro·pho·tom·e·ter [ˌ-ˌspektrəfəʊˈtɑmɪtər] n Mikrospektrophotometer nt.
mi·cro·spec·tro·pho·tom·e·try [ˌ-ˌspektrəfəʊˈtɑmɪtrɪ] n Mikrospektrophotometrie f.
mi·cro·spec·tro·scope [ˌ-ˈspektrəskəʊp] n Mikrospektroskop nt.
mi·cro·sphere [ˈ-sfɪər] n 1. Zentrosom nt, Zentriol nt, Zentralkörperchen nt. 2. Mikrozentrum nt, Zentrosphäre f.
mi·cro·sphe·ro·cyte [ˌ-ˈsfɪərəsaɪt] n hema. Kugelzelle f, Sphärozyt m.
mi·cro·sphe·ro·cy·to·sis [ˌ-ˌsfɪərəsaɪˈtəʊsɪs] n Sphärozytose f.
mi·cro·sphyg·mia [ˌ-ˈsfɪgmɪə] n radiol. kleiner Puls m, Mikrosphygmie f.
mi·cro·sphyg·my [ˌ-ˈsfɪgmɪ] n → microsphygmia.
mi·cro·sphyx·ia [ˌ-ˈsfɪksɪə] n → microsphygmia.
mi·cro·sple·nia [ˌ-ˈspliːnɪə] n Mikrosplenie f.
mi·cro·spo·ran·gi·um [ˌ-spəˈrændʒɪəm, -spəʊ-] n micro. Mikrosporangium nt.
mi·cro·spore [ˈ-spəʊər, -spɔːr] n micro. Mikrospore f, Androspore f.
Mi·cros·po·ron [maɪˈkrɑspərən] n → Microsporum.
Mi·cros·po·rum [maɪˈkrɑspərəm] n micro. Microsporon nt, Microsporum nt.
mi·cro·sto·mia [ˌmaɪkrəˈstəʊmɪə] n Mikrostomie f.
mi·cro·sur·ger·y [ˌ-ˈsɜrdʒərɪ] n Mikrochirurgie f.
mi·cro·sur·gi·cal [ˌ-ˈsɜrdʒɪkl] adj mikrochirurgisch.
mi·cro·the·lia [ˌ-ˈθiːlɪə] n Mikrothelie f.
mi·cro·throm·bo·sis [ˌ-θrɑmˈbəʊsɪs] n Mikrothrombose f.
mi·cro·throm·bus [ˌ-ˈθrɑmbəs] n, pl **-bi** [-baɪ] Mikrothrombus m.
mi·cro·tia [maɪˈkrəʊʃɪə] n Mikrotie f.
mi·cro·ti·ter [ˌmaɪkrəʊˈtaɪtər] n immun. Mikrotiter m.
mi·cro·tome [ˈ-təʊm] n Mikrotom nt.
mi·crot·o·my [maɪˈkrɑtəmɪ] n Mikrotomie f.
mi·cro·to·nom·e·ter [ˌmaɪkrətəʊˈnɑmɪtər] n Mikrotonometer nt.
mi·cro·trans·fu·sion [ˌ-trænzˈf(j)uːʒn] n gyn. Mikrotransfusion f.
mi·cro·trau·ma [ˌ-ˈtrɔːmə, -ˈtraʊmə] n Mikrotrauma nt.
mi·cro·tu·bule [ˌ-ˈt(j)uːbjuːl] n Mikrotubulus m.
mi·cro·vil·li pl → microvillus.
mi·cro·vil·lus [ˌ-ˈvɪləs] n, pl **-vil·li** [-ˈvɪlaɪ] Kleinzotte f, Mikrovillus m.
mi·cro·vis·co·sim·e·ter [ˌ-ˌvɪskəˈsɪmətər] n lab. Mikroviskosimeter nt.
mi·cro·volt [ˈ-vəʊlt] n abbr. **µV** Mikrovolt nt abbr. µV.
mi·cro·watt [ˈ-wɑt] n abbr. **µW** Mikrowatt nt abbr. µW.
mi·cro·wave [ˈ-weɪv] n phys. Mikrowelle f.
mi·cro·zoa [ˌ-ˈzəʊə] pl, sing **-zo·on** [-ˈzəʊɑn] zoo. Mikrozoen pl.
mi·cro·zone [ˈ-zəʊn] n Mikrozone f.
mic·tion [ˈmɪkʃn] n Harnen nt, Harnlassen nt, Blasenentleerung f, Urinieren nt, Miktion f, Mictio f..
mic·tu·rate [ˈmɪktʃəreɪt] vi harnen, Harn lassen, urinieren.
mic·tu·ri·tion [ˌmɪkʃəˈrɪʃn] n → miction.
micturition center spinales Blasenzentrum nt.
micturition reflex Blasenentleerungsreflex m.
mid·ax·il·lar·y line [mɪdˈæksəlerɪ] mittlere Axillarlinie f, Linea axillaris media, Linea medio-axillaris.
mid·brain [ˈmɪdbreɪn] n Mittelhirn nt, Mesenzephalon nt, Mesencephalon nt.
midbrain tegmentum Mittelhirnhaube f, Tegmentum mesencephalicum.
midbrain vesicle embryo. Mittelhirnbläschen nt.
mid·car·pal joint [mɪdˈkɑːrpl] → mediocarpal articulation.
mid·cer·vi·cal fracture of neck of femur [mɪdˈsɜrvɪkl] mediale/intermediäre Schenkelhalsfraktur f.
mid·cla·vic·u·lar line [mɪdkləˈvɪkjələr] → medioclavicular line.
mid·cy·cle pain [mɪdˈsaɪkl] gyn. Mittelschmerz m, Intermenstrualschmerz m.
mid·dle [ˈmɪdl] I n 1. Mitte f. **in the ~** in der Mitte. **in the ~ of** (a. zeitlich) mitten in/

auf, inmitten; in der Mitte (von). **2.** Mittelstück *nt*, -teil *nt*, mittlerer Teil; Innere(s) *nt*. **3.** Bauch *m*, Taille *f*. **II** *adj* **4.** (*a. fig. u. zeitlich*) mittlere(r, s), Mittel-. **5.** medial.
middle-aged *adj* mittleren Alters, in den mittleren Jahren.
middle carpal joint → mediocarpal articulation.
middle cells Sinus medii.
middle commissure of cerebrum Adhesio interthalamica.
middle concha mittlere Nasenmuschel *f*, Concha nasalis media.
middle ear Mittelohr *nt*, Auris media.
middle ear bones Mittelohrknochen *pl*, Gehörknöchelchen *pl*, Ossicula auditoria/auditus.
middle ear carcinoma Mittelohrkarzinom *nt*.
middle ear cholesteatoma *HNO* Mittelohrcholesteatom *nt*.
  secondary m. Tensacholesteatom, sekundäres Mittelohrcholesteatom.
middle ear deafness *HNO* Mittelohrschwerhörigkeit *f*, -taubheit *f*, Schalleitungsstörung *f*, -schwerhörigkeit *f*.
middle ear fibrosis *HNO* Paukenfibrose *f*, adhäsive Otitis media (chronica).
middle ear injury Mittelohrverletzung *f*.
middle ear lesion *HNO* Mittelohrschädigung *f*.
middle ear syphilis *HNO* Mittelohrsyphilis *f*.
middle ear trauma *HNO* Mittelohrverletzung *f*.
middle ear tuberculosis Mittelohrtuberkulose *f*.
middle finger Mittelfinger *m*, Digitus medius/tertius.
middle head of triceps brachii muscle langer Trizepskopf *m*, Caput longum m. tricipitis brachii.
middle kidney → mesonephros.
middle layer of myometrium Vaskulärschicht *f* des Myometriums, Stratum vasculare (myometrii).
middle life mittleres Lebensalter *nt*.
middle lobe: m. of cerebellum kaudaler (Kleinhirn-)Lappen/-Abschnitt *m*, Lobus caudalis/posterior cerebelli.
  m. of prostate (*Prostata*) Mittellappen *m*, Lobus medius prostatae.
middle lobe syndrome (*Lunge*) Mittellappensyndrom *nt*.
middle mediastinum mittleres Mediastinalraum *m*, mittleres Mediastinum *nt*, Mediastinum medium, Cavum mediastinale medius.
mid·dle·most ['mɪdlməʊst] *adj* ganz in der Mitte (liegend).
middle name zweiter Vorname *m*.
middle neurogenic potentials mittlere neurogene Potentiale *pl*, schnelle Rindenpotentiale *pl*.
middle pain *gyn.* Mittelschmerz *m*, Intermenstrualschmerz *m*.
middle phalanx mittleres Glied *nt*, Mittelglied *nt*, -phalanx *f*, Phalanx media.
middle piece Mittelstück *nt* des Spermiums.
middle plate *embryo.* Nephrotom *nt*.
middle sinuses mittlere Siebbeinzellen *pl*, Cellulae mediae, Sinus medii.
middle-sized *adj* von mittlerer Größe.
middle trunk of brachial plexus mittlerer Primärfaszikel *m* des Plexus brachialis, Truncus medius (plexus brachialis).
mid·foot ['mɪdfʊt] *n* Mittelfuß *m*.
mid·for·ceps delivery [mɪd'fɔːrsəps, -seps] *gyn.* Zangengeburt *f* aus der Beckenmitte.

midg·et ['mɪdʒɪt] *n* proportionierter Zwerg *m*.
mid·gut ['mɪdɡʌt] *n embryo.* Mitteldarm *m*, Mesenteron *nt*.
mid·life ['mɪdlaɪf] **I** *n* Lebensmitte *f*, mittlere Jahre *pl*. **II** *adj* → middle-aged.
midlife crisis Midlife-crisis *f*, Krise *f* in der Lebensmitte.
mid·line granuloma ['mɪdlaɪn] letales Mittelliniengranulom *nt*, Granuloma gangraenescens nasi.
midline incision Medianschnitt *m*.
mid·nod·al rhythm [,-'nəʊdl] mittlerer Knotenrhythmus *m*.
mid·pain ['mɪdpeɪn] *n gyn.* Mittelschmerz *m*, Intermenstrualschmerz *m*.
mid·part of telencephalic vesicle ['mɪdpɑːrt] Telencephalon impar.
mid·piece ['mɪdpiːs] *n* → middle 2.
  m. of spermatozoon Mittelstück *nt* des Spermiums.
mid·riff ['mɪdrɪf] *n* **1.** Zwerchfell *nt*, Diaphragma *nt*. **2.** Obertaille *f*.
midriff bulge *inf.* (Hüft-, Taillen-)Fettpolster *nt*.
mid·sag·it·tal plane [mɪd'sædʒɪtl] *anat.* Medianebene *f*, Mediansagittale *f*, Mediansagittalebene *f*.
mid·sec·tion [mɪd'sekʃn] *n* **1.** → middle 2. **2.** → midriff.
midst [mɪdst] *n* Mitte *f*. **from the ~** aus der Mitte. **in the ~ of** inmitten, mitten in.
mid·ster·num [mɪd'stɜːrnəm] *n* → mesosternum.
mid·tar·sal fractures [mɪd'tɑːrsl] Frakturen *pl* im Fußwurzelbereich.
midtarsal joint Chopart'-Gelenklinie *f*, Artic. tarsi transversa.
mid·wife ['mɪdwaɪf] **I** *n*, *pl* **-wives** [-waɪvz] Hebamme *f*, Geburtshelferin *f*. **II** *vt* entbinden.
mid·wife·ry [mɪd'wɪfərɪ, 'mɪdwaɪf(ə)rɪ] *n* Geburtshilfe *f*.
Miescher ['miːʃər]: **M.'s tubes/tubules** *micro.* Rainey-Körperchen *pl*, Miescherschläuche *pl*.
MIF *abbr.* **1.** → melanocyte stimulating hormone inhibiting factor. **2.** → migration inhibiting factor.
MIF fixative → methiolate-iodine-formaline fixative.
MIF test → migration inhibiting factor test.
mi·graine ['maɪɡreɪn; *Brit.* 'miː-] *n* Migräne *f*, Migraine *f*.
migraine headache → migraine.
migraine phosphene *neuro.* Migränephosphen *nt*.
mi·grain·oid [maɪ'ɡreɪnɔɪd] *adj* migräneartig.
mi·grain·ous [maɪ'ɡreɪnəs] *adj* migräneartig, Migräne-.
migrainous neuralgia Bing-Horton-Syndrom *nt*, -Neuralgie *f*, Horton-Syndrom *nt*, -Neuralgie *f*, Histaminkopfschmerz *m*, -kephalgie *f*, Erythroprosopalgie *f*, Cephalaea histaminica, cluster headache (*nt*).
mi·grate ['maɪɡreɪt] *vi* wandern, migrieren; ziehen.
mi·grat·ing abscess ['maɪɡreɪtɪŋ] Senkungsabszeß *m*.
migrating cheilitis/cheilosis Perlèche *f*, Faulecken *pl*, Mundwinkelcheilitis *f*, -rhagaden *pl*, Cheilitis/Stomatitis angularis, Angulus infectiosus oris/candidamycetica.
migrating neuritis Neuritis migrans.
mi·gra·tion [maɪ'ɡreɪʃn] *n* **1.** Wanderung *f*, Migration *f*; Abwandern *nt*, Fortziehen *nt*, Zug *m*. **2.** → m. of leukocytes.
  m. of leukocytes Leukozytenmigration,

(Leukozyten-)Diapedese *f*.
migration inhibiting factor *abbr.* **MIF** Migrationsinhibitionsfaktor *m abbr.* MIF.
migration inhibiting factor test Migrationsinhibitionsfaktortest *m*, MIF-Test *m*.
mi·gra·to·ry ['maɪɡrətɔːriː, -təʊ-] *adj* wandernd, migratorisch, Zug-, Wander-.
migratory cell 1. amöboid-bewegliche Zelle *f*. **2.** Wanderzelle *f*.
migratory ophthalmia sympathische Ophthalmie *f*, Ophthalmia sympathica.
migratory pneumonia wandernde Pneumonie *f*, Pneumonia migrans.
Mikulicz ['mɪkjəlɪtʃ]: **M.'s angle** *ortho.* (*Femur*) Anteversionswinkel *m*.
  M.'s aphthae Mikulicz-Aphthen *pl*, habituelle Aphthen *pl*, chronisch rezidivierende Aphthen *pl*, rezidivierende benigne Aphthosis *f*, Periadenitis mucosa necrotica recorrens.
  M.'s cells Mikulicz-Zellen *pl*.
  M.'s clamp Mikulicz-Klemme *f*.
  M.'s colostomy Mikulicz-Operation *f*.
  M.'s disease Mikulicz-Krankheit *f*.
  M.'s drain Mikulicz-Tampon *nt*.
  M.'s forceps Mikulicz-Klemme *f*.
  M.'s operation 1. Mikulicz-Operation *f*. **2.** *chir.* Heineke-Mikulicz-Operation *f*, -Pyloroplastik *f*.
  M.'s peritoneal clamp/forceps Mikulicz-Klemme *f*.
  M.'s syndrome *HNO* Mikulicz-Krankheit *f*.
mil [mɪl] *n* → milliliter.
mil·am·me·ter [mɪl'æmiːtər] *n phys.* Milliamperemeter *nt*.
mil·dew ['mɪl'd(j)uː] *n* **1.** Schimmel *m*, Moder *m*. **2.** Mehltau *m*, Meltau *m*.
Miles [maɪlz]: **M.' operation/resection** *chir.* Miles-Operation *f*, abdominoperineale Rektumamputation *f*.
mil·i·ar·ia [mɪlɪ'eərɪə] *pl derm.* Schweißfrieseln *pl*, Hitzepickel *pl*, Hitzeblattern *pl*, Schweiß-, Schwitzbläschen *pl*, Miliaria *f*.
mil·i·a·ry ['mɪlɪˌerɪ, 'mɪljərɪ] *adj* hirsekorngroß, miliar, Miliar-.
miliary abscess Miliarabszeß *m*.
miliary aneurysm Miliaraneurysma *nt*.
miliary carcinosis Miliarkarzinose *f*.
miliary papular syphilid kleinpapulöses/miliares/lichenoides Syphilid *nt*, Lichen syphiliticus.
miliary tubercle Miliartuberkel *nt*.
miliary tuberculosis Miliartuberkulose *f*, miliare Tuberkulose *f*, Tuberculosis miliaris.
mi·lieu [mɪl'jɔ, miː'l-] *n*, *pl* **-lieus** *physiol.*, *patho.* Milieu *nt*, Umgebung *f*.
mil·i·um ['mɪlɪəm] *n*, *pl* **mil·ia** ['mɪlɪə] Hautgrieß *m*, Milium *nt*, Milie *f*.
milk [mɪlk] *n* **1.** Milch *f*. **2.** (*a. chem.*) Milch *f*, milchige *od.* milchähnliche Flüssigkeit *f*. **3.** *bot.* (Pflanzen-)Milch *f*.
  m. of almonds Mandelmilch *f*.
  m. of calcium bile Kalkgalle *f*, Kalkmilchgalle *f*.
  m. of lime *chem.* Kalkmilch *f*.
  m. of sulfur *chem.* Schwefelmilch *f*.
milk agent Mäuse-Mamma-Tumorvirus *nt abbr.* MMTV.
milk-alkali syndrome Burnett-Syndrom *nt*, Milch-Alkali-Syndrom *nt*.
milk anemia Kuhmilchanämie *f*.
milk bank Milchbank *f*.
milk bud *embryo.* Brustknospe *f*.
milk corpuscles Milchkügelchen *pl*, -partikel *pl*.
milk crust Milchschorf *m*, frühexsudatives Ekzematoid *nt*, konstitutionelles Säuglingsekzem *nt*, Crusta lactea, Eccema infantum.

milk cure Milchdiät *f*, -kur *f*.
milk cyst Laktations-, Milchzyste *f*.
milk diet Milchdiät *f*, -kur *f*.
milk ducts Milchgänge *pl*, Ductus lactiferi.
milk-ejection reflex *gyn.* Milchejektionsreflex *m*.
milk·er's node ['mɪlkər] Melkerknoten *m*, -pocken *pl*, Nebenpocken *pl*, Paravakzineknoten *m*, Paravaccinia *f*.
milker's node virus Melkerknotenvirus *nt*, Paravacciniavirus *nt*, Paravakzinevirus *nt*.
milker's nodule → milker's node.
milk factor Mäuse-Mamma-Tumorvirus *nt abbr.* MMTV.
milk fat Milchfett *nt*.
milk fever Milch-, Laktationsfieber *nt*, Galaktopyra *f*.
milk glass Milchglas *nt*, milchiges Glas *nt*.
milk-glass cell Milchglaszelle *f*.
milk globules Milchkügelchen *pl*.
milk·i·ness ['mɪlkɪnɪs] *n* Milchigkeit *f*.
milk leg Milchbein *nt*, Leukophlegmasie *f*, Phlegmasia alba dolens.
milk let-down reflex → milk-ejection reflex.
milk line *embryo.* Milchleiste *f*.
Milkman ['mɪlkmən]: **M.'s syndrome** Milkman-Syndrom *nt*, Looser-Syndrom *nt*, Looser-Milkman-Syndrom *nt*.
milk ridge *embryo.* → milk line.
milk plasma *bio., chem.* Milchplasma *nt*.
milk powder Trockenmilch *f*, Milchpulver *nt*.
milk pox Alastrim *nt*, weiße Pocken *pl*, Variola minor.
milk ring test Abortus-Bang-Ringprobe *f*, ABR-Probe *f*.
milk scall → milk crust.
milk streak *embryo.* Milchstreifen *m*.
milk sugar Milchzucker *m*, Laktose *f*, Lactose *f*, Laktobiose *f*.
milk tetter Milchschorf *m*, frühexsudatives Ekzematoid *nt*, konstitutionelles Säuglingsekzem *nt*, Crusta lactea, Eccema infantum.
milk tooth Milchzahn *m*, Dens deciduus.
milk-white *adj* milchweiß.
milk·y ['mɪlkɪ] *adj* 1. milchig, milchartig, Milch-. 2.
milky ascites fettiger/adipöser Aszites *m*.
milky tetter → milk tetter.
milky urine chylöser Urin *m*; Chylurie *f*.
Millar ['mɪlər]: **M.'s asthma** Stimmritzenkrampf *m*, Laryngismus stridulus.
Millard-Gubler ['gu:blər]: **M.-G. paralysis/syndrome** Millard-Gubler-Syndrom *nt*, Gubler-Lähmung *f*, Brücken-Mittelhirn-Syndrom *nt*, Hemiplegia alternans inferior.
Miller ['mɪlər]: **M.'s disease** Knochenerweichung *f*, Osteomalazie *f*, -malacia *f*.
Miller-Abbott ['æbət]: **M.-A. tube** Miller--Abbott-Sonde *f*.
mill·er's asthma ['mɪlər] Müller-, Mehlasthma *nt*.
Miller-Kurzrok ['kʊrtsrɔk]: **M.-K. test** *gyn.* Kurzrok-Miller-Test *m*, Invasionstest *m*.
Milles [mɪlz]: **M.' syndrome** Milles-Syndrom *nt*.
mil·let seed ['mɪlɪt] Hirsekorn *nt*.
mill fever [mɪl] *pulmo.* Baumwollfieber *nt*, Baumwoll(staub)pneumokoniose *f*, Byssinose *f*.
milli- *pref. abbr.* **m** Milli- *abbr.* m.
mil·li·am·me·ter [,mɪlɪ'æmɪtər] *n phys.* Milliamperemeter *nt*.
mil·li·am·pere [,-'æmpɪər, -æm'pɪər] *n abbr.* **mA** Milliampere *nt abbr.* mA.
mil·li·bar ['-bɑːr] *n abbr.* **mb, mbar** Millibar *nt abbr.* mbar.
mil·li·cou·lomb [,-'kuːlɑm, -kuː'lɑm, -lɑʊm] *n abbr.* **mC** Millicoulomb *nt abbr.* mC.
mil·li·cu·rie ['-kjʊəri, -kjʊə,rɪ] *n abbr.* **mCi** Millicurie *nt abbr.* mCi.
mil·li·e·quiv·a·lent [,-ɪ'kwɪvələnt] *n abbr.* **mEq., meq.** Milliäquivalent *nt abbr.* mäq, meq, mVal.
mil·li·gam·ma [,-'gæmə] *n old* → nanogram.
mil·li·gram ['-græm] *n abbr.* **mg** Milligramm *nt abbr.* mg.
Millikan ['mɪlɪkən]: **M. rays** *phys.* kosmische Strahlung *f*.
mil·li·li·ter ['mɪləlɪtər] *n abbr.* **ml** Milliliter *nt*/*m abbr.* ml.
mil·li·me·ter ['-miːtər] *n abbr.* **mm** Millimeter *nt*/*m abbr.* mm.
millimicro- *pref. old* → nano-.
mil·li·mo·lar [,-'məʊlər] *adj abbr.* **mM** millimolar *abbr.* mM.
mil·li·mole ['-məʊl] *n abbr.* **mmol** Millimol *nt abbr.* mmol.
mil·lion·fold ['mɪljən'fəʊld] *adj* millionenfach.
mil·li·os·mol(e) [,mɪlɪ'ɑsməʊl, -mɑl] *n abbr.* **mOsm** Milliosmol *nt abbr.* mOsm.
mil·li·rad ['-ræd] *n abbr.* **mrad** Millirad *nt abbr.* mrad.
mil·li·rem ['-rem] *n abbr.* **mrem** Millirem *nt abbr.* mrem.
mil·li·sec·ond ['-sekənd] *n abbr.* **ms, msec** Millisekunde *f abbr.* ms.
mil·li·volt ['-vəʊlt] *n abbr.* **mV** Millivolt *nt abbr.* mV.
Millon ['mɪlɑn; mɪ'lɔ̃]: **M.'s reaction/test** Millon-Probe *f*.
Mills [mɪlz]: **M.' disease** Mills-Syndrom *nt*, -Lähmung *f*.
Milroy ['mɪlrɔɪ]: **M.'s disease/edema** Lymphödem/Trophödem *nt* Typ Nonne-Milroy.
Milton ['mɪltn]: **M.'s disease/edema** Quincke-Ödem *nt*, angioneurotisches Ödem *nt*.
Mil·wau·kee brace [mɪl'wɔːki] Milwaukee-Korsett *nt*.
milz·brand ['mɪltsbrɑnt] *n* Milzbrand *m*, Anthrax *m*.
mi·me·sis [mɪ'miːsɪs, maɪ-] *n bio.* Mimese *f*.
mi·met·ic [mɪ'metɪk, maɪ-] *adj* bewegend, erregend, mimetisch.
mimetic convulsion → mimic spasm.
mimetic paralysis Lähmung *f* der mimischen Muskulatur.
mim·ic ['mɪmɪk] *adj* 1. Mimik betr., mimisch. 2. mimetic.
mimic convulsion → mimic spasm.
mim·ic·ry ['mɪmɪkrɪ] *n bio.* Mimikry *f*.
mimic spasm mimischer Gesichtskrampf *m*, Bell-Spasmus *m*, Fazialiskrampf *m*, Gesichtszucken *nt*, Fazialis-Tic *m*, Tic convulsif/facial.
mimic tic → mimic spasm.
mi·mo·sis [mɪ'məʊsɪs, maɪ-] *n* → mimesis.
Min·a·ma·ta disease [mɪnə'mɑːtə] Minamata-Krankheit *f*.
mind [maɪnd] *n* 1. Sinn *m*, Gemüt *nt*; Seele *f*, Verstand *m*, Geist *m*. **to be of sound ~** bei (vollem) Verstand sein. **of unsound ~** geistesgestört, unzurechnungsfähig. **to lose one's ~** den Verstand verlieren. 2. Meinung *f*, Ansicht *f*. 3. Neigung *f*, Lust *f*, Absicht *f*.
mind blindness zerebrale/zerebralbedingte/organbedingte Blindheit *f*.
miner ['maɪnər]: **m.'s anemia** Anämie *f* bei Hakenwurmbefall.
m.'s asthma Asthma *nt* bei Anthrakose.
m.'s cramp Heizerkrampf *m*.
m.'s disease Hakenwurmbefall *m*, -infektion *f*, Ankylostomiasis *f*, Ankylostomatosis *f*, Ankylostomatidose *f*.
m.'s elbow Entzündung *f* des Ellenbogenschleimbeutels, Bursitis olecrani.
m.'s lung Kohlenstaublunge *f*, Lungenanthrakose *f*, Anthracosis pulmonum.
m.'s nystagmus Bergarbeiternystagmus *m*.
m.'s phthisis → m.'s lung.
min·er·al ['mɪn(ə)rəl] **I** *n* Mineral *nt*. **II** *adj* **1.** Mineral(ien) betr. enthaltend, mineralisch, Mineral-. **2.** *chem.* anorganisch, mineralisch.
mineral acid Mineralsäure *f*, anorganische Säure *f*.
mineral chemistry anorganische Chemie *f*.
min·er·al·i·za·tion [,mɪn(ə)rəlaɪ'zeɪʃn, -lɪ'z-] *n* **1.** Einlagerung *f* von Mineralstoffen in organische Grundsubstanz, Mineralisation *f*. **2.** *bio.* Umwandlung *f* organischer Substanzen in anorganische, Mineralbildung *f*, Mineralisation *f*. **3.** **~s** *pl Brit.* → mineral water.
min·er·al·ize ['mɪn(ə)rəlaɪz] *vt* mineralisieren, in ein Mineral umwandeln; Mineralstoffe einlagern.
min·er·al·o·coid ['mɪn(ə)rələʊkɔɪd] *n* → mineralocorticoid.
min·er·al·o·cor·ti·coid [,-'kɔːrtɪkɔɪd] *n* Mineralokortikoid *nt*, -corticoid *nt*.
mineralocorticoid system Mineralokortikoidsystem *nt*.
mineral salt Mineralsalz *nt*, Mineral *nt*.
mineral water Mineralwasser *nt*.
min·i·a·ture stomach ['mɪnɪətʃər, 'mɪnətʃər] Pawlow-Magen *m*, -Tasche *f*.
min·i·fy ['mɪnəfaɪ] *vt* vermindern, verkleinern.
min·i·mal ['mɪnɪməl] *adj* → minimum II.
minimal alveolar concentration *abbr.* **MAC** *anes.* minimale alveoläre Konzentration *f abbr.* MAC.
minimal bactericidal concentration *abbr.* **MBC** minimale bakterizide Konzentration *f abbr.* MBK.
minimal brain dysfunction hyperkinetisches Syndrom *nt* des Kindesalters.
minimal change glomerulonephritis Minimal-change-Glomerulonephritis *f*, Lipoidnephrose *f*.
minimal dose *pharm.* Minimaldosis *f*.
minimal glomerulonephritis → minimal change glomerulonephritis.
minimal hepatitis Minimalhepatitis *f*, reaktive Hepatitis *f*.
minimal inhibitory concentration *abbr.* **MIC** minimale Hemmkonzentration *f abbr.* MHK.
minimal lethal concentration *abbr.* **MLC** → minimal bactericidal concentration.
min·i·mize ['mɪnəmaɪz] *vt* auf das Minimum herabsetzen *od.* reduzieren, das Minimum anstreben, minimieren.
min·i·mum ['mɪnəməm] **I** *n, pl* **-mums, -ma** [-mə] Minimum *nt*, Mindestmaß *nt*, -betrag *m*, -wert *m*. **at a ~** auf dem Tiefststand. **II** *adj* minimal, mindeste(r, s), kleinste(r, s), geringste(r, s), Minimal-, Mindest-.
minimum age Mindestalter *nt*.
minimum dose → minimal dose.
minimum free-energy form *biochem.* Form/Konformation *f* mit minimaler freier Energie.
minimum separable angle → minimum separable angle.
minimum separable angle *ophthal.* Grenzwinkel *m*, kleinster Sehwinkel *m*, Minimum separabile.
minimum thermometer Minimumthermometer *nt*.
minimum visible/visual angle → minimum separable angle.

min·i·pill ['mɪnɪpɪl] *n gyn.* Minipille *f.*
Minkowski-Chauffard [mɪn'kɔvskɪ ʃɔ'fɑːr]: **M.-C. syndrome** Minkowski--Chauffard(-Gänsslen)-Syndrom *nt*, hereditäre Sphärozytose *f*, konstitutionelle hämolytische Kugelzellanämie *f*, familiärer hämolytischer Ikterus *m*, Morbus Minkowski-Chauffard *m*.
mi·no·cy·cline [,mɪnəʊ'saɪkliːn, -klɪn] *n pharm.* Minocyclin *nt*.
mi·nor ['maɪnər] *adj* **1.** kleiner, geringer, weniger bedeutend; *anat.* minor. **2.** Unter-, Neben-, Hilfs-.
minor agglutinin Neben-, Minoragglutinin *nt*.
minor base *biochem.* seltene Base *f.*
minor cartilages Cartilagines nasales accessoriae.
minor chain *biochem.* schwere Kette *f*, H-Kette *f.*
minor circulation kleiner Kreislauf *m*, Lungenkreislauf *m.*
minor curve *ortho.* (*Skoliose*) Neben-, Minorkrümmung *f*, Minorkurve *f.*
minor epilepsy 1. Epilepsie *f* mit Absence--Symptomatik. **2.** Petit-mal(-Epilepsie *f*) *nt abbr.* PM.
minor histocompatibility complex minor Histokompatibilitätsantigene *pl.*
minor nucleoside *biochem.* seltenes Nukleosid *n.*
minor periodicity *biochem.* Neben-, Unterperiodizität *f.*
Minor ['miːnɔːr]: **M.'s sign** Minor-Zeichen *nt.*
minor test *immun.* Minortest *m*, -probe *f.*
minor wing of sphenoid bone kleiner Keilbeinflügel *m*, Ala minor (ossis sphenoidalis).
Minot-von Willebrand ['maɪnət fɔn 'vɪləbrant]: **M.-v.W. syndrome** (von) Willebrand-Jürgens-Syndrom *nt*, konstitutionelle Thrombopathie *f*, hereditäre/vaskuläre Pseudohämophilie *f*, Angiohämophilie *f.*
min·ox·i·dil [mɪ'nɑksɪdɪl] *n pharm.* Minoxidil *nt.*
mint [mɪnt] *n* Minze *f*, Mentha *f.*
mint camphor *pharm.* Menthakampfer *m*, Menthol *nt.*
mint oil Pfefferminzöl *nt.*
mi·nus ['maɪnəs] **I** *adj* negativ, minus, unter null, Minus-. **II** *prep mathe.* minus, weniger, abzüglich; ohne.
minus cyclophoria *ophthal.* Inzyklophorie *f.*
minus cyclotropia *ophthal.* Inzyklotropie *f.*
minus lens Konkavlinse *f*, (Zer-)Streuungslinse *f.*
min·ute ['mɪnɪt] **I** *n* **1.** Minute *f.* **for a ~** eine Minute (lang). **to the ~** auf die Minute. **2. ~s** *pl* Protokoll *nt.* **to take/keep the ~s** das Protokoll führen. **II** *adj* **3.** winzig. **4.** *fig.* unbedeutend, geringfügig. **5.** minuziös, (peinlich) genau. **III** *vt* **6.** die Zeit nehmen *od.* messen, mitstoppen. **7.** protokollieren, notieren.
minute anatomy → microscopical anatomy.
mi·nute·ness ['-nɪs] *n* **1.** Winzigkeit *f.* **2.** Genauigkeit *f.*
minute output *card.* Herzminutenvolumen *nt abbr.* HMV, Minutenvolumen *nt.*
minute ventilation → minute volume 1.
minute volume *physiol.* **1.** *abbr.* **MV** (*Lunge*) Atemzeitvolumen *nt*, Atemminutenvolumen *nt abbr.* AMV. **2.** Minutenvolumen *nt*, Herzminutenvolumen *nt abbr.* HMV.
mi·o·car·dia [,maɪə'kɑːrdɪə] *n* Systole *f.*
mi·o·did·y·mus [,ɪ-'dɪdəməs] *n embryo.* Mio(di)dymus *m.*

mi·od·y·mus [maɪ'ɑdɪməs] *n* → miodidymus.
mi·o·lec·i·thal [,maɪə'lesɪθəl] *adj bio.* miolezithal.
mi·o·pap·o·va·vi·rus [,-,pæpəʊvæ'vaɪrəs] *n micro.* Polyomavirus *nt*, Miopapovavirus *nt.*
mi·o·pus ['maɪəpəs] *n embryo.* Miopus *m.*
mi·o·sis [maɪ'əʊsɪs] *n*, *pl* **-ses** [-siːz] **1.** Pupillenverengung *f*, -engstellung *f*, Miosis *f.* **2.** → meiosis.
mi·ot·ic [maɪ'ɑtɪk] **I** *n pharm.* pupillenverengendes Mittel *nt*, Miotikum *nt*, Mioticum *nt.* **II** *adj* **1.** Miosis betr. *od.* auslösend, miotisch. **2.** → meiotic.
mi·ra·cid·i·um [,maɪrə'sɪdɪəm] *n*, *pl* **-dia** [-dɪə] *micro.* Mirazidium *nt*, -cidium *nt*, -zidie *f.*
MIRF *abbr.* → macrophage Ia recruting factor.
Mirizzi [mɪ'rɪzɪ]: **M.'s syndrome** Mirizzi--Syndrom *nt.*
mir·ror ['mɪrər] **I** *n* **1.** Spiegel *m.* **2.** *phys., techn.* Reflektor *m*, Rückstrahler *m.* **II** *vt* spiegeln, widerspiegeln; reflektieren.
mirror image Spiegelbild *n.*
mirror laryngoscopy indirekte Kehlkopfspiegelung/Laryngoskopie *f.*
MIS *abbr.* → müllerian inhibiting substance.
mis·an·thrope ['mɪsnθrəʊp] *n* Menschenfeind *m*, -hasser *m*, Misanthrop *m.*
mis·an·thro·pia [,-'θrəʊpɪə] *n* → misanthropy.
mis·an·throp·ic [,-'θrɑpɪk] *adj* menschenfeindlich, -scheu, misanthropisch.
mis·an·throp·i·cal [,-'θrɑpɪkl] *adj* → misanthropic.
mis·an·thro·pist [mɪs'ænθrəpɪst] *n* → misanthrope.
mis·an·thro·py [mɪs'ænθrəpɪ] *n* Menschenscheu *m*, -haß *m*, Misanthropie *f.*
mis·car·riage [mɪs'kærɪdʒ, 'mɪskærɪdʒ] *n* **1.** *gyn.* Spontanabort *m*, Fehlgeburt *f.* **2.** Fehlschlag *m*, Mißlingen *nt.*
mis·car·ry [mɪs'kærɪ, 'mɪskærɪ] *vi* **1.** *gyn.* eine Fehlgeburt haben. **2.** mißlingen, fehlschlagen, scheitern.
mis·ce·ge·na·tion [mɪ,sedʒə'neɪʃn, ,mɪsədʒə-] *n bio., genet.* Rassenmischung *f.*
mis·ci·bil·i·ty [,mɪsə'bɪlətɪ] *n* Mischbarkeit *f.*
mis·ci·ble ['mɪsəbl] *adj* mischbar.
mis·di·ag·nose [mɪs'daɪəgnəʊs] *vt* eine Fehldiagnose stellen.
mis·di·ag·no·sis [,mɪsdaɪəg'nəʊsɪs] *n*, *pl* **-ses** [-siːz] Fehldiagnose *f.*
mi·sog·a·my [mɪ'sɑgəmɪ] *n psychia.* Ehescheu *f*, Misogamie *f.*
mi·sog·y·nis·tic [mɪ,sɑdʒə'nɪstɪk] *adj* frauenfeindlich, misogyn.
mi·sog·y·nous [mɪ'sɑdʒənəs] *adj* → misogynistic.
mi·sog·y·ny [mɪ'sɑdʒənɪ] *n* Frauenhaß *m*, -feindlichkeit *f*, Misogynie *f.*
missed abortion [mɪst] *gyn.* verhaltener Abort *m*, missed abortion (*f*).
mis·sense mutation [mɪs'sens] Missense--Mutation *f*, Falsch-Sinn-Mutation *f.*
MIT *abbr.* → monoiodotyrosine.
Mitchell ['mɪtʃl]: **M.'s disease** Gerhardt--Syndrom *nt*, Mitchell-Gerhardt-Syndrom *nt*, Weir-Mitchell-Krankheit *f*, Erythromelalgie *f*, Erythralgie *f*, Erythermalgie *f*, Akromelalgie *f.*
M.'s operation *ortho.* Mitchell-Operation *f.*
mite [maɪt] *n micro.* Milbe *f.*
mite-borne typhus → mite typhus.
mi·tel·la [mɪ'telə] *n ortho.* Armtragetuch *nt*, Mitella *f.*

mite typhus japanisches Fleckfieber *nt*, Milbenfleckfieber *nt*, Scrub-Typhus *m*, Tsutsugamushi-Fieber *nt.*
mith·ra·my·cin [mɪθrə'maɪsɪn] *n pharm.* Mithramycin *nt.*
mit·i·ci·dal [,maɪtə'saɪdl] *adj* milben(ab)tötend, mitizid.
mit·i·cide ['-saɪd] *n* milbentötendes Mittel *nt*, Mitizid *nt.*
mit·i·gate ['mɪtɪgeɪt] *vt* mildern, abschwächen, mitigieren; (*Schmerzen*) lindern.
mit·i·gat·ed ['-geɪtɪd] *adj* abgeschwächt, gemildert, mitigiert.
mit·i·ga·tion [,-'geɪʃn] *n* Linderung *f*, Milderung *f*, Abschwächung *f.*
mit·i·ga·tive ['-geɪtɪv] *adj* lindernd, mildernd, abschwächend, mitigierend.
mit·i·ga·to·ry ['-gə,tɔːriː, -təʊ-] *adj* → mitigative.
mi·to·chon·dria *pl* → mitochondrion.
mi·to·chon·dri·al [,maɪtə'kɑndrɪəl] *adj* Mitochondrien betr., von Mitochondrien stammend, mitochondrial, Mitochondrien-.
mitochondrial antibodies (Anti-)Mitochondrienantikörper *pl.*
mitochondrial chromosome Mitochondrienchromosom *nt.*
mitochondrial DNA *abbr.* **mtDNA** mitochondriale DNS *f*, mitochondriale DNA *f*, Mitochondrien-DNA *f abbr.* mtDNA.
mitochondrial inheritance extrachromosomale Vererbung *f.*
mitochondrial matrix Mitochondrienmatrix *f.*
mitochondrial membrane Mitochondrienmembran *f.*
mitochondrial mutant Mitochondrienmutante *f.*
mitochondrial ribosome mitochondriales Ribosom *nt.*
mi·to·chon·dri·on [,-'kɑndrɪən] *n*, *pl* **-dria** [-drɪə] Mitochondrie *f*, -chondrion *nt*, -chondrium *nt*, Chondriosom *nt.*
mit·o·gen [-'dʒən] *n* Mitogen *nt.*
mit·o·ge·ne·sia [,-dʒɪ'niːʒ(ɪ)ə] *n* → mitogenesis.
mit·o·gen·e·sis [,-'dʒenəsɪs] *n* Mitogenese *f.*
mit·o·ge·net·ic [,-dʒə'netɪk] *adj* Mitogenese betr. *od.* induzierend, mitogenetisch.
mit·o·gen·ic [,-'dʒenɪk] *adj* mitoseauslösend, -stimulierend, mitogen.
mitogenic agent → mitogen.
mitogenic factor Lymphozytenmitogen *nt*, Lymphozytentransformationsfaktor *m abbr.* LTF.
mi·to·my·cin [,-'maɪsɪn] *n pharm.* Mitomycin *nt.*
mi·to·schi·sis [mɪ'tɑskəsɪs] *n* → mitosis.
mi·to·sis [maɪ'təʊsɪs] *n*, *pl* **-ses** [-siːz] Mitose *f*, mitotische Zellteilung *f*, indirekte Kernteilung *f*; Karyokinese *f.*
mit·o·some ['mɪtəsəʊm, 'maɪt-] *n* Mitosom *nt.*
mi·tot·ic [maɪ'tɑtɪk, mɪ-] *adj* Mitose betr., mitotisch, Mitose(n)-.
mitotic index Mitoseindex *m.*
mitotic period *bio.* M-Phase *f.*
mitotic poison Mitosegift *nt.*
mitotic rate *bio.* Mitoserate *f.*
mitotic spindle Kern-, Mitosespindel *f.*
mitotic stability Mitosestabilität *f.*
mi·tral ['maɪtrəl] *adj* **1.** *anat.* (bischofs-)mützen-, mitralförmig, mitral. **2.** Mitralklappe betr., mitral, Mitral(klappen)-.
mitral area *card.* Mitralisauskultationspunkt *m.*
mitral atresia Mitral(klappen)atresie *f.*
mitral buttonhole → mitral stenosis, buttonhole.
mitral cells Mitralzellen *pl.*

mitral facies *card.* Mitralgesicht *nt*, Facies mitralis.
mitral incompetence → mitral insufficiency.
mitral insufficiency *card.* Mitral(klappen)insuffizienz *f*.
mi·tral·i·za·tion [ˌmaɪtrəlaɪˈzeɪʃn, -lɪ-] *n card.* Mitralisation *f*.
mitral layer of olfactory bulb Lamina mitralis bulbi olfactorii.
mitral murmur *card.* Mitral(klappen)geräusch *nt*.
mitral orifice Ostium atrioventriculare sinistrum.
mitral regurgitation → mitral insufficiency.
mitral stenosis Mitral(klappen)stenose *f*.
 buttonhole m. Knopflochstenose, Fischmaulstenose.
 congenital m. Duroziez-Syndrom *nt*, -Erkrankung *f*, angeborene Mitral(klappen)stenose.
 fishmouth m. → buttonhole m.
mitral valve Mitralklappe *f*, Mitralis *f*, Valvula bicuspidalis/mitralis, Valva atrioventricularis sinistra.
mitral valve prolapse syndrome Barlow-Syndrom *nt*, Klick-Syndrom *nt*, Mitralklappenprolapssyndrom *nt*, Floppy-valve-Syndrom *nt*.
mi·tro·tri·cus·pid facies [ˌmaɪtrətraɪˈkʌspɪd] → mitral facies.
Mitsuda [mɪtˈsuːdə]: **M. antigen** Lepromin *nt*, Mitsuda-Antigen *nt*.
 M. reaction Mitsuda-Reaktion *f*, Leprominreaktion *f*.
 M. test Lepromintest *m*.
mit·tel·schmerz [ˈmɪtlʃmɛrts] *n gyn.* Mittelschmerz *m*, Intermenstrualschmerz *m*.
mit·ten hand [ˈmɪtn] Flossenhand *f*.
mix [mɪks] (*v* **mixed**; **mixt**) **I** *n* Gemisch *nt*, Mischung *f*. **II** *vt* mixen, (ver-)mischen, vermengen, versetzen (*with* mit). **III** *vi* **1.** s. (ver-)mischen; s. mischen lassen. **2.** *bio.* s. kreuzen.
mix into *vt* beimischen.
mix up *vt* (ver-)mischen; verrühren.
mixed [mɪkst] *adj* ge-, vermischt, unterschiedlich, Misch-.
mixed agglutination → mixed agglutination reaction.
mixed agglutination reaction Mischzellagglutination *f*.
mixed anesthesia Kombinationsanästhesie *f*, -narkose *f*.
mixed aneurysm kombiniertes Aneurysma *nt*.
mixed aphasia *neuro.* Total-, Globalaphasie *f*.
mixed articulation Artic. composita/complexa.
mixed astigmatism *ophthal.* Astigmatismus mixtus.
mixed beat *card.* Kombinationssystole *f*.
mixed blood 1. Mischling *m*. **2.** gemischtes Blut *nt*, gemischte Abstammung *f*.
mixed cell sarcoma → malignant mesenchymoma.
mixed connective tissue disease Sharp-Syndrom *nt*, Mischkollagenose *f*, gemischte Bindegewebserkrankung *f*, mixed connective tissue disease (*nt*).
mixed culture gemischte Kultur *f*, Mischkultur *f*.
mixed dentition Übergangsgebiß *nt*.
mixed fermentation heterolaktische/heterofermentative/gemischte Milchsäuregärung *f*.
mixed-function oxygenase mischfunktionelle Oxygenase *f*.
mixed gland 1. seromuköse (Misch-)Drüse *f*, Gl. seromucosa. **2.** gemischt endokrin-exokrine Drüse *f*.
mixed hemorrhoids *chir.* intermediäre Hämorrhoiden *pl*.
mixed hyperlipemia 1. (primäre/essentielle) Hyperlipoproteinämie *f* Typ IIb, (familiäre) kombinierte Hyperlipidämie *f*. **2.** (primäre/essentielle) Hyperlipoproteinämie *f* Typ V, fett- u. kohlenhydratinduzierte Hyperlipidämie/Hyperlipoproteinämie *f*, exogen-endogene Hyperlipoproteinämie *f*, kalorisch-induzierte Hyperlipoproteinämie *f*, Hyperchylomikronämie *f* u. Hyperpräbetalipoproteinämie.
mixed hyperlipidemia → mixed hyperlipemia 1.
mixed hyperlipoproteinemia → mixed hyperlipemia.
mixed infection Mischinfektion *f*.
mixed joint → mixed articulation.
mixed lymphocyte culture *abbr.* **MLC** gemischte Lymphozytenkultur *f*, Lymphozytenmischkultur *f*, mixed lymphocyte culture *abbr.* MLC, MLC-Assay *m*, MLC-Test *m*.
mixed lymphocyte culture assay/test → mixed lymphocyte culture.
mixed lymphocyte reaction *abbr.* **MLR** → mixed lymphocyte culture.
mixed marriage Mischehe *f*.
mixed nerve gemischter Nerv *m*, N. mixtus.
mixed paralysis gemischte Lähmung *f*.
mixed porphyria gemischte (hepatische) Porphyrie *f*, südafrikanische genetische Porphyrie *f*, (hereditäre) Protokoproporphyrie *f*, Porphyria variegata *abbr.* PV.
mixed thrombus *patho.* Abscheidungsthrombus *m*.
mixed tumor Mischtumor *m*.
 m. of salivary gland Speicheldrüsenmischtumor, pleomorphes Adenom *nt*.
mixed vaccine polyvalenter Impfstoff *m*.
mix·ing [ˈmɪksɪŋ] *adj* Misch-.
mix·o·sco·pia [mɪksəˈskəʊpɪə] *n psychia.* Mixoskopie *f*.
mix·ture [ˈmɪkstʃər] *n* **1.** Mischung *f*, Gemisch *nt* (*of ... and* aus ... und). **2.** *chem.* Gemisch *nt*. **3.** *pharm.* Mixtur *f*, Mixtura *f*. **4.** *bio.* Kreuzung *f*.
mi·ya·ga·wa bodies [ˈmɪəgɑːwə] Miyagawa-Körper *pl*.
Mi·ya·ga·wa·nel·la [ˌmɪəgɑːwəˈnelə] *n micro.* Chlamydie *f*, Chlamydia *f*, PLT-Gruppe *f*, *old* Bedsonia *f*, *old* Miyagawanella *f*.
ml *abbr.* → milliliter.
µl *abbr.* → microliter.
MLC *abbr.* **1.** [minimal lethal concentration] → minimal bactericidal concentration. **2.** → mixed lymphocyte culture.
MLC test → mixed lymphocyte culture test.
M.L.D. *abbr.* → lethal dose, minimal.
M-line protein M-Linien-Protein *nt*.
MLM *abbr.* → malignant lentigo melanoma.
MLNS *abbr.* → mucocutaneous lymph node syndrome.
MLR *abbr.* [mixed lymphocyte reaction] → mixed lymphocyte culture.
MLV *abbr.* → murine leukemia virus.
MM *abbr.* → malignant melanoma.
mM *abbr.* → millimolar.
mm *abbr.* → millimeter.
µM *abbr.* → micromolar.
µm *abbr.* → micrometer 1.
M-mode *n radiol.* M-mode *m*, TM-mode *m*.
mmol *abbr.* → millimole.
MMR *abbr.* → measles, mumps, and rubella vaccine live.
MMTV *abbr.* → mouse mammary tumor virus.
Mn *abbr.* → manganese.
MN blood group (system) MNSs-Blutgruppe *f*, -Blutgruppensystem *nt*.
mne·me [ˈniːmiː] *n* Gedächtnis *nt*, Erinnerung *f*, Mneme *f*.
mne·men·ic [niːˈmenɪk] *adj* → mnemic.
mne·mic [ˈniːmɪk] *adj* Gedächtnis betr., mnemisch, mnestisch.
mne·mon·ic [niːˈmɒnɪk] *adj* **1.** → mnemic. **2.** Mnemotechnik betr., mnemonisch, mnemotechnisch.
mne·mon·ics [niːˈmɒnɪks] *pl* Mnemonik *f*, Mnemotechnik *f*.
MNSs blood group (system) MNSs-Blutgruppe *f*, -Blutgruppensystem *nt*.
Mo *abbr.* → molybdenum.
Moberg [ˈməʊbɜːrg]: **M. arthrodesis** *ortho.* Spanbolzung *f* nach Moberg.
mo·bile [ˈməʊbəl, -biːl; *Brit.* -baɪl] *adj* **1.** beweglich, mobil; (*a. fig.*) wendig. **2.** *chem.* leicht-, dünnflüssig. **3.** *socio.* mobil.
mobile cecum C(a)ecum mobile.
mobile gallbladder flottierende Gallenblase *f*.
mobile spasm Athetose *f*.
mo·bil·i·ty [məʊˈbɪlətɪ] *n* **1.** Beweglichkeit *f*, Bewegungsfähigkeit *f*, Mobilität *f*; (*a. fig.*) Wendigkeit *f*. **2.** *chem.* Leichtflüssigkeit *f*. **3.** *socio.* Mobilität *f*.
mo·bi·li·za·tion [ˌməʊbəlɪˈzeɪʃn] *n* Beweglichmachung *f*, Mobilisierung *f*, Mobilisation *f*.
mo·bi·lize [ˈməʊbəlaɪz] *vt* mobilisieren, (wieder) beweglich machen.
Mobitz [ˈməʊbɪts]: **M. (heart) block** Mobitz-Typ *m*, -Block *m*, AV-Block *m* II. Grades Typ II.
Möbius [ˈmiːbɪəs; ˈmøːbiʊs]: **M.' disease 1.** Möbius'-Krankheit *f*, ophthalmoplegische Migräne *f*. **2.** Möbius'-Krankheit *f*, periodische Okulomotoriuslähmung *f* mit Neuralgie.
 M.' sign Moebius-Zeichen *nt*.
 M.' syndrome Möbius-Syndrom *nt*, -Kernaplasie *f*.
mock-up *n* Modell *nt*, Attrappe *f*.
mo·dal·i·ty [məʊˈdælətɪ] *n*, *pl* **-ties 1.** Anwendung(smethode *f*) *f*, Modalität *f*. **2.** *physiol.* (Empfindungs-)Modalität *f*.
mod·al value [ˈməʊdl] *physiol.* Modalwert *m*.
mode [məʊd] *n* **1.** Art u. Weise *f*, Regel *f*, Form *f*, Modus *m*; Erscheinungsform *f*. **2.** *stat.* Modus *m*, häufigster *od.* dichtester Wert *m*.
 m. of action Wirkungsweise, -mechanismus *m*.
 m. of application Anwendungsmodus *m*.
 m. of life Lebensweise, -gewohnheiten *pl*, -art.
 m. of taste Geschmacksqualität *f*.
mod·el [ˈmɒdl] **I** *n* Modell *nt*, Muster *nt*, Vorlage *f*, Schema *nt*, Vorbild *nt* (*of* für); *fig.* (Denk-)Modell *nt*; *anat.* Phantom *nt*. **II** *adj* vorbildlich, musterhaft, Muster-. **III** *vt* formen, nachbilden, modellieren. **IV** *vi* Modell(e) herstellen.
mod·er·ate [*adj* ˈmɒd(ə)rɪt; *v* -dəreɪt] **I** *adj* mäßig, gemäßigt, mittelgradig; maßvoll; mittelmäßig, bescheiden. **II** *vt* mäßigen; beruhigen; *techn.* dämpfen. **III** *vi* s. mäßigen; s. beruhigen, nachlassen, s. abschwächen.
moderate deafness mittelgradige Schwerhörigkeit *f*.
mod·er·a·tion [ˌmɒdəˈreɪʃn] *n* Mäßigung *f*, Maß(halten *nt*) *nt*. **in ~** mit Maß(en).

mod·er·a·tor ['mɑdəreɪtər] *n phys. chem.* Moderator *m*.
moderator band Trabecula septomarginalis.
mod·i·fi·a·bil·i·ty [,mɑdəfaɪə'bɪlətɪ] *n* Modifizierbarkeit *f*.
mod·i·fi·a·ble ['mɑdəfaɪəbl] *adj* modifizierbar.
mod·i·fi·ca·tion [,mɑdəfɪ'keɪʃn] *n* (Ab-, Ver-)Änderung *f*, Ab-, Umwandlung *f*, Modifizierung *f*; (*a. genet.*) Modifikation *f*.
modification enzyme Modifikationsenzym *nt*.
modification methylase Modifikationsmethylase *f*.
modification reaction Modifikationsreaktion *f*.
mod·i·fied scattering ['mɑdəfaɪd] *phys.* Quantenstreuung *f*, Compton-Streuung *f*.
modified Thayer-Martin medium *abbr.* **MTM** modifiziertes Thayer-Martin-Medium *nt*.
mod·i·fy ['mɑdəfaɪ] *vt* 1. modifizieren, (ver-, ab-)ändern, ab-, umwandeln. 2. mildern, abschwächen.
mo·di·o·lus [məʊ'daɪələs, mə-] *n* Schneckenachse *f*, -spindel *f*, Modiolus *f*.
mod·u·lar ['mɑdʒələr] *adj* Modul betr., modular.
mod·u·late ['mɑdʒəleɪt] *vt* abwandeln, abstimmen, regulieren, ab-, umwandeln.
mod·u·la·tion [,mɑdʒə'leɪʃn] *n* Abwandlung *f*, Veränderung *f*, Abstimmung *f*, Regulierung *f*, Modulation *f*.
mod·u·la·tor ['mɑdʒəleɪtər] *n genet.* Modulator *m*.
mod·u·la·to·ry ['mɑdʒələ,tɔːrɪ, -,təʊ-] *adj* modulatorisch, Modulations-.
mod·u·lus of elasticity ['mɑdʒələs] *phys.* Elastizitätsmodul *m*.
MODY *abbr.* → maturity-onset diabetes of youth.
Moe [məʊ]: **M.'s method** *ortho.* (*Skoliose*) Bestimmung *f* der Rotation nach Moe u. Nash.
M.'s operation/technique *ortho.* Skoliosekorrektur *f* nach Moe.
Moe and Nash [næʃ]: **M.a.N. method** → Moe's method.
Moebius → Möbius.
Moeller ['mɪlər; 'mœlər]: **M.'s glossitis** Möller-Glossitis *f*, Glossodynia exfoliativa.
M.'s grass bacillus Mycobacterium phlei.
Moeller-Barlow ['bɑːrloʊ]: **M.-B. disease** subperiostales Hämatom *nt* bei Rachitis.
Moenckeberg → Mönckeberg.
mo·fe·bu·ta·zone [mɑfɪ'bjuːtəzəʊn] *n pharm.* Mofebutazon *nt*.
mog·i·ar·thria [,mɑdʒɪ'ɑːrθrɪə] *n HNO* Mogiarthrie *f*.
mog·i·graph·ia [,-'græfɪə] *n* Schreibkrampf *m*, Mogigraphie *f*, Graphospasmus *m*.
mog·i·la·lia [,-'leɪlɪə, -jə] *n* Sprachstörung *f*, Mogilalie *f*.
mog·i·pho·nia [,-'fəʊnɪə] *n* Mogiphonie *f*.
Mohr [mɔːr]: **M. syndrome** Mohr--Claussen-Syndrom *nt*.
Mohrenheim ['moːrənhaɪm]: **M.'s fossa** Mohrenheim'-Grube *f*, Trigonum deltoideo-pectorale, Fossa infraclavicularis.
M.'s space/triangle → M.'s fossa.
Mohs [məʊz]: **M. hardness number** → M. scale.
M. scale Mohs-Härteskala *f*.
moi·e·ty ['mɔɪətɪ] *n, pl* **-ties** Teil *m*; Hälfte *f*; Einheit *f*, Untereinheit *f*; *socio.* Moiety *f*.
moist [mɔɪst] *adj* 1. feucht. 2. *patho.* nässend.

mois·ten ['mɔɪsn] **I** *vt* an-, befeuchten, benetzen. **II** *vi* feucht werden.
mois·ten·ing ['mɔɪsənɪŋ] *n* Benetzung *f*.
moist gangrene feuchte Gangrän *f*.
moist heat sterilization Dampfsterilisation *f*.
moist necrosis feuchte Nekrose *f*.
moist·ness ['mɔɪstnɪs] *n* Feuchtheit *f*, Feuchte *f*.
moist papule 1. (spitze) Feig-, Feuchtwarze *f*, spitzes Kondylom *nt*, Condyloma acuminatum, Papilloma acuminatum/venereum. 2. breites Kondylom *nt*, Condyloma latum.
moist rales feuchte Rasselgeräusche *pl*.
mois·ture ['mɔɪstʃər] *n* Feuchtigkeit *f*.
mois·tur·ize ['mɔɪstʃəraɪz] *vt* 1. (*Luft*) an-, befeuchten. 2. (*Haut*) mit einer Feuchtigkeitscreme behandeln.
mois·tur·iz·er ['mɔɪstʃəraɪzər] *n* 1. Luftbefeuchter *m*. 2. *derm.* Feuchtigkeitscreme *f*.
mois·tur·iz·ing cream ['mɔɪstʃəraɪzɪŋ] *derm.* Feuchtigkeitscreme *f*.
moist wart → moist papule 1.
mol [məʊl] *abbr.* → mole 1.
mo·lal ['məʊlal] *adj abbr.* **m** *chem.* molal *abbr.* m.
mo·lal·i·ty [məʊ'lælətɪ] *n chem.* Molalität *f*.
mo·lar ['məʊlər] **I** *n* Mahlzahn *m*, großer Backenzahn *m*, Molar *m*, Dens molares. **II** *adj* 1. Molar(en) betr., molar, Backen-, Molar-, Mahl-. 2. *phys.* Massen-. 3. *abbr.* **M** *chem.* molar, Mol(ar)- *abbr.* M.
molar activity molare/molekulare Aktivität *f*, *old* Wechselzahl *f*.
molar concentration *abbr.* **c** molare Konzentration *f*.
molar glands Gll. molares.
mo·lar·i·ty [məʊ'lærətɪ] *n chem.* Molarität *f*.
molar number Molzahl *f*.
molar ratio molares Verhältnis *f*.
molar tooth → molar I.
third m. Weisheitszahn *m*, dritter Molar *m*, Dens serotinus.
molar weight Mol(ar)gewicht *nt*.
mold[1] [məʊld] **I** *n* 1. (Gieß-, Guß-)Form *f*. 2. Abdruck *m*, Guß *m*. 3. (Körper-)Bau *m*, Gestalt *f*; Form *f*. 4. Art *f*, Natur *f*, Wesen *nt*. **II** *vt* 5. gießen; formen, modellieren. 6. (*a. fig.*) formen, bilden, gestalten. **III** *vi* s. formen (lassen).
mold[2] **I** *n* Schimmel *m*, Moder *m*; Schimmelpilz *m*. **II** *vi* schimm(e)lig werden, (ver-)schimmeln.
mold·ing ['məʊldɪŋ] *n* Formen *nt*, Formung *f*, Formgebung *f*.
mole [məʊl] 1. *chem. abbr.* **mol** Grammolekül *n*, -mol *nt*, Mol *nt abbr.* mol, Grammolekulargewicht *nt*. 2. *patho., gyn.* Mole *f*, Mola *f*. 3. (kleines) Muttermal *nt*, Mal *nt*, Leberfleck *m*, Pigmentfleck *m*, Nävus *m*, Naevus *m*.
mo·lec·u·lar [mə'lekjələr] *adj* Molekül betr., molekular, Molekular-.
molecular activity → molar activity.
molecular anemia molekuläre Anämie *f*, Anämie *f* durch pathologisches Hämoglobin.
molecular basis molekulare Grundlage *f*.
molecular biology Molekularbiologie *f*.
molecular dimension molekulare Dimension *f*.
molecular disease Molekularkrankheit *f*, molekulare Krankheit *f*.
molecular dissociation theory *ophthal.* Ladd-Franklin-Theorie *f*.
molecular-exclusion chromatography molekulare Ausschlußchromatographie *f*, Molekularsiebfiltration *f*, Molekularsiebchromatographie *f*.

molecular formula *chem.* Summenformel *f*.
molecular genetics Molekulargenetik *f*, molekulare Genetik *f*.
molecular layer: **m. of cerebellum** Stratum moleculare/plexiforme (cerebelli).
m. of cerebral cortex Molekularschicht *f*, Lamina molecularis/plexiformis (corticis cerebralis).
external m. äußere retikuläre Schicht *f*.
m. of hippocampus Stratum moleculare hippocampi.
inner/internal m. innere retikuläre Schicht *f*.
outer m. → external m.
molecular movement *phys.* Brown'-Molekularbewegung *f*.
molecular nitrogen molekularer Stickstoff *m*.
molecular orderliness *phys.* molekularer Ordnungsgrad *m*.
molecular oxygen *abbr.* O_2 molekularer Sauerstoff *m abbr.* O_2.
molecular pathology Molekularpathologie *f*.
molecular sieve *chem.* Molekularsieb *nt*.
molecular-sieve chromatography → molecular-exclusion chromatography.
molecular solution *phys.* molekulare Lösung *f*.
molecular substance Nervenfilz *m*, Neuropil *nt*.
molecular weight *abbr.* **Mol. wt.** Molekulargewicht *nt*.
mol·e·cule ['mɑləkjuːl] *n* Molekül *nt*, Molekel *f*/*nt*.
mol·i·la·lia [,mɑlə'leɪlɪə, -jə] *n* → mogilalia.
mo·li·men [mə'laɪmən] *n, pl* **mo·lim·i·na** [mə'lɪmɪnə] *gyn.* Molimina *pl*.
Moll [mɑl]: **M.'s glands** Moll'-Drüsen *pl*, Gll. ciliares.
Mol·li·cu·tes [,mɑlɪ'kjuːtiːz] *pl micro.* Mollicutes *pl*.
mol·li·ti·es [mɑ'lɪʃɪ,iːz] *n* Weichheit *f*; *patho.* Erweichung *f*, Malazie *f*, Malacia *f*.
mol·lusc *n* → mollusk.
Mol·lus·ca [mə'lʌskə] *pl bio.* Weichtiere *pl*, Mollusken *pl*, Mollusca *pl*.
mol·lus·ca·ci·dal [mə,lʌskə'saɪdl] *adj* → molluscicide.
mol·lus·ca·cide [mə'lʌskəsaɪd] *n* Molluskizid *nt*.
mol·lus·ci·cide [mə'lʌskəsaɪd] *adj* molluskizid.
mol·lus·cous [mə'lʌskəs] *adj derm.* Molluscum betr., molluscumartig, -ähnlich.
mol·lus·cum [mə'lʌskəm] *n, pl* **-ca** [-kə] *derm.* 1. weicher Hauttumor *m*, Molluscum *nt*. 2. molluscum contagiosum.
molluscum bodies Molluskumkörperchen *pl*.
molluscum conjunctivitis *ophthal.* Konjunktivitis *f* bei Molluscum contagiosum.
molluscum contagiosum Dellwarze *f*, Molluscum contagiosum, Epithelioma contagiosum/molluscum.
molluscum contagiosum virus Molluscum contagiosum-Virus *nt*.
molluscum corpuscles → molluscum bodies.
mol·lusk ['mɑləsk] *n* Weichtier *nt*, Molluske *f*.
Moloney [mə'ləʊnɪ]: **M. reaction** Moloney-Underwood-Test *m*.
M. test Moloney-Test *m*.
M. virus Moloney-Virus *nt*.
molt [məʊlt] **I** *n* Mauser *f*; Federwechsel *m*; Häutung *f*; Haarwechsel *m*. **II** *vt* (*Federn*, *Haare*, *Haut*) abwerfen, verlieren. **III** *vi* s. mausern; s. häuten.
molt·ing ['məʊltɪŋ] *n* → molt I.

Mol. wt. abbr. → molecular weight.
mo·lyb·date [məˈlɪbdeɪt] n Molybdat nt.
mo·lyb·de·num [məˈlɪbdənəm] n abbr. **Mo** Molybdän nt abbr. Mo.
mo·men·tum [moʊˈmentəm] n, pl **-ta** [-tə] phys. Impuls m, Moment nt.
m. of inertia Trägheitsmoment.
m. of torsion Drehmoment.
Momp abbr. → membrane protein, major outer.
mon- pref. → mono-.
mon·ac·id [mɒnˈæsɪd] n, adj → monoacid.
mon·a·cid·ic [mɒnəˈsɪdɪk] adj → monoacid II.
mon·ad [ˈmɒnæd, ˈmoʊ-] n **1.** bio. Einzeller m, Monade f. **2.** chem. einwertiges Element od. Atom od. Radikal nt. **3.** genet. Monade f.
Monakow [ˈmɒnˈækəf]: **M.'s bundle** Monakow'-Bündel nt, Tractus rubrospinalis.
M.'s fasciculus → M.'s bundle.
M.'s nucleus Monakow'-Kern m, Nc. cuneatus lateralis.
M. syndrome Monakow-Syndrom nt.
M.'s tract → M.'s bundle.
mon·am·ide [mɒnˈæmaɪd, -ɪd] n → monoamide.
mon·a·mine [ˌ-ˈæmiːn, -mɪn] n → monoamine.
mon·am·i·ner·gic [ˌ-ˌæmɪˈnɜrdʒɪk] adj → monoaminergic.
mon·ar·thrit·ic [ˌ-ɑːrˈθrɪtɪk] adj nur ein Gelenk betr., mon(o)artikulär.
mon·ar·thri·tis [ˌ-ɑːrˈθraɪtɪs] n ortho. mon(o)artikuläre Gelenkentzündung f, Monarthritis f.
mon·ar·tic·u·lar [ˌ-ɑːrˈtɪkjələr] adj → monarthritic.
mon·as·ter [ˌ-ˈæstər] n Monaster f.
mon·ath·e·to·sis [ˌ-æθəˈtoʊsɪs] n neuro. Mon(o)athetose f.
mon·a·tom·ic [ˌ-əˈtɑmɪk] adj → monoatomic.
mon·au·ral [ˌ-ˈɔːrəl] adj nur ein Ohr betr., monaural.
monaural diplacusis HNO monaurale Diplakusis f, Diplacusis monauralis.
mon·a·va·lent [ˌ-əˈveɪlənt] adj → monovalent.
mon·ax·i·al [ˌ-ˈæksɪəl] adj einachsig, monaxial, uniaxial.
Mönckeberg [ˈmɛŋkəbɜrg; ˈmæŋkəbɜrk]: **M.'s arteriosclerosis/calcification/degeneration** → M.'s medial calcification.
M.'s medial calcification Mönckeberg-Sklerose f, -Mediaverkalkung f, -Mediasklerose f.
M.'s mesarteritis/sclerosis → M.'s medial calcification.
Monday fever [ˈmʌndeɪ, -dɪ] Baumwollfieber nt, Baumwoll(staub)pneumokoniose f, Byssinose f.
Mondini [mɒnˈdɪni]: **M.'s deafness** Mondini-Schwerhörigkeit f, Mondini-Typ m der angeborenen Taubheit.
M.'s syndrome isolierte Schneckendysplasie f, Mondini-Syndrom nt.
Mondonesi [ˌmɒndəˈnɛsi]: **M.'s reflex** bulbomimischer Reflex m, Mondonesi-Reflex m.
Mondor [mɔ̃ˈdɔːr]: **M.'s disease** Mondor'-Krankheit f.
mo·ne·cious [məˈniːʃəs, moʊ-] adj → monoecious.
Mo·ne·ra [məˈnɪərə] pl bio. niedere Protisten pl, Moneren pl, Monera pl.
mon·es·thet·ic [mænɛsˈθɛtɪk] adj physiol., neuro. monästhetisch.
mon·es·trous [mɒnˈɛstrəs] adj bio. monoöstrisch.
Monge [ˈmɑŋɡə]: **M.'s disease** Monge'-Krankheit f, chronische Höhenkrankheit f.
mon·go·li·an [mɑŋˈɡoʊliən, mɑn-] adj **1.** mongolisch. **2.** old → mongoloid II.
mongolian fold Mongolenfalte f, Epikanthus m, Plica palpebronasalis.
mongolian macula n mongolian spot.
mongolian spot Mongolenfleck m.
mon·gol·ism [ˈmɑŋɡəlɪzəm, ˈmɑn-] n old → Down's disease.
mon·gol·oid [ˈmɑŋɡəlɔɪd, ˈmɑn-] old **I** n an Down Syndrom Leidende(r), Mongoloide(r) m) f. **II** adj mongoloid.
mon·i·lat·ed [ˈmɑnɪleɪtɪd] adj → moniliform.
mo·nil·e·thrix [məˈnɪləθrɪks] n derm. Spindelhaare pl, Monilethrichie f, Monilethrix(-Syndrom nt) f, Aplasia pilorum intermittens.
Mo·nil·ia [məˈnɪliə] n **1.** bio. Monilia f. **2.** micro. Candida f, Monilia f, Oidium nt.
Mo·nil·i·a·ce·ae [məˌnɪliˈeɪsiˌiː] pl micro. Moniliaceae f.
mo·nil·i·al [məˈnɪliəl] adj Candida betr., durch Candida verursacht, Candida-, Soor-.
Mo·nil·i·a·les [məˌnɪliˈeɪliːz] pl micro. Moniliformis m.
monilial granuloma Candida-, Soorgranulom nt.
mo·nil·i·a·sis [ˌmɑnɪˈlaɪəsɪs] n, pl **-ses** [-siːz] Kandida-, Candida-, Soormykose f, Candidiasis f, Candidose f, Moniliasis f, Moniliose f.
mo·nil·i·form [moʊˈnɪləˌfɔːrm] adj moniliform.
moniliform hair → monilethrix.
Mo·nil·i·for·mis [məˌnɪləˈfɔːrmɪs] n micro. Moniliformis m.
mo·nil·i·id [məˈnɪlɪaɪd] n Candidid nt.
mo·nil·i·o·sis [məˌnɪliˈoʊsɪs] n → moniliasis.
mon·i·tor [ˈmɑnɪtər] **I** n Monitor m; Kontrollgerät nt; Warn-, Anzeigegerät nt. **II** vt überwachen, kontrollieren, überprüfen.
mon·i·tor·ing [ˈmɑnɪtərɪŋ] n Kontrolle f, Beobachtung f, Überwachung f, Monitoring nt.
mon·key hand [ˈmʌŋki] neuro. Affenhand f.
monkey kidney cell culture Affennierenzellkultur f.
monkey-paw n neuro. Affenhand f.
mon·key·pox [ˈmʌŋkipɑks] pl Affenpocken pl.
monkeypox virus Affenpockenvirus nt.
mono- pref. Einfach-, Mon(o)-.
mon·o·a·cid [ˌmɑnoʊˈæsɪd] **I** n einbasische od. -wertige Säure f. **II** adj einbasisch.
mon·o·ac·yl·glyc·er·ol [ˌ-ˈæsɪlˈɡlɪsərɔl, -rɑl] n Monoacylglycerin nt, old Monoglycerid nt.
mon·o·am·ide [ˌ-ˈæmaɪd, -ɪd] n Monoamid nt.
mon·o·a·mine [ˌ-ˈæmiːn, -mɪn] n Monoamin nt.
monoamine oxidase abbr. **MAO** Monoamin(o)oxidase f abbr. MAO.
monoamine oxidase inhibitor abbr. **MAOI** Monoamin(o)oxidase-Hemmer m, MAO-Hemmer m abbr. MAOH.
mon·o·am·i·ner·gic [ˌ-ˌæmɪˈnɜrdʒɪk] adj monoaminerg.
monoaminergic system monoaminerges System nt.
mon·o·am·i·no·di·phos·pha·tide [ˌ-ˌæmɪnoʊdaɪˈfɑsfətaɪd] n Monoaminodiphosphatid nt.
mon·o·am·i·no·mon·o·phos·pha·tide [ˌ-ˌæminoʊˌmɑnəˈfɑsfətaɪd] n Monoaminomonophosphatid nt.
mon·o·am·i·nu·ria [ˌ-ˌæmɪˈn(j)ʊəriə] n Monoaminausscheidung f im Harn, Monoaminurie f.
mon·o·an·es·the·sia [ˌ-ˌænəsˈθiːʒə] n neuro. Monoanästhesie f.
mon·o·ar·tic·u·lar [ˌ-ɑːrˈtɪkjələr] adj → monarthritic.
mon·o·a·tom·ic [ˌ-əˈtɑmɪk] adj **1.** chem. einatomig. **2.** chem. einbasisch. **3.** → monovalent.
mon·o·ba·sic [ˌ-ˈbeɪsɪk] adj chem. einbasisch, -basig.
monobasic acid → monoacid I.
monobasic phosphate primäres Phosphat nt.
mon·o·ben·zone [ˌ-ˈbenzoʊn] n pharm. Monobenzon nt.
mon·o·blast [ˈ-blæst] n Monoblast m.
mon·o·brach·ia [ˌ-ˈbreɪkiə] n embryo. Monobrachie f.
mon·o·bra·chi·us [ˌ-ˈbreɪkiəs] n embryo. Monobrachius m.
mon·o·celled [ˈ-seld] adj → monocellular.
mon·o·cel·lu·lar [ˌ-ˈseljələr] adj bio. einzellig, mono-, unizellulär.
mon·o·ceph·a·lus [ˌ-ˈsefələs] n embryo. Monozephalus m.
mon·o·chlo·ride [ˌ-ˈklɔːraɪd, -ˈkloʊr-] n Monochlorid nt.
mon·o·chlor·phen·a·mide [ˌ-klɔːrˈfenəˌmaɪd, -kloʊr-] n pharm. Clofenamid nt.
mon·o·cho·rea [ˌ-kəˈriə] n neuro. Monochorea f.
mon·o·cho·ri·al [ˌ-ˈkɔːriəl, -ˈkoʊ-] adj embryo. monochorial.
monochorial twins → monochorionic twins.
mon·o·cho·ri·on·ic [ˌ-ˌkɔːriˈɑnɪk, -ˌkoʊ-] adj → monochorial.
monochorionic twins erbgleiche/eineiige/identische/monozygote/monovuläre Zwillinge pl.
mon·o·chro·ic [ˌ-ˈkroʊɪk] adj → monochromatic.
mon·o·chro·ma·sia [ˌ-kroʊˈmeɪziə, -ʒə] → monochromasy.
mon·o·chro·ma·sy [ˌ-ˈkroʊməsi] n ophthal. (totale) Farbenblindheit f, Einfarbensehen nt, Monochromasie f, Achromatopsie f.
mon·o·chro·mat [ˌ-ˈkroʊmæt] n Patient(in f) m mit Monochromasie, Monochromate(r) m) f.
mon·o·chro·mat·ic [ˌ-kroʊˈmætɪk, -krə-] adj **1.** einfarbig, monochrom, monochromatisch. **2.** ophthal. Monochromasie betr., monochromatisch.
monochromatic light monochromatisches Licht nt.
monochromatic radiation → monochromatic light.
mon·o·chro·ma·tism [ˌ-ˈkroʊmətɪzəm] n → monochromasy.
mon·o·chro·mat·o·phil [ˌ-krəˈmætəfɪl] **I** n monochromatophile Zelle od. Struktur f. **II** adj histol. monochromatophil.
mon·o·chro·mat·o·phile [ˌ-krəˈmætəfaɪl], adj → monochromatophil.
mon·o·chro·ma·tor [ˌ-ˈkroʊmeɪtər] n ophthal. Monochromator m.
mon·o·chro·mo·phil·ic [ˌ-ˌkroʊməˈfɪlɪk] adj → monochromatophil.
mon·o·cle [ˈmɑnəkəl] n Monokel nt.
mon·o·clo·nal [ˌmɑnəˈkloʊnl] adj von einer Zelle od. einem Zellklon abstammend, monoklonal.
monoclonal antibody abbr. **MAb** monoklonaler Antikörper m.
monoclonal gammopathy monoklonale Gammopathie f.
monoclonal immunoglobulin monoklonales Immunglobulin nt.

monoclonal protein monoklonaler Antikörper *m*.
mon·o·cra·ni·us [-'kreɪnɪəs] *n* → monocephalus.
mon·o·crot·ic [ˌ-'krɑtɪk] *adj* card. monokrot.
monocrotic pulse Monokrotie *f*, monokroter Puls *m*, Pulsus monocrotus.
mo·noc·ro·tism [mə'nɑkrətɪzəm] *n* card. Monokrotie *f*.
mon·oc·u·lar [mɑn'ɑkjələr] **I** *n* monokulares Instrument *nt*. **II** *adj* **1.** nur ein Auge betr., nur für ein Auge, einäugig, monokular, monokulär. **2.** (*Mikroskop*) monokular.
monocular diplopia → monodiplopia.
monocular strabismus *ophthal*. einseitiges/unilaterales Schielen *nt*, Strabismus unilateralis.
mon·oc·u·lus [mɑn'ɑkjələs] *n* **1.** *ophthal*. einseitiger Augenverband *m*, Monoculus *m*. **2.** *embryo*. Zyklop *m*, Zyklozephalus *m*, Synophthalmus *m*.
mon·o·cy·clic [ˌmɑnə'saɪklɪk, -'sɪk-] *adj chem., phys*. monozyklisch.
mon·o·cyte ['-saɪt] *n* mononukleärer Phagozyt *m*, Monozyt *m*.
monocyte series *hema*. monozytäre Reihe *f*.
mon·o·cyt·ic [ˌ-'sɪtɪk] *adj* Monozyt(en) betr., monozytär, Monozyten-.
monocytic angina Monozytenangina *f*.
monocytic leukemia (akute) Monozytenleukämie *f abbr*. AMOL.
monocytic leukocytosis → monocytosis.
monocytic leukopenia Monozytopenie *f*.
monocytic series → monocyte series.
mon·o·cy·toid [ˌ-'saɪtɔɪd] *adj* monozytenartig, -förmig, monozytoid.
mon·o·cy·to·pe·nia [ˌ-saɪtə'piːnɪə] *n* Monozytenverminderung *f*, Monozytopenie *f*.
mon·o·cy·to·poi·e·sis [ˌ-saɪtəpɔɪ'iːsɪs] *n* Monozytenbildung *f*, Monozytopo(i)ese *f*.
mon·o·cy·to·sis [ˌ-saɪ'təʊsɪs] *n* Monozytenvermehrung *f*, Monozytose *f*.
mon·o·dac·tyl·ia [ˌ-dæk'tiːlɪə] *n* → monodactyly.
mon·o·dac·tyl·ism [ˌ-'dæktəlɪzəm] *n* → monodactyly.
mon·o·dac·ty·lous [ˌ-'dæktɪləs] *adj* einfingrig, -zehig, monodaktyl.
mon·o·dac·ty·ly [ˌ-'dæktɪlɪ] *n* Einfingrigkeit *f*, -zehigkeit *f*, Monodaktylie *f*.
mon·o·di·plo·pia [ˌ-dɪ'pləʊpɪə] *n ophthal*. monokuläre Diplopie *f*, Monodiplopie *f*.
mon·o·dis·perse ['-dɪspərs] *adj phys*. monodispers.
mo·noe·cious [mə'nɪʃəs] *adj bio*. einhäusig, monözisch.
mon·o·en·er·get·ic [ˌmɑnəˌenər'dʒetɪk] *adj* monoenergetisch.
monoenergetic radiation monoenergetische Strahlung *f*.
mon·o·e·no·ic [ˌ-'nəʊɪk] *adj chem*. einfachungesättigt, Monoen-.
mon·o·eth·a·nol·a·mine [ˌ-eθə'nɑləmiːn] *n* (Mono-)Äthanolamin *nt*, Ethanolamin *nt*.
mon·o·fac·to·ri·al [ˌ-fæk'tɔːrɪəl, -'təʊ-] *adj* mono-, unifaktoriell.
monofactorial inheritance monofaktorielle Vererbung *f*.
mon·o·fil·a·ment suture [ˌ-'fɪləmənt] *chir*. monofiles/nicht-geflochtenes Nahtmaterial *nt*.
mon·o·film ['-fɪlm] *n chem., phys*. monomolekulare Schicht *f*.
mon·o·gam·ic [ˌ-'gæmɪk] *adj* → monogamous.

mo·nog·a·mist [mə'nɑgəmɪst] *n* Monogamist(in *f*) *m*.
mo·nog·a·mous [mə'nɑgəməs] *adj* monogam, monogamisch.
mo·nog·a·my [mə'nɑgəmɪ] *n* Monogamie *f*, Einehe *f*.
mon·o·gen·e·sis [ˌmɑnə'dʒenəsɪs] *n* Monogenese *f*, Monogenie *f*.
mon·o·ge·net·ic [ˌ-dʒə'netɪk] *adj* monogenetisch.
mon·o·gen·ic [ˌ-'dʒenɪk] *adj* nur ein Gen betr., durch ein Gen bedingt, monogen.
mon·o·ger·mi·nal [ˌ-'dʒɜrmɪnl] *adj* → monozygotic.
mon·o·glyc·er·ide [ˌ-'glɪsəraɪd, -ɪd] *n* → monoacylglycerol.
mo·nog·o·ny [mə'nɑgənɪ] *n bio*. Monogonie *f*.
mon·o·gyn·ic [ˌmɑnə'dʒɪnɪk] *adj* → monogynous.
mo·nog·y·nous [mə'nɑdʒɪnəs] *adj bio*. einweibig, monogyn.
mo·nog·y·ny [mə'nɑdʒɪnɪ] *n bio*. Einweibigkeit *f*, Monogynie *f*.
mon·o·hap·loid [ˌmɑnə'hæplɔɪd] *adj genet*. monohaploid.
mon·o·hap·loi·dy [ˌ-'hæplɔɪdɪ] *n genet*. Monohaploidie *f*.
mon·o·hy·brid [ˌ-'haɪbrɪd] **I** *n* Monohybride *f*. **II** *adj* monohybrid.
mon·o·hy·brid·ism [ˌ-'haɪbrədɪzəm] *n* Monohybridie *f*.
mon·o·hy·drate [ˌ-'haɪdreɪt] *n* Monohydrat *nt*.
mon·o·hy·drat·ed [ˌ-'haɪdreɪtɪd] *adj chem*. monohydriert.
mon·o·hy·dric [ˌ-'haɪdrɪk] *adj chem*. einwertig.
monohydric alcohol einwertiger Alkohol *m*.
mon·o·ide·ism [ˌ-aɪ'diːɪzəm] *n psycho*. Monoideismus *m*.
mon·o·in·fec·tion [ˌ-ɪn'fekʃn] *n* Rein-, Monoinfektion *f*.
mon·o·i·o·do·ty·ro·sine [ˌ-aɪˌəʊdə'taɪrəsiːn] *n abbr*. **MIT** Monojodtyrosin *nt*, -iodtyrosin *nt abbr*. MIT.
mon·o·kar·y·on [ˌ-'kærɪɑn] *n micro*. Monokaryon *nt*.
mon·o·kine ['-kaɪn] *n* Monokin *nt*.
mon·o·lat·er·al strabismus [ˌ-'lætərəl] *ophthal*. einseitiges/unilaterales Schielen *nt*, Strabismus unilateralis.
mon·o·lay·er [ˌ-'leɪər] **I** *n* monomolekulare Schicht *f*, Monolayer *m*. **II** *adj* einlagig, -schichtig.
mon·o·loc·u·lar [ˌ-'lɑkjələr] *adj* einkamm(e)rig, unilokular.
mon·o·ma·nia [ˌ-'meɪnɪə, -jə] *n psycho*. Einzelwahn *m*, Monomanie *f*, fixe Idee *f*.
mon·o·ma·ni·ac [ˌ-'meɪnɪæk] **I** *n* Monomane *m*, Monomanin *f*. **II** *adj* monoman(isch).
mon·o·mas·ti·gote [ˌ-'mæstɪgəʊt] *n bio*. Monomastigote *f*.
mon·o·mer [ˌ-mər] *n chem*. Monomer(e) *nt*.
mon·o·mer·ic [ˌ-'merɪk] *adj* monomer.
ε-N-mon·o·meth·yl·ly·sine [ˌ-meθəl'laɪsiːn] *n* ε-N-Monomethyllysin *nt*.
mon·o·meth·yl·mor·phine [ˌ-meθəl'mɔːrfiːn] *n* Kodein *nt*, Codein *nt*, Methylmorphin *nt*.
mon·o·meth·yl·xan·thine [ˌ-meθəl'zænθiːn, -θɪn] *n* → methylxanthine.
mon·o·mo·lec·u·lar [ˌ-mə'lekjələr] *adj* monomolekular.
mon·o·mor·phic [ˌ-'mɔːrfɪk] *adj* → monomorphous.
mon·o·mor·phism [ˌ-'mɔːrfɪzəm] *n* Eingestaltigkeit *f*, Monomorphie *f*, Monomorphismus *m*.

mon·o·mor·phous [ˌ-'mɔːrfəs] *adj* gleichgestaltet, monomorph.
mon·om·pha·lus [mɑn'ɑmfələs] *n embryo*. Monomphalus *m*.
mon·o·my·o·ple·gia [ˌ-ˌmaɪə'pliːdʒ(ɪ)ə] *n neuro*. Monomyoplegie *f*.
mon·o·my·o·si·tis [ˌ-ˌmaɪə'saɪtɪs] *n* Monomyositis *f*.
mon·o·neph·rous [ˌ-'nefrəs] *adj* nur eine Niere betr., monorenal.
mon·o·neu·ral [ˌ-'njʊərəl, -'nʊ-] *adj* nur einen Nerv(en) betr., mononeural.
mon·o·neu·ral·gia [ˌ-njʊə'rældʒ(ɪ)ə, -njə-] *n neuro*. Mononeuralgie *f*.
mon·o·neu·ric [ˌ-'njʊərɪk, -'nʊ-] *adj* → mononeural.
mon·o·neu·ri·tis [ˌ-njʊə'raɪtɪs, -nʊ-] *n* Entzündung *f* eines einzelnen Nerven, Mononeuritis *f*.
mon·o·neu·rop·a·thy [ˌ-njʊə'rɑpəθɪ, -nʊ-] *n* Erkrankung *f* eines einzelnen Nerven, Mononeuropathie *f*, -pathia *f*.
mon·o·nu·cle·ar [ˌ-'n(j)uːklɪər] **I** *n* einkernige Zelle *f*. **II** *adj* **1.** nur einen Kern besitzend, mononukleär. **2.** → monocyclic.
mononuclear leukocyte, large *old* → monocyte.
mononuclear leukocytosis → mononucleosis 1.
mononuclear phagocyte → macrophage.
mononuclear phagocytic system *abbr*. **MPS** mononukleäres Phagozytensystem *nt abbr*. MPS.
mon·o·nu·cle·ate [ˌ-'n(j)uːklɪeɪt] *adj* → mononuclear 1.
mon·o·nu·cle·o·sis [ˌ-ˌn(j)uːklɪ'əʊsɪs] *n* **1.** Mononukleose *f*, Mononucleosis *f*. **2.** infektiöse Mononukleose *f*, Pfeiffer'-Drüsenfieber *nt*, Monozytenangina *f*, Mononucleosis infectiosa.
mon·o·nu·cle·o·tide [ˌ-'n(j)uːklɪətaɪd] *n* Mononukleotid *nt*, -nucleotid *nt*.
mono-ovular *adj* → monovular.
mono-ovular twins → monochorionic twins.
mon·o·ox·y·gen·ase [ˌ-'ɑksɪdʒəneɪz] *n* Mon(o)oxygenase *f*.
mon·o·pa·re·sis [ˌ-pə'riːsɪs] *n neuro*. Monoparese *f*.
mon·o·par·es·the·sia [ˌ-pæres'θiːʒ(ɪ)ə] *n neuro*. Monoparästhesie *f*.
mo·nop·a·thy [mə'nɑpəθɪ] *n* Monopathie *f*.
mon·o·pe·nia [ˌmɑnə'piːnɪə] *n* → monocytopenia.
mon·o·pha·gia [ˌ-'feɪdʒ(ɪ)ə] *n bio*. Monophagie *f*.
mo·noph·a·gism [mə'nɑfədʒɪzəm] *n bio*. Monophagie *f*.
mo·noph·agous [mə'nɑfəgəs] *adj bio*. monophag.
mon·o·pha·sia [ˌmɑnə'feɪzɪə] *n neuro*. Monophasie *f*.
mon·o·pha·sic [ˌ-'feɪzɪk] *adj* ein-, monophasisch.
monophasic complex (*EKG*) monophasischer Komplex *m*, monophasische Deflektion *f*.
mon·o·phe·nol monooxygenase [ˌ-'fiːnɒl, -nəl] Monophenolmonooxygenase *f*, Monophenyloxidase *f*.
mon·o·phen·yl oxidase [ˌ-'fenl, -'fiːnl] → monophenol monooxygenase.
mon·o·pho·bia [ˌ-'fəʊbɪə] *n psycho*. (krankhafte) Furcht *f* vor dem Alleinsein, Monophobie *f*.
mon·o·phos·phate [ˌ-'fɑsfeɪt] *n* Monophosphat *nt*.
mon·oph·thal·mus [ˌmɑnɑf'θælməs] *n embryo*. Zyklop *m*, Zyklozephalus *m*, Synophthalmus *m*.

monophyletic

mon·o·phy·let·ic [ˌmɒnəfaɪˈletɪk] *adj bio.* monophyletisch.
monophyletic theory Monophylie *f*, Monophyletismus *m*.
mon·o·phy·le·tism [ˌ-ˈfaɪlətɪzəm] *n* → monophyletic theory.
mon·o·pia [mɒnˈəʊpɪə] *n embryo.* Zyklopie *f*, Zyklozephalie *f*.
mon·o·ple·gia [ˌmɒnəˈpliːdʒ(ɪ)ə] *n neuro.* Monoparalyse *f*, -plegie *f*.
mon·o·po·dia [ˌ-ˈpəʊdɪə] *n embryo.* Monopodie *f*, monopodale Symmelie *f*.
mon·o·po·di·al [ˌ-ˈpəʊdɪəl] *adj* Monopodie betr., von ihr betroffen, monopodal.
mon·o·poi·e·sis [ˌ-pɔɪˈiːsɪs] *n* → monocytopoiesis.
mon·ops [ˈmɒnɒps] *n* → monophthalmus.
mon·o·pty·chi·al [ˌmɒnəˈtaɪkɪəl] *adj histol.* monoptych.
monoptychial glands monoptyche Drüsen *pl*.
mon·or·chia [mɒnˈɔːrkɪə] *n* → monorchism.
mon·or·chid [mɒnˈɔːrkɪd] I *n* → monorchis. II *adj* → monorchidic.
mon·or·chid·ic [ˌmɒnɔːrˈkɪdɪk] *adj* Monorchie betr., monorchid.
mon·or·chid·ism [mɒnˈɔːrkədɪzəm] *n* → monorchism.
mon·or·chis [mɒnˈɔːrkɪs] *n* Patient *m* mit Monorchie, Monorchider *m*.
mon·or·chism [mɒnˈɔːrkɪzəm] *n* Monorchie *f*, Monorchidie *f*, Monorchidismus *m*, Monorchismus *m*.
mon·o·sac·cha·ride [ˌmɒnəˈsækəraɪd, -rɪd] *n* Einfachzucker *m*, Monosaccharid *nt*.
mon·o·sac·cha·rose [ˌ-ˈsækərəʊs] *n* → monosaccharide.
mon·ose [ˈmɒnəʊz, ˈmɒn-] *n* → monosaccharide.
mon·o·so·di·um glutamate [ˌmɒnəˈsəʊdɪəm] Natriumglutamat *nt*.
monosodium urate Natriumurat *nt*.
mon·o·some [ˈ-səʊm] *n* 1. ungepaartes Sexchromosom *nt*. 2. einzelnes Chromosom *nt* bei Monosomie, Monosom *nt*.
mon·o·so·mia [ˌ-ˈsəʊmɪə] *n embryo.* Monosomie *f*.
mon·o·so·mic [ˌ-ˈsəʊmɪk] *adj* Monosomie betr., von ihr gekennzeichnet, monosom.
mon·o·so·mous [ˌ-ˈsəʊməs] *adj* → monosomic.
mon·o·so·my [ˈ-səʊmɪ] *n* Monosomie *f*.
mon·o·spasm [ˈ-spæzəm] *n neuro.* Monospasmus *m*.
mon·o·spe·cif·ic [ˌ-spəˈsɪfɪk] *adj immun.* monospezifisch.
mon·o·sper·my [ˈ-spɜːmɪ] *n embryo.* Monospermie *f*.
Mon·o·spo·ri·um [ˌ-ˈspɔːrɪəm, -ˈspɔː-] *n micro.* Monosporium *nt*.
mon·os·tot·ic [ˌmɒnəsˈtɒtɪk] *adj* nur einen Knochen betr., auf einen Knochen beschränkt, monostotisch.
mon·o·stra·tal [ˌmɒnəˈstreɪtəl] *adj* nur aus einer Schicht bestehend, einschichtig.
mon·o·strat·i·fied [ˌ-ˈstrætɪfaɪd] *adj* → monostratal.
mon·o·sub·sti·tut·ed [ˌ-ˈsʌbstɪt(j)uːtɪd] *adj chem.* einfach substituiert.
mon·o·symp·tom [ˈ-sɪm(p)təm] *n* Mono-, Einzelsymptom *nt*.
mon·o·symp·to·mat·ic [ˌ-sɪm(p)təˈmætɪk] *adj* nur ein Symptom aufweisend, monosymptomatisch.
mon·o·syn·ap·tic [ˌ-sɪˈnæptɪk] *adj* monosynaptisch.
monosynaptic reflex monosynaptischer Reflex *m*.
mon·o·ter·pene [ˌ-ˈtɜːpiːn] *n* Monoterpen *nt*.

mon·o·ther·mia [ˌ-ˈθɜːmɪə] *n patho.* gleichbleibende Temperatur *f*, Monothermie *f*.
mon·ot·ic [mɒnˈɒtɪk] *adj* → monaural.
mo·not·o·nous [məˈnɒtnəs] *adj* eintönig, (ermüdend) ein-, gleichförmig, monoton.
monotonous work monotone Arbeit *f*.
Mon·o·trem·a·ta [ˌmɒnəˈtremətə] *pl bio.* Kloakentiere *pl*, Monotremen *pl*, Monotremata *pl*.
mon·o·treme [ˈ-triːm] *n* → Monotremata.
mo·not·ri·chate [məˈnɒtrɪkət] *adj* → monotrichous.
mon·o·trich·ic [ˌ-ˈtrɪkɪk] *adj* → monotrichous.
mo·not·ri·chous [məˈnɒtrɪkəs] *adj bio.* monotrich.
mon·o·un·sat·u·rat·ed [ˌmɒnəʌnˈsætʃəreɪtɪd] *adj chem.* einfach ungesättigt.
mon·o·va·lence [ˌ-ˈveɪləns] *n chem.* Einwertigkeit *f*.
mon·o·va·lent [ˌ-ˈveɪlənt] *adj chem.* mit nur einer Valenz, einwertig, mono-, univalent.
monovalent serum monovalentes/spezifisches Serum *nt*.
mon·ov·u·lar [mɒnˈɒvjələr, -ˈəʊvjə-, məʊn-] *adj embryo.* eineiig, monovular, monovulär.
monovular twins → monochorionic twins.
mon·ox·ide [mɒnˈɒksaɪd, məˈnɒk-] *n chem.* Monoxid *nt*.
mon·ox·y·gen·ase [mɒnˈɒksɪdʒəneɪz] *n* → monooxygenase.
mon·o·zy·got·ic [ˌmɒnəzaɪˈɡɒtɪk] *adj embryo.* eineiig, monozygot.
monozygotic twins → monochorionic twins.
mon·o·zy·gous [ˌ-ˈzaɪɡəs] *adj* → monozygotic.
Monro [mənˈrəʊ]: **M.'s bursa** Bursa intratendinea olecrani.
fissure of M. Sulcus hypothalamicus.
M.'s foramen Monro-Foramen *nt*, For. Monroi, For. interventriculare.
M.'s line Monro'-Linie *f*.
M.'s sulcus Hypothalamusrinne *f*, Sulcus hypothalamicus.
Monro-Richter [ˈrɪktər, ˈrɪçtər]: **M.-R. line** Monro-Richter-Linie *f*.
mons [mɒnz] *n, pl* **mon·tes** [ˈmɒntɪz] *anat.* Hügel *m*, Berg *m*, Vorbuchtung *f*, Mons *m*.
mons pubis Schamhügel *m*, -berg *m*, Venushügel *m*, Mons pubis/veneris.
mon·ster [ˈmɒnstər] *n embryo.* Mißbildung *f*, Mißgeburt *f*, Monstrum *nt*, Monstrositas *f*.
mon·stros·i·ty [mɒnˈstrɒsətɪ] *n* → monster.
mon·strum [ˈmɒnstrəm] *n, pl* **-stra** [-strə] → monster.
mons veneris → mons pubis.
Monteggia [mɒnˈtedʒə]: **M.'s dislocation** *ortho.* Monteggia-Hüftluxation *f*, Luxatio coxae iliaca.
M.'s fracture/fracture-dislocation/injury Monteggia-(Subluxations)-Fraktur *f*.
month·ly period [ˈmʌnθlɪ] Monats-, Regelblutung *f*, Menstruation *f*, Menses *pl*, Periode *f*.
Montenegro [ˌmɒntəˈniːɡrəʊ, -ˈneɡ-]: **M. reaction/test** Montenegro-Test *m*, Leishmanin-Test *m*.
Montgomery [mɒntˈɡʌm(ə)rɪ]: **M.'s follicles** Naboth'-Eier *pl*, Ovula Nabothi.
M.'s glands Montgomery-Knötchen *pl*, Warzenvorhofdrüsen *pl*, Gll. areolares.
M.'s tubercles → M.'s glands.
mood [muːd] *n* Stimmung *f*, Laune *f*; Gemüt *nt*.
mood disorder *psychia.* affektive Psychose *f*, *old* Gemütskrankheit *f*.
moon face [muːn] (Voll-)Mondgesicht *nt*, Facies lunata.

moon facies → moon face.
moon-shaped face → moon face.
moor bath [mʊər] Moorbad *nt*.
Moore [mʊər, mɔːr, məʊr]: **M.'s pin** Moore-Nagel *m*.
Mooren [ˈmʊərən, ˈmɔːrən]: **M.'s ulcer** *ophthal.* Mooren-Ulkus *nt*.
Morand [mɔˈrɑ̃]: **M.'s spur** Calcar avis.
Morax-Axenfeld [ˈmɔːræks ˈæksənfelt, ˈaksən-]: **M.-A. bacillus** → diplococcus of M.-A.
M.-A. conjunctivitis Diplobazillenkonjunktivitis *f*, Conjunctivitis/Blepharoconjunctivitis angularis.
diplobacillus of M.-A. → diplococcus of M.-A.
diplococcus of M.-A. Diplobakterium *nt* Morax-Axenfeld, Moraxella (Moraxella) lacunata.
Mor·ax·el·la [ˌmɔːrækˈselə] *n micro.* Moraxella *f*.
M. (Moraxella) lacunata Diplobakterium Morax-Axenfeld *nt*, Moraxella (Moraxella) lacunata.
mor·bid [ˈmɔːrbɪd] *adj* 1. erkrankt, krankhaft, krank, pathologisch, kränklich, morbid. 2. *psycho.* abartig, abnormal, anormal, morbid.
morbid anatomy pathologische Anatomie *f*.
morbid fear *psychia.* krankhafte/pathologische Angst/Furcht *f*.
mor·bid·i·ty [mɔːrˈbɪdətɪ] *n* Krankheitshäufigkeit *f*, Erkrankungsrate *f*, Morbidität *f*.
morbidity rate → morbidity.
morbid obesity krankhafte Fettleibigkeit/Adipositas *f*.
morbid thirst pathologischer/krankhafter Durst *m*, krankhaftes Durstgefühl *nt*.
mor·bif·ic [mɔːrˈbɪfɪk] *adj* → morbigenous.
mor·big·e·nous [mɔːrˈbɪdʒənəs] *adj* pathogen, krankmachend, krankheitserregend, -verursachend.
mor·bil·i·ty [mɔːrˈbɪlətɪ] *n* → morbidity.
mor·bil·li [mɔːrˈbɪlaɪ] *pl* Masern *pl*, Morbilli *pl*.
mor·bil·li·form [mɔːrˈbɪləfɔːrm] *adj* masernähnlich, morbilliform.
Mor·bil·li·vi·rus [mɔːrˌbɪlɪˈvaɪrəs] *n micro.* Morbillivirus *nt*.
mor·bil·lous [mɔːrˈbɪləs] *adj* Masern betr., Masern-.
mor·bus [ˈmɔːrbəs] *n, pl* **-bi** [-baɪ] Krankheit *f*, Morbus *m*.
mor·cel·la·tion [ˌmɔːrsəˈleɪʃn] *n* → morcellement.
mor·celle·ment [mɔrsɛlˈmɑ̃] *n French chir.* Zerstückelung *f*, Morcellement *nt*.
mor·dant [ˈmɔːrdnt] I *n* Beize *f*; Ätzwasser *nt*. II *adj* beißend; brennend; beizend; ätzend.
Morel [mɔˈrɛl]: **M. ear** Morel-Ohr *nt*.
M.'s syndrome Morgagni-Morel-Syndrom *nt*, Morgagni-Morel-Stewart-Syndrom *nt*, Hyperostosis frontalis interna.
Morgagni [mɔːrˈɡɑːnjɪ]: **M.'s appendices** Morgagni-Hydatiden *pl*, Appendices vesiculosae (epoophorontis).
M.'s appendix 1. Morgagni'-Hydatide *f*, Appendix testis. 2. Lobus pyramidalis (gl. thoroideae).
M.'s cartilage Morgagni'-Knorpel *m*, Wrisberg'-Knorpel *m*, Cartilago cuneiformis.
M.'s caruncle Lobus medius prostatae.
M.'s cataract Morgagni-Katarakt *f*, Cataracta liquida/fluida.
columns of M. Analsäulen *pl*, -papillen *pl*, Morgagni'-Papillen *pl*, Columna anales/rectales.

crypts of M. Morgagni'-Krypten *pl*, Analkrypten *pl*, Sinus anales.
M.'s disease 1. → Morgagni-Adams-Stokes syndrome. **2.** Morgagni-Syndrom *nt*, Morgagni-Morel-Stewart-Syndrom *nt*, Hyperostosis frontalis interna.
M.'s foramen 1. For. singulare. **2.** For. Morgagnii, For. caecum linguae.
fossa of M. Fossa navicularis urethrae.
fovea of M. → fossa of M.
frenulum of M. → M.'s frenum.
M.'s frenum Bändchen *nt* der Bauhin'-Klappe, Frenulum valvae ilealis.
M.'s glands Littre'-Drüsen *pl*, Urethraldrüsen *pl*, Gll. urethrales.
M.'s globules *ophthal.* Morgagni-Kügelchen *pl*.
M.'s hernia Morgagni-Hernie *f*.
M.'s hydatid → M.'s appendix 1.
hydatids of M. → M.'s appendices.
M.'s hyperostosis → M.'s disease 2.
M.'s retinaculum → M.'s frenum.
semilunar valves of M. → crypts of M.
sinus of M. 1. Aortensinus *m*, Sinus aortae. **2.** → ventricle of M.
M.'s spheres → M.'s globules.
M.'s syndrome → M.'s disease.
M.'s tubercle 1. Riechkolben *m*, -kegel *m*, Bulbus olfactorius. **2.** → M.'s cartilage.
urethral lacunes of M. Urethrallakunen *pl*, -buchten *pl*, Lacunae urethrales.
M.'s valves Valvulae anales.
M.'s ventricle → ventricle of M.
ventricle of M. Morgagni'-Ventrikel *m*, -Tasche *f*, Ventriculus laryngis.
Morgagni-Adams-Stokes ['ædəmz stəʊks]: **M.-A.-S. syndrome** Adams-Stokes-Syndrom *nt*, -Synkope *f*, -Anfall *m abbr.* ASA.
mor·ga·gni·an [mɔːr'gæniən, -'gɑːn-]: **m. caruncle** → Morgagni's caruncle.
m. cataract → Morgagni's cataract.
m. cyst → Morgagni's appendix 1.
m. cysts → Morgagni's appendices.
m. foramen → Morgagni's foramen.
Morgagni-Stewart-Morel ['st(j)uːərt mə'rɛl]: **M.-S.-M. syndrome** → Morgagni's disease 2.
Morgan ['mɔːrgən]: **M.'s bacillus** Morganella morganii, Proteus morganii.
Mor·ga·nel·la [mɔːrgə'nɛlə] *n micro.* Morganella *f*.
morgue [mɔːrg] *n* Leichenschauhaus *nt*.
mor·i·bund ['mɔːrəbʌnd, 'mɑr-] *adj* sterbend, im Sterben liegend, moribund.
Morison ['mɒrɪsən, 'mɑr-]: **M.'s pouch** hepatorenale Peritonealgrube *f*, Rec. hepatorenalis.
Moritz ['mɔrits]: **M. reaction/test** Moritz-Probe *f*.
morn·ing sickness (of pregnancy) ['mɔːrnɪŋ] morgendliche Übelkeit *f* der Schwangeren, Nausea gravidarum.
morning stiffness *ortho.* morgendliche Steifheit *f*.
Moro ['mɔːroʊ; 'moroː]: **M.'s embrace reflex** Moro-Reflex *m*.
M.'s reflex Moro-Reflex *m*.
M.'s test Moro-Test *m*, -Probe *f*.
mo·ron ['mɔːrɑn, 'moʊ-] *n old* Schwachsinnige(r *m*) *f*.
mo·ron·ic [mə'rɑnɪk] *adj old* schwachsinnig.
mo·ron·i·ty [mə'rɑnəti] *n old* Schwachsinn *m*, Moronität *f*.
morph- *pref.* → morpho-.
mor·phal·lax·is [ˌmɔːrfə'læksɪs] *n bio.* Morphallaxis *f*, Morpholaxis *f*.
mor·phea ['mɔːrfɪə] *n derm.* zirkumskripte/lokalisierte Sklerodermie *f*, Sclerodermia circumscripta, Morphea *f*, Morphoea *f*.

mor·pheme ['mɔːrfiːm] *n* Morphem *nt*.
mor·phia ['mɔːrfɪə] *n* → morphine.
mor·phine ['mɔːrfiːn] *n* Morphin *nt*, Morphium *nt*, Morphineum *nt*.
morphine addiction → morphinism.
morphine receptor Morphinrezeptor *m*.
mor·phin·ic [mɔːr'fɪnɪk] *adj* Morphin betr., Morphin-.
mor·phin·ism ['mɔːrfənɪzəm] *n* Morphinsucht *f*, Morphinismus *m*, Morphiumsucht *f*; (chronische) Morphinvergiftung *f*.
mor·phin·ist ['mɔːrfənɪst] *n* Morphin-, Morphiumsüchtige(r *m*) *f*, Morphinist(in *f*) *m*.
mor·phi·nis·tic [mɔːrfə'nɪstɪk] *adj* Morphinismus betr.
mor·phin·i·um [mɔːr'fɪnɪəm] *n* → morphine.
mor·phi·um ['mɔːrfɪəm] *n* → morphine.
morpho- *pref.* Form-, Gestalt-, Morph(o)-.
mor·pho·gen ['mɔːrfədʒən] *n* Morphogen *nt*.
mor·pho·ge·ne·sia [ˌ-dʒə'niːʒ(ɪ)ə] *n* → morphogenesis.
mor·pho·gen·e·sis [ˌ-'dʒɛnəsɪs] *n embryo.* Gestalt- u. Formentwicklung *f*, Morphogenese *f*, -genie *f*.
mor·pho·ge·net·ic [ˌ-dʒə'nɛtɪk] *adj* Morphogenese betr., auf Morphogenese beruhend, morphogenetisch.
mor·phog·e·ny [mɔːr'fɑdʒənɪ] *n* → morphogenesis.
mor·pho·log·ic [ˌmɔːrfə'lɑdʒɪk] *adj* → morphological.
mor·pho·log·i·cal [ˌ-'lɑdʒɪkl] *adj* Form/Gestalt/Morphologie betr., morphologisch, Form-.
mor·phol·o·gist [mɔːr'fɑlədʒɪst] *n* Morphologe *m*, -login *f*.
mor·phol·o·gy [mɔːr'fɑlədʒɪ] *n* **1.** Gestalten-, Formenlehre *f*, Morphologie *f*. **2.** Gestalt *f*, Form *f*.
mor·pho·met·ric [ˌmɔːrfə'mɛtrɪk] *adj* morphometrisch.
mor·pho·me·try [mɔːr'fɑmətrɪ] *n* Morphometrie *f*.
mor·phon ['mɔːrfən] *n* Morphon *nt*.
mor·pho·sis [mɔːr'foʊsɪs] *n, pl* **-ses** [-siːz] Gestaltbildung *f*, Morphose *f*.
mor·pio ['mɔːrpɪoʊ] *n micro.* Filzlaus *f*, Phthirus pubis/inguinalis.
mor·pi·on ['mɔːrpɪən] *n* → morpio.
Morquio [mɔːr'kiːoʊ]: **M.'s disease** → Morquio-Ullrich disease.
M.'s syndrome → Morquio-Ullrich disease.
M.'s syndrome, type A Morquio-Syndrom Typ A *nt*.
M.'s syndrome, type B Morquio-Syndrom Typ B *nt*.
Morquio-Brailsford ['breɪlsfɔːrd]: **M.-B. disease** → Morquio-Ullrich disease.
Morquio-Ullrich ['ʊlrɪç]: **M.-U. disease/syndrome** Morquio-Syndrom *nt*, Morquio-Ullrich-Syndrom *nt*, Morquio-Brailsford-Syndrom *nt*, spondyloepiphysäre Dysplasie *f*, Mukopolysaccharidose *f* Typ IV *abbr.* MPS IV.
Morris ['mɒrɪs, 'mɑr-]: **M.'s syndrome** Goldberg-Maxwell-Morris-Syndrom *nt*, testikuläre Feminisierung *f*.
mors [mɔːrz] *n* Tod *m*, Mors *f*, Exitus letalis.
mor·sus ['mɔːrsəs] *n* Biß(wunde *f*) *m*, Morsus *m*.
mor·tal ['mɔːrtl] *adj* tödlich, todbringend (*to* für); Tod-, Todes-; sterblich, Sterbe-.
mor·tal·i·ty [mɔːr'tælətɪ] *n* **1.** Sterblichkeit *f*, Mortalität *f*. **2.** → mortality rate.

mortality rate Sterberate *f*, -ziffer *f*, Mortalitätsrate *f*, -ziffer *f*.
infant m. Säuglingssterblichkeit, Erstjahressterblichkeit.
maternal m. maternale Sterblichkeit/Mortalität *f*.
neonatal m. neonatale Sterblichkeit/Mortalität *f*.
perinatal m. perinatale Sterblichkeit/Mortalität *f*.
puerperal m. → maternal m.
mortality table Sterblichkeitstabelle *f*.
mor·tar ['mɔːrtər] *n* Mörser *m*.
mortar kidney Kitt-, Mörtelniere *f*.
mor·ti·fi·ca·tion [mɔːrtəfɪ'keɪʃn] *n* Gangrän *f*, Brand *m*, gangräne Nekrose *f*, Gangraena *f*.
mor·ti·fied ['mɔːrtɪfaɪd] *adj* Gangrän betr., mit *od.* in Form einer Gangrän, gangränös.
mor·tise joint ['mɔːrtɪs] oberes Sprunggelenk *nt*, Talokruralgelenk *nt*, Artic. talocruralis.
Morton ['mɔːrtn]: **M.'s disease** → M.'s neuroma.
M.'s foot → M.'s neuroma.
M.'s interdigital neuroma → M.'s neuroma.
M.'s neuralgia → M.'s neuroma.
M.'s neuroma Morton-Syndrom *nt*, -Neuralgie *f*.
M.'s syndrome → M.'s neuroma.
M.'s toe → M.'s neuroma.
mor·tu·ar·y ['mɔːrtʃʊɛrɪ] **I** *n* Leichenhalle *f*. **II** *adj* Tod-, Todes-, Begräbnis-.
mor·u·la ['mɔːr(j)ʊlə, 'mɑr-] *n, pl* **-las, -lae** [-liː] *embryo.* Morula *f*.
morula cell *hema.* Morula-, Traubenzelle *f*.
mor·u·lar ['mɔːr(j)ʊlər] *adj embryo.* Morula betr., Morula-.
mor·u·la·tion [mɔːrə'leɪʃn, mɑr-] *n embryo.* Morulabildung *f*.
mor·u·loid fat ['mɔːr(j)ʊlɔɪd] braunes Fettgewebe *nt*.
Morvan [mɔr'vã]: **M.'s disease/syndrome 1.** Syringomyelie *f*. **2.** Morvan-Syndrom *nt*, Panaritium analgicum.
mo·sa·ic [moʊ'zeɪɪk] *n genet., embryo.* Mosaik *m*.
mo·sa·i·cism [moʊ'zeɪəsɪzəm] *n genet.* Mosaizismus *m*, Mosaik *nt*.
Moschcowitz ['mɑʃkəwɪts]: **M.'s disease** Moschcowitz-Syndrom *nt*, thrombotisch-thrombozytopenische Purpura *f*, Moschcowitz-Singer-Symmers-Syndrom *nt*, thrombotische Mikroangiopathie *f*, Purpura thrombotica (thrombocytopenica), Purpura Moschcowitz).
M.'s operation *chir.* Moschcowitz-Operation *f*.
M.'s sign Moszkowicz-Kollateralzeichen *nt*.
M. test → M.'s sign.
Mos·cow typhus ['mɑskoʊ] → murine typhus.
Mosher-Toti ['moʊʃər 'toʊtɪ; 'mɒ-]: **M.-T. operation** *HNO* Tränensacköffnung *f*, -inzision *f*, Dakryozystotomie *f*.
mOsm *abbr.* → milliosmol(e).
mos·qui·to [mə'skiːtoʊ] *n, pl* **-toes, -tos** *micro.* Stechmücke *f*, Moskito *m*.
mosquito clamp *chir.* Moskitoklemme *f*.
mosquito forceps *chir.* Moskitoklemme *f*.
moss [mɔs, mɑs] *n* Moos *nt*.
Mosse ['mɑsə, 'mɔsə]: **M.'s syndrome** Mosse-Syndrom *nt*.
moss fibers Moosfasern *pl*.
Mossman ['mɑsmən, 'mɑs-]: **M. fever** Tsutsugamushi-Fieber *nt*, japanisches Fleckfieber *nt*, Milbenfleckfieber *nt*, Scrub-Typhus *m*.

moss·y ['mɒsɪ, 'mɑsɪ] *adj* moosartig, moosig, Moos-.
mossy cell 1. protoplasmatischer/fibrillenarmer Astrozyt *m*. **2.** Mikrogliazelle *f*, Oligodendrogliazelle *f*.
mossy-fiber projections (*ZNS*) Moosfaserprojektionen *pl*.
mossy fibers → moss fibers.
Moszkowicz → Moschcowitz.
Motais [mɔ'tɛ]: **M.' operation** *ophthal*. Motais-Operation *f*.
moth [mɒθ, mɑθ] *n zoo*., *micro*. Motte *f*.
moth dermatitis Insektendermatitis *f*.
moth-eaten alopecia *derm*. Alopecia specifica diffusa.
moth·er ['mʌðər] **I** *n* (*a. fig.*) Mutter *f*; *zoo*. Muttertier *nt*. **II** *adj* Mutter-. **III** *vt* bemuttern; groß-, aufziehen.
mother cell Mutterzelle *f*.
mother cyst Eltern-, Mutterzyste *f*, primäre Zyste *f*.
mother fixation *psycho*. Mutterbindung *f*, -fixierung *f*.
moth·er·hood ['mʌðərhʊd] *n* Mutterschaft *f*.
mother-in-law *n* Schwiegermutter *f*.
moth·er·less ['mʌðərlɪs] *adj* mutterlos.
moth·er·li·ness ['-lɪnɪs] *n* Mütterlichkeit *f*.
moth·er·ly ['-lɪ] *adj* mütterlich, Mutter-.
motherly instinct *psycho*. Mutterinstinkt *m*.
mother-of-pearl I *n* Perlmutter *f*, Perlmutt *nt*. **II** *adj* perlmuttern, Perlmutt-.
mother's milk Muttermilch *f*.
mother tongue Muttersprache *f*.
mother yaw *derm*. Muttereffloreszenz *f*, Primärläsion *f*, Frambösiom *nt*.
moth patch *derm*. Chloasma *nt*, Melasma *nt*.
mo·tile ['məʊtɪl, -tɪl, -taɪl] **I** *n psychia*. Motilitätspsychotiker *m*. **II** *adj bio*. (frei) beweglich, bewegungsfähig.
mo·til·in [məʊ'tɪlɪn] *n* Motilin *nt*.
mo·til·i·ty [məʊ'tɪlətɪ] *n* Bewegungsvermögen *nt*, Beweglichkeit *f*, Motilität *f*.
motility study Motilitätsuntersuchung *f*, -prüfung *f*.
mo·tion ['məʊʃn] *n* **1.** Bewegung *f*. **in ~** in Bewegung, s. bewegend; *techn*. laufend, funktionierend. **2.** Bewegungsablauf *f*, Gang *m*. **3.** Stuhlgang *m*; Stuhl *m*. **to have a ~** Stuhlgang haben. **4.** Antrieb *m*. **of one's own ~** aus eigenem Antrieb. **5.** Geste *f*, Gebärde *f*, (Körper-)Bewegung *f*.
mo·tion·al ['məʊʃnl] *adj* Bewegungs-.
mo·tion·less ['məʊʃnlɪs] *adj* unbeweglich, reg(ungs)los, bewegungslos.
motion sickness Bewegungs-, Reisekrankheit *f*, Kinetose *f*.
motion therapy Bewegungstherapie *f*.
mo·ti·vate ['məʊtɪveɪt] *vt* **1.** jdn. motivieren, anregen. **2.** motivieren, begründen.
mo·ti·va·tion [,məʊtɪ'veɪʃn] *n* **1.** Anregung *f*, Motivation *f*, Motivierung *f*. **2.** Motivation *f*, (innere) Bereitschaft *f*, Interesse *nt*.
mo·ti·va·tion·al [,-'veɪʃnl] *adj* motivational, Motiv-, Motivations-.
motivational research → motivation research.
motivation area *physiol*. Motivationsareal *nt*.
motivation research *psycho*. Motivationsforschung *f*; *socio*. Motivforschung *f*.
mo·tive ['məʊtɪv] **I** *n* Motiv *nt*, Beweggrund *m*, Antrieb *m* (*for* zu). **II** *adj* treibend, bewegend, Antriebs-, Trieb-.
motive power Triebkraft *f*.
mo·tiv·i·ty [məʊ'tɪvətɪ] *n* Bewegungsfähigkeit *f*, -kraft *f*.
mo·to·neu·ron [,məʊtə'njʊərɑn, -'nʊr-] *n* motorische Nervenzelle *f*, Motoneuron *nt*.
mo·tor ['məʊtər] **I** *n* **1.** Motor *m*. **2.** *fig*. Motor *m*, treibende Kraft *f*. **II** *adj* **3.** bewegend, (an-)treibend, Motor-. **4.** *physiol*. motorisch, Bewegungs-.
motor agraphia *neuro*. motorische Agraphie *f*.
motor amusia *neuro*. motorische Amusie *f*.
motor aphasia *neuro*. motorische Aphasie *f*, Broca-Aphasie *f*.
motor apraxia *neuro*. motorische Apraxie *f*.
motor area → motor cortex.
motor ataxia *neuro*. motorische Ataxie *f*.
motor aura *neuro*. motorische Aura *f*.
motor cell → motoneuron.
motor center motorisches Zentrum *nt*.
motor complex, interdigestive myoelectric interdigestiver myoelektrischer Motorkomplex *m*.
motor cortex *abbr*. **MC** motorischer Cortex *m*, motorischer Kortex *m*, motorische Rinde(nregion *f*) *f*, Motokortex *m*, -cortex *m*.
motor decussation Pyramiden(bahn)kreuzung *f*, Decussatio pyramidum/motoria.
motor disorder motorische Störung *f*, Störung *f* der Motorik.
motor dysfunction motorische Dysfunktion *f*.
motor end-plate motorische Endplatte *f*.
motor fasciculus, extrapyramidal Monakow'-Bündel *nt*, Tractus rubrospinalis.
motor fiber motorische (Nerven-)Faser *f*.
motor hemiparesis *neuro*. motorische Hemiparese *f*.
mo·to·ri·al [məʊ'tɔːrɪəl] *adj* **1.** motorisch, Bewegungs-. **2.** bewegend, (an-)treibend.
mo·tor·ic [məʊ'tɔːrɪk] *adj* motorisch, Bewegungs-.
mo·to·ric·i·ty [məʊtə'rɪsətɪ] *n physiol*. Motorik *f*.
motor innervation motorische Innervation *f*.
motor learning motorisches Lernen *nt*.
motor nerve motorischer Nerv *m*, N. motorius.
m. of tongue Hypoglossus *m*, XII. Hirnnerv *m*, N. hypoglossus [XII].
motor nerve fiber motorische (Nerven-)Faser *f*.
motor neuron → motoneuron.
motor neuron disease Motoneuronerkrankung *f*.
motor nucleus motorischer Kern *m*.
m. of trigeminal nerve motorischer Trigeminuskern, Nc. motorius (n.) trigeminalis.
motor paralysis motorische Lähmung *f*.
motor point *physiol*. motorischer Nervenpunkt *m*, Reizpunkt *m*.
motor reflex motorischer Reflex *m*, Bewegungsreflex *m*.
motor region → motor cortex.
motor root: m. of ciliary ganglion Radix oculomotoria/parasympathica ggl. ciliares.
m. of spinal nerves vordere/motorische Spinalnervenwurzel *f*, Radix anterior/motoria/ventralis n. spinalium.
m. of trigeminal nerve motorische Trigeminuswurzel *f*, Portio minor n. trigemini, Radix motoria n. trigemini.
motor-sensory region motorisch-sensorische Region *f*.
motor speech area motorisches Sprachzentrum *nt*, motorische Sprachregion *f*, Broca'-Feld *nt*.
motor system motorisches System *nt*, Motorik *f*.
goal-directed m. Zielmotorik.
higher m. höhere Motorik.
postural m. Haltungs-, Stützmotorik.
spinal m. Spinalmotorik.
motor thalamus motorischer Thalamus *m*.
motor unit motorische Einheit *f*.
MOTT *abbr*. → mycobacteria other than tuberkle bacilli.
Mott [mɒt]: **M. bodies** Mott-Körperchen *pl*. **M. cell** Mott-Zelle *f*.
mot·tle ['mɒtl] **I** *n* **1.** (Farb-)Fleck *m*. **2.** Sprenkelung *f*. **II** *adj* → mottled.
mot·tled ['mɒtld] *adj* gefleckt, gesprenkelt, bunt.
mot·tling ['mɒtlɪŋ] *n* Tüpfelung *f*, Sprenkelung *f*.
mould [məʊld] *n*, *v Brit*. → mold.
mould·ing ['məʊldɪŋ] *n* → molding.
mound·ing ['maʊndɪŋ] *n* idiomuskuläre Kontraktion *f*.
Mounier-Kuhn [muni'e kyn]: **M.-K. syndrome** *embryo*. Tracheobronchomegalie *f*, Mounier-Kuhn-Syndrom *nt*.
mount [maʊnt] **I** *n* (*Mikroskop*) Objektträger *m*. **II** *vt* **1.** (*Präparat*) fixieren. **2.** montieren.
moun·tain fever ['maʊntn] Felsengebirgsfleckfieber *nt*, amerikanisches Zeckenbißfieber *nt*, Rocky Mountain spotted fever (*nt*) *abbr*. RMSF.
mountain sickness 1. Berg-, Höhenkrankheit *f*. **2.** → acute mountain sickness. **3.** → chronic mountain sickness.
acute m. (akute) Bergkrankheit *f*, d'Acosta-Syndrom *nt*, Mal di Puna.
chronic m. Monge'-Krankheit *f*, chronische Höhenkrankheit *f*.
mountain tick fever Colorado-Zeckenfieber *nt*, amerikanisches Gebirgszeckenfieber *nt*.
mountain tobacco *pharm*. Bergwohlverleih *m*, Arnika *f*, Arnica montana.
mountain wood tick *micro*. Dermacentor andersoni.
moun·tant ['maʊntnt] *n* (*Mikroskop*) Fixiermittel *nt*, Fixativ *nt*.
mount·ing ['maʊntɪŋ] *n* **1.** (*Präparat*) Fixieren *nt*, Fixierung *f*, Fixation *f*. **2.** Montage *f*, Ein-, Aufbau *nt*; Gestell *nt*; Fassung *f*.
mounting medium → mountant.
mourn [mɔːrn, məʊrn] **I** *vt* jdn. betrauern, beklagen, trauern um. **II** *vi* trauern, klagen (*at*, *over* über; *for*, *over* um).
mourn·er ['mɔːrnər, 'məʊrnər] *n* Trauernde(r *m*) *f*.
mourn·ing ['mɔːrnɪŋ, 'məʊrn-] **I** *n* Trauer *f*, Trauern *nt*. **II** *adj* trauernd, traurig, trauervoll, Trauer-.
mouse [maʊs] *n*, *pl* **mice** [maɪs] *zoo*. Maus *f*.
mouse antialopecia factor Inosit *nt*, Inositol *nt*.
mouse leprosy Rattenlepra *f*.
mouse mammary tumor factor → mouse mammary tumor virus.
mouse mammary tumor virus *abbr*. **MMTV** Mäuse-Mamma-Tumorvirus *nt abbr*. MMTV.
mouse mite *micro*. Allodermanyssus sanguineus.
mouse-pox ['maʊspɒks] *pl* Mäusepocken *pl*.
mousepox virus Mäusepockenvirus *nt*.
mouse-tail pulse ['maʊsteɪl] Pulsus myurus.
mouth [maʊθ] *n*, *pl* **mouths** [maʊðz] **1.** Mund *m*; *anat*. Os *nt*, Ostium *nt*. **2.** *zoo*. Maul *nt*, Schnauze *f*. **3.** (*a. techn*.) Ein-, Ausgang *m*, Mündung *f*, Öffnung *f*.

mouth breather *ped.* Mundatmer *m.*
mouth breathing Mundatmung *f.*
mouth gag Mundöffner *m,* -sperrer *m.*
mouth mirror Mundspiegel *m.*
mouth piece Mundstück *n.*
mouth respiration Mundatmung *f.*
mouth-to-mouth respiration Mund-zu-Mund-Beatmung *f.*
mouth-to-mouth resuscitation → mouth-to-mouth respiration.
mouth wash Mund-, Zahnwasser *nt,* Collutorium *nt.*
mov·a·bil·i·ty [ˌmuːvəˈbɪlətɪ] *n* Beweglichkeit *f,* Bewegbarkeit *f.*
mov·a·ble [ˈmuːvəbl] *adj* beweglich, bewegbar; *techn.* verschieb-, verstellbar.
movable joint 1. ~*s pl* Articc. cartilagineae. **2.** echtes Gelenk *nt,* Diarthrose *f,* Artic./Junctura synovialis.
mov·a·ble·ness [ˈmuːvəblnɪs] *n* → movability.
movable kidney Wanderniere *f,* Ren mobilis/migrans.
movable spleen Wandermilz *f,* Lien migrans/mobilis.
move [muːv] **I** *n* **1.** *fig.* Schritt *m,* Maßnahme *f.* **2.** (Fort-)Bewegung *f.* **II** *vt* **3.** (fort-)bewegen, (an-)treiben, in Bewegung setzen *od.* halten. **4.** (*Verdauung, Appetit*) anregen. **to ~ the bowels** abführen. **III** *vi* **5.** *s.* bewegen; *s.* fortbewegen, gehen, fahren; (*Maschine*) laufen. **6.** (*Darm*) entleeren.
move·a·bil·i·ty *n* → movability.
move·a·ble *adj* → movable.
move·a·ble·ness [ˈmuːvəblnɪs] *n* → movability.
move·ment [ˈmuːvmənt] *n* **1.** Bewegung *f.* **2.** *fig.* Bewegung *f,* Entwicklung *f,* Trend *m,* Tendenz *f* (*towards* zu). **3.** *physiol.* Stuhlgang *m;* Stuhl *m.* **4.** Rythmus *m.* **5.** *techn.* Antrieb(smechanismus *m*) *m,* Bewegung *f.* **6.** ~*s pl* Maßnahmen *pl,* Handeln *nt.*
movement design *physiol.* Bewegungsentwurf *m.*
movement pattern *physiol.* Bewegungsmuster *nt.*
movement perception *physiol.* Bewegungswahrnehmung *f,* -perzeption *f.*
movement program *physiol.* Bewegungsprogramm *nt.*
movement sensitivity *physiol.* Bewegungsempfindlichkeit *f.*
movement synergy *physiol.* Bewegungssynergie *f.*
mov·ing [ˈmuːvɪŋ] *adj* beweglich, (s.) bewegend, Bewegungs-; (*Kraft*) treibend, Antriebs-; fließend.
moving pattern *physiol.* bewegliches (Reiz-)Muster *n.*
moving phase *phys.* bewegliche Phase *f.*
mow·er's mite [ˈməʊər] *micro.* Chigger *m,* Trombicula-Larve *f.*
mox·a [ˈmɒksə] *n* Moxa *f,* Moxabrennen *nt,* Moxibustion *f.*
mox·i·lac·tam [ˌmɒksəˈlæktæm] *n pharm.* Lamoxactam *nt,* Latamoxef *nt.*
mox·i·bus·tion [ˌmɒksɪˈbʌstʃn] *n* → moxa.
m.p. *abbr.* → melting point.
6-MP *abbr.* → 6-mercaptopurine.
M.P.D. *abbr.* → maximal permissible dose.
M period *bio.* M-Phase *f.*
MPO *abbr.* → myeloperoxidase.
M protein 1. monoklonaler Antikörper *m.* **2.** *micro.* M-Protein *nt.*
MPS *abbr.* **1.** → mononuclear phagocytic system. **2.** → mucopolysaccharide. **3.** → mucopolysaccharidosis.
MPS I H *abbr.* → mucopolysaccharidosis I H.

MPS I H/S *abbr.* → mucopolysaccharidosis I H/S.
MPS I S *abbr.* → mucopolysaccharidosis I S.
MPS II *abbr.* → mucopolysaccharidosis II.
MPS III *abbr.* → mucopolysaccharidosis III.
MPS IV *abbr.* → mucopolysaccharidosis IV.
MPS V *abbr.* [mucopolysaccharidosis V] *old* → mucopolysaccharidosis I S.
MPS VI *abbr.* → mucopolysaccharidosis VI.
MPS VII *abbr.* → mucopolysaccharidosis VII.
MR *abbr.* → mumps and rubella vaccine live.
mrad *abbr.* → millirad.
mrem *abbr.* → millirem.
MRF *abbr.* **1.** → melanocyte stimulating hormone releasing factor. **2.** → mesencephalic reticular formation.
MRI *abbr.* → magnet resonance imaging.
mRNA *abbr.* → messenger RNA.
MR test → milk-ring test.
MS *abbr.* → multiple sclerosis.
ms *abbr.* → millisecond.
µs *abbr.* → microsecond.
msec *abbr.* → millisecond.
MSF *abbr.* → macrophage slowing factor.
MSH *abbr.* → melanocyte stimulating hormone.
MSH cells MSH(-bildende)-Zellen *pl.*
MS-1 hepatitis (Virus-)Hepatitis A *f abbr.* HA, epidemische Hepatitis *f,* Hepatitis epidemica.
MS-2 hepatitis (Virus-)Hepatitis B *f abbr.* HB, Serumhepatitis *f.*
MSH inhibiting factor → melanocyte stimulating hormone inhibiting factor.
MSH-RF *abbr.* → melanocyte stimulating hormone releasing factor.
MSIF *abbr.* → macrophage spreading inhibitory factor.
MSUD *abbr.* → maple syrup urine disease.
MSV *abbr.* → murine sarcoma virus.
mtDNA *abbr.* → mitochondrial DNA.
MTM *abbr.* → modified Thayer-Martin medium.
MTP *abbr.* → metatarsophalangeal.
MTPJ *abbr.* → metatarsophalangeal joint.
MTP joint → metatarsophalangeal joint.
MTT *abbr.* → malignant trophoblastic teratoma.
MTU *abbr.* → methylthiouracil.
muc- *pref.* → muco-.
Mucha [ˈmuːkə; mɒtʃa]: **M.'s disease** → Mucha-Habermann disease.
Mucha-Habermann [ˈhɑːbərman]: **M.-H. disease** Mucha-Habermann-Syndrom *nt,* Pityriasis lichenoides et varioliformis acuta (Mucha-Habermann).
mu chain disease [m(j)uː] µ-Kettenkrankheit *f,* µ-Schwerekettenkrankheit *f.*
muci- *pref.* Schleim-, Muzi-, Muci-, Muko-, Muco-, Myxo-.
mu·cid [ˈmjuːsɪd] *adj* → mucilaginous.
mu·cif·er·ous [mjuːˈsɪfərəs] *adj* → muciparous.
muciferous cell muköseröse Zelle *f.*
mu·ci·form [ˈmjuːsɪfɔːrm] *adj* → mucoid II.
mu·cig·e·nous [mjuːˈsɪdʒənəs] *adj* → muciparous.
mu·ci·lage [ˈmjuːsɪlɪdʒ] *n pharm.* Gummischleim *m,* Mucilaginosum *nt,* Mucilago *f.*
mu·ci·lag·i·nous [ˌ-ˈlædʒɪnəs] *adj* schleimig, klebrig, muzilaginös.
mu·ci·la·go [mjuːsɪˈleɪɡəʊ] *n, pl* **-lag·i·nes** [-ˈlædʒɪniːz] *v* → mucilage.
mu·cin [ˈmjuːsɪn] *n* Muzin *nt,* Mukoid *nt,* Mukoproteid *nt.*

mu·ci·nase [ˈmjuːsɪneɪz] *n* Muzinase *f,* Mucinase *f,* Mukopolysaccharidase *f.*
mucin clot Muzingerinnsel *nt.*
mu·ci·ne·mia [ˌ-ˈniːmɪə] *n* Muzinämie *f.*
mu·cin·o·gen [mjuːˈsɪnədʒən] *n* Muzinogen *nt,* Mucinogen *nt.*
mu·ci·noid [ˈmjuːsɪnɔɪd] *adj* **1.** muzinartig. **2.** → mucoid II.
mucinoid carcinoma verschleimendes Karzinom *nt.*
mucinoid degeneration → mucinous degeneration.
mu·ci·no·sis [ˌmjuːsɪˈnəʊsɪs] *n* Muzinose *f,* Myxodermie *f,* Mucinosis *f.*
mu·ci·nous [ˈmjuːsɪnəs] *adj* **1.** Muzin betr., muzinartig, -ähnlich, muzinös. **2.** → mucoid II.
mucinous adenocarcinoma → mucinous carcinoma.
mucinous cancer → mucinous carcinoma.
mucinous carcinoma Gallertkrebs *m,* -karzinom *nt,* Schleimkrebs *m,* -karzinom *nt,* Kolloidkrebs *m,* -karzinom *nt,* Ca. colloides/gelatinosum/mucoides/mucosum.
mucinous cystadenoma muzinöses Zystadenom *nt,* Kystadenom *nt.*
mucinous degeneration muzinöse Degeneration *f.*
mucinous pancreatitis Speichelödem *nt* des Pankreas.
mucinous plaque → mucous plaque.
mu·ci·nu·ria [ˌmjuːsɪˈn(j)ʊərɪə] *n* Muzinausscheidung *f* im Harn, Muzinurie *f.*
mu·cip·a·rous [mjuːˈsɪpərəs] *adj* schleimbildend, -produzierend, -sezernierend, muciparus.
muciparous gland → mucous gland.
mu·ci·tis [mjuːˈsaɪtɪs] *n* → mucositis.
Muckle-Wells [ˈmʌkl welz]: **M.-W. syndrome** Muckle-Wells-Syndrom *nt.*
muco- *pref.* **1.** Schleim-, Muzi-, Muci-, Muko-, Muco-, Myxo-. **2.** Schleimhaut-, Mukosa-.
mu·co·al·bu·mi·nous cell [ˌmjuːkəʊælˈbjuːmɪnəs] muköseröse Zelle *f.*
mu·co·cele [ˈ-siːl] *n* **1.** Schleimzyste *f,* Mukozele *f.* **2.** → mucous polyp.
m. of appendix Mukozele der Appendix, Appendicitis myxoglobulosa.
mu·co·cil·i·ar·y insufficiency [ˌ-ˈsɪlɪˌeriː, ˈsɪlɪəri] (*Lunge*) mukoziliäre Insuffizienz *f.*
mu·coc·la·sis [mjuːˈkɒkləsɪs] *n* Mukoklase *f.*
mu·co·co·li·tis [ˌmjuːkəkəˈlaɪtɪs] *n* Colica mucosa/mucomembranacea, Colitis mucosa.
mu·co·col·pos [ˌ-ˈkɒlpəs] *n gyn.* Mukokolpos *m.*
mu·co·cu·ta·ne·ous [ˌ-kjuːˈteɪnɪəs] *adj* Haut u. Schleimhaut betr., mukokutan.
mucocutaneous candidiasis Schleimhautcandidose *f.*
mucocutaneous hemorrhoids intermediäre Hämorrhoiden *pl.*
mucocutaneous leishmaniasis amerikanische/mukokutane Leishmaniose *f,* Haut-Schleimhaut-Leishmaniase (Südamerikas) *f,* Leishmaniasis americana, Espundia *f.*
mucocutaneous lymph node syndrome *abbr.* MLNS Kawasaki-Syndrom *nt,* Morbus Kawasaki *m,* mukokutanes Lymphknotensyndrom *nt abbr.* MCLS, akutes febriles mukokutanes Lymphadenopathiesyndrom *nt.*
mu·co·cys·tic degeneration of cartilage [ˌ-ˈsɪstɪk] *patho.* mukoidzystische (Knorpel-)Degeneration *f.*
mu·co·en·ter·i·tis [ˌ-entəˈraɪtɪs] *n old* → irritable bowel syndrome.

mucoepidermoid

mu·co·ep·i·der·moid [ˌ-epɪˈdɜrmɔɪd] *adj patho.* mukoepidermoid, Mukoepidermoid-.
mucoepidermoid carcinoma mukoepidermoides Karzinom *nt*.
mucoepidermoid tumor Mukoepidermoidtumor *m*.
mu·co·fi·brous [ˌ-ˈfaɪbrəs] *adj* mukofibrös.
mu·co·glob·u·lin [ˌ-ˈglɑbjəlɪn] *n* Mukoglobulin *nt*.
mu·coid [ˈmjuːkɔɪd] **I** *n* Mukoid *nt*, Mucoid *nt*. **II** *adj* schleimähnlich, -artig, schleimig, mukoid, mukös.
mucoid colony *micro.* M-Kolonie *f*, M-Form *f*, mukoide Form *f*.
mucoid degeneration mukoide Degeneration *f*.
mucoid gland mukoide Drüse *f*.
mucoid medial degeneration Erdheim-Gsell-Krankheit *f*, Gsell-Erdheim-Syndrom *nt*, Medionecrosis *f* Erdheim-Gsell.
mu·co·i·tin sulfate [mjuːˈkɔʊətɪn] Mukoitinsulfat *nt*.
mu·co·i·tin·sul·fu·ric acid [mjuːˌkɔʊətɪnsʌlˈfjʊərɪk] Mukoitinschwefelsäure *f*.
mu·co·lip·id [ˌmjuːkəˈlɪpɪd] *n* Muko-, Mucolipid *nt*.
mu·co·lip·i·do·sis [ˌ-ˌlɪpɪˈdəʊsɪs] *n* Mukolipidose *f*, Mucolipidosis *f*.
mucolipidosis I Mukolipidose I *f*, Lipomukopolysaccharidose *f*.
mucolipidosis II I-Zellen-Krankheit *f*, Mukolipidose II *f*.
mucolipidosis III *f* Mukolipidose III *f*, Pseudo-Hurler-Dystrophie *f*.
mu·col·y·sis [mjuːˈkɑləsɪs] *n* Schleimauflösung *f*, -verflüssigung *f*, Mukolyse *f*.
mu·co·lyt·ic [ˌmjuːkəˈlɪtɪk] **I** *n* schleimlösendes Mittel *nt*, Mukolytikum *nt*, Mucolyticum *nt*. **II** *adj* schleimlösend, mukolytisch.
mucolytic agent → mucolytic I.
mu·co·mem·bra·nous [ˌ-ˈmembrənəs] *adj* Schleimhaut betr., Schleimhaut-, Mukosa-.
mu·co·pep·tide [ˌ-ˈpeptaɪd] *n* Muko-, Mucopeptid *nt*; Peptidoglykan *nt*, Murein *nt*.
mu·co·per·i·chon·dri·al [ˌ-ˌperɪˈkɑndrɪəl] *adj* Mukoperichondrium betr.
mu·co·per·i·chon·dri·um [ˌ-ˌperɪˈkɑndrɪəm] *n* Mukoperichondrium *nt*.
mu·co·per·i·os·te·al [ˌ-ˌperɪˈɑstɪəl] *adj* Mukoperiost betr.; aus Mukosa u. Periost bestehend, mukoperiostal.
mu·co·per·i·os·te·um [ˌ-ˌperɪˈɑstɪəm] *n* mit Schleimhaut überzogenes Periost *nt*, muköses Periost *nt*, Mukoperiost *nt*.
mu·co·pol·y·sac·cha·ri·dase [ˌ-ˌpɑlɪˈsækəraɪdeɪz] *n* → mucinase.
mu·co·pol·y·sac·cha·ride [ˌ-ˌpɑlɪˈsækəraɪd, -rɪd] *n abbr.* **MPS** Muko-, Mucopolysaccharid *nt abbr.* MPS, Glykosaminoglykan *nt*.
mu·co·pol·y·sac·cha·ri·do·sis [ˌ-ˌpɑlɪˌsækərɪˈdəʊsɪs] *n*, *pl* **-ses** [-siːz] *abbr.* **MPS** Muko-, Mucopolysaccharidose *f abbr.* MPS, Mukopolysaccharid-Speicherkrankheit *f*.
mucopolysaccharidosis I H *n abbr.* **MPS I H** Hurler-Krankheit *f*, -Syndrom *nt*, von Pfaundler-Hurler-Krankheit *f*, -Syndrom *nt*, Lipochondrodystrophie *f*, Dysostosis multiplex, Mukopolysaccharidose I-H *f abbr.* MPS I-H.
mucopolysaccharidosis I H/S *n abbr.* **MPS I H/S** Hurler-Scheie-Variante *f*, Mukopolysaccharidose I-H/S *f abbr.* MPS I-H/S.
mucopolysaccharidosis I S *abbr.* **MPS I S** Morbus Scheie *m*, Scheie-Krankheit *f*, -Syndrom *nt*, Ullrich-Scheie-Krankheit *f*, -Syndrom *nt*, Mukopolysaccharidose I-S *f abbr.* MPS I-S.
mucopolysaccharidosis II *n abbr.* **MPS II** Morbus Hunter *m*, Hunter-Syndrom *nt*, Mukopolysaccharidose II *f abbr.* MPS II.
mucopolysaccharidosis III *n abbr.* **MPS III** Sanfilippo-Syndrom *nt*, Morbus Sanfilippo *m*, polydystrophische Oligophrenie *f*, Mukopolysaccharidose III *f abbr.* MPS III.
mucopolysaccharidosis IV *n abbr.* **MPS IV** Morquio-Syndrom *nt*, Morquio-Ullrich-Syndrom *nt*, Morquio-Brailsford-Syndrom *nt*, spondyloepiphysäre Dysplasie *f*, Mukopolysaccharidose *f* Typ IV *abbr.* MPS IV.
mucopolysaccharidosis V *n abbr.* **MPS V** *old* → mucopolysaccharidosis I S.
mucopolysaccharidosis VI *n abbr.* **MPS VI** Maroteaux-Lamy-Syndrom *nt*, Morbus Maroteaux-Lamy *m*, Mukopolysaccharidose VI *f abbr.* MPS VI.
mucopolysaccharidosis VII *n abbr.* **MPS VII** Sly-Syndrom *nt*, Mukopolysaccharidose VII *f abbr.* MPS VII.
mu·co·pol·y·sac·cha·ri·du·ria [ˌ-ˌpɑlɪsækərɪˈd(j)ʊərɪə] *n* Mukopolysaccharidausscheidung *f* im Harn, Mukopolysaccharidurie *f*.
mu·co·pro·tein [ˌ-ˈprəʊtiːn] *n* Mukoprotein *nt*, -proteid *nt*, Mucoprotein *nt*, -proteid *nt*.
mu·co·pu·ru·lent [ˌ-ˈpjʊər(j)ələnt] *adj patho.* schleimig-eitrig, mukopurulent.
mucopurulent bronchitis schleimig-eitrige Bronchitis *f*.
mucopurulent conjunctivitis *ophthal.* akute Konjunktivitis *f*, Conjunctivitis acuta.
Mu·cor [ˈmjuːkər, -kɔːr] *n micro.* Köpfchenschimmel *m*, Mucor *m*.
M. mucedo gemeiner Köpfchenschimmel, Mucor mucedo.
M. pusillus kleiner Köpfchenschimmel, Mucor pusillus.
M. racemosus Traubenkopfschimmel, Mucor racemosus.
Mu·co·ra·ce·ae [ˌmjuːkəˈreɪsɪˌiː] *pl micro.* Mucoraceae *pl*.
mu·co·ra·ceous [ˌ-ˈreɪʃəs] *adj micro.* Mucorales betr.
Mu·co·ra·les [ˌ-ˈreɪliːz] *pl micro.* Mucorales *pl*.
mu·co·rin [ˈmjuːkərɪn] *n* Mukorin *nt*, Mucorin *nt*.
mu·cor·my·co·sis [ˌmjuːkərmaɪˈkəʊsɪs] *n* Mukor-, Mucormykose *f*.
mu·co·sa [mjuːˈkəʊzə] *n*, *pl* **-sae** [-ziː] Schleimhaut *f*, Mukosa *f*, Tunica mucosa.
m. of auditory tube Tubenschleimhaut, Tunica mucosa tubae auditivae.
m. of bladder → m. of urinary bladder.
m. of colon Kolonschleimhaut, Tunica mucosa coli.
m. of esophagus Speiseröhren-, Ösophagusschleimhaut, Tunica mucosa (o)esophagi.
m. of gallbladder Gallenblasenschleimhaut, Tunica mucosa vesicae biliaris/felleae.
m. of larynx Kehlkopfschleimhaut, Tunica mucosa laryngis.
m. of mouth Mundschleimhaut, Tunica mucosa oris.
m. of rectum Rektumschleimhaut, Tunica mucosa recti.
m. of small intestine Dünndarmschleimhaut, Tunica mucosa intestini tenuis.
m. of stomach Magenschleimhaut, Tunica mucosa gastris/ventriculi.
m. of tongue Zungenschleimhaut, Tunica mucosa linguae.
m. of trachea Trachealschleimhaut, Tunica mucosa tracheae.
m. of tympanic cavity Paukenhöhlenschleimhaut, Tunica mucosa cavi tympani, Tunica mucosa cavitatis tympanicae.
m. of ureter Harnleiterschleimhaut, Tunica mucosa ureteris.
m. of urinary bladder (Harn-)Blasenschleimhaut, Tunica mucosa vesicae urinariae.
m. of uterine tube (*Uterus*) Tubenschleimhaut, Tunica mucosa tubae uterinae.
m. of uterus Uterusschleimhaut, Endometrium *nt*, Tunica mucosa uteri.
m. of vagina Vagina(l)schleimhaut, Tunica mucosa vaginae.
mu·co·sal [mjuːˈkəʊzl] *adj* Schleimhaut/Mukosa betr., Schleimhaut-, Mukosa-.
mucosal atrophy Schleimhautatrophie *f*.
mucosal barrier Schleimhautbarriere *f*.
gastric m. Magenschleimhautbarriere.
mucosal catarrh Schleimhautkatarrh *m*.
mucosal cell Schleimhaut-, Mukosazelle *f*.
mucosal cellular injury Schädigung *f* der Schleimhautzellen.
mucosal edema Schleimhautödem *nt*.
mucosal erythema Schleimhautrötung *f*, -erythem *nt*.
mucosal fistula Schleimhautfistel *f*.
mucosal fold Schleimhautfalte *f*.
m.s of gall bladder (*Gallenblase*) Schleimfalten *pl od.* -relief *nt*, Plicae mucosae (vesicae felleae).
mucosal inflammation Schleimhautentzündung *f*, Mukositis *f*.
mucosal ischemia Schleimhautischämie *f*.
mucosal involution (*Magen*) Schleimhaut-, Mukosainvolution *f*.
mucosal neuroma syndrome MMN-Syndrom *nt*, MEN-Typ III *m*, MEA-Typ III *m*.
mucosal pathogen pathogener Schleimhautparasit *m*.
mucosal prolapse Schleimhautprolaps *m*, -vorfall *m*, Mukosaprolaps *m*, -vorfall *m*.
mucosal relief radiography *radiol.* Doppel-, Bikontrastmethode *f*.
mucosal tear Schleimhaut(ein)riß *m*.
mucosal ulcer Schleimhautgeschwür *nt*, -ulkus *nt*.
mucosal ulceration Schleimhautulzeration *f*.
mu·co·san·guin·e·ous [ˌmjuːkəʊsæŋˈgwɪnɪəs] *adj* blutig-schleimig.
mu·co·san·guin·o·lent [ˌ-sæŋˈgwɪnlənt] *adj* blutig-schleimig.
mu·co·se·rous [ˌ-ˈsɪərəs] *adj* mukös-serös, mukoserös.
mu·co·si·tis [ˌ-ˈsaɪtɪs] *n* Mukosa-, Schleimhautentzündung *f*, Mukositis *f*.
mu·co·so·cu·ta·ne·ous [mjuːˌkəʊsəʊkjuːˈteɪnɪəs] *adj* → mucocutaneous.
mu·co·sul·fa·ti·do·sis [ˌmjuːkəʊˌsʌlfətaɪˈdəʊsɪs] *n* Mukosulfatidose *f*, Lipomukopolysaccharidose *f*, Galaktosidase-β-positive Krankheit *f*.
mu·cous [ˈmjuːkəs] *adj* **1.** Schleim/Mucus betr., schleimartig, mukoid, mukös, Schleim-. **2.** schleimbedeckt, schleimig. **3.** schleimbildend, -haltig, -absondernd, mukös.
mucous bursa Schleimbeutel *m*, Bursa synovialis.
mucous cancer → mucinous carcinoma.
mucous carcinoma → mucinous carcinoma.
mucous cast (*Harn*) Pseudozylinder *m*, Zylindroid *nt*.
mucous-catarrhal *adj* schleimig-katarrhalisch.

mucous cell muköse/schleimsezernierende Zelle *f*.
mucous coat → mucosa.
mucous colitis → mucocolitis.
mucous crypts of duodenum Brunner'-Drüsen *pl*, Duodenaldrüsen *pl*, Gll. duodenales.
mucous cyst Schleim(retentions)zyste *f*.
mucous degeneration muköse Degeneration *f*.
mucous diarrhea Diarrhoea mucosa.
mucous edema → myxedema.
mucous fold Schleimhautfalte *f*.
m.s of rectum Analsäulen *pl*, -papillen *pl*, Morgagni'-Papillen *pl*, Columnae anales/rectales.
mucous gland schleimbildende/muköse/muzinöse Drüse *f*, Schleimdrüse *f*, Gl. mucosa.
m.s of auditory tube muköse Tubendrüsen *pl*, Gll. tubariae.
m.s of duodenum → mucous crypts of duodenum.
mucous layer Regenerationsschicht *f*, Stratum germinativum epidermidis.
m. of tympanic membrane (Platten-)Epithel *nt* der Trommelfellinnenseite, Stratum mucosum membranae tympani.
mucous membrane → mucosa.
m. of colon Kolonschleimhaut *f*, Tunica mucosa coli.
m. of esophagus Speiseröhren-, Ösophagusschleimhaut *f*, Tunica mucosa (o)esophagi.
m. of gallbladder Gallenblasenschleimhaut *f*, Tunica mucosa vesicae biliaris.
m. of mouth Mundschleimhaut *f*, Tunica mucosa oris.
m. of pharynx Pharynxschleimhaut *f*, Tunica mucosa pharyngis.
proper m. *histol.* Propria *f* mucosae, Lamina propria mucosae.
m. of rectum Rektumschleimhaut *f*, Tunica mucosa recti.
m. of small intestine Dünndarmschleimhaut *f*, Tunica mucosa intestini tenuis.
m. of stomach Magenschleimhaut *f*, Tunica mucosa gastris/ventriculi.
m. of tongue Zungenschleimhaut *f*, Tunica mucosa linguae.
m. of ureter Harnleiterschleimhaut *f*, Tunica mucosa ureteris.
m. of urinary bladder (Harn-)Blasenschleimhaut *f*, Tunica mucosa vesicae urinariae.
mucous membrane barrier Schleimhautbarriere *f*.
mucous membrane carcinoma Schleimhautkrebs *m*, -karzinom *nt*.
mucous membrane defect Schleimhautdefekt *m*.
mucous membrane infarct Schleimhautinfarkt *m*.
mucous membrane prolapse → mucosal prolapse.
mucous membrane wart Schleimhautwarze *f*.
mucous neck cell (*Magen*) Nebenzelle *f*.
mucous ophthalmia katarrhalische/muköse Ophthalmie *f*.
mucous papule → moist papule.
mucous plaque *dent.* (Zahn-)Plaque *f*.
mucous plug Schleimpfropf *m*.
mucous polyp schleimbildender/muköser Polyp *m*.
mucous-producing *adj* schleimbildend.
mucous retention cyst Schleimretentionszyste *f*.
mucous-secretory cell → mucous cell.
mucous sheaths of tendons of fingers 1. Sehnenscheiden *pl* der Beugersehnen, Vaginae synoviales tendinum digitorum pedis. **2.** Vaginae tendinum digitorum pedis.
mucous tissue gallertartiges/gallertiges Bindegewebe *nt*.
mucous tumor → myxoma.
mucous tunic → mucosa.
mu·co·vis·ci·do·sis [ˌmjuːkəʊˌvɪsɪˈdəʊsɪs] *n* Mukoviszidose *f*, zystische (Pankreas-)Fibrose *f*, Fibrosis pancreatica cystica.
mu·cus [ˈmjuːkəs] *n histol.* Schleim *m*, Mukus *m*, Mucus *m*.
mud bath [mʌd] Schlammbad *nt*.
mud fever Feld-, Ernte-, Schlamm-, Sumpffieber *nt*, Erbsenpflückerkrankheit *f*, Leptospirosis grippotyphosa.
Mueller-Hinton [ˈmjuːlər ˈhɪntn; ˈmyːlər]: **M.-H. agar** Mueller-Hinton-Agar *m/nt*.
mul·ber·ry cell [ˈmʌlberiː, -bəri] Maulbeerzelle *f*.
mulberry fat braunes Fettgewebe *nt*.
Mules [mjuːlz]: **M.' operation** *ophthal.* Mules-Operation *f*.
Müller [ˈmjuːlə(r), ˈmɪl-; ˈmyːlər]: **arteries of M.** Rankenarterien (des Penis), Aa. helicinae (penis).
blood dust of M. → M.'s dust bodies.
M.'s canal Müller'-Gang *m*, Ductus paramesonephricus.
M.'s capsule Bowman'-Kapsel *f*, Capsula glomerularis.
cells of M. Müller'-Stützzellen *pl*, -Stützfasern *pl*.
duct of M. → M.'s canal.
M.'s dust bodies Hämokonien *pl*, -konia *pl*, Blutstäubchen *pl*.
M.'s experiment *physiol.* Müller'-Atemversuch *m*.
M.'s fibers → cells of M.
ganglion of M. Müller'-Ganglion *nt*, Ehrenritter'-Ganglion *nt*, oberes Glossopharyngeusganglion *nt*, Ggl. rostralis/superius n. glossopharyngei.
M.'s law Müller'-Gesetz *nt* (der spezifischen Reizbarkeit).
M.'s law of specific nerve energies → M.'s law.
M.'s maneuver → M.'s experiment.
M.'s muscle 1. Müller'-Muskel *m*, Fibrae circulares m. ciliaris. **2.** M. orbitalis.
radial cells of M. → cells of M.
M.'s sign *card.* Müller-Zeichen *nt*.
supporting cells of M. → cells of M.
M.'s tubercle *embryo.* Müller'-Hügel *m*.
mül·le·ri·an [mjuˈlɪərɪən, mɪ-, mə-; myˈl-]:
m. capsule Bowman'-Kapsel *f*, Capsula glomerularis.
m. duct Müller'-Gang *m*, Ductus paramesonephricus.
m. duct-inhibiting factor → m. inhibiting substance.
m. inhibiting substance *abbr.* **MIS** *embryo.* Anti-Müller-Hormon *nt abbr.* **AMH.**
m. regression factor → m. inhibiting substance.
m. tubercle *embryo.* Müller'-Hügel *m*.
mul·tan·gu·lar [mʌlˈtæŋɡjələr] *adj* vielwink(e)lig, vieleckig.
multangular bone: accessory m. Os centrale.
greater m. Os trapezium.
larger m. → greater m.
lesser m. → smaller m.
smaller m. Os trapezoideum.
multi- *pref.* Viel-, Vielfach-, Multi-.
mul·ti·an·gu·lar [ˌmʌltɪˈæŋɡjələr] *adj* → multangular.
mul·ti·ar·tic·u·lar [ˌ-ɑːrˈtɪkjələr] *adj* mehrere Gelenke betr., multi-, polyartikulär.
mul·ti·ax·i·al [ˌ-ˈæksɪəl] *adj* mehrere Achsen habend, mehrachsig, multiaxial.
multiaxial articulation Kugelgelenk *nt*, Artic. sph(a)eroidea/cotylica.
multiaxial joint → multiaxial articulation.
mul·ti·cap·su·lar [ˌ-ˈkæpsələr] *adj* mehrere/viele Kapseln (besitzend), multikapsular, -kapsulär.
mul·ti·cel·lu·lar [ˌ-ˈseljələr] *adj* mehr-, vielzellig, multizellular, -zellulär.
mul·ti·cel·lu·lar·i·ty [ˌ-seljəˈleərətɪ] *n* Vielzelligkeit *f*.
mul·ti·cen·tric [ˌ-ˈsentrɪk] *adj* polyzentrisch.
multicentric mitosis multipolare Mitose *f*.
multicentric reticulohistocytosis multiple Retikulohistiozytome *pl*, multizentrische Retikulohistiozytose *f*, Lipoiddermatoarthritis *f*, Reticulohistiocytosis disseminata.
Mul·ti·ceps [ˈ-seps] *n micro.* Multiceps *m*.
M. multiceps Quesenbandwurm *m*, Multiceps multiceps.
mul·ti·col·ored [ˌ-ˈkʌlərd] *adj* mehrfarbig, Mehrfarben-.
mul·ti·cys·tic [ˌ-ˈsɪstɪk] *adj* aus mehreren Zysten bestehend, polyzystisch.
mul·ti·en·zyme complex [ˌ-ˈenzaɪm] Multienzymkomplex *m*.
multienzyme system Multienzymsystem *nt*.
dissociated/soluble m. lösliches/dissoziiertes Multienzymsystem.
mul·ti·fac·to·ri·al [ˌ-fækˈtɔːrɪəl, -ˈtəʊr-] *adj* **1.** aus mehreren Faktoren bestehend, multifaktoriell. **2.** *genet.* durch eine Vielzahl von Faktoren bedingt, multifaktoriell.
multifactorial disorder multifaktorielle Erkrankung *f*.
multifactorial inheritance multifaktorielle Vererbung *f*.
mul·tif·i·dus (muscle) [mʌlˈtɪfɪdəs] Multifidus *m*, M. multifidus.
mul·ti·fo·cal [ˌ-ˈfəʊkl] *adj* mehrere Fokus betr., von mehreren Fokus ausgehend, multifokal.
multifocal progressive leukoencephalopathy progressive multifokale Leukoenzephalopathie *f abbr.* **PML.**
mul·ti·fold [ˈ-fəʊld] *adj* viel-, mehrfach.
mul·ti·form [ˈ-fɔːrm] *adj* vielförmig, -gestaltig, multiform, polymorph.
mul·ti·for·mi·ty [ˌ-ˈfɔːrmətɪ] *n* Vielförmigkeit *f*, -gestaltigkeit *f*.
multiform layer of cerebral cortex multiforme Schicht *f*, Lamina multiformis (corticis cerebralis).
multiform neuron → multipolar neuron.
mul·ti·ges·ta [ˌ-ˈdʒestə] *n* → multigravida.
mul·ti·glan·du·lar [ˌ-ˈɡlændʒələr] *adj* multi-, pluriglandulär.
mul·ti·grav·i·da [ˌ-ˈɡrævɪdə] *n, pl* **-das, dae** [-diː] Multi-, Plurigravida *f*.
mul·ti·hand·i·capped [ˌ-ˈhændɪkæpt] *adj* mehrfach behindert.
multi-infarct dementia Multiinfarktenzephalopathie *f*, -demenz *f*.
mul·ti·la·mel·lar body [ˌ-ləˈmelər, -ˈlæmələr] Zytosom *nt*.
mul·ti·lat·er·al [ˌ-ˈlætərəl] *adj* mehrseitig, multilateral.
mul·ti·lay·ered [ˌ-ˈleɪərd] *adj histol.* mehrschichtig, mehrreihig.
mul·ti·lin·gual [ˌ-ˈlɪŋɡwəl] *adj* mehrsprachig.
mul·ti·lo·bar [ˌ-ˈləʊbər, -bɑːr] *adj* multilobär.
mul·ti·lo·bate placenta [ˌ-ˈləʊbeɪt] Placenta multilobata.
mul·ti·lobed placenta [ˌ-ˈləʊbd] Placenta multilobata.
mul·ti·lob·u·lar [ˌ-ˈlɒbjələr] *adj* mehr-, viellappig, multilobulär.

multilobular cirrhosis postnekrotische/ ungeordnete/großknotige Leberzirrhose *f*.
mul·ti·loc·u·lar [ˌ-ˈlɑkjələr] *adj patho.* vielkamm(e)rig, multilokulär.
multilocular cyst multilokuläre Zyste *f*.
multilocular cystoma multilokuläres Kystom/Cystom *nt*.
mul·ti·loc·u·late cyst [ˌ-ˈlɑkjəleɪt] → multilocular cyst.
mul·ti·mam·mae [ˌ-ˈmæmɪ] *pl* Polymastie *f*, akzessorische Mammae *f*, Mammae accessoriae.
mul·ti·mod·al [ˌ-ˈmoʊdl] *adj* multimodal.
mul·ti·neu·ron·al circuit of Papez [ˌ-ˈn(j)ʊərənl, -n(j)ʊːˈrəʊnl] Neuronenkreis *m* von Papez.
mul·ti·nod·u·lar [ˌ-ˈnɑdʒələr] *adj* multinodulär.
multinodular goiter multinoduläre (Knoten-)Struma *f*.
mul·ti·nu·cle·ar [ˌ-ˈn(j)uːkliər] *adj* mehr-, vielkernig, mit mehreren/vielen Kernen versehen, multinukleär, -nuklear.
mul·ti·nu·cle·ate [ˌ-ˈn(j)uːklɪt, -eɪt] *adj* → multinuclear.
mul·ti·or·gan donation [ˌ-ˈɔːrgən] Multiorganspende *f*.
multiorgan failure (syndrome) multiples Organversagen *nt*.
mul·tip·a·ra [mʌlˈtɪpərə] *n, pl* **-ras, -rae** [-riː] Mehrgebärende *f*, Multi-, Pluripara *f*.
mul·tip·a·rous [mʌlˈtɪpərəs] *adj* multipar.
mul·ti·pen·nate muscle [ˌmʌltɪˈpeneɪt] vielseitig/vielfach gefiederter Muskel *m*, M. multipennatus.
mul·ti·phase [ˈ-feɪz] *adj* mehrphasig.
mul·ti·pha·sic [ˌ-ˈfeɪsɪk] *adj* → multiphase.
mul·ti·ple [ˈmʌltɪpl] **I** *n* Vielfache *nt*. **II** *adj* **1.** viel-, mehrfach, vielfältig, mehrere, viele, multipel, multiple, multiplex, vielfach-. **2.** vielseitig.
multiple alleles *genet.* multiple Allele *pl*.
multiple birth Mehrlingsgeburt *f*.
multiple cartilaginous exostoses → multiple exostoses.
multiple-choice *adj* Multiple-choice-.
multiple chondromas multiple Chondrome *pl*, Chondromatose *f*.
multiple congenital enchondroma → multiple enchondromatosis.
multiple enchondromatosis Ollier'-Erkrankung *f*, -Syndrom *nt*, Enchondromatose *f*, multiple kongenitale Enchondrome *pl*, Hemichondrodystrophie *f*.
multiple endocrine adenomatosis *abbr.* **MEA** → multiple endocrine neoplasia.
multiple endocrine neoplasia *abbr.* **MEN** multiple endokrine Adenopathie *f abbr.* MEA, multiple endokrine Neoplasie *f abbr.* MEN, pluriglanduläre Adenomatose *f*.
multiple endocrine neoplasia I Wermer'-Syndrom *nt*, MEN-Typ I *m*, MEA-Typ I *m*.
multiple endocrine neoplasia IIa Sipple'-Syndrom *nt*, MEN-Typ IIa *m*, MEA-Typ IIa *m*.
multiple endocrine neoplasia III MMN-Syndrom *nt*, MEN-Typ III *m*, MEA-Typ III *m*.
multiple endocrinomas → multiple endocrine neoplasia.
multiple endocrinopathy → multiple endocrine neoplasia.
multiple exostoses multiple kartilaginäre Exostosen *pl*, hereditäre multiple Exostosen *pl*, multiple Osteochondrome *pl*, Ekchondrosis ossificans.
multiple familial polyposis familiäre Polypose/Polyposis *f*, Polyposis familiaris, Adenomatosis coli.
multiple fissions Sporenbildung *f*, Sporulation *f*.
multiple fracture 1. Mehretagenfraktur *f*. **2.** ~s *pl* multiple Frakturen *pl*.
multiple hamartoma syndrome Cowden'-Krankheit *f*, -Syndrom *nt*, multiple Hamartome-Syndrom *nt*.
multiple idiopathic hemorrhagic sarcoma Kaposi-Sarkom *nt*, Morbus Kaposi *m*, Retikuloangiomatose *f*, Angioretikulomatose *f*, idiopathisches multiples Pigmentsarkom Kaposi *nt*, Sarcoma idiopathicum multiplex haemorrhagicum.
multiple labor Mehrlingsgeburt *f*.
multiple lentigines syndrome Lentiginosis-Syndrom *nt*, LEOPARD-Syndrom *nt*.
multiple lipoprotein-type hyperlipidemia 1. (primäre/essentielle) Hyperlipoproteinämie *f* Typ II, kombinierte Hyperlipoproteinämie *f*. **2.** (primäre/essentielle) Hyperlipoproteinämie *f* Typ IV, endogene/kohlenhydratinduzierte Hyperlipidämie/Triglyzeridämie *f*, familiäre Hypertriglyzeridämie *f*.
multiple myeloma Kahler-Krankheit *f*, Huppert-Krankheit *f*, Morbus Kahler *m*, multiples Myelom *nt*, Plasmozytom *nt*, plasmozytisches Immunozytom *nt*, plasmozytisches Lymphom *nt*.
multiple myositis Polymyositis *f*.
multiple neuritis Polyneuritis *f*.
multiple neurofibroma (von) Recklinghausen-Krankheit *f*, Neurofibromatosis generalisata.
multiple organ failure multiples Organversagen *m*.
multiple osteocartilaginous exostoses → multiple exostoses.
multiple personality *psycho.* multiple/gespaltene Persönlichkeit *f*.
multiple plasmacytoma of bone → multiple myeloma.
multiple pregnancy Mehrlingsschwangerschaft *f*.
monovular m. eineiige Mehrlingsschwangerschaft.
polyovular m. mehreiige Mehrlingsschwangerschaft.
multiple rib fractures Rippenserienfraktur *f*.
multiple root *mathe.* mehrwertige Wurzel *f*.
multiple sclerosis *abbr.* **MS** *patho.* multiple Sklerose *f abbr.* MS, Polysklerose *f*, Sclerosis multiplex, Encephalomyelitis disseminata.
multiple self-healing squamous epithelioma Keratoakanthom *nt*, selbstheilendes Stachelzellkarzinom *nt*, selbstheilender Stachelzell(en)krebs *m*, Molluscum sebaceum/pseudocarcinomatosum.
multiple serositis Polyserositis *f*.
multiple vision *ophthal.* Mehrfachsehen *nt*, Polyopie *f*, Polyopsie *f*.
mul·ti·plex [ˈmʌltɪpleks] *adj* zahlreich, mehrfach, vielfach, -fältig, multipel, multiplex, Mehr(fach)-, Multiplex-.
mul·ti·pli·a·ble [ˈmʌltɪplaɪəbl] *adj* multiplizierbar.
mul·ti·pli·ca·ble [ˌ-ˈplɪkəbl] *adj* → multipliable.
mul·ti·pli·cand [ˌ-plɪˈkænd] *n* Multiplikand *m*.
mul·ti·pli·ca·tion [ˌ-plɪˈkeɪʃn] *n* **1.** Multiplikation *f*; Multiplizieren *nt*. **2.** *fig.* Vervielfachung *f*; *bio.* Vermehrung *f*.
multiplication period Vermehrungs-, Multiplikationsperiode *f*.
mul·ti·plic·i·ty [ˌ-ˈplɪsɪtɪ] *n, pl* **-ties 1.** Vielfältigkeit *f*, Vielfalt *f*. **2.** Vielzahl *f*, Fülle *f*.

mul·ti·plier [ˈ-plaɪər] *n* **1.** *mathe.* Multiplikator *m*. **2.** *phys.* Verstärker *m*, Vervielfacher *m*, Multiplier *m*; Vergrößerungsglas *nt*.
mul·ti·ply [ˈ-plaɪ] **I** *vt* **1.** *bio.* vermehren. **2.** vervielfältigen, vervielfachen; *mathe.* multiplizieren (*by* with). **II** *vi* **3.** *bio.* s. vermehren. **4.** s. vervielfachen; *mathe.* multiplizieren.
mul·ti·ply·ing glass [ˈ-plaɪɪŋ] Vergrößerungsglass *nt*, -linse *f*.
mul·ti·po·lar [ˌ-ˈpəʊlər] *adj* **1.** (*Nervenzelle*) multi-, pluripolar. **2.** viel-, mehrpolig, multipolar.
multipolar cell → multipolar neuron.
multipolar mitosis multipolare Mitose *f*.
multipolar neuroblast *embryo.* multipolarer Neuroblast *m*.
multipolar neuron multipolares Neuron *nt*.
mul·ti·re·cep·tive neuron [ˌmʌltɪrɪˈseptɪv] multirezeptives Neuron *nt*.
mul·ti·sen·so·ry [ˌ-ˈsensərɪ] *adj phys.* multisensorisch.
mul·ti·stage [ˈ-steɪdʒ] *adj* mehrstufig, -phasig, Mehrstufen-.
mul·ti·syn·ap·tic [ˌ-sɪˈnæptɪk] *adj* mehrere Synapsen umfassend, multi-, polysynaptisch.
multisynaptic reflex poly-/multisynaptischer Reflex *m*.
mul·ti·vac·u·o·lar [ˌ-ˌvækjuˈəʊlər, -ˈvækjuə-, -ˈvækjələr] *adj* pluriglandulär.
mul·ti·va·lence [ˌ-ˈveɪləns] *n* Mehr-, Vielwertigkeit *f*, Multivalenz *f*.
mul·ti·va·lent [ˌ-ˈveɪlənt, mʌlˈtɪvələnt] *adj* **1.** *chem.* mehrwertig, multivalent. **2.** *immun.* multi-, polyvalent.
multivalent vaccine polyvalenter Impfstoff *m*.
mul·ti·var·i·ate analysis [ˌ-ˈveərɪɪt] *stat.* Multivarianzanalyse *f*.
mul·ti·ve·sic·u·lar body [ˌ-vəˈsɪkjələr] multivesikuläres Körperchen *nt*.
mum·mi·fi·ca·tion [ˌmʌməfɪˈkeɪʃn] *n* **1.** Mummifikation *f*, Mummifizierung *f*. **2.** trockene Gangrän *f*, Mummifikation *f*, Mummifizierung *f*.
mummification necrosis → mummification 2.
mum·mi·fied [ˈmʌməfaɪd] *adj* **1.** mummifiziert. **2.** vertrocknet, eingetrocknet.
mum·mi·fy [ˈmʌməfaɪ] **I** *vt* mummifizieren. **II** *vi* vertrocknen, verdorren.
mumps [mʌmps] *n* Mumps *m/f*, Ziegenpeter *m*, Parotitis epidemica.
mumps and rubella vaccine live *abbr.* **MR** Mumps-Röteln-Lebendvakzine *f*, MR-Lebendvakzine *f*.
mumps meningitis Mumps-Meningitis *f*.
mumps meningoencephalitis Mumps-Meningoenzephalitis *f*.
mumps orchitis Mumps-Orchitis *f*.
mumps vaccine → mumps virus vaccine.
mumps virus Mumpsvirus *nt*.
mumps virus vaccine Mumpsimpfstoff *m*, -vakzine *f*.
mumps virus vaccine live Mumpsviruslebendvakzine *f*.
Munchausen [ˈmʌntʃaʊzən]: **M. syndrome** Münchhausen-Syndrom *nt*.
Münchmeyer [ˈmɪntʃmaɪər; ˈmʏnç-]: **M.'s disease** Münchmeyer-Syndrom *nt*.
Munro [mənˈrəʊ]: **M. abscess/microabscess** Munro'-Mikroabszeß *m*.
M.'s point Munro'-Punkt *m*.
mu·ral [ˈmjʊərəl] *adj* die Wand eines Hohlorgans betr., mural; intramural.
mural aneurysm (*Herz*) Kammerwandaneurysma *nt*.
mural endocarditis Endocarditis parietalis.

mural pregnancy intramurale/interstitielle Schwangerschaft *f*, Graviditas interstitialis.
mural salpingitis *patho.*, *gyn.* parenchymatöse Salpingitis *f*.
mural thrombus *patho.* Parietalthrombus *m*.
mu·ram·ic acid [mjʊəˈræmɪk] Muraminsäure *f*.
mu·ram·i·dase [mjʊəˈræmɪdeɪz] *n* Lysozym *nt*.
Murand [məˈrænd]: **M.'s foramen** For. caecum linguae.
Murchison-Pel-Ebstein [ˈmɜrtʃɪsən pel ˈebstaɪn]: **M.-P.-E. fever** Pel-Ebstein-Fieber *nt*.
Murchison-Sanderson [ˈsændərsən]: **M.-S. syndrome** Hodgkin-Krankheit *f*, -Lymphom *nt*, Morbus Hodgkin *m*, (Hodgkin-)Paltauf-Steinberg-Krankheit *f*, (maligne) Lymphogranulomatose *f*, Lymphogranulomatosis maligna.
mu·rein [ˈmjʊəriːn] *n* Murein *nt*, Mukopeptid *nt*, Peptidoglykan *nt*.
mu·rex·ide [mjʊəˈreksaɪd, -sɪd] *n* Murexid *nt*.
murexide test Murexidprobe *f*.
mu·rine [ˈmjʊəraɪn, -rɪn] *adj* Mäuse *od.* Ratten betr., murin, Mäuse-, Ratten-.
murine leprosy Rattenlepra *f*.
murine leukemia virus *abbr.* **MLV**. Mäuse-Leukämie-Virus *nt*, murine leukemia virus *abbr.* MLV.
murine sarcoma virus *abbr.* **MSV** Mäuse-Sarkom-Virus *nt*, murine sarcoma virus *abbr.* MSV.
murine typhus endemisches/murines Fleckfieber *nt*, Ratten-, Flohfleckfieber *nt*.
mur·mur [ˈmɜrmər] *n* **1.** *patho.* (Herz-)Geräusch *nt*. **2.** Rauschen, Murmeln *nt*, Geräusch *nt*.
Murphy [ˈmɜrfɪ]: **M.'s sign/test** Murphy--Zeichen *nt*.
Mur·ray Valley [ˈmʌrɪ]: **M. V. disease** → M.-V. encephalitis.
M. V. encephalitis *abbr.* **MVE** Murray--Valley-Enzephalitis *f* *abbr.* MVE, Australian-X-Enzephalitis *f*.
M. V. encephalitis virus Murray-Valley--Enzephalitis-Virus *nt*.
Mus [mʌs] *n zoo.* Maus *f*, Mus *m*.
M. musculus Hausmaus, Mus musculus.
M. rattus Hausratte *f*, Mus rattus.
Mus·ca [ˈmʌskə] *n zoo.* Musca *f*.
M. domestica Haus-, Stubenfliege *f*, Musca domestica.
mus·ca [ˈmʌskə] *n zoo.* Fliege *f*, Musca *f*.
muscae volitantes *ophthal.* Mückensehen *nt*, Mouches volantes.
mus·ca·rine [ˈmʌskərɪn, -riːn] *n* Muskarin *nt*, Muscarin *nt*.
mus·ca·rin·ic [mʌksəˈrɪnɪk] *adj* muskarinartig.
muscarinic receptor Muskarinrezeptor *m*.
mus·car·in·ism [ˈmʌskərɪnɪzəm] *n* Muscarinvergiftung *f*, Muscarianismus *m*.
Mus·ci·dae [ˈmʌsədiː] *pl bio.* Muscidae *pl*.
mus·cle [ˈmʌsəl] *n* Muskel *m*, Muskelgewebe *nt*; *anat.* Musculus *m*.
m.s of abdomen Bauchmuskeln *pl*, -muskulatur *f*, Mm. abdominis.
m.s of auditory ossicles Muskeln der Gehörknöchelchen, Mm. ossiculorum auditus.
m.s of buttock Gesäßmuskeln *pl*, -muskulatur *f*.
m.s of (facial) expression Gesichtsmuskeln *pl*, -muskulatur *f*, mimische Muskulatur *f*, Mm. faciales.
m.s of head Kopfmuskeln *pl*, -muskulatur *f*, Mm. capitis.

m.s of larynx Kehlkopfmuskeln *pl*, -muskulatur *f*, Mm. laryngis.
m.s of lower limb Muskeln *pl*/Muskulatur *f* der unteren Gliedmaße, Mm. membri inferioris.
m.s of mastication Kaumuskeln *pl*, -muskulatur *f*, Mm. masticatorii.
m.s of perineum Dammuskulatur *f*, Mm. perinei/perineales.
m.s of tongue Zungenmuskeln *pl*, -muskulatur *f*, Mm. linguae.
m. of tragus M. tragicus.
m.s of upper limb Muskeln *pl*/Muskulatur *f* der oberen Gliedmaße, Mm. membri superioris.
m. of uvula Zäpfchenmuskel, M. uvulae.
muscle adenylate deaminase → myoadenylate deaminase.
muscle belly Muskelbauch *m*, Venter musculi.
mus·cle-bound [ˈmʌsəlbaʊnd] *adj* **1.** **to be** ~ Muskelkater haben. **2.** *fig.* starr.
muscle bundle Muskelbündel *nt*.
muscle cell Muskelzelle *f*, (einzelne) Muskelfaser *f*.
smooth m. glatte Muskelzelle.
muscle cement → myoglia.
muscle clamp Muskelklemme *f*.
muscle contraction Muskelkontraktion *f*.
muscle curve → myogram.
muscle energetics Muskelenergetik *f*.
muscle fascicle Muskelfaserbündel *nt*.
muscle fiber Muskelzelle *f*, (einzelne) Muskelfaser *f*.
cardiac m. Herzmuskel-, Myokardfaser *f*.
red m. rote Muskelfaser.
white m. weiße Muskelfaser.
muscle fibril → myofibril.
muscle giant cell Muskelriesenzelle *f*.
muscle glycogen Muskelglykogen *nt*.
muscle heat Muskelwärme *f*.
muscle hemoglobin → myoglobin.
muscle insertion Muskelansatz *m*.
muscle massage Muskelmassage *f*.
muscle mechanics Muskelmechanik *f*.
muscle metabolism Muskelstoffwechsel *m*, -metabolismus *m*.
muscle perfusion Muskeldurchblutung *f*, -perfusion *f*.
muscle phosphofructokinase deficiency Tarui-Krankheit *f*, Muskelphosphofruktokinaseinsuffizienz *f*, Glykogenose *f* Typ VII.
muscle phosphorylase Muskelphosphorylase *f*.
muscle phosphorylase deficiency (glycogenosis) McArdle-Krankheit *f*, -Syndrom *nt*, muskuläre Glykogenose *f*, Muskelphosphorylasemangel *m*, Myophosphorylaseinsuffizienz *f*, Glykogenose *f* Typ V.
muscle physiology Muskelphysiologie *f*.
muscle plate Myotom *nt*.
muscle pump *physio.* Muskel(venen)pumpe *f*.
muscle receptor Muskelrezeptor *m*.
muscle relaxant *pharm.*, *anes.* Muskelrelaxans *nt*.
depolarizing m. depolarisierendes Muskelrelaxans.
nondepolarizing m. nicht-polarisierendes/stabilisierendes Muskelrelaxans.
muscle relaxation Muskelerschlaffung *f*, -entspannung *f*, -relaxation *f*.
muscles [ˈmʌsəlz] *pl* Muskeln *pl*, Muskulatur *f*.
muscle sense → myesthesia.
muscle sensibility → myesthesia.
muscle spasm Muskelkrampf *m*.
muscle spindle Muskelspindel *f*.
muscle-spindle ending, primary anulospiralige Endigung *f*, Anulospiralendigung *f*.
muscle stiffness Muskelsteifheit *f*.
muscle sugar Inosit *nt*, Inositol *nt*.
muscle tendon (Muskel-)Sehne *f*.
muscle tissue Muskelgewebe *nt*.
muscle tone Muskeltonus *m*.
muscle twitching Muskelzuckung *f*.
muscle wasting → muscular atrophy.
muscle weakness → myoparesis.
mus·cu·lar [ˈmʌskjələr] *adj* **1.** Muskel(n) betr., muskulär, Muskel-. **2.** stark, kräftig, muskulös.
muscular arteries Arterien *pl* vom muskulären Typ.
muscular asthenopia *ophthal.* muskuläre Asthenopie *f*.
muscular atrophy Muskelatrophie *f*, -schwund *m*, Myatrophie *f*.
Aran-Duchenne m. Aran-Duchenne--Krankheit *f*, -Syndrom *nt*, Duchenne--Aran-Krankheit *f*, -Syndrom *nt*, adult-distale Form *f* der spinalen Muskelatrophie, spinale progressive Muskelatrophie.
denervated m. Muskelatrophie nach Denervierung.
Duchenne-Aran m. → Aran-Duchenne m.
facioscapulohumeral m. Landouzy--Déjérine-Krankheit *f*, -Syndrom *nt*, -Typ *m*, fazio-skapulo-humerale Muskeldystrophie *f*.
familial spinal m. → Hoffmann's m.
Hoffmann's m. Werdnig-Hoffmann--Krankheit *f*, -Syndrom *nt*, infantile Form *f* der spinalen Muskelatrophie, infantile spinale Muskelatrophie (Werdnig-Hoffmann).
idiopathic m. → muscular dystrophy, progressive.
infantile m. → Hoffmann's m.
infantile progressive spinal m. → Hoffmann's m.
ischemic m. Volkmann-Kontraktur *f*.
juvenile m. Kugelberg-Welander-Krankheit *f*, -Syndrom *nt*, juvenile Form *f* der spinalen Muskelatrophie, Atrophia musculorum spinalis pseudomyopathica (Kugelberg-Welander).
myelopathic m. myelopathische Muskelatrophie *f*.
neuritic m. neurogene Muskelatrophie.
peroneal m. → progressive neuropathic m.
progressive m. → spinal m.
progressive neural m. → progressive neuropathic m.
progressive neuropathic m. Charcot--Marie-Tooth-HoffmannKrankheit *f*, -Syndrom *nt*, Charcot-Marie-Krankheit *f*, -Syndrom *nt*.
progressive neuropathic peroneal m. → progressive neuropathic m.
progressive spinal m. Cruveilhier'-Krankheit *f*, spinale progressive Muskelatrophie.
pseudohypertrophic m. Duchenne--Krankheit *f*, -Muskeldystrophie *f*, Duchenne-Typ *m* der progressiven Muskeldystrophie, pseudohypertrophe pelvifemorale Form *f*, Dystrophia musculorum progressiva Duchenne.
spinal m. spinale Muskelatrophie.
Werdnig-Hoffmann m. → Hoffmann's m.
muscular branch Muskelast *m*, Ramus muscularis.
m.es of accessory nerve Muskeläste *pl* des N. accessorius, Rami musculares n. accessorii.
m.es of axillary nerve Muskeläste *pl* des N. axillaris, Rami musculares n. axillaris.

m.es of deep peroneal nerve Muskeläste pl des N. peron(a)eus profundus, Rami musculares n. fibularis/peron(a)ei profundi.
m.es of femoral nerve Muskeläste pl des N. femoralis, Rami musculares n. femoralis.
m.es of iliohypogastric nerve Muskeläste pl des N. iliohypogastricus, Rami musculares n. iliohypogastrici.
m.es of intercostal nerves Muskeläste pl der Interkostalnerven, Rami musculares nn. intercostalium.
m.es of median nerve Muskeläste pl des N. medianus, Rami musculares n. mediani.
m.es of musculocutaneous nerve Muskeläste pl des N. musculocutaneus, Rami musculares n. musculocutanei.
m.es of obturator nerve Muskeläste pl des N. obturatorius, Rami musculares n. obturatorii.
m.es of radial nerve Muskeläste pl des N. radialis, Rami musculares n. radialis.
m.es of sciatic nerve Muskeläste pl des N. ischiadicus, Rami musculares n. ischiadici.
m.es of superficial peroneal nerve Muskeläste pl des N. peron(a)eus superficialis, Rami musculares n. fibularis/peron(a)ei superficialis.
m.es of tibial nerve Muskeläste pl des N. tibialis, Rami musculares n. tibialis.
m.es of ulnar nerve Muskeläste pl des N. ulnaris, Rami musculares n. ulnaris.
m.es of vertebral artery Muskeläste pl der A. vertebralis, Rami musculares a. vertebralis.
muscular clubfoot muskulärer Klumpfuß m.
muscular coat → muscularis.
m. of pharynx Muskelschicht f der Pharynxwand, Tunica muscularis pharyngis.
muscular compartment anat. Lacuna musculorum.
muscular contracture muskuläre/myogene Kontraktur f.
muscular diaphragm anat. Zwerchfell nt, Scheidewand f, Diaphragma nt.
muscular dystrophy Muskel-, Myodystrophie f.
 adult pseudohypertrophic m. → Becker's m.
 Becker's m. Becker-Muskeldystrophie f.
 childhood m. → Duchenne (type) m.
 Duchenne (type) m. Duchenne-Krankheit f, -Muskeldystrophie, Duchenne-Typ m der progressiven Muskeldystrophie, pseudohypertrophe pelvifemorale Form f, Dystrophia musculorum progressiva Duchenne.
 facioscapulohumeral m. Landouzy-Déjérine-Krankheit f, -Syndrom nt, -Typ m, fazio-skapulo-humerale Muskeldystrophie.
 Leyden-Möbius m. Leyden-Möbius--Krankheit f, -Syndrom nt, Gliedgürtelform f der progressiven Muskeldystrophie.
 limb-girdle m. → Leyden-Möbius m.
 pelvofemoral m. → Leyden-Möbius m.
 progressive m. abbr. **PMD** progressive Muskeldystrophie abbr. PMD, Dystrophia musculorum progressiva.
 pseudohypertrophic m. → Duchenne (type) m.
muscular fasciae of eye Fasciae musculares (bulbi).
muscular fatigue 1. Muskelermüdung f. 2. körperliche/physische Ermüdung f.
muscular fibril → myofibril.
muscular force Muskelkraft f.
muscular hypotonia Muskelhypotonie f.

muscular irritabiality physiol. muskuläre Erregbarkeit f.
mus·cu·la·ris [ˌmʌskjəˈlɛərɪs] n histol. Muskularis f, Tunica muscularis.
muscularis mucosae histol. Muscularis/Muskularis f mucosae, Lamina muscularis mucosae.
mus·cu·lar·i·ty [ˌmʌskjəˈlærətɪ] n muskulöser Körperbau m.
muscular layer: m. of fallopian tube Tunica muscularis tubae uterinae.
m. of mucosa Lamina muscularis mucosae.
muscular line of scapula Linea muscularis scapulae.
muscular paralysis → myoparalysis.
 pseudohypertrophic m. Duchenne--Krankheit f, -Muskeldystrophie f, Duchenne-Typ m der progressiven Muskeldystrophie, pseudohypertrophe pelvifemorale Form f, Dystrophia musculorum progressiva Duchenne.
muscular part of interventricular septum muskulärer Teil m des Kammerseptums, Pars muscularis septi interventricularis cordis.
muscular process of arytenoid process Muskelfortsatz m des Arynknorpels, Proc. muscularis cartilaginis aryt(a)enoideae.
muscular reflex Muskeldehnungsreflex m.
muscular rheumatism Weichteil-, Muskelrheumatismus m, Fibrositis-Syndrom nt.
muscular spasm → myospasm.
muscular strabismus ophthal. 1. Begleitschielen nt, Strabismus concomitans. 2. Lähmungsschielen nt, Strabismus paralyticus.
muscular strength Muskelkraft f, -stärke f.
muscular subaortic stenosis idiopathische hypertrophische subaortale Stenose f abbr. IHSS, Subaortenstenose f.
muscular substance of prostate glatte Prostatamuskulatur f, Substantia muscularis (prostatae).
muscular sulcus of tympanic cavity Semicanalis m. tensoris tympani.
muscular system muskuläres System nt, Muskulatur f.
muscular tension Muskelspannung f.
muscular tissue Muskelgewebe nt.
muscular torticollis ortho., neuro. muskulärer Schiefhals/Torticollis m.
muscular trabeculae of heart Herztrabekel pl, Herzmuskelbälkchen pl, Trabeculae carneae cordis.
muscular triangle Trigonum musculare/omotracheale.
muscular trichinosis Muskeltrichinose f.
muscular trigone → muscular triangle.
muscular trochlea Trochlea muscularis.
muscular trophoneurosis → muscular atrophy, progressive.
muscular tumor → myoma.
muscular tunic → muscularis.
muscular wryneck → muscular torticollis.
mus·cu·la·ture [ˈmʌskjʊlətʃər, -ˌtʃʊər] n Muskulatur f, Muskelapparat m.
m. of larynx Kehlkopfmuskeln pl, -muskulatur, Mm. laryngis.
mus·cu·lo·cu·ta·ne·ous [ˌmʌskjəlˌoʊkjuːˈteɪnəs, -nɪəs] adj Haut- u. Muskel(gewebe) betr., Haut-Muskel-.
musculocutaneous amputation chir. Amputation f mit Hautmuskellappendeckung.
musculocutaneous flap chir. Hautmuskellappen m.
musculocutaneous nerve N. musculocutaneus.

m. of foot Fibularis/Peronäus m superficialis, N. fibularis/peron(a)eus superficialis.
m. of leg Fibularis/Peronäus m profundus, N. fibularis/peron(a)eus profundus.
mus·cu·lo·der·mic [ˌ-ˈdɜrmɪk] adj → musculocutaneous.
mus·cu·lo·phren·ic artery [ˌ-ˈfrɛnɪk] A. musculophrenica.
musculophrenic veins Vv. musculophrenicae.
mus·cu·lo·skel·e·tal [ˌ-ˈskɛlɪtl] adj Knochenskelett u. Muskulatur betr., Skelettmuskulatur betr.
musculoskeletal graft Muskel-Knochen--Transplantat nt.
musculoskeletal system (Stütz- u.) Bewegungsapparat m.
mus·cu·lo·spi·ral groove [ˌ-ˈspaɪərəl] Radialisrinne f, Sulcus (n.) radialis.
musculospiral nerve old → radial nerve.
mus·cu·lo·ten·di·nous cuff [ˌ-ˈtɛndɪnəs] 1. Muskel-Sehnen-Manschette f. 2. (Schulter) Rotatorenmanschette f.
mus·cu·lo·tub·al canal [ˌ-ˈt(j)uːbl] (Semi-)Canalis musculotubarius.
mush·room poisoning [ˈmʌʃruːm, -rʊm] Pilzvergiftung f, Myzetismus m.
mu·si·cal agraphia [ˈmjuːzɪkl] neuro. musikalische Agraphie f.
musical alexia neuro. musikalische Alexie f.
musical murmur musikalisches Geräusch nt.
mu·sic blindness [ˈmjuːzɪk] neuro. musikalische Alexie f.
mu·si·co·gen·ic epilepsy [ˌmjuːzɪkoʊˈdʒɛnɪk] musikogene Epilepsie f.
mu·si·co·ther·a·py [ˌ-ˈθɛrəpɪ] n Musiktherapie f.
mus·ky [ˈmʌskɪ] adj moschusartig, Moschus-; nach Moschus riechend.
Musset [myˈsɛ]: **M.'s sign** (de) Musset-Zeichen nt.
Mustard [ˈmʌstərd]: **M.'s operation** HTG Mustard-Operation f.
mus·tard [ˈmʌstərd] n Senf m, Mostrich m.
mustard gas Senfgas nt, Gelbkreuz nt.
mustard oil chem. (ätherisches) Senföl nt.
mustard plaster Senfpflaster nt.
mu·ta·bil·i·ty [mjuːtəˈbɪlɪtɪ] n Veränderlichkeit f; bio. Mutationsfähigkeit f, Mutabilität f.
mu·ta·ble [ˈmjuːtəbəl] adj wandelbar, veränderlich; bio. mutationsfähig, mutabel.
mu·ta·gen [ˈmjuːtədʒən] n Mutagen nt, mutagenes Agens nt.
mu·ta·gen·e·sis [ˌmjuːtəˈdʒɛnəsɪs] n Mutagenese f.
mu·ta·gen·ic [ˌ-ˈdʒɛnɪk] adj Mutation verursachend, mutagen.
mutagenic agent → mutagen.
mu·ta·ge·nic·i·ty [ˌ-dʒəˈnɪsətɪ] n Mutationsfähigkeit f, Mutagenität f.
mu·tant [ˈmjuːtnt] I n Mutante f. II adj durch Mutation entstanden, mutiert, mutant.
mutant gene mutiertes Gen nt.
mutant virus mutiertes Virus nt.
mu·ta·ro·tase [ˌmjuːtəˈraʊteɪz] n Aldose-1--epimerase f, Mutarotase f.
mu·ta·ro·ta·tion [ˌ-raʊˈteɪʃn] n chem. Mutarotation f.
mu·tase [ˈmjuːteɪz] n Mutase f.
mu·tate [ˈmjuːteɪt] I vt verändern; bio. zu einer Mutation führen. II vi s. (ver-)ändern; bio. mutieren (to zu).
mu·ta·tion [mjuːˈteɪʃn] n (Ver-)Änderung f, Umwandlung f; bio. Erbänderung f, Mutation f.
m. of energy phys. Energieumformung f.

mu·ta·tion·al [mju:'teɪʃnl] *adj* Mutation betr., Mutations-; Änderungs-.
mutational unit mutierbare Einheit *f*.
mutation rate Mutationsrate *f*.
mute [mju:t] **I** *n* Stumme(r *m*) *f*. **II** *adj* **1.** stumm. **2.** still, schweigend, stumm; wort-, sprachlos.
mute·ness ['mju:tnɪs] *n* **1.** Stummheit *f*. **2.** Lautlosigkeit *f*.
mu·ti·late ['mju:tleɪt] *vt* verstümmeln.
mu·ti·lat·ing keratoderma ['mju:tleɪtɪŋ] Keratoma hereditaria mutilans.
mu·ti·la·tion [ˌmju:tɪ'leɪʃn] *n* Verstümmelung *f*, Mutilation *f*.
mu·tism ['mju:tɪzəm] *n psychia.* Mutismus *m*.
mu·ton ['mju:tɒn] *n genet.* Muton *nt*.
mut·ter·ing delirium ['mʌtərɪŋ] mussitierendes Delirium *nt*, Delirium mussitans.
mu·tu·al ['mju:tʃʊəl, -tʃəl] *adj* gegen-, wechselseitig, mutuell.
mu·tu·al·ism ['mju:tʃ(ə)wəlɪzəm] *n bio.* Mutualismus *m*.
MV *abbr.* **1.** → megavolt. **2.** → minute volume 1.
mV *abbr.* → millivolt.
µV *abbr.* → microvolt.
MVE *abbr.* → Murray Valley encephalitis.
MVV *abbr.* [maximum voluntary ventilation] → maximum breathing capacity.
µW *abbr.* → microwatt.
MWC *abbr.* → maximal work place concentration.
MWC value *physiol.* MAK-Wert *m*.
My. *abbr.* → myopia.
my- *pref.* → myo-.
my·al·gia [maɪ'ældʒ(ɪ)ə] *n* Muskelschmerz(en *pl*) *m*, Myalgie *f*, Myodynie *f*.
my·a·sis ['maɪəsɪs] *n*, *pl* **-ses** [-siːz] → myiasis.
my·as·the·nia [ˌmaɪəs'θiːnɪə] *n neuro., ortho.* Myasthenie *f*, Myasthenia *f*.
myasthenia gravis → myasthenia gravis syndrome.
myasthenia gravis syndrome Erb-Goldflam-Syndrom *nt*, -Krankheit *f*, Erb-Oppenheim-Goldflam-Syndrom *nt*, -Krankheit *f*, Hoppe-Goldflam-Syndrom *nt*, Myasthenia gravis pseudoparalytica.
my·as·then·ic [ˌmaɪəs'θɜɛnɪk] *adj* Myasthenie betr., myasthenisch.
myasthenic crisis myasthenische Krise *f*.
myasthenic reaction Jolly-Reaktion *f*, myasthenische Reaktion *f*.
myasthenic syndrome Lambert-Eaton-Rooke-Syndrom *nt*, pseudomyasthenisches Syndrom *nt*.
my·a·to·nia [ˌmaɪə'təʊnɪə] *n neuro.* Myatonie *f*, Myatonia *f*.
my·at·o·ny [maɪ'ætənɪ] *n* → myatonia.
my·at·ro·phy [maɪ'ætrəfɪ] *n* → muscular atrophy.
myc- *pref.* → myco-.
my·ce·li·al [maɪ'siːlɪəl] *adj micro.* Myzel betr., Myzel-.
mycelial fungi *micro.* Fadenpilze *pl*, Hyphomyzeten *pl*, Hyphomycetes *pl*.
my·ce·li·an [maɪ'siːlɪən] *adj* → mycelial.
my·ce·li·oid [maɪ'siːlɪɔɪd] *adj micro.* myzelähnlich, -artig.
my·ce·li·um [maɪ'siːlɪəm] *n*, *pl* **-lia** [-lɪə] *micro.* Pilzgeflecht *nt*, Myzel *nt*, Myzelium *nt*.
mycet- *pref.* → myco-.
my·ce·tes [maɪ'siːtiːz] *pl micro.* Pilze *f*, Fungi *pl*, Myzeten *pl*, Mycota *pl*.
my·ce·the·mia [ˌmaɪsə'θiːmɪə] *n* Pilzsepsis *f*, Fungämie *f*, Mykämie *f*, Myzet(h)ämie *f*.
my·ce·tism ['maɪsətɪzəm] *n* → mycetismus.

my·ce·tis·mus [maɪsə'tɪzməs] *n* Pilzvergiftung *f*, Myzetismus *m*.
myceto- *pref.* → myco-.
my·ce·to·ge·net·ic [maɪˌsiːtə'dʒənetɪk] *adj* durch Pilze verursacht, myzetogen, Pilz-.
my·ce·to·gen·ic [ˌ-'dʒenɪk] *adj* → mycetogenetic.
my·ce·tog·e·nous [maɪsɪ'tɒdʒənəs] *adj* → mycetogenetic.
my·ce·to·ma [maɪsə'təʊmə] *n*, *pl* **-mas**, **-ma·ta** [-mətə] Madurafuß *m*, -mykose *f*, Myzetom *nt*, Mycetoma *nt*.
my·cid ['maɪsɪd] *n* Mykid *f*.
myco- *pref.* Pilz-, Myko-, Myzeto-.
my·co·bac·te·ria *pl* → mycobacterium.
my·co·bac·te·ri·al adjuvant [ˌmaɪkəʊbæk-'tɪərɪəl] komplettes Freund-Adjuvans *nt*.
My·co·bac·te·ri·a·ce·ae [ˌ-bækˌtɪərɪ'eɪsɪˌiː] *pl micro.* Mycobacteriaceae *pl*.
my·co·bac·te·ri·o·sis [ˌ-bækˌtɪərɪ'əʊsɪs] *n* Mykobakteriose *f*.
My·co·bac·te·ri·um [ˌ-bæk'tɪərɪəm] *n micro.* Mycobacterium *nt*.
M. leprae Hansen-Bazillus *m*, Leprabazillus *m*, -bakterium *nt*, Mycobacterium leprae.
M. paratuberculosis Johne-Bazillus *m*, Mycobacterium paratuberculosis.
M. tuberculosis Tuberkel-, Tuberkulosebazillus *m*, -bakterium *nt*, TB-Bazillus *m*, TB-Erreger *m*, Mycobacterium tuberculosis, Mycobacterium tuberculosis var. hominis.
my·co·bac·te·ri·um [ˌ-bæk'tɪərɪəm] *n*, *pl* **-ria** [-rɪə] *micro.* Mykobakterium *nt*, Mycobacterium *nt*.
group I m.a photochromogene Mykobakterien *pl*, Mykobakterien *pl* der Runyon-Gruppe I.
group II m.a skotochromogene Mykobakterien *pl*, Mykobakterien *pl* der Runyon-Gruppe II.
group III m.a nicht-chromogene Mykobakterien *pl*, Mykobakterien *pl* der Runyon-Gruppe III.
group IV m.a schnellwachsende (atypische) Mykobakterien *pl*, Mykobakterien *pl* der Runyon-Gruppe IV.
m.a other than tubercle bacilli *abbr.* MOTT atypische/nicht-tuberkulöse Mykobakterien *pl*.
my·co·bac·tin [ˌ-'bæktɪn] *n micro.* Mykobaktin *nt*, Mycobactin *nt*.
my·co·der·ma [ˌ-'dɜːmə] *n micro.* Mycoderma *nt*.
my·col·ic acid [maɪ'kɒlɪk] Mykol-, Mycolsäure *f*.
my·col·o·gy [maɪ'kɒlədʒɪ] *n* Mykologie *f*.
my·co·myr·in·gi·tis [ˌmaɪkəʊˌmɪrən'dʒaɪtɪs] *n* → myringomycosis.
my·co·phage ['-feɪdʒ] *n micro.* Pilz-, Mykophage *m*.
My·coph·y·ta [maɪ'kɒfɪtə] *pl micro.* Pilze *pl*, Fungi *pl*, Myzeten *pl*, Mycetes *pl*, Mycophyta *pl*, Mycota *pl*.
My·co·plas·ma [ˌmaɪkə'plæzmə] *n micro.* Mycoplasma *nt*.
M. pneumoniae Eaton-agent *nt*, Mycoplasma pneumoniae.
my·co·plas·ma [ˌ-'plæzmə] *n*, *pl* **-mas**, **-ma·ta** [-mətə] *micro.* Mykoplasma *nt*, Mycoplasma *nt*.
my·co·plas·mal [ˌ-'plæzməl] *adj* Mykoplasma betr., durch Mykoplasma verursacht, Mykoplasma-, Mykoplasmen-.
mycoplasmal pneumonia Mykoplasmapneumonie *f*.
Mycoplasma pneumoniae pneumonia Mycoplasma-pneumoniae-Pneumonie *f*, Mykoplasmapneumonie *f*.
My·co·plas·mas [ˌ-'plæzməs] *pl* → Mycoplasmatales.

My·co·plas·ma·ta·ce·ae [ˌ-ˌplæzmə'teɪsɪˌiː] *pl* Mycoplasmataceae *pl*.
My·co·plas·ma·ta·les [ˌ-ˌplæzmə'teɪləs] *pl micro.* Mycoplasmatales *pl*.
my·co·plas·mo·sis [ˌ-plæz'məʊsɪs] *n* Mykoplasmainfektion *f*.
my·cose ['maɪkəʊs] *n* Trehalose *f*, Mykose *f*.
my·co·side ['maɪkəsaɪd] *n* Mykosid *nt*.
my·co·sis [maɪ'kəʊsɪs] *n* Pilzerkrankung *f*, Mykose *f*, Mycosis *f*.
mycosis cell Mycosis-fungoides-Zelle *f*.
mycosis fungoides cell → mycosis cell.
my·co·stat ['maɪkəstæt] *n pharm.* fungistatisches Mittel *nt*, Fungistatikum *nt*.
my·co·stat·ic [ˌ-'stætɪk] *adj* Pilzwachstum hemmend, fungistatisch.
my·cos·ter·ol [maɪ'kɒstərɒl, -rəʊl] *n* Mycosterol *nt*.
my·co·ta [maɪ'kəʊtə] *pl* → mycetes.
my·cot·ic [maɪ'kɒtɪk] *adj* **1.** Mykose betr., mykotisch, Mykose-. **2.** durch Pilze verursacht, mykotisch, Pilz-.
mycotic abscess mykotischer Abszeß *m*.
mycotic aneurysm mykotisches Aneurysma *nt*.
mycotic arthritis Gelenkfungus *m*, Arthritis fungosa.
mycotic endocarditis Pilzendokarditis *f*, Endocarditis mycotica.
mycotic infection → mycosis.
mycotic keratitis Keratomykosis *f*.
mycotic stomatitis Mundsoor *m*, Candidose *f* der Mundschleimhaut.
my·co·tox·i·co·sis [ˌmaɪkəˌtɒksɪ'kəʊsɪs] *n*, *pl* **-ses** [-siːz] Mykotoxikose *f*.
my·co·tox·in [ˌ-'tɒksɪn] *n* Pilz-, Mykotoxin *nt*.
my·dri·a·sis [mɪ'draɪəsɪs, maɪ-] *n* Pupillenweitstellung *f*, -vergrößerung *f*, Mydriasis *f*.
my·dri·at·ic [mɪdrɪ'ætɪk, maɪ-] **I** *n* pupillenerweiternde Substanz *f*, Mydriatikum *nt*, Mydriaticum *nt* **II** *adj* pupillenerweiternd, mydriatisch.
my·ec·to·my [maɪ'ektəmɪ] *n chir.* operative Muskel(teil)entfernung *f*, Myektomie *f*.
my·ec·to·pia [maɪek'təʊpɪə] *n patho.* Muskelverlagerung *f*.
my·ec·to·py [maɪ'ektəpɪ] *n* → myectopia.
myel- *pref.* → myelo-.
my·el·ap·o·plex·y [ˌmaɪel'æpəpleksɪ] *n* Rückenmarks(ein)blutung *f*, Hämatomyelie *f*.
my·el·a·te·lia [ˌmaɪelə'tiːlɪə] *n embryo.* entwicklungsbedingter Rückenmarksdefekt *m*.
my·el·at·ro·phy [ˌmaɪel'ætrəfɪ] *n* Rückenmark(s)atrophie *f*.
my·e·le·mia [maɪə'liːmɪə] *n* → myelocytosis.
my·e·len·ceph·a·li·tis [ˌmaɪəlenˌsefə'laɪtɪs] *n* → myeloencephalitis.
my·el·en·ceph·a·lon [ˌmaɪəlen'sefələn] *n* **1.** *embryo.* Markhirn *nt*, Myelenzephalon *nt*, Myelencephalon *nt*. **2.** Markhirn *nt*, verlängertes Mark *nt*, Medulla oblongata, Bulbus *m* (medullae spinalis), Myelencephalon *nt*.
my·e·let·er·o·sis [ˌmaɪəˌletə'rəʊsɪs] *n* pathologische Rückenmark(s)veränderung *f*.
my·el·ic [maɪ'elɪk] *adj* **1.** Rückenmark betr., Rückenmark(s)-. **2.** Knochenmark betr., Knochenmark(s)-.
my·e·lin ['maɪəlɪn] *n* Myelin *nt*.
my·e·li·nat·ed ['maɪəlɪneɪtɪd] *adj* markhaltig, myelinisiert.
myelinated matter weiße Hirn- u. Rückenmarkssubstanz *f*, Substantia alba.
m. of spinal cord weiße Rückenmarkssubstanz, Substantia alba medullae spinalis.

myelinated nerve

myelinated nerve markhaltige Nervenfaser f.
myelinated substance → myelinated matter.
m. of spinal cord → myelinated matter of spinal cord.
my·e·li·na·tion [ˌmaɪəlɪ'neɪʃn] n → myelogenesis 2.
my·e·lin·ic [maɪə'lɪnɪk] adj Myelin betr., Myelin-.
my·e·lin·i·za·tion [ˌmaɪəlɪnə'zeɪʃn] n → myelogenesis 2.
my·e·li·noc·la·sis [ˌmaɪəlɪ'nɑkləsɪs] n patho. Myelinzerstörung f.
my·e·lin·o·gen·e·sis [ˌmaɪəlɪnəʊ'dʒenəsɪs] n → myelogenesis 2.
my·e·lin·o·ge·net·ic [ˌmaɪəlɪnə'dʒənetɪk] adj 1. myelinbildend, myelinogen. 2. myelinisierend.
my·e·lin·og·e·ny [maɪəlɪ'nɑdʒənɪ] n → myelogenesis 2.
my·e·li·nol·y·sis [maɪəlɪ'nɑləsɪs] n Myelinauflösung f, Myelinolyse f.
my·e·li·nop·a·thy [maɪəlɪ'nɑpəθɪ] n Myelinopathie f.
my·e·li·no·tox·ic [ˌmaɪəlɪnə'tɑksɪk] adj myelinschädigend, -toxisch.
myelin sheath Mark-, Myelinscheide f.
myelin stain Markscheiden-, Myelinfärbung f.
my·e·lit·ic [maɪə'lɪtɪk] adj Myelitis betr., myelitisch.
my·e·li·tis [maɪə'laɪtɪs] n 1. Rückenmark(s)entzündung f, Myelitis f. 2. Knochenmark(s)entzündung f, Myelitis f, Osteomyelitis f.
myelo- pref. Mark-, Rückenmark(s)-, Knochenmark(s)-, Myelo-.
my·e·lo·ar·chi·tec·ton·ics [ˌmaɪəloʊˌɑːrkɪtek'tɑnɪks] pl Myeloarchitektonik f.
my·e·lo·blast ['-blæst] n Myeloblast m.
my·e·lo·blas·te·mia [ˌ-blæs'tiːmɪə] n hema. Myeloblastämie f.
my·e·lo·blas·tic leukemia [ˌ-'blæstɪk] Myeloblastenleukämie f.
my·e·lo·blas·to·ma [ˌ-blæs'toʊmə] n Myeloblastom nt.
my·e·lo·blas·to·ma·to·sis [ˌ-ˌblæstoʊmə'toʊsɪs] n Myeloblastomatose f.
my·e·lo·blas·to·sis [ˌ-blæs'toʊsɪs] n Myeloblastose f.
my·e·lo·cele ['-siːl] n Myelozele f.
my·e·lo·cys·to·cele [ˌ-'sɪstəsiːl] n Myelozystozele f.
my·e·lo·cys·to·me·nin·go·cele [ˌ-ˌsɪstəmɪ'nɪŋɡəsiːl] n Myelozystomeningozele f.
my·e·lo·cyte ['-saɪt] n Myelozyt m.
my·e·lo·cy·the·mia [ˌ-saɪ'θiːmɪə] n Myelozyt(h)ämie f.
my·e·lo·cyt·ic [ˌ-'sɪtɪk] adj Myelozyt(en) betr., Myelozyten-.
myelocytic crisis hema. Myelozytenkrise f.
myelocytic leukemia myeloische/granulozytäre Leukämie f.
myelocytic series → myeloid series.
my·e·lo·cy·to·ma [ˌ-saɪ'toʊmə] n Myelozytom nt.
my·e·lo·cy·to·sis [ˌ-saɪ'toʊsɪs] n Myelozytose f; Myelose f.
my·e·lo·dys·pla·sia [ˌ-dɪs'pleɪʒ(ɪ)ə, -zɪə] n Rückenmark(s)fehlbildung f, Myelodysplasie f.
my·e·lo·en·ce·phal·ic [ˌ-ˌensɪ'fælɪk] adj Rückenmark u. Gehirn betr., spinozerebral, zerebrospinal.
my·e·lo·en·ceph·a·li·tis [ˌ-enˌsefə'laɪtɪs] n Entzündung f von Rückenmark u. Gehirn, Myeloenzephalitis f, Enzephalo-, Encephalomyelitis f.
my·e·lo·fi·bro·sis [ˌ-faɪ'broʊsɪs] n Knochenmark(s)fibrose f, Myelofibrose f, -sklerose f, Osteomyelofibrose f abbr. OMF, Osteomyelosklerose f.
my·e·lof·u·gal [maɪə'lɑfjəɡəl] adj vom Rückenmark weg, myelofugal.
my·e·lo·gen·e·sis [ˌmaɪəloʊ'dʒenəsɪs] n 1. Rückenmarksentwicklung f, Myelogenese f. 2. Markscheidenbildung f, Markreifung f, Myelinisation f, Myel(in)ogenese f.
my·e·lo·gen·ic [ˌ-'dʒenɪk] adj → myelogenous.
myelogenic leukemia → myelocytic leukemia.
my·e·log·e·nous [maɪə'lɑdʒənəs] adj im Knochenmark entstanden, aus dem Knochenmark stammend, myelogen, osteomyelogen.
myelogenous callus ortho. zentraler/innerer Kallus m.
myelogenous leukemia → myelocytic leukemia.
my·e·log·e·ny [maɪə'lɑdʒənɪ] n → myelogenesis 2.
my·e·lo·gram ['maɪəlɑɡræm] n 1. radiol. Myelogramm nt. 2. hema. Myelogramm nt, Hämatomyelogramm nt.
my·e·log·ra·phy [maɪə'lɑɡrəfɪ] n radiol. Kontrastdarstellung f des Wirbelkanals, Myelographie f.
my·e·loid ['maɪəlɔɪd] adj 1. Knochenmark betr., vom Knochenmark stammend, knochenmarkähnlich, markartig, myeloid, Knochenmark(s)-. 2. Rückenmark betr., Rückenmark(s)-. 3. hema. myelozytenähnlich, myeloid, myeloisch.
myeloid cell hema. (hämopoetische) Knochenmark(s)zelle f.
my·e·loi·din [maɪə'lɔɪdɪn] n Myeloidin nt.
myeloid leukemia → myelocytic leukemia.
myeloid metaplasia myeloische Metaplasie f.
myeloid series hema. myeloide/myelozytäre Reihe f.
myeloid tissue rotes Knochenmark nt, Medulla ossium rubra.
my·e·lo·li·po·ma [ˌmaɪəloʊlɪ'poʊmə] n Myelolipom nt.
my·e·lol·y·sis [maɪə'lɑləsɪs] n → myelinolysis.
my·e·lo·ma [maɪə'loʊmə] n, pl -mas, -mata [-mətə] Myelom nt, Myeloma nt.
myeloma kidney Myelomniere f.
my·e·lo·ma·la·cia [ˌmaɪəloʊmə'leɪʃ(ɪ)ə] n patho. Rückenmark(s)erweichung f, Myelomalazie f.
my·e·lo·ma·to·sis [maɪəˌloʊmə'toʊsɪs] n, pl -ses [-siːz] → multiple myeloma.
my·e·lo·men·in·gi·tis [ˌmaɪəloʊˌmenɪn'dʒaɪtɪs] n Entzündung f des Rückenmarks u. seiner Häute, Myelomeningitis f, Meningomyelitis f.
my·e·lo·me·nin·go·cele [ˌ-mɪ'nɪŋɡəsiːl, -'nɪndʒə-] n Myelomeningozele f, Meningomyelozele f.
my·e·lo·mon·o·cyt·ic leukemia [ˌ-ˌmɑnə'sɪtɪk] f abbr. AMML, (akute) Myelomonozytenleukämie f.
my·e·lom·y·cis [maɪə'lɑməsɪz] n → medullary carcinoma.
my·e·lo·neu·ri·tis [ˌmaɪəloʊnjʊə'raɪtɪs, -nʊ-] n Neuromyelitis f.
myelo-opticoneuropathy n Myelooptikoneuropathie f.
my·e·lo·path·ic [ˌ-'pæθɪk] adj Myelopathie betr., myelopathisch.
myelopathic anemia leukoerythroblastische Anämie f, idiopathische/primäre myeloische Metaplasie f, Leukoerythroblastose f.
myelopathic polycythemia Morbus Osler-Vaquez m, Vaquez-Osler-Syndrom nt, Osler-Vaquez-Krankheit f, Osler-Krankheit f, Erythrämie f, Polycythaemia (rubra) vera.
my·e·lop·a·thy [maɪə'lɑpəθɪ] n 1. Rückenmark(s)erkrankung f, Myelopathie f, -pathia f. 2. Knochenmark(s)erkrankung f, Myelopathie f, -pathia f.
my·e·lo·per·ox·i·dase [ˌmaɪəloʊpə'rɑksɪdeɪz] n abbr. **MPO** Myeloperoxidase f abbr. MPO.
my·e·lo·pe·tal [maɪə'lɑpətəl] adj in Richtung auf das Rückenmark, myelopetal.
my·e·lo·phage ['maɪəloʊfeɪdʒ] n Myelophage m.
my·e·lo·phthi·sic anemia [ˌmaɪəloʊ'tɪzɪk] → myelopathic anemia.
my·e·lo·phthi·sis [ˌ-'tiːsɪs, -'tɪs-, -'taɪ-, -'θaɪ-] n 1. Rückenmark(s)schwund m, Myelophthise f. 2. hema. Knochenmark(s)schwund m, Panmyelophthise f.
my·el·o·plaque ['-plæk] n Knochenmark(s)riesenzelle f.
my·el·o·plast ['-plæst] n Myeloplast m.
my·el·o·plax ['-plæks] n, pl -plaxes [-plæksɪz] → myeloplaque.
my·e·lo·ple·gia [ˌ-'pliːdʒ(ɪ)ə] n Spinalparalyse f.
my·e·lo·poi·e·sis [ˌ-pɔɪ'iːsɪs] n Myelopoese f.
my·e·lo·poi·et·ic hemopoiesis [ˌ-pɔɪ'etɪk] medulläre/myelopoetische Blutbildung f.
my·e·lo·pro·lif·er·a·tive [ˌ-prəʊ'lɪfəreɪtɪv] adj myeloproliferativ.
myeloproliferative disease/syndrome myeloproliferative Erkrankung f, myeloproliferatives Syndrom nt abbr. MPS.
my·e·lo·ra·dic·u·li·tis [ˌ-rəˌdɪkjə'laɪtɪs] n Entzündung f von Rückenmark- u. Nervenwurzeln, Myeloradikulitis f.
my·e·lo·ra·dic·u·lo·dys·pla·sia [ˌ-rəˌdɪkjəlоʊdɪs'pleɪʒ(ɪ)ə, -zɪə] n Myeloradikulodysplasie f.
my·e·lo·ra·dic·u·lop·a·thy [ˌ-rəˌdɪkjə'lɑpəθɪ] n Erkrankung f von Rückenmark- u. Nervenwurzeln, Myeloradikulopathie f.
my·e·lor·rha·gia [ˌ-'reɪdʒ(ɪ)ə] n Rückenmarks(ein)blutung f, Hämatomyelie f.
my·e·lo·sar·co·ma·to·sis [ˌ-ˌsɑːrkəmə'toʊsɪs] n → multiple myeloma.
my·e·los·chi·sis [maɪə'lɑskəsɪs] n embryo. Myeloschisis f.
my·e·lo·scin·ti·gram [ˌmaɪələ'sɪntəɡræm] n radiol. Myeloszintigramm nt.
my·e·lo·scin·tig·ra·phy [ˌ-sɪn'tɪɡrəfɪ] n radiol. Myeloszintigraphie f.
my·e·lo·scle·ro·sis [ˌ-sklɪ'roʊsɪs] n 1. → myelofibrosis. 2. Myelosklerose f.
my·e·lo·sis [maɪə'loʊsɪs] n 1. hema. Myelose f; Myelozytose f. 2. neuro. degenerativer Rückenmarksprozeß m, Myelose f.
my·e·lo·sup·pres·sion [ˌmaɪəloʊə'preʃn] n Knochenmark(s)depression f, -hemmung f.
my·e·lo·sup·pres·sive [ˌ-sə'presɪv] I n myelodepressive Substanz f. II adj knochenmark(s)hemmend, myelodepressiv.
myelosuppressive agent → myelosuppressive.
my·e·lo·syph·i·lis [ˌ-'sɪf(ə)lɪs] n Rückenmark(s)syphilis f.
my·e·lo·sy·rin·go·sis [ˌ-sɪrɪŋ'ɡoʊsɪs] n Syringomyelie f, -myelia f.
my·e·lo·tome ['-toʊm] n neurochir. Myelotom nt.
my·e·lo·to·mog·ra·phy [ˌ-tə'mɑɡrəfɪ] n radiol. Myelotomographie f.
my·e·lot·o·my [maɪə'lɑtəmɪ] n neurochir. Rückenmark(s)schnitt m, Myelotomie f.
my·e·lo·tox·ic [maɪəloʊ'tɑksɪk] adj knochenmark(s)schädigend, -toxisch, myelotoxisch.

my·e·lo·tox·ic·i·ty [,-tak'sısətı] n Knochenmark(s)schädlichkeit f, Myelotoxizität f.
my·en·ter·ic plexus [,maıən'terık] Auerbach'-Plexus m, Plexus myentericus.
my·es·the·sia [maıes'θi:ʒ(ı)ə] n Muskelsensibilität f, -sinn m, Myästhesie f.
my·ia·sis ['maı(j)əsıs, maı'aıəsıs] n, pl -ses [-si:z] derm. Myiasis f.
my·io·ceph·a·lon [,maıjəʊ'sefələn, maı,aıə-] n ophthal. Irisprolaps m, -hernie f, Iridozele f.
my·io·ceph·a·lum [,-'sefələm] n → myiocephalon.
my·io·des·op·sia [,-des'ɑpsıə] n → muscae volitantes.
my·io·sis [maı'jəʊsıs, ,maıaı'əʊsıs] n, pl -ses [-si:z] → myiasis.
my·i·tis [maı'aıtıs] n → myositis.
myk(o)- pref. → myco-.
my·kol ['maıkɒl, -kəl] n → mycolic acid.
my·lo·hy·oid [,maıləʊ'haıɔıd] adj Kiefer u. Zungenbein betr.
mylohyoid artery Ramus mylohyoideus a. alveolaris inferioris.
mylohyoid branch of inferior alveolar artery → mylohyoid artery.
my·lo·hy·oi·de·an [,-haı'ɔıdıən] adj → mylohyoid.
mylohyoidean line (of mandible) Linea mylohyoidea (mandibulae).
my·lo·hy·oi·de·us (muscle) [,-haı'ɔıdıəs] Mylohyoideus m, M. mylohyoideus.
mylohyoid line (of mandible) Linea mylohyoidea (mandibulae).
mylohyoid muscle → mylohyoideus (muscle).
mylohyoid nerve N. mylohyoideus.
mylohyoid sulcus of mandible Sulcus mylohyoideus (mandibulae).
my·lo·pha·ryn·ge·al muscle [,-fə'rındʒ(ı)əl] → mylopharyngeus (muscle).
my·lo·pha·ryn·ge·us (muscle) [,-fə'rındʒ(ı)əs] old M. mylopharyngeus, Pars mylopharyngea m. constrictoris pharyngis superioris.
myo- pref. Muskel-, My(o)-.
my·o·a·den·yl·ate deaminase [,maıəʊə'denlıt, -eıt] Myoadenylatdeaminase f, Muskeladenylatdeaminase f.
myoadenylate deaminase deficiency Myoadenylatdeaminase-Mangel m.
myo·al·bu·min [,-æl'bju:mın] n Myoalbumin nt.
my·o·as·the·nia [,-æs'θi:nıə] n Muskelschwäche f, Myasthenie f.
my·o·at·ro·phy [,-'ætrəfı] n → muscular atrophy.
my·o·blast ['-blæst] n embryo. Myoblast m.
my·o·blas·tic [,-'blæstık] adj Myoblast(en) betr., Myoblasten-.
my·o·blas·to·ma [,-blæs'təʊmə] n Myoblastom nt, Abrikossoff-Geschwulst f, -Tumor m, Myoblastenmyom nt, Granularzelltumor m.
my·o·blas·to·my·o·ma [,-,blæstəmaı'əʊmə] n → myoblastoma.
my·o·car·di·ac [,-'kɑ:rdıæk] adj → myocardial.
my·o·car·di·al [,-'kɑ:rdıəl] adj Herzmuskel(gewebe) betr., myokardial, Herzmuskel-, Myokard-.
myocardial abscess Herzmuskel-, Myokardabszeß m.
myocardial amyloidosis Herz(muskel)-, Myokardamyloidose f.
myocardial aneurysm Herzwand-, Kammerwand-, Ventrikelaneurysma nt, Aneurysma cordis.
myocardial anoxia Herzmuskel-, Myokardanoxie f.
myocardial atrophy Herzmuskel-, Myokardatrophie f.
myocardial calcification Herzmuskel-, Myokardverkalkung f.
myocardial cell Herzmuskel-, Myokardzelle f.
myocardial contusion Herzmuskel-, Myokardprellung f.
myocardial degeneration Herzmuskel-, Myokarddegeneration f.
myocardial depressant factor abbr. **MDF** Myocardial-Depressant-Faktor m abbr. MDF.
myocardial fiber Herzmuskel-, Myokardfaser f.
myocardial hypertrophy Herzmuskel-, Myokardhypertrophie f.
myocardial hypoxia Herzmuskel-, Myokardhypoxie f.
myocardial infarct Herzinfarkt m, infarziertes Myokardareal nt.
myocardial infarction abbr. **MI** Herz(muskel)infarkt m, Myokardinfarkt m, inf. Infarkt m.
  anterior m. Vorderwandinfarkt.
  anteroinferior m. Vorderwandspitzeninfarkt.
  anterolateral m. anterolateraler (Myokard-)Infarkt.
  anteroseptal m. anteroseptaler (Myokard-)Infarkt.
  diaphragmatic m. → inferior m.
  inferior m. diaphragmaler/inferiorer (Myokard-)Infarkt.
  inferolateral m. inferolateraler (Myokard-)Infarkt.
  lateral m. Seitenwandinfarkt, Lateralinfarkt.
  posterior m. Hinterwandinfarkt.
  posterolateral m. posterolateraler (Myokard-)Infarkt.
  recurrent m. Infarktrezidiv nt, rezidivierender (Myokard-)Infarkt.
  septal m. Septuminfarkt.
  silent m. stummer (Myokard-)Infarkt.
  subendocardial m. subendokardialer (Myokard-)Infarkt.
  through-and-through m. → transmural m.
  transmural m. transmuraler (Myokard-)Infarkt.
myocardial inflammation → myocarditis.
myocardial injury Herzmuskel-, Myokardverletzung f.
myocardial insufficiency Herzinsuffizienz f, -versagen nt, Myokardinsuffizienz f, Herzmuskelschwäche f, Insufficientia cordis.
myocardial metastasis Herzmuskel-, Myokardmetastase f.
myocardial necrosis Herzmuskel-, Myokardnekrose f.
myocardial rupture Herzmuskelriß m, -ruptur f, Myokardriß m, -ruptur f.
myocardial scar Herzmuskelschwiele f, -narbe f, Myokardschwiele f, -narbe f.
myocardial siderosis Herzmuskel-, Myokardsiderose f.
myocardial trauma Herzmuskel-, Myokardverletzung f.
my·o·car·di·op·a·thy [,-kɑ:rdı'ɑpəθı] n abbr. **MCP** Myokardiopathie f abbr. MKP, Kardiomyopathie f, Cardiomyopathie f abbr. CM.
my·o·car·di·or·rha·phy [,-kɑ:rdı'ɔrəfı] n HTG Herzmuskel-, Myokardnaht f.
my·o·car·di·o·sis [,-kɑ:rdı'əʊsıs] n → myocardosis.
my·o·car·dit·ic [,-kɑ:r'dıtık] adj Myokarditis betr., myokarditisch, Myokarditis-.
my·o·car·di·tis [,-kɑ:r'daıtıs] n Herzmuskel-, Myokardentzündung f, Myokarditis f, Myocarditis f.
my·o·car·do·sis [,-kɑ:r'dəʊsıs] n nichtentzündliche Herzmuskelerkrankung f, Myokardose f.
my·o·car·di·um [,-'kɑ:rdıəm] n, pl -dia [-dıə] Herzmuskulatur f, Myokard nt, Myocardium nt.
my·o·cele ['maıəsi:l] n Muskelhernie f, Myozele f.
my·o·ce·li·al·gia [,-,si:lı'ældʒ(ı)ə] n Bauchmuskelschmerz(en pl) m.
my·o·ce·li·tis [,-sı'laıtıs] n Bauchmuskelentzündung f.
my·o·cep·tor ['-septər] n motorische Endplatte f.
my·o·ce·ro·sis [,-sı'rəʊsıs] n wachsartige Muskeldegeneration f.
my·o·chor·di·tis [,-kɔ:r'daıtıs] n HNO Stimmuskelentzündung f, Myochorditis f.
my·o·chrome ['-krəʊm] n Myochrom nt.
my·o·cin·e·sim·e·ter [,-,sınə'sımıtər] n → myokinesimeter.
my·o·clo·nia [,-'kləʊnıə] n neuro. Myoklonie f, Myoclonia f.
my·o·clon·ic [,-'klɑnık, -'kləʊ-] adj Myoklonus betr., myoklonisch.
myoclonic encephalopathy of childhood Kinsbourne-Syndrom nt, myoklonisch--infantile Enzephalopathie f.
my·oc·lo·nus [maı'ɑklənəs] n neuro. Myoklonus m.
myoclonus epilepsy Lafora-Syndrom nt, Unverricht-Syndrom nt, Myoklonusepilepsie f, myoklonische Epilepsie f.
my·o·col·pi·tis [maıəkɑl'paıtıs] n gyn. Myokolpitis f.
my·oc·u·la·tor [maı'ɑkjəleıtər] n Myokulator m.
my·o·cu·ta·ne·ous flap [,maıəkju:'teınıəs] chir. Hautmuskellappen m.
my·o·cyte ['-saıt] n Muskelzelle f, Myozyt m.
my·o·cy·tol·y·sis [,-saı'tɑləsıs] n patho. Muskelfaserauflösung f, Myozytolyse f.
my·o·cy·to·ma [,-saı'təʊmə] n Myozytom nt.
my·o·de·gen·er·a·tion [,-dı,dʒenə'reıʃn] n Muskeldegeneration f.
my·o·de·mia [,-'di:mıə] n patho. fettige Muskeldegeneration f.
my·o·de·sis [,-'di:sıs] n ortho. Myodese f.
my·o·des·op·sia [,-des'ɑpsıə] n → muscae volitantes.
my·o·di·as·ta·sis [,-daı'æstəsıs] n embryo. Muskeldiastase f.
my·o·dy·na·mom·e·ter [,-,daınə'mɑmıtər] n physiol. Myodynamometer nt.
my·o·dyn·ia [,-'di:nıə] n Muskelschmerz(en pl) m, Myodynie f, Myalgie f.
my·o·dys·to·nia [,-dıs'təʊnıə] n neuro. Myodystonie f.
my·o·dys·to·ny [,-'dıstənı] n → myodystonia.
my·o·dys·tro·phia [,-dıs'trəʊfıə] n → muscular dystrophy.
my·o·dys·tro·phy [,-'dıstrəfı] n → muscular dystrophy.
my·o·e·de·ma [,-ı'di:mə] n 1. Muskelödem nt. 2. idiomuskuläre Kontraktion f.
my·o·e·las·tic [,-ı'læstık] adj myoelastisch.
my·o·e·lec·tric [,-ı'lektrık] adj myoelektrisch.
my·o·e·lec·tri·cal [,-ı'lektrıkl] adj myoelektrisch.
my·o·en·do·car·di·tis [,-,endəʊkɑ:r'daıtıs] n kombinierte Myokarditis f u. Endokarditis, Myoendokarditis f.
my·o·ep·i·the·li·al cell [,-,epı'θi:lıəl] Myoepithelzelle f.
my·o·ep·i·the·li·oid cell [,-,epı'θi:lıɔıd] (myo-)epitheloide Zelle f.
my·o·ep·i·the·li·o·ma [,-,epı,θılı'əʊmə] n Myoepitheliom(a) nt.

myoepithelium

my·o·ep·i·the·li·um [ˌ-epɪˈθiːlɪəm] *n* Myoepithel *nt*.

my·o·fa·cial pain dysfunction (syndrome) [ˌ-feɪʃl] Costen-Syndrom *nt*, temporomandibuläres Syndrom *nt*.

my·o·fas·ci·tis [ˌ-fəˈsaɪtɪs] *n* Myositis fibrosa.

my·o·fi·bril [ˌ-ˈfaɪbrəl, -fɪb-] *n* Muskelfaser *f*, Myofibrille *f*.

my·o·fi·bril·la [ˌ-ˈfaɪbrɪlə, -ˈfɪb-] *n, pl* **-lae** [-liː] → myofibril.

my·o·fi·bril·lar [ˌ-ˈfaɪbrələr, -ˈfɪb-] *adj* Myofibrille(n) betr., myofibrillär, Myofibrillen-, Muskelfaser-.

my·o·fi·bro·blast [ˌ-ˈfaɪbrəblæst] *n* Myofibroblast *m*.

my·o·fi·bro·ma [ˌ-faɪˈbrəʊmə] *n patho.* Myofibrom *nt*, Fibromyom *nt*.

my·o·fi·bro·sis [ˌ-faɪˈbrəʊsɪs] *n patho.* Myofibrose *f*, -fibrosis *f*.

myofibrosis-osteosclerosis syndrome Knochenmark(s)fibrose *f*, Myelofibrose *f*, -sklerose *f*, Osteomyelofibrose *f abbr.* OMF, Osteomyelosklerose *f*.

my·o·fi·bro·si·tis [ˌ-faɪbrəˈsaɪtɪs] *n patho.* Myofibrositis *f*, Perimysitis *f*.

my·o·fil·a·ment [ˌ-ˈfɪləmənt] *n* Myofilament *nt*.

my·o·ge·lo·sis [ˌ-dʒɪˈləʊsɪs] *n* Myogelose *f*.

my·o·gen [ˈ-dʒən] *n* Myogen *nt*.

my·o·gen·e·sis [ˌ-ˈdʒenəsɪs] *n* Muskelentwicklung *f*, Myogenese *f*.

my·o·ge·net·ic [ˌ-dʒəˈnetɪk] *adj* Myogenese betr., myogenetisch.

my·o·gen·ic [ˌ-ˈdʒenɪk] *adj* **1.** muskel(gewebe)bildend, myogen. **2.** vom Muskel(gewebe) ausgehend, myogen.

myogenic autoregulation myogene/mechanogene Autoregulation *f*.

myogenic contracture muskuläre/myogene Kontraktur *f*.

myogenic paralysis (epidemische/spinale) Kinderlähmung *f*, Heine-Medin-Krankheit *f*, Poliomyelitis (epidemica) anterior acuta.

myogenic torticollis myogener Schiefhals/Torticollis *m*.

myogenic wryneck → myogenic torticollis.

my·og·e·nous [maɪˈɑdʒənəs] *adj* vom Muskel(gewebe) ausgehend, myogen.

my·og·lia [maɪˈɑglɪə] *n* Myoglia *f*.

my·o·glo·bin [ˌmaɪəˈglɔʊbɪn] *n abbr.* **Mb** Myoglobin *nt abbr.* Mb.

myoglobin cast *urol.* Myoglobinpräzipitat *nt*, -zylinder *m*.

myoglobin precipitate *urol.* Myoglobinpräzipitat *nt*, -zylinder *m*.

my·o·glo·bin·u·ria [ˌ-ˌglɔʊbɪˈn(j)ʊərɪə] *n* Myoglobinausscheidung *f* im Harn, Myoglobinurie *f*.

my·o·glo·bin·u·ric nephrosis [ˌ-ˌglɔʊbɪˈn(j)ʊərɪk] myoglobinurische Nephrose *f*.

my·o·glob·u·lin [ˌ-ˈglɑbjəlɪn] *n* Myoglobulin *nt*.

my·o·glob·u·lin·e·mia [ˌ-ˌglɑbjəlɪˈniːmɪə] *n* Myoglobulinämie *f*.

my·o·glob·u·lin·u·ria [ˌ-ˌglɑbjəlɪˈn(j)ʊərɪə] *n* Myoglobulinausscheidung *f* im Harn, Myoglobulinurie *f*.

my·o·gram [ˈ-græm] *n* Myogramm *nt*.

my·o·graph [ˈ-græf] *n* Myograph *m*.

my·og·ra·phy [maɪˈɑgrəfɪ] *n* **1.** *physiol.* Myographie *f*. **2.** *radiol.* Myographie *f*.

my·o·he·ma·tin [ˌmaɪəˈhiːmətɪn, -ˈhem-] *n* **1.** Myohämatin *nt*. **2.** → myoglobin.

my·o·he·mo·glo·bin [ˌ-ˈhiːməglɔʊbɪn, -ˈhem-] *n* → myoglobin.

my·o·hy·per·pla·sia [ˌ-ˌhaɪpərˈpleɪʒ(ɪ)ə, -zɪə] *n* Muskelhyperplasie *f*, Myohyperplasie *f*, Myohyperplasia *f*.

my·o·hy·per·tro·phia [ˌ-ˌhaɪpərˈtrəʊfɪə] *n* Muskelhypertrophie *f*.

my·oid [ˈmaɪɔɪd] *adj* muskel(zellen)ähnlich, myoid.

myoid cells Myoidzellen *pl*.

my·oi·dem [maɪˈɔɪdem] *n* → myoedema.

my·oi·de·ma [ˌmaɪɔɪˈdiːmə] *n* → myoedema.

my·o·id·ism [maɪəˈɪdɪzəm] *n* → myoedema 2.

myo-inositol *n* meso-Inositol *nt*, -Inosit *nt*, myo-Inositol *nt*, -Inosit *nt*.

my·o·is·che·mia [ˌmaɪɔrˈskiːmɪə, -mjə] *n* Muskelischämie *f*.

my·o·ke·ro·sis [ˌ-keˈrəʊsɪs] *n* → myocerosis.

my·o·ki·nase [ˌ-ˈkaɪneɪz, -kɪ-] *n* Adenylatkinase *f*, Myokinase *f*, AMP-Kinase *f*, A-Kinase *f*.

my·o·kin·e·sim·e·ter [ˌ-ˌkɪnəˈsɪmətər] *n physiol.* Myokinesimeter *nt*.

my·o·ki·ne·sis [ˌ-kɪˈniːsɪs, -kaɪ-] *n* Muskelbewegung *f*, Myokinese *f*.

my·o·kin·in [ˌ-ˈkaɪnɪn, -ˈkɪ-] *n* Myokinin *nt*.

my·o·kym·ia [ˌ-ˈkɪmɪə, -ˈkaɪ-] *n neuro.* Myokymie *f*.

my·o·lem·ma [ˌ-ˈlemə] *n* Myolemm *nt*, Sarkolemm *nt*.

my·o·li·po·ma [ˌ-aɪˈpəʊmə] *n* Myolipom(a) *nt*.

my·ol·y·sis [maɪˈɑləsɪs] *n* Muskel(faser)degeneration *f*, -nekrose *f*, -auflösung *f*, Myolyse *f*.

my·o·ma [maɪˈəʊmə] *n, pl* **-ma·ta** [-mətə] Myom(a) *nt*.

my·o·ma·la·cia [ˌmaɪəməˈleɪʃ(ɪ)ə] *n patho.* Muskelerweichung *f*, Myomalazie *f*, Myomalacia *f*.

my·o·mas·toid artery [ˌ-ˈmæstɔɪd] Ramus occipitalis a. auricularis posterioris.

my·o·ma·tec·to·my [ˌ-məˈtektəmɪ] *n* → myomectomy 1.

my·o·ma·to·sis [ˌ-məˈtəʊsɪs] *n patho., gyn.* Myomatose *f*.

my·om·a·tous [maɪˈɑmətəs] *adj patho., gyn.* myomatös.

my·o·mec·to·my [maɪəˈmektəmɪ] *n chir., gyn.* **1.** Myomentfernung *f*, Myomektomie *f*. **2.** → myectomy.

my·o·mel·a·no·sis [ˌ-ˌmeləˈnəʊsɪs] *n* Myomelanose *f*.

my·o·mere [ˈ-mɪər] *n embryo.* Muskelsegment *nt*, Myomere *f*.

my·om·e·ter [maɪˈɑmɪtər] *n physiol.* Myometer *nt*.

my·o·me·tri·tis [ˌmaɪəmɪˈtraɪtɪs] *n gyn.* Myometriumentzündung *f*, Myometritis *f*.

my·o·me·tri·um [ˌ-ˈmiːtrɪəm] *n* Muskelschicht *f* der Gebärmutter, Uterusmuskulatur *f*, Myometrium *nt*, Tunica muscularis uteri.

my·on [ˈmaɪɑn] *n* Myon *nt*.

my·o·ne·cro·sis [ˌmaɪəɪˈkrəʊsɪs] *n* Muskel-, Myonekrose *f*.

my·o·neme [ˈ-niːm] *n micro., bio.* Stielfaden *m*, Myoneme *f*.

my·o·neu·ral [ˌ-ˈnjʊərəl, -ˈnʊr-] *adj* Muskel u. Nerv betr. *od.* verbindend, myoneural, neuromuskulär.

my·o·neu·ral·gia [ˌ-njʊˈrældʒ(ɪ)ə] *n* **1.** → myalgia. **2.** Muskelneuralgie *f*.

myoneural junction neuromuskuläre Verbindung(sstelle *f*) *f*.

myoneural synapse myoneurale/myoneuronale Synapse *f*.

my·on·o·sus [maɪˈɑnəsəs] *n* → myopathy.

my·o·pa·chyn·sis [ˌmaɪəpəˈkɪnsɪs] *n* Muskelhypertrophie *f*.

my·o·pal·mus [ˌ-ˈpælməs] *n* Muskelzuckung *f*.

my·o·pa·ral·y·sis [ˌ-pəˈræləsɪs] *n* Muskellähmung *f*, Myoparalyse *f*.

my·o·pa·re·sis [ˌ-pəˈriːsɪs, -ˈpærə-] *n* unvollständige Muskellähmung *f*, Muskelschwäche *f*, Myoparese *f*.

my·o·path·ia [ˌ-ˈpæθɪə] *n* → myopathy.

my·o·path·ic [ˌ-ˈpæθɪk] *adj* Myopathie betr., von Myopathie betroffen *od.* gekennzeichnet, myopathisch.

myopathic atrophy myogene/myopathische Muskelatrophie *f*.

myopathic dilation of stomach myopathische Magendilatation *f*.

myopathic facies Sphinxgesicht *nt*, Facies myopathica.

myopathic paralysis myopathische/myogene Lähmung *f*.

myopathic scoliosis *ortho.* myopathische Skoliose *f*.

my·op·a·thy [maɪˈɑpəθɪ] *n* Muskelerkrankung *f*, Myopathie *f*, Myopathia *f*.

my·ope [ˈmaɪəʊp] *n* Kurzsichtige(r *m*) *f*, Myope(r *m*) *f*.

my·o·per·i·car·di·tis [maɪəˌperɪkɑːrˈdaɪtɪs] *n* kombinierte Myokarditis *f* u. Perikarditis, Myoperikarditis *f*.

my·o·phos·pho·ry·lase deficiency (glycogenosis) [ˌ-fɑsˈfɔrəleɪz, -ˈfɑrə-] McArdle-Krankheit *f*, -Syndrom *nt*, muskuläre Glykogenose *f*, Muskelphosphorylasemangel *m*, Myophosphorylaseinsuffizienz *f*, Glykogenose *f* Typ V.

my·o·pia [maɪˈəʊpɪə] *n abbr.* **My.** Kurzsichtigkeit *f*, Myopie *f*.

my·op·ic [maɪˈɑpɪk, -ˈəʊp-] *adj* Myopie betr., von ihr betroffen, kurzsichtig, myop.

myopic astigmatism *abbr.* **am** *ophthal.* kombinierte Myopie u. Astigmatismus.

myopic conus *ophthal.* Conus myopicus.

myopic crescent *ophthal.* Conus myopicus.

my·o·plasm [ˈmaɪəplæzəm] *n* Myoplasma *nt*.

my·o·plas·tic [ˌ-ˈplæstɪk] *adj chir.* Myoplastik betr., myoplastisch.

my·o·plas·ty [ˈ-plæstɪ] *n chir., ortho.* **1.** Muskel-, Myoplastik *f*. **2.** Myoplastik *f*, myoplastische Deckung *f*.

my·o·pro·tein [ˌ-ˈprəʊtiːn, -tiːn] *n* Muskel-, Myoprotein *nt*.

my·op·sis [maɪˈɑpsɪs] *n* → muscae volitantes.

my·o·re·cep·tor [ˌmaɪərɪˈseptər] *n* Muskel-, Myorezeptor *m*.

my·or·rha·phy [maɪˈɔrəfɪ] *n chir., ortho.* Muskelnaht *f*, Myorrhaphie *f*.

my·or·rhex·is [maɪəˈreksɪs] *n* Muskelriß *m*, -ruptur *f*, Myorrhexis *f*.

my·o·sal·gia [ˌ-ˈsældʒ(ɪ)ə] *n* → myalgia.

my·o·sal·pin·gi·tis [ˌ-ˌsælpɪnˈdʒaɪtɪs] *n gyn.* Myosalpingitis *f*.

my·o·sal·pinx [ˌ-ˈsælpɪŋks] *n* Myosalpinx *f*.

my·o·san [ˈ-sæn] *n* Myosan *nt*.

my·o·sar·co·ma [ˌ-sɑːrˈkəʊmə] *n patho.* Myosarkom *nt*, -sarcoma *nt*.

my·o·schwan·no·ma [ˌ-ʃwɑˈnəʊmə] *n* Schwannom *nt*, Neurinom *nt*, Neurilem(m)om *nt*.

my·o·scle·ro·sis [ˌ-sklɪˈrəʊsɪs] *n* Muskelverhärtung *f*, Myosklerose *f*.

my·o·se·rum [ˌ-ˈsɪərəm] *n* Muskelsaft *m*, -serum *nt*.

my·o·sin [ˈmaɪəsɪn] *n* Myosin *nt*.

myosin adenosine triphosphatase reaction Myosin-ATPase-Reaktion *f*.

myosin ATPase Myosin-ATPase *f*.

myosin ATPase reaction Myosin-ATPase-Reaktion *f*.

myosin filament Myosinfilament *nt*.

myosin head Myosinköpfchen *nt*.

my·o·sin·o·gen [ˌmaɪəˈsɪnədʒən] *n* Myogen *nt*.
my·o·sin·u·ria [ˌ-sɪˈn(j)ʊərɪə] *n* Myosinausscheidung *f* im Harn, Myosinurie *f*.
my·o·sis [maɪˈəʊsɪs] *n* Pupillenverengung *f*, -engstellung *f*, Miosis *f*.
my·o·sit·ic [ˌmaɪəˈsɪtɪk] *adj* Myositis betr., myositisch, Myositis-.
my·o·si·tis [ˌ-ˈsaɪtɪs] *n* Muskelentzündung *f*, Myositis *f*.
my·o·spasm [ˈ-spæzəm] *n* Muskelkrampf *m*, -spasmus *m*, Myospasmus *m*.
my·o·spas·mus [ˌ-ˈspæzməs] *n* → myospasm.
my·o·su·ria [ˌ-ˈs(j)ʊərɪə] *n* → myosinuria.
my·o·su·ture [ˌ-ˈsuːtʃər] *n* → myorrhaphy.
my·o·syn·i·ze·sis [ˌ-ˌsɪnəˈziːsɪs] *n patho.* Muskelverklebung *f*.
my·ot·a·sis [maɪˈɑtəsɪs] *n* Muskeldehnung *f*.
my·o·tat·ic contraction [ˌ-ˈtætɪk] myotatische (Muskel-)Kontraktion *f*.
myotatic reflex Muskeldehnungsreflex *m*.
my·o·ten·on·to·plas·ty [ˌmaɪətenˈɑntəplæstɪ] *n ortho., chir.* Sehnen-Muskel--Plastik *f*, Tenomyoplastik *f*.
my·o·ten·o·si·tis [ˌ-ˌtenəˈsaɪtɪs] *n* kombinierte Muskel- u. Sehnenentzündung, Myotendinitis *f*.
my·o·te·not·o·my [ˌ-təˈnɑtəmɪ] *n ortho.* Myotenotomie *f*.
my·ot·ic [maɪˈɑtɪk] *n* → miotic I.
my·o·til·i·ty [ˌmaɪəˈtɪlətɪ] *n* Muskelkontraktilität *f*.
my·o·tome [ˈ-təʊm] *n* **1.** *embryo.* Myotom *nt*. **2.** *chir.* Myotom *nt*.
my·ot·o·my [maɪˈɑtəmɪ] *n ortho.* Muskeldurchtrennung *f*, Myotomie *f*.
my·o·tone [ˈmaɪətəʊn] *n* → myotonus.
my·o·to·nia [ˌ-ˈtəʊnɪə] *n* → myotony.
my·o·ton·ic [ˌ-ˈtɑnɪk] *adj* Myotonie betr., myotonisch.
myotonic atrophy → myotonic dystrophy.
myotonic cataract Katarakt *f* bei Muskeldystrophie, Cataracta myotonica.
myotonic dystrophy Curschmann--(Batten-)Steinert-Syndrom *nt*, myotonische Dystrophie *f*, Dystrophia myotonica.
my·o·to·nom·e·ter [ˌ-təˈnɑmɪtər] *n* Myotonometer *nt*.
my·ot·o·nus [maɪˈɑtənəs] *n* tonischer Muskelkrampf *m*; Myotonie *f*, Myotonia *f*.
my·ot·o·ny [maɪˈɑtənɪ] *n* (erhöhte) Muskelspannung *f*, Myotonie *f*, Myotonia *f*.
my·ot·ro·phy [maɪˈɑtrəfɪ] *n* Muskelernährung *f*, Myotrophie *f*.
my·o·trop·ic [ˌmaɪəˈtrɑpɪk, -ˈtrəʊp-] *adj* mit besonderer Affinität zu Muskelgewebe, myotrop.
my·o·tu·bu·lar myopathy [ˌ-ˈt(j)uːbjələr] zentronukleäre Myopathie *f*.
Myr·i·ap·o·da [ˌmɪrɪˈæpədə] *pl zoo.* Vielfüßler *pl*, Myriapoden *pl*, Myriopoden *pl*.
myring- *pref.* → myringo-.
my·rin·ga [mɪˈrɪŋgə] *n* Trommelfell *nt*, Membrana tympanica.

myr·in·gec·to·my [ˌmɪrənˈdʒektəmɪ] *n HNO* Trommelfellentfernung *f*, Myringektomie *f*.
myr·in·gi·tis [ˌ-ˈdʒaɪtɪs] *n* Trommelfellentzündung *f*, Myringitis *f*.
myringo- *pref.* Trommelfell-, Myring(o)-.
my·rin·go·dec·to·my [mɪˌrɪŋgəʊˈdektəmɪ] *n* → myringectomy.
my·rin·go·der·ma·ti·tis [ˌ-ˌdɜrməˈtaɪtɪs] *n HNO* Myringodermatitis *f*.
my·rin·go·my·co·sis [ˌ-maɪˈkəʊsɪs] *n HNO* Myringomykose *f*.
my·rin·go·plas·ty [ˈ-plæstɪ] *n HNO* Trommelfell-, Myringoplastik *f*.
my·rin·go·rup·ture [ˌ-ˈrʌptʃər] *n* Trommelfellriß *m*, -ruptur *f*.
my·rin·go·sta·pe·di·o·pex·y [ˌ-stəˈpɪdɪəʊpeksɪ] *n HNO* Myringostapediopexie *f*.
my·rin·go·tome [ˈ-təʊm] *n HNO* Parazentesemesser *nt*.
myr·in·got·o·my [mɪrənˈgɑtəmɪ] *n HNO* Trommelfellschnitt *m*, Myringotomie *f*, Parazentese *f*.
myringotomy drain tube *HNO* Paukenröhrchen *nt*.
myringotomy knife → myringotome.
myringotomy tube *HNO* Paukenröhrchen *nt*.
my·rinx [ˈmaɪrɪŋks, ˈmɪr-] *n* → myringa.
myr·is·tate [ˈmɪərɪsteɪt] *n* Myristat *nt*.
my·ris·tic acid [mɪˈrɪstɪk] Myristinsäure *f*.
my·ris·ti·cene [mɪˈrɪstəsiːn] *n* Myristicin *nt*.
myr·ti·form caruncles [ˈmɜrtɪfɔːrm] Fleischwärzchen *pl* (der Scheide), Hymenalkarunkeln *pl*, Carunculae hymenales (myrtiformes).
my·so·phil·ia [ˌmaɪsəˈfɪlɪə] *n psychia.* Mysophilie *f*.
my·so·pho·bia [ˌ-ˈfəʊbɪə] *n psychia.* Mysophobie *f*.
myth·o·ma·nia [ˌmɪθəˈmeɪnɪə, -jə] *n psychia.* Mythomanie *f*.
myth·o·pho·bia [ˌ-ˈfəʊbɪə] *n psychia.* Mythophobie *f*.
myx- *pref.* → myxo-.
myx·ad·e·ni·tis [mɪksˌædəˈnaɪtɪs] *n* Schleimdrüsenentzündung *f*, Myxadenitis *f*.
myx·ad·e·no·ma [mɪksˌædəˈnəʊmə] *n* Myxadenom(a) *nt*.
myx·a·me·ba [mɪksəˈmiːbə] *n bio.* Myxamöbe *f*.
myx·an·gi·tis [ˌmɪksænˈdʒaɪtɪs] *n* Myxangitis *f*.
myx·an·go·i·tis [ˌmɪksæŋgəˈwaɪtɪs] *n* → myxangitis.
myx·e·de·ma [mɪksəˈdiːmə] *n* Myxödem *nt*, Myxoedema *nt*, Myxodermia diffusa.
myx·e·dem·a·toid [mɪksəˈdemətɔɪd] *adj* myxödemähnlich, -artig.
myx·e·dem·a·tous [mɪksəˈdemətəs, -ˈdiːm-] *adj* Myxödem betr., myxödematös, Myxödem-.
myxedematous infantilism Kretinismus *m*.

myxo- *pref.* Schleim-, Myx(o)-, Muk(o)-, Muc(o)-, Muz(i)-, Muc(i)-.
myx·o·ad·e·no·ma [ˌmɪksəʊˌædɪˈnəʊmə] *n* Myxadenom(a) *nt*.
myx·o·bac·te·ria [ˌ-bækˈtɪərɪə] *pl micro.* Schleimbakterien *pl*, Myxobakterien *pl*.
myx·o·blas·to·ma [ˌ-blæsˈtəʊmə] *n* → myxoma.
myx·o·chon·dro·fi·bro·sar·co·ma [ˌ-ˌkɑndrəʊˌfaɪbrəsɑːrˈkəʊmə] *n* malignes Mesenchymom *nt*.
myx·o·chon·dro·ma [ˌ-kɑnˈdrəʊmə] *n* Myxochondrom(a) *nt*.
myx·o·chon·dro·os·te·o·sar·co·ma [ˌ-kɑndrəʊˌɑstɪəʊsɑːrˈkəʊmə] *n* → myxochondrofibrosarcoma.
myx·o·chon·dro·sar·co·ma [ˌ-ˌkɑndrəʊsɑːrˈkəʊmə] *n* → myxochondrofibrosarcoma.
myx·o·cys·ti·tis [ˌ-sɪsˈtaɪtɪs] *n* Entzündung *f* der Blasenschleimhaut.
myx·o·cys·to·ma [ˌ-sɪsˈtəʊmə] *n* Myxokystom *nt*, -zystom *nt*.
myx·o·cyte [ˈ-saɪt] *n* Schleimzelle *f*, Myxozyt *f*.
myx·o·en·chon·dro·ma [ˌ-enkɑnˈdrəʊmə] *n* Myxoenchondrom(a) *nt*.
myx·o·en·do·the·li·o·ma [ˌ-endəʊˌθɪlɪˈəʊmə] *n* Myxoendotheliom(a) *nt*.
myx·o·fi·bro·ma [ˌ-faɪˈbrəʊmə] *n* Fibromyxom *nt*, Myxofibrom(a) *nt*, Myxoma fibrosum.
myx·o·fi·bro·sar·co·ma [ˌ-ˌfaɪbrəsɑːrˈkəʊmə] *n* Myxofibrosarkom *nt*.
myxoid cyst [ˈmɪksɔɪd] *ortho.* Synovialzyste *f*, Ganglion *nt*, Überbein *nt*.
myx·o·in·o·ma [ˌmɪksəʊɪnˈəʊmə] *n* → myxofibroma.
myx·o·li·po·ma [ˌ-lɪˈpəʊmə] *n* Myxolipom(a) *nt*, Myxoma lipomatosum.
myx·o·ma [mɪkˈsəʊmə] *n, pl* **-mas**, **-ma·ta** [-mətə] Myxom(a) *nt*.
myx·o·ma·to·sis [ˌmɪksəʊməˈtəʊsɪs] *n* **1.** Myxomatose *f*, Myxomatosis *f*. **2.** myxomatöse Degeneration *f*.
myx·om·a·tous [mɪkˈsɑmətəs] *adj* schleimig, schleimbildend, -ähnlich, myxomartig, myxomatös.
myxomatous degeneration myxomatöse Degeneration *f*.
myx·o·mem·bra·nous colitis [ˌmɪksəʊˈmembrənəs] → mucocolitis.
Myx·o·my·ce·tes [ˌ-maɪˈsiːtɪːz] *pl micro.* Schleimpilze *pl*, Myxomyzeten *pl*, Myxomycetes *pl*, Myxophyta *pl*, Myxomykota *pl*.
myx·o·poi·e·sis [ˌ-pɔɪˈiːsɪs] *n* Schleimbildung *f*.
myx·or·rhea [ˌ-ˈrɪə] *n* Schleimfluß *m*, Myxorrhoe *f*.
myx·o·sar·co·ma [ˌ-sɑːrˈkəʊmə] *n* Myxosarkom *nt*, -sarcoma *nt*, Myxoma sarcomatosum.
myx·o·sar·com·a·tous [ˌ-sɑːrˈkɑmətəs] *adj* myxosarkomatös.
myx·o·vi·rus [ˌ-ˈvaɪrəs] *n micro.* Myxovirus *nt*.

N

N *abbr.* **1.** → neutron number. **2.** → newton. **3.** → nitrogen. **4.** → normal 5.
n *abbr.* **1.** → nano-. **2.** → normal 5.
ν *abbr.* → kinematic viscosity.
NA *abbr.* **1.** → neuraminidase. **2.** → Nomina Anatomica.
N.A. *abbr.* → numerical aperture.
Na *abbr.* → natrium.
Naboth ['neɪbəʊθ, -baθ]: **N.'s cysts/follicles/glands/ovules/vesicles** Naboth'-Eier *pl*, Ovula Nabothi.
na·bo·thi·an [neɪ'bəʊθɪən]: **n. cysts/follicles/glands/ovules/vesicles** Naboth'-Eier *pl*, Ovula nabothi.
Na channel *physiol.* Natriumkanal *m*, Na+-Kanal *m*.
NaCl *abbr.* → sodium chloride.
NaCl solution Kochsalzlösung *f*.
na·cre·ous ['neɪkrɪəs] *adj histol.* perlmuttartig.
na·crous ['neɪkrəs] *adj* → nacreous.
NAD *abbr.* → nicotinamide-adenine dinucleotide.
NAD+ *abbr.* oxidiertes Nicotinsäureamid-adenin-dinukleotid *nt abbr.* NAD+.
NADH *abbr.* reduziertes Nicotinsäureamid-adenin-dinucleotid *nt abbr.* NADH.
NADH cytochrome b₅-reductase Cytochrom b₅-Reduktase *f*.
NADH dehydrogenase NADH-Dehydrogenase *f*.
NADH-ferredoxin reductase NADH-Ferredoxin-reduktase *f*.
NADH-methemoglobin reductase NADH-abhängige Methämoglobinreduktase *f*, NADH-Methämoglobinreduktase *f*.
NADH oxidase NADH-Oxidase *f*.
NADH shuttle NADH-Shuttle *m*.
Na·di reaction ['nædaɪ] Nadi-Reaktion *f*.
nad·ide ['nædaɪd] *n pharm.* Nadid *nt*, Nicotinamidadenindinucleotid *nt*.
NAD-linked dehydrogenase NAD-abhängige Dehydrogenase *f*.
na·do·lol [neɪ'dəʊlɒl, -lal] *n pharm.* Nadolol *nt*.
NADP *abbr.* → nicotinamide-adenine dinucleotide phosphate.
NADP+ *abbr.* oxidiertes Nicotinamid-adenin-dinucleotid-phosphat *nt abbr.* NADP+.
NADPH *abbr.* reduziertes Nicotinamid-adenin-dinucleotid-phosphat *nt abbr.* NADPH.
NADPH-cytochrome reductase NADPH-Cytochromreduktase *f*, Cytochrom-P₄₅₀-Reduktase *f*.
NADPH-ferrihemoprotein reductase → NADPH-cytochrome reductase.
NADPH-methemoglobin reductase Methämoglobinreduktase (NADPH) *f*, NADPH-abhängige Methämoglobinreduktase *f*.
NADPH oxidase NADPH-Oxidase *f*.
NAD(P)+-transhydrogenase NAD(P)+-Transhydrogenase *f*, Pyridinnucleotid-transhydrogenase *f*.
Naegele ['neɪgəlɪ; 'nɛːgələ]: **N.'s pelvis** Naegele-Becken *nt*.
N.'s rule *gyn.* Naegele-Regel *f*.
Naegeli ['neɪgəlɪ; 'nɛːgəlɪ]: **chromatophore nevus of N.** → N. syndrome.
N.'s incontinentia pigmenti → N. syndrome.
N. leukemia (akute) myelomonozytäre Leukämie *f abbr.* AMML, (akute) Myelomonozytenleukämie *f, old* Naegeli-Typ *m* der Monozytenleukämie.
N. syndrome Franceschetti-Jadassohn-Syndrom *nt*, Naegeli-Syndrom *nt*, Naegeli-Bloch-Sulzberger-Syndrom *nt*, retikuläre Pigmentdermatose *f*, Melanophorennaevus *m*, familiärer Chromatophorennaevus *m*, Incontinentia pigmenti Typ Franceschetti-Jadassohn.
Nae·gle·ria [neɪ'glɪərɪə] *n micro.* Naegleria *nt*.
N. fowleri Naegleria fowleri.
nae·gle·ri·a·sis [,neɪglə'raɪəsɪs] *n* Naegleria-Infektion *f*.
Naffziger ['næfzɪgər]: **N.'s operation** *ophthal.* Naffziger-Operation *f*.
N.'s syndrome Naffziger-Syndrom *nt*, Skalenus-anterior-Syndrom *nt*, Scalenus-anterior-Syndrom *nt*.
N.'s test Naffziger-Test *m*.
na·ga·na [nə'gɑːnə] *n micro.* Nagana *f*.
nag·a·nol ['nægənɒl, -nɒl] *n* Germanin *nt*, Suramin-Natrium *nt*.
Na+ gate Natriumschleuse *f*.
Nagel ['naːgəl]: **N.'s test** *ophthal.* Nagel-Test *m*.
Nageotte [naː'ʒɔt]: **N.'s cells** Nageotte-Zellen *pl*.
Nager ['naːgər]: **N.'s acrofacial dysostosis** Nager-Reynier-Syndrom *nt*, Reynier-Nager-Syndrom *nt*, Dysostosis mandibularis.
NAG vibrios *micro.* nicht-agglutinable Vibrionen *pl*, NAG-Vibrionen *pl*, Vibrio cholerae non-01.
nail [neɪl] **I** *n* **1.** Finger-, Zehennagel *m*, Nagel *m*, Unguis *m*. **2.** Nagel *m*. **II** *vt* (an-)nageln (*to* an).
nail bed → nail matrix 2.
nail-biting *n* Nägelkauen *nt*.
nail brush Nagelbürste *f*.
nail extension *ortho.* Nagelextension *f*.
nail file Nagelfeile *f*.
nail fold Nagelfalz *m*, Sulcus matricis unguis.
nail infection Nagelinfektion *f*.
nail·ing ['neɪlɪŋ] *n ortho.* Nagelung *f*, Nageln *nt*.
nail matrix 1. Nagelbettepithel *nt*, Hyponychium *nt*. **2.** Nagelbett *nt*, Matrix unguis.
nail-patella syndrome Nagel-Patella-Syndrom *nt*, Osteoonychodysplasie *f*, Osteoonychodysostose *f*, Onycho-osteodysplasie *f*.
nail plate Nagelplatte *f*, Corpus unguis.
nail pulse Nagelpuls *m*.
nail root Nagelwurzel *f*, Radix unguis.
nail scissors Nagelschere *f*.
nail sinus Nageltasche *f*, Sinus unguis.
nail wall Nagelwall *m*, Vallum unguis.
Na+-K+-ATPase Natrium-Kalium-ATPase *f*, Na+-K+-ATPase *f*.
na·ked axon ['neɪkɪd] markloses Axon *nt*.
naked virus *micro.* nacktes Virus *nt*.
Na·ki·wo·go virus [nækɪ'wəʊgəʊ] *micro.* Semunya-Virus *nt*.
Na+-K+-pump Natrium-Kalium-Pumpe *f*, Na+-K+-Pumpe *f*.
nal·i·dix·ic acid [næl'dɪksɪk] *pharm.* Nalidixinsäure *f*.
nal·or·phine ['nælɔrfiːn, næl'ɔːrfiːn] *n* Nalorphin *nt*.
nal·ox·one [næl'ɒksəʊn, 'nælək-] *n pharm.* Naloxon *nt*.
nan- *pref.* → nano-.
NANA *abbr.* → N-acetylneuraminic acid.
NANB *abbr.* → Non-A,non-B hepatitis.
nan·dro·lone ['nændrələʊn] *n pharm.* Nandrolon *nt*.
na·nism ['neɪnɪzəm, 'næn-] *n* Minder-, Zwergwuchs *m*, Nan(n)ismus *m*, Nan(n)osomie *f*.
Nan·niz·zia [nə'nɪzɪə] *n micro.* Nannizzia *f*.
nano- *pref. abbr.* **n** Nano- *abbr.* n.
nan·o·ce·pha·lia [,nænəsɪ'feɪlɪə, ,neɪnə-] *n* → nanocephaly.
nan·o·ce·phal·ic [,-sɪ'fælɪk] *adj* mikrozephal, -kephal.
nanocephalic dwarf nanozephaler Zwerg *m*.
nan·o·ceph·a·lous [,-'sefələs] *adj* → nanocephalic.
nan·o·ceph·a·lus [,-'sefələs] *n* Mikrozephalus *m*.
nan·o·ceph·a·ly [,-'sefəlɪ] *n embryo.* Mikrozephalie *f*, -kephalie *f*, Mikrozephalus *m*.
nan·o·cor·mia [,-'kɔːrmɪə] *n* Kleinwuchs *m*, Mikrosomie *f*.
nan·o·cu·rie [,-'kjʊərɪ, -kjʊə'rɪ] *n abbr.* **nCi** Nanocurie *nt abbr.* nCi.
nan·o·gram ['-græm] *n abbr.* **ng** Nanogramm *nt abbr.* ng.
nan·oid ['nænɔɪd, 'neɪn-] *adj* zwergenhaft.
nan·o·kat·al [,nænə'kætæl, ,neɪnə-] *n abbr.* **nkat** Nanokatal *nt abbr.* nkat.
nan·o·li·ter [,-'liːtər] *n abbr.* **nl** Nanoliter *m abbr.* nl.
nan·o·me·lia [,-'miːlɪə] *n embryo.* Nano-, Mikromelie *f*.
na·nom·e·lous [nə'nɒmələs] *adj embryo.* nanomel, mikromel.
na·nom·e·lus [nə'nɒmələs] *n* Nano-, Mikromelus *m*.
nan·o·me·ter [,nænə'miːtər, ,neɪnə-] *n abbr.* **nm** Nanometer *nt/m abbr.* nm.
nan·oph·thal·mia [,nænəf'θælmɪə] *n* → nanophthalmos.
nan·oph·thal·mos [,nænəf'θælmɒs] *n ophthal.* Mikrophthalmie *f*, Mikrophthalmus *m*.
nan·oph·thal·mus [,nænəf'θælməs] *n* → nanophthalmos.

nan·o·sec·ond [ˌnænə'sekənd, ˌneɪnə-] *n abbr.* **ns, nsec** Nanosekunde *f abbr.* ns, nsec.
na·no·so·ma [ˌ-'səʊmə] *n* → nanism.
na·no·so·mia [ˌ-'səʊmɪə] *n* → nanism.
na·nous ['nænəs, 'neɪ-] *adj* zwergenhaft.
na·nu·ka·ya·mi [ˌnɑːnukɑ'jɑːmɪ] *n* Nanukayami(-Krankheit *f*) *nt*, (japanisches) Siebentagefieber *nt*, japanisches Herbstfieber *nt*.
nanukayami fever/disease → nanukayami.
na·nus ['nænəs, 'neɪ-] *n* Zwerg *m*.
NaOH *abbr.* → sodium hydroxide.
nape nevus [neɪp] Storchenbiß *m*, Unna--Politzer-Nackennävus *m*, Nävus Unna *m*.
na·phaz·o·line [nə'fæzəliːn] *n pharm.* Naphazolin *nt*.
naph·ta·lin ['næftəlɪn] *n* → naphthalene.
naph·tha ['næfθə] *n chem.* Naphtha *nt*.
naph·tha·lene ['næfθəliːn] *n* Naphthalin *nt*.
2-naphthalene sulfonate 2-Naphthalinsulfonat *nt*, β-Naphthalinsulfonat *nt*.
2-naphthalene sulfonic acid 2-Naphthalinsulfonsäure *f*, β-Naphthalinsulfonsäure *f*.
naph·thol ['næfθɒl, 'næp-] *n* Naphthol *nt*.
naph·thyl ['næfθɪl, 'næp-] *n* Naphthyl-(Radikal *nt*).
naph·thyl·a·mine [ˌnæfθɪlə'miːn, -'æmɪn, ˌnæp-] *n* Naphthylamin *nt*.
naph·tol ['næfθɒl] *n* → naphthol.
nap·kin dermatitis ['næpkɪn] *derm., ped.* Windeldermatitis *f*, posterosives Syphiloid *nt*, Dermatitis ammoniacalis, Dermatitis glutaealis infantum, Erythema glutaeale, Erythema papulosum posterosivum.
nap·py ['næpɪ] *n, pl* -**pies** Windel *f*.
nappy rash → napkin dermatitis.
na·prox·en [nə'prɒksən] *n pharm.* Naproxen *nt*.
Na+ pump Natriumpumpe *f*.
Narath [nə'ræθ]: **N.'s hernia** Narath--Hernie *f*.
nar·cism ['nɑːrsɪzəm] *n* → narcissism.
nar·cis·sism ['nɑːrsəsɪzəm] *n psychia.* Narzißmus *m*.
nar·cis·sis·tic [ˌnɑːrsə'sɪstɪk] *adj psychia.* Narzißmus betr., narzißtisch.
narcissistic personality disorder narzißtische Persönlichkeit(sstörung *f*) *f*.
narco- *pref.* Lähmungs-, Narko-, Narkose-.
nar·co·a·nal·y·sis [ˌnɑːrkəʊə'næləsɪs] *n psychia.* Narkoanalyse *f*.
nar·co·hyp·nia [ˌ-'hɪpnɪə] *n* Narkohypnie *f*.
nar·co·hyp·no·sis [ˌ-hɪp'nəʊsɪs] *n psychia.* Narkohypnose *f*.
nar·co·lep·sy ['-lepsɪ] *n neuro.* Narkolepsie *f*.
nar·co·lep·tic [ˌ-'leptɪk] *adj* Narkolepsie betr., *od.* auslösend, narkoleptisch.
nar·co·ma·nia [ˌ-'meɪnɪə, -jə] *n neuro., psychia.* Narkomanie *f*.
nar·cose ['nɑːrkəʊs] *adj* stuporartig, stuporös.
nar·co·sine ['nɑːrkəsiːn, -sɪn] *n pharm.* Noscapin *nt*.
nar·co·sis [nɑːr'kəʊsɪs] *n, pl* -**ses** [-siːz] Narkose *f*, Voll-, Allgemeinnarkose *f*, -anästhesie *f*.
nar·co·syn·the·sis [ˌnɑːrkə'sɪnθəsɪs] *n* → narcoanalysis.
nar·co·ther·a·py [ˌ-'θerəpɪ] *n psychia.* Narkotherapie *f*.
nar·cot·ic [nɑːr'kɒtɪk] **I** *n* **1.** Betäubungsmittel *nt*, Narkotikum *nt*. **2.** Rauschgift *nt*. **II** *adj* **3.** Narkose betr., eine Narkose herbeiführend, narkotisch, Narkose-. **4.** berauschend, betäubend, narkotisch.
narcotic addict Betäubungsmittelabhängige(r *m*) *f*, -süchtige(r *m*) *f*, Rauschgiftabhängige(r *m*) *f*, -süchtige(r *m*) *f*.
narcotic addiction Betäubungsmittel-, Rauschgiftsucht *f*.
narcotic agent → narcotic 1.
nar·co·tine ['nɑːrkətiːn, -tɪn] *n* → narcosine.
nar·co·tism ['-tɪzəm] *n* **1.** *old* → narcosis. **2.** Narkotismus *m*.
nar·co·tize ['-taɪz] *vt* betäuben, narkotisieren.
nar·cous ['nɑːrkəs] *adj* → narcose.
na·ris ['neərɪs, 'neɪ-] *n, pl* -**res** [-riːz] *anat.* Nasenloch *nt*, Naris *f*.
nar·row-angle glaucoma ['nærəʊ] akutes Winkelblockglaukom/Engwinkelglaukom *nt*, Glaucoma acutum (congestivum).
chronic n. chronisches Winkelblockglaukom/Engwinkelglaukom, chronisch--kongestives Glaukom, Glaucoma chronicum congestivum.
narrow-chested *adj* engbrüstig.
nas- *pref.* → naso-.
na·sal ['neɪzl] **I** *n* Nasal(laut *m*) *m*. **II** *adj* Nase betr., nasal, Nasen-, Nasal-.
nasal aperture, anterior vordere Öffnung *f* der (knöchernen) Nasenhöhle, Apertura piriformis, Apertura nasalis anterior.
nasal arteriole of retinae: inferior n. untere nasale/mediale Netzhautarteriole *f*, Arteriola nasalis retinae inferior.
superior n. obere nasale/mediale Netzhautarteriole *f*, Arteriola nasalis retinae superior.
nasal artery: dorsal n. Nasenrückenarterie *f*, A. dorsalis nasi, A. nasalis externa.
external n. → dorsal n.
posterior and lateral n.ies hintere seitliche Nasenarterien *pl*, Aa. nasales posteriores et laterales.
nasal bleeding Nasenbluten *nt*, -blutung *f*, Epistaxis *f*.
nasal bone Nasenbein *nt*, Os nasale.
supreme n. oberste Nasenmuschel *f*, Concha nasalis suprema.
nasal branch: n. of anterior ethmoidal nerve Nasenast *m* des N. ethmoidalis anterior.
anterior n.es of anterior ethmoidal nerve Rami nasales anteriores n. ethmoidalis anterioris.
external n. of anterior ethmoidal nerve Ramus nasalis externus n. ethmoidalis anterioris.
external n.es of infraorbital nerve (äußere) Nasenflügeläste *pl* des N. infraorbitalis, Rami nasales externi n. infraorbitalis.
inferior n.es of greater palatine nerve, posterior Rami nasales posteriores inferiores n. palatini majoris.
internal n.es of anterior ethmoidal nerve Rami nasales interni n. ethmoidalis anterioris.
internal n.es of infraorbital nerve (innere) Nasenäste *pl* des N. infraorbitalis, Rami nasales interni n. infraorbitalis.
lateral n.es of anterior ethmoidal artery, anterior Rami nasales anteriores laterales a. ethmoidalis anterioris.
lateral n.es of anterior ethmoidal nerve Rami nasales mediales n. ethmoidalis anterioris.
lateral n. of facial artery Ramus lateralis nasi a. facialis.
medial n.es of anterior ethmoidal nerve Rami nasales mediales n. ethmoidalis anterioris.
posterior n.es of pterygopalatine ganglion, (lateral) inferior Rami nasales posteriores inferiores (laterales) ggl. pterygopalatini.
posterior n.es of pterygopalatine ganglion, lateral superior Rami nasales posteriores superiores laterales ggl. pterygopalatini.
posterior n.es of pterygopalatine ganglion, medial superior Rami nasales posteriores superiores mediales ggl. pterygopalatini.
n.es of pterygopalatine ganglion Nasenäste *pl* des Ggl. pyterygopalatinum, Rami nasales ggl. pterygopalatini.
nasal breathing Nasenatmung *f*.
nasal bridge Nasenbrücke *f*.
nasal calculus Nasenstein *m*, Rhinolith *m*.
nasal canal → nasolacrimal canal.
nasal cartilage: n.s *pl* Nasenknorpel *pl*, Cartilagines nasales.
accessory n.s akzessorische Nasenknorpel *pl*, Cartilagines nasales accessoriae.
lateral n. Cartilago nasi lateralis.
nasal catarrh Nasenkatarrh *m*, (akute) Rhinitis *f*.
nasal cavity Nasenhöhle *f*, Cavitas nasi/nasalis.
nasal chamber → nasal cavity.
primitive n. *embryo.* primitive Nasenhöhle *f*.
nasal commissure of eye lid mediale Augenlidkommissur *f*, Commissura palpebrarum medialis.
nasal concha Nasenmuschel *f*, Concha nasalis.
inferior n. untere Nasenmuschel, Concha nasalis inferior.
middle n. mittlere Nasenmuschel, Concha nasalis media.
superior n. obere Nasenmuschel, Concha nasalis superior.
supreme n. oberste Nasenmuschel, Concha nasalis suprema.
nasal concrement → nasal calculus.
nasal crest: n. of maxilla Crista nasalis maxillae.
n. of palatine bone Crista nasalis ossis palatini.
nasal diphtheria Nasendiphtherie *f*.
nasal douche Nasendusche *f*, -spülung *f*.
nasal drops Nasentropfen *pl*.
nasal duct → nasolacrimal duct.
nasal eczema Nasenekzem *nt*.
nasal endoscopy endoskopische Nasenspiegelung *f*, Nasen-, Rhinoendoskopie *f*.
nasal feeding Ernährung *f* über eine Magensonde.
nasal foramen Forr. nasalia.
nasal foramina Forr. nasalia.
nasal furuncle Nasenfurunkel *m/nt*.
nasal glands Nasen(schleimhaut)drüsen *pl*, Gll. nasales.
nasal groove Sulcus ethmoidalis (ossis nasalis).
nasal hemorrhage → nasal bleeding.
nasal hydrorrhea Nasen(aus)fluß *m*, Rhinorrhoe *f*.
nasal incisure: n. of frontal bone Margo nasalis ossis frontalis.
n. of maxilla → nasal notch of maxilla.
nasal intubation nasale Intubation *f*.
na·sa·lis [neɪ'zælɪs, -'zeɪ-] *n* → nasalis muscle.
nasalis muscle Nasenmuskel *m*, Nasalis *m*, M. nasalis.
na·sal·i·ty [neɪ'zælɪtɪ, næ-] *n* Nasalität *f*.
na·sal·i·za·tion [ˌneɪzəlaɪ'zeɪʃn, ˌnæ-] *n* **1.** Näseln *nt*, Näselung *f*. **2.** Nasalierung *f*, nasale Aussprache *f*.
na·sal·ize ['neɪzəlaɪz, 'næ-] **I** *vt* nasalieren. **II** *vi* näseln, durch die Nase sprechen, nasal sprechen.
nasal margin of frontal bone Margo nasalis (ossis frontalis).

nasal meatus

nasal meatus Nasengang *m*, Meatus nasi.
inferior n. unterer Nasengang, Meatus nasi inferior.
middle n. mittlerer Nasengang, Meatus nasi medius.
superior n. oberer Nasengang, Meatus nasi superior.
nasal mucosa Nasenschleimhaut *f*, Tunica mucosa nasi.
nasal muscle → nasalis muscle.
nasal notch of maxilla Inc. nasalis (maxillae).
nasal ointment Nasensalbe *f*.
nasal pit *embryo.* Riechgrube *f*.
nasal placode *embryo.* Riechplakode *f*.
nasal polyp Nasenpolyp *m*.
nasal probe Nasensonde *f*.
nasal prominence *embryo.* Nasenhöcker *m*, -wulst *m*.
  lateral n. lateraler Nasenwulst.
  medial n. medialer Nasenwulst.
nasal region Nasengegend *f*, -region *f*, Regio nasalis.
nasal resistance *physiol.* Nasenwiderstand *m*.
nasal respiration Nasenatmung *f*.
nasal root Nasenwurzel *f*, Radix nasalis/nasi.
nasal septum Nasenscheidewand *f*, Nasenseptum *nt*, Septum nasi/nasale.
  cartilaginous n. knorpeliger Abschnitt/Teil *m* des Nasenseptums, Pars cartilaginea septi nasi.
  fibrous n. bindegewebiger Abschnitt/Teil *m* des Nasenseptums, Pars fibrosa septi nasi.
  membranous n. membranöser Abschnitt/Teil *m* des Nasenseptums, Pars membranacea septi nasi.
  osseous n. knöcherner Abschnitt/Teil *m* des Nasenseptums, Pars ossea septi nasi.
nasal sinuses (Nasen-)Nebenhöhlen *pl*, Sinus paranasales.
nasal speculum Nasenspekulum *nt*, -spiegel *m*, Rhinoskop *nt*.
nasal spine → n. of frontal bone.
  anterior n. (of maxilla) Spina nasalis anterior (maxillae).
  n. of frontal bone Spina nasalis ossis frontalis.
  n. of palatine bone Spina nasalis posterior.
nasal spray *pharm.* Nasenspray *m/nt*.
nasal stone Nasenstein *m*, Rhinolith *m*.
nasal swab Nasenabstrich *m*.
nasal tip Nasenspitze *f*, Apex nasi.
nasal-tracheal intubation nasotracheale Intubation *f*.
nasal tuberculosis Nasentuberkulose *f*.
nasal veins, external äußere Nasenvenen *pl*, Vv. nasales externae.
nasal venule of retina: inferior n. untere mediale/nasale Netzhautvene *f*, Venula nasalis retinae inferior.
  superior n. obere mediale/nasale Netzhautvene *f*, Venula nasalis retinae superior.
nasal vestibule Nasenvorhof *m*, -eingang *m*, Vestibulum nasi/nasale.
nasal wing Nasenflügel *m*, Ala nasi.
nas·cent ['næsənt, 'neɪsənt] *adj bio., chem.* entstehend, freiwerdend, naszierend.
nascent condition → nascent state.
nascent state *chem.* Status nascendi.
na·si·on ['neɪzɪən] *n anat.* Nasion *nt*.
na·si·tis [neɪ'zaɪtɪs] *n* Nasenentzündung *f*.
Nasmyth ['næsmɪθ]: **N.'s membrane** Nasmyth-Membran *f*, Cuticula dentalis.
naso- *pref.* Nasen-, Nas(o)-, Rhin(o)-.
na·so·an·tral [ˌneɪzəʊ'æntrəl] *adj* Nase u. Kieferhöhle betr., nasoantral.
na·so·an·tri·tis [ˌ-æn'traɪtɪs] *n HNO* Ent-

zündung *f* von Nase u. Kieferhöhle, Nasoantritis *f*.
na·so·an·tros·to·my [ˌ-æn'trɒstəmɪ] *n HNO* transnasale Kieferhöhlenfensterung *f*.
na·so·cil·i·ar·y branch of ciliary ganglion [ˌ-'sɪlɪərɪ] → nasociliary root of ciliary ganglion.
nasociliary nerve Nasoziliaris *m*, N. nasociliaris.
nasociliary neuralgia Nasoziliarisneuralgie *f*.
nasociliary root of ciliary ganglion sensorische Wurzel *f* des Ggl. ciliare, Ramus communicans ggl. ciliaris cum n. nasociliaris, Radix sensoria/nasociliaris ggl. ciliare.
na·so·fron·tal vein [ˌ-'frʌntl] V. nasofrontalis.
na·so·fu·gal [ˌ-'fjuːgl] *adj* von der Nase weg, nasofugal.
na·so·gas·tric feeding [ˌ-'gæstrɪk] Ernährung *f* über eine Magensonde.
nasogastric tube Nasensonde *f*, Nasen-Magen-Sonde *f*.
na·so·la·bi·al [ˌ-'leɪbɪəl] *adj* Nase u. Lippe betr. *od.* verbindend, nasolabial, Nasolabial-.
nasolabial reflex *ped.* Nasolabialreflex *m*.
nasolabial sulcus Nasolabialfurche *f*, Sulcus nasolabialis.
na·so·lac·ri·mal [ˌ-'lækrɪməl] *adj* Nase u. Tränendrüse betr., nasolakrimal.
nasolacrimal canal Kanal *m* des Ductus nasolacrimalis, Canalis nasolacrimalis.
nasolacrimal duct Tränen-Nasen-Gang *m*, Ductus nasolacrimalis.
nasolacrimal groove *embryo.* Tränen-Nasenfurche *f*.
na·so·max·il·lar·y [ˌ-'mæksəˌlerɪ·, -mæk'sɪlərɪ] *adj* Nase u. Oberkiefer betr., nasomaxillär.
nasomaxillary suture Sutura nasomaxillaris.
na·so·men·tal reflex [ˌ-'mentl] Nasomentalreflex *m*.
naso-oral *adj* Nase u. Mund betr. *od.* verbindend, oronasal.
naso-oral leishmaniasis mukokutane Leishmaniase Südamerikas *f*, südamerikanische Haut-Schleimhautleishmaniase *f*, Espundia *f*.
na·so·pal·a·tine artery [ˌ-'pælətaɪn, -tɪn] Sphenopalatina *f*, A. sphenopalatina.
nasopalatine canal Canalis incisivus.
nasopalatine nerve N. nasopalatinus.
  long n. N. nasopalatinus longus.
  short n.s Nn. nasopalitini breves.
na·sop·e·tal [neɪ'zɒpətəl] *adj* zur Nase hin, nasopetal.
na·so·pha·ryn·ge·al [ˌneɪzəʊfə'rɪndʒ(ɪ)əl, -ˌfærən'dʒiːəl] *adj* Nasopharynx betr., nasopharyngeal, Nasopharyngeal-.
nasopharyngeal airway Nasopharyngealtubus *m*, -katheter *m*.
nasopharyngeal angiofibroma (juveniles) Nasenrachenfibrom *nt*, Schädelbasisfibrom *nt*, Basalfibroid *nt*, -fibrom *nt*.
nasopharyngeal carcinoma nasopharyngeales Karzinom *nt*, Nasopharyngealkarzinom *nt*.
nasopharyngeal diphtheria Nasenrachendiphtherie *f*.
nasopharyngeal fibroangioma → nasopharyngeal angiofibroma.
nasopharyngeal fibromatosis nasopharyngeales Fibrom *nt*.
nasopharyngeal fold Tubenwulst *m*, Plica salpingopalatina/palatotubalis.
nasopharyngeal intubation nasopharyngeale Intubation *f*.
nasopharyngeal leishmaniasis amerikanische/mukokutane Leishmaniose *f*,

Haut-Schleimhaut-Leishmaniase (Südamerikas) *f*, Leishmaniasis americana.
nasopharyngeal meatus Meatus nasopharyngeus.
nasopharyngeal space → nasopharynx.
nasopharyngeal tubus → nasopharyngeal airway.
na·so·phar·yn·gi·tis [ˌ-ˌfærən'dʒaɪtɪs] *n HNO* Entzündung *f* des Nasenrachenraums, Naso-, Rhino-, Epipharyngitis *f*.
na·so·pha·ryn·go·la·ryn·go·scope [ˌ-fəˌrɪŋɡəʊlə'rɪŋɡəskəʊp] *n HNO* Nasopharyngolaryngoskop *nt*.
na·so·pha·ryn·go·scope [ˌ-fə'rɪŋɡəskəʊp] *n HNO* Nasopharyngoskop *nt*.
na·so·phar·ynx [ˌ-'færɪŋks] *n*, *pl* **-pha·ryn·ges** [-fə'rɪndʒiːz], **-phar·ynx·es** Nasenrachenraum *m*, Naso-, Rhino-, Epipharynx *m*, Pars nasalis pharyngei.
na·so·scope ['-skəʊp] *n* Nasenspiegel *m*, Rhinoskop *nt*.
na·so·sep·tal [ˌ-'septəl] *adj* Nasenseptum betr., Septum-.
na·so·sep·ti·tis [ˌ-sep'taɪtɪs] *n HNO* Entzündung *f* des Nasenseptums.
na·so·si·nus·i·tis [ˌ-ˌsaɪnə'saɪtɪs] *n HNO* Entzündung *f* der Nasennebenhöhlen, Nebenhöhlenentzündung *f*, Sinusitis *f*.
na·so·tra·che·al airway [ˌ-'treɪkɪəl] Nasotrachealtubus *m*, -katheter *m*.
nasotracheal aspiration nasotracheale Aspiration *f*.
nasotracheal intubation nasotracheale Intubation *f*.
nasotracheal tubus → nasotracheal airway.
na·so·tur·bi·nal concha [ˌ-'tɜrbɪnl] Agger nasi.
na·sus ['neɪzəs] *n*, *pl* **-si** [-saɪ] *anat.* (äußere) Nase *f*, Nasus (externus) *m*.
na·tal ['neɪtl] *adj* **1.** Geburt betr., natal, Geburts-, Geburten-. **2.** Gesäß betr., Gesäß-, After-.
natal cleft Gesäßspalte *f*, Afterfurche *f*, Crena ani, Rima ani.
na·tal·i·ty [neɪ'tælətɪ, nə-] *n* Geburtenziffer *f*, -häufigkeit *f*, Natalität *f*.
Na·tal sore [nə'tæl, -tɑl, 'neɪtl] kutane Leishmaniose/Leishmaniase *f*, Hautleishmaniose *f*, Orientbeule *f*, Leishmaniasis cutis.
nat·a·my·cin [nætə'maɪsn] *n pharm.* Natamycin *nt*.
na·tes ['neɪtiːz] *pl* Hinterbacken *pl*, Gesäß *nt*, Clunes *pl*, Nates *pl*.
na·tive ['neɪtɪv] **I** *n* **1.** Eingeborene(r *m*) *f*, Ureinwohner(in *f*) *m*. **2.** Einheimische(r *m*) *f*. **3.** *bot.* einheimische Pflanze *f*; *zoo.* einheimisches Tier *nt*. **II** *adj* **4.** *chem.* natürlich, unverändert, nativ, Nativ-. **5.** angeboren (*to s.o.* jdm.). **6.** eingeboren, Eingeborenen-. **7.** (ein-)heimisch; Mutter-, Heimat-; gebürtig. **8.** ursprünglich, eigentlich.
native-born *adj* gebürtig.
native conformation *chem.* native Konformation *f*.
native form *chem.* native Form *f*.
native immunity angeborene Immunität *f*.
native language Muttersprache *f*.
native protein natives Protein *nt*.
native speaker Muttersprachler(in *f*) *m*.
na·tre·mia [nə'triːmɪə] *n* erhöhter Natriumgehalt *m* des Blutes, Hypernatriämie *f*.
na·tri·e·mia [neɪtrɪ'iːmɪə] *n* → natremia.
nat·ri·um ['neɪtrɪəm] *n abbr.* **Na** Natrium *nt abbr.* Na.
na·tri·u·re·sis [ˌneɪtrɪə'riːsɪs, ˌnæ-] *n* (erhöhte) Natriumausscheidung *f* im Harn, Natriurese *f*, Natriurie *f*.
na·tri·u·ret·ic [ˌ-jə'retɪk] **I** *n pharm.* Natri-

uretikum *nt*. II *adj* Natriurese betr. *od*. fördernd, natriuretisch.
na·tron ['neɪtrən, -trɒn, 'næt-] *n* **1.** Natriumkarbonat *nt*, Soda *f*/*nt*. **2.** Natriumbikarbonat *nt*, doppeltkohlensaures Natron *nt*. **3.** Natriumhydroxid *nt*, kaustisches Natron *nt*.
na·trum ['neɪtrəm] *n* → natrium.
nat·ru·re·sis [,nætrə'riːsɪs] *n* → natriuresis.
nat·ru·ret·ic [,-'retɪk] *n*, *adj* → natriuretic.
nat·u·ral ['nætʃ(ə)rəl] **I** *n* natürliche *od*. naturreine Substanz *f*. **II** *adj* **1.** Natur betr., natürlich, naturgegeben, Natur-. **to die a ~ death** eines natürlichen Todes sterben. **2.** angeboren, natürlich (*to*). **3.** unehelich. **a ~ child**. **4.** natürlich, ungekünstelt. **5.** physisch, wirklich, real. **6.** fleischfarben. **7.** *mathe*. natürlich.
natural amputation *embryo*., *ped*. kongenitale/intrauterine Amputation *f*.
natural antibody natürlicher/regulärer Antikörper *m*.
natural-born *adj* **1.** von Geburt, geboren. **2.** gebürtig.
natural childbirth natürliche Geburt *f*.
natural death natürlicher Tod *m*.
natural dentition Zahnreihe *f*, (natürliches) Gebiß *nt*.
natural frequency *phys*. Eigenfrequenz *f*.
natural immunity natürliche Immunität *f*.
nat·u·ral·ist ['nætʃ(ə)rəlɪst] *n* Naturwissenschaftler(in *f*) *m*, -forscher(in *f*) *m*; Zoologe *m*, Zoologin *f*; Botaniker(in *f*) *m*.
natural killer cells NK-Zellen *pl*, natürliche Killerzellen *pl*, Natural-Killer-Zellen *pl*.
natural resistance → natural immunity.
natural rubber Naturkautschuk *m*.
natural science Naturwissenschaft(en *pl*) *f*.
natural scientist Naturwissenschaftler(in *f*) *m*.
natural selection *bio*. natürliche Auslese *f*.
na·ture ['neɪtʃər] *n* **1.** Natur *f*, Schöpfung *f*. **against ~** gegen die Natur. **2.** (*Person*) Wesen(sart *f*) *nt*, Charakter *m*, Natur *f*; (*Objekt*) Beschaffenheit *f*. **by ~** von Natur aus.
nature cure Naturheilverfahren *nt*.
na·tur·o·path ['neɪtʃərəpæθ, 'nætʃ-] *n* Naturheiler(in *f*) *m*; Naturheilkundige(r *m*) *f*.
na·tu·rop·a·thy [,neɪtʃə'rɒpəθɪ, ,nætʃ-] *n* **1.** Naturheilverfahren *nt*. **2.** Naturheilkunde *f*, Physiatrie *f*, biologische Medizin *f*.
nau·path·ia [nɔː'pæθɪə] *n* Seekrankheit *f*, Naupathia *f*.
nau·sea ['nɔːzɪə, -ʒə, -ʃə] *n* Übelkeit *f*, Brechreiz *m*, Nausea *f*.
nau·se·ant ['nɔːzɪənt, -ʒɪ-, -sɪ-, -ʃɪ-] **I** *n* Brechmittel *nt*. II *adj* Übelkeit/Brechreiz erregend.
nau·se·ate ['nɔːzɪeɪt, -ʒɪ-, -sɪ-, -ʃɪ-] *vt* Übelkeit/Brechreiz hervorrufen.
nau·se·ous ['nɔːʃəs, -zɪəs] *adj* Übelkeit/Brechreiz erregend.
na·vel ['neɪvl] *n* **1.** Nabel *m*, Umbilikus *m*; *anat*. Umbilicus *m*, Umbo *m*. **2.** *fig*. Nabel *m*, Mittelpunkt *m*.
navel string Nabelstrang *m*, -schnur *f*, Chorda/Funiculus umbilicalis.
na·vic·u·lar [nə'vɪkjələr] **I** *n* Kahnbein *nt*, Os naviculare. II *adj* boot-, kahnförmig, navikular.
navicular abdomen Kahnbauch *m*.
navicular bone → navicular I.
n. of foot *old* → navicular I.
n. of hand *old* → scaphoid I.
navicular fossa: n. of Cruveilhier Fossa scaphoidea.
n. of (male) urethra Fossa navicularis urethrae.

Nb *abbr*. → niobium.
NBT *abbr*. → nitroblue tetrazolium.
NBT test → nitroblue tetrazolium test.
NCF *abbr*. → neutrophil chemotactic factor.
nCi *abbr*. → nanocurie.
NCVs *abbr*. → noncholera vibrios.
Nd *abbr*. → neodymium.
NDP *abbr*. → nucleoside(-5'-)diphosphate.
NDP kinase → nucleoside diphosphate kinase.
NDP sugar → nucleoside diphosphate sugar.
NDV *abbr*. → Newcastle disease virus.
Ne *abbr*. → neon.
ne- *pref*. → neo-.
near [nɪər] *adj* **1.** (*örtlich*) nahe, in der Nähe; (*zeitlich*) nahe. **2.** nahe (verwandt); vertraut. **3.** (*Problem*) akut, brennend. **4.** knapp, beinahe, fast.
near point *ophthal*. Nahpunkt *m*, Punctum proximum.
absolute n. absoluter Nahpunkt.
n. of convergence *ophthal*., *physiol*. Konvergenznahpunkt.
relative n. relativer Nahpunkt.
near-point reaction → near reflex.
near reaction → near reflex.
near reflex *ophthal*. Naheinstellungsreaktion *f*, -reflex *m*, Konvergenzreaktion *f*, Akkommodationsreflex *m*.
near sight → nearsightedness.
near·sight·ed ['nɪərsaɪtɪd] *adj* kurzsichtig, myop.
near·sight·ed·ness [,-nɪs] *n* Kurzsichtigkeit *f*, Myopie *f*.
near-threshold *adj* schwellennah.
ne·ar·thro·sis [nɪəˈθrəʊsɪs] *n* ortho. **1.** Gelenkneubildung *f*, Nearthrose *f*; Pseudarthrose *f*. **2.** Gelenkprothese *f*, -ersatz *m*, künstliches Gelenk *nt*.
near-vision response *ophthal*. Naheinstellungsreaktion *f*, -reflex *m*, Konvergenzreaktion *f*, Akkommodationsreflex *m*.
neb·u·la ['nebjələ] *n*, *pl* **-lae** [-liː], **-las 1.** *ophthal*. leichte Hornhauttrübung *f*, Nubekula *f*, Nubecula *f*, Nebula *f*. **2.** (*Harn*) Trübung *f*, Nubekula *f*.
neb·u·li·za·tion [,nebjəlaɪ'zeɪʃn] *n* **1.** Vernebeln *nt*, Zerstäuben *nt*. **2.** Aerosoltherapie *f*.
neb·u·lize ['nebjəlaɪz] **I** *vt* zerstäuben, vernebeln. **II** *vi* zerstäubt werden.
neb·u·liz·er ['nebjəlaɪzər] *n* Zerstäuber *m*, Vernebler *m*.
neb·u·lous urine ['nebjələs] trüber/getrübter Urin *m*, Urina jumentosa.
NEC *abbr*. → neonatal necrotizing enterocolitis.
Ne·ca·tor [nɪ'keɪtər] *n* micro. Necator *m*.
N. americanus Todeswurm *m*, Necator americanus.
ne·ca·to·ri·a·sis [nɪ,keɪtəˈraɪəsɪs] *n* **1.** Necator-Befall *m*, -Infektion *f*. **2.** Hakenwurmbefall *m*, -infektion *f*, Ankylostomiasis *f*, -stomatosis *f*, -stomatidose *f*.
Neck [nek]: **N.'s disease** (van) Neck--Odelberg-Syndrom *nt*, Osteochondrosis ischiopubica.
neck [nek] *n* **1.** Hals *m*; *anat*. Collum *nt*, Zervix *f*, Cervix *f*. **a stiff ~** ein steifer Nacken *od*. Hals. **2.** *allg*. Hals(teil *nt*) *m*; (Flaschen-)Hals *m*.
n. of ankle bone → n. of talus.
n. of condyloid process of mandible → n. of mandible.
n. of dorsal horn of spinal cord Hinterhornhals, Cervix cornus dorsalis/posterioris medullae spinalis, Cervix columnae posterioris medullae spinalis.

n. of femur (Ober-)Schenkelhals, Collum femoris.
n. of fibula Wadenbeinhals, Collum fibulae.
n. of gallbladder Gallenblasenhals, Collum vesicae felleae/biliaris.
n. of glans (penis) Ringfurche *f* der Eichel, Collum glandis.
n. of humerus Humerushals, Collum humeri.
n. of malleus Hammerhals, Collum mallei.
n. of mandible Collum mandibulae.
n. of posterior horn of spinal cord → n. of dorsal horn of spinal cord.
n. of radius Radiushals, Collum radii.
n. of rib Rippenhals, Collum costae.
n. of scapula Schulterblatthals, Collum scapulae.
n. of spermatozoon Spermienhals.
n. of talus Talushals, Collum tali.
n. of thigh bone → n. of femur.
n. of tooth Zahnhals, Cervix/Collum dentis.
n. of urinary bladder (Harn-)Blasenhals, Cervix vesicae.
n. of uterus Uterus-, Gebärmutterhals, Zervix (uteri), Cervix uteri.
n. of womb → n. of uterus.
neck bend *embryo*. Nackenbeuge *f*.
neck cell, mucous (*Magen*) Nebenzelle *f*.
neck dissection HNO Halsdissektion *f*, -ausräumung *f*, neck dissection *f*.
neck fracture *ortho*. subkapitale Fraktur *f*.
neck injury Halsverletzung *f*, -trauma *nt*.
neck ligament Nackenband *nt*, Lig. nuchae.
neck muscles Halsmuskeln *pl*, Nackenmuskulatur *f*, Mm. colli/cervicis.
deep n. tiefe Nackenmuskulatur.
short n. kurze Nackenmuskulatur.
neck organs Halsorgane *f*.
neck pain Nackenschmerz *m*, Zervikodynie *f*.
neck radiation (*Schmerzen*) Ausstrahlung *f* in den Nacken.
neck region Nackengegend *f*, -region *f*, Regio cervicalis posterior, Regio nuchalis.
lateral n. seitliches Halsdreieck *nt*, Regio cervicalis lateralis, Trigonum cervicale posterius.
neck sign Brudzinski'-Nackenzeichen *nt*, Brudzinski-Zeichen *nt*.
neck stiffness Nackensteifigkeit *f*.
neck trauma Halsverletzung *f*, -trauma *nt*.
necr- *pref*. → necro-.
nec·rec·to·my *n* [nek'rektəmɪ] *n chir*., *ortho*. Nekroseexzision *f*, -entfernung *f*.
necro- *pref*. Nekrose-, Nekr(o)-.
nec·ro·bi·o·sis [,nekrəʊbaɪ'əʊsɪs] *n derma*., *patho*. Nekrobiose *f*, Necrobiosis *f*.
nec·ro·bi·ot·ic [,-baɪ'ɒtɪk] *adj* Nekrobiose betr., von ihr gekennzeichnet, nekrobiotisch.
nec·ro·cy·to·sis [,-saɪ'təʊsɪs] *n* Zelltod *m*, -untergang *m*, Zytonekrose *f*.
nec·ro·gen·ic [,-'dʒenɪk] *adj* Nekrose hervorrufend, nekrogen.
necrogenic wart Wilk'-Krankheit *f*, warzige Tuberkulose *f* der Haut, Leichentuberkel *m*, Schlachtertuberkulose *f*, Tuberculosis cutis verrucosa, Verruca necrogenica, Tuberculum anatomicum.
ne·crog·e·nous [nɪ'krɒdʒənəs] *adj* → necrogenic.
ne·crol·o·gy [nɪ'krɒlədʒɪ] *n* Nekrologie *f*.
ne·crol·y·sis [nɪ'krɒləsɪs] *n* Nekrolyse *f*, Nekrolysis *f*.
nec·ro·lyt·ic migratory erythema [,nekrə'lɪtɪk] Erythema migrans necrolytica.

necromania

nec·ro·ma·nia [ˌ-'meɪnɪə, -jə] *n psychia.* Nekromanie *f.*
nec·ro·nec·to·my [ˌ-'nektəmɪ] *n* → necrectomy.
ne·croph·a·gous [nɪ'krɒfəgəs] *adj* **1.** *bio.* aasfressend, nekrophag. **2.** → necrophilous.
nec·ro·phil·ia [ˌnekrə'fɪlɪə] *n psychia.* Nekrophilie *f.*
nec·ro·phil·ic [ˌ-'fɪlɪk] *adj* **1.** *psychia.* Nekrophilie betr., nekrophil. **2.** → necrophilous.
ne·croph·i·lism [nɪ'krɒfəlɪzəm] *n* → necrophilia.
ne·croph·i·lous [nɪ'krɒfɪləs] *adj bio.* mit besonderer Affinität zu nekrotischem Gewebe, nekrophil.
ne·croph·i·ly [nɪ'krɒfəlɪ] *n* → necrophilia.
nec·ro·pho·bia [ˌnekrə'fəʊbɪə] *n psychia.* Nekrophobie *f.*
nec·ro·pneu·mo·nia [ˌ-n(j)uː'məʊnɪə] *n* Lungengangrän *f.*
nec·rop·sy ['nekrəpsɪ] *n* Autopsie *f*, Obduktion *f*, Nekropsie *f.*
nec·ro·sad·ism [ˌnekrə'seɪdɪzəm, -'sæd-] *n psychia.* Nekrosadismus *m.*
ne·cros·co·py [nɪ'krɒskəpɪ] *n* → necropsy.
ne·crose [ne'krəʊs, 'ne-] **I** *vt* nekrotisieren. **II** *vi* absterben, brandig werden, nekrotisieren.
ne·cro·sis [nɪ'krəʊsɪs, ne-] *n, pl* **-ses** [-siːz] lokaler Zell-/Gewebstod *m*, Nekrose *f*, Necrosis *f.*
  n. of the femoral head Hüftkopfnekrose.
  n. of the head of femur Hüftkopfnekrose.
necrosis bacillus Fusobacterium necrophorum.
nec·ro·sper·mia [ˌnekrə'spɜːmɪə] *n* Nekrospermie *f*, Nekrozoospermie *f.*
ne·cros·te·on [nɪ'krɒstɪən] *n* Knochen-, Osteonekrose *f.*
ne·cros·te·o·sis [nɪˌkrɒstɪ'əʊsɪs] *n* Knochen-, Osteonekrose *f.*
ne·crot·ic [nɪ'krɒtɪk, ne-] *adj* Nekrose betr., in Nekrose übergegangen, nekrotisch, nekrotisierend, Nekro-, nekrose-.
necrotic angina *HNO* nekrotisierende Angina *f.*
necrotic caries nekrotischer Knochenfraß *m.*
necrotic cirrhosis postnekrotische/ungeordnete/großknotige Leberzirrhose *f.*
necrotic cyst nekrotische Zyste *f.*
necrotic infectious conjunctivitis *ophthal.* Pascheff-Konjunktivitis *f*, Conjunctivitis necroticans infectiosa.
necrotic inflammation nekrotisierende Entzündung *f.*
necrotic osteitis Knochenmark(s)entzündung *f*, Osteomyelitis *f.*
nec·ro·tize ['nekrətaɪzɪŋ] **I** *vt* Nekrose verursachen. **II** *vi* nekrotisieren.
nec·ro·tiz·ing ['nekrətaɪzɪŋ] *adj* Nekrose auslösend, nekrotisierend.
necrotizing angiitis nekrotisierende Angiitis/Vaskulitis *f.*
necrotizing arteriolitis Arteriolo-, Arteriolennekrose *f.*
necrotizing cellulitis → necrotizing fasciitis.
necrotizing cystitis nekrotisierende Blasenentzündung/Zystitis *f*, Cystitis necroticans.
necrotizing encephalomyelopathy → necrotizing encephalopathy.
necrotizing encephalopathy Leigh-Syndrom *nt*, -Enzephalomyelopathie *f*, nekrotisierende Enzephalomyelopathie *f.*
necrotizing enteritis Darmbrand *m*, Enteritis necroticans.
necrotizing enterocolitis pseudomembranöse Enteritis/Enterokolitis/Kolitis *f.*

necrotizing erysipelas → necrotizing fasciitis.
necrotizing factor → necrotoxin.
necrotizing fasciitis Erysipelas gangraenosum.
necrotizing infection nekrotisierende Infektion *f.*
necrotizing inflammation → necrotic inflammation.
necrotizing myocarditis nekrotisierende Myokarditis *f.*
necrotizing papillitis (*Niere*) Papillennekrose *f*, Papillitis necroticans.
necrotizing renal papillitis → necrotizing papillitis.
necrotizing scleritis nekrotisierende Skleritis *f*, Scleritis necroticans.
necrotizing tonsillitis nekrotisierende Tonsillitis *f.*
necrotizing ulcerative gingivitis/gingivostomatitis *abbr.* **NUG** Plaut-Vincent-Angina *f*, Fusospirillose *f*, Fusospirochätose *f*, Angina ulcerosa/ulceromembranacea.
necrotizing vasculitis nekrotisierende Angiitis/Vaskulitis *f.*
ne·crot·o·my [nɪ'krɒtəmɪ] *n* **1.** *chir.* Zerschneidung *f*, Aufspaltung *f*, Dissektion *f*, Dissectio *f*. **2.** *ortho.* Sequesterentfernung *f*, Nekrotomie *f*, Sequesterotomie *f.*
nec·ro·tox·in [ˌnekrə'tɒksɪn] *n* Nekrotoxin *nt.*
nec·ro·zo·o·sper·mia [ˌ-ˌzəʊə'spɜːmɪə] *n* → necrospermia.
need [niːd] **I** *n* **1.** Bedarf *m* (*of, for* an); Bedürfnis *nt* (*of, for* nach). **to be/stand in ~ of** etw. dringend benötigen. **2.** Mangel *m* (*of, for* an). **3.** **~s** *pl* Bedürfnisse *pl*, Erfordernisse *pl*. **II** *vt* brauchen, benötigen, nötig haben.
nee·dle ['niːdl] **I** *n* **1.** Nadel *f*. **2.** Zeiger *m*; (*Waage*) Zunge *f*. **II** *vt* (mit einer Nadel) nähen; durchstechen; *med.* punktieren.
needle aspiration Nadelaspiration *f.*
needle aspiration biopsy Nadelaspiration(sbiopsie *f*) *f.*
needle aspiration cytology Nadelaspirationszytologie *f*, Nadelpunktionszytologie *f.*
needle bath Strahldusche *f.*
needle biopsy Nadelbiopsie *f.*
needle culture *micro.* Stabkultur *f.*
needle electrode Nadelelektrode *f.*
needle holder *chir.* Nadelhalter *m.*
ne·en·ceph·a·lon [ˌniːən'sefəlɒn] *n* Neenzephalon *nt.*
Neer [nɪər]: **N.'s classification** *ortho.* Neer--Klassifikation *f* der proximalen Humerusfrakturen.
NEFA *abbr.* → fatty acid, nonesterified.
ne·fluor·o·pho·tom·e·ter [nɪˌflʊərəfəʊ'tɒmɪtər] *n* Fluoronephelometer *nt.*
nef·o·pam ['nefəpæm] *n anes., pharm.* Nefopam *nt.*
ne·gate [nɪ'geɪt, 'negeɪt] *vt* verneinen, leugnen, negieren.
ne·ga·tion [nɪ'geɪʃn] *n* Verneinung *f*, Verneinen *nt*, Verleugnen *nt*, Negieren *nt.*
neg·a·tive ['negətɪv] **I** *n* **1.** negative Eigenschaft *f*, Negativfaktor *m*, Negativum *nt*. **2.** *mathe.* Minuszeichen *nt*; negative Zahl *f*. **3.** *photo.* Negativ *nt*. **4.** Verneinung *f*. **5.** negativer Pol *m*. **II** *adj* negativ, erfolg-, ergebnislos; ohne Befund; fehlend, nicht vorhanden. **III** *vt* **6.** neutralisieren. **7.** negieren, verneinen.
negative acceleration negative Beschleunigung *f.*
negative accommodation *physiol.* Fernakkommodation *f.*
negative afterimage *ophthal.* negatives Nachbild *nt.*
negative charge negative Ladung *f.*

negative-contrast staining *histol.* Negativkontrastierung *f*, Negativkontrastfärbung *f.*
negative convergence *ophthal.* Auswärtsdrehung *f* der Sehachse.
negative cyclophoria *ophthal.* Inzyklophorie *f.*
negative cyclotropia *ophthal.* Inzyklotropie *f.*
negative declination *ophthal.* Inzyklovergenz *f*, Konklination *f.*
negative electrode Kathode *f abbr.* K.
negative image *ophthal., psycho.* Nachbild *nt.*
negative lens *opt.* Zerstreuungslinse *f.*
negative meniscus Konvexokonkavlinse *f.*
negative modulator *biochem.* hemmender/negativer Modulator *m.*
negative reinforcement *psycho.* negative Verstärkung *f.*
negative reinforcer *psycho.* negativer Verstärker *m.*
negative rheotaxis Bewegung *f* mit einem Flüssigkeitsstrom, negative Rheotaxis *f.*
negative scotoma *ophthal.* negatives/objektives Skotom *nt.*
negative-sense RNA *genet.* Minus--Strang-RNA *f.*
negative-sense RNA viruses *micro.* Minus-Strang-RNA-Viren *pl.*
negative sign *mathe.* Minuszeichen *nt*, negatives Vorzeichen *nt.*
negative stain Negativfärbung *f.*
negative staining → negative-contrast staining.
negative-strand RNA → negative-sense RNA.
neg·a·tiv·ism ['negətɪvɪzəm] *n psycho.* Negativismus *m.*
neg·a·tron ['negətrɒn] *n* Negatron *nt*, negatives/negativgeladenes Elektron *nt.*
Negri ['neɪgrɪ]: **N. bodies/corpuscles** Negri-Körperchen *pl.*
Negro ['neɪgrəʊ]: **N.'s phenomenon/sign** *neuro.* Zahnradphänomen *nt.*
Neisser ['naɪsər]: **N.'s coccus** → diplococcus of N.
  diplococcus of N. Gonokokkus *m*, Gonococcus *m*, Neisseria gonorrhoeae.
  N.'s stain Neisser-Färbung *f.*
Neis·se·ria [naɪ'sɪərɪə] *n micro.* Neisseria *f.*
  N. gonorrhoeae Gonokokkus *m*, Gonococcus *m*, Neisseria gonorrhoeae.
  N. gonorrhoeae, penicillinase-producing *abbr.* **PPNG** Penicillinase-produzierende Neisseria gonorrhoeae *abbr.* PPNG.
  N. meningitidis Meningokokkus *m*, Neisseria meningitidis.
neis·se·ri·a·ce·ae [naɪˌsɪərɪ'eɪsiː] *pl micro.* Neisseriaceae *pl.*
neis·se·ri·al [naɪ'sɪərɪəl] *adj* Neisseria betr., durch Neisseria verursacht, Neisserien-.
neis·se·ri·an [naɪ'sɪərɪən] *adj* → neisserial.
Neisser-Wechsberg ['weksbɜːg]: **N.-W. phenomenon** Neisser-Wechsberg-Phänomen *nt.*
nekr(o)- *pref.* → necro-.
Nélaton [nela'tɔ̃]: **N.'s catheter** Nélaton--Katheter *m.*
  N.'s dislocation *ortho.* Nélaton'-Luxation *f.*
  N.'s line (Roser-)Nélaton'-Linie *f.*
  N.'s sphincter Nélaton-Fasern *pl.*
Nelson ['nelsən]: **N.'s syndrome** Nelson--Syndrom *nt.*
  N.'s tumor Nelson-Tumor *m.*
ne·ma ['niːmə] *n* → nematode.
nem·a·line myopathy ['neməlaɪn, -lɪn] Nemalinmyopathie *f.*

nemat- pref. → nemato-.
nem·a·thel·minth [‚nemə'θelmɪnθ] n micro. Schlauch-, Rundwurm m, Aschelminth m, Nemathelminth m.
Nem·a·thel·min·thes [‚-θel'mɪnθi:z] pl micro. Schlauch-, Rundwürmer pl, Nemathelminthes pl, Aschelminthes pl.
nem·a·thel·min·thi·a·sis [‚-'θelmɪn'θaɪəsɪs] n Nemathelmintheninfektion f.
ne·mat·i·cide [nə'mætəsaɪd] n, adj → nematocide.
nem·a·ti·za·tion [‚nemətaɪ'zeɪʃn] n → nematodiasis.
nemato- pref. 1. rund-, nemat(o)-. 2. micro. Rundwurm-, Nemato-.
nem·a·to·blast ['nemətəblæst] n Spermatide f, Spermatidium nt.
nem·a·to·cide ['-saɪd] I n Nematozid nt. II adj nematoden(ab)tötend, nematozid.
nem·a·to·cyst ['-sɪst] n bio. Nesselkapsel f, Nematozyste f, Knide f.
Nem·a·to·da [‚nemə'təʊdə] pl micro. Faden-, Rundwürmer pl, Nematoden pl, Nematodes pl.
nem·a·tode ['-təʊd] n micro. Rund-, Fadenwurm m, Nematode f.
nem·a·to·di·a·sis [‚nemətəʊ'daɪəsɪs] n Nematodeninfektion f, Nematodiasis f, Nematosis f.
Nem·a·to·mor·pha [‚-'mɔ:rfə] pl micro. Saitenwürmer pl, Nematomorpha pl.
nem·a·to·sis [‚nemə'təʊsɪs] n → nematodiasis.
Ne·mer·tea [nɪ'mɜrtɪə] pl micro. Schnurwürmer pl.
ne·mer·te·an [nɪ'mɜrtɪən] micro. I n Schnurwurm m. II adj Schnurwürmer betr.
Nem·er·ti·na [nemər'taɪnə, -'tɪnə] pl → Nemertea.
nem·ic ['nemɪk] adj Nematoden betr., Nematoden-.
neo- pref. Neu-, Jung-, Ne(o)-.
ne·o·an·ti·gen [‚ni:əʊ'æntɪdʒən] n immun. Neoantigen nt; Tumorantigen nt.
ne·o·an·ti·mo·san [‚-‚æntɪ'məʊsən] n pharm. Stibophen nt.
ne·o·ar·thro·sis [‚-ɑ:r'θrəʊsɪs] n → nearthrosis.
ne·o·cer·e·bel·lar [‚-serə'belər] adj Neozerebellum betr., neozerebellar, neozerebellär.
ne·o·cer·e·bel·lum [‚-serə'beləm] n Neozerebellum nt, Neocerebellum nt.
ne·o·cor·tex [‚-'kɔ:rteks] n Neokortex m, Neocortex m.
ne·o·cor·ti·cal [‚-'kɔ:rtɪkl] adj Neokortex betr., neokortikal.
ne·o·cy·to·sis [‚-saɪ'təʊsɪs] n Neozytose f.
ne·o·di·a·ther·my [‚-'daɪəθɜrmɪ] n Kurzwellendiathermie f.
ne·o·dym·i·um [‚-'dɪmɪəm] n abbr. Nd Neodym nt abbr. Nd.
ne·o·en·ceph·a·lon [‚-en'sefəlɒn] n Neencephalon nt.
ne·o·for·ma·tion [‚-fɔ:r'meɪʃn] n patho. Neubildung f, Neoplasma nt; Neoplasie f.
ne·o·gen·e·sis [‚-'dʒenəsɪs] n Neubildung f, Regeneration f, Neogenese f.
ne·o·ge·net·ic [‚-dʒɪ'netɪk] adj Neogenese betr., neogenetisch, regeneratorisch.
ne·o·gly·co·gen·e·sis [‚-‚ɡlaɪkəʊ'dʒenəsɪs] n Gluko-, Glyko-, Gluconeogenese f.
ne·o·ki·net·ic [‚-kɪ'netɪk] adj physiol. neokinetisch.
ne·o·la·lia [‚-'leɪlɪə] n psychia. Neolalie f.
ne·o·lal·ism [‚-'læhzəm] n → neolalia.
ne·ol·o·gism [nɪ'ɒlədʒɪzəm] n psychia. Wortneubildung f, Neologismus m.
ne·o·mem·brane [ni:əʊ'membreɪn] n Pseudomembran f.

ne·o·min ['-mɪn] n → neomycin.
ne·o·morph ['-mɔ:rf] n embryo. neomorphes Teil nt.
ne·o·mor·phic [‚-'mɔ:rfɪk] adj embryo. neomorph.
ne·o·mor·phism ['-mɔ:rfɪzəm] n embryo. Neomorphismus m.
ne·o·my·cin [‚-'maɪsɪn] n pharm. Neomycin nt.
neomycin B pharm. Neomycin B nt, Framycetin nt.
ne·on ['ni:ɒn] n abbr. **Ne** Neon nt abbr. Ne.
ne·o·na·tal [ni:əʊ'neɪtl] adj Neugeborenen-/Neonatalperiode betr., neonatal, Neonatal-, Neugeborenen-.
neonatal acne Neugeborenenakne f, Akne/Acne neonatorum.
neonatal apoplexy Neugeborenenapoplexie f.
neonatal asphyxia Neugeborenenasphyxie f, Atemdepressionszustand m des Neugeborenen, Asphyxia neonatorum.
neonatal death Neugeborenentod m, Tod m in der Neugeborenenperiode.
neonatal diarrhea infektiöse Säuglingsenteritis/Säuglingsdyspepsie f.
neonatal giant cell hepatitis (neonatale) Riesenzellhepatitis f.
neonatal hepatitis → neonatal giant cell hepatitis.
neonatal herpes neonataler Herpes m, Herpes neonatorum.
neonatal hyperbilirubinemia physiologische Neugeborenhyperbilirubinämie f.
neonatal lines Owen'-Linien pl.
neonatal mortality Neugeborenensterblichkeit f, Sterblichkeit f in der Neugeborenenperiode.
neonatal necrotizing enterocolitis abbr. **NEC** Enterocolitis necroticans neonatorum.
neonatal tetanus Neugeborenentetanus m, Tetanus neonatorum.
neonatal tetany Neugeborenentetanie f.
neonatal tyrosinemia transitorische Tyrosinämie f des Neugeborenen.
ne·o·nate ['ni:əʊneɪt] I n Neugeborene nt. II adj neugeboren.
ne·o·na·tol·o·gist [‚-neɪ'tɒlədʒɪst] n Neonatologe m, -login f.
ne·o·na·tol·o·gy [‚-neɪ'tɒlədʒɪ] n Neonatologie f.
ne·o·pal·li·um [‚-'pælɪəm] n Neopallium nt.
ne·op·a·thy [nɪ'ɒpəθɪ] n Neopathie f.
ne·o·phre·nia [ni:əʊ'fri:nɪə] n psychia. old Neophrenie f.
ne·o·pla·sia [‚-'pleɪʒ(ɪ)ə, -ʒɪə] n patho. Gewebeneubildung f, Neoplasie f.
ne·o·plasm ['-plæzəm] n Neubildung f, Neoplasma nt; Tumor m.
ne·o·plas·tic [‚-'plæstɪk] adj Neoplasie od. Neoplasma betr., neoplastisch.
neoplastic disease Tumorleiden nt.
neoplastic fibrosis proliferative Fibrose f.
ne·o·ru·brum [‚-'ru:brəm] n Neorubrum f.
ne·o·stig·mine [‚-'stɪɡmi:n, -mɪn] n pharm., anes. Neostigmin nt.
ne·o·stri·a·tum [‚-straɪ'eɪtəm] n Neostriatum nt.
ne·ot·e·ny [nɪ'ɒt(ə)nɪ] n embryo., bio. Neotenie f.
ne·o·thal·a·mus [‚ni:əʊ'θæləməs] n Neothalamus m.
ne·o·type ['-taɪp] n micro. Neostandard m.
ne·o·vas·cu·lar·i·za·tion [‚-‚væskjələrɪ'zeɪʃn, -raɪ-] n patho. **1.** (Tumor) Gefäßneubildung f. **2.** Kapillareinsprossung f, Revaskularisierung f, Revaskularisation f.

neph·e·lom·e·ter [‚nefə'lɒmɪtər] n Trübungsmesser m, Nephelometer nt.
neph·e·lo·met·ric [‚nefələ'metrɪk] adj Nephelometrie betr., nephelometrisch.
neph·e·lom·e·try [‚nefə'lɒmətrɪ] n Nephelometrie f.
nephr- pref. → nephro-.
neph·rad·e·no·ma [nefrædɪ'nəʊmə] n Nierenadenom nt.
ne·phral·gia [nɪ'frældʒ(ɪ)ə] n Nierenschmerz(en pl) m, Nephralgie f.
ne·phral·gic [nɪ'frældʒɪk] adj Nephralgie betr.
neph·ra·pos·ta·sis [‚nefrə'pɒstəsɪs] n Nierenabszeß m.
neph·ra·to·nia [‚-'təʊnɪə] n Nierenatonie f.
ne·phrat·o·ny [nɪ'frætənɪ] n → nephratonia.
neph·rauxe [nef'rɔ:ksɪ] n → nephromegaly.
neph·rec·ta·sia [nefrek'teɪʒ(ɪ)ə] n Nierendilatation f, Nephrektasie f; Sackniere f.
ne·phrec·ta·sis [nɪ'frektəsɪs] n → nephrectasia.
ne·phrec·ta·sy [nɪ'frektəsɪ] n → nephrectasia.
ne·phrec·to·mize [nɪ'frektəmaɪz] vt chir. eine Nephrektomie durchführen, nephrektomieren.
ne·phrec·to·my [nɪ'frektəmɪ] n chir. Nierenentfernung f, -exstirpation f, Nephrektomie f.
neph·re·de·ma [nefrɪ'di:mə] n **1.** Nierenstauung f. **2.** Stauungsniere f. **3.** nephrogenes Ödem nt.
neph·rel·co·sis [nefrel'kəʊsɪs] n Nierenulzeration f.
ne·phre·mia [nɪ'fri:mɪə] n → nephredema.
neph·rem·or·rha·gia [nefremə'reɪdʒ(ɪ)ə] n **1.** Nieren(ein)blutung f, Nephrorrhagie f. **2.** Blutung f aus der Niere.
neph·ric ['nefrɪk] adj Niere/Ren betr., renal, Nieren-.
nephric colic Nierenkolik f, Colica renalis.
nephric duct Harnleiter m, Ureter m.
ne·phrit·ic [nɪ'frɪtɪk] adj **1.** → nephric. **2.** Nierenentzündung/Nephritis betr., von Nephritis betroffen, nephritisch, Nephritis-.
nephritic calculus → nephrolith.
nephritic retinitis renale Retinopathie f.
nephritic syndrome nephritisches Syndrom nt.
ne·phri·tis [nɪ'fraɪtɪs] n Nierenentzündung f, Nephritis f.
n. of pregnancy Schwangerschaftsnephritis, -nephropathie f, Nephritis gravidarum.
neph·rit·o·gen·ic [nɪ‚frɪtəʊ'dʒenɪk] adj Nephritis verursachend, nephritogen.
nephro- pref. Niere(n), Reno-, Nephr(o)-.
neph·ro·ab·dom·i·nal [‚nefræb'dɒmɪnl] adj Niere(n) u. Bauch(wand) betr., nephroabdominal, renoabdominal.
neph·ro·an·gi·op·a·thy [‚-‚ændʒɪ'ɒpəθɪ] n Nephroangiopathie f.
neph·ro·an·gi·o·scle·ro·sis [‚-‚ændʒɪəʊsklɪ'rəʊsɪs] n patho. Nephroangiosklerose f.
neph·ro·blas·to·ma [‚-blæs'təʊmə] n Wilms-Tumor m, embryonales Adeno(myo)sarkom nt, Adenomyohidrosarkom nt der Niere, Nephroblastom nt.
neph·ro·cal·ci·no·sis [‚-‚kælsɪ'nəʊsɪs] n patho. Nephrokalzinose f.
neph·ro·cap·sec·to·my [‚-kæp'sektəmɪ] n chir. Entfernung f der Nierenkapsel, Nierendekapsulation f, Nephrokapsulektomie f.
neph·ro·car·di·ac [‚-'kɑ:rdɪæk] adj Herz u. Niere(n) betr., renokardial, kardiorenal.

nephrocele

neph·ro·cele ['-siːl] *n* 1. *patho.* Nephrozele *f.* 2. *bio.* Nephrozöl *nt.*
neph·ro·ce·lom [ˌ-'siːləm] *n bio.* Nephrozöl *nt.*
neph·ro·col·ic [ˌ-'kɑlɪk] **I** *n* Nierenkolik *f*, Colica renalis. **II** *adj* Niere(n) u. Kolon betr., kolorenal.
neph·ro·co·lop·to·sis [ˌ-ˌkəʊləp'təʊsɪs] *n patho.* Senkung *f* von Niere u. Kolon.
neph·ro·cyst·a·nas·to·mo·sis [ˌ-ˌsɪstəˌnæstə'məʊsɪs] *n urol.* Nieren-Blasen-Fistel *f.*
neph·ro·cys·ti·tis [ˌ-sɪs'taɪtɪs] *n* Entzündung *f* von Niere(n) u. Blase.
neph·ro·gas·tric [ˌ-'gæstrɪk] *adj* Magen u. Niere(n) betr., gastrorenal.
neph·ro·gen·ic [ˌ-'dʒenɪk] *adj* → nephrogenous.
nephrogenic cord *embryo.* nephrogener Strang *m.*
ne·phrog·e·nous [nə'frɑgənəs, ne-] *adj* aus der Niere stammend, durch die Niere bedingt, nephrogen, renal.
nephrogenous proteinuria echte/renale Proteinurie/Albuminurie *f.*
neph·ro·gram ['nefrəgræm] *n radiol.* Nephrogramm *nt.*
ne·phrog·ra·phy [nə'frɑgrəfɪ] *n radiol.* Kontrastdarstellung *f* der Niere, Nephrographie *f.*
neph·ro·he·mia [ˌnefrə'hiːmɪə] *n* Nierenstauung *f*; Stauungsniere *f.*
neph·ro·hy·dro·sis [ˌ-haɪ'drəʊsɪs] *n* Harnstauungs-, Wassersackniere *f*, Hydronephrose *f*, Uronephrose *f.*
neph·ro·hy·per·tro·phy [ˌ-haɪ'pɜrtrəfɪ] *n* Nierenhypertrophie *f.*
neph·roid ['nefrɔɪd] *adj* nierenförmig, -artig, nephroid.
neph·ro·lith ['nefrəlɪθ] *n* Nierenstein *m*, Nephrolith *m*, Calculus renalis.
neph·ro·li·thi·a·sis [ˌ-lɪ'θaɪəsɪs] *n* Nierensteinleiden *nt*, -krankheit *f*, Nephrolithiasis *f.*
neph·ro·li·thot·o·my [ˌ-lɪ'θɑtəmɪ] *n urol., chir.* operative Nierensteinentfernung *f*, Nephrolithotomie *f.*
ne·phrol·o·gist [nə'frɑlədʒɪst] *n* Nephrologe *m*, -login *f.*
ne·phrol·o·gy [nə'frɑlədʒɪ] *n* Nephrologie *f.*
ne·phrol·y·sis [nə'frɑləsɪs] *n* 1. *patho.* Nephrolyse *f.* 2. *chir., urol.* Nierenlösung *f*, Nephrolyse *f*, Nephroliberation *f.*
ne·phro·ma [nə'frəʊmə] *n* Nierengeschwulst *f*, Nephrom(a) *nt.*
neph·ro·ma·la·cia [ˌnefrəmə'leɪ(ɪ)ə] *n patho.* Nierenerweichung *f*, Nephromalazie *f.*
neph·ro·meg·a·ly [ˌ-'megəlɪ] *n* Nierenvergrößerung *f*, Nephromegalie *f.*
neph·ro·mere ['-mɪər] *n* nephrotome.
neph·ron ['nefrɑn] *n* Nephron *nt.*
neph·ron·cus [nef'rɑŋkəs] *n* → nephroma.
neph·rone ['nefrəʊn] *n* Nephron *nt.*
ne·phron·ic loop [nɪ'frɑnɪk] Henle'-Schleife *f.*
neph·ro·noph·thi·sis [ˌnefrə'nɑfθəsɪs] *n patho.* Nephronophthise *f*, Nephronophthisis *f.*
neph·ro·path·ia [ˌ-'pæθɪə] *n* → nephropathy.
neph·ro·path·ic [ˌ-'pæθɪk] *adj* Nephropathie betr., die Niere schädigend, nephropathisch.
nephropathic cardiopathy nephropathische Kardiopathie *f.*
ne·phrop·a·thy [nə'frɑpəθɪ] *n* Nierenerkrankung *f*, -schädigung *f*, Nephropathie *f*, -pathia *f.*
neph·ro·path·o·gen·ic [ˌnefrəˌpæθə'dʒenɪk] *adj* nieren-, nephropathogen.
neph·ro·pex·y ['-peksɪ] *n chir.* Nierenfixation *f*, -anheftung *f*, Nephropexie *f.*
ne·phroph·thi·sis [nə'frɑfθəsɪs] *n* 1. → nephronophthisis. 2. → nephrotuberculosis.
neph·ro·poi·e·tin [ˌnefrəʊ'pɔɪətɪn] *n embryo.* Nephropo(i)etin *nt.*
neph·rop·to·sia [ˌnefrɑp'təʊsɪə] *n* → nephroptosis.
neph·rop·to·sis [ˌnefrɑp'təʊsɪs] *n patho.* Nierensenkung *f*, Nephroptose *f*; Senkniere *f.*
neph·ro·py·e·li·tis [ˌnefrəʊˌpaɪə'laɪtɪs] *n* Pyelonephritis *f abbr.* PN.
neph·ro·py·e·log·ra·phy [ˌ-ˌpaɪə'lɑgrəfɪ] *n radiol., urol.* Kontrastdarstellung *f* von Niere u. Nierenbecken, Nephropyelographie *f.*
neph·ro·py·e·lo·li·thot·o·my [ˌ-ˌpaɪələlɪ'θɑtəmɪ] *n chir., urol.* Nephropyelolithotomie *f.*
neph·ro·py·e·lo·plas·ty [ˌ-ˌpaɪələplæstɪ] *n chir., urol.* Nierenbeckenplastik *f.*
neph·ro·py·o·sis [ˌ-paɪ'əʊsɪs] *n* Niereneiterung *f*, Nephropyose *f.*
neph·ror·rha·gia [ˌ-'reɪdʒ(ɪ)ə] *n* Nierenblutung *f*, Nephrorrhagie *f.*
ne·phror·rha·phy [ne'frɔːrəfɪ] *n chir.* Nierennaht *f*, Nephrorrhaphie *f.*
neph·ro·scle·ria ['nefrəsklerɪə] *n* → nephrosclerosis.
neph·ro·scle·ro·sis [ˌ-sklɪ'rəʊsɪs] *n patho.* Nephrosklerose *f.*
ne·phro·sis [nə'frəʊsɪs] *n, pl* **-ses** [-siːz] 1. Nephrose *f*, Nephrosis *f.* 2. → nephropathy. 3. → nephrotic syndrome.
ne·phro·so·ne·phri·tis [nəˌfrəʊsəʊnɪ'fraɪtɪs] *n* Nephrosonephritis *f.*
neph·ro·so·nog·ra·phy [ˌnefrəsə'nɑgrəfɪ] *n radiol.* Nierensonographie *f.*
ne·phros·to·my [nə'frɑstəmɪ] *n chir., urol.* Nephrostomie *f.*
ne·phrot·ic [nə'frɑtɪk] *adj* Nephrose betr., nephrotisch.
nephrotic edema nephrotisches Ödem *nt.*
nephrotic syndrome nephrotisches Syndrom *nt*; Nephrose *f.*
neph·ro·tome ['nefrətəʊm] *n embryo.* Nephrotom *nt.*
neph·ro·to·mo·gram [ˌ-'təʊməgræm] *n radiol.* Nephrotomogramm *nt.*
neph·ro·to·mog·ra·phy [ˌ-tə'mɑgrəfɪ] *n radiol.* Nephrotomographie *f.*
ne·phrot·o·my [nə'frɑtəmɪ] *n chir., urol.* Nephrotomie *f.*
neph·ro·tox·ic [ˌnefrə'tɑksɪk] *adj* nierenschädigend, -giftig, nephrotoxisch.
nephrotoxic cardiopathy nephrotoxische Kardiopathie *f.*
neph·ro·tox·ic·i·ty [ˌ-tɑk'sɪsətɪ] *n* Nierenschädlichkeit *f*, -giftigkeit *f*, Nieren-, Nephrotoxizität *f.*
nephrotoxic serum nephritis Masugi-Nephritis *f*, nephrotoxische Serumnephritis *f.*
neph·ro·tox·in [ˌ-'tɑksɪn] *n* Nierengift *nt*, nephrotoxische Substanz *f*, Nephrotoxin *nt.*
neph·ro·trop·ic [ˌ-'trɑpɪk, -'trəʊp-] *adj* mit besonderer Affinität zur Niere, nephrotrop.
neph·ro·tu·ber·cu·lo·sis [ˌ-təˌbɜrkjə'ləʊsɪs] *n* Nierentuberkulose *f*, Nephrophthisis *f.*
neph·ro·u·re·ter·ec·to·my [ˌ-jəˌriːtə'rektəmɪ] *n urol.* Nephroureterektomie *f.*
neph·ro·u·re·ter·o·cys·tec·to·my [ˌ-jəˌriːtərəsɪs'tektəmɪ] *n urol.* Nephroureterozystektomie *f.*
neph·ry·dro·sis [nefrɪ'drəʊsɪs] *n* → nephrohydrosis.
nep·tu·ni·um [nep't(j)uːnɪən] *n abbr.* **Np** Neptunium *nt abbr.* Np.

Neri ['neərɪ]: **N.'s sign** Neri-Zeichen *nt.*
Nernst [neərnst, nɜrnst]: **N. equation** *phys.* Nernst'-Gleichung *f.*
   N. potential Nernst-Potential *nt.*
nerv·al ['nɜrvl] *adj* → nervous 1.
nerve [nɜrv] *n* 1. Nerv *m*; *anat.* Nervus *m.* 2. ~**s** *pl* Nervosität *f.* 3. *bot.* (*Blatt*) Nerv *m*, Ader *f.*
   n. of Cotunnius Nasopalatinus *m*, N. nasopalatinus.
   n. of external acoustic meatus N. meatus acustici externi.
   n. of pterygoid canal Radix facialis, N. Vidianus/Vidii, N. canalis pterygoidei.
   n. of quadrate muscle of thigh N. musculi quadrati femoris, N. quadratus femoris.
   n.s of smell Riechfäden *pl*, Fila olfactoria, I. Hirnnerv, Nn. olfactorii [I].
   n. of tensor tympani muscle N. musculi tensoris tympani.
   n. of tensor veli palatini muscle N. musculi tensoris veli palatini.
   n. of Willis Akzessorius *m*, XI. Hirnnerv, N. accessorius [XI].
nerve accommodation Akkommodation *f* des Nervs.
nerve-action current (Nerven-)Aktionsstrom *m.*
nerve block 1. *neuro.* Nervenblock(ade *f*) *m.* 2. *anes.* Nervenblockade *f*, Leitungs-, Regionalanästhesie *f.*
nerve block anesthesia → nerve block 2.
nerve calix Nervenkelch *m.*
nerve cavity (*Zahn*) Pulpahöhle *f*, Cavitas dentis/pulparis.
nerve cell Nervenzelle *f*, Neuron *nt.*
   neurosecretory n. neurosekretorische Nervenzelle, neurosekretorisches Neuron.
   primitive n. *embryo.* Neuroblast *m.*
   pseudounipolar n. pseudounipolare Nervenzelle.
nerve cement Neuroglia *f.*
nerve center Nervenzentrum *nt.*
nerve cord *anat.* Nervenstrang *m.*
nerve corpuscles, terminal sensible Endorgane *pl*, Terminal-, Nervenendkörperchen *pl*, Corpuscula nervosa terminalia.
nerve damage Nervenschädigung *f*, -schaden *m.*
nerve deafness retrokochleäre Schwerhörigkeit *f.*
nerve decompression Nervendekompression *f.*
nerve end corpuscles Nervenendkörperchen *pl.*
nerve ending: encapsulated n. sensibles Endorgan *nt*, Terminal-, Nervenendkörperchen *nt*, Corpusculum nervosum terminale.
   free n. freie Nervenendigung *f.*
   non-corpuscular n. → free n.
nerve excitability test Nervenerregbarkeitstest *m*, Nerve-excitability-Test *m.*
nerve fascicle Nervenfaserbündel *nt.*
nerve fiber → neurofiber.
   myelinated n. markhaltige Nervenfaser *f.*
nerve fiber layer (*Auge*) Schicht *f* der Nervenfasern.
nerve fibril Achsenzylinder *m*, Axon *nt*, Neuraxon *nt.*
nerve ganglion *anat.* (Nerven-)Knoten *m*, Ganglion *nt.*
nerve gas Nervengas *nt.*
nerve graft 1. Nerventransplantat *nt.* 2. Nerventransplantation *f.*
nerve grafting Nerventransplantation *f.*
   interfascicular n. sekundäre Nervennaht *f*, autologe interfaszikuläre Transplantation.
nerve growth factor *abbr.* **NGF** Nervenwachstumsfaktor *m abbr.* NGF.

nerve hook *chir.*, *neurochir.* Nervenhaken *m.*
nerve impulse Nervenimpuls *m.*
nerve injury Nervenverletzung *f*, -schädigung *f*, -trauma *nt.*
nerve-less ['nɜrvlɪs] *adj* **1.** *anat.* nervenlos, ohne Nerven; *bot.* ohne Adern, ungeädert. **2.** kraft-, energielos, schwach.
nerve plexus Nervengeflecht *nt*, -plexus *m.*
nerve poison Nervengift *nt.*
nerve-racking *adj* nervenaufreibend.
nerve regeneration Nervenregeneration *f.*
nerve root Nervenwurzel *f.*
nerve stimulation Nervenstimulation *f*, -stimulierung *f.*
   transcutaneous electrical n. *abbr.* **TENS** transkutane elektrische Nervenstimulation *abbr.* TENS.
nerve stretching → neurotony.
nerve supply Nervenversorgung *f.*
   motor n. motorische Nervenversorgung.
   sensory n. sensible Nervenversorgung.
nerve tissue Nervengewebe *nt.*
nerve trauma Nervenverletzung *f*, -trauma *nt*, -schädigung *f.*
nerve trunk Nervenstamm *m.*
nerve-wracking *adj* nervenaufreibend.
ner·von ['nɜrvɑn] *n* → nervone.
ner·vone ['nɜrvəʊn] *n* Nervon *nt.*
ner·von·ic acid [nɜr'vɑnɪk] Nervonsäure *f.*
ner·vos·i·ty [nɜr'vɑsəti] *n* Nervosität *f*, Aufgeregtheit *f.*
ner·vous ['nɜrvəs] *adj* **1.** *anat.* Nerv/Nervus betr., nerval, nervös (bedingt), neural, nervlich, Nerven-. **2.** nervös, aufgeregt; überempfindlich.
nervous asthenopia 1. hysterische Asthenopie *f.* **2.** nervöse Asthenopie *f.*
nervous asthma streßbedingtes Asthma *nt.*
nervous bladder *inf.* nervöse Blase *f.*
nervous breakdown Nervenzusammenbruch *m.*
nervous chill nervöses Zittern *nt.*
nervous collapse Nervenzusammenbruch *m.*
nervous coat of eye Netzhaut *f*, Retina *f.*
nervous discharge *physiol.* Nervenentladung *f.*
nervous dyspepsia nervöse Dyspepsie *f.*
nervous energy Vitalität *f.*
nervous exhaustion → neurasthenia.
nervous gas Nervengas *nt.*
nervous indigestion nervöse Dyspepsie *f.*
nervous layer of retina Stratum cerebrale, Pars nervosa (retinae).
ner·vous·ness ['nɜrvəsnɪs] *n* → nervosity.
nervous part of retina → nervous layer of retina.
nervous plexus nervöser Plexus *m.*
nervous pregnancy psychogene Scheinschwangerschaft *f.*
nervous prostration → neurasthenia.
nervous respiration Corrigan-Atmung *f.*
nervous stratum of retina Stratum cerebrale, Pars nervosa (retinae).
nervous system Nervensystem *nt*, Systema nervosum.
   autonomic n. *abbr.* **ANS** autonomes/vegetatives Nervensystem *abbr.* ANS, Pars autonomica systematis nervosi, Systema nervosum autonomicum.
   central n. *abbr.* **CNS** Zentralnervensystem *abbr.* ZNS, Gehirn u. Rückenmark, Systema nervosa centrale, Pars centralis systematis nervosi.
   enteric n. Darmnervensystem.
   exteroceptive n. extero(re)zeptives System.
   interoceptive n. intero(re)zeptives System.
   involuntary n. → autonomic n.
   parasympathetic n. parasympathischer Teil *m* des vegetativen Nervensystems, Parasympathikus *m*, parasympathisches System, Pars parasympathetica/parasympathica systematis nervosi autonomici.
   peripheral n. *abbr.* **PNS** peripheres Nervensystem *abbr.* PNS, Systema nervosa peripherium, Pars peripherica systematis nervosi.
   proprioceptive n. proprio(re)zeptives System.
   somatic n. somatisches Nervensystem.
   sympathetic n. 1. → autonomic n. **2.** sympathischer Teil *m* des vegetativen Nervensystems, Sympathikus *m*, sympathisches System, Pars sympathetica/sympathica systematis nervosi autonomici.
   vegetative/visceral n. → autonomic n.
nervous tension Nervenanspannung *f.*
nervous tissue Nervengewebe *nt.*
nervous tunic of eye, internal innere Augenhaut *f*, Tunica interna/sensori bulbi.
ner·vus ['nɜrvəs] *n*, *pl* **-vi** [-vaɪ, -viː] → nerve 1.
ne·sid·i·ec·to·my [nə,sɪdɪ'ektəmi] *n chir.* (*Pankreas*) Exzision *f* des Inselgewebes.
ne·sid·i·o·blast [nə'sɪdɪəblæst] *n* (*Pankreas*) Inselzelle *f.*
ne·sid·i·o·blas·to·ma [,-blæs'təʊmə] *n* Inselzelladenom *nt*, Nesidioblastom *nt*, Nesidiom *nt*, Adenoma insulocellulare.
ne·sid·i·o·blas·to·sis [,-blæs'təʊsɪs] *n* (*Pankreas*) diffuse Inselzellhyperplasie *f.*
net [net] **I** *n* → network. **II** *adj* netto, Netto-; End-; *techn.* Nutz-.
net current *phys.* Nettostrom *m.*
net efficiency Nutzleistung *f.*
net flow *phys.* Nettostrom *m*, -strömung *f.*
Netherton ['neθərtən]: **N.'s syndrome** Netherton-Syndrom *nt.*
net·il·mi·cin [netl'maɪsn] *n pharm.* Netilmicin *nt.*
net knot Karyosom *nt.*
net-like ['netlaɪk] *adj* netzartig.
net result Endresultat *nt.*
net shift *physiol.* Nettoverschiebung *f.*
net·ted ['netɪd] *adj* netzförmig, maschig.
net·ting ['netɪŋ] *n* Netz(werk *nt*) *nt*, Netzgewebe *nt*, Geflecht *nt.*
net·tle ['netl] *n* **1.** *bot.* Nessel *f.* **2.** *derm.* Quaddel *f*, Urtika *f*, Urtica *f.*
nettle cell *n* nematocyst.
nettle rash *patho.* Nesselausschlag *m*, -fieber *nt*, -sucht *f*, Urtikaria *f*, Urticaria *f.*
Nettleship ['netlʃɪp]: **N.'s disease** Nettleship'-Erkrankung *f*, -Syndrom *nt*, kutane Mastozytose *f*, Mastozytose-Syndrom *nt*, Urticaria pigmentosa.
net transport *physiol.* Nettotransport *m.*
net·work [netwɜrk] *n* (*a. fig.*) Netz *nt*; Netz-, Maschenwerk *nt*, Netzgewebe *nt*, Geflecht *nt*; *anat.* Rete *nt.*
   n. of terminal bars *histol.* Schlußleistennetz.
network fibrosis *patho.* Maschendrahtfibrose *f.*
Neubauer ['nɔ(j)uːbaʊər; 'nɔy-]: **N.'s artery** unterste Schilddrüsenarterie *f*, Thyroidea *f* ima, A. thyroidea ima.
Neuberg ['n(j)uːbɜrg; 'nɔybɛrk]: **N. ester** Fructose-6-phosphat *nt abbr.* F-6-P, Neuberg-Ester *m.*
Neufeld ['n(j)uːfeld; 'nɔyfelt]: **N. capsular swelling** *micro.* Neufeld-Reaktion *f*, Kapselquellungsreaktion *f.*
   N.'s reaction/test → N. capsular swelling.
Neumann ['n(j)uːmən; 'nɔymən]: **N.'s cells** *hema.* Neumann-Zellen *pl.*
   N.'s disease Neumann'-Krankheit *f*, Pemphigus vegetans, Erythema bullosum vegetans, Pyostomatitis vegetans.
   N.'s sheath Neumann'-Scheide *f.*
neur- *pref.* → neuro-.
neu·rag·mia [njʊə'rægmɪə, nʊ-] *n neuro.* Nervendehnung *f*, -zerrung *f*, -riß *m.*
neu·ral ['njʊərəl, 'nʊ-] *adj* **1.** → nervous 1. **2.** in der Nähe des Rückenmarks liegend.
neural arch of vertebra Wirbelbogen *m*, Arcus vertebralis/vertebrae.
neural atrophy neurogene Muskelatrophie *f.*
neural axis → nervous system, central.
neural blockade Nervenblockade *f.*
neural canal Wirbel(säulen)-, Vertebralkanal *m*, Canalis vertebralis.
neural crest *embryo.* Neuralleiste *f.*
neural crest cell *embryo.* Neurallistenzelle *f.*
neural cyst Neuralzyste *f.*
neural deafness retrokochleäre Schwerhörigkeit *f.*
neural ectoderm Neuroderm *nt*, neurales Ektoderm *nt.*
neural folds *embryo.* Neuralfalten *pl.*
neural ganglion Nervenknoten *m*, Ganglion *nt.*
neu·ral·gia [njʊə'rældʒ(ɪ)ə, nʊ-] *n neuro.* Neuralgie *f*, Neuralgia *f.*
   n. of the sphenopalatine ganglion Sluder--Neuralgie, -Syndrom *nt*, Neuralgia sphenopalatina.
neu·ral·gic [njʊə'rældʒɪk, nʊ-] *adj* Neuralgie betr., neuralgisch.
neuralgic pain neuralgischer Schmerz *m.*
neur·al·gi·form [njʊə'rældʒɪfɔːrm, nʊ-] *adj* neuralgieartig, neuralgiform.
neural groove *embryo.* Neuralrinne *f.*
neural impulse Nervenimpuls *m.*
neural layer of retina Stratum cerebrale, Pars nervosa (retinae).
neural lobe. → n. of hypophysis **1.** → neurohypophysis. **2.** → n. of neurohypophysis.
   n. of neurohypophysis Neurallappen *m* der Neurohypophyse, Lobus nervosus neurohypophyseos.
   n. of pituitary (gland) 1. → neurohypophysis. **2.** → n. of neurohypophysis.
neural part of retina → neural layer of retina.
neural plate *embryo.* Neuralplatte *f.*
neural presbyacusis neurale Altersschwerhörigkeit/Presbyakusis *f.*
neural stalk Hypophysenstiel *m*, Infundibulum hypothalami.
neural stratum of retina → neural layer of retina.
neural tube *embryo.* Neuralrohr *nt.*
neur·a·min·ic acid [,njʊərə'mɪnɪk, -əˈmiːn-, ˌnʊ-] Neuraminsäure *f.*
neur·a·min·i·dase [,njʊərə'mɪnɪdeɪz, -nʊ-] *n abbr.* **NA** Neuraminidase *f abbr.* NA, Sialidase *f.*
neur·an·a·gen·e·sis [,njʊəræn·ə'dʒenəsɪs, ˌnʊ-] *n* Nervenregeneration *f.*
neu·ra·prax·ia [njʊərə'præksɪə, ˌnʊ-] *n* Neurapraxie *f*, Neuropraxie *f.*
neur·ar·throp·a·thy [,njʊərɑːr'θrɑpəθi, ˌnʊ-] *n* → neuroarthropathy.
neur·as·the·nia [,njʊərəs'θiːnɪə, ˌnʊ-] *n* Beard-Syndrom *nt*, Nervenschwäche *f*, nervöse Übererregbarkeit *f*, Neurasthenie *f*, Neurasthenia *f.*
neur·as·the·ni·ac [,-'θiːnɪæk] *n* → neurasthenic I.
neur·as·then·ic [,-'θenɪk] **I** *n* Neurastheniker(in *f*) *m.* **II** *adj* Neurasthenie betr., neurasthenisch.
neurasthenic asthenopia 1. hysterische Asthenopie *f.* **2.** retinale Asthenopie *f.*
neurasthenic neurosis → neurasthenia.
neur·ax·i·al [njʊə'ræksɪəl, ˌnʊ-] *adj* (Neur-)Axon betr., Axon-, Achsen-.

neuraxis

neur·a·xis [njʊəˈræksɪs, nʊ-] *n* 1. → neuraxon. 2. → nervous system, central.
neur·a·xon [njʊəˈræksən, nʊ-] *n* Achsenzylinder *m*, Neuraxon *nt*, Axon *nt*, Neurit *m*.
neur·ec·ta·sia [ˌnjʊərekˈteɪʒ(ɪ)ə, ˌnʊ-] *n* → neurotony.
neur·ec·ta·sis [njʊəˈrektəsɪs, nʊ-] *n* → neurotony.
neur·ec·ta·sy [njʊəˈrektəsɪ, nʊ-] *n* → neurotony.
neur·ec·to·my [njʊəˈrektəmɪ, nʊ-] *n neurochir*. Nerventeilentfernung *f*, -resektion *f*, Neurektomie *f*.
neur·ec·to·pia [ˌnjʊərekˈtəʊpɪə, ˌnʊ-] *n patho*. Nervenektopie *f*, Neurektopie *f*, Neurectopia *f*.
neur·ec·to·py [njʊəˈrektəpɪ, nʊ-] *n* → neurectopia.
neur·en·ter·ic canal [njʊərenˈterɪk, nʊ-] *embryo*. Canalis neurentericus.
neur·ep·i·the·li·al [njʊərˌepɪˈθiːlɪəl, nʊ-] *adj* → neuroepithelial.
neur·ep·i·the·li·um [ˌ-ˌepɪˈθiːlɪəm] *n* → neuroepithelium.
neur·ex·er·e·sis [njʊərekˈserəsɪs, nʊ-] *n neurochir*. Neurexhärese *f*, Neurexhairese *f*.
neu·ri·at·ria [njʊərˈætrɪə, nʊ-] *n* Behandlung *f* von Nervenleiden.
neu·ri·a·try [njʊəˈraɪətrɪ, nʊ-] *n* → neuriatria.
neu·ri·lem·ma [njʊərɪˈlemə, nʊ-] *n* Schwann'-Scheide *f*, Neuri-, Neurolemm *nt*, Neurilemma *nt*.
neurilemma cell Schwann-Zelle *f*.
neu·ri·lem·mal sheath [ˌ-ˈleml] → neurilemma.
neu·ri·lem·mi·tis [ˌ-leˈmaɪtɪs] *n* Entzündung *f* der Schwann'-Scheide, Neuri-, Neurolemmitis *f*.
neu·ri·lem·mo·ma *n* → neurilemoma.
neu·ri·le·mo·ma [ˌ-ləˈməʊmə] *n* Neurilem(m)om *nt*, Neurinom *nt*, Schwannom *nt*.
neu·rin [ˈnjʊərɪn, ˈnʊ-] *n* → neurine.
neu·rine [ˈnjʊərɪn, ˈnʊ-] *n* Neurin *nt*.
neu·ri·no·ma [ˌnjʊərɪˈnəʊmə, ˌnʊ-] *n* → neurilemoma.
neu·rite [ˈnjʊəraɪt, ˈnʊ-] *n* → neuraxon.
neu·rit·ic [njʊəˈrɪtɪk, nʊ-] *adj* Neuritis betr., neuritisch.
neu·ri·tis [ˌ-ˈraɪtɪs] *n* Nervenentzündung *f*, Neuritis *f*.
neuro- *pref*. Nerven-, Neur(o)-.
neu·ro·al·ler·gic polyradiculitis [ˌnjʊərəʊəˈlɜːdʒɪk, ˌnʊ-] neuroallergische Polyradikulitis *f*.
neu·ro·al·ler·gy [ˌ-ˈælərdʒɪ] *n* Neuroallergie *f*.
neu·ro·am·e·bi·a·sis [ˌ-ˌæməˈbaɪəsɪs] *n* Amöbenneuritis *f*.
neu·ro·a·nas·to·mo·sis [ˌ-əˌnæstəˈməʊsɪs] *n neurochir*. Nervenanastomose *f*.
neu·ro·an·a·tom·i·cal [ˌ-ˌænəˈtɒmɪkl] *adj* Neuroanatomie betr., neuroanatomisch.
neu·ro·a·nat·o·my [ˌ-əˈnætəmɪ] *n* Neuroanatomie *f*.
neu·ro·ar·throp·a·thy [ˌ-ɑːˈθrɒpəθɪ] *n* Neuroarthropathie *f*.
neu·ro·bi·ol·o·gist [ˌ-baɪˈɒlədʒɪst] *n* Neurobiologe *m*, -biologin *f*.
neu·ro·bi·ol·o·gy [ˌ-baɪˈɒlədʒɪ] *n* Neurobiologie *f*.
neu·ro·bi·o·tax·is [ˌ-ˌbaɪəʊˈtæksɪs] *n* Neurobiotaxis *f*.
neu·ro·blast [ˈ-blæst] *n* Neuroblast *m*.
neu·ro·blas·to·ma [ˌ-blæsˈtəʊmə] *n patho*. Neuroblastom(a) *nt*.
neu·ro·buc·cal pouch [ˌ-ˈbʌkl] *embryo*. Rathke'-Tasche *f*.
neu·ro·ca·nal [ˌ-kəˈnæl] *n* Rückenmarks-, Spinal-, Wirbelkanal *m*, Canalis vertebralis.
neu·ro·car·di·ac [ˌ-ˈkɑːdɪæk] *adj* Herz u. Nervensystem betr., neurokardial, kardioneural.
neu·ro·cer·a·tin [ˌ-ˈserətɪn] *n* → neurokeratin.
neu·ro·chem·i·cal [ˌ-ˈkemɪkl] *adj* Neurochemie betr., neurochemisch.
neurochemical transmission *physiol*. neurochemische Erregungsübertragung *f*.
neu·ro·chem·is·try [ˌ-ˈkemɪstrɪ] *n* Neurochemie *f*.
neu·ro·chi·tin [ˌ-ˈkaɪtɪn] *n* → neurokeratin.
neu·ro·cho·ri·o·ret·i·ni·tis [ˌ-ˌkɔːrɪəʊretɪˈnaɪtɪs] *n ophthal*. Neurochorioretinitis *f*.
neu·ro·cho·roid·i·tis [ˌ-ˌkɔːrɔɪˈdaɪtɪs, -ˌkəʊ-] *n* Neurochorioiditis *f*.
neu·ro·cir·cu·la·to·ry [ˌ-ˈsɜːkjələˌtəʊrɪ, -ˌtɔː-] *adj* neurozirkulatorisch.
neurocirculatory asthenia neurozirkulatorische Asthenie *f*, Effort-Syndrom *nt*, DaCosta-Syndrom *nt*, Soldatenherz *nt*, Phrenikokardie *f*.
neu·ro·cra·ni·al [ˌ-ˈkreɪnɪəl] *adj* Neurokranium betr., neurokranial.
neu·ro·cra·ni·um [ˌ-ˈkreɪnɪəm] *n* Hirnschädel *m*, Neurokranium *nt*, Neurocranium *nt*.
neu·ro·crine [ˈ-kraɪn] *adj* → neuroendocrine.
neu·ro·cu·ta·ne·ous [ˌ-kjuːˈteɪnɪəs] *adj* Nerv(en) u. Haut betr., neurokutan.
neurocutaneous melanosis neurokutane Melanose *f*, neurokutanes Melanoblastosesyndrom *nt*, Melanosis neurocutanea.
neurocutaneous syndrome Phakomatose *f*, neurokutanes Syndrom *nt*.
neu·ro·cyte [ˈ-saɪt] *n* Nervenzelle *f*, Neurozyt *m*, Neuron *nt*.
neu·ro·cy·tol·o·gy [ˌ-saɪˈtɒlədʒɪ] *n* Neurozytologie *f*.
neu·ro·cy·tol·y·sin [ˌ-saɪˈtɒləsɪn] *n* Neurocytolysin *nt*, -zytolysin *nt*.
neu·ro·cy·tol·y·sis [ˌ-saɪˈtɒləsɪs] *n* Neuronauflösung *f*, Neurozytolyse *f*.
neu·ro·cy·to·ma [ˌ-saɪˈtəʊmə] *n* 1. Neurozytom *nt*, Ganglioneurom *nt*. 2. Neuroepitheliom(a) *nt*.
neu·ro·de·al·gia [ˌ-dɪˈældʒ(ɪ)ə] *n ophthal*. Netzhautschmerz *m*.
neu·ro·de·a·tro·phia [ˌ-dɪəˈtrəʊfɪə] *n ophthal*. Netzhautatrophie *f*.
neu·ro·de·gen·er·a·tive [ˌ-dɪˈdʒenərətɪv, -ˌreɪt-] *adj* neurodegenerativ.
neu·ro·den·drite [ˌ-ˈdendraɪt] *n* Dendrit *m*.
neu·ro·den·dron [ˌ-ˈdendrən] *n* Dendrit *m*.
neu·ro·derm [ˈ-dɜːm] *n* Neuroderm *nt*, neurales Ektoderm *nt*.
neu·ro·der·ma·ti·tis [ˌ-ˌdɜːməˈtaɪtɪs] *n* 1. Neurodermitis *f*, Neurodermatose *f*. 2. atopisches/endogenes/exsudatives/neuropathisches/konstitutionelles Ekzem *nt*, atopische Dermatitis *f*, neurogene Dermatose *f*, Neurodermitis disseminata/diffusa/constitutionalis/atopica, Morbus Besnier *m*, Prurigo Besnier. 2. Vidal'-Krankheit *f*, Lichen Vidal *m*, Lichen simplex chronicus (Vidal), Neurodermitis circumscriptus.
neu·ro·der·ma·to·sis [ˌ-ˌdɜːməˈtəʊsɪs] *n* → neurodermatitis 1.
neu·ro·di·ag·no·sis [ˌ-ˌdaɪəɡˈnəʊsɪs] *n* Neurodiagnose *f*.
neu·ro·di·ag·nos·tic [ˌ-ˌdaɪəɡˈnɒstɪk] *adj* neurodiagnostisch.
neu·ro·dy·nam·ic [ˌ-daɪˈnæmɪk] *adj* neurodynamisch.
neu·ro·dyn·ia [ˌ-ˈdiːnɪə] *n* → neuralgia.
neu·ro·ec·to·derm [ˌ-ˈektədɜːm] *n embryo*. Neuroektoderm *nt*.
neu·ro·ec·to·der·mal [ˌ-ˌektəʊˈdɜːml] *adj* Neuroektoderm betr., neuroektodermal.
neu·ro·ec·to·my [ˌ-ˈektəmɪ] *n* → neurectomy.
neu·ro·ef·fec·tor [ˌ-ɪˈfektər] *n* Neuroeffektor *m*.
neu·ro·en·ceph·a·lo·my·e·lop·a·thy [ˌ-enˌsefələʊmaɪəˈlɒpəθɪ] *n* Neuroenzephalomyelopathie *f*.
neu·ro·en·do·crine [ˌ-ˈendəkrɪn, -kraɪn, -kriːn] *adj* neuroendokrines System betr., neuroendokrin, neurokrin.
neuroendocrine cell neuroendokrine Zelle *f*.
neuroendocrine response neuroendokrine Antwort/Anpassung/Reaktion *f*.
neuroendocrine system neuroendokrines System *nt*, Neuroendokrinium *f*.
neu·ro·en·do·cri·nol·o·gy [ˌ-ˌendəkrɪˈnɒlədʒɪ, -kraɪ-] *n* Neuroendokrinologie *f*.
neu·ro·en·ter·ic canal [ˌ-enˈterɪk] → neurenteric canal.
neu·ro·ep·i·der·mal [ˌ-epɪˈdɜːml] *adj* neuroepidermal.
neu·ro·ep·i·the·li·al [ˌ-epɪˈθiːlɪəl] *adj* Neuroepithel betr., aus Neuroepithel bestehend, neuroepithelial, Neuroepithel-.
neuroepithelial cell 1. *embryo*. Neuroepithelzelle *f*. **2.** → neuroglia cell.
neuroepithelial layer of retina Schicht *f* der Stäbchen u. Zapfen, Stratum neuroepitheliale retinae.
neuroepithelial stratum of retina → neuroepithelial layer of retina.
neuroepithelial tumor neuroepithelialer Tumor *m*.
neu·ro·ep·i·the·li·o·ma [ˌ-epɪˌθiːlɪˈəʊmə] *n* Neuroepitheliom(a) *nt*.
neu·ro·ep·i·the·li·um [ˌ-epɪˈθiːlɪəm] *n* 1. Sinnes-, Neuroepithel *nt*, Neuroepithelium *nt*. 2. *embryo*. Neuroepithelium *nt*.
n. of ampullary crest Sinnes-/Neuroepithel der Crista ampullaris, Neuroepithelium cristae ampullaris.
n. of maculae Sinnes-/Neuroepithel der Maculae, Neuroepithelium macularum.
neu·ro·fi·ber [ˌ-ˈfaɪbər] *n* Nervenfaser *f*, Neurofibra *f*.
neu·ro·fi·bra [ˌ-ˈfaɪbrə] *n*, *pl* **-brae** [-briː] → neurofiber.
neu·ro·fi·bril [ˌ-ˈfaɪbrɪl] *n* Neurofibrille *f*.
neu·ro·fi·bril·lar [ˌ-faɪˈbrɪlər] *adj* Neurofibrille betr., neurofibrillär.
neu·ro·fi·bril·lar·y [ˌ-ˈfaɪbrələrɪ] *adj* → neurofibrillar.
neurofibrillary tangels *patho*. Alzheimer'-Fibrillenveränderungen *pl*, Fädchenplaque *f*.
neu·ro·fi·bro·ma [ˌ-faɪˈbrəʊmə] *n* Neurofibrom(a) *nt*.
neu·ro·fi·bro·ma·to·sis [ˌ-ˌfaɪbrəməˈtəʊsɪs] *n* (von) Recklinghausen-Krankheit *f*, Neurofibromatosis generalisata.
neu·ro·fi·bro·sar·co·ma [ˌ-ˌfaɪbrəsɑːˈkəʊmə] *n* Neurofibrosarkom *nt*.
neu·ro·fil·a·ment [ˌ-ˈfɪləmənt] *n* Neurofilament *nt*.
neu·ro·gan·gli·it·is [ˌ-ˌɡæŋɡlɪˈaɪtɪs] *n old* Ganglionentzündung *f*, Gangliitis *f*.
neu·ro·gan·gli·on [ˌ-ˈɡæŋɡlɪən] *n* Nervenknoten *m*, Ganglion *nt*.
neu·ro·gen [ˈ-dʒən] *n embryo*. Neurogen *nt*.
neu·ro·gen·e·sis [ˌ-ˈdʒenəsɪs] *n* Neurogenese *f*.
neu·ro·ge·net·ic [ˌ-dʒəˈnetɪk] *adj* Neurogenese betr., neurogenetisch.
neu·ro·gen·ic [ˌ-ˈdʒenɪk] *adj* in Nerven(zellen) entstehend, Nerven(gewebe) bildend, neurogen.
neurogenic arthritis neurogene/neuropathische Arthropathie *f*, Arthropathia neuropathica.

neurogenic arthropathy → neurogenic arthritis.
neurogenic atrophy neurogene Muskelatrophie f.
neurogenic bladder neurogene Blase f.
atonic n. neurogene atonische Blase.
uninhibited n. neurogene Überlaufblase.
neurogenic clubfoot ortho. neurogener Klumpfuß m.
neurogenic contracture neurogene Kontraktur f.
neurogenic fracture neurogene Fraktur f.
neurogenic joint → neuropathic joint.
neurogenic shock neurogener Schock m.
neurogenic torticollis neurogener Schiefhals/Torticollis m.
neurogenic tumor neurogener Tumor m.
neurogenic ulcer → neurotrophic ulcer.
neurogenic wryneck → neurogenic torticollis.
neu·rog·e·nous [njʊə'rɒdʒənəs, nʊ-] adj im Nervensystem entstehend, vom Nervensystem stammend, neurogen.
neu·ro·glan·du·lar [njʊərə'glændʒələr, nʊ-] adj neuroglandulär.
neuroglandular synapse neuroglanduläre Synapse f.
neu·rog·li·a [njʊə'rɒglɪə, nʊ-] n Neuroglia f, Glia f.
neuroglia cell Neurogliazelle f, Neurogliozyt m.
neu·rog·li·al [njʊə'rɒglɪəl] adj Neuroglia betr., (neuro-)glial.
neuroglial cell → neuroglia cell.
neu·rog·li·ar [njʊə'rɒglɪər, nʊ-] adj → neuroglial.
neu·rog·li·form cell [njʊə'rɒglɪfɔːrm, nʊ-] Neurogliformzelle f.
neu·rog·li·o·cyte [njʊə'rɒglɪəsaɪt, nʊ-] n → neuroglia cell.
neu·rog·li·o·cy·to·ma [njʊə,rɒglɪəsaɪ'təʊmə, nʊ-] n → neuroglioma.
neu·ro·gli·o·ma [,njʊərəʊglaɪ'əʊmə, ,nʊ-] n Neurogliom nt, Gliom nt, Neuroma verum.
neu·ro·gli·o·ma·to·sis [-,glaɪəmə'təʊsɪs] n Gliomatose f.
neu·rog·li·o·sis [njʊə,rɒglɪ'əʊsɪs, nʊ-] n Gliomatose f.
neu·ro·he·mal [,njʊərəʊ'hiːməl, ,nʊ-] adj neurohämal.
neurohemal zone neurohämale Zone f.
neu·ro·his·tol·o·gy [,-hɪs'tɒlədʒɪ] n Neurohistologie f.
neu·ro·hor·mo·nal [,-'hɔːrməʊnl] adj neurohormonal.
neu·ro·hor·mone [,-'hɔːrməʊn] n Neurohormon nt.
neu·ro·hu·mor·al [,-'(h)juːmərəl] adj neurohumoral.
neurohumoral transmission → neurochemical transmission.
neu·ro·hy·poph·y·se·al [,-haɪ,pɒfə'siːəl, -,haɪpə'fiːzɪəl] adj Neurohypophyse betr., neurohypophysär, Neurohypophysen-.
neu·ro·hy·po·phys·ec·to·my [,-,haɪpɒfɪ'sektəmɪ] n neurochir. Entfernung f der Neurohypophyse, Neurohypophysektomie f.
neu·ro·hy·poph·y·si·al adj → neurohypophyseal.
neurohypophysial hormone Neurohypophysenhormon nt, Hormon nt der Neurohypophyse, (Hypophysen-)Hinterlappenhormon nt, HHL-Hormon nt.
neu·ro·hy·poph·y·sis [,-haɪ'pɒfəsɪs] n Neurohypophyse f, Hypophysenhinterlappen m abbr. HHL, Neurohypophysis f, Lobus posterior hypophyseos.
neu·roid ['njʊərɔɪd, 'nʊ-] adj nervenähnlich, -artig.
neu·ro·im·mu·no·log·ic [,njʊərəʊ,ɪmjənə'lɒdʒɪk, ,nʊ-] adj Neuroimmunologie betr., neuroimmunologisch.
neu·ro·im·mu·nol·o·gy [,-,ɪmjə'nɒlədʒɪ] n Neuroimmunologie f.
neu·ro·ker·a·tin [,-'kerətɪn] n Neurokeratin nt.
neu·ro·lab·y·rin·thi·tis [,-læbərɪn'θaɪtɪs] n HNO, neuro. Neurolabyrinthitis f.
neu·ro·lath·y·rism [,-'læθərɪzəm] n Kichererbsenvergiftung f, Lathyrismus m, Lathyrismus-Syndrom nt.
neu·ro·lem·ma [,-'lemə] n → neurilemma.
neurolemma cell Schwann-Zelle f.
neu·ro·lem·mi·tis [,-lə'maɪtɪs] n → neurilemmitis.
neu·ro·lem·mo·ma [,-lə'məʊmə] n → neurilemoma.
neu·ro·lept·an·al·ge·si·a [,-,leptænl'dʒiːzɪə] n anes. Neuroleptanalgesie f abbr. NLA.
neu·ro·lept·an·al·ge·sic [,-,leptænl'dʒiːzɪk] I n neuroleptanalgetisches Mittel nt. II adj neuroleptanalgetisch.
neu·ro·lept·an·es·the·sia [,-,leptænəs'θiːʒə] n anes. Neuroleptanästhesie f, -narkose f.
neu·ro·lept·an·es·thet·ic [,-,leptænəs'θetɪk] adj neuroleptanästhetisch.
neu·ro·lep·tic [,-'leptɪk] I n Neuroleptikum nt, Antipsychotikum nt. II adj neuroleptisch.
neuroleptic agent/drug → neuroleptic I.
neu·ro·li·po·ma·to·sis [,-laɪ,pəʊmə'təʊsɪs] n Neurolipomatose f, -lipomatosis f.
neu·ro·log·ic [,-'lɒdʒɪk] adj → neurological.
neu·ro·log·i·cal [,-'lɒdʒɪkl] adj neurologisch.
neurologic assessment neurologische Untersuchung f.
neurologic disorder neurologische Störung/Erkrankung f.
neu·rol·o·gist [njʊə'rɒlədʒɪst, nʊ-] n Neurologe m, -login f.
neu·rol·o·gy [njʊə'rɒlədʒɪ, nʊ-] n Neurologie f.
neu·ro·lu·es [,njʊərəʊ'luːiːz, ,nʊ-] n → neurosyphilis.
neu·ro·lymph ['-lɪmf] n Liquor cerebrospinalis.
neu·ro·lym·pho·ma·to·sis [,-,lɪmfəmə'təʊsɪs] n patho. Neurolymphomatose f.
neu·rol·y·sin [njʊə'rɒləsɪn, nʊ-] n Neurolysin nt.
neu·rol·y·sis [njʊə'rɒləsɪs, nʊ-] n 1. operative Nervendekompression f, Neurolyse f. 2. Exoneurolyse f. 3. Endoneurolyse f. 4. Neurolepsis f. 5. Nervenauflösung f, Neurolyse f.
neu·ro·lyt·ic [,njʊərə'lɪtɪk, ,nʊ-] adj neurolytisch.
neu·ro·ma [njʊə'rəʊmə, nʊ-] n Neurom(a) nt.
neu·ro·ma·la·cia [,njʊərəʊmə'leɪʃ(ɪ)ə, ,nʊ-] n patho. Nervenerweichung f, Neuromalazie f, -malacia f.
neu·ro·ma·la·kia [,-mə'leɪkɪə] n → neuromalacia.
neu·ro·ma·to·sis [,-mə'təʊsɪs] n → neurofibromatosis.
neu·ro·mel·a·nin [,-'melənɪn] n Neuromelanin nt.
neu·ro·mi·met·ic [,-mɪ'metɪk] I n neuromimetische Substanz f. II adj neuromimetisch.
neu·ro·mod·u·la·tor [,-'mɒdʒəleɪtər] n Neuromodulator m.
neu·ro·mus·cu·lar [,-'mʌskjələr] adj Muskel(n) u. Nerv(en) betr. od. verbindend, neuromuskulär.
neuromuscular atrophy, progressive Charcot-Marie-Krankheit f, -Syndrom nt, Charcot-Marie-Tooth-Hoffmann-Krankheit f, -Syndrom nt.
neuromuscular block/blockade neuromuskulärer Block m.
neuromuscular blocking agent Muskelrelaxans nt.
neuromuscular compartment Lacuna musculorum.
neuromuscular excitability neuromuskuläre Erregbarkeit f.
neuromuscular junction neuromuskuläre Verbindung(sstelle f) f.
neuromuscular scoliosis ortho. neuromuskuläre Skoliose f.
neuromuscular spindle Muskelspindel f.
neuromuscular transmission neuromuskuläre Erregungsübertragung f.
neuromuscular weakness neuromuskuläre Schwäche f.
neu·ro·my·al ['-maɪəl] adj → neuromuscular.
neu·ro·my·as·the·nia [,-,maɪəs'θiːnɪə] n neuro. Neuromyasthenie f.
neu·ro·my·e·li·tis [,-maɪə'laɪtɪs] n Neuromyelitis f.
neu·ro·my·ic [,-'maɪɪk] adj → neuromuscular.
neu·ro·my·o·ep·i·the·li·al [,-,maɪə,epɪ'θiːlɪəl] adj neuromyoepithelial.
neu·ro·my·o·path·ic [,-maɪə'pæθɪk] adj neuromyopathisch.
neu·ro·my·o·si·tis [,-maɪə'saɪtɪs] n Neuromyositis f.
neu·ron ['njʊərɒn, 'nʊ-] n Nervenzelle f, Neuron n.
n. of latency class I Y-Neuron, Neuron der Latenzklasse I.
n. of latency class II X-Neuron, Neuron der Latenzklasse II.
n. of latency class III W-Neuron, Neuron der Latenzklasse III.
neu·ro·nal ['njʊərənl, njʊə'rəʊnl, nʊ-] adj Neuron betr., neuronal, Neuronen-.
neuronal ceroid lipofuscinosis Stock-Vogt-Spielmeyer-Syndrom nt, Batten-Spielmeyer-Vogt-Syndrom nt, neuronale/juvenile Zeroidlipofuszinose/Ceroidlipofuscinose f, juvenile Form f der amaurotischen Idiotie.
neuronal circuit physiol. Neuronenschaltung f, -kreis m.
neuronal layer, piriform Purkinje-(Zell-)Schicht f, Stratum neurium piriformium.
neuronal memory neuronales Gedächtnis nt.
neuron chain Neuronenkette f.
neuron circuit → neuronal circuit.
neu·rone ['njʊərəʊn, 'nʊ-] n → neuron.
neuro-neuronal synapse neuro-neuronale Synapse f.
neu·ron·ic [njʊə'rɒnɪk, nʊ-] adj Neuron betr., Neuron(en)-, Neuro-.
neu·ron·in [njʊərə'nɪn, 'nʊ-] n Neuronin nt.
neu·ron·i·tis [,njʊərə'naɪtɪs, nʊ-] n 1. Neuron(en)entzündung f, Neuronitis f. 2. old Guillain-Barré-Syndrom nt, (Poly-)Radikuloneuritis f, Neuronitis f.
neu·ro·nog·ra·phy [,-'nɒgrəfɪ] n Neuronographie f.
neu·ron·o·phage [njʊə'rɒnəfeɪdʒ, nʊ-] n Neuro(no)phage m.
neu·ron·o·pha·gia [,njʊərənəʊ'feɪdʒ(ɪ)ə, ,nʊ-] n Neuronophagie f.
neu·ron·oph·a·gy [,njʊərə'nɒfədʒɪ, nʊ-] n → neuronophagia.
neu·ron·o·trop·ic [,njʊərənəʊ'trɒpɪk, -'trəʊp-, ,nʊ-] adj mit besonderer Affinität zu Neuronen, neuronotrop.
neuro-ophthalmologic adj neuroophthalmologisch.
neuro-ophthalmology n Neuroophthalmologie f.

neuro-optic myelitis Devic-Syndrom *nt*, -Krankheit *f*, Neuromyelitis optica.
neuro-otologic *adj* neurootologisch.
neuro-otology *n* Neurootologie *f*.
neu·ro·pap·il·li·tis [ˌnjʊərəʊˌpæpəˈlaɪtɪs, ˌnʊ-] *n* Optikusneuritis *f*, Neuritis n. optici.
neu·ro·pa·ral·y·sis [ˌ-pəˈræləsɪs] *n* neurogene Lähmung/Paralyse *f*, Neuroparalyse *f*.
neu·ro·par·a·lyt·ic [ˌ-ˌpærəˈlɪtɪk] *adj* neuroparalytisch.
neuroparalytic keratitis Keratitis/Keratopathia neuroparalytica.
neu·ro·path·ic [ˌ-ˈpæθɪk] *adj* Neuropathie betr., durch sie bedingt, neuropathisch.
neuropathic amyloidosis neuropathische Amyloidose *f*.
neuropathic arthritis → neuropathic joint.
neuropathic arthropathy → neuropathic joint.
neuropathic atrophy neurogene Muskelatrophie *f*.
neuropathic joint neurogene/neuropathische Arthropathie *f*, Arthropathia neuropathica.
neuropathic scoliosis neuropathische Skoliose *f*.
neuropathic ulcer neurogenes Ulkus *nt*.
neu·ro·path·o·gen·e·sis [ˌ-ˌpæθəˈdʒenəsɪs] *n* Neuropathogenese *f*.
neu·ro·path·o·ge·nic·i·ty [ˌ-ˌpæθədʒəˈnɪsətɪ] *n* Neuropathogenität *f*.
neu·ro·path·o·log·i·cal [ˌ-ˌpæθəˈlɒdʒɪkl] *adj* neuropathologisch.
neu·ro·pa·thol·o·gist [ˌ-pəˈθɒlədʒɪst] *n* Neuropathologe *m*, -login *f*.
neu·ro·pa·thol·o·gy [ˌ-pəˈθɒlədʒɪ] *n* Neuropathologie *f*.
neu·rop·a·thy [njʊəˈrɒpəθɪ, nʊ-] *n* **1.** nicht-entzündliche Nervenerkrankung *f*, Neuropathie *f*. **2.** Nervenleiden *nt*, Neuropathie *f*.
neu·ro·pep·tide [ˌnjʊərəʊˈpeptaɪd, ˌnʊ-] *n* Neuropeptid *nt*.
neu·ro·phage [ˈ-feɪdʒ] *n* Neuro(no)phage *m*.
neu·ro·phar·ma·co·log·ic [ˌ-ˌfɑːməkəˈlɒdʒɪk] *adj* Neuropharmakologie betr., neuropharmakologisch.
neu·ro·phar·ma·co·log·i·cal [ˌ-ˌfɑːməkəˈlɒdʒɪkl] *adj* → neuropharmacologic.
neu·ro·phar·ma·col·o·gy [ˌ-ˌfɑːrməˈkɑlədʒɪ] *n* Neuropharmakologie *f*.
neu·ro·phil·ic [ˌ-ˈfɪlɪk] *adj* → neurotropic.
neu·roph·thal·mol·o·gy [ˌ-fθælˈmɒlədʒɪ, ˌnʊ-] *n* → neuro-ophthalmology.
neu·ro·phy·sin [ˌnjʊərəʊˈfaɪsɪn, ˌnʊ-] *n* Neurophysin *nt*.
neu·ro·phys·i·o·log·ic [ˌ-ˌfɪzɪəˈlɒdʒɪk] *adj* Neurophysiologie betr., neurophysiologisch.
neu·ro·phys·i·o·log·i·cal [ˌ-ˌfɪzɪəˈlɒdʒɪkl] *adj* → neurophysiologic.
neu·ro·phys·i·ol·o·gist [ˌ-ˌfɪzɪˈɒlədʒɪst] *n* Neurophysiologe *m*, -physiologin *f*.
neu·ro·phys·i·ol·o·gy [ˌ-ˌfɪzɪˈɒlədʒɪ] *n* Neurophysiologie *f*.
neu·ro·pil [ˈ-pɪl] *n* Nervenfilz *m*, Neuropil *nt*.
neu·ro·pile [ˈ-paɪl] *n* → neuropil.
neu·ro·plasm [ˈ-plæzəm] *n* Neuroplasma *nt*.
neu·ro·plas·mic [ˌ-ˈplæzmɪk] *adj* Neuroplasma betr., neuroplasmatisch.
neu·ro·plas·ty [ˈ-plæstɪ] *n neurochir.* Nerven-, Neuroplastik *f*.
neu·ro·plex·us [ˌ-ˈpleksəs] *n* Nervenplexus *m*.
neu·ro·ple·gic [ˌ-ˈpliːdʒɪk] *adj* neuroplegisch.

neu·ro·po·di·on [ˌ-ˈpəʊdɪˌɒn] *n* → neuropodium.
neu·ro·po·di·um [ˌ-ˈpəʊdɪəm] *n*, *pl* **-dia** [-dɪə] Endfüßchen *nt*.
neu·ro·pore [ˈ-pɔːr] *n embryo.* Neuroporus *m*.
neu·ro·po·ten·tial [ˌ-pəˈtentʃl] *n* Nervenpotential *nt*.
neu·ro·psy·chi·at·ric [ˌ-ˌsaɪkɪˈætrɪk] *adj* neuropsychiatrisch.
neu·ro·psy·chi·a·trist [ˌ-sɪˈkaɪətrɪst, -saɪ-] *n* Neuropsychiater(in *f*) *m*.
neu·ro·psy·chi·a·try [ˌ-sɪˈkaɪətrɪ, -saɪ-] *n* Neuropsychiatrie *f*, Neurologie u. Psychiatrie *f*.
neu·ro·psy·chic [ˌ-ˈsaɪkɪk] *adj* neuropsychisch.
neu·ro·psy·cho·log·i·cal [ˌ-ˌsaɪkəˈlɒdʒɪkl] *adj* neuropsychologisch.
neu·ro·psy·chol·o·gy [ˌ-saɪˈkɒlədʒɪ] *n* Neuropsychologie *f*.
neu·ro·psy·cho·phar·ma·col·o·gy [ˌ-ˌsaɪkəˌfɑːrməˈkɒlədʒɪ] *n* Psychopharmakologie *f*.
neu·ro·ra·di·o·log·ic [ˌ-ˌreɪdɪəˈlɒdʒɪk] *adj* Neuroradiologie betr., neuroradiologisch.
neu·ro·ra·di·ol·o·gy [ˌ-ˌreɪdɪˈɒlədʒɪ] *n* Neuroradiologie *f*.
neu·ro·ret·i·ni·tis [ˌ-ˌretɪˈnaɪtɪs] *n neuro., ophthal.* Neuroretinitis *f*.
neu·ro·ret·i·nop·a·thy [ˌ-ˌretɪˈnɒpəθɪ] *n ophthal.* Neuroretinopathie *f*.
neu·ro·roent·gen·og·ra·phy [ˌ-ˌrentɡəˈnɒɡrəfɪ] *n* → neuroradiology.
neu·ror·rha·phy [njʊəˈrɒːrəfɪ, nʊ-] *n neurochir.* Nervennaht *f*, Neurorrhaphie *f*.
neu·ro·sar·co·ma [ˌnjʊərəsɑːrˈkəʊmə, ˌnʊ-] *n* Neurosarkom *nt*.
neu·ro·schwan·no·ma [ˌ-ʃwæˈnəʊmə] *n* → neurilemoma.
neu·ro·scle·ro·sis [ˌ-sklɪˈrəʊsɪs] *n* Nervensklerose *f*.
neu·ro·se·cre·tion [ˌ-sɪˈkriːʃn] *n* **1.** Neurosekretion *f*. **2.** Neurosekret *nt*.
neu·ro·se·cre·to·ry [ˌ-sɪˈkriːtərɪ] *adj* Neurosekretion betr., neurosekretorisch.
neurosecretory cell neurosekretorische (Nerven)Zelle *f*, neurosekretorisches Neuron *nt*.
neurosecretory neuron → neurosecretory cell.
neu·ro·sen·so·ry [ˌ-ˈsensərɪ] *adj* neurosensorisch.
neu·ro·sis [njʊəˈrəʊsɪs, nʊ-] *n*, *pl* **-ses** [-siːz] Neurose *f*, Neurosis *f*.
neu·ro·skel·e·ton [ˌ-ˈskelətn, ˌnʊ-] *n* Innen-, Endo-, Entoskelett *nt*.
neu·ro·spasm [ˈ-spæzəm] *n* neurogener Muskelkrampf *m*.
neu·ro·splanch·nic [ˌ-ˈsplæŋknɪk] *adj* → neurovisceral.
neu·ro·spon·gi·o·ma [ˌ-spʌndʒɪˈəʊmə] *n* Gliageschwulst *f*, -tumor *m*, Gliom(a) *nt*.
Neu·ros·po·ra [njʊəˈrɒspərə, nʊ-] *n micro.* Brotschimmel *m*, Neurospora *f*.
neu·ro·sta·tus [ˌ-ˈsteɪtəs, ˌnʊ-] *n* Neurostatus *m*.
neu·ro·sur·geon [ˌ-ˈsɜːdʒən] *n* Neurochirurg(in *f*) *m*.
neu·ro·sur·ger·y [ˌ-ˈsɜːdʒərɪ] *n* Neurochirurgie *f*.
neu·ro·sur·gi·cal [ˌ-ˈsɜːdʒɪkl] *adj* neurochirurgisch.
neu·ro·su·ture [ˌ-ˈsuːtʃər] *n* → neurorrhaphy.
neu·ro·syph·i·lis [ˌ-ˈsɪf(ə)lɪs] *n* Neurosyphilis *f*, Neurolues *f*.
neu·ro·ten·di·nal spindle [ˌ-ˈtendɪnl] Golgi'-Sehnenorgan *nt*, -Sehnenspindel *f*.
neu·ro·ten·di·nous [ˌ-ˈtendɪnəs] *adj* Nerv(en) u. Sehne(n) betr., neurotendinös.
neurotendinous spindle Golgi'-Sehnenorgan *nt*, -Sehnenspindel *f*.
neu·ro·ten·sin [ˌ-ˈtensɪn] *n* Neurotensin *nt*.
neu·ro·ten·sion [ˌ-ˈtenʃn] *n* → neurotony.
neu·ro·ther·a·peu·tics [ˌ-ˌθerəˈpjuːtɪks] *pl* Behandlung *f* von Nervenleiden, Neurotherapie *f*.
neu·ro·ther·a·py [ˌ-ˈθerəpɪ] *n* → neurotherapeutics.
neu·rot·ic [njʊəˈrɒtɪk, nʊ-] **I** *n* Neurotiker(in *f*) *m*, Nervenkranke(r *m*) *f*. **II** *adj* **1.** *psychia.* an einer Neurose leidend, auf einer Neurose beruhend, neurotisch, Neurosen-. **2.** *old patho.* nervenleidend, -krank, Nerven-.
neurotic atrophy neurogene Muskelatrophie *f*.
neurotic depression *psychia.* depressive Neurose *f*, neurotische Depression *f*.
neu·rot·i·cism [njʊəˈrɒtəsɪzəm, nʊ-] *n psychia.* Neurotizismus *m*.
neu·rot·i·gen·ic [njʊəˌrɒtɪˈdʒenɪk, nʊ-] *psychia.* eine Neurose hervorrufend, neurotigen.
neu·rot·me·sis [ˌnjʊərɒtˈmiːsɪs, ˌnʊ-] *n patho.* Neurotmesis *f*.
neu·ro·tol·o·gy [njʊərəˈtɒlədʒɪ, ˌnʊ-] *n* → neuro-otology.
neu·ro·tome [ˈ-təʊm] *n neurochir.* Neurotom *nt*.
neu·ro·to·mog·ra·phy [ˌ-təˈmɒɡrəfɪ] *n radiol.* Neurotomographie *f*.
neu·rot·o·my [njʊəˈrɒtəmɪ, nʊ-] *n neurochir.* Nervenschnitt *m*, -durchtrennung *f*, Neurotomie *f*.
neu·ro·to·nia [ˌnjʊərəˈtəʊnɪə, ˌnʊ-] *n neuro., psychia.* Neurotonie *f*.
neu·ro·ton·ic [ˌ-ˈtɒnɪk] *adj* neurotonisch.
neurotonic reaction neurotonische Reaktion *f*.
neu·rot·o·ny [njʊəˈrɒtənɪ, nʊ-] *n* therapeutische Nervendehnung *f*, Neurotonie *f*.
neu·ro·tox·ic [ˌnjʊərəˈtæksɪk, ˌnʊ-] *adj* neurotoxisch.
neu·ro·tox·ic·i·ty [ˌ-tækˈsɪsətɪ] *n* Nervengiftigkeit *f*, Neurotoxizität *f*.
neu·ro·tox·in [ˌ-ˈtæksɪn] *n* Nervengift *nt*, Neurotoxin *nt*.
neu·ro·trans·mit·ter [ˌ-ˈtrænzmɪtər] *n* Neurotransmitter *m*.
neu·ro·trau·ma [ˌ-ˈtrɔːmə, -ˈtraʊmə] *n* Nervenverletzung *f*, -trauma *nt*.
neu·ro·trip·sy [ˌ-ˈtrɪpsɪ] *n neurochir.* operative Nervenquetschung *f*, Neurotripsie *f*.
neu·ro·troph·ic [ˌ-ˈtrɒfɪk, -ˈtrəʊ-] *adj* Neurotrophie betr., neurotroph(isch).
neurotrophic atrophy neurotroph(isch)e Atrophie *f*.
neurotrophic ulcer neurotrophische Ulzeration *f*, trophoneurotisches Ulkus *nt*, Ulcus trophoneuroticum.
neu·rot·ro·phy [njʊəˈrɒtrəfɪ, nʊ-] *n* Neurotrophie *f*.
neu·ro·trop·ic [ˌnjʊərəˈtrɒpɪk, -ˈtrəʊ-, ˌnʊ-] *adj* auf Nerven(gewebe) wirkend, mit besonderer Affinität zu Nerven(gewebe), neurotrop.
neurotropic virus neurotropes Virus *nt*.
neu·rot·ro·pism [njʊəˈrɒtrəpɪzəm, nʊ-] *n* Neurotropie *f*.
neu·rot·ro·py [njʊəˈrɒtrəpɪ, nʊ-] *n* → neurotropism.
neu·ro·tro·sis [ˌnjʊərəˈtrəʊsɪs, ˌnʊ-] *n* → neurotrauma.
neu·ro·tu·bule [ˌ-ˈt(j)uːbjuːl] *n* Neurotubulus *m*.
neu·ro·vac·cine [ˌ-ˈvæksiːn] *n* Neurovakzine *f*.
neu·ro·var·i·co·sis [ˌ-ˌværɪˈkəʊsɪs] *n neuro.* Neurovarikose *f*.

neu·ro·var·i·cos·i·ty [ˌ-ˌværɪ'kɑsətɪ] *n* neuro. Neurovarikose *f*.
neu·ro·va·ri·o·la [ˌ-və'raɪələ] *n* → neurovaccine.
neu·ro·vas·cu·lar [ˌ-'væskjələr] *adj* neurovaskulär.
neurovascular bundle Gefäßnervenbündel *nt*.
neurovascular trunk Gefäßnervenstamm *m*.
neu·ro·veg·e·ta·tive [ˌ-'vedʒəteɪtɪv] *adj* das vegetative Nervensystem betr., neurovegetativ.
neu·ro·vir·u·lence [ˌ-'vɪr(j)ələns] *n* Neurovirulenz *f*.
neu·ro·vir·u·lent [ˌ-'vɪr(j)ələnt] *adj* neurovirulent.
neu·ro·vi·rus [ˌ-'vaɪrəs] *n micro.* Neurovirus *nt*.
neu·ro·vis·cer·al [ˌ-'vɪsərəl] *adj* Nervensystem u. Eingeweide betr., neuroviszeral.
neu·ru·la ['njʊərələ, 'nʊ-] *n, pl* **-las, -lae** [-liː, -laɪ] *embryo.* Neurula *f*.
neu·ru·la·tion [ˌnjʊərə'leɪʃn, ˌnʊ-] *n embryo.* Neurulation *f*.
neu·tral ['n(j)uːtrəl] *adj* neutral; unbestimmt, indifferent (*to* gegenüber).
neutral axis *mathe., phys.* Nullinie *f*, neutrale Achse *f*.
neutral fat Neutralfett *nt*.
neutral β-galactosidase deficiency Lactosylceramidose *f*, neutrale β-Galaktosidase-Defekt *m*.
neu·tral·i·ty [n(j)uː'trælətɪ] *n* Neutralität *f*.
neu·tral·i·za·tion [ˌn(j)uːtrəlɪ'zeɪʃn, -laɪ-] *n* Neutralisierung *f*, Neutralisation *f*, Ausgleich *m*, Aufhebung *f*.
neutralization test *micro.* Neutralisationstest *m abbr.* NT.
neu·tral·ize ['n(j)uːtrəlaɪz] *vt* ausgleichen, aufheben, unwirksam *od.* unschädlich machen, neutralisieren.
neu·tra·liz·ing antibody ['n(j)uːtrəlaɪzɪŋ] neutralisierender Antikörper *m*.
neutral range Indifferenzbereich *m*.
neutral reaction *chem.* neutrale Reaktion *f*.
neutral red Neutralrot *nt*.
neutral salt *chem.* Neutralsalz *nt*.
neu·tri·no [n(j)uː'triːnəʊ] *n, pl* **-nos** *phys.* Neutrino *nt*.
neu·tro·cyte ['n(j)uːtrəsaɪt] *n* → neutrophil 1.
neu·tro·cy·to·pe·nia [ˌ-ˌsaɪtə'piːnɪə] *n* → neutropenia.
neu·tro·cy·to·sis [ˌ-saɪ'təʊsɪs] *n* → neutrophilia.
neu·tron ['n(j)uːtrɒn] *n phys.* Neutron *nt*.
neutron activation (analysis) *phys.* Neutronenaktivierungsanalyse *f*.
neutron number *phys. abbr.* **N** Neutronenzahl *f*.
neu·tro·pe·nia [ˌn(j)uːtrə'piːnɪə] *n* Neutropenie *f*, Neutrozytopenie *f*.
neu·tro·pe·nic [ˌ-'piːnɪk] *adj* neutropenisch.
neutropenic angina Agranulozytose *f*.
neu·tro·phil ['-fɪl] I *n* 1. neutrophiler/polymorphkerniger Granulozyt *m abbr.* PNG, neutrophiler Leukozyt *m*; *inf.* Neutrophiler *m*. 2. neutrophile Zelle *od.* Substanz *f*. II *adj* neutrophil.
neutrophil chemotactic factor *abbr.* **NCF** Neutrophilen-chemotaktischer Faktor *m abbr.* NCF.
neu·tro·phile ['-faɪl] *n, adj* → neutrophil.
neu·tro·phil·ia [ˌ-'fɪlɪə] *n* Neutrophilie *f*, Neutrozytose *f*.
neu·tro·phil·ic [ˌ-'fɪlɪk] *adj* → neutrophil II.
neutrophilic cell → neutrophil 1.
neutrophilic granulocyte → neutrophil 1.
neutrophilic leukocyte → neutrophil 1.
neutrophilic leukocytosis Neutrophilie *f*.
neutrophilic leukopenia Neutropenie *f*.
neutrophilic myelocyte neutrophiler Myelozyt *m*.
neutrophilic series → neutrophil series.
neutrophil series *hema.* neutrophile Reihe *f*.
neu·tro·pism ['-pɪzəm] *n* → neurotropism.
neu·tro·tax·is [ˌ-'tæksɪs] *n* Neutrotaxis *f*.
nev- *pref.* → nevo-.
ne·vi *pl* → nevus.
nevo- *pref.* Nävus-, Nävo-.
ne·vo·cel·lu·lar nevus [ˌniːvəʊ'seljələr] → nevus cell nevus.
ne·vo·cyte ['-saɪt] *n* → nevus cell.
ne·vo·cyt·ic [ˌ-'sɪtɪk] *adj* aus Nävuszellen bestehend, nävozytisch.
nevocytic nevus → nevus cell nevus.
ne·void ['niːvɔɪd] *adj* nävusähnlich, -artig, nävoid.
nevoid amentia Brushfield-Wyatt-Syndrom *nt*.
nevoid basal cell carcinoma syndrome → nevoid basalioma syndrome.
nevoid basalioma syndrome Gorlin-Goltz-Syndrom *nt*, Basalzellnävus-Syndrom *nt*, nävoides Basalzell(en)karzinom-Syndrom *nt*, nävoide Basaliome *pl*, Naevobasaliome *pl*, Naevobasaliomatose *f*.
nevoid cyst nävoide Zyste *f*.
nevoid hypertrichosis naevoide Hypertrichose *f*.
nevoid lipoma Angiolipom(a) *nt*.
ne·vo·li·po·ma [ˌniːvəʊlaɪ'pəʊmə, -lɪ-] *n* Nävolipom *nt*, Naevus lipomatosus.
ne·vose ['niːvəʊs] *adj* 1. mit Nävi besetzt, Nävus-. 2. → nevoid.
ne·vous ['niːvəs] *adj* 1. → nevose. 2. → nevoid.
ne·vo·xan·tho·en·do·the·li·o·ma [ˌniːvəˌzænθəʊˌendəʊˌθiːlɪ'əʊmə] *n* juveniles Riesenzellgranulom *nt*, juveniles Xanthom/Xanthogranulom *nt*, Naevoxanthoendotheliom *nt*, Naevoxanthom *nt*.
ne·vus ['niːvəs] *n, pl* **-vi** [-vaɪ] 1. (Mutter-)Mal *nt*, Nävus *m*, Naevus *m*. 2. → nevus cell nevus.
nevus cell Nävuszelle *f*, Nävozyt *m*.
nevus cell nevus Nävuszell(en)nävus *m abbr.* NZN, Naevus naevocellularis.
nevus elasticus of Lewandowsky Naevus elasticus Lewandowsky.
nevus sebaceus of Jadassohn Talgdrüsennävus Jadassohn *m*, Nävolipom *nt*, Naevus sebaceus/lipomatosus.
new·born ['n(j)uːbɔːrn] I *n* Neugeborene(s) *nt*. II *adj* neugeboren.
newborn infant Neugeborene(s) *nt*.
newborn pneumonitis virus *micro.* Sendai-Virus *nt*.
new candle ['n(j)uː] *phys.* Candela *f abbr.* cd.
New·cas·tle disease ['n(j)uːkæsl, -kɑːsl] atypische Geflügelpest *f*, Newcastle disease (*nt*).
Newcastle disease virus *abbr.* **NDV** Newcastle-disease-Virus *nt abbr.* NDV.
new growth Neubildung *f*, Neoplasma *nt*, Geschwulst *f*.
Newton ['n(j)uːtn]: **N.'s disk** *phys.* Newton-Scheibe *f*.
N.'s law Newton'-Gravitationsgesetz *nt*.
N.'s rings Newton'-Ringe *pl*.
new·ton ['n(j)uːtn] *n abbr.* **N** Newton *nt abbr.* N.
New·to·ni·an [n(j)uː'təʊnɪən]: **N. aberration** chromatische Aberration *f*, Newton-Aberration *f*.
N. constant of gravitation Gravitationskonstante *f*.
N. fluid *phys.* Newton'-Flüssigkeit *f*, homogene Flüssigkeit *f*.
N. force Newton'-Kraft *f*.
N. mechanics Newton'-Mechanik *f*.
non-N. fluid heterogene Flüssigkeit *f*, nicht-Newton'-Flüssigkeit *f*.
New World hookworm *micro.* Todeswurm *m*, Necator americanus.
New World leishmaniasis amerikanische/mukokutane Leishmaniose *f*, Haut--Schleimhaut-Leishmaniase (Südamerikas) *f*, Leishmaniasis americana.
New York City medium → NYC medium.
nex·us ['neksəs] *n, pl* **nex·us** *histol.* Nexus *m*, gap junction (*f*).
Nezelof [nɛzə'lɒf]: **N. syndrome** Nézelof--Krankheit *f*, -Syndrom *nt*, Immundefekt *m* vom Nézelof-Typ.
ng *abbr.* → nanogram.
NGF *abbr.* → nerve growth factor.
NG tube Nasensonde *f*, Nasen-Magen--Sonde *f*.
NH$_2$-terminal *adj biochem.* N-terminal, aminoterminal.
Ni *abbr.* → nickel.
ni·a·cin ['naɪəsɪn] *n* Niacin *nt*, Nikotin-, Nicotinsäure *f*.
ni·a·cin·a·mide [ˌnaɪə'sɪnəmaɪd] *n* → nicotinamide.
nic·co·lum ['nɪkələm] *n* → nickel.
ni·cer·go·line [naɪ'sɜːrgəliːn] *n pharm.* Nicergolin *nt*.
niche [nɪtʃ, niːʃ] *n (a. radiol.)* Nische *f*.
niche cell Nischenzelle *f*, Alveolarzelle *f* Typ II, Pneumozyt *m* Typ II.
niche sign *radiol.* Haudek-Nische *f*.
nick·el ['nɪkl] *n abbr.* **Ni** Nickel *nt abbr.* Ni.
nickel dermatitis Kontaktdermatitis *f* bei Nickelallergie.
Nickerson-Kveim ['nɪkərsən k(ə)'veɪm]: **N.-K. test** Kveim-Hauttest *m*, Kveim--Nickerson-Test *m*.
ni·clo·sa·mide [nɪ'kləʊsəmaɪd] *n pharm.* Niclosamid *nt*.
Nicol ['nɪkəl]: **N. prism** Nicol'-Prisma *nt*.
Nicoladoni [nɪkələ'dəʊnɪ]: **N.'s sign** Nicoladoni-Branham-Zeichen *nt*.
N.'s suture/technique Nicoladoni-Sehnennaht *f*.
Nicolaier ['nɪkəlaɪər]: **N.'s bacillus** Tetanusbazillus *m*, -erreger *m*, Wundstarrkrampfbazillus *m*, -erreger *m*, Clostridium/Plectridium tetani.
Nicolas-Favre [nɪkɔ'la 'faːvrə]: **N.-F. disease** Morbus Durand-Nicolas-Favre *m*, klimatischer Bubo *m*, vierte Geschlechtskrankheit *f*, Lymphogranuloma inguinale/venereum *abbr.* LGV, Lymphopathia venerea, Poradenitis inguinalis.
nic·o·tin·a·mide [ˌnɪkə'tɪnəmaɪd] *n* → Nicotin(säure)amid *nt*.
nicotinamide-adenine dinucleotide *abbr.* **NAD** Nicotinamid-adenin-dinucleotid *nt abbr.* NAD, Diphosphopyridinnucleotid *nt abbr.* DPN, Cohydrase I *f*, Coenzym I *nt*.
nicotinamide-adenine dinucleotide phosphate *abbr.* **NADP** Nicotinamid--adenin-dinucleotid-phosphat *nt abbr.* NADP, Triphosphopyridinnucleotid *nt abbr.* TPN, Cohydrase II *f*, Coenzym II *nt*.
nicotinamide mononucleotide *abbr.* **NMN** Nicotinamid-mononucleotid *nt abbr.* NMN.
nic·o·tine ['nɪkətiːn] *n* Nikotin *nt*, Nicotin *nt*.
nicotine content Nikotingehalt *m*.
nic·o·tine·less ['-lɪs] *adj* nikotinfrei.
nicotine-stained *adj* (*Finger*) nikotingelb.
nic·o·tin·ic [nɪkə'tiːnɪk] *adj* nikotinartig, -haltig, nikotinerg, Nikotin-.

nicotinic acid

nicotinic acid → niacin.
nicotinic acid mononucleotide Nicotinsäuremononucleotid *nt*.
nicotinic receptor nikotinerger Rezeptor *m*.
nic·o·tin·ism ['nɪkətɪnɪzəm] *n* Nikotinvergiftung *f*, Nikoti(a)nismus *m*, Nicotinismus *m*.
nic·o·tin·ize ['nɪkətɪnaɪz] *vt chem*. mit Nikotin vergiften *od*. sättigen.
nic·ta·tion [nɪk'teɪʃn] *n* → nictitation.
nic·ti·tat·ing spasm ['nɪktɪteɪtɪŋ] Blinzelkrampf *m*, Spasmus nictitans.
nic·ti·ta·tion [‚nɪktə'teɪʃn] *n* Blinzeln *nt*, Niktation *f*, Nictitatio *f*, Nictatio *f*.
ni·dal ['naɪdl] *adj* Nidus betr., Nidus-.
ni·da·tion [naɪ'deɪʃn] *n* Einnistung *f* des Eies, Nidation *f*, Implantation *f*.
NIDD *abbr*. → non-insulin-dependent diabetes.
NIDDM *abbr*. [non-insulin-dependent diabetes mellitus] → non-insulin-dependent diabetes.
ni·dus ['naɪdəs] *n*, *pl* **-di** [-daɪ] **1.** Nest *nt*, Nidus *m*. **2.** *patho*. Fokus *m*, Nidus *m*. **3.** Kern *m*, Zentrum *nt*.
Niemann ['niːmən; -man]: **N. disease/splenomegaly** → Niemann-Pick disease.
Niemann-Pick [pɪk]: **N.-P. cells** Niemann-Pick-Zellen *pl*.
N.-P. disease Niemann-Pick-Krankheit *f*, Sphingomyelinose *f*, Sphingomyelinlipidose *f*.
ni·fed·i·pine [naɪ'fedəpiːn] *n pharm*. Nifedipin *nt*.
ni·fur·a·tel [naɪ'fjʊərətel] *n pharm*. Nifuratel *nt*.
ni·fur·pra·zine [naɪfərprə'zaɪn] *n pharm*. Nifurprazin *nt*.
ni·fur·ti·mox [naɪ'fjʊərtɪmɑks] *n pharm*. Nifurtimox *nt*.
night [naɪt] *n* **1.** Nacht *f*. ~ **after** ~ jede Nacht. **at ~/by ~** nachts, bei Nacht. **all ~ (long)** die ganze Nacht. **to be on ~s** Nachtdienst *od*. -schicht haben. ~ **and day** Tag u. Nacht. **to have a good ~('s sleep)** gut schlafen. **to have a bad ~('s sleep)** schlecht schlafen. **in/during the ~** in/während der Nacht. **last ~** gestern Abend; letzte *od*. heute Nacht. **late at ~** (tief) in der Nacht. **over ~** über Nacht. **to work ~s** nachts arbeiten. **2.** Abend *m*.
night bell Nachtglocke *f*.
night-blind *adj* nachtblind.
night blindness Nachtblindheit *f*, Hemeralopie *f*.
night chair Nachtstuhl *m*.
night-clothes ['naɪtkləʊ(ð)z] *pl* Nachtzeug *nt*, -wäsche *pl*.
night-dress ['naɪtdres] *n* → nightgown.
night-gown ['naɪtgaʊn] *n* (Damen-, Kinder-)Nachthemd *nt*.
night hospital Nachtklinik *f*.
night·ie ['naɪtɪ] *n inf*. → nightgown.
night-light *n* Nachtlicht *nt*.
night-long ['naɪtlɔŋ, -lɑŋ] *adj* die ganze Nacht (dauernd); nächtelang.
night·ly ['naɪtlɪ] *adj* jede Nacht, (all-)nächtlich, Nacht-; jeden Abend, (all-)abendlich, Abend-.
night·mare ['naɪtmeər] *n* Alp(drücken *nt*) *m*, Alptraum *m*; *fig*. Alptraum *m*, Grauen *nt*.
night·mar·ish ['naɪt'meərɪʃ] *adj* alptraum-, grauenhaft.
night nurse Nachtschwester *f*, -pfleger *m*.
night pain nächtlicher Schmerz *m*, Nyktalgie *f*.
night porter Nachtportier *m*.
night robe → nightgown.
night·shade ['naɪtʃeɪd] *n bot*. Nachtschatten(gewächs *nt*) *m*, Solanum *nt*.

night shift Nachtschicht *f*. **to be/work on ~** Nachtschicht haben *od*. arbeiten.
night-shirt ['naɪtʃərt] *n* (Herren-)Nachthemd *nt*.
night sight *ophthal*. Tagblindheit *f*, Nykteralopie *f*, Nyktalopie *f*.
night splint *ortho*. Nachtschiene *f*.
night staff (*Klinik*) Nachtpersonal *nt*.
night·stand ['naɪtstænd] *n* → night table.
night·stool ['naɪtstuːl] *n* Nachtstuhl *m*.
night table Nachttisch *m*.
night terror(s) *ped*. Nachtangst *f*, Pavor nocturnus.
night-time *n* Nacht(zeit *f*) *f*. **at ~** nachts, zur Nachtzeit. **in the ~** nachts, in der Nacht.
night vision skotopes Sehen *nt*, Dämmerungs-, Nachtsehen *nt*, Skotop(s)ie *f*.
night work Nachtarbeit *f*.
ni·gra ['naɪgrə] *n anat*. Substantia nigra.
ni·gral ['naɪgrəl] *adj* Substantia nigra betr.
ni·gri·cans ['naɪgrɪkæns, 'nɪg-] *adj* schwärzlich.
ni·gri·ti·es [naɪ'grɪʃɪˌiːz] *n* Schwarzfärbung *f*, Nigrities *f*.
ni·gro·pal·li·dal fibers [‚naɪgrəʊ'pælɪdl] nigropallidale Fasern *pl*.
ni·gro·sin ['-sɪn] *n* Nigrosin *nt*.
ni·gro·sine ['-siːn] *n* → nigrosin.
ni·gro·stri·a·tal fibers [‚-strɪ'eɪtl] nigrostriatale Fasern *pl*, Fibrae nigrostriatales.
nigrostriatal system nigrostriatales System *nt*.
ni·hil·ism ['naɪəlɪzəm] *n* Nihilismus *m*.
ni·hil·is·tic delusion [naɪə'lɪstɪk] nihilistischer Wahn *m*.
Nikolsky [nɪ'kɑlskɪ]: **N.'s sign** Nikolski-Phänomen *nt*.
nine-mile fever [naɪn] Balkangrippe *f*, Q-Fieber *nt*.
nin·hy·drin [nɪn'haɪdrɪn] *n* Ninhydrin *nt*, Triketohydrindenhydrat *nt*.
ninhydrin reaction Ninhydrinreaktion *f*.
ninhydrin test Ninhydrintest *m*, Moberg-Test *m*.
ninth nerve [naɪnθ] Glossopharyngeus *m*, IX. Hirnnerv *m*, N. glossopharyngeus [IX].
ni·o·bi·um [naɪ'əʊbɪəm] *n abbr*. **Nb** Niob *nt* *abbr*. Nb.
ni·per·yt ['naɪpərɪt] *n pharm*. Pentaerythrityl-Tetranitrat *nt*.
nip·ple ['nɪpl] *n* **1.** Brustwarze *f*, Mamille *f*, Mamilla *f*, Papilla mammaria. **2.** (*Saugflasche*) (Gummi-)Sauger *m*.
nipple bud *embryo*. Warzenknospe *f*.
nipple discharge 1. Ausfluß *m* aus der Brustwarze. **2.** Brustwarzensekret *nt*.
nipple inversion (Brust-)Warzeneinziehung *f*.
nipple line Mamillarlinie *f*, Linea mamillaris.
Nisbet ['nɪsbet]: **N.'s chancre** Bubonulus *m*, Lymphangiitis dorsalis penis.
Nissen ['nɪsn]: **N. fundoplication** Fundoplikation *f* nach Nissen, Fundoplicatio *f*.
N. operation → N. fundoplication.
N. total fundoplication → N. fundoplication.
Nissl ['nɪsl]: **N. bodies** Nissl-Schollen *pl*, -Substanz *f*, -Granula *pl*, Tigroidschollen *pl*.
N. degeneration Nissl-Degeneration *f*.
N. granules → N. bodies.
N.'s method → N.'s stain.
N.'s stain Nissl-Färbung *f*.
N. substance → N. bodies.
nit [nɪt] *n micro*. Nisse *f*.
Nitabuch ['niːtəbʊk; 'niːtabuːx]: **N.'s layer/stria/zone** *embryo*. Nitabuch'-Fibrinstreifen *m*.

ni·ta·vi·rus [‚naɪtə'vaɪrəs] *n micro*. Nitavirus *nt*.
ni·ter ['naɪtər] *n* Kaliumnitrat *nt*, Kalisalpeter *m*.
ni·ton ['naɪtɑn] *n* Radon *nt abbr*. Rn.
ni·tra·tase ['naɪtrəteɪz] *n* → nitrate reductase.
ni·trate ['naɪtreɪt] **I** *n* Nitrat *nt*. **II** *vt* **1.** mit Salpetersäure behandeln. **2.** in ein Nitrat umwandeln.
nitrate broth *micro*. Nitratboullion *f*.
nitrate reductase Nitratreduktase *f*.
nitrate reduction test *micro*. Nitratreduktionstest *m*.
nitrate respiration *bio*. Nitratatmung *f*.
ni·tra·tion [naɪ'treɪʃn] *n chem*. Nitrierung *f*.
ni·tra·ze·pam [naɪ'træzɪpæm, -'treɪ-] *n pharm*. Nitrazepam *nt*.
ni·tre ['naɪtər] *n* → niter.
ni·tre·mia [naɪ'triːmɪə] *n* Azot(h)ämie *f*.
ni·tric ['naɪtrɪk] *adj* Stickstoff/Nitrogen betr. *od*. enthaltend, Salpeter-, Stickstoff-.
nitric acid Salpetersäure *f*.
fuming n. rauchende Salpetersäure.
nitric oxide → nitrogen monoxide.
ni·tri·da·tion [naɪtrɪ'deɪʃn] *n* Nitritbildung *f*.
ni·tride ['naɪtraɪd, -trɪd] *n* Nitrid *nt*.
ni·tri·fi·ca·tion [‚naɪtrɪfɪ'keɪʃn] *n bio*. Nitrifizierung *f*.
ni·tri·fi·er ['-faɪər] *n bio*. nitrifizierender Mikroorganismus *m*.
ni·tri·fy·ing ['-faɪɪŋ] *adj bio*. nitrifizierend.
nitrifying bacteria *bio*. nitrifizierende Bakterien *pl*.
ni·trile ['naɪtrɪl, -traɪl] *n* Nitril *nt*.
ni·trite ['naɪtraɪt] *n* Nitrit *nt*.
nitrite reductase Nitritreduktase *f*.
ni·tri·tu·ria [‚naɪtrɪ't(j)ʊərɪə] *n* Nitritausscheidung *f* im Harn, Nitriturie *f*.
nitro- *pref*. Nitro-.
ni·tro·ben·zene [‚naɪtrəʊ'benziːn] *n* Nitrobenzol *nt*.
ni·tro·ben·zol [‚-'benzɔl, -zɑl] *n* → nitrobenzene.
ni·tro·blue tetrazolium ['-bluː] *abbr*. **NBT** Nitroblau-Tetrazolium *nt abbr*. NBT.
nitroblue tetrazolium test Nitroblau-Tetrazolium-Test *m*, NBT-Test *m*.
ni·tro·cel·lu·lose [‚-'seljələʊs] *n* Nitrozellulose *f*, Zellulosenitrat *nt*, Schießbaumwolle *f*.
ni·tro·chlo·ro·form [‚-'klɔːrəfɔːrm] *n* Chlorpikrin *nt*, Trichlornitromethan *nt*.
ni·tro·fu·ran [‚-'fjʊəræn] *n pharm*. Nitrofuran *nt*.
ni·tro·fu·ran·to·in [‚-fjʊə'ræntəwɪn] *n pharm*. Nitrofurantoin *nt*.
ni·tro·fu·ra·zone [‚-'fjʊərəzəʊn] *n pharm*. Nitrofurazon *nt*.
ni·tro·gen ['-dʒən] *n abbr*. **N** Stickstoff *m*, Nitrogen *nt*; *chem*. Nitrogenium *nt abbr*. N.
ni·trog·en·ase [naɪ'trɑdʒəneɪz, 'naɪtrədʒə-] *n* Nitrogenase *f*.
nitrogenase system *biochem*. Nitrogenasesystem *nt*.
nitrogen balance Stickstoffbilanz *f*.
nitrogen cycle *biochem*. Stickstoffkreislauf *m*, -zyklus *m*.
nitrogen dioxide Stickstoffdioxid *nt*.
nitrogen equilibrium Stickstoffbilanz *f*.
nitrogen fixation *biochem*. Stickstofffixierung *f*.
nonsymbiotic n. nichtsymbiontische Stickstofffixierung.
symbiotic n. symbiontische Stickstofffixierung.
nitrogen-fixing *adj biochem*. stickstoffbindend, -fixierend.

nitrogen-fixing bacteria stickstoffbindende Bakterien *pl*.
nitrogen monoxide Stickoxid *nt*, Stickstoffmonoxid *nt*.
nitrogen mustard *abbr*. **HN2** Stickstoff-Lost *nt*, N-Lost *nt*, Chlormethin *nt*.
ni·trog·e·nous [naɪ'trɑdʒənəs] *adj* stickstoffhaltig.
nitrogenous base stickstoffhaltige Base *f*.
nitrogenous equilibrium → nitrogen equilibrium.
nitrogen source Stickstoffquelle *f*.
nitrogen washout method *physiol*. Stickstoffauswaschmethode *f*.
ni·tro·glyc·er·in [ˌnaɪtrə'glɪsərɪn] *n pharm*. Glyceroltrinitrat *nt*, Nitroglyzerin *nt*.
ni·tro·hy·dro·chlo·ric acid [ˌ-ˌhaɪdrə'klɔːrɪk, -'klaʊr-] *chem*. Königswasser *nt*.
ni·tro·meth·ane [ˌ-'meθeɪn] *n* Nitromethan *nt*.
ni·tro·phe·nol [ˌ-'fiːnɔl, -nɑl] *n* Nitrophenol *nt*.
p-ni·tro·phe·nyl acetate [ˌ-'fenl, -'fiːnl] p-Nitrophenylacetat *nt*.
ni·tro·prus·side [ˌ-'prʌsaɪd] *n* Nitroprussid *nt*.
ni·tros·am·ine [ˌnaɪtrəʊs'æmɪn] *n* Nitrosamin *nt*.
nitroso- *pref*. Nitroso-.
ni·tro·so·u·rea [naɪˌtrəsəʊ'(j)ʊərɪə] *n* Nitrosoharnstoff(verbindung *f*) *m*.
ni·tro·sug·ars [ˌnaɪtrə'ʃʊgərz] *pl* Nitrozucker *pl*, -körper *pl*.
ni·tro·syl ['naɪtrəsɪl] *n* Nitrosyl-(Radikal *nt*).
ni·trous ['naɪtrəs] *adj* nitros, salpetrig, Salpeter-.
nitrous acid salpetrige Säure *f*.
nitrous gases nitrose Gase *pl*.
nitrous oxide Lachgas *nt*, Distickstoffmonoxid *nt*.
ni·tro·xan·thic acid [ˌnaɪtrə'zænθɪk] Pikrinsäure *f*, Trinitrophenol *nt*.
ni·trox·o·line [naɪ'trɑksəliːn] *n pharm*. Nitroxolin *nt*.
niv·e·my·cin [ˌnɪvə'maɪsɪn] *n* → neomycin.
nkat *abbr*. → nanokatal.
NK cells → natural killer cells.
nl *abbr*. → nanoliter.
NM *abbr*. → nodular melanoma.
nm *abbr*. → nanometer.
NMN *abbr*. → nicotinamide mononucleotide.
NMP *abbr*. → nucleoside(-5'-)monophosphate.
NMP kinase → nucleoside monophosphate kinase.
NMR *abbr*. → nuclear magnetic resonance.
NMR spectroscopy → nuclear magnetic resonance spectroscopy.
No *abbr*. → nobelium.
Noack ['nəʊæk]: **N.'s syndrome** Noack-Syndrom *nt*.
no·bel·i·um [nəʊ'bɪlɪəm] *n abbr*. **No** Nobelium *nt abbr*. No.
no·ble gas ['nəʊbl] Edelgas *nt*.
No·car·dia [nəʊ'kɑːrdɪə] *n micro*. Nocardia *f*.
No·car·di·a·ce·ae [nəʊˌkɑːrdɪ'eɪsɪˌiː] *pl micro*. Nocardiaceae *pl*.
no·car·di·al [nəʊ'kɑːrdɪəl] *adj* Nokardien betr., durch Nokardien hervorgerufen, Nokardien-.
no·car·di·a·sis [nəʊkɑːr'daɪəsɪs] *n* → nocardiosis.
no·car·di·o·sis [nəʊˌkɑːrdɪ'əʊsɪs] *n* Nokardieninfektion *f*, Nokardiose *f*, Nocardiosis *f*.
no·ci·cep·tive [ˌnəʊsɪ'septɪv] *adj* nozi(re)zeptiv.
nociceptive fiber nozizeptive Faser *f*.

nociceptive system nozizeptives System *nt*.
no·ci·cep·tor [ˌ-'septər] *n* Nozi(re)zeptor *m*.
no·ci·per·cep·tion [ˌ-pər'sepʃn] *n* Nozi(re)zeption *f*, Noziperzeption *f*.
no·ci·re·cep·tor [ˌ-rɪ'septər] *n* → nociceptor.
no·ci·sen·si·tive neuron [ˌ-'sensətɪv] nozisensitives Neuron *nt*.
no·ci·sen·sor [ˌ-'sensər, -sɔr] *n* → nociceptor.
noc·tam·bu·la·tion [nɑkˌtæmbjə'leɪʃn] *n* Schlafwandeln *nt*, Noktambulismus *m*, Somnambulismus *m*.
noc·tam·bu·lism [nɑk'tæmbjəlɪzəm] *n* → noctambulation.
noc·tu·ria [nɑk't(j)ʊərɪə] *n* verstärkte nächtliche Harnproduktion *f*, Nykturie *f*.
noc·tur·nal [nɑk'tɜrnl] *adj* während der Nacht, nächtlich, Nacht-.
nocturnal amblyopia *ophthal*. Nachtblindheit *f*, Hemeralopie *f*.
nocturnal burning pain Brachialgia par(a)esthetica nocturna.
nocturnal dyspnea nächtliche Dyspnoe *f*.
nocturnal enuresis nächtliches Einnässen *nt*, Bettnässen *nt*, Enuresis nocturna.
nocturnal epilepsy Epilepsia nocturna.
nod·al ['nəʊdl] *adj* Knoten/Nodus betr., nodal, Knoten-.
nodal arrhythmia → nodal rhythm.
nodal artery Ast *m* der rechten *od*. linken Kranzarterie zum Sinusknoten, Ramus nodi sinu-atrialis a. coronariae dextrae sive sinistrae.
atrioventricular n. Ast *m* der rechten *od*. linken Kranzarterie zum Nodus atrioventricularis, Ramus nodi atrioventricularis a. coronariae dextrae sive sinistrae.
sinoatrial/sinuatrial n. → nodal artery.
nodal bigeminy *card*. Knotenbigeminie *f*.
nodal bradycardia *card*. Knotenbradykardie *f*.
nodal branch: atrioventricular n. of left coronary artery Ast *m* der linken Kranzarterie zum Nodus atrioventricularis, Ramus nodi atrioventricularis a. coronariae sinistrae.
atrioventricular n. of right coronary artery Ast *m* der rechten Kranzarterie zum Nodus atrioventricularis, Ramus nodi atrioventricularis a. coronariae dextrae.
sinoatrial n. of left coronary artery Ast *m* der linken Kranzarterie zum Sinusknoten, Ramus nodi sinuatrialis a. coronariae sinistrae.
sinoatrial n. of right coronary artery Ast *m* der rechten Kranzarterie zum Sinusknoten, Ramus nodi sinuatrialis a. coronariae dextrae.
nodal disease (*Tumor*) Lymphknotenbefall *m*, -metastase *f*, -metastasierung *f*.
regional n. regionaler Lymphknotenbefall, regionale Lymphknotenmetastasierung.
nodal dissection *chir*. Lymphknotenentfernung *f*, -dissektion *f*.
nodal extrasystole *card*. nodale Extrasystole *f*, Extrasystole *f* mit Ursprung im AV-Knoten.
nodal fever Knotenrose *f*, Erythema nodosum.
nodal point *mathe.*, *phys*. Knotenpunkt *m*.
nodal rhythm *physiol*. Knotenrhythmus *m*, AV-Rhythmus *m*.
lower n. unterer Knotenrhythmus.
midnodal n. mittlerer Knotenrhythmus.
upper n. oberer Knotenrhythmus.
nodal tachycardia AV-Knoten-Tachykardie *f*.

nodular myxedema

nod·ding spasm ['nɑdɪŋ] Salaamkrampf *m*, Nickkrampf *m*, Spasmus nutans.
node [nəʊd] *n* **1.** *anat*. Knoten *m*, Knötchen *nt*, knotige Struktur *f*, Nodus *m*, Nodulus *m*. **2.** *allg*. Knoten *m*.
n. of anterior border of epiploic foramen Lymphknoten am For. epiploicum, Nodus foraminalis.
n. of epiploic foramen → n. of anterior border of epiploic foramen.
n. of ligamentum arteriosum Lymphknoten am Lig. arteriosum, Nodus lig. arteriosi.
n. of neck of gallbladder Lymphknoten am Gallenblasenhals, Nodus cysticus.
n.s of Ranvier Ranvier'-Schnürringe *pl*, -knoten *pl*.
n. of Tawara Atrioventrikularknoten, AV-Knoten, Aschoff-Tawara'-Knoten, Nodus atrioventricularis.
node dissection *chir*. Lymphknotenentfernung *f*, -dissektion *f*.
no·dose ['nəʊdəʊs, nəʊ'dəʊs] *adj* knotig, voller Knoten.
nodose arteriosclerosis noduläre Arteriosklerose *f*.
nodose ganglion unteres Vagusganglion *nt*, Ggl. caudalis/inferius n. vagi.
no·dos·i·ty [nəʊ'dɑsətɪ] *n anat*. Knoten *m*, Knötchen *nt*, knotige Struktur *f*, Nodus *m*.
no·dous ['nəʊdəs] *adj* → nodose.
nod·u·lar ['nɑdʒələr] *adj* **1.** Knoten betr., knoten-, knötchenförmig, nodulär, Knoten-. **2.** mit Knoten besetzt, knotig.
nodular arteriosclerosis → nodose arteriosclerosis.
nodular circumscribed lipomatosis multiple symmetrische Lipomatose *f*.
nodular colloid goiter knotige Kolloidstruma *f*, Struma colloides nodosa.
nodular conjunctivitis *ophthal*. Raupenhaarkonjunktivitis *f*, Conjunctivitis/Ophthalmia nodosa.
nodular disease Oesophagostomum-Infektion *f*, Oesophagostomiasis *f*.
nodular elastoidosis (of Favre-Racouchot) Favre-Racouchot-Krankheit *f*, Elastoidosis cutanea nodularis et cystica.
nodular fasciitis noduläre Fasziitis *f*, Fasciitis nodularis.
pseudosarcomatous n. pseudosarkomatöse (noduläre) Fasziitis, Fasciitis nodularis pseudosarcomatosa.
nodular glomerulonephritis membranoproliferative Glomerulonephritis *f*.
nodular glomerulosclerosis Kimmelstiel-Wilson-Syndrom *nt*, diabetische Glomerulosklerose *f*.
nodular goiter Knotenkropf *m*, -struma *f*, Struma nodosa.
toxic n. hyperthyreote Knotenstruma.
nodular headache Knötchenkopfschmerz *m*, Cephalaea nodularis.
nodular hidradenoma noduläres Hidradenom *nt*, Hidradenoma solidum.
nodular leprosy tuberkuloide Lepra *f abbr*. TL, Lepra tuberculoides.
nodular lymphoma zentroblastisch-zentrozytischen (malignes) Lymphom *nt*, Brill-Symmers-Syndrom *nt*, Morbus Brill-Symmers *m*, großfollikuläres Lymphom/Lymphoblastom *nt*.
nodular melanoma *abbr*. **NM** noduläres Melanom *nt abbr*. NM, knotiges malignes Melanom *nt*, primär knotiges Melanom *nt*, nodöses Melanomalignom *nt*.
nodular myxedema prätibiales Myxödem *nt*, Myxoedema circumscriptum tuberosum, Myxoedema praetibiale symmetricum.

nodular nonsuppurative panniculitis (Pfeiffer-)Weber-Christian-Syndrom *nt*, rezidivierende fieberhafte nicht-eitrige Pannikulitis *f*, Panniculitis nodularis nonsuppurativa febrilis et recidivans.
nodular panencephalitis Enzephalitis Pette-Döring *f*, einheimische Panenzephalitis *f*.
nodular-papillary *adj* nodulär-papillär.
nodular poorly-differentiated lymphocytic lymphoma *abbr*. **NPDL** nodular poorly-differentiated lymphocytic lymphoma *abbr*. NPDL.
nodular poorly-differentiated lymphoma → nodular lymphoma.
nodular prurigo *derm*. nodulöse Prurigo *f*, Prurigo nodularis Hyde.
nodular scleritis noduläre Skleritis *f*.
nodular sclerosis Atherosklerose *f*.
nodular subepidermal fibrosis Fibrosis subepidermalis nodularis.
nodular synovitis noduläre Synovialitis/Synovi(i)tis *f*.
nodular syphilid Gummiknoten *m*, Syphilom *nt*, Gumma (syphiliticum) *nt*.
nodular tenosynovitis pigmentierte villonoduläre Synovitis *f abbr*. PVNS, benignes Synovialom *nt*, Riesenzelltumor *m* der Sehnenscheide, Tendosynovitis nodosa.
nodular tuberculid *derm*. Knotenrose *f*, nodöses Tuberkulid *nt*, Erythema nodosum.
nodular vasculitis noduläre Vaskulitis *f*, Vasculitis nodularis, Phlebitis nodularis.
nodular well-differentiated lymphocytic lymphoma *abbr*. **NWDL** nodular well-differentiated lymphocytic lymphoma *abbr*. NWDL.
nodular worm *micro*. 1. Knäuelfilarie *f*, Onchocerca volvulus. 2. Oesophagostomum columbianum.
nod·u·lat·ed ['nɑdʒəleɪtɪd] *adj* → nodular 2.
nod·ule ['nɑdʒuːl] *n anat*. Knötchen *nt*, Nodulus *m*.
n.s of aortic valve → n.s of Arantius.
n.s of Arantius Arantius-Knötchen *pl* der Aortenklappe, Noduli valvularum semilunarium.
n. of cerebellum → nodulus 2.
n.s of pulmonary trunk valve Arantius-Knötchen *pl* der Pulmonal(is)klappe.
n. of vermis → nodulus 2.
nod·u·lous ['nɑdʒələs] *adj* → nodose.
nod·u·lus ['nɑdʒələs] *n, pl* -li [-laɪ] 1. → nodule. 2. medialer Kleinhirnhöcker *m*, Nodulus *m*, Nodulus cerebelli/vermis.
no·dus ['nəʊdəs] *n, pl* -di [-daɪ] → node 1.
noise [nɔɪz] *n* 1. Geräusch *nt*. 2. Lärm *m*, Krach *m*. 3. (störendes) Rauschen *nt*.
noise box HNO Lärmtrommel *f*.
noise control Lärmbekämpfung *f*.
noise deafness HNO (chronische) Lärmschwerhörigkeit *f*.
noise·less ['nɔɪzlɪs] *adj* geräuschlos; lautlos, still.
noise·less·ness ['-nɪs] *n* Geräuschlosigkeit *f*.
noise level Lärm-, Störpegel *m*.
noise nuisance Lärmbelästigung *f*.
no·ma ['nəʊmə] *n* Noma *f*, Wangenbrand *m*, Wasserkrebs *m*, infektiöse Gangrän *f* des Mundes, Cancer aquaticus, Chancrum oris, Stomatitis gangraenosa.
no·men·cla·ture ['nəʊmənkleɪtʃər, nəʊˈmenklə-, -tʃʊər] *n* Nomenklatur *f*.
no·mi·fen·sine [ˌnəʊmɪˈfensiːn] *n pharm*. Nomifensin *nt*.
Nom·i·na An·a·to·mi·ca ['nɑmɪnə ænəˈtɑmɪkə, 'nəʊm-] *abbr*. **NA** anatomische

Nomenklatur *f*, Nomina Anatomica *abbr*. NA.
nom·i·nal ['nɑmɪnl] *adj* 1. (nur) dem Namen nach, nominal, nominell, Nominal-, Namen-. 2. *techn*. Soll-, Nenn-, Nominal-.
nominal aphasia anomische Aphasie *f*, Anomie *f*.
nominal current *electr*. Nennstrom *m*.
nominal frequency *electr*. Sollfrequenz *f*.
nominal scale *mathe*. Nominalskala *f*.
nom·o·gram ['nɑməgræm] *n* Nomogramm *nt*.
nom·o·graph ['-græf] *n* → nomogram.
nom·o·top·ic [ˌ-'tɑpɪk] *adj* am regelrechten Ort, nomotop.
non- *pref*. Un-, Nicht-, Non-.
non-absorbable suture *chir*. nicht-absorbierbares Nahtmaterial *nt*.
non·a·co·sane [ˌnɑnəˈkəʊseɪn] *n* Nonacosan *nt*.
non·ad·dict [nɑnˈædɪkt] *n* nicht-abhängiger Drogenkonsument *m*.
non·ad·her·ent [ˌnɑnædˈhɪərənt, -ˈher-] *adj* nicht-adhärent.
non-adrenergic *adj* nicht-adrenerg.
non·age ['nɑnɪdʒ, 'nəʊnɪdʒ] *n* 1. Minderjährigkeit *f*, Unmündigkeit *f*. 2. Unreife *f*, unreifes Stadium *nt*.
non·agglutinating *adj* nicht-agglutinierend.
non-agglutinating antibodies blockierende/inkomplette/nicht-agglutinierende Antikörper *pl*.
non-agglutinating vibrios *micro*. nicht-agglutinable Vibrionen *pl*, NAG-Vibrionen *pl*, Vibrio cholerae non-01.
non·al·co·hol·ic [ˌnɑnælkəˈhɑlɪk, -ˈhɑl-] *adj* alkoholfrei.
non·al·ler·gic vasomotor rhinitis [ˌnɑnəˈlɜrdʒɪk] Rhinitis vasomotorica nonallergica.
non-A,non-B hepatitis *abbr*. **NANB** Nicht-A-Nicht-B-Hepatitis *f*, Non-A-Non-B-Hepatitis *f abbr*. NANB, NANBH.
non-A,non-B hepatitis virus Hepatits-C-Virus *nt*, Non-A-Non-B-Hepatitis-Virus *nt*, NANB-Hepatitisvirus *nt*.
non·an·ti·gen·ic [nɑnˌæntɪˈdʒenɪk] *adj immun*. keine Immunantwort auslösend, nicht-antigen.
non·a·pep·tide [nɑnəˈpeptaɪd] *n* Nonapeptid *nt*.
non·a·que·ous [nɑnˈeɪkwɪəs, -ˈækwɪ-] *adj phys*. nicht-wäßrig.
non·ar·o·mat·ic [nɑnˌærəˈmætɪk] *adj chem*. nicht-aromatisch.
non·as·so·ci·at·ing [nɑnəˈsəʊʃɪeɪtɪŋ, -sɪ-] *adj phys*. nicht-assoziierend.
non·as·so·ci·a·tive learning [nɑnəˈsəʊʃɪeɪtɪv, -sɪ-, -ʃətɪv] nicht-assoziatives Lernen *nt*.
non·bac·te·ri·al pneumonia [nɑnbækˈtɪərɪəl] abakterielle Pneumonie *f*.
nonbacterial pneumonitis → nonbacterial pneumonia.
nonbacterial regional lymphadenitis Katzenkratzkrankheit *f*, cat-scratch disease (*nt*), benigne Inokulationslymphoretikulose *f*, Miyagawanellose *f*.
nonbacterial thrombotic endocarditis → nonbacterial verrucous endocarditis.
nonbacterial verrucous endocarditis atypische verruköse Endokarditis *f*, Libman-Sacks-Syndrom *nt*, Endokarditis Libman-Sacks *f*, Endocarditis thrombotica.
non-beta islet cell tumor Nicht-Betazell-Pankreastumor *m*.
non·cel·lu·lar [nɑnˈseljələr] *adj* nicht-zellulär.
non-cholera vibrios [nɑnˈkɑlərə] *abbr*.

NCVs *micro*. NC-Vibrionen *pl*, Non-cholera-Vibrionen *pl abbr*. NCV.
non-cholinergic *adj* nicht-cholinerg.
non·chro·maf·fin [nɑnˈkrəʊməfɪn] *adj histol*. nichtchromaffin.
nonchromaffin paraganglioma nicht-chromaffines Paragangliom *nt*, Chemodektom *nt*.
non·chro·mo·gens [nɑnˈkrəʊmədʒəns] *pl* → nonphotochromogens.
non-cleaved follicular center cell [nɑnˈkliːvd] Germino-, Zentroblast *m*.
non·clot·ta·ble fibrinogen [nɑnˈklɑtəbl] nicht-gerinnbares Fibrinogen *nt*, Dysfibrinogen *nt*.
non·com·i·tant strabismus [nɑnˈkɑmɪtənt] → nonconcomitant strabismus.
non·com·mu·ni·cat·ing hydrocephalus [nɑnkəˈmjuːnɪkeɪtɪŋ] obstruktiver Hydrozephalus *m*, Hydrocephalus occlusus.
non·com·mu·ni·ca·tion hydrocephalus [nɑnkəˌmjuːnɪˈkeɪʃn] → noncommunicating hydrocephalus.
non·com·pet·i·tive inhibition [ˌnɑnkəmˈpetətɪv] *biochem*. nicht-kompetitive Hemmung *f*.
non·con·com·i·tant strabismus [nɑnkənˈkɑmɪtənt] *ophthal*. Lähmungsschielen *nt*, Strabismus paralyticus.
non·con·duc·tor [ˌnɑnkənˈdʌktər] *n electr*. Nichtleiter *m*.
non·con·ges·tive glaucoma [nɑnkənˈdʒestɪv] Simplex-, Weitwinkelglaukom *nt*, Glaucoma simplex.
non·co·op·er·a·tion [nɑnkəʊˌɑpəˈreɪʃn] *n* Verweigerung *f* der Mit- od. Zusammenarbeit.
non·co·va·lent [nɑnkəʊˈveɪlənt] *adj chem*. nicht-kovalent.
noncovalent interaction *chem*. nicht-kovalente Wechselwirkung *f*.
non·crush·ing clamp [nɑnˈkrʌʃɪŋ] *chir*. atraumatische Klemme *f*.
non·cyc·lic phosphorylation [nɑnˈsaɪklɪk, -ˈsɪk-] nichtzyklische Phosphorylierung *f*.
non·cy·to·path·o·gen·ic [nɑnˌsaɪtəˌpæθəˈdʒenɪk] *adj* nicht-zytopathogen.
non·de·po·lar·iz·er [nɑndiːˈpəʊləraɪzər] *n pharm*., *anes*. nicht-depolarisierendes Muskelrelaxans *nt*.
non·di·a·bet·ic glycosuria [nɑndaɪəˈbetɪk] renale Glukosurie/Glycosurie *f*.
non·dis·junc·tion [nɑndɪsˈdʒʌŋkʃn] *n genet*. Non-Disjunction *f*.
non·dis·placed fracture [nɑndɪsˈpleɪst] nicht-dislozierte Fraktur *f*.
non·dis·so·ci·at·ing [nɑndɪˈsəʊʃɪeɪtɪŋ, -sɪ-] *adj phys*. nicht-dissoziierend.
non·dys·troph·ic [nɑndɪsˈtrɑfɪk, -ˈtrəʊ-] *adj* nicht-dystrophisch.
non·e·las·tic resistance [nɑnɪˈlæstɪk] nichtelastischer/viskoser Widerstand *m*.
non·e·lec·tro·lyte [nɑnɪˈlektrəlaɪt] *n phys*. Nichtelektrolyt *m*.
non·en·ter·o·coc·cal group D streptococci [ˌnɑnˌentərəʊˈkɑkəl] Nichtenterokokken *pl* der Gruppe D.
non·e·qui·lib·ri·um thermodynamics [nɑnˌiːkwəˈlɪbrɪəm, ˌekwə-] Thermodynamik *f* offener Systeme.
non·es·sen·tial [nɑnɪˈsenʃl] *adj* nichtessentiell, unwesentlich.
non·ex·ist·ence [ˌnɑnɪgˈzɪstəns] *n* Fehlen *nt*, Nichtvorhandensein *nt*.
non·ex·ist·ent [nɑnˈzɪstənt] *adj* nicht existierend, fehlend.
non·fa·mil·ial hyperlipoproteinemia [nɑnfəˈmɪlɪəl] nichtfamiliäre/symptomatische Hyperlipoproteinämie *f*.
non·fatiguing *adj* nicht-ermüdend.
non·fis·sion·a·ble [nɑnˈfɪʃənəbl] *adj chem*. nicht spaltbar.

non-flam·ma·ble [nɑnˈflæməbl] *adj* nicht--entflammbar, nicht-brennbar.
non-freez·ing [nɑnˈfriːzɪŋ] *adj* kältebeständig.
nonfreezing mixture Frostschutzmittel *nt*.
non-ge·net·ic interactions [nɑndʒɪˈnetɪk] *micro*. (*Virus*) nicht-genetische Wechselwirkungen *pl*.
non-glandotropic hormone nicht-glandotropes Hormon *nt*.
non-gon·o·coc·cal urethritis [nɑnˌɡɑnəˈkɑkəl] unspezifische/nicht-gonorrhoische Urethritis *f abbr*. NGU.
non-he·mo·lyt·ic [nɑnˌhiːməˈlɪtɪk, -ˌhemə-] *adj micro*. γ-hämolytisch, gamma-hämolytisch, nicht-hämolytisch, nicht-hämolysierend.
nonhemolytic jaundice nicht-hämolytischer Ikterus *m*.
nonhemolytic streptococci gamma-hämolytische/nicht-hämolysierende Streptokokken *pl*.
non-his·tone protein [nɑnˈhɪstəʊn] Nicht-Histon-Protein *nt*.
non-Hodgkin's lymphoma non-Hodgkin--Lymphom *nt abbr*. NHL.
non-ho·mol·o·gous recombination [nɑnhəˈmɑləɡəs, -həʊ-] *genet*. illegitime/nicht-homologe Rekombination *f*.
non-hy·per·gly·ce·mic glycosuria [nɑnˌhaɪpərɡlaɪˈsiːmɪk] renale Glukosurie/Glycosurie *f*.
non-i·den·ti·cal [nɑnaɪˈdentɪkl, -ɪˈden-] *adj* nicht identisch, ungleich.
nonidentical twins binovuläre/dissimilare/dizygote/erbungleiche/heteroovuläre/zweieiige Zwillinge *pl*.
non-in·fec·tious [nɑnɪnˈfekʃəs] *adj* nicht-infektiös.
non-in·flam·ma·ble [nɑnɪnˈflæməbl] *adj* nicht entflammbar, nicht brennbar.
non-in·flam·ma·to·ry arthropathy [nɑnɪnˈflæmətɔːriː, -təʊ-] nichtentzündliche Arthropathie *f*.
noninflammatory edema nicht-entzündliches Ödem *nt*.
non-in·for·ma·tion·al biomolecule [nɑnˌɪnfərˈmeɪʃənl] nicht-informatives Biomolekül *nt*.
non-insulin-dependent diabetes *abbr*. NIDD nicht-insulinabhängiger Diabetes mellitus *m*, Typ-II-Diabetes mellitus *m*, non-insulin-dependent diabetes (mellitus) *abbr*. NIDD(M).
non-in·va·sive [nɑnɪnˈveɪsɪv] *adj patho*. nicht-invasiv.
non-ion·ic [nɑnaɪˈɑnɪk] *adj phys*. nicht--ionisch.
non-ke·tot·ic hyperglycinemia [nɑnkiːˈtɑtɪk] nicht-ketotische Hyperglycinämie *f*.
non-lactating breast ruhende/nicht-laktierende Brustdrüse *f*.
non-leu·ke·mic myelosis [nɑnluːˈkiːmɪk] idiopathische/primäre myeloische Metaplasie *f*, Leukoerythroblastose *f*, leukoerythroblastische Anämie *f*.
non-lin·e·ar [nɑnˈlɪniər] *adj* nicht-linear.
non-lip·id-containing viruses [nɑnˈlɪpɪd] *micro*. nicht-lipidhaltige Viren *pl*.
nonlipid histiocytosis Letterer-Siwe--Krankheit *f*, Abt-Letterer-Siwe-Krankheit *f*, maligne/akute Säuglingsretikulose *f*, maligne generalisierte Histiozytose *f*.
non-liv·ing [nɑnˈlɪvɪŋ] *adj bio*. unbelebt.
non-lym·pho·cyt·ic leukemia, acute [nɑnˌlɪmfəˈsɪtɪk] *abbr*. ANLL akute myeloische Leukämie *f abbr*. AML, akute nicht-lymphatische Leukämie *f abbr*. ANLL.
non-me·di·at·ed transport [nɑnˈmiːdɪeɪtɪd] nicht-vermittelter/nicht-katalysierter Transport *m*.

non-med·ul·lat·ed [nɑnˈmedleɪtɪd, -ˈmedʒə-] *adj* → nonmyelinated.
nonmedullated fibers marklose (Nerven-)Fasern *pl*, Remak-Fasern *pl*.
non-met·al [nɑnˈmetl] *n chem*. Nichtmetall *nt*.
non-me·tal·lic [nɑnməˈtælɪk] *adj* nichtmetallisch.
non-my·e·li·nat·ed [nɑnˈmaɪələneɪtɪd] *adj* mark(scheiden)los, markfrei.
nonmyelinated matter graue Gehirn- u. Rückenmarkssubstanz *f*, graue Substanz *f*, Substantia grisea.
n. of spinal cord graue Rückenmarkssubstanz *f*, Substantia grisea medullae spinalis.
nonmyelinated substance → nonmyelinated matter.
n. of spinal cord → nonmyelinated matter of spinal cord.
non-myotonic *adj* nicht-myotonisch.
Nonne [ˈnɑnɪ; ˈnɔnə]: **N.'s syndrome** Nonne-Marie-Krankheit *f*, Marie--Krankheit *f*, Pierre Marie-Krankheit *f*, zerebellare Heredoataxie *f*, Heredoataxia cerebellaris.
Nonne-Apelt [ˈɑpəlt]: **N.-A. reaction/test** Nonne-Apelt(-Schumm) Reaktion *f*.
Nonne-Milroy [ˈmɪlrɔɪ]: **N.-M. disease** Lymphödem/Trophödem *nt* Typ Nonne--Milroy.
Nonne-Milroy-Meige [mɛːʒ]: **N.-M.-M. syndrome** Nonne-Milroy-Meige-Syndrom *nt*, chronisch hereditäres Trophödem *nt*, chronisch kongenitales Lymphödem *nt*, Elephantiasis congenita hereditaria.
non-neuronal *adj* nicht-neuronal.
non-Newtonian fluid heterogene Flüssigkeit *f*, nicht-Newton'-Flüssigkeit *f*.
non-nucleated *adj* kernlos, ohne Kern, anukleär.
non-ol·fac·to·ry cortex [nɑnalˈfækt(ə)rɪ, -əʊl-] → neocortex.
non-on·co·gen·ic [nɑnˌɑŋkəʊˈdʒenɪk] *adj* nicht-onkogen.
non-or·gan·ic [nɑnɔːrˈɡænɪk] *adj* 1. *chem*. anorganisch. 2. unorganisch.
non-ose [ˈnɑnəʊs] *n* Nonose *f*.
non-osmotic diuretic nicht-osmotisches Diuretikum *nt*.
non-ossifying fibroma of bone nicht--osteogenes/nicht-ossifizierendes Knochenfibrom *nt*, xanthomatöser/faseriger Riesenzelltumor *m* des Knochens, Xanthogranuloma *nt* des Knochens.
non-os·te·o·gen·ic fibroma [nɑnˌɑstiːəˈdʒenɪk] nicht-ossifizierendes Fibrom *nt*, fibröser Kortikalisdefekt *m*, fibröser metaphysärer Defekt *m*, benignes fibröses Histiozytom *nt* des Knochens.
non-ov·u·la·tion·al menstruation [nɑnˌɑvjəˈleɪʃnl, -əʊv-] anovulatorische Menstruation *f*.
non-ox·i·da·tive decarboxylation [nɑnˈɑksɪdeɪtɪv] *biochem*. nicht-oxidative Decarboxylierung *f*.
non-ox·y·nol [nɑnˈɑksɪnɔl] *n pharm*. Nonoxinol *nt*.
non-par·a·lyt·ic poliomyelitis [nɑnˌpærəˈlɪtɪk] aparalytische Poliomyelitis *f*.
non-par·ous [nɑnˈpærəs] *adj* → nulliparous.
non-path·o·gen [nɑnˈpæθədʒən] *n* apathogener Mikroorganismus *m*.
non-path·o·ge·net·ic [nɑnˌpæθədʒəˈnetɪk] *adj* → nonpathogenic.
non-path·o·gen·ic [nɑnˌpæθəˈdʒenɪk] *adj* apathogen.
non-pe·dun·cu·lat·ed hydatid [nɑnpɪˌdʌŋkjəleɪtɪd] Morgagni-Hydatide *f*, Appendix testis.

non-per·ish·a·ble [nɑnˈperɪʃəbl] *adj* (*Lebensmittel*) haltbar.
non-per·mis·sive [nɑnpərˈmɪsɪv] *adj micro*. nicht-permissiv.
nonpermissive conditions *micro*. nicht--permissive Bedingungen *pl*.
non-pho·to·chro·mo·gens [ˌnɑnfəʊtəˈkrəʊmədʒəns] *pl micro*. nichtchromogene Mykobakterien *pl*, Mykobakterien *pl* der Runyon-Gruppe III.
non-pho·to·syn·thet·ic [nɑnˌfəʊtəsɪnˈθetɪk] *adj bio*. nicht-photosynthetisch aktiv.
non-piliated *adj histol*. nicht-pilitragend.
non-poi·son·ous [nɑnˈpɔɪzənəs] *adj* ungiftig.
non-po·lar [nɑnˈpəʊlər] *adj* nichtpolar, unpolar; apolar.
nonpolar compound *chem*. apolare Verbindung *f*.
non-pre·cip·i·ta·ble antibody [nɑnprɪˈsɪpətəbl] nichtpräzipitierender Antikörper *m*.
non-pre·ci·pi·tat·ing antibody [nɑnprɪˈsɪpəteɪtɪŋ] nichtpräzipitierender Antikörper *m*.
non-pro·duc·tive cough [nɑnprəˈdʌktɪv] unproduktiver/nichtproduktiver Husten *m*.
non-pro·lif·er·a·tive disease of the breast [nɑnprəˈlɪfəˌreɪtɪv] einfache nicht-proliferative Mastopathie *f*.
non-pro·pri·e·ta·ry drugs [nɑnprəˈpraɪəteriː] Fertigarzneimittel *pl*, Generika *pl*.
nonproprietary name *pharm*. Freiname *m*, generic name (*m*).
non-pro·pul·sive peristalsis [nɑnprəˈpʌlsɪv] nichtpropulsive Peristaltik *f*.
non-pro·tein nitrogen [nɑnˈprəʊtiːn, -tiːɪn] *abbr*. NPN Reststickstoff *m*, Rest-N *m/nt abbr*. RN, nicht-proteingebundener Stickstoff *m abbr*. NPN.
non-pu·ru·lent myocarditis [nɑnˈpjʊər(j)ələnt] nicht-eitrige Myokarditis *f*.
non-pyramidal system extrapyramidal--motorisches System *nt*.
non-ra·chit·ic bowleg [nɑnrəˈkɪtɪk] Blount'-Krankheit *f*, Osteochondrosis deformans tibiae.
non-rapid eye movement sleep → non--REM sleep.
non-re·flex bladder [nɑnˈrɪfleks] autonome Blase *f*.
non-re·flux·ing anastomosis [nɑnrɪˈflʌksɪŋ] (*Blase*) refluxverhindernde Anastomose *f*, Anti-Reflux-Anastomose *f*.
non-reg·u·la·to·ry enzyme [nɑnˈreɡjələtɔːrɪ, -təʊ-] nicht-regulatorisches Enzym *nt*.
non-REM sleep non-REM-Schlaf *m*, NREM-Schlaf *m*, orthodoxer/synchronisierter Schlaf *m*.
non-re·nal [nɑnˈriːnl] *adj* nicht-nierenbedingt, nicht-nephrogen, nicht-renal.
non-re·pet·i·tive [nɑnrɪˈpetɪtɪv] *adj genet*. nichtrepetitiv.
non-res·pi·ra·to·ry acidosis [nɑnrɪˈspaɪrətɔːrɪ, -təʊ-] metabolische/stoffwechselbedingte Azidose *f*.
nonrespiratory alkalosis metabolische/stoffwechselbedingte Alkalose *f*.
non-responder *n* Non-Responder *m*.
non-ro·ta·tion [nɑnrəʊˈteɪʃn] *n embryo*. Nonrotation *f*.
non-sa·pon·i·fi·a·ble [nɑnsəˈpəʊnɪfaɪəbl] *adj chem*. nicht-verseifbar.
nonsaponifiable lipid einfaches/nicht-verseifbares Lipid *nt*.
non-sea·son·al allergic rhinitis [nɑnˈsiːznəl] perenniale (allergische) Rhinitis *f*.
non-se·cre·tor [nɑnsɪˈkriːtər] *n immun*. Nichtausscheider *m*, Nonsekretor *m*.
non-se·lec·tive [nɑnsɪˈlektɪv] *adj* nicht--selektiv.

nonself

non·self [nɑn'self] *adj immun.* nicht-selbst, nonself.
non·sense codon ['nɑnsens, -səns] Abbruchs-, Kettenabbruchs-, Terminationskodon *nt.*
nonsense mutation Nonsense-, Unsinn--Mutation *f.*
nonsense syndrome Ganser-Syndrom *nt*, Pseudodemenz *f*, Scheinblödsinn *m*, Zweckpsychose *f.*
non·sep·tate [nɑn'septeɪt] *adj* ohne Septum, nicht-septiert, unseptiert.
non·sex·u·al generation [nɑn'sekʃəwəl] *bio.* ungeschlechtliche/vegetative Fortpflanzung *f.*
non·shi·ver·ing thermogenesis [nɑn-'ʃɪvərɪŋ] zitterfreie Wärmebildung *f.*
non·smok·er [nɑn'sməʊkər] *n* Nichtraucher(in *f*) *m.*
non-smoking *adj* Nichtraucher-.
non·spe·cif·ic [nɑnspə'sɪfɪk] *adj* **1.** *patho.* unspezifisch. **2.** (*Behandlung*) unspezifisch.
nonspecific cholinesterase unspezifische/unechte Cholinesterase *f abbr.* ChE, Pseudocholinesterase *f*, Typ II-Cholinesterase *f*, β-Cholinesterase *f*, Butyrylcholinesterase *f.*
nonspecific system aufsteigendes retikuläres aktivierendes System *nt abbr.* ARAS.
nonspecific therapy unspezifische Therapie *f.*
non-staphylococcal scalded skin syndrome (medikamentöses) Lyell-Syndrom *nt*, Syndrom *nt* der verbrühten Haut, Epidermolysis acuta toxica, Epidermolysis necroticans combustiformis.
non-steroidal anti-inflammatory drugs *abbr.* **NSAIDs** nicht-steroidale Antirheumatika *pl abbr.* NSAR, nicht-steroidale antiinflammatorisch-wirkende Medikamente *pl abbr.* NSAIM.
non·ste·roi·dals [nɑnstɪ'rɔɪdlz] *pl* → non--steroidal anti-inflammatory drugs.
non·stri·at·ed muscles [nɑn'straɪeɪtɪd] glatte *od.* unwillkürliche Muskeln *pl*/Muskulatur *f.*
non·struc·tur·al curve [nɑn'strʌktʃərəl] *ortho.* (*Skoliose*) nicht-strukturelle Krümmung *f.*
non·sup·press·ible insulin-like activity [nɑnsə'presɪbl] *abbr.* **NSILA** insulinähnliche Wachstumsfaktoren *pl*, insulin-like growth factors *abbr.* IGF, insulinähnliche Aktivität *f.*
non·sup·pu·ra·tive cholangitis [nɑn'sʌpjəreɪtɪv] akute Cholangitis *f.*
nonsuppurative myocarditis nicht-eitrige Myokarditis *f.*
non·syn·o·vi·al articulation/joint [nɑnsɪ-'nəʊvɪəl] kontinuierliche Knochenverbindung *f*, Synarthrose *f.*
non·throm·bo·cy·to·pe·nic purpura [nɑn-,θrɑmbəʊ,saɪtə'piːnɪk] Purpura simplex.
non·tox·ic [nɑn'tɑksɪk] *adj* nicht-, ungiftig.
nontoxic goiter blande Struma *f.*
non·tox·ic·i·ty [nɑntɑk'sɪsətɪ] *n* Ungiftigkeit *f.*
non·tu·ber·cu·lous mycobacteria [nɑn-t(j)uː'bɜːrkjələs] atypische/nicht-tuberkulöse Mykobakterien *pl.*
non·ul·cer·a·tive blepharitis [nɑn'ʌlsəreɪtɪv, -'ʌlsərətɪv] *ophthal.* Blepharitis squamosa.
non·un·ion [nɑn'juːnjən] *n ortho.* Pseudoarthrose(nbildung *f*) *f.*
non·u·ni·form [nɑn'juːnɪfɔːrm] *adj* ungleichmäßig.
non·va·lent [nɑn'veɪlənt] *adj chem., phys.* nullwertig.
non·ve·ne·re·al syphilis [nɑnvɪ'nɪərɪəl] Bejel *f*, endemische Syphilis *f.*
non·ver·bal [nɑn'vɜrbəl] *adj* nicht-, nonverbal.
nonverbal learning nonverbales Lernen *nt.*
non·vi·a·ble [nɑn'vaɪəbl] *adj* nicht lebensfähig, lebensunfähig.
non·vi·tal [nɑn'vaɪtl] *adj* nicht von vitaler Bedeutung, nicht-vital.
non·vol·a·tile acid [nɑn'vɑlətl, -tɪl] nichtflüchtige Säure *f.*
non·yl ['nɑnɪl, 'nəʊ-, -iːl] *n* Nonyl-(Radikal *nt*).
Noon [nuːn] *N.* **pollen unit** Noon-Einheit *f.*
Noonan ['nuːnən] *N.'s* **syndrome** Noonan--Syndrom *nt*, Pseudo-Ullrich-Turner--Syndrom *nt.*
nor- *pref. chem.* Nor-.
nor·a·dren·a·lin [,nɔːrə'drenlɪn] *n* → norepinephrine.
nor·a·dren·a·line [,nɔːrə'drenliːn] *n* → norepinephrine.
nor·a·dren·er·gic [nɔːr,ædrə'nɜrdʒɪk] *adj* noradrenerg.
noradrenergic fiber *physiol.* noradrenerge Faser *f.*
noradrenergic neuron noradrenerges Neuron *nt.*
noradrenergic system noradrenerges System *nt.*
nor·an·dro·sten·o·lone [,nɔːrændrəʊ'stenəlɔʊn] *n pharm.* Nandrolon *nt.*
nor·ep·i·neph·rine [nɔːr,epɪ'nefrɪn, -rɪːn] *n* Noradrenalin *nt*, Norepinephrin *nt*, Arterenol *nt*, Levarterenol *nt.*
nor·eth·in·drone [nɔːr'eθɪndrəʊn] *n pharm.* Norethisteron *nt.*
nor·eth·is·ter·one [,nɔːrəˈθɪstərəʊn] *n pharm.* Norethisteron *nt.*
nor·flox·a·cin [nɔːr'flɑksəsɪn] *n pharm.* Norfloxacin *nt.*
nor·ges·trel [nɔːr'dʒestrəl] *n pharm.* Norgestrel *nt.*
nor·leu·cine [nɔːr'luːsiːn, -sɪn] *n* Norleucin *nt*, α-Amino-n-capronsäure *f.*
norm- *pref.* → normo-.
norm [nɔːrm] *n* **1.** Norm *f*, Richtschnur *f*, Regel *f*, Normwert *m.* **2.** (Durchschnitts-)Leistung *f.*
nor·ma ['nɔːrmə] *n anat.* Norma *f.*
nor·mal ['nɔːrml] **I** *n* **1.** Normalzustand *m*, das Normale. **2.** Normalwert *m*, Durchschnitt *m.* **3.** *mathe.* Senkrechte *f*, Normale *f.* **II** *adj* **4.** normal, üblich, gewöhnlich, Normal-. **5.** *chem.* dekadisch, **N, n** normal *abbr.* N, n. **6.** *mathe.* senkrecht, normal.
normal acceleration *phys.* Normalbeschleunigung *f.*
normal antibody natürlicher/regulärer Antikörper *m.*
normal breathing normale/freie/ungestörte Atmung *f*, normale Ruheatmung *f*, Eupnoe *f.*
normal curve (of distribution) *stat.* Glockenkurve *f*, Gauss-Kurve *f.*
nor·mal·cy ['nɔːrməlsɪ] *n* normality.
normal distribution *stat.* Gauss'-Normalverteilung *f.*
normal gingantism proportionierter Riesenwuchs *m.*
normal hearing Normalhörigkeit *f.*
nor·mal·i·ty [nɔːr'mælətɪ] *n* (*a. chem., mathe.*) Normalität *f*, normaler Zustand *m.* **to return to** ~ **s.** (*wieder*) normalisieren.
nor·mal·i·za·tion [,nɔːrməlɪ'zeɪʃn] *n* Normalisierung *f.*
nor·mal·ize ['nɔːrməlaɪz] *vt* normalisieren.
normal range Normalbereich *m.*
normal respiration → normal breathing.
normal saline (solution) *pharm.* physiologische Kochsalzlösung *f.*
normal salt Neutralsalz *nt.*
normal solution Normal-, Standard-, Bezugs-, Vergleichslösung *f.*
normal value Normalwert *m.*
normal weight Normalgewicht *nt.*
nor·mer·gia [nɔːr'mɜrdʒɪə] *n* Normergie *f.*
nor·mer·gic [nɔːr'mɜrdʒɪk] *adj* normergisch, normerg.
nor·met·a·neph·rine [nɔːr,metə'nefrɪːn] *n* Normetanephrin *nt.*
normo- *pref.* Normal-, Norm(o)-.
nor·mo·blast ['nɔːrməblæst] *n* Normoblast *m.*
nor·mo·blas·tic [,-'blæstɪk] *adj* Normoblast(en) betr., normoblastisch, Normoblasten-.
nor·mo·blas·to·sis [,-blæs'təʊsɪs] *n* Normoblastose *f.*
nor·mo·cal·ce·mi·a [,-kæl'siːmɪə] *n* Normokalz(i)ämie *f.*
nor·mo·cal·ce·mic [,-kæl'siːmɪk] *adj* Normokalzämie betr., normokalz(i)ämisch.
normocalcemic hyperparathyroidism normokalzämischer Hyperparathyreoidismus *m.*
nor·mo·cap·nia [,-'kæpnɪə] *n* normale Kohlendioxidspannung *f* des Blutes, Normokapnie *f*, Normokarbie *f.*
nor·mo·ce·pha·lia [,-sɪ'feɪlɪə] *n* Normozephalie *f.*
nor·mo·cho·les·ter·ol·e·mia [,-kə,lestərə-'liːmɪə] *n* normaler Cholesteringehalt *m* des Blutes, Normocholesterinämie *f.*
nor·mo·chro·ma·sia [,-krəʊ'meɪʒɪə] *n hema.* Normochromie *f.*
nor·mo·chro·mia [,-'krəʊmɪə] *n* → normochromasia.
nor·mo·chro·mic [,-'krəʊmɪk] *adj* **1.** von normaler Farbe, normochrom. **2.** *hema.* normochromic.
normochromic anemia normochrome Anämie *f.*
nor·mo·cyte ['-saɪt] *n* (reifer) Erythrozyt *m*, Normozyt *m.*
nor·mo·cyt·ic anemia [,-'sɪtɪk] normozytäre Anämie *f.*
nor·mo·e·ryth·ro·cyte [,-ɪ'rɪθrəsaɪt] *n* → normocyte.
nor·mo·gly·ce·mia [,-glaɪ'siːmɪə] *n* normaler Glukosegehalt *m* des Blutes, Normoglykämie *f.*
nor·mo·gly·ce·mic [,-glaɪ'siːmɪk] *adj* normoglykämisch.
normoglycemic glycosuria renale Glukosurie/Glycosurie *f.*
nor·mo·ka·le·mia [,-kə'liːmɪə] *n* normaler Kaliumgehalt *m* des Blutes, Normokal(i)ämie *f.*
nor·mo·ka·le·mic [,-kə'liːmɪk] *adj* normokal(i)ämisch.
nor·mo·ka·li·e·mia [,-,kælɪ'iːmɪə, -,keɪ-] *n* → normokalemia.
nor·mo·phos·phat·e·mia [,-fɑsfə'tiːmɪə] *n* Normophosphatämie *f.*
nor·mo·sper·mat·o·gen·ic sterility [,-spɜr-,mætə'dʒenɪk] *urol.* normospermatogene Sterilität *f.*
nor·mo·sper·mia [,-'spɜrmɪə] *n* Normo(zoo)spermie *f.*
nor·mo·sper·mic [,-'spɜrmɪk] *adj* Normo(zoo)spermie betr., normo(zoo)sperm.
nor·mos·then·u·ria [,-sθe'n(j)ʊərɪə] *n* Normosthenurie *f.*
nor·mo·ten·sion [,-'tenʃn] *n* Normaltonus *m*, -spannung *f*; Normaldruck *m.*
nor·mo·ten·sive [,-'tensɪv] *adj* mit normalem Blutdruck, normotensiv.
nor·mo·ther·mia [,-'θɜrmɪə] *n* Normothermie *f.*
nor·mo·ther·mic [,-'θɜrmɪk] *adj* normotherm.
nor·mo·to·nia [,-'təʊnɪə] *n* Normaltonus *m*, Normotonie *f.*

nor·mo·ton·ic [ˌ-'tɑnɪk] *adj* 1. mit Normaltonus, normoton. 2. → normotensive.
nor·mo·to·pia [ˌ-'təʊpɪə] *n embryo.* Normotopie *f*.
nor·mo·top·ic [ˌ-'tɑpɪk] *adj embryo.* am regelrechten Ort, normotop.
nor·mo·u·ri·ce·mia [ˌ-ˌjʊərɪ'siːmɪə] *n* normaler Harnsäuregehalt *m* des Blutes, Normourikämie *f*.
nor·mo·u·ri·cu·ria [ˌ-ˌjʊərɪ'kjʊərɪə] *n* normale Harnsäureausscheidung *f*, Normourikurie *f*.
nor·mo·ven·ti·la·tion [ˌ-ˌventə'leɪʃn] *n* Normoventilation *f*.
nor·mo·vo·le·mia [ˌ-vəʊ'liːmɪə] *n* Normovolämie *f*.
nor·mo·vo·le·mic [ˌ-vəʊ'liːmɪk] *adj* Normovolämie betr., normovolämisch.
norm·ox·ia [nɔːr'mɑksɪə] *n* Normoxie *f*.
nor·pseu·do·e·phed·rine [nɔːrˌsuːdəʊɪ'fedrɪn, -'efidriːn] *n* Norpseudoephedrin *nt*.
Norrie ['nɔrɪs, 'nɑr-]: **N.'s disease** Norrie-Warburg-Syndrom *nt*, Atrophia bulborum hereditaria.
nor·sul·fa·zole [nɔːr'sʌlfəzəʊl] *n pharm.* Sulfathiazol *m*.
North African relapsing fever [nɔːrθ] nordafrikanisches Rückfallfieber *nt*.
North American blastomycosis nordamerikanische Blastomykose *f*, Gilchrist-Krankheit *f*.
North Asian tick typhus nordasiatisches Zeckenbißfieber *nt*.
North·ern fowl mite ['nɔːrðərn] *micro.* Ornithonyssus sylviarum.
North Queensland tick fever/typhus Queensland-, Nordqueensland-Zeckenfieber *nt*.
nor·trip·ty·line [nɔːr'trɪptəliːn] *n pharm.* Nortriptylin *nt*.
Norum-Gjone ['nɔːrəm 'jɔːn 'dʒ-]: **N.-G. disease** Norum-Krankheit *f*, familiärer primärer LCAT-Mangel *m*.
Norwalk ['nɔːrwɔːk]: **N. agent/virus** Norwalk-Agens *nt*, -Virus *nt*.
nor·we·gian scabies [nɔːr'wiːdʒən] Borkenkrätze *f*, norwegische Skabies *f*, Scabies crustosa/norvegica.
nos- *pref.* → noso-.
nos·az·on·tol·o·gy [nɑsˌæzən'tɑlədʒɪ] *n* Ätiologie *f*.
nos·ca·pine [nɑskəpiːn] *n pharm.* Noscapin *nt*.
nose [nəʊz] **I** *n* **1.** Nase *f*; *anat.* Nasus *m.* **to bleed at the ~** aus der Nase bluten. **my ~ is bleeding** ich habe Nasenbluten. **2.** *techn.* Nase *f*, Schnabel *m*; Schnauze *f*, Bug *m.* **II** *vt* **3.** riechen; beschnüffeln. **4.** durch die Nase sprechen, näseln.
nose·bleed ['nəʊzbliːd] *n* Nasenbluten *nt*, -blutung *f*, Epistaxis *f*. **to have a ~** Nasenbluten haben.
nose-bridge-lid reflex Orbicularis-oculi-Reflex *m*.
nose drops *pharm.* Nasentropfen *pl*.
decongestant n. abschwellende Nasentropfen.
nose-eye reflex Orbicularis-oculi-Reflex *m*.
nose·piece ['nəʊzpiːs] *n* **1.** *techn.* Mundstück *nt*. **2.** (*Mikroskop*) Revolver *m*. **3.** (Brillen-)Steg *m*.
nose spray *pharm.* Nasenspray *m/nt*.
nos·e·ti·ol·o·gy [ˌnɑsɪtɪ'ɑlədʒɪ] *n* Ätiologie *f*.
no-smoking *adj* Nichtraucher-.
noso- *pref.* Krank-, Krankheit-, Nos(o)-.
nos·och·tho·nog·ra·phy [nɑsˌɑkθəʊ'nɑgrəfɪ] *n* Geomedizin *f*.
nos·o·co·mi·al [ˌnɑsə'kəʊmɪəl] *adj* mit Bezug zum Krankenhaus, nosokomial.

nosocomial infection nosokomiale Infektion *f*, nosokomialer Infekt *m*, Nosokomialinfektion *f*.
nos·o·gen·e·sis [ˌnɑsə'dʒenəsɪs] *n* Pathogenese *f*.
nos·o·gen·ic [ˌ-'dʒenɪk] *adj* Pathogenese betr., pathogen.
no·sog·e·ny [nəʊ'sɑdʒənɪ] *n* Pathogenese *f*.
nos·o·ge·og·ra·phy [ˌnɑsədʒɪ'ɑgrəfɪ] *n* Geomedizin *f*.
no·sog·ra·phy [nəʊ'sɑgrəfɪ] *n* Nosographie *f*.
nos·o·log·ic [ˌnɑsə'lɑdʒɪk] *adj* Nosologie betr., nosologisch.
no·sol·o·gy [nəʊ'sɑlədʒɪ] *n* Krankheitslehre *f*, Nosologie *f*.
nos·o·ma·nia [ˌnɑsə'meɪnɪə, -jə] *n psychia.* Krankheitsfurcht *f*, Nosomanie *f*; hypochondrischer Wahn *m*.
nos·o·my·co·sis [ˌmaɪ'kəʊsɪs] *n* Pilzerkrankung *f*, Mykose *f*, Mycosis *f*.
no·son·o·my [nəʊ'sɑnəmɪ] *n* → nosology.
nos·o·par·a·site [ˌnɑsə'pærəsaɪt] *n* Nosoparasit *m*.
nos·o·phil·ia [ˌ-'fɪlɪə] *n psychia.* Nosophilie *f*.
nos·o·pho·bia [ˌ-'fəʊbɪə] *n psychia.* Nosophobie *f*.
nos·o·phyte ['faɪt] *n bio.* Nosophyt *m*.
nos·o·poi·et·ic [ˌ-pɔɪ'etɪk] *adj* eine Krankheit verursachend, pathogen.
Nos·o·psyl·lus [ˌ-'sɪləs] *n micro.* Nosopsyllus *m*.
N. fasciatus Rattenfloh *m*, Nosopsyllus fasciatus.
nos·o·tax·y ['tæksɪ] *n* → nosology.
nos·o·tox·i·co·sis [ˌ-ˌtɑksɪ'kəʊsɪs] *n* Nosotoxikose *f*, Toxikose *f*.
nos·o·tox·in [ˌ-'tɑksɪn] *n* Nosotoxin *nt*.
nos·tal·gia [nɑ'stældʒ(ɪ)ə, nə-] *n psycho.*, *psychia.* Heimweh *nt*, Nostalgie *f*.
nos·to·ma·nia [ˌnɑstə'meɪnɪə, -jə] *n psychia.* krankhaftes Heimweh *nt*, Nostomanie *f*.
nos·to·pho·bia [ˌ-'fəʊbɪə] *n psychia.* Nostophobie *f*.
nos·tril ['nɑstrəl] *n* Nasenloch *nt*; *anat.* Naris *f*.
no·tal ['nəʊtl] *adj* Rücken betr., dorsal, Rücken-.
no·tal·gia [nəʊ'tældʒ(ɪ)ə] *n old* → dorsalgia.
notch [nɑtʃ] **I** *n* Kerbe *f*, Scharte *f*, Einschnitt *m*, Fissur *f*, Inzisur *f*; *anat.* Incisura *f.* **II** *vt* (ein-)kerben, (ein-)schneiden.
n. of Rivinus Inc. tympanica.
n. for round ligament Lebereinschnitt durch das Lig. teretis hepatis, Inc. lig. teretis.
note blindness [nəʊt] musikalische Alexie *f*.
Nothnagel ['nɔːtnɑːɡəl]: **N.'s syndrome** Nothnagel-Syndrom *nt*, oberes Syndrom *nt* des Nc. ruber, oberes Nc. ruber-Syndrom *nt*.
no·ti·fi·a·ble disease ['nəʊtəfaɪəbl] anzeigepflichtige/meldepflichtige Erkrankung/Krankheit *f*.
no·to·chord ['nəʊtəkɔːrd] *n anat.* Rückensaite *f*, -strang *m*, Chorda dorsalis/vertebralis.
no·to·chord·al canal [ˌ-'kɔːrdl] *embryo.* Chordakanal *m*.
notochordal plate *embryo.* Chordafortsatz *m*.
notochordal process *embryo.* → notochordal plate.
no·to·chor·do·ma [ˌ-kɔːr'dəʊmə] *n* Chordom *nt*, Notochordom *nt*.
no·tom·e·lus [nəʊ'tɑmələs] *n* Notomelus *m*.

no-touch technique *chir.* No-touch-Technik *f*.
no·vo·bi·o·cen [ˌnəʊvəʊ'baɪəsɪn] *n pharm.* Novobiocen *nt*.
nox·a ['nɑksə] *n, pl* **-ae** [-siː] Schadstoff *m*, schädigendes *od.* krankheitserregendes Agens *nt*, Noxe *f*.
nox·ious ['nɑkʃəs] *adj* schädigend, schädlich, ungesund (*to für*).
nox·ious·ness ['-nɪs] *n* Schädlichkeit *f*.
noxious substance → noxa.
NP *abbr.* → nucleoprotein.
Np *abbr.* → neptunium.
NPDL *abbr.* → nodular poorly-differentiated lymphocytic lymphoma.
NPN *abbr.* → nonprotein nitrogen.
N.R.C. *abbr.* → retinal correspondence, normal.
NREM sleep → non-REM sleep.
nRNA *abbr.* → nuclear RNA.
ns *abbr.* → nanosecond.
NSAIDs *abbr.* → non-steroidal anti-inflammatory drugs.
nsec *abbr.* → nanosecond.
NSILA *abbr.* → nonsuppressible insulin-like activity.
N-terminal *adj chem.* aminoterminal, N-terminal.
NTP *abbr.* → nucleoside(-5'-)triphosphate.
nu·bec·u·la [n(j)uː'bekjələ] *n, pl* **-lae** [-liː] **1.** *ophthal.* leichte Hornhauttrübung *f*, Nubekula *f*, Nubecula *f*, Nebula *f*. **2.** (*Harn*) Trübung *f*, Nubekula *f*.
nu·cha ['n(j)uːkə] *n, pl* **-chae** [-kiː] *anat.* Nacken *m*, Nucha *f*.
nu·chal ['n(j)uːkl] *adj* Nacken betr., zum Nacken gehörend, nuchal, Nacken-.
nuchal fascia Fascia nuchae.
nuchal flexure *embryo.* Nackenbeuge *f*.
nuchal ligament Nackenband *nt*, Lig. nuchae.
nuchal line Linea nuchalis.
highest n. Linea nuchalis suprema.
inferior n. Linea nuchalis inferior.
median n. Crista occipitalis externa.
middle n. → median n.
superior n. Linea nuchalis superior.
supreme n. → highest n.
nuchal nevus Storchenbiß *m*, Unna-Politzer-Nackennävus *m*, Nävus Unna *m*.
nuchal region Nackengegend *f*, -region *f*, Regio cervicalis posterior, Regio nuchalis.
nuchal tubercle Vertebra prominens.
Nuck [nɔk]: **canal of N.** Proc. vaginalis peritonei.
N.'s diverticulum → canal of N.
N.'s hydrocele Nuck-Zyste *f*, Hydrocele feminae/muliebris.
nucle- → nucleo-.
nu·cle·ar ['n(j)uːklɪər] *adj* **1.** (Zell-)Kern *od.* Nukleus betr., nukleär, nuklear, Zellkern-, Kern-. **2.** *phys.* Atomkern betr., nuklear, (Atom-)Kern-, Nuklear-.
nuclear agenesia Möbius-Syndrom *nt*, -Kernaplasie *f*.
nuclear agenesis → nuclear agenesia.
nuclear antigen *immun.* Kernantigen *nt*, nukleäres Antigen *nt*.
Epstein-Barr n. *abbr.* **EBNA** Epstein-Barr nukleäres Antigen *abbr.* EBNA, Epstein-Barr nuclear antigen.
nuclear aplasia → nuclear agenesia.
nuclear atom Rutherford'-Atom(modell *nt*) *nt*.
nuclear bag fiber Kernhaufenfaser *f*.
nuclear cataract Kernstar *m*, Cataracta nuclearis.
nuclear chain fiber Kernkettenfaser *f*.
nuclear charge *phys.* Kernladung *f*.
nuclear chemistry Kernchemie *f*.

nuclear decay *phys.* Kernzerfall *m*, radioaktiver Zerfall *m*.
nuclear disintegration *phys.* Kernzerfall *m*, radioaktiver Zerfall *m*.
nuclear DNA Kern-DNA, Kern-DNS *f*.
nuclear electron *phys.* Kernelektron *nt*.
nuclear energy *phys.* Atom-, Kernenergie *f*.
nuclear envelope → nuclear membrane.
nuclear-fast red *histol.* Kernechtrot *nt*.
nuclear fission *phys.* Kernspaltung *f*.
nuclear fusion *phys.* Kernfusion *f*, -verschmelzung *f*.
nuclear groups of thalamus Kerngruppen *od.* -komplexe *pl* des Thalamus.
nuclear hyaloplasma Kernsaft *m*, Karyolymphe *f*.
nuclear icterus → nuclear jaundice.
nuclear jaundice Kernikterus *m*, Bilirubinenzephalopathie *f*.
nuclear layer: n. of cerebellum innere Körnerschicht *f* der Kleinhirnrinde, Stratum granulare/granulosum cerebelli.
external n. äußere Körnerschicht *f*.
inner/internal n. innere Körnerschicht *f*.
outer n. → external n.
nuclear magnetic resonance *abbr.* **NMR** Kern(spin)resonanz *f*.
nuclear magnetic resonance spectroscopy Kern(spin)resonanzspektroskopie *f*, NMR-Spektroskopie *f*.
nuclear medicine Nuklearmedizin *f*.
nuclear membrane *histol.* Kernmembran *f*, -wand *f*, -hülle *f*.
nuclear model *phys.* Kernmodell *nt*.
nuclear ophthalmoplegia nukleäre Ophthalmoplegie *f*.
nuclear particle 1. *phys.* Kernteilchen *nt*. **2.** ~s *pl* (Howell-)Jolly-Körperchen *pl*.
nuclear physicist Kernphysiker(in *f*) *m*.
nuclear physics Kernphysik *f*.
nuclear polymerism *chem.* Kernpolymerie *f*.
nuclear polymorphism Kernpolymorphie *f*.
nuclear pore Kernpore *f*.
nuclear power *phys.* Atomkraft *m*, Kernenergie *f*.
nuclear radiation Radioaktivität *f*, Kernstrahlung *f*.
nuclear reaction *phys.* Kernreaktion *f*.
Feulgen's n. *histol.* Feulgen'-Nuklealreaktion.
nuclear reactor *phys.* Kernreaktor *m*.
nuclear receptor nukleärer Rezeptor *m*.
nuclear resonance scanning *radiol.* Kernspinresonanztomographie *f*, NMR--Tomographie *f*, MR-Tomographie *f* *abbr.* MRT.
nuclear RNA *abbr.* **nRNA** Kern-RNA *f* *abbr.* nRNA, Kern-RNS *f*.
nuclear sclerosis *ophthal.* Linsensklerosierung *f*.
nuclear sex Kerngeschlecht *nt*.
nuclear spindle Kern-, Mitosespindel *f*.
nuclear stain Kernfärbung *f*.
nuclear swelling Kernschwellung *f*.
nuclear zone 1. (*ZNS*) Kerngebiet *nt*. **2.** *bio.* Kernäquivalent *nt*. **3.** *anat.* Vortex lentis.
nu·cle·ase ['n(j)u:klieɪz] *n* Nuklease *f*, Nuclease *f*.
nu·cle·at·ed ['n(j)u:klieɪtɪd] *adj* kernhaltig.
nucleated cell kernhaltige Zelle *f*.
nucleated red (blood) cell kernhaltige Erythrozytenvorläuferzelle *f*.
nu·cle·ic acid [nʊ'kli:ɪk] Nuklein-, Nucleinsäure *f*.
nucleic acid core *micro.* Nukleinsäure--haltiger Innenkörper/Kern *m*, Core *m*.
nucleic base Purinbase *f*.
nu·cle·ide ['n(j)u:klіaɪd] *n* Nukleid *nt*.

nu·cle·in ['n(j)u:kli:n] *n* Nuklein *nt*.
nuclein base Purinbase *f*.
nu·cle·in·ic acid [ˌn(j)u:klɪ'ɪnɪk] → nucleic acid.
nucleo- *pref.* Kern-, Nukle(o)-, Nucle(o)-.
nu·cle·o·cap·sid [ˌn(j)u:klіəʊ'kæpsɪd] *n* *micro.* Nukleokapsid *nt*.
nu·cle·o·cer·e·bel·lar tract [ˌ-serə'belər] Tractus nucleocerebellaris.
nu·cle·o·chy·le·ma [ˌ-kaɪ'li:mə] *n* Kernsaft *m*, Karyolymphe *f*.
nu·cle·o·chyme ['-kaɪm] *n* Kernsaft *m*, Karyolymphe *f*.
nu·cle·o·cy·to·plas·mic ratio [ˌ-ˌsaɪtəʊ'plæzmɪk] Kern-Zytoplasma-Relation *f*.
nu·cle·of·u·gal [n(j)u:'klɪ'ʌfjəɡəl] *adj* vom Kern weg, nukleofugal.
nu·cle·o·glu·co·pro·tein [ˌn(j)u:klіəʊˌɡluːkəʊ'prəʊti:n, -ti:ɪn] *n* Nukleoglukoprotein *nt*.
nu·cle·o·his·tone [ˌ-'hɪstəʊn] *n* Nukleo-, Nucleohiston *nt*.
nu·cle·oid ['n(j)u:klɔɪd] **I** *n* Nukleoid *nt*, Nucleoid *nt*. **II** *adj* kernartig, -ähnlich, nukleoid.
nu·cle·o·ker·a·tin [ˌn(j)u:klіəʊ'kerətɪn] *n* Nukleo-, Nucleokeratin *nt*.
nu·cle·o·lar [n(j)u:'klɪələr] *adj* Nukleolus betr., Nukleolen-, Nukleolus-.
nu·cle·ole ['n(j)u:klɪəʊl] *n* → nucleolus.
nu·cle·ol·i·form [n(j)u:'klɪəlɪfɔːrm] *adj* nukleolusartig, -förmig.
nu·cle·o·loid ['n(j)u:klɪəlɔɪd] *adj* → nucleoliform.
nu·cle·o·lo·ne·ma [n(j)u:klɪˌəʊlə'ni:mə] *n* *histol.* Nukleolonema *nt*, Nucleolonema *nt*.
nu·cle·o·lo·neme [ˌn(j)u:klɪ'əlɑni:m] *n* → nucleolonema.
nu·cle·o·lus [n(j)u:'klɪələs] *n*, *pl* **-li** [-laɪ] Kernkörperchen *nt*, Nukleolus *m*, Nucleolus *m*.
nucleolus organizer *histol.* Nukleolusorganisator *m*.
nu·cle·o·lymph ['n(j)u:klɪəlɪmf] *n* Kernsaft *m*, Karyolymphe *f*.
nu·cle·on ['n(j)u:klɑn] *n* *phys.* Nukleon *nt*.
nu·cle·on·ic [ˌn(j)u:klɪ'ɑnɪk] *adj* Kern/Nukleus betr., Kern-.
nu·cle·on·ics [ˌ-'ɑnɪks] *pl* Kernphysik *f*.
nu·cle·op·e·tal [n(j)u:klɪ'ɑpətəl] *adj* zum Kern hin, nukleopetal.
nu·cle·o·phile ['n(j)u:klɪəfaɪl] *n* *chem.* nukleophile Substanz *f*.
nu·cle·o·phil·ic [ˌ-'fɪlɪk] *adj* *chem.* nukleophil.
nu·cle·o·phos·pha·tase [ˌ-'fɑsfəteɪz] *n* → 5'-nucleotidase.
nu·cle·o·plasm ['-plæzəm] *n* (Zell-)Kernprotoplasma *nt*, Karyo-, Nukleoplasma *nt*.
nu·cle·o·pro·tein [ˌ-'prəʊti:n, -ti:ɪn] *n* *abbr.* **NP** Nukleo-, Nucleoprotein *nt* *abbr.* NP.
nu·cle·o·sid·ase [ˌ-'saɪdeɪz] *n* Nukleo-, Nucleosidase *f*.
nu·cle·o·side ['-saɪd] *n* Nukleosid *nt*, Nucleosid *nt*.
nucleoside analogues Nukleosidanaloga *pl*.
nucleoside(-5'-)diphosphate *n* *abbr.* **NDP** Nucleosid(-5'-)diphosphat *nt* *abbr.* NDP.
nucleoside diphosphate kinase Nucleosiddiphosphatkinase *f*, NDP-Kinase *f*.
nucleoside diphosphate sugar Nucleosiddiphosphatzucker *m*, NDP-Zucker *m*.
nucleoside kinase Nukleosidkinase *f*.
nucleoside(-5'-)monophosphate *n* *abbr.* **NMP** Nucleosid(-5'-)monophosphat *nt* *abbr.* NMP.

nucleoside monophosphate kinase Nucleosidmonophosphatkinase *f*, NMP-Kinase *f*.
nucleoside pair *biochem.* Basenpaar *nt*.
nucleoside phosphorylase Nucleosidphosphorylase *f*.
nucleoside(-5'-)triphosphate *n* *abbr.* **NTP** Nucleosid(-5'-)triphosphat *nt* *abbr.* NTP.
nu·cle·o·sin ['n(j)u:klіəsɪn] *n* Thymopo(i)etin *nt*, Thymin *nt*.
nu·cle·o·sis [ˌn(j)u:klɪ'əʊsɪs] *n* Kernproliferation *f*.
nu·cle·o·some ['n(j)u:klіəsəʊm] *n* Nukleosom *nt*.
nu·cle·o·tid·ase [ˌn(j)u:klіə'taɪdeɪz] *n* Nukleo-, Nucleotidase *f*.
5'-nucleotidase *n* 5'-Nukleotidase *f*, 5'-Nucleotidase *f*.
nu·cle·o·tide ['n(j)u:klіətaɪd] *n* Nukleotid *nt*, Nucleotid *nt*.
nucleotide coenzyme Nukleotidcoenzym *nt*.
nucleotide cyclase Nukleotid(yl)zyklase *f*, -cyclase *f*.
nucleotide pair *biochem.* Basenpaar *nt*.
nucleotide polymerase Nukleotidpolymerase *f*.
nucleotide sequence Nukleotidsequenz *f*.
nu·cle·o·tid·yl [ˌn(j)u:klіə'taɪdɪl] *n* Nukleotidyl-(Rest *m*).
nucleotidyl cyclase → nucleotide cyclase.
nu·cle·o·tid·yl·trans·fer·ase [n(j)u:klіəˌtaɪdɪl'trænsfəreɪz] *n* Nukleotidyltransferase *f*.
nu·cle·us ['n(j)u:klіəs] *n*, *pl* **-cle·us·es**, **-cle·i** [-klaɪ] **1.** *anat.*, *bio.* (Zell-)Kern *m*, Nukleus *m*, Nucleus *m*; *phys.* (Atom-)Kern *m*. **2.** (*ZNS*) Kern *m*, Kerngebiet *nt*, Nucleus *m*. **3.** *allg.* Kern *m*, Zentrum *nt*, Mittelpunkt *m*.
n. of abducens nerve Abducenskern, Nc. abducens, Nc. n. abducentis.
n. of accessory nerve Akzessoriuskern, Nc. n. accessorii, Nc. accessorius.
n.i of acoustic nerve Vestibulariskerne *pl*, Ncc. vestibulares.
n. of ansa lenticularis Kern der Linsenschleife, Nc. ansae lenticularis.
n.i of areas H/H1/H2 Kerne *pl* der Forel'-Felder H/H1/H2, Ncc. regionum H/H1/H2.
n. of Burdach's column/tract Burdach'--Kern, Nc. cuneatus.
n. of caudal colliculus Nc. colliculi caudalis/inferioris.
n.i of cerebellum Kleinhirnkerne *pl*, Ncc. cerebellaris.
n.i of cochlear nerve Cochleariskerne *pl*, Ncc. cochleares.
n.i of cranial nerves Hirnnervenkerne *pl*, Ncc. nn. cranialium/encephalicorum.
n. of facial nerve motorischer Fazialiskern, Nc. (n.) facialis.
n. of Goll's column/tract Nc. gracilis.
n.i of habenula Ncc. habenulares mediales et laterales.
n. of hypoglossal nerve Hypoglossuskern, Nc. n. hypoglossi, Nc. hypoglossalis.
n.i of hypothalamus Hypothalamuskerne *pl*, Ncc. hypothalamici.
n. of inferior colliculus → n. of caudal colliculus.
n. of internal geniculate body Kern des medialen Kniehöckers, Nc. geniculatus medialis.
n. of lateral geniculate body Kern des lateralen Kniehöckers, Nc. geniculatus lateralis.
n.i of lateral lemniscus Ncc. lemnisci lateralis.
n. of lens (*Auge*) Linsenkern, Nc. lentis.

nutritional deficiency

n. of lenticular loop → n. of ansa lenticularis.
n. of Luys Luys'-Kern, -Körper *m*, Corpus Luys, Nc. subthalamicus.
n. of medial geniculate body Kern des medialen Kniehöckers, Nc. geniculatus medialis.
n.i of median raphe Ncc. raphae.
n. of mesencephalic tract of trigeminal nerve oberer Trigeminuskern, Mittelhirnkern des N. trigeminus, Nc. tractus mesencephalici n. trigeminalis, Nc. mesencephalicus trigeminalis, Nc. mesencephalicus n. trigeminalis.
n. of oculomotor nerve Okulomotoriuskern, Nc. n. oculomotorii, Nc. oculomotorius.
n. of Perlia Perlia'-Kern.
n. of phrenic nerve Phrenikuskern, Kern des N. phrenicus, Nc. n. phrenici, Nc. phrenicus.
n.i of pons Brückenkerne *pl*, Ncc. pontis.
n.i of rhombencephalon Rautenhirnkerne *pl*.
n. of solitary tract Nc. tractus solitarius, Nc. solitarius.
n.i of spinal cord Rückenmarkskerne *pl*.
n. of superior olive Nc. olivaris rostralis/superioris.
n.i of termination Endkerne *pl*, Ncc. terminatorius.
n.i of thalamus Thalamuskerne *pl*, Ncc. thalami.
n.i of trigeminal nerve Trigeminuskerne *pl*, Ncc. trigemini.
n. of trochlear nerve Trochleariskern, Nc. (n.) trochlearis.
nucleus caeruleus Nc. caeruleus.
nucleus icterus Kernikterus *m*, Bilirubinenzephalopathie *f*.
nucleus jaundice → nucleus icterus.
nucleus magnus Nc. magnus.
nucleus obscurus Nc. obscurus.
nucleus proprius Nc. proprius.
nucleus reticularis intermedius: n. gigantocellularis Nc. reticularis intermedius gigantocellularis.
n. medullae oblongatae Nc. reticularis intermedius medullae oblongatae.
n. pontis inferioris Nc. reticularis intermedius pontis inferioris.
n. pontis superioris Nc. reticularis intermedius pontis superioris.
nucleus reticularis lateralis: n. medullae oblongatae Nc. reticularis lateralis medullae oblongatae.
n. pontis Nc. reticularis lateralis pontis.
n. precerebelli Nc. reticularis lateralis pr(a)ecerebelli.
nucleus reticularis paramedianus (precerebelli) Nc. reticularis paramedianus pr(a)ecerebelli.
nucleus reticularis tegmentalis: n. pedunculo-pontinus Nc. reticularis tegmentalis pedunculo-pontinus.
n. pontinus Nc. reticularis tegmentalis pontinus.
nucleus reuniens Nc. reuniens.
nucleus reuniens thalami Nc. reuniens thalami.
nucleus ruber roter Kern *m*, Nc. ruber.
nucleus subc(a)eruleus Nc. subcaeruleus.
nu·clide ['n(j)u:klaɪd] *n chem.* Nuklid *nt*.
nu·do·pho·bia [nu:dəʊ'fəʊbɪə] *n psychia.* Nudophobie *f*.
Nuel [ny'ɛl]: **N.'s space** Nuel'-Raum *m*.
NUG *abbr.* → necrotizing ulcerative gingivitis.
Nuhn [nu:n]: **N.'s gland** Nuhn'-Drüse *f*, Gl. lingualis anterior.
null [nʌl] **I** *n mathe.* Null *f*. **II** *adj* 1. fehlend,

nicht vorhanden. 2. *mathe.* leer.
null cells *immun.* Nullzellen *pl*.
null hypothesis *abbr.* **H₀** Nullhypothese *f abbr.* H₀.
nul·li·grav·i·da [nʌlɪ'grævɪdə] *n gyn.* Nulligravida *f*.
nul·lip·a·ra [nʌ'lɪpərə] *n, pl* -ras, -rae [-ri:] *gyn.* Nullipara *f*.
nul·lip·a·rous [nʌ'lɪpərəs] *adj gyn.* nullipar.
nulliparous woman *gyn.* Nullipara *f*.
numb [nʌm] **I** *adj* 1. starr, erstarrt, taub. 2. abgestumpft, betäubt. **II** *vt* 3. betäuben, abstumpfen. 4. starr *od.* taub machen, erstarren lassen.
num·ber ['nʌmbər] **I** *n* 1. *mathe.* Zahl *f*, Ziffer *f*. 2. (Telefon-, Zimmer-)Nummer *f*. 3. (An-)Zahl *f (of an)*. **II** *vt* 4. rechnen, zählen; (zusammen-)zählen, aufrechnen. 5. numerieren. **III** *vi* zählen.
number comprehension *HNO (Gehör)* Zahlenverständnis *nt*.
num·ber·ing ['nʌmbərɪŋ] *n* Numerierung *f*.
numb·ness ['nʌmnɪs] *n* 1. Taubheit *f*, Betäubung *f*. 2. Erstarrung *f*, Starrheit *f*, Taubheit *f*.
nu·mer·i·cal [n(j)u:'merɪkl] *adj* numerisch, Zahlen-.
numerical aperture *abbr.* **N.A.** *phys.* numerische Apertur *f*.
numerical atrophy numerische Atrophie *f*.
numerical classification → numerical taxonomy.
numerical hypertrophy numerische Hypertrophie *f*, Hyperplasie *f*.
numerical taxonomy *micro.* numerische Taxonomie *f*.
num·mu·lar ['nʌmjələr] *adj* münzenförmig, nummulär.
nummular eczema nummuläres/mikrobielles/nummulär-mikrobielles/parasitäres/diskoides Ekzem *nt*, bakterielles Ekzematoid *nt*, Dermatitis nummularis, Eccema nummularis.
nummular eczematous dermatitis → nummular eczema.
nummular neurodermatitis → nummular eczema.
nummular psoriasis *derm.* Psoriasis nummularis.
nummular sputum Sputum nummulare.
nun's murmur [nʌn] *card.* Nonnensausen *nt*, -geräusch *nt*, Kreiselgeräusch *nt*, Bruit de diable.
Nunn [nʌn]: **N.'s gorged corpuscles** Nunn-Körperchen *pl*.
nurse [nɜrs] **I** *n* 1. (Kranken-)Schwester *f*, (Kranken-)Pfleger(in *f*) *m*. 2. Kindermädchen *nt*, -frau *f*. 3. Amme *f*. 4. Säuglings-, Kinderschwester *f*. **II** *vt* 5. (*Kranke*) pflegen; hegen, schonen. 6. (eine Krankheit) auskurieren. **to ~ a cold.** 7. (*Säugling*) stillen. 8. (*Kind*) auf-, großziehen. **III** *vi* 9. stillen; (*Säugling*) saugen, die Brust nehmen. 10. als Krankenschwester *od.* -pfleger tätig sein.
nurse's aid Schwesternhelfer(in *f*) *m*.
nurse cells Sertoli'Zellen *pl*, Stütz-, Ammen-, Fußzellen *pl*.
nurse child Pflege-, Ziehkind *nt*.
nurse·ling ['nɜrslɪŋ] *n* → nursling.
nurse-maid's elbow ['nɜrsmeɪd] *ortho.* Chassaignac-Lähmung *f*, Subluxation *f* des Radiusköpfchens, Pronatio dolorosa, Subluxatio radii peranularis.
nurs·er·y ['nɜrsərɪ] *n* 1. Kinderzimmer *nt*. 2. Kindertagesstätte *f*, Kindergarten *m*.
nursery nurse Kindergärtnerin *f*.
nursery school Kindergarten *m*.
nurs·ing ['nɜrsɪŋ] **I** *n* 1. Säugen *nt*, Stillen *nt*. 2. Krankenpflege *f*. **II** *adj* Pflege-, Kranken-; Nähr-.

nursing auxiliary *Brit.* Schwesternhelfer(in *f*) *m*.
nursing bottle (Saug-, Säuglings-)Flasche *f*, Fläschchen *nt*.
nursing care Krankenpflege *f*.
nursing cells → nurse cells.
nursing father Pflegevater *m*.
nursing home 1. Pflegeheim *nt*. 2. *Brit.* Privatklinik *f*.
nursing mother 1. stillende Mutter *f*. 2. Pflegemutter *f*.
nursing period Stillzeit *f*.
nursing personal Pflegepersonal *nt*.
nursing staff Pflegepersonal *nt*.
nursing treatment Pflege(behandlung *f*) *f*.
nurs·ling ['nɜrslɪŋ] *n* 1. Pflegekind *nt*. 2. Säugling *m*.
nut [nʌt] *n* Nuß *f*.
nu·ta·tion [n(j)u:'teɪʃn] *n* 1. Nicken *nt*, Nutation *f*. 2. *phys.* Nutation *f*.
nut·gall ['nʌtgɔ:l] *n* Gallapfel *m*.
nut·meg liver ['nʌtmeg] Muskatnußleber *f*.
nu·tri·ent ['n(j)u:trɪənt] **I** *n* Nährstoff *m*; *bio.* Baustoff *m*. **II** *adj* 1. nahrhaft; (er-)nährend, mit Nährstoffen versorgend. 2. Ernährungs-, Nähr-.
nutrient agar Nähragar *m/nt*.
nutrient artery A. nutricia/nutriens.
n.s of femur Aa. nutriciae/nutrientes femoris.
n. of fibula A. nutricia/nutriens fibulae.
n.s of humerus Aa. nutriciae/nutrientes humeri.
n.s of kidney Aa. capsularis/perirenales.
n. of tibia A. nutricia/nutriens tibialis.
nutrient base Nährsubstrat *nt*.
nutrient bouillon *micro.* Nährbrühe *f*, -bouillon *f*, Bouillon *f*.
nutrient broth → nutrient bouillon.
nutrient canal (*Knochen*) Canalis nutriens.
nutrient circulation Nährstoffkreislauf *m*.
nutrient consumption Nährstoffverbrauch *m*.
nutrient content Nährstoffgehalt *m*.
nutrient deficiency Nährstoffmangel *m*.
nutrient-dense *adj* nahrhaft, nährstoffreich.
nutrient density Reichhaltigkeit *f* an Nährstoffen.
nutrient foramen (*Knochen*) For. nutricium/nutriens.
nutrient medium Nährboden *m*, -medium *nt*, -substanz *f*.
nutrient molecule Nährstoffmolekül *nt*.
nutrient needs Nährstoffbedarf *m*.
nutrient requirement Nährstoffbedarf *m*.
nutrient solution Nährlösung *f*.
nutrient vessels of lung ernährende Vasa privata der Lunge.
nu·tri·ment ['n(j)u:trɪmənt] *n* Nahrung *f*, Nährstoff *m*, Nahrungsmittel *nt*, Nutriment *nt*.
nu·tri·men·tal [,-'mentl] *adj* → nutritious.
nu·tri·tion [n(j)u:'trɪʃn] *n* 1. Ernährung *f*, Nutrition *f*. 2. → nutriment. 3. Nahrungsaufnahme *f*, Ernähren *nt*.
nu·tri·tion·al [n(j)u:'trɪʃnl] *adj* Ernährungs-, Nähr-.
nutritional amblyopia *ophthal.* ernährungsbedingte/nutritive Amblyopie *f*.
nutritional amenorrhea *gyn.* Notstandsamenorrhoe *f*, ernährungsbedingte/nutritive Amenorrhoe *f*.
nutritional anemia Mangelanämie *f*, nutritive/alimentäre Anämie *f*.
nutritional cataract nutritive Katarakt *f*.
nutritional cirrhosis nutritive/ernährungsbedingte Leberzirrhose *f*.
nutritional deficiency Nährstoffmangel *m*.

nutritional deficiency cataract → nutritional cataract.
nutritional deficit Nährstoffmangel *m*.
nutritional disorder Ernährungsstörung *f*.
nutritional dropsy → nutritional edema.
nutritional edema Hungerödem *nt*.
nutritional factor → nutritive factor.
nutritional state Ernährungszustand *m*, -lage *f*.
nutrition cycle Nahrungskreislauf *m*.
nu·tri·tion·ist [n(j)u:'trɪʃənɪst] *n* Ernährungswissenschaftler(in *f*) *m*, Trophologe *m*, -login *f*.
nu·tri·tious [n(j)u:'trɪʃəs] *adj* nahrhaft, nährend, nutritiv.
nu·tri·tious·ness [n(j)u:'trɪʃəsnɪs] *n* Nahrhaftigkeit *f*.
nu·tri·tive ['n(j)u:trətɪv] **I** *n* Nahrung *f*, Diätetikum *nt*. **II** *adj* **1.** nahrhaft, nährend, nutritiv. **2.** ernährend, Nähr-, Ernährungs-.
nutritive behavior nutritives Verhalten *nt*.
nutritive deficiency Nährstoffmangel *m*.
nutritive factor Ernährungs-, Nahrungsfaktor *m*.
nutritive gelatin Nährgelatine *f*.
nutritive medium Nährboden *m*, -medium *nt*, -substanz *f*.
nutritive needs Nährstoffbedarf *m*.
nu·tri·tive·ness ['n(j)u:trətɪvnɪs] *n* Nahrhaftigkeit *f*.
nutritive plasma Trophoplasma *nt*, Nährplasma *nt*.
nutritive requirement Nährstoffbedarf *m*.
nutritive substance → nutrient I.
nutritive substrate Nährsubstrat *nt*.
nutritive tissue Nährgewebe *nt*.
nutritive value Nährwert *m*.
nu·trix ['n(j)u:trɪks] *n* Amme *f*, Nutrix *f*.

Nut·tal·lia [nə'tælɪə] *n old* → Babesia.
nux [nʌks] *n pharm*. Nuß *f*, Nux *f*.
NWDL *abbr*. → nodular well-differentiated lymphocytic lymphoma.
ny·a·cyne ['naɪəsaɪn] *n* → neomycin.
NYC medium NYC-Medium *nt*, New York City-Medium *nt*.
nyct- *pref*. → nycto-.
nyc·tal·gia [nɪk'tældʒ(ɪ)ə] *n* nächtlicher Schmerz *m*, Nyktalgie *f*.
nyc·ta·lope ['nɪktələʊp] *n* Nachtblinde(r *m*) *f*.
nyc·ta·lo·pia [ˌ-'ləʊpɪə] *n ophthal*. Nachtblindheit *f*, Hemeralopie *f*.
nyc·ta·no·pia [ˌ-'nəʊpɪə] *n* → nyctalopia.
nyc·ter·ine ['-raɪn] *adj* **1.** während der Nacht auftretend, nachts, nächtlich. **2.** unklar, obskur.
nyc·ter·o·hem·er·al [ˌnɪktərəʊ'hemərəl] *adj* → nyctohemeral.
nycto- *pref*. Nacht-, Nykt(o)-.
nyc·to·hem·er·al [ˌnɪktəʊ'hemərəl] *adj* Tag u. Nacht betr., nykt(o)hemeral.
nyc·to·phil·ia [ˌ-'fɪlɪə] *n psychia*. Nyktophilie *f*.
nyc·to·pho·bia [ˌ-'fəʊbɪə] *n psychia*. Nyktophobie *f*.
nyc·tu·ria [nɪk't(j)ʊərɪə] *n* vermehrtes nächtliches Wasserlassen *nt*, Nykturie *f*.
NYHA classification [New York heart association] NYHA-Einteilung *f*, -Klassifikation *f*.
ny·lon ['naɪlən] *n* Nylon *nt*.
nymph [nɪmf] *n bio*. Nymphe *f*, Nympha *f*.
nym·pha ['nɪmfə] *n, pl* **-phae** [-fi:] kleine Schamlippe *f*, Labium minus pudendi, Nympha *f*.
n. of Krause Kitzler *m*, Klitoris *f*, Clitoris *f*.

nym·phec·to·my [nɪm'fektəmɪ] *n gyn*. Nymphektomie *f*.
nym·phi·tis [nɪm'faɪtɪs] *n gyn*. Entzündung *f* der kleinen Schamlippen.
nym·pho·cus ['nɪmfəkəs] *n* Schwellung *f* der kleinen Schamlippen.
nym·pho·ma·nia [ˌnɪmfə'meɪnɪə, -jə] *n psychia*. Mannstollheit *f*, Nymphomanie *f*, Andromanie *f*, Hysteromanie *f*.
nym·pho·ma·ni·ac [ˌ-'meɪnɪæk] **I** *n* Nymphomanin *f*. **II** *adj* Nymphomanie betr., an Nymphomanie leidend, mannstoll, nymphoman(isch).
nym·phot·o·my [nɪm'fɑtəmɪ] *n gyn*. Nymphotomie *f*.
nys·tag·mic [nɪ'stægmɪk] *adj* Nystagmus betr., durch Nystagmus gekennzeichnet, nystagtisch, Nystagmus-.
nys·tag·mi·form [nɪ'stægmɪfɔ:rm] *adj* nystagmusähnlich, -artig, nystagmoid.
nys·tag·mo·gram [nɪ'stægməgræm] *n* Nystagmogramm *nt*.
nys·tag·mo·graph [nɪ'stægməgræf] *n* Nystagmograph *m*.
nys·tag·moid [nɪ'stægmɔɪd] *adj* → nystagmiform.
nys·tag·mus [nɪ'stægməs] *n* Nystagmus *m*.
nystagmus-myoclonus Nystagmus-Myoklonie *f*.
nystagmus test Bárány-Versuch *m*, -Kalorisation *f*.
nys·ta·tin ['nɪstətɪn] *n pharm*. Nystatin *nt*.
nys·tax·is [nɪ'stæksɪs] *n* → nystagmus.
Nysten [nɪ'stɛ̃]: **N.'s law** *forens*. Nysten--Regel *f*.
nyx·is ['nɪksɪs] *n, pl* **-es** [-si:z] *chir*. Punktion *f*; Parazentese *f*.

O

O *abbr.* → oxygen.
o- *abbr.* → ortho-.
O₂ *abbr.* → molecular oxygen.
O₃ *abbr.* → ozone.
Ω *abbr.* **1.** → ohm. **2.** → omega.
ω *abbr.* → omega.
OA *abbr.* **1.** → ocular albinism. **2.** → osteoarthritis.
OAF *abbr.* → osteoclast activating factor.
O agglutination O-Agglutination *f.*
Oakley-Fulthorpe ['əʊklɪ 'fʊlθɔːrp]: **O.-F. technique/test** *lab.* Oakley-Fulthorpe-Technik *f*, eindimensionale Immunodiffusion *f* nach Oakley-Fulthorpe.
O antigen 1. *micro.* O-Antigen *nt*, Körperantigen *nt.* **2.** *hema.* Antigen O *nt.*
oa·ri·al·gia [əʊeərɪ'ældʒ(ɪ)ə] *n* → oophoralgia.
oa·ri·ot·o·my [əʊeərɪ'ɒtəmɪ] *n* → ovariotomy.
oa·ri·tis [əʊə'raɪtɪs] *n* → oophoritis.
oa·ri·um [əʊ'eərɪəm] *n* → ovary.
oast-house urine disease ['əʊsthaʊs] Methioninmalabsorptionssyndrom *nt.*
oat cell carcinoma [əʊt] **1.** Haferzellkarzinom *nt*, oat-cell-Karzinom *nt*, Ca. avenocellulare. **2.** kleinzelliges/kleinzellig-anaplastisches Bronchialkarzinom *nt*, *inf.* Kleinzeller *m.*
oat cells *patho.* Haferzellen *pl*, Oat-cells *pl.*
oat-shaped cells → oat cells.
OAV dysplasia/syndrome → oculoauriculovertebral dysplasia.
ob·dor·mi·tion [əbdɔːr'mɪʃn] *n neuro.* (*Glieder*) Einschlafen *nt*, Obdormtio *f.*
ob·du·cent cartilage [əb'd(j)uːsnt] Gelenkknorpel *m*, Cartilago articularis.
ob·duc·tion [əb'dʌkʃn] *n forens.* Obduktion *f*, Autopsie *f*, Nekropsie *f*, Sektion *f.*
o·be·li·ac [əʊ'bilɪæk] *adj* Obelion betr.
o·be·li·on [əʊ'bilɪən] *n anat.* Obelion *nt.*
Obermeier ['oːbərmaɪər]: **O.'s spirillum** Borrelia recurrentis, Spirochaeta obermeieri.
Oberst ['oːbərst]: **O.'s method** *anes.* Oberst-Anästhesie *f.*
Obersteiner-Redlich ['oːbərstaɪnər 'reːdlɪç]: **O.-R. area/space/zone** Redlich-Obersteiner'-Zone *f.*
o·bese [əʊ'biːs] *adj* fett(leibig), korpulent, adipös.
o·bese·ness ['-nɪs] *n* → obesity.
o·be·si·ty [əʊ'biːsətɪ] *n* Fettleibigkeit *f*, Fettsucht *f*, Korpulenz *f*, Obesität *f*, Adipositas *f*, Obesitas *f.*
o·bex ['əʊbeks] *n* (*ZNS*) Marklamelle *f*, -blatt *nt*, Obex *m.*
ob·fus·cate ['əbfəskeɪt, əb'fʌskeɪt] *vt* **1.** verdunkeln, trüben; verfinstern. **2.** *fig.* trüben, verwirren; (*Sinne*) benebeln.
ob·fus·ca·tion [ˌəbfʌs'keɪʃn] *n* **1.** Trübung *f*, Verdunkelung *f.* **2.** *fig.* Verwirrung *f.*
o·bi·dox·ime chloride [əbɪ'dɒksiːm] *pharm.* Obidoximchlorid *nt.*
ob·ject ['əbdʒɪkt, -dʒekt] *n* **1.** Objekt *nt*, Ding *nt*, Gegenstand *m.* **2.** Zweck *m*, Ziel *nt.*

object agnosia Objektagnosie *f.*
object choice *psycho.* Objektwahl *f.*
object glass → objective I.
ob·jec·tive [əb'dʒektɪv] **I** *n opt.* Objektiv-(linse *f*) *nt.* **II** *adj* sachlich, unpersönlich, objektiv.
objective lens → objective I.
ob·jec·tive·ness ['-nɪs] *n* → objectivity.
objective sign objektives Zeichen *nt.*
objective symptom objektives Symptom *nt.*
objective vertigo objektiver Schwindel *m.*
ob·jec·tiv·i·ty [ˌəbdʒɪk'tɪvətɪ] *n* Okjektivität *f.*
ob·jec·tiv·ize [əb'dʒektɪvaɪz] *vt* objektivieren.
object lens → objective I.
object lesson Anschauungsunterricht *m.*
object plate (*Mikroskop*) Objektträger *m*, -glas *nt*, Deckglas *nt.*
object slide → object plate.
object teaching → object lesson.
ob·li·gate ['əblɪgɪt, -geɪt] *adj* unerlässlich, unbedingt, obligat, Zwangs-.
obligate aerobe *micro.* obligater Aerobier *m.*
obligate anaerobe *micro.* obligater Anaerobier *m.*
o·blig·a·to·ry [ə'blɪgətɔːrɪ, -təʊ-] *adj* obligatorisch, verpflichtend (*on, upon* für); Zwangs-, Pflicht-.
obligatory parasite *micro.* obligater Parasit *m.*
o·blique [əʊ'bliːk, -'blaɪk] *adj* schief, schräg, quer, geneigt. **at an ~ angle to** im spitzen Winkel zu.
oblique amputation *ortho., chir.* Amputation *f* mit Ovalärschnitt.
oblique aponeurosis Obliquusaponeurose *f*, Aponeurosis *m.* obliquus abdominis.
external o. Externusaponeurose, Aponeurosis *m.* obliquus externus abdominis.
internal o. Internusaponeurose, Aponeurosis *m.* obliquus internus abdominis.
oblique astigmatism *ophthal.* Astigmatismus *m* mit schiefen Achsen, Astigmatismus obliquus.
oblique cord (of elbow joint) Chorda obliqua (membranae interosseae antebrachii).
oblique diameter (of pelvis) schräger Beckendurchmesser *m*, Diameter obliqua (pelvis).
oblique fibers: o. of ciliary muscle radiäre Ziliarmuskelfasern *pl*, Fibrae radiales m. ciliares.
o. of stomach schräge Muskel(faser)züge *pl* der Magenwand, Fibrae obliquae (gastricae/ventriculi).
oblique fissure of lung schräger Interlobärspalt *m*, Fissura obliqua (pulmonis).
oblique fracture Schrägbruch *m*, -fraktur *f.*
oblique head of adductor hallucis muscle Caput obliquum m. adductoris hallucis.

oblique hernia äußerer/seitlicher/indirekter/schräger Leistenbruch *m*, Hernia inguinalis externa/indirecta/lateralis/obliqua.
oblique incision Ovalärschnitt *m.*
oblique ligament: o. of elbow joint → oblique cord (of elbow joint).
o.s of knee Kreuzbänder *pl*, Ligg. cruciata genus/genualia.
posterior o. (of knee) Lig. popliteum obliquum.
o. of scapula Lig. transversum scapulae superius.
oblique line: o. of femur Linea intertrochanterica.
o. of mandible Linea obliqua mandibulae.
o. of thyroid (cartilage) Linea obliqua cartilaginis thyroideae.
oblique muscle: o. of auricle → obliquus auriculae (muscle).
external o. of abdomen → obliquus externus abdominis (muscle).
inferior o. of eye → obliquus inferior (muscle).
inferior o. of head → obliquus capitis inferior (muscle).
internal o. of abdomen → obliquus internus abdominis (muscle).
superior o. of eye → obliquus superior (muscle).
superior o. head → obliquus capitis superior (muscle).
o·blique·ness [əʊ'bliːknɪs, -'blaɪk-] *n* → obliquity.
oblique pelvis Nägele-Becken *nt.*
oblique presentation *gyn.* Querlage *f.*
oblique sinus of pericardium Sinus obliquus pericardii.
oblique transverse lie → oblique presentation.
oblique triangle *mathe.* schiefwinkliges Dreieck *nt.*
oblique vein of left atrium Marshall'-Vene *f*, V. obliqua atrii sinistri.
ob·liq·ui·ty [əb'lɪkwətɪ] *n* Schrägheit *f*, Schiefe *f*, schräge/schiefe Lage *od.* Richtung *f*, Obliquität *f.*
ob·li·quus auriculae/auricularis (muscle) [əb'lɪkwəs] M. obliquus auricularis.
obliquus capitis inferior (muscle) Obliquus *m* capitis inferior, M. obliquus capitis inferior.
obliquus capitis superior (muscle) Obliquus *m* capitis superior, M. obliquus capitis superior.
obliquus externus abdominis (muscle) Obliquus *m* externus abdominis, Externus *m* abdominis, M. obliquus externus abdominis.
obliquus inferior (muscle) Obliquus *m* inferior, M. obliquus inferior (bulbi).
obliquus internus abdominis (muscle) Obliquus *m* internus abdominis, Internus *m* abdominis, M. obliquus internus abdominis.
obliquus superior (muscle) Obliquus *m* superior, M. obliquus superior (bulbi).

ob·lit·er·ate [ə'blɪtəreɪt] *vt* verschließen, veröden, obliterieren.
ob·lit·er·at·ing [ə'blɪtəreɪtɪŋ] *adj* verschließend, obliterierend.
obliterating arteritis Arteritis/Endarteritis obliterans.
obliterating pericarditis obliterierende Perikarditis *f*, Pericarditis obliterans.
ob·lit·er·a·tion [ə,blɪtə'reɪʃn] *n* Verschluß *m*, Verödung *f*, Obliteration *f*, Obliteratio *f*.
ob·lit·er·a·tive bronchitis [ə'blɪtəreɪtɪv, -ərətɪv] Bronchitis obliterans.
ob·long ['ɒblɒŋ, -lɑŋ] **I** *n mathe.* Rechteck *nt*. **II** *adj* länglich; *mathe.* rechteckig.
ob·long·a·ta [,ɒblɒŋ'gɑːtə] *n* Medulla oblongata, *inf.* Oblongata *f*.
ob·long·a·tal [,ɒblɒŋ'gɑːtl] *adj* Medulla oblongata betr., Oblongata-.
oblong fovea (of arytenoid cartilage) Fovea oblonga (cartilaginis aryt(a)enoideae).
oblong pit (of arytenoid cartilage) → oblong fovea (of arytenoid cartilage).
ob·nu·bi·la·tion [ɑb,n(j)uːbə'leɪʃn] *n* Bewußtseinseintrübung *f*.
ob·serv·ance [əb'zɜrvəns] *n* **1.** Vorschrift *f*, Regel *f*. **2.** (*Regel*) Einhaltung *f*, Befolgung *f*.
ob·serv·ant [əb'zɜrvənt] *adj* beachtend, verfolgend (*of*).
ob·ser·va·tion [,ɑbzɜr'veɪʃn] **I** *n* **1.** Beobachtung *f*, Überwachung *f*; Wahrnehmung *f*. **2.** Beobachtungsgabe *f*, -vermögen *nt*. **II** *adj* Beobachtungs-.
ob·serve [əb'zɜrv] **I** *vt* **1.** beobachten, überwachen; betrachten, verfolgen. **2.** wahrnehmen, erkennen. **3.** etw. befolgen *od.* beachten. **4.** sagen, äußern. **II** *vi* **5.** aufmerksam sein. **6.** Beobachtungen machen.
ob·serv·er [əb'zɜrvər] *n* Beobachter(in *f*) *m*.
ob·serv·ing [əb'zɜrvɪŋ] *adj* → observant.
ob·sess [əb'ses] *vt* jdn. quälen, verfolgen, heimsuchen. **to be ~ed by/with** besessen sein von.
ob·ses·sion [əb'seʃn] *n psycho.* Besessenheit *f*, Zwangsvorstellung *f*, fixe Idee *f*, Obsession *f*.
ob·ses·sion·al neurosis [əb'seʃnl] Zwangsneurose *f*, Anankasmus *m*, anankastisches Syndrom *nt*, obsessiv-kompulsive Reaktion *f*.
ob·ses·sive [əb'sesɪv] *adj psychia.* zwanghaft, obsessiv, Zwangs-.
obsessive-compulsive *adj psychia.* obsessiv-kompulsiv.
obsessive-compulsive neurosis → obsessional neurosis.
obsessive-compulsive reaction zwanghafte/anankastische Persönlichkeit(sstörung *f*) *f*, Zwangscharakter *m*.
ob·so·lete [ɑbsə'liːt, 'ɑbsəliːt] *adj* veraltet, überholt, nicht mehr gebräuchlich, obsolet.
ob·stet·ric [əb'stetrɪk] *adj* Geburtshilfe betr., geburtshilflich, Geburts-, Geburtshelfer-, Entbindungs-.
ob·stet·ri·cal [əb'stetrɪkl] *adj* → obstetric.
obstetrical forceps Geburtszange *f*, Forceps *f*.
obstetrical paralysis Geburtslähmung *f*, geburtstraumatische Lähmung *f*.
obstetrical position *gyn.* Sims-Lage *f*.
obstetric canal *gyn.* Geburtskanal *m*.
obstetric conjugate Conjugata anatomica vera obstetrica.
ob·ste·tri·cian [,ɑbstɪ'trɪʃn] *n* Geburtshelfer *m*, -helferin *f*.
obstetrician's hand Geburtshelferhand *f*.
obstetric paralysis Geburtslähmung *f*, geburtstraumatische Lähmung *f*.
ob·stet·rics [əb'stetrɪks] *pl* Geburtshilfe *f*, Obstetrik *f*.
ob·sti·pa·tion [,ɑbstə'peɪʃn] *n* (Stuhl-)Verstopfung *f*, Obstipation *f*, Konstipation *f*, Obstructio alvi.
ob·struct [əb'strʌkt] *vt* versperren, verstopfen, blockieren.
ob·struc·tion [əb'strʌkʃn] *n* Blockierung *f*, Verstopfung *f*, Verlegung *f*, Verschluß *m*, Obstruktion *f*, Obstructio *f*.
ob·struc·tive [əb'strʌktɪv] *adj* blockierend, versperrend, verstopfend, verschließend, obstruktiv, Obstruktions-.
obstructive anuria Obstruktionsanurie *f*.
obstructive appendicitis obstruktive Appendizitis *f*.
obstructive atelectasis (*Lunge*) Absorptions-, Obstruktionsatelektase *f*.
obstructive bronchiectasis Stenosebronchiektas(i)e *f*.
obstructive cholestasis Stauungscholestase *f*.
obstructive dysmenorrhea *gyn.* obstruktive Dysmenorrhö *f*.
obstructive emphysema obstruktives Lungenemphysem *nt*.
obstructive glaucoma akutes Winkelblockglaukom/Engwinkelglaukom *nt*, Glaucoma acutum (congestivum).
obstructive hydrocephalus obstruktiver Hydrozephalus *m*, Hydrocephalus occlusus.
obstructive icterus Obstruktions-, Verschlußikterus *m*.
obstructive ileus *chir.* Obstruktionsileus *m*.
obstructive jaundice Verschlußikterus *m*, mechanischer Ikterus *m*.
obstructive uropathy Harnwegsobstruktion *f*.
ob·stru·ent ['ɑbstrʊənt] **I** *n* verstopfendes Mittel *nt*. **II** *adj* verstopfend; blockierend.
ob·tu·ra·tion [,ɑbt(j)ə'reɪʃn] *n* Verlegung *f*, Verstopfung *f*, Obturation *f*, Obturatio *f*.
ob·tu·ra·tor ['ɑbt(j)əreɪtər] *n* **1.** Verschluß *m*, Verlegung *f*. **2.** *dent.* Verschlußprothese *f*, künstliche Gaumenplatte *f*, Obturator *m*. **3.** *techn.* (Ab-)Dichtung *f*.
obturator artery Obturatoria *f*, A. obturatoria.
accessory o. Obturatoria *f* accessoria, A. obturatoria accessoria.
obturator branch of inferior epigastric artery Ramus obturatorius a. epigastricae inferioris.
obturator canal Obturatorkanal *m*, Canalis obturatorius.
obturator crest Crista obturatoria.
obturator externus (muscle) Obturatorius *m* externus, M. obturator externus.
obturator fascia Obturatorfaszie *f*, Fascia obturatoria.
obturator foramen For. obturatorium.
obturator groove (of pubis) Sulcus obturatorius (ossis pubis).
obturator hernia Obturatorhernie *f*, Hernia obturatoria.
obturator internus (muscle) Obturatorius *m* internus, M. obturator internus.
ob·tu·ra·to·ri·us externus (muscle) [,ɑbt(j)ʊrə'tɔːriəs, -'toʊ-] → obturator externus (muscle).
obturatorius internus (muscle) → obturator internus (muscle).
obturator ligament of pelvis → obturator membrane.
obturator membrane Membrana obturatoria.
anterior o. of atlas Membrana atlanto-occipitalis anterior.
posterior o. of atlas Membrana atlanto-occipitalis posterior.
obturator nerve Obturatorius *m*, N. obturatorius.
accessory o. Obturatorius accessorius, N. obturatorius accessorius.
internal o. N. musculi obturatorii interni.
obturator pouch seitlicher Abschnitt *m* der Excavatio vesicouterina.
obturator sign *chir.* (*Appendizitis*) Obturatorzeichen *nt*.
obturator sulcus (of pubis) → obturator groove (of pubis).
obturator test *chir.* Psoaszeichen *nt*, Cope-Zeichen *nt*.
obturator tubercle: anterior o. Tuberculum obturatorium anterius.
posterior o. Tuberculum obturatorium posterius.
obturator veins Obturatorvenen *pl*, Vv. obturatoriae.
ob·tuse [əb't(j)uːs] *adj* **1.** stumpf, abgestumpft; begriffsstutzig, beschränkt. **2.** (*Schmerz*) dumpf.
obtuse angle *mathe.* stumpfer Winkel *m*.
obtuse margin of spleen unterer Milzrand *m*, Margo inferior lienis/splenis.
obtuse pain dumpfer Schmerz *m*.
ob·tu·sion [əb't(j)uːʒn] *n psycho.*, *psychia.* Obtusion *f*.
OCA *abbr.* → oculocutaneous albinism.
oc·cip·i·tal [ɑk'sɪpɪtl] **I** *n* → occipital bone. **II** *adj* Hinterhaupt(sbein) betr., okzipital, Hinterhaupt(s)-.
occipital angle of parietal bone Angulus occipitalis (ossis parietalis).
occipital artery Hinterhauptschlagader *f*, Occipitalis *f*, A. occipitalis.
lateral o. Occipitalis lateralis, A. occipitalis lateralis.
medial/middle o. Occipitalis medialis, A. occipitalis medialis.
occipital articulation oberes Kopfgelenk *nt*, Atlantookzipitalgelenk *nt*, Artic. atlanto-occipitalis.
occipital bone Hinterhauptsbein *nt*, Os occipitale.
occipital branch: o.es of occipital artery Hinterhauptsäste *pl* der A. occipitalis, Rami occipitales a. occipitalis.
o. of posterior auricular artery Hinterhauptsast *m* der A. auricularis posterior, Ramus occipitalis a. auricularis posterioris.
o. of posterior auricular nerve Ramus occipitalis n. auricularis posterioris.
occipital condyle Hinterhauptskondyle *f*, Condylus occipitalis.
occipital crest: external o. Crista occipitalis externa.
internal o. Crista occipitalis interna.
occipital fasciculus, vertical Fasciculus occipitalis verticalis.
occipital fissure Sulcus parieto-occipitalis.
occipital fontanelle kleine/hintere Fontanelle *f*, Hinterhauptsfontanelle *f*, Fonticulus posterior.
occipital foramen, (great) For. (occipitale) magnum.
occipital genu of optic radiation okzipitales Knie *nt* der Sehstrahlung, Genu occipitale.
occipital horn of lateral ventricle Hinterhorn *nt* des Seitenventrikels, Cornu occipitale/posterius (ventriculi lateralis).
oc·cip·i·ta·lis [ɑk,sɪpɪ'teɪləs] *n* → occipital muscle.
occipitalis minor (muscle) Transversus *m* nuchae, M. transversus nuchae.
occipitalis muscle → occipital muscle.
oc·cip·i·tal·i·za·tion [ɑk,sɪpɪtælə'zeɪʃn] *n*

embryo. Okzipitalisation *f*, Atlasassimilation *f*.
occipital joint → occipital articulation.
occipital lobe Okzipital-, Hinterhauptslappen *m*, Lobus occipitalis.
occipital margin: o. of parietal bone Margo occipitalis ossis parietalis.
o. of temporal bone Margo occipitalis ossis temporalis.
occipital muscle Okzipitalis *m*, M. occipitalis, Venter occipitalis m. occipitofrontalis.
occipital nerve: greater o. Okzipitalis *m* major, N. occipitalis major.
least o. → third o.
lesser o. Okzipitalis *m* minor, N. occipitalis minor.
third o. Okzipitalis *m* tertius, N. occipitalis tertius.
occipital plane Planum occipitale.
occipital plexus vegetativer Plexus *m* der A. occipitalis.
occipital pole of cerebral hemisphere Okzipitalpol *m* einer Großhirnhemisphäre, Polus occipitalis (hemisph(a)erii cerebri).
occipital protuberance Protuberantia occipitalis.
external o. Protuberantia occipitalis externa.
internal o. Protuberantia occipitalis interna.
occipital region Hinterhauptsgegend *f*, Okzipitalregion *f*, Regio occipitalis.
occipital sinus Sinus occipitalis.
occipital sulcus: anterior o. Sulcus occipitalis anterior.
lateral o.i Sulci occipitales laterales.
superior o.i Sulci occipitales superiores.
transverse o. Sulcus occipitalis transversus.
occipital triangle/trigone seitliches Halsdreieck *nt*, Regio cervicalis lateralis, Trigonum cervicale posterius.
occipital vein 1. Hinterhauptsvene *f*, V. occipitalis. **2.** *~s pl* Hinterhauptslappenvenen *pl*, Vv. occipitales.
oc·cip·i·to·an·te·ri·or [ˌakˌsɪpɪtəʊænˈtɪərɪər] *adj gyn.* okzipitoanterior.
occipito-atlantal *adj* Hinterhaupt(sbein) u. Atlas betr., atlantookzipital.
occipito-atlantal articulation → occipital articulation.
occipito-atlantal joint → occipital articulation.
oc·cip·i·to·at·loid [ˌ-ˈætlɔɪd] *adj* → occipito-atlantal.
oc·cip·i·to·ax·i·al [ˌ-ˈæksɪəl] *adj* Os occipitale u. Dens axis betr.
occipitoaxial ligament Membrana tectoria.
oc·cip·i·to·ax·oid [ˌ-ˈæksɔɪd] *adj* → occipitoaxial.
oc·cip·i·to·cer·vi·cal [ˌ-ˈsɜrvɪkl] *adj* Hinterhaupt u. Nacken betr., okzipitozervikal.
oc·cip·i·to·fa·cial [ˌ-ˈfeɪʃl] *adj* okzipitofazial.
oc·cip·i·to·fron·tal [ˌ-ˈfrʌntl] *adj* Hinterhaupt u. Stirn betr., okzipitofrontal.
occipitofrontal diameter *gyn., ped.* frontookzipitaler/okzipitofrontaler Durchmesser *m*, Diameter frontooccipitalis/occipitofrontalis.
occipitofrontal fasciculus: inferior o. Fasciculus occipitofrontalis inferior.
superior o. Fasciculus occipitofrontalis superior, Fasciculus subcallosus.
oc·cip·i·to·fron·ta·lis [ˌ-franˈteɪlɪs] *n* Okzipitofrontalis *m*, M. occipitofrontalis.
occipitofrontalis muscle → occipitofrontalis.

occipitofrontal muscle → occipitofrontalis.
oc·cip·i·to·mas·toid [ˌ-ˈmæstɔɪd] *adj* Os occipitale u. Proc. mastoideus betr.
occipitomastoid suture Sutura occipitomastoidea.
oc·cip·i·to·men·tal [ˌ-ˈmentl] *adj* okzipitomental.
occipitomental diameter *gyn., ped.* okzipitomentaler/mentookzipitaler Durchmesser *m*, Diameter occipitomentalis/mentooccipitalis.
occipito-odontoid *adj* Os occipitale u. Dens axis betr.
occipito-odontoid ligaments Flügelbänder *pl*, Ligg. alaria.
oc·cip·i·to·pa·ri·e·tal [ˌ-pəˈraɪɪtl] *adj* okzipitoparietal.
oc·cip·i·to·pon·tine fibers [ˌ-ˈpɑntɪn, -tiːn] okzipitopontine Fasern *pl*.
occipitopontine tract → occipitopontine fibers.
oc·cip·i·to·pos·te·ri·or [ˌ-pəˈstɪərɪər] *adj gyn.* okzipitoposterior.
oc·cip·i·to·sphe·noi·dal fissure [ˌ-sfiːˈnɔɪdl] Fissura spheno-occipitalis.
oc·cip·i·to·tem·po·ral [ˌ-ˈtemp(ə)rəl] *adj* okzipitotemporal.
occipitotemporal branch of medial occipital artery Okzipitotemporalast *m* der A. occipitalis medialis, Ramus occipitotemporalis a. occipitalis medialis.
occipitotemporal convolution Gyrus occipitotemporalis lateralis.
occipitotemporal gyrus: lateral o. Gyrus occipitotemporalis lateralis.
medial/middle o. Gyrus occipitotemporalis medialis.
occipitotemporal sulcus Sulcus occipitotemporalis.
oc·cip·i·to·tha·lam·ic [ˌ-θəˈlæmɪk] *adj* Hinterhauptslappen u. Thalamus betr. *od.* verbindend, okzipitothalamisch, thalamookzipital.
occipitothalamic radiation → optic radiation.
oc·ci·put [ˈɑksɪpʌt] *n, pl* **-puts, oc·cip·i·ta** [akˈsɪpɪtə] *anat.* Hinterhaupt *nt*, Okziput *nt*, Occiput *nt*.
oc·clude [əˈkluːd] **I** *vt* **1.** ab-, verschließen, versperren, verstopfen, ein-, ausschließen. **2.** *chem.* absorbieren, okkludieren. **II** *vi dent.* schließen.
oc·clud·ent junction [əˈkluːdənt] *histol.* Verschlußkontakt *m*, Zonula occludens.
oc·clud·ing junction [əˈkluːdɪŋ] → occludent junction.
oc·clu·sal [əˈkluːzl] *adj dent.* Kaufläche *od.* Okklusion betr., okklusal, Biß-, Okklusions-.
occlusal plane *dent.* Biß-, Okklusionsebene *f*.
occlusal surface (*Zahn*) Kaufläche *f*, Facies occlusalis/masticatoria (dentis).
oc·clu·sion [əˈkluːʒn] *n* **1.** Verschließung *f*, Verstopfung *f*; Ein-, Ausschließung *f*, Umschließung *f*. **2.** *patho.* Verschluß *m*, Okklusion *f*. **3.** *dent.* Zahnreihenschluß *m*, Okklusion *f*. **4.** *chem.* Absorption *f*, Okklusion *f*.
occlusion compound *chem.* Klathrat *nt*.
oc·clu·sive [əˈkluːsɪv] *adj* Okklusion betr., durch Okklusion verursacht, ab-, verschließend, hemmend, okklusiv, Verschluß-.
occlusive ileus Okklusionsileus *m*.
oc·cult [əˈkʌlt, ˈakʌlt] *adj* verborgen, okkult.
occult bleeding okkulte Blutung *f*.
occult blood okkultes Blut *nt*.
occult blood test Test *m* für okkultes Blut.
occult cancer → occult carcinoma.

occult carcinoma okkultes Karzinom *nt*.
occult cholesteatoma *HNO* okkultes/kongenitales Cholesteatom *nt*.
occult disease okkulte/nicht-manifeste Erkrankung *f*.
occult hemorrhage → occult bleeding.
occult injury okkulte Verletzung/Schädigung *f*.
occult jaundice okkulter/latenter Ikterus *m*.
occult sinusitis okkulte/latente Sinusitis *f*.
oc·cu·pa·tion [ˌakjəˈpeɪʃn] *n* Beruf *m*, Gewerbe *nt*; Beschäftigung *f*.
oc·cu·pa·tion·al [ˌakjəˈpeɪʃnl] *adj* beruflich, Berufs-, Arbeits-; Beschäftigungs-.
occupational accident Arbeitsunfall *m*.
occupational acne Berufsakne *f*, Akne/Acne occupationalis.
occupational deafness chronische Lärmschwerhörigkeit *f*.
occupational dermatitis berufsbedingte Kontaktdermatitis *f*.
occupational disease Berufskrankheit *f*.
occupational medicine Arbeitsmedizin *f*.
occupational psychology Arbeitspsychologie *f*.
occupational therapist Beschäftigungstherapeut(in *f*) *m*.
occupational therapy Beschäftigungstherapie *f*.
o·cel·lus [əʊˈseləs] *n, pl* **-li** [-laɪ, -liː] *bio.* **1.** Punkt-, Neben-, Stirnauge *nt*, Ozelle *f*. **2.** Facette *f*. **3.** Augenfleck *m*.
o·chrom·e·ter [əʊˈkrɑmɪtər] *n* Ochrometer *nt*.
o·chro·no·sis [ˌəʊkrəˈnəʊsɪs] *n, pl* **-ses** [-siːz] *derm.* Ockerfarbenkrankheit *f*, Ochronose *f*.
o·chro·no·sus [ˌ-ˈnəʊsəs] *n* → ochronosis.
o·chro·not·ic [ˌ-ˈnɑtɪk] *adj* Ochronose betr.
O colony *micro.* (*Kolonie*) O-Form *f*.
OCT *abbr.* → ornithine carbamoyltransferase.
oc·ta·dec·a·no·ate [ˌaktəˌdekəˈnəʊeɪt] *n* Stearat *nt*.
oc·ta·dec·a·no·ic acid [ˌ-ˌdekəˈnəʊɪk] *adj*, n-Octadecansäure *f*.
oc·ta·myl·a·mine [ˌ-ˈmɪləmiːn] *n pharm.* Octamylamin *nt*.
oc·tane [ˈɑkteɪn] *n* Oktan *nt*, Octan *nt*.
oc·ta·no·ic acid [ˌaktəˈnəʊɪk] Caprylsäure *f*, Oktansäure *f*.
oc·ta·pep·tide [ˌ-ˈpeptaɪd] *n* Oktapeptid *nt*.
oc·ta·va·lent [ˌ-ˈveɪlənt] *adj chem.* achtwertig, oktavalent.
OCT deficiency → ornithine carbamoyl phosphate deficiency.
oc·tet(te) [akˈtet] *n chem.* Oktett *nt*.
oc·to·drine [ˈɑktədriːn] *n pharm.* Octodrin *nt*.
oc·to·pam·ine [ˌ-ˈpæmiːn] *n pharm.* Octopamin *nt*.
oc·tose [ˈɑktəʊs] *n* Oktose *f*, Octose *f*, C_8-Zucker *m*.
ocul- *pref.* → oculo-.
oc·u·lar [ˈɑkjələr] **I** *n phys.* Okular *nt*, Okularlinse *f*. **II** *adj* **1.** Auge betr., okular, Augen-, Okulo-. **2.** augenähnlich. **3.** sichtbar.
ocular albinism *abbr.* **OA** okulärer Albinismus *m*.
autosomal recessive o. *abbr.* **AROA** autosomal rezessiver okulärer Albinismus *m*.
ocular angle Augenwinkel *m*.
ocular ataxia Nystagmus *m*.
ocular bulb Augapfel *m*, Bulbus oculi.
ocular capsule Tenon'-Kapsel *f*, Vagina bulbi.
ocular cone Sehkegel *m*.
ocular conjunctiva Bindehaut *f* des Augapfels, Tunica conjunctiva bulbaris.
ocular crisis *neuro., ophthal.* Augenkrise *f*.

ocular cup

ocular cup *embryo.* Augenbecher *m*, Caliculus ophthalmicus.
ocular dominance *ophthal.* monokuläre Dominanz *f*.
ocular hypertelorism Greig-Syndrom *nt*, okulärer Hypertelorismus *m*.
ocular lens Okular *nt*, Okularlinse *f*.
ocular motor apraxia Balint-Syndrom *nt*.
ocular muscles, (extrinsic) äußere Augenmuskeln *pl*, Mm. bulbi.
ocular nystagmus okulärer Nystagmus *m*.
ocular paralysis totale/komplette Okulomotoriuslähmung *f*, totale/komplette Augenmuskellähmung *f*.
 periodic o. Möbius-Krankheit *f*, periodische Okulomotoriuslähmung *f* mit Neuralgie.
ocular pemphigoid vernarbendes Pemphigoid *nt*, benignes Schleimhautpemphigoid *nt*, okulärer Pemphigus *m*, Dermatitis pemphigoides mucocutanea chronica.
ocular phthisis → ophthalmomalacia.
ocular region Orbitaregion *f*, Regio orbitalis.
ocular scoliosis *ortho.* okuläre Skoliose *f*.
ocular torticollis okulärer Schiefhals *m*.
ocular toxoplasmosis Toxoplasmose-Chorioretinitis *f*.
ocular trichiasis Trichiasis oculi.
ocular vertigo Augen-, Gesichtsschwindel *m*, Vertigo ocularis.
ocular vesicle *embryo.* Augenbläschen *nt*, Vesicula ophthalmica.
ocular wryneck → ocular torticollis.
oc·u·len·tum [akjəˈlentəm] *n, pl* **-ta** [-tə] *pharm.* Augensalbe *f*, Oculentum *nt*, Unguentum ophthalmicum.
oc·u·list [ˈakjəlɪst] *n* **1.** → ophthalmologist. **2.** → optometrist.
oculo- *pref.* Augen-, Okul(o)-.
oc·u·lo·au·ric·u·lar [ˌakjələʊːˈrɪkjələr] *adj* okuloaurikulär.
oculoauricular dysplasia → oculoauriculovertebral dysplasia.
oc·u·lo·au·ric·u·lo·ver·te·bral [ˌ-ɔːˌrɪkjələʊˈvɜːtəbrəl] *adj* okuloaurikulovertebral.
oculoauriculovertebral dysplasia Goldenhar-Syndrom *nt*, okuloaurikuläres/okulo-aurikulo-vertebrales Syndrom *nt*, okulo-aurikulo-vertebrale Dysplasie *f*, Dysplasia oculo-auricularis, Dysplasia oculo-auriculo-vertebralis.
oc·u·lo·bu·co·gen·i·tal syndrome [ˌ-ˌbʌkəʊˈdʒenɪtl] Behçet-Krankheit *f*, -Syndrom *nt*, bipolare/große/maligne Aphthose *f*, Gilbert-Syndrom *nt*, Aphthose Touraine/Behçet.
oc·u·lo·car·di·ac [ˌ-ˈkɑːrdiˌæk] *adj* Auge(n) u. Herz betr., okulokardial.
oculocardiac reflex okulokardialer Reflex *m*, Bulbusdruckreflex *m*, Aschner-Dagnini-Bulbusdruckversuch *m*.
oc·u·lo·ce·phal·ic [ˌ-sɪˈfælɪk] *adj* Auge(n) u. Gehirn betr., okulozephal.
oculocephalic reflex okulozephaler Reflex *m*.
oc·u·lo·ce·re·bral [ˌ-səˈriːbrəl, -ˈserə-] *adj* Auge(n) u. Großhirn betr., okulozerebral.
oculocerebral-hypopigmentation syndrome Cross-McKusick-Breen-Syndrom *nt*.
oc·u·lo·cer·e·bro·re·nal dystrophy [ˌ-ˌserəbrəʊˈriːnl] → oculocerebrorenal syndrome.
oculocerebrorenal syndrome Lowe-Syndrom *nt*, Lowe-Terrey-MacLachlan-Syndrom *nt*, okulo-zerebro-renales Syndrom *nt*.

oc·u·lo·cu·ta·ne·ous [ˌ-kjuːˈteɪnɪəs] *adj* okulokutan.
oculocutaneous albinism *abbr.* **OCA** okulokutaner Albinismus *m*.
 autosomal dominant o. autosomal dominanter okulokutaner Albinismus.
 brown o. brauner okulokutaner Albinismus.
 ty-neg o. → tyrosinase-negative o.
 ty-pos o. → tyrosinase-positive o.
 tyrosinase-negative o. Tyrosinase-negativer okulokutaner Albinismus.
 tyrosinase-positive o. Tyrosinase-positiver okulokutaner Albinismus.
 yellow mutant o. Yellow-Typ *m* des okulokutanen Albinismus.
oculocutaneous melanosis → Ota's nevus.
oculocutaneous syndrome okulokutanes Syndrom *nt*, Vogt-Koyanagi(-Harada)-Syndrom *nt*.
oc·u·lo·den·to·dig·i·tal [ˌ-ˌdentəʊˈdɪdʒɪtl] *adj* okulodentodigital.
oculodentodigital dysplasia Meyer-Schwickerath-Weyers-Syndrom *nt*, okulodentodigitales Syndrom *nt*.
oculodentodigital syndrome → oculodentodigital dysplasia.
oc·u·lo·den·to·os·se·ous dysplasia/syndrome [ˌ-ˌdentəʊˈɒsɪəs] → oculodentodigital dysplasia.
oc·u·lo·der·mal [ˌ-ˈdɜːrml] *adj* → oculocutaneous.
oculodermal melanocytosis → Ota's nevus.
oc·u·lo·en·ce·phal·ic angiomatosis [ˌ-ˌensɪˈfælɪk] Krabbe-Syndrom *nt*, okuloenzephalische/enzephalookulare Angiomatose *f*, Angiomatosis encephalo-cutanea.
oc·u·lo·fa·cial [ˌ-ˈfeɪʃl] *adj* Auge(n) u. Gesicht betr., okulofazial.
oc·u·lo·glan·du·lar tularemia [ˌ-ˈglændʒələr] okuloglanduläre Tulärämie *f*.
oc·u·log·ra·phy [akjəˈlɑgrəfi] *n ophthal.* Okulographie *f*.
oc·u·lo·gy·ric crisis [ˌakjələʊˈdʒaɪrɪk] *neuro.* Crisis oculogyris.
oc·u·lo·man·dib·u·lo·dys·ceph·a·ly [ˌ-ˌmænˌdɪbjələʊdɪsˈsefəli] *n* Hallermann-Streiff(-Francois)-Syndrom *nt*, Dysmorphia mandibulo-oculo-facialis.
oc·u·lo·man·dib·u·lo·fa·cial syndrome [ˌ-ˌmænˌdɪbjələʊˈfeɪʃl] → oculomandibulodyscephaly.
oc·u·lo·mo·tor center [ˌ-ˈməʊtər] blickmotorisches/okulomotorisches Zentrum *nt*.
oc·u·lo·mo·to·ri·us [ˌ-məʊˈtɔːriəs] *n* → oculomotor nerve.
oculomotor loop *physiol.* okulomotorische Schleife *f*.
oculomotor nerve Okulomotorius *m*, III. Hirnnerv *m*, N. oculomotorius.
oculomotor nerve nucleus → oculomotor nucleus.
oculomotor nucleus Okulomotoriuskern *m*, Nc. n. oculomotorii, Nc. oculomotorius.
 accessory o. Edinger-Westphal-Kern, Nc. oculomotorius accessorius.
oculomotor paralysis Okulomotorius-, Oculomotoriuslähmung *f*.
oculomotor root of ciliary ganglion Radix oculomotoria/parasympathetica (ggl. ciliaris).
oc·u·lo·my·co·sis [ˌ-maɪˈkəʊsɪs] *n ophthal.* Pilzerkrankung *f* des Auges.
oc·u·lo·na·sal [ˌ-ˈneɪzl] *adj* Auge(n) u. Nase betr., okulonasal.
oc·u·lop·a·thy [akjəˈlɑpəθi] *n* → ophthalmopathy.
oc·u·lo·pha·ryn·ge·al reflex [ˌ-fəˈrɪndʒ(ɪ)əl] okulopharyngealer Reflex *m*.

oculopharyngeal syndrome okulopharyngeales Syndrom *nt*.
oc·u·lo·pu·pil·lar·y [ˌ-ˈpjuːpəˌleri:, -ləri] *adj* Pupille betr., pupillar, okulopupillar, Pupillen-.
oculopupillary reflex Trigeminusreflex *m*.
oc·u·lo·ro·ta·to·ry muscles [ˌ-ˈrəʊtətəˌri:, -təʊ-] äußere Augenmuskeln *pl*, Mm. bulbi.
oc·u·lo·sen·so·ry cell reflex [ˌ-ˈsensəri] Trigeminusreflex *m*.
oc·u·lo·spi·nal [ˌ-ˈspaɪnl] *adj* okulospinal.
oc·u·lo·ver·te·bral [ˌ-ˈvɜːrtəbrəl] *adj* okulovertebral.
oculovertebral dysplasia → oculovertebral syndrome.
oculovertebral syndrome okulovertebrales Syndrom *nt*.
oc·u·lo·ves·tib·u·lar reflex [ˌ-vəˈstɪbjələr] okulovestibulärer Reflex *m*, okulovestibuläre Reaktion *f*.
oculovestibulo-auditory syndrome Cogan-Syndrom *nt*.
oc·u·lus [ˈakjələs] *n, pl* **-li** [-laɪ] Auge *nt*; *anat.* Oculus *nt*.
o·cy·to·cin [əʊsɪˈtəʊsɪn] *n* → oxytocin.
OD *abbr.* → optical density.
ODC *abbr.* → orotidylic acid decarboxylase.
ODD dysplasia → oculodentodigital dysplasia.
Oddi [ˈɑdiː]: **O.'s muscle/sphincter** Sphinkter *m* Oddi/ampullae, Sphincter *m* Oddi/ampullae, M. sphincter Oddi, Sphincter *m*, M. sphincter ampullae hepatopancreaticae.
od·di·tis [ɑˈdaɪtɪs] *n* Entzündung *f* des Sphinkter Oddi, Odditis *f*.
ODD syndrome → oculodentodigital dysplasia.
odont- *pref.* → odonto-.
o·don·tal·gia [ˌɑdɑnˈtældʒ(i)ə] *n dent.* Zahnschmerz(en *pl*) *m*, Odontalgie *f*.
o·don·tal·gic [ˌ-ˈtældʒɪk] *adj* Odontalgie betr.
o·don·tec·to·my [ˌ-ˈtektəmi] *n dent.* Zahnentfernung *f*, -extraktion *f*.
o·don·ti·a·sis [ˌ-ˈtaɪəsɪs] *n dent.* Zahnen *nt*, Zahndurchbruch *m*, Dentition *f*, Dentitio *f*.
o·don·tic [əʊˈdɑntɪk] *adj* Zahn od. Zähne betr., dental, Odont(o)-, Dent(o)-, Dental-, Zahn-.
odonto- *pref.* Zahn-, Dental-, Dent(o)-, Odont(o)-.
o·don·to·am·e·lo·blas·to·ma [əʊˌdɑntəʊˌæmələʊˈblæsˈtəʊmə] *n* Odontoadamantinom *nt*, Odontoameloblastom *nt*, ameloblastisches (Fibro-)Odontom *nt*.
o·don·to·am·e·lo·blas·to·sar·co·ma [ˌ-ˌæmələʊˌblæstəsɑːrˈkəʊmə] *n* Odontoameloblastosarkom *nt*.
o·don·to·blast [ˈ-blæst] *n* Odontoblast *m*, Dentinoblast *m*.
o·don·to·blas·to·ma [ˌ-blæsˈtəʊmə] *n* Odontoblastom *nt*.
o·don·to·both·ri·on [ˌ-ˈbɑθrɪɑn] *n* Zahnalveole *f*, Alveolus dentalis.
o·don·to·both·ri·tis [ˌ-bɑˈθraɪtɪs] *n dent.* Entzündung *f* der Zahnalveole, Alveolitis *f*.
o·don·to·clast [ˈ-klæst] *n* Odontoklast *m*, -clast *m*.
o·don·to·dyn·ia [ˌ-ˈdiːnɪə] *n* → odontalgia.
o·don·to·gen·e·sis [ˌ-ˈdʒenəsɪs] *n* Zahnentwicklung *f*, -bildung *f*, Odontogenese *f*.
o·don·to·ge·net·ic [ˌ-dʒəˈnetɪk] *adj* Zahnentwicklung/Odontogenese betr., odontogenetisch.
o·don·to·gen·ic [ˌ-ˈdʒenɪk] *adj* **1.** von den Zähnen ausgehend, odontogen, dentogen. **2.** zahnbildend.

odontogenic cyst dentogene Zyste *f*.
o·don·tog·e·ny [,ɔʊdan'tadʒənɪ] *n* → odontogenesis.
o·don·toid [ɔʊ'dantɔɪd] *adj* zahnförmig, -ähnlich, dentoid, odontoid.
odontoid apophysis Dens axis.
odontoid bone Dens axis.
odontoid process of axis Dens axis.
o·don·to·lith [ɔʊ'dantəlɪθ] *n* Zahnstein *m*, Calculus dentis/dentalis.
o·don·to·log·i·cal [,-'ladʒɪkl] *adj* odontologisch.
o·don·tol·o·gist [ɔʊdan'talədʒɪst] *n* Zahnarzt *m*, -ärztin *f*.
o·don·tol·o·gy [,ɔʊdan'talədʒɪ] *n* Zahn-(heil)kunde *f*, Zahnmedizin *f*, Dentologie *f*, Odontologie *f*.
o·don·to·ma [ɔʊdan'tɔʊmə] *n* 1. Odontom *nt*. 2. odontogener Tumor *m*.
o·don·top·a·thy [ɔʊdan'tapəθɪ] *n* Zahnerkrankung *f*, Odontopathie *f*.
o·don·to·per·i·os·te·um [ɔʊ,dantə,perɪ'astɪəm] *n* Zahnbett *nt*, Parodont *nt*, Parodontium *nt*.
o·dor ['ɔʊdər] *n* 1. Geruch *m*, Odor *m*. 2. Duft *m*, Wohlgeruch *m*.
o·dor·ant ['ɔʊdərənt] **I** *n* Duftstoff *m*. **II** *adj* duftend, wohlriechend.
odor classes *physiol*. Geruchsklassen *pl*.
o·dor·if·er·ous [ɔʊdə'rɪfərəs] *adj* → odorant II.
odoriferous crypts of prepuce präputiale (Talg-)Drüsen *pl*, Präputialdrüsen *pl*, Gll. pr(a)eputiales.
o·do·rim·e·ter [ɔʊdə'rɪmɪtər] *n* Odorimeter *nt*.
o·do·rim·e·try [ɔʊdə'rɪmɪtrɪ] *n* Odorimetrie *f*.
o·dor·less ['ɔʊdərlɪs] *adj* geruchlos.
o·dor·ous ['ɔʊdərəs] *adj* → odorant II.
o·dor·ous·ness ['-nɪs] *n* odor 2.
odor quality *physiol*. Geruchsqualität *f*.
odor stimulus *physiol*. Geruchsreiz *m*.
odor substance → odorant I.
odyn- *pref*. → odyno-.
o·dyn·a·cu·sis [,ɔʊdɪnə'kjuːsɪs] *n* schmerzhaftes Hören *nt*, Hyperakusis dolorosa.
odyno- *pref*. Schmerz-, Odyn(o)-.
o·dy·nom·e·ter [ɔʊdɪ'namɪtər] *n* Algesimeter *nt*.
o·dyn·o·pha·gia [ɔʊ,dɪnɔʊ'feɪdʒ(ɪ)ə] *n* schmerzhaftes Schlucken *nt*, Odynophagie *f*.
o·dyn·pha·gia [ɔʊdɪn'feɪdʒ(ɪ)ə] *n* → odynophagia.
oed·i·pal period ['edɪpəl, 'iːdɪ-] → oedipal phase.
oedipal phase *psycho*. ödipale Phase *f*.
Oedipus ['edɪpəs, 'iːdə-]: **O. complex** *psycho.*, *psychia*. Ödipus-Komplex *m*.
oesophag(o)- *pref*. → esophago-.
oe·soph·a·go·sto·mi·a·sis [ɪ,safəgɔʊstə'maɪəsɪs] *n* Oesophagostomum-Infektion *f*, Oesophagostomiasis *f*.
Oe·soph·a·gos·to·mum [ɪ,safə'gastəməm] *n micro*. Oesophagostomum *m*.
oe·soph·a·gus *n* → esophagus.
Oes·tri·dae ['estrədɪ] *pl bio.*, *micro*. Oestridae *pl*.
oes·trone ['estrɔʊn] *n* Estron *nt*, Östron *nt*, Follikulin *nt*, Folliculin *nt*.
oes·trous ['estrəs] *adj bio*. Östrus betr., Östral-, Brunst-.
oes·tru·al ['estrʊəl] *adj* → oestrous.
Oes·trus ['estrəs] *n bio.*, *micro*. Oestrus *m*.
oes·trus ['estrəs] *n bio*. Brunst *f*, Östrus *m*.
OFA *abbr*. → oncofetal antigen.
OFD syndrome → oral-facial-digital syndrome.
off-bipolar cells *physiol*. Off-Bipolarzellen *pl*.

of·fen·sive breath [ə'fensɪv] (übler) Mund-/Atemgeruch *m*, Kakostomie *f*, Halitosis *f*, Halitose *f*, Foetor ex ore.
of·fi·cial [ə'fɪʃl] *adj* 1. amtlich, dienstlich, behördlich, offiziell, Amts-, Dienst-. 2. formell, förmlich, offiziell. 3. *pharm*. als Heilmittel anerkannt, arzneilich, offizinell, offizinal.
of·fic·i·nal [ə'fɪʃənl] **I** *n* 1. offizinelles Heilmittel *nt*. 2. Arzneimittel *nt*, -droge *f*; Heilkraut *nt*, Heilpflanze *f*. **II** *adj* als Heilmittel anerkannt, arzneilich, offizinell, offizinal, Arznei-, Heil-.
OF medium OF-Medium *nt*, Oxidations--Fermentationsmedium *nt* nach Hugh.
Ogilvie ['ɔʊgəlvɪ]: **O.'s syndrome** Ogilvie--Syndrom *nt*, Pseudo-Obstruktionsileus *m*.
Ogino-Knaus [ɔʊ'dʒiːnɔʊ nɔːz; (k)naʊs]: **O.-K. method/rule** *gyn*. Knaus-Ogino-Methode *f*.
oGTT *abbr*. → oral glucose tolerance test.
Oguchi [ɔʊ'guːtʃɪ]: **O.'s disease** Oguchi--Krankheit *f*, -Syndrom *nt*.
Ohara [ɔʊ'hɛərə]: **O.'s disease** Francis--Krankheit *f*, Ohara-Krankheit *f*, Hasen-, Nagerpest *f*, Lemming-Fieber *nt*, Tularämie *f*.
17-OH-corticoid test Porter-Silber-Methode *f*.
17-OH-CS *abbr*. → 17-hydroxycorticosteroid.
OHF *abbr*. → Omsk hemorrhagic fever.
Ohm [ɔʊm]: **O.'s law** Ohm'-Gesetz *nt*.
ohm [ɔʊm] *n abbr*. Ω *nt abbr*. Ω.
ohm·age ['ɔʊmɪdʒ] *n* Ohmzahl *f*.
ohm·ic ['ɔʊmɪk] *adj* Ohm'-.
ohmic resistance Ohm'-Widerstand *m*.
ohm·me·ter ['ɔʊmiːtər] *n* Widerstandsmesser *m*, Ohmmeter *nt*.
OI *abbr*. → osteogenesis imperfecta.
OIC *abbr*. → osteogenesis imperfecta congenita.
oid-oid disease [ɔɪd] exsudative diskoide lichenoide Dermatitis *f*, oid-oid disease (*nt*).
oid·i·o·my·co·sis [ɔʊ,ɪdɪɔʊmaɪ'kɔʊsɪs] *n old* → candidiasis.
Oid·i·um [ɔʊ'ɪdɪəm] *n old* → Candida.
oid·i·um [ɔʊ'ɪdɪəm] *n bio.*, *micro*. Oidium *nt*.
oi·ko·ma·nia [,ɔɪkə'meɪnɪə, -jə] *n psychia*. Oikomanie *f*.
oi·ko·pho·bia [,-'fɔʊbɪə] *n psychia*. Oikophobie *f*.
oi·ko·trop·ic [,-'trapɪk, -'trɔʊp-] *adj* oikotrop.
oil [ɔɪl] **I** *n* Öl *nt*, Oleum *nt*. **II** *vt* (ein-)ölen, einfetten, schmieren.
o. of geranium Geraniënöl.
oil-aspiration pneumonia Ölaspirations-, Fettaspirationspneumonie *f*, Lipidpneumonie *f*.
oil-based *adj* auf Ölbasis.
oil bath *techn*. Ölbad *nt*.
oil cloth 1. Wachstuch *nt*. 2. → oil skin.
oil cyst Ölzyste *f*.
oil embolism Fettembolie *f*.
oil glands Talgdrüsen *pl*, Gll. sebaceae.
oil immersion Ölimmersion *f*.
oil-immersion lens Ölimmersionsobjektiv *nt*.
oil-immersion objective → oil-immersion lens.
oil·i·ness ['ɔɪlɪnɪs] *n* fettige *od*. ölige Beschaffenheit *f*, Fettigkeit *f*, Öligkeit *f*.
oil phase *phys*. Ölphase *f*.
oil pneumonia Öl-, Fettaspirationspneumonie *f*, Lipidpneumonie *f*.
oil skin Öltuch *nt*, Ölhaut *f*.
oil tumor Lipogranulom *nt*, Oleogranulom *nt*.

oil·y ['ɔɪlɪ] *adj* 1. ölig, ölhaltig, Öl-. 2. fettig, schmierig, voller Öl.
oint·ment ['ɔɪntmənt] *n* Salbe *f*; *pharm*. Unguentum *nt*.
ointment base *pharm*. Salbengrundlage *f*.
OIT *abbr*. → osteogenesis imperfecta tarda.
Okazaki [ɔːkə'zaːkɪ]: **O. fragments** Okazaki-Fragmente *pl*, -stückchen *pl*.
Oken ['ɔʊkən]: **O.'s body** *embryo*. Urniere *f*, Wolff-Körper *m*, Mesonephron *nt*, Mesonephros *m*.
canal of O. Wolff-Gang *m*, Urnierengang *m*, Ductus mesonephricus.
O.'s corpus → O.'s body.
OKN *abbr*. → optokinetic nystagmus.
ol·a·mine ['alɔmiːn] *n* Äthanol-, Ethanolamin *nt*, Colamin *nt*, Monoethanolamin *nt*.
old [ɔʊld] **I** *the* ~ *pl* die Alten. **II** *adj* alt, betagt.
old age hohes Alter *nt*, Greisenalter *nt*, Senium *nt*, Senilität *f*.
old brain Urhirn *nt*, Althirn *nt*, Palaeencephalon *nt*.
Oldfield ['ɔʊldfiːld]: **O.'s syndrome** Oldfield-Krankheit *f*, -Syndrom *nt*.
old sight Alterssichtigkeit *f*, Presbyopie *f*.
old thalamus Paläothalamus *m*.
old tuberculin *abbr*. **OT** Alttuberkulin *nt abbr*. AT, Tuberkulin-Original-Alt *nt abbr*. TOA.
Old World hookworm (europäischer) Hakenwurm *m*, Grubenwurm *m*, Ancylostoma duodenale.
Old World leishmaniasis kutane Leishmaniose/Leishmaniase *f*, Hautleishmaniose *f*, Orientbeule *f*, Leishmaniasis cutis.
ole- *pref*. → oleo-.
o·le·ag·i·nous [,ɔʊlɪ'ædʒənəs] *adj* ölhaltig, -artig, ölig, Öl-.
o·le·an·do·my·cin [,ɔʊlɪ,ændɔʊ'maɪsɪn] *n pharm*. Oleandomycin *nt*.
o·le·an·drin [ɔʊlɪ'ændrɪn] *n* Oleandrin *nt*.
o·le·ate [ɔʊlɪeɪt] *n* Oleat *nt*.
o·lec·ra·nal [ɔʊ'lekrənl] *adj* Olekranon betr., Olekranon-.
o·lec·ra·non [ɔʊ'lekrənan, ɔʊlɪ'kreɪnan] *n* Ell(en)bogenfortsatz *m*, -höcker *m*, Olekranon *nt*, Olecranon *nt*.
olecranon bursa Bursa subcutanea olecrani.
olecranon bursitis Entzündung *f* des Ellenbogenschleimbeutels, Bursitis olecrani.
olecranon fossa Fossa olecrani.
olecranon process of ulna → olecranon.
o·le·fin ['ɔʊlɪfɪn] *n* olefine.
o·le·fine ['ɔʊləfiːn] *n* Olefin *nt*, Alken *nt*.
o·le·ic acid [ɔʊ'liːɪk] Ölsäure *f*.
o·le·in ['ɔʊliːɪn] *n* Olein *nt*, Triolen *nt*.
oleo- *pref*. Ole(o)-, Öl-.
o·le·o·gran·u·lo·ma [,ɔʊlɪɔʊ,grænjə'lɔʊmə] *n* Öleo-, Lipogranulom *nt*.
o·le·o·ma [ɔʊlɪ'ɔʊmə] *n* Oleom *nt*, Oleosklerom *nt*, Oleogranulom *nt*, Elaiom *nt*.
o·le·o·pal·mi·tate [,ɔʊlɪɔʊ'pælmɪteɪt, -'paː(l)m-] *n* Oleopalmitat *nt*.
o·le·o·ste·a·rate [,-'stɪəreɪt] *n* Oleostearat *nt*.
o·le·o·tho·rax [,-'θɔːræks] *n histor*. Oleothorax *m*.
o·le·um ['ɔʊlɪəm] *n, pl* **o·lea** [ɔʊlɪə] Öl *nt*, Oleum *nt*.
o·le·yl [ɔʊ'liːɪl] *n* Oleyl-(Radikal *nt*).
ol·fac·tion [al'fækʃn, ɔʊl-] *n* 1. Riechen *nt*. 2. Geruchssinn *m*; *anat*. Olfactus *m*.
ol·fac·to·gen·i·tal dysplasia [al'fæktɔʊ-'dʒenɪtl, ɔʊl-] (Gauthier-)Kallmann-Syndrom *nt*, olfaktogenitales Syndrom *nt*.
olfacto-hypothalamo-tegmental fibers

olfactometer

olfakto-hypothalamo-tegmentale Fasern *pl*, Fibrae olfacto-hypothalamo-tegmentales.
ol·fac·tom·e·ter [ˌɒlfækˈtɒmɪtər, ˌoʊl-] *n* Olfaktometer *nt*.
ol·fac·tom·e·try [ˌ-ˈtɒmətrɪ] *n* Olfaktometrie *f*.
ol·fac·to·pho·bia [ɒlˌfæktəʊˈfəʊbɪə, ˌoʊl-] *n* → osmophobia.
ol·fac·to·ry [ɒlˈfækt(ə)rɪ, ˌoʊl-] *adj* Geruchssinn betr., olfaktorisch, Riech-, Geruchs-.
olfactory amnesia olfaktorische Amnesie *f*.
olfactory anesthesia *neuro*. Anosmie *f*.
olfactory area basale Riechrinde *f*, Area olfactoria, Substantia perforata anterior/rostralis.
olfactory aura *neuro*. olfaktorische Aura *f*.
olfactory brain Riechhirn *nt*, Rhinencephalon *nt*.
olfactory bulb Riechkolben *m*, -kegel *m*, Bulbus olfactorius.
olfactory cells Riechzellen *pl*.
olfactory centers Riechzentren *pl*.
olfactory cilia Riechhäärchen *pl*, -geißeln *pl*.
olfactory cleft Riechspalte *f*.
olfactory cortex 1. → olfactory brain. 2. Archäo-, Archaeo-, Archicortex *m*.
olfactory epithelium Riechepithel *nt*.
olfactory fibers → olfactory nerve 2.
olfactory field → olfactory mucosa.
olfactory glands Bowman'-Spüldrüsen *pl*, Gll. olfactoriae.
olfactory glomeruli Glomeruli olfactorii.
olfactory gyri, medial and lateral Gyri olfactorii mediales et laterales.
olfactory hairs → olfactory cilia.
olfactory hallucination *psychia*. olfaktorische Halluzination *f*, Geruchshalluzination *f*.
olfactory hyperesthesia gesteigertes Geruchsvermögen *nt*, olfaktorische Hyperästhesie *f*, Hyperosmie *f*.
olfactory hypesthesia → olfactory hypoesthesia.
olfactory hypoesthesia *neuro*. vermindertes Geruchsvermögen *nt*, olfaktorische Hypästhesie *f*, Hyposmie *f*.
olfactory knob → olfactory bulb.
olfactory lobe Riechlappen *m*, Lobus olfactorius.
olfactory mucosa Riechschleimhaut *f*, -feld *nt*, Regio olfactoria (tunicae mucosae nasi).
olfactory nerve 1. Riechnerv *m*, Olfaktorius *m*, N. olfactorius, I. Hirnnerv *m*. 2. ‿s *pl* Riechfäden *pl*, Fila olfactoria, Nn. olfactorii.
olfactory organ Riechorgan *nt*, Organum olfactorium/olfactus.
olfactory part of amygdaloid body kortikomediale Kerngruppe *f* des Mandelkerns, Pars corticomedialis/olfactoria corporis amygdaloidei.
olfactory pit *embryo*. Riechgrube *f*.
olfactory placode *embryo*. Riechplakode *f*.
olfactory region Riechschleimhaut *f*, -feld *nt*, Regio olfactoria (tunicae mucosae nasi).
olfactory stria: lateral o. Stria olfactoria lateralis.
   medial o. Stria olfactoria medialis.
olfactory sulcus: o. of frontal lobe Olfaktoriusrinne *f* des Frontallappens, Sulcus olfactorius lobi frontalis.
   o. of nose Sulcus olfactorius nasi.
olfactory tract Riechbahn *f*, Tractus olfactorius.
olfactory trigone Trigonum olfactorium.
olfactory tubercle → olfactory bulb.
olfactory vesicle → olfactory bulb.
olig- *pref*. → oligo-.
ol·ig·ak·i·su·ria [ˌɒlɪɡækɪˈs(j)ʊərɪə] *n* seltenes Harnlassen *nt*, Oligakisurie *f*.
ol·ig·am·ni·os [ɒlɪˈɡæmnɪəs] *n* → oligoamnios.
ol·ig·e·mia [ɒlɪˈɡiːmɪə] *n* Hypovolämie *f*, Oligämie *f*.
ol·ig·e·mic [ɒlɪˈɡiːmɪk] *adj* Hypovolämie betr., hypovolämisch.
oligemic shock Volumenmangelschock *m*, hypovolämischer Schock *m*.
ol·ig·hid·ria [ɒlɪɡˈhɪdrɪə] *n* verminderte Schweißsekretion *f*, Oligohidrosis *f*.
ol·ig·id·ria [ɒlɪɡˈɪdrɪə] *n* → olighidria.
oligo- *pref*. Klein-, Olig(o)-.
ol·i·go·am·ni·os [ˌɒlɪɡəʊˈæmnɪəs] *n* *gyn*. Oligoamnion *nt*, Olaminion *nt*, Oligohydramnie *f*.
ol·i·go·car·dia [ˌ-ˈkɑːrdɪə] *n* *card*. Bradykardie *f*.
ol·i·go·cho·lia [ˌ-ˈkəʊlɪə] *n* verminderte/mangelhafte Galle(n)sekretion *f*, Hypocholie *f*, Oligocholie *f*.
ol·i·go·chro·ma·sia [ˌ-krəʊˈmeɪʒɪə] *n* 1. Hypochromasie *f*. 2. Hypochromie *f*.
ol·i·go·chy·lia [ˌ-ˈkaɪlɪə] *n* verminderte Magensaftbildung *f*, Hypochylie *f*, Oligochylie *f*.
ol·i·go·cys·tic [ˌ-ˈsɪstɪk] *adj* oligozystisch.
ol·i·go·cy·the·mia [ˌ-saɪˈθiːmɪə] *n* *hema*. Oligozythämie *f*.
ol·i·go·cy·to·sis [ˌ-saɪˈtəʊsɪs] *n* → oligocythemia.
ol·i·go·dac·tyl·ia [ˌ-dækˈtɪlɪə] *n* → oligodactyly.
ol·i·go·dac·ty·ly [ˌ-ˈdæktəlɪ] *n* *embryo*. Oligodaktylie *f*.
ol·i·go·den·dria [ˌ-ˈdendrɪə] *n* → oligodendroglia.
ol·i·go·den·dro·blas·to·ma [ˌ-ˌdendrəʊblæsˈtəʊmə] *n* Oligodendrogliom *nt*.
ol·i·go·den·dro·cyte [ˌ-ˈdendrəsaɪt] *n* Oligodendrogliazelle *f*, Oligodendrozyt *m*.
ol·i·go·den·drog·lia [ˌ-denˈdrɒɡlɪə] *n* Oligodendroglia *f*.
oligodendroglia cell Oligodendrogliazelle *f*.
ol·i·go·den·drog·li·al cell [ˌ-denˈdrɒɡlɪəl] → oligodendroglia cell.
ol·i·go·den·dro·gli·o·ma [ˌ-ˌdendrəʊɡlaɪˈəʊmə] *n* Oligodendrogliom *nt*.
ol·i·go·dip·sia [ˌ-ˈdɪpsɪə] *n* pathologisch verminderter Durst *m*, Durstmangel *m*, Oligodipsie *f*.
ol·i·go·don·tia [ˌ-ˈdɒnʃ(ɪ)ə] *n* *dent*. 1. Oligodontie *f*. 2. Hypodontie *f*.
ol·i·go·dy·nam·ia [ˌ-daɪˈnæmɪə] *n* *micro*. Oligodynamie *f*.
ol·i·go·dy·nam·ic [ˌ-daɪˈnæmɪk] *adj* *micro*. oligodynamisch.
ol·i·go·ga·lac·tia [ˌ-ɡəˈlækʃɪə] *n* *gyn*. Oligogalaktie *f*.
ol·i·go·gene [ˈ-dʒiːn] *n* *genet*. Oligogen *nt*, Hauptgen *nt*.
ol·i·go·gen·ic [ˌ-ˈdʒenɪk] *adj* *genet*. oligogen.
ol·i·gog·lia [ɒlɪˈɡɒɡlɪə] *n* Oligodendroglia *f*.
oligo-1,6-α-glucosidase α-Dextrinase *f*, Oligo-1,6-α-glukosidase *f*.
ol·i·go·he·mia [ˌɒlɪɡəʊˈhiːmɪə] *n* → oligemia.
ol·i·go·hy·dram·ni·os [ˌ-haɪˈdræmnɪəs] *n* → oligoamnios.
ol·i·go·hy·per·men·or·rhea [ˌ-ˌhaɪpərmenəˈriːə] *n* *gyn*. Oligohypermenorrhoe *f*.
ol·i·go·hy·po·men·or·rhea [ˌ-ˌhaɪpəʊmenəˈriːə] *n* *gyn*. Oligohypomenorrhoe *f*.
ol·i·go·lec·i·thal [ˌ-ˈlesɪθəl] *adj* *bio*. dotterarm, oligolezithal.

oligolecithal ovum *bio*. oligolezithales Ei *nt*.
ol·i·go·men·or·rhea [ˌ-menəˈriːə] *n* *gyn*. Oligomenorrhoe *f*.
o·lig·o·mer [ˈɒlɪɡəʊmər] *n* Oligomer *nt*.
o·lig·o·mer·ic [ˌ-ˈmerɪk] *adj* oligomer.
oligomeric protein oligomeres Protein *nt*.
ol·i·go·mor·phic [ˌ-ˈmɔːrfɪk] *adj* *micro*. oligomorph.
ol·i·go·my·cin-sensitivity-conferring factor [ˌ-ˈmaɪsɪn] *abbr*. F_O, OSCF *biochem*. oligomycinempfindlichkeitsübertragender Faktor *m* *abbr*. F_O, OSCF.
ol·i·go·nu·cle·o·tide [ˌ-ˈn(j)uːklɪətaɪd] *n* Oligonukleotid *nt*.
ol·i·go·pep·sia [ˌ-ˈpepsɪə] *n* mangelhafte Verdauung *f*, Hypopepsie *f*, Oligopepsie *f*.
ol·i·go·phre·nia [ˌ-ˈfriːnɪə] *n old* → mental retardation.
ol·i·go·pep·tide [ˌ-ˈpeptaɪd] *n* Oligopeptid *nt*.
ol·i·gop·nea [ɒlɪɡəpˈniːə, ɒlɪˈɡɒpnɪə] *n* verlangsamte Atmung *f*, Oligopnoe *f*.
ol·i·go·po·sia [ˌɒlɪɡəʊˈpəʊzɪə] *n* pathologisch verminderte Flüssigkeitsaufnahme *f*.
ol·i·gop·o·sy [ɒlɪˈɡɒpəsɪ] *n* → oligoposia.
ol·i·gop·ty·a·lism [ɒlɪɡəʊˈtaɪəlɪzəm, ɒlɪˈɡɒp-] *n* → oligosialia.
ol·i·go·sac·cha·ride [ˌɒlɪɡəʊˈsækəraɪd, -rɪd] *n* Oligosaccharid *nt*.
ol·i·go·si·a·lia [ˌ-saɪˈeɪlɪə] *n* verminderte Speichelsekretion *f*, Oligosialie *f*.
ol·i·go·sper·ma·tism [ˌ-ˈspɜːrmətɪzəm] *n* → oligospermia.
ol·i·go·sper·mia [ˌ-ˈspɜːrmɪə] *n* Oligo(zoo)spermie *f*.
ol·i·go·sper·mic [ˌ-ˈspɜːrmɪk] *adj* Oligo(zoo)spermie betr., oligo(zoo)sperm.
ol·i·go·symp·to·mat·ic [ˌ-ˌsɪmptəˈmætɪk] *adj* oligosymptomatisch.
ol·i·go·syn·ap·tic [ˌ-sɪˈnæptɪk] *adj* oligosynaptisch.
ol·i·go·trich·ia [ˌ-ˈtrɪkɪə] *n* → oligotrichosis.
ol·i·go·tri·cho·sis [ˌ-trɪˈkəʊsɪs] *n* spärliche Behaarung *f*, Haarmangel *m*, Hypotrichose *f*, -trichosis *f*, -trichia *f*.
ol·i·go·zo·o·sper·ma·tism [ˌ-ˌzəʊəˈspɜːrmətɪzəm] *n* → oligospermia.
ol·i·go·zo·o·sper·mia [ˌ-ˌzəʊəˈspɜːrmɪə] *n* → oligospermia.
ol·i·gu·re·sia [ˌɒlɪɡjʊəˈriːsɪə] *n* → oliguria.
ol·i·gu·re·sis [ˌ-ˈriːsɪs] *n* → oliguria.
ol·i·gu·ria [ɒlɪˈɡ(j)ʊərɪə] *n* verminderte Harnausscheidung *f*, Oligurie *f*.
ol·i·gu·ric [ɒlɪˈɡ(j)ʊərɪk] *adj* Oligurie betr., oligurisch.
oliguric shock hypovolämischer Schock *m*, Volumenmangelschock *m*.
o·li·va [əʊˈlaɪvə] *n, pl* -vae [-viː] olive 1.
ol·i·va·ry [ˈɒləverɪ] *adj* 1. olivenartig, -förmig. 2. *anat*. Olive betr., Oliven-.
olivary body → olive 1.
olivary nucleus *anat*. 1. → olive 1. 2. *anat*. Olivenkern *m*, Nc. olivaris.
   accessory o., dorsal Nc. olivarius accessorius dorsalis/posterior.
   accessory o., medial Nc. olivarius accessorius medialis.
   accessory o., posterior → accessory o., dorsal.
   caudal o. Olivenhauptkern, Nc. olivaris caudalis/inferior.
   inferior o. → caudal o.
   main o. → caudal o.
   superior o. 1. Nc. dorsalis corporis trapezoidei. 2. Nc. olivaris rostralis.
   superior o., medial Nc. medialis olivae superioris.
   rostral o. Nc. olivaris rostralis.

ol·ive ['ɑlɪv] I *n* 1. (*ZNS*) Olive *f*, Oliva *f*. 2. Olive(nfrucht *f*) *f*; Oliven-, Ölbaum *m*. 3. Oliv(grün *nt*) *nt*. II *adj* oliv, oliv(en)farben, -farbig, Oliven-; olivenartig.
olive oil Olivenöl *nt*.
Oliver ['ɑləvər]: **O.'s sign** Oliver-Cardarelli-Zeichen *nt*.
ol·i·vif·u·gal [ɑlɪ'vɪfjəgəl] *adj* von der Olive weg(gerichtet), olivifugal, olivofugal.
ol·i·vip·e·tal [ɑlɪ'vɪpətəl] *adj* auf die Olive zu, olivipetal, olivopetal.
ol·i·vo·cer·e·bel·lar fibers [,ɑlɪvəʊserə-'belər] → olivocerebellar tract.
olivocerebellar tract Oliven-Kleinhirn-Bahn *f*, Tractus olivocerebellaris.
ol·i·vo·coch·le·ar fasciculus [,-'kɑklɪər] → olivocochlear tract.
olivocochlear tract Tractus olivocochlearis.
ol·i·vo·pon·to·cer·e·bel·lar atrophy [,-,pɑntəʊ,serə'belər] Déjérine-Thomas-Syndrome *nt*, olivopontozerebelläre Atrophie *f*.
olivopontocerebellar degeneration → olivopontocerebellar atrophy.
ol·i·vo·spi·nal tract [,-'spaɪnl] Helweg'-Dreikantenbahn *f*, Tractus olivospinalis.
Ollier [ɔl'je]: **O.'s disease** Ollier-Erkrankung *f*, -Syndrom *nt*, Enchondromatose *f*, Hemichondrodystrophie *f*, multiple kongenitale Enchondrome *pl*.
O. graft Thiersch-Lappen *m*.
O.'s (osteogenetic) layer (*Periost*) Ollier'-Schicht *f*.
Ollier-Thiersch [tɪərʃ]: **O.-T. graft** Thiersch-Lappen *m*.
O-locus *n* → operator locus.
O·lym·pi·an brow [ə'lɪmpɪən, əʊ-] *patho*. Olympierstirn *f*.
o·lym·pic brow [ə'lɪmpɪk, əʊ-] *patho*. Olympierstirn *f*.
om- *pref*. → omo-.
o·ma·ceph·a·lus [,əʊmə'sefələs] *n embryo*. Omazephalus *m*, -cephalus *m*, -kephalus *m*.
o·ma·gra [əʊ'mægrə, -'meɪ-] *n* gichtbedingte Schulterschmerzen *pl*, Gicht *f* im Schultergelenk, Omagra *f*.
o·mal·gia [əʊ'mældʒ(ɪ)ə] *n* Schulterschmerz(en *pl*) *m*, Omalgie *f*, Omalgia *f*.
o·mar·thri·tis [əʊmɑr'θraɪtɪs] *n* Schultergelenkentzündung *f*, Omarthritis *f*.
o·ma·sum [əʊ'meɪsəm] *n bio*. Blättermagen *m*, Psalter *m*.
Ombrédanne [ɔ̃brə'dan]: **O.'s operation** *urol*. Ombrédanne-Operation *f*, transskrotale Orchidopexie *f*.
om·bro·pho·bia [,ɑmbrəʊ'fəʊbɪə] *n psychia*. krankhafte Angst *f* vor Regen, Ombrophobie *f*.
o·me·ga [əʊ'miːgə, -'megə, -'meɪ-] *n abbr*. Ω, ω Omega *nt abbr*. Ω, ω.
omega loop hypermobiles Sigma *nt*, Omega-Schleife *f*.
omega oxidation ω-Oxidation *f*, omega--Oxidation *f*.
oment- *pref*. → omento-.
o·men·tal [əʊ'mentl] *adj* (Bauch-)Netz/Omentum betr., omental, epiploisch, Omento-.
omental appendages/appendixes Appendices epiploicae/omentales.
omental band → omental tenia.
omental branches: o. of left gastroepiploic/gastro-omental artery Netzbeuteläste *pl* der A. gastroepiploica sinistra, Rami epiploici/omentales a. gastroepiploicae/gastro-omentalis sinistrae.
o. of right gastroepiploic/gastro-omental artery Netzbeuteläste *pl* der A. gastroepiploica dextra, Rami epiploici/omentales

a. gastroepiploicae/gastro-omentalis dextrae.
omental bursa Netzbeutel *m*, Bauchfellsche *f*, Bursa omentalis.
omental cyst Netz-, Omentalzyste *f*.
omental enterocleisis *chir*. Netzdeckung *f* einer Darmperforation.
omental foramen Winslow'-Foramen *nt*, -Loch *nt*, For. epiploicum/omentale.
omental graft Omentum-, Netzlappen *m*.
omental hernia Hernia omentalis.
omental patch *chir*. Netzzipfel *m*, -läppchen *nt*.
omental patch closure *chir*. Deckung *f* mit einem Netzzipfel, Netzdeckung *f*.
omental recess Rec. omentalis.
inferior o. Rec. inferior omentalis.
superior o. Rec. superior omentalis.
omental sac Netzbeutel *m*, Bauchfellsche *f*, Bursa omentalis.
omental taenia → omental tenia.
omental tenia omentale Tänie *f*, T(a)enia omentalis.
omental transplant → omental graft.
omental tuber: o. of liver Leberhöcker *m*, Tuber omentale hepatis.
o. of pancreas Tuber omentale pancreatis.
o·men·tec·to·my [,əʊmen'tektəmɪ] *n chir*. Omentumresektion *f*, Omentektomie *f*.
o·men·ti·tis [,-'taɪtɪs] *n* Bauchnetzentzündung *f*, Omentitis *f*.
omento- *pref*. Netz-, Omentum-, Oment(o)-.
o·men·to·fix·a·tion [əʊ,mentəʊfɪk'seɪʃn] *n* → omentopexy.
o·men·to·mec·to·my [,-'mektəmɪ] *n* → omentectomy.
o·men·to·pex·y ['-peksɪ] *n chir*. Omentopexie *f*, Epiplopexie *f*.
o·men·to·plas·ty ['-plæstɪ] *n chir*. Netz-, Omentum-, Omentoplastik *f*.
o·men·tor·rha·phy [,əʊmen'tɔːrəfɪ] *n chir*. Omentum-, Netznaht *f*, Omentorrhaphie *f*.
o·men·tot·o·my [,əʊmen'tɑtəmɪ] *n chir*. Omentotomie *f*.
o·men·tum [əʊ'mentəm] *n*, *pl* **-ta** [-tə] (Bauch-)Netz *nt*, Omentum *nt*, Epiploon *nt*.
o·mi·tis [əʊ'maɪtɪs] *n* 1. Schulterentzündung *f*, Omitis *f*. 2. → omarthritis.
Ommaya [əʊ'maɪə]: **O. reservoir** Ommaya-Reservoir *nt*.
om·mo·chrome ['ɑməkrəʊm] *n biochem*. Ommochrom *nt*.
om·ni·vore ['ɑmnəvɔːr, -vəʊr] *n bio*. Allesfresser *m*, Omnivore *m*, Pantophage *m*.
om·niv·o·rous [ɑm'nɪvərəs] *adj bio*. allesfressend, omnivor, pantophag.
omo- *pref*. Schulter-, Om(o)-.
o·mo·ceph·a·lus [,əʊməʊ'sefələs] *n embryo*. Omozephalus *m*, -kephalus *m*, -cephalus *m*.
o·mo·cla·vic·u·lar triangle/trigone [,-klə-'vɪkjələr] große Schlüsselbeingrube *f*, Fossa supraclavicularis major, Trigonum omoclaviculare.
o·mo·dyn·ia [,-'diːnɪə] *n* Schulterschmerz(en *pl*) *m*, Omodynie *f*.
o·mo·hy·oid [,-'haɪɔɪd] *n* → omohyoideus muscle.
o·mo·hy·oi·de·us [,-haɪ'ɔɪdɪəs] *n* → omohyoideus muscle.
omohyoideus muscle Omohyoideus *m*, M. omohyoideus.
omohyoid muscle omohyoideus muscle.
o·mo·tra·che·al triangle/trigone [,-'treɪkɪəl] Trigonum musculare/omotracheale.
Omp *abbr*. → membrane protein, outer.
omphal- *pref*. → omphalo-.

om·phal·ec·to·my [ɑmfə'lektəmɪ] *n chir*. Nabelexzision *f*, Omphalektomie *f*.
om·phal·el·co·sis [,ɑmfælel'kəʊsɪs] *n* Nabelulzeration *f*.
om·phal·ic [ɑm'fælɪk] *adj* Nabel betr., umbilikal, Nabel-, Omphalo(-)-.
om·pha·li·tis [,ɑmfə'laɪtɪs] *n* Nabelentzündung *f*, Omphalitis *f*.
omphalo- *pref*. Nabel-, Omphal(o)-.
om·pha·lo·cele ['ɑmfələʊsiːl] *n* Nabelschnurbruch *m*, Omphalozele *f*, -cele *f*.
omphalocele sac Bruchsack *m* bei Omphalozele.
om·pha·lo·en·ter·ic [,-en'terɪk] *adj* Nabel u. Darm betr., omphaloenterisch.
om·pha·lo·ma [ɑmfə'ləʊmə] *n* → omphaloncus.
om·pha·lo·mes·a·ra·ic [,ɑmfələʊmesə'reɪ-ɪk] *adj* → omphalomesenteric.
om·pha·lo·mes·en·ter·ic [,-mesən'terɪk] *adj* Nabel/Umbilicus u. Darmgekröse/Mesenterium betr. *od*. verbindend, omphalomesenterisch.
omphalomesenteric canal Darmstiel *m*, Dotter(sack)gang *m*, Ductus omphalo-(mes)entericus.
omphalomesenteric circulation *embryo*. Dottersackkreislauf *m*.
omphalomesenteric duct → omphalomesenteric canal.
omphalomesenteric fistula Dottergangsfistel *f*, Fistula omphaloenterica.
omphalomesenteric vessels Dottergefäße *pl*, Vasa omphalomesentericae.
om·pha·lon·cus [ɑmfə'lɑŋkəs] *n* Nabelschwellung *f*, -tumor *m*.
om·pha·lop·a·gus [ɑmfə'lɑpəgəs] *n embryo*. Omphalopagus *m*.
om·pha·lo·phle·bi·tis [,ɑmfələʊflɪ'baɪtɪs] *n* Nabelvenenentzündung *f*, Omphalophlebitis *f*, Thrombophlebitis umbilicalis.
om·pha·lor·rha·gia [,-'reɪdʒ(ɪ)ə] *n* Nabelblutung *f*, Omphalorrhagie *f*.
om·pha·lor·rhea [,-'rɪə] *n* Omphalorrhoe *f*.
om·pha·lor·rhex·is [,-'reksɪs] *n* Nabelschnurriß *m*, Omphalorrhexis *f*.
om·pha·los ['ɑmfələs, -las] *n*, *pl* **-li** [-laɪ, -liː] *anat*. Nabel *m*, Umbilikus *m*, Umbilicus *m*, Omphalos *m*, Umbo *m*.
om·pha·lot·o·my [ɑmfə'lɑtəmɪ] *n gyn*. Abnabelung *f*, Omphalotomie *f*.
Omsk hemorrhagic fever [ɔmsk] *abbr*. **OHF** Omsk hämorrhagisches Fieber *nt abbr*. OHF.
Omsk hemorrhagic fever virus Omsk-hämorrhagisches-Fieber-Virus *nt*.
o·nan·ism ['əʊnənɪzəm] *n* 1. Selbstbefriedigung *f*, Onanie *f*, Masturbation *f*. 2. Koitus/Coitus interruptus.
on-bipolar cells On-Bipolarzellen *pl*.
onc- *pref*. → onco-.
On·cho·cer·ca [,ɑŋkəʊ'sɜrkə] *n micro*. Onchocerca *m*.
O. volvulus Knäuelfilarie *f*, Onchocerca volvulus.
on·cho·cer·ci·a·sis [,-sɜr'kaɪəsɪs] *n* Onchozerkose *f*, Onchocercose *f*, Onchocerciasis *f*, Knotenfilariose *f*, Onchocerca-volvulus-Infektion *f*.
on·cho·cer·co·sis [,-sɜr'kəʊsɪs] *n* → onchocerciasis.
onco- *pref*. Tumor-, Geschwulst-, Onko-.
On·co·cer·ca *n* → Onchocerca.
on·co·cyte ['ɑŋkəsaɪt] *n* Onkozyt *m*.
on·co·cyt·ic [-'sɪtɪk] *adj* aus Onkozyten bestehend, onkozytär.
oncocytic adenoma onkozytäres Adenom *nt*.
oncocytic carcinoma onkozytäres Karzinom *nt*, Ca. oncocyticum.

oncocytoma

on·co·cy·to·ma [ˌ-saɪ'təʊmə] *n* **1.** Onkozytom *nt*, Hürthle-Tumor *m*, -Zelladenom *nt*, -Struma *f*, oxyphiles Schilddrüsenadenom *nt*. **2.** Hürthle-Zell-Karzinom *nt*, malignes Onkozytom *nt*.
on·co·dna·vi·rus [ɑŋ'kadnəvaɪrəs] *n micro.* Oncodnavirus *nt*.
on·co·fe·tal antigen [ˌɑŋkəʊ'fiːtl] *abbr.* OFA onkofötales/onkofetales Antigen *nt abbr.* OFA.
on·co·gene ['-dʒiːn] *n* Onkogen *nt*.
on·co·gen·e·sis [ˌ-'dʒenəsɪs] *n* Tumorbildung *f*, Onkogenese *f*.
on·co·ge·net·ic [ˌ-dʒə'netɪk] *adj* Onkogenese betr., onkogenetisch.
on·co·gen·ic [ˌ-'dʒenɪk] *adj* einen Tumor erzeugend, geschwulsterzeugend, onkogen.
on·co·ge·nic·i·ty [ˌ-dʒə'nɪsəti] *n* Fähigkeit *f* zur Tumorbildung, Onkogenität *f*.
oncogenic viruses *micro.* onkogene Viren *pl.*
on·cog·e·nous [ɑŋ'kadʒənəs] *adj* von einem Tumor (ab-)stammend, onkogen.
on·coi·des [ɑŋ'kɔɪdiːz] *n* Anschwellung *f*, Intumeszenz; Turgeszenz *f*.
on·co·log·ic [ˌɑŋkə'ladʒɪk] *adj* Onkologie betr., onkologisch.
on·col·o·gist [ɑŋ'kalədʒɪst] *n* Onkologe *m*, Onkologin *f*.
on·col·o·gy [ɑŋ'kalədʒɪ] *n* Geschwulstlehre *f*, Onkologie *f*.
on·col·y·sis [ɑŋ'kaləsɪs] *n* Geschwulstauflösung *f*, Onkolyse *f*.
on·co·lyt·ic [ˌɑŋkə'lɪtɪk] *adj* Onkolyse betr. *od.* auslösend, onkolytisch.
on·co·ma [ɑŋ'kəʊmə] *n* Geschwulst *f*, Tumor *m*.
on·com·e·ter [ɑŋ'kamɪtər] *n lab.* Onkometer *nt*.
on·cor·na·vi·rus [ɑŋ'kɔːrnəvaɪrəs] *n micro.* Oncornavirus *nt*.
on·co·sis [ɑŋ'kəʊsɪs] *n* Onkose *f*.
on·co·sphere ['ɑŋkəsfɪər] *n micro.* Hakenlarve *f*, Onkosphäre *f*.
on·co·ther·a·py [ˌ-'θerəpɪ] *n* Tumor-, Onkotherapie *f*.
on·cot·ic [ɑŋ'katɪk] *adj* Schwellung *od.* Geschwulst betr., durch eine Schwellung verursacht, onkotisch.
oncotic pressure kolloidosmotischer/onkotischer Druck *m abbr.* KOD.
on·co·trop·ic [ˌɑŋkə'trapɪk] *adj* mit besonderer Affinität zu Tumorzellen, onkotrop.
On·co·vir·i·nae [ˌ-'vɪərəniː] *pl micro.* Oncoviren *pl*, Oncovirinae *pl*.
on·co·vi·rus [ˌ-'vaɪrəs] *n micro.* Onko-, Oncovirus *nt*.
Ondine [ɑn'diːn]: **O.'s curse** Schlafapnoe-(syndrom *nt*) *f*.
one-armed [wʌn] *adj* einarmig.
one-digit *adj mathe.* (*Zahl*) einstellig.
one-dimensional *adj* eindimensional.
one-eyed *adj* einäugig.
one-fold *adj, adv* einzeln, einfach.
one gene-one enzyme hypothesis *biochem.* Ein Gen-ein Enzym-Hypothese *f*, Ein Gen-ein(e) Polypeptid(kette)-Hypothese *f*.
one gene-one polypeptide (chain) hypothesis → one gene-one enzyme hypothesis.
one-handed *adj* **1.** einhändig. **2.** *techn.* mit nur einer Hand zu bedienen.
one-horned uterus Uterus unicornis.
oneir- *pref.* → oneiro-.
o·nei·ric [əʊ'naɪrɪk] *adj* Traum *od.* Träumen betr., Traum-.
oneiric image Traumbild *nt*.
o·nei·rism [əʊ'naɪrɪzm] *n psycho.*, *psychia.* Traumzustand *m*, Oneirismus *m*.

oneiro- *pref.* Traum-, Oneir(o)-.
o·nei·ro·crit·ic [əʊˌnaɪrə'krɪtɪk] *n* Traumdeuter(in *f*) *m*.
o·nei·ro·crit·i·cal [ˌ-'krɪtɪkl] *adj* traumdeutend, -deuterisch.
o·nei·ro·crit·i·cism [ˌ-'krɪtəsɪzəm] *n* Traumdeutung *f*.
o·nei·ro·dyn·ia [ˌ-'diːnɪə] *n* Oneirodynia *f*, Alptraum *m*.
o·nei·ro·gen·ic [ˌ-'dʒenɪk] *adj* Träume auslösend, oneirogen.
o·nei·roid [əʊ'naɪrɔɪd] *adj* traumartig, -ähnlich, oneiroid.
o·nei·rol·o·gy [ˌəʊnaɪ'ralədʒɪ] *n* (wissenschaftliche) Traumdeutung *f*, Oneirologie *f*.
o·nei·ro·phre·nia [əʊˌnaɪrə'friːnɪə] *n psychia.* Oneirophrenie *f*.
o·nei·ros·co·py [əʊnaɪ'raskəpɪ] *n* Traumanalyse *f*, -deutung *f*.
one-legged *adj* einbeinig.
one·ness ['wʌnɪs] *n* **1.** Einheit *f*. **2.** Gleichheit *f*, Identität *f*.
one-parent child Kind, das mit nur einem Elternteil aufwächst.
one-place *adj mathe.* einstellig, -gliedrig.
one-sided *adj* (*a. fig.*) einseitig; halbseitig.
one-sided chorea *neuro.* Hemichorea *f*.
one-sided dominance *physiol.* Seitendominanz *f*.
one-sided epilepsy halbseitige/einseitige Epilepsie *f*, Hemiepilepsie *f*.
one-sidedness *n* (*a. fig.*) Einseitigkeit *f*.
one-substrate reaction *biochem.* Ein-Substrat-Reaktion *f*.
one-syllable comprehension *HNO* (*Gehör*) Einsilbenverständnis *nt*.
o·ni·o·ma·nia [ˌəʊnɪəʊ'meɪnɪə, -jə] *n psychia.* krankhafter/zwanghafter Kauftrieb *m*, Oniomanie *f*.
onion bodies ['ʌnjən] *patho.* Epithel-, Hornperlen *pl*.
onion mite *micro.* Acarus rhyzoglypticus hyacinthi.
onion-peel appearance/reaction *radiol.* (*Periost*) Zwiebelschalenstruktur *f*, zwiebelschalenartige Reaktion *f*.
onion-scale lesion (*Milz*) Zwiebelschalenläsion *f*.
onion-skin appearance → onion-peel appearance.
onion-skin periostitis *ortho.*, *radiol.* Zwiebelschalenperiostitis *f*.
onion-skin reaction → onion-peel appearance.
o·ni·um ion ['əʊnɪəm, 'əʊnjəm] *chem.* Oniumion *nt*.
on·lay ['ɑnleɪ, 'ɔn-] *n ortho.* Anlegespan *m*, Onlay-Span *m*.
on-off phenomenon On-Off-Effekt *m*.
on·o·ma·to·ma·nia [ˌɑnəˌmætə'meɪnɪə, -jə] *n neuro.*, *psychia.* Onomatomanie *f*.
on·o·mat·o·pho·bia [ˌ-'fəʊbɪə] *n neuro.*, *psychia.* Onomatophobie *f*.
on·o·mat·o·poi·e·sis [ˌ-pɔɪ'iːsɪs] *n psychia.* Onomatopoese *f*.
on·to·gen·e·sis [ˌɑntə'dʒenəsɪs] *n* ontogeny.
on·to·ge·net·ic [ˌ-dʒə'netɪk] *adj* → ontogenic.
on·to·ge·net·i·cal [ˌ-dʒə'netɪkl] *adj* → ontogenic.
on·to·gen·ic [ˌ-'dʒenɪk] *adj* Ontogenese betr., entwicklungsgeschichtlich, ontogenetisch.
onych- *pref.* → onycho-.
on·y·chal·gia [ɑnɪ'kældʒ(ɪ)ə] *n* Nagelschmerz(en *pl*) *m*, Onychalgie *f*.
on·y·cha·tro·phia [ˌɑnɪkə'trəʊfɪə] *n* Nagel-

on·y·chat·ro·phy [ˌɑnɪ'kætrəfɪ] *n* → onychatrophia.
on·y·ch·aux·is [ɑnɪ'kɔːksɪs] *n* Nagelverdickung *f*, -hypertrophie *f*, Onychauxis *f*; Pachyonychie *f*, Pachyonyxie *f*.
on·y·chec·to·my [ɑnɪ'kektəmɪ] *n chir.* Nagelexzision *f*, Onychektomie *f*.
o·nych·ia [əʊ'nɪkɪə] *n* Nagelbettentzündung *f*, Onychie *f*, Onychia *f*, Onychitis *f*, Onyxitis *f*.
on·y·chi·tis [ɑnə'kaɪtɪs] *n* → onychia.
onycho- *pref.* Nagel-, Onych(o)-.
on·y·choc·la·sis [ɑnɪ'kakləsɪs] *n* Onychoklasie *f*.
on·y·cho·cryp·to·sis [ˌɑnɪkəʊkrɪp'təʊsɪs] *n* eingewachsener Nagel *m*, Onychokryptosis *f*.
on·y·cho·dys·tro·phy [ˌ-'dɪstrəfɪ] *n* Nageldystrophie *f*, Onychodystrophie *f*, Dystrophia unguium.
on·y·cho·gry·pho·sis [ˌ-grɪ'fəʊsɪs, -graɪ-] *n* → onychogryposis.
on·y·cho·gry·po·sis [ˌ-grɪ'pəʊsɪs, -graɪ-] *n* Krumm-, Krallen-, Krallnagel *m*, Onychogrypose *f*, Onychogryposis *f*.
on·y·cho·het·er·o·to·pia [ˌ-ˌhetərə'təʊpɪə] *n* Nagelheterotopie *f*, Onychoheterotopie *f*.
on·y·chol·y·sis [ɑnɪ'kaləsɪs] *n* Onycholyse *f*, Onycholysis *f*.
on·y·cho·ma [ɑnɪ'kəʊmə] *n* Nagelbettgeschwulst *f*, -tumor *m*.
on·y·cho·ma·de·sis [ˌɑnɪkəʊmə'diːsɪs] *n* Onychomadesis *f*, Onychomadose *f*, Onycholysis totalis.
on·y·cho·ma·la·cia [ˌ-mə'leɪʒ(ɪ)ə] *n* Nagelerweichung *f*, Onychomalazie *f*.
on·y·cho·my·co·sis [ˌ-maɪ'kəʊsɪs] *n* Nagelmykose *f*, Onychomykose *f*, -mycosis *f*, Tinea unguium.
on·y·cho·no·sus [ˌ-'nəʊsəs] *n* → onychopathy.
onycho-osteodysplasia *n* Nagel-Patella-Syndrom *nt*, Osteoonychodysplasie *f*, Osteoonychodysostose *f*, Onycho-osteodysplasie *f*.
on·y·chop·a·thy [ɑnɪ'kɑpəθɪ] *n* Nagelerkrankung *f*, Onychopathie *f*, Onychose *f*, Onychosis *f*.
on·y·cho·pha·gia [ˌɑnɪkəʊ'feɪdʒ(ɪ)ə] *n* → onychophagy.
on·y·choph·a·gy [ɑnɪ'kɑfədʒɪ] *n* Nägelkauen *nt*, Onychophagie *f*.
on·y·cho·phy·ma [ˌɑnɪkəʊ'faɪmə] *n* Nagelhypertrophie *f*, Onychophym *nt*.
on·y·cho·pto·sis [ˌɑnɪkɑp'təʊsɪs] *n* → onychomadesis.
on·y·cho·plas·ty ['ɑnɪkəʊplæstɪ] *n chir.*, *derm.* Nagelplastik *f*.
on·y·chor·rhex·is [ˌ-'reksɪs] *n* Onychorrhexis *f*.
on·y·cho·schiz·ia [ˌ-'skɪzɪə] *n* Onychoschisis *f*.
on·y·cho·sis [ɑnɪ'kəʊsɪs] *n* → onychopathy.
on·y·cho·til·lo·ma·nia [ˌɑnɪkəʊˌtɪlə'meɪnɪə, -jə] *n psychia.* Nägelreißen *nt*, Onychotillomanie *f*.
on·y·chot·o·my [ɑnɪ'kɑtəmɪ] *n derm.*, *chir.* Onychotomie *f*.
O'nyong-nyong [əʊ'njɑŋ njɑŋ] *n* O'nyong-nyong-Fieber *nt*.
O'nyong-nyong fever → O'nyong-nyong.
O'nyong-nyong virus *micro.* O'nyong-nyong-Virus *nt*.
on·yx ['ɑnɪks, 'əʊ-] *n* **1.** Nagel *m*, Ungus *m*, Onyx *m*. **2.** *ophthal.* Onyx *m*.
o·nyx·is [əʊ'nɪksɪs] *n* → onychocryptosis.
on·yx·i·tis [əʊnɪk'saɪtɪs] *n* → onychia.
oo- *pref.* → ovi-.
o·o·blast ['əʊəblæst] *n* Ooblast *m*.

o·o·cen·ter [ˌ-'sentər] *n* Oozentrum *nt*, Ovozentrum *nt*.
o·o·ceph·a·lus [ˌ-'sefələs] *n* Oozephalus *m*, -kephalus *m*.
o·o·ci·ne·sia [ˌ-sɪ'niːʒ(ɪ)ə] *n* → ookinesis.
o·o·cy·e·sis [ˌ-saɪ'iːsɪs] *n* → ovarian pregnancy.
o·o·cyst ['-sɪst] *n* Oozyste *f*.
o·o·cyte ['-saɪt] *n* Eizelle *f*, Oozyt(e *f*) *m*, Ovozyt *m*, Ovocytus *m*.
o·og·a·mous [əʊ'ɒgəməs] *adj* 1. oogam. 2. hetero-, anisogam.
o·og·a·my [əʊ'ɒgəmɪ] *n* Eibefruchtung *f*, Oogamie *f*.
o·o·gen·e·sis [ˌəʊə'dʒenəsɪs] *n* Eireifung *f*, Oogenie *f*, Ovo-, Oogenese *f*.
o·o·ge·net·ic [ˌ-dʒə'netɪk] *adj* Eireifung/Oogenese betr., oogenetisch.
oogenetic cycle → ovarian cycle.
o·o·gen·ic [ˌ-'dʒenɪk] *adj* → oogenetic.
o·og·e·nous [əʊ'ɒdʒenəs] *adj* → oogenetic.
o·o·go·ni·um [ˌəʊə'gəʊnɪəm] *n*, *pl* **-nia** [-nɪə] Urei(zelle *f*) *n*, Oogonie *f*, Oogonium *nt*.
o·o·ki·ne·sis [ˌ-kɪ'niːsɪs, -kaɪ-] *n* Ookinese *f*.
o·o·ki·nete [ˌ-'kaɪniːt, -kɪ'niːt] *n micro*. Ookinet *m*.
o·o·lem·ma [ˌ-'lemə] *n* Eihülle *f*, Oolemma *nt*, Zona/Membrana pellucida.
O·o·my·ce·tes [ˌ-maɪ'sɪtiːz] *pl micro*. Oomyzeten *pl*, Oomycetes *pl*.
oophor- *pref*. → oophoro-.
o·o·pho·ral·gia [ˌəʊəfə'rældʒ(ɪ)ə] *n* Eierstockschmerz(en *pl*) *m*, Ovarialgie *f*.
o·o·pho·rec·to·mize [ˌ-'rektəmaɪz] *vt gyn*. eine Eierstockentfernung/Oophorektomie durchführen, die Eierstöcke entfernen, oophorektomieren.
o·o·pho·rec·to·my [ˌ-'rektəmɪ] *n gyn*. Eierstockentfernung *f*, Oophorektomie *f*, Ovar(i)ektomie *f*.
o·o·pho·rit·ic cyst [ˌ-'rɪtɪk] → ovarian cyst.
o·o·pho·ri·tis [ˌ-'raɪtɪs] *n* Eierstockentzündung *f*, Oophoritis *f*.
oophoro- *pref*. Eierstock-, Ovarial-, Oophor(o)-.
o·oph·o·ro·cys·tec·to·my [əʊˌɒfərəʊsɪs'tektəmɪ] *n gyn*. Exzision *f* einer Eierstockzyste, Oophorozystektomie *f*.
o·oph·o·ro·hys·ter·ec·to·my [ˌ-hɪstə'rektəmɪ] *n gyn*. Entfernung *f* von Gebärmutter u. Eierstöcken, Oophorohysterektomie *f*, Ovariohysterektomie *f*.
o·o·pho·ro·ma [əʊˌɒfə'rəʊmə] *n* Ovarialschwellung *f*, -tumor *m*, Eierstockschwellung *f*, -tumor *m*, Oophorom *nt*.
oph·o·ron [əʊ'ɒrɒn] *n* → ovary.
o·oph·or·op·a·thy [əʊˌɒfə'rɒpəθɪ] *n* Eierstockerkrankung *f*, Oophoropathie *f*, Ovariopathie *f*.
o·oph·or·o·pel·i·o·pex·y [əʊˌɒfərəʊ'pelɪəʊpeksɪ] *n* → ovariopexy.
o·oph·or·o·pex·y [əʊˌɒfə'rɒpeksɪ] *n* → ovariopexy.
o·oph·or·o·plas·ty ['-plæstɪ] *n gyn*. Eierstockplastik *f*.
o·oph·o·ro·sal·pin·gec·to·my [ˌ-ˌsælpɪŋ'dʒektəmɪ] *n* → ovariosalpingectomy.
o·oph·o·ro·sal·pin·gi·tis [ˌ-ˌsælpɪŋ'dʒaɪtɪs] *n* → ovariosalpingitis.
o·oph·o·ros·to·my [əʊˌɒfə'rɒstəmɪ] *n gyn*. Oophorostomie *f*, Ovariostomie *f*.
o·oph·o·rot·o·my [əʊˌɒfə'rɒtəmɪ] *n* → ovariotomy.
o·oph·or·rha·gia [əʊˌɒfə'reɪdʒ(ɪ)ə] *n* Eierstock-, Ovarialblutung *f*.
o·o·plasm ['əʊəʊplæzəm] *n* Eiplasma *nt*, Ovo-, Ooplasma *nt*.
o·o·sphere ['-sfɪər] *n* Oosphäre *f*.
O·os·po·ra [əʊ'ɒspərə] *n micro*. Oospora *f*.
o·o·spo·ran·gi·um [ˌəʊəspə'rændʒɪəm, -spəʊ-] *n* Oosporangium *nt*.
o·o·spore ['-spəʊər, -spɔːr] *n* Ei-, Oospore *f*.
o·o·the·ca [ˌ-'θiːkə] *n* 1. *bio*. Eikapsel *f*. 2. → ovary.
o·o·tid ['-tɪd] *n* Reifei *nt*, Ootide *f*.
o·o·type ['-taɪp] *n micro*. Ootyp(us *m*) *m*.
ooze [uːz] **I** *n* Sickern *nt*. **II** *vt* ausströmen, (aus-)schwitzen. **III** *vi* sickern.
ooze away *vi* versickern.
ooze in *vi* einsickern, eindringen.
ooze out *vt* → ooze II.
ooze through *vi* durchsickern, durchdringen.
o·o·zo·oid [ˌəʊə'zəʊɔɪd] *n bio*. Oozoid *nt*.
o·pac·i·fi·ca·tion [əʊˌpæsəfɪ'keɪʃn] *n ophthal*. Opakifikation *f*.
o·pac·i·ty [əʊ'pæsətɪ] *n* 1. *phys*. Opazität *f*. 2. *phys*. (Licht-, Strahlen-)Undurchlässigkeit *f*, Absorptionsvermögen *nt*. 3. Undurchsichtigkeit *f*, Opazität *f*. 4. Trübung *f*.
o·pal·gia [əʊ'pældʒ(ɪ)ə] *n* Trigeminusneuralgie *f*, Neuralgia trigeminalis.
o·paque [əʊ'peɪk] *adj* 1. undurchsichtig, nicht durchscheinend, opak. 2. (strahlen-, licht-)undurchlässig. 3. *fig*. unklar, dunkel, unverständlich.
o·paque·ness [əʊ'peɪknɪs] *n* → opacity.
O₂ partial pressure → oxygen partial pressure.
o·pal·esce [əʊpə'liːs] *vi* opalisieren, opaleszieren.
o·pal·es·cence [ˌ-'lesəns] *n* Opaleszenz *f*.
o·pal·es·cent [ˌ-'lesənt] *adj* Opaleszenz aufweisend, opaleszierend, opalisierend, opaleszent.
OPD *abbr*. → out-patients department.
o·pen ['əʊpən] **I** *adj* 1. *allg*. offen, geöffnet; *med*. offen. 2. offen, frei, zugänglich (*to* für). 3. *fig*. aufgeschlossen, offen (*to* für). 4. (*Gebiß*) lückenhaft. **II** *vt* 5. (er-)öffnen, aufmachen; beginnen. 6. *chir*. aufschneiden, -stechen, -bohren, (er-)öffnen. **to ~ the bowels** Stuhlgang haben; abführen. **III** *vi* 7. aufgehen, s. (er-)öffnen. 8. anfangen, beginnen.
open out I *vt* ausbreiten, ausdehnen; weitern, vergrößern. **II** *vi* s. ausbreiten, verbreitern (*into* zu); s. (aus-)weiten, s. öffnen, s. erweitern.
open up I *vt* größer *od*. weiter machen, vergrößern; (er-)öffnen, aufmachen. **II** *vi* s. (er-)öffnen, aufgehen.
open amputation *ortho*., *chir*. offene Amputation *f*, Amputation *f* ohne Stumpfdeckung.
open anesthesia offene Narkose *f*, offenes Narkosesystem *nt*.
open-angle glaucoma Simplex-, Weitwinkelglaukom *nt*, Glaucoma simplex.
open biopsy offene Biopsie *f*.
open chain *chem*. offene Kette *f*; offene Form *f*.
open-chain compound → open chain.
open dislocation *ortho*. offene Luxation *f*.
open form *chem*. offene/gestreckte Form *f*.
open fracture *ortho*. offene/komplizierte Fraktur *f*, offener/komplizierter (Knochen-)Bruch *m*, Wundfraktur *f*, Fractura complicata.
open-heart ['əʊpənhɑːrt] *adj* am offenen Herzen.
openheart surgery offene Herzchirurgie *f*.
o·pen·ing ['əʊpənɪŋ] **I** *n* 1. Öffnung *f*, (Ein-)Mündung *f*, Spalt *m*, Lücke *f*, Loch *nt*; *anat*. Ostium *nt*, Orificium *nt*; Erweiterung *f*. 2. Eröffnung *f*; Öffnen *nt*, Aufmachen *nt*, -stechen *nt*, -bohren *nt*. **II** *adj* (Er-)Öffnungs-.
o. of bladder innere Harnröhrenöffnung, Harnröhrenanfang *m*, Ostium urethrae internum.

o. of coronary sinus Ostium sinus coronarii.
o. of external acoustic meatus äußere Öffnung des Gehörganges, Porus acusticus externus.
o. of inferior vena cava Mündung der unteren Hohlvene, Ostium venae cavae inferioris.
o. of orbital cavity Aditus orbitalis.
o. of pulmonary trunk Pulmonalisöffnung des rechten Ventrikels, Ostium trunci pulmonalis.
o.s of pulmonary veins Ostia vv. pulmonarium.
o. of superior vena cava Mündung der oberen Hohlvene, Ostium venae cavae superioris.
o. of uterus (äußerer) Muttermund *m*, Ostium uteri.
o. of vermiform appendix Wurmfortsatzöffnung, Ostium appendicis vermiformis.
opening contraction *physiol*. Öffnungskontraktion *f*.
open pneumothorax offener Pneu(mothorax *m*) *m*.
open reduction and internal fixation *abbr*. **ORIF** *ortho*. offene Reposition u. Osteosynthese.
open rhinolalia *HNO* offenes Näseln *nt*, Rhinophasie *f*, -phasia *f*, Rhinolalia aperta.
open system *physiol*. offenes System *nt*, steady-state-System *nt*.
nonequilibrium o. nicht im Gleichgewicht stehendes offenes System.
open tuberculosis offene (Lungen-)Tuberkulose *f*.
open wound offene Wunde *f*.
op·er·a·bil·i·ty [ˌɒpərə'bɪlətɪ] *n* 1. *patho*. Operabilität *f*. 2. Operationsfähigkeit *f*, Operabilität *f*.
op·er·a·ble ['ɒp(ə)rəbl] *adj* 1. *chir*. operierbar, operabel. 2. durchführbar. 3. *techn*. betriebsfähig.
op·er·and ['ɒpərænd] *n* (*Computer*) Operand *m*, Rechengröße *f*.
op·er·ant ['ɒpərənt] *adj psycho*. operant, nicht reizgebunden.
operant conditioning operante/instrumentelle Konditionierung *f*.
op·er·ate ['ɒpəreɪt] **I** *vt* 1. bewirken, verursachen, schaffen. 2. (*Gerät*) handhaben, bedienen, betätigen. **II** *vi chir*. operieren (*upon/on s.o.* jdn.).
op·er·at·ing ['ɒpəreɪtɪŋ] *adj* 1. *chir*. Operations-. 2. in Betrieb, Betriebs-, Arbeits-.
operating microscope Operationsmikroskop *nt*, Op-Mikroskop *nt*.
operating room *abbr*. **O.R.** Operationssaal *m*, Operationsraum *m abbr*. OP.
operating suite Operationstrakt *m*.
operating surgeon Operateur *m*.
operating table Operationstisch *m*.
operating team Operationsteam *nt*, Op-Team *nt*.
operating theatre *Brit*. → operating room.
op·er·a·tion [ɒpə'reɪʃn] *n* 1. *chir*. (chirurgischer) Eingriff *m*, Operation *f abbr*. Op. 2. *chir*. Operation *f*, Technik *f*, Verfahren *nt*. 3. *techn*. Betrieb *m*, Tätigkeit *f*, Lauf *m*.
op·er·a·tive ['ɒpərətɪv, 'ɒprə-, -ˌreɪtɪv] *adj* 1. *chir*. operativ, chirurgisch, Operations-, Operativ-. 2. wirkend, wirksam, operativ. **to be ~** wirksam sein. **to become ~** zur Wirkung kommen, wirksam werden; in Kraft treten.
operative cholangiography intraoperative Cholangiographie *f*.
operative dentistry Zahn- u. Kieferchirurgie *f*.

operative mortality operative Mortalität *f.*
operative myxedema postoperatives Myxödem *nt.*
operative pancreatography *chir.* intraoperative Pankreat(ik)ographie *f.*
operative permit Einwilligung/Einverständniserklärung *f* zur Operation.
operative repair operativer Verschluß *m*, operative Versorgung *f.*
operative risk Operationsrisiko *nt.*
operative technique Operationstechnik *f.*
operative temperature *physiol.* Operativtemperatur *f.*
operative treatment operative Behandlung *f.*
op·er·a·tor ['ɒpəreɪtər] *n* **1.** Operateur(in *f*) *m*, operierender Arzt *m*, operierende Ärztin *f.* **2** *techn., mathe.* Operator *m.* **3.** *genet.* → operator locus.
operator-constitutive mutant Operator-konstitutive-Mutante *f.*
operator gene → operator locus.
operator locus Operatorgen *nt*, O-Gen *nt.*
o·per·cu·lar part of inferior frontal gyrus [əʊ'pɜːkjələr] Operculum frontale, Pars opercularis.
o·per·cu·lum [əʊ'pɜːkjələm] *n, pl* **-lums, -la** [-lə] *anat.* Operculum *nt.*
op·er·on ['ɒpə,rɒn] *n genet.* Operon *nt.*
operon model Operonmodell *nt.*
o·phi·a·sis [əʊ'faɪəsɪs] *n derm.* Ophiasis *f.*
o·phi·di·a·sis [əʊfɪ'daɪəsɪs] *n* → ophidism.
o·phi·dism ['əʊfɪdɪzəm] *n* Schlangengiftvergiftung *f*, Ophidismus *m.*
oph·ry·on ['ɒfrɪən] *n anat.* Ophryon *nt.*
ophthalm- *pref.* → ophthalmo-.
oph·thal·ma·gra [,ɒfθæl'mægrə, -'meɪ-] *n ophthal.* plötzlicher Augenschmerz *m*, Ophthalmagra *f.*
oph·thal·mal·gia [,-'mældʒ(ɪ)ə] *n* Augenschmerz(en *pl*) *m*, Ophthalmalgie *f*, Ophthalmodynie *f.*
oph·thal·mi·a [ɒf'θælmɪə] *n ophthal.* Augenentzündung *f*, Ophthalmie *f*, Ophthalmia *f*; Ophthalmitis *f.*
oph·thal·mic [ɒf'θælmɪk] *adj* Auge betr., zum Auge gehörend, ophthalmisch, Augen-, Ophthalm(o)-, Okul(o)-.
ophthalmic artery Augenschlagader *f*, Ophthalmika *f*, A. ophthalmica.
ophthalmic cup → optic cup 2.
ophthalmic division of trigeminal nerve → ophthalmic nerve.
ophthalmic nerve Ophthalmikus *m*, I. Trigeminusast *m*, N. ophthalmicus.
ophthalmic ointment → oculentum.
ophthalmic plexus vegetativer Plexus *m* der A. ophthalmica.
ophthalmic reaction → ophthalmic test.
ophthalmic scoliosis *ortho.* okuläre Skoliose *f.*
ophthalmic test *derm., immun.* Konjunktivalprobe *f*, -test *m*, Ophthalmoreaktion *f*, -test *m.*
ophthalmic vein: inferior o. untere Augen(höhlen)vene *f*, V. ophthalmica inferior. **superior o.** obere Augen(höhlen)vene *f*, V. ophthalmica superior.
ophthalmic vesicle Augenbläschen *nt*, Vesicula ophthalmica/optica.
ophthalmic zoster Zoster ophthalmicus, Herpes zoster ophthalmicus.
oph·thal·mit·ic [,ɒfθæl'mɪtɪk] *adj* Ophthalmitis betr., ophthalmitisch.
oph·thal·mi·tis [,-'maɪtɪs] *n* Augenentzündung *f*, Ophthalmitis *f.*
ophthalmo- *pref.* Augen-, Ophthalm(o)-, Okul(o)-.
oph·thal·mo·blen·nor·rhea [ɒfθælmə-,blenə'rɪə] *n ophthal.* Augentripper *m*, Ophthalmoblennorrhoe *f*, Conjunctivitis gonorrhoica.
oph·thal·mo·cele ['-siːl] *n ophthal.* Exophthalmos *m*, Exophthalmus *m*, Exophthalmie *f*, Ophthalmoptose *f*, Protrusio/Protopsis bulbi.
oph·thal·mo·co·pi·a [,-'kəʊpɪə] *n ophthal.* Asthenopie *f.*
oph·thal·mo·des·mi·tis [,-dez'maɪtɪs] *n ophthal.* Entzündung *f* der Augenmuskelsehnen.
oph·thal·mo·di·a·phan·o·scope [,-daɪə-'fænəskəʊp] *n ophthal.* Ophthalmodiaphanoskop *nt.*
oph·thal·mo·dy·na·mom·e·ter [,-,daɪnə-'mɑmɪtər] *n ophthal.* Ophthalmodynamometer *nt.*
oph·thal·mo·dy·na·mom·e·try [,-,daɪnə-'mɑmətrɪ] *n ophthal.* Ophthalmodynamometrie *f.*
oph·thal·mo·dyn·ia [,-'diːnɪə] *n* → ophthalmalgia.
oph·thal·mo·gram ['-græm] *n ophthal.* Ophthalmogramm *nt.*
oph·thal·mo·graph ['-græf] *n ophthal.* Ophthalmograph *m.*
oph·thal·mog·ra·phy [,ɒfθæl'mɑgrəfɪ] *n ophthal.* Ophthalmographie *f.*
oph·thal·mo·lith [ɒf'θælməlɪθ] *n* Tränenstein *m*, Dakryolith *m.*
oph·thal·mo·log·ic [ɒf,θælmə'lɑdʒɪk] *adj* Ophthalmologie betr., ophthalmologisch.
oph·thal·mo·log·i·cal [,-'lɑdʒɪkl] *adj* → ophthalmologic.
oph·thal·mol·o·gist [,ɒfθæl'mɑlədʒɪst] *n* Augenarzt *m*, -ärztin *f*, Ophthalmologe *f*, -login *f.*
oph·thal·mol·o·gy [ɒfθæl'mɑlədʒɪ] *n* Augenheilkunde *f*, Ophthalmologie *f.*
oph·thal·mo·ma·la·cia [ɒfθælməmə'leɪʃ(ɪ)ə] *n ophthal.* Augapfel-, Bulbuserweichung *f*, Ophthalmomalazie *f.*
oph·thal·mo·mel·a·no·sis [,-melə'nəʊsɪs] *n ophthal.* Ophthalmomelanose *f.*
oph·thal·mo·me·nin·ge·al vein [,-mɪ'nɪn-dʒɪəl] V. ophthalmomeningea.
oph·thal·mom·e·ter [,ɒfθæl'mɑmɪtər] *n ophthal.* Ophthalmometer *nt.*
oph·thal·mom·e·try [,-'mɑmətrɪ] *n ophthal.* Ophthalmometrie *f.*
oph·thal·mo·my·co·sis [ɒfθælməmaɪ-'kəʊsɪs] *n* Pilzerkrankung *f* des Auges, Ophthalmomykose *f.*
oph·thal·mo·my·ia·sis [,-maɪ(j)əsɪs] *n ophthal.* Madenkrankheit *f* des Auges, Ophthalmomyiasis *f.*
oph·thal·mo·my·i·tis [,-maɪ'aɪtɪs] *n ophthal.* Entzündung *f* der äußeren Augenmuskeln, Ophthalmomyitis *f.*
oph·thal·mo·my·ot·o·my [,-maɪ'ɑtəmɪ] *n ophthal.* Ophthalmomyotomie *f.*
oph·thal·mo·neu·ri·tis [,-njʊə'raɪtɪs, -nʊ-] *n ophthal., neuro.* Entzündung *f* des N. ophthalmicus.
oph·thal·mo·neu·ro·my·e·li·tis [,-,njʊərə-maɪə'laɪtɪs, -,nʊ-] *n* → optic neuromyelitis.
oph·thal·mop·a·thy [,ɒfθæl'mɑpəθɪ] *n ophthal.* Augenleiden *nt*, -erkrankung *f*, Ophthalmopathie *f*, Ophthalmopathia *f.*
oph·thal·moph·thi·sis [,ɒfθæl'mɑfθəsɪs] *n ophthal.* Augapfelschwund *m*, Ophthalmophthisis *f*, Phthisis bulbi.
oph·thal·mo·plas·ty [ɒf'θælməplæstɪ] *n ophthal.* Augenplastik *f.*
oph·thal·mo·ple·gia [,-'pliːdʒ(ɪ)ə] *n ophthal.* Augenmuskellähmung *f*, Ophthalmoplegie *f*, Ophthalmoplegia *f.*
oph·thal·mo·ple·gic [,-'pliːdʒɪk] *adj* Ophthalmoplegie betr., ophthalmoplegisch.
ophthalmoplegic migraine Möbius'-Krankheit *f*, ophthalmoplegische Migräne *f.*
oph·thal·mop·to·sis [ɒf,θælmɑp'təʊsɪs] *n ophthal.* Exophthalmos *m*, Exophthalmus *m*, Ophthalmie *f*, Ophthalmoptose *f*, Protrusio/Protopsis bulbi.
oph·thal·mo·re·ac·tion [ɒf,θælməʊrɪ'æk-ʃn] *n* → ophthalmic test.
oph·thal·mor·rha·gia [,-'reɪdʒ(ɪ)ə] *n ophthal.* Augenblutung *f*, Blutung *f* aus dem Auge, Ophthalmorrhagie *f.*
oph·thal·mor·rhea [,-'rɪə] *n ophthal.* Sickerblutung *f* aus dem Auge, Ophthalmorrhoe *f.*
oph·thal·mor·rhex·is [,-'reksɪs] *n ophthal.* Augapfel-, Bulbuszerreißung *f*, -ruptur *f*, Ophthalmorrhexis *f.*
oph·thal·mos·cope ['-skəʊp] *n ophthal.* Augenspiegel *m*, Ophthalmoskop *m*, Funduskop *nt.*
oph·thal·mos·co·py [ɒfθæl'mɑskəpɪ] *n ophthal.* Augenspiegelung *f*, Ophthalmoskopie *f*, Funduskopie *f.*
oph·thal·mo·spec·tro·scope [ɒf,θælməʊ-'spektrəskəʊp] *n ophthal.* Ophthalmospektroskop *nt.*
oph·thal·mo·spec·tros·co·py [,-spek'trɑs-kəpɪ] *n ophthal.* Ophthalmospektroskopie *f.*
oph·thal·mo·stat ['-stæt] *n ophthal.* Ophthalmostat *m.*
oph·thal·mo·sta·tom·e·ter [,-stə'tɑmɪtər] *n* Exophthalmometer *nt.*
oph·thal·mot·o·my [,ɒfθæl'mɑtəmɪ] *n ophthal.* Augapfel-, Bulbusinzision *f*, Ophthalmotomie *f.*
oph·thal·mo·to·nom·e·ter [ɒf,θælməʊtəʊ-'nɑmɪtər] *n ophthal.* Ophthalmotonometer *nt*, Tonometer *nt.*
oph·thal·mo·to·nom·e·try [,-təʊ'nɑmətrɪ] *n ophthal.* Ophthalmotonometrie *f*, Tonometrie *f.*
oph·thal·mo·tro·pom·e·ter [,-trəʊ'pɑmɪ-tər] *n ophthal.* Strabismometer *nt*, Strabometer *nt.*
oph·thal·mo·tro·pom·e·try [,-trəʊ'pɑmə-trɪ] *n ophthal.* Strabismometrie *f*, Strabometrie *f.*
oph·thal·mo·vas·cu·lar [,-'væskjələr] *adj* Augengefäße betr.
oph·thal·mo·xe·ro·sis [,-zɪ'rəʊsɪs] *n ophthal.* Xerophthalmie *f.*
o·pi·an ['əʊpɪən] *n pharm.* Noscapin *nt.*
o·pi·a·nine [əʊ'paɪənɪn] *n pharm.* Noscapin *nt.*
o·pi·ate ['əʊpɪɪt, -eɪt] **I** *n* **1.** Opiat *nt*, Opiumpräparat *nt*, Opioid *nt.* **2.** Schlafmittel *nt*, Hypnotikum *nt*, Beruhigungsmittel *nt*, Sedativum *nt*; Betäubungsmittel *nt*, Narkotikum *nt.* **II** *adj* **3.** opiumhaltig. **4.** einschläfernd; beruhigend; sedierend; betäubend.
opiate analgesia Opiatanalgesie *f.*
opiate analgesics/analgetics Opiatanalgetika *pl.*
opiate receptor Opiatrezeptor *m.*
opiate sensitivity Opiatempfindlichkeit *f.*
o·pi·oid ['əʊpɪɔɪd] *n* **1.** Opioid *nt.* **2.** (endogenes) Opioid *nt*, Opioid-Peptid *nt.*
o·pip·ra·mol [əʊ'pɪprəməʊl] *n pharm.* Opipramol *nt.*
o·pis·the·nar [əʊ'pɪsθɪnɑːr] *n* Handrücken *m.*
o·pis·thi·on [əʊ'pɪsθɪən] *n anat.* Opisthion *nt.*
o·pis·tho·ge·nia [əʊ,pɪsθə'dʒiːnɪə] *n* Opisthogenie *f.*
o·pis·thog·na·thism [əʊpɪs'θɑgnəθɪzəm] *n* Opisthognathie *f.*
o·pis·tho·mas·ti·gote [ə,pɪsθə'mæstɪgəʊt] *n micro.* opisthomastigote Form *f*, Herpetomonas-Form *f.*

opisthomastigote stage → opisthomastigote.
o·pis·tho·po·reia [ˌɪ-pəʊˈraɪə] *n neuro.* unwillkürliches Rückwärtslaufen *nt.*
o·pis·thor·chi·a·sis [əˌpɪsθɔːrˈkaɪəsɪs] *n* Opisthorchis-Befall *m,* -Infektion *f,* Opisthorchiasis *f,* Opisthorchiose *f.*
O·pis·thor·chi·i·dae [əˌpɪsθɔːrˈkaɪədiː] *pl micro.* Opisthorchiidae *pl.*
Op·is·thor·chis [ˌɒpɪsˈθɔːrkɪs] *n micro.* Opisthorchis *m.*
O. felineus Katzenleberegel *m,* Opisthorchis felineus.
O. sinensis chinesischer Leberegel *m,* Clonorchis/Opisthorchis sinensis.
O. viverrini hinterindischer Leberegel *m,* Opisthorchis viverrini.
o·pis·thor·cho·sis [əˌpɪsθɔːrˈkəʊsɪs] *n* → opisthorchiasis.
op·is·thot·ic [ɒpɪsˈθɒtɪk] *adj* hinter dem Ohr (liegend), postaural.
o·pis·tho·ton·ic [əˌpɪsθəˈtɒnɪk] *adj* Opisthotonus betr.
op·is·thot·o·noid [ɒpɪsˈθɒtənɔɪd] *adj neuro., psychia.* opisthotonusähnlich, -artig, opisthotonoid.
op·is·thot·o·nos *n* → opisthotonus.
o·pis·thot·o·nus [ɒpɪsˈθɒtənəs] *n neuro., psychia.* Opisthotonus *m.*
Opitz [ˈɒpɪts]: **O.'s disease** Opitz'-Krankheit *f,* -Syndrom *nt,* thrombophlebitische Splenomegalie *f.*
o·pi·um [ˈəʊpɪəm] *n* Opium *nt,* Laudanum *nt,* Meconium *nt.*
op·o·ceph·a·lus [ˌɒpəʊˈsefələs] *n embryo.* Opozephalus *m,* -kephalus *m.*
op·o·did·y·mus [ˌ-ˈdɪdəməs] *n embryo.* Opo(di)dymus *m.*
o·pod·y·mus [əˈpɒdɪməs] *n* → opodidymus.
Oppenheim [ˈɒpənhaɪm]: **O.'s disease** Oppenheim-Krankheit *f,* -Syndrom *nt,* Myotonia congenita (Oppenheim).
O.'s reflex → O.'s sign.
O.'s sign Oppenheim-Zeichen *nt.*
O.'s syndrome → O.'s disease.
op·plo·ten·tes [ˌɒpləˈtentəs] *pl ophthal.* Mückensehen *nt,* Mouches volantes.
op·po·nens digiti minimi (muscle) [əˈpəʊnənz] Opponens *m* digiti minimi, M. opponens digiti minimi.
opponens pollicis (muscle) Opponens *m* pollicis, M. opponens pollicis.
op·po·nent [əˈpəʊnənt] **I** *n* Gegner *m,* Gegenspieler *m,* Opponent *m.* **II** *adj* → opposing 2.
opponent colors theory Hering'-Farbentheorie *f,* Gegenfarbentheorie *f.*
opponent-process theory → opponent colors theory.
op·por·tun·is·tic infection [ˌɒpərt(j)uːˈnɪstɪk] opportunistische Infektion *f.*
opportunistic pathogen opportunistisch-pathogener Erreger *m.*
op·pos·ing [əˈpəʊzɪŋ] *adj* 1. gegnerisch, feindlich, opponierend. 2. gegenüberstehend, -liegend. 3. *phys., anat.* entgegenwirkend, Gegen-. 4. entgegengesetzt, gegensätzlich, unvereinbar.
opposing muscle: o. of little finger → opponens digiti minimi (muscle).
o. of thumb → opponens pollicis (muscle).
OPRT *abbr.* → orotate phosphoribosyltransferase.
OPSI *abbr.* [overwhelming post-splenectomy infection] → overwhelming post-splenectomy sepsis (syndrome).
op·si·al·gia [ɒpsɪˈældʒ(ɪ)ə] *n neuro.* Genikulatumneuralgie *f,* Ramsay Hunt-Syndrom *nt,* Neuralgia geniculata, Zoster oticus, Herpes zoster oticus.

op·sin [ˈɒpsɪn] *n* Opsin *nt.*
op·sin·o·gen [ɒpˈsɪnədʒən] *n* → opsogen.
op·si·om·e·ter [ɒpsɪˈɒmɪtər] *n* → optometer.
op·si·u·ria [ɒpsɪˈ(j)ʊərɪə] *n* Opsiurie *f.*
op·so·clo·nia [ˌɒpsəˈkləʊnɪə] *n* → opsoclonus.
op·so·clo·nus [ˌ-ˈkləʊnəs] *n neuro.* Opsoklonus *m,* Opsoklonie *f.*
op·so·gen [ˈ-dʒən] *n* Opsinogen *nt,* Opsogen *nt.*
op·so·ma·nia [ˌ-ˈmeɪnɪə, -jə] *n psychia., gyn.* Opsomanie *f.*
op·son·ic [ɒpˈsɒnɪk] *adj* Opsonin(e) betr., opsonisch.
opsonic index opsonischer Index *m.*
op·so·nin [ˈɒpsənɪn] *n* Opsonin *nt.*
op·so·ni·za·tion [ˌɒpsənaɪˈzeɪʃn] *n* Opsonisierung *f.*
op·so·nom·e·try [ɒpsəˈnɒmətrɪ] *n* Opsonometrie *f.*
op·so·no·phil·ia [ˌɒpsənəʊˈfɪlɪə] *n* Opsonophilie *f.*
op·so·no·phil·ic [ˌ-ˈfɪlɪk] *adj immun.* opsonophil.
OPSS *abbr.* → overwhelming post-splenectomy sepsis (syndrome).
op·tic [ˈɒptɪk] **I** *n* 1. Auge *nt.* 2. Optik *f,* optisches System *nt;* Objektiv *nt.* **II** *adj* Auge betr., zum Auge gehörend, Sehen betr., visuell, okulär, okular, Gesichts-, Augen-, Seh-.
optic agnosia → optical agnosia.
optic agraphia *neuro.* optische Agraphie *f.*
op·ti·cal [ˈɒptɪkl] *adj* 1. Optik betr., optisch. 2. → optic II.
optical activity *chem.* optische Aktivität *f.*
optical agnosia Seelenblindheit *f,* optische/visuelle Agnosie *f.*
optical alexia Leseunfähigkeit *f,* -unvermögen *nt,* Alexie *f.*
optical allachesthesia *neuro.* visuelle Allästhesie *f.*
optical aphasia *neuro.* optische Aphasie *f.*
optical density *abbr.* **OD** *phys.* Absorption *f.*
optical fiber Glasfaser *f,* -fiber *f.*
optical flat → optical plane.
optical illusion optische Täuschung *f.*
optical iridectomy *ophthal.* optische Iridektomie *f.*
optical isomer *chem.* optisches Isomer *nt.*
optical isomerism *chem.* optische Isomerie *f,* Spiegelbildisomerie *f,* Enantiomerie *f.*
optical maser Laser *m.*
optical microscope Lichtmikroskop *nt.*
optical plane optische Ebene *f.*
optical properties *chem.* optische Eigenschaften *pl.*
optical resolution *phys.* Auflösung(svermögen *nt*) *f,* Resolution *f.*
optical rotation *chem.* optische Drehung *f.*
optical screen *phys.* Filter *nt/m,* Blende *f.*
optical specificity *chem.* optische Spezifität *f.*
optic angle Seh-, Gesichts(feld)winkel *m.*
optic atrophy Optikusatrophie *f.*
primary o. einfache Optikusatrophie (*mit scharfen Grenzen*).
secondary o. graue/sekundäre Optikusatrophie *f.*
optic aura *neuro.* optische/visuelle Aura *f.*
optic axis 1. → o. of eye. 2. *phys.* optische Achse *f.*
o. of eye optische Augenachse *f,* Sehachse *f,* Axis opticus (bulbi oculi).
optic canal Optikuskanal *m,* Canalis opticus.
optic chiasm(a) Sehnervenkreuzung *f,* Chiasma opticum.

optic cortex Sehrinde *f,* visueller Kortex *m.*
optic cup 1. Papillenexkavation *f,* Excavatio papillae/disci n. optici. 2. *embryo.* Augenbecher *m,* Caliculus ophthalmicus.
optic decussation → optic chiasm(a).
optic disk → optic nerve disk.
optic glioma Optikusgliom *nt.*
optic grooves *embryo.* Augenfurchen *pl.*
op·ti·cian [ɒpˈtɪʃn] *n* Optiker(in *f*) *m.*
optic iridectomy → optical iridectomy.
optic nerve Sehnerv *m,* Optikus *m,* II. Hirnnerv *m,* N. opticus.
optic nerve disk (Sehnerven-)Papille *f,* Discus/Papilla n. optici.
optic nerve fibers: crossed o. gekreuzte Optikusfasern *pl.*
uncrossed o. ungekreuzte Optikusfasern *pl.*
optic nerve head → optic nerve disk.
optic nerve papilla → optic nerve disk.
optic neuritis Optikusneuritis *f,* Neuritis n. optici.
optic neuroencephalomyelopathy → optic neuromyelitis.
optic neuromyelitis Devic-Syndrom *nt,* -Krankheit *f,* Neuromyelitis optica.
op·ti·co·chi·as·mat·ic [ˌɒptɪkəʊˌkaɪəzˈmætɪk] *adj* N. opticus u. Chiasma opticum betr.
op·ti·co·cil·i·ar·y [ˌ-ˈsɪlɪərɪ] *adj* N. opticus u. Nn. ciliari betr.
op·ti·co·fa·cial reflex [ˌ-ˈfeɪʃl] Blinzelreflex *m.*
op·ti·co·ki·net·ic nystagmus [ˌ-kɪˈnetɪk, -kaɪ-] → optokinetic nystagmus.
optic papilla → optic nerve disk.
optic part of retina lichtempfindlicher Netzhautteil *m,* Pars optica retinae.
optic pathway Sehbahn *f.*
optic pit *embryo.* Augentrichter *m.*
optic placode *embryo.* Linsenplatte *f,* -plakode *f.*
optic radiation Gratiolet'-Sehstrahlung *f,* Radiatio optica.
central o. zentrale Sehstrahlung.
optic recess Rec. opticus.
optic reflex optischer Reflex *m.*
optic reflex tract optische Reflexbahn *f.*
op·tics [ˈɒptɪks] *pl* Optik *f,* Lehre *f* vom Licht.
optic stalk *embryo.* Augenbecherstiel *m.*
optic sulcus Chiasma opticus-Rinne *f,* Sulcus pr(a)echiasmatis/pr(a)echiasmaticus.
optic surgery Augenchirurgie *f.*
optic thalamus Sehhügel *m,* Thalamus *m* (opticus).
optic tract Tractus opticus.
optic ventricle *embryo.* Ventriculus opticus.
optic vesicle *embryo.* Augenbläschen *nt,* Vesicula ophthalmica/optica.
op·ti·mal [ˈɒptɪml] *adj* → optimum II.
optimal dose *pharm., radiol.* Optimaldosis *f.*
op·tim·e·ter [ɒpˈtɪmətər] *n* → optometer.
op·ti·mism [ˈɒptɪmɪzəm] *n* Optimismus *m.*
op·ti·mist [ˈ-mɪst] *n* Optimist(in *f*) *m.*
op·ti·mis·tic [ˌ-ˈmɪstɪk] *adj* zuversichtlich, optimistisch.
op·ti·mis·ti·cal [ˌ-ˈmɪstɪkl] *adj* → optimistic.
op·ti·mi·za·tion [ˌ-mɪˈzeɪʃn] *n* Optimierung *f.*
op·ti·mize [ˈ-maɪz] *vt* optimieren.
op·ti·mum [ˈ-məm] **I** *n, pl* **-ma** [-mə] das Beste, das Bestmögliche, Höchstmaß *nt,* Optimum *nt.* **II** *adj* bestmöglich, optimal, Best-.
optimum dose → optimal dose.
optimum pH pH-Optimum *nt.*

optimum temperature Temperaturoptimum *nt*.
op·to·chi·as·mic [ˌɒptəʊkaɪˈæzmɪk] *adj* → opticochiasmatic.
op·to·chin [ˈ-kɪn] *n* Optochin *nt*, Äthylhydrocuprein *nt*.
optochin test Optochin-Test *m*.
op·to·gram [ˈ-græm] *n physiol.* Optogramm *nt*.
op·to·ki·net·ic nystagmus [ˌ-kɪˈnetɪk, -kaɪ-] *abbr.* OKN optokinetischer Nystagmus *m abbr.* OKN.
optokinetic test optokinetische Prüfung *f*.
op·to·me·ninx [ˌ-ˈmiːnɪŋks] *n* Netzhaut *f*, Retina *f*.
op·tom·e·ter [ɒpˈtɒmɪtər] *n ophthal.* Optometer *nt*; Refraktometer *nt*.
op·tom·e·trist [ɒpˈtɒmətrɪst] *n* Optometrist(in *f*) *m*.
op·tom·e·try [ɒpˈtɒmətrɪ] *n ophthal.* 1. Sehprüfung *f*, -test *m*, Augenuntersuchung *f*. 2. Optometrie *f*, Sehkraft-, Sehweitemessung *f*. 3. Optometrie *f*.
op·to·mo·tor control [ɒptəˈməʊtər] blickmotorische/optomotorische Kontrolle *f*.
op·to·type [ˈ-taɪp] *n ophthal.* Optotype *f*, Sehzeichen *nt*.
OPV *abbr.* → poliovirus vaccine live oral.
O.R. *abbr.* → operating room.
o·ra¹ [ˈɔːrə, ˈəʊrə] *n, pl* **o·ras**, **o·rae** [ˈɔːriː, ˈəʊriː] *anat.* Rand *m*, Saum *m*, Ora *f*.
o·ra² [ˈɔːrə, ˈəʊrə] *pl* → os¹.
o·ral [ˈɔːrəl, ˈəʊrəl] *adj* 1. Mund(höhle) betr., zum Mund *nt.* zur Mundhöhle gehörend, durch den Mund, vom Mund her, oral, Oral-, Mund-. **for ~ use** zum Einnehmen. 2. mündlich.
oral alimentation orale Nahrungsaufnahme/Ernährung *f*.
oral arch Gaumenbogen *m*.
oral candidiasis Mundsoor *m*, Candidose *f* der Mundschleimhaut.
oral cavity Mundhöhle *f*, Cavitas/Cavum oris.
 external o. Mundvorhof *m*, Cavum oris externum, Vestibulum oris.
 primitive o. *embryo.* primitive Mundhöhle.
 proper o. (eigentliche) Mundhöhle, Cavitas/Cavum oris propria.
oral cholecystogram orales Cholezystogramm *nt*, orale Galle *f*.
oral coitus Oralverkehr *m*, Fellatio *f*, Coitus oralis.
oral contraceptive orales Verhütungsmittel *nt*, orales Kontrazeptivum *nt*, Anti-Baby-Pille *f*, *inf.* Pille *f*.
 combination o. Kombinationspräparat *nt*.
 sequential o. Sequenzpräparat *nt*.
oral diaphragm M. mylohyoideus.
oral epithelial nevus *derm.* weißer Schleimhautnävus *m*, Naevus spongiosus albus mucosae.
oral eroticism/erotism Oralerotik *f*.
oral examination mündliche Prüfung *f*, mündlicher Test *m*.
oral-facial-digital syndrome orofaziodigitales Syndrom *nt*, linguofaziale Dysplasie *f*, Dysplasia linguofacialis.
 type II o. Mohr-Claussen-Syndrom *nt*.
oral fissure Mundspalte *f*, Rima oris.
oral flora Mundflora *f*.
oral glucose tolerance test *abbr.* oGTT oraler Glukosetoleranztest *m abbr.* oGTT.
oral herpes Herpes simplex (febrilis); *inf.* Fieberbläschen *pl*.
oral hygiene Zahnhygiene *f*, Mundpflege *f*.
oral hypothalamus oraler Hypothalamus *m*.

oral intercourse Oralverkehr *m*, Fellatio *f*, Coitus oralis.
oral intubation orale Intubation *f*.
o·ral·i·ty [ɔːˈrælətɪ, əʊ-] *n psycho.* orale Fixierung *f*.
oral leukoplakia orale Leukoplakie *f*, Leukoplakie *f* der Mundschleimhaut, Leukoplakia oris.
oral medicine Zahn(heil)kunde *f*, Zahnmedizin *f*, Dentologie *f*, Odontologie *f*.
oral membrane 1. Fascia pharyngobasilaris. 2. *embryo.* Mundbucht *f*, -nische *f*, Stoma(to)deum *nt*.
oral mucosa Mundschleimhaut *f*, Tunica mucosa oris.
oral neuropore oraler/vorderer Neuroporus *m*.
oral penicillin Oralpenicillin *nt*, oralverabreichbares Penicillin *nt*.
oral period → oral phase.
oral phase *psycho.* orale Phase *f*.
oral plate *embryo.* Mundbucht *f*, -nische *f*, Stoma(to)deum *nt*.
oral region Mundgegend *f*, -region *f*, Regio oralis.
oral stage *psycho.* orale Phase *f*.
oral stereotypy *psychia.* Verbigeration *f*.
oral surgeon Gesichts- u. Kieferchirurg(in *f*) *m*.
oral surgery Gesichts- u. Kieferchirurgie *f*.
oral temperature Mundhöhlen-, Sublingualtemperatur *f*.
oral vaccine Schluckimpfstoff *m*, Oralvakzin(e *f*) *nt*.
oral vestibule → oral cavity, external.
or·ange skin [ˈɒrɪndʒ, ˈɑr-] Orangen(schalen)haut *f*, Apfelsinen(schalen)haut *f*, Peau d'orange.
o·ra ser·ra·ta [ˌɔːrə səˈreɪtə] Ora serrata retinae.
or·bic·u·lar [ɔːˈbɪkjələr] *adj* 1. rund, kreisförmig, zirkulär. 2. kugelförmig. 3. ringförmig, Ring-.
or·bic·u·la·re [ɔːrˌbɪkjəˈleərɪ] *n anat.* Proc. lenticularis.
or·bi·cu·la·ris oculi (muscle) [ɔːˌrbɪkjəˈleərɪs] Ringmuskel *m* des Auges, Orbikularis *m* okuli, M. orbicularis oculi.
orbicularis oculi reflex Orbicularis-oculi--Reflex *m*.
orbicularis oris (muscle) Ringmuskel *m* des Mundes, Orbikularis *m* oris, M. orbicularis oris.
orbicularis phenomenon → orbicularis pupillary reflex.
orbicularis pupillary reflex Westphal-Piltz-Phänomen *nt*, Orbikularisphänomen *nt*, Lid-Pupillen-Reflex *m*.
orbicularis reaction → orbicularis pupillary reflex.
orbicularis reflex → orbicularis pupillary reflex.
orbicular ligament of radius Lig. a(n)nulare radii.
orbicular muscle ring-/kreisförmiger Muskel *m*, Orbikularis *m*, M. orbicularis.
 o. of eye → orbicularis oculi (muscle).
 o. of mouth → orbicularis oris (muscle).
orbicular zone of hip joint Zona orbicularis (artic. coxae).
or·bic·u·lus [ɔːˈbɪkjələs] *n, pl* **-li** [-laɪ] *anat.* Orbiculus.
or·bit [ˈɔːbɪt] *n* 1. *anat.* Augenhöhle *f*, Orbita *f*, Cavitas orbitalis. **2.** → orbital I.
or·bi·ta [ˈɔːbɪtə] *n, pl* **-tae** [-tiː] → orbit 1.
or·bit·al [ˈɔːbɪtl] I *n phys., chem.* Orbital *nt*, Bahn *f*. II *adj* Augenhöhle betr., orbital, Augenhöhlen-, Orbita-.
orbital abscess Augenhöhlen-, Orbita(l)abszeß *m*.

orbital aneurysm intraorbitales Aneurysma *nt*.
orbital aperture Orbitaeingang *m*, Aditus orbitalis.
orbital apex fracture Orbitaspitzenfraktur *f*.
orbital apex syndrome Orbitaspitzensyndrom *nt*, Malatesta-Syndrom *nt*, Apex--orbitae-Syndrom *nt*.
orbital area Augenregion *f*, Regio orbitalis.
orbital bone *old* → zygomatic bone.
orbital branch: o. of middle meningeal artery Orbitaast *m* der A. meningea media, Ramus orbitalis a. meningeae mediae.
o.es of pterygopalatine ganglion Orbitaäste *pl* des Ggl. pterygopalatinum, Rami orbitales ggl. pterygopalatini.
orbital cavity → orbit 1.
orbital cortex (*Gehirn*) orbitale Rinde *f*.
orbital crest Margo orbitalis (ossis frontalis).
or·bi·tale [ɔːrbəˈteɪlɪ, -ˈtɑː-] *n anat.* Orbitale *f*.
orbital edema *ophthal.* Orbitaödem *nt*.
orbital eminence of zygomatic bone Eminentia orbitalis (ossis zygomatici).
orbital fasciae Orbitafaszien *pl*, Fasciae orbitales.
orbital fissure: inferior o. Augenhöhlenbodenspalte *f*, untere Orbitaspalte *f*, Fissura orbitalis inferior.
 superior o. Augenhöhlendachspalte *f*, obere Orbitaspalte *f*, Fissura orbitalis superior.
orbital floor Augenhöhlen-, Orbitaboden *m*.
orbital gyri Gyri orbitales.
orbital hypertelorism → ocular hypertelorism.
orbital injury Orbitaverletzung *f*.
or·bi·ta·lis [ɔːrbɪˈteɪlɪs] *n* → orbitalis muscle.
orbitalis muscle Müller'-Muskel *m*, Orbitalis *m*, M. orbitalis.
orbital lamina (of ethmoid bone) *old* Lamina papyracea, Lamina orbitalis (ossis ethmoidalis).
orbital margin Orbitarand *m*, Margo orbitalis.
orbital muscle → orbitalis muscle.
orbital myositis Pseudotumor orbitae.
orbital opening Aditus orbitalis.
orbital optic neuritis Retrobulbärneuritis *f*, Neuritis optica retrobulbaris.
orbital part: o. of inferior frontal gyrus Pars orbitalis gyri frontalis inferioris.
 o. of lacrimal gland oberer Hauptteil *m* der Tränendrüse, Gl. lacrimalis superior, Pars orbitalis gl. lacrimalis.
 o. of optic nerve Orbita-Abschnitt *m* des N. opticus, Pars orbitalis n. optici.
orbital periostitis orbitale Periostitis *f*.
orbital phlegmon Orbita(l)phlegmone *f*.
orbital plane *ophthal.* Sehebene *f*.
orbital plate: o. of ethmoid bone Lamina orbitalis (ossis ethmoidalis).
 o. of frontal bone Pars orbitalis ossis frontalis.
orbital process of palatine bone Proc. orbitalis (ossis palatini).
orbital pseudotumor Pseudotumor orbitae.
orbital region Orbitaregion *f*, Regio orbitalis.
orbital roof Augenhöhlen-, Orbitadach *nt*.
orbital septum Orbitaseptum *nt*, Septum orbitale.
orbital steering *biochem.* Orbitalausrichtung *f*.
orbital sulci of frontal lobe Sulci orbitales (lobi frontalis).

orbital syndrome Orbitaspitzensyndrom *nt*, Malatesta-Syndrom *nt*, Apex-orbitae--Syndrom *nt*.
orbital trauma Orbitaverletzung *f*.
orbital veins Vv. orbitae.
orbital wall Augenhöhlen-, Orbitawand *f*.
orbital wall fracture Orbitawandfraktur *f*.
orbital wing of sphenoid bone kleiner Keilbeinflügel *m*, Ala minor (ossis sphenoidalis).
or·bi·to·fron·tal branch of anterior cerebral artery, medial [ˌɔːrbɪtəʊˈfrʌntl] A. frontobasalis medialis, Ramus orbitofrontalis medialis a. cerebri anterioris.
orbitofrontal cortex orbitofrontaler Kortex *m*.
orbitofrontal fasciculus orbitofrontales Bündel *nt*, Fasciculus orbitofrontalis.
or·bi·tog·ra·phy [ˌɔːrbɪˈtɑɡrəfɪ] *n* radiol. Orbitographie *f*.
or·bi·to·na·sal [ˌɔːrbɪtəʊˈneɪzl] *adj* Orbita u. Nase betr. *od.* verbindend, orbitonasal.
or·bi·to·sphe·noi·dal bone [ˌ-sfɪˈnɔɪdl] → orbital wing of sphenoid bone.
or·bi·tot·o·my [ˌɔːrbɪˈtɑtəmɪ] *n ophthal.* Orbitotomie *f*, -tomia *f*.
Or·bi·vi·rus [ˈɔːrbɪvaɪrəs] *n micro.* Orbivirus *nt*.
or·ce·in [ˈɔːrsɪɪn, -siːn] *n* Orzein *nt*, Orcein *nt*.
or·chec·to·my [ɔːrˈkektəmɪ] *n* → orchiectomy.
orchi- *pref.* → orchio.
or·chi·al·gia [ˌ-ˈældʒ(ɪ)ə] *n* Hodenschmerz(en *pl*) *m*, -neuralgie *f*, Orchialgie *f*.
or·chi·at·ro·phy [ˌ-ˈætrəfɪ] *n* Hodenatrophie *f*.
or·chic [ˈɔːrkɪk] *adj* → orchidic.
orchid- *pref.* → orchido-.
or·chi·dal·gia [ˌ-ˈdældʒ(ɪ)ə] *n* → orchialgia.
or·chi·dec·to·my [ˌ-ˈdektəmɪ] *n* → orchiectomy.
or·chid·ic [ɔːrˈkɪdɪk] *adj* Hoden/Testis betr., Hoden-, Orchid(o)-, Orchi(o)-.
or·chi·di·tis [ˌɔːrkɪˈdaɪtɪs] *n* → orchitis.
orchido- *pref.* Hoden-, Orchid(o)-, Orchi(o)-.
or·chi·do·ep·i·did·y·mec·to·my [ˌ-dəʊˌepɪdɪdəˈmektəmɪ] *n urol.* Orchidoepididymektomie *f*.
or·chi·don·cus [ˌ-ˈdɑŋkəs] *n* Hodenschwellung *f*, -tumor *m*.
or·chi·dop·a·thy [ˌ-ˈdɑpəθɪ] *n* → orchiopathy.
or·chi·do·pex·y [ˈɔːrkɪdəpeksɪ] *n* → orchiopexy.
or·chi·do·plas·ty [ˈɔːrkɪdəplæstɪ] *n* → orchioplasty.
or·chi·dop·to·sis [ˌɔːrkɪdɑpˈtəʊsɪs] *n urol.* Hodensenkung *f*, Orchidoptose *f*.
or·chi·dor·rha·phy [ˌɔːrkɪˈdɔrəfɪ] *n* → orchiopexy.
or·chi·dot·o·my [ˌ-ˈdɑtəmɪ] *n* → orchiotomy.
or·chi·ec·to·my [ˌ-ˈektəmɪ] *n* Hodenentfernung *f*, Orchiektomie *f*, Orchidektomie *f*.
or·chi·en·ceph·a·lo·ma [ˌ-ˌensəfəˈləʊmə] *n* embryonales Hodenkarzinom *nt*, Orchi(o)blastom *nt*.
or·chi·ep·i·did·y·mi·tis [ˌ-ˌepɪdɪdəˈmaɪtɪs] *n urol.* Entzündung *f* von Hoden u. Nebenhoden, Orchiepididymitis *f*.
orchio- *pref.* → orchido-.
or·chi·o·ca·tab·a·sis [ˌɔːrkɪəʊkəˈtæbəsɪs] *n* Hodendeszensus *m*, Descensus testis.
or·chi·o·cele [ˈ-siːl] *n* 1. Hodentumor *m*. 2. Leisten-, Inguinalhoden *m*. 3. Hodenbruch *m*, Skrotalhernie *f*, Hernia scrotalis.
or·chi·o·dyn·ia [ˌ-ˈdiːnɪə] *n* → orchialgia.

or·chi·o·my·e·lo·ma [ˌ-maɪəˈləʊmə] *n* Plasmozytom *nt* des Hodens.
or·chi·on·cus [ˌɔːrkɪˈɑŋkəs] *n* Hodentumor *m*, -schwellung *f*.
or·chi·o·neu·ral·gia [ˌɔːrkɪəʊnjʊəˈrældʒ(ɪ)ə, -nʊ-] *n* → orchialgia.
or·chi·op·a·thy [ˌɔːrkɪˈɑpəθɪ] *n* Hodenerkrankung *f*, Orchio-, Orchidopathie *f*.
or·chi·o·pex·y [ˈɔːrkɪəpeksɪ] *n urol.* Hodenfixation *f*, -fixierung *f*, Orchio-, Orchidopexie *f*.
or·chi·o·plas·ty [ˈ-plæstɪ] *n urol.* Hodenplastik *f*.
or·chi·or·rha·phy [ˌɔːrkɪˈɔrəfɪ] *n* → orchiopexy.
or·chi·o·scir·rhus [ˌɔːrkɪəʊˈs(k)ɪrəs] *n urol.* Hodenverhärtung *f*, -sklerosierung *f*.
or·chi·ot·o·my [ˌɔːrkɪˈɑtəmɪ] *n urol.* Orchiotomie *f*.
or·chis [ˈɔːrkɪs] *n* Hoden *m*, Orchis *m*, Testis *m*.
or·chit·ic [ɔːrˈkɪtɪk] *adj* Orchitis betr. *od.* auslösend, orchitisch.
or·chi·tis [ɔːrˈkaɪtɪs] *n* Hodenentzündung *f*, Orchitis *f*, Didymitis *f*.
or·chot·o·my [ɔːrˈkɑtəmɪ] *n* → orchiotomy.
or·cin [ˈɔːrsɪn] *n* orcinol.
or·cin·ol [ˈɔːrsɪnɒl, -nəʊl] *n* Orcinol *nt*.
orcinol test Bial-(Pentose-)Probe *f*.
or·deal bean [ɔːrˈdiːl, -ˈdɪəl, ˈɔːrdiːl] Calabarbohne *f*.
or·der [ˈɔːrdər] *n bio.* Ordnung *f*, Ordo *m*.
or·der·li·ness [ˈɔːrdərlɪnɪs] *n* 1. *phys.* Ordnungsgrad *m*. 2. Ordnung *f*, Regelmäßigkeit *f*. 3. Ordentlichkeit *f*.
or·der·ly [ˈɔːrdərlɪ] *n* Krankenpfleger *m*; Sanitäter *m*.
or·di·nal [ˈɔːrdnəl] I *n mathe.* Ordinal-, Ordnungszahl *f*. II *adj* 1. Ordinal-, Ordnungs-. 2. *bio.* Ordnungs-.
ordinal scale Ordinalskala *f*.
or·di·nar·y [ˈɔːrdəneriː] *adj* normal, gewöhnlich, üblich; durchschnittlich, Durchschnitts-; alltäglich.
ordinary hydrogen leichter Wasserstoff *m*, Protium *nt*.
ordinary phosphorus weißer/gelber/gewöhnlicher Phosphor *m*.
or·di·nate [ˈɔːrdnɪt, -neɪt] *n mathe.* Ordinate *f*.
or·dure [ˈɔːrdʒər, ˈɔːrdjʊər] *n* 1. Ausscheidung *f*, Exkrement *nt*, Excrementum *nt*. 2. Stuhl *m*, Kot *m*, Exkremente *pl*, Fäzes *pl*, Faeces *pl*.
O$_2$-response *n physiol.* O$_2$-Antwort *f*.
o·rex·ia [əʊˈreksɪə, ə-] *n* Appetit *m*.
o·rex·i·gen·ic [əʊˌreksɪˈdʒenɪk] *adj* appetitanregend.
orf [ɔːrf] *n* Orf *f*, Ecthyma contagiosum, atypische Schafpocken *pl*, Steinpocken *pl*, Stomatitis pustulosa contagiosa.
orf virus *micro.* Orfvirus *nt*.
organ- *pref.* → organo-.
or·gan [ˈɔːrɡn] *n* 1. *anat.* Organ *nt*, Organum *nt*, Organon *nt*. 2. *allg.* Sprachrohr *nt*; Werkzeug *nt*, Instrument *nt*. 3. Stimme *f*, Organ *nt*. 4. *sl.* Penis *m*.
o. of balance Gleichgewichtsorgan.
o. of equilibrium Gleichgewichtsorgan.
o. of hearing (Ge-)Hörorgan.
o. of hearing and balance (Ge-)Gleichgewichtsorgan, Organon auditus, Organum statoacusticus/vestibulocochleare.
o. of hearing and equilibrium → o. of hearing and balance.
o.s of Ruffini Ruffini'-Endorgane *pl*.
o. of sight → o. of vision.
o. of vision Sehorgan, Organum visus/visuale.
o. of Zuckerkandl Zuckerkandl'-Organ, Paraganglion aorticum abdominale.

organ atrophy Organatrophie *f*.
organ capsule Organkapsel *f*.
organ culture Organkultur *f*.
organ donation Organspende *f*.
organ donor Organspender *m*.
or·gan·el·la [ɔːrɡəˈnelə] *n, pl* **-lae** [-liː] → organelle.
or·gan·elle [ɔːrɡəˈnel] *n* (Zell-)Organelle *f*, Organell *nt*.
organelle membrane Organellenmembran *f*.
or·gan·ic [ɔːrˈɡænɪk] I *n* organische Substanz *f*; organischer Dünger *m*; organisches Pestizid *nt*. II *adj* 1. Organ(e) *od.* Organismus betr., organisch. 2. organisch, somatisch. 3. die belebte Natur betr.; lebendig, belebt. 4. *chem.* organisch. 5. biodynamisch, organisch.
organic acid *chem.* organische Säure *f*.
organic amnesia organisch-bedingte Amnesie *f*.
organic analysis *chem.* Elementaranalyse *f*.
organic brain syndrome (hirn-)organisches Psychosyndrom *nt*, psychoorganisches Syndrom *nt*.
organic chemistry organische Chemie *f*.
organic compound *chem.* organische Verbindung/Komponente *f*.
organic contracture organisch-bedingte Kontraktur *f*.
organic deafness organisch-bedingte Schwerhörigkeit/Taubheit *f*.
organic disease organische Erkrankung *f*, organisches Leiden *nt*.
organic epilepsy symptomatische/organische Epilepsie *f*.
organic growth organisches Wachstum *nt*.
organic hallucinosis organische Halluzinose *f*.
organic headache organisch-bedingter Kopfschmerz *m*.
or·gan·i·cism [ɔːrˈɡænəsɪzəm] *n patho., socio.* Organizismus *m*.
organic lesion strukturelle Schädigung *f*.
organic mental disorder organische Psychose *f*.
organic mental syndrome → organic brain syndrome.
organic murmur *card.* organisch-bedingtes Herzgeräusch *nt*.
organic muscle Eingeweide-, Visceralmuskel *m*.
organic paralysis organische/neurogene Lähmung *f*.
organic psychosis organische Psychose *f*.
organic stricture permanente Striktur *f*.
organic vertigo organisch-bedingter Schwindel *m*.
organ injury Organschädigung *f*, -verletzung *f*.
or·gan·ism [ˈɔːrɡənɪzəm] *n* Organismus *m*.
or·gan·is·mal [ˌ-ˈnɪzml] *adj* Organismus betr., zum Organismus gehörend, wie ein Organismus (beschaffen), organismisch.
or·gan·is·mic [ˌ-ˈnɪzmɪk] *adj* → organismal.
or·gan·i·za·tion [ˌɔːrɡənəˈzeɪʃn] *n* 1. Organisation *f*, Aufbau *m*, Gliederung *f*, (An-)Ordnung *f*, Struktur *f*. 2. Organisation *f*, Organisierung *f*, Bildung *f*, Gründung *f*. 3. Organisation *f*, Verband *m*, Zusammenschluß *m*. 4. Organismus *m*, System *nt*.
organization principle Organisationsprinzip *nt*.
or·gan·ize [ˈɔːrɡənaɪz] I *vt* 1. organisieren, vorbereiten, planen. 2. organisieren, gliedern, (an-)ordnen, einteilen, aufbauen. II *vi* s. organisieren.

or·gan·ized cirrhosis ['ɔːrgənaɪzd] mikronoduläre/kleinknotige/organisierte Leberzirrhose f.
organized thrombus organisierter Thrombus m.
or·gan·iz·er ['ɔːrgənaɪzər] n embryo. Organisator m.
or·gan·iz·ing pleurisy/pleuritis ['ɔːrgənaɪzɪŋ] Pleuritis f in Organisation.
organizing pneumonia fibrös-organisierte Pneumonie f.
organizing thrombus Thrombus m in Organisation.
organo- pref. Organ(o)-.
or·ga·no·chlo·rine [ˌɔːrgənəʊˈklɔːriːn, -ɪn, -ˈklɔʊr-, ɔːrˌgænəʊ-] n organische Chlorverbindung f.
or·gan·o·gel [ɔːrˈgænədʒəl] n chem. Organogel nt.
or·ga·no·gen·e·sis [ˌɔːrgənəʊˈdʒenəsɪs] n Organentwicklung f, Organogenese f.
or·ga·no·ge·net·ic [ˌ-dʒəˈnetɪk] adj Organogenese betr., organogenetisch.
or·ga·no·gen·ic [ˌ-ˈdʒenɪk] adj von einem Organ stammend od. ausgehend, organogen.
or·ga·nog·e·ny [ˌɔːrgəˈnɒdʒənɪ] n → organogenesis.
or·ga·nog·ra·phy [ˌ-ˈnɑgrəfɪ] n radiol. Organographie f.
or·gan·oid ['ɔːrgənɔɪd] I n → organelle. II adj 1. organähnlich, -artig, organoid. 2. patho. organoid.
organoid nevus organoider Nävus m.
organoid tumor embryo., patho. teratoide/teratogene Geschwulst f, Teratom(a) nt.
or·ga·no·lep·tic [ˌɔːrgənəʊˈleptɪk] adj 1. die Sinnesorgane stimulierend, organoleptisch. 2. empfänglich für Sinnesreize, organoleptisch.
or·ga·nol·o·gy [ˌɔːrgəˈnɒlədʒɪ] n Organologie f.
or·ga·no·meg·a·ly [ˌɔːrgənəʊˈmegəlɪ] n Eingeweidevergrößerung f, Splanchno-, Viszeromegalie f.
or·ga·no·me·tal·lic compound [ˌ-məˈtælɪk] metallorganische Verbindung f.
or·ga·non ['ɔːrgənɒn] n, pl **-na** [-nə] → organ 1.
or·ga·nop·a·thy [ˌɔːrgəˈnɒpəθɪ] n → organic disease.
or·ga·no·pex·ia ['ɔːrgənəʊpeksɪə] n → organopexy.
or·ga·no·pex·y ['-peksɪ] n chir. Organopexie f.
or·ga·no·phil·ic [ˌ-ˈfɪlɪk] adj → organotropic.
or·ga·noph·i·lism [ˌɔːrgəˈnɒfəlɪzəm] n → organotropism.
or·ga·no·phos·phate [ˌɔːrgənəʊˈfɒsfeɪt, ɔːrˌgænəʊ-] n Organophosphat nt.
or·ga·no·phos·pho·rus [ˌ-ˈfɒsfərəs] n organische Phosphorverbindung f.
or·gan·o·sol [ɔːrˈgænəsɒl, -sɔl] n chem. Organosol nt.
or·ga·no·tax·is [ˌɔːrgənəʊˈtæksɪs] n Organotaxis f.
or·ga·no·ther·a·py [ˌ-ˈθerəpɪ] n Organbehandlung f, Organotherapie f.
or·ga·no·troph·ic [ˌ-ˈtrɑfɪk, -ˈtrəʊ-] adj organotroph(isch).
or·ga·no·trop·ic [ˌ-ˈtrɑpɪk, -ˈtrəʊp-] adj organotrop.
or·ga·not·ro·pism [ɔːrgəˈnɒtrəpɪzəm] n Organotropie f.
or·ga·not·ro·py [ɔːrgəˈnɒtrəpɪ] n → organotropism.
organ perfusion Organdurchblutung f, -perfusion f.
organ preservation chir. Organkonservierung f.

organ recipient chir. Organempfänger m.
organ-specific antigen organspezifisches Antigen nt.
organ specifity biochem. Organspezifität f.
organ tolerance dose abbr. **OTD** radiol. Organtoleranzdosis f abbr. OTD.
organ transplantation Organtransplantation f, -verpflanzung f, -übertragung f.
organ tuberculosis Organtuberkulose f.
organ tumor Organtumor m.
or·ga·num ['ɔːrgənəm] n, pl **-nums**, **-na** [-nə] → organ 1.
or·gasm ['ɔːrgæzəm] n (sexueller) Höhepunkt m, Orgasmus m.
O·ri·en·tal [ɔːrɪˈentl, əʊr-] O. blood fluke micro. japanischer Pärchenegel m, Schistosoma japonicum.
O. boil/button → O. sore.
O. cholangiohepatitis rezidivierende pyogene Cholangitis f.
O. ringworm orientalische/indische/chinesische Flechte f, Tinea imbricata (Tokelau), Trichophytia corporis superficialis.
O. schistosomiasis japanische Schistosomiasis/Bilharziose f, Schistosomiasis japonica.
O. sore Hautleishmaniose f, kutane Leishmaniose f, Orientbeule f, Leishmaniasis cutis.
o·ri·en·ta·tion [ˌɔːrɪənˈteɪʃn] n 1. neuro., psycho. Orientierung f. 2. chem. Orientierung f.
o·ri·ent·ing reflex ['ɔːrɪəntɪŋ] Orientierungsreaktion f.
orienting response → orienting reflex.
ORIF abbr. → open reduction and internal fixation.
or·i·fice ['ɒrɪfɪs, 'ɑr-] n Mund m, Mündung f, Öffnung f; anat. Orificium nt, Ostium nt.
o. of coronary sinus Ostium sinus coronarii.
o. of mouth Mundspalte f, Rima oris.
o. of ureter Harnleiter(ein)mündung, Ostium ureteris.
or·i·fi·cial [ɒrəˈfɪʃl, ɑr-] adj anat. Orificium betr.
orificial tuberculosis Tuberculosis cutis orificialis, Tuberculosis miliaris ulcerosa cutis.
or·i·fi·ci·um [ɒrəˈfɪʃɪəm, ɑr-] n, pl **-cia** [-ʃɪə] anat. Mündung f, Öffnung f, Orificium nt.
or·i·gin ['ɒrədʒɪn, 'ɑr-] n Ursprung m; anat. Origo f; Herkunft f, Abstammung f; Entstehung f.
o·rig·i·nal [əˈrɪdʒənl] I n Original nt; Vorlage f. II adj 1. original, ursprünglich, erste(r, s), Original-, Ur-. 2. originell.
o·rig·i·nate [əˈrɪdʒəneɪt] I vt verursachen, hervorbringen, ins Lebens rufen. II vi entstehen (from aus; in in); ausgehen, herrühren, stammen (from von).
o·rig·i·na·tion [əˌrɪdʒəˈneɪʃn] n Entstehung f, Hervorbringung f, Erzeugung f.
Ormond ['ɔːrmənd]: **O.'s disease/syndrome** (idiopathische) retroperitoneale Fibrose f, Ormond-Syndrom nt.
Orn abbr. → ornithine.
or·nid·a·zole [ɔːrˈnɪdəzəʊl] n pharm. Ornidazol nt.
or·ni·thine ['ɔːrnəθiːn, -θɪn] n abbr. **Orn** Ornithin nt.
ornithine aminotransferase Ornithinaminotransferase f, -transaminase f, Ornithinketosäureaminotransferase f.
ornithine carbamoyl phosphate deficiency Hyperammoniämie-Typ II f, Ornithintranskarbamylasedefekt m.
ornithine carbamoyltransferase abbr.

OCT Ornithincarbamyltransferase f abbr. OCT, Ornithintranscarbamylase f abbr. OTC.
ornithine cycle Harnstoff-, Ornithinzyklus m, Krebs-Henseleit-Zyklus m.
ornithine decarboxylase Ornithindecarboxylase f.
ornithine-keto-acid aminotransferase → ornithine aminotransferase.
or·ni·thi·ne·mia [ˌɔːrnəθɪˈniːmɪə] n Ornithinämie f.
ornithine-oxo-acid aminotransferase → ornithine aminotransferase.
ornithine transaminase → ornithine aminotransferase.
ornithine transcarbamoylase abbr. **OTC** → ornithine carbamoyltransferase.
ornithine-transcarbamoylase deficiency → ornithine carbamoyl phosphate deficiency.
or·ni·thi·nu·ria [ɔːrnəθɪˈn(j)ʊərɪə] n vermehrte Ornithinausscheidung f im Harn, Ornithinurie f.
Or·ni·thod·o·ros [ɔːrnɪˈθɑdərəs] n micro. Ornithodorus m.
or·ni·tho·sis [ɔːrnɪˈθəʊsɪs] n Ornithose f, Papageienkrankheit f, Psittakose f.
ornithosis virus old Chlamydia psittaci/ ornithosis.
oro- pref. Mund-, Oro-.
o·ro·dig·i·to·fa·cial [ˌɔːrəʊˌdɪdʒɪtəʊˈfeɪʃl, ˌəʊrəʊ-] adj orodigitofazial.
orodigitofacial dysostosis → orodigitofacial syndrome.
orodigitofacial syndrome orodigitofaziale Dysostose f, orofaziodigitales Syndrom nt, OFD-Syndrom nt, Papillon-Léage-Psaume-Syndrom nt.
o·ro·fa·cial [ˌ-ˈfeɪʃl] adj Mund u. Gesicht betr., orofazial.
o·ro·fa·cio·dig·i·tal [ˌ-ˌfeɪʃɪəʊˈdɪdʒɪtl] adj orofaziodigital.
orofaciodigital syndrome orofaziodigitales Syndrom nt, lingofaziale Dysplasie f, Dysplasia linguofacialis.
type II o. Mohr-Claussen-Syndrom nt.
o·ro·gas·tric tube],-ˈgæstrɪk] Mund-Magensonde f.
o·ro·lin·gual [ˌ-ˈlɪŋgwəl] adj Mund u. Zunge betr., orolingual.
or·o·men·in·gi·tis [ˌ-ˌmenɪnˈdʒaɪtɪs] n Serosaentzündung f, Serositis f.
o·ro·na·sal [ˌ-ˈneɪzl] adj Mund u. Nase betr., oronasal.
oronasal fistula oronasale Fistel f.
o·ro·pha·ryn·ge·al [ˌ-fəˈrɪndʒ(ɪ)əl] adj Oropharynx betr., oro-, mesopharyngeal, Oropharyngeal-, Mesopharyngeal-, Mundrachen-.
oropharyngeal airway Oropharyngealkatheter m, -tubus m.
oropharyngeal dysphagia oropharyngeale Dysphagie f.
oropharyngeal intubation oropharyngeale Intubation f.
oropharyngeal isthmus Schlund-, Rachenenge f, Isthmus faucium.
oropharyngeal membrane embryo. Oronasal-, Bukkonasalmembran f, Membrana bucconasalis.
oropharyngeal mucosa Mund- u. Rachenschleimhaut f.
oropharyngeal tube → oropharyngeal airway.
oropharyngeal tularemia oropharyngeale/oralglanduläre/glandulopharyngeale Tularämie f.
o·ro·phar·ynx [ˌ-ˈfærɪŋks] n Meso-, Oropharynx m, Pars oralis pharyngis.
Or·o·pouche virus ['ɔːrəʊpuːʃ] Oropouche-Virus nt.
or·o·so·mu·coid [ˌɔːrəsəʊˈmjuːkɔɪd] n

(Plasma-)Orosomukoid *nt*, saures α₁--Glykoprotein *nt*.
or·o·tate ['ɔːrəteɪt] *n* Orotat *nt*.
orotate dehydrogenase Orotsäuredehydrogenase *f*.
orotate phosphoribosyltransferase *abbr.* **OPRT** Orotsäurephosphoribosyltransferase *f abbr.* OPRT.
o·rot·ic acid [ɔː'rɑtɪk] Orotsäure *f*, 6-Carboxyuracil *nt*.
orotic aciduria Orotazidurie(-Syndrom *nt*) *f*.
o·rot·i·dine-5'-phosphate [ɔː'rɑtɪdiːn] *n* Orotidin-5'-Phosphat *nt*, Orotidinmonophosphat *nt abbr.* OMP, Orotidylsäure *f*.
orotidine-5'-phosphate decarboxylase → orotidylic acid decarboxylase.
orotidine-5'-phosphate pyrophosphorylase → orotate phosphoribosyltransferase.
o·rot·i·dy·late decarboxylase [ɔː'rɑtɪ'dɪleɪt] → orotidylic acid decarboxylase.
o·rot·i·dyl·ic acid [ɔː'rɑtɪ'dɪlɪk] → orotidine -5'-phosphate.
orotidylic acid decarboxylase *abbr.* **ODC** Orotidylsäuredecarboxylase *f abbr.* ODC.
o·ro·tra·che·al intubation [ˌɔːrəʊ'treɪkɪəl, ˌəʊrəʊ-] orotracheale Intubation *f*.
O·roy·a fever [ɔː'rɔɪə] Oroyafieber *nt*.
or·phen·a·drine [ɔːr'fenədriːn] *n pharm.* Orphenadrin *n*.
or·rho·men·in·gi·tis [ˌɔːrəʊˌmenɪn'dʒaɪtɪs, ˌəʊrəʊ-] *n* Serosaentzündung *f*, Serositis *f*.
Orsi-Grocco ['ɔːrsɪ 'grɑkəʊ]: **O.-G. method** palpatorische Herzperkussion *f*.
O-R system *chem.* Redoxsystem *nt*.
orth- *pref.* → ortho- 1.
or·the·sis [ɔːr'θiːsɪs] *n*, *pl* **-ses** [-siːz] *ortho.* Orthese *f*.
ortho- *pref.* **1.** Orth(o)-. **2.** *chem. abbr.* o- ortho- *abbr.* o-.
or·tho·ac·id [ˌɔːrθəʊ'æsɪd] *n chem.* Orthosäure *f*.
or·tho·ar·te·ri·ot·o·ny [ˌ-ˌɑːrtərɪ'ɑtənɪ] *n* normaler Blutdruck *m*, Normotonus *m*, Normotonie *f*.
or·tho·ce·phal·ic [ˌ-sɪ'fælɪk] *adj* orthokephal, -zephal.
or·tho·ceph·a·lous [ˌ-'sefələs] *adj* → orthocephalic.
or·tho·cho·rea [ˌ-kə'rɪə] *n neuro.* Orthochorea *f*.
or·tho·chro·mat·ic [ˌ-krəʊ'mætɪk, -krə-] *adj* orthochromatisch.
orthochromatic dye orthochromatischer Farbstoff *m*.
orthochromatic erythroblast azidophiler/ orthochromatischer/oxaphiler Normoblast *m*.
orthochromatic leukodystrophy orthochromatische Leukodystrophie *f*.
orthochromatic normoblast → orthochromatic erythroblast.
or·tho·chro·mia [ˌ-'krəʊmɪə] *n hema.* Orthochromie *f*.
or·tho·chro·mo·phil [ˌ-'krəʊməfɪl] *adj* → orthochromatic.
or·tho·chro·mo·phile [ˌ-'krəʊməfaɪl, -fɪl] *adj* → orthochromatic.
or·tho·cre·sol [ˌ-'kriːsɔl, -sɑl] *n* o-Kresol *nt*, ortho-Kresol *nt*.
or·tho·cy·to·sis [ˌ-saɪ'təʊsɪs] *n* Orthozytose *f*.
or·tho·don·tia [ˌ-'dɑnʃ(ɪ)ə] *n* → orthodontics.
or·tho·don·tics [ˌ-'dɑntɪks] *pl* Kieferorthopädie *f*.
or·tho·don·tist [ˌ-'dɑntɪst] *n* Kieferorthopäde *m*, -orthopädin *f*.
or·tho·don·tol·o·gy [ˌ-dɑn'tɑlədʒɪ] *n* → orthodontics.

or·tho·dox ['-dɑks] *adj* orthodox.
orthodox sleep non-REM-Schlaf *m*, NREM-Schlaf *m*, orthodoxer/synchronisierter Schlaf *m*.
or·tho·drom·ic [ˌ-'drɑmɪk] *adj* in normaler Richtung, orthodrom.
or·tho·gen·e·sis [ˌ-'dʒenəsɪs] *n* Orthogenese *f*.
or·tho·gen·ics [ˌ-'dʒenɪks] *pl* Erbhygiene *f*, Eugenik *f*, Eugenetik *f*.
or·tho·gly·ce·mic [ˌ-glaɪ'siːmɪk] *adj* mit normalem Blutzuckerspiegel, normoglykämisch.
orthoglycemic glycosuria renale Glukosurie/Glycosurie *f*.
or·tho·grade ['-greɪd] *adj* orthograd.
orthograde degeneration *neuro.* Waller'- -Degeneration *f*, orthograde/sekundäre Degeneration *f*.
or·tho·ker·a·tol·o·gy [ˌ-ˌkerə'tɑlədʒɪ] *n ophthal.* Orthokeratologie *f*.
or·tho·ker·a·tot·ic [ˌ-kerə'tɑtɪk] *adj* orthokeratotisch.
or·thom·e·ter [ɔːr'θɑmɪtər] *n* Exophthalmometer *nt*.
Or·tho·myx·o·vir·i·dae [ˌɔːrθəʊˌmɪksəʊ'vɪrɪdiː, -vaɪr-] *pl micro.* Orthomyxoviren *pl*, Orthomyxoviridae *pl*.
or·tho·myx·o·vi·rus [ˌ-ˌmɪksə'vaɪrəs] *n micro.* Orthomyxovirus *nt*.
or·tho·pae·dic *adj* → orthopedic.
or·tho·pae·dics *pl* → orthopedics.
or·tho·pae·dist *n* → orthopedist.
or·tho·pan·to·graph [ˌ-'pæntəgræf] *n radiol.* Orthopantomograph *m*.
or·tho·pan·tog·ra·phy [ˌ-pæn'tɑgrəfɪ] *n radiol.* Orthopantomographie *f*.
or·tho·pe·dic [ˌ-'piːdɪk] *adj* orthopädisch.
or·tho·pe·dics [ˌ-'piːdɪks] *pl* Orthopädie *f*.
orthopedic shoe orthopädischer Schuh *m*.
orthopedic surgeon Orthopäde *m*, -pädin *f*; Unfallchirurg *m*.
orthopedic surgery Orthopädie *f*.
or·tho·pe·dist [ˌ-'piːdɪst] *n* Orthopäde *m*, -pädin *f*.
or·tho·phe·nan·thro·line [ˌ-fɪ'nænθrəliːn] *n* o-Phenanthrolin *nt*.
or·tho·pho·ria [ˌ-'fɔːrɪə] *n ophthal.* Orthophorie *f*.
or·tho·phor·ic [ˌ-'fɑrɪk] *adj ophthal.* Orthophorie betr., orthophor.
or·tho·phos·phate [ˌ-'fɑsfeɪt] *n* (Ortho-)-Phosphat *nt*.
orthophosphate cleavage Orthophosphatspaltung *f*.
or·tho·phos·phor·ic acid [ˌ-fɑs'fɔrɪk, -fɑr-] (Ortho-)Phosphorsäure *f*.
or·thop·ne·a [ɔːr'θɑpnɪə, ˌɔːrˌθɑp'nɪə] *n* Orthopnoe *f*.
or·thop·ne·ic [ˌɔːrθɑp'niːɪk] *adj* Orthopnoe betr., orthopnoisch.
Or·thop·ter·a [ɔːr'θɑptərə] *pl bio.* Orthoptera *pl*, Orthopteren *pl*.
or·thop·tic [ɔːr'θɑptɪk] *adj ophthal.* Orthoptik betr., orthoptisch.
or·thop·tics [ɔːr'θɑptɪks] *pl ophthal.* Orthoptik *f*.
or·thop·to·scope [ɔːr'θɑptəskəʊp] *n* Orthoskop *nt*.
or·tho·scope ['ɔːrθəskəʊp] *n* Orthoskop *nt*.
or·tho·scop·ic [ˌ-'skɑpɪk] *adj* **1.** Orthoskopie betr., orthoskopisch. **2.** normalsichtig.
or·thos·co·py [ɔːr'θɑskəpɪ] *n* Orthoskopie *f*.

or·tho·sis [ɔːr'θəʊsɪs] *n*, *pl* **-ses** [-siːz] Orthese *f*.
or·tho·stat·ic [ˌɔːrθə'stætɪk] *adj* Orthostase betr., orthostatisch.
orthostatic albuminuria orthostatische/ lordotische Albuminurie/Proteinurie *f*.
orthostatic dyspnea orthostatische Dyspnoe *f*.
orthostatic hypotension orthostatische Hypotonie *f*.
chronic o. Shy-Drager-Syndrom *nt*.
hyperdiastolic o. hyperdiastolische orthostatische Hypotonie.
hypodiastolic o. hypodiastolische orthostatische Hypotonie.
idiopathic o. Shy-Drager-Syndrom *nt*.
orthostatic proteinuria → orthostatic albuminuria.
or·tho·stat·ism ['-stætɪzəm] *n* aufrechte Körperhaltung *f*, Orthostase *f*.
or·tho·sym·pa·thet·ic [ˌ-ˌsɪmpə'θetɪk] *adj* Sympathikus betr., sympathisch, orthosympathisch, Symphato-, Sympathiko-.
or·tho·top·ic [ˌ-'tɑpɪk] *adj* am normalen Ort, an normaler Stelle, orthotop.
orthotopic transplantation orthotope Transplantation *f*.
or·tho·volt·age therapy [ˌ-'vəʊltɪdʒ] *radiol.* Orthovolttherapie *f*.
or·thu·ria [ɔːr'θʊərɪə] *n* Orthurie *f*.
Ortner ['ɔːrtnər]: **O.'s disease** Ortner-Syndrom II *nt*, Morbus Ortner *m*, Angina abdominalis/intestinalis, Claudicatio intermittens abdominalis.
Ortolani [ɔːrtəʊ'lɑːniː]: **O.'s click/sign** *ortho.* Ortolani-Zeichen *nt*, -Click *m*.
o·ry·ze·nin [əʊ'raɪzənɪn] *n* Oryzenin *nt*, Orycenin *nt*.
o·ry·zoid [əʊ'raɪzɔɪd] *adj* reiskornähnlich, oryzoid.
oryzoid bodies Reiskörper(chen *pl*) *pl*, Corpora oryzoidea.
Os *abbr.* → osmium.
os¹ [ɑs] *n*, *pl* **o·ra** ['ɔːrə, 'əʊrə] *anat.* (Körper-)Öffnung *f*, Mündung *f*; Mund *m*, Os *nt*.
os² [ɑs] *n*, *pl* **os·sa** ['ɑsə] *anat.* Knochen *m*, (Ge-)Bein *nt*, Os *nt*.
osa·mine ['əʊsəmiːn] *n* Osamin *nt*.
osa·zone ['əʊsəzəʊn, 'ɑsə-] *n* Osazon *nt*.
os calcis Fersenbein *nt*, Kalkaneus *m*, Calcaneus *m*.
OSCF *abbr.* → oligomycin-sensitivity-conferring factor.
osche- *pref.* → oscheo-.
os·che·al ['ɑskɪəl] *adj* Skrotum betr., skrotal, Skrotum-, Skrotal-.
os·che·i·tis [ɑskɪ'aɪtɪs] *n* Skrotumentzündung *f*, Skrotitis *f*.
os·chei·e·phan·ti·a·sis [ˌɑskəlɪfən'taɪəsɪs] *n* Elephantiasis scroti, Skrotalelephantiasis *f*.
oscheo- *pref.* Skrotum-, Skrotal-.
os·che·o·cele [ɑskɪəsiːl] *n* **1.** Hodenbruch *m*, Skrotalhernie *f*, Hernia scrotalis. **2.** *old* → oscheoncus.
os·che·o·hy·dro·cele [ˌ-'haɪdrəsiːl] *n* Hydrozele *f*, Hydrocele *f*.
os·che·o·ma [ɑskɪ'əʊmə] *n old* → oscheoncus.
os·che·on·cus [ɑskɪ'ɑŋkəs] *n* Skrotaltumor *m*, -schwellung *f*.
os·che·o·plas·ty ['ɑskɪəplæstɪ] *n urol.* Skrotumplastik *f*.
os·chi·tis [ɑs'kaɪtɪs] *n* → oscheitis.
os·cil·la·te ['ɑsəleɪt] *phys.* **I** *vt* in Schwingungen versetzen. **II** *vi* schwingen, schwanken, pendeln, oszillieren.
os·cil·lat·ing ['ɑsəleɪtɪŋ] *adj* schwingend, schwankend, pendelnd, oszillierend, Schwing-.
oscillating circuit *electr.* Schwingkreis *m*.

oscillating current

oscillating current *electr.* oszillierender Strom *m*, Schwingstrom *m*.
oscillating nystagmus Pendelnystagmus *m*.
oscillating saw *ortho.* oszillierende Säge *f*.
oscillating vision Brückner-Phänomen *nt*, Oszillopsie *f*.
os·cil·la·tion [ˌɑsəˈleɪʃn] *n phys.* Schwingung *f*, Schwankung *f*, Oszillation *f*.
oscillation energy Schwingungsenergie *f*.
os·cil·la·tor [ˈɑsəleɪtər] *n electr.* Oszillator *m*.
os·cil·la·to·ry [ˈɑsələtɔːrɪ, -təʊ-] *adj* → oscillating.
oscillatory saw *ortho.* oszillierende Säge *f*.
oscillo- *pref.* Oszillo-, Oszillations-.
os·cil·lo·gram [əˈsɪləgræm] *n phys.* Oszillogramm *nt*.
os·cil·lo·graph [əˈsɪləgræf] *n* Oszillograph *m*.
os·cil·lom·e·ter [ˌɑsɪˈlɑmɪtər] *n* Oszillometer *nt*.
os·cil·lo·met·ric [ˌɑsɪləʊˈmetrɪk] *adj* Oszillometer *od.* Oszillometrie betr., oszillometrisch.
os·cil·lom·e·try [ˌɑsɪˈlɑmətrɪ] *n* Oszillometrie *f*.
os·cil·lop·sia [ˌɑsɪˈlɑpsɪə] *n* Brückner-Phänomen *nt*, Oszillopsie *f*.
os·cil·lo·scope [əˈsɪləskəʊp] *n* Oszilloskop *nt*.
os·ci·tate [ˈɑsəteɪt] **I** *n* Gähnen *nt*. **II** *vi* gähnen.
os·ci·ta·tion [ˌɑsəˈteɪʃn] *n* Gähnen *nt*.
Osgood-Schlatter [ˈɑzgʊd ˈʃlætər]: **O.-S. disease** Osgood-Schlatter-Krankheit *f*, -Syndrom *nt*, Schlatter-Osgood-Krankheit *f*, -Syndrom *nt*, Apophysitis tibialis adolescentium.
Osler [ˈɑzlər]: **O.'s disease 1.** → Osler-Vaquez disease. **2.** → Osler-Weber-Rendu disease.
O.'s nodes/sign Osler-Knötchen *pl*.
Osler-Vaquez [vaˈke]: **O.-V. disease** Morbus Vaquez-Osler *m*, Vaquez-Osler-Syndrom *nt*, Osler-Krankheit *f*, Osler-Vaquez-Krankheit *f*, Polycythaemia (rubra) vera, Erythrämie *f*.
Osler-Weber-Rendu [ˈwebər rãˈdy]: **O.-W.-R. disease** hereditäre Teleangiektasie *f*, Morbus Osler *m*, Osler-Rendu-Weber-Krankheit *f*, Osler-Rendu, Rendu-Osler-Weber-Krankheit *f*, -Syndrom *nt*, Teleangiectasia hereditaria haemorrhagica.
Osm *abbr.* → osmole.
osm- *pref.* → osmo-.
os·mate [ˈɑzmeɪt] *n* Osmat *nt*.
os·mat·ic [ɑzˈmætɪk] *adj* olfaktorisch, Riech-, Geruchs-.
os·me·sis [ɑzˈmiːsɪs] *n* Riechen *nt*.
os·mic [ˈɑzmɪk] *adj chem.* osmiumhaltig, Osmium-.
osmic acid 1. Osmiumsäure *f*. **2.** Osmiumtetroxid *nt*.
os·mi·cate [ˈɑzmɪkeɪt] *vt histol.* mit Osmium(tetroxid) behandeln.
os·mi·dro·sis [ɑzmɪˈdrəʊsɪs] *n* Brom(h)idrosis *f*.
os·mi·fi·ca·tion [ˌɑzmɪfɪˈkeɪʃn] *n histol.* Behandlung *f* mit Osmium(verbindungen).
os·mi·o·phil·ic [ˌɑzmɪəˈfɪlɪk] *adj* osmiophil.
os·mi·o·phob·ic [ˌ-ˈfəʊbɪk] *adj* osmiophob.
os·mi·um [ˈɑzmɪəm] *n abbr.* **Os** Osmium *nt abbr.* Os.
osmium tetroxide Osmiumtetroxid *nt*.
osmo- *pref.* **1.** Geruch(s)-, Osm(o)-. **2.** *physiol.* Osm(o)-.
os·mo·cep·tor [ˌɑzməˈseptər] *n* → osmoreceptor.
os·mo·gram [ˈ-græm] *n* Elektroolfaktogramm *nt abbr.* EOG.

os·mol [ɑzməʊl, -mɑl] *n* → osmole.
os·mo·lal clearance [ˈɑzmələl] osmolale Clearance *f*.
os·mo·lal·i·ty [ˌɑzməʊˈlælɪtɪ] *n* Osmolalität *f*.
os·mo·lar [ɑzˈməʊlər] *adj* osmolar.
os·mo·lar·i·ty [ˌɑzməʊˈlærɪtɪ] *n* Osmolarität *f*.
os·mole [ˈɑzməʊl] *n abbr.* **Osm** Osmol *nt abbr.* osm.
os·mol·o·gy [ɑzˈmɑlədʒɪ] *n* **1.** → osphresiology. **2.** *physiol.* Osmologie *f*.
os·mom·e·ter [ɑzˈmɑmɪtər] *n* Osmometer *nt*.
os·mom·e·try [ɑzˈmɑmətrɪ] *n* Osmometrie *f*.
os·mo·phil·ic [ˌɑzməʊˈfɪlɪk] *adj* osmophil.
os·mo·pho·bia [ˌ-ˈfəʊbɪə] *n psychia.* Osmophobie *f*, Olfaktophobie *f*.
os·mo·re·cep·tor [ˌ-rɪˈseptər] *n* **1.** Osmorezeptor *m*. **2.** Geruchs-, Osmorezeptor *m*.
os·mo·re·cep·tive sensor [ˌ-rɪˈseptɪv] → osmoreceptor.
os·mo·reg·u·la·tion [ˌ-regjəˈleɪʃn] *n* Osmoregulation *f*.
os·mo·reg·u·la·to·ry [ˌ-ˈregjələtɔːrɪ, -təʊ-] *adj* osmoregulatorisch.
os·mo·sis [ɑzˈməʊsɪs] *n* Osmose *f*.
os·mo·tax·is [ˌɑzməʊˈtæksɪs] *n* Osmotaxis *f*.
os·mo·ther·a·py [ˌ-ˈθerəpɪ] *n* Osmotherapie *f*.
os·mot·ic [ɑzˈmɑtɪk] *adj* Osmose betr., osmotisch, Osm(o)-.
osmotic diarrhea osmotische Diarrhö *f*.
osmotic diuresis osmotische Diurese *f*, Molekulardiurese *f*.
osmotic diuretic *pharm.* osmotisches Diuretikum *nt*.
osmotic fragility osmotische Erythrozytenresistenz *f*.
osmotic gradient osmotischer Gradient *m*, osmotisches Gefälle *nt*.
osmotic hemolysis (kolloid-)osmotische Hämolyse *f*.
osmotic nephrosis hypokaliämische Nephropathie *f*.
osmotic pressure osmotischer Druck *m*.
  colloid o. kolloidosmotischer/onkotischer Druck *abbr.* KOD.
  crystalloid o. kristalloidosmotischer Druck.
  effective o. effektiver osmotischer Druck.
  total o. totaler osmotischer Druck.
osmotic shock osmotischer Schock *m*.
osmotic thirst osmotischer Durst *m*.
osmotic work osmotische Arbeit *f*.
O-specific chain O-spezifische Kette *f*.
osphresi(o)- *pref.* Geruchs-, Osphresi(o)-, Osm(o)-, Olfakt(o)-.
os·phre·si·o·lag·nia [ɑzˌfriːzɪəʊˈlægnɪə] *n psychia., psycho.* Osphresiolagnie *f*.
os·phre·si·ol·o·gy [ɑzˌfriːzɪˈɑlədʒɪ] *n* Osphresiologie *f*, Osmologie *f*.
os·phre·si·o·phil·ia [ɑzˌfriːzɪəʊˈfɪlɪə] *n psychia.* Osphresiophilie *f*.
os·phre·si·o·pho·bia [ˌ-ˈfəʊbɪə] *n* → osmophobia.
os·phre·sis [ɑzˈfriːsɪs] *n* → olfaction 2.
os·phret·ic [ɑzˈfretɪk] *adj* → olfactory.
os·phy·ar·thro·sis [ˌɑsfɪɑːrˈθrəʊsɪs] *n* Hüftgelenk(s)entzündung *f*, Koxitis *f*, Koxarthritis *f*, Coxitis *f*.
os pubis Schambein *nt*, Pubis *f*, Os pubis.
os sacrum Kreuzbein *nt*, Sacrum *nt*, Os sacrum/sacrale.
os·se·in [ˈɑsɪən] *n* Kollagen *nt*.
os·se·ine *n* → ossein.
os·se·o·al·bu·moid [ˌɑsɪəʊˈælbjəmɔɪd] *n* Osseoalbumoid *nt*.
os·se·o·car·ti·lag·i·nous [ˌ-ˌkɑːrtɪˈlædʒɪnəs] *adj* → osteocartilaginous.

os·se·o·fi·brous [ˌ-ˈfaɪbrəs] *adj* osteofibrös.
os·se·o·mu·cin [ˌ-ˈmjuːsɪn] *n* Osseomuzin *nt*, -mucin *nt*.
os·se·o·mu·coid [ˌ-ˈmjuːkɔɪd] *n* Osseomukoid *nt*.
os·se·o·tym·pan·ic conduction [ˌ-tɪmˈpænɪk] → osteoacusis.
os·se·ous [ˈɑsɪəs] *adj* Knochen betr., aus Knochen, knöchern, ossär, ossal, Knochen-.
osseous ampulla (*Ohr*) knöcherne Ampulle *f* der Bogengänge, Ampulla ossea.
  anterior o. Ampulle des vorderen Bogenganges, Ampulla ossea anterior.
  lateral o. Ampulle des seitlichen Bogenganges, Ampulla ossea lateralis.
  posterior o. Ampulle des hinteren Bogenganges, Ampulla ossea posterior.
osseous ankylosis *ortho.* knöcherne Gelenkversteifung/Ankylose *f*, Ankylosis ossea.
osseous cell → osteocyte.
osseous crus: o.ra *pl* knöcherne Bogengangsschenkel *pl*, Crura ossea.
  ampullary o.ra Crura ossea ampullaria.
  common o. hinterer knöcherner Bogengangsschenkel *m*, Crus osseum commune.
  simple o. knöcherner Bogengangsschenkel *m* des seitlichen Bogenganges, Crus osseum simplex.
osseous excrescence *patho.* Knochenvorsprung *m*.
osseous graft Knochentransplantat *nt*.
osseous labyrinth knöchernes/ossäres Labyrinth *nt*, Labyrinthus osseus.
osseous lacuna Knochenzellhöhle *f*, -lakune *f*.
osseous lamella Kochenlamelle *f*.
osseous metastasis Knochenmetastase *f*, ossäre Metastase *f*.
osseous outgrowth *patho.* Knochenvorsprung *m*.
osseous palate knöcherner Gaumen *m*, Palatum osseum.
osseous part: o. of auditory tube knöcherner Tubenabschnitt *m*, Pars ossea tubae auditivae.
  o. of nasal septum → osseous septum (of nose).
osseous rheumatism rheumatoide Arthritis *f*, progrediente/primär chronische Polyarthritis *f abbr.* PCP, PcP.
osseous septum (of nose) knöcherner Abschnitt/Teil *m* des Nasenseptums, Pars ossea septi nasi.
osseous syndactyly *embryo.* ossäre Syndaktylie *f*.
osseous tissue knochenbildendes Gewebe *nt*.
osseous torticollis ossärer Schiefhals/Torticollis *m*.
osseous tuberculosis Knochentuberkulose *f*, Knochen-Tb *f*.
osseous wryneck → osseous torticollis.
os·si·cle [ˈɑsɪkl] *n* kleiner Knochen *m*, Knöchelchen *nt*, Ossiculum *nt*.
os·sic·u·lar [əˈsɪkjələr] *adj* Knöchelchen/Ossiculum *od.* Gehörknöchelchen/Ossicula auditus betr., ossikulär, Gehörknöchelchen-.
ossicular chain Gehörknöchelchenkette *f*.
os·sic·u·late [əˈsɪkjəlɪt] *adj* → ossicular.
os·si·cu·lec·to·my [ˌɑsɪkjəˈlektəmɪ] *n HNO* Ossikulektomie *f*.
os·si·cu·lot·o·my [ˌɑsɪkjəˈlɑtəmɪ] *n HNO* Ossikulotomie *f*.
os·sic·u·lum [əˈsɪkjələm] *n, pl* **-la** [-lə] → ossicle.
os·si·des·mo·sis [ˌɑsɪdesˈməʊsɪs] *n* → osteodesmosis.

os·sif·er·ous [ɒ'sɪfərəs] *adj* Knochen enthaltend; knochenbildend.
os·sif·ic [ɒ'sɪfɪk] *adj* knochenbildend; s. in Knochen umwandelnd.
os·si·fi·ca·tion [ˌɒsəfɪ'keɪʃn] *n* **1.** Knochenbildung *f*, -entwicklung *f*, Ossifikation *f*, Osteogenese *f*. **2.** *patho.* (krankhafte) Verknöcherung *f*; Verknöchern *nt*, Ossifikation *f*.
ossification center Verknöcherungs-, Knochenkern *m*, Centrum ossificationis.
primary o. diaphysärer/primärer Knochenkern, Centrum ossificationis primarum.
secondary o. epiphysärer/sekundärer Knochenkern, Centrum ossificationis secundarium.
ossification nucleus → ossification center.
ossification point → ossification center.
os·sif·lu·ence [ɒ'sɪfləwəns] *n old* → osteolysis.
os·si·form ['ɒsɪfɔːrm] *adj* knochenähnlich, -artig, osteoid.
os·si·fy ['ɒsɪfaɪ] *vt, vi* verknöchern, ossifizieren.
os·si·fy·ing ['ɒsəfaɪɪŋ] *adj* verknöchernd, ossifizierend.
ossifying cartilage Vorläuferknorpel *m*, verknöchernder Knorpel *m*.
ossifying fibroma (of bone) ossifizierendes Fibrom *nt*, osteofibröse Dysplasie *f*.
ossifying periosteal hemangioma ossifizierendes periostales Hämangiom *nt*, subperiostaler Riesenzelltumor *m*.
ossifying periostitis Periostitis ossificans.
ost- *pref.* → osteo-.
os·tal·gia [ɒs'tældʒ(ɪ)ə] *n* → ostealgia.
os·tar·thri·tis [ˌɒstɑːr'θraɪtɪs] *n* → osteoarthritis.
oste- *pref.* → osteo-.
os·te·al ['ɒstɪəl] *adj* → osseous.
os·te·al·bu·moid [ˌɒstɪ'ælbjəmɔɪd] *n* → osseoalbumoid.
os·te·al·gia [ˌɒstɪ'ældʒ(ɪ)ə] *n* Knochenschmerz(en *pl*) *m*, Ostealgie *f*, Osteodynie *f*.
os·te·an·a·bro·sis [ˌɒstɪˌænə'brəʊsɪs] *n old* Knochenatrophie *f*.
os·te·an·a·gen·e·sis [ˌɒstɪˌænə'dʒenəsɪs] *n* Knochenregeneration *f*.
os·te·a·naph·y·sis [ˌɒstɪə'næfəsɪs] *n* → osteanagenesis.
os·te·ar·thri·tis [ˌɒstɪɑːr'θraɪtɪs] *n* → osteoarthritis.
os·tec·to·my [ɒs'tektəmɪ] *n* Knochenexzision *f*, -resektion *f*.
os·te·ec·to·my [ˌɒstɪ'ektəmɪ] *n* → ostectomy.
os·te·ec·to·pia [ˌɒstɪek'təʊpɪə] *n* Knochenektopie *f*.
os·te·ec·to·py [ˌɒstɪ'ektəpɪ] *n* → osteectopia.
os·te·in ['ɒstɪɪn] *n* Kollagen *nt*.
os·te·ine *n* → ostein.
os·te·it·ic [ˌɒstɪ'ɪtɪk] *adj* Ostitis betr., ostitisch.
os·te·i·tis [ˌɒstɪ'aɪtɪs] *n* Knochen(gewebs)entzündung *f*, Ostitis *f*, Osteitis *f*.
os·tem·bry·on [ɒs'tembrɪɒn] *n old* → osteopedion.
osteo- *pref.* Knochen-, Osteo-.
os·te·o·a·cu·sis [ˌɒstɪəʊə'kjuːsɪs] *n physiol.* Knochenleitung *f*, Osteoakusis *f*, Osteophonie *f*.
os·te·o·al·bu·mi·noid [ˌɒstɪəʊæl'bjuːmɪnɔɪd] *n* → osseoalbumoid.
os·te·o·an·a·gen·e·sis [ˌɒstɪəʊˌænə'dʒenəsɪs] *n* Knochenregeneration *f*.
os·te·o·an·eu·rysm [ˌɒstɪəʊ'ænjərɪzəm] *n* Knochenaneurysma *nt*.
os·te·o·ar·thri·tis [ˌɒstɪəʊɑːr'θraɪtɪs] *n abbr.* **OA** degenerative Gelenkerkrankung *f*, Osteoarthrose *f*, Gelenk(s)arthrose *f*, Arthrosis deformans.
os·te·o·ar·throp·a·thy [ˌɒstɪəʊɑːr'θrɒpəθɪ] *n patho.* Osteoarthropathie *f*, -pathia *f*.
os·te·o·ar·thro·sis [ˌɒstɪəʊɑːr'θrəʊsɪs] *n* → osteoarthritis.
os·te·o·ar·tic·u·lar [ˌɒstɪəʊɑːr'tɪkjələr] *adj* Knochen u. Gelenk(e) betr., osteoartikulär.
os·te·o·blast ['ɒstɪəʊblæst] *n* Osteoblast *m*, Osteoplast *m*.
os·te·o·blas·tic [ˌɒstɪəʊ'blæstɪk] *adj* **1.** Osteoblasten betr., aus Osteoblasten bestehend, osteoblastisch. **2.** osteoplastisch.
osteoblastic metastasis osteoplastische Metastase *f*.
osteoblastic-osteolytic metastasis osteoplastische-osteolytische Metastase *f*.
osteoblastic osteosarcoma osteoblastisches/osteoplastisches Osteosarkom *f*.
osteoblastic sarcoma → osteosarcoma.
os·te·o·blas·to·ma [ˌɒstɪəʊblæs'təʊmə] *n* Osteoblastom(a) *nt*.
os·te·o·ca·chex·ia [ˌɒstɪəʊkə'keksɪə] *n* **1.** chronische Knochenerkrankung *f*. **2.** Kachexie *f* bei chronischer Knochenerkrankung.
os·te·o·camp·sia [ˌɒstɪəʊ'kæmpsɪə] *n* Knochenverbiegung *f*, -verkrümmung *f*.
os·te·o·camp·si [ˌɒstɪəʊ'kæmpsɪ] *n* → osteocampsia.
os·te·o·car·ci·no·ma [ˌɒstɪəʊˌkɑːrsɪ'nəʊmə] *n* Knochenkrebs *m*.
os·te·o·car·ti·lag·i·nous [ˌɒstɪəʊˌkɑːrtɪ'lædʒɪnəs] *adj* aus Knochen u. Knorpel bestehend, osteochondral, osteokartilaginär.
osteocartilaginous exostosis → osteochondroma.
os·te·o·chon·dral [ˌɒstɪəʊ'kɒndrəl] *adj* → osteocartilaginous.
os·te·o·chon·dri·tis [ˌɒstɪəʊkɒn'draɪtɪs] *n* Knochen-Knorpel-Entzündung *f*, Osteochondritis *f*.
o. of the capitellum Panner'-Krankheit *f*.
osteochondritis dissecans Osteochondrosis dissecans.
os·te·o·chon·dro·dys·pla·sia [ˌɒstɪəʊˌkɒndrəʊdɪs'pleɪʒ(ɪ)ə, -zɪə] *n* Morquio-Syndrom *nt*, Morquio-Ullrich-Syndrom *nt*, Morquio-Brailsford-Syndrom *nt*, spondyloepiphysäre Dysplasie *f*, Mukopolysaccharidose *f* Typ IV *abbr.* MPS IV.
os·te·o·chon·dro·dys·tro·phy [ˌɒstɪəʊˌkɒndrəʊ'dɪstrəfɪ] *n* **1.** → osteochondrodysplasia. **2.** Osteochondrodystrophie *f*, Chondroosteodystrophie *f*.
os·te·o·chon·dro·fi·bro·ma [ˌɒstɪəʊˌkɒndrəʊfaɪ'brəʊmə] *n* Osteochondrofibrom(a) *nt*.
os·te·o·chon·drol·y·sis [ˌɒstɪəʊkɒn'drɒləsɪs] *n* Osteochondrosis dissecans.
os·te·o·chon·dro·ma [ˌɒstɪəʊkɒn'drəʊmə] *n* Osteochondrom *nt*, knorpelige/kartilaginäre Exostose *f*, Chondroosteom *nt*.
o. of the epiphysis Trevor-Erkrankung *f*, -Syndrom *nt*, Dysplasia epiphysealis hemimelica.
os·te·o·chon·dro·ma·to·sis [ˌɒstɪəʊˌkɒndrəʊmə'təʊsɪs] *n* multiple kartilaginäre Exostosen *pl*, hereditäre multiple Exostosen *pl*, multiple Osteochondrome *pl*, Ecchondrosis ossificans.
os·te·o·chon·dro·my·o·sar·co·ma [ˌɒstɪəʊˌkɒndrəˌmaɪəsɑːr'kəʊmə] *n* Osteochondromyosarkom *nt*, -sarcoma *nt*.
os·te·o·chon·dro·myx·o·ma [ˌɒstɪəʊˌkɒndrəmɪk'səʊmə] *n* Osteochondromyxom(a) *nt*.
os·te·o·chon·dro·path·ia [ˌɒstɪəʊˌkɒndrəʊ'pæθɪə] *n* → osteochondropathy.
os·te·o·chon·drop·a·thy [ˌɒstɪəʊkɒn'drɒpəθɪ] *n* Knochen-Knorpel-Erkrankung *f*, Osteochondropathie *f*, -pathia *f*.
os·te·o·chon·dro·phyte [ˌɒstɪəʊ'kɒndrəfaɪt] *n* → osteochondroma.
os·te·o·chon·dro·sar·co·ma [ˌɒstɪəʊˌkɒndrəsɑːr'kəʊmə] *n* Osteochondrosarkom *nt*, -sarcoma *nt*.
os·te·o·chon·dro·sis [ˌɒstɪəʊkɒn'drəʊsɪs] *n* degenerative Knochen-Knorpel-Erkrankung *f*, Osteochondrose *f*, Osteochondrosis *f*.
o. of capital femoral epiphysis Perthes-Krankheit *f*, Morbus Perthes *m*, Perthes-Legg-Calvé-Krankheit *f*, Legg-Calvé-Perthes(-Waldenström)-Krankheit *f*, Osteochondropathia deformans, Coxae juveniles, Coxa plana (idiopathica).
o. of the head of humerus Hass'-Krankheit *f*, -Syndrom *nt*.
osteochondrosis dissecans Osteochondrosis dissecans.
o. of the femoral head idiopathische Hüftkopfnekrose *f* des Erwachsenen, avaskuläre/ischämische Femurkopfnekrose *f*.
os·te·o·chon·drous [ˌɒstɪəʊ'kɒndrəs] *adj* → osteocartilaginous.
os·te·o·cla·sia [ˌɒstɪəʊ'kleɪʒ(ɪ)ə] *n* → osteoclasis.
os·te·oc·la·sis [ˌɒstɪ'ɒkləsɪs] *n* **1.** *ortho.* Osteoklase *f*, Osteoklasie *f*. **2.** *patho.* vermehrte Osteoklastentätigkeit *f*, Osteoklasie *f*, Osteoklase *f*.
os·te·o·clast ['ɒstɪəklæst] *n* **1.** *histol.* Knochenfreßzelle *f*, Osteoklast *m*, Osteoclastocytus *m*. **2.** *ortho.* Osteoklast *m*.
osteoclast activating factor *abbr.* **OAF** Osteoklasten-aktivierender Faktor *m abbr.* OAF.
os·te·o·clas·tic [ˌɒstɪəʊ'klæstɪk] *adj* Osteoklast(en) betr., osteoklastisch.
os·te·o·clas·to·ma [ˌɒstɪəʊklæs'təʊmə] *n* Riesenzelltumor *m* des Knochens, Osteoklastom *nt*.
os·te·o·clas·ty ['ɒstɪəʊklæstɪ] *n* → osteoclasis.
os·te·o·cra·ni·um [ˌɒstɪəʊ'kreɪnɪəm] *n* knöcherner Schädel *m*, Osteokranium *nt*, -cranium *nt*.
os·te·o·cys·to·ma [ˌɒstɪəʊsɪs'təʊmə] *n* Knochenzyste *f*.
os·te·o·cyte ['ɒstɪəʊsaɪt] *n* Osteozyt *m*, Osteocytus *m*.
os·te·o·der·mia [ˌɒstɪəʊ'dɜːrmɪə] *n* Osteoma cutis.
os·te·o·des·mo·sis [ˌɒstɪəʊdez'məʊsɪs] *n* Sehnen-, Bandverknöcherung *f*, Osteodesmose *f*.
os·te·o·dyn·ia [ˌɒstɪəʊ'diːnɪə] *n* → ostealgia.
os·te·o·dys·tro·phia [ˌɒstɪəʊdɪ'strəʊfɪə] *n* → osteodystrophy.
os·te·o·dys·tro·phy [ˌɒstɪəʊ'dɪstrəfɪ] *n* Knochendystrophie *f*, Osteodystrophie *f*, -dystrophia *f*.
os·te·o·ec·ta·sia [ˌɒstɪəʊek'teɪʒ(ɪ)ə] *n* Knochenverbiegung *f*.
os·te·o·ec·to·my [ˌɒstɪəʊ'ektəmɪ] *n ortho.* Knochenexzision *f*, -resektion *f*.
os·te·o·en·chon·dro·ma [ˌɒstɪəʊenkɒn'drəʊmə] *n* → osteochondroma.
os·te·o·epiph·y·sis [ˌɒstɪəʊɪ'pɪfəsɪs] *n* Knochen-, Osteoepiphyse *f*.
os·te·o·fi·bro·chon·dro·sar·co·ma [ˌɒstɪəʊˌfaɪbrəˌkɒndrəsɑːr'kəʊmə] *n* malignes Mesenchymom *nt*.
os·te·o·fi·bro·ma [ˌɒstɪəʊfaɪ'brəʊmə] *n* Knochen-, Osteofibrom *nt*.
os·te·o·fi·bro·ma·to·sis [ˌɒstɪəʊˌfaɪbrəmə'təʊsɪs] *n* Osteofibromatose *f*.
os·te·o·fi·bro·sar·co·ma [ˌɒstɪəʊˌfaɪbrəsɑːr'kəʊmə] *n* Osteofibrosarkom *nt*, -sarcoma *nt*.
os·te·o·fi·bro·sis [ˌɒstɪəʊfaɪ'brəʊsɪs] *n* Knochen-, Osteofibrose *f*.
os·te·o·fi·brous dysplasia [ˌɒstɪəʊ'faɪbrəs] osteofibröse Dysplasie *f*, ossifizierendes Fibrom *nt*.

osteogenesis

os·te·o·gen·e·sis [ˌ-'dʒenəsɪs] *n* Knochenbildung *f*, -entwicklung *f*, -synthese *f*, Osteogenese *f*, Osteogenesis *f*.
osteogenesis imperfecta *abbr.* **OI** Osteogenesis imperfecta, Osteopsathyrosis *f*.
  early form o. → osteogenesis imperfecta tarda.
  lethal perinatal o. → osteogenesis imperfecta congenita.
  type I o. → osteogenesis imperfecta tarda.
  type II o. → osteogenesis imperfecta congenita.
  o. with blue sclerae → osteogenesis imperfecta tarda.
osteogenesis imperfecta congenita *abbr.* **OIC** Vrolik-Krankheit *f*, Vrolik-Typ *m* der Osteogenesis imperfecta, Osteogenesis imperfecta congenita, Osteogenesis imperfecta Typ Vrolik.
osteogenesis imperfecta tarda *abbr.* **OIT** Lobstein-Krankheit *f*, -Syndrom *nt*, Lobstein-Typ *m* der Osteogenesis imperfecta, Osteogenesis imperfecta tarda, Osteogenesis imperfecta Typ Lobstein.
os·te·o·ge·net·ic [ˌ-dʒə'netɪk] *adj* Knochenbildung/Osteogenese betr., knochenbildend, osteogenetisch.
os·te·o·gen·ic [ˌ-'dʒenɪk] *adj* **1.** von Knochen(gewebe) ausgehend *od.* stammend, osteogen. **2.** → osteogenetic.
osteogenic fibroma → osteoblastoma.
osteogenic sarcoma → osteosarcoma.
  periosteal o. periostales Osteosarkom *nt*, perossales Sarkom *nt*, periostales (osteogenes) Sarkom *nt*.
os·te·og·e·nous [ˌɑstɪ'ɑdʒənəs] *adj* → osteogenetic.
os·te·og·e·ny [ˌɑstɪ'ɑdʒənɪ] *n* → osteogenesis.
os·te·o·hal·i·ste·re·sis [ˌɑstɪəʊˌhælǝstə'riːsɪs, -hə,lɪs-] *n ortho.* Halisterese *f*, Halisteresis *f*.
os·te·o·hy·per·tro·phy [ˌ-haɪ'pɜːrtrǝfɪ] *n* Knochenhypertrophie *f*.
os·te·oid ['ɑstɪɔɪd] **I** *n* organische Grundsubstanz *f* des Knochens, Osteoid *nt*. **II** *adj* knochenähnlich, -artig, osteoid.
osteoid osteoma Osteoidosteom *nt*.
  giant o. Osteoblastom *nt*.
osteoid sarcoma → osteosarcoma.
osteoid tissue → osteoid I.
os·te·o·lip·o·chon·dro·ma [ˌɑstɪəʊˌlɪpəkɑn'drəʊmǝ] *n* Osteolipochondrom(a) *nt*.
os·te·o·li·po·ma [ˌ-lɪ'pǝʊmǝ] *n* Osteolipom(a) *nt*.
os·te·ol·o·gia [ˌ-'lǝʊdʒɪǝ] *n* → osteology.
os·te·ol·o·gist [ˌɑstɪ'ɑlǝdʒɪst] *n* Osteologe *f*, -login *f*.
os·te·ol·o·gy [ˌɑstɪ'ɑlǝdʒɪ] *n* Knochenlehre *f*, Osteologie *f*, Osteologia *f*.
os·te·ol·y·sis [ɑstɪ'ɑlǝsɪs] *n* Knochenauflösung *f*, Osteolyse *f*.
os·te·o·lyt·ic [ˌɑstɪǝʊ'lɪtɪk] *adj* Osteolyse betr. *od.* erzeugend, knochenauflösend, osteolytisch.
osteolytic metastasis osteolytische Metastase *f*.
osteolytic osteosarcoma osteolytisches Osteosarkom *nt*.
osteolytic sarcoma → osteosarcoma.
os·te·o·ma [ˌɑstɪ'ǝʊmǝ] *n* (benigne) Knochengeschwulst *f*, Osteom(a) *nt*.
os·te·o·ma·la·cia [ˌɑstɪǝʊmǝ'leɪʃ(ɪ)ǝ] *n* Knochenerweichung *f*, Osteomalazie *f*, -malacia *f*.
os·te·o·ma·la·cic [ˌ-mǝ'leɪsɪk] *adj* Osteomalazie betr., durch Osteomalazie charakterisiert, osteomalazisch.
osteomalacic pelvis osteomalazisches Becken *nt*, Pelvis osteomalacica.

os·te·o·mal·a·co·sis [ˌ-mælǝ'kǝʊsɪs] *n* → osteomalacia.
os·te·om·a·toid [ɑstɪ'ɑmǝtɔɪd] *adj* osteomähnlich, -artig.
os·te·o·ma·to·sis [ˌɑstɪǝʊmǝ'tǝʊsɪs] *n* Osteomatose *f*.
os·te·o·my·e·lit·ic [ˌ-ˌmaɪǝ'lɪtɪk] *adj* Osteomyelitis betr., osteomyelitisch.
os·te·o·my·e·li·tis [ˌ-ˌmaɪǝ'laɪtɪs] *n* Knochenmark(s)entzündung *f*, Osteomyelitis *f*.
  o. of temporal bone Schläfenbeinosteomyelitis.
os·te·o·my·e·lo·dys·pla·sia [ˌ-ˌmaɪǝlǝʊdɪs'pleɪʒ(ɪ)ǝ, -zɪǝ] *n* Osteomyelodysplasie *f*.
os·te·o·my·e·lo·fi·brot·ic syndrome [ˌ-ˌmaɪǝlǝʊfaɪ'brɑtɪk] → osteomyelofibrosis.
os·te·o·my·e·lo·fi·bro·sis [ˌ-ˌmaɪǝlǝʊfaɪ'brǝʊsɪs] *n* Myelofibrose *f*, Osteomyelofibrose *f* *abbr.* **OMF**; Osteomyelosklerose *f*, Myelosklerose *f*.
os·te·o·my·e·log·ra·phy [ˌ-maɪǝ'lɑgrǝfɪ] *n radiol.* Medullographie *f*, Osteomedullographie *f*, Osteomyelographie *f*.
os·te·o·my·e·lo·re·tic·u·lo·sis [ˌ-ˌmaɪǝlǝʊˌrɪtɪkjǝ'lǝʊsɪs] *n* Osteomyeloretikulose *f*.
os·te·o·my·e·lo·scle·ro·sis [ˌ-ˌmaɪǝlǝʊskl'rǝʊsɪs] *n* → osteomyelofibrosis.
os·te·o·myx·o·chon·dro·ma [ˌ-ˌmɪksǝkǝn'drǝʊmǝ] *n* Osteochondromyxom(a) *nt*.
os·te·on ['ɑstɪǝn] *n* Havers'-System *nt*, Osteon *nt*.
os·te·o·ne → osteon.
os·te·o·ne·cro·sis [ˌɑstɪǝʊnɪ'krǝʊsɪs] *n* Knochen-, Osteonekrose *f*.
os·te·o·neu·ral·gia [ˌ-njuǝ'rældʒ(ɪ)ǝ, nu-] *n* Knochen-, Osteoneuralgie *f*.
os·te·on·o·sus [ɑstɪ'ɑnǝsǝs] *n* Knochenerkrankung *f*, Osteopathie *f*, -pathia *f*.
osteo-odontoma *n* Odontoadamantinom *nt*, -ameloblastom *nt*, ameloblastisches (Fibro-)Odontom *nt*.
os·te·o·path ['ɑstɪǝpæθ] *n* Osteopath *m*.
os·te·o·path·ia [ˌ-'pæθɪǝ] *n* → osteopathy 1.
os·te·o·path·ic [ˌ-'pæθɪk] *adj* Osteopathie betr., osteopathisch.
osteopathic scoliosis osteopathische Skoliose *f*.
os·te·o·pa·thol·o·gy [ˌ-pǝ'θɑlǝdʒɪ] *n* → osteopathy 1.
os·te·op·a·thy [ˌɑstɪ'ɑpǝθɪ] *n* **1.** Knochenerkrankung *f*, Osteopathie *f*, -pathia *f*. **2.** (*Therapie*) Osteopathie *f*.
os·te·o·pe·cil·ia [ˌ-pǝ'sɪlɪǝ] *n* → osteopoikilosis.
os·te·o·pe·di·on [ˌ-'pɪdɪǝn] *n embryo.* Steinkind *nt*, Lithopädion *nt*.
os·te·o·pe·nia [ˌ-'pɪnɪǝ] *n* Osteopenie *f*.
os·te·o·pen·ic [ˌ-'penɪk] *adj* Osteopenie betr., osteopenisch.
os·te·o·per·i·os·te·al [ˌ-ˌperɪ'ɑstɪǝl] *adj* osteoperiostal.
os·te·o·per·i·os·ti·tis [ˌ-ˌperɪɑs'taɪtɪs] *n* Knochen-Periost-Entzündung *f*, Osteoperiostitis *f*.
os·te·o·pe·tro·sis [ˌ-pǝ'trǝʊsɪs] *n* Marmorknochenkrankheit *f*, Albers-Schönebergs-Krankheit *f*, Osteopetrose *f*, -petrosis *f*.
os·te·o·phage ['-feɪdʒ] *n* Osteoklast *m*, Osteophage *m*.
os·te·oph·o·ny [ɑstɪ'ɑfǝnɪ] *n physiol.* Knochenleitung *f*, Osteoakusis *f*, Osteophonie *f*.
os·te·o·phy·ma [ˌɑstɪǝ'faɪmǝ] *n* → osteophyte.
os·te·o·phyte ['-faɪt] *n* Osteophyt *m*.
os·te·o·phy·to·sis [ˌ-faɪ'tǝʊsɪs] *n ortho.* Osteophytenbildung *f*.
os·te·o·plast ['-plæst] *n* → osteoblast.

os·te·o·plas·tic [ˌ-'plæstɪk] *adj* **1.** → osteogenic 1. **2.** → osteogenetic. **3.** *ortho.* Osteoplastik betr., osteoplastisch.
osteoplastic amputation osteoplastische Amputation *f*.
osteoplastic craniotomy *neurochir.* osteoplastische Schädeltrepanation/Kraniotomie *f*.
osteoplastic epulis osteoplastische Epulis *f*, Epulis osteoplastica.
os·te·o·plas·ty ['-plæstɪ] *n ortho.* Knochen-, Osteoplastik *f*.
os·te·o·poi·ki·lo·sis [ˌ-ˌpɔɪkɪ'lǝʊsɪs] *n ortho.* Osteopoikilose *f*, -poikilie *f*, Osteopathia condensans disseminata.
os·te·o·poi·ki·lot·ic [ˌ-ˌpɔɪkɪ'lɑtɪk] *adj* Osteopoikilose betr., von ihr gekennzeichnet.
os·te·o·po·ro·sis [ˌ-pǝ'rǝʊsɪs] *n* Osteoporose *f*, -porosis *f*.
os·te·o·po·rot·ic [ˌ-pǝ'rɑtɪk] *adj* Osteoporose betr., von Osteoporose gekennzeichnet, osteoporotisch.
os·te·op·sath·y·ro·sis [ˌɑstɪɑpˌsæθɪ'rǝʊsɪs] *n* → osteogenesis imperfecta.
os·te·o·ra·di·o·ne·cro·sis [ˌɑstɪǝʊˌreɪdɪǝʊnɪ'krǝʊsɪs] *n* Strahlungs-, Strahlenosteonekrose *f*, Osteoradionekrose *f*, Radioosteonekrose *f*.
os·te·or·rha·gia [ˌ-'reɪdʒ(ɪ)ǝ] *n* Knochenblutung *f*, Osteorrhagie *f*.
os·te·or·rha·phy [ɑstɪ'ɔrǝfɪ] *n ortho.* Knochennaht *f*.
os·te·o·sar·co·ma [ˌɑstɪǝʊsɑːr'kǝʊmǝ] *n* Knochen-, Osteosarkom *nt*, Osteosarcoma *nt*, osteogenes/osteoplastisches Sarkom *nt*.
os·te·o·scle·ro·sis [ˌ-sklɪ'rǝʊsɪs] *n* Knochen-, Osteosklerose *f*; Eburnisation *f*, Eburneation *f*.
os·te·o·scle·rot·ic [ˌ-sklɪ'rɑtɪk] *adj* Osteosklerose betr., osteosklerotisch.
osteosclerotic anemia osteosklerotische Anämie *f*.
os·te·o·sep·tum [ˌ-'septǝm] *n* knöcherner Abschnitt/Teil *m* des Nasenseptums, Pars ossea septi nasi.
os·te·o·su·ture ['-suːtʃǝr] *n ortho.* Knochennaht *f*.
os·te·o·syn·o·vi·tis [ˌ-ˌsɪnǝ'vaɪtɪs] *n ortho.* Osteosynovitis *f*.
os·te·o·syn·the·sis [ˌ-'sɪnθǝsɪs] *n ortho.* Osteosynthese *f*.
os·te·o·tel·an·gi·ec·ta·sia [ˌ-tǝlˌændʒɪek'teɪʒ(ɪ)ǝ] *n* teleangiektatisches Osteosarkom *nt*.
os·te·o·throm·bo·phle·bi·tis [ˌ-ˌθrɑmbǝʊflɪ'baɪtɪs] *n* Osteothrombophlebitis *f*.
os·te·o·throm·bo·sis [ˌ-θrɑm'bǝʊsɪs] *n* Osteothrombose *f*.
os·te·ot·o·me ['-tǝʊm] *n ortho.* Osteotom *nt*.
os·te·ot·o·my [ˌɑstɪ'ɑtǝmɪ] *n ortho.* Knochendurchtrennung *f*, Osteotomie *f*.
os·te·ot·ro·phy [ɑstɪ'ɑtrǝfɪ] *n* Knochenernährung *f*.
os·te·o·tym·pan·ic conduction [ˌɑstɪǝʊtɪm'pænɪk] → osteophony.
os·ti·al ['ɑstɪǝl] *adj anat.* Ostium betr., Ostium-.
os·ti·tis [ɑs'taɪtɪs] *n* → osteitis.
os·ti·um ['ɑstɪǝm] *n, pl* **-tia** [-tɪǝ] *anat.* Mündung *f*, Eingang *m*, Ostium *nt*; Orificium *nt*.
ostium primum defect *card.* Foramen-primum-Defekt *m*, Ostium-primum-Defekt *m*, Primum-Defekt *m*, tiefsitzender Vorhofseptumdefekt *m*, Atriumseptumdefekt I *m abbr.* **ASD I**, Vorhofseptumdefekt *m* vom Primumtyp.
ostium secundum defect *card.* Foramen-secundum-Defekt *m*, Ostium-secundum-Defekt *m*, Secundum-Defekt *m*,

Fossa-ovalis-Defekt *m*, hochsitzender Vorhofseptumdefekt *m*, Atriumseptumdefekt II *m abbr.* ASD II, Vorhofseptumdefekt *m* vom Sekundumtyp.
os·to·my ['ɑstəmɪ] *n chir.* **1.** Stomaoperation *f.* **2.** Stoma *nt.*
os·to·sis [ɑs'təʊsɪs] *n* → osteogenesis.
os·tra·ceous psoriasis [ɑs'treɪʃəs] *derm.* Psoriasis ostracea/rupioides.
Ostrum-Furst ['ɑstrəm fʊrst]: **O.-F. syndrome** Ostrum-Furst-Syndrom *nt.*
OT *abbr.* → old tuberculin.
ot- *pref.* → oto-.
Ota ['əʊtə]: **O.'s nevus** Nävus Ota *m*, okulodermale Melanozytose *f*, Naevus fuscocoeruleus ophthalmomaxillaris.
o·tag·ra [əʊ'tægrə] *n* → otalgia.
o·tal·gia [əʊ'tældʒ(ɪ)ə] *n* Ohrenschmerz(en *pl*) *m*, Otalgie *f*, Otagra *f*, Otodynie *f*, Otalgia *f.*
o·tal·gic [əʊ'tældʒɪk] *adj* Otalgie betr., otalgisch.
OTC *abbr.* [ornithine transcarbamoylase] → ornithine carbamoyltransferase.
OTC deficiency → ornithine carbamoyl phosphate deficiency.
OTD *abbr.* → organ tolerance dose.
Othello [əʊ'θeləʊ, ə-]: **O. syndrome** Othello-Syndrom *nt.*
ot·he·ma·to·ma [əʊ'θi:mətəʊmə, əʊt'hi:mə-] *n* Othämatom *nt.*
ot·hem·or·rha·gia [əʊ'θi:məreɪdʒ(ɪ)ə, əʊt'hi:mə-] *n* Blutung *f* aus dem Ohr.
other-directed *adj* fremdbestimmt.
o·tic ['əʊtɪk, 'ɑtɪk] *adj* Ohr betr., zum Ohr gehörend, Ohr-.
otic abscess otogener Abszeß *m.*
otic depression *embryo.* Ohrgrübchen *nt.*
otic ganglion Arnold'-Ganglion *nt*, Ggl. oticum.
otic neuralgia *neuro.* Genikulatumneuralgie *f*, Ramsay Hunt-Syndrom *nt*, Neuralgia geniculata, Zoster oticus, Herpes zoster oticus.
otic pit *embryo.* Ohrgrübchen *nt.*
otic placode *embryo.* Ohrplakode *f.*
otic vesicle *embryo.* Ohrbläschen *nt.*
o·ti·o·bi·o·sis [,əʊtɪəʊbaɪ'əʊsɪs] *n* → otobiosis.
O·ti·o·bi·us [əʊtɪ'əʊbɪəs] *n* → Otobius.
o·tit·ic [əʊ'tɪtɪk] *adj* Otitis betr., otitisch.
otitic barotrauma Fliegerotitis *f*, Aer(o)otitis *f*, Baro(o)titis *f*, Otitis barotraumatica.
otitic hydrocephalus otitischer Hydrozephalus *m.*
otitic meningitis otogene Meningitis *f.*
o·ti·tis [əʊ'taɪtɪs] *n* Ohrentzündung *f*, Otitis *f.*
otitis externa Entzündung *f* des äußeren Gehörganges, Otitis externa.
 bacterial o. bakterielle Otitis externa.
 chronic o. chronische Otitis externa.
 circumscribed o. Gehörgangsfurunkel *nt/m*, Ohrfurunkel *nt/m*, Otitis externa circumscripta/furunculosa.
 diffuse o. Otitis externa diffusa.
 malignant o. progressive nekrotisierende Otitis, progrediente Otitis, Otitis externa maligna.
 swimmer's o. Bade-Otitis externa.
 viral o. virale Otitis externa.
otitis media Mittelohrentzündung *f*, Otitis media.
 acute o. akute Mittelohrentzündung *f*, akuter Mittelohrkatarrh *m*, Otitis media acuta.
 adhesive o. Pauken(höhlen)fibrose *f*, adhäsive Otitis media (chronica).
 chronic o. chronische Mittelohrentzündung/Schleimhauteiterung *f*, Otitis media chronica.

chronic seromucinous o. chronische seromuköse Otitis media, chronischer Tuben-Mittelohrkatarrh *m*, Seromukotympanum *nt.*
 latent o. latente Otitis media.
 purulent o. Mittelohreiterung *f*, Otitis media purulenta.
 swimmer's o. Bade-Otitis media.
 viral o. virale Otitis media.
oto- *pref.* Ohr-, Gehör-, Ot(o)-.
o·to·bi·o·sis [,əʊtəbaɪ'əʊsɪs] *n* Otobius-Befall *m*, Otobiosis *f.*
O·to·bi·us [əʊ'təʊbɪəs] *n micro.* Otobius *m.*
o·to·blen·nor·rhea [,əʊtəblenə'rɪə] *n* muköser Ohr(en)ausfluß *m*, Otoblennorrhoe *f.*
O·to·cen·tor [,-'sentər] *n micro.* Anocentor *m.*
o·to·ceph·a·lus [,-'sefələs] *n embryo.* Otozephalus *m*, -kephalus *m.*
o·to·ceph·a·ly [,-'sefəlɪ] *n embryo.* Otozephalie *f*, -kephalie *f.*
o·to·cer·e·bri·tis [,-,serə'braɪtɪs] *n* → otoencephalitis.
o·to·clei·sis [,-'klaɪsɪs] *n* Otokleisis *f*, Otoklisis *f.*
o·to·co·nia [,-'kəʊnɪə] *pl, sing* **-ni·um** [-nɪəm] *physiol.* Ohrkristalle *pl*, Otokonien *pl*, -lithen *pl*, Statokonien *pl*, -lithen *pl*, -conia *pl*, Otoconia *pl.*
o·toc·o·nites [əʊ'θɒkənaɪtɪs] *pl* → otoconia.
o·to·co·ni·um *sing* → otoconia.
o·to·cyst ['əʊtəsɪst] *n embryo.* Ohrbläschen *nt.*
o·to·dyn·ia [,-'dɪːnɪə] *n* → otalgia.
o·to·en·ceph·a·li·tis [,-en,sefə'laɪtɪs] *n* otogene Enzephalitis *f.*
o·to·gan·gli·on [,-'gæŋglɪən] *n* Ggl. oticum.
o·to·gen·ic [,-'dʒenɪk] *adj* vom Ohr stammend *od.* ausgehend, otogen.
otogenic abscess otogener Abszeß *m.*
otogenic dyslalia otogene/audiogene Dyslalie *f.*
otogenic meningitis otogene Meningitis *f.*
o·tog·e·nous [əʊ'tɒdʒənəs] *adj* → otogenic.
o·to·lar·yn·gol·o·gy [,əʊtəlærɪn'gɒlədʒɪ] *n* Otolaryngologie *f.*
o·to·lites ['-laɪts] *pl* **1.** → otoconia. **2.** *HNO* Otolithen *pl.*
otolith apparatus ['-lɪθ] Otolithenorgan *nt*, -apparat *m.*
o·to·li·thi·a·sis [,-lɪ'θaɪəsɪs] *n* Otolithiasis *f.*
otolith organ → otolith apparatus.
o·to·liths ['-lɪθs] *pl* **1.** → otoconia. **2.** *HNO* Otolithen *pl.*
o·to·lith·ic membrane [,-'lɪθɪk] Statolithenmembran *f.*
o·to·log·ic surgery [,-'lɒdʒɪk] Ohrchirurgie *f.*
otologic torticollis otologer Schiefhals/Torticollis *m.*
otologic wryneck → otologic torticollis.
o·tol·o·gist [əʊ'tɒlədʒɪst] *n* Ohrenarzt *m*, -ärztin *f*, Otologe *m*, -login *f.*
o·to·mas·toid·i·tis [,əʊtə,mæstɔɪ'daɪtɪs] *n HNO* Otomastoiditis *f.*
o·to·mu·cor·my·co·sis [,-,mjuːkɔːrmaɪ'kəʊsɪs] *n* Mukormykose *f* des Ohres.
o·to·my·co·sis [,-maɪ'kəʊsɪs] *n* Gehörgangs-, Ohr-, Otomykose *f.*
o·to·my·i·a·sis [,-'maɪ(j)əsɪs] *n* Myiasis *f* des Gehörgangs, Otomyiasis *f.*
o·to·neu·ral·gia [,-njʊə'rældʒ(ɪ)ə, -nʊ-] *n* neuralgischer Ohrenschmerz *m.*
o·to·pal·a·to·dig·i·tal syndrome [,-,pælətəʊ'dɪdʒɪtl] otopalatodigitales Syndrom *nt.*
o·top·a·thy [əʊ'tɒpəθɪ] *n* Ohrenerkrankung *f*, -leiden *nt*, Otopathie *f.*

o·to·pha·ryn·ge·al [,əʊtəfə'rɪndʒ(ɪ)əl] *adj* Ohr u. Pharynx betr., otopharyngeal.
otopharyngeal tube Ohrtrompete *f*, Eustach'-Kanal *m*, -Röhre *f*, Tuba auditiva/auditoria.
o·to·plas·ty ['-plæstɪ] *n* Ohrplastik *f*, plastische Chirurgie *f* des Ohrs.
o·to·pol·y·pus [,-'pɒlɪpəs] *n* Gehörgangspolyp *m*, Otopolyp *m.*
o·to·py·or·rhea [,-,paɪə'rɪə] *n* eitriger Ohrenausfluß *m*, Otopyorrhoe *f.*
o·to·rhi·no·lar·yn·gol·o·gy [,-,raɪnəʊlærɪn'gɒlədʒɪ] *n* Hals-Nasen-Ohrenheilkunde *f abbr.* HNO, Otorhinolaryngologie *f.*
o·to·rhi·nol·o·gy [,-raɪ'nɒlədʒɪ] *n* Nasen-Ohren-Heilkunde *f*, Otorhinologie *f.*
o·tor·rha·gia [,-'reɪdʒ(ɪ)ə] *n* Ohrblutung *f*, Otorrhagie *f.*
o·tor·rhea [,-'rɪə] *n* Ohren(aus)fluß *m*, Otorrhoe *f.*
o·to·sal·pinx [,-'sælpɪŋks] *n* Ohrtrompete *f*, Eustach'-Röhre *f*, -Kanal *m*, Tuba auditiva/auditoria.
o·to·scle·ro·sis [,-sklɪ'rəʊsɪs] *n HNO* Otosklerose *f.*
o·to·scle·rot·ic [,-sklɪ'rɒtɪk] *adj* Otosklerose betr., otosklerotisch.
o·to·scope ['-skəʊp] *n* Otoskop *nt*; Ohrenspekulum *nt.*
o·to·scop·ic [,-'skɒpɪk] *adj* Otoskopie *od.* Otoskop betr., otoskopisch.
o·tos·co·py [əʊ'tɒskəpɪ] *n HNO* Ohrspiegelung *f*, Otoskopie *f.*
o·to·tox·ic [,əʊtə'tɒksɪk] *adj* ototoxisch.
o·to·tox·ic·i·ty [,-tɒk'sɪsətɪ] *n* Ototoxizität *f.*
Otto ['ɑtəʊ]: **O.'s disease/pelvis** Otto-Chrobak-Becken *nt*, Protrusionsbecken *nt*, Protrusio acetabuli.
Ottoson ['ɑtəʊsən]: **O. potential** Elektroolfaktogramm *nt abbr.* EOG.
O.U. *abbr.* → Oxford unit.
oua·ba·in [wɑ'baːɪn, -beɪn] *n pharm.* Ouabain *n*, g-Strophanthin *nt.*
Ouchterlony ['ɑktərləʊnɪ]: **O. technique/test** Ouchterlony-Technik *f*, zweidimensionale Immunodiffusion *f* nach Ouchterlony.
Oudin [u'dɛ̃]: **O. technique/test** Oudin-Methode *f.*
ounce [aʊns] *n abbr.* **oz.** Unze *f*, ounce *abbr.* oz.
out [aʊt] **I** *n* Außenseite *f.* **II** *adj* Außen-; über normal, Über-. **III** *adv* **1.** außen, draußen; hinaus, (he-)raus. **2.** aus, vorbei, vorüber, zu Ende; erloschen. **3. to be ~ 1.** bewußtlos *od.* weg sein. **2.** eingeschlafen sein. **4.** nicht an der richtigen Stelle sein; (*Arm*) verrenkt; verrückt. **IV** *prep* **5.** aus, heraus/hinaus/hervor aus, **6. ~ of** aus **.** heraus; **~ of breath** außer Atem.
out·break ['aʊtbreɪk] *n* (*Epidemie*) Ausbruch *m.*
out·burst ['aʊtbɜːst] **I** *n* (*a. fig.*) Ausbruch *m.* **II** *vi* ausbrechen.
 o. of temper/anger Wutausbruch *m.*
out·come ['aʊtkʌm] *n* Ergebnis *nt*, Resultat *nt*, Folge(zustand *m*) *f.*
out·dat·ed [aʊt'deɪtɪd] *adj* veraltet, überholt.
out·er ['aʊtər] *adj* äußere(r, s), obere(r, s), Über-, Ober-, Außen-.
outer band of Baillarger äußere Baillarger-Schicht *f*, äußerer Baillarger-Streifen *m*, Stria laminae granularis interna corticis cerebri.
outer border: o. of scapula Außenrand *m* der Skapula, Margo lateralis scapulae.
 o. of spleen oberer Milzrand *m*, Margo superior lienis/splenis.
outer ear äußeres Ohr *nt*, Auris externa.
outer line of Baillarger → outer band of Baillarger.

outer malleolus

outer malleolus Außenknöchel *m*, Malleolus lateralis.
outer margin: o. of iris äußerer/ziliarer Irisrand *m*, Margo ciliaris iridis.
o. of scapula → outer border of scapula.
o. of spleen → outer border of spleen.
outer mesaxon äußeres Mesaxon *nt*.
out·er·most ['aʊtəməʊst] *adj* äußerste(r, s).
outer plate of cranial bone äußeres Blatt *nt* des knöchernen Schädeldaches, Lamina externa (ossis cranii).
outer ridge embryo. (Ohr) äußere Leiste *f*.
outer skin Oberhaut *f*, Epidermis *f*.
outer stria of Baillarger → outer band of Baillarger.
outer stripe of Baillarger → outer band of Baillarger.
outer surface Außenseite *f*, -fläche *f*, Oberfläche *f*.
outer table of skull Lamina externa.
outer tunnel 1. (Ohr) äußerer Tunnel *m*. **2.** Nuel'-Raum *m*.
out·fit ['aʊtfɪt] *n* Ausrüstung *f*; techn. Gerät(e *pl*) *nt*, Werkzeug(e *pl*) *nt*.
out·flow ['aʊtfləʊ] *n* Ab-, Ausfluß *m*; Ab-, Ausfließen *nt*; (Gas) Ausströmen *nt*.
out·go·ing [,aʊt'gəʊɪŋ] *adj* psycho. extrovertiert, aus s. herausgehend, kontaktfreudig.
out·growth ['aʊtgrəʊθ] *n* Auswuchs *m*, Exkreszenz *f*.
out·gush ['aʊtgʌʃ] *n* **1.** Ausfluß *m*. **2.** fig. Ausbruch *m*, Erguß *m*.
out knee O-Bein *nt*, Genu varum.
out·let ['aʊtlet, -lɪt] *n* **1.** Austritt *m*, Auslaß *m*, Abfluß *m*, Ausgang *m*, Öffnung *f*, Mündung *f*. **2.** fig. Ventil *nt*, Betätigungsfeld *nt*.
outlet syndrome Thoracic-outlet-Syndrom *nt*, Engpaß-Syndrom *nt*.
out·li·er ['aʊtlaɪər] *n* stat. Ausreißer *m*.
out·line ['aʊtlaɪn] **I** *n* Umriß *m*, Kontur *f*; Umrißlinie *f*; (Gesichts-)Züge *pl*. **II** *vt* umreißen, skizzieren.
out·look ['aʊtlʊk] *n* **1.** Ansicht(en *pl*) *f*, Einstellung *f*, Standpunkt *m*. **2.** (Zukunfts-)Aussichten *pl*; Prognose *f*.
out·ly·ing ['aʊtlaɪɪŋ] *adj* außerhalb gelegen, äußere(r, s), abgelegen.
out·mod·ed [aʊt'məʊdɪd] *adj* → out-of--date.
out-of-balance *adj* unausgeglichen, unausgewogen.
out-of-date *adj* veraltet, überholt.
out-of-focus *adj* außerhalb des Brennpunkts gelegen; unscharf.
out·pa·tient ['aʊtpeɪʃənt] *n* ambulanter Patient *m*, ambulante Patientin *f*.
outpatient clinic Poliklinik *f*, Ambulanz *f*, Ambulatorium *nt*.
out-patients department abbr. **OPD** Ambulanz *f*, Poliklinik *f*.
out·pock·et·ing [aʊt'pɒkɪtɪŋ] *n* Ausstülpung *f*, Evagination *f*.
out·pouch·ing [aʊt'paʊtʃɪŋ] *n* Ausstülpung *f*, Evagination *f*.
out·pour ['aʊtpɔːr, -pəʊr] *n* **1.** Aus-, Hervorströmen *nt*. **2.** Guß *m*, Strom *m*. **3.** fig. Ausbruch *m*, Erguß *m*.
out·pour·ing ['aʊtpɔːrɪŋ, -pəʊr-] *n* Erguß *m*.
out·put ['aʊtpʊt] *n* Output *m*; physiol. Abgabe *f*, (Arbeits-, Produktions-)Leistung *f*, (-)Ertrag *m*.
output capacity Leistungsfähigkeit *f*.
out·set ['aʊtset] *n* Beginn *m*, Anfang *m*. **at the ~** zu Beginn, am Anfang. **from the ~** von Anfang an.
out·side [aʊt'saɪd; adj, adv aʊt'saɪd] **I** *n* Außenseite *f*; (a. fig.) das Äußere, äußere Erscheinung *f*. **from the ~** von außen. **on**

the ~ of an der Außenseite. **II** *adj* an der Außenseite befindlich, von außen kommend, äußere(r, s), Außen-. **III** *adv* (dr-)außen, außerhalb; (von) außen, an der Außenseite.
out·size ['aʊtsaɪz] **I** *n* Übergröße *f*. **II** *adj* übergroß.
out·skirts ['aʊtskɜːts] *pl* Umgebung *f*, Rand(bezirke *pl*) *m*, Peripherie *f*.
out·spread [adj 'aʊtspred; v aʊt'spred] **I** *adj* ausgebreitet. **II** *vt* ausbreiten.
out·stand·ing [aʊt'stændɪŋ] *adj* hervorragend (for durch, wegen); außerordentlich, ausgezeichnet.
out·stretch [aʊt'stretʃ] *vt* (aus-)strecken, (aus-)dehnen.
out·stretched [aʊt'stretʃd] *adj* ausgestreckt; (Arme) ausgebreitet.
out·ward ['aʊtwərd] **I** *n* das Äußere. **II** *adj* **1.** äußerlich, äußere(r, s), Außen-; sichtbar. **for ~ application** zur äußerlichen Anwendung. **2.** nach (dr-)außen gerichtet, Aus(wärts)-.
outward angle mathe. Außenwinkel *m*.
out·wear [aʊt'weər] *vt* **1.** überdauern, länger halten als, dauerhafter sein als. **2.** abnutzen. **3.** fig. erschöpfen, aufreiben.
ov- pref. → ovi-.
o·va *pl* → ovum.
o·val ['əʊvl] *adj* eiförmig, O-förmig, ellipsenförmig, eirund, ellipsoid, oval.
oval amputation chir., ortho. Amputation *f* mit Ovalärschnitt.
ov·al·bu·min [,ævəl'bjuːmɪn, ,əʊv-] *n* Ovalbumin *nt*.
oval center, greater Centrum semiovale.
o·va·le malaria [əʊ'veɪlɪ] Ovale-Malaria *f*.
oval fossa: o. of fetus embryo. For. ovale cordis.
o. of heart → o. of fetus.
oval fossa: o. of heart Fossa ovalis cordis.
o. of thigh Hiatus saphenus.
oval incision Ovalärschnitt *m*.
o·va·lo·cy·tar·y [,əʊvələʊ'saɪtərɪ, əʊˌvæl-əʊ-] *adj* ovalocytic.
o·va·lo·cyte ['-saɪt] *n* hema. Elliptozyt *m*, Ovalozyt *m*.
o·va·lo·cyt·ic [,-'sɪtɪk] *adj* Elliptozyten betr., elliptozytär, Elliptozyten-.
ovalocytic anemia → ovalocytosis.
o·va·lo·cy·to·sis [,-saɪ'təʊsɪs] *n* hema. hereditäre Elliptozytose *f*, Ovalozytose *f*, Kamelozytose *f*, Elliptozytenanämie *f*, Dresbach-Syndrom *nt*.
oval window ovales (Vorhofs-)Fenster *nt*, Fenestra ovalis/vestibuli.
ovari- pref. → ovario-.
o·var·i·al·gia [əʊˌveərɪ'ældʒ(ɪ)ə] *n* → oophoralgia.
o·var·i·an [əʊ'veərɪən] *adj* Eierstock/Ovarium betr., ovarial, ovariell, Eierstock-, Ovarial-.
ovarian agenesis Eierstock-, Ovarialagenesie *f*, Agenesia ovarii.
ovarian amenorrhea gyn. ovarielle Amenorrhoe *f*.
ovarian appendage Nebeneierstock *m*, Rosenmüller'-Organ *nt*, Parovarium *f*, Epoophoron *f*.
ovarian artery Eierstockarterie *f*, Ovarica *f*, A. ovarica.
ovarian bleeding Eierstock-, Ovarialblutung *f*.
ovarian branch of uterine artery Eierstockast *m* der A. uterina, Ramus ovaricus a. uterinae.
ovarian canal → oviduct.
ovarian carcinoma Eierstockkrebs *m*, Ovarialkarzinom *nt*.
ovarian colic Ovarialkolik *f*.
ovarian cumulus Eihügel *m*, Discus proligerus/oophorus, Cumulus oophorus.

ovarian cycle ovarieller Zyklus *m*.
ovarian cyst Ovarial-, Eierstockzyste *f*.
ovarian cystadenocarcinoma verkrebstes Ovarialkystom *nt*, Cystadenocarcinoma ovarii.
ovarian cystadenoma Ovarialkystom *nt*, Cystadenoma ovarii.
  mucinous o. (pseudo-)muzinöses Ovarialkystom, Cystadenoma ovarii pseudomucinosum.
  pseudomucinous o. → mucinous o.
  serous o. seröses Ovarialkystom, Cystadenoma ovarii serosum.
ovarian cystoma → ovarian cystadenoma.
ovarian endometriosis gyn. Ovarialendometriose *f*, Endometriosis ovarii.
ovarian fibroma gyn. Eierstock-, Ovarialfibrom *nt*.
ovarian fimbria längste Tubenfimbrie *f*, Ovarialfimbrie *f*, Fimbria ovarica.
ovarian follicles Eierstock-, Ovarialfollikel *pl*, Folliculi ovarii.
  primary o. Primärfollikel, Folliculi ovarici primarii.
  secondary o. Sekundärfollikel, wachsende Follikel, Folliculi ovarici secundarii.
ovarian fossa Claudius'-Grube *f*, Eierstockmulde *f*, Fossa ovarica.
ovarian hemorrhage → ovarian bleeding.
ovarian hernia Ovariozele *f*, Hernia ovarialis.
ovarian hormone Eierstockhormon *nt*.
ovarian ligament Eierstockband *nt*, old Chorda utero-ovarica, Lig. ovarii proprium.
ovarian medulla embryo. Ovarialmark *nt*, Medulla ovarii.
ovarian opening of uterine tube abdominelle Tubenöffnung *f*, Ostium abdominale tubae uterinae.
ovarian pain → oophoralgia.
ovarian plexus Plexus ovaricus.
ovarian pregnancy Eierstockschwangerschaft *f*, -gravidität *f*, Ovarialschwangerschaft *f*, -gravidität *f*, Graviditas ovarica.
ovarian seminoma gyn. Seminom *nt* des Ovars, Dysgerminom(a) *nt*.
ovarian stroma Eierstockbindegewebe *nt*, Ovarialstroma *nt*.
ovarian stromal hyperplasia gyn. Thekomatose *f*.
ovarian tubular adenoma Arrhenoblastom *nt*.
ovarian tumor gyn. Eierstockgeschwulst *f*, -tumor *m*, Ovarialgeschwulst *f*, -tumor *m*.
ovarian vein: left o. linke Eierstockvene *f*, V. ovarica sinistra.
  right o. rechte Eierstockvene *f*, V. ovarica dextra.
ovarian vein syndrome Ovarika-Syndrom *nt*, Ureter-Ovarika-Kompressionssyndrom *nt*.
o·var·i·ec·to·my [əʊˌveərɪ'ektəmɪ] *n* gyn. Eierstockentfernung *f*, Oophorektomie *f*, Ovariektomie *f*, Ovarektomie *f*.
ovario- pref. Eierstock-, Ovarial-, Ovari(o)-, Oophor(o)-.
o·var·i·o·ab·dom·i·nal pregnancy [əʊˌveərɪəʊæb'dɒmɪnl] ovarioabdominale Schwangerschaft *f*.
o·var·i·o·cele ['-siːl] *n* → ovarian hernia.
o·var·i·o·cen·te·sis [,-sen'tiːsɪs] *n* gyn. Eierstockpunktion *f*, Ovariozentese *f*.
o·var·i·o·cy·e·sis [,-saɪ'iːsɪs] *n* → ovarian pregnancy.
o·var·i·o·dys·neu·ria [,-dɪs'njʊərɪə, -'nʊ-] *n* neuralgischer Eierstockschmerz *m*.
o·var·i·o·gen·ic [-'dʒenɪk] *adj* im Eierstock entstehend, aus dem Eierstock stammend, ovariogen.

o·var·i·o·hys·ter·ec·to·my [ˌ-hɪstə'rektəmɪ] *n gyn.* Entfernung *f* von Gebärmutter u. Eierstöcken, Ovariohysterektomie *f*, Oophorohysterektomie *f*.

o·var·i·on·cus [əʊˌveərɪ'aŋkəs] *n* → oophoroma.

o·var·i·op·a·thy [əʊˌveərɪ'apəθɪ] *n* Eierstockerkrankung *f*, Ovariopathie *f*.

o·var·i·o·pex·y [əʊˌveərɪəʊ'peksɪ] *n gyn.* Eierstockfixierung *f*, Ovariopexie *f*.

o·var·i·or·rhex·is [ˌ-'reksɪs] *n gyn.* Eierstockruptur *f*, Ovariorrhexis *f*.

o·var·i·o·sal·pin·gec·to·my [ˌ-ˌsælpɪŋ'dʒektəmɪ] *n gyn.* Entfernung *f* von Eierstock u. Eileiter, Ovariosalpingektomie *f*, Oophorosalpingektomie *f*.

o·var·i·o·sal·pin·gi·tis [ˌ-ˌsælpɪŋ'dʒaɪtɪs] *n gyn.* Entzündung *f* von Eierstock u. Eileiter, Ovariosalpingitis *f*, Oophorosalpingitis *f*.

o·var·i·os·to·my [əʊˌveərɪ'ɑstəmɪ] *n* → oophorostomy.

o·var·i·o·tes·tis [ˌ-'testɪs] *n* → ovotestis.

o·var·i·ot·o·my [əʊˌveərɪ'ɑtəmɪ] *n gyn.* Eierstockschnitt *m*, -inzision *f*, Ovariotomie *f*, Ovaritomie *f*.

o·va·ri·tis [əʊvə'raɪtɪs] *n gyn.* Eierstockentzündung *f*, Oophoritis *f*.

o·var·i·um [əʊ'veərɪəm] *n, pl* **-var·ia** [-'veərɪə] → ovary.

o·va·ry ['əʊvərɪ] *n, pl* **-ries** weibliche Geschlechts-/Keimdrüse *f*, Eierstock *m*, Ovarium *nt*, Ovaron *nt*, Oophoron *nt*.

o·ver ['əʊvər] **I** *n* Überschuß *m*. **II** *adj* obere(r, s), Ober-; äußere(r, s), Außen-; überzählig, übrig, Über-. **III** *adv* **1.** hinüber, darüber, herüber, über-. **2.** zu Ende, aus, vorbei. **3.** allzu, übermäßig, über-.

o·ver·ac·cu·mu·la·tion [ˌəʊvərəˌkjuːmjə'leɪʃn] *n* übermäßige Anhäufung *f*.

o·ver·a·chieve [ˌ-ə'tʃiːv] *vi* (*im Test*) mehr leisten als erwartet.

o·ver·ac·tive [ˌ-'æktɪv] *adj* übertrieben aktiv, übermäßig tätig sein, hyperaktiv.

o·ver·ac·tiv·i·ty [ˌ-æk'tɪvətɪ] *n* Hyperaktivität *f*; Überfunktion *f*.

o·ver·age ['-eɪdʒ] *adj* zu alt; älter als der Durchschnitt.

o·ver·all ['-ɔːl] **I** *n* **1.** ∼s *pl Brit.* Kittel *m*. **2.** (Arbeits-)Anzug *m*, Overall *m*. **II** *adj* gesamt, Gesamt-; allgemein. **III** *adv* insgesamt.

overall length Gesamtlänge *f*.

over-and-over suture *chir.* Knopfnaht *f*.

o·ver·anx·ious [ˌ-'æŋkʃəs] *adj* überängstlich, übermäßig besorgt; übernervös.

o·ver·bal·ance [*n* ['-ˌbæləns; *v* ˌ-'bæləns] **I** *n* Übergewicht *nt*. **II** *vt* **1.** (*a. fig.*) überwiegen, das Übergewicht haben über. **2.** umwerfen, -stoßen, (um-)kippen; aus dem Gleichgewicht bringen. **III** *vi* umkippen, aus dem Gleichgewicht kommen, das Gleichgewicht verlieren.

o·ver·bite ['-baɪt] *n dent.* Überbiß *m*.

o·ver·bur·den [*n* ['-ˌbɜːdn; *v* ˌ-'bɜːdn] **I** *n* Überladung *f*, Über(be)lastung *f*. **II** *vt* überladen, über(be)lasten.

o·ver·ca·pac·i·ty [ˌ-kə'pæsətɪ] *n* Überkapazität *f*.

o·ver·cau·tious [ˌ-'kɔːʃəs] *adj* übervorsichtig, übertrieben vorsichtig.

o·ver·cau·tious·ness [ˌ-'kɔːʃəsnɪs] *n* Eiertriebene Vorsicht *f*.

o·ver·come [ˌ-'kʌm] *vt* überstehen, überwinden, bezwingen; (*Angewohnheit*) s. abgewöhnen.

o·ver·com·pen·sate [ˌ-'kɑmpənseɪt] *vt, vi psycho.* überkompensieren.

o·ver·com·pen·sa·tion [ˌ-ˌkɑmpən'seɪʃn] *n psycho.* Überkompensation *f*, Überkompensierung *f*.

o·ver·con·fi·dence [ˌ-'kɑnfɪdəns] *n* gesteigertes Selbstbewußtsein *od.* -vertrauen *nt*.

o·ver·con·fi·dent [ˌ-'kɑnfɪdənt] *adj* übertrieben selbstsicher *od.* selbstbewußt.

o·ver·con·sump·tion [ˌ-kən'sʌmpʃn] *n* zu starker Verbrauch *m* (*of* an).

o·ver·de·vel·op [ˌ-dɪ'veləp] *vt photo.* überentwickeln, überbelichten.

o·ver·dos·age [ˌ-'dəʊsɪdʒ] *n* **1.** Überdosierung *f*, Verabreichung *f* einer Überdosis. **2.** Überdosis *f*, Überdosierung *f*.

o·ver·dose [*n* ['-dəʊs; *v* ˌ-'dəʊs] **I** *n* Überdosis *f*, Überdosierung *f*. **II** *vt* überdosieren, eine Überdosis verabreichen. **III** *vi* eine Überdosis nehmen; an einer Überdosis sterben.

o·ver·eat [ˌ-'iːt] *vi* (*a.* ∼ *o.s.*) s. überessen.

o·ver·eat·ing [ˌ-'iːtɪŋ] *n* Überessen *nt*.

o·ver·ex·cit·a·bil·i·ty [ˌ-ɪkˌsaɪtə'bɪlətɪ] *n neuro., psycho.* Übererregbarkeit *f*.

o·ver·ex·cit·a·ble [ˌ-ɪk'saɪtəbl] *adj neuro., psycho.* übererregbar.

o·ver·ex·cite [ˌ-ɪk'saɪt] *vt* überreizen, zu sehr aufregen.

o·ver·ex·cit·ed [ˌ-ɪk'saɪtɪd] *adj* überreizt, zu aufgeregt; (*Kinder*) überdreht.

o·ver·ex·er·cise [ˌ-'eksəsaɪz] **I** *vt* übertrainieren. **II** *vi* übermäßig viel trainieren.

o·ver·ex·ert [ˌ-ɪk'zɜːt] *vt* überanstrengen; **to ∼ o.s.** s. überanstrengen.

o·ver·ex·er·tion [ˌ-ɪk'zɜːʃn] *n* Überanstrengung *f*.

o·ver·ex·pose [ˌ-ɪk'spəʊz] *vt* **1.** *photo.* überbelichten. **2.** s. übermäßig Kälte, Sonne, Hitze etc. aussetzen.

o·ver·ex·po·sure [ˌ-ɪk'spəʊʒər] *n photo.* Überbelichtung *f*.

o·ver·ex·tend·ed [ˌ-ɪk'stendɪd] *adj* (*Gelenk*) überdehnt, überstreckt.

o·ver·ex·ten·sion [ˌ-ɪk'stenʃn] *n* (*Gelenk*) Überstreckung *f*.

o·ver·fa·tigue [ˌ-fə'tiːg] **I** *n* Übermüdung *f*, Überanstrengung *f*. **II** *vt* übermüden, überanstrengen.

o·ver·feed [ˌ-'fiːd] *vt* überfüttern, überernähren.

o·ver·feed·ing [ˌ-'fiːdɪŋ] *n* Überfütterung *f*, Überernährung *f*.

o·ver·flow [*n* ['-fləʊ; *v* ˌ-'fləʊ] **I** *n* Überschwemmung *f*; Überlaufen *nt*, -fließen *nt*; Überschuß *m* (*of* an); *techn.* Überlauf *m*. **II** *vt* überfluten, -schwemmen; zum Überlaufen bringen. **III** *vi* überfließen, -laufen, -strömen (*with* von); überquellen, überfüllt sein (*with* mit).

overflow incontinence paradoxe Harninkontinenz *f*, Incontinentia urinae paradoxa, Ischuria paradoxa.

o·ver·flow·ing [ˌ-'fləʊɪŋ] **I** *n* Überfließen *nt*, -strömen *nt*. **II** *adj* überfließend, -strömend, -laufend.

overflow proteinuria Überlaufproteinurie *f*, -albuminurie *f*.

overflow ventil Überlaufventil *nt*.

o·ver·grow [ˌ-'grəʊ] **I** *vt* überwachsen, -wuchern; hinauswachsen über. **II** *vi* zu groß werden.

o·ver·grown [ˌ-'grəʊn] *adj* überwuchert (*with* von); übergroß, zu groß.

o·ver·growth ['-grəʊθ] *n* (Über-)Wucherung *f*, übermäßiges Wachstum *nt*.

o·ver·head traction ['-hed] *ortho.* Overhead-Traction *f*, vertikale Überkopfextension *f*, (Überkopf-)Vertikalextension *f*.

o·ver·heat [ˌ-'hiːt] **I** *vt* überhitzen, -heizen, -temperieren. **II** *vi* heißlaufen.

o·ver·heat·ing [ˌ-'hiːtɪŋ] *n* Überheizen *nt*, -hitzen *nt*.

Overhold ['-həʊld]: **O. forceps** *chir.* Overhold-Klemme *f*.

o·ver·hy·dra·tion [ˌ-haɪ'dreɪʃn] *n* Überwässerung *f*, Hyperhydratation *f*.

o·ver·in·fla·tion [ˌ-ɪn'fleɪʃn] *n* (*Lunge*) Überblähung *f*.

o·ver·lad·en [ˌ-'leɪdn] *adj* überladen, über(be)lastet.

o·ver·lap [*n* ['-læp; *v* ˌ-'læp] **I** *n* Überschneiden *nt*, -schneidung *f*, teilweise Entsprechung *od.* Deckung *f*; *techn.* Überlapp(ung *f*) *m*; (*a. phys.*) Überlagerung *f*. **II** *vi* s. überschneiden, teilweise zusammenfallen, s. teilweise decken; *techn.* überlappen, -lagern.

o·ver·lay ['əʊvərleɪ] *n psycho.* Überlagerung *f*.

o·ver·load [*n* ['-ləʊd; *v* ˌ-'ləʊd] **I** *n* Überlast(ung *f*) *f*, Überladung *f*, Überbelastung *f*. **II** *vt* überladen, über(be)lasten.

overload capacity *electr.* Überlastbarkeit *f*.

o·ver·load·ing syndrome [ˌ-'ləʊdɪŋ] Überlastungssyndrom *nt*.

o·ver·night [ˌ-'naɪt] **I** *adj* Nacht-, Übernachtungs-. **II** *adv* die Nacht über, in der Nacht, über Nacht.

o·ver·nour·ished [ˌ-'nɜrɪʃd] *adj* überernährt.

o·ver·nour·ish·ment [ˌ-'nɜrɪʃmənt] *n* Überernährung *f*.

o·ver·nu·tri·tion [ˌ-n(j)uː'trɪʃn] *n* → overnourishment.

o·ver·plus ['-plʌs] **I** *n* Überschuß *m*, Mehr *nt* (*of* an). **II** *adj* überschüssig.

o·ver·pres·sure [ˌ-'preʃər] *n* Überanstrengung *f*; *techn.* Überdruck *m*.

overpressure valve *techn.* Überdruck-, Sicherheitsventil *nt*.

o·ver·pro·duce [ˌ-prə'd(j)uːs] *vt* überproduzieren.

o·ver·pro·duc·tion ['-prəˌdʌkʃn] *n* Überproduktion *f*.

o·ver·pro·tect [ˌ-prə'tekt] *vt* (*Kind*) überbehüten, zu sehr behüten.

o·ver·pro·tec·tive [ˌ-prə'tektɪv] *adj* (*Eltern*) überängstlich, überfürsorglich.

o·ver·re·act [ˌ-rɪ'ækt] *vi* überreagieren (*to* auf).

o·ver·re·ac·tion [ˌ-rɪ'ækʃn] *n* Überreaktion *f* (*to* auf).

o·ver·re·sponse [ˌ-rɪ'spɑns] *n* → overreaction.

o·ver·ride [ˌ-'raɪd] *vt* s. übereinander schieben, s. überlagern.

o·ver·rid·ing aorta [ˌ-'raɪdɪŋ] *cardio.* überreitende Aorta *f*.

overriding pulmonary artery überreitende Pulmonalis *f*, überreitende A. pulmonalis.

o·ver·ripe ['-raɪp] *adj* überreif.

overripe cataract überreifer Star *m*, Cataracta hypermatura.

o·ver·sat·u·ra·tion [ˌ-ˌsætʃə'reɪʃn] *n* Übersättigung *f*.

o·ver·sen·si·tive [ˌ-'sensətɪv] *adj* überempfindlich (*to* gegen).

o·ver·sen·si·tive·ness [ˌ-'sensətɪvnɪs] *n* → oversensitivity.

o·ver·sen·si·tiv·i·ty [ˌ-sensə'tɪvətɪ] *n* Überempfindlichkeit *f*.

o·ver·sew [ˌ-'səʊ] *vt chir.* übernähen.

o·ver·sexed ['-sekst] *adj* einen übermäßig starken Sexualtrieb haben, sexbesessen, nymphoman(isch).

o·ver·size [ˌ-'saɪz] **I** *n* Übergröße *f*. **II** *adj* übergroß; überdimensional.

o·ver·sized ['-saɪzd] *adj* → oversize II.

o·ver·strain [ˌ-'streɪn] **I** *n* Überanstrengung *f*, -müdung *f*, -(be)lastung *f*. **II** *vt* überanstrengen, -fordern, -(be)lasten, -beanspruchen, -strapazieren. **to ∼ o.s.** s. überanstrengen.

o·ver·stretch [ˌ-'stretʃ] *vt* überdehnen, -strecken, -spannen.

overstrung

o·ver·strung ['strʌŋ] *adj* (*Nerven, Person*) überreizt.
over-the-counter *adj* rezeptfrei, frei verkäuflich.
o·ver·tire [ˌ-'taɪər] *vt* übermüden.
o·ver·tired [ˌ-'taɪərd] *adj* übermüdet.
o·ver·tone ['-təʊn] *n phys.* Oberton *m*.
o·ver·trans·fu·sion [ˌ-trænsˈfjuːʒn] *n* Übertransfusion *f*.
o·ver·use [*n* '-juːz; *v* ˌ-'juːz] I *n* Überbeanspruchung *f*, übermäßiger Gebrauch *m*. II *vt* übermäßig gebrauchen.
o·ver·ven·ti·la·tion [ˌ-ˌventɪ'leɪʃn] *n* Überbeatmung *f*, Hyperventilation *f*.
o·ver·weight ['-weɪt] I *n* Übergewicht *nt*. II *adj* zu schwer, übergewichtig.
o·ver·whelm·ing post-splenectomy infection [ˌ-'(h)welmɪŋ] *abbr.* OPSI → overwhelming post-splenectomy sepsis (syndrome).
overwhelming post-splenectomy sepsis (syndrome) *abbr.* OPSS Post-Splenektomiesepsis(syndrom *nt*) *f*, overwhelming post-splenectomy sepsis (syndrome) *abbr.* OPSS, overwhelming post-splenectomy infection *abbr.* OPSI.
o·ver·work [*n* '-wɜrk; *v* ˌ-'wɜrk] I *n* Arbeitsüberlastung *f*; Überarbeitung *f*. II *vt* überanstrengen, überstrapazieren; mit Arbeit überlasten. III *vi s.* überarbeiten.
o·ver·wrought [ˌ-'rɔːt] *adj* überarbeitet, erschöpft; überreizt.
ovi- *pref.* Ei-, Oo-, Ov(o)-, Ov(i)-.
o·vi·cide ['əʊvɪsaɪd] *n* Ovizid *nt*.
o·vi·du·cal [ˌ-'d(j)uːkl] *adj* Eileiter betr., Eileiter-, Tuben-.
o·vi·duct ['-dʌkt] *n anat.* Eileiter *m*, Tube *f*, Ovidukt *m*, Tuba/Salpinx uterina.
o·vi·duc·tal [ˌ-'dʌktl] *adj* → oviducal.
oviductal pregnancy Eileiter-, Tuben-, Tubarschwangerschaft *f*, Tubargravidität *f*, Graviditas tubaria.
o·vi·form ['-fɔːrm] *adj* → ovoid II.
o·vi·gen·e·sis [ˌ-'dʒenəsɪs] *n* → oogenesis.
o·vi·ge·net·ic [ˌ-dʒɪ'netɪk] *adj* → oogenetic.
o·vi·gen·ic [ˌ-'dʒenɪk] *adj* → oogenetic.
o·vig·e·nous [əʊ'vɪdʒənəs] *adj* → oogenetic.
o·vine ['əʊvaɪn] *adj* Schaf-.
o·vin·ia [əʊ'vɪnɪə] *pl* Schafpocken *pl*.
o·vi·par·i·ty [ˌəʊvɪ'pærətɪ] *n bio.* Oviparie *f*.
o·vip·a·rous [əʊ'vɪpərəs] *adj bio.* eierlegend, ovipar.
ovo- *pref.* → ovi-.
o·vo·cen·ter ['əʊvəʊsentər] *n* → oocenter.
o·vo·cyte ['-saɪt] *n* → oocyte.
o·vo·gen·e·sis [ˌ-'dʒenəsɪs] *n* → oogenesis.
o·vo·glob·u·lin [ˌ-'glɒbjəlɪn] *n* Ovoglobulin *nt*.
o·vo·go·ni·um [ˌ-'gəʊnɪəm] *n* → oogonium.
o·void ['əʊvɔɪd] I *n* eiförmiger Körper *m*. II *adj* eiförmig, ovoid.
ovoid articulation Sattelgelenk *nt*, Artic. sellaris.
ovoid joint → ovoid articulation.
o·vo·mu·cin [ˌəʊvə'mjuːsɪn] *n* Ovomuzin *nt*, -mucin *nt*.
o·vo·mu·coid [ˌ-'mjuːkɔɪd] *n* Ovomukoid *nt*.
o·vo·plasm ['-plæzəm] *n* Ovo-, Ooplasma *nt*.
o·vo·tes·tis [ˌ-'testɪs] *n* Ovotestis *m*.
o·vo·vi·vi·par·i·ty [ˌ-ˌvaɪvə'pærətɪ] *n bio.* Ovoviviparie *f*.
o·vo·vi·vip·a·rous [ˌ-vaɪ'vɪpərəs] *adj bio.* ovovivipar.
ov·u·lar ['ɒvjələr, 'əʊv-] *adj* ovulär, Ovular-.
ov·u·lar·y ['ɒvjələrɪː, 'əʊv-] *adj* → ovular.
ov·u·la·tion [ˌɒvjə'leɪʃn, ˌəʊv-] *n* Ei-, Follikelsprung *m*, Ovulation *f*.

ov·u·la·to·ry ['ɒvjələtɔːriː, -təʊ-] *adj* Ovulation betr., ovulatorisch, Ovulations-.
ov·ule ['ɒvjuːl, 'əʊv-] *n anat., bio.* kleines Ei *nt*, Ovulum *nt*.
ov·u·lum ['ɒvjələm] *n, pl* **-la** [-lə] → ovule.
o·vum ['əʊvəm] *n, pl* **o·va** ['əʊvə] weibliche Keimzelle *f*, Ei(zelle *f*) *nt*, Ovum *nt*.
Owen ['əʊən]: **interglobular spaces of O.** Czermak-Räume *pl*, Interglobularräume *pl*, Spatia interglobularia.
lines of O. Owen'-Linien *pl*.
owl monkey [aʊl] *immun.* Krallenaffe *m*.
Owren ['əʊwrən]: **O.'s disease** Parahämophilie (A) *f*, Owren-Syndrom *nt*, Faktor--V-Mangel *m*, Hypoproakzelerinämie *f*, -accelerinämie *f*.
ox·ac·id [ɒksˈæsɪd] *n chem.* Oxo-, Oxysäure *f*.
ox·a·cil·lin [ɒksə'sɪlɪn] *n pharm.* Oxacillin *nt*.
ox·al·al·de·hyde [ɒksəl'ældəhaɪd] *n* Oxalaldehyd *m*, Glyoxal *nt*.
ox·a·late ['ɒksəleɪt] *n* Oxalat *nt*.
ox·a·lat·ed ['-leɪtɪd] *adj* mit Oxalat versetzt *od.* behandelt.
oxalate plasma Oxalatplasma *nt*.
oxalate stone Oxalatstein *m*.
ox·a·le·mia [ˌ-'liːmɪə] *n* erhöhter Oxalatgehalt *m* des Blutes, Oxalämie *f*, Hyperoxalämie *f*.
ox·al·ic acid [ɒk'sælɪk] Oxal-, Kleesäure *f*.
oxalic gout → oxalism.
ox·al·ism ['ɒksəlɪzəm] *n* Oxalat-, Oxalsäurevergiftung *f*.
ox·a·lo·ac·e·tate [ˌɒksələʊ'æsɪteɪt, ɒkˌsæləʊ-] *n* Oxalacetat *nt*.
oxaloacetate pathway *biochem.* Oxalacetatweg *m*.
oxaloacetate transacetase Zitratsynthase *f*.
ox·a·lo·a·ce·tic acid [ˌ-ə'siːtɪk, -'set-] Oxalessigsäure *f*.
ox·a·lo·glu·tar·ic acid [ˌ-gluː'tærɪk] Oxalglutarsäure *f*.
ox·a·lo·sis [ˌɒksə'ləʊsɪs] *n patho.* Oxalose(-Syndrom *nt*) *f*.
ox·a·lo·suc·ci·nate [ˌɒksələʊ'sʌksəneɪt, ɒkˌsæləʊ-] *n* Oxalsuccinat *nt*, -sukzinat *nt*.
ox·a·lo·suc·cin·ic acid [ˌ-sək'sɪnɪk] Oxalbernsteinsäure *f*.
ox·a·lo·u·rea [ˌ-jʊə'rɪə] *n* → oxalosuccinic acid.
ox·al·u·ria [ˌɒksəl'jʊərɪə] *n* erhöhte Oxalatausscheidung *f* im Harn, Oxalurie *f*, Hyperoxalurie *f*.
ox·amide [ɒk'sæmɪd, 'ɒksəmaɪd] *n* Oxamid *nt*.
Ox antigen [ɒks] Ox-Antigen *nt*.
ox·a·to·mide [ɒk'sætəmaɪd] *n pharm.* Oxatomid *nt*.
ox·az·e·pam [ɒk'sæzəpæm] *n pharm.* Oxazepam *nt*.
ox bile [ɒks] Ochsengalle *f*, Fel bovis/tauri.
ox·el·a·din [ɒk'selədɪn] *n pharm.* Oxeladin *nt*.
ox·eth·a·zaine [ɒk'seθəzeɪn] *n pharm., anes.* Oxetacain *nt*, Oxetazin *nt*.
Ox·ford unit ['ɒksfərd] *abbr.* **O.U.** Oxford--Einheit *f abbr.* O.E.
ox·gall [ɒks] *n* → ox bile.
ox heart Ochsenherz *nt*, Bukardie *f*, Cor bovinum.
ox·id ['ɒksɪd] *n* → oxide.
ox·i·dant ['ɒksɪdənt] *n* Oxidationsmittel *nt*, Oxidans *nt*.
oxidant injury Verletzung *f* durch Oxidationsmittel.
ox·i·dase ['ɒksɪdeɪz] *n biochem.* Oxidase *f*.
oxidase-negative *adj* oxidasenegativ.
oxidase-positive *adj* oxidasepositiv.

oxidase reaction Oxidasereaktion *f*, -test *m*.
oxidase test → oxidase reaction.
ox·i·date ['ɒksɪdeɪt] *vt*, *vi* → oxidize.
ox·i·da·tion [ɒksɪ'deɪʃn] *n* Oxidation *f*, Oxidieren *nt*.
oxidation-fermentative medium OF-Medium *nt*, Oxidations-Fermentationsmedium *nt* nach Hugh.
oxidation number *chem.* Oxidationszahl *f*.
oxidation-reduction *n* Oxidations-Reduktion *f*, Oxidations-Reduktions-Reaktion *f*, Redox-Reaktion *f*.
oxidation-reduction enzyme Redoxenzym *nt*.
oxidation-reduction potential Redoxpotential *nt*.
midpoint/standard o. Normalpotential.
oxidation-reduction reaction → oxidation-reduction.
oxidation-reduction system Redoxsystem *nt*.
oxidation state *chem.* Oxidationszahl *f*.
ox·i·da·tive [ɒksɪ'deɪtɪv] *adj* Oxidation betr., mittels Oxidation, oxidativ, oxidierend.
oxidative deamination oxidative Desaminierung *f*.
oxidative decarboxylation oxidative Decarboxylierung *f*.
oxidative degradation oxidativer Abbau *m*.
oxidative phosphorylation oxidative Phosphorylierung *f*, Atmungskettenphosphorylierung *f*.
ox·ide ['ɒksaɪd] *n* Oxid *nt*.
ox·i·diz·a·ble ['ɒksɪdaɪzəbl] *adj* oxidierbar.
ox·i·dize ['ɒksɪdaɪz] *vt*, *vi* oxidieren.
ox·i·dized ['ɒksɪdaɪzd] *adj* oxidiert.
oxidized glutathione *abbr.* **GSSG** oxidiertes Glutathion *nt abbr.* GSSG.
oxidized hemoglobin → oxyhemoglobin.
ox·i·diz·er ['ɒksɪdaɪzər] *n* → oxidant.
oxi·diz·ing agent ['ɒksɪdaɪzɪŋ] *n* oxidant.
ox·i·do·re·duc·tase [ˌɒksɪdəʊrɪ'dʌkteɪz] *n* Oxidoreduktase *f*.
ox·i·do·re·duc·tion [ˌ-rɪ'dʌkʃn] *n* Oxidation-Reduktion *f*, Oxidations-Reduktions-Reaktion *f*, Redox-Reaktion *f*.
ox·i·do·sis [ˌɒksɪ'dəʊsɪs] *n* Azidose *f*, Acidose *f*.
ox·im ['ɒksɪm] *n* → oxime.
ox·ime ['ɒksɪm] *n* Oxim *nt*.
ox·im·e·ter [ɒk'sɪmətər] *n lab.* Oximeter *nt*.
ox·im·e·try [ɒk'sɪmətrɪ] *n lab.* Oximetrie *f*.
oxo- *pref.* Oxo-, Keto-, Oxy-.
ox·o acid ['ɒksəʊ] → oxacid.
ox·o·glu·ta·rate dehydrogenase [ˌɒksəʊ'gluːtəreɪt] α-Ketoglutaratdehydrogenase *f*.
2-ox·o·glu·tar·ic acid [ˌ-gluː'tærɪk] α-Ketoglutarsäure *f*.
2-ox·o·i·so·val·er·ate dehydrogenase (lipoamide) [ˌ-ˌaɪsə'væləreɪt] α-Ketoisovaleratdehydrogenase *f*.
ox·o·lin·ic acid [ˌ-'lɪnɪk] *pharm.* Oxolinsäure *f*.
5-ox·o·pro·li·nase [ˌ-'prəʊlɪneɪz] *n* 5-Oxoprolinase *f*.
5-ox·o·pro·line [ˌ-'prəʊliːn, -lɪn] *n* 5-Oxoprolin *nt*, Pyroglutaminsäure *f*.
5-ox·o·pro·lin·u·ria [ˌ-ˌprəʊlɪ'n(j)ʊərɪə] *n* Pyroglutaminazidurie *f*, hämolytische Anämie *f* mit Glutathionsynthetasedefekt.
ox·pen·tif·yl·line [ˌɒkspen'tɪfəlɪn] *n pharm.* Pentoxifyllin *nt*.
ox·pren·o·lol [ɒks'prenəʊlɒl, -lɒl] *n pharm.* Oxprenolol *nt*.
oxy- *pref.* Sauerstoff-, Oxy-, Oxi-.
ox·y·ac·id [ˌɒksɪ'æsɪd] *n* → oxacid.

ox·y·ben·zene [ˌ-'benziːn] *n* Phenol *nt*, Karbolsäure *f*, Monohydroxybenzol *nt*.
ox·y·ce·pha·lia [ˌ-sɪ'feɪljə] *n* → oxycephaly.
ox·y·ce·phal·ic [ˌ-sɪ'fælɪk] *adj* Oxyzephalie/Akrozephalie betr., von Oxyzephalie/Akrozephalie betroffen *od.* gekennzeichnet, spitz-, turmschädelig, akrozephal, oxyzephal, hypsicephal, turricephal.
ox·y·ceph·a·lous [ˌ-'sefələs] *adj* → oxycephalic.
ox·y·ceph·a·ly [ˌ-'sefəlɪ] *n* Spitz-, Turmschädel *m*, Akrozephalie *f*, -zephalus *m*, -cephalie *f*, Oxyzephalie *f*, -cephalie *f*, Hypsizephalie *f*, -cephalie *f*, Turrizephalie *f*, -cephalie *f*.
ox·y·cho·line [ˌ-'kəʊliːn, -'kɑ-] *n* Muskarin *nt*, Muscarin *nt*.
ox·y·chro·mat·ic [ˌ-krəʊ'mætɪk] *adj histol.* azidophil.
ox·y·chro·ma·tin [ˌ-'krəʊmətɪn] *n* Oxychromatin *nt*.
ox·y·ci·ne·sia [ˌ-sɪ'niːʒ(ɪ)ə] *n* Bewegungsschmerz *m*.
ox·y·co·done [ˌ-'kəʊdəʊn] *n pharm.* Oxycodon *nt*.
ox·y·dase *n old* → oxidase.
ox·y·do·re·duc·tase [ˌ-] *n* oxidoreductase.
ox·y·es·ter bond [ˌ-'estər] Oxyester-, Sauerstoffesterbindung *f*.
ox·y·es·the·sia [ˌ-es'θiːʒ(ɪ)ə] *n neuro.* Überempfindlichkeit *f*, Hyperästhesie *f*, Hyperaesthesia *f*.
ox·y·gen ['ɑksɪdʒən] *n abbr.* **O** Sauerstoff *m*; *chem.* Oxygen *nt*, Oxygenium *nt abbr.* **O**.
oxygen acceptor *chem.* Sauerstoffakzeptor *m*.
oxygen apparatus Sauerstoff-, Atemgerät *nt*.
ox·y·gen·ase ['dʒəneɪz] *n* Oxygenase *f*, Oxigenase *f*.
ox·y·gen·ate ['dʒəneɪt] *vt* oxygenieren.
ox·y·gen·at·ed blood ['dʒəneɪtɪd] arterielles/sauerstoffreiches Blut *nt*, Arterienblut *nt*.
oxygenated hemoglobin → oxyhemoglobin.
ox·y·gen·a·tion [ˌ-dʒə'neɪʃn] *n* Oxygenisation *f*, Oxygenation *f*, Oxygenieren *nt*, Oxygenierung *f*.
oxygenation deficiency mangelhafte Oxygenation *f*.
ox·y·gen·a·tor [ˌ-dʒə'neɪtər] *n* Oxygenator *m*.
oxygen bath Sauerstoffbad *nt*.
oxygen capacity Sauerstoffbindungskapazität *f*.
oxygen consumption Sauerstoffverbrauch *m*. **basal/resting o.** Ruhesauerstoffverbrauch, Sauerstoffverbrauch in Ruhe.
oxygen consumption index Sauerstoffverbrauchsindex *m*.
oxygen cycle *biochem.* Sauerstoffkreislauf *m*.
oxygen debt *physiol.* Sauerstoffschuld *f*.
oxygen deficiency Sauerstoffmangel *m*, Hypoxie *f*.
oxygen deficit Sauerstoffdefizit *nt*, -mangel *m*.
oxygen dissociation curve *physiol.* Sauerstoffdissoziationskurve *f*, Sauerstoffbindungskurve *f*.
oxygen electrode Sauerstoffelektrode *f*.

oxygen-enriched *adj* mit Sauerstoff angereichert.
oxygen-hemoglobin dissociation curve → oxygen dissociation curve.
ox·y·gen·ic [ˌ-'dʒenɪk] *adj* sauerstoffhaltig.
oxygen mask Sauerstoffmaske *f*.
oxygen partial pressure *abbr.* P_{O_2}, pO_2 Sauerstoffpartialdruck *m*, O_2-Partialdruck *m abbr.* P_{O_2}, pO_2.
oxygen poisoning Sauerstoffvergiftung *f*.
oxygen-producing *adj* sauerstofferzeugend.
oxygen-requiring *adj* sauerstofferfordernd.
oxygen saturation *physiol.* Sauerstoffsättigung *f*.
oxygen tension *physiol.* Sauerstoffspannung *f*.
oxygen tent Sauerstoffzelt *nt*.
oxygen therapy Sauerstofftherapie *f*.
oxygen-tolerant *adj* aerotolerant.
oxygen transferase Sauerstofftransferase *f*, Dioxygenase *f*.
oxygen utilization Sauerstoffausnutzung *f*, -utilisation *f*.
oxygen utilization coefficient Sauerstoffausnutzungskoeffizient *m*, Sauerstoffutilisationskoeffizient *m*.
oxyhemoglobin dissociation curve → oxygen dissociation curve.
ox·y·lu·cif·er·in [ˌ-luː'sɪfərɪn] *n* Oxyluciferin *nt*.
ox·y·me·taz·o·line [ˌ-mə'tæzəliːn, -'metəzəʊ-] *n pharm.* Oxymetazolin *nt*.
ox·y·meth·o·lone [ˌ-'meθələʊn] *n pharm.* Oxymetholon *nt*.
ox·ym·e·try [ɑk'sɪmətrɪ] *n* → oximetry.
ox·y·my·o·glo·bin [ˌɑksɪ'maɪə'gləʊbɪn] *n* Oxymyoglobin *nt*.
ox·y·ner·von [ˌ-'nɜrvɑn] *n* Oxynervonsäure *f*.
ox·y·neu·rine [ˌ-'njʊərɪn, -'nʊ-] *n* Betain *nt*, Trimethylglykokoll *nt*, Glykokollbetain *nt*.
ox·yn·tic cell [ɑk'sɪntɪk] (*Magen*) Beleg-, Parietalzelle *f*.
ox·y·o·pia [ˌɑksɪ'əʊpɪə] *n ophthal.* extreme Scharfsichtigkeit *f*, Oxyopie *f*, Oxyopia *f*.
ox·y·o·sis [ˌ-'əʊsɪs] *n* Azidose *f*, Acidose *f*.
ox·y·os·mia [ˌ-'ɑzmɪə] *n neuro.* pathologisch gesteigertes Geruchsvermögen *nt*, olfaktorische Hyperästhesie *f*, Hyperosmie *f*.
ox·y·os·phre·sia [ˌ-ɑs'friːʒ(ɪ)ə] *n* → oxyosmia.
ox·y·per·tine [ˌ-'pertiːn] *n pharm.* Oxypertin *nt*.
ox·y·phen·bu·ta·zone [ˌ-fen'bjuːtəzəʊn] *n pharm.* Oxyphenbutazon *nt*.
ox·y·phen·cy·cli·mine [ˌ-fen'saɪkləmiːn] *n pharm.* Oxyphencyclimin *nt*.
ox·y·phen·yl·a·mi·no·pro·pi·on·ic acid

[ˌ-ˌfenləˌmiːnəʊˌprəʊpɪ'ɑnɪk, -'əʊnɪk, -ˌfiːnl-] Tyrosin *nt abbr.* Tyr.
ox·y·phen·yl·eth·yl·a·mine [ˌ-ˌfenlˌeθɪl'æmɪn] *n* Tyramin *nt*, Tyrosamin *nt*.
ox·y·phil ['-fɪl] **I** *n* oxyphile Zelle *f*. **II** *adj* oxy-, azidophil.
oxyphil cells (*Nebenschilddrüse*) Welsh'-Zellen *pl*, oxyphile Zellen *pl*.
oxyphil cell tumor Hürthle-Tumor *m*, -Zelladenom *nt*, -Struma *f*, oxyphiles Schilddrüsenadenom *nt*.
oxyphil chromatin → oxychromatin.
ox·y·phile ['-faɪl] *n, adj* → oxyphil.
oxyphil granules azidophile Granula *pl*.
ox·y·phil·ic [ˌ-'fɪlɪk] *adj* → oxyphil II.
oxyphilic cells → oxyphil cells.
oxyphilic erythroblast → oxyphilic normoblast.
oxyphilic normoblast orthochromatischer Normoblast *m*.
ox·yph·i·lous [ɑk'sɪfələs] *adj* → oxyphil II.
ox·y·pho·nia [ˌɑksɪ'fəʊnɪə] *n* Oxyphonie *f*.
ox·y·pu·rine [ˌ-'pjʊəriːn, -ɪn] *n* Oxypurin *nt*.
ox·y·te·tra·cy·cline [ˌ-ˌtetrə'saɪkliːn] *n pharm.* Oxytetracyclin *nt*.
ox·y·thi·a·mine [ˌ-'θaɪəmiːn, -mɪn] *n* Oxythiamin *nt*.
ox·y·to·cia [ˌ-'təʊʃ(ɪ)ə] *n gyn.* Sturzgeburt *f*.
ox·y·to·cic [ˌ-'təʊsɪk] **I** *n* Wehenmittel *nt*, Oxytocicum *nt*. **II** *adj* die Geburt fördernd *od.* beschleunigend.
ox·y·to·cin [ˌ-'təʊs(ɪ)n] *n* Oxytozin *nt*, Oxytocin *nt*.
ox·y·u·ria [ˌ-'(j)ʊərɪə] *n* → oxyuriasis.
ox·y·u·ri·a·sis [ˌ-jʊə'raɪəsɪs] *n* Oxyuriasis *f*; Enterobiasis *f*.
ox·y·u·ri·cide [ˌ-'jʊərəsaɪd] *n* Oxyurizid *nt*.
ox·y·u·rid [ˌ-'jʊərɪd] *n micro.* Oxyurid *m*.
Ox·y·u·ri·dae [ˌ-'jʊərɪdiː] *pl micro.* Madenwürmer *pl*, Oxyuridae *pl*.
ox·y·u·ri·o·sis [ˌ-ˌjʊərɪ'əʊsɪs] *n* → oxyuriasis.
Ox·y·u·ris [ˌ-'jʊərɪs] *n micro.* Oxyuris *f*. **O. vermicularis** Madenwurm *m*, Enterobius/Oxyuris vermicularis.
Ox·y·u·roid [ˌ-'jʊərɔɪd] *n micro.* Oxyurid *nt*.
Ox·y·u·roi·dea [ˌ-jʊərɔɪ'dɪə] *pl micro.* Oxyuroidea *f*.
oz. *abbr.* → ounce.
Oz allotypes Oz-Allotypen *pl*.
Oz antigens Oz-Antigene *pl*.
o·ze·na [əʊ'ziːnə] *n* Stinknase *f*, Ozäna *f*, Rhinitis atrophicans cum foetore.
o·ze·nous [əʊ'ziːnəs] *adj* Ozäna betr.
o·zone ['əʊzəʊn] *n abbr.* O_3 Ozon *nt abbr.* O_3.
ozone layer Ozonschicht *f*.
ozon·ic [əʊ'zɑnɪk, əʊ'zəʊ-] *adj* ozonhaltig, ozonisch, Ozon-.
o·zo·nide ['-əʊzəʊnaɪd] *n* Ozonid *nt*.
o·zon·i·za·tion [əʊˌzəʊnɪ'zeɪʃn] *n chem.* Ozonisierung *f*.
o·zon·ize [ˌ-'əʊzənaɪz] *vt* ozonisieren, mit Ozon behandeln.
o·zo·nom·e·ter [əʊzə'nɑmɪtər] *n* Ozonmesser *m*, Ozonometer *nt*.
o·zo·sto·mia [əʊzə'stəʊmɪə] *n* (übler) Mundgeruch *m*, Atemgeruch *m*, Halitosis *f*, Halitose *f*, Kakostomie *f*, Ozostomia *f*, Foetor ex ore.
Ozzard ['ɑzərd]: **O.'s filaria** Mansonella ozzardi.
O.'s filariasis/mansonelliasis Mansonella-ozzardi-Infektion *f*, Mansonelliasis *f*.

P

P *abbr.* 1. → permeability. 2. → phosphorus. 3. → poise. 4. → probability.
P₁ *abbr.* → parental generation.
p *abbr.* → pico-.
p- *abbr.* → para-.
Ψ *abbr.* → pseudouridine.
p.a. *abbr.* → posteroanterior.
Pa *abbr.* 1. → pascal. 2. → protactinium.
PAB *abbr.* → para-aminobenzoic acid.
PABA *abbr.* → para-aminobenzoic acid.
PABA test (*Pankreas*) PABA-Test *m*.
pab·u·lum ['pæbjələm] *n* Nahrung *f*.
PAC *abbr.* → premature atrial contraction.
pac·chi·o·ni·an [,pæki'əʊnjən]: **p. bodies** → p. granulations.
p. depressions Foveolae granulares.
p. (granular) foveolae → p. depressions.
p. granulations Pacchioni'-Granulationen *pl*, Arachnoidalzotten *pl*, Granulationes arachnoideae.
pace [peɪs] I *n* Schritt *m*, Gang(art *f*) *m*, Tritt *m*; Tempo *nt*. **~ for ~** Schritt für Schritt. **to make/set the ~** das Tempo angeben. **to keep ~ with** Schritt halten mit. **to stand/stay the ~ with** Schritt halten. II *vt* hin u. her gehen, auf u. abgehen; (*Raum*) ab-, durchschreiten.
pace·mak·er ['peɪsmeɪkər] *n physiol.* Reizbildungszentrum *nt*, Schrittmacher *m*, Pacemaker *m*.
p. of heart 1. *physiol.* Herzschrittmacher. 2. *card.* künstlicher Herzschrittmacher, Pacemaker *m*.
pacemaker cell *physiol.* Schrittmacherzelle *f*.
pacemaker potential *physiol.* Schrittmacherpotential *nt*.
pacemaker step *chem.* geschwindigkeitsbestimmender Schritt *m*.
pacemaker system *physiol.* Erregungsbildungs-, Schrittmachersystem *nt*.
pacemaker tissue *physiol.* Schrittmachergewebe *nt*.
pa·chom·e·ter [pə'kɒmɪtər] *n* → pachymeter.
pachy- *pref.* Dick-, Pachy-.
pach·y·bleph·a·ron [pæki'blefərɒn] *n ophthal.* Pachyblepharon *nt*; Tylosis ciliaris.
pach·y·bleph·a·ro·sis [,-blefə'rəʊsɪs] *n* → pachyblepharon.
pach·y·ce·pha·lia [,-sɪ'feɪlɪə] *n* → pachycephaly.
pach·y·ce·phal·ic [,-sɪ'fælɪk] *adj embryo.* Pachyzephalie betr., pachyzephal.
pach·y·ceph·a·lous [,-'sefələs] *adj* → pachycephalic.
pach·y·ceph·a·ly [,-'sefəlɪ] *n embryo.* Pachyzephalie *f*.
pach·y·chei·lia [,-'kaɪlɪə] *n* Pachycheilie *f*, -chilie *f*.
pach·y·chi·li·a *n* → pachycheilia.
pach·y·cho·lia [,-'kəʊlɪə] *n patho.* Pachycholie *f*.
pach·y·chro·mat·ic [,-krəʊ'mætɪk] *adj histol.* pachromatisch, pachychrom.

pach·y·dac·tyl·ia [,-dæk'tɪlɪə, -jə] *n* → pachydactyly.
pach·y·dac·ty·ly [,-'dæktəlɪ] *n embryo.* Pachydaktylie *f*.
pach·y·der·ma [,-'dɜrmə] *n derm.* Pachydermie *f*, -dermia *f*.
pach·y·der·ma·to·cele [,-'dɜrmətəsi:l] *n* 1. Fall-, Schlaffhaut *f*, Cutis-laxa-Syndrom *nt*, generalisierte Elastolyse *f*, Zuviel--Haut-Syndrom *nt*, Dermatochalasis *f*, Dermatolysis *f*, Dermatomegalie *f*, Chalazodermie *f*, Chalodermie *f*. 2. Lappenelephantiasis *f*, Elephantiasis neuromatosis.
pach·y·der·ma·to·sis [,-,dɜrmə'təʊsɪs] *n* → pachyderma.
pach·y·der·ma·tous [,-'dɜrmətəs] *adj* Pachydermie betr., dickhäutig, pachyderm.
pach·y·der·mia [,-'dɜrmɪə] *n* → pachyderma.
pach·y·der·mic [,-'dɜrmɪk] *adj* → pachydermatous.
pach·y·der·mo·per·i·os·to·sis (syndrome) [,-,dɜrmə,perɪɒs'təʊsɪs] Pachydermoperiostose *f*, Touraine-Solente-Golé-Syndrom *nt*, familiäre Pachydermoperiostose *f*, idiopathische hypertrophische Osteoarthropathie *f*, Akropachydermie *f* mit Pachydermoperiostose, Hyperostosis generalisata mit Pachydermie.
pach·y·glos·sia [,-'glɒsɪə] *n* Pachyglossie *f*; Makroglossie *f*.
pach·y·gy·ria [,-'dʒaɪrɪə] *n* Pachygyrie *f*; Makrogyrie *f*.
pach·y·hy·me·nia [,-haɪ'mi:nɪə] *n* → pachymenia.
pach·y·lep·to·men·in·gi·tis [,-,leptəmenɪn'dʒaɪtɪs] *n* Entzündung *f* der harten u. weichen Hirnhäute, Pachyleptomeningitis *f*, Meningitis *f*.
pach·y·me·nia [,-'mi:nɪə] *n* 1. *derm.* Pachydermie *f*, -dermia *f*. 2. Schleimhautverdickung *f*, Pachymenie *f*.
pach·y·men·in·gi·tis [,-menɪn'dʒaɪtɪs] *n* Entzündung *f* der Dura mater, Dura--Entzündung *f*, Dura mater-Entzündung *f*, Pachymeningitis *f*.
pach·y·men·in·gop·a·thy [,-menɪn'gɒpəθɪ] *n* Erkrankung *f* der Dura mater, Pachymeningopathie *f*.
pach·y·me·ninx [,-'mi:nɪŋks] *n, pl* **-me·nin·ges** [-mɪ'nɪndʒi:z] äußere Hirn- u. Rückenmarkshaut *f*, Dura *f*, Dura mater.
pa·chym·e·ter [pə'kɪmətər] *n* Pachymeter *nt*.
pach·y·ne·ma [,pækɪ'ni:mə] *n* → pachytene.
pa·chyn·sis [pə'kɪnsɪs] *n patho.* pathologische Verdickung *f*.
pach·y·o·nych·ia [,pækɪəʊ'nɪkɪə] *n derm.* Verdickung *f* der Nagelplatte, Pachyonychie *f*, Pachyonychia *f*, Skleronychie *f*, Onychauxis *f*.
pach·y·o·tia [,pækɪ'əʊʃɪə] *n* Pachyotie *f*.
pach·y·per·i·os·ti·tis [,-,perɪɒs'taɪtɪs] *n*

ortho. proliferative Periostitis *f*, Pachyperiostitis *f*.
pach·y·per·i·to·ni·tis [,-perɪtə'naɪtɪs] *n patho.* Pachyperitonitis *f*.
pach·y·pleu·ri·tis [,-plu:'raɪtɪs] *n patho.* 1. Fibrothorax *m*. 2. Pleuritis fibroplastica.
pach·y·sal·pin·gi·tis [,-,sælpɪn'dʒaɪtɪs] *n patho., gyn.* 1. chronisch interstitielle Salpingitis *f*. 2. parenchymatöse Salpingitis *f*.
pachysalpingo-ovaritis *n patho., gyn.* chronisch parenchymatöse Entzündung *f* von Eileiter u. Eierstock.
pach·y·tene ['-ti:n] *n* Pachytän *nt*.
Pa·cif·ic coast dog tick [pə'sɪfɪk] *micro.* Dermacentor occidentalis.
Pacini [pɑ'si:nɪ]: **P.'s corpuscles** Vater--Pacini'-(Lamellen-)Körperchen *pl*, Corpuscula lamellosa.
pa·cin·i·an [pə'si:nɪən]: **p. corpuscles** → Pacini's corpuscles.
p.-corpuscle sensor Sensor *m* der Vater--Pacini-Körperchen, PC-Sensor *m*.
pa·cin·i·tis [pæsɪ'naɪtɪs] *n* Entzündung *f* der Vater-Pacini'-Körperchen.
pack [pæk] I *n* 1. Ballen *m*, Pack(en *m*) *m*, Bündel *nt*; Packung *f*, Schachtel *f*, Päckchen *nt*, Paket *nt*. 2. Packung *f*; Wickel *m*. 3. *bio.* Rudel *nt*; Meute *f*. II *vt* 4. ein-, zusammen-, ab-, verpacken. 5. bepacken, beladen. 6. konservieren.
packed blood cells [pækt] Erythrozytenkonzentrat *nt*, Erythrozytenkonserve *f*.
packed-cell volume *abbr.* **PCV** (venöser) Hämatokrit *m*.
packed human blood cells → packed blood cells.
packed human red cells → packed blood cells.
packed red cells → packed blood cells.
pack·ing ['pækɪŋ] *n* 1. (Ver-)Packen *nt*; Verpackung *f*. 2. Konservierung *f*. 3. *radiol.* Packing *nt*, Packmethode *f*. 4. Füllmaterial *nt*, Füllung *f*.
P-A conduction time *card.* PA-Intervall *nt*.
PAD *abbr.* → primary afferent depolarization.
pad [pæd] I *n* 1. (Schutz-)Polster *nt*, Kissen *nt*; (Knie-)Schützer *m*. 2. *anat.* (Fuß-)Ballen *m*; *allg.* Fettkörper *m*, (Fett-)Polster *nt*. 3. Kompresse *f*. 4. (Schreib-)Block *m*. II *vt* (aus-)polstern, wattieren, füttern.
pad out *vt* → pad II.
pad·ded ['pædɪd] *adj* gepolstert, wattiert.
pad·ding ['pædɪŋ] *n* 1. (Aus-)Polstern *nt*, Wattieren *nt*. 2. (Aus-)Polsterung *f*, Wattierung *f*.
Padgett ['pædʒɪt]: **P.'s dermatome** *chir.* Padgett-Dermatom *nt*.
Pae·cil·o·my·ces [pɪ,sɪləʊ'maɪsi:z] *n micro.* Paecilomyces *m*.
paed(o)- *pref.* → pedo-¹.
PAF *abbr.* → platelet activating factor.
Paget ['pædʒɪt]: **P.'s cell** Paget-Zelle *f*.
P.'s disease 1. Paget-Krebs *m*, Krebsekzem *nt* der Brust, Morbus Paget *m*. 2.

extramammärer Morbus Paget *m.* 3. →
P.'s disease of bone.
P.'s disease of bone Paget-Krankheit *f*, -Syndrom *nt*, Morbus Paget *m, inf.* Knochen-Paget *m*, Osteodystrophia/Ostitis deformans.
P.'s disease of the breast → P.'s disease 1.
P.'s disease of the nipple → P.'s disease 1.
extramammary P.'s disease → P.'s disease 2.
juvenile P.'s disease juveniler Morbus Paget *m*, Hyperostosis corticalis deformans juvenilis.
P.'s sarcoma Paget-Sarkom *nt*.
pag·et·oid bone ['pædʒətɔɪd] *ortho.* pagetoider Knochen *m*.
pagetoid cell pagetoide Zelle *f*.
pagetoid deafness Schwerhörigkeit *f* bei Osteitis deformans.
pagetoid reticulosis Morbus Woringer--Kolopp *m*, pagetoide/epidermotrope Retikulose *f*.
pa·go·pha·gia [ˌpeɪɡə'feɪdʒ(ɪ)ə] *n patho.* Pagophagie *f*.
pa·go·plex·ia [ˌ-'pleksɪə] *n* Erfrierung *f*, Kongelation *f*, Congelatio *f*.
PAH *abbr.* → para-aminohippuric acid.
PAHA *abbr.* → para-aminohippuric acid.
PAH clearance *physiol.* PAH-Clearance *f*.
Pahvant Valley fever/plague ['pɑːvənt] Tularämie *f*, Hasen-, Nagerpest *f*, Lemming-Fieber *nt*, Ohara-, Francis-Krankheit *f*.
pai·dol·o·gy [peɪ'dɑləʒɪ, paɪ-] *n* → pedology.
pain [peɪn] **I** *n* 1. Schmerz(en *pl*) *m*, Schmerzempfindung *f*. **to aggravate ~** Schmerzen verschlimmern. **to be in ~** Schmerzen haben. 2. (Geburts-)Wehen *pl.* 3. *fig.* Leid *nt*, Kummer *m*, Qualen *f*; **~s** *pl* Mühen *pl.* **II** *vt* jdm. Schmerzen bereiten, jdm. weh tun.
p. on coughing Hustenschmerz, Schmerzen *pl* beim Husten.
p. in the head Kopfschmerz(en *pl*) *m*, Kopfweh *nt*, Kephalgie *f*, Kephalalgie *f*, Kephal(a)ea *f*, Cephalgia *f*, Cephalalgia *f*, Cephal(a)ea *f*, Kephalodynie *f*, Zephalgie *f*, Zephalalgie *f*.
p. on palpation Druckschmerz.
p. on percussion Klopfschmerz.
p. on sneezing Niesschmerz, Schmerzen *pl* beim Niesen.
p. on weight bearing (*Gelenk*) Belastungsschmerz.
pain-control system *physiol.* Schmerzkontrollsystem *nt*.
pain dysfunction syndrome Costen-Syndrom *nt*, temporomandibuläres Syndrom *nt*.
pained [peɪnd] *adj* (*Gesichtsausdruck*) schmerzerfüllt, gequält.
pain epicenter Schmerzzentrum *nt*.
pain fibers Schmerzfasern *pl*.
pain-free *adj* schmerzfrei.
pain·ful ['peɪnfəl] *adj* 1. schmerzend, schmerzlich, schmerzhaft. 2. beschwerlich, mühsam.
painful bruising syndrome Erythrozytenautosensibilisierung *f*, schmerzhafte Ekchymosen-Syndrom *nt*, painful bruising syndrome (*nt*).
painful hematuria schmerzhafte Hämaturie *f*.
pain·ful·ness ['peɪnfəlnɪs] *n* 1. Schmerzhaftigkeit *f*, Schmerzlichkeit *f*. 2. Beschwerlichkeit *f*.
painful paraplegia Paraplegia dolorosa.
painful points Valleix-Punkte *pl*.
painful toe Hallux dolorosus.
pain-induced reflex contracture schmerzbedingt-reflektorische Kontraktur *f*.

pain inhibition Schmerzhemmung *f*.
pain intensity Schmerzintensität *f*.
pain·kil·ler ['peɪnkɪlər] *n* Schmerzmittel *nt*, schmerzstillendes Mittel *nt*, Analgen *nt*, Analgetikum *nt*.
pain·kil·ling ['peɪnkɪlɪŋ] *adj* schmerzstillend.
pain·less ['peɪnlɪs] *adj* schmerzlos.
painless death leichter/schmerzloser Tod *m*, Euthanasie *f*.
painless hematuria schmerzlose Hämaturie *f*.
pain·less·ness ['peɪnlɪsnɪs] *n* Schmerzlosigkeit *f*.
pain point *physiol.* Schmerzpunkt *m*.
pain quality Schmerzqualität *f*.
pain reaction Schmerzreaktion *f*.
pain receptor Schmerzrezeptor *m*.
pain relief Schmerzlinderung *f*, -stillung *f*.
pain sensation *physiol.* Schmerzempfindung *f*.
pain sense Schmerzsinn *m*.
pain sensitivity Schmerzempfindsamkeit *f*.
pain spots Schmerzpunkte *pl*.
pain stimulus Schmerzreiz *m*.
paint [peɪnt] **I** *n* 1. Farbe *f*, Lack *m*. 2. *pharm., derm.* (Farbstoff-)Lösung *f*; Tinktur *f*. **II** *vt* an-, bemalen, anstreichen. **III** *vi* malen; streichen.
paint·er's colic ['peɪntər] *patho.* Bleikolik *f*, Colica saturnina.
P-A interval *card.* PA-Intervall *nt*.
pain therapy Schmerztherapie *f*.
pain threshold Schmerzschwelle *f*.
pain-tolerance threshold Schmerztoleranzschwelle *f*.
pair [peər] **I** *n allg.* Paar *nt*; Ehepaar *nt*; *zoo.* Paar *nt*, Pärchen *nt*. **II** *vt* paarweise *od.* in Paaren ordnen. **III** *vi* 1. Paare bilden, s. verbinden *od.* vereinigen (*with* mit). 2. *bio.* s. paaren.
pair off *vt, vi* → pair II, III.
paired [peərd] *adj* paarig, paarweise, gepaart.
paired beat *card.* Bigeminus *m*.
paired-pulse stimulation *physiol.* paarige Stimulation *f*.
pair·ing ['peərɪŋ] *n bio.* Paarung *f*.
pa·ja·ro·el·lo (tick) [pɑhɑrə'weɪoʊ] *micro.* Ornithodoros coriaceus.
Palade [pɛ'leɪd]: **P.'s granules** Palade--Granula *pl*, Ribosom *nt*.
pa·lae·cer·e·bel·lum [ˌpeɪlɪsərə'beləm, ˌpælɪ-] *n* → palaeocerebellum.
pa·lae·cor·tex [ˌ-'kɔːrteks] *n* → palaeocortex.
pa·lae·o·cer·e·bel·lum [ˌpeɪlɪoʊsərə'beləm, ˌpælɪoʊ-] *n* Paläozerebellum *nt*, Pal(a)eocerebellum *nt*.
pa·lae·o·cor·tex [ˌ-'kɔːrteks] *n* Paläokortex *m*, Pal(a)eocortex *m*.
pa·lae·o·cor·ti·cal [ˌ-'kɔːrtɪkl] *adj* Paläokortex betr., paläokortikal.
pa·lae·o·pal·li·um [ˌ-'pælɪəm] *n* Paläopallium *nt*, Pal(a)eopallium *nt*.
palat- *pref.* → palato-.
pal·a·tal ['pælətl] *adj* Gaumen/Palatum betr., palatal, Gaumen-.
palatal abscess Gaumenabszeß *m*.
palatal arch Gaumenbogen *m*.
palatal component of intermaxillary segment *embryo.* Gaumenanteil *m* des Zwischenkiefersegments.
palatal nystagmus Nystagmus veli palatini.
palatal reflex Gaumenreflex *m*.
palatal retraction *HNO* Velotractio *f*.
pal·ate ['pælət] *n* Gaumen *m*; *anat.* Palatum *nt*.
palate bone → palatine bone.

palate hook *HNO* Gaumensegelhaken *m*.
palate retractor → palate hook.
pa·lat·i·form [pə'lætɪfɔːrm] *adj* gaumenförmig.
pal·a·tine ['pælətaɪn, -tɪn] *adj* Gaumen betr., palatal, Gaumen-.
palatine aponeurosis Gaumenaponeurose *f*, Aponeurosis palatina.
palatine arch: anterior p. vorderer Gaumenbogen *m*, Arcus palatoglossus.
posterior p. hinterer Gaumenbogen *m*, Arcus palatopharyngeus.
palatine artery Gaumenschlagader *f*, A. palatina.
ascending p. aufsteigende Gaumenschlagader, Palatina *f* ascendens, A. palatina ascendens.
descending p. absteigende Gaumenschlagader, Palatina *f* descendens, A. palatina descendens.
greater p. große Gaumenschlagader, Palatina *f* major, A. palatina major.
lesser p.ies kleine Gaumenarterien *pl*, Aa. palatinae minores.
major p. → greater p.
minor p.ies → lesser p.ies.
palatine bone Gaumenbein *nt*, Os palatinum.
palatine canal Canalis palatinus.
accessory p.s → lesser p.s.
anterior p. 1. Canalis incisivus. 2. For. incisivum.
greater p. Canalis palatinus major.
lesser p.s Canales palatini minores.
posterior p.s → lesser p.s.
palatine crest Crista palatina.
palatine folds, (transverse) Plicae palatinae transversae.
palatine foramen For. palatinum.
accessory p.mina Forr. palatina minora.
anterior p. For. incisivum.
greater p. → posterior p.
lesser p.mina Forr. palatina minora.
posterior p. For. palatinum majus.
palatine incisure Fissura pterygoidea.
p. of Henle Inc. sphenopalatina (ossis palatini).
palatine glands Gaumen(speichel)drüsen *pl*, Gll. palatinae.
palatine grooves Sulci palatini.
palatine lamina of maxilla Proc. palatinus (maxillae).
palatine nerve N. palatinus.
anterior p. → greater p.
greater p. großer Gaumennerv *m*, Palatinus *m* major, N. palatinus major.
lesser p.s kleine Gaumennerven *pl*, Nn. palatini minores.
medial p. N. palatinus medius.
middle p. → medial p.
posterior p. N. palatinus posterior.
palatine papilla Papilla incisiva.
palatine process of maxilla Gaumenfortsatz *m* des Oberkieferknochens, Proc. palatinus (maxillae).
palatine protuberance Torus palatinus.
palatine raphe Gaumenleiste *f*, Raphe palati.
palatine reflex Gaumenreflex *m*.
palatine shelves *embryo.* Gaumenplatten *pl*.
palatine spines Spinae palatinae.
palatine sulcus Sulcus palatinus.
greater p. of maxilla Sulcus palatinus major maxillae.
greater p. of palatine bone Sulcus palatinus major ossis palatini.
p.i of maxilla Sulci palatini maxillae.
p.i of palatine bone Sulci palatini ossis palatini.
palatine suture: median p. mediane Gaumennaht *f*, Sutura palatina mediana.

palatine tonsil

transverse p. quere Gaumennaht *f*, Sutura palatina transversa.
palatine tonsil Gaumenmandel *f*, Tonsilla palatina.
palatine uvula (Gaumen-)Zäpfchen *nt*, Uvula *f* (palatina).
palatine vein, (external) (seitliche) Gaumenvene *f*, V. palatina (externa).
pa·lat·i·nose [pə'lætɪnəʊz] *n* Palatinose *f*, Isomaltulose *f*.
pal·a·ti·tis [pælə'taɪtɪs] *n* Gaumenentzündung *f*, Uranitis *f*.
palato- *pref.* Gaumen-, Palato-.
pal·a·to·eth·moi·dal suture [‚pælətəʊeθ-'mɔɪdl] Sutura palato-ethmoidalis.
pal·a·to·glos·sal [‚-'glɒsəl, -'glɔ-] *adj* Gaumen/Palatum u. Zunge/Glossa betr., palatolingual, glossopalatinal.
palatoglossal arch → palatine arch, anterior.
palatoglossal muscle → palatoglossus (muscle).
pal·a·to·glos·sus (muscle) [‚-'glɒsəs, -'glɔ-] Palatoglossus *m*, M. palatoglossus.
pal·a·to·gram ['-græm] *n* HNO Palatogramm *nt*.
pal·a·to·graph ['-græf] *n* HNO Palatograph *m*.
pal·a·tog·ra·phy [pælə'tɒgrəfɪ] *n* HNO Palatographie *f*.
pal·a·to·max·il·lar·y [‚pælətəʊ'mæksɪlərɪ] *adj* Gaumen/Palatum u. Oberkiefer/Maxilla betr. *od.* verbindend, palatomaxillär.
palatomaxillary arch Gaumenbogen *m*.
palatomaxillary suture Sutura palatomaxillaris.
pal·a·to·my·o·graph [‚-'maɪəgræf] *n* HNO Palatomyograph *m*.
pal·a·to·my·og·ra·phy [‚-maɪ'ɒgrəfɪ] *n* HNO Palatomyographie *f*.
pal·a·to·na·sal [‚-'neɪzl] *adj* Gaumen/Palatum u. Nase/Nasus betr. *od.* verbindend, palatonasal.
pal·a·top·a·gus [pælə'tɒpəgəs] *n* embryo. Palatopagus *m*.
pal·a·to·pha·ryn·ge·al [‚pælətəʊfə'rɪndʒɪəl, -‚færɪn'dʒiːəl] *adj* Gaumen/Palatum u. Rachen/Pharynx betr. *od.* verbindend, palatopharyngeal.
palatopharyngeal arch → palatine arch, posterior.
palatopharyngeal muscle → palatopharyngeus (muscle).
pal·a·to·pha·ryn·ge·us (muscle) [‚-fə'rɪndʒɪəs, -‚færɪn'dʒiːəs] Palatopharyngeus *m*, *old* M. pharyngopalatinus, M. palatopharyngeus.
pal·a·to·phar·yn·gor·rha·phy [‚-‚færɪn'gɔrəfɪ] *n* HNO Staphylouranorrhaphie *f*.
pal·a·to·plas·ty ['-plæstɪ] *n* HNO Gaumen-, Palatoplastik *f*.
pal·a·to·ple·gia [‚-'pliːdʒ(ɪ)ə] *n* Gaumensegellähmung *f*.
pal·a·tor·rha·phy [pælə'tɔrəfɪ] *n* HNO Gaumennaht *f*, Urano-, Staphylorrhaphie *f*.
pal·a·to·sal·pin·ge·us (muscle) [‚pælətəʊ-sæl'pɪndʒɪəs] Tensor *m* veli palatini, M. tensor veli palatini.
pal·a·tos·chi·sis [pælə'tɒskəsɪs] *n* embryo. Gaumenspalte *f*, Palato-, Uranoschisis *f*, Palatum fissum.
pal·a·to·vag·i·nal canal [‚pælətəʊ'vædʒ-ənl] Canalis palatovaginalis.
palatovaginal sulcus Sulcus palatovaginalis.
pa·la·tum [pə'leɪtəm, -'lɑː-] *n*, *pl* **-ta** [-tə] *n* palate.
pale- *pref.* → paleo-.
pale [peɪl] **I** *adj* blaß, bleich, fahl. **II** *vt* bleich machen, erbleichen lassen. **III** *vi* blaß *od.* bleich werden, erbleichen, erblassen.
pale cell adenocarcinoma hellzelliges Adenokarzinom *nt*.
pa·le·en·ceph·a·lon [‚peɪlɪen'sefəlɒn] *n* Urhirn *nt*, Althirn *nt*, Palaeencephalon *nt*.
pale hypertension maligne Hypertonie *f*.
pale infarct ischämischer/anämischer/weißer/blasser Infarkt *m*.
paleo- *pref.* Alt-, Ur-, Palae(o)-.
pa·le·o·cer·e·bel·lum *n* → palaeocerebellum.
pa·le·o·cor·tex *n* → palaeocortex.
pa·le·o·en·ceph·a·lon [‚peɪlɪəʊen'sefəlɒn] *n* → paleencephalon.
pa·le·o·pal·li·um *n* → palaeopallium.
pa·le·o·ru·brum [‚-'ruːbrəm, ‚pælɪ-] *n* Palaeorubrum *nt*.
pa·le·o·stri·a·tal syndrome [‚-straɪ'eɪtl] neuro. Pallidumsyndrom *nt*, progressive Pallidumatrophie *f* Hunt, Paralysis agitans juvenilis.
pa·le·o·stri·a·tum [‚-straɪ'eɪtəm] *n* → pallidum.
pa·le·o·thal·a·mus [‚-'θæləməs] *n* Paläothalamus *m*.
pale thrombus Abscheidungs-, Konglutinationsthrombus *m*, weißer/grauer Thrombus *m*.
pal·i·ci·ne·sia [‚pælɪsɪ'niːʒ(ɪ)ə] *n* → palikinesia.
pal·i·ki·ne·sia [‚-kɪ'niːʒ(ɪ)ə, -kaɪ-] *n* neuro., psychia. Palikinesie *f*.
pal·i·la·lia [‚-'leɪlɪə, -jə] *n* neuro., psychia. Palilalie *f*.
pal·in·drome ['pælɪndrəʊm] *n* genet. Palindrom *nt*.
pal·in·dro·mia [‚-'drəʊmɪə] *n* (Krankheits-)Rezidiv *nt*, Rückfall *m*.
pal·in·dro·mic [‚-'drɒmɪk] *adj* wiederauftretend, rezidivierend, palindromisch.
pal·in·es·the·sia [‚-esˈθiːʒ(ɪ)ə] *n* Palinästhesie *f*.
pal·in·gra·phia [‚-'græfɪə] *n* psychia. Palingraphie *f*.
pal·in·mne·sis [‚-'niːsɪs] *n* Palinmnese *f*.
pal·in·op·sia [‚-'ɒpsɪə] *n* ophthal. Palinopsie *f*.
pal·in·phra·sia [‚-'freɪʒ(ɪ)ə, -zɪə] *n* psychia., neuro. Palinphrasie *f*.
pal·i·phra·sia [‚pælɪ'freɪʒ(ɪ)ə, -zɪə] *n* → palinphrasia.
pal·i·sade ['pælɪseɪd] *n* patho. Palisadenstellung *f*.
palisade cells bio. Palisadenzellen *pl*.
palisade layer Palisadensaum *m*.
palisade worm micro. **1.** Palisadenwurm *m*, Strongylus equinus. **2.** Palisadenwurm *m*, Strongylus *m*.
pal·la·di·um [pəˈleɪdɪəm] *n abbr.* **Pd** Palladium *nt abbr.* Pd.
pal·lan·es·the·sia [pæl‚ænəs'θiːʒə] *n* neuro. Fehlen *nt* der Vibrationsempfindung, Pallanästhesie *f*.
pal·les·cense [pə'lesnt, peɪ-] *n* → pallor.
pal·les·the·sia [pæləs'ʒiːʒ(ɪ)ə] *n* neuro. Vibrationsempfindung *f*, Pallästhesie *f*.
pall·es·thet·ic sensibility [‚-'θetɪk] → pallesthesia.
pall·hyp·es·the·sia [‚pælhaɪpes'θiːʒ(ɪ)ə] *n* neuro. Verminderung *f* der Vibrationsempfindung, Pallhypästhesie *f*.
pal·li·al ['pælɪəl] *adj* Pallium betr., Pallium-.
pal·li·ate ['pælɪeɪt] *vt* lindern, mildern.
pal·li·a·tion [pælɪ'eɪʃn] *n* (Krankheits-, Symptom-)Milderung *f*, Linderung *f*, Palliation *f*.
pal·li·a·tive ['pælɪeɪtɪv, 'pælɪətɪv] **I** *n* Linderungsmittel *nt*, Palliativum *nt*, Palliativ *nt*. **II** *adj* mildernd, lindernd, palliativ, Palliativ-.
palliative therapy Palliativbehandlung *f*, -therapie *f*.
palliative treatment → palliative therapy.
pal·li·dal ['pælɪdl] *adj* Pallidum betr., pallidal, Pallidum-.
pallidal atrophy Pallidumsyndrom *nt*, progressive Pallidumatrophie *f* Hunt, Paralysis agitans juvenilis.
pallidal degeneration neuro. Pallidumatrophie *f*, Globus-pallidus-Atrophie *f*.
pallidal nucleus Nc. pallidus.
pallidal syndrome → pallidal atrophy.
pal·li·dec·to·my [‚pælɪ'dektəmɪ] *n* neurochir. Pallidumexzision *f*, Pallidektomie *f*.
pal·li·dof·u·gal [‚-'dʌfjəgəl, ‚pælɪdəʊ-'fjuːgl] *adj* vom Pallidum weg, pallidofugal.
pallidofugal system pallidofugales System *nt*.
pal·li·do·hy·po·tha·lam·ic fasciculus [‚pælɪdəʊ‚haɪpəʊθə'læmɪk] pallidohypothalamisches Bündel *nt*, Fasciculus pallidohypothalamicus.
pallido-olivary fibers pallido-oliväre Fasern *pl*, Fibrae pallido-olivares.
pal·li·do·ru·bral tract [‚-'ruːbrəl] Tractus pallidorubralis.
pal·li·do·sub·tha·lam·ic bundle [‚-sʌbθə-'læmɪk] pallidosubthalamisches Bündel *nt*.
pal·li·do·teg·men·tal bundle [‚-teg'mentl] pallidotegmentales Bündel *nt*.
pal·li·dot·o·my [pælɪ'dɒtəmɪ] *n* neurochir. Pallidotomie *f*.
pal·li·dum ['pælɪdəm] *n* Globus pallidus, Pallidum *nt*, Paläostriatum *nt*.
pallidum I Globus pallidus lateralis.
pallidum II Globus pallidus medialis.
pal·li·o·tha·lam·ic nuclei [‚pælɪəʊθə'læm-ɪk] → palliothalamus.
pal·li·o·thal·a·mus [‚-'θæləməs] *n* palliothalamische Kerne *pl*, Palliothalamus *m*, spezifische Thalamuskerne *pl*.
pal·li·um ['pælɪəm] *n*, *pl* **-li·ums**, **-lia** [-lɪə] anat. **1.** (Groß-)Hirnrinde *f*, Pallium *nt*, Cortex cerebri. **2.** Hirnmantel *m*, Pallium *nt*.
pal·lor ['pælər] *n* Blässe *f*, Bleichheit *f*, Pallor *m*.
palm [pɑː(l)m] *n* **1.** Handteller *m*, Hand(innen)fläche *f*, hohle Hand *f*; anat. Palma *f*. **2.** (Handschuh-)Innenfläche *f*. **3.** Handbreit *f*.
pal·ma ['pælmə, 'pɑː(l)mə] *n*, *pl* **-mae** [-miː] anat. → palm 1.
pal·man·es·the·sia [‚pælmænəs'θiːʒ(ɪ)ə] *n* → pallanesthesia.
pal·mar ['pælmər, 'pɑː(l)m-] *adj* Handfläche betr., palmar, volar, Handflächen-, Handteller-.
palmar aponeurosis Palmaraponeurose *f*, Aponeurosis palmaris.
palmar arch: deep p. Hohlhandbogen *m*, Arcus palmaris profundus.
superficial p. oberflächlicher Hohlhandbogen *m*, Arcus palmaris superficialis.
palmar branch: deep p. of ulnar artery tiefer Hohlhandast *m* der A. ulnaris, Ramus palmaris profundus a. ulnaris.
p. of median nerve Hohlhand-, Palmarast *m* des N. medianus, Ramus palmaris n. mediani.
superficial p. of radial artery oberflächlicher palmarer Handwurzelast *m* der A. radialis, Ramus palmaris superficialis a. radialis.
p. of ulnar nerve Hohlhand-/Palmarast *m* des N. ulnaris, Ramus palmaris n. ulnaris.

palmar contraction Dupuytren'-Kontraktur f, -Erkrankung f.
palmar crease Querfurche f der Handfläche.
palmar erythema Palmarerythem nt, Erythema palmare.
palmar fascia → palmar aponeurosis.
palmar fibromatosis palmare Fibromatose f, Palmarfibromatose f.
palmar flexion Palmar-, Volarflexion f.
pal·ma·ris brevis (muscle) [pæl'meərɪs] Palmaris m brevis, M. palmaris brevis.
palmaris longus (muscle) Palmaris m longus, M. palmaris longus.
palmar ligament: p.s pl Ligg. palmaria.
  p. of carpus Lig. carpi radiatum.
  p. of radiocarpal joint Lig. radiocarpale palmare.
palmar muscle: long p. → palmaris longus (muscle).
  short p. → palmaris brevis (muscle).
palmar psoriasis derm. Psoriasis palmarum.
palmar reflex Palmarreflex m.
palmar side Hohlhand-, Handflächen(innen)seite f.
pal·mate ['pælmeɪt, 'pɑː(l)-] adj handförmig.
pal·mat·ed ['-meɪtɪd] adj → palmate.
palmate folds palmartige Schleimhautfalten pl des Zervikalkanals, Plicae palmatae.
palm-chin reflex → palmomental reflex.
pal·mes·the·sia [ˌpælmes'θiː(ɪ)ə] n neuro. Vibrationsempfindung f, Pallästhesie f.
pal·mes·thet·ic sensibility [ˌpælmes'θetɪk] → palmesthesia.
pal·mic ['pælmɪk] adj klopfend, schlagend.
pal·mi·tate ['pælmɪteɪt] n Palmitat nt.
pal·mit·ic acid [pæl'mɪtɪk] Palmitinsäure f, n-Hexadecansäure f.
pal·mi·tin ['pælmɪtɪn] n Palmitin nt.
1-pal·mi·to·di·ste·a·rin [ˌpælmɪtəʊdaɪ'stɪərɪn] n 1-Palmitodistearin nt, 1-Palmityldistearylglycerin nt.
pal·mi·to·le·ic acid [ˌ-'liːɪk] Palmitoleinsäure f.
pal·mi·to·le·yl [ˌ-'liːɪl] n Palmitoleyl-(Radikal nt).
pal·mi·to·yl [pæl'mɪtəwɪl] n Palmityl-(Radikal nt).
1-pal·mi·to·yl·di·ste·a·ro·yl glycerol [ˌ-daɪstɪ'ærəwɪl] → 1-palmitodistearin.
pal·mi·tyl ['pælmɪtɪl] n Palmityl-(Radikal nt).
pal·mo·men·tal reflex [ˌpælməʊ'mentl, ˌpɑː(l)məʊ-] Palmomentalreflex m abbr. PMR.
pal·mo·plan·tar keratoderma [ˌ-'plæntər] palmoplantare Keratose f, Keratosis palmoplantaris, Keratodermia palmoplantare.
palmoplantar pustulosis derma. Psoriasis pustulosa palmaris et plantaris, Psoriasis pustulosa Typ Königsbeck-Barber.
pal·mus ['pælmʌs, n, pl -mi [-maɪ] 1.** Palpitation f, Palpitatio f. **2.** Bell-Spasmus m, Fazialiskrampf m, Fazialis-Tick m, Gesichtszucken nt, mimischer Gesichtskrampf m, Tic convulsif/facial. **3.** Herzschlag m. **4.** Bamberger-Krankheit f, saltatorischer Reflexkrampf m.
pal·pa·bil·i·ty [ˌpælpə'bɪlətɪ] n Tast-, Greif-, Fühlbarkeit f.
pal·pa·ble ['pælpəbəl] adj durch Palpation wahrnehmbar, tast-, fühlbar, palpabel, palpierbar.
pal·pate ['pælpeɪt] vt ab-, betasten, befühlen, beklopfen, palpieren.
pal·pa·tion [pæl'peɪʃn] n Be-, Abtasten nt, Palpation f, Palpieren nt.
pal·pa·to·ry albuminuria ['pælpətəʊrɪ]

palpatorische Albuminurie/Proteinurie f.
palpatory percussion Tastperkussion f, palpatorische Perkussion f.
palpatory proteinuria → palpatory albuminuria.
pal·pe·bra ['pælpɪbrə, pæl'piː-] n, pl -brae [-briː] anat. (Augen-)Lid nt, Palpebra f.
pal·pe·bral ['pælpəbrəl, pæl'piː-] adj (Augen-)Lid/Palpebra betr., palpebral, Lid-.
palpebral arch: inferior p. Arcus palpebralis inferior.
  superior p. Arcus palpebralis superior.
palpebral arteries: lateral p. seitliche Lidarterien pl, Aa. palpebrales laterales.
  medial p. mediale Lidarterien pl, Aa. palpebrales mediales.
palpebral branches: inferior p. of infraorbital nerve Unterlidäste pl des N. infraorbitalis, Rami palpebrales inferiores n. infraorbitalis.
  p. of infratrochlear nerve Augenlidäste pl des N. infratrochlearis, Rami palpebrales n. infratrochlearis.
palpebral cartilage Lidknorpel m, Tarsus m (palpebrae).
palpebral coloboma ophthal. Lidkolobom nt.
palpebral commissure: lateral p. äußere/seitliche Augenlidkommissur f, Commissura palpebralis lateralis.
  medial p. innere/mediale Augenlidkommissur f, Commissura palpebralis medialis.
palpebral conjunctiva Bindehaut f des Lids, Tunica conjunctiva palpebralis.
palpebral fissure Lidspalte f, Rima palpebrarum.
palpebral glands Meibom'-Drüsen pl, Gll. tarsales.
palpebral ligament: lateral p. laterales Lidband nt, Lig. palpebrale laterale.
  medial p. mediales Lidband nt, Lig. palpebrale mediale.
palpebral part of lacrimal gland Rosenmüller'-Drüse f, Gl. lacrimalis inferior, Pars palpebralis gl. lacrimalis.
palpebral ptosis ophthal. (Lid-)Ptose f, Ptosis (palpebrae) f, Blepharoptose f.
palpebral raphe, lateral Raphe palpebralis lateralis.
palpebral region: inferior p. Unterlidregion f, Regio palpebralis inferior.
  superior p. Oberlidregion f, Regio palpebralis superior.
palpebral veins (Augen-)Lidvenen pl, Vv. palpebrales.
  inferior p. Unterlidvenen pl, Vv. palpebrales inferiores.
  superior p. Oberlidvenen pl, Vv. palpebrales superiores.
pal·pe·brate ['pælpəbreɪt, -brɪt, pæl'piː-] **I** adj bio. mit Lidern versehen. **II** vi blinzeln, zwinkern.
pal·pe·bra·tion [ˌpælpə'breɪʃn] n Blinzeln nt.
pal·pe·bri·tis [ˌ-'braɪtɪs] n ophthal. Lidentzündung f, Blepharitis f.
pal·pe·bro·na·sal fold [ˌpælpəbrəʊ'neɪzl] Nasen-Lid-Spalte f, Mongolenfalte f, Epikanthus m, Plica palpebronasalis.
pal·pi·ta·tion [ˌpælpɪ'teɪʃn] n **1.** Palpitation f, Palpitatio f. **2.** Herzklopfen nt, Palpitatio cordis, Palpitation f, Kardiopalmus m.
PALS abbr. → periarterial lymphatic sheath.
pal·sied ['pɔːlsɪd] adj gelähmt.
pal·sy ['pɔːlzɪ] **I** n (vollständige) Lähmung f, Paralyse f, Paralysis f, Plegie f. **II** vt lähmen, paralysieren (a. fig.).
pa·lu·dal fever [pə'luː-, 'pæljədəl]

Sumpf-, Wechselfieber nt, Malaria f.
pal·u·dism ['pæljədɪzəm] n → paludal fever.
PAM abbr. → primary amebic meningoencephalitis.
pam·pin·i·form [pæm'pɪnəfɔːrm] adj anat. rankenförmig, gewunden.
pampiniform body Nebeneierstock m, Rosenmüller'-Organ nt, Parovarium nt, Epoophoron nt.
pampiniform plexus Venengeflecht nt des Samenstranges, Plexus pampiniformis.
pam·pin·o·cele [pæm'pɪnəsiːl] n Krampfaderbruch m, Varikozele f, Hernia varicosa.
pam·ple·gi·a [pæm'pliːdʒ(ɪ)ə] n vollständige Lähmung f; Paralyse f.
pan- pref. Ganz-, Pan-.
pan·a·cea [pænə'sɪə] n Allheilmittel nt.
pan·ac·i·nar emphysema [pæn'æsɪnər] panazinäres/panlobuläres/diffuses Lungenemphysem nt.
pan·ag·glu·tin·a·ble [ˌ-ə'gluːtɪnəbl] adj panagglutinierbar, panagglutinabel.
pan·ag·glu·ti·na·tion [ˌ-əˌgluːtə'neɪʃn] n Panagglutination f.
pan·ag·glu·ti·nin [ˌ-ə'gluːtənɪn] n Panagglutinin nt.
pan·an·gi·i·tis [ˌ-ændʒɪ'aɪtɪs] n Panangiitis f, Panangiitis f.
pan·a·ris ['pænərɪs, pə'nærɪs] n Panaritium nt.
pan·ar·te·ri·tis [ˌpænɑːrtə'raɪtɪs] n Panarteriitis f.
pan·ar·thri·tis [ˌ-ɑːr'θraɪtɪs] n ortho. Panarthritis f.
pan·blas·tic [ˌ-'blæstɪk] adj embryo. alle Keimschichten betr.
pan·cake kidney ['pænkeɪk] patho. Kuchen-, Klumpenniere f.
pan·car·di·tis [ˌ-kɑːr'daɪtɪs] n card. Pankarditis f, -carditis f.
pan·chrest ['-krest] n Allheilmittel nt.
pan·chro·mat·ic [ˌ-krəʊ'mætɪk] adj phys. panchromatisch.
pan·chro·mia [ˌ-'krəʊmɪə] n histol. Panchromie f.
Pancoast ['pænkəʊst]: **P.'s suture** chir. Pancoast-Naht f.
  P.'s syndrome Pancoast-Syndrom nt.
  P.'s tumor Pancoast-Tumor m, apikaler Sulkustumor m.
pan·coch·le·ar deafness [ˌpæn'kɑklɪər] pankochleärer Gehörverlust m, pankochleäre Taubheit f.
pan·col·ec·to·my [-kə'lektəmɪ] n chir. totale Kolektomie f, Pankolektomie f.
pan·co·li·tis [-kə'laɪtɪs] n Pankolitis f.
pan·cre·al·gia [ˌpæŋkrɪ'ældʒ(ɪ)ə, pæn-] n → pancreatalgia.
pan·cre·as ['pæŋkrɪəs, 'pæn-] n, pl -cre·a·ta [pæŋ'krɪətə, ˌpæŋkrɪ'eɪtə] Bauchspeicheldrüse f, Pankreas nt, Pancreas nt.
pancreas graft chir. Pankreastransplantat nt.
pancreas transplant → pancreas graft.
pancreas transplantation Pankreastransplantation f.
  segmental p. Pankreasteiltransplantation.
pancreat- pref. → pancreatico-.
pan·cre·a·tal·gia [ˌpæŋkrɪə'tældʒ(ɪ)ə, ˌpæn-] n Pankreasschmerz m, Pankrealgie f, Pankreatalgie f.
pan·cre·a·tec·to·my [ˌ-'tektəmɪ] n chir. (totale) Pankreasentfernung f, Pankreasresektion f, Pankreatektomie f.
pan·cre·at·ic [ˌpæŋkrɪ'ætɪk, ˌpæŋ-] adj Bauchspeicheldrüse/Pancreas betr., aus dem Pancreas stammend, pankreatisch, Bauchspeicheldrüsen-, Pankreas-.
pancreatic abscess Pankreasabszeß m.

pancreatic achylia

pancreatic achylia fehlende Pankreassekretion *f*, Achylia pancreatica.
pancreatic adenoma Pankreasadenom *nt*.
  acinar cell p. azinäres Pankreasadenom.
  ductular cell p. duktales Pankreasadenom.
pancreatic apoplexy Pankreasapoplexie *f*, Apoplexia pancreatis.
pancreatic artery: dorsal p. hintere Pankreas-/Bauchspeicheldrüsenarterie *f*, Pancreatica *f* dorsalis, A. pancreatica dorsalis.
  great p. große Pankreas-/Bauchspeicheldrüsenarterie *f*, Pancreatica *f* magna, A. pancreatica magna.
  inferior p. untere Pankreas-/Bauchspeicheldrüsenarterie *f*, Pancreatica *f* inferior, A. pancreatica inferior.
pancreatic ascites pankreatogener Aszites *m*.
pancreatic branches: p. of anterior superior pancreaticoduodenal artery Rami pancreatici a. pancreaticoduodenalis superioris anterioris.
  p. of posterior superior pancreaticoduodenal artery Rami pancreatici a. pancreaticoduodenalis superioris posterioris.
  p. of splenic artery Pankreasäste *pl* der Milzarterie, Rami pancreatici a. lienalis/splenicae.
pancreatic bud *embryo.* Pankreasknospe *f*.
  dorsal p. dorsale Pankreasknospe/-anlage *f*.
  ventral p. ventrale Pankreasknospe/-anlage *f*.
pancreatic calculus Pankreasstein *m*, Pankreatolith *m*.
pancreatic capsule Pankreaskapsel *f*, Capsula pancreatis.
pancreatic carcinoma Bauchspeicheldrüsenkrebs *m*, Pankreaskarzinom *nt*.
  acinar cell p. azinöses Pankreaskarzinom.
  ductular (cell) p. duktales Pankreaskarzinom.
pancreatic cholera Verner-Morrison-Syndrom *nt*, pankreatische Cholera *f*.
pancreatic cirrhosis Pankreaszirrhose *f*, -fibrose *f*.
pancreatic colic Pankreaskolik *f*, Colica pancreatica.
pancreatic contusion Pankreaskontusion *f*.
pancreatic-cutaneous fistula äußere Pankreasfistel *f*.
pancreatic cyst Pankreaszyste *f*.
pancreatic diabetes pankreatischer Diabetes (mellitus) *m*.
pancreatic diverticula *embryo.* Pankreasdivertikel *pl*.
pancreatic dornase Pankreasdornase *f*.
pancreatic drainage 1. *histol.* Pankreasabfluß *m*. **2.** *chir.* Pankreasdrainage *f*.
pancreatic duct Wirsung'-Gang *m*, -Kanal *m*, Pankreasgang *m*, Ductus pancreaticus (Wirsungi).
  accessory/minor p. Santorini'-Gang, Ductus pancreaticus accessorius.
pancreatic ductal anastomosis Pankreasganganastomose *f*.
pancreatic duct injury Pankreasgangverletzung *f*, -schädigung *f*.
pancreatic dysfunction Pankreasdysfunktion *f*.
pancreatic edema Pankreasödem *nt*, Zöpfel-Ödem *nt*.
pancreatic fibrosis Pankreasfibrose *f*.
pancreatic fistula Pankreasfistel *f*.
  internal p. innere Pankreasfistel.
pancreatic function tests Pankreasfunktionsdiagnostik *f*.

pancreatic hormones Pankreashormone *pl*.
pancreatic hydrothorax pankreatogener Hydrothorax *m*.
pancreatic injury Pankreasverletzung *f*, -trauma *nt*.
pancreatic insufficiency Pankreasinsuffizienz *f*.
pancreatic islands/islets Pankreasinseln *pl*, Langerhans'-Inseln *pl*, Inselorgan *nt*, endokrines Pankreas *nt*, Pars endocrina pancreatis.
pancreatic juice Pankreassaft *m*, -speichel *m*, Sucus prancreaticus.
pancreatic lipase Pankreaslipase *f*.
pancreatic lobule Pankreasläppchen *nt*, Lobulus pancreatis.
pancreatic necrosis Pankreasnekrose *f*.
pancreatic notch Pankreasrinne *f*, Inc. pancreatis.
pancreatico- *pref.* Bauchspeicheldrüsen-, Pankreas-, Pankreatiko-, Pankreato-.
pan·cre·at·i·co·du·o·de·nal [ˌpænkrɪˌætɪkəʊd(j)uːˈdiːnl, -d(j)uːˈədnəl, ˌpæn-] *adj* Pankreas u. Duodenum betr. *od.* verbindend, pankreatikoduodenal.
pancreaticoduodenal artery: inferior p. A. pancreaticoduodenalis inferior.
  superior p., anterior A. pancreaticoduodenalis superior anterior.
  superior p., posterior A. pancreaticoduodenalis superior posterior.
pancreaticoduodenal transplant *chir.* pankreatikoduodenales Transplantat *nt*.
pancreaticoduodenal transplantation *chir.* pankreatikoduodenale Transplantation *f*.
pancreaticoduodenal veins Vv. pancreaticoduodenales.
pan·cre·at·i·co·du·o·de·nec·to·my [ˌ-ˌd(j)uːədɪˈnektəmɪ] *n chir.* Duodenopankreatektomie *f*.
pan·cre·at·i·co·du·o·de·nos·to·my [ˌ-ˌd(j)uːədɪˈnɒstəmɪ] *n chir.* Pankreat(ik)oduodenostomie *f*.
pan·cre·at·i·co·en·ter·os·to·my [ˌ-ˌentəˈrɒstəmɪ] *n chir.* Pankreat(ik)oenterostomie *f*.
pan·cre·at·i·co·gas·tric fold [ˌ-ˈɡæstrɪk] Plica gastropancreatica.
pan·cre·at·i·co·gas·tros·to·my [ˌ-ɡæsˈtrɒstəmɪ] *n chir.* Pankreat(ik)ogastrostomie *f*.
pan·cre·at·i·co·je·ju·nos·to·my [ˌ-ˌdʒɪdʒuːˈnɒstəmɪ] *n chir.* Pankreat(ik)ojejunostomie *f*.
pancreatic oncofetal antigen *abbr.* **POA** pankreatisches onkofetales Antigen *nt abbr.* POA.
pancreatic phlegmon Pankreasphlegmone *f*.
pancreatic plexus Pankreasplexus *m*, Plexus pancreaticus.
pancreatic polypeptide *abbr.* **PP** pankreatisches Polypeptid *nt abbr.* PP.
pancreatic polypeptide cells (Pankreas) F-Zellen *pl*.
pancreatic proteases Pankreasproteasen *pl*.
pancreatic pseudocyst Pankreaspseudozyste *f*.
pancreatic ribonuclease alkalische Ribonuklease *f*, Pankreasribonuclease *f*.
pancreatic secretion Pankreassekret *nt*.
pancreatic stone → pancreatic calculus.
pancreatic stump *chir.* Pankreasstumpf *m*.
pancreatic surgery Pankreaschirurgie *f*.
pancreatic transplantation → pancreas transplantation.
pancreatic trauma → pancreatic injury.
pancreatic veins Pankreasvenen *pl*, Vv. pancreaticae.

pancreatic vessels Pankreasgefäße *pl*.
pan·cre·a·ti·tis [ˌpænkrɪəˈtaɪtɪs, ˌpæn-] *n* Bauchspeicheldrüsen-, Pankreasentzündung *f*, Pankreatitis *f*, Pancreatitis *f*.
pancreato- *pref.* → pancreatico-.
pan·cre·a·to·du·o·de·nec·to·my [ˌpænkrɪətəʊˌd(j)uːədɪˈnektəmɪ, ˌpæn-] *n chir.* Duodenopankreatektomie *f*.
pan·cre·a·to·du·o·de·nos·to·my [ˌ-ˌd(j)uːədɪˈnɒstəmɪ] *n* → pancreaticoduodenostomy.
pan·cre·a·to·en·ter·os·to·my [ˌ-ˌentəˈrɒstəmɪ] *n* → pancreaticoenterostomy.
pan·cre·at·o·gas·tros·to·my [ˌ-ɡæsˈtrɒstəmɪ] *n* → pancreaticogastrostomy.
pan·cre·a·to·gen·ic [ˌ-ˈdʒenɪk] *adj* → pancreatogenous.
pan·cre·a·tog·e·nous [pænkrɪəˈtɒdʒənəs, pæn-] *adj* vom Pankreas ausgehend, pankreatogen.
pancreatogenous diarrhea → pancreatogenous fatty diarrhea.
pancreatogenous fatty diarrhea pankreatogener Durchfall *m*, pankreatogene Diarrhö *f*.
pan·cre·at·o·gram [pænkrɪˈætəɡræm, pæn-] *n chir., radiol.* Pankreat(ik)ogramm *nt*.
pan·cre·a·tog·ra·phy [pænkrɪəˈtɒɡrəfɪ, pæn-] *n chir., radiol.* Pankreat(ik)ographie *f*.
pan·cre·at·o·lith [pænkrɪˈætəlɪθ, pæn-] *n* Pankreasstein *m*, Pankreatolith *m*.
pan·cre·a·to·li·thec·to·my [ˌpænkrɪətəʊlɪˈθektəmɪ, ˌpæn-] *n chir.* Pankreatolithektomie *f*.
pan·cre·a·to·li·thi·a·sis [ˌ-lɪˈθaɪəsɪs] *n* Pankreatolithiasis *f*.
pan·cre·a·to·li·thot·o·my [ˌ-lɪˈθɒtəmɪ] *n chir.* Pankreatolithotomie *f*.
pan·cre·a·tol·y·sis [pænkrɪəˈtɒləsɪs, pæn-] *n* pancreolysis.
pan·cre·a·to·lyt·ic [ˌpænkrɪətəʊˈlɪtɪk, pæn-] *adj* → pancreolytic.
pan·cre·at·o·my [pænkrɪˈætəmɪ, pæn-] *n* → pancreatotomy.
pan·cre·a·top·a·thy [pænkrɪəˈtɒpəθɪ, pæn-] *n* Bauchspeicheldrüsen-, Pankreaserkrankung *f*, Pankreatopathie *f*, Pankreopathie *f*.
pan·cre·a·tot·o·my [ˌ-ˈtɒtəmɪ] *n chir.* Pankreatotomie *f*.
pan·cre·a·to·trop·ic [pænkrɪətəʊˈtrɒpɪk, -ˈtrəʊp-, pæn-] *adj* mit besonderer Affinität zum Pankreas, pankreatotrop, pankreotrop.
pan·cre·a·trop·ic [pænkrɪəˈtrɒpɪk, -ˈtrəʊ-, pæn-] *adj* → pancreatotropic.
pan·cre·ec·to·my [pænkrɪˈektəmɪ, pæn-] *n* → pancreatectomy.
pan·cre·o·cy·min-secretin test [ˌpænkrɪəˈsaɪmɪn, ˌpæn-] Sekretin-Pankreozymin-Test *m*.
pan·cre·o·lith [ˈ-lɪθ] *n* → pancreatolith.
pan·cre·o·li·thot·o·my [ˌ-lɪˈθɒtəmɪ] *n* → pancreatolithotomy.
pan·cre·ol·y·sis [pænkrɪˈɒləsɪs, pæn-] *n patho.* Pankreasauflösung *f*, -selbstverdauung *f*, -autolyse *f*, Pankreatolyse *f*, Pankreolyse *f*.
pan·cre·o·lyt·ic [pænkrɪəˈlɪtɪk, pæn-] *adj* Pankreolyse betr., pankreolytisch, pankreatolytisch.
pan·cre·op·a·thy [pænkrɪˈɒpəθɪ, pæn-] *n* → pancreatopathy.
pan·cre·o·priv·ic [pænkrɪəʊˈprɪvɪk, pæŋ-] *adj* pankreopriv.
pan·cre·o·ther·a·py [ˌ-ˈθerəpɪ] *n* Behandlung *f* mit Pankreasenzymen.
pan·cre·o·trop·ic [ˌ-ˈtrɒpɪk, -ˈtrəʊp-] *adj* → pancreatotropic.
pan·cre·o·zy·min [ˌ-ˈzaɪmɪn] *n* Pankreozy-

min *nt abbr.* PZ, Cholezystokinin *nt abbr.* CCK.
pan·cu·ro·ni·um [ˌpænkjʊəˈrəʊnɪəm] *n anes.* Pancuronium *nt.*
pancuronium bromide *anes.* Pancuroniumbromid *nt.*
pan·cys·ti·tis [ˌ-sɪsˈtaɪtɪs] *n urol.* Panzystitis *f.*
pan·cy·to·pe·nia [ˌ-saɪtəˈpiːnɪə] *n hema.* Panzytopenie *f.*
pancytopenia-dysmelia syndrome Fanconi-Anämie *f*, konstitutionelle infantile Panmyelopathie *f.*
pan·de·mia [ˌ-ˈdiːmɪə] *n* → pandemic I.
pan·dem·ic [ˌ-ˈdemɪk] *epidem.* **I** *n* Pandemie *f.* **II** *adj* pandemisch.
pandemic disease → pandemic I.
pan·du·ri·form placenta [ˌ-ˈd(j)ʊərɪfɔːrm] Placenta panduraformis.
Pándy [ˈpændɪ]: **P.'s reaction/test** Pandy-Test *m.*
pan·en·ceph·a·li·tis [ˌpænenˌsefəˈlaɪtɪs] *n* Panenzephalitis *f*, Panencephalitis *f.*
pan·en·do·crine [ˌ-ˈendəʊkrɪn, -kraɪn] *adj* panendokrin.
pan·en·do·scope [ˌ-ˈendəskəʊp] *n* Panendoskop *nt.*
pan·es·the·sia [ˌ-esˈθiːʒ(ɪ)ə] *n* Panästhesie *f.*
pan·es·thet·ic [ˌ-esˈθetɪk] *adj* Panästhesie betr., panästhetisch.
Paneth [ˈpɑːneɪt; ˈpanet]: **P.'s cells** Paneth'-(Körner-)Zellen *pl*, Davidoff-Zellen *pl*.
P.'s granular cells → P.'s cells.
pang [pæŋ] *n* plötzlicher stechender Schmerz *m.*
pan·hem·a·to·pe·nia [ˌpænˌhemətəʊˈpiːnɪə, -ˌhiːm-] *n* → pancytopenia.
pan·hy·per·e·mia [ˌ-ˌhaɪpəˈriːmɪə] *n* Panhyperämie *f.*
pan·hy·po·gam·ma·glob·u·lin·e·mia [ˌ-ˌhaɪpəʊˌgæməˌglɑbjəlɪnˈiːmɪə] *n* Hypogammaglobulinämie *f.*
pan·hy·po·go·nad·ism [ˌ-ˌhaɪpəʊˈɡəʊnædɪzəm, -ˈɡa-] *n* Panhypogonadismus *m.*
pan·hy·po·pi·tu·i·tar·ism [ˌ-ˌhaɪpəʊpɪˈt(j)uːətərɪzəm] *n* Panhypopituitarismus *m.*
pan·hys·ter·ec·to·my [ˌ-ˌhɪstəˈrektəmɪ] *n gyn.* totale Gebärmutterentfernung *f*, Uterusexstirpation *f*, Hysterektomie *f.*
pan·ic [ˈpænɪk] **I** *n* Panik *f*, panischer Schrecken *m*, panische Angst *f.* **II** *adj* panisch. **III** *vt* in Panik versetzen, eine Panik auslösen. **IV** *vi* in Panik geraten, von panischer Angst erfaßt *od.* ergriffen werden.
panic attack Angstanfall *m*, Panikattacke *f.*
pan·im·mu·ni·ty [ˌpænɪˈmjuːnətɪ] *n* Panimmunität *f.*
pan·lob·u·lar emphysema [ˌ-ˈlɑbjələr] panazinäres/panlobuläres/diffuses Lungenemphysem *nt.*
pan·mix·ia [ˌ-ˈmɪksɪə] *n* → panmixis.
pan·mix·is [ˌ-ˈmɪksɪs] *n bio., genet.* Panmixie *f*, Panmixis *f.*
pan·mu·ral cystitis [ˌ-ˈmjʊərəl] chronisch interstitielle (Harn-)Blasenentzündung/Zystitis *f*, Cystitis intermuralis/interstitialis.
panmural fibrosis of the bladder → panmural cystitis.
pan·my·e·loid [ˌ-ˈmaɪəlɔɪd] *adj* alle Knochenmarkselemente betr., panmyeloid.
pan·my·e·lo·path·ia [ˌ-ˌmaɪəlɔʊˈpæθɪə] *n* → panmyelopathy.
pan·my·e·lop·a·thy [ˌ-maɪəˈlɑpəθɪ] *n hema.* Panmyelopathie *f.*
pan·my·e·loph·thi·sis [ˌ-maɪəˈlɑfθəsɪs] *n* 1. Panmyelophthise *f.* 2. aplastische Anämie *f.*

pan·my·e·lo·sis [ˌ-maɪəˈlɔʊsɪs] *n hema.* Panmyelose *f.*
Panner [ˈpænər]: **P.'s disease** Panner'-Krankheit *f.*
pan·nic·u·lal·gia [pəˌnɪkjəˈlældʒ(ɪ)ə] *n* Adiposalgie *f.*
pan·nic·u·lar hernia [pəˈnɪkjələr] Fettgewebsbruch *m*, Fetthernie *f*, Hernia adiposa.
pan·nic·u·lec·to·my [pəˌnɪkjəˈlektəmɪ] *n chir.* Exzision *f* der Fettschürze, Pannikulektomie *f.*
pan·nic·u·li·tis [pəˌnɪkjəˈlaɪtɪs] *n* Entzündung *f* des Unterhautfettgewebes, Pannikulitis *f*, Panniculitis *f.*
pan·nic·u·lus [pəˈnɪkjələs] *n, pl* **-li** [-laɪ] *anat.* Panniculus *m.*
pan·nus [ˈpænəs] *n, pl* **-ni** [-naɪ] **1.** *ophthal.* Pannus (corneae) *m.* **2.** *anat.* Unterhautfettgewebe *nt*, Panniculus adiposus. **3.** *ortho.* Pannus *m.*
pan·o·pho·bia [pænəˈfəʊbɪə] *n* → panphobia.
pan·oph·thal·mia [ˌpænɑfˈθælmɪə] *n* → panophthalmitis.
pan·oph·thal·mi·tis [ˌpænɑfθælˈmaɪtɪs] *n ophthal.* Panophthalmie *f*, Panophthalmitis *f*, Pantophthalmie *f.*
pan·op·tic [pænˈɑptɪk] *adj phys., histol.* panoptisch.
panoptic stain panoptische Färbung *f.*
pan·o·ram·ic radiograph [pænəˈræmɪk] *radiol.* **1.** Panoramaaufnahme *f*, Pantomogramm *nt.* **2.** → pantomograph.
panoramic radiography → pantomography.
pan·os·te·i·tis [ˌ-ɑstɪˈaɪtɪs] *n* → panostitis.
pan·os·ti·tis [ˌ-ɑsˈtaɪtɪs] *n patho.* Panostitis *f.*
pan·o·ti·tis [ˌ-əʊˈtaɪtɪs] *n HNO* Panotitis *f.*
pan·pho·bia [ˌ-ˈfəʊbɪə] *n psychia.* Panphobie *f.*
pan·ple·gia [ˌ-ˈpliːdʒ(ɪ)ə] *n neuro.* Lähmung *f* des ganzen Körpers, Panplegie *f.*
pan·proc·to·co·lec·to·my [ˌ-ˌprɑktəkəʊˈlektəmɪ] *n chir.* Panproktokolektomie *f.*
Pansch [pænʃ]: **P.'s fissure** Sulcus intraparietalis.
pan·scle·ro·sis [ˌpænsklɪˈrəʊsɪs] *n patho.* Pansklerose *f.*
pan·si·nu·i·tis [ˌ-saɪnəˈwaɪtɪs] *n* → pansinusitis.
pan·si·nu·si·tis [ˌ-saɪnəˈsaɪtɪs] *n HNO* Entzündung *f* aller Nebenhöhlen, Pansinusitis *f.*
Pan·stron·gy·lus [ˌ-ˈstrɑndʒələs] *n micro.* Panstrongylus *m.*
P. megistus brasilianische Schreitwanze *f*, Triatoma megista, Panstrongylus megistus.
pan·sys·tol·ic [ˌ-sɪsˈtɑlɪk] *adj card.* während der gesamten Systole, pansystolisch, holosystolisch.
pansystolic murmur *card.* pansystolisches/holosystolisches (Herz-)Geräusch *nt.*
pant- *pref.* → panto-.
pant [pænt] **I** *n* Keuchen *nt*, Japsen *nt*, Schnaufen *nt.* **II** *vi* keuchen, japsen, schnaufen.
pan·tal·gia [pænˈtældʒ(ɪ)ə] *n* Schmerzen *pl* über den gesamten Körper, Pantalgie *f.*
pan·ta·loon embolism [pæntəˈluːn] Sattelembolie *f.*
pantaloon embolus reitender Embolus *m*, Sattelembolus *m.*
pan·ta·mor·phic [ˌpæntəˈmɔːrfɪk] *adj* ohne Form, formlos.
pan·tan·en·ce·pha·lia [ˌpæntænensɪˈfeɪlɪə] *n* → pantanencephaly.
pan·tan·en·ceph·a·ly [ˌpæntænenˈsefəlɪ] *n* komplette Anenzephalie *f.*

pan·tan·ky·lo·bleph·a·ron [pænˌtæŋkɪləʊˈblefərɑn] *n ophthal.* Lidverklebung *f*, -verwachsung *f*, Blepharosynechie *f*, -symphysis *f*, Symblepharon *nt.*
pan·te·the·ine [ˌpæntəˈθiːɪn] *n* Pantethein *nt.*
pan·the·nol [ˈpænθɪnɑl, -nɔl] *n* Panthenol *nt*, Pantothenol *nt.*
panto- *pref.* All-, Pant(o)-.
pan·to·graph [ˈpæntəgræf] *n* Pantograph *m.*
pan·to·ic acid [pænˈtɔɪk] Pantoinsäure *f.*
pan·to·mo·gram [pænˈtəʊməgræm] *n radiol.* Panoramaaufnahme *f*, Pantomogramm *nt.*
pan·to·mo·graph [pænˈtəʊməgræf] *n radiol.* Pantomograph *m.*
pan·to·mog·ra·phy [ˌpæntəˈmɑgrəfɪ] *n radiol.* Pantomographie *f*, Panorama-(aufnahme)technik *f.*
pan·to·pho·bia [ˌ-ˈfəʊbɪə] *n* → panphobia.
pan·to·then [ˈ-θen] *n* → pantothenic acid.
pan·to·then·ate [ˌ-ˈθeneɪt, pænˈtæθə-] *n* Pantothenat *nt.*
pantothenate kinase Pantothenatkinase *f.*
pan·to·then·ic acid [ˌ-ˈθenɪk] Pantothensäure *f*, Vitamin B₃ *nt.*
pan·to·the·nol [ˌ-ˈθiːnɑl, -nɔl] *n* → panthenol.
pan·to·then·yl alcohol [ˌ-ˈθenɪl] → panthenol.
pan·to·trop·ic [ˌ-ˈtrɑpɪk, -ˈtrəʊp-] *adj* pantropic.
pan·to·yl·tau·rine [ˌpæntəwɪlˈtɔːriːn] *n* Pantoyltaurin *nt*, Thiopansäure *f.*
pan·trop·ic [pænˈtrɑpɪk, -ˈtrəʊp-] *adj* mit Affinität zu allen Geweben, pantotrop, pantrop.
Panum [ˈpænəm]: **P.'s areas** Panum'-Felder *f.*
pan·u·ve·i·tis [ˌpænjuːvɪˈaɪtɪs] *n ophthal.* Panuveitis *f.*
pan·zer·herz [ˈpænzərherts; ˈpantsərherts] *n* Panzerherz *nt*, Pericarditis calcarea.
PAP *abbr.* → pulmonary artery pressure.
Pap *abbr.* → Papanicolaou's stain.
pap [pæp] *n* Brei *m*, Mus *nt.*
pa·pa·in [pəˈpeɪɪn] *n* Papain *nt.*
Papanicolaou [pɑpəˌniːkəˈlɑʊ, ˌpæpəˈniːkə-]: **P.'s smear** Papanicolaou-Abstrich *m.*
P.'s stain *abbr.* **Pap** Pap-Färbung *f*, Papanicolaou-Färbung *f.*
P.'s test Papanicolaou-Test *m*, Pap-Test *m.*
Pa·pav·er [pəˈpævər, -ˈpeɪv-] *n bio., pharm.* Papaver *nt.*
P. somniferum Schlafmohn *m*, Papaver somniferum.
pa·pav·er·ine [pəˈpævərɪn, pəˈpeɪ-] *n pharm.* Papaverin *nt*, Papavereinum *nt.*
pa·pay·o·tin [pəˈpaɪətɪn] *n* → papain.
pa·pes·cent [pəˈpesnt] *adj* breiig, breiartig, musartig.
pa·per [ˈpeɪpər] **I** *n* **1.** Papier *nt.* **2.** Blatt *nt*, Papier *nt.* **3.** **~s** *pl* Dokumente *pl*, Papiere *pl*, Urkunden *pl.* **4.** (wissenschaftliche) Abhandlung *f, od.* Arbeit *f*, Referat *nt*, Vortrag *m* (*on* über). **5.** Klausur *f*, Testbogen *m.* **II** *adj* papierähnlich, hauchdünn.
paper chromatography Papierchromatographie *f.*
paper-doll fetus Fetus papyraceus.
paper plate Lamina orbitalis (ossis ethmoidalis).
paper work Schreibarbeit(en *pl*) *f.*
pa·per·y [ˈpeɪpərɪ] *adj* → paper II.
Papez [ˈpɑːpez, -peɪ]: **multineuronal circuit of P.** Neuronenkreis *m* von Papez.
pa·pil·la [pəˈpɪlə] *n, pl* **-lae** [-liː] *anat.* war-

papillar

zenförmige Hauterhebung f, Wärzchen nt, Papille f, Papilla f.
pap·il·lar ['pæpɪlər, pə'pɪlər] adj → papillary.
pap·il·lar·y ['pæpɪˌleriː, pə'pɪləri] adj **1.** Papille od. Warze betr., papillenförmig, warzenförmig, papillär, papillar, Papillen-, Warzen-. **2.** mit Papillen od. Wärzchen bedeckt, warzig.
papillary adenocarcinoma papilläres Adenokarzinom nt.
papillary adenocystoma lymphomatosum → papillary cystadenoma lymphomatosum.
papillary adenoma papilläres Adenom nt.
  p. of large intestine villöses Dickdarmadenom.
papillary carcinoma papilläres Karzinom nt, Ca. papillare/papilliferum.
papillary cystadenoma → papilloadenocystoma.
papillary cystadenoma lymphomatosum Whartin-Tumor m, Whartin-Albrecht-Arzt-Tumor m, Adenolymphom nt, Cystadenoma lymphomatosum, Cystadenolymphoma papilliferum.
papillary cystic adenoma papillär-zystisches Adenom nt.
papillary cystoma papilläres Kystom/Cystom nt.
papillary ducts (Niere) Ausführungsgänge pl der Sammelrohre, Ductus papillares.
papillary ectasia senile Angiome/Hämangiome pl, Alters(häm)angiome pl.
papillary epithelium papilläres Epithel nt.
papillary foramina (Niere) Mündungsöffnungen pl der Harnkanälchen, Forr. papillaria.
papillary hidradenoma tubuläres Adenom nt der Vulva, Hidradenom nt der Vulva, Hidradenoma papilliferum.
papillary layer of corium/dermis Papillar(körper)schicht f, Stratum papillare dermidis.
papillary line Mamillarlinie f, Linea mamillaris.
papillary muscle (Herz) Papillarmuskel m, M. papillaris.
  anterior p. of left ventricle vorderer Papillarmuskel des linken Ventrikels, M. papillaris anterior ventriculi sinistri.
  anterior p. of right ventricle vorderer Papillarmuskel des rechten Ventrikels, M. papillaris anterior ventriculi dextri.
  posterior p. of left ventricle hinterer Papillarmuskel des linken Ventrikels, M. papillaris posterior ventriculi sinistri.
  posterior p. of right ventricle hinterer Papillarmuskel des rechten Ventrikels, M. papillaris posterior ventriculi dextri.
  septal p.s of right ventricle septale Papillarmuskeln pl des rechten Ventrikels, Mm. papillares septales ventriculi dextri.
papillary muscle dysfunction → papillary muscle syndrome.
papillary muscle syndrome Papillarsyndrom nt.
papillary necrosis (Niere) Papillennekrose f.
papillary process (of liver) Papillenvorsprung m des Lobus caudatus, Proc. papillaris (hepatis).
papillary tumor → papilloma.
pap·il·late ['pæpɪleɪt, pə'pɪlət] adj → papillary.
pap·il·lat·ed ['pæpɪleɪtɪd] adj → papillary.
pap·il·lec·to·my [ˌpæpɪ'lektəmɪ] n chir. Papillenexzision f, Papillektomie f.
pap·il·le·de·ma [ˌpæpɪlɪ'diːmə] n ophthal. Stauungspapille f, Papillenödem nt.
pap·il·lif·er·ous [ˌpæpə'lɪfərəs] adj histol. mit Papillen besetzt.

pa·pil·li·form [pə'pɪləfɔːrm] adj anat. papillenähnlich, warzenförmig, papillär, papillar, papilliform.
pap·il·li·tis [ˌpæpɪ'laɪtɪs] n **1.** ophthal. Papillenentzündung f, Papillitis f. **2.** ophthal. Optikusneuritis f, Neuritis n. optici. **3.** Entzündung f der Duodenalpapille, Papillitis f. **4.** Entzündung f der Analpapillen, Papillitis f.
pa·pil·lo·ad·e·no·cys·to·ma [ˌpæpɪləʊˌædnəʊsɪs'təʊmə, pəˌpɪləʊ-] n papilläres Zystadenom/Kystadenom nt, papilläres Adenokystom nt.
pa·pil·lo·car·ci·no·ma [ˌ-ˌkɑːrsɪ'nəʊmə] n → papillary carcinoma.
pap·il·lo·ma [pæpɪ'ləʊmə] n Papillom(a) nt.
  p. of the ureter Harnleiter-, Ureterpapillom.
pa·pil·lo·mac·u·lar fasciculus [ˌpæpɪləʊ'mækjələr, pəˌpɪləʊ-] papillomakuläres Bündel nt, Fasciculus papillomacularis.
pap·il·lo·ma·to·sis [ˌpæpɪˌləʊmə'təʊsɪs] n Papillomatose f, Papillomatosis f.
pap·il·lom·a·tous [pæpɪ'lɑmətəs] adj Papillom betr., papillomartig, papillomatös.
Pap·il·lo·ma·vi·rus [ˌpæpɪˌləʊmə'vaɪrəs] n micro. Papillomavirus nt.
papilloma virus → Papillomavirus.
Papillon-Léage and Psaume [papi'jɔ̃ le'aːʒ psoːm]: **P.-L.a.P. syndrome** Papillon-Léage-Psaume-Syndrom nt, orodigitofaziale Dysostose f, orofaziodigitales Syndrom nt, OFD-Syndrom nt.
Papillon-Lefèvre [lə'fɛːvrə]: **P.-L. syndrome** Papillon-Lefèvre-Syndrom nt, Keratosis palmoplantaris mit Paradontose/Periodontose, Keratosis palmoplantaris diffusa non circumscripta nt.
pap·il·lo·ret·i·ni·tis [ˌpæpɪləʊˌretə'naɪtɪs, pəˌpɪləʊ-] n ophthal. kombinierte Papillitis f u. Retinitis, Papilloretinitis f, Retinopapillitis f.
pap·il·lo·sphinc·ter·ot·o·my [ˌ-ˌsfɪŋktə'rɑtəmɪ] n chir. Papillosphinkterotomie f, Papillotomie f, Sphinkterotomie f.
pap·il·lo·tome ['pæpɪlətəʊm] n chir. Papillotom nt.
pap·il·lot·o·my [pæpɪ'lɑtəmɪ] n → papillosphincterotomy.
pap·il·lo·tu·bu·lar adenoma [ˌpæpɪləʊ't(j)uːbjələr, pəˌpɪləʊ-] papillär-tubuläres Adenom nt.
pap·il·lose ['pæpɪləʊz] adj → papillary.
Pa·po·va·vir·i·dae [pəˌpəʊvə'vɪrɪdiː] pl micro. Papovaviren pl, Papovaviridae pl.
pap·o·va·vi·rus [ˌ-'vaɪrəs] n micro. Papovavirus nt.
pap·pa·ta·ci fever [pɑːpə'tɑːtʃɪ] Phlebotomus-, Pappataci-, Moskitofieber nt, Drei-Tage-Fieber nt.
pappataci fever virus Pappataci(fieber)virus nt.
Pappenheim ['paːpənhaɪm]: **lymphoid hemoblast of P.** Proerythroblast m.
  P.'s stain Pappenheim-Färbung f, panoptische Färbung f nach Pappenheim.
Pap test → Papanicolaou's test.
pap·u·lar ['pæpjələr] adj derm. Papel betr., mit Papelbildung, papulös.
papular acrodermatitis of childhood Gianotti-Crosti-Syndrom nt, infantile papulöse Akrodermatitis f, Acrodermatitis papulosa eruptiva infantilis.
papular dermatitis of pregnancy abbr. **PDP** papulöse Dermatitis f in der Schwangerschaft, papular dermatitis of pregnancy abbr. PDP.
papular mucinosis Lichen myxoedematosus, Mucinosis papulosa seu lichenoides, Myxodermia papulosa, Lichen fibromucinoidosus.

papular myxedema → papular mucinosis.
papular rosacea derm. lupoide Rosazea f, Rosacea granulomatosa.
papular syphilid papulöses Syphilid nt.
papular urticaria Urticaria papulosa chronica, Prurigo simplex subacuta, Prurigo simplex acuta et subacuta adultorum, Strophulus adultorum, Lichen urticatus.
pap·u·la·tion [ˌpæpjə'leɪʃn] n Papelbildung f.
pap·ule ['pæpjuːl] n derm. Knötchen nt, Papel f, Papula f.
pap·u·lo·er·y·them·a·tous [ˌpæpjələʊˌerɪ'θemətəs, -'θɪːmə-] adj papuloerythematös.
pap·u·loid ['pæpjəlɔɪd] adj papelähnlich, -artig, papuloid; papulös.
pap·u·lo·ne·crot·ic tuberculid [ˌpæpjələʊnə'krɑtɪk] derm. papulonekrotisches Tuberkulid nt, Tuberculosis cutis papulonecrotica.
papulonecrotic tuberculosis → papulonecrotic tuberculid.
pap·u·lo·pus·tu·lar [ˌ-'pʌstʃələr] adj papulopustulös.
pap·u·lo·sis [ˌpæpjə'ləʊsɪs] n derm. Papulose f, Papulosis f.
pap·u·lo·squa·mous [ˌpæpjələʊ'skeɪməs] adj papulosquamös.
papulosquamous syphilid papulosquamöses/psoriasiformes Syphilid nt.
pap·u·lo·ve·sic·u·lar [ˌ-'vesɪkjələr] adj papulovesikulär.
pap·y·ra·ceous [pæpə'reɪʃəs] adj papierartig, pergamentartig.
papyraceous fetus Fetus papyraceus.
papyraceous plate → paper plate.
par(a)- pref. **1.** neben, über ... hinaus, para(a)-, Neben-, Par(a)-. **2.** patho. fehlerhaft, gestört, abweichend, teilweise, para-.
para- pref. chem. abbr. **p-** para-, Para- abbr. p-.
par·a ['pærə] n gyn. Gebärende f.
para-aminobenzoic acid abbr. **PAB**, **PABA** p-Aminobenzoesäure f, para-Aminobenzoesäure f, Paraaminobenzoesäure f abbr. PABA, PAB.
para-aminohippuric acid abbr. **PAH**, **PAHA** p-Aminohippursäure f, para-Aminohippursäure f, Paraaminohippursäure f abbr. PAH.
para-aminosalicyclic acid abbr. **PAS** p-Aminosalizylsäure f, Paraaminosalizylsäure f abbr. PAS.
para-analgesia n neuro. Par(a)analgesie f.
para-anesthesia n neuro. Par(a)anästhesie f.
para-aortic bodies Corpora para-aortica.
para-appendicitis n Para-, Periappendizitis f.
par·a·bal·lism [ˌpærə'bælɪzəm] n neuro. Paraballismus m, doppelseitiger Ballismus m.
par·a·ban·ic acid [ˌ-'bænɪk] Parabansäure f.
par·a·ba·sal apparatus [ˌ-'beɪzl] histol. Parabasalapparat m.
parabasal body Parabasalkörper m, -körperchen nt.
par·ab·i·on [pær'æbɪɑn] n → parabiont.
par·a·bi·ont [pær'æbɪɑnt] n bio. Parabio(nt) m.
par·a·bi·o·sis [ˌpærəbaɪ'əʊsɪs] n **1.** chir., immun. Parabiose f. **2.** psycho. Parabiose f. **3.** neuro. Parabiose f.
par·a·blast ['blæst] n embryo. Parablast nt.
par·a·blas·tic [ˌ-'blæstɪk] adj embryo. parablastisch.

par·a·blep·sia [ˌ-'blepsɪə] *n ophthal.* Parablepsie *f*.
pa·rab·o·la [pə'ræbələ] *n mathe.* Parabel *f*.
par·a·bol·ic [ˌpærə'bɑlɪk] *adj mathe.*, *techn.* Parabel betr., parabelförmig, parabolisch, Parabel-.
parabolic mirror Parabolspiegel *m*.
pa·rab·o·loid [pə'ræbəlɔɪd] *n mathe.* Paraboloid *nt*.
par·a·bra·chi·al nucleus [ˌpærə'breɪkɪəl] Nc. parabrachialis (isthmorhombencephalicus).
par·a·bu·lia [ˌ-'bjuːlɪə] *n neuro.*, *psychia.* Parabulie *f*.
par·a·car·ci·no·ma·tous myelopathy [ˌ-ˌkɑːrsɪ'nəʊmətəs] paraneoplastische Myelopathie *f*.
par·a·car·di·ac [ˌ-'kɑːrdɪæk] *adj* neben dem Herzen (liegend), parakardial.
par·a·ca·sein [ˌ-'keɪsiː(ɪ)n, -keɪ'siːn] *n* Parakasein *nt*, -casein *nt*.
par·a·cel·lu·lar [ˌ-'seljələr] *adj* parazellulär.
paracellular transport parazellulärer Transport *m*.
par·a·cel·lu·lose [ˌ-'seljəloʊs] *n* Parazellulose *f*.
par·a·ce·nes·the·sia [ˌ-ˌsɪnes'θiːʒ(ɪ)ə] *n* Parazenästhesie *f*.
par·a·cen·te·sis [ˌ-sen'tiːsɪs] *n* **1.** *chir.* Stichinzision *f*, Parazentese *f*. **2.** *HNO* Trommelfellschnitt *m*, Parazentese *f*, Myringotomie *f*, Auripunktur *f*.
p. of heart Herzpunktion *f*, Kardiozentese *f*, -centese *f*.
par·a·cen·tet·ic [ˌ-sen'tetɪk] *adj* Parazentese betr., Parazentese-.
par·a·cen·tral [ˌ-'sentrəl] *adj* parazentral.
paracentral artery A. paracentralis.
paracentral gyrus Gyrus/Lobulus paracentralis.
paracentral lobule → paracentral gyrus.
paracentral nucleus of thalamus Nc. paracentralis (thalami).
paracentral scotoma *ophthal.* parazentrales Skotom *nt*.
par·a·ceph·a·lus [ˌ-'sefələs] *n embryo.* Parazephalus *m*.
par·a·cer·vi·cal block [ˌ-'sɜrvɪkl] Parazervikalblock *m*, -anästhesie *f*.
paracervical block anesthesia → paracervical block.
par·a·cer·vix [ˌ-'sɜrvɪks] *n* Parazervix *f*, Paracervix *f*.
par·ac·et·al·de·hyde [pærˌæsɪ'tældəhaɪd] *n* → paraldehyde.
par·ac·et·am·ol [ˌpærə'setəmɒl] *n pharm.* Paracetamol *nt*.
par·a·chlo·ro·phe·nol [ˌ-ˌklɔːrəʊ'fiːnɒl, -nal] *n* p-Chlor(o)phenol *nt*.
par·a·chol·era [ˌ-'kɒlərə] *n* Paracholera *f*.
paracholera vibrios *micro.* NC-Vibrionen *pl*, Non-Cholera-Vibrionen *pl abbr.* NCV.
par·a·chord·al cartilage [ˌ-'kɔːrdl] *embryo.* parachordaler Knorpel *m*.
par·a·chroi·a [ˌ-'krɔɪə] *n* → parachroma.
par·a·chro·ma [ˌ-'krəʊmə] *n derm.* abnormale/pathologische Hautverfärbung *f*.
par·a·chro·ma·tin [ˌ-'krəʊmətɪn] *n* Parachromatin *nt*.
par·a·chro·ma·tism [ˌ-'krəʊmətɪzəm] *n* → parachromatopsia.
par·a·chro·ma·top·sia [ˌ-krəʊmə'tɑpsɪə] *n ophthal.* Di-, Bichromasie *f*, Dichromatopsie *f*.
par·a·chro·ma·to·sis [ˌ-krəʊmə'təʊsɪs] *n* → parachroma.
par·a·cic·a·tri·cial emphysema [ˌ-sɪkə'trɪʃəl] (*Lunge*) Narbenemphysem *nt*.
par·a·ci·ne·sia [ˌ-sɪ'niːʒ(ɪ)ə] *n* → parakinesia.

par·a·ci·ne·sis [ˌ-sɪ'niːsɪs, -saɪ-] *n* → parakinesia.
par·a·clin·i·cal [ˌ-'klɪnɪkl] *adj* paraklinisch.
par·a·coc·cid·i·oi·dal granuloma [ˌ-kɑkˌsɪdɪ'ɔɪdl] Lutz-Splendore-Almeida--Krankheit *f*, brasialianische/südamerikanische Blastomykose *f*, Parakokzidioidomykose *f*, Granuloma paracoccidioides.
Par·a·coc·cid·i·oi·des brasiliensis [ˌ-kɑkˌsɪdɪ'ɔɪdiːz] *n micro.* Paracoccidioides/Blastomyces brasiliensis.
par·a·coc·cid·i·oi·din [ˌ-kɑkˌsɪdɪ'ɔɪdɪn] *n* Parakokzidioidin *nt*.
paracoccidioidin (skin) test Parakokzidioidin-(Haut-)Test *m*.
par·a·coc·cid·i·oi·do·my·co·sis [ˌ-kɑksɪdɪˌɔɪdəʊmaɪ'kəʊsɪs] *n* → paracoccidioidal granuloma.
par·a·col·ic [ˌ-'kɑlɪk] *adj* parakolisch.
paracolic recesses → paracolic sulci.
paracolic sulci parakolische Bauchfellnischen *pl*, Sulci paracolici.
par·a·co·li·tis [ˌ-kə'laɪtɪs] *n* Parakolitis *f*.
par·a·col·pi·tis [ˌ-kɑl'paɪtɪs] *n gyn.* Parakolpitis *f*, -vaginitis *f*.
par·a·col·pi·um [ˌ-'kɑlpɪəm] *n* Paracolpium *nt*.
par·a·cor·tex [ˌ-'kɔːrteks] *n* (*Lymphknoten*) thymusabhängiges Areal *nt*, T-Areal *nt*, thymusabhängige/parakortikale Zone *f*.
par·a·cor·ti·cal [ˌ-'kɔːrtɪkl] *adj* parakortikal.
paracortical zone parakortikale Zone *f*.
par·a·cou·sis *n* → paracusis.
par·a·cre·sol [ˌ-'kriːsɒl, -sal] *n* p-Kresol *nt*, para-Kresol *nt*.
par·a·crine ['krɪn] *adj* parakrin *nt*.
paracrine secretion parakrine Sekretion *f*; parakrines Sekret *nt*.
par·a·crys·tals [ˌ-'krɪstlz] *pl micro.* Parakristalle *pl*.
par·a·cu·sia [ˌ-'k(j)uːʒ(ɪ)ə] *n* → paracusis.
par·a·cu·sis [ˌ-'k(j)uːsɪs] *n HNO* Hörstörung *f*, Parakusis *f*, Paracusis *f*.
p. of Willis Paracusis Willisii.
par·a·cy·e·sis [ˌ-saɪ'iːsɪs] *n* Extrauterinschwangerschaft *f*, -gravidität *f abbr.* EU, EUG.
par·a·cys·tic [ˌ-'sɪstɪk] *adj* neben der Harnblase (liegend), parazystisch, paravesikal.
paracystic pouch seitlicher Abschnitt *m* der Excavatio vesicouterina.
par·a·cys·ti·tis [ˌ-sɪs'taɪtɪs] *n urol.* Parazystitis *f*.
par·a·cys·ti·um [ˌ-'sɪstɪəm] *n*, *pl* **-tia** [-tɪə] Paracystium *nt*.
par·a·den·ti·tis [ˌ-den'taɪtɪs] *n* Parodontitis *f*, Periodontitis *f*.
par·a·den·ti·um [ˌ-'dentɪəm, -tʃ(ɪ)əm] *n*, *pl* **-tia** [-tɪə, -tʃ(ɪ)ə] → periodontium 1.
par·a·den·to·sis [ˌ-den'təʊsɪs] *n* Para-, Parodontose *f*.
par·a·did·y·mis [ˌ-'dɪdəmɪs] *n*, *pl* **-di·dym·i·des** [-dɪ'dɪmədiːz] Beihoden *m*, Paradidymis *f*.
par·a·di·meth·yl·a·mi·no·benz·al·de·hyde [ˌ-daɪˌmeθəlaˌmiːnəʊben'zældəhaɪd] *n* p--Dimethylaminobenzaldehyd *nt*.
par·a·dip·sia [ˌ-'dɪpsɪə] *n psychia.* Paradipsie *f*.
par·a·dox ['dɑks] *n phys.* Paradox *nt*, Paradoxon *nt*.
par·a·dox·i·cal diarrhea [ˌ-'dɑksɪkl] Verstopfungsdurchfall *m*, uneigentlicher Durchfall *m*, Diarrhoea paradoxa/stercoralis.
paradoxical diplopia *ophthal.* gekreuzte/heteronyme/temporale Diplopie *f*.
paradoxical embolism paradoxe/gekreuzte Embolie *f*.

paradoxical incontinence paradoxe Harninkontinenz *f*, Incontinentia urinae paradoxa, Ischuria paradoxa.
paradoxical metastasis paradoxe/retrograde Metastase *f*.
paradoxical pulse paradoxer Puls *m*, Pulsus paradoxus.
paradoxical respiration paradoxe Atmung *f*.
paradoxical sleep paradoxer/desynchronisierter Schlaf *m*, REM-Schlaf *m*, Traumschlaf *m*.
par·a·du·o·de·nal [ˌ-ˌd(j)uːəʊ'diːnl, -d(j)uː'ɑdnəl] *adj* neben dem Duodenum (liegend), in der Nähe des Duodenums (liegend), paraduodenal.
paraduodenal fold Paraduodenalfalte *f*, Plica paraduodenalis.
paraduodenal fossa Rec. duodenalis inferior.
paraduodenal recess paraduodenale Bauchfelltasche *f*, Rec. paraduodenalis.
par·a·dys·en·ter·y [ˌ-'dɪsntərɪ] *n* Paradysenterie *f*.
paradysentery bacillus Flexner-Bazillus *m*, Shigella flexneri.
par·ae·qui·lib·ri·um [ˌ-ˌɪkwə'lɪbrɪəm] *n* Par(a)äquilibrium *nt*.
par·a·e·soph·a·ge·al [ˌ-ˌɪˌsɑfə'dʒiːəl] *adj* neben der Speiseröhre (liegend), paraösophageal.
paraesophageal hernia paraösophageale (Hiatus-)Hernie *f*.
par·aes·the·sia *n* → paresthesia.
par·a·fas·cic·u·lar nucleus of thalamus [ˌ-fə'sɪkjələr] Nc. parafascicularis (thalami).
par·af·fin ['-fɪn] **I** *n* **1.** Paraffin *nt*, Paraffinum *nt*. **2.** Alkan *nt*. **II** *vt* mit Paraffin behandeln, paraffinieren.
paraffin bath Paraffinbad *nt*.
paraffin cancer Paraffinkrebs *m*.
paraffin compound *chem.* aliphatische Verbindung *f*.
par·af·fine ['-fiːn] *n* → paraffin I.
par·af·fi·no·ma [ˌ-fɪ'nəʊmə] *n* Paraffinom *nt*.
paraffin tumor → paraffinoma.
par·a·floc·cu·lus [ˌ-'flɑkjələs] *n* Paraflocculus *m*.
par·a·fol·lic·u·lar cells [ˌ-fə'lɪkjələr] (*Schilddrüse*) parafollikuläre Zellen *pl*, C-Zellen *pl*.
par·a·form·al·de·hyde [ˌ-ˌfɔːr'mældəhaɪd] *n* Paraformaldehyd *m*, Paraform *nt*.
par·a·fo·ve·al region [ˌ-'foʊvɪəl] (*Auge*) parafoveale Region *f*.
par·a·fre·nal abscess [ˌ-'friːnl] (*Penis*) parafrenaler Abszeß *m*.
par·a·fuch·sin [ˌ-'f(j)uːksɪn] *n* Pararosanilin *nt*.
par·a·func·tion [ˌ-'fʌŋkʃn] *n* Funktionsstörung *f*, Fehlfunktion *f*, Dysfunktion *f*, Parafunktion *f*.
par·a·gam·ma·cism [ˌ-'gæməzɪsəm] *n* Paragammazismus *m*.
par·a·gan·gli·o·ma [ˌ-ˌgæŋglɪ'əʊmə] *n* Paragangliom(a) *nt*.
par·a·gan·gli·on [ˌ-'gæŋglɪən] *n*, *pl* **gli·ons**, **-glia** [-glɪə] Paraganglion *nt*.
par·a·gen·i·tal tubules [ˌ-'dʒenɪtl] *embryo.* Paragenitalis *f*, Tubuli paragenitales.
par·a·geu·sia [ˌ-'g(j)uːzɪə] *n neuro.* veränderte Geschmacksempfindung *f*, Parageusie *f*.
par·a·geu·sic [ˌ-'g(j)uːzɪk] *adj* Parageusie betr.
pa·rag·na·thus [pə'rægnəθəs] *n embryo.* Paragnathus *m*.
par·a·gon·i·mi·a·sis [ˌpærəˌgɑnɪ'maɪəsɪs] *n* Lungenegelbefall *m*, Paragonimiasis *f*, Paragonimose *f*.

paragonimosis

par·a·gon·i·mo·sis [ˌ-ˌgɑnɪˈməʊsɪs] n → paragonimiasis.
Par·a·gon·i·mus [ˌ-ˈgɑnɪməs] n micro. Paragonimus m.
 P. **ringeri/westermani** Lungenegel m, Paragonimus ringeri/westermani.
Par·a·gor·di·us [ˌ-ˈgɔːrdɪəs] n micro. Paragordius m.
par·a·gram·ma·tism [ˌ-ˈgræmətɪzəm] n psychia. Paragrammatismus m.
par·a·gran·u·lo·ma [ˌ-ˌgrænjəˈləʊmə] n lymphozytenreiche Form f des Hodgkin-Lymphoms, Hodgkin-Paragranulom nt, Paragranulom nt.
par·a·graph·ia [ˌ-ˈgræfɪə] n neuro., psychia. Paragraphie f.
par·a·he·mo·phil·ia [ˌ-ˌhiːməˈfɪlɪə, -ˌhem-] n Parahämophilie (A) f, Owren-Syndrom nt, Faktor-V-Mangel m, Hypoproakzelerinämie f, Hypoproaccelerinämie f.
par·a·he·pat·ic [ˌ-hɪˈpætɪk] adj neben der Leber (liegend), parahepatisch; perihepatisch.
par·a·hep·a·ti·tis [ˌ-ˌhepəˈtaɪtɪs] n Perihepatitis f.
par·a·hi·a·tal hernia [ˌ-haɪˈeɪtl] paraösophageale (Hiatus-)Hernie f.
par·a·hi·dro·sis [ˌ-haɪˈdrəʊsɪs] n Parahidrosis f, Paridrosis f.
par·a·hip·po·cam·pal gyrus [ˌ-ˌhɪpəˈkæmpəl] Gyrus hippocampi/parahippocampalis.
par·a·hor·mone [ˌ-ˈhɔːrməʊn] n Parahormon nt.
par·a·hyp·no·sis [ˌ-hɪpˈnəʊsɪs] n Parahypnose f.
par·a·in·flu·en·za virus [ˌ-ɪnfluˈenzə] micro. Parainfluenzavirus nt.
parainfluenza 1 virus Parainfluenza-1-Virus nt, Parainfluenzavirus nt Typ-1.
parainfluenza 2 virus Parainfluenza-2-Virus nt, Parainfluenzavirus nt Typ-2.
parainfluenza 3 virus Parainfluenza-3-Virus nt, Parainfluenzavirus nt Typ-3.
par·a·je·ju·nal fossa [ˌ-dʒɪˈdʒuːnl] Broesike'-Raum f, Fossa parajejunalis.
par·a·ker·a·to·sis [ˌ-kerəˈtəʊsɪs] n derm. Parakeratose f, -keratosis f.
par·a·ker·a·tot·ic [ˌ-kerəˈtɑtɪk] adj Parakeratose betr., parakeratotisch.
par·a·ki·ne·sia [ˌ-kɪˈniːʒ(ɪ)ə, -kaɪ-] n Parakinese f, -kinesis f.
par·a·ki·ne·sis [ˌ-kɪˈniːsɪs, -kaɪ-] n → parakinesia.
par·a·ki·net·ic [ˌ-kɪˈnetɪk, -kaɪ-] adj Parakinese betr., durch sie gekennzeichnet, parakinetisch.
par·a·lab·y·rin·thine cells [ˌ-ˌlæbəˈrɪnθɪn, -θiːn] paralabyrinthäre Zellen pl.
par·a·la·lia [ˌ-ˈleɪlɪə, -ˈlæl-] n neuro. Sprachstörung f, Paralalie f.
par·a·lamb·da·cism [ˌ-ˈlæmdəsɪzəm] n HNO Paralambdazismus m.
par·al·bu·min [ˌpærælˈbjuːmɪn] n Paralbumin nt.
par·al·de·hyde [pəˈrældəhaɪd] n chem. Paraldehyd m.
par·a·lex·ia [ˌpærəˈleksɪə] n Lesestörung f, Paralexie f.
par·a·lex·ic [ˌ-ˈleksɪk] adj Paralexie betr., von Paralexie betroffen, paralektisch.
par·al·ge·sia [ˌpærælˈdʒiːzɪə] n neuro. Paralgesie f.
par·al·ge·sic [ˌpærælˈdʒiːzɪk] adj Paralgesie betr., paralgetisch, paralgesisch.
par·al·gia [pærˈældʒɪə] n → paralgesia.
par·a·li·nin [ˌpærəˈlaɪnɪn] n Kernsaft m, Karyolymphe f.
par·al·lac·tic [ˌ-ˈlæktɪk] adj Parallaxe betr., parallaktisch.
parallactic shift parallaktische Verschiebung f.

par·al·lax [ˈ-læks] n phys. Parallaxe f.
par·al·lel [ˈ-ləl, -lel] I n mathe., fig. Parallele f. **in ~ with** parallel zu. II adj **1.** techn., mathe. parallel (to, with zu, mit). **2.** fig. vergleichbar; parallel verlaufend, gleichgerichtet, -laufend, parallel. III vt **3.** vergleichen (with mit). **4.** anpassen, angleichen (with, to an).
parallel-elastic element abbr. PE physiol. parallelelastisches Element nt abbr. PE.
parallel elasticity physiol. Parallelelastizität f.
parallel fibers Parallelfasern pl.
parallel grid radiol. Parallelraster nt.
par·al·lel·ism [ˈ-lelɪzəm] n mathe. Parallelität f; fig. Ähnlichkeit f, gleiche Entwicklung f, Parallelität f.
parallel rays Parallelstrahlen pl.
parallel shift Parallelverschiebung f.
parallel synapse Parallelkontakt m, Bouton en passage.
par·al·ler·gic [ˌpærəˈlɜrdʒɪk] adj Parallergie betr., parallergisch.
par·al·ler·gy [pærˈælərdʒɪ] n immun. Parallergie f; parallergische Reaktion f.
par·a·lo·gia [ˌpærəˈləʊdʒ(ɪ)ə] n psychia. Paralogie f.
pa·ral·o·gism [pəˈrælədʒɪzəm] n → paralogia.
pa·ral·o·gy [pəˈrælədʒɪ] n → paralogia.
par·a·lu·te·al cell [ˌpærəˈluːtɪəl] Thekaluteinzelle f.
par·a·lu·te·in cell [ˌ-ˈluːtɪɪn, -tiːn] Thekaluteinzelle f.
pa·ral·y·sis [pəˈrælɪsɪs] n, pl **-ses** [-siːz] **1.** (vollständige) Lähmung f, Paralyse f, Plegie f, Parese f. **2.** fig. Lähmung f.
 p. **of accommodation** Akkommodationslähmung f.
 p. **of gaze** Blicklähmung f.
paralysis tick micro. Ixodes pilosus.
par·a·lys·or [ˈpærəlaɪzər] n paralyzer.
par·a·lyt·ic [ˌ-ˈlɪtɪk] I n Gelähmte(r m) f, Paralytiker(in f) m. II adj Paralyse betr., von ihr betroffen, lähmend, gelähmt, paralytisch, Lähmungs-.
paralytic abasia neuro. paralytische Abasie f.
paralytic beriberi trockene Form f der Beriberi, paralytische Beriberi f.
paralytic bladder neurogene atonische Blase f.
 motor p. motorische Blasenlähmung f.
paralytic chest Thorax paralyticus.
paralytic clubfoot ortho. paralytischer Klumpfuß m.
paralytic dementia progressive Paralyse f abbr. PP, Paralysis progressiva.
paralytic ectropion ophthal. Ektropium paralyticum.
paralytic ileus chir. paralytischer Ileus m, Ileus paralyticus.
paralytic mydriasis ophthal. paralytische Mydriasis f, Mydriasis paralytica.
paralytic phase anes. Lähmungsstadium nt, paralytisches Stadium nt.
paralytic scoliosis ortho. paralytische Skoliose f.
paralytic stage → paralytic phase.
paralytic strabismus ophthal. Lähmungsschielen nt, Strabismus paralyticus.
par·a·ly·to·gen·ic [ˌ-laɪtəˈdʒenɪk] adj eine Paralyse verursachend. auslösend, lähmend, paralytisch, paralytogen.
par·a·ly·zant [ˈ-laɪzənt] I n eine Lähmung verursachendes Mittel nt. II adj eine Paralyse auslösend, lähmend, paralytisch.
par·a·ly·za·tion [ˌ-laɪˈzeɪʃn] n → paralysis.
par·a·lyze [ˈ-laɪz] vt lähmen, paralysieren.
par·a·lyz·er [ˈ-laɪzər] n chem. Hemmstoff m, Hemmer m, Inhibitor m.

par·a·lyz·ing vertigo [ˈ-laɪzɪŋ] Vertigo epidemica.
par·a·mag·net·ic [ˌ-mægˈnetɪk] adj phys. Paramagnetismus betr. od. zeigend, paramagnetisch.
par·a·mag·net·ism [ˌ-ˈmægnətɪzəm] n phys. Paramagnetismus m.
par·a·mas·ti·tis [ˌ-mæsˈtaɪtɪs] n gyn. Paramastitis f.
par·a·mas·toid·i·tis [ˌ-mæstɔɪˈdaɪtɪs] n HNO Paramastoiditis f.
par·a·mas·toid process [ˌ-ˈmæstɔɪd] Proc. paramastoideus.
par·a·me·a·tal [ˌ-mɪˈeɪtəl] adj parameatal.
Par·a·me·ci·um [ˌ-ˈmiːʃ(ɪ)əm] n bio. Pantoffeltierchen nt, Paramecium nt.
par·a·me·di·an [ˌ-ˈmiːdɪən] adj neben der Medianlinie od. -ebene (liegend), paramedian.
paramedian incision Paramedianschnitt m.
paramedian lobule Lobulus gracilis/paramedianus (cerebelli).
paramedian nucleus: dorsal p. Nc. paramedianus dorsalis/posterior.
 posterior p. → dorsal p.
par·a·med·ic [ˌ-ˈmedɪk] n **1.** Sanitäter m. **2.** ärztlicher Assistent m, ärztliche Assistentin f, Gehilfe m, Gehilfin f.
par·a·med·i·cal [ˌ-ˈmedɪkl] adj nichtärztlich.
par·a·me·nia [ˌ-ˈmiːnɪə] n gyn. Menstruationsstörung f, Paramenie f.
par·a·me·si·al [ˌ-ˈmiːsɪəl] adj → paramedian.
par·a·mes·o·neph·ric duct [ˌ-ˌmezəˈnefrɪk] Müller'-Gang m, Ductus paramesonephricus.
paramesonephric tubercle embryo. Müller'-Hügel m.
pa·ram·e·ter [pəˈræmɪtər] n stat., mathe. Parameter m.
par·a·meth·a·sone [ˌpærəˈmeθəsəʊn] n pharm. Parametason f.
par·a·me·tri·al [ˌ-ˈmiːtrɪəl] adj gyn. **1.** Parametrium betr., parametran, parametrisch. **2.** neben der Gebärmutter (liegend), parametran.
parametrial abscess parametraner Abszeß m.
par·a·met·ric[1] [ˌ-ˈmetrɪk] adj stat., mathe. parametrisch, Parameter-.
par·a·met·ric[2] [ˌ-ˈmetrɪk] adj → parametrial **1.**
parametric abscess → parametrial abscess.
parametric hematocele gyn. Haematocele retrouterina.
par·a·me·tris·mus [ˌ-məˈtrɪzməs] n gyn. Parametropathia spastica, Pelvipathia vegetativa.
par·a·me·trit·ic [ˌ-məˈtrɪtɪk] adj Parametritis betr., parametritisch.
par·a·me·tri·tis [ˌ-mɪˈtraɪtɪs] n gyn. Entzündung f des Parametriums, Parametriumentzündung f, Parametritis f.
par·a·me·tri·um [ˌ-ˈmiːtrɪəm] n, pl **-tria** [-trɪə] Parametrium nt, Retinaculum uteri.
par·a·mim·ia [ˌ-ˈmɪmɪə] n psychia. Paramimie f.
par·a·mi·tome [ˌ-ˈmaɪtəʊm] n → paraplasm 1.
par·a·mi·to·sis [ˌ-maɪˈtəʊsɪs] n bio. Paramitose f.
par·am·ne·si·a [ˌpæræmˈniːʒə] n neuro., psychia. Erinnerungsverfälschung f, Paramnesie f.
Par·a·moe·ba [ˌpærəˈmiːbə] n micro. Entamoeba f.
par·am·phi·sto·mi·a·sis [pærˌæmfɪstəˈmaɪəsɪs] n Paramphistomiasis f.

Par·am·phis·to·mum [ˌpæræm'fɪstəməm] *n micro.* Paramphistomum *nt.*

par·a·mu·cin [ˌpærə'mju:sɪn] *n* Paramuzin *nt.*

par·a·mu·sia [ˌ-'mju:zɪə] *n neuro.* Paramusie *f.*

par·a·my·e·lin [ˌ-'maɪəlɪn] *n* Paramyelin *nt.*

par·a·my·e·lo·blast [ˌ-'maɪələblæst] *n hema.* Paramyeloblast *m.*

par·am·y·loi·do·sis [pærˌæmɪlɔɪ'dəʊsɪs] *n* Par(a)amyloidose *f.*

par·a·my·oc·lo·nus [ˌpærəmaɪ'ɑklənəs] *n neuro.* Paramyoklonus *m,* -myoclonus *m.*

par·a·my·o·sin [ˌ-'maɪəsɪn] *n* Paramyosin *nt,* Tropomyosin A *nt.*

par·a·my·o·sin·o·gen [ˌ-ˌmaɪə'sɪnədʒən] *n* Paramyosinogen *nt.*

paramyosin strand Paramyosinstrang *m.*

par·a·my·o·tone [ˌ-'maɪətəʊn] *n* → paramyotonia.

par·a·my·o·to·nia [ˌ-ˌmaɪə'təʊnɪə] *n neuro.* Paramyotonie *f,* -tonia *f.*

par·a·my·ot·o·nus [ˌ-maɪ'ɑtənəs] *n* → paramyotonia.

Par·a·myx·o·vir·i·dae [ˌ-ˌmɪksəʊ'vɪrədi:, -'vaɪr-] *pl micro.* Paramyxoviren *pl,* Paramyxoviridae *pl.*

par·a·myx·o·vi·rus [ˌ-ˌmɪksə'vaɪrəs] *n micro.* Paramyxovirus *nt.*

par·an·al·ge·si·a [pærˌænl'dʒi:zɪə] *n* Par(a)analgesie *f.*

par·a·na·sal [ˌpærə'neɪzl] *adj* neben der Nase *od.* Nasenhöhle (liegend), paranasal.

paranasal sinuses (Nasen-)Nebenhöhlen *pl,* Sinus paranasales.

paranasal sinusitis *HNO* (Nasen-)Nebenhöhlenentzündung *f,* Sinusitis *f.*

par·a·ne·o·plas·tic [ˌ-ˌni:ə'plæstɪk] *adj* paraneoplastisch.

paraneoplastic acrokeratosis Bazex-Syndrom *nt,* Akrokeratose Bazex *f,* Akrokeratosis paraneoplastica.

paraneoplastic hyperparathyroidism paraneoplastischer Hyperparathyr(e)oidismus *m,* Pseudohyperparathyr(e)oidismus *m.*

paraneoplastic syndrome paraneoplastisches Syndrom *nt.*

par·a·neph·ric [ˌ-'nefrɪk] *adj* neben der Niere (liegend), pararenal, paranephritisch.

paranephric abscess paranephritischer Abszeß *m.*

paranephric body → pararenal fat body.

paranephric fat → pararenal fat body.

paranephric fat pad → pararenal fat body.

par·a·ne·phri·tis [ˌ-nɪ'fraɪtɪs] *n* Paranephritis *f.*

par·a·ne·phro·ma [ˌ-nɪ'frəʊmə] *n* Nebennierentumor *m,* -geschwulst *f.*

par·a·neph·ros [ˌ-'nefrɑs] *n, pl* **-roi** [-rɔɪ] Nebenniere *f,* Gl. suprarenalis/adrenalis.

par·an·es·the·sia [pærˌænəs'θi:ʒə] *n neuro.* Par(a)anästhesie *f.*

par·a·neu·ral anesthesia [ˌpærə'njʊərəl, -'nʊ-] → paraneural block.

paraneural block paraneurale Leitungsanästhesie *f,* paraneuraler Block *m.*

paraneural infiltration → paraneural block.

pa·ran·gi [pə'rændʒi] *n* Frambösie *f,* Pian *f,* Parangi *f,* Yaws *f,* Framboesia tropica.

par·a·nod·al zone [ˌpærə'nəʊdl] paranodale Zone *f.*

par·a·noia [ˌ-'nɔɪə] *n psychia.* Paranoia *f.*

par·a·noi·ac [ˌ-'nɔɪæk, -ɪk] **I** *n* an Paranoia Leidende(r), Paranoiker(in *f*) *m.* **II** *adj* Paranoia betr., auf Paranoia beruhend, paranoisch, wahnhaft.

par·a·noid ['-nɔɪd] *adj* der Paranoia ähnlich, paranoid, wahnhaft.

paranoid delusion paranoider Wahn *m.*

paranoid disorders paranoide Psychosen *pl.*

paranoid personality (disorder) paranoide Persönlichkeit(sstörung *f*) *f.*

par·a·no·mia [ˌ-'nəʊmɪə] *n neuro.* Paranomie *f.*

par·a·nor·mal [ˌ-'nɔːrml] *adj* paranormal, übersinnlich.

par·a·nu·cle·ar [ˌ-'n(j)u:klɪər] *adj* **1.** um einen Kern herum (liegend), paranukleär. **2.** Paranukleus betr.

paranuclear body Zentroplasma *nt,* Zentrosphäre *f.*

par·a·nu·cle·o·lus [ˌ-n(j)u:'klɪələs] *n* Paranukleolus *m.*

par·a·nu·cle·us [ˌ-'n(j)u:klɪəs] *n* Nebenkern *m,* Paranukleus *m.*

par·a·om·phal·ic [ˌ-ɑm'fælɪk] *adj* → paraumbilical.

par·a·o·ral [ˌ-'ɔːrəl] *adj* paraoral.

par·a·os·mia [ˌ-'ɑzmɪə] *n* → parosmia.

par·a·os·se·ous chondroma [ˌ-'ɑsɪəs] juxtakortikales/periostales/paraossales Chondrom *nt.*

par·a·pan·cre·at·ic [ˌ-ˌpæŋkr'ætɪk, -ˌpæn-] *adj* neben der Bauchspeicheldrüse (liegend), parapankreatisch.

par·a·pa·re·sis [ˌ-pə'riːsɪs, -'pærəsɪs] *n neuro.* Paraparese *f.*

par·a·pa·ret·ic [ˌ-pə'retɪk] **I** *n* Parapaketiker(in *f*) *m.* **II** *adj* Paraparese betr., paraparetisch.

par·a·pe·de·sis [ˌ-pə'di:sɪs] *n* Parapedese *f.*

par·a·per·i·to·ne·al [ˌ-ˌperətə'ni:əl] *adj* paraperitoneal.

paraperitoneal hernia Hernia paraperitonealis.

par·a·per·tus·sis [ˌ-pər'tʌsɪs] *n* Parapertussis *f.*

par·a·pes·tis [ˌ-'pestɪs] *n* Pestis minor.

par·a·pha·ryn·ge·al [ˌ-fə'rɪn'dʒ(i)əl, -ˌfærɪn'dʒiːəl] *adj* neben dem Rachen/Pharynx (liegend), parapharyngeal.

parapharyngeal space parapharyngealer Raum *m,* Spatium parapharyngeum.

par·a·pha·sia [ˌ-'feɪʒə] *n neuro.* Paraphasie *f.*

par·a·pha·sic [ˌ-'feɪzɪk] *adj* Paraphasie betr.

par·a·phe·mia [ˌ-'fi:mɪə] *n neuro.* Paraphemie *f.*

par·a·phen·yl·ene·di·am·ine [ˌ-ˌfenəlɪnˈdaɪ'æmɪn] *n* Paraphenylendiamin *nt.*

pa·ra·phia [pə'reɪfɪə, -'ræf-] *n neuro.* Störung *f* des Tastsinns, Parapsis *f.*

par·a·phil·ia [ˌpærə'fɪlɪə] *n psychia.* Paraphilie *f,* sexuelle Deviation *f;* Perversion *f.*

par·a·phil·i·ac [ˌ-'fɪlɪæk] *psychia.* **I** *n* Paraphile(r *m*) *f;* *inf.* Perverse(r *m*) *f.* **II** *adj* Paraphilie betr., paraphil; pervers.

par·a·phi·mo·sis [ˌ-faɪ'məʊsɪs, -fɪ-] *n urol.* Paraphimose *f,* Capistratio *f.*

par·a·pho·bia [ˌ-'fəʊbɪə] *n psychia.* Paraphobie *f.*

par·a·pho·nia [ˌ-'fəʊnɪə] *n HNO* Paraphonie *f,* -phonia *f.*

par·a·phra·sia [ˌ-'freɪʒ(ɪ)ə] *n neuro.* Paraphrasie *f.*

par·a·phre·nia [ˌ-'fri:nɪə] *n* **1.** *psychia.* Paraphrenie *f.* **2.** → paraphrenitis.

par·a·phren·ic [ˌ-'frenɪk] *psychia.* **I** *n* Paraphreniker(in *f*) *m.* **II** *adj* Paraphrenie betr., paraphrenisch.

par·a·phre·ni·tis [ˌ-frɪ'naɪtɪs] *n* Paraphrenitis *f.*

par·a·phys·e·al [ˌ-'fɪzɪəl] *adj* Paraphyse betr., paraphysär.

paraphyseal body → paraphysis.

pa·raph·y·sis [pə'ræfəsɪs] *n, pl* **-ses** [-si:z] Paraphyse *f.*

par·a·plasm ['pærəplæzəm] *n* **1.** Hyaloplasma *nt,* Grundzytoplasma *nt,* zytoplasmatische Matrix *f.* **2.** Paraplasma *nt,* Alloplasma *nt.*

par·a·plas·mat·ic [ˌ-plæz'mætɪk] *adj* → paraplasmic.

para·plas·mic [ˌ-'plæzmɪk] *adj* Paraplasma betr., im Paraplasma (liegend), paraplasmatisch.

par·a·plec·tic [ˌ-'plektɪk] *n, adj* → paraplegic.

par·a·ple·gia [ˌ-'pli:dʒ(ɪ)ə] *n neuro.* Paraplegie *f,* -plegia *f;* tiefe Querschnittslähmung *f.*

par·a·ple·gic [ˌ-'pli:dʒɪk, -'pledʒɪk] **I** *n* Querschnittsgelähmte(r *m*) *f,* Paraplegiker(in *f*) *m.* **II** *adj* querschnittsgelähmt, paraplegisch.

par·a·pleg·i·form [ˌ-'pledʒɪfɔːrm] *adj* in Form einer Paraplegie, paraplegiform.

par·a·pleu·ri·tis [ˌ-plʊ'raɪtɪs] *n* Parapleuritis *f.*

par·a·pneu·mo·nia [ˌ-n(j)u:'məʊnɪə] *n* Parapneumonie *f.*

par·a·pneu·mon·ic [ˌ-n(j)u:'mɑnɪk] *adj* im Verlauf einer Pneumonie auftretend, parapneumonisch.

parapneumonic pleurisy/pleuritis parapneumonische Rippenfellentzündung *f,* Pleuritis *f.*

Par·a·pox·vi·rus [ˌ-'pɑksvaɪrəs] *n micro.* Parapoxvirus *nt.*

par·a·pox·vi·rus [ˌ-'pɑksvaɪrəs] *n micro.* Parapoxvirus *nt.*

par·a·prax·ia [ˌ-'præksɪə] *n neuro.* Parapraxie *f.*

par·a·prax·is [ˌ-'præksɪs] *n* → parapraxia.

par·a·proc·ti·tis [ˌ-prɑk'taɪtɪs] *n* Paraproktitis *f.*

par·a·proc·ti·um [ˌ-'prɑktɪəm, -ʃ(ɪ)əm] *n* Paraproctium *nt.*

par·a·pros·ta·ti·tis [ˌ-ˌprɑstə'taɪtɪs] *n urol.* Paraprostatitis *f.*

par·a·pro·tein [ˌ-'prəʊti:n, -ti:ɪn] *n* Paraprotein *nt.*

par·a·pro·tein·e·mia [ˌ-ˌprəʊti'ni:mɪə] *n* Paraproteinämie *f.*

pa·rap·sia [pə'ræpsɪə] *n* → parapsis.

pa·rap·sis [pə'ræpsɪs] *n* Störung *f* des Tastsinns, Parapsis *f.*

par·a·pso·ri·a·sis [ˌpærəsə'raɪəsɪs] *n derm.* Parapsoriasis *f.*

parapsoriasis en plaques *derm.* Brocq-Krankheit *f,* Parapsoriasis en plaques, chronische superfizielle Dermatitis *f.*

par·a·psy·chic [ˌ-'saɪkɪk] *adj* → parapsychical.

par·a·psy·chi·cal [ˌ-'saɪkɪkl] *adj* übersinnlich, parapsychisch.

par·a·psy·cho·log·i·cal [ˌ-saɪkə'lɑdʒɪkl] *adj* parapsychologisch.

par·a·psy·chol·o·gist [ˌ-saɪ'kɑlədʒɪst] *n* Parapsychologe *m,* -login *f.*

par·a·psy·chol·o·gy [ˌ-saɪ'kɑlədʒi] *n* Parapsychologie *f.*

par·a·quat ['-kwɑt] *n* Paraquat *nt.*

par·a·rec·tal [ˌ-'rektl] *adj* **1.** neben dem Rektum (liegend), pararektal. **2.** neben dem M. rectus abdominis, pararektal, Pararektal-.

pararectal incision *chir.* Pararektal-, Kulissenschnitt *m.*

pararectal line Linea pararectalis.

pararectal pouch seitlicher Abschnitt *m* der Excavatio rectouterina.

par·a·rec·tus incision [ˌ-'rektəs] → pararectal incision.

par·a·re·flex·ia [ˌ-rɪ'fleksɪə] *n neuro.* Reflexstörung *f,* Parareflexie *f.*

pararenal

par·a·re·nal [ˌ-'riːnl] *adj* neben der Niere (liegend), pararenal.
pararenal body → pararenal fat body.
pararenal fat → pararenal fat body
pararenal fat body pararenales Fettpolster *nt*, pararenaler Fettkörper *m*, Corpus adiposum pararenale.
pararenal fat pad → pararenal fat body.
par·a·rho·ta·cism [ˌ-'rəʊtəsɪzəm] *n HNO*, *neuro.* Pararhotazismus *m*.
par·a·ros·an·i·line [ˌ-rəʊ'zænɪlɪn, -liːn] *n* Pararosanilin *nt*.
par·ar·rhyth·mia [ˌ-'rɪðmɪə] *n* → parasystole 2.
par·ar·thria [pæ'rɑːrθrɪə] *n HNO, neuro.* Pararthrie *f*, Pararthria *f*.
par·a·sac·cu·lar hernia [ˌpærə'sækjələr] Gleithernie *f*, -bruch *m*.
par·a·sa·cral [ˌ-'seɪkrəl] *adj* neben dem Sakrum (liegend), parasakral, Parasakral-.
parasacral block Parasakralanästhesie *f*.
par·a·sag·it·tal plane [ˌ-'sædʒɪtl] Parasagittalebene *f*.
par·a·sal·pin·gi·tis [ˌ-ˌsælpɪn'dʒaɪtɪs] *n gyn.* Parasalpingitis *f*.
par·a·scap·u·lar [ˌ-'skæpjələr] *adj* paraskapulär.
par·a·scar·la·ti·na [ˌ-ˌskɑːrlə'tiːnə] *n* Dukes'-Krankheit *f*, Dukes-Filatoff-Krankheit *f*, vierte Krankheit *f*, Parascarlatina *f*, Rubeola scarlatinosa.
par·a·scar·let [ˌ-'skɑːrlɪt] *n* → parascarlatina.
par·a·sel·lar [ˌ-'selər] *adj* neben der Sella turcica (liegend), parasellär.
parasellar tumor parasellärer Tumor *m*.
par·a·sep·tal emphysema [ˌ-'septl] paraseptales Lungenemphysem *nt*.
par·a·sex·u·al [ˌ-'sekʃəwəl] *adj bio.* parasexuell.
par·a·sex·u·al·i·ty [ˌ-ˌsekʃə'wælətɪ] *n* 1. *bio.* Parasexualität *f*. 2. *psychia.* sexuelle Perversion *f*, Parasexualität *f*.
par·a·sig·ma·tism [ˌ-'sɪɡmətɪzəm] *n neuro.*, *HNO* Parasigmatismus *m*.
par·a·si·noi·dal [ˌ-saɪ'nɔɪdl] *adj* neben einem Sinus (liegend), parasinoidal, parasinuidal.
parasinoidal lacunae Seitennischen *pl* des Sinus sagittalis superior, Lacunae laterales.
par·a·si·tal [ˌ-'saɪtl] *adj* → parasitic.
par·a·si·ta·ry [ˌ-'saɪtərɪ] *adj* → parasitic.
par·a·site ['-saɪt] *n* 1. Schmarotzer *m*, Parasit *m*. 2. *embryo.* Parasit *m*.
par·a·sit·e·mia [ˌ-saɪ'tiːmɪə] *n* Parasitämie *f*.
par·a·sit·ic [ˌ-'sɪtɪk] *adj* durch Parasiten hervorgerufen, schmarotzend, schmarotzerhaft, parasitisch, parasitär.
par·a·sit·i·cal [ˌ-'sɪtɪkl] *adj* → parasitic.
parasitic bacterium parasitäres Bakterium *nt*.
parasitic blepharitis *ophthal.* Blepharitis parasitica/parasitalis.
parasitic chylocele Elephantiasis scroti.
parasitic cyst Parasitenzyste *f*, parasitäre Zyste *f*.
parasitic disease Parasitenerkrankung *f*, Parasitose *f*.
parasitic hemoptysis parasitäre Hämoptoe/Hämoptyse *f*.
par·a·sit·i·ci·dal [ˌ-ˌsɪtɪ'saɪdl] *adj* parasiten(ab)tötend, parasitizid.
par·a·sit·i·cide [ˌ-'sɪtɪsaɪd] I *n* parasiten(ab)tötendes Mittel *nt*, Parasitizid *nt*. II *adj* → parasiticidal.
par·a·sit·i·cid·ic [ˌ-ˌsɪtɪ'sɪdɪk] *adj* → parasiticidal.
parasitic melanoderma *hema.* Vaganten-, Vagabundenhaut *f*, Cutis vagantium.
parasitic worms *micro.* parasitische Würmer *pl*, Helminthen *pl*, Helminthes *pl*.
par·a·sit·i·fer [ˌ-'sɪtɪfər] *n* Parasitenwirt *m*.
par·a·sit·ism ['-saɪtɪzm] *n* 1. (*a. fig.*) Schmarotzertum *nt*, schmarotzende Lebensweise *f*, Parasitismus *m*, Parasitie *f*. 2. → parasitization.
par·a·sit·i·za·tion [ˌ-ˌsaɪtə'zeɪʃn] *n* Parasitenbefall *m*, -infektion *f*.
par·a·si·tize ['-sɪtaɪz] *vt* schmarotzen, als Parasit leben, parasitieren.
par·a·si·to·gen·ic [ˌ-ˌsaɪtə'dʒenɪk] *adj* durch Parasiten verursacht, parasitogen, Parasiten-.
par·a·sit·oid ['-saɪtɔɪd, -sɪ-] I *n* Parasitoid *m*. II *adj* parasitenähnlich.
par·a·si·to·log·ic [ˌ-ˌsaɪtə'lɑdʒɪk] *adj* → parasitological.
par·a·si·to·log·i·cal [ˌ-ˌsaɪtə'lɑdʒɪkl] *adj* parasitologisch.
par·a·si·tol·o·gist [ˌ-ˌsaɪ'tɑlədʒɪst] *n* Parasitologe *m*, -login *f*.
par·a·si·tol·o·gy [ˌ-ˌsaɪ'tɑlədʒɪ] *n* Parasitologie *f*.
par·a·si·to·pho·bia [ˌ-ˌsaɪtə'fəʊbɪə] *n psychia.* krankhafte Angst *f* vor Parasiten, Parasitophobie *f*.
par·a·si·to·sis [ˌ-saɪ'təʊsɪs, -sɪ-] *n* Parasitenerkrankung *f*, Parasitose *f*.
par·a·si·to·trope [ˌ-'saɪtətrəʊp] *adj* → parasitotropic.
par·a·si·to·trop·ic [ˌ-ˌsaɪtə'trɑpɪk] *adj* mit besonderer Affinität zu Parasiten, parasitotrop.
par·a·si·tot·ro·pism [ˌ-saɪ'tɑtrəpɪzəm] *n* → parasitotropy.
par·a·si·tot·ro·py [ˌ-saɪ'tɑtrəpɪ] *n pharm.* Parasitotropie *f*.
par·a·sol insertion ['-sɔl, -sɑl] *gyn.* Insertio velamentosa.
par·a·sol·i·tar·y nucleus [ˌ-'sɑlɪtərɪ] Nc. solitarius.
par·a·so·ma [ˌ-'səʊmə] *n* → paranucleus.
par·a·som·nia [ˌ-'sɑmnɪə] *n neuro.*, *psychia.* Parasomnie *f*.
par·a·spa·dia [ˌ-'speɪdɪə] *n* → paraspadias.
par·a·spa·di·as [ˌ-'speɪdɪəs] *n urol.* seitlicher Harnröhrenspalt *m*, Paraspadie *f*.
par·a·spasm [ˌ-'spæzəm] *n neuro.* Paraspastik *f*.
par·a·spas·mus [ˌ-'spæzməs] *n* → paraspasm.
par·a·spe·cif·ic therapy [ˌ-spə'sɪfɪk] unspezifische Therapie *f*.
par·a·ster·nal [ˌ-'stɜrnl] *adj* neben dem Sternum (liegend), parasternal.
parasternal line Parasternallinie *f*, Linea parasternalis.
par·a·stru·ma [ˌ-'struːmə] *n* Parastruma *f*.
par·a·sym·pa·thet·ic [ˌ-ˌsɪmpə'θetɪk] *adj* parasympathisches Nervensystem betr., parasympathisch.
parasympathetic ganglion parasympathisches Ganglion *nt*, Parasympathikusganglion *nt*, Ggl. parasympathicum/parasympatheticum.
parasympathetic nerve parasympathischer Nerv *m*.
parasympathetic nervous system parasympathisches (Nerven-)System *nt*, Parasympathikus *m*, parasympathischer Teil *m* des vegetativen Nervensystems, Pars parasympathica systematis nervosi autonomici.
parasympathetic neuron parasympathisches Neuron *nt*.
parasympathetic paraganglia parasympathische Paraganglien *pl*.
parasympathetic root: p. of ciliary ganglion Radix oculomotoria/parasympathetica gg. ciliaris.
p. of pterygopalatine ganglion Radix parasympathetica.
par·a·sym·path·i·co·to·nia [ˌ-ˌsɪmˌpæθɪkəʊ'təʊnɪə] *n* Parasympathikotonie *f*, Parasympathotonie *f*, Vagotonie *f*; Vagotonus *m*.
par·a·sym·pa·tho·lyt·ic [ˌ-ˌsɪmpəθəʊ'lɪtɪk] I *n* Parasympatholytikum *nt*, Anticholinergikum *nt*, cholinerger Antagonist *m*. II *adj* parasympatholytisch, anticholinerg(isch).
par·a·sym·pa·tho·mi·met·ic [ˌ-ˌsɪmpəθəʊmɪ'metɪk, -maɪ-] I *n* Parasympathomimetikum *nt*. II *adj* parasympathomimetisch.
par·a·sym·pa·tho·par·a·lyt·ic [ˌ-ˌsɪmpəθəʊˌpærə'lɪtɪk] *n*, *adj* → parasympatholytic.
par·a·sym·pa·tho·to·nia [ˌ-ˌsɪmpəθəʊ'təʊnɪə] *n* → parasympathicotonia.
par·a·syn·ap·sis [ˌ-sɪ'næpsɪs] *n bio.* Parasynapsis *f*, Parasyndesis *f*.
par·a·syn·de·sis [ˌ-sɪn'diːsɪs] *n* → parasynapsis.
par·a·syn·o·vi·tis [ˌ-ˌsɪnə'vaɪtɪs] *n* Parasynovitis *f*.
par·a·syph·i·lis [ˌ-'sɪf(ə)lɪs] *n* Parasyphilis *f*.
par·a·syph·i·lit·ic [ˌ-ˌsɪfə'lɪtɪk] *adj* Parasyphilis betr., parasyphilitisch.
par·a·syph·i·lo·sis [ˌ-ˌsɪfə'ləʊsɪs] *n* → parasyphilis.
par·a·sys·to·le [ˌ-'sɪstəlɪ] *n card.* 1. Parasystolie *f*, parasystolischer Rhythmus *m*. 2. Pararrhythmie *f*.
par·a·sys·tol·ic beat [ˌ-sɪs'tɑlɪk] → parasystole 1.
parasystolic rhythm → parasystole.
par·a·tax·ia [ˌ-'tæksɪə] *n* → parataxis.
par·a·tax·is [ˌ-'tæksɪs] *n psycho.* Parataxie *f*.
par·a·te·ni·al nucleus of thalamus [ˌ-'tiːnɪəl] Nc. parat(a)enialis (thalami).
par·a·ten·ic host [ˌ-'tenɪk] *micro.* Hilfs-, Transport-, Wartewirt *m*, paratenischer Wirt *m*.
par·a·ten·on [ˌ-'tenən] *n* Paratenon *nt*, Paratendineum *nt*.
par·a·ter·mi·nal gyrus [ˌ-'tɜrmɪnl] Gyrus paraterminalis/subcallosus.
par·a·thi·on [ˌ-'θaɪən] *n* Parathion *nt*, E 605 *nt*.
par·a·thor·mone [ˌ-'θɔːrməʊn] *n* → parathyroid hormone.
par·a·thy·mia [ˌ-'θaɪmɪə] *n psychia.* Parathymie *f*.
par·a·thy·rin [ˌ-'θaɪrɪn] *n* → parathyroid hormone.
par·a·thy·roid [ˌ-'θaɪrɔɪd] I *n* Nebenschilddrüse *f*, Epithelkörperchen *nt*, Parathyr(e)oidea *f*, Gl. parathyroidea. II *adj* neben der Schilddrüse (liegend), parathyr(e)oidal.
parathyroid adenoma Nebenschilddrüsen-, Epithelkörperchenadenom *nt*, Parathyreoidom *nt*.
par·a·thy·roi·dal [ˌ-'θaɪrɔɪdl] *adj* Nebenschilddrüse betr., parathyr(e)oid, parathyr(e)oidal.
parathyroid carcinoma Nebenschilddrüsen-, Epithelkörperchenkarzinom *nt*, Karzinom *nt* der Nebenschilddrüse.
parathyroid cyst Nebenschilddrüsen-, Epithelkörperchenzyste *f*.
par·a·thy·roid·ec·to·mize [ˌ-ˌθaɪrɔɪ'dektəmaɪz] *vt chir.* die Nebenschilddrüsen entfernen, eine Parathyreoidektomie durchführen, parathyreoidektomieren.
par·a·thy·roid·ec·to·my [ˌ-ˌθaɪrɔɪ'dektəmɪ] *n chir.* Nebenschilddrüsen-, Epithelkörperchenentfernung *f*, Parathyr(e)oidektomie *f*.
parathyroid gland → parathyroid I.
inferior p. Gl. parathyroidea inferior.
superior p. Gl. parathyroidea superior.

parathyroid hormone abbr. **PTH** Parathormon nt abbr. PTH, Parathyrin nt.
parathyroid hyperplasia Nebenschilddrüsen-, Epithelkörperchenhyperplasie f.
parathyroid insufficiency Unterfunktion f der Nebenschilddrüsen, Hypoparathyr(e)oidismus m.
par·a·thy·roi·do·ma [ˌ-ˌθaɪrɔɪ'dəʊmə] n **1.** → parathyroid adenoma. **2.** → parathyroid carcinoma.
parathyroid osteitis Ostitis fibrosa cystica.
parathyroid resection chir. partielle Parathyreoidektomie f.
parathyroid tetany Tetania parathyreopriva.
parathyroid tumor Nebenschilddrüsentumor m, -geschwulst f, Epithelkörperchentumor m, -geschwulst f.
par·a·thy·rop·a·thy [ˌ-θaɪ'rɒpəθɪ] n Erkrankung f der Nebenschilddrüsen/Epithelkörperchen, Parathyreopathie f.
par·a·thy·ro·pri·val [ˌ-ˌθaɪrəʊ'praɪvəl] adj parathyreopriv.
parathyroprival tetany → parathyroid tetany.
par·a·thy·ro·priv·ic [ˌ-ˌθaɪrə'prɪvɪk] adj → parathyroprival.
par·a·thy·rop·ri·vous [ˌ-θaɪ'rɒprɪvəs] adj → parathyroprival.
par·a·thy·ro·troph·ic [ˌ-ˌθaɪrə'trɒfɪk, -'trəʊ-] adj → parathyrotropic.
par·a·thy·ro·trop·ic [ˌ-ˌθaɪrə'trɒpɪk, -'trəʊ-] adj parathyreotrop.
par·a·to·nia [ˌ-'təʊnɪə] n neuro. Paratonie f.
par·a·tope ['-təʊp] n immun. Paratop nt.
par·a·tra·che·al [ˌ-'treɪkɪəl] adj neben der Luftröhre/Trachea (liegend), paratracheal.
par·a·tra·cho·ma [ˌ-trə'kəʊmə] n ophthal. Paratrachom nt.
par·a·tu·ber·cu·lo·sis [ˌ-təˌbɜrkjə'ləʊsɪs] n Pseudotuberkulose f.
par·a·tu·ber·cu·lous lymphadenitis [ˌ-təˌbjɜrkjələs] Pseudotuberkulose f.
par·a·type ['-taɪp] n micro. Paratyp m, -typus m.
par·a·typh·li·tis [ˌ-tɪf'laɪtɪs] n Paratyphlitis f.
par·a·ty·phoid [ˌ-'taɪfɔɪd] n **1.** Paratyphus m. **2.** Salmonellenenteritis f; Salmonellose f.
paratyphoid fever Paratyphus m.
par·a·um·bil·i·cal [ˌ-ʌm'bɪlɪkl] adj um den Nabel/Umbilicus herum (liegend), neben dem Nabel, par(a)umbilikal.
paraumbilical veins Sappey'-Venen pl, Vv. paraumbilicales.
par·a·u·re·thral [ˌ-jʊə'riːθrəl] adj neben der Harnröhre/Urethra (liegend), paraurethral.
paraurethral canals of male urethra Paraurethralkanälchen pl der männliche Harnröhre, Canales/Ductus paraurethrales urethrae masculinae.
paraurethral ducts: p. of female urethra Skene'-Gänge pl, Ductus paraurethrales (urethrae femininae).
p. of male urethra → paraurethral canals of male urethra.
paraurethral glands of female urethra → paraureathral ducts of female urethra.
paraurethral tubules → paraurethral canals of male urethra.
par·a·u·re·thri·tis [ˌ-jʊərə'θraɪtɪs] n Paraurethritis f.
par·a·u·ter·ine [ˌ-'juːtərɪn, -raɪn] adj neben der Gebärmutter (liegend), parauterin.
par·a·vac·cin·ia [ˌ-væk'sɪnɪə] n Melkerknoten m, Neben-, Melkerpocken pl, Paravakzineknoten pl, Paravaccinia f.
paravaccinia virus Melkerknotenvirus nt, Paravacciniavirus nt, Paravakzine-Virus nt.
par·a·vag·i·nal [ˌ-'vædʒənl] adj neben der Scheide (liegend), paravaginal.
paravaginal incision Schuchardt-Schnitt m.
par·a·vag·i·ni·tis [ˌ-ˌvædʒə'naɪtɪs] n gyn. Parakolpitis f, -vaginitis f.
par·a·var·i·ce·al injection [ˌ-ˌværɪ'siːəl] chir. Varizenumspritzung f, paravasale Applikation f.
par·a·ve·nous [ˌ-'viːnəs] adj neben einer Vene (liegend), paravenös.
par·a·ven·tric·u·lar [ˌ-ven'trɪkjələr] adj um einen Ventrikel herum (liegend), paraventrikulär.
paraventricular fibers Fibrae paraventriculares.
paraventricular nucleus: anterior and posterior p.i Ncc. paraventriculares anteriores et posteriores.
p.i (of hypothalamus) Ncc. paraventriculares (hypothalami).
par·a·ven·tric·u·lo·hy·poph·y·si·al tract [ˌ-venˌtrɪkjələʊhaɪˌpɒfə'siːəl] Tractus paraventriculohypophysialis.
par·a·ven·tric·u·lo·ven·tric·u·lar fibers [ˌ-ˌventrɪkjələʊven'trɪkjələr] → paraventricular fibers.
par·a·ver·te·bral [ˌ-'vɜrtəbrəl] adj neben der Wirbelsäule (liegend), paravertebral.
paravertebral anesthesia → paravertebral block.
paravertebral block Paravertebralanästhesie f, -block m.
paravertebral line Paravertebrallinie f, Linea paravertebralis.
paravertebral triangle Grocco-Rauchfuß-Dreieck nt.
par·a·ves·i·cal [ˌ-'vesɪkl] adj neben der Harnblase (liegend), paravesikal.
paravesical fossa Fossa paravesicalis.
paravesical pouch seitlicher Abschnitt m der Excavatio vesicouterina.
par·a·ve·sic·u·lar [ˌ-və'sɪkjələr] adj → paravesical.
par·ax·i·al mesoderm [pær'æksɪəl] paraxiales Mesoderm nt.
par·a·zo·on [pærə'zəʊən] n bio. tierischer Parasit m, Parazoon nt.
parch·ment induration ['pɑːrtʃmənt] patho. schiefrige Induration f.
Paré [pɑ're]: **P.'s suture** chir. Paré-Naht f.
par·ec·ta·sia [ˌpærek'teɪʒ(ɪ)ə] n → parectasis.
par·ec·ta·sis [pær'ektəsɪs] n patho. Überdehnung f, Überblähung f.
par·ec·tro·pia [ˌpærek'trəʊpɪə] n neuro. Apraxie f.
pa·ren·chy·ma [pə'reŋkɪmə] n Parenchym nt.
p. of prostate Drüsenparenchym der Prostata, Parenchyma (gl.) prostatae.
p. of testis Hodengewebe nt, -parenchym, Parenchyma testis.
pa·ren·chy·mal [pə'reŋkɪml] adj Parenchym betr., parenchymatös, Parenchym-.
parenchymal cell (ZNS) Parenchymzelle f.
parenchymal damage patho. Parenchymschaden m, -schädigung f.
parenchymal injury Parenchymschaden m, -verletzung f.
parenchymal necrosis Parenchymnekrose f.
par·en·chym·a·ti·tis [ˌpærəŋˌkɪmə'taɪtɪs] n patho. Parenchymentzündung f, Entzündung f des Organparenchyms.
par·en·chym·a·tous [ˌpærəŋ'kɪmətəs] adj → parenchymal.
parenchymatous cartilage parenchymatöser/zellulärer Knorpel m.

parenchymatous degeneration patho. albuminöse/albuminoide/albuminoid-körnige Degeneration f, trübe Schwellung f.
parenchymatous goiter parenchymatöse Struma f, Struma parenchymatosa.
parenchymatous hemorrhage Parenchymeinblutung f.
parenchymatous keratitis interstitielle/parenchymatöse Keratitis f, Keratitis interstitialis/parenchymatosa.
parenchymatous mastitis gyn. parenchymatöse Mastitis f.
parenchymatous nephritis parenchymatöse Nephritis f.
parenchymatous neuritis parenchymatöse Neuritis f.
parenchymatous neurosyphilis → parenchymatous syphilis.
parenchymatous salpingitis patho., gyn. parenchymatöse Salpingitis f.
parenchymatous syphilis parenchymatöse (Neuro-)Syphilis f.
parenchymatous tissue → parenchyma.
par·ent ['peərənt, 'pær-] I n **1.** ∼s pl Eltern pl. **2.** bio. Elter nt/m, Elternteil m. II adj Stamm-, Mutter; ursprünglich, Ur-.
par·ent·age ['peərəntɪdʒ, 'pær-] n Herkunft f, Abstammung f.
pa·ren·tal [pə'rentl] adj elterlich, Eltern-.
parental consent Einverständniserklärung f der Eltern.
parental generation abbr. P_1 genet. Elterngeneration f abbr. P_1.
parent atom phys. Ausgangsatom nt.
parent authority elterliche Gewalt f.
parent cell Mutterzelle f.
par·en·ter·al [pæ'rentərəl] adj unter Umgehung des Magen-Darm-Kanals, parenteral.
parenteral alimentation parenterale Ernährung f.
total p. vollständige/totale parenterale Ernährung.
parenteral feeding → parenteral alimentation.
parenteral hyperalimentation → parenteral alimentation, total.
parenteral nutrition parenterale Ernährung f.
peripheral p. abbr. **PPN** parenterale Ernährung f über einen peripheren Zugang m.
total p. abbr. **TPN** vollständige/totale parenterale Ernährung.
parenteral solution Lösung f zur parenteralen Applikation.
parent form Urform f, Urgestalt f.
par·ent·hood ['peərənthʊd, 'pær-] n Elternschaft f.
parent lattice phys. Hauptgitter n.
par·ent·less ['peərəntlɪs] adj elternlos.
parent power → parent authority.
parent strand biochem. Elternstrang m.
parent tissue Muttergewebe nt.
par·ep·en·dy·mal tract [ˌpærə'pendɪməl] Tractus parependymalis.
par·ep·i·did·y·mis [pærˌepɪ'dɪdəmɪs] n → paradidymis.
par·er·ga·sia [pærər'geɪʒ(ɪ)ə] n psychia. Schizophrenie f, -phrenia f, Spaltungsirresein nt, old Dementia praecox.
pa·re·sis [pə'riːsɪs, 'pærəsɪs] n, pl **-ses** [-sɪz] leichte od. unvollständige Paralyse/Lähmung f, motorische Schwäche f, Parese f.
par·es·the·sia [pæres'θiːʒ(ɪ)ə] n neuro. Fehlempfindung f, Parästhesie f.
par·es·thet·ic [pæres'θetɪk] adj Parästhesie betr., durch sie gekennzeichnet, parästhetisch.
pa·ret·ic [pə'retɪk, -'rɪtɪk] I n an Parese Lei-

paretic analgesia

dende(r *m*) *f*, Paretiker(in *f*) *m*. **II** *adj* Parese betr., von ihr betroffen, (teilweise *od.* unvollständig) gelähmt, paretisch, Parese-.
paretic analgesia paretische Analgesie *f*.
paretic iron *patho.* Paralyseeisen *nt*.
paretic neurosyphilis progressive Paralyse *f abbr.* PP, Paralysis progressiva.
paretic nystagmus paretischer Nystagmus *m*.
pa·ri·es ['peərɪˌiːz] *n*, *pl* **par·i·e·tes** [pə-'raɪətiːz] *anat.* Wand *f*, Paries *m*.
pa·ri·e·tal [pə'raʊtl] *anat.* **I** *n* → parietal bone. **II** *adj* **1.** seitlich, wand-, randständig, parietal, Wand-, Parietal-. **2.** Scheitelbein/Os parietale betr., parietal.
parietal angle of sphenoid bone Margo parietalis alae majoris.
parietal artery: anterior p. vordere Scheitellappenarterie *f*, Parietalis *f* anterior, A. parietalis anterior.
posterior p. hintere Scheitellappenarterie *f*, Parietalis *f* posterior, A. parietalis posterior.
parietal bone Scheitelbein *nt*, Os parietale.
parietal branch: p. of medial occipital artery Scheitellappenast *m* der A. occipitalis medialis, Ramus parietalis a. occipitalis medialis.
p. of middle meningeal artery Scheitelast *od.* hinterer Endast *m* der A. meningea media, Ramus parietalis a. meningeae mediae.
p. of superficial temporal artery hinterer Scheitelast *m* der A. temporalis superficialis, Ramus parietalis a. temporalis superficialis.
parietal cell (*Magen*) Beleg-, Parietalzelle *f*.
parietal cell vagotomy *chir.* selektive proximale Vagotomie *f abbr.* SPV.
parietal convolution, ascending Gyrus postcentralis.
parietal decidua Decidua parietalis/vera.
parietale fistula parietale Fistel *f*.
parietal eminence → parietal tuber.
parietal emissary parietales Emissarium *nt*, V. emissaria parietalis.
parietal endocarditis Endocarditis parietalis.
parietal foramen For. parietale.
parietal gyri Scheitellappenwindungen *pl*.
parietal hernia Darmwandbruch *m*, Littré'-Hernie *f*.
parietal incisure of temporal bone Inc. parietalis (ossis temporalis).
parietal layer: p. of serous pericardium → parietal pericardium.
p. of tunica vaginalis testis Lamina parietalis tunicae vaginalis testis.
parietal lobe Parietal-, Scheitellappen *m*, Lobus parietalis.
parietal lobule: inferior p. unterer Scheitellappenteil *m*, unteres Parietallappchen *nt*, Lobulus parietalis inferior.
superior p. oberer Scheitellappenteil *m*, oberes Parietallappchen *nt*, Lobulus parietalis superior.
parietal margin: p. of frontal bone Margo parietalis ossis frontalis.
p. of great wing of sphenoid bone Margo parietalis alae majoris.
p. of parietal bone Margo sagittalis ossis parietalis.
p. of temporal bone Margo parietalis ossis temporalis.
parietal mesoderm *embryo.* parietales Mesoderm *nt*.
parietal notch of temporal bone → parietal incisure of temporal bone.
parietal pericardium parietales Perikard *nt*, parietales Blatt *nt* des Perikards, Lamina parietalis pericardii.
parietal peritoneum Peritoneum *nt* der Bauchwand, parietales Peritoneum *nt*, Peritoneum parietale.
anterior p. Peritoneum parietale anterius.
parietal pleura parietales Blatt *nt* der Pleura, Parietalpleura *f*, Pleura parietalis.
parietal pregnancy intramurale/interstitielle Schwangerschaft *f*, Graviditas interstitialis.
parietal region Parietal-, Scheitelregion *f*, Regio parietalis.
parietal thrombus parietaler/wandständiger Thrombus *m*, Parietalthrombus *m*.
parietal tuber Tuber parietale.
parietal veins Scheitellappenvenen *pl*, Vv. parietales.
p. of Santorini → parietal emissary.
pa·ri·e·tog·ra·phy [pəˌraɪə'tɒgrəfɪ] *n radiol.* Parietographie *f*.
pa·ri·e·to·mas·toid suture [pəˌraɪətəʊ-'mæstɔɪd] Sutura parietomastoidea.
parieto-occipital *adj* parieto-okzipital.
parieto-occipital aphasia *neuro.* kombinierte Aphasie *f* u. Aphraxie.
parieto-occipital artery A. parieto-occipitalis.
parieto-occipital branch: p. of medial occipital artery A. occipitalis medialis-Ast *m* zum Sulcus parieto-occipitalis, Ramus parieto-occipitalis a. occipitalis medialis.
p. of posterior cerebral artery Ramus parieto-occipitalis a. cerebri posterioris.
parieto-occipital fissure → parieto-occipital sulcus 1.
parieto-occipital sulcus 1. Sulcus parieto--occipitalis. **2.** Sulcus intraparietalis.
parieto-occipitopontine fasciculus Fasciculus parieto-occipitopontinus.
pa·ri·e·to·pon·tine tract [ˌ-'pɒntiːn, -taɪn] Tractus parietopontinus.
pa·ri·e·to·sphe·noid [ˌ-'sfiːnɔɪd] *adj* parietosphenoidal.
pa·ri·e·to·splanch·nic [ˌ-'splæŋknɪk] *adj* → parietovisceral.
pa·ri·e·to·tem·po·ral [ˌ-'tempərəl] *adj* parietotemporal.
pa·ri·e·to·tem·po·ro·pon·tine fibers [ˌ-ˌtempərəʊ'pɒntiːn, -taɪn] Fibrae parietotemporopontinae.
pa·ri·e·to·vis·cer·al [ˌ-'vɪsərəl] *adj* parietoviszeral.
Parinaud [parɪ'no]: **P.'s conjunctivitis** Parinaud-Konjunktivitis *f*, okuloglanduläres Syndrom *nt* nach Parinaud.
P.'s oculoglandular syndrome → P.'s conjunctivitis.
P.'s ophthalmoplegia → P.'s syndrome.
P.'s syndrome Parinaud-Syndrom *nt*.
Paris classification [ˈpærɪs] *genet.* Paris--Einteilung *f*, -Klassifikation *f*.
Paris violet Gentianaviolett *nt*.
Park [paːrk]: **P.'s aneurysm** Park-Aneurysma *nt*.
Parkinson ['pɑːrkɪnsən]: **P.'s disease** Parkinson'-Krankheit *f*, Morbus Parkinson *m*, Paralysis agitans.
P.'s facies *neuro.*, *patho.* Maskengesicht *nt*.
par·kin·so·ni·an [ˌpɑːrkɪn'səʊnɪən] **I** *n* Parkinsonpatient(in *f*) *m*. **II** *adj* Parkinson'-Krankheit betr., Parkinson-.
p. crisis Parkinsonkrise *f*.
p. facies → Parkinson's facies.
p. syndrome Parkinson-Syndrom *nt*.
par·kin·son·ism ['pɑːrkɪnsənɪzəm] *n* **1.** → Parkinson's disease. **2.** Parkinsonoid *nt*.
par·o·don·ti·tis [ˌpærədɒn'taɪtɪs] *n* → periodontitis.
par·o·don·ti·um [ˌ-'dɒnʃɪəm] *n* → periodontium 1.

par·ol·fac·to·ry area (of Broca) [ˌpærəl-'fækt(ə)rɪ, -əʊl-] Area parolfactoria/subcallosa.
par·o·mo·my·cin [ˌpærəməʊ'maɪsɪn] *n pharm.* Paromomycin *nt*.
par·om·pha·lo·cele [pær'amfələʊsiːl] *n* Paromphalozele *f*.
Parona [pa'rəʊna]: **P.'s space** Parona'--Raum *m*.
par·o·nych·ia [ˌpærəʊ'nɪkɪə] *n derm.* Nagelfalzentzündung *f*, Umlauf *m*, Paronychie *f*, Paronychia *f*.
par·o·nych·i·al [ˌ-'nɪkɪəl] *adj* **1.** Paronychie betr. **2.** Nagelfalz betr., Nagelfalz-, paronychial.
paronychial warts paronychiale Warzen *pl*, Verrucae perionychialis.
par·o·oph·o·ri·tis [ˌ-ˌafə'raɪtɪs] *n gyn.* Par(o)ophoritis *f*.
par·o·oph·o·ron [ˌ-'afərən] *n* Beieierstock *m*, Paroophoron *nt*.
par·oph·thal·mia [pæraf'θælmɪə] *n ophthal.* Parophthalmie *f*.
par·op·sia [pær'apsɪə] *n* → paropsis.
par·op·sis [pær'apsɪs] *n* Sehstörung *f*, Paropsie *f*.
par·or·chis [pær'ɔːrkɪs] *n* Nebenhoden *m*, Epididymis *f*.
par·o·rex·ia [pærə'reksɪə] *n gyn.*, *psychia.* Parorexie *f*, Pikazismus *m*, Pica-Syndrom *nt*.
par·os·mia [pær'azmɪə] *n* Fehlriechen *nt*, Geruchstäuschung *f*, Parosmie *f*, Parosphresie *f*.
par·os·phre·sia [pæraz'friːzɪə] *n* → parosmia.
par·os·phre·sis [pæraz'friːzɪs] *n* → parosmia.
par·os·te·al sarcoma [pær'astɪəl] **1.** parosteales/juxtakortikales Sarkom *nt*. **2.** periostales Osteosarkom *nt*, perossales Sarkom *nt*, periostales (osteogenes) Sarkom *nt*.
par·os·te·i·tis [pærˌastɪ'aɪtɪs] *n ortho.* Parostitis *f*.
par·os·te·o·sis [pærˌastɪ'əʊsɪs] *n ortho.* Parostosis *f*.
par·os·ti·tis [pæras'taɪtɪs] *n* → parosteitis.
par·os·to·sis [pæras'təʊsɪs] *n* → parosteosis.
pa·rot·ic [pə'rəʊtɪk, -'rat-] *adj* → parotid 1.
pa·rot·id [pə'rɒtɪd] **I** *n* Ohrspeicheldrüse *f*, Parotis *f*, Gl. parotis/parotidea. **II** *adj* **1.** in der Nähe des Ohres (liegend). **2.** Ohrspeicheldrüse/Gl. parotis betr., Parotis-, Ohrspeicheldrüsen-.
parotid abscess Parotisabszeß *m*.
parotid branch: p.es of auriculotemporal nerve Parotisäste *pl* des N. auriculotemporalis, Rami parotidei n. auriculotemporalis.
p.es of facial vein Parotisäste *pl* zur V. facialis, Rami parotidei v. facialis.
p. of posterior auricular artery Parotisast *m* der A. auricularis posterior, Ramus parotideus a. auricularis posterioris.
p. of superficial temporal artery Parotisast *m* der A. temporalis superficialis, Ramus parotideus a. temporalis superficialis.
parotid duct Parotisgang *m*, Stensen'--Gang *m*, Stenon'-Gang *m*, Ductus parotideus.
pa·rot·i·de·an [pəˌratɪ'dɪən] *adj* → parotid 2.
pa·rot·i·dec·to·my [pəˌratɪ'dektəmɪ] *n* Parotisentfernung *f*, Parotidektomie *f*.
parotid fascia Faszienhülle *f* der Parotis, Fascia parotidea.
parotid gland → parotid I.
accessory p. Parotis *f* accessoria, Gl. parotis/parotidea accessoria.

pa·rot·id·i·tis [pəˌrɑtɪˈdaɪtɪs] *n* → parotitis.
parotid nerves Parotisäste *pl* des N. auriculotemporalis, Rami parotidei n. auriculotemporalis.
parotid papilla Papilla ductus parotidei.
parotid plexus of facial nerve Parotisplexus *m* des N. facialis, Plexus intraparotideus n. facialis.
parotid saliva Parotisspeichel *m*.
parotid space Parotisloge *f*.
parotid veins Parotisvenen *pl*, Vv. parotideae.
  anterior p. Rami parotidei v. facialis.
par·o·ti·tis [ˌpærəˈtaɪtɪs] *n* Parotisentzündung *f*, Entzündung *f* der Ohrspeicheldrüse, Parotitis *f*.
par·o·var·i·an [ˌ-ˈvɛərɪən] *adj* **1.** Parovarium betr., parovarial. **2.** neben dem Eierstock (liegend), paraovarial.
par·o·var·i·um [ˌ-ˈvɛərɪəm, -ˈvɛr-] *n* Nebeneierstock *m*, Rosenmüller'-Organ *nt*, Parovarium *nt*, Epoophoron *nt*.
par·ox·ysm [ˈpærəksɪzəm] *n* **1.** (plötzlicher) Anfall *m*, Paroxysmus *m*. **2.** paroxysmaler Krampf *m*.
par·ox·ys·mal [pærəkˈsɪzməl] *adj* anfallsartig, in Anfällen auftretend, paroxysmal.
paroxysmal albuminuria paroxysmale Albuminurie/Proteinurie *f*.
paroxysmal cold hemoglobinuria paroxysmale Kältehämoglobinurie *f*.
paroxysmal nocturnal dyspnea paroxysmale nächtliche Dyspnoe *f*.
paroxysmal nocturnal hemoglobinuria *abbr.* **PNH** Marchiafava-Micheli-Anämie *f*, paroxysmale nächtliche Hämoglobinurie *f*.
paroxysmal proteinuria → paroxysmal albuminuria.
paroxysmal sleep Narkolepsie *f*.
paroxysmal tachycardia Bouveret-Syndrom *nt*, paroxysmale Tachykardie *f*.
paroxysmal trepidant abasia *neuro.* spastische Abasie *f*.
Parrot [paˈro] **P.'s atrophy of newborn** → P.'s disease 3.
  P.'s disease 1. Bednar-Parrot-Pseudoparalyse *f*, Parrot'-Krankheit *f*, -Syndrom *nt*, Parrot-Kaufmann-Syndrom *nt*, Achondroplasie *f*. **3.** Marasmus *m*.
  P.'s node Parrot-Knoten *m*.
  P.'s pseudoparalysis → P.'s disease 1.
  P.'s sign 1. Parrot-Zeichen *nt*. **2.** Parrot-Knoten *pl*.
parrot disease/fever [ˈpærət] Papageienkrankheit *f*, Psittakose *f*; Ornithose *f*.
Parry [ˈpærɪ] **P.'s disease** hyperthyreote Knotenstruma *f*.
par·ry fracture [ˈpærɪ] Monteggia-(Subluxations-)Fraktur *f*.
Parry-Romberg [ˈrɑmbɜrg] **P.-R. syndrome** Romberg-Syndrom *nt*, -Trophoneurose *f*, Romberg-Parry-Syndrom *nt*, -Trophoneurose *f*, progressive halbseitige Gesichtsatrophie *f*, Hemiatrophia progressiva faciei/facialis.
pars [pɑrz] *n*, *pl* **par·tes** [ˈpɑrtiːz] *anat.* Teil *m*, Abschnitt *m*, Pars *f*.
pars flac·ci·da [ˈflæksɪdə] Pars flaccida (membranae tympanicae).
pars ten·sa [ˈtɛnsə] Pars tensa (membranae tympanicae).
part [pɑrt] **I** *n* **1.** (An-, Bestand-)Teil *m*, (Bau-, Einzel-)Teil *m*, Abschnitt *m*, Stück *nt*. **in ~** teilweise, zum Teil. **in equal ~s** zu gleichen Teilen. **to take ~** teilnehmen (*in* an); mitmachen (*in* bei). **2.** *mathe.* Bruchteil *m*. **3.** Körperteil *m*/*nt*, Glied *nt*. **4.** (*Haar*) Scheitel *m*. **5.** Ersatzteil *nt*. **II** *adj* Teil-. **III** *adv* zum Teil, teilweise. **IV** *vt* **6.**

(ein-, zer-)teilen. **7.** (*Haar*) scheiteln. **V** *vi* s. lösen, aufgehen; s. öffnen; s. teilen, s. trennen.
par·tal [ˈpɑrtəl] *adj* Geburt/Entbindung betr., Geburts-, Entbindungs-.
part·ed [ˈpɑrtɪd] *adj* **1.** getrennt, geteilt, gespalten. **2.** (*Haar*) gescheitelt.
par·the·no·car·py [ˌpɑrθənəʊˈkɑrpɪ] *n bio.* Parthenokarpie *f*.
par·the·no·gen·e·sis [ˌ-ˈdʒɛnəsɪs] *n bio.*, *genet.* Jungfernzeugung *f*, Parthenogenese *f*.
par·the·no·ge·net·ic [ˌ-dʒəˈnɛtɪk] *adj* auf Parthenogenese beruhend, aus unbefruchteten Keimzellen entstehend, parthenogenetisch.
par·the·no·pho·bi·a [ˌ-ˈfəʊbɪə] *n psychia.* krankhafte Angst *f* vor Mädchen, Parthenophobie *f*.
par·tho·gen·e·sis [ˌpɑrθəʊˈdʒɛnəsɪs] *n* → parthenogenesis.
par·tial [ˈpɑrʃl] *adj* teilweise, partiell, Teil-, Partial-.
partial agglutinin *immun.* Neben-, Minoragglutinin *nt*.
partial albinism *derm.* partieller/umschriebener Albinismus *m*, Albinismus circumscriptus.
partial anodontia Hypodontie *f*, Hypodontia *f*.
partial antigen *immun.* Partial-, Teilantigen *nt*, Hapten *nt*.
partial aphrasia → paraphrasia.
partial charge Teil-, Partialladung *f*.
partial cleavage *bio.* partielle/meroblastische Furchung(steilung *f*) *f*.
partial colectomy *chir.* partielle Kolektomie *f*.
partial deletion *genet.* partielle Deletion *f*.
partial denture Teilgebiß *nt*, -prothese *f*.
partial dislocation *ortho.* unvollständige Verrenkung *f*, Ausrenkung *f*, Subluxation *f*.
partial dominance *genet.* Semidominanz *f*, unvollständige Dominanz *f*.
partial epilepsy fokale Epilepsie *f*.
partial excision *chir.* Teilentfernung *f*, partielle Exzision *f*, Resektion *f*.
partial fracture *mathe.* Partialbruch *m*.
partial fundoplication *chir.* (*Magen*) partielle Fundoplikation *f*.
partial gastrectomy *chir.* Magen(teil)resektion *f*, partielle Gastrektomie *f*.
partial gigantism partieller Riesenwuchs/Gigantismus *m*.
partial hepatectomy *chir.* partielle Leberresektion/Hepatektomie *f*.
partial hydrolysis Teil-, Partialhydrolyse *f*.
partial hysterectomy partielle/subtotale Gebärmutterentfernung/Hysterektomie *f*, Hysterectomia partialis.
partial lipodystrophy Simons-Syndrom *nt*, Lipodystrophia progressiva/paradoxa.
partial mastectomy *gyn.* (*Brust*) Segment-, Quadrantenresektion *f*, Lumpektomie *f*, Tylektomie *f*.
partial ophthalmoplegia Ophthalmoplegia partialis.
partial pack Teilpackung *f*.
partial pressure *phys.* Partialdruck *m*.
  carbon dioxide p. *abbr.* **Pco$_2$, PCO$_2$** Kohlendioxidpartialdruck, CO_2-Partialdruck *abbr.* Pco$_2$, pCO$_2$.
  CO$_2$ p. → carbon dioxide p.
  O$_2$ p. → oxygen p.
  oxygen p. *abbr.* **Po$_2$, pO$_2$** Sauerstoffpartialdruck, O_2-Partialdruck *abbr.* Po$_2$, pO$_2$.
  water-vapor p. Wasserdampfpartialdruck.

partial product *mathe.* Teilprodukt *nt*.
partial remission *abbr.* **PR** Teilremission *f*, partielle Remission *f abbr.* PR.
partial-thickness burn Verbrennung *f* 2. Grades.
partial thromboplastin time *abbr.* **PTT** partielle Thromboplastinzeit *f abbr.* PTT.
partial transposition of great vessels Taussig-Bing-Syndrom *nt*.
par·ti·ble [ˈpɑrtɪbl] *adj* teil-, trennbar.
par·tic·i·pant [pɑrˈtɪsəpənt] **I** *n* Teilnehmer(in *f*) *m*. **II** *adj* teilnehmend, Teilnehmer-.
par·tic·i·pate [pɑrˈtɪsəpeɪt] **I** *vt* teilen, gemeinsam haben (*with* mit). **II** *vi* s. beteiligen *od.* teilnehmen (*in* an).
par·tic·i·pa·tion [pɑrˌtɪsəˈpeɪʃn] *n* Teilnahme *f*, (Mit-)Beteiligung *f*, Mitwirkung *f*.
par·ti·cle [ˈpɑrtɪkl] *n* (*a. phys.*) Teilchen *nt*, Körperchen *nt*, Partikel *nt*.
  α particle α-Teilchen *nt*, alpha-Teilchen *nt*.
  β particle β-Teilchen *nt*, beta-Teilchen *nt*.
particle accelerator *phys.* Teilchenbeschleuniger *m*.
particle physicist Hochenergiephysiker(in *f*) *m*.
particle physics Hochenergie-, Elementarteilchenphysik *f*.
particle weight *phys.* Partikelgewicht *nt*.
par·tic·u·late [pərˈtɪkjəlɪt, -leɪt] *adj* aus Teilchen/Partikeln bestehend, Teilchen-, Partikel-, Korpuskel-.
particulate radiation Teilchen-, Korpuskel-, Korpuskularstrahlung *f*, korpuskuläre/materielle Strahlung *f*.
par·tite [ˈpɑrtaɪt] *adj* geteilt, -teilig.
par·ti·tion [pɑrˈtɪʃn, pər-] **I** *n* **1.** (Auf-, Zer-, Ver-)Teilung *f*, Trennung *f*. **2.** Abtrennung *f*, Trenn-, Scheidewand *f*; *anat.* Septum *nt*. **3.** Teil *nt*, Abschnitt *m*, Sektor *m*, Abteilung *f*. **II** *vt* (auf-, zer-, ver-)teilen, spalten, (ab-)trennen.
partition chromatography Verteilungschromatographie *f*.
partition coefficient Verteilungskoeffizient *m*.
parts per million *abbr.* **ppm**. *phys.* Teilchen *pl* pro Million, parts per million *abbr.* ppm.
par·tu·ri·ent [pɑrˈt(j)ʊərɪənt] *adj* Geburt/Entbindung betr., Geburts-, Entbindungs-, Gebär-.
parturient canal *gyn.* Geburtskanal *m*.
par·tu·ri·fa·cient [pɑrˌt(j)ʊərɪˈfeɪʃənt] **I** *n* Wehenmittel *nt*. **II** *adj* die Wehen anregend.
par·tu·ri·tion [ˌpɑrt(j)ʊəˈrɪʃn] *n* → partus.
par·tus [ˈpɑrtəs] *n* Geburt *f*, Entbindung *f*, Partus *m*.
pa·ru·lis [pəˈruːlɪs] *n dent.*, *HNO* Parulis *f*.
par·um·bil·i·cal [pɑrʌmˈbɪlɪkl] *adj* → paraumbilical.
parumbilical veins → paraumbilical veins.
par·vi·cel·lu·lar [ˌpɑrvɪˈsɛljələr] *adj* → parvocellular.
par·vo·cel·lu·lar [ˌpɑrvəʊˈsɛljələr] *adj* kleinzellig, aus kleinen Zellen bestehend.
parvocellular part of nucleus ruber kleinzelliger Abschnitt *m* des Nc. ruber, Pars parvocellularis (nc. rubri).
Par·vo·vir·i·dae [ˌ-ˈvɪrədiː, -ˈvaɪr-] *pl micro.* Parvoviren *pl*, Parvoviridae *pl*.
Par·vo·vi·rus [ˌ-ˈvaɪrəs] *n micro.* Parvovirus *nt*.
par·vule [ˈpɑrvjuːl] *n pharm.* (sehr) kleine Pille *f*.
PAS *abbr.* **1.** → para-aminosalicylic acid. **2.** → periodic acid-Schiff reaction.
Pascal [pæˈskæl; pasˈkal] **P.'s law** Pascal'-Gesetz *nt*.

pas·cal [pæ'skæl; pas'kal] *n abbr.* **Pa** Pascal *nt abbr.* Pa.
Pascheff ['paʃef]: **P.'s conjunctivitis** *ophthal.* Pascheff-Konjunktivitis *f*, Conjunctivitis necroticans infectiosa.
Paschen [paʃən]: **P. bodies/corpuscles/granules** Paschen-Körperchen *pl.*
Pasini [pa'sini]: **P.'s syndrome** *derm.* Pasini-Syndrom *nt*, Pasini-Pierini-Syndrom *nt*, Epidermolysis bullosa albopapuloidea.
Pasini and Pierini [pjɛ'rini]: **atrophoderma of P.a.P.** *derm.* Atrophodermia idiopathica Pasini-Pierini.
idiopathic atrophoderma/atrophodermia of P.a.P. → atrophoderma of P.a.P.
PAS-reaction *n* → periodic acid-Schiff reaction.
pass [pæs, pɑːs] I *vt* 1. (*Barriere*) passieren, überwinden; (*Instrument*) einführen. 2. (*Fremdkörper*) ausscheiden; (*Darm*) entleeren; (*Urin*) lassen. 3. durchseihen, passieren. 4. billigen, gutheißen, genehmigen. 5. (*Examen*) bestehen; bestehen lassen. II *vi* 6. (hin-)durchgehen, durchkommen, (*Barriere*) überwinden, passieren (*through* durch). 7. (*Fremdkörper*) abgehen; abgeführt *od.* ausgeschieden werden. 8. (*Schmerz*) vorbei-, vorübergehen, s. legen; (*Zeit*) verstreichen. 9. (*Examen*) bestehen.
pass away *vi* 1. (*Schmerz*) vorüber-, vorbeigehen. 2. sterben, entschlafen, verscheiden.
pass off *vi* (*Schmerz*) vorüber-, vorbeigehen.
pass on *vt* weiterleiten, -geben, -reichen (*to* an); (*Krankheit*) übertragen.
pass out *vi* in Ohnmacht fallen, ohnmächtig werden.
pass through *vi* passieren, hindurchgehen, -führen.
pass·a·ble ['pæsəbl, 'pɑːs-] *adj* 1. passierbar. 2. leidlich (gut), erträglich, passabel.
pas·sage ['pæsɪdʒ] *n* 1. Passage *f*, (Durch-, Verbindungs-)Gang *m*; *techn.* Durchlaß *m*. 2. *anat.* Gang *m*, Weg *m*; (~**s** *pl*) Trakt *m*, Wege *pl*. 3. Durch-, Herein-, Herausgehen *nt*; (*Sonde*) Einführen *nt*, Einbringen *nt*. 4. *physiol.* (Darm-)Entleerung *f*, (Urin-)Ausscheidung *f*. 5. (*Fremdkörper*) Abgang *m*.
pas·sage·way ['pæsɪdʒweɪ] *n* → passage 1.
Passavant ['pæsəvænt]: **P.'s bar/cushion/pad/ridge** Passavant'-(Ring-)Wulst *m*.
pas·si·bil·i·ty [,pæsə'bɪlətɪ] *n* Empfindungsvermögen *nt*.
pas·si·ble ['pæsɪbl] *adj* empfindungsfähig.
pass·ing ['pæsɪŋ, 'pɑːs-] I *n* Vorbei-, Durchgehen *nt*. II *adj* 1. vorbei-, durchgehend. 2. vorübergehend, flüchtig, vergänglich.
pas·sion ['pæʃn] *n* 1. Leidenschaft(lichkeit *f*) *f*. 2. Wut *f*, Zorn *m*.
pas·si·vate ['pæsɪveɪt] *vt chem.* passivieren.
pas·sive ['pæsɪv] *adj* 1. *allg., electr.* passiv, nicht aktiv; *psycho.* passiv, untätig, träge, teilnahmslos. 2. *chem.* Passivität aufweisend, träge, passiv.
passive agglutination *immun.* passive/indirekte Agglutination *f*.
passive-aggressive personality (disorder) passiv-aggressive Persönlichkeit(sstörung *f*) *f*.
passive algolagnia *psychia.* Masochismus *m*, Passivismus *m*.
passive anaphylaxis *immun.* passive Anaphylaxie *f*.
passive congestion venöse/passive (Blut-)Stauung *f*, venöse/passive Hyperämie *f*.

passive cutaneous anaphylaxis *abbr.* **PCA** passive cutane Anaphylaxie *f abbr.* PCA.
passive diffusion *physiol.* passive Diffusion *f*.
passive hemagglutination indirekte/passive Hämagglutination *f*.
passive hyperemia → passive congestion.
passive immunity passive Immunität *f*.
passive immunization passive Immunisierung *f*.
passive incontinence passive Harninkontinenz *f*.
passive movement passive Bewegung *f*.
pas·sive·ness ['pæsɪvnɪs] *n* Untätigkeit *f*, Teilnahmslosigkeit *f*, Trägheit *f*, Passivität *f*.
passive scopophilia *psychia.* Exhibitionismus *m*.
passive smoking passives Rauchen *nt*, Passivrauchen *nt*.
passive-tension curve *physiol.* Ruhe-Dehnungs-Kurve *f*.
passive transfer test → Prausnitz-Küstner reaction.
passive transport *physiol.* passiver Transport *m*.
passive tremor Ruhetremor *m*.
pas·siv·ism ['pæsɪvɪzəm] *n psychia.* Passivismus *m*.
pas·siv·i·ty [pæ'sɪvətɪ] *n* → passiveness.
PAS stain *histol.* periodic acid-Schiff-Färbung *f*, PAS-Färbung *f*.
past [pæst, pɑːst] I *n* Vergangenheit *f*, Vorleben *nt.* **in the ~** in der Vergangenheit. II *adj* vergangen, vorüber, frühe(r, s), vergangene(r, s).
pas·ta ['pɑːstə] *n, pl* **-tae** [-tiː] → paste 3.
paste [peɪst] I *n* 1. (teigartige *od.* breiige) Masse *f*, Salbe *f*, Paste *f*, Brei *m*. 2. Klebstoff *m*, Kleister *m*. 3. *pharm.* Paste *f*, Pasta *f*. II *vt* (zusammen-)kleben, (ein-)kleistern.
Pasteur [pæ'stɑr; pa'stœːr]: **P. effect/reaction** Pasteur-Effekt *m*.
Pas·teu·rel·la [pæstə'relə] *n micro.* Pasteurella *f*.
P. pestis Pestbakterium *nt*, Yersinia/P. pestis.
Pas·teu·rel·la·ce·ae [pæstərə'leɪsɪiː] *pl micro.* Pasteurellaceae *pl*.
pas·teu·rel·lo·sis [,-'ləʊsɪs] *n* Pasteurellainfektion *f*, Pasteurellose *f*.
pas·teur·i·za·tion [,pæstʃəraɪ'zeɪʃn, ,pæstə-] *n* Pasteurisierung *f*.
pas·teur·ize ['-raɪz] *vt* pasteurisieren.
pas·til ['pæstɪl] *n* → pastille.
pas·tille [pæ'stiːl, -stɪl] *n pharm.* Pastille *f*.
past illnesses frühere Krankheiten *pl*.
past·i·ness ['peɪstɪnɪs] *n* (*Gewebe*) teigige *od.* breiige Beschaffenheit *f*.
past·y ['peɪstɪ] *adj* 1. breiig, dickflüssig, teigig. 2. (*Haut*) teigig, gedunsen, aufgeschwemmt, pastös.
Patau [pa'taʊ]: **P.'s syndrome** Patau-Syndrom *nt*, Trisomie 13-Syndrom *nt*, D_1-Trisomiesyndrom *nt*.
patch [pætʃ] I *n* 1. Fleck(en *m*) *m*, Flicken *m*, Lappen *m*. 2. *chir.* (Gewebe-)Lappen *m*, Lappen *nt*. 3. (Heft-)Pflaster *nt*; Augenklappe *f*, -binde *f*. II *vt* (zusammen-)flicken, ausbessern.
patch graft Patchgraft *f/nt*.
patch test *derm.* Pflasterprobe *f*, Patch-Test *m*.
patch·y ['pætʃɪ] *adj* fleckig.
patchy atelectasis (*Lunge*) Fleckenatelektase *f*.
pa·tel·la [pə'telə] *n, pl* **-lae** [-liː] *anat.* Kniescheibe *f*, Patella *f*.
pa·tel·lar [pə'telər] *adj* Patella betr., patellar.

patellar bursa Bursa subcutanea tuberositatis tibiae.
deep p. Bursa subtendinea praepatellaris.
middle p. Bursa subfascialis praepatellaris.
prespinous p. Bursa subcutanea tuberositatis tibiae.
subcutaneous p. Bursa subcutanea praepatellaris.
patellar clonus Patellarklonus *m*.
patellar fossa Glaskörpermulde *f*, Fossa hyaloidea.
p. of femur → patellar surface (of femur).
p. of tibia Area intercondylaris anterior (tibiae).
patellar incisure of femur Facies patellaris femoris.
patellar ligament Kniescheibenband *nt*, Lig. patellae.
patellar reflex → patellar tendon reflex.
patellar retinaculum: lateral p. Retinaculum patellae laterale.
medial p. Retinaculum patellae mediale.
patellar surface (of femur) Facies patellaris (femoris).
patellar tap *ortho.* tanzende Patella *f*.
patellar tendon → patellar ligament.
patellar tendon reflex Patellarsehnenreflex *m abbr.* PSR, Quadrizepssehnenreflex *m abbr.* QSR.
pat·el·lec·to·my [,pætə'lektəmɪ] *n ortho.* Patellaresektion *f*, Patellektomie *f*.
pa·tel·lo·fem·o·ral [pə,teləʊ'femərəl] *adj* Patella u. Femur betr., patellofemoral.
pat·en·cy ['pætənsɪ, 'peɪ-] *n* (*Gang*) Offensein *nt*, Durchgängigkeit *f*.
pa·tent ['pætnt, 'peɪ-] I *n* Patent *nt.* II *adj* 1. (*Gang*) offen, durchgängig, nicht-verschlossen. 2. offenkundig, -sichtlich, evident. 3. patentiert. III *vt* 4. patentieren, ein Patent erteilen auf. 5. *etw.* patentieren lassen.
pa·ter·nal [pə'tɜrnl] *adj* väterlich, väterlicherseits.
pa·ter·ni·ty [pə'tɜrnətɪ] *n* Vaterschaft *f*.
paternity test Vaterschaftstest *m*, -nachweis *m*.
Paterson ['pætərsən]: **P.'s syndrome** Plummer-Vinson-Syndrom *nt*, Paterson-Brown-Syndrom *nt*, Kelly-Paterson-Syndrom *nt*, sideropenische Dysphagie *f*.
Paterson-Brown-Kelly [braʊn 'kelɪ]: **P.-B.-K. syndrome** → Paterson's syndrome.
Paterson-Kelly: P.-K. syndrome → Paterson's syndrome.
Patey ['pætɪ]: **P.'s operation** *gyn.* Patey-Operation *f*, modifizierte radikale Mastektomie *f*.
path- *pref.* → patho-.
path [pæθ, pɑːθ] *n, pl* **paths** [pæðz, pɑːðs] *anat., phys., physiol., techn.* Bahn *f*, Weg *m*; Leitung *f*.
p. of conduction Leitungsbahn.
p. of current Stromweg.
p. of discharge Entladungsstrecke *f*.
p. of electrons Elektronenbahn.
pa·ther·gia [pə'θɜrdʒɪə] *n* → pathergy.
path·er·gic ['pæθərdʒɪk] *adj* Pathergie betr., patherg(isch).
path·er·gy ['pæθərdʒɪ] *n* Pathergie *f*.
patho- *pref.* Path(o-), Krankheits-.
path·o·an·a·tom·i·cal [,pæθəʊˌænə'tɑmɪkl] *adj* pathologisch-anatomisch.
path·o·a·nat·o·my [,-ə'næto mɪ] *n* pathologische Anatomie *f*.
path·o·bi·ol·o·gy [,-baɪ'alədʒɪ] *n* Pathobiologie *f*.
path·o·clis·is [,-'klɪsɪs] *n* Pathoklise *f*.
path·o·don·tia [,-'dɑntʃ(ɪ)ə] *n* Zahnpathologie *f*.

path·o·gen ['-dʒən] *n* Krankheitserreger *m*, pathogener (Mikro-)Organismus *m*.
path·o·gen·e·sis [,-'dʒenəsɪs] *n* Krankheitsentstehung *f*, -entwicklung *f*, Pathogenese *f*.
path·o·gen·e·sy [,-'dʒenəsɪ] *n* → pathogenesis.
path·o·ge·net·ic [,-dʒə'netɪk] *adj* **1.** Pathogenese betr., pathogenetisch. **2.** pathogen, krankheitserregend, -verursachend, krankmachend.
path·o·gen·ic [,-'dʒenɪk] *adj* → pathogenetic 2.
pathogenic agent → pathogen.
pathogenic bacteria pathogene/krankheitserregende Bakterien *pl*.
path·o·ge·nic·i·ty [,-dʒə'nɪsətɪ] *n* Pathogenität *f*.
pathogenic microorganism → pathogen.
pa·thog·e·ny [pə'θadʒənɪ] *n* → pathogenesis.
pa·thog·no·mon·ic [pə,θɑ(g)nə'mɑmɪk] *adj* für eine Krankheit kennzeichnend, krankheitskennzeichnend, pathognomonisch, pathognostisch.
pathognomonic symptom pathognomonisches Zeichen/Symptom *nt*.
path·og·nos·tic [,pæθəg'nɑstɪk] *adj* → pathognomonic.
path·o·log·ic [,pæθə'lɑdʒɪk] *adj* → pathological.
path·o·log·i·cal [,-'lɑdʒɪkl] *adj* **1.** Pathologie betr., pathologisch. **2.** krankhaft, pathologisch.
pathological anatomy pathologische Anatomie *f*.
pathological finding pathologischer/pathologisch-anatomischer Befund *m*.
pathological histology Histopathologie *f*.
pathologic amenorrhea *gyn*. pathologische Amenorrhoe *f*.
pathologic anatomy → pathological anatomy.
pathologic atrophy pathologische Atrophie *f*.
pathologic dislocation *ortho*. pathologische Luxation *f*.
pathologic fracture pathologische Fraktur *f*, Spontanfraktur *f*.
pathologic glycosuria pathologische Glukosurie/Glycosurie *f*.
pathologic leukocytosis pathologische Leukozytose *f*.
pathologic myopia *ophthal*. bösartige/maligne Myopie *f*.
pathologic osteoporosis pathologische Osteoporose *f*.
pathologic physiology Pathophysiologie *f*.
pathologic presbycusis *HNO* pathologische Presbyakusis *f*.
pathologic reflex pathologischer Reflex *m*.
pathologic staging pathologisches Staging *nt*, P-Staging *nt*.
pathologic stimulus pathologischer Reiz/Stimulus *m*.
pa·thol·o·gist [pə'θɑlədʒɪst] *n* Pathologe *m*, -login *f*.
pa·thol·o·gy [pə'θɑlədʒɪ] *n* **1.** Krankheitslehre *f*, Pathologie *f*. **2.** pathologischer Befund *m*. **3.** (Abteilung für) Pathologie *f*.
path·o·mi·me·sis [,pæθəmɪ'mi:sɪs] *n* Simulation *f*, Simulieren *nt*.
path·o·mim·ia [,-'mɪmɪə] *n* → pathomimesis.
path·o·mim·ic·ry [,-'mɪməkrɪ] *n* → pathomimesis.
path·o·mor·phism [,-'mɔːrfɪzəm] *n* Pathomorphologie *f*.
path·o·pho·bia [,-'fəʊbɪə] *n psychia*. pathologische Angst *f* vor Krankheiten, Nosophobie *f*, Pathophobie *f*.
path·o·phys·i·o·log·ic [,-,fɪzɪə'lɑdʒɪk] *adj* Pathophysiologie betr., pathophysiologisch.
path·o·phys·i·o·log·i·cal [,-,fɪzɪə'lɑdʒɪkl] *adj* → pathophysiologic.
path·o·phys·i·ol·o·gy [,-,fɪzɪ'ɑlədʒɪ] *n* Pathophysiologie *f*.
path·o·psy·chol·o·gy [,-saɪ'kɑlədʒɪ] *n* Pathopsychologie *f*.
path·o·psy·cho·sis [,-saɪ'kəʊsɪs] *n* organische/symptomatische Psychose *f*.
path·way ['pæθweɪ, 'pɑː θ-] *n* → path.
p.s of hypothalamus Hypothalamusbahnen *pl*.
pa·tience ['peɪʃəns] *n* Geduld *f*. **to have (no) ~ with** (keine) Geduld haben mit.
pa·tient ['peɪʃənt] **I** *n* Patient(in *f*) *m*, Kranke(r *m*) *f*. **II** *adj* **1.** geduldig. **2.** zulassend, gestattend.
patient management Patientenversorgung *f*, -führung *f*, -management *nt*.
pat·ri·cide ['pætrɪsaɪd] *n* **1.** Vatermord *m*. **2.** Vatermörder(in *f*) *m*.
Patrick ['pætrɪk]: **P.'s sign 1.** Patrick-Probe *f*. **2.** Patrick-Phänomen *nt*.
P.'s test → P.'s sign 1.
pat·ri·lin·e·al [,pætrɪ'lɪnɪəl] *adj genet., bio*. patrilineal, patrilinear.
pat·ro·cli·nous [,pætrəʊ'klaɪnəs] *adj bio., genet*. patroklin.
pat·ro·gen·e·sis [,-'dʒenəsɪs] *n* Androgenese *f*.
pat·tern ['pætərn; *Brit*. 'pætn] **I** *n* **1.** Muster *nt*, Vorlage *f*, Modell *nt*, Pattern *nt*; (Waren-)Probe *f*; *techn*. Schablone *f*. **2.** (*Krankheitsverlauf*) Schema *nt*, Struktur *f*, Phänomen *nt*. **3.** *fig*. Vorbild *nt*, Beispiel *nt*. **4.** Verhaltensmuster *nt*, -weise *f*, -schema *nt*. **II** *vt* formen, gestalten, (nach-)bilden (*after* nach).
pat·tern·al alopecia ['pætərnəl] *derm*. androgenetische Alopezie *f*, Haarausfall *m* vom männlichen Typ, männliche Glatzenbildung *f*, androgenetisches Effluvium *nt*, Calvities hippocratica, Alopecia androgenetica.
pattern scanning *physiol*. Musterabtastung *f*.
pattern-reversal potential *physiol*. Musterwechselpotential *nt*.
pau·ci·ar·tic·u·lar [,pɔːsɪɑːr'tɪkjələr] *adj ortho*. nur wenige Gelenke betr., oligoartikulär.
pau·ci·syn·ap·tic [,-sɪ'næptɪk] *adj* oligosynaptisch.
Paul [pɔːl]: **P.'s reaction** Paul-Versuch *m*.
Paul-Bunnell [bjuː'nel]: **P.-B. reaction** Paul-Bunnell-Reaktion *f*.
P.-B. test Paul-Bunnell-Test *m*.
Paul-Bunnell-Davidsohn ['deɪvɪdsən]: **P.-B.-D. test** modifizierter Paul-Bunnell-Test *m* nach Davidsohn.
Pauling-Corey ['pɔːlɪŋ 'kɔːrɪ]: **P.-C. helix** *biochem*. α-Helix *f*.
Paul-Mixter ['mɪkstər]: **P.-M. tube** *chir*. Paul-Mixter-Rohr *nt*.
paunch [pɔːntʃ, pɑːntʃ] *n* **1.** Bauch *m*, Wanst *m*. **2.** *bio*. Pansen *m*.
paunch·y ['pɔːntʃɪ, 'pɑːn-] *adj* dickbäuchig.
pause [pɔːz] **I** *n* Pause *f*, Unterbrechung *f*. **to have/make a ~** → pause II. **II** *vi* eine Pause machen, pausieren, innehalten. **without (a) ~** pausenlos, ohne Unterbrechung.
Pautrier [potri'e]: **P.'s abscess/microabscess** Pautrier'-Mikroabszeß *m*.
pave·ment cells ['peɪvmənt] Plattenepithelzellen *pl*.

pavement epithelium einschichtiges Plattenepithel *nt*.
Pavlik ['pævlɪk]: **P. harness** *ortho*. Pavlik-Bandage *f*, -Zügel *m*.
Pavlov ['pævlɒv]: **P. pouch/stomach** Pawlow-Magen *m*, -Tasche *f*.
pa·vor ['peɪvəʊr] *n neuro., psychia*. Pavor *m*.
pavor diurnus *ped*. Tagangst *f*, Pavor diurnus.
pavor nocturnus *ped*. Nachtangst *f*, Pavor nocturnus.
PAWP *abbr*. → pulmonary artery wedge pressure.
Paxton ['pækstən]: **P.'s disease** Trichobacteriosis axillaris, Trichomycosis axillaris/palmellina, Trichonocardiosis *f*.
Payr ['paɪər]: **P.'s clamp** *chir*. Payr-Darmkompressorium *nt*.
P.'s disease Payr-Syndrom *nt*.
P.'s sign Payr-Zeichen *nt*.
PB *abbr*. → barometric pressure.
Pb *abbr*. → plumbum.
PBG *abbr*. → porphobilinogen.
PBI *abbr*. → protein-bound iodine.
P biatriale → P cardiale
PBI test → protein-bound iodine test.
P blood group (system) P-Blutgruppe *f*, P-Blutgruppensystem *nt*.
PBP *abbr*. → penicillin-binding protein.
PC *abbr*. **1.** → phosphatidylcholine. **2.** → phosphocreatine. **3.** → pyruvate carboxylase.
PCA *abbr*. → passive cutaneous anaphylaxis.
P cardiale *card*. P cardiale, P biatriale, P congenitale.
P congenitale → P cardiale.
PCB *abbr*. → polychlorinated biphenyl.
PC deficiency → pyruvate carboxylase deficiency.
PCE *abbr*. → pseudocholinesterase.
PCECV *abbr*. → purified chick embryo cell vaccine.
PCG *abbr*. → phonocardiography.
pCi *abbr*. → picocurie.
PCL *abbr*. → cruciate ligament of knee, posterior.
Pco₂ *abbr*. → partial pressure, carbon dioxide.
pCo₂ *abbr*. → partial pressure, carbon dioxide.
PC-sensor *n* → pacinian-corpuscle sensor.
PCV *abbr*. → packed-cell volume.
PD *abbr*. **1.** → primary disease. **2.** → proliferative disease (of the breast).
Pd *abbr*. → palladium.
p.d. *abbr*. → prism diopter.
PDE *abbr*. → phosphodiesterase.
P dextroatriale → P pulmonale.
P dextrocardiale → P pulmonale.
PDGF *abbr*. → platelet-derived growth factor.
PDH *abbr*. → pyruvate dehydrogenase.
PDHC *abbr*. → pyruvate dehydrogenase complex.
PDHC deficiency → pyruvate dehydrogenase complex deficiency.
PDL *abbr*. → poorly-differentiated lymphocytic lymphoma.
PDLL *abbr*. → poorly-differentiated lymphocytic lymphoma.
PDP *abbr*. → papular dermatitis of pregnancy.
PD-sensor *n* → proportional-differential sensor.
PDWA *abbr*. → proliferative disease without atypia.
PE *abbr*. **1.** → parallel-elastic element. **2.** → phosphatidylethanolamine. **3.** → physical examination. **4.** [physical education] → physical training. **5.** → pulmonary embolism.

peak [piːk] *n mathe.* Gipfel *m*, Maximum *nt*, Spitze *f*, Peak *m*.
Péan [pe'ã]: **P.'s clamp/forceps** *chir.* Péan-Klemme *f*.
pea·nut butter ['piːnʌt, -nət] Erdnußbutter *f*.
peanut oil Erdnußöl *nt*.
pearl tumor [pɜrl] *HNO* Perlgeschwulst *f*, Cholesteatom *nt*.
pearl·y bodies ['pɜrli] *patho.* Epithel-, Hornperlen *pl*.
pearly tubercle Hautgrieß *m*, Milium *nt*, Milie *f*.
pearly tumor → pearl tumor.
pea-soup stool [piː] Erbs(en)suppenstuhl *m*.
Peau de Chagrin [pəʊ; po] Chagrinleder--Haut *f*.
peau de chagrin → Peau de Chagrin.
peau d'orange Orangen(schalen)haut *f*, Apfelsinen(schalen)haut *f*, Peau d'orange.
peb·ble ['pebəl] *n* 1. Bergkristall *m*. 2. *phys., ophthal.* Bergkristallinse *f*.
PEC *abbr.* → pyrogenic exotoxin C.
pec·cant ['pekənt] *adj* krankhaft; (gesundheits-)schädlich; pathogen.
pec·ca·ti·pho·bia [ˌpekətɪ'fəʊbɪə] *n patho.* Peccatiphobie *f*.
pech·y·ag·ra [pekɪ'ægrə, -'eɪg-] *n* Ell(en)bogengicht *f*.
pecil(o)- *pref.* → poikil(o)-.
Pecquet [pe'keɪ; pe'ke]: **P.'s cistern** Cisterna chyli.
  duct of P. Brustmilchgang *m*, Milchbrustgang *m*, Ductus thoracicus.
  P.'s reservoir → P.'s cistern.
pec·ten ['pektən] *n*, *pl* **-tens, -ti·nes** [-tə‚niːz] *anat.* Pekten *m*, kammartiger Fortsatz *od.* Teil *m*, Pecten *M*.
  p. of anus Analkamm, Pecten analis.
  p. of pubis Pecten ossis pubis.
pec·te·ni·tis [ˌpektɪ'naɪtɪs] *n* Entzündung *f* des Pecten analis, Pektenitis *f*.
pec·te·no·sis [ˌ-'nəʊsɪs] *n* Pektenose *f*.
pec·te·not·o·my [ˌ-'nɒtəmɪ] *n chir.* Pektenotomie *f*.
pec·tic ['pektɪk] *adj* Pektin betr., Pektin-.
pectic acid Galakturon-, Galacturonsäure *f*.
pec·tin ['pektɪn] *n* Pektin *nt*.
pec·ti·nal ['pektɪnəl] *adj* → pectineal.
pectinal ligament of iris Hueck'-Band *nt*, Stenon'-Band *nt*, iridokorneales Balkenwerk *nt*, Reticulum trabeculare (anguli iridocornealis), Lig. pectinatum (anguli iridocornealis).
pec·ti·nate ['pektɪneɪt] *adj* → pectineal 1.
pectinate bundles → pectinate muscles.
pec·ti·nat·ed ['pektɪneɪtɪd] *adj* → pectineal 1.
pectinate ligament of iridocorneal angle → pectinal ligament of iris.
pectinate line Anokutanlinie *f*, Linea anocutanea.
pectinate muscles (*Herz*) Muskelbälkchen *pl* des rechten Vorhofes, Mm. pectinati.
pec·tin·e·al [pek'tɪnɪəl] *adj anat.* 1. kammartig, -förmig. 2. Schambein betr., pubisch, pektineal, Schambein-.
pectineal crest of femur Linea pectinea.
pectineal hernia Cloquet-Hernie *f*, Hernia femoralis pectinea.
pectineal ligament Lig. pectineale.
pectineal line 1. Pecten ossis pubis. 2. Linea pectinea (femoris).
pectineal muscle → pectineus (muscle).
pec·tin·e·us (muscle) [pek'tɪnɪəs] *old* Kammuskel *m*, Pektineus *m*, M. pectineus.
pec·tin·i·form [pek'tɪnəˌfɔːrm] *adj* kammförmig, -artig.

pec·to·ral ['pektərəl] *adj* Brust *od.* Brustkorb betr., thorakal, pektoral, Brust-.
pectoral branches of thoracoacromial artery Rami pectorales a. thoracoacromialis.
pectoral cavity Brusthöhle *f*, Brustkorbinnenraum *m*, Cavitas/Cavum thoracis.
pectoral fascia Pektoralisfaszie *f*, Fascia pectoralis.
pectoral fremitus Stimmfremitus *m*, Fremitus pectoralis.
pec·to·ral·gia [pektə'rældʒ(ɪ)ə] *n* Schmerzen *pl* in der Brust, Brustschmerz(en *pl*) *m*.
pectoral girdle Schultergürtel *m*, Cingulum membri superioris, Cingulum pectorale.
pec·to·ra·lis major fascia [ˌpektə'reɪlɪs, -'rɑː-] → pectoral fascia.
pectoralis major flap *chir.* Pectoralis--major-Lappen *m*.
pectoralis major (muscle) Pektoralis *m* major, M. pectoralis major.
pectoralis minor (muscle) Pektoralis *m* minor, M. pectoralis minor.
pectoral muscle: greater p. → pectoralis major (muscle).
  lesser/smaller p. → pectoralis minor (muscle).
pectoral nerve: lateral p. N. pectoralis lateralis.
  medial p. N. pectoralis medialis.
pectoral reflex Pektoralis-major-Reflex *m*.
pectoral region Pektoralisgegend *f*, -region *f*, Regio pectoralis.
pectoral regions Regiones pectorales.
pectoral ridge Crista tuberculi majoris.
pectoral veins Pektoralisvenen *pl*, Vv. pectorales.
pec·to·ril·o·quy [ˌpektə'rɪləkwɪ] *n* Bronchophonie *f*, Bronchialstimme *f*.
pec·to·roph·o·ny [ˌ-'rɒfənɪ] *n* → pectoriloquy.
pec·tous ['pektəs] *adj* Pektin betr., aus Pektin bestehend, pektinartig, Pektin-.
pec·tus ['pektəs] *n*, *pl* **-to·ra** [-tərə] Brust *f*, Brustkorb *m*, Pectus *nt*.
ped- *pref.* → pedo-¹, pedo-².
ped·al ['pedl, 'piːdl] *adj* Fuß betr., Fuß-.
pe·da·tro·phia [pedə'trəʊfɪə] *n* Säuglingsdystrophie *f*, Marasmus *m*.
pe·dat·ro·phy [pe'dætrəfɪ] *n* → pedatrophia.
ped·er·ast ['pedəræst, 'piː-] *n* Päderast *m*.
ped·er·as·tic [ˌpedə'ræstɪk, ˌpiː-] *adj* päderastisch.
ped·er·as·ty ['pedəræstɪ, 'piː-] *n* Päderastie *f*, Knabenliebe *f*.
pe·des *pl* → pes.
pedi- *pref.* → pedo-².
pe·di·al·gia [pedɪ'ældʒ(ɪ)ə] *n* (neuralgischer) Fußschmerz *m*.
pe·di·at·ric [piːdɪ'ætrɪk] *adj* Pädiatrie betr., pädiatrisch, Kinderheilkunde-.
pediatric audiology Pädaudiologie *f*.
pediatric audiometry Kinderaudiometrie *f*.
pe·di·a·tri·cian [ˌpiːdɪə'trɪʃn] *n* Kinderarzt *m*, -ärztin *f*, Pädiater *m*.
pediatric neurologist Neuropädiater *m*.
pediatric psychiatrist Kinderpsychiater(in *f*) *m*.
pe·di·at·rics [piːdɪ'ætrɪks] *pl* Kinderheilkunde *f*, Pädiatrie *f*.
pediatric surgeon Kinderchirurg *m*, -chirurgin *f*.
pediatric surgery Kinderchirurgie *f*.
pe·di·a·trist [piːdɪ'ætrɪst] *n* → pediatrician.
pe·di·at·ry [piː'dɪætrɪ] *n* → pediatrics.
ped·i·cel ['pedəsel] *n histol.* (*Podozyt*) Füßchen *nt*.

pe·dic·el·late [pə'dɪsəleɪt] *adj histol.* gestielt.
ped·i·cel·lat·ed [ˈpedɪsəleɪtɪd] *adj histol.* gestielt.
ped·i·cled ['pedɪkəld] *adj histol.* gestielt.
ped·i·cle ['pedɪkl] *n* 1. *anat., bio.* Füßchen *nt*, Stiel *m*, stiel- *od.* stammähnliche Basis *f*, Pediculus *m*. 2. (*Wirbel*) Bogenfuß *m*, Pediculus arcus vertebrae/vertebralis.
pedicle flap → pedicle graft.
pedicle graft Stiellappen *m*, gestielter Lappen *m*.
pe·dic·u·lar [pɪ'dɪkjələr] *adj* durch Läuse verursacht, Läuse-.
pe·dic·u·late [pɪ'dɪkjəlɪt] *adj histol.* gestielt.
pe·dic·u·la·tion [pɪˌdɪkjə'leɪʃn] *n* Läusebefall *m*, Verlausung *f*; Pedikulose *f*, Pediculosis *f*.
pe·dic·u·li·cide [pɪ'dɪkjələsaɪd] **I** *n* Pedikulizid *nt*. **II** *adj* läuse(ab)tötend, pedikulizid.
Ped·i·cu·li·dae [pedə'kjuːlədiː] *pl micro.* Menschenläuse *pl*, Pediculidae *pl*.
pe·dic·u·lo·pho·bia [pəˌdɪkjələ'fəʊbɪə] *n psychia.* krankhafte Angst *f* vor Läusen, Pedikulophobie *f*.
pe·dic·u·lo·sis [pəˌdɪkjə'ləʊsɪs] *n* Läusebefall *m*, Verlausung *f*, Pedikulose *f*, Pediculosis *f*.
pediculosis capitis Kopflausbefall *m*, Pediculosis capitis.
pediculosis corporis Körper-, Kleiderlausbefall *m*, Pediculosis corporis/vestimentorum.
pediculosis pubis Filzlausbefall *m*, Pediculosis pubis, Phthiriase *f*, Phthiriasis *f*.
pediculosis vestimentorum → pediculosis corporis.
pe·dic·u·lous [pɪ'dɪkjələs] *adj* mit Läusen infestiert, von Läusen befallen.
pediculous blepharitis *ophthal.* Blepharitis parasitica bei Läusebefall.
Pe·dic·u·lus [pɪ'dɪkjələs] *n micro.* Pediculus *m*.
  P. humanus Menschenlaus *f*, Pediculus humanus.
  P. humanus capitis Kopflaus *f*, Pediculus (humanus) capitis.
  P. humanus corporis Kleider-, Körperlaus *f*, Pediculus (humanus) corporis, Pediculus humanus vestimentorum, Pediculus vestimenti.
pe·dic·u·lus [pɪ'dɪkjələs] *n*, *pl* **-li** [-laɪ] 1. *micro.* Laus *f*, Pediculus *m*. 2. *anat.* Stiel *m*, Pediculus *m*.
ped·i·cure ['pedɪkjʊər] *n* 1. Fußpflege *f*, Pediküre *f*. 2. → podiatrist.
ped·i·gree ['pedəgriː] *n genet.* Stammbaum *m*.
ped·i·lu·vi·um [pedɪ'luːvɪəm] *n* Fußbad *nt*.
pedo-¹ *pref.* Kind-, Kinder-, Päd(o)-.
pedo-² *pref.* Fuß-, Pedi-.
pe·dog·a·my [pɪ'dɒgəmɪ] *n* Pädogamie *f*.
pe·do·gen·e·sis [ˌpiːdəʊ'dʒenəsɪs] *n bio.* Pädogenese *f*.
ped·o·gram ['pedəʊgræm] *n* Pedigramm *nt*, -graph *m*.
ped·o·graph ['-græf] *n* Pedigraph *m*.
pe·dog·ra·phy [pɪ'dɒgrəfɪ] *n* Pedigraphie *f*.
pe·dol·o·gy [pɪ'dɒlədʒɪ] *n* Pädologie *f*.
pe·dop·a·thy [pɪ'dɒpəθɪ] *n* Fußerkrankung *f*.
pe·do·phil·ia [ˌpiːdə'fɪlɪə] *n psychia.* Pädophilie *f*.
pe·do·phil·ic [ˌ-'fɪlɪk] *adj* Pädophilie betr., pädophil.
pe·do·pho·bia [ˌ-'fəʊbɪə] *n psychia.* krankhafte Angst *f* vor Kindern, Pädophobie *f*.
pe·dun·cle [pɪ'dʌŋkl] *n anat., bio.* stiel- *od.* stammartige Struktur *f*, Stiel *m*, Stamm *m*, Pedunculus *m*.

p. of cerebellum Kleinhirnstiel, Pedunculus cerebellaris.
p. of cerebrum Hirnstiel, Pedunculus cerebralis/cerebri.
p. of flocculus Pedunculus flocculi/flocculi.
p. of mamillary body Pedunculus corporis mamillaris.
pe·dun·cled [pɪ'dʌŋkəld] *adj anat., bio.* gestielt.
pe·dun·cu·lar [pɪ'dʌŋkjələr] *adj anat., bio.* gestielt, stielförmig, Stiel-.
peduncular loop Hirnschenkelschlinge *f*, Ansa pedunculares.
p. and bundle Ansa et fasciculus pedunculares.
peduncular veins Hirnschenkelvenen *pl*, Vv. pedunculares.
pe·dun·cu·lat·ed polyp [pɪ'dʌŋkjəleɪtɪd] *patho.* gestielter Polyp *m*.
pe·dun·cu·lot·o·my [pɪˌdʌŋkjə'lɒtəmɪ] *n neurochir.* Pedunkulotomie *f*.
pe·dun·cu·lus [pɪ'dʌŋkjələs] *n, pl* **-li** [-laɪ] → peduncle.
peel [piːl] **I** *n* Rinde *f*, Schale *f*, Haut *f*. **II** *vt* abschälen, -ziehen, -lösen. **III** *vi s.* (ab-)schälen, s. (ab-)lösen; *(Haut)* (ab-)schilfern, abblättern, s. schuppen.
peel off *vt, vi* → peel II, III.
peel·ing ['piːlɪŋ] *n* **1.** *(Haut)* (Ab-)Schälen *nt*; Schuppung *f*, Schuppen *nt*. **2.** (abgeschälte) Haut *f*, Schale *f*, Rinde *f*.
PEEP *abbr.* → positive end-expiratory pressure.
PEG *abbr.* → pneumoencephalography.
peg [peg] **I** *n* Nagel *m*, Stift *m*, Dübel *m*, Keil *m*, Splint *m*; *(a. anat.)* Zapfen *m*. **II** *vt techn.* festnageln, pflocken; (an-, ver-)dübeln.
peg-and-socket articulation/joint 1. Einkeilung *f*, Einzapfung *f*, Gomphosis *f*. **2.** Artic. dentoalveolaris, Gomphosis *f*.
pe·jo·ra·tive [pɪ'dʒɔːrətɪv, 'pedʒərɪtɪv] *adj* verschlechternd, pejorativ.
Pel [pel]: **P.'s crises** Pel'-Krisen *pl*, tabische Augenkrisen *pl*.
pe·lade [pə'lɑːd] *n derm.* Pelade *f*, kreisrunder Haarausfall *m*, Alopecia areata, Area celsi.
pel·age ['pelɪdʒ] *n bio.* Fell *nt*, Haarkleid *nt*.
Pel-Ebstein [pel 'ebstaɪn; 'epʃtaɪn]: **P.-E. disease** Pel-Ebstein-Krankheit *f*.
P.-E. fever/pyrexia/symptom Pel-Ebstein-Fieber *nt*.
Pelger ['pelgər]: **P.'s nuclear anomaly** Pelger-Huët-Kernanomalie *f*.
Pelger-Huët ['hjuːet]: **P.-H. anomaly** → P.-H. nuclear anomaly 1.
P.-H. nuclear anomaly 1. Pelger-Huët-Kernanomalie *f*. **2.** Pseudopelgeranomalie *f*.
pe·lid·no·ma [pɪlɪd'nəʊmə] *n derm.* Pelioma *nt*.
pe·li·o·ma [ˌpɪlɪ'əʊmə] *n derm.* Pelioma *nt*.
pe·li·o·sis [ˌ-'əʊsɪs] *n* → purpura.
Pelizaeus-Merzbacher [pælɪ'zaɪəs, 'mertsbækər; peːlɪ'tseʊs, 'mertsbaxər]: **P.-M. disease/sclerosis** Pelizaeus-Merzbacher-Krankheit *f*, -Syndrom *nt*, orthochromatische Leukodystrophie *f*, sudanophile Leukodystrophie *f* Typ Pelizaeus-Merzbacher.
pel·la·gra [pə'lægrə, -'leɪ-] *n* Pellagra *f*, Vitamin-B₂-Mangelsyndrom *nt*, Niacinmangelsyndrom *nt*.
pel·lag·ra·gen·ic [pəˌleɪgrə'dʒenɪk, -læg-] *adj* Pellagra verursachend.
pel·lag·ral [pə'leɪgrəl, -'læg-] *adj* Pellagra betr., durch Pellagra hervorgerufen, Pellagra-.

pel·lag·ra·min [pə'lægrəmɪn] *n* Niacin *nt*, Nikotin-, Nicotinsäure *f*.
pellagra-preventing factor → pellagramin.
pel·lag·roid [pə'lægrɔɪd] **I** *n* Pellagroid *nt*. **II** *adj* pellagraähnlich, pellagroid.
pel·lag·rose [pə'lægrəʊs] *adj* → pellagrous.
pel·la·gro·sis [peləˈgrəʊsɪs] *n derm.* Hauterscheinungen *pl* bei Pellagra.
pel·lag·rous [pə'leɪgrəs, -'læg-] *adj* von Pellagra betroffen, Pellagra-.
Pellegrini [ˌpelə'griːniː]: **P.'s disease** → Pellegrini-Stieda disease.
Pellegrini-Stieda ['stiːdə]: **P.-S. disease/syndrome** *ortho.* Stieda-Pellegrini-Schatten *m*, Pellegrini-Schatten *m*.
pel·let ['pelɪt] *n pharm.* Mikrodragée *nt*, Pellet *nt*.
pel·li·cle ['pelɪkl, 'peliː-] *n* **1.** Film *m*, Häutchen *nt*. **2.** *bio.* Pellikula *f*, Pellicula *f*.
Pellizzi [pe'liːzi]: **P.'s syndrome** Pellizzi-Syndrom *nt*, Macrogenitosomia praecox.
pel·lo·te [pə'ləʊtə, pə'jəʊ-] *n* → peyote.
pel·lu·cid [pə'luːsɪd] *adj* durchscheinend, durchsichtig, klar.
pellucid septum Septum pellucidum/lucidum.
pellucid zone 1. Eihülle *f*, Oolemma *nt*, Zona/Membrana pellucida. **2.** *bio.* Area pellucida.
pel·oid ['pelɔɪd] *n* Peloid *nt*, (Heil-)-Schlamm *m*.
pe·lop·a·thy [pe'lɒpəθɪ] *n* → pelotherapy.
pe·lo·ther·a·py [ˌpiːlə'θerəpɪ] *n* Behandlung/Therapie *f* mit Heilschlamm.
pel·tate ['pelteɪt] *adj* schildförmig.
Peltier ['peltjeɪ]: **P. element** Peltier-Element *nt*.
pel·vic ['pelvɪk] *adj* Becken betr., pelvin, Becken-.
pelvic abscess Beckenabszeß *m*, Abszeß *m* im Beckenbereich.
pelvic actinomycosis Beckenaktinomykose *f*.
pel·vi·cal·i·ce·al [ˌpelvɪˌkælə'sɪəl] *adj (Niere)* Becken u. Kelche betr.
pel·vi·cal·y·ce·al *adj* → pelvicaliceal.
pelvic aneurysm intrapelvines Aneurysma *nt*.
pelvic aperture Beckenöffnung *f*, Apertura pelvis/pelvica.
inferior p. Beckenausgang *m*, Apertura pelvis/pelvica inferior.
superior p. Beckeneingang *m*, Apertura pelvis/pelvica superior.
pelvic artery, posterior innere Hüftarterie *f*, Hypogastrika *f*, Iliaka *f* interna, *old* A. hypogastrica, A. iliaca interna.
pelvic axis Beckenachse *f*, Axis pelvis.
pelvic bone Hüftbein *nt*, Hüftknochen *m*, Os coxae/pelvicum.
pelvic brim Beckenrand *m*, Apertura pelvis/pelvica superior.
pelvic cast calculus (Nieren-)Beckenausgußstein *m*.
pelvic cavity Beckenhöhle *f*, Cavitas pelvis/pelvica.
pelvic cellulitis → parametritis.
pelvic colon Sigma *nt*, Sigmoid *nt*, Colon sigmoideum.
pelvic diameter Beckendurchmesser *m*.
pelvic diaphragm 1. Diaphragma pelvicum. **2.** muskulärer Beckenboden *m*, Diaphragma pelvis.
pel·vi·cel·lu·li·tis [ˌpelvɪˌseljə'laɪtɪs] *n* → parametritis.
pelvic extremity of ovary unterer Eierstockpol *m*, Uteruspol *m*, Extremitas uterina (ovarii).
pelvic fascia Beckenfaszie *f*, Fascia pelvis.

parietal p. parietale Beckenfaszie, Fascia pelvis parietalis.
visceral p. viszerale Beckenfaszie, Fascia endopelvina, Fascia pelvis visceralis.
pelvic fracture 1. Beckenbruch *m*, -fraktur *f*. **2.** Beckenringbruch *m*, -fraktur *f*. **3.** Beckenrandbruch *m*, -fraktur *f*.
pelvic ganglia Beckenganglien *pl*, Ggll. pelvica.
pelvic girdle Beckengürtel *m*, Cingulum membri inferioris, Cingulum pelvicum.
pelvic hematocele Haematocele retrouterina.
pelvic hematoma Blutansammlung *f* im Becken, Hämatopelvis *f*.
pelvic inclination → pelvic incline.
pelvic incline *gyn.* Beckenneigung *f*, Inclinatio pelvis.
pelvic inflammatory disease *abbr.* **PID** *gyn.* (aszendierende) Adnexitis *f*.
pelvic inlet Beckeneingang *m*, Apertura pelvis/pelvica superior.
pelvic kidney Beckenniere *f*.
pelvic ligament: posterior p., great Lig. sacrotuberale.
posterior p., short Lig. sacrospinale.
pelvic limbs untere Gliedmaßen/Extremitäten *pl*, Beine *pl*.
pelvic mesocolon Meso(kolon *nt*) *nt* des Sigmas, Mesosigma *nt*, Mesocolon sigmoideum.
pelvic osteotomy *ortho.* Becken(ring)-osteotomie *f*.
pelvic outlet Beckenausgang *m*, Apertura pelvis/pelvica inferior.
pelvic part: p. of autonomic nervous system Beckenabschnitt *m* des vegetativen Nervensystems, Pars pelvica autonomica.
p. of ureter Beckenabschnitt *m* des Harnleiters, Pars pelvina ureteris.
pelvic peritonitis → pelvioperitonitis.
pelvic plane Beckenebene *f*.
p. of inlet Beckeneingangsebene *f*.
p. of outlet Beckenausgangsebene *f*.
pelvic plexus Beckenplexus *m*, Plexus pelvinus, Plexus hypogastricus inferior.
pelvic presentation *gyn.* Beckenendlage *f abbr.* BEL; Steißlage *f*.
pelvic ring Beckenring *m*.
pelvic sling *ortho.* Beckenschwebe *f*.
pelvic sonography Beckensonographie *f*.
pelvic strait: inferior p. Beckenausgang *m*, Apertura pelvis inferior.
superior p. Beckeneingang *m*, Apertura pelvis superior.
pelvic ultrasonography Beckensonographie *f*.
pelvic veins Beckenvenen *pl*.
pelvic venous thrombosis Beckenvenenthrombose *f*.
pelvic viscera Organe/Eingeweide *pl* des kleinen Beckens, Beckeneingeweide *pl*, -organe *pl*.
pel·vi·fem·o·ral [ˌpelvɪ'femərəl] *adj* Becken/Hüft u. Oberschenkel(knochen)/Femur betr., pelvifemoral.
pel·vi·li·thot·o·my [-lɪ'θɒtəmɪ] *n* → pyelolithotomy.
pel·vim·e·ter [pel'vɪmɪtər] *n gyn.* Pelvimeter *nt*.
pel·vim·e·try [pel'vɪmɪtrɪ] *n gyn.* Beckenmessung *f*, Pelvimetrie *f*.
pel·vi·og·ra·phy [ˌpelvɪ'ɒgrəfɪ] *n* → pelviradiography.
pel·vi·o·il·e·o·ne·o·cys·tos·to·my [ˌpelvɪəʊˌɪlɪəʊˌniːəʊsɪs'tɒstəmɪ] *n urol.* Pelvioileoneozystostomie *f*.
pel·vi·o·li·thot·o·my [-lɪ'θɒtəmɪ] *n* → pyelolithotomy.
pel·vi·o·ne·os·to·my [ˌ-nɪ'ɒstəmɪ] *n urol.* Ureteropyeloneostomie *f*, Uretero(neo)pyelostomie *f*.

pelvioperitonitis

pel·vi·o·per·i·to·ni·tis [ˌ-ˌperɪtəʊˈnaɪtɪs] n Beckenbauchfellentzündung f, Pelvioperitonitis f.
pel·vi·o·plas·ty [ˈ-plæstɪ] n → pyeloplasty.
pel·vi·o·ra·di·og·ra·phy [ˌ-ˌreɪdɪˈɑgrəfɪ] n → pelviradiography.
pel·vi·os·co·py [ˌpelvɪˈɑskəpɪ] n 1. Beckenuntersuchung f. 2. → pyeloscopy.
pel·vi·os·to·my [ˌ-ˈɑstəmɪ] n → pyelostomy.
pel·vi·ot·o·my [ˌ-ˈɑtəmɪ] n 1. ortho. Pelviotomie f, Pubeotomie f. 2. → pyelotomy.
pel·vi·per·i·to·ni·tis [ˌ-ˌperɪtəˈnaɪtɪs] n → pelvioperitonitis.
pel·vi·pros·tat·ic fascia [ˌ-prɑˈstætɪk] → prostatic fascia.
pel·vi·ra·di·og·ra·phy [ˌ-ˌreɪdɪˈɑgrəfɪ] n radiol. Pelvigraphie f.
pel·vi·rec·tal [ˌ-ˈrektəl] adj Becken/Pelvis u. Mastdarm/Rektum betr., pelvirektal.
pelvirectal abscess pelvirektaler Abszeß m.
pelvirectal achalasia aganglionäres/kongenitales Megakolon nt, Hirschsprung-Krankheit f, Morbus Hirschsprung m, Megacolon congenitum.
pel·vi·roent·gen·og·ra·phy [ˌ-ˌrentgəˈnɑgrəfɪ] n → pelviradiography.
pel·vis [ˈpelvɪs] n, pl -ves [-viːz], -vis·es Becken nt, Pelvis f.
p. of the gallbladder Hartmann-Sack m.
p. of the ureter Nierenbecken, Pyelon nt, Pelvis renalis.
pel·vi·sa·cral [ˌpelvɪˈsækrəl, -ˈseɪ-] adj Becken/Pelvis u. Kreuzbein/Sakrum betr., pelvisakral.
pel·vi·scope [ˈ-skəʊp] n Pelviskop nt.
pel·vit·o·my [pelˈvɪtəmɪ] n gyn., chir. Pelvi(o)tomie f.
pel·vi·u·re·ter·ic junction [ˌpelvɪˌjʊərəˈterɪk] Nierenbecken-Uretergrenze f, Nierenbecken-Ureterübergang m.
pel·vi·u·re·te·rog·ra·phy [ˌ-jə-ˌriːtəˈrɑgrəfɪ] n → pyelography.
pel·vi·ver·te·bral angle [ˌ-ˈvɜːrtəbrəl] Beckenneigung f, Inclinatio pelvis.
Pemberton [ˈpembərtən]: **P.'s osteotomy** ortho. Azetabulumplastik f nach Pemberton.
pem·o·line [ˈpeməliːn] n pharm. Pemolin nt.
pem·phi·goid [ˈpem(p)fɪgɔɪd] derm. I n 1. Pemphigoid nt. 2. bullöses Pemphigoid nt, Alterspemphigus m, Parapemphigus m. II adj pemphigusartig, pemphigoid.
pemphigoid syphilid bullöses Syphilid nt; Pemphigus syphiliticus.
pem·phi·gus [ˈpem(p)fɪgəs, pemˈfaɪgəs] n derm. 1. Blasensucht f, Pemphigus m. 2. Pemphigus vulgaris.
pemphigus neonatorum Schälblasenausschlag m, Pemphigoid nt der Neugeborenen, Impetigo bullosa, Pemphigus (acutus) neonatorum.
pen·bu·to·lol [penˈbjuːtəlɒl, -ləʊl] n pharm. Penbutolol nt.
pen·cil [ˈpensl] I n 1. phys., mathe. Büschel nt, (Strahlen-)Bündel nt. 2. (Blei-, Farb-)Stift m; (Kostmetik-)Stift m. 3. zoo. Büschel nt. II vt (auf-)zeichnen, skizzieren; markieren.
pen·del·luft [ˈpendəlɔft] n Pendelluft f.
Pendred [ˈpendrɪd]: **P.'s syndrome** Pendred-Syndrom nt.
pen·du·lar movement [ˈpendələr, ˈpendʒ-] Pendelbewegung f.
pendular nystagmus Pendelnystagmus m.
congenital/hereditary p. Fixationsnystagmus, kongenitaler/hereditärer Pendelnystagmus.
pendular osteotomy ortho. Pendelosteotomie f.

pen·du·lous [ˈpendələs, ˈpendʒə-] adj (herab-)hängend, pendelnd.
pendulous abdomen Hängebauch m.
pendulous heart Tropfenherz nt, Cor pendulum.
pendulous palate (Gaumen-)Zäpfchen nt, Uvula f (palatina).
pen·du·lum rhythm [ˈpendələn, ˈpendʒə-] card. Pendel-Rhythmus m, Tick-Tack-Rhythmus m, Embryokardie f.
pe·nec·to·my [pɪˈnektəmɪ] n chir., urol. Penisentfernung f, -exstirpation f, Penektomie f, Phallektomie f, Exphallatio f.
pen·e·tra·bil·i·ty [ˌpenɪtrəˈbɪlətɪ] n Durchdringbarkeit f, Durchdringlichkeit f.
pen·e·tra·ble [ˈpenɪtrəbl] adj durchdringbar, durchdringlich.
pen·e·trance [ˈpenɪtrəns] n genet. Penetranz f.
pen·e·trate [ˈpenɪtreɪt] I vt 1. durch-, eindringen (into in); durchstoßen, -stechen, penetrieren. 2. penetrieren, einführen (des Penis). 3. fig. (seelisch) durchdringen, ergreifen. II vi eindringen (into, in in).
pen·e·trat·ing [ˈpenɪtreɪtɪŋ] adj durchdringend, penetrierend; (a. fig.) durchbohrend; (Geruch) penetrant; (Geschwür) perforierend; (Schmerz) stechend.
penetrating glance durchdringender Blick m.
penetrating injury perforierende/penetrierende Verletzung f.
penetrating intellect scharfer Verstand m.
penetrating odor penetranter Geruch m.
penetrating ulcer penetrierendes Ulkus nt, Ulcus penetrans.
penetrating wound penetrierende Wunde f.
pen·e·tra·tion [ˌpenɪˈtreɪʃn] n 1. Ein-, Durchdringen nt (into in); Durchstoßen nt, -stechen nt, Penetration f, Penetrierung f. 2. Einführung f (des Penis), Penetration f. 3. fig. Eindringungsvermögen nt. 4. phys. Schärfe f, Auflösungsvermögen nt. 5. patho. (Tumor) Einwachsen nt, Durchbrechen nt, Penetration f. 6. micro. Penetration f.
pen·e·tra·tive [ˈpenɪtreɪtɪv] adj 1. durchdringend, Eindringungs-. 2. → penetrating.
PENG abbr. → photoelectronystagmography.
pe·ni·al [ˈpiːnɪəl] adj → penile.
pen·i·cil·la·mine [ˌpenəˈsɪləmiːn] n pharm. Penizillamin nt, Penicillamin nt.
pen·i·cil·lar arteries [ˌ-ˈsɪlər] (Milz) Pinselarterien pl, Endbäumchen pl, Penicilli pl, Penicilli a. lienalis/splenicae.
pen·i·cil·lic acid [ˌ-ˈsɪlɪk] Penizillin-, Penicillinsäure f.
pen·i·cil·li of spleen [ˌ-ˈsɪlaɪ] → penicillar arteries.
pen·i·cil·lin [ˌ-ˈsɪlɪn] n Penizillin nt, Penicillin nt.
penicillin I → penicillin F.
penicillin II → penicillin G.
penicillin III → penicillin X.
penicillin IV → penicillin K.
penicillin V Penicillin V nt, Phenoxymethylpenicillin nt.
penicillin X Hydroxybenzylpenicillin nt, Penicillin X nt.
penicillin amide-β-lactamhydrolase → penicillinase.
pen·i·cil·lin·ase [ˌ-ˈsɪləneɪz] n Penizillinase f, Penicillinase f, Penicillin-Beta-Lactamase f.
penicillinase-producing Neisseria gonorrhoeae abbr. **PPNG** Penizillinase-produzierende Neisseria gonorrhoeae f abbr. PPNG.

penicillinase-resistent adj penicillinasefest.
penicillin-binding protein abbr. **PBP** penicillinbindendes Protein nt abbr. PBP.
penicillin F 2-Pentenylpenicillin nt, Penicillin F nt, Penicillin I nt.
penicillin-fast adj penicillinfest.
penicillin G Penicillin G nt, Benzylpenicillin nt.
penicillin G benzathine Benzathin-Penicillin G nt, Benzathin-Benzylpenicillin nt.
penicillin G procaine Procain-Penicillin G nt, Procain-Benzylpenicillin nt.
penicillin K Heptylpenicillin nt, Penicillin K nt, Penicillin IV nt.
penicillin N Adicillin nt, Penicillin N nt, Cephalosporin N nt.
penicillin O Penicillin O nt, Allylmercaptomethylpenicillinsäure f, Almecillin nt, Penicillin AT nt.
penicillin-resistant adj penicillinresistent.
pen·i·cil·li·o·sis [ˌ-ˌsɪlɪˈəʊsɪs] n Penicillium-Infektion f.
Pen·i·cil·li·um [ˌ-ˈsɪlɪəm] n micro. Pinselschimmel m, Penicillium nt.
P. glaucum grüner Pinselschimmel, Penicillium glaucum.
pen·i·cil·lo·ic acid [ˌ-sɪˈləʊɪk] Penizilloin-, Penicilloinsäure f.
pen·i·cil·loyl-polylysine test [ˌ-ˈsɪləwɪl] Penicilloyl-Polylysin-Test m, PPL-Test m.
pe·nile [ˈpiːnl, ˈpiːnaɪl] adj Penis betr., penil, phallisch, Penis-.
penile epispadias urol. penile Epispadie f.
penile fibromatosis Penisfibromatose f.
penile hypospadias urol. penile Hypospadie f.
penile induration Peyronie-Krankheit f, Penisfibromatose f, Induratio penis plastica, Sclerosis fibrosa penis.
penile reflex Bulbocavernosus-Reflex m.
penile urethra Penisabschnitt m der Urethra.
pe·nis [ˈpiːnɪs] n (männliches) Glied nt, Penis m, Phallus m, Membrum virile.
pe·nis·chi·sis [pɪˈnɪskəsɪs] n embryo. Harnröhren-, Penisspalte f.
penis envy psycho., psychia. Penisneid m.
penis reflex Bulbocavernosus-Reflex m.
pe·ni·tis [pɪˈnaɪtɪs] n Penisentzündung f, Penitis f.
Pen·je·deh sore [ˈpendʒədeɪ] kutane Leishmaniose/Leishmaniase f, Hautleishmaniose/-leishmaniase f, Orientbeule f, Leishmaniasis cutis.
pen·nate [ˈpeneɪt] adj → penniform.
pen·ni·form [ˈpenɪfɔːrm] adj federförmig, federartig; gefiedert.
pe·no·scro·tal [ˌpiːnəʊˈskrəʊtl] adj Penis u. Skrotum betr., penoskrotal.
penoscrotal hypospadias urol. penoskrotale Hypospadie f.
Penrose [ˈpenrəʊz]: **P. drain** chir. Penrose-Drain m.
pen·sion neurosis [ˈpenʃn] Renten-, Unfall-, Entschädigungsneurose f, Rentenbegehren nt, -tendenz f, traumatische Neurose f, tendenziöse Unfallreaktion f.
pen·ta·ba·sic [ˌpentəˈbeɪsɪk] adj chem. fünfbasisch.
pen·ta·cyc·lic [ˌ-ˈsaɪklɪk, -ˈsɪk-] adj chem. pentazyklisch.
pen·tad [ˈpentæd] n 1. Pentade f. 2. chem. fünfwertiges Element od. Radikal nt.
pen·ta·dac·tyl [ˌpentəˈdæktɪl] adj fünffingrig, fünfzehig, pentadaktyl.
pen·ta·ene [ˈpentəwiːn] n chem. Pentaen nt.
pen·ta·e·ryth·ri·tol [ˌpentərˈrɪθrətɒl, -tɑl] n pharm. Pentaerythrityl nt.
pentaerythritol tetranitrate abbr. **PTEN** pharm. Pentaerythrityl-Tetranitrat nt.

pen·ta·e·ryth·ri·tyl [ˌ-ɪˈrɪθrətɪl] *n* → pentaerythritol.
pentaerythrityl tetranitrate → pentaerythritol tetranitrate.
pen·ta·gas·trin [ˌ-ˈgæstrɪn] *n* Pentagastrin *nt*.
pentagastrin test Pentagastrintest *m*.
pen·ta·gly·cine [ˌ-ˈglaɪsiːn] *n* Pentaglycin *nt*.
pen·tal·o·gy [penˈtælədʒɪ] *n* Pentalogie *f*.
pen·ta·mer [ˈpentəmər] *n* Pentamer *nt*.
pen·ta·me·tho·ni·um [ˌ-mɪˈθəʊnɪəm] *n pharm*. Pentamethonium *nt*.
pen·ta·meth·yl·ene·di·am·ine [ˌ-ˌmeθɪliːnˈdaɪəmiːn, -daɪˈæmɪn] *n* Kadaverin *nt*, Cadaverin *nt*, Pentamethylendiamin *nt*, 1,5-Diaminopentan *nt*.
pen·ta·meth·yl violet [ˌ-ˈmeθəl] Gentianaviolett *nt*.
pen·tam·i·dine [penˈtæmədiːn] *n pharm*. Pentamidin *nt*.
pen·tane [ˈpenteɪn] *n* Pentan *nt*.
pen·ta·no·ic acid [ˌpentəˈnəʊɪk] Valeriansäure *f*.
pen·ta·pep·tide [ˌ-ˈpeptaɪd] *n* Pentapeptid *nt*.
pen·ta·sac·cha·ride [ˌ-ˈsækəraɪd, -rɪd] *n* Pentasaccharid *nt*.
pen·ta·so·my [ˌ-ˈsəʊmɪ] *n genet*. Pentasomie *f*.
Pen·tas·to·ma [penˈtæstəmə] *n micro*. Pentastomum *nt*.
pen·ta·sto·mi·a·sis [ˌpentəstəʊˈmaɪəsɪs] *n* Zungenwurmbefall *m*, Pentastomiasis *f*.
pen·ta·sto·mid [ˌ-ˈstəʊmɪd] *n micro*. Zungenwurm *m*, Pentastomid *nt*.
Pen·ta·stom·i·da [ˌ-ˈstɒmɪdə] *pl micro*. Zungenwürmer *pl*, Pentastomida *pl*, Linguatulida *pl*, Pentastomiden *pl*.
pen·ta·tom·ic [ˌ-ˈtɒmɪk] *adj chem*. **1.** aus fünf Atomen bestehend, fünfatomig. **2.** → pentabasic.
Pen·ta·trich·o·mon·as [ˌ-ˌtrɪkəˈməʊnəs, -trɪˈkɒmə-] *n micro*. Pentatrichomonas *f*.
pen·ta·va·lent [ˌ-ˈveɪlənt] *adj chem*. fünfwertig, pentavalent.
pen·taz·o·cine [penˈtæzəsiːn, -sɪn] *n pharm*., *anes*. Pentazocin *nt*.
pent·dy·o·pent [pentˈdaɪəpent] *n lab*. Pentdyopent *nt*.
pen·tene [ˈpentiːn] *n chem*. Penten *nt*, Amylen *nt*.
2-pen·te·nyl·pen·i·cil·lin [ˌpentənɪlˌpenɪˈsɪlɪn] *n pharm*. 2-Pentenylpenicillin *nt*, Penicillin F *nt*, Penicillin I.
pen·thrit [ˈpenθrɪt] *n* → pentaerythritol tetranitrate.
pen·to·bar·bi·tal [ˌpentəʊˈbɑːrbɪtɔl, -tæl] *n pharm*. Pentobarbital *nt*.
pen·to·bar·bi·tone [ˌ-ˈbɑːrbɪtəʊn] *n* → pentobarbital.
pen·tone [ˈpentəʊn] *n micro*. Penton *nt*.
pen·to·san [ˈpentəsæn] *n* Pentosan *nt*.
pen·to·sa·zone [ˌpentəʊsəzəʊn, ˌpentəʊˈsaɪzəʊn] *n* Pentosazon *nt*.
pen·tose [ˈpentəʊs] *n* Pentose *f*, C₅-Zucker *m*.
pen·to·se·mia [ˌpentəʊˈsiːmɪə] *n* Pentosämie *f*.
pentose nucleic acid Ribonukleinsäure *f abbr*. RNA, RNS.
pentose phosphate pathway Pentosephosphatzyklus *m*, Phosphogluconatweg *m*.
pentose shunt → pentose phosphate pathway.
pen·to·side [ˈpentəsaɪd] *n* Pentosid *nt*.
pen·to·su·ria [ˌ-ˈs(j)ʊərɪə] *n* Pentosurie *f*.
pen·to·su·ric [ˌ-ˈsʊərɪk] *adj* Pentosurie betr., pentosurisch.
pen·to·syl [ˌ-sɪl] *n* Pentosyl-(Radikal *nt*).
pent·ox·ide [pentˈɒksaɪd] *n* Pentoxid *nt*.

pen·tox·i·fyl·line [pentɒkˈsɪfəlɪn] *n pharm*. Pentoxifyllin *nt*.
pen·tri·ni·trol [ˌpentraɪˈnaɪtrəʊl] *n* → pentaerythritol tetranitrate.
pe·o·til·lo·ma·nia [ˌpɪəˌtɪləˈmeɪnɪə, -jə] *n psychia*. Peotillomanie *f*, Pseudomasturbation *f*.
pe·ot·o·my [pɪˈɒtəmɪ] *n* → penectomy.
PEP *abbr*. → phosphoenolpyruvate.
pep·lo·mer [ˈpepləmər] *n micro*. Peplomer *nt*.
pep·los [ˈpeplɒs] *n micro*. Peplos *nt*.
Pepper [ˈpepər]: **P.'s syndrome/type** Pepper-Syndrom *nt*, -Typ *m*.
pepper and salt fundus Pfeffer- u. Salzfundus *m*.
pep·per·mint [ˈpepərmɪnt] *n* **1.** Pfefferminze *f*. **2.** → peppermint oil.
peppermint camphor Menthol *nt*, Mentholeum *nt*, Pfefferminzkampfer *m*.
peppermint oil Pfefferminzöl *nt*.
pep·sase [ˈpepseɪz] *n* → pepsin.
pep·sic [ˈpepsɪk] *adj* → peptic.
pep·sin [ˈpepsɪn] *n* Pepsin *nt*.
pepsin A Pepsin A *nt*.
pep·sin·ate [ˈpepsɪneɪt] *vt* mit Pepsin behandeln.
pepsin B Pepsin B *nt*.
pepsin C Pepsin C *nt*, Gastrizin *nt*.
pep·sin·ia [pepˈsɪnɪə] *n* Pepsinsekretion *f*.
pep·si·nif·er·ous [pepsɪˈnɪfərəs] *adj* Pepsin produzierend *od*. sezernierend.
pep·sin·o·gen [pepˈsɪnədʒən] *n* Pepsinogen *nt*.
pep·si·nu·ria [pepsɪˈn(j)ʊərɪə] *n* Pepsinausscheidung *f* im Harn, Pepsinurie *f*.
pep·tic [ˈpeptɪk] *adj* verdauungsfördernd, -anregend, peptisch, Verdauungs-.
peptic cells (*Magen*) Hauptzellen *pl*.
peptic digestion Magenverdauung *f*, peptische Verdauung *f*.
peptic esophagitis peptische Speiseröhrenentzündung/Ösophagitis *f*.
 chronic p. chronisch-peptische Ösophagitis, Refluxösophagitis *f*.
peptic glands Magendrüsen *f*, Fundus- u. Korpusdrüsen *pl*, Gll. gastricae propriae.
peptic stricture peptische Striktur *f*.
peptic theory of ulcer formation Theorie *f* der peptischen Ulkusentstehung.
peptic ulcer peptisches Ulkus *nt*, Ulcus pepticum.
peptic ulcer disease *abbr*. **PUD** Ulkuskrankheit *f*.
pep·tid [ˈpeptɪd] *n* → peptide.
pep·ti·dase [ˈpeptɪdeɪz] *n* Peptidase *f*, Peptidhydrolase *f*.
pep·tide [ˈpeptaɪd] *n* Peptid *nt*.
peptide antibiotic Peptidantibiotikum *nt*.
peptide bond *chem*. Peptidbindung *f*.
peptide chain *biochem*. Peptidkette *f*.
peptide hormone Peptidhormon *nt*.
peptide hydrolase → peptidase.
peptide map *biochem*. Peptidmuster *nt*, peptide map.
pep·ti·der·gic [ˌpeptɪˈdɜrdʒɪk] *adj* peptiderg.
peptidergic neuron peptiderges Neuron *nt*.
peptidergic synapse peptiderge Synapse *f*.
peptidergic system peptiderges System *nt*.
peptide transmitter Peptidtransmitter *m*.
pep·ti·do·gly·can [ˌpeptɪdəʊˈglaɪkæn] *n* Peptidoglykan *nt*, Murein *nt*, Mukopeptid *nt*.
pep·ti·dyl site [ˈpeptədɪl] *biochem*. P-Bindungsstelle *f*, Peptid(bindungs)stelle *f*.
peptidyl transferase Peptidyltransferase *f*.
peptidyl-tRNA *n* Peptidyl-tRNA *f*, Peptidyl-tRNS *f*.

pep·ti·za·tion [ˌpeptɪˈzeɪʃn] *n chem*. Peptisation *f*.
pep·tize [ˈpeptaɪz] *vt chem*. peptisieren.
Pep·to·coc·ca·ce·ae [ˌpeptəʊkəˈkeɪsɪˌiː] *pl micro*. Peptococcaceae *pl*.
Pep·to·coc·cus [ˌ-ˈkɒkəs] *n micro*. Peptococcus *m*.
pep·to·gen·ic [ˌ-ˈdʒenɪk] *adj* **1.** pepsinbildend, peptogen. **2.** peptonbildend, peptogen. **3.** die Verdauung fördernd.
pep·tog·e·nous [pepˈtɒdʒənəs] *adj* → peptogenic.
pep·tol·y·sis [pepˈtɒləsɪs] *n* Peptonhydrolyse *f*, Peptolyse *f*.
pep·to·lyt·ic [ˌpeptəˈlɪtɪk] *adj* Peptone hydrolysierend, peptolytisch.
pep·tone [ˈpeptəʊn] *n* Pepton *nt*.
peptone water Peptonwasser *nt*.
peptone-yeast extract-glucose medium Pepton-Hefeextrakt-Glucose-Medium *nt*.
peptone-yeast extract medium Pepton-Hefeextrakt-Medium *nt*.
pep·ton·ic [pepˈtɒnɪk] *adj* Pepton betr., Pepton-.
pep·to·noid [ˈpeptənɔɪd] *n* peptonartige Substanz *f*.
Pep·to·strep·to·coc·cus [ˌpeptəˌstreptəʊˈkɒkəs] *n micro*. Peptostreptococcus *m*.
per·ac·e·tate [pərˈæsɪteɪt] *n* Peroxyacetat *nt*.
per·a·ce·tic acid [pərəˈsiːtɪk] Peroxiessigsäure *f*.
per·ac·id [pərˈæsɪd] *n chem*. Peroxisäure *f*, Persäure *f*.
per·a·cute [pərəˈkjuːt] *adj* sehr akut, perakut; hyperakut.
per·am·bu·lat·ing ulcer [pərˈæmbjəleɪtɪŋ] Ulcus phagedaenicum.
per anum beim After, peranal.
per·ar·tic·u·la·tion [pərɑːrˌtɪkjəˈleɪʃn] *n* echtes Gelenk *nt*, Diarthrose *f*, Artic. synovialis.
per·ceiv·a·ble [pərˈsiːvəbl] *adj* → perceptive.
per·ceive [pərˈsiːv] *vt* **1.** wahrnehmen, empfinden, perzipieren. **2.** verstehen, erkennen, begreifen.
per·cent [pərˈsent] **I** *n abbr*. **%** Prozent *nt abbr*. p.c., %. **II** *adj* -prozentig.
per·cent·age [pərˈsentɪdʒ] *n* **1.** Prozentsatz *m*. **2.** (An-)Teil *m*, Gehalt *nt* (*of* an); Rate *f*. **3.** Prozentgehalt *m*.
per·cent·al [pərˈsentl] *adj* prozentual, in Prozenten (gerechnet *od*. ausgedrückt), prozentisch, Prozent-.
per·cen·tile [pərˈsentɪl, -taɪl] *n* Perzentile *f*, Percentile *f*.
per·cep·ti·bil·i·ty [pərˌseptəˈbɪlətɪ] *n* Wahrnehmbarkeit *f*, Perzeptibilität *f*.
per·cep·ti·ble [pərˈseptɪbl] *adj* wahrnehmbar, spür-, fühlbar, merklich, deutlich, perzeptibel.
per·cep·tion [pərˈsepʃn] *n* **1.** (Reiz-)Wahrnehmung *f*, Empfindung *f*, Perzeption *f*. **2.** Wahrnehmungsvermögen *nt*, Auffassungsgabe *f*, Perzeptibilität *f*.
 p. of light Lichtempfindung *f*.
perception psychology Wahrnehmungspsychologie *f*.
perception threshold *physiol*. Wahrnmungsschwelle *f*.
per·cep·tive [pərˈseptɪv] *adj* **1.** Perzeption betr., auf ihr beruhend, durch sie bewirkt, wahrnehmend, perzeptorisch, perzeptiv, Perzeptions-, Wahrnehmungs-. **2.** auffassungsfähig.
perceptive deafness *HNO* Schallempfindungsstörung *f*, Schallempfindungsschwerhörigkeit *f*.
per·cep·tive·ness [pərˈseptɪvnɪs] *n* → perception 2.

per·cep·tiv·i·ty [ˌpərsep'tɪvətɪ] *n* **1.** → perception 2. **2.** Fähigkeit zur Perzeption, Perzeptivität *f*.
per·cep·to·ri·um [pərsep'tɔːrɪəm, -'toʊr-] *n* Bewußtsein *nt*, Sensorium *nt*.
per·chlo·rate [pər'klɔːreɪt, -'kloʊr-] *n* Perchlorat *nt*.
per·chlor·ic acid [pər'klɔːrɪk, -'kloʊr-] Perchlorsäure *f*.
per·chlo·ride [pər'klɔːraɪd, -ɪd, -'kloʊr-] *n* Perchlorid *nt*.
per·chlor·meth·ane [pərˌklɔːr'meθeɪn] *n* Tetrachlorkohlenstoff *m*, Kohlenstofftetrachlorid *nt*.
per·chlor·meth·yl·for·mate [pərklɔːrˌmeθɪl'fɔːrmeɪt, -ˌkloʊr-] *n* Diphosgen *nt*.
per·chlo·ro·eth·yl·ene [pərˌklɔːroʊ'eθəliːn, -ˌkloʊr-] *n* Tetrachloräthylen *nt*, -ethylen *nt*, Perchloräthylen *nt*, Äthylentetrachlorid *nt*.
per·cip·i·ence [pər'sɪpɪəns] *n* **1.** Wahrnehmung *f*, Perzeption *f*. **2.** Wahrnehmungsvermögen *nt*, Perzeptibilität *f*.
per·cip·i·ent [pər'sɪpɪənt] **I** *n* Wahrnehmer(in *f*) *m*, Wahrnehmende(r *m*) *f*. **II** *adj* → perceptive 1.
per·co·late [*n* 'pərkəlɪt, -leɪt; *v* -leɪt] **I** *vt* Filtrat *nt*, Perkolat *nt*. **II** *vt* filtern, filtrieren, perkolieren. **III** *vi* **1.** durchsickern, -laufen, versickern. **2.** gefiltert werden.
per·co·la·tion [ˌpərkə'leɪʃn] *n* Filtration *f*, Perkolation *f*; Perkolieren *nt*.
per·co·la·tor ['pərkəleɪtər] *n* Filtrierapparat *m*, Perkolator *m*.
per·con·dy·lar fracture [pər'kɒndɪlər]: **p. of the femur** perkondyläre Oberschenkelfraktur/Femurfraktur *f*.
p. of humerus perkondyläre Humerusfraktur *f*.
per·cuss [pər'kʌs] *vt* mittels Perkussion untersuchen, be-, abklopfen, perkutieren.
per·cus·sion [pər'kʌʃn] **I** *n* **1.** Be-, Abklopfen *nt*, Perkutieren *nt*, Perkussion *f*. **2.** Klopfmassage *f*. **3.** Schlag *m*, Stoß *m*, Erschütterung *f*. **II** *adj* Schlag-, Stoß-; Perkussions-.
percussion sound Perkussionsgeräusch *nt*.
per·cus·sive [pər'kʌsɪv] *adj* schlagend, perkussiv.
per·cus·sor [pər'kʌsər] *n* Perkussionsinstrument *m*, Hammer *m*.
per·cu·ta·ne·ous [pərkjuː'teɪnɪəs] *adj* durch die Haut hindurch (wirkend), perkutan.
percutaneous biopsy perkutane Biopsie *f*.
percutaneous cystostomy *urol*. perkutane Blasenfistel/Zystostomie *f*.
percutaneous pinning *ortho*. perkutane (Draht-)Spickung *f*.
percutaneous pyelostomy *urol*. perkutane Pyelostomie *f*.
percutaneous suture *chir*. perkutane Naht *f*.
percutaneous transhepatic biliary drainage/intubation perkutane transhepatische Cholangiodrainage/Gallendrainage *f*.
percutaneous transhepatic cholangiography *abbr*. **PTC** perkutane transhepatische Cholangiographie *f abbr*. PTC.
percutaneous transhepatic coronary vein occlusion perkutane transhepatische Obliteration *f* der V. coronaria ventriculi.
percutaneous transhepatic venous sampling *abbr*. **PTVS** (*Pankreas*) perkutane transhepatische Venenblutentnahme *f*.
percutaneous transjugular cholangiography *abbr*. **PTJC** perkutane transjugulare Cholangiographie *f abbr*. PTJC.
percutaneous transluminal angioplasty *abbr*. **PTA** perkutane transluminale Angioplastie *f abbr*. PTA.
per·en·ceph·a·ly [perən'sefəlɪ] *n* → porencephaly.
per·en·ni·al [pə'renɪəl] *adj* **1.** (alljährlich) wiederkehrend, unaufhörlich, ständig, immerwährend; das ganze Jahr über (andauernd), perennial. **2.** *bot*. perennierend, mehrjährig.
perennial rhinitis perenniale (allergische) Rhinitis *f*.
per·fect [*adj* 'pɜːfɪkt; *v* pər'fekt] **I** *adj* vollkommen, vollendet, tadellos, makellos, ideal, perfekt. **II** *vt* vervollständigen, vervollkommnen, perfektionieren.
per·fec·tion·ism [pər'fekʃənɪzəm] *n psychia*. Perfektionismus *m*.
perfect stage *bio*., *micro*. geschlechtliche/generative Phase *f*.
perfect state *micro*. perfektes Stadium *nt*.
perfect yeast *micro*. echte/perfekte Hefe *f*.
per·fo·rate [*adj* 'pərfərɪt, -reɪt; *v* -reɪt] **I** *adj* perforiert, mit Löchern versehen, durchbohrt, durchlöchert; gezähnt. **II** *vt* durchbohren, -löchern, lochen, perforieren. **III** *vi* s. durchbohren, penetrieren, durchbrechen.
per·fo·rat·ed ['pərfəreɪtɪd] *adj* → perforate I.
perforated appendicitis perforierende Appendizitis *f*, Appendicitis perforans/perforata.
perforated substance: anterior p. basale Riechrinde *f*, Area olfactoria, Substantia perforata anterior/rostralis.
interpeduncular p. Substantia perforata interpeduncularis.
posterior p. Substantia perforata posterior.
rostral p. → anterior p.
perforated ulcer perforiertes Ulkus *nt*, Ulcus perforans.
per·fo·rat·ing abscess ['pərfəreɪtɪŋ] perforierender Abszeß *m*.
perforating appendicitis → perforated appendicitis.
perforating arteries perforierende (Oberschenkel-)Arterien *pl*, Aa. perforantes.
perforating branch: p. of fibular artery Perforansast *m* der A. fibularis, Ramus perforans a. peron(a)eae/fibularis.
p.es of internal thoracic artery Perforansäste *pl* der A. thoracica interna, Rami perforantes a. thoracicae internae.
p.es of palmar metacarpal arteries Perforansäste *pl* der palmaren Metakarpalarterien, Rami perforantes aa. metacarpalium palmarium.
p.es of plantar metatarsal arteries Perforansäste *pl* der plantaren Metatarsalarterien, Rami perforantes aa. metatarsalium plantarium.
perforating elastosis *derm*. perforierendes Elastom *nt*, Elastosis perforans serpiginosa, Elastoma intrapapillare perforans verruciforme, Keratosis follicularis serpiginosa.
perforating fibers Sharpey-Fasern *pl*.
perforating tract Tractus perforans.
perforating veins Verbindungs-, Perforansvenen *pl*, Vv. perforantes.
perforating wound perforierende Wunde *f*.
per·fo·ra·tion [ˌpərfə'reɪʃn] *n* **1.** Perforieren *nt*, Durchbohren *nt*, -löchern *nt*; Lochung *f*, Durchbohrung *f*, Durchlöcherung *f*. **2.** *patho*. Durchbruch *m*, Perforation *f*. **3.** *gyn*. Perforation *f*.
per·fo·ra·tive appendicitis ['pərfəreɪtɪv] → perforated appendicitis.
per·fo·ra·tor ['pərfəreɪtər] *n chir*., *gyn*. Perforatorium *nt*.
per·form [pər'fɔːrm] **I** *vt* (*Operation*) aus-, durchführen (*on* bei); vornehmen, verrichten, leisten; (*Pflicht*) erfüllen. **II** *vi* **1.** etw. erfüllen *od*. leisten *od*. ausführen. **2.** *techn*. (*Maschine*) funktionieren.
per·form·a·ble [pər'fɔːrməbl] *adj* aus-, durchführbar.
per·for·mance [pər'fɔːrməns] *n* **1.** Aus-, Durchführung *f*, Verrichtung *f*, Erfüllung *f*; (*a. physiol*.) Leistung *f*. **2.** *techn*. (*Maschine*) (Arbeits-)Leistung *f*.
performance capacity *physiol*. Leistungsfähigkeit *f*.
maximal p. Höchstleistungsfähigkeit.
performance chart Leistungsdiagramm *nt*.
performance limit *physiol*. Grenzleistung *f*.
performance-limiting *adj* leistungsbegrenzend.
performance maximum *physiol*. Endleistung *f*.
performance-pulse index *abbr*. **PPI** *physiol*. Leistungspulsindex *m abbr*. LPI.
performance test Leistungsprüfung *f*, -test *m*.
per·for·mic acid [pər'fɔːrmɪk] Perameisensäure *f*.
per·frig·er·a·tion [pərˌfrɪdʒə'reɪʃn] *n* Erfrierung *f*, Kongelation *f*, Congelatio *f*.
per·fume dermatitis ['pərfjuːm, pər'fjuːm] Berloque-Dermatitis *f*, Kölnisch-Wasser-Dermatitis *f*.
per·fu·sate [pər'fjuːzeɪt, -zɪt] *n* Perfusionsflüssigkeit *f*, Perfusat *nt*.
per·fuse [pər'fjuːz] *vt* **1.** durchspülen, -strömen, perfundieren. **2.** übergießen, -strömen, besprengen (*with* mit).
per·fu·sion [pər'fjuːʒn] *n* **1.** Durchspülung *f*, -strömung *f*, Durchblutung *f*, Perfusion *f*. **2.** Perfusionsflüssigkeit *f*.
perfusion cannula Perfusionskanüle *f*.
perfusion chemotherapy Perfusionschemotherapie *f*.
perfusion weight *physiol*. Durchblutung *f*, Durchblutungsgröße *f*.
per·hex·i·line [pər'heksəliːn] *n pharm*. Perhexilin *f*.
peri- *pref*. Peri-.
per·i·ac·i·nal [ˌperɪ'æsɪnæl] *adj histol*. um einen Azinus herum (liegend), periazinär, periazinös.
per·i·ac·i·nous [ˌ-'æsɪnəs] *adj* → periacinal.
per·i·ad·e·ni·tis [ˌ-ˌædɪ'naɪtɪs] *n* Periadenitis *f*.
per·i·ad·ven·ti·tial [ˌ-ˌædven'tɪʃ(ɪ)əl] *adj* periadventitial.
per·i·am·pul·la·ry [ˌ-æm'pʌlərɪ, -'pʊl-] *adj* periampullär.
per·i·a·myg·da·loid cortex [ˌ-ə'mɪgdəlɔɪd] periamygdaläre Rinde *f*, periamygdalärer Cortex *m*.
periamygdaloid region Regio periamygdalaris.
per·i·a·nal [ˌ-'eɪnl] *adj* um den Anus/After herum (liegend), perianal, zirkumanal.
perianal abscess perianaler Abszeß *m*.
perianal fistula perianale Fistel *f*, Perianalfistel *f*.
perianal hematoma perianales Hämatom *nt*.
perianal reflex Analreflex *m*.
per·i·a·nas·to·mot·ic abscess [ˌ-ə,næstə'mɒtɪk] perianastomotischer Abszeß *m*.
per·i·an·gi·itis [ˌ-ændʒɪ'aɪtɪs] *n* Periangi(i)tis *f*; Perivaskulitis *f*.
per·i·an·gi·o·cho·li·tis [ˌ-ˌændʒɪoʊkoʊ'laɪtɪs] *n* Pericholangitis *f*.
per·i·an·gi·tis [ˌ-æn'dʒaɪtɪs] *n* → periangiitis.

per·i·a·or·tic [ˌ-eɪˈɔːrtɪk] *adj* um die Aorta herum (liegend), periaortal.
per·i·a·or·ti·tis [ˌ-ˌeɪɔːrˈtaɪtɪs] *n* Periaortitis *f*.
per·i·ap·i·cal [ˌ-ˈeɪpɪkl, -ˈæp-] *adj* periapikal.
periapical abscess 1. (*Lunge*) Spitzenabszeß *m*. **2.** (*Zahn*) Wurzelspitzenabszeß *m*.
acute p. akuter Wurzelspitzenabszeß.
chronic p. chronischer Wurzelspitzenabszeß.
periapical cyst (*Zahn*) radikuläre Zyste *f*.
periapical periodontal abscess (*Zahn*) Wurzelspitzenabszeß *m*.
per·i·ap·pen·di·ce·al [ˌ-ˌæpənˈdɪʃl, -ˌəˌpendɪˈsiːəl] *adj* um die Appendix vermiformis herum (liegend), periappendikal, periappendizeal.
periappendiceal abscess appendizealer/periappendizealer Abszeß *m*.
per·i·ap·pen·di·ci·tis [ˌ-ˌəˌpendɪˈsaɪtɪs] *n* Periappendizitis *f*.
per·i·ap·pen·dic·u·lar [ˌ-ˌæpənˈdɪkjələr] *adj* → periappendiceal.
periappendicular abscess periappendizitischer Abszeß *m*.
per·i·aq·ue·duc·tal [ˌ-ˌækwɪˈdʌktl] *adj* periaquäduktal.
periaqueductal gray zentrales Höhlengrau *nt*, Griseum centrale, Stratum griseum centrale cerebri, Substantia grisea centralis cerebri.
per·i·ar·chi·cor·tex [ˌ-ˌɑːrkɪˈkɔːrteks] *n* Periarchikortex *m*.
per·i·a·re·o·lar abscess [ˌ-əˈrɪələr] (*Brust*) periareolarer Abszeß *m*.
periareolar incision *gyn.* Warzenhofrandschnitt *m*, periareolärer Schnitt *m*.
per·i·ar·te·ri·al [ˌ-ˌɑːrˈtɪəriəl] *adj* um eine Arterie herum (liegend), eine Arterie umgebend, periarteriell.
periarterial lymphatic sheath *abbr.* **PALS** (*Milz*) periarterielle Lymphscheide *f abbr.* PALS.
periarterial lymphoid sheath → periarterial lymphatic sheath.
periarterial plexus vegetatives Adventitiageflecht *nt* der Arterien, Plexus periarterialis.
periarterial sympathectomy Leriche--Operation *f*, periarterielle Sympatektomie *f*.
per·i·ar·te·ri·tis [ˌ-ˌɑːrtəˈraɪtɪs] *n* Periarteriitis *f*.
per·i·ar·thric [ˌ-ˈɑːrθrɪk] *adj* → periarticular.
per·i·ar·thri·tis [ˌ-ɑːrˈθraɪtɪs] *n ortho.* Periarthritis *f*.
p. of shoulder schmerzhafte Schultersteife *f*, Periarthritis/Periarthropathia humeroscapularis *abbr.* PHS.
per·i·ar·tic·u·lar [ˌ-ɑːrˈtɪkjələr] *adj* um ein Gelenk herum (liegend), periartikulär, zirkumartikulär.
periarticular abscess periartikulärer Abszeß *m*.
periarticular fracture periartikuläre Fraktur *f*.
per·i·a·tri·al [ˌ-ˈeɪtriəl] *adj* periatrial, periaurikulär.
per·i·au·ric·u·lar [ˌ-ɔːˈrɪkjələr] *adj* **1.** → periatrial. **2.** um die Ohrmuschel herum (liegend), periaurikulär.
per·i·ax·i·al [ˌ-ˈæksiəl] *adj* um eine Achse herum (liegend), periaxial.
periaxial neuritis Neuritis periaxialis.
periaxial neuropathy segmentale/periaxiale Neuropathie *f*.
per·i·ax·il·la·ry [ˌ-ˈæksɪleri:] *adj* periaxillär, zirkumaxillär.
per·i·ax·on·al cleft [ˌ-ˈæksənl] Periaxonalspalt *m*.

per·i·blast [ˈperɪblæst] *n* Periblast *m*.
per·i·bron·chi·al [ˌ-ˈbrɑŋkɪəl] *adj* um einen Bronchus herum (liegend), peribronchial.
per·i·bron·chi·o·lar [ˌ-ˌbrɑŋkɪˈəʊlər] *adj* um eine Bronchiole herum (liegend), peribronchiolar, peribronchiolär.
per·i·bron·chi·ol·i·tis [ˌ-ˌbrɑŋkɪəʊˈlaɪtɪs] *n* Peribronchiolitis *f*.
per·i·bron·chi·tis [ˌ-brɑŋˈkaɪtɪs] *n* Peribronchitis *f*.
per·i·bul·bar [ˌ-ˈbʌlbər] *adj* um einen Bulbus herum (liegend), um den Augapfel herum (liegend), peribulbär, zirkumbulbär.
per·i·cal·lo·sal artery [ˌ-kæˈləʊsəl] Pars postcommunicalis a. cerebri anterioris, A. pericallosa.
per·i·can·a·lic·u·lar [ˌ-ˌkænəˈlɪkjələr] *adj* perikanalikulär.
pericanalicular fibroadenoma *gyn.* kanalikuläres/kanalikulär-wachsendes Fibroadenom *nt* der Brust, Fibroadenoma pericanaliculare.
per·i·cap·il·la·ry [ˌ-kəˈpɪləri, -ˈkæpəˌleri:] *adj* um eine Kapillare herum (liegend), perikapillär.
pericapillary cell → pericyte.
pericapillary coloboma perikapilläres Kolobom *nt*.
per·i·cap·su·lar [ˌ-ˈkæpsələr] *adj* um eine Kapsel herum (liegend), perikapsulär.
per·i·car·dec·to·my [ˌ-kɑːrˈdektəmɪ] *n* → pericardiectomy.
per·i·car·di·ac [ˌ-ˈkɑːrdɪæk] *adj* → pericardial.
pericardiac arteries, posterior → pericardiac branches of thoracic aorta.
pericardiac branch: p. of phrenic nerve Herzbeutelast *m* des N. phrenicus, Ramus pericardiacus n. phrenici.
p.es of thoracic aorta Herzbeuteläste *pl* der Aorta thoracica, Rami pericardiaci aortae thoracicae.
pericardiac veins Perikardvenen *pl*, Vv. pericardiacae.
per·i·car·di·al [ˌ-ˈkɑːrdɪəl] *adj* **1.** Herzbeutel/Perikard betr., in der Umgebung des Herzens (liegend), perikardial, Perikard-. **2.** in der Umgebung des Magenmundes/der Kardia (liegend), perikardial.
pericardial adhesion Perikardverwachsung *f*.
pericardial carcinomatosis Herzbeutel-, Perikardkarzinose *f*.
pericardial cavity Perikardhöhle *f*, Cavitas pericardialis.
pericardial decompression Herzdekompression *f*.
pericardial disease Perikarderkrankung *f*.
pericardial effusion Perikarderguß *m*.
pericardial fremitus Perikardreiben *nt*.
pericardial friction sound → pericardial fremitus.
pericardial murmur *card.* Perikardreiben *nt*.
pericardial pleura Perikardpleura *f*, Pleura pericardiaca.
pericardial rub Perikardreiben *nt*.
pericardial sac → pericardium 1.
pericardial serum Perikardflüssigkeit *f*, Liquor pericardii.
pericardial tamponade *card.* Herz(beutel-), Perikardtamponade *f*.
pericardial villi Perikardzotten *pl*.
per·i·car·di·o·cen·te·sis [ˌ-ˌkɑːrdɪsənˈtiːsɪs] *n* → pericardiocentesis.
per·i·car·di·ec·to·my [ˌ-ˌkɑːrdɪˈektəmɪ] *n* HTG Herzbeutel-, Perikardexzision *f*, Perikardektomie *f*.
per·i·car·di·o·cen·te·sis [ˌ-ˌkɑːrdɪəʊsən-

ˈtiːsɪs] *n* Herzbeutel-, Perikardpunktion *f*.
per·i·car·di·co·phren·ic artery [ˌ-ˌkɑːrdɪkəʊˈfrenɪk] A. pericardiacophrenica.
pericardicophrenic veins Begleitvenen *pl* der A. pericardicophrenica, Vv. pericardicophrenicae.
per·i·car·di·ol·y·sis [ˌ-ˌkɑːrdɪˈɑləsɪs] *n* HTG Perikardiolyse *f*.
per·i·car·di·o·me·di·as·ti·ni·tis [ˌ-ˌkɑːrdəʊmɪdɪˌæstɪˈnaɪtɪs] *n* kombinierte Perikarditis *f* u. Mediastinitis, Perikardiomediastinitis *f*.
per·i·car·di·o·per·i·to·ne·al canal [ˌ-ˌkɑːrdɪəʊˌperɪtəʊˈniːəl] *embryo.* Pleuroperikardkanal *m*.
per·i·car·di·o·pleu·ral [ˌ-ˌkɑːrdɪəʊˈplʊərəl] *adj* Perikard u. Pleura betr., perikardiopleural.
pericardiopleural membrane → pleuropericardial membrane.
per·i·car·di·or·rha·phy [ˌ-ˌkɑːrdɪˈɔrəfɪ] *n* HTG Herzbeutel-, Perikardnaht *f*, Perikardiorrhaphie *f*.
per·i·car·di·os·to·my [ˌ-ˌkɑːrdɪˈɑstəmɪ] *n* HTG Herzbeutel-, Perikardfensterung *f*, Perikardiostomie *f*.
per·i·car·di·ot·o·my [ˌ-ˌkɑːrdɪˈɑtəmɪ] *n* HTG Herzbeutel-, Perikarderöffnung *f*, Perikardiotomie *f*.
per·i·car·dit·ic [ˌ-kɑːrˈdɪtɪk] *adj* Perikarditis betr., perikarditisch.
per·i·car·di·tis [ˌ-kɑːrˈdaɪtɪs] *n* Herzbeutelentzündung *f*, Perikardentzündung *f*, Perikarditis *f*, Pericarditis *f*.
per·i·car·di·um [ˌ-ˈkɑːrdɪəm] *n, pl* **-dia** [-dɪə] **1.** Herzbeutel *m*, Perikard *nt*, Pericardium *nt*. **2.** *bio.* perikardialer Sinus *m*, Perikardium *nt*.
per·i·car·dot·o·my [ˌ-kɑːrˈdɑtəmɪ] *n* → pericardiotomy.
per·i·car·y·on *n* → perikaryon.
per·i·ce·cal [ˌperɪˈsiːkəl] *adj* um das Zäkum herum (liegend), perizäkal, perizökal.
per·i·cel·lu·lar [ˌ-ˈseljələr] *adj* um eine Zelle herum (liegend), perizellulär.
per·i·ce·men·ti·tis [ˌ-ˌsɪmənˈtaɪtɪs] *n dent.* Perizementitis *f*, Pericementitis *f*.
per·i·ce·men·tum [ˌ-sɪˈmentəm] *n* Wurzelhaut *f*, Desmodont *nt*, Periodontium *nt*.
per·i·cen·tral [ˌ-ˈsentrəl] *adj* um ein Zentrum herum (liegend), perizentral.
pericentral scotoma *ophthal.* perizentrales Skotom *nt*.
per·i·chol·an·gi·o·lar abscess [ˌ-ˈkəʊlænˈdʒɪələr] pericholangiolärer Abszeß *m*.
per·i·cho·lan·gi·tis [ˌ-ˌkəʊlænˈdʒaɪtɪs] *n* Pericholangitis *f*.
per·i·cho·le·cys·tic abscess [ˌ-ˌkəʊləˈsɪstɪk, -ˌkal-] pericholezystischer Abszeß *m*.
per·i·cho·le·cys·ti·tis [ˌ-ˌkəʊləsɪsˈtaɪtɪs, -ˌkal-] *n* Pericholezystitis *f*.
per·i·chon·dral [ˌ-ˈkɑndrəl] *adj* **1.** Knorpelhaut/Perichondrium betr., perichondral. **2.** in Knorpelnähe (liegend), perichondral.
perichondral ossification perichondrale Verknöcherung/Knochenbildung/Ossifikation *f*.
per·i·chon·dri·al [ˌ-ˈkɑndrɪəl] *adj* → perichondral 1.
per·i·chon·dri·tis [ˌ-kɑnˈdraɪtɪs] *n ortho.* Perichondriumentzündung *f*, Perichondritis *f*.
per·i·chon·dri·um [ˌ-ˈkɑndrɪəm] *n* Knorpelhaut *f*, Perichondrium *nt*.
per·i·chon·dro·ma [ˌ-kɑnˈdrəʊmə] *n* Perichondrom(a) *nt*.
per·i·chord [ˈpɔːrd] *n embryo.* Chordascheide *f*, Perichord *nt*.
per·i·cho·ri·oi·dal [ˌ-kɔːrɪˈɔɪdl, kəʊr-] *adj* → perichoroidal.

perichoroidal

per·i·cho·roi·dal [ˌ-kəˈrɔɪdl] *adj* perichoroidal, perichorioidal.
perichoroidal space perichoroidaler Spaltraum *m*, Spatium perichoroideale.
per·i·claus·tral lamina [ˌ-ˈklɔːstrəl] Capsula extrema.
per·i·co·lic [ˌ-ˈkɑlɪk] *adj* um das Kolon herum (liegend), perikolisch.
per·i·co·li·tis [ˌ-kəˈlaɪtɪs] *n* Perikolitis *f*.
per·i·co·lon·i·tis [ˌ-ˌkɔʊləˈnaɪtɪs] *n* → pericolitis.
per·i·col·pi·tis [ˌ-kɑlˈpaɪtɪs] *n* → perivaginitis.
per·i·co·lum·nar inhibition [ˌ-kəˈlʌmnər] perikolumnare Hemmung *f*.
per·i·con·chal [ˌ-ˈkɑŋkəl] *adj* 1. periconchal. 2. → periauricular 2.
per·i·cor·ne·al [ˌ-ˈkɔːrnɪəl] *adj* um die Hornhaut herum (liegend), perikorneal, zirkumkorneal, Perikorneal-.
per·i·cor·o·nal [ˌ-kəˈrəʊnl, -ˈkɔːrənl] *adj* (*Zahn*) perikoronal.
per·i·cox·i·tis [ˌ-kɑkˈsaɪtɪs] *n* Perikoxitis *f*, -coxitis *f*.
per·i·cra·ni·al [ˌ-ˈkreɪnɪəl] *adj* Perikranium betr., perikranial.
per·i·cra·ni·tis [ˌ-kreɪˈnaɪtɪs] *n* Perikranitis *f*.
per·i·cra·ni·um [ˌ-ˈkreɪnɪəm] *n, pl* **-nia** [-nɪə] Periost *nt* der Schädelaußenfläche, Perikranium *nt*, Pericranium *nt*.
per·i·cy·a·zine [ˌ-ˈsaɪəziːn] *n pharm.* Periciazin *nt*.
per·i·cys·tec·to·my [ˌ-sɪsˈtektəmɪ] *n urol.*, *chir.* Perizystektomie *f*.
per·i·cys·tic [ˌ-ˈsɪstɪk] *adj* um eine Zyste herum (liegend), perizystisch.
per·i·cys·ti·tis [ˌ-sɪsˈtaɪtɪs] *n* Perizystitis *f*.
per·i·cyte [ˈ-saɪt] *n* Perizyt *m*, Adventitiazelle *f*.
per·i·cy·tial [ˌ-ˈsɪʃ(ɪ)əl, -ˈsɪtɪəl] *adj* → pericellular.
per·i·dec·to·my [ˌ-ˈdektəmɪ] *n ophthal.* Peridektomie *f*, Periektomie *f*, Peritomie *f*.
per·i·def·er·en·ti·tis [ˌ-ˌdefərənˈtaɪtɪs] *n* Perideferentitis *f*.
per·i·den·drit·ic [ˌ-denˈdrɪtɪk] *adj* peridendritisch.
per·i·den·tal [ˌ-ˈdentl] *adj* → periodontal 1.
peridental branches: p. of inferior alveolar artery Rami peridentales a. alveolaris inferioris.
p.es of infraorbital artery Rami peridentales a. infraorbitalis.
p.es of posterior superior alveolar artery Rami peridentales a. alveolaris superioris posterioris.
peridental membrane → periodontium 2.
per·i·den·ti·um [ˌ-ˈdentʃɪəm, -tɪəm] *n* → periodontium 1.
per·i·derm [ˈ-dɜrm] *n embryo.* Periderm *nt*, Epitrichium *nt*.
per·i·der·mal [ˌ-ˈdɜrməl] *adj* Periderm betr., perideramal.
per·i·der·mic [ˌ-ˈdɜrmɪk] *adj* → peridermal.
per·i·des·mic [ˌ-ˈdezmɪk] *adj* 1. Peridesmium betr. 2. → periligamentous.
per·i·des·mi·tis [ˌ-dezˈmaɪtɪs] *n* Peridesmitis *f*, Peridesmitis *f*.
per·i·des·mi·um [ˌ-ˈdezmɪəm] *n* Peridesmium *nt*.
per·i·di·as·to·le [ˌ-daɪˈæstəlɪ] *n* → prediastole.
per·i·di·as·tol·ic [ˌ-ˌdaɪəˈstɑlɪk] *adj* → prediastolic.
per·i·did·y·mis [ˌ-ˈdɪdəmɪs] *n* Perididymis *f*, Tunica vaginalis testis.
per·i·did·y·mi·tis [ˌ-ˌdɪdəˈmaɪtɪs] *n urol.* Perididymisentzündung *f*, Perididymitis *f*, Vaginitis testis.

pe·rid·i·um [pəˈrɪdɪəm] *n, pl* **-dia** [-dɪə] *micro.* Peridie *f*, Peridium *nt*.
per·i·di·ver·tic·u·li·tis [ˌperɪˌdaɪvərˌtɪkjəˈlaɪtɪs] *n* Peridivertikulitis *f*.
per·i·duc·tal [ˌ-ˈdʌktəl] *adj* um einen Gang/Ductus herum (liegend), periduktal.
periductal abscess (*Brust*) periduktaler Abszeß *m*.
periductal mastitis *gyn.* periduktale Brustdrüsenentzündung/Mastitis *f*.
per·i·duc·tile [ˌ-ˈdʌktaɪl] *adj* → periductal.
per·i·du·o·de·ni·tis [ˌ-ˌd(j)uːədɪˈnaɪtɪs] *n* Periduodenitis *f*.
per·i·du·ral [ˌ-ˈd(j)ʊərəl] *adj* in der Nähe der Dura mater, außerhalb der Dura mater, peridural, epidural, Peridural-, Epidural-.
peridural anesthesia Epidural-, Periduralanästhesie *f*, *inf.* Epidurale *f*, *inf.* Peridurale *f*.
per·i·en·ceph·a·li·tis [ˌ-enˌsefəˈlaɪtɪs] *n* Perienzephalitis *f*, -encephalitis *f*.
per·i·en·ter·ic [ˌ-enˈterɪk] *adj* um den Darm herum (liegend), perienteral, periintestinal, zirkumintestinal.
per·i·en·ter·i·tis [ˌ-ˌentəˈraɪtɪs] *n* Perienteritis *f*.
per·i·en·ter·on [ˌ-ˈentərɑn] *n embryo.* Perienteron *nt*.
per·i·ep·en·dy·mal [ˌ-əˈpendɪməl] *adj* periependymal.
per·i·ep·i·the·li·o·ma [ˌ-ˌepɪˌθɪlɪˈəʊmə] *n* Nebennierenrindenkarzinom *nt*, NNR-Karzinom *nt*.
per·i·e·soph·a·ge·al [ˌ-ɪˌsɑfəˈdʒiːəl] *adj* um die Speiseröhre herum (liegend), periösophageal.
per·i·e·soph·a·gi·tis [ˌ-ɪˌsɑfəˈdʒaɪtɪs] *n* Periösophagitis *f*.
per·i·fas·cic·u·lar [ˌ-fəˈsɪkjələr] *adj* um einen Faszikel herum (liegend), perifaszikulär.
per·i·fo·cal [ˌ-ˈfəʊkl] *adj* um einen Krankheitsherd/Fokus herum (liegend), perifokal.
per·i·fol·lic·u·lar [ˌ-fəˈlɪkjələr] *adj* um einen Follikel herum (liegend), perifollikulär.
per·i·fol·lic·u·li·tis [ˌ-fəˌlɪkjəˈlaɪtɪs] *n derm.* Perifollikulitis *f*, -folliculitis *f*.
per·i·fo·vea [ˌ-ˈfəʊvɪə] *n* Perifovea *f*.
per·i·gan·gli·on·ic [ˌ-ˌgæŋglɪˈɑnɪk] *adj* um ein Ganglion herum (liegend), periganglionär.
per·i·gas·tric [ˌ-ˈgæstrɪk] *adj* um den Magen herum (liegend), perigastrisch, -gastral, -ventral.
per·i·gas·tri·tis [ˌ-gæsˈtraɪtɪs] *n* Perigastritis *f*.
per·i·gem·mal [ˌ-ˈdʒeml] *adj* zirkum-, perigemmal.
per·i·glan·du·lar [ˌ-ˈglændʒələr] *adj* um eine Drüse herum (liegend), periglandulär.
per·i·glan·du·li·tis [ˌ-ˌglændʒəˈlaɪtɪs] *n* Periglandulitis *f*.
per·i·gli·al [ˌ-ˈglaɪəl] *adj* periglial.
per·i·glo·mer·u·lar cells [-gləʊˈmer(j)ələr, -glə-] periglomeruläre Zellen *pl*.
per·i·glos·si·tis [ˌ-gləˈsaɪtɪs] *n* Periglossitis *f*.
per·i·glot·tic [ˌ-ˈglɑtɪk] *adj* um die Zunge herum (liegend), periglottisch, -lingual.
per·i·glot·tis [ˌ-ˈglɑtɪs] *n* Zungenschleimhaut *f*, Periglottis *f*.
per·i·he·pat·ic [ˌ-hɪˈpætɪk] *adj* um die Leber herum (liegend), perihepatisch.
per·i·hep·a·ti·tis [ˌ-ˌhepəˈtaɪtɪs] *n* Entzündung *f* der Leberkapsel, Perihepatitis *f*.
per·i·her·ni·al [ˌ-ˈhɜrnɪəl] *adj chir.* um eine Hernie herum (liegend), perihernial.
per·i·hi·lar [ˌ-ˈhaɪlər] *adj* um einen Hilus herum (liegend), perihilär.
peri-insular *adj* periinsulär.

peri-islet *adj* (*Pankreas*) periinsulär.
per·i·je·ju·ni·tis [ˌ-ˌdʒɪdʒuːˈnaɪtɪs] *n* Perijejunitis *f*.
per·i·kar·y·on [ˌ-ˈkærɪˌɑn, -ən] *n, pl* **-kar·ya** [ˌ-ˈkærɪə] Zellkörper/-leib *m* der Nervenzelle, Perikaryon *nt*.
per·i·ke·rat·ic [ˌ-kəˈrætɪk] *adj* → pericorneal.
per·i·lab·y·rin·thi·tis [ˌ-ˌlæbərɪnˈθaɪtɪs] *n* HNO Perilabyrinthitis *f*.
per·i·la·ryn·ge·al [ˌ-ləˈrɪndʒ(ɪ)əl] *adj* um den Larynx herum (liegend), perilaryngeal.
per·i·lar·yn·gi·tis [ˌ-ˌlærɪnˈdʒaɪtɪs] *n* Perilaryngitis *f*.
per·i·len·tic·u·lar [ˌ-lenˈtɪkjələr] *adj ophthal.* um die Linse herum (liegend), zirkum-, perilental, zirkum-, perilentikulär.
per·i·lig·a·men·tous [ˌ-ˌlɪgəˈmentəs] *adj* um ein Band/Ligament herum (liegend), periligamentär.
per·i·lo·bar [ˌ-ˈləʊbər] *adj* um einen Lappen/Lobus herum (liegend), perilobär, -lobar.
per·i·lob·u·lar [ˌ-ˈlɑbjələr] *adj* um einen Lobulus herum (liegend), perilobulär, -lobular.
per·i·lob·u·li·tis [ˌ-ˌlɑbjəˈlaɪtɪs] *n* Perilobulitis *f*.
per·i·lu·nar dislocation [ˌ-ˈluːnər] *ortho.* perilunäre Luxation *f*.
per·i·lymph [ˈ-lɪmf] *n* Cotunnius'-Flüssigkeit *f*, Perilymphe *f*, Perilympha *f*, Liquor cotunnii.
per·i·lym·pha [ˌ-ˈlɪmfə] *n* → perilymph.
per·i·lymph·ad·e·ni·tis [ˌ-lɪmˌfædɪˈnaɪtɪs] *n* Perilymphadenitis *f*.
per·i·lym·phan·ge·al [ˌ-lɪmˈfændʒɪəl] *adj* → perilymphatic 2.
per·i·lym·phan·gi·tis [ˌ-ˌlɪmfænˈdʒaɪtɪs] *n* Perilymphangitis *f*.
per·i·lym·phat·ic [ˌ-lɪmˈfætɪk] *adj* 1. Perilymphe betr., perilymphatisch. 2. um ein Lymphgefäß herum (liegend), perilymphatisch.
perilymphatic duct Ductus perilymphaticus.
perilymphatic labyrinth → perilymphatic space.
perilymphatic space perilymphatischer Raum *m*, Spatium perilymphaticum.
per·i·mas·ti·tis [ˌ-mæsˈtaɪtɪs] *n gyn.* Perimastitis *f*.
per·i·ma·trix [ˌ-ˈmeɪtrɪks, -ˈmæ-] *n* Perimatrix *f*.
per·i·med·ul·lar·y [ˌ-ˈmedəˌlerɪ] *adj* perimedullär.
per·i·mem·bra·nous glomerulonephritis [ˌ-ˈmembrənəs] membranöse Glomerulonephritis *f*.
per·i·men·in·gi·tis [ˌ-ˌmenɪnˈdʒaɪtɪs] *n* → pachymeningitis.
pe·rim·e·ter [pəˈrɪmɪtər] *n* 1. *mathe.* Umfang *m*, Perimeter *m*. 2. *ophthal.* Perimeter *nt*.
per·i·met·ric [ˌperɪˈmetrɪk] *adj* 1. Perimeter betr., perimetrisch. 2. in der Umgebung des Uterus (liegend), Perimetrium betr., Perimetrium-.
per·i·me·tri·tis [ˌ-ˈmaɪtrɪtɪs] *n gyn.* Perimetriumentzündung *f*, Perimetritis *f*.
per·i·me·tri·um [ˌ-ˈmiːtrɪəm] *n, pl* **-tria** [-trɪə] Perimetrium *nt*, Tunica serosa uteri.
per·i·met·ro·sal·pin·gi·tis [ˌ-ˌmetrəʊˌsælpɪnˈdʒaɪtɪs] *n* Perimetrosalpingitis *f*.
pe·rim·e·try [pəˈrɪmɪtrɪ] *n ophthal.* Gesichtsfeldbestimmung *f*, Perimetrie *f*.
per·i·my·e·li·tis [ˌperɪˌmaɪəˈlaɪtɪs] *n* 1. *ortho.*

Endostentzündung f, Endostitis f. 2. Rückenmarkshautentzündung f, Meningitis spinalis.
per·i·my·o·car·di·tis [ˌɪ-ˌmaɪəkɑːrˈdaɪtɪs] n card. kombinierte Perikarditis f u. Myokarditis, Myoperikarditis f.
per·i·my·o·en·do·car·di·tis [ˌɪ-ˌmaɪəˌendəʊkɑːrˈdaɪtɪs] n card. Endoperimyokarditis f, Pankarditis f.
per·i·my·o·si·tis [ˌɪ-ˌmaɪəˈsaɪtɪs] n ortho. Perimyositis f.
per·i·my·si·al [ˌɪ-ˈmɪzɪəl] adj Perimysium betr., perimysial.
per·i·my·si·i·tis [ˌɪ-ˌmɪsɪˈaɪtɪs] n ortho. **1.** Perimysiumentzündung f, Perimys(i)itis f. **2.** → perimyositis.
per·i·my·si·tis [ˌɪ-mɪˈsaɪtɪs] n **1.** → perimysiitis 1. **2.** → perimyositis.
per·i·my·si·um [ˌɪ-ˈmɪːzɪəm, -ˈmɪːʒ-] n, pl **-sia** [-zɪə] Muskelhüllgewebe nt, Perimysium nt.
per·i·na·tal [ˌɪ-ˈneɪtl] adj um die Zeit der Geburt herum, perinatal, Perinatal-.
perinatal death perinataler Tod m, Tod m in der Perinatalperiode.
perinatal infection perinatale Infektion f.
perinatal listeriose Neugeborenenlisteriose f, Granulomatosis infantiseptica.
perinatal mortality perinatale Sterblichkeit f, Sterblichkeit f in der Perinatalperiode.
perinatal period Perinatalperiode f.
per·i·na·tol·o·gist [ˌɪ-ˌneɪˈtɑlɪdʒɪst] n Perinatologe m, -login f.
per·i·na·tol·o·gy [ˌɪ-ˌneɪˈtɑlədʒɪ] n Perinatologie f.
per·i·ne·al [ˌɪ-ˈniːəl] adj Damm/Perineum betr., perineal, Damm-, Perineal-.
perineal artery Dammarterie f, Perinealis f, A. perinealis.
perineal body Sehnenplatte f des Damms, Centrum tendineum perinei.
perineal branches of posterior femoral cutaneous nerve Dammäste pl des N. cutaneus femoris posterior, Rami perineales n. cutanei femoris posterioris.
perineal fascia, superficial Fascia perinei superficialis.
perineal fistula Damm-, Beckenbodenfistel f, Fistula perinealis.
perineal flexure of rectum Perinealflexur f des Rektums, Flexura perinealis (recti).
perineal fossa Fossa ischio-analis.
perineal hernia Dammbruch m, Perineozele f, Hernia perinealis/ischiorectalis.
perineal hypospadias urol. perineale Hypospadie f.
perineal ligament: p. of Carcassone → transverse p.
transverse p. Lig. transversum perinei.
perineal membrane Membrana perinei.
perineal muscles Dammuskulatur f, -muskeln pl, Mm. perinei/perineales.
perineal nerves Dammnerven pl, Nn. perineales.
perineal pouch: deep p. Spatium perinei profundum.
superficial p. Spatium perinei superficiale.
perineal prostatectomy urol. perineale Prostatektomie f.
perineal raphe, (median) Perinealraphe f, -naht f, Raphe perinealis.
perineal region Damm m, Dammgegend f, -region f, Regio perinealis.
perineal space: deep p. Spatium perinei profundum.
superficial p. Spatium perinei superficiale.
perineal urethrotomy Urethrotomia externa.

per·i·ne·o·cele [ˌɪ-ˈniːəʊsiːl] n → perineal hernia.
per·i·ne·om·e·ter [ˌɪ-nɪˈɑmɪtər] n Perineometer nt.
per·i·ne·o·plas·ty [ˌɪ-ˈniːəplæstɪ] n gyn. Dammplastik f, Perineoplastik f.
per·i·ne·or·rha·phy [ˌɪ-nɪˈɔrəfɪ] n gyn. Dammnaht f, Perineorrhaphie f.
per·i·ne·o·scro·tal [ˌɪ-ˌniːəˈskrəʊtl] adj Damm/Perineum u. Skrotum betr., perineoskrotal.
per·i·ne·ot·o·my [ˌɪ-nɪˈɑtəmɪ] n chir., gyn. Perineotomie f.
per·i·ne·o·vag·i·nal [ˌɪ-niːəʊˈvædʒɪnl] adj Damm/Perineum u. Scheide/Vagina betr. od. verbindend, perineovaginal.
perineovaginal fistula Scheiden-Damm-Fistel f, perineovaginale Fistel f.
per·i·ne·o·vag·i·no·rec·tal [ˌɪ-niːəʊˌvædʒɪnəʊˈrektəl] adj perineovaginorektal.
per·i·ne·o·vul·var [ˌɪ-ˌniːəʊˈvʌlvər] adj Damm/Perineum u. Vulva betr., perineovulvar, -vulvär.
per·i·neph·ri·al [ˌɪ-ˈnefrɪəl] adj Perinephrium betr., um die Niere herum, perinephrial.
per·i·neph·ric [ˌɪ-ˈnefrɪk] adj **1.** → perinephrial. **2.** um die Niere herum (liegend), perinephral.
perinephric abscess perirenaler Abszeß m.
perinephric capsule 1. Capsula adiposa (renis). **2.** Capsula fibrosa renis.
perinephric fat Nierenfettkapsel f, perirenale Fettkapsel f, Capsula adiposa renis.
per·i·neph·rit·ic [ˌɪ-nɪˈfrɪtɪk] adj Perinephritis betr., perinephritisch.
per·i·neph·ri·tis [ˌɪ-nɪˈfraɪtɪs] n Perinephritis f.
per·i·neph·ri·um [ˌɪ-ˈnefrɪəm] n, pl **-ria** [-rɪə] Perinephrium nt.
per·i·ne·um [ˌɪ-ˈniːəm] n, pl **-nea** [-ˈniːə] Damm m, Perineum nt.
per·i·neu·ral [ˌɪ-ˈnjʊərəl, -ˈnʊ-] adj um einen Nerv herum (liegend), perineural, Perineural-.
perineural anesthesia → perineural block.
perineural block perineurale Leitungsanästhesie f, perineuraler Block m.
perineural sheath Perineuralscheide f.
per·i·neu·ri·al [ˌɪ-ˈnjʊərɪəl, -ˈnʊ-] adj **1.** Perineurium betr., perineur(i)al. **2.** → perineural.
perineurial cyst Perineuralzyste f.
per·i·neu·rit·ic [ˌɪ-njʊəˈrɪtɪk, -nʊ-] adj Perineuritis betr., perineuritisch.
per·i·neu·ri·tis [ˌɪ-njʊəˈraɪtɪs, -nʊ-] n Perineumentzündung f, Perineuritis f.
per·i·neu·ri·um [ˌɪ-ˈnjʊərɪəm, ˈnʊ-] n, pl **-ria** [-rɪə] Perineurium nt.
per·i·nod·u·lar emphysema [ˌɪ-ˈnɑdʒələr] perinoduläres Lungenemphysem nt.
per·i·nu·cle·ar [ˌɪ-ˈn(j)uːklɪər] adj um einen Kern/Nukleus herum (liegend), perinuklear, perinukleär.
perinuclear cataract perinukleäre Katarakt f.
perinuclear cistern perinukleäre Zisterne f, perinukleärer Spaltraum m, Cisterna caryothecae/nucleolemmae.
perinuclear space → perinuclear cistern.
per·i·oc·u·lar [ˈnɑdʒələrˈakjələr] adj um das Auge herum (liegend), zirkum-, periokular, zirkum-, periokulär.
periocular dermatitis periokuläre Dermatitis f.
pe·ri·od [ˈpɪərɪəd] n **1.** Periode f, Zyklus m; Zeitspanne f, -dauer f, -raum m. **for the ~ of** für die Dauer von. **2.** patho. (s. wiederholender) Schub m. **3.** Monats-, Regelblutung f, Menstruation f, Menses pl, Periode f. **4.** chem., mathe., phys. Periode f.

p. of exposure photo., radiol. Belichtungszeit f.
p. of isometric contraction card. isometrische Kontraktionsphase f, Phase f der isometrischen Anspannung.
p. of isometric relaxation card. Phase f der isometrischen Entspannung.
per·i·o·date [pəˈraɪədeɪt] n Perjodat nt, Periodat nt.
pe·ri·od·ic [1 ˌpɪərɪˈɑdɪk; 2 ˌpaɪərɪˈɑdɪk] adj **1.** periodisch, regelmäßig (wiederkehrend), phasenhaft (ablaufend), zyklisch; in Schüben verlaufend. **2.** chem. aus Perjodsäure bestehend od. abstammend, perjodsauer.
periodic acid Perjod-, Periodsäure f.
periodic acid-Schiff reaction abbr. **PAS** PAS-Reaktion f, PAS-Schiff-Reaktion f.
periodic acid-Schiff stain PAS-Färbung f.
periodic afterimage ophthal. periodisches Nachbild n.
pe·ri·od·i·cal [ˌpɪərɪˈɑdɪkl] adj → periodic 1.
periodical disease periodische Krankheit f, Krankheit/Erkrankung f mit Periodizität.
periodic breathing Cheyne-Stokes-Atmung f, periodische Atmung f.
periodic edema Quincke-Ödem nt, angioneurotisches Ödem nt.
periodic fever periodisches Fieber nt, Febris periodica.
pe·ri·o·dic·i·ty [ˌpɪərɪəˈdɪsətɪ] n **1.** regelmäßige Wiederkehr f, Periodizität f, Periodik f. **2.** chem. Stellung f eines Elements im periodischen System. **3.** phys. elektrische Frequenz f.
periodicity analysis biochem. Periodizitätsanalyse f.
periodic law Mendelejew-Regel f, Periodenregel f.
periodic neutropenia periodische/zyklische Leukozytopenie/Neutropenie f.
periodic paralysis: hyperkalemic p. Gamstorp-Syndrom nt, Adynamia episodica hereditaria.
hypokalemic p. familiäre paroxysmale hypokalämische Lähmung f.
normokalemic p. normokalämische periodische Lähmung f.
sodium-responsive p. → normokalemic p.
type I p. → hypokalemic p.
type II p. → hyperkalemic p.
type III p. → normokalemic p.
periodic parasite periodischer Parasit m.
periodic peritonitis → periodic polyserositis.
periodic polyserositis familiäres Mittelmeerfieber nt, familiäre rekurrente Polyserositis f.
periodic respiration Cheyne-Stokes-Atmung f, periodische Atmung f.
periodic system chem. Periodensystem nt (der Elemente).
periodic table chem. Atomtafel f; Periodensystem n der Elemente.
periodic vomiting periodisches/zyklisches/rekurrierendes Erbrechen nt.
per·i·o·don·tal [ˌperɪəʊˈdɑntl] adj **1.** um einen Zahn herum (liegend), peridental, periodontal. **2.** Wurzelhaut/Periodontium betr., periodontal.
periodontal ligament/membrane → periodontium 2.
per·i·o·don·ti·tis [ˌɪ-dɑnˈtaɪtɪs] n Periodontitis f, Parodontitis f.
per·i·o·don·ti·um [ˌɪ-ˈdɑnʃ(ɪ)əm] n, pl **-tia** [-ʃ(ɪ)ə] **1.** Zahnbett nt, -halteapparat m, Parodont nt, Parodontium nt. **2.** Wurzelhaut f, Desmodontium nt, Periodontium nt.

periodontosis

per·i·o·don·to·sis [ˌ-dɑnˈtəʊsɪs] *n* Parodontose *f*, Parodontose *f*.
per·i·om·phal·ic [ˌperɪəmˈfælɪk] *adj* um den Nabel herum (liegend), periumbilikal.
per·i·o·nych·ia [ˌ-əʊˈnɪkɪə] *n derm.* Nagelfalzentzündung *f*, Umlauf *m*, Paronychie *f*, Paronychia *f*.
per·i·o·nych·i·um [ˌ-əʊˈniːkɪəm] *n, pl* **-nych·ia** [-ˈniːkɪə] Nagelhaut *f*, Perionychium *nt*.
per·i·o·nyx·is [ˌ-əʊˈnɪksɪs] *n* → perionychia.
per·i·o·pho·ri·tis [ˌ-əʊəfəˈraɪtɪs] *n gyn.* Perioophoritis *f*.
per·i·o·oph·o·ro·sal·pin·gi·tis [ˌ-əʊˌɑfərəʊˌsælpɪnˈdʒaɪtɪs] *n gyn.* Perioophorosalpingitis *f*.
per·i·o·o·the·ci·tis [ˌ-əʊθɪˈsaɪtɪs] *n* → perioophoritis.
per·i·op·er·a·tive [ˌ-ˈɑp(ə)rətɪv] *adj* perioperativ.
perioperative risk perioperatives Risiko *nt*.
per·i·oph·thal·mia [ˌ-ɑfˈθælmɪə] *n* → periophthalmitis.
per·i·oph·thal·mic [ˌ-ɑfˈθælmɪk] *adj* → periocular.
per·i·oph·thal·mi·tis [ˌ-ɑfθælˈmaɪtɪs] *n ophthal.* Periophthalmitis *f*.
per·i·op·tom·e·try [ˌ-ɑpˈtɑmətrɪ] *n* → perimetry.
per·i·o·ral [ˌ-ˈɔːrəl, -ˈəʊrəl] *adj* um den Mund herum (liegend), perioral, zirkumoral.
perioral dermatitis perorale Dermatitis *f*, Rosazea-artige Dermatitis *f*, Stewardessen-Krankheit *f*, Dermatitis perioralis.
per·i·or·bit [ˌ-ˈɔːrbɪt] *n* → periorbita.
per·i·or·bi·ta [ˌ-ˈɔːrbɪtə] *n* Periorbita *f*, Orbitaperiost *nt*.
per·i·or·bit·al [ˌ-ˈɔːrbɪtl] *adj* um die Orbita herum (liegend), periorbital.
periorbital edema periorbitales Ödem *nt*.
periorbital membrane → periorbita.
per·i·or·bi·ti·tis [ˌ-ˌɔːrbəˈtaɪtɪs] *n ophthal.* Periorbititis *f*.
per·i·or·chi·tis [ˌ-ɔːrˈkaɪtɪs] *n urol.* Entzündung *f* der Hodenhüllen, Periorchitis *f*, *inf.* Vaginalitis *f*.
per·i·or·chi·um [ˌ-ˈɔːrkɪəm] *n* Periorchium *nt*, Lamina parietalis tunicae vaginalis testis.
per·i·ost [ˈperɪɑst] *n* → periosteum.
per·i·os·te·al [ˌperɪˈɑstɪəl] *adj* Knochenhaut/Periost betr., periostal, Periost-.
periosteal chondroma juxtakortikales/periostales/parossales Chondrom *nt*.
periosteal desmoid periostales Desmoid *nt*.
periosteal elevator *chir., ortho.* Periostelevatorium *nt*; Rasparatorium *nt*.
periosteal lining of alveolar socket → periodontium 2.
periosteal ossification periostale Verknöcherung/Knochenbildung/Ossifikation *f*.
periosteal osteosarcoma periostales Osteosarkom *nt*, perossales Sarkom *nt*, periostales (osteogenes) Sarkom *nt*.
periosteal sarcoma → periosteal osteosarcoma.
per·i·os·te·i·tis [ˌ-ˌɑstɪˈaɪtɪs] *n* → periostitis.
periosteo- *pref.* Knochenhaut-, Periost-.
per·i·os·te·o·de·ma [ˌ-ˌɑstɪəʊˈdiːmə] *n* → periosteoedema.
per·i·os·te·o·e·de·ma [ˌ-ˌɑstɪəʊɪˈdiːmə] *n* Periost-, Knochenhautödem *nt*.
per·i·os·te·o·ma [ˌ-ˌɑstɪˈəʊmə] *n* Periosteom *nt*.
per·i·os·te·o·med·ul·li·tis [ˌ-ˌɑstɪəʊmedə'laɪtɪs] *n* → periosteomyelitis.
per·i·os·te·o·my·e·li·tis [ˌ-ˌɑstɪəʊmaɪəˈlaɪtɪs] *n* Periosteomyelitis *f*, Panosteitis *f*, Panostitis *f*.
per·i·os·te·op·a·thy [ˌ-ɑstɪˈɑpəθɪ] *n* Periosterkrankung *f*, Periostopathie *f*.
per·i·os·te·o·phyte [ˌ-ˈɑstɪəfaɪt] *n* → periosteoma.
per·i·os·te·o·plas·tic amputation [ˌ-ˌɑstɪəʊˈplæstɪk] *chir., ortho.* Amputation *f* mit Periostlappendeckung.
per·i·os·te·o·sis [ˌ-ˌɑstɪˈəʊsɪs] *n* → periostosis.
per·i·os·te·o·tome [ˌ-ˈɑstɪətəʊm] *n* Periosteotom *nt*.
per·i·os·te·ot·o·my [ˌ-ˌɑstɪˈɑtəmɪ] *n chir., ortho.* Periosteotomie *f*.
per·i·os·te·ous [ˌ-ˈɑstɪəs] *adj* **1.** → periosteal. **2.** aus Periost bestehend od. entstehend, periostal.
per·i·os·te·um [ˌ-ˈɑstɪəm] *n, pl* **-tea** [-tɪə] (äußere) Knochenhaut *f*, Periost *nt*, Periosteum *nt*.
periosteum elevator *chir., ortho.* Periostelevatorium *nt*; Rasparatorium *nt*.
per·i·os·ti·tis [ˌ-ɑsˈtaɪtɪs] *n* Knochenhaut-, Periostentzündung *f*, Periostitis *f*.
per·i·os·to·ma [ˌ-ɑsˈtəʊmə] *n* → periosteoma.
per·i·os·to·med·ul·li·tis [ˌ-ˌɑstəʊˌmedəˈlaɪtɪs] *n* → periosteomyelitis.
per·i·os·to·sis [ˌ-ɑsˈtəʊsɪs] *n* Periostose *f*.
per·i·os·tos·te·i·tis [ˌ-ɑsˌtɑstɪˈaɪtɪs] *n* Knochen-Periost-Entzündung *f*, Osteoperiostitis *f*.
per·i·os·to·tome [ˌ-ˈɑstətəʊm] *n* → periosteotome.
per·i·os·tot·o·my [ˌ-ɑsˈtɑtəmɪ] *n* → periosteotomy.
per·i·o·tic [ˌ-ˈəʊtɪk] *adj* um das (Innen-) Ohr herum (liegend).
per·i·o·va·ri·tis [ˌperɪˌəʊvəˈraɪtɪs] *n gyn.* Perioophoritis *f*.
per·i·o·vu·lar [ˌ-ˈɑvjələr] *adj* um ein Ovum herum (liegend), periovulär.
per·i·pach·y·men·in·gi·tis [ˌ-ˌpækɪˌmenɪnˈdʒaɪtɪs] *n* Peripachymeningitis *f*.
per·i·pal(a)e·o·cor·tex [ˌ-ˌpeɪlɪəʊˈkɔːrteks, -ˌpælɪ-] *n* Peripalaeokortex *m*.
per·i·pan·cre·at·ic [ˌ-ˌpænkrɪˈætɪk, -ˌpæŋ-] *adj* um das Pankreas herum (liegend), peripankreatisch.
per·i·pan·cre·a·ti·tis [ˌ-ˌpænkrɪəˈtaɪtɪs, -ˌpæŋ-] *n* Peripankreatitis *f*.
per·i·pap·il·lar·y [ˌ-ˈpæpɪlərɪ] *adj* peripapillär.
peripapillary scotoma *ophthal.* peripapilläres Skotom *nt*.
per·i·par·tal [ˌ-ˈpɑːrtl] *adj* um die Geburt herum (auftretend), peripartal.
peripartal cardiomyopathy peripartale Kardiomyopathie/Myokardiopathie *f*.
peripartal myocardiopathy → peripartal cardiomyopathy.
per·i·par·tum [ˌ-ˈpɑːrtəm] *adj* → peripartal.
peripartum cardiomyopathy → peripartal cardiomyopathy.
peripartum myocardiopathy → peripartal cardiomyopathy.
per·i·pa·tel·lar [ˌ-pəˈtelər] *adj* um die Kniescheibe herum (liegend), peripatellär.
per·i·pha·ci·tis [ˌ-fəˈsaɪtɪs] *n ophthal.* Periphakitis *f*.
per·i·pha·ki·tis [ˌ-fəˈkaɪtɪs] *n* → periphacitis.
per·i·pha·ryn·ge·al [ˌ-fəˈrɪndʒ(ɪ)əl] *adj* um den Rachen/Pharynx herum (liegend), peripharyngeal.
peripharyngeal space peripharyngealer Raum *m*, Spatium peripharyngeum.
pe·riph·er·al [pəˈrɪfərəl] *adj* **1.** am Rand/an der Peripherie (liegend), peripher(isch); *phys., techn.* peripher(isch). **2.** *anat.* im äußeren (Körper-)Bereich (liegend), zur Körperoberfläche hin, peripher.
peripheral anesthesia *neuro.* periphere Sensibilitätsstörung/Anästhesie *f*.
peripheral aneurysm peripheres Aneurysma *nt*.
peripheral chondroma peripheres Chondrom *nt*, Ekchondrom *nt*.
peripheral cyanosis periphere Zyanose *f*.
peripheral fibroma *ortho.* peripheres verknöcherndes Fibrom *nt*.
peripheral giant cell epulis/granuloma Riesenzellepulis *f*, Epulis gigantocellularis.
peripheral glioma Schwannom *nt*, Neurinom *nt*, Neurilem(m)om *nt*.
peripheral iridectomy *ophthal.* periphere Iridektomie *f*.
peripheral lesion periphere Nervenschädigung *f*.
peripheral necrosis periphere Lebernekrose *f*.
peripheral nerve peripherer Nerv *m*.
peripheral nerve injury Verletzung/Schädigung *f* eines peripheren Nerven.
peripheral nervous system *abbr.* **PNS** peripheres Nervensystem *nt abbr.* PNS, Pars peripherica systematis nervosi, Systema nervosum periphericum.
peripheral neuralgia periphere Neuralgie *f*.
peripheral neuritis periphere Neuritis *f*.
peripheral neuropathy periphere Neuropathie *f*.
peripheral occlusive disease periphere (arterielle) Verschlußkrankheit *f*.
peripheral osteosarcoma → periosteal osteosarcoma.
peripheral paralysis periphere Lähmung *f*.
peripheral paraplegia periphere Paraplegie *f*.
peripheral resistance *physiol.* periphärer Widerstand *m*.
peripheral scotoma *ophthal.* peripheres Skotom *nt*.
peripheral tabes → pseudotabes.
peripheral vascular disease → peripheral occlusive disease.
peripheral vertigo Vestibularisschwindel *m*, Vertigo vestibularis.
peripheral vision indirektes/periphäres Sehen *nt*.
per·i·pher·ic [ˌperɪˈferɪk] *adj* → peripheral.
per·i·phle·bit·ic [ˌ-flɪˈbɪtɪk] *adj* Periphlebitis betr., periphlebitisch.
per·i·phle·bi·tis [ˌ-flɪˈbaɪtɪs] *n* Periphlebitis *f*.
pe·riph·er·y [pəˈrɪfərɪ] *n* Rand *m*, Randgebiet *nt*, Randzone *f*, Peripherie *f*.
per·i·pho·ria [ˌperɪˈfəʊrɪə] *n ophthal.* Zyklophorie *f*.
per·i·phre·ni·tis [ˌ-frɪˈnaɪtɪs] *n* Periphrenitis *f*.
per·i·plasm [ˈ-plæzəm] *n* Periplasma *nt*.
per·i·plas·mic [ˌ-ˈplæzmɪk] *adj* periplasmatisch.
periplasmic protein periplasmatisches Protein *nt*.
periplasmic space *bio.* periplasmatischer Raum *m*.
per·i·pleu·ral [ˌ-ˈplʊərəl] *adj* um die Pleura herum (liegend), peripleural.
per·i·pleu·rit·ic abscess [ˌ-plʊəˈrɪtɪk] peripleuritischer Abszeß *m*.
per·i·pleu·ri·tis [ˌ-plʊəˈraɪtɪs] *n* Peripleuritis *f*.
per·i·pneu·mo·nia [ˌ-n(j)uːˈməʊnɪə] *n* **1.** Pleuropneumonie *f*. **2.** Lungenentzündung *f*, Pneumonie *f*, Pneumonia *f*.

per·i·pneu·mo·ni·tis [ˌ-ˌn(j)uːməˈnaɪtɪs] *n* → peripneumonia.
per·i·po·lar cell [ˌ-ˈpəʊlər] (*Glomerulum*) peripolare Zelle *f*.
per·i·po·le·sis [ˌ-pəʊˈliːsɪs] *n* Peripolese *f*, Peripolesis *f*.
per·i·po·ri·tis [ˌ-pəˈraɪtɪs] *n* Periporitis *f*.
per·i·por·tal [ˌ-ˈpɔːrtl, -ˈpəʊr-] *adj* 1. im Bereich der Leberpforte (liegend), periportal. 2. um die Pfortader herum (liegend), periportal.
periportal carcinoma periportales Leberkarzinom *nt*.
periportal cirrhosis postnekrotische/ungeordnete/großknotige Leberzirrhose *f*.
per·i·proc·tic [ˌ-ˈpraktɪk] *adj* um den Anus/After herum (liegend), zirkum-, perianal.
per·i·proc·ti·tis [ˌ-prakˈtaɪtɪs] *n* Periproktitis *f*.
per·i·pros·tat·ic [ˌ-prasˈtætɪk] *adj* um die Prostata herum (liegend), periprostatisch.
per·i·pros·ta·ti·tis [ˌ-ˌprastəˈtaɪtɪs] *n* Periprostatitis *f*.
per·i·py·le·phle·bi·tis [ˌ-ˌpaɪləflɪˈbaɪtɪs] *n* Peripylephlebitis *f*.
per·i·py·lor·ic [ˌ-paɪˈlɔːrɪk] *adj* um den Pylorus herum (liegend), peripylorisch.
per·i·ra·dic·u·lar [ˌ-rəˈdɪkjələr] *adj* um eine Wurzel herum (liegend), periradikulär.
per·i·rec·tal [ˌ-ˈrektəl] *adj* um das Rektum herum (liegend), perirektal.
perirectal abscess perirektaler Abszeß *m*, Perirektalabszeß *m*.
perirectal fistula perirektale Fistel *f*, Perirektalfistel *f*.
per·i·rec·ti·tis [ˌ-rekˈtaɪtɪs] *n* → periproctitis.
per·i·re·nal [ˌ-ˈriːnl] *adj* um die Niere herum (liegend), perirenal.
perirenal fat Nierenfettkapsel *f*, perirenale Fettkapsel *f*, Capsula adiposa renis.
per·i·rhi·nal [ˌ-ˈraɪnl] *adj* um die Nase *od.* Nasenhöhle herum (liegend), perinasal.
per·i·sal·pin·gi·tis [ˌperɪˌsælpɪnˈdʒaɪtɪs] *n gyn.* Perisalpingitis *f*.
perisalpingo-ovaritis *n gyn.* Perisalpingoovaritis *f*.
per·i·sal·pinx [ˌ-ˈsælpɪŋks] *n* Perisalpinx *f*.
per·i·scaph·o·lu·nar dislocation [ˌ-ˌskæfəˈluːnər] *ortho.* periskapholunäre Luxation *f*.
per·i·scop·ic [ˌ-ˈskapɪk] *adj* periskopisch.
periscopic lens periskopisches Glas *nt*.
periscopic concave lens konvexokonkave Linse *f*, Konvexokonkavlinse *f*.
periscopic convex lens konkavokonvexe Linse *f*, Konkavokonvexlinse *f*.
per·i·sig·moi·di·tis [ˌ-ˌsɪgmɔɪˈdaɪtɪs] *n* Perisigmoiditis *f*.
per·i·si·nu·i·tis [ˌ-ˌsaɪnəˈwaɪtɪs] *n* → perisinusitis.
per·i·sin·u·ous abscess [ˌ-ˈsɪnjəwəs] perisinuöser Abszeß *m*.
per·i·si·nu·si·tis [ˌ-ˌsaɪnəˈsaɪtɪs] *n* Perisinusitis *f*.
per·i·si·nus·oi·dal space [ˌ-ˌsaɪnəˈsɔɪdl] (*Leber*) Disse'-Raum *m*, perisinusoidaler Raum *m*.
per·i·sper·ma·ti·tis [ˌ-ˌspɜrməˈtaɪtɪs] *n* Perispermatitis *f*.
per·i·splanch·nic [ˌ-ˈsplæŋknɪk] *adj* perivisceral.
per·i·splanch·ni·tis [ˌ-splæŋkˈnaɪtɪs] *n* Perisplanchnitis *f*.
per·i·splen·ic [ˌ-ˈsplɪnɪk, -ˈsplen-] *adj* um die Milz herum (liegend), perisplenisch, perilienal.
per·i·sple·ni·tis [ˌ-splɪˈnaɪtɪs] *n* Perisplenitis *f*.
per·i·spon·dyl·ic [ˌ-spanˈdɪlɪk] *adj* um einen Wirbel herum (liegend), perivertebral.
per·i·spon·dy·li·tis [ˌ-spandəˈlaɪtɪs] *n* Perispondylitis *f*.
per·i·stal·sis [ˌ-ˈstɔːlsɪs, -ˈstæl-, -ˈstɑːl-] *n, pl* -ses [-siːz] Peristaltik *f*.
per·i·stal·tic [ˌ-ˈstɔːltɪk, -ˈstæl-, -ˈstɑːl-] *adj* Peristaltik betr., peristaltisch.
peristaltic contractions peristaltische Kontraktionswellen *pl*.
peristaltic movement → peristalsis.
peristaltic rush 1. Holzknecht'-Massenbewegung *f*. 2. Widerstandsperistaltik *f*.
peristaltic unrest Hyperperistaltik *f*.
per·i·staph·y·line [ˌ-ˈstæfəliːn] *adj* um die Uvula herum (liegend), perivulär.
per·i·staph·y·li·tis [ˌ-ˌstæfəˈlaɪtɪs] *n* Peristaphylitis *f*.
pe·ris·ta·sis [pəˈrɪstəsɪs] *n* 1. *genet.* Peristase *f*, Peristasis *f*. 2. *patho.* peristatische Hyperämie *f*, Peristase *f*.
per·i·stat·ic hyperemia [ˌperɪˈstætɪk] *patho.* peristatische Hyperämie *f*, Peristase *f*.
per·i·ster·nal perichondritis [ˌ-ˌstɜrnl] Tietze-Syndrom *nt*.
pe·ris·to·le [pəˈrɪstəʊlɪ] *n* Peristole *f*.
per·i·stol·ic [ˌperɪˈstalɪk] *adj* Peristole betr., peristolisch.
per·i·sto·ma [pəˈrɪstəmə, perɪˈstəʊmə] *n* → peristome.
per·i·stom·al [ˌperɪˈstəʊməl] *adj chir.* um ein Stoma herum (liegend), peristomal.
peristomal hernia peristomale Hernie *f*.
peristomal stenosis *chir.* peristomale Stenose *f*.
per·i·sto·ma·tous [ˌ-ˈstəʊmətəs] *adj* 1. → peristomal. 2. → perioral.
per·i·stome [ˈ-stəʊm] *n bio.* Peristom *nt*, Peristomfeld *nt*, -scheibe *f*, Mundfeld *nt*, -scheibe *f*.
per·i·sto·mi·al [ˌ-ˈstəʊmɪəl] *adj bio.* Peristom betr., Peristom-.
per·i·stru·mi·tis [ˌ-struˈmaɪtɪs] *n* → perithyroiditis.
per·i·stru·mous [ˌ-ˈstruːməs] *adj* um eine Struma herum (liegend), peristrumal.
per·i·syn·o·vi·al [ˌ-sɪˈnəʊvɪəl] *adj* perisynovial.
per·i·sy·rin·gi·tis [ˌ-ˌsɪrɪnˈdʒaɪtɪs] *n* Perisyringitis *f*.
per·i·sys·to·le [ˌ-ˈsɪstəlɪ] *n* → presystole.
per·i·sys·tol·ic [ˌ-sɪsˈtalɪk] *adj* → presystolic.
per·i·tec·to·my [ˌperɪˈtektəmɪ] *n ophthal.* Peritektomie *f*, Periektomie *f*, Peritomie *f*.
per·i·ten·din·e·um [ˌ-tenˈdɪnɪəm] *n, pl* -nea [-nɪə] Sehnengleitgewebe *nt*, Peritendineum *nt*, Peritenonium *nt*.
per·i·ten·di·ni·tis [ˌ-ˌtendɪˈnaɪtɪs] *n ortho.* Sehnenscheidenentzündung *f*, Tendovaginitis *f*, Tendosynovitis *f*, Tenosynovitis *f*.
per·i·ten·di·nous [ˌ-ˈtendɪnəs] *adj* um eine Sehne herum (liegend), peritendinös.
per·i·ten·on [ˌ-ˈtenən] *n* → peritendineum.
per·i·ten·o·ni·tis [ˌ-ˌtenəˈnaɪtɪs] *n* → peritendinitis.
per·i·ten·on·ti·tis [ˌ-ˌtenənˈtaɪtɪs] *n* → peritendinitis.
per·i·the·ci·um [ˌ-ˈθiːsɪəm, -ʃɪəm] *n micro.* Perithezium *nt*, -thecium *nt*.
per·i·the·li·al cells [ˌ-ˈθiːlɪəl] Adventitialzellen *pl*, Makrophagen *pl* der Gefäßwand.
perithelial endothelioma Hämangioperizytom *nt*.
per·i·the·li·o·ma [ˌ-ˌθɪlɪˈəʊmə] *n* Peritheliom(a) *nt*.
per·i·the·li·um [ˌ-ˈθiːlɪəm] *n, pl* -lia [-lɪə] Perithelium *nt*.
per·i·tho·rac·ic [ˌ-θəˈræsɪk] *adj* um den Brustkorb/Thorax herum (liegend), perithorakal.
per·i·thy·re·oid·i·tis [ˌ-θaɪrɔɪˈdaɪtɪs] *n* → perithyroiditis.
per·i·thy·roid·i·tis [ˌ-ˌθaɪrɔɪˈdaɪtɪs] *n* Perithyr(e)oiditis *f*.
pe·rit·o·my [pəˈrɪtəmɪ] *n* 1. *urol.* Beschneidung *f*, Zirkumzision *f*. 2. → peritectomy.
peritone- *pref.* → peritoneo-.
per·i·to·ne·al [ˌperɪtəʊˈniːəl] *adj* Bauchfell/Peritoneum betr., aus Peritoneum bestehend, peritoneal, Bauchfell-, Peritoneal-.
peritoneal abscess Bauchfell-, Peritonealabszeß *m*.
peritoneal carcinomatosis Peritonealkarzinose *f*, Peritonitis carcinomatosa.
peritoneal carcinosis → peritoneal carcinomatosis.
peritoneal cavity Peritoneal-, Bauchfellhöhle *f*, Cavitas peritonealis.
greater p. → peritoneal cavity.
lesser p. Netzbeutel *m*, Bauchfelltasche *f*, Bursa omentalis.
peritoneal dialysis Peritonealdialyse *f*.
continuous ambulatory p. *abbr.* CAPD kontinuierliche ambulante Peritonealdialyse *f abbr.* CAPD.
peritoneal drainage *chir.* Peritonealdrainage *f*.
peritoneal dropsy Bauchwassersucht *f*, Aszites *m*.
peritoneal epithelium Peritoneal-/Keimepithel *nt* des Ovars, Epithelium germinale.
peritoneal fasciitis 1. Ormond-Syndrom *nt*, (idiopathische) retroperitoneale Fibrose *f*. 2. symptomatische retroperitoneale Fibrose *f*.
per·i·to·ne·al·gia [ˌperɪˌtəʊnəˈældʒ(ɪ)ə] *n* Bauchfell-, Peritonealschmerz(en *pl*) *m*.
peritoneal irritation Bauchfell-, Peritonealreizung *f*.
peritoneal lavage Peritoneallavage *f*, -spülung *f*.
peritoneal lining Peritonealüberzug *m*.
per·i·to·ne·al·ize [ˌperɪtəˈnɪəlaɪz] *vt chir.* mit Peritoneum bedecken *od.* abdecken.
peritoneal metastasis Bauchfell-, Peritonealmetastase *f*.
peritoneal pseudomyxoma Gallertbauch *m*, Pseudomyxoma peritonei.
peritoneal reflection peritoneale Umschlag(s)falte *f*.
peritoneal sepsis Peritonealsepsis *f*.
peritoneal tuberculosis Peritonealtuberkulose *f*, Peritonitis tuberculosa.
peritoneo- *pref.* Bauchfell-, Peritoneal-, Peritone(o)-.
per·i·to·ne·o·cen·te·sis [perɪtəˌnɪəsənˈtiːsɪs] *n* 1. Bauchhöhlenpunktion *f*, Zöliozentese *f*. 2. Peritoneozentese *f*.
per·i·to·ne·o·cly·sis [ˌperɪtənɪəˈklɪsɪs] *n* Bauchhöhlenspülung *f*, Abdominallavage *f*.
per·i·to·ne·op·a·thy [ˌperɪtənɪˈɑpəθɪ] *n* Bauchfellerkrankung *f*, Peritoneopathie *f*.
per·i·to·ne·o·per·i·car·di·al [perɪtəˌnɪəˌperɪˈkɑːrdɪəl] *adj* Peritoneum u. Perikard betr., peritoneoperikardial.
per·i·to·ne·o·per·i·ne·al fascia [perɪtəˌniːəʊˌperɪˈniːəl] Fascia peritoneoperinealis.
per·i·to·ne·o·pex·y [ˌperɪˈtəʊnɪəpeksɪ] *n chir., gyn.* Peritoneopexie *f*.
per·i·to·ne·o·plas·ty [ˈ-plæstɪ] *n chir.* Bauchfell-, Peritoneoplastik *f*.
per·i·to·ne·o·scope [ˈ-skəʊp] *n* Peritoneoskop *nt*.
per·i·to·ne·os·co·py [perɪˌtəʊnɪˈɑskəpɪ] *n* Peritoneoskopie *f*.

peritoneotomy

per·i·to·ne·ot·o·my [ˌ-'ɑtəmɪ] *n chir.* Peritoneotomie *f*.

per·i·to·ne·o·ve·nous shunt [perɪtəˌnɪə'viːnəs] peritoneovenöser Shunt *m*.

per·i·to·ne·um [ˌperɪtə'niːəm] *n, pl* **-neums, -nea** [-'niːə] Bauchfell *nt*, Peritoneum *nt*.

per·i·to·nism ['perɪtəʊnɪzəm] *n* **1.** *patho., chir.* Peritonismus *m*. **2.** *psychia.* Pseudoperitonitis *f*.

per·i·to·ni·tis [ˌperɪtə'naɪtɪs] *n* Bauchfellentzündung *f*, Peritonitis *f*.

per·i·to·ni·za·tion [ˌperɪtəʊnaɪ'zeɪʃn] *n chir.* Bauchfelldeckung *f*, Bauchfell-, Peritoneoplastik *f*.

per·i·to·nize ['perɪtənaɪz] *vt chir.* mit Bauchfell bedecken *od.* abdecken.

per·i·ton·sil·lar abscess [ˌperɪ'tɑn(t)sɪlər] Peritonsillarabszeß *m*.

per·i·ton·sil·li·tis [ˌ-ˌtɑn(t)sə'laɪtɪs] *n* Peritonsillitis *f*.

per·i·tra·che·al [ˌ-'treɪkɪəl] *adj* um die Trachea herum (liegend), peritracheal.

pe·rit·ri·chal [pə'rɪtrɪkl] *adj* → peritrichous.

pe·rit·ri·chate [pə'rɪtrɪkɪt, -keɪt] *adj* → peritrichous.

per·i·trich·ic [ˌperɪ'trɪkɪk] *adj* → peritrichous.

Per·i·trich·ia [ˌ-'trɪkɪə] *pl bio.* Peritrichia *pl*.

Per·i·trich·i·da [ˌ-'trɪkədə] *pl bio.* Peritrichida *pl*.

pe·rit·ri·chous [pə'rɪtrɪkəs] *adj micro., bio.* peritrich.

per·i·tro·chan·ter·ic [ˌperɪˌtrəʊkən'terɪk] *adj* um einen Trochanter herum (liegend), peritrochantär.

per·i·tu·ber·cu·lo·sis [ˌ-təˌbərkjə'ləʊsɪs] *n* Pseudotuberkulose *f*.

per·i·tu·bu·lar capillary [ˌ-'t(j)uːbjələr] peritubuläre Kapillare *f*.

peritubular contractile cells Myoidzellen *pl*.

per·i·typh·lic [ˌ-'tɪflɪk] *adj* um das Zäkum herum (liegend), perizäkal, -zökal.

per·i·typh·li·tis [ˌ-tɪf'laɪtɪs] *n* **1.** Perityphlitis *f*. **2.** Periappendizitis *f*.

per·i·um·bil·i·cal [ˌ-ʌm'bɪlɪkl] *adj* um den Nabel herum (liegend), periumbilikal.

periumbilical pain paraumbilikaler Schmerz *m*.

per·i·un·gual [ˌ-'ʌŋgwəl] *adj* um einen Nagel herum (liegend), periungual.

periungual fibroma Koenen-Tumor *m*, periunguales Fibrom *nt*.

per·i·u·re·ter·al [ˌ-jə'riːtərəl] *adj* um einen Ureter/Harnleiter herum (liegend), periureteral.

per·i·u·re·ter·ic [ˌ-jʊərə'terɪk] *adj* → periureteral.

per·i·u·re·ter·i·tis [ˌ-jəˌriːtə'raɪtɪs] *n urol.* Periureteritis *f*.

per·i·u·re·thral [ˌ-jə'riːθrəl] *adj* um die Harnröhre/Urethra herum (liegend), periurethral.

periurethral abscess periurethraler Abszeß *m*.

periurethral cellulitis → periurethral phlegmon.

periurethral phlegmon periurethrale Phlegmone *f*.

per·i·u·re·thri·tis [ˌ-jʊərə'θraɪtɪs] *n* Periurethritis *f*.

per·i·u·ter·ine [ˌ-'juːtərɪn, -raɪn] *adj* um die Gebärmutter herum (liegend), perimetral, -metrisch, periuterin.

per·i·vag·i·nal [ˌ-'vædʒənl] *adj* um die Scheide/Vagina herum (liegend), perivaginal.

per·i·vag·i·ni·tis [ˌ-ˌvædʒə'naɪtɪs] *n gyn.* Perivaginitis *f*, Perikolpitis *f*.

per·i·vas·cu·lar [ˌ-'væskjələr] *adj* um ein Gefäß herum (liegend), perivaskulär, perivasal.

perivascular edema perivaskuläres Ödem *nt*.

perivascular gliosis perivaskuläre Gliose *f*.

perivascular space Perivaskulärraum *m*.

per·i·vas·cu·li·tis [ˌ-ˌvæskjə'laɪtɪs] *n* Perivaskulitis *f*, -vasculitis *f*.

peri-Vaterian diverticulum periampulläres Duodenaldivertikel *nt*.

per·i·ve·nous [ˌ-'viːnəs] *adj* um eine Vene herum (liegend), perivenös.

per·i·ven·tric·u·lar [ˌ-ven'trɪkjələr] *adj* um einen Ventrikel herum (liegend), periventrikular.

periventricular fibers periventrikuläre Fasern *pl*, Fibrae periventriculares.

periventricular nucleus, posterior Nc. periventricularis posterior.

per·i·ver·te·bral [ˌ-'vɜːrtəbrəl] *adj* um einen Wirbel herum (liegend), perivertebral.

perivertebral abscess perivertebraler Abszeß *m*.

per·i·ves·i·cal [ˌ-'vesɪkl] *adj* um die (Harn-)Blase herum (liegend), perivesikal.

per·i·ve·sic·u·lar [ˌ-və'sɪkjələr] *adj* um die Bläschendrüse herum (liegend), perivesikulär.

per·i·ve·sic·u·li·tis [ˌ-vəˌsɪkjə'laɪtɪs] *n urol.* Perivesikulitis *f*.

per·i·vis·cer·al [ˌ-'vɪsərəl] *adj* periviszeral.

per·i·vis·cer·i·tis [ˌ-ˌvɪsə'raɪtɪs] *n* Perisplanchnitis *f*.

per·i·vi·tel·line [ˌ-vaɪ'telɪn, -liːn] *adj* perivitellin.

per·lèche [per'leʃ, pər-] *n* Perlèche *f*, Faulecken *pl*, Mundwinkelcheilitis *f*, -rhagaden *pl*, Cheilitis/Stomatitis angularis, Angulus infectiosus oris/candidamycetica.

Perlia ['perlɪə]: **nucleus of P.** Perlia'-Kern *m*.

Perls [pɜːrlz, perlz]: **P.' stain/test** Berliner--Blau-Reaktion *f*.

per·ma·nence ['pɜːrmənəns] *n* Dauerhaftigkeit *f*, Beständigkeit *f*, Permanenz *f*.

per·ma·nen·cy ['pɜːrmənənsɪ] *n* **1.** → permanence. **2.** etw. Dauerhaftes *od.* Bleibendes.

per·ma·nent ['pɜːrmənənt] *adj* (fort-)dauernd, anhaltend, dauerhaft, (be-)ständig, bleibend, permanent, Dauer-.

permanent address → permanent residence.

permanent callus *ortho.* Intermediärkallus *m*.

permanent carrier Dauerausscheider *m*.

permanent cartilage permanenter/nicht--verknöcherender Knorpel *m*.

permanent condition Dauerzustand *m*.

permanent deformation bleibende Verformung *f*.

permanent dentition bleibende/zweite Zähne *pl*, Dauergebiß *nt*, Dentes permanentes.

permanent effect Dauerwirkung *f*.

permanent hardness bleibende (Wasser-)Härte *f*.

permanent magnet *phys.* Permanentmagnet *m*.

permanent parasite stationärer Parasit *m*.

permanent residence fester Wohnsitz *m*.

permanent stricture permanente Striktur *f*.

permanent threshold shift *abbr.* **PTS** *HNO* permanente Schwellenabwanderung *f*, permanent threshold shift *abbr.* PTS.

permanent tooth bleibender Zahn *m*, Dauerzahn *m*, Dens permanens.

permanent white *chem.* Permanent-, Berylweiß *nt*.

per·man·ga·nate [pər'mæŋgəneɪt] *n* Permanganat *nt*.

per·man·gan·ic acid [ˌpɜːrmæn'gænɪk] Permangansäure *f*.

per·me·a·bil·i·ty [ˌpɜːrmɪə'bɪlətɪ] *n abbr.* **P** Durchlässigkeit *f*, Durchdringlichkeit *f*, Permeabilität *f abbr.* P.

permeability barrier Permeabilitätsbarriere *f*, -schranke *f*.

per·me·a·ble ['pɜːrmɪəbl] *adj* durchlässig, durchdringbar, permeabel (*to* für).

per·me·ance ['pɜːrmɪəns] *n* **1.** → permeation. **2.** *phys.* magnetischer Leitwert *m*.

per·me·ant ['pɜːrmɪənt] *adj* durchdringend.

per·me·ase ['pɜːrmɪeɪz] *n* Permease *f*, Permeasesystem *nt*.

per·me·ate ['pɜːrmɪeɪt] **I** *n* Permeat *nt*. **II** *vt* (hin-)durchdringen, permeieren, penetrieren. **III** *vi* (durch-)sickern (*through* durch); (ein-)dringen (*into* in); *s.* verbreiten (*among* unter).

per·me·a·tion [ˌpɜːrmɪ'eɪʃn] *n* Ein-, Durchdringen *nt*, Permeieren *nt*, Permeation *f*, Penetration *f*.

permeation analgesia/anesthesia Oberflächenanästhesie *f*.

per·mis·sive [pər'mɪsɪv] *adj* erlaubend, gewährend, permissiv; erlaubt, zulässig.

permissive conditions *micro.* permissive Bedingungen *f*.

per·mit·tiv·i·ty [ˌpɜːrmɪ'tɪvətɪ] *n* Dielektrizitätskonstante *f abbr.* D, Dielektrizitätszahl *f*.

perm·se·lec·tiv·i·ty [ˌpɜːrmˌsɪlek'tɪvətɪ] *n* Permselektivität *f*.

per·mu·ta·tion [ˌpɜːrmjuː'teɪʃn] *n* Austausch *m*, Umstellung *f*, Vertauschung *f*, Permutation *f*.

permutation theory Permutationstheorie *f*.

per·mute [pər'mjuːt] *vt* aus-, vertauschen, permutieren.

per·mut·ed [pər'mjuːtɪd] *adj* permutiert.

per·na ['pɜːrnə] *n* Perna *nt*, Perchlornaphthalin *nt*.

perna acne/disease Perna-Krankheit *f*, -Akne *f*, Perchlornaphthalinkrankheit *f*.

per·na·sal [pər'neɪzl] *adj* durch die Nase, pernasal.

per·ni·cious [pər'nɪʃəs] *adj patho.* gefährlich, schwer, bösartig, perniziös.

pernicious anemia perniziöse Anämie *f*, Biermer-Anämie *f*, Addison-Anämie *f*, Morbus Biermer *m*, Perniciosa *f*, Perniziosa *f*, Anaemia perniciosa, Vitamin B_{12}-Mangelanämie *f*.

juvenile p. juvenile perniziöse Anämie.

pernicious leukopenia Agranulozytose *f*, maligne/perniziöse Neutropenie *f*.

pernicious malaria Falciparum-Malaria *f*, Tropenfieber *nt*, Malaria tropica.

pernicious myopia *ophthal.* bösartige/maligne Myopie *f*.

per·nio ['pɜːrnɪəʊ] *n, pl* **per·ni·o·nes** [pɜːrnɪ'əʊniːz] Frostbeule *f*, Pernio *m*.

per·ni·o·sis [ˌpɜːrnɪ'əʊsɪs] *n* Frostbeulen *pl*, Pernionen *pl*, Perniones *pl*, Perniosis *f*.

pero- *pref.* Pero-.

pe·ro·bra·chi·us [ˌpɪərəʊ'breɪkɪəs] *n embryo.* Perobrachius *m*.

pe·ro·ceph·a·lus [ˌ-'sefələs] *n embryo.* Perozephalus *m*, -kephalus *m*, -cephalus *m*.

pe·ro·chi·rus [ˌ-'kaɪrəs] *n embryo.* Perochirus *m*.

pe·ro·cor·mus [ˌ-'kɔːrməs] *n* → perosomus.

pe·ro·dac·ty·lus [ˌ-'dæktɪləs] *n embryo.* Perodaktylus *m*.

pe·ro·dac·ty·ly [ˌ-'dæktəlɪ] *n embryo.* Stummelfingrigkeit *f*, Perodaktylie *f*.

pe·rom·e·ly [pəˈrɑməlɪ] *n* → peromelia.
pe·ro·me·lia [ˌpɪərəˈmiːlɪə] *n embryo.* Stummelgliedrigkeit *f*, Peromelie *f*.
pe·ro·me·lic [-ˈmelɪk] *adj* stummelgliedrig, peromel.
pe·rom·e·lus [pəˈrɑmələs] *n embryo.* Peromelus *m*.
per·o·ne [pərˈəʊnɪ] *n old* → fibula.
per·o·ne·al [ˌperəˈniːəl] *adj* Wadenbein od. Peronäusnerv betr., peronäal, Wadenbein-, Peronäus-.
peroneal artery Wadenbeinschlagader *f*, -arterie *f*, Fibularis *f*, A. fibularis.
peroneal atrophy Charcot-Marie-Krankheit *f*, -Syndrom *nt*, Charcot-Marie--Tooth-Hoffmann-Krankheit *f*, -Syndrom *nt*.
peroneal incisure of tibia Inc. fibularis tibiae.
peroneal muscle: long p. → peroneus longus (muscle).
short p. → peroneus brevis (muscle).
third p. → peroneus tertius (muscle).
peroneal nerve: common p. Fibularis/Peronäus *m* communis, N. fibularis/peron(a)eus communis.
deep p. Fibularis/Peronäus *m* profundus, N. fibularis/peron(a)eus profundus.
superficial p. Fibularis/Peronäus *m* superficialis, N. fibularis/peron(a)eus superficialis.
peroneal-nerve phenomenon → peroneal phenomenon.
peroneal node Lymphknoten *m* an der A. fibularis, Nodus fibularis.
peroneal notch of tibia Inc. fibularis tibiae.
peroneal paralysis Fibularis-, Peronäuslähmung *f*.
peroneal phenomenon Lust-Phänomen *nt*, Fibularisphänomen *nt*.
peroneal retinaculum Halteband *nt* der Peronäussehnen, Retinaculum mm. peron(a)eorum.
inferior p. Retinaculum mm. peron(a)eorum/fibularium inferius.
superior p. Retinaculum mm. peron(a)eorum/fibularium superius.
peroneal septum: anterior p. Septum intermusculare cruris anterius.
posterior p. Septum intermusculare cruris posterius.
peroneal trochlea (of calcaneus) Trochlea peron(a)ealis/fibularis calcanei.
peroneal veins Wadenbeinvenen *pl*, Vv. fibulares/peron(a)eae.
pe·ro·ne·o·tib·i·al [perəˌnɪəˈtɪbɪəl] *adj* Fibula u. Tibia betr., peroneotibial, tibiofibular.
pe·ro·ne·us accessorius (muscle) [ˌperəˈnɪəs] Peronäus *m* accessorius, M. peron(a)eus accessorius.
peroneus brevis (muscle) Peronäus *m* brevis, M. peron(a)eus/fibularis brevis.
peroneus longus (muscle) Peronäus *m* longus, M. peron(a)eus/fibularis longus.
peroneus quartus (muscle) Peronäus *m* quartus, M. peron(a)eus quartus.
peroneus tertius (muscle) Peronäus *m* tertius, M. peron(a)eus/fibularis tertius.
pe·ro·pus [ˈpɪərəʊpəs] *n embryo.* Peropus *m*.
per·o·ral [pərˈɔːrəl, -ˈrəʊr-] *adj* durch den Mund, durch die Mundhöhle, peroral, per os.
per os → peroral.
per·os·mic anhydride [pərˈɑzmɪk] Osmiumtetroxid *nt*.
pe·ro·so·mus [ˌpɪərəˈsəʊməs] *n embryo.* Perosomus *m*.
per·ox·i·dase [pərˈɑksɪdeɪz] *n* Peroxidase *f*.

peroxidase reaction Peroxidasreaktion *f*.
peroxidase stain *histol.* Peroxidasefärbung *f*.
Goodpasture's p. Peroxidasefärbung nach Goodpasture.
Graham's p. Peroxidasefärbung nach Graham.
peroxidase test Peroxidase-Test *m*.
per·ox·ide [pərˈɑksaɪd] *n* Peroxid *nt*.
per·ox·i·dize [pərˈɑksɪdaɪz] *vt, vi chem.* peroxidieren.
per·ox·i·some [pərˈɑksɪsəʊm] *n* Peroxisom *nt*, Microbody *m*.
peroxy- *pref. chem.* Peroxi-, Peroxy-.
per·ox·y·a·ce·tic acid [pəˌrɑksɪəˈsiːtɪk, -əˈset-] Peroxiessigsäure *f*.
per·pen·dic·u·lar [ˌpɜːrpənˈdɪkjələr] I *n* 1. Senkrechte *f*. **out of (the) ~** nicht senkrecht, schief. 2. aufrechte Haltung od. Stellung *f*. II *adj* 3. lot-, senkrecht, vertikal, perpendikular, perpendikulär (*to* zu). 4. aufrecht. 5. rechtwink(e)lig (*to* zu).
per·pen·dic·u·lar·i·ty [ˌpɜːrpənˌdɪkjəˈlærətɪ] *n* senkrechte Richtung od. Haltung *f*, Senkrechtstehen *nt*.
perpendicular lamina of ethmoid bone Lamina perpendicularis ossis ethmoidale.
perpendicular layer of ethmoid bone Lamina perpendicularis ossis ethmoidale.
perpendicular plate: p. of ethmoid bone Lamina perpendicularis ossis ethmoidale.
p. of palatine bone Lamina perpendicularis ossis palatini.
per·pet·u·al [pərˈpetʃəwəl] *adj* fort-, immerwährend, unaufhörlich, andauernd, beständig, ständig, perpetuell.
perpetual arrhythmia absolute Arrhythmie *f*, Arrhythmia absoluta/perpetua.
per·phen·a·zine [pərˈfenəziːn, -zɪn] *n pharm.* Perphenazin *nt*.
Perrin-Ferraton [pɛˈrɛ̃ fɛrɑˈtɔ̃]: **P.-F. disease** schnappende/schnellende Hüfte *f*, Coxa saltans.
per·se·cu·tion·al mania [ˌpɜːrsɪˈkjuːʃənl] *psychia.* persekutorischer Wahn *m*, Verfolgungswahn *m*.
per·se·cu·tion complex/mania [ˌ-ˈkuːʃn] *psychia.* persekutorischer Wahn *m*, Verfolgungswahn *m*.
per·se·cu·to·ry delusion [ˈ-kjuːtərɪ, -kjəˌtɔːrɪ] *psychia.* persekutorischer Wahn *m*, Verfolgungswahn *m*.
per·sev·er·ate [pərˈsevəreɪt] *vi psychia.* perseverieren, ständig wiederkehren.
per·sev·er·a·tion [pərˌsevəˈreɪʃn] *n psychia.* Perseveration *f*.
Persian relapsing fever [ˈpɜːrʒn, -ʃn] persisches Rückfallfieber *nt*.
Persian tick *micro.* Argas persicus.
per·sist [pərˈsɪst] *vi* 1. anhalten, fortdauern, fort-, weiterbestehen, persistieren 2. be-, verharren (*in* auf, bei); bleiben (*in* bei); bestehen (*in* auf).
per·sist·ence [pərˈsɪstəns] *n* → persistency.
per·sist·en·cy [pərˈsɪstənsɪ] *n* 1. Anhalten *nt*, Fortdauern *nt*, Fortbestehen *nt*. 2. Beharrlichkeit *f*, Hartnäckigkeit *f*, Beharren *nt* (*in* auf); Persistenz *f*; Ausdauer *f*.
p. of follicle *gyn.* Follikelpersistenz *f*.
per·sist·ent [pərˈsɪstənt] *adj* 1. anhaltend, dauernd. 2. beharrlich, hartnäckig, ausdauernd, persistierend. 3. *bio.* ausdauernd.
persistent acantholytic dermatosis *derm.* Morbus Grove *m*, transitorische akantholytische Dermatose *f*.
persistent cloaca *embryo., patho.* Cloaca congenitalis/persistens.
persistent hyperphenylalaninemia Hyperphenylalaninämie *f* Typ II, persistierende Hyperphenylalaninämie *f*.
p. and tyrosinemia Hyperphenylalaninämie *f* Typ VI, persistierende Hyperphenylalaninämie *f* mit Tyrosinämie.
persistent infection persistierende Infektion *f*.
persistent nystagmus persistierender Nystagmus *m*.
persistent pain anhaltender Schmerz *m*, Dauerschmerz *m*.
persistent thymus persistierender Thymus *m*, Thymuspersistenz *f*.
persistent tremor kontinuierlicher Tremor *m*.
per·sis·ter [pərˈsɪstər] *n pharm., micro.* Persister *m*.
per·son [ˈpɜːrsn] *n* 1. Person *f*, Mensch *m*. 2. **~s** *pl* Körper *m*, Äußere(s) *nt*. **in ~** persönlich.
per·son·al [ˈpɜːrsnəl] *adj* 1. persönlich, Personen-, Personal-. 2. vertraulich, privat, persönlich. 3. äußere(r, s), körperlich.
personal audit *psycho.* Persönlichkeitstest *m*, -analyse *f*.
personal damage Körperverletzung *f*.
personal data Personalien *pl*.
personal hygiene Körperpflege *f*.
personal injury → personal damage.
per·son·al·i·ty [ˌpɜːrsəˈnælətɪ] *n* 1. Persönlichkeit *f*, Person *f*; Charakter *m*; persönliche Ausstrahlung *f*; Individualität *f*. 2. → personality disorder.
personality changes Wesens-, Persönlichkeitsveränderungen *pl*.
personality development *psycho.* Persönlichkeitsentwicklung *f*, -entfaltung *f*.
personality disorder Persönlichkeit(störung *f*) *f*, Psychopathie *f*, Charakterneurose *f*.
affective p. → cyclothymic p.
antisocial p. antisoziale Persönlichkeit(störung).
borderline p. Borderline-Persönlichkeit(störung).
cyclothymic p. *psychia.* zyklothymes Temperament *nt*, zyklothyme Persönlichkeit, Zyklothymie *f*.
cycloid p. → cyclothymic p.
histrionic p. hysterische/histrionische Persönlichkeit(störung).
narcissistic p. narzißtische Persönlichkeit(störung).
obsessive-compulsive p. zwanghafte/anankastische Persönlichkeit(störung), Zwangscharakter *m*.
paranoid p. paranoide Persönlichkeit(störung).
passive-aggressive p. passiv-aggressive Persönlichkeit(störung).
sadistic p. sadistische Persönlichkeit(störung).
schizoid p. schizoide Persönlichkeit(störung).
schizotypal p. schizotypische Persönlichkeit(störung).
personality inventory *psycho.* Persönlichkeitsfragebogen *m*.
personality structure *psycho.* Persönlichkeitsstruktur *f*.
personality test *psycho.* Persönlichkeitstest *m*.
personality trait Persönlichkeitsmerkmal *nt*.
personality type *psycho.* Persönlichkeitstyp *m*.
personal life Privatleben *nt*.
personal status Familien-, Personenstand *m*.
per·spec·tive [pərˈspektɪv] I *n* (*a. mathe., fig.*) Perspektive *f*; (*a. fig.*) Aussicht *f*, Ausblick *m*. II *adj* perspektivisch.

perspective formula *chem.* perspektivische Formel *f*.
per·spi·ra·tion [ˌpɜrspəˈreɪʃn] *n* **1.** Hautatmung *f*, Perspiration *f*, Perspiratio *f*. **2.** Schwitzen *nt*, funktionelle Schweißsekretion *f*. **3.** Schweiß *m*, Sudor *m*.
per·spir·a·to·ry [pərˈspaɪrətɔːrɪ, -təʊ-, ˈpɜrspə-] *adj* **1.** Perspiration betr., perspiratorisch. **2.** Schweiß *od.* Schwitzen betr., Schwitzen anregend *od.* verursachend.
per·spire [pərˈspaɪər] *vi* schwitzen, perspirieren, transpirieren.
per·sua·sion [pərˈsweɪʒn] *n psychia.* Persuasion *f*.
per·sul·fate [pərˈsʌlfeɪt] *n* Persulfat *nt*.
per·sul·fide [pərˈsʌlfaɪd, -fɪd] *n* Persulfid *nt*.
per·sul·fu·ric acid [ˌpɜrsʌlˈfjʊərɪk] Peroxyschwefelsäure *f*.
Perthes [ˈpɜrtiːz]: **P.' disease** Perthes-Krankheit *f*, Morbus Perthes *m*, Perthes-Legg-Calvé-Krankheit *f*, Legg-Calvé-Perthes(-Waldenström)-Krankheit *f*, Osteochondropathia deformans coxae juvenilis, Coxa plana (idiopathica).
P.' test Perthes-Versuch *m*.
per·troch·an·ter·ic fracture [pərˌtrəʊkənˈterɪk] pertrochantäre Oberschenkel-/Femurfraktur *f*.
per·tu·ba·tion [ˌpɜrtjuːˈbeɪʃn] *n gyn.* Pertubation *f*, Persufflation *f*, Tubenperflation *f*, Insufflation *f*.
per·tus·si·gen [pərˈtʌsɪdʒən] *n old* → pertussis toxin.
per·tus·sis [pərˈtʌsɪs] *n* Keuchhusten *m*, Pertussis *f*, Tussis convulsiva.
pertussis immune globulin Keuchhusten-Immunglobulin *nt*.
pertussis toxin Pertussistoxin *nt abbr.* PT.
pertussis vaccine Pertussisvakzine *f*, -impfstoff *m*, Keuchhustenvakzine *f*, -impfstoff *m*.
per·tus·soid [pərˈtʌsɔɪd] **I** *n* Pertussoid *m*. **II** *adj* keuchhusten-, pertussisartig, pertussoid.
Pe·ru·vi·an [pəˈruːvɪən]: **P. balsam** *pharm.* Perubalsam *m*, Balsamum peruvianum.
P. bark *pharm.* Chinarinde *f*.
P. wart Peruwarze *f*, Verruca peruana.
per·vade [pərˈveɪd] *vt* durchdringen, ziehen.
per·va·sion [pərˈveɪʒn] *n* Durchdringung *f*.
per·va·sive [pərˈveɪzɪv] *adj* durchdringend.
per·verse [pərˈvɜrs] *adj* **1.** verkehrt, falsch; verstockt, querköpfig. **2.** *psycho.* pervers.
per·verse·ness [pərˈvɜrsnɪs] *n* → perversity.
per·ver·sion [pərˈvɜrʒn, -ʃn] *n* **1.** *psycho.* (sexuelle) Perversion *f*. **2.** Verdrehung *f*, (Ver-)Fälschung *f*, Irreleitung *f*, Verzerrung *f*, Entstellung *f*, Pervertierung *f*.
per·ver·si·ty [pərˈvɜrsətɪ] *n* **1.** Verkehrtheit *f*, Verstocktheit *f*, Querköpfigkeit *f*. **2.** *psycho.* Perversität *f*.
per·vert [*n* ˈpɜrvərt; *v* pərˈvɜrt] **I** *n* perverser Mensch *m*. **II** *vt* verdrehen, (ver-)fälschen, verzerren, entstellen, pervertieren.
per·vi·gil·i·um [ˌpɜrvɪˈdʒɪlɪəm] *n* Schlaflosigkeit *f*, Pervigilium *nt*.
per·vi·ous [ˈpɜrvɪəs] *adj* **1.** (*a. tech., phys.*) durchlässig (*to* für); permeabel. **2.** *fig.* zugänglich (*to* für).
per·vi·ous·ness [ˈpɜrvɪəsnɪs] *n* Durchlässigkeit *f*; *fig.* Zugänglichkeit *f*, Empfänglichkeit *f* (*to* für).
pes [piːs, peɪs] *n*, *pl* **pe·des** [ˈpiːdiːz, ˈpediːz] *anat.* Fuß *m*, fußähnliche Struktur *f*, Pes *m*.
pes abductus *ortho.* **1.** Pes abductus. **2.** → pes valgus.

pes adductus *ortho.* Sichelfuß *m*, Pes adductus, Metatarsus varus.
pes anserinus *anat.* **1.** Pes anserinus. **2.** Plexus intraparotideus.
pes calcaneocavus *ortho.* Hackenhohlfuß *m*, Pes calcaneocavus.
pes calcaneus *ortho.* Hackenfuß *m*, Pes calcaneus.
acquired p. erworbener Hackenfuß.
congenital p. angeborener Hackenfuß, Pes calcaneus congenitus.
pes cavus *ortho.* Hohlfuß *m*, Pes cavus.
pes equinocavus *ortho.* Ballenhohlfuß *m*, Pes equinocavus.
pes equinovalgus *ortho.* Pes equinovalgus.
pes equinovarus *ortho.* Klumpfuß *m*, Pes equinovarus (excavatus et adductus).
pes equinus *ortho.* Spitzfuß *m*, Pes equinus.
pes hippocampi: (major) p. (eigentliches) Ammonshorn *nt*, Cornu Ammonis, Pes hippocampi.
minor p. Calcar avis.
pes metatarsus *ortho.* Spreizfuß *m*, Pes metatarsus.
pes planovalgus *ortho.* Knickplattfuß *m*, Pes planovalgus.
adolescent p. Adoleszentenknickplattfuß.
adult p. Knickplattfuß des Erwachsenen.
childhood p. kindlicher Knickplattfuß.
ligamental p. ligamentärer Knickplattfuß.
muscular p. muskulärer Knickplattfuß.
osseous p. ossärer Knickplattfuß.
pes planus *ortho.* Plattfuß *m*, Pes planus.
pes·sa·ry [ˈpesərɪ] *n*, *pl* **-ries** *gyn.* **1.** Pessar *nt*. **2.** Vaginalzäpfchen *nt*, -suppositorium *nt*.
pessary cell *hema.* (*Erythrozyt*) Ring-, Pessarform *f*.
pessary corpuscle → pessary cell.
pest [pest] *n* **1.** Pest *f*, Pestis *f*; *histor.* schwarzer Tod *m*. **2.** *fig.* Seuche *f*, Plage *f*.
pes·ti·ce·mia [ˌpestɪˈsiːmɪə] *n* Pestsepsis *f*, -septikämie *f*, septische/septikämische Pest *f*.
pes·ti·cid·al [ˌ-ˈsaɪdl] *adj* schädlingsbekämpfend, pestizid.
pes·ti·cide [ˈ-saɪd] *n* Schädlingsbekämpfungsmittel *nt*, Pestizid *nt*, Biozid *nt*.
pes·tif·er·ous [peˈstɪfərəs] *adj* → pestilential.
pes·ti·lence [ˈpestləns] *n* **1.** → pest. **2.** Seuche *f*, Plage *f*, Pest *f*, Pestilenz *f*.
pes·ti·lent [ˈpestlənt] *adj* → pestilential.
pes·ti·len·tial [ˌpestəˈlenʃl] *adj* **1.** pestbringend, verpestend, ansteckend. **2.** verderblich, schädlich.
pes·tis [ˈpestɪs] *n* → pest.
pes·tle [ˈpesl, ˈpestl] **I** *n* **1.** *chem.* Pistill *nt*. **2.** (*Mörser*) Stößel *m*. **II** *vt* zerstoßen, zerreiben, zermahlen.
pes valgus *ortho.* Knickfuß *m*, Pes valgus.
PET *abbr.* → positron-emission tomography.
pe·te·chia [pɪˈtiːkɪə, pɪˈtekɪə] *n*, *pl* **-te·chiae** [-ˈtiːkɪiː, -ˈtekɪiː] Punktblutung *f*, Petechie *f*.
pe·te·chi·al [pɪˈtiːkɪəl, -ˈtekɪəl] *adj* punkt-, fleckförmig, petechienartig, petechial.
petechial angioma petechiales/petechienartiges Angiom *nt*.
petechial bleeding → petechia.
petechial fever *old* → cerebrospinal meningitis.
petechial hemorrhage → petechia.
Peters [ˈpiːtərs]: **P.' anomaly** Peters-Anomalie *f*, -Syndrom *nt*.

peth·i·dine [ˈpeθədiːn] *n pharm., anes.* Pethidin *nt*.
pet·i·o·late [ˈpetɪəleɪt] *adj* gestielt.
pet·i·o·lat·ed [ˈpetɪəleɪtɪd] *adj* gestielt.
pet·i·ole [ˈpetɪəʊl] *n anat.* Stiel *m*, Petiolus *m*.
pet·i·oled [ˈpetɪəʊld] *adj* gestielt.
pe·ti·o·lus [pɪˈtaɪələs] *n* → petiole.
Petit [p(ə)ˈti]: **P.'s canal** Petit'-Kanal *m*, Spatia zonularia.
P.'s hernia Petit'-Hernie *f*.
P.'s law Dulong-Petit-Gesetz *nt*.
P.'s ligament Sakrouteralband *nt*, Lig. sacrouterinum.
P.'s sinus Aortensinus *m*, Sinus aortae.
P.'s triangle Lenden-, Lumbaldreieck *nt*, Petit'-Dreieck *nt*, Trigonum lumbale, Trigonum Petiti.
pet·it mal [ˈpetiː; p(ə)ˈti] → petit mal epilepsy.
petit mal attacks → petit mal epilepsy.
petit mal epilepsy Petit-mal(-Epilepsie *f*) *nt abbr.* PM.
petit mal seizures → petit mal epilepsy.
Petragnani [ˌpetra(g)ˈnɑːni]: **P. (culture) medium** Petragnani-Medium *nt*.
Petri [ˈpiːtrɪː; ˈpeːtrɪ]: **P. dish** Petrischale *f*.
P. plate Petri-Platte *f*.
pet·ri·fac·tion [ˌpetrəˈfækʃn] *n patho.* Petrifikation *f*.
pé·tris·sage [peɪtrɪˈsɑːʒ; petriˈsaːʒ] *n* Kneten *nt*, Knetmassage *f*, Pétrissage *f*.
pet·ro·bas·i·lar fissure [ˌpetrəʊˈbæsɪlər] → petro-occipital fissure.
pe·troc·cip·i·tal [pəˌtrɒkˈsɪpɪtl] *adj* → petro-occipital.
pet·ro·mas·toid [ˌpetrəʊˈmæstɔɪd] *adj* Felsenbein u. Warzenfortsatz betr., petromastoid.
petromastoid fissure Fissura tympanomastoidea.
petro-occipital *adj* Felsenbein u. Os occipitale betr., petrookzipital.
petro-occipital articulation Synchondrosis petro-occipitalis.
petro-occipital fissure Fissura petrooccipitalis.
petro-occipital joint Synchondrosis petro-occipitalis.
petro-occipital synchondrosis Synchondrosis petro-occipitalis.
pe·tro·sal [pɪˈtrəʊsl] *adj* Felsenbein betr., Felsenbein-.
petrosal bone → petrous pyramid.
petrosal branch of middle meningeal artery Felsenbeinast *m* der A. meningea media, Ramus petrosus a. meningeae mediae.
petrosal foramen → petrous foramen.
petrosal fossa/fossula Fossula petrosa.
petrosal ganglion (inferior) unteres Glossopharyngeusganglion *nt*, Ggl. caudalis/inferius n. glossopharyngei.
petrosal nerve N. petrosus.
deep p. N. petrosus profundus.
greater p. N. petrosus major.
lesser p. N. petrosus minor.
middle p. → lesser p.
superficial p. → lesser p.
petrosal part of internal carotid artery Felsenbeinabschnitt *m* der A. carotis interna, Pars petrosa a. carotidis internae.
pet·ro·sal·pin·go·staph·y·li·nus [ˌpetrəʊsælˌpɪŋgəʊˌstæfəˈlaɪnəs] *n* M. levator veli palatini.
petrosal sinus: inferior p. Sinus petrosus inferior.
superior p. Sinus petrosus superior.
petrosal vein Felsenbeinvene *f*, V. petrosa.
pet·ro·sec·to·my [ˌ-ˈsektəmɪ] *n HNO* Felsenbeinspitzenresektion *f*.

pet·ro·si·tis [ˌ-'saɪtɪs] *n HNO* Felsenbeinentzündung *f*, Petrositis *f*.
pet·ro·so·mas·toid [pəˌtrəʊsə'mæstɔɪd] *adj* → petromastoid.
pet·ro·sphe·noid [ˌpetrəʊ'sfiːnɔɪd] *adj* Felsenbein u. Keilbein betr., petrosphenoidal.
pet·ro·sphe·noi·dal syndrome [ˌ-sfiːˈnɔɪdl] petrosphenoidales Syndrom *nt*.
petrosphenoid fissure Fissura sphenopetrosa.
petrosphenoid ligament 1. Synchondrosis sphenopetrosa. **2.** Synchondrosis spheno-occipitalis.
pet·ro·squa·mo·sal [ˌ-skwə'məʊzl] *adj* Pars petrosa u. squamosa des Schläfenbeins betr.
petrosquamosal fissure Fissura petrosquamosa.
pet·ro·squa·mous [ˌ-'skweɪməs] *adj* → petrosquamosal.
petrosquamous fissure Fissura petrosquamosa.
pet·ro·staph·y·li·nus [ˌ-ˌstæfə'laɪnəs] *n* M. levator veli palatini.
pet·ro·tym·pan·ic [ˌ-tɪm'pænɪk] *adj* Felsenbein u. Paukenhöhle betr.
petrotympanic fissure Glaser'-Spalte *f*, Fissura petrotympanica.
pet·rous ['petrəs, 'piː-] *adj* **1.** felsig, (stein-)hart, steinig. **2.** → petrosal.
petrous bone → petrous pyramid.
petrous foramen For. petrosum.
petrous ganglion unteres Glossopharyngeusganglion *nt*, Ggl. caudalis/inferius n. glossopharyngei.
inferior p. → petrous ganglion.
pet·rous·i·tis [ˌpetrə'saɪtɪs] *n* → petrositis.
petrous part of temporal bone → petrous pyramid.
petrous pyramid Felsenbein(pyramide *f*) *nt*, Pyramis ossis temporalis, Pars petrosa ossis temporalis.
Pette-Döring ['pɛtə 'dœrɪŋ]: **P.-D. disease/panencephalitis** Enzephalitis Pette-Döring *f*, einheimische Panenzephalitis *f*.
Pettenkofer ['pɛtənkoːfər]: **P.'s test** von Pettenkofer-Reaktion *f*.
Peutz [pɔʏts]: **P.' syndrome** → Peutz-Jeghers syndrome.
Peutz-Jeghers ['dʒegərs]: **P.-J. intestinal polyposis** → P.-J. syndrome.
P.-J. syndrome Peutz-Jeghers-Syndrom *nt*, Polyposis intestini Peutz-Jeghers.
pex·ia ['peksɪə] *n* → pexis.
pex·ic ['peksɪk] *adj histol.*, *biochem.* einlagernd, fixierend.
pex·in ['peksɪn] *n* Chymosin *nt*, Rennin *nt*, Labferment *nt*.
pex·is ['peksɪs] *n* **1.** *chir.* Anheftung *f*, Fixierung *f*. **2.** *patho.*, *biochem.* Einlagerung *f*, Fixierung *f*.
Peyer ['paɪər]: **P.'s glands/insulae/patches/plaques** Peyer'-Plaques *pl*, Folliculi lymphatici aggregati.
pe·yo·te [peɪ'(j)əʊtɪ] *n* **1.** Peyotel-Kaktus *m*. **2.** Peyotel *nt*.
pe·yotl [peɪ'(j)əʊtl] *n* → peyote.
Peyronie [pɛrɔ'niː]: **P.'s disease** Peyronie-Krankheit *f*, Penisfibromatose *f*, Induratio penis plastica, Sclerosis fibrosa penis.
Pezzer [pe'zeː]: **P.'s catheter** Pezzer-Katheter *m*.
PF₁ *abbr.* → platelet factor 1.
PF₂ *abbr.* → platelet factor 2.
PF₃ *abbr.* → platelet factor 3.
PF₄ *abbr.* → platelet factor 4.
Pfannenstiel ['pfanənʃtiːl]: **P.'s incision** *gyn.* Pfannenstiel-Schnitt *m*.
Pfaundler-Hurler ['(p)fɔːndlər 'hərlər;

'pfaʊn-, 'huːr-]: **P.-H. syndrome** von Pfaundler-Hurler-Syndrom *nt*, -Krankheit *f*, Hurler-Syndrom *nt*, -Krankheit *f*, Dysostosis multiplex, Lipochondrodystrophie *f*, Mukopolysaccharidose I-H *f abbr.* MPS I-H.
PFC *abbr.* → plaque-forming cells.
Pfeiffer ['(p)faɪfər]: **P.'s bacillus** Pfeiffer'-(Influenza-)Bazillus *m*, Haemophilus influenzae, Bact. influenzae.
P.'s blood agar Pfeiffer'-(Blut-)Agar *m/nt*.
P.'s disease Pfeiffer'-Drüsenfieber *nt*, infektiöse Mononukleose *f*, Monozytenangina *f*, Mononucleosis infectiosa.
P.'s glandular fever → P.'s disease.
P.'s phenomenon Pfeiffer-Phänomen *nt*.
P.'s reaction Pfeiffer-Versuch *m*.
P.'s syndrome Pfeiffer-Syndrom *nt*, Akrosyndaktylie *f* Typ V.
P. type acrocephalosyndactyly Noack-Syndrom *nt*.
Pfeif·fer·el·la [(p)faɪfə'relə] *n micro.* Pfeifferella *f*.
PFK *abbr.* → (6-)phosphofructokinase.
Pflüger ['pflyːgər]: **P.'s cords** *old* Eileiter *pl*.
P.'s law Pflüger'-Zuckungsgesetz *nt*.
PFU *abbr.* → plaque-forming unit.
PG *abbr.* → prostaglandin.
pg *abbr.* → picogram.
PGD₂ *abbr.* → prostaglandin D₂.
PGE₁ *abbr.* → prostaglandin E₁.
PGE₂ *abbr.* → prostaglandin E₂.
PGF₂α *abbr.* → prostaglandin F₂α.
PGH₂ *abbr.* → prostaglandin H₂.
PGI₂ *abbr.* [prostaglandin I₂] → prostacyclin.
PGL *abbr.* → progressive generalized lymphadenopathy.
PGR *abbr.* → psychogalvanic response.
pH *abbr.* [pondus Hydrogenii] *chem.* pH (-Wert *m*) *m*.
PHA *abbr.* → phytohemagglutinin.
phac- *abbr.* → phaco-.
pha·ci·tis [fə'saɪtɪs] *n* → phakitis.
phaco- *pref.* Augenlinsen-, Linsen-, Phak(o)-, Phac(o)-.
phac·o·an·a·phy·lac·tic endophthalmitis [ˌfækəʊˌænəfɪ'læktɪk] *ophthal.* phakoantigene Uveitis *f*.
phac·o·an·ti·gen·ic uveitis [ˌ-ˌæntɪ'dʒenɪk] *ophthal.* phakoantigene Uveitis *f*.
phac·o·cele ['-siːl] *n ophthal.* Linsenvorfall *m*, Phakozele *f*, Hernia lentis.
phac·o·cyst ['-sɪst] *n* Linsenkapsel *f*, Capsula lentis.
phac·o·cys·tec·to·my [ˌ-sɪs'tektəmɪ] *n ophthal.* Linsenkapselresektion *f*, Phakozystektomie *f*.
phac·o·cys·ti·tis [ˌ-sɪs'taɪtɪs] *n ophthal.* Linsenkapselentzündung *f*, Phakozystitis *f*.
phac·o·e·mul·si·fi·ca·tion [ˌ-ˌmʌlsəfɪ'keɪʃn] *n ophthal.* Phakoemulsifikation *f*.
phac·o·er·y·sis [ˌ-'erəsɪs, -ə'riː-] *n ophthal.* Linsenextraktion *f*, Phakoeresis *f*.
phac·o·hy·me·ni·tis [ˌ-ˌhaɪmə'naɪtɪs] *n* → phacocystitis.
phac·oid ['fækɔɪd] *adj* linsenförmig, phakoid.
phac·oi·di·tis [ˌfækɔɪ'daɪtɪs] *n* → phakitis.
pha·coi·do·scope [fə'kɔɪdəskəʊp] *n* → phacoscope.
pha·col·y·sis [fə'kɒləsɪs] *n ophthal.* Linsenauflösung *f*, Phakolyse *f*.
phac·o·lyt·ic [ˌfækə'lɪtɪk] *adj* phakolytisch.
pha·co·ma [fə'kəʊmə] *n* → phakoma.
phac·o·ma·la·cia [ˌ-mə'leɪʃ(ɪ)ə] *n ophthal.* Linsenerweichung *f*, Phakomalazie *f*.
phac·o·ma·to·sis *n* → phakomatosis.
phac·o·met·a·cho·re·sis [ˌ-ˌmetəkɔː'riːsɪs] *n ophthal.* Linsenverlagerung *f*, -luxation *f*.

phac·o·met·e·ce·sis [ˌ-ˌmetə'siːsɪs] *n* → phacometachoresis.
phac·o·pla·ne·sis [ˌ-plə'niːsɪs] *n ophthal.* pathologische Mobilität *f* der Linse.
phac·o·scle·ro·sis [ˌ-sklɪ'rəʊsɪs] *n ophthal.* Linsenverhärtung *f*.
phac·o·scope ['-skəʊp] *n ophthal.* Phakoskop *nt*.
pha·cos·co·py [fæ'kɒskəpɪ] *n ophthal.* Phakoskopie *f*.
phac·o·sco·tas·mus [ˌfækəskəʊ'tæzməs] *n ophthal.* Linsentrübung *f*.
phac·o·tox·ic uveitis [ˌ-'tɒksɪk] *ophthal.* phakotoxische Uveitis *f*.
phag- *pref.* → phago-.
phage [feɪdʒ] *n* Bakteriophage *m*, Phage *m*, bakterienpathogenes Virus *nt*.
phage coat *micro.* Phagenhülle *f*.
phag·e·de·na [ˌfædʒə'diːnə] *n patho.*, *derm.* Phagedaena *f*.
phag·e·den·ic [ˌ-'denɪk] *adj* phagedänisch.
phagedenic balanitis Corbus'-Krankheit *f*, gangränöse Balanitis *f*, Balanitis gangraenosa.
phagedenic gingivitis → Plaut's angina.
phagedenic ulcer 1. Ulcus phagedaenicum. **2.** Tropen-, Wüstengeschwür *nt*, Ulcus tropicum.
phage infection *micro.* Phageninfektion *f*.
phage type → phagovar.
phage typing *micro.* Lysotypie *f*.
phago- *pref.* Freß-, Phage(n)-, Phag(o)-.
phag·o·cyt·able [ˌfægə'saɪtəbl] *adj* durch Phagozytose aufnehmbar *od.* abbaubar, phagozytierbar.
phag·o·cyte ['-saɪt] *n* Freßzelle *f*, Phagozyt *m*, Phagocyt *m*.
phag·o·cyt·ic [ˌ-'sɪtɪk] *adj* Phagozyt *od.* Phagozytose betr., phagozytär, phagozytisch, Phagozyt-.
phag·o·cyt·ize ['-sɪtaɪz] *vt* durch Phagozytose abbauen, durch/mittels Phagozytose aufnehmen, phagozytieren.
phag·o·cy·tol·y·sis [ˌ-saɪ'tɒləsɪs] *n* Phago(zyto)lyse *f*.
phag·o·cy·to·lyt·ic [ˌ-ˌsaɪtə'lɪtɪk] *adj* Phago(zyto)lyse betr., phago(zyto)lytisch.
phag·o·cy·tose ['-saɪtəʊz] *vt* → phagocytize.
phag·o·cy·to·sis [ˌ-saɪ'təʊsɪs] *n*, *pl* **-ses** [-siːz] Phagozytose *f*, Phagozyteinschluß *m*.
phagocytosis factor Phagozytosefaktor *m*.
phag·o·cy·tot·ic [ˌ-saɪ'tɒtɪk] *adj* Phagozytose betr., phagozytotisch.
phagocytotic vesicle Phagosom *m*.
pha·gol·y·sis [fə'gɒləsɪs] *n*, *pl* **-ses** [-siːz] Phago(zyto)lyse *f*.
phag·o·ly·so·some [ˌfægə'laɪsəsəʊm] *n* Phagolysosom *m*.
phag·o·lyt·ic [ˌ-'lɪtɪk] *adj* → phagocytolytic.
phag·o·ma·nia [ˌ-'meɪnɪə, -jə] *n psychia.* Phagomanie *f*.
phag·o·pho·bia [ˌ-'fəʊbɪə] *n psychia.* Phagophobie *f*.
phag·o·some ['-səʊm] *n* Phagosom *m*.
phag·o·type ['-taɪp] *n* → phagovar.
phag·o·var ['-vɑːr] *n micro.* Lysotyp *m*, Phagovar *m*.
phak- *pref.* → phaco-.
pha·ki·tis [fə'kaɪtɪs] *n ophthal.* Linsenentzündung *f*, Phakitis *f*, Phacitis *f*, Lentitis *f*.
phako- *pref.* → phaco-.
pha·ko·ma [fə'kəʊmə] *n derm.* Phakom(a) *nt*.
phak·o·ma·to·sis [ˌfækəmə'təʊsɪs, ˌfeɪ-] *n* Phakomatose *f*, neurokutanes Syndrom *nt*.
phalang- *pref.* → phalango-.
phal·ange ['fælændʒ, 'feɪ-, fə'lændʒ] *n*, *pl* **-lan·ges** [fəˈlændʒiːz, fæ-] → phalanx.

phalangeal

pha·lan·ge·al [fə'lændʒɪəl] *adj* Finger- *od.* Zehenglied betr., phalangeal.
phalangeal articulation (Finger-, Zehen-)Mittel-, Endgelenk *nt*, Interphalangealgelenk *nt*, Artic. interphalangealis/interphalangea.
phalangeal bones: p. of foot Zehenknochen *pl*, Ossa digitorum pedis.
p. of hand Fingerknochen *pl*, Ossa digitorum manus.
phalangeal cells Phalangenzellen *pl*.
outer p. Deiters'-Stützzellen *pl*.
phalangeal fracture Phalangenfraktur *f*.
phalangeal joint → phalangeal articulation.
phalangeal process (*Ohr*) Außenruder *nt*.
phal·an·gec·to·my [ˌfælən'dʒektəmɪ] *n ortho.* Phalangenexzision *f*, Phalangektomie *f*.
phal·an·gi·tis [ˌfælən'dʒaɪtɪs] *n* Phalangenentzündung *f*, Phalangitis *pl*.
phalango- *pref.* Phalangen-, Phalango-.
pha·lan·go·pha·lan·ge·al amputation [fəˌlæŋɡəʊfə'lændʒɪəl] *ortho.* Amputation *f* im Interphalangealgelenk.
pha·lanx ['feɪlæŋks, 'fæ-] *n, pl* **-lanx·es, -lan·ges** [fə'lændʒiːz, fæ-] Phalanx *f*, Finger-, Zehenglied *nt*.
phall- *pref.* → phallo-.
phal·lal·gia [fæ'læld(ɪ)ə] *n* → phallodynia.
phal·lec·to·my [fæ'lektəmɪ] *n* → penectomy.
phal·lic ['fælɪk] *adj* phallisch.
phallic phase → phallic stage.
phallic stage *psycho.* phallische Phase *f*.
phallic symbol *psycho.* Phallussymbol *nt*.
phal·li·form ['fælɪfɔːrm] *adj* → phalloid.
phal·li·tis [fæ'laɪtɪs] *n* Penisentzündung *f*, Phallitis *f*.
phallo- *pref.* Glied-, Penis-, Phallus-, Phall(o)-.
phal·lo·dyn·ia [ˌfælə'di:nɪə] *n* Penisschmerz *m*, Phallodynie *f*.
phal·loid ['fælɔɪd] *adj* phallusartig, -förmig, phallisch, phalloid.
phal·loi·din [fæ'lɔɪdn] *n* Phalloidin *nt*.
phal·loi·dine [fæ'lɔɪdiːn, -dɪn] *n* → phalloidin.
phal·lon·cus [fæ'lɑŋkəs] *n* Penisschwellung *f*, Penistumor *m*.
phal·lo·plas·ty ['fæləplæstɪ] *n* Penis-, Phalloplastik *f*.
phal·lor·rha·gia [ˌ-'reɪd(ɪ)ə] *n* Penis-, Phallusblutung *f*.
phal·lot·o·my [fæ'lɑtəmɪ] *n urol.* Phallotomie *f*.
phal·lo·tox·in [ˌfæləʊ'tɑksɪn] *n* Phallotoxin *nt*.
phal·lus ['fæləs] *n, pl* **-lus·es, -li** [-laɪ] (erigiertes) männliches Glied *nt*, Phallus *m*, Phallos *m*.
phan·er·o·ge·net·ic [ˌfænərəʊdʒɪ'netɪk] *adj* → phanerogenic.
phan·er·o·gen·ic [ˌ-'dʒenɪk] *adj* (*Krankheit*) mit bekannter Ursache; spezifisch.
phan·er·o·scope ['-skəʊp] *n* Phaneroskop *nt*.
phan·er·os·co·py [fænə'rɑskəpɪ] *n* Phaneroskopie *f*.
phan·er·o·sis [fænə'rəʊsɪs] *n* Phanerose *f*, Phanerosis *f*.
phan·tasm ['fæntæzəm] *n* Wahn-, Trugbild *nt*, Hirngespinst *nt*, Sinnestäuschung *f*, Phantasma *n*.
phan·tas·mal [fæn'tæzməl] *adj* 1. halluzinatorisch, Phantasie-. 2. unwirklich, trügerisch, imaginär.
phan·tas·mat·ic [ˌfæntæz'mætɪk] *adj* phantasmal.
phan·tas·mic [fæn'tæzmɪk] *adj* → phantasmal.

phan·tast ['fæntæst] *n* Träumer *m*, Phantast *m*.
phan·ta·sy ['fæntəsɪ] **I** *n* 1. Einbildung(skraft *f*) *f*, Vorstellungsvermögen *nt*, Phantasie *f*. 2. Phantasie *f*, Phantasievorstellung *f*, -gebilde *nt*; Hirngespinst *nt*, Trugbild *nt*. 3. Tag-, Wachtraum *m*. 4. Phantasieren *nt*. **II** *vt s.* jdn. *od.* etw. vorstellen. **III** *vi* 5. phantasieren (*about* von). 6. (tag-)träumen.
phan·tom ['fæntəm] **I** *n* 1. (anatomisches) Modell *nt*, Phantom *nt*. 2. Sinnestäuschung *f*, Schein-, Trugbild *nt*; Hirngespinst *nt*. **II** *adj* 3. eingebildet, scheinbar. 4. falsch, fiktiv.
phantom bone Gorham(-Staut)-Erkrankung *f*.
phantom corpuscle Halbmondkörper *m*, Achromozyt *m*, Achromoretikulozyt *m*.
phantom hand Phantomhand *f*.
phantom limb 1. Phantomglied *nt*. 2. → phantom limb pain.
phantom limb pain Amputationstäuschung *f*, Phantomschmerz(en *pl*) *m*, -empfinden *nt*.
phantom pregnancy *gyn.* Scheinschwangerschaft *f*, Pseudokyesis *f*, Pseudograviditat *f*.
phantom tumor *radiol.* Scheingeschwulst *f*, Phantomtumor *m*.
phar·a·on·ic circumcision [færeɪ'ɑnɪk] *gyn.* weibliche Beschneidung *f*, Klitoridektomie *f*, Klitorisektomie *f*.
phar·ma·cal ['fɑːrməkəl] *adj* → pharmaceutic.
phar·ma·ceu·tic [ˌfɑrmə'sjuːtɪk] *adj* arzneikundlich, pharmazeutisch.
phar·ma·ceu·ti·cal [ˌ-'suːtɪkl] **I** *n* Arzneimittel *nt*, Pharmazeutikum *nt*. **II** *adj* → pharmaceutic.
pharmaceutical chemistry pharmazeutische Chemie *f*.
phar·ma·ceu·tics [ˌ-'suːtɪks] *pl* Arzneikunde *f*, -lehre *f*, Pharmazeutik *f*, Pharmazie *f*.
phar·ma·ceu·tist [ˌ-'suːtɪst] *n* → pharmacist.
phar·ma·cist ['-sɪst] *n* 1. Pharmazeut(in *f*) *m*, Apotheker(in *f*) *m*. 2. pharmazeutischer Chemiker *m*.
pharmaco- *pref.* Arzneimittel-, Pharma-, Pharmako-.
phar·ma·co·chem·is·try [ˌfɑrməkəʊ'kemɪstrɪ] *n* pharmazeutische Chemie *f*.
phar·ma·co·di·ag·no·sis [ˌ-,daɪəɡ'nəʊsɪs] *n* Pharmakodiagnostik *f*.
phar·ma·co·dy·nam·ic [ˌ-,daɪ'næmɪk] *adj* Pharmakodynamik betr., pharmakodynamisch.
phar·ma·co·dy·nam·ics [ˌ-,daɪ'næmɪks] *pl* Pharmakodynamik *f*.
phar·ma·co·en·do·cri·nol·o·gy [ˌ-,endəʊkrɪ'nɑlədʒɪ] *n* Pharmakoendokrinologie *f*.
phar·ma·co·ge·net·ics [ˌ-dʒɪ'netɪks] *pl* Pharmakogenetik *f*.
phar·ma·cog·nos·tics [ˌfɑrməkɑɡ'nɑstɪks] *pl* → pharmacognosy.
phar·ma·cog·no·sy [ˌfɑrmə'kɑɡnəsɪ] *n* Drogenkunde *f*, Pharmakognosie *f*, Pharmakognosis *f*.
pharm·a·co·ki·net·ic [ˌfɑrməkəʊkɪ'netɪk] *adj* Pharmakokinetik betr., pharmakokinetisch.
phar·ma·co·ki·net·ics [ˌ-kɪ'netɪks] *pl* Pharmakokinetik *f*.
phar·ma·co·log·ic [ˌ-'lɑdʒɪk] *adj* → pharmacological.
phar·ma·co·log·i·cal [ˌ-'lɑdʒɪkl] *adj* pharmakologisch.
pharmacologic reversal pharmakologische Umkehr *f*.

phar·ma·col·o·gist [ˌfɑrmə'kɑlədʒɪst] *n* Pharmakologe *m*, -login *f*.
phar·ma·col·o·gy [ˌ-'kɑlədʒɪ] *n* Arzneimittellehre *f*, -forschung *f*, Pharmakologie *f*.
phar·ma·co·ma·ni·a [ˌfɑrməkəʊ'meɪnɪə, -jə] *n* Arzneimittelsucht *f*, Pharmakomanie *f*.
phar·ma·con ['fɑːrməkɑn] *n* Arzneistoff *m*, Arzneimittel *nt*, Wirkstoff *m*, Pharmakon *nt*.
phar·ma·co·peia [ˌfɑrməkə'peɪ(j)ə] *n* Arzneibuch *nt*, Pharmakopoe *f*.
phar·ma·co·pei·al [ˌ-'peɪ(j)əl] *adj* Pharmakopoe betr.
phar·ma·co·phil·ia [ˌ-'fɪlɪə] *n psychia., pharm.* Pharmakophilie *f*.
phar·ma·co·pho·bi·a [ˌ-'fəʊbɪə] *n* Pharmakophobie *f*.
phar·ma·co·phore ['-fəʊər, -fɔːr] *n* pharmakophore Gruppe *f*.
phar·ma·co·poeia *n* → pharmacopeia.
phar·ma·co·psy·cho·sis [ˌ-,saɪ'kəʊsɪs] *n* Pharmakopsychose *f*.
phar·ma·co·ra·di·og·ra·phy [ˌ-,reɪdɪ'ɑɡrəfɪ] *n* Pharmakoradiographie *f*.
phar·ma·co·roent·gen·og·ra·phy [ˌ-,rentɡə'nɑɡrəfɪ] *n* → pharmacoradiography.
phar·ma·co·ther·a·py [ˌ-'θerəpɪ] *n* Pharmakotherapie *f*.
phar·ma·cy ['fɑːrməsɪ] *n, pl* **-cies** 1. → pharmaceutics. 2. Apotheke *f*.
pharyng- *pref.* → pharyngo-.
pha·ryn·gal [fə'rɪŋɡl] *adj* → pharyngeal.
phar·yn·gal·gia [færɪn'ɡæld(ɪ)ə] *n* Rachen-, Pharynxschmerz *m*, Pharyngalgie *f*, Pharyngodynie *f*.
pha·ryn·ge·al [fə'rɪndʒ(ɪ)əl, færɪn'dʒiːəl] *adj* Rachen/Pharynx betr., pharyngeal, Schlund-, Rachen-, Pharynx-.
pharyngeal anesthesia Anästhesie *f* der Rachenschleimhaut.
pharyngeal aponeurosis → pharyngobasilar fascia.
pharyngeal arch *embryo.* Schlund-, Kiemen-, Pharyngialbogen *m*.
pharyngeal arch musculature branchiogene Muskulatur *f*, Kiemenbogenmuskulatur *f*.
pharyngeal artery, ascending Pharyngea *f* ascendens, A. pharyngea ascendens.
pharyngeal branch: p. of artery of pterygoid canal Ramus pharyngeus a. canalis pterygoidei.
p.es of ascending pharyngeal artery Rami pharyngei a. pharyngeae ascendentis.
p.es of glossopharyngeal nerve Pharynxäste *pl* des N. glossopharyngei, Rami pharyngeales/pharyngei n. glossopharyngei.
p.es of inferior thyroid artery Pharynxäste *pl* der A. thyroidea inferior, Rami pharyngeales a. thyroideae inferioris.
p. of pterygopalatine ganglion Pharynxast *m* des Ggl. pterygopalatinum, Ramus pharyngeus ggl. pterygopalatini.
p.es of superior thyroid artery Pharynxäste *pl* der A. thyroidea superior, Rami pharyngeales a. thyroideae superioris.
p.es of vagus nerve Pharynxäste *pl* des N. vagus, Rami pharyngeales/pharyngei n. vagi.
pharyngeal bursa Bursa pharyngealis.
pharyngeal bursitis Entzündung *f* der Bursa pharyngealis, Bursitis pharyngealis.
pharyngeal calculus → pharyngolith.
pharyngeal canal → palatovaginal canal.
pharyngeal cavity Schlund-, Rachenhöhle *f*, Cavitas pharyngis.
pharyngeal cleft Schlundfurche *f*, Kiemenspalte *f*.

pharyngeal crisis *neuro.* (tabische) Pharynxkrise *f.*
pharyngeal diphtheria Rachen-, Pharynxdiphtherie *f.*
pharyngeal edema Pharynxödem *nt.*
pharyngeal fistula Rachen-, Pharynxfistel *f.*
pharyngeal glands Rachen-, Pharynx(speichel)drüsen *pl*, Gll. pharyngis.
pharyngeal gut *embryo.* Schlunddarm *m.*
pharyngeal membrane → pharyngobasilar fascia.
pharyngeal muscles Schlundmuskeln *pl*, -muskulatur *f*, Pharynxmuskeln *pl*, -muskulatur *f.*
pharyngeal musculature → pharyngeal muscles.
pharyngeal nerve N. pharyngeus.
pharyngeal opening of auditory tube Rachenöffnung *f* der Ohrtrompete, Ostium pharyngeum tubae auditivae/auditoriae.
pharyngeal orifice of auditory tube → pharyngeal opening of auditory tube.
pharyngeal part of adenohypophysis → pharyngeal pituitary.
pharyngeal pituitary Pars pharyngea lobi anterioris hypophyseos.
pharyngeal plexus Venengeflecht *nt* des Pharynx, Plexus pharyngeus/pharyngealis.
  p. of vagus nerve Plexus pharyngealis n. vagi.
pharyngeal pouch *embryo.* Schlundtasche *f.*
pharyngeal pouch syndrome DiGeorge--Syndrom *nt*, Schlundtaschensyndrom *nt*, Thymusaplasie *f.*
pharyngeal raphe Raphe pharyngis.
pharyngeal recess Rosenmüller'-Grube *f*, Rec. pharyngeus (Rosenmülleri).
pharyngeal reflex 1. Würg(e)reflex *m.* 2. Schluckreflex *m.*
pharyngeal ridge Passavant'-(Ring-)-Wulst *m.*
pharyngeal tonsil Rachenmandel *f*, Tonsilla pharyngealis/adenoidea.
pharyngeal tubercle Tuberculum pharyngeum.
pharyngeal veins Pharynxvenen *pl*, Vv. pharyngeales.
pharyngeal wall Rachenwand *f.*
phar·yn·gec·ta·sia [ˌfærɪndʒek'teɪʒ(ɪ)ə] *n* → pharyngocele.
phar·yn·gec·to·my [færɪn'dʒektəmɪ] *n* HNO Pharyngektomie *f.*
phar·yn·gem·phrax·is [ˌfærɪndʒem'fræksɪs] *n* Pharynxobstruktion *f.*
phar·yn·gism ['færɪndʒɪzəm] *n* → pharyngismus.
phar·yn·gis·mus [ˌfærɪn'dʒɪzməs] *n* Schlundkrampf *m*, Pharyngismus *m*, Pharyngospasmus *m.*
phar·yn·git·ic [ˌ-'dʒɪtɪk] *adj* Pharyngitis betr., pharyngitisch.
phar·yn·gi·tis [ˌ-'dʒaɪtɪs] *n* Rachenschleimhautentzündung *f*, Pharyngitis *f.*
pharyngo- *pref.* Rachen-, Schlund-, Pharyng(o)-, Pharynx-.
pha·ryn·go·bas·i·lar aponeurosis [fəˌrɪŋgəʊ'bæsɪlər] → pharyngobasilar fascia.
pharyngobasilar coat → pharyngobasilar fascia.
pharyngobasilar fascia Fascia pharyngobasilaris.
pharyngobasilar membrane → pharyngobasilar fascia.
pha·ryn·go·cele ['-si:l] *n* Pharynxdivertikel *nt.*
pha·ryn·go·cer·a·to·sis [ˌ-ˌserə'təʊsɪs] *n* Pharynxkeratose *f.*
pha·ryn·go·con·junc·ti·val fever [ˌ-ˌkɑn-

dʒʌŋk'taɪvl] Pharyngokonjunktivalfieber *nt.*
pharyngoconjunctival fever virus *micro.* Adenovirus *nt* Typ 3.
pha·ryn·go·con·junc·ti·vi·tis [ˌ-kənˌdʒʌŋktə'vaɪtɪs] *n* Pharyngokonjunktivitis *f.*
pha·ryn·go·dyn·ia [ˌ-'di:nɪə] *n* → pharyngalgia.
pha·ryn·go·ep·i·glot·tic [ˌ-ˌepɪ'glɑtɪk] *adj* Rachen/Pharynx u. Kehldeckel/Epiglottis betr., pharyngoepiglottisch.
pharyngoepiglottic arch hinterer Gaumenbogen *m*, Arcus palatopharyngeus.
pharyngoepiglottic fold Plica glossoepiglottica lateralis.
pha·ryn·go·ep·i·glot·tid·e·an [ˌ-ˌepɪgla-'ti:dɪən] *adj* → pharyngoepiglottic.
pha·ryn·go·e·soph·a·ge·al [ˌ-ɪˌsɑfə'dʒi:əl, -ˌɪsə'fædʒɪəl] *adj* Rachen/Pharynx u. Speiseröhre/Oesophagus betr., pharyngoösophageal, ösophagopharyngeal.
pharyngoesophageal carcinoma pharyngoösophageales Karzinom *nt*, hohes Speiseröhrenkarzinom *nt.*
pharyngoesophageal diverticulum Zenker'-Divertikel *nt*, pharyngoösophageales Divertikel *nt.*
pharyngoesophageal junction pharyngoösophagealer Übergang *m*, pharyngoösophageale Übergangszone *f.*
pha·ryn·go·e·soph·a·go·plas·ty [ˌ-ɪ'sɑfəgəʊplæstɪ] *n chir.* Pharynx-Ösophagus--Plastik *f.*
pha·ryn·go·glos·sal [ˌ-'glɑsl, -'glɔs-] *adj* Rachen/Pharynx u. Zunge/Glossa betr., glossopharyngeal.
pha·ryn·go·glos·sus (muscle) [ˌ-'glɑsəs, -'glɔs-] → glossopharyngeus (muscle).
pha·ryn·go·ker·a·to·sis [ˌ-ˌkerə'təʊsɪs] *n* Pharynxkeratose *f.*
pha·ryn·go·la·ryn·ge·al [ˌ-ləˈrɪndʒɪəl, -ˌlærɪn'dʒi:əl] *adj* Rachen/Pharynx u. Kehlkopf/Larynx betr. *od.* verbindend, Laryngopharynx betr., pharyngolaryngeal, laryngopharyngeal.
pharyngolaryngeal cavity Hypo-, Laryngopharynx *m*, Pars laryngea pharyngis.
pha·ryn·go·lar·yn·gi·tis [ˌ-ˌlærɪn'dʒaɪtɪs] *n* Pharyngolaryngitis *f.*
pha·ryn·go·lith ['-lɪθ] *n patho.* Pharyngolith *m.*
pha·ryn·go·max·il·lar·y [ˌ-'mæksəˌlerɪ, -ˌmæk'sɪlərɪ] *adj* Rachen/Pharynx u. Oberkiefer/Maxilla betr. *od.* verbindend, pharyngomaxillär, -maxillar.
pha·ryn·go·my·co·sis [ˌ-maɪ'kəʊsɪs] *n* Rachen-, Pharynxmykose *f*, Pharyngomykose *f.*
pha·ryn·go·na·sal [ˌ-'neɪzl] *adj* Rachen/Pharynx u. Nase betr. *od.* verbindend, Nasopharynx betr., pharyngonasal, nasopharyngeal.
pharyngonasal cavity Nasenrachen(raum *m*) *m*, Epi-, Naso-, Rhinopharynx *m*, Pars nasalis pharyngis.
pha·ryn·go·oe·soph·a·ge·al *adj* → pharyngoesophageal.
pha·ryn·go·o·ral [ˌ-'ɔːrəl, -'əʊr-] *adj* Rachen/Pharynx u. Mund/Os betr. *od.* verbindend, Oropharynx betr., pharyngo--oral, oropharyngeal.
pharyngooral cavity Meso-, Oropharynx *m*, Pars oralis pharyngis.
pharyngooral isthmus Schlund-, Rachenenge *f*, Isthmus faucium.
pha·ryn·go·pal·a·tine [ˌ-'pælətaɪn, -tɪn] *adj* Rachen/Pharynx u. Gaumen/Palatinum betr. *od.* verbindend, pharyngopalatinal, palatopharyngeal.
pharyngopalatine arch hinterer Gaumenbogen *m*, Arcus palatopharyngeus.

pharyngopalatine muscle → palatopharyngeus (muscle).
pha·ryn·go·pa·ral·y·sis [ˌ-pə'rælǝsɪs] *n* Schlund(muskel)lähmung *f*, Pharyngoplegie *f.*
phar·yn·gop·a·thy [færɪn'gɑpəθɪ] *n* Rachen-, Pharynxerkrankung *f*, Pharyngopathie *f.*
pha·ryn·go·plas·ty [fəˈrɪŋgəʊplæstɪ] *n* Rachen-, Pharynx-, Pharyngoplastik *f.*
pha·ryn·go·ple·gia [ˌ-'pli:dʒ(ɪ)ə] *n* → pharyngoparalysis.
pha·ryn·go·rhi·ni·tis [ˌ-raɪ'naɪtɪs] *n* Pharyngorhinitis *f.*
pha·ryn·go·rhi·nos·co·py [ˌ-raɪ'nɑskəpɪ] *n* Pharyngorhinoskopie *f.*
pha·ryn·gor·rha·gia [ˌ-'reɪdʒ(ɪ)ə] *n* Rachen-, Pharynxblutung *f*, Pharyngorrhagie *f.*
pha·ryn·gor·rhea [ˌ-'rɪə] *n* Pharyngorrhoe *f.*
pha·ryn·go·sal·pin·gi·tis [ˌ-ˌsælpɪn'dʒaɪtɪs] *n* Pharyngosalpingitis *f.*
pha·ryn·go·scle·ro·ma [ˌ-sklɪ'rəʊmə] *n* Pharynx-, Pharyngosklerom *nt.*
pha·ryn·go·scope ['-skəʊp] *n* Pharyngoskop *nt.*
phar·yn·gos·co·py [færɪn'gɑskəpɪ] *n* Pharyngoskopie *f.*
pha·ryn·go·spasm [fə'rɪŋgəspæzəm] *n* → pharyngismus.
pha·ryn·go·ste·no·sis [ˌ-stɪ'nəʊsɪs] *n* Rachen-, Pharynx-, Pharyngostenose *f.*
phar·yn·gos·to·ma [færɪn'gɑstəmə] *n* HNO, *chir.* Pharyngostoma *nt.*
phar·yn·gos·to·my [færɪn'gɑstəmɪ] *n chir.*, HNO Pharyngostomie *f.*
pha·ryn·go·tome [fə'rɪŋgətəʊm] *n* Pharyngotom *nt.*
phar·yn·got·o·my [færɪn'gɑtəmɪ] *n* Pharyngotomie *f.*
pha·ryn·go·ton·sil·li·tis [fəˌrɪŋgəˌtɑnsə'laɪtɪs] *n* Pharyngotonsillitis *f.*
pha·ryn·go·tym·pan·ic cephalalgia [ˌ-tɪm-'pænɪk] Cephal(al)gia pharyngotympanica.
pharyngotympanic tube Ohrtrompete *f*, Eustach'Kanal *m*, -Röhre *f*, Tuba auditiva/auditoria.
pha·ryn·go·xe·ro·sis [ˌ-zɪ'rəʊsɪs] *n* pathologische Trockenheit *f* der Rachenschleimhaut.
phar·ynx ['færɪŋks] *n, pl* **phar·ynx·es**, **-ryn·ges** [fə'rɪndʒi:z] Rachen *m*, Schlund *m*, Pharynx *m.*
phase [feɪz] I *n* Phase *f*, Abschnitt *m*; (Entwicklungs-)Stufe *f*, Stadium *nt.* **out of ~** *electr.* phasenverschoben; *fig.* unkoordiniert. **in ~** *electr.* phasengleich, in Phase; *fig.* koordiniert. II *vt* 1. schrittweise durchführen *od.* planen; aufeinander abstimmen, gleichschalten, synchronisieren. 2. *electr.* in Phase bringen.
  phase in I *vt* schrittweise einführen. II *vi* schrittweise eingeführt werden.
  phase out I *vt* auslaufen lassen. II *vi* schrittweise aufhören.
p. of decline *micro.* Absterbephase.
p.s of menstrual cycle Zyklusphasen *pl.*
p.s of mitosis Mitosephasen *pl.*
phase-contrast microscope → phase microscope.
phase-contrast microscopy Phasenkontrastverfahren *nt*, -bild *nt*, -mikroskopie *f.*
phase difference *phys.* Phasendifferenz *f.*
phase microscope Phasenkontrastmikroskop *nt.*
phase microscopy → phase-contrast microscopy.
phase rule *chem., phys.* (Gibb'-)Phasenregel *f.*

phase shift

phase shift *techn.* Phasenverschiebung *f.*
phase shifting → phase shift.
pha·sic ['feɪsɪk] *adj* phasisch, Phasen-.
phasic arrhythmia respiratorische Arrhythmie *f.*
phasic reflex phasischer Reflex *m.*
phasic response *physiol.* dynamische/phasische Antwort *f*, Differentialantwort *f.*
phas·ing ['feɪzɪŋ] *n* Gleichschaltung *f*, Synchronisierung *f.*
Ph[1] chromosome → Philadelphia chromosome.
P-H conduction time *card.* PH-Intervall *nt.*
PHC syndrome [premolar aplasia, hyperhidrosis, canities] Böök-Syndrom *nt*, PHC-Syndrom *nt.*
pH-dependence *n* pH-Abhängigkeit *f*, pH-Wert-Abhängigkeit *f.*
Phe *abbr.* → phenylalanine.
Phemister ['femɪstər]: **P. graft** Phemister-Span *m.*
P. onlay bone graft → P. graft.
P. operation *ortho.* Epiphyseodese *f* nach Phemister.
phen- *pref.* → pheno-.
phe·nac·e·mide [fɪ'næsəmaɪd] *n pharm.* Phenacemid *nt.*
phe·nac·e·tin [fɪn'æsətɪn] *n pharm.* Phenazetin *nt*, Phenacetin *nt.*
phenacetin kidney Analgetika-, Phenacetinniere *f.*
phe·nan·threne [fə'nænθriːn] *n* Phenanthren *nt.*
phe·nan·thro·lene [fə'nænθrəliːn] *n* o-Phenanthrolin *nt.*
phe·nate ['fiːneɪt] *n, vt* → phenolate.
phen·a·zone ['fenəzəʊn] *n pharm.* Phenazon *nt*, Phenyldimethylpyrazolon *nt.*
phen·az·o·pyr·i·dine [fen,æzəʊ'pɪrədiːn] *n pharm.* Phenazopyridin *nt.*
phen·eth·i·cil·lin [fen,eθə'sɪlɪn] *n pharm.* Pheneticillin *nt.*
phen·for·min [fen'fɔːrmɪn] *n pharm.* Phenformin *nt.*
phen·go·pho·bia [,fengəʊ'fəʊbɪə] *n* → photophobia.
phe·nic acid ['fiːnɪk, 'fen-] → phenol 1.
phen·i·din ['fenədɪn] *n old* → phenacetin.
phe·nin ['fiːnɪn] *n old* → phenacetin.
phe·nin·da·mine [fə'nɪndəmiːn] *n pharm.* Phenindamin *nt.*
phen·ir·a·mine [fen'ɪərəmiːn] *n pharm.* Pheniramin *nt.*
phen·met·ra·zine [fen'metrəziːn] *n pharm.* Phenmetrazin *nt.*
pheno- *pref.* **1.** Phen(o)-. **2.** Phän(o)-.
phe·no·bar·bi·tal [,fiːnəʊ'bɑːrbɪtɔl, -tæl] *n pharm.* Phenobarbital *nt.*
phe·no·bar·bi·tone [,-'bɑːrbɪtəʊn] *n* → phenobarbital.
phe·no·cop·y ['-kɑpɪ] *n* Phänokopie *f.*
phe·no·din ['-dɪn] *n* Hämatin *nt*, Oxyhämin *nt.*
phe·no·ge·net·ics [,-dʒɪ'netɪks] *pl* Phänogenetik *f.*
phe·nol ['fiːnɔl, -nɑl] *n* **1.** Phenol *nt*, Karbolsäure *f*, Monohydroxybenzol *nt.* **2.** ~s *pl* Phenole *pl.*
phe·no·lase ['fiːnəleɪz] *n* Phenoloxidase *f*, Phenolase *f.*
phe·no·late ['-leɪt] **I** *n* Phenolat *nt.* **II** *vt* mit Phenol behandeln *od.* sterilisieren.
phe·no·le·mia [,fiːnəʊ'liːmɪə] *n* Phenolämie *f.*
phenol glucuronoside Phenolglucuronosid *nt.*
phe·no·lic [fɪ'nəʊlɪk, -'nɑl-] *adj* Phenol betr. *od.* enthaltend, phenolisch, Phenol-.

phe·nol·i·za·tion [,fiːnəlaɪ'zeɪʃn] *n* Behandlung *f* mit Phenol, Phenolisieren *nt.*
phe·no·log·ic [fiːnə'lɑdʒɪk] *adj* Phänologie betr., phänologisch.
phe·nol·o·gy [fɪ'nɑlədʒɪ] *n* Phänologie *f.*
phe·nol·phthal·e·in [,fiːnɔl'(f)θæliːn, -liːɪn] *n* Phenolphthalein *nt.*
phenol poisoning Phenolvergiftung *f*, -intoxikation *f*, Karbolismus *m.*
phenol red → phenolsulfonephthalein.
phenol red medium Phenolrotmedium *nt.*
phenol sulfatase Arylsulfatase *f.*
phe·nol·sul·fone·phthal·ein [,-,sʌlfəʊn-'(f)θæliːn, -liːɪn] *n abbr.* **PSP** Phenolrot *nt*, Phenolsulfo(n)phthalein *nt abbr.* PSP.
phe·nol·u·ria [,-(j)ʊərɪə] *n* Phenolausscheidung *f* im Harn, Phenolurie *f.*
phe·nom·e·no·log·ic [fɪ,nɑmənə'lɑdʒɪk] *adj* Phänomenologie betr., zu Phänomenologie gehörend, phänomenologisch.
phe·nom·e·no·log·i·cal [,-'lɑdʒɪkl] *adj* → phenomenologic.
phe·nom·e·nol·o·gy [fɪ,nɑmə'nɑlədʒɪ] *n* Phänomenologie *f.*
phe·nom·e·non [fɪ'nɑmə,nɑn, -nən] *n, pl* **-na** [nə] **1.** Erscheinung *f*, Zeichen *nt*, (objektives) Symptom *nt*, Phänomen *nt.* **2.** außergewöhnliches Ereignis *nt*, Vorkommnis *nt*, Phänomen *nt.*
phe·no·thi·a·zine [,fiːnə'θaɪəziːn] *n pharm.* **1.** Phenothiazin *nt.* **2.** Phenothiazinderivat *nt.*
phe·no·type ['-taɪp] *n* (äußeres) Erscheinungsbild *nt*, Phänotyp *m*, -typus *m.*
phe·no·typ·ic [,-'tɪpɪk] *adj* Phänotyp betr., phänotypisch.
phenotypic adaptation phänotypische Adaptation *f.*
phenotypic masking *micro.* Transkapsidation *f.*
phenotypic mixing *genet., micro.* phänotypische Mischung *f*, Phenotypic-mixing *nt.*
phenotypic reversion *genet.* phänotypische Rückmutation/Reversion *f.*
phenotypic variation phänotypische Variation *f.*
phe·nox·ide [fɪ'nɑksaɪd] *n* → phenolate I.
phenoxy- *pref.* Phenoxy-.
phe·noxy·ben·za·mine [fɪ,nɑksɪ'benzəmiːn] *n pharm.* Phenoxybenzamin *nt.*
phe·nox·y·meth·yl penicillin [,-'meθl] → phenoxymethylpenicillin.
phe·nox·y·meth·yl·pen·i·cil·lin [,-,meθlpenə'sɪlɪn] *n pharm.* Phenoxymethylpenicillin *nt*, Penicillin V *nt.*
phen·pro·ba·mate [fen'prəʊbəmeɪt] *n pharm.* Phenprobamat *nt.*
phen·pro·cou·mon [,fenprəʊ'kuːmən] *n pharm.* Phenprocoumon *nt.*
phen·tol·a·mine [fen'tɑləmiːn] *n pharm.* Phentolamin *nt.*
phentolamine test Phentolamin-Test *m.*
phen·yl [fenl, 'fiːnl] *n* Phenyl-(Radikal *nt*), Benzolrest *m.*
phen·yl·a·ce·tic acid [,fenlə'siːtɪk, -'setɪk] Phenylessigsäure *f.*
phen·yl·a·ce·tyl·u·rea [,-ə,siːtɪljʊə'rɪə] *n* → phenacemide.
phen·yl·al·a·nine [,-'æləniːn] *n abbr.* **Phe** Phenylalanin *nt abbr.* Phe.
phenylalanine agar Phenylalaninagar *m/nt.*
phenylalanine-4-hydroxylase *n* Phenylalanin-4-hydroxylase *f*, Phenylalanin-4--monooxygenase *f*, Phenylalaninase *f.*
phenylalanine hydroxylase deficiency → phenylketonuria.
phen·yl·al·a·ni·ne·mia [,-æləni'niːmɪə] *n* erhöhter Phenylalaningehalt *m* des Blutes, Hyperphenylalaninämie *f*, Phenylalaninämie *f.*

phenylalanine-4-monooxygenase *n* → phenylalanine-4-hydroxylase.
phen·yl·al·a·nyl [,-'æləɪnl] *n* Phenylalanyl--(Radikal *nt*).
phenylalanyl chain (*Insulin*) B-Kette *f.*
phen·yl·a·mine [,-ə'miːn, -'æmɪn] *n* Anilin *nt.*
phen·yl·bu·ta·zone [,-'bjuːtəzəʊn] *n pharm.* Phenylbutazon *nt.*
phen·yl·car·bi·nol [,-'kɑːrbɪnɔl, -nɑl] *n* Benzylalkohol *m*, Phenylcarbinol *nt.*
phen·yl·di·meth·yl·py·ra·zo·lon [,-daɪ,meθlpaɪ'ræzəlɑn] *n* → phenazone.
phen·yl·eph·rine [,-'efriːn, -rɪn] *n pharm.* Phenylephrin *nt.*
phen·yl·eth·a·nol·a·mine-*N*-methyltransferase [,-,eθə'nɑləmiːn] *n abbr.* **PNMT** Phenyläthanolamin-*N*-methyltransferase *f abbr.* PNMT.
phen·yl·eth·yl·bar·bi·tu·ric acid [,-,eθl-,bɑːrbɪ'tjʊərɪk] *n* → phenobarbital.
phen·yl·gly·col·ic acid [,-glaɪ'kɑlɪk] Mandelsäure *f.*
phen·yl·hy·dra·zine [,-'haɪdrəziːn, -zɪn] *n* Phenylhydrazin *nt.*
phenylhydrazine anemia hämolytische Anämie *f* durch Phenylhydrazin.
phe·nyl·ic [fə'nɪlɪk] *adj* phenylisch, Phenyl-.
phenylic acid → phenol 1.
phenylic alcohol → phenol 1.
phen·yl·i·so·thi·o·cy·a·nate [,fenl,aɪsəθaɪ-əʊ'saɪəneɪt] *n abbr.* **PITC** *biochem.* Phenylisothiocyanat *nt abbr.* PITC, Edman--Reagenz *nt.*
phen·yl·ke·to·nu·ria [,-,kiːtə'n(j)ʊərɪə] *n abbr.* **PKU** Fölling-Krankheit *f*, Morbus Fölling *m*, Phenylketonurie *f abbr.* PKU, Brenztraubensäureschwachsinn *m*, Oligophrenia phenylpyruvica.
phenylketonuria II Dihydropteridinreduktase-Mangel *m*, DHPR-Mangel *m*, maligne Hyperphenylalaninämie *f*, Hyperphenylalaninämie Typ IV.
phenylketonuria III Dihydrobiopterinreduktase-Mangel *m*, atypische Phenylketonurie *f*, Hyperphenylalaninämie Typ *f* V.
phen·yl·lac·tic acid [,-'læktɪk] Phenylmilchsäure *f.*
phen·yl·mer·cu·ric acetate [,-mər'kjʊərɪk] *pharm.* Phenylmercuriacetat *nt.*
phen·yl·meth·a·nol [,-'meθənɔl, -nɑl] *n* Benzylalkohol *m*, Phenylcarbinol *nt.*
phen·yl·o·sa·zone [,-'əʊsəzəʊn] *n* Phenylosazon *nt.*
phen·yl·py·ru·vate [,-paɪ'ruːveɪt, -pɪ-] *n* Phenylpyruvat *nt.*
phen·yl·py·ru·vic acid [,-paɪ'ruːvɪk, -pɪ-] *n* Phenylbrenztraubensäure *f.*
phen·yl·py·ru·vic·ac·i·du·ria [,-paɪ'ruːvɪk-æsɪ'd(j)ʊərɪə] *n* → phenylketonuria.
phen·yl·thi·o·car·ba·mide [,-,θaɪəʊ'kɑːrbəmaɪd, -kɑːr'bæm-] *n abbr.* **PTC** → phenylthiourea.
phen·yl·thi·o·car·bam·o·yl peptide [,-,θaɪəkɑːr'bæməʊɪl] PTC-Peptid *nt*, Phenylthiocarbamid-Peptid *nt.*
phen·yl·thi·o·u·rea [,-,θaɪəʊjʊə'rɪə] *n* Phenylthiocarbamid *nt abbr.* PTC, Phenylthioharnstoff *m.*
phen·yl·tol·ox·a·mine [,-tɑl'ɑksəmiːn] *n pharm.* Phenyltoloxamin *nt.*
phen·y·to·in [fenɪ'təʊɪn, fə'nɪtəʊɪn] *n pharm.* Phenytoin *nt*, Diphenylhydantoin *nt.*
phe·o·chrome ['fiːəkrəʊm] *adj* chromaffin, phäochrom.
pheochrome body Paraganglion *nt.*
pheochrome cells phäochrome/chromaffine Zellen *pl.*
phe·o·chro·mo·blast [,-'krəʊməblæst] *n* Phäochromoblast *m.*

phe·o·chro·mo·blas·to·ma [ˌ-ˌkrəʊməblæs'təʊmə] *n* → pheochromocytoma.
phe·o·chro·mo·cytes [ˌ-'krəʊməsaɪts] *pl* → pheochrome cells.
phe·o·chro·mo·cy·to·ma [ˌ-ˌkrəʊməsaɪ'təʊmə] *n* Phäochromozytom *nt*.
phe·o·mel·a·nin [ˌ-'melənɪn] *n* Phäomelanin *nt*.
phe·re·sis [fə'riːsɪs, 'ferə-] *n lab.*, *hema.* Pherese *f*, Apherese *f*.
pher·o·mone ['ferəməʊn] *n bio.* Pheromon *nt*.
phi·al ['faɪəl] *n* Phiole *f*.
phi·a·lide ['faɪəlaɪd] *n micro.* Phialide *f*.
Phi·a·loph·o·ra [faɪə'lɒfərə] *n micro.* Phialophora *nt*.
phi·a·lo·phore ['faɪələfəʊər, -fɔːr] *n micro.* Phialophore *f*.
phi·a·lo·spore ['-spɔʊər, -spɔːr] *n micro.* Phialospore *f*.
Phil·a·del·phia chromosome [fɪlə'delfɪə] Philadelphia-Chromosom *nt abbr.* Ph₁.
Philippe-Gombault [fiˈlip gɔ̃'bo]: **P.-G. triangle/tract** Philippe-Gombault'-Triangel *f*, Gombault-Philippe'-Triangel *f*.
Phil·ip·pine dengue ['fɪləpiːn, fɪlə'piːn] Dengue-hämorrhagisches Fieber *nt*.
Philippine hemorrhagic fever → Philippine dengue.
phil·trum ['fɪltrəm] *n, pl* **-tra** [-trə] *anat.* Oberlippenrinne *f*, Philtrum *nt*.
phi·mo·sis [faɪ'məʊsɪs, fɪ-] *n ped.*, *urol.* Phimose *f*.
phi·mot·ic [faɪ'mɒtɪk, fɪ-] *adj* Phimose betr., Phimosen-.
phleb- *pref.* → phlebo-.
phleb·al·gia [flɪ'bældʒ(ɪ)ə] *n* Venen-, Varizenschmerz *m*, Phlebalgie *f*, Phlebalgia *f*; phlebogener Schmerz *m*.
phleb·an·es·the·sia [fleb,ænəs'θiːʒ(ɪ)ə] *n* intravenöse Anästhesie *f*.
phleb·an·gi·o·ma [ˌ-ændʒɪ'əʊmə] *n* Venenaneurysma *nt*, venöses Aneurysma *nt*.
phleb·ar·te·ri·ec·ta·sia [ˌ-ˌɑːrtɪərɪek'teɪʒ(ɪ)ə] *n* Phlebarteriektasie *f*.
phleb·as·the·nia [ˌ-æs'θiːnɪə] *n* Phlebasthenie *f*.
phleb·ec·ta·sia [ˌ-ek'teɪʒ(ɪ)ə] *n* Venenerweiterung *f*, Phlebektasie *f*, Venektasie *f*, Phlebectasia *f*.
phleb·ec·ta·sis [flɪ'bektəsɪs] *n* → phlebectasia.
phle·bec·to·my [flɪ'bektəmɪ] *n chir.* Venenresektion *f*, Phlebektomie *f*, Venektomie *f*.
phleb·ec·to·pia [ˌflebek'təʊpɪə] *n* → phlebectopy.
phleb·ec·to·py [flɪ'bektəpɪ] *n* Venenektopie *f*.
phleb·em·phrax·is [ˌflebem'fræksɪs] *n* Venenverschluß *m*, -obstruktion *f*; Venenthrombose *f*.
phleb·ex·air·e·sis [ˌ-ek'saɪrəsɪs] *n chir.* Phlebex(h)airese *f*, Venenexhärese *f*, -ex(h)airese *f*.
phle·bit·ic [flɪ'bɪtɪk] *adj* Phlebitis betr., phlebitisch.
phle·bi·tis [flɪ'baɪtɪs] *n* Venenentzündung *f*, Phlebitis *f*.
phlebo- *pref.* Venen-, Phleb(o)-, Ven(o)-.
phle·boc·ly·sis [flɪ'bɒkləsɪs] *n* intravenöse Infusion/Injektion *f*.
phleb·o·dy·nam·ics [ˌflebəʊdaɪ'næmɪks] *pl* Phlebodynamik *f*.
phleb·o·fi·bro·sis [ˌ-faɪ'brəʊsɪs] *n* Phlebofibrose *f*.
phle·bog·e·nous [flɪ'bɒdʒənəs] *adj* aus einer Vene stammend, von einer Vene ausgehend, phlebogen.
phleb·o·gram ['flebəgræm] *n* **1.** *radiol.* Phlebogramm *nt*. **2.** *card.*, *physiol.* Phlebogramm *nt*.

phleb·o·graph ['-græf] *n card.*, *physiol.* Phlebograph *m*.
phle·bog·ra·phy [flə'bɒgrəfɪ] *n* **1.** *radiol.* Phlebographie *f*, Venographie *f*. **2.** *card.*, *physiol.* Phlebographie *f*.
phleb·oid ['flebɔɪd] *adj* **1.** venenartig, -förmig. **2.** venös.
phleb·o·lite ['flebəlaɪt] *n* → phlebolith.
phleb·o·lith ['-lɪθ] *n* Venenstein *m*, Phlebolith *m*.
phleb·o·li·thi·a·sis [ˌ-lɪ'θaɪəsɪs] *n* Phlebolithiasis *f*.
phleb·o·ma·nom·e·ter [ˌ-mə'nɒmɪtər] *n* Phlebomanometer *nt*.
phleb·o·me·tri·tis [ˌ-mɪ'traɪtɪs] *n gyn.* Entzündung *f* der Uterusvenen, Phlebometritis *f*.
phleb·o·my·o·ma·to·sis [ˌ-ˌmaɪəmə'təʊsɪs] *n* Phlebomyomatose *f*.
phleb·o·nar·co·sis [ˌ-nɑːr'kəʊsɪs] *n* intravenöse Anästhesie *f*.
phleb·o·phle·bos·to·my [ˌ-flɪ'bɒstəmɪ] *n chir.* Venen-Venen-Anastomose *f*, Phlebophlebostomie *f*, Venovenostomie *f*.
phleb·o·pi·e·zom·e·try [ˌ-ˌpɪə'zɒmətrɪ, -ˌpaɪə-] *n* Venendruckmessung *f*, Bestimmung *f* des venösen Blutdrucks.
phleb·o·plas·ty ['-plæstɪ] *n chir.* Venen-, Phleboplastik *f*.
phleb·or·rha·gia [ˌ-'reɪdʒ(ɪ)ə] *n* venöse Blutung *f*.
phle·bor·rha·phy [flə'bɒrəfɪ] *n chir.* Venennaht *f*, Phleborrhaphie *f*.
phleb·or·rhex·is [ˌflebə'reksɪs] *n* Venenruptur *f*, Phleborrhexis *f*.
phleb·o·scle·ro·sis [ˌ-sklɪ'rəʊsɪs] *n* Phlebosklerose *f*.
phleb·o·sta·sia [ˌ-'steɪʒ(ɪ)ə] *n* → phlebostasis.
phle·bos·ta·sis [flɪ'bɒstəsɪs] *n* **1.** Venostase *f*. **2.** Venenstauung *f*, Venostase *f*. **3.** unblutiger Aderlaß *m*.
phleb·o·ste·no·sis [ˌflebəʊstɪ'nəʊsɪs] *n* Venenstenose *f*.
phleb·o·throm·bo·sis [ˌ-θrɒm'bəʊsɪs] *n* Phlebothrombose *f*.
phleb·o·tome ['-təʊm] *n* Phlebotom *nt*.
Phle·bot·o·mus [flə'bɒtəməs] *n bio.*, *micro.* Phlebotomus *m*.
phlebotomus fever Phlebotomus-, Pappataci-, Moskitofieber *nt*, Drei-Tage-Fieber *nt*.
phlebotomus fever virus *micro.* Pappataci(fieber)virus *nt*.
phle·bot·o·my [flə'bɒtəmɪ] *n* **1.** Venenschnitt *m*, Phlebotomie *f*, Venaesectio *f*. **2.** Venenpunktion *f*. **3.** Veneneröffnung *f*, Venaesectio *f*.
phleb·o·vi·rus [ˌflebəʊ'vaɪrəs] *n micro.* Phlebovirus *m*.
phlegm [flem] *n* **1.** Schleim *m*, Phlegma *nt*. **2.** *fig.* Phlegma *nt*, Trägkeit *f*, Schwerfälligkeit *f*.
phleg·ma·sia [fleg'meɪʒ(ɪ)ə, -ʒɪə] *n patho.* Entzündung *f*, Fieber *nt*, Phlegmasie *f*, Phlegmasia *f*.
phleg·mat·ic [fleg'mætɪk] *adj* phlegmatisch, träge, schwerfällig.
phleg·mon ['flegmən] *n* **1.** Phlegmone *f*, phlegmonöse Entzündung *f*. **2.** Pankreasphlegmone *f*.
p. of the colon Dickdarmphlegmone.
p. of the floor of the mouth Mundbodenphlegmone.
p. of the gastric wall Magenwandphlegmone.
phleg·mo·no·sis [ˌflegmə'nəʊsɪs] *n* → phlegmasia.
phleg·mon·ous ['flegmənəs] *adj* Phlegmone betr., phlegmonös.
phlegmonous abscess Phlegmone *f*.
phlegmonous appendicitis phlegmonöse Appendizitis *f*, Appendicitis phlegmonosa.
phlegmonous cellulitis → phlegmon.
phlegmonous erysipelas Erysipelas phlegmonosum.
phlegmonous gastritis phlegmonöse Gastritis *f*, Gastritis phlegmonosa.
phlegmonous laryngitis phlegmonöse Laryngitis *f*.
phlegmonous mastitis *gyn.* phlegmonöse Mastitis *f*.
phlegmonous pharyngitis Pharynxphlegmone *f*.
phlegmonous ulcer phlegmonöses Geschwür *nt*.
phlo- *pref.* → phlogo-.
phlo·gis·tic [fləʊ'dʒɪstɪk] *adj* Entzündung betr., entzündlich, phlogistisch, Entzündungs-.
phlo·gis·ton [fləʊ'dʒɪstən] *n histor.* Phlogiston *nt*.
phlogiston theory *histor.* Phlogistontheorie *f*.
phlogo- *pref.* Entzündung(s)-.
phlog·o·cytes ['flɒgəsaɪts] *pl* Entzündungszellen *pl*.
phlog·o·gen·ic [ˌ-'dʒenɪk] *adj* eine Entzündung verursachend, phlogogen.
phlo·gog·e·nous [fləʊ'gɒdʒənəs] *adj* → phlogogenic.
phlo·got·ic [fləʊ'gɒtɪk] *adj* → phlogistic.
phlor·e·tin ['flɔːrətɪn, 'flɑ-, flə'riːtɪn] *n* Phloretin *nt*.
phlo·rhi·zin ['flɑrzɪn, fləʊ'raɪzɪn] *n* Phlorizin *nt*, Phlorrhidzin *nt*.
phlorhizin glycosuria → phloridzin glycosuria.
phlo·rid·zin [flə'rɪdzɪn] *n* → phlorhizin.
phloridzin diabetes Phlorizindiabetes *m*.
phloridzin glycosuria Phlorizinglucosurie *f*, -glykosurie *f*.
phlor·i·zin *n* → phlorhizin.
phlorizin diabetes → phloridzin diabetes.
phlorizin glycosuria → phloridzin glycosuria.
phlor·o·glu·cin [ˌflɔːrəʊ'gluːsɪn, ˌflɑr-] *n* Phloroglucin *nt*, 1,3,5-Trihydroxybenzol *nt*.
phlor·o·glu·cin·ol [ˌ-'gluːsənɒl, -nɑl] *n* → phloroglucin.
phlor·rhi·zin *n* → phlorhizin.
phlyc·ten ['flɪktən] *n* → phlyctena.
phlyc·te·na [flɪk'tiːnə] *n, pl* **-nae** [-niː] *ophthal.* Phlyktäne *f*, Phlyktaena *f*.
phlyc·te·noid [flɪk'tiːnɔɪd, 'flɪktə-] *adj ophthal.* phlyktän-ähnlich.
phlyc·ten·u·lar conjunctivitis [flɪk'tenjələr] → phlyctenular keratitis.
phlyctenular keratitis Conjunctivitis/Keratitis/Keratoconjunctivitis eccematosa/eczematosa/scrufulosa/phlyctaenulosa.
phlyctenular keratoconjunctivitis → phlyctenular keratitis.
phlyctenular ophthalmia → phlyctenular keratitis.
pho·bia ['fəʊbɪə] *n psycho.*, *psychia.* Phobie *f*, Phobia *f*.
pho·bic ['fəʊbɪk] *adj* Phobie betr., phobisch.
phobic neurosis → phobia.
pho·bo·pho·bia [ˌfəʊbəʊ'fəʊbɪə] *n psycho.*, *psychia.* Phobophobie *f*.
pho·co·me·lia [ˌfəʊkəʊ'miːlɪə, -ljə] *n* Robbengliedrigkeit *f*, Phokomelie *f*.
pho·co·me·lic [ˌ-'miːlɪk] *adj* robbengliedrig, phokomel.
phocomelic dwarf phokomeler Zwerg *m*.
pho·com·e·lus [fəʊ'kɒmələs] *n* Phokomelus *m*.
pho·com·e·ly [fəʊ'kɒməlɪ] *n* → phocomelia.
pho·ko·me·lia *n* → phocomelia.

phol·co·dine ['fɑlkəʊdiːn] *n pharm.* Pholcodin *nt.*
phol·e·drine ['fəʊlədriːn] *n pharm.* Pholedrin *nt.*
phon- *pref.* → phono-.
phon [fɑn] *n phys.* Phon *nt.*
pho·nal ['fəʊnl] *adj* Stimm-, Phon-.
phon·as·the·nia [ˌfəʊnæs'θiːnɪə] *n* Stimmschwäche *f*, Phonasthenie *f.*
pho·nate ['fəʊneɪt] *vi* Laute bilden, phonieren.
pho·na·tion [fəʊ'neɪʃn] *n* Laut-, Stimmbildung *f*, Phonation *f.*
pho·na·to·ry ['fəʊnətɔːriː, -təʊ-] *adj* Phonation betr., Phonations-.
phon·au·to·graph [fəʊ'nɔːtəɡræf] *n* Phonautograph *m.*
pho·neme ['fəʊniːm] *n* 1. Phonem *nt.* 2. *psychia.* akustische Sinnestäuschung *f*, Stimmenhören *nt*, Phonem *nt.*
pho·ne·mic [fə'niːmɪk, fəʊ-] *adj* phonemisch, phonematisch, Phonem-.
phon·en·do·scope [fəʊ'nendəskəʊp] *n* Phonendoskop *nt.*
pho·net·ic [fə'netɪk, fəʊ-] *adj* → phonetical.
pho·net·i·cal [fə'netɪkl, fəʊ-] *adj* Phonetik betr., phonetisch.
pho·net·ics [fə'netɪks, fəʊ-] *pl* Laut(bildungs)lehre *f*, Phonetik *f.*
pho·ni·at·rics [ˌfəʊnɪ'ætrɪks] *pl* Phoniatrie *f.*
phon·ic ['fɑnɪk, 'fəʊ-] *adj* Stimme betr., phonisch, Stimm-, Phon-.
pho·nism ['fəʊnɪzəm] *n* Phonismus *m.*
phono- *pref.* Stimm-, Schall-, Phon(o)-.
pho·no·an·gi·og·ra·phy [ˌfəʊnəʊændʒɪ'ɑɡrəfɪ] *n* Phonoangiographie *f.*
pho·no·aus·cul·ta·tion [-ˌɔːskəl'teɪʃn] *n* Phonoauskultation *f.*
pho·no·car·di·o·gram [-'kɑːrdɪəɡræm] *n* Phonokardiogramm *nt.*
pho·no·car·di·o·graph [-'kɑːrdɪəɡræf] *n* Phonokardiograph *m.*
pho·no·car·di·o·graph·ic [-ˌkɑːrdɪə'ɡræfɪk] *adj* Phonokardiographie *od.* Phonokardiogramm betr., phonokardiographisch.
pho·no·car·di·og·ra·phy [-ˌkɑːrdɪ'ɑɡrəfɪ] *n abbr.* **PCG** Phonokardiographie *f abbr.* PKG.
pho·no·cath·e·ter [ˌ-'kæθɪtər] *n* Phonokatheter *m.*
pho·no·gram ['-ɡræm] *n* Phonogramm *nt.*
pho·nol·o·gy [fəʊ'nɑlədʒɪ] *n* 1. Phonologie *f.* 2. Phonetik *f.*
pho·no·ma·nia [ˌfəʊnəʊ'meɪnɪə, -jə] *n psychia.* Phonomanie *f.*
pho·nom·e·ter [fəʊ'nɑmɪtər] *n* Phonometer *nt.*
pho·no·my·oc·lo·nus [ˌfəʊnəmaɪ'ɑklənəs] *n* Phonomyoklonus *m.*
pho·no·my·o·gram [ˌ-'maɪəɡræm] *n* Phonomyogramm *nt.*
pho·no·my·og·ra·phy [-ˌmaɪ'ɑɡrəfɪ] *n* Phonomyographie *f.*
pho·no·pho·bia [ˌ-'fəʊbɪə] *n psychia.* Phonophobie *f.*
pho·nop·si·a [fəʊ'nɑpsɪə] *n neuro.* Phonopsie *f*; Auditio colorata.
pho·no·scope ['fəʊnəskəʊp] *n* Phonoskop *nt.*
pho·nos·co·py [fəʊ'nɑskəpɪ] *n* Phonoskopie *f.*
phon scale *physiol.* Phonskala *f.*
pho·re·sis [fə'riːsɪs] *n* 1. Elektrophorese *f.* 2. *bio.* Phoresie *f.*
phor·e·sy ['fɔːrəsɪ] *n bio.* Phoresie *f.*
pho·ria ['fɔːrɪə, 'fɔːr-] *n ophthal.* Neigung *f* zum Schielen, Heterophorie *f.*
phor·o·blast ['fɔːrəblæst] *n* Fibroblast *m.*

phor·o·cyte ['-saɪt] *n* Bindegewebszelle *f*, Fibrozyt *m.*
phor·om·e·ter [fə'rɑmɪtər] *n ophthal.* Phorometer *nt.*
pho·rom·e·try [fə'rɑmətrɪ] *n ophthal.* Phorometrie *f.*
phor·o·plast ['fɔːrəplæst] *n* Bindegewebe *nt.*
pho·rop·ter [fə'rɑptər] *n ophthal.* Phoropter *nt.*
phose [fəʊz] *n ophthal., physiol.* Phose *f.*
phos·gene ['fɑzdʒiːn] *n* Phosgen *nt.*
phos·pha·gen ['fɑsfədʒən] *n* 1. Phosphatbildner *m*, Phosphagen *nt.* 2. → phosphocreatine.
phos·pha·gen·ic [ˌ-'dʒenɪk] *adj* phosphatbildend.
phos·pha·tase ['fɑsfəteɪz] *n* Phosphatase *f.*
phos·phate ['fɑsfeɪt] *n* Phosphat *nt.*
phosphate acyltransferase Phosphat-acyltransferase *f.*
phosphate-ATP-exchange *n biochem.* Phosphat-ATP-Austausch *m.*
phosphate balance *biochem.* Phosphathaushalt *m.*
phosphate binder phosphatbindende Substanz *f*, Phosphatbinder *m.*
phosphate bond Phosphatbindung *f.*
high-energy p. energiereiche Phosphatbindung.
phosphate-bond energy Phosphatbindungsenergie *f*, Energie *f* der Phosphatbindung, phosphatgebundene Energie *f.*
phosphate buffer Phosphatpuffer *m.*
phosphate buffer system *physiol.* Phosphatpuffer(system *nt*) *m.*
phosphate calculus *urol.* Phosphatstein *m.*
phosphate carrier *biochem.* Phosphatcarrier *m.*
phos·phat·ed ['fɑsfeɪtɪd] *adj* phosphathaltig, phosphatisch.
phosphate diabetes Phosphatdiabetes *m.*
phosphate donor *biochem.* Phosphatdonor *m.*
phosphate ester Phosphatester *m.*
phosphate group Phosphatgruppe *f.*
phosphate-group transfer potential *biochem.* Phosphatgruppenübertragungspotential *nt.*
phos·pha·te·mia [ˌfɑsfə'tiːmɪə] *n* erhöhter Phosphatgehalt *m* des Blutes, Phosphatämie *f.*
phosphate-water-exchange *n biochem.* Phosphat-Wasser-Austausch *m.*
phos·phat·ic [fɑs'fætɪk] *adj* Phosphat betr., phosphathaltig, Phosphat-.
phosphatic calculus *urol.* Phosphatstein *m.*
phos·pha·ti·dase [ˌ-'taɪdeɪz] *n* Phosphatidase *f*, Phospholipase A₂ *f.*
phos·pha·ti·date phosphatase [ˌ-'taɪdeɪt] Phosphatidsäurephosphatase *f.*
phos·pha·tide ['-taɪd, -tɪd] *n* 1. → phospholipid 2. *inf.* → phosphoglycerid.
phos·pha·tid·ic acid [ˌ-'tɪdɪk] Phosphatidsäure *f.*
phos·pha·ti·do·li·pase [ˌ-taɪdəʊ'lɪpeɪz] *n* → phosphatidase.
phos·pha·ti·do·sis [ˌ-tɪ'dəʊsɪs] *n* Phosphatidspeicherkrankheit *f*, Phospholipidose *f.*
phos·pha·ti·dyl·cho·line [ˌ-ˌtaɪdl'kəʊliːn, -'kɑl-] *n abbr.* **PC** Phosphatidylcholin *nt.* PC, Cholinphosphoglycerid *nt*, Lecithin *nt.*
phosphatidylcholine-cholesterol acyltransferase → phosphatidylcholine-sterol acyltransferase.
phosphatidylcholine-sterol acyltransferase Phosphatidylcholin-Cholesterin-Acyltransferase *f*, Lecithin-Cholesterin-Acyltransferase *f abbr.* LCAT.

phos·pha·ti·dyl·eth·a·nol·a·mine [ˌ-ˌtaɪdlˌeθə'nɑləmiːn] *n abbr.* **PE** Phosphatidyl-äthanolamin *nt*, Äthanolaminphosphoglycerid *nt.*
phos·pha·ti·dyl·glyc·er·ol [ˌ-ˌtaɪdl'ɡlɪsərɒl, -rəl] *n* Phosphatidylglycerin *nt.*
phos·pha·ti·dyl·in·o·sine diphosphate [ˌ-ˌtaɪdl'ɪnəsiːn, -sɪn] *abbr.* **PIP₂** Phosphatidylinosindiphosphat *nt abbr.* PIP₂.
phos·pha·ti·dyl·in·o·si·tol [ˌ-ˌtaɪdl'ɪnəsɪtɒl, -təʊl] *n abbr.* **PI** Phosphatidylinosit(ol) *nt.*
phosphatidylinositol diphosphate → phosphatidylinosine diphosphate.
phos·pha·ti·dyl·ser·ine [ˌ-ˌtaɪdl'serɪn, -'sɪər-] *n abbr.* **PS** Phosphatidylserin *nt abbr.* PS.
phosphatidyl sugar Glykophosphoglycerid *nt.*
phos·pha·tu·ria [ˌ-'t(j)ʊərɪə] *n* erhöhte Phosphatausscheidung *f* im Harn, Kalkariurie *f*, Phosphaturie *f.*
phos·phene ['fɑsfiːn] *n ophthal., neuro.* Phosphen *nt.*
phos·phide ['fɑsfaɪd] *n* Phosphid *nt.*
phos·phine ['fɑsfiːn, -fɪn] *n* Phosphin *nt*, Phosphorwasserstoff *m.*
phos·phite ['fɑsfaɪt] *n* Phosphit *nt.*
phos·pho·am·i·dase [ˌfɑsfəʊ'æmɪdeɪz] *n* Phosphoamidase *f.*
phos·pho·am·ide bond [ˌ-'æmaɪd, -ɪd] Phosphoamidbindung *f.*
phos·pho·ar·gi·nine [ˌ-'ɑːrdʒəniːn] *n* Arginin(o)phosphat *nt.*
phos·pho·cho·line [ˌ-'kəʊliːn, 'kɑl-] *n* Phosphocholin *nt.*
phosphocholine cytidylyltransferase Phosphocholincytidyl(yl)transferase *f.*
phosphocholine transferase Phosphocholintransferase *f.*
phos·pho·cre·a·tine [ˌ-'kriːətiːn, -tɪn] *n abbr.* **PC** Phosphokreatin *nt*, Kreatin-, Creatinphosphat *nt.*
phos·pho·di·es·ter·ase [ˌ-daɪ'estəreɪz] *n abbr.* **PDE** Phosphodiesterase *f abbr.* PDE.
phos·pho·di·es·ter bridge [ˌ-daɪ'estər] Phosphodiesterbrücke *f.*
phos·pho·e·nol·pyr·u·vate [ˌ-ˌiːnɑlpaɪ'ruːveɪt, -pɪ-] *n abbr.* **PEP** Phosphoenolpyruvat *nt abbr.* PEP.
phosphoenolpyruvate carboxykinase (GTP) Phosphoenolpyruvatcarboxykinase (GTP) *f*, Phosphopyruvatcarboxykinase *f.*
phos·pho·e·nol·py·ru·vic acid [ˌ-ˌiːnɑlpaɪ'ruːvɪk, -pɪ-] Phosphoenolbrenztraubensäure *f.*
phos·pho·en·zyme [ˌ-'enzaɪm] *n* Phosphoenzym *nt.*
phos·pho·eth·a·nol·a·mine [ˌ-ˌeθə'nɑləmiːn, -'nɒl-, -nə'læmɪn] *n* Phosphoäthanolamin *nt.*
phosphoethanolamine cytidylyltransferase Phosphoäthanolamincytidyl(yl)transferase *f.*
phosphoethanolamine transferase Phosphoäthanolamintransferase *f.*
phos·pho·fruc·to·al·dol·ase [ˌ-ˌfrʌktəʊ'æl-dəleɪz] *n* Fructosediphosphataldolase *f*, -bisphosphataldolase *f*, Aldolase *f abbr.* ALD.
(6-)phos·pho·fruc·to·ki·nase [ˌ-ˌfrʌktə'kaɪneɪz] *n abbr.* **PFK** (6-)Phosphofruktokinase *f abbr.* PFK.
6-phosphofructo-2-kinase *n* 6-Phosphofrukto-2-kinase *f.*
phos·pho·glob·u·lin [ˌ-'ɡlɑbjəlɪn] *n* Phosphoglobulin *nt.*
phos·pho·glu·co·ki·nase [ˌ-ˌɡluːkəʊ'kaɪneɪz] *n* Phosphoglukokinase *f*, -glucokinase *f.*

phos·pho·glu·co·mu·tase [ˌ-ˌgluːkəʊ-'mjuːteɪz] n Phosphoglukomutase f, -glucomutase f abbr. PGluM.
6-phos·pho·glu·co·nate [ˌ-'gluːkəneɪt] n 6-Phosphogluconat nt.
6-phosphogluconate dehydrogenase 6-Phosphogluconatdehydrogenase f abbr. 6-PGD.
phosphogluconate pathway → pentose phosphate pathway.
6-phos·pho·glu·co·no·lac·tone [ˌ-ˌgluːkənəʊ'læktəʊn] n 6-Phosphogluconolacton nt.
phos·pho·glu·co·pro·tein [ˌ-ˌgluːkəʊ'prəʊtiːn, -tiːɪn] n Phosphoglykoprotein nt.
phos·pho·glu·cose isomerase [ˌ-'gluːkəʊz] Glukose(-6-)phosphatisomerase f, Phosphohexoseisomerase f abbr. PHI, Phosphoglucoseisomerase f abbr. PGI.
3-phos·pho·glyc·er·al·de·hyde [ˌ-ˌɡlɪsər-'ældəhaɪd] n Glyzerinaldehyd-3-phosphat nt abbr. GAP, 3-Phosphoglyzerinaldehyd m.
3-phosphoglyceraldehyde dehydrogenase Glyzerinaldehyd(-3-)dehydrogenase f abbr. GAPD(H), 3-Phosphoglyzerinaldehydrogenase f.
phos·pho·glyc·er·ate [ˌ-'ɡlɪsəreɪt] n Phosphoglycerat nt.
phosphoglycerate dehydrogenase Phosphoglyceratdehydrogenase f.
phosphoglycerate kinase Phosphoglyceratkinase f abbr. PGK.
phosphoglycerate mutase Phosphoglyceratmutase f, Phosphoglyceromutase f abbr. PGM, Phosphoglyceratphosphomutase f.
phos·pho·glyc·er·ic acid [ˌ-ɡlɪ'sərɪk] Phosphoglycerinsäure f.
phos·pho·glyc·er·ide [ˌ-'ɡlɪsəraɪd, -ɪd] n Phosphoglycerid nt, Glycerophosphatid nt, inf. Phospholipid nt, inf. Phosphatid nt.
phos·pho·glyc·er·o·mu·tase [ˌ-ˌɡlɪsərəʊ-'mjuːteɪz] n → phosphoglycerate mutase.
3-phos·pho·glyc·er·o·yl phosphate [ˌ-'ɡlɪsərəwɪl] Negelein-Ester m 1,3-Diphosphoglycerat nt abbr. 1,3-DIPG, 3-Phosphoglyceroylphosphat nt.
phospho-glycogen synthase Phosphoglykogensynthase f.
phos·pho·gly·co·late [ˌ-'glaɪkəleɪt] n Phosphoglykolat nt.
phos·pho·gly·col·ic acid [ˌ-glaɪ'kɑlɪk] Phosphoglykolsäure f.
phos·pho·guan·i·dine [ˌ-'gwænɪdiːn] n Phosphoguanidin nt, Guanidinphosphat nt.
phos·pho·hex·o·i·som·er·ase [ˌ-ˌhɛksəaɪ-'sɑmǝreɪz] n Glukose(-6-)phosphatisomerase f, Phosphohexoseisomerase f abbr. PHI, Phosphoglucoseisomerase f abbr. PGI.
phos·pho·hex·o·ki·nase [ˌ-ˌhɛksəʊ'kaɪneɪz] n → 6-)phosphofructokinase.
phos·pho·hex·ose deficiency [ˌ-'hɛksəʊs] Glucosephosphat-isomerase-Mangel m, -Defekt m.
3-phos·pho·hy·drox·y·py·ru·vic acid [ˌ-haɪˌdrɑksɪpaɪ'ruːvɪk, -pɪ-] 3-Phosphohydroxybrenztraubensäure f.
phos·pho·in·o·si·tol [ˌ-ɪ'nəʊsɪtɒl, -təʊl] n Phosphoinositol nt, Inosittriphosphat nt abbr. IP₃.
phos·pho·ke·tol·ase [ˌ-'ketleɪz] n Phosphoketolase f.
phos·pho·li·pase [ˌ-'laɪpeɪz, -lɪ-] n Phospholipase f, Lezithinase f, Lecithinase f.
phospholipase A₁ Phospholipase A₁ f, Lecithinase A f.
phospholipase A₂ Phospholipase A₂ f, Lecithinase A f.

phospholipase B Lysophospholipase f, Phospholipase B f, Lecithinase B f.
phospholipase C Phospholipase C f, Lecithinase C f, Lipophosphodiesterase I f.
phospholipase D Phospholipase D f, Lecithinase D f.
phos·pho·lip·id [ˌ-'lɪpɪd, -'laɪ-] n 1. Phospholipid nt; Phosphatid nt. 2. inf. → phosphoglyceride.
phos·pho·lip·in [ˌ-'lɪpɪn] n 1. Phospholipid nt, Phosphatid nt. 2. inf. → phosphoglyceride.
phos·pho·li·po·pro·tein [ˌ-ˌlɪpə'prəʊtiːn, -tiːɪn] n Phospholipoprotein nt.
phos·pho·man·nose isomerase [ˌ-'mænəʊs] Mannose-6-phosphatisomerase f, Mannosephosphatisomerase f.
phos·pho·mev·a·lon·ate [ˌ-ˌmevə'lɒneɪt] n Phosphomevalonat nt.
phosphomevalonate kinase Phosphomevalonatkinase f.
phos·pho·mev·a·lon·ic acid [ˌ-ˌmevə'lɒnɪk] Phosphomevalonsäure f.
phos·pho·mon·o·es·ter·ase [ˌ-ˌmɒnə'estəreɪz] n 1. alkalische Phosphatase f abbr. AP. 2. saure Phosphatase f abbr. SP.
phos·pho·mu·tase [ˌ-'mjuːteɪz] n Phosphomutase f.
phos·pho·ne·cro·sis [ˌ-nɪ'krəʊsɪs] n Phosphornekrose f.
phos·pho·nu·cle·ase [ˌ-'njuːklɪeɪz] n Nukleo-, Nucleotidase f.
4'-phos·pho·pan·te·the·ine [ˌ-ˌpæntə'θiːɪn, -pæn'teθ-] n 4'-Phosphopantethein nt.
phos·pho·pe·nia [ˌ-'piːnɪə] n Phosphormangel m.
phospho-phosphorylase kinase Phospho-Phosphorylasekinase f.
phos·pho·pro·tein [ˌ-'prəʊtiːn, -tiːɪn] n Phosphoprotein nt.
phosphoprotein phosphatase Phosphoproteinphosphatase f.
phos·pho·py·ru·vate carboxykinase [ˌ-paɪ'ruːveɪt] → phosphoenolpyruvate carboxykinase (GTP).
phosphopyruvate carboxylase 1. → phosphoenolpyruvate carboxykinase (GTP). 2. bio. Phosphopyruvatcarboxilase f.
phos·pho·rate ['fɑsfəreɪt] vt phosphorisieren.
phos·pho·rat·ed ['-reɪtɪd] adj phosphorhaltig.
phos·pho·res·cence [ˌ-'resəns] n Phosphoreszenz f.
phos·pho·res·cent [ˌ-'resənt] adj Phosphoreszenz betr. od. zeigend, phosphoreszierend.
phos·pho·ret·ted ['-retɪd] adj → phosphorated.
phos·pho·ri·bo·i·som·er·ase [ˌ-ˌraɪbəaɪ-'sɑmǝreɪz] n Ribosephosphatisomerase f, Phosphoriboisomerase f.
(5-)phos·pho·ri·bo·syl·a·mine [ˌ-ˌraɪbə'sɪləmiːn] n (5-)Phosphoribosylamin nt.
phos·pho·ri·bo·syl-AMP-cyclohydrolase [ˌ-'raɪbəsɪl] n Phosphoribosyl-AMP-cyclohydrolase f.
phos·pho·ri·bo·syl·py·ro·phos·phate [ˌ-ˌraɪbəsɪlˌpaɪrə'fɑsfeɪt] n abbr. PRPP Phosphoribosylpyrophosphat nt abbr. PRPP.
phosphoribosylpyrophosphate synthetase Ribosephosphatpyrophosphokinase f, Phosphoribosylpyrophosphatsynthetase f.
phos·pho·ri·bo·syl·trans·fer·ase [ˌ-ˌraɪbəsɪl'trænsfəreɪz] n Phosphoribosyltransferase f.
phos·pho·ri·bu·lo·ki·nase [ˌ-ˌraɪbjələʊ-'kaɪneɪz] n Phosphoribulokinase f.

phos·phor·ic acid [fɑs'fɔːrɪk, -'fɑr-] Phosphorsäure f, Orthophosphorsäure f.
glacial p. Metaphosphorsäure.
phos·pho·rize ['fɑsfəraɪz] vt phosphorisieren.
phos·pho·rized ['-raɪzd] adj phosphorhaltig.
phos·pho·ro·clas·tic cleavage [ˌfɑsfərəʊ-'klæstɪk] biochem. → phosphorolysis.
phos·pho·rol·y·sis [ˌfɑsfə'rɑləsɪs] n Phosphorolyse f.
phos·pho·ro·lyt·ic [ˌfɑsfərəʊ'lɪtɪk] adj Phosphorolyse betr., mittels Phosphorolyse, phosphorolytisch.
phosphorolytic cleavage phosphorolytische Spaltung f.
phos·phor·o·scope [fɑs'fɔrəskəʊp] n Phosphoroskop nt.
phos·pho·rous ['fɑsf(ə)rəs] adj Phosphor betr. od. enthaltend, phosphorhaltig.
phosphorous acid phosphorige Säure f.
phos·phor·pe·nia [ˌfɑsfər'pɪnɪə] n Phosphormangel m.
phos·phor·u·ria [ˌ-'(j)ʊərɪə] n → phosphaturia.
phos·pho·rus ['fɑsf(ə)rəs] n abbr. P Phosphor m abbr. P.
phosphorus burn Phosphorverbrennung f.
phosphorus poisoning Phosphorvergiftung f.
phos·pho·ryl ['fɑsfərɪl] n Phosphoryl-(Radikal nt).
phos·pho·ryl·ase [fɑs'fɒrəleɪz, -'fɑrə-, 'fɑsfərə-] n 1. Phosphorylase f. 2. Glykogen-, Stärkephosphorylase f.
α-phosphorylase n Phosphorylase a f.
β-phosphorylase n Phosphorylase b f.
phosphorylase (B) kinase Phosphorylasekinase f.
phosphorylase kinase kinase Phosphorylasekinase-kinase f, Proteinkinase f.
phosphorylase phosphatase Phosphorylasephosphatase f.
phosphorylase reaction Phosphorylase-Reaktion f.
phosphorylase rupturing enzyme Phosphorylasephosphatase f.
phos·pho·ryl·ate ['fɑsfəreɪt] vt chem. phosphorylieren.
phos·pho·ryl·at·ed thiamin ['fɑsfərəleɪtɪd] Thiaminpyrophosphat nt abbr. TPP.
phos·pho·ryl·at·ion [ˌfɑsfɔːrə'leɪʃn] n Phosphorylierung f.
phosphorylation potential Phosphorylierungspotential nt.
phos·pho·ryl·dol·i·chol [ˌfɑsfərɪl'dɑlɪkəl, -kɑl] n Dolicholphosphat nt.
phos·pho·ryl·y·sis [ˌfɑsfə'rɪləsɪs] n → phosphorolysis.
phos·pho·ser·ine [ˌfɑsfə'seriːn, -ɪn, -'sɪər-] n Phosphoserin nt.
phosphoserine phosphatase Phosphoserinphosphatase f.
phosphoserine transaminase Phosphoserintransaminase f.
phos·pho·sug·ar [ˌ-'ʃʊgər] n Phosphatzucker m.
phos·pho·trans·fer·ase [ˌ-'trænsfəreɪz] n Phosphotransferase f.
phosphotransferase system abbr. PTS Phosphotransferasesystem nt abbr. PTS.
phos·pho·tri·ose [ˌ-'traɪəʊz] n Triosephosphat nt.
phos·phu·re·sis [ˌfɑsfjə'riːsɪs] n Phosphorausscheidung f im Harn, Phosphurese f.
phos·phu·ret·ed ['fɑsfjəretɪd] adj → phosphorated.
phos·phu·ria [fɑs'fjʊərɪə] n → phosphaturia.
phot- pref. → photo-.
phot [fɑt, fəʊt] n Phot nt.

photalgia

pho·tal·gia [fəʊˈtældʒ(ɪ)ə] n → photodynia.
pho·tau·gi·a·pho·bia [ˌfəʊˌtɔːdʒɪəˈfəʊbɪə] n psychia. Photaugiaphobie f.
pho·te·ryth·rous [fəʊtɪˈrɪθrəs] adj deuteranop.
pho·tes·the·sia [fəʊtesˈθiːʒ(ɪ)ə] n Phot(o)ästhesie f.
pho·tic [ˈfəʊtɪk] adj Licht betr., Licht-, Phot(o)-.
pho·tism [ˈfəʊtɪzəm] n Photismus m.
photo- pref. Licht-, Phot(o)-.
pho·to [ˈfəʊtəʊ] n → photograph I.
pho·to·ac·tin·ic [ˌfəʊtəʊækˈtɪnɪk] adj photoaktinisch.
pho·to·ac·tive [ˌ-ˈæktɪv] adj chem. photoaktiv.
pho·to·al·ler·gic [ˌ-əˈlɜːdʒɪk] adj photoallergisch.
photoallergic contact dermatitis Photokontaktallergie f, photoallergische (Kontakt-)Dermatitis f, photoallergisches Ekzem nt.
pho·to·al·ler·gy [ˌ-ˈælədʒɪ] n Photoallergie f, Lichtallergie f.
pho·to·au·to·troph [ˌ-ˈɔːtətrɒf, -trəʊf] n photoautotropher Organismus m, Photoautotroph m.
pho·to·au·to·troph·ic [ˌ-ˌɔːtəˈtrɒfɪk, -trəʊf-] adj photoautotroph.
photoautotrophic bacterium photoautotrophes Bakterium nt.
pho·to·bac·te·ria [ˌ-bækˈtɪərɪə] pl micro. Photobakterien pl.
Pho·to·bac·te·ri·um [ˌ-bækˈtɪərɪəm] n micro. Photobacterium nt.
pho·to·bi·o·log·ic [ˌ-baɪəˈlɒdʒɪk] adj photobiologisch.
pho·to·bi·o·log·i·cal [ˌ-baɪəˈlɒdʒɪkl] adj → photobiologic.
pho·to·bi·ol·o·gy [ˌ-baɪˈɒlədʒɪ] n Photobiologie f.
pho·to·cat·a·ly·sis [ˌ-kəˈtæləsɪs] n Photo-, Lichtkatalyse f.
pho·to·cat·a·lyst [ˌ-ˈkætlɪst] n Photokatalysator m.
pho·to·cat·a·lyt·ic [ˌ-ˌkætəˈlɪtɪk] adj Photokatalyse betr. od. verursachend, photokatalytisch.
pho·to·cat·a·lyz·er [ˌ-ˈkætlaɪzər] n photocatalyst.
pho·to·cep·tor [ˌ-ˈseptər] n → photoreceptor.
pho·to·chem·i·cal [ˌ-ˈkemɪkl] adj Photochemie betr., photochemisch.
photochemical reaction photochemische Reaktion f.
photochemical spectrum photochemisches Spektrum n.
pho·to·chem·is·try [ˌ-ˈkemɪstrɪ] n Photochemie f.
pho·to·che·mo·ther·a·py [ˌ-ˌkiːməˈθerəpɪ] n Photochemotherapie f.
pho·to·chro·mo·gen·ic [ˌ-ˌkrəʊməˈdʒenɪk] adj micro. photochromogen.
pho·to·chro·mo·gens [ˌ-ˈkrəʊmədʒənz] pl micro. 1. photochromogene Mykobakterien pl, Mykobakterien pl der Runyon-Gruppe I. 2. photochromogene Mikroorganismen pl.
pho·to·co·ag·u·la·tion [ˌ-kəʊˌægjəˈleɪʃn] n Licht-, Photokoagulation f.
pho·to·co·ag·u·la·tor [ˌ-kəʊˈægjəleɪtər] n Licht-, Photokoagulator m.
pho·to·con·tact dermatitis [ˌ-ˈkɒntækt] → photoallergic contact dermatitis.
pho·to·der·ma·ti·tis [ˌ-ˌdɜːməˈtaɪtɪs] n Photodermatitis f.
pho·to·der·ma·to·sis [ˌ-ˌdɜːməˈtəʊsɪs] n Licht-, Photodermatose f.
pho·to·de·tec·tor [ˌ-dɪˈtektər] n Photodetektor m.

pho·tod·ro·my [fəʊˈtɒdrəmɪ] n Photodromie f.
pho·to·dy·nam·ic [ˌfəʊtəʊdaɪˈnæmɪk] adj photodynamisch.
pho·to·dy·nam·ics [ˌ-daɪˈnæmɪks] pl Photodynamik f.
pho·to·dyn·ia [ˌ-ˈdiːnɪə] n Photodynie f.
pho·to·dys·pho·ria [ˌ-dɪsˈfɔːrɪə, -ˈfɒː-] n Photodysphorie f, (extreme) Photophobie f.
pho·to·e·lec·tric [ˌ-ɪˈlektrɪk] adj photoelektrisch.
pho·to·e·lec·tri·cal [ˌ-ɪˈlektrɪkl] adj → photoelectric.
photoelectrical effect photoelektrischer/ lichtelektrischer Effekt m, Photoeffekt m.
pho·to·e·lec·tric·i·ty [ˌ-ˌɪlekˈtrɪsətɪ] n Photoelektrizität f.
pho·to·e·lec·tron [ˌ-ɪˈlektrən] n Photoelektron nt.
pho·to·e·lec·tro·nys·tag·mo·gram [ˌ-ɪˌlektrəʊnɪsˈtægməgræm] n Photoelektronystagmogramm nt.
pho·to·e·lec·tro·nys·tag·mog·ra·phy [ˌ-ɪˌlektrəʊnɪˈstægməgrəfɪ] n abbr. PENG Photoelektronystagmographie f abbr. PENG.
pho·to·el·e·ment [ˌ-ˈeləmənt] n Photoelement nt, Solarzelle f.
pho·to·e·mis·sion [ˌ-ɪˈmɪʃn] n phys. Photoemission f.
pho·to·e·mul·sion [ˌ-ɪˈmʌlʃn] n Photoemulsion f.
pho·to·er·y·the·ma [ˌ-erəˈθiːmə] n Licht-, Photoerythem nt.
pho·to·es·thet·ic [ˌ-esˈθetɪk] adj lichtempfindlich, phot(o)ästhetisch.
pho·to·fluo·rog·ra·phy [ˌ-flʊəˈrɒgrəfɪ] n radiol. (Röntgen-)Schirmbildverfahren nt.
pho·to·gen [ˈ-dʒən] n bio., micro. photogener Mikroorganismus m.
pho·to·gene [ˈ-dʒiːn] n ophthal. Nachbild nt.
pho·to·gen·ic [ˌ-ˈdʒenɪk] adj 1. durch Licht verursacht, photogen. 2. Licht ausstrahlend, photogen, Leucht-.
photogenic epilepsy photogene/photosensible Epilepsie f.
pho·to·graph [ˈ-græf] I n Bild nt, Aufnahme f, Photographie f, Fotografie f, Photo nt. to take a ~ → photograph II. II vt eine Aufnahme machen, photographieren, fotografieren (of von). III vi fotografiert werden.
pho·tog·ra·pher [fəˈtɒgrəfər] n Photograph(in f) m, Fotograf(in f) m.
pho·to·graph·ic [ˌfəʊtəˈgræfɪk] adj photographisch, fotografisch, Bild-, Photo-, Foto-.
photographic library Bildarchiv nt.
photographic memory photographisches Gedächtnis nt.
pho·tog·ra·phy [fəˈtɒgrəfɪ] n Photographie f, Fotografie f.
pho·to·het·er·o·troph [ˌfəʊtəʊˈhetərətrɒf, -trəʊf] n bio. photoheterotropher Organismus m.
pho·to·het·er·o·troph·ic [ˌ-ˌhetərəˈtrɒfɪk, -trəʊf-] adj bio. photoheterotroph.
photoheterotrophic bacterium photoheterotrophes Bakterium nt.
pho·to·in·ac·ti·va·tion [ˌ-ɪnˌæktəˈveɪʃn] n Photoinaktivierung f.
pho·to·ki·ne·sis [ˌ-kɪˈniːsɪs, -kaɪ-] n Photokinese f.
pho·to·ki·net·ic [ˌ-kɪˈnetɪk] adj Photokinese betr., photokinetisch.
pho·to·ky·mo·graph [ˌ-ˈkaɪməgræf] n Photokymograph m.
pho·to·lith·o·troph [ˌ-ˈlɪθətrɒf, -trəʊf] n

photolithotropher Organismus m, Photolithotroph m.
pho·to·lith·o·troph·ic [ˌ-ˌlɪθəˈtrɒfɪk, -ˈtrəʊ-] adj photolithotroph.
pho·to·lu·mi·nes·cence [ˌ-ˌluːmɪˈnesəns] n Photolumineszenz f.
pho·tol·y·sis [fəʊˈtɒləsɪs] n chem. Photolyse f.
pho·to·lyt·ic [ˌfəʊtəʊˈlɪtɪk] adj Photolyse betr., photolytisch.
pho·to·ma [fəʊˈtəʊmə] n Photom nt.
pho·to·mag·net·ism [ˌfəʊtəʊˈmægnɪtɪzəm] n Photomagnetismus m.
pho·to·ma·nia [ˌ-ˈmeɪnɪə, -jə] n psychia. Photomanie f.
pho·tom·e·ter [fəʊˈtɒmɪtər] n Photometer nt.
pho·tom·e·try [fəʊˈtɒmətrɪ] n Photometrie f.
pho·to·mi·cro·graph [ˌfəʊtəˈmaɪkrəgræf] n Mikrophotographie f.
pho·to·mi·cro·graph·ic [ˌ-ˌmaɪkrəˈgræfɪk] adj mikrophotografisch.
pho·to·mi·crog·ra·phy [ˌ-maɪˈkrɒgrəfɪ] n Mikrophotografie f.
pho·to·mul·ti·plier [ˌ-ˈmʌltəplaɪər] n Photomultiplier m, Sekundärelektronenvervielfacher m abbr. SEV.
pho·ton [ˈfəʊtɒn] n Photon nt, Licht-, Strahlungsquant nt, Quant nt.
photon beam Photonenstrahl m.
pho·ton·o·sus [fəʊˈtɒnəsəs] n → photopathy.
pho·to·or·ga·no·troph [ˌfəʊtəʊɔːrˈgænətrɒf, -trəʊf] n photoorganotropher Organismus m, Photoorganotroph m.
pho·to·or·ga·no·troph·ic [ˌ-ˌɔːrgənəʊˈtrɒfɪk, -trəʊf-] adj photoorganotroph.
pho·top·a·thy [fəʊˈtɒpəθɪ] n durch Lichteinwirkung hervorgerufene Erkrankung f, Photopathie f.
pho·to·per·cep·tion [ˌfəʊtəpərˈsepʃn] n Lichtwahrnehmung f, Photoperzeption f.
pho·to·phil·ic [ˌ-ˈfɪlɪk] adj bio. photophil.
pho·to·pho·bia [ˌ-ˈfəʊbɪə] n Lichtscheu f, Photophobie f.
pho·to·pho·bic [ˌ-ˈfəʊbɪk] adj Photophobie betr., lichtscheu, photophob(isch).
pho·to·phos·pho·ryl·a·tion [ˌ-ˌfɒsfɔːrəˈleɪʃn] n photosynthetische Phosphorylierung f, Photophosphorylierung f.
pho·to·pia [fəʊˈtəʊpɪə] n → photopic vision.
pho·top·ic [fəʊˈtɒpɪk, -ˈtəʊp-] adj photopisch.
photopic adaptation physiol. Helladaptation f, -anpassung f.
photopic vision physiol. Tages(licht)sehen nt, photopisches Sehen nt.
pho·to·prod·uct [ˈfəʊtəʊprɒdʌkt, -dəkt] n Photoprodukt nt.
pho·top·sia [fəʊˈtɒpsɪə] n Photopsie f.
pho·top·sin [fəʊˈtɒpsɪn] n Photopsin nt.
pho·top·sy [fəʊˈtɒpsɪ] n → photopsia.
pho·top·tom·e·ter [fəʊtɒpˈtɒmɪtər] n ophthal. Photoptometer nt.
pho·top·tom·e·try [fəʊtɒpˈtɒmətrɪ] n Photoptometrie f.
pho·to·ra·di·om·e·ter [ˌfəʊtəʊˌreɪdɪˈɒmɪtər] n Photoradiometer nt.
pho·to·re·ac·tion [ˌ-rɪˈækʃn] n Photoreaktion f, photochemische Reaktion f.
pho·to·re·ac·ti·va·tion [ˌ-ˌrɪæktɪˈveɪʃn] n bio. Photoreaktivierung f.
pho·to·re·cep·tion [ˌ-rɪˈsepʃn] n physiol. Photorezeption f.
pho·to·re·cep·tive [ˌ-rɪˈseptɪv] adj physiol. photorezeptiv.
pho·to·re·cep·tor [ˌ-rɪˈseptər] n Photorezeptor m.
photoreceptor cell Photorezeptor-, Sehzelle f.

pho·to·re·duc·tion [ˌ-rɪ'dʌkʃn] *n* Photoreduktion *f*.
pho·to·res·pi·ra·tion [ˌ-ˌrespɪ'reɪʃn] *n bio.* Lichtatmung *f*, Photorespiration *f*.
pho·to·ret·i·ni·tis [ˌ-retə'naɪtɪs] *n ophthal.* aktinische Retinopathie *f*.
pho·to·ret·i·nop·a·thy [ˌ-ˌretɪ'nɑpəθɪ] *n* → photoretinitis.
pho·to·re·ver·sal [ˌ-rɪ'vɜrsl] *n* → photoreactivation.
photo reversal *radiol., photo.* Umkehrung *f*.
pho·to·scope ['fəʊtəskəʊp] *n radiol.* Fluoroskop *nt*.
pho·tos·co·py [fəʊ'tɑskəpɪ] *n radiol.* (Röntgen-)Durchleuchtung *f*, Fluoroskopie *f*.
pho·to·sen·si·tive [-'sensɪtɪv] *adj* lichtempfindlich.
pho·to·sen·si·tiv·i·ty [fəʊtəˌsensə'tɪvətɪ] *n* Lichtempfindlichkeit *f*.
pho·to·sen·si·ti·za·tion [fəʊtəˌsensətaɪ'zeɪʃn, -taɪ-] *n derm.* Photosensibilisierung *f*.
pho·to·sen·so·ry [-'sensərɪ] *adj* photo-, lichtsensibel.
photosensory layer of retina Schicht *f* der Stäbchen u. Zapfen, Stratum neuroepitheliale retinae.
pho·to·sta·ble ['fəʊtəsteɪbl] *adj* lichtstabil.
pho·to·syn·the·sis [-'sɪnθəsɪs] *n* Photosynthese *f*.
pho·to·syn·thet·ic [ˌfəʊtəsɪn'θetɪk] *adj* Photosynthese betr., mittels Photosynthese, photosynthetisch, Photosynthese(n)-.
photosynthetic bacteria photosynthetisch-aktive Bakterien *pl*, Photobakterien *pl*.
photosynthetic cell photosynthetisch-aktive Zelle *f*.
photosynthetic phosphorylation → photophosphorylation.
photosynthetic pigment Photosynthesepigment *nt*.
photosynthetic unit *bio.* photosynthetische Einheit *f*.
pho·to·tax·is [fəʊtə'tæksɪs] *n bio.* Photo-, Heliotaxis *f*.
pho·to·ther·a·py [ˌfəʊtə'θerəpɪ] *n* Licht-, Phototherapie *f*.
pho·to·tox·ic [fəʊtə'tɑksɪk] *adj* phototoxisch.
phototoxic dermatitis phototoxische Dermatitis *f*, phototoxisches Ekzem *nt*.
pho·to·trans·duc·tion [-trænz'dʌkʃn] *n* Phototransduktion *f*.
pho·to·troph ['fəʊtətrɑf, -trəʊf] *n* phototropher Organismus *m*, Phototroph *m*.
pho·to·troph·ic [ˌfəʊtə'trɑfɪk, -'trəʊf-] *adj* phototroph.
phototrophic bacteria Photobakterien *pl*.
pho·to·trop·ic [fəʊtə'trɑpɪk, -'trəʊ-] *adj* Phototropismus betr., phototrop(isch); heliotrop(isch).
pho·tot·ro·pism [fəʊ'tɑtrəpɪzəm] *n* Phototropismus *m*, Heliotropismus *m*.
pho·to·tur·bi·do·met·ric [-ˌtɜrbɪdə'metrɪk] *adj* phototurbidometrisch.
phrag·mo·plast ['frægməplæst] *n bio.* Phragmoplast *m*.
phren- *pref.* → phreno-.
phren ['fren, 'friːn] *n* 1. Zwerchfell *nt*, Phren *f*, Diaphragma *nt*. 2. Geist *m*, Verstand *m*; Seele *f*, Gemüt *nt*.
phre·nal·gia [frɪ'nældʒ(ɪ)ə] *n* Zwerchfellschmerz *m*, Phrenalgie *f*, Phrenikodynie *f*.
phre·nec·to·my [frɪ'nektəmɪ] *n chir.* Zwerchfellresektion *f*, Phrenektomie *f*.
phren·em·phrax·is [ˌfrenem'fræksɪs] *n* → phrenicotripsy.
phre·net·ic [frɪ'netɪk] I *n* 1. Maniker(in *f*)

m. 2. Wahnsinnige(r *m*) *f*, Rasende(r *m*) *f*, Verrückte(r *m*) *f*. II *adj* 3. an einer Manie leidend, manisch. 4. wahnsinnig, verrückt, irr(e).
phren·ic ['frenɪk] *adj* 1. Zwerchfell betr., diaphragmal, Zwerchfell-, Phreniko-. 2. Geist *od.* Seele betr., Geistes-, Seelen-, Phren(o)-, Psycho-.
phrenic artery: great p.ies untere Zwerchfellarterien *pl*, Aa. phrenicae inferiores.
inferior p.ies → great a.ies.
superior p. 1. A. pericardiacophrenica. 2. ˷s *pl* obere Zwerchfellarterien *pl*, Aa. phrenicae superiores.
phren·i·cec·to·my [frenɪ'sektəmɪ] *n* Phrenikusresektion *f*, -exhärese *f*, -ex(h)airese *f*, Phrenikektomie *f*.
phrenic center Centrum tendineum.
phrenic ganglia Ggll. phrenica.
phren·i·cla·sia [ˌfrenɪ'kleɪʒ(ɪ)ə] *n* → phrenicotripsy.
phren·i·cla·sis [ˌ-'kleɪsɪs] *n* → phrenicotripsy.
phrenic nerve Phrenikus *m*, N. phrenicus.
accessory p.s Nn. phrenici accessorii.
phrenic nucleus (of ventral column of spinal cord) Phrenikuskern *m*, Kern *m* des N. phrenicus, Nc. n. phrenici, Nc. phrenicus columnae ventralis medullae spinalis.
phrenico- *pref.* Zwerchfell-, Phrenik(o)-, Phren(o)-.
phren·i·co·ab·dom·i·nal branches of phrenic nerve [ˌfrenɪkəʊæb'dɑmɪnl] → phrenicoabdominal nerves.
phrenicoabdominal nerves Rami phrenicoabdominales n. phrenici.
phren·i·co·col·ic [ˌ-'kɑlɪk] *adj* Zwerchfell u. Kolon betr. *od.* verbindend, zwerchfellkolisch.
phrenicocolic ligament Lig. phrenicocolicum.
phren·i·co·cos·tal [ˌ-'kɑstl, -'kɔs-] *adj* Zwerchfell u. Rippen betr. *od.* verbindend, phrenikokostal, kostodiaphragmal.
phrenicocostal recess/sinus Kostodiaphragmalsinus *m*, -spalte *f*, Sinus phrenicocostalis, Rec. costodiaphragmaticus.
phren·i·co·e·soph·a·ge·al [ˌ-ɪˌsɑfə'dʒiːəl, -ˌɪsə'fædʒɪəl] *adj* Zwerchfell u. Ösophagus betr. *od.* verbindend, phrenikoösophageal.
phren·i·co·ex·ai·re·sis [ˌ-ek'saɪriːsɪs] *n* → phrenicectomy.
phren·i·co·ex·er·e·sis [ˌ-ek'serəsɪs] *n* → phrenicectomy.
phren·i·co·gas·tric [ˌ-'gæstrɪk] *adj* Zwerchfell u. Magen betr. *od.* verbindend, phrenikogastral, gastrodiaphragmal.
phren·i·co·col·ic ligament [ˌfrenɪ'kɑlɪk] → phrenicocolic ligament.
phren·i·co·li·e·nal [ˌfrenɪkəʊlaɪ'iːnl, -'laɪə-nl] *adj* → phrenicosplenic.
phrenicolienal ligament Lig. splenorenale/lienorenale/phrenicosplenicum.
phren·i·co·me·di·as·ti·nal [ˌ-ˌmɪdɪə'staɪnl] *adj* Zwerchfell u. Mediastinum betr. *od.* verbindend, phrenikomediastinal.
phrenicomediastinal recess Phrenikomediastinalsinus *m*, -spalte *f*, Rec. phrenicomediastinalis.
phren·i·co·neu·rec·to·my [ˌ-njʊə'rektəmɪ, -nɔ-] *n* → phrenicectomy.
phren·i·co·pleu·ral [ˌ-'plʊərəl] *adj* Zwerchfell u. Pleura betr. *od.* verbindend, phrenikopleural, pleurodiaphragmal.
phrenicopleural fascia Fascia phrenicopleuralis.
phren·i·co·splen·ic [ˌ-'spliːnɪk, -'splen-]

adj Zwerchfell u. Milz betr., phrenikolienal.
phrenicosplenic ligament Lig. splenorenale/lienorenale/phrenicosplenicum.
phren·i·cot·o·my [frenɪ'kɑtəmɪ] *n chir.* Phrenikusdurchtrennung *f*, Phrenikotomie *f*.
phren·i·co·trip·sy [ˌfrenɪkəʊ'trɪpsɪ] *n chir.* Phrenikusquetschung *f*, Phrenikotripsie *f*.
phrenic phenomenon Litten-Phänomen *nt*.
phrenic plexus Plexus phrenicus.
phrenic-pressure point Phrenikusdruckpunkt *m*.
phrenic veins: inferior p. untere Zwerchfellvenen *pl*, Vv. phrenicae inferiores.
superior p. obere Zwerchfellvenen *pl*, Vv. phrenicae superiores.
phrenic wave Litten-Phänomen *nt*.
phre·ni·tis [frɪ'naɪtɪs] *n* 1. Zwerchfellentzündung *f*, Diaphragmitis *f*. 2. *old* → delirium.
phreno- *pref.* Zwerchfell-, Phren(o)-, Phrenik(o)-; Phrenikus-.
phren·o·car·dia [ˌfrenəʊ'kɑːrdɪə] *n* DaCosta-Syndrom *nt*, Effort-Syndrom *nt*, Phrenikokardie *f*, neurozirkulatorische Asthenie *f*, Soldatenherz *nt*.
phren·o·col·ic [ˌ-'kɑlɪk] *adj* → phrenicocolic.
phren·o·cos·tal [ˌ-'kɑstl, -'kɔs-] *adj* → phrenicocostal.
phren·o·dyn·ia [ˌ-'dɪːnɪə] *n* → phrenalgia.
phren·o·e·soph·a·ge·al [ˌ-ɪˌsɑfə'dʒiːəl, -ˌɪsə'fædʒɪəl] *adj* → phrenicoesophageal.
phrenoesophageal membrane Membrana phrenico(e)osophagealis.
phren·o·gas·tric [ˌ-'gæstrɪk] *adj* → phrenicogastric.
phren·o·glot·tic [ˌ-'glɑtɪk] *adj* Zwerchfell u. Glottis betr., phrenikoglottisch.
phren·o·graph ['-græf] *n* Phrenograph *m*.
phren·o·he·pat·ic [ˌ-hɪ'pætɪk] *adj* Zwerchfell u. Leber betr. *od.* verbindend, phrenikohepatisch, hepatodiaphragmal.
phren·o·per·i·car·di·tis [ˌ-ˌperɪkɑr'daɪtɪs] *n* Phrenoperikarditis *f*.
phren·o·ple·gia [ˌ-'pliːdʒ(ɪ)ə] *n* Zwerchfelllähmung *f*.
phren·op·to·sia [ˌfrenɑp'təʊsɪə] *n* Zwerchfellsenkung *f*, -tiefstand *m*.
phren·o·sin ['frenəsɪn] *n* Phrenosin *nt*, Cerebron *nt*.
phren·o·sin·ic acid [ˌfrenəʊ'sɪnɪk] Cerebronsäure *f*.
phren·o·spasm ['-spæzəm] *n* Zwerchfellkrampf *m*, -spasmus *m*.
phren·o·splen·ic [ˌ-'spliːnɪk, -'splen-] *adj* → phrenicosplenic.
pH response *physiol.* pH-Antwort *f*.
phryg·i·an cap ['frɪdʒɪən] *radiol.* phrygische Mütze *f*.
phryn·o·der·ma [ˌfrɪnə'dɜrmə, ˌfraɪ-] *n derm.* Krötenhaut *f*, Phrynoderm *nt*, -dermie *f*, Hyperkeratosis follicularis (metabolica).
pH scale pH-Skala *f*.
phthal·ate ['(f)bæleɪt] *n* Phthalat *nt*.
phthal·ein ['(f)θæliːn, -lɪːn] *n* Phthalein *nt*.
phthal·ic acid ['(f)θælɪk] Phthalsäure *f*.
phthal·yl·sul·fa·thi·a·zole [θælɪlˌsʌlfə'θaɪəzəʊl] *n pharm.* Phthalylsulfathiazol *nt*.
phthin·oid chest ['θɪnɔɪd] langer flacher Thorax *m*.
phthi·o·ic acid [θaɪ'əʊɪk] Phthionsäure *f*.
phthi·ri·a·sis [θaɪ'raɪəsɪs] *n*, *pl* **-ses** [-siːz] Filzlausbefall *m*, Phthiriasis *f*, Phthiriase *f*, Pediculosis pubis.
Phthi·rus ['θaɪrəs] *n micro.* Phthirus *m*.
P. pubis Filzlaus *f*, Phthirus/Pediculus pubis.

phthisis

phthi·sis ['θaɪsɪs, 'taɪ-] *n*, *pl* **-ses** [-siːz] **1.** (Parenchym-)Schwund *m*, Schrumpfung *f*, Phthise *f*, Phthisis *f*. **2.** Schwindsucht *f*, Auszehrung *f*, Phthise *f*, Phthisis *f*. **3.** Lungenschwindsucht *f*, -tuberkulose *f*, Phthisis pulmonum.
phy·co·bi·lin [ˌfaɪkəʊ'baɪlɪn, -'bɪl-] *n* Phykobilin *nt*, Phycobilin *nt*.
phycobilin pigment Phycobilinpigment *nt*.
phy·co·cy·a·nin [ˌ-'saɪənɪn] *n* Phykozyanin *nt*, Phycocyanin *nt*.
phy·co·cy·an·o·gen [ˌ-saɪ'ænədʒən] *n* Phykozyanogen *nt*, Phycocyanogen *nt*.
phy·co·er·y·thrin [ˌ-'erəθrɪn, ɪ'rɪθ-] *n* Phyko-, Phycoerythrin *nt*.
phy·co·e·ryth·ro·bi·lin [ˌ-ˌɪˌrɪθrə'bɪliːn] *n* (Phyco-)Erythrobilin *nt*.
Phy·co·my·ce·tae [ˌ-maɪ'siːtiː] *pl* → Phycomycetes.
Phy·co·my·ce·tes [ˌ-maɪ'siːtiːz] *pl bio.*, *micro.* niedere Pilze *pl*, Algenpilze *pl*, Phykomyzeten *pl*, Phycomycetes *pl*.
phy·co·my·ce·to·sis [ˌ-maɪsɪ'təʊsɪs] *n* Phykomyzetose *f*.
phy·co·my·ce·tous [ˌ-maɪ'siːtəs] *adj* Phykomyzeten betr., Phykomyzeten-.
phy·co·my·co·sis [ˌ-maɪ'kəʊsɪs] *n* Phykomykose *f*, Mukormykose *f*.
phycomycosis entomophthorae Entomophthorose *f*, Entomophthora-Phykomykose *f*, Rhinophykomykose *f*.
phy·go·ga·lac·tic [ˌfaɪɡəʊɡə'læktɪk] *gyn*. **I** *n* die Milchsekretion hemmendes Mittel *nt*, Lakti-, Lactifugum *nt*. **II** *adj* die Milchsekretion hemmend, milchvermindernd, milchhemmend.
phy·la *n* → phylum.
phy·lac·tic [fɪ'læktɪk] *adj* schützend, phylaktisch.
phy·lax·is [fɪ'læksɪs] *n* Phylaxis *f*.
phy·let·ic [faɪ'letɪk] *adj* Phylum *od.* Phylogenese betr., phyletisch.
phyl·lode ['fɪləʊd] *adj* blattförmig, -ähnlich.
phyl·lo·qui·none [ˌfɪləʊkwɪ'nəʊn] *n* → phytonadione.
phy·lo·gen·e·sis [ˌ-'dʒenəsɪs] *n* → phylogeny.
phy·lo·ge·net·ic [ˌ-dʒə'netɪk] *adj* → phylogenic.
phy·lo·gen·ic [ˌ-'dʒenɪk] *adj* Phylogenese betr., stammesgeschichtlich, phylogenetisch.
phy·log·e·ny [faɪ'lɒdʒənɪ] *n* Stammesgeschichte *f*, Phylogenie *f*, Phylogenese *f*.
phy·lum ['faɪləm] *n*, *pl* **-la** [-lə] *bio.* Stamm *m*, Phylum *nt*.
phy·ma ['faɪmə] *n*, *pl* **-mas**, **-ma·ta** [-mətə] Geschwulst *f*, Gewächs *nt*, Knolle *f*, Phyma *nt*.
phys·a·lif·er·ous [ˌfɪsə'lɪfərəs, -ˌfaɪ-] *adj* blasig, blasenhaltig.
phy·sal·i·form [fɪ'sæləfɔːrm] *adj* blasenförmig, blasig.
phy·sal·i·phore [fɪ'sæləfəʊər, -fɔːr] *n patho.* Physaliphore *f*.
phys·a·liph·o·rous [ˌfɪsə'lɪfərəs, faɪ-] *adj* blasig, blasenhaltig.
phys·a·lis ['fɪsəlɪs] *n patho.* Wasserblase *f*, Physalis *f*.
Phys·a·lop·ter·a [faɪsə'lɒptərə] *pl micro.* Darmfadenwürmer *pl*, Physaloptera *pl*.
phys·a·lop·ter·i·a·sis [faɪsəˌlɒptə'raɪəsɪs] *n* Physaloptera-Infektion *f*, Physalopteriasis *f*.
phys·i·a·tri·cian [fɪzɪə'trɪʃn] *n* → physiatrist.
phys·i·at·rics [ˌfɪzɪ'ætrɪks] *pl* Naturheilkunde *f*, Physiatrie *f*.
phys·i·at·rist [fɪzɪ'ætrɪst, fɪ'zaɪə-] *n* Naturheilkundige(r *m*) *f*, Physiater(in *f*) *m*.

phy·si·a·try [fɪ'zaɪətrɪ] *n* → physiatrics.
phys·ic ['fɪzɪk] **I** *n* **1.** Abführmittel *nt*, Laxans *nt*, Laxativ(um) *nt*. **2.** Arznei(mittel *nt*) *f*, Medikament *nt*. **II** *vt* **3.** jdm. ein Abführmittel verabreichen. **4.** mit Medikamenten behandeln.
phys·i·cal ['fɪzɪkl] **I** *n* → physical examination. **II** *adj* **1.** Körper betr., physisch, körperlich, Körper-, Physio-. **2.** Physik betr., physikalisch; naturwissenschaftlich.
physical allergy physikalische Allergie *f*.
physical anthropology biologische Anthropologie *f*.
physical chemistry physikalische Chemie *f*, Physikochemie *f*.
physical condition körperliche/physische Verfassung *f*, Gesundheitszustand *m*.
physical deformity körperliche Entstellung *f*.
physical dependence körperliche Abhängigkeit *f*.
physical diagnosis Diagnose *f* durch körperliche Untersuchung.
physical education *abbr.* **PE** → physical training.
physical examination *abbr.* **PE** körperliche Untersuchung *f*.
physical fatigue körperliche/physische Ermüdung *f*.
physical findings körperlicher Untersuchungsbefund *m*.
physical geography Physiogeographie *f*, physische Geographie *f*.
physical handicap Körperbehinderung *f*.
physical jerks *Brit. inf.* gymnastische Übungen *pl*, Gymnastik *f*.
physical load physische/körperliche Belastung *f*.
phys·i·cal·ly-handicapped ['fɪzɪklɪ] *adj* körperlich behindert.
physical medicine → physiatrics.
physical mutagen physikalisches Mutagen *nt*.
physical performance physische/körperliche Leistung *f*.
physical properties physikalische Eigenschaften *pl*.
physical science Naturwissenschaft(en *pl*) *f*.
physical scientist Naturwissenschaftler(in *f*) *m*.
physical sign objektives Zeichen *nt*.
physical solution physikalische Lösung *f*.
physical status Allgemeinzustand *m*, Status *m*.
physical therapist Heilgymnastiker(in *f*) *m*, Physiotherapeut(in *f*) *m*.
physical therapy 1. Bewegungstherapie *f*, Kranken-, Heilgymnastik *f*. **2.** physikalische Therapie *f*, Physiotherapie *f*.
physical training *abbr.* **PT** Sport *m*; (*Schule*) Leibeserziehung *f*.
physical treatment physikalische Behandlung/Therapie *f*.
physical work körperliche/physische Arbeit *f*.
physical work capacity *abbr.* **PWC₁₇₀**, **W₁₇₀** Arbeitskapazität *f* *abbr.* PCW₁₇₀, W₁₇₀.
phy·si·cian [fɪ'zɪʃn] *n* **1.** (praktischer) Arzt *m*, (praktische) Ärztin *f*. **2.** Arzt/Ärztin für Innere Krankheiten, Internist(in *f*) *m*.
phys·i·cist ['fɪzəsɪst] *n* Physiker(in *f*) *m*.
phys·i·co·chem·i·cal [ˌfɪzɪkəʊ'kemɪkl] *adj* physikalische Chemie betr., physikochemisch.
phys·i·co·ther·a·peu·tics [ˌ-ˌθerə'pjuːtɪks] *pl* → physical therapy.
phys·i·co·ther·a·py [ˌ-'θerəpɪ] *n* → physical therapy.
phys·ics ['fɪzɪks] *pl* Physik *f*.

phys·i·o·chem·i·cal [ˌfɪzɪəʊ'kemɪkl] *adj* Biochemie betr., biochemisch.
phys·i·o·chem·is·try [ˌ-'kemɪstrɪ] *n* **1.** physiologische Chemie *f*, Biochemie *f*. **2.** klinische Chemie *f*.
phys·i·o·gen·e·sis [ˌ-'dʒenəsɪs] *n* Embryologie *f*.
phys·i·og·no·my [fɪzɪ'ɒɡnəmɪ] *n* **1.** Physiognomie *f*. **2.** → physiognosis.
phys·i·og·no·sis [fɪzɪəɡ'nəʊsɪs] *n* Physiognomik *f*.
phys·i·o·log·ic [ˌfɪzɪə'lɒdʒɪk] *adj* **1.** normal, natürlich, physiologisch. **2.** Physiologie betr., physiologisch.
phys·i·o·log·i·cal [ˌ-'lɒdʒɪkl] *adj* → physiologic.
physiological anatomy physiologische Anatomie *f*.
physiological anemia *ped.* physiologische Anämie *f*, Drei-Monats-Anämie *f*.
physiological antidote physiologisches Antidot *nt*.
physiological buffer *biochem.*, *physiol.* physiologischer Puffer *m*.
physiologic albuminuria 1. physiologische Albuminurie/Proteinurie *f*. **2.** funktionelle Albuminurie/Proteinurie *f*.
physiological chemistry physiologische Chemie *f*, Biochemie *f*.
physiological cup Pupillenexkavation *f*, Excavatio pupillae/disci n. optici *f*.
physiological dependence körperliche Abhängigkeit *f*.
physiological diplopia *ophthal.* physiologische/stereoskopische Diplopie *f*.
physiological scotoma → physiological scotoma.
physiologic amenorrhea *gyn.* physiologische Amenorrhoe *f*.
physiologic astigmatism *ophthal.* physiologischer Astigmatismus *m*.
physiologic atrophy physiologische Atrophie *f*.
physiologic congestion physiologische Hyperämie *f*.
physiologic cup → physiological cup.
physiologic hypertrophy physiologische Hypertrophie *f*.
physiologic hypogammaglobulinemia physiologische Hypogammaglobulinämie *f*.
physiologic icterus physiologischer Neugeborenenikterus *m*.
physiologic jaundice physiologischer Neugeborenenikterus *m*.
physiologic leukocytosis physiologische Leukozytose *f*.
phys·i·o·log·i·co·a·nat·om·i·cal [fɪzɪəˌlɒdʒɪkəʊˌænə'tɒmɪkl] *adj* physiologisch-anatomisch.
physiologic presbycusis *ophthal.* physiologische Altersschwerhörigkeit *f*, Presbyakusis *f*.
physiologic proteinuria → physiologic albuminuria.
physiologic saline (solution) physiologische Kochsalzlösung *f*.
physiologic scotoma *ophthal.* physiologisches Skotom *nt*.
physiologic strain physiologische Belastung *f*.
phys·i·ol·o·gist [ˌfɪzɪ'ɒlədʒɪst] *n* Physiologe *m*, -login *f*.
phys·i·ol·o·gy [ˌ-'ɒlədʒɪ] *n* Physiologie *f*.
phys·i·o·pa·thol·o·gy [ˌfɪzɪəʊpə'θɒlədʒɪ] *n* Pathophysiologie *f*.
phys·i·o·ther·a·peu·tist [ˌ-ˌθerə'pjuːtɪst] *n* → physical therapist.
phys·i·o·ther·a·pist [ˌ-'θerəpɪst] *n* → physical therapist.
phys·i·o·ther·a·py [ˌ-'θerəpɪ] *n* → physical therapy 1.

phy·sique [fɪ'ziːk] n Körperbau m, Konstitution f, Statur f.
physo- pref. Luft-, Gas-, Physo-.
phy·so·cele ['faɪzəsiːl] n Phyozele f.
phy·so·hem·a·to·me·tra [ˌ-ˌheməto'miːtrə] n gyn. Physohämatometra f.
phy·so·hy·dro·me·tra [ˌ-haɪdrə'miːtrə] n gyn. Physohydrometra f.
phy·so·me·tra [ˌ-'miːtrə] n gyn. Physometra f, Uterustympanie f, Tympania uteri.
phy·so·py·o·sal·pinx [ˌ-ˌpaɪə'sælpɪŋks] n gyn. Physopyosalpinx f.
phy·so·stig·mine [ˌ-'stɪgmiːn] n Physostigmin nt, Eserin nt.
phy·so·stig·min·ism [ˌ-'stɪgmənɪzəm] n Physostigminvergiftung f, Physostigminismus m, Eserismus m.
phyt- pref. → phyto-.
phyt·ag·glu·ti·nin [ˌfaɪtə'gluːtɪnɪn] n Phytagglutinin nt.
phy·tan·ic acid [faɪ'tænɪk] Phytansäure f.
phytanic acid α-hydroxylase Phytansäureoxidase f, Phytansäure-α-hydroxylase f.
phytanic acid storage disease Refsum--Syndrom nt, Heredopathia atactica polyneuritiformis.
phy·tase ['faɪteɪz] n Phytase f.
phy·tic acid ['faɪtɪk] Phytinsäure f.
phy·tin ['faɪtn] n Phytin nt.
phyto- pref. Pflanzen-, Phyt(o)-.
phy·to·be·zoar [ˌfaɪtəʊ'biːzɔːr, -zəʊr] n Phytobezoar m.
phy·to·chem·is·try [ˌ-'kemɪstrɪ] n Phytochemie f.
phy·to·cho·les·ter·ol [ˌ-kə'lestərəʊl, -rɒl] n → phytosterol.
phy·to·hem·ag·glu·ti·nin [ˌ-ˌhiːmə'gluːtənɪn] n abbr. **PHA** Phytohämagglutinin nt abbr. PHA.
phy·to·hor·mone [ˌ-'hɔːrməʊn] n Pflanzenhormon nt, Phytohormon nt.
phy·toid ['faɪtɔɪd] adj pflanzenähnlich, -artig, phytoid.
phy·tol ['faɪtɒl, -tɒl] n Phytol nt.
Phy·to·mas·ti·goph·o·ra [ˌ-ˌmæstɪ'gɒf(ə)rə] pl → Phytomastigophorea.
Phy·to·mas·ti·goph·o·rea [ˌ-ˌmæstɪˌgɒfə'rɪə] pl bio. Phytomastigophorea pl.
phy·to·mel·in [ˌ-'melɪn] n Rutin nt, Rutosid nt.
phy·to·men·a·di·one [ˌ-ˌmenə'daɪəʊn] n → phytonadione.
phy·to·mi·to·gen [ˌ-'maɪtədʒən] n Phytomitogen nt.
phy·ton·o·sis [faɪ'tɒnəsɪs] n Phytonose f.
phy·to·na·di·one [ˌfaɪtəʊnə'daɪəʊn] n Phyto(me)nadion nt, Vitamin K₁ nt.
phy·to·par·a·site [ˌ-'pærəsaɪt] n pflanzlicher Parasit m, Phytoparasit m.
phy·toph·a·gous [faɪ'tɒfəgəs] adj pflanzenfressend, phytophag; vegetarisch.
phy·to·pho·to·der·ma·ti·tis [ˌfaɪtəˌfəʊtəʊˌdɜrmə'taɪtɪs] n 1. Phytophotodermatitis f. 2. → phytophototoxic dermatitis.
phy·to·pho·to·tox·ic dermatitis [ˌ-ˌfəʊtəʊ'tɒksɪk] Wiesengräserdermatitis f, Wiesengrasdermatitis f, Pflanzendermatitis f, Phyto-, Photodermatitis f, Dermatitis (bullosa) pratensis, Photodermatitis phytogenica.
phy·to·plank·ton [ˌ-'plæŋktən] n Phytoplankton nt.
phy·to·sphin·go·sine [ˌ-'sfɪŋgəsiːn, -sɪn] n Phytosphingosin nt, 4-Hydroxysphinganin nt.
phy·tos·te·rin [faɪ'tɒstərɪn] n → phytosterol.
phy·tos·te·rol [faɪ'tɒstərɒl, -rɒl] n Phytosterol nt, -sterin nt.
phy·to·ther·a·py [ˌfaɪtə'θerəpɪ] n Phytotherapie f.

phy·to·tox·in [ˌ-'tɒksɪn] n Phytotoxin nt.
phy·to·trich·o·be·zoar [ˌ-ˌtrɪkə'biːzɔːr, -zəʊr] n Phytotrichobezoar m.
PI abbr. → phosphatidylinositol.
pi- pref. → pio-.
pia ['paɪə, 'piːə] I n → pia mater. II adj anat. weich.
pia-arachnitis n Entzündung f von Pia u. Arachnoidea, Leptomeningitis f.
pia-arachnoid n weiche Hirn- u. Rückenmarkshaut f, Leptomeninx f.
pia-glial barrier Pia-Glia-Barriere f, -Schranke f.
pi·al ['paɪəl, 'piː-] adj Pia mater betr., pial, Pia-.
pial sheath Piascheide f des N. opticus.
pia ma·ter ['meɪtər] Pia f, Pia mater.
cranial p. Pia mater cranialis/encephali.
spinal p. Pia mater spinalis.
pi·a·ma·tral [ˌpaɪə'meɪtrəl] adj → pial.
pi·an [pɪ'ɑːn, 'piːæn] n Frambösie f, Pian f, Parangi f, Yaws f, Framboesia tropica.
pian bois derm. südamerikanische Hautleishmaniase f, kutane Leishmaniase Südamerikas f, Chiclero-Ulkus nt.
pi·a·rach·ni·tis [ˌpaɪəˌræk'naɪtɪs] n → pia-arachnitis.
pi·a·rach·noid [ˌ-'ræknɔɪd] n → pia-arachnoid.
pi·ca ['paɪkə, 'piː-] n Pica-Syndrom nt, Pikazismus m.
Pi·chin·de virus [pɪ'tʃɪndɪ] Pichinde-Virus nt.
Pick [pɪk] **P.'s bodies** → P.'s inclusion bodies.
P.'s cells Niemann-Pick-Zellen pl.
P.'s cirrhosis Pick'-Zirrhose f, perikarditische Pseudoleberzirrhose f.
P.'s disease 1. Pick'-(Hirn-)Atrophie f, -Krankheit f, -Syndrom nt. **2.** Niemann--Pick-Krankheit f, Sphingomyelinose f, Sphingomyelinlipidose f. **3.** → P.'s cirrhosis.
P.'s inclusion bodies Pick'-Einschlußkörper pl.
P.'s syndrome → P.'s disease 1.
P.'s tubular adenoma Androblastom nt.
pick·er's acne ['pɪkər] derm. Akne/Acne excoriée des jeunes filles.
pick·wick·i·an syndrome [pɪk'wɪkɪən] Pickwick-Syndrom nt, Pickwickier-Syndrom nt, kardiopulmonales Syndrom nt der Adipösen.
pico- pref. abbr. **p** Piko-, Pico- abbr. p.
pi·co·cu·rie [ˌpaɪkə'kjʊərɪ, -kjʊə'rɪ] n abbr. **pCi** Picocurie nt abbr. pCi.
pi·cod·na·vi·rus [paɪˌkɒdnə'vaɪrəs] n → Parvovirus.
pi·cod·na·vi·rus·es [paɪˌkɒdnə'vaɪrəsəs] pl → Parvoviridae.
pi·co·gram ['paɪkəgræm] n abbr. **pg** Picogramm nt abbr. pg.
pi·co·kat·al [ˌ-'kætæl] n abbr. **pkat** Picokatal nt abbr. pkat.
pic·o·lin·ic acid [ˌpɪkə'lɪnɪk] Picolinsäure f.
Pi·cor·na·vir·i·dae [paɪˌkɔːrnə'vɪrɪdiː, -'vaɪr-] pl micro. Picornaviren pl, Picornaviridae pl.
pi·cor·na·vi·rus [paɪˌkɔːrnə'vaɪrəs] n micro. Picornavirus nt.
pic·rate ['pɪkreɪt] n Pikrat nt.
pic·ric acid ['pɪkrɪk] Pikrinsäure f, Trinitrophenol nt.
pic·ro·geu·sia [ˌpɪkrəʊ'gjuːʒ(ɪ)ə] n neuro. Pikrogeusie f.
pic·ro·tox·in [ˌ-'tɒksɪn] n Pikrotoxin nt, Cocculin f.
pic·ro·tox·i·nism [ˌ-'tɒksɪnɪzəm] n Pikrotoxinvergiftung f.
pic·to·ri·al aphasia [pɪk'tɔːrɪəl, -'tɔʊr-] neuro. Total-, Globalaphasie f.

pigmental degeneration

pic·ture ['pɪktʃər] I n 1. Bild nt; photographische Aufnahme f; Illustration f. 2. Vorstellung f; (geistiges) Bild nt. 3. fig. Schilderung f, Darstellung f. II vt 4. abbilden; darstellen, beschreiben. 5. s. vorstellen.
PID abbr. → pelvic inflammatory disease.
pie·bald·ism ['paɪbɔːldɪzəm] n derm. partieller/umschriebener Albinismus m, Albinismus circumscriptus, Piebaldismus m.
pie·bald·ness ['paɪbɔːldnɪs] n → piebaldism.
pie·bald skin ['paɪbɔːld] derm. Weißfleckenkrankheit f, Scheckhaut f, Vitiligo f.
piece [piːs] n Stück nt; Teil m/nt; Einzelteil nt. **to go to ~s** inf. (Person) zusammenbrechen, "durchdrehen". **in ~s** in Stücken, kaputt. **to take to ~s** auseinandernehmen, (in Einzelteile) zerlegen.
piece·meal necrosis ['piːsmiːl] patho. Mottenfraßnekrose f.
pi·e·dra [pɪ'eɪdrə, 'pjeɪ-] n derm. Haarknötchenkrankheit f, Piedra f, Trichosporie f, Trichosporose f.
Pi·e·drai·a [pɪ'eɪdraɪə] n micro. Piedraia f. **P. hortai** Piedraia/Trichosporon/Microsporon hortai.
Pi·e·drai·a·ce·ae [ˌpaɪdraɪ'eɪsiːɪ] pl micro. Piedraiaceae pl.
pierce [pɪərs] I vt durchbohren, -stechen, -stoßen; fig. durchdringen; techn. durchlöchern, perforieren. II vi (ein-)dringen (into in).
pierc·er ['pɪərsər] n techn. Bohrer m.
pierc·ing ['pɪərsɪŋ] adj durchdringend, stechend, schneidend.
piercing pain stechender Schmerz m, stechende Schmerzen pl.
Pierre Robin [pjɛːr rɔ'bɛ̃]: **P. R. anomalad/syndrome** Pierre Robin-Syndrom nt, Robin-Syndrom nt.
pi·es·es·the·sia [paɪˌiːzes'θiːʒ(ɪ)ə] n Druckempfindlichkeit f, Drucksinn m.
pi·e·sim·e·ter [paɪɪ'sɪmətər] n phys. Piezometer nt.
pi·e·sis ['paɪəsɪs] n Blutdruck m.
pi·e·som·e·ter [paɪɪ'sɒmɪtər] n → piesimeter.
pi·ez·es·the·sia [ˌpaɪɪzes'θiːʒ(ɪ)ə] n → piesesthesia.
pi·e·zo·car·di·o·gram [pɪˌeɪzəʊ'kɑːrdɪəgræm, paɪˌiːzəʊ-] n Piezokardiogramm nt.
pi·e·zo·chem·is·try [ˌ-'kemɪstrɪ] n Piezochemie f.
pi·e·zo·e·lec·tric [ˌ-ɪ'lektrɪk, ˌiːzəʊ-] adj phys. piezoelektrisch, druckelektrisch.
piezoelectric effect Piezoeffekt m, Piezoelektrizität f.
pi·e·zo·e·lec·tric·i·ty [ˌ-ɪlek'trɪsətɪ] n → piezoelectric effect.
pi·e·zom·e·ter [paɪɪ'zɒmɪtər] n → piesimeter.
PIF abbr. → prolactin inhibiting factor.
pig·bel ['pɪgbel] n Darmbrand m, Enteritis necroticans.
pi·geon breast ['pɪdʒən] Kiel-, Hühnerbrust f, Pectus gallinatum/carinatum.
pigeon-breasted adj hühnerbrüstig.
pigeon-breeder's lung Vogel-, Taubenzüchterlunge f.
pigeon chest → pigeon breast.
pigeon tick micro. Argas reflexus.
pig·ment ['pɪgmənt] I n Farbe f, Farbstoff m, -körper m, farbgebende Substanz f, Pigment nt. II vt pigmentieren, färben. III vi s. pigmentieren, s. färben.
pig·men·tal [pɪg'mentl] adj → pigmentary.
pigmental degeneration → pigmentary degeneration.

pigmentary

pig·men·tar·y ['pɪgmən‚teri:, -tərɪ] *adj* Pigment betr., pigmentär, Pigment-.
pigmentary cirrhosis Pigmentzirrhose *f*, Cirrhosis pigmentosa.
pigmentary degeneration Pigmentdegeneration *f*.
  primary p. of retina *ophthal*. tapetoretinale Degeneration.
pigmentary epithelium → pigmented epithelium.
pigmentary glaucoma Pigmentglaukom *nt*.
pigmentary retinopathy Retinitis/Retinopathia pigmentosa.
pig·men·ta·tion [‚pɪgmən'teɪʃn] *n* Färbung *f*, Pigmentierung *f*, Pigmentation *f*.
pigment calculus Pigmentstein *m*.
pigment cell pigmenthaltige Zelle *f*.
pigment cirrhosis → pigmentary cirrhosis.
pig·ment·ed ['pɪgmentɪd] *adj* pigmentiert, pigmenthaltig.
pigmented ameloblastoma Melanoameloblastom *nt*.
pigmented epithelium pigmenthaltiges Epithel *nt*.
  p. of iris pigmenthaltiges Irisepithel, Epithelium pigmentosum iridis.
pigmented epulis Melanoameloblastom *nt*.
pigmented hairy epidermal nevus Becker-Nävus *m*, -Melanose *f*, Melanosis naeviformis.
pigmented layer: p. of ciliary body → pigmented stratum of ciliary body.
  p. of iris Stratum pigmenti iridis.
  p. of retina → pigmented stratum of retina.
pigmented line of the cornea *ophthal*. Stähli'-Linie.
pigmented mole → pigmented nevus.
pigmented nevus Pigmentnävus *m*, Naevus pigmentosis.
pigmented part of retina → pigmented stratum of retina.
pigmented purpuric lichenoid dermatitis (Gougerot-)Blum-Syndrom *nt*, lichenoide Purpura *f*, Gougerot-Dermatitis *f*, Dermatitis lichenoides purpurica et pigmentosa, Dermatite lichénoïde purpurique et pigmentée.
pigmented purpuric lichenoid dermatosis → pigmented purpuric lichenoid dermatitis.
pigmented stratum: p. of ciliary body Pigmentepithel *nt* des Ziliarkörpers, Stratum pigmenti coporis ciliaris.
  p. of retina Pigmentepithel *nt* der Netzhaut, Stratum pigmenti, Pars pigmentosa (retinae).
pigmented tumor Pigmenttumor *m*.
pigmented villonodular arthritis → pigmented villonodular synovitis.
pigmented villonodular synovitis *abbr*. PVNS pigmentierte villonoduläre Synovitis *f abbr*. PVNS, benignes Synovialom *nt*, Riesenzelltumor *m* der Sehnenscheide, Tendosynovitis nodosa, Arthritis villonodularis pigmentosa.
pigment granules Pigmentgranula *pl*.
pigment metastasis Pigmentmetastase *f*.
pig·men·to·gen·e·sis [pɪg‚mentəʊ'dʒenəsɪs] *n* Pigmentbildung *f*.
pig·men·tol·y·sin [pɪgmən'tɒləsɪn] *n immun*. Pigmentolysin *nt*.
pig·men·tol·y·sis [‚-'tɒləsɪs] *n* Pigmentauflösung *f*, -zerstörung *f*, Pigmentolyse *f*.
pig·men·to·phage [pɪg'mentəfeɪdʒ] *n* Pigmentophage *m*.
pigment stone Pigmentstein *m*.
pig·my ['pɪgmɪ] → pygmy.
PIH *abbr*. [prolactin inhibiting hormone]

→ prolactin inhibiting factor.
pi·i·tis [paɪ'aɪtɪs] *n* Entzündung *f* der Pia mater, Piaentzündung *f*.
pil- *pref*. → pilo-.
pi·lar ['paɪlər] *adj* Haar betr., haarig, pilär, pilar, Haar-, Pilo-, Tricho-.
pilar cyst piläre Hautzyste *f*.
pi·la·ry ['paɪlərɪ] *adj* → pilar.
pi·las·ter of Broca [pɪ'læstər] *anat*. Linea aspera.
pile [paɪl] *n* **1.** Haufen *m*, Stapel *m*, Stoß *m*. **2.** *phys*. (galvanische/voltaische) Säule *f*. **3.** *phys*. (Atom-)Meiler *m*, (Kern-)Reaktor *m*. **4.** *sing*. → piles.
piles [paɪlz] *pl* Hämorrhoiden *pl*.
pi·li ['paɪlaɪ] *pl* **1.** → pilus. **2.** *bio*. Pili *pl*, Fimbrien *pl*.
pi·li·al ['paɪlɪəl] *adj* Pilus betr., Pilus-.
pi·li·ate ['paɪlɪeɪt, -ɪt] *adj bio.*, *micro*. pilitragend.
pi·lif·e·rous cyst [paɪ'lɪfərəs] Pilonidalzyste *f*.
pil·i·form ['pɪləfɔːrm] *adj* haarförmig, -artig.
pi·lin ['paɪlɪn] *n* Pilusprotein *nt*.
pilin protein → pilin.
pill [pɪl] *pharm*. I *n* **1.** *pharm*. Pille *f*; Dragee *nt*, Pilula *f*. **2. the ~** die (Antibaby-)Pille *f*. **to be/go on the ~** die Pille nehmen. II *vt* Pillen drehen.
pil·lar ['pɪlər] *n* Säule *f*, Pfeiler *m*; (Wasser-, Rauch-)Säule *f*.
  p.s of Corti's organ → pillar cells (of Corti).
  p. of fauces Gaumenbogen *m*.
pillar cells (of Corti) (*Ohr*) Pfeilerzellen *pl*, Corti'-Pfeilerzellen *pl*.
  external p. äußere Pfeilerzellen.
  internal p. innere Pfeilerzellen.
pill-box ['pɪlbɒks] *n* Pillenschachtel *f*.
pil·let ['pɪlət] *n pharm*. kleine Pille *f*.
pill-head ['pɪlhed] *n sl*. Tablettensüchtige(r *m*) *f*.
pill-rolling *n neuro*. Pillendrehen *nt*, Münzenzählen *nt*.
pilo- *pref*. Haar-, Tricho-, Pil(o)-.
pi·lo·be·zoar [‚paɪləʊ'biːzɔːr, -zəʊr] Trichobezoar *m*.
pi·lo·car·pine [‚-'kɑːrpiːn] *n pharm*. Pilocarpin *nt*.
pi·lo·e·rec·tion [‚-ɪ'rekʃn] *n* Piloarrektion *f*, -erektion *f*, Pilo(motoren)reaktion *f*.
pi·loid ['paɪlɔɪd] *adj* haarähnlich, -artig, -förmig.
pi·lo·ma·tri·co·ma [‚paɪlə‚mætrɪ'kəʊmə] *n* → pilomatrixoma.
pi·lo·ma·trix·o·ma [‚-meɪtrɪk'səʊmə] *n derm*. Pilomatrixom *nt*, Pilomatricoma *nt*, verkalktes Epitheliom *nt*, Epithelioma calcificans (Malherbe).
pi·lo·mo·tor·func·tion [‚-‚məʊtər'fʌŋkʃn] *n* Pilomotorik *f*.
pi·lo·mo·tor reflex [‚-'məʊtər] Pilomotorenreaktion *f*.
pi·lo·ni·dal cyst [‚-'naɪdl] Pilonidalzyste *f*.
pilonidal fistula Pilonidalsinus *m*, -fistel *f*, Fistula pilonidalis.
pilonidal sinus → pilonidal fistula.
pi·lose ['paɪləʊs] *adj* mit Haaren bedeckt, haarig.
pi·lo·se·ba·ceous [‚paɪləʊsɪ'beɪʃəs] *adj* Haarfollikel u. Talgdrüsen betr.
Piltz-Westphal [pɪlts vɛstfɑːl]: **P.-W. phenomenon** Westphal-Piltz-Phänomen *nt*, Orbikularisphänomen *nt*, Lid-Pupillen-Reflex *m*.
pil·u·la ['pɪljələ] *n*, *pl* **-lae** [-liː] → pill 1.
pil·u·lar ['pɪljələr] *adj pharm*. Pille betr., pillenartig, -ähnlich, Pillen-, Tabletten-.
pil·ule ['pɪljuːl] *n* kleine Pille *f*.
pi·lus ['paɪləs] *n*, *pl* **-li** [-laɪ] **1.** *anat*. Haar *nt*, Pilus *m*. **2.** *sing*. → pili 2.

pi·mar·i·cin [pɪ'mærɪsɪn, paɪ-] *n pharm*. Pimaricin *nt*, Natamycin *nt*.
pimel- *pref*. → pimelo-.
pi·mel·ic acid [pə'melɪk] Pimelinsäure *f*.
pim·e·li·tis [‚pɪmə'laɪtɪs] *n* Fettgewebsentzündung *f*, Pimelitis *f*; Panniculitis *f*.
pimelo- *pref*. Fett-, Pimel(o)-, Lip(o)-.
pim·e·lo·ma [‚-'ləʊmə] *n* Fett(gewebs)geschwulst *f*, -tumor *m*, Lipom(a) *nt*.
pim·e·lop·te·ryg·i·um [‚pɪmələʊtə'rɪdʒɪəm] *n ophthal*. Pimelopterygium *nt*.
pim·e·lor·rhea [‚-'rɪə] *n* Fettdurchfall *m*, -diarrhoe *f*, Steatorrhoe *f*.
pim·e·lo·sis [‚pɪmə'ləʊsɪs] *n* **1.** *patho*. degenerative Verfettung *f*, fettige Degeneration *f*, Degeneratio adiposa. **2.** Fettleibigkeit *f*, Fettsucht *f*, Adipositas *f*, Obesitas *f*.
pim·e·lu·ria [‚-'l(j)ʊərɪə] *n* Fettausscheidung *f* im Harn; Lipidurie *f*.
pi·mo·zide ['paɪməsaɪd] *n pharm*. Pimozid *nt*.
pim·ple ['pɪmpəl] I *n* Pickel *m*, Pustel *f*. II *vi* pick(e)lig werden.
pim·pled ['pɪmpəld] *adj* pick(e)lig, pustelig.
pim·ply ['pɪmplɪ] *adj* → pimpled.
pin [pɪn] I *n* **1.** (Steck-)Nadel *f*. **2.** *ortho*. Nagel *m*; Spickdraht *m*. II *vt* **3.** heften, stecken, festmachen, befestigen. **4.** *ortho*. nageln.
Pinard [pi'nɑːr]: **P.'s maneuver** *gyn*. Pinard'-Handgriff *m*.
Pinaud [pi'no]: **P.'s triangle** Pirogoff'-Dreieck *nt*.
pinc·er nail syndrome ['pɪnsər] Pincernail-Syndrom *nt*.
pin·cers ['pɪnsərz] *pl* (Kneif-, Beiß-)Zange *f*; Pinzette *f*.
pinch [pɪntʃ] I *n* Kneifen *nt*, Zwicken *nt*, Quetschen *nt*. II *vt* **1.** zwicken, kneifen, quetschen, klemmen. **2.** *fig*. drücken, beengen, beschränken. **3.** *fig*. (*Kälte*) beißen; (*Durst*, *Hunger*) plagen, quälen. III *vi* **4.** drücken, kneifen, zwicken. **5.** *fig*. quälen.
pinch graft Reverdin-Läppchen *nt*, -Lappen *m*, Hautinseln *pl*.
pin·do·lol ['pɪndəlɒl, -lɑl] *n pharm*. Pindolol *nt*.
pi·ne·al ['pɪnɪəl, 'paɪ-] I *n* Zirbel-, Pinealdrüse *f*, Pinea *f*, Corpus pineale, Gl. pinealis, Epiphyse *f*, Epiphysis cerebri. II *adj* Zirbeldrüse betr., pineal, Pineal(o)-.
pineal body → pineal I.
pineal cell Pinealozyt *m*, Pinealzelle *f*.
pi·ne·al·ec·to·my [‚pɪnɪə'lektəmɪ] *n neurochir*. Entfernung *f* der Zirbeldrüse, Pinealektomie *f*.
pineal gland → pineal I.
pi·ne·a·lo·blas·to·ma [‚pɪnɪələʊblæs'təʊmə] *n* Pinealoblastom *nt*.
pi·ne·a·lo·cyte [‚-saɪt] *n* → pineal cell.
pi·ne·a·lo·cy·to·ma [‚-saɪ'təʊmə] *n* → pinealoma.
pi·ne·a·lo·ma [pɪnɪə'ləʊmə] *n* Pinealom *nt*, Pinealozytom *nt*.
pi·ne·a·lop·a·thy [pɪnɪə'lɒpəθɪ] *n* Erkrankung *f* der Zirbeldrüse, Pinealopathie *f*.
pineal peduncle Zirbeldrüsen-, Epiphysenstiel *m*, Habenula *f*.
pineal recess Rec. pinealis.
pineal syndrome → Pellizzi's syndrome.
pin·e·o·blas·to·ma [‚pɪnɪəʊblæs'təʊmə] *n* → pinealoblastoma.
pin·e·o·cy·to·ma [‚-saɪ'təʊmə] *n* → pinealoma.
p-I neuron → postinspiratory neuron.
ping-pong mechanism/reaction ['pɪŋpɒŋ] *biochem*. doppelte Verdrängungsreaktion *f*, Ping-Pong-Mechanismus *m*, -Reaktion *f*.

pin·guec·u·la [pɪŋ'gwekjələ] n, pl **-lae** [-liː, -laɪ] ophthal. Pinguecula f.
pin·guic·u·la [pɪŋ'gwɪkjələ] n → pinguecula.
pin-hole pupil ['pɪnhəʊl] Stecknadelpupille f.
pin·i·form ['pɪnəfɔːrm, 'paɪ-] adj konusförmig, konisch.
pink disease [pɪŋk] Feer'-Krankheit f, Rosakrankheit f, vegetative Neurose f der Kleinkinder, Swift-Syndrom nt, Selter-Swift-Feer'-Krankheit f, Feer-Selter-Swift-Krankheit f, Akrodynie f, Acrodynia f.
pink-eye ['pɪŋkaɪ] n ophthal. Koch-Weeks-Konjunktivitis f, akute kontagiöse Konjunktivitis f, Konjunktivitis f durch Haemophilus aegyptius.
pink puffer patho. Pink puffer m, PP-Typ m.
Pinkus ['pɪŋkəs]: **P. tumor** Pinkus-Tumor m, prämalignes Fibroepitheliom nt, fibroepithelialer Tumor m (Pinkus), Fibroepithelioma Pinkus.
pin·na (of ear) ['pɪnə] Ohrmuschel f, Aurikel f, Auricula f.
pin·ning ['pɪnɪŋ] n ortho. 1. Nagelung f. 2. Spickung f, Drahtfixierung f.
pi·no·cyte ['paɪnəsaɪt, 'pɪnə-] n Pinozyt m.
pi·no·cyt·ic [-'sɪtɪk] adj 1. Pinozyt betr., pinozytär, Pinozyten-. 2. → pinocytotic.
pinocytic vesicle → pinosome.
pi·no·cy·to·sis [-,saɪ'təʊsɪs] n Pinozytose f.
pi·no·cy·tot·ic [-,saɪ'tɒtɪk] adj Pinozytose betr., pinozytotisch, Pinozytose-.
pinocytotic vesicle → pinosome.
pi·no·some ['-səʊm] n Pinozytosebläschen nt, pinozytäres Bläschen n.
Pins [pɪnz]: **P.' sign** Ewart-Zeichen nt, Pins-Zeichen nt.
pint [paɪnt] n abbr. **pt** Pint nt.
pin·ta ['pɪntə] n Pinta f, Mal del Pinto, Carate f.
pinta fever Felsengebirgsfleckfieber nt, amerikanisches Zeckenbißfieber nt, Rocky Mountain spotted fever (nt) abbr. RMSF.
pin·tid ['pɪntɪd] n derm. Pintid nt.
pi·nus ['paɪnəs] n → pineal I.
pin·worm ['pɪnwɜrm] n micro. Madenwurm m, Enterobius vermicularis, Oxyuris vermicularis.
pio- pref. Fett-, Lip(o)-.
pi·on ['paɪɒn] n phys. Pion nt.
pi·o·ne·mia [paɪə'niːmɪə] n Lipämie f, Lipaemia f, Hyperlipämie f.
Pi·oph·i·la [paɪ'ɒfɪlə] n micro., bio. Piophila f.
P. casei Käsefliege f, Piophila casei.
PIP$_2$ abbr. → phosphatidylinosine diphosphate.
pi·pam·pe·rone [pɪ'pæmpərəʊn] n pharm. Pipamperon nt.
pi·paz·e·thate [pɪ'pæzɪθeɪt] n pharm. Pipazetat nt.
pip·e·col·ic acid [,pɪpə'kɒlɪk] Pipecolinsäure f, Homoprolin nt.
pip·e·co·lin·ic acid [,-kə'lɪnɪk] → pipecolic acid.
pi·pen·zo·late bromide [paɪ'penzəleɪt] pharm. Pipenzolatbromid nt.
pi·per·a·cil·lin [paɪ,perə'sɪlɪn] n pharm. Piperacillin nt.
pip·er·az·i·dine [pɪpə'ræzɪdiːn] n → piperazine.
pi·per·a·zine [pɪ'perəziːn, paɪ-] n pharm. Piperazin nt, Diäthylendiamin nt.
pipe-smoker's cancer [paɪp] Pfeifenraucherkrebs m.
pipet n → pipette.
pi·pette [paɪ'pet, pɪ-] **I** n Pipette f. **II** vt pipettieren.

PIP joint → interphalangeal joint, proximal.
pi·pox·o·lan [pɪ'pɒksəlæn] n pharm., anes. Pipoxolan nt.
pi·pra·drol [paɪprədrɒl, -drɒl] n pharm. Pipradrol nt.
pip·rin·hy·dri·nate [pɪprɪn'haɪdrɪneɪt] n pharm. Piprinhydrinat nt.
pip·ro·zo·lin [,pɪprə'zəʊlɪn] n pharm. Piprozolin nt.
pi·qûre [pi'kyːr] n 1. chir. Einstich m, Punktion f, Piqûre f. 2. Bernard-Zuckerstich m.
piqûre diabetes Bernard-Zuckerstich m.
pir·i·form ['pɪərɪfɔːrm] adj birnenförmig; anat. piriform.
piriform aperture vordere Öffnung f der (knöchernen) Nasenhöhle, Apertura piriformis, Apertura nasalis anterior.
piriform area piriforme Rinde f, piriformer Kortex m.
piriform bursa Bursa m. piriformis.
piriform cortex piriforme Rinde f, piriformer Kortex m.
piriform fossa → piriform recess.
pir·i·for·mis (muscle) [,pɪrɪ'fɔːrmɪs] Piriformis m, M. piriformis.
piriform lobe Lobus piriformis.
piriform muscle → piriformis (muscle).
piriform nerve Piriformis m, N. musculi piriformis.
piriform opening Apertura piriformis.
piriform recess Rec. piriformis.
Piringer ['pɪərɪŋər]: **P.'s lymphadenitis** Piringer-Kuchinka-Syndrom nt, zervikonuchale Lymphadenitis f, subakute Lymphadenitis nuchalis et cervicalis.
pir·i·ni·tra·mide [,pɪrɪ'naɪtrəmaɪd] n → piritramide.
pi·rit·ra·mide [paɪ'rɪtrəmaɪd] n pharm. Piritramid nt.
Pirogoff [pɪrə'ɡɒf]: **P. amputation** → P. operation.
P.'s angle Venenwinkel m, Angulus venosus.
P. operation ortho. Amputation f nach Pirogoff.
P.'s triangle Pirogoff-Dreieck nt.
Pir·o·plas·ma ['paɪrəplæzmə] n old micro. Babesia f.
pir·o·plas·mo·sis [,-plæz'məʊsɪs] n Piroplasmose f, Babesiose f, Babesiasis f.
pi·rox·i·cam [pɪ'rɒksɪkæm, paɪ-] n pharm. Piroxicam nt.
pir·pro·fen [pɪr'prəʊfen] n pharm. Pirprofen nt.
Pirquet [pɜr'keɪ; pɪr'kɛ]: **P.'s cutireaction/reaction/test** Pirquet-Reaktion f, -Tuberkulinprobe f.
Piry ['paɪrɪ, 'pɪə-]: **P. virus** Piry-Virus nt.
pis·ci·form cataract ['pɪsəfɔːrm] Fischflossenstar m, Cataracta pisciformis.
pi·si·form ['pɪsɪfɔːrm, 'paɪ-] **I** n Erbsenbein nt, Os pisiforme. **II** adj erbsenförmig, Erbsen-; anat. pisiform.
pisiform bone → pisiform I.
pi·so·ham·ate ligament [,pɪsəʊ'heɪmeɪt] Lig. pisohamatum.
pi·so·met·a·car·pal ligament [,-,metə'kɑːrpəl] Lig. pisometacarpale.
pi·so·tri·que·tral joint [,-traɪ'kwiːtrəl] Artic. ossis pisiformis.
pi·so·un·ci·form [,-'ʌnsəfɔːrm] adj Os pisiforme u. Os hamatum betr. od. verbindend.
pisounciform articulation/joint Artic. ossis pisiformis.
pisounciform ligament Lig. pisohamatum.
pi·so·un·ci·nate [,-'ʌnsənɪt, -neɪt] adj → pisounciform.

pisouncinate ligament → pisounciform ligament.
pis·til ['pɪstl] n 1. bio. Stempel m, Pistill(um) nt. 2. Pistill nt.
pis·tol-shot pulse ['pɪstl] card. Wasserhammerpuls m.
pistol-shot sound card. Traube-Doppelton m.
pis·ton pulse ['pɪstən] card. 1. Corrigan-Puls m, Pulsus celer et altus. 2. Wasserhammerpuls m.
pit [pɪt] **I** n 1. (a. anat.) Grube f, Vertiefung f, Einsenkung f, Loch nt. 2. (Pocken-)Narbe f. **II** vt mit Narben bedecken. **III** vi 3. (pocken-)narbig werden. 4. s. aushöhlen. 5. (auf Fingerdruck) eine Druckstelle/Delle hinterlassen.
p. of head of femur Fovea capitis ossis femoris.
p. of stomach Magengrube.
PITC abbr. → phenylisothiocyanate.
pitch [pɪtʃ] n 1. phys. Tonhöhe f. 2. biochem. Ganghöhe f. 3. chem. Teer m, Pech nt, Pix f. 4. fig. Gipfel m, höchster Punkt m, Höhepunkt m.
pitch-black adj pech(raben)schwarz, kohlrabenschwarz.
pitch level Ton-, Stimmlage f.
pitch·y ['pɪtʃɪ] adj pech-, teerartig; pechschwarz; teerig, voller Teer.
pith [pɪθ] n 1. bio. Mark nt. 2. (Rücken-, Knochen-)Mark nt.
Pitres [piː'tres; piː'trɛ]: **P.'s sign** 1. Pitres'-Zeichen nt. 2. neuro. Berührungsempfindlichkeit f der Haut, Haphalgesie f.
pit·ted keratolysis ['pɪtɪd] grübchenförmige Keratolysen pl, Keratoma (plantaris) sulcatum.
Pitts·burgh pneumonia ['pɪtsbɜrɡ] Pittsburgh-Pneumonie f.
Pittsburgh pneumonia agent abbr. **PPA** micro. Legionella micdadei, Pittsburgh pneumonia agent abbr. PPA.
pi·tu·i·cyte [pɪ't(j)uɪsaɪt] n Pituizyt m.
pi·tu·i·cy·to·ma [pɪ,t(j)uːsaɪ'təʊmə] n Pituizytom nt.
pi·tu·i·ta [pɪ't(j)uːɪtə] n patho. wäßrig-fadenziehender Schleim m, Pituita f.
pi·tu·i·tar·ism [pɪ't(j)uːɪtərɪzm] n Hypophysenfehlfunktion f, -dysfunktion f, Pituitarismus m.
pi·tu·i·ta·ri·um [pɪ,t(j)uːə'teərɪəm] n → pituitary I.
pi·tu·i·tar·y [pɪ't(j)uːəˌteriː] **I** n Hirnanhangdrüse f, Hypophyse f, Hypophysis f, Hypophysis f, Gl. pituitaria. **II** adj Hypophyse betr., hypophysär, pituitär, Hypophysen-.
pituitary adamantinoma Erdheim-Tumor m, Kraniopharyngeom nt.
pituitary adenoma Hypophysenadenom nt.
basophilic p. basophiles (Hypophysen-)-Adenom.
chromophobic p. chromophobes (Hypophysen-)Adenom.
eosinophilic p. eosinophiles (Hypophysen-)Adenom.
pituitary adiposity hypophysärbedingte Fettsucht/Adipositas f.
pituitary-adrenocortical system Hypophysen-Nebennierenrindensystem nt.
pituitary ameloblastoma → pituitary adamantinoma.
pituitary amenorrhea gyn. hypophysäre Amenorrhoe f.
pituitary apoplexy Hypophysenapoplexie f.
pituitary atrophy Hypophysenatrophie f.
pituitary basophilism Cushing-Syndrom nt.
pituitary body → pituitary I.

pituitary cachexia

pituitary cachexia Simmonds'-Kachexie f.
pituitary diverticulum embryo. Rathke-Tasche f.
pituitary dwarfism → pituitary infantilism.
pituitary dysfunction → pituitarism.
pituitary enlargement Hypophysenvergrößerung f.
pituitary fossa Fossa hypophysialis.
pituitary gigantism hypophysärer Riesenwuchs m.
pituitary gland → pituitary I.
pituitary hormone: ~s pl Hypophysenhormone pl.
 anterior p. Hormon nt der Adenohypophyse, (Hypophysen-)Vorderlappenhormon nt, HVL-Hormon nt.
 posterior p.s (Hypophysen-)Hinterlappenhormone pl, HHL-Hormone pl, Neurohypophysenhormone pl.
pituitary hyperfunction Hypophysenüberfunktion f, Hyperpituitarismus m.
pituitary infantilism Lorain-Syndrom nt, hypophysärer Zwergwuchs/Minderwuchs m.
pituitary infarct → hypophysial infarct.
pituitary membrane (of nose) Nasenschleimhaut f, Tunica mucosa nasi.
pituitary microadenoma Mikroadenom nt der Hypophyse.
pituitary myxedema sekundäres/hypophysär-bedingtes Myxödem nt.
pituitary tumor Hypophysentumor m.
pituitary portal system hypophysärer Pfortader-/Portalkreislauf m, hypophysäres Pfortader-/Portalsystem nt.
pituitary stalk Hypophysenstiel m, Infundibulum hypothalami.
pi·tu·i·tec·to·my [pɪ,t(j)uːəˈtektəmɪ] n neurochir. Hypophysenentfernung f, Hypophysektomie f.
pi·tu·i·tous [pɪˈt(j)uːətəs] adj Schleim betr., schleimig, pituitös, Schleim-.
pit·y·ri·as·ic [,pɪtəˈraɪəsɪk] adj derm. Pityriasis betr.
pit·y·ri·a·sis [,-ˈraɪəsɪs] n derm. Kleieflechte f, Pityriasis f.
pityriasis versicolor Kleienpilzflechte f, Eichstedt-Krankheit f, Willan-Krankheit f, Pityriasis/Tinea versicolor.
pit·y·roid [ˈ-rɔɪd] adj kleienartig, -förmig.
Pit·y·ros·po·ron [,-ˈrɑspərən] n → Pityrosporum.
Pit·y·ros·po·rum [,-ˈrɑspərəm] n micro. Pityrosporon m, Pityrosporum f.
piv·a·late [ˈpɪvəleɪt] n Trimethylacetat nt.
pi·val·ic acid [pɪˈvælɪk] Trimethylessigsäure f.
piv·am·pi·cil·lin [pɪv,æmpɪˈsɪlɪn] n pharm. Pivampicillin nt.
piv·ot [ˈpɪvət] n (Dreh-)Zapfen m; Achse f, Spindel f; Stift m.
piv·ot·al [ˈpɪvətl] adj Zapfen-, Angel-.
pivotal point Dreh-, Angelpunkt m.
pivot articulation Dreh-, Rad-, Zapfengelenk nt, Artic. trochoidea.
pivot joint → pivot articulation.
pivot tooth dent. Stiftzahn m.
pix [pɪks] n → pitch 3.
pix·el [ˈpɪksəl, -sel] n radiol. Bild-, Rasterpunkt m, Pixel nt.
PK abbr. → pyruvate kinase.
pK abbr. pK(-Wert m) m.
P-K antibodies → Prausnitz-Küstner antibodies.
pkat abbr. → picokatal.
PK deficiency → pyruvate kinase deficiency.
PKR abbr. → Prausnitz-Küstner reaction.
P-K reaction → Prausnitz-Küstner reaction.

P-K test → Prausnitz-Küstner reaction.
PKU abbr. → phenylketonuria.
pla·ce·bo [pləˈsiːbəʊ] n, pl -bos, -boes Plazebo nt, Placebo nt.
placebo effect Plazeboeffekt m.
pla·cen·ta [pləˈsentə] n, pl -tas, -tae [-tiː] Mutterkuchen m, Plazenta f, Placenta f; inf. Nachgeburt f.
pla·cen·tal [pləˈsentəl] adj Plazenta betr., plazental, plazentar, Plazenta-.
placental barrier Plazentaschranke f, -barriere f.
placental circulation Plazentakreislauf m.
placental cyst Plazentazyste f.
placental dysfunction syndrome Plazentainsuffizienzsyndrom nt.
placental edema Plazentaödem nt.
placental giant cell Plazentariesenzelle f.
placental growth hormone humanes Plazenta-Laktogen nt abbr. HPL, Chorionsomatotropin nt.
placental hormones Plazentahormone pl.
Plac·en·ta·lia [plæsenˈteɪlɪə] pl bio. Plazentatiere pl, Plazentalier pl, Placentalia f.
placental mammals → Placentalia.
placental polyp gyn. Plazentarpolyp m.
placental presentation gyn. Placenta pr(a)evia.
placental stage gyn. Nachgeburtsperiode f, -phase f.
placental transfusion syndrome fetofetale Transfusion f.
placental villus Plazentazotte f.
 definitive p. Tertiärzotte f.
placenta previa Placenta praevia.
 central p. Placenta praevia centralis.
 complete p. → central p.
 incomplete p. → partial p.
 lateral p. → marginal p.
 marginal p. Placenta praevia marginalis.
 partial p. Placenta praevia partialis.
 total p. → central p.
placenta protein → placental growth hormone.
plac·en·tar·y [ˈplæsən,terɪ; pləˈsentərɪ] adj → placental.
pla·cen·ta·scan [pləˈsentəskæn] n Plazentascan m, -szintigraphie f.
plac·en·ta·tion [plæsənˈteɪʃn] n Plazentabildung f, Plazentation f.
plac·en·ti·tis [,plæsənˈtaɪtɪs] n Plazentaentzündung f, Plazentitis f, Placentitis f.
pla·cen·to·gram [pləˈsentəgræm] n radiol., gyn. Plazentogramm n.
plac·en·tog·ra·phy [,plæsənˈtɑgrəfɪ] n radiol., gyn. Plazentographie f.
plac·en·to·ma [,-ˈtəʊmə] n Plazentom nt, Placentoma nt.
plac·en·top·a·thy [,-ˈtɑpəθɪ] n Plazentaerkrankung f, Plazentopathie f.
place pattern [pleɪs] physiol. Ortsmuster nt.
Plácido [plaˈsiːdəʊ, ˈplɑsɪ-]: **P.'s disk** ophthal. Placido-Scheibe f.
plac·ode [ˈplækəʊd] n embryo. Plakode f.
plagio- pref. Schief-, Plagio-.
pla·gi·o·ce·phal·ic [,pleɪdʒɪəʊsɪˈfælɪk] adj schiefköpfig.
pla·gi·o·ceph·a·lism [,-ˈsefəlɪzəm] n → plagiocephaly.
pla·gi·o·ceph·a·ly [,-ˈsefəlɪ] n Schiefköpfigkeit f, Plagiozephalie f.
plague [pleɪg] n 1. Pest f, Pestis f; histor. schwarzer Tod m. 2. Seuche f, Pest f, Plage f, Pestilenz f, Pestis f.
plague bacillus Pestbakterium nt, Yersinia/Pasteurella pestis.
plague pneumonia Lungenpest f, Pestpneumonie f.
plague septicemia septische/septikämische Pest f, Pestsepsis f, Pestseptikämie f, Pestikämie f.

plain film [pleɪn] radiol. Leeraufnahme f.
plain radiograph/roentgenogram → plain film.
plain thrombus weißer/grauer Thrombus m, Abscheidungsthrombus m.
plain x-ray → plain film.
pla·nar [ˈpleɪnər] adj eben, flächenhaft, planar, Planar-.
Planck [plɑŋk]: **P.'s constant** abbr. h Planck'-Wirkungsquantum nt abbr. h.
 P.'s quantum → P.'s constant.
 P.'s theory Planck'-Quantentheorie f.
plane [pleɪn] I n 1. (ebene) Fläche f, Ebene f; anat. Planum nt. 2. fig. Ebene f, Niveau nt, Stufe f, Bereich m. **on the same ~ as** auf gleichem Niveau wie. II adj eben, flach, plan, Plan-. III vt glätten, ebnen; (ab-, glatt-)hobeln.
 p. of incidence phys. Einfallsebene f.
 p. of inlet gyn. Beckeneingangsebene f.
 p. of occlusion dent. Biß-, Okklusionsebene f.
 p.s for orientation anat. Orientierungsebenen pl.
 p. of outlet gyn. Beckenausgangsebene f.
 p. of reference mathe. Bezugsebene.
 p. of refraction phys. Brechungsebene f.
plane angle mathe. Flächenwinkel m.
plane articulation Artic. plana.
plane joint → plane articulation.
plane mirror Planspiegel m.
plane polarization lineare Polarization f.
plane-polarized adj phys. linear polarisiert.
plane-polarized light linear polarisiertes Licht nt.
plane suture anat. Knochennaht f mit ebenen Flächen, Sutura plana.
plane verruca derm. Flachwarze f, Verruca plana (juvenilis).
plane wart → plane verruca.
pla·ni·gram [ˈpleɪnəgræm, ˈplæ-] n radiol. Schichtaufnahme f, Tomogramm n.
pla·nig·ra·phy [pleɪˈnɪgrəfɪ] n Schichtaufnahmetechnik f, Tomographie f, Planigraphie f.
pla·nim·e·ter [pləˈnɪmɪtər] n Planimeter nt.
pla·nim·e·try [pləˈnɪmətrɪ] n Planimetrie f.
plank·ton [ˈplæŋktən] n Plankton nt.
plank·ton·ic [plæŋkˈtɑnɪk] adj Plankton betr., planktonisch, planktisch, planktontisch, Plankton-.
plan·ning [ˈplænɪŋ] n Planung f, Planen nt.
pla·no·cel·lu·lar [pleɪnəʊˈseljələr] adj aus flachen Zellen bestehend, flachzellig.
pla·no·con·cave [,-ˈkɑŋkeɪv] adj plan(o)konkav.
planoconcave lens Planokonkavlinse f.
pla·no·con·vex [,-ˈkɑnveks] adj plan(o)konvex.
planoconvex lens Planokonvexlinse f.
plan·o·cyte [ˈplænəsaɪt] n Planozyt m; Leptozyt m.
pla·no·gram [ˈpleɪnəgræm, ˈplæ-] n → planigram.
pla·nog·ra·phy [pləˈnɑgrəfɪ] n → planigraphy.
pla·nont [ˈplænənt] n → planospore.
plan·o·spore [ˈplænəspəʊər, -spɔːr] n bio. Schwärmspore f, -zelle f, Schwärmer m, Plano-, Zoospore f.
plant [plænt, plɑːnt] I n 1. bot. Pflanze f, Gewächs nt. 2. Anlage(n pl) f, Einrichtung(en pl) f. II vt (ein-, an-)pflanzen.
plant out vt um-, verpflanzen.
plan·tal·gia [plænˈtældʒ(ɪ)ə] n (Fuß-)Sohlenschmerz m, Plantalgie f.
plan·ta pedis [ˈplæntə] anat. Fußsohle f, Planta pedis, Regio plantaris pedis.
plan·tar [ˈplæntər] adj Fußsohle betr., plantar, (Fuß-)Sohlen-.

plantar aponeurosis Fußsohlen-, Plantaraponeurose *f*, Aponeurosis plantaris.
plantar arch Fußsohlenbogen *m*, Arcus plantaris.
plantar artery: deep p. tiefe Fußsohlenarterie *f*, Plantaris *f* profunda, A. plantaris profunda.
  external p. seitliche/laterale Fußsohlenarterie, Plantaris *f* lateralis, A. plantaris lateralis.
  lateral p. → external p.
  medial p. innere/mediale Fußsohlenarterie, Plantaris *f* medialis, A. plantaris medialis.
plantar fascia → plantar aponeurosis.
plantar fibromatosis Ledderhose-Syndrom I *nt*, Morbus Ledderhose *m*, plantare Fibromatose *f*, Plantaraponeurosenkontraktur *f*, Dupuytren-Kontraktur *f* der Plantarfaszie, Fibromatosis plantae.
plantar flexors Plantarflexoren *pl*.
plan·tar·is (muscle) ['plæn'tɛərɪs] *n* Plantaris *m*, M. plantaris.
plantar ligaments Ligg. plantaria.
  long p. Lig. plantare longum.
  p.s of tarsus Ligg. tarsi plantaria.
plantar muscle → plantaris (muscle).
plantar muscle reflex Zehenbeugereflex *m*, Rossolimo-Reflex *m*, -Zeichen *nt*, Plantarmuskelreflex *m*.
plantar nerve: lateral p. seitlicher Fußsohlennerv *m*, N. plantaris lateralis.
  medial p. mittlerer Fußsohlennerv *m*, N. plantaris medialis.
plantar pitting grübchenförmige Keratolysen *pl*, Keratoma (plantaris) sulcatum.
plantar reflex Plantarreflex *m*, Fußsohlen(haut)reflex *m*.
plantar verruca Sohlen-, Dornwarze *f*, Verruca plantaris.
plantar wart → plantar verruca.
plant cell Pflanzenzelle *f*.
plant cytochrome pflanzliches Cytochrom *nt*, Pflanzencytochrom *nt*.
plant hormone Pflanzenhormon *nt*, Phytohormon *nt*.
plant parasite pflanzlicher Parasit *m*, Phytoparasit *m*.
plant pigment Pflanzenpigment *nt*.
plant toxin Pflanzentoxin *nt*, Phytotoxin *nt*.
plant viruses Pflanzenviren *pl*.
plan·u·la ['plænjələ] *n, pl* **-lae** [-liː] Planula *f*.
pla·num ['pleɪnəm] *n, pl* **-na** [-nə] → plane 1.
plaque [plæk; *Brit.* plɑːk] *n* 1. *anat., patho.* Fleck *m*, Plaque *f*. 2. *dent.* Zahnbelag *m*. 3. *micro.* Plaque *f*, Phagenloch *nt*.
plaque assay *micro.* Plaque-Test *m*.
plaque-forming cells *abbr.* **PFC** *micro.* plaque-bildende Zellen *pl*.
plaque-forming unit *abbr.* **PFU** *micro.* plaque-bildende Einheit *f abbr.* PBE.
plaque test *micro.* Plaque-Test *m*.
plasm- *pref.* → plasmo-.
plasm ['plæzəm] *n* → plasma.
plasma- *pref.* → plasmo-.
plas·ma ['plæzmə] *n* 1. Blutplasma *nt*, Plasma *nt*. 2. Zell-, Zytoplasma *nt*. 3. zellfreie Lymphe *f*. 4. *phys.* Plasma *nt*.
plasma albumin Plasmaalbumin *nt*.
plasma bicarbonate Plasmabikarbonat *nt*.
plasma cell Plasmazelle *f*, Plasmozyt *m*.
plasma cell balanitis Balanitis chronica circumscripta benigna plasmacellularis (Zoon).
plasma cell granuloma Plasmazellgranulom *nt*.
plasma cell hepatitis chronisch-aktive/chronisch-aggressive Hepatitis *f abbr.* CAH.
plasma cell leukemia Plasmazellenleukämie *f*.
plasma cell mastitis *gyn.* Plasmazell-, Komedomastitis *f*.
plasma cell myeloma → plasmacytoma 2.
plasma cell pneumonia Pneumocystis-Pneumonie *f*, interstitielle Plasmazellpneumonie *f*, Pneumocystose *f*.
plasma cell tumor → plasmacytoma.
plasma cell vulvitis Vulvitis chronica plasmacellularis, Vulvitis circumscripta chronica plasmacellularis (Zoon).
plas·ma·cyte ['-saɪt] *n* → plasma cell.
plasmacyte series *hema.* plasmazytäre Reihe *f*.
plas·ma·cyt·ic [ˌ-'sɪtɪk] *adj* → plasmacellular.
plasmacytic immunocytoma → plasmacytoma 2.
plasmacytic leukemia → plasma cell leukemia.
plasmacytic series → plasmacyte series.
plas·ma·cy·toid lymphocytic lymphoma [ˌ-'saɪtɔɪd] Immunozytom *nt*, lymphoplasmozytisches Lymphom *nt*, lympho-plasmozytoides Lymphom *nt*.
plas·ma·cy·to·ma [ˌ-saɪ'təʊmə] *n* 1. solitärer Plasmazelltumor *m*. 2. Kahler-Krankheit *f*, Huppert-Krankheit *f*, Morbus Kahler *m*, Plasmozytom *nt*, multiples Myelom *nt*, plasmozytisches Immunozytom/Lymphom *nt*.
plas·ma·cy·to·sis [ˌ-saɪ'təʊsɪs] *n* Plasmazellvermehrung *f*, Plasmozytose *f*.
plasma electrolyte Plasmaelektrolyt *m*.
plasma exchange Plasmaaustausch *m*.
plasma expander Plasmaexpander *m*.
plas·ma·gel ['-dʒel] *n* Plasmagel *nt*.
plas·ma·gene ['-dʒiːn] *n* Plasmagen *nt*, Plasmafaktor *m*.
plasma globulines Plasmaglobuline *pl*.
plasma iron clearance (half time) (Plasma-)Eisenclearance *f*.
plasma kallikrein Plasma-, Serumkallikrein *n*.
plasma labile factor Proakzelerin *nt*, Proaccelerin *nt*, Acceleratorglobulin *nt*, labiler Faktor *m*, Faktor V *m abbr.* F V.
plas·ma·lem·ma [ˌ-'lemə] *n* Zellmembran *f*, -wand *f*, Plasmalemm *nt*.
plas·ma·lem·mal [ˌ-'leməl] *adj* Plasmalemm betr., aus Plasmalemm bestehend.
plasmalemmal vesicle *histol.* Caveola intracellularis.
plasma lipoproteins Plasmalipoproteine *pl*.
plas·mal·o·gen [plæz'mælədʒɪn] *n* Plasmalogen *nt*, Acetalphosphatid *nt*.
plasma membrane → plasmalemma.
plasma orosomucoid (Plasma-)Orosomucoid *nt*, saures α_1-Glykoprotein *nt*.
plasma osmolality Plasmaosmolalität *f*.
plas·ma·pher·e·sis [ˌ-fə'riːsɪs, -fə'rɛsɪs] *n lab.* Plasmapherese *f*.
plas·ma·phe·ret·ic [ˌ-fə'rɛtɪk] *adj* Plasmapherese betr.
plasma protein Plasmaprotein *nt*.
plasma renin activity *abbr.* **PRA** Plasmareninaktivität *f abbr.* PRA.
plasma skimming Plasma-Skimming *nt*.
plasma substitute Plasmaersatz *m*, -expander *m*.
plas·ma·ther·a·py [ˌ-'θɛrəpɪ] *n* Therapie/Behandlung *f* mit (Blut-)Plasma, Plasmatherapie *f*.
plasma thromboplastin antecedent *abbr.* **PTA** Faktor XI *m abbr.* F XI, Plasmathromboplastinantecedent *m abbr.* PTA, antihämophiler Faktor C *m*, Rosenthal-Faktor *m*.
plasma thromboplastin component *abbr.* **PTC** Faktor IX *m abbr.* F IX, Christmas-Faktor *m*, Autothrombin II *nt*.
plasma thromboplastin factor *abbr.* **PTF** antihämophiles Globulin *nt abbr.* AHG, Antihämophiliefaktor *m abbr.* AHF, Faktor VIII *m abbr.* F VIII.
plasma thromboplastin factor B → plasma thromboplastin component.
plas·mat·ic [plæz'mætɪk] *adj* Plasma betr., im Plasma liegend, plasmatisch, Plasma-.
plasmatic canal Havers'-Kanal *m*, Canalis nutriens.
plas·ma·to·fi·brous astrocyte [ˌplæzmæt-əʊ'faɪbrəs] plasmatofibrillärer Astrozyt *m*.
plas·ma·tog·a·my [ˌplæzmə'tɑgəmɪ] *n* → plasmogamy.
plasma volume *abbr.* **PV** Plasmavolumen *nt abbr.* PV.
plasma volume expander Plasmaexpander *m*.
plas·mic ['plæzmɪk] *adj* → plasmatic.
plas·mid ['plæzmɪd] *n* Plasmid *nt*.
plas·min ['plæzmɪn] *n* Plasmin *nt*, Fibrinolysin *nt*.
α_2-plasmin inhibitor α_2-Plasmininhibitor *m*.
plas·min·o·gen [plæz'mɪnədʒən] *n* Plasminogen *nt*, Profibrinolysin *nt*.
plasminogen activator Plasminaktivator *m*, Urokinase *f*.
plasminogen proactivator Plasminogenproaktivator *m*.
plasmin prothrombin conversion factor *abbr.* **PPCF** Proakzelerin *nt*, Proaccelerin *nt*, Acceleratorglobulin *nt*, labiler Faktor *m*, Faktor V *m abbr.* F V.
plasmo- *pref.* Plasma-, Plasm(o)-.
plas·mo·cyte ['plæzməsaɪt] *n* → plasma cell.
plasmocyte nephrosis Plasmozytomnephrose *f*.
plas·mo·cy·to·ma [ˌ-saɪ'təʊmə] *n* → plasmacytoma.
plas·mo·desm ['-dezəm] *n bio.* Plasmabrücke *f*, Plasmodesma *nt*.
plas·mo·des·ma [ˌ-'dezmə] *n, pl* **-ma·ta** [-mətə] → plasmodesm.
plas·mo·di·al [plæz'məʊdɪəl] *adj* Plasmodien betr., Plasmodien-.
plas·mo·di·blast [plæz'məʊdɪblæst] *n* Synzytiotrophoblast *m*.
plas·mo·di·ci·dal [ˌplæzməʊdɪ'saɪdl] *adj* plasmodien(ab)tötend, plasmodizid.
plas·mo·di·cide [plæz'məʊdəsaɪd] *n* Plasmodizid *nt*.
plas·mo·di·troph·o·blast [plæzˌməʊdaɪ'trɑfəblæst] *n* Synzytiotrophoblast *m*.
Plas·mo·di·um [plæz'məʊdɪəm] *n, pl* **-dia** [-dɪə] *micro.* Plasmodium *nt*.
plas·mo·di·um [plæz'məʊdɪəm] *n, pl* **-dia** [-dɪə] 1. *histol.* Plasmodium *nt*, vielkernige Zytoplasmamasse *f*. 2. *micro.* Plasmodium *nt*.
plas·mog·a·my [plæz'mɑgəmɪ] *n* Plasmaverschmelzung *f*, Plasmogamie *f*.
plas·mo·gen ['plæzmədʒən] *n* → protoplasm.
plas·mo·ki·nin [ˌ-'kaɪnɪn] *n* antihämophiles Globulin *nt abbr.* AHG, Antihämophiliefaktor *m abbr.* AHF, Faktor VIII *m abbr.* F VIII.
plas·mo·lem·ma [ˌ-'lemə] *n* → plasmalemma.
plas·mol·y·sis [plæz'mɑləsɪs] *n* Plasmolyse *f*.
plas·mo·lyt·ic [ˌplæzmə'lɪtɪk] *adj* Plasmolyse betr., plasmolytisch.

plasmoma

plas·mo·ma [plæz'məʊmə] *n* → plasmacytoma.
plas·mon ['plæzmɒn] *n* Plasmon *nt*, Plasmotyp *m*, -typus *m*.
plas·mo·nu·cle·ic acid [‚plæzməʊnʊ'kliːɪk, -'kleɪ-, -'n(j)uːklɪɪk] Ribonukleinsäure *f abbr*. RNA, RNS.
plas·mo·some ['-səʊm] *n* 1. Kernkörperchen *nt*, Nukleolus *m*, Nucleolus *m*. 2. Mitochondrie *f*, -chondrion *nt*, -chondrium *nt*, Chondriosom *nt*. 3. *bio*. Plasmosom *nt*.
plas·mot·o·my [plæz'mɒtəmɪ] *n bio*. Plasmotomie *f*.
plas·mo·troph·o·blast [‚plæzmə'trɒfəblæst] *n* Synzytiotrophoblast *m*.
plas·mo·type ['-taɪp] *n* → plasmon.
plas·mo·zyme ['-zaɪm] *n* → prothrombin.
plas·ter ['plɑːstər, 'plɑːs-] **I** *n* **1**. *pharm*. (Heft-)Pflaster *nt*. **2**. → p. of Paris. **II** *vt* **3**. (*a.* **to put in ~**) (ein-)gipsen, in Gips legen, einen Gipsverband anlegen. **4**. ein (Heft-)Pflaster auflegen. **5**. (*Salbe*) dick auftragen.
p. of Paris 1. Gips *m*, Calciumsulfat(-dihydrat *nt*) *nt*. **2.** *Brit. abbr*. **POP** *ortho*. Gips(verband *m*) *m*.
plaster bandage 1. Gipsbinde *f*. **2.** Gips(verband *m*) *m*.
plaster bed *ortho*. Gipsbett *nt*.
plaster cast 1. Gips(verband *m*) *m*. **2.** Gipsabdruck *m*, -abguß *m*. **complete p.** zirkulärer Gips(verband) *m*.
plaster jacket *ortho*. Gipsmieder *nt*.
plaster-of-Paris disease Immobilisationsatrophie *f*.
plaster-of-Paris jacket *ortho*. Gipsmieder *nt*.
plaster shell Gipsschale *f*. **corrective p.** Umkrümmungsgipsliegeschale *f*.
plaster splint Gipsschiene *f*.
sugar tong p. U-Gips(schiene *f*) *m*.
plaster technique Gipstechnik *f*.
plas·tic ['plæstɪk] **I** *n* → plastics. **II** *adj* **1**. aus Plastik, Plastik-, Kunststoff-. **2**. plastisch, formgebend, gestaltend. **3**. (ver-)formbar, modellier-, knetbar. **4**. *chir., bio*. plastisch. **5**. *fig*. anschaulich, plastisch.
plastic bronchitis krupppöse/membranöse/pseudomembranöse Bronchitis *f*, Bronchitis crouposa/fibrinosa/plastica/pseudomembranacea.
plastic induration Peyronie-Krankheit *f*, Penisfibromatose *f*, Induratio penis plastica.
plas·ti·cine ['plæstəsiːn] *n* Knetmasse *f*, Plastilin *nt*.
plastic inflammation → proliferative inflammation.
plas·tic·i·ty [plæs'tɪsətɪ] *n* **1**. (Ver-)Formbarkeit *f*, Modellier-, Knetbarkeit *f*, Plastizität *f*. **2**. *fig*. Anschaulichkeit *f*, Bildhaftigkeit *f*, Plastizität *f*.
plas·ti·ciz·er ['plæstɪsaɪzər] *n chem*. Weichmacher *m*, Plastifikator *m*.
plastic operation Plastik *f*, plastische Chirurgie *f*.
plastic pleurisy proliferative Brustfellentzündung/Pleuritis *f*.
plastic prosthesis Kunststoffprothese *f*.
plas·tics ['plæstɪks] **I** *pl* Kunst-, Plastikstoff(e *pl*) *m*, Plastik *nt*. **II** *adj* Kunststoff-, Plastik-.
plastic surgeon Facharzt *m od*. -ärztin *f* für plastische Chirurgie *f*.
plastic surgery plastische Chirurgie *f*.
plas·tid ['plæstɪd] *n bio*. Plastid *nt*.
plas·to·cy·a·nin [‚plæstəʊ'saɪənɪn] *n* Plastocyanin *nt*.

plas·tog·a·my [plæs'tɒgəmɪ] *n* → plasmogamy.
plas·to·gel ['plæstədʒel] *n* Plastogel *nt*.
plas·to·quin·one [‚-kwɪ'nəʊn] *n* Plastochinon *nt*.
plate [pleɪt] *n* **1**. (Glas-, Metall-)Platte *f*; *photo*. Platte *f*. **2**. *anat*. Platte *f*. **3**. *dent*. (Gebiß-, Gaumen-)Platte *f*. **4**. Schild *nt*; (Bild-)Tafel *f*, Abbildung *f*. **5**. Teller *m*.
p. of modiolus Endplatte der Lamina spiralis ossea, Lamina modioli.
pla·teau [plæ'təʊ] *n, pl* **-teaux, -teaus** [-təʊz] *psycho., bio*. Plateau *nt*, Plateauphase *f*.
plateau phase *physiol*. Plateauphase *f*.
plateau pulse Plateaupuls *m*.
plateau speech monotone Sprache *f*.
plate culture Plattenkultur *f*.
plate·let ['pleɪtlɪt] *n* **1**. Plättchen *nt*. **2**. *hema*. (Blut-)Plättchen *nt*, Thrombozyt *m*, -cyt *m*.
platelet activating factor *abbr*. **PAF** Plättchen-aktivierender Faktor *m abbr*. PAF, platelet activating factor, platelet aggregating factor.
platelet adhesion Plättchen-, Thrombozytenadhäsion *f*.
platelet agglutination Plättchen-, Thrombozytenagglutination *f*.
platelet agglutinin Plättchen-, Thrombozytenagglutinin *nt*.
platelet aggregate Plättchen-, Thrombozytenaggregat *nt*.
platelet aggregating factor → platelet activating factor.
platelet aggregation Plättchen-, Thrombozytenaggregation *f*.
platelet aggregation test Plättchen-, Thrombozytenaggregationstest *m*.
platelet aggregometry Bestimmung *f* der Plättchenaggregation.
platelet cofactor (I) antihämophiles Globulin *nt abbr*. AHG, Antihämophiliefaktor *m abbr*. AHF, Faktor VIII *m abbr*. F VIII.
platelet cofactor II Faktor IX *m abbr*. F IX, Christmas-Faktor *m*, Autothrombin II *nt*.
platelet count 1. Thrombozytenzahl *f*. **2.** Thrombozytenzählung *f*.
platelet-derived growth factor *abbr*. **PDGF** Thrombozyten-, Plättchenwachstumsfaktor *m*, platelet-derived growth factor *abbr*. PDGF.
platelet drop *hema*. Plättchensturz *m*.
platelet factor *hema*. Plättchenfaktor *m*.
platelet factor 1 *abbr*. **PF₁** Plättchenfaktor 1 *m abbr*. PF$_1$.
platelet factor 2 *abbr*. **PF₂** Plättchenfaktor 2 *m abbr*. PF$_2$.
platelet factor 3 *abbr*. **PF₃** Plättchenfaktor 3 *m abbr*. PF$_3$.
platelet factor 4 *abbr*. **PF₄** Plättchenfaktor 4 *m abbr*. PF$_4$, Antiheparin *nt*.
platelet inhibitor Plättchenaggregationshemmer *m*.
platelet metamorphosis visköse Metamorphose *f*.
plate·let·pher·e·sis [‚pleɪtlɪt'ferəsɪs, -fə'riːsɪs] *n* Thrombo(zyto)pherese *f*.
platelet plug weißer Abscheidungsthrombus *m*, Thrombozytenpfropf *m*.
platelet thrombus → plate thrombus.
platelet tissue factor Thrombokinase *f*, -plastin *nt*, Prothrombinaktivator *m*.
plate thrombus Plättchen-, Thrombozytenthrombus *m*.
plat·ing ['pleɪtɪŋ] *n* **1**. *micro*. Anlegen *nt* einer Plattenkultur, Übertragung *f* auf eine Plattenkultur. **2**. *ortho*. Stabilisierung *f* mit einer Platte(nosteosynthese) *f*.

plat·i·num ['plætnəm] *n abbr*. **Pt** Platin *nt abbr*. Pt.
platinum electrode Platinelektrode *f*.
Platner ['plætnər]: **P.'s crystals** Platner-Kristalle *pl*.
platy- *pref*. Breit-, Platt-, Platy-.
plat·y·ba·sia [‚plætɪ'beɪsɪə] *n* Platybasie *f*, basilare Impression *f*.
plat·y·ce·phal·ic [‚-sɪ'fælɪk] *adj* platyzephal, -kephal, -kranial.
plat·y·ceph·a·lous [‚-'sefələs] *adj* → platycephalic.
plat·y·ceph·a·ly [‚-'sefəlɪ] *n* Platt-, Breitköpfigkeit *f*, Platt-, Breitkopf *m*, Platyzephalie *f*, -kephalie *f*, -kranie *f*.
plat·yc·ne·mia [‚plætɪ(k)'niːmɪə] *n ortho*. Platyknemie *f*.
plat·yc·ne·mic [‚plætɪ(k)'niːmɪk] *adj* Platyknemie betr.
plat·yc·ne·mism [‚plætɪ(k)'niːmɪzəm] *n* → platycnemia.
plat·y·cra·nia [‚plætɪ'kreɪnɪə] *n* → platycephaly.
plat·y·cyte ['-saɪt] *n* Platyzyt *m*.
plat·y·glos·sal [‚-'glɒsl] *adj* platyglossal.
plat·y·hel·minth [‚-'helmɪnθ] *n micro*. Plattwurm *m*, Plathelminth *m*.
Plat·y·hel·min·thes [‚-hel'mɪnθiːz] *pl micro*. Plattwürmer *pl*, Plathelminthes *pl*.
plat·yk·ne·mia [‚-'niːmɪə] *n* → platycnemia.
plat·y·mor·phia [‚-'mɔːrfɪə] *n ophthal*. Platymorphie *f*.
plat·y·mor·phic [‚-'mɔːrfɪk] *adj ophthal*. Platymorphie betr.
plat·y·pel·lic pelvis [‚-'pelɪk] gerad-verengtes Becken *nt*.
plat·y·pel·loid pelvis [‚-'pelɔɪd] → platypellic pelvis.
pla·typ·nea [plə'tɪpnɪə] *n* Platypnoe *f*.
pla·tys·ma [plə'tɪzmə] *n* Hautmuskel *m* des Halses, Platysma *nt*.
pla·tys·mal [plə'tɪzməl] *adj* Platysma betr., Platysma-.
plat·y·spon·dyl·ia [‚plætɪspɒn'dɪlɪə] *n* → platyspondylisis.
plat·y·spon·dyl·i·sis [‚-span'dɪləsɪs] *n ortho*. (kongenitale) Flachwirbel *m*, (kongenitale) Flachwirbelbildung *f*, Platyspondylie *f*.
plau·si·bil·i·ty [‚plɔːzə'bɪlətɪ] *n* Wahrscheinlichkeit *f*, Plausibilität *f*.
plau·si·ble ['plɔːzɪbl] *adj* glaubhaft, einleuchtend, möglich, plausibel.
Plaut [plaʊt]: **P.'s angina** Plaut-Vincent-Angina *f*, Vincent-Angina *f*, Fusospirillose *f*, Fusospirochätose *f*, Angina ulcerosa/ulceromembranacea.
pleat [pliːt] **I** *n* Falte *f*. **II** *vt* falten, fälteln.
pleat·ed sheet ['pliːtɪd] *biochem*. Faltblatt(struktur *f*) *nt*.
β-pleated sheet → pleated sheet.
pleated sheets arrangement/conformation/structure → pleated sheet.
plec·trid·i·um [plek'trɪdɪəm] *n micro*. Plectridium-Form *f*.
plec·tron ['plektrɒn] *n, pl* **-tra** [-trə] → plectridium.
plec·trum ['plektrəm] *n, pl* **-trums, tra** [-trə] **1**. Zäpfchen *nt*, zapfenförmige Struktur *f*, Uvula *f*. **2**. (Gaumen-)Zäpfchen *nt*, Uvula *f* (palatina). **3**. *micro*. Maliasmus *m*, Rotz *m*, Malleus *m*. **4**. Proc. styloideus ossis temporalis.
pledg·et ['pledʒɪt] *n* Tupfer *m*, (Watte-)Bausch *m*.
pleio- *pref*. → pleo-.
plei·o·tro·pia [‚plaɪə'trəʊpɪə] *n* → pleiotropy.
plei·o·trop·ic [‚-'trɒpɪk, -'trəʊp-] *adj* Pleiotropie betr., pleiotrop, polyphän.
plei·ot·ro·pism [plaɪ'ɒtrəpɪzəm] *n* → pleiotropy.

plei·ot·ro·py [plaɪ'ɑtrəpɪ] *n genet.* Pleiotropie *f*, Polyphänie *f*.
plek·tron ['plektrən] *n, pl* **-tra** [-trə] → plectridium.
pleo- *pref.* Viel-, Mehr-, Pleo-, Pleio-, Poly-.
ple·o·car·y·o·cyte *n* → pleokaryocyte.
ple·o·chro·ic [ˌpliːə'krəʊɪk] *adj* → pleochromatic.
ple·och·ro·ism [plɪ'ɑkrəwɪzəm] *n* → pleochromatism.
ple·o·chro·mat·ic [ˌpliːəkrə'mætɪk] *adj* pleochrom, pleiochrom.
ple·o·chro·ma·tism [ˌ-'krəʊmətɪzəm] *n phys.* Pleochroismus *m*.
ple·o·cy·to·sis [ˌ-saɪ'təʊsɪs] *n* erhöhte Zellzahl *f*, Pleozytose *f*.
ple·o·kar·y·o·cyte [ˌ-'kærɪəsaɪt] *n* Pleo-, Polykaryozyt *m*.
ple·o·mas·tia [ˌ-'mæstɪə] *n* → polymastia.
ple·o·mas·tic [ˌ-'mæstɪk] *adj* → polymastic.
ple·o·ma·zia [ˌ-'meɪʒ(ɪ)ə, -zɪə] *n* → polymastia.
ple·o·mor·phic [ˌ-'mɔːfɪk] *adj* mehrgestaltig, pleomorph, polymorph.
pleomorphic adenoma Speicheldrüsenmischtumor *m*, pleomorphes Adenom *nt*.
ple·o·mor·phism [ˌ-'mɔːfɪzəm] *n* Mehrgestaltigkeit *f*, Pleo-, Polymorphismus *m*.
ple·o·mor·phous [ˌ-'mɔːfəs] *adj* → pleomorphic.
ple·on·os·te·o·sis [plɪɑnˌɑstɪ'əʊsɪs] *n ortho.* Pleonostose *f*.
ple·op·tics [plɪ'ɑptɪks] *pl ophthal.* Pleoptik *f*.
ple·ro·cer·coid [plɪərə'sɜrkɔɪd] *n micro.* Vollfinne *f*, Plerozerkoid *nt*.
plesio- *pref.* Plesio-.
Ple·si·o·mo·nas [ˌpliːsɪəʊ'məʊnæs] *n micro.* Plesiomonas *f*.
P. shigelloides Plesiomonas/Aeromonas shigelloides.
ple·si·o·mor·phic [ˌ-'mɔːfɪk] *adj* von gleicher Form, plesiomorph.
ple·si·o·mor·phism [ˌ-'mɔːfɪzəm] *n* Plesiomorphismus *m*.
ple·si·o·mor·phous [ˌ-'mɔːfəs] *adj* → plesiomorphic.
ples·ses·the·sia [pleses'θiːʒ(ɪ)ə] *n* Tastperkussion *f*, palpatorische Perkussion *f*.
ples·sim·e·ter [ple'sɪmətər] *n* Klopfblättchen *nt*, Plessimeter *nt*.
ples·si·met·ric [ˌplesɪ'metrɪk] *adj* Plessimeter betr., mittels Plessimeter, plessimetrisch.
ples·sor ['plesər] *n* → plexor.
pleth·o·ra ['pleθərə] *n* (Blut-)Überfüllung *f*, Plethora *f*.
pleth·o·ric ['pleθərɪk, plə'θɔːrɪk] *adj* Plethora betr., Plethora-.
ple·thys·mo·gram [plə'θɪzməgræm] *n* Plethysmogramm *nt*.
ple·thys·mo·graph ['-græf] *n* Plethysmograph *m*.
pleth·ys·mog·ra·phy [pleθɪz'mɑgrəfɪ] *n* Plethysmographie *f*.
pleur- *pref.* → pleuro-.
pleu·ra ['plʊərə] *n, pl* **-rae** [-riː] *anat.* Brustfell *nt*, Pleura *f*.
pleu·ra·cen·te·sis [ˌplʊərəsen'tiːsɪs] *n* Pleurapunktion *f*, Thorakozentese *f*.
pleu·ra·cot·o·my [ˌ-'kɑtəmɪ] *n HTG* Pleurotomie *f*; Thorakotomie *f*.
pleu·ral ['plʊərəl] *adj* Pleura betr., pleural, Pleura-, Rippenfell-, Brustfell-.
pleural adhesion Pleuraverwachsung *f*.
pleural calculus → pleurolith.
pleural carcinomatosis/carcinosis Pleurakarzinose *f*, -karzinomatose *f*, Carcinosis pleurae.

pleural cavity Pleurahöhle *f*, -spalt *m*, -raum *m*, Cavitas pleuralis.
primitive p.ies *embryo.* primitive (Ur-)Pleurahöhlen *pl*.
pleural crackles Lederknarren *nt*.
pleural effusion Pleuraerguß *m*.
pancreatic p. pankreatogener Pleuraerguß.
pleural empyema Pleuraempyem *nt*.
pleural fibroma Pleurafibrom *nt*.
pleural fibrosis Pleuraschwarte *f*, -schwiele *f*.
pleural flap *chir.* Pleuralappen *m*.
pleural fluid Flüssigkeit *f* im Pleuraraum.
pleural fremitus Pleurafremitus *m*.
pleur·al·gia [plʊə'rældʒ(ɪ)ə] *n* Pleuraschmerz *m*, Pleuralgie *f*, Pleurodynie *f*.
pleur·al·gic [plʊə'rældʒɪk] *adj* Pleuralgie betr., pleuralgisch.
pleural hyalinose Pleurahyalinose *f*.
pleural mesothelioma Pleuramesotheliom *nt*.
pleural peel Pleuraschwarte *f*, -schwiele *f*.
pleural rales Pleurareibegeräusche *pl*.
pleural recesses Pleurasinus *pl*, -buchten *pl*, Recc. pleurales.
pleural rub Pleurareiben *nt*.
pleural sac → pleural cavity.
pleural scarring Pleuravernarbung *f*.
pleural sinuses → pleural recesses.
pleural space → pleural cavity.
pleural space infection Pleuralspaltinfektion *f*.
pleural tuberculosis Pleuratuberkulose *f*.
pleural tumor Rippenfell-, Pleuratumor *m*.
pleural villi Pleurazotten *pl*, Villi pleurales.
pleur·ec·to·my [plʊə'rektəmɪ] *n HTG* Rippenfell-, Pleuraresektion *f*, Pleurektomie *f*.
pleu·ri·sy ['plʊərəsɪ] *n* Brust-, Rippenfellentzündung *f*, Pleuritis *f*.
pleu·rit·ic [plʊə'rɪtɪk] *adj* Pleuritis betr., pleuritisch.
pleuritic pain pleuritischer Schmerz *m*.
pleuritic pneumonia kombinierte Pleuritis *f* u. Pneumonie, Pleuropneumonie *f*.
peuritic rub Pleurareiben *nt*.
pleu·ri·tis [plʊə'raɪtɪs] *n* → pleurisy.
pleuro- *pref.* Brustfell-, Rippenfell-, Pleura-, Pleur(o)-; Rippen-.
pleu·ro·bron·chi·tis [ˌplʊərəʊbrɑŋ'kaɪtɪs] *n* Pleurobronchitis *f*.
pleu·ro·cele ['-siːl] *n* → pneumonocele.
pleu·ro·cen·te·sis [ˌ-sen'tiːsɪs] *n* Pleurapunktion *f*, Thorakozentese *f*.
pleu·rod·e·sis [plʊə'rɑdəsɪs] *n HTG* Pleurodese *f*.
pleu·ro·dyn·ia [ˌplʊərəʊ'diːnɪə] *n* **1.** Pleurodynie *f*. **2.** → pleuralgia.
pleu·ro·gen·ic [ˌ-'dʒenɪk] *adj* → pleurogenous.
pleu·rog·e·nous [plʊə'rɑdʒənəs] *adj* von der Pleura stammend, pleurogen.
pleu·rog·ra·phy [plʊə'rɑgrəfɪ] *n radiol.* Pleurographie *f*.
pleu·ro·hep·a·ti·tis [ˌplʊərəʊhepə'taɪtɪs] *n* Pleurohepatitis *f*.
pleu·ro·lith ['-lɪθ] *n* Pleurastein *m*, Pleurolith *m*.
pleu·rol·y·sis [plʊə'rɑləsɪs] *n HTG* Pleuralösung *f*, Pleurolyse *f*.
pleu·ro·me·lus [ˌplʊərəʊ'miːləs] *n embryo.* Pleuromelus *m*.
pleu·ro·pa·ri·e·to·pex·y [ˌ-pə'raɪətəʊpeksɪ] *n HTG* Pleuroparietopexie *f*.
pleu·ro·per·i·car·di·al [ˌ-ˌperɪ'kɑːdɪəl] *adj* Pleura u. Perikard betr., pleuroperikardial.
pleuropericardial fold Pleuroperikardialfalte *f*.

pleuropericardial membrane Pleuroperikardialmembran *f*.
pleu·ro·per·i·car·di·tis [ˌ-ˌperɪkɑːr'daɪtɪs] *n* kombinierte Pleuritis *f* u. Perikarditis, Pleuroperikarditis *f*, Pericarditis externa.
pleu·ro·per·i·to·ne·al [ˌ-ˌperɪtəʊ'niːəl] *adj* pleuroperitoneal.
pleuroperitoneal cavity *embryo.* Pleuroperitonealhöhle *f*.
pleuroperitoneal fistula Pleuroperitonealfistel *f*.
pleuroperitoneal fold Pleuroperitonealfalte *f*.
pleuroperitoneal foramen → pleuroperitoneal hiatus.
pleuroperitoneal hiatus Bochdalek'-Foramen *nt*, Hiatus pleuroperitonealis.
pleuroperitoneal membrane *embryo.* Pleuroperitonealmembran *f*.
pleu·ro·pneu·mo·nia [ˌ-n(j)uː'məʊnɪə] *n* kombinierte Pleuritis *f* u. Pneumonie, Pleuropneumonie *f*.
pleuropneumonia-like organism *abbr.* **PPLO** *old* → mycoplasma.
pleu·ro·pneu·mo·nol·y·sis [ˌ-ˌn(j)uːmə'nɑləsɪs] *n HTG* Pleuropneumonolyse *f*.
pleu·ro·pul·mo·nar·y [ˌ-'pʌlmənerɪ, -nərɪ] *adj* Pleura u. Lunge(n) betr., pleuropulmonal.
pleuropulmonary regions Regiones pleuropulmonales.
pleu·ror·rhea [ˌ-'rɪə] *n* **1.** Pleuraerguß *m*, Pleurorrhoe *f*. **2.** Hydrothorax *m*.
pleu·ros·co·py [plʊə'rɑskəpɪ] *n* Pleuroskopie *f*.
pleu·ro·so·ma [ˌplʊərə'səʊmə] *n* → pleurosomus.
pleu·ro·so·mus [ˌ-'səʊməs] *n embryo.* Pleurosomus *m*.
pleu·ro·thot·o·nos [ˌ-'θɑtənəs] *n neuro., psychia.* Pleurothotonos *m*, -tonus *m*.
pleu·ro·thot·o·nus *n* → pleurothotonos.
pleu·ro·tome ['-təʊm] *n neuro., pulmo.* Pleurotom *nt*.
pleu·rot·o·my [plʊə'rɑtəmɪ] *n HTG* Pleurotomie *f*; Thorakotomie *f*.
pleu·ro·vis·cer·al [ˌplʊərəʊ'vɪsərəl] *adj* pleuroviszeral.
plex·al ['pleksəl] *adj* Plexus betr., Plexus-.
plex·ec·to·my [plek'sektəmɪ] *n chir., neuro. chir.* Plexusresektion *f*, Plexektomie *f*.
plex·i·form ['pleksɪfɔːrm] *adj anat.* geflechtartig, plexusartig, plexiformis.
plexiform angioma plexiformes Angiom *nt*.
plexiform layer: p. of cerebellum Stratum moleculare/plexiforme (cerebelli).
p. of cerebral cortex Molekularschicht *f*, Lamina molecularis/plexiformis corticis cerebri.
external p. äußere retikuläre Schicht *f*.
inner/internal p. innere retikuläre Schicht *f*.
outer p. → external p.
plex·im·e·ter [plek'sɪmətər] *n* **1.** Klopfblättchen *nt*, Plessimeter *nt*. **2.** *derm.* Glasspatel *m*.
plex·i·met·ric [ˌpleksɪ'metrɪk] *adj* Plessimeter betr., mittels Plessimeter, plessimetrisch.
pleximetric percussion Plessimeter-Perkussion *f*.
plex·im·e·try [plek'sɪmətrɪ] *n* Plessimetrie *f*.
plex·i·tis [plek'saɪtɪs] *n neuro.* Plexusentzündung *f*.
plex·o·gen·ic pulmonary arteriopathy [ˌpleksə'dʒenɪk] primäre Pulmonalsklerose *f*, Ayerza-Krankheit *f*.
plex·om·e·ter [plek'sɑmətər] *n* → pleximeter.
plex·op·a·thy [plek'sɑpəθɪ] *n* Plexuserkrankung *f*, Plexopathie *f*.

plexor

plex·or ['pleksər] *n* Perkussionshammer *m*.
plex·us ['pleksəs] *n, pl* **-us, -us·es 1.** *anat.* Plexus *m*, Geflecht *nt*. **2.** *fig.* Komplex *m*, Netz *nt*.
p. of facial artery vegetativer Plexus der A. facialis.
plexus anesthesia *anes.* Plexusanästhesie *f*.
plexus epithelium Plexusepithel *nt*.
plexus formation Netzbildung/-formation *f*, Plexusbildung/-formation *f*.
plexus hemorrhage (*ZNS*) Plexusblutung *f*.
plexus papilloma (*ZNS*) Plexuspapillom *nt*.
pli·ca ['plaɪkə] *n, pl* **-cae** [-si:] *anat.* Falte *f*, Plica *f*.
pli·cate ['plaɪkeɪt, -kɪt] *adj* faltig; gefaltet.
pli·cat·ed ['plaɪkeɪtɪd] *adj* → plicate.
plicated tongue Faltenzunge *f*, Lingua plicata/scrotalis.
pli·ca·tion [plɪ'keɪʃn, plaɪ-] *n* **1.** Falte *f*; Faltenbildung *f*, Faltung *f*. **2.** *chir.* Plikation *f*, Plicatio *f*.
plic·a·ture ['plɪkətʃər] *n* → plication.
pli·cot·o·my [plaɪ'kɑtəmɪ] *n HNO* Plikotomie *f*.
pli·ers ['plaɪərs] *pl chir., ortho.* (Draht-, Kneif-)Zange *f*.
Plimmer ['plɪmər]: **P.'s bodies** Plimmer--Körperchen *pl*.
plom·bage [pləm'bɑːʒ] *n chir.* Plombierung *f*.
plo·sive ['pləʊsɪv] **I** *n* Verschluß-, Explosions-, Plosivlaut *m*, Plosiv *m*. **II** *adj* Verschluß-, Explosions-, Plosiv-.
plot [plɑt] **I** *n* graphische Darstellung *f*, Diagramm *nt*, Schema *nt*. **II** *vt* (*Kurve*) aufzeichnen, auftragen.
PLT *abbr.* → primed lymphocyte typing.
PLT group [psittacosis, lymphogranuloma venereum, trachoma] *micro.* PLT-Gruppe *f*, Chlamydia *f*, Chlamydie *f*.
plug [plʌg] **I** *n* **1.** Pfropf(en *m*) *m*. **2.** *dent.* (Zahn-)Plombe *f*. **3.** Stöpsel *m*, Stecker *m*. **to pull the ~ on** aktive Sterbehilfe leisten. **II** *vt* **4.** ver-, zustopfen, zupfropfen. **to ~ one's ears** s. die Ohren zustopfen. **5.** *dent.* plombieren. **III** *vi* verstopfen.
plug in *vt* einstöpseln, (hin-)einstecken.
plug up I *vt* → plug 4. **II** *vi* → plug III.
plug·ger ['plʌgər] *n dent.* Stopfer *m*.
plum·ba·go [plʌm'beɪgəʊ] *n* Graphit *m*.
plumb·er's itch ['plʌmər] *derm.* Hautmaulwurf *m*, Larva migrans, Myiasis linearis migrans, creeping disease (*nt*).
plum·bic ['plʌmbɪk] *adj* Blei betr. *od.* enthaltend, bleihaltig, Blei-.
plum·bism ['plʌmbɪzəm] *n* Bleivergiftung *f*.
plum·bo·ther·a·py [ˌplʌmbəʊ'θerəpɪ] *n* Behandlung *f* mit Bleiverbindungen.
plum·bum ['plʌmbəm] *n abbr.* **Pb** *chem.* Plumbum *nt abbr.* Pb, Blei *nt*.
Plummer ['plʌmər]: **P.'s disease** Plummer--Krankheit *f*.
P.'s iodine therapy Plummer'-Jodbehandlung *f*, Plummern *nt*, Plummerung *f*.
Plummer-Vinson ['vɪnsən]: **P.-V. syndrome** Plummer-Vinson-Syndrom *nt*, Paterson-Brown-Syndrom *nt*, Kelly--Paterson-Syndrom *nt*, sideropenische Dysphagie *f*.
plu·mose ['pluːməʊs] *adj* federartig.
plung·ing goiter ['plʌndʒɪŋ] Tauchkropf *m*.
plu·ral pregnancy ['plʊərəl] Mehrlingsschwangerschaft *f*.
pluri- *pref.* Viel-, Pluri-, Multi-, Poly-.
plu·ri·caus·al [ˌplʊərɪ'kɔːzəl] *adj patho.* plurikausal.
plu·ri·glan·du·lar [ˌ-'glændʒələr] *adj* mehrere Drüsen betr., pluri-, multi-, polyglandulär.
pluriglandular adenomatosis multiple endokrine Adenopathie *f abbr.* MEA, multiple endokrine Neoplasie *f abbr.* MEN, pluriglanduläre Adenomatose *f*.
plu·ri·grav·i·da [ˌ-'grævɪdə] *n gyn.* Pluri-, Multigravida *f*.
plu·ri·loc·u·lar [ˌ-'lɑkjələr] *adj patho.* vielkamm(e)rig, multilokulär.
plu·ri·men·or·rhea [ˌ-ˌmenə'rɪə] *n* Polymenorrhoe *f*.
plu·ri·nu·cle·ar [ˌ-'n(j)uːklɪər] *adj* mehr-, vielkernig, mit mehreren/vielen Kernen versehen, multinukleär, -nuklear.
plu·rip·a·ra [plu'rɪpərə] *n gyn.* Viel-, Mehrgebärende *f*, Multi-, Pluripara *f*.
plu·ri·po·lar [ˌplʊərɪ'pəʊlər] *adj* multi-, pluripolar.
pluripolar mitosis multipolare Mitose *f*.
plu·ri·po·tent [ˌ-'pəʊtnt, plʊə'rɪpətənt] *adj* pluripotent; omnipotent.
pluripotent cell *embryo.* omnipotente/pluripotente Zelle *f*.
plu·ri·po·ten·tial [ˌ-pə'tentʃl] *adj* → pluripotent.
plu·ri·po·ten·ti·al·i·ty [ˌ-pəˌtentʃɪ'ælətɪ] *n* Pluripotenz *f*.
plur·i·vac·u·o·lar [ˌ-ˌvækjuː'əʊlər, -'vækjuːə-, -'vækjələr] *adj* plurivakulär.
plus cyclophoria [plʌs] *ophthal.* Exzyklophorie *f*.
plus cyclotropia *ophthal.* Exzyklotropie *f*.
plus lens konvexe Linse *f*, Konvexlinse *f*, Sammellinse *f*.
plu·to·ni·um [pluː'təʊnɪəm] *n abbr.* **Pu** Plutonium *nt abbr.* Pu.
Pm *abbr.* → promethium.
p.m. *abbr.* → postmortal.
PMB *abbr.* → polymorphonuclear basophil leukocyte.
PMC *abbr.* → premotor cortex.
PMD *abbr.* → progressive muscular dystrophy.
PME *abbr.* → polymorphonuclear eosinophil leukocyte.
P mitrale *card.* P mitrale, P sinistroatriale, P sinistrocardiale.
PML *abbr.* → progressive multifocale leukoencephalopathy.
PMLE *abbr.* → polymorphic light eruption.
PMMA *abbr.* → polymethyl methacrylate.
PMN *abbr.* → polymorphonuclear neutrophil leukocyte.
PMS *abbr.* → premenstrual syndrome.
PMT *abbr.* [premenstrual tension] → premenstrual syndrome.
PN *abbr.* → pyelonephritis.
pne·o·dy·nam·ics [ˌniːəʊdaɪ'næmɪks] *pl* → pneumodynamics.
pne·o·gram [ˈ-græm] *n* Spirogramm *nt*.
pne·o·graph ['-græf] *n* Spirograph *m*.
pne·om·e·ter [nɪ'ɑmɪtər] *n* Spirometer *nt*.
pneum(a)- *pref.* → pneumo-.
pneu·mal ['njuːməl, 'nʊ-] *adj* Lunge betr., pulmonal, Lungen-, Pulmonal-.
pneu·mar·thro·gram [n(j)uː'mɑːrθrəɡræm] *n radiol., ortho.* Pneumarthrogramm *nt*.
pneu·mar·throg·ra·phy [ˌn(j)uːmɑːr'θrɑgrəfɪ] *n radiol., ortho.* Pneumarthrographie *f*.
pneu·mar·thro·sis [ˌn(j)uːmɑːr'θrəʊsɪs] *n ortho.* Pneumarthrose *f*, -arthrosis *f*.
pneu·ma·the·mia [ˌn(j)uːmə'θiːmɪə] *n* → pneumatohemia.
pneu·mat·ic [njuː'mætɪk, nʊ-] *adj* Pneumatik betr.; (Druck-)Luft *od.* Gas *od.* Atmung betr., lufthaltig, pneumatisch.

608

pneumatic bone Knochen *m* mit lufthaltigen Zellen, pneumatischer Knochen *m*, Os pneumaticum.
pneumatic cuff pneumatische Manschette *f*.
pneumatic dilatation *chir.* pneumatische Dilatation *f*.
pneu·mat·ics [njuː'mætɪks, nʊ-] *pl phys.* Pneumatik *f*.
pneumatic sign *HNO* Hennebert'-Fistelsymptom *nt*.
pneumatic test → pneumatic sign.
pneumatic tourniquet pneumatische Manschette *f*.
pneu·ma·ti·nu·ria [ˌn(j)uːməti'n(j)ʊərɪə] *n* → pneumaturia.
pneu·ma·ti·za·tion [ˌ-'zeɪʃn] *n* (*Knochen*) Pneumatisation *f*.
pneu·ma·tized ['n(j)uːmətaɪzd] *adj* lufthaltig.
pneumato- *pref.* → pneumo-.
pneu·ma·to·car·dia [ˌn(j)uːmətəʊ'kɑːrdɪə] *n* Pneumatokardie *f*.
pneu·ma·to·cele ['-siːl] *n* **1.** Luftgeschwulst *f*, Pneumatozele *f*. **2.** Lungenhernie *f*, Pneumatozele *f*, Pneumozele *f*. **3.** Aerozele *f*.
pneu·ma·to·ceph·a·lus [ˌ-'sefələs] *n* → pneumocephalus.
pneu·ma·to·gram ['-græm] *n* Spirogramm *nt*.
pneu·ma·to·graph ['-græf] *n* Spirograph *m*.
pneu·ma·to·he·mia [ˌ-'hiːmɪə] *n* Luftembolie *f*, Pneumo-, Pneumatohämie *f*.
pneu·ma·tom·e·ter [ˌn(j)uːmə'tɑmɪtər] *n* **1.** Spirometer *nt*. **2.** Pneumatometer *nt*.
pneu·ma·tom·e·try [ˌ-'tɑmətrɪ] *n* **1.** Spirometrie *f*. **2.** Pneumatometrie *f*.
pneu·ma·tor·rha·chis [ˌ-'tɔːrəkɪs] *n* → pneumorrhachis.
pneu·ma·to·sis [ˌ-'təʊsɪs] *n* Pneumatose *f*, Pneumatosis *f*.
pneu·ma·to·tho·rax [ˌn(j)uːmətəʊ'θɔːræks] *n* → pneumothorax.
pneu·ma·tu·ria [ˌn(j)uːmə't(j)ʊərɪə] *n* Luftharnen *nt*, Pneumaturie *f*.
pneu·mec·to·my [n(j)uː'mektəmɪ] *n* → pneumonectomy.
pneum·en·ceph·a·log·ra·phy [ˌn(j)uːmenˌsefə'lɑgrəfɪ] *n* → pneumoencephalography.
pneumo- *pref.* Luft-, Gas-, Atem-, Atmungs-, Lungen-, Pneumo-, Pulmo-.
pneu·mo·ar·throg·ra·phy [ˌn(j)uːməʊɑːr'θrɑgrəfɪ] *n* → pneumarthrography.
pneu·mo·ba·cil·lus [ˌ-bə'sɪləs] *n micro.* Friedländer-Bakterium *nt*, -Bazillus *m*, Klebsiella pneumoniae, Bact. pneumoniae Friedländer.
pneu·mo·bi·lia [ˌ-'bɪlɪə] *n* Pneumobilie *f*.
pneu·mo·bul·bar [ˌ-'bʌlbər, -bɑːr] *adj* pneumobulbär.
pneu·mo·bul·bous [ˌ-'bʌlbəs] *adj* → pneumobulbar.
pneu·mo·car·di·al [ˌ-'kɑːrdɪəl] *adj* Herz u. Lunge(n) betr., pneumokardial, kardiopulmonal.
pneu·mo·cele ['-siːl] *n* → pneumatocele.
pneu·mo·cen·te·sis [ˌ-sen'tiːsɪs] *n* → pneumonocentesis.
pneu·mo·ceph·a·lus [ˌ-'sefələs] *n* Pneumo-, Pneumatozephalus *m*.
pneu·mo·cho·le·cys·ti·tis [ˌ-ˌkəʊləsɪs'taɪtɪs] *n* emphysematöse Gallenblasenentzündung/Cholezystitis *f*, Cholecystitis emphysematosa.
pneu·mo·cis·ter·nog·ra·phy [ˌ-ˌsɪstər'nɑgrəfɪ] *n radiol.* Pneumozisternographie *f*, -cisternographie *f*.
pneu·mo·coc·cal [ˌ-'kɑkl] *adj* Pneumokokken betr., Pneumokokken-.

pneumococcal angina Pneumokokkenangina f.
pneumococcal infection Pneumokokkeninfektion f, Pneumokokkose f.
pneumococcal meningitis Pneumokokkenmeningitis f.
pneumococcal pneumonia Pneumokokkenpneumonie f.
pneumococcal polysaccharide Pneumokokkenpolysaccharid nt.
pneumococcal vaccine Pneumokokkenvakzine f.
pneu·mo·coc·ce·mia [ˌ-kɑkˈsiːmɪə] n Pneumokokkensepsis f, Pneumokokkämie f.
pneu·mo·coc·ci pl → pneumococcus.
pneu·mo·coc·cic [ˌ-ˈkɑksɪk] adj → pneumococcal.
pneu·mo·coc·ci·dal [ˌ-kɑkˈsaɪdl] adj Pneumokokken zerstörend.
pneu·mo·coc·co·sis [ˌ-kəˈkəʊsɪs] n Pneumokokkeninfektion f, Pneumokokkose f.
pneu·mo·coc·co·su·ria [ˌ-ˌkɑkəˈs(j)ʊərɪə] n Pneumokokkenausscheidung f im Harn, Pneumokokkosurie f.
pneu·mo·coc·cus [ˌ-ˈkɑkəs] n, pl **-coc·ci** [-kaɪ, -kiː, -saɪ, -siː] (Fränkel-)Pneumokokkus m, Pneumococcus m, Streptococcus/Diplococcus pneumoniae.
pneumococcus nephritis Pneumokokkennephritis f.
pneumococcus ulcer Ulcus corneae serpens.
pneu·mo·co·lon [ˌ-ˈkəʊlən] n Pneumokolon nt.
pneu·mo·co·ni·o·sis [ˌ-ˌkəʊnɪˈəʊsɪs] n Staublunge f, Staublungenerkrankung f, Pneumokoniose f.
p. of coal workers Kohlenstaublunge f, Lungenanthrakose f, Anthracosis pulmonum.
pneu·mo·cra·nia [ˌ-ˈkreɪnɪə] n → pneumocephalus.
pneu·mo·cra·ni·um [ˌ-ˈkreɪnɪəm] n → pneumocephalus.
pneu·mo·cys·tic [ˌ-ˈsɪstɪk] adj Pneumocystis betr., durch Pneumocystis hervorgerufen, Pneumocystis-.
Pneu·mo·cys·tis [ˌ-ˈsɪstɪs] n micro. Pneumocystis f.
pneumocystis carinii pneumonitis Pneumocystis-Pneumonie f, interstitielle Plasmazellpneumonie f, Pneumocystose f.
Pneumocystis pneumonia Pneumocystis-Pneumonie f, interstitielle Plasmazellpneumonie f, Pneumocystose f.
pneu·mo·cys·tog·ra·phy [ˌ-sɪsˈtɑgrəfɪ] n urol., radiol. Pneumozystographie f.
pneu·mo·cys·to·sis [ˌ-sɪsˈtəʊsɪs] n → Pneumocystis pneumonia.
pneu·mo·cyte [ˈ-saɪt] n → pneumonocyte.
pneu·mo·der·ma [ˌ-ˈdɜrmə] n Hautemphysem nt, subkutanes Emphysem nt.
pneu·mo·dy·nam·ics [ˌ-daɪˈnæmɪks] pl Atem-, Pneumodynamik f.
pneu·mo·em·py·e·ma [ˌ-empaɪˈiːmə] n Pyopneumothorax m.
pneu·mo·en·ceph·a·li·tis [ˌ-enˌsefəˈlaɪtɪs] n atypische Geflügelpest f, Newcastle disease (nt).
pneu·mo·en·ceph·a·lo·gram [ˌ-enˈsefələgræm] n radiol. Pneum(o)enzephalogramm n.
pneu·mo·en·ceph·a·log·ra·phy [ˌ-enˌsefəˈlɑgrəfɪ] n abbr. **PEG** radiol. Pneum(o)enzephalographie f.
pneu·mo·en·ceph·a·lo·my·el·o·gram [ˌ-enˌsefələʊˈmaɪələgræm] n radiol. Pneum(o)enzephalomyelogramm nt.
pneu·mo·en·ceph·a·lo·my·e·log·ra·phy [ˌ-enˌsefələʊˌmaɪəˈlɑgrəfɪ] n radiol.

Pneum(o)enzephalomyelographie f.
pneu·mo·en·ter·i·tis [ˌ-entəˈraɪtɪs] n Pneumoenteritis f.
pneu·mo·fas·ci·o·gram [ˌ-ˈfæsɪəgræm] n radiol. Pneumofasziogramm nt.
pneu·mo·ga·lac·to·cele [ˌ-gəˈlæktəsiːl] n gyn. Pneumogalaktozele f.
pneu·mo·gas·tric [ˌ-ˈgæstrɪk] adj Magen u. Lunge(n) betr., pneumogastral, gastropulmonal.
pneu·mo·gas·trog·ra·phy [ˌ-gæsˈtrɑgrəfɪ] n radiol. Pneumogastrographie f.
pneu·mo·gram [ˈ-græm] n **1.** Spirogramm nt. **2.** radiol. Pneumogramm nt.
pneu·mo·graph [ˈ-græf] n Spirograph m.
pneu·mog·ra·phy [n(j)uːˈmɑgrəfɪ] n radiol. Pneumographie f, Pneumoradiographie f, Pneumoröntgengraphie f.
pneu·mo·he·mia [ˌn(j)uːməˈhiːmɪə] n → pneumatohemia.
pneu·mo·he·mo·per·i·car·di·um [ˌhiːməˌperɪˈkɑrdɪəm] n Pneumohämoperikard nt, Hämopneumoperikard nt.
pneu·mo·he·mo·tho·rax [ˌ-ˌhiːməˈθɔːræks] n Pneumohämothorax m, Hämopneumothorax m.
pneu·mo·hy·dro·me·tra [ˌ-ˌhaɪdrəˈmiːtrə] n gyn. Pneumohydrometra f.
pneu·mo·hy·dro·per·i·car·di·um [ˌ-ˌhaɪdrəˌperɪˈkɑrdɪəm] n Pneumohydroperikard nt, Hydropneumoperikard nt.
pneu·mo·hy·dro·per·i·to·ne·um [ˌ-ˌhaɪdrəˌperɪtnˈiːəm] n Pneumohydroperitoneum nt, Hydropneumoperitoneum nt.
pneu·mo·hy·dro·tho·rax [ˌ-ˌhaɪdrəˈθɔːræks] n Pneumohydrothorax m, Hydropneumothorax m.
pneu·mo·hy·po·der·ma [ˌ-ˌhaɪpəˈdɜrmə] n → pneumoderma.
pneu·mo·ko·ni·o·sis n → pneumoconiosis.
pneu·mo·lip·oi·do·sis [ˌ-ˌlɪpɔɪˈdəʊsɪs] n Lipidpneumonie f, Öl-, Fettaspirationspneumonie f.
pneu·mo·lith [ˈ-lɪθ] n Lungenstein m, Pneumolith m.
pneu·mo·li·thi·a·sis [ˌ-lɪˈθaɪəsɪs] n Pneumolithiasis f.
pneu·mol·o·gy [n(j)uːˈmɑlədʒɪ] n Pneumologie f, Pneumonologie f, Pulmonologie f, Pulmologie f.
pneu·mol·y·sis [n(j)uːˈmɑləsɪs] n → pneumonolysis.
pneu·mo·ma·la·cia [ˌn(j)uːməˈleɪʃ(ɪ)ə] n patho. Lungenerweichung f, Pneumomalazie f, -malacia f.
pneu·mo·me·di·as·ti·no·gram [ˌ-ˌmɪdɪəˈstaɪnəgræm] n radiol. Pneumomediastinogramm nt.
pneu·mo·me·di·as·ti·nog·ra·phy [ˌ-ˌmɪdɪæstaɪˈnɑgrəfɪ] n radiol. Pneumomediastinographie f.
pneu·mo·me·di·as·ti·num [ˌ-ˌmɪdɪəˈstaɪnəm] n (spontanes) Mediastinalemphysem nt, Hamman-Syndrom nt, Pneumomediastinum nt.
pneu·mo·mel·a·no·sis [ˌ-ˌmelæˈnəʊsɪs] n Pneumo-, Pneumonomelanose f.
pneu·mom·e·ter [n(j)uːˈmɑmɪtər] n **1.** Pneumatometer nt. **2.** Spirometer nt.
pneu·mo·my·co·sis [ˌn(j)uːməmaɪˈkəʊsɪs] n Pilzerkrankung f der Lunge, Lungen-, Pneumo-, Pneumonomykose f.
pneu·mo·my·e·log·ra·phy [ˌ-maɪəˈlɑgrəfɪ] n radiol. Pneumomyelographie f.
pneu·mon·ec·ta·sia [ˌn(j)uːmənekˈteɪʒ(ɪ)ə] n → pneumonectasis.
pneu·mo·nec·ta·sis [ˌn(j)uːməˈnektəsɪs] n Lungenüberblähung f; Lungenemphysem nt.
pneu·mo·nec·to·my [ˌ-ˈnektəmɪ] n chir., HTG **1.** Lungenresektion f, Pneumektomie f, Pneumonektomie f. **2.** Entfernung

f eines Lungenflügels, Pneumektomie f, Pneumonektomie f.
pneu·mo·ne·de·ma [ˌn(j)uːmɑnɪˈdiːmə] n Lungenödem nt.
pneu·mo·ne·mia [ˌn(j)uːməˈniːmɪə] n Lungenstauung f.
pneu·mo·nia [n(j)uːˈməʊnɪə, -njə] n Lungen(parenchym)entzündung f, Pneumonie f, Pneumonia f.
pneu·mon·ic [n(j)uːˈmɑnɪk] adj **1.** Lunge betr., pulmonal, Lungen-. **2.** Lungenentzündung/Pneumonie betr., pneumonisch.
pneumonic fever old → pneumonia.
pneumonic plague Lungenpest f, Pestpneumonie f.
pneu·mo·ni·tis [ˌn(j)uːməˈnaɪtɪs] n (interstitielle) Lungenentzündung/Pneumonie f, Pneumonitis f.
pneumono- pref. → pneumo-.
pneu·mo·no·cele [ˈn(j)uːmənəʊsiːl] n Lungenhernie f, Pneumatozele f, Pneumozele f.
pneu·mo·no·cen·te·sis [ˌ-senˈtiːsɪs] n Lungenpunktion f, Pneumozentese f.
pneu·mo·no·cir·rho·sis [ˌ-sɪˈrəʊsəs] n Lungenfibrose f, -zirrhose f.
pneu·mo·no·coc·cus [ˌ-ˈkɑkəs] n → pneumococcus.
pneu·mo·no·co·ni·o·sis [ˌ-ˌkəʊnɪˈəʊsɪs] n → pneumoconiosis.
pneu·mon·o·cyte [n(j)uːˈmɑnəsaɪt] n Alveolarzelle f, Pneumozyt m, -cyt m.
pneu·mo·no·en·ter·i·tis [ˌn(j)uːmənəʊˌentəˈraɪtɪs] n Pneumoenteritis f.
pneu·mo·nog·ra·phy [ˌn(j)uːməˈnɑgrəfɪ] n → pneumography.
pneu·mo·no·ko·ni·o·sis [ˌn(j)uːmənəʊˌkəʊnɪˈəʊsɪs] n → pneumoconiosis.
pneu·mo·no·lip·oi·do·sis [ˌ-lɪpɔɪˈdəʊsɪs] n Lipidpneumonie f, Öl-, Fettaspirationspneumonie f.
pneu·mo·nol·y·sis [ˌn(j)uːməˈnɑləsɪs] n HTG Pneumolyse f, Pleurolyse f.
pneu·mo·no·mel·a·no·sis [ˌn(j)uːmənəʊmeləˈnəʊsɪs] n → pneumomelanosis.
pneu·mo·no·mil·i·a·sis [ˌ-ˌmɑnɪˈlaɪəsɪs] n Lungencandidose f.
pneu·mo·no·my·co·sis [ˌ-maɪˈkəʊsɪs] n → pneumomycosis.
pneu·mo·no·pal·u·dism [ˌ-ˈpæljədɪzəm] n Bruns'-Krankheit f.
pneu·mo·nop·a·thy [ˌn(j)uːməˈnɑpəθɪ] n Lungenerkrankung f, Pneumopathie f.
pneu·mo·no·pex·y [n(j)uːˈmɑnəpeksɪ] n HTG Pneumo-, Pneumonopexie f.
pneu·mon·oph·thi·sis [ˌn(j)uːməˈnɑfˈθaɪsɪs] n → pulmonary tuberculosis.
pneu·mo·no·pleu·ri·tis [ˌn(j)uːmənəʊplʊəˈraɪtɪs] n → pneumopleuritis.
pneu·mo·no·re·sec·tion [ˌ-rɪˈsekʃn] n → pneumoresection.
pneu·mo·nor·rha·gia [n(j)uːˌmənəˈreɪdʒ(ɪ)ə] n → pneumorrhagia.
pneu·mo·nor·rha·phy [ˌn(j)uːməˈnɔrəfɪ] n HTG Lungennaht f, Pneumorrhaphie f.
pneu·mo·no·sis [ˌ-ˈnəʊsɪs] n Pneumonose f, Pneumonosis f.
pneu·mo·not·o·my [ˌ-ˈnɑtəmɪ] n HTG Lungenschnitt m, Pneumotomie f.
pneu·mo·pal·u·dism [ˌ-ˈpæljədɪzəm] n Bruns'-Krankheit f.
pneu·mop·a·thy [n(j)uːˈmɑpəθɪ] n Lungenerkrankung f, Pneumopathie f.
pneu·mo·per·i·car·di·um [ˌn(j)uːməˌperɪˈkɑrdɪəm] n Pneumoperikard nt.
pneu·mo·per·i·to·ne·um [ˌ-ˌperɪtəˈniːəm] n Pneumoperitoneum nt.
pneu·mo·per·i·to·ni·tis [ˌ-ˌperɪtəˈnaɪtɪs] n Pneumoperitonitis f.
pneu·mo·pex·y [ˈ-peksɪ] n → pneumonopexy.

pneu·mo·pha·gia [ˌ-ˈfeɪdʒ(ɪ)ə] n (krankhaftes) Luft(ver)schlucken nt, Aerophagie f.
pneu·mo·pleu·ri·tis [ˌ-pluːˈraɪtɪs] n Entzündung f von Lunge u. Pleura, Pneumopleuritis f, Pleuropneumonie f.
pneu·mo·py·e·log·ra·phy [ˌ-paɪəˈlɑgrəfɪ] n urol., radiol. Pneumopyelographie f.
pneu·mo·py·o·per·i·car·di·um [ˌ-ˌpaɪəˌperɪˈkɑːrdɪəm] n Pneumopyoperikard nt.
pneu·mo·py·o·tho·rax [ˌ-ˌpaɪəˈθɔːræks] n Pneumopyothorax m.
pneu·mo·ra·di·og·ra·phy [ˌ-ˌreɪdɪˈɑgrəfɪ] n radiol. Pneumographie f, Pneumoradiographie f, Pneumoröntgengraphie f.
pneu·mo·re·sec·tion [ˌ-rɪˈsekʃn] n HTG Lungenteilentfernung f, resektion f.
pneu·mo·ret·ro·per·i·to·ne·um [ˌ-ˌretrəʊperɪtəˈniːəm] n Pneumoretroperitoneum nt, Retropneumoperitoneum nt.
pneu·mo·roent·gen·og·ra·phy [ˌ-rentgəˈnɑgrəfɪ] n → pneumoradiography.
pneu·mor·rha·chis [n(j)uːˈmɔːrəkɪs] n Pneumorrhachis f.
pneu·mor·rha·gia [ˌn(j)uːməˈreɪdʒ(ɪ)ə] n Lungenblutung f, Pneumorrhagie f.
pneu·mo·se·ro·tho·rax [ˌ-ˌsɪərəˈθɔːræks] n Pneumoserothorax m, Hydropneumothorax m.
pneu·mo·sil·i·co·sis [ˌ-ˌsɪlɪˈkəʊsɪs] n (Lungen-)Silikose f.
pneu·mo·tach·o·gram [ˌ-ˈtækəgræm] n Pneumotachogramm nt.
pneu·mo·tach·o·graph [ˌ-ˈtækəgræf] n Pneumotachograph m.
pneu·mo·ta·chom·e·ter [ˌ-tæˈkɑmɪtər] n Pneumotachometer nt.
pneu·mo·tach·y·gram [ˌ-ˈtækɪgræm] n → pneumotachogram.
pneu·mo·tach·y·graph [ˌ-ˈtækɪgræf] n → pneumotachograph.
pneu·mo·tho·rax [ˌ-ˈθɔːræks] n Gasbrust f, Pneumothorax m; inf. Pneu m.
pneu·mot·o·my [n(j)uːˈmɑtəmɪ] n → pneumonotomy.
pneu·mo·trop·ic [ˌn(j)uːməˈtrɑpɪk, -ˈtrəʊ-] adj auf die Lunge einwirkend, mit besonderer Affinität zur Lunge, pneumotrop.
pneu·mot·ro·pism [n(j)uːˈmɑtrəpɪzəm] n Pneumotropismus m, Pneumotropie f.
pneu·mo·tym·pa·num [ˌn(j)uːməˈtɪmpənəm] n Pneumotympanum nt.
pneu·mo·u·ria [ˌ-ˈ(j)ʊərɪə] n → pneumaturia.
pneu·mo·ven·tri·cle [ˌ-ˈventrɪkl] n Pneumoventrikel m.
pneu·mo·ven·tric·u·log·ra·phy [ˌ-venˌtrɪkjəˈlɑgrəfɪ] n radiol. Pneumoventrikulographie f.
Pneu·mo·vi·rus [ˌ-ˈvaɪrəs] n micro. Pneumovirus nt.
pneu·sis [ˈn(j)uːsɪs] n Atmung f.
PNH abbr. → paroxysmal nocturnal hemoglobinuria.
PNH cells PNH-Erythrozyten pl.
PNMT abbr. → phenylethanolamine-N-methyltransferase.
PNPB abbr. [positive-negative pressure breathing] → positive-negative pressure ventilation.
PNPV abbr. → positive-negative pressure ventilation.
PNS abbr. → peripheral nervous system.
Po abbr. → polonium.
Po₂ abbr. → partial pressure, oxygen.
pO₂ abbr. → partial pressure, oxygen.
POA abbr. → pancreatic oncofetal antigen.
pock [pɑk] n derm. Pocke f.
pock·et [ˈpɑkɪt] n 1. Tasche f. 2. anat. Tasche f, Sack m, Beutel m.
pocket calculus urol. verkapselter (Harn-)Blasenstein m.

pock·mark [ˈpɑkmɑːrk] n Pockennarbe f.
pod- pref. → podo-.
po·dag·ra [pəʊˈdægrə, ˈpædəgrə] n Podagra f.
po·dag·ral [pəʊˈdægrəl] adj Podagra betr., an Podagra leidend, podagrisch, Podagra-.
po·dag·ric [pəʊˈdægrɪk] adj → podagral.
po·dag·rous [pəʊˈdægrəs] adj → podagral.
po·dal·gia [pəʊˈdældʒ(ɪ)ə] n Schmerzen pl im Fuß, Fußschmerz(en pl) m, Podalgie f, Pododynie f.
po·dal·ic [pəʊˈdældʒɪk] adj Fuß od. Füße betr., Pod(o)-, Fuß-.
pod·ar·thri·tis [ˌpɑdɑːrˈθraɪtɪs] n Fußgelenk(s)entzündung f, Podarthritis f.
pod·e·de·ma [pɑdɪˈdiːmə] n Fuß- u. Knöchelödem m.
pod·en·ceph·a·lus [ˌpɑdenˈsefələs] n embryo. Podenzephalus m.
po·di·at·ric [pəʊdɪˈætrɪk] adj Fußpflege betr.
po·di·a·trist [pəˈdaɪətrɪst, pəʊ-] n Fußpfleger(in f) m, Pediküre f, Podologe m, -login f.
po·di·a·try [pəˈdaɪətrɪ, pəʊ-] n Fußpflege f, Pediküre f.
po·dis·mus [pəʊˈdɪzməs] n → podospasm.
po·di·tis [pəʊˈdaɪtɪs] n entzündliche Fußerkrankung f.
podo- pref. Fuß-, Pod(o)-.
pod·o·cyte [ˈpɑdəsaɪt] n Füßchen-, Deckzelle f, Epizyt m, Podozyt m.
pod·o·dyn·ia [ˌ-ˈdɪnɪə] n → podalgia.
pod·o·gram [ˈ-græm] n Podogramm nt.
pod·o·graph [ˈ-græf] n Podograph m.
po·dol·o·gist [pəˈdɑlədʒɪst] n → podiatrist.
po·dol·o·gy [pəˈdɑlədʒɪ] n → podiatry.
pod·o·phyl·lin [ˌpɑdəˈfɪlɪn] n pharm. Podophyllin(um) nt, Resina podophylli.
pod·o·phyl·lo·tox·in [ˌ-ˌfɪləˈtɑksɪn] n Podophyllotoxin nt.
pod·o·phyl·lum [ˌ-ˈfɪləm] n pharm. Podophyllum nt.
podophyllum resin → podophyllin.
pod·o·spasm [ˈ-spæzəm] n Fuß(muskel)krampf m, Podospasmus m.
pod·o·spas·mus [ˌ-ˈspæzməs] n → podospasm.
pOH abbr. chem. pOH(-Wert m) m.
poikil(o)- pref. Bunt-, Poikil(o)-.
poi·ki·lo·blast [ˈpɔɪkɪləʊblæst, pɔɪˈkɪlə-] n Poikiloblast m.
poi·ki·lo·cyte [ˈ-saɪt] n Poikilozyt m.
poi·ki·lo·cy·the·mia [ˌ-saɪˈθiːmɪə] n → poikilocytosis.
poi·ki·lo·cy·to·sis [ˌ-saɪˈtəʊsɪs] n Poikilozytose f, -zythämie f.
poi·ki·lo·der·ma [ˌ-ˈdɜːrmə] n derm. Poikilodermie f, -dermia f, -derma nt.
 p. of Civatte Civatte²-Krankheit f, -Poikilodermie.
poi·ki·lo·der·ma·tous parapsoriasis [ˌ-ˈdɜːrmətəs] → poikilodermic parapsoriasis.
poi·ki·lo·der·mic parapsoriasis [ˌ-ˈdɜːrmɪk] 1. derm. großherdig-entzündliche Form f der Parapsoriasis en plaques, prämaligne Form f der Parapsoriasis en plaques, Parapsoriasis en plaques simples. 2. Parapsoriasis lichenoides, Parakeratosis variegata, Lichen variegatus.
poi·ki·los·mo·sis [ˌpɔɪkɪlɑzˈməʊsɪs] n bio. Poikilosmose f.
poi·ki·los·mot·ic [ˌ-ˈmɑtɪk] adj bio. poikilosmotisch.
poi·ki·lo·therm [pɔɪˈkɪləθɜːrm, ˈpɔɪkɪləʊ-] n bio. wechselwarmes/poikilothermes Lebewesen nt, Wechselblüter m.
poi·ki·lo·ther·mal [pɔɪˌkɪləˈθɜːrml, ˌpɔɪkɪləʊ-]] adj → poikilothermic.

poi·ki·lo·ther·mic [ˌ-ˈθɜːrmɪk] adj bio. wechselwarm, poikilotherm.
poi·ki·lo·ther·mism [ˌ-ˈθɜːrmɪzəm] n → poikilothermy.
poi·ki·lo·ther·my [ˌ-ˈθɜːrmɪ] n Poikilothermie f
poi·kil·o·throm·bo·cyte [ˌ-ˈθrɑmbəsaɪt] n Poikilothrombozyt m.
point [pɔɪnt] I n 1. (Messer-, Nadel-)Spitze f; spitzes Instrument od. Werkzeug nt, Nadel f. 2. mathe. (Dezimal-)Punkt m, Komma nt; (geometrischer) Punkt m. 3. phys. (Thermometer) Grad m. 4. (Anschluß-, Verbindungs-)Punkt m, (bestimmte) Stelle f, Berührungspunkt m; anat. Punctum m. 5. Grenze f, Grenz-, Höhepunkt m. 6. (kritischer) (Zeit-)Punkt m, (entscheidender) Augenblick m. 7. Ansicht f, Stand-, Gesichtspunkt m. II vt 8. (an-, zu-)spitzen. 9. hinweisen, zeigen, deuten (to auf); richten (at auf). III vi 10. (Abszeß) reifen, reif werden. 11. hinweisen, hindeuten (to auf).
 point out vt → point 9.
 p. of action → p. of application.
 p. of application phys. Angriffspunkt (der Kraft).
 p. of congelation phys. Gefrierpunkt.
 p. of convergence phys. Konvergenzpunkt.
 p. of divergence phys. Divergenzpunkt.
 p. of elbow Ell(en)bogenfortsatz m, -höcker m, Olekranon nt, Olecranon nt.
 p. of fixation Blick-, Fixierpunkt.
 p. of incidence phys. Einfallspunkt.
 p. of intersection Schnitt-, Kreuzungspunkt.
 p. of regard Blick-, Fixierpunkt.
 p. of time → point 6.
 p. of view → point 7.
point analysis Punkt-, Ortsanalyse f.
point·ed [ˈpɔɪntɪd] adj spitz, zugespitzt; fig. scharf, spitz.
pointed condyloma (spitze) Feig-, Feuchtwarze f, spitzes Kondylom nt, Condyloma acuminatum, Papilloma acuminatum/venereum.
point·ed·ness [ˈpɔɪntɪdnɪs] n Spitzigkeit f; (a. fig.) Schärfe f.
pointed wart → pointed condyloma.
point·er [ˈpɔɪntər] n 1. (Meßgerät) Zeiger m. 2. Fingerzeig m, Tip m, Hinweis m; Anzeichen nt.
point·less [ˈpɔɪntlɪs] adj 1. ohne Spitze, stumpf. 2. sinnlos.
point mutation genet. Punktmutation f.
point system Punktschrift f (für Blinde).
point tenderness Punktschmerz m, Punktschmerzhaftigkeit f.
Poirier [pwaˈrje]: **P.'s orange** Methylorange nt, Helianthin f.
poise [pɔɪz] n phys. abbr. **P** Poise nt abbr. P.
Poiseuille [pwaˈsœj]: **P.'s law** phys. Hagen-Poiseuille'-Gesetz nt.
poi·son [ˈpɔɪzn] I n (a. fig.) Gift nt. II adj gift-, Gift-. III vt 1. vergiften. **to ~ o.s.** s. vergiften. 2. infizieren.
poison cabinet Giftschrank m.
poison gas Giftgas nt.
poi·son·ing [ˈpɔɪzənɪŋ] n 1. Vergiftung f, Vergiften nt. 2. Giftmord m.
poison ivy Giftefeu nt, Rhus radicans.
poison ivy dermatitis Rhusdermatitis f.
poi·son·less [ˈpɔɪznlɪs] adj keine Gifte enthaltend, giftfrei.
poison oak Gifteiche f, Rhus diversiloba.
poison oak dermatitis → poison ivy dermatitis.
poi·son·ous [ˈpɔɪzənəs] adj als Gift wirkend, Gift(e) enthaltend, giftig, toxisch, Gift-.

poison sumac Giftsumach *m*, Rhus vernix.
poison sumac dermatitis → poison ivy dermatitis.
poison tobacco *pharm.* Bilsenkraut *nt*, Hyoscyamus niger.
Poisson [pwa'zɔ̃]: **P. distribution** *stat.* Poisson-Verteilung *f.*
Poitou colic [pwa'tu] Bleikolik *f*, Colica saturnina.
pok·er back ['pəʊkər] Bechterew-Krankheit *f*, Morbus Bechterew *m*, Bechterew--Strümpell-Marie-Krankheit *f*, Marie--Strümpell-Krankheit *f*, Spondylarthritis/Spondylitis ankylopoetica/ankylosans.
pol I DNA-abhängige DNA-Polymerase *f*, DNS-abhängige DNS-Polymerase *f*, DNS-Nukleotidyltransferase *f*, DNS--Polymerase I *f*, Kornberg-Enzym *nt.*
pol II RNS-abhängige DNS-Polymerase *f*, RNA-abhängige DNA-Polymerase *f*, reverse Transkriptase *f abbr.* RT.
Poland ['pəʊlənd]: **P.'s anomaly/syndrome** *ortho.*, *embryo.* Poland-Anomalie *f*, -Syndrom *nt.*
po·lar [pəʊlər] *adj* **1.** *fig.* entgegengesetzt (wirkend). **2.** Pol betr., polar, Pol-, Polar-.
polar body Polkörper *m*, -körperchen *nt*, -körnchen *nt.*
polar cataract Polstar *m*, Cataracta polaris.
polar cell → polar body.
polar compound *chem.* polare Verbindung *f.*
polar coordinates *mathe.* Polarkoordinaten(system *nt*) *pl.*
polar cortex polare Rinde *f.*
polar cortical region polare Rindenregion *f.*
polar curve *mathe.* Polarkurve *f.*
polar globule → polar body.
polar granule → polar body.
po·la·rim·e·ter [ˌpəʊlə'rımıtər] *n phys.* Polarimeter *nt.*
po·lar·i·met·ric [pəʊˌlærə'metrık] *adj* Polarimeter betr., polarimetrisch.
po·la·rim·e·try [pəʊlə'rımətrı] *n* Polarimetrie *f.*
po·lar·i·scope [pəʊ'lærıskəʊp] *n* Polariskop *nt.*
po·lar·i·scop·ic [ˌ-'skɑpık] *adj* Polariskop *od.* Polariskopie betr., polariskopisch.
polariscopic analysis → polariscopy.
po·la·ris·co·py [pəʊlə'rıskəpı] *n* Polariskopie *f.*
po·lar·i·ty [pəʊ'lærətı, pə-] *n phys.* Polarität *f*; *fig.* Gegensätzlichkeit *f.*
po·lar·i·za·tion [ˌpəʊlərı'zeıʃn] *n* **1.** *phys.*, *physiol.*, *fig.* Polarisation *f*; Polarisieren *nt.* **2.** *embryo.* Polarisation *f.*
po·lar·ize ['pəʊləraız] **I** *vt phys.* polarisieren, ausrichten. **II** *vi fig.* s. polarisieren, s. spalten (*into* in).
po·lar·ized light ['pəʊləraızd] *phys.* polarisiertes Licht *nt.*
po·lar·iz·er ['pəʊləraızər] *n phys.* Polarisator *m.*
po·lar·iz·ing angle ['pəʊləraızıŋ] *opt.* Polarisationswinkel *m*, Brewster'-Winkel *m.*
polarizing filter (*Mikroskop*) Polfilter *m.*
polarizing microscope Polarisationsmikroskop *nt.*
polar lipid polares/amphipatisches Lipid *nt.*
polar molecule polares Molekül *nt.*
po·lar·o·gram [pəʊ'lærəgræm] *n* Polarogramm *nt.*
po·lar·o·graph·ic [ˌpəʊlərə'græfık] *adj* Polarographie betr., polarographisch.
po·la·rog·ra·phy [ˌpəʊlə'rɑgrəfı] *n* Polarographie *f.*
polar ray *histol.* Polarstrahl *m.*
polar region → polar cortical region.
polar zone Polarzone *f.*
pole [pəʊl] *n* Pol *m*; *anat.* Polus *m.*
p. of eye ball Augenpol, Polus bulbi oculi.
p. of kidney Nierenpol, Extremitas renis.
p. of lens Linsenpol, Polus lentis.
p. of testis Hodenpol, Extremitas testis.
Polhemus-Schafer-Ivemark [pə'hi:məs 'ʃɑ:fər, 'i:vmɑ:rk]: **P.-S.-I. syndrome** Ivemark-Syndrom *nt.*
poli- *pref.* → polio-.
pol·i·clin·ic [ˌpɑlı'klınık] *n* Poliklinik *f.*
pol·i·en·ceph·a·li·tis [ˌ-enˌsefə'laıtıs] *n* → polioencephalitis.
pol·i·en·ceph·a·lo·my·e·li·tis [ˌ-enˌsefələʊˌmaıə'laıtıs] *n* → polioencephalomyelitis.
polio- *pref.* Poli(o)-.
po·li·o ['pəʊlıˌəʊ] *n* → poliomyelitis.
po·li·o·clas·tic [ˌpəʊlıəʊ'klæstık] *adj* die graue Substanz zerstörend, polioklastisch.
po·li·o·dys·tro·phia [ˌ-dıs'trəʊfıə] *n* → poliodystrophy.
po·li·o·dys·tro·phy [ˌ-'dıstrəfı] *n* Poliodystrophie *f*, -dystrophia *f.*
po·li·o·en·ceph·a·li·tis [ˌ-enˌsefə'laıtıs] *n* Polioenzephalitis *f*, Polioencephalitis *f.*
po·li·o·en·ceph·a·lo·me·nin·go·my·e·li·tis [ˌ-enˌsefələʊmıˌnıŋgəʊˌmaıə'laıtıs] *n* Polioenzephalomeningomyelitis *f.*
po·li·o·en·ceph·a·lo·my·e·li·tis [ˌ-enˌsefələʊˌmaıə'laıtıs] *n* Polioenzephalomyelitis *f.*
po·li·o·en·ceph·a·lop·a·thy [ˌ-enˌsefə'lɑpəθı] *n* Polioenzephalopathie *f*, Polioencephalopathia *f.*
po·li·o·my·el·en·ceph·a·li·tis [ˌ-ˌmaıəlenˌsefə'laıtıs] *n* Poliomyeloenzephalitis *f.*
po·li·o·my·e·li·tis [ˌ-ˌmaıə'laıtıs] *n* Poliomyelitis *f*; *inf.* Polio *f.*
poliomyelitis vaccine Polio(myelitis)-impfstoff *m*, -vakzine *f.*
poliomyelitis virus *micro.* Poliomyelitis--Virus *nt*, Polio-Virus *nt.*
po·li·o·my·e·lo·en·ceph·a·li·tis [ˌ-ˌmaıələʊenˌsefə'laıtıs] *n* Poliomyeloenzephalitis *f.*
po·li·o·my·e·lop·a·thy [ˌ-ˌmaıə'lɑpəθı] *n* Poliomyelopathie *f.*
pol·i·o·sis [pɑlı'əʊsıs] *n derm.* Poliose *f*, Poliosis (circumscripta) *f.*
po·li·o·vi·rus [ˌpəʊlıəʊ'vaıərəs] *n micro.* Poliomyelitis-Virus *nt*, Polio-Virus *nt.*
poliovirus vaccine inactivated *abbr.* **IPV** Salk-Impfstoff *m*, Salk-Vakzine *f.*
poliovirus vaccine live oral *abbr.* **OPV** oraler Lebendpolioimpfstoff *m*, Sabin--Impfstoff *m*, Sabin-Vakzine *f.*
poliovirus vaccine live oral trivalent *abbr.* **TOPV** → poliovirus vaccine live oral.
Politzer ['pɑlıtsər]: **P.'s (air) bag** Politzer--Ballon *m.*
P.'s cone Trommelfell-, Lichtreflex *m.*
P.'s ear speculum Politzer-Ohrtrichter *m.*
P.'s luminous cone → P.'s cone.
P.'s method *HNO* Politzer-Luftdusche *f*, -Verfahren *nt.*
P.'s otoscope Politzer-Otoskop *nt.*
P.'s speculum Politzer-Ohrtrichter *m.*
P.'s test Politzer-Versuch *m.*
pol·it·zer·i·za·tion [ˌpɑlıtsəraı'zeıʃn] *n* → Politzer's method.
pol·ka fever ['pəʊ(l)kə] Dengue *nt*, Dengue-Fieber *nt*, Dandy-Fieber *nt.*
pol·kis·sen [pəʊl'kısən] *n* (*Niere*) Polkissen *nt.*

polyangiitis

pol·la·ki·su·ria [ˌpɑləkı's(j)ʊərıə] *n* → pollakiuria.
pol·la·ki·u·ria [ˌpɑləkı'(j)ʊərıə] *n* häufige Blasenentleerung *f*, Pollakisurie *f*, Pollakiurie *f.*
pol·len ['pɑlən] *n* Blütenstaub *m*, Pollen *m.*
pollen allergen → pollen antigen.
pollen allergy Heufieber *nt*, -schnupfen *m.*
pollen antigen Pollenantigen *nt*, -allergen *nt.*
pollen asthma Heufieber *nt*, -schnupfen *m.*
pollen coryza allergische Rhinitis *f*, Rhinopathia vasomotorica allergica.
pol·le·no·gen·ic [ˌpɑlınəʊ'dʒenık] *adj* durch Pollen hervorgerufen, Pollen-.
pol·le·no·sis [pɑlı'nəʊsıs] *n* → pollinosis.
pol·lex ['pɑleks] *n*, *pl* **pol·li·ces** ['pɑləsi:z] Daumen *m*, Pollex *m.*
pol·li·ci·za·tion [ˌpɑlısı'zeıʃn] *n ortho.* plastischer Daumenersatz *m*, Pollizisation *f.*
pol·li·no·sis [ˌpɑlı'nəʊsıs] *n* → Pollinose *f*, Pollinosis *f*; Pollenallergie *f*; Heuschnupfen *m*, Heufieber *nt.*
pol·lu·tant [pə'lu:tənt] *n* Schad-, Schmutzstoff *m.*
pol·lute [pə'lu:t] *vt* verunreinigen, verschmutzen, verpesten.
pol·lut·ed [pə'lu:tıd] *adj* verschmutzt, verunreinigt, verseucht.
pol·lut·er [pə'lu:tər] *n* (Umwelt-)Verschmutzer *m.*
pol·lu·tion [pə'lu:ʃn] *n* **1.** (*Luft*, *Wasser*, *Umwelt etc.*) Verschmutzung *f*, Verseuchung *f*, Verunreinigung *f.* **2.** Verschmutzen *nt*, Verseuchen *nt*, Verunreinigen *nt.*
po·lo·cyte ['pəʊləsaıt] *n* → polar body.
po·lo·ni·um [pə'ləʊnıəm] *n abbr.* **Po** Polonium *nt abbr.* Po.
pol·ox·a·mer [pə'lɑksəmər] *n* Poloxamer *nt.*
poly- *pref.* Viel-, Poly-.
pol·y ['pɑlı] *n inf.* → polymorphonuclear leukocyte.
Pólya ['pəʊlja]: **P. gastrectomy** → P.'s operation.
P.'s operation *chir.* Polya-Operation *f*, -Gastrektomie *f.*
polyA *abbr.* → polyadenylate.
pol·y·a·cryl·a·mide [ˌpɑlıə'krıləmaıd, -ˌækrə'læmaıd, -mıd] *n* Polyacrylamid *nt.*
pol·y·a·de·nia [ˌ-ə'di:nıə] *n* Polyadenie *f*, -adenia *f.*
pol·y·ad·e·ni·tis [ˌ-ˌædə'naıtıs] *n* Polyadenitis *f.*
pol·y·ad·e·no·ma [ˌ-ˌædə'nəʊmə] *n* Polyadenom *nt.*
pol·y·ad·e·no·ma·to·sis [ˌ-ˌædənəʊmə'təʊsıs] *n* Polyadenomatose *f*, -adenomatosis *f.*
pol·y·ad·e·nop·a·thy [ˌ-ˌædə'nɑpəθı] *n* Polyadenopathie *f.*
pol·y·ad·e·no·sis [ˌ-ˌædə'nəʊsıs] *n* Polyadenose *f*, -adenosis *f.*
pol·y·ad·e·nous [ˌ-'ædənəs] *adj* mehrere/viele Drüsen betr., polyglandulär, Polyadeno-.
pol·y·a·den·yl·ate [ˌ-ə'denlıt, -eıt, -'ædnl-] *n abbr.* **polyA** Polyadenylat *nt abbr.* polyA.
polyadenylate nucleotidyltransferase → polynucleotide adenylyltransferase.
pol·y·am·ide [ˌ-'æmaıd, -ıd] *n* Polyamid *nt.*
pol·y·a·mine [ˌ-ə'mi:n, -'æmın] *n* Polyamin *nt.*
pol·y·a·mi·no acid [ˌ-ə'mi:nəʊ -'æmınəʊ] Polyaminosäure *f.*
pol·y·an·drous [ˌ-'ændrəs] *adj* polyandrisch.
pol·y·an·dry ['-ændrı] *n* Polyandrie *f.*
pol·y·an·gi·i·tis [ˌ-ˌændʒı'aıtıs] *n* Polyangiitis *f*, -vaskulitis *f.*

polyangular

pol·y·an·gu·lar [ˌ-ˈæŋgjələr] *adj* vieleckig, Vielecks-.
pol·y·ar·te·ri·tis [ˌ-ˌɑːrtəˈraɪtɪs]-*n* Polyarteriitis *f*; Panarteriitis *f*.
pol·y·ar·thric [ˌ-ˈɑːrθrɪk] *adj* → polyarticular.
pol·y·ar·thri·tis [ˌ-ɑːrˈθraɪtɪs] *n ortho.* Entzündung *f* mehrerer Gelenke, Polyarthritis *f*.
pol·y·ar·tic·u·lar [ˌ-ɑːrˈtɪkjələr] *adj* mehrere/viele Gelenke betr., polyartikulär.
polyarticular gout polyartikuläre Gicht *f*.
pol·y·a·tom·ic [ˌ-əˈtɑmɪk] *n chem.* aus mehreren Atomen bestehend.
pol·y·aux·o·troph·ic [ˌ-ˌɔːksəˈtrɑfɪk] *adj bio.* polyauxotroph.
pol·y·a·vi·ta·min·o·sis [ˌ-eɪˌvaɪtəmɪˈnəʊsɪs] *n* Polyavitaminose *f*.
pol·y·ax·i·al [ˌ-ˈæksɪəl] *adj* mehr-, vielachsig.
polyaxial articulation Kugelgelenk *nt*, Artic. spheroidea.
polyaxial joint → polyaxial articulation.
pol·y·ax·on [ˌ-ˈæksɑn] *n* Polyaxon *nt*.
pol·y·ax·on·ic [ˌ-ækˈsɑnɪk] *adj* polyaxonal.
pol·y·ba·sic [ˌ-ˈbeɪsɪk] **I** *n* mehrbasische Säure *f*. **II** *adj* mehrbasisch.
pol·y·blen·nia [ˌ-ˈblenɪə] *n* übermäßige Schleimsekretion *f*.
pol·y·car·dia [ˌ-ˈkɑrdɪə] *n card.* Herzjagen *nt*, Tachykardie *f*.
pol·y·cel·lu·lar [ˌ-ˈseljələr] *adj* aus vielen Zellen bestehend, poly-, multizellulär.
pol·y·cen·tric [ˌ-ˈsentrɪk] *adj* polyzentrisch.
polycentric chromosome polyzentrisches Chromosom *nt*.
pol·y·chei·ria [ˌ-ˈkaɪrɪə] *n embryo.* Polych(e)irie *f*.
pol·y·che·mo·ther·a·py [ˌ-ˌkiːməˈθerəpɪ] *n* Polychemotherapie *f*.
pol·y·chlo·rin·at·ed biphenyl [ˌ-ˈklɔːrəneɪtɪd, -ˈklɔːr-] *abbr.* **PCB** polychloriertes Biphenyl *nt abbr.* PCB.
pol·y·cho·lia [ˌ-ˈkəʊlɪə] *n* übermäßige Gallensekretion *f*.
pol·y·chon·dri·tis [ˌ-kənˈdraɪtɪs] *n* Polychondritis *f*.
pol·y·chon·dro·path·ia [ˌ-ˌkɑndrəˈpæθɪə] *n* → polychondropathy.
pol·y·chon·drop·a·thy [ˌ-kənˈdrɑpəθɪ] *n* (von) Meyenburg-Altherr-Uehlinger--Syndrom *nt*, rezidivierende Polychondritis *f*, systematisierte Chondromalazie *f*.
pol·y·chro·ma·sia [ˌ-krəʊˈmeɪʒɪə] *n* **1.** *hema.* Polychromasie *f*. **2.** *histol.* Polychromatophilie *f*, Polychromasie *f*.
pol·y·chro·ma·tia [ˌ-krəʊˈmeɪʃɪə] *n* → polychromasia 2.
pol·y·chro·mat·ic [ˌ-krəʊˈmætɪk, -krə-] *adj* vielfarbig, bunt, polychromatisch.
polychromatic cells polychromatische Erythrozyten *pl*.
polychromatic erythroblast → polychromatic normoblast.
polychromatic normoblast polychromatischer Normoblast *m*.
pol·y·chro·mat·o·cyte [ˌ-krəʊˈmætəsaɪt] *n* polychromatische Zelle *f*.
pol·y·chro·mat·o·cy·to·sis [ˌ-ˌkrəʊmətəʊsaɪˈtəʊsɪs] *n* → polychromasia 2.
pol·y·chro·mat·o·phil [ˌ-krəʊˈmætəfɪl] *histol.* **I** *n* polychromatische Zelle *f*. **II** *adj* → polychromatophile.
polychromatophil cells polychromatische Erythrozyten *pl*.
pol·y·chro·mat·o·phile [ˌ-krəʊˈmætəfaɪl] *n, adj* → polychromatophil.
pol·y·chro·ma·to·phil·ia [ˌ-ˌkrəʊmətəʊˈfɪlɪə] *n* → polychromasia 2.
pol·y·chro·ma·to·phil·ic [ˌ-ˌkrəʊmətəʊˈfɪlɪk] *adj* → polychromatophil II.

pol·y·chro·ma·to·sis [ˌ-ˌkrəʊməˈtəʊsɪs] *n* → polychromasia 2.
pol·y·chro·mic [ˌ-ˈkrəʊmɪk] *adj* vielfarbig, bunt, polychrom.
pol·y·chro·mo·phil [ˌ-ˈkrəʊməfɪl] *n, adj* → polychromatophil.
pol·y·chro·mo·phil·ia [ˌ-krəʊməˈfɪlɪə] *n* → polychromasia 2.
pol·y·chy·lia [ˌ-ˈkaɪlɪə] *n* übermäßige Chylusbildung *f*.
pol·y·clo·nal [ˌ-ˈkləʊnl] *adj* polyklonal.
polyclonal antibody polyklonaler Antikörper *m*.
polyclonal gammopathy polyklonale Gammopathie *f*.
pol·y·co·ria [ˌ-ˈkɔːrɪə, -ˈkəʊ-] *n ophthal., embryo.* Polykorie *f*.
pol·y·crot·ic [ˌ-ˈkrɑtɪk] *adj card.* polykrot.
polycrotic pulse Polykrotie *f*, polykroter Puls *m*, Pulsus polycrotus.
po·lyc·ro·tism [pəˈlɪkrətɪzəm] *n* → polycrotic pulse.
pol·y·cy·clic [ˌpɑlɪˈsaɪklɪk] *adj* polyzyklisch.
pol·y·cy·e·sis [ˌ-saɪˈiːsɪs] *n* Mehrlingsschwangerschaft *f*.
pol·y·cys·tic [ˌ-ˈsɪstɪk] *adj* aus mehreren Zysten bestehend, polyzystisch.
polycystic biliary disease polyzystische Choledochuszysten *pl*.
polycystic disease: p. of kidneys polyzystische Nieren *pl*.
p. of the liver Zystenleber *f*.
polycystic kidneys polyzystische Nieren *pl*.
polycystic liver angeborene Zystenleber *f*.
polycystic ovary *gyn.* polyzystisches Ovar *nt*.
polycystic ovary disease/syndrome Stein-Leventhal-Syndrom *nt*, Syndrom *nt* der polyzystischen Ovarien.
pol·y·cy·the·mia [ˌ-saɪˈθiːmɪə] *n* **1.** Polyzythämie *f*, Polycythaemia *f*. **2.** Polyglobulie *f*.
pol·y·dac·tyl·ia [ˌ-dækˈtiːlɪə] *n* → polydactyly.
pol·y·dac·tyl·ism [ˌ-ˈdæktəlɪzəm] *n* → polydactyly.
pol·y·dac·ty·lous [ˌ-ˈdæktɪləs] *adj* Polydaktylie betr., polydaktyl.
pol·y·dac·ty·ly [ˌ-ˈdæktəlɪ] *n* Vielfingrigkeit *f*, Vielzehigkeit *f*, Poly-, Hyperdaktylie *f*.
pol·y·de·oxy·ri·bo·nu·cle·o·tide [ˌ-ˌdiːˌɑksɪˌraɪbəʊˈn(j)uːkliətaɪd] *n* Polydesoxyribonukleotid *nt*.
polydeoxyribonucleotide ligase → polydeoxyribonucleotide synthase (ATP).
polydeoxyribonucleotide synthase (ATP) DNA-Ligase *f*, DNS-Ligase *f*, Polydesoxyribonukleotidsynthase (ATP) *f*, Polynukleotidligase *f*.
pol·y·di·men·sion·al [ˌ-dɪˈmenʃənl, -daɪ-] *adj* mehrdimensional.
pol·y·dip·sia [ˌ-ˈdɪpsɪə] *n* krankhaft gesteigerter Durst *m*, Vieltrinken *nt*, Polydipsie *f*.
pol·y·dys·pla·sia [ˌ-dɪsˈpleɪʒ(ɪ)ə, -ʒɪə] *n* Polydysplasie *f*, -dysplasia *f*.
pol·y·dys·tro·phia [ˌ-dɪsˈtrəʊfɪə] *n* → polydystrophy.
pol·y·dys·troph·ic [ˌ-dɪsˈtrɑfɪk] *adj* Polydystrophie betr., polydystrophisch.
polydystrophic oligophrenia Sanfilippo--Syndrom *nt*, Morbus Sanfilippo *m*, polydystrophische Oligophrenie *f*, Mukopolysaccharidose *f* III *abbr.* MPS III.
pol·y·dys·tro·phy [ˌ-ˈdɪstrəfɪ] *n* Polydystrophie *f*, Polydystrophia *f*.
pol·y·em·bry·o·ny [ˌ-ˈembraɪənɪ] *n* Polyembryonie *f*.
pol·y·en·do·crine [ˌ-ˈendəʊkraɪn, -krɪn] *adj* polyendokrin.

polyendocrine adenomatosis multiple endokrine Adenopathie *f abbr.* MEA, multiple endokrine Neoplasie *f abbr.* MEN, pluriglanduläre Adenomatose *f*.
pol·y·en·do·cri·no·ma [ˌ-ˌendəkraɪˈnəʊmə] *n* → polyendocrine adenomatosis.
pol·y·en·do·cri·nop·a·thy [ˌ-ˌendəʊkrɪˈnɑpəθɪ] *n* Polyendokrinopathie *f*.
pol·y·ene [ˈpɑlɪˌiːn] *n chem.* Polyen *nt*.
polyene antibiotic Polyenantibiotikum *nt*.
pol·y·en·oic [ˌ-ɪˈnəʊɪk] *adj chem.* mehrfach ungesättigt.
pol·y·es·ter [ˈ-estər, ˌ-ˈestər] *n chem.* Polyester *m*.
pol·y·es·the·sia [ˌ-esˈθiːʒ(ɪ)ə] *n neuro.* Polyästhesie *f*.
pol·y·es·tra·di·ol phosphate [ˌ-ˌestrəˈdaɪɑl, -ɑl] *pharm.* Polyestradiolphosphat *nt*.
pol·y·eth·yl·ene [ˌ-ˈeθəliːn] *n* Polyäthylen *nt*.
polyethylene glycol Polyäthylenglykol *nt*.
pol·y·fruc·tose [ˌ-ˈfrʌktəʊs] *n* Fruktosan *nt*, Fructosan *nt*, L(a)evulan *nt*.
pol·y·ga·lac·tia [ˌ-gəˈlækʃɪə] *n gyn.* übermäßige Milchsekretion *f*, Poly-, Hypergalaktie *f*.
po·lyg·a·mous [pəˈlɪgəməs] *adj* Polygamie betr., polygam.
po·lyg·a·my [pəˈlɪgəmɪ] *n* **1.** *socio.* Vielehe *f*, Polygamie *f*. **2.** *bio.* Polygamie *f*.
pol·y·gan·gli·on·ic [ˌpɑlɪˌgæŋglɪˈɑnɪk] *adj* mehrere Ganglien betr., polyganglionär.
pol·y·gene [ˈ-dʒiːn] *n* Polygen *nt*.
pol·y·ge·nia [ˌ-ˈdʒiːnɪə] *n* Polygenie *f*.
pol·y·gen·ic [ˌ-ˈdʒenɪk] *adj* Polygenie betr., polygen(isch).
polygenic inheritance polygene Vererbung *f*.
po·lyg·e·ny [pəˈlɪdʒənɪ] *n* → polygenia.
pol·y·glan·du·lar [ˌpɑlɪˈglændʒələr] *adj* mehrere Drüsen betr., poly-, pluriglandulär.
pol·y·gly·col [ˌ-ˈglaɪkɑl, -kəl] *n* Polyglykol *nt*.
pol·y·gly·col·ic acid [ˌ-glaɪˈkɑlɪk] Polyglykolsäure *f*.
pol·y·gram [ˈ-græm] *n* Polygramm *nt*.
pol·y·graph [ˈ-græf] *n* **1.** *physiol.* Polygraph *m*. **2.** Lügendetektor *m*.
po·lyg·y·nous [pəˈlɪdʒənəs] *adj* polygyn.
po·lyg·y·ny [pəˈlɪdʒənɪ] *n* Polygynie *f*.
pol·y·gy·ria [ˌpɑlɪˈdʒaɪrɪə] *n* Polygyrie *f*.
pol·y·he·dral [ˌ-ˈhiːdrəl, -ˈhe-] *adj* polyedrisch, Polyeder-.
pol·y·he·dric [ˌ-ˈhiːdrɪk, -ˈhe-] *adj* → polyhedral.
pol·y·he·dron [ˌ-ˈhiːdrən] *n, pl* **-drons, -dra** [-drə] Vielflächner *m*, Polyeder *nt*.
pol·y·hex·ose [ˌ-ˈheksəʊs] *n* Polyhexose *f*.
pol·y·hi·dro·sis [ˌ-haɪˈdrəʊsɪs, -hɪ-] *n* übermäßiges Schwitzen *nt*, Hyperhidrose *f*, Polyhidrose *f*, Hyper(h)idrosis *f*, Poly(h)idrosis *f*.
pol·y·hy·dram·ni·os [ˌ-haɪˈdræmnɪəs] *n gyn.* Polyhydramnie *f*, Polyhydramnion *nt*, Hydramnion *nt*.
pol·y·hy·drox·y acetal [ˌ-haɪˈdrɑksɪ] Polyhydroxyacetal *nt*.
polyhydroxy aldehyde Polyhydroxyaldehyd *m*.
polyhydroxy ketal Polyhydroxyketal *nt*.
polyhydroxy ketone Polyhydroxyketon *nt*.
pol·y·hy·per·men·or·rhea [ˌ-ˌhaɪpərmenəˈrɪə] *n gyn.* Polyhypermenorrhoe *f*.
pol·y·hy·po·men·or·rhea [ˌ-ˌhaɪpəʊmenəˈrɪə] *n gyn.* Polyhypomenorrhoe *f*.
pol·y·id·ro·sis [ˌ-ɪdˈrəʊsɪs] *n* → polyhidrosis.
pol·y·i·on·ic [ˌ-aɪˈɑnɪk] *adj* viel-, mehrionisch.

pol·y·kar·y·o·cyte [ˌ-'kærɪəsaɪt] *n* Polykaryozyt *m*.
pol·y·lec·i·thal [ˌ-'lesɪθəl] *adj bio.* poly-, makrolezithal.
pol·y·lep·tic [ˌ-'leptɪk] *adj* (*Krankheit*) in mehreren Schüben verlaufend.
pol·y·ly·sine [ˌ-'laɪsiːn, -sɪn] *n* Polylysin *nt*.
pol·y·mas·tia [ˌ-'mæstɪə] *n* Polymastie *f*, akzessorische Mammae *f*, Mammae accessoriae.
pol·y·mas·tic [ˌ-'mæstɪk] *adj* Polymastie betr., von ihr betroffen *od.* gekennzeichnet.
Pol·y·mas·ti·gi·da [ˌ-mæs'tɪdʒɪdə] *pl micro.* mehrgeißelige Flagellaten *pl*, Polymastigida *pl*.
pol·y·mas·ti·gote [ˌ-'mæstɪgəʊt] *n micro.* Polymastigote *f*.
pol·y·mas·ty [ˌ-'mæstɪ] *n* → polymastia.
pol·y·me·lia [ˌ-'miːlɪə, -ljə] *n embryo.* Polymelie *f*.
po·lym·e·lus [pə'lɪmələs, ˌpalɪ'miːləs] *n embryo.* Polymelus *m*.
po·lym·e·ly [pə'lɪməlɪ, ˌpalɪ'miːlɪ] *n* → polymelia.
pol·y·me·nia [ˌpalɪ'miːnɪə] *n* → polymenorrhea.
pol·y·men·or·rhea [ˌ-menə'rɪə] *n gyn.* Polymenorrhoe *f*.
pol·y·mer ['-mər] *n* Polymer(e) *nt*.
pol·ym·er·ase [pə'lɪmərēɪz] *n* Polymerase *f*.
polymer fume fever Polymerenfieber *nt*.
pol·y·me·ria [ˌpalɪ'mɪərɪə] *n embryo.* Polymerie *f*.
pol·y·mer·ic [ˌ-'merɪk] *adj* polymer.
po·lym·er·id [pə'lɪmərɪd, -raɪd] *n* → polymer.
po·lym·er·ism [pə'lɪmərɪzəm, 'paləmə-] *n* Polymerisieren *nt*, Polymerisierung *f*.
po·lym·er·i·za·tion [pəˌlɪmərɪ'zeɪʃn] *n* Polymerisation *f*.
po·lym·er·ize [pə'lɪməraɪz, 'palɪm-] *vt, vi* polymerisieren, in Polymer bilden.
pol·y·met·a·phos·phate [ˌpalɪˌmetə'fasfeɪt] *n* Poly(meta)phosphat *nt*.
pol·y·meth·yl methacrylate [ˌ-'meθəl] *abbr.* **PMMA** Polymethylmethacrylat *nt abbr.* PMMA.
pol·y·mi·cro·bi·al [ˌ-maɪ'krəʊbɪəl] *adj* durch mehrere Mikroorganismen hervorgerufen.
pol·y·mi·cro·bic [ˌ-maɪ'krəʊbɪk] *adj* → polymicrobial.
pol·y·mi·cro·gy·ria [ˌ-ˌmaɪkrə'dʒaɪrɪə] *n* Polymikrogyrie *f*.
pol·y·morph ['-mɔːrf] *n* **1.** *inf.* → polymorphonuclear leukocyte. **2.** *chem., bio.* polymorpher Körper *m*.
pol·y·mor·phic [ˌ-'mɔːrfɪk] *adj* vielgestaltig, multi-, pleo-, polymorph.
polymorphic layer of cerebral cortex multiforme Schicht *f*, Lamina multiformis corticis cerebri.
polymorphic light eruption *abbr.* **PMLE** polymorpher Lichtausschlag *m*, polymorphe Lichtdermatose (Haxthausen) *f*, Sommerprurigo *f*, Prurigo aestivalis, Lupus-erythematodes-artige Lichtdermatose *f*, Lichtekzem *nt*, Eccema solare, Dermatopathia photoelectrica.
polymorphic neuron multipolares Neuron *nt*.
pol·y·mor·phism [ˌ-'mɔːrfɪzəm] *n* Vielförmig-, Vielgestaltigkeit *f*; *genet.* Polymorphismus *m*, Polymorphie *f*.
pol·y·mor·pho·cel·lu·lar [ˌ-ˌmɔːrfəʊ'seljələr] *adj* polymorphzellig.
polymorphocellular immunocytoma polymorphzelliges Immunozytom *nt*.
pol·y·mor·pho·nu·cle·ar [ˌ-ˌmɔːrfə'n(j)uːklɪər] **I** *n* → polymorphonuclear leuko-

cyte. **II** *adj histol.* polymorphkernig.
polymorphonuclear basophil leukocyte *abbr.* **PMB** *hema.* basophiler Leukozyt/ Granulozyt *m*; *inf.* Basophiler *m*.
polymorphonuclear eosinophil leukocyte *abbr.* **PME** eosinophiler Leukozyt/ Granulozyt *m*; *inf.* Eosinophiler *m*.
polymorphonuclear granulocyte → polymorphonuclear leukocyte.
polymorphonuclear leukocyte polymorphkerniger neutrophiler Granulozyt *m abbr.* **PNG**, neutrophiler Leukozyt *m*, *inf.* Neutrophiler *m*.
polymorphonuclear neutrophil leukocyte *abbr.* **PMN** → polymorphonuclear leukocyte.
pol·y·mor·phous [ˌ-'mɔːrfəs] *adj* → polymorphic.
polymorphous cell sarcoma polymorphzelliges Sarkom *nt*.
polymorphous sarcoma malignes Mesenchymom *nt*.
pol·y·my·al·gia [ˌ-maɪ'ældʒ(ɪ)ə] *n* Polymyalgie *f*, -myalgia *f*.
pol·y·my·op·a·thy [ˌ-maɪ'ɑpəθɪ] *n* Polymyopathie *f*.
pol·y·my·o·si·tis [ˌ-maɪə'saɪtɪs] *n* Polymyositis *f*.
pol·y·myx·in [ˌ-'mɪksɪn] *n pharm.* Polymyxin *nt*, Polymyxinantibiotikum *nt*.
polymyxin B Polymyxin B *nt*.
polymyxin E Polymyxin E *nt*, Colistin *nt*.
pol·y·neu·ral [ˌ-'njʊərəl, -nʊ-] *adj* mehrere Nerven betr., von mehreren Nerven versorgt, polyneural.
pol·y·neu·ral·gia [ˌ-njʊə'rældʒ(ɪ)ə, -nʊ-] *n* Polyneuralgie *f*.
pol·y·neu·ric [ˌ-'njʊərɪk, -nʊ-] *adj* → polyneural.
pol·y·neu·rit·ic [ˌ-ˌnjʊə'rɪtɪk, -nʊ-] *adj* Polyneuritis betr., polyneuritisch.
polyneuritic psychosis Korsakow-Psychose *f*, -Syndrom *nt*.
pol·y·neu·ri·tis [ˌ-ˌnjʊə'raɪtɪs, -nʊ-] *n* Polyneuritis *f*.
pol·y·neu·ro·my·o·si·tis [ˌ-ˌnjʊərəˌmaɪə'saɪtɪs, -nʊ-] *n* Polyneuromyositis *f*.
pol·y·neu·ro·ni·tis [ˌ-ˌnjʊərə'naɪtɪs, -nʊ-] *n* Polyneuronitis *f*.
pol·y·neu·rop·a·thy [ˌ-njʊə'rɑpəθɪ, -nʊ-] *n* Polyneuropathie *f*.
pol·y·neu·ro·ra·dic·u·li·tis [ˌ-ˌnjʊərərəˌdɪkjə'laɪtɪs, -nʊ-] *n* Polyneuroradikulitis *f*.
pol·y·nu·cle·ar [ˌ-'n(j)uːklɪər] *adj* vielkernig, polynuclear.
polynuclear leukocyte 1. Granulozyt *m*, granulärer Leukozyt *m*. **2.** → polymorphonuclear leukocyte.
polynuclear neutrophilic leukocyte → polymorphonuclear leukocyte.
pol·y·nu·cle·ate [ˌ-'n(j)uːklɪɪt, -eɪt] *adj* → polynuclear.
pol·y·nu·cle·at·ed [ˌ-'n(j)uːklɪeɪtɪd] *adj* → polynuclear.
pol·y·nu·cle·o·tid·ase [ˌ-ˌn(j)uːklɪəʊ'taɪdēɪz] *n* → polynucleotide phosphatase.
pol·y·nu·cle·o·tide [ˌ-'n(j)uːklɪətaɪd] *n* Polynukleotid *nt*, -nucleotid *nt*.
polynucleotide adenylyltransferase Polynukleotidadenyl(yl)transferase *f*.
polynucleotide chain Polynukleotidkette *f*.
polynucleotide ligase → polydeoxyribonucleotide synthase (ATP).
polynucleotide phosphatase Polynukleotidphosphatase *f*.
polynucleotide phosphorylase → polyribonucleotide nucleotidyltransferase.
Pol·y·o·ma·vi·rus [ˌpalɪˌəʊmə'vaɪrəs] *n micro.* Polyomavirus *nt*, Miopapovavirus *nt*.

pol·y·o·ma virus [ˌ-'əʊmə] → Polyomavirus.
pol·y·o·nych·ia [ˌ-əʊ'nɪkɪə] *n* Polyonychie *f*.
pol·y·o·pia [ˌ-'əʊpɪə] *n ophthal.* Mehrfachsehen *nt*, Polyopie *f*, Polyopsie *f*.
pol·y·op·sia [ˌ-'ɑpsɪə] *n* → polyopia.
pol·y·o·py ['-əʊpɪ] *n* → polyopia.
pol·y·or·chi·dism [ˌ-'ɔːrkədɪzəm] *n* Polyorchidie *f*, Polyorchie *f*.
pol·y·or·chism [ˌ-'ɔːrkɪzəm] *n* → polyorchidism.
pol·y·os·tot·ic [ˌ-ɑs'tɑtɪk] *adj* mehrere Knochen betr., polyostotisch.
polyostotic fibrous dysplasia Albright--Syndrom *nt*, Albright-McCune-Syndrom *nt*, McCune-Albright-Syndrom *nt*, polyostotische fibröse Dysplasie *f*.
pol·y·o·tia [ˌ-'əʊʃɪə] *n embryo.* Polyotie *f*.
pol·y·ov·u·lar [ˌ-'ɑvjələr, -'əʊv-] *adj embryo.* polyovulär.
pol·y·ov·u·la·tion [ˌ-ˌɑvjə'leɪʃn, -ˌəʊv-] *n embryo.* Polyovulation *f*.
pol·y·ov·u·la·to·ry [ˌ-'ɑvjələtɔːriː] *adj embryo.* polyovulatorisch, polyzygot.
pol·yp ['pɑlɪp] *n patho.* Polyp *m*, Polypus *m*.
pol·y·pap·il·lo·ma tropicum [ˌpɑlɪˌpæpə'ləʊmə] Frambösie *f*, Pian *f*, Parangi *f*, Yaws *f*, Frambœsia tropica.
pol·y·pa·re·sis [ˌ-pə'riːsɪs] *n old* → general paralysis of the insane.
pol·y·path·ia [ˌ-'pæθɪə] *n* Mehrfachleiden *nt*, Multimorbidität *f*, Polypathie *f*.
pol·y·pec·to·my [ˌ-'pektəmɪ] *n chir.* Polypenabtragung *f*, Polypektomie *f*.
pol·y·pep·ti·dase [ˌ-'peptɪdeɪz] *n* → peptidase.
pol·y·pep·tide [ˌ-'peptaɪd, -tɪd] *n* Polypeptid *nt*.
polypeptide chain Polypeptidkette *f*.
polypeptide fraction Polypeptidfraktion *f*.
polypeptide hormone → proteohormone.
pol·y·pep·ti·de·mia [ˌ-ˌpeptɪ'diːmɪə] *n* Polypeptidämie *f*.
pol·y·pep·ti·dor·rha·chia [ˌ-ˌpeptɪdəʊ'reɪkɪə] *n* Polypeptidorrhachie *f*.
pol·y·per·i·os·ti·tis [ˌ-ˌperɪɑs'taɪtɪs] *n* Polyperiostitis *f*.
polyp forceps *chir.* Polypenfaßzange *f*.
polyp grasper *chir.* Polypenfaßzange *f*.
pol·y·pha·gia [ˌ-'feɪdʒ(ɪ)ə] *n psychia.* krankhafte Gefräßigkeit *f*, Polyphagie *f*.
pol·y·pha·lan·gia [ˌ-fə'lændʒ(ɪ)ə] *n embryo.* Vielgliedrigkeit *f*, Poly-, Hyperphalangie *f*.
pol·y·pha·lan·gism [ˌ-fə'lændʒɪzəm] *n* → polyphalangia.
pol·y·phar·ma·cy [ˌ-'fɑːrməsɪ] *n* **1.** gleichzeitige Verabreichung *f* vieler/mehrerer Arzneimittel, Polypragmasie *f*. **2.** Verabreichung *f* einer größeren Dosis.
pol·y·phase ['-feɪz] *adj phys.* mehr-, viel-, verschiedenphasig, Mehrphasen-.
pol·y·pha·sic [ˌ-'feɪzɪk] *adj* → polyphase.
pol·y·phen·ic [ˌ-'fenɪk] *adj* → pleiotropic.
pol·y·phe·nol·ox·i·dase [ˌ-ˌfiːnəl'ɑksɪdeɪz] *n* o-Diphenoloxidase *f*, Cathecholoxidase *f*, Polyphenoloxidase *f*.
pol·y·pho·bia [ˌ-'fəʊbɪə] *n psychia.* Polyphobie *f*.
pol·y·phos·phate [ˌ-'fɑsfeɪt] *n* Polyphosphat *nt*.
pol·y·phos·phor·ic acid [ˌ-fɑs'fɔːrɪk] Polyphosphorsäure *f*.
pol·y·phy·let·ic [ˌ-faɪ'letɪk] *adj bio.* polyphyletisch.
po·lyp·i·form [pəʊ'lɪpəfɔːrm] *adj* → polypoid.
pol·y·plas·mia [ˌpalɪ'plæzmɪə] *n* Verdünnungsanämie *f*, Hydrämie *f*, Hydroplasmie *f*.

polyplastic

pol·y·plas·tic [,-'plæstɪk] *adj* polyplastisch.
pol·y·ple·gia [,-'pliːdʒ(ɪ)ə] *n* Polyplegie *f*.
pol·y·ploid ['-plɔɪd] *genet*. **I** *n* polyploide Zelle *f*, polyploider Organismus *m*. **II** *adj* polyploid.
pol·y·ploi·dy ['-plɔɪdɪ] *n genet*. Polyploidie *f*, Polyploidisierung *f*.
pol·yp·nea [palɪp'nɪə] *n* Tachypnoe *f*.
pol·y·po·dia [,palɪ'pəʊdɪə] *n embryo*. Polypodie *f*.
pol·y·poid ['-pɔɪd] *adj* polyp(en)ähnlich, -förmig, polypös.
polypoid adenocarcinoma papilläres Adenokarzinom *nt*.
polypoid adenoma adenomatöser Polyp *m*.
polypoid sinusitis polypöse Sinusitis *f*.
po·lyp·o·rous [pə'lɪpərəs] *adj* siebartig, siebförmig, Sieb-.
Po·lyp·o·rus [pə'lɪpərəs] *n micro*. Polyporus *m*.
pol·y·po·sia [,-'pəʊzɪə] *n* anhaltendes übermäßiges Trinken *nt*.
pol·y·po·sis [,-'pəʊsɪs] *n patho*. Polyposis *f*.
po·lyp·o·tome [pə'lɪpətəʊm] *n chir*. Polypotom *nt*.
pol·y·pous ['palɪpəs] *adj* Polyp(en) betr., in Polypenform, polypös, Polyp-.
polypous gastritis Gastritis polyposa.
pol·y·prag·ma·sy [,-'prægməsɪ] *n* → polypharmacy 1.
pol·y·pro·pyl·ene [,-'prəʊpəliːn] *n* Polypropylen *nt*.
pol·y·pus ['-pəs] *n, pl* **-pi** [-paɪ, -piː] → polyp.
pol·y·ra·dic·u·li·tis [,-rə,dɪkjə'laɪtɪs] *n neuro*. Polyradikulitis *f*.
pol·y·ra·dic·u·lo·my·op·a·thy [,-rə,dɪkjələʊmaɪ'apəθɪ] *n* Polyradikulomyopathie *f*.
pol·y·ra·dic·u·lo·neu·ri·tis [,-rə,dɪkjələʊnjʊə'raɪtɪs, -nʊ-] *n* Polyradikuloneuritis *f*.
pol·y·ra·dic·u·lo·neu·rop·a·thy [,-rə,dɪkjələʊnjʊə'rapəθɪ] *n* Guillain-Barré-Syndrom *nt*, (Poly-)Radikuloneuritis *f*, Neuronitis *f*.
pol·y·ri·bo·nu·cle·o·tide [,-,raɪbəʊ'n(j)uːklɪətaɪd] *n* Polyribonukleotid *nt*.
polyribonucleotide nucleotidyltransferase Polynukleotidphosphorylase *f*, Polyribonukleotidnukleotidyltransferase *f*.
polyribonucleotide strand Polyribonukleotidstrang *m*.
pol·y·ri·bo·some [,-'raɪbəsəʊm] *n* Poly(ribo)som *nt*, Ergosom *nt*.
pol·yr·rhea [,-'rɪə] *n* Polyrrhoe *f*.
pol·yr·rhi·nia [,-'rɪnɪə] *n embryo*. Polyrrhinie *f*.
pol·y·sac·cha·ride [,-'sækəraɪd, -rɪd] *n* Polysaccharid *nt*, hochmolekulares Kohlenhydrat *nt*.
pol·y·sac·cha·rose [,-'sækərəʊs] *n* → polysaccharide.
pol·y·scope ['-skəʊp] *n* Diaphanoskop *nt*.
pol·y·se·ro·si·tis [,-,sɪrəʊ'saɪtɪs, -,serə-] *n* Polyserositis *f*.
pol·y·si·a·lia [,-saɪ'eɪlɪə] *n* vermehrter Speichelfluß *m*, Polysialie *f*, Ptyalismus *m*.
pol·y·sin·u·i·tis [,-,sɪnjə'waɪtɪs] *n* → polysinusitis.
pol·y·si·nu·sec·to·my [,-,saɪnə'sektəmɪ] *n HNO* Polysinusektomie *f*.
pol·y·si·nu·si·tis [,-,saɪnə'saɪtɪs] *n HNO* Polysinusitis *f*.
pol·y·some ['-səʊm] *n* → polyribosome.
pol·y·so·mic [,-'səʊmɪk] *adj genet*. polysom.
pol·y·so·my [,-'səʊmɪ] *n genet*. Polysomie *f*.
pol·y·sper·mia [,-'spɜrmɪə] *n* **1.** *embryo*. Polyspermie *f*. **2.** Polyspermie *f*, Polyse-

mie *f*. **3.** Polyzoospermie *f*, Polyspermie *f*. **4.** Spermatorrhoe *f*, Polyspermie *f*.
pol·y·sper·mism [,-'spɜrmɪzəm] *n* → polyspermia.
pol·y·sper·my [,-'spɜrmɪ] *n* → polyspermia 1.
pol·y·sple·nia [,-'spliːnɪə] *n embryo*. Polysplenie *f*.
pol·y·stich·ia [,-'stɪkɪə] *n* Polystichiasis *f*.
pol·y·sty·rene [,-'staɪriːn] *n* Polystyrol *nt*.
pol·y·syn·ap·tic [,-sɪ'næptɪk] *adj* poly-, multisynaptisch.
polysynaptic reflex polysynaptischer Reflex *m*, Fremdreflex *m*.
pol·y·syn·dac·tyl·y [,-sɪn'dæktəlɪ] *n embryo*. Polysyndaktylie *f*.
pol·y·syn·o·vi·tis [,-,sɪnə'vaɪtɪs] *n* Polysynovitis *f*.
pol·y·ten·di·ni·tis [,-,tendɪ'naɪtɪs] *n* Polytendinitis *f*.
pol·y·ten·di·no·bur·si·tis [,-,tendɪnəʊbɜr'saɪtɪs] *n* Polytendinobursitis *f*.
pol·y·tene ['-tiːn] *n genet*. Polytän *nt*.
polytene chromosome Riesenchromosom *nt*.
pol·y·ten·o·syn·o·vi·tis [,-,tenəʊ,sɪnə'vaɪtɪs] *n* Polytenosynovitis *f*.
pol·y·te·ny [,-'tiːnɪ] *n genet*. Polytänie *f*.
pol·y·ter·pene [,-'tɜrpiːn] *n* Polyterpen *nt*.
pol·y·the·lia [,-'θiːlɪə] *n* Polythelie *f*.
pol·y·the·lism [,-'θiːlɪzəm] *n* → polythelia.
pol·y·the·ne ['-θiːn] *n* → polyethylene.
pol·y·thi·a·zide [,-'θaɪəzaɪd] *n pharm*. Polythiazid *nt*.
pol·y·to·mo·gram [,-'təʊməgræm] *n radiol*. Polytomogramm *nt*.
pol·y·to·mo·graph·ic [,-,təʊmə'græfɪk] *adj* Polytomographie betr., polytomographisch.
pol·y·to·mog·ra·phy [,-tə'magrəfɪ] *n radiol*. Tomographie *f* in mehreren Ebenen, Polytomographie *f*.
pol·y·trich·ia [,-'trɪkɪə] *n* übermäßige Behaarung *f*, Polytrichie *f*, Hypertrichie *f*, Hypertrichose *f*.
pol·y·tri·cho·sis [,-trɪ'kəʊsɪs] *n* → polytrichia.
pol·y·trop·ic [,-'trapɪk, -'trəʊp-] *adj* polytrop.
pol·y·un·guia [,-'ʌŋgwɪə] *n* → polyonychia.
pol·y·un·sat·u·rat·ed [,-ʌn'sætʃəreɪtɪd] *adj* → polyenoic.
polyunsaturated fat/lipid Lipid *nt* mit mehrfach ungesättigten Fettsäuren.
pol·y·u·ria [,-'(j)ʊərɪə] *n* übermäßige Harnausscheidung *f*, Polyurie *f*.
pol·y·u·ric [,-'(j)ʊərɪk] *adj* Polyurie betr., polyurisch.
polyuric phase polyurische Phase *f*.
pol·y·va·lence [,-'veɪləns] *n* Mehr-, Vielwertigkeit *f*, Polyvalenz *f*.
pol·y·va·lent [,-'veɪlənt, pə'lɪvələnt] *adj* mehr-, vielwertig, multi-, polyvalent.
polyvalent allergy polyvalente Überempfindlichkeit/Allergie *f*.
polyvalent antiserum polyvalentes Antiserum *nt*.
polyvalent serum polyvalentes Serum *nt*.
polyvalent vaccine polyvalenter Impfstoff *m*.
pol·y·vi·nyl acetat [,-'vaɪnl] *n* Polyvinylazetat *nt*.
polyvinyl alcohol *abbr*. **PVA** Polyvinylalkohol *m abbr*. PVA.
polyvinyl benzene → polystyrene.
polyvinyl chloride *n abbr*. **PVC** Polyvinylchlorid *nt abbr*. PVC.
pol·y·vi·nyl·pyr·rol·i·done [,-,vaɪnlpɪ'rəʊlɪdəʊn, -'ral-] *n abbr*. **PVP** Polyvinylpyrrolidon *nt abbr*. PVP, Polyvidon *nt*.
polyvinylpyrrolidone-iodine *n abbr*. **PVP-I**

Polyvinylpyrrolidon-Jod *nt*, Polyvidon-Jod *nt*, Polyvidon-Iod *nt*.
pol·y·zy·got·ic [,-zaɪ'gatɪk] *adj* → polyovulatory.
POM *abbr*. → prescription only medicine.
po·made acne [pəʊ'meɪd, -'maːd] *derm*. Pomadenakne *f*.
POMC *abbr*. → proopiomelanocortin.
POMC cells → proopiomelanocortin cells.
Pomeroy ['paməroɪ] : **P.'s operation** *gyn*. Pomeroy-Methode *f*.
Po·mo·na fever [pə'əʊnə] Pomona-Fieber *nt*.
Pompe ['pampɪ]: **P.'s disease** Pompe-Krankheit *f*, generalisierte maligne Glykogenose *f*, Glykogenose *f* Typ II.
pom·pho·lyx ['pam(p)falɪks] *n derm*. Pompholyx *f*, dyshidrotisches Ekzem *nt*, Dyshidrose *f*, Dyshidrosis *f*, Dyshidrose-Syndrom *nt*.
Poncet [pɔ̃'seː]: **P.'s disease/rheumatism** Poncet-Krankheit *f*.
Ponfick ['panfɪk]: **P.'s shadows** *hema*. Achromo(retikulo)zyt *m*, Halbmondkörper *m*, Schilling-Halbmond *m*.
Pon·go·la virus ['paŋgələ] Pongola-Virus *nt*.
pons [panz] *n, pl* **pon·tes** ['pantiːz] **1.** *anat*. (Gewebs-)Brücke *f*. **2.** (*ZNS*) Brücke *f*, Pons *m* (cerebri).
Pon·ti·ac fever ['pantɪæk] Pontiac-Fieber *nt*.
pon·til [pantl] *adj* → pontine.
pon·tile ['pantaɪl] *adj* → pontine.
pontile apoplexy Apoplexia bulbaris.
pon·tine ['pantiːn, -taɪn] *adj* Brücke/Pons betr., pontin, Brücken-, Pons-.
pontine angle Kleinhirnbrückenwinkel *m*, Angulus pontocerebellaris.
pontine angle tumor Akustikusneurinom *nt*.
pontine arteries Brückenarterien *pl*, Aa. pontis, Rami ad pontem (a. basilaris).
pontine apoplexy Apoplexia bulbaris.
pontine branches of basilar artery → pontine arteries.
pontine bulb Brückenfuß *m*.
pontine cistern Cisterna pontocerebellaris.
pontine fibers: longitudinal p. longitudinale Brückenfasern *pl*, Fibrae pontis longitudinales.
transverse p. transverse Brückenfasern *pl*, Fibrae pontis transversae.
pontine flexure *embryo*. Brückenbeuge *f*.
pontine nucleus 1. Nc. pontis. **2.** *pl* Brückenkerne *pl*, Ncc. pontis.
p. of trigeminal nerve sensibler Haupt-/Brückenkern *m* des N. trigeminus, Nc. pontinus n. trigeminalis.
pontine raphe, median Raphe (mediana) pontis.
pontine syndrome Raymond-Cestan-Syndrom *nt*.
pontine tegmentum Tegmentum pontis, Pars dorsalis pontis.
pon·to·bul·bar [,pantəʊ'bʌlbər, -baːr] *adj* Brücke/Pons u. Medulla oblongata betr., pontobulbär.
pon·to·bul·bia [,-'bʌlbɪə] *n neuro*. Syringobulbie *f*.
pon·to·cer·e·bel·lar [,-serə'belər] *adj* Brücke/Pons u. Kleinhirn/Cerebellum betr. *od*. verbindend, pontozerebellar, -zerebellär.
pontocerebellar fibers pontozerebelläre Fasern *pl*, Fibrae pontocerebellares.
pontocerebellar trigone Kleinhirnbrückenwinkel *m*, Trigonum pontocerebellare.
pon·to·cer·e·bel·lum [,-serə'beləm] *n* Pontozerebellum *nt*.

pon·to·med·ul·lar·y [ˌ-'medəleriː, -mə'dʌləri] *adj* Brücke/Pons u. Medulla oblongata betr. *od.* verbindend, pontomedullär.
pon·to·mes·en·ce·phal·ic [ˌ-mesənsə'fælɪk] *adj* Brücke/Pons u. Mittelhirn/Mesencephalon betr. *od.* verbindend, pontomesenzephal.
pontomesencephalic vein, anterior Brücken-Mittelhirnvene *f*, V. pontomesencephalica anterior.
pon·toon [pɑn'tuːn] *n* Dünndarmschlinge *f*.
pon·to·re·tic·u·lo·spi·nal tract [ˌpɑntəʊriˌtɪkjələʊ'spaɪnl] Tractus pontoreticulospinalis.
Pool [puːl]: **P.'s phenomenon 1.** Pool-Beinphänomen *nt*, Pool-Schlesinger-Phänomen *nt*. **2.** Pool-Armphänomen *nt*.
pool [puːl] **I** *n* **1.** *bio.*, *biochem.* Pool *m*; *serol.* Pool *m*, Mischplasma *nt*, -serum *nt*. **2.** (Blut-, Flüssigkeits-)Ansammlung *f*. **3.** (Daten-, Informations-)Pool *m*. **II** *vt* einen Pool bilden *od.* mischen, poolen. **III** *vi* s. ansammeln.
pool·ing ['puːlɪŋ] *n serol.* Sammlung *od.* Mischung *f* von Blutplasma *od.* -serum, Poolen *nt*, Poolung *f*.
Pool-Schlesinger [ˌʃlesɪndʒər, 'ʃleɪzɪŋər]: **P.-S. sign** Pool-Phänomen *nt*, Pool-Schlesinger-Phänomen *nt*.
poor [pʊər] **I** *n* **the** ~ die Armen *pl*. **II** *adj* **1.** *fig.* arm (*in* an); mangelhaft, schlecht, schwach, unzulänglich. **2.** mittellos, arm.
poor·ly ['pʊərli] **I** *adj inf.* kränklich, unwohl. **II** *adv* mangelhaft, schlecht; dürftig.
poorly-differentiated carcinoma mittelgradig differenziertes Karzinom *nt*.
poorly-differentiated lymphocytic lymphoma *abbr.* **PDLL, PDL** poorly-differentiated lymphocytic lymphoma *abbr.* PDLL, PDL.
poorly-myelinated *adj histol.* mark-, myelinarm.
POP *abbr.* → plaster of Paris 2.
pop·les ['pɑpliːz] *n* Kniekehle *f*.
pop·lit·e·al [pɑp'lɪtɪəl, ˌpɑplə'tiː-] *adj* Kniekehle betr., popliteal, Kniekehlen-.
popliteal arch Lig. popliteum arcuatum.
popliteal artery Kniekehlenarterie *f*, Poplitea *f*, A. poplitea.
popliteal artery disruption Popliteal(ab)riß *m*.
popliteal bursa Rec. subpopliteus, Bursa m. popliteï.
popliteal bursitis Baker-Zyste *f*.
popliteal cavity → popliteal fossa.
popliteal fossa Kniekehle *f*, Fossa poplitea.
  anterior p. of tibia Area intercondylaris anterior (tibiae).
  posterior p. of tibia Area intercondylaris posterior (tibiae).
popliteal groove Sulcus popliteus.
popliteal incisure Fossa intercondylaris (femoris).
popliteal ligament: arcuate p. Lig. popliteum arcuatum.
  oblique p. Lig. popliteum obliquum.
popliteal line: p. of femur Linea intercondylare.
  p. of tibia Linea m. solei.
popliteal muscle → popliteus (muscle).
popliteal nerve: external p. *old* Fibularis/Peronäus *m* communis, N. fibularis/peron(a)eus communis.
  internal p. *old* Tibialis *m*, N. tibialis.
  lateral p. *old* → external p.
  medial p. *old* → internal p.
popliteal notch Fossa intercondylaris (femoris).

popliteal pterygium syndrome 1. → popliteal web syndrome. **2.** Fèvre-Languepin-Syndrom *nt*.
popliteal space → popliteal fossa.
popliteal sulcus Sulcus popliteus.
popliteal trifurcation *chir.*, *radiol.* Trifurkation *f*.
popliteal vein Kniekehlenvene *f*, V. poplitea.
popliteal web syndrome popliteales Flügelfellsyndrom *nt*.
pop·lit·e·us (muscle) [pɑp'lɪtɪəs] Popliteus *m*, M. popliteus.
pop·py ['pɑpi] *n* → Papaver.
pop·u·la·tion [ˌpɑpjə'leɪʃn] *n* **1.** Bevölkerung *f*. **2.** *stat.* Bevölkerungs-, Einwohnerzahl *f*; Gesamtzahl *f*, Bestand *m*, Population *f*.
population analysis Populationsanalyse *f*.
population density Bevölkerungs-, Populationsdichte *f*.
population dynamics Populationsdynamik *f*.
population explosion Bevölkerungsexplosion *f*.
population genetics Populationsgenetik *f*.
population growth Bevölkerungs-, Populationswachstum *nt*.
population growth rate Populationswachstumsrate *f*.
population movement Populationsbewegung *f*, Abundanzdynamik *f*.
population pressure Bevölkerungs-, Populationsdruck *m*.
population pyramid Bevölkerungs-, Alterspyramide *f*.
population size Populationsgröße *f*.
population structure Populationsstruktur *f*.
por·a·de·nia [ˌpɔːrə'diːnɪə] *n* → poradenitis.
por·ad·e·ni·tis [pɔːrˌædə'naɪtɪs] *n* Poradenitis *f*.
poradenitis nostras/venerea → poradenolymphitis.
por·ad·e·no·lym·phi·tis [pɔːrˌædnəʊlɪm'faɪtɪs] *n* Lymphogranuloma inguinale/venereum *nt abbr.* LGV, Lymphopathia venerea, Morbus Durand-Nicolas-Favre *m*, klimatischer Bubo *m*, vierte Geschlechtskrankheit *f*, Poradenitis inguinalis.
por·al ['pɔʊrəl, 'pɔːr-] *adj* Pore(n) betr., Poren-.
por·ce·lain ['pɔːrs(ə)lɪn, 'pɔʊr-] **I** *n* Porzellan *nt*. **II** *adj* Porzellan-.
porcelain gallbladder *patho.* Porzellangallenblase *f*.
por·cine ['pɔːrsaɪn, -sɪn] *adj* Schweine-.
por·cu·pine skin ['pɔːrkjəpaɪn] Erythrodermia congenitalis ichthyosiformis bullosa.
pore [pɔːr, pɔʊr] *n* kleine Öffnung *f*, Pore *f*; *anat.* Porus *m*.
  p. of sweat duct Schweißdrüsenpore, Porus sudoriferus.
pore-forming protein → porin.
por·en·ce·pha·lia [ˌpɔːrensɪ'feɪlɪə, pɔʊ-] *n* → porencephaly.
por·en·ce·phal·ic [ˌ-sɪ'fælɪk] *adj* Porenzephalie betr.
porencephalic cyst Zyste *f* bei Porenzephalie.
por·en·ceph·a·li·tis [ˌ-, sefə'laɪtɪs] *n* Porenzephalitis *f*.
por·en·ceph·a·lous [ˌ-'sefələs] *adj* → porencephaly.
por·en·ceph·a·ly [ˌ-'sefəli] *n* Porenzephalie *f*.
pore protein → porin.
po·rif·er·ous [pɔː'rɪfərəs, pəʊ-] *adj* mit Poren (versehen), porig.

po·rin ['pɔːrɪn, 'pəʊ-] *n* porenbildendes Protein *nt*, Porin *nt*.
po·ri·o·ma·nia [ˌpɔːrɪəʊ'meɪnɪə, -jə, pɔː-] *n psychia.* krankhafter Wandertrieb *m*, Poriomanie *f*.
pork tapeworm [pɔːrk, pɔʊrk] *micro.* Schweine(finnen)bandwurm *m*, Taenia solium.
pork worm *micro.* Trichine *f*, Trichina/Trichinella spiralis.
po·ro·ceph·a·li·a·sis [ˌpɔʊrəʊˌsefə'laɪəsɪs] *n* Porocephalusinfektion *f*, Porozephalose *f*.
Po·ro·ce·phal·i·da [ˌ-sɪ'fælɪdə] *pl micro.* Porocephalida *pl*.
Po·ro·ce·phal·i·dae [ˌ-sɪ'fælədiː] *pl micro.* Porocephalidae *pl*.
po·ro·ce·pha·lo·sis [ˌ-ˌsefə'ləʊsɪs] *n* → porocephaliasis.
Po·ro·ceph·a·lus [ˌ-'sefələs] *n micro.* Porocephalus *m*.
po·ro·ker·a·to·sis (of Mibelli) [ˌ-kerə'təʊsɪs] *derm.* Mibelli'-Krankheit *f*, Porokeratosis/Parakeratosis Mibelli *f*, Keratoatrophodermie *f*, Hyperkeratosis concentrica, Hyperkeratosis figurata centrifugata atrophicans, Keratodermia excentrica.
po·ro·ker·a·tot·ic [ˌ-kerə'tɑtɪk] *adj* Porokeratosis betr., porokeratotisch.
po·ro·ma [pə'rəʊmə] *n* **1.** Porom(a) *nt*. **2.** Verhornung *f*, Hornschwiele *f*, Porom *nt*. **3.** Exostose *f*.
po·ro·sis [pə'rəʊsɪs] *n*, *pl* **-ses** [-siːz] **1.** Kallusbildung *f*, Porose *f*, Porosis *f*. **2.** Höhlenbildung *f*, Porose *f*, Porosis *f*.
po·ros·i·ty [pɔː'rɑsətɪ, pəʊ-] *n* **1.** Pore *f*, poröse Stelle *f*. **2.** (Luft-, Gas-, Wasser-)Durchlässigkeit *f*, Porosität *f*.
po·rot·o·my [pə'rɑtəmɪ] *n HNO*, *urol.* Meatotomie *f*.
po·rous ['pɔːrəs, 'pəʊ-] *adj* **1.** (gas-, luft-, wasser-)durchlässig, porös. **2.** mit Poren versehen, porös.
po·rous·ness ['pɔːrəsnɪs, 'pəʊ-] *n* → porosity.
por·phin ['pɔːrfɪn] *n chem.* Porphin *nt*.
por·pho·bi·lin·o·gen [ˌpɔːrfəʊbaɪ'lɪnədʒən] *n abbr.* **PBG** Porphobilinogen *nt abbr.* PBG.
porphobilinogen deaminase Porphobilinogendeaminase *f*.
porphobilinogen synthase Porphobilinogensynthase *f*.
porphobilinogen test Watson-Schwartz-Test *m*.
por·pho·bi·lin·o·gen·u·ria [ˌ-baɪˌlɪnədʒə-'n(j)ʊərɪə] *n* Porphobilinogenausscheidung *f* im Harn, Porphobilinogenurie *f*.
por·phy·ran ['pɔːrfɪræn] *n* Metalloporphyrin *nt*.
por·phyr·ia [pɔːr'fɪərɪə] *n* Porphyrie *f*, Porphyria *f*.
por·phy·rin ['pɔːrfərɪn] *n* Porphyrin *nt*.
por·phy·rin·e·mia [ˌpɔːrfərɪ'niːmɪə] *n* Porphyrinämie *f*.
por·phy·rin·o·gen [ˌ-'rɪnədʒən] *n* Porphyrinogen *nt*.
por·phyr·in·op·a·thy [ˌ-rɪ'nɑpəθɪ] *n* Störung *f* des Porphyrinstoffwechsels, Porphyrinopathie *f*.
porphyrin ring *chem.* Porphyrinring *m*.
por·phy·rin·u·ria [ˌ-rɪ'n(j)ʊərɪə] *n* erhöhte Porphyrinausscheidung *f* im Harn, Porphyrinurie *f*.
por·phy·rism ['-rɪzəm] *n* → porphyria.
por·phy·ris·mus [ˌ-'rɪzməs] *n* Porphyrismus *m*.
por·phy·ri·za·tion [ˌ-raɪ'zeɪʃn] *n* Pulverisieren *nt*, Pulverisierung *f*.
por·phyr·u·ria [ˌ-'(j)ʊərɪə] *n* → porphyrinuria.

porphyry spleen

por·phy·ry spleen ['pɔːrfərɪ] Bauernwurstmilz f, Porphyrmilz f.
por·ri·go [pəʊ'raɪgəʊ] n derm. Porrigo m.
Porro ['pɔrəʊ]: **P.'s cesarean section** → P.'s operation.
P. hysterectomy → P. operation.
P. operation gyn. Hysterectomia c(a)esarea.
por·ta·ca·val [ˌpɔːrtə'keɪvl] adj Pfortader u. Vena cava betr., portokaval.
portacaval shunt chir. portokavaler Shunt m, portokavale Anastomose f.
por·tal ['pɔːrtl, 'pəʊr-] I n 1. Ein-, Ausgang m, Tor nt, Pforte f, Portal nt; anat. Porta f. 2. → portal vein (of liver). II adj 3. Pforte/Porta betr., portal. 4. Pfortader/Vena portae betr., portal, Portal-. 5. Leberpforte/Porta hepatis betr., portal, Portal-.
portal blood Pfortaderblut nt.
portal circulation Pfortader-, Portalkreislauf m, Pfortader-, Portalsystem nt.
portal cirrhosis mikronoduläre/kleinknotige/organisierte Leberzirrhose f.
portal fissure Leberpforte f, Porta hepatis.
portal hypertension portale Hypertonie f.
portal lobule funktionelles Leberläppchen nt, Zentralvenenläppchen nt.
portal pressure Pfortaderdruck m.
portal system → portal circulation.
  pituitary p. hypophysärer Pfortader-/Portalkreislauf m, hypophysäres Pfortader-/Portalsystem nt.
portal-systemic encephalopathy hepatische/portosystemische Enzephalopathie f, hepatozerebrales Syndrom nt, Encephalopathia hepatica.
portal tract (Leber) Periportalfeld nt, Glisson'-Dreieck nt.
portal triad → portal tract.
portal triaditis chir. Entzündung f von A. hepatica, V. portae u. Ductus hepaticus communis.
portal vein (of liver) Pfortader f, Porta f, Vena portae (hepatis).
portal vein pressure → portal pressure.
portal vein thrombosis Pfortaderthrombose f.
portal venography → portography.
por·ta·sys·tem·ic encephalopathy [ˌpɔːrtəsɪs'temɪk] → portal-systemic encephalopathy.
Porter ['pɔːrtər, 'pəʊ-]: **P.'s sign** Oliver--Cardarelli-Zeichen nt.
Porter-Silber ['sɪlbər]: **P.-S. chromagens** Porter-Silber-Chromogene pl.
P.-S. chromagens test → P.-S. test.
P.-S. reaction Porter-Silber-Farbreaktion f.
P.-S. test Porter-Silber-Methode f.
por·tio ['pɔːrʃɪəʊ] n anat. Teil m, Anteil m, Portio f; Pars m.
por·tion ['pɔːrʃn, 'pəʊ-] I n 1. (An-)Teil m (of an); Abschnitt m, Stück nt. 2. Menge f, Quantum nt; (Essen) Portion f. II vt auf-, zuteilen.
  portion out vt auf-, verteilen (among unter).
por·to·en·ter·os·to·my [ˌpɔːrtəʊˌentə'rɒstəmɪ, ˌpəʊr-] n chir. Hepato(porto)enterostomie f, intrahepatische Cholangiojejunostomie f.
por·to·gram ['-græm] n radiol. Portogramm nt.
por·tog·ra·phy [pɔːr'tɒgrəfɪ, pəʊr-] n radiol. Kontrastdarstellung f der Pfortader, Portographie f.
por·to·je·ju·nos·to·my [ˌpɔːrtəˌdʒɪdʒʊ-'nɒstəmɪ, pəʊr-] n → portoenterostomy.
por·to·sys·tem·ic anastomosis [ˌ-sɪs'temɪk] portokavale Anastomose f, portokavaler Shunt m.

portosystemic shunt → portosystemic anastomosis.
por·to·um·bil·i·cal circulation [ˌ-ʌm'bɪlɪkl] Cruveilhier(-von)-Baumgarten-Syndrom nt.
por·to·ve·no·gram [ˌ-'viːnəgræm] n → portogram.
por·to·ve·nog·ra·phy [ˌ-vɪ'nɒgrəfɪ] n → portography.
Por·tu·guese-Azorean disease [ˌpɔːrtʃə-'giːz, ˌpəʊr-] Machado-Joseph-Syndrom nt, Azorenkrankheit f.
port-wine mark derm. Feuer-, Gefäßmal nt, Portwein-, Weinfleck m, Naevus flammeus.
port-wine nevus/stain → port-wine mark.
po·rus ['pɔːrəs, 'pəʊ-] n, pl **-ri** [-raɪ] anat. Öffnung f, Porus m.
Posada [pəʊ'saːda]: **P.'s disease/mycosis** → Posada-Wernicke disease.
Posada-Wernicke ['vernɪkə]: **P.-W. disease** Posada-Mykose f, Wüstenfieber nt, Kokzidioidomykose f, Coccioidomycose f, Granulom coccioides.
pose [pəʊz] I n Haltung f, Stellung f, Pose f, Positur f. II vi posieren, eine Pose einnehmen u. einhalten.
po·si·tion [pə'zɪʃn] I n 1. Lage f, Anordnung f, Stellung f, Haltung f, Position f; anat. Positio f. **to be in ~ of** in der richtigen Lage sein; an der richten Stelle sein. **to be out of ~** nicht in der richtigen Lage sein; an der falschen Stelle sein. 2. gyn. Stellung f, Positio f. 3. chir. Lage f, Lagerung f, Stellung f, Position f. 4. techn. (Schalt-)Stellung f. 5. Platz m, Stelle f, (Stand-)Ort m. 6. (soziale) Stellung f, Position f. 7. (Sach-)Lage f, Situation f. 8. Standpunkt m, Haltung f, Einstellung f. II vt auf-, einstellen, anbringen, in die richtige Lage bringen.
position agnosia neuro. Stellungs-, Positionsagnosie f.
po·si·tion·al [pə'zɪʃnəl] adj Lage-, Stellungs-, Positions-.
position ametropia ophthal. Positionsametropie f.
positional nystagmus Lage-, Lagerungsnystagmus m.
  direction changing p. richtungswechselnder Lagenystagmus.
  direction-determined p. richtungsbestimmter Lagenystagmus.
  dynamic p. dynamischer Lagenystagmus.
  irregular p. regelloser Lagenystagmus.
  paroxysmal p. paroxysmaler Lagenystagmus.
  regular p. regelmäßiger Lagenystagmus.
  static p. statischer Lagenystagmus.
position-dependent adj lage-, positionsabhängig.
position effect genet. Positionseffekt m.
pos·i·tive ['pɒzɪtɪv] I n 1. positive Eigenschaft f, positiver Sachverhalt od. Faktor m, Positivum nt. 2. photo. Positiv nt. II adj 3. bio., electr., mathe., phys. positiv. 4. (Befund) positiv. 5. (Antwort) positiv, bejahend; allg. eindeutig, sicher, feststehend; definitiv.
positive accommodation physiol. Nahakkommodation f.
positive afterimage positives Nachbild nt.
positive charge positive Ladung f.
positive convergence ophthal. Einwärtsdrehung f der Sehachse.
positive cyclophoria ophthal. Exzyklophorie f.
positive cyclotropia ophthal. Exzyklotropie f.
positive electrode Anode f, positive Elektrode f, positiver Pol m.
positive electron → positron.

positive end-expiratory pressure abbr. **PEEP** positive-endexspiratorische Druckbeatmung f, positive end-expiratory pressure abbr. PEEP.
positive feedback Mitkopplung f, positive Rückkopplung f.
positive lens konvexe Linse f, Konvexlinse f, Sammellinse f.
positive meniscus Konkavokonvexlinse f.
positive modulator biochem., genet. positiver/fördernder/stimulierender Modulator m.
positive-negative pressure breathing abbr. **PNPB** → positive-negative pressure ventilation.
positive-negative pressure ventilation abbr. **PNPV** Wechseldruckbeatmung f, positive-negative Druckbeatmung f, positive-negative pressure breathing abbr. PNPB, positive-negative pressure ventilation abbr. PNPV.
positive pole 1. Pluspol m. **2.** Anode f, positive Elektrode f, positiver Pol m.
positive pressure Überdruck m.
positive pressure breathing CPAP-(Be-)Atmung f, kontinuierliche (Be-)Atmung f gegen erhöhten Druck.
positive pressure respiration → positive pressure breathing.
positive pressure ventilation abbr. **PPV** Überdruckbeatmung f.
positive rays Anodenstrahlen pl, -strahlung f.
positive reinforcement psycho. positive Verstärkung f.
positive reinforcer psycho. positiver Verstärker m.
positive rheotaxis Bewegung f gegen einen Flüssigkeitsstrom, positive Rheotaxis f.
positive scotoma ophthal. positives/subjektives Skotom f.
positive-sense RNA Plus-Strang-RNA f, Plus-Strang-RNS f.
positive-sense RNA viruses Plus-Strang--RNA-Viren pl.
positive sign mathe. positives Vorzeichen nt, Pluszeichen nt.
positive stain Positivfärbung f.
pos·i·tron [pɒsɪtrən] n abbr. **e+**, **β+** phys. Antielektron nt, positives Elektron nt, Positron nt abbr. e+, β+.
positron-emission tomography abbr. **PET** Positronenemissionstomographie f abbr. PET.
post- pref. Nach-, Post-.
post·ab·sorp·tive [ˌpəʊstæb'sɔːrptɪv] adj postabsorptiv, -resorptiv.
post·a·do·les·cence [ˌ-ædə'lesəns] n Postadoleszenz f, Postpubertät f.
post·ag·gres·sion metabolism [ˌ-ə'greʃn] Postaggressionsstoffwechsel m.
post·a·nal dimple [ˌ-'eɪnl] → postanal pit.
postanal pit Steißbeingrübchen nt, Foveola coccygea.
post·an·es·thet·ic [ˌ-ænəs'θetɪk] adj nach einer Narkose/Anästhesie (auftretend), postanästhetisch.
post·ap·o·plec·tic [ˌ-æpə'plektɪk] adj nach einem apoplektischen Anfall (auftretend), postapoplektisch.
post·au·ric·u·lar [ˌ-ɔː'rɪkjələr] adj hinter der Ohrmuschel (liegend), postaurikulär.
post·ax·i·al [ˌ-'æksɪəl] adj hinter einer Achse (liegend), postaxial.
post·ax·il·lar·y line [ˌ-'æksəˌlerɪ, -æk-'sɪlərɪ] hintere Axillarlinie f, Linea axillaris posterior.
post·bra·chi·al [ˌ-'breɪkɪəl] adj auf der Rückseite des Oberarms (liegend), postbrachial.

post·bran·chi·al body [,-'bræŋkɪəl] *embryo.* Ultimobranchialkörper *m*, ultimobranchialer Körper *m*.
post·bul·bar [,-'bʌlbər, -bɑːr] *adj* postbulbär.
post·cal·ca·ne·al bursa [,-kæl'keɪnɪəl] Bursa subcutanea calcanea.
post·cap·il·lar·y [,-'kæpə,lerɪ] **I** *n* venöse Kapillare *f*, venöser Teil *m* der Kapillarschlinge. **II** *adj* postkapillär.
post·car·di·ot·o·my (psychosis) syndrome [,-,kɑːrdɪ'ɑtəmɪ] Postkardiotomie-Syndrom *nt*.
post·ca·va [,-'keɪvə] *n* untere Hohlvene *f*, V. cava inferior.
post·ca·val [,-'keɪvl] *adj* retrocaval, -kaval.
postcaval shunt *chir.* portokavaler Shunt *m*, portokavale Anastomose *f*.
post·cen·tral [,-'sentrəl] *adj* post-, retrozentral.
postcentral area sensibler/sensorischer Cortex *m*, sensible/sensorische Rinde *f*.
postcentral artery A. sulci postcentralis.
postcentral fissure Sulcus postcentralis.
postcentral gyrus Gyrus postcentralis.
postcentral sulcus Sulcus postcentralis.
post·cho·le·cys·tec·to·my syndrome [,-,kaʊləsɪs'tektəmɪ] *chir.* Postcholezystektomie-Syndrom *nt abbr.* PCHES.
post·ci·bal [,-'caɪbl] *adj* → postprandial.
post·cis·ter·na [,-sɪs'tɜrnə] *n* Cisterna cerebellomedularis/magna.
post·com·mis·su·ral [,-kə'mɪʃərəl, -,kamə-'ʃʊərəl] *adj* hinter einer Kommissur (liegend), postkommissural.
postcommissural fibers postkommissurale Fasern *pl*.
postcommissural fornix → postcommissural part of fornix.
postcommissural part of fornix postkommissuraler Teil *m* des Fornix, Fornix cerebri.
post·com·mis·sur·ot·o·my syndrome [,-,kamɪʃə'rɑtəmɪ] Postkommissurotomie-Syndrom *nt*.
post·com·mu·ni·cal part [,-kə'mjuːnɪkl]: **p. of anterior cerebral artery** Pars postcommunicalis (a. cerebri anteriores), A. pericallosa.
p. of posterior cerebral artery Pars postcommunicalis a. cerebri posterioris.
post·con·cus·sion·al syndrome [,-kən-'kʌʃənl] postkommotionelles Syndrom *nt*, posttraumatische Hirnleistungsschwäche *f*.
post·con·vul·sive stupor [,-kən'vʌlsɪv] postkonvulsiver Stupor *m*.
post·cor·nu [,-'kɔːrn(j)uː] *n* Hinterhorn *nt* des Seitenventrikels, Cornu occipitale/posterius.
post·di·as·tol·ic [,-,daɪə'stɑlɪk] *adj* nach der Diastole (auftretend), postdiastolisch.
post·di·crot·ic [,-daɪ'krɑtɪk] *adj card.* postdikrot.
post·diph·ther·ic paralysis [,-dɪfˈθerɪk] (post-)diphtherische Lähmung *f*.
post·diph·the·rit·ic paralysis [,-dɪfθə'rɪtɪk] → postdiphtheric paralysis.
post·dor·mi·tal [,-'dɔːrmɪtæl] *adj* Postdormitium betr.
post·dor·mi·tum [,-'dɔːrmɪtəm] *n* Postdormitium *nt*.
post·em·bry·on·ic [,-,embrɪ'ɑnɪk] *adj* nach dem Embryonalstadium (auftretend), postembryonal.
post·en·ceph·a·lit·ic [,-en,sefə'lɪtɪk] *adj* nach einer Enzephalitis (auftretend), postenzephalitisch.
postencephalitic parkinsonism → parkinsonian syndrome.
post·e·pi·lep·tic [,-epɪ'leptɪk] *adj* nach einem epileptischen Anfall (auftretend), postepileptisch.

pos·te·ri·or [pɑ'stɪərɪər, pəʊ-] **I** *n* Hintern *m*, Hinterteil *nt*. **II** *adj* **1.** *anat.* hinten (liegend), hintere(r, s), posterior, Hinter-. **2.** hinter, später (*to* als).
posterior arch of atlas hinterer Atlasbogen *m*, Arcus posterior atlantis.
posterior belly of digastric muscle hinterer Digastrikusbauch *m*, Venter posterior m. digastrici.
posterior border: p. of radius Radiushinterkante *f*, Margo posterior radii.
p. of spleen unterer Milzrand *m*, Margo inferior lienis/splenis.
p. of ulna Ulnahinterrand *m*, Margo posterior ulnae.
posterior branch: p.es of cervical nerves hintere/dorsale Halsnervenäste *pl*, Rami dorsales/posteriores nn. cervicalium.
p. of coccygeal nerve Ramus dorsalis n. coccygei.
p. of great auricular nerve hinterer Ast *m* des N. auricularis magnus, Ramus posterior n. auricularis magni.
p. of inferior laryngeal nerve hinterer Ast *m* des N. laryngealis inferior, Ramus posterior n. laryngeali inferioris.
p. of inferior pancreaticoduodenal artery Ramus posterior a. pancreaticoduodenalis inferioris.
p. of lateral cerebral sulcus Ramus posterior sulci lateralis (cerebri).
p. of left pulmonary artery Ramus posterior a. pulmonalis sinistrae.
p.es of lumbar nerves Rückenäste *pl* der Lendennerven, Rami dorsales/posteriores nn. lumbalium.
p. of medial cutaneous nerve of forearm Ramus posterior n. cutanei antebrachii medialis.
p. of obturator artery hinterer (End-)Ast *m* der A. obturatoria, Ramus posterior a. obturatoriae.
p. of obturator nerve hinterer Ast *m* des N. obturatorius, Ramus posterior n. obturatorii.
p. of recurrent ulnar artery hinterer Ast *m* der A. recurrens ulnaris, Ramus posterior a. recurrentis ulnaris.
p. of renal artery hinterer Ast *m* der Nierenarterie, Ramus posterior a. renalis.
p. of right hepatic duct Ramus posterior ductus heptici dextri.
p.es of sacral nerves dorsale/hintere Äste *pl* der Sakralnerven, Rami dorsales/posteriores nn. sacralium.
p. of spinal nerves hinterer Ast *od.* Rückenast *m* der Spinalnerven, Ramus dorsalis/posterior nn. spinalium.
p. of superior thyroid artery hinterer Drüsenast *m* der A. thyroidea superior, Ramus glandularis posterior a. thyroideae superioris.
p.es of thoracic nerves Rückenäste *pl* der Brust-/Thorakalnerven, Rami dorsales/posteriores nn. thoracicorum.
posterior bronchus, anterior Bronchus anterior posterior.
posterior cells Sinus posteriores.
posterior chamber of eye hintere Augenkammer *m*, Camera oculi posterior, Camera posterior (bulbi).
posterior cistern Cisterna magna/cerebellomedullaris.
posterior colpotomy *gyn.* Kuldotomie *f*.
posterior column: p. of fauces hinterer Gaumenbogen *m*, Arcus palatopharyngeus.
p. of rugae of vagina Columna rugarum posterior.
p. of spinal cord Hintersäule *f* (der grauen Substanz), Columna dorsalis/posterior medullae spinalis.
posterior commissure: p. of cerebrum hintere Kommissur *f*, Commissura epithalamica, Commissura posterior cerebri.
p. of labia hintere Verbindung *f* der großen Schamlippen, Commissura labiorum posterior.
posterior cord of brachial plexus hinteres Bündel *nt* des Plexus brachialis, Fasciculus posterior (plexus brachialis).
posterior cord syndrome Hinterstrangsyndrom *nt*.
posterior crus: p. of internal capsule hinterer Kapselschenkel *m*, Crus posterius capsulae internae.
p. of stapes hinterer Steigbügelschenkel *m*, Crus posterius stapedis.
p. of superficial inguinal ring Crus laterale anuli inguinalis superficialis.
posterior divisions of trunks of brachial plexus hintere Äste *pl* der Trunci plexus brachialis, Divisiones dorsales/posteriores truncorum plexus brachialis.
posterior edges of eye lids hintere Lidkanten *pl*, Limbi palpebrales posteriores.
posterior embryotoxon (of Axenfeld) Embryotoxon posterius.
posterior epithelium of cornea inneres Korneaepithel *nt*, Korneaendothel *nt*, Endothelium corneae, Epithelium posterius (corneae).
posterior extremity of spleen oberer Milzpol *m*, Extremitas posterior (lienis/splenis).
posterior fissure of auricle Antitragus-Helix-Trennfurche *f*, Fissura antitragohelicina.
posterior fontanelle kleine/hintere Fontanelle *f*, Hinterhauptsfontanelle *f*, Fonticulus posterior.
posterior fornix hinteres Scheidengewölbe *nt*, Pars posterior fornicis vaginae.
posterior funiculus (of spinal cord) Hinterstrang *m*, Funiculus dorsalis/posterior medullae spinalis.
posterior head of rectus femoris muscle hinterer Kopf *m* des M. rectus femoris, Caput reflexum m. recti femoris.
posterior horn: p. of lateral ventricle Hinterhorn *nt* des Seitenventrikels, Cornu occipitale/posterius ventriculi lateralis.
p. of spinal cord Hinterhorn *nt* des Rückenmarks, Cornu dorsalis/posterius medullae spinalis.
posterior horn cell (*ZNS*) Hinterhornzelle *f*.
posterior inferior cerebellar artery syndrome Wallenberg-Syndrom *nt*, dorsolaterales Oblongata-Syndrom *nt*.
posterior ligament: p. of incus hinteres Incusband *nt*, Lig. incudis posterius.
p. of radiocarpal joint Lig. radiocarpale dorsale.
posterior limb: p. of internal capsule → posterior crus of internal capsule.
p. of stapes Crus posterius stapedis.
posterior lip: p. of cervix of uterus hintere Lippe des äußeren Muttermundes, Labium posterius (ostii uteri).
p. of ostium of uterus → p. of cervix of uterus.
posterior lobe: p. of cerebellar body Lobus posterior corporis cerebelli.
p. of cerebellum kaudaler (Kleinhirn-)Lappen/-Abschnitt *m*, Lobus caudalis/posterior cerebelli.
p. of hypophysis Neurohypophyse *f*, Hypophysenhinterlappen *m abbr.* HHL, Neurohypophysis *f*, Lobus posterior hypophyseos.
p. of pituitary (gland) → p. of hypophysis.

posterior margin

posterior margin: p. of fibula Fibulahinterrand *m*, Margo posterior fibulae.
p. of radius → posterior border of radius.
p. of spleen → posterior border of spleen.
p. of testis hinterer/konkaver Hodenrand *m*, Margo posterior testis.
p. of ulna → posterior border of ulna.
posterior mediastinum hinterer Mediastinalraum *m*, hinteres Mediastinum *nt*, Mediastinum posterius, Cavum mediastinale posterius.
posterior nephrectomy *urol*., *chir*. hintere Nephrektomie *f*.
posterior neuropore *embryo*. hinterer/kaudaler Neuroporus *m*.
posterior nucleus Nc. posterior.
p.i of thalamus hintere Kerngruppe *f* des Thalamus, Ncc. posteriores thalami.
p. of trapezoid body Nc. corporis trapezoidei posterior.
posterior part: p. of cerebral peduncle Mittelhirnhaube *f*, Tegmentum *nt* (mesencephali), Pars dorsalis/posterior pedunculi cerebri.
p. of trabecular retinaculum hinterer Abschnitt des Hueck'-Bandes, Pars uvealis.
posterior pillar of fornix Crus fornicis.
posterior pituitary *abbr*. PP Hypophysenhinterlappen *m abbr*. HHL, Neurohypophyse *f*, Neurohypophysis *f*.
posterior pituitary hormones (Hypophysen-)Hinterlappenhormone *pl*, HHL--Hormone *pl*, Neurohypophysenhormone *pl*.
posterior pituitary system Hypophysenhinterlappensystem *nt*, HHL-System *nt*.
posterior pole: p. of eye ball hinterer Augenpol *m*, Polus posterior bulbi oculi.
p. of lens hinterer Linsenpol *m*, Polus posterior lentis.
posterior pouch of Tröltsch → posterior recess of tympanic membrane.
posterior process: p. of cartilage of nasal septum Proc. posterior/sphenoidalis.
p. of talus Proc. posterior tali.
posterior recess of tympanic membrane hintere Schleimhauttasche *f* des Trommelfells, Rec. (membranae tympanicae) posterior.
posterior rhinoscopy Postrhinoskopie *f*, Epipharyngoskopie *f*, Rhinoscopia posterior.
posterior rhizotomy *neuro*. Dana-Operation *f*, Rhizotomia posterior.
posterior root hintere/sensible Spinal(nerven)wurzel *f*, Radix dorsalis/posterior/sensoria nn. spinalium.
p. of spinal nerves → posterior root.
posterior root fibers Hinterwurzelfasern *pl*.
posterior scleritis Scleritis posterior.
posterior sclerosis Rückenmark(s)schwindsucht *f*, Rückenmarksdarre *f*, Ducchenne-Syndrom *nt*, Tabes dorsalis.
posterior segment: p. of kidney Segmentum posterius.
p. of right lobe of liver Segmentum posterius.
p. of right lung Dorsalsegment *nt* des rechten Oberlappens, Segmentum posterius [S. II].
p. of thalamus hinterer Teil *m* des Thalamus, Pulvinar thalami.
posterior sinus. p.es *pl* hintere Siebbeinzellen *pl*, Cellulae/Sinus posteriores.
p. of tympanic cavity Sinus posterior cavi tympani.
posterior staphyloma Staphyloma verum posticum.
posterior sulcus of auricle Sulcus auricularis posterior.
posterior surface: p. of cornea Hornhauthinterfläche *f*, Facies posterior corneae.
p. of eyelid innere/hintere Lidfläche *f*, Facies posterior palpebrarum.
p. of iris Irisrückfläche *f*, Facies posterior iridis.
p. of lens Linsenrückfläche *f*, Facies posterior lentis.
p. of sacral bone Facies dorsalis (ossis sacri).
p. of scapula Rückfläche *f* des Schulterblattes, Facies posterior scapulae.
p. of uterus Darmfläche *f* des Uterus, Facies intestinalis uteri.
posterior synechia *ophthal*. hintere Synechie *f*, Synechia posterior.
posterior triangle of neck seitliches Halsdreieck *nt*, Regio cervicalis lateralis, Trigonum cervicale posterius.
posterior tubercle: p. of atlas Tuberculum posterius (atlantis).
p. of cervical vertebrae Tuberculum posterius vertebrarum cervicalium.
p. of humerus Tuberculum major humeri.
posterior urethritis Urethritis posterior.
posterior uveitis *ophthal*. hintere Uveitis *f*, Uveitis posterior.
posterior vein: p. of corpus callosum hintere Balkenvene *f*, V. posterior corporis callosi.
p. of left ventricle V. ventriculi sinistri posterior.
p. of septum pellucidum V. posterior septi pellucidi.
posterior wall: p. of stomach Hinterwand *f* des Magens, Paries posterior ventriculi.
p. of tympanic cavity Hinterwand *f* der Paukenhöhle, Paries mastoideus cavitatis tympanicae.
postero- *pref*. postero-.
pos·ter·o·an·te·ri·or [ˌpɑstərəʊænˈtɪərɪər] *adj abbr*. **p.a.** von hinten nach vorne (verlaufend), posterior-anterior *abbr*. PA, posteroanterior *abbr*. p.a.
pos·ter·o·ex·ter·nal [ˌ-ɪkˈstɜrnl] *adj* → posterolateral.
pos·ter·o·in·fe·ri·or [ˌ-ɪnˈfɪərɪər] *adj* hinten u. unten (liegend), posterior-inferior, posteroinferior.
pos·ter·o·in·ter·me·di·ate groove/sulcus of spinal cord [ˌ-ɪntərˈmiːdɪɪt] Sulcus intermedius dorsalis/posterior medullae spinalis.
pos·ter·o·in·ter·nal [ˌ-ɪnˈtɜrnl] *adj* → posteromedial.
pos·ter·o·lat·er·al [ˌ-ˈlætərəl] *adj* hinten u. außen (liegend), posterior-lateral, posterolateral.
posterolateral branch of right coronary artery, right Ast *m* zur Hinterwand des rechten Ventrikels, Ramus posterolateralis dexter.
posterolateral fissure of cerebellum Fissura dorsolateralis/posterolateralis cerebelli.
posterolateral fontanelle hintere Seitenfontanelle *f*, Warzenfontanelle *f*, Fonticulus mastoideus/posterolateralis.
posterolateral groove: p. of medulla oblongata Hinterseitenfurche *f* der Medulla, Sulcus dorsolateralis/posterolateralis medullae oblongatae.
p. of spinal cord Hinterseitenfurche *f* des Rückenmarks, Sulcus dorsolateralis/posterolateralis medullae spinalis.
posterolateral sclerosis Lichtheim-Syndrom *nt*, Dana-Lichtheim-Syndrom *nt*, Dana-Syndrom *nt*, Dana-Lichtheim--Putnam-Syndrom *nt*, funikuläre Spinalerkrankung/Myelose *f*.
posterolateral sulcus: p. of medulla oblongata → posterolateral groove of medulla oblongata.

p. of spinal cord → posterolateral groove of spinal cord.
pos·ter·o·me·di·al [ˌ-ˈmiːdɪəl] *adj* hinten u. in der Mitte (liegend), posterior-medial, posteromedial.
pos·ter·o·me·di·an [ˌ-ˈmiːdɪən] *adj* hinten u. in der Mittellinie (liegend), posterior-median, posteromedian.
posteromedian column: p. of medulla oblongata Fasciculus gracilis medullae oblongatae.
p. of spinal cord Goll'-Strang, Fasciculus gracilis (medullae spinalis).
pos·ter·o·pa·ri·e·tal [ˌ-pəˈraɪɪtl] *adj* posteroparietal.
pos·ter·o·su·pe·ri·or [ˌ-səˈpɪərɪər, -suː-] *adj* hinten u. oben (liegend), posterior-superior, posterosuperior.
pos·ter·o·tem·po·ral [ˌ-ˈtemp(ə)rəl] *adj* posterotemporal.
posterotemporal fontanelle → posterolateral fontanelle.
post·ex·po·sure prophylaxis [ˌpəʊstɪkˈspəʊzər] postexpositionelle Prophylaxe *f*, Postexpositionsprophylaxe *f*.
post·ex·tra·sys·tol·ic pause [ˌ-ˌekstrəsɪˈstɑlɪk] *card*. postextrasystolische Pause *f*.
postextrasystolic potentiation *physiol*. postextrasystolische Potenzierung *f*.
post·gan·gli·on·ic [ˌ-ˌgæŋglɪˈɑnɪk] *adj* distal eines Ganglions (liegend), postganglionär.
postganglionic fibers → postganglionic neurofibers.
postganglionic neurofibers postganglionäre Nervenfasern *pl*, Neurofibrae postganglionares.
postganglionic neuron postganglionäres Neuron *nt*.
post·gas·trec·to·my syndrome [ˌ-gæsˈtrektəmɪ] *chir*. **1.** Postgastrektomiesyndrom *nt*. **2.** Dumpingsyndrom *nt*.
post·glo·mer·u·lar [ˌ-gləʊˈmerjələr, -glə-] *adj* (*Niere*) postglomerulär.
postglomerular arteriole abführende/efferente Glomerulusarterie *f*, abführende/efferente Glomerulusarteriole *f*, Arteriola glomerularis efferens, Vas efferens (glomeruli).
post·gon·o·coc·cal urethritis [ˌ-gɑnəˈkɑkəl] postgonorrhoische Urethritis *f abbr*. PGU.
post·hem·or·rha·gic [ˌ-heməˈrædʒɪk] *adj* nach einer Blutung (auftretend), posthämorrhagisch.
posthemorrhagic anemia posthämorrhagische Anämie *f*.
post·he·pat·ic [ˌ-hɪˈpætɪk] *adj* hinter der Leber (auftretend), posthepatisch.
posthepatic cholestasis posthepatische Gallestauung/Cholestase *f*.
posthepatic cirrhosis chronisch-persistierende Hepatitis *f abbr*. CPH.
posthepatic icterus posthepatischer Ikterus *m*.
post·her·pet·ic neuralgia [ˌ-hɜrˈpetɪk] Post-Herpes-Neuralgie *f*.
pos·thet·o·my [pɑsˈθetəmɪ] *n urol*. Beschneidung *f*, Zirkumzision *f*.
pos·thi·o·plas·ty [ˈpɑsθaɪəplæstɪ] *n urol*. Vorhautplastik *f*.
pos·thi·tis [pɑsˈθaɪtɪs] *n urol*. Vorhautentzündung *f*, Posthitis *f*.
pos·tho·lith [ˈpəʊsθəlɪθ] *n urol*. Vorhaut-, Präputialstein *m*, Postholith *m*, Balanolith *m*, Smegmolith *m*.
post·hu·mous [ˈpɑstʃəmɑs, -tʃʊ-] *adj* nach dem Tod erfolgend; nach dem Tod des Vaters geboren, posthum, postum.
post·hy·oi·de·an cleft [ˌpəʊsthaɪˈɔɪdɪən] *embryo*. Hyobranchialspalt *m*, -furche *f*.

post·hyp·not·ic amnesia [ˌ-hɪp'nɒtɪk] posthypnotische Amnesie *f*.
pos·ti·cus palsy [pɑs'taɪkəs] Postikuslähmung *f*, -paralyse *f*.
posticus paralysis → posticus palsy.
post·in·fec·tious encephalitis [ˌpəʊstɪn-'fekʃəs] → postinfectious encephalomyelitis.
postinfectious encephalomyelitis Impfenzephalitis *f*, -enzephalomyelitis *f*, -enzephalopathie *f*, Vakzinationsenzephalitis *f*, Encephalomyelitis postvaccinalis.
postinfectious polyneuritis Guillain-Barré-Syndrom *nt*, Polyradikuloneuritis *f*, Radikuloneuritis *f*, Neuronitis *f*.
post·in·fec·tive bradycardia [ˌ-ɪn'fektɪv] postinfektiöse Bradykardie *f*.
post·in·flam·ma·to·ry cataract [ˌ-ɪn'flæmətɔːriː, -təʊ-] postentzündliche Katarakt *f*.
postinflammatory clubfoot *ortho.* entzündungsbedingter Klumpfuß *m*.
post·in·spi·ra·tion [ˌ-ˌɪnspə'reɪʃn] *n physiol.* Postinspiration *f*.
post·in·spir·a·to·ry neuron [ˌ-ɪn'spaɪərəˌtɔːriː, -təʊ-] postinspiratorisches Neuron *nt*, p-I-Neuron *nt*.
post-kala-azar dermal leishmaniasis Post-Kala-Azar-Hautleishman(o)id *nt*, Post-Kala-Azar-Dermatose *f*, Post-Kala-Azar dermale Leishmaniose *f*, Post-Kala-Azar dermale Leishmanoide *pl*.
post·lam·i·nar part of optic nerve [ˌ-'læmɪnər] postlaminärer Abschnitt *m* des N. opticus, Pars postlaminaris n. optici.
post·ma·ture [ˌ-mə'tʃʊər] *adj gyn.* übertragen, überreif.
postmature delivery *gyn.* Entbindung *f* eines übertragenen Säuglings.
postmature infant übertragener Säugling *m*.
post·me·di·as·ti·num [ˌ-mɪdiæ'staɪnəm] *n* hinterer Mediastinalraum *m*, hinteres Mediastinum *nt*, Mediastinum posterius, Cavum mediastinale posterius.
post·mei·ot·ic [ˌ-maɪ'ɒtɪk] *adj* nach der Meiose (auftretend), postmeiotisch.
postmeiotic phase postmeiotische Phase *f*.
post·men·in·git·ic hydrocephalus [ˌ-ˌmenɪn'dʒɪtɪk] postmeningitischer Hydrozephalus *m*.
post·men·o·pau·sal [ˌ-ˌmenə'pɔːzl] *adj* nach der Menopause (auftretend), postmenopausal, Postmenopausen-.
postmenopausal atrophy postmenopausale Atrophie *f*, Postmenopausenatrophie *f*.
postmenopausal osteoporosis postmenopausale/klimakterische Osteoporose *f*, präsenile Involutionsosteoporose *f*.
post·mes·en·ter·ic [ˌ-mesən'terɪk] *adj* post-, retromesenterial.
post·men·stru·al [ˌ-'menstr(ʊ)əl, -strəwəl] *adj* nach der Menstruation, postmenstruell, postmenstrual.
postmenstrual stage → postmenstruum.
post·men·stru·um [ˌ-'menstr(ʊ)əm, -strəwəm] *n, pl* **-stru·ums, -stru·a** [-str(ʊ)ə, -strəwə] Postmenstrualphase *f*, -stadium *nt*, Postmenstruum *nt*.
post·mi·ot·ic *adj* → postmeiotic.
post·mi·tot·ic [ˌ-maɪ'tɒtɪk] *adj* nach der Mitose (auftretend), postmitotisch.
post·mor·tal [ˌ-'mɔːrtl] *adj abbr.* **p.m.** nach dem Tode (auftretend), postmortal, post mortem *abbr.* p.m.
post·mor·tem [ˌ-'mɔːrtəm] **I** *n* Leichen(er)öffnung *f*, Obduktion *f*, Autopsie *f*, Nekropsie *f*. **to hold a ~** eine Obduktion durchführen. **II** *adj* nach dem Tode (eintretend), postmortal, post mortem *abbr.* p.m.

postmortem clot Leichengerinnsel *nt*.
postmortem delivery *gyn.* Entbindung *f* eines Säuglings aus einer verstorbenen Mutter.
postmortem examination → postmortem I.
postmortem hypostasis → postmortem lividity.
postmortem livedo → postmortem lividity.
postmortem lividity Totenflecke *pl*, Livor mortis, Livores *pl*.
postmortem rigidity Totenstarre *f*, Rigor mortis.
postmortem suggillation → postmortem lividity.
postmortem thrombus Post-mortem-Thrombus *m*.
postmortem wart Wilk'-Krankheit *f*, warzige Tuberkulose *f* der Haut, Leichentuberkel *m*, Schlachtertuberkulose *f*, Tuberculosis cutis verrucosa, Verruca necrogenica, Tuberculum anatomicum.
post·my·o·car·di·al infarction syndrome [ˌ-ˌmaɪəʊ'kɑːrdɪəl] *card.* Dressler-Myokarditis *f*, -Syndrom *nt*, Postmyokardinfarktsyndrom *nt abbr.* PMI.
post·na·sal [ˌ-'neɪzl] *adj* hinter der Nase (liegend), postnasal.
postnasal catarrh chronische Rhinopharyngitis *f*.
post·na·tal [ˌ-'neɪtl] *adj* nach der Geburt (eintretend), nachgeburtlich, postnatal.
postnatal dimple Steißbeingrübchen *nt*, Foveola coccygea.
postnatal hemopoiesis postnatale Blutbildung/Hämopoese *f*.
postnatal infection postnatale Infektion *f*.
postnatal life Postnatalperiode *f*.
postnatal pit → postnatal dimple.
postnatal toxoplasmosis postnatale Toxoplasmose *f*.
post·ne·crot·ic cirrhosis [ˌ-nə'krɒtɪk, -ne-] postnekrotische/ungeordnete/großknotige Leberzirrhose *f*.
post·ob·struc·tive diuresis [ˌpəʊstəb-'strʌktɪv] postobstruktive Diurese *f*.
post·oc·u·lar neuritis [ˌ-'ɒkjələr] Retrobulbärneuritis *f*, Neuritis optica retrobulbaris.
post·op·er·a·tive [ˌ-'ɒp(ə)rətɪv, -reɪtɪv] *adj* nach der Operation (eintretend *od.* erfolgend), postoperativ.
postoperative hemolysis postoperative Hämolyse *f*.
postoperative hypoparathyroidism postoperativer Hypoparathyreoidismus *m*.
postoperative irradiation → postoperative radiation.
postoperative mortality postoperative Mortalität *f*.
postoperative pneumonia postoperative Pneumonie *f*.
postoperative psychosis postoperative Psychose *f*.
postoperative radiation *radiol.* Nachbestrahlung *f*, postoperative Bestrahlung *f*.
post·par·tal [ˌ-'pɑːrtl] *adj* nach der Geburt (auftretend), postpartal, post partum *f*.
postpartal cardiomyopathy/myocardiopathy → postpartum cardiomyopathy.
post·par·tum [ˌ-'pɑːrtəm] *adj* → postpartal.
postpartum alopecia postpartale Alopezie *f*, Alopecia postpartalis.
postpartum amenorrhea *gyn.* postpartale Amenorrhoe *f*.
postpartum cardiomyopathy postpartale Kardiomyopathie/Myokardiopathie *f*.

postpartum hemorrhage postpartale Blutung *f*.
postpartum hypertension postpartale Hypertonie *f*.
postpartum myocardiopathy → postpartum cardiomyopathy.
postpartum pituitary necrosis (syndrome) Scheehan-Syndrom *nt*, postpartale Hypophysenvorderlappeninsuffizienz *f*.
postpartum psychosis Wochenbett-, Puerperalpsychose *f*.
post·per·fu·sion syndrome [ˌ-pər'fjuːʒn] Postperfusionssyndrom *nt*, Posttransfusionssyndrom *nt*.
post·per·i·car·di·ot·o·my syndrome [ˌ-ˌperiˌkɑːrdɪ'ɒtəmɪ] Postperikardiotomie-Syndrom *nt*.
post·phle·bit·ic syndrome [ˌ-flɪ'bɪtɪk] postthrombotisches Syndrom *nt*, postthrombotischer Symptomenkomplex *m*.
post·pneu·mo·nec·to·my empyema [ˌ-ˌn(j)uːmə'nektəmɪ] *chir.* Postpneumonektomieempyem *nt*.
post·pneu·mon·ic [ˌ-nju:'mɒnɪk] *adj* nach einer Pneumonie (auftretend), postpneumonisch, metapneumonisch.
post·pran·di·al [ˌ-'prændɪəl] *adj* nach der Mahlzeit/Nahrungsaufnahme, postprandial.
postprandial lipemia alimentäre/postprandiale Lipämie *f*.
postprandial pain postprandialer Schmerz *m*.
post·pri·ma·ry stage [ˌ-'praɪmeriː, -məri] (*Tuberkulose*) Postprimärstadium *nt*.
postprimary tuberculosis postprimäre Tuberkulose *f*.
post·pu·ber·al [ˌ-'pjuːbərəl] *adj* → postpubertal.
post·pu·ber·tal [ˌ-'pjuːbərtəl] *adj* nach der Pubertät (auftretend), postpubertär, postpuberal, postpubertal.
post·pu·ber·ty [ˌ-'pjuːbərtɪ] *n* Postpubertät *f*.
post·pu·bes·cence [ˌ-pjuː'besns] *n* → postpuberty.
post·pu·bes·cent [ˌ-pjuː'besnt] *adj* → postpubertal.
post·py·ram·i·dal fissure [ˌ-pɪ'ræmɪdl] Fissura secunda (cerebelli).
post·re·duc·tion phase [ˌ-rɪ'dʌkʃn] *n* postmeiotische Phase *f*.
pos·tre·mal area [pɑs'triːml] Area postrema.
post·re·nal albuminuria [ˌpəʊst'riːnl] postrenale Albuminurie/Proteinurie *f*.
postrenal anuria postrenale Anurie *f*.
postrenal azotemia postrenale Azot(h)ämie *f*.
postrenal obstruction postrenale (Harnwegs-)Obstruktion *f*.
postrenal proteinuria → postrenal albuminuria.
post·ro·lan·dic area [ˌ-rəʊ'lændɪk] sensibler/sensorischer Cortex *m*, sensible/sensorische Rinde *f*.
post·ro·ta·to·ry nystagmus [ˌ-'rəʊtətɔːriː, -təʊ-] postrotatorischer Nystagmus *m*.
post·si·nous abscess [ˌ-'saɪnəs] postsinuöser Abszeß *m*.
post·sphyg·mic [ˌ-'sfɪgmɪk] *adj card.* nach der Pulswelle.
postsphygmic interval/period → period of isometric relaxation.
post·spi·nal headache [ˌ-'spaɪnl] Kopfschmerz(en *pl*) *m* nach einer Lumbalpunktion.
post·splen·ic [ˌ-'spliːnɪk] *adj* hinter der Milz (liegend), postsplenisch.
post·ste·not·ic [ˌ-stɪ'nɒtɪk] *adj* hinter einer Stenose (liegend), poststenotisch.

poststreptococcal diseases

post·strep·to·coc·cal diseases [ˌ-strepˈtəˈkɑkəl] Poststreptokokkenerkrankungen pl.
poststreptococcal glomerulonephritis Poststreptokokkenglomerulonephritis f.
post·sur·gi·cal [ˌ-ˈsɜrdʒɪkl] adj nach einer Operation, postoperativ.
post·syn·ap·tic [ˌ-sɪˈnæptɪk] adj hinter einer Synapse (liegend), postsynaptisch.
postsynaptic current physiol. postsynaptischer Strom m.
  excitatory p. abbr. **EPSC** erregender postsynaptischer Strom, excitatory postsynaptic current abbr. EPSC.
  inhibitory p. abbr. **IPSC** hemmender/inhibitorischer postsynaptischer Strom, inhibitory postsynaptic current abbr. IPSC.
postsynaptic facilitation physiol. postsynaptische Bahnung f.
postsynaptic inhibition postsynaptische Hemmung/Inhibition f.
postsynaptic membrane postsynaptische Membran f.
postsynaptic potential physiol. postsynaptisches Potential nt.
  excitatory p. abbr. **EPSP** erregendes postsynaptisches Potential abbr. EPSP.
  inhibitory p. abbr. **IPSP** hemmendes/inhibitorisches postsynaptisches Potential abbr. IPSP.
post-term adj gyn. (Schwangerschaft) übertragen.
post-term infant → postmature infant.
post·te·tan·ic potentiation [ˌpoʊstəˈtænɪk] physiol. posttetanische Potenzierung f.
post-thrombotic syndrome postthrombotisches Syndrom nt, postthrombotischer Symptomenkomplex m.
post·tran·scrip·tion·al [ˌ-trænˈskrɪpʃənl] adj posttranskriptional.
posttranscriptional processing biochem. posttranskriptionales Processing nt, posttranskriptionaler Reifungsprozess m.
post-transfusion hepatitis Posttransfusionshepatitis f.
post-transfusion mononucleosis → postperfusion syndrome.
post-transfusion purpura posttransfusionelle Purpura f.
post-transfusion syndrome → postperfusion syndrome.
post·trans·la·tion·al [ˌ-trænsˈleɪʃənl] adj posttranslational.
posttranslational modification biochem. posttranslationale Modifizierung f.
post-traumatic adj nach einem Unfall (auftretend), durch eine Verletzung hervorgerufen, als Folge eines Unfalls, posttraumatisch; traumatisch.
post-traumatic amnesia posttraumatische Amnesie f.
post-traumatic arthritis posttraumatische Arthrose f.
post-traumatic atrophy of bone → post-traumatic osteoporosis.
post-traumatic bowleg ortho. posttraumatisches Crus varum.
post-traumatic brain syndrome → postconcussional syndrome.
post-traumatic cholesteatoma HNO posttraumatisches Cholesteatom nt.
post-traumatic clubfoot ortho. posttraumatischer Klumpfuß m.
post-traumatic delirium posttraumatisches Delir(ium) nt.
post-traumatic epilepsy (post-)traumatische Epilepsie f.
post-traumatic hydrocephalus posttraumatischer Hydrozephalus m.
post-traumatic neck syndrome posttraumatisches Halswirbelsäulensyndrom nt.

post-traumatic osteoporosis Sudeck'-Dystrophie f, -Syndrom nt, Morbus Sudeck m.
post-traumatic pancreatitis posttraumatische Pankreatitis f.
post-traumatic psychosis posttraumatische Psychose f.
post-traumatic respiratory insufficiency syndrome Schocklunge f, adult respiratory distress syndrome abbr. ARDS.
post-traumatic scoliosis ortho. posttraumatische Skoliose f.
post-traumatic stress disorder akute Belastungsreaktion f.
post-traumatic syndrome posttraumatisches Syndrom nt.
pos·tu·late [n ˈpɑstʃəleɪt; v -lɪt, -leɪt] I n Forderung f, Gebot nt, (Grund-)Bedingung f, Postulat nt. II vt fordern, verlangen; voraussetzen, behaupten, postulieren.
pos·tur·al [ˈpɑstʃərəl] adj postural, Haltungs-, Stellungs-, Lage-.
postural albuminuria orthostatische/lordotische Albuminurie/Proteinurie f.
postural apparatus Haltungsapparat m.
postural drainage chir. Lagerungsdrainage f.
postural hypotension orthostatische Hypotonie f.
postural muscles Haltemuskeln pl, -muskulatur f.
postural proteinuria → postural albuminuria.
postural reflex Halte-, Haltungsreflex m.
postural scoliosis ortho. haltungsbedingte Skoliose f.
postural tachycardia card. orthostatische/lageabhängige Tachykardie f.
pos·ture [ˈpɑstʃər] I n (Körper-)Haltung f, Stellung f; (a. fig.) Lage f; Pose f, Positur f. II vt in eine Stellung od. Haltung bringen. III vi eine Haltung einnehmen od. einhalten; posieren.
post·vac·ci·nal [ˌpoʊstˈvæksənəl] adj nach einer Impfung (auftretend), als Folge einer Impfung, postvakzinal.
postvaccinal encephalitis/encephalomyelitis → postinfectious encephalomyelitis.
post·va·got·o·my diarrhea [ˌ-veɪˈgɑtəmɪ] Postvagotomiesyndrom nt.
post·val·var [ˌ-ˈvælvər] adj → postvalvular.
post·val·vu·lar [ˌ-ˈvælvjələr] adj hinter einer Klappe/Valva (liegend), postvalvulär.
post·ve·sic·u·lar [ˌ-vɪˈsɪkjələr] adj postvesikal.
post·vi·tal [ˌ-ˈvaɪtəl] adj histol. postvital.
post-zone [ˈ-zoʊn] n immun. Postzone f, Zone f des Antigenüberschusses.
post·zy·got·ic [ˌ-zaɪˈgɑtɪk] adj embryo. postzygotisch.
pot [pɑt] n Topf m; (Tee-, Kaffee-)Kanne f, Krug m; Tiegel m; (Kind) "Töpfchen" nt.
po·ta·ble [ˈpoʊtəbl] I ~s pl Getränke pl. II adj trinkbar, Trink-.
potable water Trinkwasser nt.
pot·ash [ˈpɑtæʃ] n Pottasche f, Kaliumkarbonat nt.
potash soap Kali(schmier)seife f, Sapo kalinus/mollis.
pot·as·se·mia [pɑtəˈsiːmɪə] n erhöhter Kaliumgehalt m des Blutes, Hyperkali(i)ämie f.
po·tas·sic [pəˈtæsɪk] adj kaliumhaltig, Kalium-, Kali-.
po·tas·si·um [pəˈtæsɪəm] n Kalium nt abbr. K.
potassium balance physiol. Kaliumhaushalt m.

potassium carbonate → potash.
potassium channel physiol. Kalium-Kanal m, K⁺-Kanal m.
potassium chloride abbr. **KCl** Kaliumchlorid nt abbr. KCl.
potassium contracture physiol. Kaliumkontraktur f.
potassium cyanide Kaliumcyanid nt, Zyankali nt, Cyankali nt.
potassium depletion Kaliummangel m.
potassium ferricyanide Kaliumferricyanid nt.
potassium gymnemate Kaliumgymnemat nt.
potassium iodide Kaliumjodid nt, -iodid nt.
potassium-losing nephritis Kaliumverlustniere f, kaliumverlierende Nephropathie f.
potassium-losing nephropathy → potassium-losing nephritis.
potassium oxalate Kaliumoxalat nt.
potassium permanganate Kaliumpermanganat nt.
potassium-sparing diuretic kaliumsparendes Diuretikum nt.
potassium tellurite Kaliumtellurit nt.
potassium thiocyanate Kaliumthiocyanat nt.
po·ta·tion [poʊˈteɪʃn] n 1. Trinken nt; Schluck m. 2. (alkoholisches) Getränk nt.
po·ta·to blood agar [pəˈteɪtoʊ, -tə] micro. Bordet-Gengou-Agar m/nt, -Medium nt.
potato dextrose agar micro. Kartoffel-Dextrose-Agar m/nt.
potato nose Kartoffel-, Säufer-, Pfund-, Knollennase f, Rhinophym nt, Rhinophyma nt.
potato tumor Glomus-caroticum-Tumor m.
pot·bel·lied [ˈpɑtbeliːd] adj dick-, schmerbäuchig.
pot·bel·ly [ˈpɑtbelɪ] n Dick-, Schmerbauch m.
po·tence [ˈpoʊtəns] n 1. physiol. Potenz f, Potentia coeundi. 2. Wirksamkeit f, Stärke f, Kraft(entfaltung f) f; (a. pharm., chem.) Wirkung f. 3. fig. Stärke f, Macht f.
po·ten·cy [ˈpoʊtənsɪ] n → potence.
po·tent [ˈpoʊtənt] adj 1. physiol. potent. 2. wirksam, stark. 3. fig. mächtig, stark.
po·ten·tial [pəˈtenʃəl] I n 1. phys., chem. Potential nt; electr. Spannung f. 2. Reserven pl, (Kraft-)Vorrat m, Potential nt; Leistungsfähigkeit f. 3. → potentiality. II adj möglich, potentiell, Potential-; phys. potentiell.
potential-dependent adj potentialabhängig.
potential difference phys. Potentialdifferenz f.
potential energy potentielle Energie f.
potential equation mathe. Potentialgleichung f.
potential flow phys. Potentialströmung f.
potential fluctuation Potentialschwankung f.
potential function mathe. Potentialfunktion f.
po·ten·ti·al·i·ty [pəˌtenʃɪˈælətɪ] n (Entwicklungs-)Möglichkeit f, Potentialität f.
po·ten·ti·a·tion [pəˌtentʃəlˈzeɪʃn] n → potentiation.
po·ten·tial·ize [pəˈtentʃəlaɪz] vt → potentiate.
po·ten·ti·ate [pəˈtentʃɪeɪt] vt pharm. steigern, verstärken, wirksam(er) machen, potenzieren.
po·ten·ti·a·tion [pəˌtentʃɪˈeɪʃn] n pharm., phys. Potenzierung f.

po·ten·ti·om·e·ter [pəˌtentʃɪˈɒmɪtər] *n phys.* Potentiometer *nt.*
po·tion [ˈpəʊʃn] *n* (Arznei-, Gift-)Trank *m.*
po·to·ma·nia [ˌpəʊtəˈmeɪnɪə, -jə] *n* 1. Trunksucht *f*, Potomanie *f.* 2. Dilirium tremens.
Pott [pɒt]: **P.'s abscess** Pott'-Abszeß *m.*
P.'s aneurysm Aneurysmaknoten *m.*
P.'s caries → P.'s disease.
P.'s curvature Pott-Buckel *m*, Pott--David-Syndrom *nt.*
P.'s disease Wirbeltuberkulose *f*, Spondylitis tuberculosa.
first degree P.'s fracture Knöchelbruch *m*, -fraktur *f.*
P.'s fracture distale Fibulafraktur *f*, Außenknöchelfraktur *f.*
P.'s gangrene Altersgangrän *f*, senile Gangrän *f.*
P.' operation *HTG* Potts-Operation *f*, -Anastomose *f.*
P.'s paraplegia Pott-Lähmung *f*, -Paraplegie *f.*
P.'s paralysis → P.'s paraplegia.
second degree P.'s fracture bimalleoläre (Knöchel-)Fraktur *f.*
third degree P.'s fracture trimalleoläre (Knöchel-)Fraktur *f.*
P.'s trias Pott-Trias *f.*
Potter [ˈpɒtər]: **P.'s disease/facies** Potter--Syndrom *I nt*, reno-faziale Dysplasie *f.*
P.'s syndrome Potter-Syndrom *nt.*
Potter-Bucky [ˈbʌkɪ]: **P.-B. diaphragm/grid** *radiol.* Bucky-Blende *f*, Streustrahlenraster *nt.*
pouch [paʊtʃ] *n* (*a. anat.*) Beutel *m*, Tasche *f*, (kleiner) Sack *m.*
p. of Douglas Douglas'-Raum *m*, Excavatio rectouterina.
pouched [paʊtʃt] *adj* beutelig, beutel-, sackförmig, Beutel-, Sack-; ausgebuchtet.
pou·drage [puːˈdrɑːʒ] *n French* Einpudern *nt.*
poul·tice [ˈpəʊltɪs] **I** *n* Brei-, Kräuterpackung *f*, -umschlag *m*, Kataplasma *nt.* **II** *vt* mit Breiumschlägen behandeln, einen Breiumschlag auflegen.
poul·try mite [ˈpəʊltrɪ] *micro.* Vogelmilbe *f*, Dermanyssus avium.
pound¹ [paʊnd] **I** *n* Stampfen *nt.* **II** *vt* 1. (zer-)stoßen, (-)stampfen. 2. hämmern, schlagen, (fest-)stampfen. **III** *vi* hämmern, trommeln, schlagen (*on, against* gegen); (*Herz*) pochen.
pound² [paʊnd] *n* 1. *abbr.* **lb** (*Gewicht*) Pfund *nt.* 2. (*Währung*) Pfund *nt.*
pound·er [ˈpaʊndər] *n* (*Mörser*) Stößel *m*, Stößer *m.*
pound·ing pain [ˈpaʊndɪŋ] klopfender Schmerz *m.*
Poupart [puːˈpɑːr]: **P.'s ligament** Leistenband *nt*, Lig. inguinale, Arcus inguinalis.
P. lines Poupart-Linie *f.*
pour plate [pɔːr, pəʊr] *micro.* Gießplatte *f.*
pov·er·ty [ˈpɒvərtɪ] *n* Armut *f*, Mangel *m* (*of, in* an).
p. of movement Bewegungsarmut.
p. in vitamins Vitaminmangel.
poverty line Armutsgrenze *f.*
po·vi·done [ˈpəʊvɪdəʊn] *n* → polyvinylpyrrolidone.
povidone-iodine *n* → polyvinylpyrrolidone-iodine.
Po·was·san encephalitis [ˈpəʊwəsæn] Powassan-Enzephalitis *f.*
Powassan virus *micro.* Powassan-Virus *nt.*
pow·der [ˈpaʊdər] **I** *n* Pulver *nt*, Puder *m*; *pharm.* Pulvis *m*; Staub *m.* **II** *vt* pulverisieren, zu Puder zerkleinern; (be-, über-,

ein-)pudern. **III** *vi* zu Pulver werden, zu Staub zerfallen.
powder burn *forens.* Pulverschmauch *m.*
pow·dered milk [ˈpaʊdərt] Trockenmilch *f*, Milchpulver *nt.*
pow·der·y [ˈpaʊdərɪ] *adj* pulv(e)rig, puderig, Pulver-, Puder-; staubig; gepudert.
pow·er [ˈpaʊər] *n* 1. (*a. phys.*) Kraft *f*, Stärke *f*, Energie *f.* 2. *mathe.* Potenz *f.* 3. *opt.* Vergrößerung(skraft *f*) *f*, (Brenn-)Stärke *f.* 4. Macht *f*, Gewalt *f*, Autorität *f.* 5. (juristische) Vollmacht *f*, Befugnis *f.*
p. of concentration Konzentrationsfähigkeit *f.*
power factor *phys.* Leistungsfaktor *m.*
pow·er·ful [-fəl] *adj* stark, kraftvoll, kräftig, gewaltig; wirkungsvoll; *fig.* einflußreich.
powerful lens *opt.* starke Linse *f.*
powerful solvent starkes Lösungsmittel *nt.*
power function *mathe.* Potenzfunktion *f.*
power generation *electr.* Stromerzeugung *f.*
power loss *phys.* 1. Leistungs-, Energieverlust *m.* 2. Verlustleistung *f.*
power-loss factor *phys.* Verlustfaktor *m.*
power transmission Leistungs-, Kraftübertragung *f.*
pox [pɒks] *n* 1. pockenähnliche Erkrankung *f.* 2. *old* → syphilis.
Pox·vir·i·dae [pɒksˈvɪrɪdiː] *pl micro.* Pockenviren *pl*, Poxviridae *pl.*
pox·vi·rus [pɒksˈvaɪrəs] *n micro.* Pockenvirus *nt*, Poxvirus *nt.*
pox viruses Poxviridae *pl.*
PP *abbr.* 1. → pancreatic polypeptide. 2. → posterior pituitary.
PPA *abbr.* → Pittsburgh pneumonia agent.
PP-cells *n* → pancreatic polypeptide cells.
PPCF *abbr.* → plasmin prothrombin conversion factor.
P.P.D. tuberculin gereinigtes Tuberkulin *nt abbr.* GT, PPD-Tuberkulin *nt.*
P.-P. factor Niacin *nt*, Nikotin-, Nicotinsäure *f.*
PPI *abbr.* → performance pulse index.
P-P interval *card.* PP-Intervall *nt.*
PPLO *abbr.* [pleuropneumonia-like organism] *old* → mycoplasma.
PPL test Penicilloyl-Polylysin-Test *m*, PPL-Test *m.*
ppm. *abbr.* → parts per million.
PPN *abbr.* → parenteral nutrition, peripheral.
PPNG *abbr.* → penicillinase-producing Neisseria gonorrhoeae.
PPRF *abbr.* → reticular formation, paramedian pontine.
P pulmonale *card.* P pulmonale, P dextroatriale, P dextrocardiale.
PPV *abbr.* → positive pressure ventilation.
P-Q interval *card.* PQ-Intervall *nt.*
PQ segment *card.* PQ-Strecke *f*, PQ-Segment *nt.*
PR *abbr.* 1. → partial remission. 2. → pulse rate.
Pr *abbr.* → praseodymium.
PRA *abbr.* → plasma renin activity.
prac·ti·ca·bil·i·ty [ˌpræktɪkəˈbɪlətɪ] *n* 1. Anwendbar-, Brauchbarkeit *f*, Praktikabilität *f.* 2. Aus-, Durchführbarkeit *f.*
prac·ti·ca·ble [ˈpræktɪkəbl] *adj* 1. anwendbar, brauchbar, praktikabel. 2. aus-, durchführbar.
prac·ti·ca·ble·ness [ˈ-nɪs] *n* → practicability.
prac·ti·cal [ˈpræktɪkl] *adj* 1. angewandt, praktisch. 2. praktisch (veranlagt), geschickt. 3. praktisch, nützlich, brauchbar, zweckmäßig, nutzbringend.

practical chemistry angewandte Chemie *f.*
prac·ti·cal·i·ty [ˌpræktɪˈkælətɪ] *n* praktische Anwendung *od.* Veranlagung *f*, das Praktische.
prac·ti·cal·ness [ˈpræktɪklnɪs] *n* → practicality.
prac·tice [ˈpræktɪs] **I** *n* 1. (Arzt-)Praxis *f.* **to be in ~** praktizieren. 2. Übung *f*, Training *nt.* **to be in ~** in Übung sein. **to be out of ~** aus der Übung sein. **to keep in ~** in Übung bleiben. 3. Praxis *f.* **in ~** in der Praxis. **to put in(to) ~** in die Tat umsetzen. 4. *techn.* Verfahren *nt*, Technik *f.* 5. Brauch *m*, (An-)Gewohnheit *f*, Praktik *f.* **it is common ~** es ist allgemein üblich. **II** *vt* 6. (*Arzt*) praktizieren; (*Beruf*) ausüben, tätig sein als *od.* in. 7. (ein-)üben, probieren, proben. 8. jdn. ausbilden. **III** *vi* praktizieren; (s.) üben.
prac·ticed [ˈpræktɪst] *adj* geübt (*in* in); erfahren.
prac·tic·ing [ˈpræktɪsɪŋ] *adj* praktizierend.
prac·ti·tion·er [prækˈtɪʃənər] *n* Praktiker *m.*
prac·to·lol [ˈpræktəlɒl, -ləʊl] *n pharm.* Practolol *n.*
Prader-Willi [ˈprɑːdər ˈwɪlɪ]: **P.-W. syndrome** Prader-Willi-Syndrom *nt*, Prader--Labhart-Willi-Syndrom *nt.*
prae- *pref.* → pre-.
prag·mat·ag·no·sia [ˌprægmætæɡˈnəʊ-ʒ(ɪ)ə, -zɪə] *n neuro.* Pragmatagnosie *f.*
prag·mat·am·ne·si·a [ˌprægmætæmˈniːʒə] *n neuro.* Pragmatamnesie *f.*
prag·mat·ic [præɡˈmætɪk] **I** *n* Pragmatiker(in *f*) *m.* **II** *adj* sachlich, den Tatsachen/Erfahrungen entsprechend, pragmatisch.
prag·ma·tism [ˈprægmətɪzəm] *n* Pragmatismus *m.*
Prague maneuver [prɑːɡ] *gyn.* Prager--Handgriff *m.*
Prague pelvis Wirbelgleitbecken *nt*, spondylisthetisches Becken *nt*, Pelvis spondylolisthetica.
prai·rie itch [ˈpreərɪ] *derm.* Gerstenkrätze *f*, Acarodermatitis urticaroides.
pral·i·dox·ime [ˌprælɪˈdɒksiːm] *n pharm.* Pralidoxim *n.*
pran·di·al [ˈprændɪəl] *adj* Essen *od.* Mahlzeit betr., Essens-, Tisch-.
Pr antigen Pr-Antigen *nt.*
pra·se·o·dym·i·um [ˌpreɪzɪəʊˈdɪmɪəm] *n abbr.* **Pr** Praseodym *nt abbr.* Pr.
PRAS medium *micro.* PRAS-Medium *nt.*
Prausnitz-Küstner [ˈpraʊsnɪts ˈkɪstnər]: **P.-K. antibodies** Prausnitz-Küstner-Antikörper *pl*, PK-Antikörper *pl.*
P.-K. reaction *abbr.* **PKR** Prausnitz--Küstner-Reaktion *f abbr.* PKR.
P.-K. test → P.-K. reaction.
pra·ze·pam [ˈpræzɪpæm] *n pharm.* Prazepam *nt.*
pra·zi·quan·tel [ˌpræzɪˈkwɒntəl] *n pharm.* Praziquantel *nt.*
pra·zo·sin [ˈpræzəsɪn] *n pharm.* Prazosin *nt.*
pre- *pref.* (zeitlich, räumlich) Vor-, Prä-.
preach·er's hand [ˈpriːtʃər] Predigerhand *f.*
pre·ad·o·les·cence [ˌpriːədəˈlesəns] *n* Präadoleszenz *f*, späte Kindheit *f.*
pre·ad·o·les·cent [-ˈlesənt] **I** *n* Jugendliche(r *m*) *f* in der Präadoleszenz. **II** *adj* präadoleszent, Präadoleszenten-, Präadoleszenz-.
pre·al·bu·min [ˌpriːælˈbjuːmən] *n* Präalbumin *nt.*
pre·am·pli·fi·er [priːˈæmplɪfaɪər] *n* Vorverstärker *m.*

preanesthetic medication

pre·an·es·thet·ic medication [ˌpriænəs-'θetɪk] *anes.* Prämedikation *f.*
pre·aor·tic [ˌpriei'ɔːrtɪk] *adj* vor der Aorta (liegend), präaortal.
pre·ar·thrit·ic [ˌpriɑːr'θrɪtɪk] *adj* präarthritisch, präarthrotisch.
pre·au·ric·u·lar [ˌpriɔː'rɪkjələr] *adj* vor der Ohrmuschel (liegend), präaurikulär.
preauricular fistula, congenital kongenitale präaurikuläre Fistel *f*, Fistula auris congenita.
pre·ax·i·al [prɪ'eɪksɪəl] *adj* vor einer Achse (liegend), präaxial.
pre·ax·il·lar·y line [prɪ'æksəˌleriː, -æk'sɪlərɪ] vordere Axillarlinie *f*, Linea axillaris anterior.
pre-B cells Prä-B-Lymphozyten *pl.*
pre·be·ta-lipoprotein [prɪ'beɪtə] *n* Lipoprotein *nt* mit sehr geringer Dichte, very low-density lipoprotein *abbr.* VLDL, prä-β-Lipoprotein *nt.*
pre·be·ta·lip·o·pro·tein·e·mia [prɪˌbiːtəˌlɪpəˌprəʊtɪ'niːmɪə] *n* Erhöhung *f* der Präbetalipoproteine im Blut, Hyperpräbetalipoproteinämie *f.*
pre·bi·ot·ic [ˌprɪbaɪ'ɑtɪk] *adj* bio. präbiotisch.
prebiotic evolution *bio.* präbiotische Evolution *f.*
pre·blad·der [prɪ'blædər] *n urol.* Vorblase *f.*
pre·can·cer [prɪ'kænsər] *n patho.* Präkanzerose *f*, prämaligne Läsion *f.*
pre·can·cer·o·sis [ˌprɪkænsə'rəʊsɪs] *n* → precancer.
pre·can·cer·ous [prɪ'kænsərəs] *adj* präkanzerös, präkarzinomatös, prämaligne.
precancerous condition → precancer.
precancerous dermatitis Bowen-Krankheit, -Dermatose *f*, Morbus Bowen *m*, Dyskeratosis maligna.
precancerous dermatosis präkanzeröse Hautveränderung *f.*
precancerous melanosis of Dubreuilh Dubreuilh-Krankheit *f*, -Erkrankung *f*, Dubreuilh-Hutchinson-Krankheit *f*, -Erkrankung *f*, prämaligne Melanose *f*, melanotische Präkanzerose *f*, Lentigo maligna, Melanosis circumscripta praeblastomatosa/praecancerosa (Dubreuilh).
pre·cap·il·lar·y [prɪ'kæpəˌleriː, -kə'pɪlərɪ] I *n* Präkapillare *f*, End-, Metarteriole *f.* II *adj* präkapillar, präkapillär.
precapillary anastomosis *anat.* präkapilläre Anastomose *f.*
precapillary artery kleine Arterie *f*, Arteriole *f*, Arteriola *f.*
precapillary sphincter präkapillärer Sphincter *m.*
pre·car·ci·no·ma·tous [prɪˌkɑːrsɪ'nəʊmətəs] *adj* → precancerous.
pre·car·di·ac [prɪ'kɑːrdɪæk] *adj* vor dem Herzen (liegend), präkardial, präkordial, Präkordial-.
pre·car·di·um [prɪ'kɑːrdɪəm] *n* → precordium.
pre·car·i·ous [prɪ'keərɪəs] *adj* 1. unsicher, bedenklich, prekär. 2. riskant, gefährlich.
pre·car·i·ous·ness [prɪ'keərɪəsnɪs] *n* Unsicherkeit *f*; Gefährlichkeit *f.*
pre·car·ti·lage [prɪ'kɑːrtlɪdʒ] *n embryo.* Vorknorpel *m.*
pre·car·ti·lag·i·nous [prɪˌkɑːrtɪ'lædʒənəs] *adj embryo.* aus Vorknorpel bestehend, präkartilaginär.
pre·cau·tion [prɪ'kɔːʃn] *n* Vorsicht *f*; Vorsichtsmaßnahme *f*, -regel *f*, (Sicherheits-)Vorkehrung *f.* **as a ~** vorsorglich, vorsichtshalber. **to take ~s** Vorsorge treffen.
pre·cau·tion·ar·y [prɪ'kɔːʃəˌnerɪ] *adj* vorbeugend, Sicherheits-, Vorsichts-.

pre·ca·va [prɪ'keɪvə] *n* obere Hohlvene *f*, V. cava superior.
pre·ca·val [prɪ'keɪvl] *adj* präkaval.
pre·ce·cal [prɪ'siːkl] *adj* präzäkal.
pre·cen·tral [prɪ'sentrəl] *adj* präzentral.
precentral area → precentral cortex.
precentral artery A. sulci pr(a)ecentalis.
precentral cortex präzentrale Rinde *f*, präzentraler Kortex *m*, Rinde *f* des Gyrus pr(a)ecentralis.
precentral fissure Sulcus pr(a)ecentralis.
precentral gyrus Gyrus pr(a)ecentralis.
precentral region Präzentralregion *f.*
precentral sulcus Sulcus pr(a)ecentralis.
precentral vein (of cerebellum) Präzentralvene *f*, V. pr(a)ecentralis (cerebelli).
pre·chi·as·mat·ic [prɪˌkaɪæz'mætɪk] *adj* vor dem Chiasma opticum (liegend), prächiasmatisch, prächiasmal.
prechiasmatic sulcus Chiasma opticus-Rinne *f*, Sulcus pr(a)echiasmatis/pr(a)echiasmaticus.
pre·chord·al plate [prɪ'kɔːrdl] Prächordalplatte *f.*
pre·cip·i·ta·bil·i·ty [prɪˌsɪpɪtæ'bɪlətɪ] *n* Ausfällbarkeit *f*, Präzipitationsfähigkeit *f.*
pre·cip·i·ta·ble [prɪ'sɪpɪtəbl] *adj* niederschlagbar, (aus-)fällbar, abscheidbar, präzipitierbar.
pre·cip·i·tant [prɪ'sɪpɪtənt] *chem.* I *n* Fällmittel *nt*, (Aus-)Fällungsagens *nt*. II *adj* s. als Niederschlag absetzend.
pre·cip·i·tate [*n, adj* prɪ'sɪpɪtət, -teɪt; *v* -teɪt] I *n chem.* Präzipitat *nt*, Niederschlag *m*, Kondensat *nt.* II *adj fig.* kopfüber, hastig, (über-)eilig, überstürzt, jäh, plötzlich. III *vt* 1. *fig.* herbeiführen, beschleunigen, heraufbeschwören. 2. *chem.* (aus-)fällen, niederschlagen, präzipitieren. IV *vi chem.* ausfällen, s. niederschlagen.
precipitate labor überstürzte Geburt *f*, Partus praecipitatus.
pre·cip·i·tat·ing antibody [prɪ'sɪpɪteɪtɪŋ] → precipitin.
pre·cip·i·ta·tion [prɪˌsɪpɪ'teɪʃn] *n* 1. *chem.* (Aus-)Fällung *f*, Ausflockung *f*, Präzipitation *f*; Ausfallen *nt*, Präzipitieren *nt.* 2. *fig.* Hast *f*, Eile *f*, Überstürzung *f.*
pre·cip·i·ta·tive [prɪ'sɪpɪteɪtɪv] *adj* ausfällend, präzipitierend.
pre·cip·i·ta·tor [prɪ'sɪpɪteɪtər] *n* 1. → precipitant I. 2. Ausfällapparat *m.*
pre·cip·i·tin [prɪ'sɪpɪtɪn] *n* Präzipitin *nt.*
pre·cip·i·tin·o·gen [prɪˌsɪpə'tɪnədʒən] *n* Präzipitinogen *nt.*
precipitin test Präzipitationstest *m.*
pre·cip·i·to·gen [prɪ'sɪpɪtəʊdʒən] *n* → precipitinogen.
pre·cise [prɪ'saɪs] *adj* genau, exakt, präzis(e).
pre·cise·ness [prɪ'saɪsnɪs] *n* Genauigkeit *f*, Exaktheit *f.*
pre·ci·sion [prɪ'sɪʒn] I *n* Präzision *f*, Genauigkeit *f*, Exaktheit *f.* II *adj* Präzisions-, Fein-.
precision adjustment Feineinstellung *f.*
precision balance Präzisions-, Feinwaage *f.*
precision instrument Präzisionsinstrument *nt.*
precision mechanics Feinmechanik *f.*
precision tool Präzisionswerkzeug *nt.*
precision work Präzisionsarbeit *f.*
pre·clin·i·cal [prɪ'klɪnɪkl] I *n inf.* Vorklinik *f*, vorklinischer Studienabschnitt *m.* II *adj* präklinisch, vorklinisch.
preclinical diabetes Prädiabetes *m.*
pre·co·cious [prɪ'kəʊʃəs] *adj* 1. vorzeitig, verfrüht, früh. 2. frühreif vorzeitig *od.* frühzeitig (entwickelt).

precocious dentition vorzeitige Zahnung/Dentition *f*, Dentitio praecox.
pre·co·cious·ness [prɪ'kəʊʃəsnɪs] *n* → precocity.
precocious pseudopuberty Pseudopubertas praecox.
precocious puberty Pubertas praecox.
pre·coc·i·ty [prɪ'kɑsətɪ] *n* 1. Vor-, Frühzeitigkeit *f.* 2. (*Person*) Frühreife *f.*
pre·cog·ni·tion [ˌprɪkɑg'nɪʃn] *n* Hellsehen *nt*, Präkognition *f.*
pre·col·la·ge·nous [prɪkə'lædʒənəs] *adj* präkollagenös.
pre·co·ma [prɪ'kəʊmə] *n* drohendes Koma *nt*, Präkoma *nt*, Praecoma *nt.*
pre·com·mis·su·ral fornix [prɪkə'mɪʃərəl, -ˌkəmə'ʃʊərəl] → precommissural part of fornix.
precommissural part of fornix präkommissuraler Teil *m* des Fornix, Fornix cerebri.
precommissural septum Septum pr(a)ecommissurale.
pre·com·mu·ni·cal part [prɪkə'mjuːnɪkl]: **p. of anterior cerebral artery** Pars pr(a)ecommunicalis a. cerebri anterioris. **p. of posterior cerebral artery** Pars pr(a)ecommunicalis a. cerebri posterioris.
pre·con·di·tion [prɪkən'dɪʃn] I *n* Vorbedingung *f*, Voraussetzung *f.* **on ~ that** unter der Voraussetzung, daß. II *vt* (*Material etc.*) vorbehandeln.
pre·con·scious [prɪ'kɑnʃəs] *psycho.* I *n* the ~ das Vorbewußte. II *adj* vorbewußt.
pre·con·vul·sive [prɪkən'vʌlsɪv] *adj* präkonvulsiv.
pre·cor·dia *pl* → precordium.
pre·cor·dial [prɪ'kɔːrdɪəl] *adj* 1. → precardiac. 2. Praecordium betr., präkordial, Präkordial-.
pre·cor·di·al·gia [ˌprɪkɔːrdɪ'ældʒ(ɪ)ə] *n* Präkordialschmerz *m.*
precordial lead *physiol. (EKG)* Brustwandableitung *f.* **Wilson's p.s** Brustwandableitungen *pl* nach Wilson.
pre·cor·di·um [prɪ'kɔːrdɪəm] *n, pl* **-dia** [-dɪə] Praecordium *nt*, Präkordialregion *f.*
pre·cor·nu [prɪ'kɔːrn(j)uː] *n* Vorderhorn *nt* des Seitenventrikels, Cornu frontale/anterius.
pre·cos·tal [prɪ'kɑstl, -'kɔstl] *adj* vor den Rippen (liegend), präkostal.
pre·cu·ne·al artery [prɪ'kjuːnɪəl] A. pr(a)ecunealis.
pre·cu·ne·ate [prɪ'kjuːnɪɪt, -nɪeɪt] *adj* Präcuneus betr.
pre·cu·ne·us [prɪ'kjuːnɪəs] *n* Präcuneus *m*, Pr(a)ecuneus *m.*
pre·cur·sive [prɪ'kɜrsɪv] *adj* → precursory.
pre·cur·sor [prɪ'kɜrsər] *n* (erstes) Anzeichen *nt*, Vorzeichen *nt*, Vorbote *nt*; *bio., chem.* Vorläufer *m*, Vorstufe *f*, Präkursor *m.*
precursor cell Vorläuferzelle *f.*
pre·cur·so·ry [prɪ'kɜrsərɪ] *adj* 1. vorhergehend, voraus-. 2. einleitend, vorbereitend.
precursory cartilage Vorläuferknorpel *m*, verknöcherter Knorpel *m.*
precursory symptom Frühsymptom *nt.*
pre·cyst [prɪ'sɪst] *n* Präzyste *f.*
pre·den·tin [prɪ'dentn, -tɪn] *n* unverkalkte Dentinmatrix *f*, Prädentin *nt*, Odontoid *nt.*
pre·di·a·be·tes [prɪˌdaɪə'biːtəs] *n* Prädiabetes *m.*
pre·di·as·to·le [ˌprɪdaɪ'æstəlɪ] *n* Prädiastole *f.*
pre·di·a·stol·ic [prɪˌdaɪə'stɑlɪk] *adj* vor der Diastole, prädiastolisch.

prediastolic murmur *card.* prädiastolisches (Herz-)Geräusch *nt.*
pre·di·crot·ic [ˌprɪdaɪˈkrɑtɪk] *adj card.* prädikrot.
pre·di·gest [ˌprɪdɪˈdʒest, -daɪ-] *vt* vorverdauen.
pre·di·ges·tion [ˌprɪdɪˈdʒestʃn, -daɪ-] *n* Vorverdauung *f.*
pre·dis·po·si·tion [prɪˌdɪspəˈzɪʃn] *n* Veranlagung *f*, Neigung *f*, Empfänglichkeit *f*, Anfälligkeit *f.*
pred·ni·mus·tine [ˌprednəˈmʌstiːn] *n pharm.* Prednimustin *nt.*
pred·nis·o·lone [predˈnɪsələʊn] *n pharm.* Prednisolon *nt.*
pred·ni·sone [ˈprednɪsəʊn] *n pharm.* Prednison *nt.*
pred·nyl·i·dene [priːdˈnɪlədiːn] *n pharm.* Prednyliden *nt.*
pre·dor·mi·tal [prɪˈdɔːrmɪtæl] *adj* Prädormitium betr.
pre·dor·mi·tum [prɪˈdɔːrmɪtəm] *n* Prädormitium *nt.*
pre·duc·tal [prɪˈdʌktəl] *adj* präduktal.
pre·ec·lamp·sia [prɪɪˈklæmpsɪə] *n* **1.** Präeklampsie *f.* **2.** EPH-Gestose *f.*
pre·ec·lamp·tic toxemia [prɪɪˈklæmptɪk] → preeclampsia.
pre·ep·i·glot·ic [prɪˌepɪˈɡlɑtɪk] *adj* vor der Epiglottis (liegend), präepiglottisch.
pre·e·rup·tive [prɪˈrʌptɪv] *adj* präeruptiv.
preeruptive phase präeruptive Phase *f.*
pre·e·ryth·ro·cyt·ic cycle/phase [prɪɪˌrɪθrəˈsɪtɪk] *micro.* präerythrozytärer Zyklus *m*, präerythrozytäre Phase *f.*
pre·ex·ci·ta·tion [prɪˌeksaɪˈteɪʃn] *n card.* **1.** Präexzitation *f.* **2.** → preexcitation syndrome.
preexcitation syndrome WPW-Syndrom *nt*, Wolff-Parkinson-White-Syndrom *nt.*
pre·ex·po·sure prophylaxis [prɪɪkˈspəʊʒər] präexpositionelle Prophylaxe *f*, Präexpositionsprophylaxe *f.*
pre·fol·li·cle cells [prɪˈfɑlɪkl] → prefollicular cells.
pre·fol·lic·u·lar cells [prɪfəˈlɪkjələr] präfollikuläre Zellen *pl*, primitive Granulosazellen *pl.*
pre·fron·tal area [prɪˈfrʌntl] präfrontale Rinde *f*, präfrontaler Kortex *m*, Präfrontalkortex *m.*
prefrontal bone Pars nasalis (ossis frontalis).
prefrontal cortex → prefrontal area.
prefrontal lobotomy *neurochir.* Leukotomie *f*, Lobotomie *f.*
prefrontal veins Stirnpolvenen *pl*, Vv. pr(a)efrontales.
pre·gan·gli·on·ic [prɪˌɡæŋɡlɪˈɑnɪk] *adj* vor einem Ganglion (liegend), präganglionär.
preganglionic fibers → preganglionic neurofibers.
preganglionic neurofibers präganglionäre Nervenfasern *pl*, Neurofibrae pr(a)eganglionares.
preganglionic neuron präganglionäres Neuron *nt.*
pre·gen·i·tal [prɪˈdʒenɪtl] *adj psycho.*, *psychia.* prägenital.
pregenital phase *psychia.* prägenitale Phase *f.*
pre·germ layer stage [ˈprɪdʒɜrm] *embryo.* Vorkeimblattperiode *f.*
pre·glo·mer·u·lar arteriole [ˌprɪɡləʊˈmerjələr, -ɡlə-] zuführende Glomerulusarterie/-arteriole *f*, Arteriola glomerularis afferens, Vas afferens (glomeruli).
preg·nan·cy [ˈpreɡnənsɪ] *n*, *pl* **-cies** Schwangerschaft *f*, Gravidität *f*, Graviditas *f.*
pregnancy cells (*Hypophyse*) Schwangerschaftszellen *pl.*

pregnancy diabetes Gestationsdiabetes *m.*
pregnancy gingivitis Schwangerschaftsgingivitis *f*, Gingivitis gravidarum.
pregnancy luteoma Luteoma gravidarum.
pregnancy osteomalacia Schwangerschafts-, Graviditätsosteomalazie *f.*
pregnancy rhinitis Schwangerschaftsrhinopathie *f.*
pregnancy test Schwangerschaftstest *m.*
preg·nane [ˈpreɡneɪn] *n* Pregnan *nt.*
preg·nane·di·ol [ˌpreɡneɪnˈdaɪɒl, -ɑl] *n* Pregnandiol *nt.*
preg·nane·tri·ol [ˌ-ˈtraɪɒl, -ɑl] *n* Pregnantriol *nt.*
preg·nant [ˈpreɡnənt] *adj* schwanger, in anderen Umständen, Schwangerschafts-, Graviditäts-.
preg·nen·o·lone [preɡˈniːnələʊn] *n* Pregnenolon *nt.*
pre·hal·lux [prɪˈhæləks] *n ortho.* Prähallux *m.*
pre·hen·sion [prɪˈhenʃn] *n* **1.** (Er-)Greifen *nt*, Fassen *nt*, Aufnehmen *nt*, Aufheben *nt.* **2.** *fig.* Begreifen *nt*, Erfassen *nt*, Verstehen *nt.*
pre·he·pat·ic [ˌprɪhɪˈpætɪk] *adj* vor der Leber (liegend), prähepatisch, antehepatisch.
prehepatic cholestasis prähepatische Gallestauung/Cholestase *f.*
prehepatic jaundice prähepatischer/antehepatischer Ikterus *m.*
Prehn [priːn, preɪn]: **P.'s sign** Prehn-Zeichen *nt.*
pre·in·farc·tion angina [ˌprɪɪnˈfɑːrkʃn] Status anginosus.
preinfarction syndrome Präinfarkt(-Syndrom *nt*) *m.*
pre·in·su·lar gyri [prɪˈɪns(j)ələr] kurze Inselwindungen *pl*, Gyri breves insulae.
pre·in·va·sive [ˌprɪɪnˈveɪzɪv] *adj patho.* präinvasiv.
preinvasive carcinoma Oberflächenkarzinom *nt*, präinvasives/intraepitheliales Karzinom *nt*, Carcinoma in situ *abbr.* CIA.
Preiser [ˈpraɪzər]: **P.'s disease** Preiser'-Krankheit *f.*
Preisz-Nocard [praɪz nəʊˈkɑːrd]: **P.-N. bacillus** Preisz-Nocard-Bazillus *m*, Corynebacterium pseudotuberculosis.
pre·kal·li·kre·in [prɪˌkæləˈkriːɪn] *n* Präkallikrein *n*, Fletscher-Faktor *m.*
pre·lam·i·nar part of optic nerve [prɪˈlæmɪnər] laminärer Abschnitt *m* des N. opticus, Pars pr(a)elaminaris n. optici.
pre·lar·val stage [prɪˈlɑːrvəl] *micro.* Prälarvenstadium *nt.*
pre·la·ryn·ge·al [prɪləˈrɪndʒ(ɪ)əl, ˌlærɪnˈdʒɪəl] *adj* prälaryngeal.
pre·leu·ke·mia [prɪluːˈkiːmɪə] *n hema.* Präleukämie *f*, präleukämisches Syndrom *nt.*
pre·leu·ke·mic [prɪluːˈkiːmɪk] *adj* präleukämisch.
pre·load [ˈprɪləʊd] *n physiol.* Last *f*, Vorbelastung *f*, Preload (*f*).
pre·ma·lig·nant [ˌprɪməˈlɪɡnənt] *adj* präkanzerös, präkarzinomatös, prämaligne.
premalignant fibroepithelial tumor → premalignant fibroepithelioma.
premalignant fibroepithelioma Pinkus-Tumor *m*, prämalignes Fibroepitheliom *nt*, fibroepithelialer Tumor (Pinkus) *m*, Fibroepithelioma Pinkus.
pre·ma·mil·lar·y nucleus [prɪˈmæməˌlerɪː, -ˈmæmɪləˌrɪ] Nc. pr(a)emamillaris.
pre·mam·ma·ry abscess [prɪˈmæmərɪ] präglandulärer Brustabszeß *m.*
pre·ma·ture [ˌprɪməˈtʃʊər, -ˈt(j)ʊər; *Brit.* ˈpre-] **I** *n* Frühgeborene *nt*, Frühgeburt *f*, Frühchen *nt.* **II** *adj* **1.** früh-, vorzeitig, verfrüht. **2.** frühreif, nicht ausgereift, prämatur.
premature alopecia Alopecia praematura.
premature atrial beat → premature atrial contraction.
premature atrial contraction *abbr.* **PAC** *card.* Vorhofextrasystole *f*, atriale Extrasystole *f.*
premature atrial systole → premature atrial contraction.
premature beat → premature contraction.
premature birth Frühgeburt *f.*
premature child Frühgeborene *nt*, Frühgeburt *f*, Frühchen *nt.*
premature contraction *card.* Extrasystole *f abbr.* **ES**, vorzeitige Herz(muskel)kontraktion *f.*
premature death frühzeitiger Tod *m.*
premature delivery *gyn.* Frühgeburt *f*, Entbindung *f* einer Frühgeburt.
premature dentition Dentes natales/connatales.
premature detachment of the placenta *gyn.* vorzeitige Plazentalösung *f*, Ablatio placentae.
premature infant → premature child.
premature labor vorzeitige Geburt *f*, Frühgeburt *f.*
pre·ma·ture·ness [ˌprɪməˈtʃʊərnɪs, -ˈt(j)ʊər-; *Brit.* ˈpre-] *n* → prematurity.
premature senility syndrome → progeria.
premature systole → premature contraction.
premature ventricular beat → premature ventricular contraction.
premature ventricular contraction *abbr.* **PVC** *card.* Kammerextrasystole *f*, ventrikuläre Extrasystole *f.*
premature ventricular systole → premature ventricular contraction.
pre·ma·tu·ri·ty [ˌprɪməˈtʃʊərətɪ, -ˈt(j)ʊər-; *Brit.* ˈpre-] *n* **1.** Früh-, Vorzeitigkeit *f.* **2.** Frühreife *f*, Prämaturität *f.*
pre·max·il·la [ˌprɪmækˈsɪlə] *n embryo.* Prämaxilla *f.*
pre·max·il·lar·y [prɪˈmæksəlerɪː, -mækˈsɪlərɪ] **I** *n* Zwischenkiefer *m*, Os incisivum. **II** *adj* prämaxillär.
premaxillary bone Prämaxilla *f.*
pre·med·i·ca·tion [ˌprɪmedɪˈkeɪʃn] *n anes.* Prämedikation *f.*
pre·mei·ot·ic [ˌprɪmaɪˈɑtɪk] *adj* vor der Meiose, prämeiotisch.
premeiotic phase prämeiotische Phase *f.*
pre·men·o·pau·sal [prɪˌmenəˈpɔːzl] *adj* vor der Menopause, prämenopausal, präklimakterisch.
pre·men·stru·al [prɪˈmenstr(u)əl, -strəwəl] *adj* vor der Menstruation, prämenstruell, prämenstrual.
premenstrual acne prämenstruelle Akne *f.*
premenstrual stage → premenstruum.
premenstrual syndrome *abbr.* **PMS** prämenstruelles (Spannungs-)Syndrom *nt abbr.* **PMS.**
premenstrual tension *abbr.* **PMT** → premenstrual syndrome.
premenstrual tension syndrome → premenstrual syndrome.
pre·men·stru·um [prɪˈmenstr(u)əm, -strəwəm] *n*, *pl* **-stru·ums**, **-stru·a** [-str(u)ə, -strəwə] Prämenstrualstadium *nt*, -phase *f*, Prämenstruum *nt.*
pre·mi·tot·ic [ˌprɪmaɪˈtɑtɪk] *adj* vor der Mitose (ablaufend), prämitotisch.
pre·mo·lar [prɪˈməʊlər] **I** *n* vorderer/kleiner Backenzahn *m*, Prämolar(zahn *m*) *m*, Dens praemolaris. **II** *adj* prämolar.

premolar tooth

premolar tooth → premolar I.
pre·mo·ni·tion [ˌprɪməˈnɪʃn, ˌpremə-] n 1. (Vor-)Warnung f. 2. (Vor-)Ahnung f, (Vor-)Gefühl nt.
pre·mon·i·to·ry [prɪˈmɑnɪtɔːriː, -təʊ-] adj (vor-)warnend, prämonitorisch.
premonitory symptom Frühsymptom nt.
pre·mon·o·cyte [prɪˈmɑnəsaɪt] n → promonocyte.
pre·mor·bid [prɪˈmɔːrbɪd] adj prämorbid.
pre·mor·tal [prɪˈmɔːrtl] adj vor dem Tod, prämortal.
pre·mo·tor area [prɪˈməʊtər] → premotor cortex.
premotor cortex abbr. **PMC** prämotorische Rinde f, prämotorischer Kortex m.
premotor positivity physiol. prämotorische Positivität f.
premotor region prämotorische Rindenregion f.
pre·mu·cin [prɪˈmjuːsɪn] n Prämuzin nt.
pre·mu·ni·tion [ˌprəmjuːˈnɪʃn] n immun. begleitende Immunität f, Prämunität f, Prämmunität f, Prämunition f.
pre·my·e·lo·blast [prɪˈmaɪələblæst] n hema. Prämyeloblast m.
pre·my·e·lo·cyte [prɪˈmaɪələsaɪt] n hema. Promyelozyt m.
pre·nar·co·sis [ˌprɪnɑːrˈkəʊsɪs] n Pränarkose f.
pre·nar·cot·ic [ˌprɪnɑːrˈkɑtɪk] adj pränarkotisch.
pre·na·tal [prɪˈneɪtl] adj vor der Geburt, vorgeburtlich, pränatal.
prenatal care Schwangerschaftsvorsorge f.
prenatal clinic Schwangerenberatungsstelle f.
prenatal dislocation of hip ortho., embryo. teratologische/pränatale Hüftgelenk(s)dislokation f.
prenatal examination Mutterschaftsvorsorgeuntersuchung f.
prenatal exercises Schwangerschaftsgymnastik f.
prenatal hemopoiesis pränatale Blutbildung/Hämopoese f.
prenatal life Pränatalperiode f.
PR enzyme Phosphorylasephosphatase f.
pre·oc·cip·i·tal incisure/notch [ˌprɪɑkˈsɪpɪtl] Inc. pr(a)eoccipitalis.
pre-oedipal phase psychia. präödipale Phase f.
pre·op·er·a·tive [prɪˈɑpərətɪv, -ˈɑprə-] adj vor einer Operation, präoperativ.
preoperative irradiation Vorbestrahlung f, präoperative Bestrahlung f.
preoperative radiation → preoperative irradiation.
pre·op·tic [prɪˈɑptɪk] adj vor dem Chiasma opticum (liegend), präoptisch.
preoptic area Area pr(a)e-optica.
preoptic nuclei, lateral and medial Ncc. pr(a)e-optici lateralis et medialis.
preoptic recess Rec. pr(a)e-opticus.
preoptic region → preoptic area.
pre·os·te·o·blast [prɪˈɑstɪəblæst] n Präosteoblast m.
pre·o·tic [prɪˈəʊtɪk, -ˈɑtɪk] adj embryo. präotisch.
pre·ovu·la·to·ry [prɪˈɑvjələtɔːriː, -təʊ-] adj vor der Ovulation (ablaufend), präovulatorisch.
pre·o·vum [prɪˈəʊvəm] n sekundäre Oozyte f.
pre·par·a·lyt·ic [prɪˌpærəˈlɪtɪk] adj präparalytisch.
prep·a·ra·tion [ˌprepəˈreɪʃn] n 1. Vorbereitung f (for für). **in ~ for** als Vorbereitung für. **to make ~s** Vorbereitungen treffen (for für). 2. (a. pharm.) (Zu-)Bereitung f, Herstellung f, Preparation f. 3. pharm.

Präparat nt, (Arznei-)Mittel nt; bio. (mikroskopisches) Präparat nt. 4. Präparieren nt, Haltbarmachen nt, Imprägnieren nt. 5. Bereitschaft f.
preparation phase Vorbereitungsphase f.
pre·par·a·tive [prɪˈpærətɪv] I n Vorbereitung f (for für, auf); vorbereitende Maßnahme f (to zu). II adj → preparatory.
pre·par·a·tor [prɪˈpærətər, -ˈpeər-] n Präparator m.
pre·par·a·to·ry [prɪˈpærətɔːriː, -təʊ-, ˈprepərə-] adj als Vorbereitung dienen (to für, auf, zu); vorbereitend, Vorbereitungs-.
preparatory pathway biochem. vorbereitender Stoffwechselweg m.
pre·pare [prɪˈpeər] I vt 1. (vor-, zu-)bereiten. 2. bearbeiten, anfertigen; präparieren; chem. darstellen; techn. herstellen. 3. jdn. (seelisch) vorbereiten (to do zu tun; for auf). II vi s. vorbereiten (for auf); Vorbereitungen treffen (for für).
pre·pared [prɪˈpeərd] adj 1. vorbereitet, bereit, fertig; (Person) gefaßt, bereit, gewillt (for auf). 2. anat. präpariert, seziert, zerlegt; imprägniert. 3. zubereitet, hergestellt.
pre·par·tal [prɪˈpɑːrtl] adj vor der Entbindung/Geburt, präpartal.
pre·pa·tel·lar [ˌprɪpəˈtelər] adj vor der Kniescheibe/Patella (liegend), präpatellar.
prepatellar bursa vor der Kniescheibe liegender Schleimbeutel m, Bursa pr(a)epatellaris.
  subcutaneous p. Bursa subcutanea pr(a)epatellaris.
  subfascial p. Bursa subfascialis pr(a)epatellaris.
  subtendinous p. Bursa subtendinea pr(a)epatellaris.
prepatellar bursitis ortho. Bursitis pr(a)epatellaris.
pre·pat·ent period [prɪˈpætnt, -ˈpeɪ-] micro. Präpatentperiode f, Präpatenz f.
pre·pep·sin [prɪˈpepsɪn] n → pepsinogen.
pre·per·i·car·di·al [prɪˌperɪˈkɑːrdɪəl] adj präperikardial.
pre·per·i·to·ne·al [ˌprɪperɪtəˈniːəl] adj präperitoneal.
pre·phe·nate dehydratase [prɪˈfiːneɪt, -ˈfen-] Prephensäuredehydratase f.
prephenate dehydrogenase Prephensäuredehydrogenase f.
pre·phe·nic acid [prɪˈfiːnɪk, -ˈfen-] Prephensäure f.
pre·pir·i·form cortex [prɪˈpɪrəfɔːrm] präpiriforme Rinde f, präpiriformer Kortex m.
prepiriform region Regio pr(a)epiriformis.
pre·pon·der·ance [prɪˈpɑndərəns] n Vorherrschaft f, Übergewicht nt, Präponderanz f.
pre·pon·der·an·cy [prɪˈpɑndərənsiː] n → preponderance.
pre·pon·der·ant [prɪˈpɑndərənt] adj vorwiegend, überwiegend, entscheidend.
pre·po·tence [prɪˈpəʊtns] n 1. Vorherrschaft f, Übermacht f, Überlegenheit f. 2. genet. Individualpotenz f, Präpotenz f.
pre·po·ten·cy [prɪˈpəʊtnsiː] n → prepotence.
pre·po·tent [prɪˈpəʊtnt] adj 1. vorherrschend, überlegen, stärker. 2. genet. präpotent.
pre·po·ten·tial [ˌprɪpəˈtenʃl] n physiol. Präpotential nt.
pre·pran·di·al [prɪˈprændɪəl] adj vor der Mahlzeit/Nahrungsaufnahme, präprandial.
pre·pro·hor·mone [ˌprɪprəʊˈhɔːrməʊn] n Präprohormon nt.

pre·pro·phage [prɪˈprəʊfeɪdʒ] n Präprophage m.
pre·pro·pro·tein [ˌprɪprəʊˈprəʊtiːn, -tiːɪn] n Präproprotein nt.
pre·pros·thet·ic [ˌprɪprɑsˈθetɪk] adj chir. präprothetisch.
pre·pro·tein [prɪˈprəʊtiːn, -tiːɪn] n Präprotein nt.
pre·psy·chot·ic schizophrenia [ˌprɪsaɪˈkɑtɪk] latente Schizophrenie f, Borderline-Psychose f, Borderline-Schizophrenie f.
pre·pu·ber·al [prɪˈpjuːbərəl] adj → prepubertal.
pre·pu·ber·tal [prɪˈpjuːbərtəl] adj vor der Pubertät (auftretend), präpubertär, präpuberal, präpubertal.
pre·pu·ber·ty [prɪˈpjuːbərtiː] n Präpubertät f.
pre·pu·bes·cence [ˌprɪpjuːˈbesəns] n → prepuberty.
pre·pu·bes·cent [ˌprɪpjuːˈbesnt] adj → prepubertal.
pre·puce [ˈpriːpjuːs] n 1. bedeckende Hautfalte f, Präputium nt. 2. Vorhaut f, Präputium nt, Praeputium penis.
  p. of clitoris Klitorisvorhaut, Praeputium clitoridis.
  p. of penis → prepuce 2.
pre·pu·tial [prɪˈpjuːʃl] adj Vorhaut/Praeputium betr., präputial, Präputial-, Vorhaut-.
preputial calculus urol. Vorhaut-, Präputialstein m, Postholith m, Balanolith m, Smegmolith m.
preputial concretion → preputial calculus.
preputial glands präputiale (Talg-)Drüsen pl, Präputialdrüsen pl, Gll. pr(a)eputiales.
pre·pu·ti·um [prɪˈpjuːʃ(ɪ)əm] n, pl **-tia** [-ʃ(ɪ)ə] → prepuce.
pre·py·lo·ric [ˌprɪpaɪˈlɔrɪk, -ˈlɑr-] adj vor dem Pylorus (liegend), präpylorisch.
prepyloric ulcer präpylorisches Ulkus nt.
prepyloric vein Pylorusvene f, V. pr(a)epylorica.
pre·re·duced and anaerobically sterilized medium [prɪrɪˈd(j)uːst] → **PRAS medium**.
pre·re·duc·tion phase [ˌprɪrɪˈdʌkʃn] → premeiotic phase.
pre·re·nal [prɪˈriːnl] adj vor der Niere (liegend), prärenal.
prerenal albuminuria prärenale Albuminurie/Proteinurie f.
prerenal anuria prärenale Anurie f.
prerenal azotemia prärenale Azot(h)ämie f.
prerenal proteinuria → prerenal albuminuria.
pre·req·ui·site [prɪˈrekwəzɪt] I n Voraussetzung f, Vorbedingung f (for, to für). II adj vorausssetzend, erforderlich, notwendig (for, to für).
pre·ro·lan·dic sulcus [ˌprɪrəʊˈlændɪk] → precentral sulcus.
pre·ru·bral fields [prɪˈruːbrəl] Forel'-Felder pl.
pre·sa·cral [prɪˈseɪkrəl, -ˈsæk-] adj vor dem Kreuzbein (liegend), präsakral.
presacral anesthesia → presacral block.
presacral block Präsakralanästhesie f, -block(ade) f m.
presacral nerve Plexus hypogastricus superior.
presacral plexus sakraler Venenplexus m, Plexus venosus sacralis.
presby- pref. Alters-, Presby-.
pres·by·a·cou·sia [ˌprezbɪəˈkjuːʒ(ɪ)ə] n → presbycusis.

pres·by·a·cu·sia [ˌ-əˈkjuːʒ(ɪ)ə] *n* → presbycusis.
pres·by·a·cu·sis [ˌ-əˈkjuːsɪs] *n* → presbycusis.
pres·by·at·rics [ˌ-ˈætrɪks] *pl* Alters-, Greisenheilkunde *f*, Geriatrie *f*, Presbyatrie *f*.
pres·by·car·dia [ˌ-ˈkɑːrdɪə] *n card.* Altersherz *nt*, senile Herzkrankheit *f*, Presbykardie *f*.
pres·by·cu·sis [ˌ-ˈkjuːsɪs] *n* Altersschwerhörigkeit *f*, Presbyakusis *f*.
pres·by·e·soph·a·gus [ˌ-ɪˈsɑfəɡəs] *n* Presbyösophagus *m*.
pres·by·ope [ˈ-əʊp] *n* Presbyope(r *m*) *f*.
pres·by·o·phre·nia [ˌ-əˈfriːnɪə] *n* senile Demenz *f*, Altersdemenz *f*, Presbyophrenie *f*.
pres·by·o·pia [ˌ-ˈəʊpɪə] *n* Alterssichtigkeit *f*, Presbyopie *f*.
pres·by·op·ic [ˌ-ˈɑpɪk] *adj* Presbyopie betr., presbyop(isch).
pres·by·phre·nia [ˌ-ˈfriːnɪə] *n* → presbyophrenia.
pres·by·tia [prezˈbɪʃɪə] *n* → presbyopia.
pres·by·tism [ˈprezbətɪzəm] *n* → presbyopia.
pre·school child [ˈprɪskuːl] Kind *nt* im Vorschulalter.
pre·scle·rot·ic [ˌprɪskləˈrɑtɪk] *adj* präsklerotisch.
pre·scribe [prɪˈskraɪb] I *vt* 1. verschreiben, verordnen. ~ sth. for s.o. jdm. etw. verschreiben/verordnen. ~ sth. for sth. jdn. etw. gegen etw. verschreiben. 2. vorschreiben, anordnen. II *vi* etw. verschreiben *od.* verordnen (*to, for*); ein Rezept ausstellen.
pre·scrip·tion [prɪˈskrɪpʃn] *n* 1. Rezept *nt*, Verordnung *f*. 2. verordnete Medizin *f*. 3. Vorschrift *f*, Verordnung *f*.
prescription drug rezeptpflichtiges Medikament *nt*.
prescription only medicine *abbr.* **POM** *Brit.* rezeptpflichtiges Medikament *nt*.
pre·se·cre·tin [ˌprɪsɪˈkriːtɪn] *n* → prosecretin.
pre·se·cre·to·ry [ˌprɪsɪˈkriːtərɪ] *adj* vor der Sekretion/Abgabe, präsekretorisch.
pre·se·nile [prɪˈsɪnaɪl, -nɪl] *adj* vor dem Greisenalter (auftretend), im Präsenium, präsenil.
presenile arteriosclerosis präsenile Arteriosklerose *f*.
presenile cataract präseniler Katarakt *f*.
presenile dementia 1. präsenile Demenz *f*. 2. Alzheimer-Krankheit *f*, präsenile Alzheimer-Demenz *f*, Demenz *f* vom Alzheimer-Typ.
presenile osteoporosis präsenile Osteoporose *f*.
pre·se·nil·i·ty [ˌprɪsɪˈnɪlətɪ] *n* vorzeitige Alterung *f*, Präsenilität *f*.
pre·se·ni·um [prɪˈsiːnɪəm] *n* Präsenium *nt*.
pre·sen·ta·tion [ˌprezn̩ˈteɪʃn] *n* 1. *gyn.* (Frucht-)Einstellung *f*, Praesentatio (fetus) *f*. 2. *immun.* Präsentation *f*.
pres·er·va·tion [ˌprezərˈveɪʃn] *n* Bewahrung *f*, Schutz *m* (*from* vor); Erhaltung *f*, Konservierung *f*.
pre·serv·a·tive [prɪˈzɜrvətɪv] I *n* Konservierungsmittel *nt*. II *adj* 1. schützend, bewahrend, Schutz-. 2. erhaltend, konservierend, Konservierungs-.
pre·serve [prɪˈzɜrv] *vt* 1. bewahren, (be-)schützen (*from* vor). 2. erhalten, konservieren.
pre·si·nu·ous abscess [prɪˈsɪnjəwəs] präsinuöser Abszeß *m*.
pre·so·mite [prɪˈsəʊmaɪt] *adj* Präsomitenstadium betr., Präsomiten-.
presomite embryo Präsomitenembryo *m*.

pre·sper·ma·tid [prɪˈspɜrmətɪd] *n* sekundärer Spermatozyt *m*, Präspermatide *f*.
pre·sphyg·mic [prɪˈsfɪɡmɪk] *adj card.* vor der Pulswelle.
presphygmic interval → presphygmic period.
presphygmic period *card.* isometrische Kontraktionsphase *f*, Phase *f* der isometrischen Anspannung.
pre·spon·dy·lo·lis·the·sis [prɪˌspɑndɪləʊlɪsˈθiːsɪs] *n ortho.* Präspondylolisthese *f*.
pre·squal·ene pyrophosphate [prɪˈskweɪliːn] Präsqualenpyrophosphat *nt*.
presqualene synthase Präsqualensynthase *f*.
pres·som·e·ter [preˈsɑmɪtər] *n* Druckmesser *m*, Manometer *nt*.
pres·so·re·cep·tive [ˌpresəʊrɪˈseptɪv] *adj* presso(re)zeptiv, pressosensorisch.
pres·so·re·cep·tor [ˌ-rɪˈseptər] *n* Presso(re)zeptor *m*, -sensor *m*.
pressoreceptor reflex Karotissinussyndrom *nt*, Charcot-Weiss-Baker-Syndrom *nt*, hyperaktiver Karotissinusreflex *m*.
pres·so·sen·si·tive [ˌ-ˈsensətɪv] *adj* → pressoreceptive.
pres·so·sen·sor [ˌ-ˈsensər, -sɔr] *n* → pressoreceptor.
pres·sure [ˈpreʃər] I *n* 1. *phys.* Druck *m*; *fig.* Druck *m*, Streß *m*, Last *f*; Zwang *m*. **to put/place ~ (up)on s.o.** jdn. unter Druck setzen. **under ~** unter Druck. 2. Drücken *nt*, Pressen *nt*, Druck *m*. **to apply ~ to a part** auf ein Körperteil drücken *od.* Druck ausüben. II *vt* → pressurize.
p. of the respiratory system intraalveolärer/intrapulmonaler Druck.
pressure alopecia mechanische Alopezie *f*, Alopecia mechanica.
pressure atrophy Druckatrophie *f*.
pressure bandage Druck-, Kompressionsverband *m*.
pressure chamber *phys.* Druckkammer *f*.
pressure diverticulum Pulsionsdivertikel *nt*.
pressure dressing Druck-, Kompressionsverband *m*.
pressure enhancement Druckerhöhung *f*, -verstärkung *f*.
pressure equalization Druckausgleich *m*.
pressure gangrene Wundliegen *nt*, Dekubitalulkus *nt*, -geschwür *nt*, Dekubitus *m*, Decubitus *m*.
pressure gradient Druckgradient *m*, -gefälle *nt*.
pressure head *phys.* Staudruck(messer *m*) *m*, Druckgefälle *nt*, -höhe *f*.
pressure-increase phase *physiol.* Druckanstiegsphase *f*, -zeit *f*.
pressure injury Druckverletzung *f*, Barotrauma *nt*.
pressure load Druckbelastung *f*.
pressure necrosis Drucknekrose *f*.
pressure pack Druck-, Kompressionsverband *m*.
pressure paralysis Druck-, Kompressionslähmung *f*.
pressure phosphene Druckphosphen *nt*.
pressure pneumothorax Spannungspneu(mothorax *m*) *m*.
pressure point *neuro.* Druckpunkt *m*.
pressure pulse *physiol.* Druckpuls *m*.
pressure receptor Druck-, Berührungsrezeptor *m*.
pressure reservoir function *physiol.* Windkesselfunktion *f*.
pressure sensation Druckempfindung *f*. **crude p.** grobe Druckempfindung.
pressure sense Druck-, Gewichtssinn *m*, Barästhesie *f*.

pressure sensibility Druckempfindlichkeit *f*, Drucksinn *m*.
pressure-sensitive *adj* druckempfindlich.
pressure sore Wundliegen *nt*, Dekubitus *m*, Decubitus *m*, Dekubitalulkus *nt*, -geschwür *nt*.
pressure spot → pressure point.
pressure syncope vasovagale Synkope *f*.
pressure transducer *techn.* Druckwandler *m*.
pressure transformation *phys.* Druckumwandlung *f*, Drucktransformation *f*.
pressure ulceration Druckulzeration *f*.
pressure urticaria Druckurtikaria *f*, Urticaria mechanica.
pressure valve Druckventil *nt*.
pressure-volume diagram Druck-Volumen-Diagramm *nt*.
pressure-volume work Druck-Volumen--Arbeit *f*.
pressure wave Druckwelle *f*.
pres·sur·ize [ˈpreʃəraɪz] *vt fig., chem., techn.* unter Druck setzen.
pre·ster·nal region [prɪˈstɜrnl] Brustbeingegend *f*, -region *f*, Regio pr(a)esternalis.
pre·ster·num [prɪˈstɜrnəm] *n* Manubrium sterni.
Preston [ˈprestn]: **P. salt** Seignettesalz *nt*, Natrium-Kalium-Tartrat *nt*.
pre·stretch·ing [prɪˈstretʃɪŋ] *n physiol.* Vordehnung *f*.
pre·su·bic·u·lum [prɪsəˈbɪkjələm] *n* Pr(a)esubiculum *nt*.
pre·sume [prɪˈzuːm] *vt* annehmen, vermuten, voraussetzen.
pre·sump·tion [prɪˈzʌmpʃn] *n* 1. Vermutung *f*, Annahme *f*, Präsumtion *f*. 2. Wahrscheinlichkeit *f*.
presumption diagnosis Verdachts-, Wahrscheinlichkeitsdiagnose *f*.
pre·sump·tive [prɪˈzʌmptɪv] *adj* wahrscheinlich, voraussichtlich, vermutlich, präsumtiv.
pre·sur·gi·cal [prɪˈsɜrdʒɪkl] *adj* vor einer Operation, präoperativ.
pre·syn·ap·tic [prɪˈsɪnæptɪk] *adj* vor einer Synapse (liegend), präsynaptisch.
presynaptic facilitation präsynaptische Bahnung *f*.
presynaptic inhibition präsynaptische Hemmung/Inhibition *f*.
presynaptic membrane präsynaptische Membran *f*.
pre·syn·thet·ic [ˌprɪsɪnˈθetɪk] *adj* vor der Synthese, präsynthetisch.
pre·sys·to·le [prɪˈsɪstəlɪ] *n card.* Präsystole *f*.
pre·sys·tol·ic [ˌprɪsɪsˈtɑlɪk] *adj card.* vor der Systole (auftretend), präsystolisch.
presystolic gallop *card.* Atrial-, Aurikular-, Vorhofgalopp(rhythmus *m*) *m*, präsystolischer Galopp(rhythmus *m*) *m*.
presystolic murmur präsystolisches/spät-diastolisches (Herz-)Geräusch *nt*.
presystolic thrill *card.* präsystolisches Schwirren *nt*.
pre·tar·sal [prɪˈtɑrsl] *adj* prätarsal.
pre-T cells prä-T-Lymphozyten *pl*.
pre·tec·tal area [prɪˈtektl] Area pr(a)etectalis.
pretectal nuclei Ncc. pr(a)etectales.
pretectal region → pretectal area.
pre·tec·tum [prɪˈtektəm] *n* → pretectal area.
pre-term infant [ˈprɪtɜrm] Frühgeborene *nt*, Frühgeburt *f*, Frühchen *nt*.
pre·ter·nat·u·ral anus [ˌprɪtərˈnætʃərəl] künstlicher Darmausgang *m*, Kunstafter *m*, Stoma *nt*, Anus praeter (naturalis).
pre·thy·roid [prɪˈθaɪrɔɪd] *adj* vor der Schilddrüse *od.* dem Schildknorpel (liegend), präthyr(e)oidal.

prethyroideal

pre·thy·roi·de·al [ˌpriːθaɪ'rɔɪdɪəl] adj → prethyroid.
pre·thy·roi·de·an [ˌpriːθaɪ'rɔɪdɪən] adj → prethyroid.
pre·tib·i·al [prɪ'tiːbɪəl] adj vor der Tibia (liegend), prätibial.
pretibial bursa Bursa subcutanea tuberositatis tibiae.
pretibial fever Fort-Bragg-Fieber *nt*.
pretibial myxedema prätibiales Myxödem *nt*, Myxoedema circumscriptum tuberosum, Myxoedema praetibiale symmetricum.
pre·tra·che·al [prɪ'treɪkɪəl; *Brit.* -trə'kiːəl] adj vor der Luftröhre/Trachea (liegend), prätracheal.
pretracheal fascia mittlere Halsfaszie *f*, Fascia colli media, Lamina pr(a)etrachealis fasciae cervicalis.
pre·treat [prɪ'triːt] vt vorbehandeln.
pre·treat·ment [prɪ'triːtmənt] *n* Vorbehandlung *f*.
pre·u·re·thral ligament of Waldeyer [ˌpriːjʊə'riːθrəl] Lig. transversum perinei.
prev·a·lence ['prevələns] *n* 1. Vorherrschen *nt*, Überwiegen *nt*, weite Verbreitung *f*. 2. *epidem.* Prävalenz *f*.
prevalence rate Prävalenzrate *f*.
pre·vent [prɪ'vent] vt verhindern, verhüten, vorbeugen.
pre·vent·a·ble [prɪ'ventəbl] adj verhütbar, abwendbar.
pre·vent·a·tive [prɪ'ventətɪv] *n, adj* → preventive.
pre·vent·i·ble [prɪ'ventɪbl] adj → preventable.
pre·ven·tion [prɪ'venʃn] *n* 1. Verhinderung *f*, Verhütung *f*. 2. Vorbeugung *f*, Verhütung *f*, Prävention *f*; Prophylaxe *f*.
pre·ven·tive [prɪ'ventɪv] **I** *n* 1. Vorbeugungs-, Schutzmittel *nt*, Präventivmittel *nt*. 2. Schutz-, Vorsichtsmaßnahme *f*. **II** adj verhütend, vorbeugend, präventiv, Vorbeugungs-, Schutz-; prophylaktisch.
preventive treatment Präventivbehandlung *f*, vorbeugende Behandlung *f*, Prophylaxe *f*.
pre·ver·te·bral [prɪ'vɜrtəbrəl] adj vor der Wirbelsäule *od.* einem Wirbelkörper (liegend), prävertebral.
prevertebral fascia tiefe Halsfaszie *f*, Fascia colli profunda, Lamina pr(a)evertebralis fasciae cervicalis.
prevertebral ganglia prävertebrale Ganglien *pl*.
prevertebral part of vertebral artery prävertebraler Abschnitt *m* der A. vertebralis, Pars pr(a)evertebralis (a. vertebralis).
prevertebral space Holzknecht-Raum *m*, Retrokardialraum *m*.
pre·ves·i·cal [prɪ'vesɪkl] adj vor der Harnblase (liegend), prävesikal.
prevesical space Retzius'-Raum *m*, Spatium retropubicum.
pre·ve·sic·u·lar [ˌpriːvə'sɪkjələr] adj prävesikal.
pre·vil·lous chorion [prɪ'vɪləs] *gyn.* primitives Chorion *nt*.
pre·zone ['priːzəʊn] *n* → prozone.
pre·zy·got·ic [ˌpriːzaɪ'gɒtɪk] adj vor der Befruchtung, präzygot.
PRF *abbr.* → prolactin releasing factor.
PRH *abbr.* [prolactin releasing hormone] → prolactin releasing factor.
pri·a·pism ['praɪəpɪzəm] *n* Priapismus *m*.
pri·a·pi·tis [ˌpraɪə'paɪtɪs] *n andro.* Penisentzündung *f*, Penitis *f*.
pri·a·pus ['praɪeɪpəs] *n* → penis.
Price-Jones [praɪs dʒəʊnz]: **P.-J. curve/ method** *hema.* Price-Jones-Kurve *f*.
prick [prɪk] **I** *n* 1. (Insekten-, Nadel-)Stich *m*. 2. Stechen *nt*, stechender Schmerz *m*. 3. (*a. fig.*) Dorn *m*, Stachel *m*. **II** vt (ein-, auf-, durch-)stechen; punktieren. **to ~ one's finger** s. in den Finger stechen. **III** vi stechen, schmerzen.
prick·ing ['prɪkɪŋ] *n* (*Schmerz*) Stechen *nt*.
prick·le ['prɪkl] **I** *n* 1. Stachel *m*, Dorn *m*. 2. Stechen *nt*, Jucken *nt*, Kribbeln *nt*, Prickeln *nt*. **II** vi stechen, jucken, kribbeln.
prickle cell (*Haut*) Stachelzelle *f*.
prickle cell carcinoma Plattenepithelkarzinom *nt*, Ca. planocellulare/platycellulare.
prickle cell layer Stachelzellschicht *f*, Stratum spinosum epidermidis.
prick·ly ['prɪklɪ] adj 1. dornig, stachlig. 2. juckend, stechend, prickelnd.
prickly heat *derm.* Roter Hund *m*, tropische Flechte *f*, Miliaria rubra.
prick test *derm.* Prick-, Stichtest *m*.
Priesel ['priːzl]: **P. tumor** Priesel-Tumor *m*, Loeffler-Priesel-Tumor *m*, Thekom *nt*, Thekazelltumor *m*, Fibroma thecacellulare xanthomatosum.
pril·o·caine ['prɪləʊkeɪn] *n anes.* Prilocain *nt*.
pri·ma·cy ['praɪməsɪ] *n* Primat *nt*.
pri·ma·quine ['praɪməkwiːn, 'prɪmə-] *n pharm.* Primaquin *nt*.
primaquine sensitive anemia Anämie *f* durch Glukose-6-phosphatdehydrogenasemangel.
pri·ma·ry ['praɪˌmerɪ, -mərɪ] adj 1. wichtigste(r, s), wesentlich, primär, Haupt-; elementar, Grund-. 2. erste(r, s), ursprünglich, Ur-, Erst-, Anfangs-. 3. *chem.* primär, Primär-.
primary adhesion → primary healing.
primary afferent depolarization *abbr.* **PAD** *physiol.* primäre afferente Depolarisation *f abbr.* PAD.
primary alcohol primärer Alkohol *m*.
primary amebic meningoencephalitis *abbr.* **PAM** primäre Amöben-Meningoenzephalitis *f abbr.* PAM.
primary amenorrhea *gyn.* primäre Amenorrhoe *f*.
primary amine primäres Amin *nt*.
primary amyloidosis primäre/idiopathische (System-)Amyloidose *f*, Paramyloidose *f*.
primary anemia essentielle/primäre/idiopathische Anämie *f*.
primary assimilation *biochem.* Chylusbildung *f*, primäre Fettassimilation *f*.
primary atelectasis (*Lunge*) primäre Atelektase *f*.
primary attic cholesteatoma *HNO* primäres Kuppelraumcholesteatom *nt*, Flaccidacholesteatom *nt*.
primary atypical pneumonia atypische/primär-atypische Pneumonie *f*.
primary bronchus Primär-, Haupt-, Stammbronchus *m*, Bronchus principalis.
primary bubo primärer Bubo *m*, Bubon d'emblée.
primary bundle (*Muskel*) Primärbündel *nt*.
primary carcinoma primäres Karzinom *nt*.
p. of liver cells (primäres) Leberzellkarzinom, hepatozelluläres Karzinom, malignes Hepatom *nt*, Ca hepatocellulare.
p. of lung primäres Lungenkarzinom, primärer Lungenkrebs *m*.
primary cardiomyopathy primäre/idiopathische Kardiomyopathie *f*.
primary coccidioidomycosis Wüsten-, Talfieber *nt*, San Joaquin-Valley-Fieber *nt*, Primärform *f* der Kokzidioidomykose.

primary color Primär-, Grundfarbe *f*.
primary complex *pulmo.* Ghon'-Primärkomplex *m*, -Herd *m*.
primary component → primary ingredient.
primary constriction Zentromer *nt*, Kinetochor *nt*.
primary contact *immun.* Primärkontakt *m*.
primary culture Primärkultur *f*.
primary dentition Milchzähne *pl*, -gebiß *nt*, Dentes decidui.
primary disease *abbr.* **PD** Grundleiden *nt abbr.* GL, Primärerkrankung *f*.
primary drinking *psychia.* primäres Trinken *nt*.
primary dysmenorrhea *gyn.* primäre/essentielle Dysmenorrhö *f*.
primary epitympanic cholesteatoma → primary attic cholesteatoma.
primary extrapulmonary coccidioidomycosis primär-extrapulmonale Kokzidioidomykose *f*.
primary familial xanthomatosis Wolman--Krankheit *f*.
primary fissure Fissura prima (cerebelli).
p. of lung schräger Interlobärspalt *m*, Fissura obliqua (pulmonis).
primary follicles 1. *gyn.* Primärfollikel *pl*, Folliculi ovarici primarii. 2. (*Lymphknoten*) Primärfollikel *pl*.
primary gain *psycho.* primärer Krankheitsgewinn *m*.
primary generalized epilepsy generalisierte Epilepsie *f*.
primary glaucoma primäres Glaukom *nt*.
primary gout primäre Gicht *f*.
primary group *socio.* Primärgruppe *f*.
primary healing Primärheilung *f*, primäre Wundheilung *f*, Heilung per primam intentionem, p.p.-Heilung *f*.
primary hematuria primäre Hämaturie *f*.
primary host *micro.* Endwirt *m*.
primary hydrocephalus kongenitaler/primärer Hydrozephalus *m*, Hydrocephalus congenitalis.
primary hyperaldosteronism primärer Hyperaldosteronismus *m*, Conn-Syndrom *nt*.
primary hyperoxaluria primäre Hyperoxalurie *f*, Oxalose *f*.
type 1 p. Glykolazidurie *f*, Oxalose Typ I.
type 2 p. L-Glyzerinazidurie *f*, Oxalose Typ II.
primary hyperparathyroidism primärer Hyperparathyreoidismus *m abbr.* pHPT.
primary hypertension essentielle/idiopathische/primäre Hypertonie *f*.
primary hypertrophic osteoarthropathy Pachydermoperiostose *f*, Touraine--Solente-Golé-Syndrom *nt*, familiäre Pachydermoperiostose *f*, idiopathische hypertrophische Osteoarthropathie *f*, Akropachydermie *f* mit Pachydermoperiostose, Hyperostosis generalisata mit Pachydermie.
primary hypogonadism primärer/hypergonadotroper Hypogonadismus *m*.
primary hypotension essentielle/primäre/konstitutionelle Hypotonie *f*.
primary infection Erstinfektion *f*.
primary ingredient Grund-, Hauptbestandteil *m*.
primary instinct Urinstinkt *m*.
primary irritant dermatitis nicht-allergische Kontaktdermatitis *f*, toxische Kontaktdermatitis *f*, toxisches Kontaktekzem *nt*.
primary lesion 1. Primärläsion *f*. 2. *pulmo.* Ghon'-Primärkomplex *m*, -Herd *m*.
primary lysosome Primärlysosom *nt*.
primary memory primäres Gedächtnis *nt*.

primary mesoderm extraembryonales Mesoderm *nt.*
primary oocyte primäre Oozyte *f,* Primäroozyte *f,* Ovocytus primarius.
primary oxidase Oxi-, Oxygenase *f.*
primary pacemaker *physiol.* primärer Schrittmacher *m.*
primary palate *embryo.* primärer Gaumen *m.*
primary pentosuria benigne essentielle Pentosurie *f,* Xylulosurie *f.*
primary phosphate primäres Phosphat *nt.*
primary polycythemia Osler-Krankheit *f,* Osler-Vaquez-Krankheit *f,* Vaquez--Osler-Syndrom *nt,* Morbus Vaquez--Osler *m,* Erythrämie *f,* Polycythaemia (rubra) vera.
primary process Primärprozess *m.*
primary progressive cerebellar degeneration *neuro.* zerebellooliväre Atrophie *f* Typ Holmes.
primary ramus: dorsal p. *embryo.* primärer Dorsal-/Rückenast *m,* Ramus dorsalis primarii.
   ventral p. *embryo.* primärer Ventral-/Bauchast *m,* Ramus ventralis primarii.
primary rays Primärstrahlen *pl.*
primary reaction → primary response.
primary refractory anemia primär-refraktäre Anämie *f.*
primary reinforcement *psycho.* Primärverstärkung *f.*
primary reinforcer *psycho.* Primärverstärker *m.*
primary response Primärreaktion *f,* -antwort *f.*
primary-retroperitoneal *adj* primär retroperitoneal.
primary sclerosing cholangitis primär--sklerosierende Cholangitis *f.*
primary spermatocyte *embryo.* primärer Spermatozyt *m,* Spermiozyt *m,* Spermatozyt *m* I. Ordnung, Spermatocytus primarius.
primary splenic neutropenia hypersplenie-bedingte Neutropenie *f.*
primary splenic pancytopenia hypersplenie-bedingte Panzytopenie *f.*
primary stage Primärstadium *nt.*
primary structure *chem.* Primärstruktur *f.*
primary sulcus Primärfurche *f,* -sulcus *m.*
primary suture primäre Naht *f,* Pirmärnaht *f.*
primary syphilis Primärstadium *nt.*
primary therapy Primärtherapie *f.*
primary thrombocythemia hämorrhagische/essentielle Thrombozythämie *f,* Megakaryozytenleukämie *f,* megakaryozytäre Myelose *f.*
primary tuberculosis Primärtuberkulose *f.*
primary tumor Primärtumor *m,* -geschwulst *f.*
primary villi *embryo.* Primärzotten *pl.*
pri·mate ['praɪmeɪt] *n bio.* Primat *m.*
Pri·ma·tes [praɪ'meɪtiːz] *pl bio.* Herrentiere *pl,* Primaten *pl.*
primed lymphocyte typing [praɪmd] *abbr.* **PLT** *immun.* Primed-lymphocyte-Typing *nt abbr.* PLT.
prim·er ['praɪmər] *n chem., biochem.* Primer *m,* Starter *m.*
primer strand Starterstrang *m.*
prim·i·done ['prɪmədəʊn] *n pharm.* Primidon *nt.*
pri·mi·grav·id [ˌpraɪmɪ'grævɪd] *adj gyn.* zum ersten Mal schwanger.
pri·mi·grav·i·da [ˌ-'grævɪdə] *n, pl* **-das, -dae** [-diː] *gyn.* erstmals Schwangere *f,* Primigravida *f.*
prim·ing reaction ['praɪmɪŋ] Starter-, Initialreaktion *f.*

priming RNA Starter-RNA *f,* Starter-RNS *f,* priming-RNA *f.*
priming terminus *genet.* Startterminus *m.*
pri·mip·a·ra [praɪ'mɪpərə] *n, pl* **-ras, -rae** [-riː] Erstgebärende *f,* Primipara *f.*
pri·mip·a·rous [praɪ'mɪpərəs] *adj* erstgebärend, primipar.
primiparous woman → primipara.
prim·i·tive ['prɪmətɪv] *adj allg., bio.* erste(r, s), ursprünglich, primitiv, Ur-, Primitiv-.
primitive axon *embryo.* primitives Axon *nt.*
primitive bone Geflechtknochen *m.*
primitive brain Urhirn *nt.*
primitive choanae *embryo.* primitive Choanen *pl.*
primitive chorion *gyn.* primitives Chorion *nt.*
primitive dendrite *embryo.* primitiver Dendrit *m.*
primitive gut *embryo.* primitiver Darmkanal *m,* Urdarm *m,* Archenteron *nt.*
primitive knot *embryo.* Primitivknoten *m.*
primitive line *embryo.* Primitivstreifen *m.*
primitive node *embryo.* Primitivknoten *m.*
primitive segment *embryo.* Ursegment *nt.*
primitive streak *embryo.* Primitivstreifen *m.*
primitive ventricle of heart *embryo.* embryonale Herzkammer *f,* primitiver Ventrikel *m.*
pri·mor·di·al [praɪ'mɔːrdɪəl, -djəl] *adj* **1.** von Anfang an, ursprünglich, primordial, Ur-. **2.** *bio., embryo.* im Ansatz vorhanden, im Keim angelegt, primordial, Ur-.
primordial biomolecule ursprüngliches Biomolekül *nt,* Urbiomolekül *nt.*
primordial cyst Primordialzyste *f.*
primordial duct → paramesonephric duct.
primordial follicle Primordialfollikel *m,* früher Primärfollikel *m.*
primordial kidney *embryo.* Vorniere *f,* Pronephros *m.*
pri·mor·di·um [praɪ'mɔːrdɪəm] *n, pl* **-dia** [-dɪə] *embryo.* Embryonalanlage *f,* Primordium *nt.*
prin·ci·pal ['prɪnsɪpl] *adj* wichtigste(r, s), erste(r, s), hauptsächlich, Haupt-.
principal angle *phys.* Haupt-, Brechungswinkel *m.*
principal artery of thumb Hauptschlagader *f* des Daumens, A. princeps pollicis.
principal axis 1. *mathe.* Hauptachse *f.* **2.** *phys.* optische Achse *f.*
principal bronchus *embryo.* → primary bronchus.
principal cell Hauptzelle *f.*
principal nucleus Hauptkern *m.*
principal point *opt.* Hauptpunkt *m.*
principal visual ray *phys.* Sehstrahl *m.*
prin·ci·ple ['prɪnsəpl] *n* **1.** Prinzip *nt,* (Grund-)Satz *m,* (-)Regel *f,* (-)Lehre *f,* Gesetz *nt,* Gesetzmäßigkeit *f.* **in/on** ~ in/aus Prinzip. **2.** *pharm., chem.* Wirkstoff *m,* wirksamer Bestandteil *m;* Grundbestandteil *m.* **3.** Grundzug *m,* Charakteristikum *nt.*
   p. of causality Kausalitätsprinzip.
   p. of function Funktionsprinzip.
   p. of relativity Relativitätstheorie *f,* -lehre.
Pringle ['prɪŋgl]: **P.'s disease** Pringle-Tumor *m,* Naevus Pringle *m,* Adenoma sebaceum Pringle.
   P.'s maneuver vorübergehende Kompression *f* des Lig. hepatoduodenale.
   P.'s sebaceous adenoma → P.'s disease.
Pringle-Bourneville [burn'vɪl]: **P.-B. disease/syndrome** Bourneville-Pringle-Syndrom *nt,* Pringle-Bourneville-Syndrom *nt,* Pringle-Bourneville'-Phakomatose *f.*

P-R interval *card.* PR-Intervall *nt.*
print·out ['prɪntaʊt] *n* (Computer-)Ausdruck *m.*
Prinzmetal ['prɪntsmetl]: **P.'s angina** *card.* Prinzmetal-Angina *f.*
pri·on ['praɪɒn] *n micro.* Prion *nt.*
prism ['prɪzəm] *n* Prisma *nt.*
pris·mat·ic [prɪz'mætɪk] *adj* durch ein Prisma verursacht, prismenförmig, primatisch, Prismen-.
prismatic colors Spektralfarben *pl.*
prismatic ligament of Weitbrecht Lig. capitis femoris.
prismatic spectrum Prismaspektrum *nt.*
prism diopter *abbr.* **p.d.** Prismendioptrie *f, abbr.* pdpt, prdr, prdptr.
pris·moid ['prɪzmɔɪd] *adj* prismaähnlich, prismoid.
prism spectrum Prismenspektrum *nt.*
pris·on fever ['prɪzn] epidemisches/klassisches Fleckfieber *nt,* Läusefleckfieber *nt,* Fleck-, Hunger-, Kriegstyphus *m,* Typhus exanthematicus.
pri·vate ['praɪvɪt] *adj* privat, eigene(r, s), Privat-, Eigen-.
private antigens 1. seltene/private Antigene *pl.* **2.** Individualantigene *pl.*
private practice Privatpraxis *f.*
prize·fight·er ear [praɪzfaɪtər] Blumenkohl-, Boxerohr *nt.*
PRL *abbr.* → prolactin.
Prl *abbr.* → prolactin.
Pro *abbr.* → proline.
pro·ac·cel·er·in [ˌprəʊæk'selərɪn] *n* Proakzelerin *nt,* Proaccelerin *nt,* Acceleratorglobulin *nt,* labiler Faktor *m,* Faktor V *m abbr.* F V.
pro·ac·tin·i·um [ˌprəʊæk'tɪnɪəm] *n* → protactinium.
pro·ac·ti·va·tor [prəʊ'æktɪveɪtər] *n biochem.* Proaktivator *m.*
pro·ac·tive inhibition [prəʊ'æktɪv] *biochem.* proaktive Hemmung *f.*
pro·az·a·mine [prəʊ'æzəmiːn] *n* → promethazine.
prob·a·bil·i·ty [prɒbə'bɪlətɪ] *n abbr.* **P** Wahrscheinlichkeit *f abbr.* P. **in all** ~ aller Wahrscheinlichkeit nach, höchstwahrscheinlich.
probability curve *stat.* Kurve *f* der Wahrscheinlichkeitsverteilung.
probability distribution *mathe.* Wahrscheinlichkeitsverteilung *f.*
prob·a·ble ['prɒbəbl] *adj* wahrscheinlich.
pro·bac·te·ri·o·phage [ˌprəʊbæk'tɪərɪəfeɪdʒ] *n micro.* Prophage *m.*
pro·band ['prəʊbænd] *n* Test-, Versuchsperson *f,* Proband(in *f*) *m.*
probe [prəʊb] **I** *n* **1.** Sonde *f.* **2.** Gensonde *f,* Probe (*f*). **3.** Untersuchung *f.* **II** *vt* **4.** sondieren, mit einer Sonde untersuchen. **5.** erforschen, untersuchen.
pro·ben·e·cide [prəʊ'benəsaɪd] *n pharm.* Probenecid *nt.*
pro·bos·cis [prəʊ'bɒsɪs, -kɪs] *n, pl* **-bos·cis·es, -bos·ci·des** [-'bɒsɪdiːz] *bio.* Rüssel *m,* Proboscis *f.*
Probst [prabst]: **P.'s commissure** Probst'-Kommissur *f.*
pro·bu·col ['prəʊbjukɒl] *n pharm.* Probucol *nt.*
pro·cain·am·ide [ˌprəʊkeɪn'æmaɪd, prəʊ-'keɪnəmaɪd] *n pharm.* Procainamid *nt.*
pro·caine [prəʊ'keɪn, 'prəʊkeɪn] *n pharm., anes.* Prokcain *nt,* Procain *nt.*
procaine amide → procainamide.
pro·cal·lus [prəʊ'kæləs] *n ortho.* Prokallus *m.*
pro·cap·sid [prəʊ'kæpsɪd] *n micro.* Prokapsid *nt,* Procapsid *nt.*
pro·car·ba·zine [prəʊ'kɑːrbəziːn] *n pharm.* Procarbazin *nt.*

procarboxypeptidase

pro·car·box·y·pep·ti·dase [ˌprəʊkɑːrˌbaksɪ'peptɪdeɪz] n Procarboxypeptidase f.
pro·car·cin·o·gen [ˌprəʊkɑːr'sɪnədʒən] n Prokarzinogen nt.
Pro·car·y·o·tae [prəʊˌkærɪˌəʊtiː] pl bio. Prokaryo(n)ten pl, Procaryotae pl.
pro·car·y·ote n → prokaryote.
pro·car·y·ot·ic adj → prokaryotic.
pro·ce·dur·al [prə'siːdʒərəl] adj verfahrensmäßig, prozedural, Verfahren-, Prozedur-.
procedural learning prozedurales Lernen nt.
procedural memory prozedurales Langzeitgedächtnis nt.
pro·ce·dure [prə'siːdʒər] n Vorgehen nt; (a. techn.) Verfahren nt, Technik f.
pro·ceed [prə'siːd] vi 1. fig. Fortschritte machen, vorankommen; weitermachen, fortfahren (in, with in, mit). 2. vorgehen, verfahren. 3. (Krankheit, Geräusch) kommen, ausgehen (from von). 4. prozessieren, einen Prozeß anstrengen (against gegen).
pro·cen·tri·ole [prəʊ'sentrɪəʊl] n Prozentriole f.
pro·ce·phal·ic [ˌprəʊsɪ'fælɪk] adj Vorderkopf betr.
pro·cer·coid [prəʊ'sɜrkɔɪd] n micro. Prozerkoid nt.
pro·ce·rus (muscle) [prəʊ'sɪərəs] Prozerus m, M. procerus.
proc·ess ['prəses; Brit. 'prəʊ-] I n, pl **-es** ['prəsesɪz, -ə,siːz; Brit. 'prəʊ-] 1. anat. Fortsatz m, Vorsprung m, Processus m. 2. (a. techn., chem., phys.) Prozeß m, Verfahren nt; Vorgang m, Verlauf m. II vt be-, verarbeiten, behandeln, einem Verfahren unterwerfen.
p. of combustion Verbrennungsvorgang.
p. of Folius vorderer Hammerfortsatz, Proc. anterior (mallei).
p. of selection bio. Ausleseprozeß.
pro·chi·ral [prəʊ'kaɪrəl] adj chem. prochiral.
pro·chi·ral·i·ty [ˌprəʊkaɪ'rælətɪ] n chem. Prochiralität f.
prochiral molecule chem. prochirales Molekül nt.
pro·chord·al plate [prəʊ'kɔːrdl] embryo. Prächordalplatte f.
pro·chro·mo·some [prəʊ'krəʊməsəʊm] n Prochromosom nt.
pro·chy·mo·sin [prəʊ'kaɪməsɪn] n Prochymosin nt, Prorennin nt.
pro·col·la·gen [prəʊ'kɒlədʒən] n Prokollagen nt.
pro·col·la·gen·ase [prəʊkə'lædʒəneɪz] n Prokollagenase f.
procollagen filament Prokollagenfilament nt.
procollagen peptidase Prokollagenpeptidase f, -protease f.
procollagen-proline, 2-oxoglutarate 4-dioxygenase Prolinhydroxylase f, Prolylhydroxylase f.
procollagen protease → procollagen peptidase.
procollagen N-proteinase → procollagen peptidase.
pro·con·ver·tin [ˌprəʊkən'vɜrtɪn] n Prokonvertin nt, -convertin nt, Faktor VII m abbr. F V II, Autothrombin I nt, Serum--Prothrombin-Conversion-Accelerator m abbr., SPCA, stabiler Faktor m.
proct- pref. → procto-.
proc·tag·ra [prɒk'tægrə] n → proctalgia.
proc·tal·gia [prɒk'tældʒɪə] n Schmerzen pl im unteren Mastdarm, Proktalgie f, Proctalgia f.
proc·ta·tre·sia [ˌprɒktə'triːʒɪə] n Analatresie f, Atresia ani.

proc·tec·ta·sia [ˌprɒktek'teɪʒ(ɪ)ə] n Anus-, Rektum-, Mastdarmdehnung f, Proktektasie f.
proc·tec·to·my [prɒk'tektəmɪ] n chir. Rektumamputation f, -resektion f, Proktektomie f.
proc·ten·clei·sis [ˌprɒktən'klaɪsəs] n Anus-, Rektum-, Mastdarmstenose f, Proktostenose f.
proc·ten·cli·sis n → proctencleisis.
proc·ti·tis [prɒk'taɪtɪs] n Rektum-, Mastdarmentzündung f, Proktitis f, Proctitis f, Rektitis f.
procto- pref. Enddarm-, Mastdarm-, Ano-, Anus-, Procto-, Rektum-, Rekto-.
proc·to·cele ['prɒktəʊsɪl] n Rekto-, Proktozele f; Mastdarmbruch m, Hernia rectalis.
proc·to·coc·cy·pex·y [ˌ-'kɒksɪpeksɪ] n chir. Proktokokzygopexie f.
proc·to·co·lec·to·my [ˌ-kə'lektəmɪ] n chir. Proktokolektomie f.
proc·to·co·li·tis [ˌ-kəʊ'laɪtɪs] n Proktokolitis f, Koloproktitis f.
proc·to·co·lon·os·co·py [ˌ-ˌkəʊlən'ɒskəpɪ] n Proktokoloskopie f.
proc·to·col·po·plas·ty [ˌ-'kɒlpəplæstɪ] n chir., gyn. Rektum-Scheiden-Plastik f.
proc·to·cys·to·plas·ty [ˌ-'sɪstəplæstɪ] n chir., gyn. Rektum-Blasen-Plastik f.
proc·to·cys·tot·o·my [ˌ-sɪs'tɒtəmɪ] n chir., urol. transrektale Zystotomie f.
proc·to·dae·um n → proctodeum.
proc·to·de·um [ˌ-'diːəm] n embryo. Aftergrube f, Proctodaeum nt.
proc·to·dyn·ia [ˌ-'dɪːnɪə] n Enddarm-, Anusschmerz(en pl) m, Proktodynie f.
proc·to·el·y·tro·plas·ty [ˌ-'elɪtrəʊplæstɪ] n → proctocolpoplasty.
proc·tol·o·gy [prɒk'tɒlədʒɪ] n Proktologie f.
proc·to·me·nia [ˌprɒktəʊ'miːnɪə] n gyn. rektale Endometriose f.
proc·to·pa·ral·y·sis [ˌ-pə'rælɪsɪs] n Lähmung/Paralyse f der Analmuskulatur.
proc·to·per·i·ne·o·plas·ty [ˌ-ˌperɪ'niːəʊplæstɪ] n gyn., chir. Rektum-Damm-Plastik f.
proc·to·per·i·ne·or·rha·phy [ˌ-ˌperɪnɪ'ɔrəfɪ] n gyn., chir. Rektum-Damm-Plastik f, -Naht f.
proc·to·pex·y ['-peksɪ] n chir. Mastdarmanheftung f, Proktopexie f.
proc·to·plas·ty ['-plæstɪ] n Rektum-, Proktoplastik f.
proc·to·ple·gia [ˌ-'pliːdʒɪə] n → proctoparalysis.
proc·to·pol·y·pus [ˌ-'pɒlɪpəs] n Rektumpolyp m.
proc·top·to·sia [ˌprɒktəp'təʊsɪə] n Prolapsus ani et recti.
proc·top·to·sis [ˌprɒktəp'təʊsɪs] n → proctoptosia.
proc·tor·rha·gia [ˌprɒktəʊ'reɪdʒɪə] n Mastdarm-, Enddarm-, Rektumblutung f.
proc·tor·rha·phy [prɒk'tɒrəfɪ] n chir. Rektumnaht f.
proc·to·scope ['prɒktəskəʊp] n Proktoskop nt, Rektoskop nt.
proc·tos·co·py [prɒk'tɒskəpɪ] n Mastdarmspiegelung f, Proktoskopie f, Rektoskopie f.
proc·to·sig·moid·ec·to·my [ˌprɒktəʊˌsɪgmɔɪ'dektəmɪ] n chir. Proktosigmoidektomie f.
proc·to·sig·moi·di·tis [ˌ-ˌsɪgmɔɪ'daɪtɪs] n Entzündung f von Mastdarm u. Sigmoid, Proktosigmoiditis f.
proc·to·sig·moid·o·scope [ˌ-sɪg'mɔɪdəskəʊp] n Proktosigmoid(e)oskop nt, Rektosigmoid(e)oskop nt.

proc·to·sig·moi·dos·co·py [ˌ-ˌsɪgmɔɪ'dɒskəpɪ] n Proktosigmoid(e)oskopie f, Rektosigmoid(e)oskopie f.
proc·to·spasm ['-spæzəm] n Proktospasmus m.
proc·to·ste·no·sis [ˌ-stɪ'nəʊsɪs] n → proctencleisis.
proc·tos·to·my [prɒk'tɒstəmɪ] n chir. Rekto-, Proktostomie f.
proc·tot·o·my [prɒk'tɒtəmɪ] n chir. Rekto-, Proktotomie f.
pro·cum·bent [prəʊ'kʌmbənt] adj auf dem Bauch liegend.
pro·cur·sive [prəʊ'kɜrsɪv] adj prokursiv, Prokursiv-.
procursive chorea neuro. Chorea festinans.
pro·cur·va·tion [ˌprəʊkɜr'veɪʃn] n Beugung/Biegung f nach vorne, Vorwärtsbeugung f.
pro·cy·cli·dine [prəʊ'saɪklədiːn] n pharm. Procyclidin n.
pro·dig·i·o·sin [ˌprəʊdɪdʒɪ'əʊsɪn] n Prodigiosin nt.
pro·dro·ma [prə'drəʊmə, 'prɒdrəmə] n, pl **-mas, -ma·ta** [-mətə] → prodrome.
pro·dro·mal [prə'drəʊməl, 'prɒdrəməl] adj ankündigend, vorangehend, prodromal, Prodromal-.
prodromal glaucoma latentes Winkelblockglaukom nt, Glaucoma prodromale.
prodromal period Prodromalstadium nt, -phase f, Vorläuferstadium nt.
prodromal phase/stage → prodromal period.
pro·drome ['prəʊdrəʊm] n Prodromalerscheinung f, Prodrom nt, Vorzeichen nt, Frühsymptom nt.
pro·drom·ic [prə'drɒmɪk] adj → prodromal.
prod·ro·mous ['prɒdrəməs] adj → prodromal.
prod·ro·mus ['prɒdrəməs] n → prodrome.
pro·drug ['prəʊdrʌg] n pharm. Prodrug (f).
pro·duce [prə'd(j)uːs] vt erzeugen, hervorbringen, hervorrufen, bewirken, schaffen; (Wirkung) erzielen.
prod·uct ['prɒdʌkt] n 1. Erzeugnis nt, Produkt nt. 2. Ergebnis nt, Resultat nt, Werk nt, Produkt nt. 3. chem., mathe. Produkt nt.
pro·duc·tive [prə'dʌktɪv] adj 1. ertragreich, fruchtbar, produktiv. 2. patho. produktiv, Produktions-.
productive bronchitis produktive Bronchitis f, Bronchitis f mit Auswurf, Bronchitis productiva.
productive cough produktiver Husten m, Husten m mit Auswurf.
productive inflammation → proliferative inflammation.
productive nephritis produktive Nephritis f.
productive osteitis Ostitis condensans.
productive peritonitis Peritonitis productiva.
productive phlebitis Phlebosklerose f.
productive tuberculosis produktive Lungentuberkulose f.
pro·e·las·tin [ˌprəʊɪ'læstɪn] n Proelastin nt.
pro·e·mi·al [prəʊ'iːmɪəl] adj → prodromal.
pro·en·ceph·a·lon [ˌprəʊen'sefələn] n → prosencephalon.
pro·en·ceph·a·lus [ˌprəʊen'sefələs] n embryo. Proenzephalus m.
pro·en·zyme [prəʊ'enzaɪm] n Enzymvorstufe f, Proenzym nt, Zymogen nt.
pro·e·ryth·ro·blast [prəʊɪ'rɪθrəblæst] n Proerythroblast m, Pronormoblast m.
pro·e·ryth·ro·cyte [prəʊɪ'rɪθrəsaɪt] n Erythrozytenvorläufer(zelle f) m.

pro·es·tro·gen [prəʊ'estrədʒən] *n* Proöstrogen *nt*.
pro·fer·ment [prəʊ'fɜrment] *n* → proenzyme.
pro·fes·sor angles [prə'fesər] *derm.* Geheimratsecken *pl.*
pro·fi·bri·nol·y·sin [ˌprəʊfaɪbrə'nɒləsɪn] *n* Plasminogen *nt*, Profibrinolysin *nt*.
Profichet [prɔfi'ʃe]: **P.'s disease/syndrome** Profichet-Krankheit *f*, -Syndrom *nt*, Kalkgicht *f*, Calcinosis circumscripta.
pro·file ['prəʊfaɪl] **I** *n* **1.** Seitenansicht *f*, Profil *nt*; Umriß *m*, Kontur *f*. **2.** Profil *nt*; Längsschnitt *m*; Durchschnitt *m*; Querschnitt *m*. **3.** (Persönlichkeits-, Leistungs-)Diagramm *nt*, Kurve *f*. **II** *vt* im Profil darstellen, profilieren.
pro·fla·vine [prəʊ'fleɪviːn] *n* Proflavin *nt*, Diaminoacridin *nt*.
pro·fun·da·plas·ty [prəʊ'fʌndəplæstɪ] *n* HTG Profundaplastik *f*, A.-profunda-femoris-Plastik *f*.
pro·fun·do·plas·ty [prəʊˌfʌndəplæstɪ] *n* → profundaplasty.
pro·gam·ic [prəʊ'gæmɪk] *adj bio.* vor der Befruchtung, progam.
prog·a·mous ['prɑgəməs] *adj* → progamic.
pro·gas·trin [prəʊ'gæstrɪn] *n* Progastrin *nt*.
pro·gen·e·sis [prəʊ'dʒenəsɪs] *n* Progenese *f*.
pro·ge·nia [prəʊ'dʒiːnɪə] *n* → prognathism.
pro·gen·i·tive [prəʊ'dʒenətɪv] *adj* zeugungsfähig, Zeugungs-.
pro·gen·i·tor [prəʊ'dʒenɪtər] *n* **1.** Vorläufer *m*; Vorfahr *m*. **2.** *histol.*, *hema.* Vorläuferzelle *f*.
prog·e·ny ['prɑdʒənɪ] *n* Nachkommen(schaft *f*) *pl*, Abkömmlinge *pl*, Kinder *pl*, Progenitur *f*.
pro·ge·ria [prəʊ'dʒɪərɪə] *n* Hutchinson-Gilford-Syndrom *nt*, Gilford-Syndrom *nt*, Progerie *f*, greisenhafter Zwergwuchs *m*, Progeria Hutchinson-Gilford, Progeria infantilis.
p. with cataract/microphthalmia Hallermann-Streiff-Syndrom *nt*, Hallermann-Streiff-Francois-Syndrom *nt*, Dyskephaliesyndrom *nt* von Francois, Dysmorphia mandibulo-oculo-facialis.
progeria syndrome → progeria.
pro·ges·ta·gen [prəʊ'dʒestədʒən] *n* → progestogen.
pro·ges·ta·tion·al [prəʊdʒe'steɪʃənl] *adj* Lutealphase betr.
progestational hormone → progesterone.
progestational phase → progestational stage.
progestational stage *gyn.* gestagene/sekretorische Phase *f*, Sekretions-, Lutealphase *f*.
pro·ges·te·roid [prəʊ'dʒestərɔɪd] *n* progesteron-ähnliche Substanz *f*, Progesteroid *nt*.
pro·ges·ter·one [prəʊ'dʒestərəʊn] *n* Gelbkörperhormon *nt*, Progesteron *nt*, Corpus-luteum-Hormon *nt*.
progesterone receptor Progesteronrezeptor *m*.
progesterone receptor activity Progesteronrezeptorbindungskapazität *f*.
progesterone-receptor complex Progesteronrezeptor-Komplex *m*.
progesterone unit Progesteron-Einheit *f*.
pro·ges·tio·nal stage [prəʊ'dʒestʃənl] → progestational stage.
pro·ges·to·gen [prəʊ'dʒestədʒən] *n* Progestagen *nt*, Progestogen *nt*.
pro·glos·sis [prəʊ'glɒsɪs] *n* Zungenspitze *f*.

pro·glot·tid [prəʊ'glɒtɪd] *n micro.* Bandwurmglied *nt*, Proglottid *m*.
pro·glot·tis [prəʊ'glɒtɪs] *n*, *pl* **-ti·des** [-tədiːz] → proglottid.
pro·glu·ca·gon [prəʊ'gluːkəgən] *n* Proglukagon *nt*.
pro·glu·mide [prəʊ'gluːmaɪd] *n pharm.* Proglumid *nt*.
prog·na·thia [prəʊ'neɪθɪə, -'næθ-, prɑg-] *n* → prognathism.
prog·nath·ic [prəʊ'neɪθɪk, -'næθ-, prɑg-] *adj* → prognathous.
prog·na·thism ['prɑgnəθɪzəm] *n* Prognathie *f*, Progenie *f*.
prog·na·thous ['prɑgnəθəs] *adj* prognath.
prog·nose [prɑg'nəʊz] *vt*, *vi* eine Prognose stellen, prognostizieren.
prog·no·sis [prɑg'nəʊsɪs] *n*, *pl* **-ses** [-siːz] Voraus-, Vorhersage *f*, Prognose *f*. **to make a ~** eine Prognose stellen.
prog·nos·tic [prɑg'nɒstɪk] **I** *n* **1.** (An-)Zeichen *nt*, Prognostikum *nt*. **2.** Voraus-, Vorhersage *f*. **II** *adj* voraus-, vorhersagend, prognostisch.
prog·nos·ti·cate [prɑg'nɒstɪkeɪt] *vt* **1.** voraus-, vorhersagen, prognostizieren. **2.** anzeigen.
prog·nos·ti·ca·tion [prɑgnɒstɪ'keɪʃn] *n* → prognosis.
pro·grade urethrography [prəʊ'greɪd] *urol.* prograde Urethrographie *f*.
pro·gram ['prəʊgræm, -grəm] **I** *n* **1.** Programm *nt*, Plan *m*. **2.** (Computer-)Programm *nt*. **II** *vt* **3.** planen, ein Programm aufstellen. **4.** (*Computer*) programmieren.
program-controlled *adj techn., physiol.* programmgesteuert.
pro·gram·ma·ble ['prəʊgræməbl, prəʊ'græm-] *adj* (*Computer*) programmierbar.
pro·gramme *n Brit.* → program.
pro·gram·mer ['prəʊgræmər] *n* (*Computer*) Programmierer(in *f*) *m*.
pro·gram·ming ['prəʊgræmɪŋ, -grəmɪŋ] *n* Programmieren, *nt*, Programmierung *f*.
programming language Programmier-, Computersprache *f*.
pro·gran·u·lo·cyte [prəʊ'grænjələsaɪt] *n* → promyelocyte.
prog·ress [*n* 'prɑgres, 'prəʊ-; *v* prə'gres] **I** *n* Fortschritt *m*, -schritte *pl*, Fortgang *m*, Lauf *m*. **in ~** im Werden (begriffen), im Gange. **II** *vi* Fortschritte machen, fortschreiten, seinen Fortgang nehmen, s. (fort-, weiter-)entwickeln.
pro·gres·sion [prə'greʃn] *n* **1.** Vorwärts-, Fortbewegung *f*. **2.** Weiterentwicklung *f*, Verlauf *m*.
pro·gres·sive [prə'gresɪv] *adj* fortschreitend, zunehmend, s. weiterentwickelnd, progressiv.
progressive bacterial synergistic gangrene Meleney-Geschwür *nt*, Pyoderma gangraenosum, Dermatitis ulcerosa, Pyodermia ulcerosa serpiginosa.
progressive bulbar paralysis in children familiäre progressive Bulbärparalyse *f*, Fazio-Londe-Syndrom *nt*.
progressive cerebral poliodystrophy Alpers-Syndrom *nt*, Poliodystrophia cerebri progressiva infantilis.
progressive choroidal atrophy Chorioiderämie *f*, Degeneratio chorioretinalis progressiva.
progressive coccidioidomycosis sekundäre/progressive Kokzidioidomykose *f*, Sekundärform *f* der Kokzidioidomykose.
progressive congenital lipodystrophy Lawrence-Syndrom *nt*, lipatrophischer Diabetes *m*.

progressive dialysis encephalopathy chronisch-progressive dialysebedingte Enzephalopathie *f*, Dialyseenzephalopathie *f*.
progressive dystrophic hyperkeratosis Vohwinkel-Syndrom *nt*, Pseudoainhumartige Dermatose *f*, Keratoma hereditarium mutilans, Keratosis palmoplantaris mutilans.
progressive emphysematous necrosis *patho.* Gasbrand *m*, -gangrän *f*, -ödem *nt*, -ödemerkrankung *f*, malignes Ödem *nt*, Gasphlegmone *f*, Gangraena emphysematosa.
progressive epilepsy Dromolepsie *f*, Epilepsia cursiva.
progressive familial myoclonic epilepsy Lafora-Syndrom *nt*, Unverricht-Syndrom *nt*, Myoklonusepilepsie *f*, myoklonische Epilepsie *f*.
progressive generalized lymphadenopathy *abbr.* **PGL** progressive generalisierte Lymphadenopathie *f abbr.* PGL.
progressive hypertrophic interstitial neuropathy Déjérine-Sottas-Syndrom *nt*, -Krankheit *f*, hypertrophische Neuropathie *f* (Déjérine-Sottas), hereditäre motorische u. sensible Neuropathie *f* Typ III.
progressive lingual hemiatrophy halbseitiger Zungenschwund *m*, Hemiatrophia linguae.
progressive lipodystrophy Simons-Syndrom *nt*, Lipodystrophia progressiva/paradoxa.
progressive multifocale leukoencephalopathy *abbr.* **PML** progressive multifokale Leukoenzephalopathie *f abbr.* PML.
progressive multiple hyaloserositis progressive maligne Polyserositis *f*.
progressive muscular dystrophy *abbr.* **PMD** progressive Muskeldystrophie *f abbr.* PMD, Dystrophia musculorum progressiva.
progressive myopia *ophthal.* progressive Myopie *f*.
progressive nonsuppurative cholangitis primär biliäre Zirrhose *abbr.* PBZ, nicht-eitrige destruierende Cholangitis *f*.
progressive ossifying myositis progressive/generalisierte Myositis ossificans, Myositis ossificans progressiva.
progressive partial lipodystrophy → progressive lipodystrophy.
progressive pigmentary dermatosis Schamberg-Krankheit *f*, -Syndrom *nt*, Morbus Schamberg *m*, progressive Pigmentpurpura *f*, progressive pigmentöse Dermatose *f*, Purpura pigmentosa progressiva, Purpura Schamberg *f*, Dermatosis pigmentaria progressiva, Capillaritis haemorrhagica maculosa.
progressive rubella panencephalitis *abbr.* **PRP** progressive Rötelnpanenzephalitis *f abbr.* PRP.
progressive spinal muscular atrophy Cruveilhier'-Krankheit *f*, spinale progressive Muskelatrophie *f*.
progressive subcortical encephalopathy Schilder'-Krankheit *f*, Encephalitis periaxialis diffusa.
progressive supranuclear palsy progressive supranukleäre Lähmung *f*.
progressive synergistic (bacterial) gangrene → progressive bacterial synergistic gangrene.
progressive systemic sclerosis systemische Sklerose *f*, Systemsklerose *f*, progressive/diffuse/systemische Sklerodermie *f*, Sclerodermia diffusa/progressiva.
progressive tapetochoroidal dystrophy → progressive choroidal atrophy.

progressive torsion spasm of childhood Ziehen-Oppenheim-Krankheit f, -Syndrom nt, Torsionsneurose f, -dystonie f, Dysbasia lordotica.
pro·guan·il [prəʊˈgwænɪl] n pharm. Proguanil nt.
pro·hor·mone [prəʊˈhɔːrməʊn] n Prohormon nt.
pro·in·su·lin [prəʊˈɪnsəlɪn, -ˈɪns(j)u-] n Proinsulin nt.
pro·i·so·cor·tex [prəʊˈaɪsəkɔːrteks] n Proisocortex nt.
proj·ect [n ˈprɑdʒekt, -ɪkt; v prəˈdʒekt] **I** n Plan m, Entwurf m, Vorhaben nt, Unternehmen nt, Projekt nt. **II** vt **1.** psycho., mathe., opt. projizieren. **2.** (voraus-)planen, entwerfen, (ein-)schätzen, projektieren; stat. hochrechnen, überschlagen. **III** vi **3.** hervorspringen, -stehen, vorragen (from aus). **4.** psycho. projizieren.
pro·ject·ed pain [prəˈdʒektɪd] projizierter Schmerz m.
pro·jec·tile vomiting [prəˈdʒektɪl, -taɪl] explosionsartiges Erbrechen nt, Erbrechen nt im Strahl.
pro·ject·ing staphyloma [prəˈdʒektɪŋ] Hornhautstaphylom nt, Staphyloma corneae.
pro·jec·tion [prəˈdʒekʃn] n **1.** Vorsprung m, Überhang m, Fortsatz m. **2.** (Her-)Vorspringen nt, Vorstehen nt. **3.** mathe., opt., psycho. Projektion f. **4.** Planung f, Entwurf m, (Ein-)Schätzung f; stat. Hochrechnung f.
pro·jec·tion·al [prəˈdʒekʃənl] adj Projektions-.
projection area physiol. Projektionsareal nt, -feld nt.
projection fibers → projection neurofibers.
projection field → projection area.
projection focus Projektionsherd m, -fokus m.
projection formula chem. Projektionsformel f.
projection neurofibers Projektionsfasern pl, Neurofibrae projectionis.
projection tract Projektionsbahn f.
pro·jec·tive [prəˈdʒektɪv] adj projektiv, Projektions-; (a. psycho.) projizierend.
projective geometry projektive Geometrie f.
projective test psycho. Projektionstest m, projektiver Test m.
pro·kal·li·kre·in [prəʊˌkæləˈkriːɪn] n → prekallikrein.
Pro·kar·y·o·tae pl → Procaryotae.
pro·kar·y·ote [prəʊˈkærɪəʊt, -ɪət] n bio. Prokaryo(n)t m.
pro·kar·y·ot·ic [prəʊˌkærɪˈɒtɪk] adj bio. Prokaryo(n)ten betr., prokaryontisch, prokaryotisch.
prokaryotic cell prokaryo(n)tische Zelle f.
prokaryotic protist bio. niederer Protist m, Prokaryo(n)t m.
pro·lac·tin [prəʊˈlæktɪn] n abbr. **PRL, Prl** Prolaktin nt abbr. PRL, Prolactin nt, laktogenes Hormon nt.
prolactin cell (Adenohypophyse) Prolaktin-Zelle f, mammotrope Zelle f.
prolactin inhibiting factor abbr. **PIF** Prolactin-inhibiting-Faktor m abbr. PIF, Prolactin-inhibiting-Hormon nt abbr. PIH.
prolactin inhibiting hormone abbr. **PIH** → prolactin inhibiting factor.
pro·lac·ti·no·ma [prəʊˌlæktɪˈnəʊmə] n Prolaktinom nt, Prolactinom(a) nt.
prolactin-producing tumor → prolactinoma.
prolactin releasing factor abbr. **PRF** Prolactin-releasing-Faktor m abbr. PRF, Prolactin-releasing-Hormon nt abbr. PRH.
prolactin releasing hormone abbr. **PRH** → prolactin releasing factor.
pro·lam·in [prəʊˈlæmɪn, ˈprəʊləmɪn] n Prolamin nt.
pro·lam·ine [prəʊˈlæmiːn, -mɪn, ˈprəʊləmɪn] n → prolamin.
pro·lapse [n ˈprəʊlæps; v prəʊˈlæps] patho. **I** n Vorfall m, Prolaps m, Prolapsus m. **II** vi vorfallen, hervortreten, prolabieren.
p. of the anus Analprolaps, Prolapsus ani.
p. of the rectum Mastdarmvorfall, Rektumprolaps, -vorfall, Prolapsus recti.
p. of the uterus Gebärmuttervorfall, -prolaps, Uterusprolaps, Prolapsus uteri.
pro·lapsed hemorrhoids [prəʊˈlæpst] prolabierte Hämorrhoiden pl, Hämorrhoidalprolaps m.
pro·lap·sus [prəʊˈlæpsəs] n, pl -sus·es → prolapse **I**.
pro·leu·ko·cyte [prəʊˈluːkəsaɪt] n hema. Leukozytenvorläufer(zelle f) m.
pro·li·dase [ˈprɑlɪdeɪz] n → proline dipeptidase.
prolidase deficiency Prolidasemangel m.
pro·lif·er·ate [prəˈlɪfəreɪt, prəʊ-] vi wuchern, proliferieren; s. (rasch) ausbreiten od. vermehren.
pro·lif·er·at·ing retinitis [prəʊˈlɪfəreɪtɪŋ] Retinitis/Retinopathia proliferans.
pro·lif·er·a·tion [prəˌlɪfəˈreɪʃn] n **1.** Wucherung f, Proliferation f. **2.** Wuchern nt, Proliferieren nt, (rasche) Vermehrung od. Ausbreitung f.
proliferation cyst proliferierende Zyste f.
pro·lif·er·a·tive [prəˈlɪfəˌreɪtɪv] adj proliferativ, proliferierend, wuchernd, Vermehrungs-, Proliferations-.
proliferative arthritis rheumatoide Arthritis f, progrediente/primär chronische Polyarthritis f abbr. PCP, PcP.
proliferative cyst → proliferation cyst.
proliferative disease abbr. **PD** proliferative Mastopathie f.
p. of the breast → proliferative disease.
p. without atypia abbr. **PDWA** proliferative Mastopathie f ohne Atypien.
proliferative endophlebitis → phlebosclerosis.
proliferative fasciitis noduläre Fasziitis f, Fasciitis nodularis.
proliferative fibrosis proliferative Fibrose f.
proliferative glomerulonephritis proliferative Glomerulonephritis f.
proliferative inflammation proliferative/produktive Entzündung f.
proliferative intra-extracapillary glomerulonephritis intra-extrakapilläre proliferative Glomerulonephritis f.
proliferative phase gyn. östrogene/proliferative Phase f, Proliferations-, Follikelreifungsphase f.
proliferative retinopathy Retinopathia diabetica haemorrhagica proliferans.
proliferative stage → proliferative phase.
proliferative synovitis proliferative Synovitis f.
pro·lif·er·ous [prəʊˈlɪfərəs] adj → proliferative.
proliferous cyst → proliferation cyst.
proliferous inflammation → proliferative inflammation.
pro·lif·ic [prəʊˈlɪfɪk] adj fruchtbar.
pro·lig·er·ous cyst [prəʊˈlɪdʒərəs] old → cystadenocarcinoma.
proligerous disk Eihügel m, Discus proligerus/oophorus, Cumulus oophorus.
proligerous membrane → proligerous disk.

pro·li·nase [ˈprɑlɪneɪz] n → prolyl dipeptidase.
pro·line [ˈprəʊliːn, -lɪn] n abbr. **Pro** Prolin nt abbr. Pro.
proline dehydrogenase Prolindehydrogenase f, Prolin(-5-)oxidase f.
proline dehydrogenase deficiency Hyperprolinämie f Typ I, Prolinoxidasemangel m.
proline dipeptidase Prolidase f, Prolindipeptidase f.
proline hydxroxylase → prolyl hydroxylase.
pro·li·ne·mia [ˌprəʊlɪˈniːmɪə] n erhöhter Prolingehalt m des Blutes, Hyperprolinämie f.
proline-4-monooxygenase n Prolin-4--monooxygenase f.
proline(-5-)oxidase n → proline dehydrogenase.
pro·lin·tane [prəʊˈlɪnteɪn] n pharm. Prolintan nt.
pro·longed labor [prəˈlɔːŋt, -ˈlɒŋt] protrahierte Geburt f.
pro·lyl [ˈprəʊlɪl] n Prolyl-(Radikal nt).
prolyl dipeptidase Prolinase f, Prolyldipeptidase f.
prolyl hydroxylase Prolinhydroxylase f, Prolylhydroxylase f.
pro·lym·pho·cyte [prəʊˈlɪmfəsaɪt] n Prolymphozyt m.
pro·mas·ti·gote [prəʊˈmæstɪgəʊt] n micro. promastigote Form f, Leptomonas--Form f.
promastigote stage → promastigote.
pro·ma·zine [ˈprəʊməziːn] n pharm. Promazin f.
pro·meg·a·kar·y·o·cyte [prəʊˌmegəˈkærɪəsaɪt] n Promegakaryozyt m.
pro·meg·a·lo·blast [prəʊˈmegələblæst] n Promegaloblast m.
pro·met·a·phase [prəʊˈmetəfeɪz] n Prometaphase f.
pro·meth·a·zine [prəʊˈmeθəziːn] n pharm. Promethazin f.
pro·me·thi·um [prəʊˈmiːθɪəm] n abbr. **Pm** Promethium nt abbr. Pm.
prom·i·nence [ˈprɑmɪnəns] n **1.** anat. Vorsprung m, (Vor-)Wölbung f, Prominentia f. **2.** (Her-)Vorragen nt, -stehen nt; deutliche Sichtbarkeit f.
p. of facial canal Prominentia canalis facialis.
p. of lateral semicircular canal Prominentia canalis semicircularis lateralis.
prom·i·nent [ˈprɑmɪnənt] adj **1.** vorstehend, -springend, prominent. **2.** auffallend, markant, hervorstechend.
prom·i·nen·tia [ˌprɑmɪˈnenʃɪə] n, pl -tiae [-ʃɪˌiː] → prominence 1.
prominent vertebra VII. Halswirbel m, Prominens m, Vertebra prominens.
prom·is·cu·i·ty [ˌprɑmɪˈskjuːəti, ˌprəʊ-] n Promiskuität f.
pro·mis·cu·ous [prəˈmɪskjuwəs] adj promiskuitiv, promiskuos, promiskuös.
pro·mi·to·sis [ˌprəʊmaɪˈtəʊsɪs] n Promitose f.
pro·mon·o·cyte [prəʊˈmɒnəsaɪt] n Promonozyt m.
pro·mon·to·ri·um [ˌprɒmənˈtɔːrɪəm, -ˈtəʊ-] n, pl -ria [-rɪə] → promontory.
prom·on·to·ry [ˈprɑmənˌtɔːriː, -təʊ-] n anat. vorspringender (Körper-)Teil m, Promontorium nt.
p. of tympanic cavity Promontorium tympani.
promontory sulcus (of tympanic cavity) Sulcus promontorii (cavi tympani).
pro·mote [prəˈməʊt] vt fördern, unterstützen, begünstigen, anregen.

pro·mot·er [prə'məutər] *n genet., biochem.* Promotor *m*, Aktivator *m*.
pro·mo·tion [prə'məuʃn] *n* **1.** Förderung *f*, Unterstützung *f*, Begünstigung *f*, Anregung *f*. **2.** Beförderung *f*.
pro·my·e·lo·cyte [prəu'maɪələsaɪt] *n* Promyelozyt *m*.
pro·my·e·lo·cyt·ic leukemia [prəu,maɪələu'sɪtɪk] (akute) Promyelozytenleukämie *f abbr.* APL, (akute) promyelozytäre Leukämie *f*.
pro·nase ['prəuneɪz] *n* Pronase *f*.
pro·nate ['prəuneɪt] *vt* einwärtsdrehen um die Längsachse, pronieren.
pro·na·tion [prəu'neɪʃn] *n* Einwärtsdrehung *f* um die Längsachse, Pronation *f*.
pro·na·tor [prə'neɪtər, 'prəuneɪ-] *n* Pronator *m*, M. pronator.
pronator muscle → pronator.
   quadrate p. → pronator quadratus (muscle).
   round p. → pronator teres (muscle).
pronator quadratus (muscle) Pronator *m* quadratus, M. pronator quadratus.
pronator teres (muscle) Pronator *m* teres, M. pronator teres.
pronator teres syndrome Pronator-teres--Syndrom *nt*.
prone [prəun] *adj* **1.** proniert, auf dem Bauch liegend, mit dem Gesicht nach unten liegend; (flach) hingestreckt liegend. **2.** *fig.* tendierend *od.* neigend (*to* zu). **3.** geneigt, gebeugt. **4.** mit nach unten gedrehter Handfläche.
prone·ness ['prəunɪs] *n* Neigung *f*, Hang *m*, Veranlagung *f* (*to* zu).
pro·neph·ric [prəu'nefrɪk] *adj embryo.* Vorniere/Pronephros betr., pronephrogen, Vornieren-.
pronephric duct *embryo.* Vornierengang *m*.
pronephric system *embryo.* Vornierensystem *nt*.
pro·neph·ron [prəu'nefrən, -rɑn] *n* → pronephros.
pro·neph·ros [prəu'nefrəs, -rɑs] *n, pl* **-ra** [-rə], **-roi** [-rɔɪ] *embryo.* Vorniere *f*, Pronephros *m*.
prone position Bauchlagerung *f*, -lage *f*.
pro·nor·mo·blast [prəu'nɔːrməblæst] *n* Proerythroblast *m*, Pronormoblast *m*.
pro·nu·cle·us [prəu'n(j)uːklɪəs] *n, pl* **-cle·i** [-klɪaɪ] *embryo.* Vorkern *m*, Pronukleus *m*, Pronucleus *m*.
pro·o·pi·o·me·lan·o·cor·tin [prəu,əupɪəu,melənəu'kɔːrtɪn, -mə,læn-] *n abbr.* POMC Proopiomelanocortin *nt abbr.* POMC.
proopiomelanocortin cells Proopiomelanocortinzellen *pl*, POMC-Zellen *pl*.
prop [prɑp] **I** *n* (*a. fig.*) Stütze *f*, Halt *m*. **II** *vt* (ab-)stützen, halten.
   prop up *vt* → prop II.
prop·a·gate ['prɑpəgeɪt] **I** *vt* **1.** (*Lehre*) verbreiten, propagieren. **2.** (*Krankheit*) übertragen. **3.** (*Schall, Licht*) weiter-, fortleiten, übertragen. **4.** ~ **o.s.** *s.* vermehren *od.* fortpflanzen. **II** *vi* **5.** *s.* fortpflanzen *od.* vermehren. **6.** *s.* aus- *od.* verbreiten.
prop·a·ga·tion [,prɑpə'geɪʃn] *n* **1.** *allg.* Vermehrung *f*, Ausbreitung *f*; (*Lehre*) Propagierung *f*. **2.** (*Seuche*) Übertragung *f*, Verbreitung *f*, Propagation *f*. **3.** (*Licht, Schall*) Fort-, Weiterleitung *f*, Übertragung *f*. **4.** Vermehrung *f*, Fortpflanzung *f*.
propagation velocity Weiter-, Fortleitungsgeschwindigkeit *f*.
prop·a·ga·tive ['prɑpəgeɪtɪv] *adj* ver-, ausbreitend; weiter-, fortleitend; (s.) fortpflanzend, Fortpflanzungs-.
propagative body *micro.* Brutkörper *m*.
prop·a·gule ['prɑpəgjuːl] *n* → propagative body.
pro·pag·u·lum [prəu'pægjələm] *n* → propagative body.
pro·pane ['prəupeɪn] *n* Propan *nt*.
pro·pan·i·did [prəu'pænədɪd] *n anes.* Propanidid *nt*.
pro·pa·no·ic acid [,prəupə'nəuɪk] → propionic acid.
pro·pan·the·line bromide [prəu'pænθəliːn] *pharm.* Propanthelinbromid *nt*.
prop cell → Purkinje's cell.
pro·pe·deu·tic [,prəupɪ'd(j)uːtɪk] *adj* vorbereitend, einführend, propädeutisch.
pro·pe·deu·tics [,-'d(j)uːtɪks] *pl* vorbereitende Einführung *f*, Propädeutik *f*.
pro·pene ['prəupiːn] *n* → propylene.
pro·pep·sin [prəu'pepsɪn] *n* → pepsinogen.
prop·er [prɑpər] *adj* **1.** eigen (*to*); *anat.* proprius. **2.** richtig, passend, ordnungsgemäß. **3.** wirklich, echt, richtig. **4.** korrekt, einwandfrei; genau, exakt.
proper coat → propria.
   p. of corium/dermis Geflechtschicht *f*, Stratum reticulare corii/dermidis.
prop·er·din [prəu'pɜrdɪn, 'prəupərdɪn] *n* Properdin *nt*.
properdin pathway/system Properdin--System *nt*, alternativer Weg *m* der Komplimentaktivierung.
proper fasciculi Grundbündel *pl*, Fasciculi proprii.
   p. of spinal cord Binnen-, Elementar-, Grundbündel *pl* des Rückenmarks, Intersegmentalfaszikel *pl*, Fasciculi proprii (medullae spinalis).
   anterior p. of spinal cord Fasciculi proprii anteriores/ventrales (medullae spinalis).
   dorsal p. of spinal cord Fasciculi proprii dorsales/posteriores (medullae spinalis).
   lateral p. of spinal cord Fasciculi proprii laterales (medullae spinalis).
   posterior p. of spinal cord → dorsal p. of spinal cord.
   ventral p. of spinal cord → anterior p. of spinal cord.
proper fungi *micro.* echte Pilze *pl*, Eumyzeten *pl*, Eumycophyta *pl*.
pro·per·i·to·ne·al [,prəupɛrɪtə'niːəl] *adj* präperitoneal.
proper ligament of ovary Eierstockband *nt*, *old* Chorda utero-ovarica, Lig. ovarii proprium.
proper membrane of semicircular duct äußere Bogengangsmembran *f*, Membrana propria ductus semicircularis.
proper substance: p. of cornea Grund-/Hauptschicht *f* der Hornhaut, Substantia propria corneae.
   p. of sclera Hauptschicht *f* der Sklera, Substantia propria sclerae.
proper tunic → propria.
prop·er·ty ['prɑpərtɪ] *n, pl* **-ties 1.** Eigentum *nt*, Besitz *m*. **2.** *phys.* Eigenschaft *f*. **3.** Fähigkeit *f*, Vermögen *nt*.
pro·phage ['prəufeɪdʒ] *n micro.* Prophage *m*.
pro·phase ['prəufeɪz] *n* Prophase *f*.
prophase banding *genet.* hochauflösendes Banding *nt*.
pro·phen·py·rid·a·mine [,prəufenpaɪ'rɪdəmiːn] *n* → pheniramine.
pro·phy·lac·tic [,prəufə'læktɪk, ,prɑfə-] **I** *n* **1.** vorbeugendes Mittel *nt*, Prophylaktikum *nt*. **2.** vorbeugende Maßnahme *f*. **3.** Präservativ *nt*, Kondom *nt*. **II** *adj* vorbeugend, prophylaktisch, Vorbeugungs-, Schutz-.
prophylactic antibiotics Antibiotikaprophylaxe *f*.
prophylactic treatment vorbeugende/prophylaktische Behandlung *f*.

pro·phy·lax·is [,prəufə'læksɪk, ,prɑfə-] *n* vorbeugende Behandlung *f*, Präventivbehandlung *f*, Vorbeugung *f*, Prophylaxe *f*.
pro·pi·cil·lin [,prəupɪ'sɪlɪn] *n pharm.* Propicillin *nt*, Phenoxypropylpenicillin *nt*.
pro·pi·o·nate ['prəupɪəneɪt] *n* Propionat *nt*.
propionate carboxylase → propionyl--CoA carboxylase.
Pro·pi·on·i·bac·te·ri·a·ce·ae [,prəupɪɑnɪbæk,tɪərɪ'eɪsɪ,iː, -əuni,-] *pl micro.* Propionibacteriaceae *pl*.
Pro·pi·on·i·bac·te·ri·um [,-bæk'tɪərɪəm] *n micro.* Propionibacterium *nt*.
pro·pi·on·ic acid [,prəupɪ'ɑnɪk, -'əunɪk] Propionsäure *f*, Propansäure *f*.
propionic acidemia Propionazidämie *f*.
pro·pi·o·ni·trile [,prəupɪəu'naɪtrɪl, -triːl, -traɪl] *n* Propionitril *nt*, Äthylzyanid *nt*, Ethylcyanid *nt*.
pro·pi·o·nyl ['prəupɪənɪl, -niːl] *n* Propionyl-(Radikal *nt*).
propionyl-CoA carboxylase Propionyl--CoA-carboxylase *f*.
pro·plas·min [prəu'plæzmɪn] *n* → plasminogen.
pro·plas·tid [prəu'plæstɪd] *n bio.* Proplastide *f*.
pro·por·phy·rin·o·gen oxidase [prəu,pɔːrfə'rɪnədʒən] → protoporphyrinogen oxidase.
pro·por·tion [prə'pɔːrʃn, -'pəur-] *n* **1.** (*a. chem., mathe.*) Verhältnis *nt*, Proportion *f*. **in ~ to** im Verhältnis zu. **to be in ~** im Verhältnis stehen (*to, with* zu; *to one another* zueinander). **to be out of ~** in keinem Verhältnis stehen (*to, with* zu; *to one another* zueinander). **2.** (verhältnismäßiger) Anteil *m*. **in ~ anteilig. 3.** Symmetrie *f*, Ebenmaß *nt*. **4.** **~s** *pl* Ausmaße *pl*, Dimentionen *pl*.
pro·por·tion·al [prə'pɔːrʃnəl, -'pəur-] *adj* proportional (*to* zu); anteilmäßig (*to* zu); verhältnismäßig, Proportions-, Proportional-, Verhältnis-.
proportional-differential sensor *physiol.* Proportional-Differentialsensor *m*, PD--Sensor *m*.
pro·por·tion·al·i·ty [prə,pɔːrʃə'nælətɪ, -,pəur-] *n* Verhältnis(mäßigkeit *f*) *nt*, Proportionalität *f*.
proportionality constant Proportionalitätskonstante *f*.
proportional number *stat.* Verhältniszahl *f*.
proportional response *physiol.* proportionale/statische/tonische Antwort *f*.
proportional sensor *physiol.* Proportionalsensor *m*, P-Sensor *m*.
pro·por·tion·ate [prə'pɔːrʃənɪt, -'pəur-] *adj* proportional, proportioniert, im richtigen Verhätnis stehend (*to* zu); angemessen.
proportionate infantilism proportionierter Zwergwuchs/Minderwuchs *m*.
pro·pran·o·lol [prəu'prænəlɒl, -əul] *n pharm.* Propranolol *nt*.
pro·pria ['prɑprɪə] *n* Propria *f*, Tunica propria.
propria mucosa Propria *f* mucosae, Lamina propria mucosae.
pro·pri·e·tar·y [prə'praɪəterɪ] **I** *n pharm.* Markenartikel *m*. **II** *adj* gesetzlich geschützt, Marken-.
proprietary name Markenname *m*.
pro·pri·o·cep·tion [,prəuprɪə'sepʃn] *n* proprio(re)zeptive/kinästhetische Sensibilität *f*, Tiefensensibilität *f*, Proprio(re)zeption *f*.
pro·pri·o·cep·tive [,-'septɪv] *adj* Körpereigenempfindungen aufnehmend, proprio(re)zeptiv.

proprioceptive nervous system

proprioceptive nervous system proprio(re)zeptives System *nt*.
proprioceptive reflex propriozeptiver Reflex *m*, Eigenreflex *m*.
proprioceptive sense → proprioception.
proprioceptive sensibility → proprioception.
proprioceptive stimuli proprio(re)zeptive Reize/Stimuli *pl*.
pro·pri·o·cep·tor [ˌ-'septər] *n* Proprio(re)zeptor *m*.
pro·pri·o·spi·nal tract [ˌ-'spaɪnl] propriospinale Bahn *f*.
pro·pro·tein [prəʊ'prəʊtiːn, -tiːɪn] *n* Proprotein *nt*.
prop·tom·e·ter [prap'tamɪtər] *n* ophthal. Exophthalmometer *nt*.
prop·to·sis [prap'təʊsɪs] *n* ophthal. Glotzauge *nt*, Exophthalmus *m*, Exophthalmos *m*, Exophthalmie *f*, Ophthalmoptose *f*, Proptosis/Protrusio bulbi.
pro·pul·sion [prə'pʌlʃn] *n* 1. (*a. fig.*) Antrieb *m*; Antriebskraft *f*; Vorwärts-, Fortbewegung *f*. 2. *patho.* Propulsion *f*.
pro·pul·sive [prə'pʌlsɪv] *adj* (*a. fig.*) vorantreibend, vorwärtsdrängend, -treibend, propulsiv.
propulsive peristalsis propulsive Peristaltik *f*.
pro·pyl ['prəʊpɪl] *n* Propyl-(Radikal *nt*).
pro·pyl·ene ['prəʊpəliːn] *n* Propylen *nt*, Propen *nt*.
pro·pyl·i·o·done [ˌprəʊpɪl'aɪədəʊn] *n* radiol. Propyliodon *nt*.
2-propyl-pentanoic acid *pharm.* Valproinsäure *f*, Dipropylessigsäure *f*.
pro·pyl·thi·o·ur·a·cil [ˌ-ˌθaɪəʊ'jʊərəsɪl] *n abbr.* **PTU** *pharm.* Propylthiouracil *nt*.
pro·qua·zone ['prəʊkwəzəʊn] *n pharm.* Proquazon *nt*.
pro·ren·nin [prəʊ'renɪn] *n* Prorennin *nt*.
pro·ru·bri·cyte [prəʊ'ruːbrəsaɪt] *n* basophiler Normoblast *m*.
pros·cil·lar·i·din [prəʊsɪl'ærədɪn] *n pharm.* Proscillaridin *nt*.
pro·se·cre·tin [ˌprəʊsɪ'kriːtɪn] *n* Prosekretin *nt*.
pro·se·cre·to·ry [ˌprəʊsɪ'kriːtəri] *adj* → presecretory.
pro·sec·tor's wart [prəʊ'sektər] Wilk'-Krankheit *f*, warzige Tuberkulose *f* der Haut, Leichentuberkel *m*, Schlachtertuberkulose *f*, Tuberculosis cutis verrucosa, Verruca necrogenica, Tuberculum anatomicum.
pros·en·ceph·a·lic fasciculus, medial [ˌprasənse'fælɪk] mediales Vorderhirnbündel *nt*, Fasciculus prosencephalicus medialis.
pros·en·ceph·a·lon [ˌprasən'sefələn, -lan] *n, pl* **-la** [-lə] Vorderhirn *nt*, Prosenzephalon *nt*, Prosencephalon *nt*.
prosencephalon vesicle *embryo.* Vorderhirnbläschen *nt*.
pros·o·gas·ter ['prasəgæstər] *n embryo.* Kopf-, Vorderdarm *m*.
prosop- *pref.* → prosopo-.
pros·op·ag·no·sia [ˌprasəpæg'nəʊʒ(ɪ)ə, -zɪə] *n neuro.* Prosopagnosie *f*.
pro·sop·a·gus [prəʊ'sapəgəs] *n* → prosopopagus.
pros·o·pal·gia [ˌprasə'pældʒ(ɪ)ə] *n* Gesichtsneuralgie *f*, Prosopalgie *f*; Trigeminusneuralgie *f*.
pros·o·phe·no·sia [ˌprasəfɪ'nəʊsɪə] *n* → prosopagnosia.
prosopo- *pref.* Gesichts-, Prosop(o)-.
pros·o·po·a·nos·chi·sis [ˌprasəpəʊə'naskɪsɪs] *n embryo.* Wangenspalte *f*, Meloschisis *f*.
pros·o·po·di·ple·gia [ˌ-daɪ'pliːdʒ(ɪ)ə] *n* beidseitige Gesichtslähmung/Fazialislähmung *f*, Prosopodiplegie *f*.
pros·o·po·dys·mor·phia [ˌ-dɪs'mɔːrfɪə] *n neuro.* Romberg(-Parry)-Syndrom *nt*, Romberg-Trophoneurose *f*, progressive halbseitige Gesichtsatrophie *f*, Hemiatrophia faciei/facialis progressiva, Atrophia (hemi-)facialis.
pros·o·po·neu·ral·gia [ˌ-njʊə'rældʒ(ɪ)ə, -nʊ-] *n* → prosopalgia.
pros·o·pop·a·gus [prasə'papəgəs] *n embryo.* Prosopopagus *m*.
pros·o·po·ple·gia [ˌprasəpəʊ'pliːdʒ(ɪ)ə] *n* Fazialislähmung *f*, -parese *f*, Fazioplegie *f*, Prosopoplegie *f*.
pros·o·pos·chi·sis [prasə'paskəsɪs] *n embryo.* Gesichtsspalte *f*, Prosoposchisis *f*, Fissura facialis.
pros·o·po·spasm ['prasəpəʊspæzəm] *n* Bell-Spasmus *m*, Fazialiskrampf *m*, Gesichtszucken *nt*, mimischer Gesichtskrampf *m*, Fazialis-Tic *m*, Tic convulsif/facial.
pros·o·pos·ter·no·dy·mus [ˌ-ˌstɜrnəʊ'daɪməs] *n embryo.* Prosoposternodymus *m*.
pros·o·po·tho·ra·cop·a·gus [ˌ-ˌθɔːrə'kapəgəs, -ˌθɔː-] *n embryo.* Prosopothorakopagus *m*.
pros·pect ['praspekt] *n fig.* Aussicht *f* (*of* auf).
pro·spec·tive [prə'spektɪv] *adj* voraussichtlich, (zu-)künftig, Prospektiv-.
prospective study/trial *stat.* Prospektivstudie *f*.
pros·ta·cy·clin [ˌprastə'saɪklɪn] *n* Prostazyklin *nt*, -cyclin *nt*, Prostaglandin I₂ *f abbr.* PGI₂.
prostacyclin synthetase Prostazyklinsynthetase *f*.
pros·ta·glan·din [ˌ-'glændɪn] *n abbr.* **PG** Prostaglandin *nt abbr.* PG.
prostaglandin D₂ *abbr.* **PGD₂** Prostaglandin D₂ *nt abbr.* PGD₂.
prostaglandin E₁ *abbr.* **PGE₁** Prostaglandin E₁ *nt abbr.* PGE₁, Alprostadil *nt*.
prostaglandin E₂ *abbr.* **PGE₂** Prostaglandin E₂ *nt abbr.* PGE₂, Dinoproston *nt*.
prostaglandin endoperoxide synthase Prostaglandinsynthase *f*, Prostaglandinendoperoxidsynthase *f*.
prostaglandin F₂α *abbr.* **PGF₂α** Prostaglandin F₂α *nt abbr.* PGF₂α, Dinoprost *nt*.
prostaglandin H₂ *abbr.* **PGH₂** Prostaglandin H₂ *nt abbr.* PGH₂.
prostaglandin I₂ *abbr.* **PGI₂** → prostacyclin.
prostaglandin synthase → prostaglandin endoperoxide synthase.
pros·ta·no·ic acid [ˌprastə'nəʊɪk] Prostansäure *f*.
pro·sta·ta ['prastətə] *n* → prostate I.
pros·ta·tal·gia [ˌprastə'tældʒ(ɪ)ə] *n* → prostatodynia.
pros·ta·taux·e [ˌ-'tɔːksɪ] *n* Prostatavergrößerung *f*.
pros·tate ['prasteɪt] **I** *n* Vorsteherdrüse *f*, Prostata(drüse *f*) *f*, Gl. prostatica. **II** → prostatic.
pros·ta·tec·to·my [ˌprastə'tektəmɪ] *n urol.* Prostataentfernung *f*, Prostatektomie *f*.
prostate gland Vorsteherdrüse *f*, Prostata(drüse *f*) *f*, Gl. prostatica.
external p. äußere Prostatadrüse.
inner/periurethral p. innere/periurethrale Prostatadrüse.
prostate tuberculosis Prostatatuberkulose *f*, Prostatitis tuberculosa.
pros·tat·ic [pras'tætɪk] *adj* Prostata betr., von ihr ausgehend, prostatisch, Prostat(a)-.
prostatic adenocarcinoma Adenokarzinom *nt* der Prostata.
prostatic adenoma (benigne) Prostatahypertrophie *f*, -hyperplasie *f*, Prostataadenom *nt*, Blasenhalsadenom *nt*, Blasenhalskropf *m*, Adenomyomatose *f* der Prostata.
prostatic branches of inferior vesical artery Prostataäste *pl* der A. vesicalis inferior, Rami prostatici a. vesicalis inferioris.
prostatic calculus Prostatastein *m*, -konkrement *nt*, Prostatolith *m*.
prostatic carcinoma Prostatakrebs *m*, -karzinom *nt*.
prostatic capsule Prostatakapsel *f*, Capsula prostatica.
surgical p. chirurgische Prostatakapsel, Pseudokapsel der Prostata.
prostatic catheter gebogener (Harn-)Blasenkatheter *m*.
prostatic concrement → prostatic calculus.
prostatic concretions Amyloidkörperchen *pl*, Corpora amylacea.
prostatic ducts → prostatic ductules.
postatic ductules Ausführungsgänge *pl* der Prostatadrüsen, Ductuli prostatici.
prostatic fascia Prostatafaszie *f*, Fascia prostatae.
prostatic hyperplasia → prostatic hypertrophy.
prostatic hypertrophy Prostatavergrößerung *f*.
adenomatous/benign/nodular p. → prostatic adenoma.
pros·tat·i·co·ves·i·cal [pras,tætɪkəʊ'vesɪkl] *adj* Prostata u. (Harn-)Blase betr.
prostatic part of urethra Prostataabschnitt *m* der Harnröhre, Pars prostatica.
prostatic plexus 1. Prostataplexus *m*, Plexus prostaticus. **2.** venöser Prostataplexus *m*, Plexus venosus prostaticus.
prostatic secretion Prostatasekret *nt*.
prostatic sinus Prostatasinus *m*, -rinne *f*, Sinus prostaticus.
prostatic stone → prostatic calculus.
pros·ta·tit·ic [ˌprastə'tɪtɪk] *adj* Prostatitis betr., prostatitisch.
prostatic utricle Prostatablindsack *m*, Utrikulus *m*, Utriculus prostaticus.
pros·ta·ti·tis [ˌ-'taɪtɪs] *n* Prostataentzündung *f*, Prostatitis *f*.
pros·ta·to·cys·ti·tis [ˌprastətəʊsɪs'taɪtɪs] *n* Entzündung *f* von Prostata u. Harnblase, Prostatozystitis *f*.
pros·ta·to·cys·tot·o·my [ˌ-sɪs'tatəmɪ] *n chir., urol.* Prostatozystotomie *f*.
pros·ta·to·dyn·ia [ˌ-'diːnɪə] *n* Prostataschmerz *m*, Prostatodynie *f*.
pros·ta·to·lith [pras'tætəlɪθ] *n* Prostatastein *m*, -konkrement *nt*, Prostatolith *m*.
pros·ta·to·li·thot·o·my [ˌprastətəʊlɪ'θatəmɪ] *n* Prostatolithotomie *f*.
pros·ta·to·meg·a·ly [ˌ-'megəlɪ] *n* → prostatic hypertrophy.
pros·tat·o·my [pras'tætəmɪ] *n* → prostatotomy.
pros·ta·tor·rhe·a [ˌprastətə'rɪə] *n urol.* Prostatorrhoe *f*.
pros·ta·tot·o·my [prastə'tatəmɪ] *n urol.* Prostatotomie *f*.
pros·the·sis [pras'θɪsɪs, 'prasθɪsɪs] *n, pl* **-ses** [-siːz] Prothese *f*, Gliedersatz *m*, Kunstglied *nt*.
pros·thet·ic [pras'θetɪk] *adj* Prothese od. Prothetik betr., prothetisch, Prothesen-.
prosthetic dentistry → prosthodontics.
prosthetic group *chem.* prosthetische Gruppe *f*.
pros·thet·ics [pras'θetɪks] *pl* Prothetik *f*, Zahnersatz-, Gliederersatzkunde *f*.
prosthetic valve *HTG* Herzklappenprothese *f*, -ersatz *m*, künstliche Herzklappe *f*.

pros·the·tist ['prɒsθɪtɪst] *n* Orthopädietechniker(in *f*) *m*.
pros·tho·don·tia [ˌprɒsθə'dɒnʃ(ɪ)ə] *n* → prosthodontics.
pros·tho·don·tics [ˌ-'dɒntɪks] *pl* Zahntechnik *f*, Zahnersatzkunde *f*, zahnärztliche Prothetik *f*.
pros·tho·don·tist [ˌ-'dɒntɪst] *n* Zahnprothetiker(in *f*) *m*.
pros·tra·tion [prɒʊ'streɪʃn] *n* extreme Erschöpfung *f*, extreme Kraftlosigkeit *f*, Prostration *f*.
prot- *pref.* → proto-.
prot·ac·tin·i·um [ˌprɒʊtæk'tɪnɪəm] *n abbr.* Pa Protactinium *nt abbr.* Pa.
pro·ta·gon ['prɒʊtəgæn] *n* Protagon *nt*.
pro·tam·i·nase [prɒʊ'tæmɪneɪz] *n* Carboxypeptidase B *f*.
prot·a·mine ['prɒʊtəmiːn, prɒ'tæmɪn] *n* Protamin *nt*.
protamine chloride Protaminchlorid *nt*.
protamine sulfate Protaminsulfat *nt*.
pro·tan ['prɒʊtæn] *ophthal.* **I** *n* **1.** Protanomale(r *m*) *f*. **2.** Protanope(r *m*) *f*. **II** *adj* **3.** Protanomalie betr., protanomal. **4.** Protanopie betr., rotblind, protanop.
prot·an·drous [prɒʊt'ændrəs] *adj bio.* vormännlich, protandrisch, proterandrisch.
prot·an·dry [prɒʊt'ændrɪ] *n bio.* Vormännlichkeit *f*, Protandrie *f*, Proterandrie *f*.
prot·a·nom·al [ˌprɒʊtə'nɒməl] *n ophthal.* Protanomale(r *m*) *f*.
prot·a·nom·a·lous [ˌ-'nɒmələs] *adj* Protanomalie betr., protanomal.
prot·a·nom·a·ly [ˌ-'nɒməlɪ] *n ophthal.* Rotschwäche *f*, Protanomalie *f*.
pro·ta·nope ['-nɒʊp] *n ophthal.* Rotblinde(r *m*) *f*, Protanope(r *m*) *f*.
pro·ta·no·pia [ˌ-'nɒʊpɪə] *n ophthal.* Rotblindheit *f*, Protanopie *f*, Protanopsie *f*.
pro·ta·nop·ic [ˌ-'nɒpɪk] *adj ophthal.* Protanopie betr., rotblind, protanop.
pro·ta·nop·sia [ˌ-'nɒpsɪə] *n* → protanopia.
prote- *pref.* → proteo-.
pro·te·ase ['prɒʊtɪeɪz] *n* → proteinase.
protease sensitive antigen Pr-Antigen *nt*.
pro·tect [prɒ'tekt] **I** *vt* (be-)schützen (*from* vor; *against* gegen); (ab-)sichern. **II** *vi* schützen (*against* vor).
pro·tect·ing reagent [prɒ'tektɪŋ] *biochem.* Schutz-, Blockierungsreagenz *nt*.
pro·tec·tion [prɒ'tekʃn] *n* Schutz *m*, Beschützung *f* (*from* vor; *against* gegen).
protection test Neutralisationstest *m*.
pro·tec·tive [prɒ'tektɪv] *adj* **1.** (be-)schützend, Schutz-. **2.** beschützerisch (*towards* gegenüber).
protective antibody protektiver Antikörper *m*.
protective appendicitis obliterierende Appendizitis *f*, Appendicitis obliterans.
protective clothing Schutzkleidung *f*.
protective goggles Schutzbrille *f*.
protective instinct Beschützerinstinkt *m*.
protective protein Schutzprotein *nt*.
protective reflex *physiol.* Schutzreflex *m*.
protective spectacles Schutzbrille *f*.
pro·tec·tor [prɒ'tektər] *n* Schutz *m*, Schutzvorrichtung *f*, -mittel *nt*, Schützer *m*.
pro·teid ['prɒʊtiːd, -tiːɪd] *n* → protein I.
pro·te·id·ic [prɒʊtɪ'ɪdɪk] *adj* Protein(e) betr., Protein-.
pro·tein ['prɒʊtiːn, -tiːɪn] **I** *n* Eiweiß *nt*, Protein *nt*. **II** *adj* eiweiß-, proteinartig, eiweiß-, proteinhaltig, Protein-, Eiweiß-.
protein A Protein A *nt*.
pro·te·in·a·ceous [ˌprɒʊtɪ(ɪ)'neɪʃəs] *adj* Protein betr., proteinartig, Protein-, Eiweiß-.
pro·tein·ase ['prɒʊtɪ(ɪ)neɪz] *n* Proteinase *f*, Protease *f*.
pro·tein·ate buffer (system) ['prɒʊtɪ(ɪ)neɪt] Protein(at)puffer *m*, Protein(at)puffersystem *nt*.
protein balance Proteinbilanz *f*, -haushalt *m*, Eiweißbilanz *f*, -haushalt *m*.
protein biosynthesis Proteinbiosynthese *f*.
protein-bound iodine *abbr.* **PBI** proteingebundenes Jod/Iod *nt abbr.* PBI.
protein-bound iodine test PBI-Test *m*.
protein breakdown Eiweißabbau *m*.
protein buffer (system) Protein(at)puffer *m*, Protein(at)puffersystem *nt*.
protein C Protein C *nt*.
protein-caloric malnutrition Protein--Energie-Mangelsyndrom *nt abbr.* PEM.
protein cast *urol.* Protein-, Eiweißzylinder *m*.
protein coat *micro.* Proteinhülle *f*.
protein electrophoresis *lab.* Proteinelektrophorese *f*.
pro·tein·e·mia [ˌprɒʊtɪ(ɪ)'niːmɪə] *n* erhöhter Proteingehalt *m* des Blutes, Proteinämie *f*.
protein fraction *biochem.* Protein-, Eiweißfraktion *f*.
protein-glutamine γ-glutamyltransferase Faktor XIIIa *m*.
protein hormone Proteinhormon *nt*.
pro·tein·ic [prɒʊ'tiːnɪk, ˌprɒʊtɪ'ɪnɪk] *adj* Protein betr., Eiweiß-, Protein-.
protein kinase *old* Phosphorylasekinase--kinase *f*, Proteinkinase *f*.
protein-losing enteropathy eiweißverlierende/exsudative Enteropathie/Gastroenteropathie *f*, Eiweißverlustsyndrom *nt*.
protein malabsorption Eiweiß-, Proteinmalabsorption *f*.
protein malnutrition *ped.* Kwashiorkor *nt*.
protein matrix Protein-, Eiweißmatrix *f*.
protein metabolism → proteometabolism.
pro·te·in·o·chrome [ˌprɒʊtɪ'ɪnəkrɒʊm] *n* Proteinochrom *nt*.
pro·tei·nog·e·nous [ˌprɒʊtɪ(ɪ)'nɒdʒənəs] *adj* von Proteinen abstammend, aus Proteinen gebildet, proteinogen.
pro·tei·noid ['-nɔɪd] *n* Proteinoid *nt*.
pro·tei·no·sis [ˌ-'nɒʊsɪs] *n* Proteinose *f*.
protein-polysaccharide *n* Proteinpolysaccharid *nt*.
protein-shell *n* Proteinhülle *f*.
protein structure Proteinstruktur *f*.
protein synthesis Protein-, Eiweißsynthese *f*.
protein synthesis inhibitor Proteinsynthesehemmer *m*.
pro·tein·u·ria [ˌ-'n(j)ʊərɪə] *n* Eiweißausscheidung *f* im Harn, Proteinurie *f*, Albuminurie *f*.
pro·tein·u·ric [ˌ-'n(j)ʊərɪk] *adj* Proteinurie betr., proteinurisch, albuminurisch.
proteo- *pref.* Protein-, Prote(o)-.
pro·te·o·clas·tic [ˌprɒʊtɪɒ'klæstɪk] *adj* eiweißspaltend, proteoklastisch.
pro·te·o·gly·can [ˌ-'glaɪkæn] *n* Proteoglykan *nt*.
pro·te·o·hor·mone [ˌ-'hɔːrmɒʊn] *n* Proteo-, Polypeptidhormon *nt*.
pro·te·o·lip·id [ˌ-'lɪpɪd, -'laɪ-] *n* Proteolipid *nt*.
pro·te·o·lip·in [ˌ-'lɪpɪn] *n* → proteolipid.
pro·te·ol·y·sis [ˌprɒʊtɪ'ɒləsɪs] *n* Protein-, Eiweißspaltung *f*, Proteolyse *f*.
pro·te·o·lyt·ic [ˌprɒʊtɪɒ'lɪtɪk] **I** *n* proteolytisches Enzym *nt*; Proteinase *f*, Protease *f*. **II** *adj* Proteolyse betr., eiweißspaltend, proteolytisch.
proteolytic enzyme proteolytisches Enzym *nt*; Proteinase *f*, Protease *f*.
pro·te·o·me·tab·o·lic [ˌ-ˌmetə'bɒlɪk] *adj* Eiweißstoffwechsel betr.
pro·te·o·me·tab·o·lism [ˌ-mə'tæbəlɪzəm] *n* Proteinstoffwechsel *m*, -metabolismus *m*, Eiweißstoffwechsel *m*, -metabolismus *m*.
Pro·te·o·my·ces [ˌ-'maɪsiːz] *n micro.* Trichosporon *nt*.
pro·te·o·pec·tic [ˌ-'pektɪk] *adj* → proteopexic.
pro·te·o·pep·sis [ˌ-'pepsɪs] *n* Eiweißverdauung *f*.
pro·te·o·pep·tic [ˌ-'peptɪk] *adj* eiweißverdauend, proteopeptisch.
pro·te·o·pex·ic [ˌ-'peksɪk] *adj biochem.* eiweißeinlagernd, -fixierend.
pro·te·o·pex·y ['-peksɪ] *n biochem.* Fixierung/Einlagerung *f* von Eiweiß.
pro·te·ose ['prɒʊtɪɒʊs] *n* Proteose *f*.
pro·ter·an·drous [ˌprɒʊtər'ændrəs, ˌprɒ-] *adj* → protandrous.
pro·ter·an·dry [ˌ-'ændrɪ] *n* → protandry.
pro·te·rog·y·nous [ˌprɒtə'rɒdʒənəs] *adj* → protogynous.
pro·te·rog·y·ny [ˌprɒtə'rɒdʒənɪ] *n* → protogyny.
pro·te·u·ria [ˌprɒʊtɪ'(j)ʊərɪə] *n* → proteinuria.
pro·te·u·ric [ˌ-'(j)ʊərɪk] *adj* → proteinuric.
Pro·te·us ['prɒʊtɪəs, -tjuːs] *n micro.* Proteus *m*.
pro·te·us ['prɒʊtɪəs, -tjuːs] *n, pl* **-tei** [-tɪaɪ] *micro.* Proteus *m*.
pro·thion·am·ide [prɒʊˌθaɪən'æmaɪd] *n pharm.* Prothionamid *m*.
pro·thi·pen·dyl [prɒʊ'θaɪpendɪl] *n pharm.* Prothipendyl *m*.
pro·throm·bin [prɒʊ'θræmbɪn] *n* Prothrombin *nt*, Faktor II *m abbr.* FII.
prothrombin activator Thrombokinase *f*, -plastin *nt*, Prothrombinaktivator *m*.
pro·throm·bin·ase [prɒʊ'θræmbɪneɪz] *n* → prothrombin activator.
prothrombinase complex Prothrombinasekomplex *m*.
prothrombin-consumption test Prothrombin-Konsumptionstest *m*.
prothrombin conversion factor Prokonvertin *nt*, -convertin *nt*, Faktor VII *m abbr.* F V II, Autothrombin I *nt*, Serum--Prothrombin-Conversion-Accelerator *m abbr.* SPCA, stabiler Faktor *m*.
prothrombin converting factor → prothrombin conversion factor.
pro·throm·bi·no·pe·nia [prɒʊˌθræmbɪnɒʊ'piːnɪə] *n* Faktor-II-Mangel *m*, Hypoprothrombinämie *f*.
prothrombin test → prothrombin time.
prothrombin time *abbr.* **PT** Thromboplastinzeit *f*, Quickwert *m*, -zeit *f*, *inf.* Quick *m*, Prothrombinzeit *f*.
pro·throm·bo·ki·nase [prɒʊˌθræmbɒʊ'kaɪneɪz, -kɪ-] *n* → prothrombin conversion factor.
pro·tide ['prɒʊtaɪd] *n* → protein I.
pro·ti·de·mia [ˌprɒʊtɪ'diːmɪə] *n* → proteinemia.
pro·tin·i·um [prɒʊ'tɪnɪəm] *n* → protium.
pro·tion·a·mide [ˌprɒʊtɪ'ɒnəmaɪd] *n pharm.* Prothionamid *m*.
pro·ti·re·lin [prɒʊ'taɪrɪlɪn] *n pharm.* Protirelin *nt*.
pro·tist ['prɒʊtɪst] *n bio.* Einzeller *m*, Protist *m*.
Pro·tis·ta [prɒʊ'tɪstə] *pl bio.* Einzeller *pl*, Protisten *pl*, Protista *pl*.
pro·ti·um ['prɒʊtɪəm, -ʃɪəm] *n* leichter Wasserstoff *m*, Protium *nt*.
proto- *pref.* Erst-, Ur-, Prot(o)-.
pro·to·ac·tin·i·um [ˌprɒʊtɒʊæk'tɪnɪəm] *n* → protactinium.
pro·to·cell ['-sel] *n* Proto-, Urzelle *f*.
pro·to·chor·dal knot [ˌ-'kɔːrdl] → primitive knot.
pro·to·col ['-kɒl, -kəl] *n* Protokoll *nt*.

protocoproporphyria

pro·to·cop·ro·por·phyr·ia [ˌ-ˌkɑprəpɔːr-ˈfɪərɪə] *n derm.* Protokoproporphyrie *f.*
pro·to·di·a·stol·ic [ˌ-ˌdaɪəˈstɑlɪk] *adj card.* früh-, protodiastolisch.
protodiastolic gallop *card.* protodiastolischer/diastolischer Galopp *m*, Ventrikelgalopp *m.*
pro·to·du·o·de·num [ˌ-ˌd(j)uːəˈdiːnəm] *n* Protoduodenum *nt.*
pro·to·fi·bril [ˌ-ˈfaɪbrəl, -ˈfɪb-] *n* Elementar-, Protofibrille *f.*
pro·to·gene [ˈ-dʒən] *n* Urgen *nt*, Protogen *nt.*
pro·to·gy·nous [ˌ-ˈdʒaɪnəs] *adj bio.* vorweiblich, protogyn, proterogyn.
pro·tog·y·ny [prəʊˈtɑdʒənɪ] *n bio.* Vorweiblichkeit *f*, Protogynie *f*, Proterogynie *f.*
pro·to·heme [ˈprəʊtəhiːm] *n* Protohäm *nt*, Häm *nt.*
pro·to·hy·dro·gen [ˌ-ˈhaɪdrədʒən] *n* → protium.
Pro·to·mas·tig·i·da [ˌ-mæsˈtɪdʒɪdə] *pl micro.* Kinetoplastida *pl.*
pro·to·mer [ˈ-mər] *n* Protomer *nt.*
pro·tom·e·ter [prəʊˈtɑmɪtər] *n* Exophthalmometer *nt.*
Pro·to·mon·a·di·na [ˌprəʊtəˌmɑnəˈdaɪnə, -ˈdiːnə] *pl micro.* Kinetoplastida *pl.*
pro·ton [ˈprəʊtɑn] *n phys.* Proton *nt.*
proton-absorbing *adj* protonenaufnehmend, -absorbierend.
proton acceptor *chem.* Protonenakzeptor *m.*
proton affinity *chem.* Protonenaffinität *f.*
pro·ton·at·ed [ˈprəʊtneɪtɪd] *adj chem.* protoniert.
pro·to·na·tion [ˌprəʊtəˈneɪʃn] *n chem.* Protonierung *f.*
proton beam Protonenstrahl *m.*
proton beam radiotherapy Protonenstrahltherapie *f.*
proton donor *chem.* Protonendonor *m*, -spender *m.*
pro·to·neph·ron [ˌprəʊtəˈnefrɑn] *n* → pronephros.
pro·to·neph·ros [ˌ-ˈnefrɑs] *n* → pronephros.
proton jump *phys.* Protonensprung *m.*
proton-motive force *biochem.* protonentreibende Kraft *m.*
proton-motive gradient *biochem.* protonentreibender Gradient *m.*
proton number Protonenzahl *f.*
proton pump Protonenpumpe *f.*
proton ray Protonenstrahl *m.*
proton transfer *biochem.* Protonenübertragung *f.*
proton-yielding *adj biochem.* protonenliefernd.
proto-oncogene *n* Protoonkogen *nt.*
pro·to·path·ic [ˌprəʊtəˈpæθɪk] *adj* **1.** ohne erkennbare Ursache (entstanden), unabhängig von anderen Krankheiten, selbständig, idiopathisch; essentiell, primär, genuin. **2.** gestört, entdifferenziert; protopathisch.
protopathic sensibility protopathische Sensibilität *f.*
pro·to·plasm [ˈ-plæzəm] *n* Protoplasma *nt.*
pro·to·plas·mal [ˌ-ˈplæzməl] *adj* → protoplasmic.
pro·to·plas·mat·ic [ˌ-plæzˈmætɪk] *adj* → protoplasmatic.
pro·to·plas·mic [ˌ-ˈplæzmɪk] *adj* Protoplasma betr. *od.* enthaltend, aus Protoplasma bestehend, protoplasmatisch, Protoplasm(a)-.
protoplasmic astrocyte protoplasmatischer/fibrillenarmer Astrozyt *m.*
protoplasmic astrocytoma faserarmes/

protoplasmatisches Astrozytom *nt*, Astrocytoma protoplasmaticum.
protoplasmic streaming (Zyto-)Plasmazirkulation *f*, Zyklosis *f.*
pro·to·plast [ˈ-plæst] *n bio.* Protoplast *m.*
pro·to·por·phyr·ia [ˌ-pɔːrˈfɪərɪə] *n derm.* Protoporphyrie *f*, Protoporphyria *f.*
pro·to·por·phy·rin [ˌ-ˈpɔːrfɪrɪn] *n* Protoporphyrin *nt.*
pro·to·por·phy·rin·o·gen oxidase [ˌ-pɔːrfəˈrɪnədʒən] Protoporphyrinogenoxidase *f.*
pro·to·por·phy·rin·u·ria [ˌ-ˌpɔːrfɪrɪˈn(j)ʊərɪə] *n* Protoporphyrinausscheidung *f* im Harn, Protoporphyrinurie *f.*
pro·to·spasm [ˈ-spæzəm] *n neurol.* Protospasmus *m.*
pro·to·sto·ma [ˌ-ˈstəʊmə] *n embryo.* Urmund *m*, Urdarmöffnung *f*, Blastoporus *m.*
Pro·to·sto·mia [ˌ-ˈstəʊmɪə] *pl bio.* Erst-, Alt-, Urmünder *pl*, Protostomier *pl.*
pro·to·troph·ic [ˌ-ˈtrɑfɪk, -ˈtrəʊ-] *adj bio.* prototroph.
pro·to·type [ˈ-taɪp] *n* Urform *f*, Urtyp *m*, Prototyp *m.*
Pro·to·zoa [ˌ-ˈzəʊə] *pl bio.* Urtierchen *pl*, tierische Einzeller *pl*, Protozoen *pl*, Protozoa *pl.*
pro·to·zoa *pl* → protozoon.
pro·to·zo·al [ˌ-ˈzəʊəl] *adj* Protozoen betr., Protozoen-.
protozoal dysentery Protozoendysenterie *f.*
pro·to·zo·an [ˌ-ˈzəʊən] **I** *n* → protozoon. **II** *adj* → protozoal.
protozoan cyst Protozoenzyste *f.*
pro·to·zo·i·a·sis [ˌ-zəʊˈaɪəsɪs] *n* Protozoeninfektion *f.*
pro·to·zo·on [ˌ-ˈzəʊən, -ˈzəʊɑn] *n*, *pl* **-zoa** [-ˈzəʊə] *bio.* Urtierchen *nt*, Protozoon *nt.*
pro·to·zo·o·sis [ˌ-zəʊˈəʊsɪs] *n* Protozoeninfektion *f.*
pro·tract [prəʊˈtrækt, prə-] *vt* in die Länge ziehen, hinausziehen, hinauszögern, verschleppen, verzögern, verlängern, protrahieren.
pro·tract·ed [prəʊˈtræktɪd, prə-] *adj* verzögert, verlängert, aufgeschoben, protrahiert.
protracted labor → prolonged labor.
pro·trac·tion [prəʊˈtrækʃn, prə-] *n* Hinausschieben *nt*, Hinausziehen *nt*, Hinauszögern *nt*, Verschleppen *nt*, Verzögern *nt*, Verzögerung *f*, Protrahieren *nt*, Protrahierung *f*, Protraktion *f.*
pro·trip·ty·line [prəʊˈtrɪptəliːn] *n pharm.* Protriptylin *nt.*
pro·trude [prəʊˈtruːd, prə-] **I** *vt* herausstrecken. **II** *vi* vorstehen, -ragen, -treten.
pro·trud·ed disk [prəʊˈtruːdɪd, prə-] *ortho.*, *neurochir.* Bandscheibenvorfall *m*, -prolaps *m*, -hernie *f.*
pro·trud·ing (intervertebral) disk [prəʊˈtruːdɪŋ, prə-] Bandscheibenprotrusion *f.*
pro·tru·sion [prəʊˈtruːʒn] *n* **1.** Vorstrecken *nt*, -treten *nt*, Herausragen *nt*. **2.** Vorsprung *m*, Vorwölbung *f*, *anat.* Protrusion *f*, Protrusio *f.*
p. of the acetabulum Protrusio acetabuli.
p. of the bulb *ophthal.* Glotzauge *nt*, Exophthalmus *m*, Exophthalmos *m*, Exophthalmie *f*, Ophthalmoptose *f*, Proptosis/Protrusio bulbi.
p. of the disk Bandscheibenprotrusion.
p. of the eyeball → p. of the bulb.
pro·tru·sive [prəˈtruːsɪv] *adj* hervortretend, vorstehend.
pro·tryp·sin [prəʊˈtrɪpsɪn] *n* Trypsinogen *nt.*
pro·tu·ber·ance [prəʊˈt(j)uːbərəns, prə-] *n* **1.** Vorsprung *m*, (her-)vorstehende Stelle

f. **2.** *anat.* Höcker *m*, Beule *f*, Protuberanz *f*, Protuberantia *f*; (*Knochen*) Apophyse *f.* **3.** (Her-)Vorstehen *nt*, (Her-)Vortreten *nt.*
p. of chin Protuberantia mentalis.
pro·tu·ber·ant [prəʊˈt(j)uːbərənt, prə-] *adj* (her-)vorstehend, -tretend.
pro·tu·ber·an·tia [prəʊˌt(j)uːbəˈrænʃɪə] *n* → protuberance 2.
proud flesh [praʊd] wildes Fleisch *nt*, Caro luxurians.
Proust [ˈpruːst]: **P.'s law** Gesetz *nt* der konstanten Proportionen, Proust-Gesetz *nt*.
P.'s space Proust-Raum *m*, Excavatio rectovesicalis.
Prov·i·den·cia [prɑvəˈdensɪə] *n micro.* Providencia *f.*
pro·vi·ral [prəʊˈvaɪrəl] *adj* proviral.
pro·vi·rus [prəʊˈvaɪrəs] *n micro.* Provirus *nt.*
pro·vi·sion·al [prəˈvɪʒənl] *adj* vorläufig, vorübergehend, provisorisch, Behelfs-.
provisional callus *ortho.* provisorischer Kallus *m.*
pro·vi·ta·min [prəʊˈvaɪtəmɪn; *Brit.* -ˈvɪtə-] *n* Provitamin *nt.*
pro·voc·a·tive test [prəˈvɑkətɪv] Provokation *f*, Provokationstest *m*, -probe *f.*
pro·voked nystagmus [prəʊˈvəʊkt] Provokationsnystagmus *m.*
Prowazek [prɑˈvɑːtsek]: **P.'s bodies** Halberstädter-Prowazek-(Einschluß-)-Körperchen *pl*, Prowazek-(Einschluß-)-Körperchen *pl.*
Prowazek-Greeff [greɪf; greːf]: **P.-G. bodies** → Prowazek's bodies.
prox·i·mal [ˈprɑksɪməl] *adj* rumpfwärts liegend, zur Körpermitte, proximal.
proximal convolution (*Niere*) proximales Konvolut *nt.*
proximal dysphagia oropharyngeale Dysphagie *f.*
proximal fracture of the femur proximale/ hüftgelenksnahe Oberschenkelfraktur *f*, Femurfraktur *f.*
proximal margin of nail Hinterrand *m* des Nagels, Margo occultus unguis.
proximal phalanx proximales Glied *nt*, Grundglied *nt*, -phalanx *f*, Phalanx proximalis.
proximal tubule *histol.* Hauptstück *nt*, proximaler Tubulus *m.*
pro·zone [ˈprəʊzəʊn] *n immun.* Prozone *f.*
prozone reaction Prozonenphänomen *nt.*
PRP *abbr.* → progressive rubella panencephalitis.
PRPP *abbr.* → phosphoribosylpyrophosphate.
prune-belly syndrome [pruːn] ventrales Defektsyndrom *nt*, Bauchdeckenaplasie *f*, Pflaumenbauchsyndrom *nt*, prune-belly syndrome (*nt*).
pru·rig·i·nous [prəˈrɪdʒənəs] *adj* Prurigo betr., prurigoartig, pruriginös; juckend, mit Jucken einhergehend.
pru·ri·go [prəˈraɪɡəʊ] *n derm.* Juckblattersucht *f*, Prurigo *f.*
prurigo gestationis of Besnier Prurigo gestationis/gravidarum.
pru·rit·ic [prəˈrɪtɪk] *adj* Pruritus betr., mit Juckreiz verbunden, juckend.
pru·ri·tus [prəˈraɪtəs] *n* (Haut-)Jucken *nt*, Juckreiz *m*, Pruritus *m.*
Prussak [ˈpruːsɑk]: **P.'s pouch/space** Prussak'-Raum *m*, Rec. (membranae tympanicae) superior.
Prussian blue [ˈprʌʃn] Berliner-Blau *nt*, Ferriferrocyanid *nt.*
Prussian blue reaction Berliner-Blau--Reaktion *f*, Ferriferrocyanid-Reaktion *f.*
Prussian blue stain/test → Prussian blue reaction.

prus·si·ate ['prʌʃɪeɪt, -ɪt, 'prʌs-] n Zyanid nt, Cyanid nt.
prus·sic acid ['prʌsɪk] Blausäure f, Zyan-, Cyanwasserstoff m.
PS abbr. → phosphatidylserine.
psal·te·ri·al cord [sɔːl'tɪərɪəl] Stria vascularis (ductus cochlearis).
psal·te·ri·um [sɔːl'tɪərɪəm] n, pl **-te·ria** [-'tɪərɪə] Fornix-, Hippocampuskommissur, Commissura hippocampi/fornicis.
psamm(o)- pref. Sand-, Psamm(o)-.
psam·mo·car·ci·no·ma [ˌsæmə̩kɑːrsɪ'nəʊmə] n Psammokarzinom nt.
psam·mo·ma [sæ'məʊmə] n, pl **-mas, -mata** [-mətə] Sandgeschwulst f, Psammom nt.
psammoma bodies Sand-, Psammomkörperchen pl.
psam·mom·a·tous [sæ'məʊmətəs, -'mɑm-] adj durch Psammomkörperchen gekennzeichnet.
psam·mo·sar·co·ma [ˌsæməsɑːr'kəʊmə] n Psammosarkom nt.
psam·mo·ther·a·py [ˌ-'θerəpɪ] n Psammotherapie f.
psam·mous ['sæməs] adj sandig.
psel·a·phe·sia [ˌselə'fiːzɪə, -ʒə] n Tastsinn m, Pselaphesie f.
psel·a·phe·sis [ˌ-'fiːsɪs] n → pselaphesia.
psel·lism ['selɪzəm] n Stammeln nt, Stottern nt, Psellismus m.
P sensor → proportional sensor.
pseud- pref. → pseudo-.
pseud·a·cou·sis [ˌsuːdə'kjuːsɪs] n → pseudacousma.
pseud·a·cous·ma [ˌ-'kəʊzmə] n Pseudakusie f.
pseud·ac·ro·meg·a·ly [suːˌdækrə'meɡəlɪ] n Pseudoakromegalie f.
pseud·a·graph·ia [suːdə'ɡræfɪə] n neurol. Pseudoagraphie f.
pseud·al·bu·min·u·ria [ˌsuːdælˌbjuːmɪ'n(j)ʊərɪə] n zyklische/intermittierende Albuminurie f.
pseud·an·gi·na [ˌsuːdæn'dʒaɪnə] n → pseudoangina.
pseud·an·ky·lo·sis [suːˌdæŋkə'ləʊsɪs] n ortho. Pseud(o)ankylose f.
pseud·aph·ia [suː'dæfɪə] n neuro. Störung f des Tastsinns, Parapsis f.
pseud·ar·thro·sis [ˌsuːdɑːr'θrəʊsɪs] n ortho. Falsch-, Schein-, Pseudogelenk nt, Pseudarthrose f.
pseud·en·ceph·a·lus [ˌsuːden'sefələs] n embryo. Pseudenzephalus m.
pseud·es·the·sia [ˌsuːdes'θiːʒ(ɪ)ə] n 1. neuro. Störung f des Tastsinns, Parapsis f. 2. Scheinempfindung f, Pseudästhesie f. 3. Amputationstäuschung f, Phantomschmerz(en pl) m.
pseudo- pref. Falsch-, Schein-, Pseud(o)-.
pseu·do·ac·an·tho·sis [ˌsuːdəˌækən'θəʊsɪs] n derm. Pseudoakanthose f, Pseudoacanthosis f.
pseu·do·a·ceph·a·lus [ˌ-eɪ'sefələs] n embryo. Pseudoazephalus m.
pseu·do·a·chon·dro·pla·sia [ˌ-eɪˌkɒndrəʊ'pleɪʒ(ɪ)ə, -zɪə] n Pseudoachondroplasie f.
pseu·do·ac·i·nus [ˌ-'æsɪnəs] n histol. Pseudoazinus m, -acinus m.
pseu·do·ag·glu·ti·na·tion [ˌ-əˌɡluːtɪ'neɪʃn] n 1. Pseudoagglutination f. 2. Geldrollenbildung f, Pseudo(häm)agglutination f.
pseu·do·a·graph·ia [ˌ-eɪ'ɡræfɪə] n neuro. Pseudoagraphie f.
pseu·do·al·bu·min·u·ri·a [ˌ-ælˌbjuːmɪ'n(j)ʊərɪə] n → pseudalbuminuria.
pseu·do·al·leles [ˌ-ə'liːlz] pl genet. Pseudoallele pl.
pseu·do·al·lel·ic [ˌ-ə'liːlɪk] adj Pseudoallele betr., pseudoallel.

pseu·do·al·le·lism [ˌ-'ælɪlɪzəm] n genet. Pseudoallelie f.
pseu·do·al·ler·gic reaction [ˌ-ə'lɜrdʒɪk] pseudoallergische Reaktion f; Pseudoallergie f.
pseudo-alopecia areata derm. Pseudo--Alopezie f.
pseu·do·an·a·phy·lax·is [ˌ-ænəfɪ'læksɪs] n anaphylaktoide Reaktion f.
pseu·do·a·ne·mia [ˌ-ə'niːmɪə] n Pseudoanämie f.
pseu·do·an·eu·rysm [ˌ-'ænjərɪzəm] n Pseudoaneurysma nt.
pseu·do·an·gi·na [ˌ-æn'dʒaɪnə] n card. Pseudoangina f, Angina pectoris vasomotoria.
pseu·do·an·ky·lo·sis [ˌ-æŋkɪ'ləʊsɪs] n Pseud(o)ankylose f.
pseu·do·an·tag·o·nist [ˌ-æn'tæɡənɪst] n physiol. Pseudoantagonist m.
pseu·do·ap·o·plex·y [ˌ-'æpəpleksɪ] n neuro. Pseudoapoplexie f.
pseu·do·ap·pen·di·ci·tis [ˌ-əˌpendə'saɪtɪs] n Pseudoappendizitis f.
pseu·do·ar·thro·sis [ˌ-ɑːr'θrəʊsɪs] n → pseudarthrosis.
pseu·do·asth·ma [ˌ-'æzmə] n paroxysmale Dyspnoe f.
pseu·do·a·tax·ia [ˌ-ə'tæksɪə] n → pseudotabes.
pseu·do·ath·e·to·sis [ˌ-ˌæθə'təʊsɪs] n neuro. Pseudoathetose f.
pseu·do·bas·e·dow [ˌ-'bɑːzədəʊ] n Basedoid nt.
pseu·do·blep·sia [ˌ-'blepsɪə] n → pseudoblepsia.
pseu·do·blep·sis [ˌ-'blepsɪs] n → pseudoblepsia.
pseu·do·bul·bar [ˌ-'bʌlbər, -bɑːr] adj pseudobulbär.
pseudobulbar palsy/paralysis Pseudobulbärparalyse f.
pseu·do·cap·il·lar·y [ˌ-kə'pɪlərɪ, -'kæpəleriː] adj pseudokapillär.
pseu·do·cap·sule [ˌ-'kæpsəl, -s(j)uːl] n Schein-, Pseudokapsel f.
p. of prostate chirurgische Prostatakapsel f, Pseudokapsel der Prostata.
pseu·do·cast ['-kæst, -kɑːst] n (Harn) Pseudozylinder m.
pseu·do·cele ['-siːl] n Cavum septi pellucidi.
pseu·do·ceph·a·lo·cele [ˌ-'sefələsiːl] n Pseudozephalozele f.
pseu·do·cho·le·cys·ti·tis [ˌ-ˌkəʊləsɪs'taɪtɪs, -ˌkɒlə-] n Pseudocholezystitis f.
pseu·do·cho·les·te·a·to·ma [ˌ-kəʊˌlestɪə'təʊmə] n HNO Pseudocholesteatom nt.
pseu·do·cho·lin·es·ter·ase [ˌ-kəʊlɪn'estəreɪz, -ˌkɒl-] n abbr. PCE unspezifische/unechte Cholinesterase f abbr. ChE, Pseudocholinesterase f, Typ II-Cholinesterase f, β-Cholinesterase f, Butyrylcholinesterase f.
pseudocholinesterase deficiency Pseudocholinesterasemangel m.
pseu·do·cho·rea [ˌ-kə'rɪə] n neuro. Pseudochorea f.
pseu·do·chrom·es·the·sia [ˌ-ˌkrəʊmes'θiːʒ(ɪ)ə, -zɪə] n neuro. Pseudochromästhesie f.
pseu·do·chrom·hi·dro·sis [ˌ-ˌkrəʊmhaɪ'drəʊsɪs, -hɪ-] n Pseudochrom(h)idrose f.
pseu·do·chro·mi·dro·sis [ˌ-ˌkrəʊmɪ'drəʊsɪs] n → pseudochromhidrosis.
pseu·do·chy·lous [ˌ-'kaɪləs] adj pseudochylös.
pseudochylous ascites pseudochylöser Aszites m.
pseu·do·cir·rho·sis [ˌ-sɪ'rəʊsɪs] n Stauungsinduration f der Leber, Cirrhose cardiaque f.

pseu·do·clau·di·ca·tion [ˌ-ˌklɔːdɪ'keɪʃn] n Claudicatio intermittens des Rückenmarks/der Cauda equina.
pseu·do·clo·nus [ˌ-'kləʊnəs] n Pseudoklonus m.
pseu·do·co·arc·ta·tion (of the aorta) [ˌ-ˌkəʊɑːrk'teɪʃn] radiol. Pseudocoarctatio aortae.
pseu·do·coele n → pseudocele.
pseu·do·col·loid [ˌ-'kɑlɔɪd] n Pseudokolloid nt.
pseu·do·col·o·bo·ma [ˌ-ˌkɑlə'bəʊmə] n ophthal. Pseudokolobom nt.
pseu·do·cow·pox [ˌ-'kaʊpɑks] n Melkerknoten m, Nebenpocken pl, Paravaccinia f, Melkerpocken pl, Paravakzineknoten pl.
pseudocowpox virus micro. Melkernotenvirus nt, Paravakzinevirus nt, Paravacciniavirus nt.
pseu·do·cox·al·gia [ˌ-kɑk'sældʒ(ɪ)ə] n → Perthes' disease.
pseu·do·cri·sis [suː'dɑkrɪsɪs] n (Fieber) Pseudokrise f.
pseu·do·croup ['suːdəkruːp] n falscher Krupp m, Pseudokrupp m, subglottische Laryngitis f, Laryngitis subglottica.
pseu·do·cy·e·sis [ˌ-saɪ'iːsɪs] n Scheinschwangerschaft f, Pseudokyesis f, Pseudogravidität f.
pseu·do·cy·lin·droid [ˌ-sɪlɪn'drɔɪd] n (Harn) Pseudozylindroid nt.
pseu·do·cyst ['-sɪst] n Pseudozyste f.
p.s of lung Zystenlunge f.
pseu·do·cys·tic [ˌ-'sɪstɪk] adj Pseudozyste betr., pseudozystisch.
pseu·do·de·fi·cien·cy rickets [ˌ-dɪ'fɪʃənsɪ] familiäre Hypophosphatämie f, Vitamin D-resistente Rachitis f, (Vitamin D-)refraktäre Rachitis f.
pseu·do·de·men·tia [ˌ-dɪ'menʃ(ɪ)ə] n psychia. Pseudodemenz f.
pseu·do·dex·tro·car·dia [ˌ-ˌdekstrəʊ'kɑːrdɪə] n Pseudodextrokardie f.
pseu·do·di·a·be·tes [ˌ-daɪə'biːtɪs] n subklinischer Diabetes (mellitus) m.
pseu·do·di·as·tol·ic [ˌ-daɪə'stɑlɪk] adj card. pseudodiastolisch.
pseu·do·diph·the·ri·a [ˌ-dɪf'θɪərɪə, -dɪp-] n diphtheroide Erkrankung f, Diphtheroid nt.
pseu·do·di·ver·tic·u·lum [ˌ-daɪvər'tɪkjələm] n Pseudodivertikel nt.
pseu·do·dom·i·nant [ˌ-'dɑmɪnənt] adj quasidominant.
pseu·do·dys·en·ter·y [ˌ-'dɪsntrɪ] n Pseudodysenterie f.
pseu·do·e·de·ma [ˌ-ɪ'diːmə] n Pseudoödem nt.
pseu·do·em·bry·on·ic [ˌ-ˌembrɪ'ɑnɪk] adj pseudoembryonal.
pseu·do·em·phy·se·ma [ˌ-ˌemfə'siːmə] n Pseudoemphysem nt.
pseu·do·en·do·cri·nop·a·thy [ˌ-ˌendəkrɪ'nɑpəθɪ] n Pseudoendokrinopathie f.
pseu·do·e·phed·rine [ˌ-'efɪdrɪn, -ɪ'fedrɪn] n Pseudoephedrin nt.
pseu·do·e·piph·y·sis [ˌ-ɪ'pɪfəsɪs] n ortho. Pseudoepiphyse f.
pseu·do·ep·i·the·li·o·ma·tous hyperplasia [ˌ-ˌepɪˌθiːlɪ'əʊmətəs] pseudoepitheliomatöse Hyperplasie f.
pseu·do·e·ro·sion [ˌ-ɪ'rəʊʒn] n gyn. Pseudoerosion f.
pseu·do·er·y·sip·e·las [ˌ-ˌerɪ'sɪpələs] n Schweinerotlauf m, Pseudoerysipel nt, Erysipeloid nt, Rosenbach-Krankheit f, Erythema migrans.
pseu·do·es·the·sia [ˌ-es'θiːʒ(ɪ)ə] n → pseudesthesia.
pseu·do·ex·o·pho·ria [ˌ-ˌeksə'fɔːrɪə] n ophthal. Pseudoexophorie f.

pseu·do·fis·tu·la symptom [ˌ-'fɪstʃələ] *HNO* Pseudofistelsymptom *nt*.
pseu·do·fol·lic·u·li·tis [ˌ-fəˌlɪkjə'laɪtɪs] *n derm*. Pseudofollikulitis/Pseudofolliculitis barbae, Pili incarnati/recurvati.
pseu·do·frac·ture [ˌ-'fræktʃər] *n radiol*. Schein-, Pseudofraktur *f*.
pseu·do·gan·gli·on [ˌ-'gæŋglɪən] *n* Pseudoganglion *nt*.
pseu·do·ges·ta·tion [ˌ-dʒe'steɪʃn] *n gyn*. Scheinschwangerschaft *f*, Pseudokyese *f*, Pseudogravidität *f*.
pseu·do·geu·ses·the·sia [ˌ-ˌgjuːzes'θiːʒ(ɪ)ə] *n neuro*. Pseudogeusästhesie *f*.
pseu·do·geu·sia [ˌ-'gjuːʒ(ɪ)ə] *n neuro*. Pseudogeusie *f*.
pseu·do·glan·ders [ˌ-'glændərs] *n* Pseudomalleus *m*, Whitmore'-Krankheit *f*, Pseudorotz *m*, Melioidose *f*, Malleoidose *f*, Melioidosis *f*.
pseu·do·gli·o·ma [ˌ-glaɪ'əʊmə] *n ophthal*. Pseudogliom(a) *nt*.
pseu·do·glo·mer·u·lar [ˌ-gləʊ'mer(j)ələr] *adj* pseudoglomerulär.
pseu·do·gon·or·rhea [ˌ-ˌgɑnə'rɪə] *n* unspezifische/nicht-gonorrhoische Urethritis *f abbr*. NGU.
pseu·do·gout ['gaʊt] *n* Pseudogicht *f*, Chondrokalzinose *f*, -calcinosis *f*.
pseu·do·graph·ia [ˌ-'græfɪə] *n neuro*. Pseudographie *f*.
pseu·do·gyn·e·co·mas·tia [ˌ-ˌdʒɪnɪkəʊ'mæstɪə, -ˌdʒaɪnɪ, -ˌgaɪnɪ-] *n* unechte Gynäkomastie *f*, Pseudogynäkomastie *f*.
pseu·do·hal·lu·ci·na·tion [ˌ-həˌluːsɪ'neɪʃn] *n psychia*. Pseudohalluzination *f*.
pseu·do·hau·stra·tion [ˌ-hɔː'streɪʃn] *n* Pseudohaustrierung *f*.
pseu·do·he·mag·glu·ti·na·tion [ˌ-hiːməˌgluːtn'eɪʃn, -ˌhemə-] *n* Geldrollenbildung *f*, Pseudo(häm)agglutination *f*.
pseu·do·he·ma·tu·ria [ˌ-hiːmə't(j)ʊərɪə] *n* Pseudohämaturie *f*.
pseu·do·he·mo·phil·ia [ˌ-hiːmə'fɪlɪə, -ˌhem-] *n* (von) Willebrand-Jürgens-Syndrom *nt*, konstitutionelle Thrombopathie *f*, hereditäre/vaskuläre Pseudohämophilie *f*, Angiohämophilie *f*.
pseu·do·he·mop·ty·sis [ˌ-hɪ'mɑptəsɪs] *n* Pseudohämoptoe *f*.
pseu·do·he·red·i·tar·y [ˌ-hə'redɪtərɪ] *adj* pseudohereditär.
pseu·do·her·maph·ro·dism [ˌ-hɜr'mæfrədɪzəm] *n* → pseudohermaphroditism.
pseu·do·her·maph·ro·dite [ˌ-ˌhɜrmæfrədaɪt] *n* Pseudohermaphrodit *m*, Scheinzwitter *m*.
pseu·do·her·maph·ro·di·tism [ˌ-hɜr'mæfrədaɪtɪzəm] *n* Pseudohermaphroditismus *m*, Pseudohermaphrodismus *m*, Scheinzwittertum *nt*, falscher Hermaphroditismus *m*, Hermaphroditismus spurius.
pseu·do·her·nia [ˌ-'hɜrnɪə] *n chir*. Pseudohernie *f*, Scheinbruch *m*, Hernia spuria.
pseu·do·het·er·o·to·pia [ˌ-ˌhetərə'təʊpɪə] *n patho*. Pseudoheterotopie *f*.
pseudo-Hurler polydystrophy Mukolipidose *f* III, Pseudo-Hurler-Dystrophie *f*.
pseu·do·hy·dro·ceph·a·lus [ˌ-ˌhaɪdrə'sefələs] *n* Pseudohydrozephalus *m*.
pseu·do·hy·dro·ne·phro·sis [ˌ-ˌhaɪdrənɪ'frəʊsɪs] *n urol*. Pseudohydronephrose *f*, pararenale/paranephritische Zyste *f*.
pseu·do·hy·per·ka·le·mia [ˌ-ˌhaɪpərkə'liːmɪə] *n* Pseudohyperkal(i)ämie *f*.
pseu·do·hy·per·par·a·thy·roid·ism [ˌ-ˌhaɪpərˌpærə'θaɪrɔɪdɪzəm] *m*, paraneoplastischer Hyperparathyreoidismus *m*.
pseu·do·hy·per·troph·ic [ˌ-ˌhaɪpər'trɑfɪk, -'trəʊf-] *adj* pseudohypertroph(isch).
pseudohypertrophic muscular atrophy Duchenne-Krankheit *f*, -Muskeldystrophie *f*, Duchenne-Typ *m* der progressiven Muskeldystrophie, pseudohypertrophe pelvifemorale Form *f*, Dystrophia musculorum progressiva Duchenne.
pseudohypertrophic muscular dystrophy → pseudohypertrophic muscular atrophy.
pseudohypertrophic muscular paralysis → pseudohypertrophic muscular atrophy.
pseu·do·hy·per·tro·phy [ˌ-haɪ'pɜrtrəfɪ] *n* Pseudohypertrophie *f*.
pseu·do·hy·phae [ˌ-'haɪfiː, -faɪ] *pl micro*. Pseudohyphen *pl*.
pseu·do·hy·po·al·dos·ter·on·ism [ˌ-ˌhaɪpəʊæl'dɑstərəʊnɪzəm] *n* Pseudohypoaldosteronismus *m*.
pseu·do·hy·po·na·tre·mia [ˌ-ˌhaɪpəʊneɪ'triːmɪə] *n* Pseudohyponatr(i)ämie *f*.
pseu·do·hy·po·par·a·thy·roid·ism [ˌ-ˌhaɪpəʊˌpærə'θaɪrɔɪdɪzəm] *n* Pseudohypoparathyreoidismus *m*.
pseu·do·hy·po·phos·pha·ta·sia [ˌ-ˌhaɪpəfɑsfə'teɪzɪə] *n* Pseudohypophosphatasie *f*.
pseu·do·hy·po·thy·roid·ism [ˌ-ˌhaɪpəʊ'θaɪrɔɪdɪzəm] *n* Pseudohypothyreoidismus *m*.
pseu·do·ic·ter·us [ˌ-'ɪktərəs] *n* Pseudogelbsucht *f*, Pseudoikterus *m*.
pseu·do·il·e·us [ˌ-'ɪlɪəs] *n* Pseudoileus *m*.
pseu·do·in·farc·tion [ˌ-ɪn'fɑrkʃn] *n card*. Pseudoinfarkt *m*.
pseu·do·i·so·chro·mat·ic color [ˌ-ˌaɪsəkrəʊ'mætɪk] *ophthal*. pseudoisochromatische Farbe *f*.
pseu·do·jaun·dice [ˌ-'dʒɔːndɪz] *n* → pseudoicterus.
pseudo-Kaposi sarcoma Pseudo-Kaposi-Syndrom *nt*, Akroangiodermatitis *f*, Pseudosarcoma Kaposi.
pseu·do·ker·a·tin [ˌ-'kerətɪn] *n* Pseudokeratin *nt*.
pseu·do·la·mel·lar [ˌ-lə'melər, -'læmə-] *adj* pseudolamellär.
pseu·do·lep·rom·a·tous leishmaniasis [ˌ-le'prɑmətəs] leproide Leishmaniasis *f*, Leishmaniasis cutis/tegumentaria diffusa.
pseu·do·leu·ke·mi·a [ˌ-luː'kiːmɪə] *n* Pseudoleukämie *f*.
pseu·do·li·po·ma [ˌ-lɪ'pəʊmə, -laɪ-] *n* Pseudolipom(a) *nt*.
pseu·do·li·thi·a·sis [ˌ-lɪ'θaɪəsɪs] *n* Pseudolithiasis *f*.
pseu·dol·o·gy [suː'dɑlədʒɪ] *n psychia*. Lügen *nt*, Pseudologie *f*, Pseudologia *f*.
pseu·do·lu·te·in body [ˌsuːdəʊ'luːtiːɪn, -tɪɪn] atretischer Follikel *m*, Corpus atreticum.
pseu·do·lux·a·tion [ˌ-lʌk'seɪʃn] *n ortho*. Pseudoluxation *f*.
pseu·do·lym·pho·ma [ˌ-lɪm'fəʊmə] *n* Pseudolymphom *nt*.
pseu·do·mam·ma [ˌ-'mæmə] *n* Pseudomamma *f*.
pseu·do·ma·nia [ˌ-'meɪnɪə, -jə] *n* Pseudomanie *f*.
pseu·do·mas·toi·di·tis [ˌ-ˌmæstɔɪ'daɪtɪs] *n HNO* Pseudomastoiditis *f*.
pseu·do·mas·tur·ba·tion [ˌ-ˌmæstər'beɪʃn] *n psychia*. Peotillomanie *f*, Pseudomasturbation *f*.
pseu·do·meg·a·co·lon [ˌ-'megəkəʊlən] *n* Pseudomegakolon *nt*.
pseu·do·mel·a·no·ma [ˌ-melə'nəʊmə] *n* Pseudomelanom *nt*.
pseu·do·mel·a·no·sis [ˌ-melə'nəʊsɪs] *n patho*. Pseudomelanose *f*.
pseu·do·me·lia [ˌ-'miːlɪə] *n* Phantomglied *nt*.
pseu·do·mem·brane [ˌ-'membraɪn] *n* Pseudomembran *f*.
pseu·do·mem·bra·nous [ˌ-'membrənəs] *adj* pseudomembranös.
pseudomembranous angina Plaut-Vincent-Angina *f*, Fusospirillose *f*, Fusospirochätose *f*, Angina ulcerosa/ulceromembranacea.
pseudomembranous bronchitis kruppöse/membranöse/pseudomembranöse Bronchitis *f*, Bronchitis crouposa/fibrinosa/plastica/pseudomembranacea.
pseudomembranous colitis pseudomembranöse Kolitis/Enteritis/Enterokolitis *f*.
pseudomembranous conjunctivitis Bindehautkrupp *m*, kruppöse/pseudomembranöse Konjunktivitis *f*, Conjunctivitis pseudomembranacea.
pseudomembranous croup echter Krupp *m* bei Diphtherie, Kehlkopfdiphtherie *f*.
pseudomembranous enteritis → pseudomembranous colitis.
pseudomembranous enterocolitis → pseudomembranous colitis.
pseudomembranous gastritis pseudomembranöse Gastritis *f*.
pseudomembranous inflammation pseudomembranöse Entzündung *f*.
pseudomembranous-necrotizing *adj* pseudomembranös-nekrotisierend.
pseudomembranous-necrotizing inflammation diphtherische Entzündung *f*, pseudomembranös-nekrotisierende Entzündung *f*.
pseudomembranous rhinitis pseudomembranöse/fibrinöse Rhinitis *f*, Rhinitis pseudomembranacea.
pseudomembranous tracheitis pseudomembranöse Luftröhrenentzündung/Tracheitis *f*.
pseu·do·men·in·gi·tis [ˌ-ˌmenɪn'dʒaɪtɪs] *n* Pseudomeningitis *f*, Meningismus *m*.
pseu·do·men·stru·a·tion [ˌ-ˌmenstrʊ'eɪʃn, -'streɪ-] *n gyn*. Pseudomenstruation *f*.
pseu·do·mes·en·chy·mal [ˌ-mes'eŋkɪməl] *adj* pseudomesenchymal.
pseu·do·met·a·pla·sia [ˌ-ˌmetə'pleɪʒ(ɪ)ə, -zɪə] *n* histologische Anpassung *f*, Pseudometaplasie *f*.
pseu·do·met·he·mo·glo·bin [ˌ-metˌhiːmə'gləʊbɪn, -ˌhemə-] *n* Methämalbumin *nt*.
pseu·do·mi·cro·ceph·a·lus [ˌ-ˌmaɪkrə'sefələs] *n* Pseudomikrozephalus *m*.
pseu·dom·ne·sia [ˌsuːdɑm'niːzɪə] *n neuro*. positive Erinnerungstäuschung *f*, Pseudomnesie *f*.
pseu·do·mo·nad [ˌsuːdə'məʊnæd, suː'dɑmənæd] *n micro*. Pseudomonade *f*.
Pseu·dom·o·na·da·ce·ae [suːˌdɑmənə'deɪsɪˌiː, ˌsuːdəˌmɑnə'd-] *pl micro*. Pseudomonadaceae *pl*.
Pseu·do·mo·nas [ˌsuːdə'məʊnəs, suː'dɑmənəs] *n micro*. Pseudomonas *f*.
P. aeruginosa Pseudomonas aeruginosa, Pyozyaneus *m*, *old* Pseudomonas pyocyanea, *old* Bact. pyocyaneum.
Pseu·do·mo·nil·ia [ˌsuːdəmə'nɪlɪə] *n micro*. Candida *f*, Monilia *f*, Oidium *nt*.
pseu·do·mor·phine [ˌ-'mɔːrfiːn] *n* Pseudomorphin *nt*, Dehydromorphin *nt*.
pseu·do·mu·cin [ˌ-'mjuːsɪn] *n* Pseudomuzin *nt*, -mucin *nt*, Metalbumin *nt*.
pseu·do·mu·ci·nous [ˌ-'mjuːsənəs] *adj* pseudomuzinös.
pseudomucinous cyst pseudomuzinöse Zyste *f*.
pseudomucinous cystoma pseudomuzinöses Kystom/Zystom *nt*, Pseudomuzinkystom *nt*.
pseudomucinous epithelium pseudomuzinöses Epithel *nt*.
pseu·do·mus·cu·lar hypertrophy [ˌ-'mʌskjələr] → pseudohypertrophic muscular atrophy.

pseu·do·my·ce·li·um [ˌ-maɪˈsiːlɪəm] *n micro.* Pseudomyzel *nt.*
pseu·do·my·co·sis [ˌ-maɪˈkəʊsɪs] *n* Pseudomykose *f.*
pseu·do·my·cot·ic infection [ˌ-maɪˈkɑtɪk] Pseudomykose *f.*
pseu·do·my·ia·sis [ˌ-ˈmaɪ(j)əsɪs] *n* Pseudomyiasis *f.*
pseu·do·my·o·pia [ˌ-maɪˈəʊpɪə] *n ophthal.* Pseudomyopie *f.*
pseu·do·myx·o·ma [ˌ-mɪkˈsəʊmə] *n* Pseudomyxom(a) *nt.*
p. peritonei Gallertbauch *m*, Pseudomyxoma peritonei, Hydrops spurius.
pseu·do·nar·cot·ic [ˌ-nɑːrˈkɑtɪk] *adj* pseudonarkotisch.
pseu·do·ne·o·plasm [ˌ-ˈniːəplæzəm] *n* Pseudoneoplasma *nt.*
pseu·do·neu·ri·tis [ˌ-njʊəˈraɪtɪs, -nʊ-] *n ophthal.* Pseudoneuritis (optica) *f.*
pseu·do·neu·ro·ma [ˌ-njʊəˈrəʊmə, -nʊ-] *n* Pseudoneurom(a) *nt.*
pseu·do·neu·rot·ic schizophrenia [ˌ-njʊəˈrɑtɪk, -nʊ-] pseudoneurotische Schizophrenie *f.*
pseu·do·nu·cle·o·lus [ˌ-n(j)uːˈklɪələs] *n* Karyosom *nt.*
pseu·do·nys·tag·mus [ˌ-nɪˈstægməs] *n* Endstellungs-, Pseudonystagmus *m.*
pseudo-obstruction *n* Pseudoobstruktion *f*, Pseudookklusion *f.*
pseudo-osteomalacia *n* Pseudoosteomalazie *f.*
pseudo-osteomalacic pelvis pseudo-osteomalazisches Becken *nt.*
pseu·do·pap·il·lar·y proliferation [ˌsuːdəpəˈpɪləri] pseudopapilläre Wucherung *f.*
pseu·do·pap·il·le·de·ma [ˌ-ˌpæpəlˈdiːmə] *n ophthal.* Pseudostauungspapille *f*, Pseudopapillitis vascularis.
pseu·do·pa·ral·y·sis [ˌ-pəˈræləsɪs] *n* Scheinlähmung *f*, Pseudoparalyse *f*, -paralysis *f.*
pseu·do·par·a·ple·gia [ˌ-ˌpærəˈpliːdʒ(ɪ)ə] *n* Pseudoparaplegie *f.*
pseu·do·par·a·site [ˌ-ˈpærəsaɪt] *n* Pseudoparasit *m.*
pseu·do·pa·re·sis [ˌ-pəˈriːsɪs] *n* 1. → pseudoparalysis. 2. psychogene Parese *f*, Pseudoparese *f.*
pseu·do·pe·lade [ˌ-pɪˈlɑːd, -ˈpiːleɪd] *n derm.* Pseudopelade (Brocq) *f*, Alopecia (areata) atrophicans.
pseu·do·per·i·car·di·al [ˌ-ˌperɪˈkɑːrdɪəl] *adj* pseudoperikardial.
pseu·do·per·i·car·di·tis [ˌ-ˌperɪkɑːrˈdaɪtɪs] *n* pseudoperikardiales Geräusch *nt.*
pseu·do·per·i·to·ni·tis [ˌ-ˌperɪtəˈnaɪtɪs] *n* Pseudoperitonitis *f*, Peritonismus *m.*
pseu·do·ple·gia [ˌ-ˈpliːdʒ(ɪ)ə] *n* 1. psychogene Paralyse *f*. 2. → pseudoparalysis. 3. → pseudoapoplexie.
pseu·do·pod [ˈ-pɑd] *sing* → pseudopodia.
pseu·do·po·dia [ˌ-ˈpəʊdɪə] *pl, sing* **-di·um** [-dɪəm] Scheinfüßchen *pl*, Pseudopodien *pl.*
pseu·do·po·di·al [ˌ-ˈpəʊdɪəl] *adj* Pseudopodien betr., pseudopodienähnlich.
pseu·do·po·di·um *sing* → pseudopodia.
pseu·do·pol·y·cy·the·mia [ˌ-ˌpɑlɪsaɪˈθiːmɪə] *n* Pseudopolyglobulie *f*, relative Polyglobulie *f.*
pseu·do·pol·yp [ˌ-ˈpɑlɪp] *n* Pseudopolyp *m.*
pseu·do·pol·y·po·sis [ˌ-ˌpɑlɪˈpəʊsɪs] *n* entzündliche Polypose *f*, Pseudopolyposis *f.*
pseu·do·preg·nan·cy [ˌ-ˈpregnənsɪ] *n* → pseudocyesis.
pseu·do·hy·po·par·a·thy·roid·ism [ˌ-ˌsuːdəˌhaɪpəʊˌpærəˈθaɪrɔɪdɪzəm] *n* Pseudo-Pseudohypoparathyroidismus *m.*

pseu·dop·sia [suːˈdɑpsɪə] *n* visuelle Halluzination *f*, Pseudop(s)ie *f.*
pseu·do·psy·cho·sis [ˌsuːdəʊsaɪˈkəʊsɪs] *n* Ganser-Syndrom *nt*, Pseudodemenz *f*, Scheinblödsinn *m*, Zweckpsychose *f.*
pseu·do·pte·ryg·i·um [ˌ-təˈrɪdʒɪəm] *n ophthal.* Pseudopterygium *nt.*
pseu·do·pto·sis [ˌsuːdɑpˈtəʊsɪs] *n ophthal.* Pseudoptose *f.*
pseu·do·pu·ber·ty [ˌ-ˈpjuːbərtɪ] *n* Pseudopubertät *f*, Pseudopubertas *f.*
pseu·do·ra·bies [ˌ-ˈreɪbiːz] *n* Pseudowut *f*, -lyssa *f*, -rabies *f*, Aujeszky'-Krankheit *f.*
pseudorabies virus *micro.* Pseudowut-Virus *nt.*
pseu·do·re·ac·tion [ˌ-rɪˈækʃn] *n derm.* Pseudoreaktion *f.*
pseu·do·re·duc·tion [ˌ-rɪˈdʌkʃn] *n genet.* Pseudoreduktion *f.*
pseu·do·rheu·ma·tism [ˌ-ˈruːmətɪzəm] *n* Pseudorheumatismus *m.*
pseu·do·rick·ets [ˌ-ˈrɪkɪts] *pl* renale Rachitis *f.*
pseu·do·ro·sette [ˌ-rəʊˈzet] *n immun.* Pseudorosette *f.*
pseu·do·ru·bel·la [ˌ-ruːˈbelə] *n* Pseudorubella *f*, Dreitagefieber *nt*, sechste Krankheit *f*, Exanthema subitum, Roseola infantum.
pseu·do·sar·co·ma [ˌ-sɑːrˈkəʊmə] *n* Pseudosarkom *nt.*
pseu·do·sar·co·ma·to·sis [ˌ-sɑːrˌkəʊməˈtəʊsɪs] *n* Pseudosarkomatose *f.*
pseu·do·sar·co·ma·tous [ˌ-sɑːrˈkɑmətəs] *adj* pseudosarkomatös.
pseudosarcomatous (nodular) fasciitis pseudosarkomatöse (noduläre) Fasziitis *f*, Fasciitis nodularis pseudosarcomatosa.
pseu·do·scle·re·ma [ˌ-sklɪˈriːmə] *n* Adiponecrosis subcutanea neonatorum.
pseu·do·scle·ro·sis [ˌ-sklɪəˈrəʊsɪs] *n* 1. Pseudosklerose *f*, -sklerosierung *f*. 2. Westphal-Strümpell-Pseudosklerose *f*, -Syndrom *nt.*
pseu·do·se·rous membrane [ˌ-ˈsɪərəs] pseudoseröse Membran *f.*
pseu·do·small·pox [ˌ-ˈsmɔːlpɑks] *n* weiße Pocken *pl*, Alastrim *nt*, Variola minor.
pseu·dos·mia [suːˈdɑzmɪə] *n* osmische Halluzination *f*, Geruchshalluzination *f*, Pseudosmie *f.*
pseu·do·stra·bis·mus [ˌsuːdəstrəˈbɪzməs] *n ophthal.* Scheinschielen *nt*, Pseudostrabismus *m.*
pseu·do·ta·bes [ˌsuːdəˈteɪbiːz] *n* Pseudotabes *f.*
pseu·do·tet·a·nus [ˌ-ˈtetənəs] *n* Pseudotetanus *m.*
pseu·do·trun·cus arteriosus [ˌ-ˈtrʌŋkəs] *card.* Pseudotruncus arteriosus (communis).
pseu·do·tu·ber·cle [ˌ-ˈt(j)uːbərkl] *n* Pseudotuberkel *nt.*
pseu·do·tu·ber·cu·lo·ma [ˌ-t(j)uːˌbɜːrkjəˈləʊmə] *n* Pseudotuberkulom *nt*, -tuberculoma *nt.*
pseu·do·tu·ber·cu·lo·sis [ˌ-t(j)uːˌbɜːrkjəˈləʊsɪs] *n* Pseudotuberkulose *f.*
pseu·do·tu·ber·cu·lous ophthalmia [ˌ-t(j)uːˈbɜːrkjələs] Ophthalmia nodosa/pseudotuberculosa.
pseudotuberculous thyroiditis subakute nicht-eitrige Thyreoiditis *f*, de Quervain-Thyreoiditis *f*, granulomatöse Thyreoiditis *f*, Riesenzellthyreoiditis *f.*
pseu·do·tu·bu·lar [ˌ-ˈt(j)uːbjələr] *adj* pseudotubulär.
pseudotubular degeneration (*Nebenniere*) pseudotubuläre Degeneration *f.*
pseu·do·tu·mor [ˌ-ˈt(j)uːmər] *n* Scheingeschwulst *f*, falsche Geschwulst *f*, Pseudotumor *m.*
pseudo-Turner's syndrome Bonnevie-Ullrich-Syndrom *nt*, Pterygium-Syndrom *nt.*
pseu·do·type [ˈ-taɪp] *n micro.* (*Virus*) Pseudotyp *m.*
pseu·do·u·ni·po·lar [ˌ-ˌjuːnɪˈpəʊlər] *adj* pseudounipolar.
pseudounipolar cell/neuron pseudounipolare Nervenzelle *f*, pseudounipolare Ganglienzelle *f*, pseudounipolarer Neurozyt/Gangliozyt *m*, pseudounipolares Neuron *nt.*
pseu·do·u·re·mia [ˌ-jəˈriːmɪə] *n* Pseudourämie *f.*
pseu·do·u·ri·dine [ˌ-ˈjʊərədiːn, -dɪn] *n abbr.* ψ Pseudouridin *nt abbr.* ψ.
pseu·do·u·ri·dyl·ic acid [ˌ-ˌjʊərəˈdɪlɪk] Pseudouridylsäure *f.*
pseu·do·vac·u·ole [ˌ-ˈvækjəwəʊl] *n* Pseudovakuole *f.*
pseu·do·vag·i·nal hypospadias [ˌ-ˈvædʒɪnl] *urol.* perineale Hypospadie *f.*
pseu·do·valve [ˈ-vælv] *n card.* Pseudoklappe *f.*
pseu·do·ven·tri·cle [ˌ-ˈventrɪkl] *n* Cavum septi pellucidi.
pseu·do·vi·ri·on [ˌ-ˈvaɪrɪɑn, -ˈvɪrɪ-] *n micro.* Pseudovirion *nt.*
pseu·do·vi·ta·min B₁₂ [ˌ-ˈvaɪtəmɪn; Brit. -ˈvɪtə-] Pseudovitamin B_{12} *nt.*
pseu·do·vom·it·ing [ˌ-ˈvɑmɪtɪŋ] *n* Scheinerbrechen *nt.*
pseu·do·xan·tho·ma cell [ˌ-zænˈθəʊmə] Pseudoxanthomzelle *f.*
pseudoxanthoma elasticum *derm.* Darier-Grönblad-Strandberg-Syndrom *nt*, Grönblad-Strandberg-Syndrom *nt*, systematische Elastorrhexis *f*, Pseudoxanthoma elasticum.
psi·cose [ˈsaɪkəʊz] *n* Psicose *f.*
psil·o·cy·bin [saɪləˈsaɪbɪn, -ˈsɪb-] *n* Psilocybin *nt.*
psi·lo·sis [saɪˈləʊsɪs] *n* 1. Sprue *f*, tropische Aphthen *pl*, Psilosis linguae. 2. Kahlheit *f*, Psilosis *f.*
P sinistroatriale → P mitrale.
P sinistrocardiale → P mitrale.
P site *n* peptidyl site.
psit·ta·co·sis [sɪtəˈkəʊsɪs] *n* Psittakose *f*, Papageienkrankheit *f*, Ornithose *f.*
psittacosis virus *old* → Chlamydia psittaci.
pso·as [ˈsəʊəs] *n* Psoas *m*, M. psoas.
psoas abscess Psoasabszeß *m.*
psoas major (muscle) Psoas *m* major, M. psoas major.
psoas minor (muscle) Psoas *m* minor, M. psoas minor.
psoas muscle → psoas.
 greater p. → psoas major (muscle).
 smaller p. → psoas minor (muscle).
psoas shadow *radiol.* Psoasschatten *m.*
psoas sign/test *chir.* Cope-Zeichen *nt*, Psoaszeichen *nt.*
pso·i·tis [səʊˈaɪtɪs] *n* Psoitis *f.*
pso·ra·len [ˈsɔːrələn, ˈsəʊr-] *n* Psoralen *nt.*
pso·ri·a·si·form [səʊˈraɪəsɪfɔːrm, ˌsəʊraɪˈæsɪ-] *adj* Psoriasis-artig, -ähnlich, psoriasiform.
pso·ri·a·sis [səˈraɪəsɪs] *n* Schuppenflechte *f*, Psoriasis (vulgaris) *f.*
pso·ri·at·ic [sɔːrɪˈætɪk, səʊ-] **I** *n* Patient(in *f*) *m* mit Psoriasis, Psoriatiker(in *f*) *m.* **II** *adj* Psoriasis betr., von ihr betroffen, Psoriasis-artig, -ähnlich, psoriatisch.
psoriatic arthritis/arthropathy Arthritis/Arthropathia psoriatica.
PSP *abbr.* → phenolsulfonephthalein.
P substances P-Substanzen *pl.*
psych- *pref.* → psycho-.

psychalgalia

psy·chal·ga·lia [ˌsaɪkæl'geɪlɪə] *n* → psychalgia.
psy·chal·gia [saɪ'kældʒ(ɪ)ə] *n* psychogener (Kopf-)Schmerz *m*, Psychalgie *f*.
psy·cha·nal·y·sis [ˌsaɪkə'næləsɪs] *n* → psychoanalysis.
psy·cha·nop·sia [ˌ-'nɑpsɪə] *n* → psychic blindness.
psych·as·the·nia [ˌsaɪkæs'θiːnɪə] *n* Psychasthenie *f*.
psy·che ['saɪkiː] *n* Psyche *f*.
psych·e·del·ic [ˌsaɪkɪ'delɪk] **I** *n* Psychedelikum *nt*. **II** *adj* psychedelisch, psychodelisch.
psy·chi·at·ric [ˌ-'ætrɪk] *adj* Psychiatrie betr., psychiatrisch.
psychiatric disturbances psychiatrische Störungen *pl*.
psychiatric medicine → psychiatry.
psy·chi·at·rics [ˌ-'ætrɪks] *pl* → psychiatry.
psy·chi·a·trist [saɪ'kaɪətrɪst] *n* Psychiater(in *f*) *m*, Arzt *m*/Ärztin *f* für Psychiatrie.
psy·chi·a·try [saɪ'kaɪətrɪ] *n* Psychiatrie *f*.
psy·chic ['saɪkɪk] *adj* Psyche betr., seelisch, psychisch, psychogen; mental.
psychic blindness zerebralbedingte/organbedingte Blindheit *f*.
psychic deafness psychogene Schwerhörigkeit/Taubheit *f*.
psychic epilepsy psychogene Epilepsie *f*, Affektepilepsie *f*.
psychic pain → psychogenic pain.
psycho- *pref.* Psych(o)-, Seele(n)-.
psy·cho·ac·tive drugs [ˌsaɪkəʊ'æktɪv] psychotrope Substanzen *pl*, Psychopharmaka *pl*.
psychoactive substance abusus Mißbrauch *m* von psychotropen Substanzen.
psychoactive substance dependence Substanzabhängigkeit *f*, Abhängigkeit *f* von psychotropen Substanzen.
psychoactive substances → psychoactive drugs.
psy·cho·an·a·lep·tic [ˌ-ˌænə'leptɪk] **I** *n pharm.* Psychoanaleptikum *nt*. **II** *adj* psychoanaleptisch.
psy·cho·a·nal·y·sis [ˌ-ə'næləsɪs] *n* Psychoanalyse *f*.
psy·cho·an·a·lyst [ˌ-'ænlɪst] *n* Psychoanalytiker(in *f*) *m*.
psy·cho·an·a·lyt·ic [ˌ-ˌænə'lɪtɪk] *adj* psychoanalytisch.
psy·cho·an·a·lyt·i·cal [ˌ-ˌænə'lɪtɪkl] *adj* → psychoanalytic.
psychoanalytic psychiatry psychoanalytische Psychiatrie *f*.
psy·cho·an·a·lyze [ˌ-'ænəlaɪz] *vt* psychologisch untersuchen *od.* behandeln, psychoanalysieren.
psy·cho·bi·ol·o·gy [ˌ-baɪ'ɑlədʒɪ] *n* Psychobiologie *f*.
psy·cho·car·di·ac reflex [ˌ-'kɑːrdɪæk] psychokardialer Reflex *m*.
psy·cho·ca·thar·sis [ˌ-kə'θɑːrsɪs] *n* psycho. Katharsis *f*.
psy·cho·chem·i·stry [ˌ-'kemɪstrɪ] *n* Psychochemie *f*.
psy·cho·del·ic [ˌ-'delɪk] *n, adj* → psychedelic.
psy·cho·di·ag·no·sis [ˌ-ˌdaɪəg'nəʊsɪs] *n* Psychodiagnostik *f*.
psy·cho·di·ag·nos·tics [ˌ-ˌdaɪəg'nɑstɪks] *pl* → psychodiagnosis.
Psy·chod·i·dae [saɪ'kɑdɪdiː, -'kəʊdə-] *pl bio.* Schmetterlingsmücken *pl*, Psychodidae *pl*.
psy·cho·dra·ma [ˌsaɪkəʊ'drɑːmə, -'dræmə] *n psychia.* Psychodrama *nt*.
psy·cho·dy·nam·ics [ˌ-daɪ'næmɪks] *pl* Psychodynamik *f*.

psy·cho·dys·lep·tic [ˌ-dɪs'leptɪk] *pharm.* **I** *n* Halluzinogen *nt*, Psychodysleptikum *nt*, Psychomimetikum *nt*, Psychotomimetikum *nt*. **II** *adj* halluzinogen, psychodysleptisch, psychomimetisch.
psy·cho·en·do·cri·nol·o·gy [ˌ-ˌendəʊkrɪ'nɑlədʒɪ] *n* Psychoendokrinologie *f*.
psy·cho·gal·van·ic [ˌ-gæl'vænɪk] *adj* psychogalvanisch.
psychogalvanic reaction → psychogalvanic response.
psychogalvanic reflex → psychogalvanic response.
psychogalvanic response *abbr.* **PGR** psychogalvanischer (Haut-)Reflex *m*.
psychogalvanic skin reaction → psychogalvanic response.
psychogalvanic skin reflex → psychogalvanic response.
psychogalvanic skin response → psychogalvanic response.
psy·cho·gal·va·nom·e·ter [ˌ-ˌgælvə'nɑmɪtər] *n* Psychogalvanometer *nt*.
psy·cho·gen·e·sis [ˌ-'dʒenəsɪs] *n* **1.** geistige Entwicklung *f*. **2.** Psychogenie *f*.
psy·cho·gen·e·tic [ˌ-dʒɪ'netɪk] *adj* **1.** → psychogenic. **2.** die geistige Entwicklung betr., psychogenetisch.
psy·cho·gen·ic [ˌ-'dʒenɪk] *adj* psychisch/seelisch bedingt, in der Psyche begründet, seelisch, psychisch, psychogen.
psychogenic alopecia streßbedingte Alopezie *f*, Alopecia neurotica.
psychogenic amnesia psychogene Amnesie *f*.
psychogenic deafness psychogene Schwerhörigkeit/Taubheit *f*.
psychogenic dysmenorrhea *gyn.* psychogene/psychosomatisch-bedingte Dysmenorrhö *f*.
psychogenic glossitis Zungenbrennen *nt*, Glossopyrosis *f*, -pyrie *f*.
psychogenic overlay *psycho.* psychogene Überlagerung *f*.
psychogenic pain psychogener Schmerz *m*.
psychogenic polydipsia *psychia.* psychogene Polydipsie *f*.
psy·chog·e·ny [saɪ'kɑdʒənɪ] *n* Psychogenie *f*.
psy·cho·ger·i·at·rics [ˌsaɪkəʊˌdʒɪərɪ'ætrɪks] *pl* Psychogeriatrie *f*.
psy·cho·gram ['-græm] *n* Psychogramm *nt*.
psy·cho·graph ['-græf] *n* → psychogram.
psy·chog·ra·phy [saɪ'kɑgrəfɪ] *n* Psychographie *f*.
psy·cho·ki·ne·sia [ˌsaɪkəʊkɪ'niːʒ(ɪ)ə, -kaɪ-] *n* → psychokinesis.
psy·cho·ki·ne·sis [ˌ-kɪ'niːsɪs, -kaɪ-] *n* Psychokinese *f*.
psy·cho·lag·ny ['-lægnɪ] *n* Psycholagnie *f*.
psy·cho·log·ic [ˌ-'lɑdʒɪk] *adj* Psychologie betr., auf ihr beruhend, psychologisch.
psy·cho·log·i·cal [ˌ-'lɑdʒɪkl] *adj* → psychologic.
psychological dependence psychische Abhängigkeit *f*.
psychological fatique psychische/zentrale Ermüdung *f*.
psychological load psychische Belastung *f*.
psychological performance psychische Leistung *f*.
psychological terror Psychoterror *m*.
psychological test psychologischer Test *m*.
psy·chol·o·gist [saɪ'kɑlədʒɪst] *n* Psychologe *m*, -login *f*.
psy·chol·o·gy [saɪ'kɑlədʒɪ] *n* **1.** Psychologie *f*. **2.** Psyche *f*, Seelenleben *nt*, Mentalität *f*.

638

psy·cho·met·rics [ˌsaɪkə'metrɪks] *pl* → psychometry.
psy·chom·e·try [saɪ'kɑmətrɪ] *n* Psychometrie *f*.
psy·cho·mo·tor [ˌsaɪkə'məʊtər] *adj* psychomotorisch.
psychomotor area motorische Rinde *f*, motorischer Kortex *m*, Motorkortex *m*.
psychomotor epilepsy psychomotorische Epilepsie *f*.
psychomotor test psychomotorischer Test *m*.
psy·cho·neu·ro·sis [ˌ-njʊə'rəʊsɪs, -'nʊ-] *n* **1.** Psychoneurose *f*. **2.** Neurose *f*.
psy·cho·path ['-pæθ] *n* Psychopath(in *f*) *m*.
psy·cho·path·ic [ˌ-'pæθɪk] *adj* seelisch-charakterlich gestört, psychopathisch.
psychopathic personality → psychopath.
psy·cho·pa·thol·o·gy [ˌ-pə'θɑlədʒɪ] *n* Psychopathologie *f*.
psy·chop·a·thy [saɪ'kɑpəθɪ] *n* Psychopathie *f*.
psy·cho·phar·ma·col·o·gy [ˌsaɪkəˌfɑːrmə'kɑlədʒɪ] *n* Psychopharmakologie *f*.
psy·cho·phys·i·cal [ˌ-'fɪzɪkl] *adj* seelisch-leiblich, seelisch-körperlich, psychophysisch.
psychophysical law Weber-Fechner-Gesetz *nt*.
psy·cho·phys·ics [ˌ-'fɪzɪks] *pl* Psychophysik *f*.
psy·cho·phys·i·o·log·ic [ˌ-ˌfɪzɪə'lɑdʒɪk] *adj* psychophysiologisch; psychosomatisch.
psychophysiological disorder psychosomatische Störung *f*.
psy·cho·phys·i·ol·o·gy [ˌ-ˌfɪzɪ'ɑlədʒɪ] *n* physiologische Psychologie *f*, Psychophysiologie *f*.
psy·cho·ple·gic [ˌ-'pliːdʒɪk] *n* Psychoplegikum *nt*.
psy·cho·pro·phy·lax·is [ˌ-ˌprəʊfɪ'læksɪs] *n* Psychoprophylaxe *f*.
psy·cho·sed·a·tive [ˌ-'sedətɪv] *n* Psychosedativum *nt*, Tranquilizer *m*, Ataraktikum *nt*.
psy·cho·sen·so·ri·al [ˌ-sen'sɔːrɪəl, -'səʊ-] *adj* → psychosensory.
psy·cho·sen·so·ry [ˌ-'sensərɪ] *adj* psychosensorisch.
psychosensory aphasia sensorische Aphasie *f*, Wernicke-Aphasie *f*.
psy·cho·sex·u·al [ˌ-'sekʃəwəl] *adj* psychosexuell.
psy·cho·sin [saɪ'kəʊsɪn] *n* Psychosin *nt*.
psy·cho·sis [saɪ'kəʊsɪs] *n, pl* **-ses** [-siːz] Psychose *f*.
psy·cho·so·cial [ˌsaɪkə'səʊʃəl] *adj* psychosozial.
psy·cho·so·mat·ic [ˌ-sə'mætɪk, -səʊ-] *adj* psychosomatisch.
psychosomatic disorder psychosomatische Störung *f*.
psychosomatic factor psychosomatischer Faktor *m*.
psychosomatic illness → psychosomatic disorder.
psychosomatic medicine psychosomatische Medizin *f*.
psy·cho·so·mi·met·ic [ˌ-səmɪ'metɪk] *n, adj* → psychotomimetic.
psy·cho·stim·u·lant [ˌ-'stɪmjələnt] **I** *n* Psychostimulans *nt*, Psychotonikum *nt*. **II** *adj* die Psyche anregend, psychotonisch.
psy·cho·sur·ger·y [ˌ-'sɜːrdʒərɪ] *n* Psychochirurgie *f*.
psy·cho·ther·a·peu·tic [ˌ-ˌθerə'pjuːtɪk] *adj* psychotherapeutisch.
psy·cho·ther·a·peu·tics [ˌ-ˌθerə'pjuːtɪks] *pl* Psychotherapeutik *f*.
psy·cho·ther·a·pist [ˌ-'θerəpɪst] *n* Psychotherapeut(in *f*) *m*.

psy·cho·ther·a·py [ˌ-'θerəpɪ] *n* Psychotherapie *f*.
psy·chot·ic [saɪ'kɑtɪk] **I** *n* Psychotiker(in *f*) *m*. **II** *adj* Psychose betr., an einer Psychose leidend, psychotisch.
psy·chot·o·mi·met·ic [saɪˌkɑtəʊmɪ'metɪk] *pharm*. **I** *n* Psychodysleptikum *nt*, Halluzinogen *nt*, Psychomimetikum *nt*, Psychotomimetikum *nt*. **II** *adj* die Psyche anregend, psychomimetisch.
psy·cho·trop·ic [ˌsaɪkə'trəʊpɪk] *adj* psychotrop.
psychotropic drugs psychotrope Substanzen *pl*, Psychopharmaka *pl*.
psychr(o)- *pref.* Kälte-, Psychro-, Kry(o)-.
psy·chro·al·gia [ˌsaɪkrə'ældʒ(ɪ)ə] *n* schmerzhafte Kälteempfindung *f*, Psychroalgie *f*, Psychrohyperästhesie *f*.
psy·chro·es·the·sia [ˌ-es'θiːʒ(ɪ)ə] *n* Psychroästhesie *f*.
psy·chro·phile ['-faɪl] *n* kälteliebender/psychrophiler Mikroorganismus *m*.
psy·chro·phil·ic [ˌ-'fɪlɪk] *adj* kälteliebend, psychrophil.
psychrophilic bacteria kälteliebende/psychrophile Bakterien *pl*.
psy·chro·ther·a·py [ˌ-'θerəpɪ] *n* Kälte-, Kryotherapie *f*.
PT *abbr.* 1. → physical training. 2. → prothrombin time.
Pt *abbr.* → platinum.
pt *abbr.* → pint.
PTA *abbr.* 1. → percutaneous transluminal angioplasty. 2. → plasma thromboplastin antecedent.
PTA deficiency PTA-Mangel *m*, Faktor XI-Mangel *m*.
PTA factor → plasma thromboplastin antecedent.
ptar·mus ['tɑːrməs] *n* Nieskrampf *m*, Ptarmus *m*.
PTC *abbr.* 1. → percutaneous transhepatic cholangiography. 2. → plasma thromboplastin component. 3. [phenylthiocarbamide] → phenylthiourea.
PTC factor → plasma thromboplastin component.
PTC peptide → phenylthiocarbamoyl peptide.
Pt electrode Platinelektrode *f*.
PTEN *abbr.* → pentaerythritol tetranitrate.
pter·i·dine ['terədiːn, -dɪn] *n* Pteridin *nt*.
pter·in ['terɪn] *n* Pterin *nt*.
pte·ro·ic acid [tə'rəʊɪk] Pteroinsäure *f*.
pter·op·ter·in [ter'ɑptərɪn] *n* → pteroyltriglutamic acid.
pter·o·yl·glu·ta·mate [ˌterəwɪl'gluːtəmeɪt] *n* Folinat *nt*.
pter·o·yl·glu·tam·ic acid [ˌ-gluː'tæmɪk] Fol(in)säure *f*, Folacin *nt*, Pteroylglutaminsäure *f*, Vitamin B$_c$ *nt*.
pter·o·yl·tri·glu·tam·ic acid [ˌ-traɪglu'tæmɪk] Pteroyltriglutaminsäure *f*.
pte·ryg·i·um [tə'rɪdʒɪəm] *n, pl* **-gi·ums, -gia** [-dʒɪə] 1. *ophthal*. Flügelfell *nt*, Pterygium *nt*. 2. *bio*. Schwimm-, Flughaut *f*, Pterygium *nt*. 3. Nagelhäutchen *nt*, Pterygium *nt*.
pterygium colli syndrome Bonnevie--Ullrich-Syndrom *nt*, Pterygium-Syndrom *nt*.
pter·y·goid ['terɪɡɔɪd] *adj* flügelähnlich, -förmig, Flügel-; Proc. pterygoideus betr.
pter·y·goi·dal ['terɪɡɔɪdl] *adj* → pterygoid.
pterygoid arteries Rami pterygoidei a. maxillaris.
pterygoid bone Proc. pterygoideus (ossis sphenoidalis).
pterygoid branches of maxillary artery → pterygoid arteries.
pterygoid canal Canalis pterygoideus/Vidii.

pterygoid chest flacher langer Thorax *m*.
pterygoid depression → pterygoid fovea (of mandible).
pter·y·goi·de·us [ˌterɪ'gɔɪdɪəs] *n* Pterygoideus *m*, M. pterygoideus.
pterygoideus lateralis (muscle) Pterygoideus *m* lateralis/externus, M. pterygoideus lateralis/externus.
pterygoideus medialis (muscle) Pterygoideus *m* medialis/internus, M. pterygoideus medialis/internus.
pterygoid fissure → pterygoid notch.
pterygoid fossa (of sphenoid bone) Fossa pterygoidea.
pterygoid fovea (of mandible) Fovea pterygoidea.
pterygoid hamulus Hamulus pterygoideus.
pterygoid incisure Inc. pterygoidea.
pterygoid muscle → pterygoideus.
 lateral p. → pterygoideus lateralis (muscle).
 medial p. → pterygoideus medialis (muscle).
pterygoid nerve: external p. → lateral p.
 internal p. → medial p.
 lateral p. Pterygoideus *m* lateralis, N. pterygoideus lateralis.
 medial p. Pterygoideus *m* medialis, N. pterygoideus medialis.
pterygoid notch Inc. pterygoidea.
pterygoid pit → pterygoid fovea (of mandible).
pterygoid plate: external p. Lamina lateralis proc. pterygoidei.
 lateral p. → external p.
pterygoid plexus Venengeflecht *nt* auf den Mm. pterygoidei, Plexus (venosus) pterygoideus.
pterygoid process Flügelfortsatz *m* des Keilbeins, Proc. pterygoideus.
pterygoid tubercle Tuberositas pterygoidea.
pterygoid tuberosity Tuberositas pterygoidea.
 p. of mandible Tuberositas pterygoidea mandibulae.
pter·y·go·man·dib·u·lar raphe [ˌterɪɡəʊmæn'dɪbjələr] Raphe pterygomandibularis.
pter·y·go·max·il·lar·y fissure [ˌ-mæk'sɪlərɪ, -'mæksəˌleri] Fissura pterygomaxillaris.
pterygomaxillary fossa → pterygopalatine fossa.
pter·y·go·pal·a·tine fissure [ˌ-'pælətaɪn, -tɪn] → pterygomaxillary fissure.
pterygopalatine foramen For. palatinum majus.
pterygopalatine fossa Flügelgaumengrube *f*, Fossa pterygopalatina.
pterygopalatine ganglion Meckel'-Ganglion *nt*, Ggl. pterygopalatinum.
pterygopalatine nerves Nn. pterygopalatini.
pterygopalatine sulcus: p. of palatine bone 1. Sulcus palatinus major ossis palatini. 2. Sulcus pterygopalatinus ossis palatini.
 p. of pterygoid process Sulcus pterygopalatinus proc. pterygoidei.
pter·y·go·pha·ryn·ge·al muscle [ˌ-fə'rɪndʒ(ɪ)əs, ˌfærɪn'dʒiːəl] → pterygopharyngeus (muscle).
pter·y·go·pha·ryn·ge·us (muscle) [ˌ-fə'rɪndʒ(ɪ)əs, ˌfærɪn'dʒiːəs] *old* M. pterygopharyngeus, Pars pterygopharyngea m. constrictoris pharyngis superioris.
pter·y·go·spi·nal ligament [ˌ-'spaɪnl] Lig. pterygospinale.
pter·y·go·spi·nous process [ˌ-'spaɪnəs] Proc. pterygospinosus.

pter·y·go·tym·pan·ic fissure [ˌ-tɪm'pænɪk] → petrotympanic fissure.
PTF *abbr.* → plasma thromboplastin factor.
PTH *abbr.* → parathyroid hormone.
Pthir·us ['θɪrəs] *n* → Phthirus.
pti·lo·sis [tə'ləʊsɪs, taɪ-] *n, pl* **-ses** [-siːz] *ophthal*. Verlust *f* der Wimpern, Ptilosis *f*.
PTJC *abbr.* → percutaneous transjugular cholangiography.
pto·maine ['təʊmeɪn, təʊ'meɪn] *n* Ptomain *nt*, Leichengift *nt*, Leichenalkaloid *nt*.
pto·ma·tine ['təʊmətɪn] *n* → ptomaine.
pto·ma·top·sia [ˌtəʊmə'tɑpsɪə] *n* → ptomatopsy.
pto·ma·top·sy [ˌ-'tɑpsɪ] *n* Autopsie *f*, Obduktion *f*, Nekropsie *f*.
pto·mat·ro·pine [təʊ'mætrəpiːn] *n* Ptomatropin *nt*.
ptosed [təʊst] *adj* von Ptose betroffen, ptotisch, herabhängend; prolabiert.
pto·sis ['təʊsɪs] *n* 1. (Organ-)Senkung *f*, Ptose *f*, Ptosis *f*. 2. *ophthal*. Oberlidptose *f*, Ptosis (palpebrae) *f*, Blepharoptose *f*.
ptot·ic ['tɑtɪk] *adj* Ptose betr., von Ptose betroffen, ptotisch.
PTS *abbr.* 1. → permanent threshold shift. 2. → phosphotransferase system.
PTT *abbr.* → partial thromboplastin time.
PTT-test *n* PTT-Bestimmung *f*, Bestimmung *f* der partiellen Thromboplastinzeit.
PTU *abbr.* → propylthiouracil.
PTVS *abbr.* → percutaneous transhepatic venous sampling.
ptyal- *pref.* → ptyalo-.
pty·al·a·gogue [taɪ'æləɡɑɡ] **I** *n* Sialagogum *nt*. **II** *adj* den Speichelfluß anregend, sialagog.
pty·a·lec·ta·sis [taɪə'lektəsɪs] *n, pl* **-ses** [-siːz] Sialektasie *f*.
pty·a·lin ['taɪəlɪn] *n* Ptyalin *nt*, Speicheldiastase *f*.
pty·a·lism ['taɪəlɪzəm] *n pathol*. übermäßiger Speichelfluß *m*, Ptyalismus *m*, Sialorrhoe *f*, Hypersalivation *f*.
ptyalo- *pref.* Speichel-, Ptyal(o)-, Sial(o)-.
pty·a·log·ra·phy [taɪə'lɑɡrəfɪ] *n* HNO, *radiol*. Sialographie *f*.
pty·a·lo·lith ['taɪəlɑlɪθ] *n* Speichelstein *m*, Sialolith *m*.
pty·a·lo·li·thi·a·sis [ˌtaɪəlɑʊlɪ'θaɪəsɪs] *n* Sialolithiasis *f*.
pty·a·lo·li·thot·o·my [ˌ-lɪ'θɑtəmɪ] *n* HNO Sialolithotomie *f*.
pty·a·lor·rhea [ˌ-'rɪə] *n* → ptyalism.
pty·a·lose ['taɪəloʊs] *n* Maltose *f*.
Pu *abbr.* → plutonium.
pu·bar·che [pjuː'bɑːrkɪ] *n* Pubarche *f*.
pu·ber·al ['pjuːbərəl] *adj* Pubertät betr., während der Pubertät auftretend, puberal, pubertierend, Pubertäts-.
pu·ber·tal ['pjuːbərtl] *adj* → puberal.
pu·ber·tas ['pjuːbərtæs] *n* → puberty.
pu·ber·ty ['pjuːbərtɪ] *n* Geschlechtsreife *f*, Pubertät *f*, Pubertas *f*.
puberty involution Pubertätsinvolution *f*.
puberty vocal change Stimmwechsel *m* in der Pubertät, Stimmbruch *m*, Mutation *f*.
pu·bes ['pjuːbiːz] *n, pl* **pu·bes** *anat.* 1. → pubic region. 2. → pubic hair(s).
pu·bes·cence [pjuː'besəns] *n f*. 1. Geschlechtsreifung *f*, Pubeszenz *f*. 2. *bio*. (flaumige) Behaarung *f*.
pu·bes·cent [pjuː'besənt] *adj* 1. heranwachsend, pubeszent. 2. *bio*. flaumhaarig.
pu·bic ['pjuːbɪk] *adj* Schambein *od.* Schamgegend betr., pubisch, Scham(bein)-.
pubic angle Schambogen *m*, Angulus subpubicus.

pubic arch

pubic arch Schambogen *m*, Arcus pubicus.
pubic arcuate ligament Lig. arcuatum pubis.
pubic artery Schambeinast *m* der A. epigastrica inferior, Ramus pubicus a. epigastricae inferioris.
pubic body Schambeinkörper *m*, Corpus ossis pubis.
pubic bone → pubis.
pubic branch: p. of inferior epigastric artery → pubic artery.
p. of obturator artery Schambeinast *m* der A. obturatoria, Ramus pubicus a. obturatoriae.
pubic crest Crista pubica.
pubic hair(s) Schamhaare *pl*, Pubes *f*.
pubic ligament: p. of Cowper Leistenband *nt*, Lig. inguinale, Arcus inguinale.
 inferior p. 1. → pubic arcuate ligament. **2.** Lig. suspensorium ovarii.
 superior p. Lig. pubicum superius.
pubic louse *micro*. Filzlaus *f*, Phthirus pubis, Pediculus pubis.
pubic ramus Schambeinast *m*, Ramus ossis pubis.
 inferior p. unterer Schambeinast, Ramus inferior ossis pubis.
 superior p. oberer Schambeinast, Ramus superior ossis pubis.
pubic region Scham *f*, Schambeinregion *f*, Pubes *f*, Hypogastrium *nt*, Regio pubica.
pubic symphysis Scham(bein)fuge *f*, Symphysis pubica.
pubic synchondrosis → pubic symphysis.
pubic tubercle Tuberculum pubicum.
pu·bi·o·plas·ty ['pjuːbɪəʊplæstɪ] *n chir.*, *gyn.* Pubeo-, Pubioplastik *f*.
pu·bi·ot·o·my [ˌpjuːbɪˈɒtəmɪ] *n gyn.*, *chir.* Pubeo-, Pubiotomie *f*, Hebotomie *f*, Beckenringosteotomie *f*.
pu·bis ['pjuːbɪs] *n, pl* **-bes** [-biːz] Schambein *nt*, Pubis *f*, Os pubis.
pub·lic antigens ['pʌblɪk] *hema.* obiquitäre (Blutgruppen-)Antigene *pl*.
public name *pharm.* Freiname *m*, Generic name (*m*).
pu·bo·cap·su·lar ligament [ˌpjuːbəʊˈkæps(j)ələr] → pubocapsularis (muscle).
pu·bo·coc·cyg·e·al muscle [ˌ-kɒkˈsɪdʒɪəl] → pubococcygeus (muscle).
pu·bo·coc·cy·ge·us (muscle) [ˌ-kɒkˈsɪdʒɪəs] Pubokokzygeus *m*, M. pubococcygeus.
pu·bo·fem·o·ral [ˌ-ˈfemərəl] *adj* Schambein/Os pubis u. Oberschenkel/Femur betr. *od.* verbindend, pubofemoral.
pubofemoral ligament Lig. pubofemorale.
pu·bo·pros·tat·ic [ˌ-prɒˈstætɪk] *adj* Schambein/Os pubis u. Prostata betr. *od.* verbindend, puboprostatisch.
puboprostatic ligament Lig. puboprostaticum.
puboprostatic muscle → puboprostaticus (muscle).
pu·bo·pro·sta·ti·cus (muscle) [ˌ-prɒˈstætɪkəs] Puboprostaticus *m*, M. puboprostaticus.
pu·bo·rec·tal [ˌ-ˈrektl] *adj* Schambein/Os pubis u. Rektum betr. *od.* verbindend, puborektal.
pu·bo·rec·ta·lis (muscle) [ˌ-rekˈteɪlɪs] Puborektalis *m*, M. puborectalis.
puborectalis sling Puborektalisschlinge *f*.
puborectal ligament 1. → puboprostatic ligament. **2.** → pubovesical ligament.
puborectal muscle → puborectalis (muscle).
pu·bo·sa·cral diameter [ˌ-ˈseɪkrəl, -ˈsæk-] Conjugata anatomica.
pu·bo·vag·i·nal [ˌ-ˈvædʒənl] *adj* Schambein/Os pubis u. Scheide/Vagina betr. *od.* verbindend, pubovaginal.
pu·bo·vag·i·na·lis (muscle) [ˌ-ˌvædʒəˈneɪlɪs] Pubovaginalis *m*, M. pubovaginalis.
pubovaginal muscle → pubovaginalis (muscle).
pu·bo·ves·i·cal [ˌ-ˈvesɪkl] *adj* Schambein/Os pubis u. Harnblase betr. *od.* verbindend, pubovesikal.
pu·bo·ve·si·ca·lis (muscle) [ˌ-ˌvesɪˈkeɪlɪs] Pubovesicalis *m*, M. pubovesicalis.
pubovesical ligament Lig. pubovesicale.
pubovesical muscle → pubovesicalis (muscle).
PUD *abbr.* → peptic ulcer disease.
pu·den·dal [pjuːˈdendl] *adj* Scham(gegend) betr., zur Scham(gegend) gehörend, pudendal, pubisch, Scham-, Pudendal-.
pudendal anesthesia → pudendal block.
pudendal artery: external p.ies äußere Schamarterien *pl*, Pudendae *pl* externae, A. pudendae externae.
 internal p. innere Schamarterie *f*, Pudenda *f* interna, A. pudenda interna.
pudendal block Pudendusanästhesie *f*, -block *m*.
pudendal canal Alcock'-Kanal *m*, Canalis pudendalis.
pudendal cleavage → pudendal fissure.
pudendal fissure Schamspalte *f*, Rima pudendi.
pudendal hernia Levatorhernie *f*.
pudendal labia Schamlippen *pl*, Labia pudendi.
 greater p. große Schamlippen, Labia majora pudendi.
 lesser p. kleine Schamlippen, Labia minora pudendi.
pudendal nerve Pudendus *m*, N. pudendus.
pudendal plexus venöser Prostataplexus *m*, Plexus venosus prostaticus.
pudendal slit → pudendal fissure.
pudendal ulcer Lymphogranuloma inguinale/venereum *nt abbr.* LGV, Lymphopathia venerea, klimatischer Bubo *m*, Morbus Durand-Nicolas-Favre *m*, vierte Geschlechtskrankheit *f*, Poradenitis inguinalis.
pudendal vein: external p.s äußere Schamvenen *pl*, Vv. pudendae externae.
 internal p. innere Scham(bein)vene *f*, V. pudenda interna.
pu·den·dum [pjuːˈdendəm] *n, pl* **-da** [-də] (weibliche) Scham(gegend *f*) *f*, Vulva *f*, äußere weibliche Geschlechtsorgane/Genitalien *pl*, Pudendum *nt*.
pu·dic ['pjuːdɪk] *adj* → pudendal.
pudic nerve → pudendal nerve.
pu·er·ile ['pjuːərɪl, 'pjʊərɪl, -aɪl] *adj* **1.** kindlich, pueril. **2.** zurückgeblieben, kindisch, pueril.
pu·er·i·lism ['pjuːərəlɪzəm, 'pjʊər-] *n* Puerilismus *m*, Puerilität *f*.
pu·er·per·a [pjuːˈɜrpərə] *n, pl* **-per·ae** [-pəriː] Wöchnerin *f*, Puerpera *f*.
pu·er·per·al [pjuːˈɜrpərəl] *adj* Wochenbett betr., puerperal, Wochenbett-, Kindbett-, Puerperal-.
puerperal convulsions → puerperal eclampsia.
puerperal eclampsia Spätgestose *f* im Wochenbett.
puerperal endometritis *gyn.* Endometritis *f* im Wochenbett, Endometritis puerperalis.
puerperal fever Wochenbett-, Kindbettfieber *nt*, Puerperalfieber *nt*, -sepsis *f*, Febris puerperalis.
puerperal mastitis Mastitis *f* der Wöchnerinnen, Mastitis puerperalis.
puerperal metritis *gyn.* Gebärmutterentzündung *f* während der Puerperalperiode; Metritis puerperalis.
puerperal phlebitis *gyn.* Phlegmasia puerperalis.
puerperal psychosis Wochenbett-, Puerperalpsychose *f*.
puerperal scarlatina puerperaler Scharlach *m*, Scarlatina puerperalis.
puerperal sepsis → puerperal fever.
puerperal septicemia → puerperal fever.
pu·er·per·ant [pjuːˈɜrpərənt] **I** *n* → puerpera. **II** *adj* → puerperal.
pu·er·pe·ri·um [pjuːˈpɪərɪəm] *n gyn.* Wochenbett *nt*, Kindbett *nt*, Puerperium *nt*.
Puestow ['puːstəʊ]: **P.'s procedure I** longitudinale laterolaterale Pankreatikojejunostomie *f*, Puestow-Mercadier I-Operation *f*.
 P.'s procedure II longitudinale lateroterminale Pankreatikojejunostomie *f*, Puestow-Mercadier II-Operation *f*.
puff [pʌf] **I** *n* **1.** *genet.* Puff *m*. **2.** (kurzer) Atemzug *m*; Schnauben *nt*, Schnaufen *nt*. **3.** Schwellung *f*, Beule *f*. **II** *vi* **4.** blasen, pusten. **5.** aufblasen, (auf-)blähen. ~**ed eyes** geschwollene Augen. **III** *vi* **6.** keuchen, blasen, pusten, schnaufen, schnauben. **to ~ and blow** keuchen u. schnaufen. **7.** *s.* (auf-)blähen.
puff out *vi* → puff 7.
puff up I *vt* → puff 5. **II** *vi* → puff 7.
puffed [pʌft] *adj* → puffy 1.
puff·er poisoning ['pʌfər] Tetrodotoxinvergiftung *f*, Tetrodotoxismus *m*.
puff·i·ness ['pʌfɪnɪs] *n* **1.** Aufgeblähtsein *nt*, Aufgeblasenheit *f*, Gedunsenheit *f*; Schwellung *f*. **2.** Kurzatmigkeit *f*.
puff·ing ['pʌfɪŋ] *n genet.* Puffing *nt*.
puff·y ['pʌfɪ] *adj* **1.** aufgebläht, (auf-)gedunsen, aufgeschwemmt, pastös; geschwollen. **2.** kurzatmig, keuchend, außer Atem.
Pu·lex ['pjuːleks] *n micro.* Pulex *m*.
 P. cheopis Pestfloh *m*, Xenopsylla cheopis.
 P. dugesi → P. irritans.
 P. irritans Menschenfloh *m*, Pulex irritans.
 P. penetrans Sandfloh *m*, Tunga/Dermatophilus penetrans.
pu·lex ['pjuːleks] *n micro.* Pulex *m*; Floh *m*.
pu·lic·i·cide [pjuːˈlɪsəsaɪd] *n* → pulicide.
Pu·lic·i·dae [pjuːˈlɪsədiː] *pl micro.* Pulicidae *pl*.
pu·li·cide ['pjuːlɪsaɪd] *n pharm.* Pulizid *nt*.
pull [pʊl] **I** *n* Ruck *m*, Zug *m*; Ziehen *nt*; (*a. fig.*) Anziehungskraft *f*. **II** *vt* **1.** ziehen, zerren. **to ~ a muscle** s. einen Muskel zerren. **2.** (her-)ausziehen, (-)ausreißen; (*Zahn*) extrahieren. **III** *vi* **3.** ziehen, zerren, reißen (*at* an). **4.** saugen (*at* an).
pull out *vt* → pull 2.
pulled elbow [pʊlt] *ortho.* Chassaignac--Lähmung *f*, Subluxation *f* des Radiusköpfchens, Pronatio dolorosa, Subluxatio radii peranularis.
pulled tendon Sehnenzerrung *f*.
pul·ley ['pʊlɪ] *n, pl* **-leys** Ringband *nt*.
pull·ing force ['pʊlɪŋ] Zug(kraft *f*) *m*, Zugspannung *f*.
pull-out suture *chir.*, *ortho.* Ausziehnaht *f*, Bunnell-Naht *f* mit Ausziehdraht.
pull-through procedure *chir.* Durchzugsverfahren *nt*.
pul·lu·late ['pʌljəleɪt] *vi* keimen, sprossen, knospen.
pul·lu·la·tion [ˌpʌljəˈleɪʃn] *n* Sprossen *nt*, Keimen *nt*, Knospen *nt*.
pulmo- *pref.* Lungen-, Pulmonal-, Pulmo-.
pul·mo ['pʌlməʊ] *n, pl* **-mo·nes** [-ˈməʊniːz] Lunge *f*, Lungenflügel *m*; *anat.* Pulmo *m*.

pul·mo·a·or·tic [ˌpʌlməʊeɪˈɔːrtɪk] *adj* Lunge/Pulmo u. Aorta betr. *od.* verbindend, aortopulmonal.
pulmoaortic canal Ductus Botalli, Ductus arteriosus.
pul·mo·lith [ˈ-lɪθ] *n* Lungenstein *m*, Pulmolith *m*, Pneumolith *m*.
pulmon- *pref.* → pulmo-.
pul·mo·nal [ˈpʌlmənl] *adj* → pulmonary.
pulmonal disease Lungenkrankheit *f*.
pul·mo·nar·y [ˈpʌlməˌnerɪː, -nərɪ, ˈpʊl-] *adj* Lunge/Pulmo betr., pulmonal, Lungen-, Pulmonal-, Pulmo-.
pulmonary abscess Lungenabszeß *m*.
pulmonary acid aspiration syndrome *gyn.* Mendelson-Syndrom *nt*.
pulmonary adenomatosis → pulmonary carcinoma, bronchoalveolar.
pulmonary alveolar proteinosis pulmonale alveoläre Proteinose *f*, Lungen-, Alveolarproteinose *f*.
pulmonary alveoli Lungenalveolen *pl*, -bläschen *pl*, Alveoli pulmonis.
pulmonary amebiasis Lungenamöbiasis *f*.
pulmonary anthracosis Lungenanthrakose *f*, Kohlenstaublunge *f*, Anthracosis pulmonum.
pulmonary anthrax Lungenmilzbrand *m*, Wollsortierer-, Lumpensortierer-, Hadernkrankheit *f*.
pulmonary arch *embryo.* Pulmonalbogen *m*.
pulmonary area Pulmonalisauskultationspunkt *m*.
pulmonary artery Truncus pulmonalis.
 left p. linke Lungenschlagader *f*, Pulmonalis *f* sinistra, A. pulmonalis sinistra.
 overriding p. überreitende Pulmonalis *f*, überreitende A. pulmonalis.
 right p. rechte Lungenschlagader *f*, Pulmonalis *f* dextra, A. pulmonalis dextra.
pulmonary artery banding *HTG* Drosselung/Bändelung *f* der A. pulmonalis.
pulmonary artery catheter Pulmonalarterienkatheter *m*.
pulmonary artery pressure *abbr.* **PAP** Pulmonalarteriendruck *m*, Pulmonalisdruck *m*.
pulmonary artery wedge pressure *abbr.* **PAWP, PWP** pulmonaler Kapillardruck *m*, pulmonary artery/capillary wedge pressure *abbr.* PAWP, PWP.
pulmonary aspergilloma Aspergillom *nt* der Lunge, Lungenaspergillose *f*.
pulmonary atresia Pulmonalatresie *f*.
pulmonary auscultation Lungenauskultation *f*.
pulmonary bleeding Lungen(ein)blutung *f*.
pulmonary branches of autonomic nervous system Lungenfasern *pl* des autonomen Nervensystems, Rami pulmonales systematis autonomici.
pulmonary calcinosis, metastatic metastatische Lungenkalzinose *f*, Bimsstein-, Tuffsteinlunge *f*.
pulmonary capillary wedge pressure → pulmonary artery wedge pressure.
pulmonary carcinoma Lungenkrebs *m*, -karzinom *nt*.
 bronchoalveolar p. bronchiolo-alveoläres Lungenkarzinom, Alveolarzellenkarzinom, Lungenadenomatose *f*, Ca. alveolocellulare/alveolare.
pulmonary carcinosis → pulmonary carcinoma, bronchoalveolar.
pulmonary cavity Lungenkaverne *f*.
pulmonary channel *embryo.* Pulmonalkanal *m*.
pulmonary circulation kleiner Kreislauf *m*, Lungenkreislauf *m*.

pulmonary cirrhosis Lungenzirrhose *f*, diffuse interstitielle Lungenfibrose *f*.
pulmonary collapse Lungenkollaps *m*.
pulmonary cone Conus arteriosus, Infundibulum *nt*.
pulmonary congestion Lungenstauung *f*.
pulmonary contusion Kontusionslunge *f*, Lungenkontusion *f*, -quetschung *f*.
pulmonary cyanosis pulmonale/pulmonal-bedingte Zyanose *f*.
pulmonary denervation Lungendenervierung *f*.
pulmonary disease Lungenerkrankung *f*, -krankheit *f*, -leiden *nt*.
 chronic obstructive p. *abbr.* **COPD** chronisch-obstruktive Lungenerkrankung/Atemwegserkrankung.
 obstructive p. obstruktive Lungenerkrankung.
 restrictive p. restriktive Lungenerkrankung.
pulmonary distomiasis Lungenegelbefall *m*, Paragonimiasis *f*, Paragonimose *f*.
pulmonary dysmaturity (syndrome) Wilson-Mikity-Syndrom *nt*, bronchopulmonale Dysplasie *f*.
pulmonary dystomiasis Lungenegelbefall *m*, Paragonimiasis *f*, Paragonimose *f*.
pulmonary edema Lungenödem *nt*.
 interstitial p. interstitielles Lungenödem.
 intra-alveolar p. intraalveoläres Lungenödem.
 inveterate p. inveteriertes Lungenödem.
pulmonary embolism *abbr.* **PE** Lungenembolie *f*.
pulmonary embolus Lungenembolus *m*.
pulmonary emphysema Lungenemphysem *nt*, -blähung *f*, Emphysema pulmonum.
 acute p. akutes Lungenemphysem.
 alveolar p. alveoläres Lungenemphysem.
 bullous p. bullöses Lungenemphysem.
 centriacinar p. zentroazinäres/zentriaziäres (Lungen-)Emphysem.
 centrilobular p. zentrilobuläres (Lungen-)Emphysem.
 centroacinar p. → centriacinar p.
 chronic p. chronisches Lungenemphysem.
 compensating/compensatory p. kompensatorisches Lungenemphysem.
 constitutional p. → senile p.
 destructive p. chronisch-destruktives Lungenemphysem.
 diffuse p. → panacinar p.
 interstitial p. interstitielles Lungenemphysem.
 kinetic p. kinetisches Lungenemphysem.
 marginal p. Randemphysem.
 obstructive p. obstruktives Lungenemphysem.
 panacinar p. panazinäres/panlobuläres/diffuses Lungenemphysem.
 panlobular p. → panacinar p.
 paracicatricial p. → scar p.
 paraseptal p. paraseptales Lungenemphysem.
 perinodular p. perinoduläres Lungenemphysem.
 scar p. (*Lunge*) Narbenemphysem.
 senile p. Altersemphysem, konstitutionelles/seniles Lungenemphysem.
 subpleural p. subpleurales Lungenemphysem.
pulmonary fat embolism syndrome Schocklunge *f*, adult respiratory distress syndrome *abbr.* ARDS.
pulmonary fever *old* → pneumonia.
pulmonary fibrosis 1. Lungenfibrose *f*. **2.** → pulmonary cirrhosis.
 idiopathic p. → pulmonary cirrhosis.

 diffuse interstitial p. → pulmonary cirrhosis.
pulmonary fistula Lungenfistel *f*.
pulmonary function study/test Lungenfunktionsprüfung *f*.
pulmonary graft Lungentransplantat *nt*.
pulmonary heart Rechtsherz *nt*.
pulmonary hemorrhage → pulmonary bleeding.
pulmonary hemosiderosis Lungenhämosiderose *f*.
 idiopathic/primary p. Ceelen-Gellerstedt-Syndrom *nt*, primäre/idiopathische Lungenhämosiderose.
pulmonary hilum Lungenhilus *m*, Hilum pulmonis.
pulmonary hypertension pulmonale Hypertonie *f*.
pulmonary hypoplasia Lungenhypoplasie *f*.
pulmonary hypostasis Lungenhypostase *f*.
pulmonary incompetence → pulmonary regurgitation.
pulmonary infarction Lungeninfarkt *m*.
 anemic p. anämischer Lungeninfarkt.
 hemorrhagic p. hämorrhagischer Lungeninfarkt.
pulmonary infiltration Lungeninfiltrat *nt*.
pulmonary infection Lungeninfektion *f*.
pulmonary insufficiency 1. respiratorische Insuffizienz *f*. **2.** → pulmonary regurgitation.
pulmonary ligament Lig. pulmonale.
pulmonary lobe Lungenlappen *m*, Lobus pulmonis.
 inferior p., left linker Unterlappen, Lobus inferior pulmonis sinistri.
 inferior p., right rechter Unterlappen, Lobus inferior pulmonis dextri.
 middle p., (right) Mittellappen, Lobus medius pulmonis dextri.
 superior p., left linker Oberlappen, Lobus superior pulmonis sinistri.
 superior p., right rechter Oberlappen, Lobus superior pulmonis dextri.
pulmonary metastasis Lungenmetastase *f*.
pulmonary murmur Pulmonal(klappen)geräusch *nt*.
pulmonary osteoarthropathy Marie-Bamberger-Syndrom *nt*, Bamberger-Marie-Syndrom *nt*, Akropachie *f*, hypertrophische pulmonale Osteoarthropathie *f*.
pulmonary perfusion Lungendurchblutung *f*, -perfusion *f*.
pulmonary phthisis Lungenschwindsucht *f*, -tuberkulose *f*, Phthisis pulmonum.
pulmonary physiotherapy Atemgymnastik *f*.
pulmonary pleura Lungenfell *nt*, Viszeralpleura *f* der Lunge, Pleura visceralis/pulmonalis.
pulmonary pleurisy Lungenfellentzündung *f*.
pulmonary plexus vegetatives Lungengeflecht *nt*, Plexus pulmonalis.
 anterior p. vorderer Teil *m* des Lungengeflechts, Plexus pulmonalis anterior.
 posterior p. hinterer Teil *m* des Lungengeflechts, Plexus pulmonalis posterior.
pulmonary pressure → pulmonary artery pressure.
pulmonary pseudocysts Zystenlunge *f*.
pulmonary regurgitation *card.* Pulmonalisinsuffizienz *f*, Pulmonal(klappen)insuffizienz *f*.
pulmonary resection → pneumonectomy.
pulmonary respiration Lungenatmung *f*, (äußere) Atmung *f*, Atmen *nt*, Respiration *f*.

pulmonary schistosomiasis Lungenbilharziose f, Schistosomiasis pulmonalis.
pulmonary sclerosis Lungensklerose f.
  emphysematous p. emphysematöse Lungensklerose.
pulmonary siderosis Eisen(staub)lunge f, Lungensiderose f, Siderosis pulmonum.
pulmonary stenosis Pulmonalis-, Pulmonal(klappen)stenose f.
  infundibular p. card. Infundibulumstenose f, subvalvuläre/infundibuläre Pulmonalstenose f.
  subvalvular p. → infundibular p.
  supravalvular p. supravalvuläre Pulmonalisstenose.
  valvular p. valvuläre Pulmonalisstenose.
pulmonary sulcus (of thorax) Sulcus pulmonalis thoracis.
pulmonary sulcus tumor Pancoast-Tumor m, apikaler Sulkustumor m.
pulmonary surface of heart (*Herz*) Seiten-, Lungenfläche f, Facies pulmonalis/lateralis (cordis).
pulmonary talcosis Talkumlunge f, -pneumokoniose f, Talkose f.
pulmonary toilet Bronchialtoilette f.
pulmonary transplant Lungentransplantat nt.
pulmonary transplantation Lungentransplantation f.
pulmonary trunk Tuncus pulmonalis.
pulmonary trunk valve → pulmonary valve.
pulmonary tuberculosis Lungentuberkulose f, Lungen-Tb f.
  acinonodular p. azino-noduläre Lungentuberkulose.
  apical p. (Lungen-)Spitzentuberkulose.
  exudative p. exsudative Lungentuberkulose.
  productive p. produktive Lungentuberkulose.
  progressive p. progressive Lungentuberkulose.
pulmonary tularemia pulmonale Tularämie f, Lungentularämie f.
pulmonary valve Pulmonal(is)klappe f, Valva trunci pulmonalis.
pulmonary vein Lungenvene f, V. pulmonalis.
  left p.s linke Lungenvenen pl, Vv. pulmonales sinistrae.
  left p., inferior untere linke Lungenvene, V. pulmonalis sinistra inferior.
  left p., superior obere linke Lungenvene, V. pulmonalis sinistra superior.
  right p.s rechte Lungenvenen pl, Vv. pulmonales dextrae.
  right p., inferior untere rechte Lungenvene, V. pulmonalis dextra inferior.
  right p., superior obere rechte Lungenvene, V. pulmonalis dextra superior.
pulmonary vesicles → pulmonary alveoli.
pulmonary vessels Lungengefäße pl.
pul·mo·nec·to·my [ˌpʌlməˈnɛktəmɪ] n → pneumonectomy.
pul·mon·ic [pʌlˈmɑnɪk, pʊl-] adj → pulmonary.
pulmonic incompetence → pulmonary regurgitation.
pulmonic murmur → pulmonary murmur.
pulmonic plague Lungenpest f, Pestpneumonie f.
pulmonic regurgitation → pulmonary regurgitation.
pulmonic tularemia → pulmonary tularemia.
pul·mo·ni·tis [ˌpʌlməˈnaɪtɪs] n **1.** → pneumonia. **2.** → pneumonitis.
pulmono- pref. → pulmo-.

pul·mo·nol·o·gy [ˌ-ˈnɑlədʒɪ] n → pneumology.
pul·mo·no·per·i·to·ne·al [ˌpʌlmənəʊˌperɪtəˈniːəl] adj Lunge(n) u. Peritoneum betr., pulmo-, pneumoperitoneal.
pulp [pʌlp] I n **1.** anat. (*Organ*) Mark nt, Parenchym nt, Pulpa f. **2.** bio. gefäßreiches weiches Gewebe nt. **3.** Fruchtfleisch nt; Brei m, breiige Masse f. II vt zu Brei verarbeiten. III vi breiig werden.
  p. of spleen rote Pulpa, Milzpulpa, Pulpa splenica/lienis.
pul·pa [ˈpʌlpə] n → pulp.
pulp abscess 1. dent. Pulpaabszeß m. **2.** ortho. Fingerbeerenabszeß m.
pul·pal [ˈpʌlpəl] adj Mark/Pulpa betr., Pulpa-, Mark-.
pulpal abscess → pulp abscess.
pulpal cells (*Milz*) Pulpazellen pl.
pul·pal·gia [pʌlˈpældʒ(ɪ)ə] n dent. Pulpalgie f.
pulp amyloidosis (*Milz*) Pulpaamyloidose f.
pulp arteries (*Milz*) Pulpaarterien pl.
pulp canal (Zahn-)Wurzelkanal m, Canalis radicis dentis.
pulp cavity Zahn-, Pulpahöhle f, Cavitas dentis/pulparis.
pulp chamber Kronenabschnitt m der Zahn-/Pulpahöhle, Cavitas coronalis.
pulp·i·ness [ˈpʌlpɪnɪs] n Weichheit f, Breiigkeit f, Fleischigkeit f.
pul·pi·tis [pʌlˈpaɪtɪs] n dent. Pulpaentzündung f, Zahnmarkentzündung f, Pulpitis f.
pulp veins (*Milz*) Pulpavenen pl.
pulp·y [ˈpʌlpɪ] adj weich, breiig, fleischig, markartig, markig, pulpös.
pulpy swelling patho. markige Schwellung f.
pul·sate [ˈpʌlseɪt] vi **1.** (rhythmisch) schlagen od. pochen, pulsieren. **2.** vibrieren.
pul·sa·tile [ˈpʌlsətɪl, -taɪl] adj (rhythmisch) schlagend od. klopfend, pochend, pulsierend, pulsatil.
pulsatile flow pulsierende Strömung f.
pul·sat·ing exophthalmus [ˈpʌlseɪtɪŋ] pulsierender Exophthalmus m, Exophthalmus pulsans.
pulsating pain pulsierender Schmerz m.
pul·sa·tion [pʌlˈseɪʃn] n **1.** Schlagen m, Pochen nt, Pulsieren nt, Pulsation f, Pulsatio f. **2.** Pulsschlag m. **3.** Vibrieren nt.
pul·sa·tive [ˈpʌlsətɪv] adj → pulsatile.
pul·sa·to·ry [ˈpʌlsətɔːriː, -təʊ-] adj → pulsatile.
pulse [pʌls] I n **1.** Puls m, Pulsschlag m; Pulsus m. **to feel/take s.o.'s ~** jdm. den Puls fühlen od. messen; inf. pulsen. **2.** Pulsieren nt. **3.** phys. Impuls m. II vi → pulsate.
pulse-beat [ˈpʌlsbiːt] n Pulsschlag m.
pulse curve Pulskurve f, Sphygmogramm nt.
pulse deficit Pulsdefizit nt.
pulse generator physiol., card. Impulsnerator m.
pulse·less disease [ˈpʌlslɪs] Martorell-Krankheit f, -Syndrom nt, Takayasu-Krankheit f, -Syndrom nt, Pulslos-Krankheit f, pulseless disease (nt).
pulse·less·ness [ˈpʌlslɪsnɪs] n Pulslosigkeit f.
pulse pressure Pulsdruck m.
pulse quality Pulsqualität f.
pulse rate abbr. **PR** Pulsfrequenz f; inf. Puls m.
pulse wave Pulswelle f.
pulse wave transmission time, central physiol. zentrale Pulswellenlaufzeit f.
pulse wave velocity abbr. **PWV** physiol. Pulswellengeschwindigkeit f abbr. PWG.

pul·sim·e·ter [pʌlˈsɪmətər] n Pulsmesser m.
pul·sion diverticulum [ˈpʌlʃn] Pulsionsdivertikel nt.
pulsion hernia Pulsionshernie f.
pul·som·e·ter [pʌlˈsɑmɪtər] n → pulsimeter.
pul·sus [ˈpʌlsəs] n → pulse 1.
pul·ver·a·ble [ˈpʌlvərəbl] adj pulverisierbar.
pul·ver·iz·a·ble [ˈpʌlvəraɪzəbl] adj → pulverable.
pul·ver·i·za·tion [ˌpʌlvərɪˈzeɪʃn] n Pulverisierung f, Pulverisieren nt.
pul·ver·ize [ˈpʌlvəraɪz] vt zerreiben, zerstoßen, zermahlen, pulverisieren.
pul·ver·u·lent [pʌlˈverjələnt, -ˈverə-] adj pulv(e)rig; staubig.
pul·vi·nar [pʌlˈvaɪnər] n, pl **-nar·ia** [ˌpʌlvəˈneərɪə] anat. **1.** Polster nt, Pulvinar nt. **2.** hinterer Teil m des Thalamus, Pulvinar thalami.
pulvinar nuclei Ncc. pulvinares.
pul·vi·nate [ˈpʌlvɪneɪt] adj kissenförmig.
pul·vis [ˈpʌlvɪs] n pharm. Pulver nt, Pulvis m; Puder m.
pu·mex [ˈpjuːmɛks] n → pumice.
pum·ice [ˈpʌmɪs] n Bimsstein m.
pumice lung Bimsstein-, Tuffsteinlunge f, metastatische Lungenkalzinose f.
pump [pʌmp] I n Pumpe f. II vt, vi pumpen.
pump dry vt (her-)auspumpen, leerpumpen.
pump out vt auspumpen.
pump up vt auf-, hochpumpen.
pump-and-leak mechanism physiol. Pump-und-Leck-Mechanismus m.
pump current physiol. Pumpstrom m.
pump·ing rate [ˈpʌmpɪŋ] physiol. Pumprate f.
pump-oxygenator n Herz-Lungen-Maschine f.
pump room Trinkhalle f, Brunnenhaus nt (in Kurorten).
pu·na [ˈpuːnɑ] n Höhenkrankheit f.
punch biopsy [pʌntʃ] Stanzbiopsie f.
punch-drunk adj → punch-drunk syndrome.
punch-drunk encephalopathy → punch-drunk syndrome.
punch-drunk syndrome Boxerenzephalopathie f, Encephalopathia traumatica.
punch graft Stanzläppchen nt.
punc·tate [ˈpʌŋkteɪt] adj **1.** punktiert, getüpfelt. **2.** punktförmig, Punkt-.
punctate bleeding Punktblutung f, punktförmige Blutung f.
punctate cataract punktförmige Linsentrübung f, Cataracta punctata.
punc·tat·ed [ˈpʌŋkteɪtɪd] adj → punctate.
punctate hemorrhage → punctate bleeding.
punc·ta·tion [pʌŋkˈteɪʃn] n **1.** Tüpfelung f, Punktierung f. **2.** Punkt m, Tüpfel m.
punc·tum [ˈpʌŋktəm] n, pl **-ta** [-tə] anat. Punkt m, Punctum nt.
punc·ture [ˈpʌŋktʃər] I n **1.** Stich m, Einstich m, Loch nt. **2.** Punktion f, Punktur f, Punctio f. II vt **3.** durchstechen, durchbohren. **4.** punktieren, eine Punktion vornehmen od. durchführen. III vi ein Loch bekommen, platzen.
puncture biopsy Punktionsbiopsie f, Punktion f.
puncture diabetes Bernard-Zuckerstich m.
puncture headache Kopfschmerz(en pl) m nach einer Lumbalpunktion.
pun·gen·cy [ˈpʌndʒənsɪ] n Schärfe f; Stechen nt, Beißen nt.
pun·gent [ˈpʌndʒənt] adj (*Geruch*) stechend, beißend; (*Schmerz*) stechend; (*Geschmack*) scharf.

pu·pa ['pju:pə] *n*, *pl* -pas, -pae [-pi:] *bio.* Puppe *f*, Pupa *f*.
pu·pal ['pju:pəl] *adj bio.* Puppen-.
pu·pil ['pju:pl, -pɪl] *n* 1. (*Auge*) Pupille *f*, Pupilla *f*. 2. Schüler(in *f*) *m*, Praktikant(in *f*) *m*.
pupil dilation Pupillenvergrößerung *f*, -dilatation *f*.
pupill- *pref.* → pupillo-.
pu·pil·la [pjuːˈpɪlə] *n*, *pl* -lae [-liː] → pupil 1.
pu·pil·lar·y ['pjuːpəˌleriː, -ləri] *adj* Pupille betr., pupillär, Pupillen-.
pupillary accommodation reflex Akkommodationsreaktion *f*, -reflex *m*, Naheinstellungsreaktion *f*, -reflex *m*.
pupillary athetosis Pupillenzittern *nt*, Irisblinzeln *nt*, Hippus *m* (pupillae), Athetosis pupillaris.
pupillary block glaucoma akutes Winkelblockglaukom/Engwinkelglaukom *nt*, Glaucoma acutum (congestivum).
pupillary light reflex (*Pupille*) Lichtreaktion *f*, -reflex *m*.
pupillary margin of iris innerer Rand *od.* Pupillenrand *m* der Iris, Margo pupillaris iridis.
pupillary membrane *embryo.* Membrana pupillaris.
pupillary phenomenon → pupillary reflex 1.
  paradoxical p. → pupillary reflex, paradoxical.
pupillary reaction Pupillenreaktion *f*, -reflex *m*.
  hemiopic p. Wernicke-Phänomen *nt*.
pupillary reflex 1. Pupillenreflex *m*, -reaktion *f*. 2. (*Pupille*) Lichtreaktion *f*, -reflex *m*.
  paradoxical p. Bechterew-Pupillenreflex, paradoxer Pupillenreflex.
  reversed p. → paradoxical p.
pupillary-skin reflex ziliospinaler Reflex *m*.
pu·pil·la·to·nia [ˌpju:pɪləˈtəʊnɪə] *n* Adie'-Pupille *f*, Pupillotonie *f*.
pupillo- *pref.* Pupillen-, Pupill(o)-, Pupillar-.
pu·pil·lo·graph [pjuːˈpɪləgræf] *n* Pupillograph *m*.
pu·pil·log·ra·phy [ˌpju:pɪˈlagrəfi] *n* Pupillographie *f*.
pu·pil·lom·e·ter [ˌ-ˈlamɪtər] *n* Pupillometer *nt*.
pu·pil·lom·e·try [ˌ-ˈlamətri] *n* Pupillometrie *f*.
pu·pil·lo·mo·tor [ˌpju:pɪləʊˈməʊtər] *adj* pupillomotorisch.
pupillomotor muscles pupillomotorische Muskeln *pl*.
pu·pil·lo·ple·gia [ˌ-ˈpli:dʒ(ɪ)ə] *n* Pupillotonie *f*.
pu·pil·los·co·py [ˌpju:pɪˈlaskəpɪ] *n ophthal.* Retinoskopie *f*, Skiaskopie *f*.
pu·pil·lo·sta·tom·e·ter [pjuːˌpɪləʊstəˈtamɪtər] *n* Pupillostatometer *nt*.
pu·pil·lo·to·nia [ˌpju:pɪləˈtəʊnɪə] *n* Adie'-Pupille *f*, Pupillotonie *f*.
pu·pil·lo·ton·ic pseudotabes [ˌ-ˈtanɪk] Adie-Syndrom *nt*.
pupil response *physiol.* Pupillenreaktion *f*.
pure [pjʊər] *adj* rein, unvermischt, pur.
pure color reine Farbe *f*, reiner Farbton *m*, Farbton *m* einer Wellenlänge.
pure culture *micro.* Reinkultur *f*.
pure leukocytosis Granulozytose *f*.
pure red cell anemia → pure red cell aplasia.
pure red cell aplasia 1. aregenerative Anämie *f*. 2. chronische kongenitale aregenerative Anämie *f*, Blackfan-Diamond--Anämie *f*, pure red cell aplasia.

pure tone audiometry *HNO* Reintonaudiometrie *f abbr.* RTA.
pur·ga·tion [pərˈgeɪʃn] *n* (Darm-)Reinigung *f*, (Darm-)Entleerung *f*.
pur·ga·tive ['pərgətɪv] I *n* Abführmittel *nt*, Purgativ *nt*, Purgativum *nt*. II *adj* reinigend, abführend, purgierend, Abführ-.
purge [pɜrdʒ] I *n* 1. Reinigung *f*, Säuberung *f*. 2. Darmentleerung *f*, -reinigung *f*. II *vt* 3. reinigen, säubern, befreien (*of, from* von); (*Flüssigkeit*) klären. 4. (*Darm*) entleeren, reinigen, entschlacken; ein Abführmittel geben. III *vi* Stuhlgang haben; (*Medikament*) abführen.
pu·ric ['pjʊərɪk] *adj* 1. Eiter betr., Eiter-. 2. Purin betr., Purin-.
pu·ri·fi·ca·tion [ˌpjʊərɪfɪˈkeɪʃn] *n phys., chem.* Reinigung *f*; Klärung *f*.
pu·ri·fied ['pjʊərəfaɪd] *adj* gereinigt, geklärt, raffiniert.
purified chick embryo cell vaccine *abbr.* PCECV. purified chick embryo cell vaccine *abbr.* PCECV.
purified placental protein humanes Plazenta-Laktogen *nt abbr.* HPL, Choriosomatotropin *nt*.
purified protein derivative tuberculin gereinigtes Tuberkulin *nt abbr.* GT, PPD-Tuberkulin *nt*.
pu·ri·fier ['pjʊərɪfaɪər] *n* Reiniger *m*, Reinigungsmittel *nt od.* -apparat *m*.
pu·ri·form ['pjʊərɪfɔːrm] *adj* eiterartig, eitrig, purulent.
puriform softening *patho.* puriforme Erweichung *f*.
pu·ri·fy ['pjʊərɪfaɪ] *vt phys., chem.* reinigen, klären, aufbereiten (*of, from* von); raffinieren.
pu·ri·fy·ing plant ['pjʊərɪfaɪɪŋ] Reinigungsanlage *f*.
pu·rine ['pjʊəriːn, -rɪn] *n* Purin *nt*.
purine antagonist Purinantagonist *m*.
purine base Purinbase *f*.
purine body → purine base.
purine degradation Purinabbau *m*.
purine derivative Purinderivat *nt*.
pu·ri·ne·mia [pjʊərɪˈniːmɪə] *n* Purinämie *f*.
purine-nucleoside phosphorylase Purinnukleosidphosphorylase *f*.
purine-5'-nucleotidase *n* 5'-Nukleotidase *f*, 5'-Nucleotidase *f*.
purine nucleotide cycle Purinnukleotidzyklus *m*.
purine ribonucleotide Purinribonukleotid *nt*.
pu·ri·ty ['pjʊərətɪ] *n* Reinheit *f*, Reinheitsgrad *m*.
Purkinje [pərˈkɪnjiː]: **P.'s afterimages** Purkinje'-Nachbilder *pl*.
  P.'s cell Purkinje-Zelle *f*.
  P.'s cell layer (of cerebellum) Purkinje-(Zell-)Schicht *f*, Stratum neurium piriformium.
  P.'s conduction *card.* Erregungsleitung *f* in den Purkinje'-Fasern.
  P.'s corpuscle → P.'s cell.
  P.'s effect → P.'s phenomenon.
  P. fibers Purkinje-Fasern *pl*.
  P.'s figures → P.'s afterimages.
  P.'s layer (of cerebellum) → P.'s cell layer (of cerebellum).
  P.'s network Rami subendocardiales.
  P.'s phenomenon Purkinje-Phänomen *nt*.
  P.'s shadows → P.'s afterimages
  P.'s shift → P.'s phenomenon.
  P.'s vesicle Keimbläschen *nt*.
pur·pu·ra ['pɜrpjʊərə] *n* Purpura *f*.
pur·pu·ric [pərˈpjʊərɪk] *adj* Purpura betr., purpurisch, Purpura-.
pur·pu·rin [pərˈpjʊərɪn] *n* Uroerythrin *f*.
purr [pɜr] *n card.* (*Auskultation*) Schnurren *nt*, Summen *nt*.

purse-string suture [pɜrsˈstrɪŋ] *chir.* Tabaksbeutelnaht *f*.
pur·suit movement [pərˈs(j)uːt] (*Auge*) Folgebewegung *f*.
Purtscher ['pʊərtʃər]: **P.'s angiopathic retinopathy** → P.'s syndrome.
  P.'s disease → P.'s syndrome.
  P.'s syndrome Purtscher-Syndrom *nt*, -Netzhautschädigung *f*.
pu·ru·hep·a·ti·tis [pjʊərəˌhepəˈtaɪtɪs] *n* Leberabszeß *m*.
pu·ru·lence ['pjʊər(j)ələns] *n* 1. Eitrigkeit *f*. 2. Eiter *m*.
pu·ru·len·cy ['pjʊər(j)ələnsɪ] *n* → purulence.
pu·ru·lent ['pjʊər(j)ələnt] *adj* eitrig, eiternd, purulent, suppurativ.
purulent appendicitis eitrige Appendizitis *f*, Appendicitis purulenta.
purulent balanitis eitrige/purulente Balanitis *f*, Balanorrhoe *f*; Balanoblennorrhoe *f*.
purulent catarrh eitriger Katarrh *m*.
purulent conjunctivitis eitrige Konjunktivitis *f*, Conjunctivitis purulenta.
purulent cyclitis eitrige/purulente Zyklitis *f*.
purulent effusion eitriger Erguß *m*.
purulent encephalitis eitrige Enzephalitis *f*, Encephalitis purulenta; Hirnabszeß *m*.
purulent expectoration Eiterspucken *nt*, Pyoptyse *f*.
purulent inflammation eitrige Entzündung *f*.
purulent iritis *ophthal.* eitrige Iritis *f*, Iritis purulenta.
purulent keratitis eitrige Keratitis *f*, Keratitis purulenta/suppurativa.
purulent meningitis eitrige Meningitis *f*, Meningitis purulenta.
purulent myocarditis eitrige Myokarditis *f*.
purulent ophthalmia eitrige Konjunktivitis/Ophthalmie *f*.
purulent pericarditis eitrige Herzbeutelentzündung/Perikarditis *f*, Pericarditis purulenta.
purulent peritonitis eitrige Bauchfellentzündung/Peritonitis *f*, Peritonitis purulenta.
purulent pleurisy 1. eitrige Brustfellentzündung/Pleuritis *f*, Pleuritis purulenta. 2. Thoraxempyem *nt*.
purulent pneumonia eitrige Pneumonie *f*.
purulent rhinitis eitrige Rhinitis *f*, Rhinitis purulenta.
purulent salpingitis eitrige Salpingitis *f*, Salpingitis purulenta, Pyosalpingitis *f*.
purulent sinusitis eitrige Sinusitis *f*, Sinusitis purulenta.
purulent synovitis akute eitrige Arthritis *f*, Gelenkeiterung *f*, -empyem *nt*, Pyarthrose *f*, Arthritis purulenta.
pu·ru·loid [pjʊərˈpjɔɪd] *adj* eiterartig, -ähnlich, eitrig, puriform.
pu·ru·mu·cous [ˌpjʊərəˈmjuːkəs] *adj* schleimig-eitrig, mukopurulent.
pus [pʌs] *n* Eiter *m*.
pus cast *urol.* Leukozytenzylinder *m*.
pus cells Eiterzellen *pl*, -körperchen *pl*.
pus corpuscles → pus cells.
pus focus Eiterherd *m*.
push-back procedure [pʊʃ] *HNO* Gaumenrückverlagerung *f*, Push-back-Operation *f*.
pus tube → pyosalpinx.
pus·tu·la ['pʌstʃələ] *n*, *pl* -lae [-liː] → pustule.
pus·tu·lar ['pʌstʃələr] *adj* Pustel/Pustula betr., mit Pustelbildung einhergehend, pustulös, Pustel-.

pustular blepharitis *ophthal.* Blepharitis follicularis.
pustular miliaria *derm.* Miliaria pustulosa.
pustular psoriasis *derm.* **1.** pustulöse Psoriasis vulgaris, Psoriasis pustulosa. **2.** → generalized p.
generalized p. Psoriasis pustulosa vom Typ Zumbusch, Psoriasis pustulosa generalisata, Psoriasis pustulosa gravis Zumbusch.
localized p. Psoriasis pustulosa Typ Königsbeck-Barber, Psoriasis pustulosa palmaris et plantaris.
pustular syphilid pustulöses Syphilid *nt.*
pus·tu·la·tion [ˌpʌstʃəˈleɪʃn] *n* Pustelbildung *f.*
pus·tule [ˈpʌstʃʊl] *n derm.* Eiterbläschen *nt*, Pustel *f*, Pustula *f.*
pus·tu·li·form [ˈpʌstʃəlɪfɔːrm] *adj* pustelartig, pustuliform.
pus·tu·lo·sis [ˌpʌstʃəˈləʊsɪs] *n derm.* Pustulose *f*, Pustulosis *f.*
put [pʊt] (**put; put**) *vt* **1.** setzen, stellen, legen; stecken; (*zu Bett*) bringen; (*in Ordnung*) bringen; (*in Gang*) setzen; (*Vorschlag*) vorbringen. **2. to ~ o.s. under s.o.'s care** s. in jds. Obhut begeben. **3.** anbringen (*on* an); befestigen *od.* machen (*on* an). **4.** schreiben, malen, zeichnen.
put across *vt* jdm. etw. verständlich machen, jdm. etw. vermitteln (*to sb.*).
put away *vt* **1.** ein-, weg-, aufräumen, weglegen, -stecken, beiseite tun. **2.** *inf.* jdn. in eine Anstalt stecken. **3.** (*Tier*) einschläfern.
put back *vt* **1.** zurückschieben, -stellen, -tun, -setzen, -legen; (*Uhr*) zurückstellen. **2.** *fig.* aufhalten, hemmen. **3.** etw. auf-, verschieben.
put down *vt* **1.** weglegen, -tun, -setzen, -stellen. **2.** (*Tier*) einschläfern. **3.** (auf-, nieder-)schreiben. **4.** heruntersetzen, reduzieren; beschränken. **5.** zuschreiben (*to*); zurückführen (*to* auf).
put in *vt* herein-, hineinlegen, -stellen, -setzen; einbauen.
put off *vt* **1.** etw. ver-, aufschieben; hinauszögern. **2.** jdn. hinhalten (*with* mit). **3.** jdm. abraten (*from* von); jdn. abbringen (*from* etc.) **4.** jdm. etw. verleiden. **5.** (*Licht etc.*) ausschalten.
put on *vt* **1.** (*Kleidung*) anziehen; (*Brille*) aufsetzen. **2.** (*Gewicht*) zunehmen. **3.** (*Makeup*) auftragen, auflegen. **4.** vortäuschen, heucheln, so tun als ob, übertreiben. **5.** auf eine bestimmte Therapie/Diät setzen. **to ~ a diet auf** Diät setzen. **to ~ a splint** (*Bruch*) schienen.
put out *vt* **1.** (*Hand, Zunge*) aus-, herausstrecken. **2.** (*Gliedmaße*) auskugeln, aus-, verrenken. **3.** (*Feuer*) löschen, ausmachen. **4.** bewußtlos machen, betäuben. **5.** verstimmen, verärgern. **to be ~ about sth.** über etw. verärgert sein.
put over *vt* → put across.
put up *vt* **1.** jdn. unterbringen. **2.** (*Arm*) hochheben. **3.** aufstellen, errichten, aufhängen. **4.** (*Preis*) erhöhen, heraufsetzen.
put up with *vi* s. abfinden mit, s. gefallen lassen.
pu·ta·men [pjuːˈteɪmɪn] *n, pl* **-tam·i·na** [-ˈtæmɪnə] *anat., bot.* Schale *f*, Hülse *f*, Putamen *nt.*
Putnam [ˈpʌtnəm]: **P.'s disease/type** → Putnam-Dana syndrome.
Putnam-Dana [ˈdænə]: **P.-D. syndrome** Lichtheim-Syndrom *nt*, Dana-Syndrom *nt*, Dana-Lichtheim-Krankheit *f*, Dana-Lichtheim-Putnam-Syndrom *nt*, funikuläre Spinalerkrankung/Myelose *f.*

pu·tre·fa·cient [ˌpjuːtrəˈfeɪʃnt] *adj* → putrefactive.
pu·tre·fac·tion [ˌ-ˈfækʃn] *n* **1.** Fäulnis *f*, Verwesung *f*, Zersetzung *f*, Putrefaktion *f*; Faulen *nt*, Putreszieren *nt.* **2.** Verfall *m.*
pu·tre·fac·tive [ˌ-ˈfæktɪv] *adj* fäulniserregend, Fäulnis-.
putrefactive alkaloid Leichengift *nt*, -alkaloid *nt*, Ptomain *nt.*
putrefactive bacterium Fäulnisbakterium *nt*, -bakterie *f*, -erreger *m.*
putrefactive fermentation Fäulnisgärung *f.*
pu·tre·fy [ˈ-faɪ] *vt* zum (Ver-)Faulen bringen. **II** *vi* in Fäulnis übergehen, (ver-)faulen, verwesen, putreszieren.
pu·tres·cence [pjuːˈtresns] *n* Faulen *nt*, Fäulnis(vorgang *m*) *f*; Putreszenz *f.*
pu·tres·cen·cy [pjuːˈtresnsɪ] *n* → putrescence.
pu·tres·cent [pjuːˈtresnt] *adj* (ver-)faulend, verwesend; faulig, Fäulnis.
pu·tres·cine [pjuːˈtresiːn, -sɪn] *n* Putreszin *nt*, Putrescin *nt*, 1,4-Diaminobutan *nt*, Tetramethylendiamin *nt.*
pu·trid [ˈpjuːtrɪd] *adj* **1.** faulig, übelriechend, putrid. **2.** zersetzt, verwest, verfault, Fäulnis-, Faul-.
putrid bronchitis eitrige/putride Bronchitis *f*, Bronchitis foetida/putrida.
Putti-Platt [ˈpʌtɪ plæt]: **P.-P. arthroplasty** → P.-P. operation.
P.-P. operation *ortho.* Putti-Platt-Operation *f.*
P.-P. procedure/repair → P.-P. operation.
put·ty kidney [ˈpʌtɪ] Kitt-, Mörtelniere *f.*
Puusepp [ˈpjuːəsep]: **P.'s reflex** Puusepp-Reflex *m.*
PV *abbr.* → plasma volume.
PVA *abbr.* → polyvinyl alcohol.
PVC *abbr.* **1.** → polyvinyl chloride. **2.** → premature ventricular contraction.
PV diagram → pressure-volume diagram.
PVNS *abbr.* → pigmented villonodular synovitis.
PVP *abbr.* → polyvinylpyrrolidone.
PVP-I *abbr.* → polyvinylpyrrolidone-iodine.
P wave *physiol.* P-Welle *f*, P-Zacke *f.*
PWC$_{170}$ *abbr.* → physical work capacity.
PWC-test *n physiol.* W$_{170}$-Test *m.*
PWP *abbr.* → pulmonary artery wedge pressure.
PWV *abbr.* → pulse wave velocity.
py- *pref.* → pyo-.
py·ar·thro·sis [ˌpaɪɑːˈθrəʊsɪs] *n* **1.** eitrige Gelenkentzündung *f*, Pyarthrose *f.* **2.** Gelenkeiterung *f*, -empyem *nt*, Pyarthrose *f*, Pyarthros *m.*
pyc·no·sis *n* → pyknosis.
pyc·not·ic *adj* → pyknotic.
pyel- *pref.* → pyelo-.
py·el·ec·ta·sia [ˌpaɪəlekˈteɪʒ(ɪ)ə] *n* → pyelectasis.
py·el·ec·ta·sis [ˌpaɪəlˈektəsɪs] *n* Nierenbeckenerweiterung *f*, Pyelektasie *f*, Pyelokaliektasie *f.*
py·el·ic [paɪˈelɪk] *adj* Nierenbecken betr., Nierenbecken-, Pyel(o)-.
py·e·lit·ic [ˌpaɪəˈlɪtɪk] *adj* Pyelitis betr., pyelitisch.
py·e·li·tis [ˌpaɪəˈlaɪtɪs] *n* Nierenbeckenentzündung *f*, Pyelitis *f.*
pyelo- *pref.* Nierenbecken-, Pyel(o)-; Becken-.
py·e·lo·cal·i·ec·ta·sis [ˌpaɪəlʊˌkælɪˈektəsɪs] *n* **1.** → pyelectasis. **2.** Nierenkelchdilatation *f*, Kalikektasie *f.*
py·e·lo·cys·ti·tis [ˌ-sɪsˈtaɪtɪs] *n* Entzündung *f* von Nierenbecken u. Blase, Pyelozystitis *f.*

py·e·lo·gram [ˈ-græm] *n urol., radiol.* Pyelogramm *nt.*
py·e·lo·graph [ˈ-græf] *n* → pyelogram.
py·e·log·ra·phy [paɪəˈlɒgrəfɪ] *n urol., radiol.* Pyelographie *f.*
p. by elimination Ausscheidungspyelographie, intravenöse Pyelographie.
py·e·lo·li·thot·o·my [ˌpaɪəlʊlɪˈθɒtəmɪ] *n urol.* Pyelolithotomie *f.*
py·e·lo·neph·rit·ic [ˌ-nɪˈfrɪtɪk] *adj* Pyelonephritis betr., pyelonephritisch.
pyelonephritic dwarf kidney pyelonephritische Zwergniere *f.*
py·e·lo·ne·phri·tis [ˌ-nɪˈfraɪtɪs] *n abbr.* **PN** Pyelonephritis *f abbr.* **PN.**
p. of pregnancy Pyelonephritis der Schwangeren, Pyelonephritis gravidarum.
py·e·lo·ne·phro·sis [ˌ-nɪˈfrəʊsɪs] *n* Pyelonephrose *f.*
py·e·lop·a·thy [paɪəˈlɒpəθɪ] *n* Nierenbeckenerkrankung *f*, Pyelopathie *f.*
py·e·lo·phle·bit·ic abscess [ˌpaɪəlʊflɪˈbɪtɪk] pyelophlebitischer Abszeß *m.*
py·e·lo·phle·bi·tis [ˌ-flɪˈbaɪtɪs] *n* Pyelophlebitis *f.*
py·e·lo·plas·ty [ˈ-plæstɪ] *n urol.* Nierenbecken-, Pyeloplastik *f.*
py·e·los·co·py [paɪəˈlɒskəpɪ] *n urol.* Pyeloskopie *f.*
py·e·los·to·my [paɪəˈlɒstəmɪ] *n urol.* Pyelostomie *f.*
py·e·lot·o·my [paɪəˈlɒtəmɪ] *n urol.* Pyelotomie *f.*
py·e·lo·u·re·ter·ec·ta·sis [ˌpaɪəlʊjʊəˌrɪtərˈektəsɪs] *n* Pyeloureterektasie *f.*
py·e·lo·u·re·te·rog·ra·phy [ˌ-jʊə,rɪtəˈrɒgrəfɪ] *n* → pyelography.
py·e·lo·u·re·te·rol·y·sis [ˌ-jʊəˌrɪtəˈrɒləsɪs] *n urol.* Pyeloureterolyse *f.*
py·e·lo·u·re·te·ro·plas·ty [ˌ-jʊəˈriːtərəplæstɪ] *n urol.* Nierenbecken-Ureter-Plastik *f*, Pyeloureteroplastik *f.*
py·em·e·sis [paɪˈeməsɪs] *n* Eitererbrechen *nt.*
py·e·mia [paɪˈiːmɪə] *n* Pyämie *f.*
py·e·mic [paɪˈiːmɪk] *adj* Pyämie betr., durch Pyämie gekennzeichnet, pyämisch.
pyemic abscess pyämischer Abszeß *m.*
pyemic embolism infektiöse/septische Embolie *f.*
py·en·ceph·a·lus [ˌpaɪenˈsefələs] *n* Pyozephalus *m.*
py·e·sis [paɪˈiːsɪs] *n* Eiterung *f*, Suppuration *f.*
pyg- *pref.* → pygo-.
py·gal [ˈpaɪgəl] *adj* Gesäß betr., Gesäß-, Pygo-.
PYG medium → peptone-yeast extract-glucose medium.
pyg·my [ˈpɪgmɪ] *n* (physiologischer) Zwerg *m*; Pygmäe *m.*
pygo- *pref.* Gesäß-, Pyg(o)-.
py·go·a·mor·phus [ˌpaɪgəəˈmɔːrfəs] *n embryo.* Pygoamorphus *m.*
py·go·did·y·mus [ˌ-ˈdɪdəməs] *n embryo.* Pygodidymus *m.*
py·go·me·lus [paɪˈgɒmələs] *n embryo.* Pygomelus *m.*
py·gop·a·gus [paɪˈgɒpəgəs] *n embryo.* Pygopagus *m.*
py·ic [ˈpaɪɪk] *adj* Eiter betr., eitrig, Eiter-.
pyk·nic [ˈpɪknɪk] **I** *n* Pykniker(in *f*) *m.* **II** *adj* untersetzt, stämmig, pyknisch.
pyk·no·cyte [ˈpɪknəsaɪt] *n* Pyknozyt *m.*
pyk·no·cy·to·ma [ˌ-saɪˈtəʊmə] *n* Onkozytom *nt*, Hürthle-Tumor *m*, -Zelladenom *nt*, -Struma *f*, oxyphiles Schilddrüsenadenom *nt.*
pyk·no·cy·to·sis [ˌ-saɪˈtəʊsɪs] *n* Pyknozytose *f.*

pyk·no·dys·os·to·sis [ˌ-dɪsɑs'təʊsɪs] *n ortho.* Pyknodysostose *f.*
pyk·no·ep·i·lep·sy [ˌ-'epɪlepsɪ] *n* **1.** Pyknoepilepsie *f.* **2.** → petit mal epilepsy.
pyk·nom·e·ter [pɪk'nɑmɪtər] *n phys.* Pyknometer *nt.*
pyk·nom·e·try [pɪk'nɑmətrɪ] *n phys.* Pyknometrie *f.*
pyk·no·mor·phic [ˌpɪknə'mɔːrfɪk] *adj histol.* pyknomorph.
pyk·no·mor·phous [ˌ-'mɔːrfəs] *adj* → pyknomorphic.
pyk·no·sis [pɪk'nəʊsɪs] *n histol.* (Kern-)Verdichtung *f,* Verdickung *f,* Pyknose *f,* Karyo-, Kernpyknose *f.*
pyk·not·ic [pɪk'nɑtɪk] *adj histol.* Pyknose betr., verdichtet, pyknotisch.
Pyle [paɪl]: **P.'s disease** Pyle'-Krankheit *f,* familäre metaphysäre Dysplasie *f.*
pyle- *pref.* Pfortader-, Pyle-.
py·le·phleb·ec·ta·sia [ˌpaɪləˌflebek'teɪʒ(ɪ)ə] *n* Pfortaderdilatation *f,* -ektasie *f.*
py·le·phle·bec·ta·sis [ˌ-flɪ'bektəsɪs] *n* → pylephlebectasia.
py·le·phle·bi·tis [ˌ-flɪ'baɪtɪs] *n* Pfortaderentzündung *f,* Pylephlebitis *f.*
py·le·throm·bo·phle·bi·tis [ˌ-ˌθrɑmbəʊflɪ-'baɪtɪs] *n* Pylethrombophlebitis *f.*
py·le·throm·bo·sis [ˌ-θrɑm'bəʊsɪs] *n* Pfortaderthrombose *f.*
py·lic ['paɪlɪk] *adj* Pfortader betr., Pfortader-, Pyle-.
pylor- *pref.* → pyloro-.
py·lo·ral·gia [ˌpaɪlə'ræld(ɪ)ə] *n* Schmerz(en *pl*) *m* in der Pylorusregion.
py·lo·rec·to·my [ˌ-'rektəmɪ] *n chir.* Pylorusresektion *f,* Pylorektomie *f.*
py·lo·ric [paɪ'lɔːrɪk, -'lɑr-] *adj* Pylorus od. Pars pylorica betr., pylorisch, Pyloro-, Pylorus-, Magenausgangs-.
pyloric antrum präpylorischer Magenabschnitt *m,* Antrum *nt* (pyloricum).
pyloric artery rechte Magen(kranz)arterie *f,* Gastrica *f* dextra, A. gastrica dextra.
pyloric canal Pyloruskanal *m,* Canalis pyloricus.
pyloric cap Pars superior duodeni.
pyloric carcinoma (*Magen*) Pyloruskarzinom *nt.*
pyloric exclusion *chir.* Pylorusausschaltung *f.*
pyloric glands Pylorusdrüsen *pl,* Gll. pyloricae.
pyloric obstruction Pylorusobstruktion *f.*
pyloric opening Öffnung *f* des Magenpförtners, Ostium pyloricum.
pyloric orifice → pyloric opening.
pyloric region Pylorusregion *f.*
pyloric sphincter (muscle) Schließmuskel *m* des Magenausgangs, Sphinkter/Sphincter *m* pylori, M. sphincter pylori.
pyloric stenosis Magenausgangs-, Pylorusstenose *f.*
 congenital p. kongenitale Pylorusstenose, Pylorusstenose der Säuglinge.
 hypertrophic p. hypertrophe Pylorusstenose.
pyloric ulcus pylorusnahes Magengeschwür *nt,* Ulcus ventriculi ad pylorum, Ulcus pyloricum.
pyloric vein rechte Magenkranzvene *f,* V. gastrica dextra.
py·lo·ri·ste·no·sis [paɪˌlɔːrɪstɪ'nəʊsɪs] *n* → pyloric stenosis.
py·lo·ri·tis [ˌpaɪlə'raɪtɪs] *n* Pylorusentzündung *f,* Pyloritis *f.*
pyloro- *pref.* Magenausgangs-, Pylorus-, Pylor(o)-.
py·lo·ro·du·o·de·ni·tis [paɪˌlɔːrəˌd(j)uːədɪ-'naɪtɪs] *n* Pyloroduodenitis *f.*
py·lo·ro·gas·trec·to·my [ˌ-gæs'trektəmɪ] *n chir.* Gastropylorektomie *f;* Pylorektomie *f.*
py·lo·ro·my·ot·o·my [ˌ-maɪ'ɑtəmɪ] *n chir.* Weber-Ramstedt-Operation *f,* Pyloro(myo)tomie *f,* Ramstedt-Operation *f.*
py·lo·ro·plas·ty ['-plæstɪ] *n chir.* Pyloroplastik *f.*
py·lo·ro·spasm ['-spæzəm] *n* Magenpförtnerkrampf *m,* Pylorospasmus *m.*
py·lo·ro·ste·no·sis [ˌ-stɪ'nəʊsɪs] *n* → pyloric stenosis.
py·lo·ros·to·my [ˌpaɪlə'rɑstəmɪ] *n chir.* Pylorostomie *f.*
py·lo·rot·o·my [ˌ-'rɑtəmɪ] *n chir.* Pylorotomie *f.*
py·lo·rus [paɪ'lɔːrəs, -'lɔʊr-, pɪ-] *n, pl* **-rus·es, -ri** [-raɪ] *anat.* **1.** (Magen-)Pförtner *m,* Magenausgang *m,* Pylorus *m.* **2.** → pyloric canal. **3.** → pyloric opening.
Pym [pɪm]: **P.'s fever** Phlebotomus-, Pappataci-, Moskitofieber *nt,* Drei-Tage-Fieber *nt.*
PY medium → peptone-yeast extract medium.
pyo- *pref.* Eiter-, Py(o)-.
py·o·ar·thro·sis [ˌpaɪəʊɑːr'θrəʊsɪs] *n* → pyarthrosis.
py·o·cele ['-siːl] *n urol.* Pyozele *f,* eitrige Hydrozele *f.*
py·o·ce·lia [ˌ-'siːlɪə] *n* Pyoperitoneum *nt.*
py·o·ceph·a·lus [ˌ-'sefələs] *n* Pyozephalus *m.*
py·o·che·zi·a [ˌ-'kiːzɪə] *n* eitriger Stuhl *m.*
py·o·cin ['-sɪn] *n* Pyozin *nt,* Pyocin *nt.*
py·o·coc·cic [ˌ-'kɑksɪk] *adj* Pyokokken betr.
py·o·coc·cus [ˌ-'kɑkəs] *n* Eiter-, Pyokokkus *m.*
py·o·col·po·cele [ˌ-'kɑlpəsiːl] *n gyn.* Pyokolpozele *f.*
py·o·col·pos [ˌ-'kɑlpəs] *n gyn.* Pyokolpos *m.*
py·o·cy·an·ic [ˌ-saɪ'ænɪk] *adj* Pseudomonas aeruginosa betr., Pyozyaneus-.
py·o·cy·a·nin [ˌ-'saɪənɪn] *n* Pyozyanin *nt,* Pyocyanin *nt.*
py·o·cy·a·no·gen·ic [ˌ-ˌsaɪənəʊ'dʒenɪk] *adj* Pyozyanin-bildend.
py·o·cy·a·no·sis [ˌsaɪə'nəʊsɪs] *n* Pyozyaneus-Infektion *f,* Pseudomonas-aeruginosa-Infektion *f.*
py·o·cyst ['-sɪst] *n* Eiter-, Pyozyste *f.*
py·o·cys·tis [ˌ-'sɪstɪs] *n* eitrige (Harn-)Blasenentzündung *f,* Eiterblase *f.*
py·o·cytes ['-saɪts] *pl* Eiterzellen *pl,* -körperchen *pl.*
py·o·der·ma [ˌ-'dɜrmə] *n derm.* Eiter-, Grindausschlag *m,* Pyodermie *f,* -dermitis *f,* -dermia *f.*
py·o·der·ma·ti·tis [ˌ-ˌdɜrmə'taɪtɪs] *n* → pyoderma.
py·o·der·ma·to·sis [ˌ-ˌdɜrmə'təʊsɪs] *n* → pyoderma.
py·o·der·mia [ˌ-'dɜrmɪə] *n* → pyoderma.
py·o·fe·cia [ˌ-'fiːsɪə] *n* eitriger Stuhl *m.*
py·o·gen·e·sis [ˌ-'dʒenəsɪs] *n* Eiterbildung *f,* Pyogenese *f.*
py·o·gen·ic [ˌ-'dʒenɪk] *adj* eiterbildend, pyogen, pyogenetisch.
pyogenic abscess pyogener/metastatisch-pyämischer Abszeß *m.*
pyogenic bacteria *micro.* pyogene/eiterbildende Bakterien *pl.*
pyogenic encephalitis → purulent encephalitis.
pyogenic fever → pyemia.
pyogenic granuloma teleangiektatisches Granulom *nt,* Granuloma pediculatum/pyogenicum/teleangiectaticum.
pyogenic infection pyogene Infektion *f.*
py·o·gen·in [paɪ'ɑdʒənɪn] *n* Pyogenin *nt.*

py·og·e·nous [paɪ'ɑdʒənəs] *adj* durch Eiter verursacht, pyogen.
py·o·he·mia [ˌpaɪəʊ'hiːmɪə] *n* Pyämie *f.*
py·o·he·mo·tho·rax [ˌ-ˌhiːmə'θɔːræks, -ˌhem-] *n* Pyohämothorax *m.*
py·o·hy·dro·ne·phro·sis [ˌ-ˌhaɪdrəˌnɪ'frəʊsɪs] *n urol.* Pyohydronephrose *f.*
py·oid ['paɪɔɪd] *adj* eiterartig, -ähnlich, pyoid.
py·o·lab·y·rin·thi·tis [ˌpaɪəʊˌlæbərɪn'θaɪtɪs] *n HNO* eitrige/suppurative Labyrinthitis *f.*
py·o·mel·a·nin [ˌ-'melənɪn] *n* Pyomelanin *nt.*
py·o·me·tra [ˌ-'miːtrə] *n gyn.* Pyometra *f.*
py·o·me·tri·tis [ˌ-mɪ'traɪtɪs] *n gyn.* eitrige/suppurative Gebärmutterentzündung/Metritis *f,* Pyometritis *f.*
py·o·me·tri·um [ˌ-'miːtrɪəm] *n gyn.* Pyometra *f.*
py·o·my·o·ma [ˌ-maɪ'əʊmə] *n gyn.* Pyomyom *nt.*
py·o·my·o·si·tis [ˌ-ˌmaɪə'saɪtɪs] *n* eitrige/suppurative Muskelentzündung/Myositis *f,* Myositis purulenta.
py·o·ne·phri·tis [ˌ-nɪ'fraɪtɪs] *n* Pyonephritis *f.*
py·o·neph·ro·li·thi·a·sis [ˌ-ˌnefrəʊlɪ'θaɪəsɪs] *n urol.* Pyonephrolithiasis *f.*
py·o·ne·phro·sis [ˌ-nɪ'frəʊsɪs] *n urol.* Pyonephrose *f.*
py·o·neph·rot·ic [ˌ-nɪ'frɑtɪk] *adj* Pyonephrose betr., pyonephrotisch.
pyo-ovarium *n gyn.* Pyoovar(ium *nt*) *nt,* Pyovar *nt.*
py·o·per·i·car·di·tis [ˌpaɪəʊˌperɪkɑːr'daɪtɪs] *n* eitrige Perikarditis *f,* Pyoperikarditis *f.*
py·o·per·i·car·di·um [ˌ-perɪ'kɑːrdɪəm] *n* Pyoperikard *nt.*
py·o·per·i·to·ne·um [ˌ-ˌperɪtəʊ'niːəm] *n* Pyoperitoneum *nt.*
py·o·per·i·to·ni·tis [ˌ-ˌperɪtə'naɪtɪs] *n* eitrige Peritonitis *f,* Pyoperitonitis *f.*
py·oph·thal·mia [paɪɑf'θælmɪə] *n ophthal.* Pyophthalmie *f.*
py·oph·thal·mi·tis [ˌpaɪɑfθæl'maɪtɪs] *n* → pyophthalmia.
py·o·phy·so·me·tra [ˌpaɪəʊˌfaɪsə'miːtrə] *n gyn.* Pyophysometra *f.*
py·o·pneu·mo·cho·le·cys·ti·tis [ˌ-ˌn(j)uːməˌkɑʊlɔsɪs'taɪtɪs, -ˌkɑlə-] *n* Pyopneumocholezystitis *f.*
py·o·pneu·mo·cyst [ˌ-'n(j)uːməsɪst] *n* Pyopneumozyste *f.*
py·o·pneu·mo·hep·a·ti·tis [ˌ-ˌn(j)uːməˌhepə'taɪtɪs] *n* luft- u. eiterhaltiger Leberabszeß *m.*
py·o·pneu·mo·per·i·car·di·um [ˌ-ˌn(j)uːməˌperɪ'kɑːrdɪəm] *n* Pyopneumoperikard *nt.*
py·o·pneu·mo·per·i·to·ne·um [ˌ-ˌn(j)uːməˌperɪtəʊ'niːəm] *n* Pyopneumoperitoneum *nt.*
py·o·pneu·mo·per·i·to·ni·tis [ˌ-ˌn(j)uːməˌperɪtə'naɪtɪs] *n* Pyopneumoperitonitis *f.*
py·o·pneu·mo·tho·rax [ˌ-ˌn(j)uːmə'θɔːræks] *n* Pyopneumothorax *m.*
py·o·poi·e·sis [ˌ-pɔɪ'iːsɪs] *n* Eiterbildung *f,* Pyogenese *f;* Eiterung *f,* Suppuration *f.*
py·o·poi·et·ic [ˌ-pɔɪ'etɪk] *adj* eiterbildend, pyogen, pyogenetisch.
py·op·ty·sis [paɪ'ɑptəsɪs] *n* Eiterspucken *nt,* Pyoptyse *f.*
py·or·rhea [ˌpaɪəʊ'rɪə] *n* **1.** Eiterfluß *m,* Pyorrhoe *f.* **2.** Alveolarpyorrhoe *f,* Parodontitis marginalis.
pyorrhea alveolaris → pyorrhea 2.
py·o·ru·bin [ˌ-'ruːbɪn] *n* Pyorubin *nt.*
py·o·sal·pin·gi·tis [ˌ-ˌsælpɪn'dʒaɪtɪs] *n* eitrige Salpingitis *f,* Salpingitis purulenta, Pyosalpingitis *f.*

pyosalpingo-oophoritis *n gyn.* Pyosalpingo-Oophoritis *f.*
pyosalpingo-oothecitis *n* → pyosalpingo-oophoritis.
py·o·sal·pinx [,-'sælpɪŋks] *n gyn.* Pyosalpinx *f.*
py·o·sep·ti·ce·mia [,-,septɪ'siːmɪə] *n* Pyoseptikämie *f,* Pyosepsis *f.*
py·o·sin ['-sɪn] *n* Pyosin *nt.*
py·o·sis [paɪ'əʊsɪs] *n* Eiterung *f,* Pyosis *f.*
py·o·sper·mia [,paɪəʊ'spɜrmɪə] *n* Pyospermie *f,* eitriges Sperma *m.*
py·o·sto·ma·ti·tis [,-,stəʊmə'taɪtɪs] *n* eitrige/purulente Stomatitis *f,* Stomatitis purulenta, Pyostomatitis *f.*
py·o·tho·rax [,-'θɔːræks] *n* Pyothorax *m,* Thorax-, Pleuraempyem *nt,* eitrige Pleuritis *f.*
py·o·tox·i·ne·mia [,-,tɑksɪ'niːmɪə] *n* Pyotoxinämie *f.*
py·o·um·bil·i·cus [,-ʌm'bɪləkəs] *n ped.* eitrige/purulente Nabelentzündung *f.*
py·o·u·ra·chus [,-'jʊərəkəs] *n ped.* Pyourachus *m.*
py·o·u·re·ter [,-jʊə'riːtər] *n urol.* Pyoureter *m.*
py·o·ver·din [,-'vɜrdɪn] *n* Pyoverdin *nt.*
py·o·xan·thin [,-'zænθɪn] *n* Pyoxanthin *nt.*
pyr- *pref.* → pyro-.
pyr·a·cin [ˈpɪərəsɪn] *n* Pyrazin *nt.*
pyr·a·mid ['pɪrəmɪd] *n* Pyramide *f,* pyramidenähnliche Struktur *f; anat.* Pyramis *f.*
 p. of cerebellum → p. of vermis.
 p.s of Ferrein (*Niere*) Markstrahlen *pl,* Radii medullares.
 p.s of Malpighi Nierenpyramiden *pl,* Pyramides renales.
 p. of medulla oblongata Pyramide, Pyramis medullae oblongatae.
 p. of thyroid Pyramidenlappen *m* der Schilddrüse, Lobus pyramidalis (gl. thyroideae).
 p. of vermis Pyramis vermis.
 p. of vestibule oberer Teil *m* der Crista vestibuli, Pyramis vestibuli.
py·ram·i·dal [pɪ'ræmɪdl] *adj* pyramidenartig, -förmig, pyramidal, Pyramiden-.
pyramidal bone Dreiecksbein *nt,* Os triquetrum.
pyramidal cartilage Stell-, Gießbecken-, Aryknorpel *m,* Cartilago aryt(a)enoidea.
pyramidal cataract Pyramidenstar *m,* Cataracta pyramidalis.
pyramidal cell Pyramidenzelle *f.*
 giant p.s Betz'-Riesenzellen *pl.*
pyramidal cell layer Meynert-Schicht *f,* Pyramidenzellschicht *f.*
pyramidal decussation Pyramiden(bahn)kreuzung *f,* Decussatio pyramidum/motoria.
py·ram·i·da·le [pɪ,ræmɪ'deɪli:] *n* → pyramidal bone.
pyramidal eminence Eminentia pyramidalis.
pyramidal fasciculus of medulla oblongata Fasciculus pyramidalis (medullae oblongatae).
pyramidal fracture LeFort II-Fraktur *f.*
 longitudinal p. Pyramidenlängsfraktur.
 transverse p. Pyramidenquerfraktur.
py·ram·i·dalis auriculae (muscle) [pɪ,ræmɪ'deɪlɪs] → pyramidalis auriculares (muscle).
pyramidalis auricularis (muscle) M. pyramidalis auricularis.
pyramidalis (muscle) Pyramidenmuskel *m,* M. pyramidalis.
pyramidal layer of cerebral cortex: external p. äußere Pyramidenzellschicht *f,* Lamina pyramidalis externa (corticis cerebralis).
 ganglionic/internal p. innere Pyramidenzellschicht *f,* Lamina pyramidalis ganglionaris/interna (corticis cerebralis).
pyramidal lobe of thyroid Pyramidenlappen *m* der Schilddrüse, Lobus pyramidalis (gl. thyroideae).
pyramidal muscle → pyramidalis (muscle).
 p. of auricle → pyramidalis auricularis (muscle).
pyramidal neuron → pyramidal cell.
pyramidal nucleus Nc. olivarius accessorius medialis.
pyramidal process of palatine bone Proc. pyramidalis (ossis palatini).
pyramidal signs *neuro.* Pyramiden(bahn)zeichen *pl.*
pyramidal stratum Stratum pyramidale.
pyramidal system pyramidales/pyramidal-motorisches System *f.*
pyramidal tract: anterior p. Pyramidenvorderstrangbahn *f,* direkte/vordere Pyramidenbahn *f,* Tractus pyramidalis anterior, Tractus corticospinalis anterior.
 crossed p. seitliche/gekreuzte Pyramidenbahn *f,* Tractus corticospinalis/pyramidalis lateralis.
 direct p. → anterior p.
 lateral p. → crossed p.
 p. of spinal cord Pyramidenbahn *f* des Rückenmarks.
pyramidal-tract lesion Pyramidenbahnschädigung *f,* -läsion *f.*
py·ram·i·dot·o·my [pɪ,ræmɪ'dɑtəmɪ] *n neurochir.* Pyramidenbahndurchtrennung *f,* Pyramidotomie *f.*
pyramid signs → pyramidal signs.
py·ra·mis ['pɪrəmɪs] *n, pl* **py·ra·mi·des** [pɪ'ræmɪdiːz] → pyramid.
pyr·an ['paɪræn, paɪ'ræn] *n* Pyran *nt.*
pyr·a·nin ['pɪrənɪn] *n* Pyranin *nt.*
py·ra·nis·a·mine [,paɪrə'nɪsəmiːn] *n pharm.* Mepyramin *nt.*
py·ra·nose ['paɪrənəʊz] *n chem.* Pyranose *f.*
pyranose form *chem.* Pyranoseform *f.*
pyranose ring *chem.* Pyranosering *m.*
pyran ring *chem.* Pyranring *m.*
py·ran·tel [pɪ'ræntəl] *n pharm.* Pyrantel *f.*
pyr·a·zin·a·mide [pɪərə'zɪnəmaɪd, -mɪd] *n pharm.* Pyrazinamid *nt.*
pyr·a·zine ['pɪərəziːn] *n* Pyrazin *nt.*
py·raz·o·lone [pɪ'ræzəlɒʊn, paɪ-] *n* Pyrazolon *nt.*
py·rec·tic [paɪ'rektɪk] *n, adj* → pyretic.
pyret- *pref.* → pyreto-.
py·ret·ic [paɪ'retɪk] **I** *n* fiebererzeugendes Mittel *nt,* Pyretikum *nt,* Pyreticum *nt.* **II** *adj* fiebererzeugend, pyretisch.
pyreto- *pref.* Fieber-, Pyret(o)-.
py·ret·o·gen [paɪ'retəʊdʒən] *n* → pyretic I.
pyr·e·to·gen·e·sis [,pɪrətəʊ'dʒenəsɪs, ,paɪ-] *n* Fieberauslösung *f,* Pyretogenese *f.*
pyr·e·to·ge·net·ic [,-dʒə'netɪk] *adj* → pyretogenic.
pyr·e·to·gen·ic [,-'dʒenɪk] *adj* fieberauslösend, pyrogen, pyretogen.
pyretogenic stage Stadium *nt* des Fieberanstiegs, Stadium incrementi.
py·re·tog·e·nous [pɪrə'tɑdʒənəs, paɪrə-] *adj* **1.** → pyretogenic. **2.** durch Fieber verursacht.
pyr·e·to·ther·a·py [,pɪrətəʊ'θerəpɪ, ,paɪ-] *n* **1.** Fiebertherapie *f.* **2.** Behandlung *f* von Fieber.
pyr·e·to·ty·pho·sis [,-taɪ'fəʊsɪs] *n* Fieberdelir(ium *nt*) *nt.*
py·rex·ia [paɪ'reksɪə] *n* Fieber *nt,* fieberhafte Erkrankung *f,* Pyrexie *f.*
py·rex·i·al [paɪ'reksɪəl] *adj* Fieber/Pyrexie betr., Fieber-.
pyrexial headache Fieberkopfschmerz *m.*
py·rex·i·o·gen·ic [paɪ,reksɪəʊ'dʒenɪk] *adj* → pyretogenic.
py·rex·y ['paɪreksɪ] *n* → pyrexia.
pyr·i·dine ['pɪrɪdiːn, -dɪn] *n* Pyridin *nt.*
4-pyridine carboxylic acid hydrazide *pharm.* Isoniazid *nt,* Isonicotinsäurehydrazid *nt abbr.* INH, Pyridin-4-carbonsäurehydrazid *nt.*
pyridine coenzyme Pyridincoenzym *nt.*
pyridine-linked dehydrogenase pyridinabhängige Dehydrogenase *f.*
pyridine nucleotide Pyridinnukleotid *nt.*
pyridine nucleotide dehydrogenase Pyridinnukleotiddehydrogenase *f.*
pyridine nucleotide reductase Pyridinnukleotidreduktase *f.*
 photosynthetic p. *bio.* photosynthetische Pyridinnukleotidreduktase.
pyridine nucleotide transhydrogenase Pyridinnukleotidtranshydrogenase *f,* NAD(P)+-Transhydrogenase *f.*
pyridine ring *chem.* Pyridinring *m.*
pyr·i·do·stig·mine [,pɪrədəʊ'stɪgmiːn] *n pharm.* Pyridostigmin *nt.*
pyridostigmine bromide *pharm.* Pyridostigminbromid *nt.*
pyr·i·dox·al [,pɪrə'dɑksəl, -sæl] *n* Pyridoxal *nt.*
pyridoxal phosphate Codecarboxylase *f,* Pyridoxalphosphat *nt abbr.* PLP, PLAP.
pyr·i·dox·a·mine [,pɪrɪ'dɑksəmiːn] *n* Pyridoxamin *nt.*
pyridoxamine phosphate Pyridoxaminphosphat *nt.*
pyr·i·dox·ic acid [pɪrɪ'dɑksɪk] Pyridoxinsäure *f.*
pyr·i·dox·ine [,pɪrɪ'dɑksiːn, -sɪn] *n* Pyridoxin *nt,* Vitamin B₆ *nt.*
pyridoxine coenzyme Pyridoxincoenzym *nt.*
pyr·i·form *adj* → piriform.
pyr·il·a·mine [pɪ'rɪləmiːn, paɪ-] *n pharm.* Mepyramin *nt.*
pyr·i·meth·a·mine [pɪrɪ'meθəmiːn, rɪ-] *n pharm.* Pyrimethamin *nt.*
py·rim·i·dine [paɪ'rɪmɪdiːn, pɪ-, 'pɪrəmɪdiːn] *n* Pyrimidin *nt.*
pyrimidine antagonist Pyrimidinantagonist.
pyrimidine base Pyrimidinbase *f.*
pyrimidine degradation Pyrimidinabbau *m.*
pyrimidine derivative Pyrimidinderivat *nt.*
pyrimidine nucleotide Pyrimidinnukleotid *nt.*
pyr·i·thi·a·mine [,pɪrə'θaɪəmiːn] *n* Pyrithiamin *nt.*
pyro- *pref.* **1.** *chem.* Pyro-. **2.** Feuer-, Pyr(o)-.
py·ro·bo·rate [,paɪrəʊ'bɔːreɪt, -ɪt, -'bəʊr-] *n* Tetraborat *nt.*
py·ro·bo·ric acid [,-'bɔːrɪk, -'bəʊr-] Tetraborsäure *f.*
py·ro·cat·e·chin [,-'kætɪtʃɪn, -kɪn] *n* → pyrocatechol.
py·ro·cat·e·chol [,-'kætɪkɑl, -kɒl] *n* Brenzkatechin *nt,* -catechin *nt.*
py·ro·gal·lic acid [,-'gælɪk, -'gɒl-] *n* pyrogallol.
py·ro·gal·lol [,-'gælɒl, -gə'lɑl] *n* Pyrogallol *nt,* 1,2,3,-Trihydroxybenzol *nt.*
py·ro·gen ['-dʒən] *n* pyrogene Substanz *f,* Pyrogen *nt.*
py·ro·ge·net·ic [,-dʒɪ'netɪk] *adj* → pyretogenic.
pyrogenetic stage → pyretogenic stage.
py·ro·gen·ic [,-'dʒenɪk] *adj* → pyretogenic.
pyrogenic exotoxin C *abbr.* **PEC** Toxisches-Schock-Syndrom-Toxin-1 *nt abbr.* TSST-1, toxic shock-syndrome toxin 1

abbr. TSST-1, *old* pyrogenes Exotoxin C *nt abbr.* PEC, *old* Staphylokokkenenterotoxin F *nt abbr.* SEF.
py·rog·e·nous [paɪˈrɒdʒənəs] *adj* **1.** → pyretogenous **2. 2.** → pyretogenic.
py·ro·glob·u·lin [ˌpaɪrəʊˈglɒbjəlɪn] *n* Pyroglobulin *nt.*
py·ro·glu·ta·mase [ˌ-ˈgluːtəmeɪz] *n* 5-Oxoprolinase *f.*
py·ro·glu·ta·mate [ˌ-ˈgluːtəmeɪt] *n* 5-Oxoprolin *nt*, Pyroglutaminsäure *f.*
pyroglutamate hydrolase → pyroglutamase.
py·ro·glu·tam·ic acid [ˌ-gluːˈtæmɪk] → pyroglutamate.
pyroglutamic aciduria Pyroglutaminazidurie *f*, hämolytische Anämie *f* mit Glutathionsynthetasedefekt.
py·ro·lag·nia [ˌ-ˈlægnɪə] *n psychia.* Pyrolagnie *f.*
py·rol·y·sis [paɪˈrɒləsɪs] *n chem.* Pyrolyse *f.*
py·ro·ma·nia [ˌpaɪrəˈmeɪnɪə, -jə] *n psychia.* Pyromanie *f.*
py·rom·e·ter [paɪˈrɒmɪtər] *n phys.* Pyrometer *nt.*
py·ro·nin [ˈpaɪrənɪn] *n histol.* Pyronin *nt.*
py·ro·nin·o·phil·ia [ˌpaɪrəˌnɪnəˈfɪlɪə] *n histol.* Pyroninophilie *f.*
py·ro·nin·o·phil·ic [ˌ-ˌnɪnəˈfɪlɪk] *adj* pyroninophil.
py·ro·pho·bia [ˌ-ˈfəʊbɪə] *n psychia.* krankhafte Angst *f* vor Feuer, Pyrophobie *f.*
py·ro·phos·pha·tase [ˌ-ˈfɒsfəteɪz] *n* Pyrophosphatase *f.*
py·ro·phos·phate [ˌ-ˈfɒsfeɪt] *n* Pyrophosphat *nt.*
pyrophosphate bond *chem.* Pyrophosphatbindung *f.*
pyrophosphate ribose-P-synthetase Ribosephosphatpyrophosphokinase *f*, Phosphoribosylpyrophosphatsynthetase *f.*

py·ro·phos·pho·ki·nase [ˌ-ˌfɒsfəʊˈkaɪneɪz, -ˈkɪ-] *n* Diphosphotransferase *f*, Pyrophosphokinase *f*, -transferase *f.*
py·ro·phos·pho·me·val·o·nate [ˌ-ˌfɒsfəʊməˈvæləneɪt] *n* Pyrophosphomevalonat *nt.*
pyrophosphomevalonate decarboxylase Pyrophosphomevalonatdecarboxylase *f.*
5-py·ro·phos·pho·mev·a·lon·ic acid [ˌ-ˌfɒsfəʊmevəˈlɒnɪk] 5-Pyrophosphomevalonsäure *f.*
py·ro·phos·phor·ic acid [ˌ-fɒsˈfɒrɪk] Pyrophosphorsäure *f.*
py·ro·phos·pho·rol·y·sis [ˌ-ˌfɒsfəˈrɒləsɪs] *n* Pyrophosphorolyse *f.*
py·ro·phos·pho·ryl·ase [ˌ-fɒsˈfɒrəleɪz, -ˈfɑːr-] *n* Pyrophosphorylase *f*, Glykosyl--1-phosphatnukleotidyltransferase *f.*
py·ro·phos·pho·trans·fer·ase [ˌ-ˌfɒsfəʊˈtrænsfəreɪz] *n* → pyrophosphokinase.
py·ro·sis [paɪˈrəʊsɪs] *n* Sodbrennen *nt*, Pyrosis *f.*
py·rot·ic [paɪˈrɒtɪk] *adj* brennend, ätzend.
py·ro·tox·in [ˌpaɪrəˈtɒksɪn] *n* Pyrotoxin *nt.*
py·rox·y·lin [paɪˈrɒksəlɪn, pɪ-] *n* Schießbaumwolle *f*, Nitrozellulose *f.*
pyr·role [pɪˈrəʊl, ˈpɪrəʊl] *n* Pyrrol *nt.*
pyrrole ring *chem.* Pyrrolring *m.*
pyr·rol·i·dine [pɪˈrəʊlɪdiːn, -dɪn, -ˈrɒlɪ-] *n* Pyrrolidin *nt.*
pyr·ro·line [ˈpɪrəliːn, -lɪn] *n* Pyrrolin *nt.*
Δ¹-pyrroline-5-carboxylate *n* Δ¹-Pyrrolin-5-carboxylat *nt.*
Δ¹-pyrroline-5-carboxylate dehydrogenase Δ¹-Pyrrolin-5-carboxylat-dehydrogenase *f.*
Δ¹-pyrroline-5-carboxylate dehydrogenase deficiency Hyperprolinämie *f* Typ II, Pyrrolin-5-carboxylat-dehydrogenasemangel *m.*
pyrroline-5-carboxylate reductase Pyrrolin-5-carboxylat-reduktase *f.*

pyrroline-2-carboxylic acid reductase Pyrrolin-2-carbonsäurereduktase *f.*
pyr·ro·lo·por·phyr·ia [ˌpɪərələʊpɔːˈfɪərɪə] *n* akute intermittierende Porphyrie *f*, Schwedischer Typ *m* der Porphyrie, Porphyria acuta intermittens.
pyr·u·vate [paɪˈruːveɪt, pɪ-] *n* Pyruvat *nt.*
pyruvate carboxylase *abbr.* **PC** Pyruvatcarboxylase *f abbr.* PC.
pyruvate carboxylase deficiency Pyruvatcarboxylasemangel *m.*
pyruvate decarboxylase 1. Pyruvatdecarboxylase *f.* **2.** *old* → pyruvate dehydrogenase lipoamide.
pyruvate dehydrogenase *abbr.* **PDH** Pyruvatdehydrogenase *f abbr.* PDH.
pyruvate dehydrogenase complex *abbr.* **PDHC** Pyruvatdehydrogenasekomplex *m.*
pyruvate dehydrogenase complex deficiency Pyruvatdehydrogenasemangel *m*, -defekt *m.*
pyruvate dehydrogenase kinase Pyruvatdehydrogenasekinase *f.*
pyruvate dehydrogenase lipoamide Pyruvatdehydrogenase (Lipoamid) *f.*
pyruvate dehydrogenase phosphatase Pyruvatdehydrogenasephosphatase *f.*
pyruvate kinase *abbr.* **PK** Pyruvatkinase *f abbr.* PK.
pyruvate kinase deficiency Pyruvatkinasemangel *m.*
pyruvate orthophosphate dikinase Pyruvat(ortho)phosphatdikinase *f.*
pyruvate oxidation factor Liponsäure *f*, Thiooctansäure *f.*
py·ru·vic acid [paɪˈruːvɪk, pɪ-] Brenztraubensäure *f*, Acetylameisensäure *f*, α-Ketopropionsäure *f.*
pyr·vin·i·um pamoate [pɪərˈvɪnɪəm] *pharm.* Pyrvinium-Pamoat *nt.*
py·u·ria [paɪˈjʊərɪə] *n* Eiterharn *m*, Pyurie *f.*

Q

Q *abbr.* 1. → quantity of electric charge. 2. → quantity of heat.
q *abbr.* 1. → quantity of electric charge. 2. → quantity of heat.
Q band *genet.* (*Chromosom*) Q-Bande *f*.
Q banding → quinacrine banding.
Q disk *histol.* A-Band *nt*, A-Streifen *m*, A-Zone *f*, anisotrope Bande *f*.
Q fever Balkangrippe *f*, Q-Fieber *nt*.
Q-R interval *card.* QR-Intervall *nt*.
QRS complex *card.* QRS-Komplex *m*.
QRS interval *card.* QRS-Intervall *nt*.
QRST interval *card.* QT-Intervall *nt*.
Q-T interval *card.* QT-Intervall *nt*.
QT syndrome QT-Syndrom *nt*.
quack [kwæk] **I** *n* Quacksalber *m*, Kurpfuscher *m*. **II** *adj* quacksalberisch, kurpfuscherisch. **III** *vt* herumpfuschen an. **IV** *vi* quacksalbern.
quack doctor → quack I.
quack·er·y ['kwækərɪ] *n* Quacksalberei *f*, Kurpfuscherei *f*.
quack·sal·ver ['kwæksælvər] *n* → quack I.
quad·ran·gu·lar [kwɒd'ræŋɡjələr] *adj* viereckig, quadrangulär.
quadrangular cartilage Nasenseptumknorpel *m*, Cartilago septi nasi.
quadrangular fontanelle vordere/große Fontanelle *f*, Stirnfontanelle *f*, Fonticulus anterior.
quadrangular lobe/lobule of cerebellum Lobulus quadrangularis cerebelli, Pars anterior lobuli cerebelli.
quadrangular membrane viereckige Kehlkopfmembran *f*, Membrana quadrangularis.
quad·rant ['kwɒdrənt] *n* Quadrant *m*.
quad·ran·tal [kwɒ'dræntl] *adj* Quadranten-.
quad·ran·ta·no·pia [ˌkwɒdræntə'nəʊpɪə] *n* → quadrant hemianopia.
quad·ran·ta·nop·sia [ˌ-'nɒpsɪə] *n* → quadrant hemianopia.
quadrant hemianopia *ophthal.* Quadrantenhemianop(s)ie *f*, Quadrantenanop(s)ie *f*.
quadrant hemianopsia → quadrant hemianopia.
quad·ran·tic hemianopia [kwɒ'dræntɪk] → quadrant hemianopia.
quadrantic hemianopsia → quadrant hemianopia.
quadrantic scotoma *ophthal.* Quadrantenskotom *nt*.
quad·rate ['kwɒdrɪt, -reɪt] **I** *n* Vier-, Rechteck *nt*. **II** *adj* vier-, rechteckig, quadratisch, Quadrat-, Viereck-, Rechteck-.
quadrate ligament Lig. quadratum.
quadrate lobe (of liver) viereckiger Leberlappen *m*, Lobus quadratus (hepatis).
quadrate lumbar muscle → quadratus lumborum (muscle).
quadrate muscle: q. of sole → quadratus plantae (muscle).
q. of thigh → quadratus femoris (muscle).
quadrate pronator (muscle) Pronator *m* quadratus, M. pronator quadratus.

qua·dra·tus femoris (muscle) [kwɑ'dreɪtəs] Quadratus *m* femoris, M. quadratus femoris.
quadratus lumborum (muscle) Quadratus *m* lumborum, M. quadratus lumborum.
quadratus plantae (muscle) Quadratus *m* plantae, M. quadratus plantae, M. flexor accessorius.
quad·ren·ni·al [kwɑ'drenɪəl] *adj* vierjährig.
quadri- *pref.* Vier-, Quadri-, Tetra-.
quad·ri·ba·sic [ˌkwɒdrɪ'beɪsɪk] *adj* *chem.* vierbasisch.
quad·ri·ceps ['-seps] **I** *n*, *pl* **-ceps**, **-ceps·es** [-ˌsepsɪz] Quadrizeps *m*, M. quadriceps femoris. **II** *adj* *anat.* vierköpfig.
q. of thigh → quadriceps I.
quadriceps jerk Patellarsehnenreflex *m* *abbr.* PSR, Quadrizepssehnenreflex *m* *abbr.* QSR.
quadriceps muscle of thigh → quadriceps I.
quad·ri·ceps·plas·ty [ˌ-'sepsplæstɪ] *n* *ortho.* Quadrizepsnaht *f*, -versorgung *f*.
quadriceps reflex → quadriceps jerk.
quad·ri·cip·i·tal [ˌkwɒdrɪ'sɪpɪtl] *adj* Quadrizeps betr.
quad·ri·cus·pid [ˌ-'kʌspɪd] *adj* tetrakuspid.
quad·ri·den·tate [ˌ-'denteɪt] *adj* *chem.* vierzähnig.
quad·ri·dig·i·tate [ˌ-'dɪdʒəteɪt] *adj* vierfingrig, vierzehig, tetradaktyl.
quad·ri·gem·i·nal plate [ˌ-'dʒemɪnl] Vierhügelplatte *f*, Lamina quadrigemina, Lamina tecti/tectalis (mesencephali).
quadrigeminal pulse Quadrigeminus *m*, Quadrigeminuspuls *m*, -rhythmus *m*, Pulsus quadrigeminus.
quadrigeminal rhythm → quadrigeminy.
quad·ri·gem·i·nus [ˌ-'dʒemɪnəs] *n* → quadruplet 1.
quad·ri·gem·i·ny [ˌ-'dʒemɪnɪ] *n* Quadrigeminus *m*, Quadrigeminusrhythmus *m*.
quad·ri·lat·er·al [ˌ-'lætərəl] **I** *n* Viereck *nt*, Vierseit *nt*. **II** *adj* vierseitig.
quadrilateral fracture (*Becken*) Schmetterlingsbruch *m*, doppelseitige vordere Ringfraktur *f*.
quad·ri·nu·cle·ate [ˌ-'n(j)u:klɪɪt] *adj* vierkernig.
quad·ri·par·tite [ˌ-'pɑ:rtaɪt] *adj* viergeteilt.
qua·drip·e·dal extensor reflex [kwɑ'trɪpədəl] Brain-Reflex *m*.
quad·ri·ple·gia [ˌkwɒdrɪ'pli:dʒ(ɪ)ə] *n* *neuro.* hohe Querschnittslähmung *f*, Tetra-, Quadriplegie *f*.
qua·dri·ple·gic [ˌ-'pli:dʒɪk] **I** *n* Patient(in *f*) *m* mit Tetraplegie, Tetraplegiker(in *f*) *m*. **II** *adj* Tetraplegie betr., quadri-, tetraplegisch.
quad·ri·po·lar [ˌ-'pəʊlər] *adj* vierpolig.
quad·ri·sect [ˌ-'sekt] *vt* vierteilen.
quad·ri·sec·tion [ˌ-'sekʃn] *n* Vierteilung *f*.
quad·ri·va·lence [ˌ-'veɪləns, kwɑ'drɪvələns] *n* *chem.* Vierwertigkeit *f*.
quad·ri·va·len·cy [ˌ-'veɪlənsɪ] *n* → quadrivalence.

quad·ri·va·lent [ˌ-'veɪlənt, kwɑ'drɪvələnt] *adj* *chem.* vierwertig, tetravalent.
quad·roon [kwɑ'dru:n] *n* Kind *nt* eines Weißen u. einer Mulattin, Terzerone *m*, Terzeronin *f*.
quad·ru·ped ['kwɑdrəped] **I** *n* *bio.* Vierfüß(l)er *m*, Quadrupede *m*, Tetrapode *m*. **II** *adj* vierfüßig, quadruped, tetrapod.
quad·ru·ple [kwɑ'dru:pl, -'drʌpl, 'kwɑdrʊpl] **I** *n* das Vierfache. **II** *adj* vierfach, Vierer-. **III** *vt* vervierfachen. **IV** *vi* s. vervierfachen.
quad·ru·plet [kwɑ'drʌplɪt, -'dru:p-, 'kwɑdrʊplɪt] *n* 1. Vierling *m*. 2. **~s** *pl* Vierlinge *pl*.
quad·ru·plex ['kwɑdrʊpleks, kwɑ'dru:-] *adj* vierfach, Vierfach-.
quak·er button ['kweɪkər] *pharm.* Brechnuß *f*, Nux vomica.
qual·i·ta·tive ['kwɑlɪteɪtɪv] *adj* Qualität betr., qualitativ, Qualitäts-.
qualitative analysis *chem.* qualitative Analyse/Bestimmung *f*.
qualitative test → qualitative analysis.
qual·i·tive ['kwɑlətɪv] *adj* → qualitative.
qualitive analysis → qualitative analysis.
qual·i·ty ['kwɑlətɪ] *n* 1. Eigenschaft *f*, (Eigen-)Art *f*, Beschaffenheit *f*, Qualität *f*. **in ~** qualitativ. 2. Talent *nt*, Fähigkeit *f*, Qualität *f*.
q. of life Lebensqualität.
q.ies of taste Geschmacksqualitäten *pl*.
quality control Qualitätskontrolle *f*.
quality dimension *physiol.* Qualitätsdimension *f*.
quan·tal ['kwɑntl] *adj* *phys.* Quant betr., Quanten-.
quantal current *phys.* Quantenstrom *m*.
quan·ti·fi·a·ble ['kwɑntɪfaɪəbl] *adj* quantitativ bestimmbar, meßbar, quantifizierbar.
quan·ti·fi·ca·tion [ˌkwɑntəfɪ'keɪʃn] *n* Quantifizierung *f*, Quantitätsbestimmung *f*, Messung *f*.
quan·ti·fy ['kwɑntɪfaɪ] *vt* quantitativ bestimmen, messen, quantifizieren.
quan·ti·ta·tive ['kwɑntɪteɪtɪv] *adj* quantitativ, mengenmäßig, Mengen-.
quantitative analysis quantitative/mengenmäßige Bestimmung *f*, Gewichtsanalyse *f*, Gravimetrie *f*.
quantitative assay → quantitative analysis.
quantitative hypertrophy numerische Hypertrophie *f*, Hyperplasie *f*.
quantitative inheritance polygene Vererbung *f*.
quantitative ratio Mengenverhältnis *nt*.
quan·ti·tive ['kwɑntətɪv] *adj* → quantitative.
quantitive analysis → quantitative analysis.
quan·ti·ty ['kwɑntətɪ] *n* Menge *f*, Größe *f*, Quantität *f*; Quantum *nt*; große Menge *f*, Unmenge *f*, Masse *f*; *mathe.*, *phys.* Größe *f*.

q. of electric charge *abbr.* Q, q Elektrizitätsmenge *abbr.* Q.
q. of heat *abbr.* Q, q Wärmemenge *abbr.* Q.
quan·ti·za·tion [ˌkwɑntɪ'zeɪʃn] *n phys.* Quantelung *f.*
quan·tum ['kwɑntəm] *n, pl* **-ta** [-tə] **1.** (bestimmte) Menge *f*, Quantum *nt.* **2.** *phys.* Licht-, Strahlungsquant *nt*; Photon *nt*, Quant *nt.*
quantum constant Planck'-Wirkungsquantum *nt abbr.* h.
quantum efficiency *phys.* Quantenausbeute *f.*
quantum electronics Quantenelektronik *f.*
quantum field theory Quantenfeldtheorie *f.*
quantum mechanics Quantenmechanik *f.*
quantum number Quantenzahl *f.*
quantum physics Quantenphysik *f.*
quantum theory (Planck'-)Quantentheorie *f.*
quantum yield → quantum efficiency.
Quar·an·fil virus ['kwɔːrənfɪl] Quaranfil-Virus *nt.*
quar·an·tine ['kwɔːrəntiːn, 'kwɑr-] **I** *n* **1.** Quarantäne *f.* **in ~** unter Quarantäne (sein *od.* stehen). **to put sb. in ~** → quarantine II. **2.** Quarantäne-, Isolierstation *f.* **II** *vt* jdn. unter Quarantäne stellen.
quar·tan fever ['kwɔːrtn] **1.** Febris quartana. **2.** → quartan malaria.
quartan malaria Malariae-Malaria *f*, Malaria quartana.
quar·tile ['kwɔːrtaɪl, -tɪl] *n stat.* Viertelswert *m*, Quartil *nt.*
quar·ti·sect ['kwɔːrtɪsekt] *vt* vierteilen, in vier Teile teilen.
quartz [kwɔːrts] *n chem.* Quarz *m.*
quartz crystal Quarzkristall *m.*
quartz dust Quarzstaub *m.*
quartz glass Quarzglas *nt.*
quartz·if·er·ous ['kwɔːrtˈsɪfərəs] *adj* quarzig, quarzhaltig, Quarz-.
quartz lamp Quartzlampe *f.*
qua·si·dom·i·nant [ˌkweɪzɪ'dɑmɪnənt] *adj* quasidominant.
quasidominant inheritance quasidominante Vererbung *f.*
quat·er·nar·y ['kwɑtərniːr, kwə'tɜrnərɪ] *adj chem.* vier Elemente *od.* Gruppen enthaltend, quarternär, Quartär-.
quaternary compound quartäre/quatenäre Verbindung *f.*
quaternary structure *chem.* Quartärstruktur *f.*
quaternary syphilis Quartärstadium *nt*, Lues *f* IV.
quea·si·ness ['kwiːzɪnɪs] *n* **1.** Übelkeit *f.* **2.** (Über-)Empfindlichkeit *f.*
quea·sy ['kwiːzɪ] *adj* **1.** unwohl. **2.** (*Magen*) (über-)empfindlich.
Queckenstedt ['kwekənstet]: **Q.'s phenomenon** → Q.'s sign.
Q.'s sign Queckenstedt-Zeichen *nt.*
Q.'s test → Q.'s sign.
Queckenstedt-Stookey ['stuːkɪ]: **Q.-S. test** Queckenstedt-Zeichen *nt.*

Queens·land fever ['kwiːnzlænd] Queensland-Zeckenfieber *nt*, Nordqueensland-Zeckenfieber *nt.*
Queensland tick typhus → Queensland fever.
queer [kwɪər] **I** *n* Homosexuelle(r *m*) *f*; *inf.* Schwule(r *m*) *f.* **II** *adj* **1.** komisch, seltsam, eigenartig. **2.** homosexuell; *inf.* schwul.
quel·lung phenomenon ['kvelʊŋ] Kapselquellungsreaktion *f*, Neufeld-Reaktion *f.*
quellung reaction/test → quellung phenomenon.
quench [kwentʃ] *vt* **1.** (*Feuer*) (aus-)löschen. **2.** (*Durst*) löschen; (*Verlangen*) stillen. **3.** *phys.* (*Schwingung*) abdämpfen, löschen.
Quénu [ke'ny]: **Q.'s hemorrhoidal plexus** Quénu-Plexus *m.*
Quervain → de Quervain.
que·ry fever ['kwɪərɪ] → Q fever.
Quetelet [kɛtə'lɛ]: **Q. index** *physiol.* Körpermasseindex *m*, Quetelet-Index *m*, body mass index *abbr.* BMI.
Queyrat [ke'rɑ]: **erythroplasia of Q.** Erythroplasie *f* Queyrat *f*, Queyrat-Syndrom *nt.*
Quick [kwɪk]: **Q.'s method** → Q. test.
Q. test Thromboplastinzeit *f*, Quickwert *m*, -zeit *f*, *inf.* Quick *m*, Prothrombinzeit *f.*
Q. value → Q. test.
quick [kwɪk] **I** *n* **1.** Nagelhäutchen *nt*, Eponychium *nt.* **2.** Nagelhaut *f*, Cuticula *f*, Perionychium *nt*, Perionyx *m.* **II** *adj* **3.** schnell, sofort, umgehend, rasch, prompt. **4.** schnell, flink, geschwind. **5.** (*Temperament*) hitzig, aufbrausend. **6.** (*Auge*) scharf; (*Ohr*) fein. **7.** *gyn.* (hoch-)schwanger.
quick-acting *adj* schnellwirkend.
quick·en ['kwɪkən] **I** *vt* **1.** anregen, beleben, stimulieren. **2.** (*Puls*) beschleunigen. **II** *vi* **3.** (*Fetus*) s. bewegen; (*Schwangere*) Kindsbewegungen spüren. **4.** (*Puls*) s. beschleunigen.
quick·en·ing ['kwɪkənɪŋ] *n gyn.* erste Kindsbewegungen *pl.*
quick-freeze **I** *n* → quick freezing. **II** *vt* tiefkühlen, einfrieren.
quick freezing Tiefkühl-, Gefrierverfahren *nt.*
quick-frozen *adj* tiefgekühlt, Tiefkühl-, Gefrier-.
quick·lime ['kwɪklaɪm] *n* Kalziumoxid *nt.*
quick·ly formed clot ['kwɪklɪ] Kruorgerinnsel *nt.*
quick pulse **1.** kurzer Puls *m.* **2.** schneller Puls *m.*
quick·sil·ver ['kwɪksɪlvər] *n* Quecksilber *nt*; *chem.* Hydrargyrum *nt abbr.* Hg.
quick-tempered *adj* reizbar, leicht aufbrausend, hitzig.
qui·es·cent [kwiː'esnt] *adj* ruhig, still; bewegungslos.
quiescent state Ruhezustand *m.*
qui·et hip disease [kwaɪɪt] Perthes-Krankheit *f*, Morbus Perthes *m*, Legg-Calvé-Perthes-Krankheit *f*, Perthes-Legg-Calvé-Krankheit *f*, Legg-Calve-

-Perthes-Waldenström-Krankheit *f*, Osteochondropathia deformans coxae juvenilis, Coxa plana (idiopathica).
quiet sleep non-REM-Schlaf *m*, NREM-Schlaf *m*, orthodoxer/synchronisierter Schlaf *m.*
quilt·ed suture ['kwɪltɪd] *chir.* Matratzennaht *f.*
qui·na ['kiːnə] *n pharm.* Chinarinde *f.*
quin·a·crine ['kwɪnəkriːn, -krɪn] *n* Quinacrin *nt*, Chinacrin *nt.*
quinacrine banding *genet.* Quinacrinbanding *nt*, Q-Banding *nt.*
quin·al·bar·bi·tone [ˌkwɪnæl'bɑːrbɪtəʊn] *n pharm.* Secobarbital *nt.*
qui·na·qui·na [kiːnə'kiːnə] *n* → quina.
Quincke ['kwɪŋkə]: **Q.'s disease/edema** Quincke-Ödem *nt*, angioneurotisches Ödem *nt.*
Q.'s pulse Kapillarpuls *m*, Quincke'-Zeichen *nt.*
Q.'s puncture Lumbalpunktion *f.*
Q.'s sign → Q.'s pulse.
quin·es·trol [kwɪn'estrəʊl] *n pharm.* Quinestrol *nt.*
quin·i·dine ['kwɪnɪdiːn, -dɪn] *n* Chinidin *nt*, Quinidine *nt.*
qui·nine ['kwɪnɪn, kwɪ'niːn, 'kwaɪnaɪn] *n* Chinin *nt*, Quinine *nt.*
quinine amblyopia Chininamblyopie *f.*
qui·nin·ism ['kwaɪnɪnɪzəm, 'kwɪn-] *n* Chininvergiftung *f*, Chinchonismus *f*, Cinchonismus *f.*
quin·o·line ['kwɪnəliːn] *n pharm.* Chinolin *nt.*
quin·o·lone ['kwɪnələʊn] *n* Chinolon *nt*, Quinolon *nt*, Chinolon-Antibiotikum *nt.*
qui·none [kwɪ'nəʊn, 'kwɪnəʊn] *n* Chinon *nt.*
Quinquaud [kẽ'ko]: **Q.'s disease** Quinquaud'-Krankheit *f*, Folliculitis decalvans/depilans.
quin·que·va·lent [ˌkwɪŋkwə'veɪlənt, kwɪn'kwevələnt] *adj chem.* fünfwertig.
quin·qui·na [kwɪn'kwaɪnə] *n* → quina.
quin·qui·va·lent *adj* → quinquevalent.
quin·sy ['kwɪnzɪ] *n patho.* Peritonsillarabszeß *m.*
quin·tan fever ['kwɪntən] Wolhyn'-Fieber *nt*, Fünftagefieber *nt*, Wolhynienfieber *nt*, Febris quintana.
Quinton and Scribner ['kwɪntn'skraɪbnər]: **Q. and S. shunt** Quinton-Scribner-Shunt *m*, Scribner-Shunt *m.*
quin·tu·ple [kwɪn't(j)uːpl, -'tʌpl, 'kwɪnt(j)ʊpl] **I** *n* das Fünffache. **II** *adj* fünffach. **III** *vt* verfünffachen. **IV** *vi* s. verfünffachen.
quin·tu·plet [kwɪn'tʌplɪt, -'t(j)uːp-, 'kwɪnt(j)ʊ-] *n* **1.** Fünfling *m.* **2.** **~s** *pl* Fünflinge *pl.*
quo·tid·i·an [kwəʊ'tɪdɪən] **I** *n* → quotidian fever. **II** *adj* täglich.
quotidian fever **1.** Febris quotidiana. **2.** → quotidian malaria.
quotidian malaria Febris quotidiana bei Malaria (tropica), Malaria quotidiana.
quo·tient [kwəʊʃnt] *n* Quotient *m.*
Q wave (*EKG*) Q-Zacke *f*, Q-Welle *f.*

R

R *abbr.* 1. → gas constant. 2. → roentgen I.
RA *abbr.* → rheumatoid arthritis.
Ra *abbr.* → radium.
RAAS *abbr.* → renin-angiotensin-aldosterone system.
rab·bit ['ræbɪt] *n* Kaninchen *nt*; Hase *m*.
rabbit fever Tularämie *f*, Hasen-, Nagerpest *f*, Lemming-Fieber *nt*, Ohara- -Krankheit *f*, Francis-Krankheit *f*.
rab·bit·pox ['ræbɪtpɑks] *n* Kaninchenpocken *pl*.
rabbitpox virus *micro.* Kaninchenpockenvirus *nt*.
rabbit tick *micro.* Haemaphysalis leporis- -palustris.
rab·id ['ræbɪd] *adj* 1. von Tollwut befallen, tollwütig. 2. *fig.* rasend, wütend.
ra·bies ['reɪbiːz] *n* Tollwut *f*, Rabies *f*, Lyssa *f*.
rabies antigen Rabiesantigen *nt*.
rabies immune globulin Tollwut-Immunglobulin *nt*, Rabiesimmunglobulin *nt*.
human r. *abbr.* **RIG** humanes Rabiesimmunglobulin *abbr.* **RIG**.
rabies vaccine Tollwut-, Rabiesvakzine *f*.
rabies virus *micro.* Tollwut-, Rabies-, Lyssavirus *nt*.
ra·bi·form ['reɪbɪfɔːrm] *adj* tollwutähnlich, -artig, rabiform.
race [reɪs] *n bio.* Rasse *f*; Gattung *f*, Unterart *f*.
RA cell RA-Zelle *f*, R(h)agozyt *m*.
ra·ce·mase ['ræsəmeɪz] *n* Razemase *f*, Racemase *f*.
ra·ce·mate ['-meɪt] *n chem.* Razemat *nt*, Racemat *nt*.
ra·ceme [reɪˈsiːm, rə-] *n* 1. *bio.* Traube *f*. 2. → racemate.
ra·ce·mic [reɪˈsiːmɪk, -ˈsem-] *adj chem.* razemisch, racemisch.
racemic form/mixture/modification → racemate.
ra·ce·mi·za·tion [ˌræsɪmɪˈzeɪʃn, ˌreɪsɪ-] *n chem.* Razemisierung *f*, Racemisierung *f*, Racemisierungsreaktion *f*.
racemization reaction → racemization.
rac·e·mize ['ræsəmaɪz, reɪˈsiː-] *vt* razemisieren, racemisieren.
rac·e·mose ['ræsəmoʊz] *adj histol.* traubenförmig, Trauben-.
racemose aneurysm Traubenaneurysma *nt*, Aneurysma cirsoideum/racemosum.
rachi- *pref.* → rachio-.
ra·chi·al ['reɪkɪəl] *adj* → rachidial.
ra·chi·al·gia [ˌreɪkɪˈældʒ(ɪ)ə] *n* Wirbelsäulenschmerz *m*, Rhachi(o)algie *f*, Rhachiodynie *f*.
ra·chi·an·al·ge·sia [ˌ-ˌænlˈdʒiːzɪə] *n anes.* Spinalanästhesie *f*; *inf.* Spinale *f*.
ra·chi·an·es·the·sia [ˌ-ˌænəsˈθiːʒə] *n* → rachianalgesia.
ra·chi·cen·te·sis [ˌ-senˈtiːsɪs] *n* Lumbalpunktion *f*.
ra·chid·i·al [rəˈkɪdɪəl] *adj* Wirbelsäule betr., Wirbelsäulen-, Rückgrat-, Spinal-, Rachi(o)-, Rhachi(o)-.
ra·chid·i·an [rəˈkɪdɪən] *adj* → rachidial.

rachidian quotient *neuro.* Ayala-Quotient *m*, -Gleichung *f*.
ra·chil·y·sis [rəˈkɪləsɪs] *n, pl* **-ses** [-siːz] *ortho.* Rhachi(o)lyse *f*.
rachio- *pref.* Rückgrat-, Wirbelsäulen-, Spinal-, Rachi(o)-, Rhachi(o)-.
ra·chi·o·camp·sis [ˌreɪkɪoʊˈkæmpsɪs] *n* Wirbelsäulenkrümmung *f*, -biegung *f*.
ra·chi·o·cen·te·sis [ˌ-senˈtiːsɪs] *n* Lumbalpunktion *f*.
ra·chi·o·cy·pho·sis [ˌ-saɪˈfoʊsɪs] *n* Kyphose *f*.
ra·chi·o·dyn·ia [ˌ-ˈdiːnɪə] *n* → rachialgia.
ra·chi·o·ky·pho·sis [ˌ-kaɪˈfoʊsɪs] *n* Kyphose *f*.
ra·chi·o·my·e·li·tis [ˌ-ˌmaɪəˈlaɪtɪs] *n* Rückenmark(s)entzündung *f*.
ra·chi·op·a·gus [ˌreɪkɪˈɑpəgəs] *n embryo.* R(h)achiopagus *m*.
ra·chi·op·a·thy [ˌ-ˈɑpəθɪ] *n* Wirbelsäulenerkrankung *f*, Spondylopathie *f*.
ra·chi·o·ple·gia [ˌreɪkəʊˈpliːdʒ(ɪ)ə] *n* Spinalparalyse *f*.
ra·chi·o·sco·li·o·sis [ˌ-skəʊlɪˈəʊsɪs] *n* Skoliose *f*.
ra·chi·o·tome ['-təʊm] *n neurochir., ortho.* Rhachi(o)tom *nt*.
ra·chi·ot·o·my [ˌreɪkɪˈɑtəmɪ] *n neurochir., ortho.* 1. Kolumnotomie *f*, Rhachi(o)tomie *f*. 2. Laminektomie *f*.
ra·chip·a·gus [rəˈkɪpəgəs] *n embryo.* R(h)achipagus *m*.
ra·chis ['reɪkɪs] *n, pl* **-es, rach·i·des** ['rækədiːz] Wirbelsäule *f*, Columna vertebralis.
ra·chis·ag·ra [ˌreɪkɪsˈægrə] *n* gichtbedingte Wirbelsäulenschmerzen *pl*, Rhachisagra *f*.
ra·chis·chi·sis [rəˈkɪskəsɪs] *n embryo.* R(h)achischisis *f*.
ra·chit·ic [rəˈkɪtɪk] *adj* Rachitis betr., von ihr betroffen, durch sie gekennzeichnet, rachitisch.
rachitic beads rachitischer Rosenkranz *m*.
rachitic bowleg rachitisches Crus varum.
rachitic craniotabes rachitische Kraniotabes *f*.
rachitic dwarf rachitischer Zwerg *m*.
rachitic pelvis rachitisches Becken *nt*, Pelvis rachitica.
rachitic rosary rachitischer Rosenkranz *m*.
rachitic scoliosis rachitische Skoliose *f*.
ra·chi·tis [rəˈkaɪtɪs] *n* 1. Rachitis *f*. 2. entzündliche Wirbelsäulenerkrankung *f*.
rach·i·to·gen·ic [ˌrækɪtəʊˈdʒenɪk] *adj* Rachitis verursachend *od.* auslösend, rachitogen.
rach·i·tome ['rækɪtəʊm] *n neurochir., ortho.* Rhachi(o)tom *nt*.
ra·chit·o·my [rəˈkɪtəmɪ] *n* → rachiotomy.
ra·cial ['reɪʃl] *adj* Rasse betr., rassisch, Rassen-.
rack·et amputation ['rækɪt] *chir., ortho.* Amputation *f* mit Racketschnitt.
racket cut *chir.* Racketschnitt *m*.
racket incision → racket cut.
racket-shaped *adj histol.* tennisschlägerförmig.

rad *abbr.* 1. → radiation absorbed dose. 2. → radian.
ra·di·a·bil·i·ty [ˌreɪdɪəˈbɪlətɪ] *n radiol.* (Röntgen-)Strahlendurchlässigkeit *f*.
ra·di·a·ble ['reɪdɪəbl] *adj radiol.* (röntgen-)strahlendurchlässig.
ra·di·al ['reɪdɪəl, -jəl] *adj* 1. *anat.* Radius betr., zur Radialseite hin, radial, Radial-, Radius-, Speichen-. 2. Radius betr., radial, strahlenförmig, strahlig, Strahlen-, Radial-. 3. *bio.* radiär.
radial abduction Radialabduktion *f*.
radial aplasia Radiusaplasie *f*.
radial aplasia-thrombocytopenia syndrome Radiusaplasie-Thrombozytopenie-Syndrom *nt*.
radial artery Radialis *f*, A. radialis.
collateral r. A. collateralis radialis.
r. of index (finger) seitliche Zeigefingerarterie *f*, Radialis *f* indicis, A. radialis indicis.
radial bone → radius 2.
radial border of forearm Außenseite *f* des Unterarms, Margo lateralis/radialis antebrachii.
radial clubhand Manus valga.
radial crest Margo interosseus radii.
radial depression → radial fossa (of humerus).
radial deviation Radialdeviation *f*, -abduktion *f*.
radial diffusion *immun.* Radialdiffusion *f*.
single r. → radial diffusion method.
radial diffusion method *immun.* radiale Diffusionsmethode *f*, Radialimmundiffusion *f*.
radial ectromelia *embryo.* radiale Ektromelie *f*.
radial eminence of wrist Eminentia carpi radialis.
radial fibers of ciliary muscle radiäre Ziliarmuskelfasern *pl*, Fibrae radiales (m. ciliaris).
radial fossa (of humerus) Fossa radialis (humeri).
radial fracture Speichenbruch *m*, Radiusfraktur *f*.
radial groove → radial sulcus.
radial head: r. of flexor digitorum superficialis (muscle) Caput radiale m. flexoris digitorum superficialis.
r. of humerus Capitulum humeri.
radial head fracture Radiusköpfchenfraktur *f*.
radial head prosthesis *ortho.* Radiusköpfchenprothese *f*.
radial hemimelia Radiushemimelie *f*.
radial humeral joint Humeroradialgelenk *nt*, Artic. humeroradialis.
radial immunodiffusion *abbr.* **RID** → radial diffusion method.
radial incisure of ulna → radial notch (of ulna).
radial ligament: annular r. Lig. a(n)nulare radii.
lateral r. Lig. collaterale carpi radiale.
radial malleolus Proc. styloideus radii.

radial margin of forearm → radial border of forearm.
radial neck fracture Halsfraktur f des Radiusköpfchens.
radial nerve Radialis m, N. radialis.
  deep r. Ramus profundus n. radialis.
  superficial r. Ramus superficialis n. radialis.
radial notch (of ulna) Inc. radialis (ulnae).
radial palsy → radial paralysis.
radial paralysis Radialislähmung f, -parese f, -paralyse f.
radial phenomenon Radialisphänomen nt.
radial pulse Radialispuls m.
radial reflex Radius(periost)reflex m abbr. RPR.
  inverted r. dissoziierter Radius(periost)reflex m.
radial styloid tendovaginitis de Quervain-Krankheit f, Tendovaginitis sclerosans de Quervain.
radial sulcus Radialisrinne f, Sulcus (n.) radialis.
radial symmetry bio. Radiärsymmetrie f.
radial tuberosity Tuberositas radii.
radial-ulnar joint 1. unteres/distales Radioulnargelenk nt, Artic. radioulnaris distalis. 2. oberes/proximales Radioulnargelenk nt, Artic. radioulnaris proximalis.
radial veins Begleitvenen pl der A. radialis, Vv. radiales.
ra·di·an ['reɪdɪən] n abbr. **rad** mathe. Radiant m abbr. rad.
ra·di·ant ['reɪdɪənt] I n mathe., phys. Strahl m, Strahlungspunkt m. II adj (aus-)strahlend, aussendend, Strahlungs-.
radiant energy Strahlungsenergie f.
radiant flux Strahlungsfluß m.
radiant heat Strahlungswärme f.
radiant intensity Strahlungsintensität f.
radiant temperature Strahlungstemperatur f.
ra·di·ate [adj 'reɪdɪɪt, -eɪt; v -eɪt] I adj strahlen-, sternförmig, radial, Radial-, Strahl(en)-. II vt ab-, ausstrahlen. III vi 1. ausstrahlen (from von); ausgestrahlt werden; Strahlen aussenden, strahlen. 2. strahlen- od. sternförmig ausgehen (from von).
radiate arteries of kidney (Niere) Radial-, Interlobulararterien pl, Aa. interlobulares renis.
radiate crown Corona radiata.
radiate layer of tympanic membrane äußere radiäre Trommelfellfasern pl, Stratum radiatum membranae tympani.
radiate ligament Lig. capitis costae radiatum.
  r. of carpus Lig. carpi radiatum.
  r. of head of rib Lig. capitis costae radiatum.
  lateral r. Lig. collaterale carpi ulnare.
  r. of Mayer Lig. carpi radiatum.
radiate part of renal cortex (Niere) Pars radiata.
ra·di·a·ther·my [ˌreɪˌdaɪə'θɜrmɪ] n Kurzwellendiathermie f.
ra·di·a·tio [reɪdɪ'eɪʃɪəʊ, ˌræd-] n, pl **-ti·o·nes** [-ʃɪ'əʊniːz] anat. Strahlung f, Radiatio f.
ra·di·a·tion [reɪdɪ'eɪʃn] n 1. (Aus-)Strahlung f, (Aus-)Strahlen nt, Radiation f. **contaminated with ~** strahlenverseucht. 2. radiol. Bestrahlung f, Strahlentherapie f, -behandlung f, Radiotherapie f. 3. anat. Strahlung f, Radiatio f. 4. fig. Ausstrahlung f.
  r. of corpus callosum Balkenstrahlung, Radiatio corporis callosi.
  r. of Gratiolet Gratiolet'-Sehstrahlung, Radiatio optica.
  r. of pain Schmerzausstrahlung.
  r. of thalamus Thalamusstrahlung, Radiatio thalamica.
radiation absorbed dose abbr. **rad** Rad nt abbr. rd.
ra·di·a·tion·al [reɪdɪ'eɪʃnl] adj Strahlung betr., Strahlungs-.
radiation anemia Strahlenanämie f.
radiation biology → radiobiology.
radiation burn Strahlenverbrennung f.
radiation cataract Strahlenstar m, Cataracta radiationis.
radiation chemistry Strahlenchemie f.
radiation colitis Strahlenkolitis f, aktinische Kolitis f.
radiation dermatitis Strahlen-, Radium-, Radiodermatitis f.
radiation dermatosis Strahlendermatose f.
radiation dose Strahlendosis f.
radiation energy Strahlungsenergie f.
radiation enteritis Strahlenenteritis f.
radiation fibromatosis Strahlenfibromatose f.
radiation gastritis Strahlengastritis f.
radiation heat transfer coefficient abbr. h_r phys., physiol. Wärmeübergangszahl f für Strahlung abbr. h_r.
radiation hepatitis Strahlenhepatitis f.
radiation illness → radiation sickness.
radiation injury 1. Strahlenschädigung f, -schaden m. 2. **~ies** pl Strahlenschäden pl.
radiation load Strahlenbelastung f, -exposition f.
radiation myelitis Strahlenmyelitis f.
radiation necrosis Strahlennekrose f.
radiation neuritis → radioneuritis.
radiation osteonecrosis Strahlungs-, Radioosteonekrose f, Osteoradionekrose f.
radiation pneumonitis Strahlenpneumonitis f, -pneumonie f.
radiation proctitis Strahlenproktitis f, aktinische Proktitis f.
radiation protection Strahlenschutz m.
radiation rectitis → radiation proctitis.
radiation sickness Strahlenkrankheit f.
radiation source Strahlenquelle f.
radiation syndrome → radiation sickness.
radiation therapy → radiation 2.
  short distance r. Brachytherapie f.
radiation treatment → radiation 2.
ra·di·a·tive ['reɪdɪeɪtɪv] adj → radiatory.
ra·di·a·to·ry ['reɪdɪəˌtɔːrɪ, -təʊ-] adj ab-, ausstrahlend, Strahlungs-.
rad·i·cal ['rædɪkl] I n 1. chem. Radikal nt. 2. mathe. Wurzel f; Wurzelzeichen nt. 3. fig. Grundlage f, Basis f. II adj 4. drastisch, extrem, radikal, Radikal-; fundamental, grundlegend, Grund-. 5. bot., mathe. Wurzel-. 6. chem. Radikal-.
radical axis mathe. Potenzlinie f.
radical chain (reaction) chem. Radikalkette f.
radical cure Roß-, Radikalkur f.
radical expression mathe. Wurzelausdruck m.
radical hypophysectomy neurochir. radikale Hypophysenentfernung/Hypophysektomie f.
radical hysterectomy gyn. radikale Gebärmutterentfernung/Hysterektomie f.
radical mastectomy gyn. Halstedt-Operation f, radikale Mastektomie f, Mammaamputation f, Ablatio mammae f.
  extended r. erweiterte radikale Mastektomie, superradikale Mastektomie.
  modified r. Patey-Operation f, modifizierte radikale Mastektomie.
radical operation chir. Radikaloperation f.
radical sign mathe. Wurzelzeichen nt.

ra·dic·i·form [rə'dɪsəfɔːrm] adj wurzelförmig.
rad·i·cle ['rædɪkl] n 1. anat. (kleine) (Nerven-, Gefäß-)Wurzel f. 2. bot. Würzelchen nt. 3. chem. Radikal nt.
rad·i·cot·o·my [rædɪ'kɑtəmɪ] n → rhizotomy.
radicul- pref. → radiculo-.
ra·dic·u·ia [rə'dɪkjələ] n → radicle 1.
ra·dic·u·lal·gia [rəˌdɪkjə'lældʒ(ɪ)ə] n (Spinalnerven-)Wurzelneuralgie f.
ra·dic·u·lar [rə'dɪkjələr] adj 1. anat. Wurzel/Radix betr., von einer Wurzel ausgehend, radikulär, Wurzel-, Radikul(o)-. 2. chem. Radikal betr. 3. bot., mathe. Wurzel/Radix betr.
radicular abscess dent. Wurzelspitzenabszeß m.
radicular arteries Rückenäste pl der A. vertebralis, Rami spinales/radiculares a. vertebralis.
radicular branches of vertebral artery → radicular arteries.
radicular cyst (Zahn) radikuläre Zyste f.
radicular fibers (ZNS) Wurzelfasern pl.
radicular innervation radikuläre Innervation f.
radicular neuritis → radiculitis.
radicular pain (Nerv) radikulärer Schmerz m.
radicular pulp Wurzelabschnitt m der (Zahn-)Pulpa, Pulpa radicularis.
radicular syndrome Wurzelsyndrom nt, radikuläres Syndrom nt.
ra·dic·u·lec·to·my [rəˌdɪkjə'lektəmɪ] n neurochir. 1. Wurzelresektion f, Radikulektomie f. 2. → rhizotomy.
ra·dic·u·li·tis [rəˌdɪkjə'laɪtɪs] n Entzündung f der Spinalnervenwurzel, Wurzelneuritis f, Radikulitis f.
radiculo- pref. Wurzel-, Radikul(o)-.
ra·dic·u·lo·gan·gli·on·i·tis [rəˌdɪkjələʊˌgæŋglɪə'naɪtɪs] n Radikuloganglionitis f.
ra·dic·u·lo·me·nin·go·my·e·li·tis [ˌ-mɪˌnɪŋgəʊmaɪə'laɪtɪs] n Radikulomeningomyelitis f.
ra·dic·u·lo·my·e·lop·a·thy [ˌ-maɪə'lɑpəθɪ] n Radikulomyelopathie f.
ra·dic·u·lo·neu·ri·tis [ˌ-njʊə'raɪtɪs, -nʊ-] n 1. Entzündung f der Spinalnervenwurzel, Wurzelneuritis f, Radikulitis f. 2. Landry-Lähmung f, -Paralyse f, -Typ m, Paralysis spinalis ascendens acuta. 3. Guillain-Barré-Syndrom nt, Neuronitis f, (Poly-)Radikuloneuritis f.
ra·dic·u·lo·neu·rop·a·thy [ˌ-njʊə'rɑpəθɪ, -nʊ-] n Radikuloneuropathie f.
ra·dic·u·lop·a·thy [rəˌdɪkjə'lɑpəθɪ] n Erkrankung f der Spinalnervenwurzel, Radikulopathie f.
ra·dif·er·ous [reɪ'dɪf(ə)rəs] adj radiumhaltig.
radio- pref. 1. allg., anat. Radio-, Radius-, Radial-, Speichen-. 2. radiol. Strahl(en-), Strahlungs-, Radio-. 3. chem., phys. Radioaktivität betr., Radium-, Radio-.
ra·di·o·ac·tion [ˌreɪdɪəʊ'ækʃn] n → radioactivity.
ra·di·o·ac·ti·vate [ˌ-'æktɪveɪt] vt phys. radioaktiv machen.
ra·di·o·ac·tive [ˌ-'æktɪv] adj Radioaktivität betr. od. aufweisend, radioaktiv.
radioactive atom radioaktives Atom nt.
radioactive carbon → radiocarbon.
radioactive chain → radioactive series.
radioactive decay radioaktiver Zerfall m.
radioactive disintegration radioaktiver Zerfall m.
radioactive iodide uptake test Radiojodtest m.
radioactive iodine → radioiodine.

radioactive iodine therapy → radioiodine therapy.
radioactive iron → radioiron.
radioactive isotope → radioisotope.
radioactive nuclide → radionuclide.
radioactive phosphorus → radiophosphorus.
radioactive pollution Strahlenverseuchung f.
radioactive series phys. Zerfallsreihe f.
radioactive strontium → radiostrontium.
radioactive sulfur → radiosulfur.
radioactive tracer radioaktiver Marker m, Tracer m.
ra·di·o·ac·tiv·i·ty [ˌ-æk'tɪvɪtɪ] n Radioaktivität f.
ra·di·o·al·ler·go·sor·bent test [ˌ-ˌælərgəʊ-'sɔːrbənt] abbr. **RAST** Radio-Allergen--Sorbent-Test m abbr. RAST.
ra·di·o·au·to·gram [ˌ-'ɔːtəgræm] n → radioautograph.
ra·di·o·au·to·graph [ˌ-'ɔːtəgræf] n Autoradiogramm nt.
ra·di·o·au·tog·ra·phy [ˌ-ɔː'tɑgrəfɪ] n Auto(histo)radiographie f.
ra·di·o·bi·o·log·ic [ˌ-baɪə'lɑdʒɪk] adj strahlen-, radiobiologisch.
ra·di·o·bi·o·log·i·cal [ˌ-baɪə'lɑdʒɪkl] adj → radiobiologic.
ra·di·o·bi·ol·o·gy [ˌ-baɪ'ɑlədʒɪ] n Strahlen-, Strahlungsbiologie f, Radiobiologie f, Strahlenforschung f.
ra·di·o·cal·ci·um [ˌ-'kælsɪəm] n Radiokalzium nt.
ra·di·o·car·bon [ˌ-'kɑːrbən] n Radiokohlenstoff m, Radiokarbon nt.
radiocarbon test Radiocarbon-, Radiokarbontest m.
ra·di·o·car·di·o·gram [ˌ-'kɑːrdɪəgræm] n Radiokardiogramm m.
ra·di·o·car·di·og·ra·phy [ˌ-ˌkɑːrdɪ'ɑgrəfɪ] n Radiokardiographie f.
ra·di·o·car·pal [ˌ-'kɑːrpl] adj Radius u. Handwurzel betr., radiokarpal, Radiokarpal-.
radiocarpal articulation/joint proximales Handgelenk nt, Radiokarpalgelenk nt, Artic. radiocarpalis.
radiocarpal ligament: anterior r. → palmar r.
  dorsal Lig. radiocarpale dorsale.
  palmar r. Lig. radiocarpale palmare.
  volar r. → palmar r.
ra·di·o·car·pus [ˌ-'kɑːrpəs] n anat. M. flexor carpi radialis.
ra·di·o·ce·phal·ic (arteriovenous) fistula/shunt [ˌ-sɪ'fælɪk] chir. A. radialis-V. cephalica-Shunt m.
ra·di·o·chem·i·cal [ˌ-'kemɪkl] adj Radio-/Strahlenchemie betr., radio-, strahlenchemisch.
ra·di·o·chem·is·try [ˌ-'kemɪstrɪ] n Radio-, Strahlenchemie f.
ra·di·o·cur·a·bil·i·ty [ˌ-ˌkjʊərə'bɪlətɪ] n Heilbarkeit f durch Strahlenbehandlung.
ra·di·o·cur·a·ble [ˌ-'kjʊərəbl] adj durch Strahlentherapie heilbar.
ra·di·o·cys·ti·tis [ˌ-sɪs'taɪtɪs] n Strahlen-, Radiozystitis f.
ra·di·o·dense ['-dens] adj strahlendicht.
ra·di·o·den·si·ty [ˌ-'densətɪ] n Strahlendichte f, -undurchlässigkeit f.
ra·di·o·der·ma·ti·tis [ˌ-ˌdɜːrmə'taɪtɪs] n Strahlen-, Radio-, Radiumdermatitis f.
ra·di·o·di·ag·no·sis [ˌ-ˌdaɪəg'nəʊsɪs] n Radiodiagnose f.
ra·di·o·di·ag·nos·tics [ˌ-ˌdaɪəg'nɑstɪks] pl Radiodiagnostik f.
ra·di·o·dig·i·tal [ˌ-'dɪdʒɪtl] adj Radius u. Finger betr., radiodigital.
ra·di·o·e·col·o·gy [ˌ-ɪ'kɑlədʒɪ] n Radioökologie f.

ra·di·o·e·lec·tro·car·di·o·gram [ˌ-ɪˌlektrə-'kɑːrdɪəgræm] n Radioelektrokardiogramm nt.
ra·di·o·e·lec·tro·car·di·og·ra·phy [ˌ-ɪˌlektrəˌkɑːrdɪ'ɑgrəfɪ] n Radioelektrokardiographie f.
ra·di·o·el·e·ment [ˌ-'eləmənt] n Radioelement nt.
ra·di·o·en·ceph·a·lo·gram [ˌ-en'sefələgræm] n abbr. **REG** Radioenzephalogramm nt.
ra·di·o·en·ceph·a·log·ra·phy [ˌ-enˌsefə-'lɑgrəfɪ] n Radioenzephalographie f.
ra·di·o·ep·i·der·mi·tis [ˌ-epɪdɜr'maɪtɪs] n → radiodermatitis.
ra·di·o·ep·i·the·li·tis [ˌ-epɪθɪ'laɪtɪs] n → radiodermatitis.
radio-frequency spectroscopy Radiofrequenzspektroskopie f.
ra·di·o·gene ['-dʒiːn] n radioaktive Substanz f, Radiogen nt.
ra·di·o·gen·ic [ˌ-'dʒenɪk] adj chem., phys. von radioaktiver Herkunft, radiogen.
ra·di·o·gold ['-gəʊld] n Radiogold nt.
ra·di·o·gram ['-græm] n → radiograph I.
ra·di·o·graph ['-græf] **I** n Röntgenbild nt, -aufnahme f, Radio-, Röntgenogramm nt. **II** vt ein Radiogramm machen; röntgen.
ra·di·o·graph·ic [ˌ-'græfɪk] adj Radiographie betr., mittels Radiographie, radiographisch, Röntgen-; radiologisch.
radiographic examination radiologische Untersuchung f.
ra·di·og·ra·phy [ˌ-reɪdɪ'ɑgrəfɪ] n Röntgen(untersuchung f) nt, Radio-, Röntgenographie f.
ra·di·o·hu·mer·al [ˌreɪdɪəʊ'(h)juːmərəl] adj Radius u. Humerus betr., radiohumeral.
radiohumeral bursitis → radiohumeral epicondylitis.
radiohumeral epicondylitis Tennisell(en)bogen m, Epicondylitis radialis humeri.
ra·di·o·im·mu·no·as·say [ˌ-ˌɪmjənəʊ'æseɪ, -æ'seɪ] n abbr. **RIA** Radioimmunoassay m abbr. RIA.
ra·di·o·im·mu·no·de·tec·tion [ˌ-ˌɪmjənəʊdɪ'tekʃn] n abbr. **RAID** Radioimmundetektion f.
ra·di·o·im·mu·no·dif·fu·sion [ˌ-ˌɪmjənəʊdɪ'fjuːʒn] n Radioimmun(o)diffusion f.
ra·di·o·im·mu·no·e·lec·tro·pho·re·sis [ˌ-ˌɪmjənəʊɪˌlektrəʊfə'riːsɪs] n Radioimmunoelektrophorese f.
ra·di·o·im·mu·no·lo·cal·i·za·tion [ˌ-ˌɪmjənəʊˌləʊkəlaɪ'zeɪʃn] n Radioimmunlokalisation f.
ra·di·o·im·mu·no·sor·bent test [ˌ-ˌɪmjənəʊ'sɔːrbənt] abbr. **RIST** Radioimmunosorbenttest m abbr. RIST.
ra·di·o·i·o·din·at·ed serum albumin [ˌ-'aɪədəneɪtɪd] abbr. **RISA** Radioiod-Serumalbumin m abbr. RISA.
ra·di·o·i·o·dine ['-aɪədaɪn, -dɪn] n Radiojod nt, -iod nt.
radioiodine therapy Radiojod-, Radioiodtherapie f.
ra·di·o·i·ron ['-aɪərn] n radioaktives Eisen nt, Radioeisen nt.
ra·di·o·i·so·tope [ˌ-'aɪsətəʊp] n radioaktives Isotop nt, Radioisotop nt.
radioisotope scanning Szintigraphie f.
ra·di·o·ky·mog·ra·phy [ˌ-kaɪ'mɑgrəfɪ] n → roentgenkymography.
ra·di·o·log·ic [ˌ-'lɑdʒɪk] adj Radiologie betr., auf ihr beruhend, radiologisch.
ra·di·o·log·i·cal [ˌ-'lɑdʒɪkl] adj → radiologic.
radiological anatomy radiologische Anatomie f.

ra·di·ol·o·gist [ˌreɪdɪ'ɑlədʒɪst] n Radiologe m, -login f, Arzt m/Ärztin f für Radiologie.
ra·di·ol·o·gy [ˌ-'ɑlədʒɪ] n Strahlen(heil)kunde f, Radiologie f.
ra·di·o·lu·cen·cy [ˌreɪdɪəʊ'luːsnsɪ] n Strahlendurchlässigkeit f.
ra·di·o·lu·cent [ˌ-'luːsənt] adj strahlendurchlässig.
radiolucent medium radiol. strahlendurchlässiges Medium nt.
ra·di·o·lu·mi·nes·cence [ˌ-ˌluːmɪ'nesəns] n phys. Radiolumineszenz f.
ra·di·ol·y·sis [ˌreɪdɪ'ɑləsɪs] n chem. Radiolyse f.
ra·di·om·e·ter [ˌ-'ɑmɪtər] n phys. Strahlungsmesser m, Radiometer nt.
ra·di·om·e·try [ˌ-'ɑmətrɪ] n phys. Radiometrie f.
ra·di·o·mi·crom·e·ter [ˌreɪdɪəʊmaɪ'krɑmɪtər] n Radiomikrometer nt.
ra·di·o·mi·met·ic [ˌ-mɪ'metɪk] **I** n Radiomimetikum nt. **II** adj radiomimetisch.
ra·di·o·mus·cu·lar [ˌ-'mʌskjələr] adj anat. radiomuskulär.
ra·di·o·ne·cro·sis [ˌ-nɪ'krəʊsɪs] n Radionekrose f.
ra·di·o·neu·ri·tis [ˌ-njʊə'raɪtɪs, -nʊ-] n Strahlen-, Radioneuritis f.
ra·di·o·nu·clide [ˌ-'n(j)uːklaɪd] n radioaktives Nuklid nt, Radionuklid nt.
radionuclide angiography Radionuklidangiographie f.
radionuclide generator radiol. (Radio-)Nuklidgenerator m.
radionuclide imaging Szintigraphie f.
radionuclide scan Radionuklid-Scan m.
radionuclide scanning Radionuklid--Scanning nt.
radio-opacity n → radiopacity.
ra·di·o·pac·i·ty [ˌ-'pæsətɪ] n Strahlendichte f, -undurchlässigkeit f.
ra·di·o·paque [ˌ-'peɪk] adj strahlendicht, -undurchlässig; röntgendicht.
radiopaque dye strahlendichter Farbstoff m.
radiopaque medium radiol. röntgendichtes/strahlendichtes Medium nt.
ra·di·o·par·en·cy [ˌ-'pærənsɪ] n Strahlendurchlässigkeit f.
ra·di·o·par·ent [ˌ-'pærənt] adj strahlendurchlässig.
ra·di·o·pa·thol·o·gy [ˌ-pə'θɑlədʒɪ] n Strahlenpathologie f.
ra·di·o·pen·e·tra·ble [ˌ-'penətrəbl] adj strahlendurchlässig.
ra·di·o·per·i·os·te·al reflex [ˌ-ˌperɪ'ɑstɪəl] Radius-, Radiusperiostreflex m abbr. RPR.
ra·di·o·phar·ma·ceu·ti·cals [ˌ-ˌfɑrmə'suːtɪkls] pl Radiopharmaka pl.
ra·di·o·pho·bia [ˌ-'fəʊbɪə] n psychia. krankhafte Angst f vor Röntgenstrahlen, Radiophobie f.
ra·di·o·phos·pho·rus [ˌ-'fɑsfərəs] n Radiophosphor m.
ra·di·o·phys·ics [ˌ-'fɪzɪks] pl Strahlenphysik f.
ra·di·o·pill ['-pɪl] n Telemetriesonde f, -kapsel f.
ra·di·o·po·tas·si·um [ˌ-pə'tæsɪəm] n Radiokalium nt.
ra·di·o·re·sis·tance [ˌ-rɪ'zɪstəns] n Strahlenunempfindlichkeit f, -resistenz f.
ra·di·o·re·sis·tant [ˌ-rɪ'zɪstənt] adj strahlenunempfindlich, -resistent.
ra·di·o·scope ['-skəʊp] n Radioskop nt.
ra·di·o·scop·ic [ˌ-'skɑpɪk] adj röntgenoskopisch.
ra·di·o·scop·i·cal [ˌ-'skɑpɪkl] adj → radioscopic.
ra·di·os·co·py [ˌreɪdɪ'ɑskəpɪ] n Röntgen-

untersuchung f, -durchleuchtung f, Röntgeno-, Radioskopie f.
ra·di·o·sen·si·bil·i·ty [ˌreɪdɪəʊˌsensəˈbɪlətɪ] n Strahlenempfindlichkeit f.
ra·di·o·sen·si·tive [ˌ-ˈsensətɪv] adj strahlenempfindlich.
ra·di·o·sen·si·tive·ness [ˌ-ˈsensətɪvnɪs] n → radiosensibility.
ra·di·o·sen·si·tiv·i·ty [ˌ-sensɪˈtɪvətɪ] n → radiosensibility.
ra·di·o·so·di·um [ˌ-ˈsəʊdɪəm] n Radionatrium nt.
radio spectrum phys. Strahlenspektrum nt.
ra·di·o·stron·ti·um [ˌ-ˈstrɒnʃ(ɪ)əm, -tɪəm] n chem. Radiostrontium nt; Strontium 90 nt.
ra·di·o·sul·fur [ˌ-ˈsʌlfər] n radioaktiver Schwefel m, Radioschwefel m.
ra·di·o·tel·e·me·ter·ing capsule [ˌ-ˌteləˈmiːtərɪŋ] Telemetriesonde f, -kapsel f.
ra·di·o·te·lem·e·try [ˌ-təˈlemətrɪ] n Radiotelemetrie f; Biotelemetrie f.
ra·di·o·ther·a·peu·tics [ˌ-ˌθerəˈpjuːtɪks] pl 1. → radiology. 2. → radiotherapy.
ra·di·o·ther·a·pist [ˌ-ˈθerəpɪst] n Strahlen-, Röntgentherapeut(in f) m.
ra·di·o·ther·a·py [ˌ-ˈθerəpɪ] n Bestrahlung f, Strahlentherapie f, -behandlung f, Radiotherapie f.
ra·di·o·ther·my [ˈ-θɜrmɪ] n 1. Wärmestrahlenbehandlung f. 2. Kurzwellenbehandlung f.
ra·di·o·tho·ri·um [ˌ-ˈθɔːrɪəm, -ˈθəʊ-] n Radiothorium nt; Thorium 228 nt.
ra·di·o·trac·er [ˈ-treɪsər] n radioaktiver Tracer m, Radiotracer m.
ra·di·o·trans·par·en·cy [ˌ-trænsˈpeərənsɪ] n Strahlendurchlässigkeit f.
ra·di·o·trans·par·ent [ˌ-trænsˈpærənt] adj → radiolucent.
ra·di·o·ul·nar [ˌ-ˈʌlnər] adj Radius u. Ulna betr., radioulnar, Radioulnar-.
radioulnar articular disk → radioulnar disk.
radioulnar articulation: distal/inferior r. unteres/distales Radioulnargelenk nt, Artic. radioulnaris distalis.
proximal/superior r. oberes/proximales Radioulnargelenk nt, Artic. radioulnaris proximalis.
radioulnar disk Discus artic. radioulnaris.
radioulnar joint: distal/inferior r. → radioulnar articulation, distal/inferior.
proximal/superior r. → radioulnar articulation, proximal/superior.
radioulnar synarthrosis/syndesmosis Syndesmosis radioulnaris.
radioulnar synostosis radioulnäre/radioulnare Synostose f.
ra·di·um [ˈreɪdɪəm] n abbr. **Ra** Radium nt abbr. Ra.
ra·di·us [ˈreɪdɪəs] n, pl **-di·us·es, -di·i** [-dɪaɪ] 1. Radius m. 2. anat. Speiche f, Radius m. 3. Umkreis m; (Einfluß-, Wirkungs-)Bereich m, Aktionsradius m.
radius aplasia Radiusaplasie f.
radius hypoplasia Radiushypoplasie f.
ra·dix [ˈreɪdɪks] n, pl **rad·i·ces** [ˈrædəsiːz, ˈreɪdə-] 1. anat., bot. Wurzel f, Radix f. 2. mathe. Grundzahl f, Basis f.
ra·don [ˈreɪdɒn] n abbr. **Rn** Radon nt abbr. Rn.
raf·fi·nose [ˈræfɪnəʊs] n Raffinose f, Melitriose f, Melitose f.
rage [reɪdʒ] I n Wut f, Raserei f, Zorn m, Rage f, Wutanfall m. II vi (Krankheit) wüten.
rag·o·cyte [ˈrægəsaɪt] n R(h)agozyt m, RA-Zelle f.
rag·pick·er's disease [ˈrægpɪkər] → ragsorter's disease.

rag·sort·er's disease [ˈrægsɔːrtər] Wollsortierer-, Lumpensortierer-, Hadernkrankheit f, Lungenmilzbrand m.
RAID abbr. → radioimmunodetection.
Rail·li·e·ti·na [ˌraɪlɪəˈtaɪnə] n micro. Raillietina f.
rail·lie·ti·ni·a·sis [ˌraɪlɪətɪˈnaɪəsɪs] n Raillietina-Befall m.
railroad nystagmus [ˈreɪlrəʊd] 1. Eisenbahnnystagmus m. 2. optokinetischer Nystagmus m.
rainbow symptom [ˈreɪnbəʊ] ophthal. Halo glaucomatosus.
rainbow vision ophthal. Halosehen nt.
Rainey [ˈreɪnɪ]: **R.'s corpuscles/tubes/tubules** micro. Rainey-Körperchen pl, Miescherschläuche pl.
RAI test → radioactive iodide uptake test.
Raji [ˈrɑːdʒɪ]: **R. cells** immun. Raji-Zellen pl.
rales [rælz, rɑːlz] pl (Lunge) Rasselgeräusche pl abbr. RG, Rasseln nt, Rhonchi pl.
Ra·ma·chan·dran plot [ˌrɑːməˈtʃʌndrən] biochem. Ramachandran-Auftragung f, -Darstellung f, -Diagramm nt.
ra·mal [ˈreɪməl] adj anat. Ramus/Zweig betr.
Raman [ˈrɑːmən]: **R. effect** radiol. Raman-Effekt m.
ram·i·cot·o·my [ˌræmɪˈkɒtəmɪ] n → ramisection.
ram·i·fi·ca·tion [ˌræmɪfɪˈkeɪʃn] n 1. Verzweigung f, Verästelung f, Aufzweigung f. 2. Zweig m, Sproß m.
ram·i·fy [ˈræmɪfaɪ] I vt verzweigen. II vi s. verzweigen, s. verästeln.
Ramirez [rəˈmɪərəz]: **ashy dermatosis of R.** Erythema dyschromicum perstans.
ram·i·sec·tion [ˌræmɪˈsekʃn] n neurochir. Ramikotomie f, Ramisektion f.
ram·i·sec·to·my [ˌ-ˈsektəmɪ] n → ramisection.
ra·mose [ˈreɪməʊz] adj verzweigt.
ra·mous [ˈreɪməs] adj → ramose.
Ramsey Hunt [ˈræmzɪ hʌnt]: **R. H. disease** → R. H. syndrome 1.
R. H. paralysis progressive Pallidumatrophie Hunt f, Pallidumsyndrom nt, Paralysis agitans juvenilis.
R. H. syndrome 1. Genikulatumneuralgie f, Ramsey Hunt-Syndrom nt, Zoster oticus, Herpes zoster oticus, Neuralgia geniculata. **2.** Hunt-Syndrom nt, Dyssynergia cerebellaris myoclonica. **3.** Hunt-Syndrom nt, Dyssynergia cerebellaris progressiva.
Ramstedt [ˈrɑːmstet; ˈramʃtet]: **R.'s operation** chir. Weber-Ramstedt-Operation f, Ramstedt-Operation f, Pyloro(myo)tomie f.
ram·u·lus [ˈræmjələs] n, pl **-li** [-laɪ] anat. Ramulus m.
ra·mus [ˈreɪməs] n, pl **-mi** [-maɪ] anat. Ast m, Zweig m, Abzweigung f, Ramus m.
r. of ischium Sitzbeinast m, Ramus ossis ischii.
r. of mandible Unterkieferast, Ramus mandibulae.
r. of pubis Schambeinast m, Ramus ossis pubis.
ran·cid [ˈrænsɪd] adj (Butter) ranzig.
ran·cid·i·ty [rænˈsɪdətɪ] n Ranzigkeit f.
ran·dom [ˈrændəm] adj zufällig, wahllos, willkürlich, Zufalls-; **at ~** blindlings, wahl-, ziellos, auf gut Glück.
random check stat. Stichprobe f.
random genetic drift genet. Gendrift f, genetische Drift.
ran·dom·i·za·tion [ˌrændəmaɪˈzeɪʃn] n stat. Randomisierung f.
ran·dom·ize [ˈrændəmaɪz] vt stat. eine Zufallsauswahl treffen, randomisieren.

random mating bio., genet. Panmixie f, Panmixis f.
random mating equilibrium bio., genet. Hardy-Weinberg-Gesetz nt.
ran·dom·ness [ˈrændəmnɪs] n phys., mathe. Unordnung f, Ungeordnetheit f, zufallsbedingte Verteilung f.
random number stat. Zufallszahl f, beliebige Zahl f.
random pattern Zufallsmuster nt.
random sample stat. (Zufall-)Stichprobe f.
random sampling stat. (Zufalls-)Stichprobenerhebung f.
random variable stat. Zufallsvariable f.
range [reɪndʒ] I n 1. fig. (Aktions-)Radius m; Reichweite f; techn. (Meß-, Skalen-)Bereich m; (Gelenk) Spiel-, Freiraum m; (Stimmen-)Umfang m. 2. stat. Toleranz-, Streuungsbreite f, Bereich m. 4. bio. Verbreitung(sgebiet nt) f. II vt (an-, ein-)ordnen, einteilen, klassifizieren. III vi 5. variieren; schwanken, s. bewegen, liegen (from ... to zwischen ... und); gehen (from ... to von ... bis). 6. bio. vorkommen, verbreitet sein, s. erstrecken (over über).
r. of accommodation physiol. Akkommodationsbreite f.
r. of action Aktionsbereich, -radius.
r. of activities Aktionsbereich, Betätigungsfeld nt.
r. of application Anwendungsbereich.
r. of atom phys. Atombezirk m.
r. of convergence ophthal. Konvergenzbreite f, -amplitude f.
r. of knowledge Wissensbereich.
r. of motion abbr. **ROM** (Gelenk) Bewegungsfreiraum m, -spielraum m.
r. of movement abbr. **ROM** → r. of motion.
r. of normal Normalbereich.
r. of uses Anwendungsmöglichkeiten pl, Verwendungsbereich.
ra·nine artery [ˈreɪnaɪn] tiefe Zungenschlagader/-arterie f, A. profunda linguae.
ra·ni·ti·dine [reɪˈnaɪtədiːn] n pharm. Ranitidin nt.
rank [ræŋk] I n Rang m, Stand m; Aufstellung f; Reihe f, Kette f; **to form into ~s** s. ordnen, s. formieren. II vt (ein-)ordnen, einreihen. III vi s. ordnen, s. formieren.
rank correlation stat. Rangkorrelation f.
Ranke [ˈraŋkiː]: **R. complex** pulmo. Ghon'-Primärkomplex m, -Herd m.
R.'s formula Ranke-Formel f.
R.'s stages Ranke-Stadien pl, Ranke-Dreistadienlehre f.
Rankine [ˈræŋkaɪn]: **R. scale** Rankine-Skala f.
R. thermometer Rankine-Thermometer nt, Thermometer nt mit Rankine-Skala.
rank order stat. Rangordnung f.
rank sum test stat. Wilcoxon-Test m, Rangsummentest m.
R antigen R-Antigen nt.
ran·u·la [ˈrænjələ] n HNO Ranula f.
Ranvier [ˈrɑːvɪ-e]: **R.'s crosses** Ranvier'-Kreuze pl.
internode of R. → R.'s segment.
nodes of R. Ranvier'-Schnürringe pl, -Knoten pl.
R.'s segment Internodalsegment nt.
Raoult [rɑːˈuːl]: **R.'s law** Raoult-Gesetz nt.
rape [reɪp] I n Vergewaltigung f. II vt vergewaltigen.
ra·phe [ˈreɪfɪ] n, pl **-phae** [-fiː] anat. Naht f, Verwachsungsnaht f, Raphe f, Raphé f, Rhaphe f.
r. of medulla oblongata Raphe (mediana) medullae oblongatae.

rapheal nuclei

r. of palate Gaumenleiste *f*, Raphe palati.
r. of penis Penisnaht, -raphe, Raphe penis.
r. of perineum Perinealraphe, -naht, Raphe perinealis.
r. of pharynx Raphe pharyngis.
r. of pons Raphe (mediana) pontis.
r. of scrotum Skrotalnaht, -raphe, Raphe scroti/scrotalis.
ra·pheal nuclei ['reɪfɪəl] Ncc. raphae.
raphe penis Penisnaht *f*, -raphe *f*, Raphe penis.
rap·id ['ræpɪd] *adj* schnell, rasch, rapide, Schnell-.
rapid breathing beschleunigte/schnelle Atmung *f*, Tachypnoe *f*.
rapid decompression explosive/rapide Dekompression *f*.
rapid eating hastiges/überstürztes Essen *nt*, Tachyphagie *f*.
rapid eye movements *abbr*. REM *physiol*. rapid eye movements *abbr*. REM.
rapid eye movement sleep paradoxer/ desynchronisierter Schlaf *m*, Traumschlaf *m*, REM-Schlaf *m*.
rapid eye movement state → rapid eye movement sleep.
rap·id·ly-adapting receptor ['ræpɪdlɪ] *physiol*. schnell adaptierender Rezeptor/ Sensor *m*, RA-Rezeptor *m*, RA-Sensor *m*.
rapidly-adapting sensor → rapidly-adapting receptor.
rapidly growing mycobacteria *micro*. schnellwachsende (atypische) Mykobakterien *pl*, Mykobakterien *pl* der Runyon-Gruppe IV.
rapidly progressive glomerulonephritis maligne Glomerulonephritis *f*, rasch progrediente Glomerulonephritis *f*, rapidly progressive glomerulonephritis.
rapidly progressive osteoarthritis entzündliche/rapid-progressive Arthrose *f*.
rapid metabolism Tachymetabolismus *m*.
rapid plasma reagin test rapid plasma reagin test (*m*), RPR-Test *m*.
rapid speech *neuro*., *psychia*. Tachylalie *f*.
Rapoport [rapo'pɔːr]: **R. test** *urol*. Rapoport-Test *m*.
rap·port [ræ'pɔːr, -'pəʊr, rə-] *n* **1.** (persönliches) Verhältnis *nt*, Beziehung *f*, Verbindung *f*. **2.** *psycho*. Rapport *m*.
rap·ture ['ræptʃər] *n* Entzückung *nt*, Verzückung *f*, Begeisterung *f*; Begeisterungstaumel *m*, Ekstase *f*.
r. of the deep Tiefenrausch *m*.
rare [reər] *adj* selten, rar; (*Atmosphäre*) dünn; (*Materie*) porös; (*Strahlung*) schwach.
rare base *biochem*. seltene Base *f*.
RA receptor → rapidly-adapting receptor.
rare earth elements → rare earths.
rare earths *chem*. seltene Erden *pl*.
rar·e·fac·tion [reərə'fækʃn] *n* **1.** *phys*. Verdünnung *f*. **2.** *patho*. Rarefizierung *f*, Rarefactio *f*, Rareficatio *f*.
rare gas Edelgas *nt*.
rare mutant *genet*. seltene Mutante *f*.
rare pulse langsamer Puls *m*, Pulsus rarus.
rar·i·ty ['reərətɪ] *n* Seltenheit *f*, Rarität *f*.
RAS *abbr*. **1.** → renin-angiotensin system. **2.** → reticular activating system.
RA sensor → rapidly-adapting receptor.
rash [ræʃ] *n* **1.** *derm*. (Haut-)Ausschlag *m*, Exanthem(a) *nt*. **2.** Vorexanthem *nt*, Rash *m/nt*.
Rasin [rə'siːn; ra'sɛ̃]: **R.'s sign** Jellinek-Zeichen *nt*.
Rasmussen ['ræsmʊsən]: **R.'s aneurysm** Rasmussen-Aneurysma *nt*.
rasp [ræsp] **I** *n* Raspel *f*; (Grob-)Feile *f*. **II** *vt*, *vi* raspeln, feilen, schaben.

ras·pa·to·ry ['ræspətɔːriː, -təʊ-] *n* *chir*., *ortho*. Knochenschaber *m*, Raspatorium *nt*.
rasp·ber·ry tongue ['ræzberɪ, -bərɪ, 'rɑːz-] Himbeerzunge *f*, rote Zunge *f*.
rasp·ing ['ræspɪŋ] **I** *n* Raspeln *nt*. **II** *adj* kratzend; (*Stimme*) rauh, krächzend.
RAST *abbr*. → radioallergosorbent test.
Rastelli [rɑs'telɪ]: **R.'s operation/procedure** HTG Rastelli-Operation *f*.
rat [ræt] *n* Ratte *f*.
rat-bite disease 1. Rattenbißkrankheit *f*, Rattenbiß-Fieber I *nt*, Sodoku *nt*. **2.** Rattenbißkrankheit *f*, Rattenbiß-Fieber II *nt*, atypisches Rattenbiß-Fieber *nt*, Haverhill-Fieber *nt*, Bakterienrattenbißfieber *nt*, Streptobazillenrattenbißfieber *nt*, Erythema arthriticum epidemicum.
rat-bite fever → rat-bite disease.
rate [reɪt] **I** *n* Quote *f*, Rate *f*; Geschwindigkeit *f*, Tempo *nt*. **at the ~ of** im Verhältnis von. **II** *vt* (ein-)schätzen, einstufen, bewerten, beurteilen.
r. of change Änderungsgeschwindigkeit.
r. of consumption Verbrauch(sgeschwindigkeit *f*) *m*.
r. of flow Durchflußgeschwindigkeit, -menge *f*, Fluß *m*.
r. of formation Bildungsgeschwindigkeit.
r. of respiratory metabolism respiratorische Stoffwechselrate.
rate constant Geschwindigkeitskonstante *f*.
rate-determining step → rate-limiting step.
rate enhancement *phys*. Geschwindigkeitserhöhung *f*, -beschleunigung *f*.
rate equation *phys*. Geschwindigkeitsgleichung *f*.
rate-limiting *adj* geschwindigkeitsbestimmend, -begrenzend.
rate-limiting step *chem*., *biochem*. geschwindigkeitsbestimmender *od*. -begrenzender Schritt *m*.
rate-zonal centrifugation Zonenzentrifugation *f*.
rat flea *micro*. Rattenfloh *m*.
Rathke ['ratkə]: **R.'s cyst** Rathke'-Zyste *f*.
R.'s diverticulum *embryo*. Rathke'-Tasche *f*.
R.'s duct Rathke'-Gang *m*.
R.'s pouch → R.'s diverticulum.
R.'s pouch tumor Erdheim-Tumor *m*, Kraniopharyngeom *nt*.
R.'s tumor → R.'s pouch tumor.
ra·tio ['reɪʃ(ɪ)əʊ] *n*, *pl* **-tios** *mathe*. Verhältnis *nt*; Verhältniszahl *f*; Quotient *m*. **in the/a ~ of 2 to 1** im Verhältnis 2 zu 1. **in inverse ~** umgekehrt proportional.
ra·tion·al ['ræʃənl] *adj* **1.** vernünftig, verständig, rational. **2.** rationell, praktisch. **3.** *mathe*. rational.
ra·tion·ale [ræʃə'næl] *n* logische Grundlage *f*, Grundprinzip *nt*.
rational formula *chem*. Strukturformel *f*.
ra·tio·nal·i·za·tion [ˌræʃənəlɪ'zeɪʃn] *n* *psycho*. Rationalisierung *f*.
rational scale *mathe*. Rationalskala *f*.
rat·i·zide ['rætɪsaɪd] *n* *hyg*. Ratizid *nt*.
rat leprosy *micro*. Rattenlepra *f*.
rat lungworm *micro*. Rattenlungenwurm *m*, Angiostrongylus cantonensis.
rat stomach worm *micro*. Magenwurm *m* der Ratte, Gnathostoma spinigerum.
rat tapeworm *micro*. Ratten-, Mäusebandwurm *m*, Hymenolepis diminuta.
Rau [raʊ]: **R.'s process** vorderer Hammerfortsatz *m*, Proc. anterior mallei.
Rauber ['raʊbər]: **hepatic funiculus of R.** *old* → hepatic artery.
spinal crest of R. Dornfortsatz *m*, Proc. spinosis.

tubopharyngeal ligament of R. Plica salpingopharyngea.
Rauchfuss ['raʊxfʊs]: **R.' triangle** Grocco-Rauchfuß-Dreieck *nt*.
Rauscher ['raʊʃər]: **R.'s (leukemia) virus** Rauscher-Leukämievirus *nt*.
Rau·wol·fia [rɔː'wʊlfɪə, raʊ-] *n* *pharm*., *bio*. Rauwolfia *f*.
RAV *abbr*. → Rous-associated virus.
ra·vi·an process ['reɪvɪən] vorderer Hammerfortsatz *m*, Proc. anterior mallei.
ray [reɪ] **I** *n* Strahl *m*; Lichtstrahl *m*. **II** *vt* **1.** ausstrahlen. **2.** bestrahlen. **3.** *inf*. röntgen. **III** *vi* Strahlen aussenden, strahlen; s. strahlenförmig ausbreiten.
ray out *vt* → ray 1.
ray filter *photo*. Farbfilter *m*.
Rayleigh ['reɪlɪ]: **R. test** *ophthal*. Rayleigh-Test *m*.
ray·less ['reɪlɪs] *adj* strahlenlos; lichtlos, dunkel.
Raymond [rɛ'mɔ̃ː]: **R.'s (type of) apoplexy** Raymond'-Apoplexie *f*.
Raymond-Cestan [sɛs'tɑ̃]: **R.-C. syndrome** Raymond-Cestan-Syndrom *nt*.
Raynaud [rɛ'no]: **R.'s disease 1.** echte/essentielle/primäre Raynaud-Krankheit *f*. **2.** Raynaud-Syndrom *nt*, sekundäre Raynaud-Krankheit *f*.
R.'s phenomenon 1. Raynaud-Phänomen *nt*. **2.** → R.'s disease 1.
secondary R.'s disease → R.'s disease 2.
R.'s sign Akrozyanose *f*, Akroaspyxie *f*.
R.'s syndrome → R.'s disease 2.
ray resection *radiol*. (*Hand*) Strahlenamputation *f*, -resektion *f*.
ray treatment *radiol*. Bestrahlung *f*, Strahlentherapie *f*, -behandlung *f*, Radiotherapie *f*.
Rb *abbr*. → rubidium.
RBA *abbr*. → recurrent benign aphthosis.
R bacteria *micro*. R-Form *f*, R-Stamm *m*.
R-band *n* (*Chromosom*) R-Bande *f*.
R banding *genet*. R-Banding *nt*.
RBBB *abbr*. → bundle-branch block, right.
RBC *abbr*. → red blood count 1.
RBE *abbr*. → relative biological effectiveness.
RBF *abbr*. → renal blood flow.
RCC *abbr*. → red cell count 1.
RCM *abbr*. **1.** → red cell mass. **2.** → restrictive cardiomyopathy.
R colony *micro*. (*Kolonie*) R-Form *f*.
R.D. *abbr*. → reaction of degeneration.
RDS *abbr*. → respiratory distress syndrome (of the newborn).
Re *abbr*. → rhenium.
re·ab·sorb [riːəb'zɔːrb] *vt* → resorb.
re·ab·sorb·ing [riːəb'zɔːrbɪŋ] *adj* → resorbent.
re·ab·sorp·tion [riːəb'zɔːrpʃn] *n* **1.** Reabsorption *f*. **2.** → resorption.
reabsorption atelectasis (*Lunge*) Absorptions-, Obstruktionsatelektase *f*.
reabsorption pressure *physiol*. Re(ab)sorptionsdruck *m*.
re·act [rɪ'ækt] **I** *vt chem*. zur Reaktion bringen. **II** *vi* **1.** (negativ) reagieren (*to* auf); entgegenwirken (*against*). **slow to ~** *chem*. reaktionsträge. **2.** *chem*. reagieren, eine Reaktion bewirken.
re·ac·tance [rɪ'æktəns] *n* *phys*. Blindwiderstand *m*, Reaktanz *f*.
re·ac·tant [rɪ'æktənt] *n* Reaktionspartner *m*, Reaktant *m*.
re·ac·tion [rɪ'ækʃn] *n* (*a. chem*., *phys*.) Reaktion *f* (*to* auf; *against* gegen); Rück-, Gegenwirkung *f* (*on* auf).
r. of degeneration *abbr*. **R.D., D.R.** Entartungsreaktion *abbr*. EAR, EaR.
r. of exhaustion Erschöpfungsreaktion.

r. of identity *immun.* Identitätsreaktion.
r. of nonidentity *immun.* Nichtidentitätsreaktion.
r. of partial identity *immun.* Teilidentitätsreaktion.
reaction center Keim-, Reaktionszentrum *nt.*
reaction-formation *n psycho.* Reaktionsbildung *f.*
reaction kinetics *chem.* Reaktionskinetik *f.*
reaction mechanism *chem.* Reaktionsmechanismus *m.*
reaction order *chem.* Reaktionsordnung *f.*
reaction pathway *chem.* Reaktionsweg *m.*
reaction rate Reaktionsgeschwindigkeit *f,* -rate *f,* Umsatzgeschwindigkeit *f,* -rate *f.*
specific r. → reaction rate constant.
reaction rate constant Reaktionsgeschwindigkeitskonstante *f.*
reaction time Reaktionszeit *f.*
reaction velocity Reaktionsgeschwindigkeit *f.*
re·ac·ti·vate [rɪ'æktəveɪt] *vt* reaktivieren.
re·ac·ti·va·tion [rɪˌæktɪ'veɪʃn] *n* Reaktivierung *f,* Reaktivieren *nt.*
re·ac·tive [rɪ'æktɪv] *adj* reaktiv, rück-, gegenwirkend; empfänglich (*to* für); Reaktions-.
reactive depression *psychia.* reaktive Depression *f,* depressive Reaktion *f.*
reactive hepatitis Minimalhepatitis *f,* reaktive Hepatitis *f.*
reactive hyperemia reaktive Hyperämie *f.*
reactive hypoglycemia *chir.* reaktive Hypoglykämie *f,* Spät-Dumping *nt,* postalimentäres Spätsyndrom *nt.*
reactive lymphadenopathy reaktive Lymphknotenschwellung *f.*
reactive nonspecific hepatitis reaktiv-unspezifische Hepatitis *f.*
reactive schizophrenia schizophrene Reaktion *f.*
reactive systemic amyloidosis reaktiv-sekundäre Amyloidose *f.*
re·ac·tiv·i·ty [ˌriæk'tɪvətɪ] *n* Reaktivität *f.*
re·ac·tor [rɪ'æktər] *n* 1. *immun.* positiv Reagierende(r *m*) *f.* 2. *phys.* (Kern-)Reaktor *m.* 3. *chem.* Reaktionsgefäß *nt;* Reaktionsmittel *nt.*
read·i·ness [ˈrɛdɪnɪs] *n* Bereitschaft *f.* **in ~** bereit, in Bereitschaft.
readiness level (of metabolism) *physiol.* Bereitschaftsumsatz *m.*
readiness potential *physiol.* Bereitschaftspotential *nt.*
read·ing [ˈriːdɪŋ] *n* 1. Lesen *nt.* 2. *techn.* Stand *m,* Wert *m,* Anzeige *f;* Ablesung *f.* 3. Deutung *f,* Auslegung *f.*
reading chart *ophthal.* Lese(proben)tafel *f.*
reading glass Vergrößerungsglas *nt,* Lupe *f.*
reading glasses Lesebrille *f.*
re·ad·just [ˌriːəˈdʒʌst] *vt techn.* neu einstellen, nachstellen, -richten, anpassen, korrigieren.
re·ad·just·ment [ˌriːəˈdʒʌstmənt] *n techn.* Neueinstellung *f,* Nachstellung *f,* Anpassung *f,* Korrektur *f.*
re·ad·mis·sion [ˌriːədˈmɪʃn] *n* Wiederaufnahme *od.* -einweisung *f (ins Krankenhaus).*
re·ad·mit [ˌriːədˈmɪt] *vt* wieder aufnehmen *od.* einweisen (*ins Krankenhaus*).
re·ad·mit·tance [ˌriːədˈmɪtəns] *n* → readmission.
read·out [ˈriːdaʊt] *n* 1. → reading 2. 2. (Computer-)Ausdruck *m.*
re·a·gent [rɪˈeɪdʒənt] *n* 1. Reagenz *nt,* Reagens *nt.* 2. *psycho.* Versuchs-, Testperson *f.*

re·a·gin [riːˈeɪdʒɪn, -gɪn] *n* 1. Reagin *nt,* IgE-Antikörper *m.* 2. *old immun.* Reagin *nt.*
re·a·gin·ic [rɪəˈdʒɪnɪk] *adj* Reagin betr., Reagin-.
reaginic antibody → reagin 1.
reagin titer *immun.* Reagintiter *m.*
real image [rɪəl, ˈriːəl] wirkliches/reelles Bild *nt.*
real thirst echter Durst *m.*
ream [riːm] *vt ortho., techn.* (auf-, aus-)bohren, (auf-, aus-)räumen.
ream·er [ˈriːmər] *n ortho., techn.* Reibahle *f,* Räumahle *f;* Fräse *f;* Raspel *f.*
re·ap·pear [ˌriːəˈpɪər] *vi* wiedererscheinen.
re·ap·pli·ca·tion [ˌriːæplɪˈkeɪʃn] *n* 1. wiederholte/erneute Anwendung *f.* 2. wiederholte Bewerbung *f.*
re·ap·ply [ˌriːəˈplaɪ] **I** *vt* wieder *od.* erneut anwenden. **II** *vi* 1. wieder Anwendung finden. 2. s. erneut bewerben (*for* um).
re·as·sess [ˌriːəˈsɛs] *vt* (*Situation, Verlauf*) neu beurteilen, nochmals (ab-)schätzen.
re·as·sess·ment [ˌriːəˈsɛsmənt] *n* (*Situation, Verlauf*) erneute (Ab-)Schätzung *f,* neue Beurteilung *f.*
re·as·sort·ant [ˌriːəˈsɔːrtənt] *n micro.* (*Virus*) Reassortante *f.*
re·as·sort·ment [ˌriːəˈsɔːrtmənt] *n micro.* (*Virus*) Reassortment *nt.*
Réaumur [ˈreɪəmjʊər, reoˈmyːr]: **R.'s scale** Réaumur-Skala *f.*
R.'s thermometer Réaumur-Thermometer *nt,* Thermometer *nt* mit Réaumur-Skala.
re·bound [*n* ˈriːbaʊnd; *v* rɪˈbaʊnd] **I** *n* Rückprall *m,* Zurückprallen *nt;* Rebound *m/nt.* **II** *vt* zurückprallen lassen. **III** *vi* zurückprallen, abprallen (*from* von).
rebound phenomenon *neuro.* Holmes-Phänomen *nt,* Holmes-Stewart-Phänomen *nt,* Rückstoß *m,* Rückschlag *m,* Reboundphänomen *nt.*
rebound tenderness *chir.* Blumberg-Zeichen *nt,* -Symptom *nt,* Loslasschmerz *m.*
re·breath·ing technique [rɪˈbriːðɪŋ] Rückatmungsmethode *f.*
re·cal·ci·fi·ca·tion [ˌriːkælsɪfɪˈkeɪʃn] *n* Rekalzifizierung *f,* Rekalzifikation *f.*
recalcification time *hema.* Rekalzifizierungszeit *f.*
re·call [rɪˈkɔːl, rɪˈkɔːl; *v* rɪˈkɔːl] **I** *n* (*Erinnerung*) Wachrufen *nt.* **II** *vt* s. erinnern an, s. ins Gedächtnis zurückrufen.
re·can·al·i·za·tion [ˌkænəlɪˈzeɪʃn] *n patho.* Rekanalisation *f,* Rekanalisierung *f.*
re·ceiv·er [rɪˈsiːvər] *n* 1. *lab.* (Aufnahme-, Auffang-)Gefäß *nt,* (Sammel-)Behälter *m; phys.* Glasglocke *f,* Rezipient *m.* 2. Empfänger(in *f*) *m.*
re·cep·ta·cle [rɪˈsɛptəkl] *n* 1. *lab.* Behälter *m,* Gefäß *nt.* 2. Steckdose *f.*
re·cep·tion [rɪˈsɛpʃn] *n* 1. An-, Aufnahme *f,* Empfang *m.* 2. *physiol.* (Reiz-)Aufnahme *f,* (Reiz-)Empfindung *f,* Wahrnehmung *f,* Rezeption *f.*
r. of taste Geschmacksempfindung, -wahrnehmung.
reception desk Empfang *m,* Rezeption *f,* Anmeldung *f.*
re·cep·tive [rɪˈsɛptɪv] *adj* 1. aufnahmefähig, empfänglich (*to, of* für). 2. *anat.* Rezeptor(en) *od.* Rezeption betr., rezeptiv, sensorisch, Rezeptoren-, Reiz-, Sinnes-. 3. *obst.* empfängisbereit, Empfängnis-.
receptive aphasia sensorische Aphasie *f,* Wernicke-Aphasie *f.*
receptive field *abbr.* **RF** rezeptives Feld *nt abbr.* RF.

excitatory r. *abbr.* **ERF** exzitatorisches rezeptives Feld *abbr.* ERF.
inhibitory r. *abbr.* **IRF** inhibitorisches rezeptives Feld *abbr.* IRF.
re·cep·tive·ness [rɪˈsɛptɪvnɪs] *n* → receptivity.
re·cep·tiv·i·ty [ˌriːsɛpˈtɪvətɪ] *n* Aufnahmefähigkeit *f,* Empfänglichkeit *f,* Rezeptivität *f; obst.* Empfängisbereitschaft *f.*
re·cep·tor [rɪˈsɛptər] *n* Rezeptor *m.*
receptor blockade Rezeptor(en)block *m,* -blockade *f.*
receptor density Rezeptordichte *f.*
receptor-mediated *adj* rezeptor-gesteuert, rezeptor-vermittelt.
receptor membrane Rezeptormembran *f.*
receptor molecule Rezeptormolekül *nt.*
receptor potential *physiol.* Rezeptorpotential *nt.*
early r. *abbr.* **ERP** frühes/primäres Rezeptorpotential, early receptor potential *abbr.* ERP.
late r. *abbr.* **LRP** spätes/sekundäres Rezeptorpotential, late receptor potential *abbr.* LRP.
primary r. → early r.
secondary r. → late r.
receptor protein Rezeptorprotein *nt.*
receptor site Rezeptorstelle *f.*
receptor specifity Rezeptorspezifität *f.*
re·cess [rɪˈsɛs, ˈriːsɛs] *n* 1. *anat.* kleine Ausbuchtung/Höhlung/Vertiefung *f,* Nische *f,* Recessus *m.* 2. Pause *f,* Unterbrechung *f.*
r. of infundibulum Rec. infundibularis/infundibuli.
re·ces·sion [rɪˈsɛʃn] *n* Rückgang *m;* Zurückweichen *nt,* -gehen *nt,* treten *nt.*
re·ces·sive [rɪˈsɛsɪv] *adj* zurücktretend, -gehend; *genet.* rezessiv.
recessive gene rezessives Gen *nt.*
recessive inheritance rezessive Vererbung *f.*
re·ces·sive·ness [rɪˈsɛsɪvnɪs] *n genet.* Rezessivität *f.*
re·ces·sus [rɪˈsɛsəs] *n, pl* **-sus** *anat.* → recess 1.
re·cid·i·va·tion [rɪˌsɪdəˈveɪʃn] *n* → recidivism.
re·cid·i·vism [rɪˈsɪdəvɪzəm] *n* 1. *patho.* Rückfall *m,* Rezidiv *nt.* 2. *forens.* Rückfall *m,* Rückfälligkeit *f.*
rec·i·pe [ˈrɛsəpɪ] *n* 1. *old* Verschreibung *f,* Rezept *nt.* 2. Rezept *nt,* Zubereitungsvorschrift *f.*
re·cip·i·ence [rɪˈsɪpɪəns] *n* → recipiency.
re·cip·i·en·cy [rɪˈsɪpɪənsɪ] *n* 1. Aufnahme *nt;* Aufnahmefähigkeit *f,* Empfänglichkeit *f.*
re·cip·i·ent [rɪˈsɪpɪənt] **I** *n* Empfänger(in *f*) *m.* **to be ~ of sth.** etw. empfangen. **II** *adj* empfänglich, aufnahmefähig (*of, to* für); aufnehmend.
recipient antigen Empfängerantigen *nt.*
recipient blood Empfängerblut *nt.*
recipient cell Empfängerzelle *f.*
recipient serum Empfängerserum *nt.*
re·cip·ro·cal [rɪˈsɪprəkl] **I** *n mathe.* Kehrwert *m.* **II** *adj* wechsel-, gegenseitig, Gegen-; *mathe.* reziprok.
reciprocal genes Komplementärgene *pl.*
re·cip·ro·cal·ly proportional [rɪˈsɪprəkəlɪ] umgekehrt proportional.
reciprocal ratio umgekehrtes Verhältnis *nt.*
reciprocal relationship Wechselbeziehung *f.*
reciprocal translocation *genet.* reziproke Translokation *f.*
re·cip·ro·cate [rɪˈsɪprəkeɪt] **I** *vt* (gegenseitig) austauschen. **II** *vi* in Wechselbeziehung stehen, s. gegenseitig beeinflussen, gegenseitig aufeinander einwirken.

rec·i·proc·i·ty [ˌresɪ'prɑsətɪ] n Austausch m; Wechselwirkung f, Wechselseitigkeit f, Reziprozität f.
reciprocity law Bunsen-Roscoe-Gesetz nt.
re·cir·cu·la·tion [rɪˌsɜrkjə'leɪʃn] n Rezirkulation f.
Recklinghausen ['rɛklɪŋhaʊzn]: **R.'s disease** (von) Recklinghausen-Krankheit f, Neurofibromatosis generalisata.
R.'s disease of bone Engel-(von) Recklinghausen-Syndrom nt, (von) Recklinghausen-Krankheit f, Osteodystrophia fibrosa cystica generalisata, Ostitis fibrosa cystica (generalisata).
R.'s tumor Adenomatoidtumor m.
Recklinghausen-Applebaum ['æplbaʊm]: **R.-A. disease** (von) Recklinghausen--Applebaum-Krankheit f, idiopathische Hämochromatose f.
re·cline [rɪ'klaɪn] **I** vt **1.** (an-, zurück-)lehnen (on, upon an). **2.** hinlegen (on auf). **II** vi **3.** s. (an-, zurück-)lehnen (on, upon an). **4.** ruhen, liegen (on, upon an, auf).
re·clin·ing brace [rɪ'klaɪnɪŋ] Reklinationskorsett nt.
re·clot·ting phenomenon [rɪ'klɑtɪŋ] Thixotropie f.
Reclus [rə'kly]: **R.' disease** gyn. Reclus'--Krankheit f.
rec·og·ni·tion [ˌrekəg'nɪʃn] n (Wieder-)Erkennen nt, (-)Erkennung f.
recognition site Erkennungsstelle f.
enzyme r. Enzymerkennungsstelle.
recognition threshold physiol. Erkennungsschwelle f.
rec·og·nize ['rekəgnaɪz] vt (wieder-)erkennen.
re·col·lect [ˌriːkə'lekt] **I** vt s. erinnern (an); s. besinnen auf, s. ins Gedächtnis zurückrufen. **II** vi s. erinnern.
re·col·lec·tion [ˌriːkə'lekʃn] n **1.** Erinnerungsvermögen nt, Gedächtnis nt, Erinnerung f. **2.** Erinnerung f (of an).
re·com·bi·nant [rɪˈkɑmbɪnənt] **I** n genet. Rekombinante f. **II** adj genet. rekombinant abbr. r.
recombinant plasmid Rekombinationsplasmid nt.
re·com·bi·na·tion [ˌriːkɑmbɪ'neɪʃn] n chem., genet. Rekombination f.
recombination repair genet. Rekombinationsreparatur f.
re·com·bine [ˌriːkəm'baɪn] vt chem., genet. rekombinieren.
re·con·sti·tu·ent [ˌriːkən'stɪtʃəwənt] **I** n Kräftigungs-, Stärkungsmittel nt, Roborans nt. **II** adj kräftigend, stärkend.
re·con·sti·tute [riː'kɑnstɪt(j)uːt] vt **1.** wiederherstellen, rekonstruieren, rekonstituieren. **2.** chem. aus einem Konzentrat herstellen; in Wasser auflösen.
re·con·sti·tut·ed erythrocyte [riː'kɑnstɪt(j)uːtɪd] hema. rekonstituierter Erythrozyt m.
reconstituted hyalin Rekonstitutionshyalin nt.
re·con·sti·tu·tion [riːˌkɑnstɪ't(j)uːʃn] n **1.** Wiederherstellung f, Neubildung f, Rekonstitution f. **2.** chem. Zubereitung f aus einem Konzentrat; Auflösung f in Wasser.
re·con·struct [ˌriːkən'strʌkt] vt wieder aufbauen od. herstellen; umbauen, rekonstruieren.
re·con·struc·tion [ˌriːkən'strʌkʃn] n Umbau m; Wiederaufbau m, -herstellung f; Rekonstruktion f.
reconstruction phase physiol. Rekonstruktionsphase f.
reconstruction zone histol. Umbauzone f, Transformationsfeld nt.

re·con·struc·tive [ˌriːkən'strʌktɪv] adj wiederaufbauend, rekonstruktiv.
reconstructive arthroplasty ortho. rekonstruktive Gelenkplastik/Arthroplastik f.
reconstructive surgery rekonstruktive Chirurgie f; plastische Chirurgie f.
re·cord [n, adj 'rekərd; v rɪ'kɔːrd] **I** n **1.** Niederschrift f, (schriftlicher) Bericht m. **2.** Dokument nt, Akte f, Unterlage f. **on ~** aktenkundig, in den Akten. **3.** Verzeichnis nt, Register nt, Liste f. **4.** Registrierung f, Aufzeichnung f. **II** vt **5.** auf-, niederschreiben, aufnehmen; protokollieren, dokumentieren. **6.** (Daten) registrieren, erfassen, aufnehmen. **III** vi registrieren, aufzeichnen.
re·cord·er [rɪ'kɔːrdər] n Registrier-, Aufnahmegerät nt, Bild-, Kurvenschreiber m.
re·cord·ing [rɪ'kɔːrdɪŋ] **I** n **1.** (a. techn.) Aufzeichnung f, Registrierung f; Protokollierung f; (Band-)Aufnahme f. **2.** physiol. (EKG) Ableitung f. **II** adj aufzeichnend, registrierend.
recording electrode Meßelektrode f.
recording instrument aufzeichnendes od. registrierendes Meßgerät nt.
re·cov·er [rɪ'kʌvər] vt **1.** wiederbekommen, -finden, zurückgewinnen; (Bewußtsein) wiedererlangen; (Zeit) wiederaufholen. **to ~ one's breath/strength** wieder zu Atem/Kräften kommen. **2.** techn., chem. rück-, wiedergewinnen. **II** vi **3.** genesen, gesunden; s. erholen (from, of von). **to be ~ing** auf dem Weg der Besserung sein. **4.** (Bewußtsein) wiedererlangen, wieder zu s. kommen. **5.** entschädigt werden.
re·cov·er·y [rɪ'kʌvərɪ] n **1.** Zurückgewinnung f, Wiederherstellung f, Wiedergutmachung f; (Bewußtsein) Wiedererlangung f. **2.** Genesung f, Gesundung f, Rekonvaleszenz f; Erholung f. **to make a quick ~** s. schnell erholen (from von). **past/beyond ~** unheilbar. **3.** techn., chem. Rück-, Wiedergewinnung f.
recovery area Aufwachraum m.
recovery heat physiol. Erholungswärme f.
recovery nystagmus physiol. Erholungsnystagmus m.
recovery phase physiol. Erholungsphase f; Erregungsrückbildungsphase f.
recovery pulse sum physiol. Erholungspulssumme f.
recovery room Aufwachraum m.
recovery time physiol. Erholungszeit f.
rec·re·a·tion center [ˌrekrɪ'eɪʃn] Freizeit-, Erholungszentrum nt.
re·cru·des·cence [ˌriːkruː'desəns] n **1.** Wiederverschlimmerung f, Rekrudeszenz f. **2.** Rückfall m, Rezidiv f.
re·cru·des·cent [ˌriːkruː'desənt] adj **1.** rekrudeszent. **2.** rezidivierend.
recrudescent typhus (fever) Brill-Krankheit f, Brill-Zinsser-Krankheit f.
re·cruit [rɪ'kruːt] **I** vt **1.** wieder stärken; jdn. (gesundheitlich) wiederherstellen. **to ~ o.s.** s. stärken. **2.** (an-)werben, heranziehen, ein-, anstellen. **to be ~ed** (Testpersonen) s. rekrutieren (from aus). **II** vi **3.** s. erholen, genesen, wieder gesund werden. **4.** (Testpersonen) werben.
re·cruit·ing response [rɪ'kruːtɪŋ] → recruitment 3.
re·cruit·ment [rɪ'kruːtmənt] n **1.** Stärkung f, Erholung f. **2.** Verstärkung f, Auffrischung f; Werbung f, Einstellung f, Rekrutierung f. **3.** physiol., HNO Lautheitsausgleich m, Rekrutierung f, Rekrutierungsphänomen nt, Recruitment nt.
rect- pref. → recto-.
rec·tal ['rektl] adj Enddarm/Rektum betr.;

zum Rektum gehörend, im Rektum befindlich, rektal, Rektal-, Rektum-, Rekto-; Mastdarm-.
rectal abscess rektaler Abszeß m.
rectal adenoma Rektumadenom nt.
rectal ampulla (Rektum-)Ampulle f, Ampulla recti.
rectal anesthesia rektale Anästhesie f.
rectal artery Mastdarm-, Rektumarterie f.
inferior r. untere Mastdarm-/Rektumarterie, Rektalis f inferior, A. rectalis inferior.
middle r. mittlere Mastdarm-/Rektumarterie, Rektalis f media, A. rectalis media.
superior r. obere Mastdarm-/Rektumarterie, Rektalis f superior, A. rectalis superior.
rectal atresia Mastdarm-, Rektumatresie f, Atresia recti.
rectal biopsy Rektumbiopsie f.
rectal bleeding rektale Blutung f, Blutung f aus dem After, Rektum-, Mastdarmblutung f.
rectal columns Morgagni'-Papillen pl, Analsäulen pl, -papillen pl, Columnae anales/rectales.
rectal continence Darm-, Stuhlkontinenz f.
rectal crisis neuro. Mastdarm-, Rektumkrise f.
rectal drainage Rektum-, Rektaldrainage f.
rectal examination rektale Untersuchung f.
rectal fascia Fascia diaphragmatis pelvis superior.
rectal fistula Mastdarm-, Rektalfistel f, Fistula rectalis.
rectal folds, transverse zirkuläre Enddarmfalten pl, Plicae transversae recti.
rec·tal·gia [rek'tældʒ(ɪ)ə] n Schmerzen pl im unteren Mastdarm, Proktalgie f, Proctalgia f.
rectal hemorrhage → rectal bleeding
rectal incontinence Stuhl-, Darminkontinenz f, Incontinentia alvi.
rectal injury Rektum-, Mastdarmverletzung f.
rectal intussusception inkompletter Rektumprolaps m.
rectal nerves, inferior untere Rektal-, Analnerven pl, Nn. anales/rectales inferiores.
rectal plexus: inferior r. Plexus rectalis inferior.
middle r. Plexus h(a)emorrhoidalis medius, Plexus rectalis medius.
superior r. Plexus h(a)emorrhoidalis superior, Plexus rectalis superior.
rectal pouch Rektumblindsack m.
rectal prolapse Mastdarmprolaps m, -vorfall m, Rektumprolaps m, -vorfall m, Prolapsus recti.
rectal reflex Defäkationsreflex m.
rectal resection chir. Rektumresektion f, -amputation f.
abdominoperineal r. Miles-Operation f, abdominoperineale Rektumamputation f.
anterior r. anteriore Rektumresektion f.
anteroposterior r. → abdominoperineal r.
rectal sinuses Morgagni'-Krypten pl, Analkrypten pl, Sinus anales.
rectal smear → rectal swab.
rectal swab Rektal-, Rektumabstrich m.
rectal syringe Klistierspritze f.
rectal temperature Rektaltemperatur f.
rectal tenesmus schmerzhafter Stuhldrang m, Tenesmus alvi/ani.
rectal tube Rektumsonde f.
rectal vein Mastdarm-, Rektumvene f.
inferior r.s untere Mastdarm-/Rektumvenen pl, Vv. rectales inferiores.

middle r. s mittlere Mastdarm-/Rektumvenen pl,Vv. rectales mediae.
superior r. obere Rektumvene, V. rectalis superior.
rec·tan·gle ['rektæŋgl] n mathe. Rechteck nt.
rec·tan·gu·lar [rek'tæŋgjələr] adj mathe. rechteckig; rechtwinklig.
rec·tec·to·my [rek'tektəmɪ] n chir. Rektumamputation f, -resektion f, Proktektomie f.
rec·ti·fi·ca·tion [ˌrektəfɪ'keɪʃn] n 1. Berichtigung f, Korrektur f, Richtigstellung f; Beseitigung f, Behebung f. 2. chem. Rektifikation f; phys. Gleichrichtung f.
rec·ti·fi·er ['rektəfaɪər] n chem. Rektifizierapparat m; phys. Gleichrichter m.
rec·ti·fy ['rektəfaɪ] vt 1. berichtigen, korrigieren, richtigstellen. 2. chem. rektifizieren; phys. gleichrichten.
rec·ti·tis [rek'taɪtɪs] n Mastdarm-, Rektumentzündung f, Proktitis f, Rektitis f, Proctitis f.
recto- pref. Enddarm-, Anus-, Ano-, Prokt(o)-, Mastdarm-, Rekt(o)-, Rektal-, Rektum-.
rec·to·ab·dom·i·nal [ˌrektəʊæb'dɒmɪnl] adj Rektum u. Abdomen betr., rektoabdominal.
rec·to·a·nal junction [ˌ-'eɪnl] Anorektalübergang m, -linie f, Linea anorectalis.
rec·to·cele ['-siːl] n Rektozele f, Hernia rectovaginalis.
rec·to·coc·cyg·e·al [ˌ-kɑk'siːdʒɪəl] adj Enddarm/Rektum u. Steißbein/Os coccygis betr. od. verbindend, rektokokzygeal.
rectococcygeal muscle → rectococcygeus (muscle).
rec·to·coc·cy·ge·us (muscle) [ˌ-kɑk'siːdʒɪəs] Rektokokzygeus m, Rectococcygeus m, M. rectococcygeus.
rec·to·coc·cy·pex·y [ˌ-'kɑksɪpeksɪ] n chir. Proktokokzygopexie f.
rec·to·co·li·tis [ˌ-kə'laɪtɪs] n Entzündung f von Rektum u. Kolon, Rektokolitis f, Proktokolitis f.
rec·to·cys·tot·o·my [ˌ-sɪs'tɒtəmɪ] n chir., urol. transrektale Zystotomie f.
rec·to·four·chette fistula [ˌ-foər'ʃet] → rectovestibular fistula.
rec·to·is·chi·ad·ic excavation [ˌ-ɪskɪ'ædɪk] Fossa ischioanalis.
rec·to·la·bi·al fistula [ˌ-'leɪbɪəl] rektolabiale Fistel f.
rec·to·per·i·ne·al [ˌ-ˌperɪ'niːəl] adj Rektum u. Perineum betr., rektoperineal.
rec·to·per·i·ne·or·rha·phy [ˌ-ˌperɪnɪ'ɔrəfɪ] n gyn., chir. Rektum-Damm-Plastik f, -Naht f.
rec·to·pex·y ['-peksɪ] n chir. Mastdarmanheftung f, Proktopexie f.
rec·to·plas·ty ['-plæstɪ] n chir. Rektum-, Proktoplastik f.
rec·to·ro·man·o·scope [ˌ-rəʊ'mænəskəʊp] n Rektosigmoid(e)oskop nt.
rec·to·ro·ma·nos·co·py [ˌ-rəʊmə'nɒskəpɪ] n Rektosigmoid(e)oskopie f.
rec·tor·rha·phy [rek'tɔrəfɪ] n chir. Rektumnaht f.
rec·to·scope ['rektəskəʊp] n Rektoskop nt.
rec·tos·co·py [rek'tɒskəpɪ] n Mastdarmspiegelung f, Rektoskopie f.
rec·to·sig·moid [ˌrektəʊ'sɪɡmɔɪd] I n Rektum u. Sigma, Rektosigma nt. II adj Enddarm/Rektum u. Sigma betr. od. verbindend, rektosigmoidal.
rec·to·sig·moid·ec·to·my [ˌ-ˌsɪɡmɔɪ'dektəmɪ] n chir. Resektion f von Sigma u. Rektum, Rektumsigmoidektomie f.
rectosigmoid junction rektosigmoidale Übergangszone f.

rec·to·ste·no·sis [ˌ-stɪ'nəʊsɪs] n Mastdarm-, Enddarm-, Rektumstenose f.
rec·tos·to·my [rek'tɒstəmɪ] n chir. Rekto-, Proktostomie f.
rec·tot·o·my [rek'tɒtəmɪ] n chir. Rekto-, Proktotomie f.
rec·to·u·re·thral [ˌrektəʊjʊə'riːθrəl] adj Enddarm/Rektum u. Harnröhre/Urethra betr., rektourethral.
rectourethral fistula Mastdarm-Harnröhren-Fistel f, Rektourethralfistel f, Fistula rectourethralis.
rec·to·u·re·thra·lis (muscle) [ˌ-jʊərɪ'θreɪlɪs] Rektourethralis m, M. rectourethralis.
rectourethral muscle → rectourethralis (muscle).
rec·to·u·ter·ine [ˌ-'juːtərɪn, -raɪn] adj Enddarm/Rektum u. Gebärmutter/Uterus betr. od. verbindend, rektouterin.
rectouterine excavation Douglas'-Raum m, Excavatio recto-uterina.
rectouterine fold Plica recto-uterina.
rectouterine ligament → rectouterinus (muscle).
rectouterine muscle → rectouterinus (muscle).
rectouterine pouch → rectouterine excavation.
rec·to·u·te·ri·nus (muscle) [ˌ-ˌjuːtə'raɪnəs] Rektouterinus m, M. rectouterinus.
rec·to·vag·i·nal [ˌrektəʊ'vædʒənl, -və'dʒaɪnl] adj Enddarm/Rektum u. Scheide/Vagina betr. od. verbindend, rektovaginal.
rectovaginal fistula Rektovaginalfistel f, Mastdarm-Scheiden-Fistel f, Fistula rectovaginalis.
rectovaginal hernia Rektozele f, Hernia rectovaginalis.
rectovaginal pouch → rectouterine excavation.
rectovaginal septum rektovaginale Scheidewand f, rektovaginales Septum nt, Septum rectovaginale.
rec·to·ves·i·cal [ˌ-'vesɪkl] adj Enddarm/Rektum u. Harnblase betr. od. verbindend, rektovesikal.
rectovesical center rektovesikales Reflexzentrum nt, Centrum rectovesicale.
rectovesical excavation Proust'-Raum m, Excavatio rectovesicalis.
rectovesical fascia Fascia diaphragmatis pelvis superior.
rectovesical fistula Rektovesikalfistel f, Mastdarm-Blasen-Fistel f, Fistula rectovesicalis.
rectovesical fold → rectouterine fold.
rec·to·ves·i·ca·lis (muscle) [ˌ-ˌvesɪ'keɪlɪs] Rektovesikalis m, Rectovesicalis m, M. rectovesicalis.
rectovesical muscle → rectovesicalis (muscle).
rectovesical pouch → rectovesical excavation.
rectovesical septum Harnblasen-Rektum-Scheidewand f, rektovesikales Septum nt, Septum rectovesicale.
rec·to·ves·tib·u·lar fistula [ˌ-ves'tɪbjələr] Mastdarm-Scheidenvorhof-Fistel f, Rektovestibulärfistel f, Fistula rectovestibularis.
rec·to·vul·var [ˌ-'vʌlvər] adj Rektum u. Vulva betr., rektovulvär, rektovulvar.
rectovulvar fistula Rektum-Vulva-Fistel f, rektovulväre Fistel f.
rec·tum ['rektəm] n, pl -tums, -ta [-tə] Enddarm m, Rektum nt, Rectum nt, Intestinum rectum.
rec·tus ['rektəs] n, pl -ti [-taɪ] 1. gerader Muskel m, Rektus m, M. rectus. 2. → rectus abdominis (muscle).

rectus abdominis (muscle) Rektus m abdominis, M. rectus abdominis.
rectus capitis anterior (muscle) Rektus m capitis anterior, M. rectus capitis anterior.
rectus capitis lateralis (muscle) Rektus m capitis lateralis, M. rectus capitis lateralis.
rectus capitis posterior major (muscle) Rektus m capitis posterior major, M. rectus capitis posterior major.
rectus capitis posterior minor (muscle) Rektus m capitis posterior minor, M. rectus capitis posterior minor.
rectus femoris (muscle) Rektus m femoris, M. rectus femoris.
rectus inferior (muscle) Rektus m inferior, M. rectus inferior.
rectus lateralis (muscle) Rektus m lateralis, M. rectus lateralis.
rectus medialis (muscle) Rektus m medialis, M. rectus medialis.
rectus muscle (of eye): inferior r. → rectus inferior (muscle).
lateral r. → rectus lateralis (muscle).
medial r. → rectus medialis (muscle).
superior r. → rectus superior (muscle).
rectus sheath Rektusscheide f, Vagina m. recti abdominis.
rectus superior (muscle) Rektus m superior, M. rectus superior.
re·cum·ben·cy [rɪ'kʌmbənsɪ] n liegende Stellung f, Liegen nt; Ruhestellung f, Ruhelage f.
re·cum·bent [rɪ'kʌmbənt] adj liegend, ruhend (on auf); s. lehnend (on auf).
recumbent position liegende Stellung f, (im) Liegen nt.
re·cu·per·ate [rɪ'k(j)uːpəreɪt] I vt (Gesundheit) wiedererlangen. II vi s. erholen.
re·cu·per·a·tion [rɪˌk(j)uːpə'reɪʃn] n Erholung f.
re·cu·per·a·tive [rɪ'k(j)uːpərətɪv, -ˌreɪtɪv] adj stärkend, kräftigend; Erholungs-.
re·cur [rɪ'kɜr] vi wiederkehren, wieder auf- od. eintreten. s. wiederholen, rezidivieren; mathe. s. periodisch wiederholen.
re·cur·rence [rɪ'kɜrəns, -'kʌr-] n Wiederkehr f, Wiederauftreten nt, -auftauchen nt; Rückfall m, Rezidiv nt; mathe. Rekursion f.
re·cur·rent [rɪ'kɜrənt, -'kʌr-] adj regelmäßig od. ständig wiederkehrend, s. wiederholend, rekurrent, rezidivierend; habituell; anat. rückläufig; mathe. periodisch.
recurrent abortion gyn. habitueller Abort m, habituelle Fehlgeburt f.
recurrent albuminuria zyklische/intermittierende Albuminurie f.
recurrent aphthous stomatitis rezidivierende aphthöse Stomatitis f.
recurrent appendicitis rezidivierende Appendizitis f.
recurrent artery A. centralis longa, A. recurrens.
radial r. Recurrens f radialis, A. recurrens radialis.
tibial r., anterior Recurrens f tibialis anterior, A. recurrens tibialis anterior.
tibial r., posterior Recurrens f tibialis posterior, A. recurrens tibialis posterior.
ulnar r. Recurrens f ulnaris, A. recurrens ulnaris.
recurrent attacks s. wiederholende Anfälle pl, immer wiederkehrende Anfälle pl.
recurrent benign aphthosis abbr. RBA Mikulicz-Aphthen pl, habituelle Aphthen pl, chronisch rezidivierende Aphthen pl, rezidivierende benigne Aphthosis f, Periadenitis mucosa necrotica recurrens.

recurrent carcinoma Krebs-, Karzinomrezidiv *nt*, rezidivierendes Karzinom *nt*.
recurrent digital fibroma of childhood infantile digitale Fibromatose *f*, juvenile Fibromatose *f*.
recurrent dislocation of the patella *ortho.* habituelle/chronisch-rezidivierende Patellaluxation *f*.
recurrent fever Rückfallfieber *nt*, Febris recurrens.
recurrent infarction Infarktrezidiv *nt*, rezidivierender (Myokard-)Infarkt *m*.
recurrent laryngeal nerve → recurrent nerve.
recurrent laryngeal nerve palsy → recurrent nerve palsy.
recurrent laryngeal paralysis → recurrent nerve palsy.
recurrent nerve Rekurrens *m*, N. laryngeus recurrens.
 ophthalmic r. Ramus tentorii n. ophthalmici.
recurrent nerve palsy Rekurrenslähmung *f*, -parese *f*, -paralyse *f*.
recurrent pain (immer) wiederkehrender Schmerz *m*.
recurrent polyserositis familiäres Mittelmeerfieber *nt*, familiäre rekurrente Polyserositis *f*.
recurrent pyogenic cholangitis rezidivierende pyogene Cholangitis *f*.
recurrent scarring aphthae → recurrent benign aphthosis.
recurrent ulcer Rezidivulkus *nt*.
recurrent ulcer disease → recurrent ulcer.
recurrent vomiting periodisches/zyklisches/rekurrierendes Erbrechen *nt*.
re·cur·ring digital fibrous tumors of childhood [rɪˈkɜrɪŋ] infantile digitale Fibromatose *f*, juvenile Fibromatose *f*.
recurring hemorrhage intermittierende/rezidivierende Blutung *f*.
re·cur·vate [rɪˈkɜrvɪt, -veɪt] *adj* nach hinten gebogen *od.* gebeugt, zurückgebogen.
re·cur·va·tion [ˌrikarˈveɪʃn] *n* Beugung/Biegung *f* nach hinten.
red [red] **I** *n* Rot *nt*, rote Farbe *f*, roter Farbstoff *m*. **II** *adj* **1.** rot. **2.** rot, gerötet. **3.** rot(haarig); rot(häutig); rot(glühend).
red atrophy *patho.* rote Leberatrophie *f*.
red blindness Rotblindheit *f*, -schwäche *f*, Protanop(s)ie *f*.
red blood cells rote Blutzellen *pl*, -körperchen *pl*, Erythrozyten *pl*.
red blood clot roter Abscheidungsthrombus *m*.
red blood corpuscles → red blood cells.
red blood count 1. *abbr.* **RBC** Erythrozytenzahl *f abbr.* Z_E. **2.** Bestimmung *f* der Erythrozytenzahl, Erythrozytenzählung *f*.
red body of ovary Rotkörper *m*, Corpus rubrum.
red bug *micro.* Trombicula-Larve *f*, Chigger *m*.
red cell cast *urol.* Erythrozytenzylinder *m*.
red cell count 1. *abbr.* **RCC** Erythrozytenzahl *f abbr.* Z_E. **2.** Bestimmung *f* der Erythrozytenzahl, Erythrozytenzählung *f*.
red cell ghost *herm.* (Erythrozyten-)-Ghost *m*, Schattenzelle *f*, Blutkörperchenschatten *m*.
red cell mass *abbr.* **RCM** Erythrozytenmasse *f*.
red cells → red blood cells.
red cell series *hema.* rote Reihe *f*.
red cell volume totales Erythrozytenvolumen *nt*.
red corpuscles → red blood cells.
red·den [ˈrednˌ] **I** *vt* röten, rot färben. **II** *vi* rot werden, erröten; s. röten.

red·den·ing [ˈrednɪŋ] *n* Rötung *f*.
red dermatographism *derm.* roter Dermographismus *m*, Dermographismus ruber.
red·dish [ˈredɪʃ] *adj* rötlich.
red-drop phenomenon *biochem.* Red--drop-Phänomen *nt*.
red-eyed *adj* mit geröteten Augen.
red-faced *adj* rotgesichtig, mit rotem Kopf/Gesicht.
red fever (of the Congo) endemisches/murines Fleckfieber *nt*, Ratten-, Flohfleckfieber *nt*.
red filter Rotfilter *m*/*nt*.
red-green blindness Rotgrünblindheit *f*, -anomalie *f*.
red-green-system neuron *physiol.* Neuron *nt* des Rot-Grün-Systems.
red hepatization *patho.* rote Hepatisation *f*.
red hypertension benigne Hypertonie *f*.
re·dia [ˈriːdɪə] *n*, *pl* **-di·ae** [dɪˌiː] *micro.* Redia *f*, Redie *f*, Stablarve *f*.
red induration *patho.* rote Induration *f*.
red infarct hämorrhagischer/roter Infarkt *m*.
red·in·te·grate [redˈɪntɪɡreɪt, rɪˈdɪn-] *vt* **1.** wieder herstellen. **2.** erneuern.
red·in·te·gra·tion [ˌredˌɪntɪˈɡreɪʃn, rɪˌdɪn-] *n* **1.** Wiederherstellung *f*, Redintegration *f*. **2.** Erneuerung *f*, Redintegration *f*.
re·dis·tri·bute [ˌriːdɪsˈtrɪbjuːt] *vt* neu-, umverteilen.
re·dis·tri·bu·tion [ˌriːˌdɪstrəˈbjuːʃn] *n* Neu-, Umverteilung *f*.
red lead Bleitetroxid *nt*, Bleimennige *f*, rotes Bleioxid *nt*.
Redlich-Obersteiner [ˈreːdlɪç ˈoːbərstaɪnər]: **R.-O. zone** Redlich-Obersteiner--Zone *f*.
red marrow rotes blutbildendes Knochenmark *nt*, Medulla ossium rubra.
red muscle rote Muskelfaser *f*, rotes Muskelgewebe *nt*.
red·ness [ˈrednɪs] *n* Röte *f*; Rötung *f*.
red neuralgia Gerhardt-Syndrom *nt*, Mitchell-Gerhardt-Syndrom *nt*, Weir--Mitchell-Krankheit *f*, Erythromelalgie *f*, Erythralgie *f*, Erythermalgie *f*, Akromelalgie *f*.
red nucleus roter Kern *m*, Nc. ruber.
Redon [rəˈdɔn]: **R. drain** Redondrain *m*.
re·dox [ˈriːdɔks] *n chem.* Oxidation-Reduktion *f*, Redox(-Reaktion *f*).
redox couple *chem.* Redoxpaar *f*.
redox enzyme Redoxenzym *nt*, Oxidoreduktase *f*.
 flavin-linked r. flavinabhängiges Redoxenzym.
redox pair *chem.* Redoxpaar *nt*.
 conjugate r. konjugiertes Redoxpaar.
redox potential *abbr.* E_h Redoxpotential *nt abbr.* E_h.
 midpoint/standard r. Normalpotential.
redox reaction Oxidations-Reduktionsreaktion *f*, Redoxreaktion *f*.
redox system *chem.* Redoxsystem *nt*.
red phosphorus roter/amorpher Phosphor *m*.
red pulp (*Milz*) rote Pulpa *f*, Milzpulpa *f*, Pulpa splenica/lienis.
red pulp cords Milzstränge *pl*.
red reflex *ophthal.* Fundusreflex *m*.
re·dress [rɪˈdres] **I** *vt* **1.** wieder anziehen, wieder ankleiden. **2.** (*Wunde*) neu verbinden. **II** *vi* s. wieder ankleiden.
re·dresse·ment [rɪdresˈmɑ̃] *n ortho.* Redression *f*, Redressement *f*.
red shock warmer/roter Schock *m*.
red substance of spleen → red pulp.
red-tailed botfly [ˈredteɪld] *micro.* Gasterophilus haemorrhoidalis.

red thrombus roter Thrombus *m*, Gerinnungs-, Schwanzthrombus *m*.
re·duce [rɪˈd(j)uːs] **I** *vt* **1.** herabsetzen, verringern, vermindern, verkleinern, reduzieren (*by* um; *to* auf); drosseln, senken; (*Schmerz*) lindern; (*Lösung*) schwächen, verdünnen. **2.** *chir. ortho.* reponieren, reduzieren, einrichten, einrenken. **3.** (*Zelle*) reduzieren. **4.** *mathe., chem., phys.* reduzieren. **5.** etw. verwandeln (*to* in, zu). **to ~ to powder** zermahlen, pulverisieren. **6.** zurückführen, reduzieren (*to* auf). **II** *vi* **7.** abnehmen, eine Schlankheitskur machen. **8.** *bio.* s. meiotisch teilen.
re·duced glutathione [rɪˈd(j)uːst] *abbr.* **GSH** reduziertes Glutathion *nt abbr.* GSH.
reduced hematin Häm *nt*, Protohäm *nt*.
reduced hemoglobin reduziertes/desoxygeniertes Hämoglobin *nt*, Desoxyhämoglobin *nt*.
re·duc·i·ble [rɪˈd(j)uːsɪbl] *adj* **1.** zerlegbar, verkleinerbar, verkürzbar; *chem., mathe., phys.* reduzibel, reduzierbar. **2.** *chir., ortho.* einrenkbar, reponierbar, reponibel.
reducible hernia reponible/reponierbare Hernie *f*.
re·duc·ing agent [rɪˈd(j)uːsɪŋ] *chem.* → reductant.
reducing diet Abmagerungskur *f*.
reducing equivalent *chem.* Reduktionsäquivalent *nt*.
reducing glass Verkleinerungsglas *nt*.
reducing sugar *chem.* reduzierender Zucker *m*.
re·duc·tant [rɪˈdʌktənt] *n* Reduktionsmittel *nt*, Reduktor *m*.
re·duc·tase [rɪˈdʌkteɪz] *n* Reduktase *f*.
5α-reductase *n* 5α-Reduktase *f*.
re·duc·tion [rɪˈdʌkʃn] *n* **1.** Herabsetzung *f*, Verringerung *f*, Verminderung *f*, Verkleinerung *f*, Reduzierung *f* (*by* um; *to* auf); Drosselung *f*, Senkung *f*; (Ab-)Schwächung *f*; (*Schmerz-*)Linderung *f*. **2.** *chir., ortho.* Reposition *f*, Einrichtung *f*, Einrenkung *f*. **3.** *bio.* Reduktion(steilung *f*) *f*, Meiose *f*. **4.** *chem.* Reduktion *f*; *mathe.* Reduktion *f*, Auflösung *f*, Zerlegung *f* (*to* in). **5.** Zurückführung *f*, Reduzierung *f* (*to* auf).
reduction (cell) division 1. Reduktion(steilung *f*) *f*, Meiose *f*. **2.** erste Reifeteilung *f*.
re·duc·tive [rɪˈdʌktɪv] **I** *n chem.* Reduktionsmittel *nt*. **II** *adj* Reduktion bewirkend, reduzierend, vermindernd (*of*); reduktiv.
re·dun·dance [rɪˈdʌndəns] *n* → redundancy.
re·dun·dan·cy [rɪˈdʌndənsɪ] *n* **1.** *phys., genet.* Redundanz *f*. **2.** *allg.* Überfluß *m*, Übermaß *nt*, -fülle *f*; Überflüssigkeit *f*.
re·du·pli·cate [rɪˈd(j)uːplɪkeɪt] *vt* verdoppeln, wiederholen, reduplizieren.
re·du·pli·ca·tion [rɪˌd(j)uːplɪˈkeɪʃn] *n bio.* Verdopp(e)lung *f*, Wiederholung *f*, Reduplikation *f*.
re·du·pli·ca·tive [rɪˈd(j)uːplɪkeɪtɪv] *adj* verdoppelnd, wiederholend, reduplizierend, Reduplikations-.
re·du·vi·id [rɪˈd(j)uːvɪɪd] *n micro.* Raubwanze *f*.
Red·u·vi·i·dae [red(j)uːˈvaɪɪdiː] *pl micro.* Raubwanzen *pl*, Reduviiden *pl*, Reduviidae *pl*.
red vision Rotsehen *nt*, Erythrop(s)ie *f*.
red-wa·ter (fever) [ˈredwɔːtər] Texas-Fieber *nt*.
Reed [riːd]: **R.'s cell** Sternberg-Riesenzelle *f*, Sternberg-Reed-Riesenzelle *f*..
Reed-Hodgkin [ˈhɒdʒkɪn]: **R.-H. disease**

Hodgkin-Krankheit f, -Lymphom nt, Morbus Hodgkin m, (Hodgkin-)Paltauf--Steinberg-Krankheit f, (maligne) Lymphogranulomatose f, Lymphogranulomatosis maligna.
Reed-Sternberg ['stɜrnbɜrg]: **R.-S. cell** Sternberg-Riesenzelle f, Sternberg-Reed--Riesenzelle f.
re·ed·u·cate [riː'edʒʊkeɪt] vt umerziehen, umschulen.
re·ed·u·ca·tion [riːˌedʒʊ'keɪʃn] n Umerziehung f, Umschulung f, Reedukation f.
reef knot [riːf] richtiger Knoten m, Schifferknoten m.
reel foot [riːl] ortho. (angeborener) Klumpfuß m, Pes equinovarus (excavatus et adductus).
re-entrant mechanism → reentry.
re·en·try [riː'entrɪ] n card. Reentry(-Mechanismus m) nt.
reentry phenomenon → reentry.
reentry theory Reentry-Theorie f.
re·ep·i·the·li·al·i·za·tion [riːˌepɪˌθɪlɪæli'zeɪʃn] n Reepithelialisation f, Reepithelisierung f.
Rees [riːs]: **R. dermatome** Rees-Dermatom nt.
re·es·tab·lish [rɪə'stæblɪʃ] vt wiederherstellen.
re·ex·am·i·na·tion [riːɪgˌzæmɪ'neɪʃn] n Nachprüfung f, -untersuchung f, erneute Untersuchung f.
re·ex·am·ine [riːɪg'zæmɪn] vt nachuntersuchen, erneut untersuchen.
re·fer [rɪ'fɜr] vt 1. verweisen, weiterleiten (to an); (Patient) überweisen (to an). 2. zuschreiben, zurückführen (to auf). 3. s. wenden (to an); konsultieren.
ref·er·ence ['ref(ə)rəns] n 1. Weiterleitung f, Übergabe f (to an). 2. Referenz f, Zeugnis nt. 3. Verweis m, Hinweis m, Bezug m (to auf).
reference cell phys. Referenz-, Bezugszelle f.
reference electrode Referenz-, Bezugselektrode f.
reference potential Referenz-, Bezugspotential nt.
reference signal physiol., techn. Sollwert m.
reference state physiol. Referenz-, Standardzustand m.
reference tone Referenzton m.
referred value Referenz-, Bezugswert m.
referred pain [rɪ'fɜrd] übertragener Schmerz m.
re·fine [rɪ'faɪn] vt techn., chem. reinigen, klären, veredeln, raffinieren.
re·fined [rɪ'faɪnd] adj techn., chem. raffiniert, Fein-.
re·fine·ment [rɪ'faɪnmənt] n Verfeinerung f, Reinigung f, Klärung f, Raffinierung f, Raffination f.
re·flect [rɪ'flekt] I vt 1. (Strahlen, Licht) zurückwerfen, reflektieren; spiegeln. 2. anat. zurückbiegen, reflektieren. II vi 3. reflektieren. 4. nachdenken (upon über).
re·flect·ance [rɪ'flektəns] n → reflection coefficient.
re·flect·ed head of rectus femoris muscle [rɪ'flektɪd] hinterer Kopf m des M. rectus femoris, Caput reflexum m. recti femoris.
reflected ligament Lig. reflexum.
reflected light reflektiertes Licht nt.
reflected ray reflektierter Strahl m.
reflected wave reflektierte Welle f, Echowelle f.
re·flect·ing microscope [rɪ'flektɪŋ] Spiegelmikroskop nt.
re·flec·tion [rɪ'flekʃn] n 1. Zurückwerfung f, -strahlung f, Reflexion f, Reflektierung f; (Wieder-)Spiegelung f; Spiegelbild nt.

2. anat. Zurückbiegung f, -beugung f. 3. anat. Umschlagsfalte f, Duplikatur f. 4. Nachdenken nt, Reflexion f.
reflection coefficient phys. Reflektionskoeffizient m, Reflektanz f, Reflexion f.
re·flec·tive [rɪ'flektɪv] adj 1. zurückstrahlend, -werfend, reflektierend, (wieder)-spiegelnd. 2. nachdenklich.
re·flec·tor [rɪ'flektər] n Beleuchtungs-, Reflektorspiegel m, Reflektor m.
re·flex [n, adj 'riːfleks; v rɪ'fleks] I n 1. physiol. Reflex m. 2. → reflection 1. II adj 3. physiol. Reflex(e) betr., durch einen Reflex bedingt, reflektorisch, Reflex-. 4. (Licht) zurückgeworfen, gespiegelt, reflektiert. 5. anat. zurückgebogen, reflektiert. III vt zurückbiegen.
reflex act Reflexhandlung f.
reflex amaurosis ophthal. reflektorische Blindheit/Amaurose f.
reflex amblyopia ophthal. reflektorische Amblyopie f.
reflex angina Angina (pectoris) vasomotoria.
reflex anosmia reflektorische Anosmie f.
reflex arch neuro., physiol. Reflexbogen m.
 monosynaptic r. monosynaptischer Reflexbogen.
 multisynaptic r. multisynaptischer Reflexbogen.
reflex bladder neuro. Reflexblase f.
reflex center neuro. Reflexzentrum nt.
reflex circuit neuro. Reflexbogen m.
reflex-controlled adj reflexgesteuert.
reflex cough Reflexhusten m.
reflex decidua Decidua capsularis/reflexa.
reflex dyspepsia reflektorische Dyspepsie f.
reflex epilepsy Reflexepilepsie f.
reflex eye movement reflektorische Augenbewegung f.
reflex headache reflektorischer/symptomatischer Kopfschmerz m.
reflex hypersensitivity reflektorische Überempfindlichkeit f.
re·flex·ion in Brit. → reflection.
reflex latency physiol. Reflexlatenz f.
reflex ligament of Gimbernat Lig. reflexum.
reflex movement Reflexbewegung f.
re·flex·o·gen·ic [ˌrɪfleksə'dʒenɪk] adj physiol. Reflexe auslösend, eine Reflexaktion verstärkend, reflexogen.
reflexogenic zone reflexogene Zone f.
re·flex·og·e·nous [riːflek'sɑdʒənəs] adj → reflexogenic.
re·flex·o·phil [rɪ'fleksəfɪl] adj neuro. mit gesteigerten Reflexen (einhergehend).
re·flex·o·phile ['-faɪl] adj → reflexophil.
reflex otalgia reflektorische Otalgie f, Otalgia reflectoria.
re·flex·o·ther·a·py [ˌ-'θerəpɪ] n Reflextherapie f.
reflex paralysis reflektorische Lähmung f.
reflex paraplegia reflektorische Paraplegie f.
reflex path physiol. Reflexweg m, -bahn f.
reflex respiratory arrest reflektorischer Atemstillstand m.
reflex response Reflexwirkung f.
reflex sympathetic dystrophy Sudeck'--Dystrophie f, -Syndrom nt, Morbus Sudeck m.
reflex therapy Reflextherapie f.
reflex time physiol. Reflexzeit f.
reflex tonus physiol. Reflextonus m.
reflex torticollis reflektorischer Schiefhals/Torticollis m.
reflex tract neuro., physiol. Reflexbahn f.
 optic r. optische Reflexbahn.
reflex wryneck → reflex torticollis.

re·flux ['riːflʌks] n Zurückfließen nt, Rückfluß m, Reflux m.
reflux esophagitis Refluxösophagitis f, chronisch peptische Ösophagitis f.
reflux gastritis Refluxgastritis f.
 alkaline r. alkalische Refluxgastritis.
reflux ulcer Refluxulkus nt.
re·fract [rɪ'frækt] vt 1. phys. (Licht, Wellen) brechen. 2. ophthal. Refraktionsanomalien erkennen u. behandeln.
re·fract·ed light [rɪ'fræktɪd] gebrochenes Licht nt.
refracted ray gebrochener Strahl m.
re·fract·ing [rɪ'fræktɪŋ] adj (Licht, Wellen) brechend, Brechungs-, Refraktions-.
refracting angle phys. (Prisma) Haupt-, Brechungswinkel m.
re·frac·tion [rɪ'frækʃn] n 1. (Licht, Wellen) Brechung f, Refraktion f. 2. opt. Brechkraft f des Auges, Refraktion(svermögen nt) f. 3. ophthal. Erkennung u. Behandlung von Refraktionsfehlern.
re·frac·tive [rɪ'fræktɪv] adj Refraktion betr., brechend, refraktiv, Brech(ungs)-, Refraktions-.
refractive ametropia ophthal. Brechungsametropie f.
refractive anomalies ophthal. Refraktionsanomalien pl.
refractive dose fraktionierte Dosis f, Dosis refracta.
refractive index Brechungs-, Refraktionsindex m.
refractive medium phys. brechendes Medium nt.
refractive power → refractivity.
re·frac·tiv·i·ty [ˌriːfræk'tɪvətɪ] n phys., physiol. Brech(ungs)kraft f, -vermögen nt, Refraktionskraft f, -vermögen nt.
re·frac·tom·e·ter [ˌ-'tɑmɪtər] n 1. Refraktionsophthalmoskop nt, Refraktometer nt. 2. Refraktionsmesser m, Refraktometer nt.
re·frac·tom·e·try [ˌ-'tɑmətrɪ] n Bestimmung f von Brechungsindizes, Refraktometrie f.
re·frac·tor [rɪ'fræktər] n phys. brechendes Medium nt, Refraktor m.
re·frac·to·ri·ness [rɪ'fræktərɪnɪs] n 1. physiol. (Reiz-)Unempfindlichkeit f (to für); Refraktärität f. 2. (Krankheit) Hartnäckigkeit f, Widerstandsfähigkeit f, Refraktärität f. 3. (Kind) Eigensinn m, Störrisch-, Halsstarrigkeit f. 4. chem., techn. Hitzebeständigkeit f, Feuerfestigkeit f.
re·frac·to·ry [rɪ'fræktərɪ] adj 1. physiol., neuro. (reiz-)unempfindlich, refraktär. 2. (Krankheit) hartnäckig; widerstandsfähig, nicht reagierend (to auf); refraktär. 3. (Kind) eigensinnig, störrisch, halsstarrig. 4. chem., techn. hitzebeständig, feuerfest.
refractory anemia aplastische Anämie f.
 secondary r. sekundär-refraktäre Anämie.
refractory period physiol. Refraktärphase f, -stadium nt, -periode f.
 absolute r. absolute Refraktärperiode.
 effective r. effektive Refraktärperiode.
 functional r. funktionelle Refraktärperiode.
 relative r. relative Refraktärperiode.
 total r. totale Refraktärperiode.
refractory rickets familiäre Hypophosphatämie f, Vitamin D-resistente Rachitis f, Vitamin D-refraktäre Rachitis f, refraktäre Rachitis f.
refractory shock refraktärer Schock m.
refractory state Refraktärstadium nt, -phase f.
re·frac·ture [rɪ'fræktʃər] n ortho. 1. Refraktur f. 2. Refrakturierung f.

refrangibility

re·fran·gi·bil·i·ty [rɪˌfrændʒə'bɪlətɪ] *n phys.* (Strahlen) Brechbarkeit *f*.
re·fran·gi·ble [rɪ'frændʒɪbl] *adj phys.* (Strahlen) brechbar.
re·fresh [rɪ'freʃ] I *vt* erfrischen, frisch machen. II *vi s.* erfrischen.
re·frig·er·ant [rɪ'frɪdʒərənt] I *n techn.* Kühl-, Kältemittel *nt; pharm.* kühlendes Mittel *nt*, Refrigerans *nt*. II *adj* (ab-)kühlend, kühl-; erfrischend.
re·frig·er·ate [rɪ'frɪdʒəreɪt] *vt* kühlen, tiefkühlen; vereisen.
re·frig·er·a·tion [rɪˌfrɪdʒə'reɪʃn] *n* 1. Kühlung *f*, Tiefkühlung *f*. 2. (*Therapie*) (Ab-)Kühlung *f*, Kühlen *nt*, Refrigeration *f*.
refrigeration anesthesia Kryo-, Kälteanästhesie *f*.
re·frig·er·at·ive [rɪ'frɪdʒərətɪv] *adj* → refrigerary.
re·frig·er·a·tor [rɪ'frɪdʒəreɪtər] *n* Kühlschrank *m*, -raum *m*, -kammer *f*, -anlage *f*, -vorrichtung *f*.
re·frig·er·a·to·ry [rɪ'frɪdʒərətɔːriː, -təʊ-] *adj* kälteerzeugend, (ab-)kühlend, Kühl-, Kälte-.
re·frin·gence [rɪ'frɪndʒəns] *n* → refractivity.
re·frin·gent [rɪ'frɪndʒənt] *adj* → refractive.
Refsum ['refsum]: **R. disease/syndrome** Refsum-Syndrom *nt*, Heredopathia atactica polyneuritiformis.
re·fu·sion [rɪ'fjuːʒn] *n* Wiederdurchblutung *f*, Refusion *f*, Reperfusion *f*.
REG *abbr.* → radioencephalogram.
re·gain [rɪ'geɪn] *vt* zurück-, wiedergewinnen, -erlangen; (*Bewußtsein*) wiedererlangen. **to ~ one's breath/strength** wieder zu Atem/Kräften kommen. **to ~ one's health** wieder gesund werden.
Regaud [rə'gəʊ]: **R.'s tumor** Schmincke-Tumor *m*, Lymphoepitheliom *nt*, lymphoepitheliales Karzinom *nt*.
re·gen·er·ate [*adj* rɪ'dʒenərɪt; *v* -reɪt] I *adj* regeneriert. II *vt* erneuern, neubilden, regenerieren. III *vi s.* neubilden, s. erneuern, s. regenerieren.
re·gen·er·a·tion [rɪˌdʒenə'reɪʃn] *n* (*a. bio.*) Neubildung *f*, Erneuerung *f*, Regeneration *f; techn.* Wiedergewinnung *f*, Regenerierung *f*.
regeneration process Regenerationsprozess *m*.
re·gen·er·a·tive [rɪ'dʒenərətɪv, -ˌreɪtɪv] *adj* Regeneration betr., regenerationsfähig, s. regenerierend; s. erneuernd, regenerativ, Regenerativ-, Regenerations-.
regenerative capacity Regenerationskapazität *f*, Regenerationsvermögen *nt*, -fähigkeit *f*.
regenerative layer of epidermis Regenerationsschicht *f*, Stratum germinativum epidermidis.
regenerative metaplasia indirekte Metaplasie *f*.
regenerative node *patho.* Regeneratknoten *m*.
regenerative phase Regenerationsphase *f*.
re·gen·er·a·tor [rɪ'dʒenəreɪtər] *n* Regenerator *m*.
re·gio ['redʒɪəʊ, 'riː-] *n, pl* **-gi·o·nes** [ˌ-dʒɪ-'əʊniːz] → region 1.
re·gion ['riːdʒn] *n* 1. *anat.* Region *f*, (Körper-)Gegend *f*, (-)Bereich *m*, Regio *f*. 2. Gebiet *nt*, Region *f*, Bereich *m*.
r.s of the inferior limb Regiones membri inferioris.
r. of nape Nackengegend, -region, Regio cervicalis posterior, Regio nuchalis.
r.s of the superior limb Regiones membri superioris.
re·gion·al ['riːdʒnl] *adj* regional, regionär,

lokal, örtlich (begrenzt), Regional-.
regional anesthesia *anes.* Regional-, Leitungsanästhesie *f*.
regional chemotherapy lokale/regionale Chemotherapie *f*.
regional colitis Colitis regionalis, Enteritis regionalis des Dickdarms.
regional enteritis Crohn'-Krankheit *f*, Morbus Crohn *m*, Enteritis regionalis, Ileitis/Ileocolitis regionalis/terminalis.
regional enterocolitis → regional enteritis.
regional hypothermia Kryo-, Kälteanästhesie *f*.
regional ileitis → regional enteritis.
regional lymphadenitis Katzenkratzkrankheit *f*, cat-scratch disease (*nt*), benigne Inokulationslymphoretikulose *f*, Miyagawanellose *f*.
regional reflex segmentaler Reflex *m*.
reg·is·ter ['redʒɪstər] I *n* Register *nt*, Verzeichnis *nt*, Liste *f*. II *vt* registrieren, eintragen *od.* einschreiben (lassen), anmelden, (amtlich) erfassen. III *vi s.* einschreiben (für *für*); s. anmelden (at, with bei).
reg·is·tered ['redʒɪstərd] *adj* 1. registriert, eingetragen. 2. (*Arzt*) approbiert; (*Krankenschwester*) staatlich geprüft, examiniert.
registered nurse *abbr.* **R.N.** examinierte Krankenschwester *f*.
re·gress [rɪ'gres] I *n* → regression 1. II *vi s.* rückläufig entwickeln, s. zurückbilden, s. zurückentwickeln.
re·gres·sion [rɪ'greʃn] *n* 1. *patho., bio.* Rückbildung *f*, Rückentwicklung *f*, rückläufige Entwicklung *f*, Regression *f*. 2. *psycho.* Regression *f*. 3. Rückwärtsbewegung *f*, Regression *f*.
regression saccade *physiol.* Regressionssakkade *f*.
re·gres·sive [rɪ'gresɪv] *adj* 1. *patho., bio.* s. zurückbildend, s. zurückentwickelnd, regressiv, Regressions-. 2. zurückgehend, rückläufig.
regressive behavior *psychia.* regressives Verhalten *nt*.
reg·u·lar ['regjələr] *adj* regelmäßig, genau, pünktlich, regulär, normal, gewohnt; (*Atmung, Puls*) regel-, gleichmäßig; (*Lebensweise*) geordnet, geregelt; (*Zähne*) regelmäßig; (*Gesichtszüge*) ebenmäßig; *mathe.* (*Dreieck*) gleichseitig; (*Arzt*) approbiert. **at ~ intervals** regelmäßig, in regelmäßigen Abständen.
regular astigmatism *ophthal.* regulärer Astigmatismus *m*.
regular gout Gelenkgicht *f*, reguläre Gicht *f*.
reg·u·lar·i·ty [ˌregjə'lærətɪ] *n* Regelmäßigkeit *f*; Genauigkeit *f*; Pünktlichkeit *f*; Gewohnheit *f*; Gleichmäßigkeit *f*; Richtigkeit *f*, Ordnung *f*; Ebenmäßigkeit *f*; Gleichseitigkeit *f*.
regular pulse regelmäßiger Puls *m*, Pulsus regularis.
reg·u·late ['regjəleɪt] *vt* (*a. physiol.*) regeln, einstellen, steuern, regulieren.
reg·u·lat·ing ['regjəleɪtɪŋ] *adj* regelnd, steuernd, regulierend, Regulier-, Steuer-.
reg·u·la·tion [ˌregjə'leɪʃn] *n* 1. (*a. physiol.*) Regelung *f*, Einstellung *f*, Steuerung *f*, Regulierung *f*. 2. Vorschrift *f*, Bestimmung *f*.
reg·u·la·tive ['regjəleɪtɪv, -lətɪv] *adj* regelnd, ordnend, regulierend, regulativ.
reg·u·la·tor ['regjəleɪtər] *n techn.* Regler *m*.
reg·u·la·to·ry ['regjələtɔːriː, -təʊ-] *adj* regulatorisch, Regulations-, Regulator-, Steuer-, Ausführungs-, Durchführungs-.
regulatory cell Regulatorzelle *f*.

regulatory circuit *physiol., biochem.* Regelkreis *m*.
regulatory DNA spacer-DNA *f*, Regulator-DNA *f*.
regulatory enzyme regulatorisches Enzym *nt*, Regulatorenzym *nt*.
regulatory gene *genet.* Regulatorgen *nt*.
regulatory hormone Steuer-, Regulationshormon *nt*.
regulatory process Regelungsvorgang *m*.
regulatory subunit regulatorische Untereinheit *f*.
re·gur·gi·tant [rɪ'gɜːdʒɪtənt] *adj* zurückfließend, zurückströmend.
regurgitant disease Herzklappeninsuffizienz *f*.
regurgitant murmur *card.* Strömungsgeräusch *nt* bei Klappeninsuffizienz.
re·gur·gi·tate [rɪ'gɜːdʒɪteɪt] I *vt* 1. zurückfließen lassen. 2. (*Essen*) erbrechen. II *vi* zurückfließen.
re·gur·gi·ta·tion [rɪˌgɜːdʒɪ'teɪʃn] *n* 1. *card.* Rückströmen *nt*, Rückstau *m*, Regurgitation *f*. 2. *chir.* Regurgitation *f*; Reflux *m*.
re·ha·bil·i·tate [ˌriː(h)ə'bɪlɪteɪt] *vt* eine Rehabilitierung durchführen, (wieder-)eingliedern, rehabilitieren.
re·ha·bil·i·ta·tion [ˌriː(h)əˌbɪlə'teɪʃn] *n* (Wieder-)Eingliederung *f*, Rehabilitation *f*, Rehabilitierung *f*.
rehabilitation center Rehabilitationszentrum *nt*.
Rehfuss ['reɪfəs]: **R.' method** → R.' test.
R.' stomach tube Rehfuss-Sonde *f*.
R.' test Rehfuss-Probe *f*, -Test *m*.
R.' tube → R.' stomach tube.
re·hy·dra·tion [ˌriːhaɪ'dreɪʃn] *n* Rehydratation *f*, Rehydrierung *f*.
Reichert ['raɪkərt, 'raɪç-]: **R.'s canal** Hensen'-Gang *m*, -Kanal *m*, Ductus reuniens.
R.'s cartilage *embryo.* Reichert-Knorpel *m*.
R.'s recess Rec. cochlearis (vestibuli).
substantia innominata of R. Meynert'-Ganglion *nt*, Substantia innominata.
Reichmann ['raɪkmən, 'raɪç-]: **R.'s disease/syndrome** Reichmann-Syndrom *nt*, Gastrosukorrhoe *f*.
Reichstein ['raɪkʃtaɪn, 'raɪç-]: **R.'s substance Fa** Kortison *nt*, Cortison *nt*.
R.'s substance G Adrenosteron *nt*.
R.'s substance H Kortiko-, Corticosteron *nt*, Compound B Kendall.
R.'s substance M Kortisol *nt*, Cortisol *nt*, Hydrocortison *nt*.
R.'s substance Q (11-)Desoxycorticosteron *nt abbr.* DOC, Desoxykortikosteron *nt*, Cortexon *nt*.
R.'s substance S 11-Desoxycortisol *nt*.
Reifenstein ['raɪfnstaɪn]: **R.'s syndrome** Reifenstein-Syndrom *nt*.
Reil ['raɪl]: **band of R.** Reil'-Bündel *nt*.
insula of R. Insel *f*, Inselrinde *f*, Insula *f*, Lobus insularis.
island of R. → insula of R.
limiting sulcus of R. Sulcus circularis insulae.
substantia innominata of R. Meynert'-Ganglion *nt*, Substantia innominata.
R.'s sulcus Sulcus circularis insulae.
R.'s triangle Reil-Dreieck *nt*, Trigonum lemnisci.
Reilly ['raɪlɪ]: **R. granulations** *hema.* (Alder-)Reilly-Granulationsanomalie *f*.
re·im·plant [ˌriːɪm'plænt] I *n* Reimplantat *nt*. II *vt* wieder einpflanzen, reimplantieren.
re·im·plan·ta·tion [ˌriːɪmplæn'teɪʃn] *n chir.* Wiedereinpflanzung *f*, Reimplantation *f*; Replantation *f*.

re·in·fec·tion [riːɪnˈfekʃn] *n* 1. Reinfektion *f*. 2. Reinfekt *m*, Reinfektion *f*.
reinfection tuberculosis 1. postprimäre Tuberkulose *f*. 2. Reinfektionstuberkulose *f*.
re·in·force [ˌriːɪnˈfɔːrs] *vt* (*a. fig., psycho.*) verstärken; stärken, stützen.
re·in·force·ment [riːɪnˈfɔːrsmənt] *n* (*a. fig., psycho.*) Verstärkung *f*; Stärkung *f*, Stützung *f*.
re·in·forc·er [riːɪnˈfɔːrsər] *n psycho.* Verstärker *m*.
Reinke [ˈraɪnkə]: **R.'s crystalloids/crystals** Reinke-Kristalle *pl*.
re·in·ner·va·tion [ˌriːˌɪnərˈveɪʃn] *n* Reinnervierung *f*, Reinnervation *f*.
re·in·oc·u·la·tion [riːɪˌnɑkjəˈleɪʃn] *n* Reinokulation *f*.
re·in·tu·ba·tion [rɪˌɪnt(j)uːˈbeɪʃn] *n* Reintubation *f*.
Reissner [ˈraɪznər]: **R.'s fiber** Reissner'-Faden *m*.
R.'s membrane Reissner'-Membran *f*, Membrana vestibularis, Paries vestibularis ductus cochlearis.
Reiter [ˈraɪtər]: **R.'s disease** Reiter'-Krankheit *f*, -Syndrom *nt*, Fiessinger-Leroy-Reiter-Syndrom *nt*, venerische Arthritis *f*, Okulourethrosynovitis *f*, urethro-okulo-synoviales Syndrom *nt*.
R.'s spirochete *micro.* Reiter-Spirochäte *f*, Treponema forans.
R.'s syndrome → R.'s disease.
R. test Reiter-Komplementbindungsreaktion *f*.
re·ject [rɪˈdʒekt] *vt* 1. *immun.* (*Transplantat*) abstoßen. 2. zurückweisen, abschlagen, ablehnen.
re·jec·tion [rɪˈdʒekʃn] *n* 1. *immun.* Abstoßung *f*, Abstoßungsreaktion *f*. 2. Ablehnung *f*, Zurückweisung *f*, Verwerfung *f*. 3. ~s *pl* Exkremente *pl*.
rejection process Abstoßungsprozess *m*.
rejection reaction → rejection response.
rejection response *immun.* Abstoßung *f*, Abstoßungsreaktion *f*.
re·lapse [*n* rɪˈlæps, ˈriːlæps; *v* rɪˈlæps] **I** *n* Rückfall *m*, Rezidiv *m*; Rückfall *m*. **II** *vi* 1. einen Rückfall erleiden. 2. *forens.* rückfällig werden.
re·laps·ing [rɪˈlæpsɪŋ] *adj* rezidivierend, Rückfall-.
relapsing appendicitis rezidivierende Appendizitis *f*.
relapsing febrile nodular nonsuppurative panniculitis (Pfeiffer-)Weber-Christian-Syndrom *nt*, rezidivierende fieberhafte nicht-eitrige Pannikulitis *f*, Panniculitis nodularis nonsuppurativa febrilis et recidivans.
relapsing fever Rückfallfieber *nt*, Febris recurrens.
 cosmopolitan r. → epidemic r.
 Dutton's r. Dutton-(Rückfall-)Fieber, Rückfallfieber durch Borrelia duttoni.
 endemic r. endemisches Rückfallfieber, Zeckenrückfallfieber.
 epidemic r. epidemisches (europäisches) Rückfallfieber, Läuserückfallfieber.
 European r. → epidemic r.
 Indian r. indisches Rückfallfieber.
 louse-borne r. → epidemic r.
 North African r. nordafrikanisches Rückfallfieber.
 Persian r. persisches Rückfallfieber.
 Spanish r. spanisches Rückfallfieber.
 tick-borne r. → endemic r.
relapsing perichondritis → relapsing polychondritis.
relapsing polychondritis rezidivierende Polychondritis *f*, (von) Meyenburg-Altherr-Uehlinger-Syndrom *nt*, systematisierte Chondromalazie *f*.
re·lat·ed [rɪˈleɪtɪd] *adj* 1. verwandt (*to, with* mit); Verwandten-. 2. verbunden, verknüpft (*to* mit).
related donation Verwandten(organ)spende *f*, Organspende *f* durch Verwandte.
related transplant Verwandtentransplantat *nt*.
re·la·tion [rɪˈleɪʃn] *n* 1. Beziehung *f*, Verhältnis *nt*; Bezug *m*, Bezogenheit *f*; ~s *pl* Beziehungen *pl*. **to bear a ~ to** in Beziehung stehen zu. **in ~ to** im Verhältnis zu, in bezug auf. 2. Verwandte(r *m*) *f*. 3. *mathe.* Relation *f*.
re·la·tion·ship [rɪˈleɪʃnʃɪp] *n* Beziehung *f*, Verbindung *f*, Verhältnis *nt* (*to* zu); Verwandtschaft *f* (*to* mit).
rel·a·tive [ˈrelətɪv] **I** *n* 1. Verwandte(r *m*) *f*. 2. *chem.* (verwandtes) Derivat *nt*. **II** *adj* 3. vergleichsweise, ziemlich, verhältnismäßig, relativ, Verhältnis-. 4. bezüglich, (s.) beziehend (*to* auf); Bezugs-.
relative accommodation *ophthal.* relative Akkommodation *f*.
relative amblyopia *ophthal.* relative Amblyopie *f*.
relative amenorrhea *gyn.* Oligomenorrhoe *f*.
relative atomic mass *phys., chem.* relative Atommasse *f*.
relative biological effectiveness *abbr.* **RBE** *radiol.* relative biologische Wirksamkeit *f abbr.* RBW.
relative density *phys.* relative Dichte *f*.
relative hemianopia/hemianopsia *ophthal.* relative Hemianop(s)ie *f*.
relative humidity relative Feuchtigkeit *f*.
relative hyperopia *ophthal.* relative Weitsichtigkeit/Hyperopie *f*.
relative immunity *immun.* begleitende Immunität *f*, Prämunität *f*, Präimmunität *f*, Prämunition *f*.
relative index of refraction → refractive index.
relative leukocytosis relative Leukozytose *f*.
relative movement Relativbewegung *f*.
relative number *mathe.* Verhältniszahl *f*.
relative proportions Mengen-, Größenverhältnis *nt*.
relative refractoriness *physiol.* relative Refraktärität *f*.
relative scotoma *ophthal.* relatives Skotom *nt*.
relative sterility relative Sterilität *f*.
relative value *mathe.* Bezugswert *m*.
rel·a·tiv·i·ty [reləˈtɪvətɪ] *n* Relativität *f*.
relativity theory Relativitätstheorie *f*.
re·lax [rɪˈlæks] **I** *vt* entspannen, lockern. **to ~ one's muscles** die Muskeln lockern. **to ~ the bowels** den Stuhlgang fördern. **II** *vi s.* entspannen, ausspannen, s. erholen; s. lockern; erschlaffen, schlaff werden.
re·lax·ant [rɪˈlæksənt] **I** *n pharm.* entspannungsförderndes Mittel *nt*, Relaxans *nt*. **II** *adj* entspannend, relaxierend.
re·lax·a·tion [ˌrɪlækˈseɪʃn] *n* Ent-, Ausspannung *f*, Erholung *f*; Lockerung *f*, Erschlaffung *f*, Relaxation *f*.
relaxation period *physiol.* Entspannungsphase *f*.
re·laxed [rɪˈlækst] *adj* entspannt, locker, ruhig; (*Atmosphäre*) zwanglos, gelockert.
relaxed control *biochem.*, *chir.* entspannte Kontrolle *f*, relaxed control (*f*).
re·lax·in [rɪˈlæksɪn] *n* Relaxin *nt*.
re·lax·ing [rɪˈlæksɪŋ] *adj* entspannend, erholsam, Erholungs-.
re·lay neuron [ˈriːleɪ] Schalt-, Relaisneuron *nt*.
relay nucleus Relaiskern *m*.

re·lease [rɪˈliːs] **I** *n* 1. Befreiung *f*, Erlösung *f* (*from* von). 2. *physiol.* Ausschüttung *f*, Abgabe *f*; Freisetzung *f*, Freigabe *f*; Auslösung *f*. **II** *vt* 3. befreien, erlösen (*from* von). 4. *physiol.* ausschütten, abgeben; freigeben, -setzen; *techn.* auslösen.
re·leas·ing factor [rɪˈliːsɪŋ] *abbr.* **RF** Releasingfaktor *m abbr.* RF, Releasinghormon *nt abbr.* RH.
releasing hormone *abbr.* **RH** → releasing factor.
re·li·a·bil·i·ty [rɪˌlaɪəˈbɪlətɪ] *n* Zuverlässigkeit *f*, Verläßlichkeit *f*; *stat.* Reliabilität *f*.
re·lief¹ [rɪˈliːf] *n* 1. Erleichterung *f*, Entlastung *f*; Unterstützung *f*, Hilfe *f*. 2. Entspannung *f*, Abwechslung *f*. 3. Vertretung *f*, Aushilfe *f*.
re·lief² [rɪˈliːf] *n* Relief *nt*.
re·lieve [rɪˈliːv] *vt* 1. (*Schmerzen*) erleichtern, lindern. 2. jdn. entlasten *od.* unterstützen, jdm. von etw. befreien. 3. jdn. erleichtern; beruhigen.
re·luc·tance [rɪˈlʌktəns] *n* 1. Widerstreben *nt*, Abneigung *f* (*to* gegen). 2. *phys.* Reluktanz *f*, Permeanzer Widerstand *m*.
rel·uc·tiv·i·ty [ˌrelʌkˈtɪvətɪ] *n phys.* Reluktivität *f*, spezifischer magnetischer Widerstand *m*.
REM *abbr.* → rapid eye movements.
rem [rem] *n* [roentgen equivalent man] Rem *nt abbr.* rem.
Remak [ˈreɪmæk; ˈremaːk]: **R.'s fibers** marklose (Nerven-)Fasern *pl*, Remak-Fasern *pl*.
R.'s ganglia Bidder-Haufen *pl*, -Ganglien *pl*, Remak-Haufen *pl*, Bidder-Remak-Ganglien *pl*.
R.'s plexus *old* → Meissner's plexus.
R.'s paralysis Bleilähmung *f*.
R.'s reflex → R.'s sign.
R.'s sign Remak-Zeichen *nt*, Femoralisreflex *m*.
R.'s symptom Remak-Symptom *nt*, Polyästhesie *f*.
R.'s type → R.'s paralysis.
rem·a·nence [ˈremənəns] *n phys.* → residual magnetism.
rem·a·nent [ˈremənənt] *adj phys.* zurückbleibend, übrig, restlich, remanent.
re·me·di·a·ble [rɪˈmiːdɪəbl] *adj* heilend, kurativ.
re·me·di·al [rɪˈmiːdɪəl] *adj* heilend, kurativ, Heil-.
rem·e·dy [ˈremɪdɪ] **I** *n, pl* **-dies** (Heil-)Mittel *nt*, Arzneimittel *nt*, Arznei *f*, Remedium *nt*, Kur *f* (*for, against* gegen). **II** *vt* heilen, kurieren (*for, against* gegen).
re·min·er·al·i·za·tion [rɪˌmɪn(ə)rəlaɪˈzeɪʃn, -lɪˈz-] *n* Remineralisation *f*.
rem·i·nis·cence [reməˈnɪsəns] *n* Erinnerung *f*, Reminiszenz *f*.
re·mis·sion [rɪˈmɪʃn] *n* vorübergehende Besserung *f*, Remission *f*.
re·mit·tence [rɪˈmɪtns] *n* vorübergehende Besserung *f*.
re·mit·tent [rɪˈmɪtnt] *adj* (vorübergehend) nachlassend, abklingend, remittierend.
remittent fever remittierendes Fieber *nt*, Febris remittens.
rem·nant [ˈremnənt] **I** *n* 1. Überrest *m*, Rest *m*, Überbleibsel *nt*. 2. *phys.* Rest *m*, Residuum *nt*. **II** *adj* Rest-.
re·mote control [rɪˈməʊt] Fernbedienung *f*, Fernsteuerung *f*, Fernlenkung *f*.
remote-controlled *adj* 1. ferngelenkt, ferngesteuert. 2. mit Fernbedienung.
re·mov·a·ble [rɪˈmuːvəbl] *adj* abnehmbar, auswechselbar, abbaubar.
re·mov·al [rɪˈmuːvəl] *n* 1. Fort-, Wegschaffen *nt*, Entfernen *nt*, Beseitigung *f*, Abfuhr *f*, Abtransport *m*. 2. *chir.* Entnahme *f*, Entfernung *f*; Amputation *f*. 3. Entlas-

sung *f*, Ab-, Versetzung *f*. **4.** Beseitigung *f*, Behebung *f*. **5.** Umzug *m*.
re·move [rɪ'muːv] **I** *vt* **1.** entfernen, wegnehmen; abnehmen, abmontieren, ausbauen. **2.** *chir.* entnehmen, entfernen. **3.** (*Kleidung*) ablegen, abnehmen. **4.** wegräumen, wegbringen, abtransportieren. **5.** entlassen, absetzen, versetzen. **II** *vi* aus-, um-, verziehen.
REM sleep paradoxer/desynchronisierter Schlaf *m*, Traumschlaf *m*, REM-Schlaf *m*.
ren- *pref.* → reno-.
ren [ren] *n*, *pl* **re·nes** ['riːniːz] *anat.* Niere *f*, Ren *m*, Nephros *m*.
re·nal ['riːnl] *adj* Niere/Ren betr., von der Niere ausgehend, renal, Nephr(o)-, Nieren-, Reno-.
renal abscess Nierenabszeß *m*.
renal adenocarcinoma → renal cell carcinoma.
renal agenesis Nierenagenesie *f*.
renal anemia renale/nephrogene Anämie *f*.
renal aneurysm intrarenales Aneurysma *nt*.
renal angiography Nierenangiographie *f*, renale Angiographie *f*, Renovasographie *f*.
renal anomaly Nierenfehlbildung *f*, Nierenanomalie *f*.
renal anuria renale Anurie *f*.
renal aplasia Nierenaplasie *f*.
renal apoplexy Nierenapoplexie *f*.
renal arteriogram *radiol.* Arteriogramm *nt* der A. renalis u. ihrer Äste.
renal artery 1. Nierenarterie *f*, -schlagader *f*, Renalis *f*, A. renalis. **2.** ... *ies pl* Nierenarterien *pl*, Aa. renales.
renal artery angiography → renal angiography.
renal artery embolism Nierenarterienembolie *f*.
renal artery injury Nierenarterienverletzung *f*.
renal artery stenosis Nierenarterienstenose *f*.
renal artery thrombosis Nierenarterienthrombose *f*.
renal artery trauma → renal artery injury.
renal atrophy Nierenatrophie *f*.
renal azotemia renale Azot(h)ämie *f*.
renal biopsy Nierenbiopsie *f*, -punktion *f*.
renal blood flow *abbr.* **RBF** renaler Blutfluß *m abbr.* RBF.
renal branch: r. of lesser/minor splanchnic nerve Nierenast *m* des N. splanchnicus minor, Ramus renalis n. splanchnici minoris.
r.es of vagus nerve Vagusäste *pl* zum Plexus renalis, Rami renales n. vagi.
renal calculus Nierenstein *m*, Nephrolith *m*, Calculus renalis.
primary r. primärer Nierenstein.
secondary r. sekundärer Nierenstein, Infektstein.
renal calices Nierenkelche *pl*, Calices renales.
major r. primäre Nierenkelche, Calices renales majores.
minor r. sekundäre Nierenkelche, Calices renales minores.
renal capsule 1. Capsula adiposa (renis). **2.** Capsula fibrosa renis.
renal capsulectomy *urol.* Nierenkapselresektion *f*.
renal carbuncle Nierenkarbunkel *m*.
renal carcinoma, hypernephroid → renal cell carcinoma.
renal carcinosarcoma Wilms-Tumor *m*, embryonales Adeno(myo)sarkom *nt*, Nephroblastom *nt*, Adenomyorhabdosarkom *nt* der Niere.
renal cast *urol.* **1.** Harnzylinder *m*. **2.** Nierenzylinder *m*.
renal cell carcinoma hypernephroides (Nieren-)Karzinom *nt*, klarzelliges Nierenkarzinom *nt*, (maligner) Grawitz-Tumor *m*, Hypernephrom *nt*.
renal circulation Nierenkreislauf *m*, -durchblutung *f*.
renal clamp *urol.* Nierenfaßzange *f*.
renal colic Nierenkolik *f*, Colica renalis.
renal columns Bertin'-Säulen *pl*, Columnae renales.
renal congestion Nierenstauung *f*.
renal corpuscle Nierenkörperchen *nt*, Malpighi'-Körperchen *nt*, Corpusculum renalis.
renal cortex Nierenrinde *f*, Cortex renis.
renal cortical abscess Nierenrindenabszeß *m*.
renal cortical adenoma Nierenrindenadenom *nt*.
renal cortical fatty degeneration Nierenrindenverfettung *f*.
renal cortical laceration Nierenrinden(ein)riß *m*.
renal cortical necrosis Nierenrindennekrose *f*.
renal crisis *neuro.* Nierenkrise *f*.
renal cyst Nierenzyste *f*.
renal decortication *urol.* Nierenkapselentfernung *f*, Dekapsulation *f*.
renal diabetes renale Glukosurie/Glykosurie *f*.
renal dialysis (Nieren-)Dialyse *f*.
renal disease Nierenerkrankung *f*, -leiden *nt*.
end-stage r. *abbr.* **ESRD** terminale Niereninsuffizienz *f*.
polycystic r. polyzystische Nieren *pl*.
renal disorder Nierenerkrankung *f*, -leiden *nt*.
renal duct Harnleiter *m*, Ureter *m*.
renal dwarfism renaler Zwergwuchs *m*.
renal ectopia Nierenektopie *f*, Ectopia renis.
renal edema renales Ödem *nt*.
renal failure Nierenversagen *nt*.
acute r. *abbr.* **ARF** akutes Nierenversagen.
high-output r. → polyuric r.
non-oliguric r. nicht-oligurisches Nierenversagen.
oliguric r. oligurisches Nierenversagen.
polyuric r. polyurisches Nierenversagen.
renal fascia Fascia renalis.
renal function Nierenfunktion *f*.
renal function test Nierenfunktionsprüfung *f*.
renal ganglia Ggll. renalia.
renal glomerulus (Nieren-)Glomerulus *m*, Glomerulus renalis.
renal glycosuria renale Glukosurie/Glykosurie *f*.
renal glycosuric rickets renale glykosurische Rachitis *f*, Fanconi-Syndrom *nt*.
renal graft → renal transplant.
renal hematuria renale Hämaturie *f*.
renal hemorrhage Nierenblutung *f*.
renal hyperchloremic acidosis renal-tubuläre Azidose *f*.
renal hypertension renale Hypertonie *f*.
renal hypoperfusion Mangeldurchblutung/Minderdurchblutung *f* der Niere.
renal hypoplasia *patho.* Nierenhypoplasie *f*.
renal impairment Beeinträchtigung *f* der Nierenfunktion.
renal impression of liver Nierenabdruck *m* auf der Leberoberfläche, Impressio renalis (hepatis).
renal infantilism renaler Infantilismus *m*.
renal infarct Niereninfarkt *m*.
renal injury Nierenverletzung *f*, -schädigung *f*, -trauma *nt*.
renal insufficiency Niereninsuffizienz *f*.
renal ischemia renale Ischämie *f*, Nierenischämie *f*.
renal lipoidosis Lipoidnephrose *f*, Lipidnephrose *f*, Minimal-change-Glomerulonephritis *f*.
renal lobes *embryo.* Nierenlappen *pl*, Lobi renales.
renal malformation Nierenmißbildung *f*.
renal medulla Nierenmark *nt*, Medulla renalis.
renal medullary abscess Nierenmarkabszeß *m*.
renal osteodystrophy renale Osteodystrophie *f*.
renal pain Nierenschmerzen *pl*.
renal papillae (Nieren-)Papillen *pl*, Papillae renales.
renal papillary necrosis (*Niere*) Papillennekrose *f*.
renal parenchyma Nierenparenchym *nt*.
renal pedicle Nierenstiel *m*.
renal pedicle clamp *chir.*, *urol.* Nierenstielklemme *f*.
renal pedicle injury Verletzung *f* des Nierenstiels.
renal pelvic papilloma Nierenbeckenpapillom *nt*.
renal pelvis Nierenbecken *nt*, Pelvis renalis, Pyelon *nt*.
renal perfusion Nierendurchblutung *f*, -perfusion *f*.
renal plasma flow *abbr.* **RPF** renaler Plasmafluß *m abbr.* RPF, Nierenplasmafluß *m*.
renal plexus Plexus renalis.
renal primordium *embryo.* Nierenanlage *f*.
renal proteinuria echte/renale Proteinurie/Albuminurie *f*.
renal pyramids Nierenpyramiden *pl*, Pyramides renales.
renal retinitis → renal retinopathy.
renal retinopathy renale Retinopathie *f*.
renal rickets renale Rachitis *f*.
renal scintigraphy Nieren-, Renoszintigraphie *f*.
renal segments Nierensegmente *pl*, Segmenta renalia.
renal sinus Nierensinus *m*, Sinus renalis.
renal stone → renal calculus.
renal threshold *physiol.* Nierenschwelle *f*, renale Schwelle *f*.
renal toxicity Nierengiftigkeit *f*, -schädlichkeit *f*, Nephrotoxizität *f*.
renal transplant Nierentransplantat *nt*.
cadaveric r. Leichenniere(ntransplantat *nt*) *f*.
related r. Verwandtenniere(ntransplantat *nt*) *f*.
renal transplantation Nierenverpflanzung *f*, -transplantation *f*.
renal trauma Nierenverletzung *f*, -schädigung *f*, -trauma *nt*.
renal tuberculosis Nierentuberkulose *f*.
renal tubular acidosis renal-tubuläre Azidose *f*.
primary r. primäre renal-tubuläre Azidose.
secondary r. sekundäre renal-tubuläre Azidose.
renal tubular osteomalacia renal-tubuläre Osteomalazie *f*.
renal tubules Nierenkanälchen *pl*, -tubuli *pl*, Tubuli renales.
convoluted r. gewundene Nierentubuli, (Nieren-)Konvolut *nt*, Tubuli renales contorti.

convoluted r., distal distales (Nieren-)-Konvolut *nt.*
convoluted r., proximal proximales (Nieren-)Konvolut *nt.*
straight r. gerade Abschnitte *pl* der Nierentubuli, Tubuli renales recti.
renal tuft (Nieren-)Glomerulus *m,* Glomerulus renalis.
renal vascular injury Nierengefäßverletzung *f.*
renal vein 1. Nierenvene *f,* V. renalis. **2.** ~s *pl* (intrarenale) Nierenvenen *pl,* Vv. renales/renis.
renal vein injury Nierenvenenverletzung *f.*
renal vein thrombosis Nierenvenenthrombose *f.*
renal vein trauma → renal vein injury.
renal vesicle *embryo.* Nierenbläschen *nt.*
renal vessels Nierengefäße *pl.*
re·na·tur·a·tion [rɪˌneɪtʃəˈreɪʃn] *n chem.* Renaturierung *f.*
re·na·ture [rɪˈneɪtʃər] *vt chem.* renaturieren.
ren·cu·lus [ˈrenkjələs] *n, pl* **-li** [-laɪ] → reniculus.
Rendu-Osler-Weber [rãˈdy ˈɑzlər ˈwebər]: **R.-O.-W. disease/syndrome** hereditäre Teleangiektasie *f,* Morbus Osler *m,* Osler-Rendu-Weber-Krankheit *f,* -Syndrom *nt,* Rendu-Osler-Weber-Krankheit *f,* -Syndrom *nt,* Teleangiectasia hereditaria haemorrhagica.
ren·i·cap·sule [ˈrenɪˌkæpsəl, -s(j)uːl] *n* **1.** Nierenkapsel *f.* **2.** Nebenniere *f.*
re·nic·u·lus [rɪˈnɪkjələs] *n, pl* **-li** [-laɪ] *embryo.* Nierenläppchen *nt,* Renculus *m.*
ren·i·form [ˈrenɪfɔːrm] *adj* nierenförmig, reniform.
reniform pelvis nierenförmiges Becken *nt.*
ren·i·pel·vic [ˌ-ˈpelvɪk] *adj* Nierenbecken betr., Nierenbecken-.
re·nin [ˈriːnɪn] *n* Renin *nt.*
renin-angiotensin-aldosterone system *abbr.* **RAAS** Renin-Angiotensin-Aldosteron-System *nt abbr.* RAAS.
renin-angiotensin system *abbr.* **RAS** Renin-Angiotensin-System *nt abbr.* RAS.
ren·net [ˈrenɪt] *n* → rennin.
ren·nin [ˈrenɪn] *n* Labferment *nt,* Rennin *nt,* Chymosin *nt.*
reno- *pref.* Nieren-, Nephr(o)-, Ren(o)-.
re·no·cor·ti·cal [ˌriːnəʊˈkɔːrtɪkl] *adj* Nierenrinde betr., Nierenrinden-.
re·no·cu·ta·ne·ous [ˌ-kjuːˈteɪnɪəs] *adj* Niere(n) u. Haut betr.
re·no·cys·to·gram [ˌ-ˈsɪstəgræm] *n* → renogram.
re·no·fa·cial dysplasia [ˌ-ˈfeɪʃl] renofaziale Dysplasie *f,* Dysplasia renofacialis.
re·no·gas·tric [ˌ-ˈgæstrɪk] *adj* Niere(n) u. Magen betr., renogastral, gastrorenal.
re·no·gen·ic [ˌ-ˈdʒenɪk] *adj* von der Niere ausgehend, nephrogen, renal.
re·no·gram [ˈ-græm] *n radiol.* Renogramm *nt.*
re·nog·ra·phy [rɪˈnɑgrəfɪ] *n radiol.* Renographie *f,* Nephrographie *f.*
re·no·in·tes·ti·nal [ˌriːnəʊɪnˈtestɪnl] *adj* Niere(n) u. Darm betr., renointestinal.
renointestinal reflex renointestinaler Reflex *m.*
re·no·pa·ren·chy·mal hypertension [ˌriːnəʊpəˈreŋkɪml] renoparenchymale Hypertonie *f.*
re·nop·a·thy [rɪˈnɑpəθɪ] *n* Nierenerkrankung *f,* Renopathie *f,* Nephropathie *f.*
re·no·pri·val [ˌ-ˈpraɪvl] *adj* renopriv, nephropriv.
re·no·re·nal reflex [ˌ-ˈriːnl] renorenaler Reflex *m.*
re·no·trop·ic [ˌ-ˈtrɑpɪk, -ˈtrəʊ-] *adj* mit besonderer Affinität für Nierengewebe, renotrop.
re·no·vas·cu·lar [ˌ-ˈvæskjələr] *adj* Nierengefäße betr., renovaskulär.
renovascular hypertension renovaskuläre Hypertonie *f.*
Renshaw [ˈrenʃɔː]: **R. cell** Renshaw-Zelle *f.*
 R. inhibition Renshaw-Hemmung *f.*
re·nun·cu·lus [rɪˈnʌŋkjələs] *n* → reniculus.
re·op·er·a·tion [rɪɑpəˈreɪʃn] *n* Reoperation *f.*
Re·o·vir·i·dae [ˌriːəʊˈvɪrədiː, -ˈvaɪr-] *pl micro.* Reoviridae *pl.*
Re·o·vi·rus [ˌ-ˈvaɪrəs] *n micro.* Reovirus *nt.*
re·o·vi·rus [ˌ-ˈvaɪrəs] *n micro.* Reovirus *nt.*
re·ox·i·da·tion [rɪˌɑksɪˈdeɪʃn] *n chem.* Reoxidation *f.*
re·ox·i·dize [rɪˈɑksɪdaɪz] *vt, vi chem.* reoxidieren.
re·pair [rɪˈpeər] **I** *n* **1.** *chir., ortho.* operative Versorgung *f,* Operation *f;* Technik *f;* Naht *f.* **2.** Wiederherstellung *f,* Reparatur *f;* Instandsetzung *f,* Ausbesserung *f.* **II** *vt* **3.** operativ versorgen. **4.** reparieren, ausbessern, instandsetzen.
re·peat [rɪˈpiːt] **I** *vt* wiederholen. **II** *vi* **1.** (s.) wiederholen. **2.** *(Magen)* aufstoßen.
re·pel·lent [rɪˈpelənt] **I** *n* Abschreck-, Abwehrmittel *nt,* Repellent *nt.* **II** *adj* abstoßend.
repellent substance → repellent I.
rep·e·ti·tion [ˌrepɪˈtɪʃn] *n* Wiederholung *f,* Repetition *f.*
rep·e·ti·tious [ˌrepɪˈtɪʃəs] *adj* (s.) (dauernd) wiederholend; monoton, eintönig, gleichbleibend.
re·pet·i·tive [rɪˈpetɪtɪv] *adj* (s.) wiederholend, repetitiv.
repetitive sequence *biochem., genet.* repetitive Sequenz *f.*
re·phos·pho·ryl·ate [rɪfɑsˈfɔːrəleɪt] *vt biochem.* rephosphorylieren.
re·phos·pho·ryl·a·tion [rɪfɑsˌfɔːrəˈleɪʃn] *n biochem.* Rephosphorylierung *f.*
re·place [rɪˈpleɪs] *vt* **1.** ersetzen *(by,* with durch); austauschen; wieder einsetzen. **2.** jdn. ersetzen od. ablösen, an die Stelle treten von. **3.** (zurück-)erstatten, ersetzen.
re·place·a·ble [rɪˈpleɪsəbl] *adj* ersetzbar, austauschbar.
re·place·ment [rɪˈpleɪsmənt] *n* **1.** *ortho., chir.* Prothese *f.* **2.** Ersetzen *nt,* Austauschen *nt;* Ersatz *m.* **3.** Vertretung *f.*
replacement bone Ersatzknochen *m.*
replacement parts Ersatzteile *pl.*
replacement steroid therapy Steroidersatztherapie *f.*
replacement therapy Ersatztherapie *f.*
replacement tissue Ersatzgewebe *nt.*
replacement transfusion (Blut-)Austauschtransfusion *f,* Blutaustausch *m.*
re·plant [riːˈplænt] *chir.* **I** *n* Replantat *nt.* **II** *vt* ver-, umpflanzen, replantieren.
re·plan·ta·tion [ˌriːplænˈteɪʃn] *n chir.* Replantation *f;* Reimplantation *f.*
re·plen·ish [rɪˈplenɪʃ] *vt* (wieder) auffüllen, nachfüllen, ergänzen.
re·plen·ish·ment [rɪˈplenɪʃmənt] *n* (Wieder-)Auffüllung *f,* Ergänzung *f.*
rep·li·case [ˈreplɪkeɪz] *n* Replicase *f,* Replicase *f.*
rep·li·cate [*adj* ˈreplɪkɪt; *v* -keɪt] **I** *n* Wiederholung *f.* **II** *adj* zurückgebogen, -geschlagen. **III** *vt* **1.** zurück-, umbiegen, -schlagen. **2.** verdoppeln, kopieren, wiederholen; *biochem., genet.* replizieren. **IV** *vi biochem., genet.* replizieren, s. verdoppeln.
rep·li·cat·ed [ˈreplɪkeɪtɪd] *adj* → replicate II.
rep·li·ca·tion [ˌreplɪˈkeɪʃn] *n* **1.** *genet.* Replikation *f,* Autoduplikation *f.* **2.** *allg.* Verdoppelung *f;* Kopie *f.* **3.** Echo *nt.* **4.** Erwiderung *f,* Antwort *f.*
replication process Replikationsprozess *m.*
replication unit → replicon.
rep·li·ca·tive [ˈreplɪkeɪtɪv] *adj* Replikation betr., replikativ, Replikations-.
replicative cycle Replikations-, Vermehrungszyklus *m.*
replicative form *biochem.* Replikationsform *f.*
rep·li·con [ˈreplɪkɑn] *n* Replikationseinheit *f,* Replikon *nt,* Replicon *nt.*
re·po·lar·i·za·tion [rɪˌpəʊlərɪˈzeɪʃn] *n physiol.* Repolarisation *f.*
repolarization phase Repolarisationsphase *f.*
re·port·a·ble disease [rɪˈpɔːrtəbl, -ˈpəʊrt-] anzeigepflichtige/meldepflichtige Erkrankung/Krankheit *f.*
re·po·si·tion·ing [riːpəˈzɪʃənɪŋ] *n chir., ortho.* Reposition *f.*
re·press [rɪˈpres] *vt* eindämmen, hemmen, unterdrücken, beschränken, reprimieren; *fig.* (*Gefühle*) unterdrücken; *psychia.* verdrängen.
re·pres·sion [rɪˈpreʃn] *n* **1.** *allg.* Unterdrückung *f,* Hemmung *f,* Eindämmung *f; fig.* (Gefühls-)Unterdrückung *f; biochem.* Repression *f.* **2.** *psychia.* Verdrängung *f,* Repression *f.* **3.** *genet.* (Gen-)Repression *f.*
repression mechanism Repressionsmechanismus *m.*
re·pres·sive [rɪˈpresɪv] *adj* hemmend, unterdrückend, Unterdrückungs-, repressiv.
re·pres·sor [rɪˈpresər] *n biochem., genet.* Repressor *m.*
repressor gene Regulatorgen *nt.*
repressor molecule Repressormolekül *nt.*
re·pro·duce [ˌriːprəˈd(j)uːs] **I** *vt* **1.** züchten, fortpflanzen. **2.** (wieder-)erzeugen; wiedergeben, wiederholen; *bio.* neu bilden, regenerieren. **3.** *photo.* reproduzieren, vervielfältigen. **II** *vi* s. vermehren, s. fortpflanzen.
re·pro·duc·i·ble [ˌriːprəˈd(j)uːsɪbl] *adj* reproduzierbar.
re·pro·duc·tion [ˌriːprəˈdʌkʃn] *n* **1.** Fortpflanzung *f,* Vermehrung *f,* Reproduktion *f.* **2.** Wiedererzeugung *f;* Wiedergabe *f,* Reproduktion *f.* **3.** Replikation *f,* Duplikation *f,* Reproduktion *f;* Vervielfältigung *f;* Kopie *f.*
re·pro·duc·tive [ˌriːprəˈdʌktɪv] *adj* Fortpflanzung betr., reproduzierend, (s.) fortpflanzend, (s.) vermehrend, Fortpflanzungs-, Reproduktions-; Regenerations-.
reproductive behavior *bio.* reproduktives Verhalten *nt.*
reproductive organs Geschlechts-, Genitalorgane *pl,* Genitalien *pl,* Genitale *pl,* Organa genitalia.
re·pro·ter·ol [rɪprəʊˈterəʊl] *n pharm.* Reproterol *nt.*
rep·til·ase [ˈreptɪleɪz] *n* Reptilase *f.*
reptilase clotting time Reptilase-Zeit *f.*
reptilase test Reptilase-Test *nt.*
rep·tile [ˈreptaɪl, -tɪl] *n bio.* Reptil *nt.*
Rep·til·ia [repˈtɪlɪə] *pl bio.* Kriechtiere *pl,* Reptilien *pl.*
re·pulse [rɪˈpʌls] **I** *n phys.* Rückstoß *m.* **II** *vt* zurückschlagen, zurückwerfen.
re·pul·sion [rɪˈpʌlʃn] *n phys.* Abstoßung *f,* Rückstoß *m.*
R-ER *abbr.* → endoplasmic reticulum, rough.
re·rout·ing [rɪˈruːtɪŋ] *n chir.* Rerouting *nt.*

RES

RES *abbr.* → reticuloendothelial system.
re·scin·na·mine [rɪ'sɪnəmɪn] *n pharm.* Rescinnamin *m*.
re·sealed erythrocyte [rɪ'siːlt] *hema.* rekonstituierter Erythrozyt *m*.
re·search [rɪ'sɜrtʃ, 'riːsɜrtʃ] **I** *n* **1.** Forschung *f*; Forschungsarbeit *f*, (wissenschaftliche) Untersuchung *f* (*into, on* über). **to do ~/carry out ~** forschen, Forschung betreiben. **2.** (genaue) Untersuchung *f*, Nachforschung *f* (*after, for* nach). **II** *adj* Forschungs-. **III** *vt* erforschen, untersuchen. **IV** *vi* forschen, Forschung(en) betreiben (*on* über).
research assignment Forschungsauftrag *m*.
research center Forschungszentrum *nt*.
re·search·er [rɪ'sɜrtʃər] *n* Forscher(in *f*) *m*.
research laboratory Forschungslabor *nt*.
research program Forschungsprogramm *nt*.
research team Forscherteam *nt*.
research work → research 1.
research worker → researcher.
re·sect [rɪ'sɛkt] *vt chir.* weg-, ausschneiden, operativ entfernen, reserzieren.
re·sec·ta·bil·i·ty [rɪˌsɛktə'bɪlətɪ] *n chir.* Reserzierbarkeit *f*.
re·sec·ta·ble [rɪ'sɛktəbl] *adj chir.* reserzierbar.
re·sec·tion [rɪ'sɛkʃn] *n chir.* operative (Teil-)Entfernung *f*, Resektion *f*.
re·sec·to·scope [rɪ'sɛktəskoʊp] *n urol.* Resektoskop *nt*, Resektionszystoskop *nt*.
res·er·pine ['rɛsərpɪn, -piːn, rɪ'sɜr-] *n pharm.* Reserpin *nt*.
re·serve [rɪ'zɜrv] **I** *n* **1.** Reserve *f*, Vorrat *m*. **in ~** vorrätig, in Reserve. **2.** Ersatz *m*. **3.** Zurückhaltung *f*, Verschlossen-, Reserviertheit *f*. **II** *vt* aufsparen, aufheben.
r. of energy Kraftreserven *pl*.
r. of strength → r. of energy.
reserve air *physiol.* Reserveluft *f*.
reserve carbohydrate Speicher-, Reservekohlenhydrat *nt*.
re·served [rɪ'zɜrvd] *adj* zurückhaltend, verschlossen, reserviert; Reserve-.
reserve food *bio.* Nährstoffvorrat *m*.
reserve volume *abbr.* **RV** *physiol.* **1.** (*Herz*) Reserve-, Restvolumen *nt abbr.* RV. **2.** (*Lunge*) Reserve-, Residualvolumen *nt abbr.* RV, Residualluft *f*.
expiratory r. *abbr.* **ERV** exspiratorisches Reservevolumen *abbr.* ERV.
inspiratory r. *abbr.* **IRV** inspiratorisches Reservevolumen *abbr.* IRV.
res·er·voir ['rɛzə(r)vwɑːr] *n* **1.** Behälter *m*, Reservoir *nt*; (*a. anat.*) Becken *nt*. **2.** Vorrat *m*, Bestand *m*, Reserve *f* (*of* an). **3.** Speicher *m*, Lager *nt*. **4.** *micro.* Parasitenreservoir *nt*.
reservoir host *micro.* Parasitenreservoir *nt*.
res·i·dent ['rɛzɪdənt] *n* Assistenzarzt *m*, -ärztin *f*.
resident flora *bio., micro.* Residentflora *f*.
re·sid·u·al [rɪ'zɪdʒəwəl, -dʒəl] **I** *n* **1.** Rückstand *m*, Rest *m*, Überbleibsel *nt*, Residuum *nt*. **2.** *mathe.* Rest(wert *m*) *m*; Abweichung *f*, Variation *f*. **II** *adj* übrig, übriggeblieben, restlich, Residual-, Rest-.
residual abscess Residualabszeß *m*.
residual air → residual volume.
residual body *histol.* Rest-, Residualkörper *m*.
residual magnetism *phys.* Remanenz *f*, Restmagnetismus *m*.
residual product *chem., techn.* Nebenprodukt *nt*.
residual urine Restharn *m*.
residual volume *abbr.* **RV** *physiol.* (*Lunge*) Reserve-, Residualvolumen *nt abbr.* RV, Residualluft *f*.
res·i·due ['rɛzɪd(j)uː] *n chem., techn., mathe.* Rest *m*, Überbleibsel *nt*, Rückstand *m*, Residuum *nt*.
re·sid·u·um [rɪ'zɪdʒəwəm] *n, pl* **-dua** [-dʒəwə] → residue.
re·sil·ience [rɪ'sɪljəns, -'zɪlɪəns] *n* → resiliency.
re·sil·ien·cy [rɪ'sɪljənsɪ, -'zɪlɪənsɪ] *n* **1.** *phys.* Elastizität *f*. **2.** Spannkraft *f*, Elastizität *f*.
re·sil·ient [rɪ'sɪljənt, -'zɪlɪənt] *adj* **1.** elastisch. **2.** *fig.* elastisch.
resilient nystagmus Rucknystagmus *m*.
re·sil·in [rə'zɪlɪn] *n bio.* Resilin *nt*.
res·in ['rɛz(ɪ)n] *n* **1.** Harz *nt*, Resina *f*. **2.** Ionenaustauscher(harz *nt*) *m*, Resin *nt*.
res·in·ous ['rɛzɪnəs] *adj* harzig, Harz-.
re·sist·ance [rɪ'zɪstəns] *n* **1.** Widerstand *m* (*to* gegen). **2.** Widerstandskraft *f*, -fähigkeit *f*, Abwehr(kraft *f*) *f* (*to* gegen); Resistenz *f*. **3.** *physiol.* Atemwegswiderstand *m*, Resistance *f*. **4.** *micro., pharm.* Resistenz *f*. **5.** *techn.* Beständig-, Haltbarkeit *f*, Festigkeit *f*.
r. to flow Fließ-, Strömungswiderstand.
r. to heat Hitzebeständigkeit.
r. to stretch Dehnungswiderstand.
r. to wear Verschleißfähigkeit.
resistance factor Resistenzplasmid *nt*, -faktor *m*, R-Plasmid *nt*, R-Faktor *m*.
resistance hypertension Widerstandshochdruck *m*, -hypertonie *f*.
resistance plasmid Resistenzplasmid *nt*, Resistenzfaktor *m*, R-Plasmid *nt*, R-Faktor *m*.
resistance reflex Babinski-Zeichen *nt*, -Reflex *m*, (Groß-)Zehenreflex *m*.
resistance thermometer Widerstandsthermometer *nt*.
resistance transfer factor *abbr.* **RTF** Resistenztransferfaktor *m abbr.* RTF.
resistance vessel Widerstandsgefäß *nt*.
re·sist·ant [rɪ'zɪstənt] *adj* **1.** *immun.* widerstandsfähig, resistent, nicht anfällig, immun (*to* gegen). **2.** *techn.* beständig, haltbar (*to* gegen).
r. to light lichtecht.
res·o·lu·tion [ˌrɛzə'luːʃn] *n* **1.** *opt.* Auflösung(svermögen *nt*) *f*, Resolution *f*. **2.** *chem.* Auflösung *f*, Zerlegung *f* (*into* in). **3.** *patho.* (Auf-)Lösung *f*, Rückbildung *f*, Resolution *f*. **4.** Beschluß(fassung *f*) *m*, Resolution *f*; Entschluß *m*; Entschlossenheit *f*.
resolution phase *physiol.* Rückbildungsphase *f*.
re·sol·u·tive [rɪ'zɑljətɪv, 'rɛzəluː-] *adj* (auf-)lösend.
re·solve [rɪ'zɑlv] **I** *vt chem., mathe., opt.* auflösen (*into* in); *patho.* (auf-)lösen, zerteilen. **II** *vi* s. auflösen (*into* in).
re·sol·vent [rɪ'zɑlvənt] **I** *n chem.* Lösungsmittel *nt*; *pharm.* Lösemittel *nt*, (Re-)Solvens *nt*, (Re-)Solventium *nt*. **II** *adj* (auf-)lösend; *patho.* auflösend, zerteilend.
re·solv·ing power [rɪ'zɑlvɪŋ] *opt.* Auflösungsvermögen *nt*.
res·o·nance ['rɛzənəns] *n phys.* Mitschwingen *nt*, Nach-, Widerhall *m*, Resonanz *f*.
resonance energy Resonanzenergie *f*.
resonance frequency Resonanzfrequenz *f*.
resonance hybrid Resonanzhybrid *nt*.
resonance neutron Resonanzneutron *nt*.
resonance radiation Resonanzstrahlung *f*.
resonance stabilization Resonanzstabilisierung *f*.
resonance stabilization energy Resonanzstabilisierungsenergie *f*.
resonance theory of hearing Resonanzhypothese *f*, Helmholtz-Hörtheorie *f*.
res·o·nant ['rɛzənənt] *adj* mitschwingend, widerhallend (*with* von); resonant, Resonanz-.
resonant circuit *electr.* Resonanz-, Schwingkreis *m*.
res·o·nate ['rɛzəneɪt] *vi phys.* mitschwingen.
res·o·na·tor ['rɛzəneɪtər] *n* Resonator *m*; Resonanzkasten *m*.
re·sorb [rɪ'zɔːrb] *vt* aufnehmen, (wieder) aufsaugen, re(ab)sorbieren.
re·sorb·ence [rɪ'zɔːrbəns] *n* → resorption.
re·sorb·ent [rɪ'zɔːrbnt] *adj* ein-, aufsaugend, aufnehmend, resorbierend.
re·sor·cin [rɪ'zɔːrsɪn] *n* → resorcinol.
re·sor·cin·ol [rɪ'zɔːrsɪnɒl, -nəʊl] *n* Resorcin *nt*, Resorzin *nt*, (*m*-)Dihydroxybenzol *nt*.
re·sor·cin·ol·phthal·ein [rɪˌzɔːrsənɒl-'(f)θæliːn, -liːn] *n* Fluorescein *nt*, -zein *nt*, Resorcinphthalein *nt*.
re·sorp·tion [rɪ'zɔːrpʃn] *n* (Flüssigkeits-)Aufnahme *f*, Aufsaugung *f*, Resorption *f*, Reabsorption *f*.
resorption lacunae Howship'-Lakunen *pl*.
resorption tissue Resorptionsgewebe *nt*.
res·pi·ra·ble ['rɛspɪrəbl, rɪ'spaɪə-] *adj* **1.** zum Einatmen geeignet, atembar, respirabel. **2.** atemfähig.
res·pi·ra·tion [ˌrɛspɪ'reɪʃn] *n* **1.** Lungenatmung *f*, (äußere) Atmung *f*, Atmen *nt*, Respiration *f*. **2.** (innere) Atmung *f*, Zell-, Gewebeatmung *f*.
respiration-dependent *adj* atmungsabhängig.
respiration-independent *adj* atmungsunabhängig.
respiration rate Atemfrequenz *f*.
res·pi·ra·tor ['rɛspəreɪtər] *n* **1.** Beatmungs-, Atemgerät *nt*, Respirator *m*. **2.** Atemfilter *m*.
res·pi·ra·to·ry ['rɛspɪrətɔːriː, -təʊ-, rɪ-'spaɪərə-] *adj* Atmung/Respiration betr., respiratorisch, Atmungs-, Atem-, Respirations-.
respiratory acidosis respiratorische/atmungsbedingte Azidose *f*.
respiratory air Atemluft *f*.
respiratory alkalosis respiratorische/atmungsbedingte Alkalose *f*.
respiratory and circulatory center Atem- u. Kreislaufzentrum *nt*.
respiratory anosmia respiratorische/mechanische Anosmie *f*.
respiratory apparatus Atmungsorgane *pl*, Atemwege *f*, Respirationssystem *nt*, -trakt *m*, Apparatus respiratorius, Systema respiratorium.
respiratory arrest Atemstillstand *m*, Apnoe *f*.
reflex r. reflektorischer Atemstillstand.
respiratory arrhythmia respiratorische Arrhythmie *f*.
respiratory brain *patho.* Respiratorhirn *nt*.
respiratory bronchioles Alveolarbronchiolen *pl*, Bronchioli alveolares/respiratorii.
respiratory capacity (*Lunge*) Vitalkapazität *f abbr.* VK, VC.
respiratory center Atemzentrum *nt*.
respiratory chain *biochem.* Atmungskette *f*.
respiratory-chain phosphorylation *biochem.* Atmungskettenphosphorylierung *f*, oxidative Phosphorylierung *f*.
respiratory coefficient → respiratory quotient.
respiratory depression Atemdepression *f*.

respiratory disease Atemwegserkrankung f.
  acute r. abbr. **ARD** akute Atemwegserkrankung, akute respiratorische Erkrankung f abbr. **ARE**.
  chronic r. abbr. **CRD** chronische Atemwegserkrankung.
respiratory distress syndrome (of the newborn) abbr. **RDS** Atemnotsyndrom nt des Neugeborenen abbr. **ANS**, Respiratory-distress-Syndrom nt des Neugeborenen abbr. **RDS**.
respiratory diverticulum embryo. Lungendivertikel nt.
respiratory drive Atem-, Atmungsantrieb m.
respiratory enzyme Cytochrom a_3 nt, Cytochrom(c)oxidase f, old Warburg'-Atmungsferment nt, Ferrocytochrom c--Sauerstoff-Oxidoreduktase f.
respiratory epithelium respiratorisches Flimmerepithel nt.
respiratory exchange respiratorischer Gasaustausch m.
respiratory exchange ratio → respiratory quotient.
respiratory failure akute respiratorische Insuffizienz f.
  r. in the newborn Neugeborenenasphyxie f, Atemdepressionszustand m des Neugeborenen, Asphyxia neonatorum.
respiratory frequency Atemfrequenz f.
respiratory gases Atemgase pl.
respiratory infection Atemwegsinfekt m, -infektion f, -erkrankung f.
  acute r. akute Atemwegserkrankung, akuter Atemwegsinfekt, akute Atemwegsinfektion.
respiratory insufficiency respiratorische Insuffizienz f.
respiratory mechanics Atmungs-, Atemmechanik f.
respiratory metabolism Atmungsstoffwechsel m, respiratorischer Stoffwechsel m.
respiratory minute volume Atemminutenvolumen nt abbr. **AMV**.
respiratory muscles/musculature Atemmuskeln pl, -muskulatur f.
  accessory r. Atemhilfsmuskeln, -muskulatur.
respiratory neuron physiol. respiratorisches Neuron nt.
respiratory organ Atmungsorgan nt.
respiratory passages Luft-, Atemwege pl, Respirationstrakt m, Apparatus respiratorius, Systema respiratorium.
  lower r. untere Luftwege.
  upper r. obere Luftwege.
respiratory pigment Atmungspigment nt.
respiratory primordium embryo. Anlage f des Respirationstraktes.
respiratory pump physiol. Saug-Druck--Pumpeneffekt m der Atmung.
respiratory pyelography urol. Veratmungspyelographie f.
respiratory quotient abbr. **RQ** physiol. respiratorischer Austauschquotient m; respiratorischer Quotient m abbr. **RQ**.
respiratory region (Nasenschleimhaut) Regio respiratoria.
respiratory resistances Atmungswiderstände pl.
respiratory rhythm Atem-, Atmungsrhythmus m.
respiratory sound respiratorisches Geräusch nt, Atemgeräusch nt.
respiratory spasm respiratorischer Spasmus m, Spasmus respiratorius.
respiratory substrate Atmungs(ketten)substrat nt.
respiratory syncytial virus micro. RS-Virus nt, Respiratory-Syncytial-Virus nt.
respiratory system → respiratory passages.
respiratory tract → respiratory passages.
respiratory volume per minute Atemminutenvolumen nt abbr. **AMV**.
respiratory zone Respirationszone f.
re·spire [rɪ'spaɪər] vt, vi (ein-)atmen, respirieren.
res·pi·rom·e·ter [respɪ'rɑmɪtər] n physiol. Respirometer nt.
re·spond [rɪ'spɑnd] vi antworten (to auf); reagieren, ansprechen (to auf). **to ~ poorly** nicht ansprechen od. reagieren (to auf).
re·sponse [rɪ'spɑns] n **1.** Antwort f (to auf). **in ~ to** als Antwort auf. **2.** physiol., psycho. Reaktion f, Reizantwort f, Response f, Antwort f (to auf); Ansprechen nt, Reagieren nt (to auf).
response cycle Reaktionszyklus m.
re·spon·sive [rɪ'spɑnsɪv] adj **1.** antwortend, als Antwort (to auf); Antwort-. **2.** (leicht) reagierend od. ansprechend (to auf); empfänglich (to für).
re·spon·sive·ness [rɪ'spɑnsɪvnɪs] n Ansprechbarkeit f, Rekationsfähigkeit f, Empfänglichkeit f (to für).
rest¹ [rest] I n **1.** Ruhe f; Nachtruhe f. **to have a good night's ~** gut schlafen. **2.** (Ruhe-)Pause f, Erholung f; Ausruhen nt, Ausspannen nt. **to take a ~** (s.) ausruhen. **to be at ~** ruhig sein. **3.** Ruhelage f. **to be at ~** s. in Ruhelage od. -stellung befinden. **4.** Stütze f, Halt m, Lehne f, Auflage f; (Brillen-)Steg m. II vt **5.** ruhen lassen, ausruhen, schonen. **to ~ o.s.** s. ausruhen. **6.** legen, lagern (on auf); lehnen, stützen (against gegen; on auf). III vi **7.** ruhen, (s.) ausruhen. **8.** s. stützen od. lehnen (on an; against gegen); ruhen (on auf).
rest² [rest] n Rest m.
rest contact electr. Ruhekontakt m.
rest cure Erholung f; Ruhe-, Liegekur f.
rest·ed ['restɪd] adj erholt, ausgeruht.
re·ste·no·sis [rɪstɪ'nəʊsɪs] n patho. Restenose f.
rest·ful ['restfəl] adj erholsam.
rest home Alten-, Alters-, Pflegeheim nt.
res·ti·form ['restɪfɔːrm] adj seil-, strangförmig, schnurartig.
restiform body → restiform process of Henle.
restiform process of Henle unterer Kleinhirnstiel m, Pedunculus cerebellaris caudalis/inferior.
rest·ing ['restɪŋ] adj ruhend, inaktiv, Ruhe-.
resting activity physiol. Ruheaktivität f.
resting breast ruhende/nicht-laktierende Brustdrüse f.
resting conditions physiol. Ruhebedingungen pl.
resting follicle Ruhefollikel m, ruhender Follikel m.
resting level Ruhewert m, -niveau nt.
resting phase 1. old → interphase. **2.** → resting stage.
resting potential Ruhepotential nt.
resting pressure Ruhedruck m.
resting stage embryo. Ruhestadium nt.
resting tension curve physiol. Ruhedehnungskurve f.
resting tone physiol. Ruhetonus m.
res·ti·tu·tio [ˌrestɪ't(j)uːʃɪəʊ] n → restitution.
res·ti·tu·tion [ˌ-'t(j)uːʃn] n patho. Wiederherstellung f, Restitution f, Restitutio f.
rest·less ['restlɪs] adj nervös, unruhig, rast-, ruhelos; schlaflos.
restless legs syndrome Ekbom-Syndrom nt, Wittmaack-Ekbom-Syndrom nt, Syndrom nt der unruhigen Beine.
rest·less·ness ['restlɪsnɪs] n Nervosität f, (nervöse) Unruhe f, Unrast f, Ruhelosigkeit f; Schlaflosigkeit f.
rest mass phys. Ruhemasse f.
rest nitrogen Reststickstoff m, Rest-N m/nt abbr. **RN**, nicht-proteingebundener Stickstoff m abbr. **NPN**.
re·stor·a·ble [rɪ'stɔːrəbl] adj wiederherstellbar.
res·to·ra·tion [ˌrestə'reɪʃn] n **1.** Wiederherstellung f. **2.** Instandsetzung f; Rekonstruktion f. **3.** dent. Plombieren nt.
  r. of health gesundheitliche Wiederherstellung f, Genesung.
  r. from sickness → r. of health.
re·stor·a·tive [rɪ'stɔːrətɪv, -'stɔʊr-] I n Aufbau-, Stärkungsmittel nt. II adj **1.** stärkend, aufbauend, Stärkungs-. **2.** wiederherstellend.
re·store [rɪ'stɔːr, -'stɔʊr] vt **1.** wiederherstellen. **~ s.o.** jdn. (gesundheitlich) wiederherstellen. **2.** techn. instand setzen; rekonstruieren.
re·strain [rɪ'streɪn] vt **1.** zurückhalten, hindern; (Gefühle) unterdrücken. **2.** einsperren, einschließen, in einer Anstalt unterbringen.
re·straint [rɪ'streɪnt] n **1.** Ein-, Beschränkung f; Zwang m. **2.** Freiheitsbeschränkung f, Haft f; Unterbringung f in einer Anstalt.
re·strict [rɪ'strɪkt] vt ein-, beschränken, begrenzen (to auf).
re·strict·ed [rɪ'strɪktɪd] adj ein-, beschränkt, begrenzt.
re·stric·tion [rɪ'strɪkʃn] n **1.** Ein-, Beschränkung f (to auf); Vorbehalt m, Restriktion f. **without ~s** uneingeschränkt. **2.** genet. Restriktion f.
restriction endonuclease Restriktionsendonuklease f.
restriction enzyme → restrictive enzyme.
restriction fragment Restriktionsfragment nt.
re·stric·tive [rɪ'strɪktɪv] adj ein-, beschränkend, begrenzend, restriktiv, Restriktions-.
restrictive cardiomyopathy abbr. **RCM** restriktive Kardiomyopathie f abbr. **RCM**, obliterative Kardiomyopathie f abbr. **OCM**.
restrictive enzyme 1. Restriktionsenzym nt. **2.** Restriktionsendonuklease f.
rest tremor Ruhetremor m.
re·sult [rɪ'zʌlt] I n **1.** Ergebnis nt, Resultat nt; **~s** pl (Test) Werte pl. **without ~s** ergebnislos, negativ. **2.** Erfolg m, (gutes) Ergebnis nt. **to get ~s** gute Ergebnisse erzielen (from mit). **3.** Nach-, Auswirkung f, Folge f. **as a ~** folglich. II vi s. ergeben, resultieren (from aus).
result in vi enden mit, zur Folge haben führen zu.
re·sult·ant [rɪ'zʌltnt] I n **1.** mathe., phys. Resultante f, Resultierende f. **2.** Ergebnis nt, Resultat nt. II adj s. ergebend, resultierend (from aus).
re·sus·ci·tate [rɪ'sʌsɪteɪt] I vt wiederbeleben, reanimieren. II vi das Bewußtsein wiedererlangen.
re·sus·ci·ta·tion [rɪˌsʌsɪ'teɪʃn] n **1.** Wiederbelebung f, Reanimation f. **2.** Notfalltherapie f, Reanimationstherapie f.
resuscitation cart Notfall-, Reanimationswagen m.
resuscitation limit Wiederbelebungs-, Strukturerhaltungszeit f.
re·sus·ci·ta·tive [rɪ'sʌsɪteɪtɪv] adj wiederbelebend, reanimierend, Wiederbelebungs-, Reanimations-.
re·sus·ci·ta·tor [rɪ'sʌsɪteɪtər] n Reanimator m.

resynthesis

re·syn·the·sis [rɪ'sɪnθəsɪs] *n* Resynthese *f*.
re·tained menstruation [rɪ'teɪnd] *gyn.* Hämatokolpos *m*, Hämokolpos *m*.
retained placenta Plazentaretention *f*, Retentio placentae.
retained testicle/testis Hodenretention *f*, Kryptorchismus *m*, Retentio/Maldescensus testis.
re·tard [rɪ'tɑːrd] **I** *vt* (*a. bio., phys., physiol.*) verlangsamen, hemmen, aufhalten, verzögern, retardieren. **II** *vi* s. verzögern, zurückbleiben.
re·tar·date [rɪ'tɑːrdeɪt] *n* (geistig) zurückgebliebener Mensch *m*.
re·tar·da·tion [ˌrɪtɑːr'deɪʃn] *n* Verlangsamung *f*, (Entwicklungs-)Hemmung *f*, Verzögerung *f*, Retardierung *f*, Retardation *f*.
retardation phase Verzögerungsphase *f*.
retardation period → retardation phase.
re·tar·da·tive [rɪ'tɑːrdətɪv] *adj* verlangsamend, hemmend, verzögernd, retardierend.
re·tar·da·to·ry [rɪ'tɑːrdətɔːrɪ, -təʊ-] *adj* → retardative.
re·tard·ed [rɪ'tɑːrdɪd] **I** *n the ~ pl* geistig *od.* körperlich Zurückgebliebene *pl*. **II** *adj* (geistig *od.* körperlich) zurückgeblieben, retardiert, Spät-.
retarded dentition verspätete Zahnung/Dentition *f*, Dentitio tarda.
re·tard·ee [ˌrɪtɑːr'diː] *n* → retardate.
retch·ing ['retʃɪŋ] *n* Brechreiz *m*, Würgen *nt*.
retching reflex Würg(e)reflex *m*.
re·te ['riːtɪ] *n*, *pl* **re·tia** ['riːʃ(ɪ)ə, -tɪə] *anat.* Netz *nt*, Netzwerk *nt*, Rete *nt*.
  r. of Haller Haller'-Netz, Rete testis.
  r. of patella patelläres Arteriengeflecht *nt*, Rete patellare.
rete chords *embryo.* Hodenstränge *pl*.
rete mi·ra·bi·le [mɪ'reɪbəliː] *anat.* Wundernetz *nt*, Rete mirabile.
  arterial r. Arteriennetz, Rete arteriosum.
  venous r. Venennetz, Rete venosum.
re·ten·tion [rɪ'tenʃn] *n* **1.** Zurückhaltung *f*, Zurückhalten *nt*, Verhaltung *f*, Retention *f*, Retentio *f*. **2.** *chir.* Ruhigstellung *f*, Retention *f*.
retention cyst Retentionszyste *f*.
retention toxicosis Retentionstoxikose *f*.
rete o·va·rii [əʊ'veərɪaɪ] Rete ovarii.
rete testis → rete of Haller.
re·te·the·li·o·ma [ˌriːtəˌθɪlɪ'əʊmə] *n* **1.** Hodgkin-Krankheit *f*, -Lymphom *nt*, Morbus Hodgkin *m*, (Hodgkin-)Paltauf-Steinberg-Krankheit *f*, (maligne) Lymphogranulomatose *f*, Lymphogranulomatosis maligna. **2.** non-Hodgkin-Lymphom *nt abbr.* NHL.
re·ti·al ['riːʃɪəl] *adj anat.* Rete betr.
reticul- *pref.* → reticulo-.
re·tic·u·lar [rɪ'tɪkjələr] *adj anat., techn.* netzförmig, -artig, retikular, retikulär, Netz-.
reticular activating system *abbr.* **RAS** aufsteigendes retikuläres aktivierendes System *nt abbr.* ARAS.
reticular cartilage elastischer Knorpel *m*, Cartilago elastica.
reticular cell Retikulumzelle *f*.
  dendritic r. dendritische Retikulumzelle.
reticular dysgenesis retikuläre Dysgenesie *f*.
reticular fiber Retikulum-, Retikulinfaser *f*, Gitterfaser *f*, argyrophile Faser *f*.
reticular formation Formatio/Substantia reticularis.
  r. of medulla oblongata Formatio/Substantia reticularis medullae oblongatae.
  mesencephalic r. *abbr.* **MRF** → r. of mesencephalon.

r. of mesencephalon mesencephale Formatio reticularis *abbr.* **MRF**, Formatio reticularis mesencephali.
paramedian pontine r. *abbr.* **PPRF** paramediane pontine Formatio reticularis *abbr.* PPRF.
r. of pons Formatio reticularis pontis.
r. of spinal cord Formatio reticularis medullae spinalis.
r. of thalamus Nc. reticularis thalami.
reticular layer of corium/dermis Geflechtschicht *f*, Stratum reticulare corii/dermidis.
reticular membrane of cochlear duct Membrana reticularis (ductus cochlearis).
reticular nucleus: large-cell r.i Ncc. reticulares magnocellulares.
  small-cell r.i Ncc. reticulares parvocellulares.
  rapheal i. Ncc. reticulares raphae.
reticular part of substantia nigra Pars reticularis.
reticular sarcoma of bone Ewing-(Knochen-)Sarkom *nt*, endotheliales Myelom *nt*.
reticular substance Substantia reticulo-granulofilamentosa.
  r. of medulla oblongata → reticular formation of medulla oblongata.
reticular tissue retikuläres Bindegewebe *nt*.
reticular zone (*NNR*) Zona reticularis.
re·tic·u·late [rɪ'tɪkjəleɪt] *adj* → reticular.
reticulate body Retikular-, Initialkörperchen *nt*.
re·tic·u·lat·ed [rɪ'tɪkjəleɪtɪd] *adj* → reticular.
reticulated membrane of cochlear duct → reticular membrane of cochlear duct.
reticulated tissue retikuläres Bindegewebe *nt*.
re·tic·u·la·tion [rɪˌtɪkjə'leɪʃn] *n* Netz *nt*, Netzwerk *nt*, Geflecht *nt*.
re·tic·u·lin [rɪ'tɪkjəlɪn] *n* Retikulin *nt*, Reticulin *nt*.
reticulo- *pref.* Netz-, Retikul(o)-, Retikulum-.
re·tic·u·lo·cer·e·bel·lar tract [rɪˌtɪkjələʊˌserə'belər] Tractus reticulocerebellaris.
re·tic·u·lo·cyte ['-saɪt] *n* Retikulozyt *m*.
re·tic·u·lo·cyt·ic sarcoma [ˌ-'sɪtɪk] → reticulum cell sarcoma.
  r. of bone → reticulum cell sarcoma of bone.
re·tic·u·lo·cy·to·pe·nia [ˌ-ˌsaɪtə'piːnɪə] *n* Retikulo(zyto)penie *f*.
re·tic·u·lo·cy·to·sis [ˌ-ˌsaɪ'təʊsɪs] *n* Retikulozytose *f*.
re·tic·u·lo·en·do·the·li·al [ˌ-ˌendəʊ'θiːlɪəl] *adj* retikuloendotheliales Gewebe *od.* System betr., retikuloendothelial.
reticuloendothelial cell Zelle *f* des retikuloendothelialen Systems.
reticuloendothelial sarcoma → reticulum cell sarcoma.
  r. of bone → reticulum cell sarcoma of bone.
reticuloendothelial system *abbr.* **RES** retikuloendotheliales System *nt abbr.* RES, retikulohistiozytäres System *nt abbr.* RHS.
reticuloendothelial tissue retikuloendotheliales Gewebe *nt*.
re·tic·u·lo·en·do·the·li·o·ma [ˌ-ˌendəʊˌθiːlɪ'əʊmə] *n* → retethelioma.
re·tic·u·lo·en·do·the·li·o·sis [ˌ-ˌendəʊˌθiːlɪ'əʊsɪs] *n* Retikuloendotheliose *f*.
re·tic·u·lo·en·do·the·li·um [ˌ-ˌendəʊ'θiːlɪəm] *n* retikuloendotheliales Gewebe *nt*.
re·tic·u·lo·his·ti·o·cyt·ic [ˌ-ˌhɪstɪə'sɪtɪk] *adj* retikulohistiozytär.

reticulohistiocytic granuloma → reticulohistiocytoma.
reticulohistiocytic system *abbr.* **RHS** → reticuloendothelial system.
re·tic·u·lo·his·ti·o·cy·to·ma [ˌ-ˌhɪstɪəʊsaɪ'təʊmə] *n* **1.** retikulohistiozytisches Granulom *nt*, Riesenzellhistiozytom *nt*, Retikulohistiozytom (Cak) *nt*. **2.** ~mata *pl* multiple Retikulohistiozytome *pl*, multizentrische Retikulohistiozytose *f*, Lipoiddermatoarthritis *f*, Retikulohistiocytosis disseminata.
re·tic·u·lo·his·ti·o·cy·to·sis [ˌ-ˌhɪstɪəʊsaɪ'təʊsɪs] *n* Retikulohistiozytose *f*.
re·tic·u·loid [rɪ'tɪkjəlɔɪd] **I** *n* Retikuloid *nt*. **II** *adj* Retikulose-ähnlich, retikuloid.
reticulo-olivary fibers retikulo-oliväre Fasern *pl*, Fibrae reticulo-olivarii.
re·tic·u·lo·pe·nia [rɪˌtɪkjələʊ'piːnɪə] *n* Retikulo(zyto)penie *f*.
reticulo-reticular fibers retikulo-retikuläre Fasern *pl*, Fibrae reticuloreticulares.
re·tic·u·lo·sis [rɪˌtɪkjə'ləʊsɪs] *n* Retikulose *f*.
re·tic·u·lo·spi·nal tract [rɪˌtɪkjələʊ'spaɪnl] Tractus reticulospinalis.
re·tic·u·lo·tha·lam·ic fasciculus [ˌ-θə'læmɪk] retikulothalamisches Bündel *nt*, Fasciculus reticulothalamicus.
re·tic·u·lo·the·li·um [ˌ-'θiːlɪəm] *n* Retothel *nt*.
re·tic·u·lum [rɪ'tɪkjələm] *n*, *pl* **-la** [-lə] **1.** Retikulum *nt*. **2.** retikuläres Bindegewebe *nt*.
reticulum cell Retikulumzelle *f*.
reticulum cell sarcoma Retikulosarkom *nt*, Retikulumzell(en)sarkom *nt*, Retothelsarkom *nt*.
  r. of bone Retikulumzell(en)sarkom/Retikulosarkom/Retothelsarkom des Knochens, malignes Lymphom *nt* des Knochens.
reticulum plasma Retikulumplasma *nt*.
re·ti·form ['riːtəfɔːrm, 'retə-] *adj* netzförmig.
retiform parapsoriasis Parapsoriasis lichenoides, Parakeratosis variegata, Lichen variegatus.
ret·i·na ['retɪnə] *n*, *pl* **-nas, -nae** [-niː] Netzhaut *f*, Retina *f*.
ret·i·nac·u·lum [ˌretə'nækjələm] *n*, *pl* **-la** [-lə] *anat.* Halteband *nt*, Retinakulum *nt*, Retinaculum *nt*.
  r.la of nail Retinacula unguis.
  r.la of skin Retinacula cutis.
ret·i·nal¹ ['retɪnəl] *n* Retinal *nt*, Vitamin A₁-Aldehyd *m*.
ret·i·nal² ['retɪnəl] *adj* Netzhaut/Retina betr., retinal, Netzhaut-, Retina-.
retinal₂ *n* Dehydroretinal *nt*, Retinal₂ *nt*.
retinal abiotrophy *ophthal.* retinale Abiotrophie *f*.
retinal adaptation *ophthal.* Netzhautadaptation *f*, -anpassung *f*, Empfindlichkeitsanpassung *f* der Netzhaut.
retinal anlage *embryo.* Retinaanlage *f*.
retinal anlage tumor Melanoameloblastom *nt*.
retinal aplasia *ophthal.* Netzhautaplasie *f*, -dysplasie *f*.
  hereditary r. angeborene Blindheit *f*, Amaurosis congenita.
retinal asthenopia *ophthal.* retinale Asthenopie *f*.
retinal cones (*Auge*) Zapfen(zellen *pl*) *pl*.
retinal correspondence *ophthal.* Korrespondenz *f* der Netzhaut.
  anomalous r. *abbr.* **A.R.C.** anomale Korrespondenz der Netzhaut.
  normal r. *abbr.* **N.R.C.** normale Korrespondenz der Netzhaut.

retinal detachment *ophthal.* Netzhautablösung *f*, Ablatio/Amotio retinae.
retinal dysplasia Netzhautdysplasie *f*.
retinal embolism *ophthal.* (*Retina*) Zentralarterienembolie *f*.
retinal gliocytes Müller'-Stützzellen *pl*, -Stützfasern *pl*.
retinal image *ophthal.* Netzhautbild *nt*.
retinal isomerase Retinalisomerase *f*.
retinal receptor Netzhautrezeptor *m*.
retinal reductase Retinalreduktase *f*.
retinal rivalry *ophthal.* Netzhautrivalität *f*.
retinal rods (*Auge*) Stäbchen(zellen *pl*) *pl*.
ret·i·nene ['retniːn] *n* → retinal[1].
ret·i·ni·tis [retə'naɪtɪs] *n ophthal.* Netzhautentzündung *f*, Retinitis *f*.
ret·i·no·blas·to·ma [ˌretɪnəʊblæs'təʊmə] *n ophthal.* Retinoblastom *nt*, Glioma retinae.
ret·i·no·ce·re·bral angiomatosis [ˌ-'serəbrəl, -sə'riːbrəl] Netzhautangiomatose *f*, (von) Hippel-Lindau-Syndrom *nt*, Angiomatosis retinae cystica, Angiomatosis cerebelli et retinae.
ret·i·no·cho·roid [ˌ-'kɔːrɔɪd, -'kəʊr-] *adj* Aderhaut/Choroidea u. Netzhaut/Retina betr., chorioretinal.
ret·i·no·cho·roi·dal coloboma [ˌ-kə'rɔɪdl] *ophthal.* Funduskolobom *nt*.
ret·i·no·cho·roid·i·tis [ˌ-ˌkɔːrɔɪ'daɪtɪs, -ˌkəʊ-] *n* Entzündung *f* von Netz- u. Aderhaut, Retinochorioiditis *f*, Chorioretinitis *f*.
ret·i·no·graph ['-græf] *n ophthal.* Retinograph *m*.
ret·i·nog·ra·phy [retɪ'nɑgrəfɪ] *n ophthal.* Retinographie *f*.
ret·i·no·hy·po·tha·lam·ic fibers [ˌretɪnəʊˌhaɪpəʊθə'læmɪk] retinohypothalamische Fasern *pl*.
ret·i·no·ic acid [ˌretɪ'nəʊɪk] Retinsäure *f*, Vitamin A_1-Säure *f*, Tretinoin *nt*.
ret·i·noid ['retɪnɔɪd] I *n* Retinoid *nt*. II *adj* 1. *ophthal.* retinoid. 2. *chem.* harzartig, Harz-.
ret·i·nol ['retnɒl, -nəl] *n* Retinol *nt*, Vitamin A_1 *nt*, Vitamin-A-Alkohol *m*.
retinol$_1$ *n* → retinol.
retinol$_2$ *n* (3-)Dehydroretinol *nt*, Vitamin A_2 *nt*.
ret·i·no·ma·la·cia [ˌretɪnəʊmə'leɪʃ(ɪ)ə] *n ophthal.* Netzhauterweichung *f*, Retinomalazie *f*, -malacia *f*.
ret·i·no·pap·il·li·tis [ˌ-pæpə'laɪtɪs] *n ophthal.* Entzündung *f* von Netzhaut u. Papille, Retinopapillitis *f*, Papilloretinitis *f*.
r. of premature infants → retinopathy of prematurity.
ret·i·nop·a·thy [ˌretɪ'nɑpəθɪ] *n* (nicht-entzündliche) Netzhauterkrankung *f*, Retinopathie *f*, Retinopathia *f*, Retinose *f*.
r. of prematurity *ped.* retrolentale Fibroplasie *f*, Frühgeborenenretinopathie *f*, Terry-Syndrom *nt*, Retinopathia praematurorum *f*.
ret·i·nos·chi·sis [ˌ-'nɑskəsɪs] *n ophthal.* Netzhautspalt *m*, -spalte *f*, -spaltung *f*, Retinoschisis *f*.
ret·i·no·scope ['retɪnəskəʊp] *n ophthal.* Retinoskop *nt*, Skiaskop *nt*.
ret·i·nos·co·py [ˌretɪ'nɑskəpɪ] *n ophthal.* Retinoskopie *f*, Skiaskopie *f*.
ret·i·no·sis [ˌ-'nəʊsɪs] *n* → retinopathy.
ret·i·no·top·ic [ˌretɪnə'tɑpɪk] *adj* retinotop.
ret·i·no·tox·ic [ˌ-'tɑksɪk] *adj* netzhautschädlich, -schädigend, retinotoxisch.
re·tort [rɪ'tɔːt] *n chem.* Retorte *f*.
Re·tor·ta·mo·nad·i·da [rɪˌtɔːrtəməʊ'nædɪdə] *pl micro.* Retortamonadida *pl*.
Re·tor·tam·o·nas [ˌrɪtɔːr'tæmənæs] *n micro.* Retortamonas *f*.

re·to·thel ['riːtəʊθel] *adj* → reticuloendothelial.
re·to·the·li·al [ˌ-'θiːlɪəl] *adj* Retothel betr., retothelial, Retothel-.
retothelial sarcoma → reticulum cell sarcoma.
r. of bone → reticulum cell sarcoma of bone.
ret·o·the·li·um [ˌretəʊ'θiːlɪəm] *n* Retothel *nt*.
re·tract [rɪ'trækt] I *vt* zurück-, zusammen-, einziehen, kontrahieren. II *vi* s. zurückod. zusammenziehen, kontrahieren.
re·tract·a·bil·i·ty [rɪˌtræktə'bɪlətɪ] *n* Retraktionsfähigkeit *f*.
re·tract·a·ble [rɪ'træktəbl] *adj* zurück-, einziehbar, retraktionsfähig, retraktil.
re·trac·ta·tion [ˌrɪtræk'teɪʃn] *n* → retraction.
re·tract·ed [rɪ'træktɪd] *adj* eingezogen.
retracted nipple Hohl-, Schlupfwarze *f*.
re·tract·i·bil·i·ty *adj* → retractability.
re·tract·i·ble *adj* → retractable.
re·trac·tile [rɪ'træktɪl] *adj* → retractable.
re·trac·til·i·ty [ˌriːtræk'tɪlətɪ] *n* → retractability.
re·trac·tion [rɪ'trækʃn] *n* Zurück-, Zusammen-, Einziehen *nt*, Einziehung *f*; Schrumpfung *f*, Verkürzung *f*, Retraktion *f*.
retraction nystagmus Retraktionsnystagmus *m*, Nystagmus retractorius.
retraction pocket *HNO* (*Ohr*) Retraktionstasche *f*.
retraction ring *gyn.* Kontraktionsring *m*.
pathologic r. *gyn.* Bandl-Kontraktionsring.
retraction syndrome *ophthal.* Duane-Syndrom *nt*, Stilling-Türk-Duane-Syndrom *nt*.
re·trac·tor [rɪ'træktər] *n* 1. *chir.* (Wund-)-Haken *m*; Wundspreizer *m*, -sperrer *m*. 2. *anat.* Retraktionsmuskel *m*.
re·trans·plan·ta·tion [rɪˌtrænsplæn'teɪʃn] *n* Retransplantation *f*.
retro- *pref.* Zurück-, Retro-, Rück-, Rückwärts-.
ret·ro·act ['retrəʊækt] *vi* zurückwirken, entgegengesetzt wirken.
ret·ro·ac·tion [ˌ-'ækʃn] *n* Rückwirkung *f*.
ret·ro·ac·tive [ˌ-'æktɪv] *adj* (zu-)rückwirkend, umgekehrt wirkend, retroaktiv.
retroactive inhibition *physiol.* retroaktive Hemmung *f*.
ret·ro·au·ric·u·lar [ˌ-ɔː'rɪkjələr] *adj* hinter der Ohrmuschel (liegend), retroaurikulär.
retroauricular atheroma retroaurikuläres Atherom *nt*.
ret·ro·buc·cal [ˌ-'bʌkəl] *adj* retrobukkal.
ret·ro·bul·bar [ˌ-'bʌlbər, -baːr] *adj* 1. hinter dem Auge/Bulbus oculi (liegend), retrobulbär. 2. (*ZNS*) hinter der Brücke (liegend), retrobulbär.
retrobulbar abscess retrobulbärer Abszeß *m*.
retrobulbar anesthesia retrobulbäre Anästhesie *f*.
retrobulbar neuritis Retrobulbärneuritis *f*, Neuritis optica retrobulbaris.
retrobulbar space Retrobulbärraum *m*.
ret·ro·cal·ca·ne·al bursitis [ˌ-kæl'keɪnɪəl] Achillobursitis *f*.
ret·ro·cal·ca·ne·o·bur·si·tis [ˌ-kælˌkeɪnɪəʊbər'saɪtɪs] *n* Achillobursitis *f*.
ret·ro·car·di·ac space [ˌ-'kɑːrdɪæk] Holzknecht-Raum *m*, Retrokardialraum *m*.
ret·ro·ce·cal [ˌ-'siːkəl] *adj* hinter dem Blinddarm/Zäkum (liegend), retrozäkal, -zökal.
retrocecal abscess retrozäkaler Abszeß *m*.

retrognathic

retrocecal appendicitis retrozäkale Appendizitis *f*.
retrocecal fossa Rec. retrocaecalis.
retrocecal hernia Rieux'-Hernie *f*, retrozäkale Hernie *f*.
retrocecal recess Retrozäkalgrube *f*, Rec. retrocaecalis.
ret·ro·cede [ˌ-'siːd] *vi* zurückgehen, -weichen; (*Ausschlag*) nach innen schlagen.
ret·ro·ced·ence [ˌ-'siːdəns] *n* → retrocession.
ret·ro·cen·tral sulcus [ˌ-'sentrəl] Sulcus postcentralis.
ret·ro·cer·vi·cal [ˌ-'sɜrvɪkl, -sɜr'vaɪkl] *adj* hinter der Zervix (liegend), retrozervikal.
ret·ro·ces·sion [ˌ-'seʃn] *n* Zurückgehen *nt*, -weichen *nt*, Rückgang *m*; (*Ausschlag*) Nachinnenschlagen *nt*; *epidem.* Retrozession *f*.
ret·ro·ces·sive [ˌ-'sesɪv] *adj* zurückgehend, -weichend; (*Ausschlag*) nach innen schlagend.
ret·ro·coch·le·ar [ˌ-'kɑklɪər, -'kəʊ-] *adj* hinter der Kochlea (liegend), retrokochleär.
retrocochlear deafness retrokochleäre Schwerhörigkeit/Taubheit *f*.
ret·ro·col·ic [ˌ-'kɑlɪk] *adj* hinter dem Kolon (liegend), retrokolisch.
retrocolic appendicitis retrokolische Appendizitis *f*.
ret·ro·col·ic spasm [ˌ-'kɑlɪk] → retrocollis.
ret·ro·col·lis [ˌ-'kɑlɪs] *n neuro.* Retrocollis (spasmodicus) *m*.
ret·ro·con·duc·tion [ˌ-kən'dʌkʃn] *n* → retrograde conduction.
ret·ro·cos·tal artery [ˌ-'kɑstl, -'kɒs-] Ramus costalis lateralis a. thoracicae internae.
ret·ro·cur·sive [ˌ-'kɜrsɪv] *adj* retrokursiv.
ret·ro·de·vi·a·tion [ˌ-dɪvɪ'eɪʃn] *n* Rückwärtsbiegung *f*, -beugung *f*, Retrodeviation *f*.
ret·ro·dis·place·ment [ˌ-dɪs'pleɪsmənt] *n* Verlagerung *f* nach hinten.
ret·ro·dor·so·lat·er·al nucleus of ventral column of spinal cord [ˌ-ˌdɔːrsəʊ'lætərəl] Nc. retroposterolateralis.
ret·ro·du·o·de·nal [ˌ-ˌdjuːəʊ'diːnl, -d(j)uː'ɑdnəl] *adj* hinter dem Zwölffingerdarm/ Duodenum (liegend), retroduodenal.
retroduodenal arteries Retroduodenalarterien *pl*, Aa. retroduodenales.
retroduodenal fossa → retroduodenal recess.
retroduodenal recess retroduodenale Bauchfelltasche *f*, Rec. retroduodenalis.
ret·ro·e·soph·a·ge·al [ˌ-ɪˌsɑfə'dʒiːəl] *adj* hinter der Speiseröhre/dem Ösophagus (liegend), retroösophageal.
ret·ro·fa·cial nucleus [ˌ-'feɪʃl] Nc. retrofacialis.
ret·ro·flect·ed ['-flektɪd] *adj* → retroflex I.
ret·ro·flec·tion *n* → retroflexion.
ret·ro·flex ['-fleks] I *adj* nach hinten/rückwärts gebeugt, zurückgebogen, retroflektiert. II *vt* nach hinten biegen od. wenden. III *vi* s. nach hinten biegen od. wenden.
ret·ro·flexed ['-flekst] *adj* → retroflex I.
ret·ro·flex·ion [ˌ-'flekʃn] *n* 1. Rückwärtsbiegung *f*, -beugung *f*, Retroflexion *f*. 2. Retroflexion *f* des Uterus, Retroflexio uteri.
ret·ro·gas·se·ri·an neurectomy [ˌ-gə'sɪərɪən] *neurochir.* retroganglionäre Neurotomie *f*.
retrogasserian neurotomy/rhizotomy → retrogasserian neurectomy.
ret·ro·gnath·ia [ˌ-'næθɪə] *n* Retrognathie *f*.
ret·ro·gnath·ic [ˌ-'næθɪk] *adj* Retrognathie betr., retrognath.

retrognathism

ret·ro·gnath·ism [ˌ-'næθɪzəm] *n* → retrognathia.
ret·ro·gra·da·tion [ˌ-greɪ'deɪʃn] *n* Zurückgehen *nt*, Abnahme *f*, Rückgang *m*; Verschlechterung *f*.
ret·ro·grade ['-greɪd] **I** *adj* rückläufig, -gängig, von hinten her, retrograd, Rückwärts-; rückwirkend, zeitlich/örtlich zurückliegend. **II** *vi* entarten, degenerieren.
retrograde amnesia retrograde Amnesie *f*.
retrograde aortography *radiol*. retrograde Aortographie *f*.
retrograde block *card*. retrograder Block *m*.
retrograde chromatolysis retrograde/zentrale Chromatolyse *f*.
retrograde conduction *cardio*. retrograde Erregungsleitung *f*.
retrograde degeneration *neuro*. retrograde/aufsteigende Degeneration *f*.
retrograde embolism retrograde Embolie *f*.
retrograde extrasystole → return extrasystole.
retrograde hernia retrograde Hernie *f*, Hernie en W.
retrograde metamorphosis retrograde Metamorphose *f*.
retrograde metaplasia retrograde Metaplasie *f*, Retroplasie *f*.
retrograde metastasis paradoxe/retrograde Metastase *f*.
retrograde peristalsis → reversed peristalsis.
retrograde pyelography *radiol.*, *urol*. retrograde Pyelographie *f*.
retrograde transport *physiol*. retrograder Transport *m*.
retrograde urethrography *urol.*, *radiol*. retrograde Urethrographie *f*.
retrograde urography *urol.*, *radiol*. retrograde Urographie *f*.
ret·ro·gress ['-gres] *vi* zurückentwickeln; zurückgehen, -weichen.
ret·ro·gres·sion [ˌ-'greʃn] *n* rückläufige Entwicklung *f*, Degeneration *f*, Kataplasie *f*, Rückbildung *f*, Regression *f*.
ret·ro·gres·sive [ˌ-'gresɪv] *adj* rückentwickelnd, in Rückbildung begriffen, rückschreitend, -gehend, retrogressiv, regressiv.
retrogressive metamorphosis retrograde Metamorphose *f*.
ret·ro·hy·oid bursa [ˌ-'haɪɔɪd] Bursa retrohyoidea.
ret·ro·il·e·al appendicitis [ˌ-'ɪliəl] retroileale Appendizitis *f*.
re·tro·in·fec·tion [ˌ-ɪn'fekʃn] *n gyn*. Retroinfektion *f*.
ret·ro·in·gui·nal space [ˌ-'ɪŋgwɪnl] Doors'-Raum *m*, Retroinguinalraum *m*.
ret·ro·in·hi·bi·tion [ˌ-ɪn(h)ɪ'bɪʃn] *n biochem*. Endprodukt-, Rückkopplungshemmung *f*, Feedback-Hemmung *f*.
ret·ro·jec·tion [ˌ-'dʒekʃn] *n* Retrojektion *f*.
re·tro·ien·tal [ˌ-'lentl] *adj* hinter der Linse (liegend), retrolental, retrokristallin.
retrolental fibroplasia *abbr*. RLF *ped*. retrolentale Fibroplasie *f*, Frühgeborenenretinopathie *f*, Terry-Syndrom *nt*, Retinopathia praematurorum.
ret·ro·len·tic·u·lar part of internal capsule [ˌ-len'tɪkjələr] retrolentikulärer Kapselabschnitt *m*, Pars retrolenticularis/retrolentiformis (capsulae internae).
ret·ro·len·ti·form part of internal capsule [ˌ-'lentɪfɔːrm] → retrolenticular part of internal capsule.
ret·ro·lin·gual [ˌ-'lɪŋgwəl] *adj* retrolingual.
ret·ro·mam·ma·ry [ˌ-'mæməri] *adj* hinter der Brust(drüse)/Mamma (liegend), retromammär.
retromammary abscess (*Brust*) retroglandulärer/retromammärer Abszeß *m*.
retromammary bursa (*Brust*) retroglandulärer Spaltraum *m*.
retromammary mastitis *gyn*. Paramastitis *f*.
ret·ro·man·dib·u·lar vein [ˌ-mæn'dɪbjələr] V. retromandibularis.
ret·ro·mor·pho·sis [ˌ-mɔːr'fəʊsɪs] *n* retrograde Metamorphose *f*.
retro-ocular space → retrobulbar space.
retro-olivary area Area retro-olivaris.
retro-olivary sulcus Sulcus retro-olivaris.
ret·ro·pa·tel·lar chondropathy/osteoarthritis [ˌ-pə'telər] Büdinger-Ludloff-Löwen-Syndrom *nt*, Chondromalacia patellae.
ret·ro·per·i·to·ne·al [ˌ-ˌperɪtə'niːəl] *adj* hinter dem Bauchfell/Peritoneum (liegend), im Retroperitonealraum (liegend), retroperitoneal.
retroperitoneal abscess retroperitonealer Abszeß *m*.
retroperitoneal air *radiol*. retroperitoneale Luft(ansammlung *f*) *f*.
retroperitoneal bleeding retroperitoneale Blutung *f*.
retroperitoneal fibrosis 1. Ormond-Syndrom *nt*, (idiopathische) retroperitoneale Fibrose *f*. **2.** symptomatische retroperitoneale Fibrose *f*.
retroperitoneal hemorrhage → retroperitoneal bleeding.
retroperitoneal hernia Treitz'-Hernie *f*, Hernia duodenojejunalis.
retroperitoneal space Retroperitonealraum *m*, Spatium retroperitoneale.
ret·ro·per·i·to·ne·um [ˌ-ˌperɪtə'niːəm] *n* → retroperitoneal space.
ret·ro·per·i·to·ni·tis [ˌ-ˌperɪtə'naɪtɪs] *n* Entzündung *f* des Retroperitonealraums, Retroperitonitis *f*.
ret·ro·pha·ryn·ge·al [ˌ-fə'rɪn(d)ʒ(ɪ)əl, -ˌfærɪn'dʒiːəl] *adj* hinter dem Rachen/Pharynx (liegend), retropharyngeal, Retropharyngeal-.
retropharyngeal abscess retropharyngealer Abszeß *m*, Retropharyngealabszeß *m*.
retropharyngeal space retropharyngealer Raum *m*, Retropharyngealraum *m*, Spatium retropharyngeum.
ret·ro·phar·yn·gi·tis [ˌ-ˌfærɪn'dʒaɪtɪs] *n* Retropharyngitis *f*.
ret·ro·pla·cen·tal [ˌ-plə'sentəl] *adj* hinter der Plazenta (liegend), retroplazentar.
ret·ro·pla·sia [ˌ-'pleɪzɪə] *n* retrograde Metaplasie *f*, Retroplasie *f*.
ret·ro·posed ['-pəʊzd] *adj* nach hinten verlagert.
ret·ro·po·si·tion [ˌretrəpə'zɪʃn] *n anat., patho*. Rückwärtsverlagerung *f*, Retroposition *f*, Retropositio *f*.
r. of uterus Retroposition des Uterus, Retropositio uteri.
ret·ro·pu·bic [ˌ-'pjuːbɪk] *adj* hinter dem Schambein/Os pubis (liegend), retropubisch.
retropubic prevesical prostatectomy *urol*. retropubische prävesikale Prostatektomie *f*.
retropubic space Retzius'-Raum *m*, Spatium retropubicum.
ret·ro·pul·sion [ˌ-'pʌlʃn] *n* Retropulsion *f*.
ret·ro·py·lor·ic [ˌ-paɪ'lɔːrɪk, -'lɑr-] *adj* retropylorisch.
ret·ro·spect ['-spekt] *n* Rückblick *m*, Rückschau *f*. **in ~** rückschauend, im Rückblick.
ret·ro·spec·tion [ˌ-'spekʃn] *n* Rückblick *m*, Rückschau *f*; Zurückblicken *nt*, -schauen *nt*, Retrospektion *f*.
ret·ro·spec·tive [ˌ-'spektɪv] *adj* zurückschauend, zurückblickend, nach rückwärts gerichtet, retrospektiv.
retrospective study *stat*. retrospektive Studie *f*.
ret·ro·spon·dy·lo·lis·the·sis [ˌ-ˌspɒndɪləʊlɪs'θiːsɪs] *n ortho*. Retrospondylolisthese *f*.
ret·ro·ster·nal [ˌ-'stɜːrnl] *adj* hinter dem Sternum (liegend), retrosternal.
ret·ro·ton·sil·lar abscess [ˌ-'tɑnsɪlər] retrotonsillärer Abszeß *m*, Retrotonsillarabszeß *m*.
ret·ro·u·re·thral catheterization [ˌ-jʊə'riːθrəl] posteriore/retrourethrale (Blasen-)Katheterisierung *f*.
ret·ro·u·ter·ine [ˌ-'juːtərɪn, -raɪn] *adj* hinter der Gebärmutter/dem Uterus (liegend), retrouterin.
retrouterine hematocele *gyn*. Haematocele retrouterina.
retrouterine hematoma retrouterines Hämatom *nt*.
ret·ro·vas·cu·lar hernia [ˌ-'væskjələr] Serafini-Hernie *f*, retrovaskuläre Schenkelhernie *f*.
ret·ro·verse ['-vɜːrs] *adj* → retroverted.
ret·ro·ver·si·o·flex·ion [ˌ-ˌvɜːsɪəʊ'flekʃn, ˌ-ˌvɜːʒəʊ-] *n* Retroversion u. -flexion *f*, Retroversioflexion *f*.
ret·ro·ver·sion [ˌ-'vɜːʒn, -ʃn] *n* **1.** Rückwärtsneigung *f*, -beugung *f*, Retroversion *f*. **2.** Retroversio *f* des Uterus, Retroversio uteri.
r. of uterus → retroversion 2.
ret·ro·vert·ed [ˌ-'vɜːrtɪd] *adj* nach hinten *od*. rückwärts geneigt, rückwärtsverlagert, retrovertiert.
Ret·ro·vir·i·dae [ˌ-'vɪrədiː] *pl micro*. Retroviren *pl*, Retroviridae *pl*.
ret·ro·vi·rus [ˌ-'vaɪrəs] *n micro*. Retrovirus *nt*.
re·tru·sion [rɪ'truːʃn, -ʒn] *n* Zurückverlagerung *f*, Retrusion *f*.
Rett [ret]: **R. syndrome** Rett-Syndrom *nt*.
re·turn extrasystole [rɪ'tɜːrn] *card*. Umkehrextrasystole *f*, Echophänomen *nt*.
Retzius ['retsɪəs]: **body of R.** Retzius'-Körperchen *nt*.
R.' cavity → R.' space.
R.' fibers Retzius'-Fasern *pl*.
R.' foramen Apertura lateralis.
lines of R. Retzius'-Streifung *f*.
R.' space Retzius'-Raum *m*, Spatium retropubicum.
R.' striae → lines of R.
R.' veins Retzius'-Venen *pl*.
re·vac·ci·na·tion [rɪˌvæksə'neɪʃn] *n* Wiederholungsimpfung *f*, Wiederimpfung *f*, Revakzination *f*.
re·vas·cu·lar·i·za·tion [rɪˌvæskjələrɪ'zeɪʃn] *n* **1.** *patho*. Kapillareinsprossung *f*, Revaskularisierung *f*, Revaskularisation *f*. **2.** *chir*. Revaskularisation *f*, Revaskularisierung *f*.
re·ver·ber·ant [rɪ'vɜːrbərənt] *adj phys*. nach-, widerhallend; reflektierend.
re·ver·ber·ate [*adj* rɪ'vɜːrbərɪt; *v* -reɪt] **I** *adj* → reverberant. **II** *vt* (*Licht, Hitze*) zurückwerfen, reflektieren. **III** *vi* nach-, widerhallen; (*Hitze, Licht*) reflektieren.
re·ver·ber·at·ing excitation [rɪ'vɜːrbəreɪtɪŋ] *physiol*. reverberatorische/kreisende Erregung *f*.
re·ver·ber·a·tion [rɪˌvɜːrbə'reɪʃn] *n* Nach-, Widerhall *m*; (*Licht, Hitze*) Zurückstrahlen *nt*, -werfen *nt*, Reflexion *f*.
re·ver·ber·a·to·ry [rɪ'vɜːrbərətɔːriː, -təʊ-] *adj* zurückgeworfen, reflektiert, reverberatorisch, Reverberier-.

reverberatory circuit *physiol.* Erregungskreis *m*.
Reverdin [rəvɛr'dɛ̃]: **R. graft** Reverdin--Läppchen *nt*, -Lappen *m*, Hautinseln *pl*.
re·ver·sal [rɪ'vɜrsl] *n* Umkehrung *f*, Umkehren *nt*, -drehen *nt*, -stellen *nt*, Wenden *nt*; Umschlag *m*.
  r. of polarity Umpolung *f*.
  reversal potential *physiol.* Umkehrpotential *nt*.
  reversal process Umkehrentwicklung *f*.
re·verse [rɪ'vɜrs] **I** *n* **1.** Gegenteil *nt*, das Umgekehrte. **2.** Rückschlag *m*, Niederlage *f*. **3.** Rückseite *f*. **II** *adj* **4.** umgekehrt, verkehrt, entgegengesetzt (*to*); Gegen-; *opt.* seitenverkehrt. **5.** rückwärts, rückläufig, Rückwärts-. **III** *vt* umkehren, -drehen, wenden, herumdrehen; *electr.* umpolen.
  reverse banding *genet.* R-Banding *nt*.
  re·versed coarctation [rɪ'vɜrsd] Pulslos--Krankheit *f*, Martorell-Krankheit *f*, -Syndrom *nt*, Takayasu-Krankheit *f*, -Syndrom *nt*, pulseless disease (*nt*).
  reversed peristalsis (*Darm*) retrograde Peristaltik *f*.
  reversed shunt Rechts-Links-Shunt *m*.
  reverse T₃ → reverse triiodothyronine.
  reverse transcriptase → RNA-directed DNA polymerase.
  reverse transcription *biochem.*, *genet.* reverse Transkription *f*.
  reverse triiodothyronine *abbr.* **rT₃** reverses/inaktives Triiodothyronin *nt* *abbr.* rT₃, reverses/inaktives T₃ *nt*.
re·vers·i·bi·li·ty [rɪˌvɜrsə'bɪlətɪ] *n* Umkehrbarkeit *f*, Reversibilität *f*.
re·vers·i·ble [rɪ'vɜrsɪbl] *adj* umkehrbar, reversibel; heilbar, reversibel.
  reversible colloid stabiles Kolloid *nt*.
  reversible inhibition reversible Hemmung *f*.
  reversible reaction *chem.* reversible/umkehrbare Reaktion *f*.
re·ver·sion [rɪ'vɜrʒn, -ʃn] *n* (*a. genet.*) Umkehrung *f*, Umkehr *f* (*to zu*); Reversion *f*; *bio.* Rückmutation *f*, Reversion *f*.
re·ver·tant [rɪ'vɜrtnt] *n genet.* Revertante *f*.
Revinus ['revɪnəs]: **R.' ducts** Ductus sublinguales minores.
re·viv·i·fi·ca·tion [rɪˌvɪvəfɪ'keɪʃn] *n ortho.* (*Wundrand*) Auffrischung *f*, Auffrischen *nt*.
re·viv·i·fy [rɪ'vɪvəfaɪ] *vt ortho.* (*Wundrand*) auffrischen.
rev·o·lute ['revəluːt] *adj* zurückgerollt.
re·vul·sant [rɪ'vʌlsənt] *adj* → revulsive.
re·vul·sion [rɪ'vʌlʃn] *n* Ableitung *f*, Revulsion *f*.
re·vul·sive [rɪ'vʌlsɪv] *adj* ableitend, revulsiv.
Reye [raɪ, reɪ]: **R.'s syndrome** Reye-Syndrom *nt*.
Reynold ['reɪnəld]: **R.'s number** Reynold'--Zahl *f*.
RF *abbr.* **1.** → receptive field. **2.** → releasing factor. **3.** → rheumatic fever. **4.** → rheumatoid factors.
R factor Resistenzplasmid *nt*, -faktor *m*, R-Plasmid *nt*, R-Faktor *m*.
RF-center *n physiol.* RF-Zentrum *nt*.
RF latex → rheumatoid factor latex agglutination test.
RF-periphery *n physiol.* RF-Peripherie *f*.
RH *abbr.* [releasing hormone] → releasing factor.
Rh *abbr.* **1.** → rhesus factor. **2.** → rhodium.
rhabd- *pref.* → rhabdo-.
rhab·dit·ic [ræb'dɪtɪk] *adj micro.* Rhabditis *od.* Rhabditoidea betr.
rhab·dit·i·form [ræb'dɪtəfɔːrm] *adj* → rhabdoid.

Rhab·di·tis [ræb'daɪtɪs] *n micro.* Rhabditis *f*.
rhab·di·toid ['ræbdɪtɔɪd] *adj* → rhabdoid.
Rhab·di·toi·dea [ræbdɪ'tɔɪdɪə] *pl micro.* Rhabditoidea *pl*.
rhabdo- *pref.* Stab-, Rhabd(o)-.
rhab·do·cyte ['ræbdəsaɪt] *n* Metamyelozyt *m*.
rhab·doid ['ræbdɔɪd] *adj* stabförmig.
Rhab·do·mo·na·di·na [ˌræbdəˌmɔʊnə'daɪnə] *pl micro.* Rhabdomonadina *pl*.
Rhab·do·mo·nas [ˌ-'mɔʊnæs] *n micro.* Rhabdomonas *f*.
rhab·do·my·o·blas·to·ma [ˌ-ˌmaɪəblæs'tɔʊmə] *n* Rhabdo(myo)sarkom *nt*.
rhab·do·my·o·chon·dro·ma [ˌ-ˌmaɪəkɒn'drɔʊmə] *n* benignes Mesenchymom *nt*.
rhab·do·my·o·fi·bril [ˌ-ˌmaɪə'fɪbrɪl, -'faɪ-] *n* Rhabdomyofibrille *f*.
rhab·do·my·ol·y·sis [ˌ-ˌmaɪ'ɒləsɪs] *n* Rhabdomyolyse *f*.
rhab·do·my·o·ma [ˌ-maɪ'əʊmə] *n* Rhabdomyom *nt*.
rhab·do·my·o·myx·o·ma [ˌ-ˌmaɪəmɪk'sɔʊmə] *n* benignes Mesenchymom *nt*.
rhab·do·my·o·sar·co·ma [ˌ-ˌmaɪəsɑːr'kɔʊmə] *n* Rhabdo(myo)sarkom *nt*.
Rhab·do·ne·ma [ˌ-'niːmə] *n* → Rhabditis.
rhab·do·sar·co·ma [ˌ-sɑːr'kɔʊmə] *n* Rhabdo(myo)sarkom *nt*.
Rhab·do·vir·i·dae [ˌ-'vɪrɪdiː] *pl micro.* Rhabdoviridae *pl*, Rhabdoviren *pl*.
rhab·do·vi·rus [ˌ-'vaɪrəs] *n micro.* Rhabdovirus *nt*.
rhae·bo·cra·nia [ˌriːbəʊ'kreɪnɪə] *n ortho.* Schiefhals *m*, Torticollis *m*.
rhag·a·des ['rægədiːz] *pl* Hautschrunden *pl*, Hautfissuren *pl*, Rhagaden *pl*.
rha·gad·i·form [rə'gædɪfɔːrm] *adj* rhagadenähnlich, -förmig.
rhag·i·o·crine cell ['reɪdʒɪəkrɪn] → reticuloendothelial cell.
(L-)rham·nose ['ræmnəʊz] *n* Isodulcit *nt*, (L-)Rhamnose *f*, 6-Desoxy-L-mannose *f*.
rham·no·side ['ræmnəsaɪd] *n* Rhamnosid *nt*.
Rh antibodies Rh-Antikörper *pl*, Rhesus--Antikörper *pl*.
Rh antigen Rh-Antigen *nt*, Rhesus-Antigen *nt*.
rha·phe ['reɪfɪ] *n* → raphe.
rheg·ma ['regmə] *n* Riß *m*, Fissur *f*, Bruch *f*.
rhe·ni·um ['riːnɪəm] *n abbr.* **Re** Rhenium *nt* *abbr.* Re.
rheo- *pref.* Fluß-, Rheo-.
rhe·o·base ['riːəbeɪs] *n phys.*, *physiol.* Rheobase *f*.
rhe·o·car·di·og·ra·phy [ˌ-ˌkɑːrdɪ'ɒgrəfɪ] *n* Rheokardiographie *f*.
rhe·o·cord [ˌ-kɔːrd] *n* Rheostat *m*.
rhe·o·en·ceph·a·lo·gram [ˌ-en'sefələgræm] *n* Rheoenzephalogramm *nt*.
rhe·o·en·ceph·a·log·ra·phy [ˌ-ˌensefə'lɒgrəfɪ] *n* Rheoenzephalographie *f abbr.* REG.
rhe·o·gram ['-græm] *n* Rheogramm *nt*.
rhe·og·ra·phy [rɪ'ɒgrəfɪ] *n* Rheographie *f*.
rhe·ol·o·gy [rɪ'ɒlədʒɪ] *n* Fließlehre *f*, Rheologie *f*.
rhe·om·e·ter [rɪ'ɒmɪtər] *n* **1.** Rheometer *nt*. **2.** Galvanometer *nt*.
rhe·om·e·try [ˌ-'ɒmətrɪ] *n* Rheometrie *f*.
rhe·o·pex·y ['riːəpeksɪ] *n* Rheopexie *f*, Dilatanz *f*.
rhe·o·stat ['-stæt] *n* Rheostat *m*.
rhe·os·to·sis [ˌriːɒs'tɔʊsɪs] *n ortho.*, *radiol.* Rheostose *f*, Melorheostose *f*.
rhe·o·tach·y·gra·phy [ˌriːətæ'kɪgrəfɪ] *n* Rheotachygraphie *f*.
rhe·o·tac·tic [ˌ-'tæktɪk] *adj* Rheotaxis betr., mittel Rheotaxis, rheotaktisch.

rhe·o·tax·is [ˌ-'tæksɪs] *n* Bewegung *f* in einem Flüssigkeitsstrom, Rheotaxis *f*.
rhe·ot·ro·pism [riː'ɒtrəpɪzəm] *n* Rheotropismus *m*.
rhe·sus antibodies ['riːsəs] Rh-Antikörper *pl*, Rhesus-Antikörper *pl*.
rhesus antigen Rh-Antigen *nt*, Rhesus--Antigen *nt*.
rhesus factor *abbr.* **Rh** Rhesusfaktor *m abbr.* Rh.
rhesus monkey Rhesusaffe *m*.
rhesus system Rhesussystem *nt*, Rh-System *nt*.
rheum [ruːm] *n* wäßrige *od.* seröse Flüssigkeit *f*, Schleim *m*.
rheu·ma ['ruːmə] *n* → rheum.
rheu·ma·py·ra [ˌruːmə'paɪrə] *n* → rheumatic fever.
rheu·mar·thri·tis [ˌruːmɑːr'θraɪtɪs] *n* → rheumatoid arthritis.
rheu·ma·tal·gia [ˌruːmə'tældʒɪə] *n* (chronischer) Rheumaschmerz *m*, (chronische) Rheumaschmerzen *pl*.
rheu·mat·ic [ruː'mætɪk] **I** *n* Rheumatiker(in *f*) *m*. **II** *adj* auf Rheumatismus beruhend, an Rheumatismus leidend, rheumatisch, Rheuma-.
  rheumatic aortitis rheumatische Aortitis *f*, Aortitis rheumatica.
  rheumatic arteritis rheumatische Arteriitis *f*, Arteriitis rheumatica.
  rheumatic arthritis, acute → rheumatic fever.
  rheumatic carditis rheumatische Karditis *f*, Carditis rheumatica.
  rheumatic chorea Sydenham-Chorea *f*, Chorea minor (Sydenham), Chorea juvenilis/rheumatica/infectiosa/simplex.
  rheumatic disease rheumatische Erkrankung *f*, Erkrankung *f* des rheumatischen Formenkreises, Rheumatismus *m*, Rheuma *nt*.
  rheumatic endocarditis rheumatische Endokarditis *f*, Bouillaud'-Krankheit *f*.
  rheumatic fever *abbr.* **RF** rheumatisches Fieber *nt abbr.* RF, Febris rheumatica, akuter Gelenkrheumatismus *m*, Polyarthritis rheumatica acuta.
  rheumatic gout → rheumatoid arthritis.
  rheumatic myocarditis rheumatische Myokarditis *f*, Myocarditis rheumatica.
  rheumatic neuritis rheumatische Neuritis *f*.
  rheumatic nodule Rheumaknötchen *nt*, Nodulus rheumaticus.
  rheumatic pericarditis rheumatische Herzbeutelentzündung/Perikarditis *f*, Pericarditis rheumatica.
  rheumatic polyarthritis, acute → rheumatic fever.
  rheumatic scar rheumatische Narbe *f*.
  rheumatic scoliosis *ortho.* rheumatische Skoliose *f*.
  rheumatic valvulitis → rheumatic endocarditis.
rheu·ma·tid ['ruːmətɪd] *n* Rheumatid *n*.
rheu·ma·tism ['ruːmətɪzəm] *n* → rheumatic diesase.
rheu·ma·tis·mal [ˌ-'tɪzməl] *adj* → rheumatic.
rheu·ma·to·ce·lis [ˌruːmətəʊ'siːlɪs] *n* Schoenlein-Henoch-Syndrom *nt*, (anaphylaktoide) Purpura Schoenlein--Henoch *f*, rheumatoide/athrombopenische Purpura *f*, Immunkomplexpurpura *f*, -vaskulitis *f*, Purpura anaphylactoides (Schoenlein-Henoch), Purpura rheumatica (Schoenlein-Henoch).
rheu·ma·to·gen·ic [ˌ-'dʒenɪk] *adj* Rheumatismus verursachend, rheumatogen.
rheu·ma·toid ['ruːmətɔɪd] *adj* **1.** rheuma-

rheumatoid arthritis

ähnlich, rheumatoid, Rheuma-. **2.** → rheumatic.
rheumatoid arthritis *abbr.* RA rheumatoide Arthritis *f*, progrediente/primär chronische Polyarthritis *f* *abbr.* PCP, PcP.
  juvenile r. juvenile Form *f* der chronischen Polyarthritis, Morbus Still *m*, Still-Syndrom *nt*, Chauffard-Ramon-Still-Krankheit *f*.
rheumatoid arthritis test Rheumatest *m*.
rheumatoid disease Rheumatoid *nt*, rheumatoide Erkrankung *f*.
rheumatoid factor latex agglutination test Latex-Rheumafaktor-Test *m*.
rheumatoid factors *abbr.* RF Rheumafaktoren *pl abbr.* RF.
rheumatoid nodule → rheumatic nodule.
rheumatoid pneumoconiosis Caplan-Syndrom *nt*, Caplan-Colinet-Petry-Syndrom *nt*, Silikoarthritis *f*.
rheumatoid spondylitis Bechterew-Krankheit *f*, Morbus Bechterew *m*, Bechterew-Strümpell-Marie-Krankheit *f*, Marie-Strümpell-Krankheit *f*, Spondylarthritis/Spondylitis ankylopoetica/ankylosans.
rheumatoid synovitis rheumatoide Synovitis *f*.
rheumatoid torticollis rheumatischer Schiefhals/Torticollis *m*.
rheumatoid wryneck → rheumatoid torticollis.
rheu·ma·tol·o·gist [ˌruːməˈtalədʒɪst] *n* Rheumatologe *m*, -login *f*.
rheu·ma·tol·o·gy [ˌ-ˈtalədʒɪ] *n* Rheumatologie *f*.
rheu·ma·to·py·ra [ˌruːmətəʊˈpaɪrə] *n* → rheumatic fever.
rheum·ic [ˈruːmɪk] *adj* → rheumy.
rheum·y [ˈruːmɪ] *adj* Schnupfen hervorrufen, verschnupft; katarrhalisch; *(Augen)* (vom Schnupfen) wäßrig u. gerötet.
rhex·is [ˈreksɪs] *n*, *pl* **rhex·es** [ˈreksiːz] Zerreißen *nt*, Zerreißung *f*, Riß *m*, Rhexis *f*.
Rh factor → rhesus factor.
rhi·go·sis [rɪˈgəʊsɪs] *n* Kaltempfindung *f*, -empfindsamkeit *f*.
rhin- *pref.* → rhino-.
rhi·nal [ˈraɪnl] *adj* Nase betr., nasal, Nasen-, Naso-, Rhino-.
rhin·al·gia [raɪˈnældʒɪə] *n* Nasenschmerz(en *pl*) *m*, Rhinalgie *f*, Rhinodynie *f*.
rhin·al·ler·go·sis [ˌraɪnælərˈgəʊsɪs] *n* allergische Rhinitis/Rhinopathie *f*, Rhinitis/Rhinopathia allergica, Rhinallergose *f*.
rhinal sulcus Sulcus rhinalis.
Rh incompatibility Rhesus-Blutgruppenunverträglichkeit *f*, Rhesus-Inkompatibilität *f*, Rh-Inkompatibilität *f*.
rhin·e·de·ma [raɪnɪˈdiːmə] *n* Ödem *nt* der Nasenschleimhaut, Nasenschleimhautödem *nt*.
rhin·en·ce·pha·lia [ˌraɪnɛnsɪˈfeɪljə] *n* → rhinocephaly.
rhin·en·ceph·a·lon [ˌraɪnɛnˈsefələn] *n*, *pl* **-lons**, **-la** [-lə] Riechhirn *nt*, Rhinenzephalon *nt*, Rhinencephalon *nt*.
rhin·en·ceph·a·lus [ˌ-ˈsefələs] *n* → rhinocephalus.
rhin·en·chy·sis [raɪˈnɛnkəsɪs] *n* Nasendusche *f*.
rhin·es·the·sia [ˌraɪnɛsˈθiːʒə] *n* Geruchssinn *m*.
rhi·ni·tis [raɪˈnaɪtɪs] *n* Nasenschleimhautentzündung *f*, Rhinitis *f*; Schnupfen *m*, Nasenkatarrh *m*, Koryza *f*, Coryza *f*.
rhino- *pref.* Nasen-, Naso-, Rhin(o)-.
rhi·no·an·tri·tis [ˌraɪnəʊænˈtraɪtɪs] *n* HNO Entzündung *f* von Nasen- u. Kieferhöhle(n).

rhi·no·by·on [raɪˈnəʊbɪən] *n* HNO Nasentampon *m*.
rhi·no·ce·pha·lia [ˌraɪnəʊsɪˈfeɪljə] *n* → rhinocephaly.
rhi·no·ceph·a·lus [ˌ-ˈsefələs] *n* embryo. Rhinencephalus *m*, Rhinenzephalus *m*.
rhi·no·ceph·a·ly [ˌ-ˈsefəlɪ] *n* embryo. Rhinozephalie *f*, Rhinenzephalie *f*.
rhi·no·chei·lo·plas·ty [ˌ-ˈkaɪləplæstɪ] *n* HNO Lippen-Nasen-Plastik *f*.
rhi·no·chi·lo·plas·ty *n* → rhinocheiloplasty.
rhi·no·clei·sis [ˌ-ˈklaɪsɪs] *n* → rhinostenosis.
rhi·no·dac·ry·o·lith [ˌ-ˈdækrɪəlɪθ] *n* Rhinodakryolith *m*.
rhi·no·dyn·ia [ˌ-ˈdiːnɪə] *n* Nasenschmerz(en *pl*) *m*, Rhinodynie *f*, Rhinalgie *f*.
rhi·no·en·to·moph·tho·ro·my·co·sis [ˌ-ˌentəʊˌmafθərəʊmaɪˈkəʊsɪs] *n* → rhinophycomycosis.
Rhin·oes·trus [raɪnˈestrəs] *n* micro. Rhinoestrus *f*.
rhi·no·gen·ic [ˌraɪnəˈdʒɛnɪk] *adj* → rhinogenous.
rhi·nog·e·nous [raɪˈnadʒənəs] *adj* von der Nase ausgehend, rhinogen.
rhinogenous headache rhinogener Kopfschmerz *m*.
rhi·no·la·lia [ˌraɪnəʊˈleɪlɪə] *n* näselnde Sprache *f*, Näseln *nt*, Rhinolalie *f*, Rhinolalia *f*.
rhinolalia aperta offenes Näseln *nt*, Rhinophasie *f*, Rhinophasia *f*, Rhinolalia aperta.
rhinolalia clausa geschlossenes Näseln *nt*, Hyporhinolalie *f*, Rhinolalia clausa.
rhi·no·lar·yn·gi·tis [ˌ-ˌlærɪnˈdʒaɪtɪs] *n* HNO Nasen-Rachen-Katarrh *m*, Rhinolaryngitis *f*.
rhi·no·lar·yn·gol·o·gy [ˌ-ˌlærɪnˈgalədʒɪ] *n* Rhinolaryngologie *f*.
rhi·no·lite [ˈ-laɪt] *n* → rhinolith.
rhi·no·lith [ˈ-lɪθ] *n* Nasenstein *m*, Rhinolith *m*.
rhi·no·li·thi·a·sis [ˌ-lɪˈθaɪəsɪs] *n* HNO Rhinolithiasis *f*.
rhi·nol·o·gist [raɪˈnalədʒɪst] *n* Rhinologe *m*, -login *f*.
rhi·nol·o·gy [raɪˈnalədʒɪ] *n* Nasenheilkunde *f*, Rhinologie *f*.
rhi·no·ma·nom·e·ter [ˌraɪnəməˈnamɪtər] *n* Rhinomanometer *nt*.
rhi·no·ma·nom·e·try [ˌ-məˈnamətrɪ] *n* Rhinomanometrie *f*, Rhinorheographie *f*.
rhi·no·mu·cor·my·co·sis [ˌ-ˌmjuːkərmaɪˈkəʊsɪs] *n* → rhinophycomycosis.
rhi·no·my·co·sis [ˌ-maɪˈkəʊsɪs] *n* Pilzerkrankung *f* der Nase(nschleimhaut), Rhinomykose *f*.
rhi·no·ne·cro·sis [ˌ-nɪˈkrəʊsɪs] *n* Nekrose *f* der Nasenknochen.
rhi·no·path·ia [ˌ-ˈpæθɪə] *n* → rhinopathy.
rhi·nop·a·thy [raɪˈnapəθɪ] *n* Nasenerkrankung *f*, Rhinopathie *f*, -pathia *f*.
rhi·no·pha·ryn·ge·al [ˌraɪnəʊfəˌrɪnˈdʒɪəl] *adj* Nasopharynx betr., nasopharyngeal, Nasopharyngeal-.
rhi·no·phar·yn·gi·tis [ˌ-ˌfærɪnˈdʒaɪtɪs] *n* Nasopharynxentzündung *f*, Rhinopharyngitis *f*.
rhi·no·pha·ryn·go·cele [ˌ-fəˈrɪŋgəsiːl] *n* Rhinopharyngocele *f*.
rhi·no·pha·ryn·go·lith [ˌ-fəˈrɪŋgəlɪθ] *n* Rhinopharyngolith *m*.
rhi·no·phar·ynx [ˌ-ˈfærɪŋks] *n* Nasenrachen *m*, Epi-, Naso-, Rhinopharynx *m*, Pars nasalis pharyngis.
rhi·no·pho·nia [ˌ-ˈfəʊnɪə] *n* **1.** → rhinolalia. **2.** → rhinolalia aperta.
rhi·no·phy·co·my·co·sis [ˌ-ˌfaɪkəʊmaɪˈkəʊsɪs] *n* Entomophthorose *f*, Entomophthora-Phykomykose *f*, Rhinophykomykose *f*.
rhi·no·phy·ma [ˌ-ˈfaɪmə] *n* Kartoffel-, Säufer-, Pfund-, Knollennase *f*, Rhinophym *nt*, Rhinophyma *nt*.
rhi·no·plas·tic [ˌ-ˈplæstɪk] *adj* Nasenplastik betr., rhinoplastisch.
rhi·no·plas·ty [ˌ-ˈplæstɪ] *n* HNO Nasen-, Rhinoplastik *f*.
rhi·no·pol·y·pus [ˌ-ˈpalɪpəs] *n* Nasenpolyp *m*.
rhi·nor·rha·gia [ˌ-ˈreɪdʒ(ɪ)ə] *n* (starkes) Nasenbluten *nt*, Rhinorrhagie *f*, Epistaxis *f*.
rhi·nor·rha·phy [raɪˈnɔrəfɪ] *n* HNO Rhinorrhaphie *f*.
rhi·nor·rhea [ˌraɪnəˈrɪə] *n* Nasen(aus)fluß *m*, Rhinorrhoe *f*.
rhi·no·sal·pin·gi·tis [ˌ-ˌsælpɪnˈdʒaɪtɪs] *n* Rhinosalpingitis *f*.
rhi·no·scle·ro·ma [ˌ-sklɪˈrəʊmə] *n* Rhinosklerom *nt*.
rhi·no·scope [ˈ-skəʊp] *n* HNO Nasenspiegel *m*, -spekulum *nt*, Rhinoskop *nt*.
rhi·no·scop·ic [ˌ-ˈskapɪk] *adj* Rhinoskopie betr., rhinoskopisch.
rhi·nos·co·py [raɪˈnaskəpɪ] *n* HNO Nasen(höhlen)spiegelung *f*, Rhinoskopie *f*, -scopia *f*.
rhi·no·spo·rid·i·o·sis [ˌraɪnəʊspəˌrɪdɪˈəʊsɪs] *n* Rhinosporidiose *f*.
Rhi·no·spo·rid·i·um seeberi [ˌ-spəˈrɪdɪəm] *micro.* Rhinosporidium seeberi.
rhi·no·ste·no·sis [ˌ-stɪˈnəʊsɪs] *n* Verlegung/Obstruktion *f* der Nasenwege, Rhinostenose *f*.
rhi·not·o·my [raɪˈnatəmɪ] *n* HNO Rhinotomie *f*.
rhi·no·tra·che·i·tis [ˌraɪnəʊˌtreɪkɪˈaɪtɪs] *n* Rhinotracheitis *f*.
rhi·no·vi·ral [ˌ-ˈvaɪrəl] *adj* Rhinoviren betr., Rhinovirus-, Rhinoviren-.
rhi·no·vi·rus [ˌ-ˈvaɪrəs] *n* micro. Rhinovirus *nt*.
Rhi·pi·cen·tor [ˌraɪpɪˈsentər] *n* micro. Rhipicentor *m*.
Rhi·pi·ceph·a·lus [ˌ-ˈsefələs] *n* micro. Rhipicephalus *m*.
rhiz(o)- *pref.* Wurzel-, Rhiz(o)-.
Rhi·zo·bi·a·ce·ae [raɪˌzəʊbɪˈeɪsɪˌiː] *pl micro.* Rhizobiaceae *pl*.
Rhi·zo·bi·um [raɪˈzəʊbɪəm] *n* micro. Rhizobium *nt*.
Rhi·zog·ly·phus [raɪˈzaglɪfəs] *n* micro. Rhizoglyphus *m*.
rhi·zoid [ˈraɪzɔɪd] **I** *n* Rhizoid *nt*. **II** *adj* wurzelähnlich, rhizoid.
rhi·zoi·dal [raɪˈzɔɪdl] *adj* → rhizoid II.
rhi·zol·y·sis [raɪˈzalɪsɪs] *n* neurochir. Rhizolyse *f*.
rhi·zome [ˈraɪzəʊm] *n* bio. Wurzelstock *m*, Rhizoma *nt*.
rhi·zo·mel·ic [ˌraɪzəˈmelɪk] *adj* rhizomel(isch).
rhizomelic dwarf rhizomel(isch)er Zwerg *m*.
rhizomelic spondylosis → rheumatoid spondylitis.
rhi·zo·me·nin·go·my·e·li·tis [ˌ-mɪˌnɪŋgəʊmaɪəˈlaɪtɪs] *n* Radikulomeningomyelitis *f*.
rhi·zo·neure [ˈ-n(j)ʊər, -nʊr] *n* Rhizoneuron *n*.
rhi·zo·plast [ˈ-plæst] *n* Rhizoplast *m*.
Rhi·zo·po·da [raɪˈzapədə] *pl bio.* Wurzelfüßler *pl*, Rhizopoden *pl*, Rhizopoda *pl*.
Rhi·zo·po·di·um [ˌraɪzəˈpəʊdɪəm] *n bio.* Wurzelfüßchen *nt*, Rhizopodium *nt*.
Rhi·zo·pus [ˈ-pəs] *n* micro. Wurzelkopfschimmel *m*, Rhizopus *m*.
rhi·zot·o·my [raɪˈzatəmɪ] *n* neurochir. Rhizotomie *f*, Rhizotomia *f*, Radikulotomie *f*.

rhod- pref. → rhodo-.
rho·da·mine ['rəʊdəmiːn, -mɪn, rəʊ'dæm-ɪn] n Rhodamin nt.
rho·da·nate ['rəʊdəneɪt] n Rhodanat nt, Thiozyanat nt.
rho·dan·ic acid [rəʊ'dænɪk] 1. Thiozyansäure f. 2. → rhodanine.
rho·da·nine ['rəʊd(ə)niːn, rəʊ'dænɪn] n Rhodanin nt.
Rho·de·sian [rəʊ'diːʒən]: **R. fever** East--Coast-Fieber nt, bovine Piroplasmose/Theileriose f.
 R. redwater fever → R. fever.
 R. sleeping sickness → R. trypanosomiasis.
 R. tick fever → R. fever.
 R. trypanosomiasis ostafrikanische Schlafkrankheit/Trypanosomiasis f.
rho·di·um ['rəʊdɪəm] n abbr. **Rh** Rhodium nt abbr. Rh.
Rhod·ni·us pro·lix·us ['rɒdnɪəs prəʊ'lɪksəs] micro. venezolanische Schreitwanze f, Rhodnius prolixus.
rhodo- pref. Rot-, Rhod(o)-.
rho·do·gen·e·sis [ˌrəʊdəʊ'dʒenəsɪs] n physiol. Rhodogenese f.
rho·dop·sin [rəʊ'dɒpsɪn] n Sehpurpur nt, Rhodopsin nt.
rhodopsin-retinin cycle Rhodopsin-Retinin-Zyklus m.
Rho·do·tor·u·la [ˌrəʊdəʊ'tɔr(j)ələ, -'tɑr-] pl micro. rote Hefen pl, Rhodotorula pl.
rhom·ben·ce·phal·ic [ˌrɒmbənsɪ'fælɪk] adj Rautenhirn/Rhombencephalon betr., rhombenzephalisch.
rhombencephalic isthmus embryo. Isthmus rhombencephali.
rhom·ben·ceph·a·lon [ˌrɒmbən'sefələn] n, pl **-lons, -la** [-lə] Rautenhirn nt, Rhombenzephalon nt, Rhomencephalon nt.
rhombencephalon vesicle Rautenhirnbläschen nt.
rhom·bic ['rɒmbɪk] adj → rhomboid II.
rhombic lip embryo. Rautenlippe f.
rhom·boid ['rɒmbɔɪd] **I** n mathe. Rhomboid nt. **II** adj Rhombus od. Rhomboid betr., rauten-, rhombenförmig, rhombisch, rhomboidisch, Rauten-.
rhom·boi·dal [rɒm'bɔɪdl] adj → rhomboid II.
rhomboidal nucleus Rautenkern m des Thalamus, Nc. rhomboidalis (thalami).
rhom·boi·de·us major (muscle) [rɒm'bɔɪdɪəs] Rhomboideus m major, M. rhomboideus major.
rhomboideus minor (muscle) Rhomboideus m minor, M. rhomboideus minor.
rhomboid fossa Rautengrube f, Fossa rhomboidea.
rhomboid impression of clavicle Impressio lig. costoclavicularis.
rhomboid ligament: r. of clavicle Lig. costoclaviculare.
 r. of wrist Lig. radiocarpeum dorsale.
rhomboid muscle: greater r. → rhomboideus major (muscle).
 lesser r. → rhomboideus minor (muscle).
rhomboid muscle flap chir. Musculus--rhomboideus-Lappen m.
rhom·bus ['rɒmbəs] n, pl **-bus·es, -bi** [-baɪ] Raute f, Rhombus m.
rhon·chal ['rɒŋkəl] adj Rhonchus betr.
rhonchal fremitus Bronchialfremitus m, Fremitus bronchialis.
rhon·chi·al ['rɒŋkɪəl] adj Rhonchus betr.
rhon·chus ['rɒŋkəs] n, pl **-chi** [-kaɪ, -kiː] (Rassel-)Geräusch nt, Rhonchus m.
rho·ta·cism ['rəʊtəsɪzəm] n Rhotazismus m.
RHS abbr. [reticulohistiocytic system] → reticuloendothelial system.
Rh system → rhesus system.

Rhus ['rʌs, 'ruːs] n Rhus m.
rhus dermatitis Rhusdermatitis f.
rhythm ['rɪðəm] n **1.** Rhythmus m; Takt m. **2.** physiol. Pulsschlag m, -folge f; Menstruations-, Monatszyklus m.
rhythm-generating adj rhythmusbildend.
rhyth·mic ['rɪðmɪk] adj gleichmäßig, regelmäßig, rhythmisch.
rhyth·mi·cal ['rɪðmɪkl] adj → rhythmic.
rhythmical nystagmus Rucknystagmus m.
rhythm-inhibiting adj rhythmushemmend.
rhythm·less ['rɪðəmlɪs] adj ohne Rhythmus, unrhythmisch; arhythmisch, arrhythmisch.
rhythm method (Kontrazeption) Knaus--Ogino-Methode f.
rhyth·mo·gen·e·sis [ˌrɪðmə'dʒenəsɪs] n Rhythmusbildung f, -entstehung f, Rhythmogenese f.
rhyt·i·dec·to·my [rɪtɪ'dektəmɪ] n chir. Face--Lifting f, Rhytidektomie f.
rhyt·i·do·plas·ty ['rɪtɪdəʊplæstɪ] n → rhytidectomy.
RIA abbr. → radioimmunoassay.
rib [rɪb] n Rippe f; anat. Costa f.
Ribas-Torres ['riːbəs 'tɔːrez]: **R.-T. disease** Milchpocken pl, weiße Pocken/Blattern pl, Alastrim nt, Variola minor.
ri·ba·vi·rin [ˌraɪbə'vaɪrɪn, ˌrɪb-] n pharm. Ribavirin nt, Virazol nt.
rib·bon ['rɪbən] n Band nt, Strang m; Streifen m.
ribbon-like keratitis bandförmige Keratitis f.
rib cage Brustkorb m, (knöcherner) Thorax m.
rib cartilage Rippenknorpel m, Cartilago costalis.
 slipping r. Subluxation f eines Rippenknorpels.
rib elevator (muscle) Levator m costae, M. levator costae.
rib fracture Rippenbruch m, -fraktur f.
 multiple r.s Rippenserienfraktur f.
rib hump ortho. Rippenbuckel m.
ri·bi·tol ['raɪbətɒl, -təʊl] n Ribitol nt, Ribit nt.
ribitol teichoic acid Ribitolteichonsäure f.
ri·bo·fla·vin [ˌraɪbəʊ'fleɪvɪn, ˌrɪb-] n Ribo-, Laktoflavin nt, Vitamin B_2 nt.
riboflavin deficiency Ariboflavinose(-Syndrom nt) f.
riboflavin kinase Riboflavinkinase f.
riboflavin-5'-phosphate n Flavinmononukleotid nt abbr. FMN, Riboflavin-(5'-)-phosphat nt.
ri·bo·nu·cle·ase [ˌ-'n(j)uːklɪeɪz] n abbr. **RNase** Ribonuklease f, -nuclease f abbr. RNase (f).
ribonuclease I alkalische Ribonuklease f, Pankreasribonuklease f.
ri·bo·nu·cle·ic acid [ˌ-nəʊ'kliːɪk] abbr. **RNA** Ribonukleinsäure f abbr. RNA, RNS.
 activator r. Aktivator-RNA f, Aktivator--RNS f.
 double-stranded r. abbr. **dsRNA** Doppelstrang-RNA f abbr. dsRNA, Doppelstrang-RNS f abbr. dsRNS.
 heterogenous nuclear r. abbr. **hnRNA** heterogene Kern-RNA f abbr. hnRNA, heterogene Kern-RNS f.
 informational r. → messenger r.
 initiator t r. Initiator-tRNA f, Starter--tRNA f.
 messenger r. abbr. **mRNA** Boten-RNA f, Matrizen-RNA f abbr. mRNA, Boten--RNS f, Matrizen-RNS f abbr. mRNS.
 nuclear r. abbr. **nRNA** Kern-RNA f abbr. nRNA, Kern-RNS f.
 priming r. Starter-RNA f, Starter-RNS f, priming-RNA.

ribosomal r. abbr. **rRNA** ribosomale RNA f, ribosomale RNS f, Ribosomen--RNA f abbr. rRNA, Ribosomen-RNS f.
 soluble r. → transfer r.
 template r. → messenger r.
 transfer r. abbr. **tRNA** Transfer-RNA f abbr. tRNA, Transfer-RNS f.
 viral r. Virus-RNA f, Virus-RNS f, virale RNA f, virale RNS f.
ri·bo·nu·cle·o·pro·tein [ˌ-ˌn(j)uːklɪəʊ-'prəʊtiːn, -tiːn] n Ribonukleoprotein nt.
ri·bo·nu·cle·o·side [ˌ-'n(j)uːklɪəsaɪd] n Ribonukleosid nt, -nucleosid nt.
ribonucleoside 2',3'-cyclic phosphate zyklisches Ribonukleosid-2',3'-phosphat nt.
ribonucleoside diphosphate reductase Ribonukleosiddiphosphatreduktase f, RDP-Reduktase f, Ribonukleotidreduktase f.
ribonucleoside monophosphate Ribonukleosidmonophosphat nt.
ribonucleoside-2'-phosphate n Ribonukleosid-2'-phosphat nt.
ribonucleoside-3'-phosphate n Ribonukleosid-3'-phosphat nt.
ri·bo·nu·cle·o·tide [ˌ-'n(j)uːklɪətaɪd] n Ribonukleotid nt, -nucleotid nt.
ribonucleotide reductase → ribonucleoside diphosphate reductase.
ri·bo·py·ra·nose [ˌ-'paɪrənəʊz] n Ribopyranose f.
ri·bose ['raɪbəʊs] n Ribose f.
ribose nucleic acid → ribonucleic acid.
ribose-5-phosphate n Ribose-5-phosphat nt.
ribose(-5-)phosphate isomerase Ribosephosphatisomerase f, Phosphoriboisomerase f.
ribose-phosphate pyrophosphokinase Ribosephosphatpyrophosphokinase f, Phosphoribosylpyrophosphatsynthetase f.
ri·bo·so·mal [ˌraɪbə'səʊml] adj Ribosom(en) betr., ribosomal, Ribosomen-.
ribosomal apparatus histol. Ribosomenapparat m, ribosomaler Apparat m.
ribosomal RNA abbr. **rRNA** ribosomale RNA f, ribosomale RNS f, Ribosomen--RNA f abbr. rRNA, Ribosomen-RNS f.
ri·bo·some ['-səʊm] n Ribosom nt, Palade--Granula pl.
ri·bo·su·ria [ˌ-'s(j)ʊərɪə] n erhöhte Riboseausscheidung f im Harn, Ribosurie f.
ri·bo·syl ['-sɪl] n Ribosyl(-Radikal) nt.
5-ri·bo·syl·u·ri·dine [ˌ-sɪl'jʊərɪdiːn, -dɪn] n Pseudouridin nt abbr. ψ.
ri·bo·thy·mi·dyl·ic acid [ˌ-ˌθaɪmə'dɪlɪk] Ribothymidylsäure f.
ri·bo·vi·rus [ˌ-'vaɪrəs] n → RNA virus.
rib prominence ortho. Rippenbuckel m.
rib rudiment Rippenrest m, -rudiment nt.
rib shears chir. Rippenresektionsschere f.
rib spreader chir. Rippensprenger m, -sperrer m.
ri·bu·lose ['raɪbjəʊz] n Ribulose f.
ribulose diphosphate carboxydismutase Ribulosediphosphatcarboxydismutase f.
ribulose diphosphate carboxylase Ribulosediphosphatcarboxylase f.
ribulose-5-phosphate n Ribulose-5-phosphat nt.
ribulose-phosphate 3-epimerase Ribulosephosphat-3-epimerase f.
Ricard [ri'kɑːr]: **R.'s amputation** ortho. Fußamputation f nach Ricard, Ricard--Amputation f.
rice [raɪs] n Reis m.
rice agar Reisagar m/nt.
rice bodies Reiskörper(chen pl) pl, Corpora oryzoidea.
rice disease Beriberi f, Vitamin B_1-Man-

rice-field fever

gel(krankheit f) m, Thiaminmangel-(krankheit f) m.
rice-field fever Batavia-, Reisfeldfieber nt, Leptospirosis bataviae.
rice-water stools Reiswasserstühle pl.
rich [rɪtʃ] adj **1.** reich (in, with an); reichhaltig. **2.** schwer, nahrhaft, fett, kräftig; (Aroma) schwer, stark; (Farbe) kräftig, voll, satt; (Ton) voll, satt; (Stimme) voll, klangvoll. **3.** chem., techn. schwer, fett, reich.
Richard ['rɪtʃərd]: **R.'s fringes** Eileiterfransen pl, Fimbriae tubae.
Richet [ri'ʃe]: **R.'s aneurysm** fusiformes Aneurysma nt, Aneurysma fusiforme.
rich·ly-myelinated ['rɪtʃlɪ] adj myelin-, markreich.
Richner-Hanhart ['rɪtʃnər 'hænhɑːrt]: **R.-H. syndrome** Richner-Hanhart-Syndrom nt, Tyrosinaminotransferasemangel m, TAT-Mangel m.
rich·ness ['rɪtʃnɪs] n **1.** Reichtum m, Reichhaltigkeit f, Fülle f. **2.** Nahrhaftigkeit f; Gehalt m, Schwere f; Sattheit f; Klangfülle f. **3.** Gehalt m, Schwere f, Ergiebigkeit f.
Richter ['rɪktər, 'rɪçtər]: **R.'s hernia** Darmwandbruch m, Littré-Hernie f.
R.'s syndrome hema. Richter-Syndrom nt.
Richter-Monro [mən'roʊ]: **R.-M. line** Monro-Richter-Linie f.
ri·cin ['raɪsn, 'rɪ-] n Rizin nt, Ricin nt.
ric·in·ism ['rɪsənɪzəm] n Ricinvergiftung f, Rizinismus m.
ric·in·o·le·ic acid [ˌrɪsɪnoʊ'liːɪk, -'noʊliːɪk] Rizinolsäure f.
rick·ets ['rɪkɪts] pl Rachitis f.
rick·ett·se·mia [rɪkət'siːmɪə] n Rickettsiensepsis f.
Rick·ett·sia [rɪ'ketsɪə] n micro. Rickettsia f.
rick·ett·sia [rɪ'ketsɪə] n, pl **-si·ae** [-sɪˌiː] micro. Rickettsie f, Rickettsia f.
Rick·ett·si·a·ce·ae [rɪˌketsɪ'eɪsɪˌiː] pl micro. Rickettsiaceae pl.
Rick·ett·si·ae [rɪ'ketsɪˌiː] pl micro. Rickettsieae pl.
rick·ett·si·al [rɪ'ketsɪəl] adj Rickettsien betr., durch Rickettsien hervorgerufen, Rickettsien-.
rickettsial disease Rickettsieninfektion f, -erkrankung f, Rickettsiose f.
rickettsial endocarditis Rickettsienendokarditis f.
Rick·ett·si·a·les [rɪˌketsɪ'eɪlɪːz] pl micro. Rickettsiales f.
rickettsial infection → rickettsial disease.
rick·ett·si·al·pox [rɪ'ketsɪəlpɑks] pl Rickettsienpocken pl, Pockenfleckfieber nt.
rickettsial toxin Rickettsientoxin nt.
rick·ett·si·ci·dal [rɪˌketsɪ'saɪdl] adj rickettsien(ab)tötend, rickettsizid.
Rick·ett·si·e·ae [ˌrɪket'saɪəˌiː] pl micro. Rickettsieae pl.
rick·ett·si·o·sis [rɪˌketsɪ'oʊsɪs] n Rickettsienerkrankung f, -infektion f, Rickettsiose f.
rick·ett·si·o·stat·ic [rɪˌketsɪə'stætɪk] **I** n Rickettsiostatikum nt. **II** adj das Rickettsienwachstum hemmend, rickettsiostatisch.
rick·et·y ['rɪkətɪ] adj Rachitis betr., rachitisch.
RID abbr. [radial immunodiffusion] → radial diffusion method.
Rideal-Walker ['rɪdɪəl 'wɔːkər]: **R.-W. method** Rideal-Walker-Methode f.
R.-W. test Rideal-Walker-Test m.
rid·er's bone ['raɪdər] ortho. Reitknochen m.
rider's spur ortho. Reitersporn m.

riders' vertigo Bewegungs-, Reisekrankheit f, Kinetose f.
ridge [rɪdʒ] n (a. anat.) Kamm m, Grat m, Kante f, Rücken m; Leiste f, Wulst m.
r. of nose Nasenwall m, Agger nasi.
rid·ing embolus ['raɪdɪŋ] reitender Embolus m, Sattelembolus m.
Ridley ['rɪdlɪ]: **R.'s circles/sinuses** Sinus intercavernosi.
Rieckenberg ['riːkənbɜrɡ]: **R.'s test** Rieckenberg-Beladungsphänomen nt.
Riedel ['riːdl]: **R.'s disease** eisenharte Struma Riedel f, Riedel-Struma f, chronische hypertrophische Thyreoiditis f.
R.'s lobe (Leber) Riedel'-Lappen m.
R.'s struma/thyroiditis → R.'s disease.
Rieder ['riːdər]: **R.'s cell** hema. Rieder-Form f.
Rieger ['riːɡər]: **R.'s anomaly** ophthal. Rieger-Anomalie f.
R.'s syndrome Rieger-Syndrom nt.
Riehl [riːl]: **R.'s melanosis** Riehl-Melanose f, -Syndrom nt, Civatte-Krankheit f, Kriegsmelanose f, Melanosis toxica lichenoides.
Rieux [rjø]: **R.'s hernia** Rieux'-Hernie f, retrozäkale Hernie f.
rif·am·pi·cin ['rɪfæmpəsɪn] n pharm. Rifampizin nt, Rifampicin nt.
rif·am·pin ['rɪfæmpɪn] n → rifampicin.
rif·a·my·cin [rɪfə'maɪsɪn] n pharm. Rifamycin nt.
rif·o·my·cin n old → rifamycin.
Rift Valley fever [rɪft 'vælɪ] Rift-Valley-Fieber nt.
Rift Valley fever virus micro. Rift-Valley-Fieber-Virus nt.
RIG abbr. → rabies immune globulin, human.
Riga-Fede ['riːɡɑ 'fiːdɪ]: **R.-F. disease** Riga-Geschwür f, Fede-Riga-Geschwür nt.
Riggs [rɪɡs]: **R.' disease** Alveolarpyorrhoe f, Parodontitis marginalis.
right [raɪt] **I** n **1.** Recht nt; Anrecht nt, Anspruch m. **in the ~** im Recht. **of ~/by ~s** von Rechts wegen. **2.** das Richtige. **3.** rechte Seite f; rechte Hand f. **at/on/to the ~** rechts, auf der rechten Seite (of von). **II** adj **4.** richtig, recht; korrekt; wahr; geeignet; in Ordnung. **5.** rechte(r, s), Rechts-. **on/to the ~ side** rechts, rechter Hand. **6.** rechtwink(e)lig; (Linie) gerade; senkrecht. **III** adv **7.** rechts (from von; to nach); auf der rechten Seite. **8.** direkt, sofort, gerade(wegs); genau; richtig, korrekt. **IV** vi s. (wieder) aufrichten.
right-angled adj rechtwink(e)lig.
right atrium rechter (Herz-)Vorhof m, Atrium cordis dextrum.
right auricle/auricula of heart rechtes Herzohr nt, Auricula dextra.
right branch: r. of av-bundle rechter Tawara-Schenkel m, rechter Schenkel des His'-Bündels, Crus dextrum fasciculi atrioventricularis.
r. of portal vein Ramus dexter v. portae hepatis.
r. of proper hepatic artery A. hepatica propria-Ast m zum rechten Leberlappen, Ramus dexter a. hepaticae propriae.
right crus of diaphragm rechter Zwerchfellschenkel m, Crus dextrum diaphragmatis.
right duct of caudate lobe Ductus lobi caudati dexter.
right flexure of colon rechte Kolonflexur f, Flexura hepatica coli, Flexura coli dextra.
right-hand adj **1.** rechte(r, s), Rechts-; phys. rechtsdrehend. **2.** rechtshändig, mit der rechten Hand.
right-handed adj → right-hand 2.

right-handedness n Rechtshändigkeit f.
right-handed person Rechthänder(in f) m.
right-hander n Rechtshänder(in f) m.
right-hand side rechte Seite f.
right heart Rechtsherz nt, rechte Herzkammer f, rechter Ventrikel m.
right heart bypass HTG Rechtsbypass m.
right heart dilatation card. Rechtsherzdilatation f, rechtsventrikuläre Dilatation f.
right heart hypertrophy Rechts(herz)hypertrophie f, rechtsventrikuläre Hypertrophie f.
right hemicolectomy chir. rechtsseitige Hemikolektomie f.
right·ing reflex ['raɪtɪŋ] physiol. Stellreflex m.
right leg of av-bundle → right branch of av-bundle.
right lobe of liver rechter Leberlappen m, Lobus hepatis dexter.
right lung rechte Lunge f, rechter Lungenflügel m, Pulmo dexter.
right margin of uterus Margo uteri dexter.
right mesocolon Meso nt des aufsteigenden Kolons, Mesocolon ascendens.
right rotation Rechtsdrehung f.
right side Oberseite f, rechte Seite f.
right-to-left shunt card. Rechts-Links-Shunt m.
right trisegmentectomy chir. radikale Leberresektion f, Dreiviertelresektion f.
right ventricle of heart rechte Herzkammer f, rechter Ventrikel m, Ventriculus cordis dexter.
right ventricular dilatation → right heart dilatation.
right-ventricular failure Rechts(herz)insuffizienz f.
right ventricular hypertrophy → right heart hypertrophy.
right-ward ['raɪtwərd] adj nach rechts (gerichtet), Rechts-.
rightward shift Rechtsverschiebung f.
rig·id ['rɪdʒɪd] adj **1.** starr, steif, unbiegsam; unbeweglich, rigid(e). **2.** fig. streng, strikt, unbeugsam, rigid(e).
rigid bacteria micro. Bakterien pl mit starrer Zellwand.
ri·gid·i·ty [rɪ'dʒɪdətɪ] n **1.** Starre f, Starrheit f, Steifheit f, Unbiegsamkeit f, Rigidität f, Rigiditas f. **2.** fig. Strenge f, Härte f, Unnachgiebigkeit f, Unbeugsamkeit f, Rigidität f. **3.** psycho. Rigidität f. **4.** neuro. Rigor m, Rigidität f.
Rigler ['rɪɡlər]: **R.'s sign** radiol. Rigler'-Zeichen nt.
rig·or ['rɪɡər] n neuro. Rigor m, Rigidität f.
Riley-Day ['raɪlɪ deɪ]: **R.-D. syndrome** Riley-Day-Syndrom nt, Dysautonomie f.
rim [rɪm] **I** n Rand m, Kante f; (Brille) Fassung f. **II** vt (ein-)fassen, umranden.
ri·ma ['raɪmə] n, pl **-mae** [-miː] anat., bio. Ritze f, Spalt(e f) m, Furche f, Rima f.
ri·mal ['raɪməl] adj anat. Rima betr.
ri·man·ta·dine [raɪ'mæntədiːn] n pharm. Rimantadin nt.
rim·less ['rɪmlɪs] adj ohne Rand, randlos.
ri·mose ['raɪmoʊs, raɪ'moʊs] adj rissig, zerklüftet, furchig.
ri·mous ['raɪməs] adj → rimose.
rim·u·la ['rɪmjʊlə] n, pl **-lae** [-liː] kleinste Spalte f, kleinster Riß m.
Rindfleisch ['rɪntflaɪʃ]: **R.'s cell** old eosinophiler Granulozyt m, Eosinophiler m.
ring [rɪŋ] **I** n **1.** ring- od. kreisförmige Struktur f, Ring m, Kreis m; anat. A(n)nulus m. **to have (livid) ~s round one's eyes** (dunkle) Ringe unter den Augen haben. **2.** chem. Ring m, geschlossene od. kontinuierliche Kette f. **3.** techn. Ring m,

Öse *f*, Glied *nt*. **4.** *mathe*. Ringfläche *f*. **II** *vt* **5.** umkreisen, umgeben, umringen. **6.** einen Ring bilden aus.
ring about *vt* → ring 5.
ring around *vt* → ring 5.
ring bleeding Ringblutung *f*.
ring chromosome Ringchromosom *nt*.
ring compound *chem*. Ringverbindung *f*.
ringed [rɪŋd] *adj* **1.** ringförmig, Ring-. **2.** eingeschlossen, umringt. **3.** beringt.
ringed hairs Ringelhaare *pl*, Pili anulati.
Ringer ['rɪŋər]: **R.'s bicarbonate (solution)** Ringer-Bikarbonat(lösung *f*) *nt*.
 R.'s glucose (solution) Ringer-Glukose-(lösung *f*) *f*.
 R.'s irrigation Ringer-Lösung *f*.
 R.'s lactate (solution) Ringer-Laktat(lösung *f*) *nt*.
 R.'s mixture Ringer-Lösung *f*.
 R.'s solution Ringer-Lösung *f*.
ring finger Ringfinger *m*, Digitus anularis/quartus.
ring foramen For. obturatorium.
ring forceps *chir*. Ringfaßzange *f*.
ring hemorrhage → ring bleeding.
ring pessary *gyn*. Ringpessar *nt*.
ring precipitin test → ring test.
ring scotoma *ophthal*. Ringskotom *nt*.
ring test Ringtest *m*.
ring-worm ['rɪŋwɜrm] *n derm*. Tinea *f*; Trichophytie *f*, Trichophytia *f*.
 r. of the beard (tiefe) Bartflechte *f*, Tinea barbae, Trichophytia (profunda) barbae, *old* Sycosis (barbae) parasitaria.
 r. of the body oberflächliche Trichophytie *f* des Körpers, Tinea/Trichophytia/Epidermophytia corporis.
 r. of the face oberflächliche Tinea *f* des Gesichts, Tinea faciei.
 r. of the feet Athleten-, Sportlerfuß *m*, Fußpilz *m*, Fußpilzerkrankung *f*, Fußmykose *f*, Tinea *f* der Füße, Tinea/Epidermophytia pedis/pedum.
 r. of the genitocrural region Tinea inguinalis, Epidermophytia inguinalis, Eccema marginatum, Ekzema marginatum Hebra.
 r. of the groin → r. of the genitocrural region.
 r. of the hand Fadenpilzerkrankung/Tinea *f* der Hände, Tinea/Epidermophytia manus/manuum.
 r. of the nail Tinea *f* des Nagels, Nagel-, Onychomykose *f*, Onychomycosis *f*, Tinea unguium.
 r. of the scalp Tinea *f* der Kopfhaut, Tinea capitis/capillitii, Trichophytia capillitii.
Rinne ['rɪnə]: **R.'s test** *HNO, physiol*. Rinne-Test *m*, -Versuch *m*.
rinse [rɪns] **I** *n* (Aus-)Spülung *f*. **to give sth. a ~** etw. (ab-, aus-)spülen. **Have a ~ please!** (*beim Zahnarzt*) Bitte ausspülen. **II** *vt* (ab-, aus-, nach-)spülen. **to ~ one's hands** s. die Hände waschen.
rinse out *vt* (*Mund*) ausspülen.
rins-ing ['rɪnsɪŋ] **I** *n* **1.** (Aus-)Spülen *nt*, (Aus-)Spülung *f*. **2. ~s** *pl* Spülwasser *nt*. **II** *adj* (aus-)spülend, Spül-.
rinsing glands Spüldrüsen *pl*.
Riolan [riːoˈlɑ̃]: **R.'s anastomosis** *anat*. Riolan'-Anastomose *f*.
 R.'s arch Riolan'-Bogen *m*.
 R.'s muscle 1. M. cremaster. **2.** Riolan'-Muskel *m*.
ripe cataract [raɪp] reifer Star *m*, Cataracta matura.
RISA *abbr*. → radioiodinated serum albumin.
risk [rɪsk] *n* **1.** Risiko *nt*. **2.** Risiko *nt*, Gefahr *f*, Wagnis *nt*.
risk factor Risikofaktor *m*.

ri·so·ri·us (muscle) [rɪˈsɔːrɪəs] Lachmuskel *m*, Risorius *m*, M. risorius.
Risser ['rɪsər]: **R.'s jacket** *ortho*. Risser-Gipskorsett *nt*.
 R.'s operation *ortho*. Risser-Operation *f*, Skoliosekorrektur *f* nach Risser.
 R.'s technique → R.'s operation.
 R.'s wedging jacket → R.'s jacket.
Risser-Ferguson [ˈfɜrgəsən]: **R.-F. method** *ortho*. Ferguson-Methode *f*.
RIST *abbr*. → radioimmunosorbent test.
Ritgen ['rɪtgən]: **R.'s maneuver/method** *gyn*. Ritgen-Handgriff *m*.
rit·o·drine ['rɪtədriːn] *n pharm., gyn*. Ritodrin *nt*.
Ritter ['rɪtər]: **R.'s bougie** Ritter-Bougie *f*.
 R.'s disease 1. Ritter-Krankheit *f*, -Dermatitis *f*, Morbus Ritter von Rittershain *m*, Pemphigoid *nt* der Säuglinge, Syndrom *nt* der verbrühten Haut, staphylogenes Lyell-Syndrom *nt*, Dermatitis exfoliativa neonatorum, Epidermolysis toxica acuta. **2.** (medikamentöses) Lyell-Syndrom *nt*, Syndrom *nt* der verbrühten Haut, Epidermolysis acuta toxica, Epidermolysis necroticans combustiformis.
rit·u·al ['rɪtʃuːəl] *n psycho., psychia*. Ritual *nt*.
Rivalta [rɪˈvɑːltə]: **R.'s reaction/test** Rivalta-Probe *f*.
Riva-Rocci [ˈriːvə ˈrɔtʃi]: **R.-R. method** Riva-Rocci-Methode *f*, Blutdruckbestimmung *f* nach Riva-Rocci.
riv·er blindness ['rɪvər] Onchozerkose *f*, -cercose *f*, -cerciasis *f*, Knotenfilariose *f*, Onchocerca-volvulus-Infektion *f*.
riv·i·an incisure [rɪˈviːən] Inc. tympanica.
rivian notch Inc. tympanica.
Rivière [rɪˈvjɛːr]: **S.'s salt** Kaliumzitrat *nt*.
ri·vin·i·an foramen [rɪˈvɪnɪən] Inc. tympanica.
rivinian segment Inc. tympanica.
Rivinus [rɪˈviːnəs]: **canals of R.** Ductus sublinguales minores.
 R.' foramen Inc. tympanica.
 R.'s gland Unterzungen(speichel)drüse *f*, Gl. sublingualis.
 incisure of R. Inc. tympanica.
 notch of R. Inc. tympanica.
riz·i·form ['rɪzəfɔːrm] *adj* reiskornartig.
RKY *abbr*. → roentgenkymography.
RLF *abbr*. → retrolental fibroplasia.
RMSF *abbr*. → Rocky Mountain spotted fever.
R.N. *abbr*. → registered nurse.
Rn *abbr*. → radon.
RNA *abbr*. → ribonucleic acid.
RNA-containing virus *micro*. RNA-Virus *nt*.
RNA-directed DNA polymerase RNS-abhängige DNS-Polymerase *f*, RNA-abhängige DNA-Polymerase *f*, reverse Transkriptase *f abbr*. RT.
RNA-directed RNA polymerase RNS-abhängige RNS-Polymerase *f*, RNA-abhängige RNA-Polymerase *f*.
RNA nucleotidyltransferase DNA-abhängige RNA-Polymerase *f*, DNS-abhängige RNS-Polymerase *f*, Transkriptase *f*.
RNA polymerase RNA-Polymerase *f*, RNS-Polymerase *f*.
RNA primer RNA-primer *m*, RNA-Starterstrang *m*.
RNA-priming *n* RNA-priming *nt*.
RNA replicase → RNA-directed RNA polymerase.
RNase *abbr*. → ribonuclease.
RNA virus *micro*. RNA-Virus *nt*.
road traffic accident [rəʊd] *abbr*. **RTA** *Brit*. Verkehrsunfall *m*.

Robert ['rɑbərt]: **R.'s pelvis** Robert-Becken *nt*.
 R.'s syndrome Robert-Syndrom *nt*.
Robertson ['rɑbərtsən]: **R. pupil** Argyll-Robertson-Phänomen *nt*, -Zeichen *nt*, Robertson-Zeichen *nt*.
 R.'s sign 1. Robertson-Zeichen *nt*. **2.** → R. pupil.
rob·ert·son·i·an translocation [rɑbərtˈsoʊnɪən] *genet*. Robertson-Translokation *f*.
Robin [rɔˈbɛ̃]: **R.'s anomalad/syndrome** Robin-Syndrom *nt*, Pierre Robin-Syndrom *nt*.
Robinow ['rɑbɪnoʊ]: **R.'s dwarfism/syndrome** Robinow-Syndrom *nt*.
Robison ['rɑbɪsən]: **R. ester** Glukose-6-phosphat *nt abbr*. G-6-P, Robison-Ester *m*.
 R. ester dehydrogenase Glukose-6-phosphatdehydrogenase *f abbr*. G-6-PDH, GPP.
Robles ['rɑblz]: **R.' disease** → river blindness.
Robner ['rɑb(ə)nər]: **R.'s law 1.** Robner-Energiegesetz *nt*. **2.** Robner-Wachstumsgesetz *nt*.
rob·o·rant ['rɑbərənt, 'rəʊ-] **I** *n* Stärkungsmittel *nt*, Roborans *nt*, Roborantium *nt*. **II** *adj* stärkend.
ro·bo·vi·ru·ses [rəʊbəʊˈvaɪrəsəs] *pl micro*. durch Nager/Rodentia übertragene Viren *pl*, rodent-borne viruses *pl*.
Ro·cha·li·maea [ˌrəʊkəlaɪˈmiːə] *n micro*. Rochalimaea *f*.
Ro·chelle salt [rəʊˈʃel] Seignettesalz *nt*, Natrium-Kalium-Tartrat *nt*.
Rocher [rɔˈʃe]: **R.'s sign** *ortho*. Schubladenphänomen *nt*, -zeichen *nt*.
rock crystal [rɑk] Bergkristall *nt*.
rocker bottom flat foot ['rɑkər] → rocker bottom foot 2.
rocker bottom foot 1. Schaukelfuß *m*, angeborener konvexer Klumpfuß *m*. **2.** Schaukelfuß *m*, konvexer Knick-Plattfuß *m*.
Rockwell ['rɑkwel]: **R. hardness number** Rockwell-Härte *f*.
Rocky-Davis ['rɑki 'deɪvɪs]: **R.-D. incision** Bauchdeckenschnitt *m* nach Rocky-Davis.
Rock·y Moun·tain ['rɑki 'maʊntn]: **R. M. spotted fever** *abbr*. **RMSF** Felsengebirgsfleckfieber *nt*, amerikanisches Zeckenbißfieber *nt*, Rocky Mountain spotted fever (*nt*) *abbr*. RMSF.
 R. M. spotted fever tick *micro*. Dermacentor andersoni.
 R. M. wood tick *micro*. Dermacentor andersoni.
rod [rɑd] *n* **1.** Zapfen *m*; Stab *m*, Stange *f*. **2. ~s** *pl* (*Auge*) Stäbchen(zellen *pl*) *pl*. **3.** *sl*. Penis *m*.
rod achromatopsy → rod monochromasy.
rod bacterium → rod-shaped bacterium.
rod cells → rod 2.
ro·dent ['rəʊdnt] **I** *n bio*. Nager *m*, Nagetier *nt*. **II** *adj* **1.** *bio*. nagend. **2.** *patho*. (*Ulcus*) fressend, exulzerierend.
rodent-borne viruses *micro*. durch Nager/Rodentia übertragene Viren *pl*, rodent-borne viruses *pl*.
rodent cancer → rodent ulcer.
Ro·den·tia [rəʊˈden(t)ɪə, -tɪə] *pl bio*. Nager *pl*, Nagetiere *pl*, Rodentia *pl*.
ro·den·ti·cide [rəʊˈdentɪsaɪd] **I** *n* Rodentizid *nt*. **II** *adj* rodentizid.
rodent ulcer knotiges/solides/noduläres, nodulo-ulzeröses Basaliom *nt*, Basalioma exulcerans, Ulcus rodens.
rod monochromasy *ophthal*. Stäbchen(farben)blindheit *f*.

rod myopathy *patho.* Nemalinmyopathie *f.*
rod nuclear cell *hema.* stabkerniger Granulozyt *m*; *inf.* Stabkerniger *m.*
ro·do·nal·gia ['rəʊdan'ældʒɪə] *n* (Mitchell-)Gerhardt-Syndrom *n*, Weir--Mitchell-Krankheit *f*, Erythromelalgie *f*, Erythralgie *f*, Erythermalgie *f*, Akromelalgie *f.*
rod-shaped bacterium *micro.* stäbchenförmiges Bakterium *nt*, Stäbchen *nt.*
rod vision Dämmerungs-, Nachtsehen *nt*, skotopes Sehen *nt*, Skotop(s)ie *f.*
Roederer ['rəʊdərər; 'rœ-]: **R.'s spontaneous evolution** *gyn.* Roederer-Selbstentwicklung *f.*
roent·gen ['rentgən] *I n abbr.* **R** Röntgen *nt*, Röntgeneinheit *f abbr.* R. *II adj* Röntgen-.
roentgen equivalent man → rem.
roentgen intoxication → radiation sickness.
roent·gen·ize ['rentgənaɪz] *vt* mit Röntgenstrahlen behandeln, bestrahlen; eine Röntgenuntersuchung durchführen, durchleuchten, röntgen.
roent·gen·ky·mo·graph [,rentgən'kaɪməgræf] *n* Röntgenkymograph *m.*
roent·gen·ky·mog·ra·phy [,-kaɪ'mɑgrəfɪ] *n abbr.* **RKY** Röntgenkymographie *f.*
roent·gen·o·cin·e·ma·tog·ra·phy [,rentgənəʊ,sɪnəmə'tɑgrəfɪ] *n* Röntgenkinematographie *f.*
roent·gen·o·gram ['-græm] *n* Roentgenaufnahme *f*, -bild *nt.*
roent·gen·o·graph ['-græf] *n* → roentgenogram.
roent·gen·o·graph·ic [,-'græfɪk] *adj* Radiographie betr., mittels Radiographie, radiographisch, Röntgen-; radiologisch.
roentgenographic film *I* Röntgenfilm *m.* 2. Röntgenaufnahme *f*, -bild *nt.*
roent·gen·og·ra·phy [,rentgə'nɑgrəfɪ] *n* 1. Röntgenphotografie *f.* 2. Röntgenuntersuchung *f*, Röntgen *nt.*
roent·gen·o·ky·mo·graph [,rentgənəʊ'kaɪməgræf] *n* Röntgenkymograph *m.*
roent·gen·o·log·ic [,-'lɑdʒɪk] *adj* → roentgenological.
roent·gen·o·log·i·cal [-'lɑdʒɪkl] *adj* Röntgenologie betr., auf Röntgenologie beruhend, röntgenologisch, Röntgen-.
roent·gen·ol·o·gist [,rentgə'nɑlədʒɪst, -dʒə-] *n* Röntgenologe *m*, -login *f.*
roent·gen·ol·o·gy [-'nɑlədʒɪ] *n* Röntgenologie *f.*
roent·gen·o·lu·cent [,rentgənəʊ'luːsnt] *adj* → radiolucent.
roent·gen·o·nom·e·ter [,rentgə'nɑmɪtər] *n* → radiometer.
roent·gen·o·paque [,rentgənəˈpeɪk] *adj* → radiopaque.
roent·gen·o·par·ent [,-'peərənt] *adj* → radioparent.
roent·gen·o·scope ['-skəʊp] *n* Röntgen-, Durchleuchtungsapparat *m*, Fluoroskop *nt*; Bestrahlungsgerät *nt.*
roent·gen·os·co·py [,rentgə'nɑskəpɪ] *n* Röntgenuntersuchung *f*, -durchleuchtung *f*, Röntgenoskopie *f*, Fluoroskopie *f.*
roent·gen·o·ther·a·py [,rentgənəʊ'θerəpɪ] *n* Röntgentherapie *f*; Strahlentherapie *f.*
roentgen-ray dermatitis Strahlen-, Radio-, Radiumdermatitis *f.*
roentgen rays Röntgenstrahlen *pl*, -strahlung *f.*
roentgen therapy → roentgenotherapy.
roet·eln ['retəln] *pl* → rubella.
Roger [rɔ'ʃe]: **R.'s bruit** → R.'s murmur.
R.'s disease Roger-Syndrom *nt*, Morbus Roger *m.*

maladie de R. → R.'s disease.
R.'s murmur *card.* Roger'-Geräusch *nt.*
R.'s reflex Roger-Reflex *m.*
Rohr [rɔʊr]: **R.'s layer/stria** Rohr'-Fibrinoidstreifen *m*, Rohr'-Fibrinoid *nt.*
Rokitansky [rəʊkɪ'tænskɪ]: **R.'s diverticulum** Rokitansky-Divertikel *nt.*
R.'s kidney Amyloid(schrumpf)niere *f*, Wachs-, Speckniere *f.*
R.'s pelvis Wirbelgleitbecken *nt*, spondylolisthetisches Becken *nt*, Pelvis spondylolisthetica.
Rokitansky-Aschoff ['ɑʃɔf]: **R.-A. ducts/sinus** Rokitansky-Aschoff-Sinus *pl.*
Rokitansky-Küster-Hauser ['kɪstər 'haʊsər; 'kystər]: **R.-K.H. syndrome** Mayer-Rokitansky-Küster-Syndrom *nt*, MRK-Syndrom *nt*, Rokitansky-Küster--Syndrom *nt.*
ro·lan·dic area [rəʊ'lændɪk] → Rolando's area.
rolandic epilepsy rolandische Epilepsie *f.*
rolandic region → Rolando's area.
Rolando [rəʊ'lændəʊ]: **R.'s area** motorischer Cortex *m*, motorischer Kortex *m*, motorische Rinde(nregion *f*) *f*, Motokortex *m*, -cortex *m.*
R.'s cells Rolando-Zellen *pl.*
fissure of R. Rolando'-Fissur *f*, Zentralfurche *f* des Großhirns, Sulcus centralis (cerebri).
R.'s substance Substantia gelatinosa.
role [rəʊl] *n psycho.* Rolle *f.*
role conflict *psycho.* Rollenkonflikt *m.*
role-playing *psycho.* Rollenspiel *nt.*
ro·li·tet·ra·cy·cline [rəʊlɪ,tetrə'saɪkliːn] *n pharm.* Rolitetracyclin *nt.*
roll [rəʊl] *I n* 1. Wulst *m*, Rolle *f.* 2. *techn.* Rolle *f*, Walze *f.*
Roller ['rəʊlər]: **R.'s nucleus** Roller'-Kern *m*, Nc. vestibularis caudalis/inferior.
Rolleston ['rɑlstəns]: **R.'s rule** Rolleston--Regel *f.*
roll·ing hernia ['rəʊlɪŋ] paraösophageale (Hiatus-)Hernie *f.*
roll tube *micro.* Rollröhrchen *nt.*
ROM *abbr.* → range of motion/movement.
Romaña [rəʊ'mɑnjɑ]: **R.'s sign** Romaña--Zeichen *nt.*
Ro·man chamomile ['rəʊmən] echte Kamille *f*, Chamomilla *f*, Matricaria chamomilla/officinalis.
Romanovsky [rəʊmə'nɔfskɪ]: **R.'s stain** Romanowsky-Färbung *f.*
Romano-Ward ['rəʊmənəʊ 'wɔːrd]: **R.-W. syndrome** *card.* Romano-Ward-Syndrom *nt.*
Romanowsky → Romanovsky.
Romberg ['rɑmbɜrg]: **R.'s disease** Romberg-Syndrom *nt*, -Trophoneurose *f*, Romberg-Parry-Syndrom *nt*, -Trophoneurose *f*, progressive halbseitige Gesichtsatrophie *f*, Hemiatrophia progressiva faciei/facialis.
R.'s sign Romberg-Zeichen *nt.*
R.'s symptom 1. Romberg-Zeichen *nt*, -Phänomen *nt.* 2. → Romberg-Howship symptom.
R.'s syndrome → R.'s disease.
R.'s test Romberg-Versuch *m.*
R.'s trophoneurosis → R.'s disease.
Romberg-Howship ['haʊʃɪp]: **R.-H. symptom** Howship-von Romberg-Zeichen *nt.*
rom·berg·ism ['rɑmbɜrgɪzəm] *n* Romberg--Zeichen *nt.*
ron·geur [rəʊ'ʒɜr; rɔ̃'ʒœːr] *n French chir.* Knochenzange *f*, Knochenschneider *m.*
rönt·gen·og·ra·phy *n* → roentgenography.
R-on-T phenomenon *card.* R-auf-T-Phänomen *nt.*
roof [ruːf] *I n* Dach *nt*, dachähnliche Struktur *f*; Gewölbe *nt.* *II vt* mit einem Dach versehen, überdachen; bedecken.
r. of fourth ventricle Dach des IV. Ventrikels, Tegmen ventriculi quarti.
r. of mouth Gaumen *m*, Palatum *nt.*
r. of orbit Orbitadach, Paries superior orbitae.
r. of skull knöchernes Schädeldach, Kalotte *f*, Calvaria *f.*
r. of tympanic cavity Paukenhöhlendach, Tegmen tympani.
r. of tympanum → r. of tympanic cavity.
roof nuclei Kleinhirnkerne *pl*, Ncc. cerebellaris.
roof plate *embryo.* Deckplatte *f.*
room [ruːm, rʊm] *n* 1. Raum *m*, Zimmer *nt*; Saal *m.* 2. Platz *m*, Raum *m.* **to make ~ Platz machen** (*for* für).
room air Raumluft *f.*
room divider Trennwand *f*, Raumaufteiler *m.*
rooming-in *n gyn.* Rooming-in *nt.*
room temperature Raum-, Zimmertemperatur *f.*
room·y ['ruːmɪ, 'rʊmɪ] *adj* geräumig.
root [ruːt] *I n* 1. *anat., bot., mathe.* Wurzel *f*, Radix *f.* **to pull out by the ~** mit der Wurzel herausziehen. 2. *fig.* Wurzel *f*, Ursache *f*, Kern *m.* *II vt* tief einpflanzen, einwurzeln lassen. *III vi* 3. Wurzeln schlagen, wurzeln. 4. *fig.* wurzeln (*in* in); seinen Ursprung haben (*in* in).
root out *vt* mit der Wurzel ausreißen, ausrotten.
root up *vt* → root out.
r. of iris Iriswurzel.
r. of lung Lungenwurzel, Radix/Pediculus pulmonis.
r. of mesentery Mesenterial-, Gekrösewurzel, Radix mesenterii.
r. of nose Nasenwurzel, Radix nasalis/nasi.
r. of penis Peniswurzel, Radix penis.
r. of tongue Zungenwurzel, Radix linguae.
root abscess Wurzelspitzenabszeß *m.*
root-and-branch *adj* restlos, radikal.
root canal (Zahn-)Wurzelkanal *m*, Canalis radicis dentis.
root cell (*ZNS*) Wurzelzelle *f.*
parasympathetic r. Parasympathikuswurzelzelle.
somatomotor r. motorische Nervenzelle *f*, Motoneuron *nt.*
sympathetic r. Sympathikuswurzelzelle.
root·ed ['ruːtɪd] *adj* (fest) verwurzelt.
root·ed·ness ['ruːtɪdnɪs] *n* Verwurzelung *f.*
root entry zone (*ZNS*) Wurzeleintrittszone *f.*
root filaments of spinal nerves (Spinal-)-Wurzelfasern *pl*, Fila radicularia.
root·less ['ruːtlɪs] *adj* wurzellos; *fig.* entwurzelt.
root·let ['ruːtlɪt] *n* kleine Wurzel *f*, Wurzelfaser *f.*
root part of pulp → radicular pulp.
root resection *dent.* (Zahn-)Wurzelspitzenresektion *f*, Apikoektomie *f.*
root sheath (*Haar*) Wurzelscheide *f.*
connective tissue r. bindegewebige Wurzelscheide.
dermal r. → connective tissue r.
epithelial r. epitheliale Wurzelscheide.
root treatment *dent.* Wurzelbehandlung *f.*
rope burn [rəʊp] Verbrennung *f* durch Reibung(shitze).
roped flap [rəʊpt] → rope flap.
rope flap Rundstiellappen *m.*
Rorschach ['rɔːrʃɑx]: **R. test** *psycho.* Rorschach-Test *m.*
ro·sa·cea [rəʊ'zeɪʃɪə, -zɪə] *n derm.* Kupferrotfinne *f*, Rosazea *f*, Rosacea *f*, Akne rosacea.

rosacea keratitis Akne-rosacea-Keratitis *f*, Rosazea-Keratitis *f*.
rosacea-like tuberculid *derm.* lupoide Rosazea *f*, Rosacea granulomatosa.
Roscoe-Bunsen ['rɑskəʊ 'bʌnsən]: **R.-B. law** Bunsen-Roscoe-Gesetz *nt*.
rose [rəʊz] *n* **1.** → rose disease 1. **2.** Rose *f*.
rose bengal test Rose-Bengal-Probe *f*.
rose disease 1. Wundrose *f*, Erysipel *nt*, Erysipelas *nt*, Streptodermia cutanea lymphatica. **2.** Rosenbach'-Krankheit *f*, Rotlauf *m*, Schweinerotlauf *m*, Erysipeloid *nt*, Pseudoerysipel *nt*, Erythema migrans.
Rosenbach ['rəʊznbax]: **R.'s disease 1.** Heberden'-Polyarthrose *f*. **2.** Rosenbach'-Krankheit *f*, Rotlauf *m*, Schweinerotlauf *m*, Erysipeloid *nt*, Pseudoerysipel *nt*, Erythema migrans.
R.'s syndrome *card.* Rosenbach-Syndrom *nt*.
Rosenbach-Semon ['si:mən]: **R.-S. law** Rosenbach-Semon-Gesetz *nt*.
Rosenmüller ['rəʊz(ə)nmʌlər, -mju-, mɪl-]: **R.'s body** Nebeneierstock *m*, Parovarium *nt*, Rosenmüller'-Organ *nt*, Epoophoron *nt*.
R.'s cavity → R.'s recess.
R.'s fossa → R.'s recess.
R.'s gland 1. oberster tiefer Leistenlymphknoten *m*. **2.** Cloquet-Drüse *f*, Rosenmüller-Cloquet-Drüse *f*, Rosenmüller-Drüse *f*.
R.'s lymph node → R.'s gland.
R.'s node → R.'s gland.
R.'s organ → R.'s body.
R.'s recess Rosenmüller'-Grube *f*, Rec. pharyngeus.
R.'s valve Hasner'-Klappe *f*, Plica lacrimalis.
Rosenthal ['rəʊzənθɔl, -tɑl]: **R.'s canal** Rosenthal'-Kanal *m*, Schneckenspindelkanal *m*, Canalis ganglionaris, Canalis spiralis modioli.
R.'s fibers *patho.* Rosenthal-Fasern *pl*.
R. syndrome *hema.* Rosenthal-Krankheit *f*.
R.'s vein Rosenthal'-Vene *f*, Basalis *f*, V. basalis.
ro·se·o·la [rəʊ'zɪələ, rəʊzɪ'əʊlə] *n derm.* **1.** Roseola *f*. **2.** → roseola infantum.
roseola infantum Dreitagefieber *nt*, sechste Krankheit *f*, Exanthema subitum, Roseola infantum.
Roser ['rəʊzər]: **R.'s line** Roser-Nélaton'-Linie *f*, Nélaton'-Linie *f*..
ro·set [rəʊ'zet] *n* Rosette *f*.
ro·sette *n* → roset.
rosette assay *immun., hema.* Rosettentest *m*.
E r. E-Rosettentest.
EAC r. EAC-Rosettentest.
erythrocyte r. E-Rosettentest.
erythrocyte, antibody, complement r. EAC-Rosettentest.
Rose-Waaler [rəʊz 'wɔ:lər]: **R.-W. test** Rose-Waaler-Test *m*, Waaler-Rose-Test *m*.
Rosin ['rəʊzɪn]: **R.'s test** Rosin-Probe *f*.
Ross [rɒs, rɑs]: **R.'s bodies** Ross'-Körperchen *pl*.
Rossolimo [rɒsəʊ'li:məʊ]: **R.'s reflex/sign 1.** Zehenbeugereflex *m*, Rossolimo-Reflex *m*, -Zeichen *nt*, Plantarmuskelreflex *m*. **2.** Rossolimo-Fingerzeichen *nt*.
Ross river virus [rɒs] Ross-river-Virus *nt*.
Rostan [rɒs'tɑ̃]: **R.'s asthma** Herzasthma *nt*, Asthma cardiale.
ros·tel·lum [rɒ'steləm] *n, pl* **-la** [-lə] *micro.* Rostellum *nt*.
ros·tral ['rɒstrəl] *adj* **1.** *anat.* kopfwärts,

zum Körperende *od.* Kopf hin liegend, rostral. **2.** (*ZNS*) Rostrum betr., rostral.
rostral branch of vestibular nerve oberer Teil *m* des N. vestibularis, Pars rostralis/ superior n. vestibularis.
rostral colliculus oberer/vorderer Hügel *m* der Vierhügelplatte, Colliculus cranialis/rostralis/superior.
rostral commissure (of cerebrum) Commissura anterior/rostralis cerebri.
rostral ganglion: r. of glossopharyngeal nerve Müller'-Ganglion *nt*, Ehrenritter'- -Ganglion *nt*, oberes Glossopharyngeusganglion *nt*, Ggl. rostralis/superius n. glossopharyngei.
r. of vagus nerve oberes Vagusganglion *nt*, Ggl. rostralis/superius n. vagi.
rostral lamina Lamina rostralis.
rostral lobe of cerebellum kranialer (Kleinhirn-)Lappen/Abschnitt *m*, Lobus anterior/cranialis/rostralis cerebelli.
ros·trate pelvis ['rɒstreɪt] osteomalazisches Becken *nt*, Pelvis osteomalacica.
ros·tri·form ['rɒstrɪfɔ:rm] *adj* schnabelförmig.
ros·trum ['rɒstrəm] *n, pl* **-trums, -tra** [-trə] *anat.* **1.** Schnabel *m*, schnabelförmiges Gebilde *f*, Rostrum *nt*. **2.** Rostrum sphenoidale.
r. of corpus callosum Balkenvorderende *m*, -schnabel, Rostrum corporis callosi.
ro·sux·a·cin [rəʊ'sʌksəsɪn] *n pharm.* Rosuxacin *nt*.
ros·y-cheeked ['rəʊzɪ] *adj* rotbäckig.
Rot [rɒt]: **R.'s disease/syndrome** → Roth-Bernhardt disease.
rot [rɒt] **I** *n* Fäulnis *f*, Verwesung *f*. **II** *vt* (ver-)faulen lassen. **III** *vi* (ver-)faulen, (ver-)modern.
ro·tar·y ['rəʊtərɪ] *adj* rotierend, (s.) drehend, kreisend, umlaufend, Dreh-, Umlauf-, Rotations-, Kreis-.
rotary articulation Dreh-, Rad-, Zapfengelenk *nt*, Artic. trochoidea.
rotary current *electr.* Drehstrom *m*.
rotary joint → rotary articulation.
rotary motion → rotary movement.
rotary movement Rotations-, Drehbewegung *f*, Rotation *f*.
rotary vertigo Drehschwindel *m*, Vertigo rotatoria.
ro·tate ['rəʊteɪt; *Brit.* rəʊ'teɪt] **I** *vt* **1.** drehen *od.* rotieren lassen. **2.** turnusmäßig abwechseln. **II** *vi* **3.** rotieren, kreisen, s. drehen. **4.** s. (turnusmäßig) abwechseln.
ro·tat·ed fracture ['rəʊteɪtɪd] Fraktur *f* mit Rotationsfehlstellung.
ro·tat·ing disk oxygenator ['rəʊteɪtɪŋ] Scheibenoxygenator *m*.
ro·ta·tion [rəʊ'teɪʃn] *n* **1.** (Um-)Drehung *f*, Drehbewegung *f*, Rotation *f*. **2.** Wechsel *m*. **~** turnusmäßig, abwechselnd.
ro·ta·tion·al acceleration [rəʊ'teɪʃənl] *phys.* Drehbeschleunigung *f*.
rotational isomerism *chem.* Rotationsisomerie *f*.
rotational movement → rotary movement.
rotation flap Rotationslappen *m*.
ro·ta·tor ['rəʊteɪtər] *n, pl* **-tors, -to·res** [ˌrəʊteɪ'tɔ:ri:z, -'tɔ:r-] **1.** *anat.* Drehmuskel *m*, Rotator *m*, M. rotator. **2.** *techn.* s. drehender Apparat *od.* Maschinenteil *m*.
rotator cuff (*Schulter*) Rotatorenmanschette *f*.
rotatores breves (muscles) kurze Wirbeldreher *pl*, Rotatores *pl* breves, Mm. rotatores breves.
rotatores cervicis (muscles) zervikale Wirbeldreher *pl*, Rotatores *pl* cervicis, Mm. rotatores cervicis.
rotatores longi (muscles) lange Wirbel-

dreher *pl*, Rotatores *pl* longi, Mm. rotatores longi.
rotatores lumborum (muscles) lumbale Wirbeldreher *pl*, Rotatores *pl* lumborum, Mm. rotatores lumborum.
rotatores thoracis (muscles) thorakale Wirbeldreher *pl*, Rotatores *pl* thoracis, Mm. rotatores thoracis.
rotator muscles: lumbar r. → rotatores lumborum (muscles).
r. of neck → rotatores cervicis (muscles).
r. of thorax → rotatores thoracis (muscles).
ro·ta·to·ry ['rəʊtətɔ:rɪ, -təʊ-] *adj* **1.** → rotary. **2.** turnusmäßig, abwechselnd.
rotatory deformity *ortho.* (*Fraktur*) Rotationsfehlstellung *f*, -deformität *f*.
rotatory dispersion, optical *phys., biochem.* optische Rotationsdispersion *f*.
rotatory joint → rotary articulation.
rotatory malalignment *ortho.* (*Fraktur*) Verheilung *f* in Rotationsfehlstellung.
rotatory malunion → rotatory malalignment.
rotatory movement → rotary movement.
rotatory nystagmus Drehnystagmus *m*, rotatorischer Nystagmus *m*.
rotatory spasm Drehkrampf *m*, Spasmus rotatorius.
rotatory test HNO (*Ohr*) Drehprüfung *f*.
rotatory tic → rotatory spasm.
rotatory vertigo → rotary vertigo.
Ro·ta·vi·rus ['rəʊtəvaɪrəs] *n micro.* Rotavirus *nt*.
Rot-Bernhardt [rɒt 'bɛrnhɑ:rt]: **R.-B. disease/syndrome** → Roth-Bernhardt disease.
rö·teln ['reɪtəln] *pl* → rubella.
Roth [rɒθ]: **R.'s disease/syndrome** → Roth-Bernhardt disease.
Roth-Bernhardt ['bɛrnhɑ:rt]: **R.-B. disease** Bernhardt-Roth-Syndrom *nt*, Myalgia paraesthetica.
R.-B. syndrome → R.-B. disease.
Roth·ia ['rɒθɪə] *n micro.* Rothia *f*.
R. dentocariosus Rothia dentocariosus.
Rothmann-Makai ['rɑθmən 'mɔ:kɔɪ]: **R.-M. syndrome** Rothmann-Makai-Syndrom *nt*, Lipogranulomatosis subcutanea, Spontanpannikulitis *f* Rothmann-Makai.
Rothmund ['rɑθmənd]: **R.'s syndrome** Rothmund-Syndrom *nt*, Rothmund- -Thomson-Syndrom *nt*.
Rothmund-Thomson ['tɑmsən]: **R.-T. syndrome** → Rothmund's syndrome.
rot·lauf ['rɑtlaʊf] *n* Rosenbach'-Krankheit *f*, Rotlauf *m*, Schweinerotlauf *m*, Erysipeloid *nt*, Pseudoerysipel *nt*, Erythema migrans.
rot·ten ['rɑtn] *adj* verfault, faulig.
Rotor ['rəʊtər]: **R.'s syndrome** Rotor-Syndrom *nt*.
Rouget [ru'ʒɛ]: **R.'s cells** Rouget-Zellen *pl*.
R.'s muscle Müller'-Muskel *m*, Fibrae circulares m. ciliaris.
rough [rʌf] **I** *n* Rauheit *f*, Unebenheit *f*, Rauhe *nt*, Unebene *nt*; Rohzustand *m*. **in the ~** im Rohzustand. **II** *adj* **1.** rauh, uneben; zerklüftet; unfertig, roh; (*Haare*) struppig; (*Haut*) rauh. **2.** *fig.* roh, grob, ungehobelt, Roh-. **3.** (*Schätzungen*) grob, ungefähr. **III** *adv* roh, rauh, hart. **IV** *vt* **4.** an-, aufrauhen. **5.** (*Person*) mißhandeln. **V** *vi* rauh werden.
roug up *vt* → rough 5.
rough·age ['rʌfɪdʒ] *n* Ballaststoffe *pl*.
rough analysis Rohanalyse *f*.
rough bacteria *micro.* R-Form *f*, R-Stamm *m*.
rough calculation Überschlagsrechnung *f*.
rough colony *micro.* (*Kolonie*) R-Form *f*.

rough crest of femur Linea aspera (femoris).
rough·en ['rʌfn] I vt an-, aufrauhen, rauh machen. II vi rauh(er) werden.
rough line of femur Linea aspera (femoris).
rough·ness ['rʌfnɪs] n 1. Rauheit f, Unebenheit f; rauhe Stelle f. 2. fig. Roheit f, Grobheit f, Härte f.
rough ridge of femur Linea aspera (femoris).
rough strain → rough bacteria.
Rougnon-Heberden [ru'njõ 'hebərdən]: **R.-H. disease** Herzbräune f, Stenokardie f, Angina pectoris.
rou·leaux formation [ru:'ləʊ] hema. Geldrollenbildung f, -agglutination f, Rouleau-Bildung f, Pseudoagglutination f.
round [raʊnd] I n 1. Kreis m, Ring m, Rundung f, runde kreisförmige Struktur f. **out of ~** unrund. 2. Kreislauf m, Runde f. 3. Runde f, Rundgang m. 4. (Personen-)Kreis m, Runde f. II adj 5. (kreis-, kugel-)rund, zylindrisch; ringförmig; (ab-)gerundet. 6. fig. rund, voll. 7. mathe. ganz (ohne Bruch); auf-, abgerundet; annähernd, ungefähr. III vt rund machen, abrunden. IV vi 8. rund werden, s. (ab-)runden. 9. umgeben, umschließen; umkreisen. 10. (Visite) die Runde machen. **round off** vt (Kante) abrunden; (Zahl) auf-, abrunden (to auf).
round angle mathe. Vollwinkel m.
round back Rundrücken m.
round cell sarcoma rundzelliges Sarkom nt, Rundzellensarkom nt.
round cells Rundzellen pl.
round·ed ['raʊndɪd] adj (ab-)gerundet, rundlich, rund, Rund-; fig. abgerundet.
rounded number ab- od. aufgerundete Zahl f.
round foramen (of sphenoid bone) For. rotundum.
round heart Kugelherz nt.
round·ing ['raʊndɪŋ] I n (Ab-)Rundung f. II adj rund(lich), Rund-.
round·ish ['raʊndɪʃ] adj rundlich.
round ligament: r. of acetabulum Lig. capitis femoris.
r. of Cloquet Lig. capitis costae intraarticulare.
r. of elbow joint Chorda obliqua.
r. of femur → r. of acetabulum.
r. of liver Lig. teres hepatis.
r. of uterus rundes Mutter-/Uterusband nt, Lig. teres uteri.
round·ness ['raʊndnɪs] n Rundung f, Rundheit f, das Runde.
round pelvis rundes Becken nt.
round pronator muscle Pronator m teres, M. pronator teres.
round-the-clock adj rund um die Uhr, 24stündig.
round window rundes Fenster nt, Fenestra cochleae/rotunda.
round·worm ['raʊndwɜrm] n micro. Rund-, Fadenwurm m, Nematode f.
Rous [raʊs, ru:s]: **R.-associated virus** abbr. **RAV** Rous-assoziiertes Virus nt abbr. RAV.
R. sarcoma Rous-Sarkom nt.
R. sarcoma virus abbr. **RSV** Rous-Sarkom-Virus nt abbr. RSV.
R. tumor → R. sarcoma.
Roussy-Déjérine [ru'sɪ deʒe'rin]: **R.-D. syndrome** neuro. Déjérine-Roussy-Syndrom nt, Thalamussyndrom nt.
Roussy-Lévy [le'vi]: **R.-L. disease** Roussy--Lévy-Syndrom nt, erbliche areflektorische Dysstasie f.
R.-L. hereditary areflexic dystasia → R.-L. disease.

R.-L. hereditary ataxic dystasia → R.-L. disease.
R.-L. syndrome → R.-L. disease.
Roux [ru]: **R.'s anastomosis** Roux-Y--Schlinge f, Roux-Y-Anastomose f, Y--Schlinge f, Y-Anastomose f, Y--Roux-Schlinge f, Y-Roux-Anastomose f.
R. retractor Roux-Haken m.
Roux-en-Y [ru ã i]: **R. anastomosis** → Roux's anastomosis.
R. choledochojejunostomy Choledochojejunostomie f mit Roux-Y-Anastomose.
R. cystojejunostomy Zystojejunostomie f mit Roux-Y-Schlinge.
R. operation → Roux's anastomosis.
R. pancreaticojejunostomy Pankreat(ik)ojejunostomie f mit Roux-Y-Schlinge.
Rovsing ['rɔvsɪŋ]: **R.'s sign** Rovsing-Zeichen nt, -Symptom nt.
R.'s syndrome Rovsing-Syndrom nt.
RPF abbr. → renal plasma flow.
R plasmid Resistenzplasmid nt, -faktor m, R-Plasmid nt, R-Faktor m.
R protein R-Protein nt.
RPR test hema. RPR-Test m, rapid plasma reagin test m.
RQ abbr. → respiratory quotient.
R-R interval card. RR-Intervall nt.
rRNA abbr. → ribosomal RNA.
RSSE abbr. → Russian spring-summer encephalitis.
RSSE virus micro. RFSE-Virus nt, RSSE-Virus nt, russische Frühsommerenzephalitis-Virus nt.
RS system biochem. Cahn-Ingold-Prelog--System nt, RS-System nt.
R strain micro. R-Form f, R-Stamm m.
RSV abbr. → Rous sarcoma virus.
RS virus micro. RS-Virus nt, Respiratory-syncitial-Virus nt.
RS virus disease RS-Virus-Erkrankung f.
RS virus infection RS-Virus-Infektion f.
rT$_3$ abbr. → reverse triiodothyronine.
RTA abbr. → road traffic accident.
RTF abbr. → resistance transfer factor.
R-type n micro. (Kolonie) R-Form f.
Ru abbr. → ruthenium.
rub [rʌb] I n 1. (Ab-)Reiben nt, Abreibung f. 2. card. Reibegeräusch nt, Reiben nt. II vt 3. reiben. to ~ one's hands s. die Hände reiben. 4. reiben, streichen. III vi reiben, streifen (against, upon, on an).
rub·ber ['rʌbər] I n 1. (Natur-)Kautschuk m, Gummi nt/m. 2. (Radier-)Gummi m/ nt. 3. Gummiring m, -band m, Gummi m. 4. sl. Kondom nt. II vt → rubberize.
rub·ber·ize ['rʌbəraɪz] vt mit Gummi überziehen, gummieren.
rubber pelvis Gummibecken nt.
rub·bing ['rʌbɪŋ] n phys. Reibung f, Friktion f.
ru·be·fa·cient [ru:bə'feɪʃənt] I n hyperämisierendes Mittel nt, Hyperämikum nt, Rubefaciens nt. II adj hautrötend, hyperämisierend.
ru·bel·la [ru:'belə] n Röteln pl, Rubella f, Rubeola f.
rubella cataract Katarakt f bei Rötelnembryopathie f.
rubella embryopathy Röteln-, Rubeolaembryopathie f, Embryopathia rubeolosa.
rubella syndrome kongenitale Röteln pl, kongenitales Rötelnsyndrom nt.
rubella vaccination Röteln(schutz)impfung f.
rubella vaccine Röteln(virus)-Lebendimpfstoff m.
rubella virus micro. Rötelnvirus nt.

rubella virus live vaccine Röteln(virus)--Lebendimpfstoff m.
rubella virus vaccine live Röteln(virus)--Lebendimpfstoff m.
ru·be·o·la [ru:'bɪələ, ˌru:bɪ'əʊlə] n Masern pl, Morbilli pl.
ru·be·o·sis [ˌru:bɪ'əʊsɪs] n Rötung f, Rubeosis f, Rubeose f.
ru·bes·cent [ru:'besənt] adj rötlich; rötend.
ru·bid·i·um [ru:'bɪdɪəm] n abbr. **Rb** Rubidium nt abbr. Rb.
ru·bid·o·my·cin [ru:'bɪdəʊmaɪsɪn] n pharm. Rubidomycin nt, Daunomycin nt.
ru·big·i·nose [ru:'bɪdʒənəʊs] adj → rubiginous.
ru·big·i·nous [ru:'bɪdʒənəs] adj rostfarben, rubiginös.
ru·bin ['ru:bɪn] n Fuchsin nt.
Rubinstein ['ru:bɪnstaɪn, -ʃtaɪn]: **R.'s syndrome** → Rubinstein-Taybi syndrome.
Rubinstein-Taybi ['teɪbɪ]: **R.-T. syndrome** Rubinstein-Taybi-Syndrom nt.
Ru·bi·vi·rus [ru:bə'vaɪrəs] n micro. Rubivirus nt.
ru·bri·blast ['ru:brɪblæst] n Proerythroblast m.
ru·bri·cyte ['-saɪt] n polychromatischer Normoblast m.
rubro-olivary bundle → rubro-olivary fasciculus.
rubro-olivary fasciculus Probst-Gamper'--Bündel nt, Fasciculus rubro-olivaris.
rubro-olivary fibers rubro-olivare Fasern pl, Fibrae rubro-olivares.
ru·bro·re·tic·u·lo·spi·nal tract [ˌru:brəʊrɪˌtɪkjələʊ'spaɪnl] Tractus rubroreticulospinalis.
ru·bro·spi·nal cerebellar peduncle syndrome [ˌ-'spaɪnl] Claude-Syndrom nt, unteres Ruber-Syndrom nt, unteres Syndrom nt des Nc. ruber.
rubrospinal tract Monakow'-Bündel nt, Tractus rubrospinalis.
ru·by spots ['ru:bɪ] senile (Häm-)Angiome pl, Alters(häm)angiome pl.
ruck·sack paralysis ['rʌksæk] Rucksacklähmung f.
ruc·tus ['rʌktəs] n Aufstoßen nt, Rülpsen nt, Ruktation f, Ruktus m, Ructus m, Eruktation f.
Rud [rʊd]: **R.'s syndrome** Rud-Syndrom nt.
rude respiration [ru:d] bronchovesikuläres/vesikobronchiales Atmen/Atmungsgeräusch nt.
ru·di·ment ['ru:dɪmənt] n 1. Rudiment nt, Überbleibsel nt. 2. ~s pl Grundlagen pl, Anfangsgründe pl; Ansatz m.
ru·di·men·tal [ˌru:dɪ'mentl] adj → rudimentary.
ru·di·men·ta·ry [ˌru:dɪ'mentərɪ] adj 1. zurückgebildet, verkümmert, rudimentär. 2. elementar, rudimentär, Anfangs-.
Ruffini [ru'fi:nɪ]: **brushes of R.** → R.'s end-organs.
R.'s corpuscles Ruffini'-Körperchen pl.
R.'s cylinders → R.'s corpuscles.
R.'s end-organs Ruffini'-Endorgane pl.
organs of R. → R.'s end-organs.
ru·ga ['ru:gə] n, pl **-gae** [-dʒi:] anat. Runzel f, Falte f, Ruga f.
r.e of stomach Magenfalten pl, -runzeln pl, Rugae gastricae.
r.e of vagina Querfalten pl der Vaginalschleimhaut, Rugae vaginalis.
ru·gate ['ru:geɪt, -gɪt] adj faltig, runz(e)lig, gerunzelt.
rug·by knee ['rʌgbɪ] Osgood-Schlatter--Krankheit f, Schlatter--Osgood-Krankheit f, -Syndrom nt, Apophysitis tibialis adolescentium.

ru·gine [ruː'ʒiːn] n chir. Raspatorium nt.
ru·gose ['ruːgəʊs] adj faltig, runz(e)lig.
ru·gos·i·ty [ruː'gɒsɪtɪ] n 1. Faltigkeit f, Runz(e)ligkeit f. 2. → ruga.
ru·gous ['ruːgəs] adj → rugose.
rule [ruːl] I n 1. Regel f, das Übliche. as a ~ in der Regel, normalerweise. 2. Gesetz nt, Vorschrift f, Richtlinie f, Richtschnur f, Bestimmung f, Norm f. by ~ laut Vorschrift. II vt anordnen, bestimmen, entscheiden.
r.s of conduct Richtlinien pl.
r. of thumb Daumen-, Faustregel.
rum-blossom [rʌm] n → rum nose.
ru·men ['ruːmɪn] n, pl -mens, -mi·na [-mɪnə] bio. Pansen m.
ru·mi·nant ['ruːmɪnənt] n bio. Wiederkäuer m.
ru·mi·nate ['ruːmɪneɪt] vt, vi 1. bio. wiederkäuen. 2. psycho., psychia. ruminieren. 3. ped. wiederkäuen, ruminieren.
ru·mi·na·tion [ruːmɪ'neɪʃn] n 1. bio. Wiederkäuen nt, Rumination f. 2. psycho., psychia. Rumination f. 3. ped. Rumination f.
rum nose [rʌm] Kartoffel-, Säufer-, Pfund-, Knollennase f, Rhinophym nt, Rhinophyma nt.
Rumpel-Leede ['rʌmpl 'liːdɪ]: R.-L. phenomenon → R.-L. sign.
R.-L. sign Rumpel-Leede-Phänomen nt.
R.-L. test Rumpel-Leede-Test m.
run [rʌn] (v run; run) I n 1. (Sport) Lauf m. to go for/take a ~ laufen, einen Lauf machen. 2. Laufen nt, Rennen nt; Laufschritt m. at/on the ~ im Lauf(schritt), im Dauerlauf. 3. fig. (Ver-)Lauf m, Fortgang m; Tendenz f. in the long ~ auf lange Sicht, auf die Dauer, langfristig. in the short ~ kurzfristig. to come down with a ~ (Temperatur) plötzlich fallen. 4. techn. Durchlauf m; lab. (Beschickungs-)Menge f, Charge f. 5. techn. (Arbeits-)Gang m. 6. Folge f, Reihe f, Serie f. 7. techn. Rinne f, Kanal m. 8. Länge f, Ausdehnung f. II adj geschmolzen.
III vi 9. rennen, laufen; (a. fig.) (durch-)laufen, zurücklegen. 10. befördern, transportieren. 11. (Fieber) haben, fiebern. to ~ a temperature. 12. (Test, Experimente) durchführen. 13. (Bad) einlaufen lassen. 14. schieben, stechen, stoßen, (through durch).
IV vi 15. laufen, rennen, eilen; davonweglaufen. 16. techn. laufen; arbeiten, funktionieren, gehen, in Gang sein. 17. (Blut) fließen, strömen; (Nase) laufen; (Augen) tränen; (Tränen) laufen; (Abszeß) eitern. 18. (Zeit) vergehen; dauern. 19. werden. to ~ dry austrocken; fig. (Vorrat) ausgehen, leer werden.
run down vi 1. heruntern-, herab-, hinunterlaufen, -rennen. 2. (Zeit) ablaufen; (Batterie) leer werden. 3. to be ~ erschöpft od. ausgepumpt od. abgespannt sein.

run out vi 1. (Flüssigkeit) herauslaufen. 2. (Zeit) ablaufen, zu Ende gehen. 3. (Vorrat) knapp werden (of an), ausgehen.
run over vt (mit dem Auto) überfahren.
run through vt (Infektion) durchlaufen, s. hindurchziehen durch ein Gebiet.
run to vi neigen zu. to ~ fat Fett ansetzen.
run-down I n Analyse f, Zusammenfassung f, Bericht m, Übersicht f (on über). II adj 1. abgespannt, erschöpft; (Batterie) verbraucht, leer; (Zeit) abgelaufen. 2. heruntergekommen.
run·let ['rʌnlɪt] n Rinnsal nt.
run·nel ['rʌnl] n 1. Rinnsal nt. 2. Rinne f.
run·ning ['rʌnɪŋ] I n 1. Laufen nt, Rennen nt; Wettlauf m. 2. Laufen nt (einer Maschine). 3. (Lauf-)Kraft f. 4. Bedienung f (einer Maschine). 5. Management nt, Führung f, Leitung f. II adj 6. laufend. 7. (Wasser) fließend; (Wunde) eiternd; (Nase) laufend. 8. (Blick) flüchtig. 9. (Monat) laufend. 10. wässrig, flüssig. 11. (fort-)laufend; aufeinanderfolgend.
running cold schwerer Schnupfen m.
running sore eiternde Wunde f.
runt disease [rʌnt] immun. Runt-Krankheit f, runt disease (nt).
Runyon ['rʌnjən]: R. classification micro. Runyon-Einteilung f, -Klassifikation f.
R. group I micro. photochromogene Mykobakterien pl, Mykobakterien pl der Runyon-Gruppe I.
R. group II micro. skotochromogene Mykobakterien pl, Mykobakterien pl der Runyon-Gruppe II.
R. group III micro. nicht-chromogene Mykobakterien pl, Mykobakterien pl der Runyon-Gruppe III.
R. group IV micro. schnellwachsende (atypische) Mykobakterien pl, Mykobakterien pl der Runyon-Gruppe IV.
ru·pia ['ruːpɪə] n derm. Rupia f, Rhypia f.
ru·pi·al ['ruːpɪəl] adj derm. Rupia betr.
rupial syphilid frambösiformes Syphilid nt.
ru·pi·oid ['ruːpɪɔɪd] adj rupiaähnlich.
rup·ture ['rʌptʃər] I n 1. Bruch m, Riß m, Ruptur f. 2. Brechen nt, Zerplatzen nt, Zerreißen nt. 3. Bruch m, Hernie f, Hernia f. II vt brechen, zersprengen, zerreißen, rupturieren. III vi 4. zerspringen, zerreißen, einen Riß bekommen, bersten, rupturieren. 5. s. einen Bruch heben.
r. of the Achilles tendon Achillessehnenruptur.
r. of the myocardial wall Herz(wand)ruptur.
r. of the papillary muscles Papillarmuskelruptur, -abriß m.
r. of the symphysis pubis Symphysenruptur, Ruptur der Symphysis pubis.
rup·tured disk ['rʌptʃərd] ortho., neurochir. Bandscheibenvorfall m, -prolaps m, -hernie f.

Rusconi [rusˈkəʊnɪ]: R.'s anus embryo. Urmund m, Urdarmöffnung f, Blastoporus m.
Rush [rʌʃ]: R. pin ortho. Rush-Nagel m.
Russell ['rʌsl]: R.'s bodies Russell'-Körperchen pl.
R. dwarf → R.'s syndrome.
R.'s syndrome Silver-Syndrom nt, Russell-Silver-Syndrom nt.
rus·set tick ['rʌsɪt] micro. Ixodes pilosus.
Rus·sian ['rʌʃən]: R. autumn(al) encephalitis japanische B-Enzephalitis f abbr. JBE, Encephalitis japonica B.
R. autumn(al) encephalitis virus japanische B-Enzephalitis-Virus nt, JBE-Virus nt.
R. endemic encephalitis → R. spring-summer encephalitis.
R. forest-spring encephalitis → R. spring-summer encephalitis.
R. influenza russischer Schnupfen m, russische Grippe f.
R. spring-summer encephalitis abbr. RSSE russische Früh(jahr-)Sommer-Enzephalitis f abbr. RSSE, russische Zeckenenzephalitis f.
R. spring-summer encephalitis virus RSSE-Virus nt, RFSE-Virus nt, russische Frühsommer-Enzephalitis-Virus nt.
R. tick-borne encephalitis → R. spring-summer encephalitis.
R. vernal encephalitis → R. spring-summer encephalitis.
Rust [ruːst]: R.'s disease Rust-Krankheit f.
R.'s syndrome Rust-Syndrom nt.
rust [rʌst] I n 1. Rost m. 2. bio. Rost m, Brand m. II vt verrosten lassen, rostig machen. III vi (ein-, ver-)rosten, rostig werden.
rust·y sputum ['rʌstɪ] rostfarbenes/rubiginöses Sputum nt, Sputum rubiginosum.
rut [rʌt] n bio. Brunft f; Brunst f; Brunft-, Brunstzeit f.
ru·the·ni·um [ruːˈθiːnɪəm, -jəm] n abbr. Ru Ruthenium nt abbr. Ru.
Rutherford ['rʌðərfərd, 'rʌθ-]: R. atom phys. Rutherford'-Atom nt, -Atommodell nt.
ru·tin ['ruːtn] n Rutin nt, Rutosid nt.
ru·ti·nose ['ruːtɪnəʊs] n Rutinose f.
ru·to·side ['ruːtəsaɪd] n → rutin.
Ruysch ['rɔɪʃ]: R.'s disease aganglionäres/kongenitales Megakolon nt, Hirschsprung-Krankheit f, Morbus Hirschsprung m, Megacolon congenitum.
R.'s membrane Choriokapillaris f, Lamina choroidocapillaris.
R.'s muscle Ruysch-Muskel m.
R.'s veins hintere Ziliarvenen pl, Vv. vorticosae, Vv. choroideae oculi.
RV abbr. 1. → reserve volume. 2. → residual volume.
R wave (EKG) R-Zacke f.
rye [raɪ] n bio. Roggen m.
Ryle [raɪl]: R.'s tube Ryle-Sonde f.

S

S *abbr.* **1.** → entropy. **2.** → siemens. **3.** → sulfur. **4.** → Svedberg unit.
s *abbr.* **1.** → second 1. **2.** → sedimentation coefficient.
SA *abbr.* → sinoatrial.
SAB agar → Sabouraud's agar.
sa·ber shin ['seɪbər] *ortho.* Säbelscheidentibia *f*.
Sabhi ['sɑːbɪ]: **S. agar** → Sabouraud's agar.
Sabin ['sæbɪn]: **S.'s vaccine** Sabin-Impfstoff *m*, -Vakzine *f*, oraler Lebendpolioimpfstoff *m*.
Sabin-Feldman ['feldmən]: **S.-F. dye test** Sabin-Feldman-Test *m*.
sab·i·nism ['sæbənɪzəm] *n* Sabinaölvergiftung *f*, Sabinismus *m*.
sab·i·nol ['sæbɪnɒl, -nɔl] *n* Sabinol *nt*.
S-A block → sinoatrial block.
sabot heart ['sæboʊ; sa'bo] *French card.* Holzschuhform *f* des Herzens, Coeur en sabot.
Sabouraud ['sæbjəroʊ; sabu'ro]: **S.'s agar** Sabouraud-Agar *m/nt*, Sabouraud-Glucose-Agar *m/nt*.
S. dextrose agar → S.'s agar.
S. dextrose and brain heart infusion agar Sabouraud-Glucose-Pepton-Agar *m/nt*.
Sab·ou·rau·dia [sæbjəˈroʊdɪə] *n micro.* Trichophyton *nt*.
Sab·ou·rau·di·tes [sæbjəroʊˈdaɪtiːz] *n micro.* Microsporon *nt*, Microsporum *nt*.
sab·u·lous ['sæbjələs] *adj* sandig, grießig, Sand-.
sa·bur·ra [sə'bʌrə] *n* Saburra *f*.
sa·bur·ral [sə'bʌrəl] *adj* Saburra betr., saburrös.
sac [sæk] *n anat., bio.* Sack *m*, Aussackung *f*, Beutel *m*, Saccus *m*.
sac·cade [sæ'kɑːd, sə-] *n physiol.* (Blick-)Sakkade *f*.
sac·cad·ic [sæ'kɑːdɪk, sə-] *adj* ruck-, stoßartig, ruckartig unterbrochen, sakkadisch, sakkadiert.
sac·cate ['sækɪt, -eɪt] *adj* sackförmig, -artig, beutelförmig, -artig.
sacchar- *pref.* → sacchro-.
sac·cha·rase ['sækəreɪz] *n* Saccharase *f*, β-Fructofuranosidase *f*.
sac·cha·rate ['-reɪt] *n* Sa(c)charat *nt*.
sac·cha·rat·ed ['-reɪtɪd] *adj* zucker-, sa(c)charosehaltig.
sac·char·eph·i·dro·sis [ˌsækərˌefɪ'droʊsɪs] *n* Zuckerausscheidung *f* im Schweiß.
sac·char·ic acid [sə'kærɪk] Aldar-, Zuckersäure *f*.
sac·cha·ride ['sækəraɪd, -rɪd] *n* Kohlenhydrat *nt*, Sa(c)charid *nt*.
sac·cha·rif·er·ous [ˌ-'rɪfərəs] *adj* zuckerhaltig; zuckerbildend.
sac·cha·ri·fi·ca·tion [səˌkærəfɪ'keɪʃn] *n chem.* Umwandlung *f* in einen Zucker.
sac·cha·ri·fy [sə'kærɪfaɪ] *vt* **1.** verzuckern, saccharifizieren. **2.** reagieren, süßen.
sac·cha·rim·e·ter [ˌsækə'rɪmɪtər] *n* Sa(c)charimeter *nt*.

sac·cha·rim·e·try [ˌ-'rɪmɪtrɪ] *n* Sa(c)charimetrie *f*.
sac·cha·rin ['sækərɪn] *n* Sa(c)charin *nt*.
sac·cha·rine ['sækərɪn, -riːn, -raɪn] *adj* süß, zuck(e)rig, Zucker-.
sac·char·i·nol [sə'kærɪnɒl, -əʊl] *n* → saccharin.
sac·cha·ri·num [ˌsækə'raɪnəm] *n* → saccharin.
saccharo- *pref.* Sa(c)char(o)-, Zucker-.
sac·cha·ro·bi·ose [ˌsækəroʊ'baɪoʊs] *n* Sa(c)charobiose *f*.
sac·cha·ro·ga·lac·tor·rhea [ˌ-gəˌlæktə'riə] *n gyn.* Saccharogalaktorrhoe *f*.
sac·cha·ro·lyt·ic [ˌ-'lɪtɪk] *adj* Zucker spaltend, sa(c)charolytisch.
sac·cha·ro·met·a·bol·ic [ˌ-ˌmetə'bɒlɪk] *adj* Zuckerstoffwechsel betr.
sac·cha·ro·me·tab·o·lism [ˌ-mə'tæbəlɪzəm] *n* Zuckerstoffwechsel *m*, -metabolismus *m*.
sac·cha·rom·e·ter [ˌsækə'rɒmɪtər] *n* → saccharimeter.
Sac·cha·ro·my·ces [ˌsækəroʊ'maɪziːz] *n micro.* Saccharomyces *m*.
S. cerevisiae Back-, Bierhefe *f*, Saccharomyces cerevisiae.
sac·cha·ro·my·ces [ˌ-'maɪziːz] *n* Saccharomycete *f*, Saccharomyces *m*.
Sac·cha·ro·my·ce·ta·ce·ae [ˌ-ˌmaɪsə'teɪsɪˌiː] *pl micro.* Saccharomycetaceae *pl*.
sac·cha·ro·my·cet·ic [ˌ-maɪ'setɪk] *adj* Saccharomyceten betr., durch sie hervorgerufen, Saccharomyceten-.
sac·cha·ro·pine ['-piːn] *n* Saccharopin *nt*.
saccharopine dehydrogenase (NAD+, L-glutamate forming) Saccharopindehydrogenase (NAD+, L-Glutamat-bildend) *f*.
saccharopine dehydrogenase (NADP+, L-lysine forming) Saccharopindehydrogenase (NADP+, L-Lysin-bildend) *f*.
sac·cha·ror·rhea [ˌ-'riə] *n* (Trauben-)Zuckerausscheidung *f* im Harn, Glukosurie *f*, Glucosurie *f*, Glykosurie *f*, Glykurie *f*, Glukurese *f*, Glucurese *f*.
sac·cha·rose ['sækəroʊz] *n* Rüben-, Rohrzucker *m*, Saccharose *f*.
sac·cha·ro·su·ria [ˌsækəroʊ's(j)ʊərɪə] *n* übermäßige Saccharoseausscheidung *f* im Harn, Saccharosurie *f*, Sucrosuria *f*.
sac·cha·rum ['sækərəm] *n* **1.** Zucker *m*, Saccharum *nt*. **2.** → saccharose.
sac·cha·ria [sækə'r(j)ʊərɪə] *n* → saccharorrhea.
sac·ci·form ['sæk(s)ɪfɔːrm] *adj anat.* sackförmig, -artig.
sacciform kidney Sackniere *f*.
sacciform recess: s. of (articulation of) elbow Rec. sacciformis artic. cubiti.
s. of distal radioulnar articulation Rec. sacciformis artic. radioulnaris distalis.
sac·cu·lar ['sækjələr] *adj* sackförmig, -artig.
saccular aneurysm sackartiges Aneurysma *nt*, Aneurysma sacciforme.

saccular bronchiectasis sackförmige Bronchiektas(i)e *f*.
saccular kidney Sackniere *f*.
saccular lung Sacklunge *f*.
saccular nerve N. saccularis.
saccular part/portion of otic vesicle *embryo.* Sacculus-Abschnitt *m* des Ohrbläschens.
saccular spot Macula sacculi.
sac·cu·lat·ed ['sækjəleɪtɪd] *adj* → saccular.
sacculated aneurysm → saccular aneurysm.
sacculated bronchiectasis → saccular bronchiectasis.
sacculated pleurisy Pleuritis saccata.
sac·cu·la·tion [ˌsækjə'leɪʃn] *n* Aussackung *f*, Sacculation *f*, Sacculatio *f*.
s.s of colon Kolon-, Dickdarmhaustren *pl*, Haustra/Sacculationes coli.
sac·cule ['sækjuːl] *n* **1.** *anat.* kleine Aussackung *f*, Säckchen *nt*, Sacculus *m*. **2.** (Ohr) Sakkulus *m*, Sacculus *m*.
sac·cu·lo·coch·le·ar [ˌsækjəloʊ'kɒklɪər, -'koʊ-] *adj* Sacculus u. Cochlea betr., sacculokochlear.
sac·cu·lo·u·tric·u·lar canal/duct [ˌ-juː'trɪkjələr] Ductus utriculosaccularis.
sac·cu·lus ['sækjələs] *n, pl* **-li** [-laɪ] *anat.* kleiner Sack *m*, Säckchen *nt*, Sacculus *m*.
sac·cus ['sækəs] *n, pl* **-ci** [-kaɪ, -saɪ, -kiː] *anat.* Sack *m*, Saccus *m*.
sac fungi *micro.* Schlauchpilze *pl*, Askomyzeten *pl*, Ascomycetes *pl*, Ascomycotina *pl*.
Sachs [zaks]: **S.' bacillus** Pararauschbrandbazillus *m*, Clostridium septicum.
S.' disease Tay-Sachs-Erkrankung *f*, -Syndrom *nt*, infantile amaurotische Idiotie *f*, GM$_2$-Gangliosidose *f* Typ I.
Sachs-Georgi ['dʒɔːrdʒɪ]: **S.-G. reaction/test** Sachs-Georgi-Reaktion *f*, Lentochol-Reaktion *f*.
sacr- *pref.* → sacro-.
sa·cral ['sækrəl, 'seɪ-] *adj* Kreuzbein betr., sakral, Kreuzbein-, Sakral-.
sacral agenesis sakrokokzygeale Agenesie *f*, Syndrom *nt* der kaudalen Regression.
sacral ala Kreuzbeinflügel *m*, Ala sacralis.
sacral anesthesia Sakralanästhesie *f*, -blockade *f*.
sacral artery, median mittlere Kreuzbeinarterie *f*, Sakralis *f* mediana, A. sacralis mediana.
sacral block Sakralanästhesie *f*, -blockade *f*.
sacral branches of median sacral artery, lateral Rami sacrales laterales a. sacralis medianae.
sacral bone → sacrum.
sacral canal Kreuzbeinkanal *m*, Canalis sacralis.
sacral cord → sacral part of spinal cord.
sacral crest Crista sacralis mediana.
 articular s. → intermediate s.
 external s. → lateral s.
 intermediate s. Crista sacralis intermedia.

lateral s. Crista sacralis lateralis.
medial s. Crista sacralis mediana.
sacral dermoid Sakraldermoid *nt*.
sacral flexure of rectum Sakralflexur *f* des Rektums, Flexura sacralis (recti).
sacral foramina: anterior s. Forr. sacralia anteriora/pelvica.
dorsal s. Forr. sacralia dorsalia/posteriora.
internal s. → anterior s.
posterior s. → dorsal s.
sacral ganglia Sakralganglien *pl* des Grenzstrangs, Ggll. sacralia.
sa·cral·gia [seɪˈkrældʒ(ɪ)ə] *n* Kreuzbeinschmerz *m*, Sakralgie *f*, Sakrodynie *f*.
sacral hiatus untere Öffnung *f* des Kreuzbeinkanals, Hiatus sacralis.
sa·cral·i·za·tion [ˌseɪkrəlɪˈzeɪʃn] *n* ortho., embryo. Sakralisation *f*.
sacral nerves sakrale Spinalnerven *pl*, Sakral-, Kreuzbeinnerven *pl*, Nn. sacrales.
sacral nuclei, parasympathetic Kerne *pl* des sakralen Parasympathikus, Ncc. parasympathici sacrales.
sacral parasite *patho.* Sakralparasit *m*.
sacral part of spinal cord Sakralabschnitt *m* des Rückenmarks, Sakralmark *nt*, Kreuzbein-, Sakralsegmente *pl*, Pars sacralis (medullae spinalis), Sacralia *pl*.
sacral plexus 1. Kreuzbein-, Sakralplexus *m*, Plexus sacralis. **2.** Plexus venosus sacralis.
sacral region Kreuzbeinregion *f*, -gegend *f*, Regio sacralis.
sacral segments of spinal cord → sacral part of spinal cord.
sacral spot Mongolenfleck *m*.
sacral tuberosity Tuberositas sacralis.
sacral vein: lateral s.s *pl* seitliche Kreuzbeinvenen *pl*, Vv. sacrales laterales.
middle s. mittlere Kreuzbeinvene *f*, V. sacralis mediana.
sacral vertebrae Kreuz(bein)-, Sakralwirbel *pl*, Vertebrae sacrales.
sa·crec·to·my [seɪˈkrektəmɪ] *n* ortho., chir. Kreuzbeinresektion *f*, Sakrektomie *f*.
sacro- *pref.* Sakral-, Sakr(o)-, Kreuzbein-.
sac·ro·car·di·nal veins [ˌseɪkrəʊˈkɑːrdɪnl, ˌsæk-] *embryo.* Sakrokardinalvenen *pl*.
sac·ro·coc·cyg·e·al [ˌ-kɑkˈsɪdʒ(ɪ)əl] *adj* Kreuzbein/Os sacrum u. Steißbein/Os coccygis betr., sakrokokzygeal.
sacrococcygeal artery → sacral artery, median.
sacrococcygeal articulation/joint Kreuzbein-Steißbein-Gelenk *nt*, Sakrokokzygealgelenk *nt*, Artic. sacrococcygea.
sacrococcygeal ligament Lig. sacrococcygeum.
anterior s. Lig. sacrococcygeum anterius.
dorsal s., deep Lig. sacrococcygeum posterius profundum.
dorsal s., superficial Lig. sacrococcygeum posterius superficiale.
lateral s. Lig. sacrococcygeum laterale.
posterior s., deep → dorsal s., deep.
posterior s., superficial → dorsal s., superficial.
sacrococcygeal muscle: anterior s. → sacrococcygeus ventralis (muscle).
posterior s. → sacrococcygeus dorsalis (muscle).
sacrococcygeal sinus Pilonidalsinus *m*, -fistel *f*, Fistula pilonidalis.
sacrococcygeal symphysis → sacrococcygeal articulation.
sacrococcygeal teratoma Steiß-, Sakralteratom *nt*.
sa·cro·coc·cy·ge·us dorsalis (muscle) [ˌ-kɑkˈsɪdʒɪəs] hinterer/dorsaler Sakrokokzygeus *m*, M. sacrococcygeus dorsalis.
sacrococcygeus ventralis (muscle) vorderer/ventraler Sakrokokzygeus *m*, M. sacrococcygeus ventralis.
sa·cro·coc·cyx [ˌ-ˈkɑksɪks] *n* Kreuzbein u. Steißbein *nt*, Sacrococcyx *f*.
sa·cro·cox·al·gia [ˌ-kɑkˈsældʒ(ɪ)ə] *n* Schmerz(en *pl*) *m* im Iliosakralgelenk, Sakrokoxalgie *f*.
sa·cro·cox·i·tis [ˌ-kɑkˈsaɪtɪs] *n* Entzündung *f* des Iliosakralgelenk, Sakrokoxitis *f*, Sacrocoxitis *f*.
sa·cro·dyn·ia [ˌ-ˈdiːnɪə] *n* → sacralgia.
sac·ro·gen·i·tal fold [ˌ-ˈdʒenɪtl] Plica recto-uterina.
sac·ro·il·i·ac [ˌ-ˈɪlɪæk] *adj* Kreuzbein/Os sacrum u. Ilium betr., sakroiliakal, iliosakral.
sacroiliac articulation Kreuzbein-Darmbein-Gelenk *nt*, Iliosakralgelenk *nt abbr.* ISG, Artic. sacroiliaca.
sacroiliac joint → sacroiliac articulation.
sacroiliac ligaments Ligg. sacroiliaca.
anterior s. Ligg. sacroiliaca anteriora.
dorsal s. → posterior s.
interosseous s. Ligg. sacroiliaca interossea.
posterior s. Ligg. sacroiliaca posteriora.
ventral s. → anterior s.
sacroiliac symphysis → sacroiliac articulation.
sa·cro·il·i·i·tis [ˌ-ˌɪlɪˈaɪtɪs] *n* → sacrocoxitis.
sa·cro·lis·the·sis [ˌ-lɪsˈθiːsɪs] *n* → spondylolisthesis.
sac·ro·lum·ba·lis (muscle) [ˌ-lʌmˈbeɪlɪs] Iliokostalis *m* lumborum, M. iliocostalis lumborum.
sa·cro·lum·bar [ˌ-ˈlʌmbər] *adj* Kreuzbein u. Lende betr., lumbosakral.
sa·cro·per·i·ne·al [ˌ-ˌperɪˈniːəl] *adj* Kreuzbein/Os sacrum u. Damm/Perineum betr., sakroperineal, perineosakral.
sa·cro·pu·bic diameter [ˌ-ˈpjuːbɪk] *gyn.* Distantia sacropubica.
sac·ro·sci·at·ic [ˌ-saɪˈætɪk] *adj* Kreuzbein/Os sacrum u. Ischium betr., ischiosakral.
sacrosciatic foramen: greater s. For. ischiadicum majus.
lesser s. For. ischiadicum minus.
sacrosciatic ligament → sacrospinal ligament.
great s. → sacrotuberal ligament.
sacrosciatic notch: greater s. Inc. ischiadica major.
lesser s. Inc. ischiadica minor.
sac·ro·spi·nal [ˌ-ˈspaɪnl] *adj* Kreuzbein/Os sacrum u. Wirbelsäule betr., sakrospinal, spinosakral.
sac·ro·spi·na·lis muscle [ˌ-spaɪˈneɪlɪs] → sacrospinal muscle.
sacrospinal ligament Lig. sacrospinale.
sacrospinal muscle Erektor *m* spinae, Sakrospinalis *m*, *old* M. sacrospinalis, M. erector spinae.
sac·ro·spi·nous [ˌ-ˈspaɪnəs] *adj* → sacrospinal.
sacrospinous ligament → sacrospinal ligament.
sa·crot·o·my [seɪˈkrɑtəmɪ] *n* ortho. Sakrotomie *f*.
sac·ro·tu·ber·al [ˌseɪkrəʊˈt(j)uːbərəl, ˌsæk-] *adj* Kreuzbein/Os sacrum u. Tuber ischiadicum betr., sakrotuberal, tuberosakral.
sacrotuberal ligament Lig. sacrotuberale.
sac·ro·tu·ber·ous [ˌ-ˈt(j)uːbərəs] *adj* → sacrotuberal.
sacrotuberous ligament → sacrotuberal ligament.
sa·cro·u·ter·ine [ˌ-ˈjuːtərɪn, -raɪn] *adj* Kreuzbein/Os sacrum u. Gebärmutter/Uterus betr., sakrouterin, uterosakral.
sa·cro·ver·te·bral angle [ˌ-ˈvɜrtəbrəl] Lumbosakral-, Sakrovertebralwinkel *m*.
sa·crum [ˈseɪkrəm, ˈsæk-] *n*, *pl* **sac·ra** [-krə] Kreuzbein *nt*, Sakrum *nt*, Sacrum *nt*, Os sacrum/sacrale.
sac·to·sal·pinx [ˌsæktəʊˈsælpɪŋks] *n gyn.* Sakto-, Sactosalpinx *f*.
sad·dle [ˈsædl] *n* Sattel *m*, sattelähnliche Struktur *f*.
saddle anesthesia *neuro.* Reithosenanästhesie *f*.
saddle articulation Sattelgelenk *nt*, Artic. sellaris.
saddle back Hohl(rund)rücken *m*, Hohlkreuz *nt*.
saddle-back nose Sattelnase *f*.
saddle block (anesthesia) Sattelblock-(anästhesie *f*) *m*.
saddle embolism Sattelembolie *f*.
saddle embolus reitender Embolus *m*, Sattelembolus *m*.
saddle head Sattelkopf *m*, Klinokephalie *f*, -zephalie *f*.
saddle joint → saddle articulation.
saddle nose Sattelnase *f*.
saddle-shaped uterus Uterus arcuatus.
sa·dism [ˈseɪdɪzəm, ˈsæd-] *n* Sadismus *m*.
sa·dist [ˈ-dɪst] *n* Sadist(in *f*) *m*.
sa·dis·tic [-ˈdɪstɪk] *adj* Sadismus betr., sadistisch.
sadistic personality (disorder) sadistische Persönlichkeit(sstörung *f*) *f*.
sad·o·mas·o·chism [ˌseɪdəʊˈmæsəkɪzəm, ˌsæd-] *n* Sadomasochismus *m*.
sad·o·mas·o·chis·tic [ˌ-ˌmæsəˈkɪstɪk] *adj* Sadomasochismus betr., sadomasochistisch.
Saemisch [ˈseɪmɪʃ; ˈzɛː-]: **S.'s ulcer** Ulcus corneae serpens.
Saenger [ˈzɛŋər]: **S.'s operation** *gyn.* Saenger-Methode *f*.
Saethre-Chotzen [ˈsæθrɪ ˈʃɔtsən, ˈsɛːtrə ˈkɔː-]: **S.-C. syndrome** Chotzen-(-Saethre)-Syndrom *nt*, Akrozephalosyndaktylie *f* Typ III.
safe·ty [ˈseɪftɪ] **I** *n* **1.** Sicherheit *f*; Gefahrlosigkeit *f*. **2.** Sicherheit *f*, Zuverlässigkeit *f*, Verlässlichkeit *f*. **3.** Schutz-, Sicherheitsvorrichtung *f*, Sicherung *f*. **II** *adj* Sicherheits-.
safety belt Sicherheitsgürtel *m*, -gurt *m*.
safety fuse (Schmelz-)Sicherung *f*.
safety glass Sicherheitsglas *nt*.
safety glasses Schutzbrille *f*.
safety lens Schutzbrille *f*.
safety limit Sicherheitsgrenze *f*.
safety measure Sicherheitsmaßnahme *f*, -vorkehrung *f*.
safety provisions Sicherheitsvorkehrungen *pl*.
safety rules Sicherheits-, Unfallverhütungsvorschriften *pl*.
safety spectacles Schutzbrille *f*.
safety switch Sicherheitsschalter *m*.
safety valve Überdruck-, Sicherheitsventil *nt*.
SAF fixative [sodium acetate formaline] SAF-Fixierlösung *f*.
saf·fron liver [ˈsæfrən] Safranleber *f*, Hepar crocatum.
saf·ra·nin [ˈsæfrənɪn] *n* → safranine.
saf·ra·nine [ˈsæfrəniːn, -nɪn] *n* Safranin *nt*.
sag·it·tal [ˈsædʒɪtl] *adj* sagittal, pfeilartig, Pfeil-.
sagittal axis of eye optische Augenachse *f*, Sehachse *f*, Axis opticus (bulbi oculi).
sagittal diameter sagittaler Durchmesser *m*, Diameter sagittalis.
sagittal groove → sagittal sulcus.
sagittal margin of parietal bone Margo sagittalis (ossis parietalis).

sagittal plane

sagittal plane Sagittalebene *f*, Sagittale *f*.
sagittal section Sagittalschnitt *m*.
sagittal sinus: inferior s. Sinus sagittalis inferior.
superior s. Sinus sagittalis superior.
sagittal sulcus Sinus sagittalis superior--Rinne *f*, Sulcus sinus sagittalis superioris.
sagittal suture Pfeilnaht *f*, Sutura sagittalis.
sagittal synostosis → scaphocephaly.
sa·go liver ['seɪgəʊ] Sagoleber *f*.
sago spleen Sagomilz *f*.
sail·or's skin ['seɪlər] Farmer-, Landmanns-, Seemannshaut *f*.
Saint [seɪnt; sɛ̃]: **S.'s triad** Saint'-Trias *f*, -Syndrom *nt*.
St. Anthony ['æntənɪ, 'ænθə-]: **St. A.'s dance** → Sydenham's chorea.
St. A.'s fire 1. *derm*. Wundrose *f*, Rose *f*, Erysipel *nt*, Erysipelas *nt*, Streptodermia cutanea lymphatica. **2.** Vergiftung *f* durch Mutterkornalkaloide, Ergotismus *m*.
St. Guy [gaɪ]: **St. G.'s dance** → Sydenham's chorea.
St. John [dʒɑn]: **St. J.'s dance** → Sydenham's chorea.
St. Louis encephalitis ['luːɪs] *abbr*. **SLE** St. Louis-Enzephalitis *f abbr*. SLE.
St. Louis encephalitis virus St. Louis--Enzephalitis-Virus *nt*.
St. Vitus ['vaɪtəs]: **St. V.' dance** → Sydenham's chorea.
Sakati-Nyhan [sɑˈkɑːtɪ 'naɪhæn]: **S.-N. syndrome** Sakati-Nyhan-Syndrom *nt*.
sa·ku·shu fever [sɑˈkuːʃu] Sakushu-, Akiyami-, Hasamiyami-Fieber *nt*.
sal [sæl] *n* Salz *nt*, Sal *nt*.
Sala ['sælə]: **S.'s cells** Sala-Zellen *pl*.
sa·laam attack [səˈlɑːm] → salaam spasm.
salaam convulsion → salaam spasm.
salaam spasm Salaamkrampf *m*, Nickkrampf *m*, Spasmus nutans.
sal·a·zo·sul·fa·pyr·i·dine [ˌsæləzoʊˌsʌlfəˈpɪrɪdiːn] *n pharm*. Salazosulfapyridin *nt*.
sal·bu·ta·mol [sælˈbjuːtəmɑl, -mɔl] *n pharm*. Salbutamol *nt*.
sal·i·cyl ['sælɪsɪl] *n* Salizyl-, Salicyl-(Radikal *nt*).
sal·i·cyl·al·de·hyde [ˌ-ˈældəhaɪd] *n* → salicylic aldehyde.
sal·i·cyl·am·ide [ˌ-ˈæmaɪd, sæləˈsɪləmaɪd] *n pharm*. Salizylamid *nt*, Salicylamid *nt*, Salicylsäureamid *nt*, *o*-Hydroxybenzamid *nt*.
sa·lic·y·late [səˈlɪsəleɪt, -lɪt] **I** *n* Salizylat *nt*, Salicylat *nt*. **II** *vt* mit Salizylsäure behandeln.
sa·lic·y·lat·ed [səˈlɪsəleɪtɪd] *adj* mit Salizylsäure behandelt; Salizylsäure-haltig.
sal·i·cyl·a·zo·sul·fa·pyr·i·dine [sæləsɪlˌeɪzoʊˌsʌlfəˈpɪrɪdiːn] *n pharm*. Salazosulfapyridin *nt*.
sal·i·cyl·e·mia [ˌ-ˈiːmɪə] *n* Salizylämie *f*.
sal·i·cyl·ic acid [sæləˈsɪlɪk] Salizylsäure *f*, Salicylsäure *f*, *o*-Hydroxybenzoesäure *f*.
salicylic aldehyde Salizylaldehyd *nt*.
sal·i·cyl·ism ['sæləsɪlɪzəm] *n* Salicyl(säure)-vergiftung *f*, Salizylismus *m*, Salicylismus *m*.
sal·i·cyl·ize ['sæləsɪlaɪz, səˈlɪsə-] *vt* → salicylate II.
sal·i·cyl·sul·fon·ic acid [ˌsæləsɪlsʌlˈfɑnɪk] → sulfosalicylic acid.
sal·i·cyl·u·ric acid [ˌ-ˈ(j)ʊərɪk] Salicylursäure *f*.
sa·li·ent ['seɪljənt, -lɪənt] *adj* (her-)vorspringend, herausragend.
sa·lif·er·ous [səˈlɪfərəs] *adj* salzbildend; salzhaltig.

sal·i·fi·a·ble ['sælɪfaɪəbl] *adj chem*. salzbildend.
sal·i·fy ['sælɪfaɪ] *vt chem*. **1.** in ein Salz umwandeln. **2.** ein Salz bilden mit.
sa·lim·e·ter [səˈlɪmɪtər] *n* Salimeter *nt*.
sa·line ['seɪliːn, -laɪn] **I** *n* Salzlösung *f*; physiologische Kochsalzlösung *f*. **II** *adj* salzig, salzhaltig, -artig, salinisch, Salz-.
saline agglutinin → saline antibody.
saline antibody kompletter/agglutinierender Antikörper *m*.
Sal·i·nem fever/infection ['sælɪnem] Salinem-Fieber *nt*.
saline solution Salzlösung *f*.
isotonic s. isotone (Koch-)Salzlösung.
normal/physiologic s. physiologische Kochsalzlösung.
sa·lin·i·ty [səˈlɪnətɪ] *n* Salzigkeit *f*, Salzhaltigkeit *f*; Salzgehalt *m*.
sal·i·nom·e·ter [sælɪˈnɑmɪtər] *n* Salinometer *nt*.
sa·li·va [səˈlaɪvə] *n* Speichel(flüssigkeit *f*) *m*, Saliva *f*.
sal·i·vant ['sælɪvənt] **I** *n* den Speichelfluß anregendes Mittel *nt*. **II** *adj* den Speichelfluß anregend.
sal·i·var·y ['sæləˌverɪ, -vərɪ] *adj* **1.** Speichel/Saliva betr., Speichel-, Sial(o)-. **2.** Speichel produzierend.
salivary calculus 1. Speichelstein *m*, Sialolith *m*. **2.** → supragingival calculus.
salivary corpuscle Speichelkörperchen *nt*.
salivary fistula Speichelfistel *f*.
salivary gland disease Zytomegalie(-Syndrom *nt*) *f*, Zytomegalievirusinfektion *f*, zytomegale Einschlußkörperkrankheit *f*.
salivary gland granuloma Speicheldrüsengranulom *nt*.
salivary gland mixed tumor Speicheldrüsenmischtumor *m*.
salivary glands Speicheldrüsen *pl*, Gll. salivariae.
large s. große Speicheldrüsen, Gll. salivariae majores.
major s. → large s.
minor s. → small s.
small s. kleine Speicheldrüsen, Gll. salivariae minores.
salivary gland tumor Speicheldrüsentumor *m*.
salivary gland virus Zytomegalievirus *nt*, Cytomegalievirus *nt abbr*. CMV.
salivary stone → sialolith.
sal·i·vate ['sælɪveɪt] **I** *vt* vermehrten Speichelfluß hervorrufen. **II** *vi* Speichel/Saliva produzieren.
sal·i·va·tion [ˌsælɪˈveɪʃn] *n* **1.** Speichelbildung *f*, -absonderung *f*, Salivation *f*. **2.** übermäßiger Speichelfluß *m*, Hypersalivation *f*, Salivation *f*.
sal·i·va·tor ['sælɪveɪtər] *n* → salivant I.
sal·i·va·to·ry ['sælɪvətɔːriː, -təʊ-] *adj* die Speichelsekretion betr. *od*. fördernd.
salivatory nucleus: caudal s. Nc. salivarius caudalis/inferior.
cranial s. Nc. salivarius cranialis/rostralis/superior.
inferior s. → caudal s.
rostral s. → cranial s.
superior s. → cranial s.
sal·i·vo·li·thi·a·sis [ˌsælɪvoʊlɪˈθaɪəsɪs] *n* → sialolithiasis.
Salk ['sɔː(l)k]: **S. vaccine** Salk-Impfstoff *m*, -Vakzine *f*.
sal·mi·ac ['sælmɪˌæk] *n* Ammoniumchlorid *nt*, Salmiak *nt*.
Sal·mo·nel·la [ˌsælməˈnelə] *n micro*. Salmonella *f*.
S. enteritidis Gärtner-Bazillus *m*, Salmonella enteritidis.

S. typhi Typhusbazillus *m*, -bacillus *m*, Salmonella typhi.
S. typhosa → S. typhi.
sal·mo·nel·la [ˌ-ˈnelə] *n*, *pl* **-lae** [-liː] Salmonelle *f*, Salmonella *f*.
sal·mo·nel·lal [ˌ-ˈnelə] *adj* Salmonellen betr., durch Salmonellen verusacht, Salmonellen-.
salmonellal infection Salmonelleninfektion *f*.
Salmonella-Shigella agar Salmonella--Shigella-Agar *m/nt*.
sal·mo·nel·lo·sis [ˌ-nəˈloʊsɪs] *n* Salmonellose *f*.
salm·on patch ['sæmən] **1.** *ophthal*. Hornhautfleck(en *pl*) *m* bei konnataler Lues. **2.** *derm*. Feuer-, Gefäßmal *nt*, Portwein-, Weinfleck *m*, Naevus flammeus.
sal·ol ['sælɔl, -al] *n* Phenylsalicylat *nt*.
salping- *pref*. → salpingo-.
sal·pin·gec·to·my [ˌsælpɪnˈdʒektəmɪ] *n gyn*. Eileiterentfernung *f*, -resektion *f*, Salpingektomie *f*.
sal·pin·gem·phrax·is [ˌsælpɪndʒəmˈfræksɪs] *n* **1.** HNO Verlegung/Obstruktion *f* der Ohrtrompete. **2.** *gyn*. Eileiterverlegung *f*, -obstruktion *f*.
sal·pin·gi·an [sælˈpɪndʒɪən] *adj* **1.** HNO Ohrtrompete betr., Salping(o)-, Syring(o)-. **2.** *gyn*. Eileiter betr., Eileiter-, Salping(o)-, Tuben-.
salpingian dropsy Hydrosalpinx *f*, Hydrops tubae, Sactosalpinx serosa.
sal·pin·gi·o·ma [ˌsælpɪndʒɪˈəʊmə] *n gyn*. Eileitertumor *m*.
sal·pin·git·ic [ˌsælpɪnˈdʒɪtɪk] *adj* Salpingitis betr., von Salpingitis gekennzeichnet, salpingitisch.
sal·pin·gi·tis [ˌ-ˈdʒaɪtɪs] *n* **1.** *gyn*. Eileiterentzündung *f*, Salpingitis *f*. **2.** HNO → syringitis.
salpingo- *pref*. **1.** HNO Salping(o)-, Syring(o)-. **2.** *gyn*. Eileiter-, Tuben-, Salping(o)-.
sal·pin·go·cele [sælˈpɪŋɡəʊsiːl] *n gyn*. Salpingozele *f*.
sal·pin·go·cy·e·sis [ˌ-saɪˈiːsɪs] *n* Eileiter-, Tuben-, Tubarschwangerschaft *f*, Tubargravidität *f*, Graviditas tubaria.
sal·pin·gog·ra·phy [ˌsælpɪŋˈɡɑɡrəfɪ] *n gyn*., *radiol*. Salpingographie *f*.
sal·pin·go·li·thi·a·sis [sælˌpɪŋɡəʊlɪˈθaɪəsɪs] *n gyn*. Salpingolithiasis *f*.
sal·pin·gol·y·sis [ˌsælpɪŋˈɡɑləsɪs] *n gyn*. Eileiterlösung *f*, Salpingolyse *f*, -lysis *f*.
salpingo-oophorectomy *n gyn*. Entfernung *f* von Eileiter u. Eierstock, Salpingo-Oophorektomie *f*, Salpingo-Ovariektomie *f*.
salpingo-oophoritis *n gyn*. Entzündung *f* von Eileiter u. Eierstock, Salpingo--Oophoritis *f*.
salpingo-oophorocele *n gyn*., *chir*. Salpingo-Oophorozele *f*.
salpingo-oothecitis *n* → salpingo-oophoritis.
salpingo-oothecocele *n* → salpingo-oophorocele.
salpingo-ovariectomy *n* → salpingo-oophorectomy.
salpingo-ovariotomy *n* → salpingo-oophorectomy.
sal·pin·go·pal·a·tine [sælˌpɪŋɡəʊˈpælətaɪn] *adj* Ohrtrompete/Tuba auditiva u. Gaumen/Palatum betr. *od*. verbindend.
salpingopalatine fold Tubenwulst *m*, Plica salpingopalatina/palatotubalis.
sal·pin·go·per·i·to·ni·tis [ˌ-ˌperɪtəˈnaɪtɪs] *n gyn*. Salpingoperitonitis *f*.
sal·pin·go·pex·y ['-peksɪ] *n gyn*. Eileiterfixation *f*, Salpingopexie *f*.
sal·pin·go·pha·ryn·ge·al [ˌ-fəˈrɪnˈdʒ(ɪ)əl]

adj Ohrtrompete/Tuba auditiva u. Rachen/Pharynx betr. *od.* verbindend.
salpingopharyngeal fold Plica salpingopharyngea.
salpingopharyngeal ligament Plica salpingopharyngea.
salpingopharyngeal muscle → salpingopharyngeus (muscle).
sal·pin·go·pha·ryn·ge·us (muscle) [ˌfə-ˈrɪndʒ(ɪ)əs] Salpingopharyngeus *m*, M. salpingopharyngeus.
sal·pin·go·plas·ty [ˈ-ˌplæstɪ] *n gyn.* Eileiter-, Tuben-, Salpingoplastik *f.*
sal·pin·gor·rha·gia [ˌ-ˈreɪdʒ(ɪ)ə] *n gyn.* Eileiterblutung *f*, Salpingorrhagie *f.*
sal·pin·gor·rha·phy [ˌsælpɪŋˈɡɔrəfɪ] *n gyn.* Eileiter-, Tubennaht *f*, Salpingorrhaphie *f.*
sal·pin·gos·co·py [ˌsælpɪŋˈɡɒskəpɪ] *n* 1. *gyn., radiol.* Salpingoskopie *f*. 2. *HNO* Salpingoskopie *f.*
sal·pin·go·sto·mat·o·my [sælˌpɪŋɡəʊstəʊ-ˈmætəmɪ] *n gyn.* Salpingostoma(to)tomie *f*, Salpingostomatoplastik *f.*
sal·pin·go·sto·mat·o·plas·ty [ˌ-stəʊˈmætəplæstɪ] *n* → salpingostomatomy.
sal·pin·gos·to·my [ˌsælpɪŋˈɡɒstəmɪ] *n* 1. → salpingostomatotomy. 2. Salpingostomie *f.*
sal·pin·got·o·my [ˌsælpɪŋˈɡɒtəmɪ] *n gyn.* Eileitereröffnung *f*, -schnitt *m*, Salpingotomie *f.*
sal·pinx [ˈsælpɪŋks] *n* 1. *anat.* Salpinx *f*. 2. *gyn.* Eileiter *m*, Salpinx *f*, Tube *f*, Tuba uterina. 3. *HNO* Ohrtrompete *f*, Tuba auditiva/auditoria, Salpinx *f.*
salt [sɔːlt] **I** *n* 1. *chem.* Salz *nt*. 2. Koch-, Tafelsalz *nt*, Natriumchlorid *nt*. 3. ˷s *pl* (Abführ-)Salz *nt*. 4. *fig.* Würze *f*, Salz *nt*. **II** *adj* 5. salzig, Salz-. 6. (ein-)gesalzen, (ein-)gepökelt. **III** *vt* (ein-)salzen, würzen, mit Salz bestreuen; *chem.* mit Salz behandeln.
salt in *vt chem., phys.* einsalzen.
salt out *vt chem., phys.* aussalzen.
salt agglutination Salzagglutination *f.*
salt and pepper fundus *ophthal.* Pfeffer- u. Salzfundus *m.*
sal·ta·tion [sælˈteɪʃn] *n* 1. Springen *nt*, Tanzen *nt*. 2. *neuro.* Veitstanz *m*, Chorea *f.* 3. saltatorische Erregungsleitung *f*. 4. *genet.* (sprunghafte) Mutation *f.*
sal·ta·to·ri·al [ˌsæltəˈtɔːrɪəl, -ˈtɔːr-] *adj* → saltatory.
sal·ta·to·ric [ˌ-ˈtɔːrɪk, -ˈtəʊ-] *adj* → saltatory.
sal·ta·to·ry [ˈ-təʊrɪ, -ˌtɔː-] *adj* sprunghaft, (über-)springend, hüpfend, saltatorisch, Sprung-, Spring-.
saltatory conduction *physiol.* saltatorische Erregungsleitung/-fortleitung *f.*
saltatory spasm/tic Bamberger-Krankheit *f*, saltatorischer Reflexkrampf *m.*
saltatory variation sprunghafte Variation *f*, Haematogenese *f*, -genesis *f.*
salt bridge *phys.* Salzbrücke *f.*
salt cake *chem.* (technisches) Natriumsulfat *nt.*
salt depletion Salzverlust *m*, -mangel *m.*
salt-depletion crisis/syndrome Salzmangelsyndrom *nt.*
salt·ed [ˈsɔːltɪd] *adj* (ein-)gesalzen.
Salter [ˈsɔːltər]: **S. classification** *ortho.* Einteilung *f* der Epiphysenfrakturen nach Salter u. Harris.
  S. innominate osteotomy → S. operation.
  S.'s lines Owen-Linien *pl.*
  S. operation *ortho.* Beckenosteotomie *f* nach Salter.
  S. osteotomy → S. operation.
Salter and Harris [ˈhærɪs]: **S.a.H. classification** *ortho.* Einteilung *f* der Epiphysenfrakturen nach Salter u. Harris.
salt fever Salzfieber *nt.*
salt-free *adj (Diät)* salzfrei; salzarm.
salt-graving *n patho., gyn.* Salzhunger *m.*
salt·i·ness [ˈsɔːltɪnɪs] *n* Salzigkeit *f*, Salzgeschmack *m*; Salzgehalt *m.*
salting-in *n chem., phys.* Einsalzen *nt.*
salting-out *n chem., phys.* Aussalzen *nt.*
salt intoxication Salzvergiftung *f*, -intoxikation *f.*
salt·less [ˈsɔːltlɪs] *adj* salzlos, -frei.
salt-losing *adj* salzverlierend, Salzverlust-.
salt-losing crisis Salzverlustsyndrom *nt.*
salt-losing defect Salzverlustsyndrom *nt.*
salt-losing nephritis Thorn-Syndrom *nt*, Salzverlustnephritis *f.*
salt-losing nephropathy salzverlierende Nephropathie *f*, renales Salzverlustsyndrom *nt.*
salt-losing syndrome Salzverlustsyndrom *nt.*
salt loss Salzverlust *m.*
salt·ness [ˈsɔːltnɪs] *n* → saltiness.
salt·pe·ter [ˈsɔːltˈpiːtər] *n chem.* Salpeter *m*, Kaliumnitrat *nt.*
salt retention Salzeinlagerung *f*, -retention *f.*
salt solution 1. Salzlösung *f*. 2. Kochsalzlösung *f.*
  normal/physiologic s. physiologische Kochsalzlösung.
salt wasting Salzverlust *m.*
salt·y [ˈsɔːltɪ] *adj* salzig.
sa·lu·bri·ous [səˈluːbrɪəs] *adj* gesund, bekömmlich, heilsam, saluber.
sa·lu·bri·ty [səˈluːbrətɪ] *n* Heilsamkeit *f*, Bekömmlichkeit *f*, Salubrität *f.*
sa·lu·re·sis [ˌsæljəˈriːsɪs] *n* Salurese *f*, Salidiurese *f.*
sal·u·ret·ic [ˌ-ˈretɪk] **I** *n* Saluretikum *nt.* **II** *adj* Salurese betr. *od.* fördernd, saluretisch.
sa·lu·tar·y [ˈsæljətərɪ] *adj* heilsam, gesund, bekömmlich, Heil-.
salve [sæv, sɑːv] *n pharm.* Salbe *f*, Unguentum *nt.*
sa·mar·i·um [səˈmeərɪəm] *n abbr. Sm* Samarium *nt abbr.* Sm.
sam·ple [ˈsæmpəl, ˈsɑːm-] **I** *n* 1. Probe *f.* 2. Probepackung *f*, Probe *f.* 3. *stat.* Stichprobe *f*, Probeerhebung *f*, Sample *nt.* 4. Musterbeispiel *nt*, typisches Exemplar *nt.* **II** *adj* Muster-, Probe-. **III** *vt* 5. eine Stichprobe machen, eine Auswahl erheben von. 6. als Muster dienen für, ein Beispiel sein für.
sam·pling [ˈsæmplɪŋ, ˈsɑːm-] *n stat.* 1. Stichprobenerhebung *f.* 2. Muster *nt*, Probe *f.*
Sampson [ˈsæmpsən]: **S.'s cyst** *old* → chocolate cyst.
Sanarelli [sanaˈreli]: **S.'s phenomenon** Sanarelli-Shwartzman-Phänomen *nt*, -Reaktion *f.*
Sanarelli-Shwartzman [ʃwɔːrtsmən]: **S.-S. phenomenon** Sanarelli-Shwartzman-Phänomen *nt*, -Reaktion *f.*
san·a·tive [ˈsænətɪv] *adj* heilend, heilsam, heilungsfördernd, kurativ, Heil(ungs)-.
san·a·to·ri·um [ˌsænəˈtɔːrɪəm, -ˈtəʊ-] *n, pl* **-ri·ums, -ri·a** [-rɪə] 1. Sanatorium *nt*; Erholungsheim *nt.* 2. Lungenheilstätte *f*, Sanatorium *nt.* 3. (Höhen-, Luft-)Kurort *m.*
san·a·to·ry [ˈ-tɔːriː, -təʊ-] *adj* → sanative.
sand [sænd] *n* Sand *m*; ˷s *pl* Sand(körner *pl*) *m.*
sand·bag [ˈsændbæɡ] *n* Sandsack *m.*
sand bath 1. *chem.* Sandbad *nt.* 2. Sandbad *nt*, Balneum arenae.
sand bodies Hirnsand *m*, Acervulus *m* (cerebri).

Sanders [ˈsændərs]: **S.' disease** epidemische Keratokonjunktivitis *f*, Keratoconjunctivitis epidemica.
sand flea *micro.* Sandfloh *m*, Tunga/Dermatophilus penetrans.
sand-fly [ˈsændflaɪ] *n micro.* Sandfliege *f*, Stechfliege *f*; Sandmücke *f*; Kriebelmücke *f*, Phlebotomus *f.*
sandfly fever Phlebotomus-, Pappataci-, Moskitofieber *nt*, Drei-Tage-Fieber *nt.*
sandfly fever virus *micro.* Pappataci(fieber)virus *nt.*
Sandhoff [ˈsændhɔf]: **S.'s disease** GM_2-Gangliosidose *f* Typ II, Sandhoff-Jatzekewitz-Syndrom *nt*, -Variante *f.*
Sandström [ˈzantstreɪm; -strøːm]: **S.'s body/gland** Nebenschilddrüse *f*, Epithelkörperchen *nt*, Parathyr(e)oidea *f*, Gl. parathyroidea.
sand·wich arrangement [ˈsæn(d)wɪtʃ] *histol.* Sandwichpackung *f.*
sand·worm disease [ˈsændwɜːrm] creeping disease (*nt*), Hautmaulwurf *m*, Larva migrans, Myiasis linearis migrans.
sand tumor Sandgeschwulst *f*, Psammom *nt.*
sand·y [ˈsændɪ] *adj* 1. sandig, Sand-; sandartig, körnig. 2. sandfarben, rotblond.
sane [seɪn] *adj* (geistig) normal, gesund; *forens.* zurechnungsfähig.
Sanfilippo [sænfiˈlɪpəʊ]: **S.'s syndrome** Sanfilippo-Syndrom *nt*, Morbus Sanfilippo *m*, polydystrophische Oligophrenie *f*, Mukopolysaccharidose *f* III *abbr.* MPS III.
Sanger [ˈsæŋər]: **S. reaction** *biochem.* Sanger-Reaktion *f.*
  S. reagent 2,4-Dinitrofluorbenzol *nt abbr.* DNFB, Sanger-Reagenz *f.*
Sanger Brown [braʊn]: **S. B. ataxia** *neuro.* Brown-Ataxie *f.*
sangui- *pref.* Blut-, Sangui-, Häma-, Hämat(o)-, Häm(o)-.
san·gui·fa·cient [ˌsæŋɡwəˈfeɪʃnt] *adj* → sanguinopoietic.
san·guif·er·ous [sæŋˈɡwɪfərəs] *adj* bluthaltig, -führend, blutig.
san·gui·fi·ca·tion [ˌsæŋɡwɪfɪˈkeɪʃn] *n* Blutbildung *f*, Hämatopo(i)ese *f*, Hämopo(i)ese *f.*
san·guine [ˈsæŋɡwɪn] *adj* 1. (blut-)rot. 2. *(Temperament)* sanguinisch.
san·guin·e·ous [sæŋˈɡwɪnɪəs] *adj* 1. Blut betr., blutig, Blut-. 2. (blut-)rot.
sanguineous cyst hämorrhagische Zyste *f.*
san·guin·o·lent [sæŋˈɡwɪnələnt] *adj* Blut enthaltend, mit Blut vermischt, blutig, sanguinolent.
san·gui·no·poi·et·ic [ˌsæŋɡwɪnəʊpɔɪˈetɪk] *adj* Blut(zell)bildung betr. *od.* anregend, hämopoietisch.
san·gui·no·pu·ru·lent [ˌ-ˈpjʊər(j)ələnt] *adj* blutig-eitrig.
san·gui·nous [ˈsæŋɡwɪnəs] *adj* → sanguineous.
san·guis [ˈsæŋɡwɪs] *n* Blut *nt*, Sanguis *f.*
san·guiv·or·ous [sæŋˈɡwɪvərəs] *adj micro., bio.* blutsaugend, -fressend.
sa·ni·es [ˈseɪniːz] *n* blutig-eitriger Ausfluß *m.*
san·i·tar·y [ˈsænɪterɪ] *adj* 1. hygienisch, gesundheitlich, sanitär, Gesundheits-. 2. hygienisch (einwandfrei), gesund.
sanitary towel *hyg.* (Monats-, Damen-)Binde *f.*
san·i·ti·za·tion [ˌsænɪtɪˈzeɪʃn] *n hyg.* Sanitizing *nt*, Sanitization *f*, Sanitation *f.*
san·i·tize [ˈsænɪtaɪz] *vt* keimfrei machen, sterilisieren.
san·i·ty [ˈsænətɪ] *n* (geistige) Gesundheit *f*; *forens.* Zurechnungsfähigkeit *f.*

San Joaquin Valley fever

San Joa·quin Valley fever [sæn wɑˈkiːn] San-Joaquin-Valley-Fieber *nt*, Wüsten-, Talfieber *nt*, Primärform *f* der Kokzidioidomykose.
Santorini [ˌsæntəˈriːnɪ, sɑn-]: **S.'s canal** → S.'s duct.
S.'s cartilage Santorini-Knorpel *m*, Cartilago corniculata.
S.'s clefts → S.'s fissures.
S.'s concha oberste Nasenmuschel *f*, Concha nasalis suprema.
S.'s duct Santorini'-Gang *m*, Ductus pancreaticus accessorius.
S.'s fissures Spalten *pl* des Gehörgangsknorpels, Incc. cartilaginis meatus acustici.
S.'s ligament Santorini'-Band *nt*, Lig. cricopharyngeum.
S.'s major caruncle → S.'s papilla.
S.'s minor caruncle Papilla duodeni minor.
S.'s muscle M. risorius.
S.'s papilla Vater'-Papille *f*, Papilla Vateri, Papilla duodeni major.
parietal vein of S. → S.'s vein.
S.'s plexus 1. Prostataplexus *m*, Plexus prostaticus. **2.** venöser Prostataplexus *m*, Plexus venosus prostaticus.
tubercle of S. Tuberculum corniculatum.
S.'s vein V. emissaria parietalis.
São Pau·lo fever [ˈsaʊn ˈpaʊlʊ] Felsengebirgsfleckfieber *nt*, amerikanisches Zeckenbißfieber *nt*, Rocky Mountain spotted fever (*nt*) *abbr*. RMSF.
sap [sæp] *n bio*. Gewebe-, Zell-, Pflanzensaft *m*.
saph·e·nec·to·my [ˌsæfɪˈnektəmɪ] *n chir*. Saphenaexzision *f*, -resektion *f*, Saphenektomie *f*.
sa·phe·nous [səˈfiːnəs] **I** *n* V. saphena. **II** *adj* V. saphena betr.
saphenous branch of descending genicular artery Ramus saphenus a. descendentis genicularis.
saphenous hiatus Hiatus saphenus.
saphenous nerve N. saphenus.
saphenous opening Hiatus saphenus.
saphenous vein V. saphena.
 accessory s. Saphena *f* accessoria, V. saphena accessoria.
 great s. Saphena *f* magna, *inf*. Magna *f*, V. saphena magna.
 small s. Saphena *f* parva, *inf*. Parva *f*, V. saphena parva.
sap·id [ˈsæpɪd] *adj* schmackhaft, einen Geschmack habend.
sa·po [ˈseɪpəʊ] *n* Seife *f*, Sapo *m*.
sa·pog·e·nin [səˈpædʒənɪn, ˌsæpəˈdʒenɪn] *n* Sapogenin *nt*.
sap·o·na·ceous [ˌsæpəˈneɪʃəs] *adj* seifenartig, wie Seife, seifig.
sa·pon·i·fi·a·ble [səˈpɑnɪfaɪəbl] *adj chem*. verseifbar.
saponifiable lipid *chem*. verseifbares/kompliziertes Lipid *nt*.
sa·pon·i·fi·ca·tion [səˌpɑnɪfɪˈkeɪʃn] *n chem*. Verseifung *f*, Saponifikation *f*.
saponification number Verseifungszahl *f*.
sa·pon·i·fi·er [səˈpɑnɪfaɪər] *n chem*. Verseifungsmittel *nt*.
sa·pon·i·fy [səˈpɑnɪfaɪ] *vt, vi chem*. verseifen, saponifizieren.
sap·o·nin [ˈsæpənɪn] *n* Saponin *nt*.
Sappey [ˈsæpɪ]: **S.'s fibers** Sappey-Fasern *pl*.
S.'s nucleus Nc. ruber.
S.'s plexus Sappey-Plexus *m*.
S.'s subareolar plexus → S.'s plexus.
veins of S. Sappey'-Venen *pl*, Vv. paraumbilicales.
sap·phism [ˈsæfɪzəm] *n* weibliche Homosexualität *f*, Lesbianismus *m*, Sapphismus *m*.
sapr(o)- *pref*. Faul-, Fäulnis-, Sapr(o)-.
sap·robe [ˈsæprəʊb] *n* → saprobiont.
sa·pro·bic [səˈprəʊbɪk] *adj bio*. Saprobiont betr., saprobisch.
sap·ro·bi·ont [ˌsæprəʊˈbaɪɒnt, səˈprəʊbɪɒnt] *n bio*. Fäulnisbewohner *m*, Saprobiont *m*, Saprobie *f*.
sap·ro·gen·ic [ˌsæprəʊˈdʒenɪk] *adj bio*. fäulniserregend, saprogen, Fäulnis-.
sa·prog·e·nous [səˈprɒdʒənəs] *adj* → saprogenic.
sap·ro·no·sis [ˌsæprəˈnəʊsɪs] *n* Sapronose *f*.
sap·ro·phile [ˈ-faɪl] *adj bio*. fäulnisliebend, saprophil.
sa·proph·i·lous [səˈprɑfɪləs] *adj* **1.** → saprophile. **2.** → saprophytic.
sap·ro·phyte [ˈsæprəfaɪt] *n bio*. Moder-, Fäulnispflanze *f*, Saprophyt *m*.
sap·ro·phyt·ic [ˌ-ˈfɪtɪk] *adj bio*. saprophytisch, saprophytär, Saprophyten-.
saprophytic bacterium saprophytäres Bakterium *nt*.
saprophytic organism → saprophyte.
sap·ro·zo·ic [ˌ-ˈzəʊɪk] *adj bio*. saprozoisch.
saprozoic organism Saprozoon *nt*.
sar·al·a·sin [særˈæləsɪn] *n pharm*. Saralasin *nt*.
sarc- *pref*. → sarco-.
Sar·ci·na [ˈsɑːrsɪnə, -kɪnə] *n micro*. Sarcina *f*.
sar·ci·na [ˈsɑːrsɪnə, -kɪnə] *n micro*. Sarcine *f*, Sarcina *f*.
sarco- *pref*. Fleisch-, Sark(o)-, Sarc(o)-.
sar·co·blast [ˈsɑːrkəʊblæst] *n* Sarkoblast *m*.
sar·co·car·ci·no·ma [ˌ,-ˌkɑːrsɪˈnəʊmə] *n* Sarcocarcinoma *nt*, Carcinosarcoma *nt*.
sar·co·cele [ˈ-siːl] *n urol*. Sarkozele *f*, Hernia carnosa.
sar·co·cyst [ˈ-sɪst] *n* **1.** → Sarcocystis. **2.** → sarcosporidian cysts.
sar·co·cys·tin [ˌ,-ˈsɪstɪn] *n* Sarcozystin *nt*, Sarkocystin *nt*.
Sar·co·cys·tis [ˌ,-ˈsɪstɪs] *n micro*. Sarcocystis *f*.
sar·co·cys·to·sis [ˌ,-sɪsˈtəʊsɪs] *n* Sarcocystis-Infektion *f*, Sarkozystose *f*, Sarcocystosis *f*, Sarkosporidiose *f*.
Sar·co·di·na [ˌ,-ˈdaɪnə, -ˈdiːnə] *pl micro*. Sarcodina *pl*.
sar·co·en·chon·dro·ma [ˌ,-ˌenkɑnˈdrəʊmə] *n* Chondrosarkom *nt*, -sarcoma *nt*.
sar·co·gen·ic [ˌ,-ˈdʒenɪk] *adj* sarkogen.
sarcogenic cell *embryo*. Myoblast *m*.
sar·co·glia [sɑːrˈkɑːglɪə, ˌsɑːrkəʊˈglaɪə] *n* Sarkoglia *f*, Sarcoglia *f*.
sar·co·hy·dro·cele [ˌsɑːrkəʊˈhaɪdrəsiːl] *n urol*. kombinierte Sarko- u. Hydrozele *f*, Sarkohydrozele *f*.
sar·coid [ˈsɑːrkɔɪd] **I** *n* **1.** → sarcoidosis. **2.** sarkomähnlicher Tumor *m*, Sarkoid *nt*. **II** *adj* fleischartig, sarkoid.
sar·coi·do·sis [ˌsɑːrkɔɪˈdəʊsɪs] *n* Sarkoidose *f*, Morbus Boeck *m*, Boeck'-Sarkoid *nt*, Besnier-Boeck-Schaumann-Krankheit *f*, Lymphogranulomatosa benigna.
sar·co·lac·tic acid [ˌsɑːrkəˈlæktɪk] *old* → lactic acid.
sar·co·lem·ma [ˌ,-ˈlemə] *n* Plasmalemm *nt* der Muskelfaser, Sarkolemm *nt*.
sar·co·lem·mal [ˌ,-ˈleməl] *adj* Sarkolemm betr., sarkolemmal, Sarkolemm-.
sarcolemmal fold Sarkolemmfalte *f*.
sar·co·lem·mic [ˌ,-ˈlemɪk] *adj* → sarkolemmal.
sar·co·lem·mous [ˌ,-ˈleməs] *adj* → sarcolemmal.
sar·col·y·sis [sɑːrˈkɑləsɪs] *n* Sarkolyse *f*, Sarcolysis *f*.

sar·co·ma [sɑːrˈkəʊmə] *n, pl* **-mas, -ma·ta** [-mətə] Sarkom *nt*, Sarcoma *nt abbr*. Sa.
sarcoma-like *adj* → sarcomatoid.
Sar·co·mas·ti·goph·o·ra [ˌsɑːrkəʊˌmæstɪˈgɑfərə] *pl micro*. Sarcomastigophora *pl*.
sar·co·ma·toid [sɑːrˈkəʊmətɔɪd] *adj* sarkomartig, in Form eines Sarkoms, sarkomatös.
sarcomatoid carcinoma spindelzelliges Karzinom *nt*, Spindelzellkarzinom *nt*, Ca. fusocellulare.
sar·co·ma·to·sis [sɑːrˌkəʊməˈtəʊsɪs] *n* Sarkomatose *f*, Sarcomatosis *f*.
sar·co·ma·tous [sɑːrˈkɑmətəs] *adj* Sarkom betr., sarkomatös, Sarkom-.
sar·co·mere [ˈsɑːrkəmɪər] *n* Sarkomer *nt*.
sar·com·phal·o·cele [sɑːrkɑmˈfæləsiːl] *n* Sarkomphalozele *f*.
Sar·coph·a·ga [sɑːrˈkɑfəgə] *n micro*. Fleischfliege *f*, Sarcophaga *f*.
Sar·co·phag·i·dae [ˌsɑːrkəˈfædʒədiː] *pl micro*. Fleischfliegen *pl*, Sarcophagidae *pl*, Sarcophaginae *pl*.
sar·coph·a·gous [sɑːrˈkɑfəgəs] *adj bio*. fleischfressend, sarkophag.
sar·co·plasm [ˈsɑːrkəplæzəm] *n* Protoplasma *nt* der Muskelzelle, Sarkoplasma *nt*.
sar·co·plas·mic [ˌ,-ˈplæzmɪk] *adj* Sarkoplasma betr., aus Sarkoplasma bestehend, sarkoplasmatisch, Sarkoplasma-.
sarcoplasmic membrane Sarkoplasmamembran *f*.
sarcoplasmic reticulum *abbr*. **SR** sarkoplasmatisches Retikulum *nt abbr*. SR.
sar·co·plast [ˈ-plæst] *n* interstitielle Muskelzelle *f*, Sarkoplast *m*.
Sar·cop·syl·la [ˌsɑːrkɑpˈsɪlə, ˌsɑːrkəʊ-] *n micro*. Sarcopsylla *f*, Tunga *f*.
S. penetrans Sandfloh *m*, Sarcopsylla/Tunga penetrans.
Sar·cop·tes [sɑːrˈkɑptiːz] *n micro*. Sarcoptes *f*.
S. scabiei Krätzmilbe *f*, Sarcoptes/Acarus scabiei.
sar·cop·tic [sɑːrˈkɑptɪk] *adj* Sarcoptes betr., durch Sarcoptes verursacht, Krätzmilben-.
sar·cop·ti·do·sis [sɑːrˌkɑptɪˈdəʊsɪs] *n* Sarcoptes-, Krätzmilbenbefall *m*.
sar·co·sine [ˈsɑːrkəsiːn, -sɪn] *n* Sarkosin *nt*, Methylglykokoll *nt*, -glycin *nt*.
sarcosine dehydrogenase Sarkosindehydrogenase *f*.
sar·co·si·ne·mia [ˌsɑːrkəsɪˈniːmɪə] *n* (Hyper-)Sarkosinämie *f*.
sar·co·some [ˈ-səʊm] *n* Mitochondrion *nt* der Muskelfaser, Sarkosom *nt*.
sar·co·spo·rid·ian [ˌ,-spəʊˈrɪdɪən] *micro*. Rainey-Körperchen *pl*, Miescher-Schläuche *pl*.
sar·co·spo·rid·i·a·sis [ˌ,-spəʊrɪˈdaɪəsɪs] *n* → sarcocystosis.
sar·co·spo·rid·i·o·sis [ˌ,-spəˌrɪdɪˈəʊsɪs] *n* → sarcocystosis.
sar·co·tu·bules [ˌ,-ˈt(j)uːbjuːlz] *pl* Sarkotubuli *pl*.
sar·cous [ˈsɑːrkəs] *adj* von fleischiger Konsistenz, fleischig, Fleisch-; Muskel-.
sar·don·ic laugh [sɑːrˈdɑnɪk] *neuro*. sardonisches Lachen *nt*, Risus sardonicus.
SA receptor → slowly-adapting receptor.
SA rhythm → sinus rhythm.
sar·to·ri·us (muscle) [sɑːrˈtɔːrɪəs] Sartorius *m*, M. sartorius.
SA sensor → slowly-adapting receptor.
SAT-chromosome *n old* → satellite chromosome.
sat·el·lite [ˈsætlaɪt] *n* **1.** *genet*. Satellit *m*. **2.** *anat*. Begleitvene *f*. **3.** Satellit *m*.
satellite cell 1. Satelliten-, Mantel-, Hüllzelle *f*, Amphizyt *m*, Lemnozyt *m*. **2.** (*Muskel*) Satellitenzelle *f*.

satellite chromosome *genet.* Satelliten-, Trabantenchromosom *nt.*
satellite colony *micro.* Satellitenkolonie *f.*
satellite DNA Satelliten-DNA *f,* Satelliten-DNS *f.*
satellite phenomenon *micro.* Ammenphänomen *nt,* -wachstum *nt,* Satellitenphänomen *nt,* -wachstum *nt.*
satellite virus *micro.* Satellitenvirus *nt.*
sat·el·li·tism ['sætlɪtɪzəm] *n* → satellite phenomenon.
sat·el·lit·osis [ˌsætlɪ'təʊsɪs] *n* Satellitose *f.*
sa·ti·ate [*adj* 'seɪʃɪɪt, -eɪt; *v* -eɪt] **I** *adj* gesättigt, gestillt, befriedigt; übersättigt. **II** *vt* (*Hunger*) sättigen; (*Durst*) stillen; befriedigen; übersättigen.
sa·ti·a·tion [seɪʃɪ'eɪʃn] *n* Befriedigung *f;* Übersättigung *f.*
sa·ti·e·ty [sə'taɪətɪ, seɪ'ʃɪətɪ] *n* **1.** (*Hunger*) Sättigung *f;* (*Durst*) Stillung *f.* **2.** Übersättigung *f* (*of* mit).
sat·u·rant ['sætʃərənt] **I** *n* sättigendes Mittel *nt.* **II** *adj chem.* (ab-)sättigend.
sat·u·rate [*adj, n* 'sætʃərət, -rɪt; *v* -reɪt] **I** *n* → saturated. **II** *adj* → saturated. **III** *vt* **1.** *chem.* (ab-)sättigen, saturieren. **2.** (durch-)tränken.
sat·u·rat·ed ['sætʃəreɪtɪd] *adj* **1.** *chem.* (ab-)gesättigt, saturiert. **2.** durchtränkt.
saturated compound *chem.* gesättigte Verbindung *f.*
saturated fat *chem.* Fett *nt* aus gesättigten Fettsäuren.
saturated hydrocarbon *chem.* gesättigter Kohlenwasserstoff *m.*
saturated lipid *chem.* Lipid *nt* aus gesättigten Fettsäuren.
saturated solution gesättigte Lösung *f.*
sat·u·ra·tion [ˌsætʃə'reɪʃn] *n* **1.** *chem.* (Ab-, Auf-)Sättigung *f,* Saturation *f.* **2.** (Ab-, Auf-)Sättigen *nt,* Saturieren *nt.* **3.** (Durch-)Tränkung *f.*
saturation analysis *lab.* kompetitiver Bindungstest/-assay *m.*
saturation curve Sättigungskurve *f.*
saturation deficit Sättigungsdefizit *nt.*
saturation effect Sättigungseffekt *m.*
saturation kinetics Sättigungskinetik *f.*
saturation level Sättigungsniveau *nt.*
saturation point Sättigungspunkt *m.*
sat·ur·nine ['sætərnaɪn] *adj* Blei-.
saturnine cachexia Kachexie *f* bei chronischer Bleivergiftung.
saturnine cerebritis Enzephalitis *f* bei Bleivergiftung.
saturnine colic Bleikolik *f,* Colica saturnina.
saturnine encephalopathy Bleienzephalopathie *f,* Encephalopathia saturnina.
saturnine nephritis Bleischrumpfniere *f,* Nephritis saturnina.
saturnine poisoning → saturnism.
sat·urn·ism [sætər'nɪzəm] *n* (chronische) Bleivergiftung *f,* Saturnismus *m,* Saturnialismus *m.*
sa·ty·ri·a·sis [seɪtə'raɪəsɪs, sæ-] *n psychia.* Satyriasis *f,* Satyrismus *m.*
sa·ty·ro·ma·nia [ˌseɪtɪrəʊ'meɪnɪə, -jə, ˌsæ-] *n* → satyriasis.
sau·ri·a·sis [sɔː'raɪəsɪs] *n* → sauriderma.
sau·ri·der·ma [ˌsɔːrɪ'dɜːrmə] *n* **1.** Fischschuppenkrankheit *f,* Ichthyosis vulgaris. **2.** Saurier-, Krokodil-, Alligatorhaut *f,* Sauriasis *f.*
sau·ri·o·sis [ˌ-'əʊsɪs] *n* → sauriderma.
sau·ro·der·ma [ˌsɔːrə'dɜːrmə] *n* → sauriderma.
sau·sage poisoning ['sɒsɪdʒ] Wurstvergiftung *f,* Allantiasis *f.*
Savary ['sævərɪ]: **S. bougie** Savary-Bougie *f.*

Savill ['sævɪl]: **S.'s pinch test** Pinch-Test *m* nach Savill.
SA virus *micro.* SA-Virus *nt.*
saw [sɔː] **I** *n* Säge *f.* **II** *vt, vi* sägen.
sax·i·tox·in [ˌsæksɪ'tɒksɪn] *n* Saxitoxin *nt.*
Sb *abbr.* → stibium.
S bacteria *micro.* S-Form *f,* S-Stamm *m.*
Sc *abbr.* → scandium.
scab [skæb] **I** *n* (Wund-)Schorf *m,* Grind *m,* Kruste *f.* **II** *vi* verschorfen, (s.) verkrusten.
scab·bard trachea ['skæbərd] Säbelscheidentrachea *f.*
sca·bet·ic [skə'betɪk] *adj* → scabietic.
sca·bi·ci·dal [skeɪbɪ'saɪdl] *adj* gegen Krätzmilben wirkend.
sca·bi·cide ['skeɪbɪsaɪd] **I** *n* Antiskabiosum *nt,* gegen Krätzmilben wirkendes Mittel *nt.* **II** *adj* → scabicidal.
sca·bies ['skeɪbiːz] *n* Krätze *f,* Skabies *f,* Scabies *f,* Akariasis *f,* Acariasis *f.*
sca·bi·et·ic [ˌskeɪbɪ'etɪk] *adj* Skabies betr., von Skabies betroffen, skabiös, krätzig, Skabies-.
sca·bi·et·i·cide [ˌ-'etɪsaɪd] *n* → scabicide I.
sca·bi·ous ['skeɪbɪəs] *adj* → scabietic.
sca·bri·ti·es [skeɪ'brɪʃɪˌiːz] *n* (*Haut*) Rauhigkeit *f,* Scabrities *f.*
sca·brous ['skæbrəs, 'skeɪ-] *adj* (*Haut*) rauh, schuppig.
sca·la ['skeɪlə] *n, pl* **-lae** [-liː] *anat.* Treppe *f,* Stufe *f,* treppen- *od.* leiterförmige Struktur *f,* Scala *f.*
s. of Löwenberg (häutiger) Schneckengang *m,* Ductus cochlearis.
sca·lar ['skeɪlər] *mathe.* **I** *n* Skalar *m,* skalare Größe *f.* **II** *adj* ungerichtet, skalar.
sca·lar·i·form [skə'lærɪfɔːrm] *adj bio.* leiterförmig.
scald [skɔːld] **I** *n* Verbrühung *f,* Verbrühungsverletzung *f.* **II** *vt* verbrühen.
scald·ed skin syndrome ['skɔːldɪd] (medikamentöses) Lyell-Syndrom *nt,* Syndrom *nt* der verbrühten Haut, Epidermolysis acuta toxica, Epidermolysis necroticans combustiformis.
scald injury Verbrühung *f,* Verbrühungsverletzung *f.*
scale¹ [skeɪl] *n* **1.** Schuppe *f,* schuppige Struktur *f.* **2.** Zahn-, Kesselstein *m.* **II** *vt* **3.** (ab-)schuppen, (-)schälen, (-)häuten. **4.** Zahnstein entfernen. **III** *vi* **5.** s. abschuppen *od.* -lösen, s. schälen, sich abschilfern; abblättern. **6.** Kessel- *od.* Zahnstein ansetzen.
scale² [skeɪl] **I** *n* **1.** *mathe., techn.* Skala *f,* Grad-, Maßeinteilung *f;* (Stufen-)Leiter *f,* Staffelung *f.* **2.** Maßstab *m;* Größenordnung *f,* Umfang *m.* **on a large ~ in** großem Umfang/Stil. **3.** Waagschale *f;* (**a pair of**) **~s** *pl* Waage *f.* **II** *vt* **4.** erklettern, -ersteigen, erklimmen. **5.** (ab-)wiegen. **6.** mit einer Skala versehen; einstufen. **III** *vi* auf einer Skala klettern *od.* steigen.
s. of sound intensity Schallintensitätsskala, Schallstärkeskala.
scaled [skeɪld] *adj* mit Schuppen bedeckt, voller Schuppen, schuppig.
scale·like *adj* schuppenförmig, -ähnlich, schuppig.
sca·lene [skeɪ'liːn] *adj* **1.** *mathe.* ungleichseitig; schief. **2.** Skalenusmuskel betr., Skalenus-.
sca·le·nec·to·my [ˌskeɪlɪ'nektəmɪ] *n chir., ortho.* Skalenusresektion *f,* Skalenektomie *f.*
scalene muscle: anterior s. → scalenus anterior (muscle)
middle s. → scalenus medius (muscle)
posterior s. → scalenus posterior (muscle)
smallest s. → scalenus minimus (muscle).

scalene node biopsy Skalenusbiopsie *f,* Daniels (präskalenische) Biopsie *f.*
scalene tubercle Tuberculum *m.* scaleni anterioris.
sca·le·not·o·my [ˌ-'nɒtəmɪ] *n chir., ortho.* Skalenusdurchdrennung *f,* Skalenotomie *f.*
sca·le·nus [skeɪ'liːnəs] *n* → scalenus muscle.
scalenus anterior (muscle) Skalenus *m* anterior, M. scalenus anterior.
scalenus anticus syndrome Skalenus--Syndrom *nt,* Scalenus-anterior-Syndrom *nt,* Naffziger-Syndrom *nt.*
scalenus medius (muscle) Skalenus *m* medius, M. scalenus medius.
scalenus minimus (muscle) Skalenus *m* minimus, M. scalenus minimus.
scalenus muscle Skalenus *m,* M. scalenus.
scalenus posterior (muscle) Skalenus *m* posterior, M. scalenus posterior.
scalenus syndrome → scalenus anticus syndrome.
scal·er ['skeɪlər] *n* **1.** *dent.* Zahnsteinschaber *m.* **2.** *phys.* Frequenzteiler *m.*
scal·i·ness ['skeɪlɪnɪs] *n* Schuppigkeit *f.*
scal·ing ['skeɪlɪŋ] *n* **1.** (Ab-)Schuppen *nt,* (Ab-)Schuppung *f,* Abschilfern *nt,* Abblättern *nt.* **2.** Zahnsteinentfernung *f.*
scall [skɔːl] *n derm.* (Kopf-)Grind *m,* Schorf *m.*
scal·loped ['skɒləpt, 'skæl-] *adj* muschelartig, -förmig.
scalp [skælp] **I** *n* Skalp *m,* Kopfschwarte/Galea aponeurotica u. Kopfhaut. **II** *vi* skalpieren, die Kopfhaut abziehen.
scal·pel ['skælpəl] *n chir.* Skalpell *nt;* chirurgisches Messer *nt.*
scal·per ['skælpər] *n* Knochenschaber *m.*
scalp hairs Kopfhaare *pl,* Capilli *pl.*
scalp infection Kopfhautinfektion *f.*
scal·pri·form ['skælprɪfɔːrm] *adj* meißelförmig.
scal·y ['skeɪlɪ] *adj* **1.** schuppig, geschuppt, Schuppen-; schuppenartig; squamös. **2.** s. (ab-)schuppend, abschilfernd, abblätternd.
scaly ringworm orientalische/indische/chinesische Flechte *f,* Tinea imbricata (Tokelau), Trichophytia corporis superficialis.
scan [skæn] **I** *n radiol.* **1.** Abtastung *f,* Scan *m,* Scanning *nt.* **2.** Szintigramm *nt,* Scan *m.* **II** *vt* **3.** *radiol.* abtasten, scannen. **4.** *neuro.* (*Sprache*) skandieren.
scan·di·um ['skændɪəm] *n abbr.* **Sc** Scandium *nt abbr.* **Sc.**
scan·ner ['skænər] *n radiol.* Abtastgerät *nt,* Abtaster *m,* Scanner *m;* Szintiscanner *m.*
scan·ning ['skænɪŋ] *n phys.* Abtasten *nt,* Abtastung *f,* Scanning *nt,* Szintigraphie *f;* Scan *m.*
scanning electron microscope *abbr.* **SEM** Elektronenrastermikroskop *nt,* Rasterelektronenmikroskop *nt.*
scanning microscope → scanning electron microscope.
scanning speech *neuro.* skandierende Sprache *f.*
scan·sion ['skænʃn] *n* → scanning.
Scanzoni [skæn'zəʊnɪ]: **S.'s maneuver/operation** *gyn.* Scanzoni-Manöver *nt.*
scaph- *pref.* → scapho-.
sca·pha ['skeɪfə] *n anat.* Skapha *f,* Scapha *f.*
scapho- *pref.* Kahn-, Skaph(o)-, Scaph(o)-.
scaph·o·ce·pha·lia [ˌskæfəsɪ'feɪljə] *n* → scaphocephaly.
scaph·o·ce·phal·ic [ˌ-sɪ'fælɪk] *adj* Skapho-

scaphocephalism

zephalie betr., von Skaphozephalie gekennzeichnet, skaphozephal, -kephal.
scaph·o·ceph·a·lism [ˌ-'sefəlɪzəm] *n* → scaphocephaly.
scaph·o·ceph·a·lous [ˌ-'sefələs] *adj* → scaphocephalic.
scaph·o·ceph·a·ly [ˌ-'sefəlɪ] *n* Kahn-, Leistenschädel *m*, Skaphokephalie *f*, -zephalie *f*.
scaph·o·hy·dro·ceph·a·lus [ˌ-ˌhaɪdrə'sefələs] *n* Skaphohydrozephalus *m*, Skaphohydrozephalie *f*.
scaph·oid ['skæfɔɪd] **I** *n* Kahnbein *nt*, Os scaphoideum. **II** *adj* boot-, kahnförmig, navikular.
scaphoid abdomen Kahnbauch *m*.
scaphoid bone Kahnbein *nt*, Os scaphoideum.
 s. of hand *old* → scaphoid bone.
 s. of foot *old* → navicular I.
scaphoid cast *ortho.* Navikularegips *m*.
scaphoid fossa 1. → scaphoid fossa of sphenoid bone. 2. → scapha.
 s. of sphenoid bone Fossa scaphoidea (ossis sphenoidalis).
scaphoid fracture Kahnbeinbruch *m*, -fraktur *f*, Skaphoidfraktur *f*.
scaphoid tubercle Tuberculum ossis scaphoidei.
scaphoid tuberosity 1. Tuberculum ossis scaphoidei. 2. Tuberositas ossis navicularis.
scap·u·la ['skæpjələ] *n*, *pl* **-las, -lae** [-liː] Schulterblatt *nt*, Skapula *f*, Scapula *f*.
scap·u·lal·gia [skæpjə'lældʒ(ɪ)ə] *n* → scapulodynia.
scap·u·lar ['skæpjələr] *adj* Schulter(blatt) betr., skapular, Skapular-.
scapular artery: descending s. A. scapularis descendens, Ramus profundus a. transversae colli.
 dorsal s. 1. A. scapularis dorsalis, A. dorsalis scapulae. 2. → descending s.
 transverse s. → suprascapular artery.
scapular bone *old* → scapula.
scapular extremity of clavicle Extremitas acromialis.
scapular incisure (of scapula) → scapular notch (of scapula).
scapular line Skapularlinie *f*, Linea scapularis.
scapular notch (of scapula) Inc. scapulae/scapularis.
scapular region Schulterblattregion *f*, -gegend *f*, Regio scapularis.
scapular spine Spina scapulae.
scapular tuberosity of Henle Proc. coracoideus.
scapular vein, dorsal Begleitvene *f* der A. scapularis dorsalis, V. scapularis dorsalis.
scap·u·lec·to·my [skæpjə'lektəmɪ] *n ortho.* Schulterblattentfernung *f*, Skapulektomie *f*.
scap·u·lo·cla·vic·u·lar [ˌskæpjələoklə'vɪkjələr] *adj* Schulterblatt/Scapula u. Schlüsselbein/Clavicula betr.
scapuloclavicular articulation/joint äußeres Schlüsselbeingelenk *nt*, Akromioklavikulargelenk *nt*, Artic. acromioclavicularis.
scap·u·lo·cos·tal syndrome [ˌ-'kɒstl, -'kɔstl] Skapulokostales Syndrom *nt*.
scap·u·lo·dyn·ia [ˌ-'diːnɪə] *n* Schmerzen *pl* in der Schulterblattgegend, Skapulodynie *f*, Skapulalgie *f*.
scap·u·lo·hu·mer·al [ˌ-'(h)juːmərəl] *adj* Schulterblatt/Scapula u. Humerus betr., skapulohumeral.
scapulohumeral atrophy Vulpian-Atrophie *f*, -Syndrom *nt*, Vulpian-Bernhard-Atrophie *f*, -Syndrom *nt*, adult-proxi-

male/skapulohumerale Form *f* der spinalen Muskelatrophie.
scapulohumeral bursitis Bursitis/Tendinitis scapulohumeralis.
scapulohumeral reflex Skapulohumeralreflex *m*.
scapulohumeral tendinitis → scapulohumeral bursitis.
scapulohumeral type of spinal muscular atrophy → scapulohumeral atrophy.
scap·u·lo·per·i·os·te·al reflex [ˌ-ˌperɪ'ɒstɪəl] → scapulohumeral reflex.
scap·u·lo·pex·y ['-peksɪ] *n ortho.* Schulterblattfixierung *f*, Skapulopexie *f*.
sca·pus ['skeɪpəs] *n*, *pl* **-pi** [-paɪ] Schaft *m*, Stamm *m*, Scapus *m*.
scar [skɑːr] *n* 1. Narbe *f*, Cicatrix *f*. 2. *fig.*, *psycho.* Narbe *f*; Makel *nt*.
scar over *vi* eine Narbe bilden, vernarben, verheilen.
scar bronchiectasis Bronchiektas(i)e *f* durch Narbenzug.
scar carcinoma Narbenkarzinom *nt*.
scar emphysema (*Lunge*) Narbenemphysem *nt*.
scarf bandage [skɑːrf] Dreieckstuch *nt*.
scar formation Narbenbildung *f*.
scar·i·fi·ca·tion [skærəfɪ'keɪʃn] *n immun.* Hautritzung *f*, Skarifikation *f*.
scarification test Kratztest *m*, Skarifikationstest *m*.
scar·i·fy ['skærəfaɪ] *vt immun.* (*Haut*) ritzen, skarifizieren.
scar·la·ti·na [ˌskɑːrlə'tiːnə] *n* Scharlach *m*, Scharlachfieber *nt*, Scarlatina *f*.
scar·la·ti·nal [ˌ-'tiːnəl] *adj* Scharlach betr., Scharlach-.
scarlatinal nephritis Scharlachnephritis *f*.
scar·la·ti·nel·la [ˌ-tɪ'nelə] *n* Dukes'-Krankheit *f*, Dukes-Filatoff-Krankheit *f*, vierte Krankheit *f*, Filatow-Dukes-Krankheit *f*, Parascarlatina *f*, Rubeola scarlatinosa.
scar·la·ti·ni·form [ˌ-'tɪnəfɔːrm] *adj* dem Scharlach(exanthem) ähnlich, skarlatiniform, skarlatinös, skarlatinoid.
scarlatiniform erythema Erythema scarlatiniforme.
scar·la·ti·noid [ˌ-'tɪnɔɪd, skɑːr'lætnɔɪd] **I** *n* → scarlatinella. **II** *adj* scarlatiniform.
scar·let ['skɑːrlət] **I** *n* Scharlach(rot *nt*) *m*. **II** *adj* scharlachrot, -farben.
scarlet fever Scharlach *m*, Scharlachfieber, Scarlatina *f*.
scarlet fever myocarditis Scharlachmyokarditis *f*.
scarlet fever rash Scharlachexanthem *nt*.
scarlet red → scarlet I.
scarlet red phase *histol.* Scharlachrotphase *f*, -stadium *nt*.
Scar·pa ['skɑːrpə]: **S.'s fluid** Endolymphe *f*, Endolympha *f*.
 S.'s ganglion Scarpa'-Ganglion *nt*, Rosenthal-Ferré'-Ganglion *nt*, Ggl. vestibulare.
 greater fossa of S. → S.'s trigone.
 S.'s hiatus Breschet-Hiatus *m*, Schneckenloch *nt*, Helicotrema *nt*.
 liquor of S. → S.'s fluid.
 S.'s membrane Membrana tympani secundaria.
 S.'s nerve N. nasopalatinus.
 S.'s sheath Fascia cremasterica.
 S.'s staphyloma Staphyloma verum posticum.
 S.'s trigone Scarpa'-Dreieck *nt*, Trigonum femorale.
scarred [skɑːrd] *adj* voller Narben, mit Narben bedeckt, narbig.
scarred kidney Narbenniere *f*, narbige Schrumpfniere *f*.

scar·ring ['skɑːrɪŋ] *n* Vernarbung *f*, Narbenbildung *f*.
 s. of tissue Gewebsvernarbung.
scarring alopecia narbige Alopezie *f*, Alopecia cicatricans.
scarring aphthae, recurrent Mikulicz--Aphthen *pl*, habituelle Aphthen *pl*, chronisch rezidivierende Aphthen *pl*, rezidivierende benigne Aphthosis *f*, Periadenitis mucosa necrotica recurrens.
scar stage *patho.* Narbenstadium *nt*.
scar stricture narbige Striktur *f*, Narbenstriktur *f*.
scar tissue Narbengewebe *nt*.
SCAT *abbr.* → sheep cell agglutination test.
scat- *pref.* → scato-.
scat·a·cra·tia [ˌskætə'kreɪʃ(ɪ)ə] *n* Skat(o)akratie *f*, Stuhl-, Darminkontinenz, Incontinentia alvi.
sca·te·mia [skeɪ'tiːmɪə] *n* intestinale Autointoxikation *f*.
scato- *pref.* Stuhl-, Skat(o)-.
sca·tol ['skætɒl, -əʊl] *n* → skatole.
scat·o·log·ic [ˌskætə'lɒdʒɪk] *adj* Stuhl-, Skat(o)-.
scat·ol·o·gy [skə'tɒlədʒɪ] *n* Skatologie *f*.
sca·to·ma [skə'təʊmə] *n* Kotgeschwulst *f*, Sterkorom *nt*, Koprom *nt*, Fäkalom *nt*.
sca·toph·a·gy [skə'tɒfədʒɪ] *n psychia.* Koprophagie *f*.
sca·tos·co·py [skə'tɒskəpɪ] *n* Skatoskopie *f*.
scat·ter ['skætər] **I** *n* (Ver-, Aus-, Zer-)Streuen *nt*; *phys.*, *stat.* Streuung *f*. **II** *vt* ver-, ausstreuen; *phys.* (zer-)streuen. **III** *vi* s. ver-, zerstreuen, s. verteilen, s. verbreiten.
scatter diagram → scatterplot.
scat·tered ['skætərd] *adj* vereinzelt; zerstreut *od.* verstreut *od.* gestreut liegend.
scattered rays Streustrahlung *f*.
scat·ter·gram ['skætərgræm] *n* → scatterplot.
scat·ter·graph ['-græf] *n* → scatterplot.
scat·ter·ing ['skætərɪŋ] **I** *n phys.* Streuung *f*. **II** *adj* → scattered.
scat·ter·plot ['skætərplɒt] *n* Streuungsdiagramm *nt*.
scat·u·la ['skætʃələ] *n*, *pl* **-lae** [-liː] *pharm.* Schachtel *f*, Scatula *f*.
scav·en·ger cell ['skævɪndʒər] *histol.* Abraumzelle *f*.
sce·lal·gia [skɪ'lældʒ(ɪ)ə] *n* Beinschmerz(en *pl*) *m*.
scel·o·tyr·be [selə'tɜːrbɪ] *n* spastische Beinparalyse *f*.
scent [sent] **I** *n* 1. Geruch *m*; Duft *m*. 2. Geruchssinn *m*. **II** *vt* etw. riechen.
scent·less ['sentlɪs] *adj* geruchlos.
scent molecule Duft(stoff)molekül *nt*.
Schacher [ˈʃɑːkər, -xər]: **S.'s ganglion** Schacher'-Ganglion *nt*, Ziliarganglion *nt*, Ggl. ciliare.
Schachowa [ˈʃɑːkəʊva]: **S.'s spiral tube** (*Niere*) proximales Konvolut *nt*.
Schaffer [ˈʃæfər]: **S.'s collaterals** Schaffer'-Kollateralen *pl*.
Schamberg [ˈʃæmbɜːrg]: **S.'s dermatitis** Schamberg-Krankheit *f*, -Syndrom *nt*, Morbus Schamberg *m*, progressive Pigmentpurpura *f*, progressive pigmentöse Dermatose *f*, Purpura pigmentosa progressiva, Purpura Schamberg, Dermatosis pigmentaria progressiva, Capillaritis haemorrhagica maculosa.
 S.'s dermatosis/disease → S.'s dermatitis.
 S.'s progressive pigmented purpuric dermatosis → S.'s dermatitis.
Schanz [ʃænts]: **S. operation/osteotomy** *ortho.* subtrochantäre Amputationsosteotomie *f* nach Schanz.

Schardinger ['ʃɑːrdɪŋər]: S.'s enzyme Schardinger'-Enzym nt, Xanthinoxidase f abbr. XO.
S. reaction Schardinger-Reaktion f.
Schatzki ['ʃætskɪ]: S.'s ring Schatzki-Ring m.
Schaumann ['ʃɔːmən; 'ʃaʊ-]: S.'s bodies Schaumann'-Körperchen pl.
S.'s disease Sarkoidose f, Morbus Boeck m, Boeck'-Sarkoid nt, Besnier-Boeck-Schaumann-Krankheit f, Lymphogranulomatosa benigna.
S.'s sarcoid/syndrome → S.'s disease.
Schauta ['ʃɔːtɑ; 'ʃaʊtə]: S.'s (vaginal) operation gyn. Schauta-Operation f, Schauta-Stoeckel-Operation f, vaginale Hysterektomie f.
sched·u·lar ['skedʒələr; 'ʃedjʊ-] adj Tabellen-, Listen-.
sched·ule ['skedʒuːl; 'ʃedjuːl] I n 1. Liste f, Tabelle f, Aufstellung f, Verzeichnis nt. 2. (Lehr-, Arbeits-, Stunden-, Zeit-)Plan m. 3. Formblatt nt, Formular nt. II vt 4. (in eine Liste) einfügen, eintragen; in einer Liste zusammenstellen. 5. festlegen, -setzen; planen, vorsehen.
Scheibe ['ʃeɪbə; 'ʃaɪbə]: S.'s deafness Scheibe-Schwerhörigkeit f, Scheibe-Typ m der angeborenen Taubheit.
Scheie ['ʃeɪə]: S.'s syndrome/type Morbus Scheie m, Scheie-Krankheit f, -Syndrom nt, Ullrich-Scheie-Krankheit f, -Syndrom nt, Mukopolysaccharidose f I-S abbr. MPS I-S.
Schellong ['ʃɛlɔŋ; 'ʃɛ-]: S. test Schellong-Test m.
Schellong-Strisower ['strɪsəʊər]: S.-S. phenomenon Schellong-Phänomen nt.
sche·ma ['skiːmə] n, pl -ma·ta [-mətə] 1. Schema nt, System nt, Plan m, Programm nt. 2. Schema nt, Aufstellung f, Tabelle f; Übersicht f, schematische Darstellung f.
sche·mat·ic [skɪ'mætɪk] I n schematische Darstellung f. II adj schematisch.
scheme ['skiːm] n → schema.
Schenck [ʃeŋk]: S.'s disease Sporotrichose f, De Beurmann-Gougerot-Krankheit f.
sche·ro·ma [skɪ'rəʊmə] n ophthal. Xerophthalmie f.
Scheuermann ['ʃɔɪərmən]: S.'s disease/kyphosis Scheuermann'-Krankheit f, Morbus Scheuermann m, Adoleszentenkyphose f, Osteochondritis/Osteochondrosis deformans juvenilis.
Schick [ʃɪk]: S.'s method → S.'s test.
S. reaction Schick-Probe f.
S.'s test Schick-Test m.
S. test toxin Schick-Test-Toxin nt.
Schiff [ʃɪf]: S.'s base chem. Schiff'-Base f.
S.'s biliary cycle (Gallensäuren) enterohepatischer Kreislauf m.
S.'s reagent Schiff'-Reagenz nt.
Schilder ['ʃɪldər]: S.'s diffuse inflammatory sclerosis of S. → S.'s disease.
S.'s disease Schilder'-Krankheit f, Encephalitis periaxialis diffusa.
S.'s encephalitis → S.'s disease.
Schilling ['ʃɪlɪŋ]: S.'s band cell stabkerniger Granulozyt m, inf. Stabkerniger m.
S.'s leukemia Schilling-Typ m der Monozytenleukämie, reine Monozytenleukämie f.
S. test Schilling-Test m.
Schimmelbusch ['ʃɪməlbʊʃ]: S.'s disease Schimmelbusch-Krankheit f, proliferierende Mastopathie f.
schin·dy·le·sis [ˌskɪndə'liːsɪs] n anat. Nut-u. Kammverbindung f, Schindylesis f.
Schlötz [ʃɪˈɪts]: S. tonometer ophthal. Schiötz-Tonometer nt.

Schirmer ['ʃɜrmər; 'ʃɪr-]: S.'s syndrome Schirmer-Syndrom nt.
S.'s test Schirmer-Test m.
schist(o)- pref. Spalt-, Schist(o)-, Schiz(o)-.
schis·to·ce·lia n → schistocoelia.
schis·to·ceph·a·lus [ˌskɪstəʊ'sefələs] n embryo. Schisto-, Schizozephalus m.
schis·to·coe·lia [ˌ-'siːlɪə] n embryo. Bauchspalte f, Schistocoelia f.
schis·to·cor·mia [ˌ-'kɔːrmɪə] n embryo. Schistokormie f, -somie f.
schis·to·cys·tis [ˌ-'sɪstɪs] n embryo., urol. Blasenspalte f, Schistozystis f; Spaltblase f.
schis·to·cyte ['-saɪt] n hema. Schistozyt m.
schis·to·cy·to·sis [ˌ-saɪ'təʊsɪs] n hema. Schistozytose f.
schis·to·glos·sia [ˌ-'glɒsɪə] n embryo. Zungenspalte f, Schistoglossia f.
schis·to·me·lia [ˌ-'miːlɪə] n embryo. Schistomelie f, -melia f.
schis·to·mel·us [skɪs'tɑmələs] n embryo. Schistomelus m.
schis·to·pro·so·pia [ˌskɪstəprəʊ'səʊpɪə] n embryo. Gesichtsspalte f, Schistoprosopie f, Schizoprosopie f.
schis·tor·a·chis [skɪs'tɔrəkɪs] n embryo. R(h)achischisis f.
Schis·to·so·ma [ˌskɪstə'səʊmə] n micro. Pärchenegel m, Schistosoma nt, Bilharzia f.
S. haematobium Blasenpärchenegel, Schistosoma haematobium.
S. intercalatum Darmpärchenegel, Schistosoma intercalatum.
S. japonicum japanischer Pärchenegel, Schistosoma japonicum.
schis·to·so·ma·ci·dal [ˌ-ˌsəʊmə'saɪdl] adj → schistosomicidal.
schis·to·so·ma·cide [ˌ-'səʊməsaɪd] n → schistosomicide.
schis·to·so·mal [ˌ-'səʊməl] adj Schistosomen betr., durch Schistosomen verursacht, Schistosomen-.
schis·to·some ['-səʊm] n micro. Pärchenegel m, Schistosoma nt, Bilharzia f.
schistosome dermatitis Schwimmbadkrätze f, Weiherhippel m, Bade-, Schistosomen-, Zerkariendermatitis f.
schistosome granuloma Schistosomen-, Schistosomagranulom nt.
schis·to·so·mia [ˌ-'səʊmɪə] n embryo. → schistocormia.
schis·to·so·mi·a·sis [ˌ-səʊ'maɪəsɪs] n Schistosomiasis f, Bilharziose f.
schis·to·so·mi·ci·dal [ˌ-ˌsəʊmɪ'saɪdl] adj schistosomen(ab)tötend, schistosomizid.
schis·to·so·mi·cide [ˌ-'səʊmɪsaɪd] n Schistosomenmittel nt, Schistosomizid nt.
Schis·to·so·mum [ˌ-'səʊməm] n → Schistosoma.
schis·to·ster·nia [ˌ-'stɜrnɪə] n embryo. Schisto-, Schizosternia f; Schisto-, Schizothorax m.
schis·to·tho·rax [ˌ-'θɔːræks] n → schistosternia.
schiz- pref. → schizo-.
schiz·a·cu·sis [ˌskɪzə'kjuːsɪs] n Schizakusis f.
schiz·am·ni·on [skɪz'æmnɪɒn] n embryo. Schizamnion nt.
schiz·ax·on [skɪz'æksɑn] n Schizaxon nt.
schiz·en·ceph·a·ly [ˌskɪzen'sefəlɪ] n embryo. Schizenzephalie f.
schizo- pref. Spalt-, Schiz(o)-, Schist(o)-.
schiz·o·af·fec·tive [ˌskɪzəʊæ'fektɪv] adj psychia. schizoaffektiv.
schizoaffective disorder → schizoaffective schizophrenia.
schizoaffective psychosis → schizoaffective schizophrenia.

schizoaffective schizophrenia schizoaffektive Psychose f.
schiz·o·cyte ['-saɪt] n → schistocyte.
schiz·o·cy·to·sis [ˌ-saɪ'təʊsɪs] n → schistocytosis.
schi·zog·a·my [skɪ'zɒgəmɪ] n Schizogamie f.
schiz·o·gen·e·sis [ˌskɪzə'dʒenəsɪs] n Schizogenese f.
schiz·o·gen·ic cycle [ˌ-'dʒenɪk] micro. (Protozoen) asexueller/schizogamer Vermehrungszyklus m.
schi·zog·e·nous [skɪ'zɒdʒənəs] adj Schizogenie betr., schizogen.
schizogenous cycle → schizogenic cycle.
schi·zog·o·ny [skɪ'zɒgənɪ] n bio., micro. Zerfallsteilung f, Schizogonie f.
schiz·o·gy·ria [ˌskɪzə'dʒaɪrɪə] n embryo. Schizogyrie f.
schiz·oid ['skɪtsɔɪd] psychia. I n Schizoide(r m) f. II adj schizophrenie-ähnlich, schizoid.
schizoid personality (disorder) schizoide Persönlichkeit(sstörung) f.
schiz·o·ki·ne·sis [ˌ-kɪ'niːsɪs, -kaɪ-] n Schizokinese f.
schiz·o·my·cete [ˌ-'maɪsiːt] n micro. Spaltpilz m, Schizomyzet m.
Schiz·o·my·ce·tes [ˌ-maɪ'siːtiːz] pl micro. Spaltpilze pl, Schizomyzeten pl, Schizomycetes pl.
schiz·o·my·cet·ic [ˌ-maɪ'setɪk] adj Spaltpilze betr., Schizomyzeten-.
schiz·ont ['skɪzɑnt] n micro. Schizont m.
schi·zon·ti·cide [skɪ'zɑntɪsaɪd] n Schizontizid nt.
schiz·o·nych·ia [ˌskɪzə'nɪkɪə] n Nagelzersplitterung f, Schizo(o)nychie f.
schiz·o·pha·sia [ˌ-'feɪzɪə] n psychia. Wortsalat, Schizophasie f, -phrasie f.
schiz·o·phre·nia [ˌ-'friːnɪə, -jə] n psychia. Schizophrenie f, -phrenia f, Spaltungsirresein nt, old Dementia praecox.
schiz·o·phren·ic [ˌ-'frenɪk] I n Schizophrene(r m) f. II adj Schizophrenie betr., an Schizophrenie leidend, für Schizophrenie kennzeichnend, schizophren, spaltungsirre.
schiz·o·phren·i·form [ˌ-'frenɪfɔːrm] adj schizophrenie-ähnlich, schizoid.
schiz·o·phyte ['-faɪt] n bio. Spaltpflanze f, Schizophyt m.
schiz·o·pro·so·pia [ˌ-prə'səʊpɪə] n → schistoprosopia.
schiz·o·thy·mia [ˌ-'θaɪmɪə] n psychia. Schizothymie f.
schiz·o·thy·mic [ˌ-'θaɪmɪk] psychia. I n Schizothyme(r m) f. II adj Schizothymie betr., von Schizothymie gekennzeichnet, schizothym.
schiz·o·to·nia [ˌ-'təʊnɪə] n Schizotonie f.
schiz·o·trich·ia [ˌ-'trɪkɪə] n Schizotrichie f, -trichia f.
schiz·o·tryp·a·no·so·mi·a·sis [ˌ-ˌtrɪpənəʊsəʊ'maɪəsɪs] n Chagas-Krankheit f, amerikanische Trypanosomiasis f.
Schiz·o·tryp·a·num cruzi [ˌ-'trɪpənəm] Trypanosoma cruzi, Schizotrypanum cruzi.
schiz·o·ty·pal personality (disorder) [ˌskɪzə'taɪpl] schizotypische Persönlichkeit(sstörung) f.
schiz·o·zo·ite [ˌ-'zəʊaɪt] n Schizozoit m, Merozoit m.
Schlatter ['ʃlætər]: S.'s disease/sprain → Schlatter-Osgood disease.
Schlatter-Osgood ['ɑzgʊd]: S.-O. disease Osgood-Schlatter-Krankheit f, -Syndrom nt, Schlatter-Osgood-Krankheit f, -Syndrom nt, Apophysitis tibialis adolescentium.
Schlemm [ʃlem]: S.'s canal Schlemm'-Kanal m, Sinus venosus sclerae.

Schlesinger ['ʃlesɪndʒər, 'ʃleɪzɪŋər]: **S.'s sign** Poole-Schlesinger-Phänomen nt, Poole-Phänomen nt.
schlie·ren ['ʃlɪərən] pl phys. Schlieren pl.
schlieren pattern phys. Schlierenmuster nt.
Schmidt [ʃmɪt]: **S.'s syndrome 1.** HNO Schmidt-Syndrom nt. **2.** Schmidt-Syndrom nt, thyreosuprarenales Syndrom nt.
Schmidt-Lanterman ['læntərmən]: **S.-L. clefts/incisures** Schmidt-Lanterman'-Einkerbungen pl, -Inzisuren pl.
S.-L. segment Marksegment nt.
Schmiedel ['ʃmiːdl]: **S.'s ganglion** Schmiedel'-Ganglion.
Schmincke ['ʃmɪŋkɪ]: **S. tumor** lymphoepitheliales Karzinom nt, Schmincke-Tumor m, Lymphoepitheliom nt.
Schmitz ['ʃmɪts]: **S. bacillus** Shigella schmitzii/ambigua, Shigella dysenteriae Typ 2.
Schmorl [ʃmɔrl]: **S.'s bacillus** Fusobacterium necrophorum.
S.'s bodies Schmorl'-Knötchen pl.
S.'s jaundice Kernikterus m, Bilirubinenzephalopathie f.
S.'s nodes Schmorl'-Knötchen pl.
S.'s nodules → S.'s nodes.
Schneider ['ʃnaɪdər]: **S.'s first rank symptoms** psychia. Symptome pl ersten Ranges.
schnei·de·ri·an membrane [ʃneɪ'dɪərɪən] Nasenschleimhaut f, Tunica mucosa nasi.
Schoemaker ['ʃiːmakər]: **S.'s line** Shoemaker-Linie f.
Scholander [ʃoʊ'lændər]: **S. apparatus** Scholander-Apparat m.
schol·ar ['skalər] n Gelehrte(r m) f, (Geistes-)Wissenschaftler(in f) m; Gebildete(r m) f.
schol·ar·ly ['skalərlɪ] adj gelehrt, wissenschaftlich, Wissenschafts-.
Scholz [ʃoʊlts, ʃɒl-]: **S.'s disease** Scholz-Bielschowsky-Henneberg-Sklerosetyp m, Scholz-Syndrom nt.
Schönlein ['ʃeɪnlaɪn; 'ʃøːn-]: **S.'s disease/purpura** → Schönlein-Henoch disease.
Schönlein-Henoch ['henəʊk; 'hɛnɔx]: **S.-H. disease** Schoenlein-Henoch-Syndrom nt, (anaphylaktoide) Purpura f Schoenlein-Henoch, rheumatoide/athrombopenische Purpura f, Immunkomplexpurpura f, -vaskulitis f, Purpura anaphylactoides (Schoenlein-Henoch), Purpura rheumatica (Schoenlein-Henoch).
S.-H. purpura/syndrome → S.-H. disease.
school¹ [skuːl] **I** n **1.** Schule f. **2.** Schule f, Schulhaus nt, -gebäude nt. **3.** Kurs m, Lehrgang m. **4.** Fachbereich m, Fakultät f. **II** vt schulen, ausbilden (in in).
school² [skuːl] n bio. Schwarm m, Schule f, Zug m.
school age schulpflichtiges Alter nt.
school-age adj schulpflichtig.
school child Kind nt im Grundschulalter.
Schottmüller ['ʃatmɪlər]: **S. bacillus** Salmonella schottmuelleri, Salmonella paratyphi B, Salmonella enteritidis serovar schottmuelleri.
S.'s disease/fever Paratyphus m.
Schramm [ʃræm, ʃram]: **S.'s phenomenon** urol. Schramm-Sphinkterphänomen nt.
Schreger ['ʃreɪgər; 'ʃreː-]: **lines of S.** → **S.'s striae**.
S.'s striae Schreger-Hunter'-Linien pl.
Schuchardt ['ʃukərt; 'ʃuxart]: **S.'s incision** gyn. Schuchardt-Schnitt m.
S.'s operation gyn. Schuchardt-Operation f.

Schüffner ['ʃɪfnər; 'ʃyf-]: **S.'s dots/granules/punctuation/stippling** Schüffner-Tüpfelung f.
Schüller ['ʃɪlər; 'ʃyl-]: **S. disease 1.** Hand-Schüller-Christian-Krankheit f, Schüller-Hand-Christian-Krankheit f, Schüller-Krankheit f. **2.** Osteoporosis circumscripta cranii.
S.'s ducts Skene'-Gänge pl, -Drüsen pl, Ductus paraurethrales (urethrae feminiae).
S.'s glands → S.'s ducts.
S.'s syndrome → S. disease 1.
S.'s (x-ray) view HNO Aufnahme nt nach Schüller.
Schüller-Christian ['krɪstʃən]: **S.-C. disease/syndrome** → Schüller disease 1.
Schultz [ʃʊlts]: **S.'s angina/disease/syndrome** Agranulozytose f, maligne/perniziöse Neutropenie f.
Schultz-Charlton ['tʃaːrltn]: **S.-C. phenomenon** Schultz-Charlton(-Auslösch)-Phänomen nt.
S.-C. reaction/test → S.-C. phenomenon.
Schultz-Dale [deɪl]: **S.-D. reaction** Schultz-Dale-Reaktion f.
Schultze ['ʃʊltsə, 'ʃul-]: **S.'s bundle** → S.'s fasciculus.
S.'s cells Riechzellen pl.
comma bundle of S. → S.'s fasciculus.
comma tract of S. → S.'s fasciculus.
S.'s fasciculus Schultze'-Komma nt, Fasciculus interfascicularis/semilunaris.
S.'s mechanism gyn. Schultze-Mechanismus m, -Modus m.
S. placenta Schultze-Plazenta f.
S.'s sign neuro. Chvostek-Zeichen nt.
S.'s tract → S.'s fasciculus.
Schultze-Chvostek ['vastek]: **S.-C. sign** neuro. Chvostek-Zeichen nt.
Schutz [ʃʊts]: **S.' bundle** → Schütz' bundle.
Schütz [ʃɪts, ʃyts]: **S.' bundle** Schütz'-(Längs-)Bündel nt, dorsales Längsbündel nt, Fasciculus longitudinalis dorsalis.
Schwabach ['ʃvaːbak, -bax]: **S.'s test** Schwabach-Versuch m.
Schwalbe [ʃvalbə]: **S.'s corpuscle** Geschmacksknospe f, Caliculus gustatorius, Gemma gustatoria.
S.'s fissure Fissura choroidea.
S.'s nucleus Schwalbe'-Kern m, Nc. vestibularis medialis.
S.'s ring Schwalbe'-Grenzring m.
S.'s space Spatium intervaginale (n. optici).
Schwann [ʃwan, ʃv-; ʃwan]: **S. cell** Schwann'-Zelle f.
S.-cell tumor → schwannoma.
S.'s membrane Schwann'-Scheide f, Neuri-, Neurolemm nt, Neurilemma nt.
S.'s sheath → S.'s membrane.
schwan·ni·tis [ʃwaˈnaɪtɪs] n → schwannosis.
schwan·no·gli·o·ma [ʃwanəglaɪˈəʊmə] n → schwannoma.
schwan·no·ma [ʃwaˈnəʊmə] n Schwannom nt, Neurinom nt, Neurilem(m)om nt.
schwan·no·sis [ʃwaˈnəʊsɪs] n Hypertrophie f der Schwann'-Zellen.
Schwediauer ['ʃveɪdɪaʊər; 'ʃveː-]: **S.'s disease** Albert-Krankheit f, Entzündung f der Bursa tendinis calcanei.
Schweigger-Seidel [ʃvalbə; 'ʃvaɪgər 'saɪdl]: **S.-S. sheath** Schweigger-Seidel'-Hülse f, Ellipsoid nt.
sci·at·ic [saɪˈætɪk] adj **1.** Ischiasnerv betr., ischiatisch, Ischias-. **2.** Sitzbein betr., zum Sitzbein gehörend, Ischias-, Sitzbein-.
sci·at·i·ca [saɪˈætɪkə] n **1.** Ischiassyndrom nt, Cotunnius-Syndrom nt. **2.** Ischias f,

Ischiasbeschwerden pl, Ischialgie f.
sciatica-induced scoliosis → sciatic scoliosis.
sciatic artery Begleitarterie f des N. ischiadicus, A. commitans n. ischiadici/sciatici.
sciatic bursa: s. of gluteus maximus muscle Bursa ischiadica/sciatica m. glut(a)ei maximi.
s. of obturator internus muscle Bursa ischiadica/sciatica m. obturatoris interni.
sciatic foramen: greater s. For. ischiadicum/sciaticum majus.
lesser s. For. ischiadicum/sciaticum minus.
sciatic hernia Beckenhernie f, Ischiozele f, Hernia ischiadica.
sciatic nerve Ischiasnerv m, N. ischiadicus/sciaticus.
small s. N. cutaneus femoris posterior.
sciatic neuralgia → sciatica.
sciatic neuritis → sciatica.
sciatic notch: greater s. Inc. ischiadica major.
lesser s. Inc. ischiadica minor.
sciatic scoliosis ortho. ischialgie-bedingte Skoliose f.
sciatic spine Spina ischiadica/ischialis.
sciatic tuber Tuber ischiadicum/ischiale.
SCID abbr. → severe combined immunodeficiency (disease).
sci·ence ['saɪəns] n Wissenschaft f; Naturwissenschaft f.
sci·en·tif·ic [saɪənˈtɪfɪk] adj **1.** (natur-)wissenschaftlich. **2.** systematisch, exakt.
sci·en·tism ['saɪəntɪzəm] n Wissenschaftlichkeit f.
sci·en·tist ['saɪəntɪst] n Wissenschaftler(in f) m, Forscher(in f) m.
scil·la ['sɪlə] n Meerzwiebel f, Scilla f.
scil·la·bi·ose [ˌsɪləˈbaɪəʊs] n Scillabiose f.
scil·la·ren ['sɪlərən] n Scillaren nt.
scil·lism ['sɪlɪzəm] n Scillavergiftung f, Scillismus m.
scim·i·tar syndrome ['skɪmɪtər] Scimitar-Syndrom nt.
scin·ti·gram ['sɪntɪɡræm] n → scintiscan.
scin·ti·graph·ic [ˌsɪntɪˈɡræfɪk] adj Szintigraphie betr., szintigraphisch.
scin·tig·ra·phy [sɪnˈtɪɡrəfɪ] n radiol. Szintigraphie f; Scanning nt.
scin·til·la·scope [sɪnˈtɪləskəʊp] n → scintillator.
scin·til·late ['sɪntɪleɪt] vi phys. aufblitzen, flimmern, funkeln, szintillieren.
scin·til·lat·ing scotoma ['sɪntɪleɪtɪŋ] ophthal. Flimmerskotom nt, Scotoma scintillans.
scin·til·la·tion [ˌsɪntəˈleɪʃn] n **1.** Funkeln nt, Aufblitzen nt, Szintillation f. **2.** phys. Szintillation f.
scintillation counter → scintillator.
scintillation scanner radiol. Szintiscanner m.
scintillation scanning → scintiscanning.
scin·til·la·tor ['sɪntɪleɪtər] n Szintillationszähler m, -detektor m, Szintillator m.
scin·til·lom·e·ter [ˌsɪntəˈlamɪtər] n → scintillator.
scin·ti·scan ['sɪntɪskæn] n radiol. Szintigramm nt, Scan m.
scin·ti·scan·ner [ˌ-ˈskænər] n Szintiscanner m.
scin·ti·scan·ning [ˌ-ˈskænɪŋ] n radiol. Szintigraphie f, Scanning nt.
scir·rho·ma [skɪəˈrəʊmə] n → scirrhous carcinoma.
scir·rhous ['skɪrəs] adj derb, verhärtet, szirrhös.
scirrhous cancer → scirrhous carcinoma.
scirrhous carcinoma szirrhöses Karzinom nt, Faserkrebs m, Szirrhus m, Skirrhus m, Ca. scirrhosum.

scir·rhus ['skɪrəs] *n* → scirrhous carcinoma.
scis·sion ['sɪʒn, 'sɪʃn] *n* **1.** Schneiden *nt*, Spalten *nt*; Schnitt *m*. **2.** *chem.* Spaltung *f*.
scis·sor ['sɪzər] *vt* (mit der Schere) schneiden, zer-, zuschneiden.
scissor gait *neuro.* Scherengang *m*.
scis·sors ['sɪzərz] *pl* (*a.* pair of ~) Schere *f*.
scis·su·ra [sɪ'sʊərə] *n, pl* **-rae** [-riː] Spalte *f*, Fissur *f*, Scissura *f*.
scis·sure ['sɪʒər, 'sɪʃ-] *n* → scissura.
scler- *pref.* → sclero-.
scle·ra ['sklɪərə] *n, pl* **-ras, -rae** [-riː, -raɪ] (*Auge*) Lederhaut *f*, Sklera *f*, Sclera *f*.
scler·ad·e·ni·tis [ˌsklɪræm'naɪtɪs] *n* Skleradenitis *f*.
scle·ral ['sklɪərəl, 'skle-] *adj* Lederhaut/Sklera betr., skleral, Lederhaut-, Sklera-.
scleral ectasia → sclerectasia.
scleral furrow → scleral sulcus.
scleral spur Sklerasporn *m*.
scleral staphyloma Sklerastaphylom *nt*.
scleral sulcus sklerokorneale Furche *f*, Sulcus sclerae.
scleral veins Skleravenen *pl*, Vv. sclerales.
scle·ra·ti·tis [ˌsklɪərə'taɪtɪs] *n* → scleritis.
scle·ra·tog·e·nous [ˌ-'tɑdʒənəs] *adj* → sclerogenous.
scle·rec·ta·sia [sklɪrek'teɪʒ(ɪ)ə] *n ophthal.* Sklerektasie *f*.
scle·rec·to·ir·i·dec·to·my [sklɪ'rektəʊˌɪrɪ-'dektəmɪ] *n ophthal.* Lagrange-Operation *f*, Sklerektoiridektomie *f*.
scle·rec·to·my [sklɪ'rektəmɪ] *n ophthal.* Sklerektomie *f*.
scler·e·de·ma [ˌsklɪərə'diːmə] *n* Buschke-Sklerödem *nt*, Scleroedema adultorum (Buschke), Scleroedema Buschke.
scle·re·ma [sklɪ'riːmə] *n* **1.** Sklerem *nt*, Sklerema *nt*, Sclerema *nt*. **2.** Underwood-Krankheit *f*, Fettsklerem *nt* der Neugeborenen, Sclerema adiposum neonatorum.
scler·en·ce·pha·lia [ˌsklɪərensɪ'feɪljə, -lɪə] *n* Sklerenzephalie *f*, Sclerencephalia *f*.
scler·en·ceph·a·ly [ˌsklɪəren'sefəlɪ] *n* → sclerencephalia.
scle·ri·a·sis [sklɪ'raɪəsɪs] *n* Skleriasis *f*, Scleriasis *f*.
scle·ri·rit·o·my [ˌsklɪərɪ'rɪtəmɪ] *n ophthal.* Skleriritomie *f*.
scle·ri·tis [sklɪ'raɪtɪs] *n ophthal.* Lederhaut-, Skleraentzündung *f*, Skleritis *f*, Scleritis *f*.
sclero- *pref.* **1.** *ophthal.* Lederhaut-, Sklera-, Skler(o)-. **2.** *patho.* Skler(o)-.
scle·ro·blas·te·ma [ˌsklɪərəʊblæs'tiːmə, ˌskleroʊ-] *n embryo.* Skleroblastem *nt*.
scle·ro·cho·roid·i·tis [ˌ-ˌkɔːrɔɪ'daɪtɪs, -ˌkɔʊ-] *n ophthal.* Sklerochorioiditis *f*.
scle·ro·con·junc·ti·val [ˌ-ˌkəndʒʌŋk'taɪvl] *adj* Sklera u. Konjunktiva betr., sklerokonjunktival.
scle·ro·con·junc·ti·vi·tis [ˌ-ˌkənˌdʒʌŋktə-'vaɪtɪs] *n ophthal.* Entzündung *f* von Sklera u. Konjunktiva, Sklerokonjunktivitis *f*.
scle·ro·cor·nea [ˌ-'kɔːrnɪə] *n ophthal.* Sklerokornea *f*.
scle·ro·cor·ne·al [ˌ-'kɔːrnɪəl] *adj* Lederhaut/Sklera u. Hornhaut/Kornea betr. *od.* verbindend, sklerokorneal, korneoskleral.
sclerocorneal junction Perikornealring *m*, Limbus corneae.
sclerocorneal sulcus → scleral sulcus.
scle·ro·dac·tyl·ia [ˌ-dæk'tɪlɪə] *n* → sclerodactyly.
scle·ro·dac·ty·ly [ˌ-'dæktəlɪ] *n* Sklerodaktylie *f*.

scler·o·der·ma [ˌ-'dɜrmə] *n* Sklerodermie *nt*, Sclerodermia *f*.
scler·o·der·ma·ti·tis [ˌ-ˌdɜrmə'taɪtɪs] *n* Sklerodermatitis *f*.
scle·ro·der·ma·tous [ˌ-'dɜrmətəs] *adj* Skleroderm(ie) betr.
scle·ro·gen·ic [ˌ-'dʒenɪk] *adj* → sclerogenous.
scle·rog·e·nous [sklɪ'rɑdʒənəs] *adj* Sklerose verursachend, sklerogen.
scler·oid ['sklɪərɔɪd] *adj* hart, verhärtet, sklerotisch.
scle·ro·i·ri·tis [ˌsklɪərəʊ'raɪtɪs, ˌskle-] *n ophthal.* Entzündung *f* von Sklera u. Iris, Skleroiritis *f*, Iridoskleritis *f*.
scle·ro·ker·a·ti·tis [ˌ-ˌkerə'taɪtɪs] *n ophthal.* Entzündung *f* von Sklera u. Kornea, Sklerokeratitis *f*, Korneoskleritis *f*.
scle·ro·ker·a·to·i·ri·tis [ˌ-ˌkerətəʊaɪ'raɪtɪs] *n ophthal.* Sklerokeratoiritis *f*.
scle·ro·ker·a·to·sis [ˌ-ˌkerə'təʊsɪs] *n* → sclerokeratitis.
scle·ro·ma [sklɪ'rəʊmə] *n* Sklerom *nt*, Scleroma *nt*.
scle·ro·ma·la·cia [ˌsklɪərəʊmə'leɪʃ(ɪ)ə, ˌskle-] *n ophthal.* Skleraerweichung *f*, Skleromalazie *f*, Scleromalacia (perforans) *f*.
scle·ro·me·ninx [ˌ-'miːnɪŋks, -'men-] *n* Dura mater.
scle·ro·mere ['-mɪər] *n* Skleromer *nt*.
scle·ro·mite ['-maɪt] *n embryo.* Skleromit *m*.
scle·ro·myx·e·de·ma [ˌ-mɪksə'diːmə] *n derm.* **1.** Arndt-Gottron-Syndrom *nt*, Skleromyxödem *nt*. **2.** Lichen myxoedematosus/fibromucinoidosus, Mucinosis papulosa/lichenoides, Myxodermia papulosa.
scler·o·nych·ia [ˌ-'nɪkɪə] *n* Skleronychie *f*, Scleronychia *f*.
scle·ro·nyx·is [ˌ-'nɪksɪs] *n ophthal.* Sklerapunktion *f*, Skleronyxis *f*.
sclero-oophoritis *n* sklerosierende Eierstockentzündung *f*/Oophoritis *f*.
sclero-oothecitis *n* → sclero-oophoritis.
scle·roph·thal·mia [ˌsklɪrɑf'θælmɪə] *n ophthal.* Sklerophthalmie *f*.
scle·ro·pro·tein [ˌsklɪərə'prəʊtiːn, -tiːɪn, ˌskle-] *n* Gerüsteiweiß *nt*, Skleroprotein *nt*.
scle·ro·sal [sklɪ'rəʊsl] *adj* → scleroid.
scle·ro·sant [sklɪ'rəʊsnt] *n* sklerosierendes Mittel *nt*.
scle·rose [sklɪ'rəʊs] *vt, vi* (ver-)härten, sklerosieren.
scle·rosed [sklɪ'rəʊst, 'sklɪərəʊzd] *adj* von Sklerose betroffen, sklerotisch.
scle·ros·ing [sklɪə'rəʊsɪŋ] *adj* Sklerose verursachend, sklerosierend.
sclerosing adenosis sklerosierende Adenose *f*, Korbzellenhyperplasie *f*.
sclerosing agent sklerosierendes Mittel *nt*.
sclerosing cholangitis primär-sklerosierende Cholangitis *f*.
sclerosing hemangioma sklerosierendes Hämangiom *nt*.
s. of Wolbach Histiozytom *nt*, Histiocytoma *nt*.
sclerosing inflammation sklerosierende Entzündung *f*.
sclerosing keratitis sklerosierende Keratitis *f*, Sklerokeratitis *f*.
sclerosing nonsuppurative osteomyelitis nicht-eitrige Osteomyelitis *f*, sklerosierende Osteomyelitis *f*, Garré-Osteomyelitis *f*, -Krankheit *f*, Osteomyelitis sicca Garré.
sclerosing osteitis → sclerosing nonsuppurative osteomyelitis.
sclerosing periphlebitis Mondor'-Krankheit *f*.

scle·ro·sis [sklɪə'rəʊsɪs] *n, pl* **-ses** [-siːz] Sklerose *f*, Sclerosis *f*.
s. of the arteries *inf.* Arterienverkalkung *f*, Arteriosklerose *f*, -sclerosis *f*.
scle·ro·ste·no·sis [ˌsklɪrəʊstɪ'nəʊsɪs, ˌskle-] *n* Sklerostenose *f*.
scle·ros·to·my [sklɪ'rɑstəmɪ] *n ophthal.* Sklerostomie *f*.
scle·ro·ther·a·py [ˌsklɪərəʊ'θerəpɪ, ˌskle-] *n* Verödung *f*, Sklerosierung *f*, Sklerotherapie *f*.
scle·rot·ic [sklɪ'rɑtɪk] *adj* **1.** *anat.* → scleral. **2.** *patho.* Sklerose betr., an Sklerose erkrankt, sklerotisch.
scle·rot·i·ca [sklɪ'rɑtɪkə] *n* → sclera.
sclerotic acid Sklerotinsäure *f*.
sclerotic coat → sclera.
scle·rot·i·co·cho·roid·i·tis [sklɪˌrɑtɪkəʊ-ˌkɔːrɔɪ'daɪtɪs, -ˌkəʊ-] *n* → sclerochoroiditis.
sclerotic stomach Brinton-Krankheit *f*, entzündlicher Schrumpfmagen *m*, Magenszirrhus *m*, Linitis plastica.
scle·ro·tin ['sklɪərətɪn, 'skler-] *n bio.* Sklerotin *f*.
Scle·ro·tin·ia [ˌsklɪərə'tɪnɪə] *n micro.* Sclerotinia *f*.
Scle·ro·tin·i·ace·ae [ˌ-tɪnaɪ'eɪsiː] *pl micro.* Sclerotiniaceae *pl*.
scle·ro·tin·ic acid [ˌsklɪərə'tɪnɪk, ˌskler-] → sclerotic acid.
scle·ro·ti·tis [ˌ-'taɪtɪs] *n* → scleritis.
scle·ro·ti·um [sklɪ'rəʊʃɪəm] *n, pl* **-tia** [-ʃɪə] *micro.* Dauermyzel *nt*, Sklerotium *nt*, Sclerotium *nt*.
scle·ro·tome ['sklerətəʊm, 'sklɪr-] *n* **1.** *embryo.* Sklerotom *nt*. **2.** *neuro.* Sklerotom *nt*. **3.** *ophthal.* Sklerotomiemesser *nt*, Sklerotom *nt*.
sclerotome cells *embryo.* Sklerotomzellen *pl*.
sclerotome segment *embryo.* Sklerotomsegment *nt*.
scle·ro·tom·ic diverticulum [ˌ-'tɑmɪk] *embryo.* Sklerotomdivertikel *nt*.
sclerotomic fissure *embryo.* Sklerotomfissur *f*.
scle·rot·o·my [sklɪ'rɑtəmɪ] *n ophthal.* Sklerotomie *f*.
scle·rous ['sklɪərəs] *adj* → scleroid.
sco·le·ci·a·sis [skəʊlɪ'saɪəsɪs] *n patho.* Scoleciasis *f*.
sco·lec·i·form [skəʊ'lesɪfɔːrm] *adj micro.* scolex-artig, -ähnlich.
scoleco- *pref.* Wurm-.
sco·le·coid ['skəʊlɪkɔɪd] *adj* **1.** → scoleciform. **2.** wurmartig, wurmähnlich, Wurm-. **3.** hydatid.
sco·le·col·o·gy [ˌskəʊlɪ'kɑlədʒɪ] *n* Helminthologie *f*.
sco·lex ['skəʊleks] *n, pl* **sco·le·ces** [skəʊ-'liːsiːz], **scol·i·ces** ['skɑləsiːz, 'skəʊ-] *micro.* Bandwurmkopf *m*, Skolex *m*, Scolex *m*.
scolio- *pref.* Skolio-, Scolio-.
sco·li·o·ky·pho·sis [ˌskəʊlɪəʊkaɪ'fəʊsɪs] *n ortho.* Skoliokyphose *f*.
sco·li·o·si·om·e·try [ˌ-sɪ'ɑmətrɪ] *n ortho.* Skoliosimetrie *f*.
sco·li·o·sis [ˌskəʊlɪ'əʊsɪs, ˌskɑ-] *n, pl* **-ses** [-siːz] *patho.* Skoliose *f*, Scoliosis *f*.
sco·li·ot·ic [ˌskəʊlɪ'ɑtɪk] *adj* Skoliose betr., durch Skoliose gekennzeichnet, skoliotisch, Skoliose-.
scoliotic nose Schiefnase *f*.
scoliotic pelvis Skoliosebecken *nt*.
S colony *micro.* (*Kolonie*) S-Form *f*.
scoop [skuːp] *n chir.* Löffel *m*.
sco·pin ['skəʊpɪn, -pɪn] *n* Scopin *nt*.
sco·pol·a·mine [skə'pɑləmiːn, ˌskəʊpə-'læmɪn] *n* Scopolamin *nt*.

scopophilia

sco·po·phil·ia [ˌskəʊpə'fılıə] *n psychia.* Skopophilie *f*, Skoptophilie *f*.
sco·po·pho·bia [ˌ-'fəʊbıə] *n psychia.* Skopophobie *f*, Skoptophobie *f*.
scop·to·phil·ia [ˌskɑptə'fılıə] *n* → scopophilia.
scop·to·pho·bia [ˌ-'fəʊbıə] *n* → scopophobia.
Scop·u·lar·i·op·sis [ˌskɑpjəˌleərı'ɑpsıs] *n micro.* Scopulariopsis *f*.
scop·u·lar·i·op·so·sis [ˌ-ˌleərıɑp'səʊsıs] *n* Scopulariopsidosis *f*, Scopulariopsosis *f*.
scor·a·cra·tia [ˌskɔːrə'kreıʃıə] *n* → scatacratia.
scor·bu·tic [skɔːr'bjuːtık] *adj* Skorbut betr., von Skorbut gekennzeichnet, skorbutisch, Skorbut-.
scorbutic anemia Vitamin C-Mangelanämie *f*.
scor·bu·ti·gen·ic [skɔːrˌbjuːtı'dʒenık] *adj* Skorbut verursachend, skorbutigen.
score [skɔːr] *n* Score *m*.
scor·ings ['skɔːrıŋs] *pl radiol.* Wachstumslinien *pl*.
scor·pi·on ['skɔːrpıən, pjən] *n* Skorpion *m*.
Scor·pi·on·i·da [skɔːrpı'ɑnıdə] *pl* Skorpione *pl*, Scorpionidae *pl*.
scot(o)- *pref.* Dunkel-, Skot(o)-.
sco·to·chro·mo·gen·ic [ˌskəʊtəˌkrəʊmə-'dʒenık, ˌskɑtə-] *adj micro.* skotochromogen.
sco·to·chro·mo·gens [ˌ-'krəʊmədʒəns] *pl micro.* **1.** skotochromogene Mykobakterien *pl*, Mykobakterien *pl* der Runyon--Gruppe II. **2.** skotochromogene Mikroorganismen *pl*.
sco·to·ma [skə'təʊmə] *n, pl* **-mas, -ma·ta** [-mətə] *ophthal.* Gesichtsfeldausfall *m*, Skotom *nt*, Scotoma *nt*.
sco·to·ma·graph [skə'təʊməgræf] *n* Skotomagraph *m*.
sco·tom·a·tous [skə'tɑmətəs] *adj* Skotom betr., Skotom-.
sco·tom·e·ter [skə'tɑmıtər] *n ophthal.* Skotometer *m*.
sco·tom·e·try [skə'tɑmıtrı] *n ophthal.* Skotometrie *f*.
sco·to·phil·ia [ˌskəʊtə'fılıə] *n psychia.* Nyktophilie *f*.
sco·to·pho·bia [ˌ-'fəʊbıə] *n psychia.* Nyktophobie *f*.
sco·to·pia [skə'təʊpıə] *n* Dämmerungs-, Nachtsehen *nt*, skotopes Sehen *nt*, Skotop(s)ie *f*.
sco·top·ic [skə'tɑpık] *adj* Skotop(s)ie betr., Dunkel-.
scotopic adaptation *physiol.* Dunkeladaptation *f*, -anpassung *f*.
scotopic vision → scotopia.
sco·top·sin [skə'tɑpsın] *n* Skotopsin *nt*, Scotopsin *nt*.
sco·tos·co·py [skəʊ'tɑskəpı] *n* → skiascopy.
scratch [skrætʃ] **I** *n* Kratzer *m*, Schramme *f*, Riß *m*. **II** *vt* (zer-)kratzen, ritzen. **III** *vi* s. kratzen, s. scheuern.
scratch test Scratch-, Kratz-, Skarifikationstest *m*.
screen [skriːn] **I** *n* **1.** (Schutz-)Schirm *m*. **2.** *phys.* Filter *nt/m*, Blende *f*. **3.** *radiol., techn.* Schirm *m*, Screen *nt*. **II** *vt* (be-)schirmen, (be-)schützen (*from vor*).
screen off *vt* abschirmen (*from gegen*).
screen·ing ['skriːnıŋ] *n* **1.** Screening *nt*. **2.** *Brit. radiol.* (Röntgen-)Durchleuchtung *f*, Fluoroskopie *f*. **3.** → screening test.
screening test Vor-, Such-, Siebtest *m*, Screeningtest *m*.
screen test *ophthal.* **1.** alternierender Abdecktest *m*. **2.** Abdeck-Aufdecktest *m*.
screw [skruː] **I** *n* Schraube *f*. **II** *vt* schrauben.

screw down *vt* einschrauben, festschrauben.
screw on *vt* anschrauben.
screw driver Schraubenzieher *m*.
screw driver teeth Hutchinson-Zähne *pl*.
screwed [skruːd] *adj* mit Gewinde.
screw fixation *ortho.* Verschraubung *f*, Verschrauben *nt*, Schraubenosteosynthese *f*.
screw tap Gewindebohrer *m*.
screw wire Gewindestift *m*.
Scribner ['skraıbnər]: **S. shunt** Scribner--Shunt *m*, Quinton-Scribner-Shunt *m*.
scrib·o·ma·nia [ˌskrıbə'meınıə, -jə] *n psychia.* Kritzelsucht *f*, Graphorrhoe *f*.
scrive·ners' palsy ['srıvnərs] Schreibkrampf *m*, Graphospasmus *m*, Mogigraphie *f*.
scrof·u·la ['skrɑfjələ] *n* Skrofulose *f*, Scrofulosis *f*.
scrof·u·lar conjunctivitis ['skrɑfjələr] → scrofulous keratitis.
scrof·u·lo·der·ma [ˌskrɑfjələ'dɜrmə] *n* Skrophuloderm *nt*, tuberkulöses Gumma *nt*, Tuberculosis cutis colliquativa.
scrof·u·lous ['skrɑfjələs] *adj* skrofulös; tuberkulös.
scrofulous abscess tuberkulöser Abszeß *m*.
scrofulous keratitis Conjunctivitis/Keratitis/Keratoconjunctivitis eccematosa/eczematosa/scrufulosa/phlyctaenulosa.
scrofulous ophthalmia → scrofulous keratitis.
scro·tal ['skrəʊtəl] *adj* Hodensack/Skrotum betr., skrotal, Skrotal-.
scrotal arteries: anterior s. Skrotumäste *pl* der A. femoralis, Rami scrotales anteriores a. femoralis.
posterior s. Skrotumäste *pl* der A. pudenda interna, Rami scrotales posteriores a. pudendae internae.
scrotal branch: anterior s. of femoral artery → scrotal arteries, anterior.
posterior s.es of internal pudendal artery → scrotal arteries, posterior.
scrotal edema Skrotal-, Skrotumödem *nt*.
scrotal hernia Hodenbruch *m*, Skrotalhernie *f*, Hernia scrotalis.
scrotal hydrocele Hydrocele scrotalis.
scrotal nerves Skrotalnerven *pl*, Nn. scrotales.
anterior s. vordere Skrotalnerven, Nn. scrotales anteriores.
posterior s. hintere Skrotalnerven, Nn. scrotales posteriores.
scrotal pruritus Pruritus scroti.
scrotal raphe Skrotalnaht, -raphe, Raphe scroti.
scrotal reflex Skrotalreflex *m*.
scrotal septum Mediansept um *nt* des Skrotums, Skrotal-, Skrotumseptum *nt*, Septum scroti/scrotale.
scrotal swellings *embryo.* Skrotalwülste *pl*.
scrotal tongue Faltenzunge *f*, Lingua plicata/scrotalis.
scrotal veins Skrotal-, Skrotumvenen *pl* Vv. scrotales.
anterior s. vordere Skrotalvenen, Vv. scrotales anteriores.
posterior s. hintere Skrotalvenen, Vv. scrotales posteriores.
scro·tec·to·my [skrəʊ'tektəmı] *n urol.* Hodensack, Skrotumexzision *f*, Skrotektomie *f*.
scro·ti·tis [skrəʊ'taıtıs] *n urol.* Hodensack-, Skrotumentzündung *f*, Skrotitis *f*, Scrotitis *f*.
scro·to·cele ['skrəʊtəsiːl] *n* → scrotal hernia.

scro·to·plas·ty ['-plæstı] *n urol.* Skrotumplastik *f*.
scro·tum ['skrəʊtəm] *n, pl* **-tums, -ta** [-tə] Hodensack *m*, Skrotum *nt*, Scrotum *nt*.
scrub[1] [skrʌb] **I** *n* Scheuern *nt*, Schrubben *nt*. **II** *vt* schrubben, scheuern, (ab-)reiben. **III** *vi* scheuern, schrubben, reiben.
scrub up *vt chir.* s. die Hände desinfizieren.
scrub[2] ['skrʌb] *n* Gestrüpp *nt*, Buschwerk *nt*.
scrub nurse *chir.* Instrumentierschwester *f*.
scrub tick *micro.* Ixodes holocyclus.
scrub typhus japanisches Fleckfieber *nt*, Scrub-Typhus *m*, Milbenfleckfieber *nt*, Tsutsugamushi-Fieber *nt*.
scru·ple ['skruːpl] *n* **1.** *pharm.* Skrupel *m*. **2.** Skrupel *m*, Zweifel *m*, Bedenken *pl*.
scru·pu·los·i·ty [skruːpjə'lɑsətı] *n* (übertriebene) Gewissenhaftigkeit *f*, Genauigkeit *f*, (Über-)Ängstlichkeit *f*.
scru·pu·lous ['skruːpjələs] *adj* **1.** (über-)gewissenhaft, (über-)vorsichtig, (peinlich) genau. **2.** voller Skrupel *od.* Bedenken.
scru·pu·lous·ness ['skruːpjələsnıs] *n* → scrupulosity.
scum [skʌm] **I** *n* Schaum *m*. **II** *vi* schäumen, Schaum bilden.
scurf [skɜrf] *n* **1.** Schorf *m*, Grind *m*. **2.** *derm.* (*Kopf*) Schuppen *pl*, Pityriasis simplex capitis.
scurf·y ['skɜrfı] *adj* schorfig, grindig; schuppig, verkrustet.
scur·vy ['skɜrvı] *n* Scharbock *m*, Skorbut *m*.
scurvy rickets rachitischer Säuglingsskorbut *m*, Moeller-Barlow-Krankheit *f*.
scu·tate ['skjuːteıt] *adj* → scutiform.
scute [skjuːt] *n bio.* Schild *n*.
scu·ti·form ['sk(j)uːtıfɔːrm] *adj anat.* schildförmig.
scutiform cartilage Schildknorpel *m*, Cartilago thyroidea.
scu·tu·lar ['skjuːtjələr] *adj derm.* Skutulum betr.
scu·tu·lum ['skjuːtjələm, -tʃələm] *n, pl* **-la** [-lə] *derm.* (Favus-)Skutulum *nt*, Scutulum *nt*, Favusschildchen *nt*.
scu·tum ['sk(j)uːtəm] *n micro.* Schild *m*, Scutum *nt*.
scyb·a·lous ['sıbələs] *adj* Skybala betr.
scyb·a·lum ['sıbələm] *n, pl* **-la** [-lə] harter Kotballen *m*, Skybalon *nt*, Scybalum *nt*.
scy·phi·form ['saıfıfɔːrm] *adj* becher-, kelch-, tassenförmig.
scy·phoid ['saıfɔıd] *adj* → scyphiform.
SD *abbr.* → streptodornase.
S.D. *abbr.* → standard deviation.
S.D.A. *abbr.* → specific dynamic action.
SD antigens → serologically defined antigens.
S.D.E. *abbr.* [specific dynamic effect] → specific dynamic action.
SDS *abbr.* → sodium dodecyl sulfate.
SDT *abbr.* → signal detection theory.
SE *abbr.* **1.** → series-elastic element. **2.** → standard error (of median).
Se *abbr.* → selenium.
sea bath [siː] Salzwasser-, Seewasserbad *nt*.
sea-blue histiocyte seeblauer Histiocyt *m*.
sea-blue histiocyte syndrome seeblaue Histiozytose *f*.
sea-blue histiocytoma seeblaues Histiozytom *nt*.
Seabright ['siːbraıt]: **S. bantam syndrome** Seabright-bantam-Syndrom *nt*, Pseudohypoparathyreoidismus *m*.
seal [siːl] **I** *n* **1.** Siegel *nt*. **2.** (wasserdichter/luftdichter) Verschluß *m*; (Ab-)Dichtung *f*; Versiegelung *f*. **II** *vt* (ver-)siegeln.

seal up vt (wasserdicht od. luftdicht) verschließen, abdichten, versiegeln.
seal·ant ['siːlənt] n Dichtungsmittel nt.
seam [siːm] n Saum m, Naht f.
seam·less prosthesis ['siːmlɪs] chir. nahtlose Gefäßprothese f.
search·er ['sɜrtʃər] n Sonde f.
sea scurvy Scharbock m, Skorbut m.
sea·sick·ness ['siːˌsɪknɪs] n Seekrankheit f, Naupathie f, Nausea marina.
sea·son ['siːzn] n (Jahres-)Zeit f, Saison f.
seat·worm ['siːtwɜrm] n micro. Madenwurm m, Enterobius vermicularis, Oxyuris vermicularis.
sea water Salz-, See-, Meerwasser nt.
sea-water bath Salzwasser-, Seewasserbad nt.
seb- pref. → sebo-.
se·ba·ceous [sɪ'beɪʃəs] adj 1. talgartig, talgig, Talg-. 2. talgbildend, -absondernd.
sebaceous adenoma 1. Pringle-Tumor m, Naevus Pringle m, Adenoma sebaceum Pringle. 2. Adenoma sebaceum Balzer.
sebaceous cyst 1. Epidermiszyste f, epidermale Zyste f, Epidermoid nt, Atherom nt. 2. piläre Hautzyste f.
sebaceous glands Talgdrüsen pl, Gll. sebaceae.
s. of conjunctiva Zeis'-Drüsen pl, Gll. sebaceae conjunctivales.
sebaceous nevus Talgdrüsennävus m Jadassohn m, Naevus sebaceous.
sebaceous tubercle Hautgrieß m, Milium nt, Milie f.
sebi- pref. → sebo-.
seb·i·a·gog·ic [ˌsebɪə'gɑdʒɪk] adj → sebiparous.
se·bif·e·rous [sɪ'bɪfərəs] adj → sebiparous.
se·bip·a·rous [sɪ'bɪpərəs] adj Fett od. fettige Substanzen bildend, sebipar.
sebo- pref. Talg-, Seb(o)-.
seb·o·lith ['sebəlɪθ] n Sebolith m.
seb·or·rhea [ˌ-'rɪə] n 1. Seborrhoe f, Seborrhö f, Seborrhoea f. 2. Unna'-Krankheit f, seborrhoisches Ekzem m, seborrhoische/dysseborrhoische Dermatitis f, Morbus Unna m, Dermatitis seborrhoides.
seb·or·rhe·al [ˌ-'rɪəl] adj → seborrheic 1.
seb·or·rhe·ic [ˌ-'rɪɪk] adj 1. Seborrhoe betr., seborrhoisch. 2. mit gesteigerter Talgproduktion, seborrhoisch.
seborrheic blepharitis Blepharitis squamosa.
seborrheic dermatitis → seborrhea 2.
s. of the scalp (Kopf-)Schuppen pl, Pityriasis simplex capitis.
seborrheic dermatosis → seborrhea 2.
seborrheic eczema → seborrhea 2.
seborrheic keratosis seborrhoische Alterswarze/Keratose f, Verruca sebborrhoica/senilis.
seborrheic psoriasis derm. Psoriasis inversa.
seborrheic verruca → seborrheic keratosis.
seb·or·rhi·a·sis [ˌ-'raɪəsɪs] n derm. 1. Seborrhiasis f. 2. Psoriasis inversa.
seb·o·trop·ic [ˌ-'trɑpɪk] adj sebotrop.
se·bum ['siːbəm] n (Haut-)Talg m, Sebum nt.
se·ca·le cor·nu·tum [sɪ'keɪlɪ kɔr'nuːtəm] Mutterkorn nt, Secale cornutum.
Seckel ['sekl]: **S.'s syndrome** Seckel-Syndrom nt.
se·clu·sive personality [sɪ'kluːsɪv] schizoide Persönlichkeit(sstörung f) f.
sec·o·bar·bi·tal [ˌsekoʊ'bɑːrbɪtɔl, -tæl] n pharm. Secobarbital nt.
sec·ond ['sekənd] I n 1. abbr. **s** Sekunde f abbr. s. 2. Sekunde f, Moment m, Augenblick m. 3. (der, die, das) Zweite. 4. Helfer m, Beistand m. II adj 5. zweite(r, s), zweit-. **a ~ time** noch einmal. **every ~ day** jeden zweiten Tag. 6. zweitklassig, -rangig. III adv zweitens, an zweiter Stelle. IV vt unterstützen, beistehen.
sec·ond·ar·y ['sekənˌderiː, -dərɪ] I n 1. (etw.) Untergeordnetes; Untergeordnete(r m) f, Stellvertreter(in f) m. 2. phys. sekundärer (Strom-)Kreis m. II adj 3. nächstfolgend, sekundär, Sekundär-; (nach-)folgend (to auf). 4. zweitrangig, -klassig, sekundär; neben-, untergeordnet, begleitend, Nach-, Neben-, Sekundär-.
secondary adhesion sekundäre Wundheilung f, Sekundärheilung f, Heilung f per secundam intentionem, p.s.-Heilung f.
secondary alcohol sekundärer Alkohol m.
secondary amenorrhea gyn. sekundäre Amenorrhoe f.
secondary amine sekundäres Amin nt.
secondary amyloidosis sekundäre Amyloidose f.
secondary anemia erworbene/sekundäre Anämie f.
secondary atelectasis (Lunge) erworbene/sekundäre Atelektase f.
secondary buffering physiol. Hamburger-Phänomen nt, Chloridverschiebung f.
secondary bundle (Muskel) Sekundärbündel nt.
secondary cancer → secondary carcinoma.
secondary carcinoma Karzinommetastase f, -absiedlung f, metastatisches/sekundäres Karzinom nt.
secondary cardiomyopathy sekundäre Kardiomyopathie f.
secondary cataract 1. komplizierter Star m, Cataracta complicata. 2. Nachstar m, Cataracta secundaria.
secondary coccidioidomycosis sekundäre/progressive Kokzidioidomykose f, Sekundärform f der Kokzidioidomykose.
secondary contact immun. Sekundärkontakt m.
secondary cord of cervical plexus Sekundärstrang m des Halsgeflechts, Fasciculus plexus brachialis.
secondary culture Sekundärkultur f.
secondary cuticle Schmelzoberhäutchen nt, Cuticula dentis.
secondary cyst Tochterzyste f, sekundäre Zyste f.
secondary degeneration neuro. Waller'-Degeneration f, sekundäre/orthograde Degeneration f.
secondary dentition bleibende Zähne pl, Dauergebiß nt, Dentes permanentes.
secondary diaphragm Urogenitaldiaphragma nt, Diaphragma urogenitale.
secondary disease 1. Sekundärerkrankung f, -krankheit f, Zweiterkrankung f, -krankheit f. 2. hema. Sekundärkrankheit f.
secondary division of trigeminal nerve zweiter Trigeminusast m, Maxillaris m, N. maxillaris.
secondary drinking sekundäres Trinken nt.
secondary dysmenorrhea gyn. erworbene/sekundäre Dysmenorrhö f.
secondary electron phys. Sekundärelektron nt.
secondary emission phys. Sekundäremission f.
secondary fissure Fissura secunda (cerebelli).
s. of lung horizontaler Interlobärspalt m, Fissura horizontalis (pulmonis dextris).

secondary follicle 1. (Ovar) Sekundärfollikel m, wachsender Follikel m. 2. (Lymphknoten) Sekundärfollikel m.
secondary fracture pathologische Fraktur f, Spontanfraktur f.
secondary gain psycho. sekundärer Krankheitsgewinn m.
secondary gangrene sekundäre Gangrän f.
secondary generalized epilepsy sekundär generalisierte Epilepsie f.
secondary glaucoma sekundäres Glaukom nt.
secondary gout sekundäre Gicht f.
secondary hemorrhage patho. Nachblutung f.
secondary host micro. Zwischenwirt m.
secondary hydrocephalus sekundärer Hydrozephalus m.
secondary hyperaldosteronism sekundärer Hyperaldosteronismus m.
secondary hyperparathyroidism reaktiver/sekundärer Hyperparathyreoidismus m abbr. sHPT.
secondary hypertension sekundäre/symptomatische Hypertonie f.
secondary hypertrophic osteoarthropathy Marie-Bamberger-Syndrom nt, Bamberger-Marie-Syndrom nt, Akropachie f, hypertrophische pulmonale Osteoarthropathie f.
secondary hypoaldosteronism sekundärer Hypoaldosteronismus m.
secondary hypogonadism sekundärer/hypogonadotroper Hypogonadismus m.
secondary hypotension sekundäre/symptomatische Hypotonie f.
secondary infection Sekundärinfektion f, Sekundärinfekt m.
secondary keratitis sekundäre Keratitis f.
secondary lysosome Sekundärlysosom nt.
secondary memory Sekundärgedächtnis nt.
secondary mesoderm intraembryonales Mesoderm nt.
secondary myocardiopathy sekundäre Kardiomyopathie/Myokardiopathie f.
secondary myxedema sekundäres/hypophysenbedingtes Myxödem nt.
secondary oocyte sekundäre Oozyte f, Ovocytus secundarius.
secondary pacemaker physiol. sekundärer Schrittmacher m.
secondary palate embryo. sekundärer Gaumen m.
secondary phosphate sekundäres Phosphat nt.
secondary pneumonia sekundäre Pneumonie f.
secondary reaction immun. Sekundärreaktion f, -antwort f.
secondary reinforcement psycho. Sekundärverstärkung f.
secondary reinforcer psycho. Sekundärverstärker m.
secondary repair chir., ortho. Sekundärversorgung f, -verschluß m.
secondary response → secondary reaction.
secondary-retroperitoneal adj sekundär retroperitoneal.
secondary spermatocyte sekundärer Spermatozyt m, Spermatozyt m II. Ordnung, Präspermatide f, Spermatocytus secundarius.
secondary structure biochem. Sekundärstruktur f.
secondary suture Sekundärnaht f, sekundäre Naht f.
secondary sulci embryo. Sekundärfurchen pl.

secondary syphilis Sekundärstadium *nt*, Lues *f* II.
secondary tuberculosis postprimäre Tuberkulose *f*.
secondary villus *embryo.* Sekundärzotte *f*.
second degree burn Verbrennung *f* zweiten Grades.
second finger Zeigefinger *m*, Index *m*, Digitus secundus.
second hand (*Uhr*) Sekundenzeiger *m*.
second head of triceps brachii muscle lateraler/äußerer Trizepskopf *m*, Caput laterale m. tricipitis brachii.
second intention → secondary adhesion.
second law of thermodynamics *phys.* zweiter Hauptsatz *m* der Thermodynamik.
second-look operation Second-look-Operation *f*.
second messenger *biochem.* sekundäre Botensubstanz *f*, second messenger (*m*).
second nerve Sehnerv *m*, Optikus *m*, II. Hirnnerv *m*, N. opticus.
second-order reaction *chem.* Reaktion *f* zweiter Ordnung.
second sound zweiter Herzton *m*, II. Herzton *m*.
second stage (of labor) *gyn.* Austreibungsphase *f*, -periode *f*.
second substrate *biochem.* zweites Substrat *nt*, Folgesubstrat *nt*.
second teeth bleibende/zweite Zähne *pl*, Dauergebiß *nt*, Dentes permanentes.
se·cre·ta·gogue [sɪ'kriːtəgɑg] I *n* Sekretagogum *nt*, Sekretogogum *nt*. II *adj* die Sekretion anregend, sekretorisch, sekretagog.
se·crete [sɪ'kriːt] *vt* absondern, sezernieren.
se·cre·tin [sɪ'kriːtɪn] *n* Sekretin *nt*.
secretin test Sekretin-Test *m*.
se·cre·tion [sɪ'kriːʃn] *n* 1. Absondern *nt*, Sezernieren *nt*. 2. Absonderung *f*, Sekretion *f*. 3. Absonderung *f*, Sekret *nt*, Secretum *nt*.
se·cre·tive ['siːkrətɪv, sɪ'kriː-] *adj* → secretory II.
se·cre·to·gogue *n, adj* → secretagogue.
se·cre·to·in·hib·i·to·ry [sɪˌkriːtəʊɪn'hɪbətɔːriː, -təʊ-] *adj* die Sekretion hemmend, antisekretorisch.
se·cre·to·mo·tor [ˌ-'məʊtər] *adj* die Sekretion stimulierend, sekretomotorisch.
se·cre·to·mo·tor·y [ˌ-'məʊtəriː] *adj* → secretomotor.
se·cre·tor [sɪ'kriːtər] *n genet.* Sekretor *m*, Ausscheider *m*.
se·cre·to·ry [sɪ'kriːtəriː] I *n, pl* **-ries** sekretorisches Organ *od.* Gefäß *nt*. II *adj* Sekret *od.* Sekretion betr., sekretorisch, Sekret-, Sekretions-.
secretory cell sezernierende Zelle *f*, Drüsenzelle *f*.
 mucous s. muköse Drüsenzelle.
 serous s. seröse Drüsenzelle.
secretory cyst Retentionszyste *f*.
secretory droplet Sekrettröpfchen *nt*.
secretory duct (*Drüse*) Ausführungsgang *m*.
secretory granules Sekretgranula *pl*.
secretory phase gestagene/sekretorische Phase *f*, Sekretions-, Lutealphase *f*.
secretory unit Drüsenendstück *nt*.
sec·tile ['sektɪl, -taɪl] *adj* schneidbar.
sec·tion ['sekʃn] I *n* 1. (Einzel-, Bestand-)Teil *m*; Ab-, Ausschnitt *m*; Bezirk *m*. 2. *chir.* (Ein-)Schnitt *m*, Inzision *f*; Ein-, Durchschneiden *nt*. 3. (mikroskopischer) Schnitt *m*. II *vt* 4. ab-, unter-, einteilen. 5. *chir.* einen Schnitt machen, durch Inzision eröffnen, inzidieren.

sec·tor ['sektər] *n* Sektor *m*, Abschnitt *m*.
sec·to·ri·al [sek'tɔːrɪəl, -'təʊ-] *adj* Sektor-, Sektoren-.
sector iridectomy *ophthal.* komplette/totale/vollständige Iridektomie *f*.
se·cun·di·grav·i·da [sɪˌkʌndɪ'grævɪdə] *n gyn.* Secundigravida *f*.
sec·un·di·na [ˌsekən'daɪnə] *n, pl* **-nae** [-niː] *gyn.* Nachgeburt *f*.
se·cun·di·nes ['-daɪnz, -diːnz] *pl gyn.* Nachgeburt *f*.
sec·un·dip·a·ra [ˌ-'dɪpərə] *n gyn.* Zweitgebärende *f*, Secundipara *f*.
sec·un·dip·a·rous [ˌ-'dɪpərəs] *adj gyn.* zweitgebärend, sekundipar, secundipara.
se·date [sɪ'deɪt] *vt* ein Beruhigungsmittel verabreichen, sedieren.
se·da·tion [sɪ'deɪʃn] *n* Sedieren *nt*, Sedierung *f*.
sed·a·tive ['sedətɪv] I *n* → sedative agent. II *adj* beruhigend, sedierend, sedativ; einschläfernd.
sedative agent Beruhigungsmittel *nt*, Sedativ *nt*, Sedativum *nt*, Temperans *nt*.
sed·en·tar·y ['sednˌteriː] *adj* 1. sitzend. 2. *bio.* sitzend, seßhaft, ansässig.
sed·i·ment ['sedɪmənt] *n* Niederschlag *m*, (Boden-)Satz *m*, Sediment *nt*.
sed·i·men·tal [ˌ-'mentl] *adj* → sedimentary.
sed·i·men·ta·ry [ˌ-'mentərɪ] *adj* sedimentär, Sediment-.
sedimentary cataract Morgagni-Katarakt *f*, Cataracta liquida/fluida.
sed·i·men·ta·tion [ˌ-mən'teɪʃn] *n* Ablagerung *f*, Sedimentbildung *f*, Sedimentation *f*, Sedimentieren *nt*.
sedimentation analysis Sedimentationsanalyse *f*.
sedimentation coefficient *abbr.* **s** Sedimentationskoeffizient *m* *abbr.* s.
sedimentation constant → sedimentation coefficient.
sedimentation equilibrium Sedimentationsgleichgewicht *nt*.
sedimentation-equilibrium method Sedimentationsgleichgewichtsmethode *f*.
sedimentation reaction → sedimentation time.
sedimentation time Blutkörperchensenkung *f* *abbr.* BKS, Blutkörperchensenkungsgeschwindigkeit *f* *abbr.* BSG, *inf.* Blutsenkung *f*.
sedimentation velocity Sedimentationsgeschwindigkeit *f*.
sedimentation-velocity method Sedimentationsgeschwindigkeitsmethode *f*.
se·do·hep·tu·lose-1,7-diphosphate [siːdəʊ'heptəˌləʊz] *n* Sedoheptulose-1,7-diphosphat *nt*.
sedoheptulose-7-phosphate *n* Sedoheptulose-7-phosphat *nt*.
seed [siːd] I *n* 1. *bot.* Same(n *pl*) *m*. 2. → spermatozoon. 3. *radiol.* Seed *nt*. II *vt micro.* eine Kultur ansetzen.
seed protein *bio.* Samenprotein *nt*.
seed wart *derm.* gemeine/gewöhnliche Warze *f*, Stachelwarze *f*, Verruca vulgaris.
SEF *abbr.* [staphylococcal enterotoxin F] → toxic shock-syndrome toxin-1.
seg·ment [*n* 'segmənt; *v* 'segment, seg'ment] I *n* Teil *m*, Abschnitt *m*, Segment *nt*; *anat.* Segmentum *nt*. II *vt* in Segmente teilen, segmentieren.
 s.s of kidney Nierensegmente *pl*, Segmenta renalia.
 s.s of liver Lebersegmente *pl*, Segmenta hepatis.
 s. of Rivinus Inc. tympanica.
seg·men·tal [seg'mentl] *adj* Segment *od.* Segmentation betr., segmental, segmentär, segmentar, Segment-.
segmental anesthesia *neuro.* segmentale Sensibilitätsstörung/Anästhesie *f*.
segmental appendicitis segmentale Appendizitis *f*.
segmental artery (*Leber, Niere*) Segmentarterie *f*, A. segmenti.
 anterior s. A. segmenti anterioris.
 inferior s. A. segmenti inferioris.
 inferior s., anterior A. segmenti anterioris inferioris.
 lateral s. A. segmenti lateralis.
 medial s. A. segmenti medialis.
 posterior s. A. segmenti posterioris.
 superior s. A. segmenti superioris.
 superior s., anterior A. segmenti anterioris superioris.
segmental atelectasis (*Lunge*) Segmentatelektase *f*.
segmental bronchus → segment bronchus.
segmental colitis Colitis regionalis, Enteritis regionalis Crohn des Dickdarms.
segmental demyelination neuropathy → segmental neuropathy.
segmental enteritis Crohn'-Krankheit *f*, Morbus Crohn *m*, Enteritis regionalis, Ileocolitis/Ileitis regionalis/terminalis.
segmental fracture Zweietagenfraktur *f*.
segmental glomerulonephritis segmentale Glomerulonephritis *f*.
segmental innervation segmentale/segmentäre Innervation *f*.
segmental mastectomy *gyn.* Segment-, Quadrantenresektion *f*, Lumpektomie *f*, Tylektomie *f*.
segmental neuritis segmentale Neuritis/Neuropathie *f*.
segmental neuropathy segmentale/periaxiale Neuropathie *f*.
segmental reflex segmentaler Reflex *m*.
seg·men·tar·y ['segmənˌteriː- ˌtəriː] *adj* → segmental.
seg·men·tate ['segməntˌeɪt] *adj* aus Segmenten bestehend.
seg·men·ta·tion [ˌsegmən'teɪʃn] *n* 1. Unterteilung *f* *od.* Gliederung *f* (in Segmente), Segmentierung *f*. 2. Furchung(steilung *f*) *f*, (Zell-)Teilung *f*.
segmentation cavity *embryo.* Furchungs-, Keimhöhle *f*, Blastozöl *nt*.
segmentation sphere *embryo.* 1. Furchungszelle *f*, Blastomere *f*. 2. Morula *f*.
segment bronchus Segmentbronchus *m*, Bronchus segmentalis.
 anterior s. Bronchus segmentalis anterior.
 apical s. Bronchus segmentalis apicalis.
 apicoposterior s. Bronchus segmentalis apicoposterior.
 basal s., anterior Bronchus segmentalis basalis anterior.
 basal s., lateral Bronchus segmentalis basalis lateralis.
 basal s., medial Bronchus segmentalis basalis medialis, Bronchus cardiacus.
 basal s., posterior Bronchus segmentalis basalis posterior.
 cardiac s. → basal s., medial.
 lateral s. Bronchus segmentalis lateralis.
 medial s. Bronchus segmentalis medialis.
 posterior s. Bronchus segmentalis posterior.
 superior s. Bronchus segmentalis superior.
seg·ment·ed cell ['segməntɪd] → segmented granulocyte.
segmented granulocyte segmentkerniger Granulozyt *m*.
segmented intestine Kolon *nt*, Colon *nt*, Intestinum colon.

seg·men·ter ['segmentər] *n micro.* Segmenter *m*, reifer Schizont *m*.
segment long-spacing collagen *abbr.*
SLSC segment long spacing collagen *nt abbr.* SLSC.
seg·re·ga·tion [segrɪ'geɪʃn] *n genet.* **1.** (Auf-)Spaltung *f*, Auftrennung *f*, Segregation *f*. **2.** Abtrennung *f*, Separation *f*.
Seidel ['saɪdəl]: **S.'s scotoma** *ophthal.* Seidel-Skotom *nt*.
Seignette [sɛ'nɛt]: **S.'s salt** Seignettesalz *nt*, Natrium-Kalium-Tartrat *nt*.
sei·zure ['siːʒər] *n* **1.** (plötzlicher) Anfall *m*, Iktus *m*, Ictus *m*. **2.** epileptischer Anfall *m*.
seizure disorder Krampfanfall-auslösende Erkrankung *f*.
seizure potential Krampfpotential *nt*.
Seldinger ['seldɪŋər]: **S. technique** Seldinger-Technik, -Methode *f*.
se·lect·ing mechanism [sɪ'lektɪŋ] Selektions-, Auslesemechanismus *m*.
se·lec·tion [sɪ'lekʃn] *n* **1.** *bio.* Auslese *f*, Selektion *f*. **2.** Wahl *f*; Auswahl *f* (*of* an).
selection pressure *bio.* Selektionsdruck *m*.
se·lec·tive [sɪ'lektɪv] *adj* auswählend, abgetrennt, selektiv, Selektions-.
selective amnesia selektive Amnesie *f*.
selective angiography selektive Angiographie *f*.
selective arteriography selektive Arteriographie *f*.
selective culture *micro.* Selektivkultur *f*.
selective embolization selektive Embolisation *f*.
selective factor *micro.* Selektions-, Auslesefaktor *m*.
selective hypoaldosteronism selektiver/ isolierter Hypoaldosteronismus *m*.
selective inhibition kompetitive Hemmung *f*.
selective medium Selektivnährboden *m*, -medium *nt*.
selective stain Selektivfärbung *f*.
selective toxicity selektive Toxizität *f*.
selective vagotomy selektiv gastrale Vagotomie *f*.
se·lec·tiv·i·ty [sɪlek'tɪvətɪ] *n* Selektivität *f*.
sel·e·nite broth ['selənaɪt, 'siːlnaɪt] *micro.* Selenitbouillon *f* nach Leifson.
se·le·ni·um [sɪ'liːnɪəm] *n abbr.* Se Selen *nt abbr.* Se.
selenium poisoning → selenosis.
sel·e·noid body ['selənɔɪd] Achromo(retikulo)zyt *m*, Schilling-Halbmond *m*, Halbmondkörper *m*.
sel·e·no·sis [selə'nəʊsɪs] *n* Selenvergiftung *f*, Selenose *f*, Selenosis *f*.
self [self] *n, pl* **selves 1.** Selbst *nt*, Ich *nt*. **2.** Selbstsucht *f*.
self-abasement *n* Selbsterniedrigung *f*.
self-abuse *n* **1.** Mißbrauch *m* mit der eigenen Gesundheit. **2.** Masturbation *f*, Onanie *f*.
self-actualization *n psycho.* Selbstverwirklichung *f*.
self-adjusting *adj* selbstregulierend, -einstellend.
self-affirmation *n* Selbstbewußtsein *nt*.
self-analysis *n psycho.* Selbstanalyse *f*.
self-antigen *n* Autoantigen *nt*.
self-assembly *n* → Spontanaggregation *f*, Self-assembly *nt*.
self-assembly process *biochem.* Spontanaggregationsprozess *m*.
self-assessment *n* Selbsteinschätzung *f*.
self-assurance *n* Selbstsicherheit *f*.
self-assured *adj* selbstsicher, -bewußt.
self-awareness *n* Selbstbewußtsein *nt*.
self-centered *adj* ichbezogen, egozentrisch.

self-centeredness *n* Ichbezogenheit *f*, Egozentrik *f*.
self-compressing plate *ortho.* selbstspannende Kompressionsplatte *f*.
self-confidence *n* Selbstbewußtsein *nt*, -vertrauen *nt*.
self-confident *adj* selbstbewußt.
self-conscious *adj psycho.* **1.** gehemmt, unsicher, befangen. **2.** selbstbewußt.
self-consciousness *n* **1.** Gehemmtheit *f*, Unsicherheit, Befangenheit *f*. **2.** *psycho.* Selbstbewußtsein *nt*.
self-control *n* Selbstbeherrschung *f*.
self-controlled *adj* selbstbeherrscht.
self-destruction *n* Autodestruktion *f*, Selbstzerstörung *f*; Selbstmord *m*.
self-destructive *adj* → suicidal.
self-digestion *n* Selbstverdauung *f*, Autodigestion *f*.
self-excitation *n* Selbst-, Eigenerregung *f*.
self-fermentation *n* **1.** Autolyse *f*. **2.** → self-digestion.
self-fertilization *n* Selbstbefruchtung *f*, Autogamie *f*.
self-fertilized *adj* selbstbefruchtet.
self-hypnosis *n* Autohypnose *f*.
self-image *n psycho.* Selbstbild *nt*.
self-induced *adj* **1.** *phys.* selbstinduziert. **2.** selbstverursacht, -zugefügt, -beigebracht.
self-induction *n phys.* Selbst-, Autoinduktion *f*.
self-infection *n* Selbstansteckung *f*, -infizierung *f*, Autoinfektion *f*.
self-inflicted *adj* selbstzugefügt, -beigebracht.
self-inflicted injury s. selbst zugefügte Verletzung *f*, selbst verursachte Verletzung *f*.
self-inhibition *n* autogene Hemmung *f*, Selbsthemmung *f*, Autoinhibition *f*.
self·ish ['selfɪʃ] *adj* ichbezogen, egozentrisch, selbstsüchtig; egoistisch.
self-love *n* **1.** Eigenliebe *f*, Selbstliebe *f*. **2.** *psychia.* Narzißmus *m*.
self-mutilation *n* Selbstverstümmelung *f*.
self-organizing *adj* selbstorganisierend.
self-poisoning *n* Selbstvergiftung *f*, Autointoxikation *f*.
self-possessed *adj* selbstbeherrscht.
self-possession *n* Selbstbeherrschung *f*.
self-preservation *n* Selbsterhaltung *f*.
self-preservative instinct *psycho.* Selbsterhaltungstrieb *m*.
self-protection *n* Selbstschutz *m*.
self-regulating *adj* selbstregelnd, -regulierend.
self-regulation *n* Selbst-, Autoregulation *f*.
self-replicating *adj* selbst-, autoreplizierend.
self-replication *n* Selbst-, Autoreplikation *f*.
self-respect *n* Selbstachtung *f*.
self-restraint *n* Selbstbeherrschung *f*.
self-retaining retractor *ortho.* selbsthaltender (Wund-)Spreizer *m*.
self-stimulation *n* Selbstreizung *f*, Auto-, Eigenstimulation *f*.
self-sufficiency *n* Unabhängigkeit *f*, Autarkie *f*.
self-sufficient *adj* selbständig, unabhängig, autark.
self-suggestion *n* Autosuggestion *f*.
self-tapping screw *ortho.* selbstschneidende Schraube *f*.
self-tolerance *n immun.* Autoimmuntoleranz *f*.
self-treatment *n* Eigen-, Selbstbehandlung *f*.
sel·lar fossa ['selər] Hypophysengrube *f*, Fossa hypophysialis.

sel·la tur·ci·ca [ˌselə 'tɜrkɪkə, -sɪkə] Türkensattel *m*, Sella turcica.
Selye ['selje]: **S. syndrome** Selye-Syndrom *nt*, Adaptationssyndrom *nt*.
Selter ['seltər]: **S.'s disease** Feer'-Krankheit *f*, Feer-Selter-Swift-Krankheit *f*, Selter-Swift-Feer'-Krankheit *f*, Swift--Syndrom *nt*, Akrodynie *f*, Acrodynia *f*, Rosakrankheit *f*, vegetative Neurose *f* der Kleinkinder.
Selt·ers water ['seltərs] Selterswasser *nt*.
Selt·zer water ['seltsər] Selterswasser *nt*.
SEM *abbr.* **1.** → scanning electron microscope. **2.** → standard error (of median).
se·man·tic [sɪ'mæntɪk] *adj* Semantik betr., semantisch.
semantic aphasia semantische Aphasie *f*.
semantic memory semantisches Langzeitgedächtnis *nt*.
se·man·tics [sɪ'mæntɪks] *pl* Semantik *f*, Bedeutungslehre *f*.
se·ma·si·ol·o·gy [sɪˌmeɪsɪ'alədʒɪ] *n* → semantics.
se·mei·og·ra·phy [siːmaɪ'ɑgrəfɪ, semɪ-, siːmiː-] *n* Semiographie *f*.
se·mei·ol·o·gy [ˌ-'alədʒɪ] *n* **1.** Symptomatologie *f*, Semiologie *f*. **2.** Gesamtheit *f* der (Krankheits-)Symptome, Symptomatik *f*, Symptomatologie *f*.
se·mei·ot·ics [ˌ-'atɪks] *pl* → semeiology.
se·men ['siːmən, -men] *n, pl* **-mens, se·mi·na** ['semɪnə, 'siː-] Samen *m*, Sperma *nt*, Semen *m*.
se·me·nu·ria [ˌsiːmə'n(j)ʊərɪə] *n* → seminuria.
semi- *pref.* Halb-, Semi-.
sem·i·ca·nal [ˌsemɪkə'næl] *n* Halbkanal *m*, Rinne *f*; *anat.* Semicanalis *m*.
s. of auditory tube Semicanalis tubae auditivae/auditoriae.
s. of tensor tympani muscle Semicanalis m. tensoris tympani.
sem·i·ca·na·lis [ˌ-kə'neɪlɪs] *n, pl* **-les** [-liːz] → semicanal.
sem·i·car·ti·lag·i·nous [ˌ-ˌkɑrtɪ'lædʒɪnəs, ˌsemaɪ-] *adj* semikartilaginär.
sem·i·cir·cle ['-sɜrkl] *n* Halbkreis *m*.
sem·i·cir·cu·lar [ˌ-'sɜrkjələr] *adj* halbkreisförmig.
semicircular canal (*Ohr*) knöcherner Bogengang *m*, Canalis semicircularis osseus.
anterior s. vorderer/oberer knöcherner Bogengang, Canalis semicircularis anterior/superior.
bony s. → semicircular canal.
lateral s. seitlicher knöcherner Bogengang, Canalis semicircularis lateralis.
membranous s. → semicircular duct.
osseous s. → semicircular canal.
posterior s. hinterer knöcherner Bogengang, Canalis semicircularis posterior.
superior s. → anterior s.
semicircular duct Bogengang *m*, Ductus semicircularis.
anterior s. vorderer/oberer Bogengang, Ductus semicircularis anterior/superior.
lateral s. seitlicher Bogengang, Ductus semicircularis lateralis.
posterior s. hinterer Bogengang, Ductus semicircularis posterior.
superior s. → anterior s.
semicircular line Linea arcuata vaginae m. recti abdominis.
s. of Douglas → semicircular line.
s. of frontal bone Linea temporalis.
highest s. of occipital bone Linea nuchae suprema.
inferior s. of occipital bone Linea nuchae inferior.
superior s. of occipital bone → superior s. of occipital bone, external.

semicircular stria

superior s. of occipital bone, external Linea nuchae superior.
supreme s. of occipital bone → highest s. of occipital bone.
semicircular stria Stria terminalis.
sem·i·closed anesthesia [ˌ-'kləʊzd] *anes.* halbgeschlossene Narkose/Anästhesie *f*; halbgeschlossenes Narkosesystem *nt.*
sem·i·co·ma [ˌ-'kəʊmə] *n* Semikoma *nt.*
sem·i·com·a·tose [ˌ-'kɑmətəʊs] *adj* semikomatös.
sem·i·con·duc·tor [ˌ-kən'dʌktər] *n phys.* Halbleiter *m.*
sem·i·con·scious [ˌ-'kɑnʃəs] *adj* nicht bei vollem Bewußtsein.
sem·i·con·serv·a·tive [ˌ-kən'sɜrvətɪv] *adj* semikonservativ.
semiconservative replication *genet.* semikonservative Replikation *f.*
sem·i·dom·i·nance [ˌ-'dɑmɪnəns] *n genet.* Semidominanz *f*, unvollständige Dominanz *f.*
sem·i·flex·ion [ˌ-'flekʃn] *n* Semiflexion *f.*
sem·i·flu·id [ˌ-'fluːɪd] **I** *n* halb-/zähflüssige Substanz *f.* **II** *adj* halb-, zähflüssig.
sem·i·liq·uid [ˌ-'lɪkwɪd] *n, adj* → semifluid.
sem·i·lu·nar [ˌ-'luːnər] *adj* halbmondförmig, semilunar.
semilunar body (von) Ebner'-Halbmond *m*, Giannuzzi'-Halbmond *m*, Heidenhain'-Halbmond *m*, seröser Halbmond *m.*
semilunar bone *old* → lunate I.
semilunar cartilage: lateral s. of knee joint Außenmeniskus *m*, Meniscus lateralis (artic. genus).
medial s. of knee joint Innenmeniskus *m*, Meniscus medialis (artic. genus).
semilunar cells → semilunar body.
semilunar cusp (halbmondförmige) Taschenklappe *f*, Semilunarklappe *f*, Valvula semilunaris.
anterior s. vordere Taschen-/Semilunarklappe, Valvula semilunaris anterior.
aortic s. Taschen-/Semilunarklappe der Aortenklappe, Valvula semilunaris aortae.
left s. linke Taschen-/Semilunarklappe, Valvula semilunaris sinistra.
posterior s. hintere Taschen-/Semilunarklappe, Valvula semilunaris posterior.
pulmonary s. Taschen-/Semilunarklappe der Pulmonal(is)klappe *f*, Valvula semilunaris trunci pulmonalis.
right s. rechte Taschen-/Semilunarklappe, Valvula semilunaris dextra.
semilunar fascia Aponeurosis m. bicipitis brachii.
semilunar fasciculus Schultze'-Komma *nt*, Fasciculus interfascicularis/semilunaris.
semilunar fibrocartilage: external s. → semilunar cartilage of knee joint, lateral.
internal s. → semilunar cartilage of knee joint, medial.
semilunar fold Plica semilunaris.
s.s of colon Kontraktionsfalten *pl* des Kolons, Plicae semilunares coli.
s. of conjunctiva Plica semilunaris conjunctivae.
semilunar ganglion Ganglion trigeminale/semilunare/Gasseri.
semilunar hiatus Hiatus semilunaris.
semilunar incisure Inc. scapulae/scapularis.
greater s. of ulna Inc. trochlearis ulnae.
lesser s. of ulna Inc. radialis ulnae.
s. of mandible Inc. mandibulae.
s. of radius Inc. ulnaris radii.
s. of scapula Inc. scapulae/scapularis.
s. of sternum Inc. clavicularis sterni.
s. of tibia Inc. fibularis tibiae.

semilunar lobe: caudal s. → inferior s.
cranial s. Lobulus semilunaris cranialis/rostralis/superior.
inferior s. Lobulus semilunaris caudalis/inferior.
rostral s. → cranial s.
superior s. → cranial s.
semilunar lobule: caudal s. → semilunar lobe, inferior.
cranial s. → semilunar lobe, cranial.
inferior s. → semilunar lobe, inferior.
rostral s. → semilunar lobe, cranial.
superior s. → semilunar lobe, cranial.
semilunar notch Inc. scapulae.
greater s. of ulna Inc. trochlearis ulnae.
lesser s. of ulna Inc. radialis ulnae.
s. of mandible Inc. mandibulae.
s. of radius Inc. ulnaris radii.
s. of sternum Inc. clavicularis sterni.
s. of tibia Inc. fibularis tibiae.
semilunar nucleus Nc. semilunaris, Nc. ventralis posterior thalami.
semilunar tract Schultze'-Komma *nt*, Fasciculus interfascicularis/semilunaris.
semilunar valve 1. Aortenklappe *f*, Valva aortae; Pulmonal(is)klappe *f* Valva trunci pulmonalis. **2.** → semilunar cusp.
s.s of Morgagni Morgagni'-Krypten *pl*, Analkrypten *pl*, Sinus anales.
sem·i·lux·a·tion [ˌ-lʌk'seɪʃn] *n* → subluxation.
sem·i·ma·lig·nant [ˌ-mə'lɪgnənt] *adj* semimaligne.
sem·i·mem·bra·no·sus (muscle) [ˌ-ˌmembrə'nəʊsəs] Semimembranosus *m*, M. semimembranosus.
sem·i·mem·bra·nous [ˌ-'membrənəs] *adj anat.* teilweise aus Faszie *od.* Membran bestehend, semimembranös.
semimembranous bursa Bursa m. semimembranosi.
semimembranous muscle → semimembranosus (muscle).
sem·i·nal ['semɪnl] *adj* Samen *od.* Samenflüssigkeit betr., spermatisch, Samen-, Sperma-.
seminal capsule → seminal gland.
seminal cell Epithelzelle *f* der Tubuli seminiferi.
seminal colliculus Samenhügel *m*, Colliculus seminalis.
seminal crest → seminal colliculus.
seminal ducts Samengänge *pl.*
seminal fluid Samenflüssigkeit *f*, Sperma *nt.*
seminal gland Bläschendrüse *f*, Samenblase *f*, -bläschen *nt*, Gonecystis *f*, Spermatozystis *f*, Vesicula seminalis.
seminal hillock → seminal colliculus.
seminal passages (ableitende) Samenwege *pl.*
seminal vesicle → seminal gland.
sem·i·nar·co·sis [ˌsemɪnɑːr'kəʊsɪs] *n* Dämmerschlaf *m.*
sem·i·na·tion [ˌsemɪ'neɪʃn] *n* **1.** Befruchtung *f*, Insemination *f*. **2.** *bio.* Befruchtung *f*, Besamung *f*, Insemination *f*. **3.** (Ein-)Pflanzen *nt.*
sem·i·nif·er·ous [ˌ-'nɪfərəs] *adj anat.* Samen produzierend *od.* (ab-)leitend, samenführend, semiferös.
seminiferous tubule dysgenesis 1. Tubuli-seminiferi-Dysgenese *f.* **2.** Kleinfelter-Syndrom *nt.*
seminiferous tubules Hodenkanälchen *pl*, Tubuli seminiferi.
convoluted s. gewundene Hodenkanälchen, Tubuli seminiferi contorti.
straight s. gerade Hodenkanälchen, Tubuli seminiferi recti.
sem·i·no·ma [ˌ-'nəʊmə] *n patho.* Seminom *nt.*

seminoma cell *patho.* Seminom-Zelle *f.*
sem·i·nor·mal [ˌ-'nɔːrml] *adj* halb-, seminormal.
sem·i·nose ['-nəʊs] *n* Mannose *f.*
sem·i·nu·ria [ˌsiːmɪ'n(j)ʊərɪə, ˌsemɪ-] *n* Spermaausscheidung *f* im Harn, Spermaturie *f.*
se·mi·og·ra·phy [ˌsiːmaɪ'ɑgrəfɪ, ˌsemɪ-] *n* Semiographie *f.*
se·mi·ol·o·gy [ˌ-'ɑlədʒɪ] *n* → symptomatology.
sem·i·o·pen anesthesia [ˌsemɪ'əʊpən] *anes.* halboffene Narkose/Anästhesie *f*; halboffenes Narkosesystem *nt.*
sem·i·or·bic·u·lar [ˌ-ɔːr'bɪkjələr] *adj* halbkreisförmig.
sem·i·o·val center [ˌ-'əʊvəl] Centrum semiovale.
sem·i·par·a·site [ˌ-'pærəsaɪt] *n bio.* Halb-, Hemiparasit *m*, Halbschmarotzer *m.*
sem·i·per·me·a·bil·i·ty [ˌ-ˌpɜrmɪə'bɪlətɪ] *n* Semipermeabilität *f.*
sem·i·per·me·a·ble [ˌ-'pɜrmɪəbl] *adj* halbdurchlässig, semipermeabel.
semipermeable membrane semipermeable Membran *f.*
sem·i·ple·gia [ˌ-'pliːdʒ(ɪ)ə] *n neuro.* (vollständige) Halbseitenlähmung *f*, Hemiplegie *f*, Hemiplegia *f.*
sem·i·quan·ti·ta·tive [ˌ-'kwɑntɪteɪtɪv] *adj* semiquantitativ.
sem·i·qui·none [ˌ-kwɪ'nəʊn, -'kwɪn-] *n* Semichinon *nt.*
sem·i·sid·er·a·tio [ˌ-ˌsɪdə'reɪʃɪəʊ] *n* → semiplegia.
sem·i·sol·id [ˌ-'sɑlɪd] **I** *n* halbfeste Substanz *f.* **II** *adj* halbfest, semisolid(e).
sem·i·som·nus [ˌ-'sɑmnəs] *n* → semicoma.
sem·i·so·por [ˌ-'sɑʊpər] *n* → semicoma.
sem·i·spi·na·lis [ˌ-spaɪ'neɪlɪs] *n* → semispinalis muscle.
semispinalis capitis (muscle) Semispinalis *m* capitis, M. semispinalis capitis.
semispinalis cervicis (muscle) Semispinalis *m* cervicis, M. semispinalis cervicis.
semispinalis muscle Semispinalis *m*, M. semispinalis.
semispinalis thoracis (muscle) Semispinalis *m* thoracis, M. semispinalis thoracis.
sem·i·spi·nal muscle [ˌ-'spaɪnl] → semispinalis (muscle).
s. of head → semispinalis capitis (muscle).
s. of neck → semispinalis cervicis (muscle).
s. of thorax → semispinalis thoracis (muscle).
sem·i·syn·thet·ic [ˌ-sɪn'θetɪk] *adj* halb-, semisynthetisch.
sem·i·ten·di·no·sus (muscle) [ˌ-ˌtendɪ'nəʊsəs] Semitendinosus *m*, M. semitendinosus.
sem·i·ten·di·nous [ˌ-'tendɪnəs] *adj* teilweise aus Sehnen bestehend, halbsehnig.
semitendinous bursa Bursa m. bicipitis femoris superior.
semitendinous muscle → semitendinosus (muscle).
sem·i·trans·par·ent [ˌ-ˌtræns'peərənt] *adj* halbdurchsichtig, halbtransparent.
sem·i·vow·el ['-vaʊəl] *n* Halb-, Semivokal *m.*
Sem·li·ki Forest encephalitis [sem'laɪkɪ] Semliki-Forest-Enzephalitis *f.*
Semliki Forest virus *micro.* Semliki-Forest-Virus *nt.*
sem·o·li·na [ˌsemə'liːnə] *n* (Weizen-)Grieß *m*, Grießmehl *m.*
Semon ['siːmən] **S.'s law** → Semon-Rosenbach law.
Semon-Rosenbach ['rəʊznbax] **S.-R. law** Rosenbach-Semon-Gesetz *nt.*

Se·mun·ya virus [sɪ'mʌndʒə] *micro.* Semunya-Virus *nt.*
send [send] **(sent; sent)** *vt* **1.** jdn. senden, schicken (*to*). **to ~ s.o. to bed** jdn. ins Bett schicken. **2.** (*Hilfe*) schicken (*to* an).
send for *vi* **1.** etw. anfordern, s. kommen lassen. **2.** nach jdm. schicken, jdn. kommen/holen/rufen lassen; etw. bringen lassen.
send forth *vt* (*Geruch*) verströmen; (*Licht, Wärme*) ausstrahlen, aussenden.
send out *vt* ver-, ausströmen; austrahlen; (*Hitze*) abgeben; (*Rauch*) ausstoßen.
Sen·dai virus [sen'daɪ] Sendai-Virus *nt.*
Senear-Usher [sɪ'nɪər 'ʌʃər]**: S.-U. disease/syndrome** Senear-Usher-Syndrom *nt,* Pemphigus erythematosus/seborrhoicus, Lupus erythematosus pemphigoides.
se·nes·cence [sɪ'nesəns] *n* Altern *nt,* Altwerden *nt,* Seneszenz *f.*
se·nes·cent [sɪ'nesənt] *adj* alternd, altersbedingt, Alters-.
Sengstaken-Blakemore ['seŋzteɪkn 'bleɪkmɔːr, -məʊr]**: S.-B. tube** Sengstaken-Blakemore-Sonde *f.*
se·nile ['siːnaɪl, 'senaɪl] *adj* **1.** altersschwach, greisenhaft, senil, Alters-. **2.** Senilität betr., durch Senilität bedingt, altersschwach, senil.
senile amyloidosis Altersamyloidose *f,* senile Amyloidose *f.*
senile angiomas → senile hemangiomas.
senile ankylosing hyperostosis of spine Forestier'-Krankheit *f,* -Syndrom *nt,* Morbus Forestier *m,* Hyperostosis vertebralis senilis ankylosans.
senile arteriosclerosis senile Arteriosklerose *f.*
senile atrophoderma senile Hautatrophie *f,* Atrophoderma senile.
senile atrophy Altersatrophie *f,* senile Atrophie *f.*
s. of skin → senile atrophoderma.
senile cataract Altersstar *m,* Cataracta senilis.
senile chorea senile Chorea *f,* nicht-hereditäre Chorea *f.*
senile coxitis Koxarthrose *f,* Coxarthrosis *f,* Arthrosis deformans coxae, Malum coxae senile.
senile degeneration senile Degeneration *f,* Altersdegeneration *f.*
senile delirium seniles Delir(ium *nt*) *nt.*
senile dementia senile Demenz *f, inf.* Altersschwachsinn *m,* Dementia senilis.
senile disciform degeneration *ophthal.* Kuhnt-Junius-Krankheit *f,* scheibenförmige/disziforme senile feuchte Makuladegeneration *f.*
senile ectasia → senile hemangiomas.
senile ectropion *ophthal.* Ektropium senile.
senile elastosis aktinische/senile Elastose *f,* Elastosis actinica/senilis/solaris.
senile emphysema Altersemphysem *nt,* konstitutionelles/seniles Lungenemphysem *nt.*
senile exudative disciform degeneration → senile disciform degeneration.
senile fibroma → skin tag.
senile gangrene Altersgangrän *f,* senile Gangrän *f.*
senile glands → senile plaques.
senile guttate degeneration Altersdrusen *pl,* Chorioiditis guttata senilis.
senile halo *ophthal.* Halo senilis.
senile hemangiomas senile Angiome *pl,* Hämangiome *pl,* Alters(häm)angiome *pl.*
senile involution Altersinvolution *f.*
senile keratosis aktinische/senile/solare Keratose *f,* Keratosis actinica/solaris/senilis.

senile macular exudative choroiditis → senile disciform degeneration.
senile nephrosclerosis senile Nephrosklerose *f,* Arterionephrosklerose *f.*
senile neuritis senile Neuritis *f.*
senile osteoporosis Altersosteoporose *f,* senile Osteoporose *f.*
senile plaques senile Drusen *pl,* Alzheimer'-Drusen *pl,* -Plaques *pl.*
senile pruritus Pruritus senilis.
senile psychosis senile Psychose *f.*
senile tremor seniler Tremor *m.*
senile wart seborrhoische Alterswarze *f,* Keratose *f,* Verruca seborrhoica/senilis.
se·nil·ism ['siːnɪlɪzəm] *n* vorzeitige Alterung *f,* Vergreisung *f,* Senilismus *m.*
se·nil·i·ty [sɪ'nɪlətɪ] *n* **1.** → senium. **2.** Altern *nt,* Älterwerden *nt,* Vergreisung *f,* Altersschwäche *f,* Senilität *f,* Senilitas *f.*
se·ni·um ['sɪnɪəm] *n* (Greisen-)Alter *nt,* Senium *nt,* Senilitas *f.*
sen·na (leaves) ['senə] *pharm.* Senna-, Sennesblätter *pl,* Folia sennae.
sen·no·side ['senəsaɪd] *n* Sennosid *nt.*
sen·sate ['senseɪt] *adj* mit den Sinnen wahrgenommen, sinnlich.
sen·sa·tion [sen'seɪʃn] *n* **1.** (Sinnes-)Wahrnehmung *f,* (-)Empfindung *f,* (-)Eindruck *m,* Sensation *f,* Sensibilität *f;* Gefühl *nt.* **2.** Sinn *m,* Sinnes-, Empfindungsvermögen *nt;* Wahrnehmungsfähigkeit *f.*
s. of thirst Durstgefühl.
sen·sa·tion·al [sen'seɪʃənl] *adj* Sinn(e) *od.* Sinnesempfindung betr., sinnlich, Sinnes-.
sense [sens] **I** *n* **1.** Sinn *m,* Sinnesorgan *nt.* **2.** **~s** *pl* (klarer) Verstand *m;* Vernunft *f.*
to recover one's ~s wieder zur Besinnung kommen. **to lose one's ~s** den Verstand verlieren. **3.** Sinnes-, Empfindungsfähigkeit *f;* Empfindung *f;* Gefühl *nt* (*of* für); Gespür *nt.* **4.** Sinn *m,* Bedeutung *f.* **II** *vt* fühlen, spüren, empfinden; ahnen.
s. of balance Gleichgewichtssinn.
s. of cold Kaltsinn.
s. of direction Orientierungssinn.
s. of equilibrium Gleichgewichtssinn.
s. of force Kraftsinn.
s. of hearing Hörsinn, Gehör *nt,* Hören *nt.*
s. of movement Bewegungssinn.
s. of pain Schmerzgefühl, -empfindung.
s. of posture Stellungssinn.
s. of shame Schamgefühl.
s. of sight Gesichtssinn, Sehen *nt,* Sehvermögen *nt.*
s. of smell Geruchssinn; *anat.* Olfactus *m.*
s. of taste Geschmack *m,* Geschmackssinn, -empfindung *f.*
s. of temperature Temperatursinn, Thermorezeption *f.*
s. of warmth Warmsinn.
sense cell Sinneszelle *f.*
gustatory s.s *pl* Geschmackssinneszellen *pl,* Schmeckzellen *pl.*
sense center Sinneszentrum *nt.*
sense epithelium Sinnesepithel *nt.*
sense·less ['senslɪs] *adj* **1.** unempfindlich, gefühllos. **2.** bewußt-, besinnungslos. **3.** (*Sache*) sinnlos; (*Person*) unvernünftig.
sense·less·ness ['senslɪsnɪs] *n* **1.** Unempfindlichkeit *f,* Gefühllosigkeit *f.* **2.** Bewußtlosigkeit *f,* Besinnungslosigkeit *f.* **3.** Sinnlosigkeit *f;* Unvernunft *f.*
sense organs Sinnesorgane *pl,* Organa sensoria/sensuum.
sense perception Sinneswahrnehmung *f.*
sen·si·bil·i·ty [ˌsensɪ'bɪlətɪ] *n* **1.** Empfindung(svermögen *nt*) *f,* Empfindlichkeit *f.* **2.** (*a. phys.*) Empfindlichkeit *f* (*to* für); Sensibilität *f.* **3.** Empfänglichkeit *f*

(*to* für). **4.** Gefühl *nt,* Empfinden *nt* (*to* für).
sen·si·bil·i·za·tion [ˌsensɪˌbɪlɪ'zeɪʃn] *n* Sensibilisierung *f.*
sen·si·ble ['sensɪbl] *adj* **1.** empfänglich, (reiz-)empfindlich, sensibel (*to* für); sensuell, sensual. **2.** *old* → sensitive II. **3.** bei Bewußtsein. **4.** vernünftig. **to be ~ of** s. etw. bewußt sein. **5.** spür-, fühlbar, merklich.
sensible perspiration Schwitzen *nt,* Transpiration *f,* glandulärer Wasserverlust *m,* Wasserverlust *m* durch Schwitzen, Perspiratio sensibilis.
sensible water loss → sensible perspiration.
sen·si·tive ['sensɪtɪv] **I** *n* sensibler Mensch *m.* **II** *adj* **1.** fühlend, sensibel, empfindend, empfindsam, einfühlsam, feinfühlig, Empfindungs-. **2.** sensitiv, (über-)empfindlich (*to* gegen). **3.** *chem., bio., phys.* empfindlich (*to*); *photo.* lichtempfindlich (*to*). **4.** *physiol.* sensorisch, Sinnes-.
sen·si·tive·ness ['sensɪtɪvnɪs] *n* → sensitivity.
sen·si·tiv·i·ty [ˌsensɪ'tɪvətɪ] *n* **1.** Sensibilität *f* (*to*);, Empfindsamkeit *f,* Feinfühligkeit *f,* Feingefühl *nt.* **2.** Sensitivität *f,* (Über-)Empfindlichkeit *f* (*to* gegen). **3.** *chem., bio., phys.* Empfindlichkeit *f* (*to*); *photo.* Lichtempfindlichkeit *f,* Sensibilität *f.* **4.** *stat.* Sensitivität *f.*
s. to pain Schmerzempfindlichkeit.
s. to temperature Temperaturempfindlichkeit.
s. to touch Berührungsempfindlichkeit.
sensitivity threshold Absolutschwelle *f,* Reizschwelle *f,* Reizlimen *nt abbr.* RL.
sen·si·ti·za·tion [ˌsensətɪ'zeɪʃn] *n* **1.** *immun., psycho.* Sensibilisierung *f,* Sensibilisieren *nt.* **2.** Sensitivierung *f.* **3.** Allergisierung *f.*
sen·si·tize ['sensɪtaɪz] *vt immun., psycho.* sensibel *od.* empfindsamer machen, sensibilisieren.
sen·si·tiz·er ['sensɪtaɪzər] *n* **1.** Antikörper *m.* **2.** Allergen *nt.*
sen·so·mo·bile [ˌsensə'məʊbɪl] *adj* sensomobil.
sen·so·mo·bil·i·ty [ˌ-məʊ'bɪlətɪ] *n* Sensomobilität *f.*
sen·so·mo·tor [ˌ-'məʊtər] *adj* → sensorimotor.
sen·sor ['sensər] *n* **1.** sensorischer/sinnesphysiologischer Rezeptor *m,* Sensor *m.* **2.** *techn.* (Meß-)Fühler *m,* Sensor *m.*
sen·so·ri·al [sen'sɔːrɪəl] *adj* Sensorium betr.
sen·so·ri·glan·du·lar [ˌsensərɪ'glændʒələr] *adj* sensoriglandulär.
sen·so·ri·mo·tor [ˌ-'məʊtər] *adj* sensorisch u. motorisch, sensomotorisch, sensorisch-motorisch.
sensorimotor area → sensorimotor region.
sensorimotor cortex → sensorimotor region.
sensorimotor performance *physiol.* sensomotorische Leistung *f.*
sensorimotor region sensorisch-motorische (Rinden-)Region *f.*
sen·so·ri·neu·ral deafness [ˌ-'njʊərəl, -'nʊ-] HNO Schallempfindungsstörung *f,* Schallempfindungsschwerhörigkeit *f.*
sen·so·ri·um [sen'sɔːrɪəm] *n, pl* **-ri·ums, -ria** [-rɪə] **1.** Bewußtsein *nt,* Sensorium *nt.* **2.** sensorisches Nervenzentrum *nt,* Sensorium *nt.*
sensor potential Sensorpotential *nt.*
sen·so·ry ['sensərɪ] *adj* **1.** mit den Sinnesorganen/Sinnen wahrnehmend, sensorisch, sensoriell, Sinnes-. **2.** (*Nerv*) sensibel.

sensory amblyopia *ophthal.* sensorische Amblyopie *f.*
sensory amusia Tontaubheit *f,* sensorische Amusie *f.*
sensory aphasia sensorische Aphasie *f,* Wernicke-Aphasie *f.*
sensory apraxia ideatorische Apraxie *f.*
sensory ataxia sensorische Ataxie *f.*
sensory branch of ciliary ganglion sensorische Wurzel *f* des Ggl. ciliare, Ramus communicans ggl. ciliaris cum n. nasociliaris, Radix sensoria/nasociliaris ggl. ciliare.
sensory cell sensible Zelle *f,* Sinneszelle *f.*
sensory center sensibles/sensorisches Zentrum *nt.*
sensory cilia Sinnesgeißeln *pl.*
sensory cortex sensibler/sensorischer Cortex *m,* sensible/sensorische Rinde *f.*
sensory deaf-mutism Seelentaubheit *f,* psychogene/sensorische Hörstummheit *f,* akustische Agnosie *f.*
sensory deafness → sensorineural deafness.
sensory decision theory → signal detection theory.
sensory deprivation sensorische Deprivation *f.*
sensory epilepsy sensorische Epilepsie *f.*
sensory epithelium Sinnesepithel *nt.*
sensory ganglia Spinalganglien *pl* der Hirn- u. Rückenmarksnerven, Ggll. craniospinalia/encephalospinalia/sensoria.
s. of cranial/encephalic nerves Ggll. encephalica, Ggll. sensoria neurium cranialium.
sensory ganglion → spinal ganglion.
sensory hairs Sinneshaare *pl.*
sensory impression Sinneseindruck *m.*
sensory innervation sensorische/sensible Innervation *f.*
sensory lemniscus Lemniscus medialis.
sensory memory sensorisches Gedächtnis *nt.*
sensory modality *physiol.* Sinnesmodalität *f.*
sensory nerve sensibler/sensorischer Nerv *m,* N. sensorius.
sensory neuron sensibles Neuron *nt,* sensibler Nerv *m.*
sensory nucleus of trigeminal nerve, principal sensibler Haupt-/Brückenkern *m* des N. trigeminus, Nc. pontinus n. trigeminalis.
sensory organs Sinnesorgane *pl,* Organa sensoria/sensuum.
cutaneous s. Hautsinnesorgane *pl.*
sensory paralysis sensorische Lähmung *f;* Anästhesie *f.*
sensory paralytic bladder neurogene atonische Blase *f.*
sensory pathway sensorische Bahn *f.*
sensory-physiological receptor → sensor 1.
sensory physiology Sinnesphysiologie *f,* Physiologie *f* der Sinnesorgane.
sensory placode *embryo.* Sinnesplakode *f.*
sensory presbyacusis sensorische Presbyakusis *f.*
sensory quality Sinnesqualität *f.*
sensory receptor → sensor 1.
sensory root → s. of spinal nerves.
s. of ciliary ganglion sensorische Wurzel *f* des Ggl. ciliare, Ramus communicans ggl. ciliaris cum n. nasociliaris, Radix sensoria/nasociliaris ggl. ciliare.
s. of pterygopalatine ganglion Radix sensoria.
s. of spinal nerves hintere/sensible Spinal(nerven)wurzel *f,* Radix dorsalis/posterior/sensoria n. spinalium.

s. of trigeminal nerve sensible Trigeminuswurzel *f,* Portio major n. trigemini, Radix sensoria n. trigemini.
sensory selectivity sensorische Trennschärfe/Selektivität *f.*
sensory stimulus Sinnesreiz *m.*
sensory system sensorisches System *nt,* Sinnessystem *nt.*
sensory thalamus sensorischer Thalamus *m.*
sensory threshold sensorische (Reiz-)Schwelle *f.*
sensory tract sensible/sensorische Bahn *f.*
sen·su·al ['senʃəwəl, -ʃəl] *adj* 1. sinnlich, sensual, sensuell, Sinnes-. 2. sinnlich, wollüstig, sensual, sensuell.
sen·su·al·ism ['senʃəwælɪzəm] *n* 1. Empfindungsvermögen *nt,* Sinnlichkeit *f,* Sensualität *f.* 2. Sinnlichkeit *f,* Sensualismus *m,* Sensualität *f.*
sen·tience ['sentʃ(ɪ)əns] *n* → sentiency.
sen·tien·cy ['sentʃ(ɪ)ənsɪ] *n* 1. Empfindung *f.* 2. Empfindungsvermögen *nt.*
sen·tient ['sent(ɪ)ənt] *adj* empfindungsfähig, empfindend, fühlend.
sen·ti·nel cell ['sent(ə)nəl] Goormaghtigh'-Zelle *f.*
sentinel loop sign *radiol.* Sentinel loop--Zeichen *nt.*
sentinel node Virchow'-Knötchen *nt,* -Knoten *m,* -Drüse *f,* Klavikulardrüse *f.*
SEP *abbr.* → somatic evoked potential.
sep·a·ra·bil·i·ty [ˌsep(ə)rə'bɪlətɪ] *n* Trennbarkeit *f,* Separabilität *f.*
sep·a·ra·ble ['sep(ə)rəbl] *adj* trennbar, separabel.
sep·a·ra·ble·ness ['sep(ə)rəblnɪs] *n* → separability.
sep·a·rate [*adj* 'sepərɪt; *v* -reɪt] I *adj* getrennt, (ab-)gesondert, isoliert (*from* von); separat; einzeln, Einzel-. II *vt* 1. trennen, (ab-)sondern, isolieren (*from* von). 2. spalten, auf-, zerteilen (*into* in). 3. *chem., techn.* scheiden, trennen, (ab-)spalten, aufteilen (*into* in); zentrifugieren. 4. *chir.* ab- od. durchtrennen. III *vi* s. trennen, s. scheiden, s. lösen (*from* von); *chem.* s. absondern.
sep·a·rat·ing ['sepəreɪtɪŋ] *n* Trenn-, Scheide-.
separating funiculus Funiculus separans.
sep·a·ra·tion [ˌsepə'reɪʃn] *n* Trennung *f,* Absonderung *f; chem., techn.* (Ab-)Scheidung *f,* Spaltung *f;* Separation *f.*
separation anxiety (disorder) Trennungsangst *f.*
sep·a·ra·tor ['sepəreɪtər] *n* Separator *m,* (Ab-)Scheider *m,* Zentrifuge *f.*
sep·sis ['sepsɪs] *n* Blutvergiftung *f,* Sepsis *f;* Septikämie *f,* septikämisches Syndrom *nt.*
sept- *pref.* → septo-.
sep·tal ['septl] *adj* Scheidewand/Septuma betr., septal, Septal-, Septum-.
septal arteries: (interventricular) s., anterior Septumäste *pl* der vorderen Interventrikulararterie, Rami interventriculares septales a. coronariae sinistrae.
(interventricular) s., posterior Septumäste *pl* der hinteren Interventrikulararterie, Rami interventriculares septales (rami interventriculares posteriores) a. coronariae dextrae.
septal branches: anterior s. of anterior ethmoidal artery Septumäste *pl* der A. ethmoidalis anterior, Rami septales anteriores a. ethmoidalis anterioris.
interventricular s.es of left coronary artery Septumäste *pl* der vorderen Interventrikulararterie, Rami interventriculares septales a. coronariae sinistrae.
interventricular s.es of right coronary artery Septumäste *pl* der hinteren Interventrikulararterie, Rami interventriculares septales (rami interventriculares posteriores) a. coronariae dextrae.
s. of sphenopalatine artery Septumäste *pl* der A. sphenopalatina, Rami septales posteriores a. sphenopalatine.
septal cartilage of nose Scheidewand-, Septumknorpel *m,* Cartilago septi nasi.
septal cells Septumzellen *pl,* Makrophagen *pl* des Lungenbindegewebes.
septal chisel *HNO* Septummeißel *m.*
septal cirrhosis mikronoduläre/kleinknotige/organisierte Leberzirrhose *f.*
septal cusp septales Klappensegel *nt,* Cuspis medialis/septalis.
septal defect Septumdefekt *m.*
septal deviation *HNO* (*Nase*) Septumdeviation *f.*
septal elevator *HNO* Septumelevatorium *nt.*
septal forceps *HNO* Septumzange *f.*
septal spur *HNO* Septumdorn *m.*
sep·ta·nose ['septənəʊs] *n* Septanose *f.*
sep·tate ['septeɪt] *adj* durch ein Septum abgetrennt, septiert.
septate hymen *gyn.* Hymen septus.
septate hypha *micro.* septierte Hyphe *f.*
septate uterus *gyn.* Uterus septus.
sep·ta·tion [sep'teɪʃn] *n* Septierung *f.*
sep·ta·tome ['septətəʊm] *n* → septotome.
sep·ta·va·lent [ˌseptə'veɪlənt] *adj* → septivalent.
sep·tec·to·my [sep'tektəmɪ] *n HNO* Septumexzision *f,* -resektion *f,* Septektomie *f.*
sep·te·mia [sep'tiːmɪə] *n* → septicemia.
sep·tic ['septɪk] *adj* 1. Sepsis betr., eine Sepsis verursachend, septisch. 2. nicht--keimfrei, septisch.
septic abortion *gyn.* septischer Abort *m.*
septic arthritis eitrige Arthritis *f,* Gelenkeiterung *f,* Arthritis purulenta.
septic coagulopathy septische (Verbrauchs-)Koagulopathie *f.*
septic embolus septischer Embolus *m.*
sep·ti·ce·mia [ˌseptɪ'siːmɪə] *n* Septikämie *f,* Septikhämie *f,* Blutvergiftung *f;* Sepsis *f.*
sep·ti·ce·mic [ˌ-'siːmɪk] *adj* Septikämie betr., septikämisch; septisch.
septicemic abscess pyemischer Abszeß *m.*
septicemic plague Pestsepsis *f,* Pestseptikämie *f,* Pestikämie *f,* septische/septikämische Pest *f.*
septic endocarditis septische Endokarditis *f.*
septic fever 1. septisches Fieber *nt,* Febris septica. 2. → septicemia.
septic infarct septischer Infarkt *m.*
septic intoxication → septicemia.
septic knee eitrige Kniegelenk(s)entzündung *f.*
septic necrosis septische Nekrose *f.*
sep·ti·co·py·e·mia [ˌseptɪkəʊpaɪ'iːmɪə] *n* Septikopyämie *f.*
sep·ti·co·py·e·mic [ˌ-paɪ'iːmɪk] *adj* Septikopyämie betr., septikopyämisch.
septic peritonitis septische Bauchfellentzündung/Peritonitis *f.*
septic phlebitis eitrige Venenentzündung/Phlebitis *f.*
septic plague septische/septikämische Pest *f,* Pestsepsis *f,* Pestseptikämie *f,* Pestikämie *f.*
septic retinitis septische Retinitis *f.*
septic shock septischer Schock *m.*
septic tuberculosis Landouzy-Sepsis *f,* -Typhobazillose *f,* Sepsis tuberculosa acutissima.
septic wound infizierte/septische Wunde *f.*

sep·ti·grav·i·da [ˌseptɪˈgrævɪdə] *n gyn.* Septigravida *f.*
sep·tile [ˈseptaɪl] *adj* → septal.
sep·ti·me·tri·tis [ˌseptɪmɪˈtraɪtɪs] *n gyn.* septische Uterusentzündung/Metritis *f*, Septimetritis *f.*
sep·tip·a·ra [sepˈtɪpərə] *n gyn.* Septipara *f.*
sep·ti·va·lent [ˌseptɪˈveɪlənt] *adj chem.* siebenwertig.
septo- *pref.* Septum-, Sept(o)-, Septal-.
sep·to·mar·gin·al band [ˌseptəʊˈmɑːrdʒɪnl] Trabecula septomarginalis.
septomarginal fasciculus Fasciculus septomarginalis.
septomarginal trabecula Trabecula septomarginalis.
septomarginal tract → septomarginal fasciculus.
sep·to·na·sal [ˌ-ˈneɪzl] *adj* Nasenseptum betr., Septum-.
sep·to·plas·ty [ˈ-plæstɪs] *n HNO (Nase)* Septumplastik *f.*
sep·tos·to·my [sepˈtɒstəmɪ] *n chir.*, *HTG* Septostomie *f.*
sep·to·tome [ˈseptətəʊm] *n HNO* Septotom *nt.*
sep·tot·o·my [sepˈtɒtəmɪ] *n HNO* Septotomie *f.*
sep·tu·lum [ˈseptjələm] *n, pl* **-la** [-lə] *anat.* kleines Septum *nt*, Septulum *nt.*
sep·tum [ˈseptəm] *n, pl* **-ta** [-tə] Trennwand *f*, (Scheide-)Wand *f*, Septum *nt.*
s. of auditory tube → s. of musculotubal canal.
s. of cavernous body of clitoris Trennwand der Klitorisschwellkörper, Septum corporum cavernosorum (clitoridis).
s. of frontal sinuses Sinus frontalis-Trennwand, Septum intersinuale frontale.
s. of glans penis Eichelseptum, Septum glandis.
s. of musculotubal canal Septum canalis musculotubarii.
s. of penis Penistrennwand, -septum, *old* Septum pectiniforme corporis callosi, Septum penis.
s. of scrotum Skrotalseptum, Mediansepturm des Skrotums, Septum scroti/scrotale.
s. of sphenoidal sinuses Trennwand der Keilbeinhöhlen, Septum intersinuale sphenoidale.
s. of testis 1. Mediastinum testis, Corpus Highmori. 2. **~ta of testis** *pl* Hodenscheidewände *pl*, -septen *pl*, Septula testis.
sep·tup·let [sepˈtʌplɪt, ˈseptəplɪt] *n ped.* 1. Siebenling *m*. 2. **~s** *pl* Siebenlinge *pl.*
se·quel [ˈsiːkwəl] *n* 1. (Aufeinander-)Folge *f*. 2. Folgeerscheinung *f*, (Aus-)Wirkung *f*, Konsequenz *f.*
se·que·la [sɪˈkwelə] *n, pl* **-lae** [-liː] *patho.* Folge *f*, Folgeerscheinung *f*, -zustand *m.*
se·quence [ˈsiːkwəns] *n* 1. Reihe *f*, Folge *f*, Aufeinander-, Reihenfolge *f*, Sequenz *f*. 2. → sequel 2.
sequence analysis *biochem.* Sequenzanalyse *f.*
sequence homology *biochem.* Sequenzhomologie *f.*
sequence isomer Sequenzisomer *nt.*
sequence isomerism Sequenzisomerie *f.*
se·quenc·ing [ˈsiːkwənsɪŋ] *n biochem.* Sequenzierung *f.*
se·quen·tial [sɪˈkwenʃl] *adj* Sequenz betr., (aufeinander)folgend, (nach-)folgend (*to, upon* auf); sequentiell, Sequenz-.
sequential analysis *biochem.* Sequenzanalyse *f.*
sequential degradation *biochem.* sequentieller/schrittweiser Abbau *m.*
sequential model *biochem.* Sequenzmodell *nt.*

sequential multichannel autoanalyzer *abbr.* **SMA** *lab.* sequentieller Multikanalautoanalyzer *m abbr.* SMA.
se·ques·ter [sɪˈkwestər] *vt patho.* abstoßen, absondern, sequestrieren.
se·ques·tered antigens [sɪˈkwestərd] *immun.* sequestrierte Antigene *pl.*
se·ques·tral [sɪˈkwestrəl] *adj* Sequester betr., Sequester-.
se·ques·tra·tion [ˌsɪkwəsˈtreɪʃn] *n* 1. *patho.* Sequesterbildung *f*, Sequestrierung *f*, Sequestration *f*, Dissektion *f*, Demarkation *f*. 2. (*Patient*) Absonderung *f*, Isolation *f.*
sequestration dermoid Epidermal-, Epidermoid-, Epidermiszyste *f*, epidermale Zyste *f.*
se·ques·trec·to·my [ˌ-ˈtrektəmɪ] *n ortho.* Sequesterentfernung *f*, Sequestrektomie *f.*
se·ques·trot·o·my [ˌ-ˈtrɒtəmɪ] *n* → sequestrectomy.
se·ques·trum [sɪˈkwestrəm] *n, pl* **-tra** [-trə] 1. Sequester *nt*. 2. Knochensequester *nt.*
S-ER *abbr.* → endoplasmic reticulum, smooth.
Ser *abbr.* → serine.
se·ra *pl* → serum.
Serafini [serəˈfiːnɪ]: **S.'s hernia** Serafini-Hernie *f*, retrovaskuläre Schenkelhernie *f.*
ser·al [ˈsɪərəl] *adj bio.* Sukzessionsserie betr., Serien-.
ser·al·bu·min [ˌsɪərælˈbjuːmɪn] *n* Serumalbumin *nt.*
ser·an·gi·tis [ˌsɪərænˈdʒaɪtɪs] *n urol.* Entzündung *f* der Penisschwellkörper, Kavernitis *f*, Cavernitis *f.*
sere [sɪər] *n bio.* Sukzessionsserie *f*, -folge *f*, Serie *f.*
ser·e·tin [ˈserətɪn] *n* Kohlenstofftetrachlorid *nt*, Tetrachlorkohlenstoff *m.*
se·ri·al [ˈsɪərəl] **I** *n* (Veröffentlichungs-)Reihe *f*, Serie *f*. **II** *adj* Serien-, Reihen-.
serial dilution Reihen-, Serienverdünnung *f.*
serial dilution test Reihenverdünnungstest *m.*
serial section *histol.* Serienschnitt *m.*
serial study Serienstudie *f.*
ser·i·cine [ˈserəsiːn] *n* Serizin *nt.*
se·ries [ˈsɪəriːz, -riːz] *n, pl* **-ries** Serie *f*, Reihe *f*, Folge *f*; *mathe.* Reihe *f*; *chem.* homologe Reihe *f.*
s. of experiments Versuchsreihe *f.*
series-elastic element *abbr.* **SE** *physiol.* serienelastisches Element *nt abbr.* SE.
ser·i·flux [ˈserɪflʌks, ˈsɪər-] *n* wässriger Ausfluß *m.*
ser·ine [ˈseriːn, -ɪn, ˈsɪər-] *n abbr.* **Ser** Serin *nt abbr.* Ser.
serine acetyltransferase Serinacetyltransferase *f.*
serine carboxypeptidase Serincarboxipeptidase *f.*
serine dehydratase Serindehydratase *f.*
serine enzyme Serinenzym *nt.*
serine glyoxylate aminotransferase Serin-Glyoxylat-Aminotransferase *f.*
serine hydroxymethyl transferase Serinhydroxymethyltransferase *f.*
serine protease Serinprotease *f.*
serine protease inhibitor Serinproteaseinhibitor *m.*
serine proteinase Serinproteinase *f.*
serine-pyruvate-aminotransferase Serin-Pyruvat-Aminotransferase *f.*
sero- *pref.* Serum-, Sero-.
se·ro·al·bu·mi·nous [ˌsɪərəʊælˈbjuːmɪnəs] *adj* seroalbuminös.
se·ro·co·li·tis [ˌ-kəˈlaɪtɪs] *n* Perikolitis *f.*
se·ro·con·ver·sion [ˌ-kənˈvɜːrʒn] *n immun.* Serokonversion *f.*

se·ro·cul·ture [ˈ-kʌltʃər] *n micro.* Serumkultur *f.*
sero-defined antigens → serologically defined antigens.
se·ro·di·ag·no·sis [ˌ-daɪəgˈnəʊsɪs] *n* Sero-, Serumdiagnostik *f.*
se·ro·di·ag·nos·tic [ˌ-daɪəgˈnɒstɪk] *adj* Serodiagnostik betr., serodiagnostisch.
se·ro·en·ter·i·tis [ˌ-entəˈraɪtɪs] *n* Perienteritis *f.*
se·ro·epi·de·mi·ol·o·gy [ˌ-epɪˌdiːmɪˈɒlədʒɪ] *n* Seroepidemiologie *f.*
se·ro·fast [ˈ-fæst] *adj micro.* serum-fest.
se·ro·fi·brin·ous [ˌ-ˈfaɪbrɪnəs] *adj* serös-fibrinös, serofibrinös.
serofibrinous inflammation serofibrinöse Entzündung *f.*
serofibrinous pericarditis serofibrinöse Herzbeutelentzündung/Perikarditis *f*, Pericarditis serofibrinosa.
serofibrinous pleurisy/pleuritis serofibrinöse Rippenfellentzündung/Pleuritis *f.*
se·ro·fi·brous [ˈ-faɪbrəs] *adj* serofibrös.
se·ro·flu·id [ˌ-ˈfluːɪd] *n* seröse Flüssigkeit *f.*
se·ro·glob·u·lin [ˌ-ˈglɒbjəlɪn] *n* Seroglobulin *nt.*
se·ro·group [ˈ-gruːp] *n micro.* Serogruppe *f.*
se·ro·log·ic [ˌ-ˈlɒdʒɪk] *adj* Serologie betr., auf Serologie beruhend, serologisch.
se·ro·log·i·cal [ˌ-ˈlɒdʒɪkl] *adj* → serologic.
se·ro·log·i·cal·ly defined antigens [ˌ-ˈlɒdʒɪk(ə)lɪ] serologisch definierte Antigene *pl abbr.* SDA.
serologically negativ seronegativ.
serologically positive seropositiv.
serological reaction Seroreaktion *f.*
serologic grouping serologisches Gruppieren *nt.*
serologic test serologischer Test *m.*
s.s for syphilis *abbr.* **STS** serologische Syphilisdiagnostik *f*, serologische Syphilistests *pl.*
serologic typing serologisches Typisieren *nt.*
se·rol·o·gist [sɪˈrɒlədʒɪst] *n* Serologe *m.*
se·rol·o·gy [sɪˈrɒlədʒɪ] *n* Serumkunde *f*, Serologie *f.*
se·rol·y·sin [sɪˈrɒləsɪn] *n* Sero-, Serumlysin *nt.*
se·ro·ma [sɪˈrəʊmə] *n* Serom *nt.*
se·ro·mem·bra·nous [ˌsɪərəʊˈmembrənəs] *adj* serös u. membranös, seromembranös, serös-membranös.
se·ro·mu·coid [ˌ-ˈmjuːkɔɪd] *adj* → seromucous.
se·ro·mu·cous [ˌ-ˈmjuːkəs] *adj* gemischt serös u. mukös, mukoserös, mukomukös.
seromucous catarrh seromuköser Katarrh *m.*
seromucous cell seromuköse Zelle *f.*
seromucous gland seromuköse Mischdrüse *f*, gemischte Drüse *f*, Gl. seromucosa.
se·ro·mu·cus [ˌ-ˈmjuːkəs] *n* seromuköses Sekret *nt.*
se·ro·mus·cu·lar [ˌ-ˈmʌskjələr] *adj* seromuskulär.
seromuscular tear *chir. (Darm)* seromuskulärer (Ein-)Riß *m.*
se·ro·neg·a·tive [ˌ-ˈnegətɪv] *adj* seronegativ.
se·ro·neg·a·tiv·i·ty [ˌ-ˌnegəˈtɪvətɪ] *n* Seronegativität *f.*
se·ro·phil·ic [ˌ-ˈfɪlɪk] *adj micro.* serophil.
se·ro·plas·tic [ˌ-ˈplæstɪk] *adj* → serofibrinous.
se·ro·pneu·mo·tho·rax [ˌ-ˌn(j)uːməˈθɔːræks] *n* Seropneumothorax *m.*
se·ro·pos·i·tive [ˌ-ˈpɒsɪtɪv] *adj* seropositiv.
se·ro·pos·i·tiv·i·ty [ˌ-ˌpɒsəˈtɪvətɪ] *n* Seropositivität *f.*

se·ro·pu·ru·lent [,-'pjʊər(j)ələnt] *adj* serös u. eitrig, seropurulent, eitrig-serös.
se·ro·pus ['-pʌs] *n* eitriges Serum *nt*, seröser Eiter *m*.
se·ro·re·ac·tion [,-rɪ'ækʃn] *n* Seroreaktion *f*.
se·ro·re·sist·ance [,-rɪ'zɪstəns] *n* Seroresistenz *f*.
se·ro·re·sist·ant [,-rɪ'zɪstənt] *adj* seroresistent.
se·ro·sa [sɪə'rəʊsə, -zə] *n*, *pl* **-sas**, **-sae** [-siː] seröse Haut *f*, Serosa *f*, Tunica serosa.
se·ro·sal [sɪə'rəʊsl] *adj* Serosa betr., Serosa-.
serosal cyst Serosazyste *f*.
serosal fold Serosafalte *f*.
serosal patch *chir.* Serosapatch *m*, -flicken *m*.
serosal tear Serosa(ein)riß *m*.
se·ro·sa·mu·cin [sɪ,rəʊsə'mjuːsɪn] *n* Serosamuzin *nt*.
se·ro·san·guin·e·ous [,sɪərəʊsæŋ'ɡwɪnɪəs] *adj* serös u. blutig, serosanguinös, blutig--serös.
se·ro·se·rous [,-'sɪərəs] *adj* seroserös.
seroserous suture *chir.* seroseröse Naht *f*.
se·ro·si·tis [,-'saɪtɪs] *n* Serosaentzündung *f*, Serositis *f*.
se·ros·i·ty [sɪ'rɒsətɪ] *n* **1.** seröse Flüssigkeit *f*, Serum *nt*. **2.** seröse Eigenschaft *f*.
se·ro·syn·o·vi·al [,sɪərəʊsɪn'əʊvɪəl] *adj* serosynovial.
se·ro·syn·o·vi·tis [,-,sɪnə'vaɪtɪs] *n* seröse Synovitis *f*.
se·ro·ther·a·py [,-'θerəpɪ] *n* Sero-, Serumtherapie *f*.
se·ro·tho·rax [,-'θɔːræks] *n* Sero-, Hydrothorax *m*.
se·ro·to·ner·gic [,serətə'nɜrdʒɪk, ,sɪər-] *adj* → serotoninergic.
se·ro·to·nin [,serə'təʊnɪn, ,sɪər-] *n* Serotonin *nt*, 5-Hydroxytryptamin *nt*.
serotonin antagonist Serotoninantagonist.
se·ro·to·ni·ner·gic [serə,təʊnɪ'nɜrdʒɪk] *adj* seroton(in)erg.
serotoninergic fibers serotoninerge Fasern *pl*.
serotoninergic neuron serotoninerges Neuron *nt*.
serotoninergic system serotoninerges System *nt*.
se·ro·type ['sɪərətaɪp, 'serə-] **I** *n* → serovar. **II** *vt* in Serotypen einteilen.
se·rous ['sɪərəs] *adj* **1.** (Blut-)Serum betr., aus Serum bestehend, serumhaltig, serös, Sero-, Serum-. **2.** serumartige Flüssigkeit enthaltend *od.* produzierend *od.* absondernd, serös.
serous albuminuria intrinsische Albuminurie/Proteinurie *f*.
serous apoplexy ödem-bedingte Apoplexie *f*.
serous atrophy seröse Atrophie *f*.
serous capsule of spleen seröse Milzkapsel *f*, Tunica serosa lienis.
serous cavity seröse Höhle *f*.
serous cell seröse Drüsenzelle *f*.
serous coat → serosa.
serous crescent (von) Ebner'-Halbmond *m*, seröser Halbmond *m*, Giannuzzi'--Halbmond *m*, Heidenhain'-Halbmond *m*.
serous cyclitis seröse Zyklitis *f*.
serous cyst seröse Zyste *f*.
serous cystoma seröses Kystom/Zystom *nt*.
serous diarrhea seröser/wäßriger Durchfall *m*, Diarrhoea serosa.
serous effusion seröser Erguß *m*.
serous endocarditis seröse Endokarditis *f*, Endocarditis serosa.

serous fluid seröse *od.* serumartige Flüssigkeit/Lymphe *f*.
serous fold Serosafalte *f*.
serous gland seröse Drüse *f*, Eiweißdrüse *f*, Gl. serosa.
serous infiltration seröse Infiltration *f*.
serous inflammation seröse Entzündung *f*.
serous iritis *ophthal.* seröse Iritis *f*, Iritis serosa.
serous membrane → serosa.
serous meningitis seröse Meningitis *f*, Meningitis serosa.
serous myocarditis seröse Myokarditis *f*.
serous pericarditis seröse/exsudative Herzbeutelentzündung/Perikarditis *f*, Pericarditis exsudativa.
serous pericardium seröses inneres Perikard *nt*, Pericardium serosum.
serous peritonitis seröse Bauchfellentzündung/Peritonitis *f*, Peritonitis serosa.
serous pleurisy seröse Brustfellentzündung/Pleuritis *f*, Pleuritis serosa.
serous pneumonia seröse Pneumonie *f*.
serous proteinuria intrinsische Albuminurie/Proteinurie *f*.
serous retinitis seröse Retinitis *f*, Retinitis serosa.
serous tunic → serosa.
se·ro·vac·ci·na·tion [,-,væksə'neɪʃn] *n* Serovakzination *f*, Simultanimpfung *f*.
se·ro·var ['-vær] *n micro.* Serotyp *m*, Serovar *m*.
serovar-specific *adj* serovar-spezifisch.
se·ro·zyme ['-zaɪm] *n* Prothrombin *nt*, Faktor II *m abbr.* FII.
ser·pen·tine aneurysm ['sɜrpəntiːn, -taɪn] Rankenaneurysma *nt*, Aneurysma serpentinum.
ser·pent worm ['sɜrpənt] *micro.* Medina-, Guineawurm *m*, Dracunculus medinensis, Filaria medinensis.
ser·pig·i·nous [sər'pɪdʒɪnəs] *adj* girlanden-, schlangenförmig, serpiginös.
serpiginous keratitis Hypopyonkeratitis *f*, Ulcus corneae serpens.
serpiginous ulcer 1. Ulcus serpens. **2.** Hypopyonkeratitis *f*, Ulcus corneae serpens. **3.** Ulcus molle serpiginosum.
ser·rate ['serɪt, -eɪt] *adj* → serrated.
ser·rat·ed ['sereɪtd, sə'reɪ-] *adj anat., bio.* gesägt, gezackt.
serrated suture *anat.* Zackennaht *f*, Sutura serrata.
Ser·ra·tia [sə'reɪʃ(ɪ)ə, -tɪə] *n micro.* Serratia *f*.
ser·ra·tion [sə'reɪʃn] *n* (sägeförmige) Auszackung *f*.
ser·ra·tus anterior (**muscle**) [sə'reɪtəs] Serratus *m* anterior/lateralis, M. serratus anterior.
serratus posterior inferior (**muscle**) Serratus *m* posterior inferior, M. serratus posterior inferior.
serratus posterior superior (**muscle**) Serratus *m* posterior superior, M. serratus posterior superior.
ser·ru·late ['ser(j)əleɪt, -lɪt] *adj histol.* feingezackt.
ser·ru·lat·ed ['ser(j)əleɪtɪd] *adj* → serrulate.
Sertoli ['sɜrtlɪ, sər'təʊlɪ]: **S. cell hyperplasia** Sertoli-Zell(en)-Hyperplasie *f*.
S.-cell-only syndrome del Castillo-Syndrom *nt*, Castillo-Syndrom *nt*, Sertoli--Zell-Syndrom *nt*, Sertoli-cell-only-Syndrom *nt*, Germinal(zell)aplasie *f*.
S.'s cells Sertoli'Zellen *pl*, Stütz-, Ammen-, Fußellen *pl*.
S. cell tumor Sertoli-Zell-Tumor *m*.
Sertoli-Leydig ['laɪdɪɡ]: **S.-L. cell tumor**

Sertoli-Leydig-Zell-Tumor *m*, Arrhenoblastom *nt*.
se·rum ['sɪərəm, 'serəm] *n*, *pl* **-rums**, **-ra** [-rə] **1.** Serum *nt*. **2.** (Blut-)Serum *nt*. **3.** Anti-, Immunserum *nt*.
serum agar Serumagar *m*/*nt*.
se·rum·al ['sɪərəməl, 'ser-] *adj* Serum betr., aus Serum gewonnen, Serum-.
serum albumin Serumalbumin *n*.
serum cholinesterase unspezifische/unechte Cholinesterase *f abbr.* ChE, Pseudocholinesterase *f*, Typ II-Cholinesterase *f*, β-Cholinesterase *f*, Butyrylcholinesterase *f*.
serum diagnosis Sero-, Serumdiagnostik *f*.
serum disease Serumkrankheit *f*.
serum-fast *adj micro.* serum-fest.
serum glutamic oxaloacetic transaminase *abbr.* SGOT Aspartataminotransferase *f abbr.* AST, Aspartattransaminase *f*, Glutamatoxalacetattransaminase *f abbr.* GOT.
serum glutamic pyruvate transaminase *abbr.* SGPT Alaninaminotransferase *f abbr.* ALT, Alanintransaminase *f*, Glutamatpyruvattransaminase *f abbr.* GPT.
serum hepatitis *abbr.* SH (Virus-)Hepatitis B *f abbr.* HB, Serumhepatitis *f*.
serum hepatitis antigen Australiaantigen *nt*, Hepatitis B surface-Antigen *nt abbr.* HB$_S$Ag, HB$_S$-Antigen *nt*, Hepatits B-Oberflächenantigen *nt*.
serum nephritis Serumnephritis *f*.
serum neuritis → serum neuropathy.
serum neuropathy Serumneuropathie *f*.
serum neutralization test *micro.* Neutralisationstest *m*.
serum paralysis Serumlähmung *f*.
serum potassium Serumkalium *nt*.
serum proteins Serumproteine *pl*.
serum prothrombin conversion accelerator *abbr.* SPCA Prokonvertin *nt*, -convertin *nt*, Faktor VII *m abbr.* F V II, Autothrombin I *nt*, Serum-Prothrombin-Conversion-Accelerator *m abbr.* SPCA, stabiler Faktor *m*.
serum reaction Seroreaktion *f*.
serum sickness Serumkrankheit *f*.
serum sickness-like reaction Reaktion *f* vom Serumkrankheittyp.
serum sickness-like syndrome → serum sickness-like reaction.
serum sickness neuropathy → serum neuropathy.
serum sodium Serumnatrium *nt*.
serum therapy → serotherapy.
se·rum·u·ria [,sɪərəm'(j)ʊərɪə] *n* Albuminurie *f*, Proteinurie *f*.
ser·vo·con·trol [,sɜrvəʊkən'trəʊl] *n physiol., techn.* Servokontrolle *f*.
ser·vo·mech·a·nism [,-'mekənɪzm] *n physiol., techn.* Servomechanismus *m*.
ser·yl ['sɪərɪl, 'ser-] *n* Seryl-(Radikal *nt*).
ses·a·me oil ['sesəmɪ] Sesamöl *n*.
ses·a·moid ['sesəmɔɪd] **I** *n* → sesamoid bone. **II** *adj* sesamoidähnlich, Sesam-.
sesamoid bone Sesambein *nt*, -knochen *m*, Os sesamoideum.
sesamoid cartilage: **s. of larynx** Weizenknorpel *m*, Cartilago triticea.
s.s of nose akzessorische Nasenknorpel *pl*, Cartilagines nasales accessoriae.
s. of vocal ligament Sesamknorpel *m* des Stimmbandes, Cartilago sesamoidea lig. vocalis.
ses·qui·ox·ide [,seskwɪ'ɒksaɪd, -sɪd] *n* Sesquioxid *nt*.
ses·qui·sul·fate [,-'sʌlfeɪt] *n* Sesquisulfat *nt*.
ses·qui·sul·fide [,-'sʌlfaɪd] *n* Sesquisulfid *nt*.

ses·qui·ter·pene [ˌ-'tɜrpiːn] *pl* Sesquiterpene *pl*
ses·sile ['sesəl, -aɪl] *adj histol., bio.* festsitzend, breit aufsitzend, sessil.
sessile hydatid Morgagni'-Hydatide *f*, Appendix testis.
sessile polyp breitbasiger/sessiler Polyp *m*.
set [set] **I** *n* **1.** Serie *f*, Reihe *f*, Gruppe *f*. **2.** Satz *m*, Set *nt*, (Instrumenten-)Besteck *nt*. **3.** *fig.* Tendenz *f* (*towards* zu). **4.** *psycho.* (innere) Bereitschaft *f* (*for* zu). **II** *adj* **5.** fest, hart; geronnen; (*Färbung*) fixiert. **6.** festgesetzt, -gelegt; vorgeschrieben, vorgegeben, bestimmt. **7.** fertig, bereit. **8.** (*Meinung*) fest; (*Gesichtsausdruck*) starr. **III** *vt* **9.** setzen, stellen, legen. **10.** etw. fest werden lassen; (*Milch*) gerinnen lassen, zum Gerinnen bringen; (*Färbung*) fixieren. **11.** festsetzen, -legen, anordnen, vorschreiben, bestimmen. **12.** einrichten; einstellen (*at* auf); regulieren. **13.** (*Bruch*) (ein-)richten, reponieren; (*Verrenkung*) einrenken. **IV** *vi* **14.** fest- *od.* hartwerden; gerinnen; erstarren; s. absetzen; (*Gips*) abbinden. **15.** (*Gesichtsausdruck*) erstarren. **16.** (*Knochen*) s. einrenken; (*Bruch*) zusammenwachsen.
set back *vt* **1.** (*Uhr*) zurückstellen. **2.** jdn./etw. zurückwerfen (*by* um); verzögern, behindern.
set forward *vt* **1.** (*Uhr*) vorstellen. **2.** jdn./etw. voranbringen *od.* weiterbringen.
set in *vi* einsetzen, -treten, ausbrechen, beginnen.
set up *vt* **1.** to ~ s.o. **up** jdn. (gesundheitlich) wiederherstellen. **2.** auslösen, verursachen. **3.** etw. anfangen, anstimmen.
s. of teeth Gebiß *nt*.
se·ta·ceous [sɪ'teɪʃəs] *adj* borstig.
set·back ['setbæk] *n* Rückschlag *m*, Rückfall *m*.
se·tif·er·ous [sɪ'tɪfərəs] *adj* → setigerous.
se·ti·form ['setɪfɔːrm] *adj* borstig, borstenförmig.
se·tig·er·ous [sɪ'tɪdʒərəs] *adj* mit Borsten besetzt, Borsten tragend, borstig.
set point *physiol., techn.* Sollwert *m*.
set point shift *physiol.* Sollwertschiebung *f*.
set·ting ['setɪŋ] *n* **1.** Einrichten *nt*; Einrenken *nt*; Einstellung *f*. **2.** (*Gips*) Abbinden *nt*.
setting-sun sign Sonnenuntergangsphänomen *nt*.
set·tle ['setl] **I** *vt* **1.** festlegen, -setzen, vereinbaren; entscheiden. **2.** (*Flüssigkeit*) klären. **II** *vi* **3.** s. (ab-)setzen, s. niederschlagen, s. klären. **4.** (*Erreger*) s. ansiedeln, s. festsetzen (*on, in* in).
settle down I *vt* jdn. beruhigen; (*Nerven*) beruhigen. **II** *vi* s. beruhigen, ruhiger werden; s. legen.
set·tle·ment ['setlmənt] *n* **1.** (Bakterien-)Ansiedlung *f*. **2.** (*Sediment*) Absetzen *nt*. **3.** Regelung *f*, Vereinbarung *f*; Entscheidung *f*.
set·up ['setʌp] *n* **1.** Aufbau *m*, Organisation *f*; Anordnung *f*. **2.** (*Körper-*)Haltung *f*. **3.** Umstände *pl*, Zustände *pl*, Situation *f*.
sev·en-day fever ['sevən] **1.** Feld-, Ernte-, Schlamm-, Sumpffieber *nt*, Erbsenpflückerkrankheit *f*, Leptospirosis grippotyphosa. *f*. **3.** Nanukayami(-Krankheit *f*) *nt*, (japanisches) Siebentagefieber *nt*, japanisches Siebentagefieber *nt*, Sakushu-, Akiyami-, Hasamiyami-Fieber *nt*.
sev·enth nerve ['sevənθ] Fazialis *m*, VII. Hirnnerv *m*, N. facialis [VII]; N. intermediofacialis.

seventh sense Eingeweidesinn *m*.
Sever ['siːvər]: **S.'s disease** Sever'-Krankheit *f*, Apophysitis/Apophyseose calcanei.
se·vere [sə'vɪər] *adj* **1.** streng, scharf, hart; (*Miene*) ernst, finster; (*Klima*) rauh, hart. **2.** *patho.* (*Krankheit*) schlimm, schwer; (*Schmerz*) heftig, stark.
severe combined immunodeficiency (disease) *abbr.* **SCID** schwerer kombinierter Immundefekt *m*, Schweitzer-Typ *m* der Agammaglobulinämie.
severe deafness hochgradige Schwerhörigkeit *f*.
severe pain starker Schmerz *m*, starke Schmerzen *pl*.
se·ver·i·ty [sə'verəti] *n, pl* **-ties** Strenge *f*; Schärfe *f*, Härte *f*; Rauhheit *f*; Ernst *m*; Heftigkeit *f*, Stärke *f*.
sew [soʊ] (**sewed; sewn**) *vt, vi* nähen.
sew·age ['suːɪdʒ] *n* Abwasser *nt*.
sewage treatment *hyg.* Abwasserbehandlung *f*.
sex [seks] **I** *n* **1.** Geschlecht *nt*. **2.** Geschlechtstrieb *m*, Sexualität *f*. **3.** Sex *m*, erotische Anziehungskraft *f*. **4.** Sex *m*, Geschlechtsverkehr *m*, Koitus *m*. **to have ~ with** mit jdm. Geschlechtsverkehr haben. **5.** Geschlecht *nt*, Geschlechtsteile *pl*. **II** *adj* Sex-, Sexual-.
sex abuse sexueller Mißbrauch *m*.
sex act → sexual intercourse.
sex-an·gu·lar [seks'æŋgjələr] *adj* sechseckig.
sex·a·va·lent [ˌseksə'veɪlənt] *adj chem.* sechswertig, hexavalent.
sex cell Germinal-, Keimzelle *f*.
sex characters Geschlechtsmerkmale *pl*, geschlechtsspezifische Charakteristika *pl*.
primary s. primäre Geschlechtsmerkmale.
secondary s. sekundäre Geschlechtsmerkmale.
sex chromatin Barr-Körper *m*, Sex-, Geschlechtschromatin *nt*.
sex chromosome Sex-, Hetero-, Geschlechtschromosom *nt*, Genosom *nt*, Heterosom *nt*, Allosom *nt*.
sex cords *embryo.* Keim-, Hodenstränge *pl*.
sex cycle 1. Monats-, Genital-, Sexual-, Menstruationszyklus *m*. **2.** *micro.* sexueller Vermehrungszyklus *m*.
sex determination Geschlechtsbestimmung *f*.
sex differentation Geschlechtsdifferenzierung *f*.
sex-dig·i·tate [seks'dɪdʒɪteɪt] *adj* sechsfingrig, sechszehig.
sex dimorphism Geschlechtsdimorphismus *m*, Sexualdimorphismus *m*.
sex drive Sexual-, Geschlechtstrieb *m*, Libido *f*.
sex-duc·tion [seks'dʌkʃn] *n micro.* Sexduktion *f*, F-Duktion *f*.
sex expression Geschlechtsausprägung *f*.
sex factor Fertilitätsfaktor, F-Faktor.
sex hormone Geschlechts-, Sexualhormon *nt*.
sex-hormone-binding globulin *abbr.* **SHBG** Sexualhormon-bindendes Globulin *nt abbr.* SHBG.
sex hygiene Sexualhygiene *f*.
sex-influenced *adj genet.* geschlechtsbeeinflußt.
sex inheritance Geschlechtsvererbung *f*.
sex·i·va·lent [ˌseksɪ'veɪlənt] *adj chem.* → sexavalent.
sex·less ['sekslɪs] *adj* geschlechtslos, asexuell, ungeschlechtlich.
sex-limited *adj genet.* auf ein Geschlecht beschränkt, geschlechtsbeschränkt.

sex-linked *adj* geschlechtsgebunden.
sex-linked heredity → sex-linked inheritance.
sex-linked inheritance geschlechtsgebundene/gonosomale Vererbung *f*.
sex·o·log·i·cal [ˌseksə'lɑdʒɪkl] *adj patho.* Sexologie betr., sexualwissenschaftlich, sexologisch.
sex·ol·o·gist [sek'sɑlədʒɪst] *n* Sexualwissenschaftler(in *f*) *m*, Sexologe *m*, -login *f*.
sex·ol·o·gy [sek'sɑlədʒɪ] *n* Sexualforschung *f*, Sexualwissenschaft *f*, Sexologie *f*.
sex·op·a·thy [sek'sɑpəθɪ] *n* Sexo-, Sexualpathie *f*, Sexualpsychopathie *f*.
sex organ Geschlechts-, Genital-, Sexualorgan *nt*.
sex pili *micro.* Konjugationspili *pl*.
sex-specific *adj* geschlechtsspezifisch.
sex test Sextest *m*, Geschlechtsbestimmung *f*.
sex·ti·grav·i·da [ˌseksti'grævɪdə] *n gyn.* Sextigravida *f*.
sex·tip·a·ra [seks'tɪpərə] *n gyn.* Sextipara *f*.
sex·tu·ple [seks't(j)uːpl, -'tʌp-] **I** *n* das Sechsfache. **II** *adj* sechsfach. **III** *vt* versechsfachen. **IV** *vi* s. versechsfachen.
sex·tu·plet [seks't(j)uːplɪt, -'tʌp-] *n* **1.** Sechsling *m*. **2.** ~**s** *pl* Sechslinge *pl*.
sex·u·al ['sekʃwəl; *Brit.* 'seksjʊəl] *adj* sexuell, geschlechtlich, Sexual-, Geschlechts-.
sexual act → sexual intercourse.
sexual abuse → sex abuse.
sexual behavior Sexualverhalten *nt*.
sexual cell Germinal-, Keimzelle *f*.
sexual characteristics → sex characters.
primary s. → sex characters, primary.
secondary s. → sex characters, secondary.
sexual conjugation *bio., genet.* sexuelle Konjugation *f*.
sexual cycle → sex cycle.
sexual determination Geschlechtsbestimmung *f*.
sexual deviation *psychia.* sexuelle Deviation *f*, Paraphilie *f*.
sexual differentiation Sexualdifferenzierung *f*.
sexual dimorphism Geschlechtsdimorphismus *m*, Sexualdimorphismus *m*.
sexual generation *bio.* **1.** Geschlechtsgeneration *f*. **2.** *IV* vi s. versechsfachen.
sexual infantilism sexueller Infantilismus *m*.
sexual instinct *psycho.* Geschlechts-, Sexualtrieb *m*.
sexual intercourse Sexualverkehr *m*, Geschlechtsverkehr *m*, -akt *m*, Beischlaf *m*, Koitus *m*, Coitus *m*.
sex·u·al·i·ty [ˌsekʃə'wælətɪ] *n* Sexualität *f*.
sex·u·al·ly transmitted disease ['sekʃə-wəlɪ; *Brit.* 'seksjʊəlɪ] *abbr.* **STD** sexuell/venerisch übertragene Krankheit *f*, Geschlechtskrankheit *f*, durch Sexualkontakt übertragbare Krankheit.
sexual relation Geschlechtsbeziehung *f*.
sexual reproduction *bio.* geschlechtliche/generative/sexuelle Fortpflanzung *f*.
sexual stage geschlechtliche/generative Phase.
Sé·za·ry ['sezarɪ]: **S. cell** *hema.* Sézary-Zelle *f*.
S. erythroderma → S. syndrome.
S. syndrome Sézary-Syndrom *nt*.
SGOT *abbr.* → serum glutamic oxaloacetic transaminase.
SGPT *abbr.* → serum glutamic pyruvate transaminase.
SH *abbr.* → serum hepatitis.
shad·ow ['ʃædoʊ] **I** *n* **1.** (*a. psycho.*) Schatten *m*, Schattenbild *nt*. **2.** *radiol.* Schatten

shadow cell

m. 3. → shadow cell. **II** *vt* verdunkeln, ein Schatten werfen auf, trüben.
shadow cell 1. (Erythrozyten-)Ghost *m*, Schattenzelle *f*, Blutkörperchenschatten *m*. 2. Gumprecht'-(Kern-)Schatten *pl.* 3. Halbmondkörper *m*, Achromozyt *m*, Achromoretikulozyt *m.*
shadow corpuscle Halbmondkörper *m*, Achromozyt *m*, Achromoretikulozyt *m.*
shad·ow·gram ['ʃædəʊgræm] *n* Roentgenaufnahme *f*, -bild *nt.*
shad·ow·graph ['-græf] *n* Roentgenaufnahme *f*, -bild *nt.*
shad·ow·graph·y ['-græfɪ] *n* 1. Röntgenphotografie *f*. 2. Röntgenuntersuchung *f*, Röntgen *nt.*
shadow test *ophthal.* Retinoskopie *f*, Skiaskopie *f.*
shaft [ʃæft, ʃɑːft] *n* 1. Schaft *m*, Stiel *m*, Stamm *m*; Mittelteil *m*. 2. *anat.* Knochenschaft *m*, Diaphyse *f*. 3. (Licht-)Strahl *m.*
s. of femur Femurschaft, -diaphyse, Corpus femoris.
s. of fibula Fibulaschaft, -diaphyse, Corpus fibulae.
s. of humerus Humerusschaft, -diaphyse, Corpus humeri.
s. of penis Penisschaft, -diaphyse, Corpus penis.
s. of radius Radiusschaft, -diaphyse, Corpus radii.
s. of tibia Tibiaschaft, -diaphyse, Corpus tibiae/tibiale.
s. of ulna Ulnaschaft, -diaphyse, Corpus ulnae.
shaft reamer *ortho.* Diaphysenraspel *f.*
shag·gy ['ʃægɪ] *adj* 1. zottelig, struppig; rauhhaarig. 2. *fig.* verwahrlost, ungepflegt.
shaggy chorion Zotten-, Chorionplatte *f*, Chorion frondosum.
sha·green patch [ʃə'griːn] → shagreen skin.
shagreen skin Chagrinleder-Haut *f.*
shake [ʃeɪk] (*v* shook; shaken) **I** *n* Schütteln *nt*, Rütteln *nt*; Beben *nt*, Zittern *nt*. **II** *vt* schütteln. **III** *vi* schwanken, beben, wanken; zittern, beben.
shake culture *micro.* Schüttelkultur *f.*
shakes [ʃeɪks] *pl* Schüttelfrost *m*, Schütteln *nt*, Zittern *nt*, Beben *nt.*
shak·ing chill(s) ['ʃeɪkɪŋ] Schüttelfrost *m.*
shaking palsy Parkinson'-Krankheit *f*, Morbus Parkinson *m*, Paralysis agitans.
shaking sound Plätschergeräusch *nt.*
shal·low breathing ['ʃæləʊ] flache Atmung *f.*
shallow respiration → shallow breathing.
sham movement vertigo [ʃæm] Gyrosa *f*, Vertigo gyrosa.
shank [ʃæŋk] *n* 1. *anat.* Unterschenkel *m*; Schienbein, Tibia *f*; Bein *nt*. 2. *bio.* Stengel *m*, Stiel *m*. 3. *techn., ortho.* Schaft *m.*
SH antigen Australiaantigen *nt*, Hepatitis B surface-Antigen *nt* *abbr.* HB$_s$Ag, HB$_S$-Antigen *nt*, Hepatits B-Oberflächenantigen *nt.*
shape [ʃeɪp] **I** *n* 1. Form *f*, Gestalt *f*; Figur *f*. **to put into** ~ formen, gestalten. 2. (körperliche *od.* geistige) Verfassung *f*, Form *f*. **to be in (good)** ~ in (guter) Form sein, in gutem Zustand sein. **to be in bad** ~ in vschlechter Verfassung/Form sein, in schlechtem Zustand sein. 3. *techn.* (Guß-)Form *f*, Formstück *nt*, Modell *nt*. **II** *vt* (*a. techn., psycho.*) formen (*into* zu); (*Leben*) gestalten. **III** *vi* s. formen; s. entwickeln.
shape constancy *physiol.* Formkonstanz *f.*

shape·less ['ʃeɪplɪs] *adj* 1. unförmig. 2. form-, gestaltlos.
shape·less·ness ['ʃeɪplɪsnɪs] *n* 1. Unförmigkeit *f*. 2. Form-, Gestaltlosigkeit *f.*
shape recognition *physiol.* Form-, Gestalterkennung *f.*
shape topography *phys., chem.* Gestalttopographie *f.*
sharp [ʃɑːrp] *adj* scharf; (*Messer*) scharf; (*Nadel*) spitz; (*Konstraste*) scharf, deutlich; (*Geruch, Geschmack*) scharf, beißend; (*Schmerz*) heftig, stechend; (*Augen*) wachsam; (*Kanten*) scharf; (*Schrei*) durchdringend, schrill.
sharp curet *chir.* scharfe Kürette *f.*
sharp dissection *chir.* scharfes Präparieren *nt.*
sharp-edged *adj* (*Messer*) scharfkantig.
Sharpey ['ʃɑː(r)pɪ]: **S.'s fiber** Sharpey'-Faser *f.*
sharp-eyed *adj* scharfsichtig.
sharp hook *chir.* scharfer Haken *m.*
sharp·ness ['ʃɑːpnɪs] *n* Schärfe *f*; Spitzheit *f*; Deutlichkeit *f*; Strenge *f*; Heftigkeit *f*; Wachsamkeit *f*, Scharfsinn *m*; Schrillheit *f.*
sharp pain heller stechender Schmerz *m.*
sharp-sighted *adj* → sharp-eyed.
sharp spoon *chir.* scharfer Löffel *m.*
SHBG *abbr.* → sex-hormone-binding globulin.
shear [ʃɪər] (*v* sheared/shore; sheared/shorn) **I** *n* 1. ~s *pl* (große) Schere *f*; Blechschere *f*. 2. Scheren *nt*, Schur *f*. 3. *phys.* (Ab-)Scherung *f*. **II** *vt* (ab-)scheren, (ab-)schneiden. **III** *vi* schneiden, mähen (*through* durch).
shear force (Ab-)Scherkraft *f*, Abscherung *f.*
shear·ing [ʃɪərɪŋ] *n* 1. Scheren *nt*, Schur *f*. 2. *phys.* (Ab-)Scherung *f.*
shearing edge (*Zahn*) Schneidekante *f*, Margo incisalis.
shearing force (Ab-)Scherkraft *f*, Abscherung *f.*
shearing fracture Abscherfraktur *f.*
shear resistance *phys.* (Ab-)Scherfestigkeit *f.*
sheath [ʃiːθ] **I** *n*, *pl* sheaths [ʃiːðz] 1. Scheide *f*; Hülle *f*, Mantel *m*, Ummantelung *f*. 2. Kondom *nt*. **II** *vt* → sheathe.
s. of eyeball Tenon'-Kapsel *f*, Vagina bulbi.
s. of Key and Retzius Endoneurium *nt.*
s.s of optic nerve Meningealhüllen *pl* des N. opticus, Vaginae n. optici.
s. of rectus abdominis muscle Rektusscheide, Vagina m. recti abdominis.
sheath cells Hüll-, Scheidenzellen *pl.*
sheath cuticle (*Haar*) Scheidenkutikula *f.*
sheathe [ʃiːð] *vt* umhüllen, ummanteln.
sheathed arteries [ʃiːðd] (*Milz*) Ellipsoid *nt*, Schweiger-Seidel'-Hülse *f.*
sheathed arterioles → sheathed arteries.
sheath protein Hüllprotein *nt.*
Sheehan ['ʃiːən]: **S. syndrome** Sheehan'-Syndrom *nt*, postpartale Hypophysenvorderlappeninsuffizienz *f.*
sheep cell agglutination test [ʃiːp] *abbr.* **SCAT** Schaferythrozytenagglutinationstest *m.*
sheep-pox Schafpocken *pl.*
sheep-pox virus *micro.* Schafpockenvirus *nt.*
sheep red blood cell *abbr.* **SRBC** Schaferythrozyt *m.*
sheep tick *micro.* Melophagus ovinus.
sheet [ʃiːt] **I** *n* 1. Bettuch *nt*, (Bett-)Laken *nt*, Leintuch *nt*. 2. Bogen *m*, Blatt *nt*. 3. (dünne) Platte *f*. **II** *vt* 4. (*Bett*) beziehen. 5. mit einer dünnen Schicht bedecken.
β-sheet *n biochem.* Faltblatt(struktur *f*) *nt.*

Shekelton ['ʃeklton]: **S.'s aneurysm** dissezierendes Aneurysma *nt*, Aneurysma dissecans.
shelf operation [ʃelf] *ortho.* (*Hüftgelenk*) Azetabuloplastik *f* mit Knochenkeilinsertion.
shell [ʃel] **I** *n* 1. Schale *f*; Hülse *f*, Rinde *f*; Muschel *f*. 2. (*a. fig*) Gerüst *nt*, Gerippe *nt*. **II** *vt* (ab-)schälen, enthülsen.
shel·lac [ʃə'læk] *n* Shellack *m.*
Shenton ['ʃentn]: **S.'s arc/arch** → S.'s line. **S.'s line** *radiol.* Shenton-Linie *f*, Ménard-Shenton-Linie.
Shepherd ['ʃepərd]: **S. fracture** Shepherd-Fraktur *f.*
shep·herd's crook deformity ['ʃepərd] *radiol.* Hirtenstabdeformität *f.*
Sherrington ['ʃerɪŋtən]: **S.'s law** Sherrington-Gesetz *nt.*
shield [ʃiːld] **I** *n* 1. Schild *m*. 2. Schutzschild *m*, -schirm *m*. **II** *vt* (be-)schützen, (be-)schirmen (*from* vor); *phys.* abschirmen.
SH-IF *abbr.* [somatotropin inhibiting factor] → somatostatin.
shift [ʃɪft] **I** *n* 1. Verlagerung *f*, Verschiebung *f*; Wechsel *m*, Veränderung *f*. 2. (Arbeits-)Schicht *f*. **II** *vt* verlagern, verschieben; umstellen (*to* auf); verändern; (aus-)wechseln, (aus-)tauschen. **III** *vi* s. verlagern, s. verschieben; wechseln.
s. to the left Linksverschiebung *f.*
s. to the right Rechtsverschiebung *f.*
shift·ing ['ʃɪftɪŋ] *adj* s. verlagernd; wechselnd, veränderlich.
shifting pacemaker wandernder Schrittmacher *m.*
shift work Schichtarbeit *f*. **to do** ~ Schicht arbeiten.
shift worker Schichtarbeiter(in *f*) *m.*
Shiga ['ʃiːgə]: **S. bacillus** → Shigella dysenteriae type 1.
S. toxin Shigatoxin *nt.*
Shiga-Kruse ['kruːzə]: **S.-K. bacillus** → Shigella dysenteriae type 1.
Shi·gel·la [ʃɪ'gelə] *n micro.* Shigella *f.*
S. alkalescens Escherich-Bakterium *nt*, Colibakterium *nt*, -bazillus *m*, Kolibazillus *m*, Escherichia/Bact. coli.
S. ambigua → S. dysenteriae type 2.
S. boydii Shigella boydii.
S. ceylonsis → S. sonnei.
S. dispar → S. alkalescens.
S. dysenteriae Shigella dysenteriae.
S. dysenteriae type 1 Shiga-Kruse-Ruhrbakterium *nt*, Shigella dysenteriae Typ 1.
S. dysenteriae type 2 Shigella schmitzii/ambigua, Shigella dysenteriae Typ 2.
S. flexneri Flexner-Bazillus *m*, Shigella flexneri.
S. madampensis → S. alkalescens.
S. paradysenteriae → S. flexneri.
S. schmitzii → S. dysenteriae type 2.
S. shigae → S. dysenteriae type 1.
S. sonnei Kruse-Sonne-Ruhrbakterium *nt*, E-Ruhrbakterium *nt*, Shigella sonnei.
shi·gel·la [ʃɪ'gelə] *n*, *pl* -las, -lae [-liː] *micro.* Shigelle *f*, Shigella *f.*
shig·el·lo·sis [ʃɪgə'ləʊsɪs] *n* Shigellainfektion *f*, Shigellose *f*; Bakterienruhr *f.*
shik·i·mene ['ʃɪkəmiːn] *n* → sikimin.
shi·kim·ic acid [ʃɪ'kɪmɪk] Shikimisäure *f.*
shi·ma·mu·shi disease [ˌʃiːmə'muːʃɪ] → scrub typhus.
shin [ʃɪn] *n* Schienbein *nt*, Schienbeinregion *f.*
shin-bone ['ʃɪnbəʊn] *n* Schienbein *nt*, Tibia *f.*
shinbone fever Wolhyn'-Fieber *nt*, Fünftagefieber *nt*, Wolhynienfieber, *nt* Febris quintana.
shin·gles ['ʃɪŋgəls] *pl* Gürtelrose *f*, Zoster *m*, Zona *f*, Herpes zoster.

ship fever [ʃɪp] epidemisches/klassisches Fleckfieber *nt*, Läusefleckfieber *nt*, Fleck-, Hunger-, Kriegstyphus *m*, Typhus exanthematicus.
ship-yard eye/keratoconjunctivitis [ˈʃɪpjɑːrd] *ophthal.* epidemische Keratokonjunktivitis *f*, Keratoconjunctivitis epidemica.
Shirodkar [ˈʃɪərədkɑːr]: **S.'s operation** *gyn.* Shirodkar-Operation *f.*
shirt-stud abscess [ʃɜrt] Kragenknopfabszeß *m.*
shiv-er¹ [ˈʃɪvər] **I** *n* Schauer *m*, Zittern *nt*, Frösteln *nt*. **II** *vi* zittern, frösteln, (er-)schauern.
shiv-er² [ˈʃɪvər] **I** *n* Splitter *m*, (Bruch-)Stück *nt*. **II** *vt, vi* (zer-)splittern, (zer-)schmettern.
shiv-er-y [ˈʃɪvərɪ] *adj* fröstelnd; schauernd; zitt(e)rig; fiebrig.
shock [ʃɑk] **I** *n* **1.** (seelische) Erschütterung *f*, Schlag *m*, Schock *m* (*to* für); *patho.*, *psycho.* Schock(zustand *m*) *m*, Schockreaktion *f*. **to be in (a state of) ~** einen Schock haben, unter Schock stehen. **2.** Stoß *m*, Schlag *m*, Erschütterung *f*. **3.** elektrischer Schlag *m*; (Elektro-)Schock *m*. **II** *vt* **4.** erschüttern; *fig.* schockieren, erschüttern. **5.** *patho.* Schock(reaktion) auslösen *od.* verursachen. **6.** schocken, einer Schockbehandlung unterziehen.
shock antigen schockauslösendes/anaphylaxieauslösendes Antigen *nt.*
shocked [ʃɑkd] *adj* **1.** im Schock (befindlich). **to be ~** unter Schock stehen, in einem Schockzustand sein. **2.** erschüttert, schockiert, bestürzt.
shock kidney Schockniere *f.*
shock lung Schocklunge *f*, adult respiratory distress syndrome *abbr.* ARDS.
shock therapy Schockbehandlung *f*, -therapie *f.*
shock treatment → shock therapy.
shock waves *phys.*, *physiol.* Schock-, Stoßwellen *pl.*
Shoemaker [ˈʃiːmɑkər]: **S.'s line** Shoemaker-Linie *f.*
shoe-maker's breast [ʃuː] *ortho.* Schuhmacherbrust *f.*
shoot-ing pain [ˈʃuːtɪŋ] schießender Schmerz *m.*
short [ʃɔːrt] **I** *n phys.* Kurzschluß *m*, *inf.* Kurzer *m*. **II** *adj* **1.** (*zeitlich*) kurz, knapp. **2.** (*Gestalt*) klein, kurz. **3.** kurz angebunden, barsch. **4.** zuwenig, knapp (*of* an). **III** *vi* → short-circuit 1.
s. of breath *abbr.* S.O.B. kurzatmig; dyspnoisch.
short-acting *adj pharm.* kurzwirkend.
short-age [ˈʃɔːrtɪdʒ] *n* Knappheit *f*, Mangel *m* (*of* an).
short-arm cast *ortho.* Unterarmgips(verband *m*) *m.*
short bone kurzer Knochen *m*, Os breve.
short-bowel syndrome Kurzdarmsyndrom *m*, Short-bowel-Syndrom *nt.*
short circuit *electr.* Kurzschluß *m*, *inf.* Kurzer *m.*
short-circuit *vt* **1.** einen Kurzschluß verursachen, kurzschließen. **2.** (etw.) ausschalten, umgehen.
short-com-ing [ˈʃɔːrtkʌmɪŋ] *n* Mangel *m*, Fehler *m*; Unzulänglichkeit *f.*
short crus of incus kurzer/hinterer Amboßfortsatz/-schenkel *m*, Crus breve (incudis).
short-distance radiotherapy *radiol.* Brachytherapie *f.*
short-en [ˈʃɔːrtn] *vt* (ab-, ver-)kürzen, kürzer machen.
short-en-ing [ˈʃɔːrtnɪŋ] *n* (Ab-, Ver-)Kürzung *f.*

short-gut syndrome → short-bowel syndrome.
short gyri of insula kurze Inselwindungen *pl*, Gyri breves insulae.
short head: s. of biceps brachii muscle kurzer Kopf *m* des M. biceps brachii, Caput breve m. bicipitis brachii.
s. of biceps femoris muscle kurzer Kopf *m* des M. biceps femoris, Caput breve m. bicipitis femoris.
s. of triceps brachii muscle medialer/innerer Trizepskopf *m*, Caput mediale m. tricipitis brachii.
s. of triceps femoris muscle M. adductor brevis.
short increment sensitivity index *abbr.* SISI short increment sensitivity index *m abbr.* SISI.
short increment sensitivity index test SISI-Test *m.*
short-incubation hepatitis (Virus-)Hepatitis A *f abbr.* HA, epidemische Hepatitis *f*, Hepatitis epidemica.
short leg cast Unterschenkelgips(verband *m*) *m.*
short limb of incus → short crus of incus.
short-lived *adj* kurzlebig.
short-ness [ˈʃɔːrtnɪs] *n* **1.** Kürze *f*; Kleinheit *f*. **2.** Knappheit *f*, Mangel *m* (*of* an).
s. of breath Kurzatmigkeit *f*; Dyspnoe *f.*
s. of the neck Kurz-, Froschhals *m.*
s. of sight Kurzsichtigkeit *f.*
short pulse kurzer Puls *m*, Pulsus celer.
short root of ciliary ganglion Radix oculomotoria/parasympathica ggl. ciliaris.
short sight → shortsightedness.
short-sight-ed [ˈʃɔːrtsaɪtɪd] *adj* kurzsichtig, myop.
short-sight-ed-ness [ˈʃɔːrtsaɪtɪdnɪs] *n* Kurzsichtigkeit *f*, Myopie *f.*
short-tempered *adj* aufbrausend, reizbar, jähzornig.
short-term *adj* kurzzeitig, -fristig, Kurzzeit-.
short-term memory *abbr.* STM Kurzzeitgedächtnis *nt.*
short-term performance Kurzzeitleistung *f.*
short-term treatment Kurzzeitbehandlung *f.*
short-wave *adj* kurzwellig, Kurzwellen-.
short-wave [ˈʃɔːrtweɪv] *n phys.* Kurzwelle *f.*
short-wave diathermy Kurzwellendiathermie *f*, Hochfrequenzdiathermie *f*, Hochfrequenzwärmetherapie *f.*
short wave therapy Kurzwellentherapie *f*, -behandlung *f.*
short-winded *adj* kurzatmig.
shot-ty breast [ˈʃɑtɪ] zystische/fibrös-zystische Mastopathie *f*, Mammadysplasie *f*, Zystenmamma *f*, Mastopathia chronica cystica.
shoul-der [ˈʃoʊldər] *n* Schulter *f*; Schultergelenk *nt.*
shoulder blade Schulterblatt *nt*, Skapula *f*, Scapula *f.*
shoulder disarticulation *ortho.* Schultergelenkexartikulation *f.*
shoulder dislocation *ortho.* Schulter(gelenk)luxation *f*, Luxatio humeri.
anterior s. vordere Schulterluxation, Luxatio subcoracoidea.
posterior s. hintere Schulterluxation, Luxatio posterior/infraspinata.
recurrent s. habituelle Schulterluxation.
shoulder girdle *anat.* Schultergürtel *m*, Cingulum pectorale, Cingulum membri superioris.
shoulder girdle muscles Schultergürtelmuskulatur *f.*

shoulder hand syndrome Schulter-Arm--Syndrom *nt.*
shoulder joint Schultergelenk *nt*, Artic. humeri/glenohumeralis.
shoulder pain 1. Schulterschmerz(en *pl*) *m*, Schmerzen *pl* in der Schulter. **2.** in die Schulter ausstrahlende Schmerzen *pl.*
shoulder presentation *gyn.* Schulterlage *f.*
shoulder radiation (*Schmerz*) Ausstrahlung *f* in die Schulter.
shoulder stiffness Schultersteife *f.*
shoulder tick *micro.* Ixodes scapularis.
show [ʃoʊ] *n gyn.* Zeichnen *nt.*
Shrapnell [ˈʃræpnəl]: **S.'s membrane** Shrapnell'-Membran *f*, Pars flaccida (membranae tympanicae).
shrink [ʃrɪŋk] (*v* **shrank**; **shrunk**) **I** *n inf.* Psychiater(in *f*) *m*. **II** *vt* (ein-)schrumpfen lassen. **III** *vi* (ein-, zusammen-)schrumpfen, abnehmen, schwinden.
shrink-age [ˈʃrɪŋkɪdʒ] *n* (Ein-, Zusammen-)Schrumpfen *nt*; Schrumpfung *f*, Verminderung *f*, Schwund *m*, Abnahme *f.*
shrinkage necrosis Schrumpfnekrose *f.*
shrunk-en kidney [ˈʃrʌŋkn] Schrumpfniere *f.*
shunt [ʃʌnt] **I** *n* **1.** *chir.*, *patho.* Nebenschluß *m*, Shunt *m*; Bypass *m*. **2.** *phys.* Nebenschluß *m*, Nebenwiderstand *m*, Shunt *m*. **II** *vt* **3.** *chir.* einen Shunt anlegen, shunten. **4.** *phys.* nebenschließen, shunten.
shunt cyanosis Shunt-Zyanose *f.*
shunt fraction *physiol.*, *patho.* Shunt-Fraktion *f.*
shunt surgery *chir.* Shuntanlegung *f.*
shunt vessel Nebenschluß-, Bypass-, Shuntgefäß *nt.*
shut-in personality [ʃʌt] schizoide Personality (disorder).
shut-tle [ʃʌtl] *n biochem.*, *physiol.* Shuttle *m.*
shuttle system Shuttle-System *nt.*
Shwachman [ˈʃwækmən]: **S. syndrome** Shwachman-Syndrom *nt*, Shwachman--Blackfan-Diamond-Oski-Khaw-Syndrom *nt.*
Shwachman-Diamond [ˈdaɪ(ə)mənd]: **S.-D. syndrome** → Shwachman syndrome.
Shwartzman [ˈʃwɑrtsmən]: **generalized S. phenomenon** → S. phenomenon.
S. phenomenon Sanarelli-Shwartzman--Phänomen *nt*, -Reaktion *f*, Shwartzman-Sanarelli-Reaktion *f*, -Phänomen *nt.*
S. reaction → S. phenomenon.
Shy-Drager [ʃaɪ ˈdreɪɡər]: **S.-D. syndrome** Shy-Drager-Syndrom *nt.*
SI *abbr.* [Système International d'Unites] → SI system.
Si *abbr.* → silicon.
Sia [ˈsaɪə]: **S. test** Sia-Reaktion *f.*
SIADH *abbr.* → syndrome of inappropriate antidiuretic hormone.
SIADH-like syndrome SIADH-ähnliches Syndrom *nt.*
si-a-gon-an-tri-tis [ˌsaɪəɡənænˈtraɪtɪs] *n HNO* Kieferhöhlenentzündung *f.*
sial- *pref.* → sialo-.
si-al-a-den [saɪˈælədən] *n* Speicheldrüse *f.*
si-al-ad-e-nec-to-my [saɪəlˌædəˈnɛktəmɪ] *n* → sialoadenectomy.
si-al-ad-e-ni-tis [ˌsaɪəlædəˈnaɪtɪs] *n* Speicheldrüsenentzündung *f*, Sial(o)adenitis *f.*
si-al-ad-e-nog-ra-phy [ˌ-ˌædəˈnɑɡrəfɪ] *n HNO*, *radiol.* Sial(o)adenographie *f.*
si-al-ad-e-non-cus [ˌ-ˌædəˈnɑŋkəs] *n* Speicheldrüsenschwellung *f*, -tumor *m.*
si-al-ad-e-no-sis [ˌ-ˌædəˈnoʊsɪs] *n* **1.** → sialadenitis. **2.** Speicheldrüsenerkrankung *f*, Sialadenose *f.*

sialadenotomy

si·al·ad·e·not·o·my [ˌ-ˌædəˈnɑtəmɪ] n → sialoadenotomy.
si·al·a·gog·ic [ˌsaɪələˈgɑdʒɪk] adj → sialagogue II.
si·al·a·gogue [saɪˈæləgɔg, -gɑg] I n Sialagogum nt. II adj den Speichelfluß anregend, sialagog.
si·a·late [ˈsaɪəleɪt] n Sialat nt.
si·al·ec·ta·sia [ˌsaɪəlekˈteɪʒ(ɪ)ə] n Sialektasie f.
si·al·em·e·sis [ˌsaɪəˈeməsɪs] n Speichelerbrechen nt, Sialemesis f.
si·al·ic [saɪˈælɪk] adj 1. Speichel betr., Speichel-, Sial(o)-, Ptyal(o)-. 2. Sialinsäure betr.
sialic acid Sialinsäure f, N-Acylneuraminsäure f.
si·al·i·dase [saɪˈælɪdeɪz] n Sialidase f, Neuraminidase f.
si·a·line [ˈsaɪəlaɪn, -liːn] adj → salivary.
si·a·lism [ˈsaɪəlɪzəm] n (übermäßiger) Speichelfluß m, Sialorrhoe f, Ptyalismus m, Hypersalivation f.
si·a·lis·mus [saɪəˈlɪzməs] n → sialism.
si·a·li·tis [saɪəˈlaɪtɪs] n Sialitis f.
sialo- pref. Speichel-, Sial(o)-, Ptyal(o)-.
si·a·lo·ad·e·nec·to·my [ˌsaɪəloˌædəˈnektəmɪ] n HNO Speicheldrüsenexzision f, Sial(o)adenektomie f.
si·a·lo·ad·e·ni·tis [ˌ-ˌædəˈnaɪtɪs] n → sialadenitis.
si·a·lo·ad·e·not·o·my [ˌ-ˌædəˈnɑtəmɪ] n HNO Sial(o)adenotomie f.
si·a·lo·aer·o·pha·gia [ˌ-ˌeərəˈfeɪdʒ(ɪ)ə] n Sialoaerophagie f.
si·a·lo·aer·oph·a·gy [ˌ-eəˈrɑfədʒɪ] n Sialoaerophagie f.
si·a·lo·an·gi·ec·ta·sis [ˌ-ˌændʒɪˈektəsɪs] n Sial(o)angiektasie f.
si·a·lo·an·gi·i·tis [ˌ-ˌændʒɪˈaɪtɪs] n Sial(o)angiitis f, -dochitis f, -ductitis f.
si·a·lo·an·gi·og·ra·phy [ˌ-ˌændʒɪˈɑgrəfɪ] n radiol., HNO Sial(o)angiographie f.
si·a·lo·an·gi·tis [ˌ-ænˈdʒaɪtɪs] n → sialoangiitis.
si·a·lo·cele [ˈ-siːl] n Sialozele f.
si·a·lo·do·chi·tis [ˌ-dəʊˈkaɪtɪs] n → sialoangiitis.
si·a·lo·do·cho·plas·ty [ˌ-ˈdəʊkəplæstɪ] n HNO Sialodochoplastik f.
si·a·lo·duc·ti·tis [ˌ-dʌkˈtaɪtɪs] n → sialoangiitis.
si·a·log·e·nous [saɪəˈlɑdʒənəs] adj speichelbildend, sialogen.
si·al·o·gog·ic [ˌsaɪəlɒʊˈgɑdʒɪk] adj → sialagogue II.
si·al·o·gogue n, adj → sialagogue.
si·al·o·gram [saɪˈæləgræm] n HNO, radiol. Sialogramm nt.
si·al·o·graph [saɪˈæləgræf] n → sialogram.
si·a·log·ra·phy [saɪəˈlɑgrəfɪ] n HNO, radiol. Sialographie f.
si·a·lo·lith [ˈsaɪəlɒʊlɪθ] n Speichelstein m, Sialolith m.
si·a·lo·li·thi·a·sis [ˌ-lɪˈθaɪəsɪs] n Sialolithiasis f.
si·a·lo·li·thot·o·my [ˌ-lɪˈθɑtəmɪ] n HNO Sialolithotomie f.
si·a·lo·ma [saɪəˈlɒʊmə] n Speicheldrüsengeschwulst f, -tumor m, Sialom(a) nt.
si·a·lo·met·a·pla·sia [ˌsaɪəlɒʊˌmetəˈpleɪʒ(ɪ)ə, -ʒɪə] n Speicheldrüsenmetaplasie f.
si·a·lo·mu·cin [ˌ-ˈmjuːsɪn] n Sialomuzin nt, -mucin nt.
si·a·lo·pha·gia [ˌ-ˈfeɪdʒ(ɪ)ə] n (übermäßiges) Speichelverschlucken nt, Sialophagie f.
si·al·o·pro·tein [ˌ-ˈprəʊtiːn, -tiːɪn] n Sialoprotein nt.
si·a·lor·rhea [ˌ-ˈrɪə] n → sialism.
si·a·los·chi·sis [saɪəˈlɑskəsɪs] n Hemmung f der Speichelsekretion.

si·a·lo·sis [saɪəˈlɒʊsɪs] n 1. Speichelfluß m. 2. → sialism.
si·a·lo·ste·no·sis [ˌsaɪəlɒʊstɪˈnɒʊsɪs] n HNO Sialostenose f.
si·a·lo·sy·rinx [ˌ-ˈsɪrɪŋks] n Speichelfistel f.
si·a·lyl·ol·i·go·sac·cha·ride [ˌsaɪəlɪlˌɑlɪgəʊˈsækəraɪd] n Sialyloligosaccharid nt.
si·a·lyl·trans·fer·ase [ˌ-ˈtrænsfəreɪz] n Sialyltranferase f.
Si·a·mese twins [ˌsaɪəˈmiːz] siamesische Zwillinge pl.
sib [sɪb] I n → sibling. II adj blutsverwandt (to mit).
sib·i·lant [ˈsɪbələnt] adj card., pulmo. (Geräusch) zischend, pfeifend.
sibilant rales pfeifende Rasselgeräusche nt.
sibilant rhonchi giemende/pfeifende Rasselgeräusche pl, Giemen nt, Pfeifen nt.
Si·bi·ri·an liver fluke [saɪˈbɪərɪən] micro. Katzenleberegel m, Opisthorchis felineus.
Sibirian tick typhus nordasiatisches Zeckenbißfieber nt.
sib·ling [ˈsɪblɪŋ] n 1. Bruder m, Schwester f; ~s pl Geschwister pl. 2. bio. Nachkommenschaft f.
sib·ship [ˈsɪpʃɪp] n Blutsverwandtschaft f; Blutsverwandte pl.
Sibson [ˈsɪbsən] S.'s aponeurosis/fascia Sibson'-Membran f, -Faszie f, Membrana suprapleuralis.
S.'s muscle Skalenus m minimus, M. scalenus minimus.
Sicard [siˈkaːr] S.'s sign chir. Sicard-Zeichen nt.
S.'s syndrome neuro. Sicard-Syndrom nt, Collet-Syndrom nt.
sic·ca syndrome [ˈsɪkə] Sicca-Syndrom nt.
sic·ca·tive [ˈsɪkətɪv] I n Trockenmittel nt, Sikkativ nt. II adj trocknend.
sic·cha·sia [sɪˈkeɪzɪə] n Übelkeit f, Brechreiz m, Nausea f.
sic·co·la·bile [ˌsɪkəʊˈleɪbl] adj trocknungsunbeständig, -labil.
sic·co·sta·bile [ˌ-ˈsteɪbl, -bɪl] adj trocknungsstabil.
sick [sɪk] I n 1. the ~ pl die Kranken. 2. Übelkeit f. II adj 3. krank (of an). to fall ~ krank werden, erkranken. 4. schlecht, übel. to be ~ s. übergeben (müssen). to feel ~ einen Brechreiz verspüren. 5. Kranken-, Krankheits-.
sick bed 1. Krankenbett nt. 2. Krankenlager nt.
sick certificate Krankheitsattest nt, Krankmeldung f, -schreibung f.
sick·en [ˈsɪkn] I vt Übelkeit verursachen. II vi 1. erkranken, krank werden. 2. kränkeln. 3. s. ekeln (at vor).
sick·en·ing [ˈsɪkənɪŋ] adj Übelkeit erregend.
sick headache Migräne f, Migraine f.
sick insurance Krankenversicherung f.
sick·ish [ˈsɪkɪʃ] adj 1. kränklich, unpäßlich, unwohl. 2. Übelkeit erregend.
sick·le [ˈsɪkəl] n Sichel f.
sick leave Fehlen nt wegen Krankheit. to be on ~ krank geschrieben sein, wegen Krankheit fehlen. to request ~ s. krank melden.
sickle cell Sichelzelle f.
sickle cell anemia Sichelzell(en)anämie f, Herrick-Syndrom nt.
sickle-cell crisis Sichelzellkrise f.
sickle cell dactylitis Hand-Fuß-Syndrom nt, Sichelzelldaktylitis f.
sickle-cell disease Sichelzellerkrankung f.
sickle-cell hemoglobin abbr. HbS Sichelzellhämoglobin nt, Hämoglobin S nt abbr. HbS.

sickle-cell-hemoglobin C disease Sichelzell(en)-Hämoglobin-C-Krankheit f, HbS-HbC-Krankheit f.
sickle-cell-hemoglobin D disease Sichelzell(en)-Hämoglobin-D-Krankheit f, HbS-HbD-Krankheit f.
sickle cell syndrome → sickle cell disease.
sickle-cell-thalassemia (disease) Sichelzell(en)thalassämie f, Mikrodrepanozytenkrankheit f, HbS-Thalassämie f.
sickle-cell trait Sichelzellanlage f.
sickle forms (Malaria) Sichelkeime pl.
sick·le·mia [sɪkˈliːmɪə] n → sickle cell anemia.
sickle scotoma ophthal. Bjerrum-Zeichen nt, -Skotom nt.
sick·li·ness [ˈsɪklɪnɪs] n 1. Kränklichkeit f. 2. (Klima) Ungesundheit f.
sick·ling [ˈsɪklɪŋ] n hema. Sichelzellbildung f.
sick·ly [ˈsɪklɪ] adj 1. kränklich, schwächlich; krankhaft, kränklich, blaß. 2. (Klima) ungesund. II vt krank machen.
sick·ness [ˈsɪknɪs] n 1. Krankheit f, Erkrankung f; Leiden nt. 2. Übelkeit f, Erbrechen nt.
sickness rate Krankheitshäufigkeit f, Erkrankungsrate f, Morbidität f.
sick-nursing n Krankenpflege f.
sick sinus syndrome abbr. SSS Sick-Sinus-Syndrom nt abbr. SSS, Sinusknotensyndrom nt.
side [saɪd] n 1. Seite f; (Körper-)Seite f. 2. mathe. Seite f, Seitenlinie f, -fläche f. 3. Seite f, Teil m/nt; Rand m. 4. fig. Seite f, Charakterzug m. II adj seitlich, Seiten-.
side chain chem. Seitenkette f.
side chain theory Ehrlich-Seitenkettentheorie f.
side effect (Therapie, Medikament) Nebenwirkung f abbr. NW.
sider- pref. → sidero-.
sid·er·at·ing plague [ˈsɪdəreɪtɪŋ] Pestsepsis f, Pestseptikämie f, Pestikämie f, septische/septikämische Pest f.
sid·er·i·nu·ria [ˌsɪdərɪˈn(j)ʊərɪə] n Eisenausscheidung f im Harn.
sidero- pref. Eisen-, Sider(o)-.
sid·er·o·a·chres·tic anemia [ˌsɪdərəʊəˈkrestɪk] sideroachrestische Anämie f.
acquired s. erworbene sideroachrestische Anämie.
sid·er·o·blast [ˈ-blæst] n Sideroblast m.
sid·er·o·blas·tic anemia [ˌ-ˈblæstɪk] → sideroachrestic anemia.
refractory s. → sideroachrestic anemia, acquired.
sid·er·o·cyte [ˈ-saɪt] n Siderozyt m.
sid·er·o·der·ma [ˌ-ˈdɜrmə] n Siderodermie f, -derma nt.
sid·er·o·fi·bro·sis [ˌ-faɪˈbrəʊsɪs] n Siderofibrose f.
sid·e·rog·e·nous [sɪdəˈrɑdʒənəs] adj eisenbildend.
sid·er·o·my·cin [ˌsɪdərəʊˈmaɪsɪn] n pharm. Sideromycin f.
sid·er·o·pe·nia [ˌ-ˈpiːnɪə] n (systemischer) Eisenmangel m, Sideropenie f.
sid·er·o·pe·nic [ˌ-ˈpiːnɪk] adj Sideropenie betr., durch Sideropenie bedingt, sideropenisch.
sideropenic anemia sideropenische Anämie f, Eisenmangelanämie f.
sideropenic dysphagia Plummer-Vinson-Syndrom nt, Paterson-Brown-Syndrom nt, Kelly-Paterson-Syndrom nt, sideropenische Dysphagie f.
sid·er·o·phage [ˈ-feɪdʒ] n Siderophage m, Herzfehlerzelle f.
sid·er·o·phil [ˈ-fɪl] I n siderophile Struktur f. II adj eisenliebend, siderophil.

si·de·roph·i·lin [ˌsɪdə'rɑfəlɪn] n Transferrin nt, Siderophilin nt.
sid·e·roph·i·lous [sɪdə'rɑfɪləs] adj → siderophil II.
sid·er·o·phore ['sɪdərəfəʊər, -fɔːr] n 1. eisenbindende Substanz f. 2. → siderophage.
sid·er·o·scope ['-skəʊp] n ophthal. Sideroskop nt.
sid·er·o·sil·i·co·sis [ˌ-sɪlɪ'kəʊsɪs] n Siderosilikose f, Silikosiderose f.
sid·er·o·sis [sɪdə'rəʊsɪs] n 1. Siderose f, Siderosis f. 2. Eisen(staub)lunge f, Lungensiderose f, Siderosis pulmonum.
sid·er·ot·ic [sɪdə'rɑtɪk] adj Siderose betr., siderotisch.
siderotic nodules Gamna-Gandy-Körperchen pl, -Knötchen pl.
siderotic splenomegaly siderotische Splenomegalie f.
sid·er·ous ['sɪdərəs] adj eisenhaltig, Eisen-.
SIDES abbr. → symptomatic idiopathic diffuse esophageal spasm.
side-to-end anastomosis Seit-zu-End--Anastomose f, lateroterminale Anastomose f.
side-to-side anastomosis Seit-zu-Seit--Anastomose f, laterolaterale Anastomose f.
SIDS abbr. → sudden infant death syndrome.
Siegle ['ziːgəl]: **S.'s otoscope/speculum** Siegle-Ohrtrichter m, -Otoskop nt.
sie·mens ['siːmənz] n abbr. **S, mho** Siemens nt abbr. **S**.
sieve [sɪv] I n Sieb nt. II vt (aus-, durch-)-sieben. III vi sieben.
sieve bone → sieve plate.
sieve-like adj siebförmig, -ähnlich.
sieve plate Sieb(bein)platte f, Lamina cribrosa (ossis ethmoidalis).
sie·vert ['siːvərt] n abbr. **Sv** Sievert nt abbr. **Sv**.
sigh [saɪ] I n Seufzer m. II vi seufzen, tief (auf-)atmen.
sight [saɪt] n 1. Sehvermögen nt; Sehkraft f, Sehen nt, Augenlicht nt. 2. (An-)Blick m, Sicht f.
sig·ma effect ['sɪgmə] Sigma-Effekt m, Fahraeus-Lindqvist-Effekt m.
sig·ma·sism ['sɪgməsɪzəm] n → sigmatism.
sig·ma·tism ['sɪgmətɪzəm] n Lispeln nt, Sigmatismus m.
sigmoid- pref. → sigmoido-.
sig·moid ['sɪgmɔɪd] I n Sigma nt, Sigmoid nt, Colon sigmoideum. II adj 1. Σ-förmig, s-förmig, sigmaförmig. 2. Sigmoid betr., sigmoid, Sigma-, Sigmoid-.
sigmoid arteries Sigmaarterien pl, Aa. sigmoideae.
sigmoid colon → sigmoid I.
sigmoid colon diverticulum Sigmadivertikel nt.
sig·moid·ec·to·my [ˌsɪgmɔɪ'dektəmɪ] n chir. Sigmaresektion f, Sigmoidektomie f.
sigmoid flexure Sigma nt, Sigmoid nt, Colon sigmoideum.
sigmoid fossa Sulcus sinus transversi.
s. of temporal bone Sulcus sinus sigmoidei ossis temporalis.
s. of ulna Inc. trochlearis ulnae.
sigmoid groove Sulcus sinus sigmoidei.
sig·moi·di·tis [ˌ-'daɪtɪs] n Sigmaentzündung f, Sigmoiditis f.
sigmoid mesocolon Meso(kolon nt) nt des Sigmas, Mesosigma nt, Mesocolon sigmoideum.
sigmoid nodes Lymphknoten pl der A. sigmoidea, Nodi (lymphatici) sigmoidei.
sigmoido- pref. Sigma-, Sigmoid(o)-, Sigmoideo-.

sig·moi·do·pex·y [sɪg'mɔɪdəpeksɪ] n chir. Sigmaanheftung f, Sigmoidopexie f.
sig·moi·do·proc·tos·co·py [ˌ-prɑk'tɑskəpɪ] n Sigmoid(e)orektoskopie f.
sig·moi·do·proc·tos·to·my [ˌ-prɑk'tɑstəmɪ] n chir. Sigma-Rektum-Anastomose f, Sigmoid(e)oproktostomie f, -rektostomie f.
sig·moi·do·rec·tos·co·py [ˌ-rek'tɑskəpɪ] n Sigmoid(e)orektoskopie f.
sig·moi·do·rec·tos·to·my [ˌ-rek'tɑstəmɪ] n → sigmoidoproctostomy.
sig·moi·do·scope ['-skəʊp] n Sigmoid(e)oskop nt.
sig·moi·dos·co·py [sɪgmɔɪ'dɑskəpɪ] n Sigmoid(e)oskopie f.
sig·moi·do·sig·moi·dos·to·my [sɪgˌmɔɪdəˌsɪgmɔɪ'dɑstəmɪ] n Sigmoidosigmoid(e)ostomie f.
sig·moi·dos·to·my [sɪgmɔɪ'dɑstəmɪ] n chir. 1. Sigmoid(e)ostomie f. 2. Sigmaafter m, Sigmoid(e)ostomie f.
sig·moi·dot·o·my [sɪgmɔɪ'dɑtəmɪ] n chir. Sigmaeröffnung f, Sigmoid(e)otomie f.
sig·moi·do·ves·i·cal fistula [sɪgˌmɔɪdə'vesɪkl] Sigma-Blasen-Fistel f, sigmoid(e)ovesikale Fistel f.
sigmoid sinus Sinus sigmoideus.
sigmoid veins Sigmavenen pl, Vv. sigmoideae.
sigmoid volvulus Sigma-, Sigmoidvolvulus m.
sig·mo·scope ['sɪgməskəʊp] n Sigmoid(e)oskop nt.
sign [saɪn] n 1. Zeichen nt, Symptom nt. 2. Zeichen nt, Symbol nt, Kennzeichen nt. II vt unterzeichnen, unterschreiben, signieren. III vi unterzeichnen, unterzeichnen.
s.s of maturity Reifezeichen pl.
sig·nal ['sɪgnl] n (An-)Zeichen nt (of für); Signal nt.
signal convergence physiol. Signalkonvergenz m.
signal detection theory abbr. **SDT** physiol. sensorische Entscheidungstheorie f, signal detection theory abbr. SDT.
sig·nal·ize ['sɪgnəlaɪz] vt ankündigen, signalisieren; kennzeichnen.
signal node Klavikulardrüse f, Virchow'--Knötchen nt, -Knoten m, -Drüse f.
sig·na·ture ['sɪgnətʃər] n 1. pharm. Signatur(a) f. 2. Unterschrift f, Namenszug m, Signatur f.
sig·net ring ['sɪgnɪt] allg. Siegelring m; histol. siegelringähnliche Struktur f.
signet-ring cell 1. Siegelringzelle f. **2.** Kastrationszelle f.
signet-ring cell carcinoma Siegelringzellkarzinom nt, Ca. sigillocellulare.
sig·nif·i·cance [sɪg'nɪfɪkəns] n 1. Bedeutung f, Bedeutsamkeit f, Wichtigkeit f, Tragweite f. 2. stat. Signifikanz f.
sig·nif·i·cant [sɪg'nɪfɪkənt] adj 1. bezeichnend (of für); bedeutsam, wichtig, von Bedeutung, signifikant. 2. stat. signifikant.
sik·i·min ['sɪkəmɪn] n S(h)ikimin nt.
si·lent ['saɪlənt] adj 1. still, ruhig, leise; schweigsam, schweigend; stumm. 2. (Krankheit) latent; untätig, inaktiv, nicht aktiv; okkult.
silent electrode inaktive/indifferente/passive Elektrode f.
silent gap card. auskultatorische Lücke f.
silent mastoiditis okkulte Mastoiditis f.
silent mutation stille Mutation f.
silent period physiol. Innovationsstille f, silent period (f).
silent peritonitis asymptomatische Bauchfellentzündung/Peritonitis f.
sil·hou·ette [ˌsɪlu'et] n Umriß m, Schatten-(bild nt) m, Silhouette f.

sil·i·ca ['sɪlɪkə] n Siliziumdioxid nt.
silica gel Kieselgel nt.
sil·i·cate ['sɪlɪkeɪt, -kɪt] n Silikat nt, Silicat nt.
sil·i·ca·to·sis [ˌsɪlɪkə'təʊsɪs] n Silikatose f.
si·li·ceous [sɪ'lɪʃəs] adj siliziumhaltig, quarzhaltig.
si·lic·ic acid [sɪ'lɪsɪk] Kieselsäure f.
silicic anhydride → silica.
si·li·cious [sɪ'lɪʃəs] adj → siliceous.
si·li·ci·um [sɪ'lɪʃəm] n old → silicon.
sil·i·co·an·thra·co·sis [ˌsɪlɪkəʊˌænθrə'kəʊsɪs] n Silikoanthrakose f, Anthrasilikose f.
sil·i·con ['sɪlɪkən, -kɑn] n abbr. **Si** Silizium nt, Silicium nt abbr. Si.
silicon dioxide Siliziumdioxid nt.
sil·i·cone ['sɪlɪkəʊn] n Silikon nt.
silicon granuloma Siliziumgranulom nt.
sil·i·co·sid·er·o·sis [ˌsɪlɪkəʊˌsɪdə'rəʊsɪs] n Silikosiderose f, Siderosilikose f.
sil·i·co·sis [sɪlə'kəʊsɪs] n Quarz-, Kiesel-, Steinstaublunge f, Silikose f, Silicosis f.
sil·i·cot·ic [sɪlə'kɑtɪk] adj Silikose betr., silikotisch.
sil·i·co·tu·ber·cu·lo·sis [ˌsɪlɪkəʊtəˌbɑrkjə'ləʊsɪs] n Silikotuberkulose f.
silk [sɪlk] I n Seide f, Seidenfaser f, -faden m, -gewebe nt. II adj seiden, Seiden-.
silk·worm ['sɪlkwɑrm] n zoo. Seidenraupe f.
sil·vat·ic [sɪl'vætɪk] adj Wald-.
Silver ['sɪlvər]: **S. dwarf** → S.'s syndrome. **S.'s syndrome** Russell-Silver-Syndrom nt, Silver-Syndrom nt.
sil·ver ['sɪlvər] I n Silber nt, chem. Argentum nt abbr. **Ag**. II adj silbern, Silber-.
silver bath photo. Silberbad nt.
silver cell argentaffine Zelle f.
silver-fork deformity ortho. Bajonett-, Fourchette-, Gabelrückenstellung f.
silver-fork fracture Colles-Fraktur f mit Gabelrückenstellung.
silver impregnation histol. Silberimprägnierung f, Versilberung f.
silver nitrate Silbernitrat nt.
silver oxide Silberoxid nt.
silver stain histol. Versilberung f, Silberfärbung f, -imprägnierung f.
Silvius ['sɪlvɪəs]: **aqueduct of S.** Aqu(a)eductus mesencephalici/cerebri.
Sim·bu virus ['sɪmbuː] micro. Simbu-Virus nt.
sim·i·an ['sɪmɪən] I n (Menschen-)Affe m. II adj affenartig, Affen-.
simian crease embryo. Affenfurche f, Vierfingerfurche f.
simian line → simian crease.
simian virus abbr. **SV** micro. Simian-Virus nt abbr. SV.
sim·i·lar ['sɪmələr] adj ähnlich; (fast od. ungefähr) gleich (to); gleichartig.
sim·i·lar·i·ty [ˌsɪmə'lærətɪ] n Ähnlichkeit f (to mit); Gleichartigkeit f.
similar twins erbgleiche/eineiige/identische/monozygote/monovuläre Zwillinge pl.
Simmerlin ['sɪmərlɪn]: **S. type** Leyden--Möbius-Krankheit f, -Syndrom nt, Gliedgürtelform f der progressiven Muskeldystrophie.
Simmonds ['sɪmndz]: **S.' disease 1.** Simmonds-Kachexie f. **2.** Simmonds--Syndrom nt, Hypophysenvorderlappeninsuffizienz f, HVL-Insuffizienz f, Hypopituitarismus m.
S.' syndrome → S.' disease 2.
Simon [ˈsaɪmən]: **S.'s apical focus** → S.'s focus.
S.'s focus Simon'-Spitzenherd m.
S.'s position Simon-Lage f.

Simonart

Simonart [simɔ'naːr]: S.'s bands/ligaments/threads Simonart'-Bänder pl, amniotische Stränge pl.
Simons ['saimən; 'zimoːn]: S.' disease Simons-Syndrom nt, Lipodystrophia progressiva/paradoxa.
sim·ple ['sɪmpl] I n pharm. Heilpflanze f. II adj 1. einfach; rein, unverfälscht; unkompliziert; (Person) einfältig; (Leben) schlicht, einfach. 2. chem. unvermischt. 3. (Epithel) einschichtig. 4. (Fraktur) glatt, einfach.
simple acne derm. Akne/Acne vulgaris.
simple acute conjunctivitis ophthal. akute Bindehautentzündung/Konjunktivitis f, Conjunctivitis acuta.
simple atrophy einfache Atrophie f.
simple chorea neuro. Sydenham-Chorea f, Chorea minor (Sydenham), Chorea juvenilis/rheumatica/infectiosa/simplex.
simple conjunctivitis → simple acute conjunctivitis.
simple diplopia ophthal. direkte/gleichseitige/ungekreuzte/homonyme Diplopie f, Diplopia simplex.
simple dislocation ortho. geschlossene/einfache Luxation f.
simple epithelium einschichtiges Epithel nt.
simple flat pelvis gerad-verengtes Becken nt.
simple fracture ortho. einfache/geschlossene/unkomplizierte Fraktur f.
simple gigantism einfacher/echter Riesenwuchs m.
simple glaucoma Simplex-, Weitwinkelglaukom nt, Glaucoma simplex.
simple goiter blande Struma f.
simple hemangioma 1. Kapillarhämangiom nt, Haemangioma capillare. 2. Blutschwamm m, blastomatöses Hämangiom m, Haemangioma planotuberosum/simplex.
simple hypertrophy einfache Hypertrophie f, Hypertrophia simplex.
simple ichthyosis Fischschuppenkrankheit f, Ichthyosis simplex/vulgaris.
simple joint einfaches Gelenk nt, Artic. simplex.
simple lipid Homolipid nt.
simple lymphangioma kapilläres/einfaches Lymphangiom nt, Lymphangioma capillare/simplex.
simple mastectomy gyn. einfache Mastektomie f.
simple membranous limb of semicircular ducts Crus membranaceum simplex.
simple-minded adj 1. einfältig. 2. einfach, schlicht.
simple myopia ophthal. einfache Myopie f.
simple periodontitis Alveolarpyorrhoe f, Parodontitis marginalis.
simple protein globuläres Eiweiß/Protein nt.
simple reflex einfacher Reflex m.
simple retinitis seröse Retinitis f, Retinitis serosa.
simple schizophrenia Schizophrenia simplex.
simple sugar Einfachzucker m, Monosaccharid nt.
simple syndactyly embryo. kutane Syndaktylie f.
simple ulcer einfaches Geschwür nt, Ulcus simplex.
simple urethritis unspezifische/nicht-gonorrhoische Urethritis f abbr. NGU.
simple verrucous endocarditis Endocarditis verrucosa simplex.
Simpson ['sɪmpsən]: S. light Simpson--Licht m.
S.'s sound gyn. Simpson-Sonde f.

Sims [sɪmz]: S.' position gyn. Sims-Lage f.
S.' speculum Mastdarmspekulum nt nach Sims.
S.' test (Sims-)Huhner-Test m, postkoitaler Spermakompatibilitätstest m.
S. uterine sound gyn. Sims-Sonde f.
sim·u·late ['sɪmjəleɪt] vt 1. vortäuschen, vorspiegeln, simulieren. 2. nachahmen, imitieren, simulieren; nachbilden.
sim·u·la·tion [sɪmjə'leɪʃn] n 1. Vorspiegelung f, Vortäuschung f, Simulation f. 2. Heuchelei f, Verstellung f, Simulation f. 3. Nachahmung f, Nachbildung f, Simulation f.
sim·u·la·tor ['sɪmjəleɪtər] n 1. Heuchler(in f) m, Simulant(in f) m. 2. Nachahmer(in f) m. 3. Simulator m.
Si·mu·li·i·dae [sɪmjə'laɪə,diː] pl micro. Kriebelmücken pl, Simuliidae pl.
Si·mu·li·um [sɪ'mjuːliəm] n micro. Simulium nt.
si·mul·ta·ne·i·ty [sɪməltə'niːətɪ, saɪ-] n Gleichzeitigkeit f.
si·mul·ta·ne·ous [sɪməl'teɪniəs, saɪ-] adj gleichzeitig, simultan (with mit).
simultaneous contrast physiol. Simultankontrast m.
simultaneous insanity psychia. induziertes Irresein nt, Folie à deux.
SIMV abbr. → synchronized intermittent mandatory ventilation.
si·nal ['saɪnl] adj Sinus betr., Sinus-, Sin(o)-.
sinal x-rays HNO Sinusaufnahmen pl.
sin·ci·put ['sɪnsɪpət], pl **-puts**, **sin·cip·i·ta** [sɪn'sɪpɪtə] Vorderkopf m, Sinciput nt.
Sind·bis fever ['sɪn(d)bɪs] Sindbis-Fieber nt.
Sindbis virus micro. Sindbisvirus nt.
sin·ew ['sɪnjuː] n (Muskel-)Sehne f.
sing·er's node ['sɪŋər] Sängerknötchen nt, Nodulus vocalis.
sin·gle ['sɪŋgəl] adj einzige(r, s), einzel(n), einfach, Einzel-, Einfach-; ledig.
single-blind experiment/test Blindversuch m.
single bond chem. Einfachbindung f.
single-bond character chem. Einfachbindungscharakter m.
single-celled animal Einzeller m.
single-cell necrosis Einzelzellnekrose f.
single-chain adj chem. einkettig.
single-displacement (reaction) biochem. einfache Verdrängung(sreaktion f) f.
ordered s. geordnete Verdrängungsreaktion.
random s. zufällige Verdrängungsreaktion.
single-fiber necrosis (Muskel) Einzelfasernekrose f.
single malformation embryo. Einzelmißbildung f.
single-nephron filtration rate abbr. SNFR Einzelnephronfiltrat nt abbr. ENF.
single parent alleinerziehender Elternteil m, Alleinerzieher(in f) m.
single-phase adj einphasig, Einphasen-.
single-point mutation Punktmutation f.
single-strand → single-stranded.
single-stranded adj abbr. **ss** einstrangig, Einzelstrang- abbr. ss.
single-stranded break chem. Einzelstrangbruch m.
single-stranded DNA abbr. **ssDNA** Einzelstrang-DNA f abbr. ssDNA.
single-stranded RNA abbr. **ssRNA** Einzelstrang-RNA f abbr. ssRNA.
single twitch physiol. Einzelzuckung f.
single-valued adj mathe. einwertig, eindeutig.
single vision ophthal. Einfachsehen nt, Haplopie f.

sin·gul·ta·tion [sɪŋgəl'teɪʃn] n → singultus.
sin·gul·tous [sɪŋ'gʌltəs] adj Schluckauf betr.
sin·gul·tus [sɪŋ'gʌltəs] n, pl **-tus·es** Schluckauf m, Singultus m.
sinistr- pref. → sinistro-.
sin·is·tral ['sɪnəstrəl] I n Linkshänder(in f) m. II adj 1. linkshändig. 2. linke Seite betr., linksseitig, Links-.
sin·is·tral·i·ty [sɪnə'strælətɪ] n Linkshändigkeit f.
sinistro- pref. Links-, Sinistr(o)-.
sin·is·tro·car·dia [sɪnəstrəʊ'kɑːrdɪə] n Sinistro-, Lävokardie f.
sin·is·tro·ce·re·bral [,-sə'riːbrəl, -'serə-] adj die linke Hirnhemisphäre betr.
sin·is·troc·u·lar [sɪnə'strɑkjələr] adj ophthal. linksäugig.
sin·is·troc·u·lar·i·ty [sɪnəˌstrɑkjə'lerətɪ] n ophthal. Linksäugigkeit f.
sin·is·tro·gy·ra·tion [sɪnəstrədʒaɪ'reɪʃn] n → sinistrotorsion.
sin·is·tro·man·u·al [,-'mænjuːəl] adj linkshändig.
sin·is·trop·e·dal [sɪnə'strɑpədəl] adj linksfüßig.
sin·is·trorse ['sɪnəstrɔrs] adj nach links gedreht.
sin·is·tro·tor·sion [sɪnəstrə'tɔːrʃn] n Drehung f nach links, Linksdrehung f, Sinistrotorsion f, Lävorotation f, -torsion f.
sin·is·trous ['sɪnəstrəs, sɪ'nɪstrəs] adj die linke Seite betr., linksseitig, Links-.
sin·ka·line ['sɪŋkəlɪn] n Cholin nt, Bilineurin nt, Sinkalin nt.
si·no·a·tri·al [saɪnəʊ'eɪtrɪəl] adj abbr. **SA** sinuatrial, sinuaurikulär.
sinoatrial block sinuatrialer/sinuaurikulärer Block m, SA-Block m.
sinoatrial bradycardia card. Sinusbradykardie f.
sinoatrial bundle Keith-Flack-Bündel nt, Sinuatrialbündel nt.
sinoatrial ganglia Bidder-Haufen pl, Remak-Haufen pl, Bidder-Ganglien pl, Bidder-Remak-Ganglien pl.
sinoatrial node Sinus-, Sinuatrialknoten m, SA-Knoten m, Keith-Flack'Knoten m, Nodus sinuatrialis.
si·no·au·ric·u·lar [,-ɔː'rɪkjələr] adj → sinoatrial.
sinoauricular block → sinoatrial block.
si·no·bron·chi·al syndrome [,-'brɑŋkɪəl] → sinobronchitis.
si·no·bron·chi·tis [,-brɑŋ'kaɪtɪs] n Sino-, Sinubronchitis f, sinubronchiales/sinupulmonales Syndrom nt.
si·no·gram ['-græm] n 1. HNO, radiol. Röntgenaufnahme f der Nasennebenhöhlen, Sinogramm nt. 2. radiol. Röntgenaufnahme f eines Fistelgangs, Sinogramm nt.
si·nog·ra·phy [saɪ'nɑgrəfɪ] n 1. HNO, radiol. Sinographie f. 2. radiol. Sinographie f.
si·no·pul·mo·nar·y [saɪnəʊ'pʌlmə'nerɪ; -nərɪ, -'pʊl-] adj Nasennebenhöhlen u. Lunge(n) betr., sinupulmonal.
sinopulmonary syndrome → sinobronchitis.
si·nos·co·py [saɪ'nɑskəpɪ] n HNO Sinuskopie f.
si·no·vag·i·nal bulbs [saɪnə'vædʒənl, -və-'dʒaɪnl] embryo. Sinuvaginalhöcker pl.
si·no·ven·tric·u·lar [,-ven'trɪkjələr] adj sinuventrikulär.
si·nu·a·tri·al [sɪnə(j)uː'eɪtrɪəl] adj → sinoatrial.
sinuatrial fold embryo. Sinus-Vorhof-Falte f, Sinuatrialfalte f.
sinuatrial junction embryo. Sinuseinmündung f.

sinuatrial node → sinoatrial node.
sin·u·au·ric·u·lar [,-ɔːˈrɪkjələr] *adj* → sinoatrial.
sin·u·ous [ˈsɪnjəwəs] *adj* s. schlängelnd, s. windend, gewunden, wellenförmig.
si·nus [ˈsaɪnəs] *n, pl* **si·nus, -nus·es 1.** Höhle *f*, Höhlung *f*, Bucht *f*, Tasche *f*, Sinus *m*. **2.** *anat.* Knochenhöhle *f*, Markhöhle *f*, Sinus *m*; (*Nase*) Nebenhöhle *f*; (*Gehirn*) venöser Sinus *m*. **3.** *patho.* Fistelgang *m*, -tasche *f*, Sinus *m*.
s.es of dura mater Durasinus *pl*, Hirnsinus *pl*, Sinus der Dura mater encephali, Sinus venosi durales, Sinus durae matris.
s. of epididymis Nebenhodenspalt *m*, -sinus, Sinus epididymidis.
s. of Maier Maier-, Arlt'-Sinus.
s. of Morgagni 1. Aortinsinus, Sinus aortae. **2.** Morgagni-Ventrikel *m*, -Tasche *f*, Galen'-Ventrikel *m*, -Tasche *f*, Kehlkopf-Tasche *f*, Ventriculus laryngis.
s. of pericardium Perikardnische *f*, -sinus, Sinus pericardii.
s.es of pulmonary trunk Sinus trunci pulmonalis.
s. of spleen Milzsinus, Sinus lienis/splenicus.
s. of Valsalva Aortensinus, Sinus aortae.
s. of venae cavae Venensinus des rechten Vorhofs, Sinus venarum cavarum.
si·nus·al [ˈsaɪnəsəl] *adj* Sinus betr., Sinus-, Sino-.
sinus arrest *cardio.* Sinusarrest *m*.
sinus arrhythmia Sinusarrhythmie *f*.
phasic s. respiratorische Arrhythmie *f*.
sinus barotrauma *HNO* Aero-, Barosinusitis *f*.
sinus bradycardia *card.* Sinusbradykardie *f*.
sinus block 1. sinuatrialer/sinuaurikulärer Block *m*, SA-Block *m*. **2.** *HNO* Nebenhöhlenblockade *f*.
sinus catarrh *hema.* Sinuskatarrh *m*, -histiocytosis *f*, akute unspezifische Lymphadenitis *f*.
sinus histiocytosis → sinus catarrh.
sinus horn *embryo.* Sinushorn *nt*.
si·nus·i·tis [saɪnəˈsaɪtɪs] **1.** *n HNO* (Nasen-)Nebenhöhlenentzündung *f*, Sinusitis *f*, Sinuitis *f*. **2.** Entzündung *f* eines Hirnsinus, Sinusitis *f*.
sinus lavage *HNO* Nebenhöhlenspülung *f*, -lavage *f*, Sinusspülung *f*, -lavage *f*.
sinus nerve Ramus sinus carotici n. glossopharyngei.
sinus node → sinoatrial node.
sinus node artery Ast *m* der rechten *od.* linken Kranzarterie zum Sinusknoten, Ramus nodi sinu-atrialis a. coronariae dextrae sive sinistrae.
si·nus·oid [ˈsaɪnəsɔɪd] **I** *n* **1.** sinusartige Struktur *f*, Sinusoid *m*. **2.** → sinusoidal capillary. **II** *adj* Sinusoid betr., sinusartig, sinusoid, sinusoidal, Sinus-.
si·nus·oi·dal [saɪnəˈsɔɪdl] *adj* → sinusoid II.
sinusoidal capillary Sinusoid *nt*, Sinusoidgefäß *nt*, Vas sinusoideum.
sinusoidal circulation Sinusoidalkreislauf *m*, -zirkulation *f*.
sinusoidal oscillation *phys.* Sinusschwingung *f*.
sinusoidal vessel → sinusoidal capillary.
sinusoidal vibration Sinusschwingung *f*.
si·nus·ot·o·my [saɪnəˈsɑtəmɪ] *n HNO* Sinusotomie *f*.
sinus phlebitis Entzündung *f* eines Hirnsinus.
sinus rhythm *physiol.* Sinusrhythmus *m*.
sinus standstill *card.* Sinusarrest *m*.
sinus tachycardia *card.* Sinustachykardie *f*.

sinus thrombosis Sinusthrombose *f*.
otogenic s. otogene Sinusthrombose.
sinus tubercle *embryo.* Müller'-Hügel *m*.
si·nu·ven·tric·u·lar [,saɪnəvenˈtrɪkjələr] *adj* sinuventrikulär.
si·nu·ver·te·bral nerve [,saɪnəˈvɜrtəbrəl] Ramus meningeus nn. spinalium.
si·phon [ˈsaɪfən] *n* Siphon *m*.
Si·pho·nap·tera [,saɪfəˈnæptərə] *pl micro.* Siphonaptera *pl*.
Sipple [ˈsɪpl]: **S.'s syndrome** Sipple-Syndrom *nt*, MEN-Typ *m* IIa, MEA-Typ *m* IIa.
si·re·no·me·lia [,saɪrənəʊˈmiːlɪə] *n embryo.* Sirenenbildung *f*, Sirene *f*, Sirenomelie *f*, Sympodie *f*.
si·re·nom·e·lus [,saɪrəˈnɑmələs] *n, pl* **-li** [-laɪ] *embryo.* Sirene *f*, Sirenomelus *m*.
si·ri·a·sis [sɪˈraɪəsɪs] *n* → sunstroke.
si·ro·heme [ˈsaɪrəhiːm] *n* Sirohäm *nt*.
sir·up *n* → syrup.
SISI *abbr.* → short increment sensitivity index.
SISI test *HNO* SISI-Test *m*.
sis·o·mi·cin [sɪsəʊˈmaɪsɪn] *n pharm.* Sisomicin *nt*, Sisomycin *nt*.
sis·ter [ˈsɪstər] **I** *n* **1.** Schwester *f*. **2.** *Brit.* (Stations-)Schwester *f*. **II** *adj* Schwester(n)-.
sister chromatids Schwesterchromatiden *pl*.
SI system *abbr.* **SI** internationales Einheitensystem *nt*, Système International d'Unites, SI-System *nt*.
sit- *pref.* → sitio-.
sit·i·ol·o·gy [sɪtɪˈɑlədʒɪ] *n* Sit(i)ologie *f*.
sit·i·o·ma·nia [,sɪtɪəʊˈmeɪnɪə, -jə] *n psychia.* Sit(i)omanie *f*.
sito- *pref.* Nahrungs-, Sit(i)o-.
si·tol·o·gy [saɪˈtɑlədʒɪ] *n* → sitiology.
si·to·ma·nia [,saɪtəˈmeɪnɪə, -jə] *n* → sitiomania.
si·to·pho·bia [,-ˈfəʊbɪə] *n psychia.* krankhafte Nahrungsverweigerung *f*, Sit(i)ophobia *f*.
si·tos·ter·ol [sɪˈtɑstərəl, ˌsaɪtəʊˈstɪərəl] *n*
sit·u·at·ed [ˈsɪtʃəweɪtɪd] *adj* (*a. anat.*) gelegen; lokalisiert. **to be ~** liegen.
sit·u·a·tion [ˌsɪtʃəˈweɪʃn] *n* **1.** *fig.* Lage *f*, Zustand *m*, Situation *f*; Umstände *pl*. **2.** (örtliche) Lage *f*.
sit·u·a·tion·al [-ˈweɪʃənl] *adj* Situations-, Lage-.
situational depression *psychia.* reaktive Depression *f*, depressive Reaktion *f*.
situation-specific *adj* situationsspezifisch.
si·tus [ˈsaɪtəs] *n, pl* **-tus** *anat.* Lage *f*, Situs *m*.
sitz bath [sɪts] Sitzbad *nt*; Sitzbadewanne *f*.
SI unit SI-Einheit *f*.
sixth day [sɪksθ] Dreitagefieber *nt*, sechste Krankheit *f*, Exanthema subitum, Roseola infantum.
sixth nerve Abduzens *m*, Abducens *m*, VI. Hirnnerv *m*, N. abducens [VI].
sixth sense Zönästhesie *f*.
sixth venereal disease Morbus Durand-Nicolas-Favre *m*, klimatischer Bubo *m*, vierte Geschlechtskrankheit *f*, Lymphogranuloma inguinale/venereum *abbr.* LGV, Lymphopathia venerea, Poradenitis inguinalis.
size [saɪz] *n* Größe *f*, Maß *nt*, Format *nt*; Umfang *m*; (Schuh-, Kleider-, Körper-)Größe *f*; *fig.* Ausmaß *nt*.
size constancy *physiol.* Größenkonstanz *f*.
size lens Aniseikonieglas *nt*.
Sjögren [ˈʃəʊɡrən]: **S.'s disease/syndrome** Sjögren-Syndrom *nt*.
Sjögren-Larsson [ˈlɑːrsn]: **S.-L. syndrome** Sjögren-Larsson-Syndrom *nt*.

SK *abbr.* → streptokinase.
skat·ole [ˈskætəʊl, -ɑl] *n* Skatol *nt*.
ska·to·sin [skæˈtəʊsɪn] *n* Skatosin *nt*.
ska·tox·yl [skæˈtɑksɪl] *n* Skatoxyl *nt*.
skein [skeɪn] *n* Spirem *nt*.
skein cell *n* Retikulozyt *m*.
ske·lal·gia [skɪˈlældʒ(ɪ)ə] *n* Beinschmerz(en *pl*) *m*.
ske·las·the·nia [ˌskɪlæsˈθiːnɪə] *n* Beinschwäche *f*.
skel·e·tal [ˈskelɪtl] *adj* Skelett betr., skelettartig, skelettal, Skelett-.
skeletal deformity Skelettverformung *f*, -deformierung *f*.
skeletal dysplasia Skelettdysplasie *f*.
skeletal enchondromatosis Ollier'-Erkrankung *f*, -Syndrom *nt*, Enchondromatose *f*, Hemichondrodystrophie *f*, multiple kongenitale Enchondrome *pl*.
skeletal extension → skeletal traction.
skeletal hemangiomatosis skelettale Hämangiomatose/Lymphangiomatose *f*, Angiomatose/Lymphangiektasie *f* des Knochensyndrome
skeletal lymphangiomatosis → skeletal hemangiomatosis.
skeletal muscle cell Skelettmuskelzelle *f*.
skeletal muscles 1. an Knochen ansetzende Muskeln, Skelettmuskeln *pl*. **2.** quergestreifte willkürliche Muskulatur *f*, Skelettmuskulatur *f*.
skeletal system Skelettsystem *nt*, Systema skeletale.
skeletal traction *ortho.* Knochenzug *m*, -extension *f*.
skel·e·ti·za·tion [ˌskelətɪˈzeɪʃn] *n* **1.** *patho.* extreme Abmagerung *f*. **2.** *chir.* Skelettieren *nt*, Skelettierung *f*.
skel·e·tog·e·nous [skelɪˈtɑdʒənəs] *adj* skelettbildend, skeletogen.
skeletogenous cell Osteoblast *m*.
skel·e·tog·e·ny [skelɪˈtɑdʒənɪ] *n* Skelettentwicklung *f*, -bildung *f*, Skeletogenese *f*.
skel·e·to·mo·tor [ˌskelɪtəˈməʊtər] *adj* skeletomotorisch.
skeletomotor loop *physiol.* skeletomotorische Schleife *f*.
skel·e·ton [ˈskelɪtn] **I** *n* Skelett *nt*, Skelet *nt*, Knochengerüst *nt*, Gerippe *nt*. **II** *adj* Skelett-.
s. of thorax knöcherner Brustkorb/Thorax *m*, Thoraxskelett, Compages thoracis, Skeleton thoracicum.
Skene [skiːn]: **S.'s ducts** Skene'-Gänge *pl*, -Drüsen *pl*, Ductus paraurethrales (urethrae feminiae).
S.'s glands/tubules → S.'s ducts.
ske·nei·tis *n* → skenitis.
ske·ni·tis [skɪˈnaɪtɪs] *n* Entzündung *f* der Skene'-Gänge, Sken(e)itis *f*.
ske·no·scope [ˈskɪnəskəʊp] *n* Skenoskop *nt*.
ske·o·cy·to·sis [ˌskɪəʊsaɪˈtəʊsɪs] *n old hema.* Linksverschiebung *f*.
skep·to·phy·lax·is [ˌskeptəʊfɪˈlæksɪs] *n* Skeptophylaxie *f*.
skew [skjuː] **I** *n* Schiefe *f*, Schrägheit *f*. **2.** *mathe.* Asymmetrie *f*. **II** *adj* **3.** schief, schräg; abschüssig. **4.** *mathe.* asymmetrisch. **III** *vi* schielen.
skew deviation *ophthal.* Magendie-Hertwig-Schielstellung *f*, Magendie-Schielstellung *f*, -Zeichen *nt*, Hertwig-Magendie-Phänomen *nt*, -Syndrom *nt*.
skew·ness [ˈskjuːnɪs] *n* **1.** Schiefe *f*, Schrägheit *f*. **2.** *mathe.* Asymmetrie *f*. **3.** *stat.* Abweichung *f*.
skia- *pref.* Schatten-, Skia-; Radio-.
ski·a·gram [ˈskaɪəgræm] *n* Roentgenaufnahme *f*, -bild *nt*.
ski·a·graph [-græf] *n* → skiagram.

ski·ag·ra·phy [skaɪ'ægrəfɪ] *n* 1. Röntgenphotografie *f*. 2. Röntgenuntersuchung *f*, Röntgen *nt*.
ski·am·e·try [skaɪ'æmətrɪ] *n* → skiascopy 1.
ski·a·scope ['skaɪəskəʊp] *n ophthal*. Skiaskop *nt*, Retinoskop *nt*.
ski·as·co·py [skaɪ'ɑskəpɪ] *n* 1. *ophthal*. Retinoskopie *f*, Skiaskopie *f*. 2. *radiol*. Röntgendurchleuchtung *f*, Fluoroskopie *f*.
ski·er's thumb ['skɪər] *ortho*. Skidaumen *m*.
Skillern ['skɪlərn]: **S.'s fracture** Skillern--Fraktur *f*.
skim·ming ['skɪmɪŋ] *n* 1. (*Schaum*) Abschöpfen *nt*, Abschäumen *nt*, Skimming *nt*. 2. ~s *pl* Schaum *m*.
skin [skɪn] **I** *n* 1. Haut *f*; *anat*. Integumentum commune. 2. äußere Haut *f*; *anat*. Kutis *f*, Cutis *f*. 3. *techn*. Haut *f*, Schicht *f*; *bot*. Schale *f*, Hülse *f*, Rinde *f*; *zoo*. Fell *nt*. **II** *vt* schälen, abhäuten; (*Haut*) aufschürfen.
skin appendages Hautanhangsgebilde *pl*.
skin bacteria Hautbakterien *pl*.
skin bank Hautbank *f*.
skin biopsy Hautbiopsie *f*.
skin botfly *micro*. Dasselfliege *f*, Dermatobia hominis.
skin care Hautpflege *f*.
skin closure *chir*. Hautverschluß *m*, -naht *f*.
skin color Hautfarbe *f*, -färbung *f*.
skin defect Hautdefekt *m*.
skin disease Hautkrankheit *f*; Dermatose *f*.
skin dose *radiol*. Hautdosis *f*.
skin eruption → skin rash.
skin flap *chir*. Hautlappen *m*.
skin friction *phys*. Oberflächenreibung *f*.
skin furrows Hautfurchen *pl*, Sulci cutis.
skin graft Hauttransplantat *nt*, -lappen *m*.
free s. freies Hauttransplantat.
full-thickness s. Vollhautlappen, -transplantat.
pedicle s. gestielter Hautlappen.
skin grafting Hauttransplantation *f*, -übertragung *f*.
skin grooves Sulci cutis.
skin hook *chir*. Hauthaken *m*.
skin incision Hautschnitt *m*, -inzision *f*.
skin-less ['skɪnlɪs] *adj* ohne Haut, hautlos.
skin-muscle reflex → skin reflex.
skinned [skɪnd] *adj* häutig; enthäutet; -häutig.
Skinner ['skɪnər]: **S.'s line** *radiol*. Shenton--Linie *f*, Ménard-Shenton-Linie.
skin·ner·i·an conditioning [skɪ'nɪərɪən] *psycho*., *physiol*. operante/instrumentelle Konditionierung *f*.
skin·ny ['skɪnɪ] *adj* mager, dürr, abgemagert.
skin papillae Hautpapillen *pl*, Papillae dermatis/corii.
skin perfusion Hautdurchblutung *f*, -perfusion *f*.
skin-pupillary reflex ziliospinaler Reflex *m*.
skin rash Hautausschlag *m*, Exanthem(a) *nt*.
skin reaction Hautreaktion *f*, -test *m*.
galvanic s. → skin response, galvanic.
skin reactive factor *abbr*. SRF hautreaktiver Faktor *m*, skin reactive factor *abbr*. SRF.
skin receptor Hautrezeptor *m*.
skin reflex Hautreflex *m*, -reaktion *f*.
skin response Hautreflex *m*, -reaktion *f*.
galvanic s. *abbr*. GSR psychogalvanischer (Haut-)Reflex.

skin retraction Hauteinziehung *f*, -retraktion *f*.
skin ridges Hautleisten *pl*, Cristae cutis.
skin scale Hautschuppe *f*.
skin sensation Hautsensibilität *f*.
superficial s. oberflächliche Hautsensibilität.
skin staple *chir*. Hautklammer *f*.
skin stones Hautkalzinose *f*, Calcinosis cutis.
skin suture *chir*. Hautnaht *f*.
skin tag Stielwarze *f*, Akrochordon *nt*, Acrochordon *nt*.
skin temperature Hauttemperatur *f*.
skin test Hauttest *m*.
skin test hypersensitivity Hauttestüberempfindlichkeit *f*.
skin traction *ortho*. Hautzug *m*, -extension *f*, Heftpflasterextension *f*.
skin turgor Hautturgor *m*.
skin writing Hautschrift *f*, Dermographia *f*, -graphie *f*, -graphismus *m*.
SKSD *abbr*. → streptokinase-streptodornase.
skull [skʌl] *n* Schädel *m*; Schädeldach *nt*, -decke *f*, Hirnschale *f*.
skull cap knöchernes Schädeldach *nt*, Kalotte *f*, Calvaria *f*.
skull fracture Schädel(dach)bruch *m*, -fraktur *f*.
basal s. Schädelbasisbruch, -fraktur.
basilar s. → basal s.
closed s. geschlossene Schädel(dach)fraktur.
comminuted s. Schädeltrümmerfraktur.
compound s. offene Schädel(dach)fraktur.
depressed s. Schädelimpressionsfraktur.
linear s. lineare Schädel(dach)fraktur.
open s. → compound s.
simple s. → closed s.
skull injury Schädelverletzung *f*, -trauma *nt*.
closed s. geschlossenes Schädeltrauma.
open s. offenes Schädeltrauma.
skull pan → skull cap.
skull suture *anat*. Schädelnaht *f*, Sutura cranialis.
skull trauma → skull injury.
sky·rock·et capillary ectasis ['skaɪrɑkɪt] Besenreiser(varizen *pl*) *pl*.
slant [slænt, slɑːnt] **I** *n* 1. Schräge *f*, schräge Fläche *od*. Linie *f*. 2. → slant culture. **II** *adj* schräg, schief. **III** *vt* schräg legen, kippen. **IV** *vi* schräg liegen, schief liegen; s. neigen, kippen.
slant culture *micro*. Schrägkultur *f*.
Slaviansky [slə'vjænskɪ]: **membrane of S.** Slaviansky'-Membran *f*, (Follikel-)Glashaut *f*.
SLE *abbr*. → St. Louis encephalitis.
sleep [sliːp] (*v* slept; slept) **I** *n* Schlaf *m*. **full of ~** schläfrig, verschlafen. **to get some ~** ein wenig schlafen. **to get/go to ~** einschlafen; schlafen gehen. **to have a good night's ~** s. richtig ausschlafen. **in one's ~** im Schlaf. **to put to ~** jdn. zum Schlafen bringen; (*Tier*) einschläfern. **to talk in one's ~** im Schlaf sprechen. **to walk in one's ~** nacht-, schlafwandeln. **II** *vt* schlafen. **III** *vi* 1. schlafen. 2. schlafen (*with mit*).
sleep off *vt* s. gesund schlafen; (*Rausch*) ausschlafen.
sleep apnea (syndrome) Schlafapnoe-(syndrom *nt*) *f*.
sleep disturbances Schlafstörungen *pl*.
sleep drunkenness 1. Schlaftrunkenheit *f*. 2. → sleepiness.
sleep epilepsy Schlafepilepsie *f*.
sleep·er ['sliːpər] *n* 1. Schlafende(r *m*) *f*. **to be a light/heavy ~** einen leichten/festen

Schlaf haben. 2. *a*. ~s *pl* (Kinder-)Schlafanzug *m*.
sleep-induced apnea (syndrome) → sleep apnea (syndrome).
sleep·i·ness ['sliːpɪnɪs] *n* (krankhafte) Schläfrigkeit *f*, Verschlafenheit *f*, Müdigkeit *f*, Somnolenz *f*.
sleep·ing ['sliːpɪŋ] *adj* schlafend, Schlaf-.
sleeping disease Narkolepsie *f*.
sleeping draught Schlaftrunk *m*.
sleeping pill Schlaftablette *f*.
sleeping sickness Schlafkrankheit *f*, Hypnosie *f*.
acute s. → Rhodesian s.
African s. afrikanische Schlafkrankheit/Trypano(so)miasis *f*.
chronic s. → Gambian s.
East African s. → Rhodesian s.
Gambian s. westafrikanische Schlafkrankheit/Trypano(so)miasis *f*.
Rhodesian s. ostafrikanische Schlafkrankheit/Trypano(so)miasis *f*.
West African s. → Gambian s.
sleeping tablet Schlaftablette *f*.
sleeping-waking rhythm Schlaf-Wach--Rhythmus *m*.
sleep learning Schlaflernmethode *f*, Lernen *nt* im Schlaf, Hypnopädie *f*.
sleep·less ['sliːplɪs] *adj* schlaflos.
sleep·less·ness ['sliːplɪsnɪs] *n* Schlaflosigkeit *f*, Wachheit *f*, Insomnie *f*.
sleep spindles *neuro*., *physiol*. Schlafspindeln *pl*, β-Spindeln *pl*.
sleep stages Schlafstadien *pl*.
sleep-talk·ing ['sliːpɔːkɪŋ] *n* → somniloquism.
sleep terror disorder *ped*. Nachtangst *f*, Pavor nocturnus.
sleep·walk ['sliːpwɔːk] *vi* schlaf-, nachtwandeln.
sleep·walk·er ['sliːpwɔːkər] *n* Schlaf-, Nachtwandler(in *f*) *m*, Somnambulist *m*.
sleep·walk·ing ['sliːpwɔːkɪŋ] **I** *n* Schlaf-, Nachtwandeln *nt*, Somnambulismus *m*, Noktambulismus *m*. **II** *adj* schlaf-, nachtwandlerisch, -wandelnd.
sleepwalking disorder → sleepwalking.
sleep wear Nachtwäsche *f*.
sleep·y ['sliːpɪ] *adj* schläfrig, müde, verschlafen, eingeschläfernd.
SLE-like syndrome systemischer Lupus erythematodes *abbr*. SLE, Systemerythematodes *m*, Lupus erythematodes visceralis, Lupus erythematodes integumentalis et visceralis.
slen·der lobule ['slendər] Lobulus gracilis.
slide [slaɪd] (*v* slid; slid) **I** *n* 1. Gleiten *nt*, Rutschen *nt*. 2. Objektträger *m*. 3. Dia(positiv *nt*) *nt*. 4. *fig*. Fall *m*, Fallen *nt*, (Ab-)Sinken *nt*. **II** *vi* gleiten, rutschen.
slide out *vi* herausgleiten, -rutschen.
s. in temperature Temperaturabfall.
slid·ing ['slaɪdɪŋ] *adj* gleitend, Gleit-, Schiebe-.
sliding-filament hypothesis (*Muskel*) Gleit-(Filament-)Theorie *f*.
sliding-filament theory → sliding-filament hypothesis.
sliding flap Verschiebelappen *m*, -plastik *f*, Vorschiebelappen *m*, -plastik *f*.
sliding hernia Gleithernie *f*, -bruch *m*.
sliding microtome *bio*., *med*. Schlittenmikrotom *nt*.
slight deafness [slaɪt] geringgradige Schwerhörigkeit *f*.
slime fever [slaɪm] Feld-, Ernte-, Schlamm-, Sumpffieber *m*, Erbsenpflückerkrankheit *f*, Leptospirosis grippotyphosa.
slime fungi *micro*. Schleimpilze *pl*, Myxomyzeten *pl*.
slime molds → slime fungi.

sling [slɪŋ] *n ortho.* Schlinge *f.*
slip [slɪp] **I** *n* (Aus-)Gleiten *nt*, (Aus-)Rutschen *nt.* **II** *vi* gleiten, rutschen.
slip hernia → sliding hernia.
slipped capital femoral epiphysis [slɪpt] → slipped upper femoral epiphysis.
slipped disk *ortho., neurochir.* Bandscheibenvorfall *m*, -prolaps *m*, -hernie *f.*
slipped hernia → sliding hernia.
slipped upper femoral epiphysis *abbr.* **SUFE** *ortho.* Lösung *f* der Femurepiphyse, Epiphyseolysis/Epiphysiolysis capitis femoris, Coxa vara adolescentium.
slip·ping ['slɪpɪŋ] *n* (Aus-)Gleiten *nt*, (Aus-, Ab-)Rutschen *nt.* **s. of the upper femoral epiphysis** → slipped upper femoral epiphysis. **s. of vertebrae** → spondylolisthesis.
slipping patella gleitende Patella *f.*
slit [slɪt] (*v* slit; slit) **I** *n* Schlitz *m*, Ritz(e *f*) *m.* **II** *vt* 1. aufschlitzen, -schneiden. 2. in Streifen schneiden; spalten. 3. ritzen.
slit-lamp ['slɪtlæmp] *n ophthal.* Spaltlampe *f.*
slit lamp microscope Spaltlampenmikroskop *nt.*
slit pores of glomerulus Filtrations-, Schlitzporen *pl* des Glomerulus.
slope [sləʊp] **I** *n* Neigung *f*, Gefälle *nt*, Schräge *f*, geneigte Fläche *f*, (Ab-)Hang *m.* **II** *vt* neigen, senken. **III** *vi* s. neigen, (schräg) abfallen.
slope culture *micro.* Schrägkultur *f.*
slough [slʌf] **I** *n patho.* Schorf *m*, abgeschilferte/tote Haut *f.* **II** *vt* (*Haut*) abstreifen, abwerfen.
slough·ing ulcer ['slʌfɪŋ] Ulcus phagedaenicum.
slow [sləʊ] **I** *adj* 1. langsam; allmählich; (*Hitze*) schwach; (*Gift*) schleichend; (*Zeit*) schleppend; (*Puls*) langsam. 2. träge, schwerfällig, begriffsstutzig. **to be ~ in learning** schwer von Begriff sein. **II** *vt* verlangsamen, verzögern; hemmen, drosseln. **III** *vi* s. verlangsamen.
slow down I *vt* → slow II. **II** *vi* → slow III.
slow up I *vt* → slow II. **II** *vi* → slow III.
s. to react reaktionsträge.
slow-acting *adj* langsam (wirkend), träge, Langzeit-.
slow·down ['sləʊdaʊn] *n* Verlangsamung *f.*
slow·ly-adapting receptor/sensor ['sləʊli] langsam adaptierender Rezeptor/Sensor *m*, SA-Rezeptor *m*, SA-Sensor *m.*
slow micturition *urol.* verlangsamte Harnentleerung *f*, Bradyurie *f.*
slow·ness ['sləʊnɪs] *n* 1. Langsamkeit *f.* 2. Trägheit *f*, Schwerfälligkeit *f*, Begriffsstutzigkeit *f.*
slow pulse langsamer Puls *m*, Pulsus rarus.
slow-reacting substance of anaphylaxis *abbr.* **SRS-A** slow-reacting substance of anaphylaxis *abbr.* SRS-A.
slow respiration verlangsamte Atmung *f.*
slow wave sleep orthodoxer/synchronisierter Schlaf *m*, non-REM-Schlaf *m*, NREM-Schlaf *m.*
slow virus *micro.* Slow-Virus *nt.*
slow virus disease Slow-Virus-Infektion *f* *abbr.* SVI.
slow virus infection *abbr.* **SVI** → slow virus disease.
SLSC *abbr.* → segment long-spacing collagen.
Sluder ['sluːdər]: **S.'s neuralgia/syndrome** Sluder-Neuralgie *f*, -Syndrom *nt*, Neuralgia sphenopalatina.
sludge [slʌdʒ] *n* Schlamm *m*, Bodensatz *m*; *hema.* Sludge *m.*
sludged blood [slʌdʒt] sludged blood-

(-Phänomen *nt*), blood-sludge(-Phänomen *nt*).
sludg·ing (of blood) [slʌdʒɪŋ] *hema.* Sludge-Phänomen *nt*, Sludging *nt*; Geldrollenbildung *f.*
slurred speech [slɜːrd] *neuro.* verwaschene Sprache *f.*
slur·ry ['slɜːri] *n phys., chem.* Aufschwemmung *f.*
Sly [slaɪ]: **S. syndrome** Sly-Syndrom *nt*, Mukopolysaccharidose *f* VII *abbr.* MPS VII.
Sm *abbr.* → samarium.
SMA *abbr.* → sequential multichannel autoanalyzer.
SMAF *abbr.* → specific macrophage arming factor.
small [smɔːl] **I** *n* (das) Kleine, (etw.) Kleines. **II** *adj* klein; (*Gestalt*) klein, schmächtig; gering, wenig; unbedeutend; (*Stimme*) schwach.
small anisogamete Mikrogamet *m*, Androgamet *m.*
small bowel → small intestine.
small bowel cancer → small bowel carcinoma.
small bowel carcinoma Dünndarmkrebs *m*, -karzinom *nt.*
small bowel diverticulum Dünndarmdivertikel *nt.*
small bowel enema Dünndarmeinlauf *m*, hoher Einlauf *m*, Enteroklysma *nt.*
small bowel ischemia Dünndarmischämie *f.*
small bowel malignancy → small bowel carcinoma.
small bowel neoplasm Dünndarmgeschwulst *f*, -neoplasma *nt*, -tumor *m.*
small bowel obstruction Dünndarmverschluß *m.*
small bowel perforation Dünndarmperforation *f.*
small bowel polyposis gastrointestinale Polypose *f*, Polyposis intestinalis.
small bowel transplantation Dünndarmtransplantation *f.*
small bowel tumor → small bowel neoplasm.
small calorie *abbr.* **c, cal** kleine Kalorie *f*, Grammkalorie *f*, (Standard-)Kalorie *f* *abbr.* cal.
small-cell carcinoma 1. kleinzelliges Karzinom *nt*, Ca. parvocellulare. 2. kleinzelliges/kleinzellig-anaplastisches Bronchialkarzinom *nt*, *inf.* Kleinzeller *m.*
small intestinal cancer/carcinoma → small bowel carcinoma.
small-intestinal disaccharidase deficiency Disaccharidintoleranz *f.*
small-intestinal fistula Dünndarmfistel *f.*
small intestine Dünndarm *m*, Intestinum tenue.
small pancreas Proc. uncinatus (pancreatis).
small plaque parapsoriasis kleinherdiger Typ *m* der Parapsoriasis en plaques, benigne kleinherdige Form *f* der Parapsoriasis en plaques, Parapsoriasis digitiformis.
small·pox ['smɔːlpɒks] *n* Pocken *pl*, Blattern *pl*, Variola *pl.*
smallpox virus *micro.* Pockenvirus *nt*, Variolavirus *nt.*
small-scale *adj* klein, in kleinem Rahmen.
small-scale structure Feinbau *m*, -struktur *f.*
small stomach syndrome Syndrom *nt* des zu kleinen Restmagens.
small wing of sphenoid bone kleiner Keilbeinflügel *m*, Ala minor (ossis sphenoidalis).
Sm antigen Sm-Antigen *nt.*

smear [smɪər] **I** *n* 1. (Zell-)Ausstrich *m*; Abstrich *m.* 2. Schmiere *f.* **II** *vt* 3. (*Kultur*) ausstreichen. 4. schmieren; etw. bestreichen (*with* mit); (*Salbe*) auftragen; (*Haut*) einreiben.
smear culture Ausstrich-, Abstrichkultur *f.*
smeg·ma ['smegmə] *n* Vorhauttalg *m*, Smegma *nt* (praeputii).
s. of prepuce → smegma.
smegma bacillus *micro.* Mycobacterium smegmatis.
smeg·ma·lith ['smegməlɪθ] *n* Smegmastein *m*, -lith *m.*
smeg·mat·ic [smeg'mætɪk] *adj* Smegma betr., Smegma-.
smell [smel] (*v* smelled; smelt) **I** *n* 1. Geruchsinn *m.* 2. Geruch *m*; Duft *m*; Gestank *m.* 3. Riechen *nt.* **II** *vt* riechen an. **III** *vi* riechen (*at* an); duften; stinken; riechen (*of* nach).
smell blindness Anosmie *f.*
smell brain Riechhirn *nt*, Rhinencephalon *nt.*
Smellie ['smelɪ]: **S.'s method** *gyn.* Smellie-Handgriff *m.*
smell·y ['smelɪ] *adj* stinkend, übelriechend.
Smith [smɪθ]: **S. antigen** Sm-Antigen *nt.* **S.'s fracture** Smith-Fraktur *f.*
Smith-Lemli-Opitz ['lemlɪ 'əʊpɪts]: **S.-L.-O. syndrome** Smith-Lemli-Opitz-Syndrom *nt.*
Smith-Petersen ['piːtərsən]: **S.-P. nail** *ortho.* Smith-Petersen-(Lamellen-)Nagel *m.*
Smith-Strang [stræŋ]: **S.-S. disease** Methioninmalabsorptionssyndrom *nt.*
smog [smɒg, smɑg] *n* Smog *m.*
smoke [sməʊk] **I** *n* 1. Rauch *m.* 2. Rauchen *nt.* **II** *vt* 3. rauchen. 4. räuchern. **III** *vi* rauchen.
smok·er's patches ['sməʊkər] orale Leukoplakie *f*, Leukoplakie *f* der Mundschleimhaut, Leukoplakia oris.
smoker's respiratory syndrome Raucherrespirationssyndrom *nt.*
smoker's tongue → smoker's patches.
SMON *abbr.* → subacute myelooopticoneuropathy.
smooth [smuːð] **I** *n* 1. Glätten *nt.* 2. glatter Teil *m.* **II** *adj* 3. glatt; sanft; weich; eben. 4. reibungslos, ruhig, fließend. **III** *vt* glätten, ebnen. **IV** *vi* s. glätten, s. beruhigen.
smooth bacteria *micro.* S-Form *f*, S-Stamm *m.*
smooth colony *micro.* (*Kultur*) S-Form *f.*
smooth leprosy tuberkuloide Lepra *f* *abbr.* TL, Lepra tuberculoides.
smooth muscle glatter unwillkürlicher Muskel *m*, glattes unwillkürliches Muskelgewebe *nt.*
smooth muscle cell glatte Muskelzelle *f.*
smooth musculature glatte Muskulatur *f.*
smooth reticulum glattes/agranuläres endoplasmatisches Retikulum *nt* *abbr.* S-ER.
smooth-rough variation *immun., micro.* S-R-Formenwechsel *m.*
smooth strain *micro.* S-Form *f*, S-Stamm *m.*
smudge cell [smʌdʒ] *hema.* Gumbrecht'-Schatten *pl*, -Kernschatten *pl.*
Smyr·na gall ['smɜːrnə] Gallapfel *m.*
Sn *abbr.* → stannum.
sn *abbr.* → stereospecific numbering.
snail [sneɪl] *n bio.* Schnecke *f.*
snail fever Schistosomiasis *f*, Bilharziose *f.*
snake [sneɪk] **I** *n* Schlange *f.* **II** *adj* schlängeln.
snake bite Schlangenbiß *m.*
snake venom Schlangengift *nt.*
snap·ping finger ['snæpɪŋ] schnellender/

snapping hip

schnappender/federnder Finger m, Trigger-Finger m.
snapping hip ortho. schnappende/schnellende Hüfte f, Coxa saltans.
snapping reflex Trömner-Reflex m, -Fingerzeichen nt, Fingerbeugereflex m, Knipsreflex m.
snare [sneər] I n (Draht-)Schlinge f. II vt chir. mit einer Schlinge fassen od. abtragen.
Sneddon-Wilkinson ['snedn 'wɪlkɪnsən]: S.-W. disease Sneddon-Wilkinson-Syndrom nt, subkorneale Pustulose f, subkorneale pustulöse Dermatose f, Pustulosis subcornealis.
sneeze [sniːz] I n Niesen nt. II vi niesen.
sneez·ing reflex ['sniːzɪŋ] Niesreflex m.
Snell [snel]: S.'s law Descartes'-Brechungsgesetz nt.
Snellen ['snelən]: S.'s charts Snellen-Tabellen pl, -Sehprobentafeln pl.
S.'s sign Snellen-Zeichen nt.
S.'s test ophthal. 1. Snellen-Sehschärfentest m. 2. Snellen-Farbentest m.
S.'s test types Snellen-Haken pl, -Sehproben pl.
SNFR abbr. → single-nephron filtration rate.
snore [snɔːr, snəʊr] I n Schnarchen nt. II vi schnarchen.
snout reflex [snaʊt] Orbicularis-oris-Reflex m, Schnauzenreflex m.
snow blindness [snəʊ] Schneeblindheit f.
snow conjunctivitis ophthal. Conjunctivitis actinica/photoelectrica, Keratoconjunctivitis/Ophthalmia photoelectrica.
snow·flake cataract ['snəʊfleɪk] Schneeflockenkatarakt f.
snow·storm cataract ['snəʊstɔːrm] → snowflake cataract.
snuff box [snʌf] n Tabatière f, Fovea radialis.
soap [səʊp] I n 1. Seife f. 2. chem. Seife f, Alkalisalze pl der Fettsäuren. II vt ein-, abseifen.
soap down vt → soap II.
soap micelle Seifenmizelle f.
soap solution Seifenlösung f.
soap·y ['səʊpɪ] adj wie Seife, seifig, Seifen-.
S.O.B. abbr. → short of breath.
so·cia·bil·i·ty [ˌsəʊʃəˈbɪlətɪ] n socio. Soziabilität f, soziales Verhalten nt, Geselligkeit f, Umgänglichkeit f.
so·cia·ble ['səʊʃəbl] adj socio. soziabel, gesellig, umgänglich.
so·cial ['səʊʃəl] adj Gesellschaft betr., sozial, Sozial-, Gesellschafts-; bio. gesellig.
so·cial·i·za·tion [ˌsəʊʃəlɪˈzeɪʃn] n socio. Sozialisierung f, Sozialisation f.
social welfare Sozialfürsorge f.
social withdrawal psycho. Sichzurückziehen nt.
social worker Sozialarbeiter(in f) m, -fürsorger(in f) m.
socio- pref. Gesellschafts-, Sozio-.
so·ci·o·bi·o·log·ic [ˌsəʊsɪəʊˌbaɪəˈlɑdʒɪk, ˌsəʊʃɪəʊ-] adj Soziobiologie betr., soziobiologisch.
so·ci·o·bi·o·log·i·cal [ˌ-ˌbaɪəˈlɑdʒɪkl] adj → sociobiologic.
so·ci·o·bi·ol·o·gy [ˌ-baɪˈɑlədʒɪ] n Soziobiologie f.
so·ci·o·gen·e·sis [ˌ-ˈdʒenəsɪs] n Soziogenese f.
so·ci·o·gram ['-græm] n Soziogramm nt.
so·ci·og·ra·phy [ˌsəʊsɪˈɑɡrəfɪ, ˌsəʊʃɪ-] n Soziographie f.
so·ci·o·log·i·cal [ˌsəʊsɪəˈlɑdʒɪkl, ˌsəʊʃɪ-] adj Soziologie betr., soziologisch.
so·ci·ol·o·gist [ˌsəʊsɪˈɑlədʒɪst, ˌsəʊʃɪ-] n Soziologe m, -login f.
so·ci·ol·o·gy [ˌ-ˈɑlədʒɪ] n Soziologie f.

so·ci·o·path·ic personality [ˌsəʊsɪəʊˈpæθɪk, ˌsəʊʃɪəʊ-] antisoziale Persönlichkeit(sstörung f) f.
sock·et ['sɑkɪt] n 1. anat. Höhle f, Aushöhlung f; (Gelenk-)Pfanne f; Zahnhöhle f. 2. Steckdose f; Sockel m, Fassung f.
s. of hip (joint) Hüftgelenkspfanne f, Azetabulum nt, Acetabulum nt.
s. of tooth Zahnfach nt.
s. of tooth Gomphosis f, Artic. dentoalveolaris.
socket joint Kugelgelenk nt, Artic. spheroidea/cotylica.
SOD abbr. → superoxide dismutase.
so·da ['səʊdə] n 1. Soda f, Natriumkarbonat nt. 2. Natriumbikarbonat nt. 3. Ätznatron nt, kaustische Soda, Natriumhydroxid nt.
so·di·um ['səʊdɪəm] n Natrium nt abbr. Na.
sodium acetate Natriumacetat nt.
sodium ascorbate Natriumaskorbat nt.
sodium aurothiomalate Natriumaurothiomalat nt, Aurothiomalatnatrium nt.
sodium balance Natriumhaushalt m, -bilanz f.
sodium benzoate Natriumbenzoat nt.
sodium bicarbonate doppeltkohlensaures Natron nt, Natriumbikarbonat nt, Natriumhydrogencarbonat nt.
sodium biphosphate Natriumbiphosphat nt.
sodium borate Borax nt, Natriumtetraborat nt.
sodium channel physiol. Natriumkanal m, Na+-Kanal m.
sodium chloride abbr. NaCl Kochsalz nt, Natriumclorid nt abbr. NaCl.
sodium chloride irrigation Kochsalzlösung f.
sodium chloride solution Kochsalzlösung f.
isotonic s. isotone Kochsalzlösung.
physiologic s. physiologische Kochsalzlösung.
sodium citrate Natriumcitrat nt.
sodium dodecyl sulfate abbr. SDS Natriumlaurylsulfat nt.
sodium fluoride Natriumfluorid nt.
sodium gate phys. Natriumschleuse f.
sodium glutamate Natriumglutamat nt.
sodium hydrate → sodium hydroxide.
sodium hydroxide abbr. NaOH Natriumhydroxid nt abbr. NaOH.
sodium hypochlorite solution Natriumhypochloritlösung f.
diluted s. verdünnte Natriumhypochloritlösung.
sodium hypoiodite Natriumhypojodit nt.
sodium iodide Natriumjodid nt, -iodid nt.
sodium ion Natrium-Ion nt.
sodium lauryl sulfate → sodium dodecyl sulfate.
sodium monofluorophosphate Natriummonofluorphosphat nt.
sodium nitrate Natriumnitrat nt, Chile-Salpeter m.
sodium nitroferricyanide → sodium nitroprusside.
sodium nitroprusside Nitroprussidnatrium nt, Dinatriumpentacyanonitrosylferrat nt.
sodium oleate Natriumoleat nt.
sodium oxalate Natriumoxalat nt.
sodium phosphate Natriumphosphat nt.
sodium-potassium adenosinetriphosphatase → sodium-potassium-ATPase.
sodium-potassium-ATPase Natrium-Kalium-ATPase f, Na+-K+-ATPase f.
sodium-potassium pump Natrium-Kalium-Pumpe f, Na+-K+-Pumpe f.

sodium pump Natriumpumpe f, Na+-Pumpe f.
sodium retention Natriumretention f.
sodium silicate chem. Wasserglas nt, wasserlösliche Alkalisilikate pl.
sodium stearate Natriumstearat nt.
sodium sulfate Natriumsulfat nt, Glaubersalz nt.
sodium thiosulfate Natriumthiosulfat nt.
sodium urate Natriumurat nt.
so·do·ku ['səʊdəkuː, səˈdəʊkəʊ] n Sodoku nt, Rattenbißkrankheit f I, Rattenbißfieber nt I.
sod·o·mist ['sɑdəmɪst] n psychia. Sodomit(in f) m.
sod·o·mite ['sɑdəmaɪt] n → sodomist.
sod·o·my ['sɑdəmɪ] n psychia. 1. Sexualverkehr m mit Tieren, Sodomie f, Zoophilie f. 2. Analverkehr m, Sodomie f.
Soemmering ['semərɪŋ]: conical papillae of S. konische Papillen pl, Papillae conicae.
S.'s foramen Sehgrube f, Fovea centralis (retinae).
S.'s ganglion Substantia nigra.
S.'s muscle M. levator gl. thyroideae.
S.'s spot gelber Fleck m, Makula f, Macula (lutea/retinae).
soft [sɔːft, sɑft] adj 1. sanft, nachgiebig, -sichtig, gutmütig; mild; gefühlvoll, empfindsam. 2. alkoholfrei; (Droge) weich. 3. weich; (Geräusch) leise; (Haut) zart; (Material) weich; (Oberfläche) glatt; (Klima) mild; (Wasser) enthärtet; (Metall) ungehärtet; (Farben, Licht) gedämpft; (Kontraste) verschwommen.
soft-bodied ticks micro. Lederzecken pl, Argasidae pl.
soft cancer medulläres Karzinom nt, Ca. medullare.
soft chancre → soft ulcer.
soft·en ['sɔːfən] I vt weichmachen, erweichen; schwächen, mildern; (Licht) dämpfen; (Wasser) enthärten. II vi weich od. mild werden, erweichen.
soft·en·er ['sɔːfənər] n 1. Weichmacher; (Wasser-)Enthärter m; Enthärtungsmittel nt, Enthärter m. 2. pharm. Erweichungs-, Lösemittel nt.
soft·en·ing ['sɔːfənɪŋ] n Erweichen nt, Erweichung f; patho. Malazie f.
s. of the brain Gehirnerweichung, Enzephalomalazie f, Encephalomalacia f.
soft fibroma weiches Fibrom nt, Fibroma molle.
soft palate weicher Gaumen m, Palatum molle, Gaumensegel nt, Velum palatinum.
soft pulse weicher Puls m, Pulsus mollis.
soft rays weiche/energiearme Röntgenstrahlung f.
soft soap Kali(schmier)seife f, Sapo kalineus/mollis.
soft sore → soft ulcer.
soft ticks micro. Lederzecken pl, Argasidae pl.
soft tissue Weichteile pl.
soft tissue calcification Weichteilverkalkung f.
soft tissue drainage chir. Weichteildrainage f.
soft tissue flap chir. Weichteillappen m, -läppchen nt.
soft tissue injury Weichteilverletzung f.
soft tissue metastasis Weichteilmetastase f.
soft tissue osteosarcoma (extraossäres) Weichteilosteosarkom nt.
soft tissue rheumatism extraartikulärer Rheumatismus m, Weichteilrheumatismus m.
soft tissue sarcoma Weichteilsarkom nt.

soft tissue swelling Weichteilschwellung f.
soft tissue trauma Weichteilverletzung f.
soft tubercle patho. verkäsender Tuberkel m.
soft ulcer weicher Schanker m, Chankroid nt, Ulcus molle.
soft wart → skin tag.
soft water weiches Wasser nt.
Sohval-Soffer ['səʊvæl 'sɔfər]: **S.-S. syndrome** Sohval-Soffer-Syndrom nt.
soil¹ [sɔɪl] **I** n Verschmutzung f; Schmutz m. **II** vt beschmutzen, schmutzig machen, verunreinigen.
soil² [sɔɪl] n (Erd-)Boden m, Erde f, Grund m.
soil-borne adj durch Erde übertragen.
so·ja bean ['sɔɪ(j)ə, 'səʊjə, 'sɔːjə] → soybean.
so·ko·sho [səʊ'kəʊʃəʊ] n → sodoku.
sol [sɔl, sal] n chem. Sol nt.
So·la·na·ce·ae [,səʊlə'neɪsɪ,iː] pl Nachtschattengewächse pl, Solanaceae pl.
so·la·na·ceous [,-'neɪʃəs] adj Solanaceae betr.
so·la·nine ['-niːn, -nɪn] n Solanin nt.
solanine poisoining Solaninvergiftung f, Solanismus m.
so·la·noid carcinoma ['səʊlənɔɪd] old → scirrhous carcinoma.
so·la·no·ma [,-'nəʊmə] n old → scirrhous carcinoma.
So·la·num [sə'leɪnəm] n micro. Solanum nt.
so·lar ['səʊlər] adj solar, Sonnen-.
solar cheilitis Cheilitis actinica.
solar dermatitis Sonnenbrand m, Dermatitis solaris, Erythema solaris, Dermatitis photoelectrica.
solar elastosis aktinische/senile Elastose f, Elastosis actinica/senilis/solaris.
solar energy Sonnenenergie f.
solar fever 1. Dengue nt, Dengue-Fieber nt, Dandy-Fieber nt. **2.** → sunstroke.
so·lar·i·um [sə'leərɪəm] n Solarium nt.
so·lar·i·za·tion [,səʊlərɪ'zeɪʃn] n Lichtbehandlung f, -therapie f.
so·lar·ize ['səʊləraɪz] vt jdn. mit Lichtbädern behandeln.
solar keratosis aktinische/senile/solare Keratose f, Keratosis actinica/senilis/solaris.
solar plexus Sonnengeflecht nt, Plexus solaris, Plexus coeliacus.
solar power → solar energy.
solar spectrum Sonnenlichtspektrum nt, Spektrum nt des Sonnenlichtes.
solar treatment Behandlung f mit Sonnenlicht, Heliotherapie f.
solar urticaria Sonnen-, Sommer-, Lichturtikaria f, photoallergische Urtikaria f, Urticaria solaris/photogenica.
sol·der ['sadər] **I** n ortho., techn. Lot m, Lötmetall nt. **II** vt, vi ortho., techn. löten.
sol·dier's heart ['səʊldʒər] n neurozirkulatorische Asthenie f, Soldatenherz nt, Effort-Syndrom nt, Da Costa-Syndrom nt, Phrenikokardie f.
sole [səʊl] **I** n **1.** (Fuß-)Sohle f; anat. Planta pedis, Regio plantaris pedis. **2.** (Schuh-)Sohle f. **3.** techn. Bodenfläche f, Sohle f. **II** adj einzig, allein, Allein-.
so·le·al line (of tibia) ['səʊlɪəl] Linea m. solei.
so·le·noid ['səʊlənɔɪd] n phys. (Zylinder-)Spule f, Solenoid n.
sole reflex Plantarreflex m.
sole tap reflex Weingrow-Reflex m.
so·le·us (muscle) ['səʊlɪəs] Soleus m, M. soleus.
sol·id ['salɪd] **I** n **1.** ~s pl feste Bestandteile pl (in Flüssigkeiten). **2.** ~s pl feste Nahrung f. **to put a baby on** ~. **3.** phys. Festkörper m. **4.** mathe. Körper m. **II** adj **5.** fest, hart, kompakt; dicht. **6.** stabil (gebaut), massiv; (Körperbau) kräftig; (Essen) kräftig; **7.** mathe. räumlich, körperlich, Raum-.
solid body Festkörper m.
solid bone Kompakta f, Substantia compacta.
solid carcinoma solides Karzinom nt, Ca. solidum.
solid chemistry Festkörperchemie f.
solid edema Myxödem nt, Myxoedema nt, Myxodermia diffusa.
so·lid·i·fi·ca·tion [sə,lɪdəfɪ'keɪʃn] n Hart-, Festwerden nt; Erstarrung f, Erstarren nt.
so·lid·i·fy [sə'lɪdɪfaɪ] **I** vt fest werden lassen; erstarren lassen. **II** vi hart od. fest werden, s. festigen, erstarren.
so·lid·i·ty [sə'lɪdətɪ] n kompakte od. massive Struktur f, Festigkeit f, Dichtheit f, Dichtigkeit f.
solid phase feste Phase f.
solid-phase technique biochem. Festphasentechnik f.
solid physics Festkörperphysik f.
solid state phys. fester (Aggregat-)Zustand m.
solid teratoma embryonales/unreifes/malignes Teratom nt, Teratoma embryonale.
solid viscera parenchymatöse Organe pl.
sol·i·tar·y ['salə,terɪ; -tərɪ] adj (a. bio.) allein, abgesondert, allein-, einzellebend, vereinzelt, einzeln, solitär, Einzel-, Solitär-.
solitary bundle → solitary tract of medulla oblongata.
solitary enostosis Knocheninsel f, solitäre Enostose f.
solitary fasciculus → solitary tract of medulla oblongata.
solitary lesion Solitärläsion f.
solitary metastasis Solitärmetastase f.
solitary myeloma solitäres/lokalisiertes Myelom/Plasmozytom nt.
solitary nodule Solitärknoten m.
solitary nucleus Nc. (tractus) solitarius.
solitary tapeworm micro. Schweine(finnen)bandwurm m, Taenia solium.
solitary tract of medulla oblongata Tractus solitarius (medullae oblongatae).
sol·u·bil·i·ty [,saljə'bɪlətɪ] n chem. Löslichkeit f, Solubilität f.
solubility coefficient abbr. α phys. Bunsen'-Löslichkeitskoeffizient m abbr. α.
solubility product abbr. L Löslichkeitsprodukt nt abbr. L.
sol·u·bi·li·za·tion [,saljəbəlɪ'zeɪʃn] n Solubilisation f.
sol·u·bi·lize ['saljəbɪlaɪz] vt löslich machen.
sol·u·ble ['saljəbl] adj löslich, (auf-)lösbar, solubel.
soluble glass Wasserglas nt.
soluble-RNA n Transfer-RNS f abbr. tRNS, Tranfer-RNA f abbr. tRNA.
so·lute ['saljuːt] **I** n gelöster Stoff m, gelöste Substanz f. **II** adj (auf-)gelöst, in Lösung.
so·lu·tion [sə'luːʃn] n **1.** chem., pharm. Lösung f, Solution f, Solutio f. **2.** Auflösen nt. **3.** (Auf-)Lösung f (to, of). **4.** patho. (Ab-)Lösung f, Solutio f.
solv·a·ble ['salvəbl] adj → soluble.
solv·ate ['salveɪt] n Solvat nt.
solv·a·tion [sal'veɪʃn] n Solvatation f, Solvation f.
sol·vent ['salvənt] **I** n Lösungsmittel nt, Solvens nt. **II** adj (auf-)lösend.

solvent fractionation phys., chem. Fraktionierung f durch Lösungsmittel, Aussüßen nt.
solvent front phys. Lösungsmittelfront f.
solvent property phys. Lösungseigenschaft f.
so·ma ['səʊmə] n, pl **-mas, -ma·ta** [-mətə] **1.** Körper m, Soma nt. **2.** histol. Zellkörper m, Soma nt.
so·mal ['səʊməl] adj → somatic.
so·man ['səʊmən] n Soman nt.
so·ma·plasm ['səʊməplæzəm] n → somatoplasm.
som·as·the·nia [,səʊmæs'θiːnɪə] n Somasthenie f.
somat- pref. → somato-.
so·mat·ag·no·sia [,səʊmətæg'nəʊsɪə] n Somatagnosie f.
so·mat·al·gia [,səʊmə'tældʒ(ɪ)ə] n **1.** Körperschmerz m, somatischer Schmerz m, Somatalgie f. **2.** somatischer Schmerz m.
so·mat·es·the·nia [,səʊmətes'θiːnɪə] n → somasthenia.
so·mat·es·the·sia [,-'θiːʒ(ɪ)ə] n Somat(o)-ästhesie f.
so·mat·es·thet·ic [,-'θetɪk] adj Somat(o)ästhesie betr., somat(o)ästhetisch.
so·mat·ic [səʊ'mætɪk, sə-] adj Körper/Soma betr., zum Körper behörend, somatisch, körperlich, Soma(to)-.
somatic agglutinin Körperagglutinin nt, O-Agglutinin nt.
somatic antigen Körperantigen nt, O-Antigen nt.
somatic cell Körperzelle f, somatische Zelle f.
somatic delusion hypochondrischer Wahn m.
somatic evoked potential abbr. **SEP** somatisch/somatosensorisch evoziertes Potential nt abbr. SEP.
somatic hallucination psychia. somatische Halluzination f.
somatic mesoderm embryo. parietales Mesoderm nt.
somatic muscles → skeletal muscles 1.
somatic mutation somatische Mutation f.
somatic nervous system 1. bio. animalisches Nervensystem nt. **2.** somatisches Nervensystem nt.
somatic neurofibers somatische Nervenfasern pl, Neurofibrae somaticae.
so·mat·i·co·splanch·nic [səʊ,mætɪkəʊ-'splæŋknɪk] adj → somaticovisceral.
so·mat·i·co·vis·cer·al [,-'vɪsərəl] adj Körper/Soma u. Eingeweide/Viscera betr., somatovisceral.
somatic pain somatischer Schmerz m.
somatic sensory area/cortex → somatosensory area.
somatic system → somatic nervous system.
so·mat·i·za·tion [sə,mætə'zeɪʃn, ,səʊmətə-] n psychia. Somatisation f, Somatisierungssyndrom nt.
somato- pref. Körper, Soma(to)-.
so·mat·o·cep·tor [sə'mætəseptər] n Somatozeptor m.
so·ma·to·did·y·mus [,səʊmətəʊ'dɪdəməs] n embryo. Somatodidymus m.
so·ma·to·dym·i·a [,-'diːmɪə] n embryo. Somatodymie f.
so·ma·to·form [sə'mætəfɔːrm] adj psychia. somatoform.
so·ma·to·gen·e·sis [,səʊmətə'dʒenəsɪs] n embryo. Somatogenese f.
so·ma·to·ge·net·ic [sə,mætədʒɪ'netɪk] adj **1.** Somatogenese betr., somatogenetisch. **2.** → somatogenic.
so·ma·to·gen·ic [,səʊmətə'dʒenɪk] adj vom Körper verursacht, körperlich, somatogen.

somatogram 708

so·mat·o·gram [sə'mætəɡræm, səʊ-] n Somatogramm nt.
so·mat·o·in·tes·ti·nal reflex [ˌsəʊmətəʊɪn-'testənl] somatointestinaler Reflex m.
so·ma·tol·o·gy [ˌsəʊmə'talədʒɪ] n Körperlehre f, Somatologie f.
so·ma·to·mam·mo·tro·pine [ˌsəʊmətəʊˌmæmə'trəʊpiːn, -pɪn] n 1. Somatomammotropin nt. 2. old humanes Plazenta-Laktogen nt abbr. HPL, Chorionsomatotropin nt.
so·ma·to·me·din [ˌ-'miːdn] n Somatomedin nt, sulfation factor (m).
somatomedin C Somatomedin C nt.
so·ma·to·meg·a·ly [ˌ-'meɡəlɪ] n Riesenwuchs m, Gigantismus m, Somatomegalie f.
so·ma·tom·e·try [ˌsəʊmə'tamətrɪ] n Somatometrie f.
so·ma·to·mo·tor [ˌsəʊmətə'məʊtər] adj somatomotorisch.
somatomotor fiber somatomotorische (Nerven-)Faser f.
somatomotor nuclei somatomotorische Kerne pl.
somatomotor system somatomotorisches System nt, Somatomotorik f.
so·ma·top·a·gus [ˌsəʊmə'tapəɡəs] n embryo. Somatopagus m.
so·ma·to·path·ic [ˌsəʊmətə'pæθɪk] adj (Erkrankung) körperlich, organisch, somatisch.
so·ma·top·a·thy [ˌsəʊmə'tapəθɪ] n körperliche/somatische/organische Erkrankung f.
so·ma·to·phre·nia [ˌsəʊmətə'friːnɪə] n psychia. Somatophrenie f.
so·mat·o·plasm [sə'mætəplæzəm] n histol. Somatoplasma nt.
so·ma·to·pleur·al [ˌsəʊmətə'plʊərəl] adj embryo. Somatopleura betr., somatopleural.
so·mat·o·pleure [sə'mætəplʊər] n embryo. Somatopleura f.
so·ma·to·pleu·ric mesoderm [ˌsəʊmətəʊ-'plʊərɪk] embryo. somatopleurales Mesoderm nt.
so·ma·to·psy·chic [ˌ-'saɪkɪk] adj Körper/Soma u. Geist/Psyche betr., psychosomatisch.
so·ma·tos·co·py [ˌsəʊmə'taskəpɪ] n körperliche Untersuchung f, Untersuchung f des Körpers, Somatoskopie f.
so·ma·to·sen·so·ry [ˌsəʊmətəʊ'sensərɪ] adj somatosensorisch.
somatosensory area/cortex somatosensorische Rinde f, somatosensorischer Kortex m.
somatosensory fiber somatosensorische (Nerven-)Faser f.
somatosensory system somatosensorisches System nt, Somatosensorik f.
so·ma·to·sex·u·al [ˌ-'sekʃəwəl] adj somatosexuell.
somato-somatic synapse somato-somatische Synapse f.
so·ma·to·stat·in [ˌ-'stætɪn] n Somatostatin nt, growth hormone release inhibiting hormone abbr. GH-RIH, somatotropin inhibiting hormone/factor abbr. SH-IF, somatotropin release inhibiting hormone/factor abbr. SR-IF, growth hormone inhibiting factor abbr. GH-IF.
so·ma·to·stat·i·no·ma [ˌ-stætɪ'nəʊmə] n Somatostatinom nt, D-Zell(en)-Tumor m.
so·ma·to·sym·pa·thet·ic reflex [ˌ-ˌsɪmpə-'θetɪk] somatosympathischer Reflex m.
so·ma·to·ther·a·py [ˌ-'θerəpɪ] n Somatotherapie f.
so·ma·to·top·ic [ˌ-'tapɪk] adj somatotopisch.

so·ma·to·top·i·cal [ˌ-'tapɪkl] adj → somatotopic.
so·ma·to·top·o·py [ˌsəʊmə'tatəpɪ] n Somatotopie f.
so·mat·o·trope [səʊ'mætətrəʊp] n → somatotroph cell.
so·mat·o·troph [səʊ'mætətrəʊf] n → somatotroph cell.
somatotroph cell (Adenohypophyse) somatotrophe Zelle f.
so·ma·to·troph·ic [ˌsəʊmətəʊ'trəʊfɪk] adj → somatotropic.
so·ma·to·tro·phin [ˌ-'trəʊfɪn] n → somatotropin.
so·ma·to·trop·ic [ˌ-'trapɪk] adj somatotrop.
somatotropic cell → somatotroph cell.
somatotropic hormone abbr. **STH** → somatotropin.
so·ma·to·tro·pin [ˌ-'trəʊpɪn] n Somatotropin nt, somatotropes Hormon nt abbr. STH, Wachstumshormon nt.
somatotropin inhibiting factor abbr. **SH-IF** → somatostatin.
somatotropin release inhibiting factor abbr. **SR-IF** → somatostatin.
somatotropin releasing factor abbr. **SRF** Somatoliberin nt, Somatotropin-releasing-Faktor m abbr. SRF, growth hormone releasing hormone releasing factor abbr. GRF, GH-RF, growth hormone releasing hormone abbr. GRH, GH-RH.
somatotropin releasing hormone abbr. **SRH** → somatotropin releasing factor.
so·ma·to·vis·cer·al [ˌ-'vɪsərəl] adj somatoviszeral.
so·mat·ro·pin [səʊ'mætrəpɪn] n → somatotropin.
som·es·the·sia [ˌsəʊmes'θiːʒ(ɪ)ə] n → somatesthesia.
som·es·thet·ic [ˌsəʊmes'θetɪk] adj → somatesthetic.
somesthetic area/cortex → somatosensory area.
somesthetic sensibility proprio(re)zeptive/kinästhetische Sensibilität f, Tiefensensibilität f, Proprio(re)zeption f.
so·mite ['səʊmaɪt] n Ursegment nt, Somit m.
so·mi·to·mere [sə'mɪtəmɪər] n embryo. Somitomer nt.
som·nam·bu·lance [sam'næmbjələns] n → somnambulism.
som·nam·bu·la·tion [samˌnæmbjə'leɪʃn] n → somnambulism.
som·nam·bu·lism [sam'næmbjəlɪzəm] n Nacht-, Schlafwandeln nt, Somnambulismus m, Noktambulismus m.
som·nam·bu·list [sam'næmbjəlɪst] n Nacht-, Schlafwandler(in f) m, Somnambulist m.
somni- pref. Schlaf-, Nacht-, Somn(o)-, Somni-.
som·ni·fa·cient [ˌsamnɪ'feɪʃənt] I n Schlafmittel nt, Somniferum n, Hypnotikum nt. II adj einschläfernd, hypnotisch.
som·nif·er·ous [sam'nɪfərəs] adj → somnifacient II.
som·nif·ic [sam'nɪfɪk] adj → somnifacient II.
som·nil·o·quence [sam'nɪləkwəns] n → somniloquism.
som·nil·o·quism [sam'nɪləkwɪzəm] n Sprechen nt im Schlaf, Somniloquie f.
som·nil·o·quy [sam'nɪləkwɪ] n → somniloquism.
som·no·lence ['samnələns] n (krankhafte) Schläfrigkeit f, Benommenheit f, Somnolenz f.
som·no·lent ['samnələnt] adj 1. schläfrig, somnolent. 2. bewußtseinseingetrübt, -beeinträchtigt, somnolent.

som·no·len·tia [ˌsamnə'lenʃɪə] n 1. Schlaftrunkenheit f. 2. → somnolence.
som·no·les·cent [ˌsamnə'lesənt] adj schläfrig.
sonde [sand] n Sonde f.
sone [səʊn] n phys. Sone nt.
Son·go fever ['sɔnɡəʊ] hämorrhagisches Fieber nt mit renalem Syndrom abbr. HFRS, koreanisches hämorrhagisches Fieber nt, akute hämorrhagische Nephrosonephritis f, Nephropathia epidemica.
son·ic ['sanɪk] adj phys. Schall-.
son·i·cate ['sanɪkeɪt] vt mit Schallwellen behandeln, beschallen.
son·i·ca·tion [sanɪ'keɪʃn] n 1. Behandlung f mit Schallwellen, Beschallung f. 2. Zerstörung f durch Schallwellen, Soni(fi)kation f.
sonic wave phys. Schallwelle f.
son·i·tus ['sanɪtəs] n HNO Ohrklingen nt, Sonitus (aurium) m.
Sonne ['sanə]: **S. bacillus** Kruse-Sonne-Ruhrbakterium nt, E-Ruhrbakterium nt, Shigella sonnei.
Sonne-Duval [dy'val]: **S.-D. bacillus** → Sonne bacillus.
son·o·gram ['sanəɡræf] n radiol. Sonogramm nt.
son·o·graph ['-ɡræf] n radiol. Ultraschallgerät nt, Sonograph m.
so·no·graph·ic [ˌ-'ɡræfɪk] adj Sonographie betr., sonographisch.
sonographic examination sonographische Untersuchung f.
real-time s. Real-time-Technik f, Echt-Zeit-Verfahren nt.
so·nog·ra·phy [sə'naɡrəfɪ] n radiol. Ultraschalldiagnostik f, Sonographie f.
so·no·lu·cen·cy [sanə'luːsnsɪ] n (Ultra-)Schalldurchlässigkeit f.
so·no·lu·cent [ˌ-'luːsnt] adj radiol. (ultra-)schalldurchlässig.
so·no·rous [sə'nɔːrəs, 'sanə-] adj tönend, resonant, klangvoll, sonor.
sonorous breathing → stertor.
sonorous rales sonore Pleurageräusche pl.
sonorous rhonchi brummende Rasselgeräusche pl, Brummen nt.
soot cancer [sʊt] Kaminkehrer-, Schornsteinfegerkrebs m.
soot wart → soot cancer.
soph·o·ma·nia [safə'meɪnɪə, -jə] n psychia. Sophomanie f.
soph·o·rin ['safərɪn] n Rutin nt, Rutosid nt.
soph·o·rine ['safəriːn, -rɪn, sə'fəʊ-] n Zytisin nt, Cytisin nt.
so·por ['səʊpər, -pɔːr] n neurol. Sopor m.
so·po·rif·er·ous [ˌsapə'rɪfərəs, ˌsəʊp-] adj einschläfernd.
so·po·rif·ic [ˌ-'rɪfɪk] I n Schlafmittel nt, Somniferum nt, Hypnotikum nt. II adj einschläfernd.
sorb [sɔːb] vt ab-, adsorbieren.
sor·be·fa·cient [sɔːrbə'feɪʃnt] I n absorptionsförderndes Mittel nt. II adj absorptionsfördernd, absorbierend.
sor·bent ['sɔːbənt] n Sorptionsmittel nt, Sorbens nt.
sor·bic acid ['sɔːbɪk] 2,4-Hexadiensäure f, Sorbinsäure f.
sor·bin ['sɔːbɪn] n → sorbose.
sor·bi·nose ['sɔːbɪnəʊs] n → sorbose.
sor·bite ['sɔːbaɪt] n → sorbitol.
sor·bi·tol ['sɔːbɪtɒl, -təʊl] n Sorbit nt, Sorbitol nt, Glucit nt, Glucitol nt.
sorbitol dehydrogenase L-Iditoldehydrogenase f, Iditdehydrogenase f, Sorbitdehydrogenase f abbr. SHD.
sor·bose ['sɔːbəʊz] n Sorbose f.

sor·des ['sɔːrdiːz] *pl* **sor·des** Schmutz *m*, Abfall *m*, Sordes *pl*.
sor·did ['sɔːrdɪd] *adj* schmutzig.
sore [sɔʊr; sɔːr] **I** *n* (Haut-, Schleimhaut-)-Wunde *f*, Entzündung *f*, wunde Stelle *f*. **II** *adj* weh, wund, schmerzhaft; entzündet.
sore mouth Orf *m*, Ecthyma contagiosum/infectiosum, Steinpocken *pl*, atypische Schafpocken *pl*, Stomatitis pustulosa contagiosa.
Sörensen ['sɔːrənsen]: **S. scale** pH-Skala *f*.
Soret [sɔ'rɛ]: **S. band** Soret-Bande *f*.
sore throat Halsentzündung *f*; Angina *f*.
  croupous s. Angina crouposa.
  epidemic streptococcal s. Streptokokkenpharyngitis *f*, -angina.
  Fothergill's s. Scarlatina anginosa.
  pseudomembranous s. → croupous s.
  septic s. Streptokokkenpharyngitis *f*, -angina.
  simple s. Angina (catarrhalis) simplex.
  spotted s. Kryptentonsillitis *f*, Angina follicularis.
  streptococcal s. → septic s.
sorp·tion ['sɔːrpʃn] *n chem.* (Ab-, Re-)-Sorption *f*.
Sorsby ['sɔːrsbɪ]: **S.'s syndrome** Sorsby-Syndrom *nt*.
so·rus ['sɔʊrəs, 'sɔː-] *n*, *pl* **-ri** [-raɪ] *bio., micro.* Sporenhäufchen *nt*, Sorus *m*.
so·ta·lol ['sɔʊtəlɒl, -lɔl] *n pharm.* Sotalol *nt*.
Sotos ['sɔʊtəs]: **S.' syndrome (of cerebral gigantism)** Sotos-Syndrom *nt*.
souf·fle ['suːfl] *n card.* blasendes Geräusch *nt*.
soul blindness [sɔʊl] zerebral-/organbedingte Blindheit *f*.
sound[1] [saʊnd] **I** *n* Ton *m*, Klang *m*, Laut *m*, Schall *m*; Geräusch *nt*. **within ~** in Hörweite. **without a ~** geräuschlos. **II** *vi* 1. be-, abhorchen. 2. (er-)schallen, (er-)klingen, schallen.
sound[2] [saʊnd] *adj* 1. gesund. 2. intakt; vernünftig; (*Schlaf*) tief; (*Wissen*) fundiert; (*Geist*) gesund, normal.
sound[3] [saʊnd] **I** *n* Sonde *f*. **II** *vi* sondieren.
sound-conducting *adj* schalleitend.
sound-conducting apparatus Schalleitungsapparat *m*.
sound conduction Schalleitung *f*.
sound conductivity Schalleitfähigkeit *f*.
sound energy Schallenergie *f*.
sound frequency Schallfrequenz *f*.
sound frequency adjustment Schallfrequenzabstimmung *f*.
sound frequency coding Schallfrequenzkodierung *f*.
sound·ing ['saʊndɪŋ] *adj* schallend, tönend.
sound intensity Schallintensität *f*.
sound intensity coding Schallintensitätskodierung *f*.
sound·less ['saʊndlɪs] *adj* still, laut-, geräuschlos; klanglos.
sound·ness ['saʊndnɪs] *n* Gesundheit *f*.
sound pressure Schalldruck *m*.
sound pressure level *abbr.* **SPL** Schalldruckpegel *m*.
sound pressure transformation Schalldrucktransformation *f*.
sound spectrogram Schallspektrogramm *nt*.
sound spectrography Schallspektrographie *f*.
sound wave *phys.* Schallwelle *f*.
source ['sɔʊrs, 'sɔːrs] *n* Quelle *f*; Ursprung *m*, Ursache *f*.
  s. of disturbance Störquelle *f*.
  s. of error Fehlerquelle *f*.
  s. of infection Infektionsquelle, Herd *m*, Fokus *m*.
  s. of light Lichtquelle.
South Af·ri·can [saʊθ 'æfrɪkən]: **S. A. genetic porphyria** gemischte (hepatische) Porphyrie *f*, südafrikanische genetische Porphyrie *f*, (hereditäre) Protokoproporphyrie *f*, Porphyria variegata *abbr.* **PV**.
  S. A. tick-bite fever Boutonneusefieber *nt*, Fièvre boutonneuse.
  S. A. tick fever südafrikanisches Zeckenfieber *nt*.
South A·mer·i·can [ə'merɪkən]: **S. A. blastomycosis** Lutz-Splendore-Almeida--Krankheit *f*, brasilianische/südamerikanische Blastomykose *f*, Parakokzidioidomykose *f*, Granuloma paracoccidioides.
  S. A. cutaneous leishmaniasis südamerikanische Hautleishmaniase *f*, kutane Leishmaniase Südamerikas *f*, Chiclero--Ulkus *nt*.
  S. A. pemphigus brasilianischer Pemphigus *m*, brasilianischer Pemphigus foliaceus *m*, Pemphigus brasiliensis, Fogo Salvagem.
  S. A. trypanosomiasis Chagas-Krankheit *f*, amerikanische Trypanosomiasis *f*.
South·ern ['sʌðərn]: **S. blot technique** *immun.* Southern-Blot-Technik *f*.
soy·a ['sɔɪə] *n* → soybean.
soy·bean ['sɔɪbiːn] *n* Sojabohne *f*.
SPA *abbr.* → stimulation produced analgesia.
spa [spɑː] *n* 1. Mineralquelle *f*. 2. Bade-, Kurort *m*, Bad *nt*.
space [speɪs] **I** *n* 1. (*a. anat.*) Raum *m*, Platz *m*; Zwischenraum *m*, Abstand *m*, Lücke *f*, Spalt *m*; Zeitraum *m*. 2. (Welt-)Raum *m*, Weltall *nt*. **II** *vt* räumlich *od.* zeitlich einteilen; in Abständen verteilen.
  s.s of Fontana (*Auge*) Fontana'-Räume *pl*, Spatia anguli iridocornealis.
  s.s of iridocorneal angle → s.s of Fontana
space diet Astronautenkost *f*.
space-filling model *chem.* Raummodell *nt*, Kalottenmodell *nt*.
space lattice *phys.* Raumgitter *nt*.
space medicine Raumfahrtmedizin *f*.
spac·er ['speɪsər] *n genet.* Zwischenstück *nt*, Spacer *m*.
spacer DNA Spacer-DNA *f*, Regulator--DNA *f*.
space sense Raumsinn *m*.
Spalding ['spɔːldɪŋ]: **S.'s sign** *gyn.* Spalding-Zeichen *nt*.
span [spæn] **I** *n* Spanne *f*; (Gedächtnis-, Zeit-)Spanne *f*. **II** *vt* 1. abmessen. 2. umspannen.
Span·ish ['spænɪʃ]: **S. collar** *urol.* Paraphimose *f*, Capistratio *f*.
  S. fly Blasenkäfer *m*, spanische Fliege *f*, Lytta/Cantharis vesicatoria.
  S. influenza spanische Grippe *f*.
  S. relapsing fever spanisches Rückfallfieber *nt*.
  S. tourniquet *ortho.* Abbindung *f*.
  S. white basisches Wismutnitrat *nt*, Bismutum subnitricum.
  S. windlass *ortho.* Abbindung *f*.
spark [spɑːrk] **I** *n* 1. Funke(n *m*) *m*; (elektrischer) Funke *m*. 2. *fig.* Funke *m*; Spur *f* (*of* von). **II** *vt* → spark off.
spark off *vt fig.* etw. auslösen.
spark chamber Funkenkammer *f*.
spark coil *phys.* Funkeninduktor *m*.
spark discharge *phys.* Funkenentladung *f*.
spark·ing ['spɑːrkɪŋ] *n phys.* Funkenbildung *f*.
spar·te·ine ['spɑːrtiːn, -tiɪn] *n* Spartein *nt*.
spasm- *pref.* → spasmo-.
spasm ['spæzəm] *n* 1. Krampf *m*, Verkrampfung *f*, Spasmus *m*; Konvulsion *f*. 2. Muskelkrampf *m*.
spasmo- *pref.* Krampf-, Spasm(o)-.
spas·mod·ic [spæz'mɒdɪk] *adj* krampfartig, spasmisch, spasmodisch.
spasmodic asthma Bronchialasthma *nt*, Asthma bronchiale.
spasmodic croup falscher Krupp *m*, Pseudokrupp *m*, subglottische Laryngitis *f*, Laryngitis subglottica.
spasmodic hiccup → spasmolygmus.
spasmodic laryngitis Laryngitis stridulosa.
spasmodic mydriasis → spastic mydriasis.
spasmodic sneezing Nieskrampf *m*, Ptarmus *m*.
spasmodic stricture funktionelle/spastische Striktur *f*.
spasmodic torticollis *ortho.* intermittierender Schiefhals/Torticollis *m*.
spas·mo·gen ['spæzmədʒən] *n* krampfauslösende/spasmogene Substanz *f*.
spas·mo·gen·ic [,-'dʒenɪk] *adj* krampfauslösend, krampferzeugend, spasmogen.
spas·mol·o·gy [spæz'mɒlədʒɪ] *n* Spasmologie *f*.
spas·mo·lyg·mus [,spæzmə'lɪgməs] *n* krampfartiger Schluckauf *m*, Spasmolygmus *m*.
spas·mol·y·sant [spæz'mɒlɪsənt] **I** *n* krampflösende *od.* krampfmildernde Substanz *f*; Antispasmodikum *nt*; Spasmolytikum *nt*. **II** *adj* krampflösend, -milderd.
spas·mol·y·sis [spæz'mɒləsɪs] *n* Krampflösung *f*, Spasmolyse *f*.
spas·mo·lyt·ic [,spæzmə'lɪtɪk] *adj* krampflösend, spasmolytisch.
spas·mo·phile ['-faɪl] *adj* → spasmophilic.
spas·mo·phil·ia [,-'fɪlɪə] *n* spasmophile Diathese *f*, (latente) Spasmophilie *f*.
spas·mo·phil·ic [,-'fɪlɪk] *adj* zu Krämpfen neigend, spasmophil.
spasmophilic diathesis → spasmophilia.
spas·mus ['spæzməs] *n* → spasm.
spas·tic ['spæstɪk] **I** *n* Spastiker(in *f*) *m*. **II** *adj* Spastik *od.* Spasmen betr., spastisch, krampfend, krampfartig, Krampf-.
spastic abasia spastische Abasie *f*.
spastic aphonia spastische Aphonie *f*.
spastic bladder *neuro.* Reflexblase *f*.
spastic clubfoot *ortho.* spastischer Klumpfuß *m*.
spastic colon Reizkolon *nt*, irritables/spastisches Kolon *nt*, Kolonneurose *f*, Colon irritabile/spasticum.
spastic diplegia 1. Erb-Charcot-Syndrom *nt*, spastische Spinalparalyse *f*. 2. Little'--Krankheit *f*, Diplegia spastica infantilis.
spastic ectropion *ophthal.* Ektropium spasticum.
spastic gait *neuro.* spastischer Gang *m*.
spastic hemiplegia spastische Hemiplegie *f*, Hemiplegia spastica.
spastic ileus spastischer Darmverschluß/Ileus *m*.
spas·tic·i·ty [spæs'tɪsətɪ] *n* Spastizität *f*.
spastic mydriasis *ophthal.* spastische Mydriasis *f*, Mydriasis spastica.
spastic paraplegia spastische Paraplegie *f*.
spastic pseudoparalysis Creutzfeldt--Jakob-Syndrom *nt*, -Erkrankung *f abbr.* **CJE**, Jakob-Creutzfeldt-Syndrom *nt*, -Erkrankung *f*.
spastic pseudosclerosis → spastic pseudoparalysis.
spastic stricture funktionelle/spastische Striktur *f*.
spastic torticollis *ortho.* spastischer Schiefhals *m*, Torticollis spasticus.

spatial

spa·tial ['speɪʃl] *adj* räumlich, Raum-.
spatial arrangement räumliche Anordnung/Formation *f*.
spatial dimension Raumdimension *f*.
spatial disorientation räumliche Desorientiertheit *f*.
spatial facilitation *physiol.* räumliche Bahnung *f*.
spatial formula *chem.* Raumformel *f*, stereochemische Formel *f*.
spatial isomerism → stereoisomerism.
spatial orientation räumliche Orientierung *f*.
spatial resolution räumliche Auflösung *f*, räumliches Auflösungsvermögen *nt*.
spatial summation *physiol.* räumliche Summation *f*.
spatial vector *mathe., phys.* Raumvektor *m*.
spa·ti·um ['speɪʃɪəm] *n, pl* **-tia** [-ʃɪə] *anat.* Raum *m*, Zwischenraum *m*, Spatium *nt*.
spat·u·la ['spætʃələ] *n chir.* Spatel *m*.
spatula foot *ortho., embryo.* Löffel-, Flossenfuß *m*.
spat·u·lar ['spætʃələr] *adj, vt* → spatulate.
spat·u·late ['spætʃəleɪt, -lɪt] **I** *adj* spatelförmig, spatelig. **II** *vt* mit einem Spatel behandeln.
SPCA *abbr.* → serum prothrombin conversion accelerator.
spe·cial ['speʃəl] *adj* speziell, besonders, Spezial-, Fach-, Sonder-.
special anatomy spezielle Anatomie *f*.
spe·cial·ist ['speʃəlɪst] **I** *n* Spezialist(in *f*) *m*, Facharzt *m*, -ärztin *f*; Fachmann *m*. **II** *adj* spezialisiert, Spezial-, Fach-.
spe·cial·i·za·tion [ˌspeʃəlɪ'zeɪʃn] *n* Spezialisierung *f*.
spe·cial·ize ['speʃəlaɪz] **I** *vi* **1.** spezialisieren. **II** *vi* **3. s.** spezialisieren. **4.** *histol.* (*Organ*) s. besonders entwickeln.
spe·cial·ized transduction ['speʃəlaɪzd] spezialisierte/begrenzte Transduktion *f*.
special pathology spezielle Pathologie *f*.
spe·ci·a·tion [spi:ʃɪ'eɪʃn] *n bio.* Artbildung *f*, -entstehung *f*, Speziation *f*.
spe·cies ['spi:ʃi:z, -sɪz] *n, pl* **-cies** *bio.* **1.** Art *f*, Spezies *f*, Species *f*; Gattung *f*. **2. the ~** die Menschheit, die menschliche Rasse.
species diversity Artenvielfalt *f*.
species formation → speciation.
species immunity absolute Wirtsresistenz *f*.
species population Artenpopulation *f*.
species preservation Arterhaltung *f*.
species-preserving *adj* arterhaltend.
species protection Artenschutz *m*.
species-specific *adj* spezies-, artspezifisch.
species-specific antigen speziesspezifisches Antigen *nt*.
species specificity *bio.* Art-, Speziesspezifität *f*.
spe·cif·ic [spɪ'sɪfɪk] **I** *n* spezifisches Heilmittel *nt*, Spezifikum *nt*. **II** *adj* **1.** *bio.* Spezies betr., artspezifisch, Arten-. **2.** spezifisch (wirkend), gezielt. **3.** *phys.* spezifisch. **4.** charakteristisch, (art-)eigen, bestimmte(r, s), speziell, spezifisch.
specific activity *biochem.* spezifische Aktivität *f*.
spec·i·fi·ca·tion [ˌspesəfɪ'keɪʃn] *n* (genaue) Beschreibung *od.* Angabe *f*, Spezifikation *f*, Spezifizierung *f*.
specific character *bio.* Artmerkmal *nt*.
specific cholinesterase Azetyl-, Acetylcholinesterase *f abbr.* AChE, echte Cholinesterase *f*.
specific compliance (of lung) spezifische Compliance *f*.

specific disease spezifische Erkrankung/Krankheit/Infektion *f*.
specific dynamic action *abbr.* **S.D.A.** *biochem., physiol.* spezifisch-dynamische Wirkung *f*.
specific dynamic effect *abbr.* **S.D.E.** → specific dynamic action.
specific gravity *phys.* spezifisches Gewicht *nt*.
specific heat *phys.* spezifische Wärme *f*.
specific immunity spezifische Immunität *f*.
specific inflammation spezifische Entzündung *f*.
spec·i·fic·i·ty [ˌspesə'fɪsətɪ] *n* spezifische Eigenschaft *f*, Spezifität *f*.
specific macrophage arming factor *abbr.* **SMAF** specific macrophage arming factor *abbr.* SMAF.
spe·cif·ic·ness [spɪ'sɪfɪknɪs] *n* → specificity.
specific reaction *immun.* spezifische Immunreaktion *f*.
specific rotation *phys.* spezifische Drehung *f*.
specific serum monovalentes/spezifisches Serum *nt*.
specific therapy spezifische Behandlung *f*.
specific transduction → specialized transduction.
specific treatment → specific therapy.
specific urethritis gonorrhoische Urethritis *f*, Urethritis gonorrhoica.
specific weight *phys.* spezifisches Gewicht *nt*, Wichte *f*.
spec·i·men ['spesɪmən] *n* **1.** (Gewebs-, Blut-, Urin-)Probe *f*, Untersuchungsmaterial *nt*. **2.** Exemplar *nt*, Muster *nt*, Probe(stück *nt*) *f*.
speck·led spleen ['spekəld] Fleckenmilz *f*.
spec·ta·cle ['spektəkl] **I** *(pair of)* **~s** *pl* Brille *f*. **II** *adj* Brillen-.
spec·ta·cled ['spektəkld] *adj* mit Brille, bebrillt, brillentragend, Brillen-.
spec·ti·no·my·cin [ˌspektɪnəʊ'maɪsɪn] *n pharm.* Spectinomycin *nt*.
spec·tral ['spektrəl] *adj* Spektrum betr., spektral, Spektral-, Spektro-.
spectral analysis Spektralanalyse *f*, spektroskopische Analyse *f*.
spectral color Spektralfarbe *f*.
spectral line Spektrallinie *f*.
spectral reflectance *phys.* spektrale Reflektanz *f*.
spec·trin ['spektrɪn] *n* Spektrin *nt*, Spectrin *nt*.
spec·tro·col·o·rim·e·ter [ˌspektrəʊˌkʌlə'rɪmətər] *n* Spektrokolorimeter *nt*.
spec·tro·flu·o·rom·e·ter [ˌ-flʊə'rɒmətər] *n* Spektrofluorometer *nt*.
spec·tro·gram ['-græm] *n* Spektrogramm *nt*.
spec·tro·graph ['-græf] *n* Spektrograph *m*.
spec·trog·ra·phy [spek'tɑgrəfɪ] *n* Spektrographie *f*.
spec·trom·e·ter [spek'trɑmətər] *n* **1.** Spektralapparat *m*, Spektrometer *nt*. **2.** Spektroskop *nt*.
spec·tro·met·ric [ˌspektrə'metrɪk] *adj* spektrometrisch.
spec·trom·e·try [spek'trɑmətrɪ] *n* Spektrometrie *f*.
spec·tro·pho·to·flu·o·rom·e·ter [ˌspektrəʊˌfəʊtəʊflʊə'rɒmətər] *n* Spektrophotofluorometer *nt*.
spec·tro·pho·tom·e·ter [ˌ-fəʊ'tɑmətər] *n* Spektro-, Spektralphotometer *nt*.
spec·tro·pho·to·met·ric analysis [ˌ-ˌfəʊtə'metrɪk] spektrophotometry.
spec·tro·pho·tom·e·try [ˌ-fəʊ'tɑmətrɪ] *n* Spektrophotometrie *f*.

spec·tro·po·la·rim·e·ter [ˌ-ˌpəʊlə'rɪmətər] *n* Spektral-, Spektropolarimeter *nt*.
spec·tro·scope ['-skəʊp] *n* Spektroskop *nt*.
spec·tro·scop·ic [ˌ-'skɑpɪk] *adj* Spektroskop *od.* Spektroskopie betr., spektroskopisch, spektralanalytisch.
spec·tro·scop·i·cal [ˌ-'skɑpɪkl] *adj* → spectroscopic.
spectroscopic analysis spektroskopische Analyse *f*, Spektralanalyse *f*.
spec·tros·co·py [spek'trɑskəpɪ] *n* Spektroskopie *f*.
spec·trum ['spektrəm] *n, pl* **-trums, -tra** [-trə] **1.** *phys.* Spektrum *nt*. **2.** Spektrum *nt*, Skala *f*, Bandbreite *f*.
spectrum analysis Spektralanalyse *f*.
spec·u·lum ['spekjələn] *n, pl* **-lums, -la** [-lə] Spiegel *m*, Spekulum *nt*, Speculum *nt*.
speech [spi:tʃ] *n* **1.** Sprache *f*; Sprachvermögen *nt*. **to lose one's ~** die Sprache verlieren. **to recover one's ~** die Sprache wiedergewinnen. **2.** Sprechen *nt*; Sprechweise *f*; Rede *f*.
speech apparatus Sprechapparat *m*.
speech audiometry Sprachaudiometrie *f*.
speech center Sprachzentrum *nt*, -region *f*.
Broca's motor s. motorisches Sprachzentrum, Broca'-Feld *nt*.
central s. → Wernicke's s.
motor s. → Broca's motor s.
Wernicke's s. Wernicke'-Sprachzentrum, akustisches/sensorisches Sprachzentrum.
speech clinic Sprachklinik *f*.
speech comprehension Sprachverständnis *nt*.
speech defect Sprachfehler *m*.
speech disorder Sprachstörung *f*.
speech disturbances Sprachstörungen *pl*.
speech education Sprecherziehung *f*.
speech hearing Sprachgehör *nt*.
speech impediment Sprach-, Sprechstörung *f*.
speech intelligibility Sprachverständlichkeit *f*.
speech·less ['spi:tʃlɪs] *adj* sprachlos (*with* vor); stumm.
speech·less·ness ['spi:tʃlɪsnɪs] *n* Sprachlosigkeit *f*, Stummheit *f*, Sprachverlust *m*.
speech organ Sprechorgan *nt*.
speech·read·ing ['spi:tʃri:dɪŋ] *n* Lippenlesen *nt*.
speech sound level Sprachschallpegel *m*.
speech test Sprachtest *m*.
speech therapist Logopäde *m*, -pädin *f*.
speech therapy Logopädie *f*.
speech training Sprachtraining *f*.
spel·ter's chill fever ['speltər] Gieß(er)fieber *nt*, Zinkfieber *nt*.
Spens [spenz] **S.' syndrome** → Stokes-Adams disease.
S-peptide *n biochem.* S-Peptid *nt*.
S period *bio.* S-Phase *f*.
sperm- *pref.* → spermato-.
sperm [spɜrm] *n, pl* **sperm, sperms 1.** Samen(flüssigkeit *f*) *m*, Sperma *nt*, Semen *nt*. **2.** → spermatozoon.
sper·ma ['spɜrmə] *n* → sperm 1.
sper·ma·cra·sia [ˌspɜrmə'kreɪʒə, -zɪə] *n* verminderte Spermienzahl *f*, Oligo-, Hypozoospermie *f*.
sperm·ag·glu·ti·na·tion [ˌ-ˌglu:tə'neɪʃn] *n* Spermagglutination *f*.
spermat- *pref.* → spermato-.
sper·ma·tel·i·o·sis [ˌspɜrmətɪli'əʊsɪs] *n* → spermiogenesis.
sper·mat·ic [spɜr'mætɪk] *adj* Samen/Sperma betr., seminal, spermatisch, Samen-, Sperma-.
spermatic abscess Samenleiterabszeß *m*.

spermatic artery: external s. Kremasterarterie f, Cremasterica f, A. cremasterica. **internal s.** Hodenarterie f, Testikularis f, A. testicularis.
spermatic cord Samenstrang m, Funiculus spermaticus.
spermatic duct Samenleiter m, Ductus/Vas deferens.
spermatic fascia: external s. Fascia spermatica externa. **internal s.** Fascia spermatica interna.
spermatic filament Samenfaden m.
spermatic fluid Samenflüssigkeit f.
sper·mat·i·cide [spɜrˈmætɪsaɪd] n → spermicide.
spermatic nerve, external Genitalast m des N. genitofemoralis, Ramus genitalis n. genitofemoralis.
spermatic plexus 1. Venengeflecht nt des Samenstranges, Plexus pampiniformis. **2.** Plexus testicularis.
spermatic vein: left s. linke Hodenvene f, V. testicularis sinistra. **right s.** rechte Hodenvene f, V. testicularis/adrenalis dextra.
sper·ma·tid [ˈspɜrmətɪd] n Spermatide f, Spermide f, Spermatidium nt.
sper·ma·tin [ˈspɜrmətɪn] n Spermatin nt.
sper·ma·tism [ˈspɜrmətɪzəm] n Spermaproduktion u. -sekretion.
sper·ma·ti·tis [ˌspɜrməˈtaɪtɪs] n Samenleiterentzündung f, Spermatitis f, Funiculitis f.
spermato- pref. Samen-, Sperma-, Spermato-, Spermio-.
sper·ma·to·blast [ˈspɜrmətəblæst] n **1.** old → Sertoli's cells. **2.** → spermatid. **3.** → spermatogonium.
sper·ma·to·cele [ˈ-siːl] n Samenbruch m, Spermatozele f.
sper·ma·to·ce·lec·to·my [ˌ-sɪˈlɛktəmɪ] n urol. Spermatozelenexzision f, Spermatozelektomie f.
sper·ma·to·ci·dal [ˌ-ˈsaɪdl] adj → spermicidal.
sper·ma·to·cide [ˈ-saɪd] n → spermicide.
sper·ma·to·cyst [ˈ-sɪst] n **1.** Bläschendrüse f, Samenblase f, -bläschen nt, Gonozystis f, Spermatozystis f, Vesicula seminalis. **2.** → spermatocele.
sper·ma·to·cys·tec·to·my [ˌ-sɪsˈtɛktəmɪ] n urol. Samenblasenentfernung f, -exstirpation f, Spermatozystektomie f.
sper·ma·to·cys·ti·tis [ˌ-sɪsˈtaɪtɪs] n Samenblasenentzündung f, Spermatozystitis f, Vesikulitis f, Vesiculitis f.
sper·ma·to·cys·tot·o·my [ˌ-sɪsˈtɛktəmɪ] n urol. Spermatozystotomie f.
sper·ma·to·cy·tal [ˌ-ˈsaɪtl] adj Spermatozyt(en) betr., spermatozytisch, Spermatozyten-.
sper·ma·to·cyte [ˈ-saɪt] n Samenmutterzelle f, Spermatozyt m.
sper·ma·to·cyt·ic seminoma [ˌ-ˈsɪtɪk] spermatozytisches Seminom nt.
sper·ma·to·cy·to·gen·e·sis [ˌ-ˌsaɪtəʊˈdʒɛnəsɪs] n Spermatozytogenese f.
sper·ma·to·cy·to·ma [ˌ-saɪˈtəʊmə] n Seminom(a) nt.
sper·ma·to·gen·e·sis [ˌ-ˈdʒɛnəsɪs] n Samen(zell)bildung f, Spermatogenese f.
sper·ma·to·ge·net·ic [ˌ-dʒəˈnɛtɪk] adj spermatogenic.
sper·ma·to·gen·ic [ˌ-ˈdʒɛnɪk] adj Samen/Sperma od. Spermien produzierend, spermatogen.
sper·ma·tog·e·nous [ˌspɜrməˈtɒdʒənəs] adj → spermatogenic.
sper·ma·tog·e·ny [ˌ-ˈtɒdʒənɪ] n → spermatogenesis.
sper·ma·to·gone [ˈspɜrmətəʊgəʊn] n → spermatogonium.

sper·ma·to·go·ni·al [ˌ-ˈgəʊnɪəl] adj **1.** Spermatogonium betr., Spermatogonien-. **2.** → spermatogenic.
spermatogonial cell → spermatogonium.
sper·ma·to·go·ni·um [ˌ-ˈgəʊnɪəm] n, pl **-ni·a** [-nɪə] Ursamenzelle f, Spermatogonie f, Spermatogonium nt. **type A s.** (Typ) A-Spermatogonium. **type B s.** (Typ) B-Spermatogonium.
sper·ma·toid [ˈspɜrmətɔɪd] adj samenähnlich, spermatoid.
sper·ma·tol·i·o·sis [ˌspɜrmətəlaɪˈəʊsɪs] n old → spermatogenesis.
sper·ma·tol·o·gy [ˌspɜrməˈtɒlədʒɪ] n Spermatologie f.
sper·ma·tol·y·sin [ˌ-ˈtɒləsɪn] n Spermatolysin nt.
sper·ma·tol·y·sis [ˌ-ˈtɒləsɪs] n Spermatolyse f.
sper·ma·to·lyt·ic [ˌspɜrmətəˈlɪtɪk] adj Spermatolyse betr. od. auslösend, spermatolytisch.
sper·ma·to·o·vum [ˌ-ˈgəʊnɪəm] n, pl **-o·va** [-ˌəʊvə] Zygote f, Spermov(i)um nt.
sper·ma·to·pa·thia [ˌ-ˈpæθɪə] n → spermatopathy.
sper·ma·top·a·thy [ˌspɜrməˈtɒpəθɪ] n Spermatopathie f.
sper·ma·to·pho·bia [ˌspɜrmətəˈfəʊbɪə] n psychia. Spermatophobie f.
sper·ma·to·phore [ˈ-fɔːr, -fəʊr] n **1.** → spermatophorum. **2.** bio. Samen-, Spermatträger m, Spermatophore f.
sper·ma·to·poi·et·ic [ˌ-pɔɪˈɛtɪk] adj Spermabildung f betr. od. -sekretion fördernd, spermatopo(i)etisch.
sper·ma·tor·rhea [ˌ-ˈrɪə] n Samenfluß m, Spermatorrhoe f.
sper·ma·tos·che·sis [ˌspɜrməˈtɑskəsɪs] n Hemmung f der Samensekretion.
sper·ma·to·some [spɜrˈmætəsəʊm] n → spermatozoon.
sper·mat·o·spore [ˈ-spɔːr, -spəʊr] n → spermatozoon.
sper·ma·to·tox·in [ˌspɜrmətəˈtɑksɪn] n Spermatotoxin nt.
sper·ma·to·cyst [ˌspɜrmætˈəʊvəm] n Spermov(i)um nt, Zygote f.
sper·ma·tox·in [ˌspɜrməˈtɑksɪn] n Spermatotoxin nt.
sper·ma·to·zo·al [ˌspɜrmətəˈzəʊəl] adj Spermatozoen betr., Spermatozoen-.
sper·ma·to·zo·i·cide [ˌ-ˈzɔɪsaɪd] n → spermicide.
sper·ma·to·zo·id [ˈ-zɔɪd] n → spermatozoon.
sper·ma·to·zo·on [ˌ-ˈzəʊən, -ɑn] n, pl **-zoa** [-ˈzəʊə] männliche Keimzelle f, Spermium nt, Spermie f, Samenfaden m, Spermatozoon nt.
sper·ma·tu·ria [ˌspɜrməˈt(j)ʊərɪə] n Spermienausscheidung f im Harn, Spermaturie f, Seminurie f.
sperm bank Samenbank f.
sperm cell → spermatozoon.
sperm count Spermatozoenzahl f, Spermienzahl f.
sperm crystals Sperminkristalle pl.
sperm granuloma Samengranulom nt.
sper·mi·ci·dal [ˌspɜrmɪˈsaɪdl] adj spermienabtötend, spermizid.
sper·mi·cide [ˈ-saɪd] n spermizides Mittel nt, Spermizid nt.
sper·mid [ˈspɜrmɪd] n → spermatid.
sper·mi·dine [ˈspɜrmədiːn] n Spermidin nt.
sper·mine [ˈspɜrmiːn] n Spermin nt.
spermine crystals → sperm crystals.
sper·mi·o·cyte [ˈspɜrmɪəʊsaɪt] n primäre Spermatogonie f, primäres Spermatogonium nt, Spermiozyt m.
sper·mi·o·gen·e·sis [ˌ-ˈdʒɛnəsɪs] n Spermio(histo)genese f.

sper·mi·o·ge·net·ic [ˌ-dʒəˈnɛtɪk] adj Spermiogenese betr. od. anregend, spermiogenetisch.
sper·mi·o·go·ni·um [ˌ-ˈgəʊnɪəm] n, pl **-nia** [-nɪə] → spermatogonium.
sper·mi·o·gram [ˈ-græm] n Spermiogramm nt.
sper·mi·o·te·le·o·sis [ˌ-ˌtiːlɪˈəʊsɪs] n Spermio(histo)genese f.
sper·mi·um [ˈspɜrmɪəm] n, pl **-mia** [-mɪə] → spermatozoon.
spermo- pref. → spermato-.
sper·mo·blast [ˈspɜrməblæst] n → spermatid.
sper·mo·cy·to·ma [ˌ-saɪˈtəʊmə] n Seminom(a) nt.
sper·mo·lith [ˈ-lɪθ] n Spermolith m.
sper·mo·ly·sin [spɜrˈmɑləsɪn] n Spermatolysin nt.
sper·mol·y·sis [spɜrˈmɑləsɪs] n → spermatolysis.
sper·mo·lyt·ic [ˌspɜrməˈlɪtɪk] adj → spermatolytic.
sper·mo·plasm [ˈ-plæzəm] n Spermatidenplasma f.
sper·mo·spore [ˈ-spɔːr, -spəʊr] n → spermatogonium.
sper·mo·tox·in [ˌ-ˈtɑksɪn] n Spermatotoxin nt.
sphac·e·late [ˈsfæsəleɪt] vt gangränös/nekrotisch werden.
sphac·e·lat·ed [ˈsfæsəleɪtɪd] adj gangränös, nekrotisch.
sphac·e·la·tion [sfæsəˈleɪʃn] n **1.** Gangrän-, Phakelusbildung f. **2.** → sphacelus. **3.** lokaler Zell-/Gewebstod m, Nekrose f, Necrosis f.
sphac·e·lous [ˈsfæsələs] adj Phakelus betr., gangränös.
sphac·e·lus [ˈsfæsələs] n Phakelus m, feuchter Brand m, Gangrän f.
sphaer- pref. → sphero-.
Sphaer·i·a·les [sfɪərɪˈeɪliːz] pl micro. Sphaeriales pl.
sphaero- pref. → sphero-.
Sphae·roph·o·rus necrophorus [sfɪˈrɑfərəs] micro. Fusobacterium necrophorum.
spha·gi·as·mus [sfeɪdʒɪˈæzməs] n **1.** Sphagiasmus m. **2.** Petit-mal(-Epilepsie f) nt abbr. PM.
S phase bio. S-Phase f.
sphen- pref. → spheno-.
sphen·eth·moid [sfɛnˈɛθmɔɪd] adj → sphenoethmoid.
spheno- pref. Keil-; Keilbein-, Spheno-.
sphe·no·bas·i·lar [sfiːnəʊˈbæsɪlər] adj sphenobasilar.
sphenobasilar synchondrosis → sphenooccipital synchondrosis.
sphe·noc·ci·pi·tal [sfɪnɑkˈsɪpɪtl] adj → sphenooccipital.
sphe·no·ceph·a·lus [sfiːnəʊˈsɛfələs] n embryo. Sphenokephalus m, -zephalus m.
sphe·no·ceph·a·ly [ˌ-ˈsɛfəlɪ] n embryo. Sphenokephalie f, -zephalie f.
sphe·no·eth·moid [ˌ-ˈɛθmɔɪd] adj Keilbein/Os sphenoidale u. Siebbein/Os ethmoidale betr. od. verbindend, sphenoethmoidal.
sphe·no·eth·moi·dal [ˌ-eθˈmɔɪdl] adj → sphenoethmoid.
sphenoethmoidal recess Rec. sphenoethmoidalis.
sphenoethmoidal suture Sutura sphenoethmoidalis.
sphenoethmoidal synchondrosis Synchondrosis sphenoethmoidalis.
sphe·no·fron·tal [ˌ-ˈfrʌntl] adj Keilbein/Os sphenoidale u. Stirnbein/Os frontale betr. od. verbindend, sphenofrontal.
sphenofrontal suture Sutura sphenofrontalis.

sphenoid

sphe·noid ['sfiːnɔɪd] **I** *n* Keilbein *nt*, Flügelbein *nt*, Os sphenoidale. **II** *adj* keilförmig; Keilbein betr., sphenoid.
sphe·noi·dal [sfiːˈnɔɪdl] *adj* → sphenoid II.
sphenoidal angle → sphenoid angle.
sphenoidal concha 1. kleiner Keilbeinflügel *m*, Ala minor (ossis sphenoidalis). **2.** Concha sphenoidalis.
sphenoidal crest Crista sphenoidalis.
sphenoidal fissure Augenhöhlendachspalte *f*, obere Orbitaspalte *f*, Fissura orbitalis superior.
  inferior s. Augenhöhlenbodenspalte *f*, untere Orbitaspalte *f*, Fissura orbitalis inferior.
  superior s. → sphenoidal fissure.
sphenoidal fontanelle Keilbeinfontanelle *f*, vordere Seitenfontanelle *f*, Fonticulus anterolateralis/sphenoidalis.
sphenoidal jugum Jugum sphenoidale.
sphenoidal lingula Lingula sphenoidalis.
sphenoidal margin of temporal bone Margo sphenoidalis ossis temporalis.
sphenoidal ostium Apertura sinus sphenoidalis.
sphenoidal part of middle cerebral artery Pars sphenoidalis (a. cerebri mediae).
sphenoidal process of cartilage of nasal septum Proc. posterior/sphenoidalis.
sphenoidal rostrum Rostrum sphenoidale.
sphenoidal septum Trennwand *f* der Keilbeinhöhlen, Septum sinuum sphenoidalium.
sphenoidal sinus Keilbeinhöhle *f*, Sinus sphenoidalis.
  bony/osseous s. knöcherne Keilbeinhöhle, Sinus sphenoidalis osseus.
sphenoidal sinusitis → sphenoiditis.
sphenoidal yoke Jugum sphenoidale.
sphenoid angle Angulus sphenoidalis (ossis parietalis).
sphenoid bone → sphenoid I.
sphenoid crest Crista sphenoidalis.
sphe·noid·i·tis [ˌsfiːnɔɪˈdaɪtɪs] *n* Keilbeinhöhlenentzündung *f*, Sinusitis sphenoidalis, Sphenoiditis *f*.
sphe·noid·os·to·my [ˌ-ˈdɒstəmɪ] *n* HNO, neurochir. Sphenoidostomie *f*.
sphe·noid·ot·o·my [ˌ-ˈdɒtəmɪ] *n* HNO, neurochir. Sphenoidotomie *f*.
sphenoid process of palatine bone Proc. sphenoidalis (ossis palatini).
sphenoid rostrum Rostrum sphenoidale.
sphe·no·ma·lar [ˌsfiːnəʊˈmeɪlər] *adj* → sphenozygomatic.
sphe·no·man·dib·u·lar [ˌ-ˈmændɪbjələr] *adj* Keilbein/Os sphenoidale u. Unterkiefer/Mandibula betr., sphenomandibular.
sphenomandibular ligament Lig. sphenomandibulare.
sphe·no·max·il·lar·y [ˌ-ˈmæksəˌlerɪ, -mækˈsɪlərɪ] *adj* Keilbein/Os sphenoidale u. Oberkiefer/Maxilla betr. *od.* verbindend, sphenomaxillär.
sphenomaxillary ganglion Meckel'-Ganglion *nt*, Ggl. pterygopalatinum.
sphenomaxillary suture Sutura sphenomaxillaris.
sphe·no·oc·cip·i·tal [ˌ-ɒkˈsɪpɪtl] *adj* Keilbein/Os sphenoidale u. Hinterhauptsbein/Os occipitale betr., sphenookzipital.
sphenooccipital fissure Fissura spheno-occipitalis.
sphenooccipital synchondrosis Synchondrosis spheno-occipitalis.
sphe·nop·a·gus [sfiːˈnɒpəgəs] *n embryo.* Sphenopagus *m*.
sphe·no·pal·a·tine [ˌsfiːnəʊˈpælətaɪn, -tɪn] *adj* Keilbein/Os sphenoidale u. Gaumenbein/Palatum betr. *od.* verbindend, sphenopalatinal.

sphenopalatine artery Sphenopalatina *f*, A. sphenopalatina.
sphenopalatine canal 1. Canalis palatovaginalis. **2.** Canalis palatinus major.
sphenopalatine foramen 1. For. sphenopalatinum. **2.** For. palatinum majus.
sphenopalatine ganglion → sphenomaxillary ganglion.
sphenopalatine incisure of palatine bone → sphenopalatine notch of palatine bone.
sphenopalatine neuralgia Sluder-Neuralgie *f*, -Syndrom *nt*, Neuralgia sphenopalatina.
sphenopalatine notch of palatine bone Inc. sphenopalatina (ossis palatini).
sphe·no·pa·ri·e·tal [ˌ-pəˈraɪɪtl] *adj* Keilbein/Os sphenoidale u. Scheitelbein/Os parietale betr., sphenoparietal.
sphenoparietal sinus Sinus sphenoparietalis.
sphenoparietal suture Sutura sphenoparietalis.
sphe·no·pe·tro·sal [ˌ-pɪˈtrəʊsəl] *adj* Keilbein/Os sphenoidale u. Felsenbein/Os petrosum betr., sphenopetrosal.
sphenopetrosal fissure Fissura sphenopetrosa.
sphenopetrosal synchondrosis Synchondrosis sphenopetrosa.
sphe·no·pha·ryn·ge·al canal [ˌ-fəˈrɪndʒ(ɪ)əl] Canalis palatovaginalis.
sphe·nor·bi·tal [sfiːˈnɔːrbɪtl] *adj* Keilbein/Os sphenoidale u. Orbita betr. *od.* verbindend, spheno(o)rbital.
sphe·no·squa·mo·sal suture [ˌsfiːnəʊskwəˈməʊzl] Sutura sphenosquamosa.
sphe·no·tem·po·ral [ˌ-ˈtemp(ə)rəl] *adj* Keilbein/Os sphenoidale u. Schläfenbein/Os temporale betr. *od.* verbindend, sphenotemporal.
sphe·no·tur·bi·nal bone [ˌ-ˈtɜrbɪnl] Concha sphenoidalis.
sphe·no·vo·mer·ine suture [ˌ-ˈvəʊmərаɪn, -rɪn, 'vɒm-] Sutura sphenovomeriana.
sphe·no·zy·go·mat·ic [ˌ-zaɪgəˈmætɪk] *adj* Keilbein/Os sphenoidale u. Jochbein/Os zygomaticum betr., sphenozygomatisch.
spher- *pref.* → sphero-.
sphere [sfɪər] *n* **1.** Kugel *f*, kugelförmiger Körper *m*. **2.** Sphäre *f*, Bereich *m*, Gebiet *nt*, (Wirkungs-)Kreis *m*.
sphe·res·the·sia [ˌsfɪərɛsˈθiːʒ(ɪ)ə] *n* Globus hystericus.
spher·ic ['sferɪk, 'sfɪər-] *adj* kugelförmig, kugelig, (kugel-)rund, sphärisch, Kugel-.
spher·i·cal ['sferɪkl, 'sfɪər-] *adj* → spheric.
spherical aberration *phys., physiol.* sphärische Aberration *f*.
spherical lens sphärische Linse *f*, sphärisches Glas *nt*.
spherical nucleus Kugelkern *m*, Nc. globosus.
spherical recess (of vestibule) Rec. sphericus (vestibuli).
sphero- *pref.* Kugel-, Sphär(o)-.
sphe·ro·blast [ˈsfɪərəblæst, ˈsfer-] *n bio.* Sphäroblast *m*.
sphe·ro·cyl·in·der [ˌ-ˈsɪlɪndər] *n* → spherocylindrical lens.
sphe·ro·cy·lin·dri·cal lens [ˌ-sɪˈlɪndrɪkl] sphärozylindrisches Glas *nt*, Sphärozylinder *m*.
sphe·ro·cyte [ˈ-saɪt] *n hema.* Kugelzelle *f*, Sphärozyt *m*.
sphe·ro·cyt·ic [ˌ-ˈsɪtɪk] *adj* Sphärozyt(en) betr., Sphärozyten-.
spherocytic anemia hereditäre Sphärozytose *f*, Kugelzellenanämie *f*, -ikterus *m*, familiärer hämolytischer Ikterus *m*, Morbus Minkowski-Chauffard *m*.

sphe·ro·cy·to·sis [ˌ-saɪˈtəʊsɪs] *n* Sphärozytose *f*.
sphe·roid [ˈsfɪərɔɪd] *n* kugelförmiger Körper *m*, Sphäroid *nt*.
sphe·roi·dal [sfɪəˈrɔɪdl] *adj* kugelförmig, kugelig, sphäroidisch.
spheroidal articulation Kugelgelenk *nt*, Artic. spheroidea/cotylica.
spheroidal joint → spheroidal articulation.
sphe·roi·dic [sfɪəˈrɔɪdɪk] *adj* → spheroidal.
sphe·ro·lith [ˈsfɪərəlɪθ] *n* Sphärolith *m*.
sphe·rom·e·ter [sfɪˈrɒmɪtər] *n* Sphärometer *nt*.
sphe·ro·pha·kia [ˌsfɪərəˈfeɪkɪə] *n ophthal.* Sphärophakie *f*.
spherophakia-brachymorphia syndrome Weill-Marchesani-Syndrom *nt*, Marchesani-Syndrom *nt*.
Sphe·roph·o·rus necrophorus [sfɪˈrɒfərəs] *micro.* Fusobacterium necrophorum.
sphe·ro·plast [ˈsfɪərəplæst] *n micro.* Sphäroplast *m*.
spher·ule [ˈsfɪər(j)uːl, ˈsfer-] *n* **1.** *anat., histol.* Sphärule *f*. **2.** *micro.* Sphaerule *f*.
spher·u·lin [ˈsfɪərjəlɪn] *n micro.* Sphaerulin *nt*.
spherulin skin test *micro.* Sphaerulin-(Haut-)Test *m*.
sphinc·ter [ˈsfɪŋktər] *n* → sphincter muscle.
s. of hepatopancreatic ampulla Sphinkter Oddii/ampullae, M. sphincter Oddii, M. sphincter ampullae hepatopancreaticae, Sphincter ampullae.
sphinc·ter·al [ˈsfɪŋktərəl] *adj* Sphinkter betr., Sphinkter-.
sphincteral achalasia Sphinkterachalasie *f*.
sphinc·ter·al·gia [sfɪŋktəˈrældʒ(ɪ)ə] *n* Schmerzen *pl* im M. sphincter ani, Sphinkteralgie *f*.
sphincter ani externus (muscle) äußerer Afterschließmuskel *m*, Sphinkter *m* ani externus, M. sphincter ani externus.
sphincter ani internus (muscle) innerer Afterschließmuskel *m*, Sphinkter *m* ani internus, M. sphincter ani internus.
sphincter dilatation Sphinkterdehnung *f*.
sphincter ductus choledochi (muscle) Sphinkter *m* ductus choledochi, M. sphincter ductus choledochi.
sphincter ductus pancreatici (muscle) Sphinkter *m* ductus pancreatici, M. sphincter ductus pancreatici.
sphinc·ter·ec·to·my [sfɪŋktəˈrektəmɪ] *n chir., ophthal.* Sphinkterektomie *f*.
sphinc·te·ri·al [sfɪŋkˈtɪərɪəl] *adj* → sphincteral.
sphinc·ter·ic [sfɪŋkˈterɪk] *adj* → sphincteral.
sphincteric fibers of ciliary muscle Müller'-Muskel *m*, Fibrae circulares m. ciliaris.
sphincteric musculature Sphinktermuskulatur *f*.
sphinc·ter·is·mus [ˌsfɪŋktəˈrɪzməs] *n* Krampf/Spasmus *m* des M. sphincter ani.
sphinc·ter·i·tis [ˌ-ˈraɪtɪs] *n* Sphinkterentzündung *f*, Sphinkteritis *f*.
sphincter muscle Schließmuskel *m*, Sphinkter *m*, M. sphincter.
s. of bile duct → sphincter ductus choledochi (muscle).
external s. of anus → sphincter ani externus (muscle).
s. of hepatopancreatic ampulla → sphincter ampullae hepatopancreaticae.
internal s., smooth unwillkürlicher/glatter innerer Schließmuskel.

internal s. of anus → sphincter ani internus (muscle).
s. of pancreatic duct → sphincter ductus pancreatici (muscle).
s. of pupil → sphincter pupillae (muscle).
pyloric s. → sphincter pylori (muscle).
s. of pylorus → sphincter pylori (muscle).
s. of urethra → sphincter urethrae (muscle).
urethral s., voluntary → sphincter urethrae (muscle).
vesical s., involuntary unwillkürlicher Blasenschließmuskel.
sphinc·ter·ol·y·sis [ˌ-'rɑləsɪs] n ophthal. Sphinkterolyse f.
sphinc·ter·o·plas·ty ['sfɪŋktərəplæstɪ] n chir. Sphinkterplastik f.
sphinc·ter·o·scope ['-skəʊp] n Sphinkteroskop nt.
sphinc·ter·os·co·py [ˌsfɪŋktə'rɑskəpɪ] n Sphinkteroskopie f.
sphinc·ter·o·tome ['sfɪŋktərətəʊm] n chir. Sphinkterotomiemesser nt, Sphinkterotom nt.
sphinc·ter·ot·o·my [ˌsfɪŋktə'rɑtəmɪ] n chir. Sphinkterotomie f.
sphincter pupillae (muscle) Pupillenschließer m, Sphinkter m pupillae, M. sphincter pupillae.
sphincter pylori (muscle) Schließmuskel m des Magenausgangs, Sphinkter m pylori, M. sphincter pylori.
sphincter urethrae (muscle) Harnröhren-, Urethralsphinkter m, Sphinkter m urethrae, M. sphincter urethrae.
sphincter vessel Sphinktergefäß nt.
sphin·ga·nine ['sfɪŋgəniːn] n Sphinganin nt, Dihydrosphingosin nt.
4-sphin·gen·ine ['sfɪŋgəniːn] n → sphingosine.
sphin·go·ga·lac·to·side [ˌsfɪŋgəʊgə'læktəsaɪd, -sɪd] n Sphingogalaktosid nt.
sphin·go·gly·co·lip·id [ˌ-ˌglaɪkə'lɪpɪd] n Sphingoglykolipid nt.
sphin·go·in ['-wɪn] n Sphingoin nt.
sphin·go·lip·id [ˌ-'lɪpɪd] n Sphingolipid nt.
sphin·go·lip·o·sis [ˌ-ˌlɪpɪ'dəʊsɪs] n 1. Sphingolipidspeicherkrankheit f, Sphingolipidose f. 2. Niemann-Pick-Krankheit f, Sphingomyelinose f, Sphingomyelinlipidose f.
sphin·go·lip·o·dys·tro·phy [ˌ-ˌlɪpɪ'dɪstrəfɪ] n → sphingolipidosis.
sphin·go·my·e·lin [ˌ-'maɪəlɪn] n Sphingomyelin nt.
sphin·go·my·e·li·nase [ˌ-'maɪəlɪneɪz] n Spingomyelinase f, Spingomyelinphosphodiesterase f.
sphingomyelinase deficiency Niemann-Pick-Krankheit f, Sphingomyelinose f, Sphingomyelinlipidose f.
sphingomyelin lipidosis → sphingomyelinase deficiency.
sphin·go·my·e·li·no·sis [ˌ-ˌmaɪəlɪ'nəʊsɪs] n → sphingomyelinase deficiency.
sphingomyelin phosphodiesterase → sphingomyelinase.
sphin·go·phos·pho·lip·id [-ˌfɑsfəʊ'lɪpɪd] n Sphingophospholipid nt.
sphin·go·sine ['sfɪŋgəsiːn, -sɪn] n Sphingosin nt, 4-Sphingenin nt.
sphingosine acyltransferase Sphingosinacyltransferase f.
sphygm- pref. → sphygmo-.
sphyg·mic ['sfɪgmɪk] adj Puls betr., Puls-, Sphygm(o)-.
sphygmic interval → sphygmic period.
sphygmic period card. Austreibungsphase f.
sphygmo- pref. Puls-, Sphygm(o)-.
sphyg·mo·bo·lo·gram [ˌsfɪgmə'bəʊləgræm] n Sphygmobologramm nt.
sphyg·mo·bo·lom·e·ter [ˌ-bə'lɑmɪtər] n Sphygmobolometer nt.
sphyg·mo·bo·lom·e·try [ˌ-bə'lɑmətrɪ] n Sphygmobolometrie f.
sphyg·mo·car·di·o·gram [ˌ-'kɑːrdɪəgræm] n Sphygmokardiogramm nt.
sphyg·mo·car·di·o·graph [ˌ-'kɑːrdɪəgræf] n Sphygmokardiograph m.
sphyg·mo·car·di·o·scope [ˌ-'kɑːrdɪəskəʊp] n Sphygmokardioskop nt.
sphyg·mo·dy·na·mom·e·ter [ˌ-ˌdaɪnə'mɑmɪtər] n Sphygmodynamometer nt.
sphyg·mo·gram ['-græm] n Pulskurve f, Sphygmogramm nt.
sphyg·mo·graph ['-græf] n Pulsschreiber m, Sphygmograph m.
sphyg·mog·ra·phy [sfɪg'mɑgrəfɪ] n Pulsschreibung f, -registrierung f, Sphygmographie f.
sphyg·moid ['sfɪgmɔɪd] adj pulsartig, pulsierend.
sphyg·mo·ma·nom·e·ter [ˌsfɪgməʊmə'nɑmɪtər] n Blutdruckmeßgerät nt, Blutdruckmesser m, Sphygmomanometer nt.
sphyg·mom·e·ter [sfɪg'mɑmɪtər] n 1. Sphygmometer nt. 2. → sphygmomanometer.
sphygmo-oscillometer n Sphygmooszillometer nt.
sphyg·mo·pal·pa·tion [ˌsfɪgməpæl'peɪʃn] n Pulsfühlen nt, Pulspalpation f.
sphyg·mo·ple·thys·mo·graph [ˌ-plɪ'θɪzməgræf] n Sphygmoplethysmograph m.
sphyg·mo·scope ['-skəʊp] n Sphygmoskop nt.
sphyg·mos·co·py [sfɪg'mɑskəpɪ] n Pulsuntersuchung f, Sphygmoskopie f.
sphyg·mo·ton·o·gram [ˌsfɪgməʊ'tɑnəgræm, -'təʊ-] n Sphygmotonogramm nt.
sphyg·mo·ton·o·graph [ˌ-'tɑnəgræf, -'təʊ-] n Sphygmotonograph m.
sphyg·mo·to·nom·e·ter [ˌ-tə'nɑmɪtər] n Sphygmotonometer nt.
sphyg·mo·vis·co·sim·e·try [ˌ-ˌvɪskə'sɪmətrɪ] n Sphygmoviskosimetrie f.
spi·ca ['spaɪkə] n, pl -cas, -cae [-siː] Kornährenverband m, Spica f.
spica bandage → spica.
spic·u·lar ['spɪkjələr] adj nadelförmig.
spic·u·la·tion [ˌspɪkjə'leɪʃn] n radiol., ortho. Spikula(e)bildung f.
spic·ule ['spɪkjuːl] n Spitze f, Dorn m, Spikula f, Spicula f, Spiculum nt.
spic·u·lum ['spɪkjələm] n, pl -la [-lə] → spicule.
spi·der ['spaɪdər] n 1. bio. Spinne f. 2. → spider angioma.
spider angioma Sternnävus m, Spider naevus, Naevus araneus.
spider-burst n Besenreiser(varizen pl) pl.
spider cell 1. (fibrillärer) Astrozyt m. 2. Rouget-Zelle f. 3. Spinnenzelle f.
spider fingers 1. Spinnenfingrigkeit f, Arachnodaktylie f, Dolichostenomelie f. 2. old Marfan-Syndrom nt, Arachnodaktylie-Syndrom nt.
spider mole → spider angioma.
spider nevus → spider angioma.
spider telangiectasia → spider angioma.
spider-web clot Spinnwebsgerinnsel nt, Spinn(en)gewebsgerinnsel nt.
Spieghel ['spiːgl] 'ʃpiː-ˌ]: **S.'s line** Spieghel'-Linie f, Linea semilunaris.
Spiegler-Fendt ['spiːglər fent; 'ʃpiː-ˌ]: **S.-F. pseudolymphoma/sarcoid** multiples Sarkoid nt, Bäfverstedt-Syndrom nt, benigne Lymphoplasie f der Haut, Lymphozytom nt, Lymphocytoma cutis, Lymphadenosis benigna cutis.
Spielmeyer ['spiːlmaɪər]: **S.'s myelin stain** Markscheidenfärbung f nach Spielmeyer.

Spielmeyer-Vogt [fəʊgt; foːgt]: **S.-V. disease** Stock-Vogt-Spielmeyer-Syndrom nt, Batten-Spielmeyer-Vogt-Syndrom nt, neuronale/juvenile Zeroidlipofuszinose/Ceroidlipofuscinose f, juvenile Form f der amaurotischen Idiotie.
spi·ge·li·an [spaɪ'dʒiːlɪən]: **s. line** → Spieghel's line.
s. hernia Spieghel-Hernie f.
s. lobe → Spigelius' lobe.
Spi·ge·li·us [spaɪ'dʒiːlɪəs]: **S.' line** → Spieghel's line.
S.' lobe Spieghel'-Leberlappen m, Lobus caudatus.
spike [spaɪk] n 1. physiol. Spitze f, Kurvenzacke f, Spike m. 2. **~s** pl micro. (Virus) Spitzen pl, Spikes pl.
spike and waves complex neuro. Spike-and-waves-Komplex m, Spitze-Wellen-Komplex m.
spike potential Spike-, Spitzen-, Spitzenaktionspotential nt.
spin- pref. → spino-.
spin [spɪn] n phys. Drehimpuls m, Spin m.
spi·na ['spaɪnə] n, pl **-nae** [-niː] anat. → spine 1.
spina bifida Spina bifida.
spina bifida occulta Spina bifida occulta.
spi·nal ['spaɪnl] I n inf. → spinal anesthesia 1. II adj Rückgrat od. Rückenmark betr., spinal, Rückgrat-, Rückenmarks-, Spinal-, Wirbel-, Wirbel-.
spinal anesthesia 1. anes. Spinalanästhesie f, inf. Spinale f. 2. neuro. Sensibilitätsverlust m durch/bei Rückenmarksläsion.
continuous s. kontinuierliche Spinalanästhesie, Dauerspinalanästhesie.
fractional s. → continuous s.
high s. hohe Spinalanästhesie.
hyperbaric s. hyperbare Spinalanästhesie.
hypobaric s. hypobare Spinalanästhesie.
isobaric s. isobare Spinalanästhesie.
low s. tiefe Spinalanästhesie.
total s. totale Spinalanästhesie.
spinal anomaly Wirbelsäulenfehlbildung f, -anomalie f.
spinal apoplexy Rückenmarks(ein)blutung f, -apoplexie f, Apoplexia spinalis, Hämatorrhachis f, spinale Meningealapoplexie f.
spinal arachnoid spinale Spinnwebenhaut f, Arachnoidea (mater) spinalis.
spinal artery: s.ies pl → spinal branches of vertebral artery.
anterior s. vordere Rückenmarksarterie f, Spinalis f anterior, A. spinalis anterior.
posterior s. hintere Rückenmarksarterie f, Spinalis f posterior, A. spinalis posterior.
spinal ataxia spinale Ataxie f.
spinal block Spinalanästhesie f, inf. Spinale f.
spinal branch Rückenmarksast m, Ramus spinalis.
s.es of ascending cervical artery Rückenmarksäste pl der A. cervicalis ascendens, Rami spinales aa. cervicalis ascendentis.
s. of iliolumbar artery Wirbelkanalast der A. iliolumbalis, Ramus spinalis (rami lumbalis) a. iliolumbalis.
s.es of lateral sacral arteries Rami spinales aa. sacralium lateralium.
s. of lumbar arteries Rückenmarksast der Lumbalarterien, Ramus spinalis aa. lumbalium.
s. of posterior intercostal arteries Rückenmarksast der hinteren Interkostalarterien, Ramus spinalis (rami dorsalis) aa. intercostalium posteriorum.
s. of subcostal artery Rückenmarksast der A. subcostalis, Ramus spinalis a. subcostalis.

spinal canal

s.es of superior intercostal artery Rückenmarksäste *pl* der A. intercostalis suprema, Rami spinales a. intercostales supremae.
s.es of vertebral artery Rückenäste *pl* der A. vertebralis, Rami spinales/radiculares a. vertebralis.
spinal canal Wirbel(säulen)-, Spinal-, Vertebralkanal *m*, Canalis vertebralis.
spinal caries → spinal tuberculosis.
spinal column Wirbelsäule *f*, Rückgrat *nt*, Columna vertebralis.
spinal compression Rückenmark(s)kompression *f*, -quetschung *f*.
spinal concussion Rückenmark(s)erschütterung *f*, Commotio (medullae) spinalis.
spinal cord Rückenmark *nt*, Medulla spinalis.
spinal cord automatism *physiol., patho.* Rückenmarksautomatismus *m*.
spinal cord compression → spinal compression.
spinal cord injury Rückenmark(s)verletzung *f*, -trauma *nt*.
spinal cord swelling Rückenmark(s)schwellung *f*.
spinal cord transection Rückenmark(s)durchtrennung *f*.
spinal cord trauma Rückenmark(s)verletzung *f*, -trauma *nt*.
spinal crest of Rauber Dornfortsatz *m*, Proc. spinosus.
spinal curvature Wirbelsäulenverkrümmung *f*, -kurvatur *f*.
spinal decompression *neurochir., ortho.* Rückenmark(s)dekompression *f*.
spinal filament Filum terminale/spinale.
spinal foramen Wirbelloch *nt*, For. vertebrale.
spinal fracture Wirbelsäulenfraktur *f*.
spinal fusion *neurochir., ortho.* operative Wirbelsäulenversteifung *f*, Spondylodese *f*.
spinal ganglion (sensorisches) Spinalganglion *nt*, Ggl. spinale/sensorium.
spinal gliosis spinale Gliose *f*.
spinal headache Kopfschmerz(en *pl*) *m* nach Lumbalpunktion.
spinal hemianesthesia spinale Hemianästhesie *f*, Hemianaesthesia spinalis.
spinal hemiplegia spinale Hemiplegie *f*.
spinal injury → spinal cord injury.
spi·na·lis [spaɪ'neɪlɪs] *n* → spinalis muscle.
spinalis capitis (muscle) Spinalis *m* capitis, M. spinalis capitis.
spinalis cervicis (muscle) Spinalis *m* cervicis, M. spinalis cervicis.
spinalis muscle Spinalis *m*, M. spinalis.
spinalis thoracis (muscle) Spinalis *m* thoracis, M. spinalis thoracis.
spinal lemniscus Lemniscus spinalis.
spinal marrow → spinal cord.
spinal medulla → spinal cord.
spinal meningitis Rückenmarkshautentzündung *f*, Meningitis spinalis.
spinal meningocele spinale Meningozele *f*, Rückenmark(s)hautbruch *m*.
spinal muscle: s. of back → spinalis thoracis (muscle).
s. of head → spinalis capitis (muscle).
s. of neck → spinalis cervicis (muscle).
spinal mydriasis *ophthal.* Mydriasis spinalis.
spinal nerve Spinal-, Rückenmarksnerv *m*; N. spinalis.
cervical s.s Halsnerven *pl*, zervikale Spinalnerven *pl*, Nn. cervicales.
lumbar s.s Lenden-, Lumbalnerven *pl*, lumbale Spinalnerven *pl*, Nn. lumbales/lumbares.
sacral s.s Kreuz-, Sakralnerven *pl*, sakrale Spinalnerven *pl*, Nn. sacrales.
thoracic s.s Brust-, Thorakalnerven *pl*, thorakale Spinalnerven *pl*, Nn. thoracici.
spinal nerve sulcus Sulcus n. spinalis.
spinal nucleus: s.i *pl* Rückenmarkskerne *pl*.
s. of accessory nerve Nc. spinalis n. accessorii.
s. of trigeminal nerve spinaler/unterer Trigeminuskern *m*, Nc. inferior/spinalis n. trigemini.
spinal osteomyelitis Osteomyelitis *f* der Wirbelsäule.
spinal paralysis Spinalparalyse *f*.
acute ascending s. 1. Landry-Lähmung *f*, -Paralyse *f*, -Typ *m*, Paralysis spinalis ascendens acuta. **2.** Guillain-Barré-Syndrom *nt*, (Poly-)Radikuloneuritis *f*, Neuronitis *f*.
anterior s. (epidemische/spinale) Kinderlähmung *f*, Heine-Medin-Krankheit *f*, Poliomyelitis (epidemica) anterior acuta.
atrophic s. → anterior s.
spastic s. Erb-Charcot-Syndrom *nt*, spastische Spinalparalyse.
spinal paralytic poliomyelitis spinale Form *f* der Kinderlähmung.
spinal punction Lumbalpunktion *f*.
spinal quotient *neuro.* Ayala-Quotient *m*, -Gleichung *f*.
spinal reflex spinaler Reflex *m*.
spinal roots of accessory nerve untere/spinale Akzessoriuswurzeln *pl*, Radices spinales n. accessorii, Pars spinalis n. accessorii.
spinal shock spinaler Schock *m*.
spinal stiffness Wirbelsäuleneinsteifung *f*, -versteifung *f*.
spinal subarachnoid block Liquorblock(ade *f*) *m*.
spinal tract of trigeminal nerve Rückenmarksabschnitt *m* des N. trigeminus, Tractus spinalis n. trigeminalis.
spinal tractotomy *neurochir.* Durchtrennung *f* des Tractus spinothalamicus.
spinal trauma Rückenmark(s)verletzung *f*, -trauma *nt*.
spinal tuberculosis Wirbelsäulentuberkulose *f*, Spondylitis tuberculosa.
spinal veins Rückenmarksvenen *pl*.
anterior s. vordere Rückenmarksvenen, Vv. spinales anteriores.
posterior s. hintere Rückenmarksvenen, Vv. spinales posteriores.
spi·nate ['spaɪneɪt] *adj* mit Dornen besetzt, dornig, dornenartig, dornförmig.
spi·na·tor reflex [spaɪneɪtər] Radius-, Radiusperiostreflex *m abbr.* RPR.
spina ventosa *ortho., ped.* Winddorn *m*, Spina ventosa.
spin·dle ['spɪndl] *n* **1.** Spindel *f*. **2.** *physiol.* Spindel(form *f*) *f*. **3.** Muskelspindel *f*. **4.** Kern-, Mitosespindel *f*.
α-spindle *n physiol.* α-Spindel *f*.
spindle and epithelioid cell nevus → spindle cell nevus.
spindle apparatus Spindelapparat *m*.
spindle cataract Spindelstar *m*, Cataracta fusiformis.
spindle cell *histol.* Spindelzelle *f*.
spindle cell carcinoma spindelzelliges Karzinom *nt*, Spindelzellkarzinom *nt*, Ca. fusocellulare.
spindle-celled layer multiforme Schicht *f*, Lamina multiformis (corticis cerebralis).
spindle cell fibrosarcoma spindelzelliges Fibrosarkom *nt*, Spindelzellsarkom *nt*.
spindle cell nevus Spitz-Tumor *m*, -Nävus *m*, Allen-Spitz-Nävus *m*, Epithelioidzellnävus *m*, Spindelzellnävus *m*, benignes juveniles Melanom *nt*.
spindle cell sarcoma spindelzelliges Sarkom *nt*, Spindelzellsarkom *nt*.
spindle cell tumor Spindelzelltumor *m*.
spindle fibers Spindelfasern *pl*.
spindle pole Spindelpol *m*.
β-spindles *pl* → sleep spindles.
spine [spaɪn] *n* **1.** *anat., bio.* Dorn *m*, Fortsatz *m*, Stachel *m*, Spina *f*. **2.** → spinal column.
s. of helix Helixhöcker *m*, Spina helicis.
s. of Henle Spina suprameatica/suprameatalis.
s. of ischium Spina ischiadica/ischialis.
s. of scapula Schulterblattgräte *f*, Spina scapulae.
s. of sphenoid bone Spina ossis sphenoidalis.
s. of vertebra Dornfortsatz *m*, Proc. spinosus.
spine cell (*Haut*) Stachelzelle *f*.
spine fusion → spinal fusion.
spi·nif·u·gal [spaɪ'nɪfəgəl] *adj* vom Rückenmark weg, spini-, spinofugal.
spi·nip·e·tal [spaɪ'nɪpətəl] *adj* zum Rückenmark hin, spini-, spinopetal.
spin label *phys.* Spinmarkierung *f*, Spinlabel *m*.
spin-label technique *phys.* Spinlabel-Technik *f*.
spin·ning mite ['spɪnɪŋ] *micro.* Bryobia praetiosia.
spino- *pref.* Rückenmark(s)-, Wirbelsäulen-, Spin(o)-.
spi·no·bul·bar [,spaɪnoʊ'bʌlbər] *adj* spinobulbär, bulbospinal.
spi·no·cer·e·bel·lar [,-,serə'belər] *adj* Rückenmark/Medulla spinalis u. Kleinhirn/Cerebellum betr. *od.* verbindend, spinozerebellär, -zerebellar.
spinocerebellar ataxia *neuro.* spinobelläre Ataxie *f*.
spinocerebellar fibers spinozerebelläre Fasern *pl*.
spinocerebellar pathways spinozerebelläre Bahnen *pl*.
spinocerebellar tract: anterior s. Gowers'-Bündel *nt*, Tractus spinocerebellaris anterior/ventralis.
direct s. Flechsig'-Bündel *nt*, Tractus spinocerebellaris dorsalis/posterior.
dorsal/posterior s. → direct s.
ventral s. → anterior s.
spi·no·cer·e·bel·lum [,-,serə'beləm] *n, pl* **-lums, -la** [-lə] Spinozerebellum *nt*.
spi·no·cer·vi·co·tha·lam·ic tract [,-,sɜrvɪkoʊθə'læmɪk] Tractus spinocervicothalamicus.
spi·no·col·lic·u·lar [,-kə'lɪkjələr] *adj* → spinotectal.
spi·no·cor·ti·cal [,-'kɔrtɪkl] *adj* Hirnrinde/Cortex u. Rückenmark/Medulla spinalis betr. *od.* verbindend, kortikospinal.
spi·no·gle·noid [,-'glenɔɪd, -'gli:-] *adj* Spina scapulae u. Cavitas glenoidalis betr. *od.* spinoglenoidal.
spinoglenoid ligament Lig. transversum scapulae inferius.
spi·no·ol·i·va·ry tract [,-'ɑlɪveri:, -vərɪ] Tractus spino-olivaris.
spi·nop·e·tal [spaɪ'nɑpətəl] *adj* → spinipetal.
spi·no·re·tic·u·lar tract [,spaɪnoʊrɪ'tɪkjələr] Tractus spinoreticularis.
spi·no·sa·cral [,-'sækrəl, -'seɪ-] *adj* → sacrospinal.
spinosacral ligament Lig. sacrospinale.
spi·nose ['spaɪnoʊs] *adj* → spinous.
spi·no·tec·tal [,spaɪnoʊ'tektəl] *adj* spinotektal, tektospinal.
spinotectal tract Tractus spinotectalis.

spi·no·tha·lam·ic cordotomy [ˌ-θəˈlæmɪk] *neurochir.* Durchtrennung *f* des Tractus spinothalamicus.
spinothalamic tract: anterior s. Tractus spinothalamicus anterior/ventralis.
lateral s. Tractus spinothalamicus lateralis.
ventral s. → anterior s.
spi·nous [ˈspaɪnəs] *adj* dornig, stach(e)lig, dorn-, stachelförmig.
spinous ear tick *micro.* Otobius *m.*
spinous foramen For. spinosum.
spinous layer of epidermis Stachelzellschicht *f*, Stratum spinosum epidermidis.
spinous process Dornfortsatz *m*, Proc. spinosus.
spinous synapse Dornsynapse *f.*
spi·no·ves·tib·u·lar tract [ˌspaɪnəʊvesˈtɪbjələr] Tractus spinovestibularis.
spin·thar·i·scope [spɪnˈθærɪskəʊp] *n phys.* Spinthariskop *nt*, Spintheriskop *nt.*
spin·ther·ism [ˈspɪnθərɪzəm] *n ophthal.* Funkensehen *nt*, Spintherismus *m*, Spintheropie *f*, Glaskörperglitzern *nt*, Synchisis scintillans.
spin·ther·o·pia [ˌspɪnθəˈrəʊpɪə] *n* → spintherism.
spin·y [ˈspaɪnɪ] *adj* dornig, stach(e)lig.
spiny-headed worms *micro.* Kratzer *pl*, Kratzwürmer *pl*, Acanthocephala *pl.*
spir- *pref.* → spiro-.
spi·rad·e·ni·tis [ˌspaɪˌrædɪˈnaɪtɪs] *n* Schweißdrüsenabszeß *m*, Hidradenitis suppurativa.
spi·rad·e·no·ma [ˌspaɪˌrædɪˈnəʊmə] *n* Schweißdrüsenadenom *nt*, Spiradenom(a) *nt*, Adenoma sudoriparum.
spi·ral [ˈspaɪrəl] I *n* Spirale *f*; Windung *f*; Spiral-, Schneckenlinie *f.* II *adj* 1. gewunden, schneckenförmig, spiral(förmig), spiralig, in Spiralen, Spiral-. 2. *mathe.* spiral, Spiral-.
spiral arteries Rankenarterien *pl.*
spiral bandage *ortho.* Schrauben-, Spiral-, Schlangengang *m*, Hobelspanverband *m.*
spiral canal: s. of cochlea Schneckengang *m*, Canalis spiralis cochleae.
s. of modiolus Rosenthal'-Kanal *m*, Schneckenspindelkanal *m*, Canalis ganglionaris, Canalis spiralis modioli.
spiral crest Labium limbi vestibulare.
s. of cochlea Lig. spirale, Crista spiralis (cochleae).
spiral drill Spiralbohrer *m.*
spiral duct → spiral canal of cochlea.
spiral fold → spiral valve (of cystic duct)
spiral foraminous tract Tractus spiralis foraminosus.
spiral fracture *ortho.* Torsions-, Dreh-, Spiralbruch *m*, -fraktur *f.*
spiral ganglion (of cochlea/of cochlear nerve) Corti'-Ganglion *nt*, Ggl. (spirale) cochleare.
spiral groove Radialisrinne *f*, Sulcus (n.) radialis.
spi·ral·iza·tion [ˌspaɪrəlɪˈzeɪʃn, -ˌlaɪˈz-] *n* Speichenbildung *f*, Spiralization *f*, Spiralisierung *f.*
spiral joint Ellipsoid-, Eigelenk *nt*, Artic. ellipsoidea/condylaris.
spiral lamina: bony s. Lamina spiralis ossea.
secondary s. Lamina spiralis secundaria.
spiral ligament of cochlea → spiral crest of cochlea.
spiral line (of femur) Linea intertrochanterica.
spiral membrane of cochlear duct untere Wand *f* des Ductus cochlearis, Membrana spiralis (cochlearis), Paries tympanicus ductus cochlearis.

spiral organ Corti'-Organ *nt*, Organum spirale.
spiral plate → spiral lamina, bony.
spiral prominence Prominentia spiralis.
spiral sulcus Radialisrinne *f*, Sulcus n. radialis, Sulcus spiralis.
external s. äußere Spiralfurche, Sulcus spiralis externus.
s. of humerus → spiral sulcus.
internal s. innere Spiralfurche, Sulcus spiralis internus.
spiral valve (of cystic duct) Heister'-Klappe *f*, Plica spiralis.
spi·ra·my·cin [spaɪrəˈmaɪsɪn] *n pharm.* Spiramycin *nt.*
spi·rem(e) [ˈspaɪriːm] *n* Spirem *nt.*
spi·ril·le·mia [ˌspaɪrəˈliːmɪə] *n* Spirillum-Sepsis *f.*
spi·ril·li·ci·dal [spaɪˌrɪləˈsaɪdl] *adj* spirillen(ab)tötend, spirillizid.
spi·ril·li·cide [spaɪˈrɪləsaɪd] I *n* spirillen(ab)tötendes Mittel *nt*, Spirillizid *nt.* II *adj* → spirillicidal.
spi·ril·lo·sis [ˌspaɪrəˈləʊsɪs, ˌspɪrɪ-] *n* Spirillenkrankheit *f*, Spirillose *f.*
spi·ril·lo·xan·thin [spaɪˌrɪləˈzænθɪn] *n* Spirilloxanthin *nt.*
Spi·ril·lum [spaɪˈrɪləm] *n micro.* Spirillum *nt.*
spi·ril·lum [spaɪˈrɪləm] *n*, *pl* **-la** [-lə] *micro.* Spirillum *nt.*
s. of Finkler and Prior Vibrio cholerae biotype proteus.
s. of Vincent Treponema/Borrelia/Spirochaeta vincentii.
spirillum fever Rückfallfieber *nt*, Febris recurrens.
spir·it [ˈspɪrɪt] *n* 1. Geist *m*, Lebenshauch *m*; Seele *f.* 2. Geist *m*, Gesinnung *f*, Sinn *m*; Charakter *m.* 3. *chem.* Spiritus *m*, Destillat *nt*; Geist *m*, Spiritus *m.* 4. Weingeist *m*, Äthylalkohol *m*, Äthanol *nt*, Ethanol *nt*, Spiritus (aethylicus) *m.*
s. of turpentine Terpentinöl *n.*
spir·it·u·ous [ˈspɪrɪt(j)əwəs] *adj* alkoholhaltig, alkoholisch.
spiro- *pref.* 1. Spiral-, Spir(o)-. 2. Atem-, Spir(o)-.
Spi·ro·chae·ta [ˌspaɪrəˈkiːtə] *n micro.* Spirochaeta *f.*
S. pseudoicterogenes apathogene Leptospiren *pl*, Wasserleptospiren *pl*, Leptospira biflexa.
Spi·ro·chae·ta·ce·ae [ˌ-kɪˈteɪsɪˌiː] *pl micro.* Spirochaetaceae *pl.*
Spi·ro·chae·ta·les [ˌ-kɪˈteɪliːz] *pl micro.* Spirochaetales *pl.*
spi·ro·chet·al [ˌ-ˈkiːtl] *adj* Spirochäten betr., druch sie verursacht, Spirochäten-.
spirochetal jaundice Weil'-Krankheit *f*, Leptospirosis icterohaemorrhagica.
spi·ro·chete [ˈ-kiːt] *n micro.* 1. Spirochäte *f.* 2. schraubenförmiges Bakterium *nt.*
spi·ro·chet·e·mia [ˌ-kɪˈtiːmɪə] *n* Spirochätensepsis *f.*
spi·ro·che·ti·ci·dal [ˌ-ˌkiːtəˈsaɪdl] *adj* spirochäten(ab)tötend, spirochätizid.
spi·ro·che·ti·cide [ˌ-ˈkiːtəsaɪd] *n* spirochäten(ab)tötendes Mittel *nt*, Spirochätizid *nt.*
spi·ro·che·tog·e·nous [ˌ-kɪˈtɒdʒənəs] *adj* durch Spirochäten verursacht, Spirochäten-.
spi·ro·chet·o·sis [ˌ-kɪˈtəʊsɪs] *n* Spirochäteninfektion *f*, Spirochätose *f.*
spi·ro·chet·u·ria [ˌ-kɪˈt(j)ʊərɪə] *n* Spirochätenausscheidung *f* im Harn, Spirochäturie *f.*
spi·ro·gram [ˈspaɪrəgræm] *n* Spirogramm *nt.*
spi·ro·graph [ˈ-græf] *n* Spirograph *m.*

spi·rog·ra·phy [spaɪˈrɒgrəfɪ] *n* Spirographie *f.*
spi·roid [ˈspaɪrɔɪd] *adj* spiralartig, -förmig, spiralig.
spiroid canal Fazialiskanal *m*, Canalis facialis.
spi·ro·lac·tone [ˌspaɪrəˈlæktəʊn] *n pharm.* Spirolakton *nt*, Spirolacton *nt.*
spi·ro·ma [spaɪˈrəʊmə] *n* → spiradenoma.
spi·rom·e·ter [spaɪˈrɒmɪtər] *n* Spirometer *nt.*
Spi·ro·met·ra [ˌspaɪrəˈmetrə] *n micro.* Spirometra *nt.*
spi·ro·met·ric [ˌ-ˈmetrɪk] *adj* Spirometrie *od.* Spirometer betr., spirometrisch.
spi·rom·e·try [spaɪˈrɒmətrɪ] *n* Spirometrie *f.*
spi·ro·no·lac·tone [ˌspaɪrənəʊˈlæktəʊn] *n pharm.* Spironolakton *nt*, Spironolacton *nt.*
spironolactone test Spironolacton-Test *m.*
spis·sat·ed [ˈspɪseɪtɪd] *adj* eingedickt, eingedampft.
Spitz [spɪts]: **S. nevus** Spitz-Tumor *m*, -Nävus *m*, Allen-Spitz-Nävus *m*, Epitheloidzellnävus *m*, Spindelzellnävus *m*, benignes juveniles Melanom *nt.*
Spitz-Allen [ˈælən]: **S.-A. nevus** → Spitz nevus.
Spitzer [ˈspɪtsər, ˈʃp-]: **S.'s fasciculus** Spitzer'-Faserbündel *nt*, Fasciculus tegmentalis ventralis.
Spitzka [ˈspɪtskə]: **S.'s (marginal) tract/zone** → Spitzka-Lissauer tract.
Spitzka-Lissauer [ˈlɪsaʊər]: **column of S.-L.** → S.-L. tract.
S.-L. tract Lissauer'(-Rand)-Bündel *nt*, Tractus dorsolateralis.
SPL *abbr.* → sound pressure level.
splanchn- *pref.* → splanchno-.
splanch·nec·to·pia [ˌsplæŋknekˈtəʊpɪə] *n* Eingeweideverlagerung *f*, Splanchnektopie *f.*
splanch·nem·phrax·is [ˌsplæŋknemˈfræksɪs] *n* Darmobstruktion *f.*
splanch·nes·the·sia [ˌsplæŋknesˈθiːʒ(ɪ)ə] *n* Eingeweidesensibilität *f.*
splanch·nes·thet·ic sensibility [ˌsplæŋknesˈθetɪk] Eingeweidesinn *m*, -sensibilität *f.*
splanch·nic [ˈsplæŋknɪk] *adj* Eingeweide/Viszera betr., Splanchno-, Eingeweide-.
splanchnic anesthesia Splanchnikusanästhesie *f.*
splanchnic block Splanchnikusblock *m.*
splanch·ni·cec·to·my [ˌsplæŋknɪˈsektəmɪ] *n neurochir.* Splanchnikusresektion *f*, Splanchnikektomie *f.*
splanchnic ganglion Ggl. thoracicum splanchnicum.
splanchnic mesoderm viszerales Mesoderm *nt.*
splanchnic nerve Eingeweidenerv *m*, Splanchnikus *m*, N. splanchnicus.
greater s. großer Eingeweidenerv *m*, Splanchnikus *m* major, N. splanchnicus (thoracicus) major.
inferior s. → lesser s.
lesser s. kleiner Eingeweidenerv *m*, Splanchnikus *m* minor, N. splanchnicus (thoracicus) minor.
lowest s. unterster Eingeweidenerv *m*, Splanchnikus *m* imus, N. splanchnicus (thoracicus) imus.
lumbar s.s lumbale Eingeweidenerven *pl*, Nn. splanchnici lumbales/lumbares.
major s. → greater s.
minor s. → lesser s.
pelvic s.s Beckeneingeweidenerven *pl*, Nn. splanchnici pelvici, Nn. erigentes.
sacral s.s sakrale Eingeweidenerven *pl*, Nn. splanchnici sacrales.

splanchnic neurectomy

thoracic s., greater → greater s.
thoracic s., inferior → lesser s.
thoracic s., lesser → lesser s.
thoracic s., lowest → lowest s.
thoracic s., major → greater s.
thoracic s., minor → lesser s.
splanchnic neurectomy → splanchnicectomy.
splanch·ni·cot·o·my [ˌsplæŋknɪˈkɑtəmɪ] n neurochir. Splanchnikusdurchtrennung f, Splachnikotomie f.
splanchno- pref. Splanchn(o)-, Eingeweide-.
splanch·no·cele [ˈsplæŋknəsiːl] n Eingeweidebruch m, Splanchnozele f.
splanch·no·coele [-siːl] n embryo. Splanchnozöl nt, Pleuroperitonealhöhle f.
splanch·no·cra·ni·um [ˌ-ˈkreɪnɪəm] n Eingeweideschädel m, Viszerokranium nt, -cranium nt, Splanchnokranium nt, -cranium nt, Cranium viscerale.
splanch·no·derm [ˈ-dɜrm] n → splanchnopleure.
splanch·no·di·as·ta·sis [ˌ-daɪˈæstəsɪs] n → splanchnectopia.
splanch·no·lith [ˈ-lɪθ] n Darmstein m, -konkrement nt, Splanchnolith m.
splanch·no·lo·gia [ˌ-ləʊdʒ(ɪ)ə] n Splanchnologie f, -logia f.
splanch·nol·o·gy [splæŋkˈnɑlədʒɪ] n → splanchnologia.
splanch·no·me·ga·lia [ˌsplæŋknəmɪˈgeɪljə] n → splanchnomegaly.
splanch·no·meg·a·ly [ˌ-ˈmegəlɪ] n Eingeweidevergrößerung f, Splanchno-, Viszeromegalie f.
splanch·no·mic·ri·a [ˌ-ˈmɪkrɪə] n Splanchno-, Viszeromikrie f.
splanch·nop·a·thy [splæŋkˈnɑpəθɪ] n Eingeweideerkrankung f, Splanchnopathie f.
splanch·no·pleu·ral [ˌsplæŋknəˈplʊərəl] adj Splanchnopleura betr., splanchnopleural.
splanch·no·pleure [ˈ-plʊər] n embryo. Splanchnopleura f.
splanch·no·pleu·ric [ˌ-ˈplʊərɪk] adj → splanchnopleural.
splanchnopleuric mesoderm splanchnopleurales Mesoderm nt.
splanch·nop·to·sia [ˌsplæŋknɑpˈtəʊsɪə] n → splanchnoptosis.
splanch·nop·to·sis [ˌsplæŋknɑpˈtəʊsɪs] n Eingeweidesenkung f, Splanchno-, Enteroptose f, Viszeroptose f.
splanch·no·scle·ro·sis [ˌsplæŋknəʊsklɪˈrəʊsɪs] n Eingeweide-, Splanchnosklerose f.
splanch·no·skel·e·ton [ˌ-ˈskelɪtn] n Visceralskelett nt.
splanch·no·so·mat·ic [ˌ-səʊˈmætɪk] adj splanchno-, viszerosomatisch.
S-plasty n chir. S-Plastik f.
splay foot [spleɪ] 1. Spreizfuß m, Pes transversus. 2. Plattfuß m, Pes planus.
spleen [spliːn] n Milz f; anat. Splen m, Lien m.
spleen tumor 1. Milzgeschwulst f, -tumor m. 2. → splenomegaly.
splen- pref. → spleno-.
splen n → spleen.
splen·ad·e·no·ma [ˌsplɪˈnædɪˈnəʊmə] n Pulpahyperplasie f, Splenadenom nt.
sple·nal·gia [splɪˈnældʒ(ɪ)ə] n → splenodynia.
splen·at·ro·phy [splenˈætrəfɪ] n Milzatrophie f, Splenatrophie f.
sple·nauxe [splɪˈnɔːksɪ] n → splenomegaly.
splen·cer·a·to·sis [ˌsplensərəˈtəʊsɪs] n Milzverhärtung f.

splen·cu·lus [ˈspleŋkjələs] n Nebenmilz f, Splen/Lien accessorius.
sple·nec·ta·sis [splɪˈnektəsɪs] n → splenomegaly.
sple·nec·to·mize [splɪˈnektəmaɪz] vt chir. eine Splenektomie durchführen, splenektomieren.
sple·nec·to·my [splɪˈnektəmɪ] n chir. Milzentfernung f, -exstirpation f, Splenektomie f.
splen·ec·to·pia [splɪnekˈtəʊpɪə] n 1. Milzverlagerung f, Splenektopie f. 2. Wandermilz f, Lien migrans/mobilis.
sple·nec·to·py [splɪˈnektəpɪ] n → splenectopia.
sple·ne·mi·a [splɪˈniːmɪə] n Milzstauung f; Stauungsmilz f.
sple·nem·phrax·is [ˌsplɪnemˈfræksɪs] n Milzstauung f.
sple·ne·o·lus [splɪˈnɪələs] n → splenculus.
sple·net·ic [spləˈnetɪk] I n 1. Milzkranke(r m) f. 2. fig. mürrischer Mensch m. II adj 3. → splenic. 4. schlechtgelaunt, mürrisch, griesgrämig.
sple·ni·al [ˈspliːnɪəl] adj 1. M. splenius betr. 2. Splenium betr.
splen·ic [ˈspliːnɪk, ˈsplen-] adj Milz/Splen betr., von der Milz ausgehend, lienal, splenisch, Lienal-, Milz-, Splen(o)-.
splenic abscess Milzabszeß m.
splen·i·cal [ˈspliːnɪkl, ˈsplen-] adj → splenic.
splenic anemia Banti-Krankheit f.
  familial s. Gaucher'-Erkrankung f, -Krankheit f, -Syndrom nt, Morbus Gaucher m, Glukozerebrosidose f, Zerebrosidlipidose f, Lipoidhistiozytose f vom Kerasintyp, Glykosylzeramidlipidose f.
splenic aneurysm → splenic artery aneurysm.
splenic arteriovenous fistula 1. arteriovenöse Fistel f der A. lienalis. 2. intrasplenale arteriovenöse Fistel f.
splenic artery Milzarterie f, Lienalis f, A. lienalis/splenica.
splenic artery aneurysm Milzarterienaneurysma nt, Aneurysma nt der A. lienalis.
splenic atrophy Milzatrophie f.
splenic bleeding Milzblutung f.
splenic branches of splenic artery Milzäste pl der Milzarterie, Rami lienales/splenici a. lienalis/splenicae.
splenic capsular hyalinosis (Milz-)Kapselhyalinose f.
splenic capsule Milzkapsel f.
splenic cords Milzstränge pl.
splenic corpuscles Malpighi'-Milzknötchen pl, Folliculi lymphatici splenici.
splenic cyst Milzzyste f.
splenic enlargement → splenomegaly.
splenic fever Milzbrand m, Anthrax m.
splenic flexure of colon linke Kolonflexur f, Flexura lienalis coli, Flexura coli sinistra.
splenic flexure syndrome Payr-Syndrom nt.
splenic follicles Milzknötchen pl, -follikel pl, Folliculi lymphatici splenici/lienalis.
splenic hematopoiesis → splenic hemopoiesis.
splenic hemopoiesis extramedulläre Blutbildung f in der Milz.
splenic hemorrhage → splenic bleeding.
splenic infarct/infarction Milzinfarkt m.
splenic injury Milzschädigung f, -verletzung f.
splenic nodules → splenic follicles.
splenic plexus Plexus lienalis/splenicus.
splenic portography radiol. Splenoportographie f.

splenic pulp (Milz) rote Pulpa f, Milzpulpa f, Pulpa splenica/lienis.
splenic puncture Milzpunktion f.
splenic recess Bucht f der Netztasche zum Milzhilus, Rec. lienalis/splenicus.
splenic rupture Milzriß m, -ruptur f.
splenic sac → splenic recess.
splenic sinus Milzsinus m, Sinus lienis/splenicus.
splenic tissue → splenic pulp.
splenic trabeculae Milzbalken pl, -trabekel pl, Trabeculae lienis/splenicae.
splenic trauma Milzverletzung f, -trauma nt.
splenic tumor 1. Milzgeschwulst f, -tumor m. 2. → splenomegaly.
sple·nic·u·lus [splɪˈnɪkjələs] n Nebenmilz f, Lien/Splen accessorius.
splenic vein Milzvene f, Lienalis f, V. lienalis/splenica.
splenic vein thrombosis Milzvenenthrombose f.
splenic venography Splenoportographie f.
splenic vessel Milzgefäße pl.
splen·i·fi·ca·tion [ˌsplenəfɪˈkeɪʃn] n → splenization.
splen·i·form [ˈsplenɪfɔːrm] adj milzartig, -förmig, spleniform.
sple·ni·tis [splɪˈnaɪtɪs] n Milzentzündung f, Splenitis f, Lienitis f.
sple·ni·um [ˈspliːnɪəm] n, pl -nia [-nɪə] Wulst m, Pflaster nt, Kompresse f, Splenium nt.
  s. of corpus callosum Balkenwulst, Splenium corporis callosi.
sple·ni·us [ˈspliːnɪəs] n, pl -nii [-nɪaɪ] → splenius muscle.
splenius capitis (muscle) Splenius m capitis, M. splenius capitis.
splenius cervicis (muscle) Splenius m cervicis, M. splenius cervicis.
splenius muscle Splenius m, M. splenius.
  s. of head → splenius capitis (muscle)
  s. of neck → splenius cervicis (muscle).
splen·i·za·tion [ˌsplenɪˈzeɪʃn] n patho. Splenisation f.
spleno- pref. Milz-, Lienal-, Splen(o)-, Lien(o)-.
sple·no·cele [ˈspliːnəsiːl] n 1. Splenozele f. 2. → splenoma.
sple·no·cer·a·to·sis [ˌ-ˌserəˈtəʊsɪs] n Milzverhärtung f.
sple·no·col·ic [ˌ-ˈkɑlɪk] adj Milz/Splen u. Kolon betr. od. verbindend, splenokolisch.
sple·no·dyn·ia [ˌ-ˈdiːnɪə] n Milzschmerzen pl, Splenodynie f, Splenalgie f.
sple·no·gas·tric ligament [ˌ-ˈgæstrɪk]Magen-Milz-Band nt, Lig. gastrolienale/gastrosplenicum.
splenogastric omentum → splenogastric ligament.
sple·nog·e·nous [splɪˈnɑdʒənəs] adj aus der Milz stammend, in der Milz gebildet, splenogen.
sple·no·gram [ˈ-græm] n radiol. Splenogramm nt.
sple·nog·ra·phy [splɪˈnɑgrəfɪ] n radiol. Kontrastdarstellung f der Milz, Splenographie f.
sple·no·hep·a·to·me·ga·lia [ˌspliːnəʊˌhepətəmɪˈgeɪljə] n → splenohepatomegaly.
sple·no·hep·a·to·meg·a·ly [ˌ-ˌhepətəʊˈmegəlɪ] n Milz- u. Lebervergrößerung f, Splenohepatomegalie f, Hepatosplenomegalie f.
sple·noid [ˈsplɪnɔɪd] adj milzartig, -ähnlich, splenoid.
sple·no·ker·a·to·sis [ˌspliːnəʊkerəˈtəʊsɪs] n Milzverhärtung f.
sple·no·lap·a·rot·o·my [ˌ-ˌlæpəˈrɑtəmɪ] n chir. Laparosplenotomie f.

716

sple·no·ma [splɪ'nəʊmə] *n* Milztumor *m*, Splenom(a) *nt*.
sple·no·ma·la·cia [ˌspliːnəʊmə'leɪʃ(ɪ)ə] *n* Milzerweichung *f*, Splenomalazie *f*.
sple·no·med·ul·lar·y [ˌ-'medlərɪː] *adj* Milz/Splen u. Knochenmark betr., splenomedullär.
sple·no·me·ga·lia [ˌ-mɪ'geɪljə] *n* splenomegaly.
sple·no·me·gal·ic polycythemia [ˌ-mɪ'gælɪk] Osler-Krankheit *f*, Osler-Vaquez--Krankheit *f*, Vaquez-Osler-Syndrom *nt*, Morbus Vaquez-Osler *m*, Erythrämie *f*, Polycythaemia (rubra) vera.
sple·no·meg·a·ly [ˌ-'megəlɪ] *n* Milzvergrößerung *f*, -schwellung *f*, -tumor *m*, Splenomegalie *f*, -megalia *f*.
sple·nom·e·try [splɪ'nɑmətrɪ] *n* Splenometrie *f*.
sple·no·my·e·log·e·nous [ˌspliːnəˌmaɪə'lɑdʒənəs] *adj* splenomedullary.
sple·no·my·e·lo·ma·la·cia [ˌ-ˌmaɪələʊmə'leɪʃ(ɪ)ə] *n* Splenomyelomalazie *f*.
sple·no·n·cus [splɪ'nɑŋkəs] *n* 1. → splenoma. 2. → splenomegaly.
sple·no·neph·ric [ˌspliːnə'nefrɪk] *adj* → splenorenal.
sple·no·neph·rop·to·sis [ˌ-ˌnefrɑp'təʊsɪs] *n* Milz- u. Nierensenkung *f*, Splenonephroptose *f*.
sple·no·pan·cre·at·ic [ˌ-ˌpæŋkrɪ'ætɪk] *adj* Milz/Splen u. Bauchspeicheldrüse/Pankreas betr., lieno-, splenopankreatisch.
sple·nop·a·thy [splɪ'nɑpəθɪ] *n* Milzerkrankung *f*, Splenopathie *f*.
sple·no·pex·ia [ˌsplɪːnəʊ'peksɪə] *n* → splenopexy.
sple·no·pex·y ['-peksɪ] *n chir.* Milzfixation *f*, -anheftung *f*, Splenopexie *f*.
sple·no·phren·ic ligament [ˌ-'frenɪk] → splenorenal ligament.
sple·no·por·tal hypertension [ˌ-'pɔːrtl] splenoportale Hypertonie *f*.
sple·no·por·to·gram [ˌ-'pɔːrtəgræm] *n* Splenoportogramm *nt*.
sple·no·por·tog·ra·phy [ˌ-pɔːr'tɑgrəfɪ] *n radiol.* Splenoportographie *f*.
sple·nop·to·sia [ˌsplɪːnɑp'təʊsɪə] *n* → splenoptosis.
sple·nop·to·sis [ˌsplɪːnɑp'təʊsɪs] *n* Milzsenkung *f*, Splenoptose *f*.
sple·no·re·nal [ˌspliːnəʊ'riːnl] *adj* Milz/Splen u. Niere/Ren betr., splenorenal, lienorenal.
splenorenal ligament Lig. splenorenale/lienorenale/phrenicosplenicum.
splenorenal shunt *chir.* splenorenale Anastomose *f*, splenorenaler Shunt *m*.
  distal s. distale splenorenale Anastomose.
  proximal s. proximale/klassische splenorenale Anastomose.
sple·nor·rha·gia [ˌ-'reɪdʒ(ɪ)ə] *n* Milzblutung *f*, Splenorrhagie *f*.
sple·nor·rha·phy [splɪ'nɔːrəfɪ] *n chir.* Milznaht *f*, Splenorrhaphie *f*.
sple·no·sis [splɪ'nəʊsɪs] *n* posttraumatische Polysplenie *f*, Splenose *f*.
sple·not·o·my [splɪ'nɑtəmɪ] *n chir.* Splenotomie *f*.
splen·ule ['splenjuːl] *n* Nebenmilz *f*, Lien/Splen accessorius.
splen·u·lus ['splenjələs] *n, pl* **-li** [-laɪ] → splenule.
sple·nun·cu·lus [splɪ'nʌŋkjələs] *n, pl* **-li** [-laɪ] → splenule.
splic·ing ['splaɪsɪŋ] *n genet.* Splicing *nt*, Spleißen *nt*.
splint [splɪnt] I *n ortho.* Schiene *f*. II *vt* schienen. **to put on a ~** (*Bruch*) schienen.
splin·ter ['splɪntər] I *n* Splitter *m*, Span *m*, Bruchstück *nt*. II *vi* zersplittern.

splin·tered fracture ['splɪntərd] Splitterbruch *m*.
splint·ing ['splɪntɪŋ] *n ortho.* Schienen *nt*, Schienung *f*.
split [splɪt] (*v* **split**; **split**) I *n* 1. Spalt *m*, Riß *m*, Sprung *m*. 2. (*a. fig.*) Spaltung *f*, Bruch *m*. II *adj* zer-, gespalten, geteilt, Spalt-. III *vt* (zer-, auf-)spalten, (zer-)teilen; *chem.* aufschließen. IV *vi* s. (auf-)spalten, s. (auf-)teilen; zerspringen, (zer-)platzen, bersten.
split cloth Binde *f* mit mehreren Enden.
split foot Spaltfuß *m*.
split hand Spalthand *f*.
split pelvis Spaltbecken *nt*.
split personality *psycho.* multiple/gespaltene Persönlichkeit *f*.
split product Spaltprodukt *nt*.
  fibrinolytic s.s *pl abbr.* FSP Fibrin(ogen)spaltprodukte *pl abbr.* FSP, Fibrin(ogen)degradationsprodukte *pl abbr.* FDP.
split-protein vaccine Spaltimpfstoff *m*, -vakzine *f*.
split-skin graft Spalthautlappen *m*, -transplantat *nt*.
split-thickness flap/graft → split-skin graft.
split·ting ['splɪtɪŋ] I *n* 1. (Zer-)Teilung *f*, Spaltung *f*; Spalten *nt*. 2. *card.* Splitting *nt*. II *adj* zerreißend, (auf-)spaltend; (*Kopfschmerz*) rasend, heftig.
split tongue gespaltene Zunge *f*, Lingua bifida.
split uvula Zäpfchen-, Uvulaspalte *f*, Uvula bifida.
split-virus vaccine → split-protein vaccine.
spo·di·o·my·e·li·tis [ˌspəʊdɪəʊˌmaɪə'laɪtɪs] *n* (epidemische/spinale) Kinderlähmung *f*, Heine-Medin-Krankheit *f*, Poliomyelitis (epidemica) anterior acuta.
spo·dog·e·nous [spə'dɑdʒənəs] *adj* durch Abfallprodukte/Zersetzungsprodukte bedingt, spodogen.
spod·o·gram ['spəʊdəgræm] *n histol.* Aschenbild *nt*, Spodogramm *nt*.
spo·dog·ra·phy [spə'dɑgrəfɪ] *n* Spodographie *f*.
spoke bone [spəʊk] *old* → radius 2.
Spond·we·ni virus [spɒnd'wiːnɪ] *micro.* Spondweni-Virus *nt*.
spondyl- *pref.* → spondylo-.
spon·dyl·al·gia [ˌspɑndɪ'lældʒ(ɪ)ə] *n* Wirbelschmerz(en *pl*) *m*, Spondylalgie *f*, Spondylodynie *f*.
spon·dyl·ar·thri·tis [ˌspɑndɪlɑːr'θraɪtɪs] *n* 1. Entzündung *f* der Wirbelgelenke, Spondylarthritis *f*. 2. Spondylarthrose *f*.
spon·dyl·ar·throc·a·ce [ˌ-ɑːr'θrɑkəsiː] *n* → spondylocace.
spon·dyl·ar·throp·a·thy [ˌ-ɑːr'θrɑpəθɪ] *n* Spondylarthropathie *f*, -pathia *f*.
spon·dyl·ex·ar·thro·sis [ˌ-ˌeksɑːr'θrəʊsɪs] *n* Wirbeldislokation *f*.
spon·dy·lit·ic [ˌspɑndɪ'lɪtɪk] *adj* Spondylitis betr., spondylitisch.
spon·dy·li·tis [ˌ-'laɪtɪs] *n* Wirbelentzündung *f*, Spondylitis *f*.
spondylo- *pref.* Wirbel-, Spondyl(o)-.
spon·dy·loc·a·ce [spɑndɪ'lɑkəsiː] *n* Wirbeltuberkulose *f*, Spondylitis tuberculosa.
spon·dy·lo·dyn·ia [ˌspɑndɪləʊ'diːnɪə] *n* → spondylalgia.
spon·dy·lo·ep·i·phys·e·al dysplasia [ˌ-epɪ'fiːzɪəl] Dysplasia spondyloepiphysaria.
spon·dy·lo·lis·the·sis [ˌ-lɪs'θiːsɪs] *n ortho.* Wirbelgleiten *nt*, Spondylolisthese *f*, -listhesis *f*.
spon·dy·lo·lis·thet·ic [ˌ-lɪs'θetɪk] *adj* Spondylolisthese betr.
spondylolisthetic pelvis Wirbelgleit-

becken *nt*, spondylolisthetisches Becken *nt*, Pelvis spondylolisthetica.
spon·dy·lol·y·sis [spɑndɪ'lɑləsɪs] *n ortho.* Spondylolyse *f*.
spon·dy·lo·ma·la·cia [ˌspɑndɪləʊmə'leɪʃ(ɪ)ə] *n* Wirbelerweichung *f*, Spondylomalazie *f*, -malacia *f*.
spon·dy·lop·a·thy [ˌspɑndɪ'lɑpəθɪ] *n ortho.* Wirbelerkrankung *f*, Spondylopathie *f*.
spon·dy·lop·to·sis [ˌ-lɑp'təʊsɪs] *n ortho.* Spondyloptose *f*.
spon·dy·lo·py·o·sis [ˌspɑndɪləʊpaɪ'əʊsɪs] *n* Wirbeleiterung *f*, Spondylopyose *f*.
spon·dy·los·chi·sis [ˌspɑndɪ'lɑskəsɪs] *n* Spondyloschisis *f*, R(h)achischisis posterior.
spon·dy·lo·sis [ˌ-'ləʊsɪs] *n* 1. Wirbelsäulenversteifung *f*, Spondylose *f*, Spondylosis *f*. 2. degenerative Spondylopathie *f*.
spon·dy·lo·syn·de·sis [ˌspɑndɪləʊsɪn'diːsɪs] *n ortho.* operative Wirbelsäulenversteifung *f*, Spondylodese *f*.
spon·dy·lot·ic [ˌspɑndɪ'lɑtɪk] *adj* Spondylose betr., spondylotisch.
spondylotic osteophyte spondylotische Randzacke/Randleiste *f*.
spon·dy·lot·o·my [ˌ-'lɑtəmɪ] *n neurochir., ortho.* 1. Kolumnotomie *f*, Rhachi(o)tomie *f*. 2. Laminektomie *f*.
spon·dy·lous ['spɑndɪləs] *adj* Wirbel betr., vertebral, Wirbel-, Spondyl(o)-.
sponge [spʌndʒ] I *n* 1. Schwamm *m*. 2. Tupfer *m*. II *vt* abwaschen. III *vi* s. vollsaugen.
sponge up *vt* (mit einem Schwamm) aufsaugen *od.* aufnehmen.
sponge forceps *chir.* Tupferklemme *f*.
spon·ge·i·tis → spongitis.
sponge kidney Schwammniere *f*, Cacchi--Ricci-Syndrom *nt*.
sponge-like *adj* → spongy.
spongi- *pref.* → spongio-.
spon·gi·form ['spʌndʒɪfɔːrm] *adj* schwammartig, -förmig, spongiform.
spongiform encephalopathy spongiforme Enzephalopathie *f*.
spongiform leukodystrophy Canavan--Syndrom *nt*, (Canavan-)van Bogaert--Bertrand-Syndrom *nt*, frühinfantile spongiöse Dystrophie *f*.
spongiform pustule of Kogoj Kogoj-Pustel *f*.
spon·gi·i·tis [ˌspʌndʒɪ'aɪtɪs] *n urol.* Entzündung *f* des Corpus spongiosum, Spong(i)itis *f*, Spongiositis *f*.
spon·gi·i·ness ['spʌndʒɪnɪs] *n* Schwammigkeit *f*, Porosität *f*.
spongio- *pref.* Schwamm-, Spongi(o)-.
spon·gio·blast ['spʌndʒɪəʊblæst, 'spɑn-] *n embryo.* Spongioblast *m*.
spon·gio·blas·to·ma [ˌ-blæs'təʊmə] *n* Spongioblastom(a) *nt*.
spon·gio·cyte [-saɪt] *n* 1. (*ZNS*) Gliazelle *f*, Spongiozyt *m*. 2. (*NNR*) Spongiozyt *m*.
spon·gio·cy·to·ma [ˌ-saɪ'təʊmə] *n* Spongioblastom(a) *nt*.
spon·gi·oid [-ɔɪd] *adj* → spongy.
spon·gi·o·sa [spɑndʒɪ'əʊsə, ˌspɑn-] *n* 1. Spongiosa *f*, Lamina/Pars spongiosa, Stratum spongiosum endometrii. 2. → spongy bone.
spon·gi·o·sa·plas·ty [spʌndʒɪˌəʊsə'plæstɪ] *n ortho.* Spongiosaplastik *f*.
spon·gi·ose ['spʌndʒɪəʊs] *adj* → spongy.
spon·gi·o·sis [ˌspʌndʒɪ'əʊsɪs] *n* Spongiose *f*, Spongiosis *f*.
spon·gi·o·si·tis [ˌspʌndʒɪə'saɪtɪs] *n* → spongiitis.
spon·gy ['spʌndʒɪ] *adj* schwammig, schwammartig, -ähnlich, spongiös, Schwamm-, porös.
spongy body: s. of male urethra Harnröh-

spongy bone

renschwellkörper *m*, Corpus spongiosum penis.
s. of penis (Penis-)Schwellkörper *m*, Corpus cavernosum penis.
spongy bone Spongiosa *f*, Substantia spongiosa/trabecularis (ossium).
inferior s. untere Nasenmuschel *f*, Concha nasalis inferior.
middle s. mittlere Nasenmuschel *f*, Concha nasalis media.
superior s. obere Nasenmuschel *f*, Concha nasalis superior.
supreme s. oberste Nasenmuschel *f*, Concha nasalis suprema.
spongy bone substance → spongy bone.
spongy degeneration (of central nervous system/of white matter) Canavan-Syndrom *nt*, (Canavan-)van Bogaert- -Bertrand-Syndrom *nt*, frühinfantile spongiöse Dystrophie *f*.
spongy layer of endometrium → spongiosa 1.
spongy part of (male) urethra spongiöser Urethraabschnitt *m*, Pars spongiosa (urethrae masculinae).
spongy substance of bone → spongy bone.
spongy tunic of female urethra Schwellgewebe *nt* der weiblichen Harnröhre, Tunica spongiosa urethrae femininae.
spon·ta·ne·ous [spɒn'teɪnɪəs] *adj* von selbst (entstanden), von innen heraus (kommend), spontan, selbsttätig, unwillkürlich, Spontan-.
spontaneous abortion *gyn.* Fehlgeburt *f*, Spontanabort *m*, Abgang *m*, Abort(us) *m*.
spontaneous agglutination Spontanagglutination *f*.
spontaneous allergy atopische Allergie *f*.
spontaneous amputation *patho.* Spontanamputation *f*.
spontaneous bacterial myositis Myositis purulenta tropica.
spontaneous convulsion zentralbedingte Konvulsion *f*.
spontaneous cretinism → sporadic cretinism.
spontaneous delivery *gyn.* Spontangeburt *f*, -entbindung *f*.
spontaneous evolution *gyn.* Spontan-, Selbstentwicklung *f*.
spontaneous fracture pathologische Fraktur *f*, Spontanfraktur *f*.
spontaneous generation *bio.* Urzeugung *f*, Abiogenese *f*, Abiogenesis *f*.
spontaneous hemorrhage Spontanblutung *f*.
spontaneous labor *gyn.* Spontangeburt *f*, -entbindung *f*.
spontaneous movement Spontanbewegung *f*.
spontaneous mutation *genet.* Spontanmutation *f*.
spontaneous myoglobinuria idiopathische/familiäre Myoglobinurie *f*.
spontaneous nystagmus Spontannystagmus *m*.
spontaneous osteonecrosis spontane/aseptische Knochennekrose *f*.
spontaneous pneumothorax Spontanpneu(mothorax *m*) *m*.
spontaneous rupture of esophagus Boerhaave-Syndrom *nt*, spontane/postemetische/emetogene Ösophagusruptur *f*.
spontaneous version *gyn.* Selbstwendung *f*, Versio spontaneu.
spoon [spuːn] *n* (*a. chir.*) Löffel *m*.
spoon nail Löffel-, Hohlnagel *m*, Koilonychie *f*.
spoon-shaped foot Löffel-, Flossenfuß *m*.

spoon-shaped hand Löffelhand *f*.
spor- *pref.* → sporo-.
spo·rad·ic [spə'rædɪk] *adj* vereinzelt, verstreut (vorkommend), unregelmäßig, sporadisch.
sporadic cretinism sporadischer Kretinismus *m*.
sporadic-recessive deafness sporadisch- -rezessive Schwerhörigkeit *f*.
spo·ran·gi·al [spə'rændʒɪəl] *adj micro.* Sporangium betr., Sporangien-, Sporangio-.
spo·ran·gi·ole [spə'rændʒɪəʊl] *n micro.* Sporangiole *f*.
spo·ran·gi·o·lum [spəˌrændʒɪ'əʊləm] *n, pl* -la [-lə] *micro.* Sporangiole *f*.
spo·ran·gi·o·phore [spə'rændʒɪəfəʊər, -fɔːr] *n micro.* Sporangienträger *m*.
spo·ran·gi·o·spore ['-spəʊər, -spɔːr] *n micro.* Sporangienspore *f*, Sporangiospore *f*.
spo·ran·gi·um [spə'rændʒɪəm] *n, pl* -gia [-dʒɪə] *micro.* Sporen-, Fruchtbehälter *m*, Sporangium *nt*.
spo·ra·tion [spə'reɪʃn] *n* → sporulation.
spore [spəʊər, spɔːr] *n micro.* Spore *f*, Spora *f*.
spore-bearing *adj* sporentragend.
spore capsule *micro.* Sporenkapsel *f*.
spore case → sporangium.
spore cortex *micro.* Sporenrinde *f*.
spore dispersal *micro.* Sporenverbreitung *f*.
spore formation 1. → sporogenesis. 2. → sporulation.
spore-forming anaerobe *micro.* sporenbildender Anaerobier *m*.
spore-forming bacilli *micro.* Sporenbildner *pl*.
spore·less ['spəʊərlɪs, 'spɔːr-] *adj micro.* nicht-sporenbildend, sporenlos.
spore stain Sporenfärbung *f*.
spore wall *micro.* Sporenwand *f*.
spo·ri·ci·dal [ˌspəʊrɪ'saɪdl] *adj* sporenzerstörend, -(ab)tötend, sporizid.
spo·ri·cide ['spəʊrɪsaɪd] *n* sporizides Mittel *nt*, Sporizid *nt*.
spo·rid·i·um [spə'rɪdɪəm] *n, pl* -dia [-dɪə] *micro.* Sporidie *f*.
spo·rif·er·ous [spə'rɪfərəs] *adj micro.* sporentragend.
spo·rip·a·rous [spə'rɪpərəs] *adj micro.* sporenbildend.
sporo- *pref.* Sporen-, Spor(o)-.
spo·ro·ag·glu·ti·na·tion [ˌspəʊərəʊəˌgluːtə'neɪʃn, ˌspɔːrə-] *n* Sporoagglutination *f*.
spor·o·blast ['-blæst] *n* Sporoblast *m*.
spo·ro·carp [-kɑːrp, -kɑp] *n bio.* Sporenfrucht *f*, Sporokarp *n*.
spor·o·cyst ['-sɪst] *n* Sporozyste *f*.
spor·o·gen·e·sis [ˌ-'dʒenəsɪs] *n micro.* Sporenbildung *f*, Sporogenese *f*, Sporogenie *f*.
spo·ro·gen·ic [ˌ-'dʒenɪk] *adj micro.* sporenbildend, sporogen.
sporogenic cycle *micro.* (*Protozoen*) sexueller/sporogoner Vermehrungszyklus *m*.
spo·rog·e·nous [spə'rɒdʒənəs] *adj* s. durch Sporen vermehrend, sporenbildend, sporogen.
sporogenous cycle → sporogenic cycle.
spo·rog·e·ny [spə'rɒdʒənɪ] *n* → sporogenesis.
spo·rog·o·ny [spə'rɒgənɪ] *n* Sporogonie *f*.
spo·ront ['spɔːrɒnt] *n* Sporont *m*.
spo·ro·phore ['spəʊərəfɔːr, 'spɔːrə-, -fɔːr] *n micro.* Sporenträger *m*, Sporophor *nt*.
spo·ro·phyte ['-faɪt] *n micro.* Sporen-, Sporoplasma *nt*.
spor·o·plasm ['-plæzəm] *n micro.* Sporen-, Sporoplasma *nt*.

Spo·ro·thrix ['-θrɪks] *n micro.* Sporothrix *f*.
spo·rot·ri·chin [spə'rɒtrɪkɪn] *n* Sporotrichin *nt*.
spo·ro·tri·cho·sis [ˌspəʊərəʊtraɪ'kəʊsɪs, ˌspɔːrə-] *n* De Beurmann-Gougerot- -Krankheit *f*, Sporotrichose *f*.
Spo·rot·ri·chum [spə'rɒtrɪkəm] *n micro.* Sporotrichum *nt*, Sporotrichon *nt*.
Spo·ro·zoa [ˌspəʊərə'zəʊə, ˌspɔːrə-] *pl micro.* Sporentierchen *pl*, Sporozoen *pl*, Sporozoa *pl*.
spo·ro·zoa *pl* → sporozoon.
Spo·ro·zo·an [ˌ-'zəʊən] *micro.* I *n* → sporozoon. II *adj* Sporozoen betr., Sporozoen-.
Spo·ro·zo·ea [ˌ-'zəʊɪə] *pl* → Sporozoa.
Spo·ro·zo·ite [ˌ-'zəʊaɪt] *n micro.* Sporozoit *m*.
Spo·ro·zo·on [ˌ-'zəʊɒn] *n, pl* -zoa [-'zəʊə] *micro.* Sporozoon *nt*.
Spo·ro·zo·o·sis [ˌ-zəʊ'əʊsɪs] *n* Sporozoeninfektion *f*.
sport[1] [spɔːrt] I *n* (*a.* **~s** *pl*) Sport *m*; Sportart *f*. II *adj* sportlich, Sport-.
sport[2] [spɔːrt] *n genet.* Knospen-, Sproßmutation *f*, Sport *m*.
sports medicine Sportmedizin *f*.
spor·u·lar ['spɔːrjələr, 'spɑːr-] *adj* Spore betr., Sporen-.
spor·u·late ['-leɪt] *vt micro.* Sporen bilden.
spor·u·la·tion [ˌ-'leɪʃn] *n* Sporenbildung *f*, Sporulation *f*.
spor·ule ['spɔːrjuːl, 'spɑːr-] *n* kleine Spore *f*.
spot [spɒt] *n* 1. Fleck(en *m*) *m*. 2. (Leber-)-Fleck *m*, Hautmal *nt*; Pickel *m*, Pustel *f*. 3. Ort *m*, Stelle *f*; Punkt *m*.
spot check Stichprobe *f*.
spot-check *vt* stichprobenweise überprüfen.
spot·ted ['spɒtɪd] *adj* 1. gefleckt, fleckig, voller Flecken, Fleck-. 2. befleckt, Fleck-.
spotted fever Fleckfieber *nt*, Flecktyphus *m*.
spotted sickness Pinta *f*, Mal del Pinto, Carate *f*.
spot test Stichprobe *f*.
spot·ting ['spɒtɪŋ] *n gyn.* Schmierblutung *f*.
spot·ty ['spɒtɪ] *adj* 1. pickelig, voller Pickel. 2. → spotted 1.
spotty kidney Fleck-, Flohstichniere *f*.
spotty spleen Fleckenmilz *f*.
spous·al ['spaʊzl] *adj* Hochzeits-, Ehe-, Gatten-.
spouse [spaʊz] *n* (Ehe-)Gatte *m*, (Ehe-)-Gattin *f*.
spout cup [spaʊt] Schnabeltasse *f*.
sprain [spreɪn] *ortho.* I *n* (*Gelenk*) Verstauchung *f*; (*Band*) Dehnung *f*; (*Muskel*) Zerrung *f*. II *vt* (*Gelenk*) verstauchen; (*Band*) dehnen; (*Muskel*) zerren.
sprain fracture Ab-, Ausrißfraktur *f*.
spray [spreɪ] I *n pharm.* Spray *m/nt*; Zerstäuber *m*, Sprüh-, Spraydose *f*. II *vt* zer-, verstäuben, versprühen, sprayen.
spread [spred] (*v* spread; spread) I *n* 1. Ver-, Ausbreitung *f*. 2. Ausdehnung *f*, Breite *f*, Weite *f*, Umfang *m*. 3. *mathe.* Streuung *f*; *stat.* Abweichung *f*. II *adj* ausgebreitet, verbreitet; gespreizt, Spreiz-. III *vt* 4. ausbreiten, ausstrecken; (*Beine*) spreizen. 5. bedecken, übersäen, überziehen (*with mit*). 6. ausbreiten, verteilen, streuen. 7. (*Krankheit*) ver-, ausbreiten. IV *vi* s. verbreiten, s. ausbreiten.
spread out s. ausbreiten, s. verteilen, s. entfalten.
spread·er ['spredər] *n* 1. Streu-, Spritzgerät *nt*. 2. Zerstäuber *m*. 3. *chir.* Spreizer *m*.
spread foot Spreizfuß *m*, Pes transversus.

spread·ing factor ['spredɪŋ] Hyaluronidase f.
spree-drinking [spri:] n ε-Alkoholismus m, Dipsomanie f, inf. Quartalsaufen nt.
Sprengel ['sprenǝl]: **S.'s deformity** kongenitaler Schulterblatthochstand m, Sprengel-Deformität f.
sprew n → sprue.
spring [sprɪŋ] (v **sprang/sprung; sprung**) **I** n 1. Sprung m, Satz m. 2. Elastizität f, Federung f, Sprung-, Schnellkraft f; techn. (Sprung-)Feder f. 3. (a. fig.) Quelle f; Ursprung m. 4. Riß m, Sprung m, Spalt m. **II** vt 5. springen/zurückschnellen lassen; (ab-)federn. 6. zerbrechen, spalten. **III** vi 7. (auf-)springen. 8. (heraus-)sprühen, (-)spritzen, sprudeln. 9. (ab-)stammen, kommen, entstehen (from aus).
spring balance Federwaage f.
spring conjunctivitis Frühjahrkonjunktivitis f, -katarrh m, Conjunctivitis vernalis.
spring·ing mydriasis ['sprɪŋɪŋ] ophthal. alternierende/springende Mydriasis f, Mydriasis alternans.
spring ligament Lig. calcaneonaviculare plantare.
spring ophthalmia → spring conjunctivitis.
spring suspensium Federung f, federnde Aufhängung f.
Sprinz-Dubin [sprɪnts 'dju:bɪn]: **S.-D. syndrome** Dubin-Johnson-Syndrom nt.
Sprinz-Nelson ['nelsǝn]: **S.-N. syndrome** → Sprinz-Dubin syndrome.
S-protein n biochem. S-Protein nt, Vitronektin nt.
sprout [spraʊt] **I** n Sproß m, Sprößling m. **II** v keimen lassen, wachsen lassen, entwickeln. **III** vi sprießen, keimen, aufgehen, Knospen treiben, knospen.
sprue [spru:] n Sprue f.
Spu·ma·vir·i·nae [ˌspju:mǝ'vɪǝrǝni:, -'vɪǝ-] pl micro. Spumaviren pl, Spumavirinae pl.
Spu·ma·vi·rus [ˌ-'vaɪrǝs] n micro. Spumavirus nt.
spur [spɜr] n 1. Sporn m. 2. bio. Sporn m; Dorn m, Stachel m.
spur-cell anemia Anämie f bei Akanthozytose.
spur crusher ortho. Hohlmeißelzange f.
spur crushing clamp ortho. Hohlmeißelzange f.
spu·ri·ous ['spjʊǝrǝs] adj ver-, gefälscht, falsch, unecht, Pseudo-, Schein-.
spurious aneurysm falsches Aneurysma nt, Aneurysma spurium.
spurious ankylosis fibröse Gelenkversteifung/Ankylose f, Ankylosis fibrosa.
spurious cast (Harn) Pseudozylinder m, Zylindroid nt.
spurious hermaphroditism falscher Hermaphroditismus m, Hermaphroditismus spurius, Pseudohermaphroditismus m.
spurious meningocele traumatische Meningozele f.
spu·ri·ous·ness ['spjʊǝrǝsnɪs] n Unechtheit f, falsche od. unechte Natur f.
spurious pregnancy gyn. Scheinschwangerschaft f, Pseudokyesis f, Pseudogravidität f.
spurious ribs falsche Rippen pl, Costae spuriae.
spurious septum embryo. Septum spurium.
spurious tube cast → spurious cast.
Spurway ['spɜrweɪ]: **S. syndrome** ortho. Eddowes-Syndrom nt, Eddowes--Spurway-Syndrom nt.

spu·ta·men·tum [spju:tǝ'mentǝm] n → sputum.
spu·tum ['spju:tǝm] n, pl **-ta** [-tǝ] Auswurf m, Sputum nt, Expektoration f.
sputum cytology Sputumzytologie f.
sputum sample Sputumprobe f.
SP vaccine Spaltimpfstoff m, -vakzine f.
squal·ene ['skweɪli:n] n Squalen nt.
squalene-2,3-epoxide n Squalen-2,3--epoxid nt.
squalene epoxide lanosterol-cyclase Squalenepoxid-Lanosterincyclase f.
squalene monooxygenase Squalenmonooxigenase f.
squalene synthase Squalensynthase f.
squa·ma ['skweɪmǝ] n, pl **-mae** [-mi:] anat., bio. Schuppe f, Squama f.
s. of frontal bone Stirnbeinschuppe, Squama frontalis.
squama occipitalis Hinterhauptsschuppe f, Squama occipitalis.
squa·mate ['skweɪmeɪt] adj mit Schuppen bedeckt, schuppig.
squa·ma·ti·za·tion [ˌskweɪmǝtɪ'zeɪʃn] n patho. Squamatisation f, squamöse Metaplasie f, Plattenepithelmetaplasie f.
squame [skweɪm] n → squama.
squa·mo·cel·lu·lar [ˌskweɪmǝʊ'seljǝlǝr] adj Plattenepithel betr., Plattenepithel-.
squa·mo·fron·tal [ˌ-'frʌntl] adj squamofrontal.
squa·mo·mas·toid [ˌ-'mæstɔɪd] adj squamomastoid.
squamo-occipital adj squamookzipital.
squa·mo·pa·ri·e·tal [ˌ-pǝ'raɪǝtl] adj squamoparietal.
squa·mo·sal [skwǝ'mǝʊsl] adj → squamous.
squamosal suture Schuppennaht f, Sutura squamosa.
squa·mose ['skeɪmǝʊs, skǝ'mǝʊs] adj → squamous.
squa·mo·so·mas·toid suture [skwǝˌmǝʊ-sǝʊ'mæstɔɪd] Sutura squamosomastoidea.
squa·mo·so·pa·ri·e·tal [ˌ-pǝ'raɪǝtl] adj squamoparietal.
squa·mo·sphe·noid [ˌskeɪmǝʊ'sfɪnɔɪd] adj squamosphenoidal.
squa·mo·tem·po·ral [ˌ-'temp(ǝ)rǝl] adj squamotemporal.
squa·mo·tym·pan·ic fissure [ˌ-tɪm'pænɪk] Fissura tympanosquamosa.
squa·mous ['skweɪmǝs] adj 1. schuppig, schuppenförmig, -ähnlich, squamös. 2. mit Schuppen bedeckt, schuppig.
squamous blepharitis ophthal. Blepharitis squamosa.
squamous bone Schläfenbeinschuppe f, Pars squamosa ossis temporalis.
squamous carcinoma → squamous cell carcinoma.
squamous cell Plattenepithelzelle f.
squamous cell carcinoma Plattenepithelkarzinom nt, Ca. planocellulare/platycellulare.
squamous cell papilloma Plattenepithelpapillom nt.
squamous epithelial carcinoma → squamous cell carcinoma.
squamous epithelium Plattenepithel nt.
  keratinized s. verhorntes Plattenepithel.
  nonkeratinized s. unverhorntes Plattenepithel.
  simple s. einschichtiges Plattenepithel.
  stratified s. mehrschichtiges Plattenepithel.
squamous margin: s. of great wing of sphenoid bone Margo squamosus alae majoris.
s. of parietal bone Margo squamosus ossis parietalis.

squamous metaplasia Plattenepithelmetaplasie f, squamöse Metaplasie f.
squamous suture Schuppennaht f, Sutura squamosa.
square [skweǝr] **I** n 1. Quadrat nt, Viereck nt, viereckige Struktur f. 2. mathe. Quadrat(zahl f) nt. **in the ~** im Quadrat. **II** adj 3. (a. mathe.) im Quadrat, quadratisch, (vier-)eckig, Quadrat-, Viereck-, Vierkant-. 4. rechtwinkelig, im rechten Winkel (to zu). 5. gerade, eben. 6. (Person) breitschultrig, stämmig. **III** vt 7. quadratisch od. rechtwink(e)lig machen. 8. mathe. quadrieren.
square knot richtiger Knoten m, Schifferknoten m.
square measure Flächenmaß nt.
square muscle viereckiger/quadratischer Muskel m, M. quadratus.
squat·ting ['skɑtɪŋ] n card. Hockerstellung f, Squatting nt.
squill [skwɪl] n → scilla.
squint [skwɪnt] **I** n Schielen nt, Strabismus m. **II** vi schielen.
squint angle ophthal. Schielwinkel m.
squint deviation → squint angle.
squir·rel plague conjunctivitis ['skwɜrǝl; 'skwɪr-] ophthal. Conjunctivitis tularensis.
SR abbr. → sarcoplasmatic reticulum.
Sr abbr. → strontium.
SRBC abbr. → sheep red blood cell.
SRF abbr. 1. → skin reactive factor. 2. → somatotropin releasing factor.
SRH abbr. [somatotropin releasing hormone] → somatotropin releasing factor.
SR-IF abbr. [somatotropin release inhibiting factor] → somatostatin.
SRS-A abbr. → slow-reacting substance of anaphylaxis.
S-R variation immun., micro. S-R-Formenwechsel m.
ss abbr. → single-stranded.
SS agar → Salmonella-Shigella agar.
ssDNA abbr. → single-stranded DNA.
S-shaped scoliosis S-förmige Skoliose f.
S sleep → slow wave sleep.
SSM abbr. → superficial spreading melanoma.
SSPE abbr. [subacute sclerosing panencephalitis] → subacute inclusion body encephalitis.
ssRNA abbr. → single-stranded RNA.
SSS abbr. 1. → sick sinus syndrome. 2. → subclavian steal syndrome.
SSSS abbr. → staphylococcal scalded skin syndrome.
stab [stæb] **I** n 1. (Messer-)Stich m; Stichwunde f. 2. Stich m, scharfer Schmerz m. **II** vt 3. jdn. niederstechen od. erstechen. 4. stechen in, durchstechen, -bohren. **III** vi 5. stechen. 6. (Schmerz) stechen; (Strahlen) stechen.
stab·bing pain ['stæbɪŋ] stechender Schmerz m.
stab cell stabkerniger Granulozyt m; inf. Stabkerniger m.
stab culture Stich-, Stabkultur f.
sta·bile ['steɪbɪl; Brit. -baɪl] adj → stable.
stabile factor Prokonvertin f, V-convertin nt, Faktor VII m, F V II, Autothrombin I nt, Serum-Prothrombin-Conversion-Accelerator m abbr. SPCA, stabiler Faktor m.
sta·bil·i·ty [stǝ'bɪlǝtɪ] n 1. Stabilität f, Beständigkeit f, Unveränderlichkeit f; Dauerhaftigkeit f, Festigkeit f, Widerstandsfähigkeit f, -kraft f; chem. Reizenz f. 2. fig. (Charakter-)Festigkeit f, (seelische) Ausgeglichenheit f.
sta·bi·li·za·tion [ˌsteɪbǝlɪ'zeɪʃn] n Stabilisierung f; Einstellung f (auf ein Medikament).

sta·bi·lize ['steɪbəlaɪz] vt stabilisieren, konstant *od.* im Gleichgewicht halten; *techn.* (be-)festigen, stützen; einstellen (*auf ein Medikament*).
sta·bi·liz·er ['steɪbəlaɪzər] *n chem.* Stabilisator *m.*
sta·ble ['steɪbl] *adj* 1. stabil, beständig, unveränderlich, konstant, gleichbleibend; sicher; dauerhaft, fest; widerstandsfähig. ~ **in water** wasserbeständig. 2. (*Charakter*) gefestigt, ausgeglichen.
stable colloid *chem., phys.* stabiles Kolloid *nt.*
stable equilibrium *phys.* stabiles Gleichgewicht *nt.*
stable fracture stabiler Bruch *m,* stabile Fraktur *f.*
stable isotope stabiles Isotop *nt.*
sta·ble·ness ['steɪblnɪs] *n* → stability.
stab neutrophil stabkerniger Granulozyt *m, inf.* Stabkerniger *m.*
stab wound Stichwunde *f.*
stac·ca·to speech [stə'kɑːtəʊ] Stakkatosprache *f.*
stack [stæk] *n* Stoß *m,* Stapel *m.*
Stacke ['stækə; 'ʃtakə]: **S.'s operation** *HNO* Stacke-Operation *f.*
stacked form [stækt] *chem.* geschlossene Form *f.*
stack·ing interactions ['stækɪŋ] *biochem.* Stapelungskräfte *pl,* -wechselwirkungen *pl.*
stac·tom·e·ter [stæk'tɑmɪtər] *n* → stalagmometer.
Stader ['steɪdər]: **S. splint** *ortho.* Stader-Schiene *f.*
Staderini [stædə'riːni]: **S.'s nucleus** Nc. intercalatus.
sta·di·um ['steɪdɪəm] *n, pl* **-di·ums, -dia** [-dɪə] Stadium *nt.*
staff [stæf, stɑːf] *n, pl* **staffs, staves** [steɪvz] 1. Personal *nt,* Belegschaft *f,* (Mitarbeiter-)Stab *m.* 2. Stab *m,* Stock *m,* Stange *f.*
staff cell → stab cell.
stage [steɪdʒ] *n* 1. Stadium *nt,* Phase *f,* Stufe *f,* Grad *m;* Abschnitt *m.* **by/in ~** schritt-, stufenweise. 2. (*Mikroskop*) Objekttisch *m.*
s. of development Entwicklungsstufe.
s. of dilatation *gyn.* Eröffnungsphase, -periode *f.*
s. of expulsion *gyn.* Austreibungsphase, -periode *f.*
s. of fervescence Stadium des Fieberanstiegs, Stadium incrementi.
s. of knowledge Bildungs-, Wissensstand.
s. of life Lebensstufe.
stag·ger ['stægər] I *n* 1. Wanken *nt,* Schwanken *nt,* Taumeln *nt.* 2. ~ *s pl* Schwindel *m,* Schwindeln *nt.* II *vt* (*a. fig.*) schwankend *od.* wankend machen, ins Wanken bringen. III *vi* schwanken, wanken, taumeln.
stag·gered ['stægərd] *adj* gestaffelt, versetzt (angeordnet), gestuft.
staggered conformation *chem.* gestaffelte Konformation *f.*
stag·ger·ing ['stægərɪŋ] *adj* schwankend, wankend, taumelnd.
stag·horn calculus ['stæghɔːrn] *urol.* Korallenstein *m,* Hirschgeweihstein *m,* (Becken-)Ausgußstein *m.*
staghorn stone → staghorn calculus.
stag·ing ['steɪdʒɪŋ] *n patho.* Staging *nt.*
staging laparotomy explorative Laparotomie *f* zum Tumorstaging.
stag·nan·cy ['stægnənsi] *n* → stagnation.
stag·nant ['stægnənt] *adj* stockend, stillstehend, stagnierend, Stagnations-; Stauungs-.
stagnant anoxia → stagnant hypoxia.
stagnant hypoxia ischämische/zirkulatorische Anoxie/Hypoxie *f,* Stagnationsanoxie *f,* -hypoxie *f.*

stag·nate ['stægneɪt] *vi* stocken, stillstehen, stagnieren.
stag·na·tion [stæg'neɪʃn] *n* Stockung *f,* Stillstand *m,* Stagnation *f;* Stauung *f.*
stagnation mastitis *gyn.* Stauungsmastitis *f.*
Stähli ['steɪlɪ; 'ʃtɛːli]: **S.'s (pigment) line** *ophthal.* Stähli'-Linie *f.*
Staib ['staɪb]: **S. agar** Staib-Agar *m/nt.*
stain [steɪn] I *n* 1. Mal *nt,* Fleck *m.* 2. Farbe *f,* Farbstoff *m,* Färbemittel *nt.* 3. Färbung *f.* 4. Schmutz-, Farbfleck *m.* II *vt* 5. (an-)färben. 6. beschmutzen, beflecken. III *vi* s. (an-, ver-)färben; Flecken bekommen.
stain·a·bil·i·ty [ˌsteɪnə'bɪlətɪ] *n* (An-)Färbbarkeit *f.*
stain·a·ble ['steɪnəbl] *adj* (an-)färbbar.
stain·a·ble·ness ['steɪnəblnɪs] *n* → stainability.
stain·ing ['steɪnɪŋ] *n* 1. Färben *nt,* Färbung *f.* 2. Verschmutzung *f.*
staining method *histol.* Färbeverfahren *nt,* -technik *f,* Färbung *f.*
staining properties *histol.* Färbeeigenschaften *pl,* Anfärbbarkeit *f.*
staining technique → staining method.
stain·less ['steɪnlɪs] *adj* 1. *fig.* fleckenlos, tadellos; rein. 2. (*Stahl*) rostfrei.
stair-case phenomenon ['steərkeɪs] *physiol.* Treppenphänomen *nt.*
stal·ag·mom·e·ter [ˌstæləg'mɑmɪtər] *n* Tropfenzähler *m,* Stalagmometer *nt.*
stalk[1] [stɔːk] I *n* in steifer/stolzierender Gang *m.* II *vi* stolzieren, steifbeinig gehen.
stalk[2] [stɔːk] *n* Stengel *m,* Stiel *m,* Stamm *m.*
stalked [stɔːkt] *adj* gestielt.
stalk·less ['stɔːklɪs] *adj* ungestielt, stiellos, ohne Stiel.
stal·tic ['stɔːltɪk] *n, adj* → styptic.
stam·mer ['stæmər] I *n* Stammeln *nt,* Dyslalie *f.* II *vt* stammeln; stottern.
stam·mer·ing ['stæmərɪŋ] I *n* Stammeln *nt,* Dyslalie *f.* II *adj* stammelnd; stotternd.
stand [stænd] I *n* 1. Stehen *nt.* 2. Stillstand *m.* 3. *fig.* Standpunkt *m.* 4. Gestell *nt,* Regal *nt;* Stativ *nt,* Ständer *m;* Stütze *f.* II *vi* stehen.
stand·ard ['stændərd] I *n* 1. Standard *m,* Norm *f;* Maßstab *m;* Richtlinie *f.* 2. Richt-, Normalmaß *nt,* Standard(wert *m*) *m.* 3. *lab., chem.* Standardlösung *f.* 4. Niveau *nt,* Stand *m.* 5. (Mindest-)Anforderungen *pl.* II *adj* Norm-, Standard-; normal, Normal-; Routine-; Einheits-.
standard bicarbonate *physiol.* Standardbikarbonat *nt.*
standard calorie → small calorie.
standard candle *phys.* Candela *f abbr.* cd.
standard conditions Standardbedingungen *pl.*
standard deviation *abbr.* δ, **S.D.** *stat.* Standardabweichung *f abbr.* S, δ, Streuung *f,* mittlere (quadratische) Abweichung *f.*
standard Einthoven's triangle Standardableitung(en *pl*) *f* nach Einthoven, Einthoven-Dreieck *nt.*
standard error (of median) *abbr.* **SE, SEM** Standardabweichung *f* des Mittelwertes, Standardfehler *m.*
standard-free-energy change Änderung *f* der freien Energie unter Standardbedingungen.
stand·ard·i·za·tion [ˌstændərdɪ'zeɪʃn] *n* 1. Normung *f,* Vereinheitlichung *f,* Standardisierung *f.* 2. *chem.* Standardisierung *f,* Titrierung *f.* 3. Eichung *f.*
stand·ard·ize ['stændərdaɪz] *vt* 1. normen,

vereinheitlichen, standardisieren. 2. *chem.* standardisieren, titrieren. 3. eichen.
stand·ard·ized solution ['stændərdaɪzd] → standard solution.
standard pressure Standarddruck *m.*
standard procedure Standardmethode *f,* -prozedur *f,* -technik *f.*
standard solution Normal-, Standard-, Bezugs-, Vergleichslösung *f.*
standard state Standardzustand *m.*
standard temperature Standardtemperatur *f.*
standard weight Normalgewicht *nt;* Gewichtseinheit *f.*
stand-by ['stændbaɪ] I *n* (Alarm-)Bereitschaft *f.* **on ~** in Bereitschaft. II *adj* Hilfs-, Reserve-, Ersatz-, Not-.
standby duty/service Bereitschaftsdienst *m.*
stand·ing ['stændɪŋ] I *n* 1. Dauer *f.* 2. Stehen *nt.* II *adj* stehend, Steh-.
standing position aufrechte Körperhaltung *f,* Orthostase *f.*
standing potential Gleichspannungs-, Bestandspotential *nt.*
standing wave *phys.* stehende Welle *f.*
stand-still ['stændstɪl] *n* Stillstand *m.* **to be at a ~** (still-)stehen. **to come to a ~** zum Stillstand kommen.
Stanford-Binet ['stænfərd bɪ'neɪ; bɪ'nɛ]: **S.-B. test** *psycho.* Stanford-Binet-Test *m.*
Stanley Kent ['stænlɪ kent]: **bundle of S. K.** His'-Bündel *nt,* Fasciculus atrioventricularis.
stan·nate ['stæneɪt] *n* Stannat *nt.*
stan·nic ['stænɪk] *adj chem.* vierwertiges Zinn enthaltend, Zinn-IV-.
stannic acid Zinnsäure *f.*
stan·nif·er·ous [stə'nɪfərəs] *adj* zinnhaltig.
stan·no·sis [stə'nəʊsɪs] *n* Zinnoxidpneumokoniose *f,* Stannose *f.*
stan·nous ['stænəs] *adj chem.* zweiwertiges Zinn enthaltend, Zinn-II-.
stan·num ['stænəm] *n abbr.* **Sn** *chem.* Zinn *nt,* Stannum *nt abbr.* Sn.
stan·o·zo·lol [ˌstænəʊ'zəʊlɒl, -lɒl] *n pharm.* Stanozolol *nt.*
St. Anthony [seɪnt 'æntəni, 'ænθə-; sẽ]: **St. A.'s dance** → Sydenham's chorea.
St. A.'s fire 1. *derm.* Wundrose *f,* Rose *f,* Erysipel *nt,* Erysipelas *nt,* Streptodermia cutanea lymphatica. 2. Vergiftung *f* durch Mutterkornalkaloide, Ergotismus *m.*
sta·pe·dec·to·my [ˌsteɪpə'dektəmɪ] *n HNO* Stapesresektion *f,* Stapedektomie *f.*
sta·pe·di·al [stə'piːdɪəl] *adj* Steigbügel/Stapes betr., Steigbügel-.
stapedial ankylosis *HNO* Stapesankylose *f.*
stapedial branch of stylomastoid artery Ramus stapedialis a. stylomastoideae.
stapedial fold Plica stapedialis.
stapedial ligament Lig. anulare stapediale.
stapedial membrane Stapesmembran *f,* Membrana (obturatoria) stapedis.
stapedial nerve N. stapedius.
stapedial reflex Stapediusreflex *m.*
sta·pe·di·ol·y·sis [stəˌpiːdɪ'ɒlɪsɪs] *n HNO* Stapediolyse *f.*
sta·pe·dio·plas·ty [stə,piːdɪə'plæstɪ] *n HNO* Stapesplastik *f.*
sta·pe·dio-te·not·o·my [ˌ-tɪ'nɑtəmɪ] *n HNO* Stapediotenotomie *f.*
sta·pe·dio·ves·tib·u·lar [ˌ-ves'tɪbjələr] *adj* stapediovestibular, -vestibulär.
sta·pe·di·us muscle [stə'piːdɪəs] M. stapedius.
stapedius nerve N. stapedius.
stapedius reflex Stapediusreflex *m.*

sta·pes ['steɪpiːz] *n, pl* **sta·pes, sta·pe·des** [stæ'piːdiːz, 'steɪpə-] *anat.* Steigbügel *m*, Stapes *m*.
stapes prosthesis *HNO* Stapesprothese *f*, -ersatz *m*.
staphyl- *pref.* Zäpfchen-, Staphyl(o)-.
staph·y·lag·ra [ˌstæfɪ'lægrə] *n HNO* Zäpfchenzange *f*.
staph·y·lec·to·my [ˌ-'lektəmɪ] *n HNO* Zäpfchenentfernung *f*, Uvulektomie *f*.
staph·yl·e·de·ma [ˌ-lɪ'diːmə] *n* Zäpfchenödem *m*.
staph·y·line ['-laɪn, -liːn] *adj* 1. Zäpfchen/Uvula betr., zum Zäpfchen/zur Uvula gehörend, uvulär, Zäpfchen-, Uvulo-, Uvula(r)-, Staphyl(o)-. 2. traubenförmig.
staph·y·li·tis [ˌ-'laɪtɪs] *n* (Gaumen-)Zäpfchenentzündung *f*, Uvulitis *f*, Staphylitis *f*.
staphylo- *pref.* 1. → staphyl-. 2. Trauben-, Staphyl(o)-.
staph·y·lo·coc·cal [ˌstæfɪlo'kɑkəl] *adj* Staphylokokken betr., durch Staphylokokken verursacht, Staphylokokken-.
staphylococcal bronchitis Staphylokokkenbronchitis *f*.
staphylococcal-clumping test Staphylokokken-Clumping-Test *m*.
staphylococcal enterotoxin Staphylokokkenenterotoxin *nt*.
staphylococcal enterotoxin F *abbr.* **SEF** *old* → toxic shock-syndrome toxin-1.
staphylococcal impetigo Schälblasenausschlag *m*, Pemphigoid *nt* der Neugeborenen, Impetigo bullosa, Pemphigus (acutus) neonatorum.
staphylococcal infection Staphylokokkeninfektion *f*, Staphylokokkose *f*.
staphylococcal meningitis Staphylokokkenmeningitis *f*.
staphylococcal parotiditis → staphylococcal parotitis.
staphylococcal parotitis Staphylokokkenparotitis *f*.
staphylococcal pneumonia Staphylokokkenpneumonie *f*.
staphylococcal scalded skin syndrome *abbr.* **SSSS** Ritter-Krankheit *f*, -Dermatitis *f*, Morbus Ritter von Rittershain *m*, Pemphigoid *nt* der Säuglinge, Syndrom *nt* der verbrühten Haut, staphylogenes Lyell-Syndrom *nt*, Dermatitis exfoliativa neonatorum, Epidermolysis toxica acuta.
staphylococcal sepsis → staphylococcemia.
staphylococcal toxin Staphylokokkentoxin *nt*.
staph·y·lo·coc·ce·mia [ˌstæfɪloʊkɑk'siːmɪə] *n* Staphylokokkensepsis *f*, Staphylokokkämie *f*.
staph·y·lo·coc·ci *pl* → staphylococcus.
staph·y·lo·coc·cic [ˌ-'kɑksɪk] *adj* → staphylococcal.
staph·y·lo·coc·cin [ˌ-'kɑksɪn] *n* Staphylokokzin *nt*, Staphylococcin *nt*.
staph·y·lo·coc·col·y·sin [ˌ-kə'kɑləsɪn] *n* → staphylolysin.
staph·y·lo·coc·co·sis [ˌ-kə'koʊsɪs] *n* Staphylokokkeninfektion *f*, Staphylokokkose *f*.
Staph·y·lo·coc·cus [ˌ-'kɑkəs] *n micro.* Staphylococcus *m*.
staph·y·lo·coc·cus [ˌ-'kɑkəs] *n, pl* **-coc·ci** [-'kɑksaɪ] *micro.* Traubenkokkus *m*, Staphylokokkus *m*, Staphylococcus *m*.
staph·y·lo·der·ma [ˌ-'dɜrmə] *n* Staphylodermie *f*, -dermia *f*.
staph·y·lo·di·al·y·sis [ˌ-daɪ'æləsɪs] *n* Zäpfchensenkung *f*, -tiefstand *m*, Uvuloptose *f*, Staphyloptose *f*.

staph·y·lo·e·de·ma [ˌ-ɪ'diːmə] *n* Zäpfchenödem *nt*.
staph·y·lo·he·mia [ˌ-'hiːmɪə] *n* → staphylococcemia.
staph·y·lo·he·mol·y·sin [ˌ-hɪ'mɑləsɪn] *n* Staphylohämolysin *nt*.
staph·y·lo·ki·nase [ˌ-'kaɪneɪs] *n* Staphylokinase *f*.
staph·y·lol·y·sin [ˌstæfɪ'lɑləsɪn] *n* Staphylolysin *nt*, Staphylokokkenhämolysin *nt*.
α-staphylolysin *n* α-Staphylolysin *nt*.
β-staphylolysin *n* β-Staphylolysin *nt*.
γ-staphylolysin *n* γ-Staphylolysin *nt*.
δ-staphylolysin *n* δ-Staphylolysin *nt*.
ε-staphylolysin *n* ε-Staphylolysin *nt*.
staph·y·lo·ma [ˌstæfɪ'loʊmə] *n ophthal.* Beerengeschwulst *f*, Staphylom(a) *nt*.
staph·y·lom·a·tous [ˌ-'lɑmətəs] *adj ophthal.* Staphylom betr., staphylomartig, staphylomatös.
staph·y·lon·cus [ˌ-'lɑŋkəs] *n* Zäpfchenschwellung *f*, -tumor *m*.
staph·y·lo·phar·yn·gor·rha·phy [ˌstæfɪloˌfærɪn'gɔrəfɪ] *n HNO* Staphylopharyngorrhaphie *f*, Palatopharyngorrhaphie *f*.
staph·y·lo·plas·ty ['-plæstɪ] *n HNO* Staphyloplastik *f*.
staph·y·lo·ple·gia [ˌ-'pliːdʒ(ɪ)ə] *n* Gaumensegellähmung *f*.
staph·y·lop·to·sia [ˌstæfɪlɑp'toʊsɪə] *n* → staphylodialysis.
staph·y·lop·to·sis [ˌ-'toʊsɪs] *n* → staphylodialysis.
staph·y·lor·rha·phy [ˌstæfɪ'lɔrəfɪ] *n HNO* Gaumennaht *f*, Urano-, Staphylorrhaphie *f*.
staph·y·los·chi·sis [ˌstæfɪ'lɑskəsɪs] *n* Staphyloschisis *f*.
staph·y·lo·tome ['stæfɪlətoʊm] *n HNO* Uvulotom *nt*, Staphylotom *nt*.
staph·y·lot·o·my [stæfɪ'lɑtəmɪ] *n* 1. *HNO* Uvulotomie *f*, Staphylotomie *f*. 2. *ophthal.* Staphylotomie *f*.
staph·y·lo·tox·in [ˌstæfɪlə'tɑksɪn] *n* Staphylotoxin *nt*.
sta·ple ['steɪpl] I *n* 1. Klammer *f*; Krampe *f*. 2. Heftdraht *m*, Heftklammer *f*. II *vt* heften, klammern.
stap·ler ['steɪplər] *n* 1. *chir., ortho.* Klammer(naht)gerät *nt*, -apparat *m*. 2. *techn.* Heftmaschine *f*.
sta·pling ['steɪplɪŋ] *n* Klammern *nt*.
stapling instrument/machine → stapler.
star [stɑr] *n histol.* Stern *m*, sternförmige Struktur *f*.
star cell *patho.* Sternzelle *f*.
starch [stɑrtʃ] I *n* 1. Stärke *f*; Stärkemehl *nt*; *chem.* Amylum *n*. 2. ~**es** *pl* stärkereiche Nahrung *f*. II *vt* stärken, mit Stärke behandeln.
starch agar Stärkeagar *m/nt*.
starch phosphorylase Stärke-, Glykogenphosphorylase *f*.
starch sugar Dextrin *nt*, Dextrinum *nt*.
starch synthase/synthetase Stärkesynthase *f*, -synthetase *f*.
starch·y ['stɑrtʃɪ] *adj* stärkehaltig, kohlehydratreich, Stärke-.
Starck [stɑrk]: **S.'s dilator** Starck-Dilatator *m*.
stare [steər] I *n* Starren *nt*, starrer Blick *m*, Stieren *nt*. II *vi* starren, stieren.
stare nystagmus Stiernystagmus *m*.
Stargardt ['stɑrgɑrt]: **S.'s disease** Stargardt-Syndrom *nt*.
Starling ['stɑrlɪŋ]: **S.'s curve** (*Herz*) Starling-Kurve *f*, Druck-Volumendiagramm *nt*.
S.'s hypothesis of capillary equilibrium → theory of S.
S.'s law of the heart Starling'-Kontraktionsgesetz *nt*.

theory of S. Starling'-(Reabsorptions-)-Theorie *f*.
Starr-Edwards [stɑr 'edwərds]: **S.-E. valve** *HTG* Starr-Edwards-Prothese *f*.
star·ry sky cell ['stɑrɪ] Sternhimmelzelle *f*.
start [stɑrt] I *n* Start *m*, Anfang *m*, Beginn *m*. **at the ~** zu Beginn, am Anfang. **from the ~** von Anfang an. II *vt* in Gang setzen *od.* bringen; etw. einleiten; anfangen, beginnen; (*Reaktion*) auslösen. III *vi* anfangen, beginnen.
start·er DNA ['stɑrtər] Starter-DNA *f*, Starter-DNS *f*.
start·ing ['stɑrtɪŋ] *adj* beginnend, Anfangs-, Start-.
star·tle reaction ['stɑrtl] → startle reflex.
startle reflex Moro-Reflex *m*.
star·va·tion [stɑr'veɪʃn] *n* 1. Hungern *nt*. 2. Hungertod *m*, Verhungern *nt*.
starvation acidosis Hungerazidose *f*, nutritive (metabolische) Azidose *f*.
starvation diabetes Hungerdiabetes *m*.
starvation osteoporosis Hungerosteoporose *f*.
starve [stɑrv] I *vt* hungern lassen. **to be ~d** Hunger leiden, ausgehungert sein. II *vi* hungern, Hunger leiden. **~ to death** verhungern.
stas·i·ba·si·pho·bia [ˌstæsɪˌbeɪsɪ'foʊbɪə, ˌsteɪ-] *n psychia.* Stasobasophobie *f*.
stas·i·pho·bia [ˌ-'foʊbɪə] *n psychia.* krankhafte Angst *f* vor dem Aufstehen, Stasiphobie *f*.
sta·sis ['steɪsɪs] *n, pl* **-ses** [-siːz] Stauung *f*, Stockung *f*, Stillstand *m*, Stase *f*, Stasis *f*.
stasis cirrhosis (of liver) Stauungsinduration *f* der Leber, Cirrhose cardiaque.
stasis dermatitis → stasis eczema.
stasis eczema Stauungsekzem *nt*, -dermatitis *f*, -dermatose *f*, Dermatitis statica/hypostatica/varicosa/haemostatica.
stasis edema Stauungsödem *nt*.
stasis gallbladder Stauungsgallenblase *f*.
stasis liver Stauungsleber *f*.
stasis ulcer Stauungssulkus *nt*, Ulcus (cruris) venosum; Ulcus (cruris) varicosum.
state [steɪt] *n* 1. Zustand *m*; Status *m*. **in a solid/liquid ~** im festen/flüssigen Zustand. **in a good/bad ~** in gutem/schlechtem Zustand. 2. Lage *f*, Stand *m*, Situation *f*. 3. (Familien-)Stand *m*. 4. Stadium *nt*.
s. of aggregation *phys.* Aggregatzustand *m*.
s. of consciousness Wach-, Bewußtseinszustand.
s. of equilibrium Gleichgewichtszustand.
s. of health Gesundheitszustand.
s. of mind Geisteszustand, geistige/mentale Verfassung *f*.
s. of minimum free energy *chem.* Zustand minimaler freier Energie.
s. of training *physiol.* Trainingszustand.
s. of transition Übergangszustand.
state 3 respiration *biochem.* aktive Atmung *f*, Atmungszustand 3 *m*.
state 4 respiration *biochem.* Atmungszustand 4 *m*.
stath·mo·ki·ne·sis [ˌstæθmoʊkɪ'niːsɪs, -kaɪ-] *n* Stathmokinese *f*.
stat·ic ['stætɪk] *adj* (still-, fest-)stehend, ruhend, unbewegt; gleichbleibend, statisch.
static ataxia statische Ataxie *f*.
static compliance (of lung) statische Compliance *f*.
static friction Haftreibung *f*.
static gangrene Stauungsgangrän *f*, venöse Gangrän *f*.
static perimetry *ophthal.* statische Perimetrie *f*.
static reflex statischer Reflex *m*.
static response *physiol.* statische/tonische/proportionale Antwort *f*.

stat·ics ['stætɪks] *pl* Statik *f*.
static scoliosis statische Skoliose *f*.
static sense *physiol.* Gleichgewichtssinn *m*.
static work *physiol.* statische Arbeit *f*.
sta·tion·ar·y ['steɪʃəˌnerɪː] *adj* **1.** ortsfest, (fest-, still-)stehend, stationär. **2.** gleichbleibend, unverändert bleibend, stagnierend, stationär.
stationary period → stationary phase.
stationary phase *phys.* stationäre Phase *f*.
sta·tion test ['steɪʃn] Romberg-Versuch *m*.
sta·tis·ti·cal [stə'tɪstɪkl] *adj* statistisch.
statistical value statistischer Wert *m*.
stat·is·ti·cian [ˌstætɪ'stɪʃn] *n* Statistiker(in *f*) *m*.
sta·tis·tics [stə'tɪstɪks] *pl* Statistik *f*; Statistik(en *pl*) *f* (*about, on* über).
stat·o·a·cous·tic [ˌstætəʊə'kuːstɪk] *adj* Gleichgewichts betr. u. Gehör betr., statoakustisch, vestibulokochleär.
stat·o·co·nia ['-kəʊnɪə] *pl*, *sing* **-ni·um** [-nɪəm] *physiol.* Ohrkristalle *pl*, Otokonien *pl*, -lithen *pl*, Statokonien *pl*, -lithen *pl*, -conia *pl*, Otoconia *pl*.
stat·o·con·ic membrane of maculae [ˌ-'kɒnɪk] Makuladrehschicht *f*, Membrana statoconiorum (macularum).
stat·o·co·ni·um → statoconia.
stat·o·cyst ['-sɪst] *n* Statozyste *f*.
stat·o·ki·net·ic reflex [ˌ-kɪ'netɪk] statokinetischer Reflex *m*.
stat·o·lith·ic [ˌ-'lɪθɪk] *adj* Statolith(en) betr., Statolithen-.
statolithic membrane Statolithenmembran *f*.
statolithic organ Statolithen-, Makula-, Maculaorgan *nt*.
stat·o·liths ['-lɪθs] *pl physiol.* Ohrkristalle *pl*, Otokonien *pl*, -lithen *pl*, Statokonien *pl*, -lithen *pl*, -conia *pl*, Otoconia *pl*.
sta·tom·e·ter [stə'tɒmɪtər] *n* Exophthalmometer *nt*.
stat·o·sphere ['stætəsfɪər] *n* Zentroplasma *nt*, Zentrosphäre *f*.
stat·o·ton·ic reflex [ˌstætə'tɒnɪk] statotonischer Reflex *m*, Stellreflex *m*.
stat·u·ral ['stætʃərəl] *adj* Gestalt/Statur betr.
stat·ure ['stætʃər] *n* Statur *f*, Wuchs *m*, Gestalt *f*, Größe *f*.
sta·tus ['steɪtəs, 'stætəs] *n* Zustand *m*, Lage *f*, Situation *f*, Stand *m* (der Dinge), Status *m*.
status quo gegenwärtiger Zustand *m*, Status quo (*m*).
Staub-Traugott [staʊb 'traʊɡɔt, ʃtraʊb]: **S.-T. phenomenon** Staub-Traugott--Effekt *m*.
S.-T. test Staub-Traugott-Versuch *m*, Glucose-Doppelbelastung *f*.
stau·ro·ple·gia [ˌstɔːrə'pliːdʒ(ɪ)ə] *n* gekreuzte Hemiplegie *f*, Hemiplegia alternans/cruciata.
stax·is ['stæksɪs] *n* (Sicker-)Blutung *f*, Staxis *f*.
STD *abbr.* → sexually transmitted disease.
stead·y ['stedɪ] *adj* **1.** unveränderlich, gleichmäßig, -bleibend, stet(ig), beständig. **2.** (*Hand*) ruhig, sicher. **3.** (stand-)fest, stabil. **4.** gewohnheitsmäßig, regelmäßig.
steady potential Gleichspannungs-, Bestandspotential *nt*.
steady state Fließgleichgewicht *nt*, dynamisches Gleichgewicht *nt*, steady state (*nt*).
steady state concentration Steady-state--Konzentration *f*.
steady state system offenes System *nt*, Steady-state-System *nt*.

steal [stiːl] *n card.* Anzapf-, Entzugseffekt *m*, -syndrom *nt*, Steal-Effekt *m*, -Phänomen *nt*.
steal phenomenon → steal.
steam [stiːm] **I** *n* (Wasser-)Dampf *m*. **II** *vt* dämpfen, dünsten; (*Gas*) ausströmen. **III** *vi* dampfen; verdampfen.
steam-fitter's asthma Asthma *nt* bei Asbestose.
steam heat Dampfhitze *f*, feuchte Hitze *f*.
steam inhalation Dampfinhalation *f*.
steam sterilization Dampfsterilisation *f*.
ste·ap·sin [stɪ'æpsɪn] *n* Steapsin *nt*, Triacylglycerinlipase *f*.
stear- *pref.* → stearo-.
ste·a·rate ['stɪərert] *n* Stearat *nt*.
ste·ar·ic acid [stɪ'ærɪk, 'stɪərɪk] Stearinsäure *f*, n-Octadecansäure *f*.
ste·a·rin ['stɪərɪn] *n* Stearin *nt*.
stearo- *pref.* Fett-, Stear(o)-, Steat(o)-, Lip(o)-.
stear·o·yl-CoA desaturase [stɪ'ærəwɪl] Acyl-CoA-desaturase *f*.
ste·ar·rhea [stɪə'rɪə] *n* → steatorrhea.
steat- *pref.* → stearo-.
ste·a·ti·tis [stɪə'taɪtɪs] *n* Fettgewebsentzündung *f*, Steatitis *f*.
ste·at·o·cele [stɪ'ætəsiːl] *n* Steatozele *f*.
ste·a·to·cys·to·ma [ˌstɪətəsɪs'təʊmə] *n* **1.** Steatocystoma *nt*. **2.** → steatoma **2**.
steatocystoma multiplex Talgzysten *pl*, Talgretentionszysten *pl*, Steatocystoma multiplex.
ste·a·tog·e·nous [stɪə'tɒdʒənəs] *adj* fettbildend *od.* -produzierend, lipogen.
ste·a·tol·y·sis [stɪə'tɒləsɪs] *n* Steatolyse *f*.
ste·a·to·lyt·ic [ˌstɪətə'lɪtɪk] *adj* Steatolyse betr. *od.* Steatolyse auslösend, steatolytisch.
ste·a·to·ma [stɪə'təʊmə] *n*, *pl* **-mas**, **-ma·ta** [-mətə] **1.** Fett(gewebs)geschwulst *f*, -tumor *m*, Lipom(a) *nt*. **2.** falsches Atherom *nt*, Follikel-, Öl-, Talgretentionszyste *f*, Sebozystom *nt*, Steatom *nt*.
ste·a·to·ma·to·sis [ˌstɪətəmə'təʊsɪs] *n* **1.** → steatocystoma multiplex. **2.** Steatomatosis *f*, Sebozystomatose *f*.
ste·a·tom·er·y [stɪə'tɒmərɪ] *n* Steatomerie *f*.
ste·a·to·ne·cro·sis [ˌstɪətənɪ'krəʊsɪs] *n* Fett-, Steatonekrose *f*.
ste·a·to·py·gia [ˌ-'pɪdʒɪə] *n* Steatopygie *f*.
ste·a·tor·rhea [ˌ-'rɪə] *n* Fettdurchfall *m*, Steatorrhoe *f*, Steatorrhö *f*, Diarrhoe *f*, Diarrhö *f*.
ste·a·to·sis [stɪə'təʊsɪs] *n*, *pl* **-ses** [-siːz] **1.** Verfettung *f*, Fettsucht *f*, Adipositas *f*, Steatosis *f*. **2.** degenerative Verfettung *f*, fettige Degeneration *f*, Degeneratio adiposa.
ste·chi·om·e·try [stekɪ'ɒmətrɪ] *n* → stoichiometry.
Steele-Richardson-Olszewski [stiːl 'rɪtʃərdsən ɒl'sevskɪ]: **S.-R.-O. disease/syndrome** Steele-Richardson-Olszewski--Syndrom *nt*.
Steell [stiːl]: **S.'s murmur** Graham Steell--Geräusch *nt*, Steell-Geräusch *nt*.
steel·y hair syndrome ['stiːlɪ] Menkes--Syndrom *nt*, Stahlhaarkrankheit *f*, Kraushaarsyndrom *nt*, Trichopoliodystrophie *f*, Pili torti mit Kupfermangel, Kinky hair disease (*nt*).
stee·ple head ['stiːpl] → steeple skull.
steeple skull Spitz-, Turmschädel *m*, Akrozephalie *f*, -cephalie *f*, Oxyzephalie *f*, -cephalie *f*, Hypsizephalie *f*, -cephalie *f*, Turrizephalie *f*, -cephalie *f*.
Stefan-Boltzmann ['ʃtefən 'bəʊltsmən]: **S.-B. equation** Stefan-Boltzmann-Gleichung *f*.
Steg·o·my·ia [stegə'maɪ(j)ə] *n micro.* Stegomyia *f*.

Steinbrocker ['staɪnbrɒkər]: **S.'s syndrome** Schulter-Arm-Syndrom *nt*.
Steiner ['staɪnər; 'ʃtaɪ-]: **S.'s syndrome** Curtius-Syndrom *nt*, Hemihypertrophie *f*.
Steinert ['staɪnərt; 'ʃtaɪ-]: **S.'s disease** Curschmann-Batten-Steinert-Syndrom *nt*, myotonische Dystrophie *f*.
Stein-Leventhal [staɪn 'levənθæl, -θɑl]: **syndrome** Stein-Leventhal-Syndrom *nt*, Syndrom *nt* der polyzystischen Ovarien.
Steinmann ['staɪnmən]: **S.'s pin** *ortho.* Steinmann-Nagel *m*.
stel·lar nevus ['stelər] Sternnävus *m*, Spider naevus, Naevus araneus.
stel·late ['stelɪt, -eɪt] *adj* stern(en)förmig.
stellate block Stellatumblockade *f*.
stellate cataract sternförmige Katarakt *f*, Cataracta stellata.
stellate cell Sternzelle *f*.
 giant s.s Meynert'-Zellen *pl*, Riesensternzellen *pl*.
 inner s. Korbzelle *f*.
 s.s of liver (von) Kupffer'-(Stern-)Zellen *pl*.
 outer s.s äußere Sternzellen *pl*.
stel·lat·ed ['steleɪtɪd] *adj* → stellate.
stellate fracture sternförmige Fraktur *f*.
stellate ganglion Ggl. cervicothoracicum/stellatum.
stellate ganglionectomy → stellectomy.
stellate veins of kidney Stellatavenen *pl*, Venulae stellatae renis.
stellate venules of kidney → stellate veins of kidney.
stel·lec·to·my [ste'lektəmɪ] *n neurochir.* Stellatumresektion *f*, Stellektomie *f*.
Stellwag ['stelvæɡ]: **S.'s sign/symptom** Stellwag-Zeichen *nt*, -Phänomen *nt*.
stem [stem] **I** *n* Stamm *m*, Stengel *m*, Stiel *m*. **II** *vt* eindämmen; zum Stillstand bringen; (*Blutung*) stillen. **III** *vi* stammen, (her-)kommen (*from* von).
 s. of epiglottis Epiglottisstiel, Petiolus *m* (epiglottidis).
stem bronchus Primär-, Haupt-, Stammbronchus *m*, Bronchus principalis.
stem cell 1. Stammzelle *f*, Vorläuferzelle *f*. **2.** (Blut-)Stammzelle *f*.
 hemopoietic s. (Blut-)Stammzelle, Hämozytoblast *m*.
 lymphatic s. lymphatische Stammzelle.
 pluripotent s. pluripotente Stammzelle.
stem cell leukemia Stammzellenleukämie *f*, akute undifferenzierte Leukämie *f* *abbr.* AUL.
stem villi *histol.* Haftzotten *pl*.
Stenger ['steŋər]: **S. test** *HNO* Stenger--Versuch *m*.
sten·o·car·dia [ˌstenə'kɑːrdɪə] *n card.* Herzbräune *f*, Stenokardie *f*, Angina pectoris.
sten·o·ce·pha·lia [ˌ-sɪ'feɪljə] *n* → stenocephaly.
sten·o·ce·phal·ic [ˌ-sɪ'fælɪk] *adj* → stenocephalous.
sten·o·ceph·a·lous [ˌ-'sefələs] *adj* Stenozephalie betr., von Stenozephalie gekennzeichnet, stenokephal, -cephal.
sten·o·ceph·a·ly [ˌ-'sefəlɪ] *n embryo.* Stenokephalie *f*, -cephalie *f*, Kraniostenose *f*.
sten·o·cho·ria [ˌ-'kəʊrɪə] *n* Verengung *f*, Verengerung *f*, Stenochorie *f*, Stenose *f*.
sten·o·co·ri·a·sis [ˌ-kəʊ'raɪəsɪs] *n* Pupillenverengung *f*, Stenokorie *f*, Miosis *f*.
sten·o·cro·ta·phia [ˌ-krəʊ'teɪfɪə] *n* → stenocrotaphy.
sten·o·crot·a·phy [ˌ-'krɒtəfɪ] *n* Stenokrotaphie *f*.
Stenon ['stenɑn]: **canal of S.** Parotisgang

m, Stensen'-Gang *m*, Stenon'-Gang *m*, Ductus parotideus.
sten·o·pe·ic [ˌstenəˈpiːɪk] *adj* stenopäisch.
stenopeic iridectomy *ophthal.* periphere Iridektomie *f*.
stenopeic spectacles stenopäische Brille *f*, Schlitzbrille *f*.
ste·no·sal [stɪˈnəʊsl] *adj* → stenotic.
stenosal murmur *card.* Stenosegeräusch *nt*.
ste·nosed [stɪˈnəʊst] *adj* verengt, stenosiert.
ste·nos·ing [stɪˈnəʊsɪŋ] *adj* stenosierend.
stenosing tenosynovitis De Quervain-Krankheit *f*, Tendovaginitis stenosans.
ste·no·sis [stɪˈnəʊsɪs] *n* Einengung *f*, Verengung *f*, Enge *f*, Stenose *f*, Stenosis *f*.
s. of the nostrils Naseneingangsstenose.
s. of the papilla of Vater Papillenstenose, Sphinkterklerose *f*, -fibrose *f*, Sklerose *f* des Sphincter Oddi, Papillitis stenosans, Odditis *f*.
sten·o·ther·mal [ˌstenəˈθɜrml] *adj* stenotherm.
sten·o·ther·mic [ˌ-ˈθɜrmɪk] *adj* stenotherm.
sten·o·tho·rax [ˌ-ˈθɔːræks, -ˈθəʊər-] *n* Stenothorax *m*.
ste·not·ic [stɪˈnɑtɪk] *adj* Stenose betr., durch Stenose gekennzeichnet, stenotisch.
ste·not·o·my [stɪˈnɑtəmɪ] *n chir.* Stenotomie *f*.
sten·ox·en·ous [steˈnɑksənəs] *adj micro.* stenoxen.
stenoxenous parasite stenoxener Parasit *m*.
Stensen [ˈsten(t)sən]: **S.'s canal/duct** Parotisgang *m*, Stensen'-Gang *m*, Stenon'-Gang *m*, Ductus parotideus.
S.'s foramen For. incisivum.
S.'s veins hintere Ziliarvenen *pl*, Vv. vorticosae, Vv. choroideae oculi.
Stenvers [ˈstenvərs]: **S. protection/view** *radiol., HNO* Stenvers-Aufnahme *f*.
step- *pref.* Stief-.
step [step] **I** *n* **1.** Schritt *m*, Tritt *m*; Gang *m*. **2.** *fig.* Schritt *m*, Maßnahme *f*. **to take ~s** Maßnahmen ergreifen. **3.** *fig.* Stufe *f*, Phase *f*, Abschnitt *m*. **~ by ~** schritt-, stufenweise. **II** *vt* abstufen. **III** *vi* schreiten, gehen, treten.
step·broth·er [ˈstepbrʌðər] *n* Stiefbruder *m*.
step child Stiefkind *nt*.
step·daugh·ter [ˈstepdɔːtər] *n* Stieftochter *f*.
step·fa·ther [ˈstepfɑːðər] *n* Stiefvater *m*.
Stephen [ˈstiːvən]: **S.'s spot** *hema.* Maurer-Körnelung *f*, -Tüpfelung *f*.
step·moth·er [ˈstepˌmʌðər] *n* Stiefmutter *f*.
step·page gait [ˈstepɪdʒ] *neuro.* Steppergang *m*.
step·par·ents [ˈstepˌpeərənts] *pl* Stiefeltern *pl*.
stepped [stept] *adj* (ab-)gestuft, Stufen-.
step·ping reflex [ˈstepɪŋ] Schreitreflex *m*.
step response *physiol.* Übergangsfunktion *m*.
step·wise [ˈstepwaɪz] *adj* schritt-, stufenweise.
sterc(o)- *pref.* Kot-, Sterk(o)-, Sterc(o)-, Fäkal-, Sterkoral-.
ster·co·bi·lin [ˌstɜrkəʊˈbaɪlɪn] *n* Sterko-, Stercobilin *n*.
ster·co·bi·lin·o·gen [ˌstɜrkəbaɪˈlɪnədʒən] *n* Sterko-, Stercobilinogen *n*.
ster·co·lith [ˈ-lɪθ] *n* Kotstein *m*, Koprolith *m*.
ster·co·ra·ceous [ˌ-ˈreɪʃəs] *adj* → stercoral.
stercoraceous abscess → stercoral abscess.

stercoraceous ulcer → stercoral ulcer.
ster·co·ral [ˈstɜrkərəl] *adj* Stuhl betr., kotig, kotartig, fäkal, sterkoral, Sterkoral-, Fäkal-, Kot-.
stercoral abscess Fäkal-, Kotabszeß *m*.
stercoral appendicitis Sterkoral-, Fäkalappendizitis *f*, Appendizitis *f* durch Kotsteine.
stercoral diarrhea Verstopfungsdurchfall *m*, uneigentlicher Durchfall *m*, Diarrhoea paradoxa/stercoralis.
stercoral fistula Kotfistel *f*, Fistula stercoralis.
stercoral ulcer Sterkoralgeschwür *nt*, -ulkus *nt*.
ster·co·rin [ˈ-rɪn] *n* Koprostanol *nt*, -sterin *nt*.
ster·co·ro·lith [ˈstɜrkərəlɪθ] *n* → stercolith.
ster·co·ro·ma [ˌ-ˈrəʊmə] *n* Kotgeschwulst *f*, Fäkalom *nt*, Koprom *nt*, Sterkorom *nt*.
ster·co·rous [ˈ-rəs] *adj* → stercoral.
ster·cus [ˈstɜrkəs] *n* Kot *m*, Stercus *nt*.
stereo- *pref.* **1.** starr, fest, stereo-. **2.** räumlich, körperlich, Raum-, Körper-, Stereo-.
ster·e·o·ag·no·sis [ˌsterɪəægˈnəʊsɪs] *n neuro.* taktile Agnosie *f*, Tastlähmung *f*, Stereoagnosie *f*, Astereognosie *f*.
ster·e·o·an·es·the·sia [ˌ-ˌænəsˈθiːʒə] *n neuro.* Stereoanästhesie *f*.
ster·e·o·aus·cul·ta·tion [ˌ-ˌɔːskəlˈteɪʃn] *n* Stereoauskultation *f*.
ster·e·o·blas·tu·la [ˌ-ˈblæstʃələ, -stjʊlə] *n embryo.* Stereoblastula *f*.
ster·e·o·cam·pim·e·ter [ˌ-ˈkæmˈpɪmətər] *n ophthal.* Stereokampimeter *nt*.
ste·re·o·chem·i·cal [ˌ-ˈkemɪkl, ˌstɪə-] *adj* Stereochemie betr., stereochemisch.
stereochemical formula Raumformel *f*, stereochemische Formel *f*.
stereochemical isomerism → stereoisomerism.
ste·re·o·chem·is·try [ˌ-ˈkemɪstrɪ] *n* Stereochemie *f*.
ster·e·o·cil·i·um [ˌ-ˈsɪlɪəm] *n, pl* **-cil·i·a** [-ˈsiːlɪə] Stereozilie *f*, Stereocilium *nt*.
ster·e·o·cog·no·sy [ˌ-ˈkɑgnəsɪ] *n* → stereognosis.
ster·e·o·en·ceph·a·lom·e·try [ˌ-ˌensefəˈlɑmətrɪ] *n* Stereoenzephalometrie *f*.
ster·e·o·en·ceph·a·lot·o·my [ˌ-ˌensefəˈlɑtəmɪ] *n* Stereoenzephalotomie *f*; stereotaktische Hirnoperation *f*.
ster·e·o·fluo·ros·co·py [ˌ-ˌflʊəˈrɑskəpɪ] *n radiol.* stereoskopische Fluoroskopie *f*.
ster·e·og·no·sis [ˌsterɪəgˈnəʊsɪs] *n* Stereognosie *f*.
ster·e·og·nos·tic [ˌsterɪəgˈnɑstɪk] *adj* Stereognosie betr., stereognostisch.
ster·e·o·gram [ˈsterɪəˌgræm] *n radiol.* stereokopische Aufnahme *f*, Stereogramm *nt*, Stereoaufnahme *f*.
ster·e·o·graph [ˈ-græf] *n* → stereogram.
ster·e·o·i·so·mer [ˌ-ˈaɪsəmər] *n* Stereoisomer *nt*.
ster·e·o·i·so·mer·ic [ˌ-ˌaɪsəˈmerɪk] *adj* Stereoisomerie betr. od. besitzend, stereoisomer(isch).
ster·e·o·i·som·er·ism [ˌ-ˈaɪsəmərɪzəm] *n chem.* Raum-, Stereoisomerie *f*.
ster·e·o·i·som·er·i·za·tion [ˌ-ˌaɪˌsɑmərɪˈzeɪʃn] *n chem.* Stereoisomerisation *f*.
ster·e·om·e·ter [ˌsterɪˈɑmɪtər, stɪər-] *n* Stereometer *nt*.
ster·e·om·e·try [ˌ-ˈɑmɪtrɪ] *n* Stereometrie *f*.
stereo-ophthalmoscope *n ophthal.* binokuläres Ophthalmoskop *nt*, Stereophthalmoskop *nt*.
ster·e·op·sis [ˌ-ˈɑpsɪs] *n* → stereoscopic vision.

ster·e·o·ra·di·og·ra·phy [ˌsterɪəˌreɪdɪˈɑgrəfɪ, ˌstɪər-] *n* Stereoradiographie *f*, Röntgenstereographie *f*.
ster·e·o·roent·gen·og·ra·phy [ˌ-ˌrentgəˈnɑgrəfɪ] *n* → stereoradiography.
ster·e·o·scope [ˈsterɪəskəʊp, ˈstɪər-] *n* Stereoskop *nt*.
ster·e·o·scop·ic [ˌ-ˈskɑpɪk] *adj* **1.** räumlich wirkend *od.* sehend, stereoskopisch. **2.** Stereoskop *od.* Stereoskopie betr., stereoskopisch.
stereoscopic diplopia *ophthal.* physiologische/stereoskopische Diplopie *f*.
stereoscopic fluoroscopy *radiol.* stereoskopische Fluoroskopie *f*.
stereoscopic miscroscope Stereomikroskop *nt*.
stereoscopic view *radiol.* stereoskopische Aufnahme *f*, Stereoaufnahme *f*, Stereogramm *nt*.
stereoscopic vision stereoskopisches Sehen *nt*.
ster·e·os·co·py [ˌsterɪˈɑskəpɪ, ˌstɪər-] *n* Stereoskopie *f*.
ster·e·o·ski·ag·ra·phy [ˌsterɪəʊskaɪˈægrəfɪ] *n* → stereoradiography.
ster·e·o·spe·cif·ic [ˌ-spɪˈsɪfɪk] *adj chem.* stereospezifisch.
ster·e·o·spec·i·fic·i·ty [ˌ-ˌspesəˈfɪsətɪ] *n chem.* Stereospezifität *f*.
stereospecific numbering *abbr.* **sn** *chem.* stereospezifische Numerierung *f abbr.* sn.
ster·e·o·tac·tic [ˌ-ˈtæktɪk] *adj* **1.** *bio.* Stereotaxis betr., stereotaktisch. **2.** *neurochir.* stereotaktisch. **3.** *bio.* Thigmotaxis betr., thigmotaktisch.
ster·e·o·tax·ic [ˌ-ˈtæksɪk] *adj* → stereotactic.
stereotaxic surgery → stereoencephalotomy.
ster·e·o·tax·is [ˌ-ˈtæksɪs] *n bio.* Stereotaxis *f*.
ster·e·o·tax·y [ˌ-ˈtæksɪ] *n* → stereoencephalotomy.
ster·e·o·trop·ic [ˌ-ˈtrɑpɪk] *adj* thigmotrop.
ster·e·o·tro·pism [sterɪˈɑtrəpɪzəm, stɪər-] *n* Thigmotropismus *m*.
ster·e·o·ty·py [ˈsterɪətaɪpɪ] *n neuro., psychia.* Stereotypie *f*.
ster·ic [ˈsterɪk, ˈstɪər-] *adj chem.* räumlich, sterisch.
ste·rig·ma [stəˈrɪgmə] *n, pl* **-mas** *od.* **-ma·ta** [-mətə] *micro.* Sterigma *nt*.
Ste·rig·ma·to·cys·tis [stəˌrɪgmətəˈsɪstɪs] *n* Kolben-, Gießkannenschimmel *m*, Aspergillus *m*.
Ste·rig·mo·cys·tis [ˌ-ˈsɪstɪs] *n* → Sterigmatocystis.
ster·i·lant [ˈsterələnt] *n* sterilisierende Substanz *f*.
ster·ile [ˈsterɪl, -aɪl] *adj* **1.** *hyg.* keimfrei, steril; aseptisch. **2.** unfruchtbar, steril, infertil.
sterile abscess steriler Abszeß *m*.
sterile cyst sterile Zyste *f*.
sterile meningitis sterile Meningitis *f*.
sterile water keimfreies/sterilisiertes Wasser *nt*.
ste·ril·i·ty [stəˈrɪlətɪ] *n* **1.** *hyg.* Keimfreiheit *f*, Sterilität *f*; Asepsis *f*. **2.** Unfruchtbarkeit *f*, Sterilität *f*.
ster·il·i·za·tion [ˌsterɪləˈzeɪʃn] *n* **1.** *hyg.* Entkeimung *f*, Sterilisierung *f*, Sterilisation *f*. **2.** *gyn., urol.* Sterilisation *f*, Sterilisierung *f*.
ster·il·ize [ˈsterɪlaɪz] *vt* **1.** *hyg.* entkeimen, keimfrei machen, sterilisieren. **2.** *gyn., urol.* unfruchtbar machen, sterilisieren.
ster·i·liz·er [ˈsterɪlaɪzər] *n* Sterilisator *nt*, Sterilisierapparat *m*.
ster·nal [ˈstɜrnl] *adj* Brustbein/Sternum betr., sternal, Sternum-, Brustbein-.

sternal angle Angulus sterni/sternalis/Ludovici.
sternal arteries, posterior → sternal branches of internal thoracic artery.
sternal biopsy Sternalbiopsie *f*, -punktion *f*.
sternal branches of internal thoracic artery Sternumäste *pl* der A. thoracica interna, Rami sternales a. thoracicae internae.
sternal cartilage Rippenknorpel *m* einer echten Rippe.
sternal cleft Brustbein-, Sternumspalte *f*, Sternoschisis *f*.
sternal extremity of clavicle Extremitas sternalis.
sternal fracture Brustbein-, Sternumfraktur *f*.
ster·nal·gia [stɜrˈnældʒ(ɪ)ə] *n* **1.** Brustbeinschmerz *m*, Sternalgie *f*. **2.** → stenocardia.
sternal incisure Inc. jugularis sterni.
ster·na·lis (muscle) [stɜrˈneɪlɪs] Sternalis *m*, M. sternalis.
sternal line *anat.* Sternallinie *f*, Linea sternalis.
sternal membrane Membrana sterni.
sternal muscle → sternalis (muscle).
sternal notch Inc. jugularis sterni.
sternal puncture Brustbein-, Sternumpunktion *f*.
sternal ribs echte Rippen *pl*, Costae verae.
sternal synchondroses Synchondroses sternales.
Sternberg [ˈstɜrnbɜrg; ˈʃtɛrnbɛrk]: **S.'s disease** Morbus Hodgkin *m*, Hodgkin-Krankheit *f*, -Lymphom *nt*, (Hodgkin-)-Paltauf-Steinberg-Krankheit *f*, (maligne) Lymphogranulomatose *f*, Lymphogranulomatosis maligna.
S.'s giant cell Sternberg(-Reed)-Riesenzelle *f*.
S.'s sign Sternberg-Zeichen *nt*.
Sternberg-Reed [riːd]: **S.-R. cell** → Sternberg's giant cell.
sterno- *pref.* Brust-, Brustbein-, Sterno-, Sternal-.
ster·no·cla·vic·u·lar [ˌstɜrnəʊkləˈvɪkjələr] *adj* Sternum u. Klavikula betr., sternoklavikular *f*.
sternoclavicular angle Sternoklavikularwinkel *m*.
sternoclavicular articulation → sternoclavicular joint.
sternoclavicular disk Discus articularis sternoclavicularis.
sternoclavicular joint inneres Schlüsselbeingelenk *nt*, Sternoklavikulargelenk *nt*, Artic. sternoclavicularis.
sternoclavicular ligament Lig. sternoclaviculare.
anterior s. Lig. sternoclaviculare anterius.
posterior s. Lig. sternoclaviculare posterius.
ster·no·clei·dal [ˌ-ˈklaɪdəl] *adj* → sternoclavicular.
ster·no·clei·do·mas·toid branch [ˌ-ˌklaɪdəˈmæstɔɪd]: **s.es of occipital artery** Rami sternocleidomastoidei a. occipitalis. Rami sternocleidomastoidei a. occipitalis.
s. of superior thyroid artery Ramus sternocleidomastoideus a. thyroideae superioris.
ster·no·clei·do·mas·to·id·e·us (muscle) [ˌ-ˌklaɪdəʊmæsˈtɔɪdɪəs] Sternocleidomastoideus *m*, M. sternocleidomastoideus.
sternocleidomastoid muscle → sternocleidomastoideus (muscle).
sternocleidomastoid region *anat.* Regio sternocleidomastoidea.

sternocleidomastoid vein V. sternocleidomastoidea.
ster·no·cos·tal [ˌ-ˈkɑstl, -ˈkɔstl] *adj* Brustbein u. Rippen betr., sternokostal, kostosternal.
sternocostal articulation → sternocostal joint.
sternocostal joint Brustbein-Rippen-Gelenk *nt*, Sternokostalgelenk *nt*, Artic. sternocostalis.
sternocostal ligament Lig. sternocostale.
sternocostal surface of heart Herzvorderfläche *f*, Sternokostalfläche *f*, Facies sternocostalis/anterior (cordis).
ster·no·dym·ia [ˌ-ˈdiːmɪə] *n embryo.* Sternodymie *f*, -pagie *f*.
ster·nod·y·mus [stɜrˈnɑdɪməs] *n embryo.* Sternodymus *m*, -pagus *m*.
ster·no·dyn·ia [ˌstɜrnəˈdiːnɪə] *n* **1.** Brustbeinschmerz *m*, Sternodynie *f*, Sternalgie *f*. **2.** → stenocardia.
ster·no·hy·oid [ˌ-ˈhaɪɔɪd] *adj* Brustbein/Sternum u. Zungenbein/Os hyoideum betr., sternohyoid.
ster·no·hy·oi·de·us (muscle) [ˌ-haɪˈɔɪdɪəs] Sternohyoideus *m*, M. sternohyoideus.
sternohyoid muscle → sternohyoideus (muscle).
ster·noid [ˈstɜrnɔɪd] *adj* sternumartig, -ähnlich, sternoid.
ster·no·mas·toid muscle [ˌ-ˈmæstɔɪd] → sternocleidomastoideus (muscle).
ster·no·pa·gia [ˌ-ˈpeɪdʒɪə] *n* → sternodymia.
ster·nop·a·gus [stɜrˈnɑpəgəs] *n* → sternodymus.
ster·no·per·i·car·di·al [ˌstɜrnəʊperɪˈkɑːrdɪəl] *adj* Brustbein/Sternum u. Perikard betr. *od.* verbindend, sternoperikardial.
sternopericardial ligaments Ligg. sternopericardiaca.
ster·no·scap·u·lar [ˌ-ˈskæpjələr] *adj* Brustbein/Sternum u. Schulterblatt/Scapula betr., sternoskapular, skapulosternal.
ster·nos·chi·sis [stɜrˈnɑskəsɪs] *n* Brustbein-, Sternumspalte *f*, Sternoschisis *f*.
ster·no·thy·re·oi·de·us (muscle) [ˌstɜrnəʊθʌɪˈɔɪdɪəs] Sternothyr(e)oideus *m*, M. sternothyr(e)oideus.
ster·no·thy·roid [ˌ-ˈθaɪrɔɪd] *adj* Brustbein u. Schilddrüse *od.* Schildknorpel betr., sternothyr(e)oid.
sternothyroid muscle → sternothyreoideus (muscle).
ster·not·omy [stɜrˈnɑtəmɪ] *n chir.* Brustbeinspaltung *f*, -durchtrennung *f*, Sternotomie *f*.
ster·no·tra·che·al [ˌstɜrnəˈtreɪkɪəl] *adj* Brustbein/Sternum u. Trachea betr., sternotracheal.
ster·no·ver·te·bral [ˌ-ˈvɜrtəbrəl] *adj* Brustbein/Sternum u. Wirbel/Vertebrae betr., sternovertebral.
ster·no·xi·phop·a·gus [ˌ-zaɪˈfɑpəgəs] *n* Sternoxiphopagus *m*.
ster·num [ˈstɜrnəm] *n, pl* **-nums, -na** [-nə] Brustbein *nt*, Sternum *nt*.
ster·nu·ta·tio [ˌstɜrnjəˈteɪʃɪəʊ] *n* → sternutation.
ster·nu·ta·tion [ˌ-ˈteɪʃn] *n* Niesen *nt*, Sternutatio *f*.
stern·zel·len [ˈstɛrntsɛlən] *pl* (von) Kupffer'-Sternzellen *pl*, (von) Kupffer'-Zellen *pl*.
ste·roid [ˈstɪərɔɪd, ˈstɛr-] *n* Steroid *nt*.
steroid alcohol Steroidalkohol *m*.
steroid diabetes Steroiddiabetes *m*.
steroid fever Steroidfieber *nt*.
steroid hormone Steroidhormon *nt*.
steroid-induced *adj* steroidinduziert, Steroid-.
steroid-induced osteoporosis steroid-induzierte Osteoporose *f*, Steroidosteoporose *f*.
steroid 11β-monooxygenase Steroid-11β-monooxygenase *f*, 11β-Hydroxylase *f*.
steroid 17α-monooxygenase Steroid-17α-monooxygenase *f*, 17α-Hydroxylase *f*.
steroid 21-monooxygenase Steroid-21-monooxygenase *f*, 21-Hydroxylase *f*.
steroid nucleus *biochem.* Steroidkern *m*.
ste·roi·do·gen·e·sis [stə,rɔɪdəˈdʒenəsɪs] *n* Steroid(bio)synthese *f*.
ste·roi·do·gen·ic [ˌ-ˈdʒenɪk] *adj* Steroide bildend, steroidogen.
steroidogenic diabetes → steroid diabetes.
steroid osteoporosis steroidinduzierte Osteoporose *f*, Steroidosteoporose *f*.
steroid purpura Steroidpurpura *f*.
steroid receptor Steroidrezeptor *m*.
steroid 5α-reductase Steroid-5α-reduktase *f*, 5α-Reduktase *f*.
steroid sulfatase → steryl sulfatase.
steroid withdrawal syndrome Steroidentzugssyndrom *nt*.
ste·rol [ˈstɪərɔl, ˈstɛr-] *n* Sterin *nt*, Sterol *nt*.
sterol carrier protein Sterin-Carrier-Protein *nt*.
ster·tor [ˈstɜrtər] *n* röchelnde/stertoröse Atmung *f*, Stertor *m*; Schnarchen *nt*.
ster·to·rous [ˈstɜrtərəs] *adj* röchelnd, stertorös.
stertorous breathing → stertor.
ster·yl sulfatase [ˈstɛrɪl, ˈstɪər-] Sterylsulfatase *f*.
steth- *pref.* → stetho-.
steth·al·gia [steθˈældʒ(ɪ)ə] *n* Brust-, Brustkorb-, Brustwandschmerz(en *pl*) *m*.
steth·e·mia [steθˈiːmɪə] *n* Lungenstauung *f*.
stetho- *pref.* Brust-, Brustkorb-, Steth(o)-.
steth·o·cyr·to·graph [ˌsteθəˈsɜrtəgræf] *n* → stethokyrtograph.
steth·o·go·ni·om·e·ter [ˌ-ˌgəʊnɪˈɑmɪtər] *n* Stethogoniometer *nt*.
steth·o·graph [ˈ-græf] *n* *ortho.* Stethograph *m*.
steth·og·ra·phy [steθˈɑgrəfɪ] *n* **1.** *ortho.* Stethographie *f*. **2.** Phonokardiographie *f* *abbr.* PKG.
steth·o·kyr·to·graph [ˌsteθəˈkɜrtəgræf] *n* → *ortho.* Stethokyrtograph *m*.
steth·om·e·ter [steθˈɑmɪtər] *n* Stethometer *nt*.
steth·o·my·i·tis [ˌsteθəmaɪˈaɪtɪs] *n* → stethomyositis.
steth·o·my·o·si·tis [ˌ-maɪəˈsaɪtɪs] *n* Entzündung *f* der Brustwandmuskeln, Stethomyositis *f*.
steth·o·par·al·y·sis [ˌ-pəˈrælɪsɪs] *n* Lähmung *f* der Brustwandmuskeln.
steth·o·phone [ˈ-fəʊn] *n* Stethophon *nt*.
steth·o·scope [ˈ-skəʊp] *n* Stethoskop *nt*.
steth·o·scop·ic [ˌ-ˈskɑpɪk] *adj* Stethoskop betr., mittels Stethoskop, stethoskopisch.
ste·thos·co·py [steˈθɑskəpɪ] *n* Stethoskopie *f*, stethoskopische Untersuchung *f*.
steth·o·spasm [ˈsteθəspæzm] *n* Krampf/Spasmus *m* der Brustwandmuskeln.
Stevens [ˈstiːvənz]: **S.' power function** Stevens'-Potenzfunktion *f*.
S.' psychophysical law Stevens psychophysisches Gesetz *nt*.
S.'s psychophysics Stevens'-Psychophysik *f*.
Stevens-Johnson [ˈdʒɑnsən]: **S.-J. syndrome** Stevens-Johnson-Syndrom *nt*, Stevens-Johnson-Fuchs-Syndrom, Dermatostomatitis Baader *f*, Fiessinger-Rendue-Syndrom, Ectodermose érosive

pluriorificielle, Erythema exsudativum multiforme majus.
Stewart-Holmes ['st(j)uːərt həʊmz]: **S.-H. sign** *neuro.* Holmes-Phänomen *nt*, Holmes-Stewart-Phänomen *nt*, Rückstoß-, Rückschlag-, Reboundphänomen *nt*.
Stewart-Morel [mɔ'rɛl]: **S.-M. syndrome** Morgagni-Syndrom *nt*, Morgagni-Morel-Stewart-Syndrom *nt*, Hyperostosis frontalis interna.
Stewart-Treves [triːvs]: **S.-T. syndrome** Stewart-Treves-Syndrom *nt*.
St. Guy [seɪnt gaɪ; sɛ̃]: **St. G.'s dance** → Sydenham's chorea.
STH *abbr.* [somatotropic hormone] → somatotropin.
sthe·ni·a ['sθiːnɪə] *n* (Körper-)Kraft *f*, Stärke *f*, Sthenie *f*.
sthen·ic ['sθɛnɪk] *adj* kräftig, kraftvoll, stark, aktiv, sthenisch.
sthen·om·e·ter [sθɪ'nɑmɪtər] *n* Sthenometer *nt*.
sthen·om·e·try [sθɪ'nɑmɪtrɪ] *n* Sthenometrie *f*.
stib·i·al·ism ['stɪbɪəlɪzəm] *n* Antimonvergiftung *f*, Stibialismus *m*, Stibismus *m*.
stib·i·at·ed ['stɪbɪeɪtɪd] *adj* antimonhaltig.
stib·i·a·tion [,stɪbɪ'eɪʃn] *n* Behandlung *f* mit Antimon.
stib·i·um ['stɪbɪəm] *n abbr.* **Sb** *chem.* Antimon *nt*, Stibium *nt abbr.* Sb.
stib·o·glu·co·nate sodium [,stɪbə'gluːkəneɪt] Natrium-Stibogluconat *nt*.
stib·o·phen ['-fen] *n pharm.* Stibophen *nt*.
Sticker ['stɪkər]: **S.'s disease** Ringelröteln *pl*, Sticker-Krankheit *f*, fünfte Krankheit *f*, Morbus quintus, Erythema infectiosum, Megalerythem *nt*, Megalerythema epidemicum/infectiosum.
Stickler ['stɪklər]: **S.'s syndrome** Stickler-Syndrom *nt*, hereditäre progressive Arthroophthalmopathie *f*.
Stieda ['stiːdə; -da]: **S.'s disease** *ortho.* Stieda-Pellegrini-Schatten *m*, Pellegrini-Schatten *m*.
S.'s fracture Stieda-Fraktur *f*.
S.'s process Proc. posterior tali.
Stierlin ['stɜːrlɪn]: **S.'s sign/symptom** *radiol.* Stierlin-Zeichen *nt*.
stiff-man syndrome [stɪf] Stiff-man-Syndrom *nt*.
stiff neck *ortho.* Schiefhals *m*, Torticollis *m*, Caput obstipum.
stiff-neck fever 1. Dengue *nt*, Dengue-Fieber *nt*, Dandy-Fieber *nt*. **2.** Meningokokkenmeningitis *f*, Meningitis cerebrospinalis epidemica.
stiff pupil Argyll-Robertson-Phänomen *nt*, -Zeichen *nt*.
stiff toe Hallux rigidus.
stig·ma ['stɪgmə] *n, pl* **-mas, -ma·ta** ['stɪgmətə, stɪg'mætə] **1.** (Kenn-)Zeichen *nt*, Mal *nt*, Stigma *nt*. **2.** (typisches) Merkmal *nt*, (Kenn-)Zeichen *nt*, Symptom *nt*, Stigma *nt*. **3.** *micro.* Augenfleck *m*, Stigma *nt*. **4.** *gyn.* Stigma *nt*, Macula pellucida.
stig·mas·ter·ol [stɪg'mæstərɔl] *n* Stigmasterin *nt*.
stig·mat·ic lens [stɪg'mætɪk] anastigmatisches/stigmatisches Glas *nt*.
stig·ma·tom·e·ter [,stɪgmə'tɑmɪtər] *n ophthal.* Stigmatometer *nt*.
stil·bene ['stɪlbiːn] *n* Stilben *nt*.
stil·bes·trol [stɪl'bestrɔl] *n pharm.* Diäthylstilböstrol *nt*, Diethylstilbestrol *nt abbr.* DES.
sti·let ['staɪlɪt, stɪ'let] *n* → stylet.
sti·lette ['staɪlɪt, stɪ'let] *n* → stylet.
Still [stɪl]: **S.'s disease** Still-Syndrom *nt*, Chauffard-Ramon-Still-Krankheit *f*, Morbus Still *m*, juvenile Form *f* der chronischen Polyarthritis.
S.'s murmur Still-Geräusch *nt*.
still-birth ['stɪlbɜːθ] *n gyn.* Totgeburt *f*; intrauteriner Fruchttod *m*.
still-born ['stɪlbɔːrn] **I** *n* Totgeborene *nt*, Totgeburt *f*. **II** *adj* totgeboren.
Still-Chauffard [ʃo'faːr]: **S.-C. syndrome** → Still's disease.
Stilling ['stɪlɪŋ]: **(central) canal of S.** Cloquet-Kanal *m*, Canalis hyaloideus.
S.'s column Clarke'-Säule *f*, Clarke-Stilling-Säule *f*, Stilling'-Kern, Nc. thoracicus, Columna thoracica.
S.'s nucleus → S.'s column.
S.'s syndrome → Stilling-Türk-Duane syndrome.
Stilling-Türk-Duane [tɪrk dweɪn, duː'eɪn; tyrk]: **S.-T.-D. syndrome** *ophthal.* Duane-Syndrom *nt*, Stilling-Türk-Duane-Syndrom *nt*.
stim·u·lant ['stɪmjələnt] **I** *n* **1.** Anregungs-, Reiz-, Aufputschmittel *nt*, Stimulans *nt*. **2.** Anreiz *m*, Antrieb *m*, Anregung *f*, Stimulanz *f*. **II** *adj* → stimulating.
stim·u·late ['-leɪt] *vt, vi* anregen, beleben, aufputschen, stimulieren.
stim·u·lat·ing ['-leɪtɪŋ] *adj* anregend, (an-)reizend, belebend, aufputschend, stimulierend, Reiz-.
stimulating drug → stimulant 1.
stimulating electrode Reizelektrode *f*.
stim·u·la·tion [,-'leɪʃn] *n* **1.** Anregung *f*, Belebung *f*, Anreiz *m*, Antrieb *m*, Stimulation, Stimulieren *nt*. **2.** *physiol.* Reiz *m*, Reizung *f*, Stimulation *f*.
stimulation produced analgesia *abbr.* **SPA** stimulationsproduzierte Analgesie *f abbr.* SPA.
stim·u·la·tive ['-leɪtɪv] *adj* → stimulating.
stim·u·la·tor ['-leɪtər] *n* → stimulant I.
stim·u·la·to·ry modulator ['-lə,tɔːriː, -təʊ-] *biochem.* fördernder/stimulierender/positiver Modulator *m*.
stim·u·lus ['stɪmjələs] *n, pl* **-li** [-laɪ, -liː] **1.** *physiol.* Reiz *m*, Stimulus *m*. **2.** Anreiz *m*, Ansporn *m*. **3.** → stimulant 1.
stimulus frequency Reizfrequenz *f*.
stimulus intensity Reizintensität *f*.
stimulus limen *physiol.* Reizschwelle *f*, -limen *nt abbr.* **RL**, Absolutschwelle *f*.
stimulus pattern Reizmuster *nt*.
electrical s. elektrisches Reizmuster *nt*.
frequency s. Frequenzmuster *nt*.
temporal s. zeitliches Reizmuster *nt*.
stimulus quality Reizqualität *f*.
stimulus range Reizbereich *m*.
stimulus-secretion coupling Stimulus-Sekretionskopplung *f*.
stimulus-specific *adj* reizspezifisch.
stimulus substitution klassische Konditionierung *f*.
stimulus threshold → stimulus limen.
stimulus transformation Reizumwandlung *f*, -transformation *f*.
stimulus transport Reizweiterleitung *f*, -transport *m*.
sting [stɪŋ] (*v* **stung; stung**) **I** *n* **1.** Stachel *m*. **2.** Stich *m*, Biß *m*. **II** *vt* **3.** stechen; beißen, brennen. **4.** brennen, wehtun, peinigen. **III** *vi* stechen; brennen, beißen; schmerzen, wehtun.
stip·ple cell ['stɪpl] getüpfelter Erythrozyt *m*.
stip·pled ['stɪplt] *adj* gepunktet, getüpfelt, punktiert, Tüpfel-.
stippled epiphysis Conradi-Syndrom *nt*, Conradi-Hühnermann(-Raap)-Syndrom *nt*, Chondrodysplasia/Chondrodystrophia calcificans congenita.
stippled tongue Stippchenzunge *f*.
stip·pling ['stɪplɪŋ] *n* **1.** Tüpfelung *f*, Punktierung *f*. **2.** *ophthal.* Pfeffer-Salz-Fundus *m*.
stir·rup ['stɜːrəp, 'stɪr-] *n anat.* Steigbügel *m*, Stapes *m*.
stirrup bone → stirrup.
stitch [stɪtʃ] **I** *n* **1.** Stich *m*, Naht *f*. **2.** Stich(art *f*) *m*. **3.** (*Schmerz*) Stich *m*, Stechen *nt*. **II** *vt* nähen.
stitch up *vt* vernähen, zusammennähen.
stitch abscess Faden-, Nahtabszeß *m*.
St. John [seɪnt dʒɑn; sɛ̃]: **St. J.'s dance** → Sydenham's chorea.
St. Louis encephalitis [seɪnt 'luːɪs; sɛ̃] *abbr.* **SLE** St. Louis-Enzephalitis *f abbr.* SLE.
St. Louis encephalitis virus St. Louis-Enzephalitis-Virus *nt*.
STM *abbr.* → short-term memory.
sto·chas·tic [stə'kæstɪk] *adj* dem Zufall unterworfen, stochastisch, Zufalls-.
sto·chas·tics [stə'kæstɪks] *pl stat.* Stochastik *f*.
stock·cock [stɑk,kɑk] *n techn.* (Wasser-, Gas-, Absperr-)Hahn *m*.
stock·i·nette ['stɑkɪnet] *n ortho.* Trikotstrumpf *m*, -schlauch *m*, Schlauchbinde *f*.
stock·ing ['stɑkɪŋ] *n* Strumpf *m*.
stocking anesthesia strumpfförmige Sensibilitätsstörung/Anästhesie *f*.
stock·y ['stɑkɪ] *adj* (*Statur*) untersetzt, gedrungen.
Stoffel ['stɔfl; 'stɒf-]: **S.'s operation** *neurochir.* Stoffel-Operation *f*.
stoi·chi·o·met·ric [,stɔɪkɪə'metrɪk] *adj chem.* Stöchiometrie betr., stöchiometrisch.
stoi·chi·om·e·try [,stɔɪkɪ'ɑmətrɪ] *n chem.* Stöchiometrie *f*.
stok·er's cramp ['stəʊkər] Heizerkrampf *m*.
Stokes [stəʊks]: **S.' amputation** → S.' operation.
collar of S. Stokes'-Kragen *m*.
S.' operation *ortho.* Beinamputation *f* nach Gritti-Stokes.
S.' radius *phys.* Stokes'-Radius *m*.
S.' syndrome → Stokes-Adams disease.
stokes [stəʊks] *n phys.* Stokes *n*.
Stokes-Adams [ˈædəmz]: **S.-A. disease** Adams-Stokes-Anfall *m abbr.* **ASA**, Adams-Stokes-Synkope *f*, -Syndrom *nt*.
S.-A. syncope/syndrome → S.-A. disease.
Stokvis-Talma ['stɑkvɪs 'tælmə]: **S.-T. syndrome** Stokvis-Talma-Syndrom *nt*, autotoxische Zyanose *f*.
stom- *pref.* → stomato-.
sto·ma ['stəʊmə] *n, pl* **-mas, -ma·ta** ['stəʊmətə, stəʊ'mɑtə] **1.** *anat.* Öffnung *f*, Mund *m*, Stoma *nt*. **2.** *chir.* künstliche Öffnung *f od.* künstlicher Ausgang *m* eines Hohlorgans, Stoma *nt*. **3.** *patho.* Fistelöffnung *f*, Stoma *nt*.
sto·mac·a·ce [stəʊ'mækəsɪ] *n* → stomatocace.
stom·ach ['stʌmək] *n* **1.** Magen *m*; *anat.* Gaster *f*, Ventriculus *m*. **on an empty ~** auf leeren/nüchternen Magen. **on a full ~** mit vollem Magen. **2.** Bauch *m*.
stomach ache Bauchweh *nt*, Magenschmerzen *pl*, Gastralgie *f*, Gastrodynie *f*.
stom·ach·al·gia [,stʌmə'kældʒ(ɪ)ə] *n* → stomach ache.
stom·a·chal vertigo ['stʌməkəl] Magenschwindel *m*, Vertigo gastrica.
stomach bubble *radiol.* Magenblase *f*.
stomach clamp *chir.* Magenklemme *f*.
sto·mach·ic [stəʊ'mækɪk] **I** *n* Magenmittel *nt*, Stomachikum *nt*. **II** *adj* **1.** Magen betr., gastrisch, Magen-, Gastro-. **2.** verdauungs-, appetitfördernd.

stomachical

sto·mach·i·cal [stəʊˈmækɪkl] *adj* → stomachic II.
stom·a·cho·dy·nia [ˌstʌməkəʊˈdiːnɪə] *n* → stomach ache.
stomach pump Magenpumpe *f*.
stomach secrete Magensekret *nt*, -saft *m*.
stomach trouble Magenbeschwerden *pl*.
stomach tube Magensonde *f*.
stomach upset Magenverstimmung *f*.
stomach wall Magenwand *f*.
stomach worm *micro*. Haemonchus contortus.
sto·ma·de·um [ˌstəʊməˈdɪəm] *n* → stomodeum.
sto·mal [ˈstəʊməl] *adj* Stoma betr., Mund-, Stoma-.
sto·mal·gia [stəʊˈmældʒ(ɪ)ə] *n* → stomatalgia.
stomal ulcer *chir*. Stoma-, Randulkus *nt*.
stomat- *pref*. → stomato-.
stom·a·tal [ˈstɒmətəl, ˈstəʊ-] *adj* → stomal.
sto·ma·tal·gia [ˌstəʊməˈtældʒ(ɪ)ə] *n* Schmerzen *pl* im Mund, Stomatalgie *f*, Stomatodynie *f*.
sto·mat·ic [stəˈmætɪk] *adj* Mund betr., oral, Mund-, Stomat(o)-.
sto·ma·ti·tis [ˌstəʊməˈtaɪtɪs] *n* Mundschleimhautentzündung *f*, Stomatitis *f*.
stomato- *pref*. Mund-, Stomat(o)-.
sto·ma·toc·a·ce [ˌstəʊməˈtɒkəsɪ] *n* Stomatokake *f*, -kaze *f*, Stomatitis ulcerosa.
sto·ma·to·cyte [ˈstəʊmətəsaɪt] *n* *hema*. Stomatozyt *m*.
sto·ma·to·cy·to·sis [ˌ-saɪˈtəʊsɪs] *n* *hema*. Stomatozytose *f*.
sto·ma·to·de·um [ˌ-ˈdɪəm] *n* → stomodeum.
sto·ma·to·dy·nia [ˌ-ˈdiːnɪə] *n* → stomatalgia.
sto·ma·to·dys·o·dia [ˌ-dɪsˈəʊdɪə] *n* (übler) Mundgeruch *m*, Atemgeruch *m*, Kakostomie *f*, Halitosis *f*, Halitose *f*, Foetor ex ore.
sto·ma·to·glos·si·tis [ˌ-ɡlɒˈsaɪtɪs] *n* Entzündung *f* von Mundschleimhaut u. Zunge, Stomatoglossitis *f*.
sto·ma·to·log·i·cal [ˌ-ˈlɒdʒɪkl] *adj* Stomatologie betr., stomatologisch.
sto·ma·tol·o·gist [ˌstəʊməˈtɒlədʒɪst] *n* Stomatologe *m*, -login *f*.
sto·ma·tol·o·gy [ˌ-ˈtɒlədʒɪ] *n* Stomatologie *f*.
sto·ma·to·ma·la·cia [ˌstəʊmətəməˈleɪʃ(ɪ)ə] *n* Stomatomalazie *f*.
sto·mat·o·my [stəʊˈmætəmɪ] *n* *chir*., HNO Stomatotomie *f*, Stomatomie *f*.
sto·ma·to·my·co·sis [ˌstəʊmətəmaɪˈkəʊsɪs] *n* pilzbedingte Stomatitis *f*, Stomatitis mycotica, Stomatomykose *f*, -mykosis *f*, -mycosis *f*.
sto·ma·to·ne·cro·sis [ˌ-nɪˈkrəʊsɪs] *n* → stomatonoma.
sto·ma·to·no·ma [ˌ-ˈnəʊmə] *n* Noma *f*, Wangenbrand *m*, Wasserkrebs *m*, infektiöse Gangrän *f* des Mundes, Cancer aquaticus, Chancrum oris, Stomatitis gangraenosa.
sto·ma·to·pa·thy [ˌstəʊməˈtɒpəθɪ] *n* Munderkrankung *f*, Stomatopathie *f*.
sto·ma·to·plas·ty [ˈstəʊmətəplæstɪ] *n* HNO Mund-, Stomatoplastik *f*.
sto·ma·tor·rha·gia [ˌ-ˈreɪdʒ(ɪ)ə] *n* Blutung *f* aus dem Mund, Stomatorrhagie *f*.
sto·ma·tos·chi·sis [ˌstəʊməˈtɒskəsɪs] *n* Lippenspalte *f*, Mundspalte *f*, Hasenscharte *f*, Stomatoschisis *f*.
sto·ma·to·scope [stəʊˈmætəskəʊp] *n* Stomatoskop *nt*.
sto·ma·tot·o·my [ˌstəʊməˈtɒtəmɪ] *n* → stomatomy.
stoma ulcer *chir*. Stoma-, Randulkus *nt*.

sto·men·ceph·a·lus [ˌstəʊmenˈsefələs] *n* *embryo*. Stomozephalus *m*.
stomo- *pref*. → stomato-.
sto·mo·ceph·a·lus [ˌstəʊməʊˈsefələs] *n* *embryo*. Stomozephalus *m*.
sto·mo·de·al [ˌ-ˈdɪəl] *adj* Stoma(to)deum betr.
sto·mo·de·um [ˌ-ˈdɪəm] *n*, *pl* **-deums**, **-dea** [-ˈdɪə] *embryo*. Mundbucht *f*, -nische *f*, Stoma(to)deum *nt*.
sto·mos·chi·sis [stəʊˈmɒskəsɪs] *n* → stomatoschisis.
Sto·mox·ys [stəʊˈmɒksɪs] *n* *micro*. Stomoxys *f*.
stone [stəʊn] **I** *n* **1.** Stein *m*. **2.** *patho*. Stein *m*, Calculus *m*. **3.** *Brit*. stone (*nt*). **II** *adj* steinern, Stein-.
stone clamp → stone forceps.
stone extraction *chir*. Steinextraktion *f*.
stone forceps *chir*. Steinfaßzange *f*.
stone-grasping forceps → stone forceps.
stone-retrieving basket *chir*. Steinkörbchen *nt*; Steinfänger *m*.
stool [stuːl] *n* **1.** Kot *m*, Fäkalien *pl*, Faeces *pl*. **2.** Hocker *m*, Stuhl *m*, Schemel *m*.
stool culture Stuhlkultur *f*.
stool examination Stuhluntersuchung *f*.
stool impaction Koteinklemmung *f*.
stool-softening agent stuhlerweichendes Mittel *nt*.
stop [stɒp] **I** *n* **1.** Stillstand *m*, Ende *nt*; Stoppen *nt*. **2.** Hemmnis *nt*, Sperre *f*, Hindernis *nt*. **II** *vt* **3.** aufhören (*doing* zu tun). **4.** zum Halten/Stillstand bringen, stoppen, an-, aufhalten, ab-, einstellen; blockieren, hemmen. **5.** zu-, verstopfen; (*Zahn*) plombieren, füllen; (*Blut*) stillen; (*Gefäß*) verschließen. **6.** unterbrechen. **III** *vi* (an-)halten, stoppen, stehenbleiben; aufhören; (*Puls*) ausbleiben.
stop consonant Explosions-, Plosiv-, Verschlußlaut *m*, Plosiv *m*.
stop·page [ˈstɒpɪdʒ] *n* **1.** Stillstand *m*, (An-)Halten *nt*, Unterbrechen *nt*. **2.** Verstopfung *f*, Stau(ung *f*) *m*, Stockung *f*; Hemmung *f*.
stop·per [ˈstɒpər] **I** *n* Stopfer *m*, Pfropf(en *m*) *m*, Stöpsel *m*. **II** *vt* zu-, verstöpseln, -stopfen.
stop·ping [ˈstɒpɪŋ] *n* *dent*. Plombieren *nt*; Plombe *f*, Füllung *f*.
stop·ple [ˈstɒpl] **I** *n* Stöpsel *m*. **II** *vt* zustöpseln.
stor·age [ˈstɔːrɪdʒ, ˈstəʊr-] *n* **1.** Lagern *nt*, Speichern *nt*, (Ein-)Lagerung *f*, Speicherung *f*. **2.** Depot *nt*, Speicher *m*.
storage capacity Speicherkapazität *f*.
storage carbohydrate Speicher-, Reservekohlenhydrat *nt*.
storage disease Speicherkrankheit *f*.
brancher glycogen s. → glycogen s., type IV.
cholesterol ester s. *abbr*. CESD Cholesterinesterspeicherkrankheit *f*.
cystine s. Zystinspeicherkrankheit *f*, Zystinose *f*, Cystinose *f*, Lignac-Syndrom *nt*, Aberhalden-Fanconi-Syndrom *nt*.
debrancher glycogen s. → glycogen s., type III.
glycogen s. Glykogenspeicherkrankheit *f*, Glykogenose *f*.
glycogen s., type I (von) Gierke-Krankheit *f*, van Creveld-von Gierke-Krankheit *f*, hepatorenale Glykogenose *f*, Glykogenose Typ I *f*.
glycogen s., type II Pompe-Krankheit *f*, generalisierte maligne Glykogenose *f*, Glykogenose Typ II *f*.
glycogen s., type III Cori-Krankheit *f*, Forbes-Syndrom *nt*, hepatomuskuläre benigne Glykogenose *f*, Glykogenose Typ III *f*.

glycogen s., type IV Andersen-Krankheit *f*, Amylopektinose *f*, leberzirrhotische retikuloendotheliale Glykogenose *f*, Glykogenose Typ IV *f*.
glycogen s., type V McArdle-Krankheit *f*, muskuläre Glykogenose *f*, Myophosphorylaseinsuffizienz *f*, Glykogenose Typ V *f*.
glycogen s., type VI Hers-Erkrankung *f*, -Syndrom *nt*, -Glykogenose *f*, Leberphosphorylaseinsuffizienz *f*, Glykogenose Typ VI *f*.
glycogen s., type VII Tarui-Krankheit *f*, Muskelphosphofruktokinaseinsuffizienz *f*, Glykogenose Typ VII *f*.
glycogen s., type VIII hepatische Glykogenose *f*, Phosphorylase-b-kinase-Insuffizienz *f*, Glykogenose Typ VIII *f*.
hepatorenal glycogen s. → glycogen s., type I.
lipid s. Lipidspeicherkrankheit *f*, Lipidose *f*, Lipoidose *f*.
phytanic acid s. Refsum-Syndrom *nt*, Heredopathia atactica polyneuritiformis.
storage dystrophy Speicherungsdystrophie *f*.
storage fat Speicher-, Depotfett *nt*.
storage form Speicherform *f*.
storage gland Speicherdrüse *f*.
storage granule *histol*. Speicherkörnchen *nt*.
storage lipid Depot-, Speicherlipid *nt*.
storage protein Speicherprotein *nt*.
store [stɔːr, stəʊr] **I** *n* Vorrat *m*; Lager *nt*, Speicher *m*. **II** *vt* **1.** (ein-)lagern, speichern; (*Computer*) speichern. **2.** versorgen (*with* mit).
STPD conditions [standard temperature and pressure, dry] *physiol*. STPD-Bedingungen *pl*.
stra·bis·mal [strəˈbɪzməl] *adj* → strabismic.
stra·bis·mic [strəˈbɪzmɪk] *adj* Schielen/Strabismus betr., schielend, Schiel-.
strabismic amblyopia *ophthal*. strabismus-bedingte Amblyopie *f*.
stra·bis·mom·e·ter [ˌstrəbɪzˈmɒmɪtər] *n* *ophthal*. Strabismometer *nt*, Strabometer *nt*.
stra·bis·mom·e·try [ˌ-ˈmɒmɪtrɪ] *n* *ophthal*. Strabismometrie *f*, Strabometrie *f*.
stra·bis·mus [strəˈbɪzməs] *n* Schielen *nt*, Strabismus *m*.
strabismus scissors *ophthal*. Strabismusschere *f*.
stra·bom·e·ter [strəˈbɒmɪtər] *n* → strabismometer.
stra·bom·e·try [strəˈbɒmɪtrɪ] *n* → strabismometry.
strab·o·tome [ˈstræbətəʊm] *n* *ophthal*. Strabotomiemesser *nt*, Strabotom *nt*.
stra·bot·o·my [strəˈbɒtəmɪ] *n* *ophthal*. Schieloperation *f*, Strabotomie *f*, Strabismotomie *f*.
strad·dling embolus [ˈstrædlɪŋ] reitender Embolus *m*, Sattelembolus *m*.
straight [streɪt] **I** *adj* **1.** gerade. **2.** (*Person*) gerade, offen, ehrlich; anständig; zuverlässig, sicher. **3.** *sl*. hetero(sexuell). **II** *adv* **4.** geradeaus; direkt, gerade, unmittelbar. **5.** ehrlich, anständig. **to ~ o.s. up** *s*. aufrichten. **II** *vi* gerade werden; (*Person*) *s*. aufrichten.
straight angle gestreckter Winkel *m*.
straight arteries of kidney Vasa recta, Arteriolae rectae.
straight arterioles of kidney → straight arteries of kidney.
straight·en [ˈstreɪtn] **I** *vt* begradigen, gerademachen, -ziehen, -biegen. **to ~ o.s. up** *s*. aufrichten. **II** *vi* gerade werden; (*Person*) *s*. aufrichten.
straight gyrus Gyrus rectus.

straight head of rectus femoris muscle vorderer/gerader Kopf *m* des M. rectus femoris, Caput rectus m. recti femoris.
straight intestine End-, Mastdarm *m*, Rektum *nt*, Rectum *nt*, Intestinum rectum.
straight-line *adj mathe.*, *phys.* geradllinig, linear.
straight muscle: s. of abdomen *old* → rectus abdominis (muscle).
anterior s. of head *old* → rectus capitis anterior (muscle).
inferior s. Rektus *m* inferior, M. rectus inferior.
lateral s. Rektus *m* lateralis, M. rectus lateralis.
lateral s. of head *old* → rectus capitis lateralis (muscle).
medial s. Rektus *m* medialis, M. rectus medialis.
posterior s. of head, greater *old* → rectus capitis posterior major (muscle).
posterior s. of head, smaller *old* → rectus capitis posterior minor (muscle).
superior s. Rektus *m* superior, M. rectus superior.
s. of thigh *old* → rectus femoris (muscle).
straight scissors *chir.* gerade Schere *f.*
straight sinus Sinus rectus.
straight venules (of kidney) (*Niere*) gestreckte Venen *pl* der Marksubstanz, Venulae rectae.
strain¹ [streɪn] **I** *n* 1. (*Muskel, Sehne*) Zerrung *f*, (Über-)Dehnung *f*; (*Herz, Auge*) Überanstrengung *f.* 2. Anstrengung *f*, Anspannung *f*, Strapaze *f*, Beanspruchung *f*, Belastung *f* (*on* für). **to put/place a ~ on** beanspruchen, belasten. 3. *techn.* Spannung *f*, Beanspruchung *f*, Druck *m*, Zug *m.* **II** *vt* 4. (*Muskel*) zerren, überdehnen; (*Herz, Augen*) überanstrengen; (*Handgelenk*) verrenken, verstauchen. 5. belasten, strapazieren. 6. (an-)spannen, (an-)ziehen; *techn.* deformieren, verformen. 7. (durch-)sieben, (-)sieben, passieren; filtern, filtrieren. 8. (fest) drücken *od.* pressen. **III** *vi* 9. s. anstrengen (*to* dazu tun); s. be-, abmühen. 10. s. (an-)spannen; zerren, ziehen. 11. *techn.* s. verziehen, s. verformen. 12. (*Flüssigkeit*) durchlaufen, -tropfen, -sickern. 13. pressen, drücken (*beim Stuhlgang*).
strain off *vt* → strain out.
strain out *vt* abseihen; (*Wasser*) abgießen, abschütten.
strain² [streɪn] *n* 1. *bio.* Rasse *f*, Art *f*; (Bakterien-)Stamm *m.* 2. *micro.* Varietät *f*, Varietas *f.* 3. (Erb-)Anlage *f*, Veranlagung *f*; Charakterzug *m*, Merkmal *nt.*
strained [streɪnd] *adj* 1. überanstrengt, strapaziert, über(be)lastet; (*Muskel*) gezerrt, überdehnt. 2. durchgeseiht, filtiert, gefiltert. 3. gezwungen, unnatürlich, (an-)gespannt.
strain·er [ˈstreɪnər] *n* Sieb *nt*; Filter *m.*
strain gauge manometer Strain-gauge-Manometer *nt.*
strain response Beanspruchungsreaktion *f.*
strait [streɪt] *n* (enger) Durchgang *m*, Enge *f.*
strand [strænd] *n* Strang *m*, Faser *f.*
stran·gal·es·the·sia [ˌstræŋgælesˈθiːʒ(ɪ)ə] *n neuro.* Gürtelgefühl *nt*, Zonästhesie *f.*
stran·gle [ˈstræŋgl] **I** *vt* erwürgen, erdrosseln, strangulieren. **II** *vi* ersticken.
stran·gu·late [ˈstræŋgjəleɪt] *vt* 1. *chir.* abbinden, abschnüren. 2. erwürgen, erdrosseln, strangulieren.
stran·gu·lat·ed hernia [ˈstræŋgjəleɪtɪd] strangulierte Hernie *f.*

stran·gu·la·tion [ˌstræŋgjəˈleɪʃn] *n* 1. Erdrosselung *f*, Strangulierung *f*, Strangulation *f.* 2. *chir.* Abschnürung *f*, Abbindung *f*, Strangulation *f.*
strangulation ileus *chir.* Strangulationsileus *m.*
strangulation mark *embryo.* Schnürfurche *f.*
stran·gu·ria [strænˈg(j)ʊərɪə] *n* → stranguiry.
stran·gu·ry [ˈstræŋgjərɪ] *n urol.* (schmerzhafter) Harnzwang *m*, Strangurie *f.*
strap [stræp] **I** *n* (Anschnall-)Riemen *m*, (Anschnall-)Gurt *m*, Band *nt.* **II** *vt* 1. fest-, anschnallen (*to* an); umschnallen. 2. (*Wunde*) mit Heftpflaster versorgen.
strap up *vt* einen Heftpflasterverband anlegen.
strap muscles Mm. sternohyoideus et thyr(e)ohyoideus.
strap·ping [ˈstræpɪŋ] *n* (Heft-)Pflasterverband *m.*
Strassmann [ˈstræsmən; ˈʃtrasman]: **S.'s phenomenon** *embryo.* Strassmann-Zeichen *nt.*
strat·i·fi·ca·tion [ˌstrætɪfɪˈkeɪʃn] *n* Schichtung *f*, Schichtenbildung *f*, Stratifikation *f.*
strat·i·fied [ˈ-faɪd] *adj histol.* mehrschichtig, geschichtet, schichtförmig.
stratified cartilage fibröser Knorpel *m*, Faserknorpel *m*, Bindegewebsknorpel *m*, Cartilago fibrosa/collagenosa.
stratified epithelium mehrschichtiges Epithel *nt.*
strat·i·form [ˈ-fɔːrm] *adj* schichtenförmig.
strat·i·fy [ˈ-faɪ] **I** *vt* (auf-)schichten, stratifizieren. **II** *vi* Schichten bilden, in Schichten legen, stratifizieren.
strat·i·gram [ˈ-græm] *n radiol.* Schichtaufnahme *f*, Tomogramm *nt.*
stra·tig·ra·phy [strəˈtɪgrəfɪ] *n radiol.* Schichtaufnahmetechnik *f*, -verfahren *f*, Tomographie *f.*
strat·o·graph·ic analysis [ˌstrætəˈgræfɪk] Chromatographie *f.*
stra·tum [ˈstreɪtəm, ˈstræ-, ˈstrɑ-] *n, pl* **-tums, -ta** [-tə] *anat.* Lage *f*, Schicht *f*, Stratum *nt.*
stratum interolivare lemnisci Stratum (interolivare) lemnisci.
stratum lacunosum Stratum lacunosum.
stratum lemnisci → stratum interolivare lemnisci.
stratum opticum Stratum opticum.
stratum oriens Stratum oriens.
stratum radiatum Stratum radiatum.
Straub-Traugott [straʊb ˈtraʊgɔt; ˈʃtraʊb]: **S.-T. effect** Straub-Traugott-Effekt *m.*
straw·ber·ry gallbladder [ˈstrɔːbərɪ, -ˌberiː] Stippchen-, Erdbeergallenblase *f.*
strawberry hemangioma Blutschwamm *m*, blastomatöses Hämangiom *nt*, Haemangioma planotuberosum/simplex.
strawberry mark → strawberry nevus.
strawberry nevus 1. vaskulärer Nävus *m*, Naevus vasculosus. 2. kavernöses Hämangiom *nt*, Kavernom *nt*, Haemangioma tuberonodosum. 3. → strawberry hemangioma.
strawberry tongue Erdbeerzunge *f*, hypertrophische Zunge *f.*
red s. Himbeerzunge *f*, rote Zunge *f.*
straw itch [strɔː] Gerstenkrätze *f*, Acarodermatitis urticaroides.
straw mite *micro.* Pyemotes.
stray light [streɪ] Streulicht *nt.*
streak [striːk] **I** *n* 1. Strich *m*, Streifen *m*; (Licht-)Strahl *m.* 2. Lage *f*, Schicht *f.* 3. *micro.* Aufstrichimpfung *f.* 4. *chem.*

Schliere *f.* **II** *vt micro.*(*Kultur*) stricheln, ausstreichen.
streak culture *micro.* (Aus-)Strichkultur *f.*
streaked [striːkt] *adj* geschichtet; streifig, gestreift.
streak·y [ˈstriːkɪ] *adj* → streaked.
stream [striːm] **I** *n* Strom *m*, Strömung *f*; *fig.* Strömung *f*, Tendenz *f.* **II** *vt* aus-, verströmen. **III** *vi* strömen, fließen, rinnen; triefen (*with* vor); (*Augen*) tränen.
s. of air Luftstrom.
s. of consciousness *psycho.* Bewußtseinsstrom.
stream·ing [ˈstriːmɪŋ] **I** *n* Strömen *nt*, Fließen *nt.* **II** *adj* strömend; (*Augen*) tränend.
streb·lo·dac·ty·ly [ˌstrebləʊˈdæktəlɪ] *n ortho., embryo.* Streblodaktylie *f.*
Streeter [ˈstriːtər]: **S.'s bands** amniotische Stränge *pl*, Simonart'-Bänder *pl.*
strength [streŋθ, -ŋkθ] *n* 1. Kraft *f*, Stärke *f*; Festigkeit *f*, Stabilität *f.* 2. *phys.* (Strom-)Stärke *f*; Wirkungsgrad *m.* 3. (Säure-)Stärke *f*; (*Lösung*) Konzentration *f.*
s. of body Körperkraft.
s. of character Charakterstärke *f.*
s. of mind Geistesstärke.
s. of will Willensstärke.
strength·en [ˈstreŋθn, -ŋkθn] **I** *vt* stark machen, (ver-)stärken; verbessern; Kraft geben, kräftigen; festigen. **II** *vi* s. verstärken, stark *od.* stärker werden, erstarken.
strength·en·er [ˈstreŋθnər, -ŋkθ-] *n* Stärkungsmittel *nt.* 2. Verstärkung *f.*
strength·en·ing [ˈstreŋθnɪŋ, -ŋkθ-] **I** *n* 1. Stärkung *f*, Kräftigung *f.* 2. Verstärkung *f.* **II** *adj* 3. stärkend, kräftigend. 4. verstärkend, Verstärkungs-.
strength·less [ˈstreŋθlɪs, -ŋkθ-] *adj* kraftlos, matt; asthenisch.
strength training *physiol.* Kraftraining *nt.*
streph·e·no·po·dia [ˌstrefənəʊˈpəʊdɪə] *n* Sichelfuß *m*, Pes adductus, Metatarsus varus.
streph·ex·o·po·dia [ˌstrefˌeksəʊˈpəʊdɪə] *n* Knickfuß *m*, Pes valgus.
streph·o·po·dia [ˌstrefəˈpəʊdɪə] *n* Spitzfuß *m*, Pes equinus.
streph·o·sym·bo·li·a [ˌ-sɪmˈbəʊlɪə] *n* Strephosymbolie *f.*
strep·i·tus [ˈstrepɪtəs] *n* (Auskultations-)Geräusch *nt*, Strepitus *m.*
strep·si·te·ne [ˈstrepsɔtiːn] *n* Strepsitän *f.*
strepsitene stage → strepsitene.
strept- *pref.* → strepto-.
strep·tam·ine [strepˈtæmɪn] *n* Streptamin *nt.*
strep·ti·ce·mia [ˌstreptəˈsiːmɪə] *n* → streptococcemia.
strepto- *pref.* Strept(o)-.
Strep·to·ba·cil·lus [ˌstreptəʊbəˈsɪləs] *n micro.* Streptobacillus *m.*
strep·to·ba·cil·lus [ˌ-bəˈsɪləs] *n, pl* **-li** [-laɪ] *micro.* Streptobacillus *m.*
strep·to·bi·o·sa·mine [ˌ-baɪˈəʊsəmiːn] *n* Streptobiosamin *f.*
Strep·to·coc·ca·ce·ae [ˌ-kɑˈkeɪsɪiː] *pl micro.* Streptococcaceae *pl.*
strep·to·coc·cal [ˌ-ˈkækl] *adj* Streptokokken betr., durch Streptokokken verursacht, Streptokokken-.
streptococcal antigen Streptokokkenantigen *nt.*
streptococcal bronchitis Streptokokkenbronchitis *f.*
streptococcal carditis Streptokokkenkarditis *f.*
streptococcal deoxyribonuclease → streptodornase.
streptococcal erythrogenic toxin Scharlachtoxin *nt*, erythrogenes Toxin *nt.*

streptococcal fibrinolysin

streptococcal fibrinolysin → streptokinase.
streptococcal gangrene Streptokokkengangrän f, Erysipelas gangraenosum.
streptococcal impetigo Eiter-, Grind-, Krusten-, Pustelflechte f, feuchter Grind m, Impetigo contagiosa/vulgaris.
streptococcal infection Streptokokkeninfektion f, Streptokokkose f.
streptococcal meningitis Streptokokkenmeningitis f.
streptococcal pneumonia Streptokokkenpneumonie f.
streptococcal pyoderma → streptococcal impetigo.
streptococcal tonsillitis Streptokokkenpharyngitis f, -angina f.
streptococcal toxin Streptokokkentoxin nt.
strep·to·coc·ce·mia [ˌ-kɑk'siːmɪə] n Streptokokkensepsis f, Streptokokkämie f.
strep·to·coc·ci pl → streptococcus.
strep·to·coc·cic [ˌ-'kɑk(s)ɪk] adj → streptococcal.
strep·to·coc·col·y·sin [ˌ-kɑ'kɑləsɪn] n → streptolysin.
strep·to·coc·co·sis [ˌ-kɑ'kəʊsɪs] n Streptokokkeninfektion f, Streptokokkose f.
Strep·to·coc·cus [ˌ-'kɑkəs] n micro. Streptococcus m.
S. lacticus/lactis Milchsäurebazillus m, Streptococcus/Bacillus lactis.
S. pneumoniae Fränkel-Pneumokokkus m, Pneumokokkus m, Pneumococcus m, Streptococcus/Diplococcus pneumoniae.
S. pyogenes Streptococcus pyogenes/haemolyticus/erysipelatis, A-Streptokokken pl, Streptokokken pl der Gruppe A.
S. viridans Streptococcus viridans, vergrünende/viridans Streptokokken pl.
strep·to·coc·cus [ˌ-'kɑkəs] n, pl **-ci** [-kaɪ, -kiː, -saɪ, -siː] micro. Streptokokke f, Streptokokkus m, Streptococcus m.
group A s.ci A-Streptokokken pl, Streptokokken pl der Gruppe A, Streptococcus pyogenes/haemolyticus/erysipelatis.
group N s.ci N-Streptokokken pl, Streptokokken pl der Gruppe N.
nonenterococcal group D s.ci Nichtenterokokken pl der Gruppe D.
strep·to·der·ma [ˌ-'dɜrmə] n Streptodermie f, -dermia f.
strep·to·dor·nase [ˌ-'dɔːrneɪs] n abbr. **SD** Streptodornase f, Streptokokken-Desoxyribonuclease f.
streptodornase-streptokinase n → streptokinase-streptodornase.
strep·to·gen·in [ˌ-'dʒenɪn] n Streptogenin nt.
strep·to·he·mol·y·sin [ˌ-hɪ'mɑləsɪn] n → streptolysin.
strep·to·ki·nase [ˌ-'kaɪneɪz, -'kɪ-] n abbr. **SK** Streptokinase f.
streptokinase-streptodornase n abbr. **SKSD** Streptokinase-Streptodornase f.
strep·tol·y·sin [strep'tɑləsɪn] n Streptolysin nt abbr. **SL**.
streptolysin O Streptolysin O nt abbr. **SLO**.
streptolysin S Streptolysin S nt abbr. **SLS**.
Strep·to·my·ces [ˌstreptə'maɪsiːz] n micro. Streptomyces m.
Strep·to·my·ce·ta·ce·ae [ˌ-ˌmaɪsə'teɪsiːˌ] pl micro. Streptomycetaceae pl.
strep·to·my·cete [ˌ-'maɪsiːt] n micro. Streptomyzet m.
strep·to·my·cin [ˌ-'maɪsn] n pharm. Streptomycin nt.
strep·to·my·co·sis [ˌ-maɪ'kəʊsɪs] n Streptomyces-Infektion f, Streptomykose f.

strep·to·sep·ti·ce·mia [ˌ-ˌseptɪ'siːmɪə] n Streptokokkensepsis f.
Strep·to·spo·ran·gi·um [ˌ-spə'rændʒɪəm] n micro. Streptosporangium nt.
strep·to·thri·cho·sis [ˌ-θraɪ'kəʊsɪs] n → streptotrichosis.
strep·to·thri·co·sis [ˌ-θraɪ'kəʊsɪs] n → streptotrichosis.
Strep·to·thrix ['-θrɪks] n micro. Streptothrix f.
strep·to·tri·chi·a·sis [ˌ-traɪ'kaɪəsɪs] n → streptotrichosis.
strep·to·tri·cho·sis [ˌ-traɪ'kəʊsɪs] n **1.** Streptotrichose f. **2.** old → actinomycosis.
stress [stres] **I** n **1.** fig. (seelische) Belastung f, Anspannung f, Druck m, Streß m, Überlastung f. **2.** phys., techn. Beanspruchung f, Belastung f. **3.** Betonung f, Ton m; Akzent m. **II** vt **4.** fig. (seelisch) belasten, stressen, überlasten. **5.** phys., techn. beanspruchen, belasten. **6.** betonen.
stress alopecia streßbedingte Alopezie f, Alopecia neurotica.
stress diabetes streßbedingte Hyperglykämie f, Streßdiabetes m.
stress disease Streß-, Managerkrankheit f.
stress erosions (Magen) Streßerosionen pl.
stress erythrocytosis Gaisböck-Syndrom nt, Polycythaemia (rubra) hypertonica.
stress fracture Ermüdungs-, Streßfraktur f, -bruch m.
stress incontinence Stressinkontinenz f.
stres·sor ['stresər] n Streßfaktor m, Stressor m.
stress polycythemia → stress erythrocytosis.
stress reaction Streßreaktion f.
stress relaxation physiol. Streßrelaxation f, delayed-Compliance f.
reverse s. reverse Streßrelaxation.
stress syndrome Streß-Syndrom nt.
stress test Belastungstest m.
stress ulcer/ulceration Streßulkus nt.
stretch [stretʃ] **I** n **1.** (Aus-)Dehnen nt, Strecken nt. **to give o.s. a ~ s.** (aus-)strecken, s. dehnen, s. recken. **2.** Dehnbarkeit f, Elastizität f. **3.** Anspannung f, (Über-)Anstrengung f, Strapazierung f. **4.** Zeitraum m, -spanne f; Strecke f, Stück m. **II** adj dehnbar, Stretch-. **III** vt **5.** (aus-)strecken, recken. **to ~ o.s. out** s. (aus-)strecken, s. dehnen, s. recken. **6.** spannen (over über); straffziehen; (aus-)weiten, strecken, (über-)aus-)dehnen. **7.** (Nerven, Muskeln) anspannen. **IV** vi s. (aus-)strecken, s. dehnen, s. recken.
stretch·er ['stretʃər] n (Trag-)Bahre f, (Kranken-)Trage f.
stretcher case nicht gehfähiger Patient.
stretch marks Schwangerschaftsstreifen pl, Stria gravidarum.
stretch properties Elastizität f, Dehnungseigenschaften pl.
stretch receptor Dehnungsrezeptor m.
stretch reflex Muskeldehnungsreflex m.
monosynaptic s. monosynaptischer Dehnungsreflex, Eigenreflex.
stretch-sensitive adj dehnungsempfindlich.
stretch·y ['stretʃɪ] adj dehnbar, elastisch.
stri·a ['straɪə] n, pl **stri·ae** ['straɪˌiː] **1.** anat. Streifen m, schmale bandförmige Struktur f, Stria f. **2.** Streifen m, Linie f, Furche f.
s. of Amici Z-Linie f, Z-Streifen m, Zwischenscheibe f, Telophragma nt.
s. of external granular layer Tangentialfa-

serschicht f der äußeren Körnerschicht, Stria laminae granularis externa (corticis cerebri).
s. of ganglionic pyramidal layer → s. of internal pyramidal layer.
s. of Gennari Gennari'-Streifen f.
s. of internal granular layer äußerer Baillarger'-Streifen, Stria laminae granularis interna (corticis cerebri).
s. of internal pyramidal layer innere Baillarger'-Schicht f, Stria laminae pyramidalis ganglionaris/interna (corticis cerebri).
s. of molecular layer Tangentialfaserschicht f der Molekularschicht, Stria laminae molecularis/plexiformis (corticis cerebri).
s. of plexiform layer → s. of molecular layer.
s.e of Zahn Zahn'-Linien pl.
stri·al type of presbyacusis ['straɪəl] HNO Stria-Typ m der Presbyakusis.
stri·a·tal [straɪ'eɪtl] adj Corpus striatum betr., striatal.
stri·ate [adj 'straɪt, -eɪt; v -eɪt] **I** adj → striated. **II** vt streifen, furchen.
striate area primäre Sehrinde f, Area striata.
striate arteries Aa. centrales/thalamostriatae anteromediales.
lateral s. Rami laterales aa. centralium anterolateralium.
medial s. Rami mediales aa. centralium anterolateralium.
striate body Streifenhügel m, Striatum nt, Corpus striatum.
striate cortex → striate area.
stri·at·ed ['straɪeɪtɪd] adj gestreift, streifig, streifenförmig, striär.
striated border histol. Bürstensaum m, Kutikulasaum m.
striated membrane 1. Eihülle f, Oolemma nt, Zona/Membrana pellucida. **2.** bio. Area pellucida.
striated muscle quergestreifter unwillkürlicher Muskel m, quergestreifte unwillkürliche Muskulatur f.
striate veins Vv. thalamostriatae inferiores.
stri·a·tion [straɪ'eɪʃn] n **1.** Streifen m/pl, Furche f; Streifenbildung f, Furchung f. **2.** (Muskel) (Quer-)Streifung f.
stri·a·to·ni·gral [ˌstraɪətəʊ'naɪgrəl] adj Corpus striatum u. Substantia nigra betr., strionigral.
stri·a·tum [straɪ'eɪtəm] n, pl **-ta** [-tə] Striatum nt, Corpus striatum.
strict [strɪkt] adj strikt, streng; genau, exakt, präzise.
strict aerobe micro. obligater Aerobier m.
strict anaerobe micro. obligater Anaerobier m.
stric·ture ['strɪktʃər] n (hochgradige) Verengung f, Striktur f, Strictum f.
stric·tured ['strɪktʃərd] adj verengt, strikturiert.
stric·tur·ot·o·my [ˌstrɪktʃə'rɑtəmɪ] n chir. Strikturotomie f.
stri·dent ['straɪdnt] adj **1.** schrill, durchdringend, schneidend, grell. **2.** knirschend, knarrend.
stri·dor ['straɪdər] n Stridor m.
strid·u·lous ['strɪdʒələs] adj **1.** in Form eines Stridors, stridorös, stridulös. **2.** → strident.
strin·gent ['strɪndʒənt] adj zwingend, stringent; streng, hart.
stringent control stringente Kontrolle f, stringent control (f).
string sign [strɪŋ] radiol. Kantor'-Zeichen nt, String sign (nt).

stri·o·cer·e·bel·lar [ˌstraɪəˌserə'belər] *adj* Corpus striatum u. Kleinhirn/Cerebellum betr., striozerebellär.
stri·o·mo·tor [ˌ-'məʊtər] *adj* Skelettmuskulatur betr. *od.* versorgend.
stri·o·mus·cu·lar [ˌ-'mʌskjələr] *adj* quergestreifte Muskulatur betr.
stri·o·ni·gral [ˌ-'naɪgrəl] *adj* → striatonigral.
strionigral fasciculus Fasciculus strionigralis.
strionigral fibers strionigräre Fasern *pl*, Fibrae strionigrales.
strionigral tract Tractus strionigrales.
stri·o·pal·li·dal [ˌ-'pælɪdl] *adj* Corpus striatum u. Globus pallidus betr., striopallidär, pallidostriär.
stri·o·some ['straɪəsəʊm] *n* Striosom *nt*.
strip [strɪp] **I** *n* schmaler Streifen *m*, Strip *m*. **II** *vt chir.* (*Vene*) strippen. **III** *vi* → strip off 2.
strip off I *vt* abziehen, abstreifen, abschälen, schälen, abkratzen. **II** *vi* **1.** s. ausziehen, s. freimachen. **2.** s. schälen, s. abschälen, s. lösen; s. lockern.
stripe [straɪp] *n* Streifen *m*, Strich *m*, Strieme(n *m*) *f*.
s. of Gennari Gennari'-Streifen.
s.s of Retzius Retzius'-Streifung *f*.
striped [straɪp(ɪ)t] *adj* streifig, gestreift.
striped muscle → striated muscle.
strip·per ['strɪpər] *n chir.* (Venen-)Stripper *m*.
stripper's asthma 1. Baumwollfieber *nt*, Baumwoll(staub)pneumokoniose *f*, Byssinose *f*. **2.** Asthma *nt* bei Byssinose.
strip·ping ['strɪpɪŋ] *n chir.* (Venen-)Stripping *nt*.
stro·bi·la [strəʊ'baɪlə] *n*, *pl* **-lae** [-liː] *micro.* Strobila *f*.
stro·bile ['strəʊbaɪl, -bɪl, 'strə-] *n* → strobila.
Strob·i·lo·cer·cus [ˌstrabɪləʊ'sɜrkəs] *n micro.* Strobilocercus *m*.
stro·bo·scope ['strəʊbəskəʊp] *n* Stroboskop *nt*.
stro·bo·scop·ic [ˌ-'skapɪk] *adj* Stroboskop betr., mittels Stroboskop, stroboskopisch.
stro·bos·co·py [strə'baskəpɪ] *n* Stroboskopie *f*.
stroke [strəʊk] *n* **1.** Schlag *m*, Stoß *m*, Hieb *m*. **2.** (Herz-)Schlag *m*. **3.** → stroke syndrome.
stroke output → stroke volumen.
stroke syndrome Gehirn-, Hirnschlag *m*, Schlaganfall *m*, apoplektischer Insult *m*, Apoplexie *f*, Apoplexia cerebri.
stroke volume *abbr.* **SV** *card.* (*Herz*) Schlagvolumen *nt*, SV.
stro·ma ['strəʊmə] *n*, *pl* **-ma·ta** [-mətə] **1.** *anat.* (Stütz-)Gerüst *nt* eines Organs, Stroma *nt*. **2.** *hema.* Erythrozytenstroma *nt*. **3.** *patho.* Tumorstroma *nt*.
s. of iris Irisgrundgerüst, -stroma, Stroma iridis.
s. of ovary Eierstock-, Ovarialstroma, Stroma ovarii.
s. of thyroid (gland) Schilddrüsenstroma, Stroma gl. thyroideae.
stroma cells Stromazellen *pl*.
stro·mal ['strəʊməl] *adj* Stroma betr., stromal, Stroma-.
stromal adenomyosis → stromatosis.
stromal endometriosis *gyn.* Stromaendometriose *f*, Stromatose *f*.
stromal invasion *patho.* Stromainfiltration *f*.
stro·mat·ic [strəʊ'mætɪk] *adj* → stromal.
stro·ma·tog·e·nous [ˌstrəʊmə'tadʒənəs] *adj* vom Stroma abstammend, stromatogen.
stro·ma·tol·y·sis [ˌ-'talɪsɪs] *n* Stromaauflösung *f*, Stromatolyse *f*.
stro·ma·to·sis [ˌ-'təʊsɪs] *n gyn.* Stromatose *f*, Stromaendometriose *f*.
stro·ma·tous ['-təs] *adj* → stromal.
Strong [strɑŋ]: **S.'s bacillus** → Shigella flexneri.
strong [strɑŋ] *adj* stark, kräftig, scharf (riechend *od.* schmeckend); stabil, solid(e); (*Gesundheit*) kräftig; (*Herz, Nerven*) gut.
strong interaction starke Wechselwirkung *f*.
strong pulse starker/hoher Puls *m*, Pulsus magnus.
stron·gy·li·a·sis [ˌstrɑndʒə'laɪəsɪs] *n* → strongylosis.
stron·gy·lid ['-lɪd] *micro.* **I** *n* → strongylus. **II** *adj* Strongylidae betr.
Stron·gyl·i·dae [strɑn'dʒɪlədiː] *pl micro.* Strongylidae *pl*.
Stron·gy·loi·dea [ˌstrɑndʒə'lɔɪdɪə] *pl micro.* Strongyloidea *pl*.
Stron·gy·loi·des [ˌ-'lɔɪdiːz] *n micro.* Fadenwurm *m*, Strongyloides *m*.
S. intestinalis → S. stercoralis.
S. stercoralis Zwergfadenwurm *m*, Kotälchen *nt*, Strongyloides stercoralis, Anguillula stercoralis.
stron·gy·loi·di·a·sis [ˌ-lɔɪ'daɪəsɪs] *n* Strongyloides-Infektion *f*, Strongyloidiasis *f*, Strongyloidosis *f*.
stron·gy·loi·do·sis [ˌ-lɔɪ'dəʊsɪs] *n* → strongyloidiasis.
stron·gy·lo·sis [ˌ-'ləʊsɪs] *n* Strongylus-Infektion *f*, Strongylosis *f*.
Stron·gy·lus ['-ləs] *n micro.* Strongylus *m*.
S. equinus Palisadenwurm *m*, Strongylus equinus.
S. gigas Nierenwurm *m*, Riesenpalisadenwurm *m*, Eustrongylus gigas, Dioctophyma renale.
S. renalis → S. gigas.
stron·gy·lus ['-ləs] *n micro.* Palisadenwurm *m*, Strongylus *m*.
stron·tia ['strɑnʃ(ɪ)ə] *n* Strontiumoxid *nt*.
stron·ti·um ['strɑnʃ(ɪ)əm] *n abbr.* **Sr** Strontium *nt abbr.* Sr.
stron·ti·u·re·sis [ˌstrɑntʃəjə'riːsɪs] *n* Strontiumausscheidung *f* im Harn, Strontiurese *f*.
stro·phan·thi·din [strə'fænθədɪn] *n* Strophanthidin *nt*.
stro·phan·thin [strəʊ'fænθɪn] *n pharm.* k-Strophanthin *nt*.
strophanthin-G *n pharm.* Ouabain *nt*, g-Strophanthin *nt*.
strophanthin-K *n* → strophanthin.
stroph·o·ceph·a·lus [ˌstrafə'sefələs] *n embryo.* Strophozephalus *m*.
stroph·o·ceph·a·ly [ˌ-'sefəlɪ] *n embryo.* Strophozephalie *f*.
stroph·u·lus ['strafjələs] *n*, *pl* **-li** [-laɪ] Urticaria papulosa chronica, Prurigo simplex subacuta, Prurigo simplex acuta et subacuta adultorum, Strophulos adultorum, Lichen urticatus.
struc·tur·al ['strʌktʃərəl] *adj* Struktur betr., strukturell, baulich, Bau-, Struktur-; morphologisch, Form-.
structural analogue Strukturanaloges *nt*.
structural curve *ortho.* (*Skoliose*) strukturelle Krümmung *f*.
structural engram strukturelles Engramm *nt*.
structural fat Struktur-, Baufett *nt*.
structural formula *chem.* Strukturformel *f*.
structural gene Strukturgen *nt*.
structural isomerism *chem.* Konstitutions-, Strukturisomerie *f*.
structural lesion strukturelle Schädigung *f*.
structural metabolism Struktur-, Baustoffwechsel *m*.
structural metamorphosis visköse Metamorphose *f*.
structural myopathy Strukturmyopathie *f*.
structural protein Strukturprotein *nt*.
structural psychology Strukturpsychologie *f*.
structural scoliosis *ortho.* strukturelle Skoliose *f*.
struc·ture ['strʌktʃər] **I** *n* Struktur *f*, (Auf-)Bau *m*, Gefüge *nt*. **II** *vt* strukturieren, aufbauen, gliedern.
β-structure *n biochem.* Faltblatt(struktur *f*) *nt*.
struc·ture·less ['strʌktʃərlɪs] *adj* strukturlos.
stru·ma ['struːmə] *n*, *pl* **-mae** [-miː, -maɪ] Kropf *m*, Struma *f*.
stru·mec·to·my [struː'mektəmɪ] *n chir.* Strumaresektion *f*, Strumektomie *f*.
stru·mi·form ['struːməfɔːrm] *adj* strumaähnlich, -förmig.
stru·mi·tis [struː'maɪtɪs] *n* **1.** Kropfentzündung *f*, Strumitis *f*. **2.** Schilddrüsenentzündung *f*, Thyr(e)oiditis *f*.
stru·mous abscess ['struːməs] tuberkulöser Abszeß *m*.
strumous ophthalmia Conjunctivitis/Keratitis/Keratoconjunctivitis eccematosa/eczematosa/scrufulosa/phlyctaenulosa.
Strümpell ['strɪmpəl; 'trympəl]: **S.'s disease 1.** Bechterew-Krankheit *f*, Morbus Bechterew *m*, Bechterew-Strümpell-Marie-Krankheit *f*, Marie-Strümpell-Krankheit *f*, Spondylarthritis/Spondylitis ankylopoetica/ankylosans. **2.** Strümpell-Krankheit *f*.
S.'s phenomenon → S.'s sign.
S.'s sign (von) Strümpell-Tibialiszeichen *nt*.
Strümpell-Leichtenstern ['laɪktənstɜrn; 'laɪçtənʃtɛrn]: **S.-L. disease** hämorrhagische Enzephalitis *f*, Encephalitis haemorrhagica.
S.-L. type of encephalitis → S.-L. disease.
Strümpell-Marie [ma'riː]: **S.-M. disease** Bechterew-Krankheit *f*, Bechterew-Strümpell-Marie-Krankheit *f*, Morbus Bechterew *m*, Marie-Strümpell-Krankheit *f*, Spondylarthritis/Spondylitis ankylopoetica/ankylosans.
Strümpell-Westphal ['vɛstfaːl]: **S.-W. disease/pseudosclerosis** Westphal-Strümpell-Syndrom *nt*, -Pseudosklerose *f*.
stru·vite ['struːvaɪt] *n* Tripelphosphat *nt*, Magnesium-Ammonium-phosphat *nt*.
struvite calculus/stone Tripelphosphatstein *m*, Magnesium-Ammonium-phosphat-Stein *m*.
strych·nine ['strɪknɪn, -niːn, -naɪn] *n* Strychnin *nt*.
strychnine poisoining → strychninism.
strych·nin·ism ['strɪknɪnɪzəm] *n* Strychninvergiftung *f*, Strychninismus *m*.
strych·nism ['strɪknɪzəm] *n* → strychninism.
STS *abbr.* → serologic tests for syphilis.
ST segment *physiol.* (*EKG*) ST-Strecke *f*, ST-Segment *nt*.
Stuart ['st(j)uːərt]: **S. factor** → Stuart-Prower factor.
Stuart-Prower ['praʊər]: **S.-P. factor** Faktor X *m abbr.* F X, Stuart-Prower-Faktor *m*, Autothrombin III *nt*.
stub fingers [stʌb] Stummelfingrigkeit *f*, Perodaktylie *f*.
stuck finger [stʌk] schnellender/schnappender/federnder Finger *m*, Trigger-Finger *m*.
Student ['st(j)uːdnt]: **S.'s t-test** *stat.* Student-Test *m*, t-Test *m*.

stu·dent nurse ['st(j)u:dnt] Schwesternschülerin f.
stud·y ['stʌdɪ] **I** n, pl **stud·ies 1.** Studieren nt. **2.** (wissenschaftliches) Studium nt. **3.** Studie f, Untersuchung f (of, in über). **4.** Studienfach nt, -objekt nt, Studium nt. **5.** Studier-, Arbeitszimmer nt. **II** vt studieren; untersuchen, prüfen. **III** vi studieren; lernen.
stump [stʌmp] n **1.** chir. (Amputations-)Stumpf m. **2.** Stumpf m, Stummel m.
stump cancer chir. (*Magen*) Stumpfkarzinom nt.
stump contracture chir. Stumpfkontraktur f.
stump edema Stumpfödem nt.
stump hallucination neuro. Phantomglied nt.
stump neuralgia Stumpfneuralgie f.
stump pain Stumpfschmerz m.
stun [stʌn] vt betäuben.
stupe [st(j)u:p] **I** n Umschlag m, Wickel m. **II** vt Umschläge/Wickel machen.
stu·pe·fa·cient [,st(j)u:pə'feɪʃnt] **I** n Betäubungsmittel nt. **II** adj betäubend, abstumpfend.
stu·pe·fac·tion [,-'fækʃn] n Betäubung f, Abstumpfung f.
stu·pe·fac·tive [,-'fæktɪv] adj betäubend, abstumpfend.
stu·pid ['st(j)u:pɪd] adj **1.** dumm, stupid(e); stumpfsinnig. **2.** benommen, betäubt.
stu·por ['st(j)u:pər] n neuro. Stupor m.
stu·por·ous ['st(j)u:pərəs] adj Stupor betr., von ihm gekennzeichnet, stuporös.
stur·dy ['stɜrdɪ] adj robust, kräftig, stabil.
Sturge [stɜrdʒ]: **S.'s disease/syndrome** → Sturge-Weber disease.
Sturge-Kalischer-Weber ['kælɪʃər 'webər; 'ka:li-]: **S.-K.-W. syndrome** → Sturge-Weber disease.
Sturge-Weber: S.-W. disease Sturge-Weber(-Krabbe)-Krankheit f, -Syndrom nt, enzephalofaziale Angiomatose f, Neuroangiomatosis encephalofacialis, Angiomatosis encephalo-oculo-cutanea, Angiomatosis encephalotrigeminalis. **S.-W. syndrome** → S.-W. disease.
Sturmdorf ['stɜrmdɔ:rf; 'stʊrm-, ʃtʊrm-]: **S.'s operation** gyn. Sturmdorf-Operation f, Koniotomie f.
stut·ter ['stʌtər] **I** n Stottern nt, Balbuties f, Dysphemie f, Dysarthria/Anarthria syllabaris, Psellismus m, Ichnophonie f. **II** vt, vi stottern.
stut·ter·er ['stʌtərər] n Stotterer m, Stotterin f.
stut·ter·ing ['stʌtərɪŋ] **I** n → stutter I. **II** adj stotternd; stammelnd.
Stuttgart disease ['stʌtgart; 'ʃtʊtga:rt] Stuttgarter-Hundeseuche f, Leptospirosis canicola.
St. Vitus [seɪnt 'vaɪtəs; sɛ̃]: **St. V.' dance** → Sydenham's chorea.
sty [staɪ] n, pl **sties** → stye.
stye [staɪ] n, pl **styes** ophthal. **1.** Gerstenkorn nt, Zilienabszeß m, Hordeolum nt. **2.** Hordeolum externum.
style [staɪl] n → stylet.
sty·let ['staɪlɪt] n **1.** chir. Stilett nt. **2.** (kleine) Sonde f, Mandrin m, Sondenführer m.
sty·lette n → stylet.
sty·li·form ['staɪləfɔ:rm] adj → styloid.
sty·lo·glos·sus (muscle) [,staɪləʊ'glɒsəs, -'glɔs-] Styloglossus m, M. styloglossus.
sty·lo·hy·al [,-'haɪəl] adj → stylohyoid.
sty·lo·hy·oid [,-'haɪɔɪd] adj Proc. styloideus u. Zungenbein betr., stylohyoid.
stylohyoid branch of facial nerve Fazialisast m zum M. stylohyoideus, Ramus stylohyoideus n. facialis.

sty·lo·hy·oi·de·us (muscle) [,-haɪ'ɔɪdɪəs] Stylohyoideus m, M. stylohyoideus.
stylohyoid ligament Lig. stylohyoideum.
stylohyoid muscle → stylohyoideus (muscle).
stylohyoid nerve → stylohyoid branch of facial nerve.
sty·loid ['staɪlɔɪd] adj griffelförmig, styloid.
sty·loi·di·tis [,staɪlɔɪ'daɪtɪs] n Entzündung f des Proc. styloideus, Styloiditis f.
styloid process Griffelfortsatz m, Proc. styloideus.
s. of radius Griffelfortsatz des Radius, Proc. styloideus radii.
s. of temporal bone Proc. styloideus ossis temporalis.
s. of ulna Griffelfortsatz der Ulna, Proc. styloideus ulnae.
styloid prominence Prominentia styloidea.
sty·lo·man·dib·u·lar [,staɪləʊmæn'dɪbjələr] adj Proc. styloideus u. Unterkiefer/Mandibula betr., stylomandibulär.
stylomandibular ligament Lig. stylomandibulare.
sty·lo·mas·toid artery [,-'mæstɔɪd] A. stylomastoidea.
stylomastoid foramen For. stylomastoideum.
stylomastoid vein V. stylomastoidea.
sty·lo·max·il·lar·y [,-'mæksə,leri:, -mæk'sɪlərɪ] adj Proc. styloideus u. Oberkiefer/Maxilla betr., stylomaxillär.
stylomaxillary ligament → stylomandibular ligament.
sty·lo·my·lo·hy·oid ligament [,-,maɪlə'haɪɔɪd] → stylomandibular ligament.
sty·lo·pha·ryn·ge·al branch of glossopharyngeal nerve [,-fə'rɪndʒ(ɪ)əl] Ramus m. stylopharyngei n. glossopharyngei.
stylopharyngeal nerve → stylopharyngeal branch of glossopharyngeal nerve.
sty·lo·pha·ryn·ge·us (muscle) [,-fə'rɪndʒɪəs] Stylopharyngeus m, M. stylopharyngeus.
sty·lo·ra·di·al reflex [,-'reɪdɪəl] Radius-, Radiusperiostreflex m abbr. RPR.
sty·lus ['staɪləs] n, pl **-li** [-laɪ] **1.** → stylet. **2.** pharm. Stift m, Stylus m.
S-type n micro. (*Kolonie*) S-Form f.
stype [staɪp] n Tampon m.
styp·sis ['stɪpsɪs] n **1.** Blutstillung f, Stypsis f. **2.** Behandlung f mit einem Styptikum.
styp·tic ['stɪptɪk] **I** n **1.** blutstillendes Mittel nt, (Hämo-)Styptikum nt. **2.** Adstringens nt. **II** adj **3.** blutstillend, (hämo-)styptisch. **4.** zusammenziehend, adstringierend.
sty·rene ['staɪri:n] n Styrol nt, Vinylbenzol nt.
sty·rol ['staɪrɒl] n → styrene.
sty·ro·lene ['staɪrəli:n] n → styrene.
sub- prefix Unter-; Infra-.
sub·ab·dom·i·nal [,sʌbæb'dɒmɪnl] adj unterhalb des Abdomens (liegend), subabdominal.
sub·ab·dom·i·no·per·i·to·ne·al [,sʌbæb,dɒmɪnəʊ,perɪtəʊ'nɪəl] adj → subperitoneal.
sub·ac·e·tab·u·lar [sʌb,æsɪ'tæbjələr] adj unterhalb des Acetabulums (liegend), subazetabulär, -azetabulär.
sub·ac·e·tate [sʌb'æsɪteɪt] n basisches Acetat nt.
sub·a·chil·le·al bursa [sʌbə'kɪlɪəl] Bursa tendinis calcanei (Achillis).
sub·ac·id [sʌb'æsɪd] adj schwach sauer, subazid.
sub·a·cid·i·ty [,sʌbə'sɪdətɪ] n verminderter Säuregehalt m, Subazidität f.
sub·a·cro·mi·al [,sʌbə'krəʊmɪəl] adj unter dem Akromion (liegend), subakromial.

subacromial bursa Bursa subacromialis.
subacromial bursitis Bursitis/Tendinitis scapulohumeralis.
sub·a·cute [,sʌbə'kju:t] adj subakut.
subacute bacterial endocarditis subakute-bakterielle Endokarditis f, Endocarditis lenta.
subacute combined degeneration of the spinal cord Lichtheim-Syndrom nt, Dana-Lichtheim-Krankheit f, Dana-Syndrom nt, Dana-Lichtheim-Putnam-Syndrom nt, funikuläre Spinalerkrankung/Myelose f.
subacute glomerulonephritis subakute/perakute Glomerulonephritis f.
subacute granulomatous thyroiditis de Quervain-Thyreoiditis f, subakute nichteitrige Thyreoiditis f, granulomatöse Thyreoiditis f, Riesenzellthyreoiditis f.
subacute hepatic necrosis subakute Leberatrophie f.
subacute hepatitis chronisch-aktive/chronisch-aggressive Hepatitis f abbr. CAH.
subacute inclusion body encephalitis subakute sklerosierende Panenzephalitis f abbr. SSPE, Einschlußkörperenzephalitis f Dawson, subakute sklerosierende Leukenzephalitis f van Bogaert.
subacute infectious endocarditis → subacute bacterial endocarditis.
subacute inflammation subakute Entzündung f.
subacute inguinal poradenitis Morbus Durand-Nicolas-Favre m, klimatischer Bubo m, vierte Geschlechtskrankheit f, Poradenitis inguinalis, Lymphopathia venerea, Lymphogranuloma inguinale/venereum abbr. LGV.
subacute myelo-opticoneuropathy abbr. SMON subakute Myelooptikoneuropathie f abbr. SMON, subakute myelooptische Neuropathie f.
subacute necrotizing encephalomyelopathy Leigh-Syndrom nt, -Enzephalomyelopathie f, nekrotisierende Enzephalomyelopathie f.
subacute necrotizing encephalopathy → subacute necrotizing encephalomyelopathy.
subacute necrotizing myelitis Foix-Alajouanine-Syndrom nt, subakute nekrotisierende Myelitis f, Myelitis necroticans.
subacute nephritis → subacute glomerulonephritis.
subacute pain subakuter Schmerz m.
subacute red atrophy subakute rote Leberdystrophie/-atrophie f.
subacute sclerosing leukoencephalitis → subacute inclusion body encephalitis.
subacute sclerosing leukoencephalopathy → subacute inclusion body encephalitis.
subacute sclerosing panencephalitis abbr. SSPE → subacute inclusion body encephalitis.
subacute spongiform (virus) encephalopathy subakute spongiforme (Virus-)Enzephalopathie f.
sub·al·i·men·ta·tion [sʌb,ælɪmen'teɪʃn] n Mangelernährung f, Hypoalimentation f.
sub·a·nal [sʌb'eɪnl] adj unterhalb des Anus (liegend), subanal.
sub·aor·tic stenosis [sʌbeɪ'ɔ:rtɪk] infravalvuläre/subvalvuläre Aortenstenose f.
sub·ap·i·cal [sʌb'æpɪkl] adj unterhalb eines Apex (liegend), subapikal.
sub·ap·o·neu·rot·ic [sʌb,æpənjəʊ'rɒtɪk] adj unterhalb einer Aponeurose (liegend), subaponeurotisch, subfaszial.

subaponeurotic abscess subfaszialer Abszeß m.
sub·a·rach·noid [ˌsʌbəˈræknɔɪd] adj unter der Arachnoidea (liegend), subarachnoidal, Subarachnoidal-.
sub·ar·ach·noi·dal [sʌbˌæræk'nɔɪdl] adj → subarachnoid.
subarachnoidal cisterns Subarachnoidalzisternen pl, -liquorräume pl, Cisternae subarachnoideae.
subarachnoidal sinuses → subarachnoidal cisterns.
subarachnoidal space Subarachnoidalraum m, -spalt m, Spatium subarachnoideum.
subarachnoid anesthesia → subarachnoid block.
subarachnoid bleeding Subarachnoidalblutung f abbr. SAB.
subarachnoid block Spinalanästhesie f, inf. Spinale f.
subarachnoid cavity → subarachnoidal space.
subarachnoid cisterns → subarachnoidal cisterns.
subarachnoid hemorrhage → subarachnoid bleeding.
subarachnoid space → subarachnoidal space.
sub·ar·cu·ate [sʌb'ɑːrkjʊɪt, -jəwət, -weɪt] adj gebogen, gewölbt; unter einem Bogen od. Gewölbe (liegend).
subarcuate fossa of temporal bone Fossa subarcuata (ossis temporalis).
sub·a·re·o·lar [ˌsʌbəˈrɪələr] adj unter der Areola (liegend), subareolär, subareolar.
subareolar abscess subareolärer Abszeß m.
sub·ar·te·ri·al canal [sʌbɑːr'tɪərɪəl] Schenkel-, Adduktorenkanal m, Canalis adductorius.
sub·as·trag·a·lar [ˌsʌbæ'strægələr] adj unterhalb des Talus (liegend), subtalar.
subastragalar amputation ortho. Fußamputation f nach Malgaigne, Malgaigne'-Amputation f.
sub·a·tom·ic [ˌsʌbə'tɑmɪk] adj subatomar.
sub·au·ral [sʌb'ɔːrəl] adj unterhalb des Ohres (liegend), subaural.
sub·au·ric·u·lar [sʌb'ɔː'rɪkjələr] adj unter dem Ohrläppchen (liegend), subaurikulär.
sub·ax·i·al [sʌb'æksɪəl] adj unterhalb einer Achse (liegend), subaxial.
sub·ax·il·lar·y [sʌb'æksəˌlerɪ, -æk'sɪlərɪ] adj unterhalb der Achselhöhle (liegend), subaxillär.
sub·ba·sal [sʌb'beɪsl] adj unterhalb einer Basis (liegend), subbasal.
sub·cal·ca·ne·al [ˌsʌbkæl'keɪnɪəl] adj unterhalb des Fersenbeins/Kalkaneus (liegend), subkalkaneal.
subcalcaneal bursa Bursa subcutanea calcanea.
sub·cal·ca·rine [sʌb'kælkəraɪn] adj unterhalb der Fissura calcarina (liegend).
sub·cal·lo·sal fasciculus [ˌsʌbkæ'ləʊsl, -kə-] Fasciculus subcallosus.
subcallosal gyrus Gyrus paraterminalis/subcallosus.
sub·cap·i·tal [sʌb'kæpɪtl] adj unterhalb eines Gelenkkopfes (liegend), subkapital.
subcapital fracture subkapitale Fraktur f.
s. of humerus subkapitale Humerusfraktur.
sub·cap·su·lar [sʌb'kæpsələr] adj unter einer Kapsel (liegend), subkapsulär.
subcapsular cataract ophthal. subkapsuläre Katarakt f.
subcapsular epithelium 1. Linsenepithel nt, Epithelium lentis. **2.** Epithelauskleidung f der Ganglienkapsel, subkapsuläres Epithel nt.
subcapsular sinus Rand-, Marginalsinus m.
sub·car·bon·ate [sʌb'kɑːrbəneɪt, -nɪt] n chem. basisches Karbonat nt.
sub·car·di·nal veins [sʌb'kɑːrdɪnl] embryo. Subkardinalvenen pl.
sub·car·ti·lag·i·nous [sʌbˌkɑːrtə'lædʒɪnəs] adj **1.** unterhalb eines Knorpels (liegend), subchondral, subkartilaginär. **2.** teilweise aus Knorpel bestehend.
sub·chon·dral [sʌb'kɑndrl] adj unter Knorpel (liegend), subchondral.
subchondral bone subchondraler Knochen m.
subchondral cyst (Knochen) Geröll-, Trümmerzyste f.
subchondral fracture of the femoral head idiopathische Hüftkopfnekrose f des Erwachsenen, avaskuläre/ischämische Femurkopfnekrose f.
sub·chor·dal [sʌb'kɔːrdl] adj **1.** unter der Chorda dorsalis (liegend), subchordal. **2.** unterhalb des Stimmbandes/der Chorda vocalis (liegend), subchordal.
sub·cho·ri·on·ic [sʌbˌkɔrɪ'ɑnɪk, -ˌkəʊr-] adj unter(halb) des Chorions (liegend), subchorional, subchorial.
subchorionic space subchorialer Raum m.
subchorionic tuberous hematoma gyn. Breus'-Mole f.
sub·cho·roi·dal [ˌsʌbkə'rɔɪdl] adj unter der Choroidea (liegend).
sub·chron·ic [sʌb'krɑnɪk] adj subchronisch.
sub·cir·cu·la·tion [sʌbˌsɜːrkjə'leɪʃn] n Teil-, Unterkreislauf m.
sub·class ['sʌbklɑːs, -klæs] n bio. Unterklasse f.
sub·cla·vi·an [sʌb'kleɪvɪən] adj unter dem Schlüsselbein/der Klavikula (liegend), subklavikulär.
subclavian artery Subklavia f, A. subclavia.
subclavian artery injury Subklaviaverletzung f, Verletzung f der A. subclavia.
subclavian loop Ansa subclavia.
subclavian nerve N. subclavius.
subclavian plexus vegetatives Geflecht nt der A. subclavia, Plexus subclavius.
subclavian steal → subclavian steal syndrome.
subclavian steal syndrome abbr. SSS Subklavia-Anzapfsyndrom nt, Subclavian-Steal-Syndrom nt.
subclavian sulcus Sulcus a. subclaviae.
subclavian triangle/trigone große Schlüsselbeingrube f, Fossa supraclavicularis major, Trigonum omoclaviculare.
subclavian trunk: left s. Truncus subclavius sinister.
right s. Truncus subclavius dexter.
subclavian vein Subklavia f, V. subclavia.
sub·cla·vic·u·lar [ˌsʌbklə'vɪkjələr] adj subclavian.
sub·cla·vi·us (muscle) [sʌb'kleɪvɪəs] Subklavius m, M. subclavius.
sub·clin·i·cal [sʌb'klɪnɪkl] adj ohne klinische Symptome, subklinisch.
subclinical diabetes old pathologische Glukosetoleranz f.
subclinical infection inapparente Infektion f.
sub·com·mis·sur·al organ [sʌb'kɑməˌʃʊərl] Subkommissuralorgan nt, Organum subcommissurale.
sub·con·junc·ti·val [sʌbˌkɑndʒʌŋk'taɪvl] adj unter der Konjunktiva (liegend), subkonjunktival.
sub·con·junc·ti·vi·tis [sʌbkən,dʒʌŋktɪvaɪtɪs] n chir. Episcleritis periodica fugax.
sub·con·scious [sʌb'kɑnʃəs] **I** n Unterbewußtsein nt, das Unterbewußte. **II** adj unterbewußt; halbbewußt.
sub·con·scious·ness [sʌb'kɑnʃəsnɪs] n Unterbewußtsein nt.
sub·cor·a·coid [sʌb'kɔːrəkɔɪd, -'kɑr-] adj unterhalb des Proc. coracoideus (liegend), subkorakoid.
subcoracoid bursa Bursa m. coracobrachialis.
sub·cor·ne·al [sʌb'kɔːrnɪəl] adj unter der Kornea (liegend), subkorneal.
subcorneal pustular dermatitis/dermatosis Snedden-Wilkinson-Syndrom nt, subkorneale Pustulose f, subkorneale pustulöse Dermatose f, Pustulosis subcornealis.
sub·cor·tex [sʌb'kɔːrteks] n Subkortex m.
sub·cor·ti·cal [sʌb'kɔːrtɪkl] adj unter der Rinde/dem Kortex (liegend), subkortikal.
subcortical aphasia subkortikale Aphasie f.
subcortical arteriosclerotic encephalopathy Binswanger-Enzephalopathie f, subkortikale progressive Enzephalopathie f, Encephalopathia chronica progressiva subcorticalis.
subcortical nuclei subkortikale Kerne pl.
sub·cos·tal [sʌb'kɑstəl, -'kɔs-] adj unter(halb) einer Rippe (liegend), subkostal.
subcostal angle Angulus infrasternalis.
subcostal artery Subkostalis f, A. subcostalis.
subcostal incision Rippenbogenrandschnitt m.
subcostal line Planum subcostale.
subcostal muscles Unterrippenmuskeln pl, Subkostalmuskeln pl, Mm. subcostales.
subcostal nerve Subkostalis m, N. subcostalis.
subcostal plane anat. Subkostalebene f, Planum subcostale.
subcostal vein V. subcostalis.
sub·cra·ni·al [sʌb'kreɪnɪəl] adj unterhalb des Schädels (liegend), subkranial.
sub·cru·ral bursa [sʌb'krʊərəl] → suprapatellar bursa.
sub·cul·ture ['sʌbkʌltʃər] n **1.** micro. Unter-, Nach-, Subkultur f, Abimpfung f. **2.** micro. Abimpfen nt. **3.** socio. Subkultur f.
sub·cu·ne·i·form nucleus [sʌbkjʊ'nɪəfɔːrm] Nc. subcuneiformis (mesencephalicus).
sub·cu·ta·ne·ous [ˌsʌbkjuː'teɪnɪəs] adj unter der Haut (liegend), subkutan, subcutan.
subcutaneous abscess subkutaner Abszeß m.
subcutaneous bursa subkutan liegender Schleimbeutel m, Bursa subcutanea.
s. of lateral malleolus Bursa subcutanea malleoli lateralis.
s. of medial malleolus Bursa subcutanea malleoli medialis.
s. of olecranon Bursa subcutanea olecrani.
s. of prominence of larynx Bursa subcutanea prominentiae laryngealis.
s. of tuberosity of tibia Bursa subcutanea tuberositatis tibiae.
subcutaneous emphysema Hautemphysem nt, Emphysema subcutaneum.
subcutaneous fascia 1. → subcutis. **2.** oberflächliche Unterhautfaszie f, Fascia superficialis.
subcutaneous fat Unterhautfettgewebe nt, Panniculus adiposus.
subcutaneous fracture ortho. einfache/geschlossene/unkomplizierte Fraktur f.

subcutaneous mastectomy gyn. subkutane Mastektomie f.
subcutaneous mycosis subkutane Pilzerkrankung/Mykose f.
subcutaneous part of external sphincter (muscle) of anus Pars subcutanea.
subcutaneous phycomycetosis → subcutaneous phycomycosis.
subcutaneous phycomycosis Basidiobolose f.
subcutaneous pseudosarcomatous fibromatosis nodulöse Fasziitis f, Fasciitis nodularis.
subcutaneous suture Subkutannaht f.
subcutaneous tissue Unterhautbindegewebe nt, Subkutangewebe nt.
sub·cu·tic·u·lar [ˌsʌbkjuːˈtɪkjələr] adj unterhalb der Epidermis (liegend), subepidermal.
subcuticular suture Intrakutannaht f.
sub·cu·tis [sʌbˈkjuːtɪs] n Unterhaut f, Subkutis f, Tela subcutanea.
sub·del·toid [sʌbˈdɛltɔɪd] adj unter dem Deltamuskel (liegend), subdeltoid.
subdeltoid bursa Bursa subdeltoidea.
subdeltoid bursitis 1. Duplay-Bursitis f, Entzündung/Bursitis f der Bursa subdeltoidea. 2. Bursitis/Tendinitis scapulohumeralis.
sub·den·tal [sʌbˈdɛntl] adj unter einem Zahn (liegend), subdental.
sub·di·a·phrag·mat·ic abscess [sʌbˌdaɪəˈfrægmætɪk] → subphrenic abscess.
sub·duce [səbˈdjuːs] vt nach unten ziehen.
sub·duct [səbˈdʌkt] vt → subduce.
sub·du·ral [sʌbˈdjʊərəl] adj unter der Dura mater (liegend), subdural, Subdural-.
subdural abscess subduraler Abszeß m.
subdural bleeding Subduralblutung f.
subdural cavity → subdural space.
subdural empyema subdurales Empyem nt.
subdural hematoma subdurales Hämatom nt, Subduralhämatom nt.
subdural hematorrhachis extradurale/subdurale Hämatorrhachis f, Haematorrhachis externa.
subdural hemorrhage Subduralblutung f.
subdural space Subduralraum m, -spalt m, Spatium subdurale.
sub·en·do·car·di·al [sʌbˌɛndəʊˈkɑːrdɪəl] adj subendokardial.
subendocardial layer Subendokardialschicht f.
subendocardial sclerosis Endokardfibroelastose f, Fibroelastosis endocardii.
subendocardial terminal network Rami subendocardiales.
sub·en·do·the·li·al [sʌbˌɛndəʊˈθiːlɪəl] adj unter dem Endothel (liegend), subendothelial.
subendothelial layer Subendothelialschicht f.
sub·en·dy·mal [sʌbˈɛndɪməl] adj → subependymal.
sub·en·er·get·ic phonation [sʌbˌɛnərˈdʒɛtɪk] HNO Stimmschwäche f, Hypophonie f, Hypophonesie f, Phonasthenie f.
sub·ep·en·dy·mal [ˌsʌbəˈpɛdɪməl] adj unter dem Ependym (liegend), subependymal, subependymär.
sub·ep·i·car·di·al [sʌbˌɛpɪˈkɑːrdɪəl] adj unter dem Epikard (liegend), subepikardial.
subepicardial layer Subepikardialschicht f.
sub·ep·i·der·mal [sʌbˌɛpɪˈdɜrml] adj unter der Epidermis (liegend), subepidermal.
subepidermal abscess subepidermaler Abszeß m.
sub·ep·i·der·mic [sʌbˌɛpɪˈdɜrmɪk] adj → subepidermal.

sub·ep·i·glot·tic [sʌbˌɛpɪˈglɑtɪk] adj unterhalb der Epiglottis (liegend), subepiglottisch.
sub·ep·i·the·li·al [sʌbˌɛpɪˈθiːlɪəl, -jəl] adj unter dem Epithel (liegend), subepithelial.
subepithelial membrane Basalmembran f, -lamina f.
su·ber·o·sis [suːbəˈrəʊsɪs] n Korkstaublunge f, Suberosis f.
sub·fam·i·ly [sʌbˈfæməlɪ] n bio. Unterfamilie f.
sub·fas·cial [sʌbˈfæʃ(ɪ)əl, -ˈfeɪ-] adj unter einer Faszie (liegend), subfaszial.
subfascial abscess subfaszialer Abszeß m.
subfascial bursa subfaszialer Schleimbeutel m, Bursa (synovialis) subfascialis.
sub·feb·rile [sʌbˈfɛbrɪl, -ˈfiː-] adj leicht fieberhaft, subfebril.
sub·fer·tile [sʌbˈfɜrtl, -taɪl] adj subfertil.
sub·fer·til·i·ty [ˌsʌbfərˈtɪlɪtɪ] n verminderte Fruchtbarkeit f, Subfertilität f.
sub·fla·val ligaments [sʌbˈfleɪvl] Ligg. flava.
sub·fla·vous [sʌbˈfleɪvəs] adj gelb.
sub·fo·li·ar [sʌbˈfəʊlɪər] adj → Subfolium betr.
sub·fo·li·um [sʌbˈfəʊlɪəm] n anat. Subfolium nt.
sub·for·ni·cal organ [sʌbˈfɔːrnɪkl] Subfornikalorgan nt, Organum subfornicale.
sub·frac·tion·ate [sʌbˈfrækʃəneɪt] vt subfraktionieren.
sub·fron·tal fissure [sʌbˈfrʌntl] Sulcus frontalis inferior.
sub·ga·le·al [sʌbˈgeɪlɪəl] adj unter der Galea aponeurotica (liegend).
subgaleal abscess Abszeß m unter der Galea aponeurotica.
sub·gem·mal [sʌbˈdʒɛml] adj histol. subgemmal.
sub·ge·nus [sʌbˈdʒiːnəs] n, pl **-gen·er·a** [-ˈdʒɛnərə], **-ge·nus·es** bio. Untergattung f.
sub·ger·mi·nal cavity [sʌbˈdʒɜrmɪnl] embryo. Furchungs-, Keimhöhle f, Blastozöl nt.
sub·gin·gi·val [sʌbˈdʒɪndʒəvəl] adj unter dem Zahnfleisch (liegend), subgingival.
subgingival calculus subgingivaler Zahnstein m.
sub·gle·noid [sʌbˈglɛnɔɪd, -ˈgliː-] adj unterhalb der Fossa glenoidea (liegend).
sub·glos·sal [sʌbˈglɑsəl, -ˈglɔs-] adj → sublingual.
sub·glos·si·tis [ˌsʌbgləˈsaɪtɪs] n Subglossitis f.
sub·glot·tal [sʌbˈglɑtl] adj unterhalb der Glottis (liegend), subglottisch.
subglottal pressure subglottischer Druck m.
sub·glot·tic [sʌbˈglɑtɪk] adj → subglottal.
subglottic laryngitis falscher Krupp m, Pseudokrupp m, subglottische Laryngitis f, Laryngitis subglottica.
subglottic stenosis subglottische Stenose f.
sub·gran·u·lar [sʌbˈgrænjələr] adj subgranulär.
sub·he·pat·ic [ˌsʌbhɪˈpætɪk] adj unterhalb der Leber (liegend), subhepatisch.
subhepatic abscess subhepatischer Abszeß m.
subhepatic recesses subhepatische Peritonealspalten pl, Recc. subhepatici.
sub·hy·a·loid [sʌbˈhaɪəlɔɪd] adj unter der Membrana vitrea (liegend).
sub·hy·oid [sʌbˈhaɪɔɪd] adj unterhalb des Zungenbeins (liegend), subhyoidal.
subhyoid bursa Bursa subcutanea prominentiae laryngealis.

sub·hy·oi·de·an [ˌsʌbhaɪˈɔɪdɪən] adj → subhyoid.
sub·ic·ter·ic [ˌsʌbɪkˈtɛrɪk] adj leicht-ikterisch, subikterisch.
su·bic·u·lar [səˈbɪkjələr] adj Subiculum betr.
su·bic·u·lum [səˈbɪkjələm] n, pl **-la** [-lə] anat. Subiculum nt.
s. of Ammon's horn Subiculum hippocampi, Subiculum cornu ammonis, Gyrus parahippocampalis/hippocampi.
s. of hippocampus → s. of Ammon's horn.
s. of promontory (of tympanic cavity) Subiculum promontorii (cavi tympani).
sub·il·i·ac [sʌbˈɪlɪæk] adj unterhalb des Iliums (liegend), subilisch, subiliakal.
subiliac bursa 1. Bursa iliopectinea. 2. Bursa subtendinea iliaca.
sub·in·fec·tion [ˌsʌbɪnˈfɛkʃn] n Subinfektion f.
sub·in·flam·ma·tion [sʌbˌɪnfləˈmeɪʃn] adj leichte/abgeschwächte Entzündung f.
sub·in·gui·nal triangle [sʌbˈɪŋgwɪnl] Schenkeldreieck nt, Scarpa²-Dreieck nt, Trigonum femorale.
sub·in·ti·mal [sʌbˈɪntɪməl] adj unter der Intima (liegend), subintimal.
sub·in·vo·lu·tion [sʌbˌɪnvəˈluːʃn] n 1. unvollständige Rückbildung/Involution f, Subinvolution f, Subinvolutio f. 2. gyn. Subinvolutio uteri.
sub·ja·cent [sʌbˈdʒeɪsənt] adj darunterliegend, tiefer gelegen.
sub·ject [n, adj. ˈsʌbdʒɪkt; v səbˈdʒɛkt] I n 1. Gegenstand m, Thema nt, Stoff m. 2. (Lehr-, Schul-, Studien-)Fach nt, Fachgebiet nt. 3. (Versuchs-)Objekt nt; Versuchsperson f; Versuchstier nt; patho. Leichnam m; Patient(in f) m. II adj neigend (to zu); anfällig (to für). III vt (einer Prüfung etc.) unterwerfen, unterziehen, aussetzen.
sub·jec·tive [səbˈdʒɛktɪv] adj nichtsachlich, voreingenommen, persönlich, subjektiv.
subjective sign subjektives Zeichen nt.
subjective symptom subjektives Symptom nt.
sub·king·dom [sʌbˈkɪŋdəm] n bio. Unterreich nt.
sub·la·tion [sʌbˈleɪʃn] n Ablösung f, Abhebung f, Sublatio f.
sub·len·tic·u·lar part of internal capsule [ˌsʌblɛnˈtɪkjələr] sublentikulärer Kapselabschnitt m, Pars sublenticularis/sublentiformis (capsulae internae).
sub·len·ti·form part of internal capsule [sʌbˈlɛntɪfɔːrm] → sublenticular part of internal capsule.
sub·le·thal [sʌbˈliːθəl] adj nicht tödlich, subletal.
sub·leu·ke·mic [ˌsʌbluːˈkiːmɪk] adj hema. subleukämisch.
subleukemic leukemia subleukämische Leukämie f.
sub·lig·a·men·tous bursa [sʌbˌlɪgəˈmɛntəs] Bursa infrapatellaris profunda.
sub·li·mate [n, adj ˈsʌbləmət, -meɪt; v -meɪt] I n chem. Sublimat nt. II adj sublimiert. III vt 1. chem. sublimieren. 2. pyscho. sublimieren.
sub·li·ma·tion [ˌsʌbləˈmeɪʃn] n 1. chem. Sublimation f, Sublimierung f. 2. psycho. Sublimation f, Sublimierung f.
sub·lime [səˈblaɪm] I vt chem. sublimieren. II vi 1. chem. sublimieren. 2. phys. s. verflüchtigen.
sub·lim·i·nal [sʌbˈlɪmɪnl] adj unterschwellig, subliminal.
subliminal stimulus unterschwelliger Reiz m.

subliminal thirst (pathologisch) verminderter Durst *m*, Hypodipsie *f*.
sub·lin·gual [sʌb'lɪŋgwəl] *adj* unter der Zunge/Lingua (liegend), sublingual.
sublingual artery Unterzungenschlagader *f*, Sublingualis *f*, A. sublingualis.
sublingual caruncle Karunkel *f*, Caruncula sublingualis.
sublingual cyst Ranula *f*.
sublingual duct: greater s. Ductus sublingualis major.
   lesser s.s *pl* Ductus sublinguales minores.
sublingual fold Plica sublingualis.
sublingual fossa → sublingual fovea.
sublingual fovea Fovea sublingualis.
sublingual ganglion Ggl. sublinguale.
sublingual gland Unterzungen(speichel)drüse *f*, Gl. sublingualis.
sublingual nerve Sublingualis *m*, N. sublingualis.
sublingual papilla → sublingual caruncle.
sublingual plica → sublingual fold.
sublingual ptyalocele Ranula *f*.
sublingual ridge Zungenbändchen *nt*, Frenulum linguae.
sublingual saliva Sublingualisspeichel *m*.
sublingual temperature Mundhöhlen-, Sublingualtemperatur *f*.
sublingual vein Unterzungenvene *f*, Sublingualis *f*, V. sublingualis.
sub·lin·gui·tis [,sʌblɪŋ'gwaɪtɪs] *n* Entzündung *f* der Gl. sublingualis, Sublinguitis *f*.
sub·lob·u·lar veins of liver [sʌb'lɒbjələr] Sammelvenen *pl* der Leber.
sub·lux·ate [sʌb'lʌkseɪt] *vt ortho.* subluxieren.
sub·lux·a·tion [,sʌblʌk'seɪʃn] *n* unvollständige Verrenkung/Ausrenkung *f*, Subluxation *f*, Subluxatio *f*.
   s. of lens Subluxatio lentis.
   s. of rib cartilage Subluxation eines Rippenknorpels.
sub·lym·phe·mia [,sʌblɪm'fiːmɪə] *n hema.* Lymphozytenmangel *m*, Lympho(zyto)penie *f*.
sub·mam·ma·ry [sʌb'mæmərɪ] *adj* **1.** unter der Brustdrüse (liegend), submammär. **2.** unterhalb der Brust(drüse) (liegend), inframammär.
submammary abscess submammärer Abszeß *m*.
submammary mastitis *gyn.* Paramastitis *f*.
sub·man·dib·u·lar [,sʌbmæn'dɪbjələr] *adj* unter dem Unterkiefer/der Mandibula (liegend), submandibulär.
submandibular duct Wharton'-Gang *m*, Ductus submandibularis.
submandibular fossa Fovea submandibularis.
submandibular fovea → submandibular fossa.
submandibular ganglion Faesebeck'-Ganglion *nt*, Blandin'-Ganglion *nt*, Ggl. submandibulare.
submandibular gland Unterkieferdrüse *f*, Gl. submandibularis. *gyn.* Paramastitis *f*.
submandibular triangle/trigone Unterkieferdreieck *nt*, Trigonum submandibulare.
sub·mar·gin·al [sʌb'mɑːrdʒɪnl] *adj* submarginal.
sub·mas·sive hepatic necrosis [sʌb'mæsɪf] *n* subacute hepatic necrosis.
sub·max·il·la [,sʌbmæk'sɪlə] *n* Unterkiefer *m*, Mandibula *f*.
sub·max·il·lar·i·tis [sʌb,mæksɪlə'raɪtɪs] *n* Entzündung *f* der Gl. submaxillaris, Submaxillaritis *f*, Submaxillitis *f*.
sub·max·il·lar·y [sʌb'mæksɪ,lerɪ, -mæk'sɪlərɪ] *adj* Unterkiefer(knochen) betr., submaxillär.

submaxillary angle Unterkieferwinkel *m*, Angulus mandibulae.
submaxillary fossa → submandibular fossa.
submaxillary ganglion → submandibular ganglion.
submaxillary mucin submaxilläres Muzin *nt*.
submaxillary mucoprotein submaxilläres Mukoprotein *nt*.
submaxillary nerves Rami glandulares ggl. submandibularis.
submaxillary saliva Submandibularisspeichel *m*.
submaxillary triangle → submandibular triangle.
sub·max·il·li·tis [sʌb,mæksə'laɪtɪs] *n* → submaxillaritis.
sub·me·di·al [sʌb'miːdɪəl] *adj* submedial, -median.
sub·me·di·an [sʌb'miːdɪən] *adj* → submedial.
sub·mem·bra·nous [sʌb'membrənəs] *adj* partiell membranös.
sub·men·tal [sʌb'mentl] *adj* unterhalb des Kinns (liegend), submental.
submental artery Submentalis *f*, A. submentalis.
submental triangle/trigone Trigonum submentale.
submental vein Unterkinnvene *f*, V. submentalis.
sub·merge [səb'mɜːrdʒ] **I** *vt* ein-, untertauchen, versenken; überschwemmen. **II** *vi* untertauchen, versinken.
sub·merged [səb'mɜːrdʒd] *adj* ein-, untergetaucht, versenkt.
sub·mer·gence [səb'mɜːrdʒəns] *n* Ein-, Untertauchen *nt*, Submersion *f*, Versenken *nt*; Überschwemmung *f*.
sub·mersed [səb'mɜːrsd] *adj* → submerged.
sub·mer·sion [səb'mɜːrʒn] *n* → submergence.
sub·met·a·cen·tric [sʌb,metə'sentrɪk] *adj* submetazentrisch.
submetacentric chromosome submetazentrisches Chromosom *nt*.
sub·mi·cro·scop·ic [sʌb,maɪkrə'skɒpɪk] *adj* nicht mit dem (Licht-)Mikroskop sichtbar, submikroskopisch.
sub·mi·cro·scop·i·cal [sʌb,maɪkrə'skɒpɪkl] *adj* → submicroscopic.
sub·mi·to·chon·dri·al [,sʌb,maɪtə'kɒndrɪəl] *adj* submitochondrial.
sub·mo·lec·u·lar [,sʌbmə'lekjələr] *adj* submolekular.
sub·mor·phous [sʌb'mɔːrfəs] *adj* submorph.
sub·mu·co·sa [,sʌbmjuː'kəʊzə] *n* Submukosa *f*, Tela *f* submucosa.
sub·mu·co·sal [,sʌbmjuː'kəʊzl] *adj* Submukosa betr., unter der Mukosa (liegend), in der Submukosa (liegend), submukös.
submucosal coat → submucosa.
submucosal plexus Meissner'-Plexus *m*, Plexus submucosus.
sub·mu·cous [sʌb'mjuːkəs] *adj* → submucosal.
submucous coat → submucosa.
submucous cystitis chronisch interstitielle (Harn-)Blasenentzündung/Zystitis *f*, Cystitis intermuralis/interstitialis.
submucous layer → submucosa.
   s. of bladder Tela submucosa vesicae urinariae.
   s. of colon Tela submucosa coli.
   s. of pharynx Tela submucosa pharyngis.
   s. of small intestine Tela submucosa intestini tenuis.

   s. of stomach Tela submucosa gastris/ventriculi.
submucous membrane → submucosa.
   s. of stomach Tela submucosa ventriculi.
submucous plexus → submucosal plexus.
submucous ulcer Fenwick-Ulkus *nt*, Hunner-Ulkus *nt*, Hunner-Fenwick-Ulkus *nt*, Fenwick-Hunner-Ulkus *nt*.
sub·mus·cu·lar bursa [sʌb'mʌskjələr] submuskulärer Schleimbeutel *m*, Bursa (synovialis) submuscularis.
sub·nar·cot·ic [,sʌbnɑː'kɒtɪk] *adj* leicht narkotisch, subnarkotisch.
sub·na·sal [sʌb'neɪzl] *adj* unterhalb der Nase (liegend), subnasal.
sub·neu·ral [sʌb'nʊrəl, -'njʊə-] *adj* unterhalb eines Nervs (liegend), subneural.
subneural apparatus subneuraler/subsynaptischer (Falten-)Apparat *m*.
sub·nor·mal [sʌb'nɔːrml] **I** *n* **1.** *psycho.* Minderbegabte(r *m*) *f*. **2.** *mathe.* Subnormale *f*. **II** *adj* **3.** (*a. psycho.*) unterdurchschnittlich, subnormal; minderbegabt. **4.** *mathe.* subnormal.
sub·nor·mal·i·ty [,sʌbnɔːr'mælətɪ] *n* (*a. psycho.*) Minderbegabung *f*.
sub·no·to·chor·dal [sʌb,nəʊtə'kɔːrdl] *adj* unter der Chorda dorsalis (liegend), subchordal.
sub·nu·cle·us [sʌb'n(j)uːklɪəs] *n* Unterkern *m*, Subnukleus *m*.
sub·nu·tri·tion [,sʌbn(j)uː'trɪʃn] *n* Mangelernährung *f*.
sub·oc·cip·i·tal [,sʌbɒk'sɪpɪtl] *adj* unterhalb des Hinterhaupts (liegend), subokzipital.
suboccipital decompression *neurochir.* subokzipitale Schädeldekompression/Entlastungstrepanation *f*.
suboccipital muscles subokzipitale Muskeln *pl*/Muskulatur *f*, Mm. suboccipitales.
suboccipital nerve N. suboccipitalis.
suboccipital puncture Subokzipital-, Zisternen-, Hirnzisternenpunktion *f*.
sub·oc·cip·i·to·breg·mat·ic diameter [sʌbɒk,sɪpɪtəʊbreg'mætɪk] *gyn.*, *ped.* Diameter suboccipitobregmatica.
sub·o·don·to·blas·tic layer [sʌbə,dɒntə'blæstɪk] Weil'-Basalschicht *f*.
sub·op·ti·mal [sʌb'ɒptɪməl] *adj* unteroptimal, suboptimal.
sub·or·bit·al [sʌb'ɔːrbɪtl] *adj* unterhalb der Orbita (liegend), sub-, infraorbital.
suborbital foramen For. infraorbitale.
sub·or·der ['sʌbɔːrdər] *n bio.* Unterordnung *f*.
sub·pap·il·lar·y [sʌb'pæpə,lerɪ] *adj* subpapillär.
sub·pap·u·lar [sʌb'pæpjələr] *adj derm.* subpapulär.
sub·pa·ri·e·tal sulcus [,sʌbpə'raɪɪtl] Sulcus subparietalis.
sub·pa·tel·lar [,sʌbpə'telər] *adj* unterhalb der Patella (liegend), subpatellar.
subpatellar bursa Bursa subcutanea infrapatellaris.
sub·pec·tor·al [sʌb'pektərəl] *adj* subpektoral.
subpectoral abscess subpektoraler Abszeß *m*.
sub·per·i·car·di·al [sʌb,perɪ'kɑːrdɪəl] *adj* unter dem Perikard (liegend), subperikardial.
sub·per·i·os·te·al [sʌb,perɪ'ɒstɪəl] *adj* unter dem Periost (liegend), subperiostal.
subperiosteal abscess subperiostaler Abszeß *m*.
subperiosteal amputation *ortho.* Amputation *f* mit Periostlappendeckung.
subperiosteal bleeding subperiostale Blutung *f*.

subperiosteal giant cell tumor subperiostaler Riesenzelltumor *m*, ossifizierendes periostales Hämangiom *nt*.
subperiosteal hemorrhage → subperiosteal bleeding.
sub·per·i·to·ne·al [sʌbˌperɪtə'niːəl] *adj* unter dem Bauchfell/Peritoneum (liegend), subperitoneal.
subperitoneal abscess subperitonealer Bauchwandabszeß *m*.
subperitoneal appendicitis subperitoneale Appendizitis *f*.
subperitoneal fascia subperitoneales Bindegewebsblatt *nt*, Fascia subperitonealis.
sub·per·i·to·ne·o·ab·dom·i·nal [ˌsʌbperɪtəˌniːəʊæb'dɑmɪnl] *adj* → subperitoneal.
sub·pha·ryn·ge·al [ˌsʌbfə'rɪndʒɪəl] *adj* unterhalb des Pharynx (liegend), subpharyngeal.
sub·phren·ic [sʌb'frenɪk] *adj* unterhalb des Zwerchfells (liegend), subphrenisch, subdiaphragmal.
subphrenic abscess subphrenischer Abszeß *m*.
subphrenic empyema subphrenisches Empyem *nt*.
subphrenic recesses subphrenische Peritonealspalten *pl*, Recc. subphrenici.
subphrenic space subphrenischer Raum *m*.
sub·phy·lum [sʌb'faɪləm] *n, pl* **-la** [-lə] *bio.* Unterstamm *m*.
sub·pi·al [sʌb'paɪəl] *adj* unter der Pia (liegend), subpial.
sub·pla·cen·ta [ˌsʌbplə'sentə] *n gyn.* Decidua basalis.
sub·pla·cen·tal [ˌsʌbplə'sentl] *adj* unter der Plazenta (liegend), subplazentar.
sub·pleu·ral [sʌb'plʊərəl] *adj* unter der Pleura (liegend), subpleural.
subpleural bleeding Subpleuralblutung *f*.
subpleural emphysema subpleurales Lungenemphysem *nt*.
subpleural hemorrhage → subpleural bleeding.
sub·plex·al [sʌb'pleksəl] *adj* unter einem Plexus (liegend).
sub·pop·lit·e·al recess [ˌsʌbpɑp'lɪtɪəl, -ˌpɑpləˈtiːəl] Rec. subpopliteus.
sub·pop·u·la·tion [sʌbˌpɑpjə'leɪʃn] *n bio.* Unter-, Subpopulation *f*.
sub·pre·pu·tial [ˌsʌbprɪ'pjuːʃl] *adj* unterhalb der Vorhaut (liegend).
sub·pu·bic [sʌb'pjuːbɪk] *adj* unterhalb des Schambeins (liegend), subpubisch.
subpubic angle Schambeinwinkel *m*, -bogen *m*, Angulus subpubicus.
subpubic arch → subpubic angle.
subpubic ligament Lig. arcuatum pubis.
sub·pul·mo·nar·y [sʌb'pʌlməˌneriː, -nərɪ] *adj* unterhalb der Lungen (liegend), sub-, infrapulmonal.
sub·pul·pal [sʌb'pʌlpəl] *adj* unter der Zahnpulpa (liegend), subpulpal.
sub·py·lor·ic [ˌsʌbpaɪ'lɔːrɪk, -'lɑr-, -pɪ-] *adj* subpylorisch.
sub·rec·tal [sʌb'rektl] *adj* unterhalb des Rektums (liegend), sub-, infrarektal.
sub·ret·i·nal [sʌb'retɪnl] *adj* unter der Retina (liegend), subretinal.
sub·sar·to·ri·al canal [ˌsʌbsɑːr'tɔːrɪəl, -'təʊr-] Adduktorenkanal *m*, Canalis adductorius.
sub·scap·u·lar [sʌb'skæpjələr] *adj* unterhalb des Schulterblattes/der Skapula (liegend), subskapulär.
subscapular abscess subskapulärer Abszeß *m*.
subscapular artery Subskapularis *f*, A. subscapularis.
subscapular branches of axillary artery A. axillaris-Äste *pl* zum M. subscapularis, Rami subscapulares a. axillaris.
subcapsular cataract subkapsuläre Katarakt *f*.
subscapular fossa Fossa subscapularis.
sub·scap·u·lar·is (muscle) [sʌbˌskæpjə'leərɪs] Subskapularis *m*, M. subscapularis.
subscapular lines Lineae muscularis scapulae.
subscapular muscle → subscapularis (muscle).
subscapular nerves Nn. subscapulares.
subscapular vein V. subscapularis.
sub·scle·ral [sʌb'sklɪərəl] *adj* unter der Sklera (liegend), subskleral.
sub·scle·rot·ic [ˌsʌbsklɪ'rɑtɪk] *adj* **1.** → subscleral. **2.** partiell sklerosiert/sklerotisch.
sub·scrip·tion [səb'skrɪpʃn] *n pharm.* Subscriptio *f*.
sub·se·ro·sa [ˌsʌbsɪə'rəʊzə] *n* subseröse Bindegewebsschicht *f*, Subserosa *f*, Tela subserosa.
sub·se·ro·sal [ˌsʌbsɪə'rəʊzl] *adj* → subserous.
subserosal plexus → subserous plexus.
sub·se·rous [sʌb'sɪərəs] *adj* unter der Serosa (liegend), subserös.
subserous coat → subserosa.
subserous layer → subserosa.
s. of peritoneum Tela subserosa peritonei.
subserous plexus seröser Peritonealplexus *m*, Plexus subserosus.
sub·son·ic [sʌb'sɑnɪk] *adj phys.* subsonisch, infrasonar, Infraschall-.
sub·spe·cial·ty [sʌb'speʃəltɪ] *n* Subspezialität *f*.
sub·spe·cies ['sʌbspiːʃiːz] *n, pl* **-cies** *bio.* Unterart *f*, Subspezies *f*.
sub·spe·cif·ic [ˌsʌbspə'sɪfɪk] *adj* Subspezies betr., zu einer Subspezies gehörend, unterartlich.
sub·spi·nous [sʌb'spaɪnəs] *adj* unter einem Proc. spinosus (liegend), subspinal, infraspinal.
sub·stance ['sʌbstəns] *n* **1.** Substanz *f*, Stoff *m*, Materie *f*, Masse *f*; *anat.* Substantia *f*. **2.** *fig.* Wesentliche *nt*, Kern *m*, Essenz *f*.
s. of lens Linsensubstanz, Substantia lentis.
substance concentration *chem., phys.* molare Konzentration *f*.
substance dependence Substanzabhängigkeit *f*, Abhängigkeit *f* von psychotropen Substanzen.
substance exchange *physiol.* Stoffaustausch *m*.
substance P *biochem.* Substanz P *f*.
substance specificity Substanz-, Stoffspezifität *f*.
sub·stan·tia [səb'stænʃɪə] *n, pl* **-tiae** [-ʃɪˌiː] *anat.* → substance 1.
substantia innominata of Reil/Reichert Meynert'-Ganglion *nt*, Substantia innominata.
substantia nigra *old* schwarzer Kern *m*, Substantia nigra.
sub·ster·nal [sʌb'stɜrnl] *adj* **1.** unterhalb des Sternums (liegend), sub-, infrasternal. **2.** hinter dem Sternum (liegend), retrosternal.
substernal angle Angulus infrasternalis.
substernal goiter retrosternale Struma *f*, Struma retrosternalis.
substernal pain retrosternaler Schmerz *m*.
sub·stit·u·ent [sʌb'stɪtʃəwənt] *n chem.* Substituent *m*.
sub·sti·tute ['sʌbstɪt(j)uːt] **I** *n* **1.** Ersatz *m*, Ersatzstoff *m*, -mittel *nt*, Surrogat *nt*. **2.** Ersatz(mann *m*) *m*, (Stell-)Vertreter(in *f*) *m.* **II** *adj* Ersatz-. **III** *vt chem., mathe.* substituieren. **IV** *vi* als Ersatz dienen (*for* für).
sub·sti·tut·ed ['sʌbstɪt(j)uːtɪd] *adj* ersatzweise, Ersatz-; *chem.* substituiert.
sub·sti·tu·tion [ˌsʌbstɪ't(j)uːʃn] *n* **1.** Ersatz *m*, Austausch *m*, Substitution *f*, Substituierung *f*, Substituieren *nt*. **2.** *chem.* Substitution *f*. **3.** Stellvertretung *f*. **4.** *psycho.* Verdrängung *f*, Substitution *f*.
substitution bone Ersatzknochen *m*.
substitution product *chem.* Substitutionsprodukt *nt*.
substitution therapy Ersatztherapie *f*.
substitution transfusion Blutaustausch *m*, (Blut-)Austauschtransfusion *f*.
sub·strate ['sʌbstreɪt] *n* **1.** *biochem.* Substrat *nt*. **2.** → substratum.
substrate concentration Substratkonzentration *f*.
substrate constant *abbr.* K_S Substratkonstante *f abbr.* K_S.
substrate induction Substratinduktion *f*.
substrate-level phosphorylation *biochem.* Substratkettenphosphorilierung *f*.
substrate saturation Substratsättigung *f*.
substrate specificity Substratspezifität *f*.
sub·stra·tum [sʌb'streɪtəm, -'stræt-] *n, pl* **-tums, -ta** [-tə] **1.** Unter-, Grundlage *f*; Unterschicht *f*. **2.** *bio.* Nähr-, Keimboden *nt*, Substrat *nt*.
sub·stri·ate layer of cerebral cortex [sʌb'straɪeɪt] Lamina substriata.
sub·struc·ture [sʌb'strʌktʃər] *n* Substruktur *f*.
sub·sup·e·ri·or segment (of lung) [ˌsʌbsə'pɪərɪər] subapikales Lungensegment *nt*, Segmentum subapikale.
sub·syn·ap·tic [ˌsʌbsɪ'næptɪk] *adj* unterhalb einer Synapse (liegend), subsynaptisch.
subsynaptic membrane subsynaptische Membran *f*.
sub·syn·o·vi·al cyst [ˌsʌbsɪ'nəʊvɪəl] subsynoviale Zyste *f*.
sub·ta·lar [sʌb'teɪlər] *adj* unterhalb des Talus (liegend), subtalar.
subtalar articulation hintere Abteilung *f* des unteren Sprunggelenks, Subtalargelenk *nt*, Artic. subtalaris/talocalcanea.
subtalar joint → subtalar articulation.
sub·tar·sal [sʌb'tɑːrsl] *adj* unterhalb des Tarsus (liegend), subtarsal.
sub·tel·o·cen·tric [sʌbˌtelə'sentrɪk] *adj* subtelozentrisch.
sub·tem·po·ral [sʌb'temp(ə)rəl] *adj* unter(halb) der Schläfe (liegend), subtemporal.
subtemporal decompression *neurochir.* subtemporale Schädeldekompression/Entlastungstrepanation *f*.
sub·ten·di·nous [sʌb'tendɪnəs] *adj* unterhalb einer Sehne (liegend), subtendinös.
subtendinous bursa subtendinöser Schleimbeutel *m*, Bursa (synovialis) subtendinea.
inferior s. of biceps femoris muscle Bursa subtendinea m. bicipitis femoris inferior.
s. of infraspinatus muscle Bursa subtendinea m. infraspinati.
s. of obturator internus muscle Bursa subtendinea m. obturatoris interni.
s.e of sartorius muscle Bursae subtendineae m. sartorii.
s. of subscapularis muscle Bursa subtendinea m. subscapularis.
s. of teres major muscle Bursa subtendinea m. teretis majoris.
s. of tibialis anterior muscle Bursa subtendinea m. tibialis anterioris.
s. of tibialis posterior muscle Bursa subtendinea m. tibialis posterioris.

s. of trapezius muscle Bursa subtendinea m. trapezii.
s. of triceps muscle Bursa subtendinea m. tricipitis brachii.
subtendinous synovial bursa → subtendinous bursa.
sub·ten·to·ri·al [ˌsʌbtenˈtɔːrɪəl] *adj* unterhalb des Tentoriums (liegend), subtentorial.
sub·ter·mi·nal [sʌbˈtɜrm(ɪ)nəl] *adj* subterminal.
sub·ter·tian malaria [sʌbˈtɜrʃn] Falciparum-Malaria *f*, Tropenfieber *nt*, Malaria tropica.
sub·te·tan·ic [ˌsʌbtəˈtænɪk] *adj* leicht tetanisch, subtetanisch.
sub·tha·lam·ic [ˌsʌbθəˈlæmɪk] *adj* **1.** unterhalb des Thalamus (liegend), subthalamisch. **2.** Subthalamus betr., subthalamisch.
subthalamic fasciculus subthalamisches Bündel *nt*, Fasciculus subthalamicus.
subthalamic nucleus Luys'-Kern *m*, -Körper *m*, Corpus Luys, Nc. subthalamicus.
subthalamic pathways subthalamische Bahnen *pl*.
subthalamic region subthalamisches Gebiet *nt*, Regio subthalamica.
sub·thal·a·mus [sʌbˈθæləməs] *n* ventraler Thalamus *m*, Thalamus ventralis, Subthalamus *m*.
sub·thres·hold [sʌbˈθreʃ(h)əʊld] *adj physiol.*, *psycho.* unterschwellig.
subthreshold stimulus unterschwelliger Reiz *m*.
sub·tile [ˈsʌtl, ˈsʌbtɪl] *adj* → subtle.
sub·til·i·sin [sʌbˈtɪləsɪn] *n* Subtilisin *nt*.
sub·til·i·ty [sʌbˈtɪləti] *n* → subtlety.
sub·til·i·za·tion [ˌsʌtləˈzeɪʃn, ˌsʌbtəlaɪ-] *n* **1.** Verfeinerung *f*. **2.** *chem.* Verflüchtigung *f*.
sub·til·ize [ˈsʌtlaɪz, ˈsʌbtəlaɪz] *vt* **1.** verfeinern. **2.** *chem.* verdünnen, verflüchtigen.
sub·tle [ˈsʌtl] *adj* **1.** scharf(sinnig); geschickt; raffiniert; subtil. **2.** (*Aroma*) fein.
sub·tle·ty [ˈsʌtlti] *n*, *pl* -ties Geschicklichkeit *f*; Raffinesse *f*; Feinheit *f*.
sub·to·tal [sʌbˈtəʊtl] **I** *n* Zwischen-, Teilsumme *f*. **II** *adj* nicht vollständig, subtotal.
subtotal colectomy *chir.* subtotale Kolonresektion/Kolektomie *f*.
subtotal distal pancreatectomy Child-Operation *f*, subtotale distale/linksseitige Pankreatektomie *f*, subtotale Pankrealinksresektion *f*.
subtotal gastrectomy *chir.* subtotale Magenentfernung/Gastrektomie *f*.
subtotal hepatectomy *chir.* subtotale Leberentfernung/Hepatektomie *f*, Leberresektion *f*.
subtotal hysterectomy partielle/subtotale Gebärmutterentfernung/Hysterektomie *f*, Hysterectomia partialis.
sub·tribe [ˈsʌbtraɪb] *n bio.* Unterstamm *m*, -klasse *f*.
sub·tro·chan·ter·ic [sʌbˌtrəʊkənˈterɪk] *adj* subtrochantär.
subtrochanteric fracture of the femur subtrochantäre Oberschenkelfraktur/Femurfraktur *f*.
sub·troch·le·ar [sʌbˈtrɒklɪər] *adj* subtrochlear.
sub·tu·ber·al [sʌbˈtjuːbərəl] *adj* subtuberal.
sub·um·bil·i·cal [ˌsʌbʌmˈbɪlɪkl] *adj* unterhalb des Nabels (liegend), sub-, infraumbilikal.
sub·un·gual [sʌbˈʌŋgwəl] *adj* unter einem Finger- *od.* Zehennagel (liegend), subungual.

subungual abscess subungualer Abszeß *m*.
subungual hematoma subunguales Hämatom *nt*.
subungual melanoma subunguales Melanom *nt*.
sub·un·gui·al [sʌbˈʌŋgwɪəl] *adj* → subungual.
sub·u·nit [ˈsʌbjuːnɪt] *n* Untereinheit *f*.
subunit model *biochem.* Untereinheitenmodell *nt*, globuläres Modell *nt*.
subunit vaccine → subvirion vaccine.
sub·u·re·thral [ˌsʌbjʊəˈriːθrəl] *adj* suburethral.
sub·vag·i·nal [sʌbˈvædʒɪnl] *adj* unter(halb) der Vagina (liegend), subvaginal.
sub·val·vu·lar [sʌbˈvælvjələr] *adj* unterhalb einer Klappe/Valva (liegend), subvalvulär.
subvalvular stenosis infravalvuläre/subvalvuläre Aortenstenose *f*.
sub·vas·cu·lar layer of myometrium [sʌbˈvæskjələr] subvaskuläre Schicht *f* des Myometriums, Stratum submucosum/subvasculare (myometrii).
sub·vi·ri·on vaccine [sʌbˈvaɪrɪən] Spaltimpfstoff *m*, -vakzine *f*.
suc·ce·da·ne·ous [ˌsʌksɪˈdeɪnɪəs] *adj* nachfolgend, sukzedan.
suc·ce·da·ne·um [ˌsʌksɪˈdeɪnɪəm] *n*, *pl* -nea [-nɪə] *pharm.* Ersatz *m*, Surrogat *nt*, Succedaneum *nt*.
suc·cen·tu·ri·ate placenta [ˌsʌksənˈt(j)ʊərɪɪt, -eɪt] Nebenplazenta *f*, Placenta succenturiata.
suc·ces·sion [səkˈseʃn] *n* **1.** (Aufeinander-, Reihen-)Folge *f*. **2.** Reihe *f*, Kette *f*, Folge *f*. **3.** Nachfolger *pl*; Nachkommen(schaft *f*) *pl*.
suc·ces·sion·al [səkˈseʃənl] *adj* **1.** (nach-)folgend, Nachfolge-. **2.** aufeinanderfolgend, zusammenhängend, Folge-.
successional series *bio.* Sukzessionsserie *f*, -folge *f*, Serie *f*.
successional teeth Ersatzzähne *pl*, Zähne *f* der II. Dentition.
suc·ces·sive [səkˈsesɪv] *adj* **1.** (aufeinander-)folgend, sukzessiv. **2.** fortlaufend, stufenweise, sukzessiv.
suc·ces·sor [səkˈsesər] *n* Nachfolger(in *f*) *m*.
suc·ci·nate [ˈsʌksɪneɪt] *n* Succinat *nt*.
succinate-CoA ligase → succinyl-CoA synthetase.
succinate dehydrogenase Succinatdehydrogenase *f*.
succinate-glycine cycle Succinat-Glycin--Zyklus *m*.
suc·cin·ic acid [səkˈsɪnɪk] Bernsteinsäure *f*.
suc·ci·nous [ˈsʌksɪnəs] *adj* Bernstein-, Sukzino-.
suc·ci·nyl [ˈsʌksɪnɪl] *n* Succinyl-(Radikal *nt*).
suc·ci·nyl·cho·line [ˌsʌksɪnɪlˈkjəʊliːn] *n pharm.*, *anes.* Succinylcholin *nt*, Suxamethonium *nt*.
succinylcholine chloride *pharm.*, *anes.* Succinylcholinchlorid *nt*, Suxamethoniumchlorid *nt*.
succinyl-CoA *n* succinylcoenzyme A.
succinyl-CoA synthetase Succinyl-CoA--synthetase *f*.
suc·ci·nyl·co·en·zyme A [ˌ-kəʊˈenzaɪm] Succinyl-CoA *nt*.
O-succinyl-homoserine *n* O-Succinylhomoserin *nt*.
succinyl phosphate Succinylphosphat *nt*.
suc·cor·rhea [sʌkəˈrɪə] *n* Sukorrhoe *f*.
suc·cus [ˈsʌkəs] *n*, *pl* -ci [-saɪ] Saft *m*, Succus *m*.
suc·cus·sion sound [səˈkʌʃn] Plätscherräusch *nt*.

suck [sʌk] **I** *n* **1.** Saugen *nt*, Lutschen *nt*. **2.** Sog *m*, Saugkraft *f*. **3.** Wirbel *m*, Strudel *m*. **II** *vt* saugen (*from*, *out of* an); lutschen (an). **III** *vi* **4.** saugen, lutschen (*at* an). **5.** (*an der Brust*) trinken *od.* saugen.
suck down *vt* hinunterziehen.
suck in *vt* auf-, ansaugen.
suck·er [ˈsʌkər] *n chir.* Sauger *m*.
sucker apparatus → sucker process.
sucker foot → sucker process.
sucker process *micro.* Saugfüßchen *nt*.
suck·ing [ˈsʌkɪŋ] *adj* **1.** saugend, Saug-. **2.** (*Säugling*) noch nicht entwöhnt.
sucking cushion Bichat'-Wangenfettpfropf *m*, Corpus adiposum buccae.
sucking disk *micro.* Saugscheibe *f*.
sucking louse *micro.* Anoplura *f*.
sucking pad → sucking cushion.
sucking reflex Saugreflex *m*.
suck·le [ˈsʌkl] *vt gyn.* (*Kind*) stillen, die Brust geben.
suck·ling [ˈsʌklɪŋ] *n* Säugling *m*.
Sucquet [syˈke]: **S.' canals** Sucquet--Hoyer-Kanäle *pl*.
Sucquet-Hoyer [ˈhɔɪər]: **S.-H. canals** → Sucquet' canals.
su·cral·fate [suːˈkrælfeɪt] *n pharm.* Sucralfat *nt*.
su·crase [ˈsuːkreɪz] *n* → sucrose α-glucosidase.
sucrase-α-dextrinase deficiency, intestinal Saccharase-Isomaltase-Mangel *m*.
sucrase-isomaltase deficiency, congenital Saccharase-Isomaltase-Mangel *m*.
su·cro·clas·tic [ˌsuːkrəˈklæstɪk] *adj* zuckerspaltend.
su·crose [ˈsuːkrəʊs] *n* Rüben-, Rohrzucker *m*, Saccharose *f*.
sucrose α-D-glucohydrolase → sucrose α-glucosidase.
sucrose α-glucosidase Sucrase *f*, Saccharose-α-glucosidase *f*.
su·cro·se·mia [ˌsuːkrəˈsiːmɪə] *n* Saccharosämie *f*.
sucrose-6'-phosphate *n* Saccharose-6'--phosphat *nt*.
sucrose phosphate synthase Saccharosephosphatsynthase *f*.
sucrose phosphorylase Saccharosephosphorylase *f*.
sucrose synthase Saccharosesynthase *f*.
su·cro·su·ria [ˌ-ˈs(j)ʊərɪə] *n* übermäßige Saccharoseausscheidung *f* im Harn, Saccharosurie *f*, Sucrosuria *f*.
suc·tion [ˈsʌkʃn] **I** *n* **1.** (An-)Saugen *nt*; Saugwirkung *f*, -leistung *f*. **2.** Sog *m*, Unterdruck *m*. **3.** *phys.* Saugfähigkeit *f*. **II** *adj* Saug-.
suction catheter Saugkatheter *m*.
suction curettage *gyn.* Saug-, Vakuumkürettage *f*.
suction drainage *chir.* Saugdrainage *f*.
suc·to·ri·al [sʌkˈtɔːrɪəl, -ˈtəʊr-] *adj* Saug-.
suctorial pad → sucking cushion.
su·da·men [suːˈdeɪmən] *n*, *pl* -dam·i·na [-ˈdæmɪnə] Schweißbläschen *nt*, Sudamen *nt*.
su·dam·i·na [suːˈdæmɪnə] *pl* **1.** *derm.* Sudamina *pl*, Miliaria cristallina. **2.** → sudamen.
su·dam·i·nal [suːˈdæmɪnəl] *adj* Schweißbläschen betr., Schweißbläschen-.
Su·dan [suːˈdæn] *n* Sudan *nt*, Sudanfarbstoff *m*.
Sudan I Sudan I *nt*.
Sudan II Sudan II *nt*.
Sudan III Sudan III *nt*.
Sudan G → Sudan III.
su·dan·o·phil [suːˈdænəfɪl] **I** *n* sudanophile Struktur *f*. **II** *adj* → sudanophilic.
su·dan·o·phil·ia [suːˌdænəˈfɪlɪə] *n* Sudanophilie *f*.

sudanophilic

su·dan·o·phil·ic [ˌ-'fılık] *adj* sudanophil.
sudanophilic leukodystrophy sudanophile Leukodystrophie *f*.
su·da·noph·i·lous [ˌsuːdə'nɑfıləs] *adj* → sudanophil.
su·dan·o·pho·bic [suːˌdænə'foʊbık] *adj* sudanophob.
sudanophobic zone (*NNR*) sudanophobe Zone *f*.
Sudan red Sudanrot *nt*.
su·da·ri·um [suː'deərıəm] *n, pl* **-ria** [-rıə] Schwitzbad *nt*, Sudarium *nt*.
su·da·tion [suː'deıʃn] *n* Schwitzen *nt*, Schweißsekretion *f*, Perspiration *f*.
sud·den ['sʌdn] *adj* plötzlich, unvermutet, überraschend, jäh.
sudden deafness Hörsturz *m*, akute Ertaubung *f*.
sudden infant death syndrome *abbr*. **SIDS** plötzlicher Kindstod *m*, Krippentod *m*, sudden infant death syndrome *abbr*. SIDS, Mors subita infantum.
sudden transitory partial blindness Amaurosis partialis fugax.
Sudeck ['suːdek]: **S.'s atrophy** Sudeck'- -Dystrophie *f*, Sudeck-Syndrom *nt*, Morbus Sudeck *m*.
S.'s critical point Sudeck-Punkt *m*.
S.'s disease → S.'s atrophy.
S.'s point → S.'s critical point.
S.'s syndrome Sudek-Syndrom *nt*, -Dystrophie *f*.
Sudeck-Leriche [lə'riʃ]: **S.-L. syndrome** Sudeck-Syndrom *nt* mit Vasospasmen.
su·do·gram ['s(j)uːdəgræm] *n* Sudogramm *nt*.
su·do·mo·tor [ˌ-'moʊtər] *adj* sudomotorisch.
sudomotor fibers Nervenfasern *pl* der Schweißdrüsen, sudomotorische Fasern *pl*.
sudomotor function Sudomotorik *f*.
sudomotor system *physiol*. Sudomotorsystem *nt*.
su·dor ['s(j)uːdər] *n* Schweiß *m*, Sudor *m*.
su·do·re·sis [ˌs(j)uːdə'riːsıs] *n* Schweißsekretion *f*, Schwitzen *nt*, Diaphorese *f*.
su·do·rif·er·ous [ˌ-'rıfərəs] *adj* 1. schweißbildend. 2. schweiß(ab)leitend, Schweiß-.
sudoriferous duct Ausführungsgang *m* einer Schweißdrüse, Ductus sudoriferus.
sudoriferous glands Schweißdrüsen *pl*, Gll. sudoriferae.
sudoriferous pore Schweißdrüsenpore *f*, Porus sudoriferus.
su·do·rif·ic [ˌ-'rıfık] **I** *n* schweißtreibendes Mittel *nt*, *old* Diaphoretikum *nt*, Sudoriferum *nt*. **II** *adj* schweißtreibend, -erzeugend, sudorifer, diaphoretisch.
su·do·rip·a·rous [ˌ-'rıpərəs] *adj* schweißbildend.
sudoriparous abscess Schweißdrüsenabszeß *m*.
sudoriparous glands → sudoriferous glands.
su·dor·rhea [ˌ-'rıə] *n* übermäßiges Schwitzen *nt*, Hyperhidrose *f*, Hyper(h)idrosis *f*, Polyhidrose *f*, Poly(h)idrosis *f*.
SUFE *abbr*. → slipped upper femoral epiphysis.
suf·fo·cate ['sʌfəkeıt] **I** *vt* 1. ersticken. 2. würgen. **II** *vi* ersticken (*with* an); umkommen (*with* vor).
suf·fo·cat·ing ['sʌfəkeıtıŋ] *adj* erstickend.
suf·fo·ca·tion [ˌsʌfə'keıʃn] *n* Erstickung *f*, Ersticken *nt*, Suffokation *f*, Suffocatio *f*.
suffocation bleeding Erstickungsblutung *f*.
suffocation hemorrhage → suffocation bleeding.
suf·fo·ca·tive catarrh ['sʌfəkeıtıv] anfallsweise Atemnot *m*, Asthma *nt*.

suf·fu·sion [sə'fjuːʒn] *n* patho. Suffusion *f*, Suffusio *f*.
sug·ar ['ʃʊgər] **I** *n* (*a. chem., physiol.*) Zucker *m*. **II** *vt* 1. süßen, zuckern. 2. kristallisieren.
s. of lead Bleiazetat *nt*.
sugar acid Zuckersäure *f*.
sugar alcohol Zuckeralkohol *m*.
sugar beet Zuckerrübe *f*.
sugar breakdown Zuckerabbau *m*.
sugar cane Zuckerrohr *nt*.
sugar carrier *physiol*. Zucker-Carrier *m*.
sugar-coat *vt* mit Zucker(masse) überziehen, überzuckern, dragieren.
sugar-coated tablet Dragée *nt*, Pille *f*.
sug·ared ['ʃʊgərd] *adj* 1. gesüßt, gezuckert. 2. süß.
sugar-icing liver *patho*. Zuckergußleber *f*, Perihepatitis chronica hyperplastica.
sugar-icing spleen *patho*. Zuckergußmilz *f*.
sug·ar·less ['ʃʊgərlıs] *adj* ungezuckert, ohne Zucker.
sugar phosphate Zuckerphosphat *nt*.
sugar test Zuckertest *m*.
sugar transport *physiol*. Zuckertransport *m*.
sug·ar·y ['ʃʊgərı] *adj* aus Zucker (bestehend), zuckerhaltig, zuck(e)rig, süß, Zucker-.
sug·gest [sə'dʒest] *vt* 1. vorschlagen, empfehlen, anregen. 2. (*Idee*) eingeben, suggerieren. 3. *psycho*. durch Suggestion beeinflussen, suggerieren.
sug·gest·i·bil·i·ty [sə,dʒestə'bılətı] *n* Beeinflußbarkeit *f*, Suggestibilität *f*.
sug·gest·i·ble [sə'dʒestıbl] *adj* 1. beeinflußbar, suggerierbar.
sug·ges·tion [sə'dʒestʃn] *n* 1. Vorschlag *m*, Empfehlung *f*, Anregung *f*. 2. Eingebung *f*. 3. *psycho*. (seelische) Beeinflussung *f*, Suggestion *f*.
sug·ges·tive [sə'dʒestıv] *adj* 1. anregend, gehaltvoll. 2. *psycho*. suggestiv, Suggestiv-.
sug·gil·la·tion [sʌ(g)jə'leıʃn, ˌsʌdʒə-] *n* 1. *patho*. Suggillation *f*, Suggillatio *f*. 2. Livedo *f*. 3. Totenflecken *pl*, Leichenflecke *pl*, Livores *pl*.
su·i·cid·al [suːə'saıdl] *adj* Selbstmord/ Suizid betr., suizidal, suicidal, Selbstmord-.
su·i·cide ['suːəsaıd] **I** *n* Selbstmord *m*, Freitod *m*, Suizid *m/nt*, Suicid *m/nt*. **II** *adj* Selbstmord-, Suizid-. **III** *vi* Selbstmord begehen, Suicid begehen.
sul·cate ['sʌlkeıt] *adj* → sulcated.
sul·cat·ed ['sʌlkeıtıd] *adj* faltig, gefurcht, Falten-.
sulcated tongue Faltenzunge *f*, Lingua plicata/scrotalis.
sul·ci·form ['sʌlsəfɔːrm] *adj* furchenartig, -ähnlich, faltenartig, -ähnlich.
sul·co·mar·gin·al fasciculus [ˌsʌlkoʊ- 'mɑːdʒənl] Fasciculus sulcomarginalis.
sulcomarginal tract → sulcomarginal fasciculus.
sul·cus ['sʌlkəs] *n, pl* **-ci** [-saı] Furche *f*, Rinne *f*; *anat*. Sulkus *m*, Sulcus *m*.
s. of auditory tube Sulcus tubae auditivae/ auditoriae.
s.i of cerebrum *pl* Großhirnfurchen *pl*, Sulci cerebrales.
s. of cingulum Sulcus cinguli/cingulatus.
s. of corpus callosum Sulcus corporis callosi.
s. of crus of helix Sulcus cruris helicis.
s. of eustachian tube → s. of auditory tube.
s. of greater petrosal nerve Sulcus n. petrosi majoris.
s. of habenula Sulcus habenulae/habenularis.

s. of hippocampus Fissura hippocampi, Sulcus hippocampi/hippocampalis.
s. of inferior petrosal sinus of occipital bone Sulcus sinus petrosi inferioris ossis occipitalis.
s. of inferior petrosal sinus of temporal bone Sulcus sinus petrosi inferioris ossis temporalis.
s. of lesser petrosal nerve Sulcus n. petrosi minoris.
s. of middle temporal artery Sulcus a. temporalis mediae.
s. of nail matrix Nagelfalz *m*, Sulcus matricis unguis.
s. of occipital artery Sulcus a. occipitalis.
s. of pterygoid hamulus Sulcus hamuli pterygoidei.
s. of radial nerve Radialisrinne, Sulcus (n.) radialis, Sulcus spiralis.
s. of sigmoid sinus Sinus-sigmoideus-Rinne, Sulcus sinus sigmoidei.
s. of sigmoid sinus of occipital bone Sulcus sinus sigmoidei ossis occipitalis.
s. of sigmoid sinus of parietal bone Sulcus sinus sigmoidei ossis parietalis.
s. of sigmoid sinus of temporal bone Sulcus sinus sigmoidei ossis temporalis.
s.i of skin *pl* Hautfurchen *pl*, Sulci cutis.
s. of subclavian artery Sulcus a. subclaviae.
s. for subclavian muscle Sulcus m. subclavii.
s. of subclavian vein Sulcus v. subclaviae.
s. of talus Talusrinne, Sulcus tali.
s. of tendon of flexor hallucis longus of calcaneus Sulcus tendinis m. flexoris hallucis longi calcanei.
s. of tendon of flexor hallucis longus of talus Sulcus tendinis m. flexoris hallucis longi tali.
s. of tendon of peroneus longus muscle of cuboid bone Sulcus tendinis m. peron(a)ei/fibularis longi ossis cuboidei.
s. of tendon of peroneus longus muscle of calcaneus Sulcus tendinis m. peron(a)ei/ fibularis longi calcanei.
s. of transverse sinus Sulcus sinus transversi.
s. of ulnar nerve Sulcus n. ulnaris.
s. of umbilical vein Sulcus venae umbilicalis.
s. of vena cava Sulcus venae cavae.
s. of vertebral artery Sulcus a. vertebralis.
sulcus vomeris Sulcus vomeris.
sulf- *pref*. → sulfo-.
sul·fa-benz·a·mide [ˌsʌlfə'benzəmaıd] *n pharm*. Sulfabenzamid *nt*.
sul·fa-car·ba·mide [ˌ-'kɑːrbəmaıd] *n pharm*. Sulfacarbamid *nt*.
sul·fa·cet·a·mide [ˌ-'setəmaıd] *n pharm*. Sulfacetamid *nt*.
sulf·ac·id [sʌlf'æsıd] *n* Thiosäure *f*.
sul·fa·di·a·zine [ˌsʌlfə'daıəziːn] *n pharm*. Sulfadiazin *nt*.
sul·fa·di·cra·mide [ˌ-'daıkrəmaıd] *n pharm*. Sulfadicramid *nt*.
sul·fa·di·meth·ox·ine [ˌ-daıme'θɑksiːn] *n pharm*. Sulfadimethoxin *nt*.
sul·fa·di·me·tine [ˌ-'daımətiːn] *n* → sulfisomidine.
sul·fa·dim·i·dine [ˌ-'dımədiːn] *n* → sulfamethazine.
sul·fa·dox·ine [ˌ-'dɑksiːn] *n pharm*. Sulfadoxin *nt*.
sul·fa·eth·i·dole [ˌ-'eθıdoʊl] *n pharm*. Sulfaethidol *nt*.
sul·fa·fu·ra·zole [ˌ-'fjʊərəzoʊl] *n* → sulfisoxazole.
sul·fa·guan·i·dine [ˌ-'gwænədiːn] *n pharm*. Sulfaguanidin *nt*.
sul·fa·gua·nole [ˌ-'gwænoʊl] *n pharm*. Sulfaguanol *nt*.

sul·fa·lene ['-li:n] *n pharm*. Sulfalen *nt*.
sul·fa·lox·ic acid [,-'lɑksɪk] *pharm*. Sulfaloxinsäure *f*.
sul·fa·mer·a·zine [,-'merəzi:n] *n pharm*. Sulfamerazin *nt*.
sul·fa·meth·a·zine [,-'meθəzi:n] *n pharm*. Sulfadimidin *nt*, Sulfamethazin *nt*.
sul·fa·meth·i·zole [,-'meθɪzəʊl] *n pharm*. Sulfamethizol *nt*.
sul·fa·meth·ox·a·zole [,-meθ'ɑksəzəʊl] *n pharm*. Sulfamethoxazol *nt*.
sul·fa·meth·yl·di·a·zine [,-,meθəl'daɪəzi:n] *n* → sulfamerazine.
sul·fa·meth·yl·thi·a·di·a·zole [,-,meθəl,θaɪə'daɪəzəʊl] *n* → sulfamethizole.
sul·fa·me·trole [,-'mi:trəʊl] *n pharm*. Sulfametrol *nt*.
sulf·am·ide [sʌl'fæmaɪd, 'sʌlfəm-] *n* Sulfamid-Gruppe *f*.
sul·fam·i·do [sʌl'fæmɪdəʊ] *n pharm*. Sulfamid *nt*.
sul·fam·in(e) [sʌl'fæmɪn, -mi:n] *n* Sulfamin-(Radikal *nt*).
sul·fa·mox·ole [,sʌlfə'mɑksəʊl] *n pharm*. Sulfamoxol *nt*.
sul·fa·nil·a·mide [,-'nɪləmaɪd] *n pharm*. Sulfanilamid *nt*, *p*-Aminobenzoesulfonamid *nt*.
sul·fan·i·late [sʌl'fænɪleɪt] *n* Sulfanilat *nt*.
sul·fa·nil·ic acid [,sʌlfə'nɪlɪk] Sulfanilsäure *f*, *p*-Aminobenzolsulfonsäure *f*.
sul·fa·per·in ['-perɪn] *n pharm*. Sulfaperin *nt*.
sul·fa·sal·a·zine [,-'sæləzi:n] *n pharm*. Salazosulfapyridin *nt*.
sul·fa·tase ['sʌlfəteɪz] *n* Sulfatase *f*.
sul·fate ['sʌlfeɪt] *n* Sulfat *nt*.
sulfate-binding protein sulfatbindendes Protein *nt*.
sul·fat·e·mia [,sʌlfer'ti:mɪə] *n* Sulfatämie *f*.
sul·fa·thi·a·zole [,sʌlfə'θaɪəzəʊl] *n pharm*. Sulfathiazol *nt*.
sul·fat·i·dase [sʌl'fætɪdeɪz] *n* Arylsulfatase *f*.
sul·fa·tide ['sʌlfətaɪd] *n* Sulfatid *nt*.
sulfatide lipidosis → sulfatidosis.
sul·fa·ti·do·sis [sʌl,fætɪ'dəʊsɪs] *n* metachromatische Leukodystrophie/Leukoenzephalopathie *f*, Sulfatidlipidose *f*.
sul·fa·tion factor [sʌl'feɪʃn] → somatomedin.
sulf·he·mo·glo·bin [sʌlf'hi:məɡləʊbɪn, -'heməə-] *n* Sulfhämoglobin *nt*.
sulf·he·mo·glo·bin·e·mia [-,hi:məɡləʊbɪ'ni:mɪə] *n* Sulfhämoglobinämie *f*.
sulf·hy·dric acid [-'haɪdrɪk] Schwefelwasserstoff *m*.
sulf·hy·dryl [-'haɪdrɪl] *n* Sulfhydryl-, SH-Radikal *nt*.
sul·fide ['sʌlfaɪd] *n* Sulfid *nt*.
sul·fin·ic acid [sʌl'fɪnɪk] Sulfinsäure *f*.
sul·fin·pyr·a·zone [,sʌlfɪn'pɪərəzəʊn, -'paɪr-] *n pharm*. Sulfinpyrazon *nt*.
sul·fi·nyl ['sʌlfənɪl] *n* Sulfinyl-(Radikal *nt*).
sul·fi·som·i·dine [,sʌlfɪ'sɑmədi:n] *n pharm*. Sulfisomidin *nt*.
sul·fi·sox·a·zole [,sʌlfɪ'zɑksəzəʊl] *n pharm*. Sulfisoxazol *nt*.
sul·fite ['sʌlfaɪt] *n* Sulfit *nt*.
sulfite oxidase Sulfitoxidase *f*.
sulfite reductase Sulfitreduktase *f*.
sulf·met·he·mo·glo·bin [sʌlf,met'hi:məɡləʊbɪn, -'heməə-] *n* → sulfhemoglobin.
sulfo- *pref*. Schwefel-, Sulfon-, Sulf(o)-.
sul·fo·ac·id [,sʌlfəʊ'æsɪd] *n* → sulfonic acid.
sul·fo·bro·mo·phthal·ein [,-,brəʊməʊ-'(f)θæli:n, -li:ɪn] *n* Bromsulfalein *nt*, Bromsulphthalein *nt*, Bromthalein *nt*, Bromsulfophthalein *nt abbr*. BSP.
sul·fo·cy·a·nate [,-'saɪəneɪt, -nɪt] *n* Thiocyanat *nt*.

sul·fo·cy·an·ic acid [,-saɪ'ænɪk] Thiocyansäure *f*, Rhodanwasserstoffsäure *f*.
sul·fo·gel ['-dʒel] *n* Sulfogel *nt*.
sul·fo·id·u·ron·ate sulfatase [,-,aɪdjə-'rɑneɪt] Iduronatsulfatsulfatase *f*.
sul·fo·lip·id [,-'lɪpɪd] *n* Sulfolipid *nt*.
sul·fol·y·sis [sʌl'fɑləsɪs] *n chem*. Sulfolyse *f*.
sul·fo·mu·cin [,sʌlfə'mju:sɪn] *n* Sulfomuzin *nt*, -mucin *nt*.
sul·fon·a·mide [sʌl'fɑnəmaɪd, sʌl'fəʊ-, -mɪd] *n pharm*. Sulfonamid *nt*.
sulfonamide antagonist *p*-Aminobenzoesäure *f*, para-Aminobenzoesäure *f*, Paraaminobenzoesäure *f abbr*. PABA, PAB.
sul·fon·am·i·do·cho·lia [,sʌlfəʊn,æmɪdəʊ-'kəʊlɪə] *n* Sulfonamidausscheidung *f* in der Galle.
sul·fon·am·i·do·ther·a·py [,-,æmɪdəʊ'θerəpɪ] *n* Behandlung *f* mit Sulfonamiden.
sul·fon·am·i·du·ria [,-,æmɪ'd(j)ʊərɪə] *n* Sulfonamidausscheidung *f* im Harn.
sul·fo·nate ['sʌlfəneɪt] **I** *n* Sulfonat *nt*. **II** *vt* sulfonieren, sulfurieren.
sul·fo·nat·ed ['-neɪtɪd] *adj* sulfoniert, sulfuriert.
sulfonated bitumen Ammonium bitumosulfonicum/sulfoichthyolicum, Ichthammol *nt*.
sul·fone ['sʌlfəʊn] *n* **1.** Sulfon *nt*. **2.** Sulfon--Gruppe *f*.
sul·fon·ic acid [sʌl'fɑnɪk] Sulfonsäure *f*.
sul·fo·nyl ['sʌlfənɪl] *n* Sulfonyl-(Radikal *nt*).
sulfonyl urea *pharm*. Sulfonylharnstoff *m*.
sul·fo·sal·i·cyl·ic acid [,sʌlfəʊ,sælə'sɪlɪk] Sulfosalizylsäure *f*.
sulfosalicylic acid turbidity test Sulfosalizylsäure-Probe *f*.
sul·fo·trans·fer·ase [,-'trænsfəreɪz] *n* Sulfotransferase *f*.
sulf·ox·ide [sʌl'fɑksaɪd] *n* **1.** Sulfoxid-(Radikal *nt*). **2.** Sulfoxid *nt*.
sul·fur ['sʌlfər] *n abbr*. **S** *chem*. Schwefel *m*, Sulfur *nt abbr*. S.
sul·fu·rat·ed ['sʌlfjəreɪtɪd] *adj* schwefelhaltig.
sulfur bacteria *micro*. Schwefelbakterien *pl*.
sulfur dioxide Schwefeldioxid *nt*.
sul·fu·ret ['sʌlfjəret] *n* → sulfide.
sul·fu·ret·ed [-retɪd] *adj* schwefelhaltig.
sulfur granules *patho*. (Strahlenpilz-)Drusen *pl*.
sul·fu·ric acid [sʌl'fjʊərɪk] Schwefelsäure *f*.
sulfuric group Schwefelsäure-Rest *m*.
sul·fu·rize ['sʌlf(j)əraɪz] *vt* mit Schwefel verbinden, verschwefeln.
sul·fu·rous acid [sʌlfərəs, -fjʊərəs] schweflige Säure *f*.
sulfurous anhydride → sulfur dioxide.
sulfurous oxide → sulfur dioxide.
sul·fur·yl ['sʌlf(j)ərɪl] *n* Sulfuryl-, SO₂-Radikal *nt*.
sul·fy·dryl [sʌl'faɪdrɪl] *n* → sulfhydryl.
sul·in·dac [sʌl'ɪndæk] *n pharm*. Sulindac *nt*.
Sulkowitch ['sʌlkəʊwɪtʃ]: **S.'s test** Sulkowitch-Probe *f*.
sul·lage ['sʌlɪdʒ] *n* **1.** Abwasser *nt*, Jauche *f*. **2.** Schlamm *m*, Ablagerung *f*.
sul·oc·ti·dil [sʌl'ɑktədɪl] *n pharm*. Suloctidil *nt*.
sulph(o)- *pref*. → sulfo-.
sul·pi·ride [sʌl'pɪraɪd] *n pharm*. Sulpirid *nt*.
sul·pros·tone [sʌl'prɑstəʊn] *n pharm*. Sulproston *nt*.
sul·thi·ame [sʌl'θaɪeɪm] *n pharm*. Sultiam *nt*.
Sulzberger-Garbe [sʌlts'bɜrɡər 'ɡɑrbɪ]: **S.-G. disease/syndrome** exsudative diskoide lichenoide Dermatitis *f*, oid-oid disease (*nt*).

su·mac *n* → sumach.
su·mach ['su:mæk, 'ʃu:-] *n* Sumach *m*.
sum·ma·tion [sə'meɪʃn] *n* **1.** (Auf-)Summierung *f*, Summation *f*, Aufrechnung *f*. **2.** (Gesamt-)Summe *f*.
summation beat *card*. Kombinationssystole *f*.
summation gallop *card*. Summationsgalopp *m*.
sum·mer cholera ['sʌmər] Sommercholera *f*, Cholera aestiva.
summer complaint → summer cholera.
summer diarrhea Sommerdiarrhö *f*.
summer encephalitis japanische B-Enzephalitis *f abbr*. JBE, Encephalitis japonica B.
summer eruption → summer prurigo of Hutchinson 1.
summer minor illness Sommergrippe *f*.
summer prurigo → summer prurigo of Hutchinson 1.
s. of Hutchinson 1. polymorphe Lichtdermatose (Haxthausen) *f*, polymorpher Lichtausschlag *m*, Lichtekzem *nt*, Sommerprurigo *f*, Lupus erythematodes-artige Lichtdermatose *f*, Prurigo aestevalis, Eccema solare, Dermatopathia photoelectrica. **2.** Sommerprurigo Hutchinson *f*, Hidroa vacciniformia/aestivalia/vacciniformis, Hydroa aestivale/vacciniforme, Dermatopathia photogenica.
summer rash *derm*. Roter Hund *m*, tropische Flechte *f*, Miliaria rubra.
sum·mit ['sʌmɪt] *n* (höchster) Gipfel *m*, Spitze *f*.
s. of bladder Apex vesicae/vesicalis.
s. of nose Nasenwurzel *f*, Radix nasi/nasalis.
sump drain [sʌmp] *chir*. doppellumige Drainage *f*.
sun·burn ['sʌnbɜrn] *n* Sonnenbrand *m*, Dermatitis solaris.
sun·flow·er cataract ['sʌnflaʊər] *ophthal*. Sonnenblumenstar *m*.
sun·light ['sʌnlaɪt] *n* Sonnenlicht *nt*.
sun·ray pattern ['sʌnreɪ] *radiol*. (*Knochen*) Spikulaebildung *f*, Sonnenstrahlenprotuberanzen *pl*.
sun stroke → sunstroke.
sun·stroke ['sʌnstrəʊk] *n* Sonnenstich *m*, Heliosis *f*.
super- *pref*. Über-, Super-, Hyper-.
su·per·ab·duc·tion [,su:pəræb'dʌkʃn] *n* extreme/übermäßige Abduktion *f*.
su·per·ac·id [,-'æsɪd] *adj* übermäßig sauer, hyperazid.
su·per·a·cid·i·ty [,-ə'sɪdətɪ] *n* Hyperazidität *f*, Hyperchlorhydrie *f*.
su·per·a·cro·mi·al [,-ə'krəʊmɪəl] *adj* → supra-acromial.
su·per·ac·tiv·i·ty [,-æk'tɪvətɪ] *n* übermäßige Aktivität *f*, Hyperaktivität *f*.
su·per·a·cute [,-ə'kju:t] *adj* perakut.
su·per·al·i·men·ta·tion [,-,ælɪmen'teɪʃn] *n* **1.** Übererernährung *f*, Hyperalimentation *f*. **2.** hochkalorische Ernährung *f*, Hyperalimentation *f*.
su·per·al·ka·lin·i·ty [,-,ælkə'lɪnətɪ] *n* übermäßige Alkalität *f*, Hyperalkalität *f*.
su·per·a·nal [,-'eɪnl] *adj* → supra-anal.
su·per·car·bon·ate [,-'kɑrbəneɪt, -nɪt] Bikarbonat *nt*, Bicarbonat *nt*, Hydrogencarbonat *nt*.
su·per·cil·i·ar·y [,-'sɪlɪ,erɪ] *adj* Augenbraue/Supercilium betr., superziliär.
superciliary arch Augenbrauenbogen *m*, Arcus superciliaris.
superciliary corrugator muscle Korrugator *m* supercilii, M. corrugator supercilii.
superciliary depressor muscle Depressor *m* supercilii/glabellae, M. depressor supercilii.

supercilium

su·per·cil·i·um [ˌ-'sɪliəm] *n, pl* **-cil·ia** [-'sɪliə] 1. Augenbraue *f*, Supercilium *nt*. 2. ~lia *pl* Augenbrauenhaare *pl*, Superzilien *pl*.
su·per·class ['klɑːs, -klæs] *n bio.* Überklasse *f*.
su·per·coil ['-kɔɪl] *n genet.* Superschraube *f*, Supercoil *f*.
su·per·coil·ing]ˌ-'kɔɪlɪŋ] *n genet.* Supercoiling *nt*.
su·per·dis·ten·tion [ˌ-dɪs'tenʃn] *n* übermäßige Dehnung *f*.
su·per·e·go [ˌ-'iːgəʊ, -'egəʊ] *n, pl* **-gos** *psycho.* Über-Ich *nt*, Superego *nt*.
su·per·ex·ci·ta·tion [ˌ-eksaɪ'teɪʃn] *n* extreme/übermäßige Erregung *f*, Übererregung *f*, Hyperexzitation *f*.
su·per·ex·tend·ed [ˌ-ɪk'stendɪd] *adj* übermäßig gedehnt, überdehnt.
su·per·ex·ten·sion [ˌ-ɪk'stenʃn] *n* übermäßige Dehnung *f*, Überdehnung *f*.
su·per·fam·i·ly ['-fæməlɪ] *n bio.* Überfamilie *f*.
su·per·fe·cun·da·tion [ˌ-ˌfiːkən'deɪʃn, -ˌfe-] *n bio., embryo.* Überschwängerung *f*, Superfekundation *f*, Superfecundatio *f*.
su·per·fe·male [ˌ-'fiːmeɪl] *n genet.* Überweibchen *nt*, Superfemale *f*.
su·per·fe·ta·tion [ˌ-fi'teɪʃn] *n bio., embryo.* Überbefruchtung *f*, Superfetation *f*, Superfetatio *f*.
su·per·fi·cial [ˌ-'fɪʃl] *adj* 1. oberflächlich, oben od. außen (liegend), äußerlich, äußere(r, s), superfiziell, (Ober-)Flächen-. 2. *fig.* oberflächlich.
superficial abscess oberflächlicher Abszeß *m*.
superficial branch: s. of lateral plantar nerve oberflächlicher Ast *m* des N. plantaris lateralis, Ramus superficialis n. plantaris lateralis.
s. of medial plantar artery oberflächlicher Ast *m* der A. plantaris medialis, Ramus superficialis a. plantaris medialis.
s. of radial nerve oberflächlicher Radialisast *m*, Ramus superficialis n. radialis.
s. of superior gluteal artery oberflächlicher Ast *m* der A. glut(a)ea superior, Ramus superficialis a. glut(a)eae superioris.
s. of transverse cervcial artery oberflächliche Halsarterie *f*, Cervicalis *f* superficialis, A. cervicalis superficialis, Ramus superficialis a. transversae colli.
s. of ulnar nerve oberflächlicher Ulnarisast *m*, Ramus superficialis n. ulnaris.
superficial burn Verbrennung *f* 1. Grades.
superficial bursa of olecranon → subcutaneous bursa of olecranon.
superficial calcaneal bursitis Achillobursitis *f*.
superficial carcinoma oberflächliches Karzinom *nt*, Oberflächenkarzinom *nt*.
superficial cleavage superfizielle Furchung(steilung *f*) *f*.
superficial fascia 1. oberflächliche Unterhautfascie *f*, Fascia superficialis. **2.** Unterhaut *f*, Subkutis *f*, Tela subcutanea.
superficial head of flexor pollicis brevis muscle Caput superficiale.
superficial implantation *gyn., embryo.* oberflächliche/superfizielle Einnistung/Implantation *f*.
superficial laceration (oberflächliche) Abschürfung *f*.
superficial lamina of levator muscle of upper eye lid oberflächliches Blatt *nt* der Levatorsehne, Lamina superficialis m. levatores palpebrae superioris.
superficial layer of levator muscle of upper eye lid → superficial lamina of levator muscle of upper eye lid.
superficial line of the cornea → Stähli's (pigment) line.

superficial measure → square measure.
superficial muscles oberflächliche Muskeln *pl*/Muskulatur *f*.
superficial mycosis Pilzerkrankung *f* der Haut, oberflächliche Mykose *f*, Dermatomykose *f*, Dermatomycosis *f*.
superficial necrosis oberflächliche Knochennekrose *f*.
superficial pain Oberflächenschmerz *m*.
superficial part: s. of external sphincter (muscle) of anus Pars superficialis.
s. of parotid gland Pars superficialis gl. parotideae.
superficial portion of parotid gland → superficial part of parotid gland.
superficial punctate keratitis Keratitis superficialis punctata.
superficial pustular perifolliculitis Staphyloderma follicularis, Ostiofolliculitis/Ostiofolliculitis/Impetigo Bockhart, Impetigo follicularis Bockhart, Folliculitis staphylogenes superficialis, Folliculitis pustolosa, Staphylodermia Bockhart.
superficial reflex oberflächlicher Reflex *m*.
superficial sensation Oberflächensensibilität *f*.
superficial skin pain Oberflächenschmerz *m* der Haut.
superficial spreading melanoma *abbr.* SSM oberflächlich/superfiziell spreitendes Melanom *nt abbr.* SSM, pagetoides malignes Melanom *nt*.
superficial vein oberflächliche Vene *f*, V. superficialis.
s.s of head oberflächliche Kopfvenen *pl*.
s.s of inferior limbs Vv. superficiales membri inferioris.
s.s of superior limbs Vv. superficiales membri superioris.
su·per·flex·ion [ˌ-'flekʃn] *n* übermäßige Beugung *f*, Hyperflexion *f*.
su·per·fron·tal fissure [ˌ-'frʌntl] Sulcus frontalis superior.
su·per·func·tion [ˌ-'fʌŋkʃn] *n* Überfunktion *f*, Hyperfunktion *f*.
su·per·gen·u·al [ˌ-'dʒenjəwəl] *adj* oberhalb des Knies (liegend).
su·per·im·preg·na·tion [ˌ-ˌɪmpreg'neɪʃn] *n* → superfetation.
su·per·in·duce [ˌ-ɪn'd(j)uːs] *vt* (noch) hinzufügen, aufpfropfen.
su·per·in·fect·ed [ˌ-ɪn'fektɪd] *adj* superinfiziert.
su·per·in·fec·tion [ˌ-ɪn'fekʃn] *n* Superinfektion *f*.
su·per·in·vo·lu·tion [ˌ-ˌɪnvə'luːʃn] *n* 1. übermäßige Rückbildung/Involution *f*, Superinvolution *f*. 2. *gyn.* Superinvolutio uteri.
su·pe·ri·or [suː'pɪərɪər] *adj* 1. höhere(r, s), obere(r, s), höher- *od.* weiter oben liegend, superior, Ober-. 2. (*Qualität*) überragend; überlegen, besser (*to* als); hervoragend. 3. größer, stärker (*to* als).
superior angle: anterior s. of parietal bone Angulus frontalis (ossis parietalis).
posterior s. of parietal bone Angulus occipitalis (ossis parietalis).
s. of scapula Angulus superior (scapulae).
superior aperture: s. of minor pelvis Eingang *m* des kleinen Beckens, Apertura pelvis/pelvica superior.
s. of thorax obere Thoraxapertur *f*, Brustkorbeingang *m*, A. thoracis superior.
s. of tympanic canaliculus innere Öffnung *f* des Canaliculus tympanicus, Apertura superior canaliculi tympanici.
superior border: s. of scapula Skapulaoberrand *m*, Margo superior scapulae.
s. of spleen oberer Milzrand *m*, Margo superior lienis/splenis.

superior branch: s. of oculomotor nerve oberer Okulomotoriusast *m*, Ramus superior n. oculomotorii.
s. of superior gluteal artery oberer Ast *m* der A. glut(a)ea superior, Ramus superior a. glut(a)eae superioris.
s.es of transverse cervical nerve *pl* obere Äste *pl* des N. transversus colli, Rami superiores n. transversi colli.
s. of vestibular nerve oberer Teil *m* des N. vestibularis, Pars rostralis/superior n. vestibularis.
superior bulb of jugular vein Bulbus superius v. jugularis.
superior bursa of biceps femoris muscle Bursa m. bicipitis femoris superior.
superior cerebellar artery syndrome Arteria-superior-cerebelli-Syndrom *nt*.
superior colliculus oberer/vorderer Hügel *m* der Vierhügelplatte, Colliculus cranialis/rostralis/superior.
superior concha obere Nasenmuschel *f*, Concha nasalis superior.
superior crus: s. of cerebellum Pedunculus cerebellaris superior.
s. of subcutaneous inguinal ring Crus mediale anuli inguinalis superficialis.
superior extremity: s. of kidney oberer Nierenpol *m*, Extremitas superior renis.
s. of testis oberer Hodenpol *m*, Extremitas superior testis.
superior fascia: s. of pelvic diaphragm Fascia diaphragmatis pelvis superior.
s. of urogenital diaphragm Fascia diaphragmatis urogenitalis superior.
superior fossa of omental sac Rec. superior omentalis.
superior fovea Fovea superior.
superior ganglion: s. of glossopharyngeal nerve Müller'-Ganglion *nt*, Ehrenritter'-Ganglion *nt*, oberes Glossopharyngeusganglion *nt*, Ggl. rostralis/superius n. glossopharyngei.
s. of vagus nerve oberes Vagusganglion *nt*, Ggl. rostralis/superius n. vagi.
superior hemorrhagic polioencephalitis Wernicke-Syndrom *nt*, -Enzephalopathie *f*, Polioencephalitis haemorrhagica superior (Wernicke).
superior horn of saphenous opening Cornu superius hiatus saphenus.
su·pe·ri·or·i·ty complex [səˌpɪərɪ'ɔrətɪ] *psycho.* Überlegenheits-, Superioritätskomplex *m*.
superior ligament: s. of incus oberes Incusband *nt*, Lig. incudis superius.
s. of malleus oberes Malleusband *nt*, Lig. mallei superius.
s. of pinna Lig. auriculare superius.
superior limbs obere Gliedmaßen/Extremitäten *pl*, Arme *pl*.
superior lingular segment (of lung) (*Lunge*) oberes Lingularsegment *nt*, Segmentum lingulare superius [S. IV].
superior lip Oberlippe *f*, Labium superius oris.
s. of ileocecal valve Labium superius valvulae coli.
superior margin: s. of pancreas oberer Pankreasrand *m*, Margo superior pancreatis.
s. of parietal bone Margo sagittalis ossis parietalis.
s. of scapula → superior border of scapula.
s. of spleen → superior border of spleen.
s. of suprarenal gland Margo superior gl. suprarenalis.
superior mediastinum oberer Mediastinalraum *m*, oberes Mediastinum *nt*, Mediastinum superius, Cavum mediastinale superius.

superior mesenteric artery syndrome Arteria-mesenterica-superior-Kompressionssyndrom *nt*, arteriomesenterialer Duodenalverschluß *m*.
superior nodes, central obere Mesenteriallymphknoten *pl*, Nodi lymphatici mesenterici superiores, Nodi superiores centrales.
superior opening of pelvis Beckeneingang *m*, Apertura pelvis/pelvica superior.
superior orbital fissure syndrome Fissura-orbitalis-superior-Syndrom *nt*.
superior part of duodenum oberer horizontaler Duodenumabschnitt *m*, Pars superior duodeni.
superior pulmonary sulcus tumor Pancoast-Tumor *m*, apikaler Sulkustumor *m*.
superior ramus of pubis oberer Schambeinast *m*, Ramus superior ossis pubis.
superior recess of tympanic membrane Prussak'-Raum *m*, Rec. (membranae tympanicae) superior.
superior root: s. of ansa cervicalis obere/hintere Wurzel *f* der Ansa cervicalis, Radix superior/posterior ansae cervicalis.
s. of cervial loop → s. of ansa cervicalis.
s. of vestibulocochlear nerve oberer vestibulärer Anteil *m* des N. vestibulocochlearis, Pars superior/vestibularis n. vestibulocochlearis.
superior segment → superior segment of lung.
s. of kidney Segmentum superius.
s. of lung (*Lunge*) Spitzensegment *nt* des Unterlappens, Segmentum apicale/superius [S. VI].
superior strait Beckeneingang *m*, Apertura pelvis superior.
superior sulcus tumor Pancoast-Tumor *m*, apikaler Sulkustumor *m*.
superior sulcus tumor syndrome Pancoast-Syndrom *nt*.
superior tarsus Knorpelplatte *f* des Oberlids, Tarsus superior (palpebrae).
superior tracheotomy obere Tracheotomie *f*.
superior trunk of brachial plexus oberer Primärfaszikel *m* (des Plexus brachialis), Truncus superior (plexus brachialis).
superior tubercle of Henle Tuberculum obturatorium posterius.
superior vein: s.s of cerebellar hemisphere Vv. hemisphaerii (cerebelli) superiores, Vv. superiores cerebelli.
s. of vermis obere Kleinhirnwurm-/Vermisvene *f*, V. vermis superior, V. superior vermis.
superior vena cava syndrome Vena-cava-superior-Syndrom *nt*.
superior wing of sphenoid bone kleiner Keilbeinflügel *m*, Ala minor (ossis sphenoidalis).
su·per·ja·cent [ˌsuːpərˈdʒeɪznt] *adj* darauf-, darüberliegend.
su·per·lac·ta·tion [ˌ-lækˈteɪʃn] *n gyn.* verstärkte u. verlängerte Milchsekretion *f*, Hyper-, Superlaktation *f*.
su·per·le·thal [ˌ-ˈliːθəl] *adj* superletal.
su·per·mo·til·i·ty [ˌ-məʊˈtɪlətɪ] *n* exessive Beweglichkeit/Motilität *f*, Hypermotilität *f*.
su·per·nu·mer·ar·y [ˌ-ˈn(j)uːmərˌrerɪː, -rərɪ] **I** *n, pl* **-ar·ies** Zusatzperson *nt*, Supernumerar *m*, Hilfskraft *f*. **II** *adj* zusätzlich, überzählig, extra.
supernumerary bone überzähliger Knochen *m*.
supernumerary breast zusätzliche/akzessorische Brustdrüsen *pl*, Mammae aberrantes/accessoriae/erraticae.

supernumerary chromosome überzähliges Chromosom *nt*.
supernumerary kidney überzählige/akzessorische Niere *f*.
supernumerary nipple(s) akzessorische Brustwarze(n *pl*) *f*, Polythelie *f*.
supernumerary placenta 1. akzessorische Planzenta *f*, Placenta accessoria. **2.** Nebenplazenta *f*, Placenta succenturiata.
su·per·nu·tri·tion [ˌ-n(j)uːˈtrɪʃn] *n* Überernährung *f*, Hyperalimentation *f*.
su·per·oc·cip·i·tal [ˌ-ɑkˈsɪpɪtl] *adj* → supraoccipital.
su·per·o·lat·er·al [ˌsuːpərəʊˈlætərəl] *adj anat.* oben u. auf der Seite (liegend), superolateral.
su·per·or·der [ˈsuːpərˌɔːrdər] *n bio.* Überordnung *f*.
su·per·ov·u·la·tion [ˌ-ˌɑvjəˈleɪʃn] *n gyn.* Superovulation *f*.
su·per·ox·ide [ˌ-ˈɑksaɪd, -sɪd] *n chem.* Super-, Hyper-, Peroxid *nt*.
superoxide dismutase *abbr.* **SOD** Hyperoxiddismutase *f*, Superoxiddismutase *f abbr.* SOD, Hämocuprein *nt*, Erythrocuprein *nt*.
superoxide radical Hyperoxidradikal *nt*.
su·per·par·a·site [ˌ-ˈpærəsaɪt] *n* **1.** Superparasit *m*. **2.** Über-, Sekundär-, Hyperparasit *m*.
su·per·phos·phate [ˌ-ˈfɑsfeɪt] *n chem.* Superphosphat *nt*.
su·per·pig·men·ta·tion [ˌ-ˌpɪgmənˈteɪʃn] *n* vermehrte Pigmentierung *f*, Hyperpigmentierung *f*.
su·per·pose [ˈ-pəʊz] *vt* **1.** (auf-)legen, lagern, schichten; übereinander anordnen, übereinanderlegen, -schichten, -lagern. **2.** *mathe.* übereinander lagern, superponieren. **3.** *phys.* überlagern, superponieren.
su·per·po·si·tion [ˌ-pəˈzɪʃn] *n* **1.** Aufschichtung *f*, -lagerung *f*; Aufeinander-, Übereinandersetzen *nt*. **2.** *mathe.* Superposition *f*. **3.** *phys.* Überlagerung *f*, Superposition *f*.
su·per·sat·u·rate [ˌ-ˈsætʃəreɪt] *vt chem., physiol.* übersättigen.
su·per·sat·u·ra·tion [ˌ-ˌsætʃəˈreɪʃn] *n chem., physiol.* Übersättigung *f*.
su·per·se·cre·tion [ˌ-sɪˈkriːʃn] *n* übermäßige Sekretion *f*, Super-, Hypersekretion *f*.
su·per·sen·si·tive [ˌ-ˈsensɪtɪv] *adj* überempfindlich; allergisch.
su·per·sen·si·tiv·i·ty [ˌ-ˌsensəˈtɪvətɪ] *n* Überempfindlichkeit *f*, Hyper-, Supersensitivität *f*.
su·per·son·ic [ˌ-ˈsɑnɪk] *adj* **1.** supersonisch, Überschall-. **2.** Ultraschall-.
su·per·struc·ture [ˌ-ˈstrʌktʃər] *n* Oberbau *m*, Aufbau *m*.
su·per·tem·po·ral fissure [ˌ-ˈtemp(ə)rəl] Sulcus temporalis superior.
su·per·vi·ta·min·o·sis [ˌ-ˌvaɪtəmɪˈnəʊsɪs] *n* Hypervitaminose *f*.
su·per·volt·age [ˌ-ˈvəʊltɪdʒ] *n phys.* Hochspannung *f*.
supervoltage radiotherapy Supervolt-, Hochvolt-, Megavolttherapie *f*.
su·pi·nate [ˈs(j)uːpɪneɪt] *vt* supinieren, auswärtsdrehen (*um die Längsachse*).
su·pi·na·tion [ˌ-ˈneɪʃn] *n* Auswärtsdrehung *f* (*um die Längsachse*), Supination *f*.
supination reflex → supinator reflex.
su·pi·na·tor [ˈ-neɪtər] *n* Supinator *M*, M. supinator.
supinator crest Crista m. supinatoris.
supinator longus reflex → supinator reflex.
supinator muscle → supinator.
supinator reflex Supinatorreflex *m*.
su·pine [suːˈpaɪn, su-] *adj* supiniert, auf dem Rücken liegend.

suppurative inflammation

supine position Rückenlage *f*.
sup·port [səˈpɔːrt] **I** *n* **1.** Stütze *f*; Halter *m*, Träger *m*; Stützapparat *m*, -vorrichtung *f*; (*Schuh*) Einlage *f*. **2.** *fig.* Stütze *f*, Unterstützung *f*, Beistand *m*, Hilfe *f*. **3.** (Lebens-)Unterhalt *m*. **II** *vt* **4.** tragen, (ab-)stützen. **5.** jdn. unterstützen, jdm. beistehen. **6.** unter-, erhalten, ernähren.
sup·port·ing [səˈpɔːrtɪŋ] *adj* (unter-)stützend, tragend, Stütz-, Trag-, Unterstützungs-.
supporting cell Stützzelle *f*.
s.s of Hensen Hensen'-Zellen *pl*, -Stützzellen *pl*.
supporting reactions Stützreaktionen *pl*, -reflexe *pl*.
negative s. negative Stützreaktionen *pl*.
positive s. positive Stützreaktionen *pl*.
supporting reflexes → supporting reactions.
supporting tissue Stützgewebe *nt*.
sup·pos·i·to·ry [səˈpɑzɪtɔːrɪ, -təʊ-] *n, pl* **-ries** *pharm.* Zäpfchen *nt*, Suppositorium *nt*.
sup·press [səˈpres] *vt* **1.** (*a. Gefühle*) unterdrücken. **2.** etw. zum Stillstand bringen, hemmen, supprimieren; (*Blutung*) stillen; (*Durchfall*) stoppen; (*Harn, Stuhl*) verhalten. **3.** *psycho.* verdrängen.
sup·pres·sant [səˈpresənt] **I** *n* Hemmer *m*, Suppressor *m*. **II** *adj* hemmend, unterdrückend.
sup·press·i·ble [səˈpresɪbl] *adj* unterdrückbar.
sup·pres·sion [səˈpreʃn] *n* **1.** (*a. Gefühle*) Unterdrückung *f*, Hemmung *f*, Suppression *f*. **2.** (Blut-)Stillung *f*; Stopfung *f*; (Harn-, Stuhl-)Verhaltung *f*. **3.** *psycho.* Verdrängung *f*. **4.** *genet.* → suppression mutation.
suppression mutation *genet.* Suppressions-, Suppressormutation *f*, kompensierende Mutation *f*.
sup·pres·sive [səˈpresɪv] *adj* unterdrückend, repressiv, Unterdrückungs-; hemmend; verstopfend.
sup·pres·sor [səˈpresər] *n* Hemmer *m*, Suppressor *m*.
suppressor cells (T-)Suppressor-Zellen *pl*.
suppressor gene Suppressorgen *nt*.
sup·pu·rant [ˈsʌpjərənt] **I** *n* Eiterung-auslösendes Mittel *nt*. **II** *adj* Eiterung/Eiterbildung auslösend.
sup·pu·ran·tia [ˌ-ˈrænʃɪə] *pl* Suppurantia *pl*.
sup·pu·ra·tion [ˌ-ˈreɪʃn] *n* Eiterbildung *f*, Vereiterung *f*, Eiterung *f*, Suppuration *f*, Suppuratio *f*.
sup·pu·ra·tive [ˈ-reɪtɪv] *adj* eiterbildend, eiternd, eitrig, suppurativ, purulent.
suppurative appendicitis eitrige Appendizitis *f*, Appendicitis purulenta.
suppurative arthritis akut-eitrige Gelenkentzündung/Arthritis *f*, Gelenkeiterung *f*, Gelenkempyem *nt*, Pyarthrose *f*, Arthritis purulenta.
acute s. → suppurative arthritis.
suppurative cerebritis phlegmonöse Enzephalitis *f*.
suppurative cholangitis eitrige Cholangitis *f*.
suppurative choroiditis *ophthal.* eitrige Chorioiditis *f*, Chorioiditis purulenta/suppurativa.
suppurative coxitis *ortho.* eitrige Koxitis *f*, Coxitis purulenta.
suppurative encephalitis eitrige Enzephalitis *f*, Encephalitis purulenta; Hirnabszeß *m*.
suppurative inflammation eitrige Entzündung *f*.

suppurative keratitis

suppurative keratitis *ophthal.* eitrige Keratitis *f*, Keratitis purulenta/suppurativa.
suppurative mastitis *gyn.* eitrige Mastitis *f*.
suppurative necrosis eitrige/purulente Nekrose *f*.
suppurative nephritis eitrige Nephritis *f*.
suppurative pericarditis eitrige Herzbeutelentzündung/Perikarditis *f*, Pericarditis purulenta.
suppurative phlebitis eitrige Venenentzündung/Phlebitis *f*.
suppurative pleurisy 1. eitrige Brustfellentzündung/Pleuritis *f*, Pleuritis purulenta. **2.** Thoraxempyem *nt*.
suppurative pneumonia eitrige Pneumonie *f*.
suppurative retinitis eitrige Retinitis *f*.
suppurative synovitis → suppurative arthritis.
supra- *pref.* Über-, Ober-, Supra-.
supra-acetabular *adj* oberhalb des Azetabulums (liegend), supraazetabulär.
supra-acetabular sulcus Sulcus supraacetabularis.
supra-acromial *adj* über dem Akromion (liegend), supraakromial.
supra-anal *adj* über dem Anus (liegend), supraanal.
su·pra·an·co·ne·al [ˌsuːprænˈkəʊnɪəl] *adj* oberhalb des Ell(en)bogens (liegend), suprakubital.
supraanconeal bursa, intratendinous Bursa intratendinea olecrani.
supra-arytenoid cartilage Cartilago corniculata.
supra-auricular *adj* über dem Ohr (liegend), supraaurikulär.
supra-axillary *adj* oberhalb der Achselhöhle (liegend), supraaxillär.
su·pra·cal·lo·sal gyrus [ˌkæˈləʊsəl, -kə-] Indusium griseum.
su·pra·car·di·ac [ˌˈkɑːrdiæk] *adj* oberhalb des Herzens (liegend), suprakardial.
su·pra·car·di·al [ˌˈkɑːrdɪəl] *adj* → supracardiac.
supracardial body Paraganglion supracardiale.
supracardial paraganglion Paraganglion supracardiale.
su·pra·car·di·nal veins [ˌ-ˈkɑːrdɪnl] *embryo.* Suprakardinalvenen *pl*.
su·pra·cer·vi·cal hysterectomy [ˌ-ˈsɜːrvɪkl] → subtotal hysterectomy.
su·pra·cho·ri·oid layer [ˌ-ˈkɔːrɪɔɪd, -ˈkəʊr-] → suprachoroid lamina.
su·pra·cho·roi·dea [ˌ-kəˈrɔɪdɪə] *n* → suprachoroid lamina.
su·pra·cho·roid lamina [ˌ-ˈkəʊrɔɪd, -ˈkɔːr-] Lamina suprachoroidea.
suprachoroid layer → suprachoroid lamina.
su·pra·cil·i·ar·y [ˌ-ˈsɪlɪˌeriː, -ˈsɪlɪəri] *adj* → superciliary.
su·pra·cla·vic·u·lar [ˌ-kləˈvɪkjələr] *adj* oberhalb des Schlüsselbeins/der Klavikula (liegend), supraklavikulär.
supraclavicular fossa: greater s. große Schlüsselbeingrube *f*, Fossa supraclavicularis major.
lesser s. kleine Schlüsselbeingrube *f*, Fossa supraclavicularis minor.
supraclavicular nerves supraklavikuläre Hautnerven *pl*, Nn. supraclaviculares.
anterior s. → medial s.
intermediate s. Nn. supraclaviculares intermedii.
lateral s. Nn. supraclaviculares laterales/posteriores.
medial s. Nn. supraclaviculares mediales.
middle s. → intermediate s.
posterior s. → lateral s.

supraclavicular part of brachial plexus supraklavikulärer Teil *m* des Plexus brachialis, Pars supraclavicularis (plexus brachialis).
su·pra·cli·noid aneurysm [ˌ-ˈklaɪnɔɪd] supraclinoidales Aneurysma *nt*.
su·pra·con·dy·lar [ˌ-ˈkɑndɪlə(r)] *adj* oberhalb einer Kondyle (liegend), suprakondylär.
supracondylar crest (of humerus) Crista supracondylaris (humeri).
lateral s. Crista supracondylaris lateralis (humeri).
medial s. Crista supracondylaris medialis (humeri).
supracondylar fracture suprakondyläre Fraktur *f*.
s. of the femur suprakondyläre Oberschenkelfraktur/Femurfraktur.
s. of the humerus suprakondyläre Humerusfraktur.
supracondylar line of femur: lateral s. Linea supracondylaris lateralis (femoris).
medial s. Linea supracondylaris medialis (femoris).
supracondylar process Proc. supracondylaris.
supracondylar ridge of humerus: lateral s. Crista supracondylaris lateralis (humeri).
medial s. Crista supracondylaris medialis (humeri).
su·pra·con·dy·loid [ˌ-ˈkɑndlɔɪd] *adj* → supracondylar.
supracondyloid bursa, internal/medial Bursa subtendinea m. gastrocnemii medialis.
su·pra·cos·tal [ˌ-ˈkɑstl] *adj* über od. auf einer Rippe (liegend), suprakostal.
su·pra·cot·y·loid [ˌ-ˈkɑtlɔɪd] *adj* → supra-acetabular.
su·pra·cra·ni·al [ˌ-ˈkreɪnɪəl] *adj* über dem Schädel/Cranium (liegend), suprakranial.
su·pra·crest·al line [ˌ-ˈkrestl] → supracrestal plane.
supracrestal plane *anat.* Planum supracristale.
su·pra·di·a·phrag·mat·ic diverticulum [ˌ-ˌdaɪəfrægˈmætɪk] epiphrenisches Ösophagusdivertikel *nt*.
su·pra·duc·tion [ˌ-ˈdʌkʃn] *n* Aufwärtswendung *f*, Supraduktion *f*.
su·pra·du·o·de·nal artery [ˌ-ˌd(j)uːəʊˈdiːnl, -d(j)uːˈædnəl] A. supraduodenalis.
su·pra·ep·i·con·dy·lar [ˌ-ˌepɪˈkɑndlər] *adj* supraepikondylär.
su·pra·ep·i·troch·le·ar [ˌ-ˌepɪˈtrɑklɪər] *adj* supraepitrochleär.
su·pra·gin·gi·val calculus [ˌ-dʒɪnˈdʒaɪvl, -ˈdʒɪndʒə-] supragingivaler Zahnstein *m*.
su·pra·gle·noid [ˌ-ˈgliːnɔɪd] *adj* oberhalb der Cavitas glenoidalis (liegend), supraglenoidal.
supraglenoid tubercle/tuberosity Tuberculum supraglenoidale.
su·pra·glot·tic [ˌ-ˈglɑtɪk] *adj* oberhalb der Glottis (liegend), supraglottisch.
supraglottic fracture supraglottische (Knorpel-)Fraktur *f*.
su·pra·he·pat·ic [ˌ-hɪˈpætɪk] *adj* oberhalb der Leber (liegend), suprahepatisch.
suprahepatic abscess suprahepatischer Abszeß *m*.
su·pra·hy·oid [ˌ-ˈhaɪɔɪd] *adj* oberhalb des Zungenbeins/Os hyoideum (liegend), suprahyoidal.
suprahyoid branch of lingual artery Ramus suprahyoideus a. lingualis.
suprahyoid muscles Zungenbeinmuskeln *pl* od -muskulatur *f*, Suprahyoidalmuskulatur *f*, Mm. suprahyoidei.

su·pra·in·gui·nal [ˌ-ˈɪŋgwɪnl] *adj* oberhalb der Leiste (liegend), suprainguinal.
su·pra·in·tes·ti·nal [ˌ-ɪnˈtestɪnl] *adj* supraintestinal.
su·pra·lim·i·nal [ˌ-ˈlɪmɪnl] *adj* überschwellig.
su·pra·lum·bar [ˌ-ˈlʌmbər] *adj* über der Lende(nregion) (liegend), supralumbal.
su·pra·mal·le·o·lar [ˌ-məˈlɪələr] *adj* oberhalb des (Fuß-)Knöchels (liegend), supramalleolär.
su·pra·ma·mil·lar·y commissure [ˌ-ˈmæmɪˌleriː, -ləri] supramamilläre Kommissur *f*, Commissura supramamillaris.
su·pra·mam·ma·ry [ˌ-ˈmæməri] *adj* oberhalb der Brustdrüse (liegend), supramammär.
su·pra·man·dib·u·lar [ˌ-mænˈdɪbjələr] *adj* über dem Unterkiefer (liegend), supramandibulär.
su·pra·mar·gin·al gyrus [ˌ-ˈmɑːrdʒɪnl] Gyrus supramarginalis.
su·pra·mas·toid crest [ˌ-ˈmæstɔɪd] Crista supramastoidea.
supramastoid fossa Foveola suprameatica/supramastoidea.
su·pra·max·il·la [ˌ-mækˈsɪlə] *n* Oberkiefer *m*, Maxilla *f*.
su·pra·max·i·mal [ˌ-ˈmæksɪml] *adj* über-, supramaximal.
su·pra·me·a·tal fossa [ˌ-mɪˈeɪtəl] → supramastoid fossa.
suprameatal pit Foveola suprameatica/suprameatalis.
suprameatal spine Spina suprameatica/suprameatalis.
su·pra·men·tal [ˌ-ˈmentl] *adj* supramental.
su·pra·mo·lec·u·lar [ˌ-məˈlekjələr] *adj* supramolekular.
supramolecular assembly *biochem.* supramolekulare Anordnung *f*.
supramolecular complex supramolekularer Komplex *m*.
su·pra·na·sal [ˌ-ˈneɪzl] *adj* oberhalb der Nase (liegend), supranasal.
su·pra·nu·cle·ar [ˌ-ˈn(j)uːklɪər] *adj* supranukleär.
supranuclear paralysis supranukleäre Lähmung *f*.
su·pra·oc·cip·i·tal [ˌ-ɑkˈsɪpɪtl] *adj* supraokzipital.
su·pra·oc·u·lar [ˌ-ˈɑkjələr] *adj* oberhalb des Auges (liegend), supraokulär.
su·pra·op·tic commissure [ˌ-ˈɑptɪk]: **dorsal s.** Ganser'-Kommissur *f*, Commissura supraoptica dorsalis.
inferior s. Gudden'-Kommissur *f*, Commissura supraoptica ventralis.
superior s. → dorsal s.
ventral s. → inferior s.
supraoptic fibers Fibrae supraopticae.
supraoptic nucleus (of hypothalamus) Nc. supraopticus (hypothalami).
su·pra·op·ti·co·hy·poph·y·si·al tract [ˌ-ˌɑptɪkəʊhaɪˌpɑfəˈsiːəl, -ˌhaɪpəˈfɪːzɪəl] Tractus supraopticohypophysialis.
su·pra·op·ti·mal [ˌ-ˈɑptɪməl] *adj* supraoptimal.
su·pra·or·bit·al [ˌ-ˈɔːrbɪtl] *adj* über/oberhalb der Augenhöhle (liegend), supraorbital.
supraorbital arch of frontal bone Margo supraorbitalis ossis frontalis.
supraorbital artery Supraorbitalarterie *f*, Supraorbitalis *f*, A. supraorbitalis.
supraorbital canal → supraorbital foramen.
supraorbital foramen Inc. supraorbitalis, For. supraorbitale.
supraorbital incisure → supraorbital foramen.

supraorbital margin oberer Augenhöhlenrand *m*, Margo supra-orbitalis.
s. of frontal bone Margo supraorbitalis ossis frontalis.
s. of orbit Margo supraorbitalis orbitae.
supraorbital nerve N. supra-orbitalis.
supraorbital neuralgia Supraorbitalneuralgie *f*.
supraorbital notch → supraorbital foramen.
supraorbital reflex Supraorbitalis-Reflex *m*.
supraorbital region Supraorbitalregion *f*, Regio supraorbitalis.
supraorbital sulcus → supraorbital foramen.
supraorbital vein Supraorbitalvene *f*, V. supraorbitalis.
su·pra·pa·tel·lar [ˌ-pəˈtelər] *adj* oberhalb der Patella (liegend), suprapatellar.
suprapatellar bursa Bursa suprapatellaris.
suprapatellar pouch Rec. suprapatellaris.
suprapatellar reflex Suprapatellarreflex *m*.
su·pra·pel·vic [ˌ-ˈpelvɪk] *adj* oberhalb des Beckens (liegend), suprapelvin.
su·pra·pha·ryn·ge·al bone [ˌ-fəˈrɪndʒɪəl] Keilbein *nt*, Flügelbein *nt*, Os sphenoidale.
su·pra·pin·e·al recess [ˌ-ˈpaɪnɪəl, -ˈpɪn-] Rec. suprapinealis.
su·pra·pir·i·form foramen [ˌ-ˈpɪrəfɔːrm] For. suprapiriforme.
su·pra·pleu·ral membrane [ˌ-ˈpluərəl] Sibson'-Membran *f*, -Faszie *f*, Membrana suprapleuralis.
su·pra·pu·bic [ˌ-ˈpjuːbɪk] *adj* oberhalb des Schambeins (liegend), suprapubisch.
suprapubic cystotomy suprapubischer Blasenschnitt *m*, suprapubische Zystotomie *f*, Epizystotomie *f*.
suprapubic lithotomy hoher Blasenschnitt *m*, Sectio alta.
suprapubic transvesical prostatectomy *urol*. suprapubische transvesikale Prostatektomie *f*.
su·pra·py·lor·ic [ˌ-paɪˈlɔːrɪk, -ˈlɑr-, -pɪ-] *adj* suprapylorisch.
su·pra·re·nal [ˌ-ˈriːnl] **I** *n* Nebenniere *f*, Gl. suprarenalis/adrenalis. **II** *adj* oberhalb der Niere/Ren (liegend), suprarenal.
suprarenal artery: aortic s. → middle s.
inferior s. untere Nebennierenarterie *f*, Suprarenalis *f* inferior, A. suprarenalis inferior.
middle s. mittlere Nebennierenarterie *f*, Suprarenalis *f* media, A. suprarenalis/adrenalis media.
superior s.s obere Nebennierenschlagadern *pl*, -arterien *pl*, Aa. suprarenales/adrenales superiores.
suprarenal body *old* → suprarenal I.
suprarenal capsule → suprarenal I.
su·pra·re·nal·ec·to·my [ˌ-riːnəˈlektəmɪ] *n* Nebennierenentfernung *f*, -resektion *f*, Adrenalektomie *f*, Epinephrektomie *f*.
suprarenal gland Nebenniere *f*, Gl. suprarenalis/adrenalis.
accessory s.s versprengte Nebennierendrüsen *pl*, versprengtes Nebennierengewebe *nt*, Gll. suprarenales/adrenales accessoriae.
suprarenal impression of liver Nebennierenabdruck *m* auf der Leber, Impressio suprarenalis (hepatis).
suprarenal marrow Nebennierenmark *nt abbr*. NNM, Medulla (gl. suprarenalis).
suprarenal medulla → suprarenal marrow.
suprarenal paraganglion Paraganglion suprarenale; Nebennierenmark *nt abbr*. NNM.
suprarenal plexus Nebennierenplexus *m*, Plexus suprarenalis.
suprarenal vein Nebennierenvene *f*, V. suprarenalis.
left s. linke Nebennierenvene, V. suprarenalis sinistra.
right s. rechte Nebennierenvene, V. suprarenalis/adrenalis dextra.
su·pra·rene [ˈ-riːn] *n* → suprarenal I.
su·pra·scap·u·lar [ˌsuːprəˈskæpjələr] *adj* oberhalb der Spina scapulae (liegend), supraskapular.
suprascapular artery Suprascapularis *f*, A. suprascapularis.
suprascapular incisure Inc. scapulae/scapularis.
suprascapular ligament Lig. transversum scapulae superius.
suprascapular nerve Suprascapularis *m*, N. suprascapularis.
suprascapular notch → scapular notch (of scapula).
suprascapular vein V. suprascapularis.
su·pra·scle·ral [ˌ-ˈsklɪərəl] *adj* auf der Sklera (liegend), supraskleral.
su·pra·sel·lar [ˌ-ˈselər] *adj* oberhalb der Sella turcica (liegend), suprasellär.
suprasellar aneurysm supraselläres Aneurysma *nt*.
suprasellar cistern suprasellärer Liquorraum *m*.
suprasellar cyst Erdheim-Tumor *m*, Kraniopharyngiom *nt*.
su·pra·sep·tal [ˌ-ˈseptəl] *adj* supraseptal.
su·pra·spi·nal [ˌ-ˈspaɪnl] *adj* über od. oberhalb der Wirbelsäule (liegend), supraspinal.
supraspinal ligament Lig. supraspinale.
su·pra·spi·na·tus (muscle) [ˌ-spaɪˈneɪtəs] Supraspinatus *m*, M. supraspinatus.
supraspinatus syndrome Supraspinatussyndrom *nt*.
su·pra·spi·nous [ˌ-ˈspaɪnəs] *adj* → supraspinal.
supraspinous fossa Fossa supraspinata/supraspinosa.
supraspinous ligament → supraspinal ligament.
supraspinous muscle → supraspinatus (muscle).
su·pra·sta·pe·di·al [ˌ-stəˈpiːdɪəl] *adj* oberhalb des Stapes (liegend), suprastapedial.
su·pra·ster·nal [ˌ-ˈstɜrnl] *adj* oberhalb des Brustbeins/Sternums (liegend), suprasternal.
suprasternal bones Ossa suprasternalia.
suprasternal notch Inc. jugularis sterni.
suprasternal region Regio suprasternalis.
su·pra·tem·po·ral [ˌ-ˈtemp(ə)rəl] *adj* supratemporal.
su·pra·ten·to·ri·al [ˌ-tenˈtɔːrɪəl, -ˈtəʊ-] *adj* oberhalb des Tentoriums (liegend), supratentorial.
su·pra·tho·rac·ic [ˌ-θəˈræsɪk, -θɔː-] *adj* oberhalb des Thorax (liegend), suprathorakal.
su·pra·thresh·old [ˌ-ˈθreʃ(h)əʊld] *adj* überschwellig.
su·pra·ton·sil·lar [ˌ-ˈtɒnsɪlər] *adj* oberhalb einer Mandel/Tonsille (liegend), supratonsillär.
supratonsillar fossa Fossa supratonsillaris.
supratonsillar recess → supratonsillar fossa.
su·pra·trag·ic tubercle [ˌ-ˈtrædʒɪk] Tuberculum supratragicum.
su·pra·troch·le·ar artery [ˌ-ˈtrɒklər] innere Stirnarterie *f*, Supratrochlearis *f*, A. frontalis (medialis), A. supratrochlearis.

supratrochlear nerve Supratrochlearis *m*, N. supratrochlearis.
supratrochlear veins mediale Stirnvenen *pl*, Supratrochlearvenen *pl*, Vv. frontales.
su·pra·tur·bi·nate [ˌ-ˈtɜrbɪneɪt, -nɪt] *n* → supreme concha.
su·pra·tym·pan·ic [ˌ-tɪmˈpænɪk] *adj* oberhalb des Tympanons (liegend), supratympanal, -tympanisch.
su·pra·um·bil·i·cal [ˌ-ʌmˈbɪlɪkl] *adj* oberhalb des Nabels (liegend), supraumbilikal.
supraumbilical reflex epigastrischer Reflex *m*.
su·pra·vag·i·nal [ˌ-ˈvædʒɪnl] *adj* oberhalb der Scheide/Vagina (liegend), supravaginal.
supravaginal hysterectomy → subtotal hysterectomy.
supravaginal part of cervix uteri Portio supravaginalis cervicis.
su·pra·val·var [ˌ-ˈvælvər] *adj* → supravalvular.
su·pra·val·vu·lar [ˌ-ˈvælvjələr] *adj* oberhalb einer Klappe (liegend), supravalvulär.
su·pra·vas·cu·lar layer of myometrium [ˌ-ˈvæskjələr] supravaskuläre Schicht *f* des Myometriums, Stratum supravasculare (myometrii).
su·pra·ven·tric·u·lar [ˌ-venˈtrɪkjələr] *adj* oberhalb eines Ventrikels (liegend), supraventrikulär.
supraventricular arrhythmia supraventrikuläre Arrhythmie *f*.
supraventricular crest (*Herz*) supraventrikuläre Muskelleiste *f*, Crista supraventricularis.
supraventricular extrasystole supraventrikuläre Extrasystole *f*.
supraventricular tachycardia supraventrikuläre Tachykardie *f*.
su·pra·ver·gence [ˌ-ˈvɜrdʒəns] *n ophthal*. Supravergenz *f*.
su·pra·ver·sion [ˌ-ˈvɜrʒn] *n ophthal*. Supraversion *f*.
su·pra·ves·i·cal fossa [ˌ-ˈvesɪkl] Fossa supravesicalis.
su·pra·vi·tal [ˌ-ˈvaɪtl] *adj* überlebend, über den Tod hinaus, supravital, Supravital-.
supravital staining *histol*. Supravitalfärbung *f*.
supreme [səˈpriːm, soʊ-] *adj* **1.** höchste(r, s), größte(r, s), oberste(r, s), äußerste(r, s), Ober-. **2.** kritisch, entscheidend.
supreme concha oberste Nasenmuschel *f*, Concha nasalis suprema.
su·ra [ˈsʊrə] *n anat*. Wade *f*, Wadenregion *f*, Sura *f*, Regio suralis.
su·ral [ˈsʊrəl, ˈsjʊə-] *adj* Wade betr., sural, Waden-.
sural arteries Wadenarterien *pl*, Aa. surales.
sur·al·i·men·ta·tion [sɜrˌælɪmenˈteɪʃn] *n* → superalimentation.
sural nerve Suralis *m*, N. suralis.
sural region *anat*. Wade *f*, Wadenregion *f*, Sura *f*, Regio suralis.
sural veins Vv. surales.
sur·a·min sodium [ˈsʊərəmɪn] Germanin *nt*, Suramin-Natrium *nt*.
sur·di·mute [ˌsɜrdɪˈmjuːt] **I** *n* Taubstumme(r *m*) *f*. **II** *adj* taubstumm.
sur·di·mu·tism [ˌ-ˈmjuːtɪzəm] *n* Taubstummheit *f*, Surdomutitas *f*.
sur·di·mu·ti·tas [ˌ-ˈmjuːtɪtæs] *n* → surdimutism.
sur·di·tas [ˈsɜrdɪtæs] *n* → surdity.
sur·di·ty [ˈsɜrdɪtɪ] *n* Taubheit *f*, Surditas *f*.
sur·do·car·di·ac syndrome [ˌsɜrdəʊˈkɑːrdɪæk] Jervell-Lange-Nielsen-Syndrom *nt*.
sur·ex·ci·ta·tion [ˌsɜreksaɪˈteɪʃn] *n* über-

surface

mäßige Erregung *f*, Übererregung *f*, Hyperexzitation *f*.
sur·face ['sɜrfɪs] **I** *n* Oberfläche *f*, Außenfläche *f*, Außenseite *f*. **II** *adj* **1.** Oberflächen-. **2.** *fig.* oberflächlich, äußerlich, vordergründig. **III** *vt* eine Oberfläche behandeln *od.* bearbeiten; glätten. **IV** *vi* an die Oberfläche *od.* zum Vorschein kommen; ans Tageslicht kommen.
surface-active agent → surfactant 1.
surface analgesia → surface anesthesia.
surface anatomy Oberflächenanatomie *f*.
surface anesthesia Oberflächenanästhesie *f*.
surface antigen Oberflächenantigen *nt*.
surface biopsy Oberflächen-, Abstrichbiopsie *f*, Abstrich *m*.
surface catalysis Oberflächenkatalyse *f*.
surface charge Oberflächenladung *f*.
surface electrode Oberflächenelektrode *f*.
surface tension Oberflächenspannung *f*.
surface topography *phys., chem.* Oberflächentopographie *f*.
sur·fac·tant [sər'fæktənt] *n* **1.** *phys., chem.* oberflächenaktive/grenzflächenaktive Substanz *f*, Detergens *nt*. **2.** (*Lunge*) Surfactant *nt*, Surfactant-Faktor *m*, Antiatelektasefaktor *m*.
surfactant factor → surfactant 2.
sur·geon ['sɜrdʒən] *n* Chirurg(in *f*) *m*.
surgeon's knot chirurgischer Knoten *m*.
sur·ger·y ['sɜrdʒərɪ] *n, pl* **-ger·ies 1.** Chirurgie *f*. **2.** chirurgischer/operativer Eingriff *m*, chirurgische Behandlung *f*, Operation *f*. **3.** Operationssaal *m abbr.* OP. **4.** Sprechzimmer *nt*, Praxis *f*. **5.** *Brit.* Sprechstunde *f*.
sur·gi·cal ['sɜrdʒɪkl] *adj* **1.** Chirurgie betr., chirurgisch. **2.** operativ, Operations-.
surgical abdomen akutes Abdomen *nt*, Abdomen acutum.
surgical adrenalectomy chirurgische Adrenalektomie *f*.
surgical anatomy chirurgische Anatomie *f*.
surgical anesthesia chirurgische Anästhesie *f*.
surgical assistant Operationsassistent(in *f*) *m*.
surgical beds Betten *pl* auf chirurgischer Station; *inf.* chirurgische Betten *pl*.
surgical débridement Débridement *nt*, chirurgische Wundtoilette/Wundausschneidung *f*.
surgical diathermy chirurgische Diathermie *f*, Elektrokoagulation *f*.
surgical disease/disorder chirurgische Erkrankung *f*.
surgical dissection chirurgisches Präparieren *nt*, chirurgische Darstellung *f*.
surgical emergency chirurgischer Notfall *m*.
surgical exploration chirurgische Untersuchung/Exploration *f*.
surgical glove 1. OP-Handschuh *m*, Gummihandschuh *m*. **2.** Einweg-, Gummihandschuh *m*.
surgical infection chirurgische Infektion *f*.
surgical knife chirurgisches Messer *nt*, Skalpell *nt*.
surgical knot chirurgischer Knoten *m*.
surgical mortality chirurgische Mortalität *f*.
surgical neck fracture of humerus subkapitale Humerusfraktur *f*.
surgical oncology chirurgische Onkologie *f*.
surgical pathology chirurgische Pathologie *f*.
surgical patient chirurgischer Patient *m*, chirurgische Patientin *f*.
surgical procedure 1. Eingriff *m*, Operation *f*. **2.** Eingriff *m*, Verfahren *nt*, Technik *f*.
surgical shoe orthopädischer Schuh *m*.
surgical solution of chlorinated soda verdünnte Natriumhypochloritlösung *f*.
surgical staging *patho.* chirurgisches Staging *nt*.
surgical stress chirurgischer Streß *m*, Streß *m* durch einen chirurgischen Eingriff.
surgical toilet Débridement *nt*, chirurgische Wundtoilette/Wundausschneidung *f*.
surgical vagotomy operative Vagotomie *f*.
sur·ro·gate ['sɜrəgeɪt, -gɪt, 'sʌr-] *n* Ersatz(stoff *m*) *m*, Surrogat *n* (*of, for* für).
sur·round [sə'raʊnd] *vt* umgeben.
sur·round·ing [sə'raʊndɪŋ] *adj* **1.** umgebend, umliegend. **2.** umschließend.
sur·round·ings [sə'raʊndɪŋs] *pl* Umgebung *f*; Umwelt *f*, Umfeld *nt*; Umstände *pl*.
surround inhibition *physiol.* Umfeldhemmung *f*.
sur·sum·duc·tion [ˌsɜrsəm'dʌkʃn] *n* → supraduction.
sur·sum·ver·gence [ˌ-'vɜrdʒəns] *n* → supravergence.
sur·sum·ver·sion [ˌ-'vɜrʒn] *n ophthal.* Sursumversion *f*.
sur·veil·lance [sər'veɪl(j)əns] *n* Überwachung *f*; Aufsicht *f*.
surveillance study Übersichtsstudie *f*.
sur·vey [*n* 'sɜrveɪ, *v* sər'veɪ] **I** *n* **1.** Überblick *m*, Übersicht *f*. **2.** (sorgfältige) Prüfung *f*, (genaue) Betrachtung *f*, Musterung *f*, Begutachtung *f*; Schätzung *f*, Gutachten *nt*, (Prüfungs-)Bericht *m*. **3.** *stat.* Erhebung *f*, Umfrage *f*; Reihenuntersuchung *f*. **II** *vt* **4.** überblicken, -schauen. **5.** sorgfältig prüfen, genau betrachten, mustern, (ab-)schätzen, begutachten. **III** *vi* eine Erhebung/Umfrage vornehmen, eine Reihenuntersuchung durchführen.
sur·viv·al rate [sər'vaɪvəl] Überlebensrate *f*, -quote *f*.
sus·cep·ti·bil·i·ty [səˌseptə'bɪlətɪ] *n, pl* **-ties** Empfindlichkeit *f* (*to* gegen); Anfälligkeit *f*, Empfänglichkeit *f*, Reizbarkeit *f*, Suszeptibilität *f* (*to* für).
sus·cep·ti·ble [sə'septɪbl] *adj* empfindlich (*to* gegen); anfällig, empfänglich, suszeptibel (*to* für).
sus·pend [sə'spend] *vt* **1.** *chem.* aufschwemmen, suspendieren. **2.** (zeitweilig) aufheben, (vorübergehend) einstellen, unterbrechen, suspendieren. **3.** aufhängen, suspendieren (*from* an).
sus·pend·ed animation [sə'spendɪd]Scheintod *m*.
sus·pend·ing medium [sə'spendɪŋ] *phys., chem.* Suspensionsmedium *nt*.
sus·pen·si·ble [sə'spensɪbl] *adj chem.* suspendierbar.
sus·pen·si·om·e·ter [səˌspensɪ'ɑmɪtər] *n* Trübungsmesser *m*, Nephelometer *nt*.
sus·pen·sion [sə'spenʃn] *n* **1.** *chem.* Aufschwemmung *f*, Suspension *f*. **2.** (zeitweilige) Aufhebung *f*, Aussetzung *f*, Unterbrechung *f*, Suspension *f*. **3.** Aufhängen *nt*; Aufhängevorrichtung *f*; Aufhängung *f*.
suspension colloid Suspensionskolloid *nt*, Suspensoid *nt*.
suspension medium Suspensionsmedium *nt*.
sus·pen·soid [sə'spensɔɪd] *n* → suspension colloid.
sus·pen·so·ri·us duodeni (muscle) [səˌspen'sɔːrɪəs] Treitz'-Muskel *m*, Suspensorius *m* duodeni, M. suspensorius duodeni.
sus·pen·so·ry [sə'spensərɪ] **I** *n, pl* **-ries** *anat.* Stütze *f*; Tragvorrichtung *f*, Tragbeutel *m*, Suspensorium *nt*. **II** *adj* (ab-)stützend, hängend, Hänge-, Stütz-, Halte-.
suspensory bandage Suspensorium scroti.
suspensory ligament Stütz-, Halteband *nt*, Lig. suspensorium.
s. of axis Lig. apicis dentis.
s. of bladder Plica umbilicalis mediana.
s.s of breast Ligg. suspensoria mammaria.
s. of clitoris Lig. suspensorium clitoridis.
s. of humerus Lig. coracohumerale.
s. of lens Zonula ciliaris.
s. of liver Lig. falciforme (hepatis).
s.s of mammary gland → s.s of breast.
s. of ovary Stützband des Eierstockes, Lig. suspensorium ovarii.
s. of penis Stütz-/Halteband des Penis, Lig. suspensorium penis.
s. of spleen Lig. splenorenale/lienorenale/phrenicosplenicum.
suspensory muscle of duodenum → suspensorius duodeni (muscle).
sus·ten·tac·u·lar [ˌsʌstən'tækjələr] *adj anat.* Sustentaculum betr., stützend, Stütz-.
sustentacular cells 1. Sertoli'Zellen *pl*, Stütz-, Ammen-, Fußzellen *pl*. **2.** Stützzellen *pl*.
sustentacular fibers Müller'-Stützzellen *pl*, -Stützfasern *pl*.
sus·ten·tac·u·lum [ˌsʌstən'tækjələm] *n, pl* **-la** [-lə] *anat.* Stütze *f*, Sustentaculum *nt*.
s. of talus Sustentaculum tali.
Sutton ['sʌtn] **S.'s disease 1.** → S.'s nevus. **2.** Mikulicz-Aphthen *pl*, habituelle Aphthen *pl*, chronisch-rezidivierende Aphthen *pl*, rezidivierende benigne Aphthosis *f*, Periadenitis mucosa necrotica recurrens. **3.** Granuloma fissuratum, Acanthoma fissuratum.
S.'s nevus Sutton-Nävus *m*, Halo-Nävus *m*, perinaevische Vitiligo *f*, Leucoderma centrifugum acquisitum, Vitiligo circumnaevalis.
su·tu·ra [sə'tjʊərs] *n, pl* **-rae** [-riː] → suture 1.
su·tur·al ['suːtʃərəl] *adj* Naht betr., mit einer Naht versehen, Naht-.
sutural bones Schalt-, Nahtknochen *pl*, Ossa suturalia.
su·ture ['suːtʃər] **I** *n* **1.** *anat.* Naht *f*, Knochennaht *f*, Verwachsungslinie *f*, Sutura *f*. **2.** *chir.* Naht *f*, Wundnaht *f*. **3.** Nähen *nt*. **4.** Naht *f*, Nahtmaterial *nt*. **II** *vt* nähen, vernähen, annähen; (*Wunde*) verschließen; (*Wundrand*) vereinigen.
s. in anatomic layers *chir.* schichtweiser Wundverschluß *m*.
suture abscess *chir.* Faden-, Nahtabszeß *m*.
suture-and-tying forceps → suture forceps.
suture forceps *chir.* Knüpfpinzette *f*.
suture ligature *chir.* Umstechungsligatur *f*, -naht *f*.
suture line recurrence *chir.* Anastomosenrezidiv *nt*.
suture material Nahtmaterial *nt*.
suture repair Nahtverschluß *m*, Naht *f*, Vernähen *nt*.
suture-tying forceps → suture forceps.
sux·a·me·tho·ni·um [ˌsʌksəmə'θoʊnɪəm] *n pharm.* Suxamethonium *nt*, Succinylcholin *nt*.
suxamethonium chloride Suxamethoniumchlorid *nt*, Succinylcholinchlorid *nt*.

SV *abbr.* 1. → simian virus. 2. → stroke volume.
Sv *abbr.* → sievert.
sved·berg ['sfedbɜrg] *n* → Svedberg unit.
Svedberg ['sfedbɜrg]: **S. equation** Svedberggleichung *f*.
S. unit *abbr.* **S** Svedberg-Einheit *f abbr.* S.
SVI *abbr.* [slow virus infection] → slow virus disease.
swab [swɒb] **I** *n* 1. Tupfer *m*, Wattebausch *m*. 2. Abstrichtupfer *m*. 3. Abstrich *m*. **to take a ~** einen Abstrich machen. **II** *vt* abtupfen, betupfen.
swad·dle ['swɒdl] **I** *n* Windel *f*. **II** *vt* 1. wickeln, in Windeln legen. 2. um-, einwickeln.
swaged needle [sweɪdʒd] *chir.* atraumatische Nadel *f*.
swal·low ['swɒləʊ] **I** *n* Schluck *m*; Schlucken *nt*. **II** *vt* (ver-, hinunter-)schlucken. **III** *vi* schlucken.
swallow down *vt* → swallow II.
swal·low·ing ['swɒləʊɪŋ] *n* Schlucken *nt*, Verschlucken *nt*.
swallowing center Schluckzentrum *nt*.
swallowing reflex Schluckreflex *m*.
swamp fever [swɒmp] 1. Feld-, Ernte-, Schlamm-, Sumpffieber *nt*, Erbsenpflückerkrankheit *f*, Leptospirosis grippotyphosa. 2. Sumpf-, Wechselfieber *nt*, Malaria *f*.
swamp sumac Rhus fernix.
Swan-Ganz [swɒn gænz]: **S.-G. catheter** Swan-Ganz-Katheter *m*.
swan neck deformity [swɒn] *ortho.* Schwanenhalsdeformität *f*.
swarm [swɔːrm] **I** *n bio.* Schwarm *m*. **II** *vi* (aus-)schwärmen.
swarm cell → swarmer.
swarm·er ['swɔːrmər] *n bio.* Schwärmspore *f*, -zelle *f*, Schwärmer *m*, Plano-, Zoospore *f*.
swarm·ing ['swɔːrmɪŋ] *n bio.*, *micro.* (Aus-)Schwärmen *nt*.
swarm spore → swarmer.
swathe [swɒð, sweɪð] **I** *n* Binde *f*, Verband *m*; Umschlag *m*. **II** *vt* (um-, ein-)wickeln, einhüllen.
S wave *physiol.* (*EKG*) S-Zacke *f*.
sway·back ['sweɪbæk] *n ortho.* Hohl-(rund)rücken *m*, Hohlkreuz *nt*.
swayback nose Sattelnase *f*.
sway·ing gait ['sweɪɪŋ] *neuro.* zerebellärer Gang *m*.
sweat [swet] (*v* sweated; sweated) **I** *n* 1. Schweiß *m*, Sudor *m*. 2. Schwitzen *nt*, Schweißausbruch *m*, Perspiration *f*. 3. Schwitzkur *f*. 4. *phys.* Ausschwitzung *f*, Feuchtigkeit *f*. **II** *vt* 5. (aus-)schwitzen. 6. schwitzen lassen, in Schweiß bringen. 7. *phys.* schwitzen *od.* gären lassen. **III** *vi* schwitzen; *phys.* schwitzen, anlaufen.
sweat out *vt* (*Fieber*) (her-)ausschwitzen.
sweat bath Schwitzbad *nt*.
sweat duct Ausführungsgang *m* einer Schweißdrüse, Ductus sudoriferus.
sweat duct adenoma Adenom *nt* eines Schweißdrüsenganges.
sweat gland abscess Schweißdrüsenabszeß *m*.
sweat gland adenoma Schweißdrüsenadenom *nt*, Syringom *nt*.
sweat gland cylindroma Schweißdrüsenzylindrom *nt*.
sweat gland metaplasia Schweißdrüsenmetaplasie *f*.
sweat glands Schweißdrüsen *pl*, Gll. sudoriferae.
apocrine s. apokrine Schweißdrüsen, Gll. sudoriferae apocrinae.
eccrine s. ekkrine Schweißdrüsen, Gll. sudoriferae eccrinae.

sweat gland tumor Schweißdrüsengeschwulst *f*, -tumor *m*.
sweat·i·ness ['swetɪnɪs] *n* Verschwitztheit *f*, Schweißigkeit *f*.
sweat·ing ['swetɪŋ] **I** *n* Schwitzen *nt*; Schweißsekretion *f*, -absonderung *f*, Perspiration *f*. **II** *adj* schwitzend, Schwitz-.
sweat pore Schweißdrüsenpore *f*, Porus sudoriferus.
sweat retention syndrome 1. thermogene/tropische Anhidrose *f*, Anhidrosis tropica. 2. Schweißretentionssyndrom *nt*.
sweat test Schweißprobe *f*, Shwachman-Probe *f*.
sweat·y ['swetɪ] *adj* verschwitzt, schweißig, Schweiß-; schweißtreibend.
sweaty feet Schweißfüße *pl*.
Swediaur [ˌsweɪdɪˈaʊər, ˌswe-]: **S.'s disease** Albert-Krankheit *f*, Entzündung *f* der Bursa tendinis calcanei.
Swed·ish genetic porphyria ['swiːdɪʃ] akute intermittierende Porphyrie *f*, schwedischer Typ *m* der Porphyrie, Porphyria acuta intermittens.
Sweet [swiːt]: **S.'s disease/syndrome** Sweet-Syndrom *nt*, akute febrile neutrophile Dermatose *f*.
sweet [swiːt] **I** *n* Süße *f*. **II** *adj* süß, süßlich.
sweet·en ['swiːtn] *vt* süßen.
sweet·en·er ['swiːtnər] *n* Süßstoff *m*.
sweet·en·ing ['swiːtnɪŋ] *n* 1. Süßstoff *m*. 2. Süßen *nt*.
sweet gas Kohlenmonoxid *nt*.
sweet·ish ['swiːtɪʃ] *adj* süßlich.
swell [swel] (*v* swelled; swollen) **I** *n* (An-)Schwellen *nt*; Schwellung *f*, Geschwulst *f*; Wölbung *f*, Ausbuchtung *f*. **II** *vt* aufblähen, auftreiben; (auf-)quellen. **III** *vi* (an-)schwellen (*into, to* zu); s. (auf-)blähen.
swell out *vi* → swell III.
swell up *vi* → swell III.
swelled [sweld] *adj* (an-)geschwollen, aufgebläht.
swel·ling ['swelɪŋ] *n* 1. (An-)Schwellen *nt*, Anwachsen *nt*, Blähen *nt*; (Auf-)Quellen *nt*. 2. Schwellung *f*, Verdickung *f*, Geschwulst *f*, Beule *f*.
swelling necrosis Quellungsnekrose *f*.
Swenson ['swensn]: **S.'s operation** *chir.* Swenson-Operation *f*.
Swift [swɪft]: **S.'s disease** Feer'-Krankheit *f*, Rosakrankheit *f*, vegetative Neurose *f* der Kleinkinder, Swift-Syndrom *nt*, Selter-Swift-Feer'-Krankheit *f*, Feer-Selter-Swift-Krankheit *f*, Akrodynie *f*, Acrodynia *f*.
Swift-Feer [feːr]: **S.-F. disease** → Swift's disease.
swim·mer's dermatitis ['swɪmər] → swimmer's itch.
swimmer's ear (Bade-)Otitis externa.
swimmer's itch Schwimmbadkrätze *f*, Weiherhippel *m*, Bade-, Schistosomen-, Zerkariendermatitis *f*.
swimmer's otitis externa (Bade-)Otitis externa.
swimmer's otitis media (Bade-)Otitis media.
swim·ming pool blennorrhea ['swɪmɪŋ] Einschluß-, Schwimmbadkonjunktivitis *f*.
swimming pool conjunctivitis → swimming pool blennorrhea.
swimming pool granuloma Schwimmbadgranulom *nt*.
swine erysipelas [swaɪn] → swine rotlauf.
swine·herd's disease ['swaɪnhɜrd] Schweinehüterkrankheit *f*, Bouchet-Gsell-Krankheit *f*, Leptospirosis pomona.

swine·pox ['swaɪnpɒks] *n* Schweinepocken *pl*.
swine rotlauf Schweinerotlauf *m*, Pseudoerysipel *nt*, Erysipeloid *nt*, Rosenbach-Krankheit *f*, Erythema migrans.
swine rotlauf bacillus *micro.* Schweinerotlauf-Bakterium *nt*, Erysipelothrix insidiosa/rhusiopathiae.
Swiss tapeworm [swɪs] *micro.* (breiter) Fischbandwurm *m*, Grubenkopfbandwurm *m*, Diphyllobothrium latum, Bothriocephalus latus.
Swiss type agammaglobulinemia schwerer kombinierter Immundefekt *m*, Schweizer-Typ *m* der Agammaglobulinämie.
switch [swɪtʃ] **I** *n* 1. *phys.*, *techn.* Schalter *m*. 2. Schalten *nt*. 3. Umstellung *f*, Wechsel *m*; Austausch *m*. **II** *vt* 4. (aus-, um-)tauschen, (aus-, um-)wechseln. 5. schalten. **III** *vi* (um-)schalten.
switch on *vt* einschalten, anschalten.
switch off *vt* abschalten, ausschalten.
swol·len ankle ['swəʊlən] geschwollener (Fuß-)Knöchel *m*, Knöchelödem *nt*.
swoon [swuːn] *n* → syncope.
SW sleep → slow wave sleep.
Swyer-James ['swaɪər 'dʒeɪmz]: **S.-J. syndrome** Swyer-James-Syndrom *nt*.
sy·ceph·a·lus [saɪˈsefələs] *n* → syncephalus.
sych·nu·ria [sɪkˈn(j)ʊərɪə] *n* häufige Blasenentleerung *f*, Pollakisurie *f*, Pollakiurie *f*.
sy·co·si·form [saɪˈkəʊsəfɔːrm] *adj derm.* sykose-artig, sykosiform.
sy·co·sis [saɪˈkəʊsɪs] *n derm.* Haarfollikelentzündung *f*, Sykose *f*, Sycosis *f*.
Sydenham ['sɪdnhæm]: **S.'s chorea** Sydenham-Chorea *f*, Chorea minor (Sydenham), Chorea juvenilis/rheumatica/infectiosa/simplex.
syl·lab·ic speech [sɪˈlæbɪk] Stakkatosprache *f*.
syl·la·ble ['sɪləbl] *n* Silbe *f*.
syl·la·bus ['sɪləbəs] *n*, *pl* **-bus·es**, **-bi** [-baɪ] (Vorlesungs-)Verzeichnis *nt*, Unterrichts-, Lehrplan *m*; Abriß *m*, Auszug *m*, Inhaltsangabe *f*.
syl·van ['sɪlvən] *adj* Wald-, Waldes-, sylvatisch.
syl·vat·ic [sɪlˈvætɪk] *adj* → sylvan.
Sylvest [sɪlˈvest]: **S.'s disease** Bornholmer Krankheit *f*, epidemische Pleurodynie *f*, Myalgia epidemica.
syl·vi·an ['sɪlvɪən]: **s. aqueduct syndrome** → s. syndrome.
s. artery mittlere Gehirnarterie *f*, Cerebri *f* media, *inf.* Media *f*, A. cerebri media.
s. fissure/fossa 1. Sylvius'-Furche *f*, Sulcus lateralis. 2. Fossa lateralis cerebralis.
s. syndrome Retraktionsnystagmus *m*, Nystagmus retractorius.
s. veins Vv. mediae superficiales cerebri.
Sylvius ['sɪlvɪəs]: **cistern of S.** Cisterna fossa lateralis cerebri.
fissure/fossa of S. → sylvian fissure.
valve of S. *embryo.* Eustachio'-Klappe *f*, Sylvius'-Klappe *f*, Heister'-Klappe *f*, Valvula Eustachii, Valvula v. cavae inferioris.
ventricle of S. Cavum septi pellucidi.
sym·bi·on ['sɪmbɪɒn, -baɪ-] *n* → symbiont.
sym·bi·on·ic [ˌsɪmbɪˈɒnɪk, -baɪ-] *adj* Symbiose betr., symbiotisch, symbiontisch.
sym·bi·ont ['sɪmbɪɒnt, -baɪ-] *n* Symbiont *m*.
sym·bi·o·sis [ˌsɪmbɪˈəʊsɪs, -baɪ-] *n*, *pl* **-ses** [-siːz] 1. *bio.* Symbiose *f*. 2. *psycho.* Symbiose *f*.
sym·bi·ote ['sɪmbɪəʊt, -baɪ-] *n* → symbiont.

sym·bi·ot·ic [ˌsɪmbɪ'ɒtɪk, -baɪ-] *adj* → symbionic.
symbiotic (infantile) psychosis symbiotische Psychose *f*.
Sym·bleph·a·ron [sɪm'blefərən] *n ophthal.* Symblepharon *nt*.
sym·bleph·a·ro·pte·ryg·i·um [sɪmˌblefərətə'rɪdʒɪəm] *n ophthal.* Symblepharopterygium *nt*.
sym·bol ['sɪmbl] *n* Zeichen *nt*, Symbol *nt*.
sym·bol·ism ['sɪmbəlɪzəm] *n psychia.* Symbolophobie *f*.
sym·bol·i·za·tion [ˌsɪmbəlɪ'zeɪʃn] *n psycho.* Symbolisation *f*.
sym·brach·y·dac·tyl·ia [sɪmˌbrækɪdæk'tɪlɪə] *n* → symbrachydactyly.
sym·brach·y·dac·tyl·ism [sɪmˌbrækɪ'dæktəlɪzəm] *n* → symbrachydactyly.
sym·brach·y·dac·ty·ly [sɪmˌbrækə'dæktəlɪ] *n embryo.* Symbrachydaktylie *f*.
Syme [saɪm]: **S.'s amputation/operation** *ortho.* Fußamputation *f* nach Syme, Syme-Amputation *f*.
sym·e·lus *n* → symmelus.
Symington ['sɪmɪŋtən]: **S.'s body** Lig. anococcygeum.
sym·me·lia [sɪ'miːlɪə] *n* Symmelie *f*.
sym·me·lus ['sɪmələs] *n* Symmelus *m*.
Symmers ['sɪmərz]: **S.' disease** Brill-Symmers-Syndrom *nt*, Morbus Brill-Symmers *m*, zentroplastisch-zentrozytisches (malignes) Lymphom *nt*, großfollikuläres Lymphoblastom/Lymphom *nt*.
sym·met·ric [sɪ'metrɪk] *adj* symmetrisch.
sym·met·ri·cal [sɪ'metrɪkl] *adj* → symmetric.
symmetrical lipomatosis multiple symmetrische Lipomatose *f*.
sym·me·try ['sɪmətrɪ] *n* Symmetrie *f*.
symmetry model *biochem.* Symmetriemodell *nt*.
symmetry principle Symmetrieprinzip *nt*.
sympath- *pref.* → sympatho-.
sym·pa·thec·to·mize [ˌsɪmpə'θektəmaɪz] *vt* eine Sympathektomie durchführen, sympathektomieren.
sym·pa·thec·to·my [ˌ-'θektəmɪ] *n neurochir.* Grenzstrangresektion *f*, Sympathektomie *f*.
sym·pa·the·tec·to·my [ˌ-θɪ'tektəmɪ] *n* → sympathectomy.
sym·pa·thet·ic [ˌ-'θetɪk] *adj* 1. sympathisches Nervensystem betr., sympathisch, Sympathiko-, Sympathikus-. 2. (*Person*) mitfühlend, teilnehmend; einfühlend, verständnisvoll; sympathisch, angenehm.
sympathetic abscess sympathischer Abszeß *m*.
sympathetic blepharospasm *ophthal.* sympathischer Lidkrampf/Blepharospasmus *m*.
sympathetic block Sympathikus-, Grenzstrangblockade *f*.
sympathetic branch of ciliary ganglion Sympathikusast *m* des Ziliarganglions, Ramus sympatheticus ggl. ciliaris, Radix sympathetica ggl. ciliaris.
sympathetic chain → sympathetic trunk.
sympathetic ganglion sympathisches Ganglion *nt*, Sympathikusganglion *nt*, Ggl. sympathicum/sympatheticum.
sympathetic imbalance Vagotonie *f*, Parasympathikotonie *f*.
sympathetic iritis *ophthal.* sympathische Iritis *f*.
sympathetic nerve 1. → sympathetic trunk. 2. sympathischer Nerv *m*.
sympathetic nervous system 1. sympathisches Nervensystem *nt*, (Ortho-)Sympathikus *m*, sympathischer Teil *m* des autonomen Nervensystems, N. sympathicus,

Pars sympathetica/sympathica systematis nervosi autonomici. 2. autonomes/vegetatives Nervensystem *nt abbr.* ANS, Pars autonomica systematis nervosi, Systema nervosum autonomicum.
sympathetic neuron sympathisches Neuron *nt*.
sympathetico- *pref.* → sympatho-.
sym·pa·thet·i·co·mi·met·ic [ˌ-ˌθetɪkəʊmɪ'metɪk] *n, adj* → sympathomimetic.
sympathetic ophthalmia sympathische Ophthalmie *f*, Ophthalmia sympathica.
sym·pa·thet·i·co·to·nia [ˌ-ˌθetɪkəʊ'təʊnɪə] *n neuro.* erhöhte Erregbarkeit *f* des Sympathikus, Sympathikotonie *f*.
sympathetic paraganglia sympathische Paraganglien *pl*.
sympathetic root: s. of ciliary ganglion → sympathetic branch of ciliary ganglion.
s. of pterygopalatine ganglion Radix sympathetica.
sympathetic saliva Sympathikusspeichel *m*.
sympathetic stress reaction Alarmreaktion *f*.
sympathetic tone Sympathikustonus *m*.
sympathetic trunk Grenzstrang *m*, Truncus sympathicus/sympatheticus.
sympathetic trunk ganglia Grenzstrangganglien *pl*, Ggll. trunci sympathici.
sympathetic uveitis *ophthal.* sympathische Uveitis *f*.
sym·pa·thet·o·blast [ˌ-'θetəblæst] *n* Sympathoblast *m*.
sym·pa·thet·o·blas·to·ma [ˌ-ˌθetəblæs'təʊmə] *n* → sympathoblastoma.
sympathic- *pref.* → sympatho-.
sym·path·ic [sɪm'pæθɪk] *adj* → sympathetic.
sym·path·i·cec·to·my [sɪmˌpæθɪ'sektəmɪ] *n* → sympathectomy.
sympathic imbalance Vagotonie *f*, Parasympathikotonie *f*.
sympathico- *pref.* → sympatho-.
sym·path·i·co·ad·re·nal system [sɪmˌpæθɪkəʊə'driːnl] sympathikoadrenales System *nt*.
sym·path·i·co·ad·re·ner·gic system [ˌ-ˌædrə'nɜrdʒɪk] sympathikoadrenerges System *nt*.
sym·path·i·co·blast ['-blæst] *n* Sympathikoblast *m*.
sym·path·i·co·blas·to·ma [ˌ-blæs'təʊmə] *n* → sympathoblastoma.
sym·path·i·co·gon·i·o·ma [ˌ-gɒnɪ'əʊmə] *n* → sympathoblastoma.
sym·path·i·co·lyt·ic [ˌ-'lɪtɪk] *n, adj* → sympatholytic.
sym·path·i·co·mi·met·ic [ˌ-mɪ'metɪk] *n, adj* → sympathomimetic.
sym·path·i·cop·a·thy [sɪmpæθɪ'kɒpəθɪ] *n* Erkrankung *f* des sympathischen Nervensystems, Sympathiko-, Sympathopathie *f*.
sym·path·i·co·to·nia [sɪmˌpæθɪkəʊ'təʊnɪə] *n* → sympatheticotonia.
sym·path·i·co·trope [ˌ-'trəʊp] *n, adj* → sympathicotropic.
sym·path·i·co·trop·ic [ˌ-'trɒpɪk] I *n* sympathotrope Substanz *f*. II *adj* sympathotrop, sympathikotrop.
sym·path·i·co·tryp·sy [ˌ-'trɪpsɪ] *n neurochir.* Sympathikotripsie *f*.
sym·path·i·cus [sɪm'pæθɪkəs] *n* → sympathetic nervous system 1.
sympatho- *pref.* Sympathikus-, Sympathik(o)-, Sympath(o)-.
sym·pa·tho·ad·re·nal [ˌsɪmpəθəʊə'driːnl] *adj* sympatho-, sympathikoadrenal.
sym·path·o·blast [sɪm'pæθəblæst] *n* Sympathoblast *m*.
sym·pa·tho·blas·to·ma [ˌsɪmpəθəʊblæs-

'təʊmə] *n* Sympathikoblastom *nt*, -goniom *nt*, Sympathoblastom *nt*, -goniom *nt*.
sym·pa·tho·gone [ˌ-'gəʊn] *n* → sympathogonium.
sym·pa·tho·go·ni·o·ma [ˌ-ˌgəʊnɪ'əʊmə] *n* → sympathoblastoma.
sym·pa·tho·go·ni·um [ˌ-'gəʊnɪəm] *n, pl* **-nia** [-nɪə] Sympathogonie *f*.
sym·pa·tho·lyt·ic [ˌ-'lɪtɪk] I *n* Sympatholytikum *nt*, Antiadrenergikum *nt*. II *adj* sympatholytisch, antiadrenerg.
sym·pa·tho·mi·met·ic [ˌ-mɪ'metɪk, -maɪ-] I *n* Sympathikomimetikum *nt*, Adrenomimetikum *nt*. II *adj* sympathiko-, adrenomimetisch.
sym·pa·tho·par·a·lyt·ic [ˌ-ˌpærə'lɪtɪk] *n, adj* → sympatholytic.
sym·pa·thy ['sɪmpəθɪ] *n, pl* **-thies** 1. Sympathie *f*, Zuneigung *f* (*for* für). 2. **-s** *pl* (An-)Teilnahme *f*, Beileid *nt*. 3. Mitleidenschaft *f*. 4. *psycho., bio.* Wechselwirkung *f*, Sympathie *f*.
sym·pha·lan·gia [ˌsɪmfə'lændʒɪə] *n embryo.* Symphalangie *f*, Symphalangismus *m*.
sym·phal·an·gism [sɪm'fælændʒɪzəm] *n* → symphalangia.
sym·phys·e·al [sɪm'fiːzɪəl] *adj* Symphyse betr., Symphysen-.
sym·phys·e·or·rha·phy *n* → symphysiorrhaphy.
sym·phys·e·o·tome *n* → symphysiotome.
sym·phys·e·ot·o·my *n* → symphysiotomy.
sym·phys·i·al *adj* → symphyseal.
symphysial surface Symphysenfläche *f* des Schambeins, Facies symphysialis (ossis pubis).
sym·phys·i·ol·y·sis [sɪmˌfiːzɪ'ɒləsɪs] *n* Symphysenlösung *f*, Symphisiolyse *f*.
sym·phys·i·or·rha·phy [sɪmˌfiːzɪ'ɔrəfɪ] *n* Symphysennaht *f*, Symphysiorrhaphie *f*.
sym·phys·i·o·tome [sɪm'fiːzɪətəʊm] *n* Symphysiotomiemesser *nt*, Symphysiotom *nt*.
sym·phys·i·ot·o·my [sɪmˌfiːzɪ'ɒtəmɪ] *n gyn.* Symphysensprengung *f*, Symphysiotomie *f*, Symphyseotomie *f*.
sym·phy·sis ['sɪmfəsɪs] *n, pl* **-ses** [-siːz] Knorpelfuge *f*, Symphyse *f*.
sym·phy·so·dac·tyl·ia [sɪmfɪsəʊdæk'tɪlɪə] *n* → syndactyly.
sym·phy·so·dac·ty·ly [ˌ-'dæktəlɪ] *n* → syndactyly.
sym·plasm ['sɪmplæzəm] *n* Symplasma *nt*.
sym·plast ['sɪmplæst] *n* → symplasm.
sym·po·dia [sɪm'pəʊdɪə] *n embryo.* Sirenenbildung *f*, Sirene *f*, Sympodie *f*, Sirenomelie *f*.
sym·port [sɪm'pɔːrt] *n physiol.* gekoppelter Transport *m*, Cotransport *m*, Symport *m*.
symport system *physiol.* Symport-, Cotransportsystem *nt*.
symp·tom ['sɪmptəm] *n* (An-, Krankheits-)Zeichen *nt*, Symptom *nt* (*of* für, von).
symp·to·mat·ic [ˌsɪmptə'mætɪk] *adj* Symptom(e) betr., auf Symptomen beruhend, kennzeichnend, bezeichnend, symptomatisch (*of* für).
symp·to·mat·i·cal [ˌsɪmptə'mætɪkl] *adj* → symptomatic.
symptomatic asthma symptomatisches Asthma *nt*.
symptomatic epilepsy symptomatische/organische Epilepsie *f*.
symptomatic fever Wundfieber *nt*, Febris traumatica.
symptomatic headache reflektorischer/symptomatischer Kopfschmerz *m*.

symptomatic hypertension sekundäre/symptomatische Hypertonie *f.*
symptomatic hypotension sekundäre/symptomatische Hypotonie *f.*
symptomatic idiopathic diffuse esophageal spasm *abbr.* SIDES idiopathischer diffuser Ösophagusspasmus *m*, symptomatic idiopathic diffuse esophageal spasm *abbr.* SIDES.
symptomatic infantilism symptomatischer Infantilismus *m.*
symptomatic neuralgia symptomatische Neuralgie *f.*
symptomatic reaction symptomatische Reaktion *f.*
symptomatic torticollis symptomatischer Schiefhals/Torticollis *m.*
symptomatic treatment symptomatische Behandlung *f.*
symptomatic ulcer symptomatisches Ulkus *nt.*
symp·tom·a·tol·o·gy [ˌsɪmptəmə'talədʒɪ] *n* 1. Symptomatologie *f*, Semiologie *f.* 2. Gesamtheit *f* der (Krankheits-)Symptome, Symptomatik *f*, Symptomatologie *f.*
symp·to·mat·o·lyt·ic [ˌsɪmptəˌmætə'lɪtɪk] *adj* Symptome beseitigend.
symptom complex Symptomenkomplex *m*; Syndrom *nt.*
symptom formation *psycho.* Symptombildung *f.*
symp·to·mo·lyt·ic [ˌsɪmptəmoʊ'lɪtɪk] *adj* → symptomatolytic.
symptom substitution → symptom formation.
sym·pus ['sɪmpəs] *n embryo.* Sympus *m.*
syn·a·del·phus [ˌsɪnə'dɛlfəs] *n embryo.* Synadelphus *m.*
syn·al·gia [sɪ'nældʒ(ɪ)ə] *n* Synalgie *f.*
syn·al·gic [sɪ'nældʒɪk] *adj* Synalgie betr.
syn·an·che [sɪ'næŋkɪ] *n* → sore throat.
syn·an·them [sɪ'nænθəm] *n* → synanthema.
syn·an·the·ma [ˌsɪnæn'θiːmə] *n derm.* Synanthem(a) *nt.*
syn·an·thrin [sɪ'nænθrɪn] *n* Inulin *nt.*
syn·aph·y·men·i·tis [sɪˌnæfɪmɛ'naɪtɪs] *n ophthal.* Bindehautentzündung *f*, Konjunktivitis *f*, Conjunctivitis *f.*
syn·apse ['sɪnæps, sɪ'næps] **I** *n*, *pl* **-aps·es** [-sɪz] Synapse *f.* **II** *vi* eine Synapse bilden.
syn·ap·sis [sɪ'næpsɪs] *n*, *pl* **-ses** [-siːz] *genet.* Chromosomenpaarung *f*, Synapsis *f.*
syn·ap·tic [sɪ'næptɪk] *adj* Synapse betr., synaptisch, Synapsen-.
syn·ap·ti·cal [sɪ'næptɪkl] *adj* → synaptic.
synaptic bulb Synapsenkolben *m.*
synaptic center Schaltzentrum *nt.*
 superimposed s. übergeordnete Schaltstelle *f.*
synaptic cleft synaptischer Spalt *m*, Synapsenspalt *m.*
synaptic complex Synapsenkomplex *m.*
 glomerulus-like s. glomerulusartige Synapse *f.*
synaptic conduction synaptische Erregungsleitung/Erregungsübertragung *f.*
synaptic facilitation synaptische Bahnung *f.*
synaptic gap synaptischer Spalt *m*, Synapsenspalt *m.*
synaptic inhibition synaptische Hemmung *f.*
synaptic knobs synaptische Endknöpfchen *pl*, Boutons termineaux.
synaptic neuron Schaltneuron *nt.*
synaptic phase → synapsis.
synaptic potential synaptisches Potential *nt.*
synaptic summation synaptische Summation *f.*

synaptic terminal synaptische Nervenendigung *f.*
synaptic transmission synaptische Erregungsübertragung *f.*
synaptic transmitter synaptischer Transmitter *m*, synaptische Übertragersubstanz *f.*
synaptic vesicle synaptisches Vesikel *nt.*
syn·ap·to·some [sɪ'næptəsoʊm] *n* Synaptosom *nt.*
syn·ar·thro·dia [ˌsɪnɑːr'θroʊdɪə] *n* → synarthrosis.
syn·ar·thro·di·al joint [ˌsɪnɑːr'θroʊdɪəl] 1. → synarthrosis. 2. Synchondrose *f*, Symphyse *f*, Junctura cartilaginea.
syn·ar·thro·phy·sis [ˌsɪnɑːθrə'faɪsɪs] *n* (Gelenk-)Versteifung *f*, Ankylosierung *f.*
syn·ar·thro·sis [ˌsɪnɑːr'θroʊsɪs] *n*, *pl* **-ses** [-siːz] kontinuierliche Knochenverbindung *f*, Knochenfuge *f*, Synarthrose *f*, Synarthrosis *f*, Artic./Junctura fibrosa.
syn·ath·re·sis [ˌsɪnæ'θriːsɪs] *n* → synathrosis.
syn·ath·roi·sis [ˌ-'rɔɪsɪs] *n pharm.* lokalisierte Hyperämie *f.*
syn·ca·ine [sɪn'keɪɪn] *n anes.* Procainhydrochlorid *nt.*
syn·can·thus [sɪn'kænθəs] *n ophthal.* Synkanthus *m.*
syn·car·y·on *n* → synkaryon.
syn·ceph·a·lus [sɪn'sɛfələs] *n embryo.* Synkephalus *m*, -cephalus *m.*
syn·chei·lia [sɪn'kaɪlɪə] *n embryo.* Synch(e)ilie *f*, Synch(e)ilia *f.*
syn·chei·ria [sɪn'kaɪrɪə] *n embryo.* Synch(e)irie *f*, Synch(e)iria *f.*
syn·che·sis ['sɪnkəsɪs] *n* → synchysis.
syn·chi·lia *n* → syncheilia.
syn·chi·ria *n* → syncheiria.
syn·chon·drec·to·my [ˌsɪnkɑn'drɛktəmɪ] *n* Synchondrektomie *f.*
syn·chon·dro·di·al joint [ˌ-'droʊdɪəl] → synchondrosis.
syn·chon·dro·se·ot·o·my [ˌ-ˌdroʊsɪ'ɑtəmɪ] *n* Synchondroseotomie *f.*
syn·chon·dro·sis [ˌ-'droʊsɪs] *n*, *pl* **-ses** [-siːz] Knorpelfuge *f*, -haft *f*, Synchondrose *f*, Synchondrosis *f.*
 s.es of cranium kraniale Synchondrosen *pl*, Synchondrosen der Schädelknochen, Synchondroses cranii/craniales.
 s.es of skull → s.es of cranium.
syn·chon·drot·o·my [ˌ-'drɑtəmɪ] *n* Synchondrotomie *f.*
syn·chro·nia [sɪn'kroʊnɪə] *n* 1. → synchronism. 2. *embryo.* Synchronie *f*, Synchronismus *m.*
syn·chro·nism ['sɪŋkrənɪzm] *n* 1. Gleichzeitigkeit *f*, zeitliche Übereinstimmung *f*, Synchronismus *m.* 2. Synchronisation *f.*
syn·chro·nize ['sɪŋkrənaɪz] **I** *vt* aufeinander abstimmen, gleichstellen, synchronisieren (with mit). **II** *vi* zusammenfallen, gleichzeitig sein (with mit); synchron laufen *od.* sein, übereinstimmen (with *m*it).
syn·chro·nized culture ['sɪŋkrənaɪzd] synchrone/synchronisierte Kultur *f*, Synchronkultur *f.*
synchronized intermittent mandatory ventilation *abbr.* SIMV synchronisierte intermittierende mandatorische Beatmung *f*, synchronized intermittent mandatory ventilation *abbr.* SIMV.
synchronized sleep → slow wave sleep.
syn·chro·nous ['sɪŋkrənəs] *adj* gleichzeitig, gleichlaufend, synchron (with mit).
synchronous muscle *physiol.* synchroner Muskel *m.*
synchronous pacemaker *card.* vorhofgesteuerter Herzschrittmacher *m*, P-gesteuerter Herzschrittmacher *m.*

syn·chro·ny ['sɪŋkrənɪ] *n* → synchronism.
syn·chro·tron ['sɪŋkrətrɑn] *n phys.* Kreisbeschleuniger *m*, Synchroton *nt.*
syn·chy·sis ['sɪnkəsɪs] *n* 1. *patho.* Verflüssigung *f*, Synchisis *f.* 2. *ophthal.* Glaskörperverflüssigung *f*, Synchisis corporis vitrei.
syn·ci·ne·sis [sɪnsɪ'niːsɪs, -saɪ-] *n* → synkinesis.
syn·ci·put *n* → sinciput.
syn·cli·nal [sɪn'klaɪnəl] *adj* synklinal.
syn·clit·ic [sɪn'klɪtɪk] *adj embryo.* Synklitismus betr., achsengerecht, synklitisch.
syn·clit·i·cism [sɪn'klɪtɪsɪzəm] *n* → synclitism.
syn·clit·ism ['sɪnklɪtɪzəm] *n embryo.* Synklitismus *m.*
syn·co·pal ['sɪŋkəpəl] *adj* Synkope betr., synkopisch, Synkopen-.
syn·co·pe ['sɪŋkəpɪ] *n* Synkope *f.*
syn·cop·ic [sɪn'kɑpɪk] *adj* → syncopal.
syn·cre·tio [sɪn'krɪʃoʊ] *n* Zusammenwachsen *nt*, Verwachsen *nt*, Syncretio *f.*
syn·cy·tial [sɪn'sɪtɪəl, -'sɪ(ɪ)əl] *adj* Synzytium betr., synzytial, Synzytio-, Synzytium-.
syncytial cells Synzytiumzellen *pl.*
syncytial knot *embryo.* Synzytiumknoten *m.*
syn·cy·tio·troph·o·blast [sɪnˌsɪtɪoʊ'trɑfəˌblæst, -'troʊfə-, -ˌsɪʃ(ɪ)oʊ-] *n* Synzytiotrophoblast *m.*
syn·cy·tium [sɪn'sɪtɪəm, -'sɪʃ(ɪ)əm] *n*, *pl* **-tia** [-tɪə, -ʃ(ɪ)ə] Synzytium *nt*, Syncytium *nt.*
syn·cy·toid ['sɪnsətɔɪd] *adj* synzytiumähnlich.
syn·dac·tyl [sɪn'dæktl] *adj* → syndactylous.
syn·dac·tyl·ia [ˌsɪndæk'tɪlɪə] *n* → syndactyly.
syn·dac·tyl·ic [ˌ-'tɪlɪk] *adj* → syndactylous.
syn·dac·ty·lism [sɪn'dæktəlɪzəm] *n* → syndactyly.
syn·dac·ty·lous [sɪn'dæktɪləs] *adj* Syndaktylie betr., syndaktyl.
syn·dac·ty·lus [sɪn'dæktɪləs] *n* Syndaktylus *m.*
syn·dac·ty·ly [sɪn'dæktəlɪ] *n* Verwachsung *f* von Fingern *od.* Zehen, Syndaktylie *f.*
syn·del·phus [sɪn'dɛlfəs] *n embryo.* Synadelphus *m.*
syn·der·ma·tot·ic cataract [sɪnˌdɑrmə'tɑtɪk] Katarakt *f* bei Dermatosen, Cataracta syndermatotica.
syn·de·sis [sɪn'dɛsɪs, sɪn'diːsɪs] *n* 1. *ortho.* operative Gelenkversteifung *f*, Arthrodese *f.* 2. → synapsis.
syndesm- *pref.* → syndesmo-.
syn·des·mec·to·my [ˌsɪndɛz'mɛktəmɪ] *n chir., ortho.* Banddurchtrennung *f*, -exzision *f*, -resektion *f*, Ligamentdurchtrennung *f*, -exzision *f*, -resektion *f*, Syndesmektomie *f.*
syn·des·mec·to·pia [sɪnˌdɛzmɛk'toʊpɪə] *n* Bandverlagerung *f*, -ektopie *f*, Ligamentverlagerung *f*, -ektopie *f.*
syn·des·mi·tis [ˌsɪndɛz'maɪtɪs] *n* 1. Band-, Ligamententzündung *f*, Syndesmitis *f.* 2. *ophthal.* Bindehautentzündung *f*, Konjunktivitis *f*, Conjunctivitis *f.*
syndesmo- *pref.* Band-, Bänder-, Ligament-, Syndesm(o)-.
syn·des·mo·di·al joint [ˌsɪndɛz'moʊdɪəl] → syndesmosis.
syn·des·mo·lo·gia [ˌsɪndɛzmə'loʊdʒ(ɪ)ə] *n* → syndesmology.
syn·des·mo·lo·gy [ˌsɪndɛz'mɑlədʒɪ] *n* Gelenklehre *f*, Arthrologie *f*, -logia *f.*
syn·des·mo·pex·y [sɪn'dɛzməpɛksɪ] *n ortho.* Syndesmopexie *f.*
syn·des·mo·phyte [sɪn'dɛzməfaɪt] *n patho., ortho.* Syndesmophyt *m.*

syndesmoplasty

syn·des·mo·plas·ty [sɪn'dezməplæstɪ] *n ortho.* Bänder-, Syndesmoplastik *f*.
syn·des·mor·rha·phy [ˌsɪndez'mɔrəfɪ] *n ortho.* Band-, Bändernaht *f*, Syndesmorrhaphie *f*.
syn·des·mo·sis [ˌsɪndez'məʊsɪs] *n, pl* **-ses** [-siːz] Bandhaft *f*, Syndesmose *f*, Syndesmosis *f*.
syn·des·mot·ic joint [ˌsɪndez'mɑtɪk] → syndesmosis.
syn·des·mot·o·my [ˌsɪndez'mɑtəmɪ] *n ortho.* Band-, Bänder-, Ligamentdurchtrennung *f*, Syndesmotomie *f*.
syn·drome ['sɪndrəʊm, -drəm] *n* Syndrom *nt*, Symptomenkomplex *m*.
 s. of approximate relevant answers Ganser-Syndrom, Pseudodemenz *f*, Scheinblödsinn *m*, Zweckpsychose *f*.
 s. of corpus striatum Vogt-Syndrom, -Erkrankung *f*, Status marmoratus.
 s. of deviously relevant answers → s. of approximate relevant answers.
 s. of inappropriate antidiuretic hormone *abbr.* **SIADH** Schwartz-Bartter-Syndrom, Syndrom der inadäquaten ADH-Sekretion *abbr.* SIADH.
 s. of prolonged ventilator dependence Syndrom der verlängerten Beatmungsabhängigkeit.
 s. of retroparotid space Villaret-Syndrom.
 s. of sea-blue histiocyte seeblaue Histiozytose *f*.
syn·dromic [sɪn'drɑmɪk, -'drəʊ-] *adj* Syndrom betr., als Syndrom auftretend.
syn·ech·ia [sɪ'nekɪə, -'niːk-] *n, pl* **-ech·iae** [-kiː, -kaɪ] Verwachsung *f*, Synechie *f*, Synechia *f*.
syn·ech·i·o·tome [sɪ'nekɪətəʊm] *n ophthal.* Synech(i)otom *nt*, Synech(i)otomiemesser *nt*.
syn·ech·i·ot·o·my [sɪˌnekɪ'ɑtəmɪ] *n ophthal.* Synech(i)otomie *f*.
syn·ech·o·tome [sɪ'nekətəʊm] *n* → synechiotome.
syn·ech·ot·o·my [ˌsɪnə'kɑtəmɪ] *n* → synechiotomy.
syn·ech·ten·ter·ot·omy [ˌsɪnekˌtentə'rɑtəmɪ] *n chir.* Durchtrennung *f* von Darmverwachsungen/Darmverklebungen.
syn·e·col·o·gy [sɪnɪ'kɑlədʒɪ] *n bio.* Synökologie *f*.
syn·en·ceph·a·lo·cele [ˌsɪnen'sefələsiːl] *n* Synenzephalozele *f*.
syn·en·ceph·a·lus [ˌ-'sefələs] *n embryo.* Synenzephalus *m*.
syn·en·ceph·a·ly [ˌ-'sefəlɪ] *n embryo.* Synenzephalie *f*.
syn·er·get·ic [ˌsɪnər'dʒetɪk] *adj* zusammenwirkend, synergetisch.
syn·er·gia [sɪ'nɜrdʒɪə] *n* → synergy.
syn·er·gic [sɪ'nɜrdʒɪk] *adj* → synergetic.
syn·er·gism ['sɪnərdʒɪzəm] *n chem.* Synergismus *m*.
syn·er·gist ['sɪnərdʒɪst] *n* **1.** *pharm.* synergistische Substanz *f*, Synergist *m*. **2.** synergistisches Organ *nt*, Synergist *m*.
syn·er·gis·tic [ˌsɪnər'dʒɪstɪk] *adj* Synergismus betr., auf Synergismus beruhend, zusammenwirkend, synergistisch.
syn·er·gy ['sɪnərdʒɪ] *n* Zusammenwirken *nt*, Zusammenspiel *nt*, Synergie *f*.
syn·es·the·sia [ˌsɪnəs'θiːʒ(ɪ)ə] *n* Synästhesie *f*.
syn·es·the·si·al·gia [ˌsɪnəsˌθiːzɪ'ældʒ(ɪ)ə] *n neuro.* schmerzhafte Synästhesie *f*, Synästhesialgie *f*, Synaesthesia algica.
syn·e·ze·sis [ˌsɪnə'ziːsɪs] *n* → synizesis.
syn·gam·ic [sɪŋ'gæmɪk] *adj* syngam.
Syn·gam·i·dae [sɪŋ'gæmədiː] *pl micro.* Syngamidae *pl*.
syn·ga·mous ['sɪŋgəməs] *adj* syngam.

Syn·ga·mus ['sɪŋgəməs] *n micro.* Syngamus *m*.
syn·ga·my ['sɪŋgəmɪ] *n* Gametenverschmelzung *f*, Syngamie *f*.
syn·ge·ne·ic [ˌsɪndʒə'nɪɪk] *adj immun.* syngen, syngenetisch, isogen, isogenetisch, isolog.
syngeneic graft → syngraft.
syngeneic homograft → syngraft.
syngeneic transplantation syngene/syngenetische/isologe/isogene/isogenetische Transplantation *f*, Isotransplantation *f*.
syn·gen·e·sis [sɪn'dʒenəsɪs] *n* Syngenese *f*.
syn·ge·net·ic [ˌsɪndʒə'netɪk] *adj* **1.** Syngenese betr., syngenetisch. **2.** → syngeneic.
syng·na·thia [sɪŋ'neɪθɪə, -'næθ-] *n embryo.* Syngnathie *f*.
syn·graft ['sɪngræft] *n* syngenes/syngenetisches/isogenes/isogenetisches/isologes Transplantat *nt*, Isotransplantat *nt*.
syn·i·ze·sis [ˌsɪnə'ziːsɪs] *n* **1.** Verschluß *m*, Okklusion *f*, Synizesis *f*. **2.** *bio.* Synizesis *f*.
syn·kar·y·on [sɪn'kærɪɑn] *n* Synkaryon *nt*.
syn·ki·ne·sia [ˌsɪŋkɪ'niːʒ(ɪ)ə, -kaɪ-] *n* → synkinesis.
syn·ki·ne·sis [ˌ-'niːsɪs] *n* Mitbewegung *f*, Synkinese *f*.
syn·ki·net·ic [ˌ-'netɪk] *adj* Synkinese betr., synkinetisch.
syn·neu·ro·sis [sɪnjʊə'rəʊsɪs, -nʊ-] *n* → syndesmosis.
syn·o·cha ['sɪnəkə] *n* kontinuierliches Fieber *nt*.
syn·o·chus ['sɪnəkəs] *n* → synocha.
syn·o·nych·ia [ˌsɪnə'nɪkɪə] *n* Synonychie *f*.
syn·oph·rid·ia [ˌsɪnɑf'rɪdɪə] *n* → synophrys.
syn·oph·rys [sɪn'ɑfrɪs] *n* zusammengewachsene Augenbrauen *pl*, Synophrys *f*.
syn·oph·thal·mia [ˌsɪnɑf'θælmɪə] *n embryo.* Synophthalmie *f*.
syn·oph·thal·mus [ˌ-'θælməs] *n embryo.* Zyklop *m*, Zyklozephalus *m*, Synophthalmus *m*.
syn·op·to·phore [sɪn'ɑptəfəʊər, -fɔːr] *n ophthal.* Synoptophor *m*.
syn·or·chi·dism [sɪn'ɔːrkɪdɪzəm] *n* → synorchism.
syn·or·chism ['sɪnɔːrkɪzəm] *n urol.* Hodenverschmelzung *f*, Synorchidie *f*.
syn·os·che·os [sɪn'ɑskɪəs] *n urol., embryo.* Synoscheos *m*.
syn·os·te·o·sis [ˌsɪnɑstɪ'əʊsɪs] *n* → synostosis.
syn·os·te·ot·ic [ˌsɪnɑstɪ'ɑtɪk] *adj* → synostotic.
syn·os·te·ot·o·my [ˌsɪnɑstɪ'ɑtəmɪ] *n ortho.* Arthrostomie *f*.
syn·os·to·sis [ˌsɪnɑs'təʊsɪs] *n, pl* **-ses** [-siːz] knöcherne Vereinigung/Verbindung *f*, Synostose *f*, Synostosis *f*.
syn·os·tot·ic [ˌsɪnɑs'tɑtɪk] *adj* Synostose betr., synostotisch.
sy·no·tia [saɪ'nəʊʃɪə] *n embryo.* Synotie *f*.
sy·no·tus [saɪ'nəʊtəs] *n embryo.* Synotus *m*.
syn·o·vec·to·my [ˌsɪnə'vektəmɪ] *n ortho.* Synovialisentfernung *f*, -exzision *f*, -resektion *f*, Synovektomie *f*, Synovialektomie *f*.
synovi- *pref.* → synovio-.
syn·o·via [sɪ'nəʊvɪə] *n* Gelenkschmiere *f*, Synovia *f*.
syn·o·vi·al [sɪ'nəʊvɪəl] *adj* Synovia od. Membrana synovialis betr.; Synovia produzierend; synovial, Synovial-.
synovial articulation → synovial joint.
synovial bursa Schleimbeutel *m*, Bursa synovialis.
 subcutaneous s. Bursa (synovialis) subcutanea.

 subfascial s. subfaszialer Schleimbeutel, Bursa (synovialis) subfascialis.
 submuscular s. submuskulärer Schleimbeutel, Bursa (synovialis) submuscularis.
 subtendinous s. Bursa (synovialis) subtendinea.
 s. of trochlea Sehnenscheide *f* des N. obliquus superior, Bursa synovialis trochlearis, Vagina synovialis/tendinis m. obliqui superioris.
synovial capsule Gelenkkapsel *f*, Capsula articularis.
synovial cell Synovial(is)zelle *f*.
synovial cell sarcoma → synovial sarcoma.
synovial chondromatosis Gelenkchondromatose *f*.
synovial chondrometaplasia → synovial chondromatosis.
synovial cyst *ortho.* Synovialzyste *f*, Ganglion *nt*, Überbein *nt*.
 s. of popliteal space Baker-Zyste.
synovial diverticulum Synovialisdivertikel *nt*.
synovial fluid → synovia.
synovial fold Synovialfalte *f*, Plica synovialis.
 infrapatellar s. Plica synovialis infrapatellaris.
synovial fringes → synovial villi.
synovial glands → synovial villi.
synovial hemangioma synoviales Hämangiom *nt*.
synovial hernia Birkett-Hernie *f*, Hernia synovialis.
synovial joint echtes Gelenk *nt*, Diarthrose *f*, Artic./Junctura synovialis.
synovial layer (of articular capsule) Synovialis *f*, Membrana synovialis (capsulae articularis), Stratum synoviale.
synovial ligament of hip Lig. capitis femoris.
synovial membrane (of articular capsule) → synovial layer (of articular capsule).
sy·no·vi·a·lo·ma [sɪˌnəʊvɪə'ləʊmə] *n* → synovioma.
synovial osteochondromatosis Gelenkchondromatose *f*.
synovial sarcoma malignes Synovi(al)om *nt*, Synovialsarkom *nt*.
synovial sheath (inneres Blatt *nt* der) Sehnenscheide *f*, Vagina synovialis tendinis.
 s. of intertubercular groove Vagina tendinis intertubercularis.
 s. of tendon → synovial sheath.
synovial tuberculosis synoviale Tuberkulose *f*.
synovial villi Synovialzotten *pl*, Villi synoviales/articulares.
syn·o·vin ['sɪnəvɪn] *n* Synovin *f*.
synovio- *pref.* Synovia-, Synovialis-, Synovial(o)-, Synovi(o)-.
syn·o·vi·o·blast [sɪ'nəʊvɪəblæst] *n* Synovioblast *m*.
syn·o·vi·o·cyte [sɪ'nəʊvɪəsaɪt] *n* Synoviozyt *m*.
syn·o·vi·o·ma [sɪˌnəʊvɪ'əʊmə] *n* Synoviom *nt*, Synovialom *nt*.
syn·o·vi·or·these [sɪˌnəʊvɪ'ɔːrθeːz] *n* → synoviorthesis.
syn·o·vi·or·the·sis [sɪˌnəʊvɪɔːr'θiːsɪs] *n radiol., ortho.* Synoviorthese *f*.
syn·o·vi·o·sar·co·ma [sɪˌnəʊvɪəʊsɑːr'kəʊmə] *n* malignes Synovi(al)om *nt*, Synovialsarkom *nt*.
syn·o·vip·a·rous [sɪnə'vɪpərəs] *adj* synovia-bildend.
syn·o·vi·tis [sɪnə'vaɪtɪs] *n* Entzündung *f* der Membrana synovialis, Synovitis *f*, Synoviitis *f*, Synovialitis *f*.
syn·o·vi·um [sɪ'nəʊvɪəm] *n* Synovialis *f*,

Membrana synovialis (capsulae articularis), Stratum synoviale.
syn·phal·an·gism [sɪn'fælændʒɪzəm] *n* → symphalangia.
syn·tac·ti·cal aphasia [sɪn'tæktɪkl] *neuro.* syntaktische Aphasie *f.*
syn·tax·is [sɪn'tæksɪs] *n* Syntaxis *f.*
syn·tec·tic [sɪn'tektɪk] *adj* Syntexis betr., syntektisch.
syn·ten·ic [sɪn'tenɪk] *adj* Syntänie betr.
syn·te·ny ['sɪntəni] *n genet.* Syntänie *f.*
syn·te·re·sis [ˌsɪntə'riːsɪs] *n* prophylaktische/präventive Behandlung *f*; Prophylaxe *f.*
syn·te·ret·ic [ˌsɪntə'retɪk] *adj* prophylaktisch.
syn·tex·is [sɪn'teksɪs] *n* Syntexis *f.*
syn·thase ['sɪnθeɪz] *n* Synthase *f.*
syn·the·sis ['sɪnθəsɪs] *n, pl* **-ses** [-siːz] Synthese *f.*
synthesis inhibitor Synthesehemmer *m*, -hemmstoff *m.*
synthesis period *bio.* S-Phase *f.*
synthesis phase Synthesephase *f.*
syn·the·size ['sɪnθəsaɪz] *vt* **1.** *chem.* synthetisch herstellen, synthetisieren. **2.** zusammenfügen, verschmelzen, verbinden.
syn·the·tase ['sɪnθəteɪz] *n* Ligase *f*, Synthetase *f.*
syn·thet·ic [sɪn'θetɪk] **I** *n* Kunststoff *m.* **II** *adj* **1.** Synthese betr., synthetisch. **2.** künstlich, artifiziell, synthetisch, Kunst-.
synthetic fiber Chemie-, Synthese-, Kunstfaser *f.*
synthetic resin Kunstharz *nt.*
synthetic suture synthetisches Nahtmaterial *nt.*
syn·tho·rax [sɪn'θɔːræks, -'θʊə-] *n embryo.* Synthorax *m*, Thorakopagus *m.*
syn·ton·ic [sɪn'tɑnɪk] *adj* synton.
syn·to·nin ['sɪntənɪn] *n* Syntonin *nt*, Azidalbumin *nt.*
syn·to·py ['sɪntəpi] *n* Syntopie *f.*
syn·troph·ic [sɪn'trɑfɪk] *adj* syntroph.
syn·tro·phism ['sɪntrəfɪzəm] *n bio.* Syntrophismus *m.*
syn·troph·o·blast [sɪn'trɑfəblæst, -'troʊ-] *n* → syncytiotrophoblast.
syn·trop·ic [sɪn'trɑpɪk] *adj* Syntropie betr., syntrop(isch).
syn·tro·py ['sɪntrəpi] *n* Syntropie *f.*
syn·u·lo·sis [ˌsɪnjə'loʊsɪs] *n* Narbenbildung *f*, Synulosis *f.*
syn·u·lot·ic [ˌ-'lɑtɪk] **I** *n* die Narbenbildung förderndes Mittel *nt.* **II** *adj* die Narbenbildung fördernd *od.* auslösend.
syphil- *pref.* → syphilo-.
syph·i·lid ['sɪfəlɪd] *n* Syphilid *nt.*
syph·i·lide ['sɪfəlaɪd] *n* → syphilid.
syph·i·lis ['sɪf(ə)lɪs] *n* harter Schanker *m*, Morbus Schaudinn *m*, Schaudinn-Krankheit *f*, Syphilis *f*, Lues (venerea) *f.*
syph·i·lit·ic [ˌsɪfə'lɪtɪk] *adj* Syphilis betr., von ihr betroffen, durch sie verursacht, syphilitisch, luetisch, Syphilis-.
syphilitic abscess syphilitischer Abszeß *m.*
syphilitic aneurysm syphilitisches Aneurysma *nt.*
syphilitic aortitis Aortensyphilis *f*, Mesaortitis luetica, Aortitis syphilitica.
syphilitic arteritis luetische Arteriitis *f*, Arteriitis luetica.
syphilitic arthritis Arthritis syphilitica.
syphilitic bubo syphilitischer Bubo *m.*
syphilitic condyloma breites Kondylom *nt*, Condyloma latum/syphiliticum.
syphilitic coxitis syphilitische/luetische Koxitis *f*, Coxitis syphilitica.
syphilitic endarteriitis obliterans of cerebral vessels Heubner'-Krankheit *f*, Endarteriitis *f.*

syphilitic endocarditis syphilitische Endokarditis *f.*
syphilitic gonitis syphilitische Gonitis *f*, Gonitis syphilitica.
syphilitic laryngitis syphilitische Laryngitis *f*, Laryngitis syphilitica.
syphilitic leukoderma syphilitisches Leukoderm *nt*, Halsband *nt* der Venus.
syphilitic meningoencephalitis progressive Paralyse *f abbr.* PP, Paralysis progressiva.
syphilitic mesaortitis → syphilitic aortitis.
syphilitic nephritis syphilitische Nephritis *f.*
syphilitic osteochondritis kongenitale Knochensyphilis *f*, Osteochondritis syphilitica, Wegner'-Krankheit *f.*
syphilitic paraplegia luische Spinalparalyse *f* Erb.
syphilitic periostitis syphilitische Periostitis *f*, Periostitis syphilitica.
syphilitic pseudoparalysis Bednar-Parrot-Pseudoparalyse *f*, Parrot'-Lähmung *f.*
syphilitic retinitis Retinitis syphilitica.
syphilitic roseola *derm.* makulöses Syphilid *nt*, Roseola syphilitica.
syphilitic ulcer harte Schanker *m*, Hunter-Schanker *m*, syphilitischer Primäraffekt *m*, Ulcus durum.
syphilo- *pref.* Syphilis-, Syphil(o)-.
syph·i·lo·derm ['sɪfəloʊdɜrm] *n* → syphilid.
syph·i·lo·der·ma [ˌ-'dɜrmə] *n* → syphilid.
syph·i·loid ['sɪfəlɔɪd] *adj* syphilisähnlich, -artig, syphiloid.
syph·i·lo·ma [ˌsɪfə'loʊmə] *n, pl* **-mas**, **-mata** [-mətə] Gummiknoten *m*, Syphilom *nt*, Gumma (syphiliticum) *nt.*
syph·i·lo·ma·nia [ˌsɪfəloʊ'meɪnɪə, -jə] *n psychia.* Syphilomanie *f.*
syph·i·lo·pho·bia [ˌ-'foʊbɪə] *n psychia.* Syphilo-, Syphilidophobie *f.*
syph·i·lous ['sɪfələs] *adj* → syphilitic.
sy·rig·mus [sə'rɪgməs] *n* Ohrenklingen *nt*, -sausen *nt*, Ohrgeräusche *pl*, Tinnitus (aurium) *m.*
syring- *pref.* → syringo-.
syr·ing·ad·e·no·ma [sɪrɪŋ(g)ædɪ'noʊmə] *n* → syringoadenoma.
sy·ringe [sə'rɪndʒ, 'sɪrɪndʒ] **I** *n* Spritze *f.* **II** *vt* (ein-)spritzen.
syr·in·gec·to·my [ˌsɪrɪŋ'dʒektəmɪ] *n HNO* Syringektomie *f.*
syr·in·gi·tis [ˌsɪrɪŋ'dʒaɪtɪs] *n HNO* Entzündung *f* der Ohrtrompete, Syringitis *f*, Salpingitis *f.*
syringo- *pref.* Tuben-, Fistel-, Synring(o)-.
sy·rin·go·ad·e·no·ma [sɪˌrɪŋgoʊædɪ'noʊmə] *n* Syring(o)adenom *nt*, Hidradenom(a) *nt*, Synringozystadenom *nt.*
sy·rin·go·bul·bia [ˌ-'bʌlbɪə] *n neuro.* Syringobulbie *f.*
sy·rin·go·car·ci·no·ma [ˌ-ˌkɑrsə'noʊmə] *n* Schweißdrüsenkarzinom *nt.*
sy·rin·go·cele ['-siːl] *n* Syringozele *f.*
sy·rin·go·cyst·ad·e·no·ma [ˌ-ˌsɪstædɪ'noʊmə] *n* → syringoadenoma.
sy·rin·go·cys·to·ma [ˌ-sɪs'toʊmə] *n* Syringozystom *nt*, -cystoma *nt*, Hidrozystom *nt*, -cystoma *nt.*
sy·rin·go·en·ce·pha·lia [ˌ-ˌensɪ'feɪlɪə, -lɪə] *n* Syringoenzephalie *f*, -encephalia *f.*
sy·rin·go·en·ce·pha·lo·my·e·lia [ˌ-ˌensefəloʊmaɪ'iːlɪə] *n* Syringoenzephalomyelie *f.*
sy·rin·goid [sɪ'rɪŋgɔɪd] *adj* tubenähnlich, -artig.
syr·in·go·ma [ˌsɪrɪŋ'goʊmə] *n* Schweißdrüsenadenom *nt*, Syringom(a) *nt.*

systemic calciphylaxis

sy·rin·go·me·nin·go·cele [səˌrɪŋgoʊmɪ'nɪŋgəsiːl] *n* Syringomyelozele *f.*
sy·rin·go·my·e·lia [ˌ-maɪ'iːlɪə] *n* Syringomyelie *f*, -myelia *f.*
sy·rin·go·my·e·lic syndrome [ˌ-maɪ'iːlɪk] → syringomyelia.
sy·rin·go·my·e·li·tis [ˌ-maɪə'laɪtɪs] *n* Syringomyelitis *f.*
sy·rin·go·my·e·lo·cele [ˌ-'maɪəloʊsiːl] *n* Syringomyelozele *f.*
sy·rin·go·my·e·lus [ˌ-'maɪələs] *n* → syringomyelia.
sy·rin·go·pon·tia [ˌ-'pɑnʃɪə] *n neuro.* Syringopontia *f.*
sy·rin·go·tome [sɪ'rɪŋgətoʊm] *n chir.* Fistelmesser *nt*, Syringotom *nt.*
syr·in·got·o·my [ˌsɪrɪŋ'gɑtəmɪ] *n chir.* Fistelspaltung *f*, Syringotomie *f.*
syr·inx ['sɪrɪŋks] *n, pl* **sy·rin·ges** [sə'rɪndʒiːz] **1.** *anat.* Tube *f*, Syrinx *f.* **2.** Ohrtrompete *f*, Tuba auditoria/auditiva.
syr·up ['sɪrəp, 'sɜr-] *n pharm.* Zuckersaft *m*, (konzentrierte) Zuckerlösung *f*, Sirup *m*, Sirupus *m.*
syr·up·us ['sɪrəpəs] *n* → syrup.
sys·sar·co·sic [ˌsɪsɑr'koʊsɪk] *adj* → syssarcotic.
sys·sar·co·sis [ˌ-'koʊsɪs] *n anat.* Syssarcosis *f.*
sys·sar·cot·ic [ˌ-'kɑtɪk] *adj* Syssarcosis betr.
sys·tal·tic [sɪs'tɔltɪk, -'tæl-] *adj* s. rhythmisch zusammenziehend, rhythmisch pulsierend, systaltisch.
sys·tem ['sɪstəm] *n* **1.** System *nt*; Aufbau *m*, Gefüge *nt*; Einheit *f*; Anordnung *f.* **2.** *anat.* (Organ-)System *nt*, Systema *f.* **3.** *techn.* System *nt*, Anlage *f*; Verfahren *nt*, Methode *f.* **4.** *phys.* System *nt*, Ordnung *f.*
s. of clear cells *old* → APUD-system.
s. of macrophages retikuloendotheliales System *abbr.* RES, retikulohistiozytäres System *abbr.* RHS.
s. of transverse tubules transversales Röhrensystem, System der transversalen Tubuli, T-System.
sys·te·ma [sɪs'tiːmə] *n anat.*, *physiol.* System *nt*, Systema *f.*
sys·tem·at·ic [ˌsɪstə'mætɪk] *adj* systematisch, methodisch; plan-, zweckmäßig, -voll.
systematic anatomy beschreibende/systematische Anatomie *f.*
systematic family *bio.* Familie *f.*
sys·tem·at·ics [ˌsɪstə'mætɪks] *pl* Systematik *f*, systematische Darstellung *f*; Klassifikation *f.*
systematic vertigo Drehschwindel *m*, Vertigo rotatoria.
sys·tem·a·tism ['sɪstəmətɪzəm] *n* Systematisierung *f.*
sys·tem·a·ti·za·tion [ˌsɪstəmətɪ'zeɪʃn] *n* Systematisierung *f.*
sys·tem·a·tize ['sɪstəmətaɪz] *vt* in ein System bringen *od.* einordnen, systematisieren.
sys·tem·a·tized delusion ['sɪstəmətaɪzd] systematisierter Wahn *m.*
sys·tem·ic [sɪs'temɪk] *adj* Gesamtorganismus *od.* Organsystem betr., systemisch, generalisiert, System-.
systemic amyloidosis systemische Amyloidose *f.*
reactive s. reaktiv-sekundäre Amyloidose.
systemic anaphylaxis anaphylaktischer Schock *m*, Anaphylaxie *f.*
systemic atrophy Systematrophie *f.*
systemic blastomycosis systemische Blastomykose *f.*
systemic calciphylaxis systemische Kalziphylaxie *f.*

systemic candidiasis Systemcandidose f.
systemic chondromalacia (von) Meyenburg-Altherr-Uehlinger-Syndrom nt, rezidivierende Polychondritis f, systematisierte Chondromalazie f.
systemic circulation großer Kreislauf m, Körperkreislauf m.
systemic disease systemische Erkrankung f, System-, Allgemeinerkrankung f.
systemic emetic pharm. zentrales Emetikum nt.
systemic heart Linksherz nt.
systemic lesion systemische Schädigung f.
systemic mycosis tiefe Mykose f, Systemmykose f.
systemic myelitis systemische Myelitis f.
systemic myelopathy systemische Myelopathie f.
systemic scleroderma → systemic sclerosis.
systemic sclerosis systemische Sklerose f, Systemsklerose f, progressive/diffuse/systemische Sklerodermie f, Sclerodermia diffusa/progressiva.
systemic symptom Allgemeinsymptom nt.
systemic treatment systemische Behandlung f.
sys·to·gene ['sɪstədʒiːn] n Tyramin nt, Tyrosamin nt.
sys·to·le ['sɪstəlɪ] n Systole f.
sys·tol·ic [sɪs'tɑlɪk] adj Systole betr., systolisch, Systolen-.
systolic bruit card. systolisches (Herz-)Geräusch nt, Systolikum nt.
systolic click card. systolischer Klick/Click m.
systolic discharge card. Schlagvolumen nt.
systolic gallop card. systolischer Galopp m.
systolic murmur card. systolisches (Herz-)Geräusch nt, Systolikum nt.
systolic pressure systolischer Druck m.
systolic thrill card. systolisches Schwirren nt.
sys·trem·ma [sɪs'tremə] n Waden(muskel)krampf m.
sy·zyg·i·al [sɪ'zɪdʒɪəl] adj Syzygie betr.
sy·zyg·i·um [sɪ'zɪdʒɪəm] n → syzygy.
syz·y·gy ['sɪzədʒɪ] n Syzygie f, Syzygium nt.
Szent-Györgyi [sent 'dʒɜrdʒɪ]: **S.-G. quotient** Szent-Györgyi-Quotient m.
S.-G. reaction Szent-Györgyi-Reaktion f.

T

T *abbr.* **1.** → absolute temperature. **2.** → tera-. **3.** → tesla. **4.** → thymidine. **5.** → thymine 2.
t *abbr.* → temperature 1.
2,4,5-T *abbr.* → 2,4,5-trichlorophenoxyacetic acid.
T½ *abbr.* **1.** → half-life. **2.** → half-time.
T₃ *abbr.* → triiodothyronine.
T₄ *abbr.* → thyroxine.
t½ *abbr.* **1.** → half-life. **2.** → half-time.
TA *abbr.* → tendo Achillis.
Ta *abbr.* → tantalum.
tab·a·cism ['tæbəsɪzəm] *n* → tabacosis.
tab·a·co·sis [tæbə'kəʊsɪs] *n* Tabakvergiftung *f*.
tab·a·nid ['tæbənɪd, tə'beɪ-] *n bio., micro.* Bremse *f*, Tabanide *f*.
Ta·ban·i·dae [tə'bænədi:] *pl bio., micro.* Bremsen *pl*, Tabaniden *pl*, Tabanidae *pl*.
tabanid flies → Tabanidae.
Ta·ba·nus [tə'beɪnəs] *n bio., micro.* Tabanus *m*.
tab·ar·dil·lo [tæbə'dɪ(l)jəʊ] *n* endemisches/murines Fleckfieber *nt*, Ratten-, Flohfleckfieber *nt*.
tab·a·tière an·a·to·mique [taba'tjɛːr anatɔ'mik] *anat.* Tabatière *f*.
tab·by cat heart ['tæbɪ] → tabby cat striation.
tabby cat striation *patho.* (*Herzmuskel*) Tigerung *f*.
ta·bel·la [tə'belə] *n, pl* **-lae** [-liː] *pharm.* Tablette *f*, Tabella *f*.
ta·bes ['teɪbiːz] *n, pl* **ta·bes 1.** Auszehrung *f*, Schwindsucht *f*, Tabes *f*. **2.** Rückenmark(s)schwindsucht *f*, -darre *f*, Duchenne-Syndrom *nt*, Tabes dorsalis.
ta·bes·cence [tə'besns] *n* Tabeszenz *f*.
ta·bes·cent [tə'besnt] *adj* schwindend, auszehrend.
tabes dorsalis → tabes 2.
ta·bet·ic [tə'betɪk] **I** *n* Tabetiker(in *f*) *m*. **II** *adj* Tabes betr., tabisch.
tabetic arthropathy tabische Arthropathie *f*, Arthropathia tabica, Charcot-Gelenk *nt*, -Krankheit *f*.
tabetic crisis tabische (Organ-)Krise *f*.
tabetic cuirass Hitzig-Zone *f*.
tabetic gait *neuro.* ataktischer Gang *m*.
tabetic neuritis tabische Neuritis *f*.
tabetic neurosyphilis → tabes 2.
tabetic otalgia tabische Otalgie *f*, Otalgia tabetica.
ta·bet·i·form [tə'betɪfɔːrm] *adj* tabesartig, -ähnlich, tabetiform.
tab·ic ['tæbɪk] *n, adj* → tabetic.
tab·id ['tæbɪd] *adj* → tabetic II.
ta·ble ['teɪbl] **I** *n* **1.** Tisch *m*; Operationstisch *m*. **2.** Tafel *f*, Tisch *m*. **3.** Tabelle *f*, Liste *f*, Verzeichnis *nt*, Register *nt*. **4.** *anat.* Tafel *f*, Tabula *f*. **5.** Ebene *f*; *opt.* Bildebene *f*. **II** *vt* tabellarisieren, in einer Tabelle zusammenstellen, in eine Tabelle eintragen.
table book Tabellenbuch *nt*.
table salt Koch-, Tafelsalz *nt*, Natriumchlorid *nt*.

ta·ble·spoon ['teɪblspuːn] *n* Eßlöffel *m*.
ta·ble·spoon·ful ['-fʊl] *adj* Eßlöffel(voll *m*) *m*.
tab·let ['tæblɪt] *n* **1.** *pharm.* Tablette *f*. **2.** (Schreib-)Block *m*.
table water Tafel-, Mineralwasser *nt*.
ta·boo [tə'buː, tæ-] **I** *n, pl* **-boos** Tabu *nt*. **II** *adj* tabu, unantastbar.
ta·bo·pa·ral·y·sis [ˌteɪbəʊpə'rælɪsɪs] *n neuro.* Taboparalyse *f*.
ta·bo·pa·re·sis [ˌ-pə'riːsɪs] *n* → taboparalysis.
ta·bu *n, adj* → taboo.
tab·u·la ['tæbjələ] *n, pl* **-lae** [-liː] *anat.* Tabula *f*.
tab·u·lar ['tæbjələr] *adj* **1.** tabellarisch, Tabellen-. **2.** flach, tafelförmig, Tafel-; dünn; platt, plattenförmig. **3.** tablettenförmig.
tab·u·lar·ize ['tæbjələraɪz] *vt* → tabulate II.
tab·u·late [*adj* 'tæbjəlɪt, -leɪt; *v* -leɪt] **I** *adj* → tabular. **II** *vt* tabellarisch anordnen.
ta·bun ['tɑbʊn] *n* Tabun *nt*, Dimethylaminozyanphosphorsäureäthylester *m*.
Ta·car·i·be virus [tə'kærəbi] *micro.* Tacaribe-Virus *m*.
tache [tæʃ] *n derm.* Fleck(en *m*) *m*, Mal *nt*, Tache *f*.
tacho- *pref.* Geschwindigkeits-, Tacho-.
tach·o·gram ['tækəgræm] *n* Tachogramm *nt*.
tach·o·graph ['-græf] *n* Tachograph *m*.
ta·chog·ra·phy [tə'kɑgrəfi] *n* Tachographie *f*.
ta·chom·e·ter [tə'kɑmɪtər] *n* Geschwindigkeitsmesser *m*, Tachometer *nt*.
tachy- *pref.* Schnell-, Tachy-.
tach·y·ar·rhyth·mia [ˌtækɪə'rɪðmɪə] *n card.* Tachyarrhythmie *f*.
tach·y·car·dia [ˌ-'kɑrdɪə] *n card.* Herzjagen *nt*, Tachykardie *f*.
tach·y·car·di·ac [ˌ-'kɑrdɪæk] *adj* tachykard.
tach·y·car·dic [ˌ-'kɑrdɪk] *adj* → tachycardiac.
tach·y·gen·e·sis [ˌ-'dʒenəsɪs] *n bio.* Tachygenese *f*.
tach·y·ki·nin [ˌ-'kaɪnɪn] *n* Tachykinin *nt*.
tach·y·la·lia [ˌ-'leɪlɪə] *n neuro., psychia.* Tachylalie *f*.
tach·y·lo·gia [ˌ-'lɑdʒɪə] *n* → tachylalia.
tach·y·me·tab·o·lism [ˌ-mə'tæbəlɪzəm] *n* Tachymetabolismus *m*.
tach·y·pha·gia [ˌ-'feɪdʒɪə] *n* hastiges/überstürztes Essen *nt*, Tachyphagie *f*.
tach·y·pha·sia [ˌ-'feɪzɪə] *n* → tachylalia.
tach·y·phe·mia [ˌ-'fiːmɪə] *n* → tachylalia.
tach·y·phre·nia [ˌ-'friːnɪə] *n* Tachyphrenie *f*.
tach·y·phy·lax·is [ˌ-fɪ'læksɪs] *n* Tachyphylaxie *f*.
tach·yp·nea [ˌtækɪ(p)'niːə] *n* beschleunigte/schnelle Atmung *f*, Tachypnoe *f*.
tach·y·rhyth·mia [ˌtækɪ'rɪðmɪə] *n card.* Tachyrhythmie *f*.

tach·ys·te·rol [tə'kɪstərɔl, -əʊl] *n* Tachysterin *nt*.
tach·y·tro·phism [ˌtækɪ'trəʊfɪzəm] *n* → tachymetabolism.
tach·y·zo·ite [ˌ-'zəʊaɪt] *n* Tachyzoit *m*.
tac·tic·i·ty [tæk'tɪsəti] *n chem.* Taktizität *f*.
tac·tile ['tæktɪl, -taɪl] *adj* **1.** Tastsinn betr., taktil, Tast-. **2.** fühl-, tast-, greifbar.
tactile agnosia taktile Agnosie *f*, Stereoagnosie *f*, Astereognosie *f*.
tactile amnesia → tactile agnosia.
tactile anesthesia *neuro.* Verlust *m* od. Verminderung *f* des Tastsinns.
tactile aphasia taktile Aphasie *f*.
tactile cells → tactile corpuscles.
tactile corpuscles Meissner'-(Tast-)Körperchen *pl*, Corpuscula tactus.
tactile disks Merkel'-Tastzellen *pl*, -Tastscheibe *f*, Meniscus tactus.
tactile elevations Toruli tactiles.
tactile hallucination *psychia.* haptische/taktile Halluzination *f*.
tactile hyperesthesia taktile Hyperästhesie *f*, Hyper(h)aphie *f*.
tactile hypesthesia taktile Hypästhesie *f*, Hypopselaphesie *f*.
tactile hypoesthesia → tactile hypesthesia.
tactile menisci → tactile disks.
tactile sensation Tast-, Berührungsempfindung *f*.
tactile sense Tast-, Berührungssinn *m*.
tac·til·i·ty [tæk'tɪləti] *n* Tastfähigkeit *f*. **2.** Tast-, Greif-, Fühlbarkeit *f*.
tac·ti·log·ical [ˌtæktɪ'lɑdʒɪkl] *adj* → tactual.
tac·tion ['tækʃn] *n* **1.** Tastsinn *m*, Tactus *m*. **2.** Tasten *nt*.
tac·tom·e·ter [tæk'tɑmɪtər] *n physiol.* Taktometer *nt*.
tac·to·sen·so·ry cortex [ˌtæktəʊ'sensərɪ] taktilsensible Rinde *f*.
tac·tu·al [tæktʃəwəl, -ʃəl] *adj* **1.** tastbar. **2.** Tastsinn betr., taktil, Tast-.
tac·tus ['tæktəs] *n* → taction 1.
Tae·nia ['tiːnɪə] *n micro.* Taenia *f*.
  T. echinococcus Blasenbandwurm *m*, Hundebandwurm *m*, Echinococcus granulosus, Taenia echinococcus.
  T. lata (breiter) Fischbandwurm *m*, Grubenkopfbandwurm *m*, Diphyllobothrium latum, Bothriocephalus latus.
  T. nana Zwergbandwurm *m*, Hymenolepis nana.
  T. saginata Rinder(finnen)bandwurm *m*, Taenia saginata, Taeniarhynchus saginatus.
  T. solium Schweine(finnen)bandwurm *m*, Taenia solium.
tae·nia ['tiːnɪə] *n, pl* **-ni·as, -ni·ae** [-nɪˌiː, -nɪaɪ] **1.** *anat.* bandartige Formation *f*, Tänie *f*, T(a)enia *f*. **2.** → Taenia.
t. of fornix T(a)enia fornicis.
t. of fourth ventricle T(a)enia ventriculi quarti.
t. of third ventricle T(a)enia thalami.
t.e of Valsalva Kolontänien *pl*, T(a)eniae coli.

tae·ni·a·cide ['tiːnɪəsaɪd] **I** *n* Bandwurmmittel *nt*, Taenizid *nt*, Taenicidum *nt*. **II** *adj* taenizid, taenia(ab)tötend.
tae·ni·a·fu·gal [ˌ-'fjuːgl] *adj pharm.* Bandwürmer abtreibend.
tae·ni·a·fuge [ˌ-'fjuːdʒ] *n pharm.* Taeniafugum *nt*.
tae·ni·al ['tiːnɪəl] *adj* 1. *micro.* Taenia betr. 2. *anat.* Tänie/Taenia betr.
Tae·ni·a·rhyn·chus saginata [ˌtiːnɪə'rɪŋkəs] → Taenia saginata.
tae·ni·a·sis [tɪ'naɪəsɪs] *n* Taenienbefall *m*, Taeniasis *f*; Bandwurmbefall *m*.
Tae·ni·i·dae [tɪ'naɪədiː] *pl micro.* Taeniidae *pl.*
tag [tæg] (*v* tagged; tagged) **I** *n* 1. *patho.* Zipfel *m*, Fetzen *m*, Lappen *m*. 2. Etikett *nt*, Anhänger *m*, Plakette *f*, (Ab-)Zeichen *nt*. **II** *vt* mit einem Etikett versehen, etikettieren; markieren.
tag·a·tose ['tægətəʊz] *n* Tagatose *f*.
tagged atom [tægt] *phys.* radioaktives/radioaktiv-markiertes Atom *nt*, radioaktives Markeratom *nt*.
T agglutinin T-Agglutinin *nt*.
ta·glia·co·ti·an operation/rhinoplasty [ˌtæljə'kəʊʃɪən] HNO italienische Methode/Rhinoplastik *f*.
Ta·hy·na virus [tə'haɪnə] *micro.* Tahyna-Virus *nt*.
tai·ga tick ['taɪgə] *micro.* Ixodes persulcatus.
tail [teɪl] *n* 1. Schwanz *m*; *zoo.* Schweif *m*; *anat.* Cauda *f*. 2. Hinterteil *nt*, hinteres/unteres Ende *nt*.
t. of caudate nucleus Caudatusschwanz, Cauda nc. caudati.
t. of epididymis Nebenhodenschwanz, Cauda epididymidis.
t. of helix Helixende, Cauda *f*, Cauda helicis.
t. of pancreas Pankreasschwanz, Cauda pancreatis.
t. of spermatozoon Spermienschwanz.
t. of spleen vorderer Milzpol *m*, Extremitas anterior lienis.
t. of testis unterer Hodenpol *m*, Extremitas inferior testis.
tail·bone ['teɪlbəʊn] *n* Steißbein *nt*, Coccyx *f*, Os coccygis.
tail bud *embryo.* End-, Schwanzknospe *f*.
tailed [teɪld] *adj* geschwänzt.
tail fiber (*Virus*) Schwanzfaser *f*.
tail fold *embryo.* Schwanzfalte *f*.
tail·less ['teɪlɪs] *adj* schwanzlos, ohne Schwanz.
tai·lor ['teɪlər] *vt* nach Maß zuschneiden *od.* arbeiten; *fig.* zuschneiden (*to* für jdn./auf etw.); abstimmen (*to* auf).
tailor's muscle Schneidermuskel *m*, Sartorius *m*, M. sartorius.
Takayasu [tɑkə'jɑːzuː]: **T.'s disease** Takahara-Krankheit *f*, Akatalasämie *f*, Akatalasie *f*.
Takayasu [tɑkə'jɑːzuː]: **T.'s arteritis** Martorell-Krankheit *f*, -Syndrom *nt*, Takayasu-Krankheit *f*, -Syndrom *nt*, Pulslos-Krankheit *f*, pulseless disease (*nt*).
T.'s disease/syndrome → T.'s arteritis.
take [teɪk] (*v* took; taken) **I** *n* 1. (*Transplantat*) Anwachsen *nt*, 2. (*Impfungs-*)Reaktion *f*.
II *vt* 3. nehmen, (er-)greifen, fassen. 4. herausnehmen (*out of* aus); wegnehmen, entnehmen (*from* von). 5. (*Essen*) zu s. nehmen; (*Medikament*) (ein-)nehmen. 6. (*Krankheit*) s. zuziehen, erkranken an; (*Farbe, Geruch*) annehmen. 7. (*Arbeit*) leisten; (*Blutprobe*) entnehmen; (*Blutbild*) machen; (*Messung*) vornehmen, messen, prüfen, Maß nehmen; (*Maßnahme*) ergreifen. 8. *mathe.* abziehen, subtrahieren (*from* von). 9. **to ~ notes** niederschreiben, erfassen. 10. *photo., radiol.* eine Aufnahme machen. **to ~ an x-ray** röntgen. 11. (*Platz*) ein-, wegnehmen. 12. ein Bad nehmen.
III *vi* (*Transplantat*) anwachsen; (*Medikament*) wirken, anschlagen.
take after *vi* jdm. nachschlagen, ähnlich sehen.
take apart *vt* etw. zerlegen, auseinander nehmen.
take down *vt* 1. → take apart. 2. (*Arznei*) (hinunter-)schlucken. 3. notieren, aufschreiben; (*Meßgerät*) aufzeichnen.
take from *vt mathe.* abziehen *od.* subtrahieren von.
take in *vt* 1. (*Nahrung*) aufnehmen, zu s. nehmen. 2. *fig.* etw. in s. aufnehmen, erfassen, verstehen, begreifen. 3. etw. (her-)einlassen.
take off *vt* 1. *chir.* absetzen, amputieren. 2. (*Verband*) abnehmen. 3. (*Kleider*) ausziehen. 4. (*Gewicht*) verlieren.
take on *vt* (*Gewicht*) ansetzen; (*Farbe, Färbung*) annehmen.
take out *vt* 1. (*Fleck*) herausmachen, entfernen (*of, from* aus). 2. (*Zahn*) (heraus-)ziehen, extrahieren; (*Organ*) entfernen, herausnehmen.
take over I *vt* (*Aufgabe*) übernehmen. **II** *vi* (*Leitung*) übernehmen.
take to *vi* 1. reagieren auf; (*Krankheit*) s. legen auf. 2. s. hingezogen fühlen, Gefallen finden an jdm. 3. s. zurückziehen in, Zuflucht suchen in.
take up *vt* 1. (*Flüssigkeit*) absorbieren, auf-, einsaugen, aufnehmen. 2. (*Gefäß*) abbinden. 3. (*Platz*) ausfüllen; (*Zeit*) beanspruchen. 4. auf-, hochnehmen, -heben.
take-down ['teɪkdaʊn] **I** *n* Zerlegen *nt*. **II** *adj* zerlegbar, auseinandernehmbar.
take-off ['teɪkɒf, -əf] *n* Wegnehmen *nt*.
take-up *n* Auf-, Einsaugen *nt*, Absorbieren *nt*;, Absorption *f*.
tak·ing ['teɪkɪŋ] *I n* 1. Nehmen *nt*, An-, Ab-, Auf-, Ein-, Ent-, Hin-, Wegnehmen *nt*. 2. Anfall *m*. 3. *photo., radiol.* Aufnahme *f*. **II** *adj inf.* ansteckend.
tal·al·gia [tə'lældʒ(ɪ)ə] *n* Fersenschmerz *m*, Talalgie *f*.
tal·an·tro·pia [tælæn'trəʊpɪə] *n* Nystagmus *m*.
ta·lar ['teɪlər] *adj* Sprungbein/Talus betr., talar, Sprungbein-, Talus-.
talar fracture Sprungbein-, Talusfraktur *f*.
talar neck fracture Talushalsfraktur *f*.
talar sulcus Sulcus tali.
talc [tælk] *n* Talkum *nt*, Talcum *nt*.
tal·co·sis [tæl'kəʊsɪs] *n* Talkumlunge *f*, -pneumokoniose *f*, -staublunge *f*, Talkose *f*.
talc pneumoconiosis → talcosis.
tal·cum ['tælkəm] *n* → talc.
tal·i·ped ['tælɪped] **I** *n* Patient(in *f*) *m* mit Klumpfuß. **II** *adj* klumpfüßig.
tal·i·pe·dic [ˌ-'pedɪk] *adj* → taliped **II**.
tal·i·pes ['-piːz] *n* 1. angeborene Fußdeformität *f*. 2. → talipes equinovarus.
talipes calcaneocavus Hackenhohlfuß *m*, Pes calcaneocavus.
talipes calcaneovalgus Knick-Hackenfuß *m*, Pes calcaneovalgus.
talipes calcaneovarus Klump-Hackenfuß *m*, Pes calcaneovarus.
talipes calcaneus Hackenfuß *m*, Pes calcaneus.
acquired t. erworbener Hackenfuß.
congenital t. angeborener Hackenfuß, Pes calcaneus congenitus.
talipes cavus Hohlfuß *m*, Pes cavus.
talipes equinocavus Ballenhohlfuß *m*, Pes equinocavus.
talipes equinovalgus Pes equinovalgus.
talipes equinovarus Klumpfuß *m*, Pes equinovarus (excavatus et adductus).
talipes equinus Spitzfuß *m*, Pes equinus.
talipes planovalgus Knickplattfuß *m*, Pes planovalgus.
talipes planus Plattfuß *m*, Pes planus.
talipes valgus Knickfuß *m*, Pes valgus.
talipes varus Sichelfuß *m*, Pes adductus, Metatarsus varus.
tal·i·pom·a·nus [ˌ-'pɒmənəs] *n* angeborene Handdeformität *f*; Klumphand *m*.
tal·low ['tæləʊ] **I** *n* 1. Talg *m*. 2. *techn.* Schmiere *f*. **II** *vt* (ein-)schmieren, talgen.
Talma ['tælmə]: **T.'s disease** Talma-Syndrom *nt*, Myotonia acquisita.
T.'s operation Talma-Operation *f*.
ta·lo·cal·ca·ne·al [ˌteɪləʊkæl'keɪnɪəl] *adj* Sprungbein/Talus u. Fersenbein/Kalkaneus betr., talokalkaneal.
talocalcaneal joint hintere Abteilung *f* des unteren Sprunggelenks, Subtalargelenk *nt*, Artic. subtalaris/talocalcanea.
talocalcaneal ligament Lig. talocalcaneum.
interosseous t. Lig. talocalcaneum interosseum.
lateral t. Lig. talocalcaneum laterale.
medial t. Lig. talocalcaneum mediale.
ta·lo·cal·ca·ne·an [ˌ-kæl'keɪnɪən] *adj* → talocalcaneal.
ta·lo·cal·ca·ne·o·na·vic·u·lar articulation [ˌ-kæl.keɪnɪəʊnə'vɪkjələr] vordere Abteilung *f* des unteren Sprunggelenks, Talokalkaneonavikulargelenk *nt*, Artic. talocalcaneonavicularis.
talocalcaneonavicular joint → talocalcaneonavicular articulation.
ta·lo·cru·ral [ˌ-'krʊərəl] *adj* Sprungbein/Talus u. Unterschenkel(knochen) betr., talokrural.
talocrural articulation oberes Sprunggelenk *nt*, Talokruralgelenk *nt*, Artic. talocruralis.
talocrural joint → talocrural articulation.
talocrural region Knöchelgegend *f*, -region *f*, Regio talocruralis.
anterior t. vordere Knöchelregion, Regio talocruralis anterior.
posterior t. hintere Knöchelregion, Regio talocruralis posterior.
ta·lo·fib·u·lar [ˌ-'fɪbjələr] *adj* Sprungbein/Talus u. Wadenbein/Fibula betr., talofibular.
talofibular ligament Lig. talofibulare.
anterior t. Lig. talofibulare anterius.
posterior t. Lig. talofibulare posterius.
ta·lo·met·a·tar·sal [ˌ-ˌmetə'tɑːrsl] *adj* Talus u. Metatarsus betr., talometatarsal.
ta·lo·na·vic·u·lar [ˌ-nə'vɪkjələr] *adj* Sprungbein/Talus u. Kahnbein/Os naviculare betr., talonavikular.
talonavicular articulation Talonavikulargelenk *nt*, Artic. talonavicularis.
talonavicular joint → talonavicular articulation.
talonavicular ligament Lig. talonaviculare.
ta·lo·scaph·oid [ˌ-'skæfɔɪd] *adj* → talonavicular.
tal·ose ['tæləʊs] *n* Talose *f*.
ta·lo·tib·i·al [ˌteɪləʊ'tɪbɪəl] *adj* Sprungbein/Talus u. Schienbein/Tibia betr., talotibial.
talotibial ligament: anterior t. Pars tibiotalaris anterior lig. medialis.
posterior t. Pars tibiotalaris posterior lig. medialis.
ta·lus ['teɪləs] *n, pl* -li [-laɪ] Sprungbein *nt*, Talus *m*.

Tam·i·am·i virus ['tæmɪæmɪ] *micro.* Tamiami-Virus *nt.*
ta·mox·i·fen [tə'mɒksɪfen] *n pharm.* Tamoxifen *nt.*
tam·pan tick ['tæmpæn] *micro.* 1. Otobius megnini. 2. Argas persicus.
tam·pon ['tæmpɒn] **I** *n* Tampon *m*, (Watte-)Bausch *m*. **II** *vt* tamponieren.
tam·pon·ade [ˌtæmpə'neɪd] *n* Tamponade *f*; Tamponieren *f*.
tam·pon·age ['tæmpənɪdʒ] *n* → tamponade.
tam·pon·ing ['tæmpənɪŋ] *n* Tamponieren *nt.*
tam·pon·ment [tæm'pɒnmənt] *n* Tamponieren *nt.*
tan [tæn] **I** *n* 1. (Sonnen-)Bräune *f*. 2. *chem.* Gerbstoff *m*. **II** *vt* 3. (*Haut*) bräunen. 4. *chem.* (*Leder*) gerben; beizen. **III** *vi* (*Haut*) *s.* bräunen, braun werden.
tan·gen·tial [tæn'dʒenʃl] *adj* 1. berührend, tangential, Berührungs-, Tangential-. 2. *psychia.* (*Gedanken*) sprunghaft, abschweifend; ziellos; flüchtig.
tangential coordinate *mathe.* Linienkoordinate *f.*
tangential excision *chir.* tangentiale Exzision *f.*
tangential fibers → tangential neurofibers.
tangential force *phys.* Tangentialkraft *f.*
tangential injury tangentiale Verletzung *f.*
tan·gen·ti·al·i·ty [ˌtæn.dʒenʃɪ'ælətɪ] *n psychia.* (*Gedanken*) Sprunghaftigkeit *f*, Flüchtigkeit *f.*
tangential neurofibers tangentiale Nervenfasern/Nervenfaserschichten *pl*, Neurofibrae tangentiales.
tangential plane *mathe.* Berührungsebene *f.*
tangential tension Tangentialspannung *f.*
tan·gent screen ['tændʒənt] *ophthal.* Bjerrum-Schirm *f.*
Tan·gier disease [tæn'dʒɪər] Tangier-Krankheit *f*, Analphalipoproteinämie *f*, Hypo-Alpha-Lipoproteinämie *f.*
tan·gle ['tæŋgl] **I** *n* Gewirr *nt*, (wirrer) Knäuel *m*; Verwirrung *f*, Durcheinander *nt*. **II** *vt* verwirren, verwickeln, durcheinanderbringen.
tank [tæŋk] *n* Tank *m*, Becken *nt*; Zisterne *f*; Bad *nt.*
tan·nal ['tænəl] *n* Aluminiumtannat *nt.*
tan·nase ['tæneɪz] *n* Tannase *f.*
tan·nate ['tæneɪt] *n* Tannat *nt.*
Tanner ['tænər]: **T.'s operation** *chir.* Tanner-Operation *f.*
tan·ner's ulcer ['tænər] Chromatgeschwür *nt*, -ulkus *nt.*
tan·nic acid ['tænɪk, -niːk] → tannin.
tan·nin ['tænɪn] *n* Gerbsäure *f*, Tannin *nt*, Acidus tannicum.
tannin acyl-hydrolase → tannase.
tan·ta·lize ['tæntlaɪz] *vt* quälen, peinigen.
tan·ta·liz·ing ['tæntlaɪzɪŋ] *adj* quälend, peinigend.
T antigen 1. *micro.* T-Antigen *nt.* 2. Tumorantigen *nt*, T-Antigen *nt.*
tan·ta·lum ['tæntləm] *n abbr.* **Ta** Tantal *nt abbr.* Ta.
tan·ta·mount ['tæntəmaʊnt] *adj* gleichbedeutend (*to* mit).
tan·trum ['tæntrəm] *n* Wutanfall *m.*
tan·y·cyte ['tænɪsaɪt] *n* Tanyzyt *m.*
tap¹ [tæp] *n* 1. (Wasser-, Gas-)Hahn *m*. 2. Zapfen *m*, Spund *m*, Hahn *m*. 3. Punktion *f*. 4. *ortho., techn.* Gewindebohrer *m*, -schneider *m*. **II** *vt* 5. anzapfen, anstechen. 6. punktieren. 7. *ortho.* mit einem Gewinde versehen.
tap² [tæp] (*v* **tapped; tapped**) **I** *n* leichter Schlag, Klaps *m*. **II** *vt* beklopfen, antippen, leicht schlagen, leicht klopfen, leicht pochen an *od.* auf *od.* gegen, beklopfen. **III** *vi* klopfen, pochen (*on, at, gegen, an*).

tap drill Gewindebohrer *m*, -schneider *m.*
tape [teɪp] **I** *n* 1. (Isolier-, Meß-, Klebe-)Band *nt*, (-)Streifen *m*. 2. (Magnet-, Video-, Ton-)Band *nt*. 3. Heftpflaster *nt*, *inf.* Pflaster *nt*. **II** *vt* 4. (mit Band) umwickeln, binden. 5. mit Heftpflaster verkleben. 6. auf Band aufnehmen, aufzeichnen.
tape measure Meßband *nt*, Bandmaß *nt.*
ta·pe·to·cho·roi·dal dystrophy [təˌpiːtəʊkə'rɔɪdl] *ophthal.* Chorioideremie *f*, Degeneratio chorioretinalis progressiva.
ta·pe·to·ret·i·nal degeneration [ˌ-'retɪnl] *ophthal.* tapetoretinale Degeneration *f.*
ta·pe·to·ret·i·nop·a·thy [ˌ-ˌretɪ'nɑpəθɪ] *n* Tapetoretinopathie *f.*
ta·pe·tum [tə'piːtəm] *n*, *pl* **-ta** [-tə] 1. *anat.* bedeckende *od.* abdeckende Struktur/Schicht *f*, Tapetum *nt*. 2. Tapetum *nt*, Tapetum corporis callosi.
tape·worm ['teɪpwɜrm] *n micro.* 1. Bandwurm *m*. 2. **~s** *pl* Bandwürmer *pl*, Zestoden *pl*, Cestoda *pl*, Cestodes *pl.*
taph·o·phil·ia [ˌtæfə'fɪlɪə] *n psychia.* Taphophilie *f.*
taph·o·pho·bia [ˌ-'fəʊbɪə] *n psychia.* Taphophobie *f.*
Tapia ['tæpɪə; 'tɑpɪə]: **T.'s syndrome** Tapia-Syndrom *nt.*
ta·pir mouth ['teɪpər, tə'pɪər] Tapierlippe *f*, -schnauze *f*, -mund *m.*
tar [tɑr] **I** *n* Teer *m*. **II** *vt* teeren.
tar acne Teerakne *f*, Akne/Acne picea, Folliculitis picea.
ta·ran·tu·la [tə'ræntʃələ] *n*, *pl* **-las, -lae** [-liː] *bio.* Tarantel *f*, Lycosa tarentula.
tar·ba·dil·lo [ˌtɑr·bə'dɪ(l)jəʊ] *n* → tabardillo.
tar cancer Teerkrebs *m.*
Tardieu [tɑr'djø]: **T.'s ecchymoses** → T.'s spots.
T.'s spots *forens.* Tardieu'-Flecken *pl.*
T.'s petechiae → T.'s spots.
tar·dive ['tɑrdɪv] *adj* spät, verspätet, langsam.
tardive cyanosis Cyanose tardive *f.*
tardive dyskinesia *neuro.* dystones Syndrom *nt*, Dyskinesia tardive.
tar·dy epilepsy ['tɑrdɪ] Spätepilepsie *f*, Epilepsia tarda/tardiva.
tardy median palsy Karpaltunnelsyndrom *nt.*
tare [tɛər] **I** *n* Tara *f*. **II** *vt* tarieren.
ta·ren·tu·la *n* → tarantula.
tar·get ['tɑrɡɪt] *n* 1. Ziel *nt*; Zielscheibe *f*. 2. Ziel *nt*, Soll *nt*. 3. *phys.* Ziel *nt*, Meßobjekt *nt*; Fangelektrode *f*; Auffänger *m*; Zielkern *m.*
target area Zielbereich *m*, Zielgebiet *nt.*
target cell 1. *hema.* Target-, Schießscheiben-, Kokardenzelle *f*. 2. Zielzelle *f.*
target cell anemia Anämie *f* mit Schießscheibenzellen.
target erythrocyte → target cell 1.
target organ Zielorgan *nt.*
target theory Target-Theorie *f.*
target tissue Erfolgs-, Zielgewebe *nt.*
Tarin [tɑ'rɛ̃]: **T.'s space** Cisterna interpeduncularis.
T.'s valve Velum medulare inferius.
Tarini [tɑ'riːni]: **T.'s recess** Rec. anterior (fossae interpeduncularis).
tar keratosis Teerkeratose *f*, Teerwarzen *pl*, Pechwarzen *pl.*
Tarlov ['tɑrlɒv]: **T.'s cyst** Tarloff-Zyste *f.*
tar melanosis Hoffmann-Habermann--Pigmentanomalie *f*, Melanodermatitis/Melanodermitis toxica.

tar·ry cyst ['tɑrɪ] *gyn.* Teerzyste *f.*
tarry stool Teerstuhl *m*, Meläna *f*, Melaena *f.*
tars- *pref.* → tarso-.
tars·ad·e·ni·tis [tɑrˌsædɪ'naɪtɪs] *n ophthal.* Tarsadenitis *f.*
tar·sal ['tɑrsl] *adj* 1. Fußwurzel(knochen) betr., tarsal, Fußwurzel-, Tarsus-. 2. Lidknorpel betr., tarsal, Lidknorpel-.
tarsal artery: lateral t. seitliche Fußwurzelarterie *f*, A. tarsalis lateralis.
medial t.ies *pl* mediale Fußwurzelarterien *pl*, Aa. tarsales mediales.
tarsal bones Fußwurzel-, Tarsalknochen *pl*, Tarsalia *pl*, Ossa tarsi.
tarsal canal → tarsal sinus.
tarsal cartilage → tarsal plate.
tarsal cyst *ophthal.* Hagelkorn *nt*, Chalazion *nt.*
tar·sal·gia [tɑr'sældʒ(ɪ)ə] *n* Schmerzen *pl* in der Fußwurzel, Tarsalgie *f*; Fersenschmerz *m.*
tarsal glands Meibom'-Drüsen *pl*, Gll. tarsales.
tar·sa·lia [tɑr'seɪlɪə] *pl* → tarsal bones.
tar·sa·lis inferior (muscle) [tɑr'seɪlɪs] Tarsalis *m* inferior, M. tarsalis inferior.
tarsalis superior (muscle) Tarsalis *m* superior, M. tarsalis superior.
tarsal joint Intertarsalgelenk *nt*, Artic. intertarsalis.
tarsal membrane Orbitaseptum *nt*, Septum orbitale.
tarsal muscle: inferior t. → tarsalis inferior (muscle).
superior t. → tarsalis superior (muscle).
tarsal plate Lidknorpel *m*, Lidplatte *f*, Tarsalplatte *f*, Tarsus *m* (palpebrae).
t. of lower lid Unterlidplatte, Tarsus inferior (palpebrae).
t. of upper lid Oberlidplatte, Tarsus superior (palpebrae).
tarsal scaphoiditis *ortho.* Morbus Köhler *m* I, Köhler'-Krankheit *f*, Köhler--Müller-Weiss-Syndrom *nt.*
tarsal sinus Tarsalkanal *m*, Sinus tarsi.
tarsal tunnel syndrome Tarsaltunnel--Syndrom *nt.*
tar·sec·to·my [tɑr'sektəmɪ] *n* 1. *ortho.* Tarsektomie *f*. 2. *ophthal.* Tarsusexzision *f*, Tarsektomie *f.*
tar·si·tis [tɑr'saɪtɪs] *n ophthal.* Lidknorpel-, Tarsusentzündung *f*, Tarsitis *f*; Blepharitis *f.*
tarso- *pref.* 1. Tarso-, Fußwurzel(knochen)-, Tarsal-. 2. Tarso-, Lidknorpel-.
tar·so·chei·lo·plas·ty [ˌtɑrsəʊ'kaɪləplæstɪ] *n ophthal.* Lidrandplastik *f.*
tar·so·chi·lo·plas·ty *n* → tarsocheiloplasty.
tar·so·con·junc·ti·val glands [ˌ-ˌkʌndʒʌŋ'taɪvl] → tarsal glands.
tar·so·ep·i·phys·e·al aclasis [ˌ-ˌepɪ'fɪzɪəl] Trever-Erkrankung *f*, -Syndrom *nt*, Dysplasia epiphyseales hemimelica.
tar·so·ma·la·cia [ˌ-mə'leɪʃ(ɪ)ə] *n ophthal.* Lidknorpel-, Tarsuserweichung *f*, Tarsomalazie *f.*
tar·so·meg·a·ly [ˌ-'megəlɪ] *n embryo., ortho.* angeborene Vergrößerung *f* des Fersenbeins, Tarsomegalie *f.*
tar·so·met·a·tar·sal [ˌ-ˌmetə'tɑrsl] *adj* Fußwurzel/Tarsus u. Mittelfuß/Metatarsus betr., tarsometatarsal.
tarsometatarsal articulations Tarsometatarsalgelenke *pl*, Articc. tarsometatarsales.
tarsometatarsal joints → tarsometatarsal articulations.
tarsometatarsal ligaments Ligg. tarsometatarsalia.
dorsal t. Ligg. tarsometatarsalia dorsalia.

tarso-orbital

plantar t. Ligg. tarsometatarsalia plantaria.
tarso-orbital adj ophthal. Lidknorpel/Tarsus u. Augenhöhle/Orbita betr., tarsoorbital.
tar·so·pha·lan·ge·al [ˌ-fə'lændʒɪəl] adj Tarsus u. Phalangen betr., tarsophalangeal.
tarsophalangeal reflex Mendel-Bechterew-Reflex m.
tar·so·phy·ma [ˌ-'faɪmə] n ophthal. Lidknorpelschwellung f, -tumor m, Tarsusschwellung f, -tumor m.
tar·so·pla·sia [ˌ-'pleɪzɪə] n → tarsoplasty.
tar·so·plas·ty ['-plæstɪ] n ophthal. Lid-, Blepharoplastik f.
tar·sor·rha·phy [tɑːr'sɔrəfɪ] n ophthal. Tarso-, Blepharorrhaphie f.
tar·so·tar·sal [ˌtɑːrsə'tɑːrsl] adj tarsotarsal.
tar·so·tib·i·al [ˌ-'tɪbɪəl] adj Fußwurzel/Tarsus u. Schienbein/Tibia betr., tarsotibial.
tar·sot·o·my [tɑːr'sɑtəmɪ] n ophthal. Lidknorpel-, Tarsusdurchtrennung f, Tarsotomie f.
tar·sus ['tɑːrsəs] n, pl -si [-saɪ] 1. Fußwurzel f, Tarsus m. 2. Lidknorpel m, Lidplatte f, Tarsalplatte f, Tarsus m (palpebrae).
TAR syndrome → thrombocytopenia--absent radius syndrome.
tar·tar ['tɑːrtər] n 1. chem. Weinstein m. 2. dent. Zahnstein m, Calculus dentalis/dentis.
tar·tar·ic acid [tɑːr'tærɪk] Wein(stein)säure f.
tart cell [tɑːrt] patho. Tart-Zelle f.
tar·trate ['tɑːrtreɪt] n Tartrat nt.
Tarui [tɑ'ruɪ]: **T. disease** Tarui-Krankheit f, Muskelphosphofruktokinaseinsuffizienz f, Glykogenose f Typ VII.
task [tɑːsk, tæsk] n (schwierige) Aufgabe f; Pflicht f, Pensum nt.
task-specific training physiol. anforderungsspezifisches Training nt.
tast·a·ble ['teɪstəbl] adj schmeckbar, zu schmecken.
tas·tant ['teɪstənt] n Geschmacks-, Schmeckstoff m.
taste [teɪst] n I n 1. Geschmack m; Geschmackssinn m, Schmecken nt. 2. (Kost-)Probe f; Vorgeschmack m. 3. fig. Geschmack(srichtung f) m; Vorliebe f, Neigung f (for für). II vt kosten, (ab-)schmecken, probieren. III vi schmecken (of nach); kosten, probieren (of von).
tast·e·able adj → tastable.
taste blindness Geschmackslähmung f, -verlust m, Ageusie f.
taste bud Geschmacksknospe f, Caliculus gustatorius, Gemma gustatoria.
taste bulb → taste bud.
taste cells Geschmackssinneszellen pl, Schmeckzellen pl.
taste center Geschmackszentrum nt.
taste corpuscle → taste bud.
taste fibers Geschmacksfasern pl.
secondary t. sekundäre Geschmacksfasern.
taste·ful ['teɪstfʊl] adj 1. schmackhaft. 2. fig. geschmackvoll.
taste hairs Geschmacksstiftchen pl.
taste impulse Geschmacksreiz m.
taste·less ['teɪstlɪs] adj a. fig. geschmacklos, fade.
taste pore Geschmackspore f, Porus gustatorius.
taste quality Geschmacksqualität f.
taste receptor Geschmacksrezeptor m.
taste-specific adj geschmacksspezifisch.
taste stimulus Schmeckreiz m.
taste substance Schmeckstoff m.
taste testing Geschmacksprüfung f.

TAT abbr. 1. → thematic apperception test. 2. → tyrosine aminotransferase.
tat·too [tə'tuː, tæ-] I n Tätowierung f. II vt tätowieren.
tau·rine ['tɔːriːn] n Taurin nt, Äthanolaminsulfonsäure f, Aminoäthylsulfonsäure f.
tau·ro·che·no·de·ox·y·cho·late [ˌtɔːroʊˌkiːnoʊdɪˌɑksɪ'koʊleɪt] n Taurochenodesoxycholat nt.
tau·ro·che·no·de·ox·y·cho·lic acid [ˌ-ˌkiːnoʊdɪˌɑksɪ'koʊlɪk, -'kɑl-] Taurochenodesoxycholsäure f.
tau·ro·cho·la·ner·e·sis [ˌ-ˌkoʊlə'nɛrəsɪs, -kələ-] n erhöhte Taurocholsäureausscheidung f.
tau·ro·chol·an·o·poi·e·sis [ˌ-ˌkoʊˌlænəpɔɪ'iːsɪs] n Taurocholsäurebildung f.
tau·ro·cho·late [ˌ-'koʊleɪt] n Taurocholat nt.
tau·ro·cho·lic acid [ˌ-'koʊlɪk, -'kɑl-] Taurocholsäure f.
Taussig-Bing ['taʊsɪɡ bɪŋ]: **T.-B. disease/syndrome** Taussig-Bing-Syndrom nt.
tau·to·mer ['tɔːtəmər] n chem. Tautomer nt.
tau·tom·er·ase [tɔː'tɑmərɛɪz] n Tautomerase f.
tau·to·mer·ic [ˌtɔːtə'mɛrɪk] adj chem. tautomer.
tau·tom·er·ism [tɔː'tɑmərɪzəm] n chem. Tautomerie f.
tau·tom·er·ize [tɔː'tɑmərɑɪz] vt tautomerisieren.
Tawara [tə'wɑːrə]: **node of T.** Atrioventrikularknoten m, AV-Knoten m, Aschoff--Tawara'-Knoten m, Nodus atrioventricularis.
tax·i·met·rics [ˌtæksɪ'mɛtrɪks] pl bio. numerische Taxonomie f.
tax·ine ['tæksiːn, -sɪn] n Taxin nt.
tax·is ['tæksɪs] n, pl **tax·es** [-siːz] 1. bio. Taxis f. 2. chir., ortho. Reposition f, Taxis f.
tax·ol·o·gy [tæk'sɑlədʒɪ] n → taxonomy.
tax·on ['tæksɑn] n, pl **tax·a** [-ksə] Taxon nt.
tax·o·nom·ic [ˌtæksə'nɑmɪk] adj Taxonomie betr., taxonomisch.
tax·o·nom·i·cal [ˌ-'nɑmɪkl] adj → taxonomic.
taxonomic unit → taxon.
tax·on·o·my [tæk'sɑnəmɪ] n Taxonomie f.
Tay [teɪ]: **T.'s choroiditis/disease** Chorioiditis gutta senilis, Altersdrusen pl.
T.'s sign/spot Tay-Fleck m.
Tay-Sachs [zæks]: **T.-S. disease** abbr. **TSD** Tay-Sachs-Erkrankung f, -Syndrom nt, infantile amaurotische Idiotie f, GM_2--Gangliosidose f Typ I.
Tb abbr. → terbium.
T-band n genet. (Chromosom) T-Bande f.
TBG abbr. → thyroxine-binding globulin.
TBII abbr. [thyroid-binding inhibitory immunoglobulin] → thyroid-stimulating immunoglobulin.
TBP abbr. [thyroxine-binding protein] → thyroxine-binding globulin.
TBPA abbr. → thyroxine-binding prealbumin.
TBSA abbr. → total body surface area.
TBV abbr. 1. → total blood volume. 2. → total body volume.
TBW abbr. → total body water.
TC abbr. → transcobalamin.
Tc abbr. → technetium.
T cell T-Zelle f, T-Lymphozyt m.
cytotoxic T. zytotoxische T-Zelle.
T4 cell CD4-Zelle f, CD4-Lymphozyt m, $T4^+$-Zelle f, $T4^+$-Lymphozyt m.
T8 cell CD8-Zelle f, CD8-Lymphozyt m, $T8^+$-Zelle f, $T8^+$-Lymphozyt m.
T cell antigen T-Zellantigen nt.

T cell antigen receptor T-Zellantigenrezeptor m, T3/T-Rezeptor m.
T cell-dependent adj T-Zellen-abhängig.
T cell growth factor abbr. **TCGF** old → interleukin-2.
T cell-independent adj T-Zellen-unabhängig.
T-cell lymphoma T-Zellymphom nt, T-Zellenlymphom nt.
T cell-mediated hypersensitivity T-zellvermittelte Überempfindlichkeitsreaktion f, Tuberkulin-Typ/Spät-Typ/Typ IV m der Überempfindlichkeitsreaktion.
T cell-mediated immunity abbr. **TCMI** zellvermittelte/zelluläre Immunität f.
T cell progenitor T-Zellvorläufer(zelle f) m.
T cell receptor abbr. **TCR** T-Zell-Rezeptor m, TCR.
T3/T cell receptor → T cell antigen receptor.
T-cell system T-Zell(en)-System nt.
TCGF abbr. [T-cell growth factor] old → interleukin-2.
TCMI abbr. → T cell-mediated immunity.
TCR abbr. → T cell receptor.
t_D abbr. → doubling time.
TDA abbr. [TSH-displacing antibody] → TSH-binding inhibitory immunoglobulin.
T-dependent antigen T-Zellen-abhängiges Antigen nt.
T_{DTA} cell T_{DTA}-Zelle f, T_{DTA}-Lymphozyt m.
Te abbr. → tellurium.
TEA abbr. → tetraethylammonium.
tea [tiː] n Tee m.
TEAC abbr. → tetraethylammonium chloride.
Teale [tiːl]: **T.'s amputation/operation** ortho. Teale-Amputation f.
tear[1] [tɪər] n Träne f; Tropfen m.
tear[2] [tɛər] (v tore; torn) I n 1. Riß m. 2. (Zer-)Reißen nt. II v 3. zerreißen; einreißen; (Haut) aufreißen; (Muskel) zerren. 4. zerren an, ausreißen. III vi (zer-)reißen, zerren (at an).
tear apart vt zerreißen.
tear down vt herunterreißen; abreißen, abbrechen.
tear off vt ab-, weg-, herunterreißen.
tear out vt (her-)ausreißen (of aus).
tear up vt auf-, ausreißen, zerreißen.
tear·drop ['tɪərdrɑp] n Träne f.
tear drop fracture ortho. (Wirbelkörper) Berstungsbruch m, -fraktur f.
tear duct Tränen-Nasengang m, Ductus nasolacrimalis.
tear fluid Tränenflüssigkeit f.
tear gas Tränengas nt.
tear·ing ['tɪərɪŋ] n Tränenträufeln nt, Dakryorrhoe f, Epiphora f.
tear·ing pain ['tɛərɪŋ] ziehender Schmerz m.
tear sac Tränensack m, Saccus lacrimalis.
tear stone Tränenstein m, Dakryolith m.
tease [tiːz] vt histol. (Präparat) zerlegen, zerzupfen.
teased preparation [tiːzt] histol. Zupfpräparat nt.
tea·spoon ['tiːspuːn] n Teelöffel m.
tea·spoon·ful ['tiːspuːnfʊl] adj Teelöffel-(voll).
TEBG abbr. → testosterone-estradiol-binding globulin.
tech·ne·ti·um [tɛk'niːʃ(ɪ)əm] n abbr. **Tc** Technetium nt abbr. Tc.
technetium polyphosphate Technetiumphosphat nt.
tech·nic ['tɛknɪk; 1 tɛk'niːk] I n 1. → technique. 2. → technology. II adj → technical.

tech·ni·cal ['tɛknɪkl] *adj* 1. Technik betr., technisch; verfahrenstechnisch. 2. fachlich, fachspezifisch, -männisch, Fach-, Spezial-.
technical expression → technical term.
technical term Fachausdruck *m*, -bezeichnung *f*.
technical terminology Fachsprache *f*, Terminologie *f*.
tech·ni·cian [tɛk'nɪʃn] *n* Techniker(in *f*) *m*; Facharbeiter(in *f*) *m*.
tech·nique [tɛk'niːk] *n* Technik *f*, (Arbeits-)Verfahren *nt*; Methode *f*; *chir.* Operation(smethode *f*) *f*.
tech·no·chem·is·try [ˌtɛknəʊ'kɛməstrɪ] *n* Industriechemie *f*.
tech·nol·o·gist [tɛk'nɑlədʒɪst] *n* 1. Technologe *m*, -login *f*. 2. → technician.
tech·nol·o·gy [tɛk'nɑlədʒɪ] *n* Technologie *f*.
tec·tal ['tɛktəl] *adj* Tectum betr., tektal.
tectal lamina of mesencephalon → tectal plate.
tectal plate Vierhügelplatte *f*, Lamina quadrigemina, Lamina tecti/tectalis (mesencephali).
tec·ti·ce·phal·ic [ˌtɛktəsɪ'fælɪk] *adj* skaphozephal, -kephal.
tec·ti·form ['-fɔːrm] *adj* dachförmig.
tec·to·bul·bar tract [ˌ-'bʌlbər, -bɑːr] tektobulbärer Trakt *m*, Tractus tectobulbaris.
tec·to·ceph·a·ly [ˌ-'sɛfəlɪ] *n* → scaphocephaly.
tec·to·cer·e·bel·lar tract [ˌ-ˌsɛrə'bɛlər] Tractus tectocerebellaris.
tec·tol·o·gy [tɛk'tɑlədʒɪ] *n bio.* Tektologie *f*.
tec·to·ri·al [tɛk'tɔːrɪəl, -'tɔʊr-] *adj* als Dach *od.* Schutz dienend, (be-, ab-)deckend, Deck-, Schutz-.
tectorial membrane Membrana tectoria.
t. of cochlear duct Corti-Membran *f*, Membrana tectoria ductus cochlearis.
tec·to·ri·um [tɛk'tɔːrɪəm, -'tɔʊr-] *n, pl* **-ria** [-rɪə] → tectorial membrane of cochlear duct.
tec·to·ru·bral tract [ˌtɛktəʊ'ruːbrəl] Tractus tectorubralis.
tec·to·spi·nal tract [ˌ-'spaɪnl] Löwenthal'-Bahn *f*, Tractus tectospinalis.
tec·tum ['tɛktəm] *n, pl* **-tums, -ta** [-tə] 1. *anat.* dachähnliche Struktur *f*, Dach *nt*, Tectum *nt*. 2. → t. of mesencephalon.
t. of mesencephalon Mittelhirndach *nt*, Tectum mesencephali.
te·di·ous labor ['tiːdɪəs, 'tiːdʒəs] Wehenschwäche *f*, Bradytokie *f*.
Hülle *f*, Decke *f*.
teeth [tiːθ] *pl* → tooth.
teethe [tiːð] *vi* Zähne bekommen, zahnen.
teeth grinding (unwillkürliches) Zähneknirschen *nt*, Bruxismus *m*.
teeth·ing ['tiːðɪŋ] *n* Zahnen *nt*.
teething ring Beißring *m*.
T effector cell T-Effektorzelle *f*.
tef·lon shakes ['tɛflɑn] Polymerenfieber *nt*.
TEG *abbr.* → thromboelastogram.
teg·a·fur ['tɛgəfʊər] *n pharm.* Tegafur *nt*.
teg·men ['tɛgmən] *n, pl* **-mi·na** [-mɪnə] 1. *anat.* Decke *f*, Dach *nt*, Tegmen *nt*. 2. *allg.* Hülle *f*, Decke *f*.
teg·men·tal [tɛg'mɛntl] *adj* Tegmen *od.* Tegmentum betr., tegmental.
tegmental decussations Haubenkreuzungen *pl*, Decussationes tegmenti/tegmentales.
dorsal t. Meynert'-Haubenkreuzung, hintere Haubenkreuzung.
Forel's t. Forel'-Haubenkreuzung, vordere Haubenkreuzung.
ventral t. → Forel's t.

tegmental fasciculus, ventral Spitzer'-Faserbündel *nt*, Fasciculus tegmentalis ventralis.
tegmental field Forel'-H-Feld *nt*.
tegmental nucleus: **...i** *pl* Haubenkerne *pl*, Ncc. tegmenti/tegmentales.
dorsal t. Nc. dorsalis tegmenti.
t.i of midbrain *pl* Haubenkerne des Mittelhirns.
tegmental part of pons Tegmentum pontis, Pars dorsalis pontis.
tegmental tract, central zentrale Haubenbahn *f*, Tractus tegmentalis centralis.
tegmental wall of tympanic cavity Dach *nt* der Paukenhöhle, Tegmen tympani, Pars tegmentalis (cavitatis tympanicae).
teg·men·to·spi·nal tract [tɛgˌmɛntəʊ-'spaɪnl] Tractus reticulospinalis.
teg·men·tum [tɛg'mɛntəm] *n, pl* **-ta** [-tə] *anat.* Decke *f*, Tegmentum *nt*.
Teichmann ['taɪkmən; 'taɪçman]: **T.'s crystals** Chlorhämin(kristalle *pl*) *nt*, Chlorhämatin *nt*, Hämin(kristalle *pl*) *nt*, Teichmann-Kristalle *pl*, salzsaures Hämin *nt*.
tei·cho·ic acids [taɪ'kəʊɪk] Teichonsäuren *pl*, Teichonsäuren *pl*.
teichoic acid synthase Teichonsäuresynthase *f*.
tei·chop·sia [taɪ'kɑpsɪə] *n ophthal.* Teichopsie *f*, Teichoskopie *f*, Zackensehen *nt*.
tei·chu·ron·ic acid [ˌtaɪkə'rɑnɪk] Teichuronsäure *f*.
tei·no·dyn·ia [ˌtaɪnə'diːnɪə] *n* → tenalgia.
tel- *pref.* → telo-.
te·la ['tiːlə] *n, pl* **-lae** [-liː] *anat.* (Binde-)Gewebe *nt*, Gewebsschicht *f*, Tela *f*.
tela choroidea: t. of fourth ventricle Tela choroidea ventriculi quarti.
t. of third ventricle Tela choroidea ventriculi tertii.
tel·an·gi·ec·ta·sia [tɛlˌændʒɪɛk'teɪʒ(ɪ)ə] *n* Tel(e)angiektasie *f*, Telangiectasia *f*.
tel·an·gi·ec·ta·sis [tɛlˌændʒɪ'ɛktəsɪs] *n* → telangiectasia.
tel·an·gi·ec·tat·ic [tɛlˌændʒɪɛk'tætɪk] *adj* Tel(e)angiektasie betr., teleangiektatisch.
telangiectatic angioma teleangiektatisches Angiom *nt*, Angioma teleangiectatica.
telangiectatic cystosarcoma *gyn.* Cystosarcoma phylloides.
telangiectatic fibroma 1. teleangiektatisches Fibrom *nt*, Fibroma cavernosum/teleangiectaticum, Fibrohämangiom *nt*. 2. Angiofibrom *nt*.
telangiectatic lipoma Angiolipom(a) *nt*.
telangiectatic osteosarcoma teleangiektatisches Osteosarkom *nt*.
telangiectatic wart Blutwarze *f*, Angiokeratom(a) *nt*.
tel·ar·che [tɛ'lɑːrkɪ] *n* → thelarche.
tele- *pref.* 1. End-, Tel(e)-. 2. Fern-, Tele-.
tel·e·can·thus [ˌtɛlə'kænθəs] *n ophthal.* Telekanthus *m*.
tel·e·car·di·o·gram [ˌ-'kɑːrdɪəgræm] *n card.* Tele(elektro)kardiogramm *nt*.
tel·e·car·di·og·ra·phy [ˌ-ˌkɑːrdɪ'ɑgrəfɪ] *n card.* Tele(elektro)kardiographie *f*.
tel·e·cep·tor ['-sɛptər] *n physiol.* → teleceptor.
tel·e·co·balt [ˌ-'kəʊbɔːlt] *n radiol.* Telekobalt *nt*.
tel·e·cu·rie·ther·a·py [ˌ-ˌkjʊər'ɪθɛrəpɪ] *n radiol.* Telecurie-, Telegammatherapie *f*.
tel·e·den·drite [ˌ-'dɛndraɪt] *n* → telodendron.
tel·e·den·dron [ˌ-'dɛndrən] *n* → telodendron.
tel·e·di·ag·no·sis [ˌ-ˌdaɪəg'nəʊsɪs] *n* Ferndiagnose *f*.

tel·e·di·as·tol·ic [ˌ-ˌdaɪə'stɑlɪk] *adj card.* enddiastolisch.
tel·e·lec·tro·car·di·o·gram [ˌtɛlɪˌlɛktrə-'kɑːrdɪəgræm] *n* → telecardiogram.
tel·e·lec·tro·car·di·og·ra·phy [ˌtɛlɪˌlɛktrə-ˌkɑːrdɪ'ɑgrəfɪ] *n* → telecardiography.
tel·e·me·ter·ing capsule ['tɛləmiːtərɪŋ] Telemetriesonde *f*, -kapsel *f*.
te·lem·e·try [tə'lɛmətrɪ] *n* Telemetrie *f*.
tel·en·ce·phal [tɛl'ɛnsɪfæl] *n* → telencephalon.
tel·en·ce·phal·ic [ˌtɛlɛnsɪ'fælɪk] *adj* Endhirn/Telencephalon betr., telenzephal, Endhirn-.
telencephalic fasciculus, medial mediales Vorderhirnbündel *nt*, Fasciculus prosencephalicus medialis.
telencephalic hemisphere Großhirnhälfte *f*, -hemisphäre *f*, Endhirnhälfte *f*, -hemisphäre *f*, Hemisph(a)erium cerebralis.
telencephalic vesicle → telencephalon vesicle.
tel·en·ceph·al·i·za·tion [ˌtɛlɛnˌsɛfælɪ'zeɪʃn] *n* Telenzephalisation *f*.
tel·en·ceph·a·lon [ˌtɛlɛn'sɛfələn, -lən] *n* Endhirn *nt*, Telenzephalon *nt*, Telencephalon *nt*.
telencephalon vesicle *embryo.* Endhirnbläschen *nt*, Telencephalon *nt*.
tel·e·neu·ron [ˌtɛlə'njʊərɑn, -'nəʊ-] *n* Nervenendigung *f*.
te·le·o·log·i·cal [ˌtɛlɪə'lɑdʒɪkl, ˌtiːlɪə-] *adj* Teleologie betr., teleologisch.
te·le·ol·o·gy [ˌtɛlɪ'ɑlədʒɪ, ˌtiːlɪ-] *n* Teleologie *f*.
te·le·o·mi·to·sis [ˌtɛlɪəmaɪ'təʊsɪs, ˌtiːlɪə-] *n bio.* abgeschlossene Mitose *f*, Teleomitose *f*.
te·le·o·nom·ic [ˌ-'nɑmɪk] *adj* Teleonomie betr., teleonomisch.
te·le·on·o·my [ˌtɛlɪ'ɑnəmɪ] *n* Teleonomie *f*.
te·le·op·sia [ˌ-'ɑpsɪə] *n ophthal.* Teleopsie *f*.
te·le·or·gan·ic [ˌ-ɔːr'gænɪk] *adj* lebensnotwendig, vital.
tel·e·o·roent·gen·o·gram [ˌtɛlɪə'rɛntgənə-græm] *n* → teleoentgenogram.
tel·e·o·roent·gen·og·ra·phy [ˌ-ˌrɛntgən-'ɑgrəfɪ] *n* → teleroentgenography.
tel·e·path·ist [tə'lɛpəθɪst] *n* Telepath *m*.
tel·e·path·y [tə'lɛpəθɪ] *n* Gedankenlesen *nt*, Telepathie *f*.
tel·e·ra·di·og·ra·phy [ˌtɛləˌreɪdɪ'ɑgrəfɪ] *n* → teleroentgenography.
tel·e·ra·di·um [ˌ-'reɪdɪəm] *n radiol.* Teleradium *nt*.
tel·e·re·cep·tor [ˌ-rɪ'sɛptər] *n physiol.* Tele-, Distanzrezeptor *m*.
tel·er·gy ['tɛlərdʒɪ] *n* automatische/unwillkürliche Handlung *od.* Reaktion *f*, Automatismus *m*.
tel·e·roent·gen·o·gram [ˌtɛlə'rɛntgənə-græm] *n* Teleröntgengramm *nt*.
tel·e·roent·gen·og·ra·phy [ˌ-ˌrɛntgə'nɑg-rəfɪ] *n* Teleröntgengraphie *f*.
tel·e·roent·gen·ther·a·py [ˌ-ˌrɛntgən'θɛrə-pɪ] *n radiol.* Teleröntgentherapie *f*.
tel·es·thet·o·scope [ˌtɛlɛs'θɛtəskəʊp] *n* Telesthetoskop *nt*.
tel·e·sys·tol·ic [ˌtɛləsɪs'tɑlɪk] *adj card.* endsystolisch.
tel·e·ther·a·py [ˌ-'θɛrəpɪ] *n radiol.* Tele(strahlen)therapie *f*.
tel·lu·ric [tɛ'lʊərɪk] *adj* 1. Erde betr., tellurisch, Erd-. 2. *chem.* tellurhaltig, tellurig, tellurisch, Tellur-.
tel·lu·rite ['tɛljəraɪt] *n* Tellurit *nt*.
tellurite plate *micro.* Tellurplatte *f*.
tellurite taurocholate gelatin agar *abbr.* **TTGA** *micro.* Tellurit-Taurocholat-Gelatineagar *m/nt abbr.* TTGA.
tel·lu·ri·um [tɛ'lʊərɪəm] *n abbr.* **Te** Tellur *nt abbr.* Te.

telo-

telo- *pref.* End-, Tel(o)-.
tel·o·bi·o·sis [ˌtelǝʊbaɪˈǝʊsɪs] *n embryo.* Telobiose *f.*
tel·o·bran·chi·al body [-ˈbræŋkɪǝl] *embryo.* Ultimobranchialkörper *m*, ultimobranchialer Körper *m.*
tel·o·cen·tric [ˌ-ˈsentrɪk] *adj* telozentrisch.
telocentric chromosome telozentrisches Chromosom *nt.*
tel·o·ci·ne·sia [ˌ-sɪˈniːʒ(ɪ)ǝ] *n* → telophase.
tel·o·ci·ne·sis [ˌ-sɪˈniːsɪs, -saɪ-] *n* → telophase.
tel·o·den·dri·on]-ˈdendrɪǝn, ˌtel-] *n, pl* **-dria** [-drɪǝ] → telodendron.
tel·o·den·dron [ˌ-ˈdendrǝn] *n* Endbäumchen *nt*, Telodendrion *nt*, Telodendron *nt.*
tel·o·di·en·ce·phal·ic border [ˌ-ˌdaɪǝnsɪ-ˈfælɪk] Zwischenhirn-Endhirn-Grenze *f*, telodienzephale Grenze *f.*
telodiencephalic sulcus *embryo.* Sulcus telodiencephalicus.
tel·o·gen [ˈtelǝdʒǝn] **I** *n (Haar)* Ruhe-, Telogenphase *f.* **II** *adj* telogen.
telogen alopecia *derm.* telogene Alopezie *f*, Alopezie *f* vom Spättyp, telogener Haarausfall *m*, telogenes Effluvium *nt.*
telogen effluvium → telogen alopecia.
telogen hair loss → telogen alopecia.
tel·og·lia [telˈɒɡlɪǝ] *n* Tegolia *f.*
tel·o·ki·ne·sia [ˌtelǝkɪˈniːʒ(ɪ)ǝ, -kaɪ-] *n* → telophase.
tel·o·ki·ne·sis [ˌ-kɪˈniːsɪs, -kaɪ-] *n* → telophase.
tel·o·lec·i·thal [ˌ-ˈlesɪθǝl] *adj embryo.* telolezithal.
telolecithal ovum *bio.* telolezithales Ei *nt.*
tel·o·lem·ma [ˌ-ˈlemǝ] *n* Telolemm *nt.*
tel·o·ly·so·some [ˌ-ˈlaɪsǝsǝʊm] *n* Telolysosom *nt.*
tel·o·mere [ˈ-mɪǝr] *n genet.* Telomer *nt.*
tel·o·phase [ˈ-feɪz] *n* Telophase *f.*
tel·o·phrag·ma [ˌ-ˈfræɡmǝ] *n* Z-Linie *f*, Z-Streifen *m*, Zwischenscheibe *f*, Telophragma *nt.*
te·lo·re·cep·tor [ˌ-rɪˈseptǝr] *n* → telereceptor.
Tel·o·spo·rea [ˌ-ˈspɔːrɪǝ] *pl micro.* Sporentierchen *pl*, Sporozoa *pl*, Sporozoa *pl.*
Tel·o·spo·rid·ia [ˌ-spǝˈrɪdɪǝ] *pl* → Telosporea.
tel·o·syn·ap·sis [ˌ-sɪˈnæpsɪs] *n* Telosynapsis *f*, Telosyndese *f.*
tel·o·syn·de·sis [ˌ-ˈsɪndǝsɪs] *n* → telosynapsis.
tel·o·tax·is [ˌ-ˈtæksɪs] *n* Telotaxis *f.*
tel·son [ˈtelsǝn] *n bio.* Telson *nt.*
TEM *abbr.* → triethylenemelamine.
te·maz·e·pam [tǝˈmæzɪpæm] *n pharm.* Temazepam *nt.*
tem·per [ˈtempǝr] **I** *n* 1. Temperament *nt*, Wesen *nt*, Naturell *nt*, Gemüt(sart *f*) nt, Gemütslage *f.* 2. Laune *f*, Stimmung *f*; Wut *f*, Zorn *m*. **fit of ~** Wutanfall *m*. **in a good/bad ~** bei guter/schlechter Laune sein. **to be in a ~** gereizt *od.* wütend sein. **to keep one's ~** s. beherrschen. **to lose one's ~** die Beherrschung verlieren, in Wut geraten. 3. *(Metall)* Härte(grad *m*) *f.* **II** *vt* mildern, abschwächen *(with durch).*
tem·per·a·ment [ˈtemp(ǝ)rǝmǝnt] *n* → temper 1.
tem·per·an·tia [ˌtempǝˈrænʃɪǝ] *pl pharm.* Beruhigungsmittel *pl*, Sedativa *pl*, Temperantia *pl.*
tem·per·ate [ˈtemp(ǝ)rɪt] *adj* gemäßigt, maßvoll, temperent.
temperate bacteriophage temperenter/ gemäßigter Bakteriophage *m.*
temperate zone Zone *f* gemäßigten Klimas.
tem·per·a·ture [ˈtemprǝtʃǝr, ˈtempǝr-ˌtʃʊǝr] *n* 1. *abbr.* **t** Temperatur *f abbr.* t. 2. Körpertemperatur *f*, -wärme *f*; Fieber *nt.* **to have/run a ~** fiebern, Fieber *od.* (erhöhte) Temperatur haben. **to take s.o.'s ~** jds. Temperatur messen.
temperature coefficient *chem.* Temperaturkoeffizient *m.*
temperature curve Temperaturkurve *f*, -tabelle *f*, Fieberkurve *f*, -tabelle *f.*
temperature-dependent *adj* temperaturabhängig.
temperature gradient Temperaturgefälle *nt*, -gradient *m.*
temperature-insensitive *adj* temperaturunempfindlich.
temperature scale Temperaturskala *f.*
temperature sensation Temperaturempfindung *f.*
temperature sense Temperatursinn *m*, Thermorezeption *f.*
temperature-sensitive *adj* temperaturempfindlich, -sensitiv.
temperature-sensitive mutant *genet.* temperatursensitive Mutante *f*, ts-Mutante *f.*
temperature sensitivity Temperaturempfindlichkeit *f.*
temperature spots Temperaturpunkte *pl.*
tem·plate [ˈtemplɪt] *n* Schablone *f*; Matrize *f*; Vorlage *f*, Muster *nt.*
template-primer *n genet.* Template-primer *(m).*
template-specific *adj* matrizenspezifisch.
template specificity Matrizenspezifität *f.*
template strand Matrizenstrang *m.*
template system Matrize *f*, Matrizensystem *nt.*
tem·ple [templ] *n* 1. *anat.* Schläfe *f*, Schläfenregion *f.* 2. (Brillen-)Bügel *m.*
tem·plet *n* → template.
tem·po·ral [ˈtemp(ǝ)rǝl] **I** *n* Schläfenbein *nt*, Os temporale. **II** *adj* 1. zeitlich, vorübergehend, temporär, Zeit-. 2. Schläfe *od.* Schläfenbein betr., temporal, Schläfenbein-, Schläfen-.
temporal aponeurosis → temporal fascia.
temporal apophysis Warzenfortsatz *m*, Mastoid *nt*, Proc. mastoideus (ossis temporalis).
temporal arteriole of retina: inferior t. untere temporale Netzhautarteriole *f*, Arteriola temporalis retinae inferior.
superior t. obere temporale Netzhautarteriole *f*, Arteriola temporalis retinae superior.
temporal arteritis (senile) Riesenzellarteriitis *f*, Horton-Riesenzellarteriitis *f*, -Syndrom *nt*, Arteriitis cranialis/gigantocellularis/temporalis.
temporal artery: anterior t. vordere Schläfenlappenarterie *f*, A. temporalis anterior.
deep t.ies tiefe Schläfenschlagadern *pl*, Aa. temporales profundae.
deep t., anterior vordere tiefe Schläfenschlagader *f*, A. temporalis profunda anterior.
deep t., posterior hintere tiefe Schläfenschlagader *f*, A. temporalis profunda posterior.
intermediate t. mittlere Schläfenlappenarterie *f*, A. temporalis intermedia.
middle t. mittlere Schläfenschlagader *f*, A. temporalis media.
posterior t. hintere Schläfenlappenarterie *f*, A. temporalis posterior.
superficial t. oberflächliche Schläfenschlagader *f*, A. temporalis superficialis.
temporal bone Schläfenbein *nt*, Os temporale.
temporal bone fracture Schläfenbeinbruch *m*, -fraktur *f.*
temporal brain Temporal-, Schläfenhirn *nt.*

temporal branches: anterior t. of lateral occipital artery Rami temporales anteriores a. occipitalis lateralis.
t. of facial nerve Schläfenäste *pl* des N. facialis, Rami temporales n. facialis.
t. of lateral occipital artery Schläfenlappenäste *pl* der A. occipitalis lateralis, Rami temporales (intermedii mediales) a. occipitalis lateralis.
posterior t. of lateral occipital artery Rami temporales posteriores a. occipitalis lateralis.
superficial t. of auriculotemporal nerve Schläfenhautäste *pl* des N. auriculotemporalis, Nn. temporales superficiales.
temporal commissure of eye lid seitliche Augenlidkommissur *f*, Commissura palpebrarum lateralis.
temporal convolution: first t. obere Schläfenwindung *f*, Gyrus temporalis superior.
inferior t. untere Schläfenwindung *f*, Gyrus temporalis inferior.
middle t. mittlere Schläfenwindung *f*, Gyrus temporalis medialis.
second t. → middle t.
superior t. → first t.
third t. → inferior t.
transverse t.s Heschl'-Querwindungen *pl*, Gyri temporales transversi.
temporal dimension zeitliche Dimension *f.*
temporal facilitation *physiol.* zeitliche Bahnung *f.*
temporal fascia Fascia temporalis.
temporal fossa Schläfengrube *f*, Fossa temporalis.
temporal genu of optic radiation temporales Knie *nt* der Sehstrahlung, Genu temporale.
temporal gyrus Schläfen(lappen)windung *f.*
inferior t. untere Schläfenwindung, Gyrus temporalis inferior.
middle t. mittlere Schläfenwindung, Gyrus temporalis medialis.
superior t. obere Schläfenwindung, Gyrus temporalis superior.
transverse t.ri *pl* Heschl'-Querwindungen *pl*, Gyri temporales transversi.
transverse t., anterior Heschl'-Querwindung, Gyrus temporalis transversus anterior.
temporal horn of lateral ventricle Unterhorn *nt* des Seitenventrikels, Cornu inferius/temporale ventriculi lateralis.
tem·po·ra·lis (muscle) [ˌtempǝˈreɪlɪs] Schläfenmuskel *m*, Temporalis *m*, M. temporalis.
temporal line: t. of frontal bone Linea temporalis (ossis frontalis).
inferior t. (of parietal bone) Linea temporalis inferior (ossis parietalis).
superior t. (of parietal bone) Linea temporalis superior (ossis parietalis).
temporal lobe Temporal-, Schläfenlappen *m*, Lobus temporalis.
temporal lobe abscess Temporallappen-, Schläfenlappenabszeß *m.*
temporal lobe epilepsy 1. psychomotorische Epilepsie *f.* 2. Temporallappen-, Schläfenlappenepilepsie *f.*
temporal margin of parietal bone Margo squamosus ossis parietalis.
temporal muscle → temporalis (muscle).
temporal nerves: deep t. tiefe Schläfennerven *pl*, Nn. temporales profundi.
subcutaneous t. Schläfenhautäste *pl* des N. auriculotemporalis, Nn. temporales superficiales.
superficial t. Nn. temporales superficiales.

temporal operculum Operculum temporale.
temporal pole of cerebral hemisphere Schläfenpol *m* einer Großhirnhemisphäre, Polus temporalis (hemisph(a)erii cerebri).
temporal process of zygomatic bone Proc. temporalis.
temporal region *anat.* Schläfen-, Temporalregion *f*, Regio temporalis.
temporal speech area 1. Wernicke'-Sprachzentrum *nt*, akustisches/sensorisches Sprachzentrum *nt*. **2.** Wernicke'-Sprachregion *f*, temporale Sprachregion *f*.
temporal squama Schläfenbeinschuppe *f*, Squama ossis temporalis.
temporal sulcus: inferior t. 1. Sulcus temporalis inferior. **2.** *old* → occipitotemporal sulcus.
superior t. Sulcus temporalis superior.
transverse t.i *pl* Sulci temporales transversi.
temporal summation *physiol.* zeitliche Summation *f*.
temporal vein: deep t.s tiefe Schläfenvenen *pl*, Vv. temporales profundae.
middle t. mittlere Schläfenvene *f*, V. temporalis media.
superficial t.s oberflächliche Schläfenvenen *pl*, Vv. temporales superficiales.
temporal venule of retina: inferior t. untere temporale Netzhautvene *f*, Venula temporalis retinae inferior.
superior t. obere temporale Netzhautvene *f*, Venula temporalis retinae superior.
temporal wing of sphenoid bone großer Keilbeinflügel *m*, Ala major (ossis sphenoidalis).
tem·po·rar·y ['tempərɪ] *adj* **1.** vorübergehend, vorläufig, zeitweilig, temporär. **2.** provisorisch, Hilfs-, Aushilfs-.
temporary callus *ortho.* provisorischer Kallus *m*.
temporary cartilage Vorläuferknorpel *m*, verknöchernder Knorpel *m*.
temporary hardness transitorische (Wasser-)Härte *f*, Carbonathärte *f*.
temporary parasite temporärer Parasit *m*.
temporary stricture funktionelle/spastische Striktur *f*.
temporary threshold shift *abbr.* **TTS** (*Gehör*) vorübergehende Schwellenabwanderung *f*, temporary threshold shift *abbr.* TTS.
tem·po·ro·au·ric·u·lar [ˌtempərɔʊ:'rɪkjələr] *adj* temporoaurikulär, aurikulotemporal.
tem·po·ro·fa·cial [ˌ-'feɪʃl] *adj* Schläfe(nregion) u. Gesicht betr., temporofazial.
tem·po·ro·fron·tal [ˌ-'frʌntl] *adj* temporofrontal.
tem·po·ro·ma·lar [ˌ-'meɪlər] *adj* → temporozygomatic.
tem·po·ro·man·dib·u·lar [ˌ-mæn'dɪbjələr] *adj* Schläfenbein/Os temporale u. Unterkiefer/Mandibula betr., temporomandibular, mandibulotemporal.
temporomandibular articular disk Discus articularis temporomandibularis.
temporomandibular articular veins Venen *pl* des Kiefergelenks, Vv. articulares (temporomandibulae).
temporomandibular articulation → temporomandibular joint.
temporomandibular disk → temporomandibular articular disk.
temporomandibular dysfunction syndrome Costen-Syndrom *nt*, temporomandibuläres Syndrom *nt*.
temporomandibular joint (Unter-)Kiefergelenk *nt*, Temporomandibulargelenk *nt*, Artic. temporomandibularis.
temporomandibular joint syndrome → temporomandibular dysfunction syndrome.
temporomandibular ligament Seitenband *nt* des Kiefergelenks, Lig. laterale (artic. temporomandibularis).
tem·po·ro·max·il·lar·y [ˌ-'mæksəˌlerɪ:, -mæk'sɪlərɪ] *adj* Schläfenbein/Os temporale u. Oberkiefer/Maxilla betr., temporomaxillär.
temporomaxillary articulation → temporomandibular joint.
temporomaxillary joint → temporomandibular joint.
temporo-occipital *adj* temporookzipital.
tem·po·ro·pa·ri·e·tal [ˌ-pə'raɪɪtl] *adj* Schläfenbein/Os temporale u. Scheitelbein/Os parietale betr., temporoparietal.
temporoparietal aphasia sensorische Aphasie *f*, Wernicke-Aphasie *f*.
tem·po·ro·pa·ri·e·ta·lis (muscle) [ˌ-pəˌraɪə'teɪlɪs] Temporoparietalis *m*, M. temporoparietalis.
temporoparietal muscle → temporoparietalis (muscle).
tem·po·ro·pon·tine fibers [ˌ-'pɑntaɪn, -ti:n] temporopontine Fasern *pl*, Fibrae temporopontinae.
temporopontine tract Türck'-Bündel *nt*, Tractus temporopontinus.
tem·po·ro·sphe·noid [ˌ-'sfinɔɪd] *adj* Schläfenbein/Os temporale u. Keilbein/Os sphenoidale betr., temporosphenoidal.
tem·po·ro·zy·go·mat·ic [ˌ-ˌzaɪgoʊ'mætɪk] *adj* Schläfenbein/Os temporale u. Jochbein/Os zygomaticum betr., zygomatikotemporal.
temporozygomatic suture Sutura temporozygomatica.
TEN *abbr.* → toxic epidermal necrolysis.
ten- *pref.* → teno-.
te·na·cious [tə'neɪʃəs] *adj* **1.** zäh, hartnäckig. **2.** zäh, klebrig. **3.** *phys.* zäh, reiß-, zugfest. **4.** widerstandsfähig.
te·na·cious·ness [tə'neɪʃəsnɪs] *n* → tenacity.
te·nac·i·ty [tə'næsətɪ] *n* **1.** Zähigkeit *f*, Tenazität *f*. **2.** Klebrigkeit *f*, Zähigkeit *f*. **3.** *psycho.* Hartnäckigkeit *f*, Zähigkeit *f*, Zug-, Reißfestigkeit *f*, Tenazität *f*. **4.** *phys.* Zähigkeit *f*, Zug-, Reißfestigkeit *f*, Tenazität *f*. **5.** *pharm., micro.* Widerstandsfähigkeit *f*, Tenazität *f*.
te·nal·gia [tə'nældʒ(ɪ)ə] *n* Sehnenschmerz *m*, Tenalgie *f*, Tenodynie *f*, Tenodynie *f*, Tenalgia *f*.
tend¹ [tend] *vi* tendieren, neigen (*to, towards to*).
tend² [tend] *vt* (*Maschine*) bedienen.
ten·den·cy ['tendnsɪ] *n, pl* **-cies 1.** Tendenz *f*, Richtung *f*, Strömung *f*. **2.** Neigung *f* (*to* für); Hang *m* (*to* zu); Anlage *f*.
ten·der ['tendər] *adj* **1.** empfindlich, sensibel (*to*); schmerzhaft. **~ on pressure** druckempfindlich. **2.** (*Haut*) zart, weich. **3.** zärtlich, liebevoll.
tenderness ['tendərnɪs] *n* **1.** (Druck-, Berührungs-)Empfindlichkeit *f*, Sensibilität *f* (*to* gegen); Schmerz(haftigkeit *f*) *m*. **2.** (*Gewebe*) Zartheit *f*, Weichheit *f*. **3.** Zärtlichkeit *f*.
t. on pressure Druckschmerz.
t. to touch Berührungsschmerz, -empfindlichkeit *f*.
tender points Valleix-Punkte *pl*.
tender zones Head'-Zonen *pl*.
ten·di·ni·tis [ˌtendə'naɪtɪs] *n* Sehnenentzündung *f*, Tendinitis *f*, Tendonitis *f*.
ten·din·o·plas·ty ['tendɪnoʊplæstɪ] *n ortho.* Sehnenplastik *f*.

ten·di·no·su·ture [ˌ-'su:tʃər] *n ortho.* Sehnennaht *f*, Tenorrhaphie *f*.
ten·di·nous ['tendɪnəs] *adj* Sehne betr., sehnenartig, -förmig, sehnig, Sehnen-.
tendinous arch Sehnenbogen *m*, Arcus tendineus.
external t. of diaphragm Quadratusarkade *f*, Lig. arcuatum laterale, Arcus lumbocostalis lateralis (Halleri).
internal t. of diaphragm Psoasarkade *f*, Lig. arcuatum mediale, Arcus lumbocostalis medialis (Halleri).
t. of levator ani (muscle) Sehnenbogen *m* des M. levator ani, Arcus tendineus m. levatoris ani.
t. of lumbodorsal fascia Lig. lumbocostale.
t. of pelvic fascia Sehnenbogen *m* der Fascia pelvis, Arcus tendineus fasciae pelvis.
t. of soleus (muscle) Sehnenbogen *m* des M. soleus, Arcus tendineus m. solei.
tendinous center *anat.* Centrum tendineum.
t. of perineum Sehnenplatte *f* des Damms, Centrum tendineum perinei.
tendinous cords of heart Sehnenfäden *pl* der Papillarmuskeln, Chordae tendineae (cordis).
tendinous intersections sehnige Querstreifen *pl* des M. rectus abdominis, Intersectiones tendineae.
tendinous junctions Con(n)exus intertendineus.
tendinous membrane Sehnenhaut *f*, -platte *f*, flächenhafte Sehne *f*, Aponeurose *f*, Aponeurosis *f*.
tendinous ring, common Zinn'-Sehnenring *m*, An(n)ulus tendineus communis.
tendinous synovitis → tenosynovitis.
tendinous xanthoma 1. pigmentierte villonoduläre Synovitis *f abbr.* PVNS, benignes Synovialom *nt*, Riesenzelltumor *m* der Sehnenscheide, Tendosynovitis nodosa, Arthritis villonodularis pigmentosa. **2.** Sehnenxanthom *nt*, tendinöses Xanthom *nt*.
ten·do ['tendoʊ] *n, pl* **-di·nes** ['tendɪni:z] *anat.* Sehne *f*, Tendo *m*.
tendo Achillis *abbr.* **TA** Achillessehne *f*, Tendo Achillis, Tendo calcaneus.
ten·dol·y·sis [ten'dɑləsɪs] *n* → tenolysis.
ten·do·my·o·gen·ic contracture [ˌtendoʊˌmaɪə'dʒenɪk] tendomyogene Kontraktur *f*.
ten·don ['tendən] *n* Sehne *f*, Tendo *m*.
t. of Hector Achillessehne, Tendo Achillis, Tendo calcaneus.
t. of infundibulum Tendo infundibuli.
t. of origin (*Muskel*) Ursprungssehne.
tendon cells Flügel-, Sehnenzellen *pl*.
tendon corpuscles → tendon cells.
tendon graft 1. Sehnentransplantat *nt*. **2.** Sehnentransplantation *f*, -plastik *f*.
free t. freie Sehnentransplantation.
one-stage t. einzeitige Sehnentransplantation.
two-stage t. zweizeitige Sehnentransplantation.
tendon grafting → tendon graft 2.
ten·do·ni·tis [tendə'naɪtɪs] *n* → tendinitis.
tendon jerk → tendon reflex.
tendon organ Golgi'-Sehnenorgan *nt*, -Sehnenspindel *f*.
tendon reaction → tendon reflex.
tendon receptor Sehnenrezeptor *m*.
tendon reflex *neuro.* Sehnenreflex *m*.
tendon release *ortho.* Tenotomie *f*.
tendon repair *ortho.* Sehnennaht *f*, Tenorrhaphie *f*.
tendon retractor *ortho.* Sehnenhaken *m*.
tendon rupture Sehnenruptur *f*.

tendon sheath

tendon sheath Sehnenscheide *f*, Vagina tendinis.
fibrous t. fibröse Sehnenscheide, Vagina fibrosa tendinis.
fibrous t.s of foot Vaginae fibrosae tendinum digitorum pedis.
fibrous t.s of toes Vaginae fibrosae digitorum pedis.
tendon sheath syndrome *ophthal.* Brown--Syndrom *nt.*
tendon sheath tumor Sehnenscheidentumor *m*, -geschwulst *f.*
tendon spindle Golgi'-Sehnenorgan *nt*, -Sehnenspindel *f.*
tendon suture *chir.* Sehnennaht *f.*
tendon synovectomy → tenosynovectomy.
tendon transfer Sehnenverpflanzung *f*, -transfer *m.*
tendon tumor Sehnengeschwulst *f*, -tumor *m.*
ten·do·plas·ty ['tendəplæsti] *n ortho.* Sehnen-, Tendoplastik *f.*
ten·do·syn·o·vi·tis [ˌ-ˌsɪnə'vaɪtɪs] *n* → tenosynovitis.
ten·do·tome ['-təʊm] *n* → tenotome.
ten·dot·o·my [ten'dɒtəmɪ] *n* → tenotomy.
ten·do·vag·i·nal [ˌtendə'vædʒɪnl] *adj* Sehnenscheide betr., Sehnenscheiden-.
ten·do·vag·i·ni·tis [ˌ-ˌvædʒɪ'naɪtɪs] *n* → tenosynovitis.
ten·dril fibers ['tendrɪl] *histol.* Kletterfasern *pl.*
te·neb·ri·my·cin [təˌnebrɪ'maɪsɪn] *n* → tobramycin.
te·nec·to·my [tə'nektəmɪ] *n* Sehnenexzision *f*, -resektion *f*, Tonenektomie *f.*
ten·e·my·cen [ˌtenə'maɪsɪn] *n* → tobramycin.
te·nes·mic [tə'nezmɪk] *adj* Tenesmus betr.
te·nes·mus [tə'nezməs] *n* schmerzhafter Stuhl- *od.* Harndrang *m*, Tenesmus *m.*
ten Horn's sign [ten] *chir.* (ten) Horn-Zeichen *nt.*
te·nia ['tɪnɪə] *n, pl* **-ni·as, -ni·ae** [-nɪˌiː] → taenia.
te·ni·a·cide *n, adj* → taeniacide.
te·ni·a·fu·gal *adj* → taeniafugal.
te·ni·a·fuge *n* → taeniafuge.
te·ni·al *adj* → taenial.
te·ni·a·sis *n* → taeniasis.
te·ni·cide ['tenɪsaɪd] *n, adj* → taeniacide.
te·nif·u·gal [te'nɪfjəgəl] *adj* → taeniafugal.
te·ni·fuge ['tenɪfjuːdʒ] *n* → taeniafuge.
ten·nis elbow ['tenɪs] Tennisellenbogen *m*, Epicondylitis radialis humeri.
teno- *pref.* Sehnen-, Tendo-, Ten(o)-, Tenont(o)-.
ten·o·de·sis [ˌtenə'diːsɪs, te'nɒdəsɪs] *n ortho.* Tenodese *f.*
ten·o·dyn·ia [ˌ-'dɪnɪə] *n* → tenalgia.
ten·o·fi·bril [ˌ-'faɪbrɪl] *n* → tonofibril.
ten·ol·y·sis [te'nɒləsɪs] *n ortho.* Sehnenlösung *f*, Tendo-, Tenolyse *f.*
ten·o·my·o·plas·ty [ˌtenə'maɪəplæsti] *n chir.*, *ortho.* Sehnen-, Sehnen-Muskel-Plastik *f*, Tenomyoplastik *f.*
ten·o·my·ot·o·my [ˌ-maɪ'ɒtəmɪ] *n ortho.* Tenomyotomie *f.*
Tenon ['tenɒn; tə'nɔ̃] *T.'s capsule* Tenon'--Kapsel *f*, Vagina bulbi.
fasciae of T. Fasciae musculares (bulbi).
T.'s membrane → T.'s capsule.
T.'s space Tenon'-Raum *m*, Spatium intervaginale/episclerale.
ten·o·nec·to·my [ˌtenə'nektəmɪ] *n* → tenectomy.
ten·o·ni·tis [ˌ-'naɪtɪs] *n* **1.** → tendinitis. **2.** *ophthal.* Entzündung *f* der Tenon-Kapsel, Tenonitis *f.*
ten·o·nom·e·ter [ˌ-'nɒmɪtər] *n* → tonometer.

ten·o·nos·to·sis [ˌ-nɒs'təʊsɪs] *n* → tenostosis.
tenont- *pref.* → teno-.
ten·on·ta·gra [ˌtenɒn'tægrə] *n* Sehnengicht *f*, Tenontagra *f.*
ten·on·ti·tis [ˌ-'taɪtɪs] *n* → tendinitis.
tenonto- *pref.* → teno-.
te·non·to·dyn·ia [teˌnɒntə'dɪːnɪə] *n* → tenalgia.
te·non·to·lem·mi·tis [ˌ-le'maɪtɪs] *n* → tenosynovitis.
te·non·to·my·o·plas·ty [ˌ-'maɪəplæsti] *n* → tenomyoplasty.
te·non·to·my·ot·o·my [ˌ-maɪ'ɒtəmɪ] *n* → tenomyotomy.
te·non·to·phy·ma [ˌ-'faɪmə] *n* Sehnenschwellung *f*, -tumor *m.*
te·non·to·plas·ty [tə'nɒntəplæsti] *n* → tenoplasty.
te·non·to·the·ci·tis [ˌ-θɪ'saɪtɪs] *n* → tenosynovitis.
ten·on·tot·o·my [ˌtenɒn'tɒtəmɪ] *n* → tenotomy.
ten·o·plas·tic [ˌtenə'plæstɪk] *adj* Tenoplastik betr., tenoplastisch.
ten·o·plas·ty ['-plæsti] *n ortho.* Sehnen-, Teno-, Tendoplastik *f.*
ten·o·re·cep·tor [ˌ-rɪ'septər] *n* Sehnenrezeptor *m.*
te·nor·rha·phy [te'nɒrəfi] *n ortho.* Sehnennaht *f*, Tenorrhaphie *f.*
ten·o·si·tis [ˌtenə'saɪtɪs] *n* → tendinitis.
ten·os·to·sis [tenəs'təʊsɪs] *n* Sehnenverknöcherung *f*, Tenostose *f.*
ten·o·su·ture [ˌtenə'sjuːtʃər] *n* → tenorrhaphy.
ten·o·sy·ni·tis [ˌ-'saɪnaɪtɪs] *n* → tenosynovitis.
ten·o·syn·o·vec·to·my [ˌ-ˌsɪnə'vektəmɪ] *n ortho.* Sehnenscheidenexzision *f*, -resektion *f*, Tenosynov(ial)ektomie *f.*
ten·o·syn·o·vi·tis [ˌ-ˌsɪnə'vaɪtɪs] *n* Sehnenscheidenentzündung *f*, Teno-, Tendosynovitis *f*, Tendovaginitis *f.*
ten·o·tome ['-təʊm] *n ortho.*, *ophthal.* Tenotomiemesser *nt*, Tenotom *nt.*
te·not·o·my [te'nɒtəmɪ] *n ortho.*, *ophthal.* Tenotomie *f.*
ten·o·vag·i·ni·tis [ˌtenəˌvædʒə'naɪtɪs] *n* → tenosynovitis.
TENS *abbr.* → nerve stimulation, transcutaneous electrical.
ten·sa cholesteatoma ['tensə] *HNO* Tensacholesteatom *nt*, sekundäres Mittelohrcholesteatom *nt.*
tense [tens] **I** *adj* **1.** gespannt, straff. **2.** *fig.* (an-)gespannt, verkrampft, nervös. **II** *vt* (an-)spannen, straffen. **III** *vi* **3.** s. (an-)spannen, s. straffen. **4.** *fig.* s. verkrampfen.
tense·ness ['tensnɪs] *n* **1.** Spannung *f*, Straffheit *f.* **2.** *fig.* (An-)Spannung *f*, Verkrampftheit *f*, Gespanntheit *f*, Nervosität *f.*
tense pulse gespannter Puls *m.*
ten·si·bil·i·ty [ˌtensə'bɪlətɪ] *n* Dehnbarkeit *f.*
ten·si·ble ['tensɪbl] *adj* dehn-, spannbar.
ten·sile ['tensɪl] *adj* dehn-, streckbar, Dehnungs-, Spannungs-, Zug-.
tensile strength Zug-, Dehnfestigkeit *f.*
tensile stress Zugbeanspruchung *f*, -belastung *f*, Dehnbeanspruchung *f*, -belastung *f.*
ten·si·lon test ['tensɪlɒn] *neuro.* Tensilon--Test *m.*
ten·si·om·e·ter [ˌtensɪ'ɒmɪtər] *n phys.* Zugmesser *m.*
ten·sion ['tenʃn] *n* **1.** Tension *f*, Spannung *f*; Dehnung *f*, Zug *m*; Druck *m*; (Muskel-)Anspannung *f.* **2.** *fig.* Anspannung *f*, Belastung *f.* **3.** *phys.* (elektrische) Span-

nung *f.* **4.** (*Gas*) Partialdruck *m*, Spannung *f.*
tension band wiring *ortho.* Zuggurtung *f*, Zuggurtungsosteosynthese *f.*
tension cavity *patho.* (*Lunge*) Spannungsblase *f.*
tension-control system *physiol.* Spannungskontrollsystem *nt.*
tension headache Spannungskopfschmerz *m.*
tension hydrothorax Spannungshydrothorax *m.*
tension pneumothorax Spannungspneu(mothorax *m*) *m.*
tension-time index *physiol.* Tension-Time-Index *m.*
ten·sor ['tensər] *n* **1.** *anat.* Spannmuskel *m*, Tensor *m*, M. tensor. **2.** *mathe.* Tensor *m.*
tensor fasciae latae (muscle) Tensor *m* fasciae latae, M. tensor fasciae latae.
tensor ligament → tensor tympani (muscle).
tensor muscle: t. of fascia lata → tensor fasciae latae (muscle).
t. of palatine velum → tensor veli palatini (muscle).
t. of tympanum → tensor tympani (muscle).
tensor tympani (muscle) Trommelfellspanner *m*, Tensor *m* tympani, M. tensor tympani.
tensor veli palatini (muscle) Tensor *m* veli palatini, M. tensor veli palatini.
tent¹ [tent] *n* Zelt *nt.*
tent² [tent] **I** *n* Tampon *m.* **II** *vt* durch einen Tampon offenhalten.
ten·ta·cle ['tentəkl] *n bio.* Fangarm *m*, Tentakel *m/nt.*
ten·ta·tive ['tentətɪv] **I** *n* Versuch *m.* **II** *adj* versuchsweise, vorübergehend, probeweise, tentativ.
tenth nerve [tenθ] Vagus *m*, X. Hirnnerv *m*, N. vagus.
ten·to·ri·al [ten'tɔːrɪəl, -'təʊr-] *adj* Tentorium cerebelli betr., tentorial, tentoriell, Tentorium-.
tentorial branch: basal t. of internal carotid artery basaler Tentoriumast *m* der A. carotis interna, Ramus basalis tentorii a. carotidis internae.
marginal t. of internal carotid artery marginaler Tentoriumast *m* der A. carotis interna, Ramus marginalis tentorii a. carotidis internae.
t. of ophthalmic nerve Tentoriumast *m* des N. ophthalmicus, Ramus tentorii/meningeus n. ophthalmici.
tentorial laceration Tentoriumriß *m.*
tentorial notch Tentoriumschlitz *m*, Inc. tentorii.
ten·to·ri·um [ten'tɔːrɪəm, -'təʊr-] *n, pl* **-ria** [-rɪə] *anat.* zeltförmiges Gebilde *nt*, Zelt *nt*, Tentorium *nt.*
t. of cerebellum Kleinhirnzelt, Tentorium cerebelli.
ten·u·ous ['tenjʊəs] *adj* **1.** fein, dünn; zart. **2.** *phys.* verdünnt; (*Luft*) dünn; (*Gas*) flüchtig. **3.** *fig.* (*Beweis*) wenig stichhaltig; (*Unterschied*) schwach.
TEPA *abbr.* → triethylenethiophosphoramide.
teph·ro·ma·la·cia [ˌtefrəʊmə'leɪʃ(ɪ)ə] *n patho.* Erweichung *f* der grauen Hirn- *od.* Rückenmarkssubstanz.
teph·ro·my·e·li·tis [ˌ-ˌmaɪə'laɪtɪs] *n patho.* Entzündung *f* der grauen Hirn- *od.* Rückenmarkssubstanz.
tep·i·dar·i·um [ˌtepɪ'deərɪəm] *n* Tepidarium *nt*, Warmbad *nt*; Badezelle *f.*
TEPP *abbr.* → tetraethyl pyrophosphate.
tera- *pref. abbr.* **T** tera- *abbr.* T.

te·ras ['terəs] *n, pl* **ter·a·ta** [tə'rætə] *embryo.* Mißbildung *f*, Teras *nt*.
terat(o)- *pref.* Mißbildungs-, Terat(o)-.
ter·a·to·blas·to·ma [ˌterətəʊblæs'təʊmə] *n* Teratoblastom(a) *nt*.
ter·a·to·car·ci·no·gen·e·sis [ˌ-ˌkɑːrsɪnə'dʒenəsɪs] *n* Teratokarzinogenese *f*.
ter·a·to·car·ci·no·ma [ˌ-ˌkɑːrsɪ'nəʊmə] *n* Teratokarzinom *nt*, -carcinoma *nt*.
te·rat·o·gen [tə'rætədʒən, 'terətə-] *n* Teratogen *nt*.
ter·a·to·gen·e·sis [ˌterətəʊ'dʒenəsɪs] *n* Mißbildungsentstehung *f*, Teratogenese *f*.
ter·a·to·ge·net·ic [ˌ-dʒə'netɪk] *adj* Teratogenese betr., teratogenetisch.
ter·a·to·gen·ic [ˌ-'dʒenɪk] *adj* Mißbildungen verursachend *od.* erzeugend, teratogen.
teratogenic dislocation of the hip *ortho.* teratologische/pränatale (Hüftgelenks-)-Dislokation *f*.
ter·a·tog·e·nous [ˌterə'tɑdʒənəs] *adj* aus fetalen Restanlagen entstehend.
ter·a·tog·e·ny [ˌ-'tɑdʒənɪ] *n* → teratogenesis.
ter·a·toid ['terətɔɪd] *adj* teratoid.
teratoid tumor → teratoma.
ter·a·to·log·ic [ˌterətəʊ'lɑdʒɪk] *adj* Teratologie betr., teratologisch.
ter·a·to·log·i·cal [ˌ-'lɑdʒɪkl] *adj* → teratologic.
ter·a·tol·o·gy [ˌterə'tɑlədʒɪ] *n embryo.* Lehre *f* von den Mißbildungen, Teratologie *f*.
ter·a·to·ma [ˌ-'təʊmə] *n, pl* **-mas, -ma·ta** [-mətə] *embryo., patho.* teratoide/teratogene Geschwulst *f*, Teratom(a) *nt*.
ter·a·to·ma·tous [ˌ-'təʊmətəs] *adj* teratomartig, teratomatös.
ter·a·to·pho·bia [ˌterətəʊ'fəʊbɪə] *n psychia., gyn.* Teratophobie *f*.
ter·a·to·sper·mia [ˌ-'spɜrmɪə] *n* Teratospermie *f*.
ter·bi·um ['tɜrbɪəm] *n abbr.* **Tb** Terbium *nt abbr.* Tb.
ter·bu·ta·line [tɜr'bjuːtəliːn] *n pharm.* Terbutalin *nt*.
ter·chlo·ride [tɜr'klɔːraɪd, -ɪd, -'kləʊ-] *n* Trichlorid *nt*.
ter·e·ben·thene [ˌterə'benθiːn] *n* Terpentinöl *nt*.
ter·e·binth ['-bɪnθ] *n* 1. Terpentinpistazie *f*, Terebinthe *f*, Pistacia terebinthus. 2. → terebinthina.
ter·e·bin·thi·na [ˌ-'bɪnθɪnə] *n* Terpentin *nt*, Terebinthina *f*.
ter·e·bin·thi·nism [ˌ-'bɪnθənɪzəm] *n* Terpentinvergiftung *f*.
ter·e·brant ['terəbrənt] *adj* → terebrating.
terebrant pain bohrender/stechender Schmerz *m*.
ter·e·bra·ting ['terəbreɪtɪŋ] *adj* bohrend, stechend.
terebrating pain → terebrant pain.
te·res major (muscle) ['tɪərɪːz, 'ter-] Teres *m* major, M. teres major.
teres minor (muscle) Teres *m* minor, M. teres minor.
ter·fen·a·dine [tɜr'fenədiːn] *n pharm.* Terfenadin *nt*.
ter·gal ['tɜrɡəl] *adj* Rücken betr., Rücken-.
term [tɜrm] **I** *n* 1. (Fach-)Ausdruck *m*, (Fach-)Bezeichnung *f*. 2. Zeit *f*, Dauer *f*, Periode *f*; Frist *f*. **on/in the long ~** langfristig. **on/in the short ~** kurzfristig. 3. *gyn.* errechneter Entbindungstermin *m*. **at ~** termingerecht, zum errechneten Termin. **to carry to ~** ein Kind austragen. **to go to ~** ausgetragen werden. 4. **~s** *pl* (Vertrags-)Bestimmungen *pl*. 5. **~s** *pl* (menschliche) Beziehungen *pl*, Verhältnis *nt*. **II** *vt* (be-)nennen, bezeichnen als.

ter·mi·nal ['tɜrmɪnl] **I** *n* Ende *nt*, Endstück *nt*, -glied *nt*, Spitze *f*. **II** *adj* 1. endständig, End-; abschließend, begrenzend, terminal, Grenz-. 2. letzte(r, s); unheilbar, terminal, im Endstadium, im Sterben, Sterbe-, Terminal-.
terminal addition enzyme DNS-Nukleotidylexotransferase *f*, DNA-Nukleotidylexotransferase *f*, terminale Desoxynukleotidyltransferase *f abbr.* TdT.
terminal arteriole terminale Arteriole *f*.
terminal artery Endarterie *f*, Cohnheim'--Arterie *f*.
terminal bar *histol.* 1. Schlußleiste *f*. 2. **~s** *pl* Schlußleistennetz *nt*.
terminal branch Endast *m*; Endarterie *f*.
terminal bronchioles Terminalbronchiolen *pl*, Bronchioles terminales.
terminal bulbs of Krause Krause'-Endkolben *pl*, Corpuscula bulboidea.
terminal buttons synaptische Endknöpfchen *pl*, Boutons termineaux.
terminal cisterns (*Muskel*) Terminalzisternen *pl*.
terminal cone of spinal cord Conus medullaris.
terminal crest of right atrium Crista terminalis.
terminal cylinders Ruffini'-Endorgane *pl*.
terminal deoxynucleotidyl transferase → terminal addition enzyme.
terminal deoxyribonucleotidyl transferase → terminal addition enzyme.
terminal division Endast *m*.
terminal enteritis Crohn'-Krankheit *f*, Morbus Crohn *m*, Enteritis regionalis, Ileocolitis regionalis/terminalis, Ileitis regionalis/terminalis.
terminal filament Filum terminale/spinale.
dural t. → external t.
external t. Filum terminale durale/externum.
internal t. Filum terminale internum/pialis.
pial t. → internal t.
t. of spinal dura mater → external t.
terminal fossa of male urethra Fossa navicularis urethrae.
terminal ganglion 1. terminales Ganglion *nt*. 2. Ggl. terminale.
terminal hair Terminalhaar *nt*.
terminal hematuria terminale Hämaturie *f*.
terminal ileitis → terminal enteritis.
terminal ileum terminales Ileum *nt*.
terminal illness Erkrankung *f* im Endstadium.
terminal incisure of ear Inc. terminalis auriculares.
terminal lamina of hypothalamus Lamina terminalis hypothalami.
terminal leukocytosis terminale Leukozytose *f*.
terminal line of pelvis Linea terminalis (pelvis).
terminal nerve N. terminalis.
terminal notch of ear → terminal incisure of ear.
terminal nuclei Endkerne *pl*, Ncc. terminationis.
terminal part: t. of middle cerebral artery End-/Rindenabschnitt *m* der A. cerebri media, Pars terminalis/corticalis a. cerebri mediae.
t. of posterior cerebral artery End-/Rindenabschnitt *m* der A. cerebri posterior, Pars terminalis/corticalis a. cerebri posterioris.
terminal plate of hypothalamus Lamina terminalis hypothalami.

terminal pneumonia terminale Pneumonie *f*.
terminal repetition *biochem.* terminale Repetition *f*.
terminal ring of spermatozoon Schlußring *m* des Spermiums.
terminal sac period *embryo.* (*Lunge*) Terminalsäckchenphase *f*.
terminal stria Stria terminalis.
terminal sulcus: t. of right atrium Sulcus terminalis cordis, Sulcus terminalis atrii dextri.
t. of tongue Terminalsulkus *m*, V-Linguae *nt*, Sulcus terminalis linguae.
terminal thread of spinal cord → terminal filament.
terminal vascular bed terminale Strombahn *f*.
terminal vein Terminalvene *f*, V. thalamostriata superior, V. terminalis.
terminal ventricle of spinal cord Ventriculus terminalis (medullae spinalis).
terminal villi freie (End-)Zotten *pl*.
ter·mi·nate ['tɜrmɪneɪt] **I** *adj* **II** *vt* 1. begrenzen. 2. beenden, beendigen, be-, abschließen. **III** *vi* enden (*in* in); aufhören (*in* mit); (*Vertrag*) ablaufen.
ter·mi·na·tion [ˌtɜrmɪ'neɪʃn] *n* 1. Ende *nt*; Aufhören *nt*, Einstellung *f*; Abschluß *m*, Abbruch *m*, Beendigung *f*, Termination *f*. 2. Endung *f*, Endigung *f*, Terminatio *f*.
t. of pregnancy Schwangerschaftsabbruch, -unterbrechung *f*.
termination codon *biochem., genet.* Kettenabbruch-, Abbruch-, Terminationskodon *nt*.
termination signal *biochem., genet.* Abbruch-, Terminationssignal *nt*.
ter·mi·no·lat·er·al anastomosis [ˌtɜrmɪnəʊ'lætərəl] End-zu-Seit-Anastomose *f*, terminolaterale Anastomose *f*.
ter·mi·nol·o·gy [ˌtɜrmɪ'nɑlədʒɪ] *n, pl* **-gies** Terminologie *f*; Nomenklatur *f*.
ter·mi·no·ter·mi·nal anastomosis [ˌtɜrmɪnəʊ'tɜrmɪnl] End-zu-End-Anastomose *f*, terminoterminale Anastomose *f*.
ter·mi·nus ['tɜrmɪnəs] *n, pl* **-nus·es, -ni** [-naɪ] 1. Ende *nt*, Grenze *f*, Terminus *m*. 2. Fachbegriff *m*, -ausdruck *m*, Terminus *m*.
ter·mo·lec·u·lar [tɜrmə'lekjələr] *adj chem.* trimolekular.
ter·na·ry ['tɜrnərɪ] *adj* 1. *chem.* dreifach, dreigliedrig, ternär. 2. → tertiary.
ternary complex *biochem.* ternärer/zentraler Komplex *m*.
ternary compound *chem.* ternäre Verbindung *f*.
ter·ni·trate [tɜr'naɪtreɪt] *n* Trinitrat *nt*.
ter·ox·ide [tɜr'ɑksaɪd, -sɪd] *n* Trioxid *nt*.
ter·pene ['tɜrpiːn] *n* Terpen *nt*.
ter·pe·noid ['tɜrpənɔɪd] *adj* terpenoid.
terpenoid alcohol Terpenalkohol *m*.
ter·ra ['terə] *n* Erde *f*, Terra *f*.
ter·res·tri·al [tə'restrɪəl] *adj* irdisch, weltlich, terrestrisch, Erd-.
Terry ['terɪ]: **T.'s syndrome** *ped.* retrolentale Fibroplasie *f*, Frühgeborenenretinopathie *f*, Terry-Syndrom *nt*, Retinopathia praematurorum.
Terson [tɛr'sɔ̃]: **T.'s glands** Krause-Drüsen *pl*, Konjunktivaldrüsen *pl*, Gll. conjunctivales.
ter·sul·fide [tɜr'sʌlfaɪd, -fɪd] *n* Trisulfid *nt*.
ter·tian ['tɜrʃn] *adj* jeden dritten Tag auftretend, tertian.
tertian fever 1. Febris tertiana. 2. → tertian malaria.
tertian malaria Tertiana *f*, Dreitagefieber *nt*, Malaria tertiana.
ter·ti·ary ['tɜrʃərɪ, -ʃɪˌerɪ] *adj* dritten Grades, drittgradig, an dritter Stelle, tertiär, Tertiär-.

tertiary alcohol tertiärer Alkohol m.
tertiary amine tertiäres Amin nt.
tertiary compound → ternary compound.
tertiary cortex (Lymphknoten) thymusabhängiges Areal nt, T-Areal nt, thymusabhängige/parakortikale Zone f.
tertiary follicle Tertiärfollikel m, Graaf-Follikel m, reifer Follikel m.
tertiary hyperparathyroidism tertiärer Hyperparathyreoidismus m abbr. tHPT.
tertiary memory tertiäres Gedächtnis nt.
tertiary pacemaker physiol. tertiärer Schrittmacher m.
tertiary phosphate tertiäres Phosphat nt.
tertiary structure biochem. Tertiärstruktur f.
tertiary sulcus Tertiärfurche f, -sulcus m.
tertiary syphilis Spätsyphilis f, Tertiärstadium nt, Lues III f.
tertiary villus Tertiärzotte f.
ter·ti·grav·i·da [,tɜrʃɪ'grævɪdə] n gyn. Tertigravida f.
ter·tip·a·ra [tɜr'tɪpərə] n gyn. Drittgebärende f, Tertipara f.
Tesla ['teslə]: **T. current** phys. Tesla-Strom m, Hochfrequenzstrom m.
tes·la ['teslə] n abbr. **T** Tesla nt abbr. T.
tes·sel·lat·ed ['tesəleɪtɪd] adj gewürfelt, mosaikartig, schachbrettartig, Mosaik-.
tessellated fundus/retina Fundus tabulatus.
test [test] **I** n **1.** Test m, Probe f, Versuch m. **2.** Prüfung f, (Stich-)Probe f, Kontrolle f; chem., lab. Analyse f, Nachweis m, Untersuchung f, Test m, Probe f, Reaktion f. **3.** (Leistungs-, Eignungs-)Prüfung f, (-)Test m. **II** vt **4.** prüfen, untersuchen, einer Prüfung unterziehen; chem. analysieren, testen (for auf). **5.** jdn. testen od. prüfen. **III** vi einen Test machen, untersuchen (for auf).
test out vt ausprobieren (on bei, an).
tes·tal·gia [tes'tældʒ(ɪ)ə] n Hodenschmerz(en pl) m, -neuralgie f, Orchialgie f.
test card ophthal. Sehprobentafel f.
test criteria Testkriterien pl, Gütekriterien pl.
 primary t. Hauptgütekriterien.
 secondary t. Nebengütekriterien.
tes·tec·to·my [tes'tektəmɪ] n Hodenentfernung f, Orchiektomie f, Orchidektomie f.
test·ed ['testɪd] adj geprüft; erprobt.
test·ee [te'stiː] n Testperson f, Prüfling f.
test·er ['testər] n **1.** Prüfer(in f) m. **2.** Prüfgerät f.
tes·ti·cle ['testɪkl] n → testis.
tes·tic·u·lar [te'stɪkjələr] adj Hoden/Testis betr., testikulär, Hoden-.
testicular appendage Morgagni'-Hydatide f, Appendix testis.
testicular artery Hodenarterie f, Testikularis f, A. testicularis.
testicular atrophy Hodenatrophie f.
testicular bag Hodensack m, Skrotum nt, Scrotum nt.
testicular cancer → testicular carcinoma.
testicular carcinoma Hodenkrebs m, -karzinom nt.
 embryonal t. embryonales Hodenkarzinom.
testicular cord Samenstrang m, Funiculus spermaticus.
testicular duct Samenleiter m, Ductus/Vas deferens.
testicular feminization (syndrome) Goldberg-Maxwell-Morris-Syndrom nt, testikuläre Feminisierung f.
testicular hematocele Haematocele testis.
testicular hormone → testosterone.

testicular involution Hodeninvolution f.
testicular lobules Hodenläppchen pl, Lobuli testis.
testicular plexus Plexus testicularis.
testicular septa Hodenscheidewände pl, -septen pl, Septula testis.
testicular torsion Hodentorsion f.
testicular tubular adenoma Androblastom nt.
testicular tumor Hodengeschwulst f, -tumor m.
 germinal t. germinaler/germinativer Hodentumor.
 nongerminal t. Nicht-Keimgeschwulst.
testicular varicocele Varikozele f des Hodens.
testicular vein: **left t.** linke Hodenvene f, V. testicularis sinistra.
 right t. rechte Hodenvene f, V. testicularis/adrenalis dextra.
tes·tic·u·lo·ma [tes,tɪkjə'ləʊmə] n → testicular tumor.
tes·tic·u·lus [tes'tɪkjələs] n, pl -li [-laɪ] → testis.
tes·ti·mo·ny ['testɪməʊnɪ] n **1.** Beweis m, Zeugnis nt. **2.** (Zeugen-)Aussage f.
test·ing ['testɪŋ] **I** n Prüfung f, Test m; Untersuchen nt, Testen nt; Versuch m. **II** adj Test-, Versuchs-, Probe-, Prüf-, Meß-.
 t. of threshold of stapedius reflex HNO Stapediusreflexschwellenprüfung.
tes·tis ['testɪs] n, pl **-tes** [-tiːz] männliche Geschlechts-/Keimdrüse f, Hode(n) m, Testikel m, Testis m, Orchis m.
testis cords embryo. Hodenstränge pl.
testis hormone → testosterone.
tes·ti·tis [tes'taɪtɪs] n Hodenentzündung f, Orchitis f, Didymitis f.
test letter n test type.
test meal Probemahl nt.
tes·to·lac·tone [,testəʊ'læktəʊn] n pharm. Testolacton f.
tes·top·a·thy [tes'tɑpəθɪ] n Hodenerkrankung f, Orchio-, Orchidopathie f.
tes·tos·ter·one [tes'tɑstərəʊn] n Testosteron nt.
testosterone-estradiol-binding globulin abbr. **TEBG** testosteronbindendes Globulin nt abbr. TEBG.
test potential Testpotential nt.
test substrate Testsubstrat nt.
test tone Testton m.
test tube Reagenzglas nt, -röhrchen nt.
test-tube baby Retortenbaby nt.
test type ophthal. Optotype f, Sehzeichen nt, -probe f.
te·tan·ic [tə'tænɪk] adj **1.** physiol. Tetanus od. Tetani betr. od. auslösend, tetanisch, Tetanus-. **2.** micro., patho. Tetanus betr., tetanisch, Tetanus-.
tetanic contraction tetanische (Muskel-)Kontraktion f, Tetanus m.
tetanic potentiation physiol. tetanische Potenzierung f.
tetanic seizure tetanischer/tonisch-klonischer Krampf m.
tetanic spasm Tetanus m, Tetanie f.
te·tan·i·form [te'tænɪfɔːrm] adj tetanusartig, tetanieartig, tetaniform, tetanoid.
tet·a·nig·e·nous [tetə'nɪdʒənəs] adj physiol. Tetanus od. Tetanie hervorrufend, tetanigen.
tet·a·ni·za·tion [,tetənɪ'zeɪʃn] n physiol. Tetanisierung f.
tet·a·nize ['tetənaɪz] vt physiol. tetanisieren.
tet·a·noid ['tetənɔɪd] adj → tetaniform.
tetanoid fever kombinierte Hirnhaut- u. Rückenmarkshautentzündung f, Meningitis cerebrospinalis.
tet·a·nol·y·sin [,tetə'nɑləsɪn] n micro. Tetanolysin nt.

tet·a·nom·e·ter [,-'nɑmɪtər] n Tetanometer nt.
tet·a·no·spas·min [,tetənəʊ'spæzmɪn] n micro. Tetanospasmin nt.
tet·a·nus ['tetənəs] n **1.** physiol. Tetanus m, Tetanie f. **2.** micro. Wundstarrkrampf m, Tetanus m.
tetanus antitoxin Tetanusantitoxin nt, antitoxisches Tetanusimmunserum nt.
tetanus bacillus Tetanusbazillus m, -erreger m, Wundstarrkrampfbazillus m, -erreger m, Clostridium/Plectridium tetani.
tetanus immune globulin abbr. **TIG** Tetanusimmunglobulin nt.
tetanus immunoglobulin → tetanus immune globulin.
tetanus prophylaxis Tetanusprophylaxe f.
tetanus toxin Tetanustoxin nt.
tetanus toxoid Tetanustoxoid nt.
tetanus vaccine Tetanusvakzine f.
tet·a·ny ['tetənɪ] n **1.** → tetanus **1. 2.** neuromuskuläre Übererregbarkeit f, Tetanie f.
tetany cataract Tetaniestar m, Cataracta tetanica.
te·tar·ta·no·pia [tə,tɑːrtə'nəʊpɪə] n ophthal. Quadrantenanop(s)ie f, Quadrantenhemianop(s)ie f.
te·tar·ta·nop·ic [,-'nɑpɪk] adj Quadranten-(hemi)anop(s)ie betr.
te·tar·ta·nop·sia [,-'nɑpsɪə] n → tetartanopia.
tetra- pref. Tetr(a)-, Vier-.
tet·ra·ac·e·tate [,tetrə'æsɪteɪt] n Tetraazetat nt.
tet·ra·ba·sic [,-'beɪsɪk] adj chem. vierbasisch.
tet·ra·bor·ic acid [,-'bɔːrɪk, -'bəʊr-] Tetraborsäure f.
tet·ra·bro·mo·fluo·res·ce·in [,-,brəʊməʊflʊə'resɪn, -flɔː-] n Eosin nt.
tet·ra·caine ['-keɪn] n pharm., anes. Tetracain nt.
tet·ra·chi·rus [,-'kaɪrəs] n embryo. Tetrach(e)irus m.
tet·ra·chlor·eth·ane [,-klɔːr'eθeɪn] n Tetrachloräthan nt, -ethan nt.
tet·ra·chlo·ride [,-'klɔːraɪd, -ɪd, 'klə͜ʊ-] n Tetrachlorid nt.
tet·ra·chlor·meth·ane [,-klɔːr'meθeɪn] n Tetrachlorkohlenstoff m, Tetrachlormethan nt, inf. Tetra nt.
tet·ra·chlor·o·eth·yl·ene [,-,klɔːrəʊ'eθɪliːn] n Perchloräthylen nt, -ethylen nt, Tetrachloräthylen nt, -ethylen nt, Äthylentetrachlorid nt.
tet·ra·co·sac·tide [,-'kəʊsæktɪd] n pharm. Tetracosactid nt.
tet·ra·co·sac·tin [,-kəʊ'sæktɪn] n → tetracosactide.
tet·ra·co·sa·no·ic acid [,-kəʊsə'nəʊɪk] Lignocerinsäure f, n-Tetracosansäure f.
tet·ra·crot·ic [,-'krɑtɪk] adj card. tetrakrot.
tet·ra·cus·pid [,-'kʌspɪd] adj tetrakuspid.
tet·ra·cy·cline [,-'saɪkliːn] n pharm. **1.** Tetracyclin nt. **2.** Tetrazyklin(-Antibiotikum nt) nt.
tet·rad ['tetræd] n **1.** → tetralogy. **2.** genet. Tetrade f. **3.** chem. vierwertiges Element nt.
tet·ra·dac·ty·lous [,tetrə'dæktɪləs] adj vierfingrig, vierzehig, tetradaktyl.
tet·ra·dac·ty·ly [,-'dæktəlɪ] n Vierfingrigkeit f, Vierzehigkeit f, Tetradaktylie f.
tet·ra·de·no·ic acid [,-,dekə'nəʊɪk] Myristinsäure f.
tet·ra·ene ['tetraɪn] n chem. Tetraen nt.
tet·ra·eth·yl·am·mo·ni·um [,tetrə,eθɪlə'məʊnɪəm] n abbr. **TEA** Tetraethylammonium nt, Tetraethylammonium nt abbr. TEA.
tetraethylammonium chloride abbr. **TEAC** Tetraäthylammoniumchlorid nt,

Tetraethylammoniumchlorid *nt abbr.* TEAC.
tet·ra·eth·yl lead [ˌ-'eθɪl] Bleitetraäthyl *nt*, Tetraäthylblei *nt*.
tetraethyl pyrophosphate *abbr.* **TEPP** Teraäthylpyrophosphorsäure *nt*, Tetraethylpyrophosphat *nt abbr.* TEPP.
tet·ra·eth·yl·thi·o·per·ox·y·di·car·bon·ic diamide [ˌ-ˌeθɪlˌθaɪəʊpəˌrɒksɪdaɪkɑːr-'bɒnɪk] → tetraethylthiuram disulfide.
tet·ra·eth·yl·thi·u·ram disulfide [ˌ-ˌeθɪl-'θaɪjərəm] *pharm.* Disulfiram *nt*, Tetraäthylthiuramidsulfid *nt*.
tet·ra·gon ['-gɒn] *n* → tetragonum.
tet·ra·go·num [ˌ-'gəʊnəm] *n anat.* Viereck *nt*, Tetragonum *nt*.
tet·ra·go·nus [ˌ-'gəʊnəs] *n* Hautmuskel *m* des Halses, Platysma *nt*.
tet·ra·he·dral [ˌ-'hiːdrəl] *adj* vierflächig, tetraedrisch.
tet·ra·he·dron [ˌ-'hiːdrən] *n, pl* **-dra** [-drə] *mathe.* Tetraeder *nt*.
tet·ra·hex·o·side [ˌ-'heksəsaɪd] *n* Tetrahexosid *nt*.
tet·ra·hy·dro·bi·op·ter·in [ˌ-ˌhaɪdrəbaɪ'ɒptərɪn] *n* Tetrahydrobiopterin *nt*.
tet·ra·hy·dro·can·nab·i·nol [ˌ-ˌhaɪdrəkə-'næbɪnɒl, -nɒl] *n abbr.* **THC** Tetrahydrocannabinol *nt abbr.* THC.
tet·ra·hy·dro·cor·ti·sol [ˌ-ˌhaɪdrə'kɔːrtɪsɒl, -sɒl] *n pharm.* Tetrahydrokortisol *nt*, -cortisol *nt*.
tet·ra·hy·dro·fo·late [ˌ-ˌhaɪdrə'fəʊleɪt] *n* Tetrahydrofolat *nt*.
tetrahydrofolate dehydrogenase Dihydrofolatreduktase *f abbr.* DHFR.
tet·ra·hy·dro·fo·lic acid [ˌ-ˌhaɪdrə'fəʊlɪk, -'fɒl-] *abbr.* **FH₄** Tetrahydrofolsäure *f abbr.* FH₄.
tet·ra·hy·drox·y·bu·tane [ˌ-ˌhaɪˌdrɒksɪ-'bjuːteɪn, -bjuː'teɪn] *n* Erythrit *nt*, Erythroglucin *nt*, Erythrol *nt*, Tetrahydroxybutan *nt*.
tet·ra·i·o·do·thy·ro·nine [ˌ-aɪˌəʊdə'θaɪrəniːn, -nɪn] *n* → thyroxine.
te·tral·o·gy [te'trælədʒɪ] *n, pl* **-gies** *patho.* Tetralogie *f*, Tetrade *f*.
t. of Fallot Fallot'-Tetralogie *f*, -Tetrade *f*, Fallot IV *m*.
tet·ra·mas·tia [ˌtetrə'mæstɪə] *n embryo.* Tetramastie *f*.
tet·ra·mas·ti·gote [ˌ-'mæstɪɡəʊt] *n micro.* Tetramastigote *f*.
tet·ra·mas·tous [ˌ-'mæstəs] *adj embryo.* vierbrüstig.
tet·ra·ma·zia [ˌ-'meɪzɪə] *n* → tetramastia.
tet·ra·mer ['-mər] *n* Tetramer *nt*.
tet·ra·mer·ic [ˌ-'merɪk] *adj* tetramer.
tet·ra·meth·yl·di·ar·sine [ˌ-ˌmeθɪldaɪ'ɑːrsiːn] *n* Kakodyl *nt*, Tetramethyldiarsin *nt*.
tet·ra·meth·yl·ene·di·am·ine [ˌ-ˌmeθɪliːn-'daɪəmiːn] *n* Putreszin *nt*, Putrescin *nt*, 1,4-Diaminobutan *nt*, Tetramethylendiamin *nt*.
Te·tram·i·tus mes·ni·li [te'træmɪtəs mes-'naɪlɪ] Chilomastix mesnili *m*, Cercomonas intestinalis.
tet·ra·ni·trol [ˌtetrə'naɪtrəʊl, -nɒl] *n pharm.* Erythrityltetranitrat *nt*.
tet·ra·nop·sia [ˌ-'nɒpsɪə] *n* → tetartanopia.
tet·ra·nu·cle·o·tide [ˌ-'n(j)uːklɪəʊtaɪd] *n* Tetranukleotid *nt*.
tet·ra·o·don poisoning [tet'reɪədən] → tetrodotoxin.
tet·ra·o·don·tox·in [tetˌreɪəʊdən'tɒksɪn] *n* → tetrodotoxin.
tet·ra·o·don·tox·ism [ˌ-'tɒksɪzəm] *n* → tetrodotoxism.
tet·ra·par·e·sis [ˌtetrə'pærəsɪs] *n neuro.* Tetraparese *f*.
tet·ra·pep·tide [ˌ-'peptaɪd] *n* Tetrapeptid *nt*.

tet·ra·ple·gia [ˌ-'pliːdʒ(ɪ)ə] *n neuro.* hohe Querschnittslähmung *f*, Tetra-, Quadriplegie *f*.
tet·ra·ple·gic [ˌ-'pliːdʒɪk] **I** *n* Patient(in *f*) *m* mit Tetraplegie, Tetraplegiker(in *f*) *m*. **II** *adj* Tetraplegie betr., quadri-, tetraplegisch.
tet·ra·ploid ['-plɔɪd] *genet.* **I** *n* tetraploides Individuum *nt*. **II** *adj* tetraploid.
tet·ra·ploi·dy ['-plɔɪdɪ] *n genet.* Tetraploidie *f*.
tet·ra·pod ['-pɒd] **I** *n bio.* Vierfüß(l)er *m*, Quadrupede *m*, Tetrapode *m*. **II** *adj* vierfüßig.
tet·ra·pus ['-pəs] *n embryo.* Tetrapus *m*.
tet·ra·pyr·role compound [ˌ-pɪ'rəʊl, -'pɪrəʊl] Tretrapyrrolverbindung *f*.
tet·ra·sac·cha·ride [ˌ-'sækəraɪd] *n* Tetrasaccharid *nt*.
tet·ra·so·mic [ˌ-'səʊmɪk] *adj genet.* Tetrasomie betr., durch Tetrasomie gekennzeichnet, tetrasom.
tet·ra·so·my ['-səʊmɪ] *n genet.* Tetrasomie *f*.
tet·ra·spore ['-spəʊər, -spɔːr] *n micro.* Tetraspore *f*.
tet·ra·ter·pene [ˌ-'tɜːrpiːn] *n chem.* Tetraterpen *nt*.
tet·ra·thi·o·nate broth [ˌ-'θaɪəneɪt] *micro.* Tetrathionatbouillon *f*.
tet·ra·tom·ic [ˌ-'tɒmɪk] *adj chem.* vieratomig, aus vier Atomen bestehend.
tet·ra·va·lent [ˌ-'veɪlənt] *adj* vierwertig, tetravalent.
tet·ro·do·tox·in [ˌtetrəʊdə'tɒksɪn] *n abbr.* **TTX** Tetrodotoxin *nt abbr.* TTX.
tet·ro·do·tox·ism [ˌ-'tɒksɪzəm] *n* Tetrodotoxinvergiftung *f*, Tetrodotoxismus *m*.
tet·roph·thal·mos *n* → tetrophthalmus.
tet·roph·thal·mus [ˌtetrɒf'θælməs] *n embryo.* Tetrophthalmus *m*.
te·trose ['tetrəʊz] *n* Tetrose *f*, C₄-Zucker *m*.
te·trox·ide [te'trɒksaɪd] *n* Tetroxid *nt*.
tet·ter ['tetər] *n derm.* Flechte *f*; Ekzem *nt*; Tinea *f*.
Tex·as (cattle) fever ['teksəs] Texas-Fieber *nt*.
Texas tick fever Bullis-Fieber *nt*, Lone-Star-Fever *nt*.
text blindness [tekst] Leseunfähigkeit *f*, -unvermögen *nt*, Alexie *f*.
tex·ti·form ['tekstɪfɔːrm] *adj histol.* gewebe-, netzartig.
tex·tur·al ['tekstʃərəl] *adj* strukturell, Gewebe-, Struktur-.
tex·ture ['tekstʃər] *n* 1. Gewebe *nt*. 2. Struktur *f*, Aufbau *m*, Beschaffenheit *f*, Konsistenz *f*, Textur *f*.
TF *abbr.* → transfer factor.
TGA *abbr.* [transposition of great arteries] → transposition of great vessels.
TGV *abbr.* → transposition of great vessels.
Th *abbr.* → thorium.
Thai hemorrhagic fever [taɪ] Dengue-hämorrhagisches Fieber *nt*.
thalam- *pref.* → thalamo-.
thal·a·mec·to·my [θælə'mektəmɪ] *n* → thalamotomy.
thal·a·men·ce·phal·ic [ˌθæləmensɪ'fælɪk] *adj* Thalamencephalon betr., thalamenzephal(isch).
thal·a·men·ceph·a·lon [ˌθæləmen'sefəlɒn] *n* Thalamushirn *nt*, Thalamenzephalon *nt*, -encephalon *nt*.
tha·lam·ic [θə'læmɪk] *adj* Thalamus betr., thalamisch, Thalamus-, Thalam(o)-.
thalamic branch: t.es of posterior cerebral artery Thalamusäste *pl* der A. cerebri posterior, Rami thalamici a. cerebri posterioris.

t. of posterior communicating artery Thalamusast *m* der A. communicans posterior, Ramus thalamicus a. communicantis posterior.
thalamic eminence Eminentia thalami.
thalamic fasciculus Forel'-Bündel *nt*, Fasciculus thalamicus.
thalamic hyperesthetic anesthesia → thalamic syndrome.
thalamic nuclei Thalamuskerne *pl*, Ncc. thalami.
specific t. palliothalamische Kerne *pl*, Palliothalamus *m*, spezifische Thalamuskerne *pl*.
nonspecific t. trunkothalamische Kerne *pl*, Trunkothalamus *m*, unspezifische Thalamuskerne *pl*.
thalamic pain Thalamusschmerz *m*.
thalamic peduncle: anterior/caudal/inferior t. vorderer Thalamusstiel *m*, Pedunculus thalamicus caudalis/inferior.
posterior t. hinterer Thalamusstiel *m*, Pedunculus thalamicus posterior.
thalamic radiation Thalamusstrahlung *f*, Radiatio thalamica.
anterior t.s vordere Thalamusstrahlung, Radiationes thalamicae anteriores.
central t.s zentrale/obere Thalamusstrahlung, Radiationes thalamicae centrales.
posterior t.s hintere Thalamusstrahlung, Radiationes thalamicae posteriores.
superior t.s → central t.s.
thalamic syndrome Déjérine-Roussy-Syndrom *nt*, Thalamussyndrom *nt*.
thalamic taenia T(a)enia thalami.
thalamo- *pref.* Thalam(o)-, Thalamus-.
thal·a·mo·cele ['θæləməsiːl] *n* dritter (Hirn-)Ventrikel *m*, Ventriculus tertius.
thal·a·mo·cor·ti·cal [ˌ-'kɔːrtɪkl] *adj* Thalamus u. Hirnrinde/Cortex betr. *od.* verbindend, thalamokortikal.
thalamocortical fibers thalamokortikale Fasern *pl*, Fibrae thalamocorticales.
thal·a·mo·fu·gal [θælə'mæfjəɡəl] *adj* thalamofugal.
thal·a·mo·len·tic·u·lar part of internal capsule [ˌθæləməʊlen'tɪkjələr] Pars thalamolenticularis/thalamolentiformis (capsulae internae).
thal·a·mo·mam·il·lary bundle/fasciculus [ˌ-'mæmɪleːɪ] Vicq d'Azyr'-Bündel *nt*, Fasciculus mamillothalamicus.
thal·a·mo·oc·cip·i·tal tract [ˌ-ɒk'sɪpɪtl] Gratiolet'-Sehstrahlung *f*, Radiatio optica.
thal·a·mo·ol·i·va·ry tract [ˌ-'ɒləveərɪ] Tractus thalamo-olivaris.
thal·a·mo·pa·ri·e·tal fibers [ˌ-pə'raɪɪtl] thalamoparietale Fasern *pl*, Fibrae thalamoparietales.
thal·a·mo·pe·tal [θælə'mɒpətəl] *adj* thalamopetal.
thal·a·mo·stri·ate arteries [ˌθæləməʊ-'straɪt, -eɪt]: **anterolateral t.** Aa. centrales/thalamostriatae anterolaterales.
anteromedial t. Aa. centrales/thalamostriatae anteromediales.
thalamostriate vein: inferior t.s Vv. thalamostriatae inferiores.
superior t. Terminalvene *f*, V. thalamostriata superior, V. terminalis.
thal·a·mo·teg·men·tal [ˌ-teɡ'mentl] *adj* Thalamus u. Tegmentum betr., thalamotegmental.
thal·a·mo·tem·po·ral radiation [ˌ-'temp(ə)rəl] Hörstrahlung *f*, Radiatio acustica.
thal·a·mot·o·my [θælə'mɒtəmɪ] *n neurochir.* Thalamotomie *f*.
thal·a·mus ['θæləməs] *n, pl* **-mi** [-maɪ] Thalamus *m*.

thalassanemia

tha·las·sa·ne·mia [θəˌlæsə'niːmɪə] *n* → thalassemia.
thal·as·se·mia [ˌθælə'siːmɪə] *n* Mittelmeeranämie *f*, Thalassämie *f*, Thalassaemia *f*.
β-thalassemia *n* β-Thalassämie *f*.
thalassemia major Cooley-Anämie *f*, homozygote β-Thalassämie *f*, Thalassaemia major.
thalassemia minor heterozygote β-Thalassämie *f*, Thalassaemia minor.
thalassemia-sickle cell disease Sichelzell(en)thalassämie *f*, Mikrodrepanozytenkrankheit *f*, HbS-Thalassämie *f*.
thal·as·so·pho·bia [θəˌlæsəʊ'fəʊbɪə] *n psychia.* krankhafte Angst *f* vor dem Meer, Thalassophobie *f*.
tha·las·so·po·sia [ˌ-'pəʊzɪə] *n* Seewasseringestion *f*.
tha·las·so·ther·a·py [ˌ-'θerəpɪ] *n* Thalassotherapie *f*.
tha·lid·o·mide [θə'lɪdəmaɪd] *n pharm.* Thalidomid *nt*.
thalidomide embryopathy Thalidomidembryopathie *f*, Contergan-Syndrom *nt*.
thall- *pref.* → thallo-.
thal·li·tox·i·co·sis [ˌθælɪˌtɒksɪ'kəʊsɪs] *n* Thalliumvergiftung *f*.
thal·li·um ['θælɪəm] *n abbr.* **Tl** Thallium *nt abbr.* Tl.
thallium acetate Thalliumazetat *nt*.
thallium poisoning Thalliumvergiftung *f*.
thallo- *pref.* **1.** *bio., micro.* Thall(o)-, Thallus-. **2.** *chem.* Thallium-, Thall(o)-.
Thal·lo·bac·te·ria [ˌθæləʊbæk'tɪərɪə] *pl micro.* Thallobacteria *pl*.
thal·loid ['θæloɪd] *adj bio.* thallös.
Thal·loph·y·ta [θæ'lɒfɪtə] *pl bio.* Thallophyta *pl*.
thal·lo·phyte ['θæləfaɪt] *n bio.* Thallophyt *m*.
thal·lose ['θæləʊs] *adj bio.* thallös.
thal·lo·spore ['θæləspəʊər, -spɔːr] *n micro.* Thallospore *f*.
thal·lo·tox·i·co·sis [ˌ-ˌtɒksɪ'kəʊsɪs] *n* → thallitoxicosis.
thal·lus ['θæləs] *n, pl* **-li** [-laɪ] *bio., micro.* Thallus *m*.
thal·po·sis [θæl'pəʊsɪs] *n physiol.* Warmsinn *m*.
THAM *abbr.* → tromethamine.
tham·u·ria [θæm'(j)ʊərɪə] *n* häufige/frequente Miktion *f*.
thanat- *pref.* Tod-, Thanat(o)-.
than·a·to·bi·o·log·ic [ˌθænətəʊbaɪə'lɒdʒɪk] *adj* thanatobiologisch.
than·a·to·gno·mon·ic [ˌ-nəʊ'mɒnɪk] *adj* thanatognomonisch, thanatognostisch.
than·a·tol·o·gy [ˌθænə'tɒlədʒɪ] *n* Thanatologie *f*.
than·a·to·ma·nia [ˌθænətəʊ'meɪnɪə, -jə] *n psychia.* Thanatomanie *f*.
than·a·to·phi·dia [ˌ-'fɪdɪə] *n bio.* Giftschlangen *pl*.
than·a·to·phid·i·al [ˌ-'fɪdɪəl] *adj* Giftschlangen betr.
than·a·to·pho·bia [ˌ-'fəʊbɪə] *n psychia.* krankhafte Angst *f* vor dem Tode, Thanatophobie *f*.
than·a·to·phor·ic [ˌ-'fɒrɪk] *adj* tödlich, letal, thanatophor.
thanatophoric dwarf thanatophorer Zwerg *m*.
than·a·top·sia [ˌθænə'tɒpsɪə] *n* → thanatopsy.
than·a·top·sy ['-tɒpsɪ] *n* Autopsie *f*, Obduktion *f*, Nekropsie *f*.
than·a·to·sis [ˌ-'təʊsɪs] *n* Gangrän *f*, Nekrose *f*.
Thayer-Martin ['θaɪər 'mɑːrtɪn]: **T.-M. agar/medium** Thayer-Martin-Agar *m/nt*, -Medium *nt abbr.* TM, TM-Agar *m/nt*, -Medium *nt*.

THC *abbr.* → tetrahydrocannabinol.
the·a ['θɪə] *n* → tea.
the·a·ism ['θɪɪzəm] *n* → theinism.
the·a·ter ['θɪətər] *n* Operationssal *m abbr.* OP.
theater nurse Operations-, OP-Schwester *m*.
the·ba·ine ['θiːbəˌiːn, θɪ'beɪiːn, -ɪn] *n* Thebain *nt*.
the·be·si·an [θə'biːʒn]: **t. foramina** Mündungen *pl* der Vv. cordis minimae, Forr. vv. minimarum (cordis).
   t. valve Sinusklappe *f*, Thebesius-(Sinus-)Klappe *f*, Valvula sinus coronarii.
   t. veins Thebesi'-Venen *pl*, kleinste Herzvenen *pl*, Vv. cordis/cardiacae minimae.
Thebesius [θə'biːsɪəs]: **veins of T.** Thebesi'-Venen *pl*, kleinste Herzvenen *pl*, Vv. cordis/cardiacae minimae.
the·ca ['θiːkə] *n, pl* **-cae** [-siː] *histol.* Hülle *f*, Kapsel *f*, Theka *f*, Theca *f*.
   t. of follicle Bindegewebshülle des Sekundärfollikels, Theka, Theca folliculi.
theca cells Thekazellen *pl*.
theca cell tumor Thekazelltumor *m*, Thekom *nt*, Priesel-Tumor *m*, Loeffler--Priesel-Tumor *m*, Fibroma thecacellulare xanthomatodes.
the·cal ['θiːkl] *adj* Theka betr., von der Theka stammend, thekal, Theka-.
thecal cyst *old ortho.* Synovialzyste *f*, Ganglion *nt*, Überbein *nt*.
theca-lutein cell Thekaluteinzelle *f*.
theca-lutein cyst Theka-Lutein-Zyste *f*.
theca tumor → theca cell tumor.
the·ci·tis [θɪ'saɪtɪs] *n* → tenosynovitis.
the·co·ma [θɪ'kəʊmə] *n* → theca cell tumor.
the·co·ma·to·sis [ˌθɪkəʊmə'təʊsɪs] *n gyn.* Thekomatose *f*.
Theile ['taɪlə]: **T.'s canal** Sinus transversus pericardii.
   T.'s glands Schleimdrüsen *pl* der Gallengänge, Gll. biliares.
   T.'s muscle M. transversus perinei superficialis.
Thei·le·ria [θaɪ'lɪərɪə] *n micro.* Theileria *f*.
thei·le·ri·a·sis [ˌθaɪlɪ'raɪəsɪs] *n* Theileriainfektion *f*, Theileriasis *f*, Theileriose *f*.
thei·ler·i·o·sis [θaɪˌlɪərɪ'əʊsɪs] *n* → theileriasis.
the·ine ['θiːɪn, -iːn, 'tiː-] *n* Thein *nt*, Tein *nt*.
the·in·ism ['θiːɪnɪzəm] *n* (chronische) Theinvergiftung *f*.
thel- *pref.* → thelo-.
the·lal·gia [θɪ'lældʒ(ɪ)ə] *n gyn.* Brustwarzenschmerz(en *pl*) *m*, Thelalgie *f*.
the·lar·che [θɪ'lɑːrkɪ] *n gyn.* Thelarche *f*.
The·la·zia [θɪ'leɪzɪə] *n micro.* Thelazia *f*.
thel·a·zi·a·sis [ˌθelə'zaɪəsɪs] *n* Thelaziainfektion *f*, Thelaziasis *f*.
thele- *pref.* → thelo-.
the·le·plas·ty ['θiːlɪplæstɪ] *n gyn.* Brustwarzenplastik *f*, Mamillenplastik *f*.
the·li·tis [θɪ'laɪtɪs] *n* Brustwarzenentzündung *f*, Mamillitis *f*, Thelitis *f*.
the·li·um ['θiːlɪəm] *n, pl* **-lia** [-lɪə] **1.** *anat.* Papille *f*. **2.** Brustwarze *f*, Mamille *f*, Mamilla *f*, Papilla mammae.
thelo- *pref.* Brustwarzen-, Thel(o)-, Mamill(o)-.
the·lon·cus [θɪ'lɒŋkəs] *n* Brustwarzenschwellung *f*, -tumor *m*.
the·lor·rha·gia [θɪləʊ'reɪdʒ(ɪ)ə] *n* Blutung *f* aus der Brustwarze, Thelorrhagie *f*.
T helper cell T-Helferzelle *f*.
T helper/inductor cell T-Helfer/Induktor--Zelle *f*.
thel·y·blast ['θelɪblæst] *n embryo.* weiblicher Vorkern *m*.
the·ly·gen·ic [ˌθiːlɪ'dʒenɪk] *adj bio.* thelygen.

thel·y·ki·nin [ˌ-'kaɪnɪn, -'kɪn-] *n old* → estrone.
thel·y·to·cia [ˌθelɪ'təʊʃɪə] *n embryo.* Thelytokie *f*.
the·lyt·o·cous [θɪ'lɪtəkəs] *adj* thelytokisch.
the·lyt·o·ky [θɪ'lɪtəkɪ] *n* → thelytocia.
the·mat·ic apperception test [θɪ'mætɪk] *abbr.* **TAT** thematischer Apperzeptionstest *m abbr.* TAT.
the·nal ['θiːnl] *adj* → thenar II.
the·nar ['θiːnɑːr, -nər] **I** *n* Daumenballen *m*, Thenar *nt*, Eminentia thenaris. **II** *adj* Handfläche *od.* Daumenballen betr., Handflächen-, Daumenballen-, Thenar-.
thenar atrophy Daumenballen-, Thenaratrophie *f*.
   partial t. Ch(e)iralgia paraesthetica.
thenar eminence → thenar I.
thenar prominence → thenar I.
then·yl·di·a·mine [ˌθenl'daɪəmiːn] *n pharm.* Thenyldiamin *nt*.
the·o·bro·mine [ˌθiːə'brəʊmiːn, -mɪn] *n pharm.* Theobromin *nt*, 3,7-Dimethylxanthin *nt*.
the·o·phyl·line [ˌ-'fɪliːn, θɪ'ɒfəliːn] *n pharm.* Theophyllin *nt*, 1,3-Dimethylxanthin *nt*.
theophylline ethylenediamine *pharm.* Theophyllin-, Ethylendiamin *nt*, Aminophyllin *nt*.
the·o·rem ['θɪərəm] *n* Lehrsatz *m*, Theorem *nt*.
the·o·ret·ic [ˌθɪə'retɪk] *adj* → theoretical.
the·o·ret·i·cal [ˌθɪə'retɪkl] *adj* theoretisch.
the·o·rize ['θɪəraɪz] *vt* **1.** theoretisieren, Theorie(n) aufstellen (*about* über). **2.** annehmen (*that* daß).
the·o·ry ['θɪərɪ] *n* **1.** Theorie *f*, Lehre *f*. **to advance/present a ~ on sth.** eine Theorie über etw. aufstellen. **to disprove/prove a ~** eine Theorie widerlegen/bestätigen. **2.** Hypothese *f*. **3.** Theorie *f*, theoretischer Teil. **in ~** in der Theorie, theoretisch.
   t. of evolution Evolutionstheorie.
   t. of probability Wahrscheinlichkeitsrechnung *f*.
   t. of relativity (*Einstein*) Relativitätstheorie.
   t. of Starling Starling'-(Reabsorptions-)-Theorie.
   t. of ulcer formation Ulkus-Theorie, Theorie der Ulkusentstehung.
ther·a·peu·sis [ˌθerə'pjuːsɪs] *n* → therapeutics.
ther·a·peu·tic [ˌ-'pjuːtɪk] *adj* **1.** Therapie/Behandlung betr., therapeutisch, Behandlungs-, Therapie-. **2.** heilend, kurativ, therapeutisch.
therapeutic abortion *gyn.* indizierter Abort *m*.
ther·a·peu·ti·cal [ˌ-'pjuːtɪkl] *adj* → therapeutic.
therapeutic anesthesia *anes.* therapeutische Anästhesie *f*.
therapeutic crisis *psychia.* therapeutische Krise *f*.
therapeutic dose therapeutische Dosis *f*, Dosis therapeutica.
therapeutic electrode aktive/differente Elektrode *f*.
therapeutic embolization therapeutische Embolisation *f*, Katheterembolisation *f*.
therapeutic exercise → therapeutic training.
therapeutic fever Fiebertherapie *f*.
therapeutic index therapeutische Breite *f*, therapeutischer Index *m*.
therapeutic iridectomy *ophthal.* therapeutische Iridektomie *f*.
therapeutic level *pharm.* therapeutischer Spiegel *m*.
therapeutic nihilism therapeutischer Nihilismus *m*.

therapeutic pneumothorax therapeutischer Pneu(mothorax *m*) *m*.
therapeutic radiation therapeutische Bestrahlung *f*, Strahlentherapie *f*.
therapeutic ratio → therapeutic index.
ther·a·peu·tics [ˌ-'pjuːtɪks] *pl* Therapie(lehre *f*) *f*, Therapeutik *f*.
therapeutic training Bewegungstherapie *f*.
ther·a·peu·tist [ˌ-'pjuːtɪst] *n* → therapist.
ther·a·pia [ˌ-'piːə] *n* → therapy.
ther·a·pist ['θerəpɪst] *n* Therapeut(in *f*) *m*.
ther·a·py ['θerəpɪ] *n* (Krankheits-)Behandlung *f*, Therapie *f*, Therapia *f*; Heilverfahren *nt*.
therm- *pref.* → thermo-.
ther·ma·co·gen·e·sis [ˌθɜrməkəʊ'dʒenəsɪs] *n* Thermakogenese *f*.
ther·mae ['θɜrmiː] *pl* **1.** Thermalquellen *pl*, Thermen *pl*. **2.** Thermalbäder *pl*, Thermen *pl*.
therm·aer·o·ther·a·py [θɜrmˌeərə'θerəpɪ] *n* Warmluftbehandlung *f*.
ther·mal ['θɜrml] *adj* Wärme *od.* Hitze betr., warm, heiß, thermal, thermisch, Wärme-, Thermal-, Thermo-.
thermal analysis *chem.* thermische Analyse *f*, Thermoanalyse *f*.
thermal anesthesia → thermanesthesia.
thermal balance *physiol.* Wärmehaushalt *m*.
thermal burn thermische Verbrennung *f*.
thermal capacity Hitzekapazität *f*.
thermal cataract Feuer-, Glasbläserstar *m*, Infrarotkatarakt *f*, Cataracta calorica.
thermal conductance *abbr.* C *phys.*, *physiol.* Wärmedurchgangszahl *f abbr.* C.
thermal diffusion Thermodiffusion *f*.
thermal efficiency Wärmewirkungsgrad *m*.
thermal energy Wärmeenergie *f*, thermische Energie *f*.
thermal expansion Wärmeausdehnung *f*.
ther·mal·ge·sia [ˌθɜrmæl'dʒiːzɪə, -dʒiːʒə] *n* Thermalgesie *f*.
ther·mal·gia [θɜr'mældʒ(ɪ)ə] *n* brennender Schmerz *m*, Thermalgie *f*.
thermal injury thermische Verletzung *f*.
thermal instability → thermolability.
thermal insulation Wärmeisolation *f*.
thermal neutron thermisches Neutron *nt*.
thermal-physical *adj* thermisch-physikalisch.
thermal resistance Wärme(durchgangs)widerstand *m*.
thermal sense Temperatursinn *m*, Thermorezeption *f*.
thermal spectrum (Spektrum der) Wärmestrahlung *f*.
thermal stimulus *physiol.* thermischer Reiz *m*.
thermal stress *physiol.* thermische Belastung *f*.
thermal sweating thermisches Schwitzen *nt*.
thermal unit Wärmeeinheit *f*.
therm·an·al·ge·sia [ˌθɜrmænl'dʒiːzɪə] *n* Therm(o)analgesie *f*.
therm·an·es·the·sia [ˌθɜrmænəs'θiːʒə] *n* Verlust *m* der Temperaturempfindung, Therm(o)anästhesie *f*.
ther·ma·tol·o·gy [ˌθɜrmə'talədʒɪ] *n* Thermatologie *f*.
ther·me·lom·e·ter [ˌθɜrme'lamɪtər] *n* elektrisches Thermometer *nt*.
therm·es·the·sia [ˌθɜrmes'θiːʒ(ɪ)ə] *n physiol.* Temperatursinn *m*, Therm(o)ästhesie *f*.
therm·es·the·si·om·e·ter [ˌθɜrmesˌθiːzɪ'amɪtər] *n physiol.* Therm(o)ästhesiometer *nt*.

therm·hy·per·es·the·sia [ˌθɜrmˌhaɪpərˌes'θiːʒ(ɪ)ə] *n* → thermohyperesthesia.
therm·hyp·es·the·sia [ˌθɜrmhaɪpes'θiːʒ(ɪ)ə] *n* Verminderung *f* der Temperaturempfindung, Therm(o)hypästhesie *f*.
ther·mic ['θɜrmɪk] *adj* Hitze *od.* Wärme betr., thermisch, Hitze-, Wärme-, Therm(o)-.
thermic anesthesia → thermanesthesia.
thermic fever Hitzschlag *m*, Thermoplegie *f*.
thermic sense Temperatursinn *m*, Thermorezeption *f*.
therm·i·on ['θɜrmɪən] *n* Thermion *nt*.
therm·is·tor [θɜr'mɪstər, 'θɜrmɪstər] *n phys.* Thermistor *m*.
thermo- *pref.* Hitze-, Wärme-, Therm(o)-.
Ther·mo·ac·ti·no·my·ces [ˌθɜrməʊˌæktɪnəʊ'maɪsiːz] *n micro.* Thermoactinomyces *m*.
ther·mo·aes·the·sia [ˌ-es'θiːʒ(ɪ)ə] *n* → thermesthesia.
ther·mo·af·fer·ent fibers [ˌ-'æfərənt] *physiol.* thermoafferente Fasern *pl*.
thermoafferent pathways *physiol.* thermoafferente Bahnen *pl*.
ther·mo·al·ge·sia [ˌ-æl'dʒiːzɪə, -dʒiːʒə] *n* → thermalgesia.
ther·mo·an·al·ge·sia [ˌ-ænl'dʒiːzɪə] *n* → thermanalgesia.
ther·mo·an·es·the·sia [ˌ-ænəs'θiːʒə] *n* → thermanesthesia.
ther·mo·cau·ter·y [ˌ-'kɔːtərɪ] *n* Elektro-, Thermokauterisation *f*.
ther·mo·chem·is·try [ˌ-'kemɪstrɪ] *n* Thermochemie *f*.
ther·mo·co·ag·u·la·tion [ˌ-kəʊˌægjə'leɪʃn] *n* Thermokoagulation *f*.
ther·mo·cou·ple ['-kʌpl] *n* Thermoelement *nt*.
thermocouple thermometer → thermocouple.
ther·mo·cur·rent [ˌ-'kʌrənt, -'kɜr-] *n* → thermoelectric current.
ther·mode ['θɜrməʊd] *n* Thermode *f*.
ther·mo·dif·fu·sion [ˌθɜrməʊdɪ'fjuːʒn] *n* Thermodiffusion *f*.
ther·mo·di·lu·tion [ˌ-dɪ'luːʃn] *n physiol.* Thermodilution *f*, Thermodilutionsmethode *f*, -technik *f*.
thermodilution method/technique → thermodilution.
ther·mo·dur·ic [ˌ-'d(j)ʊərɪk] *adj* hitzebeständig.
ther·mo·dy·nam·ic [ˌ-daɪ'næmɪk] *adj* thermodynamisch.
ther·mo·dy·nam·i·cal [ˌ-daɪ'næmɪkl] *adj* → thermodynamic.
thermodynamic equilibrium thermodynamisches Gleichgewicht *nt*.
ther·mo·dy·nam·ics [ˌ-daɪ'næmɪks] *pl* Thermodynamik *f*.
ther·mo·e·lec·tric [ˌ-ɪ'lektrɪk] *adj* thermoelektrisch.
thermoelectric current thermoelektrischer Strom *m*.
ther·mo·e·lec·tric·i·ty [ˌ-ɪlek'trɪsətɪ] *n* Thermoelektrizität *f*.
ther·mo·es·the·sia [ˌ-es'θiːʒ(ɪ)ə] *n* → thermesthesia.
ther·mo·es·the·si·om·e·ter [ˌ-esˌθiːzɪ'amɪtər] *n* → thermesthesiometer.
ther·mo·ex·ci·to·ry [ˌ-ek'saɪtərɪ] *adj* die Wärmebildung anregend.
ther·mo·gen·e·sis [ˌ-'dʒenəsɪs] *n* Wärmebildung *f*, Thermogenese *f*.
ther·mo·ge·net·ic [ˌ-dʒə'netɪk] *adj* Thermogenese betr., thermogenetisch.
ther·mo·gen·ic [ˌ-'dʒenɪk] *adj* wärmebildend, thermogen.
thermogenic anhidrosis thermogene/tropische Anhidrose *f*, Anhidrosis tropica.

ther·mog·e·nous [θɜr'madʒənəs] *adj* durch Wärme *od.* Hitze verursacht, thermogen.
ther·mo·gram ['θɜrməgræm] *n* **1.** *radiol.* Wärmebild *nt*, Thermogramm *nt*. **2.** *phys.* Thermogramm *nt*.
ther·mo·graph ['-græf] *n* **1.** *radiol.* Thermograph *m*. **2.** *phys.* Temperaturschreiber *m*, Thermograph *m*. **3.** → thermogram 1.
ther·mo·graph·ic [ˌ-'græfɪk] *adj* Thermographie betr., thermographisch.
ther·mog·ra·phy [θɜr'magrəfɪ] *n radiol.*, *phys.* Thermographie *f*.
ther·mo·hy·per·al·ge·sia [ˌθɜrməˌhaɪpərˌæl'dʒiːzɪə, -dʒiːʒə] *n* exzessive Thermalgesie *f*, Thermohyperalgesie *f*.
ther·mo·hy·per·es·the·sia [ˌ-ˌhaɪpəres'θiːʒ(ɪ)ə] *n neuro.* extreme Temperaturempfindlichkeit *f*, Thermohyperästhesie *f*.
ther·mo·hy·pes·the·sia [ˌ-ˌhaɪpes'θiːʒ(ɪ)ə] *n* → thermhypesthesia.
ther·mo·hy·po·es·the·sia [ˌ-ˌhaɪpəʊes'θiːʒ(ɪ)ə] *n* → thermhypesthesia.
ther·mo·in·ac·ti·va·tion [ˌ-ɪnˌæktə'veɪʃn] *n* Wärme-, Hitzeinaktivierung *f*.
ther·mo·in·sen·si·tive cells [ˌ-ɪn'sensɪtɪv] *physiol.* thermoinsensitive Zellen *pl*.
ther·mo·in·sta·bil·i·ty [ˌ-ˌɪnstə'bɪlətɪ] *n* → thermolability.
ther·mo·junc·tion [ˌ-'dʒʌŋkʃn] *n* → thermocouple.
ther·mo·la·bile [ˌ-'leɪbɪl, -baɪl] *adj* hitze-, wärmeunbeständig, wärmeempfindlich, thermolabil.
ther·mo·la·bil·i·ty [ˌ-lə'bɪlətɪ] *n* Wärme-, Hitzeunbeständigkeit *f*, Thermolabilität *f*.
ther·mo·lu·mi·nes·cence [ˌ-ˌluːmə'nesəns] *n* Thermolumineszenz *f*.
ther·mol·y·sin [θɜr'maləsɪn] *n* Thermolysin *nt*.
ther·mol·y·sis [θɜr'maləsɪs] *n* **1.** *chem.* thermische Dissoziation *f*, Thermolyse *f*. **2.** *physiol.* Abgabe *f* von Körperwärme.
ther·mo·lyt·ic [ˌθɜrmə'lɪtɪk] *adj chem.* Thermolyse betr., thermolytisch.
ther·mo·mas·tog·ra·phy [ˌ-mæs'tagrəfɪ] *n radiol.*, *gyn.* Thermomammographie *f*.
ther·mom·e·ter [θɜr'mamɪtər] *n* Thermometer *nt*.
thermometer scale Thermometerskala *f*.
ther·mo·met·ric [ˌθɜrmə'metrɪk] *adj* thermometrisch, Thermometer-.
ther·mo·met·ri·cal [ˌ-'metrɪkl] *adj* → thermometric.
ther·mom·e·try [θɜr'mamətrɪ] *n* Temperaturmessung *f*, Thermometrie *f*.
ther·mo·neu·ro·sis [ˌθɜrmənjʊə'rəʊsɪs, -nəʊ-] *n* psychogenes Fieber *nt*.
ther·mo·neu·tral [ˌ-'n(j)uːtrəl] *adj* thermoneutral.
thermoneutral zone *physiol.* thermische Neutralzone *f*, Neutral-, Indifferenztemperatur *f*.
ther·mo·nu·cle·ar [ˌ-'n(j)uːklɪər] *adj phys.* thermonuklear.
ther·mo·pal·pa·tion [ˌ-pæl'peɪʃn] *n* Thermopalpation *f*.
ther·mo·pen·e·tra·tion [ˌ-ˌpenə'treɪʃn] *n* Thermopenetration *f*, Diathermie *f*.
ther·mo·per·cep·tion [ˌ-pər'sepʃn] *n* Thermoperzeption *f*.
ther·mo·phile ['-faɪl, -fɪl] *n* thermophiler Mikroorganismus *m*, Thermophile(r *m*) *f*.
ther·mo·phil·ic [ˌ-'fɪlɪk] *adj* wärmeliebend, thermophil.
thermophilic bacteria thermophile Bakterien *pl*.
ther·mo·phore ['-fəʊər, -fɔːr] *n* Thermophor *nt*.
ther·mo·pile ['-paɪl] *n phys.* Thermosäule *f*.

thermoplastic

ther·mo·plas·tic [ˌ-'plæstɪk] **I** n Thermoplast m. **II** adj thermoplastisch.
ther·mo·ple·gia [ˌ-'pliːdʒ(ɪ)ə] n Hitzschlag m, Thermoplegie f.
ther·mo·pre·cip·i·ta·tion [ˌ-prɪˌsɪpɪ'teɪʃn] n Thermopräzipitation f.
ther·mo·ra·di·o·ther·a·py [ˌ-ˌreɪdɪəʊ'θerəpɪ] n Thermoradiotherapie f.
ther·mo·re·cep·tion [ˌ-rɪ'sepʃn] n Temperatursinn m, Thermorezeption f.
ther·mo·re·cep·tor [ˌ-rɪ'septər] n Thermorezeptor m.
ther·mo·reg·u·la·tion [ˌ-ˌregjə'leɪʃn] n Wärme-, Temperaturregelung f, Thermoregulation f.
ther·mo·reg·u·la·tor [ˌ-'regjəleɪtər] **I** n Thermostat m. **II** adj → thermoregulatory.
ther·mo·reg·u·la·to·ry [ˌ-'regjələtɔːrɪː, -təʊ-] adj thermoregulatorisch.
thermoregulatory behavior thermoregulatorisches Verhalten nt.
thermoregulatory center thermoregulatorisches Zentrum nt.
thermoregulatory thermogenesis thermoregulatorische Wärmebildung f.
ther·mo·re·sis·tance [ˌ-rɪ'zɪstəns] n Widerstandsfähigkeit f gegen Wärme/Hitze, Wärme-, Hitzebeständigkeit f, Thermoresistenz f.
ther·mo·re·sis·tant [ˌ-rɪ'zɪstənt] adj resistent gegen Wärme/Hitze, hitze-, wärmebeständig, thermoresistent.
ther·mo·re·spon·sive cells [ˌ-rɪ'spɒnsɪv] physiol. thermoresponsive Zellen pl.
ther·mo·scope ['-skəʊp] n Differentialthermometer nt.
ther·mo·sen·si·tive cells [ˌ-'sensɪtɪv] physiol. thermosensitive Zellen pl.
thermosensitive neuron physiol. thermosensitives Neuron nt.
ther·mo·sen·si·tiv·i·ty [ˌ-sensə'tɪvətɪ] n Temperaturempfindlichkeit f, Thermosensibilität f.
ther·mo·sen·sor [ˌ-'sensər, -sɔr] n Thermosensor m.
ther·mo·sta·ble [ˌ-'steɪbl] adj wärme-, hitzebeständig, thermostabil.
ther·mo·sta·bil·i·ty [ˌ-stə'bɪlətɪ] n Wärme-, Hitzebeständigkeit f, Thermostabilität f.
ther·mo·sta·sis [ˌ-'steɪsɪs, -'stæs-] n Thermostase f.
ther·mo·stat ['-stæt] n Temperaturregler m, Thermostat m.
ther·mo·stat·ic [ˌ-'stætɪk] adj thermostatisch.
ther·mo·ste·re·sis [ˌ-stɪ'riːsɪs] n Wärmeentzug m.
ther·mo·tac·tic [ˌ-'tæktɪk] adj Thermotaxis betr., thermotaktisch.
ther·mo·tax·ic [ˌ-'tæksɪk] adj → thermotactic.
ther·mo·tax·is [ˌ-'tæksɪs] n Thermotaxis f.
ther·mo·ther·a·py [ˌ-'θerəpɪ] n Wärmebehandlung f, -therapie f, -anwendung f, Thermotherapie f.
ther·mo·tol·er·ant [ˌ-'tɒlərənt] adj micro. thermotolerant.
ther·mo·to·nom·e·ter [ˌ-tə'nɒmɪtər] physiol. Thermotonometer nt.
ther·mo·trop·ic [ˌ-'trɒpɪk, -'trəʊp-] adj thermotrop.
ther·mot·ro·pism [θɜr'mɒtrəpɪzəm] n Thermotropismus m.
the·sau·ris·mo·sis [ˌθəˌsɔːrɪz'məʊsɪs] n Speicherkrankheit f, Thesaurismose f.
the·sau·ro·sis [θəsɔːˈrəʊsɪs] n übermäßige/ pathologische Speicherung f, Thesaurose f; Speicherkrankheit f, Thesaurismose f.
the·sis ['θiːsɪs] n, pl **-ses** [-siːz] **1.** These f; Behauptung f; Satz m, Postulat nt. **2.** (Aufsatz-)Thema nt. **3.** Doktorarbeit f, Dissertation f; wissenschaftliche Arbeit f.
the·ta rhythm ['θeɪtə] θ-Rhythmus m, Thetarhythmus m.
theta toxin Thetatoxin nt, θ-Toxin nt.
theta wave physiol., neuro. theta-Welle f.
THF abbr. → thymic humoral factor.
thi- pref. → thio-.
thi·a·bu·ta·zide [ˌθaɪə'bjuːtəzaɪd] n pharm. Butizid nt, Thiabutazid nt.
thi·a·cet·a·zone [ˌ-'setəzəʊn] n pharm. Thioazetazon nt.
thi·a·di·a·zide [ˌ-'daɪəzaɪd] n → thiazide.
thi·a·di·a·zine [ˌ-'daɪəziːn] n → thiazide.
thi·am·a·zole [θaɪ'æməzəʊl] n pharm. Thiamazol nt, Methimazol nt.
thi·a·min ['θaɪəmɪn] n → thiamine.
thi·am·i·nase [θaɪ'æmɪneɪz] n Thiaminase f.
thi·a·mine ['θaɪəmiːn, -mɪn] n Thiamin nt, Vitamin B₁ nt.
thiamine diphosphate → thiamine pyrophosphate.
thiamine pyrophosphate abbr. **TPP** Thiaminpyrophosphat nt abbr. TPP.
thiamine test → thiochrome test.
thi·am·phen·i·col [ˌθaɪæm'fenɪkəʊl, -kɒl] n pharm. Thiamphenicol nt.
thi·a·zide ['θaɪəzaɪd] n pharm. Thiazid(-Diuretikum nt) nt.
thiazide diabetes Thiaziddiabetes m.
thi·a·zin [ˈθaɪəzɪn] n Thiazin nt.
thi·a·zole [ˈθaɪəzəʊl] n Thiazol nt.
thiazole ring Thiazolring m.
thi·a·zol·i·dine ring [ˌθaɪə'zəʊlədiːn, -'zɒl-] Thiazolidinring m.
Thibierge-Weissenbach [tiˈbjɛːrʒ ˈvaɪsənbaç]: **T.-W. syndrome** Thibierge-Weissenbach-Syndrom nt.
thick [θɪk] **I** n **1.** dickster Teil m, dickste Stelle f. **2.** fig. Brennpunkt m. **3.** Dummkopf m. **II** adj **4.** dick; dick, massig, korpulent. **5.** patho. geschwollen. **6.** (Haar) dicht; (Stimme) belegt, heiser; neblig; (Flüssigkeit) getrübt, trüb(e); dickflüssig. **7.** ~ **with 1.** über u. über bedeckt von. **2.** voll von, reich an. **8.** dumm.
thick·en [θɪkn] **I** vt **1.** dick(er) machen; ver-, eindicken. **2.** dicht(er) machen, verdichten. **3.** vermehren, verstärken. **4.** trüben. **II** vt **5.** dick(er) werden, s. verdicken, dickflüssig werden. **6.** dicht(er) werden, s. verdichten. **7.** s. vermehren. **8.** s. trüben, trüb werden.
thick·ened [ˈθɪkənd] adj verdickt; schwielig, schwartig.
thick·en·er [ˈθɪkənər] n **1.** Eindicker m. **2.** chem. Verdickungsmittel nt; Verdicker m.
thick·en·ing [ˈθɪkənɪŋ] n **1.** Verdickung f, verdickte Stelle f; patho. Anschwellung f, Verdickung f; Schwarte f. **2.** Eindickung f. **3.** Eindickmittel nt. **4.** Verdichtung f.
thick myofilament Myosinfilament nt.
thick·ness [ˈθɪknɪs] n **1.** Dicke f, Stärke f. **2.** patho. Verdickung f, Schwellung f. **3.** Dichte f. **4.** (Flüssigkeit) Trübheit f, Dickflüssigkeit f. **5.** (Sprache) Undeutlichkeit f.
thick pannus ophthal. Pannus crassus.
thick-set adj (Statur) untersetzt, gedrungen.
thick-skinned adj dickhäutig, -schalig, pachyderm.
thick-walled adj dickwandig.
Thiemann [ˈtiːman]: **T.'s disease/syndrome** Thiemann'-Krankheit f.
Thiersch [tɪərʃ]: **T.'s graft** Thiersch-Lappen m.
T.'s operation Thiersch-Technik f.
thi·eth·yl·per·a·zine [θaɪˌeθl'perəziːn] n pharm. Thiethylperazin nt.
thigh [θaɪ] n (Ober-)Schenkel m, Oberschenkelregion f; anat. Regio femoris.
thigh bone (Ober-)Schenkelknochen m, Femur nt, Os femoris.
thigh joint Hüftgelenk nt, Artic. coxae/iliofemoralis.
thigm- pref. → thigmo-.
thig·mes·the·sia [ˌθɪgmes'θiːʒ(ɪ)ə] n Berührungsempfindlichkeit f.
thigmo- pref. Berührungs-, Thigm(o)-.
thig·mo·tac·tic [ˌθɪgməʊ'tæktɪk] adj Thigmotaxis betr., thigmotaktisch, stereotaktisch.
thig·mo·tax·is [ˌ-'tæksɪs] n Thigmotaxis f, Stereotaxis f.
thig·mo·trop·ic [ˌ-'trɒpɪk, -'trəʊ-] adj thigmotrop.
thig·mot·ro·pism [θɪg'mɒtrəpɪzəm] n Thigmotropismus m.
thin [θɪn] adj **I** adj dünn; (Haar) spärlich, dünn; (Stimme, Verdünnung) schwach; photo. kontrastarm; (Körper) dünn, schmächtig, mager. **to become ~** abmagern. **II** vt → **thin down I. III** vi → **thin down II**.
thin down I vt dünn(er) machen, verdünnen; verringern, dezimieren. **II** vi dünn(er) werden; s. lichten; s. verringern.
thin off vt, vi → thin down.
thin out vt, vi → thin down.
thin disk Z-Linie f, Z-Streifen m, Zwischenscheibe f, Telophragma nt.
think [θɪŋk] (v **thought; thought**) **I** v **1.** etw. denken. **2.** nachdenken über; s. vorstellen, (s.) denken. **3.** etw. halten (of von). **4.** gedenken, beabsichtigen (of doing to do zu tun). **II** vi **5.** denken (of an); s. erinnern (of an). **6.** nachdenken (about, over über). **7.** denken, glauben, meinen.
think·ing [ˈθɪŋkɪŋ] **I** n **1.** Denken nt. **2.** Nachdenken nt, Überlegen nt; Gedanken(gang m) pl, Überlegung(en pl) f. **II** adj denkend, vernünftig, Denk-.
thin-layer chromatography abbr. **TLC** Dünnschichtchromatographie f abbr. DC.
thin-layer electrophoresis abbr. **TLE** lab. Dünnschichtelektrophorese f.
thin limb of Henle's loop dünnes Segment nt der Henle'-Schleife f, Überleitungsstück nt.
thin myofilament Aktinfilament nt.
thin pannus ophthal. Pannus tenuis.
thin-split graft Thiersch-Lappen m.
thio- pref. chem. Thi(o)-, Schwefel-.
thio-acid n Thiosäure f.
thi·o·al·co·hol [ˌθaɪəʊˈælkəhɒl, -hɔl] n Merkaptan nt, Mercaptan nt, Thioalkohol m.
thi·o·am·ide [ˌ-'æmaɪd] n Thioamid nt.
thi·o·ar·se·nite [ˌ-'ɑːrsənaɪt] n Thioarsenit nt.
thi·o·bar·bi·tal [ˌ-'bɑːrbɪtəl, -tæl] n pharm. Thiobarbital nt.
thi·o·bar·bi·tu·rate [ˌ-bɑːr'bɪtʃərɪt, -reɪt] n Thiobarbiturat nt.
thi·o·bar·bi·tu·ric acid [ˌ-ˌbɑːrbɪ't(j)ʊərɪk] n Thiobarbitursäure f.
THIO broth → thioglycolate broth.
thi·o·car·ba·mide [ˌ-ˌkɑːr'bæmaɪd, -'kɑːrbə-] n → thiourea.
thi·o·chrome ['-krəʊm] n Thiochrom nt.
thiochrome test Thiochromtest m.
thi·o·clas·tic [ˌ-'klæstɪk] adj chem. thioklastisch.
thioclastic cleavage chem. thioklastische Spaltung f.
thi·oc·tic acid [θaɪˈɒktɪk] Liponsäure f, Thiooctansäure f.
thi·o·cy·a·nate [ˌθaɪəʊˈsaɪəneɪt] n **1.** Thiozyanat nt, -cyanat nt, Rhodanid nt. **2.** Thiozyansäureester m, Thiozyanat

thi·o·cy·an·ic acid [ˌ-saɪˈænɪk] Thiozyansäure f, -cyansäure f, Rhodanwasserstoffsäure f.
thi·o·cy·a·nide [ˌ-ˈsaɪənaɪd] n Thiozyanid nt.
thi·o·di·phen·yl·a·mine [ˌ-daɪˌfenləˈmiːn, -ˈæmɪn] n pharm. **1.** Phenothiazin nt. **2.** Phenothiazinderivat nt.
thi·o·do·ther·a·py [ˌθaɪədəʊˈθerəpɪ] n kombinierte Schwefel- u. Jodtherapie f.
thi·o·es·ter [ˌθaɪəˈestər] n Thioester m.
thioester bond chem. Thioesterbindung f.
thi·o·e·ther [ˌ-ˈeθər] n Thioäther m, -ether m.
thioether bridge chem. Thioätherbrücke f.
thi·o·eth·yl·a·mine [ˌ-ˈeθəlemiːn, -mɪn, -ˌæmɪn] n Thioäthylamin nt.
thi·o·fla·vine [ˌ-ˈfleɪvɪn] n Thioflavin nt.
thi·o·ga·lac·to·side [ˌ-gəˈlæktəsaɪd, -sɪd] n Thiogalaktosid nt, -galactosid nt.
β-thiogalactoside acetyltransferase (β-)-Thiogalaktosidacetyltransferase f.
thi·o·glu·cose [ˌ-ˈgluːkəʊs] n Thioglucose f.
thi·o·gly·co·late [ˌ-ˈglaɪkəleɪt] n Thioglykolat nt.
thioglycolate broth Thioglykolatbouillon f.
thi·o·gua·nine [ˌ-ˈgwɑniːn] n pharm. Thioguanin nt.
thi·o·hem·i·ac·e·tal bond [ˌ-ˌhemɪˈæsɪtæl] chem. Thiohalbacetalbindung f.
thi·o·ki·nase [ˌ-ˈkaɪneɪz, -ˈkɪn-] n Thiokinase f.
thi·ol [ˈθaɪɒl, -əl] n **1.** Sulfhydryl-, SH--Gruppe f. **2.** Thiol nt, Merkaptan nt, Thioalkohol m.
thi·o·lase [ˈθaɪəleɪz] n **1.** Thiolase f. **2.** Acetyl-CoA-Acetyltransferase f, (Acetoacetyl-)Thiolase f.
thi·ol·y·sis [θaɪˈɒləsɪs] n Thiolyse f, thiolytische Spaltung f.
thi·o·lyt·ic [ˌθaɪəˈlɪtɪk] adj thiolytisch.
thiolytic cleavage → thiolysis.
thio·ne·ine [ˌ-ˈnɪˌiːn, -nɪən] n Ergothionein nt.
thi·o·nin [ˈ-nɪn] n Thionin nt, Lauth'-Violett nt.
thi·o·nyl [ˈ-nɪl] n Thionyl-(Radikal nt).
thi·o·pan·ic acid [ˌ-ˈpænɪk] Thiopansäure f, Pantoyltaurin nt.
thi·o·pec·tic [ˌ-ˈpektɪk] adj schwefelbindend, -fixierend.
thi·o·pen·tal sodium [ˌ-ˈpentl] pharm. Thiopental-Natrium nt.
thi·o·pen·tone sodium [ˌ-ˈpentəʊn] → thiopental sodium.
thi·o·pex·ic [ˌ-ˈpeksɪk] adj → thiopectic.
thi·o·pex·y [ˌ-ˈpeksɪ] n biochem. Schwefelbindung f, -fixierung f.
thi·o·phene [ˈ-fiːn] n Thiophen(ring m) nt.
thiophene ring → thiophene.
thi·o·re·dux·in [ˌθaɪərɪˈdʌksɪn] n Thioreduxin nt.
thioreduxin reductase Thioxinreduktase f.
thi·o·rid·a·zine [ˌ-ˈrɪdəziːn] n pharm. Thioridazin nt.
thi·o·sem·i·car·ba·zide [ˌ-ˌsemɪˈkɑrbəzaɪd] n Thiosemikarbamid nt, -carbamid nt.
thi·o·sem·i·car·ba·zone [ˌ-ˌsemɪˈkɑrbəzəʊn] n Thiosemikarbazon nt, -carbazon nt.
thi·o·sul·fate [ˌ-ˈsʌlfeɪt] n Thiosulfat nt.
thi·o·sul·fu·ric acid [ˌ-sʌlˈfjʊərɪk] Thioschwefelsäure f.
thi·o·tep·a [ˌ-ˈtepə] n pharm. Thiotepa nt, Triäthylenphosphorsäuretriamid nt, Triäthylenphosphoramid nt abbr. TPA.

2-thi·o·u·ra·cil [ˌ-ˈjʊərəsɪl] n 2-Thiouracil nt.
thi·o·u·rea [ˌ-jʊəˈriːə, -ˈjʊərɪə] n Thioharnstoff m, Sulfocarbamid nt.
2-thi·o·u·ri·dine [ˌ-ˈjʊərɪdiːn, -dɪn] n 2--Thiouridin nt.
thi-ram [ˈθaɪræm] n pharm. Thiram nt, Tetramethylthiuramdisulfid nt.
third [θɜrd] **I** n der/die/das Dritte; dritter Teil; Drittel nt. **II** adj **1.** dritte(r, s). **2.** drittklassig, -rangig.
third and fourth pharyngeal pouch syndrome DiGeorge-Syndrom nt, Schlundtaschensyndrom nt, Thymusaplasie f.
third degree burn Verbrennung f dritten Grades.
third disease Röteln pl, Rubella f, Rubeola f.
third division of trigeminal nerve dritter Trigeminusast m, Mandibularis m, N. mandibularis.
third finger Mittelfinger m, Digitus medius/tertius.
third law of thermodynamics dritter Hauptsatz m der Thermodynamik.
third molar (tooth) Weisheitszahn m, dritter Molar m, Dens serotinus.
third nerve Okulomotorius m, III. Hirnnerv m, N. oculomotorius.
third-order reaction chem. Reaktion f dritter Ordnung.
third sound dritter Herzton m.
third space phys., patho. dritter/transzellulärer Raum m, third space (m).
third space loss Flüssigkeitsverschiebung f in den dritten Raum.
third space sequestration → third space loss.
third stage of labor gyn. Nachgeburtsperiode f, -phase f.
third tonsil Rachenmandel f, Tonsilla pharyngealis/adenoidea.
third ventricle of brain/cerebrum dritter (Hirn-)Ventrikel m, Ventriculus tertius (cerebri).
thirst [θɜrst] **I** n **1.** Durst, Durstempfindung f. **2.** fig. Gier f, Verlangen nt (for, after nach). **II** vi Durst haben, durstig sein, dürsten.
thirst fever ped. Durstfieber nt.
thirst·i·ness [ˈθɜrstɪnɪs] n Durst(igkeit f) m.
thirst·y [ˈθɜrstɪ] adj durstig. **to be ~** durstig sein, Durst haben.
thix·o·la·bile [ˌθɪksəˈleɪbl] adj chem. thixolabil.
thix·o·trop·ic [ˌ-ˈtrɒpɪk, -ˈtrəʊ-] adj chem. Thixotropie betr., thixotrop.
thix·ot·ro·pism [θɪkˈsɒtrəpɪzəm] n → thixotropy.
thix·ot·ro·py [θɪkˈsɒtrəpɪ] n chem. Thixotropie f.
THO abbr. → tritium-labeled water.
Thomas [ˈtɒməs]: **T.' splint** ortho. Thomas-Schiene f.
Thoma-Zeiss [ˈtəʊmə zaɪs; ˈtoːma tsaɪs]: **T.-Z. counting cell** → T.-Z. counting chamber.
T.-Z. counting chamber Abbé-Zählkammer f, Thoma-Zeiss-Kammer f.
T.-Z. hemocytometer → T.-Z. counting chamber.
Thompson [ˈtɒm(p)sən]: **T. prosthesis** ortho. Thompson-Prothese f.
T.'s test urol. Tompson-Probe f, Zweigläserprobe m.
Thomsen [ˈtɒmsən]: **T.'s disease** Thomsen--Syndrom nt, Myotonia congenita/hereditaria f.
T. phenomenon Hübener-Thomsen--Friedenreich-Phänomen nt, Thomsen--Phänomen nt, T-Agglutinationsphänomen nt.

Thomson [ˈtɒmsən]: **T.'s disease** → T.'s syndrome.
T. scattering phys. klassische Streuung f, Thomson-Streuung f.
T.'s syndrome Thomson-Syndrom nt.
thorac- pref. → thoraco-.
tho·ra·cal [ˈθɔːrəkl] adj → thoracic.
tho·ra·cal·gia [ˌθɔːrəˈkældʒ(ɪ)ə, ˌθəʊ-] n → thoracodynia.
tho·ra·cec·to·my [ˌ-ˈsektəmɪ] n chir., ortho. Thorakotomie f mit Rippenresektion.
tho·ra·cen·te·sis [ˌ-senˈtiːsɪs] n → thoracocentesis.
tho·rac·ic [θɔːˈræsɪk, θə-] adj Brustkorb/Thorax betr., thorakal, Brust-, Brustkorb-, Thorax-.
thoracic actinomycosis thorakale Aktinomykose f.
thoracic aneurysm 1. intrathorakales Aneurysma nt. **2.** Aneurysma nt der Aorta thoracica.
thoracic aorta Brustschlagader f, Aorta thoracica, Pars thoracica aortae.
thoracic aperture Brustkorböffnung f, Thoraxapertur f, Apertura thoracis. **inferior t.** → lower t. **lower t.** untere Thoraxapertur, Brustkorbausgang m, Apertura thoracis inferior. **superior t.** → upper t. **upper t.** obere Thoraxapertur, Brustkorbeingang m, Apertura thoracis superior.
thoracic approach chir. (trans-)thorakaler Zugang m.
thoracic artery: highest t. oberste Brustwandarterie f, Thoracica f suprema, A. thoracica suprema. **internal t.** innere Brustwandarterie f, Mammaria/Thoracica f interna, A. thoracica interna. **lateral t.** seitliche Brustwandarterie f, Thoracica f lateralis, A. thoracica lateralis.
thoracic axis old → thoracoacromial artery.
thoracic bones Ossa thoracis.
thoracic cage (knöcherner) Brustkorb m, Brustkasten m, Thorax(skelett nt) m, Compages thoracis, Skleleton thoracicum.
thoracic cavity Brusthöhle f, Thoraxhöhle f, Brustkorbinnenraum m, Cavitas thoracis/thoracica.
thoracic chondrodystrophy, asphyxiating → thoracic dystrophy, asphyxiating.
thoracic column Clarke'-Säule f, Clarke--Stilling'-Säule f, Stilling'-Kern m, Nc. thoracicus, Columna thoracica.
thoracic crisis neuro. Thoraxkrise f.
thoracic duct Brustmilchgang m, Milchbrustgang m, Ductus thoracicus.
right t. rechter Hauptlymphgang m, Ductus lymphaticus/thoracicus dexter.
thoracic dysplasia, asphyxiating → thoracic dystrophy, asphyxiating.
thoracic dystrophy, asphyxiating abbr. ATD Jeune'-Krankheit f, asphyxierende Thoraxdysplasie f.
thoracic empyema Pyothorax m, Thorax-, Pleuraempyem nt, eitrige Pleuritis f.
thoracic esophagus → thoracic part of esophagus.
thoracic fascia Fascia thoracica.
thoracic fistula Brustkorb-, Thoraxfistel f.
thoracic ganglion: t.ia pl thorakale Grenzstrangganglien pl, Ggll. thoracica. **splanchnic t.** Ggl. (thoracicus) splanchnicus.
thoracic girdle Schultergürtel m, Cingulum membri superioris, Cingulum pectorale.

thoracic inlet → thoracic aperture, upper.
thoracic limbs obere Gliedmaßen/Extremitäten *pl*, Arme *pl*.
thoracic muscles Brust(korb)muskeln *pl*, -muskulatur *f*, Mm. thoracis.
thoracic nerve: t.s *pl* thorakale Spinalnerven *pl*, Brustnerven *pl*, Nn. thoracici.
long t. N. thoracicus longus.
thoracic nucleus → thoracic column.
tho·rac·i·co·ab·dom·i·nal [θəˌræsɪkəʊæb-'damɪnl, θəʊ-] *adj* → thoracoabdominal.
tho·rac·i·co·a·cro·mi·al [ˌ-əˈkrəʊmɪəl] *adj* → thoracoacromial.
tho·rac·i·co·hu·mer·al [ˌ-ˈ(h)juːmərəl] *adj* Thorax u. Humerus betr., thorakohumeral.
tho·rac·i·co·lum·bar [ˌ-ˈlʌmbər] *adj* → thoracolumbar.
thoracicolumbar division of autonomic nervous system sympathisches Nervensystem *nt*, (Ortho-)Sympathicus *m*, sympathischer Teil *m* des autonomen Nervensystems, N. sympathicus, Pars sympathetica/sympathica systematis nervosi autonomici.
thoracic opening: inferior t. untere Thoraxapertur *f*, Brustkorbausgang *m*, Apertura thoracis inferior.
lower t. → inferior t.
superior t. obere Thoraxapertur *f*, Brustkorbeingang *m*, Apertura thoracis superior.
upper t. → superior t.
thoracic outlet → thoracic opening, inferior.
thoracic outlet syndrome Thoracic-outlet-Syndrom *nt*, Engpaß-Syndrom *nt*.
thoracic part: t. of aorta → thoracic aorta.
t. of autonomic nervous system Thorakalabschnitt *m* des vegetativen Nervensystems, Pars thoracica autonomica.
t. of esophagus Brustabschnitt *m* der Speiseröhre, Pars thoracica (o)esophagi.
t. of spinal cord Brust-, Thorakalsegmente *pl*, Brustmark *nt*, Brustabschnitt *m* des Rückenmarks, Thoracica *pl*, Pars thoracica (medullae spinalis).
t. of thoracic duct intrathorakaler Teil *m* des Ductus thoracicus, Pars thoracica ductus thoracici.
t. of trachea intrathorakaler Abschnitt *m* der Luftröhre, Pars thoracica tracheae.
thoracic-pelvic-phalangeal dystrophy Jeune'-Krankheit *f*, asphyxierende Thoraxdysplasie *f*.
thoracic respiration Brustatmung *f*.
thoracic scoliosis *ortho*. thorakale Skoliose *f*.
thoracic segments of spinal cord Brust-, Thorakalsegmente *pl*, Brustmark *nt*, Brustabschnitt *m* des Rückenmarks, Thoracica *pl*, Pars thoracica (medullae spinalis).
thoracic skeleton knöcherner Brustkorb/Thorax *m*, Thoraxskelett *nt*, Compages thoracis, Skeleton thoracis *f*.
thoracic spine Brustwirbelsäule *f abbr*. BWS.
thoracic surgery Thoraxchirurgie *f*.
thoracic sympathectomy thorakale Sympathektomie *f*.
thoracic syndrome Thorakalsyndrom *nt*.
thoracic vein: lateral t. Begleitvene *f* der A. thoracica lateralis, V. thoracica lateralis.
internal t.s *pl* innere Brust(wand)venen *pl*, Vv. thoracicae internae.
thoracic vertebrae Thorakal-, Brustwirbel *pl abbr* BW, Vertebrae thoracicae.
thoraco- *pref*. Brust-, Brustkorb-, Thorax-, Thorak(o)-.

tho·ra·co·ab·dom·i·nal [ˌθɔːrəkəʊæb-'damɪnl] *adj* Thorax u. Abdomen betr., thorakoabdominal.
thoracoabdominal approach *chir*. thorakoabdominaler Zugang *m*.
tho·ra·co·a·cro·mi·al [ˌ-əˈkrəʊmɪəl] *adj* Thorax u. Akromion betr., thorakoakromial.
thoracoacromial artery Thorakoakromialis *f*, A. thoracoacromialis.
thoracoacromial vein Begleitvene *f* der A. thoracoacromialis, V. thoracoacromialis.
tho·ra·co·ce·los·chi·sis [ˌ-sɪˈlɒskəsɪs] *n* → thoracogastroschisis.
tho·ra·co·cen·te·sis [ˌ-senˈtiːsɪs] *n* Pleurapunktion *f*, Thorakozentese *f*.
tho·ra·co·cyl·lo·sis [ˌ-sɪˈləʊsɪs] *n* Brustkorb-, Thoraxdeformität *f*.
tho·ra·co·del·phus [ˌ-ˈdelfəs] *n embryo*. Thora(ko)delphus *m*.
tho·ra·co·did·y·mus [ˌ-ˈdɪdəməs] *n embryo*. Thorakodidymus *m*.
tho·ra·co·dor·sal artery [ˌ-ˈdɔːrsl] hintere Brustwandarterie *f*, Thorakodorsalis *f*, A. thoracodorsalis.
thoracodorsal nerve N. thoracodorsalis.
thoracodorsal vein V. thoracodorsalis.
tho·ra·co·dyn·ia [ˌ-ˈdiːnɪə] *n* Schmerzen *pl* im Brustkorb, Thorakodynie *f*, Thorakalgie *f*.
tho·ra·co·ep·i·gas·tric veins [ˌ-ˌepɪˈgæstrɪk] seitliche Rumpfwandvenen *pl*, Vv. thoraco-epigastricae.
tho·ra·co·gas·tro·did·y·mus [ˌ-ˌgæstrə-ˈdɪdəməs] *n embryo*. Thorakogastrodidymus *m*.
tho·ra·co·gas·tros·chi·sis [ˌ-gæsˈtrɒskəsɪs] *n embryo*. angeborene Brust- u. Bauchspalte *f*, Thorakogastroschisis *f*.
tho·rac·o·graph [θɔːˈrækəgræf] *n* Thorako(pneumo)graph *m*.
tho·ra·co·lap·a·rot·o·my [ˌθɔːrəkəʊˌlæpə-ˈrɒtəmɪ] *n chir*. Thorakolaparotomie *f*.
tho·ra·co·lum·bar [ˌ-ˈlʌmbər, -baːr] *adj* Brustkorb/Thorax u. Lendenwirbelsäule betr., thorakolumbal, lumbothorakal.
thoracolumbar aponeurosis → thoracolumbar fascia.
thoracolumbar division of autonomic nervous system → thoracolumbar system.
thoracolumbar fascia Fascia thoracolumbalis.
thoracolumbar scoliosis *ortho*. thorakolumbale Skoliose *f*.
thoracolumbar sympathectomy thorakolumbale Sympathektomie *f*.
thoracolumbar system sympathisches Nervensystem *nt*, (Ortho-)Sympathicus *m*, sympathischer Teil *m* des autonomen Nervensystems, N. sympathicus, Pars sympathetica/sympathica systematis nervosi autonomici.
tho·ra·col·y·sis [ˌθɔːrəˈkɒləsɪs] *n HTG* Thorakolyse *f*.
tho·ra·com·e·lus [ˌ-ˈkamələs] *n embryo*. Thorakomelus *m*.
tho·ra·com·e·ter [ˌ-ˈkamɪtər] *n* Thorakometer *nt*, Stethometer *nt*.
tho·ra·com·e·try [ˌ-ˈkamətrɪ] *n* Thorakometrie *f*.
tho·ra·co·my·o·dyn·ia [ˌθɔːrəkəʊˌmaɪə-ˈdiːnɪə] *n* Brustmuskelschmerzen *pl*, Thorakomyodynie *f*.
tho·ra·cop·a·gus [ˌθɔːrəˈkapəgəs] *n embryo*. Thorakopagus *m*, Synthorax *m*.
tho·ra·co·par·a·ceph·a·lus [ˌθɔːrəkəʊ-ˌpærəˈsefələs] *n embryo*. Thorakoparazephalus *m*.
tho·ra·cop·a·thy [ˌθɔːrəˈkapəθɪ] *n* Brustkorberkrankung *f*, Thorakopathie *f*.

tho·ra·co·plas·ty [ˈθɔːrəkəʊplæstɪ] *n HTG* Thorax-, Thorakoplastik *f*.
tho·ra·co·pneu·mo·graph [ˌ-ˈn(j)uːmə-græf] *n* Thorako(pneumo)graph *m*.
tho·ra·cos·chi·sis [ˌθɔːrəˈkaskəsɪs] *n embryo*. angeborene Brustspalte *f*, Thorakoschisis *f*.
tho·ra·co·scope [θɔːˈrækəskəʊp] *n* Thorakoskop *nt*.
tho·ra·cos·co·py [ˌθɔːrəˈkaskəpɪ] *n* Thorakoskopie *f*.
tho·ra·cos·to·my [ˌ-ˈkastəmɪ] *n HTG* Thorakostomie *f*.
tho·ra·cot·o·my [ˌ-ˈkatəmɪ] *n HTG* Brustkorberöffnung *f*, Thorakotomie *f*.
tho·ra·del·phus [ˌ-ˈdelfəs] *n* → thoracodelphus.
tho·rax [ˈθɔːræks, ˈθəʊər-] *n*, *pl* **-rax·es**, **-ra·ces** [-rəsiːz] Brust(korb *m*) *f*, Thorax *m*.
thorax injury Brustkorbverletzung *f*, -trauma *nt*, Thoraxtrauma *nt*.
blunt t. stumpfes Thoraxtrauma.
penetrating t. penetrierendes Thoraxtrauma.
thorax trauma → thorax injury.
Thorel [ˈtɔrel]: **T.'s bundle** Thorel'-Bündel *nt*.
tho·ri·um [ˈθɔːrɪəm, ˈθəʊ-] *n abbr*. **Th** Thorium *nt abbr*. Th.
thorium emanation Thoron *nt abbr*. Tn, Thoriumemanation *f*.
Thorn [θɔːrn]: **T.'s syndrome** Thorn-Syndrom *nt*, Salzverlustnephritis *f*.
T. test Thorn-Test *m*, ACTH-Eosinophilen-Test *m*.
thorn apple crystal [θɔːrn] (*Harnsediment*) Stechapfelform *f*.
Thornwaldt [ˈtɔrnvalt]: **T.'s abscess** Tornwaldt-Abszeß *m*.
T.'s bursitis → T.'s disease.
T.'s cyst Tornwaldt-Zyste *f*, -Bursa *f*, Bursa pharyngea.
T.'s disease Entzündung *f* der Bursa pharyngealis, Tornwaldt-Krankheit *f*, Bursitis pharyngealis.
thorn·y-head·ed worms [ˈθɔːrnɪ] *micro*. Kratzer *pl*, Kratzwürmer *pl*, Acanthocephala *pl*.
tho·ron [ˈθɔːran, ˈθəʊ-] *n* → thorium emanation.
Thor·o·trast liver [ˈθɔːrətræst, ˈθəʊ-] Thorotrastleber *f*.
thor·ough [ˈθɜːrəʊ, ˈθʌrəʊ] *adj* (*Untersuchung*) gründlich, sorgfältig, eingehend; (*Wissen*) umfassend.
thought [θɔːt] *n* Gedanke *m*, Einfall *m*; Gedankengang *m*; Gedanken *pl*, Denken *nt*.
thought blocking (innere/mentale) Blockierung *f*, Sperre *f*.
thought broadcasting *psychia*. Gedankenausbreitung *f*.
thought deprivation *psychia*. Gedankenentzug *m*.
thought insertion *psychia*. Gedankeneingebung *f*.
thought reading → telepathy.
thought transference → telepathy.
thought withdrawal *psychia*. Gedankenentzug *m*.
THR *abbr*. → total hip replacement.
Thr *abbr*. → threonine.
thread [θred] **I** *n* 1. Faden *m*, fadenförmige Struktur *f*, Faser *f*, Fiber *f*. 2. Faden *m*, Garn *nt*. 3. *ortho*., *techn*. (Schrauben-)Gewinde *nt*, Gewindegang *m*. 4. *fig*. dünner (Urin-)Strahl, Faden *m*. **II** *vt* einfädeln; aufreihen, auffädeln (*on* auf).
thread·ed [ˈθredɪd] *adj* Gewinde-.
threaded nail *ortho*. Gewindestift *m*.
threaded needle 1. *chir*. Nadel *f* (mit

Öhr). **2.** Hohlnagel *m*, Nagel *m* mit Führungskanal.
threaded pin → threaded nail.
thread-like ['θredlaɪk] *adj* fadenförmig, -artig.
thread-worm ['θredwɜrm] *n micro.* **1.** Fadenwurm *m*, Strongyloides *m*. **2.** Madenwurm *m*, Enterobius/Oxyuris vermicularis.
thread-y ['θredɪ] *adj* **1.** fadenartig, faserig, filiform. **2.** *fig.* (*Puls, Stimme*) schwach, dünn. **3.** Fäden ziehend; (*Flüssigkeit*) dick-, zähflüssig..
thready pulse fadenförmiger/dünner Puls *m*, Pulsus filiformis.
threat [θret] *n* Drohung *f* (*of* mit; *to* gegen); Bedrohung *f*, Gefahr *f* (*to* für). **to pose/represent a ~ to life** lebensbedrohlich sein.
threat-ened abortion ['θretnd] *gyn.* drohender Frühabort *m*.
three [θri:] **I** *n* Drei *f*. **II** *adj* drei.
three-chambered heart Cor trilocular*e*.
three-day fever Phlebotomus-, Pappataci-, Moskitofieber *nt*, Drei-Tage-Fieber *nt*.
three-day measles Röteln *pl*, Rubella *f*, Rubeola *f*.
three-dimensional *adj* dreidimensional.
three-glass test *urol.* Dreigläserprobe *f*.
three-part fracture of proximal humerus Neer Typ III-Humerusfraktur *f*, 3-Fragmentfraktur *f*.
three point brace/corset Dreipunktkorsett *nt*.
three-quarters pack Dreiviertelpackung *f*.
thre-o-nine ['θri:ənɪ:n, -nɪn] *n abbr.* Thr Threonin *nt abbr.* Thr, α-Amino-β-hydroxybuttersäure *f*.
threonine dehydratase Threonindehydratase *f*.
thre-o-nyl ['θri:ənɪl] *n* Threonyl-(Radikal *nt*).
thre-ose ['θri:əʊs] *n* Threose *f*.
thresh-er's lung ['θreʃəz] *n* Farmerlunge *f*, Drescherkrankheit *f*, Dreschfieber *nt*.
thresh-old ['θreʃəʊld, 'θreʃh-] **I** *n phys., physiol., psycho.* Grenze *f*, Schwelle *f*, Limen *nt*. **II** *adj* Schwellen-.
t. of audibility Hör(barkeits)schwelle.
t. of consciousness Bewußtseinsschwelle.
t. of disturbance Störungsschwelle.
t. of pain Schmerzgrenze, -schwelle.
t. of stapedius reflex Stapediusreflexschwelle.
threshold audiometry Schwellenaudiometrie *f*.
threshold body → threshold substance.
threshold characteristics *physiol.* Schwellencharakteristik *f*.
threshold concentration *physiol.* Schwellenkonzentration *f*.
threshold depolarization *physiol.* Schwellendepolarisation *f*.
threshold dose *radiol.* Grenz-, Schwellendosis *f*.
threshold percussion Schwellenwertperkussion *f*.
threshold potential *physiol.* Schwellenpotential *nt*.
threshold stimulus Grenz-, Schwellenreiz *m*.
threshold substance *physiol.* Schwellensubstanz *f*.
threshold thirst Durstschwelle *f*.
thrill [θrɪl] *n* **1.** Zittern *nt*, Erregung *f*; prickelndes Gefühl *nt*. **2.** Beben *nt*, Schwirren *nt*, Vibration *f*.
thrive [θraɪv] (**thrived; thrived**) *vi* (*Kind*) gedeihen (*on* mit, bei).
throat [θrəʊt] **I** *n* **1.** Rachen *m*, Schlund *m*,

Pharynx *m*. **2.** Rachenenge *f*, Schlund *m*, Fauces *f*, Isthmus faucium. **3.** Kehle *f*; Gurgel *f*. **4.** *fig.* verengte Öffnung *f*, Hals *m*, Durchgang *m*. **II** *adj* Hals-, Rachen-.
throat swab Rachenabstrich *m*.
throat-y ['θrəʊtɪ] *adj* **1.** kehlig, guttural. **2.** heiser, rauh.
throb [θrɒb] **I** *n* Klopfen *nt*, Pochen *nt*, Hämmern *nt*. **II** *vi* (heftig) klopfen, pochen, hämmern, pulsieren.
throb-bing ['θrɒbɪŋ] **I** *n* Klopfen *nt*, Pochen *nt*. **II** *adj* pochend, hämmernd, klopfend, pulsierend.
throbbing headache pochende/klopfende Kopfschmerzen *pl*.
throbbing pain klopfender/pochender Schmerz *m*.
throe [θrəʊ] *n* **1.** heftiger Schmerz *m*. **2.** *gyn.* Geburts-, Wehenschmerzen *pl*.
thromb- *pref.* → thrombo-.
throm-ba-phe-re-sis [ˌθrɒmbəfə'ri:sɪs] *n* → thrombocytapheresis.
thromb-base ['θrɒmbeɪs] *n* → thrombin.
throm-bas-the-nia [ˌθrɒmbæs'θi:nɪə] *n* Thrombasthenie *f*, Glanzmann-Naegeli--Syndrom *nt*.
throm-bec-to-my [θrɒm'bektəmɪ] *n chir.*, *HTG* Thrombusentfernung *f*, Thrombektomie *f*.
thrombectomy catheter Thrombektomiekatheter *m*.
thromb-e-las-to-gram [ˌθrɒmbɪ'læstəɡræm] *n* → thromboelastogram.
thromb-e-las-to-graph [ˌ-ɪ'læstəɡræf] *n* → thromboelastograph.
thromb-e-las-tog-ra-phy [ˌ-ɪlæs'tɒɡrəfɪ] *n* → thromboelastography.
thromb-em-bo-lia [ˌ-em'bəʊlɪə] *n* → thromboembolism.
throm-bi *pl* → thrombus.
throm-bin ['θrɒmbɪn] *n* Thrombin *nt*, Faktor IIa *m*.
thrombin clotting time → thrombin time.
throm-bin-o-gen [θrɒm'bɪnədʒən] *n* → thrombin.
throm-bin-o-gen-e-sis [ˌθrɒmbɪnə'dʒenəsɪs] *n* Thrombinbildung *f*.
thrombin time *abbr.* **TT** (Plasma-)Thrombinzeit *f abbr.* TT, TZ, Antithrombinzeit *f abbr.* ATZ.
thrombo- *pref.* Plättchen-, Thrombus-, Thromb(o)-.
throm-bo-ag-glu-ti-nin [ˌθrɒmbəʊə'glu:tənɪn] *n* Plättchen-, Thromb(o)zyten)agglutinin *nt*.
throm-bo-an-gi-i-tis [ˌ-ændʒɪ'aɪtɪs] *n* Thromb(o)angiitis *f*.
thromboangiitis obliterans Winiwarter--Buerger-Krankheit *f*, Morbus Winiwarter-Buerger *m*, Endangiitis/Thrombangiitis/Thrombandiitis obliterans.
throm-bo-ar-ter-i-tis [ˌ-ɑ:rtə'raɪtɪs] *n* Thromb(o)arteriitis *f*.
throm-bo-as-the-ni-a [ˌ-æs'θi:nɪə] *n* → thrombasthenia.
throm-bo-blast ['-blæst] *n* Knochenmarksriesenzelle *f*, Megakaryozyt *m*.
throm-boc-la-sis [θrɒm'bɒklasɪs] *n* Thrombolysis *f*.
throm-bo-clas-tic [ˌθrɒmbəʊ'klæstɪk] *n, adj* → thrombolytic.
throm-bo-cyt-a-phe-re-sis [ˌ-ˌsaɪtəfə'ri:sɪs] *n hema., lab.* Thrombo(zyto)pherese *f*.
throm-bo-cyte ['-saɪt] *n* (Blut-)Plättchen *nt*, Thrombozyt *m*, -cyt *m*.
thrombocyte adhesion Thrombozytenadhäsion *f*.
thrombocyte aggregation Thrombozytenaggregation *f*.
thrombocyte series *hema.* thrombozytäre Reihe *f*.
throm-bo-cy-the-mia [ˌ-saɪ'θi:mɪə] *n* per-

manente Erhöhung *f* der Thrombozytenzahl, Thrombozythämie *f*.
throm-bo-cyt-ic [ˌ-'sɪtɪk] *adj* thrombozytär, Thrombozyten-.
thrombocytic series → thrombocyte series.
throm-bo-cy-tin [ˌ-'saɪtɪn] *n* Serotonin *nt*, 5-Hydroxytryptamin *nt*.
throm-bo-cy-tol-y-sis [ˌ-saɪ'tɒləsɪs] *n* Plättchen-, Thrombozytenauflösung *f*, Thrombozytolyse *f*.
throm-bo-cy-to-path-ia [ˌ-ˌsaɪtə'pæθɪə] *n* Thrombo(zyto)pathie *f*.
throm-bo-cy-to-path-ic [ˌ-ˌsaɪtə'pæθɪk] *adj* Thrombo(zyto)pathie betr., thrombo(zyto)pathisch.
throm-bo-cy-top-a-thy [ˌ-saɪ'tɒpəθɪ] *n* → thrombocytopathia.
throm-bo-cy-to-pe-nia [ˌ-ˌsaɪtə'pi:nɪə] *n* verminderte Thrombozytenzahl *f*, (Blut-)Plättchenmangel *m*, Thrombo(zyto)penie *f*.
thrombocytopenia-absent radius syndrome Radiusaplasie-Thrombozytopenie-Syndrom *nt*.
throm-bo-cy-to-pe-nic purpura [ˌ-ˌsaɪtə'pi:nɪk] **1.** thrombozytopenische Purpura *f*. **2.** idiopathische thrombozytopenische Purpura *f abbr.* ITP, essentielle/idiopathische Thrombozytopenie *f*, Morbus Werlhof *m*.
throm-bo-cy-to-poi-e-sis [ˌ-ˌsaɪtəpɔɪ'i:sɪs] *n* Thrombozytenbildung *f*, Thrombo(zyto)poese *f*.
throm-bo-cy-to-poi-et-ic [ˌ-ˌsaɪtəpɔɪ'etɪk] *adj* Thrombozytenbildung betr. *od.* stimulierend, thrombo(zyto)poetisch.
throm-bo-cy-tor-rhex-is [ˌ-ˌsaɪtə'reksɪs] *n* Thrombozytorrhexis *f*.
throm-bo-cy-to-sis [ˌ-saɪ'təʊsɪs] *n* temporäre Erhöhung *f* der Thrombozytenzahl, Thrombozytose *f*.
throm-bo-e-las-to-gram [ˌ-ɪ'læstəɡræm] *n abbr.* **TEG** Thrombelastogramm *nt abbr.* TEG.
throm-bo-e-las-to-graph [ˌ-ɪ'læstəɡræf] *n* Thrombelastograph *m*.
throm-bo-e-las-tog-ra-phy [ˌ-ɪlæs'tɒɡrəfɪ] *n* Thrombelastographie *f*.
throm-bo-em-bo-lec-to-my [ˌ-ˌembə'lektəmɪ] *n chir.*, *HTG* Thromb(o)embolektomie *f*.
throm-bo-em-bo-lia [ˌ-em'bəʊlɪə] *n* → thromboembolism.
throm-bo-em-bo-lism [ˌ-'embəlɪzəm] *n* Thromb(o)embolie *f*.
throm-bo-en-dar-ter-ec-to-my [ˌ-enˌdɑ:rtə'rektəmɪ] *n chir.*, *HTG* Thromb(o)endarteriektomie *f*.
throm-bo-en-do-car-di-tis [ˌ-ˌendəʊkɑ:r'daɪtɪs] *n card.* Thromb(o)endokarditis *f*.
throm-bo-gen ['-dʒən] *n* Prothrombin *nt*, Faktor II *m abbr.* FII.
throm-bo-gene ['-dʒi:n] *n* Proakzelerin *nt*, Proaccelerin *nt*, Acceleratorglobulin *nt*, labiler Faktor *m*, Faktor V *m abbr.* F V.
throm-bo-gen-e-sis [ˌ-'dʒenəsɪs] *n* Thrombusbildung *f*, Thrombogenese *f*.
throm-bo-gen-ic [ˌ-'dʒenɪk] *adj* thrombogen.
β-throm-bo-glob-u-lin [ˌ-'ɡlɒbjəlɪn] *n* β-Thromboglobulin *f*.
throm-boid ['θrɒmbɔɪd] *adj* thrombusartig, thromboid.
throm-bo-kin-ase [ˌθrɒmbəʊ'kaɪneɪz, -'kɪn,] *n* Thrombokinase *f*, -plastin *nt*, Prothrombinaktivator *m*.
throm-bo-ki-net-ics [ˌ-kaɪ'netɪks] *pl* Thrombokinetik *f*.
throm-bo-lym-phan-gi-tis [ˌ-ˌlɪmfæn'dʒaɪtɪs] *n* Thrombolymphangitis *f*.

thrombolysis 766

throm·bol·y·sis [θrɑm'bɑləsɪs] *n* Thrombusauflösung *f*, Thrombolyse *f*.
throm·bo·lyt·ic [,θrɑmbəʊ'lɪtɪk] **I** *n* thrombolytische Substanz *f*, Thrombolytikum *nt*. **II** *adj* Thrombolyse betr. *od.* fördernd, thrombolytisch.
throm·bo·path·ia [,-'pæθɪə] *n* → thrombocytopathia.
throm·bop·a·thy [θrɑm'bɑpəθɪ] *n* → thrombocytopathia.
throm·bo·pen·ia [,θrɑmbəʊ'piːnɪə] *n* → thrombocytopenia.
throm·bo·pe·nic purpura [,-'piːnɪk] → thrombocytopenic purpura.
throm·bo·pe·ny ['-piːnɪ] *n* → thrombocytopenia.
throm·bo·phil·ia [,-'fɪlɪə] *n* Thromboseneigung *f*, Thrombophilie *f*.
throm·bo·phle·bit·ic [,-flə'bɪtɪk] *adj* Thrombophlebitis betr., thrombophlebitisch.
thrombophlebitic splenomegaly Opitz--Krankheit *f*, -Syndrom *nt*, thrombophlebitische Splenomegalie *f*.
throm·bo·phle·bi·tis [,-flə'baɪtɪs] *n* **1.** *patho.* Thrombophlebitis *f*. **2.** *clin.* blande nicht-eitrige (Venen-)Thrombose *f*.
throm·bo·plas·tic [,-'plæstɪk] *adj* eine Thrombusbildung auslösend *od.* fördernd, thromboplastisch.
thromboplastic plasma component *abbr*. **TPC** antihämophiles Globulin *nt abbr*. AHG, Antihämophiliefaktor *m abbr*. AHF, Faktor VIII *m abbr*. F VIII.
throm·bo·plas·tid [,-'plæstɪd] *n* → thrombocyte.
throm·bo·plas·tin [,-'plæstɪn] *n* → thrombokinase.
thromboplastin generation test Thromboplastingenerationstest *m abbr*. TGT, Thromboplastinbildungstest *m*.
throm·bo·plas·tin·o·gen [,-plæs'tɪnədʒən] *n* → thromboplastic plasma component.
thromboplastin time test Thromboplastinzeit *f*, Quickwert *m*, -zeit *f*, *inf.* Quick *m*, Prothrombinzeit *f*.
throm·bo·poi·e·sis [,-pɔr'iːsɪs] *n* **1.** → thrombogenesis. **2.** → thrombocytopoiesis.
throm·bo·poi·et·in [,-pɔr'etɪn] *n* Thrombopo(i)etin *nt*.
throm·bosed ['θrɑmbəʊst] *adj* **1.** geronnen, koaguliert. **2.** von Thrombose betroffen, thrombosiert.
thrombosed hemorrhoids Hämorrhoidalthrombose *f*.
throm·bo·sin ['θrɑmbəsɪn] *n* → thrombin.
throm·bo·si·nu·si·tis [,θrɑmbəʊ,saɪnə'saɪtɪs] *n* Hirnsinusthrombose *f*, Thrombosinusitis *f*.
throm·bo·sis [θrɑm'bəʊsɪs] *n*, *pl* **-ses** [-siːz] Blutpfropfbildung *f*, Thrombusbildung *f*, Thrombose *f*.
t. of the renal vein Nierenvenenthrombose.
throm·bo·spon·din [,θrɑmbəʊ'spɑndɪn] *n* Thrombospondin *nt*.
throm·bos·ta·sis [θrɑm'bɑstəsɪs] *n* Thrombostase *f*.
throm·bo·sthe·nin [,θrɑmbəʊ'sθiːnɪn] *n* Thrombosthenin *nt*.
throm·bo·test ['-test] *n* Thrombotest *m abbr*. TT.
throm·bot·ic [θrɑm'bɑtɪk] *adj* Thrombose betr., von ihr betroffen, thrombotisch.
thrombotic apoplexy thrombotische Apoplexie *f*; thrombotischer Hirninfarkt *m*.
thrombotic gangrene postthrombotische Gangrän *f*.
thrombotic infarct thrombotischer Infarkt *m*.
thrombotic microangiopathy → thrombotic thrombocytopenic purpura.
thrombotic phlegmasia Milchbein *nt*, Leukophlegmasie *f*, Phlegmasia alba dolens.
thrombotic tendency Thromboseneigung *f*, Thrombophilie *f*.
thrombotic thrombocytopenic purpura thrombotische Mikroangiopathie *f*, thrombotisch-thrombozytopenische Purpura *f*, Moschcowitz-Singer-Symmers-Syndrom *nt*, Moschcowitz-Syndrom *nt*, Purpura thrombotica (thrombocytopenica), Purpura Moschcowitz.
throm·bo·to·nin [,θrɑmbəʊ'təʊnɪn] *n* Serotonin *nt*, 5-Hydroxytryptamin *nt*.
throm·bo·ul·cer·a·tive endocarditis [,-'ʌlsəreɪtɪv, -sərət-] thromboulzeröse Endokarditis *f*, Endocarditis thromboulcerosa.
throm·box·ane [θrɑm'bɑkseɪn] *n* Thromboxan *nt*.
thromboxane synthetase Thromboxansynthetase *f*.
throm·bo·zyme ['θrɑmbəzaɪm] *n* → thrombokinase.
throm·bus ['θrɑmbəs] *n*, *pl* **-bi** [-baɪ] Blutpfropf *m*, Thrombus *m*.
through drain [θruː] *chir.* Durchlaufdrainage *f*.
through joint echtes Gelenk *nt*, Diarthrose *f*, Artic./Junctura synovialis.
through·put ['θruːpʊt] *n* Durchsatz *m*, Anzahl *f* der behandelten Patienten.
thrush [θrʌʃ] *n* **1.** Mundsoor *m*, Candidose *f* der Mundschleimhaut. **2.** *inf.* vaginaler Soor *m*.
thrush breast heart Tigerung *f* des Herzmuskels.
thrush fungus *micro.* Candida albicans.
thu·li·um ['θuːlɪəm] *n abbr*. **Tm** Thulium *nt abbr*. Tm.
thumb [θʌm] *n* Daumen *m*; *anat.* Pollex *m*.
thumb forceps Pinzette *f*.
thumb mark Daumenabdruck *m*.
thumb-nail ['θʌmneɪl] *n* Daumennagel *m*.
thumb reflex Daumenreflex *m*.
thumb-stall [θʌmstɔːl] *n* Däumling *m*, Daumenkappe *f*, -schützer *m*.
thumb-sucker *n* Daumenlutscher *m*.
thump·ing pain ['θʌmpɪŋ] klopfender/ pochender Schmerz *m*.
Thygeson ['θɪɡəsən]: **T.'s disease** Keratitis superficialis punctata.
thy·la·koid ['θaɪlɑkɔɪd] *n bio.* Thylakoid(e *f*) *nt*.
thylakoid membrane *bio.* Thylakoidmembran *f*.
thym- *pref.* → thymo-.
thyme [taɪm] *n* Thymian *m*, Thymus *m*.
thy·mec·to·mize [θaɪ'mektəmaɪz] *vt chir.* den Thymus entfernen, eine Thymektomie durchführen, thymektomieren.
thy·mec·to·my [θaɪ'mektəmɪ] *n chir.* Thymusentfernung *f*, Thymektomie *f*.
thym·i·an ['θɪmɪən, 'tɪmɪən] *n* → thyme.
thy·mic¹ [θaɪmɪk] *adj* Thymus betr., Thym(o)-, Thymus-.
thym·ic² [taɪmɪk] *adj* Thymian-.
thymic abscesses Duboi'-Abszesse *pl*.
thymic alymphoplasia schwerer kombinierter Immundefekt *m*, Schweitzer-Typ *m* der Agammaglobulinämie.
thymic aplasia Thymusaplasie *f*.
thymic arteries Thymusäste *pl* der A. thoracica interna, Rami thymici a. thoracicae internae.
thymic branches of internal thoracic artery → thymic arteries.
thymic cortex Thymusrinde *f*, Cortex thymi.
thymic factor, humoral → thymic humoral factor.
thymic humoral factor *abbr*. **THF** humoraler Thymusfaktor *m*, thymic humoral factor *abbr*. THF.
thymic hypoplasia DiGeorge-Syndrom *nt*, Schlundtaschensyndrom *nt*, Thymusaplasie *f*.
thymic lymphocyte → T-lymphocyte.
thymic lymphopoietic factor → thymopoietin.
thy·mi·co·lym·phat·ic [,θaɪmɪkəʊlɪm'fætɪk] *adj* thymikolymphatisch.
thymic-parathyroid aplasia → thymic hypoplasia.
thymic veins Thymusvenen *pl*, Vv. thymicales.
thy·mi·dine ['θaɪmədiːn, -dɪn] *n abbr*. **T 1.** Thymidin *nt abbr*. T. **2.** Desoxythymidin *nt abbr*. dT.
thymidine kinase Thymidinkinase *f*.
thymidine monophosphate *abbr*. **TMP** Thymidinmonophosphat *nt abbr*. TMP, Thymidylsäure *f*.
thy·mi·dyl·ate [,θaɪmə'dɪleɪt] *n* Thymidylat *nt*.
thymidylate synthase Thymidylatsynthase *f*.
thy·mi·dyl·ic acid [,-'dɪlɪk] → thymidine monophosphate.
thy·min ['θaɪmɪn] *n* → thymopoietin.
thy·mine ['θaɪmiːn, -mɪn] *n* **1.** *old* → thymopoietin. **2.** *abbr*. **T** Thymin *nt abbr*. T, 5-Methyluracil *nt*.
thy·mi·on ['θaɪmɪən] *n* Warze *f*.
thy·mi·o·sis [θaɪmɪ'əʊsɪs] *n* Frambösie *f*, Pian *f*, Parangi *f*, Yaws *f*, Framboesia tropica.
thy·mi·tis [θaɪ'maɪtɪs] *n* Thymusentzündung *f*, Thymitis *f*.
thymo- *pref.* **1.** Thymus-, Thym(o)-. **2.** Gemüts-, Thym(o)-.
thy·mo·cyte ['θaɪməsaɪt] *n* Thymozyt *m*.
thy·mo·gen·ic [,-'dʒenɪk] *adj* durch Gemütsbewegungen entstanden, thymogen; psychogen.
thy·mo·ki·net·ic [,-kɪ'netɪk] *adj* den Thymus anregend, thymokinetisch.
thy·mol ['θaɪmɒl, -məʊl] *n* Thymol *nt*.
thy·mo·lep·tic [,θaɪmə'leptɪk] **I** *n pharm.* Thymoleptikum *nt*. **II** *adj* thymoleptisch.
thy·mo·lize ['-laɪz] *vt* mit Thymol behandeln.
thy·mol·phthal·ein [,θaɪmɒl'(f)θæliːn, -liːɪn] *n* Thymolphthalein *nt*.
thymol turbidity test Maclagen-Test *m*, Thymoltrübungstest *m*.
thy·mo·ma [θaɪ'məʊmə] *n*, *pl* **-mas, -ma·ta** [-mətə] Thymusgeschwulst *f*, -tumor *m*, Thymom(a) *nt*.
thy·mop·a·thy [θaɪ'mɑpəθɪ] *n* Thymuserkrankung *f*, Thymopathie *f*.
thy·mo·poi·et·in [,θaɪmə'pɔɪətɪn] *n* Thymopo(i)etin *nt*, Thymin *nt*.
thy·mo·pri·val [,-'praɪvl] *adj* → thymoprivous.
thy·mo·priv·ic [,-'prɪvɪk] *adj* → thymoprivous.
thy·mop·ri·vous [θaɪ'mɑprɪvəs] *adj* durch Thymusatrophie *od.* Thymusresektion bedingt, thymopriv.
thy·mo·sin ['θaɪməsɪn] *n* Thymosin *nt*.
thy·mo·tox·in [,-'tɑksɪn] *n* Thymotoxin *nt*.
thy·mo·troph·ic [,-'trɑfɪk, -'trəʊ-] *adj* thymotroph.
thy·mus ['θaɪməs] *n*, *pl* **-mu·ses, -mi** [-maɪ] **1.** Thymus *m*. **2.** → thyme.
thymus corpuscles Hassall'-Körperchen *pl*.
thymus-dependent *adj* thymusabhängig.
thymus-dependent area (*Lymphknoten*) thymusabhängiges Areal *nt*, T-Areal *nt*, thymusabhängige/parakortikale Zone *f*.

thymus-dependent lymphocyte thymusabhängiger Lymphozyt *m*, T-Lymphozyt *m*.
thymus-dependent zone → thymus-dependent area.
thy·mus·ec·to·my [ˌθaɪməs'ektəmɪ] *n* → thymectomy.
thymus gland → thymus 1.
thymus hyperplasia Thymushyperplasie *f*.
thymus-independent *adj* thymusunabhängig.
thymus-independent lymphocyte B--Lymphozyt *m*, B-Lymphocyt *m*, B-Zelle *f*.
thyr- *pref.* → thyro-.
thy·ra·tron ['θaɪrətrən] *n phys.* Thyratron *nt*, Stromtor *nt*.
thyre(o)- *pref.* → thyro-.
thy·re·o·hy·oi·de·us (muscle) [ˌθaɪrɪəʊˌhaɪ'ɔɪdɪəs] Thyr(e)ohyoideus *m*, M. thyrohyoideus.
thy·re·o·pha·ryn·ge·us (muscle) [ˌ-fə'rɪndʒɪəs] Thyr(e)opharyngeus *m*, Pars thyropharyngea m. constrictoris pharyngis inferioris.
thyro- *pref.* Schilddrüsen-, Thyre(o)-, Thyr(o)-.
thy·ro·ad·e·ni·tis [ˌθaɪrəʊˌædɪ'naɪtɪs] *n* → thyroiditis.
thy·ro·a·pla·sia [ˌ-ə'pleɪʒ(ɪ)ə] *n* Schilddrüsenaplasie *f*, Thyreoaplasia *f*; Atyrie *f*.
thy·ro·ar·y·te·noid [ˌ-ˌærɪ'tiːnɔɪd] *adj* Schilddrüse u. Aryknorpel betr., thyreoarytänoid.
thy·ro·ar·y·te·noi·de·us (muscle) [ˌ-ˌærətɪ'nɔɪdɪəs] Thyr(e)oarytänoideus *m*, M. thyroaryt(a)enoideus.
thyroarytenoid muscle → thyroarytenoideus (muscle).
thy·ro·cal·ci·to·nin [ˌ-ˌkælsɪ'təʊnɪn] *n* (Thyreo-)Calcitonin *nt*, Kalzitonin *nt*.
thy·ro·car·di·ac [ˌ-'kɑːdɪæk] *adj* Herz u. Schilddrüse betr., thyreokardial.
thyrocardiac disease Thyreokardiopathie *f*.
thy·ro·cele ['-siːl] *n* 1. Schilddrüsentumor *m*, -vergrößerung *f*, Thyrozele *f*. 2. Kropf *m*, Struma *f*.
thy·ro·cer·vi·cal trunk [ˌ-'sɜːvɪkl] Truncus thyrocervicalis *abbr.* TTC.
thy·ro·chon·drot·o·my [ˌ-kɒn'drɒtəmɪ] *n chir.* Thyreochondrotomie *f*, Thyreotomie *f*, Schildknorpelspaltung *f*.
thy·ro·col·loid [ˌ-'kɒlɔɪd] *n* Schilddrüsenkolloid *nt*.
thy·ro·cri·cot·o·my [ˌ-kraɪ'kɒtəmɪ, -krɪ-] *n chir.* Thyreokrikotomie *f*.
thy·ro·ep·i·glot·tic [ˌ-epɪ'glɒtɪk] *adj* Schilddrüse u. Kehldeckel betr. *od.* verbindend, thyr(e)oepiglottisch.
thyroepiglottic ligament Lig. thyroepiglotticum.
thyroepiglottic muscle → thyroepiglotticus (muscle).
thy·ro·ep·i·glot·ti·cus (muscle) [ˌ-epɪ'glɒtɪkəs] Thyr(e)oepiglottikus *m*, M. thyr(e)oepiglotticus, Pars thyroepiglottica.
thy·ro·fis·sure [ˌ-'fɪʃər] *n chir., HNO* Laryngofissur *f*.
thy·ro·gen·ic [ˌ-'dʒenɪk] *adj* → thyrogenous.
thy·rog·e·nous [θaɪ'rɒdʒənəs] *adj* von der Schilddrüse ausgehend, durch Schilddrüsenhormone verursacht, thyreogen.
thy·ro·glob·u·lin [ˌ-'glɒbjəlɪn] *n* Thyreoglobulin *nt*.
thy·ro·glos·sal cyst [ˌ-'glɒsl, -'glɔs-] → thyroglossal duct cyst.
thyroglossal duct *embryo.* Ductus thyroglossalis.
thyroglossal duct cyst mediane Halszyste *f*.

thyroglossal fistula Thyroglossusfistel *f*.
thy·ro·hy·al [ˌ-'haɪəl] *n anat.* Cornu majus (ossis hyoidei). II *adj* → thyrohyoid.
thy·ro·hy·oid [ˌ-'haɪɔɪd] *adj* Schilddrüse *od.* Schildknorpel u. Zungenbein betr., thyr(e)ohyoid.
thyrohyoid branch of ansa cervicalis Ramus thyrohyoideus ansae cervicalis.
thyrohyoid bursa Bursa subcutanea prominentiae laryngealis.
thyrohyoid ligament: lateral t. Lig. thyrohyoideum laterale.
median t. Lig. thyrohyoideum medianum.
thyrohyoid membrane Membrana thyrohyoidea.
thyrohyoid muscle → thyreohyoideus (muscle).
thy·ro·hy·poph·y·si·al syndrome [ˌ-haɪˌpɒfə'ziːəl, -haɪpə'fiːz-] Sheehan-Syndrom *nt*, postpartale Hypophysenvorderlappeninsuffizienz *f*.
thy·roid ['θaɪrɔɪd] I *n* Schilddrüse *f*, Thyr(e)oidea *f*, Gl. thyroidea. II *adj* 1. schildförmig, Schild-. 2. Schilddrüse *od.* Schildknorpel betr., Schilddrüsen-, Thyro-.
thyroid adenoma Schilddrüsenadenom *nt*.
malignant/metastasizing t. → thyroid carcinoma, follicular.
thyroid antibody (Anti-)Schilddrüsenantikörper *m*.
thyroid artery: inferior t. untere Schilddrüsenarterie *f*, Thyroidea *f* inferior, A. thyroidea inferior.
lowest t. unterste Schilddrüsenarterie *f*, Thyroidea *f* ima, A. thyroidea ima.
superior t. obere Schilddrüsenarterie *f*, Thyroidea *f* superior, A. thyroidea superior.
thyroid axis Truncus thyrocervicalis *abbr.* TTC.
thyroid-binding inhibitory immunoglobulin *abbr.* TBII → thyroid-stimulating immunoglobulin.
thyroid body *old* → thyroid I.
thyroid bruit (auskultatorisches) Schwirren *nt* über der Schilddrüse.
thyroid carcinoma Schilddrüsenkrebs *m*, -karzinom *nt*.
anaplastic t. anaplastisches Schilddrüsenkarzinom.
follicular t. metastasierendes Schilddrüsenadenom *nt*, follikuläres Schilddrüsenkarzinom.
medullary t. medulläres Schilddrüsenkarzinom, C-Zellen-Karzinom.
organoid t. Langhans-Struma *f*, organoides Schilddrüsenkarzinom.
papillary t. Schilddrüsenpapillom *nt*, papilläres Schilddrüsenkarzinom.
thyroid cardiomyopathy Thyreokardiopathie *f*.
thyroid cartilage Schildknorpel *m*, Cartilago thyroidea.
thyroid colloid Schilddrüsenkolloid *nt*.
thyroid crisis Basedow-Krise *f*, thyreotoxische/hyperthyreote Krise *f*.
thyroid disease Schilddrüsenerkrankung *f*.
thy·roi·dea [θaɪ'rɔɪdɪə] *n* → thyroid I.
thy·roid·ec·to·mize [ˌθaɪrɔɪ'dektəmaɪz] *vt* die Schilddrüse entfernen, eine Thyroidektomie durchführen, thyreoidektomieren.
thy·roid·ec·to·my [ˌ-'dektəmɪ] *n chir.* Schilddrüsenentfernung *f*, -resektion *f*, Thyr(e)oidektomie *f*.
thyroidectomy cell Thyreoidektomiezelle *f*.
thyroid eminence Adamsapfel *m*, Prominentia laryngea.

thyroid enlargement Schilddrüsenvergrößerung *f*.
thyroid follicles Schilddrüsenfollikel *pl*, Speicherfollikel *pl*, Folliculi gl. thyroideae.
thyroid foramen For. thyroideum.
thyroid function test Schilddrüsenfunktionsprüfung *f*, -analyse *f*, -test *m*.
thyroid gland → thyroid I.
accessory t.s akzessorische Schilddrüsen *pl*, Gll. thyroideae accessoriae.
thyroid hormone Schilddrüsenhormon *nt*.
thyroid incisure: inferior t. → thyroid notch, inferior.
superior t. → thyroid notch, superior.
thy·roid·i·tis [ˌ-'daɪtɪs] *n* Schilddrüsenentzündung *f*, Thyr(e)oiditis *f*.
thyroid lobe Schilddrüsenlappen *m*, Lobus gl. thyroideae.
thyroid malignant disease maligne Schilddrüsenerkrankung *f*, Schilddrüsenmalignom *nt*, -krebs *m*.
thyroid nodule Schilddrüsenknoten *m*.
cold t. kalter (Schilddrüsen-)Knoten.
hot t. heißer (Schilddrüsen-)Knoten.
solitary t. Solitärknoten.
thyroid notch: inferior t. Inc. thyroidea inferior.
superior t. Inc. thyroidea superior.
thy·roid·o·ther·a·py [θaɪˌrɔɪdəʊ'θerəpɪ] *n* → thyrotherapy.
thy·roid·ot·o·my [ˌθaɪrɔɪ'dɒtəmɪ] *n* → thyrotomy.
thyroid overactivity Schilddrüsenüberfunktion *f*, Hyperthyreose *f*.
thyroid peroxidase Jodidperoxidase *f*, Jodinase *f*.
thyroid plexus: inferior t. vegetativer Plexus *m* der A. thyroidea inferior, Plexus thyroideus inferior.
superior t. vegetativer Plexus *m* der A. thyroidea superior, Plexus thyroideus superior.
unpaired t. Venengeflecht *nt* unter der Schilddrüse, Plexus thyroideus impar.
thyroid sarcoma Schilddrüsensarkom *nt*.
thyroid scan 1. Schilddrüsenszintigraphie *f*. 2. Schilddrüsenszintigramm *nt*.
thyroid-stimulating hormone *abbr.* TSH → thyrotropin.
thyroid-stimulating hormone releasing factor *abbr.* TSH-RF → thyroliberin.
thyroid-stimulating hormone test TSH-(-Stimulations)-Test *m*.
thyroid-stimulating immunoglobulin *abbr.* TSI Thyroidea-stimulierendes Immunglobulin *nt* *abbr.* TSI, thyroid-stimulating immunoglobulin *abbr.* TSI, long-acting thyroid stimulator *abbr.* LATS.
thyroid storm → thyroid crisis.
thyroid tissue Schilddrüsengewebe *nt*.
aberrant t. versprengtes Schilddrüsengewebe.
thyroid toxicosis Thyreotoxikose *f*.
thyroid tubercle: inferior t. unterer Schildknorpelhöcker *m*, Tuberculum thyroideum inferius.
superior t. oberer Schildknorpelhöcker *m*, Tuberculum thyroideum superius.
thyroid tumor Schilddrüsengeschwulst *f*, -tumor *m*.
thyroid vein: inferior t.s untere Schilddrüsenvenen *pl*, V. thyroideae inferiores.
middle t.s mittlere Schilddrüsenvenen *pl*, Vv. thyroideae mediae.
superior t. obere Schilddrüsenvene *f*, V. thyroidea superior.
thy·ro·in·tox·i·ca·tion [θaɪrəʊɪnˌtɒksə'keɪʃn] *n* → thyrotoxicosis.
thy·ro·lib·e·rin [ˌ-'lɪbərɪn] *n* Thyroliberin *nt*, Thyreotropin-releasing-Faktor *m*

thyrolingual cyst

abbr. TRF, Thyreotropin-releasing-Hormon *nt abbr.* TRH.
thy·ro·lin·gual cyst [ˌ-'lɪŋgwəl] → thyroglossal duct cyst.
thyrolingual duct → thyroglossal duct.
thy·ro·lyt·ic [ˌ-'lɪtɪk] *adj* Schilddrüsengewebe zerstörend, thyreolytisch.
thy·ro·meg·a·ly [ˌ-'megəlɪ] *n* Schilddrüsenvergrößerung *f*.
thy·ro·nine ['-niːn, -nɪn] *n* Thyronin *nt*.
thyro-oxyindole *n* → thyroxine.
thy·ro·par·a·thy·roid·ec·to·my [ˌ-ˌpærəˌθaɪrɔɪ'dektəmɪ] *n chir.* Entfernung *f* von Schilddrüse u. Nebenschilddrüsen, Thyr(e)oparathyr(e)oidektomie *f*.
thy·ro·par·a·thy·ro·priv·ic [ˌ-ˌpærəˌθaɪrə'prɪvɪk] *adj* thyreoparathyreopriv.
thy·rop·a·thy [θaɪ'rapəθɪ] *n* Schilddrüsenerkrankung *f*, Thyreopathie *f*.
thy·ro·pha·ryn·ge·al muscle [ˌθaɪrəfə'rɪndʒ(ɪ)əl] → thyreopharyngeus (muscle).
thy·ro·priv·al [ˌ-'praɪvl] *adj* durch Schilddrüsenausfall *od.* -entfernung bedingt, thyreopriv.
thy·ro·priv·ia [ˌ-'prɪvɪə] *n* Hypothyreose *f*.
thy·ro·priv·ic [ˌ-'prɪvɪk] *adj* → thyroprival.
thy·rop·ri·vous [θaɪ'rapriːvəs] *adj* → thyroprival.
thy·ro·pro·tein [ˌθaɪrə'prəʊtiːn, -tiːɪn] *n* → thyroglobulin.
thy·rop·to·sis [θaɪrap'təʊsɪs] *n* Schilddrüsensenkung *f*, Thyr(e)optose *f*.
thy·ro·ther·a·py [ˌθaɪrə'θerəpɪ] *n* Behandlung *f* mit Schilddrüsenextrakt.
thy·ro·tome ['-təʊm] *n chir.* Thyreotom *nt*.
thy·rot·o·my [θaɪ'ratəmɪ] *n* **1.** *HNO* Schildknorpelspaltung *f*, Thyreochondrotomie *f*, Thyreotomie *f*. **2.** *HNO* Laryngofissur *f*. **3.** Schilddrüsenbiopsie *f*.
thy·ro·tox·e·mia [ˌθaɪrətak'siːmɪə] *n* → thyrotoxicosis.
thy·ro·tox·ic [ˌ-'taksɪk] *adj* durch Schilddrüsenüberfunktion bedingt, thyreotoxisch.
thyrotoxic cardiopathy thyreotoxische Kardiopathie *f*.
thyrotoxic coma thyreotoxisches Koma *nt*, Coma basedowicum.
thyrotoxic crisis thyreotoxische/hyperthyreote Krise *f*, Basedow-Krise *f*.
thyrotoxic exophthalmus Exophthalmus *m* bei Hyperthyreose.
thy·ro·tox·i·co·sis [ˌ-ˌtaksɪ'kəʊsɪs] *n* Schilddrüsenüberfunktion *f*, Thyreotoxikose *f*, Hyperthyreose *f*.
thyrotoxic storm → thyrotoxic crisis.
thy·ro·tox·in [ˌ-'taksɪn] *n* Thyrotoxin *nt*.
thy·ro·trope ['-trəʊp] *n* → thyrotroph.
thy·ro·troph ['-trəʊf] *n* (*Adenohypophyse*) basophile/thyreotrope Zelle *f*.
thyrotroph cell → thyrotroph.
thy·ro·troph·ic [ˌ-'trafɪk, -'trəʊ-] *adj* → thyrotropic.
thy·ro·tro·phin [ˌ-'trəʊfɪn, θaɪ'ratrəfɪn] *n* → thyrotropin.
thy·ro·trop·ic [ˌ-'trapɪk, -'trəʊp-] *adj* Schilddrüse(nfunktion) beeinflussend, thyr(e)otrop.
thyrotropic cell → thyrotroph.
thyrotropic exophthalmus hochgradiger Exophthalmus *m* bei Hyperthyreose.
thyrotropic hormone → thyrotropin.
thy·ro·tro·pin [ˌ-'trəʊpɪn, θaɪ'ratrəpɪn] *n* Thyr(e)otropin *nt*, thyreotropes Hormon *nt abbr.* TSH.
thyrotropin releasing factor *abbr.* TRF → thyroliberin.
thyrotropin releasing hormone *abbr.* TRH → thyroliberin.
thy·rox·in [θaɪ'raksɪn] *n* → thyroxine.
thy·rox·ine [θaɪ'raksiːn, -sɪn] *n abbr.* T₄

Thyroxin *nt abbr.* T₄. (3,5,3',5'-)Tetrajodthyronin *nt*.
thyroxine-binding globulin *abbr.* **TBG** thyroxinbindendes (α-)Globulin *nt abbr.* TBG.
thyroxine-binding prealbumin *abbr.* **TBPA** thyroxinbindendes Präalbumin *nt abbr.* TBPA.
thyroxine-binding protein *abbr.* **TBP** → thyroxine-binding globulin.
thy·rox·in·ic [ˌθaɪrak'sɪnɪk] *adj* Thyroxin betr., Thyroxin-.
thyr·sus ['θɪrsəs] *n* (männliches) Glied *nt*, Penis *m*, Phallus *m*, Membrum virile.
Ti *abbr.* → titanium.
TIA *abbr.* **1.** → transient ischemic attack. **2.** → turbidimetric immunoassay.
tib·ia ['tɪbɪə] *n, pl* **-as, -ae** [-bɪˌiː] Schienbein *nt*, Tibia *f*.
tib·i·al ['tɪbɪəl] *adj* Schienbein/Tibia betr., tibial, Schienbein-, Tibia-.
tibial artery: anterior t. vordere Schienbeinschlagader *f*, Tibialis *f* anterior, A. tibialis anterior.
posterior t. hintere Schienbeinschlagader *f*, Tibialis *f* posterior, A. tibialis posterior.
tibial border of foot Fußinnenrand *m*, Margo medialis/tibialis pedis.
tibial crest, anterior Schienbein-, Tibiavorderkante *f*, Margo anterior tibiae.
tibial fracture Schienbeinbruch *m*, -fraktur *f*, Tibiafraktur *f*.
tib·i·al·gia [tɪbɪ'ældʒ(ɪ)ə] *n* Schienbein-, Tibiaschmerz *m*.
tibial hemimelia Tibiahemimelie *f*.
tib·i·a·lis anterior (muscle) [ˌtɪbɪ'eɪlɪs] Tibialis *m* anterior, M. tibialis anterior.
tibialis posterior (muscle) Tibialis *m* posterior, M. tibialis posterior.
tibialis sign (von) Strümpell-Tibialiszeichen *nt*.
tibial malleolus Innenknöchel *m*, Malleolus medialis.
tibial margin of foot → tibial border of foot.
tibial muscle: anterior t. → tibialis anterior (muscle).
posterior t. → tibialis posterior (muscle).
tibial nerve Tibialis *m*, N. tibialis.
tibial node: anterior t. Lymphknoten *m* der A. tibialis anterior, Nodus tibialis anterior.
posterior t. Lymphknoten *m* der A. tibialis posterior, Nodus tibialis posterior.
tibial phenomenon (von) Strümpell-Tibialiszeichen *nt*.
tibial plateau Schienbein-, Tibiakopf *m*.
tibial shaft fracture Schienbeinschaftfraktur *f*, Tibiaschaftfraktur *f*.
tibial veins: anterior t. vordere Schienbeinvenen *pl*, Vv. tibiales anteriores.
posterior t. hintere Schienbeinvenen *pl*, Vv. tibiales posteriores.
tibio- *pref.* Schienbein-, Tibia-, Tibio-.
tib·i·o·cal·ca·ne·al [ˌtɪbɪəʊkæl'keɪnɪəl] *adj* → tibiocalcanean.
tib·i·o·cal·ca·ne·an [ˌ-kæl'keɪnɪən] *adj* Schienbein/Tibia u. Fersenbein/Kalkaneus betr., tibiokalkanear, kalkaneotibial.
tibiocalcanean ligament Pars tibiocalcanea lig. medialis.
tib·i·o·fem·o·ral [ˌ-'femərəl] *adj* Schienbein/Tibia u. Femur betr. *od.* verbindend, tibiofemoral, femorotibial.
tib·i·o·fib·u·lar [ˌ-'fɪbjələr] *adj* Schienbein/Tibia u. Wadenbein/Fibula betr., tibiofibular, fibulotibial.
tibiofibular articulation → tibiofibular joint.
inferior a. → tibiofibular joint 2.

superior a. → tibiofibular joint 1.
tibiofibular joint 1. Schienbein-Wadenbein-Gelenk *nt*, (oberes) Tibiofibulargelenk *nt*, Artic. tibiofibularis. **2.** unteres Tibiofibulargelenk *nt*, Syndesmosis tibiofibularis.
inferior j. → tibiofibular joint 2.
superior j. → tibiofibular joint 1.
tibiofibular ligament unteres Tibiofibulargelenk *nt*, Syndesmosis tibiofibularis.
anterior t. Lig. tibiofibulare anterius.
posterior t. Lig. tibiofibulare posterius.
tibiofibular syndesmosis → tibiofibular ligament.
tib·i·o·na·vic·u·lar [ˌ-nə'vɪkjələr] *adj* Schienbein/Tibia u. Kahnbein/Os naviculare betr., tibionavikular.
tibionavicular ligament Pars tibionavicularis lig. medialis.
tib·i·o·per·o·ne·al [ˌ-perə'niːəl] *adj* → tibiofibular.
tib·i·o·scaph·oid [ˌ-'skæfɔɪd] *adj* → tibionavicular.
tib·i·o·tar·sal [ˌ-'taːrsl] *adj* Schienbein/Tibia u. Fußwurzel/Tarsus betr., tibiotarsal.
tic [tɪk] *n* Tic *m*, Tick *m*, (nervöses) Zucken *nt*; Muskel-, Gesichtszucken *nt*.
t. de Guinon Gilles-de-la-Tourette-Syndrom *nt*, Tourette-Syndrom *nt*, Maladie des tics, Tic impulsif.
ti·car·cil·lin [taɪkaːr'sɪlɪn] *n pharm.* Ticarcillin *nt*.
tic douloureux Trigeminusneuralgie *f*.
tick [tɪk] *n micro.* Zecke *f*.
tick-borne *adj* durch Zecken übertragen, Zecken-.
tick-borne encephalitis Zeckenenzephalitis *f*.
tick-borne typhus → tick typhus.
tick-borne viruses *micro.* durch Zecken übertragene Viren.
tick fever 1. Zeckenbißfieber *nt*. **2.** endemisches Rückfallfieber *nt*, Zeckenrückfallfieber *nt*. **3.** Felsengebirgsfleckfieber *nt*, amerikanisches Zeckenbißfieber *nt*, Rocky Mountain spotted fever (*nt*) *abbr.* RMSF. **4.** → Colorado t.
African t. afrikanisches Zeckenbißfieber.
Central African t. zentralafrikanisches Zeckenbißfieber.
Colombian t. Felsengebirgsfleckfieber *nt*, amerikanisches Zeckenbißfieber *nt*, Rocky Mountain spotted fever (*nt*) *abbr.* RMSF.
Colorado t. *abbr.* **CTF** Colorado-Zeckenfieber, amerikanisches Gebirgszeckenfieber.
Gulf coast t. *micro.* Amblyomma maculatum.
mountain t. → Colorado t.
North Queensland t. Queensland-, Nordqueensland-Zeckenfieber.
Rhodesian t. East-Coast-Fieber *nt*, bovine Piroplasmose/Theileriose *f*.
South African t. südafrikanisches Zeckenbißfieber.
Texas t. Bullis-Fieber *nt*, Lone-Star-Fieber *nt*.
tick·le ['tɪkl] **I** *n* **1.** Kitzeln *nt*; Titillatus *m*; Jucken *nt*; Juckreiz *m*. **2.** Kitzeln *nt*. **II** *vt* kitzeln. **III** *vi* kitzeln; jucken.
tick·ling ['tɪklɪŋ] *n* Kitzeln *nt*, Titillatio *f*.
tick-tack sounds → tic-tac sounds.
tick typhus Zeckenbißfieber *nt*.
Australian t. → Queensland t.
Indian t. Boutonneuse-Fieber *nt*, Fièvre boutonneuse.
Kenyan tick t. → Indian t.
North Asian t. nordasiatisches Zeckenbißfieber.
North Queensland t. → Queensland t.

Queensland t. Queensland-, Nordqueensland-Zeckenfieber.
Sibirian t. nordasiatisches Zeckenbißfieber.
ti·clo·pi·dine [taɪˈkləʊpədiːn] *n pharm.* Ticlopidin *nt.*
tic-tac rhythm → tic-tac sounds.
tic-tac sounds Pendelrhythmus *m*, Tick-Tack-Rhythmus *m*, Embryokardie *f.*
tid·al [ˈtaɪdl] *adj* Tide betr., Tiden-, Tidal-.
tidal air → tidal volume.
tidal respiration Cheyne-Stokes-Atmung *f*, periodische Atmung *f.*
tidal volume *abbr.* V_T (*Lunge*) Atem(zug)volumen *nt*, Atemhubvolumen *nt.*
Tietz [tiːts]: **T.'s disease/syndrome** Tietz-Syndrom *nt.*
Tietze [ˈtiːtsə]: **T.'s disease/syndrome** Tietze-Syndrom *nt.*
Tiffeneau [ˈtɪfənəʊ; tifəˈnoː]: **T.'s test** (Ein-)Sekundenkapazität *f abbr.* ESK, Atemstoßtest *m*, Tiffeneau-Test *m.*
TIG *abbr.* → tetanus immune globulin.
ti·ger heart [ˈtaɪɡər] *patho.* (*Herzmuskel*) Tigerung *f.*
tiger lily heart → tiger heart.
tiger mosquito Gelbfieberfliege *f*, Aedes aegypti.
tight [taɪt] *adj* dicht; unbeweglich, fest(sitzend); (*Kontrolle*) streng; (*Muskel, Haut*) straff; (*Zeit*) knapp; (*Kleider*) (zu) eng; prall (voll).
tight·en [ˈtaɪtn] **I** *vt* fest-, anziehen, fester machen, spannen; (*Muskel*) straffen; *techn.* (ab-)dichten. **II** *vi s.* spannen, s. straffen, s. zusammenziehen; fester werden.
tight junction *histol.* Verschlußkontakt *m*, Zonula occludens.
tight·ness [ˈtaɪtnɪs] *n* Dichte *f*, Dichtheit *f*, Festsitzen *nt*; Strenge *f*; Festigkeit *f*, Straffheit *f*; Knappheit *f*; Enge *f.*
ti·groid [ˈtaɪɡrɔɪd] *adj* gefleckt, tigroid.
tigroid bodies Nissl-Schollen *pl*, -Substanz *f*, -Granula *pl*, Tigroidschollen *pl.*
tigroid fundus Fundus tabulatus.
tigroid masses → tigroid bodies.
tigroid retina → tigroid fundus.
tigroid spindles → tigroid bodies.
tigroid striation → tiger heart.
tigroid substance → tigroid bodies.
ti·grol·y·sis [taɪˈɡrɑləsɪs] *n* Chromatinauflösung *f*, Chromato-, Chromatino-, Tigrolyse *f.*
til·i·dine [ˈtɪlədiːn] *n pharm.* Tilidin *nt.*
tilt [tɪlt] **I** *n* 1. Kippen *nt*. 2. geneigte Lage *f*. Stellung *f*, Schräglage *f.* **II** *vt* (um-)kippen, neigen, schrägstellen, -legen. **III** *vi s.* neigen, (um-)kippen; umfallen.
tilt·ing [ˈtɪltɪŋ] *adj* kippbar, Kipp-.
tilting-disk valve *HTG* Kippscheibenprothese *f.*
tilting movement Kippbewegung *f.*
tim·bre [ˈtɪmbər, ˈtæm-; ˈtɛ̃ːbrə] *n* Klang(farbe) *f*) *m*, Timbre *nt.*
time [taɪm] **I** *n* 1. Zeit *f.* **all the ~** die ganze Zeit. **between ~s** in der Zwischenzeit. **from ~ to ~** dann u. wann, von Zeit zu Zeit. 2. Uhrzeit *f.* 3. Zeit(dauer *f*) *f*; Zeitabschnitt *m.* **for a ~** eine Zeitlang. **for a long/short ~** lang/kurz. **for the ~ being** vorläufig; vorübergehend. 4. Zeit(punkt *m*) *m.* **at one ~** früher, einmal. **at some ~** irgendwann (einmal). **at the present ~** zur Zeit, gegenwärtig. **at the same ~** gleichzeitig, zur selben Zeit. **in ~** rechtzeitig. **in four weeks'~** in vier Wochen. **on ~** pünktlich. **to be near one's ~** kurz vor der Entbindung stehen. 5. Frist *f.* 6. Mal *nt.* **and again; ~ after ~** immer wieder. **many ~s** viele Male. **the first ~** das erste Mal. **this ~** diesmal. **(the)**

last ~ letztes Mal. **II** *vt* 7. (*Zeit*) messen, (ab-)stoppen. 8. timen, den (richtigen) Zeitpunkt bestimmen *od.* abwarten; die Zeit festsetzen für. 9. zeitlich abstimmen. **III** *vi* zeitlich übereinstimmen (*with* mit).
time agnosia zeitliche Agnosie *f.*
time-consuming *adj* zeitaufwendig, -raubend.
time course Zeitverlauf *m*, zeitlicher Ab-/Verlauf *m.*
timed [taɪmd] *adj* zeitlich (genau) festgelegt.
time-keep·ing [ˈtaɪmˌkiːpɪŋ] *n* Zeitmessung *f*, -kontrolle *f*, -nehmung *f.*
time-lapse *adj* Zeitraffer-.
time limit Frist *f*; zeitliche Begrenzung *f.*
time-motion *n radiol.* Time-motion-Verfahren *nt*, TM-Scan *m*, M-Scan *m*, M-Mode *m.*
time pattern Zeitmuster *nt.*
time-periodicity analysis Zeit-Periodizitätsanalyse *f.*
tim·er [ˈtaɪmər] *n* Zeitmesser *m*; Zeitschalter *m*, Schaltuhr *f*, Timer *m.*
time-sav·ing [ˈtaɪmˌseɪvɪŋ] *adj* zeit(er)sparend.
time sense Zeitsinn *m.*
time-span [ˈtaɪmˌspæn] *n* Zeitspanne *f.*
time switch Schaltuhr *f*, Zeitschalter *m.*
time-ta·ble [ˈtaɪmˌteɪbl] *n* Zeittabelle *f*, Fahrplan *m*; Programm *nt.*
time-zone syndrome Jet-Lag *m.*
ti·mo·lol [ˈtaɪməlɔl, -lɔːl] *n pharm.* Timolol *nt.*
Timothy [ˈtɪməθi]: **T. (hay) bacillus** *micro.* Mycobacterium phlei.
tin [tɪn] *n* 1. Zinn *nt, chem.* Stannum *nt abbr.* Sn. 2. Weißblech *nt.* 3. (Blech-, Konserven-)Dose *f.* **II** *adj* zinnern, Zinn-; Blech-; *Brit.* Dosen-, Konserven-.
tinc·ta·ble [ˈtɪŋkteɪbl] *adj histol.* (an-)färbbar, tingibel.
tinc·tion [ˈtɪŋkʃn] *n* 1. Färben *nt*, Anfärben *nt.* 2. Färbung *f*, Tinktion *f.* 3. Farbbeimischung *f.* 4. Farbe *f*, Farbmischung *f.*
tinc·to·ri·al [tɪŋkˈtɔːriəl, -ˈtəʊ-] *adj* Farbe betr., färbend, Farb(e)-, Färbe-.
tinc·tu·ra [tɪŋkˈtʊərə] *n, pl* **-rae** [-riː] → tincture.
tinc·tu·ra·tion [tɪŋktəˈreɪʃn] *n pharm.* Herstellung *f* einer Tinktur.
tinc·ture [ˈtɪŋktʃər] *n pharm.* Tinktur *f*, Tinctura *f.*
Tindale [ˈtɪndeɪl]: **T.'s agar** *micro.* Tindale-Agar *m.*
T-independent antigen T-Zell-unabhängiges Antigen *nt.*
T inductor cell T-Induktorzelle *f.*
tin·ea [ˈtɪniə] *n derm.* Tinea *f*; Trichophytie *f*, Trichophytia *f.*
tinea amiantacea Asbestgrind *m*, Tinea amiantacea (Alibert), Tinea asbestina, Pityriasis amiantacea, Teigne amiantacé, Keratosis follicularis amiantacea, Impetigo scapida.
tinea axillaris Tinea axillaris.
tinea barbae (tiefe) Bartflechte *f*, Tinea barbae, Trichophytia (profunda) barbae, *old* Sycosis (barbae) parasitaria.
tinea capitis Tinea *f* der Kopfhaut, Tinea capitis/capillitii, Trichophytia capillitii.
tinea circinata 1. Tinea circinata. 2. → tinea corporis.
tinea corporis oberflächliche Trichophytie *f* des Körpers, Tinea/Trichophytia *f* Epidermophytia corporis.
tinea cruris Tinea inguinalis, Epidermophytia inguinalis, Eccema marginatum, Ekzema marginatum Hebra.
tinea faciale oberflächliche Tinea *f* des Gesichts, Tinea faciei.

tinea faciei → tinea faciale.
tinea favosa Erb-, Flechten-, Kopf-, Pilzgrind *m*, Favus *m*, Tinea favosa, Tinea capitis favosa, Dermatomycosis favosa.
tinea furfuracea → tinea versicolor.
tinea glabosa Tinea *f* der haarlosen Haut.
tinea imbricata orientalische/indische/chinesische Flechte *f*, Tinea imbricata (Tokelau), Trichophytia corporis superficialis.
tinea inguinalis → tinea cruris.
tinea kerion Celsus'-Kerion *nt*, Kerion Celsi *nt*, tiefe Trichophytie *f* der Kopfhaut, Tinea capitis profunda, Trichophytia profunda.
tinea manus Fadenpilzerkrankung/Tinea *f* der Hände, Tinea manus/manuum, Epidermophytia manus/manuum.
tinea manuum → tinea manus.
tinea nigra Tinea nigra (palmaris et plantaris).
tinea nodosa 1. → tinea cruris. 2. Haarknötchenkrankheit *f*, Piedra *f*, Trichosporie *f*, Trichosporose *f.*
tinea pedis Athleten-, Sportlerfuß *m*, Fußpilz *m*, Fußpilzerkrankung *f*, Fußmykose *f*, Tinea der Füße, Tinea pedis/pedum, Epidermophytia pedis/pedum.
tinea pedum → tinea pedis.
tinea tarsi Blepharitis mycotica.
tinea tondens → tinea capitis.
tinea tonsurans → tinea capitis.
tinea unguium Tinea *f* des Nagels, Nagel-, Onychomykose *f*, Onychomycosis *f*, Tinea unguium.
tinea versicolor Kleienpilzflechte *f*, Willan-Krankheit *f*, Eichstedt-Krankheit *f*, Tinea/Pityriasis versicolor.
Tinel [tiˈnel]: **T.'s sign** Tinel-Hoffmann'-Klopfzeichen *nt.*
tine test [taɪn] Tine-Test *m*, Nadel-, Stempeltest *m*, Multipunkturtest *m.*
tine tuberculin test → tine test.
tin-foil [ˈtɪnfɔɪl] *n* Zinnfolie *f*, Stanniol *nt.*
tinge [tɪndʒ] **I** *n* leichter Farbton *m*, Tönung *f.* **II** *vt* tönen, (leicht) färben, anfärben, tingieren. **III** *vi s.* färben.
tin·gi·bil·i·ty [ˌtɪndʒəˈbɪləti] *n histol.* Anfärbbarkeit *f.*
tin·gi·ble [ˈtɪndʒəbl] *adj histol.* (an-)färbbar, tingibel.
tin·gle [ˈtɪŋɡl] **I** *n* Prickeln *nt.* **II** *vi* 1. prickeln, kribbeln, beißen, brennen. 2. klingen, summen (*with* vor).
tin·gling [ˈtɪŋɡlɪŋ] *n* nervöses/erregtes Zittern *nt*, Beben *nt.*
ti·nid·a·zole [taɪˈnɪdəzɑl, -zɔl] *n pharm.* Tinidazol *nt.*
tin·kle [ˈtɪŋkl] **I** *n* Klingen *nt*, Klingeln *nt.* **II** *vt* klingeln mit. **III** *vi* klingeln, hell klingen; klirren.
tin·ni·tus (aurium) [tɪˈnaɪtəs] Ohrenklingen *nt*, -sausen *nt*, Ohrgeräusche *pl*, Tinnitus (aurium) *m.*
tint [tɪnt] **I** *n* Farbe *f*, Farbton *m*, Tönung *f.* **II** *vt* (leicht) färben.
tip¹ [tɪp] *n* **I** *n* 1. Spitze *f*, (äußerstes) Ende *nt*, Zipfel *m.* 2. *techn.* Spitze *f*, Düse *f*, Tülle *f*, Kappe *f.* **II** *vt* 3. mit einer Spitze versehen. 4. einen Tip *od.* Wink geben; raten, tippen.
t. of the auricle Apex auricularis.
t. of cusp Zahnhöckerspitze, Apex cuspicis.
t. of ear Ohrläppchen *nt*, Lobulus auricularis.
t. of finger Fingerspitze.
t. of nose Nasenspitze, Apex nasi.
t. of root Wurzelspitze, Apex radicis dentis.
t. of tongue Zungenspitze, Apex linguae.
tip² [tɪp] *n* **I** *n* Neigung *f*, Kippung *f.* **II** *vt*

tiptoe

kippen, neigen; aus-, umkippen. **III** *vi* s. neigen, umkippen.
tip out I *vt* ausschütten, abladen, ausleeren, auskippen. **II** *vi* herauskippen, -laufen, -rutschen.
tip over *vt*, *vi* umkippen.
tip·toe ['tɪptəʊ] **I** *n* Zehenspitze *f*. **II** *adj, adv* **on ~(s)** auf Zehenspitzen. **III** *vi* auf Zehenspitzen gehen.
tire¹ [taɪər] **I** *vt* ermüden, müde machen. **II** *vi* müde werden, ermüden, ermatten (*by*, *with* durch).
tire² [taɪər] *n* Reifen *m*.
tis·sue ['tɪʃuː; *Brit.* 'tɪsjuː] *n* **1.** *bio.*, *anat.* Gewebe *nt*. **2.** Seidenpapier *nt*; Papier(taschen)tuch *nt*, Papierhandtuch *nt*; Kohlepapier *nt*.
 t. of origin Herkunfts-, Ausgangsgewebe.
 tissue adhesive *chir.* Gewebekleber *m*.
 tissue anoxia Gewebeanoxie *f*.
 tissue antibody Gewebeantikörper *m*.
 tissue atrophy Gewebeatrophie *f*.
 tissue autolysis Gewebsautolyse *f*.
 tissue cap, metanephric *embryo.* metanephrogene Blastemkappe *f*.
 tissue cell Gewebe-, Gewebszelle *f*.
 tissue conduction *physiol.* Knochenleitung *f*, Osteoakusis *f*, Osteophonie *f*.
 tissue culture 1. Gewebekultur *f*. **2.** Gewebezüchtung *f*.
 tissue-degrading enzyme gewebsschädigendes Enzym *nt*.
 tissue density Gewebsdichte *f*.
 tissue dextrin Glykogen *nt*, tierische Stärke *f*.
 tissue diagnosis Gewebsdiagnostik *f*.
 tissue dispersion *micro.* Gewebesuspension *f*.
 tissue dose Gewebedosis *f*.
 tissue ectopy Gewebe-, Gewebsektopie *f*.
 tissue factor Gewebe-, tissue thromboplastin.
 tissue fluid Gewebsflüssigkeit *f*, interstitielle Flüssigkeit *f*.
 tissue glue → tissue adhesive.
 tissue hormone Gewebshormon *nt*.
 tissue hypoxia Gewebehypoxie *f*.
 tissue immunity Gewebeimmunität *f*.
 tissue kallikrein Gewebskallikrein *nt*.
 tissue macrophage Gewebsmakrophag *m*, Histiozyt *m*.
 tissue oxidation *biochem.* Gewebsoxidation *f*.
 tissue perfusion Gewebedurchblutung *f*, -perfusion *f*, Gewebsdurchblutung *f*, -perfusion *f*.
 tissue plasminogen activator *abbr.* **TPA** Gewebeplasminogenaktivator *m*.
 tissue resistance Gewebswiderstand *m*.
 nonelastic t. nichtelastischer Gewebswiderstand.
 tissue respiration innere Atmung *f*, Zell-, Gewebeatmung *f*.
 tissue response Gewebereaktion *f*, -antwort *f*.
 tissue retraction Gewebeeinziehung *f*, -retraktion *f*, Gewebseinziehung *f*, -retraktion *f*.
 tissue-specific *adj* gewebespezifisch; organspezifisch.
 tissue-specific antigen organspezifisches Antigen *n*.
 tissue thromboplastin Gewebsfaktor *m*, -thromboplastin *nt*, Faktor III *m abbr.* F III.
 tissue tolerance Gewebeverträglichkeit *f*.
 tissue tropism Gewebe-, Gewebstropismus *m*.
 tissue turgor Gewebeturgor *m*.
 tissue typing HLA-Typing *nt*.
ti·ta·ni·um [taɪˈteɪnɪəm, tɪ-] *n abbr.* **Ti** Titan *nt abbr.* Ti.
ti·ter ['taɪtər] *n* Titer *m*.

tit·il·la·tion [ˌtɪtəˈleɪʃn] *n* Kitzeln *nt*, Titillatio *f*.
ti·tra·ble ['taɪtrəbl] *adj* → titratable.
ti·trant ['taɪtrənt] *n* Titrant *m*.
ti·tra·ta·ble ['taɪtreɪtəbl] *adj chem.* titrierbar.
titratable acid *chem.* titrierbare Säure *f*.
ti·trate ['taɪtreɪt] *vt, vi chem.* titrieren.
ti·tra·tion [taɪˈtreɪʃn] *n chem.* Titration *f*, Titrierung *f*.
titration curve Titrationskurve *f*.
ti·tre *n* → titer.
ti·tri·met·ric [ˌtaɪtrəˈmetrɪk] *adj* titrimetrisch.
ti·trim·e·try [taɪˈtɪmətrɪ] *n* Maßanalyse *f*, Titrimetrie *f*.
tit·u·bate ['tɪtʃəbeɪt] *vi* taumeln, schwanken.
tit·u·ba·tion [ˌtɪtʃəˈbeɪʃn] *n* schwankender Gang *m*, Schwanken *nt*, Titubatio *f*.
TKD *abbr.* → tokodynamometer.
TKG *abbr.* → tokodynagraph.
T killer cells T-Killerzellen *pl*.
Tl *abbr.* → thallium.
TLC *abbr.* **1.** → thin-layer chromatography. **2.** → total lung capacity.
TLE *abbr.* → thin-layer electrophoresis.
T-lymphocyte *n* T-Zelle *f*, T-Lymphozyt *m*, T-Lymphocyt *m*.
T4⁺ lymphocyte CD4-Zelle *f*, CD4-Lymphozyt *m*, T4⁺-Zelle *f*, T4⁺-Lymphozyt *m*.
T8⁺ lymphocyte CD8-Zelle *f*, CD8-Lymphozyt *m*, T8⁺-Zelle *f*, T8⁺-Lymphozyt *m*.
T lymphokine cell T-Lymphokinzelle *f*.
Tm *abbr.* **1.** → thulium. **2.** → transport maximum.
T_m *abbr.* → melting point.
TM agar → Thayer-Martin agar.
T memory cell T-Gedächtniszelle *f*.
TM medium → Thayer-Martin agar.
TM-mode *n radiol.* Time-motion-Verfahren *nt*, TM-Scan *m*, M-Scan *m*, M-Mode *m*.
TMP *abbr.* → thymidine monophosphate.
TMV *abbr.* → tobacco mosaic virus.
T-mycoplasma *n micro.* Ureaplasma *nt*.
TNF *abbr.* → tumor necrosis factor.
TNI *abbr.* → total nodal irradiation.
TNM classification *patho.* TNM-Klassifikation *f*.
TNM staging *patho.* TNM-Staging *nt*.
TNM staging system → TNM system.
TNM system TNM-System *nt*.
TNT *abbr.* → trinitrotoluene.
toad-skin ['təʊdskɪn] *n derm.* Krötenhaut *f*, Phrynoderm *nt*, -dermie *f*, Hyperkeratosis follicularis metabolica.
to·bac·co [təˈbækəʊ] *n, pl* **-co(e)s** Tabak-(pflanze *f*) *m*.
tobacco amblyopia *ophthal.* Tabakamblyopie *f*.
to·bac·co·ism [təˈbækəʊɪzəm] *n* Tabakvergiftung *f*; Nikotin-, Tabakinvergiftung *f*, Nikotinismus *m*, Nicotinismus *m*.
tobacco mosaic virus *abbr.* **TMV** *micro.* Tabakmosaikvirus *nt abbr.* TMV.
tobacco pouch stomach Beutelmagen *m*.
Tobey-Ayer ['təʊbɪ 'eɪər]: **T.-A. test** Tobey-Ayer-Test *m*.
To·bia fever ['təʊbɪə] Felsengebirgsfleckfieber *nt*, amerikanisches Zeckenbißfieber *nt*, Rocky Mountain spotted fever (*nt*) *abbr.* RMSF.
to·bra·my·cin [ˌtəʊbrəˈmaɪsɪn] *n pharm.* Tobramycin *nt*.
toc- *pref.* → toko-.
to·cai·nide [təʊˈkeɪnaɪd] *n pharm.* Tocainid *nt*.
toco- *pref.* → toko-.
to·co·dy·na·graph *n* → tokodynagraph.

to·co·dy·na·mom·e·ter *n* → tokodynamometer.
toc·o·graph *n* → tokograph.
to·cog·ra·phy *n* → tokography.
to·col·o·gy [təʊˈkɒlədʒɪ] *n* Geburtshilfe *f*, Obstetrik *f*.
to·col·y·sis [təʊˈkɒləsɪs] *n gyn.* Tokolyse *f*, Wehenhemmung *f*.
to·com·e·ter [təʊˈkɒmɪtər] *n* → tokodynamometer.
to·coph·er·ol [təʊˈkɒfərɒl, -rəl] *n* Toko-, Tocopherol *nt*.
to·co·pho·bia [ˌtəʊkəˈfəʊbɪə] *n psychia.* Tokophobie *f*.
to·cus ['təʊkəs] *n* Geburt *f*, Entbindung *f*.
Tod [tɒd]: **T.'s muscle** M. obliquus auricularis.
Todd [tɒd]: **T.'s cirrhosis** primär biliäre (Leber-)Zirrhose *f*.
 T.'s palsy → T.'s paralysis.
 T.'s paralysis Todd-Lähmung *f*.
 T.'s postepileptic paralysis → T.'s paralysis.
Todd-Hewitt ['(h)juːɪt]: **T.-H. broth** *micro.* Todd-Hewett-Bouillon *f*.
tod·dle ['tɒdl] **I** *n* wackeliger/unsicherer Gang *m*. **II** *vi* (*Kind*) wackelig/unsicher gehen.
tod·dler ['tɒdlər] *n* Kleinkind *nt*.
toe [təʊ] *n* Zeh *m*, Zehe *f*.
toe bone Zehenknochen *m*, -glied *nt*, Phalanx *f*.
toe clonus Zehenklonus *m*.
toe·nail ['təʊˌneɪl] *n* Zehennagel *m*, Unguis pedis.
toe phenomenon → toe's sign.
toe reflex 1. → toe's sign. **2.** Zehenklonus *m*.
toe's sign Babinski-Zeichen *nt*, -Reflex *m*, (Groß-)Zehenreflex *m*.
To·ga·vir·i·dae [ˌtəʊɡəˈvɪrədiː, -ˈvaɪr-] *pl micro.* Togaviren *pl*, Togaviridae *pl*.
to·ga·vi·rus [ˌ-ˈvaɪrəs] *n micro.* Togavirus *nt*.
toi·let ['tɔɪlɪt] *n* **1.** Toilette *f*; Klosett-(becken *nt*) *nt*. **to go to (the) ~** auf die/zur Toilette gehen. **2.** Toilette *f*, (Körper-)Pflege *f*.
toilet paper Toilettenpapier *nt*.
toilet room Toilette *f*.
tok- *pref.* → toko-.
To·ke·lau [təʊkəˈlaʊ] *n* → tinea imbricata.
Tokelau ringworm [təʊkəˈlaʊ] → tinea imbricata.
toko- *pref.* Geburts-, Wehen-, Tok(o)-.
to·ko·dy·na·graph [ˌ-ˈdaɪnəɡræf] *n abbr.* **TKG** *gyn.* Tokogramm *nt*.
to·ko·dy·na·mom·e·ter [ˌ-ˌdaɪnəˈmɒmɪtər] *n abbr.* **TKD** *gyn.* Tokodynamometer *nt*, Tokometer *nt*, Wehenmesser *m*.
tok·o·graph ['-ɡræf] *n gyn.* Kardio-, Cardiotokograph *m*.
to·kog·ra·phy [təʊˈkɒɡrəfɪ] *n gyn.* Wehenmessung *f*, Tokographie *f*, Tokometrie *f*.
tol·az·a·mide [tɒlˈæzəmaɪd] *n pharm.* Tolazamid *nt*.
tol·az·o·line [tɒlˈæzəʊliːn] *n pharm.* Tolazolin *nt*.
tol·bu·ta·mide [tɒlˈbjuːtəmaɪd] *n pharm.* Tolbutamid *nt*.
tolbutamide response test *abbr.* **TRT** Tolbutamid-Test *m*, Sulfonylharnstoff-Test *m*.
tolbutamide test → tolbutamide response test.
tol·ci·clate [tɒlˈsaɪkleɪt] *n pharm.* Tolciclat *nt*.
tol·er·a·ble ['tɒlərəbl] *adj* erträglich; tolerierbar.
tol·er·ance ['tɒlərəns] *n* **1.** Widerstandsfähigkeit *f*, Toleranz *f* (*for* gegen); *a. pharm.* Verträglichkeit *f*, Toleranz *f*. **2.** *techn.*

Fehlergrenze *f*, zulässige Abweichung *f*, Toleranz *f*. **3.** Toleranz *f*, Duldsamkeit *f*; Nachsicht *f* (*of, for, towards* mit, gegenüber). **4.** *immun.* Immuntoleranz *f abbr.* IT. **5.** *immun.* Immunparalyse *f*.
tolerance adaptation *physiol.* Toleranzadaptation *f*.
tolerance dose *radiol.* Toleranzdosis *f*, Dosis tolerata.
tolerance test Toleranztest *m*.
tol·er·ant ['talərənt] *adj* **1.** widerstandsfähig (*of* gegen). **2.** duldsam, tolerant (*of* gegen); geduldig, nachsichtig (*of* mit).
tol·er·ate ['taləreɪt] *vt* (er-)dulden, er-, vertragen, tolerieren; tolerant sein (*of, towards, with* gegenüber). **to be well/poorly ~d** (das Medikament) gut/schlecht vertragen.
tol·er·a·tion [,talə'reɪʃn] *n* **1.** Tolerierung *f*, Duldung *f*. **2.** Toleranz *f*, Duldsamkeit *f*; Nachsicht *f* (*of, for, towards* mit, gegenüber).
tol·er·o·gen ['talərədʒən] *n immun.* Toleranz-induzierende Substanz *f*, Tolerogen *nt*.
tol·er·o·gen·e·sis [,talərəʊ'dʒenəsɪs] *n immun.* Toleranzinduktion *f*, Tolerogenese *f*.
tol·er·o·gen·ic [,-'dʒenɪk] *adj immun.* Toleranz-induzierend, tolerogen.
Tollens ['taləns]: **T.' test** Tollens'-Probe *f*.
tol·met·in ['talmetɪn] *n pharm.* Tolmetin *nt*.
tol·naf·tate [tal'næfteɪt, tɔl-] *n pharm.* Tolnaftat *nt*.
to·lo·ni·um chloride [tə'ləʊnɪəm] Toluidinblau O *nt*, Toloniumchlorid *nt*.
Tolosa-Hunt [tə'ləʊsə hʌnt]: **T.-H. syndrome** Tolosa-Hunt-Syndrom *nt*.
tol·u·ene ['taljəwi:n] *n* Toluol *nt*, Methylbenzol *nt*.
to·lu·i·dine [tə'lu:ədi:n, -dɪn] *n* Toluidin *nt*.
toluidine blue *histol.* Toluidinblau *nt*.
toluidine blue O → tolonium chloride.
toluidine blue stain Toluidinblaufärbung *f*.
tol·u·ol ['taljəwɒl] *n* → toluene.
tol·u·yl·ene ['taljəwəli:n] *n* Stilben *nt*.
tol·y·caine [talɪkeɪn] *n pharm., anes.* Tolycain *nt*.
tom- *pref.* → tomo-.
Tomes ['təʊmz]: **T.' fibers** Tomes'-Fasern *pl*, -Fortsätze *pl*, Dentinfasern *pl*.
T.' fibrils → T.' fibers.
T.' granular layer Tomes'-Körnerschicht *f*.
tomo- *pref.* Schicht-, Tom(o)-.
to·mo·gram ['təʊməgræm] *n radiol.* Schichtaufnahme *f*, Tomogramm *nt*.
to·mo·graph ['-græf] *n radiol.* Tomograph *nt*.
to·mog·ra·phy [tə'magrəfɪ] *n radiol.* Schichtröntgen *nt*, Schichtaufnahmeverfahren *nt*, Tomographie *f*.
ton- *pref.* → tono-.
tone [təʊn] **I** *n* **1.** Ton *m*, Laut *m*, Klang *m*; Stimme *f*; Tonfall *m*, Betonung *f*; Tonhöhe *f*. **2.** (Farb-)Ton *m*, Tönung *f*; Schattierung *f*. **3.** *physiol.* Spannung(szustand *m*) *f*, Spannkraft *f*, Tonus *m*. **II** *vt* **4.** einfärben, (ab-)tönen, abstufen; kolorieren. **5.** *physiol.* Spannkraft verleihen, stärken. **III** *vi s.* abstufen, *s.* abtönen.
tone up *vt* (*Muskeln*) kräftigen.
t. of muscle Muskeltonus, -spannung.
tone-deaf *adj* tontaub.
tone deafness Tontaubheit *f*, sensorische Amusie *f*.
tone decay test *HNO* Schwellenschwundtest *m*, Carhart-Test *m*.
tone intensity-difference threshold *HNO*
Lüscher-Test *m*, Tonintensitätsunterschiedsschwelle *f*.
tone pitch *phys.* Tonhöhe *f*.
ton·ga ['taŋgə] *n* Frambösie *f*, Pian *f*, Parangi *f*, Yaws *f*, Framboesia tropica.
tongs [tɔŋz, taŋz] *pl* Zange *f*; Klemme *f*.
tongue [tʌŋ] *n* **1.** Zunge *f*; *anat.* Lingua *f*, Glossa *f*. **to bite one's ~** s. auf die Zunge beißen. **to put one's ~ out** die Zunge herausstrecken. **2.** zungenförmige Struktur *f*, *anat.* Lingula *f*. **3.** Sprache *f*.
t. of cerebellum Lingula cerebelli.
tongue bone Zungenbein *n*, Os hyoideum.
tongue depressor Mund-, Zungenspatel *m*.
tongue-tie *n* Zungenverwachsung *f*, Ankyloglossie *f*, -glosson *nt*.
tongue worm *micro.* Zungenwurm *m*, Pentastomid *m*.
ton·ic ['tanɪk] **I** *n* **1.** kräftigendes Mittel *nt*, Stärkungsmittel *nt*, Tonikum *nt*. **2.** *fig.* Stimulanz *f*. **II** *adj* **3.** Tonus betr., durch Tonus gekennzeichnet, tonisch. **4.** normalen Tonus (wieder-)herstellend, stärkend, kräftigend, tonisch, tonisierend. **5.** *pharm.* stärkend, tonisierend. **6.** betont, tontragend, Ton-.
tonic-clonic contraction tonisch-klonische Kontraktion *f*.
tonic contraction 1. tonische (An-)Spannung/Kontraktion *f*; Tonus *m*. **2.** tetanische Kontraktur *f*, Tetanus *m*.
tonic convulsion tonische Konvulsion *f*.
tonic epilepsy tonischer Krampfanfall *m*.
tonic fiber tonische (Muskel-)Faser *f*, Tonusfaser *f*.
to·nic·i·ty [təʊ'nɪsətɪ] *n* **1.** Spannung(szustand *m*) *f*, Tonus *m*. **2.** Spannkraft *f*.
ton·i·cize ['tanɪsaɪz] *vt* kräftigen, stärken, tonisieren.
tonic labyrinth *physiol.* tonisches Labyrinth *nt*, Maculaapparat *m*.
tonic labyrinth reflex tonischer Labyrinthreflex *m*.
tonic neck reflex tonischer Nacken-/Halsreflex *m*.
ton·i·co·clon·ic [,tanɪkəʊ'klanɪk] *adj* tonisch-klonisch.
tonic pupil 1. Adie'-Pupille *f*, Pupillotonie *f*. **2.** Westphal-Piltz-Phänomen *nt*, Orbikularisphänomen *nt*, Lid-Pupillen-Reflex *m*.
tonic reflex tonischer Reflex *m*.
tonic response *physiol.* tonische/statische/proportionale Antwort *f*.
tonic spasm Tetanus *m*, Tetanie *f*.
tonic stretch reflex tonischer Dehnungsreflex *m*.
tono- *pref.* Spannungs-, Ton(o)-, Tonus-.
ton·o·clon·ic [,tanə'klanɪk, ,təʊ-] *adj* tonisch-klonisch.
ton·o·fi·bril [,-'faɪbrəl, -'fɪb-] *n* Tonofibrille *f*.
ton·o·fil·a·ment [,-'fɪləmənt] *n* Tonofilament *nt*.
to·no·gram ['təʊnəgræm] *n ophthal.* Tonogramm *nt*.
to·no·graph ['-græf] *n ophthal.* Tonograph *m*.
to·nog·ra·phy [təʊ'nagrəfɪ] *n ophthal.* Tonographie *f*.
to·nom·e·ter [təʊ'namɪtər] *n* **1.** *ophthal.* Tonometer *nt*, Ophthalmotonometer *nt*. **2.** Druckmesser *m*, Tonometer *nt*. **3.** *phys.* (Aero-)Tonometer *nt*.
to·nom·e·try [təʊ'namətrɪ] *n* **1.** Spannungs-, Druckmessung *f*, Tonometrie *f*. **2.** *ophthal.* Augeninnendruckmessung *f*, Tonometrie *f*, Ophthalmotonometrie *f*.
ton·o·plast ['tanəplæst] *n histol.* Tonoplast *m*, innere Plasmahaut *f*.
ton·o·top·ic [,-'tapɪk] *adj physiol.* tonotop(isch).
tonotopic arrangement tonotope (An-)-Ordnung *f*.
to·not·o·py [tə'natəpɪ] *n* Tonotopie *f*.
ton·sil ['tansəl] *n anat.* **1.** mandelförmiges Organ *nt*, Mandel *f*, Tonsille *f*, Tonsilla *f*. **2.** Gaumenmandel *f*, Tonsilla palatina. **to have one's ~s out** s. die Mandeln herausnehmen lassen.
t. of cerebellum Kleinhirnmandel, Tonsilla, Tonsilla cerebelli.
t. of torus tubarius Tubenmandel, Tonsilla tubaria.
tonsil-holding forceps → tonsillar forceps.
tonsill- *pref.* → tonsillo-.
ton·sil·la [tan'sɪlə] *n*, *pl* **-lae** [-li:] → tonsil 1.
ton·sil·lar ['tansɪlər] *adj* Mandel/Tonsille betr., mandelförmig, tonsillär, tonsillar, Mandel-, Tonsillen-.
tonsillar artery Gaumenmandelast *m* der A. facialis, Ramus tonsillaris a. facialis.
tonsillar branch: t. of facial artery → tonsillar artery.
t.es of glossopharyngeal nerve Tonsillenäste *pl* des N. glossopharyngeus, Rami tonsillares n. glossopharyngei.
t. of posterior inferior cerebellar artery Ramus tonsillae cerebelli a. inferioris posterioris cerebelli.
tonsillar calculus → tonsillolith.
tonsillar capsule Mandelkapsel *f*, Capsula tonsillaris.
tonsillar compressor *HNO* Tonsillenschnürer *m*.
tonsillar crypts Tonsillen-, Mandelkrypten *pl*, Cryptae/Fossulae tonsillares.
t. of palatine tonsil Gaumenmandelkrypten, Cryptae tonsillares tonsillae palatinae.
t. of pharyngeal tonsil Rachenmandelkrypten, Cryptae tonsillares tonsillae pharyngeae.
tonsillar elevator *HNO* Tonsillenelevatorium *m*.
tonsillar forceps *HNO* Tonsillenfaßzange *f*.
tonsillar fossa Gaumenmandel-, Tonsillennische *f*, Fossa tonsillaris.
tonsillar fossulae Mandelkryptenöffnungen *pl*, Fossulae tonsillares.
t. of palatine tonsil Fossulae tonsillares tonsillae palatinae.
t. of pharyngeal tonsil Fossulae tonsillares tonsillae pharyngeae.
tonsillar hernia Hernia tonsillaris.
tonsillar herniation Hernia tonsillaris.
tonsillar hook *HNO* Tonsillenhaken *m*.
tonsillar nerves → tonsillar branches of glossopharyngeal nerve.
tonsillar pits → tonsillar crypts.
tonsillar ring Waldeyer'-Rachenring *m*, lymphatischer Rachenring *m*.
tonsillar sinus → tonsillar fossa.
ton·sil·lar·y ['tansɪlerɪ] *adj* → tonsillar.
ton·sil·lec·to·my [,tansə'lektəmɪ] *n HNO* Tonsillenentfernung *f*, Tonsillektomie *f abbr.* TE.
ton·sil·lith ['tansɪlɪθ] *n* → tonsillolith.
ton·sil·lit·ic [,tansə'lɪtɪk] *adj* Tonsillitis betr., tonsillitisch.
ton·sil·li·tis [,-'laɪtɪs] *n* Mandelentzündung *f*, Tonsillitis *f*; Angina *f*.
tonsillo- *pref.* Mandel-, Tonsill(o)-.
ton·sil·lo·ad·e·noid·ec·to·my [,tansɪləʊ,ædənɔɪ'dektəmɪ] *n* Tonsilloadenoidektomie *f*.
ton·sil·lo·lith [tan'sɪləlɪθ] *n* Tonsillenstein *m*, -konkrement *nt*, Tonsillolith *m*.

tonsillomycosis

ton·sil·lo·my·co·sis [tɑnˌsɪləʊmaɪˈkəʊsɪs] *n* Mandel-, Tonsillenmykose *f*.
ton·sil·lop·a·thy [ˌtɑnsɪˈlɑpəθi] *n* Mandel-, Tonsillenerkrankung *f*, Tonsillopathie *f*.
ton·sil·lo·tome [tɑnˈsɪlətəʊm] *n* Tonsillotomiemesser *nt*, Tonsillotom *nt*.
ton·sil·lot·o·my [ˌtɑnsɪˈlɑtəmɪ] *n* HNO Tonsillotomie *f*.
tonsil-seizing forceps → tonsillar forceps.
ton·so·lith [ˈtɑnsəlɪθ] *n* → tonsillolith.
to·nus [ˈtəʊnəs] *n* kontinuierliche (An-)-Spannung *f*, Spannungszustand *m*, Tonus *m*.
tonus fiber → tonic fiber.
tool [tuːl] *n* 1. Werkzeug *nt*, Gerät *nt*, Instrument *nt*. 2. *fig.* (Hilfs-)Mittel *nt*.
Tooth [tuːθ]: **T. atrophy/disease/type** Charcot-Marie-Krankheit *f*, -Syndrom *nt*, Charcot-Marie-Tooth-Hoffmann-Krankheit *f*, -Syndrom *nt*.
tooth [tuːθ] *n*, *pl* **teeth** [tiːθ] Zahn *m*; *anat.* zahnähnliche Struktur *f*, Dens *m*.
tooth·ache [ˈtuːθˌeɪk] *n* Zahnschmerzen *pl*, -weh *nt*; *dent.* Odontalgie *f*, Odontagra *f*, Dentalgie *f*, Dentagra *f*.
tooth·brush [ˈtuːθˌbrʌʃ] *n* Zahnbürste *f*.
tooth bud → tooth germ.
tooth cement *dent.* (Zahn-)Zement *m*, Cementum *nt*, Substantia ossea dentis.
tooth decay Zahnfäule *f*, (Zahn-)Karies *f*, Caries dentium.
toothed [tuːθt] *adj* mit Zähnen versehen, gezahnt, gezähnt, Zahn-; gezackt.
tooth germ 1. Zahnanlage *f*. 2. Zahnkeim *m*.
tooth·less [ˈtuːθlɪs] *adj* ohne Zähne, zahnlos.
tooth·paste [ˈtuːθpeɪst] *n* Zahnpasta *f*, -paste *f*, -creme *f*.
tooth·pick [ˈtuːθpɪk] *n* Zahnstocher *m*.
tooth powder Zahnpulver *nt*.
tooth pulp (Zahn-)Pulpa *f*, Pulpa dentis.
tooth socket Zahnfach *nt*, Alveolus dentalis.
top- *pref.* → topo-.
top·ag·no·sia [ˌtɑpægˈnəʊzɪə, -ʒ(ɪ)ə] *n* Topagnosie *f*.
top·ag·no·sis [ˌtɑpægˈnəʊsɪs] *n* → topagnosia.
to·pal·gia [təˈpældʒ(ɪ)ə] *n psychia.* Lokalschmerz *m*, Topalgie *f*, Topoalgie *f*.
to·pec·to·my [təˈpektəmɪ] *n neurochir.* Topektomie *f*.
top·er's nose [ˈtəʊpər] Kartoffel-, Säufer-, Pfund-, Knollennase *f*, Rhinophym *nt*, Rhinophyma *nt*.
top·es·the·sia [ˌtɑpesˈθiːʒ(ɪ)ə] *n* Topästhesie *f*, Topognosie *f*.
to·pha·ceous [təˈfeɪʃəs] *adj* herd-, knotenförmig.
tophaceous gout chronisches Gichtstadium *nt*, Gicht *f* mit Tophusbildung.
to·phi *pl* → tophus.
to·phus [ˈtəʊfəs] *n*, *pl* **-phi** [-faɪ] 1. Knoten *m*, Tophus *m*. 2. Gichtknoten *m*, Tophus (arthriticus) *m*.
top·ic¹ [ˈtɑpɪk] *n* Thema *nt*, Gegenstand *m*.
top·ic² [ˈtɑpɪk] *adj* → topical.
top·i·cal [ˈtɑpɪkl] *adj* topisch, örtlich, lokal, Lokal-.
topical anesthesia örtliche Betäubung *f*, (direkte) Lokalanästhesie *f*.
topical application örtliche Anwendung *f*.
topical calciphylaxis lokale/örtliche Kalziphylaxie *f*.
topic anesthetic topisches Anästhetikum *nt*, Lokalanästhetikum *nt*.
to·pis·tic [təˈpɪstɪk] *adj* örtlich, äußerlich (wirkend), topisch.
to·pis·tics [təˈpɪstɪks] *pl anat.* Topik *f*.
topo- *pref.* Orts-, Top(o)-.

top·o·al·gia [ˌtɑpəˈældʒ(ɪ)ə] *n* → topalgia.
top·o·an·es·the·sia [ˌ-ænəsˈθiːʒə] *n* → topagnosia.
top·o·chem·is·try [ˌ-ˈkemətrɪ] *n* Topochemie *f*.
top·o·dys·es·the·sia [ˌ-dɪsesˈθiːʒə] *n* lokalisierte Dysästhesie *f*, Topodysästhesie *f*.
top·og·no·sia [ˌtɑpəgˈnəʊzɪə] *n* → topesthesia.
top·og·no·sis [-ˈnəʊsɪs] *n* → topesthesia.
top·o·graph·ic [ˌtɑpəˈɡræfɪk] *adj* → topographical.
top·o·graph·i·cal [ˌ-ˈɡræfɪkl] *adj* Topographie betr., ortsbeschreibend, topographisch.
topographical diagnosis Topodiagnose *f*.
topographic anatomy topographische Anatomie *f*.
to·pog·ra·phy [təˈpɑɡrəfɪ] *n* Topographie *f*.
top·o·nar·co·sis [ˌtɑpənɑːrˈkəʊsɪs] *n* → topical anesthesia.
top·o·nym [ˈ-nɪm] *n* Toponym *nt*.
top·o·par·es·the·sia [ˌ-ˌpæresˈθiːʒ(ɪ)ə] *n* lokalisierte Parästhesie *f*, Topoparästhesie *f*.
to·po·pho·bia [ˌ-ˈfəʊbɪə] *n psychia.* Topophobie *f*; Situationsangst *f*.
top·o·therm·es·the·si·om·e·ter [ˌ-ˌθɜrmesˌθiːzɪˈɑmɪtər] *n* Topothermästhesiometer *nt*.
TOPV *abbr.* → trivalent oral poliovirus vaccine.
tor·cu·lar [ˈtɔːrkjələr] *n* Torcular *nt*.
torcular herophili Confluens sinuum, Torcular herophili.
torcular tourniquet Abbindung *f*.
to·ric [ˈtɔːrɪk, ˈtəʊ-] *adj* Torus betr., torisch.
toric lens torische Linse *f*.
Torkildsen [ˈtɔːrkɪldsən]: **T.'s operation** *neurochir.* Torkildsen-Operation *f*, Ventrikulozisternostomie *f*.
tor·mi·na [ˈtɔːrmɪnə] *pl* Bauchkrämpfe *pl*, Koliken *pl*, Tormina *pl*.
tor·mi·nal [ˈtɔːrmɪnəl] *adj* kolikartig.
Tornwaldt [ˈtɔːrnwɔlt, -vɑlt]: **T.'s abscess** Tornwaldt-Abszeß *m*.
T.'s bursa → T.'s cyst.
T.'s bursitis Entzündung *f* der Bursa pharyngealis, Tornwaldt-Krankheit *f*, Bursitis pharyngealis.
T.'s cyst Tornwaldt-Zyste *f*, -Bursa *f*, Bursa pharyngea.
T.'s disease → T.'s bursitis.
to·rose [ˈtɔːrəʊs, ˈtɔː-] *adj* wülstig.
to·rous [ˈtɔːrəs, ˈtɔː-] *adj* → torose.
tor·pent [ˈtɔːrpənt] **I** *n* betäubendes *od.* beruhigendes Mittel *nt*. **II** *adj* torpid.
tor·pid [ˈtɔːrpɪd] *adj* träge, schlaff, ohne Aktivität, langsam, apathisch, stumpf, starr, erstarrt, betäubt, torpid.
tor·pid·i·ty [tɔːrˈpɪdətɪ] *n* → torpidness.
tor·pid·ness [ˈtɔːrpɪdnɪs] *n* Trägheit *f*, Schlaffheit *f*, Apathie *f*, Stumpfheit *f*, Erstarrung *f*, Betäubung *f*, Torpidität *f*, Torpor *m*.
tor·por [ˈtɔːrpər] *n* → torpidness.
torque [tɔːrk] *n phys.* Drehmoment *nt*.
torque impulse *phys.* Drehimpuls *m*, Spin *m*.
torr [tɔːr] *n* Torr *nt*.
Torre [ˈtɔːrə]: **T.'s syndrome** Torre-Syndrom *nt*.
tor·re·fac·tion [ˌtɔːrəˈfækʃn] *n chem., techn.* Rösten *nt*, Darren *nt*.
tor·re·fy [ˈ-faɪ] *vt chem., techn.* rösten, darren.
tor·sades de pointes [tɔrˈsad də pwɛ̃ːt] *French card.* Torsades de Pointes, atypische ventrikuläre Tachykardie *f*.

tor·sion [ˈtɔːrʃn] *n* 1. (Ver-)Drehung *f*; Drehen *nt*. 2. *mathe.*, *techn.* Drehung *f*, Torsion *f*.
tor·sion·al [ˈtɔːrʃənl] *adj* Dreh-, Torsions-, (Ver-)Drehungs-.
torsional force Dreh-, Torsionskraft *f*.
torsional moment Drehmoment *nt*.
torsional stress Torsionsspannung *f*.
torsion dystonia Ziehen-Oppenheim-Syndrom *nt*, -Krankheit *f*, Torsionsneurose *f*, -dystonie *f*, Dysbasia lordotica.
torsion fracture Torsionsbruch *m*, -fraktur *f*, Drehbruch *m*, -fraktur *f*, Spiralbruch *m*, -fraktur *f*.
torsion neurosis → torsion dystonia.
torsion nystagmus Torsionsnystagmus *m*.
cervical spine t. HWS-Torsionsnystagmus.
tor·sive [ˈtɔːrsɪv] *adj* gewunden, verdreht, gekrümmt, verkrümmt.
tor·so [ˈtɔːrsəʊ] *n*, *pl* **-sos**, **-si** [-siː] Torso *m*.
tor·ti·col·lar [ˌtɔːrtɪˈkɑlər] *adj* Torticollis betr.
tor·ti·col·lis [ˌ-ˈkɑlɪs] *n ortho.* Schiefhals *m*, Torticollis *m*, Caput obstipum.
tor·ti·pel·vis [ˌ-ˈpelvɪs] *n* Tortipelvis *f*.
tor·tu·os·i·ty [ˌtɔːrtʃʊˈwɑsətɪ] *n* Krümmung *f*, Windung *f*; Gewundenheit *f*, Schlängelung *f*, Tortuositas *f*.
tor·tu·ous [ˈtɔːrtʃəwəs] *adj* gewunden, gekrümmt, verkrümmt, ver-, gedreht, geschlängelt.
Tor·u·la [ˈtɔr(j)ələ] *n micro.* Kryptokokkus *m*, Cryptococcus *m*.
tor·u·la meningitis [ˈtɔr(j)ələ] Cryptococcus-Meningitis *f*.
tor·u·lar meningitis [ˈtɔr(j)ələr] → torula meningitis.
tor·u·lin [ˈtɔr(j)əlɪn] *n* → thiamine.
tor·u·lo·ma [ˌtɔːr(j)əˈləʊmə] *n* Kryptokokkengranulom *nt*, Torulom *nt*.
Tor·u·lop·sis [ˌ-ˈlɑpsɪs] *n micro.* Torulopsis *f*.
tor·u·lop·so·sis [ˌ-ˈlɑpsəsɪs] *n* Torulopsis-Infektion *f*, Torulopsosis *f*, Torulopsidose *f*.
tor·u·lo·sis [ˌ-ˈləʊsɪs] *n* europäische Blastomykose *f*, Kryptokokkose *f*, Cryptococcose *f*, Torulose *f*, Cryptococcus-Mykose *f*, Busse-Buschke-Krankheit *f*.
tor·u·lus [ˈ-ləs] *n*, *pl* **-li** [-laɪ, -liː] *anat.* Torulus *m*.
to·rus [ˈtɔːrəs, ˈtəʊr-] *n*, *pl* **-ri** [-raɪ] *anat.* runde Erhebung *f*, Wulst *m*, Torus *m*.
torus fracture Wulstbruch *m*.
torus levatorius Levatorwulst *m*, Torus levatorius.
torus tubarius Tubenwulst *m*, Torus tubarius.
N-tos·yl-L-phenylalanylchloromethyl ketone [ˈtɑsɪl] *abbr.* **TPCK** *N*-Tosyl-L-phenylalanylchlormethylketon *nt abbr.* TPCK.
to·tal [ˈtəʊtl] **I** *n* Gesamtmenge *f*. **II** *adj* ganz, gesamt, total, völlig, absolut, total, Gesamt-, Total-.
total anesthesia *neuro.* Totalanästhesie *f*.
total aphasia Total-, Globalaphasie *f*.
total blindness totale Erblindung/Blindheit/Amaurose *f*.
total blood volume *abbr.* **TBV** totales Blutvolumen *nt abbr.* TBV.
total body irradiation → total body radiation.
total body radiation *radiol.* Ganzkörperbestrahlung *f*.
total body scintigraphy *radiol.* Ganzkörperszintigraphie *f*.
total body surface area *abbr.* **TBSA** Gesamtkörperoberfläche *f*.
total body volume *abbr.* **TBV** Gesamtkörpervolumen *nt abbr.* GKV.

total body water *abbr.* **TBW** *physiol.* Gesamtkörperwasser *nt abbr.* GKW.
total capacity → total lung capacity.
total cataract kompletter/vollständiger Star *m*, Totalstar *m*, Cataracta totalis.
total cleavage *embryo.* totale/holoblastische Furchung(steilung *f*) *f*.
total colectomy *chir.* totale Kolonentfernung/Kolektomie *f*.
total deafness völlige Taubheit *f*, Anakusis *f*.
total dose Gesamtdosis *f*.
total endoprosthesis *chir., ortho.* Totalendoprothese *f abbr.* TEP, Totalprothese *f*.
total excision *chir.* Totalentfernung *f*.
total gastrectomy *chir.* Magenentfernung *f*, totale Magenresektion *f*, Gastrektomie *f*.
total hepatectomy totale Leberentfernung *f*, Hepatektomie *f*.
total hip replacement *abbr.* **THR** *ortho.* Hüfttotalendoprothese *f*, Hüft-TEP *f*.
total hyperopia *abbr.* **Ht** *ophthal.* totale Weitsichtigkeit/Hyperopie *f*.
total hysterectomy *gyn.* totale Gebärmutterentfernung/Hysterektomie *f*, Hysterectomia totalis.
total joint replacement → total endoprosthesis.
total lipodystrophy Lawrence-Syndrom *nt*, lipatrophischer Diabetes *m*.
total lung capacity *abbr.* **TLC** (*Lunge*) Totalkapazität *f abbr.* TK.
total mastectomy *gyn.* einfache Mastektomie *f*.
total nodal field → total nodal irradiation.
total nodal irradiation *abbr.* **TNI** *radiol.* Bestrahlung *f* aller Lymphknotengruppen, total nodal irradiation (*f*) *abbr.* TNI.
total ophthalmoplegia Ophthalmoplegia totalis.
total parenteral alimentation → total parenteral nutrition.
total parenteral nutrition *abbr.* **TPN** vollständige/totale parenterale Ernährung *f*.
total peripheral resistance *abbr.* **TPR** totaler peripherer Widerstand *m abbr.* TPR.
total prosthesis → total endoprosthesis.
total transfusion (Blut-)Austauschtransfusion *f*, Blutaustausch *m*.
Toti ['tɔʊti]: **T.'s operation** *HNO* Toti-Operation *f*, Dakryozystorhinostomie *f*, Dakryorhinostomie *f*.
to·tip·o·tence [təʊ'tɪpətəns] *n* → totipotency.
to·tip·o·ten·cy [təʊ'tɪpətənsi] *n* Toti-, Omnipotenz *f*.
to·tip·o·tent [təʊ'tɪpətənt] *adj* → totipotential.
totipotent cell omnipotente/totipotente Zelle *f*.
to·ti·po·ten·tial [ˌtəʊtɪpə'tenʃl] *adj* toti-, omnipotent.
totipotential cell → totipotent cell.
touch [tʌtʃ] **I** *n* **1.** Berührung *f*; Berühren *nt*. **at a ~** beim Berühren. **2.** Tastsinn *m*, -gefühl *nt*, Gefühl *nt*. **3.** leichter Anfall *m*. **a ~ of fever** kurzer Fieberanfall, leichtes Fieber. **4.** Spur *f*, kleine Menge *f*. **5.** Verbindung *f*, Kontakt *m*. **to be in ~ with** mit jdm. in Verbindung stehen. **to get in(to) ~ with** s. mit jdm. in Verbindung setzen. **to keep in ~ with** mit jdm. Kontakt halten bleiben. **to lose ~ with** den Kontakt zu jdm. verlieren. **II** *vt* **6.** anfassen, an-, berühren, angreifen, (be-)tasten; (leicht) drücken auf. **7.** fühlen, wahrnehmen. **8.** grenzen *od.* stoßen an.
touch·a·ble ['tʌtʃəbl] *adj* tastbar.
touch bodies/cells → touch corpuscles.
touch corpuscles Meissner'-(Tast-)Körperchen *pl*, Corpuscula tactus.
touch·i·ness ['tʌtʃɪnɪs] *n* (Über-)Empfindlichkeit *f*, Reizbarkeit *f*.
touch sensation Berührungsempfindung *f*.
crude t. grobe Berührungsempfindung.
touch·y ['tʌtʃi] *adj* **1.** (über-)empfindlich, (leicht) reizbar. **2.** (druck-)empfindlich.
Touraine-Solente-Golé [tu'rɛn sɔ'lɑ̃:t gɔ'le]: **T.-S.-G. syndrome** Pachydermoperiostose *f*, Touraine-Solente-Golé-Syndrom *nt*, familiäre Pachydermoperiostose *f*, idiopathische hypertrophische Osteoarthropathie *f*, Akropachydermie *f* mit Pachydermoperiostose, Hyperostosis generalisata mit Pachydermie.
Tourette [tu'ret]: **T.'s disease/disorder** Gilles-de-la-Tourette-Syndrom *nt*, Tourette-Syndrom *nt*, Maladie des tics, Tic impulsif.
Tournay [tur'nɛ]: **T.'s sign** *ophthal.* Tournay-Zeichen *nt*.
tour·ne·sol ['tɜrnɪsɑl, -sɔl] *n* Lackmus *nt*.
tour·ni·quet ['tɜrnɪkɪt, 'tʊər-] *n* (Abschnür-)Binde *f*, Tourniquet *nt*, Torniquet *nt*; Manschette *f*.
tourniquet test 1. Kapillarresistenzprüfung *f*. **2.** Matas-Moskowicz-Test *m*. **3.** Perthes-Versuch *m*.
Tourtual ['tʊərtʃəwəl, -ʃəl; 'tu:rtu,a:l]: **T.'s membrane** Membrana quadrangularis.
T.'s sinus Fossa supratonsillaris.
Touton ['tu:tɑn, tɔn]: **T.'s giant cells** Touton'-Riesenzellen *pl*.
tow·el ['taʊəl] **I** *n* **1.** Handtuch *nt*. **2.** *chir.* Tuch *nt*. **3.** *hyg.* (Monats-, Damen-)Binde *f*. **II** *vt* (ab-)trocknen, (ab-)reiben, frottieren.
towel down *vt* (ab-)trocknen, trockenreiben.
towel clamp *chir.* Tuchklemme *f*.
towel clip (forceps) → towel clamp.
towel forceps → towel clamp.
tow·el·ing ['taʊəlɪŋ] *n* Abreibung *f*, Frottieren *nt*.
tow·er head ['taʊər] Spitz-, Turmschädel *m*, Akrozephalie *f*, Akrokephalie *f*, Oxyzephalie *f*, -cephalie *f*, Hypsizephalie *f*, -cephalie *f*, Turrizephalie *f*, -cephalie *f*.
tower skull → tower head.
Towne [taʊn]: **T. projection** *radiol., HNO* Aufnahme *f* nach Towne.
T. roentgenogram → T. projection.
T. view → T. projection.
T. x-ray view → T. projection.
tox- *pref.* → toxico-.
tox·a·ne·mia [tɑksə'ni:miə] *n* → toxic anemia.
Tox·as·ca·ris [tɑs'sæskərɪs] *n micro.* Toxascaris *f*.
tox·e·mia [tɑk'si:miə] *n* **1.** Blutvergiftung *f*, Toxikämie *f*, Toxämie *f*. **2.** Toxinämie *f*, Toxemia.
t. of pregnancy Schwangerschaftstoxikose, Gestose *f*.
tox·e·mic [tɑk'si:mɪk] *adj* Tox(ik)ämie betr., durch Tox(ik)ämie gekennzeichnet, toxikämisch, Toxiämie-, Toxikämie- *f*.
toxemic jaundice → toxic jaundice.
toxemic retinopathy of pregnancy Retinopathia eclamptica gravidarum.
toxemic vertigo → toxic vertigo.
toxi- *pref.* → toxico-.
toxic- *pref.* → toxico-.
tox·ic ['tɑksɪk] **I** *n* Gift(stoff *m*) *nt*, Toxikum *nt*, Toxikon *nt*. **II** *adj* als Gift wirkend, Gift(e) enthaltend, giftig, toxisch, Gift-.
toxic amaurosis → toxic amblyopia.
toxic amblyopia *ophthal.* toxische Amblyopie *f*.
toxic anemia (hämo-)toxische Anämie *f*.
tox·i·cant ['tɑksɪkənt] *n, adj* → toxic.
tox·i·ca·tion [ˌtɑksɪ'keɪʃn] *n* Vergiftung *f*; Intoxikation *f*; Vergiften *nt*.
toxic atrophy toxische Atrophie *f*.
toxic bullous epidermolysis → toxic epidermal necrolysis.
toxic cardiopathy toxische Kardiopathie *f*.
toxic cataract toxische Katarakt *f*.
toxic cholangitis eitrige Cholangitis *f*.
toxic cirrhosis 1. toxische Leberzirrhose *f*. **2.** postnekrotische/ungeordnete/großknotige Leberzirrhose *f*.
toxic deafness toxische/toxisch-bedingte Schwerhörigkeit *f*.
toxic delirium toxisches Delir(ium *nt*) *nt*.
toxic dementia toxische Demenz *f*.
toxic dilatation of the colon akutes/toxisches Megakolon *nt*.
toxic dose toxische Dosis *f abbr.* TD, Dosis toxica.
toxic edema toxisches Ödem *nt*.
tox·i·ce·mia [ˌtɑksɪ'si:miə] *n* → toxemia.
toxic epidermal necrolysis *abbr.* **TEN** (medikamentöses) Lyell-Syndrom *nt*, Syndrom *nt* der verbrühten Haut, Epidermolysis acuta toxica, Epidermolysis necroticans combustiformis.
toxic erythema toxisches Erythem *nt*, Erythema toxicum.
toxic glycosuria toxische Glucosurie/Glykosurie *f*.
toxic granules toxische Granula *pl*.
toxic hemoglobinuria toxische Hämoglobinurie *f*.
toxic inflammation toxische Entzündung *f*.
tox·ic·i·ty [tɑk'sɪsətɪ] *n* Giftigkeit *f*, Toxizität *f*.
toxic jaundice toxischer Ikterus *m*.
toxic leukocytosis toxische Leukozytose *f*.
toxic megacolon akutes/toxisches Megakolon *nt*.
toxic myocarditis toxische Myokarditis *f*.
toxic myolyse toxische Myolyse *f*.
toxic myopathy toxische Myopathie *f*.
toxic nephrosis toxische Nephrose/Nephropathie *f*.
toxic neuritis toxische Neuritis *f*.
toxic nodular goiter hyperthyreote Knotenstruma *f*.
toxico- *pref.* Gift-, Toxik(o)-, Tox(o)-, Toxi-.
Tox·i·co·den·dron [ˌtɑksɪkəʊ'dendrən] *n bio., pharm.* Toxicodendron *nt*.
tox·i·co·gen·ic [-'dʒenɪk] *adj* → toxigenic.
toxicogenic bacterium → toxigenic bacterium.
tox·i·co·he·mia [-'hi:miə] *n* → toxemia.
tox·i·coid ['tɑksɪkɔɪd] *adj* giftartig, -ähnlich, toxoid.
tox·i·co·log·ic [ˌtɑksɪkəʊ'lɑdʒɪk] *adj* toxikologisch.
tox·i·co·log·i·cal [-'lɑdʒɪkl] *adj* → toxicologic.
tox·i·col·o·gist [ˌtɑksɪ'kɑlədʒɪst] *n* Toxikologe *m*, -login *f*.
tox·i·col·o·gy [-'kɑlədʒi] *n* Giftkunde *f*, Toxikologie *f*.
tox·i·co·path·ic [ˌtɑksɪkəʊ'pæθɪk] *adj* toxikopathisch.
tox·i·cop·a·thy [ˌtɑksɪ'kɑpəθi] *n* Vergiftung *f*, Toxikopathie *f*.
tox·i·co·pho·bia [ˌtɑksɪkəʊ'fəʊbiə] *n psychia.* Toxi(ko)phobie *f*.
tox·i·co·sis [ˌtɑksɪ'kəʊsɪs] *n* Toxikose *f*, Toxicosis *f*.
toxic paraplegia toxische Paraplegie *f*.
toxic psychosis toxische Psychose *f*.
toxic retinopathy toxische Retinopathie *f*.
toxic rhinopathia/rhinopathy toxische Rhinopathie *f*.

toxic shock syndrome *abbr.* TSS toxisches Schocksyndrom *nt abbr.* TSS, Syndrom *nt* des toxischen Schocks.
toxic shock-syndrome toxin-1 *abbr.* TSST-1 toxisches Schocksyndrom--Toxin-1 *nt abbr.* TSST-1, toxic shock-syndrome toxin-1.
toxic tremor toxischer Tremor *m.*
toxic vertigo toxischer Schwindel *m.*
tox·i·gen·ic [ˌ-'dʒenɪk] *adj* gift-, toxinbildend, toxogen, toxigen.
toxigenic bacterium *micro.* toxinbildendes Bakterium *nt*, Toxinbildner *m.*
tox·i·ge·nic·i·ty [ˌ-dʒə'nɪsəti] *n* Toxigenität *f.*
toxigenicity test (in vitro) *micro.* Elek--Plattentest *m.*
tox·in ['tɑksɪn] *n* Gift(stoff *m*) *nt*, Toxin *nt.*
θ toxin Thetatoxin *nt*, θ-Toxin *nt.*
toxin-antitoxin reaction Toxin-Antitoxin--Reaktion *f.*
tox·i·ne·mia [ˌtɑksɪ'niːmɪə] *n* Blutvergiftung *f*, Toxinämie *f*, Toxämie *f.*
tox·i·no·gen·ic [ˌtɑksɪnəʊ'dʒenɪk] *adj* → toxigenic.
tox·i·no·sis [ˌtɑksɪ'nəʊsɪs] *n* Toxinose *f.*
tox·ip·a·thy [tɑk'sɪpəθɪ] *n* → toxicopathy.
tox·i·pho·bia [ˌtɑksɪ'fəʊbɪə] *n* → toxicophobia.
tox·is·ter·ol [tɑks'sɪstərəl, -ɔl] *n* Toxisterin *nt.*
toxo- *pref.* → toxico-.
Tox·o·ca·ra [ˌtɑksə'kærə] *n micro.* Toxocara *f.*
T. canis Hundespulwurm *m*, Toxocara canis.
T. cati Katzenspulwurm *m*, Toxocara cati/mystax.
tox·o·ca·ral [ˌ-'kærəl] *adj* Toxocara betr., Toxocara-.
tox·o·ca·ri·a·sis [ˌ-kə'raɪəsɪs] *n* Toxocarainfektion *f*, Toxocariasis *f*, Toxokarose *f.*
tox·oid ['tɑksɔɪd] *n* Toxoid *nt*, Anatoxin *nt.*
tox·on ['tɑksən] *n* Toxon *nt.*
tox·one ['tɑksəʊn] *n* → toxon.
tox·o·no·sis [ˌtɑksə'nəʊsɪs] *n* → toxicosis.
tox·o·phil [-fɪl] *adj* toxophil.
tox·o·phil·ic [ˌ-'fɪlɪk] *adj* → toxophil.
tox·oph·i·lous [tɑks'sɑfɪləs] *adj* → toxophil.
tox·o·phore ['tɑksəfɔʊər, -fɔːr] *n* toxophore Gruppe *f.*
tox·oph·o·rous [tɑk'sɑfərəs] *adj* gifttragend, -haltig, toxophor.
Tox·o·plas·ma [ˌtɑksə'plæzmə] *n micro.* Toxoplasma *nt.*
tox·o·plas·mic [ˌ-'plæzmɪk] *adj* Toxoplasma-, Toxoplasmen-, Toxoplasmose-.
toxoplasmic chorioretinitis *ophthal.* Toxoplasmose-Chorioretinitis *f.*
toxoplasmic encephalitis Toxoplasmose--Enzephalitis *f*, Encephalitis toxoplasmatica.
toxoplasmic encephalomyelitis Toxoplasma-Enzephalomyelitis *f.*
toxoplasmic retinochorioiditis → toxoplasmic chorioretinitis.
tox·o·plas·min [ˌ-'plæzmɪn] *n* Toxoplasmin *nt.*
tox·o·plas·mo·sis [ˌ-plæz'məʊsɪs] *n* Toxoplasmainfektion *f*, Toxoplasmose *f.*
tox·u·ria [tɑk'sj(j)ʊərɪə] *n* Harnvergiftung *f*, Urämie *f.*
Toynbee ['tɔɪnbiː]: **T.'s corpuscles** *ophthal.* Hornhautkörperchen *pl.*
T.'s experiment Toynbee-Versuch *m.*
T.'s ligament M. tensor tympani.
T.'s muscle → T.'s ligament.
T.'s otoscope Toynbee-Otoskop *nt.*
TPA *abbr.* → tissue plasminogen activator.
TPC *abbr.* → thromboplastic plasma component.

TPCK *abbr.* → *N*-tosyl-L-phenylalanylchloromethyl ketone.
TPHA *abbr.* → Treponema pallidum hemagglutination assay.
TPHA test → Treponema pallidum hemagglutination assay.
TPI test → Treponema pallidum immobilization test.
T-plate *n ortho.* T-Platte *f.*
TPN *abbr.* 1. → total parenteral nutrition. 2. → triphosphopyridine nucleotide.
TPP *abbr.* → thiamine pyrophosphate.
TPR *abbr.* → total peripheral resistance.
tra·bec·u·la [trə'bekjələ] *n, pl* -lae [-liː] *anat.* Bälkchen *nt*, Trabekel *f*, Trabecula *f.*
t.e of cavernous bodies *pl* Bindegewebstrabekel *pl* der Schwellkörper, Trabeculae corporum cavernosum (penis).
t.e of spongy body Trabekel *pl* des Harnröhrenschwellkörpers, Trabeculae corporis spongiosi (penis).
tra·bec·u·lar [trə'bekjələr] *adj* Trabekel betr. *od.* bildend, trabekulär.
trabecular adenoma trabekuläres Adenom *nt.*
trabecular arteries (Milz) Trabekel-, Bälkchenarterien *pl.*
trabecular bladder Trabekel-, Balkenblase *f.*
trabecular reticulum Hueck'-Band *nt*, Stenon'-Band *nt*, iridokorneales Balkenwerk *nt*, Reticulum trabeculare (anguli iridocornealis), Lig. pectinatum (anguli iridocornealis).
trabecular substance of bone Spongiosa *f*, Substantia spongiosa/trabecularis (ossium).
trabecular vein (Milz) Balkenvene *f.*
tra·bec·u·late [trə'bekjəlɪt] *adj* → trabecular.
tra·bec·u·lat·ed ['-leɪtɪd] *adj* → trabecular.
trabeculated bladder → trabecular bladder.
tra·bec·u·la·tion [ˌ-'leɪʃn] *n* Trabekelbildung *f*, Trabekulation *f.*
tra·bec·u·lec·to·my [ˌ-'lektəmɪ] *n ophthal.* Trabekulektomie *f*, Trabekulotomie *f*, Goniotomie *f*, Goniotrabekulotomie *f.*
tra·bec·u·lo·plas·ty [trə'bekjəplæsti] *n ophthal.* Gonio-, Trabekuloplastik *f.*
trace [treɪs] I *n* 1. Spur *f*, geringe Menge *f*; (Über-)Rest *m.* 2. Kurve *f*, (Auf-)Zeichnung *f.* II *vt* 3. (auf-, nach-)zeichnen; entwerfen. 4. (ver-)folgen, etw. ausfindig machen, aufspüren, erforschen.
trace out *vt* → trace II.
trace·a·ble ['treɪsəbl] *adj* nachweis-, auffindbar, aufspürbar.
trace element Spurenelement *nt.*
trac·er ['treɪsər] *n* 1. *chem.* (Radio-, Isotopen-)Indikator *m*, radioaktiver Markierungsstoff *m*, Leitisotop *nt*, Tracer *m.* 2. *electr.* Taster *m.*
trace substance Spurensubstanz *f.*
trache- *pref.* → tracheo-.
tra·chea ['treɪkiːə trə'kiːə] *n, pl* **-che·as**, **-che·ae** [-kiː] 1. *anat.* Luftröhre *f*, Trachea *f.* 2. *bio.* tracheaähnliche Struktur *f*, Tracheole *f.*
tra·che·a·ec·ta·sy [ˌtreɪkɪə'ektəsɪ] *n* Luftröhrenerweiterung *f*, -dilatation *f*, Tracheaerweiterung *f*, -dilatation *f.*
tra·che·al [ˌtreɪ'kiːəl] *adj* Luftröhre/Trachea betr., tracheal, Luftröhren-, Tracheal-, Tracheo-.
tracheal anastomosis Luftröhren-, Tracheaanastomose *f.*
tracheal branches: t. of inferior thyroid artery Tracheaäste *pl* der A. thyroidea inferior, Rami tracheales a. thyroideae inferioris.

t. of internal thoracic artery Tracheaäste *pl* der A. thoracica interna, Rami tracheales a. thoracicae internae.
t. of recurrent laryngeal nerve Tracheaäste *pl* des N. laryngealis recurrens, Rami tracheales n. laryngealis recurrentis.
tracheal cannula Trachealkanüle *f.*
tracheal cartilages Knorpelspangen *pl* der Luftröhre, Trachealknorpel *pl*, Cartilagines tracheales.
tracheal catarrh → tracheitis.
tracheal diverticula Luftröhren-, Tracheadivertikel *pl.*
tracheal fistula Trachea(l)fistel *f.*
tra·che·al·gia [ˌtreɪkɪ'ældʒ(ɪ)ə] *n* Luftröhren-, Tracheaschmerz *m*, Trachealgie *f*, Tracheodynie *f.*
tracheal glands Luftröhren-, Trachealdrüsen *pl*, Gll. tracheales.
tracheal hernia Luftröhrenbruch *m*, Trachealhernie *f*, Tracheozele *f.*
tracheal injury Luftröhren-, Tracheaverletzung *f.*
tracheal ligaments Bindegewebsverbindungen *pl* der Trachealknorpel, Ligg. anularia, trachealia.
tracheal muscle glatte Muskulatur *f* der Trachealknorpel, M. trachealis.
tracheal musculature Luftröhren-, Trachea(l)muskulatur *f.*
tracheal necrosis Tracheanekrose *f.*
tracheal obstruction Luftröhren-, Tracheaobstruktion *f.*
tracheal rings → tracheal cartilages.
tracheal transection Trachea(que)riß *m.*
tracheal tugging Oliver-Cardarelli-Zeichen *nt.*
tracheal veins Luftröhren-, Tracheavenen *pl*, Vv. tracheales.
Tra·che·a·ta [treɪkɪ'eɪtə, -'aːtə] *pl bio.* Tracheentiere *pl*, Tracheaten *pl.*
tra·che·id ['treɪkɪɪd, 'treɪkɪːd] *n bio.* Tracheide *f.*
tra·che·i·tis [ˌtreɪkɪ'aɪtɪs] *n* Luftröhren-, Tracheaentzündung *f*, Tracheitis *f.*
trachel- *pref.* → trachelo-.
tra·che·lag·ra [ˌ-'lektəmɪ] *n* Trachelagra *f.*
tra·che·lec·to·my [ˌ-'lektəmɪ] *n gyn.* Zervixresektion *f.*
tra·che·le·ma·to·ma [ˌ-lemə'təʊmə] *n* Hals-, Nackenhämatom *nt.*
tra·che·li·an [trə'kiːlɪən] *adj* 1. Hals/Cervix betr., zervikal, Hals-, Zervikal-, Nacken-. 2. Gebärmutterhals/Cervix uteri betr., zervikal, Gebärmutterhals-, Zervix-, Cervix-.
tra·che·lism ['treɪkəlɪzəm] *n* → trachelismus.
tra·che·lis·mus [ˌtreɪkə'lɪzməs] *n* 1. Halsmuskelkrampf *m*, Trachelismus *m.* 2. *neuro.* Trachelismus *m.*
tra·che·li·tis [ˌ-'laɪtɪs] *n gyn.* Zervixentzündung *f*, Zervizitis *f*, Cervicitis *f.*
trachelo- *pref.* Hals-, Zervix-, Trachel(o)-.
trach·e·lo·cele ['trækələʊsɪl] *n* → tracheal hernia.
trach·e·lo·cyl·lo·sis [ˌ-sɪ'ləʊsɪs] *n* → torticollis.
trach·e·lo·cyr·to·sis [ˌ-sər'təʊsɪs] *n* 1. *ortho.* Kyphose *f* der Halswirbelsäule, Halswirbelsäulenkyphose *f*, HWS-Kyphose *f*, Trachelokyphose *f.* 2. Wirbeltuberkulose *f*, Spondylitis tuberculosa.
trach·e·lo·cys·ti·tis [ˌ-sɪs'taɪtɪs] *n urol.* (Harn-)Blasenhalsentzündung *f*, Trachelozystitis *f*, -cystitis *f.*
trach·e·lo·dyn·ia [ˌ-'dɪnɪə] *n* Nackenschmerzen *pl*, Zervikodynie *f.*
trach·e·lo·ky·pho·sis [ˌ-kaɪ'fəʊsɪs] *n* → trachelocyrtosis.
tra·che·lol·o·gy [treɪkɪ'lɑlədʒɪ] *n* Trachelologie *f.*

trach·e·lo·my·i·tis [ˌtrækəloʊmaɪˈaɪtɪs] *n* Halsmuskelentzündung *f*, Trachelomyitis *f*.
trachelo-occipitalis *n* M. semispinalis cervicis.
trach·e·lo·pex·ia [ˌ-ˈpeksɪə] *n* → trachelopexy.
trach·e·lo·pex·y [ˈ-peksɪ] *n gyn.* Trachelo-, Zervikopexie *f.*
trach·e·lo·phy·ma [ˌ-ˈfaɪmə] *n* Halsschwellung *f*, Halstumor *m*, Trachelophym *nt.*
trach·e·lo·plas·ty [ˈ-plæstɪ] *n gyn.* Zervixplastik *f.*
tra·che·lor·rha·phy [ˌtreɪkɪˈlɔrəfɪ] *n gyn.* Zervixnaht *f*, Zervikorrhaphie *f*; Emmet-Operation *f.*
tra·che·los·chi·sis [ˌ-ˈlɑskəsɪs] *n embryo.* kongenitale Halsspalte *f*, Tracheloschisis *f.*
tra·che·lot·o·my [ˌ-ˈlɑtəmɪ] *n gyn.* Zervixschnitt *m*, -durchtrennung *f*, Zerviko-, Trachelotomie *f.*
tracheo- *pref.* Luftröhren-, Tracheal-, Tracheo-.
tra·che·o·aer·o·cele [ˌtreɪkɪoʊˈeərəsiːl] *n* lufthaltige Trachealhernie/Tracheozele *f.*
tra·che·o·bron·chi·al [ˌ-ˈbrɑŋkɪəl] *adj* Luftröhre/Trachea u. Bronchien betr. *od.* verbindend, tracheobronchial, bronchotracheal.
tracheobronchial aspiration tracheobronchiale Aspiration *f.*
tracheobronchial disruption Bronchienabriß *m.*
tracheobronchial diverticulum *embryo.* Tracheobronchialdivertikel *nt.*
tracheobronchial groove *embryo.* Tracheobronchialrinne *f.*
tracheobronchial stenosis tracheobronchiale Stenose/Stenosierung *f.*
tracheobronchial tree Tracheobronchialbaum *m.*
tra·che·o·bron·chi·tis [ˌ-ˈbrɑŋˈkaɪtɪs] *n* Entzündung *f* von Luftröhre u. Bronchien, Tracheobronchitis *f.*
tra·che·o·bron·cho·meg·a·ly [ˌ-ˌbrɑŋkoʊˈmegəlɪ] *n embryo.* Tracheobronchomegalie *f*, Mounier-Kuhn-Syndrom *nt.*
tra·che·o·bron·chos·co·py [ˌ-brɑŋˈkɑskəpɪ] *n* Tracheobronchoskopie *f.*
tra·che·o·cele [ˈ-siːl] *n* → tracheal hernia.
tra·che·o·e·soph·a·ge·al [ˌ-ˌɪˌsɑfəˈdʒiːəl, -ˌɪsəˈfædʒɪəl] *adj* Luftröhre/Trachea u. Speiseröhre/Ösophagus betr. *od.* verbindend, ösophagotracheal, tracheoösophageal.
tracheoesophageal anomaly *embryo.* tracheoösophageale Fehlbildung/Anomalie *f.*
tracheoesophageal fistula Ösophagus-Trachea-Fistel *f*, Ösophagotrachealfistel *f*, Tracheoösophagealfistel *f.*
  distal t. untere Ösophagotrachealfistel.
  H-type t. (ösophagotracheale) H-Fistel.
  proximal t. obere Ösophagotrachealfistel.
tracheoesophageal groove ösophagotracheale Grube/Rinne *f.*
tracheoesophageal septum *embryo.* ösophagotracheale Scheidewand *f*, Septum (o)esophagotracheale.
tra·che·o·fis·tu·li·za·tion [ˌ-fɪstʃəlɪˈzeɪʃn] *n chir., HNO* Luftröhrenfistelung *f.*
tra·che·o·gen·ic [ˌ-ˈdʒenɪk] *adj* aus der Luftröhre stammend, tracheogen.
tra·che·o·la·ryn·ge·al [ˌ-ləˈrɪndʒ(ɪ)əl] *adj* Luftröhre/Trachea u. Kehlkopf/Larynx betr. *od.* verbindend, tracheolaryngeal, laryngotracheal.
tra·che·ole [ˈtreɪkɪoʊl] *n bio.* Tracheole *f.*
tra·che·o·ma·la·cia [ˌtreɪkɪoʊməˈleɪʃ(ɪ)ə] *n* Luftröhrenerweichung *f*, Tracheomalazie *f*, -malacia *f.*
tra·che·o·path·ia [ˌ-ˈpæθɪə] *n* Luftröhren-, Tracheaerkrankung *f*, Tracheopathie *f.*
tracheopathia osteoplastica Tracheopathia osteoplastica.
tra·che·op·a·thy [ˌtreɪkɪˈɑpəθɪ] *n* → tracheopathia.
tra·che·o·pha·ryn·ge·al [ˌtreɪkɪoʊfəˈrɪndʒ(ɪ)əl] *adj* Luftröhre/Trachea u. Rachen/Pharynx betr. *od.* verbindend, tracheopharyngeal, pharyngotracheal.
tra·che·oph·o·ny [treɪkɪˈɑfənɪ] *n* Tracheophonie *f.*
tra·che·o·phyte [ˈtreɪkɪoʊfaɪt] *n bio.* Tracheophyt *m.*
tra·che·o·plas·ty [ˈ-plæstɪ] *n HNO* Luftröhren-, Trachea-, Tracheoplastik *f.*
tra·che·o·py·o·sis [ˌ-paɪˈoʊsɪs] *n* eitrige Luftröhrenentzündung/Tracheitis *f.*
tra·che·or·rha·gia [ˌ-ˈrɪdʒ(ɪ)ə] *n* Luftröhren-, Trachea(l)blutung *f*, Tracheorrhagie *f.*
tra·che·or·rha·phy [ˌtreɪkɪˈɔrəfɪ] *n HNO* Luftröhren-, Tracheanaht *f*, Tracheorrhaphie *f.*
tra·che·os·chi·sis [ˌ-ˈɑskəsɪs] *n embryo.* kongenitale Luftröhrenspalte *f*, Tracheoschisis *f.*
tra·che·o·scope [ˈtreɪkɪəskoʊp] *n* Tracheoskop *nt.*
tra·che·o·scop·ic [ˌ-ˈskɑpɪk] *adj* Tracheoskopie betr., tracheoskopisch.
tra·che·os·co·py [ˌtreɪkɪˈɑskəpɪ] *n* Luftröhrenspiegelung *f*, Tracheoskopie *f.*
tra·che·os·te·no·sis [ˌtreɪkɪɑstɪˈnoʊsɪs] *n* Einengung *f* der Luftröhre, Tracheal-, Tracheostenose *f.*
tra·che·os·to·ma [ˌtreɪkɪɑsˈtoʊmə] *n chir., HNO* Tracheostoma *nt.*
tra·che·os·to·mize [ˌtreɪkɪˈɑstəmaɪz] *vt* eine Tracheostomie durchführen, ein Tracheostoma anlegen, tracheostomieren.
tra·che·os·to·my [ˌ-ˈɑstəmɪ] *n chir., HNO* 1. Tracheostomie *f.* 2. Tracheostoma *nt.*
tracheostomy tube Tracheostomiekanüle *f.*
tra·che·o·tome [ˈtreɪkɪətoʊm] *n chir., HNO* Tracheotom *nt.*
tra·che·ot·o·mize [ˌtreɪkɪˈɑtəmaɪz] *vt* eine Tracheotomie durchführen, tracheotomieren.
tra·che·ot·o·my [ˌ-ˈɑtəmɪ] *n chir., HNO* Luftröhrenschnitt *m*, Tracheotomie *f*, -tomia *f.*
tra·chi·tis [trəˈkaɪtɪs] *n* → tracheitis.
tra·cho·ma [trəˈkoʊmə] *n, pl* **-ma·ta** [-mətə] Trachom(a) *nt*, ägyptische Körnerkrankheit *f*, trachomatöse Einschlußkonjunktivitis *f*, Conjunctivitis (granulosa) trachomatosa.
trachoma bodies Prowazek-(Einschluß-)Körperchen *pl*, Halberstädter-Prowazek-(Einschluß)Körperchen *pl.*
trachoma glands *ophthal.* Bruch'-Drüsen *pl*, -Follikel *pl.*
tra·chom·a·tous [trəˈkɑmətəs, -ˈkoʊmə-] *adj* Trachom betr., trachomartig, trachomatös, Trachom-.
trachomatous conjunctivitis → trachoma.
trachomatous keratitis Pannus trachomatosus.
trachoma virus *old* → Chlamydia trachomatis.
tra·chy·chro·mat·ic [ˌtreɪkɪkroʊˈmætɪk, ˌtræk-] *adj* (*Kern*) dunkelfärbend.
tra·chy·pho·nia [ˌ-ˈfoʊnɪə] *n* Rauhheit *f* der Stimme, Trachyphonie *f*; Heiserheit *f.*
trac·ing [ˈtreɪsɪŋ] *n* 1. Suchen *nt*, Nachforschung *f.* 2. (Auf-)Zeichnung *f*; Zeichnung *f*, (Auf-)Riß *m.* 3. (Auf-)Zeichnen *nt.*

tract [trækt] *n* 1. *anat.* Trakt *m*, System *nt*, Traktus *m*, Tractus *m.* 2. *anat.* Zug *m*, Strang *m*, Bahn *f*, Traktus *m*, Tractus *m.* 3. Zeitraum *m*, -spanne *f*, Intervall *nt.* 4. Fläche *f*, Strecke *f*, Gebiet *nt.*
  t.s of anterior funiculus Vorderstrangbahnen *pl.*
  t.s of anterolateral funiculus Vorderseitenstrangbahnen *pl.*
  t. of Bruce and Muir Bruce'-Faserbündel *nt*, Fasciculus septomarginalis.
  t.s of dorsal funiculus Hinterstrangbahnen *pl.*
  t.s of lateral funiculus Seitenstrangbahnen *pl.*
  t. of Münzer and Wiener Tractus tectopontinus.
  t. of Philippe-Gombault Gombault-Philippe'-Triangel *f*, Philippe-Gombault'-Triangel *f.*
  t.s of posterior funiculus → t.s of dorsal funiculus.
  t. of spiral foramen Tractus spiralis foraminosus.
  t.s of ventral funiculus → t.s of anterior funiculus.
  t. of Vicq d'Azyr Vicq d'Azyr'-Bündel *nt*, Fasciculus mamillothalamicus.
trac·tion [ˈtrækʃn] *n* 1. Ziehen *nt.* 2. *phys.* Zug *m.* 3. *physiol.* Zug *m*, Zusammenziehen *nt*, Traktion *f.* 4. *ortho.* Zug *m*, Extension *f*, Traktion *f.*
traction aneurysm Traktionsaneurysma *nt.*
traction diverticulum Traktionsdivertikel *nt.*
traction therapy *ortho.* Extensionsbehandlung *f.*
traction tongs *ortho.* Extensionsklammer *f.*
trac·tot·o·my [trækˈtɑtəmɪ] *n neurochir.* Traktusdurchtrennung *f*, Traktotomie *f.*
trac·tus [ˈtræktəs] *n, pl* **trac·tus** → tract 1., 2.
trag·a·canth [ˈtrægəkænθ, ˈtrædʒ-] *n* Tragant *m.*
trag·a·can·tha [ˈ-kænθə] *n* → tragacanth.
tra·gal [ˈtreɪgl] *adj* Tragus betr., Tragus-.
tragi [ˈtreɪdʒaɪ] *pl* Haare *pl* des äußeren Gehörgangs, Büschelhaare *pl*, Tragi *pl.*
tra·gi·cus (**muscle**) [ˈtreɪdʒɪkəs] M. tragicus.
trag·i·on [ˈtrædʒɪɑn] *n anat.* Tragion *nt.*
trag·o·mas·chal·ia [ˌtrægəmæsˈkælɪə] *n* Brom(h)idrosis *f.*
trag·o·pho·nia [ˌ-ˈfoʊnɪə] *n* → tragophony.
tra·goph·o·ny [trəˈgɑfənɪ] *n* Ziegenmeckern *nt*, Kompressionsatmen *nt*, Ägophonie *f.*
trag·o·po·dia [ˌtrægəˈpoʊdɪə] *n* X-Bein *nt*, Genu valgum.
tra·gus [ˈtreɪgəs] *n, pl* **-gi** [-dʒaɪ] 1. Tragus *m.* 2. **~gi** *pl* → tragi.
train [treɪn] **I** *n fig.* Reihe *f*, Kette *f*, Folge *f*; *phys.* Serie *f*, Reihe *f.* **II** *v* 1. jdn. erziehen *od.* aufziehen; jdn. ausbilden *od.* unterrichten; (*Tier*) abrichten. 2. (*Sport*) trainieren.
train·a·bil·i·ty [ˌtreɪnəˈbɪlətɪ] *n* Trainierbarkeit *f*; Lern-, Ausbildungsfähigkeit *f.*
train·a·ble [ˈtreɪnəbl] *adj* trainierbar; ausbildbar, erziehbar.
trained [treɪnd] *adj* ausgebildet, geschult, gelernt, Fach-, (*Tier*) dressiert.
trained nurse diplomierte/geprüfte (Kranken-)Schwester *f.*
trained reflex erworbener/bedingter Reflex *m.*
train·ee [treɪˈniː] *n* Auszubildende(r *m*) *f*; Praktikant(in *f*) *m.*
trainee nurse Krankenpflegeschüler(in *f*) *m.*

train·er ['treɪnər] *n* Ausbilder(in *f*) *m*, Lehrer(in *f*) *m*; (*Sport*) Trainer(in *f*) *m*.
train·ing ['treɪnɪŋ] **I** *n* **1.** Schulung *f*, Ausbildung *f*; Üben *nt*. **2.** (*Sport*) Training *nt*; Trainieren *nt*. **to be in ~** durchtrainiert/fit sein, gut in Form sein; trainieren. **to be out of ~** nicht in Form sein. **II** *adj* Schulungs-, Ausbildungs-, Trainings-.
training course Ausbildungskurs *m*.
trait [treɪt] *n* Merkmal *nt*, Eigenschaft *f*.
tra·ma·dol ['træmədəl, -dɔl] *n pharm.* Tramadol *nt*.
tra·maz·o·line [trə'mæzəli:n] *n pharm.* Tramazolin *nt*.
trance [træns, trɑ:ns] *n* Trance *f*.
tran·ex·am·ic acid [ˌtrænek'sæmɪk] *pharm.* Tranexamsäure *f*.
tran·quil ['træŋkwɪl] *adj* **1.** ruhig, friedlich; gelassen. **2.** heiter.
tran·quil·i·ty [træŋ'kwɪlətɪ] *n* **1.** Ruhe *f*, Frieden *m*; Gelassenheit *f*. **2.** Heiterkeit *f*.
tran·quil·i·za·tion [ˌtræŋkwəlɪ'zeɪʃn] *n* Beruhigung *f*, Sedierung *f*.
tran·quil·ize ['træŋkwəlaɪz] **I** *vt* beruhigen, sedieren. **II** *vi* s. beruhigen.
tran·quil·iz·er ['træŋkwəlaɪzər] *n pharm.* Tranquilizer *m*, Tranquillantium *nt*.
tran·quil·iz·ing agent ['træŋkwəlaɪzɪŋ] → tranquilizer.
trans- *pref. chem., genet.* trans-.
trans [trænz] *adj chem., genet.* trans.
trans·ab·dom·i·nal [ˌtrænsæb'dɑmɪnl, ˌtrænz-] *adj* durch die Bauchwand, transabdominal, -abdominell.
trans·a·cet·y·lase [-ə'setəleɪz] *n* Transacetylase *f*, Acyltransferase *f*.
trans·a·cet·y·la·tion [-əˌsetə'leɪʃn] *n chem.* Transacetylierung *f*.
trans·ac·tion·al analysis [træn'sækʃənl, -zæk-] *psychia.* Transaktionsanalyse *f*.
trans·ac·yl·ase [ˌtræns'æsəleɪz, ˌtrænz-] *n* Acyltransferase *f*, Transacylase *f*.
trans·al·do·lase [-'ældəleɪz] *n* Transaldolase *f*.
trans·am·i·nase [-'æmɪneɪz] *n* Aminotransferase *f*, Transaminase *f*.
trans·am·i·nate [-'æmɪneɪt] *vt* transaminieren.
trans·am·i·na·tion [-ˌæmɪ'neɪʃn] *n* Transaminierung *f*.
trans·an·i·ma·tion [-ˌænɪ'meɪʃn] *n* **1.** Mund-zu-Mund-Beatmung *f*. **2.** *ped.* Reanimation *f* eines totgeborenen Säuglings.
trans·aor·tic [-eɪ'ɔ:rtɪk] *adj* durch die Aorta, transaortal.
trans·a·tri·al [-'eɪtrɪəl] *adj* durch den Vorhof, transatrial.
trans·au·di·ent [-'ɔ:dɪənt] *adj* schalldurchlässig.
trans·ba·sal [-'beɪsl] *adj* durch die Basis, transbasal.
trans·ca·lent [-'keɪlənt] *adj* wärmedurchlässig, diatherman.
trans·cap·il·lar·y [-'kæpəˌlerɪ:, -kə'pɪlərɪ] *adj* transkapillär.
trans·cap·si·da·tion [-ˌkæpsə'deɪʃn] *n micro.* Transkapsidation *f*.
trans·car·bam·o·y·lase [-ˌkɑ:r'bæməwɪleɪz] *n* Carbam(o)yltransferase *f*.
trans·car·box·yl·ase [-ˌkɑ:r'bɑksɪleɪz] *n* Carboxyltransferase *f abbr.* CT, Transcarboxylase *f*.
trans·cel·lu·lar [-'seljələr] *adj* transzellulär.
transcellular fluid transzelluläre Flüssigkeit *f*.
transcellular transport transzellulärer Transport *m*.
trans·cer·vi·cal [-'sɜ:rvɪkl] *adj gyn.* durch die Zervix, transzervikal.

trans·co·bal·a·min [-ˌkoʊ'bæləmɪn] *n abbr.* **TC** Transcobalamin *nt abbr.* TC, Vitamin-B_{12}-bindendes Globulin *nt*.
trans·con·dy·lar [-'kɑndɪlər] *adj* durch die Kondylen, transkondylär.
transcondylar fracture transkondyläre Fraktur *f*.
trans·con·dy·loid [-'kɑndɪlɔɪd] *adj* → transcondylar.
trans configuration *chem., genet.* trans-Konfiguration *f*.
trans·cor·ti·cal [-'kɔ:rtɪkl] *adj* transkortikal.
transcortical aphasia transkortikale Aphasie *f*.
motor t. transkortikale motorische Aphasie.
sensory t. transkortikale sensorische Aphasie.
transcortical apraxia ideokinetische/ideomotorische Apraxie *f*.
transcortical loop *physiol.* transkortikale (Funktions-)Schleife *f*.
trans·cor·tin [-'kɔ:rtɪn] *n* Transkortin *nt*, -cortin *nt*, Cortisol-bindendes Globulin *nt abbr.* CBG.
tran·scribe [træn'skraɪb] *vt* **1.** abschreiben, kopieren. **2.** *biochem., genet.* übertragen, umschreiben, transkribieren.
trans·cript ['trænskrɪpt] *n genet.* Abschrift *f*, Kopie *f*, Transcript *f*.
tran·scrip·tase [træn'skrɪpteɪz] *n* Transkriptase *f*, DNA-abhängige RNApolymerase *f*.
tran·scrip·tion [træn'skrɪpʃn] *n genet.* Transkription *f*.
tran·scrip·tion·al [træn'skrɪpʃənl] *adj* Transkription betr., Transkriptions-.
transcriptional control Transkriptionskontrolle *f*.
transcription fork *biochem., genet.* Transkriptionsgabel *f*.
trans·cul·tu·ral psychiatry [ˌtræns'kʌltʃ(ə)rəl, ˌtrænz-] transkulturelle Psychiatrie *f*.
trans·cu·ta·ne·ous [-ˌkju:'teɪnɪəs] *adj* durch die Haut, transkutan, perkutan, transdermal.
trans·der·mal [-'dɜ:rml] *adj* → transcutaneous.
trans·der·mic [-'dɜ:rmɪk] *adj* → transcutaneous.
trans·duc·er [-'d(j)u:sər] *n phys.* (Um-)Wandler *m*, Umformer *m*, Transducer *m*; Transformator *m*.
trans·duc·i·ble [-'d(j)u:sɪbl] *adj* transduzierbar.
transducible gene transduzierbares Gen *nt*.
trans·duc·ing [-'d(j)u:sɪŋ] *adj* transduzierend.
transducing phage *micro.* transduzierender Phage *m*.
trans·duc·tion [-'dʌkʃn] *n* **1.** *genet.* Transduktion *f*. **2.** *physiol.* Transformation *f*.
transduction process *genet., biochem.* Transduktionsprozeß *m*.
trans·du·o·de·nal [-ˌd(j)u:oʊ'di:nl] *adj* durch das Duodenum, transduodenal.
transduodenal sphincteroplasty *chir.* transduodenale Plastik *f* des Sphinkter Oddii.
trans·du·ral [-'d(j)ʊərəl] *adj* durch die Dura mater, transdural.
tran·sect [træn'sekt] *vt* durchschneiden.
tran·sec·tion [træn'sekʃn] *n* **1.** Querschnitt *m*. **2.** Durchtrennung *f*.
t. of fascia Faszienspaltung *f*, -schnitt *f*, Fasziotomie *f*.
t. of the thoracic aorta Querriß *m* der Aorta thoracica.
trans·ep·i·der·mal [ˌtrænsepɪ'dɜ:rml,

ˌtrænz-] *adj* durch die Epidermis, transepidermal.
trans·eth·moi·dal [-eθ'mɔɪdl] *adj* durch das Siebbein, transethmoidal.
trans·fec·tion [-'fekʃn] *n micro., genet.* Transfektion *f*.
trans·fer [*n* 'trænsfɜr; *v* træns'fɜr] **I** *n* **1.** Übertragung *f*, Verlagerung *f*, Transfer *m* (*to* auf). **2.** (*Patient*) Verlegung *f* (*to* nach, zu; *in, into* in). **II** *vt* übertragen, verlagern, transferieren (*to* auf); (*Patient*) verlegen (*to* nach, zu; *in, into* in); überweisen (*to* an).
trans·fer·a·bil·i·ty [trænsˌfɜrə'bɪlətɪ] *n* Übertragbarkeit *f*.
trans·fer·a·ble [træns'fɜrəbl] *adj* übertragbar.
trans·fer·ase ['trænsfəreɪz] *n* Transferase *f*.
transfer coefficient: convective heat t. *abbr.* h_c konnektive Wärmeübergangszahl *f abbr.* h_c.
evaporative heat t. *abbr.* h_e Wärmeübergangszahl *f* für Evaporation *abbr.* h_e.
radiation heat t. *abbr.* h_r Wärmeübergangszahl *f* für Strahlung *abbr.* h_r.
trans·fer·ence [træns'fɜrəns, 'trænsfɜr-] *n* **1.** → transfer I. **2.** *psycho.* Übertragung *f*.
transference neurosis Übertragung *f*, Übertragungsneurose *f*.
transfer factor *abbr.* **TF** Transferfaktor *m abbr.* TF.
transfer host Hilfs-, Transport-, Wartewirt *m*, paratenischer Wirt *m*.
transfer potential Übertragungspotential *nt*.
transferred ophthalmia [træns'fɜrt] sympathische Ophthalmie *f*, Ophthalmia sympathica.
trans·fer·rin [træns'ferɪn] *n* Transferrin *nt*, Siderophilin *nt*.
trans·fer·ring enzyme [træns'fɜrɪŋ] → transferase.
transfer-RNA *n abbr.* **tRNA** Transfer-RNS *f abbr.* tRNS, Tranfer-RNA *f abbr.* tRNA.
initiator t. Initiator-tRNA, Starter-tRNA.
trans·fix [træns'fɪks] *vt* durchstechen, -bohren, -dringen.
trans·fix·ion [træns'fɪkʃn] *n* Durchstechen *nt*, -bohren *nt*, -dringung *f*, Transfixion *f*.
trans·form [træns'fɔ:rm] **I** *vt* umwandeln, -bilden, -gestalten, -formen, überführen (*from into* von in); *electr.* transformieren. **II** *vi* s. verwandeln (*into* zu).
trans·for·ma·tion [ˌtrænsfər'meɪʃn] *n* Umwandlung *f*, Umbildung *f*, Umgestaltung *f*, Umformung *f*, Umsetzung *f*; (*a. electr., mathe.*) Transformation *f*.
transformation gastritis Umbaugastritis *f*.
transformation zone Umwandlungs-, Transformationszone *f*.
trans·form·ing gene [ˌtræns'fɔ:rmɪŋ] Onkogen *nt*.
trans·fruc·to·syl·ase [-ˌfrʌktoʊ'sɪleɪz] *n* Fruktosyltransferase *f*.
trans·fuse [-'fju:z] *vt* (*Blut*) übertragen, transfundieren, eine Transfusion vornehmen.
trans·fu·sion [-'fju:ʒn] *n* (Blut-)Transfusion *f*, Blutübertragung *f*.
transfusion hepatitis 1. Posttransfusionshepatitis *f*. **2.** (Virus-)Hepatitis B *f abbr.* HB, Serumhepatitis *f*.
transfusion immunology Transfusionsimmunologie *f*.
transfusion nephritis Transfusionsnephropathie *f*.
transfusion reaction Transfusionszwischenfall *m*.

hemolytic t. hämolytischer Transfusionszwischenfall.
transfusion syndrome fetofetale Transfusion f.
trans·glu·co·syl·ase [ˌ-'gluːkəʊsɪleɪz] n Glykosyltransferase f.
trans·glu·tam·in·ase [ˌ-gluː'tæmɪneɪz] n **1.** Transglutaminase f. **2.** Faktor XIIIa m.
trans·gly·co·si·da·tion [ˌ-ˌglaɪkəsɪ'deɪʃn] n Transglykosidierung f.
trans·gly·co·syl·ase [ˌ-'glaɪkəʊsɪleɪz] n → transglucosylase.
trans·he·pat·ic [ˌ-hɪ'pætɪk] adj durch die Leber, transhepatisch.
transhepatic portography transhepatische Portographie f.
trans·hi·a·tal [ˌ-haɪ'eɪtl] adj durch einen Hiatus, transhiatal.
trans·hy·dro·gen·ase [ˌ-'haɪdrədʒəneɪz, -haɪ'drɒdʒəneɪz] n Transhydrogenase f.
tran·sient ['trænʃənt, -zɪənt] **I** n flüchtige/transiente Erscheinung f, transientes Symptom nt. **II** adj vergänglich, flüchtig, kurz(dauernd), unbeständig, vorübergehend, transient; transitorisch.
transient acantholytic dermatosis Morbus Grover m, transitorische akantholytische Dermatose f.
transient albuminuria transiente Albuminurie/Proteinurie f.
transient dendrite embryo. vorläufiger/transienter Dendrit m.
transient flora micro. Transientflora f.
transient hypogammaglobulinemia of infancy ped. vorübergehende/transitorische/transiente Hypogammaglobulinämie f des Kindesalters.
transient ischemic attack abbr. **TIA** transitorische ischämische Attacke f abbr. TIA.
transient mild hyperphenylalaninemia Hyperphenylalaninämie f Typ III, transitorische Hyperphenylalaninämie f.
transient myopia ophthal. vorübergehende/transiente Myopie f.
transient proteinuria → transient albuminuria.
transient situational disturbance akute Stressreaktion f.
trans·il·i·ac [ˌtræns'ɪlɪæk, ˌtrænz-] adj → transilial.
trans·il·i·al [ˌ-'ɪlɪəl] adj transiliakal.
transilial biopsy transiliakale (Knochen-)Biopsie f.
trans·il·lu·mi·na·tion [ˌ-ɪˌluːmə'neɪʃn] n radiol. Durchleuchten nt, Transillumination f, Diaphanie f, Diaphanoskopie f.
trans·in·su·lar [ˌ-'ɪns(j)ələr] adj transinsulär.
tran·sis·tor [træn'zɪstər] n Transistor m.
tran·sit ['trænsɪt, -zɪt] n Durchgang m, Durchtritt m, Passage f.
tran·si·tion [træn'zɪʃn] n **1.** Übertragung f (from, to von, zu; into in); Übergangszeit f, -stadium nt, Wechsel m. **2.** genet. Transition f.
tran·si·tion·al [træn'sɪʒnl, -'zɪʃn-] adj vorübergehend, Übergangs-, Überleitungs-, Zwischen-.
transitional cell Übergangszelle f.
transitional cell carcinoma Übergangszell-, Transitionalzellkarzinom nt, Ca. transitiocellulare.
transitional cell papilloma Übergangsepithelpapillom nt.
transitional cortex Übergangs-, Mesocortex m.
transitional dentition Übergangsgebiß nt.
transitional epithelium Übergangsepithel nt.
transitional leukocyte old → monocyte.
transitional mutation → transition 2.

transitional respiration bronchovesikuläres/vesikobronchiales Atmen nt.
transitional stage Übergangsstadium nt.
transitional zone Übergangszone f.
tran·si·tio·a·ry [træn'zɪʃəˌnerɪ, -'sɪʒ-, -ʃnərɪ] adj → transitional.
transition state Übergangszustand m.
tran·si·to·ry ['trænsɪtɒːriː, -təʊ-] adj (zeitlich) vorübergehend, transitorisch.
transitory functional albuminuria paroxysmale Albuminurie/Proteinurie f.
transitory functional proteinuria → transitory functional albuminuria.
transitory nystagmus transitorischer Nystagmus m.
trans·ke·to·lase [ˌtræns'kiːtəleɪz, ˌtrænz-] n Transketolase f abbr. TK.
trans·lab·y·rin·thine [ˌtrænsˌlæbə'rɪnθɪn, -θiːn, ˌtrænz-] adj translabyrinthär.
trans·la·tion [ˌ-'leɪʃn] n **1.** genet. Translation f. **2.** ophthal. Translationsbewegung f, Translation f. **3.** (a. techn.) Übertragung f, Übersetzung f (into in).
trans·la·tion·al [ˌ-'leɪʃnl] adj Übersetzungs-, Translations-.
translational acceleration Translationsbeschleunigung f.
translational control Translationskontrolle f.
translational movement Translationsbewegung f.
trans·lo·case [ˌ-'ləʊkeɪz] n Translokase f.
trans·lo·ca·tion [ˌ-ləʊ'keɪʃn] n **1.** genet. Translokation f. **2.** chir. Verlagerung f, Verpflanzung f, Translokation f.
trans·lu·cence [ˌ-'luːsns] n Lichtdurchsigkeit f, Transluzenz f, Durchsichtigkeit f; Durchscheinen nt.
trans·lu·cen·cy [ˌ-'luːsnsɪ] n → translucence.
trans·lu·cent [ˌ-'luːsnt] adj **1.** (licht-)durchlässig, durchscheinend, -sichtig, milchig, transluzent, -luzid. **2.** fig. leicht verständlich, eingängig.
translucent layer of epidermis Stratum lucidum epidermidis.
trans·lum·bar aortography [ˌ-'lʌmbər] translumbale Aortographie f.
trans·max·il·la·ry [ˌ-'mæksəˌlerɪ, -mæk'sɪlərɪ] adj transmaxillär.
trans·mem·brane potential [ˌ-'membreɪn] transmembranöses Potential nt.
trans·meth·yl·ase [ˌ-'meθɪleɪz] n Methyltransferase f, Transmethylase f.
trans·meth·yl·a·tion [ˌ-meθə'leɪʃn] n chem. Transmethylierung f.
trans·mi·gra·tion [ˌ-maɪ'greɪʃn] n Auswandern nt, Überwanderung f, Transmigration f.
trans·mis·si·bil·i·ty [ˌ-ˌmɪsə'bɪlɪtɪ] n **1.** Übertragbarkeit f. **2.** phys. Durchlässigkeit f.
trans·mis·si·ble [ˌ-'mɪsəbl] adj **1.** übertragbar (to auf); ansteckend. **2.** genet. vererblich.
transmissible spongiform encephalopathy subakute spongiforme (Virus-)Enzephalopathie f.
trans·mis·sion [ˌ-'mɪʃn] n **1.** micro., genet. Übertragung f, Ansteckung f, Transmission f. **2.** phys. Durchstrahlung f, Durchgang m, Durchlässigkeit f, Transmission f. **3.** physiol. Über-, Weiterleitung f, Fortpflanzung f; phys. Übertragung f, Transmisssion f. **4.** Übersendung f, -mittlung f, -tragung f.
transmission deafness Mittelohrschwerhörigkeit f, -taubheit f, Schalleitungsstörung f, -schwerhörigkeit f.
trans·mit [ˌ-'mɪt] vt **1.** (Krankheit) übertragen; bio. vererben. **2.** physiol. (Reflexe) fortleiten. **3.** phys. (Wärme) fort-, weiter-

leiten; (Schall) fortpflanzen; (Kraft) übertragen.
trans·mit·ta·ble [ˌ-'mɪtəbl] adj → transmissible.
trans·mit·tance [ˌ-'mɪtns] n **1.** phys. (Licht-)Durchlässigkeit f, Transmission f. **2.** micro. Übertragung f, Transmission f.
trans·mit·ter [ˌ-'mɪtər] n Übertrager m, -mittler m; physiol. Überträgersubstanz f, Transmitter m.
transmitter organelle Transmitterorganelle f.
transmitter substance Transmittersubstanz f.
trans·mit·ting [ˌ-'mɪtɪŋ] adj übertragend, transmittierend.
trans·mu·ral [ˌ-'mjʊərəl] adj transmural.
transmural granulomatous enteritis/ileocolitis Crohn'-Krankheit f, Morbus Crohn m, Enteritis regionalis, Ileocolitis regionalis/terminalis, Ileitis regionalis/terminalis.
transmural inflammatory disease of the colon Colitis regionalis, Enteritis regionalis Crohn des Dickdarms.
transmural pressure transmuraler Druck m.
trans·mut·a·ble [ˌ-'mjuːtəbl] adj chem., bio. umwandelbar.
trans·mu·ta·tion [ˌ-mjuː'teɪʃn] n bio., chem. Umbildung f, Umwandlung f, Transmutation f.
trans·mu·ta·tive [ˌ-'mjuːtətɪv] adj umwandelnd.
trans·mute [ˌ-'mjuːt] vt ver-, umwandeln, transmutieren (into in).
trans·na·sal [ˌ-'neɪzl] adj durch die Nase/Nasenhöhle, transnasal.
trans·neu·ron·al [ˌ-'njʊərənl, -njʊə'rəʊnl, -nəʊ-] adj transneuronal.
transneuronal atrophy/degeneration transneuronale/transsynaptische Degeneration f.
trans·oc·u·lar [ˌ-'ɒkjələr] adj transokulär.
trans·o·nance ['trænsənəns] n Transonanz f.
tran·son·ic [træn'sɒnɪk] adj phys. transsonisch, Überschall-.
trans·or·bit·al lobotomy [ˌtræns'ɔːrbɪtl, ˌtrænz-] transorbitale Leukotomie/Lobotomie f.
trans·o·var·i·al [ˌ-əʊ'veərɪəl] adj transovarial.
trans·o·var·i·an [ˌ-əʊ'veərɪən] adj → transovarial.
trans·par·en·cy [ˌ-'peərənsɪ] n **1.** (Licht-)Durchlässigkeit f, Durchsichtigkeit f, Transparenz f. **2.** Dia nt, Diapositiv nt.
trans·par·ent [ˌ-'peərənt] adj (licht-)durchlässig, durchsichtig, transparent.
trans·pa·ri·e·tal [ˌ-pə'raɪɪtl] adj transparietal.
trans·pep·ti·dase [ˌ-'peptɪdeɪz] n Transpeptidase f.
trans·pep·ti·da·tion [ˌ-peptɪ'deɪʃn] n Transpeptidierung f.
transpeptidation enzyme Transpeptidase f.
trans·per·i·ne·al [ˌ-perɪ'niːəl] adj transperineal.
trans·per·i·to·ne·al [ˌ-ˌperɪtəʊ'niːəl] adj durch das Peritoneum, transperitoneal.
transperitoneal approach chir. transperitonealer Zugang m.
trans·phos·pho·ryl·ase [ˌ-fɒs'fɔːreɪz, -'fɒrə-] n **1.** Phosphotransferase f. **2.** Phosphorylase f.
trans·phos·pho·ry·la·tion [ˌ-fɒsˌfɒrɪ'leɪʃn] n biochem. Transphosphorylierung f.
tran·spi·ra·tion [ˌtrænspɪ'reɪʃn] n **1.** Ausdünstung f, Diaphorese f, Transpiration

f; Schwitzen *nt*; Schweiß *m*. 2. Absonderung *f*, Ausdünstung *f*.
tran·spire [træn'spaɪər] I *vt* ausdünsten, -schwitzen. II *vi physiol.* schwitzen, transpirieren.
trans·pla·cen·tal [ˌtrænspləˈsentl, ˌtrænz-] *adj* durch die Plazenta, transplazentar, diaplazentar.
transplacental infection transplazentare/diaplazentare Infektion *f*.
trans·plant [*n* 'trænsplænt; *v* træns'plænt] I *n* 1. Transplantat *nt*. 2. → transplantation. II *vt* um-, verpflanzen, übertragen, transplantieren.
trans·plant·a·bil·i·ty [ˌtrænsˌplæntəˈbɪlətɪ] *n* Transplantierbarkeit *f*.
trans·plant·a·ble [ˌ-ˈplæntəbl] *adj* transplantabel, transplantierbar.
trans·plan·tar [ˌ-ˈplæntər] *adj* transplantar.
trans·plan·ta·tion [ˌ-plænˈteɪʃn] *n* Ein-, Um-, Verpflanzung *f*, (Gewebe-, Organ-)Transplantation *f*, (-)Übertragung *f*.
transplantation antigens Transplantationsantigene *pl*, Histokompatibilitätsantigene *pl*, human leukocyte antigens *abbr*. HLA.
transplantation immunobiology Transplantationsimmunobiologie *f*.
transplantation metastasis Transplantationsmetastase *f*.
transplant recipient Transplantatempfänger(in *f*) *m*.
transplant rejection Transplantatabstoßung *f*.
transplant surgeon Transplantationschirurg *m*, -chirurgin *f*.
trans·pleu·ral [ˌtrænsˈplʊərəl, ˌtrænz-] *adj* durch die Pleura, transpleural.
trans·port [*n* 'trænspɔːrt, -ˌpoʊrt; *v* trænˈspɔːrt] I *n* Transport *m*, Beförderung *f*. II *vt* transportieren, befördern.
trans·port·a·bil·i·ty [ˌ-ˌpɔːrtəˈbɪlətɪ] *n* Transportfähigkeit *f*.
trans·port·a·ble [ˌ-ˈpɔːrtəbl] *adj* transportfähig, transportierbar.
trans·por·ta·tion [ˌ-pərˈteɪʃn] *n* → transport I.
transport host *micro.* Hilfs-, Transport-, Wartewirt *m*, paratenischer Wirt *m*.
transport lipoprotein Transportlipoprotein *nt*.
transport maximum *abbr.* **Tm** *physiol.* Transportmaximum *nt abbr.* Tm.
transport medium *micro.* Transportmedium *nt*.
Amies t. Amies-Transportmedium.
Carry-Blair t. Carry-Blair-Transportmedium.
transport potential Transportpotential *nt*.
transport process Transportprozeß *m*.
transport protein Transportprotein *nt*.
transport system Transportsystem *nt*.
membrane t. Membrantransportsystem.
transport vesicle Transportvesikel *nt*.
transport work *physiol.* Transportarbeit *f*.
trans·po·si·tion [ˌ-pəˈzɪʃn] *n* 1. *chem.*, *genet.* Umstellung *f*, Transposition *f*. 2. *chem.* Umlagerung *f*, Transposition *f*. 3. *chir., anat.* (Gewebe-, Organ-)Verlagerung *f*, Transposition *f*, Translokation *f*.
t. of great arteries *abbr.* TGA → t. of great vessels.
t. of great vessels *abbr.* TGV card., ped. Transposition der großen Arterien/Gefäße *abbr.* TGA.
trans·po·son [ˌ-ˈpoʊzɒn] *n* Transposon *nt*.
trans·pu·bic [ˌ-ˈpjuːbɪk] *adj* durch das Schambein, transpubisch.
trans·pul·mo·nar·y pressure [ˌ-ˈpʌlməˌnerɪ, -nərɪ, ˈpʊl-] transpulmonaler Druck *m*.

trans·py·lor·ic plane [ˌtrænspaɪˈlɔːrɪk, -ˈlɑr-, ˌtrænz-] *anat.* Planum transpyloricum.
trans·sa·cral [ˌ-ˈseɪkrəl, -ˈsæk-] *adj* durch das Kreuzbein, transsakral.
transsacral approach *chir.* transsakraler Zugang *m*.
trans·scro·tal orchiopexy [ˌ-ˈskroʊtəl] *urol.* Ombrédanne-Operation *f*, transskrotale Orchidopexie *f*.
trans·sec·tion [ˌ-ˈsekʃn] *n* → transection.
trans·seg·men·tal [ˌ-segˈmentl] *adj* transsegmental.
trans·sep·tal [ˌ-ˈseptl] *adj* transseptal.
trans·sex·u·al [ˌ-ˈsekʃəwəl] I *n* Transsexuelle(r *m*) *f*. II *adj* transsexuell.
trans·sex·u·a·lism [ˌ-ˈsekʃəwælɪzəm] *n* Transsexualismus *m*.
trans·sphe·noi·dal [ˌ-sfiːˈnɔɪdl] *adj* durch das Keilbein/Os sphenoidale, transsphenoidal.
transsphenoidal hypophysectomy *neurochir.* transsphenoidale Hypophysenentfernung/Hypophysektomie *f*.
trans·ster·nal [ˌ-ˈstɜrnl] *adj* durch das Brustbein/Sternum, transsternal.
trans·suc·ci·nyl·ase [ˌ-sʌkˈsɪnəleɪz] *n* Dihydrolipoylsuccinyltransferase *f*.
trans·syn·ap·tic [ˌ-sɪˈnæptɪk] *adj* transsynaptisch.
transsynaptic chromatolysis transneuronale/transsynaptische Degeneration *f*.
transsynaptic degeneration → transsynaptic chromatolysis.
trans·tem·po·ral [ˌ-ˈtemp(ə)rəl] *adj* transtemporal.
trans·tha·lam·ic [ˌ-θəˈlæmɪk] *adj* transthalamisch.
trans·ther·mia [ˌ-ˈθɜrmɪə] *n* → thermopenetration.
trans·tho·rac·ic [ˌ-θəˈræsɪk] *adj* durch den Brustkorb/Thorax *od.* die Brusthöhle, transthorakal.
transthoracic pressure transthorakaler Druck *m*.
trans·tra·che·al [ˌ-ˈtreɪkɪəl] *adj* durch die Luftröhre/Trachea, transtracheal.
transtracheal aspiration transtracheale Aspiration *f*.
trans·tym·pan·ic [ˌ-tɪmˈpænɪk] *adj* transtympanal.
tran·su·date ['trænsʊdeɪt] *n* Transsudat *nt*.
tran·su·da·tion [ˌtrænsʊˈdeɪʃn] *n* 1. → transudate. 2. Transsudation *f*.
tran·su·da·tive ascites [trænˈsuːdətɪv] Aszites *m* durch Transsudat.
trans·u·ran·ic elements [ˌtrænsjʊəˈrænɪk, ˌtrænz-] Transurane *pl*.
trans·u·re·ter·o·u·re·ter·os·to·my [ˌ-jʊəˌriːtərəjəˌriːtəˈrɒstəmɪ] *n urol.* Transureteroureterostomie *f*.
trans·u·re·thral [ˌ-jʊəˈriːθrəl] *adj* durch die Harnröhre/Urethra, transurethral.
transurethral prostatectomy *urol.* transurethrale Prostatektomie *f*.
trans·vag·i·nal [ˌ-ˈvædʒɪnl] *adj* durch die Scheide/Vagina, transvaginal.
trans·va·te·ri·an [ˌ-fɑːˈtɪərɪən] *adj* durch die Vater'-Papille, transpapillär.
trans·vec·tor [ˌ-ˈvektər] *n* Transvektor *m*.
trans·ven·tric·u·lar [ˌ-venˈtrɪkjələr] *adj* durch die Kammer/den Ventrikel, transventrikulär.
trans·verse [ˌ-ˈvɜrs, -ˈvɜrs] *adj* quer, quer(ver)laufend, -stehend, schräg, diagonal (*to* zu); transversal, Quer-.
transverse arch of foot Fußquergewölbe *nt*.
transverse artery: t. of face Transversa *f* faciei, A. transversa faciei/facialis.
t. of neck Transversa *f* colli, A. transversa (colli).

transverse articulation of rib Kostotransversalgelenk *nt*, Artic. costotransversaria.
transverse axis *bio., mathe.* Querachse *f*.
transverse branch: t. of lateral circumflex femoral artery Ramus transversus a. circumflexae femoris lateralis.
t. of medial circumflex femoral artery Ramus transversus a. circumflexae femoris medialis.
transverse bundles of palmar aponeurosis Fasciculi transversi aponeurosis palmaris.
transverse colon Querkolon *nt*, Colon transversum.
transverse colostomy *chir.* Transversokolostomie *f*.
transverse crest 1. Crista transversa. 2. Crista transversalis.
t. of internal acoustic meatus Crista transversa.
trans·ver·sec·to·my [ˌtrænsvərˈsektəmɪ] *n neurochir., ortho.* Querfortsatzresektion *f*, Transversektomie *f*.
transverse diameter querer/transverser Durchmesser *m*, Querdurchmesser *m*, Diameter transversa.
t. of pelvis *gyn.* Beckenquerdurchmesser, Diameter transversa pelvis.
transverse ductules of epoophoron querverlaufende Urnierenkanälchenreste *pl*, Ductuli transversi epoophori/epoophorontis.
transverse facial fracture LeFort III-Fraktur *f*.
transverse fascia Fascia transversalis.
transverse fasciculi: t. of palmar aponeurosis Fasciculi transversi aponeurosis palmaris.
t. of plantar aponeurosis Fasciculi transversi aponeurosis plantaris.
transverse fibers of pons quere Brückenfasern *pl*, Fibrae pontis transversae.
transverse fissure of cerebrum Fissura transversa cerebralis.
transverse folds of rectum quere Schleimhautfalten *pl* des Rektums, Plicae transversales recti.
transverse foramen For. proc. transversi, For. vertebroarteriale, For. transversarium.
transverse fracture Querbruch *m*, -fraktur *f*.
transverse head: t. of adductor hallucis (muscle) Caput transversum m. adductoris hallucis.
t. of adductor pollicis (muscle) Caput transversum m. adductoris pollicis.
transverse hermaphroditism Hermaphroditismus (verus) transversus.
transverse humeral ligament Brodie'-Band *nt*.
transverse incision Transversalschnitt *m*.
transverse joint of rib → transverse articulation of rib.
transverse ligament: t. of ankle Retinaculum mm. extensorum pedis superius.
t. of carpus Retinaculum flexorum.
inferior t. of scapula Lig. transversum scapulae inferius.
t. of pelvis Lig. transversum perinei.
t. of scapula Lig. transversum scapulae.
superior t. of scapula Lig. transversum scapulae superius.
t. of wrist Retinaculum flexorum.
transverse lines of sacrum Lineae transversae (ossis sacralis).
transverse mesocolon Meso(kolon *nt*) *nt* des Colon transversum, Mesocolon transversum.
transverse muscle: t. of abdomen → transversus abdominis (muscle).

t. of auricle → transversus auricularis (muscle).
t. of chin → transversus menti (muscle).
deep t. of perineum → transversus perinei profundus (muscle).
t. of nape → transversus nuchae (muscle).
superficial t. of perineum → transversus perinei superficialis (muscle).
t. of thorax → transversus thoracis (muscle).
t. of tongue → transversus linguae (muscle).
transverse myelitis Querschnittsmyelitis *f*, Myelitis transversa.
transverse myelopathy Querschnittsmyelopathie *f*, Myelopathia transversa.
transverse nerve of neck N. transversus colli.
transverse oval pelvis transvers-ovales Becken *nt*.
transverse part: t. of left branch of portal vein Pars transversa.
t. of nasal muscle Kompressor *m* naris, M. compressor naris, Pars transversa m. nasalis.
t. of vertebral artery Halsabschnitt *m* der A. vertebralis, Pars transversaria/cervicalis (a. vertebralis).
transverse perineal ligament Lig. transversum perinei.
transverse plane Transversalebene *f*.
transverse presentation *gyn.* (*Fetus*) Querlage *f*.
transverse process Querfortsatz *m*, Proc. transversus.
transverse pyramidal fracture Pyramidenquerfraktur *f*.
transverse ridge Crista transversalis.
transverse section *mathe.* Querschnitt *m*.
transverse sinus Sinus transversus.
t. of dura mater Sinus transversus (durae matris).
t. of pericardium Sinus transversus pericardii.
transverse striation Querstreifung *f*.
transverse sulcus of anthelix Sulcus anthelicis transversus.
transverse system *physiol.* T-System *nt*, transversales Röhrensystem *nt*, System *nt* der transversalen Tubuli.
transverse tarsal articulation Chopart'-Gelenklinie *f*, Artic. tarsi transversa.
transverse tarsal joint → transverse tarsal articulation.
transverse tubule Transversaltubulus *m*, T-Tubulus *m*.
transverse vesical fold transversale Blasenfalte *f*, Plica vesicalis transversa.
transverse wave Transversalwelle *f*.
trans·ver·sion [ˌtræns'vɜrʒn] *n genet.* Transversion *f*.
trans·ver·sio·nal mutation [ˌ-'vɜrʒnl] → transversion.
trans·ver·so·cos·tal [ˌtrænsˌvɜrsəʊ'kɒstl] *adj* zwischen Rippen u. Querfortsatz gelegen, kostotransversal.
trans·ver·so·spi·na·lis (muscle) [ˌ-ˌvɜrsəʊspaɪ'neɪlɪs] Transversospinalis *m*, M. transversospinalis.
trans·ver·so·spi·nal muscle [ˌ-ˌvɜrsəʊ-'spaɪnl] → transversospinalis (muscle).
transversospinal (muscular) system Spinotransversalsystem *nt* des M. erector spinae.
trans·ver·sot·o·my [ˌ-vɜr'sɒtəmɪ] *n neurochir.*, *ortho.* Transversotomie *f*.
trans·ver·sus abdominis (muscle) [ˌ-'vɜrsəs] Transversus *m* abdominis, M. transversus abdominis.
transversus auriculae (muscle) → transversus auricularis (muscle).

transversus auricularis (muscle) M. transversus auricularis.
transversus linguae (muscle) Transversus *m* linguae, M. transversus linguae.
transversus menti (muscle) Transversus *m* menti, M. transversus menti.
transversus nuchae (muscle) Transversus *m* nuchae, M. transversus nuchae.
transversus perinei profundus (muscle) Transversus *m* perinei profundus, M. transversus perinei profundus.
transversus perinei superficialis (muscle) Transversus *m* perinei superficialis, M. transversus perinei superficialis.
transversus thoracis (muscle) Transversus *m* thoracis, M. transversus thoracis.
trans·ves·i·cal [ˌ-'vesɪkl] *adj* durch die Harnblase, transvesikal.
trans·ves·tic fetishism [ˌ-'vestɪk] → transvestism.
trans·ves·tism [ˌ-'vestɪzəm] *n* Transvestismus *m*, Transvestitismus *m*.
trans·ves·tite [ˌ-'vestaɪt] *n* Transvestit *m*.
trans·ves·ti·tism [ˌ-'vestɪtɪzəm] *n* → transvestism.
tran·yl·cy·pro·mine [ˌtrænɪl'saɪprəʊmiːn] *pharm.* Tranylcypromin *nt*.
tra·pe·zi·al [trə'piːzɪəl] *adj* Trapez *od.* Trapezoid betr.
tra·pez·i·form [trə'pezɪfɔːrm] *adj* → trapezoid II.
tra·pe·zi·um (bone) [trə'piːzɪəm, -zjəm] großes Vieleckbein *nt*, Os trapezium, Os multangulum majus.
lesser t. → trapezoid 1.
t. of Lyser → trapezoid 1.
tra·pe·zi·us (muscle) [trə'piːzɪəs] Trapezius *m*, M. trapezius.
trap·e·zoid ['træpɪzɔɪd] **I** *n* **1.** kleines Vieleckbein *nt*, Os trapezoideum, Os multangulum minus. **2.** *mathe.* Trapez *nt*, Trapezoid *nt*. **II** *adj* trapezförmig, trapezoid.
trap·e·zoi·dal [ˌtræpɪ'zɔɪdl] *adj* → trapezoid II.
trapezoid body Trapezkörper *m*, Corpus trapezoideum.
trapezoid bone → trapezoid 1.
trapezoid ligament Lig. trapezoideum.
trapezoid line Linea trapezoidea.
trapezoid nuclei Trapezkerne *pl*, Kerne *pl* des Corpus trapezoidei.
Traube ['traʊbə]: **T.'s bruit** *card.* Galopp(rhythmus *m*) *m*.
T.'s corpuscle Halbmondkörper *m*, Achromozyt *m*, Achromoretikulocyt *m*.
T.'s double tone *card.* Traube-Doppelton *m*.
T.'s murmur → T.'s bruit.
T.'s plugs *patho.* Dittrich-Pfröpfe *pl*.
T.'s semilunar space → T.'s space.
T.'s sign *card.* Traube-Doppelton *m*.
T.'s space Traube-Raum *m*.
trau·ma ['traʊmə, 'trɔː-] *n, pl* **-mas, -ma·ta** [-mətə] **1.** (körperliche) Verletzung *f*, Wunde *f*, Trauma *nt*. **2.** (seelisches) Trauma *nt*, seelische Erschütterung *f*, Schock *m*.
t. to the abdomen Bauchverletzung, -trauma, Abdominalverletzung, -trauma.
t. from ischemia ischämie-bedingte Schädigung, Schädigung durch Ischämie.
trauma patient → traumatized patient.
trauma-shock kidney Crush-Niere *f*, Schockniere *f* bei Trauma.
trau·mas·the·nia [ˌtrɔːmæs'θiːnɪə] *n* traumatische Neurasthenie *f*, posttraumatische nervöse Erschöpfung *f*.
traumat- pref. → traumato-.
trau·ma·ther·a·py [ˌtrɔːmə'θerəpɪ, ˌtraʊ-] *n* Wundbehandlung *f*, Traumatherapie *f*.
trau·mat·ic [trɔː'mætɪk, traʊ-] *adj* Trauma betr., durch ein Trauma hervorgerufen,

durch Gewalteinwirkung entstanden, traumatisch, posttraumatisch, Trauma-, Verletzungs-.
traumatic amblyopia (post-)traumatische Amblyopie *f*.
traumatic amenorrhea *gyn.* (post-)traumatische Amenorrhoe *f*.
traumatic amputation *ortho.* traumatische/unfallbedingte Amputation *f*.
traumatic anesthesia *neuro.* (post-)traumatische Sensibilitätsstörung *f*.
traumatic anoxia (post-)traumatische Anoxie *f*.
traumatic apnoe traumatisches Asphyxiesyndrom *nt*, traumatische Asphyxie *f*, traumatische Apnoe *f*, traumatischer Atemstillstand *m*.
traumatic arthritis posttraumatische Arthrose *f*.
traumatic asphyxia → traumatic apnoe.
traumatic cataract (post-)traumatischer Star *m*, Wundstar *m*, Cataracta traumatica.
traumatic clubfoot *ortho.* posttraumatischer Klumpfuß *m*.
traumatic degeneration (post-)traumatische Degeneration *f*.
traumatic delirium posttraumatisches Delir(ium *nt*) *nt*.
traumatic dislocation *ortho.* traumatische Luxation *f*.
traumatic emphysema posttraumatisches Emphysem *nt*.
traumatic encephalopathy Boxerenzephalopathie *f*, Encephalopathia traumatica.
traumatic epilepsy (post-)traumatische Epilepsie *f*.
traumatic experience traumatisches Erlebnis *nt*.
traumatic fever Wundfieber *nt*, Febris traumatica.
traumatic fracture traumatische Fraktur *f*.
traumatic gangrene posttraumatische Gangrän *f*.
traumatic glaucoma posttraumatisches Glaukom *nt*.
traumatic herpes Herpes simplex traumaticus.
traumatic inflammation (post-)traumatische Entzündung *f*.
traumatic injury Verletzung *f*, Wunde *f*, Schaden *m*, Schädigung *f*, Trauma *nt*.
traumatic late apoplexy Spätapoplexie *f*, verzögerte traumatische Apoplexie *f*.
traumatic meningocele traumatische Meningozele *f*.
traumatic myelitis traumatische Myelopathie *f*.
traumatic myelopathy traumatische Myelopathie *f*.
traumatic neurasthenia → traumasthenia.
traumatic neuritis (post-)traumatische Neuritis *f*.
traumatic neuroma (post-)traumatisches Neurom *nt*.
traumatic neurosis posttraumatische Neurose *f*.
traumatic peritonitis traumatische Bauchfellentzündung/Peritonitis *f*.
traumatic pneumonia (post-)traumatische Pneumonie *f*.
traumatic psychosis posttraumatische Psychose *f*.
traumatic shock traumatischer Schock *m*.
traumatic spondylopathy Kümmel-Verneuil-Krankheit *f*, -Syndrom *nt*, traumatische Kyphose *f*, Spondylopathia traumatica.

traumatic syringomyelia (post-)traumatische Syringomyelie f.
trau·ma·tin ['trɔːmətɪn, 'traʊ-] n Traumatin nt.
trau·ma·tism ['-tɪzəm] n 1. → trauma. 2. Traumatismus m.
trau·ma·tize ['-taɪz] vt schädigen, verletzen, traumatisieren, ein Trauma hervorrufen.
trau·ma·tized patient ['-taɪzt] unfallverletzter/traumatisierter Patient m, unfallverletzte/traumatisierte Patientin f, Traumapatient(in f) m.
traumato- pref. Wund-, Trauma-, Traumat(o)-, Verletzungs-.
trau·ma·to·gen·ic [ˌtrɔːmətəʊ'dʒenɪk, ˌtraʊ-] adj 1. durch eine Verletzung/ein Trauma hervorgerufen, traumatogen. 2. ein Trauma verursachend, traumatogen.
trau·ma·tol·o·gy [ˌtrɔːmə'tɒlədʒɪ, ˌtraʊ-] n Traumatologie f.
trau·ma·top·a·thy [ˌ-'tɒpəθɪ] n traumatogene Schädigung f.
trau·ma·to·phil·ia [ˌtrɔːmətəʊ'fɪlɪə, ˌtraʊ-] n psychia. Traumatophilie f.
trau·ma·to·pho·bia [ˌ-'fəʊbɪə] n psychia. krankhafte Angst f vor Traumen, Traumatophobie f.
trau·ma·top·nea [ˌtrɔːmətɒp'niːə, ˌtraʊ-] n Traumatopnoe f.
trau·ma·to·py·ra [ˌtrɔːmətə'paɪrə, ˌtraʊ-] n Wundfieber nt, Febris traumatica.
trau·ma·to·sis [ˌtrɔːmə'təʊsɪs, ˌtraʊ-] n 1. → trauma. 2. Traumatismus m.
trau·ma·to·ther·a·py [ˌtrɔːmətəʊ'θerəpɪ, ˌtraʊ-] n Wundbehandlung f, Traumatherapie f.
tra·vail [trə'veɪl, 'trævɪl] French gyn. I n (Geburts-)Wehen pl, Kreißen nt. II vi in den Wehen liegen, kreißen.
trav·el ['trævəl] vi techn., phys. s. (hin u. her) bewegen, s. fortpflanzen.
trav·el·er's diarrhea ['trævələrz] Reisediarrhö f, Turista f, Montezumas Rache f.
trav·el·ing ['trævəlɪŋ] adj (a. phys.) fortschreitend, wandernd, Wander-.
traveling wave phys., physiol. Wanderwelle f.
tra·zo·done ['træzədəʊn] n pharm. Trazodon nt.
Treacher-Collins ['triːtʃər 'kɒlɪnz]: **T.-C. syndrome** Treacher-Collins-Syndrom nt, Franceschetti-Syndrom nt, Dysostosis mandibulo-facialis.
Treacher-Collins-Franceschetti [ˌfrɑntʃə-'skeɪtɪ]: **T.-C.-F. syndrome** → Treacher-Collins syndrome.
treach·er·ous ['tretʃərəs] adj trügerisch, tückisch.
trea·cle ['triːkl] n 1. Sirup m; Mellase f. 2. Zuckerlösung f, Sirup m. 3. histor. Allheilmittel nt.
tread-mill ergometer ['tredmɪl] physiol. Laufbandergometer nt.
treat [triːt] I vt 1. behandeln (for gegen, auf; with mit). 2. chem. behandeln; (Abwasser) klären. 3. (Thema) abhandeln, behandeln u. betrachten; behandeln (as als). 4. techn. ver-, bearbeiten, behandeln. II vi → treat of.
treat of vi handeln von.
treat·a·ble ['triːtəbl] adj behandelbar, heilbar, kurabel.
trea·tise ['triːtɪs] n (wissenschaftliche) Abhandlung f (on über).
treat·ment ['triːtmənt] n 1. Behandlung f, Behandlungsmethode f, -technik f, Therapie f. 2. techn., fig. Ver-, Bearbeitung f. 3. pharm. Heilmittel nt, Arzneimittel nt. 4. (Thema) Behandlung f; Bearbeitung f.

treatment expenses Arzt- u. Arzneikosten pl, Behandlungskosten pl.
tree [triː] n 1. bio. Baum m. 2. anat. baumartige Struktur f, Baum f.
T-reflex n → tendon reflex.
tre·foil tendon ['|triːfɔɪl, 'tref-] Centrum tendineum.
tre·ha·lose ['triːhələʊs, trɪ'hæl-] n Trehalose f, Mykose f.
trehalose-6,6'-dimycolate n Cordfaktor m, Trehalose-6,6'-dimykolat nt.
Treitz ['traɪts]: **T.'s arch** Treitz-Band nt.
  T.'s fossa Treitz'-Grube f, Rec. duodenalis superior.
  T.'s hernia Treitz'-Hernie f, Hernia duodenojejunalis.
  T.'s ligament M. suspensorius duodeni.
  T.'s muscle Treitz-Muskel m, Suspensorius m duodeni, M. suspensorius duodeni.
trel·lis arrangement ['trelɪs] histol. Scherengitteranordnung f.
tre·ma ['triːmə] n anat. 1. Öffnung f, Loch nt, Foramen nt. 2. (weibliche) Scham od. Schamgegend f, äußere (weibliche) Geschlechtsorgane/Genitalien pl, Vulva f.
Trem·a·to·da [ˌtremə'təʊdə, ˌtriːmə-] pl micro. Saugwürmer pl, Trematoden pl, Trematoda pl, Trematodes pl.
trem·a·tode ['-təʊd] n micro. Saugwurm m, Trematode f.
trem·a·to·di·a·sis [ˌtremətəʊ'daɪəsɪs] n Saugwurmbefall m, Trematodiasis f.
trem·ble ['trembl] I n Zittern nt, Beben nt. II vi (er-)zittern, beben.
trem·bling palsy ['tremblɪŋ] Parkinson'-Krankheit f, Morbus Parkinson m, Paralysis agitans.
trem·el·loid ['treməlɔɪd] adj gelartig.
trem·el·lose ['treməlɒs] adj → tremelloid.
tre·men·dous [trɪ'mendəs] adj gewaltig, ungeheuer, enorm, kolossal, schrecklich, fürchterlich.
trem·or ['tremər, 'triːmər] n (unwillkürliches) Zittern nt, Tremor m.
trem·u·lous ['tremjələs] adj 1. Tremor betr., zitternd, bebend, zitt(e)rig. 2. ängstlich.
tremulous iris Irisschlottern nt, Iris tremulans.
trem·u·lous·ness ['tremjələnɪs] n Zittern nt, Sichschütteln nt.
trench [trentʃ] I n Einschnitt m;, Furche f, Rinne f. II vt furchen, einkerben; zerschneiden, zerteilen.
trench fever Wolhyn'-Fieber nt, Fünftagefieber nt, Wolhynienfieber nt, Febris quintana.
trench mouth Plaut-Vincent-Angina f, Vincent-Angina f, Fusospirillose f, Fusospirochätose f, Angina ulcerosa/ulceromembranacea.
trend [trend] I n 1. (Ver-)Lauf m, Richtung f, Entwicklung f, Tendenz f, Trend m. 2. Bestrebung f, Neigung f, Trend m, Tendenz f. 3. mathe. Trend m, Strich m, Grundbewegung f. II vi streben, tendieren, s. neigen (towards nach).
Trendelenburg [tren'deləmbɜrg, -bʊrg]:
  T.'s gait Hüfthinken nt, Trendelenburg-(Duchenne-)Hinken nt.
  T.'s limp → T.'s gait.
  T.'s operation Trendelenburg-Operation f, transthorakale pulmonale Embolektomie f.
  T.'s position chir. Trendelenburg-Lage-(rung f) f.
  T.'s sign 1. Trendelenburg-Versuch m. 2. ortho. Trendelenburg-Zeichen nt.
  T.'s symptom Hüfthinken nt, Trendelenburg(-Duchenne)-Hinken nt.
  T.'s test → T.'s sign.

tre·pan [trɪ'pæn] I n Schädelbohrer m, Trepan m. II vt den Schädel eröffnen, trepanieren.
trep·a·na·tion [trepə'neɪʃn] n chir., neurochir. Schädelbohrung f, Trepanation f, Trepanieren nt.
treph·i·na·tion [trefɪ'neɪʃn] n ophthal., dent. Trephination f, Trephinieren nt; Trepanation f, Trepanieren nt.
tre·phine [trɪ'faɪn, -'fiːn] I n 1. ophthal., dent. Trephine f. 2. → trepan I. II vt mit einer Trephine eröffnen, trepanieren.
trephine biopsy Stanzbiopsie f.
trep·i·dant ['trepɪdənt] adj (er-)zitternd, bebend.
trep·i·da·tio [ˌ-'deɪʃɪəʊ] n → trepidation.
trep·i·da·tion [ˌ-'deɪʃn] n 1. Zittern nt, Trepidatio f. 2. (nervöse) Angst f, Ängstlichkeit f, Unruhe f, Trepidation f, Trepidatio f.
trepidation sign Patellarklonus m.
Trep·o·ne·ma [ˌtrepə'niːmə] n micro. Treponema nt.
  T. forans Reiter-Spirochäte f, -Stamm m, Treponema forans.
  T. pallidum Syphilisspirochäte f, Treponema pallidum, Spirochaeta pallida.
  T. pallidum subspecies pertenue → T. pertenue.
  T. pertenue Frambösie-Spirochäte f, Treponema pertenue, Treponema pallidum subspecies pertenue, Spirochaeta pertenuis.
trep·o·ne·ma [ˌ-'niːmə] n, pl -mas, -ma·ta [-mətə] micro. Treponeme f, Treponema nt.
treponema-immobilizing antibody Treponema-immobilisierender Antikörper m.
trep·o·ne·mal [ˌ-'niːml] adj Treponemen betr., durch Treponemen hervorgerufen, Treponema-, Treponemen-.
treponemal antibody → treponema-immobilizing antibody.
Treponema pallidum hemagglutination assay abbr. **TPHA** Treponema-Pallidum--Hämagglutinationstest m abbr. TPHA, TPHA-Test m.
Treponema pallidum hemagglutination test → Treponema pallidum hemagglutination assay.
Treponema pallidum immobilization reaction → Treponema pallidum immobilization test.
Treponema pallidum immobilization test Treponema-Pallidum-Immobilisationstest m, TPI-Test m, Nelson-Test m.
trep·o·ne·ma·to·sis [ˌ-ˌniːmə'təʊsɪs] n Treponemainfektion f, Treponematose f.
trep·o·neme ['-niːm] n → treponema.
trep·o·ne·mi·a·sis [ˌ-'maɪəsɪs] n 1. → treponematosis. 2. harter Schanker m, Morbus Schaudinn m, Schaudinn--Krankheit f, Syphilis f, Lues (venerea) f.
trep·o·ne·mi·ci·dal [ˌ-nɪmə'saɪdl] adj treponemabtötend, treponemizid.
tre·tin·o·in [trɪ'tɪnəʊɪn] n Retinsäure f, Vitamin A₁-Säure f, Tretinoin nt.
Treves [triːvz]: **T.' fold** Plica ileoc(a)ecalis.
Trevor ['trevər]: **T.'s disease** Trevor-Erkrankung f, -Syndrom nt, Dysplasia epiphysealis hemimelica.
TRF abbr. [thyrotropin releasing factor] → thyroliberin.
TRH abbr. [thyrotropin releasing hormone] → thyroliberin.
TRH stimulation test (Schilddrüse) TRH--Test m.
TRH test → TRH stimulation test.
tri- pref. Drei-, Tri-.
tri·ac·e·tate [traɪ'æsɪteɪt] n Triazetat nt, -acetat nt.

tri·ac·e·tin [traɪˈæsətɪn] *n pharm.* Triacetin *nt*, Glycerintriacetat *nt*, Glyceroltriacetat *nt*.
tri·ac·yl·glyc·er·ol [ˌtraɪˌæsɪlˈglɪsərəl, -rɒl] *n* Triacylglycerin *nt*, *old* Triglycerid *nt*.
triacylglycerol lipase Triacylglycerinlipase *f*, Triglyceridlipase *f*.
tri·ad [ˈtraɪəd, -æd] *n* **1.** Dreiergruppe *f*, Trias *f*, Triade *f*. **2.** *chem.* dreiwertiges Element *nt*, Triade *f*.
  t. of skeletal muscle (Muskel-)Triade, -Trias.
  t. of symptoms Symptomtrias.
triad structure Triadenstruktur *f*.
triad system → transverse system.
tri·age [trɪˈɑːʒ] *n French* Auslese *f*, Selektion *f*, Triage *f*.
tri·al [ˈtraɪəl, traɪl] **I** *n* **1.** Versuch *m* (*of* mit); Probe *f*, Prüfung *f*, Test *m*, Erprobung *f*. **on ~** auf/zur Probe, probeweise. **by way of ~** versuchsweise. **2.** (Nerven-)Belastung *f*, Strapaze *f* (*to* für jdn.). **II** *adj* Versuchs-, Probe-.
  t. and error Ausprobieren *nt*, Herumprobieren *nt*, empirische Methode *f*.
trial lens Probeglas *nt*, -linse *f*.
trial period Probezeit *f*.
trial prosthesis *ortho.* Probeprothese *f*.
tri·am·cin·o·lone [ˌtraɪæmˈsɪnələʊn] *n pharm.* Triamcinolon *nt*.
tri·a·mine [ˌtraɪˈæmɪn] *n* Triamin *nt*.
tri·am·ter·ene [traɪˈæmtəriːn] *n pharm.* Triamteren *nt*.
tri·am·y·lose [traɪˈæmɪləʊs] *n* Triamylose *f*.
tri·an·gle [ˈtraɪæŋgl] *n* Dreieck *nt*, dreieckige Struktur *od.* Fläche *f*; *anat.* Trigonum *nt*.
  t. of Grynfeltt and Lesgaft Grynfeltt-Dreieck, Trigonum lumbale superior.
tri·an·gu·lar [traɪˈæŋgjələr] *adj* dreieckig, -wink(e)lig, -seitig, triangulär, Dreiecks-.
triangular bandage Dreieckstuch *nt*.
triangular bone Dreiecksbein *nt*, Os triquetrum.
triangular cartilage of nose Cartilago nasi lateralis.
triangular crest Crista triangularis.
triangular eminence Agger perpendicularis, Eminentia fossae triangularis auriculae.
triangular fold Plica triangularis.
triangular fontanelle kleine/hintere Fontanelle *f*, Hinterhauptsfontanelle *f*, Fonticulus posterior.
triangular fossa (of auricle) Fossa triangularis (auriculae).
triangular fovea of arytenoid cartilage Fovea triangularis (cartilaginis aryt(a)enoideae).
triangular ligament: t. of Colles Fascia diaphragmatis urogenitalis inferior.
  left t. of liver Lig. triangulare sinistrum (hepatis).
  t. of linea alba Adminiculum lineae albae.
  right t. of liver Lig. triangulare dextrum (hepatis).
triangular muscle 1. Depressor *m* anguli oris, M. depressor anguli oris, *old* M. triangularis. **2.** M. triangularis.
triangular nucleus Schwalbe'-Kern *m*, Nc. vestibularis medialis.
triangular part of inferior frontal gyrus Pars triangularis (gyri frontalis inferioris).
triangular pit of arytenoid cartilage → triangular fovea of arytenoid cartilage.
triangular ridge Crista triangularis.
triangular tract Helweg'-Dreikantenbahn *f*, Tractus olivospinalis.
Tri·at·o·ma [traɪˈætəmə] *n micro.* Triatoma *f*.

T. megista brasilianische Schreitwanze *f*, Triatoma megista, Panstrongylus megistus.
tri·a·tom·ic [ˌtraɪəˈtɒmɪk] *adj chem.* dreiatomig, aus drei Atomen bestehend, triatomar.
tri·at·o·mine bug [traɪˈætəmiːn] *micro.* Triatoma *f*.
tri·a·tri·al heart [traɪˈeɪtrɪəl] Cor triatriatum.
tri·a·zo·lam [traɪˈæzəlæm] *n pharm.* Triazolam *nt*.
trib·ade [ˈtrɪbəd] *n* Tribade *f*.
trib·a·dism [ˈtrɪbədɪzəm] *n* Tribadie *f*, Tribadismus *m*.
trib·a·dy [ˈtrɪbədi] *n* → tribadism.
trib·al [ˈtraɪbl] *adj* **1.** *bio.* Tribus-. **2.** Stammes-.
tri·ba·sic [traɪˈbeɪsɪk] *adj chem.* drei-, tribasisch.
tribasic acid *chem.* dreibasische Säure *f*.
tribasic phosphate tertiäres Phosphat *nt*.
tribe [traɪb] *n* **1.** *bio.* Tribus *f*, Klasse *f*. **2.** Stamm *m*.
tri·ben·o·side [traɪˈbenəsaɪd] *n pharm.* Tribenosid *nt*.
tri·bol·o·gy [traɪˈbɒlədʒi] *n* Tribologie *f*.
tri·bo·lu·mi·nes·cence [ˌtraɪbəʊˌluːməˈnesəns] *n phys.* Triboluminesznz *f*.
tri·bra·chia [traɪˈbreɪkɪə] *n embryo.* Tribrachie *f*.
tri·bra·chi·us [traɪˈbreɪkɪəs] *n embryo.* Tribrachius *m*.
tri·brom·eth·a·nol [traɪˌbrɒmˈeθənɒl] *n* → tribromoethanol.
tri·bro·mide [traɪˈbrəʊmaɪd] *n* Tribromid *nt*.
tri·bro·mo·eth·a·nol [traɪˌbrəʊməʊˈeθənɒl] *n* Tribromäthanol *nt*, -ethanol *nt*.
trib·u·tar·y [ˈtrɪbjətəri:] *adj* untergeordnet (*to*), Neben-.
tri·bu·tyr·in·ase [traɪˈbjuːtərɪneɪz] *n* → triacylglycerol lipase.
TRIC agent [trachoma, inclusion conjunctivitis] *micro.* Chlamydia trachomatis, TRIC-Gruppe *f*.
tri·car·box·yl·ate carrier [ˌtraɪkɑːˈbɒksɪleɪt] Tricarboxylatcarrier *m*.
tri·car·box·yl·ic acid cycle [traɪˌkɑːbɒkˈsɪlɪk] *biochem.* Zitronensäurezyklus *m*, Citratzyklus *m*, Tricarbonsäurezyklus *m*, Krebs-Zyklus *m*.
tri·cel·lu·lar [traɪˈseljələr] *adj* aus drei Zellen bestehend, dreizellig, trizellular, trizellulär.
tri·ceph·a·lus [traɪˈsefələs] *n embryo.* Trizephalus *m*, -kephalus *m*, -cephalus *m*.
tri·ceps [ˈtraɪseps] *n, pl* **-ceps, -ceps·es** dreiköpfiger Muskel *m*; M. triceps brachii.
  t. of arm → triceps brachii (muscle).
  t. of calf → triceps surae muscle.
triceps brachii (muscle) Trizeps *m* (brachii), M. triceps brachii.
triceps muscle: t. of arm → triceps brachii (muscle).
  t. of calf → triceps surae muscle.
triceps reflex Trizepssehnenreflex *m abbr.* TSR.
triceps surae → triceps surae muscle.
triceps surae jerk → triceps surae reflex.
triceps surae muscle Trizeps *m* surae, M. triceps surae.
triceps surae reflex Achillessehnenreflex *m abbr.* ASR.
TRIC group [trachoma, inclusion conjunctivitis] → TRIC agent.
trich- *pref.* → tricho-.
trich·al·gia [trɪkˈældʒ(ɪ)ə] *n* Trichalgie *f*.
trich·a·tro·phia [ˌtrɪkəˈtrəʊfɪə] *n* Haarwurzelatrophie *f*.

trich·aux·is [trɪkˈɔːksɪs] *n* übermäßiges Haarwachstum *nt*, Trichauxis *f*.
tri·chei·ria [traɪˈkaɪrɪə] *n embryo.* Trich(e)irie *f*.
trich·es·the·sia [ˌtrɪkesˈθiːʒ(ɪ)ə] *n* → trichoesthesia.
trichi- *pref.* → tricho-.
trich·i·a·sis [trɪˈkaɪəsɪs] *n* Einwärtskehrung *f* der Wimpern, Trichiasis *f*.
Tri·chi·i·da [trɪˈkaɪɪdə] *pl micro.* Trichiida *pl*.
trich·i·lem·mal cyst [ˌtrɪkəˈleml] **1.** trichilemmale Zyste *f*, Trichilemmal-, Trichilemmzyste *f*. **2.** piläre Hautzyste *f*.
trich·i·lem·mo·ma [ˌ-leˈməʊmə] *n* Trichilemmom *nt*.
Tri·chi·na [trɪˈkaɪnə] *n* → Trichinella.
tri·chi·na [trɪˈkaɪnə] *n, pl* **-nae** [-niː] *micro.* Trichine *f*, Trichinella *f*.
trichina worm → Trichinella.
Trich·i·nel·la [ˌtrɪkɪˈnelə] *n micro.* Trichinella *f*.
T. spiralis Trichine *f*, Trichinella spiralis.
trich·i·nel·li·a·sis [ˌ-neˈlaɪəsɪs] *n* → trichinosis.
trich·i·nel·lo·sis [ˌ-neˈləʊsɪs] *n* → trichinosis.
trich·i·ni·a·sis [ˌ-ˈnaɪəsɪs] *n* → trichinosis.
trich·i·nif·er·ous [ˌ-ˈnɪfərəs] *adj* trichinenhaltig.
trich·i·ni·za·tion [ˌ-nɪˈzeɪʃn] *n* → trichinosis.
trich·i·no·pho·bia [ˌtrɪkɪnəʊˈfəʊbɪə] *n psychia.* krankhafte Angst *f* vor einer Trichinenerkrankung, Trichinophobie *f*.
trich·i·no·sis [ˌtrɪkɪˈnəʊsɪs] *n* Trichinenbefall *m*, -infektion *f*, Trichinose *f*, Trichinellose *f*, Trichinelliasis *f*.
trich·i·nous [ˈtrɪkɪnəs] *adj* trichinenhaltig, von Trichinen befallen.
trichinous myositis Myositis trichinosa.
trichinous polymyositis → trichinosis.
trich·ite [ˈtrɪkaɪt] *n* → trichocyst.
tri·chi·tis [trɪˈkaɪtɪs] *n* Haarbalgentzündung *f*, Trichitis *f*.
tri·chlo·ride [traɪˈklɔːraɪd, -ɪd, -ˈkləʊ-] *n* Trichlorid *nt*.
tri·chlor·me·thi·a·zide [traɪˌklɔːrmɪˈθaɪəzaɪd] *n pharm.* Trichlormethiazid *nt*.
tri·chlor·ni·tro·meth·ane [traɪˌklɔːrˌnaɪtrəˈmeθeɪn] *n* Chlorpikrin *nt*, Trichlornitromethan *nt*.
tri·chlo·ro·ac·et·al·de·hyde [traɪˌklɔːrəʊˌæsɪlˈtældəhaɪd] *n* Chloral *nt*, Trichloracetaldehyd *m*.
tri·chlo·ro·ace·tic acid [ˌ-əˈsiːtɪk, -əˈset-] Trichloressigsäure *f*.
tri·chlo·ro·eth·yl·ene [ˌ-ˈeθəliːn] *n* Trichloräthylen *nt*, -ethylen *nt*, Äthylentrichlorid *nt*, *inf.* Tri *nt*.
tri·chlo·ro·meth·ane [ˌ-ˈmeθeɪn] *n* Chloroform *nt*, Trichlormethan *nt*.
tri·chlo·ro·phe·nol [ˌ-ˈfiːnɒl, -nəl] *n* Trichlorphenol *nt*.
2,4,5-tri·chlo·ro·phe·nox·y·a·ce·tic acid [ˌ-fɪˌnɒksɪəˈsiːtɪk, -əˈset-] *abbr.* **2,4,5-T** Trichlorphenoxyessigsäure *f abbr.* 2,4,5-T.
tricho- *pref.* Haar-, Trich(o)-.
trich·o·aes·the·sia [ˌ-iːsˈθiːʒ(ɪ)ə] *n* → trichoesthesia.
trich·o·an·es·the·sia [ˌtrɪkəʊænesˈθiːʒ(ɪ)ə] *n* Trichoanästhesie *f*.
Trich·o·bac·te·ria [ˌ-bækˈtɪərɪə] *pl micro.* Trichobakterien *pl*, Trichobacteria *pl*.
trich·o·be·zoar [ˌ-ˈbiːzɔːr, -zəʊr] *n* Haarball *m*, Trichobezoar *m*.
trich·o·car·dia [ˌ-ˈkɑːrdɪə] *n* Zottenherz *nt*, Cor villosum.
trich·o·ceph·a·li·a·sis [ˌ-sefəˈlaɪəsɪs] *n* → trichuriasis.
trich·o·ceph·a·lo·sis [ˌ-sefəˈləʊsɪs] *n* → trichuriasis.

Trichocephalus

Trich·o·ceph·a·lus [ˌ-'sefələs] *n* → Trichuris.
trich·o·cla·sia [ˌ-'kleɪsɪə] *n* → trichorrhexis nodosa.
trich·oc·la·sis [trɪk'ɑkləsɪs] *n* → trichorrhexis nodosa.
trich·o·cyst ['trɪkəsɪst] *n* Trichozyste *f*.
Trich·o·dec·tes [ˌ-'dektiːz] *n micro.* Trichodectes *m*.
Trich·o·der·ma [ˌ-'dɜrmə] *n micro.* Trichoderma *f*.
trich·o·dyn·ia [ˌ-'diːnɪə] *n* → trichalgia.
trich·o·ep·i·the·li·o·ma [ˌ-epɪˌθɪlɪ'əʊmə] *n* Trichoepitheliom *nt*, Brooke'-Krankheit *f*, multiple Trichoepitheliome *pl*, Trichoepithelioma papulosum multiplex, Epithelioma adenoides cysticum.
trich·o·es·the·sia [ˌ-es'θiːʒ(ɪ)ə] *n* Trich(o)ästhesie *f*.
trich·o·fol·lic·u·lo·ma [ˌ-fəˌlɪkjə'ləʊmə] *n* Trichofollikulom *nt*.
trich·o·gen ['-dʒən] *n* das Haarwachstum förderndes Mittel *nt*.
tri·chog·e·nous [trɪ'kɑdʒənəs] *adj* das Haarwachstum fördernd.
trich·o·glos·sia [ˌ-'glɑsɪə] *n* Haarzunge *f*, Glossotrichie *f*, Trichoglossie *f*, Lingua pilosa/villosa.
tri·chog·ra·phism [trɪ'kɑgrəfɪzəm] *n* Pilomotorenreaktion *f*.
trich·o·hy·a·lin [ˌtrɪkəʊ'haɪəlɪn] *n* Trichohyalin *nt*.
trich·oid ['trɪkɔɪd] *adj* haarartig, -ähnlich, -förmig, trichoid.
trich·o·leu·ko·cyte [ˌtrɪkəʊ'luːkəsaɪt] *n hema.* Haarzelle *f*.
trich·o·lo·gia [ˌ-'ləʊdʒ(ɪ)ə] *n* → trichotillomania.
tri·cho·ma [trɪ'kəʊmə] *n* 1. Trichiasis *f*. 2. Trichom *nt*, Trichoadenom *nt*.
tri·cho·ma·nia [ˌtrɪkə'meɪnɪə, -jə] *n* → trichotillomania.
tri·cho·ma·tose [trɪ'kəʊmətəʊs] *adj* → trichomatous.
tri·cho·ma·to·sis [ˌtrɪˌkəʊmə'təʊsɪs] *n* → trichoma.
tri·chom·a·tous [trɪ'kɑmətəs] *adj* Trichom betr., trichomartig, trichomatös.
trich·ome ['trɪkəʊm] *n* 1. *derm.* Trichom *nt*. 2. *bio.* Pflanzenhaar *nt*, Trichom *nt*. 3. *micro.* Trichom *nt*.
trich·o·meg·a·ly [ˌtrɪkə'megəlɪ] *n* Trichomegalie *f*.
trich·o·mo·na·ci·dal [ˌ-ˌmɑnə'saɪdl, -ˌməʊ-] *adj* trichomonaden(ab)tötend, trichomonazid, trichomonadizid.
trich·o·mo·na·cide [ˌ-'mɑnəsaɪd, -'məʊ-] *n* Trichomonazid *nt*, -monadizid *nt*.
trich·o·mon·ad [trɪ'mɑnæd, -'məʊ-] *n micro.* Trichomonade *f*, Trichomonas *f*.
Trich·o·mo·nad·i·da [ˌ-məʊ'nædɪdə] *pl micro.* Trichomonadida *pl*.
trich·o·mo·nal [ˌ'mɑnl, -'məʊ-] *adj* Trichomonaden betr., durch sie hervorgerufen, Trichomonas-, Trichomonaden-.
Trich·o·mon·as [ˌ-'mɑnəs, '-məʊ-] *n micro.* Trichomonas *f*.
trich·o·mo·ni·a·sis [ˌ-mə'naɪəsɪs] *n* Trichomonaden-, Trichomonasinfektion *f*, Trichomoniasis *f*, Trichomoniase *f*.
Trich·o·my·ce·tes [ˌ-maɪ'siːtiːz] *pl micro.* Trichomyzeten *pl*, -mycetes *pl*.
trich·o·my·ce·to·sis [ˌ-maɪsə'təʊsɪs] *n* → trichomycosis.
trich·o·my·co·sis [ˌ-maɪ'kəʊsɪs] *n* Pilzerkrankung *f* der Haare, Trichomykose *f*, -mycosis *f*.
trich·o·no·car·di·o·sis [ˌ-nəʊˌkɑrdɪ'əʊsɪs] *n* Trichonokardiose *f*, -cardiosis *f*.
trich·o·no·do·sis [ˌ-nəʊ'dəʊsɪs] *n* 1. Trichonodose *f*, Trichonodosis *f*. 2. Haarknötchenkrankheit *f*, Trichorrhexis nodosa, Nodositas crinium.
trich·o·no·sis [ˌ-'nəʊsɪs] *n* → trichopathy.
tri·chon·o·sus [trɪ'kɑnəsəs] *n* → trichopathy.
trich·o·path·ic [ˌtrɪkə'pæθɪk] *adj* Trichopathie betr.
tri·chop·a·thy [trɪ'kɑpəθɪ] *n* Haarerkrankung *f*, Trichopathie *f*, Trichonosis *f*, Trichose *f*, Trichosis *f*.
trich·o·pha·gia [ˌtrɪkə'feɪdʒ(ɪ)ə] *n psychia.* Haaressen *nt*, Trichophagie *f*.
tri·choph·a·gy [trɪ'kɑfədʒɪ] *n* → trichophagia.
trich·o·phyt·ic [ˌtrɪkə'fɪtɪk] *adj* Trichophytie betr.
trichophytic granuloma Granuloma trichophyticum.
tri·choph·y·tid [trɪ'kɑfətɪd] *n* Trichophytid *nt*.
tri·choph·y·tin [trɪ'kɑfətɪn] *n* Trichophytin *nt*.
trichophytin test Trichophytin-Test *m*.
trich·o·phy·to·be·zoar [ˌtrɪkəˌfaɪtə'biːzɔːr, -zəʊr] *n* Trichophytobezoar *m*.
Tri·choph·y·ton [trɪ'kɑfətən] *n micro.* Trichophyton *nt*.
trich·o·phy·to·sis [ˌtrɪkəfaɪ'təʊsɪs] *n* Trichophytie *f*, Trichophytia *f*.
trich·op·ti·lo·sis [ˌtrɪkəʊtɪ'ləʊsɪs, trɪˌkɑptɪ'ləʊsɪs] *n* Haarspaltung *f*, Trichoptilose *f*, Trichoptilosis *f*, Trichoschisis *f*.
trich·o·rhi·no·pha·lan·ge·al syndrome [ˌ-ˌraɪnəfə'lændʒɪəl] trichorhinophalangeales Syndrom *nt*.
trich·or·rhex·is [ˌ-'reksɪs] *n* Brüchigkeit *f* der Haare, Trichorrhexis *f*.
trichorrhexis nodosa Haarknötchenkrankheit *f*, Trichorrhexis nodosa, Nodositas crinium.
trich·os·chi·sis [trɪk'ɑskəsɪs] *n* 1. → trichoptilosis. 2. → trichorrhexis.
tri·chos·co·py [trɪ'kɑskəpɪ] *n* Haaruntersuchung *f*, Trichoskopie *f*.
tri·cho·sis [trɪ'kəʊsɪs] *n* → trichopathy.
Trich·o·so·ma [ˌtrɪkə'səʊmə] *n micro.* Capillaria *f*.
Tri·cho·spo·ron [ˌ-'spəʊrɑn, trɪ'kɑspərɑn] *n micro.* Trichosporon *nt*.
trich·o·spo·ro·sis [ˌ-spə'rəʊsɪs] *n* 1. Trichosporoninfektion *f*, Trichosporose *f*. 2. Haarknötchenkrankheit *f*, Peidra *f*, Trichosporose *f*.
Tri·cho·spo·rum [ˌ-'spəʊrəm, trɪ'kɑspərəm] *n* → Trichosporon.
trich·o·sta·sis [ˌ-'steɪsɪs] *n* Trichostasis *f*.
trich·o·stron·gy·li·a·sis [ˌ-ˌstrɑndʒə'laɪəsɪs] *n* Trichostrongylusinfektion *f*, Trichostrongyliasis *f*, Trichostrongylose *f*.
Trich·o·stron·gyl·i·dae [ˌ-strɑn'dʒɪlədiː] *pl micro.* Trichostrongylidae *pl*.
trich·o·stron·gy·lo·sis [ˌ-ˌstrɑndʒɪ'ləʊsɪs] *n* → trichostrongyliasis.
Trich·o·stron·gy·lus [ˌ-'strɑndʒɪləs] *n micro.* Trichostrongylus *m*.
trich·o·til·lo·ma·nia [ˌ-tɪlə'meɪnɪə, -jə] *n psychia.* Haarrupfsucht *f*, zwanghaftes Ausrupfen *nt* der Haare, Trichotillomanie *f*.
tri·chot·o·mous [traɪ'kɑtəməs] *adj* dreigeteilt, trichotom.
tri·chro·ma·sy [traɪ'krəʊməsɪ] *n* normales Farbensehen *nt*, trichromatisches Sehen *nt*, Trichromasie *f*, Euchromasie *f*.
tri·chro·mat ['traɪkrəmæt] *n* Trichromater *m*, Euchromater *m*.
tri·chro·mat·ic [ˌtraɪkrəʊ'mætɪk] *adj* → trichromic.
trichromatic color theory *physiol.* Dreifarbentheorie *f*, Young-Helmholtz-Theorie *f*.
trichromatic vision → trichromasy.
tri·chro·ma·tism [traɪ'krəʊmətɪzəm] *n* → trichromasy.
tri·chro·ma·top·sia [traɪˌkrəʊmə'tɑpsɪə] *n* → trichromasy.
tri·chrome stain ['traɪkrəʊm] Trichromfärbung *f*.
tri·chro·mic [traɪ'krəʊmɪk] *adj* 1. drei Farben betr., aus drei Farben bestehend, dreifarbig, Dreifarben-. 2. *ophthal.* (*Farbensehen*) normalsichtig, trichrom, euchrom.
trich·ter·brust ['trɪxtərbrʊst] *n ortho.* Trichterbrust *f*, Pectus excavatum/infundibulum/recurvatum.
trich·u·ri·a·sis [ˌtrɪkjə'raɪəsɪs] *n* Peitschenwurmbefall *m*, -infektion *f*, Trichurisbefall *m*, -infektion *f*, Trichuriasis *f*, Trichuriose *f*.
Trich·u·ris [trɪ'kjʊərɪs] *n micro.* Trichuris *f*. **T. trichiura** Peitschenwurm *m*, Trichuris trichiura, Trichocephalus dispar.
Trich·u·roi·dea [ˌtrɪkjə'rɔɪdɪə] *pl micro.* Trichuroidea *pl*.
tri·cip·i·tal [traɪ'sɪpɪtl] *adj anat.* 1. dreiköpfig. 2. M. triceps betr., Trizeps-, Triceps-.
tri·clo·car·ban [ˌtraɪkləʊ'kɑːrbæn] *n pharm.* Triclocarban *nt*.
tri·clo·san [traɪ'kləʊsæn] *n pharm.* Triclosan *nt*.
tri·corn ['traɪkɔːrn] *n* (*Gehirn*) Seitenventrikel *m*, Ventriculus lateralis.
tri·cre·sol [traɪ'kriːsɔl, -sɑl] *n* Kresol *nt*.
tri·crot·ic [traɪ'krɑtɪk] *adj card.* trikrot.
tricrotic pulse Trikrotie *f*, trikroter Puls *m*, Pulsus tricrotus.
tricrotic wave trikrote Welle *f*.
tri·cro·tism ['traɪkrətɪzəm] *n* → tricrotic pulse.
tri·cus·pid [traɪ'kʌspɪd] *adj* 1. *anat.* dreizipfelig, trikuspidal. 2. Trikuspidalklappe betr., Trikuspidalis-, Trikuspidalklappen-.
tricuspid area Tricuspidalisauskultationspunkt *m*.
tricuspid atresia Trikuspidal(klappen)-atresie *f*.
tricuspid incompetence → tricuspid regurgitation.
tricuspid insufficiency → tricuspid regurgitation.
tricuspid murmur *card.* Trikuspidal(klappen)geräusch *nt*.
tricuspid orifice Ostium atrioventriculare dextrum.
tricuspid regurgitation Trikuspidalisinsuffizienz *f*, Trikuspidal(klappen)insuffizienz *f*.
tricuspid stenosis Trikuspidal(klappen)stenose *f*.
tricuspid valve Trikuspidalklappe *f*, Tricuspidalis *f*, Valva/Valvula tricuspidalis, Valva atrioventricularis dextra.
tricuspid valve atresia → tricuspid atresia.
tri·cyc·lic [traɪ'saɪklɪk] *adj chem., pharm.* trizyklisch.
tricyclic antidepressants *pharm.* trizyklische Antidepressiva *pl*.
tri·dac·ty·lism [traɪ'dæktəlɪzəm] *n embryo.* Tridaktylie *f*.
tri·dac·ty·lous [traɪ'dæktɪləs] *adj* Tridaktylie betr., dreifingrig, dreizehig, tridaktyl.
tri·dent hand ['traɪdnt] Dreizackhand *f*.
tried [traɪd] *adj* erprobt, bewährt.
tri·eth·a·nol·a·mine [traɪˌeθə'nɑləmiːn] *n* Triäthanolamin *nt*, -ethanolamin *nt*.
tri·eth·yl·am·ine [traɪˌeθəl'æmiːn, -mɪn] *n* Triäthylamin *nt*.
tri·eth·yl·ene·mel·a·mine [traɪˌeθəliːn'meləmiːn] *n abbr.* **TEM** *pharm.* Triethylenmelamin *nt abbr.* TEM.

tri·eth·y·lene·thi·o·phos·phor·a·mide [traɪˌeθəliːnˌθaɪəʊfɑsˈfɔːrəmaɪd] *n abbr.* **TEPA** *pharm.* Thiotepa *nt*, Triäthylenthiophosphorsäuretriamid *nt*, Triethylenphosphoramid *nt*, Triethylenphosphoramid *nt abbr.* TPA.
tri·fa·cial [traɪˈfeɪʃl] *adj* → trigeminal II.
trifacial neuralgia → trigeminal neuralgia.
tri·flanged nail [ˈtraɪflændʒt] *ortho.* Drei(kant)lamellennagel *m*.
tri·flu·o·per·a·zine [ˌtraɪfluːəˈperəziːn] *n pharm.* Trifluoperazin *nt*.
tri·fluor·o·thy·mi·dine [traɪˌfloərəˈθaɪmədiːn] *n* → trifluridine.
tri·flu·per·i·dol [ˌtraɪfluːˈperɪdɑl, -dɔl] *n pharm.* Trifluperidol *nt*.
tri·flu·pro·ma·zine [ˌtraɪfluːˈprəʊməziːn] *n pharm.* Triflupromazin *nt*.
tri·flur·i·dine [traɪˈfloərədiːn] *n pharm.* Trifluridin *nt*.
tri·fo·cal glass [traɪˈfəʊkəl, ˈtraɪfəʊ-] → trifocal lens.
trifocal lens Dreistärkenlinse *f*, -glas *nt*, Trifokallinse *f*, -glas *nt*.
trifocal neuralgia → trigeminal neuralgia.
tri·fur·ca·tion [ˌtraɪfərˈkeɪʃn] *n* Dreiteilung *f*, Trifurkation *f*, Trifurcatio *f*.
tri·gas·tric [traɪˈgæstrɪk] *adj anat.* dreibäuchig.
tri·gem·i·nal [traɪˈdʒemɪnl] **I** *n* → trigeminal nerve. **II** *adj* dreifach; (Nervus) Trigeminus betr., trigeminal, Trigeminus-.
trigeminal and trochlear branches of internal carotid artery Rami trigeminales et trochleares.
trigeminal cavity Meckel'-Raum *m*, Cavum trigeminale, Cavitas trigeminalis.
trigeminal cisterns Cisterna trigemini.
trigeminal cough Husten *m* durch Trigeminusreizung.
trigeminal ganglion Gasser'-Ganglion *nt*, Ggl. trigeminale/semilunare/Gasseri.
trigeminal ganglion branch of internal carotid artery A. carotis interna-Ast *m* zum Ggl. trigeminale, Ramus ganglionis trigeminalis.
trigeminal hypoesthesia Trigeminushypästhesie *f*.
trigeminal impression (of temporal bone) Impressio trigeminalis.
trigeminal lemniscus Lemniscus trigeminalis, Tractus trigeminothalamicus.
trigeminal nerve N. Drillingsnerv *m*, Trigeminus *m*, V. Hirnnerv *m*, N. trigeminus.
trigeminal neuralgia Trigeminusneuralgie *f*, Neuralgia trigeminalis.
trigeminal paralysis Trigeminuslähmung *f*, -paralyse *f*.
trigeminal pulse Trigeminus *m*, Trigeminuspuls *m*, -rhythmus *m*, Pulsus trigeminus.
trigeminal rhizotomy *neurochir.* retroganglionäre Neurotomie *f*.
trigeminal rhythm → trigeminy.
tri·gem·i·no·fa·cial reflex [traɪˌdʒemɪnəʊˈfeɪʃl] Supraorbitalis-Reflex *m*.
tri·gem·i·no·tha·lam·ic tract [ˌ-θəˈlæmɪk] → trigeminal lemniscus.
tri·gem·i·nus reflex [traɪˈdʒemɪnəs] Trigeminusreflex *m*.
tri·gem·i·ny [traɪˈdʒemənɪ] *n card.* Trigeminie *f*, Trigeminus *m*.
trig·ger [ˈtrɪgər] **I** *n* Auslöser *m*, Trigger *m*. **II** *vt* → trigger off.
  trigger off *vt* auslösen, triggern.
  trigger area *neuro.* Triggerzone *f*, -punkt *m*.
  trigger finger schnellender/schnappender/federnder Finger *m*, Trigger-Finger *m*.
  trigger finger release *ortho.* Tenosynovektomie *f* bei Trigger-Finger.
  trigger point Triggerpunkt *m*.
  trigger reaction Triggerreaktion *f*.
  trigger thumb schnellender/schnappender Daumen *m*.
  trigger zone Triggerzone *f*.
tri·glyc·er·ide [traɪˈglɪsəraɪd, -ɪd] *n old* → triacylglycerol.
tri·gon [ˈtraɪgɑn, -gən] *n* **1.** → triangle. **2.** → trigone.
trig·o·nal [ˈtrɪgənl] *adj* **1.** dreieckig. **2.** *anat.* Trigonum betr.
tri·gone [ˈtraɪgəʊn] *n anat.* Dreieck *nt*, dreieckige Struktur *od.* Fläche *f*, Trigonum *nt*.
  t. of bladder (Harn-)Blasendreieck, Lieutaud'-Dreieck, Trigonum vesicae.
  t. of fellet Trigonum lemnisci.
  t. of hypoglossal nerve Trigonum hypoglossale, Trigonum n. hypoglossi.
  t. of lemniscus Trigonum lemnisci.
  t. of vagus nerve Trigonum vagale, Trigonum n. vagi.
tri·gon·ec·to·my [ˌtraɪgəʊˈnektəmɪ] *n urol.* Trigonektomie *f*.
trig·o·nel·line [ˌtrɪgəˈnelɪn] *n* Trigonellin *nt*.
tri·go·ni·tis [ˌtraɪgəˈnaɪtɪs] *n urol.* Entzündung *f* des Blasendreiecks, Trigonitis *f*.
trig·o·no·ce·pha·lia [ˌtrɪgənəʊsɪˈfeɪljə] *n* → trigonocephaly.
trig·o·no·ce·phal·ic [ˌ-sɪˈfælɪk] *adj* Trigonozephalie betr., trigonozephal.
trig·o·no·ceph·a·lus [ˌ-ˈsefələs] *n embryo.* Trigonozephalus *m*, -cephalus *m*.
trig·o·no·ceph·a·ly [ˌ-ˈsefəlɪ] *n* Dreieckschädel *m*, Trigonozephalus *m*.
tri·go·num [traɪˈgəʊnəm] *n, pl* **-na** [-nə] *anat.* → trigone.
tri·hex·o·side [traɪˈheksəsaɪd] *n* Trihexosid *nt*.
tri·hex·o·syl·cer·a·mide [traɪˌheksəsɪlˈserəmaɪd] *n* Trihexosylceramid *nt*.
trihexosylceramide galactosylhydrolase Ceramidtrihexosidase *f*, α-(D)-Galaktosidase A *f*.
tri·hex·y·phen·i·dyl [traɪˌheksɪˈfenədɪl] *n pharm.* Trihexyphenidyl.
tri·hy·brid [traɪˈhaɪbrɪd] *adj genet.* trihybrid.
tri·hy·brid·ism [traɪˈhaɪbrədɪzəm] *n genet.* Trihybridie *f*.
tri·hy·drate [traɪˈhaɪdreɪt] *n* → trihydroxide.
tri·hy·dric alcohol [traɪˈhaɪdrɪk] dreiwertiger Alkohol *m*.
tri·hy·drox·ide [ˌtraɪhaɪˈdrɑksaɪd, -sɪd] *n chem.* Trihydroxid *nt*.
tri·hy·drox·y·ace·to·phe·none [ˌtraɪhaɪˌdrɑksɪəˌsiːtəʊfəˈnəʊn, -ˈfiːnəʊn, -ˌæsɪtəʊ-] *n* Trihydroxyacetophenon *nt*.
1,2,3-tri·hy·drox·y·ben·zene [ˌ-ˈbenziːn] *n* Pyrogallol *nt*, 1,2,3-Trihydroxybenzol *nt*.
1,3,5-trihydroxybenzene *n* Phloroglucin *nt*, 1,3,5-Trihydroxybenzol *nt*.
tri·hy·drox·y·cop·ro·stane [ˌ-ˈkɑprəsteɪn] *n* Trihydroxyprostan *nt*.
tri·hy·drox·y·cop·ro·sta·no·ic acid [ˌ-ˌkɑprəstəˈnəʊɪk] Trihydroxykoprostansäure *f*.
tri·hy·drox·y·es·ter·in [ˌ-ˈestərɪn] *n* Östriol *nt*, Estriol *nt*.
tri·i·o·dide [traɪˈaɪədaɪd, -dɪd] *n* Trijodid *nt*, Triiodid *nt*.
tri·i·o·do·meth·ane [traɪˌaɪədəʊˈmeθeɪn] *n* Jodoform *nt*.
tri·i·o·do·thy·ro·nine [traɪˌaɪədəʊˈθaɪrəniːn, -nɪn] *n abbr.* **T₃** (L-3,5-3'-)Trijodthyronin *nt abbr.* T₃, Triiodthyronin *nt*.
triiodothyronine toxicosis Thyreotoxikose *f*.
triiodothyronine uptake test T_3U-Test *m*, T_3-uptake-Test *m*.

trinitrocresol

tri·ke·to·hy·drin·dene hydrate [traɪˌkiːtəʊhaɪˈdrɪndiːn] Ninhydrin *nt*, Triketohydrindenhydrat *nt*.
tri·ke·to·pu·rine [traɪˌkiːtəʊˈpjʊəriːn, -rɪn] *n* Harnsäure *f*.
tri·labe [ˈtraɪleɪb] *n urol.* Trilabe *f*.
tri·lam·i·nar [traɪˈlæmɪnər] *adj* dreischichtig, aus drei Schichten/Lagen bestehend, trilaminär.
trilaminar blastoderm/blastodisk dreiblättrige Keimscheibe *f*.
tri·lam·i·nate [traɪˈlæmɪneɪt, -nɪt] *adj* → trilaminar.
tri·lat·er·al [traɪˈlætərəl] *adj* drei Seiten betr., trilateral.
tri·li·no·le·in [traɪlɪˈnəʊlɪən] *n* Trilinolein *nt*.
tri·lo·bate [traɪˈləʊbeɪt] *adj* dreigelappt.
trilobate placenta dreigeteilte Plazenta *f*, Placenta trilobata.
tri·lobed [ˈtraɪləʊbt] *adj* → trilobate.
tri·loc·u·lar heart [traɪˈlɑkjələr] Cor triloculare.
tril·o·gy [ˈtrɪlədʒɪ] *n patho.* Trilogie *f*; Trias *f*, Triade *f*.
  t. of Fallot Fallot'-Trilogie, -Triade, Fallot III *m*.
tri·mal·le·o·lar fracture [ˌtraɪməˈlɪələr] trimalleoläre (Knöchel-)Fraktur *f*.
tri·ma·zo·sin [traɪˈmæzəsɪn] *n pharm.* Trimazosin *nt*.
tri·me·non [traɪˈmiːnɑn] *n* → trimester 1.
tri·men·su·al [traɪˈmenʃəwəl] *adj* alle drei Monate auftretend, trimensuell, trimensual.
tri·mer [ˈtraɪmər] *n* Trimer *m*.
tri·mer·ic [traɪˈmerɪk] *adj* trimer.
tri·mes·ter [traɪˈmestər] *n* **1.** *gyn.* Trimester *nt*, Trimenon *nt*. **2.** Trimester *nt*.
tri·meth·a·di·one [ˌtraɪmeθəˈdaɪəʊn] *n pharm.* Trimethadion *nt*.
tri·meth·o·prim [traɪˈmeθəprɪm] *n pharm.* Trimethoprim *nt*.
tri·meth·yl·a·ce·tic acid [traɪˌmeθələˈsiːtɪk, -əˈset-] Trimethylessigsäure *f*.
tri·meth·yl·a·mine [traɪˌmeθələˈmiːn, -ˈæmɪn] *n* Trimethylamin *nt*.
trimethylamine oxide Trimethylaminoxid *nt*.
tri·meth·yl·am·i·nur·ia [traɪˌmeθlæmɪˈn(j)ʊərɪə] *n* Trimethylaminurie *f*.
tri·meth·yl·ene [traɪˈmeθɪliːn] *n* Zyklopropan *nt*.
ε-N-tri·meth·yl·ly·sine [traɪˌmeθəlˈlaɪsiːn, -sɪn] *n* ε-N-Trimethyllysine *nt*.
tri·meth·yl·xan·thine [traɪˌmeθəlˈzænθiːn, -θɪn] *n* Koffein *nt*, Coffein *nt*, Methyltheobromin *nt*, 1,3,7-Trimethylxanthin *nt*.
tri·met·o·zine [traɪˈmetəziːn] *n pharm.* Trimetozin *nt*.
tri·mip·ra·mine [traɪˈmɪprəmiːn] *n pharm.* Trimipramin *nt*.
tri·mor·phic [traɪˈmɔːrfɪk] *adj* → trimorphous.
tri·mor·phism [traɪˈmɔːrfɪzəm] *n bio.* Dreigestaltigkeit *f*, Trimorphismus *m*.
tri·mor·phous [traɪˈmɔːrfəs] *adj bio.* dreigestaltig, trimorph.
tri·neg·a·tive [traɪˈnegətɪv] *adj* dreifach negativ.
tri·neu·ral [traɪˈnjʊərəl, -ˈnʊ-] *adj* drei Nerven betr.
tri·neu·ric [traɪˈnjʊərɪk, -ˈnʊ-] *adj* **1.** drei Nerven betr. **2.** aus drei Nerven bestehend.
tri·ni·trate [traɪˈnaɪtreɪt, -trɪt] *n* Trinitrat *nt*.
tri·ni·trin [traɪˈnaɪtrɪn] *n* → trinitroglycerin.
tri·ni·tro·cre·sol [traɪˌnaɪtrəʊˈkriːsɔl, -sɑl] *n* Trinitrokresol *nt*.

tri·ni·tro·glyc·er·in [ˌ-ˈglɪsərɪn] *n pharm.* Glyceroltrinitrat *nt*, Nitroglyzerin *nt*.
tri·ni·tro·glyc·er·ol [ˌ-ˈglɪsərɒl, -ral] *n* → trinitroglycerin.
tri·ni·tro·phe·nol [ˌ-ˈfiːnɒl, -nal] *n* Pikrinsäure *f*, Trinitrophenol *nt*.
tri·ni·tro·tol·u·ene [ˌ-ˈtaljuwiːn] *n abbr.* TNT Trinitrotoluol *nt abbr.* TNT.
tri·nu·cle·ate [traɪˈn(j)uːklɪeɪt] *adj* dreikernig, drei Kerne besitzend.
tri·nu·cle·o·tide [traɪˈn(j)uːklɪətaɪd] *n* Trinukleotid *nt*.
tri·o·le·in [traɪˈəʊliːɪn] *n* Triolein *nt*, Trioleylglycerin *nt*.
tri·ole·o·yl·glyc·er·ol [ˌtraɪəʊˌlɪəwɪlˈglɪsərɒl] *n* → triolein.
tri·o·lism [ˈtraɪəlɪzəm] *n* Triolismus *m*.
tri·oph·thal·mos [ˌtraɪɒfˈθælməs] *n embryo.* Triophthalmos *m*, Triophthalmus *m*.
tri·o·pod·y·mus [traɪəˈpɒdɪməs] *n embryo.* Triopodymus *m*.
tri·or·chid [traɪˈɔːrkɪd] *n* Patient *m* mit Triorchidie.
tri·or·chi·dism [traɪˈɔːrkədɪzəm] *n urol.* Triorchidie *f*, Triorchidismus *m*, Triorchismus *m*.
tri·or·chis [traɪˈɔːrkɪs] *n* → trichorchid.
tri·or·chism [traɪˈɔːrkɪzəm] *n* → triorchidism.
tri·ose [ˈtraɪəʊs] *n* Triose *f*, C_3-Zucker *m*.
tri·ose·phos·phate [ˌtraɪəʊsˈfɒsfeɪt] *n* Triosephosphat *nt*.
triosephosphate dehydrogenase Glyzerinaldehyd(-3-)dehydrogenase *f abbr.* GAPD(H), 3-Phosphoglyzerinaldehyd-dehydrogenase *f*.
triosephosphate isomerase Triosephosphatisomerase *f*.
tri·ox·ide [traɪˈɒksaɪd, -sɪd] *n* Trioxid *nt*.
tri·ox·y·pu·rine [traɪˌɒksɪˈpjʊərɪn, -rɪn] *f.* Harnsäure *f*.
tri·pal·mi·tin [traɪˈpælmɪtɪn, -ˈpɑː(l)-] *n* Tripalmitin *nt*, Tripalmitylglycerin *nt*.
tri·pal·mi·to·yl·glyc·er·ol [traɪˌpælmɪtəwɪlˈglɪsərɒl, -ral] *n* → tripalmitin.
tri·pa·re·sis [ˌtraɪpəˈriːsɪs] *n neuro.* Triparese *f*.
tri·par·tite [traɪˈpɑːrtaɪt] *adj* aus drei Teilen bestehend, dreiteilig, dreigeteilt.
tripartite placenta → trilobate placenta.
tri·pel·en·na·mine [ˌtraɪpelˈenəmiːn, -mɪn] *n pharm.* Tripelennamin *nt*.
tri·pep·tide [traɪˈpeptaɪd] *n* Tripeptid *nt*.
tri·pha·lan·ge·al [ˌtraɪfəˈlændʒɪəl] *adj ortho.* dreigliedrig, triphalangeal.
tri·pha·lan·gia [ˌtraɪfəˈlændʒɪə] *n* → triphalangism.
tri·phal·an·gism [traɪˈfælændʒɪzəm] *n ortho.* Dreigliedrigkeit *f*, Triphalangie *f*.
trip-hammer pulse [trɪp] 1. Corrigan-Puls *m*, Pulsus celer et altus. 2. Wasserhammerpuls *m*.
tri·pha·sic [traɪˈfeɪzɪk] *adj physiol.* dreiphasisch.
tri·phe·nyl·tet·ra·zo·li·um chloride [traɪˌfenlˌtetrəˈzəʊlɪəm] *abbr.* TTC Triphenyltetrazoliumchlorid *nt abbr.* TTC.
triphenyltetrazolium chloride reaction Triphenyltetrazoliumchloridreaktion *f*, TTC-Reaktion *f*.
tri·phos·phate [traɪˈfɒsfeɪt] *n* Triphosphat *nt*.
tri·phos·pho·pyr·i·dine nucleotide [traɪˌfɒsfəʊˈpɪrɪdiːn, -dɪn] *abbr.* TPN Nicotinamid-adenin-dinucleotid-phosphat *nt abbr.* NADP, Triphosphopyridinnucleotid *abbr.* TPN, Cohydrase II *f*, Coenzym II *nt*.
Tripier [triˈpje]: **T.'s amputation/operation** *ortho.* Fußamputation *f* nach Tripier, Tripier-Amputation *f*.

tri·ple [ˈtrɪpl] **I** *n* das Dreifache. **II** *adj* dreifach, -malig, drei-, tripel, Drei-, Tipel-. **III** *vt* verdreifachen. **IV** *vi s.* verdreifachen.
triple arthrodesis Tripelarthrodese *f*.
triple-blind *adj stat.* dreifach blind.
triple bond *chem.* Dreifachbindung *f*.
tri·ple·gia [traɪˈpliːdʒ(ɪ)ə] *n neuro.* Triplegie *f*.
triple phosphate *chem.* Tripelphosphat *nt*.
triple point *phys.* Tripelpunkt *m*.
triple salt *chem.* Tripelsalz *nt*.
triple scoliosis *ortho.* Tripelskoliose *f*.
triple sugar iron agar Dreizucker-Eisen--Agar *m/nt*.
triple symptom complex Behçet-Krankheit *f*, -Syndrom *nt*, bipolare/große/maligne Aphthose *f*, Gilbert-Syndrom *nt*, Aphthose Touraine/Behçet.
tri·plet [ˈtrɪplɪt] *n* 1. Dreiergruppe *f*, Triplett *nt*. 2. Drilling *m*.
triple vision → triplopia.
triple-X *n genet.* 1. Metafemale *f*, Patientin *f* mit Drei-X-Syndrom *nt*. 2. Drei-X-Syndrom *nt*, Triplo-X-Syndrom *nt*, XXX-Syndrom *nt*.
tri·plex [ˈtrɪpleks, ˈtraɪ-] *adj* dreifach.
trip·loid [ˈtrɪplɔɪd] **I** *n* Triploider *m*. **II** *adj* triploid.
trip·loi·dy [ˈtrɪplɔɪdɪ] *n genet.* Triploidie *f*.
trip·lo·pia [trɪpˈləʊpɪə] *n ophthal.* Dreifachsehen *nt*, Triplopie *f*.
tri·pod [ˈtraɪpɒd] *n* Dreifuß *m*.
tri·po·dia [traɪˈpəʊdɪə] *n ortho.* Tripodie *f*.
tri·pos·i·tive [traɪˈpɒzətɪv] *adj* dreifach positiv.
tri·pro·so·pus [ˌtraɪprəˈsəʊpəs, traɪˈprɒs-] *n embryo.* Triprosopus *m*.
tri·pus [ˈtraɪpəs] *n* 1. Dreifuß *m*. 2. *embryo.* Tripus *m*.
tri·que·tral bone [traɪˈkwiːtrl, -ˈkwe-] Dreiecksbein *nt*, Os triquetrum.
triquetral cartilage Stell-, Gießbecken-, Aryknorpel *m*, Cartilago aryt(a)enoidea.
triquetral fossa Fossa triangularis (auriculae).
triquetral ligament 1. Lig. coracoacromiale. 2. Lig. cricoaryt(a)enoideum posterius.
t. of foot Lig. calcaneofibulare.
t. of scapula Lig. transversum scapulae inferius.
tri·que·trous [traɪˈkwiːtrəs, -ˈkwe-] *adj* dreieckig.
triquetrous cartilage → triquetral cartilage.
tri·que·trum [traɪˈkwiːtrəm, -ˈkwe-] *n* Dreiecksbein *nt*, Os triquetrum.
TRIS *abbr.* [tris(hydroxymethyl)aminomethane] → tromethamine.
tri·sac·cha·ride [traɪˈsækəraɪd, -rɪd] *n* Dreifachzucker *m*, Trisaccharid *nt*.
TRIS buffer TRIS-Puffer *m*.
tris·hy·drox·y·meth·yl·a·mi·no·meth·ane [trɪshaɪˌdrɒksɪˌmeθələˌmiːnəʊˈmeθeɪn, -ˌæmɪnəʊ-] → tromethamine.
tris·meth·yl·a·mi·no·meth·ane [-ˌmeθələˌmiːnəʊˈmeθeɪn, -ˌæmɪnəʊ-] → tromethamine.
tris·mic [ˈtrɪzmɪk] *adj* Trismus betr.
tris·mus [ˈtrɪzməs] *n* Kieferklemme *f*, Trismus *m*.
tris·ni·trate [trɪsˈnaɪtreɪt] *n* Trinitrat *nt*.
tri·so·mia [traɪˈsəʊmɪə] *n* → trisomy.
tri·so·mic [traɪˈsəʊmɪk] *adj* Trisomie betr., von Trisomie betroffen, trisom.
tri·so·my [ˈtraɪsəʊmɪ] *n* Trisomie *f*.
trisomy C syndrome Trisomie 8(-Syndrom *nt*) *f*.
trisomy D syndrome Trisomie 13(-Syndrom *nt*) *f*, Patau-Syndrom, D_1-Trisomie-Syndrom *nt*.

trisomy E syndrome Edwards-Syndrom *nt*, Trisomie 18(-Syndrom *nt*) *f*.
trisomy syndrome Trisomie-Syndrom *nt*.
trisomy 8 syndrome Trisomie 8(-Syndrom *nt*) *f*.
trisomy 13 syndrome → trisomy D syndrome.
trisomy 14 syndrome Trisomie 14(-Syndrom *nt*) *f*.
trisomy 18 syndrome → trisomy E syndrome.
trisomy 21 syndrome Down-Syndrom *nt*, Trisomie 21(-Syndrom *nt*) *f*, Mongoloidismus *m*, Mongolismus *m*.
tri·ste·a·rin [traɪˈstɪərɪn] *n* Tristearin *nt*, Tristearylglycerin *nt*.
tri·ste·ar·o·yl·glyc·er·ol [traɪstɪˌærəwɪlˈglɪsərɒl] *n* → tristearin.
tri·stich·ia [traɪˈstɪkɪə] *n derm.* Tristichiasis *f*.
tri·sub·sti·tut·ed [traɪˈsʌbstɪt(j)uːtɪd] *adj chem.* dreifach substituiert.
tri·sul·fate [traɪˈsʌlfeɪt] *n* Trisulfat *nt*.
tri·sul·fide [traɪˈsʌlfaɪd, -fɪd] *n* Trisulfid *nt*.
tri·syn·ap·tic [ˌtraɪsɪˈnæptɪk] *adj* drei Synapsen betr. *od.* umfassend, trisynaptisch.
tri·ta·nom·al [ˌtraɪtəˈnaml] *n ophthal.* Tritanomale(r *m*) *f*.
tri·ta·nom·a·lous [ˌ-ˈnamələs] *adj* Tritanomalie betr., tritanomal.
tri·ta·nom·a·ly [ˌ-ˈnamælɪ] *n* Gelb-Blau--Schwäche *f*, Blau-Gelb-Schwäche *f*, Tritanomalie *f*.
tri·ta·nope [ˈ-nəʊp] *n* Tritanope(r *m*) *f*.
tri·ta·no·pia [ˌ-ˈnəʊpɪə] *n* Blaublindheit *f*, Tritanop(s)ie *f*.
tri·ta·nop·ic [ˌ-ˈnɒpɪk] *adj* Tritanopie betr., blaublind, tritanop.
tri·ta·nop·sia [ˌ-ˈnɒpsɪə] *n* → tritanopia.
tri·ter·pene [traɪˈtɜːrpiːn] *n* Triterpen *nt*.
trit·i·ate [ˈtrɪtɪeɪt, ˈtrɪʃ-] *vt* mit Tritium behandeln *od.* markieren.
trit·i·a·ted water [ˈtrɪtɪeɪtɪd, ˈtrɪʃɪ-] → tritium-labeled water.
tri·ti·ce·al cartilage [trəˈtiːʃ(ɪ)əl] → triticeum.
tri·ti·ceous cartilage [trəˈtɪʃəs] → triticeum.
tri·ti·ce·um [trəˈtiːʃ(ɪ)əm] *n*, *pl* **-cei** [-ʃɪaɪ] Weizenknorpel *m*, Cartilago triticea.
trit·i·um [ˈtrɪtɪəm, ˈtrɪʃ-] *n abbr.* ³H Tritium *nt abbr.* ³H.
tritium-labeled water *abbr.* THO tritiummarkiertes Wasser *nt abbr.* THO.
trit·o·cal·ine [ˌtrɪtəˈkæliːn] *n* → tritoqualine.
tri·ton [ˈtraɪtn] *n* → trinitrotoluene.
trit·o·qual·ine [ˌtrɪtəˈkwæliːn] *n pharm.* Tritoqualin *nt*.
trit·u·ra·ble [ˈtrɪtʃərəbl] *adj pharm.* verreibbar.
trit·u·rate [ˈtrɪtʃəreɪt] *vt* pulverisieren, zermahlen, zerstoßen, zerreiben.
trit·u·ra·tion [ˌtrɪtʃəˈreɪʃn] *n* Pulverisierung *f*, Zermahlung *f*, Zerreibung *f*; Verreiben *nt*, Trituration *f abbr.* T.
tri·va·lence [traɪˈveɪləns] *n chem.* Dreiwertigkeit *f*.
tri·va·lent [traɪˈveɪlənt] *adj chem.* dreiwertig, trivalent.
trivalent chromosome trivalentes Chromosom *nt*.
trivalent oral poliovirus vaccine *abbr.* TOPV trivalente orale Poliovakzine *f*.
triv·i·al [ˈtrɪvɪəl] *adj* gering(fügig), belanglos, unbedeutend, banal, trivial.
trivial name *chem., pharm.* Trivialname *m*.
tRNA *abbr.* → transfer-RNA.
tro·car [ˈtrəʊkɑːr] *n chir.* Trokar *m*, Trokart *m*, Troikart *m*, Troicart *m*.
tro·chan·ter [trəʊˈkæntər] *n* Trochanter

tro·chan·ter·i·an [ˌtrəʊkən'tɪərɪən] *adj* → trochanteric.
tro·chan·ter·ic [-'terɪk] *adj* Trochanter betr., trochantär.
trochanteric bursa: t. of gluteus maximus (muscle) Bursa trochanterica m. glut(a)ei maximi.
t.e of gluteus medius (muscle) Bursae trochantericae m. glut(a)ei medii.
t. of gluteus minimus (muscle) Bursa trochanterica m. glut(a)ei minimi.
subcutaneous t. Bursa subcutanea trochanterica.
trochanteric crest Crista intertrochanterica.
trochanteric fossa Fossa trochanterica.
tro·chan·ter·plas·ty [trəʊ'kæntərplæstɪ] *n ortho.* Trochanterplastik *f.*
trochanter reflex Trochanterreflex *m.*
tro·chan·tin [trəʊ'kæntɪn] *n* Trochanter minor.
tro·chan·tin·i·an [ˌtrəʊkæn'tɪnɪən] *adj* Trochanter minor betr.
tro·che ['trəʊkiː] *n pharm.* Pastille *f.*
tro·chis·cus [trəʊ'kɪskəs] *n, pl* **-ci** [-kaɪ] troche.
troch·lea ['trɒklɪə] *n, pl* **-le·as, -le·ae** [-liː] *anat.* Walze *f*, Rolle *f*, Trochlea *f.*
t. of humerus Gelenkwalze des Humerus, Trochlea humeri.
t. of superior oblique muscle Trochlea, Trochlea obliqui superioris bulbi.
t. of talus Talusrolle, Trochlea tali/talare.
troch·le·ar ['trɒklɪər] *adj* **1.** walzen-, rollenförmig. **2.** Trochlea betr.
trochlear bursa, synovial Sehnenscheide *f* des N. obliquus superior, Bursa synovialis trochlearis, Vagina synovialis/tendinis n. obliqui superioris.
trochlear decussation Decussatio nn. trochlearium, Decussatio trochlearis.
trochlear fossa Fovea trochlearis.
trochlear fovea Fovea trochlearis.
troch·le·ar·i·form [ˌtrɒklɪ'eərɪfɔːrm] *adj* → trochlear 1.
trochlear ligament Lig. metacarpale transversum profundum.
t.s of hand Ligg. palmaria.
trochlear nerve Trochlearis *m*, IV. Hirnnerv *m*, N. trochlearis.
trochlear nerve nucleus Trochleariskern *m*, Nc. (n.) trochlearis.
trochlear notch (of ulna) Inc. trochlearis (ulnae).
trochlear pit Fovea trochlearis.
trochlear spine Spina trochlearis.
trochlear tubercle → trochlear spine.
troch·le·i·form ['trɒklɪaɪfɔːrm] *adj* → trochlear 1.
troch·o·car·dia [ˌtrɒkə'kɑːrdɪə] *n card.* Trochokardie *f.*
troch·o·ce·pha·lia [ˌ-sɪ'feɪlɪə] *n* → trochocephaly.
troch·o·ceph·a·ly [ˌ-'sefəlɪ] *n* Trochozephalie *f*, -kephalie *f.*
tro·choid ['trəʊkɔɪd] **I** *n* → trochoidal articulation. **II** *adj* **1.** rad-, zapfenförmig. **2.** s. um eine Achse drehend.
tro·choi·dal articulation [trəʊ'kɔɪdl, trɑ-] Dreh-, Zapfen-, Radgelenk *nt*, Artic. trochoidea.
trochoidal joint → trochoidal articulation.
tro·choi·des [trəʊ'kɔɪdiːz] *n* → trochoidal articulation.
trochoid joint → trochoidal articulation.
troch·o·phore ['trɒkəfɔʊər, -fɔːr] *n bio.* Trochophora *f.*
Trog·lo·tre·ma [ˌtrɒglə'triːmə] *n micro.* Troglotrema *nt.*
troi·lism ['trɔɪlɪzəm] *n* → triolism.
Troisier [trwɑ'zje]: **T.'s ganglion** Troisier'-Knoten *m.*

T.'s node Troisier'-Knoten *m.*
T.'s syndrome Troisier-Syndrom *nt.*
tro·la·mine ['trɒləmiːn] *n* Triäthanolamin *nt*, Triethanolamin *nt.*
Trolard [trɔ'lɑːr]: **T.'s net/network** → T.'s plexus.
T.'s plexus Venengeflecht *nt* im Hypoglossuskanal, Plexus venosus canalis hypoglossi.
T.'s vein Trolard'-Vene *f*, V. anastomotica superior.
Tröltsch ['trɛltʃ; 'trœltʃ]: **anterior pouch of T.** vordere Schleimhauttasche *f* des Trommelfells, Rec. (membranae tympanicae) anterior.
posterior pouch of T. hintere Schleimhauttasche *f* des Trommelfells, Rec. (membranae tympanicae) posterior.
T.'s recesses → T.'s spaces.
T.'s spaces *HNO* Tröltsch'-Taschen *pl.*
Trom·bic·u·la [trɒm'bɪkjələ] *n micro.* Trombicula *f.*
T. autumnalis Erntemilbe *f*, Trombicula autumnalis.
trom·bic·u·li·a·sis [trɒmˌbɪkjə'laɪəsɪs] *n* Erntekrätze *f*, Heukrätze *f*, Sendlinger Beiß *m*, Giesinger Beiß *m*, Herbstbeiße *f*, Herbstkrätze *f*, Gardnerbeiß *m*, Trombidiose *f*, Trombidiosis *f*, Erythema autumnale.
trom·bi·cu·li·dae [ˌtrɒmbə'kjuːlədiː] *pl* Trombiculidae *pl.*
trom·bid·i·a·sis [trɒmˌbɪdɪ'aɪəsɪs] *n* → trombiculiasis.
trom·bid·i·o·sis [trɒmˌbɪdɪ'əʊsɪs] *n* → trombiculiasis.
trombone tremor of tongue [trɒm'bəʊn, 'trɒmbəʊn] Magnan-Zeichen *nt.*
tro·meth·a·mine [trəʊ'meθəmiːn] *n abbr.* **THAM** Trometanol *nt abbr.* THAM, TRIS(-Puffer *m*) *nt.*
Trömner ['tremnər; 'trœm-]: **T.'s reflex/sign** Trömner-Reflex *m*, -Fingerzeichen *nt*, Fingerbeugereflex *m*, Knipsreflex *m.*
trom·o·ma·nia [ˌtrɒmə'meɪnɪə, -jə] *n* Entzugssyndrom *nt*, -delir *nt*, Delirium tremens.
tro·pa·ic acid [trəʊ'peɪɪk] Tropasäure *f.*
tro·pane ['trəʊpeɪn] *n* Tropan *nt.*
tro·pate ['trəʊpeɪt] *n* Tropat *nt.*
tro·pe·ic acid [trəʊ'piːɪk] → tropaic acid.
troph- *pref.* → tropho-.
troph·ec·to·derm [trɒf'ektədɜːrm] *n embryo.* Trophektoderm *nt.*
troph·e·de·ma [trɒfɪ'diːmə] *n* Trophödem *nt.*
troph·ic ['trɒfɪk, 'trəʊ-] *adj* Nahrung/Ernährung betr., trophisch.
trophic keratitis Keratitis/Keratopathia neuroparalytica.
trophic nucleus → trophonucleus.
trophic ulcer trophisches Ulkus *nt*, Ulcus trophicum.
tropho- *pref.* Ernährungs-, Nahrungs-, Troph(o)-, Nährstoff-.
troph·o·blast ['trɒfəblæst, 'trəʊ-] *n embryo.* Trophoblast *m.*
trophoblast giant cells Trophoblastriesenzellen *pl.*
troph·o·blas·tic [ˌ-'blæstɪk] *adj* Trophoblast betr., Trophoblasten-.
trophoblastic cells *embryo.* Trophoblastenzellen *pl.*
trophoblastic lacunae *embryo.* Trophoblastenlakunen *pl.*
trophoblast maturation Trophoblastenreifung *f.*
troph·o·blas·to·ma [ˌ-blæs'təʊmə] *n patho., gyn.* Chorioblastom *nt*, (malignes) Chorio(n)epitheliom *nt*, Chorionkarzinom *nt*, fetaler Zottenkrebs *m.*

troph·o·chro·ma·tin [ˌ-'krəʊmətɪn] *n* Trophochromatin *nt.*
troph·o·chro·mid·ia [ˌ-krəʊ'mɪdɪə] *n* → trophochromatin.
troph·o·cyte ['-saɪt] *n* Nährzelle *f*, Trophozyt *m.*
troph·o·derm ['-dɜːrm] *n* → trophoblast.
troph·o·der·ma·to·neu·ro·sis [ˌ-ˌdɜːrmətənjʊə'rəʊsɪs, -nʊ-] *n* Feer'-Krankheit *f*, Rosakrankheit *f*, vegetative Neurose *f* der Kleinkinder, Swift-Syndrom *nt*, Selter-Swift-Feer'-Krankheit *f*, Feer-Selter-Swift-Krankheit *f*, Akrodynie *f*, Acrodynia *f.*
troph·o·dy·nam·ics [ˌ-daɪ'næmɪks] *pl* Ernährungs-, Trophodynamik *f.*
troph·o·e·de·ma [ˌ-ɪ'diːmə] *n* → trophedema.
tro·phol·o·gy [trəʊ'fɒlədʒɪ] *n* Ernährungslehre *f*, Trophologie *f.*
troph·o·neu·ro·sis [ˌtrɒfənjʊə'rəʊsɪs, -nʊ-, ˌtrəʊfə-] *n* Trophoneurose *f.*
troph·o·neu·rot·ic [ˌ-njʊə'rɒtɪk, -nʊ-] *adj* Trophoneurose betr., trophoneurotisch.
trophoneurotic atrophy Denervationsatrophie *f*; Trophoneurose *f.*
trophoneurotic ulcer neurotrophische Ulzeration *f*, trophoneurotisches Ulkus *nt*, Ulcus trophoneuroticum.
troph·o·nu·cle·us [ˌ-'n(j)uːklɪəs] *n* Makro-, Meganukleus *m.*
troph·o·path·ia [ˌ-'pæθɪə] *n* → trophopathy.
tro·phop·a·thy [trəʊ'fɒpəθɪ] *n* Ernährungsfehler *m*, -mangel *m*, Trophopathie *f.*
troph·o·plasm ['trɒfəplæzəm, 'trəʊfə-] *n* Trophoplasma *nt*, Nährplasma *nt.*
troph·o·plast ['-plæst] *n* Plastid *m.*
troph·o·tax·is [ˌ-'tæksɪs] *n* → trophotropism.
tro·pho·trop·ic [ˌ-'trɒpɪk] *adj* trophotrop.
trophotropic zone trophotrope Zone *f.*
tro·phot·ro·pism [trəʊ'fɒtrəpɪzəm] *n* Trophotropismus *m*, Trophotaxis *f.*
troph·o·zo·ite [ˌtrɒfə'zəʊaɪt, ˌtrəʊf-] *n micro.* Trophozoit *m.*
trop·ic ['trɒpɪk] *adj* → tropical.
tro·pic acid ['trəʊpɪk, 'trɒpɪk] Tropasäure *f.*
trop·i·cal ['trɒpɪkl] *adj* tropisch, Tropen-.
tropical abscess Amöbenabszeß *m.*
tropical acne tropische Akne *f*, Tropenakne *f*, Akne/Acne tropicalis.
tropical anemia Anämie *f* bei Hakenwurmbefall.
tropical anhidrotic asthenia thermogene/tropische Anhidrose *f*, Anhidrosis tropica.
tropical bedbug *micro.* tropische Bettwanze *f*, Cimex hemipterus/rotundatus.
tropical bubo Morbus Durand-Nicolas-Favre *m*, klimatischer Bubo *m*, vierte Geschlechtskrankheit *f*, Poradenitis inguinalis, Lymphopathia venerea, Lymphogranuloma inguinale/venereum *abbr.* LGV.
tropical diarrhea tropische Sprue *f.*
tropical disease Tropenkrankheit *f.*
tropical fowl mite *micro.* Ornithonyssus bursa.
tropical heat tropische Hitze *f.*
tropical horse tick *micro.* Dermacentor nitens.
tropical hygiene Tropenhygiene *f.*
tropical hyphemia Hakenwurmbefall *m*, -infektion *f*, Ankylostomiasis *f*, Ankylostomatosis *f*, Ankylostomatideose *f.*
tropical lichen *derm.* Roter Hund *m*, tropische Flechte *f*, Miliaria rubra.
tropical medicine Tropenmedizin *f*, -heilkunde *f.*

tropical pyomyositis

tropical pyomyositis Myositis purulenta tropica.
tropical rat mite *micro.* Ornithonyssus bacoti.
tropical splenomegaly tropische Splenomegalie *f.*
tropical swelling Calabar-Beule *f,* -Schwellung *f,* Kamerun-Schwellung *f,* Loiasis *f,* Loiase *f.*
tropical typhus japanisches Fleckfieber *nt,* Scrub-Typhus *m,* Milbenfleckfieber *nt,* Tsutsugamushi-Fieber *nt.*
tropical ulcer 1. Tropen-, Wüstengeschwür *nt,* Ulcus tropicum. **2.** Ulzeration *f* bei kutaner Leishmaniose.
tropical zone Tropen *pl.*
tro·pic·a·mide [trəʊˈpɪkəmaɪd] *n pharm.* Tropicamid *nt.*
tropic hormone tropes Hormon *nt.*
tro·pin [ˈtrəʊpɪn] *n* Opsonin *nt.*
tro·pine [ˈtrəʊpiːn] *n* Tropin *nt.*
tropine mandelate Homatropin *nt.*
tropine tropate Atropin *nt.*
tro·pism [ˈtrəʊpɪzəm] *n* Tropismus *m,* tropistische Bewegung *f.*
tro·po·chrome cell [ˈtrəʊpəkrəʊm, ˈtrɒp-] mukoseröse Zelle *f.*
tro·po·col·la·gen [ˌ-ˈkɒlədʒən] *n* Tropokollagen *nt.*
tro·po·e·las·tin [ˌ-ɪˈlæstɪn] *n* Tropoelastin *nt.*
tro·po·my·o·sin [ˌ-ˈmaɪəsɪn] *n* Tropomyosin *nt.*
tropomyosin A Tropomyosin A *nt,* Paramyosin *nt.*
tro·po·nin [ˈtrɒpənɪn, ˈtrəʊ-] *n* Troponin *nt.*
troponin A calciumbindende Untereinheit *f,* Troponin A *nt abbr.* TN-C.
tro·tyl [ˈtrəʊtl] *n* → trinitrotoluene.
trou·ble [ˈtrʌbl] **I** *n* **1.** Mühe *f,* Anstrengung *f,* Last *f,* Belästigung *f,* Störung *f.* **2.** Schwierigkeit *f,* Problem *nt.* **3.** Leiden *nt,* Störung *f,* Beschwerden *pl.* **4.** *techn.* Störung *f,* Defekt *m.* **II** *vt* **5.** jdn. beunruhigen, stören. **6.** plagen, quälen (*with* von). **to be ~d with** geplagt werden von. **III** *vi* **7.** s. aufregen (*about* über). **8.** s. die Mühe machen, s. bemühen.
trouble-free *adj* problemlos, reibungslos, ruhig; *techn.* störungsfrei.
trouble-proof *adj* → trouble-free.
trou·ble·some [ˈtrʌblsəm] *adj* **1.** störend, lästig; unangenehm. **2.** mühsam, beschwerlich.
trou·ble·some·ness [ˈtrʌblsəmnɪs] *n* **1.** Lästigkeit *f.* **2.** Beschwerlichkeit *f,* Mühsamkeit *f.*
trouble spot Schwachstelle *f.*
trough [trɒf, trɔːf] *n* Mulde *f,* Rinne *f,* Furche *f,* Graben *m.*
trou·ser [ˈtraʊzər] *adj* Hosen-.
trou·sers [ˈtraʊzərz] *pl* (*a.* pair of ~) Hosen *pl,* Hose *f.*
Trousseau [truːˈsəʊ]: **T.'s phenomenon** → T.'s sign.
T.'s points Trousseau-Punkte *pl.*
T.'s sign Trousseau'-Zeichen *nt.*
T.'s syndrome Trousseau-Syndrom *nt.*
Trousseau-Lallemand [lalˈmɑ̃]: **T.-L. bodies** Sekretkörnchen *pl* der Samenbläschen.
trox·i·done [ˈtrɒksɪdəʊn] *n pharm.* Trimethadion *nt.*
Trp *abbr.* → tryptophan.
TRT *abbr.* → tolbutamide response test.
true [truː] *adj* wahr, wahrheitsgemäß; echt, wahr; naturgetreu; legitim; *bio.* reinrassig.
true albuminuria intrinsische Albuminurie/Proteinurie *f.*
true aneurysm echtes Aneurysma *nt,* Aneurysma verum.

true ankylosis *ortho.* knöcherne Gelenkversteifung/Ankylose *f,* Ankylosis ossea.
true anodontia Anodontia vera.
true anosmia essentielle Anosmie *f.*
true anuria echte Anurie *f.*
true aphasia echte/organisch-bedingte Aphasie *f.*
true asthma primäres/essentielles Asthma *nt.*
true chancre harter Chanker *m,* Hunter--Schanker *m,* Ulcus durum, syphilitischer Primäraffekt *m.*
true cholinesterase Azetyl-, Acetylcholinesterase *f abbr.* AChE, echte Cholinesterase *f.*
true chondroma echtes/zentrales Chondrom *nt,* Enchondrom *nt.*
true conjugate Conjugata anatomica.
true cyst echte Zyste *f.*
true decidua Decidua parietalis/vera.
true denticle wahrer/echter Dentikel *m.*
true diverticulum echtes Divertikel *nt,* Diverticulum vera.
true fungi echte Pilze *pl,* Eumyzeten *pl,* Eumycetes *pl,* Eumycophyta *pl.*
true gigantism einfacher/echter Riesenwuchs *m.*
true glottis Stimmritze *f,* Rima glottidis.
true hermaphrodite (echter) Hermaphrodit *m,* Zwitter *m,* Intersex *nt.*
true hermaphroditism echter Hermaphroditismus *m,* Hermaphroditismus verus.
true intersex → true hermaphrodite.
true knot *gyn.* echter/wahrer Nabelschnurknoten *m.*
true mole *gyn.* echte Mole *f,* Mola vera.
true neck of humerus anatomischer Humerushals *m,* Collum anatomicum humeri.
true neuroma echtes Neurom *nt;* Ganglioneurom *nt.*
true pelvis kleines Becken *nt,* Pelvis minor.
true proteinuria → true albuminuria.
true ribs echte Rippen *pl,* Costae verae.
true scurvy Scharbock *m,* Skorbut *m.*
true thirst echter Durst *m.*
true twins erbgleiche/eineiige/identische/monovuläre/monozygote Zwillinge *pl.*
true vertebra Vertebra vera.
Trüm·mer·feld line [ˈtrʏmərfɛlt] Trümmerfeldzone *f.*
trun·cal [ˈtrʌŋkl] *adj* Rumpf/Truncus betr., trunkulär, Rumpf-, Stamm-, Trunkus-.
truncal ataxia Rumpfataxie *f.*
truncal obesity Stammfettsucht *f.*
truncal vagotomy *psycho.* trunkuläre Vagotomie *f.*
trun·cate [ˈtrʌŋkeɪt] **I** *adj* abgestumpft, beschnitten, gestutzt. **II** *vt* stutzen, beschneiden.
trun·cat·ed [ˈtrʌŋkeɪtɪd] *adj* → truncate I.
trun·co·nal cushion [ˌtrʌŋkəʊˈkəʊnl] *embryo.* Trunkokonalkissen *nt.*
truncoconal septum *embryo.* Konusseptum *nt.*
trun·co·tha·lam·ic nuclei [ˌ-θəˈlæmɪk] trunkothalamische Kerne *pl,* Trunkothalamus *m,* unspezifische Thalamuskerne *pl.*
trun·co·thal·a·mus [ˌ-ˈθæləməs] *n, pl* -**mi** [-maɪ] → truncothalamic nuclei.
trun·cus [ˈtrʌŋkəs] *n, pl* -**ci** [-saɪ] **1.** Stamm *m,* Rumpf, Leib *m,* Torso *m,* Trunkus *m; anat.* Truncus *m.* **2.** Gefäßstamm *m,* -strang *m,* Nervenstamm *m,* -strang *m.*
truncus arteriosus *embryo.* Truncus arteriosus.
common t. Truncus arteriosus communis.
truncus cushion *embryo.* Trunkuswulst *m.*

major t. großer Trunkuswulst.
minor t. kleiner Trunkuswulst.
truncus septum *embryo.* Trunkusseptum *nt.*
trunk [trʌŋk] *n* **1.** Stamm *m,* Rumpf, Leib *m,* Torso *m,* Trunkus *m; anat.* Truncus *m.* **2.** Gefäßstamm *m,* -strang *m,* Nervenstamm *m,* -strang *m.* **3.** *fig.* Stamm *m,* Hauptteil *m.*
t. of accessory nerve Akzessoriusstamm, Truncus n. accessorii.
t. of atrioventricular bundle Stamm des His'-Bündels, Truncus fasciculi atrioventricularis.
t.s of brachial plexus Primärstämme/-stränge/-faszikel *pl* des Plexus brachialis, Trunci plexus brachialis.
t. of corpus callosum Balkenkörper *m,* Truncus corporis callosi.
t. of spinal nerve Spinalnervenstamm, Truncus n. spinalis.
trunk ataxia Rumpfataxie *f.*
trunk musculature Rumpf-, Stammuskulatur *f.*
trunk presentation *gyn.* Querlage *f.*
truss [trʌs] *n* Bruchband *nt.*
try [traɪ] (*v* tried; tried) **I** *n* Versuch *m.* **to have a ~ at sth.** einen Versuch haben mit; es versuchen mit etw. **II** *vt* **1.** versuchen, probieren. **2.** (aus-, durch-)probieren, testen, prüfen; (einen Versuch *od.* ein Experiment machen. **3.** (*Augen*) (über-)anstrengen, angreifen; (*Nerven*) auf eine harte Probe stellen. **4.** jdn. quälen, plagen. **III** *vi* versuchen (*at*); s. bemühen (*for* um); einen Versuch machen.
try on *vt* (*Prothese*) anprobieren.
try out *vt* → try 2.
try-on *n* Anprobe *f.*
tryp·an blue [ˈtrɪpæn, ˈtraɪ-] Trypanblau *nt.*
tryp·a·nid [ˈtrɪpənɪd] *n* → trypanosomid.
try·pan·o·ci·dal [trɪˌpænəˈsaɪdl] *adj* → trypanosomicidal.
try·pan·o·cide [trɪˈpænəsaɪd] *n* → trypanosomicide I.
try·pa·nol·y·sis [ˌtrɪpəˈnɒləsɪs] *n* Trypanosomenauflösung *f,* Trypanolyse *f.*
try·pan·o·lyt·ic [ˌtrɪpənəʊˈlɪtɪk, trɪˌpænə-] *adj* trypanosomenauflösend, trypanolytisch.
Try·pan·o·so·ma [ˌ-ˈsəʊmə] *n micro.* Trypanosoma *nt.*
try·pan·o·so·mal [ˌ-ˈsəʊməl] *adj* Trypanosomen betr., durch Trypanosomen verursacht, Trypanosomen-.
trypanosomal chancre → trypanosomid.
trypanosomal sexual stage tryptomastigote Form *f,* Trypanosomenform *f.*
try·pan·o·so·ma·tid [ˌ-ˈsəʊmətɪd] **I** *n* Trypanosomatide *f.* **II** *adj* Trypanosomatiden betr.
Try·pan·o·so·mat·i·dae [ˌ-səʊˈmætədiː] *pl micro.* Trypanosomatidae *pl.*
Try·pan·o·so·ma·ti·na [ˌ-ˌsəʊməˈtaɪnə] *pl* → Trypanosomatidae.
try·pan·o·some [trɪˈpænəsəʊm, ˈtrɪpənə-] *n micro.* **1.** Trypanosome *f,* Trypanosoma *nt.* **2.** → trypanosomal sexual stage.
try·pan·o·so·mi·a·sis [ˌ-səʊˈmaɪəsɪs] *n* Trypanosomen-, Trypanosomeninfektion *f,* Trypanosomiasis *f,* Trypanomiasis *f.*
try·pan·o·so·mi·ci·dal [ˌ-səʊməˈsaɪdl] *adj* trypanosomen(ab)tötend, trypanozid.
try·pan·o·so·mi·cide [ˌ-ˈsəʊməsaɪd] **I** *n* Trypanozid *nt,* Trypanosomizid *nt.* **II** *adj* trypanosomen(ab)tötend, trypanosomizid.
try·pan·o·so·mid [trɪˈpænəsəʊmɪd] *n* Trypanosomid *nt,* Trypanid *nt.*
trypan red → trypanroth.

try·pan·roth ['trɪpənrαθ] *n* Trypanrot *nt*.
tryp·ar·sa·mide [trɪ'pɑːrsəmaɪd] *n pharm.* Tryparsamid *nt*.
tryp·o·mas·ti·gote [ˌtraɪpəʊ'mæstɪgəʊt] *n micro.* trypomastigote Form *f*, Trypanosomenform *f*.
try·po·nar·syl [ˌ-'nɑːrsɪl] *n* → tryparsamide.
try·po·tan ['-tæn] *n* → tryparsamide.
tryp·sin ['trɪpsɪn] *n* Trypsin *nt*.
trypsin inhibitor Trypsininhibitor *m*.
tryp·sin·o·gen [trɪp'sɪnədʒən] *n* Trypsinogen *nt*.
trypt·a·mine ['trɪptəmiːn, trɪp'tæmɪn] *n* Tryptamin *nt*.
tryp·tic ['trɪptɪk] *adj* (tryptische) Verdauung betr., tryptisch.
tryptic digestion tryptische Andauung/Verdauung/Spaltung *f*.
tryp·to·mas·ti·gote stage [ˌtrɪptəʊ'mæstɪgəʊt] → trypanosomal sexual stage.
tryp·to·phan ['-fæn] *n abbr.* **Trp** Tryptophan *nt abbr.* Trp.
tryp·to·pha·nase [trɪp'tɑfəneɪz, 'trɪptəfə-] *n* Tryptophanpyrrolase *f*, Tryptophan-2,3-dioxigenase *f*.
tryptophan-2,3-dioxygenase *n* → tryptophanase.
tryp·to·phane ['trɪptəfeɪn] *n* → tryptophan.
tryptophan oxygenase Tryptophanoxigenase *f*.
tryptophan pyrrolase → tryptophanase.
tryptophan reaction Tryptophantest *m*.
tryptophan synthase Tryptophansynthase *f*.
tryp·to·phan·u·ria [ˌtrɪptəfə'n(j)ʊərɪə] *n* Tryptophanurie *f*.
tryp·to·phyl ['trɪptəfɪl] *n* Tryptophyl-(Radikal *nt*).
TSA *abbr.* → tumor-specific antigen.
TSD *abbr.* → Tay-Sachs disease.
tset·se ['tsetsiː, 'tsɪ-] *n* Zungen-, Tsetsefliege *f*, Glossina *f*.
tsetse fly → tsetse.
TSH *abbr.* [thyroid-stimulating hormone] → thyrotropin.
T-shaped fracture T-förmige Fraktur *f*.
TSH-RF *abbr.* [thyroid stimulating hormone releasing factor] → thyroliberin.
TSH test → thyroid-stimulating hormone test.
TSI *abbr.* → thyroid-stimulating immunoglobulin.
TSI agar → triple sugar iron agar.
ts mutant Temperatur-sensitive Mutante *f*, ts-Mutante *f*.
TSS *abbr.* → toxic shock syndrome.
TSST-1 *abbr.* → toxic shock-syndrome toxin-1.
TSTA *abbr.* → tumor-specific transplantation antigen.
T-strain mycoplasma *micro.* Ureaplasma urealyticum.
T substance T-Substanz *f*.
T suppressor cell T-Suppressorzelle *f*.
tsu·tsu·ga·mu·shi disease/fever [ˌtsuːtsəgə'muːʃɪ] japanisches Fleckfieber *nt*, Tsutsugamushi-Fieber *nt*, Milbenfleckfieber *nt*, Scrub-Typhus *m*.
T-system T-System *nt*, transversales Röhrensystem *nt*, System *nt* der transversalen Tubuli.
TT *abbr.* → thrombin time.
TTC *abbr.* → triphenyltetrazolium chloride.
TTC reaction Triphenyltetrazoliumchloridreaktion *f*, TTC-Reaktion *f*.
t-test *n stat.* Student-Test *m*, t-Test *m*.
TTGA *abbr.* → tellurite taurocholate gelatin agar.
t₃ toxicosis Thyreotoxikose *f*.

TTS *abbr.* → temporary threshold shift.
T tube *chir.* T-Röhrchen *nt*.
T tube catheter T-Katheter *m*.
T tube cholangiogram *radiol., chir.* Cholangiogramm *nt* über einen T-Drain.
T tube drainage *chir.* T-Drainage *f*, T-Drain *m*.
T tubule Transversaltubulus *m*, T-Tubulus *m*.
TTX *abbr.* → tetrodotoxin.
TU *abbr.* → tuberculin unit.
tu·am·i·no·hep·tane [ˌtuːəmiːnəʊ'hepteɪn, tuːˌæmɪnəʊ-] *n pharm.* Tuaminoheptan *nt*.
tu·ba ['t(j)uːbə] *n, pl* **-bae** [-biː] *anat.* Röhre *f*, Trompete *f*, Tube *f*, Tuba *f*.
tu·bal ['t(j)uːbəl] *adj* Tuba auditiva *od.* uterina betr., in einer Tube liegend *od.* ablaufend, tubar, tubal, tubär, Tubar-, Tuben-.
tubal abortion *gyn.* Tubarabort *m*, tubarer Abort *m*.
tubal air cells Cellulae pneumaticae.
tubal block *HNO* Tubenblockade *f*.
tubal branch: t.es of ovarian artery *pl* Rami tubales/tubarii a. ovaricae.
t. of tympanic plexus Ramus tubalis/tubarius plexus tympanici.
t. of uterine artery Tubenast *m* der A. uterina, Ramus tubalis/tubarius a. uterinae.
tubal canal Semicanalis tubae auditivae/auditoriae.
tubal carcinoma 1. *(Ohr)* Tubenkarzinom *nt*. 2. *gyn.* Tubenkarzinom *nt*.
tubal cartilage Tuben-, Ohrtrompetenknorpel *m*, Cartilago tubae auditoriae.
tubal catheterization *HNO* *(Ohr)* Tubenkatheterismus *m*.
tubal colic *gyn.* Tubenkolik *f*.
tubal extremity (of ovary) oberer Eierstockpol *m*, Extremitas tubaria/tubalis ovarii.
tubal folds (of uterine tube) Tubenfalten *pl*, Plicae tubariae/tubales.
tubal function *HNO* *(Ohr)* Tubenfunktion *f*.
tubal infection Tubeninfektion *f*.
tubal mole *gyn.* Tubenmole *f*.
tubal occlusion *HNO* *(Ohr)* Tubenverschluß *m*.
acute t. akuter Tubenverschluß, Serotympanum *nt*.
tubal ovarian abscess *gyn.* Tubenabszeß *m*.
tubal patency *HNO* *(Ohr)* Tubendurchlässigkeit *f*.
tubal pregnancy Eileiter-, Tuben-, Tubarschwangerschaft *f*, Tubargravidität *f*, Graviditas tubaria.
tubal prominence Torus tubarius.
tubal protuberance Torus tubarius.
tubal rupture *gyn.* Tubar-, Tubenruptur *f*.
tubal tonsil Tubenmandel *f*, Tonsilla tubaria.
tu·ba·tor·sion [ˌt(j)uːbə'tɔːrʃn] *n* → tubotorsion.
Tubbs [tʌbs]: **T.' dilator** Tubbs-Dilatator *m*.
tube [t(j)uːb] *n* 1. Rohr *nt*, Röhre *f*, Röhrchen *nt*, Schlauch *m*, Kanal *m*; Tube *f*. 2. *anat.* Röhre *f*, Kanal *m*, Tuba *f*. 3. *anat.* Eileiter *m*, Tube *f*, Ovidukt *m*, Salpinx *f*, Tuba uterina. 4. Sonde *f*, Rohr *nt*, Röhre *f*, Schlauch *m*.
tube cast *urol.* 1. Harnzylinder *m*. 2. Nierenzylinder *m*.
tu·bec·to·my [t(j)uː'bektəmɪ] *n gyn.* Eileiterentfernung *f*, -resektion *f*, Salpingektomie *f*.
tubed flap [t(j)uːbt] *chir.* Rundstiellappen *m*.

tubed pedicle flap → tubed flap.
tube flap → tubed flap.
tube graft → tubed flap.
tu·ber ['t(j)uːbə(r)] *n, pl* **-bers, -be·ra** [-bərə] 1. *anat.* Höcker *m*, Wulst *m*, Vorsprung *m*, Schwellung *f*, Tuber *nt*. 2. *patho.* Tuberkel *m*.
t. of ischium Tuber ischiadicium/ischiale.
tu·ber·al nuclei ['t(j)uːbərəl] Tuberkerne *pl*, Ncc. tuberales.
tuber angle Tuber-Gelenkwinkel *m*.
tu·ber·cle ['t(j)uːbərkl] *n* 1. *anat.* Höcker *m*, Schwellung *f*, Knoten *m*, Knötchen *nt*, Tuberculum *nt*. 2. *patho.* Tuberkel *m*, Tuberkelknötchen *nt*, Tuberculum *nt*.
t. of anterior scalene muscle Tuberculum m. scaleni anterioris.
t. of calcaneus Tuberculum calcanei.
t. of cuneate nucleus Tuberculum cuneatum.
t. of iliac crest Tuberculum iliacum.
t. of Meckel Tuberculum malus (humeri).
t. of nucleus gracilis Tuberculum gracile.
t. of rib Rippenhöcker, Tuberculum costae.
t. of Rolando Tuberculum trigeminale.
t. of scaphoid bone Tuberculum ossis scaphoidei.
t. of sella turcica Sattelknopf *m*, Tuberculum sellae turcicae.
t. of trapezium Tuberculum ossis trapezii.
t. of Weber Tuberculum minus (humeri).
tubercle bacillus Tuberkelbazillus *m*, -bakterium *nt*, Tuberkulosebazillus *m*, -bakterium *nt*, TB-Bazillus *m*, TB-Erreger *m*, Mycobacterium tuberculosis, Mycobacterium tuberculosis var. hominis.
tu·ber·cu·lar [ˌt(j)uː'bɜːrkjələr] *adj* Tuberkel betr., tuberkelähnlich, tuberkular.
tubercular meningitis tuberkulöse Meningitis *f*, Meningitis tuberculosa.
tu·ber·cu·late [ˌt(j)uː'bɜːrkjəleɪt] *adj* → tubercular.
tu·ber·cu·lat·ed [ˌt(j)uː'bɜːrkjəleɪtɪd] *adj* → tubercular.
tu·ber·cu·la·tion [ˌt(j)uː'bɜːrkjə'leɪʃn] *n* Tuberkelbildung *f*.
tu·ber·cu·lid [ˌt(j)uː'bɜːrkjəlɪd] *n derm.* Tuberkulid *nt*.
tu·ber·cu·lin [ˌt(j)uː'bɜːrkjəlɪn] *n* Tuberkulin *nt*, Tuberculin *nt*.
tuberculin reaction Tuberkulinreaktion *f*.
tuberculin sensitivity Tuberkulinsensibilität *f*.
tuberculin test Tuberkulin-Test *m*.
tuberculin-type hypersensitivity T-zellvermittelte Überempfindlichkeitsreaktion *f*, Tuberkulin-Typ/Spät-Typ/Typ IV *m* der Überempfindlichkeitsreaktion.
tuberculin unit *abbr.* **TU** Tuberkulineinheit *f abbr.* TE.
tu·ber·cu·li·tis [ˌt(j)uː'bɜːrkjə'laɪtɪs] *n* Tuberkulitis *f*.
tu·ber·cu·li·za·tion [t(j)uːˌbɜːrkjəlɪ'zeɪʃn] *n* 1. → tuberculation. 2. Behandlung *f* mit Tuberkulin.
tu·ber·cu·lo·cele [t(j)uː'bɜːrkjələsiːl] *n* Hodentuberkulose *f*.
tu·ber·cu·lo·cid·al [t(j)uːˌbɜːrkjələ'saɪdl] *adj* Tuberkelbakterien-abtötend, tuberkulozid.
tu·ber·cu·lo·der·ma [ˌ-'dɜːrmə] *n* 1. tuberkulöse Hauterkrankung *f*, Tuberkuloderm *nt*. 2. → tuberculosis of skin.
tu·ber·cu·loid [ˌt(j)uː'bɜːrkjələɪd] *adj* 1. tuberkelähnlich, -artig, tuberkuloid. 2. tuberkuloseartig, tuberkuloid.
tuberculoid leprosy tuberkuloide Lepra *f abbr.* TL, Lepra tuberculoides.
tuberculoid myocarditis Riesenzellmyokarditis *f*.

tuberculoma

tu·ber·cu·lo·ma [t(j)u:ˌbɜrkjə'ləʊmə] n Tuberkulom nt, Tuberculoma nt.
tu·ber·cu·lo·pro·tein [t(j)u:ˌbɜrkjələ'prəʊti:n, -ti:ɪn] n Tuberkuloprotein nt.
tu·ber·cu·lo·sil·i·co·sis [ˌ-sɪlɪ'kəʊsɪs] n Tuberkulosilikose f.
tu·ber·cu·lo·sis [t(j)u:ˌbɜrkjə'ləʊsɪs] n Tuberkulose f abbr. Tb, Tbc, Tbk, Tuberculosis f.
 t. of the intestines Darm-, Intestinaltuberkulose.
 t. of the kidney Nierentuberkulose.
 t. of the knee joint tuberkulöse Knie(gelenk)entzündung/Gonitis f, Gonitis tuberculosa.
 t. of the larynx Larynx-, Kehlkopftuberkulose, Laryngophthise f.
 t. of the lung Lungentuberkulose, Lungen-Tb f.
 t. of the serous membranes Tuberkulose der serösen Häute.
 t. of the skin Hauttuberbukose f, Tuberculosis cutis.
 t. of the spine Wirbelsäulentuberkulose, Spondylitis tuberculosa.
tuberculosis vaccine BCG-Impfstoff m, BCG-Vakzine f.
tu·ber·cu·lo·stat [t(j)u:'bɜrkjələstæt] n → tuberculostatic I.
tu·ber·cu·lo·stat·ic [t(j)u:ˌbɜrkjələʊ'stætɪk] I n Tuberkulostatikum nt. II adj tuberkulostatisch.
tu·ber·cu·lo·stear·ic acid [ˌ-'stɪərɪk] Tuberculosteariansäure f.
tu·ber·cu·lot·ic [t(j)u:ˌbɜrkjə'lɑtɪk] adj → tuberculose.
tu·ber·cu·lous [t(j)u:'bɜrkjələs] adj Tuberkulose betr., von ihr betroffen, tuberkulös.
tuberculous abscess tuberkulöser Abszeß m.
 metastatic t. → tuberculous gumma.
tuberculous arthritis Gelenktuberkulose f, Arthritis tuberculosa.
tuberculous cavity tuberkulöse Kaverne f.
tuberculous chancre tuberkulöser Schanker m.
tuberculous coxitis tuberkulöse Koxitis f, Coxitis tuberculosa.
tuberculous dactylitis Dactylitis tuberculosa.
tuberculous endocarditis tuberkulöse Endokarditis f.
tuberculous endometritis Endometritis tuberculosa.
tuberculous epididymitis Epididymitis tuberculosa.
tuberculous gingivitis tuberkulöse Gingivitis f.
tuberculous gonarthritis tuberkulöse Knie(gelenk)entzündung/Gonitis f, Gonitis tuberculosa.
tuberculous gonitis → tuberculous gonarthritis.
tuberculous granuloma tuberkulöses Granulom nt.
tuberculous gumma tuberkulöses Gumma nt, Tuberculosis cutis colliquativa.
tuberculous ileocolitis tuberkulöse Ileokolitis f.
tuberculous infiltrate tuberkulöses Infiltrat nt.
tuberculous laryngitis Kehlkopftuberkulose f, Laryngitis tuberculosa.
tuberculous lymphadenitis Lymphknotentuberkulose f, Lymphadenitis tuberculosa.
tuberculous lymphadenopathy → tuberculous lymphadenitis.
tuberculous lymphangitis tuberkulöse Lymphangiitis f, Lymphangiitis tuberculosa.

tuberculous mastitis gyn. tuberkulöse Mastitis f.
tuberculous meningitis → tubercular meningitis.
tuberculous myocarditis tuberkulöse Myokarditis f.
tuberculous nephritis tuberkulöse Nephritis f, Nephritis tuberculosa.
tuberculous omarthritis tuberkulöse Schultergelenkentzündung/Omarthritis f, Omarthritis tuberculosa.
tuberculous osteoarthritis Gelenktuberkulose f, Arthritis tuberculosa.
tuberculous pericarditis tuberkulöse Perikarditis f, Pericarditis tuberculosa.
tuberculous peritonitis Peritonealtuberkulose f, Peritonitis tuberculosa.
tuberculous pleurisy → tuberculous pleuritis.
tuberculous pleuritis tuberkulöse Pleuritis f, Pleuritis tuberculosa.
tuberculous pneumonia tuberkulöse Pneumonie f.
tuberculous pyelitis urol. Pyelitis tuberculosa.
tuberculous reinfection tuberkulöser Reinfekt m.
tuberculous rheumatism Poncet-Krankheit f.
tuberculous salpingitis gyn. tuberkulöse Eileiterentzündung/Salpingitis f, Salpingitis tuberculosa.
tuberculous sepsis Tuberkulosesepsis f, Sepsis tuberculosa.
 fulminating t. Landouzy-Sepsis f, -Typhobazillose f, Sepsis tuberculosa acutissima.
tuberculous spondylitis Wirbeltuberkulose f, Spondylitis tuberculosa.
tuberculous syphilid Syphilom nt, Gumma nt, Gumma syphiliticum.
tuberculous ulcer tuberkulöses Geschwür nt.
tuberculous uveitis ophthal. tuberkulöse Uveitis f.
tuberculous wart Wilk'-Krankheit f, warzige Tuberkulose f der Haut, Leichentuberkel m, Schlachtertuberkulose f, Tuberculosis cutis verrucosa, Verruca necrogenica, Tuberculum anatomicum.
tu·ber·cu·lum [t(j)u:'bɜrkjələm] n, pl **-la** [-lə] anat. kleiner Höcker m, Knötchen nt, Tuberculum nt.
tu·be·rif·er·ous [ˌt(j)u:bə'rɪfərəs] adj → tuberous.
tu·ber·o·hy·poph·y·si·al system/tract [ˌt(j)u:bərəʊhaɪˌpɑfə'si:əl] → tuberoinfundibular tract.
tu·ber·o·in·fun·dib·u·lar system [ˌ-ˌɪnfən'dɪbjələr] → tuberoinfundibular tract.
tuberoinfundibular tract tuberinfundibuläres System nt, Tractus tuberoinfundibularis.
tu·ber·o·is·chi·ad·ic bursa [ˌ-ˌɪskɪ'ædɪk] Bursa ischiadica/sciatica m. obturatoris interni.
tu·ber·o·ma·mil·lar·y nucleus [ˌ-'mæməˌleri:] Nc. tuberomamillaris.
tu·ber·o·sa·cral ligament [ˌ-'sækrəl, -'seɪ-] Lig. sacrotuberale.
tu·ber·ose ['t(j)u:bərəʊs] adj → tuberous.
tu·ber·o·sis [ˌt(j)u:bə'rəʊsɪs] n Tuberosis f.
tu·ber·os·i·ty [ˌt(j)u:bə'rɑsətɪ] n, pl **-ties** anat. Vorsprung m, Protuberanz f, Vorbuchtung f, Schwellung f, Tuberositas f.
 t. for anterior serratus muscle Tuberositas m. serrati anterioris.
 t. of calcaneus Fersenbeinhöcker m, Tuber calcanei.
 t. of cuboid bone Tuberositas ossis cuboidei.

t. of distal phalanx Tuberositas phalangis distalis.
t. of fifth metatarsal Tuberositas ossis metatarsalis quinti.
t. of first metatarsal Tuberositas ossis metatarsalis primi.
t. of ischium Sitzbeinhöcker m, Tuber ischiadicum/ischiale.
t. of maxilla Tuber maxillare, Eminentia maxillaris.
t. of navicular bone Tuberositas ossis navicularis.
t. of pubic bone Tuberculum pubicum.
t. of radius Tuberositas radii.
t. for serratus anterior muscle Tuberositas m. serrati anterioris.
t. of tibia Tuberositas tibiae.
t. of ulna Tuberositas ulnae.
tu·ber·ous ['t(j)u:bərəs] adj knotig, in Knotenform, tuberös.
tuberous sclerosis (of brain) Bourneville-Syndrom nt, Morbus Bourneville m, tuberöse (Hirn-)Sklerose f, Epiloia f.
tuberous xanthoma tuberöses Xanthom nt, Xanthoma tuberosum.
tube thoracostomy HTG Thorakostomie f mit Plazierung eines Thoraxdrains.
tu·bif·er·ous [t(j)u:'bɪfərəs] adj → tuberous.
tu·bo·ab·dom·i·nal [ˌt(j)u:bəʊæb'dɑmɪnl] adj Eileiter u. Abdomen betr., tuboabdominal, -abdominell.
tuboabdominal pregnancy tuboabdominelle/tuboabdominale Schwangerschaft f.
tu·bo·cu·ra·rine [ˌ-kjʊə'rɑ:ri:n, -rɪn] n Tubocurarin nt.
tubocurarine chloride Tubocurarinchlorid nt.
tubo-ovarian adj Eileiter u. Eierstock betr., Tuboovarial-.
tubo-ovarian abscess Tuboovarialabszeß m.
tubo-ovarian artery Eierstockarterie f, Ovarica f, A. ovarica.
tubo-ovarian pregnancy Tuboovarialschwangerschaft f, -gravidität f.
tubo-ovariotomy n gyn. Entfernung f von Eileiter u. Eierstock, Salpingo-Oophorektomie f, Salpingo-Ovariektomie f.
tubo-ovaritis n gyn. Entzündung f von Eileiter u. Eierstock, Salpingo-Oophoritis f.
tu·bo·per·i·to·ne·al [ˌ-perɪtəʊ'ni:əl] adj gyn. Eileiter u. Peritoneum betr., tuboperitoneal.
tu·bo·pha·ryn·ge·al ligament of Rauber [ˌ-fə'rɪndʒi:əl] Plica salpingopharyngea.
tu·bo·plas·ty ['-plæstɪ] n gyn. Eileiter-, Tuben-, Salpingoplastik f.
tu·bor·rhea [ˌ-'rɪə] n HNO Tuborrhoe f.
tu·bo·tor·sion [ˌ-'tɔ:rʃn] n **1.** gyn. Eileiterdrehung f, Tubotorsion f. **2.** HNO Tubendrehung f, Tubotorsion f.
tu·bo·tym·pa·nal [ˌ-'tɪmpənl] adj → tubotympanic.
tu·bo·tym·pan·ic [ˌ-tɪm'pænɪk] adj Tuba auditiva u. Paukenhöhle betr. od. verbindend, tubotympanal.
tubotympanic recess embryo. tubotympanale Ausbuchtung f, Rec. tubotympanicus.
tu·bo·tym·pa·num [ˌ-'tɪmpənəm] n Tubotympanum nt.
tu·bo·u·ter·ine [ˌ-'ju:tərɪn, -raɪn] adj Eileiter u. Gebärmutter/Uterus betr., tubouterin.
tubouterine pregnancy intramurale/interstitielle Schwangerschaft f, Graviditas interstitialis.
tu·bo·vag·i·nal [ˌ-'vædʒɪnl] adj Eileiter u. Scheide/Vagina betr. od. verbindend, tubovaginal.

tu·bu·lar ['t(j)u:bjələr] *adj* röhrenförmig, tubulär, Röhren-; (*Niere*) Tubulus-.
tubular adenoma tubuläres Adenom *nt*.
t. of testis tubuläres Hodenadenom, Adenoma tubulare testis.
tubular aneurysm zylindrisches Aneurysma *nt*, Aneurysma cylindricum.
tubular atrophy (*Niere*) Tubulusatrophie *f*.
tubular bone Röhrenknochen *m*.
tubular cancer → tubular carcinoma.
tubular carcinoma tubuläres Karzinom *nt*.
tubular cast *urol.* 1. Harnzylinder *m*. 2. Nierenzylinder *m*.
tubular cells (*Niere*) Tubuluszellen *pl*, -epithelien *pl*.
tubular cyst (*Niere*) Tubuluszyste *f*.
tubular ectasia (*Niere*) Tubulusektasie *f*.
tubular gland tubuläre/röhrchenförmige Drüse *f*.
tubular necrosis (*Niere*) Tubulusnekrose *f*.
  acute t. *abbr.* ATN akute Tubulusnekrose.
  acute ischemic t. akute ischämische Tubulusnekrose.
  acute toxic t. akute toxische Tubulusnekrose.
tubular nephrosis Tubulo-, Tubulusnephrose *f*.
tubular part of adenohypophysis Trichterlappen *m*, Pars infundibularis/tuberalis adenohypophyseos.
tubular vision *ophthal.* Tunnelsehen *nt*.
tu·bule ['t(j)u:bju:l] *n* 1. Röhrchen *nt*. 2. *anat.* Röhrchen *nt*, Kanälchen *nt*, Tubulus *m*.
tubule type mitochondrion Mitochondrium *nt* vom Tubulustyp.
tu·bu·li·form ['t(j)u:bjəlifɔ:rm] *adj* → tubular.
tu·bu·lin ['t(j)u:bjəlɪn] *n* Tubulin *nt*.
tu·bu·li·za·tion [ˌt(j)u:bjəli'zeɪʃn] *n neurochir.* Tubulisation *f*.
tu·bu·lo·ac·i·nar [ˌt(j)u:bjələu'æsɪnər] *adj histol.* tubuloazinär, tubuloazinös.
tubuloacinar gland *histol.* tubuloazinöse/tubuloalveoläre Drüse *f*.
tu·bu·lo·cyst ['-sɪst] *n* → tubular cyst.
tu·bu·lop·a·thy [t(j)u:bjə'lɒpəθi] *n* (*Niere*) Tubulopathie *f*.
tu·bu·lor·rhex·is [ˌt(j)u:bjələ'reksɪs] *n* (*Niere*) Tubulorrhexis *f*.
tu·bu·lus ['t(j)u:bjələs] *n*, *pl* **-li** [-laɪ] → tubule 2.
tu·bus ['t(j)u:bəs] *n*, *pl* **-bi** [-baɪ] *anat.* Kanal *m*, Rohr *nt*, Tubus *nt*.
tu·fa lung ['t(j)u:fə] Bimsstein-, Tuffsteinlunge *f*, metastatische Lungenkalzinose *f*.
tuft [tʌft] *n* Knäuel *m*; (Haar-)Büschel *nt*; (Gefäß-)Bündel *nt*.
tuft fracture Berstungsbruch *m*, -fraktur *f*.
tu·la·re·mia [ˌtu:lə'ri:mɪə] *n* Tularämie *f*, Hasen-, Nagerpest *f*, Lemming-Fieber *nt*, Ohara-, Franciskrankheit *f*.
tu·la·re·mic conjunctivitis [ˌ-'ri:mɪk] Conjunctivitis tularensis.
tularemic pneumonia pulmonale Tularämie *f*.
tu·la·rin ['tu:lərɪn] *n* Tularin *nt*.
Tulp ['tʌlp]: **T.'s valve** Bauhin'-Klappe *f*, Ileozäkal-, Ileozökalklappe *f*, Valva ileocaecalis/ilealis.
Tulpius ['tʌlpɪəs]: **T.' valve** → Tulp's valve.
tu·me·fa·cient [ˌtju:mə'feɪʃnt] *adj* eine Schwellung verursachend, anschwellend.
tu·me·fac·tion [ˌ-'fækʃn] *n* 1. (An-)Schwellung *f*. 2. → tumescence.
tu·me·fy ['-faɪ] I *vt* (an-)schwellen lassen. II *vi* (an-, auf-)schwellen.
tu·mes·cence [tju:'mesns] *n* (diffuse) Anschwellung/Schwellung *f*, Tumeszenz *f*.
tu·mes·cent [tju:'mesnt] *adj* geschwollen.
tu·mid ['t(j)u:mɪd] *adj* geschwollen, angeschwollen, ödematös.
tu·mor ['t(j)u:mər] *n* 1. Schwellung *f*, Anschwellung *f*, Tumor *m*. 2. Geschwulst *f*, Neubildung *f*, Gewächs *nt*, Neoplasma *nt*, Tumor *m*.
  t. of testis Hodengeschwulst *f*, -tumor.
  t. of tongue Zungentumor.
tu·mor·af·fin [ˌt(j)u:mər'æfɪn] *adj* mit besonderer Affinität zu Tumoren, tumoraffin.
tumor antigen Tumorantigen *nt*, T-Antigen *nt*.
tumor-associated antigen tumorassoziiertes Antigen *nt*.
tumor biology Tumorbiologie *f*.
tumor cell Tumorzelle *f*.
tumor embolus Tumorembolus *m*.
tumor giant cell Tumorriesenzelle *f*.
tumor grading *patho.* Tumorgrading *nt*.
tumor histology Tumorhistologie *f*.
tu·mor·i·ci·dal [ˌt(j)u:mərɪ'saɪdl] *adj* krebszellenzerstörend, -abtötend, tumorizid.
tu·mor·i·gen·e·sis [ˌ-'dʒenəsɪs] *n* Tumorentstehung *f*, -bildung *f*, Tumorgenese *f*.
tumor immunity Tumorimmunität *f*.
tumor immunology Tumorimmunologie *f*.
tumor-inducing viruses *micro.*, *patho.* onkogene Viren *pl*.
tumor-like lesion *patho.* tumorähnliche Veränderung *f*, tumor-like lesion (*f*).
tumor lysis syndrome Tumorzerfallssyndrom *nt*.
tumor marker Tumormarker *m*.
tumor necrosis factor *abbr.* TNF Tumor-Nekrose-Faktor *m abbr.* TNF, Cachectin *nt*.
tu·mor·ous ['t(j)u:mərəs] *adj* tumorartig, tumorös.
tumor regression Tumorregression *f*.
tumor shrinkage Tumorschrumpfung *f*.
tumor-specific *adj* tumorspezifisch.
tumor-specific antigen *abbr.* TSA tumorspezifisches Antigen *nt*.
tumor-specific transplantation antigen *abbr.* TSTA tumorspezifisches Transplantationsantigen *nt abbr.* TSTA.
tumor staging Tumorstaging *nt*.
tumor viruses *micro.*, *patho.* Tumorviren *pl*, onkogene Viren *pl*.
tu·mour *n Brit.* → tumor 1.
Tun·ga ['tʌŋgə] *n micro.* Tunga *f*.
  T. penetrans Sandfloh *m*, Tunga/Dermatophilus penetrans.
tun·gi·a·sis [tʌŋ'gaɪəsɪs] *n* Sandflohbefall *m*, Tungiasis *f*.
tung·sten ['tʌŋstən] *n* Wolfram *nt abbr.* W.
tu·nic ['t(j)u:nɪk] *n anat.* Hüllschicht *f*, Hülle *f*, Haut *f*, Häutchen *nt*, Tunica *f*.
tu·ni·ca ['t(j)u:nɪkə] *n*, *pl* **-cae** [-si:] → tunic.
tunica albuginea: **t. of cavernous body** Bindegewebshülle *f* der Corpora cavernosa, Tunica albuginea corporum cavernosum.
  t. of spongy body Bindegewebshülle *f* des Corpus spongiosum, Tunica albuginea corporis spongiosi.
tun·ing ['t(j)u:nɪŋ] I *n* Anpassung *f* (*to* an); Abstimmung *f*, Einstellung *f*. II *adj* Stimm-, Abstimm(ungs)-.
tuning curve Tuning-, Abstimmungskurve *f*.
tuning fork Stimmgabel *f*.
tuning fork test *HNO* Stimmgabelprüfung *f*.
tun·nel ['tʌnl] *n* Gang *m*, Kanal *m*, Tunnel *m*.
tunnel cells (*Innenohr*) Corti'-Pfeilerzellen *pl*, Pfeilerzellen *pl*.
tunnel disease 1. Hakenwurmbefall *m*, -infektion *f*, Ankylostomiasis *f*, Ankylostomatosis *f*, Ankylostomatidose *f*. 2. Druckluft-, Caissonkrankheit *f*.
tunnel flap → tubed flap.
tunnel graft → tubed flap.
tun·nel·ing ['tʌnlɪŋ] *n phys.* Tunnel-Effekt *m*.
tunnel vision Tunnelsehen *nt*.
T_3 uptake test T_3U-Test *m*, T_3-uptake--Test *m*.
tur·ban tumor ['tɜrbən] Turbantumor *m*; Zylindrom *nt*, Cylindroma *nt*.
tur·bid ['tɜrbɪd] *adj* (*Flüssigkeit*) wolkig; undurchsichtig, milchig, unklar, trüb(e).
tur·bi·dim·e·ter [ˌtɜrbɪ'dɪmətər] *n* Trübungsmesser *m*, Turbidimeter *nt*.
tur·bi·di·met·ric [ˌtɜrbədɪ'metrɪk] *adj* Turbidimeter *od.* -metrie betr., turbidimetrisch.
turbidimetric immunoassay *abbr.* TIA turbidimetrischer Immunoassay *m abbr.* TIA.
tur·bi·dim·e·try [ˌtɜrbɪ'dɪmətrɪ] *n* Trübungsmessung *f*, Turbidimetrie *f*.
tur·bid·i·ty [tɜr'bɪdəti] *n* (*Lösung*) Trübung *f*, Trübheit *f*.
tur·bid·ness ['tɜrbɪdnɪs] *n* → turbidity.
tur·bi·do·stat [tɜr'bɪdəstæt] *n* Turbidostat *m*.
tur·bi·nal ['tɜrbənl] *n*, *adj* → turbinate.
turbinal crest: **inferior t. of maxilla** Crista conchalis maxillae.
  inferior t. of palatine bone Crista conchalis ossis palatini.
  superior t. of maxilla Crista ethmoidalis maxillae.
  superior t. of palatine bone Crista ethmoidalis ossis palatini.
tur·bi·nate ['tɜrbənɪt, -neɪt] I *n anat.* 1. schalenförmig-gewundene Struktur *f*. 2. → turbinate bone. II *adj* gewunden, schnecken-, muschelförmig.
turbinate bone Nasenmuschel *f*, Concha nasalis.
  fourth t. → highest t.
  highest t. oberste Nasenmuschel, Concha nasalis suprema.
  inferior t. untere Nasenmuschel, Concha nasalis inferior.
  middle t. mittlere Nasenmuschel, Concha nasalis media.
  superior t. obere Nasenmuschel, Concha nasalis superior.
  supreme t. oberste Nasenmuschel, Concha nasalis suprema.
tur·bi·nat·ed ['tɜrbɪneɪtɪd] *adj* → turbinate II.
turbinated bone → turbinate bone.
tur·bi·nec·to·my [ˌtɜrbɪ'nektəmɪ] *n HNO* Nasenmuschelresektion *f*, Turbinektomie *f*, Konchektomie *f*.
tur·bi·not·o·my [ˌ-'nɒtəmɪ] *n HNO* Turbinotomie *f*.
tur·bu·lent ['tɜrbjələnt] *adj phys.* mit Wirbeln, wirbelnd, turbulent.
turbulent flow *phys.* turbulente Strömung *f*, Wirbelströmung *f*.
Türck [tɜrk; tʏrk]: **T.'s bundle** → T.'s tract.
  T.'s column Pyramidenvorderstrangbahn *f*, Tractus corticospinalis/pyramidalis anterior.
  T.'s degeneration *neuro.* Waller'-Degeneration *f*, sekundäre/orthograde Degeneration *f*.
  fasciculus of T. → T.'s tract.
  T.'s tract Türck'-Bündel *nt*, Tractus temporopontinus.
Turcot ['tɜrkɒt]: **T. syndrome** Turcot-Syndrom *nt*.
Turek ['tjʊərek]: **T.'s operation** *urol.* Turek-Operation *f*.

tur·ges·cence [tɜr'dʒesns] *n* (An-)Schwellung *f*, Geschwulst *f*, Turgeszenz *f*.
tur·ges·cent [tɜr'dʒesnt] *adj* (an-)schwellend; (an-)geschwollen.
tur·gid ['tɜrdʒɪd] *adj* (an-)geschwollen.
tur·gor ['tɜrgər] *n* Spannungs-, Quellungszustand *m*, Turgor *m*.
tu·ris·ta [tʊə'rɪstə] *n* → traveler's diarrhea.
Türk [tɪrk]: **T.'s cells** Türk'-Reizformen *pl*. **T.'s (irritation) leukocytes** → T.'s cells.
Turlock ['tɜrlɑk]: **T. virus** *micro.* Turlock--Virus *nt*.
tur·mer·ic ['tɜrmərɪk] *n* 1. Gelbwurz *f*, Kurkume *f*, Kurkuma *f*. 2. Kurkumagelb *nt*.
turmeric paper Kurkumapapier *nt*.
turn [tɜrn] **I** *n* 1. (Um-)Drehung *f*. **to give sth. a ~** etw. drehen. 2. Turnus *m*, Reihe(nfolge *f*) *f*. **in ~** der Reihe nach. **to take ~s** (mit-)einander/s. (gegenseitig) abwechseln (*at* in, bei). 3. Drehen *nt*; Wendung *f*. 4. Biegung *f*, Kurve *f*; *mathe.* Krümmung *f*. 5. Wendung *f*, Richtung *f*, (Ver-)Lauf *m*. **to take a ~ for the better/worse** s. bessern/s. verschlimmern. 6. Wende(punkt *m*) *f*, Wechsel *m*, Umschwung *m*; Krise *f*, Krisis *f*. 7. *patho.* Anfall *m*; Taumel *m*, Schwindel *m*. 8. Ausschlag(en *nt*) *m* der Waage. 9. Form *f*, Gestalt *f*, Beschaffenheit *f*. 10. Art *f*, Charakter *m*. 11. Neigung *f*, Hang *m* (*for, to* zu); Sinn *m* (*for, to* für). **II** *vt* 12. (um eine Achse) drehen. 13. (*Patient*) (um-, herum-)drehen, wenden. 14. etw. umkehren, stülpen, drehen, wenden. **it ~s my stomach** mir dreht s. der Magen um. 15. zuwenden, zukehren (*to*). 16. richten, lenken (*against* gegen; *on* auf; *toward* auf, nach). 17. um-, ab-, weglenken, -leiten, -wenden; etw. wenden; (*Richtung*) ändern. 18. (*Waage*) zum Ausschlagen bringen. 19. verwandeln (*into* in). 20. machen, werden lassen (*into* zu). **to ~ s.o. sick** jdn. krank machen; jdm. Übelkeit verursachen. 21. **~ sour** (*Milch*) sauer werden lassen.
III *vi* 22. s. drehen (lassen); s. hin u. herbewegen (lassen); s. (im Kreis) herumdrehen; umdrehen, umwenden. 23. s. (ab-, hin-, zu-)wenden. 24. s. (um-, herum-)drehen. 25. s. krümmen, s. winden. 26. s. umdrehen *od.* umwenden (lassen), s. umstülpen. **my stomach ~s** mir dreht s. der Magen um. **I'm be**(com)**e**(ing) werden, schwindeln. **my head ~s** mir dreht s. alles. 28. s. verwandeln (*into, to* in). 29. werden. **to ~ cold** kalt werden. **to ~ pale** erblassen. **to ~ red** erröten. **to ~ blue** blau anlaufen, zyanotisch werden. **to ~ sour** (*Milch*) sauer werden.
turn against *vi* s. (feindlich) wenden gegen.
turn down *vt* 1. (*Regler*) klein(er) drehen, herunterdrehen. 2. (*Bettdecke*) aufdecken. 3. (*Vorschlag*) ablehnen; etw. zurückweisen.
turn in I *vt* einwärts/nach innen drehen *od.* biegen *od.* stellen. **II** *vi* 1. *sl.* in Bett gehen. 2. **to ~ on o.s.** s. in s. selbst zurückziehen.
turn off *vt* (*Hahn*) zu-, abdrehen; (*Gerät*) abstellen, ab-, ausschalten.
turn on *vi* 1. (*Hahn*) aufdrehen; (*Gerät*) anstellen, einschalten. 2. *sl.* (*Drogen*) "anturnen".
turn out I *vt* 1. umstülpen, -kehren. 2. auswärts/nach außen drehen *od.* biegen *od.* stellen. 3. **~** turn off. **II** *vi* 4. *sl.* (aus dem Bett) aufstehen. 5. s. entpuppen.
turn over I *vt* umdrehen; wenden; umwerfen, umkippen. **II** *vi* 1. s. drehen, rotieren.

2. (s. im Bett) umdrehen. 3. umkippen, umschlagen. 4. (*Magen*) s. umdrehen.
turn round (*Kopf, Gesicht*) **I** *vt* (herum-)drehen. **II** *vi* s. (um-)drehen.
turn to *vi* 1. s. wenden an, jdn. zu Rate ziehen. **to ~ a doctor**. 2. s. etw. zuwenden.
turn up I *vt* 1. (*Regler*) höher/größer drehen, aufdrehen. 2. nach oben kehren/wenden/drehen. 3. ausgraben, zutage fördern. 4. *sl.* jdm. den Magen umdrehen (vor Ekel). **II** *vi* erscheinen, auftauchen, zum Vorschein kommen.
t. to the left Linkswendung.
t. of life Wechseljahre *pl*, Klimakterium *nt*; Menopause *f*.
t. to the right Rechtswendung.
Turnbull ['tɜrnbʊl]: **T.'s blue** Turnbull--Blau *nt*.
T.'s blue reaction Turnbull-Blau-Reaktion *f*.
turned [tɜrnt] *adj* 1. gedreht; (um-)gebogen. 2. verdreht, verkehrt.
turned-back *adj* zurückgebogen.
turned-down *adj* nach unten gebogen.
turned-in *adj* einwärts gebogen.
turned-out *adj* nach außen gebogen.
turned-up *adj* aufgebogen.
Turner ['tɜrnər]: **male T. syndrome** Noonan-Syndrom *nt*, Pseudo-Ullrich--Turner-Syndrom *nt*.
marginal gyrus of T. Gyrus frontalis medialis.
pseudo-T.'s syndrome Bonnevie-Ullrich--Syndrom *nt*, Pterygium-Syndrom *nt*.
T.'s sign Turner'-Zeichen *nt*.
T.'s syndrome Ullrich-Turner-Syndrom *nt*.
turn·ing ['tɜrnɪŋ] *n* 1. Drehung *f*; Drehen *nt*; Biegung *f*. 2. *gyn.* Wendung *f*.
turning point *mathe., fig.* Wende(punkt *m*) *f*; *patho.* Krise *f*, Krisis *f*.
turning test HNO (*Ohr*) Drehprüfung *f*.
turn·o·ver ['tɜrnəʊvər] *n* Umsatz(rate *f*) *m*, Fluktuation(srate *f*) *f*.
turnover dynamics *biochem., chem.* Umsetzungsdynamik *f*.
turnover number molare/molekulare Aktivität *f*, old Wechselzahl *f*.
turn·sol ['tɜrnsɒl] *n* Lackmus *nt*.
tur·pen·tine ['tɜrpəntaɪn] *n* Terpentin *nt*.
turpentine oil Terpentinöl *nt*.
turpentine poisoining Terpentinvergiftung *f*.
tur·ri·ceph·a·ly [tɜrə'sefəlɪ] *n* Spitz-, Turmschädel *m*, Akrozephalie *f*, -cephalie *f*, Oxyzephalie *f*, -cephalie *f*, Hypsizephalie *f*, -cephalie *f*, Turrizephalie *f*, -cephalie *f*.
tus·sal [tʌsl] *adj* Husten betr., Husten-.
tus·sic·u·la [tə'sɪkjələ] *n* leichter Husten *m*.
tus·sic·u·lar [tə'sɪkjələr] *adj* → tussal.
tus·sic·u·la·tion [tə,sɪkjə'leɪʃn] *n* abgehackter Husten *m*.
tus·si·gen·ic [,tʌsə'dʒenɪk] *adj* hustenerregend, tussigen, tussipar.
tus·sis ['tʌsɪs] *n* Husten *m*, Tussis *f*.
tus·sive ['tʌsɪv] *adj* → tussal.
tussive syncope Hustenschlag *m*, -synkope *f*.
TWAR chlamydiae *micro.* TWAR-Chlamydien *pl*, -Stämme *pl*, Chlamydia pneumoniae.
TWAR strains → TWAR chlamydiae.
T wave (*EKG*) T-Welle *f*, -Zacke *f*.
'tween brain [twi:n] Zwischenhirn *nt*, Dienzephalon *nt*, Diencephalon *nt*.
tweez·ers ['twi:zərz] *pl* (*a.* **pair of ~**) Pinzette *f*.
twelfth nerve [twelfθ] Hypoglossus *m*, XII. Hirnnerv *m*, N. hypoglossus.
twig [twɪg] *n anat.* Endast *m*.
twi·light ['twaɪlaɪt] *n* **I** Dämmerung *f*; Zwielicht *nt*, Halbdunkel *nt*, Dämmerlicht *nt*.

II *adj* zwielichtig, dämm(e)rig, Dämmer(ungs)-, Zwielicht-.
twilight anesthesia *neuro.* Dämmerschlaf *m*.
twilight blindness Schwäche *f* des Dämmerungssehens, Aknephaskopie *f*.
twilight sleep Dämmerschlaf *m*.
twilight state Dämmerzustand *m*.
twilight thirst (pathologisch) verminderter Durst *m*, Hypodipsie *f*.
twilight vision Dämmerungssehen *nt*, skotopes Sehen *nt*, Skotop(s)ie *f*.
twin [twɪn] **I** *n* 1. Zwilling *m*, Geminus *m*. 2. *fig.* Gegenstück *nt* (*of* zu). **II** *adj* Zwillings-; doppelt, Doppel-.
twin-bedded room Zweibettzimmer *nt*.
twin-bladed *adj* (*Messer*) doppelklingig.
twin brother Zwillingsbruder *m*.
twinge [twɪndʒ] **I** *n* stechender Schmerz *m*, Stechen *nt*, Zwicken *nt*, Stich *m*. **II** *vt, vi* stechen, schmerzen; zwicken, kneifen.
twin helix Watson-Crick-Modell *nt*, Doppelhelix *f*.
twin·kle ['twɪŋkl] **I** *n* 1. (Augen-)Zwinkern *nt*, Blinzeln *nt*; 2. Blitzen *nt*, Glitzern *nt*, Funkeln *nt*. **II** *vt* (*mit den Augen*) blinzeln. **III** *vi* 3. (mit den Augen) blinzeln, zwinkern. 4. (auf-)blitzen, glitzern, funkeln.
twin monster *patho., embryo.* Doppelmißbildung *f*, Duplicitas *f*, Monstrum duplex.
twin pregnancy Zwillingsschwangerschaft *f*.
twin sister Zwillingsschwester *f*.
twist·ed hairs ['twɪstɪd] Trichokinesis *f*, Trichotortosis *f*, Pili torti.
twitch [twɪtʃ] **I** *n* 1. Zucken *nt*; Zuckung *nt*; (*Schmerz*) Stich *m*. 2. Ruck *m*. **II** *vt* 3. zucken mit. 4. zupfen, reißen (an). **III** *vi* 5. zucken (*with* vor). 6. zupfen, reißen (*at* an).
twitch contraction Muskelzuckung *f*.
twitch fiber *physiol.* Zuckungsfaser *f*.
twitch·ing ['twɪtʃɪŋ] *n* Zucken *nt*, Zuckung *f*.
two [tu:] **I** *n* 1. Zwei *f*. 2. Paar *nt*. **II** *adj* zwei; beide.
two-cell stage Zweizellenstadium *nt*.
two-component hypothesis *biochem., physiol.* Zweikomponentenhypothese *f*.
two-digit *adj* (*Zahl*) zweistellig.
two-dimensional *adj* zweidimensional.
two-dimensional chromatography zweidimensionale Chromatographie *f*.
two-edged *adj* (*Messer*) zwei-, doppelschneidig.
two-egg twins zweieiige/dizygote/binovuläre/erbungleiche/dissimiläre Zwillinge *pl*.
two-fold ['tu:fəʊld] *adj* zweifach, doppelt.
two gene-one polypeptide chain hypothesis *biochem., genet.* Zwei Gene-eine Polypeptidkettenhypothese *f*.
two-glass test *urol.* Tompson-Probe *f*, Zweigläserprobe *f*.
two-handed *adj* zweihändig; beidhändig.
two-hourly *adj* alle zwei Stunden, zweistündlich.
two-layered *adj* doppelschichtig.
two-layer film *biochem., physiol.* Doppelschicht *f*, -film *m*.
two-part fracture of proximal humerus Neer Typ II-Humerusfraktur *f*, 2-Fragmentfraktur *f*.
two-point discrimination *neuro.* Zwei--Punkte-Diskriminierung *f*, Zwei-Punkte-Diskrimination *f*.
two-point threshold *physiol.* Zweipunktschwelle *f*.
Twort [twɔːrt]: **T. phenomenon** → Twort--d'Herelle phenomenon.
Twort-d'Herelle [də'rɛl]: **T.-d'H. phenome-**

non d'Herelle-Phänomen *nt*, Twort--d'Herelle-Phänomen *nt*, Bakteriophagie *f*.
two-sided *adj* zweiseitig.
two-stage *adj* zweiphasig, -stufig, Zweiphasen-.
two-step exercise test *card*. Master-Test *m*, Zweistufentest *m*.
two-substrate reaction *biochem*. Zwei--Substrat-Reaktion *f*.
ty·le ['taɪliː] *n* → tyloma.
ty·lec·to·my [taɪ'lektəmɪ] *n gyn*. (*Brust*) Segment-, Quadrantenresektion *f*, Lumpektomie *f*, Tylektomie *f*.
ty·lo·ma [taɪ'ləʊmə] *n* Schwiele *f*, Tyloma *nt*; Kallus *m*, Callus *m*, Callositas *f*.
ty·lo·sis [taɪ'ləʊsɪs] *n*, *pl* **-ses** [-siːz] Schwielenbildung *f*, Tylosis *f*.
ty·lot·ic [taɪ'lɒtɪk] *adj* Tylosis betr., schwielig.
ty·lox·a·pol [taɪ'lɒksəpəʊl] *n pharm*. Tyloxapol *nt*.
tympan- *pref*. → tympano-.
tym·pa·nal ['tɪmpənəl] *adj* → tympanic 1.
tym·pa·nec·to·my [tɪmpə'nektəmɪ] *n HNO* Trommelfellentfernung *f*, Tympanektomie *f*.
tym·pan·ia [tɪm'pænɪə] *n* → tympanites.
tym·pan·ic [tɪm'pænɪk] *adj* **1.** Trommelfell *od*. Paukenhöhle betr., tympanal, Trommelfell-, Paukenhöhlen-, Tympano-. **2.** (*Schall*) tympanitisch, tympanisch.
tympanic annulus An(n)ulus tympanicus.
tympanic antrum Warzenfortsatzhöhle *f*, Antrum mastoideum.
tympanic aperture: t. of canaliculus of chorda tympani → t. of chorda tympani canal.
t. of chorda tympani canal Paukenhöhlenmündung *f* des Chordakanals, Apertura tympanica canaliculi chordae tympani.
tympanic artery Paukenhöhlenschlagader *f*, A. tympanica.
 anterior t. A. tympanica anterior.
 inferior t. A. tympanica inferior.
 posterior t. A. tympanica posterior.
 superior t. A. tympanica superior.
tympanic attic Kuppelraum *m*, Attikus *m*, Rec. epitympanicus.
tympanic body Glomus jugulare/tympanicum.
tympanic bone Pars tympanica (ossis temporalis).
tympanic canal Canaliculus tympanicus.
tympanic canaliculus → tympanic canal.
tympanic cavity Paukenhöhle *f*, Tympanon *nt*, Tympanum *nt*, Cavum tympani, Cavitas tympanica.
 primitive t. *embryo*. Paukenhöhlenanlage *f*.
tympanic cells Cellulae tympanicae.
tympanic cellulae Cellulae tympanicae.
tympanic enlargement *anat*. Intumescentia tympanica, Ggl. tympanicum.
tympanic fissure Glaser'-Spalte *f*, Fissura petrotympanica.
tympanic ganglion (of Valentin) Ggl. tympanicum, Intumescentia tympanica.
tympanic gland 1. Glomus jugulare/tympanicum. **2.** ~s *pl* Gll. tympanicae.
tym·pan·i·chord [tɪm'pænɪkɔːrd] *n* Chorda tympani.
tympanic incisure Inc. tympanica.
tympanic lip of limb of spiral lamina obere Lippe *f* des Limbus laminae spiralis, Labium limbi tympanicum.
tympanic membrane Trommelfell *nt*, Membrana tympanica.
 secondary t. Membran *f* des Fenestra cochleae, Membrana tympani secundaria.

tympanic membrane perforation Trommelfellperforation *f*.
tympanic nerve N. tympanicus.
tympanic notch Inc. tympanica.
tympanic opening of auditory tube Paukenhöhlenmündung/-öffnung *f* der Ohrtrompete, Ostium tympanicum tubae auditoriae.
tympanic plexus Jacobson'-Plexus *m*, Plexus tympanicus.
tympanic resonance tympanitischer/tympanischer Klopfschall *m*.
tympanic ring Trommelfellring *m*, An(n)ulus tympanicus.
tympanic scala Scala tympani.
tympanic segment of facial nerve tympanales Segment *nt* des N. facialis.
tympanic sinus Sinus tympani.
tympanic spine: anterior/greater t. Spina tympanica major.
 lesser/posterior t. Spina tympanica minor.
tympanic sulcus (of temporal bone) Sulcus tympanicus (ossis temporalis).
tympanic veins Paukenhöhlenvenen *pl*, Vv. tympanicae.
tympanic wall of cochlear duct untere Wand *f* des Ductus cochlearis, Membrana spiralis (cochlearis), Paries tympanicus ductus cochlearis.
tym·pa·nism ['tɪmpənɪzəm] *n* → tympanites.
tym·pa·ni·tes [ˌtɪmpə'naɪtiːz] *n* Tympanie *f*, Tympania *f*.
tym·pa·nit·ic [-'nɪtɪk] *adj* **1.** (*Schall*) tympanisch, tympanitisch. **2.** Tympanie betr., tympanisch, tympanitisch.
tympanitic abscess Gasabszeß *m*.
tympanitic resonance → tympanic resonance.
tym·pa·ni·tis [ˌ-'naɪtɪs] *n* Mittelohrentzündung *f*, Otitis media.
tympano- *pref*. Trommelfell-, Pauken-, Paukenhöhlen-, Tympano-.
tym·pa·no·cen·te·sis [ˌtɪmpənəʊsen'tiːsɪs] *n HNO* Myringotomie *f*, Parazentese *f*.
tym·pa·no·cer·vi·cal abscess [ˌ-'sɜːrvɪkl] tympanozervikaler Abszeß *m*.
tym·pa·no·eu·sta·chi·an [ˌ-juː'steɪʃɪən, -kɪən] *adj* Paukenhöhle u. Eustach'-Röhre betr.
tym·pa·no·gen·ic [ˌ-'dʒenɪk] *adj* aus der Paukenhöhle stammend, tympanogen.
tym·pa·no·gram [tɪm'pænəgræm] *n HNO* Tympanogramm *nt*.
tym·pa·no·mal·le·al [ˌtɪmpənəʊ'mælɪəl] *adj* Paukenhöhle u. Malleus betr., tympanomalleal.
tym·pa·no·man·dib·u·lar [ˌ-mæn'dɪbjələr] *adj* Paukenhöhle u. Unterkiefer/Mandibula betr.
tympanomandibular cartilage *embryo*. Meckel'-Knorpel *m*.
tym·pa·no·mas·toid abscess [ˌ-'mæstɔɪd] Abszeß *m* von Paukenhöhle u. Mastoid.
tympanomastoid fissure Fissura tympanomastoidea.
tym·pa·no·mas·toi·di·tis [ˌ-ˌmæstɔɪ'daɪtɪs] *n HNO* Tympanomastoiditis *f*.
tym·pa·no·me·a·to·mas·toid·ec·to·my [ˌ-mɪˌeɪtəʊˌmæstɔɪ'dektəmɪ] *n HNO* radikale Mastoidektomie *f*.
tym·pan·o·met·ric [ˌ-'metrɪk] *adj* Tympanometrie betr., tympanometrisch.
tym·pa·nom·e·try [tɪmpə'nɒmətrɪ] *n* Tympanometrie *f*.
tym·pa·no·pho·nia [ˌtɪmpənəʊ'fəʊnɪə] *n* **1.** Tympanophonie *f*, Autophonie *f*. **2.** → tinnitus (aurium).
tym·pa·noph·o·ny [tɪmpə'nɒfənɪ] *n* **1.** Tympanophonie *f*, Autophonie *f*. **2.** → tinnitus (aurium).

tym·pa·no·plas·tic [ˌtɪmpənəʊ'plæstɪk] *adj HNO* Tympanoplastik betr., tympanoplastisch.
tym·pa·no·plas·ty ['-plæstɪ] *n HNO* Paukenhöhlen-, Tympanoplastik *f*.
tym·pa·no·scle·ro·sis [ˌ-sklɪ'rəʊsɪs] *n HNO* Pauken(höhlen)sklerose *f*, Tympanosklerose *f*.
tym·pa·no·squa·mous fissure [-'skweɪməs] Fissura tympanosquamosa.
tym·pa·no·sta·pe·di·al [ˌ-stə'piːdɪəl] *adj* Paukenhöhle u. Stapes betr., tympanostapedial.
tympanostapedial syndesmosis Syndesmosis tympanostapedialis.
tym·pa·no·tem·po·ral [ˌ-'temp(ə)rəl] *adj* tympanotemporal.
tym·pa·not·o·my [tɪmpə'nɒtəmɪ] *n HNO* **1.** Pauken(höhlen)punktion *f*, Tympanotomie *f*. **2.** Myringotomie *f*, Parazentese *f*.
tym·pa·nous ['tɪmpənəs] *adj* Tympanie betr., tympanisch, tympanitisch; gebläht.
tym·pa·num ['tɪmpənəm] *n*, *pl* **-nums**, **-na** [-nə] *anat*. **1.** → tympanic cavity. **2.** *inf*. → tympanic membrane.
tym·pa·ny ['tɪmpənɪ] *n* Tympanie *f*, Tympania *f*.
Tyndall ['tɪndl]: **T. effect/phenomenon** Tyndall-Effekt *m*.
type [taɪp] **I** *n* Typ *m*, Typus *m*; *bio*. Typus *m*; Muster *nt*, Modell *nt*, Standard *m*; Art *f*, Sorte *f*. **II** *vt* (*Blutgruppe*, *Gentyp*) bestimmen.
type 1 capillary *histol*. geschlossene Kapillare *f*, Typ 1-Kapillare *f*.
type 2 capillary *histol*. gefensterte/fenestrierte Kapillare *f*, Typ 2-Kapillare *f*.
type 3 capillary diskontinuierliche Kapillare *f*, Typ 3-Kapillare *f*.
type I cell Deckzelle *f*, Alveolarzelle *f*/Pneumozyt *m* Typ I.
type II cell Nischenzelle *f*, Alveolarzelle *f*/Pneumozyt *m* Typ II.
type I dip *gyn*. Frühtief *nt*, -dezeleration *f*, frühe Dezeleration *f*, Dip I *m*.
type II dip *gyn*. Spättief *nt*, -dezeleration *f*, späte Dezeleration *f*, Dip II *m*.
type specificity Typenspezifität *f*.
ty·phia ['taɪfɪə] *n* → typhoid fever.
ty·phic ['taɪfɪk] *adj* Typhus betr., Typhus-.
typhic corpuscles Typhuszellen *pl*.
typhl- *pref*. → typhlo-.
typh·lec·ta·sis [tɪf'lektəsɪs] *n* Blinddarm-, Zäkumüberdehnung *f*.
typh·lec·to·my [tɪf'lektəmɪ] *n chir*. Blinddarm-, Zäkumresektion *f*, Typhlektomie *f*.
typh·len·ter·i·tis [tɪfˌlentə'raɪtɪs] *n* → typhlitis 1.
typh·li·tis [tɪf'laɪtɪs] *n* **1.** Blinddarm-, Zäkumentzündung *f*, Typhlitis *f*. **2.** Wurmfortsatzentzündung *f*, *inf*. Blinddarmentzündung *f*, Appendizitis *f*, Appendicitis *f*.
typhlo- *pref*. **1.** Blinddarm-, Zäko-, Zäkum-, Typhl(o)-. **2.** Blind-, Typhl(o)-.
typh·lo·co·li·tis [ˌtɪfləkə'laɪtɪs] *n* Typhlokolitis *f*.
typh·lo·dic·li·di·tis [ˌ-dɪklə'daɪtɪs] *n* Entzündung *f* der Ileozäkalklappe.
typh·lo·em·py·e·ma [ˌ-empaɪ'iːmə] *n* appendizitischer Abszeß *m*.
typh·lo·en·ter·i·tis [ˌ-entə'raɪtɪs] *n* → typhlitis 1.
typh·lo·lex·ia [ˌ-'leksɪə] *n* Leseunfähigkeit *f*, -unvermögen *nt*, Alexie *f*.
typh·lo·li·thi·a·sis [ˌ-lɪ'θaɪəsɪs] *n* Zäko-, Typhlolithiasis *f*.
typh·lo·meg·a·ly [ˌ-'megəlɪ] *n* Zäkumvergrößerung *f*, Zäko-, Typhlomegalie *f*.
typh·lon ['tɪflɒn] *n* Blinddarm *m*, Zäkum *nt*, Zökum *nt*, C(a)ecum *nt*, Intestinum c(a)ecum.

typhlopexy

typh·lo·pex·y ['tɪfləpeksɪ] *n chir.* Zäkumfixation *f*, -anheftung *f*, Zäkopexie *f*, Typhlopexie *f*.
typh·lop·to·sis [ˌtɪflɑp'təʊsɪs] *n* Zäkumsenkung *f*, Typhloptose *f*.
typh·lor·rha·phy [tɪf'lɔrəfɪ] *n chir.* Zäkumnaht *f*, Zäkorrhaphie *f*.
typh·lo·sis [tɪf'ləʊsɪs] *n* Erblindung *f*, Blindheit *f*.
typh·los·to·my [tɪf'lɑstəmɪ] *n chir.* Zäkumfistel *f*, -fistelung *f*, Zäko-, Typhlostomie *f*.
typh·lo·ter·i·tis [ˌtɪflətɛ'raɪtɪs] *n* → typhlitis l.
typh·lot·o·my [tɪf'lɑtəmɪ] *n chir.* Zäkumeröffnung *f*, Zäko-, Typhlotomie *f*.
ty·phoid ['taɪfɔɪd] **I** *n* → typhoid fever. **II** *adj* **1.** Fleckfieber betr., Fleckfieber-. **2.** typhusartig, benommen, suporös, typhös.
ty·phoi·dal [taɪ'fɔɪdl] *adj* Typhus betr., typhös, Typhus-, Typho-.
typhoid and paratyphoid vaccine Typhus-Paratyphus-Impfstoff *m*.
typhoid bacillus *micro.* Typhusbakterium *nt*, Salmonella typhi.
typhoid bacterium → typhoid bacillus.
typhoid fever Bauchtyphus *m*, Typhus (abdominalis) *m*, Febris typhoides.
typhoid pneumonia Typhuspneumonie *f*, Pneumonia typhosa.
typhoid vaccine Typhusimpfstoff *m*, -vakzine *f*.
ty·phous ['taɪfəs] *adj* Typhus betr., typhusartig, -ähnlich, typhös, Typhus-.
ty·phus ['taɪfəs] *n* Fleckfieber *nt*.
typhus fever → typhus.
typ·i·cal ['tɪpɪkl] *adj* typisch, charakteristisch, repräsentativ, ur-, vorbildlich, echt.
typical achromatopsy (totale) Farbenblindheit *f*, Achromatopsie *f*, Monochromasie *f*, Einfarbensehen *nt*.

typical coloboma typisches Kolobom *nt*.
typical monochromasy → typical achromatopsy.
typ·ing ['taɪpɪŋ] *n immun., hema.* (Blutgruppen-, Gentypen-)Bestimmung *f*, Typing *nt*, Typisierung *f*.
ty·pol·o·gy [taɪ'pɑlədʒɪ] *n* Typologie *f*.
ty·pus ['taɪpəs] *n* → type I.
Tyr *abbr.* → tyrosine.
tyr- *pref.* → tyro-.
ty·ra·mine ['taɪrəmiːn] *n* Tyramin *nt*, Tyrosamin *nt*.
tyramine oxidase Monoamin(o)oxidase *f abbr.* MAO.
tyro- *pref.* Käse-, Tyr(o)-.
ty·ro·ci·din *n* → tyrocidine.
ty·ro·ci·dine [taɪrəsaɪdn] *n pharm.* Tyrocidin *nt*.
Tyrode ['taɪrəʊd]: **T.'s solution** Tyrode-Lösung *f*.
ty·rog·e·nous [taɪ'rɑdʒənəs] *adj* aus Käse stammend, durch Käse hervorgerufen, tyrogen, Käse-.
Ty·rog·ly·phus [taɪ'rɑglɪfəs] *n* → Tyrophagus.
ty·roid ['taɪrɔɪd] *adj* käseartig, -ähnlich, käsig.
ty·ro·ma [taɪ'rəʊmə] *n* käsiger Tumor *m*, Tyrom *nt*.
ty·ro·ma·to·sis [ˌtaɪrəmə'təʊsɪs] *n patho.* Verkäsung *f*, verkäsende Degeneration *f*.
Ty·roph·a·gus [taɪ'rɑfəgəs] *n micro.* Tyrophagus *m*.
T. farinae Mehlmilbe *f*, Tyrophagus farinae.
T. longior Käsemilbe *f*, Tyrophagus longior/casei.
ty·ros·a·mine [taɪ'rɑsəmiːn] *n* → tyramine.
ty·ro·sin·ase ['taɪrəsɪneɪz, 'tɪr-] *n* Tyrosinase *f*.
ty·ro·sine ['taɪrəsiːn, -sɪn] *n abbr.* **Tyr** Tyrosin *nt abbr.* **Tyr**.
tyrosine aminotransferase *abbr.* **TAT** Tyrosinaminotransferase *f abbr.* **TAT**, Tyrosintransaminase *f*.
tyrosine aminotransferase deficiency Richner-Hanhart-Syndrom *nt*, TAT-Mangel *m*, Tyrosinaminotransferasemangel *m*.
ty·ro·sin·e·mia [ˌtaɪrəsɪ'niːmɪə] *n* (Hyper-)Tyrosinämie *f*.
type I t. hereditäre/hepatorenale Tyrosinämie, Tyrosinose *f*.
type II t. Richner-Hanhart-Syndrom *nt*, TAT-Mangel *m*, Tyrosinaminotransferasemangel *m*.
tyrosine transaminase → tyrosine aminotransferase.
tyrosine xanthine agar Tyrosin-Xanthin-Agar *m/nt*.
ty·ro·si·no·sis [ˌtaɪrəsɪ'nəʊsɪs] *n* **1.** Tyrosinose *f*. **2.** hereditäre/hepatorenale Tyrosinämie, Tyrosinose *f*.
ty·ro·si·nu·ria [ˌtaɪrəsɪ'n(j)ʊərɪə] *n* Tyrosinausscheidung *f* im Harn, Tyrosinurie *f*.
ty·ro·sis [taɪ'rəʊsɪs] *n patho.* Verkäsung *f*, Tyrosis *f*.
ty·ro·syl ['taɪrəsɪl] *n* Tyrosyl-(Radikal *nt*).
ty·ro·thri·cin [ˌ-'θraɪsɪn] *n pharm.* Tyrothricin *nt*.
ty·ro·tox·i·co·sis [ˌ-ˌtɑksɪ'kəʊsɪs] *n* Käsevergiftung *f*, Tyrotoxikose *f*.
ty·ro·tox·ism [ˌ-'tɑksɪzəm] *n* → tyrotoxicosis.
Tyrrell ['tɪrəl]: **T.'s fascia** Septum rectovesicale.
Tyson ['taɪzn]: **crypts/glands of T.** Tyson-Drüsen *f*, präputiale (Talg-)Drüsen *pl*, Präputialdrüsen *pl*, Gll. pr(a)eputiales.
ty·son·i·tis [taɪsə'naɪtɪs] *n* Entzündung *f* der Tyson-Drüsen.
Tzanck [tsæŋk]: **T. cell** Tzanck-Zelle *f*.
T. test *derm.* Tzanck-Test *m*.
tzet·ze *n* → tsetse.
tzetze fly → tsetse.
T-zone lymphoma T-Zonenlymphom *nt*.

U

U *abbr.* 1. → uracil. 2. → uranium. 3. → uridine.
u·bi·qui·nol [juːˈbɪkwɪnal, -nɔl] *n* Ubihydrochinon *nt*.
ubiquinol-cytochrome c reductase Ubi(hydro)chinon-Cytochrom-c-reduktase *f*.
ubiquinol dehydrogenase → ubiquinol-cytochrome c reductase.
u·bi·qui·none [juːˈbɪkwɪnəʊn, ˌjuːbɪkwɪˈnəʊn] *n* Ubichinon *nt*.
u·biq·ui·tous [juːˈbɪkwɪtəs] *adj* überall vorkommend, allgegenwärtig, ubiquitär.
ud·der [ˈʌdər] *n bio.* Euter *nt/m*.
UDP *abbr.* → uridine(-5'-)diphosphate.
UDPbilirubin glucuronosyltransferase Glukuronyltransferase *f*.
UDPG *abbr.* → UDPglucose.
UDPgalactose *n* Uridindiphosphat-D-Galaktose *f*, UDP-Galaktose *f*, aktive Galaktose *f*.
UDPgalactose-4-epimerase *n* → UDPglucose-4-epimerase.
UDPglucose *n abbr.* **UDPG** Uridindiphosphat-D-Glukose *f abbr.* UDPG, UDP-Glukose *f*, aktive Glukose *f*.
UDPglucose dehydrogenase Uridindiphosphatglukose-dehydrogenase *f*, UDPG-dehydrogenase *f*.
UDPglucose-4-epimerase *n* UDP-Glukose-4-epimerase *f*, UDP-Galactose-4-epimerase *f*, Galaktowaldenase *f*.
UDPglucose-hexose-1-phosphate uridylyltransferase UDPglucose-hexose-1-phosphaturidylyltransferase *f*, UDPglukose-galaktose-1-phosphaturidylyltransferase *f*, Galaktose-1-phosphat-uridyltransferase *f*.
UDPglucose pyrophosphorylase → UDPglucose-hexose-1-phosphate uridylyltransferase.
UDPglucuronate *n* UDP-glucuronat *nt*.
UDPglucuronate-bilirubin-glucuronosyltransferase *n* Glukuronyltransferase *f*.
UDP-D-glucuronic acid Uridindiphosphatglucuronsäure *f*, UDP-D-Glucuronsäure *f*, aktive Glucuronsäure *f*.
UDPglucuronyl transferase Glukuronyltransferase *f*.
UDP-D-xylose *n* UDP-D-Xylose *f*.
Uehlinger [ˈyːlɪŋər]: **U.'s syndrome** Uehlinger-Syndrom *nt*.
UES *abbr.* → esophageal sphincter, upper.
UFA *abbr.* → fatty acid, unesterified.
U-fibers *n* (*ZNS*) U-Fasern *pl*.
U·gan·da S virus [juːˈgændə, uːˈgɑndə] Uganda-S-Virus *nt*.
Uhl [uːl]: **U.'s anomaly** *card.* (*Herz*) Uhl'-Anomalie *f*.
ul·cer [ˈʌlsər] *n patho.* Geschwür *nt*, Ulkus *nt*, Ulcus *nt*.
ul·cer·ate [ˈʌlsəreɪt] **I** *vt* eitern *od.* schwären lassen. **II** *vi* geschwürig werden, schwären, eitern, eitrig werden; ulzerieren; exulzerieren.
ul·cer·at·ed [ˈʌlsəreɪtɪd] *adj* eitrig, eiternd, vereitert; ulzeriert; exulzeriert.

ul·cer·at·ing granuloma of the pudenda [ˈʌlsəreɪtɪŋ] Granuloma inguinale/venereum, Granuloma pudendum chronicum, Donovaniosis *f*.
ul·cer·a·tion [ˌʌlsəˈreɪʃn] *n* 1. (Ver-)Eiterung *f*, Geschwür(sbildung *f*) *nt*, Ulzeration *f*; Exulzeration *f*. 2. → ulcer.
ul·cer·a·tive [ˈʌlsəreɪtɪv, -sərət-] *adj* 1. geschwürig, ulzerativ, ulzerös, eitrig, eiternd, Eiter-, Geschwür(s)-. 2. Geschwüre hervorrufend *od.* verursachend, ulzerogen.
ulcerative appendicitis ulzeröse Appendizitis *f*, Appendicitis ulcerosa.
ulcerative colitis Colitis ulcerosa/gravis.
ulcerative cystitis ulzerierende (Harn-)Blasenentzündung/Zystitis *f*, Cystitis ulcerosa.
ulcerative endocarditis ulzeröse Endokarditis *f*, Endocarditis ulcerosa.
ulcerative esophagitis ulzerierende/ulzerative Ösophagitis *f*.
ulcerative gingivitis Plaut-Vincent-Angina *f*, Fusospirillose *f*, Fusospirochätose *f*, Angina ulcerosa/ulceromembranacea.
ulcerative inflammation ulzerierende/ulzerative Entzündung *f*.
ulcerative proctitis ulzerative Proktitis *f*.
ulcerative stomatitis ulzerative Stomatitis *f*, Stomatitis ulcerosa, Stomakake *f*.
ulcerative tonsillitis ulzerierende Tonsillitis *f*.
ulcerative tumor ulzerativ-wachsender/ulzerativer Tumor *m*.
ulcer carcinoma Ulkuskarzinom *nt*, Ca. ex ulcere.
ulcer disease Ulkuskrankheit *f*.
peptic u. *abbr.* **PUD** Ulkuskrankheit.
recurrent u. Rezidivulkus *nt*.
ul·cer·o·car·ci·no·ma [ˌʌlsərəʊˌkɑːrsɪˈnəʊmə] *n* → ulcer carcinoma.
ul·cer·o·gan·gre·nous [ˌ-ˈgæŋgrənəs] *adj* ulzerös-gangrenös.
ul·cer·o·gen·e·sis [ˌ-ˈdʒenəsɪs] *n* Ulkusentstehung *f*, Ulzerogenese *f*.
ul·cer·o·gen·ic [ˌ-ˈdʒenɪk] *adj* Geschwüre hervorrufend, ulzerogen.
ul·cer·o·glan·du·lar tularemia [ˌ-ˈglændʒələr] ulzeroglanduläre/kutanoglanduläre Tularämie *f*.
ul·cer·o·mem·bra·nous [ˌ-ˈmembrənəs] *adj* ulzerös-membranös, ulzeromembranös.
ulceromembranous gingivitis → ulcerative gingivitis.
ul·cer·o·phleg·mon·ous appendicitis [ˌ-ˈflegmənəs] ulzerophlegmonöse Appendizitis *f*, Appendicitis ulcerophlegmonosa.
ul·cer·ous [ˈʌlsərəs] *adj* → ulcerative.
ulcer surgery Ulkuschirurgie *f*.
ul·cus [ˈʌlkəs] *n, pl* **ul·cera** [ˈʌlsərə] → ulcer.
ule- *pref.* → ulo-.
u·lec·to·my [juːˈlektəmɪ] *n* 1. *chir., ortho.* Narbenausschneidung *f*, -exzision *f*. 2. *dent., HNO* Zahnfleischabtragung *f*,

Gingivektomie *f*, Gingivoektomie *f*.
u·le·gy·ria [juːlɪˈdʒaɪrɪə] *n* Hirnrindenvernarbung *f*, Ulegyrie *f*.
u·lem·or·rha·gia [ˌuːlemˈreɪdʒ(ɪ)ə] *n* Zahnfleischblutung *f*.
u·ler·y·the·ma [juːˌlerɪˈθiːmə] *n derm.* Ulerythema *nt*.
ulerythema ophryogenes Ulerythema ophryogenes, Keratosis pilaris (rubra) faciei.
u·lex·ine [juːˈleksiːn] *n* Zytisin *nt*, Cytisin *nt*.
u·lig·i·nous [juːˈlɪdʒənəs] *adj* sumpfig, morastig, Sumpf-.
u·li·tis [jəˈlaɪtɪs] *n* Zahnfleischentzündung *f*, Gingivitis *f*.
Ullrich-Feichtiger [ʊlrɪç ˈfaɪçtɪŋər]: **U.-F. syndrome** Ullrich-Feichtiger-Syndrom *nt*.
Ullrich-Turner [ˈtɜrnər]: **U.-T. syndrome** Noonan-Syndrom *nt*, Pseudo-Ullrich-Turner-Syndrom *nt*.
ul·na [ˈʌlnə] *n, pl* **-nas, -nae** [-niː] Ulna *f*.
ulna aplasia *embryo.* Ulnaaplasie *f*.
ulna hypoplasia *embryo.* Ulnahypoplasie *f*.
ul·nar [ˈʌlnər] *adj* auf der Ulnarseite liegend, zur Ulna gehörend, ulnar, Ellen-, Ulno-.
ulnar artery Ulnaris *f*, A. ulnaris.
ulnar artery thrombosis Thrombose *f* der A. ulnaris, Ulnaristhrombose *f*.
ulnar bone *old* → ulna.
ulnar border of forearm Ulnarseite *f* des Unterarms, Margo medialis/ulnaris antebrachii.
ulnar branch of medial cutaneous nerve of forearm Ramus posterior/ulnaris n. cutanei antebrachii medialis.
ulnar clubhand *ortho.* Manus vara.
ulnar crest Margo interosseus ulnae.
ulnar deviation *ortho.* Ulnardeviation *f*, -abduktion *f*.
ulnar ectromelia *embryo.* ulnare Ektromelie *f*.
ulnar eminence of wrist Eminentia carpi ulnaris.
ulnar fracture Ellenbruch *m*, Ulnafraktur *f*.
ulnar groove Sulcus n. ulnaris.
ulnar head: u. of flexor carpi ulnaris (muscle) Caput ulnare m. flexoris carpi ulnaris.
u. of pronator teres (muscle) Caput ulnare m. pronatoris teretis.
ulnar hemimelia Ulnahemimelie *f*.
ulnar incisure of radius Inc. ulnaris (radii).
ulnar ligament: (collateral) u. of carpus → lateral u.
lateral u. Lig. collaterale carpi ulnare.
ulnar malleolus Proc. styloideus ulnae.
ulnar margin of forearm → ulnar border of forearm.
ulnar nerve Ulnaris *m*, N. ulnaris.
ulnar notch of radius → ulnar incisure of radius.

ulnar tunnel syndrome

ulnar tunnel syndrome Ulnartunnelsyndrom *nt*.
ulnar veins Begleitvenen *pl* der A. ulnaris, Vv. ulnares.
ul·no·car·pal [ˌʌlnəˈkɑːrpəl] *adj* Elle/Ulna u. Handwurzel/Karpus betr., ulnokarpal, karpoulnar.
ul·no·ra·di·al [ˌ-ˈreɪdɪəl] *adj* Elle/Ulna u. Speiche/Radius betr., ulnoradial, radioulnar.
ulnoradial bursa Bursa cubitalis interossea.
ulo- *pref.* **1.** Narben-, Ul(o)-. **2.** Zahnfleisch-, Ul(o)-, Gingiva-.
u·lo·ca·ce [juːˈlakəsɪ] *n* Zahnfleischulzeration *f*, -ulkus *nt*.
u·lo·car·ci·no·ma [ˌjuːloʊˌkɑːrsɪˈnoʊmə] *n* Zahnfleischkarzinom *nt*.
u·lo·glos·si·tis [ˌ-glaˈsaɪtɪs] *n* Entzündung *f* von Zahnfleisch u. Zunge.
u·loid [ˈjuːlɔɪd] *adj* narbenartig, narbig.
u·lor·rha·gia [juːləˈreɪdʒ(ɪ)ə] *n* (massive) Zahnfleischblutung *f*.
u·lor·rhea [ˌ-ˈrɪə] *n* Zahnfleisch(sicker)blutung *f*.
u·lot·o·my [juːˈlɑtəmɪ] *n* **1.** *chir.* Narbendurchtrennung *f*, -revision *f*. **2.** *HNO, dent.* Zahnfleischschnitt *m*.
u·lot·ri·chous [juːˈlɑtrɪkəs] *adj* ulotrich.
ul·ti·mate [ˈʌltəmɪt] **I** *n* das Letzte, das Äußerste; Gipfel *m*. **II** *adj* äußerste(r, s), höchste(r, s), Höchst-, Grenz-.
ul·ti·mo·bran·chi·al body [ˌʌltɪməʊˈbræŋkɪəl] *embryo.* Ultimobranchialkörper *m*, ultimobranchialer Körper *m*.
ultimobranchial cells (*Schilddrüse*) parafollikuläre Zellen *pl*, C-Zellen *pl*.
ultra- *pref.* jenseits (von), (dar-)über ... hinaus, äußerst, ultra-.
ul·tra·brach·y·ce·phal·ic [ˌʌltrəˌbrækɪsəˈfælɪk] *adj* ultrabrachyzephal.
ul·tra·cen·trif·u·ga·tion [ˌ-senˌtrɪfjəˈgeɪʃn] *n* Ultrazentrifugation *f*.
ul·tra·cen·tri·fuge [ˌ-ˈsentrɪfjuːdʒ] *n* Ultrazentrifuge *f*.
ul·tra·di·an [ʌlˈtreɪdɪən] *adj bio.* ultradian.
ul·tra·dol·i·cho·ce·phal·ic [ˌʌltrəˌdɑlɪkəʊsəˈfælɪk] *adj* ultradolichozephal.
ul·tra·fil·ter [ˌ-ˈfɪltər] *n* Ultrafilter *m*; semipermeable Membran *f*.
ul·tra·fil·trate [ˌ-ˈfɪltreɪt] *n* Ultrafiltrat *nt*.
ul·tra·fil·tra·tion [ˌ-fɪlˈtreɪʃn] *n* Ultrafiltration *f*.
ul·tra·mi·cro·a·nal·y·sis [ˌ-ˌmaɪkroʊəˈnæləsɪs] *n* Ultramikroanalyse *f*.
ul·tra·mi·cro·chem·is·try [ˌ-ˌmaɪkroʊˈkemɪstrɪ] *n* Ultramikrochemie *f*.
ul·tra·mi·cro·scope [ˌ-ˈmaɪkrəskoʊp] *n* Ultramikroskop *nt*.
ul·tra·mi·cro·scop·ic [ˌ-ˌmaɪkrəˈskɑpɪk] *adj* **1.** Ultramikroskop betr., ultramikroskopisch. **2.** (*Größe*) ultramikroskopisch, submikroskopisch, ultravisibel.
ul·tra·mi·cros·co·py [ˌ-maɪˈkrɑskəpɪ] *n* Ultramikroskopie *f*.
ul·tra·mi·cro·tome [ˌ-ˈmaɪkrətoʊm] *n* Ultramikrotom *nt*.
ul·tra·red [ˌ-ˈred] **I** *n abbr.* **UR** Ultrarot *nt abbr.* UR, Infrarot *nt abbr.* IR, Ultrarot-, Infrarotlicht *nt*, IR-Licht *nt*, UR-Licht *nt*. **II** *adj* ultrarot, infrarot.
ul·tra·short [ˌ-ˈʃɔrt] *adj* Ultrakurz-.
ultrashort acting ultrakurzwirkend.
ultrashort wave *phys.* Ultrakurzwelle *f*.
ultrashort-wave diathermy Ultrakurzwellen-, Ultrahochfrequenzdiathermie *f*.
ul·tra·son·ic [ˌ-ˈsɑnɪk] *adj* Ultraschall-, Ultrasono-.
ultrasonic atomization Ultraschallvernebelung *f*.
ultrasonic cardiography Echokardiogra-

phie *f*, Ultraschallkardiographie *f abbr.* UKG.
ultrasonic flowmeter Ultraschallflußmesser *m*.
ultrasonic microscope Ultraschallmikroskop *nt*.
ultrasonic nebulization → ultrasonic atomization.
ultrasonic nebulizer Ultraschallvernebler *m*.
ultrasonic waves → ultrasound.
ul·tra·son·o·gram [ˌ-ˈsɑnəgræm] *n* Sonogramm *nt*.
ul·tra·son·o·graph·ic [ˌ-ˌsɑnəˈgræfɪk] *adj* Ultraschall betr., sonographisch, Ultraschall-, Ultrasono-.
ultrasonographic cephalometry *embryo., ped.* Ultraschallkephalometrie *f*, sonographische Kephalometrie *f*.
ul·tra·so·nog·ra·phy [ˌ-səˈnɑgrəfɪ] *n* Ultraschalldiagnostik *f*, Sonographie *f*.
ul·tra·so·nom·e·try [ˌ-səˈnɑmətrɪ] *n* (Ultra-)Sonometrie *f*.
ul·tra·sound [ˈ-saʊnd] *n abbr.* **US**, Ultraschallstrahlen *pl*, -wellen *pl*.
ultrasound cardiography → ultrasonic cardiography.
ultrasound mammography *gyn.* Ultraschallmammographie *f*.
ul·tra·struc·tur·al [ˌ-ˈstrʌktʃərəl] *adj* ultra-, feinstrukturell.
ul·tra·struc·ture [ˈ-strʌktʃər] *n* Fein-, Ultrastruktur *f*.
ul·tra·vi·o·let [ˌ-ˈvaɪəlɪt] **I** *n abbr.* **UV** Ultraviolett *nt abbr.* UV, Ultraviolettstrahlung *f*, Ultraviolettstrahlung *f*, -strahlung *f*, UV-Licht *nt*, -Strahlung *f*. **II** *adj* ultraviolett, Ultraviolett-, UV-.
ultraviolet irradiation UV-Bestrahlung *f*.
ultraviolet keratoconjunctivitis Conjunctivitis actinica/photoelectrica, Keratoconjunctivitis/Ophthalmia photoelectrica.
ultraviolet lamp Ultraviolettlampe *f*, UV-Lampe *f*.
ultraviolet light → ultraviolet I.
ultraviolet microscope Ultraviolettmikroskop *nt*, UV-Mikroskop *nt*.
ultraviolet radiation Ultraviolettstrahlung *f*, UV-Strahlung *f*.
ultraviolet ray ophthalmia → ultraviolet keratoconjunctivitis.
ultraviolet rays Ultraviolettstrahlen *pl*, -strahlung *f*, UV-Strahlen *pl*, -Strahlung *f*.
ul·tra·vis·i·ble [ˌ-ˈvɪzəbl] *adj* → ultramicroscopic 2.
ultra x-rays *phys.* kosmische Strahlung *f*.
um·bau zone [ˈʊmbaʊ] Looser'-Umbauzone *f*.
um·bel [ˈʌmbəl] *n bio.* Dolde *f*.
um·bel·late [ˈʌmbəleɪt, -lɪt] *adj* → umbellated.
um·bel·lat·ed [ˈʌmbəleɪtɪd] *adj bio.* doldenblütig, -tragend, Dolden-.
um·bel·lif·er·ous [ʌmbəˈlɪfərəs] *adj* → umbellated.
um·bel·li·form [ʌmˈbelɪfɔrm] *adj* doldenförmig.
um·ber [ˈʌmbər] **I** *n* **1.** Umber(erde *f*) *m*, Umbra *f*. **2.** Umbra(braun) *f*, Umber *m*. **II** *adj* dunkelbraun, umbrafarben, umbrabraun.
um·bil·i·cal [ʌmˈbɪlɪkl] **I** *n* → umbilical cord. **II** *adj* Nabel betr., zum Nabel gehörend, umbilikal, Nabel-, Umbilikal-.
umbilical artery Nabel-, Umbilikalarterie *f*, A. umbilicalis.
umbilical circulation Umbilikal-, Nabel-(schnur)kreislauf *m*.
umbilical cord Nabelstrang *m*, -schnur *f*, Chorda/Funiculus umbilicalis.

umbilical cyst Nabelzyste *f*.
umbilical diphtheria Nabeldiphtherie *f*.
umbilical duct Darmstiel *m*, Dotter(sack)gang *m*, Ductus omphalo(mes)entericus.
umbilical eventration → umbilical hernia.
umbilical fissure Lebereinschnitt *m* durch Lig. teretis hepatis, Inc. lig. teretis.
umbilical fistula 1. Nabelfistel *f*, Fistula umbilicalis. **2.** Dottergangsfistel *f*, Fistula omphaloenterica.
umbilical fold: lateral u. epigastrische Falte *f*, Plica umbilicalis lateralis.
medial u. Plica umbilicalis medialis.
median u. Urachusfalte *f*, Plica umbilicalis mediana.
umbilical granuloma Nabelgranulom *nt*.
umbilical hernia Nabelbruch *m*, Exomphalos *m*, Exomphalozele *f*, Hernia umbilicalis.
congenital u. Nabelschnurbruch, Exomphalos *m*, Exomphalozele *f*, Hernia funiculi umbilicalis.
physiological u. *embryo.* physiologischer Nabelbruch.
umbilical-ileal fistula → umbilical fistula 2.
umbilical incisure → umbilical fissure.
umbilical ligament: lateral u. Lig. umbilicale mediale.
medial u. Lig. umbilicale mediale.
median u. Urachus(strang *m*) *m*, *old* Chorda urachi, Lig. umbilicale medianum.
umbilical notch → umbilical fissure.
umbilical part of portal vein Pars umbilicalis.
umbilical region *anat.* Nabelregion *f*, -gegend *f*, Regio umbilicalis.
umbilical ring Nabelring *m*, An(n)ulus umbilicalis.
umbilical sinus Nabelfistel *f*, Fistula umbilicalis.
umbilical vein Nabel-, Umbilikalvene *f*, V. umbilicalis.
left u. V. umbilicalis sinistra.
umbilical vesicle Nabelbläschen *nt*, Dottersack *m*.
umbilical vessel catheter Nabelschnur-, Nabelvenenkatheter *m*.
umbilical vessels Nabel(schnur)gefäße *pl*.
um·bil·i·cate [ʌmˈbɪlɪkeɪt] *adj* nabelförmig, -artig.
um·bil·i·cat·ed [ʌmˈbɪlɪkeɪtɪd] *adj* → umbilicate.
umbilicated cataract ringförmige/scheibenförmige Katarakt *f*.
um·bil·i·ca·tion [ʌmˌbɪlɪˈkeɪʃn] *n* nabelförmige Einziehung *f*.
um·bil·i·cus [ʌmˈbɪlɪkəs, ˌʌmbɪˈlaɪkəs] *n, pl* **-cus·es, -ci** [-kaɪ, -saɪ] *anat.* Nabel *m*, Umbilikus *m*, Umbilicus *m*, Omphalos *m*, Umbo *m*.
um·bo [ˈʌmboʊ] *n, pl* **-bos, -bo·nes** [ˈ-boʊniːz] → umbilicus.
u. of tympanic membrane Trommelfellnabel *m*, Umbo membranae tympani.
um·bo·nate [ˈʌmbənɪt, -neɪt] *adj* vorgewölbt, gebuckelt.
um·bras·co·py [ʌmˈbræskəpɪ] *n ophthal.* Retinoskopie *f*, Skiaskopie *f*.
um·brel·la iris [ʌmˈbrelə] *ophthal.* Napfkucheniris *f*, Iris bombans/bombata.
UMP *abbr.* → uridine monophosphate.
un·ac·cus·tomed [ʌnəˈkʌstəmd] *adj* ungewohnt, fremd.
un·a·ble [ʌnˈeɪbl] *adj* **1.** unfähig, nicht in der Lage (*to do* zu tun). **2.** ungeeignet, untauglich (*to* für). **3.** schwach, hilflos.
un·ac·com·pa·nied [ʌnəˈkʌmpəniːd] *adj* nicht begleitet (*by* von); alleine.

un·a·dapt·a·ble [ʌnə'dæptəbl] *adj* nicht anpassungsfähig (*to* an); nicht anwendbar (*to* auf); ungeeignet (*to, for* zu, für).
un·a·dapt·ed [ʌnə'dæptɪd] *adj* nicht angepaßt/adaptiert (*to* an).
un·ad·just·ed [ʌnə'dʒʌstɪd] *adj psycho.* nicht angepaßt (*to* an).
un·a·dul·ter·at·ed [ʌnə'dʌltəreɪtɪd] *adj chem., pharm.* rein, pur, echt, unverfälscht, unverdünnt.
un·af·fect·ed [ʌnə'fektɪd] *adj* **1.** (*Organ*) nicht befallen, nicht affiziert, gesund (*by* von). **2.** unberührt, unbeeinflußt (*by* von).
un·aid·ed [ʌn'eɪdɪd] *adj* alleine, ohne Hilfe (*by* von); (*Augen*) ohne Brille.
un·al·low·a·ble [ʌnə'laʊəbl] *adj* unzulässig, unerlaubt.
u·na·nim·i·ty [ˌjuː'nɪmətɪ] *n* Einmütigkeit *f*; Einstimmigkeit *f*.
u·nan·i·mous [juː'nænɪməs] *adj* einmütig, einstimmig.
un·ap·pre·hen·sive [ʌnˌæprɪ'hensɪv] *adj* schwerfällig, schwer von Begriff.
un·ap·proach·a·ble [ʌnə'prəʊtʃəbl] *adj* **1.** unnahbar. **2.** *chir.* unzugänglich, nicht angehbar.
un·ap·proved [ʌnə'pruːvd] *adj* ungebilligt, nicht genehmigt.
un·apt [ʌn'æpt] *adj* ungeeignet, untauglich (*for* für, zu); unpassend, unangebracht; nicht geeignet.
un·armed tapeworm [ʌn'ɑːrmd] *micro.* Rinder(finnen)bandwurm *m*, Taenia saginata, Taeniarhynchus saginatus.
un·as·cer·tain·a·ble [ʌnˌæsər'teɪnəbl] *adj* nicht feststellbar.
un·as·sim·i·la·ble [ʌnə'sɪmələbl] *adj* nicht assimilierbar, nicht assimilationsfähig.
un·as·sim·i·lat·ed [ʌnə'sɪməleɪtɪd] *adj* nicht assimiliert.
un·as·sist·ed [ʌnə'sɪstɪd] *adj* ohne Hilfe, ohne Assistenz *od.* Unterstützung (*by* von).
un·at·tached [ʌnə'tætʃt] *adj anat.* nicht festgewachsen, lose, frei.
unattached gingiva → unattached gum.
unattached gum Periodontium insertionis.
un·at·tend·ed [ʌnə'tendɪd] *adj* unbeaufsichtigt, ohne Aufsicht; (*Kind*) vernachlässigt; (*Wunde*) unversorgt; (*Krankheit*) unbehandelt; *techn.* ohne Wartung.
un·au·thor·ized [ʌn'ɔːθəraɪzd] *adj* nicht autorisiert, nicht bevollmächtigt, unbefugt, unberechtigt, unerlaubt.
un·a·vail·a·ble [ʌnə'veɪləbl] *adj* **1.** nicht vorhanden, nicht verfügbar. **2.** unbrauchbar.
unavailable energy *phys.* Verlustenergie *f*.
un·az·o·tized [ʌn'æzətaɪzd] *adj* keinen Stickstoff enthaltend, stickstofffrei.
un·bal·ance [ʌn'bæləns] **I** *n* **1.** Gleichgewichtsstörung *f*. **2.** *fig.* Unausgeglichenheit *f*. **II** *vt* aus dem Gleichgewicht bringen.
un·bal·anced [ʌn'bælənst] *adj* **1.** nicht im Gleichgewicht (befindlich). **2.** *fig.* unausgeglichen.
un·band·age [ʌn'bændɪdʒ] *vt* einen Verband abnehmen/entfernen (von).
un·bear·a·ble [ʌn'beərəbl] *adj* unerträglich.
un·bi·ased [ʌn'baɪəst] *adj* unvoreingenommen, unbefangen, vorurteilsfrei.
un·block [ʌn'blɒk] *vt* entblocken.
un·block·ing [ʌn'blɒkɪŋ] *n* Entblockung *f*.
un·born [ʌn'bɔːrn] *adj* ungeboren.
un·branched [ʌn'brɑːntʃd] *adj chem.* unverzweigt.
un·bro·ken [ʌn'brəʊkn] *adj* nicht zerbrochen, heil, unversehrt, intakt, ganz.
un·bur·den [ʌn'bɜːrdn] *vt* entlasten, erleichtern.
un·blend·ed [ʌn'blendɪd] *adj* ungemischt, rein, pur.
un·cal ['ʌŋkəl] *adj anat.* Uncus betr., Unkus-.
unc·ar·thro·sis [ʌŋkɑːr'θrəʊsɪs] *n ortho.* Unkarthrose *f*.
un·cer·tain [ʌn'sɜːrtn] *adj* **1.** unsicher, ungewiß, unbestimmt. **2.** unbeständig, veränderlich, unstet, launenhaft; unzuverlässig. **3.** unsicher, verwirrt.
un·cer·tain·ty [ʌn'sɜːrtntɪ] *n* **1.** Unsicherheit *f*, Ungewißheit *f*, Unbestimmtheit *f*. **2.** Unzuverlässigkeit *f*, Unbeständigkeit *f*, Veränderlichkeit *f*.
un·cer·tif·i·cat·ed [ʌnˌsɜːr'tɪfɪkeɪtɪd] *adj* **1.** unbescheinigt, ohne Bescheinigung. **2.** ohne amtliches Zeugnis, nicht diplomiert.
un·cer·ti·fied [ʌn'sɜːrtɪfaɪd] *adj* nicht bescheinigt, unbeglaubigt.
un·changed [ʌn'tʃeɪndʒt] *adj* (*Zustand, Befinden*) unverändert, gleich.
un·char·ac·ter·is·tic leprosy [ʌnˌkærɪktə'rɪstɪk] indeterminierte Lepra *f abbr.* IL, Lepra indeterminata.
un·charged [ʌn'tʃɑːrdʒd] *adj* nicht aufgeladen, ungeladen, ohne Ladung.
uncharged molecule ungeladenes Molekül *nt*.
un·ci·form ['ʌnsɪfɔːrm] *adj* → uncinate 1.
unciform bone Hakenbein *nt*, Hamatum *nt*, Os hamatum.
un·ci·for·me [ʌnsɪ'fɔːrmɪ] *n* → unciform bone.
unciform fasciculus → uncinate fasciculus.
unciform pancreas Proc. uncinatus (pancreatis).
un·ci·nal ['ʌnsɪnl] *adj* → uncinate.
Un·ci·nar·i·a [ʌnsə'neərɪə] *n micro.* Uncinaria *f*.
U. americana Todeswurm *m*, Necator americanus.
U. duodenalis (europäischer) Hakenwurm *m*, Grubenwurm *m*, Ancylostoma duodenale.
un·ci·nar·i·a·sis [ˌ-nə'raɪəsɪs] *n* **1.** Uncinariasis *f*. **2.** Hakenwurmbefall *m*, -infektion *f*, Ankylostomiasis *f*, Ankylostomatosis *f*, Ankylostomatidose *f*.
un·ci·nate ['-nɪt, -neɪt] *adj* **1.** *anat.* hakenförmig, gekrümmt; mit Haken versehen. **2.** Uncus betr.
uncinate bone → unciform bone.
uncinate fasciculus Hakenbündel *nt*, Fasciculus uncinatus.
uncinate gyrus → uncus 2.
uncinate pancreas → unciform pancreas.
uncinate process Hakenfortsatz *m*, hakenförmiger Fortsatz *m*, Proc. uncinatus.
u. of ethmoid bone Proc. uncinatus ossis ethmoidalis.
u. of lacrimal bone Hamulus lacrimalis.
u. of pancreas Proc. uncinatus pancreatis.
un·ci·na·tum [ˌ-'neɪtəm] *n, pl* **-tums, -ta** [-tə] → unciform bone.
un·cir·cum·cised [ʌn'sɜːrkəmsaɪzd] *adj* nicht beschnitten, nicht beschnitten.
un·clas·si·fied [ʌn'klæsɪfaɪd] *adj* nicht klassifiziert, nicht eingeordnet.
un·clean [ʌn'kliːn] *adj* unrein, unsauber; (*Zunge*) belegt.
un·clean·li·ness [ʌn'klenlɪnɪs] *n* Unreinlichkeit *f*, Unsauberkeit *f*.
un·coat·ing ['ʌnkəʊtɪŋ] *n micro.* (*Virus*) Uncoating *nt*.
un·coil [ʌn'kɔɪl] **I** *vt* abwickeln, -spulen, aufrollen, entspiralisieren. **II** *vi* s. abwickeln, s. abspulen, s. aufrollen, s. entspiralisieren.
un·col·ored [ʌn'kʌlərd] *adj* ungefärbt, farblos.
un·com·mu·ni·ca·ble [ˌʌnkə'mjuːnɪkəbl] *adj* (*Krankheit*) nicht ansteckend *od.* übertragbar.
un·com·mu·ni·ca·tive [ˌʌnkə'mjuːnɪˌkeɪtɪv] *adj* verschlossen, wenig mitteilsam.
un·com·pen·sat·ed [ʌn'kɒmpənseɪtɪd] *adj* nicht kompensiert.
uncompensated acidosis nicht-kompensierte Azidose *f*.
un·com·pet·i·tive inhibition [ˌʌnkəm'petətɪv] *biochem.* unkompetitive Hemmung *f*.
un·com·ple·ment·ed [ʌn'kɒmpləmentɪd] *adj immun.* nicht an Komplement gebunden, inaktiv.
un·com·pli·cat·ed [ʌn'kɒmplɪkeɪtɪd] *adj* einfach, unkompliziert; (*Fraktur*) glatt.
un·con·di·tioned [ˌʌnkən'dɪʃənd] *adj psycho.* angeboren, unbedingt.
unconditioned reflex *abbr.* **UR** unbedingter Reflex *m abbr.* UR.
unconditioned response unbedingte Reaktion *f*.
unconditioned stimulus *abbr.* **US** *physiol.* unbedingter Reiz *m*, unconditioned stimulus *abbr.* US.
un·con·ju·gat·ed bilirubin [ʌn'kɒndʒəgeɪtɪd] freies/indirektes/unkonjugiertes Bilirubin *nt*.
unconjugated hyperbilirubinemia Erhöhung *f* des unkonjugierten Bilirubins.
un·con·scious [ʌn'kɒnʃəs] **I** *n* **the ~** das Unbewußte. **II** *adj* **1.** (*a. psycho.*) unbewußt, unwillkürlich. **2.** bewußt-, besinnungslos, ohnmächtig. **3.** (*Materie*) leblos.
un·con·scious·ness [ʌn'kɒnʃəsnɪs] *n* **1.** Unbewußtheit *f*. **2.** Bewußt-, Besinnungslosigkeit *f*, Ohnmacht *f*.
un·con·strained [ˌʌnkən'streɪnd] *adj* ungezwungen, zwanglos.
un·con·straint [ˌʌnkən'streɪnt] *n* Ungezwungenheit *f*, Zwanglosigkeit *f*.
un·con·tam·i·nat·ed [ˌʌnkən'tæmɪneɪtɪd] *adj* nicht verunreinigt *od.* verseucht *od.* infiziert *od.* vergiftet.
un·con·trol·la·ble [ˌʌnkən'trəʊləbl] *adj* **1.** unkontrollierbar; (*Seuche*) nicht einzudämmen. **2.** unbeherrscht, unkontrolliert.
un·co·op·er·a·tive [ˌʌnkəʊ'ɒp(ə)rətɪv] *adj* (*Patient*) nicht kooperativ.
un·co·or·di·nat·ed [ˌʌnkəʊ'ɔːrdneɪtɪd] *adj* unkoordiniert.
un·cor·rect·ed [ˌʌnkə'rektɪd] *adj* unkorrigiert, unberichtigt.
un·cot·o·my [ʌn'kɒtəmɪ] *n neurochir.* Unkotomie *f*.
un·cou·pler [ʌn'kʌplər] *n biochem.* Entkoppler *m*, entkoppelnde Substanz *f*.
un·cou·pling [ʌn'kʌplɪŋ] *n biochem.* Entkopplung *f*.
uncoupling agent → uncoupler.
un·cov·er [ʌn'kʌvər] *vt* aufdecken, bloßlegen, entblößen, freilegen.
un·co·ver·te·bral [ˌʌnkəʊ'vɜːrtəbrəl] *adj* unkovertebral.
uncovertebral spondylosis Unkovertebralarthrose *f*, Spondylosis intervertebralis/uncovertebralis.
un·crossed [ʌn'krɒst, -'krɑːst] *adj anat.* nicht gekreuzt, ungekreuzt.
uncrossed diplopia *ophthal.* direkte/gleichseitige/ungekreuzte/homonyme Diplopie *f*, Diplopia simplex.
unc·tion ['ʌŋkʃn] *n* **1.** Einreibung *f*, (Ein-)Salbung *f*, Unktion *f*. **2.** *pharm.* Salbe *f*. **3.** *fig.* Trost *m*, Balsam *m* (*to* für).
unc·tious ['ʌŋkʃəs] *adj* ölig, fettig.

unctuous

unc·tu·ous ['ʌŋktʃəwəs] *adj* → unctious.
un·cus ['ʌŋkəs] *n, pl* **un·ci** ['ʌnsaɪ] **1.** *anat.* Haken *m*, Häkchen *nt*, hakenförmiger Vorsprung *m*, Uncus *m*. **2.** (*ZNS*) Uncus *m*.
uncus corporis Uncus corporis.
un·dam·aged [ʌn'dæmɪdʒd] *adj* heil, unversehrt, unbeschädigt.
un·damped [ʌn'dæmpt] *adj phys.* (*Schwingung*) ungedämpft.
un·dat·ed [ʌn'deɪtɪd] *adj* **1.** undatiert, ohne Datum. **2.** unbefristet.
un·de·cane ['ʌndəkeɪn, ʌn'de-] *n* Undekan *nt*, Undecan *nt*.
un·dec·a·pre·nol [ʌn,dekə'priːnɒl, -nɑl] *n* Undecaprenol *nt*, Bactoprenol *nt*.
un·dec·a·pre·nyl alcohol [ʌn,dekə'priːnl] → undecaprenol.
undecaprenyl phosphate Undecaprenylphosphat *nt*.
un·dec·e·no·ic acid [ʌn,desə'nəʊɪk] → undecylenic acid.
un·dec·y·len·ic acid [ʌn,desə'liːnɪk, -'len-] 10-Undecensäure *f*, Undecylensäure *f*.
un·der ['ʌndər] **I** *adj* **1.** unter(r, s), nieder(r, s), Hilfs-, Unter-; untergeordnet. **for the ~twelves** für Kinder unter 12 Jahren. **2.** ungenügend, zuwenig. **II** *prep* **3.** unter. **4.** unterhalb von, unter. **5.** unter, weniger als. **girls ~ 10 (years of age)** Mädchen unter 10 (Jahre). **in ~ an hour** in weniger als einer Stunde. **6. ~ treatment** in Behandlung. **to be ~ study** untersucht/erforscht werden.
un·der·a·chieve [,ʌndərə'tʃiːv] *vi* weniger leisten als erwartet, sein Potenzial nicht ausnutzen.
under age minderjährig, unmündig.
un·der·arm ['ʌndərɑːrm] **I** *n* Achselhöhle *f*. **II** *adj* Unterarm-.
un·der·class ['-klæs] *n socio.* Unterklasse *f*, unterprivilegierte Klasse *f*.
un·der·clothes ['-kləʊz, -kləʊðz] *pl* Unterwäsche *f*, -kleidung *f*.
un·der·cloth·ing ['-kləʊðɪŋ] *n* → underclothes.
un·der·de·vel·op [,-dɪ'veləp] *vt* (*a. radiol.*) unterentwickeln.
un·der·de·vel·oped [,-dɪ'veləpt] *adj* **1.** *radiol., phys.* unterentwickelt. **2.** (körperlich *od.* geistig) zurückgeblieben, unterentwickelt, mangelhaft entwickelt.
un·der·de·vel·op·ment [,-dɪ'veləpmənt] *n* Unterentwicklung *f*, Unreife *f*.
un·der·di·ag·nose [,-'daɪəgnəʊz] *vt* **1.** (*Krankheit*) übersehen (*Diagnose*) übersehen. **2.** eine Krankheit zu selten diagnostizieren.
un·der·dose [*n* '-dəʊs; *v* ,-'dəʊs] **I** *n* zu geringe Dosis *f*, Unterdosierung *f*. **II** *vt* zu gering dosieren, unterdosieren; jdm. eine zu geringe Dosis verabreichen.
un·der·es·ti·mate [,-'estɪmeɪt] **I** *n* Unterschätzung *f*, Unterbewertung *f*. **II** *vt* unterschätzen, unterbewerten.
un·der·es·ti·ma·tion [,-estɪ'meɪʃn] *n* → underestimate 1.
un·der·ex·pose [,-ɪk'spəʊz] *vt phys., radiol.* unterbelichten.
un·der·ex·po·sure [,-ɪk'spəʊʒər] *n phys., radiol.* Unterbelichtung *f*.
un·der·fed [,-'fed] *adj* unterernährt.
un·der·feed [,-'fiːd] *vt* unterernähren, nicht ausreichend ernähren.
un·der·feed·ing [,-'fiːdɪŋ] *n* Unterernährung *f*, Mangelernährung *f*.
un·der·go [,-'gəʊ] *vt* **1.** durch-, erleben, durchmachen, erfahren. **2.** s. (*einer Operation*) unterziehen. **3.** (*Schmerz*) ertragen, erdulden. **4.** (*einem Test*) unterzogen werden.
un·der·horn ['-hɔːrn] *n anat.* Unterhorn *nt* des Seitenventrikels, Cornu inferius/temporale ventriculi lateralis.
un·der·hung [,-'hʌŋ] *adj* (*Unterkiefer*) vorstehend.
un·der·lay [*n* '-leɪ; *v* ,-'leɪ] **I** *n* Unterlage *f*. **II** *vt* (dar-)unterlegen, stützen (*with* mit).
un·der·lip ['-lɪp] *n* Unterlippe *f*.
un·der·load·ing [,-'ləʊdɪŋ] *n* unphysiologisch geringe Belastung *f*, Unterbelastung *f*.
un·der·ly·ing ['-laɪɪŋ] *adj* **1.** *fig.* zugrundeliegend, grundlegend, eigentlich. **2.** darunterliegend.
un·der·min·ing burrowing ulcer [,-'maɪnɪŋ] Meleney-Geschwür *nt*, Pyoderma gangraenosum, Dermatitis ulcerosa, Pyodermia ulcerosa serpiginosa.
un·der·nour·ished [,-'nɜrɪʃt] *adj* unter-, mangel-, fehlernährt.
un·der·nour·ish·ment [,-'nɜrɪʃmənt] *n* Unter-, Mangel-, Fehlernährung *f*.
un·der·nu·tri·tion [,-n(j)uː'trɪʃn] *n* → undernourishment.
un·der·per·fused [,-pər'fjuːzd] *adj* minderdurchblutet, hypoperfundiert.
un·der·pop·u·lat·ed [,-'pɒpjəleɪtɪd] *adj* unterbevölkert.
un·der·pop·u·la·tion [,-pɒpjə'leɪʃn] *n* Unterbevölkerung *f*.
un·der·pro·duc·tion [,-prə'dʌkʃn] *n* Unterproduktion *f*.
un·der·pro·duc·tiv·i·ty [,-prəʊdʌk'tɪvəti] *n* → underproduction.
un·der·rate [,-'reɪt] *vt* unterschätzen, unterbewerten.
un·der·re·fer·ral [,-rɪ'fɜrəl] *n* zu seltene Patientenüberweisung.
un·der·sam·ple [,-'sæmpl, -'sɑːm-] *n stat.* Unterstichprobe *f*.
un·der·sam·pling [,-'sæmplɪŋ] *n stat.* Unterstichprobenentnahme *f*.
un·der·side ['-saɪd] **I** *n* Unterseite *f*. **II** *adj* auf der Unterseite.
un·der·size ['-saɪz] *adj* unterentwickelt, unter Normalgröße *f*, zu klein.
un·der·sized ['-saɪzd] *adj* → undersize.
un·der·stand [,-'stænd] **I** *vt* **1.** verstehen, begreifen, auffassen. **2.** wissen, s. verstehen auf. **3.** erfahren, hören; entnehmen *od.* schließen (*from* aus). **II** *vi* verstehen, Verstand haben; Bescheid wissen (*about* über).
un·der·stand·ing [,-'stændɪŋ] **I** *n* **1.** Verstehen *nt*, Begreifen *nt*. **2.** Verstand *m*, Intelligenz *f*. **3.** Verständnis *nt* (*of für*). **II** *adj* **4.** verständnisvoll. **5.** verständig, gescheit.
un·der·sur·face ['-sɜrfɪs] *n* Unterseite *f*, -fläche *f*.
un·der·take [,-'teɪk] *vt* etw. übernehmen, auf s. nehmen, etw. unternehmen; (*Untersuchung, Verfahren, Forschung, Studie*) durch-, ausführen.
un·der·tak·er ['-teɪkər] *n* **1.** Leichenbestatter *m*. **2.** Bestattungs-, Beerdigungsinstitut *nt*.
un·der·time [,-'taɪm] *vt phys., radiol.* unterbelichten.
un·der·val·ue [,-'vælju:] *vt* unterschätzen, unterbewerten, zu gering ansetzen.
un·der·ven·ti·la·tion [,-ventə'leɪʃn] *n* alveoläre Minderbelüftung *f*, Mangel-, Minderventilation *f*, Hypoventilation *f*.
under way im Werden (begriffen), im Gange sein.
un·der·weight ['-weɪt] **I** *n* Untergewicht *nt*. **II** *adj* untergewichtig.
Underwood ['ʌndərwʊd]: **U.'s disease** Underwood'-Krankheit *f*, Sklerem(a) *nt*, Fettdarre *f*, Fettsklerem *nt* der Neugeborenen, Sclerema adiposum neonatorum.
un·des·cend·ed testicle [,ʌndɪ'sendɪd] Hodenretention *f*, Kryptorchismus *m*, Retentio/Maldescensus testis.
undescended testis → undescended testicle.
un·de·sir·a·ble [,ʌndɪ'zaɪərəbl] *adj* unerwünscht, nicht wünschenswert.
undesirable effects unerwünschte Wirkungen/Folgen/Konsequenzen *pl*.
un·de·tect·ed [,ʌndɪ'tektɪd] *adj* unentdeckt.
un·de·ter·mined [,ʌndɪ'tɜrmɪnd] *adj* **1.** unbestimmt, ungewiß, vage. **2.** unentschlossen, unschlüssig; unentscheiden.
un·de·vel·oped [,ʌndɪ'veləpt] *adj* unentwickelt, schlecht entwickelt, nicht ausgebildet.
un·di·ag·nosed [ʌn'daɪəgnəʊzd] *adj* unerkannt, nicht diagnostiziert.
un·dif·fer·en·ti·at·ed [ʌn'dɪfə'renʃieɪtɪd] *adj* undifferenziert, gleichartig, homogen; *patho.* entdifferenziert.
undifferentiated carcinoma entdifferenziertes Karzinom *nt*.
undifferentiated cell leukemia Stammzellenleukämie *f*, akute undifferenzierte Leukämie *f abbr.* AUL.
un·dif·fer·en·ti·a·tion [ʌn,dɪfə,renʃi'eɪʃn] *n patho.* Entdifferenzierung *f*.
un·di·gest·ed [,ʌndaɪ'dʒestɪd, -dɪ-] *adj* unverdaut.
un·di·gest·i·ble [,ʌndaɪ'dʒestɪbl, -dɪ-] *adj* unverdaulich.
un·di·lut·ed [,ʌndaɪ'luːtɪd, -dɪ-] *adj* unverdünnt; rein, pur.
un·dine [ʌn'diːn, 'ʌndaɪn] *n* Spülgefäß *nt*, -gläschen *nt*, Undine *f*.
un·dis·placed fracture [,ʌndɪs'pleɪst] nicht-dislozierte Fraktur *f*.
un·dis·solved [,ʌndɪ'zɑlvd] *adj chem.* nicht (auf-)gelöst, ungelöst.
un·drink·a·ble [ʌn'drɪŋkəbl] *adj* nicht trinkbar.
Undritz ['ʌndrɪts]: **U.'s anomaly** *hema.* Undritz-Anomalie *f*.
un·due [ʌn'd(j)uː] *adj* übertrieben, übermäßig.
un·du·lant ['ʌndʒələnt, 'ʌnd(j)ə-] *adj* → undulating.
undulant fever 1. undulierendes Fieber *nt*, Febris undulans. **2.** Brucellose *f*, Brucellosis *f*, Bruzellose *f*.
un·du·late [*adj* 'ʌndʒəlɪt, 'ʌnd(j)ə-, -leɪt; -leɪt] **I** *adj* → undulating 1. **II** *vi* in wellenförmige Bewegung versetzen. **III** *vi* s. wellenförmig bewegen, wellenförmig verlaufen, Wellen erzeugen *od.* werfen.
un·du·lat·ed ['ʌndʒəleɪtɪd, 'ʌnd(j)ə-] *adj* → undulating 1.
un·du·lat·ing ['-leɪtɪŋ] *adj* **1.** wellig, wellenförmig, gewellt, Wellen-. **2.** wellenförmig (verlaufend), undulierend; wallend, wogend.
undulating membrane *bio., micro.* undulierende Membran *f*.
undulating pulse undulierender Puls *m*, Pulsus undulosus.
un·du·la·tion [,-'leɪʃn] *n phys.* Wellengang *m*, -bewegung *f*, -linie *f*, Schwingung(sbewegung *f*) *f*, Undulation *f*.
un·du·la·to·ry ['ʌndʒələtɔːri:, -təʊ-] *adj* → undulating.
undulatory nystagmus Pendelnystagmus *m*.
undulatory theory *phys.* Wellentheorie *f*.
un·eas·i·ness [ʌn'iːzɪnɪs] *n* **1.** Unbehagen *nt*. **2.** innere Unruhe *f*.
un·eas·y [ʌn'iːzi] *adj* unbehaglich, unruhig, besorgt; ruhelos.
un·em·ploy·a·ble [,ʌnem'plɔɪəbl] **I** *n* Arbeitsunfähige(r *m*) *f*. **II** *adj* **1.** arbeitsun-

fähig, nicht beschäftigungsfähig. **2.** unbrauchbar, nicht verwendbar.
un·en·dur·a·ble [ˌʌnen'd(j)ʊərəbl] *adj* unerträglich.
un·e·qual [ʌn'iːkwəl] *adj* **1.** ungleich, unterschiedlich (groß; ungleichförmig. **2.** *mathe.* ungerade. **3.** *bio., histol.* inäqual.
unequal cleavage *bio.* inäquale Furchung(steilung *f*) *f*.
unequal pulse Pulsus inaequalis.
un·e·quiv·o·cal [ˌʌni'kwivəkl] *adj* eindeutig, unmißverständlich.
un·es·ter·i·fied [ʌne'sterəfaid] *adj chem.* unverestert.
un·even [ʌn'iːvən] *adj* **1.** nicht glatt, uneben, höckerig. **2.** *mathe.* ungerade. **3.** *fig.* unausgeglichen. **4.** ungleich, ungleichartig.
un·e·vent·ful [ˌʌni'ventfəl] *adj* ruhig, ereignislos, ohne Zwischenfall.
un·ex·pect·ed [ˌʌnik'spektid] *adj* unerwartet, unvorhergesehen.
un·ex·pired [ˌʌnik'spaiərd] *adj* noch nicht abgelaufen.
un·ex·plained [ˌʌnik'spleind] *adj* unerklärt.
un·fed [ʌn'fed] *adj* ohne Nahrung.
un·fer·tile [ʌn'fɜːtl, -tail] *adj* unfruchtbar, infertil.
unfit [ʌn'fit] *adj* **1.** untauglich, unfähig (*for* zu). ~ **for life** lebensuntüchtig. **2.** unpassend, nicht geeignet.
un·fit·ness [ʌn'fitnis] *n* Untauglichkeit *f*.
un·fit·ted [ʌn'fitid] *adj* untauglich; nicht geeignet.
un·formed [ʌn'fɔːmd] *adj* **1.** formlos, ungeformt; amorph. **2.** noch nicht fertig, unfertig.
un·fruit·ful [ʌn'fruːtfəl] *adj* **1.** *fig.* ergebnislos; enttäuschend. **2.** unfruchtbar.
ung *abbr.* [unguentum] = unguent.
un·gual ['ʌŋgwəl] *adj* Nagel betr., Nagel-.
ungual tuberosity Tuberositas phalangis distalis.
un·guent ['ʌŋgwənt] *n pharm.* Salbe *f*, Unguentum *nt abbr.* Ungt, Ung.
un·guen·tum [ʌŋ'gwentəm] *n, pl* **-ta** [-tə] *abbr.* **ung** → unguent.
un·guic·u·lar tuberosity [ˌʌŋ'gwikjələr] → ungual tuberosity.
un·guic·u·lus [ˌʌŋ'gwikjələs] *n* kleiner Nagel *m*, Unguiculus *m*.
un·guis ['ʌŋgwis] *n, pl* **-gues** [-gwiːz] *anat.* Nagel *m*, Unguis *m*.
un·gu·late ['ʌŋgjəlit, -leit] *n zoo.* Huftier *nt*, Ungulat *m*.
un·hair [ʌn'heər] *vt* enthaaren.
un·harmed [ʌn'hɑːmd] *adj* heil, unversehrt.
un·health·i·ness [ʌn'helθinis] *n* Ungesundheit *f*.
un·healthy [ʌn'helθi] *adj* **1.** ungesund, kränkelnd; krankhaft. **2.** ungesund, gesundheitsschädlich.
un·helped [ʌn'helpt] *adj* ohne Hilfe (*by* von).
uni- *pref.* Ein-, Uni-, Mon(o)-.
u·ni·ar·tic·u·lar [ˌjuːnɑːr'tikjələr] *adj* nur ein Gelenk betr., mon(o)artikulär.
u·ni·au·ral [ˌ-'ɔːrəl] *adj* nur mit einem Ohr, mon(o)aural.
u·ni·ax·i·al [ˌ-'æksiəl] *adj* einachsig.
uniaxial joint einachsiges/uniaxiales Gelenk *nt*.
u·ni·cam·er·al [ˌ-'kæm(ə)rəl] *adj* einkammrig, unikameral.
unicameral cyst einkammrige/unikamerale/unilokuläre Zyste *f*.
u·ni·cam·er·ate [ˌ-'kæmərit] *adj* → unicameral.
u·ni·cel·lu·lar [ˌ-'seljələr] *adj* einzellig, unizellulär, -zellular.

u·ni·cen·tral [ˌ-'sentrəl] *adj* monozentral, -zentrisch, unizentral, -zentrisch.
u·ni·cen·tric [ˌ-'sentrik] *adj* → unicentral.
u·ni·col·ored [ˌ-'kʌlərd] *adj* einfarbig, uni.
u·ni·con·dy·lar fracture [ˌ-'kɑndilər] monokondyläre Fraktur *f*.
u. of the femur monokondyläre Femurfraktur.
u·ni·corn uterus ['-'kɔːrn] Uterus unicornis.
u·ni·di·men·sion·al [ˌ-di'menʃnl, -dai-] *adj* eindimensional.
u·ni·di·rec·tion·al [ˌ-di'rekʃnl, -dai-] *adj* nur in eine Richtung, unidirektional.
unidirectional replication *genet., biochem.* unidirektionale Replikation *f*.
u·ni·flag·el·late [ˌ-'flædʒəlit, -leit] *adj* eingeißelig; monotrich.
u·ni·fo·cal [ˌ-'foʊkl] *adj* einen Fokus betr., von einem Herd ausgehend, unifokal.
u·ni·form ['-fɔːrm] *adj* **1.** gleichförmig, uniform; gleichbleibend, konstant. **2.** einheitlich, uniform, Einheits-. **3.** eintönig, -förmig.
u·ni·form·i·ty [ˌ-'fɔːrməti] *n* **1.** Gleichförmigkeit *f*, Uniformität *f*; Konstanz *f*. **2.** Einheitlichkeit *f*, Uniformität *f*. **3.** Eintönigkeit *f*, -förmigkeit *f*.
u·ni·gem·i·nal [ˌ-'dʒeminl] *adj* nur einen Zwilling betr.
u·ni·ger·mi·nal [ˌ-'dʒɜːrminl] *adj* **1.** einkeimig. **2.** monozygot.
u·ni·glan·du·lar [ˌ-'glændʒələr] *adj* nur eine Drüse betr., monoglandulär.
u·ni·grav·i·da [ˌ-'grævidə] *n gyn.* Primigravida *f*.
u·ni·lam·i·nar follicle [ˌ-'læminər] Primordialfollikel *m*, früher Primärfollikel *m*.
u·ni·lat·er·al [ˌ-'lætərəl] *adj* nur eine Seite betr., ein-, halbseitig, unilateral.
unilateral anesthesia *neuro.* Hemianästhesie *f*, Hemianaesthesia *f*.
unilateral deafness einseitige Schwerhörigkeit *f*.
unilateral gigantism Halbseitenriesenwuchs *m*.
unilateral gliosis unilaterale/hemisphärische Gliose *f*.
unilateral hemianopia/hemianopsia *ophthal.* einseitige/unilaterale Hemianop(s)ie *f*.
unilateral hermaphroditism Hermaphroditismus (verus) unilateralis.
unilateral hypertrophy einseitige Hypertrophie *f*.
unilateral nystagmus einseitiger/unilateraler Nystagmus *m*.
unilateral strabismus *ophthal.* einseitiges/unilaterales Schielen *nt*, Strabismus unilateralis.
u·ni·lo·bar [ˌ-'loʊbər] *adj* aus einem Lappen bestehend, unilobar.
u·ni·lob·u·lar cirrhosis [ˌ-'lɑbjələr] primär biliäre Zirrhose *f abbr.* PBZ, nicht-eitrige destruierende Cholangitis *f*.
u·ni·loc·u·lar [ˌ-'lɑkjələr] *adj* unilokulär; einkammrig, unikameral.
unilocular cyst → unicameral cyst.
unilocular cystoma unilokuläres Kystom/Zystom *nt*.
un·im·ag·i·na·tive [ˌʌni'mædʒnətiv, -nei-] *adj* phantasielos.
un·i·mod·al [ˌʌːni'moʊdl] *adj* unimodal, *stat.* eingipfelig.
un·im·paired [ˌʌnim'peərd] *adj* **1.** unvermindert, unbeeinträchtigt. **2.** unbeschädigt, intakt, nicht befallen.
un·in·flu·enced [ʌn'ɪnfluːənst] *adj* unbeeinflußt (*by* durch, von).
un·in·hib·it·ed [ˌʌnin'hibitid] *adj* ungehemmt, frei.

un·in·jured [ʌn'indʒərd] *adj* unverletzt, unverwundet.
un·in·tel·li·gent [ˌʌnin'telidʒənt] *adj* nicht intelligent, beschränkt; *inf.* dumm.
un·in·tel·li·gi·bil·i·ty [ˌʌninˌtelidʒə'biləti] *n* Unverständlichkeit *f*.
un·in·tel·li·gi·ble [ˌʌnin'telidʒəbl] *adj* unverständlich (*to* für).
un·in·tend·ed [ˌʌnin'tendid] *adj* unbeabsichtigt, unabsichtlich.
un·in·ten·tion·al [ˌʌnin'tenʃnl] *adj* → unintended.
un·in·ter·rupt·ed suture [ˌʌnintə'rʌptid] kontinuierliche/fortlaufende Naht *f*.
u·ni·nu·cle·ar [ˌ-'n(j)uːkliər] *adj* einkernig, mononukleär.
u·ni·nu·cle·at·ed [ˌ-'n(j)uːkliːeitid] *adj* → uninuclear.
u·ni·oc·u·lar [ˌ-'ɑkjələr] *adj* nur ein Auge betr., uni-, monokulär.
uniocular hemianopia/hemianopsia *ophthal.* → unilateral hemianopia.
uniocular strabismus → unilateral strabismus.
un·ion ['juːnjən] *n* **1.** Vereinigung *f*, Verbindung *f*, Verschmelzung *f*, Verfestigung *f*. **2.** *patho., ortho.* (Ver-)Heilung *f*.
u·ni·o·val [ˌjuːni'oʊvl] *adj* → uniovular.
u·ni·ov·u·lar [ˌ-'ɑvjələr, -'oʊv-] *adj* monozygot, monovulär.
uniovular twins erbgleiche/eineiige/identische/monozygote/monovuläre Zwillinge *pl*.
u·nip·a·ra [juːˈnɪpərə] *n, pl* **-ras, -rae** [-riː] Erstgebärende *f*, Primipara *f*.
u·ni·pa·ren·tal [ˌjuːnipə'rentl] *adj* nur einen Elternteil betr.
u·nip·a·rous [juːˈnɪpərəs] *adj* erstgebärend.
u·ni·pen·nate muscle [ˌ-'peneit] einseitig gefiederter Muskel *m*, M. unipennatus.
u·ni·po·lar [ˌ-'poʊlər] *adj* einpolig, unipolar, Einpol-, Unipolar-; monopolar.
unipolar cell → unipolar neuron.
unipolar lead *physiol.* (*EKG*) unipolare Ableitung *f*.
unipolar neuron unipolares Neuron *nt*, unipolare Nervenzelle *f*.
unipolar recording → unipolar lead.
u·ni·port ['-pɔːrt] *n physiol.* Uniport *m*, Uniportsystem *nt*.
uniport system → uniport.
u·ni·po·ten·cy [ˌ-'poʊtənsi] *n* Unipotenz *f*.
u·nip·o·tent [juːˈnɪpətənt] *adj* → unipotential.
u·ni·po·ten·tial [ˌjuːnipə'tenʃl] *adj* unipotent.
u·nique [juːˈniːk] *adj* **1.** außergewöhnlich. **2.** einzig; einmalig.
un·ir·ri·ta·ble [ʌn'iritəbl] *adj* nicht erregbar, nicht reizbar.
un·i·sex·u·al [juːni'sekʃwəl; -'seksjʊəl] *adj* **1.** eingeschlechtig, unisexuell. **2.** getrenntgeschlechtlich.
u·nit ['juːnit] *n* **1.** Einheit *f*; *phys., biochem.* (Grund-, Maß-)Einheit *f*. **2.** *pharm.* Einheit *f*, Dosis *f*, Menge *f*. **3.** *techn.* (Bau-)Einheit *f*; Anlage *f*, Gerät *nt*. **4.** *mathe.* Einer *m*, Einheit *f*. **5.** (*Krankenhaus*) Station *f*, Abteilung *f*.
u. of force Krafteinheit.
u. of heat Wärmeeinheit.
u. of measure Maßeinheit.
u. of power Leistungseinheit.
u. of time Zeiteinheit.
unit area Flächeneinheit *f*.
u·ni·tar·y ['juːnitəri] *adj* **1.** Einheit betr., Einheits-. **2.** einheitlich.
unitary weight Gewichtseinheit *f*.
u·nite [juːˈnait] **I** *vt* (*a. chem., techn.*) verbinden, vereinigen. **II** *vi* **1.** (*a. chem., techn.*) verbinden (*to, with* mit); s. vereini-

unit force

gen. 2. (*Wundränder*) zusammenwachsen; (*Zellen*) verschmelzen.
unit force Krafteinheit *f*.
u·nit·ing cartilage [juːˈnaɪtɪŋ] *anat*. Zwischenknorpel *m* von fibrösen Verbindungen *od*. Symphysen.
unit membrane Einheits-, Elementarmembran *f*.
unit-membrane hypothesis Einheitsmembranhypothese *f*, Unit-membrane-Hypothese *f*.
unit time Zeiteinheit *f*.
unit volume Volumeneinheit *f*.
u·ni·vac·u·o·lar [juːnɪˌvækjuːˈəʊlər, -ˈvækjuːə-, -ˈvækjələr] *adj histol*. einkammerig, univakuolär.
u·ni·va·lence [ˌ-ˈveɪləns] *n* Einwertigkeit *f*, Univalenz *f*.
u·ni·va·lent [ˌ-ˈveɪlənt, juːˈnɪvə-] *adj* einwertig, uni-, monovalent.
univalent antibody univalenter/hemmender Antikörper *m*.
u·ni·ver·sal [juːnəˈvɜːrsl] **I** *n* das Allgemeine. **II** *adj* **1.** universal, global, allumfassend, gesamt, Universal-, Gesamt-. **2.** universell, generell, allgemeingültig, General-.
universal donor *immun*. Universalspender *m*.
universal infantilism proportionierter Zwergwuchs/Minderwuchs *m*.
universal recipient *immun*. Universalempfänger *m*.
un·known [ʌnˈnəʊn] *adj* unbekannt (*to*). ~ **to the patient** ohne Wissen des Patienten.
un·law·ful [ʌnˈlɔːfəl] *adj* **1.** ungesetzlich, rechtswidrig, illegal. **2.** unerlaubt.
un·law·ful·ness [ʌnˈlɔːfəlnɪs] *n* Ungesetzlichkeit *f*, Rechtswidrigkeit *f*, Illegalität *f*.
un·leav·ened [ʌnˈlevənd] *adj* (*Brot*) ungesäuert.
unlike [unˈlaɪk] *adj* ungleich, gegensätzlich, (voneinander) verschieden, unähnlich, nicht ähnlich.
un·like·ly [ʌnˈlaɪklɪ] *adj* unwahrscheinlich; unmöglich.
unlike twins erbungleiche/dizygote/dissimiläre/heteroovuläre/binovuläre/zweieiige Zwillinge *pl*.
un·lim·it·ed [ʌnˈlɪmɪtɪd] *adj* unbegrenzt, unbeschränkt.
un·lined [ʌnˈlaɪnd] *adj* ungefüttert; *anat*. nicht mit einem Überzug versehen.
un·man·age·a·ble [ʌnˈmænɪdʒəbl] *adj* **1.** (*Patient*) schwierig, schwer zu führen. **2.** unkontrollierbar. **3.** unhandlich.
un·med·ul·lat·ed [ʌnˈmedʒəletɪd, -ˈmedl-] *adj* → unmyelinated.
un·mixed [ʌnˈmɪkst] *adj* unvermischt, rein, pur.
un·mod·i·fied [ʌnˈmɒdəfaɪd] *adj* unverändert, nicht geändert.
unmodified scattering *phys*. klassische Streuung *f*, Thomson-Streuung *f*.
un·move·a·ble [ʌnˈmuːvəbl] *adj* unbeweglich; (*Gelenk*) steif, versteift.
un·my·e·li·nat·ed [ʌnˈmaɪəlɪˌneɪtɪd] *adj histol*. mark(scheiden)los, -frei, myelinfrei.
unmyelinated axon markloses Axon *nt*.
unmyelinated fiber → unmyelinated nerve.
unmyelinated nerve marklose/myelinfreie Nervenfaser *f*.
Unna [ˈʊnə]: **U.'s boot** Unna-Pastenschuh *m*.
U.'s disease Unna'-Krankheit *f*, seborrhoisches Ekzem *nt*, seborrhoische/dysseborrhoische Dermatitis *f*, Morbus Unna *m*, Dermatitis seborrhoides.
U.'s nevus Unna-Politzer-Nackennävus *m*, Storchenbiß *m*, Nävus Unna *m*.
U.'s paste boot → U.'s boot.

Unna-Thost [tɒst]: **U.-T. disease/syndrome** Morbus Unna-Thost *m*, Keratosis palmoplantaris diffusa circumscripta, Keratoma palmare et plantare hereditaria, Ichthyosis palmaris et plantaris (Thost).
un·nat·u·ral [ʌnˈnætʃ(ə)rəl] *adj* **1.** unnatürlich; krankhaft; anomal, abnorm. **2.** widernatürlich; ungeheuerlich, abscheulich.
unnatural drowsiness krankhafte Schläfrigkeit *f*, Benommenheit *f*, Somnolenz *f*.
un·ob·tain·a·ble [ˌʌnəbˈteɪnəbl] *adj* nicht erhältlich.
un·of·fi·cial [ˌʌnəˈfɪʃəl] *adj* nicht offiziell, inoffiziell.
un·or·gan·ized [ʌnˈɔːrgənaɪzd] *adj* **1.** ohne eigentliche Organe. **2.** unorganisiert; strukturlos. **3.** *bio*. nicht von organischen Lebewesen abstammend, unorganisch, anorganisch.
un·paired [ʌnˈpeərd] *adj anat*., *bio*. unpaar, nicht paar; ungepaart, unpaarig, ungerade, in ungerader Zahl vorhanden.
unpaired allosome → unpaired chromosome.
unpaired chromosome *genet*. einzelnes Chromosom *nt* bei Monosomie, Monosom *nt*.
unpaired ganglion letztes/unteres Grenzstrangganglion *nt*, Ggl. impar.
un·pal·at·a·ble [ʌnˈpælətəbl] *adj* ungenießbar.
un·par·ent·ed [ʌnˈpeərəntɪd] *adj* elternlos; verwaist.
un·pas·teur·ized [ʌnˈpæstʃəraɪzd] *adj* nicht pasteurisiert.
un·phys·i·o·log·ic [ʌnˌfɪzɪəˈlɒdʒɪk] *adj* nicht physiologisch, unphysiologisch.
un·pleas·ant [ʌnˈplezənt] *adj* **1.** unangenehm. **2.** (*Atem*) schlecht; (*Geruch*) widerlich.
un·pro·duc·tive [ˌʌnprəˈdʌktɪv] *adj* unproduktiv.
un·pro·duc·tiv·i·ty [ʌnˌprɒdʌkˈtɪvətɪ] *n* Unproduktivität *f*.
un·pro·fes·sion·al [ˌʌnprəˈfeʃənl] *adj* **1.** unfachmännisch. **2.** standeswidrig.
un·pro·tect·ed [ˌʌnprəˈtektɪd] *adj* ungeschützt.
un·pro·voked [ˌʌnprəˈvəʊkt] *adj* **1.** nicht provoziert. **2.** nicht gereizt, durch keinen Reiz hervorgerufen. **3.** grundlos.
un·real [ʌnˈrɪəl] *adj* unwirklich, irreal.
un·re·cep·tive [ˌʌnrɪˈseptɪv] *adj* unempfänglich (für); nicht aufnahmefähig.
un·re·fined [ʌnrɪˈfaɪnd] *adj* nicht raffiniert, roh, Roh-; ungereinigt.
unrefined sugar Rohzucker *m*.
un·re·li·a·bil·i·ty [ˌʌnrɪˌlaɪəˈbɪlətɪ] *n* Unzuverlässigkeit *f*.
un·re·li·a·ble [ˌʌnrɪˈlaɪəbl] *adj* unzuverlässig.
un·re·lieved [ˌʌnrɪˈliːvd] *adj* ungemildert, nicht gemildert; (*Schmerz*) nicht nachlassend, gleichbleibend, unvermindert; (*Erbrechen*) unstillbar.
un·re·mark·a·ble [ˌʌnrɪˈmɑːrkəbl] *adj* unauffällig.
un·re·sect·a·ble tumor [ˌʌnrɪˈsektəbl] nicht-reserzierbarer Tumor *m*.
un·re·solved [ˌʌnrɪˈzɒlvd] *adj* (*Problem*) ungelöst; *chem*. unaufgelöst.
un·re·spon·sive [ˌʌnrɪˈspɒnsɪv] *adj* **1.** unempfänglich (*to* für); nicht ansprechend *od*. reagierend (*to* auf). ~ **to treatment.** **2.** teilnahmslos.
un·rest [ʌnˈrest] *n* (innere) Unruhe *f*, Nervosität *f*; Ruhelosigkeit *f*.
un·rest·ful [ʌnˈrestfəl] *adj* unruhig, ruhelos; nervös, zappelig.
un·re·strained [ˌʌnrɪˈstreɪnd] *adj* **1.** hem-

mungslos. **2.** uneingeschränkt; ungehemmt.
un·re·strict·ed [ˌʌnrɪˈstrɪktɪd] *adj* uneingeschränkt, unbeschränkt.
un·re·ward·ing [ˌʌnrɪˈwɔːrdɪŋ] *adj* frucht-, ergebnislos, enttäuschend.
un·ripe [ʌnˈraɪp] *adj* unreif.
un·ripe·ness [ʌnˈraɪpnɪs] *n* Unreife *f*.
un·safe [ʌnˈseɪf] *adj* unsicher, gefährlich.
un·safe·ness [ʌnˈseɪfnɪs] *n* → unsafety.
un·safe·ty [ʌnˈseɪftɪ] *n* Unsicherheit *f*, Gefährlichkeit *f*.
un·salt·ed [ʌnˈsɔːltɪd] *adj* ungesalzen.
un·sat·is·fac·to·ry [ʌnˌsætɪsˈfæktə(ə)rɪ] *adj* unbefriedigend, nicht zufriedenstellend; (*Mittel*) unwirksam; (*Leistung*) unzureichend.
un·sat·u·rat·ed [ʌnˈsætʃəreɪtɪd] *adj chem*., *biochem*. ungesättigt.
unsaturated bond *chem*. ungesättigte Bindung *f*.
unsaturated compound *chem*. ungesättigte Verbindung *f*.
unsaturated fat *chem*. Fett *nt* mit ungesättigten Fettsäuren.
unsaturated hydrocarbon *chem*. ungesättigter Kohlenwasserstoff *m*.
unsaturated lipid *chem*. Lipid *nt* mit ungesättigten Fettsäuren.
un·sleep·ing [ʌnˈsliːpɪŋ] *adj* schlaflos.
un·so·cia·bil·i·ty [ʌnˌsəʊʃəˈbɪlətɪ] *n* Ungeselligkeit *f*, Menschenscheu *f*.
un·so·cia·ble [ʌnˈsəʊʃəbl] *adj* ungesellig, menschenscheu, einzelgängerisch.
un·solv·a·ble [ʌnˈsɒlvəbl] *adj chem*. unauflöslich.
un·solved [ʌnˈsɒlvd] *adj* ungelöst.
un·sound [ʌnˈsaʊnd] *adj* **1.** ungesund; (*Essen*) schlecht, verdorben. **2.** ~ **of mind** unzurechnungsfähig, geisteskrank.
un·sound·ness [ʌnˈsaʊndnɪs] *n* Ungesundsein *nt*, Ungesundheit *f*; Verdorbenheit *f*.
un·spe·cif·ic [ˌʌnspɪˈsɪfɪk] *adj* unspezifisch, nicht spezifisch.
unspecific cholinesterase unspezifische/ unechte Cholinesterase *f abbr*. ChE, Pseudocholinesterase *f*, Typ II-Cholinesterase *f*, β-Cholinesterase *f*, Butyrylcholinesterase *f*.
unspecific monooxygenase Aryl-4-hydroxylase *f*, unspezifische Monooxygenase *f*.
un·sta·ble [ʌnˈsteɪbl] *adj* **1.** *chem*. instabil. **2.** schwankend, wechselnd; (*Person*) unbeständig. **3.** nicht stabil, nicht fest.
unstable colloid *chem*. instabiles/irreversibles Kolloid *nt*.
unstable fracture instabile Fraktur *f*.
un·stained [ʌnˈsteɪnd] *adj* ungefärbt.
un·stead·i·ness [ʌnˈstedɪnɪs] *n* Unsicherheit *f*, Wackeligkeit *f*, Schwanken *nt*, Unstetigkeit *f*; Unregelmäßigkeit *f*.
un·stead·y [ʌnˈstedɪ] *adj* unsicher, wackelig, schwankend, unstet, unregelmäßig.
un·strained [ʌnˈstreɪnd] *adj chem*. ungefiltert, unfiltriert.
un·stri·at·ed [ʌnˈstraɪeɪtɪd] *adj histol*. nicht gestreift.
un·suc·cess [ˌʌnsəkˈses] *n* Mißerfolg *m*, Fehlschlag *m*.
un·suc·cess·ful [ˌʌnsəkˈsesfəl] *adj* erfolg-, ergebnislos, ohne Erfolg; mißlungen.
un·suc·cess·ful·ness [ˌʌnsəkˈsesfəlnɪs] *n* Erfolglosigkeit *f*.
un·sweet·ened [ʌnˈswiːtnd] *adj* ohne Zucker, ungesüßt.
un·sym·met·ri·cal [ˌʌnsɪˈmetrɪkl] *adj* unsymmetrisch, nicht symmetrisch.
un·taint·ed [ʌnˈteɪntɪd] *adj* (*Nahrung*) unverdorben, frisch.
un·test·ed [ʌnˈtestɪd] *adj* unerprobt, ungetestet, ungeprüft.

un·to·ward [ʌn'tɔːrd, -'təʊrd] *adj* (*Ereignis*) unglücklich, bedauerlich; (*Vorzeichen*) schlecht; unerwünscht; unpassend.
untoward effect (*Therapie, Medikament*) Nebenwirkung *f abbr.* NW.
un·treat·a·ble [ʌn'triːtəbl] *adj* nicht behandelbar, unheilbar.
un·treat·ed [ʌn'triːtɪd] *adj* unbehandelt.
Unverricht ['ʊnferɪçt]: **U.'s disease/syndrome** Lafora-Syndrom *nt*, Unverricht-Syndrom *nt*, Myoklonusepilepsie *f*, myoklonische Epilepsie *f*.
un·want·ed [ʌn'wɒntɪd] *adj* unerwünscht; (*Kind*) ungewollt.
un·well [ʌn'wel] *adj* **to be/feel ~ 1.** s. unwohl/unpäßlich fühlen. **2.** menstruierend.
un·wet·ta·ble surface [ʌn'wetəbl] *phys.* nicht-benetzbare Oberfläche *f*.
un·whole·some [ʌn'həʊlsəm] *adj* ungesund.
un·wind [ʌn'waɪnd] **I** *vt* ab-, loswickeln, entwirren; (*Verband*) aufwickeln. **II** *vi* **1.** s. ab- *od.* loswickeln. **2.** *inf.* s. entspannen, abschalten.
un·wise [ʌn'waɪz] *adj* unklug, töricht.
un·wound·ed [ʌn'wuːndɪd] *adj* unverletzt, unverwundet.
up·most ['ʌpməʊst] *adj* → uppermost.
up·per ['ʌpər] **I** *n dent.* Oberzahn *m*; ~s *pl* obere (Zahn-)Prothese *f*. **II** *adj* obere(r, s), höhere(r, s), Ober-; höherliegend, -stehend, -gelegen.
upper airways obere Luftwege *pl*.
upper arm Oberarm *m*.
upper arm stub *embryo.* Oberarmstumpf *m*.
upper arm type of brachial palsy/paralysis obere Armplexuslähmung *f*, Erb--Lähmung *f*, Erb-Duchenne-Lähmung *f*.
upper brain Großhirn *m*.
upper extremity Arm *m*, obere Extremität *m*, Membrum superius.
u. of kidney oberer Nierenpol *m*, Extremitas superior renis.
upper eye lid Oberlid *nt*, oberes Augenlid *nt*, Palpebra superior.
upper ganglion Müller'-Ganglion *nt*, Ehrenritter'-Ganglion *nt*, oberes Glossopharyngeusganglion *nt*, Ggl. rostralis/superius n. glossopharyngei.
upper jaw Oberkiefer(knochen *m*) *m*, Maxilla *f*.
upper jawbone → upper jaw.
upper jaw component of intermaxillary segment *embryo.* Oberkieferanteil *m* des Zwischenkiefersegments.
upper leg Oberschenkel *m*.
upper limbs obere Gliedmaßen/Extremitäten *pl*, Arme *pl*.
upper lip Oberlippe *f*, Labium superius oris.
up·per·most ['ʌpərməʊst] *adj* höchste(r, s), größte(r, s), oberste(r, s).
upper palpebra Oberlid *nt*, Palpebra superior.
upper pole: u. of kidney oberer Nierenpol *m*, Extremitas superior renis.
u. of testis oberer Hodenpol *m*, Extremitas superior testis.
upper ramus of pubis oberer Schambeinast *m*, Ramus superior ossis pubis.
upper respiratory tract infection Infekt(ion *f*) *m* der oberen Luftwege.
upper teeth Zähne *pl od.* Zahnreihe *f* des Oberkiefers.
Upp·sa·la virus ['ʌpsələ; 'ʊpsala] Uppsala-Virus *nt*.
up·set [*n* 'ʌpset; *adj*, *v* ʌp'set] **I** *n* **1.** (Magen-)Verstimmung *f*. **2.** (leichte) Störung *f*; Ärger *m*, Verstimmung *f*; Verwirrung *f*; Unordnung *f*. **II** *adj* **3.** (*Magen*) verstimmt. **4.** bestürzt, betrübt, verletzt, gekränkt (*about* über); aufgeregt (*about* wegen); mitgenommen; (*Kind*) durcheinander. **III** *vt* **5.** (*Magen*) verstimmen. **6.** erschüttern, bestürzen, mitnehmen, aus der Fassung bringen; verletzen, weh tun; ärgern. **7.** durcheinanderbringen, stören.
up·stroke ['ʌpstrəʊk] *n physiol.* Aufstrich *m*.
up·surge ['ʌpsɜːdʒ] *n* Zunahme *f*, Eskalation *f* (*in* in).
up·take ['ʌpteɪk] *n* **1.** *physiol.* Aufnahme *f*, Aufnehmen *nt*; *radiol.* Uptake *nt/f*. **2.** Auffassungsvermögen *nt*. **3.** Annahme *f*, Akzeptierung *f*, Anerkennung *f*.
up-to-date *adj* aktuell, auf dem neuesten Stand.
UR *abbr.* **1.** → ultrared I. **2.** → unconditioned reflex.
ur- *pref.* → urino-.
u·ra·chal ['jʊərəkəl] *adj* Urachus betr., Urachus-.
urachal cyst Urachuszyste *f*.
urachal fistula Urachusfistel *f*.
urachal sinus Urachussinus *m*.
u·ra·chus ['jʊərəkəs] *n embryo.* Harngang *m*, Urachus *m*.
u·ra·cil ['jʊərəsɪl] *n abbr.* **U** Uracil *nt abbr.* U.
u·ra·gogue ['jʊərəgɒg, -gəg] *n*, *adj old* → diuretic.
u·ra·mi·no·a·cet·ic acid [jʊərə‚miːnəʊ-ə'setɪk, -‚siːtɪk] Hydantoinsäure *f*, Uraminessigsäure *f*.
uran- *pref.* → urano-.
uranisc(o)- *pref.* → urano-.
u·ra·nis·co·chasm [jʊərə'nɪskəkæzəm] *n* → uranoschisis.
u·ra·nis·co·chas·ma [-‚kæzmə] *n* → uranoschisis.
u·ra·nis·co·la·lia [-‚leɪlɪə] *n HNO* Sprachfehler *m* bei Gaumenspalte.
u·ra·nis·co·ni·tis [-‚naɪtɪs] *n* Gaumenentzündung *f*, Uranitis *f*.
u·ra·nis·co·plas·ty ['-plæstɪ] *n* → uranoplasty.
u·ra·nis·cor·rha·phy [‚jʊərənɪs'kɒrəfɪ] *n HNO* Gaumennaht *f*, Urano-, Staphylorrhaphie *f*.
u·ra·nis·cus [jʊərə'nɪskəs] *n* Gaumen *m*; *anat.* Palatum *nt*.
u·ra·ni·um [jʊ'reɪnɪəm] *n abbr.* **U** Uran *nt abbr.* U.
urano- *pref.* Gaumen-, Uran(o)-, Palat(o)-, Staphyl(o)-.
u·ra·no·plas·ty ['jʊərənəʊplæstɪ] *n HNO* Gaumenplastik *f*, Urano-, Staphyloplastik *f*.
u·ra·no·ple·gia [-‚pliːdʒ(ɪ)ə] *n* Gaumensegellähmung *f*.
u·ra·nor·rha·phy [‚jʊərə'nɔːrəfɪ] *n HNO* Gaumennaht *f*, Urano-, Staphylorrhaphie *f*.
u·ra·nos·chi·sis [-'nɒkəsɪs] *n embryo., HNO* Gaumenspalte *f*, Uranoschisis *f*, Palatoschisis *f*, Palatum fissum.
u·ran·o·schism [jʊə'rænəskɪzəm] *n* → uranoschisis.
u·ra·no·staph·y·lo·plas·ty [‚jʊərənəʊ‚stæf-ɪləʊplæstɪ] *n HNO* Uranostaphyloplastik *f*.
u·ra·no·staph·y·lor·rha·phy [-‚stæfɪ'lɒrəfɪ] *n* → uranostaphyloplasty.
u·ra·no·staph·y·los·chi·sis [-‚stæfɪ'lɒskə-sɪs] *n* Uranostaphyloschisis *f*.
u·ra·no·ve·los·chi·sis [-‚vɪ'lɒskəsɪs] *n* → uranostaphyloschisis.
u·ra·nyl ['jʊərnɪl] *n* Uranyl-(Rest *m*).
uranyl acetate Uranylacetat *nt*.
u·ar·thri·tis [‚jʊərə:r'θraɪtɪs] *n* → uratic arthritis.
u·rate ['jʊəreɪt] *n* Urat *nt*.

uremic encephalopathy

urate calculus Uratstein *m*.
urate kidney Gicht-, Uratniere *f*.
u·ra·te·mia [‚jʊərə'tiːmɪə] *n* Uratämie *f*.
urate nephropathy Gicht-, Uratnephropathie *f*.
urate oxidase Uratoxidase *f*, Urikase *f*, Uricase *f*.
urate salts Uratsalze *pl*, Urate *pl*.
urate stone → urate calculus.
urate thesaurismosis Gicht *f*.
u·rat·ic [jə'rætɪk] *adj* **1.** Urat betr., uratisch, Urat-. **2.** Gicht betr., Gicht-.
uratic arthritis Gichtarthritis *f*, Arthritis urica.
uratic conjunctivitis Conjunctivitis petrificans.
uratic iritis *ophthal.* Iritis uratica.
u·ra·to·his·tech·ia [‚jʊərətəʊhɪs'tekɪə] *n* Uratohistechie *f*.
u·ra·tol·y·sis [‚jʊərə'tɒləsɪs] *n* Uratauflösung *f*, Uratolyse *f*.
u·ra·to·lyt·ic [‚jʊərətəʊ'lɪtɪk] *adj* uratauflösend, uratolytisch.
u·ra·to·ma [‚jʊərə'təʊmə] *n* (Urat-, Gicht-)Tophus *m*.
u·ra·to·sis [-‚təʊsɪs] *n* Uratose *f*.
u·ra·tu·ria [‚-'t(j)ʊərɪə] *n* erhöhte Uratausscheidung *f* im Harn, Uraturie *f*.
Urbach-Wiethe ['ɜːrbæk-bæx 'viːtɪ]: **U.-W. disease** Urbach-Wiethe-Syndrom *nt*, Lipoidproteinose (Urbach-Wiethe) *f*, Hyalinosis cutis et mucosae.
ur·ce·i·form ['ɜːrsɪfɔːrm] *adj* urnen-, krugförmig.
ur·ce·o·late ['ɜːrsɪəlɪt] *adj* → urceiform.
ure(a)- *pref.* → ureo-.
u·rea [jʊ'riːə, 'jʊərɪə] *n* Harnstoff *m*, Karbamid *nt*, Carbamid *nt*, Urea *f*.
urea agar Harnstoffagar *m/nt* nach Christensen.
urea clearence Harnstoffclearence *f*.
urea cycle Harnstoff-, Ornithinzyklus *m*, Krebs-Henseleit-Zyklus *m*.
urea formation Harnstoffbildung *f*.
urea frost urämischer Frost *m*, Ur(h)idrosis crystallina.
u·re·a·ge·net·ic [jə‚rɪədʒɪ'netɪk] *adj* harnstoffbildend.
u·re·al [jʊ'riːəl, 'jʊərɪəl] *adj* Harnstoff-.
urea nitrogen Harnstoffstickstoff *m*.
U·re·a·plas·ma [jə'rɪəplæzmə] *n micro.* Ureaplasma *nt*.
u·re·a·poi·e·sis [jə‚rɪəpɔɪ'iːsɪs] *n* Harnstoffbildung *f*.
u·re·ase ['jʊərɪeɪz] *n* Urease *f*.
urease-negative *adj* ureasenegativ.
urease-positive *adj* ureasepositiv.
urease test Urease-Test *m*.
urea synthesis Harnstoffsynthese *f*.
u·re·ide ['jʊərɪaɪd] *n* Ureid *nt*.
β-u·re·ido·pro·pi·o·nase [jə‚riːdəʊ'prəʊ-pɪəneɪz] *n* β-Ureidopropionase *f*.
β-u·re·ido·pro·pi·on·ic acid [-‚prəʊpɪ'ɒn-ɪk, -'əʊnɪk] β-Ureidopropionsäure *f*.
u·rel·co·sis [‚jʊərel'kəʊsɪs] *n* Harnwegsgeschwür *nt*, Urelkosis *f*.
u·re·mia [jʊə'riːmɪə] *n* Harnvergiftung *f*, Urämie *f*.
u·re·mic [jə'riːmɪk] *adj* Urämie betr., durch Urämie hervorgerufen, urämisch.
uremic acidosis urämische Azidose *f*.
uremic amaurosis urämische Amaurose *f*.
uremic amblyopia urämische Amblyopie *f*.
uremic breath Foetor uraemicus.
uremic colitis urämische Kolitis *f*.
uremic coma urämisches Koma *nt*, Coma uraemicum.
uremic encephalopathy urämische Enzephalopathie *f*, Encephalopathia uraemica.

uremic fetor → uremic breath.
uremic frost → urea frost.
uremic gastritis urämische Magenschleimhautentzündung/Gastritis f.
uremic pericarditis urämische Herzbeutelentzündung/Perikarditis f, Pericarditis uraemica.
uremic pneumonia → uremic pneumonitis.
uremic pneumonitis urämische Pneumonie f, hämorrhagisch-fibrinöses Lungenödem nt bei Urämie, urämische Wasserlunge f.
uremic retinitis urämische Retinitis f.
uremic stomatitis urämische Stomatitis f.
u·re·mi·gen·ic [jʊəˌriːmɪˈdʒenɪk] adj 1. durch Urämie bedingt, urämisch. 2. eine Urämie auslösend, urämigen.
ureo- pref. Harn(stoff)-, Urea-, Ure(o)-, Uro-.
u·re·ol·y·sis [jʊərɪˈɒləsɪs] n Harnstoffspaltung f, Ureolyse f.
u·re·o·lyt·ic [jʊərəʊˈlɪtɪk] adj Ureolyse betr., harnstoffspaltend, ureolytisch.
u·re·o·tel·ic [ˌ-ˈtelɪk] adj ureotelisch.
u·re·si·es·the·sis [jəˌriːsɪesˈθiːsɪs] n Harndrang m.
u·re·sis [jəˈriːsɪs] n 1. Harnen nt, Urese f. 2. → urination.
u·re·tal [jəˈriːtl] adj → ureteric.
ureter- pref. → uretero-.
u·re·ter [ˈjʊərətər, jʊəˈriːtər] n Harnleiter m, Ureter m.
u·re·ter·al [jʊəˈriːtərəl, jə-] adj → ureteric.
ureteral branch Ureterast m, Ast m zum Harnleiter.
   u.es of artery of ductus deferens Ureteräste pl der A. ductus deferentis, Rami ureterici a. ductus deferentis.
   u.es of ovarian artery Ureteräste pl der A. ovarica, Rami ureterici a. ovaricae.
   u.es of renal artery Ureteräste pl der A. renalis, Rami ureterici a. renalis.
   u.es of testicular artery Ureteräste pl der A. testicularis, Rami ureterici a. testicularis.
ureteral colic Harnleiterkolik f.
ureteral diverticulum Harnleiter-, Ureteren-, Ureterdivertikel nt.
ureteral fistula Harnleiter-, Ureterfistel f, Fistula ureterica.
u·re·ter·al·gia [jʊˌriːtəˈrældʒ(ɪ)ə] n Harnleiterschmerz m, -neuralgie f, Ureteralgie f.
ureteral injury Harnleiter-, Ureterverletzung f.
ureteral leak Harnleiterleck nt.
ureteral obstruction Harnleiter-, Ureterobstruktion f.
ureteral reflex Harnleiter-, Ureterreflex m.
ureteral valve Harnleiter-, Ureterklappe f.
u·re·ter·ec·ta·sia [jʊˌriːtərekˈteɪʒ(ɪ)ə] n → ureterectasis.
u·re·ter·ec·ta·sis [ˌ-ˈektəsɪs] n Harnleitererweiterung f, Ureterektasie f.
u·re·ter·ec·to·my [ˌ-ˈektəmɪ] n urol. Harnleiterresektion f, Ureterektomie f.
u·re·ter·ic [jʊərəˈterɪk] adj Harnleiter/Ureter betr., ureterisch, Harnleiter-, Ureter(o)-.
ureteric branch → ureteral branch.
ureteric bud embryo. Ureterknospe f, -anlage f.
ureteric orifice Harnleiter(ein)mündung f, Ostium ureteris.
ureteric plexus Harnleitergeflecht nt, Plexus uretericus.
u·re·ter·i·tis [jʊˌriːtəˈraɪtɪs] n Harnleiterentzündung f, Ureteritis f.
uretero- pref. Harnleiter-, Ureter(o)-.

u·re·ter·o·cele [jəˈriːtərəʊsiːl] n urol. Ureterozele f.
u·re·ter·o·ce·lec·to·my [ˌ-sɪˈlektəmɪ] n urol. Resektion f einer Ureterozele.
u·re·ter·o·cer·vi·cal [ˌ-ˈsɜrvɪkl] adj Harnleiter/Ureter u. Zervix betr., ureterozervikal.
u·re·ter·o·col·ic [ˌ-ˈkɒlɪk] adj Harnleiter/Ureter u. Kolon betr. od. verbindend, ureterokolisch.
u·re·ter·o·co·los·to·my [ˌ-kəˈlɒstəmɪ] n urol. Harnleiter-Kolon-Anastomose f, Ureterokolostomie f.
u·re·ter·o·cu·ta·ne·os·to·my [ˌ-kjuːˌteɪnɪˈɒstəmɪ] n urol. Harnleiter-Haut-Fistel f, Ureterokutaneostomie f.
u·re·ter·o·cu·ta·ne·ous [ˌ-kjuːˈteɪnɪəs] adj Harnleiter/Ureter u. Haut betr. od. verbindend, ureterokutan.
ureterocutaneous fistula äußere Ureterfistel f, ureterokutane Fistel f, Fistula ureterocutanea.
u·re·ter·o·cys·ta·nas·to·mo·sis [ˌ-ˌsɪstəˌnæstəˈməʊsɪs] n → ureteroneocystostomy.
u·re·ter·o·cys·to·scope [ˌ-ˈsɪstəskəʊp] n Ureterozystoskop nt.
u·re·ter·o·cys·tos·to·my [ˌ-sɪsˈtɒstəmɪ] n → ureteroneocystostomy.
u·re·ter·o·di·al·y·sis [ˌ-daɪˈæləsɪs] n urol. Harnleiter-, Ureterruptur f.
u·re·ter·o·du·o·de·nal [ˌ-d(j)uːəʊˈdiːnl] adj Harnleiter/Ureter u. Zwölffingerdarm/Duodenum betr. od. verbindend, ureteroduodenal.
ureteroduodenal fistula patho. Harnleiter-Duodenum-Fistel f, ureteroduodenale Fistel f.
u·re·ter·o·en·ter·ic [ˌ-enˈterɪk] adj → ureterointestinal.
u·re·ter·o·en·ter·o·a·nas·to·mo·sis [ˌ-entərəʊə næstəˈməʊsɪs] n → ureteroenterostomy.
u·re·ter·o·en·ter·os·to·my [ˌ-ˌentəˈrɒstəmɪ] n chir. Harnleiter-Dünndarm-Anastomose f, Ureteroenteroanastomose f, Ureteroenterostomie f.
u·re·ter·o·gram [ˈ-græm] n patho. Ureterogramm nt.
u·re·ter·og·ra·phy [jəˌriːtəˈrɒgrəfɪ] n urol., radiol. Kontrastdarstellung f der Harnleiter, Ureterographie f.
u·re·ter·o·hy·dro·ne·phro·sis [jəˌriːtərəʊˌhaɪdrɒnɪˈfrəʊsɪs] n urol. Ureterohydronephrose f.
u·re·ter·o·il·e·o·ne·o·cys·tos·to·my [ˌ-ɪlɪəʊˌniːəʊsɪsˈtɒstəmɪ] n urol. Ureteroileoneozystostomie f.
u·re·ter·o·il·e·os·to·my [ˌ-ɪlɪˈɒstəmɪ] n chir. Harnleiter-Ileum-Anastomose f, Ureteroileostomie f.
u·re·ter·o·in·tes·ti·nal [ˌ-ɪnˈtestɪnl] adj Harnleiter/Ureter u. Darm/Intestinum betr. od. verbindend, ureterointestinal.
ureterointestinal fistula patho. Harnleiter-Darm-Fistel f, ureterointestinale Fistel f.
u·re·ter·o·lith [ˈ-lɪθ] n Harnleiterstein m, Ureterolith m.
u·re·ter·o·li·thi·a·sis [ˌ-lɪˈθaɪəsɪs] n Ureterolithiasis f.
u·re·ter·o·li·thot·o·my [ˌ-lɪˈθɒtəmɪ] n urol. operative Harnleitersteinentfernung f, Ureterolithotomie f.
u·re·ter·ol·y·sis [jəˌriːtəˈrɒləsɪs] n urol. 1. Harnleiter-, Ureterruptur f. 2. Harnleiter-, Ureterlähmung f. 3. Harnleiterlösung f, Ureterolyse f.
u·re·ter·o·me·a·tot·o·my [jəˌriːtərəʊˌmɪəˈtɒtəmɪ] n urol. Ureteromeatotomie f.
u·re·ter·o·ne·o·cys·tos·to·my [ˌ-niːəʊsɪsˈtɒstəmɪ] n urol. Ureteroneozystostomie f, Ureterozystoneostomie f.

u·re·ter·o·ne·o·py·e·los·to·my [ˌ-niːəʊˌpaɪəˈlɒstəmɪ] n → ureteropyeloneostomy.
u·re·ter·o·ne·phrec·to·my [ˌ-nɪˈfrektəmɪ] n urol. Entfernung f von Niere u. Harnleiter, Ureteronephrektomie f, Nephroureterektomie f.
u·re·ter·op·a·thy [jəˌriːtəˈrɒpəθɪ] n Harnleiter-, Uretererkrankung f, Ureteropathie f.
u·re·ter·o·pel·vic [jʊəˌriːtərəʊˈpelvɪk] adj Harnleiter/Ureter u. Nierenbecken betr. od. verbindend, ureteropelvin.
ureteropelvic junction Nierenbecken-Uretergrenze f, Nierenbecken-Ureterübergang m.
ureteropelvic obstruction ureteropelvine Obstruktion f.
u·re·ter·o·pel·vi·o·ne·os·to·my [ˌ-ˌpelvɪəʊnɪˈɒstəmɪ] n → ureteropyeloneostomy.
u·re·ter·o·pel·vi·o·plas·ty [ˌ-ˈpelvɪəʊplæstɪ] n urol. Nierenbecken-Harnleiter-Plastik f.
u·re·ter·o·plas·ty [ˈ-plæstɪ] n urol. Harnleiter-, Ureter-, Ureteroplastik f.
u·re·ter·o·proc·tos·to·my [ˌ-prɒkˈtɒstəmɪ] n urol. Ureteroproktostomie f, Ureterekto(neo)stomie f.
u·re·ter·o·py·e·li·tis [ˌ-paɪəˈlaɪtɪs] n Entzündung f von Harnleiter- u. Nierenbecken, Ureteropyelitis f, Ureteropyelonephritis f.
u·re·ter·o·py·e·log·ra·phy [ˌ-paɪəˈlɒgrəfɪ] n radiol., urol. Ureteropyelographie f.
u·re·ter·o·py·e·lo·ne·os·to·my [ˌ-paɪələʊnɪˈɒstəmɪ] n urol. Ureteropyeloneostomie f, Uretero(neo)pyelostomie f.
u·re·ter·o·py·e·lo·ne·phri·tis [ˌ-paɪələʊnɪˈfraɪtɪs] n → ureteropyelitis.
u·re·ter·o·py·e·lo·ne·phros·to·my [ˌ-paɪəlɒnɪˈfrɒstəmɪ] n urol. Ureteropyelonephrostomie f.
u·re·ter·o·py·e·lo·plas·ty [ˌ-ˈpaɪələplæstɪ] n urol. Harnleiter-Nierenbecken-Plastik f.
u·re·ter·o·py·e·los·to·my [ˌ-paɪəˈlɒstəmɪ] n → ureteropyeloneostomy.
u·re·ter·o·py·o·sis [ˌ-paɪˈəʊsɪs] n Harnleitervereiterung f, eitrige Harnleiterentzündung f.
u·re·ter·o·rec·tal [ˌ-ˈrektl] adj Harnleiter/Ureter u. Rektum betr. od. verbindend, ureterorektal.
ureterorectal fistula patho. Harnleiter-Rektum-Fistel f, ureterorektale Fistel f.
u·re·ter·o·rec·to·ne·os·to·my [ˌ-rektəʊnɪˈɒstəmɪ] n → ureteroproctostomy.
u·re·ter·o·rec·tos·to·my [ˌ-rekˈtɒstəmɪ] n → ureteroproctostomy.
u·re·ter·or·rha·gia [ˌ-ˈreɪdʒ(ɪ)ə] n Harnleiterblutung f, Ureterorrhagie f.
u·re·ter·or·rha·phy [jəˌriːtəˈrɒrəfɪ] n urol. Harnleiternaht f, Ureterorrhaphie f.
u·re·ter·o·sig·moid·os·to·my [jəˌriːtərəʊˌsɪgmɔɪˈdɒstəmɪ] n urol. Harnleiter-Sigma-Fistel f, Ureterosigmoid(e)ostomie f.
u·re·ter·o·steg·no·sis [ˌ-stegˈnəʊsɪs] n → ureterostenosis.
u·re·ter·o·ste·no·ma [ˌ-stɪˈnəʊmə] n → ureterostenosis.
u·re·ter·o·ste·no·sis [ˌ-stɪˈnəʊsɪs] n Harnleiterverengung f, -stenose f, Ureterostenose f.
u·re·ter·os·to·ma [jəˌriːtərˈɒstəmə] n 1. Ureterostium nt, Ostium ureteris. 2. patho. Harnleiter-, Ureterfistel f, Fistula ureterica. 3. urol. Harnleiter-, Ureterfistel f, Ureterostoma nt.
u·re·ter·os·to·my [ˌ-ˈɒstəmɪ] n urol. Ureterostomie f.
u·re·ter·ot·o·my [ˌ-ˈɒtəmɪ] n urol. operative Harnleiter-/Uretereröffnung f, Ureterotomie f.

u·re·ter·o·tri·go·no·en·ter·os·to·my [jə,riːtərəutrai,gəunəu,entə'rastəmɪ] *n urol.* Ureterotrigonoenterostomie *f*.
u·re·ter·o·tri·go·no·sig·moid·os·to·my [,-trai,gəunəusigmɔi'dastəmɪ] *n urol.* Ureterotrigonosigmoid(e)ostomie *f*.
u·re·ter·o·u·re·ter·al [,-jə'riːtərəl] *adj* ureteroureteral.
u·re·ter·o·u·re·ter·os·to·my [,-jə,riːtə'rastəmɪ] *n urol.* Ureteroureterostomie *f*.
u·re·ter·o·u·ter·ine [,-'juːtərɪn, -raɪn] *adj* Harnleiter/Ureter u. Gebärmutter/Uterus betr. *od.* verbindend, ureterouterin.
ureterouterine fistula *patho.* Harnleiter--Gebärmutter-Fistel *f*, ureterouterine Fistel *f*.
u·re·ter·o·vag·i·nal [,-'vædʒɪnl] *adj* Harnleiter/Ureter u. Scheide/Vagina betr. *od.* verbindend, ureterovaginal.
ureterovaginal fistula *patho.* Harnleiter--Scheiden-Fistel *f*, ureterovaginale Fistel *f*, Fistula ureterovaginalis.
u·re·ter·o·ves·i·cal [,-'vesɪkl] *adj* Harnleiter/Ureter u. Harnblase betr., ureterovesikal.
ureterovesical fistula *patho.* Harnleiter--Blasen-Fistel *f*, ureterovesikale Fistel *f*.
ureterovesical reflux ureterovesikaler Reflux *m*.
u·re·ter·o·ves·i·co·plas·ty [,-'vesɪkəuplæstɪ] *n urol.* Ureterovesikoplastik *f*.
u·re·ter·o·ves·i·cos·to·my [,-vesɪ'kastəmɪ] *n urol.* Ureterovesikostomie *f*.
u·re·than ['juərəθæn] *n* Urethan *nt*, Carbaminsäureäthylester *m*.
u·re·thane ['juərəθeɪn] *n* → urethan.
urethr- *pref.* → urethro-.
u·re·thra [juə'riːθrə] *n, pl* **-thras, -thrae** [-θriː] Harnröhre *f*, Urethra *f*.
u·re·thral [juə'riːθrəl] *adj* Harnröhre/Urethra betr., urethral, Harnröhren-, Urethra(l)-, Urethr(o)-.
urethral abscess Harnröhren-, Urethra(l)abszeß *m*.
urethral artery Harnröhrenarterie *f*, Urethralis *f*, A. urethralis.
urethral calculus Harnröhrenstein *m*.
urethral carina of vagina Harnröhrenwulst *m* der Scheide, Carina urethralis vaginae.
urethral caruncle Harnröhrenkarunkel *f*.
urethral catheter intraurethraler Blasenkatheter *m*.
urethral crest: female u. Crista urethralis feminiae.
male u. Crista urethralis masculinae.
urethral disruption *urol.* Harnröhren-, Urethraabriß *m*.
urethral fever → urinary fever.
urethral fold *embryo.* Urethrafalte *f*.
u·re·thral·gia [juə'θrældʒ(ɪ)ə] *n* Harnröhrenschmerz *m*, Urethralgie *f*, Urethrodynie *f*.
urethral glands Littre'-Drüsen *pl*, Urethraldrüsen *pl*, Gll. urethrales urethrae masculinae.
u. of female urethra Harnröhrendrüsen *pl* der weiblichen Harnröhre, Gll. urethrales urethrae feminiae.
u. of male urethra Littre'-Drüsen *pl*, Urethraldrüsen *pl*, Gll. urethrales urethrae masculinae.
urcthral groove *embryo.* Urogenitalspalte *f*.
urethral injury Harnröhren-, Urethraverletzung *f*, -trauma *nt*.
urethral lacunae (of Morgagni) Urethrallakunen *pl*, -buchten *pl*, Lacunae urethrales.
urethral obstruction Harnröhren-, Urethraobstruktion *f*.
urethral opening: external u. äußere Harnröhrenöffnung *f*, Harnröhrenmündung *f*, Ostium urethrae externum.
internal u. innere Harnröhrenöffnung *f*, Harnröhrenanfang *m*, Ostium urethrae internum.
urethral orifice: external u. → urethral opening, external.
internal u. → urethral opening, internal.
urethral plate *embryo.* Urethraplatte *f*.
urethral ridge → urethral carina of vagina.
urethral sphincter, voluntary Harnröhren-, Urethralsphinkter *m*, Sphinkter *m* urethrae, M. sphincter urethrae.
urethral stricture Harnröhren-, Urethrastriktur *f*.
urethral surface of penis Penisunterseite *f*, Facies urethralis (penis).
urethral syndrome Urethralsyndrom *nt*.
urethral utricle Prostatablindsack *m*, Utrikulus *m*, Utriculus prostaticus.
urethral valve Harnröhren-, Urethra(l)klappe *f*.
u·re·thram·e·ter [juərə'θræmɪtər] *n* → urethrometer.
u·re·thra·scope [juə'riːθrəskəup] *n* → urethroscope.
u·re·thra·tre·sia [juə,riːθrə'triːʒ(ɪ)ə] *n* Harnröhren-, Urethraatresie *f*.
u·re·threc·to·my [juərə'θrektəmɪ] *n urol.* Harnröhren-, Urethraresektion *f*.
u·re·threm·or·rha·gia [juə,rɪθremə'reɪdʒ(ɪ)ə] *n* → urethrorrhagia.
u·re·threm·phrax·is [juərəθrem'fræksɪs] *n* Harnröhren-, Urethraobstruktion *f*.
u·re·thrism ['juərəθrɪzəm] *n urol.* Urethrismus *m*; Harnröhrenkrampf *m*, -spasmus *m*.
u·re·thris·mus [juərə'θrɪzməs] *n* → urethrism.
u·re·thri·tis [juərə'θraɪtɪs] *n* Harnröhrenentzündung *f*, Urethritis *f*.
urethro- *pref.* Harnröhren-, Urethral-, Urethr(o)-.
u·re·thro·blen·nor·rhea [jə,riːθrə,blenə'rɪə] *n* Urethroblennorrhoe *f*.
u·re·thro·bul·bar [,-'bʌlbər] *adj* Harnröhre/Urethra u. Bulbus penis betr., urethrobulbär, bulbourethral.
u·re·thro·cele ['-siːl] *n* **1.** Harnröhrendivertikel *nt*, Urethrozele *f*. **2.** *gyn.* Harnröhrenprolaps *m*, Urethrozele *f*.
u·re·thro·cys·ti·tis [,-sɪs'taɪtɪs] *n urol.* Entzündung *f* von Blase u. Harnröhre, Urethrozystitis *f*.
u·re·thro·cys·to·gram [,-'sɪstəgræm] *n radiol., urol.* Urethrozystogramm *nt*.
u·re·thro·cys·tog·ra·phy [,-sɪs'tagrəfɪ] *n radiol., urol.* Kontrastdarstellung *f* von Harnblase u. Harnröhre, Urethrozystographie *f*.
u·re·thro·cys·to·me·trog·ra·phy [,-sɪstəmɪ'tragrəfɪ] *n* → urethrocystometry.
u·re·thro·cys·tom·e·try [,-sɪs'tamətrɪ] *n urol.* Urethrozystometrie *f*.
u·re·thro·cys·to·pex·y [,-'sɪstəpeksɪ] *n urol., gyn.* Urethrozystopexie *f*.
u·re·thro·dyn·ia [,-'diːnɪə] *n* → urethralgia.
u·re·throg·ra·phy [juərə'θragrəfɪ] *n radiol., urol.* Kontrastdarstellung *f* der Harnröhre, Urethrographie *f*.
u·re·throm·e·ter ['-'θramɪtər] *n urol.* Urethrometer *nt*.
u·re·throm·e·try ['-'θramətrɪ] *n urol.* Urethrometrie *f*.
u·re·thro·pe·nile [jə,riːθrə'piːnl, -naɪl] *adj* Harnröhre/Urethra u. Penis betr.
u·re·thro·per·i·ne·al [,-perɪ'niːəl] *adj* Harnröhre/Urethra u. Damm/Perineum betr., urethroperineal.
u·re·thro·per·i·ne·o·scro·tal [,-perɪ,niːə'skrəutl] *adj* urethroperineoskrotal.

u·re·thro·pex·y ['-peksɪ] *n urol.* Urethropexie *f*.
u·re·thro·phrax·is [,-'fræksɪs] *n* Harnröhren-, Urethraobstruktion *f*.
u·re·thro·phy·ma [,-'faɪmə] *n urol.* Harnröhrenschwellung *f*, -tumor *m*.
u·re·thro·plas·ty ['-plæstɪ] *n urol.* Harnröhren-, Urethro-, Urethraplastik *f*.
u·re·thro·pros·tat·ic [,-pras'tætɪk] *adj* Harnröhre/Urethra u. Prostata betr., urethroprostatisch.
u·re·thro·rec·tal [,-'rektl] *adj* Harnröhre/Urethra u. Rektum betr. *od.* verbindend, urethrorektal.
u·re·thror·rha·gia [,-'reɪdʒ(ɪ)ə] *n urol.* Harnröhrenblutung *f*, Urethrorrhagie *f*.
u·re·thror·rha·phy [juərɪ'θrɔrəfɪ] *n urol.* Harnröhrennaht *f*, Urethrorrhaphie *f*.
u·re·thror·rhea [jə,riːθrə'rɪə] *n* Harnröhrenausfluß *m*, Urethrorrhoe *f*.
u·re·thro·scope ['-skəup] *n urol.* Urethroskop *nt*.
u·re·thro·scop·ic [,-'skapɪk] *adj* Urethroskop betr., urethroskopisch.
u·re·thros·co·py [juərə'θraskəpɪ] *n urol.* Harnröhrenspiegelung *f*, Urethroskopie *f*.
u·re·thro·scro·tal [jə,riːθrə'skrəutl] *adj* Harnröhre/Urethra u. Skrotum betr. *od.* verbindend, urethroskrotal.
urethroscrotal fistula *patho.* Harnröhren--Skrotum-Fistel *f*, urethroskrotale Fistel *f*.
u·re·thro·spasm ['-spæzm] *n* → urethrism.
u·re·thro·stax·is [,-'stæksɪs] *n* Sickerblutung *f* aus der Harnröhre.
u·re·thro·ste·no·sis [,-stɪ'nəusɪs] *n* Harnröhren-, Urethrastenose *f*.
u·re·thros·to·my [juərə'θrastəmɪ] *n urol.* Urethrostomie *f*.
u·re·thro·tome [jə'riːθrətəum] *n urol.* Urethrotom *nt*.
u·re·throt·o·my [juərɪ'θratəmɪ] *n urol.* Harnröhreneröffnung *f*, -schnitt *m*, Urethrotomie *f*, -tomia *f*.
u·re·thro·vag·i·nal [jə,riːθrə'vædʒɪnl] *adj* Harnröhre/Urethra u. Scheide/Vagina betr. *od.* verbindend, urethrovaginal.
urethrovaginal fistula *patho.* Harnröhren--Scheiden-Fistel *f*, urethrovaginale Fistel *f*.
u·re·thro·ves·i·cal [,-'vesɪkl] *adj* Harnröhre/Urethra u. Harnblase betr., urethrovesikal.
u·re·thro·ves·i·co·pex·y [,-'vesɪkəupeksɪ] *n* Urethrovesikopexie *f*.
urge [ɜrdʒ] **I** *n* Drang *m*, Trieb *m*, Antrieb *m*. **II** *vt* (an-, vorwärts-)treiben, anspornen. **III** *vi* drängen, treiben.
ur·gen·cy ['ɜrdʒənsɪ] *n, pl* **-cies** (dringende) Not *f*, Druck *m*, Dringlichkeit *f*; Drang *m*; Drängen *nt*.
ur·hi·dro·sis [juərhɪ'drəusɪs] *n* Ur(h)idrosis *f*.
u·ri·an ['juərɪən] *n* → urochrome.
uric- *pref.* → urico-.
u·ric ['juərɪk] *adj* Urin betr., Urin-, Harn-.
uric acid Harnsäure *f*.
uric acid calculus Harnsäurestein *m*.
uric acid depot Harnsäureablagerung *f*, -depot *nt*.
uric acid diathesis Gichtdiathese *f*, harnsaure/uratische Diathese *f*, Diathesis urica.
u·ric·ac·i·de·mia [,(j)uərɪk,æsɪ'diːmɪə] *n* erhöhter Harnsäuregehalt *m* des Blutes, Hyperurikämie *f*, Hyperurikosurie *f*.
uric acid infarct Harnsäureinfarkt *m*.
u·ric·ac·i·du·ria [,-æsɪ'd(j)uərɪə] *n* vermehrte Harnsäureausscheidung *f*, Hyperurikurie *f*, Hyperurikosurie *f*.

u·ri·case ['jʊərɪkeɪz] *n* → urate oxidase.
u·ri·ce·mia [ˌjʊərɪ'siːmɪə] *n* → uricacidemia.
urico- *pref.* Harnsäure-, Urik(o)-, Harn-, Urin-, Uro-, Uri-.
u·ri·co·cho·lia [ˌjʊərɪkəʊ'kəʊlɪə] *n* Urikocholie *f*.
u·ri·col·y·sis [ˌjʊərɪ'kɒləsɪs] *n* Harnsäure-, Uratspaltung *f*, Urikolyse *f*.
u·ri·co·lyt·ic [ˌjʊərɪkəʊ'lɪtɪk] *adj* Urikolyse betr. *od.* fördernd, urikolytisch.
u·ri·com·e·ter [ˌjʊərɪ'kɒmɪtər] *n* Urikometer *nt*.
urico-oxidase *n* → urate oxidase.
u·ri·co·poi·e·sis [ˌjʊərɪkəpɔɪ'iːsɪs] *n* Harnsäurebildung *f*, Urikopo(i)ese *f*.
u·ri·co·su·ria [ˌ-'s(j)ʊərɪə] *n* 1. Harnsäureausscheidung *f*, Urikosurie *f*. 2. vermehrte Harnsäureausscheidung *f*, Hyperurikosurie *f*, Hyperurikurie *f*.
u·ri·co·su·ric [ˌ-'s(j)ʊərɪk] I *n* Harnsäureausscheidung förderndes Mittel *nt*, Urikosurikum *nt*. II *adj* die Harnsäureausscheidung fördernd, urikosurisch.
uricosuric agent → uricosuric I.
u·ri·co·tel·ic [ˌ-'telɪk] *adj* uricotelisch.
u·ri·dine ['jʊərɪdiːn, -dɪn] *n abbr.* **U** Uridin *nt abbr.* U.
uridine(-5'-)diphosphate *n abbr.* **UDP** Uridin(-5'-)diphosphat *nt abbr.* UDP.
uridine diphosphate D-galactose → UDPgalactose.
uridine diphosphate glucose → UDPglucose.
uridine diphosphogalactose-4-epimerase → UDPglucose-4-epimerase.
uridine diphosphoglucuronate → UDPglucuronate.
uridine monophosphate *abbr.* **UMP** Uridinmonophosphat *nt abbr.* UMP, Uridylsäure *f*.
uridine(-5'-)triphosphate *n abbr.* **UTP** Uridin(-5'-)triphosphat *nt abbr.* UTP.
u·ri·dro·sis [ˌjʊərɪ'drəʊsɪs] *n* Ur(h)idrosis *f*.
u·ri·dyl·ate [ˌ-'dɪleɪt] *n* Uridylat *nt*.
u·ri·dyl·ic acid [ˌ-'dɪlɪk] → uridine monophosphate.
u·ri·dyl·yl transferase [ˌ-'dɪlɪl] Uridyl(yl)-transferase *f*.
u·ri·es·the·sis [ˌ-'esθɪsɪs] *n* → uresiesthesis.
urin- *pref.* → urino-.
u·ri·na [jə'raɪnə] *n* → urine.
u·ri·na·ble ['jʊərənəbl] *adj* im Harn ausscheidbar.
u·rin·ac·cel·er·a·tor [ˌjʊərɪnæk'seləreɪtər] *n* M. bulbospongiosus.
u·ri·nae·mia [ˌjʊərɪ'niːmɪə] *n* → uremia.
u·ri·nal ['jʊərɪnl] *n* 1. Urinflasche *f*, Harnglas *nt*, Urinal *nt*, Urodochium *nt*. 2. Urinbecken *nt* (in Toiletten), Urinal *nt*. 3. (Männer-)Toilette *f*, Pissoir *nt*.
u·ri·nal·y·sis [ˌjʊərɪ'næləsɪs] *n* Harn-, Urinuntersuchung *f*, Urinanalyse *f*.
u·ri·nar·y ['jʊərɪˌnerɪː, -nərɪ] *adj* Harn(organe) betr., Harn produzierend *od.* ausscheidend, Harn-, Urin-.
urinary bladder (Harn-)Blase *f*, Vesica urinaria.
urinary bladder carcinoma (Harn-)Blasenkrebs *m*, -karzinom *nt*.
urinary bladder papilloma (Harn-)Blasenpapillom *nt*.
urinary calculus Harnstein *m*, -konkrement *nt*, Urolith *m*.
urinary cast *urol.* Harnzylinder *m*.
urinary catheter 1. (Harn-)Blasenkatheter *m*. **2.** Katheter *m* zur Harnableitung.
urinary continence Blasen-, Harnkontinenz *f*.
urinary cylinder → urinary cast.
urinary cyst Harnzyste *f*.
urinary duct harnabführender Kanal *m*.
urinary fever Katheter-, Urethral-, Harnfieber *nt*, Febris urethralis.
urinary fistula Harnfistel *f*.
urinary incontinence Harninkontinenz *f*, Incontinentia urinae.
urinary organs harnproduzierende u. -ausscheidende Organe *pl*, uropoetisches System *nt*, Harnorgane *pl*, Organa urinaria.
urinary output Harnausscheidung *f*, -volumen *nt*.
urinary passages, lower untere/ableitende Harnwege *pl*.
urinary pole of glomerulus (*Niere*) Harnpol *m* des Glomerulums.
urinary reflex Blasenentleerungsreflex *m*.
urinary retention Harnstauung *f*, -verhalt *m*, -verhaltung *f*.
urinary schistosomiasis Urogenital-, Blasen-, Harnblasenbilharziose *f*, Schistosomiasis urogenitalis.
urinary stone → urinary calculus.
urinary system → urinary organs.
urinary tract → urinary organs.
lower u. ableitende Harnwege *pl*.
urinary tract infection *abbr.* **UTI** Harnwegsinfekt *m*, -infektion *f abbr.* HWI.
urinary tract obstruction Harnwegsobstruktion *f*.
u·ri·nate ['jʊərɪneɪt] *vi* die (Harn-)Blase entleeren, Harn *od.* Wasser lassen, harnen, urinieren.
u·ri·na·tion [ˌjʊərɪ'neɪʃn] *n* Harn-, Wasserlassen *nt*, Urinieren *nt*, Blasenentleerung *f*, Miktion *f*.
u·ri·na·tive ['jʊərɪneɪtɪv] I *n pharm.* harntreibendes Mittel *nt*, Diuretikum *nt*. II *adj* Diurese betr., harntreibend, diuresefördernd, -anregend, diuretisch.
u·rine ['jʊərɪn] *n* Harn *m*, Urin *m*, Urina *f*.
urine analysis → urinalysis.
urine culture Harn-, Urinkultur *f*.
urine leak Urinleck *nt*.
u·ri·ne·mia [ˌjʊərɪ'niːmɪə] *n* → uremia.
urine osmolality Harnosmolalität *f*.
urine sediment Harnsediment *nt*.
u·rin·i·dro·sis [ˌjʊərɪnɪ'drəʊsɪs] *n* Ur(h)idrosis *f*.
u·ri·nif·er·ous [ˌjʊərə'nɪfərəs] *adj* Harn transportierend *od.* ableitend, harnführend, urinifer.
uriniferous tubules Nierenkanälchen *pl*, -tubuli *pl*, Tubuli renales.
u·ri·nif·ic [ˌ-'nɪfɪk] *adj* → uniparous.
u·ri·nip·a·rous [ˌ-'nɪpərəs] *adj* harnproduzierend, -bildend, ausscheidend.
uriniparous tubules → uriniferous tubules.
urino- *pref.* Harn-, Urin-, Uri-, Uro-.
u·ri·no·gen·i·tal [ˌjʊərɪnəʊ'dʒenɪtl] *adj* → urogenital.
u·ri·nog·e·nous [ˌjʊərɪ'nɒdʒənəs] *adj* aus dem Harn stammend, urinogen.
u·ri·nol·o·gist [ˌ-'nɒlədʒɪst] *n* → urologist.
u·ri·nol·o·gy [ˌ-'nɒlədʒɪ] *n* → urology.
u·ri·no·ma [ˌ-'nəʊmə] *n* harnhaltige Zyste *f*.
u·ri·nom·e·ter [ˌ-'nɒmɪtər] *n* Urinometer *nt*.
u·ri·nom·e·try [ˌ-'nɒmətrɪ] *n lab.* Bestimmung *f* der Harndichte, Urinometrie *f*.
u·ri·noph·i·lous [ˌ-'nɒfɪləs] *adj micro.* mit besonderer Affinität zu Harn, urinophil.
u·ri·nos·co·py [ˌ-'nɒskəpɪ] *n* → uroscopy.
u·ri·no·sex·u·al [ˌjʊərɪnəʊ'sekʃəwəl] *adj* → urogenital.
u·ri·nous ['jʊərɪnəs] *adj* Urin betr., harnartig, urinös, Harn-.
u·ri·po·sia [ˌjʊərɪ'pəʊzɪə] *n socio., psychia.* Harntrinken *nt*.

uro- *pref.* → urino-.
u·ro·an·the·lone [ˌjʊərəʊ'ænθələʊn] *n* Urogastron *nt*.
u·ro·ben·zo·ic acid [ˌ-ben'zəʊɪk] Hippursäure *f*, Benzoylglykokoll *nt*.
u·ro·bi·lin [ˌ-'baɪlɪn, -'bɪlɪn] *n* Urobilin *nt*.
u·ro·bil·in·e·mia [ˌ-bɪlə'niːmɪə] *n* Urobilinämie *f*.
u·ro·bi·lin·o·gen [ˌ-baɪ'lɪnədʒən] *n* Urobilinogen *nt*.
u·ro·bi·lin·o·gen·e·mia [ˌ-baɪˌlɪnədʒə'niːmɪə] *n* Urobilinogenämie *f*.
u·ro·bi·lin·o·gen·u·ria [ˌ-baɪˌlɪnədʒə-'n(j)ʊərɪə] *n* Urobilinogenausscheidung *f* im Harn, Urobilinogenurie *f*.
u·ro·bi·li·noid [ˌ-'bɪlənɔɪd, -'baɪlɪ-] *adj* urobilinartig, urobilinoid.
u·ro·bi·lin·u·ria [ˌ-bɪlə'n(j)ʊərɪə, -'baɪlɪ-] *n* vermehrte Urobilinausscheidung *f* im Harn, Urobilinurie *f*.
u·ro·ca·nase [ˌ-'kæneɪz] *n* → urocanate hydratase.
u·ro·ca·nate [ˌ-'kæneɪt] *n* Urocanat *nt*.
urocanate hydratase Urocanase *f*, Urocanathydratase *f*.
ur·o·can·ic acid [ˌ-'kænɪk] Urocan(in)säure *f abbr.* UCS.
urocanic acid hydratase → urocanate hydratase.
u·ro·cele ['-siːl] *n urol.* Urozele *f*, Uroscheozele *f*.
u·roch·er·as [jʊ'rɒkərəs] *n* Harnsediment *nt*.
u·ro·che·zia [ˌjʊərə'kiːzɪə] *n* Urochezie *f*.
u·ro·chrome ['-krəʊm] *n* Urochrom *nt*.
u·ro·chro·mo·gen [ˌ-'krəʊmədʒən] *n* Urochromogen *nt*.
u·ro·ci·net·ic [ˌ-sɪ'netɪk] *adj* → urokinetic.
u·ro·clep·sia [ˌ-'klepsɪə] *n* unwillkürliches Harnlassen *nt*.
u·ro·cop·ro·por·phyr·ia [ˌ-kɒprəpɔː'fɪərɪə] *n* Porphyria cutanea tarda symptomatica.
u·ro·cy·a·nin [ˌ-'saɪənɪn] *n* Urozyanin *nt*.
u·ro·cy·an·o·gen [ˌ-ˌsaɪ'ænədʒən] *n* Urozyanogen *nt*.
u·ro·cy·a·no·sis [ˌ-saɪə'nəʊsɪs] *n* Urozyanose *f*.
u·ro·cyst ['-sɪst] *n* (Harn-)Blase *f*, Vesica urinaria.
u·ro·cys·tic [ˌ-'sɪstɪk] *adj* Harnblase betr., Harnblasen-, Blasen-.
u·ro·cys·ti·tis [ˌ-'sɪstaɪtɪs] *n* → urocyst.
u·ro·cys·ti·tis [ˌ-'sɪstɪs] *n* → urocyst.
u·ro·cys·ti·tis [ˌ-sɪs'taɪtɪs] *n* (Harn-)Blasenentzündung *f*, Zystitis *f*, Cystitis *f*.
u·ro·do·chi·um [ˌ-'dəʊkɪəm, -dəʊ'kaɪəm] *n* → urinal 1.
u·ro·dy·nam·ics [ˌ-daɪ'næmɪks] *pl* Urodynamik *f*.
u·ro·dyn·ia [ˌ-'dɪnɪə] *n* schmerzhaftes Wasserlassen *nt*, Schmerzen *pl* beim Wasserlassen, Urodynie *f*.
u·ro·en·ter·one [ˌ-'entərən] *n* Urogastron *nt*.
u·ro·er·y·thrin [ˌ-'erəθrɪn] *n* Uroerythrin *nt*.
u·ro·fla·vin [ˌ-'fleɪvɪn] *n* Uroflavin *nt*.
u·ro·flo·me·ter *n* → uroflowmeter.
u·ro·flow·me·ter [ˌ-'fləʊmiːtər] *n* Uroflowmeter *nt*.
u·ro·gas·trone [ˌ-'gæstrəʊn] *n* Urogastron *nt*.
u·ro·gen·i·tal [ˌ-'dʒenɪtl] *adj* Harn- u. Geschlechtsorgane betr., urogenital, Urogenital-.
urogenital apparatus → urogenital tract.
urogenital cleft Schamspalte *f*, Rima pudendi.
urogenital diaphragm Urogenitaldiaphragma *nt*, Diaphragma urogenitale.
urogenital groove *embryo.* Urogenitalspalte *f*.

urogenital membrane *embryo.* Urogenitalmembran *f.*
urogenital mesentery Urogenitalmesenterium *nt,* Mesenterium urogenitale.
urogenital peritoneum Peritoneum urogenitale.
urogenital region Urogenitalgegend *f,* -region *f,* Regio urogenitalis.
urogenital ridge *embryo.* Urogenitalleiste *f.*
urogenital sinus *embryo.* Urogenitalsinus *m,* Sinus urogenitalis.
urogenital system → urogenital tract.
urogenital tract Urogenitalsystem *nt,* -trakt *m,* Harn- u. Geschlechtsorgane *pl,* Apparatus urogenitalis, Systema urogenitale.
urogenital triangle/trigone → urogenital diaphragm.
u·rog·e·nous [jʊəˈrɑdʒənəs] *adj* **1.** urinbildend. **2.** aus dem Harn stammend, vom Harn ausgeschieden, urogen.
u·ro·glau·cin [ˌjʊərəˈglɔːsɪn] *n* → urocyanin.
u·ro·gram [ˈ-græm] *n* Urogramm *nt.*
u·rog·ra·phy [jʊəˈrɑgrəfɪ] *n* *radiol., urol.* Urographie *f.*
u·ro·gra·vim·e·ter [ˌjʊərəgrəˈvɪmətər] *n* → urinometer.
u·ro·hem·a·tin [ˌ-ˈhemətɪn] *n* → urobilin.
u·ro·hem·a·to·ne·phro·sis [ˌ-ˌhemətəʊnɪˈfrəʊsɪs] *n* *urol.* Urohämatonephrose *f.*
u·ro·hem·a·to·por·phy·rin [ˌ-ˌhemətəʊˈpɔːrfərɪn] *n* → urobilin.
u·ro·hep·a·rin [ˌ-ˈhepərɪn] *n* Uroheparin *nt.*
u·ro·ki·nase [ˌ-ˈkaɪneɪz, ˈ-kɪ-] *n* Urokinase *f.*
u·ro·ki·net·ic [ˌ-kɪˈnetɪk] *adj* urokinetisch.
u·ro·lag·nia [ˌ-ˈlægnɪə] *n* *psychia.* Urolagnie *f.*
u·ro·lith [ˈ-lɪθ] *n* Harnstein *m,* -konkrement *nt,* Urolith *m.*
u·ro·li·thi·a·sis [ˌ-lɪˈθaɪəsɪs] *n* Harnsteinleiden *nt,* Urolithiasis *f.*
u·ro·lith·ic [ˌ-ˈlɪθɪk] *adj* Harnstein(e) betr., Harnstein-.
u·ro·log·ic [ˌ-ˈlɑdʒɪk] *adj* Urologie betr., urologisch.
u·ro·log·i·cal [ˌ-ˈlɑdʒɪkl] *adj* → urologic.
u·rol·o·gist [jəˈrɑlədʒɪst] *n* Urologe *m,* -login *f.*
u·rol·o·gy [jəˈrɑlədʒɪ] *n* Urologie *f.*
u·ro·lu·te·in [ˌjʊərəˈluːtiːɪn, -tɪn] *n* Urolutein *nt.*
u·ro·mel·a·nin [ˌ-ˈmelənɪn] *n* Uromelanin *nt.*
u·ro·mel·us [jəˈræmələs] *n* *embryo.* Uromelus *m,* Sirenomelus *m.*
u·rom·e·ter [jəˈræmɪtər] *n* → urinometer.
uron- *pref.* → urino-.
u·ro·ne·phro·sis [ˌjʊərənɪˈfrəʊsɪs] *n* Harnstauungs-, Wassersackniere *f,* Hydro-, Uronephrose *f.*
u·ron·ic acid [jəˈrɑnɪk] Uronsäure *f.*
urono- *pref.* → urino-.
u·ro·nol·o·gy [ˌjʊərəˈnɑlədʒɪ] *n* → urology.
u·ro·nos·co·py [ˌ-ˈnɑskəpɪ] *n* → uroscopy.
u·rop·a·thy [jəˈrɑpəθɪ] *n* Harnwegserkrankung *f,* Uropathie *f.*
u·ro·pe·nia [ˌjʊərəˈpiːnɪə] *n* mangelhafte Harnausscheidung *od.* Harnbildung *f,* Uropenie *f.*
u·ro·pep·sin [ˌ-ˈpepsɪn] *n* → urokinase.
u·ro·pep·sin·o·gen [ˌ-pepˈsɪnədʒən] *n* Uropepsinogen *nt.*
u·ro·phan·ic [ˌ-ˈfænɪk] *adj* *biochem., pharm.* urophan.
u·ro·phil·ia [ˌ-ˈfɪlɪə] *n* *psychia.* Urophilie *f.*
u·ro·pho·bia [ˌ-ˈfəʊbɪə] *n* *psychia.* Urophobie *f.*
u·ro·poi·e·sis [ˌ-pɔɪˈiːsɪs] *n* Harnbereitung *f,* -produktion *f,* -bildung *f,* Uropoese *f.*
u·ro·poi·et·ic [ˌ-pɔɪˈetɪk] *adj* Harnbildung/Uropoese betr., uropoetisch.
uropoietic system → urinary organs.
u·ro·por·phyr·ia [ˌ-pɔːrˈfɪrɪə] *n* Uroporphyrie *f,* -porphyria *f.*
u·ro·por·phy·rin [ˌ-ˈpɔːrfərɪn] *n* Uroporphyrin *nt.*
u·ro·por·phy·rin·o·gen [ˌ-pɔːrˈfərɪnədʒən] *n* Uroporphyrinogen *nt.*
uroporphyrinogen decarboxylase Uroporphyrinogendecarboxylase *f.*
uroporphyrinogen I synthase Porphobilinogendesaminase *f.*
uroporphyrinogen III synthase Uroporphyrinogen-III-synthase *f.*
u·ro·psam·mus [ˌ-ˈsæməs] *n* Harnsediment *nt.*
u·ro·py·o·ne·phro·sis [ˌ-ˌpaɪənɪˈfrəʊsɪs] *n* *urol.* Uropyonephrose *f.*
u·ro·py·o·u·re·ter [ˌ-ˌpaɪəjəˈriːtər] *n* *urol.* Uropyoureter *m.*
u·ro·rec·tal [ˌ-ˈrektl] *adj* Harnwege u. Rektum betr., urorektal.
urorectal fistula Urorektalfistel *f.*
urorectal septum *embryo.* Urorektalseptum *nt,* Septum urorectale.
u·ro·ro·se·in [ˌ-ˈrəʊziːɪn] *n* → urorrhodin.
u·ror·rhea [ˌ-ˈrɪə] *n* unwillkürlicher Harnabgang *m;* Enuresis *f.*
u·ror·rho·din [ˌ-ˈrəʊdɪn] *n* Urorosein *nt.*
u·ro·ru·bin [ˌ-ˈruːbɪn] *n* Urorubin *nt.*
u·ro·ru·bin·o·gen [ˌ-ˌruːˈbɪnədʒən] *n* Urorubinogen *nt.*
u·ro·ru·bro·hem·a·tin [ˌ-ˌruːbrəʊˈhemətɪn] *n* Urorubrohämatin *nt.*
u·ro·sa·cin [ˌjʊərəˈseɪsɪn] *n* → urorrhodin.
u·ros·che·o·cele [jʊəˈrɑskɪəsiːl] *n* → urocele.
u·ros·che·sis [jʊəˈrɑskəsɪs] *n* Harnverhalt *m,* -verhaltung *f,* -retention *f.*
u·ro·scop·ic [ˌjʊərəˈskɑpɪk] *adj* Uroskopie betr., uroskopisch.
u·ros·co·py [jəˈrɑskəpɪ] *n* (diagnostische) Harnuntersuchung *f,* Uroskopie *f.*
u·ro·sep·sis [ˌjʊərəˈsepsɪs] *n* Urosepsis *f,* Harnsepsis *f.*
u·ro·sep·tic [ˌ-ˈseptɪk] *adj* Urosepsis betr., uroseptisch.
u·ro·spec·trin [ˌ-ˈspektrɪn] *n* Urospektrin *nt.*
u·ro·ste·a·lith [ˌ-ˈstɪəlɪθ] *n* Urostealith *m.*
u·ro·the·li·al [ˌ-ˈθiːlɪəl] *adj* Urothel betr., Urothel-.
u·ro·the·li·um [ˌ-ˈθiːlɪəm] *n* Urothel *nt.*
u·ro·tho·rax [ˌ-ˈθɔːræks] *n* Urothorax *m.*
u·ro·u·re·ter [ˌ-jəˈriːtər] *n* *urol.* Hydroureter *m,* Hydrureter *m.*
u·ro·xan·thin [ˌ-ˈzænθɪn] *n* Uroxanthin *nt.*
ur·rho·din [jʊəˈrəʊdɪn] *n* → urorrhodin.
ur·so·de·ox·y·cho·late [ˌɜːrsəʊdɪˌɑksɪˈkəʊleɪt] *n* Ursodesoxycholat *nt.*
ur·so·de·ox·y·cho·lic acid [ˌ-dɪˌɑksɪˈkəʊlɪk] Ursodesoxycholsäure *f.*
ur·ti·ca [ˈɜːrtɪkə] *n* Quaddel *f,* Urtika *f,* Urtica *f.*
ur·ti·car·i·a [ˌɜːrtɪˈkeərɪə] *n* *patho.* Nesselausschlag *m,* -fieber *nt,* -sucht *f,* Urtikaria *f,* Urticaria *f.*
ur·ti·car·i·al [ˌ-ˈkeərɪəl] *adj* Urtikaria betr., urtikariell.
urticarial fever japanische Schistosomiasis/Bilharziose *f,* Schistosomiasis japonica.
ur·ti·car·i·o·gen·ic [ˌ-ˌkeərɪəˈdʒenɪk] *adj* Urtikaria hervorrufend.
ur·ti·car·i·ous [ˌ-ˈkeərɪəs] *adj* → urticarial.
ur·ti·ca·tion [ˌ-ˈkeɪʃn] *n* **1.** Nesselbildung *f,* Quaddelbildung *f.* **2.** Brennen *nt.*
Ur·u·ma virus [ˈ(j)ʊərəmə] Uruma-Virus *nt.*

US *abbr.* → unconditioned stimulus.
us·a·ble [ˈjuːzəbl] *adj* brauchbar, verwend-, verwertbar.
us·age [ˈjuːzɪdʒ] *n* → use I.
use [juːz] **I** *n* **1.** An-, Verwendung *f,* Gebrauch *m,* Benutzung *f.* **for** ~ zum Gebrauch. **in** ~ in Gebrauch, gebräuchlich. **in common** ~ allgemein gebräuchlich. **out of** ~ außer Gebrauch, nicht mehr gebräuchlich. **to come into** ~ in Gebrauch kommen. **to fall/go/pass out of** ~ ungebräuchlich werden. **to make** ~ **of** benutzen, Gebrauch machen von. **to make (a) bad** ~ **of** (einen) schlechten Gebrauch machen von. **2.** *(Drogen, Medikamente)* Einnahme *f.* **for external** ~ **(only)** (nur) zur äußerlichen Anwendung, (nur) äußerlich anzuwenden. **3.** Verwendungszweck *m;* Nutzung *f,* Verwertung *f.* **4.** Brauchbar-, Nutzbar-, Verwendbarkeit *f.* **5.** Zweck *m,* Sinn *m.* **of** ~ **to** nützlich für. **of no** ~ nutz-, zwecklos, unbrauchbar. **6.** Gewohnheit *f,* Sitte *f,* Brauch *m,* Usus *m,* Praxis *f,* Gepflogenheit *f.*
II *vt* **7.** gebrauchen, benutzen, benützen, an-, verwenden *(on* auf*)*; Gebrauch machen von, (aus-)nutzen. **to** ~ **care** Sorgfalt anwenden. **to** ~ **force** Gewalt anwenden. **8.** handhaben. **9.** → use up. **10.** *(Nahrung)* zu s. nehmen. **11.** jdn./etw. behandeln, verfahren mit.
use up *vt* auf-, verbrauchen, verwerten; jdn. auslaugen *od.* erschöpfen.
use·ful [ˈjuːzfl] *adj* nützlich, nutzbringend, brauchbar, praktisch, (zweck-)dienlich, verwendbar, zweckmäßig, Nutz-.
useful current *electr.* Wirkstrom *m.*
useful efficiency Nutzleistung *f.*
useful load Nutzlast *f.*
use·ful·ness [ˈjuːzflnɪs] *n* Nützlichkeit *f,* Brauchbarkeit *f,* Zweckmäßigkeit *f,* -dienlichkeit *f,* Nutzen *m.*
use·less [ˈjuːzlɪs] *adj* nutzlos, unnütz, zweck-, sinnlos; unwirksam, wirkungslos; unbrauchbar.
use·less·ness [ˈjuːzlɪsnɪs] *n* Nutzlosigkeit *f,* Zweck-, Sinnlosigkeit *f;* Unwirksamkeit *f,* Wirkungslosigkeit *f;* Unbrauchbarkeit *f.*
us·er [ˈjuːzər] *n* Benutzer(in *f*) *m.*
user-friendly *adj* benutzerfreundlich.
Usher [ˈʌʃər] **U.'s syndrome** Usher-Syndrom *nt.*
ush·er in [ˈʌʃər] *vt* *(Phase)* ankündigen, einleiten.
U-slab *n* *ortho.* U-Gips(schiene *f*) *m.*
us·ne·in [ˈʌsnɪɪn] *n* usnic acid.
us·nic acid [ˈʌsnɪk] Usninsäure *f.*
Us·ti·lag·i·na·les [ˌʌstɪˌlædʒəˈneɪliːz] *pl* *micro.* Ustilaginales *f.*
us·ti·lag·i·nism [ˌʌstəˈlædʒənɪzəm] *n* Ustilagismus *m.*
Us·ti·la·go [ˌʌstəˈleɪɡəʊ] *n* *micro.* Ustilago *f.*
U. maydis Maisbrand *m,* Ustilago maydis.
u·ta [ˈuːtə] *n* südamerikanische Hautleishmaniase *f,* kutane Leishmaniase *f* Südamerikas, Chiclero-Ulkus *m.*
u·ter·al·gia [juːtəˈrældʒ(ɪ)ə] *n* Gebärmutterschmerz(en *pl*) *m,* Hysteralgie *f,* Hysterodynie *f,* Metralgie *f,* Metrodynie *f.*
u·ter·ec·to·my [juːtəˈrektəmɪ] *n* *gyn.* Gebärmutterentfernung *f,* Hysterektomie *f,* Hysterectomia *f,* Uterusextirpation *f.*
u·ter·ine [ˈjuːtərɪn, -raɪn] *adj* Gebärmutter/Uterus betr., uterin, Gebärmutter-, Uterus-.
uterine adhesions *gyn.* Gebärmutterverwachsungen *pl,* -verklebungen *pl,* Uterusverwachsungen *pl,* -verklebungen *pl.*

uterine aplasia

cervical u. Zervixverwachsungen, -verklebungen.
corporeal u. Korpusverwachsungen, -verklebungen.
traumatic u. traumatische Uterusverwachsungen/-verklebungen.
uterine aplasia Gebärmutter-, Uterusaplasie *f*.
uterine apoplexy 1. hämorrhagische Endometriumnekrose *f*. **2.** Couvelaire-Syndrom *nt*, -Uterus *m*, Apoplexia uteroplacentaris, Uterusapoplexie *f*, uteroplazentare Apoplexie *f*.
uterine artery Gebärmutter-, Uterusschlagader *f*, Uterina *f*, A. uterina.
aortic u. Eierstockarterie *f*, Ovarica *f*, A. ovarica.
uterine bleeding Gebärmutter-, Uterusblutung *f*.
essential u. hämorrhagische Metropathie *f*, Metropathia haemorrhagica.
uterine calculus Gebärmutter-, Uterusstein *m*, Uterolith *m*, Hysterolith *m*.
uterine canal 1. Gebärmutterkanal *m*, -höhle *f*, Uteruskanal *m*, -höhle *f*. **2.** → uterovaginal canal.
uterine carcinoma Gebärmutterkrebs *m*, Uteruskarzinom *m*.
uterine cavity Gebärmutter-, Uterushöhle *f*, Cavitas uteri.
uterine circulation Uteruskreislauf *m*.
uterine colic Gebärmutter-, Uteruskolik *f*, Colica uterina.
uterine cycle Uteruszyklus *m*, zyklische Uterusveränderungen *pl*.
uterine extremity of ovary unterer Pol *od*. Uteruspol *m* des Ovars, Extremitas uterina ovarii.
uterine forceps *gyn*. Uterusfaßzange *f*.
uterine glands Gebärmutter-, Uterusdrüsen *pl*, Gll. uterinae.
uterine hemorrhage → uterine bleeding.
uterine hernia Hysterozele *f*, Hernia uterina.
uterine-holding forceps → uterine forceps.
uterine horn Gebärmutterzipfel *m*, Cornu uteri.
uterine hypoplasia Gebärmutter-, Uterushypoplasie *f*.
uterine inertia Wehenschwäche *f*, Inertia uteri.
uterine leiomyoma Uterus(leio)myom *nt*, Leiomyoma uteri.
uterine life Intrauterinperiode *f*.
uterine mucosa Uterusschleimhaut *f*, Endometrium *nt*, Tunica mucosa uteri.
uterine neck Uterus-, Gebärmutterhals, Zervix (uteri), Cervix uteri.
uterine opening of uterine tube Tubenmündung *f*, Ostium uterinum tubae (uterinae).
uterine orifice of uterine tube → uterine opening of uterine tube.
uterine ostium of uterine tube → uterine opening of uterine tube.
uterine pain Gebärmutterschmerz(en *pl*) *m*, Hysteralgie *f*, Hysterodynie *f*, Metralgie *f*, Metrodynie *f*.
uterine part of uterine tube Uterusabschnitt *m* der Tube, Pars uterina (tubae uterinae).
uterine plexus 1. uteriner Teil *m* des Plexus uterovaginalis. **2.** Plexus venosus uterinus.
uterine polyp Gebärmutter-, Uteruspolyp *m*.
uterine pregnancy (intra-)uterine/eutopische Schwangerschaft/Gravidität *f*.
uterine segment, lower u. unteres Uterussegment *nt*, Uterusenge *f*, Isthmus uteri.

uterine septum *embryo*. Uterusseptum *nt*.
uterine tube Eileiter *m*, Tube *f*, Ovidukt *m*, Tuba/Salpinx uterina.
uterine tympanitis *gyn*. Physometra *f*, Uterustympanie *f*, Tympania uteri.
uterine veins Gebärmutter-, Uterusvenen *pl*. Vv. uterinae.
u·ter·o·ab·dom·i·nal [ˌjuːtərəʊæb'dɒmɪnl] *adj* Gebärmutter/Uterus u. Abdomen *od*. Bauchhöhle betr., uteroabdominal, -abdominell.
u·ter·o·cer·vi·cal [ˌ-'sɜːvɪkəl] *adj* Gebärmutter/Uterus u. Gebärmutterhals/Cervix uteri betr. *od*. verbindend, uterozervikal.
uterocervical canal Zervixkanal *m*, Canalis cervicis uteri.
u·ter·o·dyn·ia [ˌ-'diːnɪə] *n* → uteralgia.
u·ter·o·fix·a·tion [ˌ-fɪk'seɪʃn] *n gyn*. Gebärmutterfixierung *f*, -anheftung *f*, Hysteropexie *f*, Uteropexie *f*.
u·ter·o·gen·ic [ˌ-'dʒenɪk] *adj* in der Gebärmutter gebildet, aus der Gebärmutter stammend, uterogen.
u·ter·o·ges·ta·tion [ˌ-dʒes'teɪʃn] *n* → uterine pregnancy.
u·ter·og·ra·phy [juːtə'rɒgrəfɪ] *n* **1.** *radiol*. Kontrastdarstellung *f* der Gebärmutterhöhle, Hysterographie *f*, Uterographie *f*. **2.** *gyn*. Hysterographie *f*.
u·ter·o·lith ['juːtərəlɪθ] *n* → uterine calculus.
u·ter·om·e·ter [ˌjuːtə'rɒmɪtər] *n gyn*. Hysterometer *nt*.
u·ter·om·e·try [ˌ-'rɒmɪtrɪ] *n gyn*. Hysterometrie *f*.
u·ter·o·o·var·i·an [ˌjuːtərəʊ'veərɪən] *adj* Gebärmutter/Uterus u. Eierstock/Ovar betr.
uteroovarian ligament Eierstockband *nt*, *old* Chorda utero-ovarica, Lig. ovarii proprium.
u·ter·o·per·i·to·ne·al fistula [ˌ-ˌperɪtəʊ'niːəl] uteroperitoneale/metroperitoneale Fistel *f*.
u·ter·o·pex·y ['-peksɪ] *n* → uterofixation.
u·ter·o·pla·cen·tal [ˌ-plə'sentl] *adj* Gebärmutter/Uterus u. Plazenta betr. *od*. verbindend, uteroplazental, -plazentär.
uteroplacental apoplexy → uterine apoplexy 2.
uteroplacental circulation uteroplazentärer Kreislauf *m*.
u·ter·o·plas·ty ['-plæstɪ] *n gyn*. Gebärmutter-, Uterusplastik *f*.
u·ter·o·rec·tal [ˌ-'rektl] *adj* Gebärmutter/Uterus u. Rektum betr. *od*. verbindend, uterorektal, rektouterin.
uterorectal fistula *patho*. Gebärmutter-Rektum-Fistel *f*, uterorektale/rektouterine Fistel *f*.
u·ter·o·sac·ral block [ˌ-'seɪkrəl] Parazervikalblock *m*, -anästhesie *f*.
uterosacral ligament: lateral u. Kardinalband *nt*, Lig. cardinale uteri.
posterior u. Sakrouteralband *nt*, Lig. sacrouterinum.
u·ter·o·sal·pin·gog·ra·phy [ˌ-ˌsælpɪŋ'gɒgrəfɪ] *n radiol., gyn*. Kontrastdarstellung *f* von Gebärmutter u. Eileiter, Utero-, Metro-, Hysterosalpingographie *f abbr*. HSG, Utero-, Metro-, Hysterotubographie *f*.
u·ter·o·scle·ro·sis [ˌ-sklɪ'rəʊsɪs] *n* Gebärmuttersklerose *f*.
u·ter·o·scope ['-skəʊp] *n* Hysteroskop *nt*.
u·te·ros·co·py [juːtə'rɒskəpɪ] *n* Gebärmutterspiegelung *f*, Hysteroskopie *f*.
u·ter·o·ther·mom·e·try [ˌ-θə'mɒmətrɪ] *n gyn*. Messung *f* der Gebärmuttertemperatur.
u·te·rot·o·my [juːtə'rɒtəmɪ] *n gyn*. Gebär-

mutterschnitt *m*, -eröffnung *f*, Hysterotomie *f*, Hysterotomia *f*.
u·ter·o·ton·ic [ˌjuːtərə'tɒnɪk] **I** *n* den Gebärmuttertonus erhöhendes Mittel *nt*. **II** *adj* den Gebärmuttertonus erhöhend.
u·ter·o·trop·ic [ˌ-'trɒpɪk, -'trəʊp-] *adj* mit besonderer Affinität zur Gebärmutter, uterotrop.
u·ter·o·tu·bal [ˌ-'tjuːbl] *adj* Gebärmutter/Uterus u. Eileiter/Tuba betr., uterotubal, tubouterin.
u·ter·o·tu·bog·ra·phy [ˌ-tjuː'bɒgrəfɪ] *n* → uterosalpingography.
u·ter·o·vag·i·nal [ˌ-'vædʒɪnl] *adj* Gebärmutter/Uterus u. Scheide/Vagina betr. *od*. verbindend, uterovaginal, Uterovaginal-.
uterovaginal canal *embryo*. Uterovaginalkanal *m*.
uterovaginal fistula *patho*. Gebärmutter-Scheiden-Fistel *f*, uterovaginale Fistel *f*, Fistula uterovaginalis.
uterovaginal plexus 1. Plexus uterovaginalis. **2.** Plexus venosus uterinis et vaginalis.
u·ter·o·ven·tral [ˌ-'ventrəl] *adj* → uteroabdominal.
u·ter·o·ves·i·cal [ˌ-'vesɪkl] *adj* Gebärmutter/Uterus u. Harnblase betr. *od*. verbindend, uterovesikal, vesikouterin.
uterovesical fistula *patho*. Gebärmutter-Blasen-Fistel *f*, Blasen-Gebärmutter-Fistel *f*, uterovesikale/vesikouterine Fistel *f*, Fistula vesicouterina.
uterovesical pouch vorderer Douglas'-Raum *m*, Excavatio vesicouterina.
u·ter·us ['juːtərəs] *n, pl* **-us·es, -teri** [-raɪ] *anat*. Gebärmutter *f*, Uterus *m*, Metra *f*.
UTI *abbr*. → urinary tract infection.
u·ti·liz·a·ble [juː'tɪlaɪzəbl] *adj* verwend-, verwertbar, brauch-, nutzbar.
u·ti·li·za·tion [juːtɪlaɪ'zeɪʃn] *n* (Aus-, Be-)Nutzung *f*, Verwendung *f*, Verwertung *f*, Nutzbarmachung *f*, Ausnutzung *f*, Utilisation *f*.
u·ti·lize ['juːtɪlaɪz] *vt* (aus-, be-)nutzen, verwenden, verwerten.
UTP *abbr*. → uridine(-5'-)triphosphate.
UTP-galactose-1-phosphate uridylyltransferase UTP-Galaktose-1-phosphaturidylyltransferase *f*.
UTP-glucose-1-phosphate uridylyltransferase UTP-Glukose-1-phosphaturidylyltransferase *f*.
u·tri·cle ['juːtrɪkl] *n anat*. **1.** (kleiner) Schlauch *m*, schlauchförmiges Gebilde *nt*, Utrikulus *m*, Utriculus *m*. **2.** (Ohr) Vorhofbläschen *nt*, Utriculus *m* (vestibuli).
u·tric·u·lar [juː'trɪkjələr] *adj* **1.** schlauch-, beutelförmig. **2.** Utriculus betr., Utrikulus-.
utricular nerve N. utricularis.
utricular part of otic vesicle *embryo*. Utriculusabschnitt *m* des Ohrbläschens.
utricular portion of otic vesicle → utricular part of otic vesicle.
utricular spot Macula utriculi.
u·tric·u·li·tis [juːˌtrɪkjə'laɪtɪs] *n* **1.** *urol*. Entzündung *f* des Utriculus prostaticus, Utrikulitis *f*, Utriculitis *f*. **2.** *HNO* Entzündung *f* des Utriculus vestibuli.
u·tric·u·lo·am·pul·lar nerve ['-æm'pʌlər, -'pʊl-] N. utriculoampullaris.
u·tric·u·lo·sac·cu·lar canal [ˌ-'sækjələr] *n* utriculosaccularis duct.
utriculosaccular duct Ductus utriculosaccularis.
u·tric·u·lus [juː'trɪkjələs] *n, pl* **-li** [-laɪ] → utricle.
u·tri·form ['juːtrəfɔːrm] *adj* flaschenförmig.
UV *abbr*. → ultraviolet I.

u·vea ['ju:vɪə] *n* mittlere Augenhaut *f*, Uvea *f*, Tunica vasculosa bulbis.
u·ve·al ['ju:vɪəl] *adj* Uvea betr., uveal, Uvea(l)-, Uveo-.
uveal coat → uvea.
uveal part of trabecular retinaculum vorderer Abschnitt *m* des Hueck'-Bands, Pars uvealis.
uveal tract → uvea.
u·ve·it·ic [ˌju:vɪ'ɪtɪk] *adj* Uveitis betr., uveitisch.
u·ve·i·tis [ˌ-'aɪtɪs] *n ophthal.* Uveaentzündung *f*, Uveitis *f*.
u·ve·o·cu·ta·ne·ous syndrome [ˌju:vɪəʊkju:'teɪnɪəs] Vogt-Koyanagi(-Harada)--Syndrom *nt*, okulokutanes Syndrom *nt*.
uveo-encephalitic syndrome Behçet--Krankheit *f*, -Syndrom *nt*, bipolare/große/maligne Aphthose *f*, Gilbert-Syndrom *nt*, Aphthose Touraine/Behçet.
u·ve·o·en·ceph·a·li·tis [ˌ-enˌsefə'laɪtɪs] *n ophthal.* Harada-Syndrom *nt*.
u·ve·o·men·in·gi·tis syndrome [ˌ-ˌmenɪn'dʒaɪtɪs] *ophthal.* Harada-Syndrom *nt*.
u·ve·o·pa·rot·id [ˌ-pə'rɑtɪd] *adj* Uvea u. Parotis betr.
uveoparotid fever Heerfordt-Syndrom *nt*, Febris uveoparotidea.
u·ve·o·par·o·ti·tis [ˌ-pærə'taɪtɪs] *n* Uveoparotitis *f*.
u·ve·o·scle·ri·tis [ˌ-sklɪ'raɪtɪs] *n ophthal.* Uveoskleritis *f*.
u·ve·ous ['ju:vɪəs] *adj* → uveal.
u·vi·form ['ju:vɪfɔ:rm] *adj* traubenförmig.
u·vi·o·fast ['ju:vɪəʊfæst] *adj* → uvioresistant.
u·vi·om·e·ter [ˌju:vɪ'ɑmɪtər] *n* UV-Strahlenmesser *m*.
u·vi·o·re·sist·ant [ˌju:vɪəʊrɪ'zɪstənt] *adj* widerstandsfähig gegen UV-Strahlen, UV-resistent.
u·vi·o·sen·si·tive [ˌ-'sensɪtɪv] *adj* empfindlich/sensibel gegen UV-Strahlen, UV--empfindlich.
UV irradiation UV-Bestrahlung *f*.
U virus Uppsala-Virus *nt*.
u·vu·la ['ju:vjələ] *n, pl* **-las, -lae** [-li:] *anat.* **1.** Zäpfchen *nt*, zapfenförmige Struktur *f*, Uvula *f*. **2.** (Gaumen-)Zäpfchen *nt*, Uvula *f* (palatina).
 u. of bladder Blasenzäpfchen, Uvula vesicae.
 u. of cerebellum Kleinhirnzäpfchen, Uvula vermis.
u·vu·lap·to·sis [ˌju:vjələp'təʊsɪs] *n* → uvuloptosis.
u·vu·lar ['ju:vjələr] *adj* Zäpfchen/Uvula betr., zum Zäpfchen/zur Uvula gehörend, uvulär, Zäpfchen-, Uvulo-, Uvula(r)-, Staphyl(o)-.
u·vu·la·tome ['ju:vjələtəʊm] *n* → uvulotome.
u·vu·lec·to·my ['ju:vjə'lektəmɪ] *n HNO* Zäpfchenentfernung *f*, Uvulektomie *f*.
u·vu·li·tis [ˌ-'laɪtɪs] *n* (Gaumen-)Zäpfchenentzündung *f*, Uvulitis *f*, Staphylitis *f*.
u·vu·lop·to·sis [ˌ-lɑp'təʊsɪs] *n* Zäpfchensenkung *f*, -tiefstand *m*, Uvuloptose *f*, Staphyloptose *f*.
u·vu·lo·tome ['-lətəʊm] *n HNO* Uvulotom *nt*, Staphylotom *nt*.
u·vu·lot·o·my [ˌ-'lɑtəmɪ] *n HNO* Uvulotomie *f*, Staphylotomie *f*.
U wave *physiol.* (*EKG*) U-Welle *f*, U--Zacke *f*.

V

V *abbr.* **1.** → vanadium. **2.** → volt.
VA *abbr.* **1.** → visual acuity. **2.** → volt-ampere.
V-A *abbr.* → ventriculoatrial.
vac·cen·ic acid [væk'senɪk] Vaccensäure *f*.
vac·ci·na [væk'saɪnə] *n* → vaccinia.
vac·ci·nal ['væksɪnl] *adj* Impfung/Vakzination *od.* Impfstoff/Vakzine betr., vakzinal, Impf-, Vakzine-.
vaccinal fever Impffieber *nt*.
vac·ci·nate ['væksɪneɪt] *vt, vi* impfen, vakzinieren (*against* gegen).
vac·ci·na·tion [,væksɪ'neɪʃn] *n* **1.** (Schutz-)Impfung *f*, Vakzination *f*. **2.** *histor.* Pockenschutzimpfung *f*, Vakzination *f*.
vac·ci·na·tor ['væksɪneɪtər] *n* **1.** Impfarzt *m*, -ärztin *f*. **2.** Impfmesser *nt*, -nadel *f*.
vac·cine [væk'siːn; 'væksiːn] **I** *n* Impfstoff *m*, Vakzine *f*, Vakzin *nt*. **II** *adj* → vaccinal.
vac·ci·nee [væksə'niː] *n* Geimpfter *m*, Impfling *m*.
vaccine virus Impfvirus *nt*.
vac·cin·ia [væk'sɪnɪə] *n* Impfpocken *pl*, Vaccinia *f*.
vaccinia growth factor Vaccinia-Wachstumsfaktor *m*.
vaccinia virus *micro.* Vaccinia-, Vakzinevirus *nt*.
vac·cin·i·al [væk'sɪnɪəl] *adj* Vaccinia betr., Vaccinia-, Vakzine-.
vac·cin·i·form [væk'sɪnɪfɔːrm] *adj* vacciniaähnlich, -artig.
vac·ci·nog·e·nous [væksɪ'nɑdʒənəs] *adj* Vakzine-bildend.
vac·ci·noid ['væksɪnɔɪd] *adj* vacciniaähnlich, vaccinoid.
vac·ci·no·pho·bia [,væksɪnəʊ'fəʊbɪə] *n psychia.* Vakzinophobie *f*.
vac·ci·num ['væksɪnəm] *n* → vaccine I.
V-A conduction *card.* retrograde Erregungsleitung *f*.
VACTERL syndrome [vertebral, anal, cardiac, tracheoesophageal, renal and limb anomalies] VACTERL-Syndrom *nt*.
vac·u·o·lar ['vækjə,əʊlər, 'vækjələr] *adj* vakuolenartig, vakuolär, Hohl-, Vakuolen-.
vacuolar degeneration vakuoläre Degeneration *f*.
vacuolar nephrosis hypokaliämische Nephropathie *f*.
vac·u·o·late ['vækjə(wə)lɪt, -leɪt] *adj* → vacuolated.
vac·u·o·lat·ed ['vækjə(wə)leɪtɪd] *adj* mit Vakuolen durchsetzt, vakuolenhaltig, vakuolär, vakuolisiert.
vacuolated cell vakuolenhaltige/vakuoläre Zelle *f*.
vac·u·o·la·tion [,vækjʊə'leɪʃn, ,vækjə-] *n* Vakuolenbildung *f*, Vakuolisierung *f*.
vac·u·ole ['vækjʊəʊl] *n* Vakuole *f*, Vakuolenhöhle *f*, -raum *m*.
vac·u·ol·i·za·tion [,vækjə,wəʊlə'zeɪʃn] *n* → vacuolation.
vac·u·um ['vækj(əw)əm] **I** *n, pl* **-u·ums**,

-ua [-jəwə] *phys.* (luft-)leerer Raum *m*, Vakuum *nt*. **II** *adj* Vakuum-.
vacuum aspiration *gyn.* Aspirations-, Saug-, Vakuumkürettage *f*.
vacuum curettage → vacuum aspiration.
vacuum distillation Vakuumdestillation *f*.
vacuum flask Dewar-Gefäß *nt*.
vacuum pump Vakuumpumpe *f*.
vacuum tube Vakuumröhrchen *nt*.
vag·a·bond's disease ['væɡəbɒnd] *derm.* Vaganten-, Vagabundenhaut *f*, Cutis vagantium.
va·gal ['veɪɡl] *adj* Vagusnerv betr., vagal, Vagus-, Vago-.
vagal attack vasovagale Synkope *f*.
vagal block Vagusblock(ade *f*) *m*.
vagal body Glomus aorticum.
vagal bradycardia *card.* vagotonische Bradykardie *f*.
vagal ganglion Vagusganglion *nt*, Ggl. n. vagi.
  caudal v. unteres Vagusganglion, Ggl. caudalis/inferius n. vagi.
  inferior v. → caudal v.
  jugular v. → superior v.
  lower v. → caudal v.
  rostral v. → superior v.
  superior v. oberes Vagusganglion, Ggl. rostralis/superius n. vagi.
vagal nerve: anterior v. vorderer Vagusstamm *m*, Truncus vagalis anterior.
  posterior v. hinterer Vagusstamm *m*, Truncus vagalis posterior.
vagal nucleus, dorsal hinterer Kern *m* des N. vagus, Nc. dorsalis n. vagi, Nc. vagalis dorsalis.
vagal phase (*Verdauung*) vagale/zephale Phase *f*.
vagal tone Vagustonus *m*.
vagal trigone Trigonum vagale, Trigonum n. vagi.
vagal trunk: anterior v. vorderer Vagusstamm *m*, Truncus vagalis anterior.
  posterior v. hinterer Vagusstamm *m*, Truncus vagalis posterior.
va·gec·to·my [veɪ'dʒektəmɪ] *n neurochir.* Vagusresektion *f*, Vagektomie *f*.
vagin- *pref.* → vagino-.
va·gi·na [və'dʒaɪnə] *n, pl* **-nas, -nae** [-niː] **1.** *anat.* Scheide *f*, Hülle *f*, Umscheidung *f*, Vagina *f*. **2.** *gyn.* Scheide *f*, Vagina *f*.
  v. of bulb Tenon'-Kapsel *f*, Vagina bulbi.
vag·i·nal ['vædʒənl; və'dʒaɪnl] *adj* Scheide/Vagina betr., vaginal, Scheiden-, Vaginal-.
vaginal artery Scheidenarterie *f*, Vaginalis *f*, A. vaginalis.
vaginal atresia Scheiden-, Vaginalatresie *f*, Atresia vaginalis.
vaginal branches: v. of middle rectal artery Vaginaäste *pl* der A. rectalis media, Rami vaginales a. rectalis mediae.
  v. of uterine artery Vaginaäste *pl* der A. uterina, Rami vaginales a. uterinae, Aa. azygoi vaginae.
vaginal bulb Schwellkörper *m* des Scheidenvorhofes, Bulbus vestibuli (vaginae).

vaginal canal Scheidenkanal *m*.
vaginal candidiasis *gyn.* Vaginalkandidose *f*, Kandidose *f* der Vagina.
vaginal celiotomy *gyn.* Kolpozöliotomie *f*, Coeliotomia vaginalis.
vaginal coat of testis Tunica vaginalis testis.
vaginal columns Längswülste *pl* der Vagina(l)wand, Columnae rugarum (vaginae).
vaginal cycle Vaginazyklus *m*, zyklische Vaginaveränderungen *pl*.
vaginal diaphragm *gyn.* Diaphragma(pessar) *nt*.
vag·i·nal·ec·to·my [,vædʒɪnə'lektəmɪ] *n* → vaginectomy.
vaginal examination vaginale Untersuchung *f*.
vaginal flora Scheidenflora *f*.
vaginal hernia Scheidenbruch *m*, Kolpozele *f*, Hernia vaginalis.
  posterior v. Enterozele *f*, Hernia vaginalis posterior.
vaginal hysterectomy *gyn.* transvaginale Gebärmutterentfernung/Hysterektomie *f*, Hysterectomia vaginalis.
vaginal introitus Scheideneingang *m*, Introitus/Ostium vaginae.
vag·i·na·li·tis [,vædʒɪnə'laɪtɪs] *n urol.* Entzündung *f* der Tunica vaginalis testis, Vaginalitis *f*.
vaginal ligament Lig. vaginale.
vaginal nerves Vaginaäste *pl* des Plexus uterovaginalis, Nn. vaginales.
vaginal opening → vaginal orifice.
vaginal orifice Scheidenöffnung *f*, -eingang *m*, Ostium vaginae.
  external v. → vaginal orifice.
vaginal pain → vaginodynia.
vaginal part: v. of cervix uteri Portio *f*, Portio vaginalis cervicis.
  v. of uterus → v. of cervix uteri.
vaginal plate *embryo.* Vaginaplatte *f*.
vaginal plexus 1. vaginaler Teil *m* des Plexus uterovaginalis. **2.** Plexus venosus vaginalis.
vaginal process: v. of peritoneum Proc. vaginalis peritonei.
  v. of testis Proc. vaginalis testis.
vaginal rugae Querfalten *pl* der Vagina(l)schleimhaut *f*, Rugae vaginales.
vaginal secretion Vagina(l)sekret *nt*.
vaginal smear Vaginal-, Scheidenabstrich *m*, Vaginalsmear *m*.
vaginal spasm Scheiden-, Vaginalkrampf *m*.
vaginal speculum → vaginoscope 1.
vaginal swab vaginaler Smear.
vaginal synovitis Sehnenscheidenentzündung *f*, Teno-, Tendosynovitis *f*, Tendovaginitis *f*.
vaginal tunic of testis seröse Hodenhülle *f*, Epi- u. Periorchium *nt*, Tunica vaginalis testis.
va·gi·na·pex·y [və'dʒaɪnəpeksɪ] *n* → vaginofixation.
vag·i·nate ['vædʒɪnɪt, -neɪt] **I** *adj* von einer

Scheide umgeben. **II** *vt* mit einer Scheide umgeben, umscheiden.
vag·i·nec·to·my [,-'nektəmɪ] *n gyn*. Kolpektomie *f*.
vag·i·ni·per·i·ne·ot·o·my [,vædʒənɪ,perɪnɪ-'atəmɪ] *n* Paravaginalschnitt *m*.
vag·i·nism ['vædʒɪnɪzəm] *n* → vaginismus.
vag·i·nis·mus [,-'nɪzməs] *n* Scheidenkrampf *m*, Vaginismus *m*.
vag·i·ni·tis [,-'naɪtɪs] *n gyn*. Scheidenentzündung *f*, Vaginitis *f*, Kolpitis *f*.
vagino- *pref.* Scheiden-, Vagin(o)-, Kolp(o)-.
vag·i·no·ab·dom·i·nal [,vædʒɪnəʊæb'dɑmɪnl] *adj* Scheide/Vagina u. Abdomen betr. *od.* verbindend, vaginoabdominal.
vag·i·no·cele ['-siːl] *n* Scheidenbruch *m*, Kolpozele *f*, Hernia vaginalis.
vag·i·no·cu·ta·ne·ous [,-kjuː'teɪnɪəs] *adj* Scheide/Vagina u. Haut betr. *od.* verbindend, vaginokutan.
vaginocutaneous fistula *patho.* äußere Scheidenfistel *f*, vaginokutane Fistel *f*.
vag·i·no·dyn·ia [,-'diːnɪə] *n* Scheidenschmerz *m*, Kolpalgie *f*, Vaginodynie *f*.
vag·i·no·fix·a·tion [,-fɪk'seɪʃn] *n gyn*. Scheidenanheftung *f*, Kolpo-, Vaginofixation *f*, -pexie *f*.
vag·i·no·gram ['-græm] *n* Vaginogramm *nt*.
vag·i·nog·ra·phy [,vædʒɪ'nɑgrəfɪ] *n radiol.* Kontrastdarstellung *f* der Scheide, Vaginographie *f*.
vag·i·no·hys·ter·ec·to·my [,vædʒɪnəʊ,hɪstə'rektəmɪ] *n* → vaginal hysterectomy.
vag·i·no·la·bi·al [,-'leɪbɪəl] *adj* Scheide/Vagina u. Schamlippen betr., vaginolabial.
vaginolabial hernia Hernia vaginolabialis, Hernia labialis posterior.
vag·i·no·my·co·sis [,-maɪ'kəʊsɪs] *n* Pilzerkrankung *f* der Scheide, Kolpo-, Vaginomykose *f*.
vag·i·nop·a·thy [,vædʒɪ'nɑpəθɪ] *n* Vaginal-, Scheidenerkrankung *f*, Vaginopathie *f*, Kolpopathie *f*.
vag·i·no·per·i·ne·al [,vædʒɪnəʊperɪ'niːəl] *adj* Scheide/Vagina u. Damm/Perineum betr. *od.* verbindend, vaginoperineal.
vag·i·no·per·i·ne·o·plas·ty [,-perɪ'niːəplæstɪ] *n gyn*. Scheiden-Damm-Plastik *f*, Kolpo-, Vaginoperineoplastik *f*.
vag·i·no·per·i·ne·or·rha·phy [,-perɪnɪ'ɔrəfɪ] *n gyn*. Scheiden-Damm-Naht *f*, Kolpo-, Vaginoperineorrhaphie *f*.
vag·i·no·per·i·ne·ot·o·my [,-perɪnɪ'atəmɪ] *n* Paravaginalschnitt *m*.
vag·i·no·per·i·to·ne·al [,-perɪtəʊ'niːəl] *adj* Scheide/Vagina u. Bauchfell/Peritoneum betr., vaginoperitoneal.
vag·i·no·pex·y ['-peksɪ] *n* → vaginofixation.
vag·i·no·plas·ty ['-plæstɪ] *n* Scheiden-, Vaginal-, Kolpo-, Vaginoplastik *f*.
vag·i·no·scope ['-skəʊp] *n* 1. Scheidenspekulum *nt*, Vaginoskop *nt*. 2. Kolposkop *nt*.
vag·i·nos·co·py [,vædʒɪ'nɑskəpɪ] *n* 1. Scheidenuntersuchung *f*, Vaginoskopie *f*. 2. Scheidenspiegelung *f*, Kolposkopie *f*.
vag·i·no·sis [,-'nəʊsɪs] *n* Scheiden-, Vaginaerkrankung *f*, Vaginose *f*, unspezifische Vulvovaginitis *f*.
vag·i·not·o·my [,-'natəmɪ] *n gyn*. Scheiden-, Vaginalschnitt *m*, Kolpo-, Vaginotomie *f*.
vag·i·no·ves·i·cal [,vædʒɪnəʊ'vesɪkl] *adj* Scheide/Vagina u. (Harn-)Blase betr. *od.* verbindend, vaginovesikal, vesikovaginal.
vaginovesical fistula *patho.* Scheiden--Blasen-Fistel *f*, Blasen-Scheiden-Fistel *f*, vaginovesikale/vesikovaginale Fistel *f*, Vesikovaginalfistel *f*, Fistula vesicovaginalis.
vag·i·no·vul·var [,-'vʌlvəl] *adj* → vulvovaginal.
va·go·ac·ces·so·ry syndrome [,veɪgəʊæk-'sesərɪ] Schmidt-Syndrom *nt*, thyreosuprarenales Syndrom *nt*.
va·go·glos·so·pha·ryn·ge·al nucleus [,-,glɑsəʊfə'rɪndʒɪəl] Nc. ambiguus.
va·go·gram ['-græm] *n* (Elektro-)Vagogramm *nt*.
va·gol·y·sis [veɪ'gɑləsɪs] *n neurochir.* Vagolyse *f*.
va·go·lyt·ic [,veɪgə'lɪtɪk] **I** *n* Vagolytikum *nt*, vagolytisches Mittel *nt*. **II** *adj* vagolytisch.
vagolytic agent → vagolytic I.
va·go·mi·met·ic [,-maɪ'metɪk] **I** *n* Vagomimetikum *nt*; Parasympathomimetikum *nt*. **II** *adj* vagomimetisch; parasympathomimetisch.
va·go·splanch·nic [,-'splæŋknɪk] *adj* → vagosympathetic.
va·go·sym·pa·thet·ic [,-sɪmpə'θetɪk] *adj* vagosympathisch.
va·got·o·my [veɪ'gɑtəmɪ] *n neurochir.* Vagusdurchtrennung *f*, -schnitt *m*, Vagotomie *f*.
va·go·to·nia [,veɪgə'təʊnɪə] *n neurochir.* Parasympathikotonie *f*.
va·go·ton·ic [,-'tɑnɪk] *adj* Vagotonie betr., durch Vagotonie gekennzeichnet, vagoton.
va·got·o·ny [veɪ'gɑtəmɪ] *n* → vagotonia.
va·go·trope ['veɪgətrəʊp] *adj* → vagotropic.
va·go·trop·ic [,-'trɑpɪk, -'trəʊ-] *adj* auf den N. vagus einwirkend, vagotrop.
va·got·ro·pism [veɪ'gɑtrəpɪzəm] *n* Vagotropie *f*, -tropismus *m*.
va·go·va·gal ['veɪgəʊ'veɪgl] *adj* vagovagal.
vagovagal reflex vagovagaler Reflex *m*.
va·grant ['veɪgrənt] *adj* (*Zelle*) wandernd; (*Gewebe*) wuchernd.
vagrant's disease → vagabond's disease.
va·gus ['veɪgəs] *n, pl* **-gi** [-dʒaɪ, -gaɪ] Vagus *m*, X. Hirnnerv *m*, N. vagus.
vagus nerve → vagus.
vagus nerve block Vagusblock(ade *f*) *m*.
vagus neuralgia Vagusneuralgie *f*.
vagus pulse Vaguspuls *m*.
vagus reflex Vagusreflex *m*.
vagus-stoff ['veɪgəstɑf] *n old* → acetylcholine.
Val *abbr.* → valine.
va·lence ['veɪləns] *n* 1. *chem., biochem., mathe., phys.* Wertigkeit *f*, Valenz *f*. 2. Vermögen *nt*, Fähigkeit *f*, Stärke *f*, Valenz *f*.
valence change *chem.* Valenzwechsel *m*.
valence electron Valenzelektron *nt*.
va·len·cy ['veɪlənsɪ] *n* → valence.
Valentin ['vælənti:n]: **V.'s pseudoganglion** Ggl. tympanicum, Intumescentia tympanica.
tympanic ganglion of V. → V.'s pseudoganglion.
Valentine ['vælənt aɪn]: **V.'s test** *urol.* Dreigläserprobe *f*.
val·er·ate ['vælər eɪt] *n* Valerat *nt*, Valerianat *nt*.
va·le·ri·an [və'lɪər ən] *n* Baldrian *nt*, Valeriana *f*.
Va·le·ri·an·a [və,lɪər ɪ'ænə] *n bio., pharm.* Valeriana *f*.
V. officinalis echter/gemeiner Baldrian *m*, Valeriana officinalis.
va·le·ri·a·nate [və'lɪər ɪən eɪt] *n* → valerate.
va·le·ri·an·ic acid [və,lɪər ɪ'ænɪk] → valeric acid.
va·le·ri·an oil [və'lɪər ɪən] Valerianöl *nt*.

valva

va·le·ric acid [və'lerɪk, -'lɪər-] Valeriansäure *f*.
val·e·tu·di·nar·i·an [,vælɪ,t(j)uːdə'neərɪən] **I** *n* 1. chronisch Kranke(r *m*) *f*, Invalide(r *m*) *f*. 2. kränkliche Person *f*; Hypochonder *m*. **II** *adj* 3. kränklich, kränkelnd. 4. hypochondrisch.
val·e·tu·di·nar·i·an·ism [,-,t(j)uːdə'neərɪənɪzəm] *n* 1. Kränklichkeit *f*, Anfälligkeit *f*. 2. Hypochondrie *f*.
val·e·tu·di·nar·y [,-'t(j)uːdənərɪ] *n, adj* → valetudinarian.
val·gus ['vælgəs] *adj* krumm, nach innen gewölbt, Valgus-, X-.
valgus osteotomy *ortho.* Valgusosteotomie *f*.
val·id ['vælɪd] *adj* 1. (*Gründe*) stichhaltig, triftig; begründet, berechtigt; (*Entscheidung*) richtig; (*Methode*) wirksam. 2. rechtskräftig, rechtsgültig; (*Vertrag*) bindend.
va·lid·i·ty [və'lɪdətɪ] *n stat.* Gültigkeit *f*, Validität *f*.
va·line ['væliːn, 'veɪl-, -ɪn] *n abbr.* **Val** Valin *nt abbr.* Val, α-Aminoisovaleriansäure *f*.
val·i·ne·mia [vælɪ'niːmɪə] *n* erhöhter Valingehalt *m* des Blutes, Hypervalinämie *f*, Valinämie *f*.
valine transaminase Valintransaminase *f*.
val·late papillae ['væleɪt] Wallpapillen *pl*, Papillae vallatae.
val·lec·u·la [və'lekjələ] *n, pl* **-lae** [-liː] *anat.* 1. kleine Ritze *f*, Spalt(e *f*) *m*, Furche *f*, Vallecula *f*. 2. Vallecula epiglottica.
vallecula cerebelli mediane Kleinhirnfurche *f*, Vallecula cerebelli.
val·lec·u·lar dysphagia [və'lekjələr] Dysphagia vallecularis.
Valleix [va'lɛj]: **V.'s points** Valleix-Punkte *pl*.
val·ley ['vælɪ] *n* Tal *nt*.
v. of cerebellum mediane Kleinhirnfurche *f*, Vallecula cerebelli.
valley fever San-Joaquin-Valley-Fieber *nt*, Wüsten-, Talfieber *nt*, Primärform *f* der Kokzidioidomykose.
val·lis ['vælɪs] *n, pl* **-les** Valley of cerebellum.
val·lum ['væləm] *n, pl* **-la** [-lə] *anat.* Wall *m*, Vallum *m*.
val·pro·ate ['vælprəʊeɪt] *n* Valproat *nt*.
val·pro·ic acid [væl'prəʊɪk] *pharm.* Valproinsäure *f*, Dipropylessigsäure *f*.
Valsalva [væl'sælvə]: **V.'s experiment** → V.'s maneuver.
ligaments of V. Ohrmuschelbänder *pl*, Ligg. auriculana.
V.'s maneuver 1. *HNO* Valsalva-Versuch *m*. **2.** *card.* Valsalva-Preßdruckversuch *m*.
V.'s muscle M. tragicus.
sinus of V. Aortensinus *m*, Sinus aortae.
taeniae of V. Kolontänien *pl*, Taeniae coli.
V.'s test → V.'s maneuver.
val·u·a·ble ['væljəbl, 'vælju:əbl] *adj* 1. nützlich, förderlich, zuträglich, hilfreich. 2. wertvoll; kostbar, teuer.
val·u·a·ble·ness ['væljəbəlnɪs, 'vælju:əbl-] *n* Nützlichkeit *f*; Wert *m*.
val·u·a·bles ['væljəblz, 'vælju:əblz] *pl* Wertsachen *pl*, Wertgegenstände *pl*.
val·u·a·tion [vælju:'eɪʃn] *n* Bewertung *f*, Wertbestimmung *f*, Veranschlagung *f*, Taxierung *f*.
val·ue ['væljuː] **I** *n* 1. *allg., fig.* Wert *m*. 2. Einschätzung *f*. 3. *phys., bio., chem.* Gehalt *m*, Grad *m*; *stat., mathe.* (Zahlen-)Wert *m*. **II** *vt* 4. (ab-)schätzen, bewerten; den Wert bestimmen *od.* festsetzen, taxieren. 5. (wert-)schätzen, Wert legen auf.
val·va ['vælvə] *n, pl* **-vae** [-viː] → valve 1.

valval

val·val ['vælvl] *adj* → valvular.
val·var ['vælvər] *adj* → valvular.
val·vate ['vælveɪt] *adj* mit Klappe(n) versehen, Klappen-.
valve [vælv] *n* **1.** *anat.* Klappe *f*, Valva *f*, Valvula *f*. **2.** *techn.* Ventil *nt*, Klappe *f*, Hahn *m*.
 v. of coronary sinus Sinusklappe, Thebesius-(Sinus-)Klappe, Valvula sinus coronarii.
 v. of foramen ovale 1. Valvula foraminis ovalis, Falx septi. **2.** Septum primum.
 v. of inferior vena cava *embryo.* Eustachio'-Klappe, Sylvius'-Klappe, Valvula venae cavae inferioris.
 v. of Macalister Bauhin'-Klappe, Ileozökal-, Ileozäkalklappe, Valva ileocaecalis/ ilealis.
 v. of pulmonary trunk Pulmonal(is)klappe, Valva trunci pulmonalis.
 v. of Sylvius → v. of inferior vena cava.
 v. of Varolius → v. of Macalister.
 v. of veins Venenklappe, Valvula venosa.
valve cusp Klappentasche *f*.
valved [vælvd] *adj* mit Klappen versehen, Klappen-, Ventil-.
valve·less ['vælvlɪs] *adj* klappen-, ventillos.
valve·like ['vælvlaɪk] *adj anat.* klappen-, ventilähnlich.
valve plane Ventilebene *f*.
valve plane mechanism *physiol.* Ventilebenenmechanismus *m*.
valve pneumothorax Ventilpneu(mothorax *m*) *m*.
valve system *anat.* Klappenapparat *m*.
val·vi·form ['vælvɪfɔːrm] *adj* klappenförmig, -artig.
val·vo·plas·ty ['vælvoʊplæstɪ] *n HTG* (Herz-)Klappenplastik *f*, Valvo-, Valvuloplastik *f*.
val·vo·tome ['-toʊm] *n HTG* Valvotom *nt*, Valvulotom *nt*.
val·vot·o·my [væl'vɑtəmɪ] *n HTG* (Herz-)Klappenspaltung *f*, Valvo-, Valvulotomie *f*.
val·vu·la ['vælvjələ] *n, pl* **-lae** [-liː] *anat.* kleine Klappe *f*, Valvula *f*.
val·vu·lar ['vælvjələr] *adj* (Herz-)Klappe(n) betr., mit Klappe(n) versehen, klappenförmig, Klappen-.
valvular cardiopathy Kardiopathie *f* bei Klappendefekt, valvuläre Kardiopathie *f*.
valvular defect (Herz-)Klappenfehler *m*, -defekt *m*.
valvular disease (Herz-)Klappenerkrankung *f*.
 stenotic v. → valvular stenosis.
valvular endocarditis Endokarditis *f* der Herzklappen, Endokarditis valvularis.
valvular incompetence Herzklappeninsuffizienz *f*.
valvular injury (Herz-)Klappenverletzung *f*.
valvular insufficiency (Herz-)Klappeninsuffizienz *f*.
valvular pneumothorax → valve pneumothorax.
valvular regurgitation (Herz-)Klappeninsuffizienz *f*.
valvular sclerosis (Herz-)Klappensklerose *f*.
valvular stenosis (Herz-)Klappenstenose *f*.
val·vule ['vælvjuːl] *n* → valvula.
val·vu·li·tis [ˌvælvjəˈlaɪtɪs] *n* **1.** Klappenentzündung *f*, Valvulitis *f*. **2.** Herzklappenentzündung *f*; Endokarditis *f*.
val·vu·lo·plas·ty ['vælvjələʊplæstɪ] *n* → valvoplasty.
val·vu·lo·tome ['-toʊm] *n* → valvotome.

val·vu·lot·o·my [ˌvælvjəˈlɑtəmɪ] *n* → valvotomy.
val·yl ['vælɪl, 'veɪlɪl] *n* Valyl-(Radikal *nt*).
van·a·date ['vænədeɪt] *n* Vanadat *nt*.
va·nad·ic acid [vəˈnædɪk, -ˈneɪd-] Vanadinsäure *f*.
va·na·di·um [vəˈneɪdɪəm] *n abbr.* **V** Vanadium *nt abbr.* V, Vanadin *nt*.
va·na·di·um·ism [vəˈneɪdɪəmɪzəm] *n* chronische Vanadiumvergiftung *f*, Vanadismus *f*.
van Bogaert [væn ˈboʊɡərt]: **v.B.'s disease** subakute sklerosierende Panenzephalitis *f abbr.* SSPE, Einschlußkörperchenenzephalitis *f* Dawson, subakute sklerosierende Leukenzephalitis *f* van Bogaert.
 v.B.'s encephalitis → v.B.'s disease.
 v.B.'s sclerosing leukoencephalitis → v.B.'s disease.
van Buchem [væn ˈbuːkəm, ˈbuːx-]: **v.B.'s syndrome** van Buchem-Syndrom *nt*, Hyperostosis corticalis generalisata.
van Buren [væn ˈbjʊərən]: **v.B.'s disease** Peyronie-Krankheit *f*, Penisfibromatose *f*, Induratio penis plastica, Sclerosis fibrosa penis.
van·co·my·cin [ˈvænkəʊmaɪsɪn] *n pharm.* Vancomycin *nt*.
van den Bergh [væn dən bɑrɡ]: **v.d.B.'s disease** Stokvis-Talma-Syndrom *nt*, autotoxische Zyanose *f*.
 v.d.B.'s reaction (van den) Bergh-Reaktion *f*.
van der Hoeve [væn dər ˈhoʊv]: **v.d.H.'s syndrome** van der Hoeve-Syndrom *nt*.
van der Waals [væn dər wɑːlz, wɔːlz]:
 v.d.W. attractions van der Waals'-Anziehungskräfte *pl*.
 v.d.W. bond van der Waals'-Bindung *f*.
 v.d.W. forces van der Waals'-Anziehungskräfte *pl*.
 v.d.W. interaction van der Waals'-Wechselwirkung *f*.
 v.d.W. radius van der Waals'-Radius *m*.
van Gehuchten [væn ɡeɪˈhʊktən]: **cell of v.G.** Neuron *nt* vom Golgi-Typ.
van Gieson [væn ˈɡiːzən]: **elastica-v.G. stain** *abbr.* E.v.G. *histol.* Elastica-van Gieson-Färbung *f*, E.v.G-Färbung *f*.
 v.G.'s stain *abbr.* v.G. van Gieson-Färbung *f*, v.G.-Färbung *f*.
van Helmont [væn ˈhelmɑnt]: **v.H.'s mirror** Centrum tendineum.
van Hoorne [væn ˈhɔːrn]: **v.H.'s canal** Brustmilchgang *m*, Milchbrustgang *m*, Ductus thoracicus.
va·nil·la [vəˈnɪlə, -ˈnelə] *n* Vanille *f*.
va·nil·lic acid [vəˈnɪlɪk] Vanillinsäure *f*.
va·nil·lin [vəˈnɪlɪn, ˈvænl-] *n* Vanillin *nt*.
va·nil·lyl·man·del·ic acid [ˌvænɪlˈmændelɪk, -ˈdiːl-, vəˌnɪlɪl-] *abbr.* **VMA** Vanillinmandelsäure *f abbr.* VMS, VMA.
van Neck [væn nek]: **v.N.'s disease** (van) Neck-Odelberg-Syndrom *nt*, Osteochondrosis ischiopubica.
van't Hoff [vænt hɔf]: **v.H.'s law/rule** van't Hoff-Gesetz *nt*, -Regel *f*.
V antigen V-Antigen *nt*.
Vanzetti [vanˈtsetɪ]: **V.'s sign** Vanzetti-Zeichen *nt*.
va·por ['veɪpər] **I** *n, pl* **-res 1.** Dampf *m*, Dunst *m*, Nebel *m*; Vapor *m*. **2.** Gas(gemisch *nt*) *nt*. **3.** *pharm.* (Inhalations-)Dampf *m*. **II** *vt, vi* → vaporize.
va·por·a·ble ['veɪpərəbl] *adj* ver-, eindampfbar.
vapor bath Dampfbad *nt*, Balneum vaporis.
va·por·if·ic [ˌveɪpəˈrɪfɪk] *adj* **1.** dampferzeugend. **2.** → vaporous.
va·por·i·za·tion [ˌveɪpərɪˈzeɪʃn] *n* Verdampfung *f*, Verdunstung *f*; Zerstäu-

bung *f*; Vaporisation *f*, Vaporisierung *f*.
va·por·ize ['veɪpəraɪz] **I** *vt* ver-, eindampfen; verdunsten lassen; zerstäuben, vernebeln; vaporisieren. **II** *vi* verdampfen, verdunsten.
va·por·iz·er ['veɪpəraɪzər] *n* Zerstäuber *m*; Verdampfer *m*, Verdampfungsgerät *nt*; Vaporizer *m*.
va·por·ous ['veɪpərəs] *adj* dunstig, dampfig, neblig.
vapor pressure *phys.* Dampfdruck *m*.
vapor pressure depression *phys.* Dampfdruckerniedrigung *f*.
vapor tension → vapor pressure.
va·por·y ['veɪpərɪ] *adj* → vaporous.
Vaquez [vaˈkeɪ]: **V.'s disease** Morbus Vaquez-Osler *m*, Vaquez-Osler-Syndrom *nt*, Osler-Krankheit, Osler-Vaquez-Krankheit, Polycythaemia (rubra) vera, Erythrämie *f*.
Vaquez-Osler [ˈɑzlər]: **V.-O. disease** → Vaquez's disease.
var. *abbr.* → variety 1.
var·i·a·bil·i·ty [ˌveərɪəˈbɪlətɪ] *n* Veränderlichkeit *f*, Variabilität *f*; Unbeständigkeit *f*, Wechselhaftigkeit *f*, Variationsfähigkeit *f*.
var·i·a·ble ['veərɪəbl] **I** *n mathe.* variable Größe *f*, Veränderliche *f*, Variable *f*. **II** *adj* **1.** veränderlich, wandelbar, variable; unbeständig, wechselhaft, schwankend, variationsfähig. **2.** *mathe., phys., bio.* wandelbar, ungleichförmig, variabel. **3.** *techn.* regel-, regulierbar, ver-, einstellbar, variabel.
variable deceleration *gyn.* variables Tief *nt*, variable Dezeleration *f*.
var·i·a·ble·ness ['veərɪəblnɪs] *n* → variability.
variable penetrance *genet.* variable Penetranz *f*.
variable region *biochem.* variable Region *f*, V-Region *f*.
var·i·ance ['veərɪəns] *n* Veränderlichkeit *f*; Abweichung *f*; Unstimmig-, Uneinigkeit *f*; *stat.* Varianz *f*. **at** → im Widerspruch *od.* Gegensatz stehen zu
var·i·ant ['veərɪənt] **I** *n* Variante *f*, Abart *f*, Spielart *f*, -form *f*. **II** *adj* andere(r, s), veränderlich, abweichend, verschieden, unterschiedlich, variant.
var·i·ate ['veərɪət, -eɪt] *n* (Zufalls-)Variable *f*.
var·i·a·tion [ˌveərɪˈeɪʃn] *n* **1.** Veränderung *f*, Abwandlung *f*, Schwankung(en *pl*) *f*, Wechsel *m*, Abweichung *f*, Variation *f*. **2.** *mathe., bio.* Variation *f*, Variante *f*.
var·i·a·tion·al [ˌveərɪˈeɪʃnl] *adj* Variations-.
varic- *pref.* → varico-.
var·i·ca·tion [ˌveərɪˈkeɪʃn] *n* **1.** Varixbildung *f*. **2.** Varikosität *f*. **3.** → varix.
var·i·ce·al [ˌ-ˈsiːəl, vəˈrɪsɪəl] *adj* Varix betr., Varizen-, Varik(o)-.
variceal bleeding Varizenblutung *f*.
variceal hemorrhage → variceal bleeding.
variceal ligation *chir.* Varizenligation *f*.
variceal node Varixknoten *m*.
var·i·cel·la [ˌ-ˈselə] *n* Wind-, Wasserpocken *pl*, Varizellen *pl*, Varicella *f*.
varicella encephalitis Varizellen-Enzephalitis *f*.
varicella pneumonia Varizellen-Pneumonie *f*.
varicella vaccine Varicella-Vakzine *f*.
varicella virus old → varicella-zoster virus.
varicella-zoster immune globulin *abbr.* **VZIG** Varicella-Zoster-Immunglobulin *nt abbr.* VZIG.
varicella-zoster virus *abbr.* **VZV** *micro.* Varicella-Zoster-Virus *nt abbr.* VZV.

var·i·cel·li·form [ˌ-'selɪfɔːrm] *adj* Windpocken-ähnlich, varicelliform.
var·i·cel·loid [ˌ-'selɔɪd] *adj* → varicelliform.
var·i·ces *pl* → varix.
va·ric·i·form [vəˈrɪsəfɔːrm] *adj* varizenähnlich, varikös.
varico- *pref.* Krampfader-, Varizen-, Varik(o)-.
var·i·co·bleph·a·ron [ˌværɪkəʊˈblefərən] *n ophthal.* Varikoblepharon *nt*.
var·i·co·cele [ˈ-siːl] *n* Krampfaderbruch *m*, Varikozele *f*, Hernia varicosa.
var·i·co·ce·lec·to·my [ˌ-sɪˈlektəmɪ] *n urol.* Varikozelenexzision *f*.
var·i·cog·ra·phy [ˌværɪˈkɑgrəfɪ] *n radiol., urol.* Kontrastdarstellung *f* von Varizen, Varikographie *f*.
var·i·coid [ˈværɪkɔɪd] *adj* → variciform.
var·i·cole [ˈværɪkəʊl] *n* → varicocele.
var·i·com·pha·lus [ˌværɪˈkɑmfələs] *n ped.* Varikomphalus *m*.
var·i·co·phle·bi·tis [ˌværɪkəʊflɪˈbaɪtɪs] *n* Krampfader-, Varizenentzündung *f*, Varikophlebitis *f*.
var·i·cose [ˈværɪkəʊs] *adj* Varize *od.* Varikose betr., varikös, Varizen-, Varik(o)-, Krampfader-.
varicose aneurysm variköses Aneurysma *nt*, Aneurysma varicosum.
varicose ulcer Ulcus (cruris) varicosum.
varicose veins Krampfadern *pl*, Varizen *pl*, Varixknoten *pl*.
var·i·co·sis [ˌværɪˈkəʊsɪs] *n* ausgedehnte Krampfaderbildung *f*, Varikose *f*, Varicosis *f*.
var·i·cos·i·ty [ˌ-ˈkɑsətɪ] *n* 1. Varikosität *f*. 2. → varix.
var·i·cot·o·my [ˌ-ˈkɑtəmɪ] *n chir.* Varikotomie *f*.
va·ric·u·la [vəˈrɪkjələ] *n ophthal.* Konjunktivalvarize *f*.
var·ied [ˈveərɪːd] *adj* 1. vielfarbig, bunt. 2. (ab-)geändert, verändert, variiert.
var·i·e·gate porphyria [ˈveərɪəgeɪt, ˈveərɪgeɪt] gemischte (hepatische) Porphyrie *f*, (hereditäre) Protokoproporphyrie *f*, südafrikanische genetische Porphyrie *f*, Porphyria variegata *abbr.* PV.
va·ri·e·ty [vəˈraɪətɪ] *n, pl* **-ties 1.** *abbr.* **var.** *micro., genet.* Varietät *f*, Varietas *f abbr.* var., Typ *m*, Stamm *m*, Rasse *f*, Variante *f*, Spielart *f*. 2. Verschiedenheit *f*, Buntheit *f*, Vielseitigkeit *f*, Mannigfaltigkeit *f*, Abwechslung *f*. 3. Vielfalt *f*, Reihe *f*, Anzahl *f*.
va·ri·o·la [vəˈraɪələ] *pl* Pocken *pl*, Blattern *pl*, Variola *f*.
variola minor weiße Pocken *pl*, Alastrim *nt*, Variola minor.
va·ri·o·lar [vəˈraɪələr] *adj* Pocken/Variola betr., Pocken-, Variola-.
va·ri·o·la·tion [ˌveərɪəˈleɪʃn] *n* Variolation *f*.
variola virus *micro.* Pockenvirus *nt*, Variolavirus *m*.
var·i·ol·ic [ˌveərɪˈɑlɪk] *adj* → variolar.
var·i·ol·i·form [ˌ-ˈɑlɪfɔːrm] *adj* → varioloid II.
varioliform syphilid pustulöses Syphilid *nt*.
var·i·o·li·za·tion [ˌveərɪəlɪˈzeɪʃn] *n* → variolation.
var·i·o·loid [ˈveərɪəlɔɪd] I *n* Variola benigna. II *adj* pockenähnlich, -artig, varioliform.
va·ri·o·lous [vəˈraɪələs] *adj* → variolar.
var·is·tor [væˈrɪstər] *n phys.* Varistor *m*.
var·ix [ˈveərɪks] *n, pl* **var·i·ces** [ˈveərəsiːz] Varix(knoten *m*) *f*, Varize *f*, Krampfader(knoten *m*) *f*.
varix bleeding Varizenblutung *f*.

varix hemorrhage → varix bleeding.
Varolius [vəˈrəʊlɪəs]: **bridge of V.** (*ZNS*) Brücke *f*, Pons cerebri.
var·us [ˈveərəs] *adj* varus, nach außen gekrümmt, Varus-, O-.
varus malposition Varusfehlstellung *f*.
varus osteotomy *ortho.* Varusosteotomie *f*.
var·y [ˈveərɪ] I *vt* (ver-, ab-)ändern; variieren, abwandeln. II *vi* 1. s. (ver-)ändern, variieren, wechseln, schwanken. 2. abweichen (*from* von); nicht übereinstimmen (*with* mit); s. unterscheiden.
var·y·ing [ˈveərɪɪŋ] *adj* veränderlich, unterschiedlich, wechselnd.
vas- *pref.* → vaso-.
vas [ˈvæs] *n, pl* **va·sa** [ˈveɪsə, -zə] Gefäß *nt*, Vas *nt*.
vasal [ˈveɪzl] *adj* Gefäß betr., Gefäß-, Vas(o)-.
va·sal·gia [vəˈsældʒ(ɪ)ə] *n* Gefäßschmerz *m*, Vasalgie *f*, Vasodynie *f*.
vasa vasorum Vasa vasorum.
vas clamp *chir.* Gefäßklemme *f*.
vas·cu·lar [ˈvæskjələr] *adj* (Blut-)Gefäß(e) betr., vaskulär, vaskular, Gefäß-, Vaskulo-, Vaso-.
vascular access *chir.* vaskulärer Zugang *m*.
vascular atrophy vaskuläre Atrophie *f*.
vascular bud *embryo.* Gefäßanlage *f*, -knospe *f*.
vascular cecal fold Plica caecalis vascularis.
vascular circle *anat.* Circulus vasculosus.
v. of optic nerve Haller'-Gefäßkranz *m*, Zinn'-Gefäßkranz *m*, Circulus vasculosus n. optici.
vascular clamp *chir.* Gefäßklemme *f*.
vascular coat: v. of eye (ball) → vascular tunic of eye (ball).
v. of stomach Tela submucosa ventriculi.
vascular compartment Lacuna vasorum.
vascular cones Coni/Lobuli epididymidis.
vascular forceps *chir.* Gefäßpinzette *f*.
vascular goiter of the newborn Struma vasculosa neonatorum.
vascular graft Gefäßtransplantat *nt*.
vascular headache Migräne *f*, Migraine *f*.
vascular hemophilia von Willebrand-Jürgens-Syndrom *nt*, konstitutionelle Thrombopathie *f*, hereditäre/vaskuläre Pseudohämophilie *f*, Angiohämophilie *f*.
vascular hyalin Gefäßhyalin *nt*.
vascular hypertension Bluthochdruck *m*, (arterielle) Hypertonie *f*, Hypertension *f*, Hypertonus *m*, Hochdruckkrankheit *f*.
vascular injury Gefäßverletzung *f*, -trauma *nt*.
vas·cu·lar·i·ty [ˌvæskjəˈlærətɪ] *n* Gefäßreichtum *m*, Vaskularität *f*.
vas·cu·lar·i·za·tion [ˌvæskjələrɪˈzeɪʃn] *n* Gefäß(neu)bildung *f*, Vaskularisation *f*, Vaskularisierung *f*.
vas·cu·lar·ize [ˈvæskjələraɪz] I *vt* mit Blutgefäßen versorgen, vaskularisieren. II *vi* Blutgefäße (aus-)bilden.
vascular keratitis Keratitis vascularis.
vascular lamina of choroid Haller'-Membran *f*, Lamina vasculosa (choroidea).
vascular layer of myometrium Vaskulärschicht *f* des Myometriums, Stratum vasculare (myometrii).
vascular leiomyoma Angiomyom(a) *nt*.
vascular malformation Gefäßfehlbildung *f*, -malformation *f*.
vascular membrane of viscera Tela submucosa.
vascular murmur Gefäßgeräusch *nt*.
vascular nevus vaskulärer Nävus *m*, Naevus vasculosus.

vasocongestion

vascular occlusion Gefäßverschluß *m*.
vascular organ of lamina terminalis Organum vasculosum laminae terminalis.
vascular permeability Gefäßpermeabilität *f*.
vascular plexus Gefäßgeflecht *nt*, -plexus *m*, Plexus vasculosus.
vascular pole of glomerulus (*Niere*) Gefäßpol *m* des Glomerulums.
vascular polyp *HNO* angiomatöser Polyp *m*.
vascular prosthesis *HTG* Gefäßprothese *f*.
vascular reconstruction *HTG* Gefäßrekonstruktion *f*.
vascular resistance Gefäßwiderstand *m*.
vascular scissors *chir.* Gefäßschere *f*.
vascular sclerosis *inf.* Arterienverkalkung *f*, Arteriosklerose *f*, -sclerosis *f*.
vascular spider Sternnävus *m*, Spider naevus, Naevus araneus.
vascular stria of cochlear duct Stria vascularis (ductus cochlearis).
vascular supply Gefäßversorgung *f*.
vascular suture *chir.* Gefäßnaht *f*.
vascular system Gefäßsystem *nt*.
vascular theory of ulcer formation Gefäßtheorie *f* der Ulkusentstehung.
vascular tone Gefäßtonus *m*.
vascular tumor Gefäßgeschwulst *f*, -tumor *m*; Angiom *nt*.
vascular tunic of eye (ball) mittlere Augenhaut *f*, Uvea *f*, Tunica vasculosa bulbis, Tractus uvealis.
vascular villi Gefäßzotten *pl*.
vas·cu·la·ture [ˈvæskjələtʃʊər] *n* Gefäßsystem *nt*, Gefäßversorgung *f*.
vas·cu·lit·ic [ˌvæskjəˈlɪtɪk] *adj* Vaskulitis/Angiitis betr., angiitisch, vaskulitisch.
vas·cu·li·tis [ˌ-ˈlaɪtɪs] *n* Gefäßentzündung *f*, Angiitis *f*, Vaskulitis *f*, Vasculitis *f*.
vasculo- *pref.* Blutgefäß-, Gefäß-, Angi(o)-, Vas(o)-, Vaskulo-.
vas·cu·lo·car·di·ac [ˌvæskjələʊˈkɑːrdɪæk] *adj* Herz- u. Kreislauf *od.* Blutgefäße betr., kardiovaskulär, Herz-Kreislauf-.
vas·cu·lo·gen·e·sis [ˌ-ˈdʒenəsɪs] *n* Entwicklung *f* des Gefäßsystems, Vaskulogenese *f*.
vas·cu·lo·gen·ic [ˌ-ˈdʒenɪk] *adj* Blutgefäße ausbildend.
vas·cu·lo·mo·tor [ˌ-ˈməʊtər] *adj* → vasomotor II.
vas·cu·lop·a·thy [ˌvæskjəˈlɑpəθɪ] *n* (Blut-)Gefäßerkrankung *f*, Vaskulopathie *f*.
vas·cu·lo·tox·ic [ˌvæskjələʊˈtɑksɪk] *adj* Blutgefäße-schädigend, vaskulotoxisch.
vas·cu·lum [ˈvæskjələm] *n* kleines Gefäß *nt*, Vasculum *nt*.
vas deferens Samenleiter *m*, Ductus/Vas deferens.
vas·ec·to·my [væˈsektəmɪ] *n, pl* **-mies** *urol.* Vasektomie *f*, Vasoresektion *f*.
vas·i·fac·tive [ˈvæsɪfæktɪv] *adj* → vasoformative.
va·si·tis [vəˈsaɪtɪs] *n urol.* Samenleiterentzündung *f*, Deferentitis *f*.
vaso- *pref.* Gefäß-, Vas(o)-, Vaskulo-; Samenleiter-, Vas(o)-.
vas·o·ac·tive [ˌvæsəʊˈæktɪv, ˌveɪzəʊ-] *adj* den Gefäßtonus beeinflußend, vasoaktiv.
vasoactive amine vasoaktives Amin *nt*.
vasoactive intestinal peptide *abbr.* **VIP** vasoaktives intestinales Peptid/Polypeptid *nt abbr.* VIP.
vasoactive intestinal polypeptide → vasoactive intestinal peptide.
vas·o·con·ges·tion [ˌ-kənˈdʒestʃn] *n* Vasokongestion *f*.

vasoconstriction

vas·o·con·stric·tion [ˌ-kənˈstrɪkʃn] *n* Engstellung *f* von Blutgefäßen, Vasokonstriktion *f*.
vas·o·con·stric·tive [ˌ-kənˈstrɪktɪv] *adj* Vasokonstriktion betr., vasokonstriktorisch.
vas·o·con·stric·tor [ˌ-kənˈstrɪktər] I *n* vasokonstriktorische Substanz *f*, Vasokonstriktor *m*. II *adj* vasokonstriktorisch.
vasoconstrictor center vasokonstriktorisches Zentrum *nt*.
vasoconstrictor nerve vasokonstriktorischer Nerv *m*.
vas·o·de·pres·sion [ˌ-dɪˈpreʃn] *n* Reduktion *f* des Gefäßwiderstandes, Vasodepression *f*.
vas·o·de·pres·sor [ˌ-dɪˈpresər] I *n* vasodepressive Substanz *f*. II *adj* den Gefäßwiderstand senkend, vasodepressiv, vasodepressorisch.
vasodepressor syncope vasovagale Synkope *f*.
vas·o·di·la·ta·tion [ˌ-dɪləˈteɪʃn] *n* → vasodilation.
vas·o·di·la·tion [ˌ-daɪˈleɪʃn] *n* Gefäßerweiterung *f*, Vasodilatation *f*.
vas·o·di·la·tive [ˌ-daɪˈleɪtɪv] *adj* Vasodilatation betr. *od.* hervorrufend, gefäßerweiternd, vasodilatatorisch.
vas·o·di·la·tor [ˌ-daɪˈleɪtər] I *n* gefäßerweiternde Substanz *f*, Vasodilatator *m*, Vasodilatans *nt*. II *adj* gefäßerweiternd, vasodilatatorisch.
vasodilator center vasodilatatorisches Zentrum *nt*.
vasodilator nerve vasodilatorischer Nerv *m*.
vas·o·ep·i·did·y·mos·to·my [ˌ-epɪˌdɪdəˈmɑstəmɪ] *n urol.* Vasoepididymostomie *f*.
vas·o·fac·tive [ˌ-ˈfæktɪv] *adj* → vasoformative.
vasofactive cell → vasoformative cell.
vas·o·for·ma·tive [ˌ-ˈfɔːrmətɪv] *adj* (Blut-)Gefäßbildung betr. *od.* fördernd, angiopoetisch.
vasoformative cell Angioblast *m*.
vas·o·gan·gli·on [ˌ-ˈgæŋglɪən] *n* Gefäßknäuel *nt*, -ganglion *nt*.
vas·o·gen·ic edema [ˌ-ˈdʒenɪk] vasogenes Ödem *nt*.
vasogenic shock vasogener Schock *m*.
va·sog·ra·phy [væˈsɑgrəfɪ, veɪ-] *n* 1. *radiol.* Kontrastdarstellung *f* von Gefäßen, Vasographie *f*; Angiographie *f*. 2. *urol.* Vasographie *f*, Vasovesikulographie *f*.
vas·o·hy·per·ton·ic [ˌvæzəʊˌhaɪpərˈtɑnɪk, ˌveɪz-] *n, adj* → vasoconstrictor.
vas·o·hy·po·ton·ic [ˌ-haɪpəʊˈtɑnɪk] *n, adj* → vasodilator.
vas·o·in·hib·i·tor [ˌ-ɪnˈhɪbɪtər] *n* vasoinhibitorisches Mittel *nt*.
vas·o·in·hib·i·to·ry [ˌ-ɪnˈhɪbɪtəːrɪ, -təʊ-] *adj* vasoinhibitorisch.
vas·o·li·ga·tion [ˌ-laɪˈgeɪʃn] *n urol.* Unterbindung *f* des Samenleiters, Vasoligatur *f*.
vas·o·mo·tion [-ˈməʊʃn] *n* Vasomotion *f*.
vas·o·mo·tor [ˌ-ˈməʊtər] I *n* Vasomotor *m*. II *adj* vasomotorisch.
vasomotor angina Angina (pectoris) vasomotorica.
vasomotor ataxia vasomotorische Ataxie *f*.
vasomotor center Vasomotorenzentrum *nt*.
vasomotor epilepsy psychomotorische Epilepsie *f*.
vasomotor function Vasomotorik *f*.
vasomotor headache vasomotorischer Kopfschmerz *m*.
vasomotor imbalance vasomotorische Dystonie *f*.

vas·o·mo·to·ri·um [ˌ-məʊˈtəʊrɪəm] *n* vasomotorisches System *nt*, Vasomotorium *nt*.
vasomotor nerve vasomotorischer Nerv *m*.
vasomotor paralysis vasomotorische Lähmung *f*, Vasoparese *f*.
vasomotor reflex vasomotorischer Reflex *m*.
vasomotor rhinitis vasomotorische Rhinitis *f*, Rhinitis vasomotorica.
vasomotor system vasomotorisches System *nt*, Vasomotorensystem *nt*.
vasomotor tone Vasomotorentonus *m*.
vas·o·mo·to·ry [ˌ-ˈməʊtərɪ] *adj* vasomotorisch.
vas·o·neu·rop·a·thy [ˌ-njʊəˈrɑpəθɪ, -nʊ-] *n* Vasoneuropathie *f*.
vas·o·neu·ro·sis [ˌ-njʊəˈrəʊsɪs, -nʊ-] *n* Gefäßneurose *f*, Angio-, Vasoneurose *f*.
vaso-orchidostomy *n urol.* Vasoorchidostomie *f*.
vas·o·pa·ral·y·sis [ˌ-pəˈrælɪsɪs] *n* Gefäßlähmung *f*, Vaso-, Angioparalyse *f*.
vas·o·pa·re·sis [ˌ-pəˈriːsɪs] *n* vasomotorische Lähmung *f*, Angio-, Vasoparese *f*.
vas·o·pres·sin [ˌ-ˈpresɪn] *n abbr.* **VP** Vasopressin *nt*, Antidiuretin *nt*, antidiuretisches Hormon *nt abbr.* **ADH**.
vas·o·pres·si·ner·gic [ˌ-ˌpresɪˈnɜrdʒɪk] *adj* vasopressinerg.
vasopressin system Vasopressinsystem *nt*, Adiuretinsystem *nt*, ADH-System *nt*.
vas·o·pres·sor [ˌ-ˈpresər] I *n* vasopressorische Substanz *f*. II *adj* den Gefäßdruck steigernd, vasopressorisch.
vasopressor reflexes Vasopressorreflexe *pl*.
vas·o·punc·ture [ˌ-ˈpʌŋktʃər] *n* 1. Gefäßpunktion *f*. 2. *urol.* Punktion *f* des Samenleiters, Vasopunktur *f*.
vas·o·re·flex [ˌ-ˈriːfleks] *n* (Blut-)Gefäßreflex *m*.
vas·o·re·lax·a·tion [ˌ-rɪlækˈseɪʃn] *n* Abnahme *f* der Gefäßspannung, Vasorelaxation *f*.
vas·o·re·sec·tion [ˌ-rɪˈsekʃn] *n* → vasectomy.
vas·or·rha·phy [væˈsɔrəfɪ] *n urol.* Naht *f* des Samenleiters, Vasorrhaphie *f*.
vas·o·sec·tion [ˌvæzəʊˈsekʃn, ˌveɪz-] *n* → vasotomy.
vas·o·sen·so·ry [ˌ-ˈsensərɪ] *adj* vasosensorisch.
vasosensory nerve vasosensorischer Nerv *m*.
vas·o·spasm [ˈ-spæzəm] *n* Gefäß-, Vaso-, Angiospasmus *m*.
vas·o·spas·tic [ˌ-ˈspæstɪk] *adj* Vasospasmus betr., angio-, vasospastisch.
vas·os·to·my [væˈsɑstəmɪ] *n urol.* Vasostomie *f*.
vas·o·to·cin [ˌvæzəʊˈtəʊsɪn, ˌveɪz-] *n* Vasotocin *nt*.
vas·ot·o·my [væˈsɑtəmɪ] *n urol.* Samenleitereröffnung *f*, -durchtrennung *f*, -schnitt *m*, Vasotomie *f*.
vas·o·to·nia [ˌvæzəʊˈtəʊnɪə, ˌveɪz-] *n* Gefäßtonus *m*, Angio-, Vasotonus *m*.
vas·o·ton·ic [ˌ-ˈtɑnɪk] I *n* vasotonische Substanz *f*, Vasotonikum *nt*. II *adj* den Gefäßtonus erhöhend, vasotonisch.
vas·o·tribe [ˈ-traɪb] *n chir.* Gefäßquetschklemme *f*, Angiotriptor *m*.
vas·o·trip·sy [ˈ-trɪpsɪ] *n chir.* Angiotripsie *f*, -thrypsie *f*.
vas·o·troph·ic [ˌ-ˈtrɑfɪk] *adj* gefäßernährend, vaso-, angiotrophisch.
vas·o·va·gal [ˌ-ˈveɪgl] *adj* Gefäße u. N. vagus betr., vasovagal.
vasovagal attack vasovagale Synkope *f*.

vasovagal epilepsy psychomotorische Epilepsie *f*.
vasovagal syncope vasovagale Synkope *f*.
vasovagal syndrome → vasovagal syncope.
vas·o·vas·os·to·my [ˌ-væˈsɑstəmɪ] *n urol.* Vasovasostomie *f*.
vas·o·ve·sic·u·lec·to·my [ˌ-vəˌsɪkjəˈlektəmɪ] *n urol.* Vasovesikulektomie *f*.
vas·o·ve·sic·u·li·tis [ˌ-vəˌsɪkjəˈlaɪtɪs] *n urol.* Entzündung *f* von Samenleiter u. Samenbläschen, Vasovesikulitis *f*.
vas·tus intermedius (muscle) [ˈvæstəs] Vastus *m* intermedius, M. vastus intermedius.
vastus lateralis (muscle) Vastus *m* lateralis, M. vastus lateralis.
vastus medialis (muscle) Vastus *m* medialis, M. vastus medialis.
Vater [ˈfɑːtər] : **V.'s ampulla** Vater'-Ampulle *f*, Ampulla hepatopancreatica.
carcinoma of the ampulla of V. Karzinom *nt* der Ampulla hepaticopancreatica.
carcinoma of the papilla of V. Papillenkarzinom *nt*, Karzinom *nt* der Papilla Vateri.
V.'s corpuscles → Vater-Pacini corpuscles.
duct of V. *embryo.* Ductus thyroglossalis.
V.'s papilla Vater'-Papille *f*, Papilla duodeni major, Papilla Vateri.
VATER complex [vertebral defects, anal atresia, tracheoesophageal fistula with esophageal atresia, renal defects and radial dysplasia] VATER-Syndrom *nt*, -Komplex *m*.
Vater-Pacini [pɑˈsiːnɪ] : **V.-P. corpuscles** Vater-Pacini'-(Lamellen-)Körperchen *pl*, Corpuscula lamellosa.
VATER syndrome → VATER complex.
vault [vɔːlt] I *n* 1. (*a. anat.*) Gewölbe *nt*, Wölbung *f*; Dach *nt*, Kuppel *f*. 2. (*Sport*) Sprung *m*. II *vt* 3. (über-)wölben. 4. überspringen. III *vi* 5. s. wölben. 6. springen (*over* über).
v. of pharynx Schlunddach, Fornix pharyngis.
vault·ed [ˈvɔːltɪd] *adj* gewölbt, Gewölbe-, Kuppel-.
VBG *abbr.* → venous blood gases.
VC *abbr.* → vital capacity.
VCA *abbr.* → virus capsid antigen.
VCG *abbr.* 1. → vectorcardiogram. 2. → vectorcardiography.
VD *abbr.* → venereal disease.
VDRL antigen VDRL-Antigen *nt*, Cardiolipin-Cholesterin-Lecitin-Antigen *nt*.
VDRL test [Venereal Disease Research Laboratory] VDRL-Test *m*.
vec·tion [ˈvekʃn] *n* (Krankheits-)Übertragung *f*, Vektion *f*.
vec·tor [ˈvektər] *n* 1. *mathe., phys.* Vektor *m*. 2. *micro.* (Über-)Träger *m*, Vektor *m*; Carrier *m*. 3. *genet.* Vektor *m*, Carrier *m*.
vector addition *phys.* Vektoraddition *f*.
vector-borne *adj* durch einen Vektor übertragen.
vec·tor·car·di·o·gram [ˌvektərˈkɑːrdɪəgræm] *n abbr.* **VCG** Vektorkardiogramm *nt abbr.* **VKG**.
vec·tor·car·di·o·graph [ˌ-ˈkɑːrdɪəgræf] *n* Vektorkardiograph *m*.
vec·tor·car·di·og·ra·phy [ˌ-ˌkɑːrdɪˈɑgrəfɪ] *n abbr.* **VCG** Vektorkardiographie *f abbr.* **VKG**.
vector diagram Vektordiagramm *nt*.
vec·to·ri·al [vekˈtɔːrɪəl, -ˈtəʊr-] *adj* Vektor(en) betr., vektoriell, Vektor-.
vectorial analysis Vektoranalyse *f*, -analysis *f*.

vectorial metabolism vektorieller Metabolismus *m*.
vector loop Vektorschleife *f*.
VEE *abbr.* → Venezuelan equine encephalitis.
VEE virus → Venezuelan equine encephalitis virus.
ve·ga·nism ['vedʒənɪzəm] *n* streng vegetarische Lebensweise *f*.
veg·e·ta·ble ['vedʒ(ɪ)təbl] I *n* (*a.* ˷s *pl*) Gemüse *nt*. II *adj* 1. Gemüse-. 2. pflanzlich, vegetabil(isch), Pflanzen-.
vegetable fat Pflanzenfett *nt*.
veg·e·tal ['vedʒɪtl] I *n* → vegetable I. II *adj* 1. → vegetable 2. 2. → vegetative 2.
veg·e·tar·i·an [ˌvedʒɪ'teərɪən] I *n* Vegetarier(in *f*) *m*. II *adj* vegetarisch.
veg·e·tar·i·an·ism [ˌvedʒɪ'teərɪənɪzəm] *n* vegetarische Lebensweise *f*, Vegetarianismus *m*, Vegetarismus *m*.
veg·e·tate ['vedʒɪteɪt] *vi* 1. (*Pflanze*) wachsen, vegetieren. 2. *fig.* (kümmerlich) dahinleben, vegetieren. 3. *patho.* wuchern.
veg·e·ta·tion [ˌvedʒɪ'teɪʃn] *n* 1. *bot.* Pflanzenwachstum *nt*, Pflanzenwelt *f*, Vegetation *f*. 2. *fig.* (kümmerliches) Dahinleben *nt*, Vegetieren *nt*. 3. *patho.* Wucherung *f*, Gewächs *nt*.
veg·e·ta·tion·al [ˌvedʒɪ'teɪʃnl] *adj* Vegetations-.
veg·e·ta·tive ['vedʒɪteɪtɪv] *adj* 1. Vegetation betr., vegetativ, Pflanzen-, Vegetations-. 2. *bio.* (*Fortpflanzung*) ungeschlechtlich, vegetativ. 3. *physiol.* unwillkürlich, autonom, vegetativ. 4. untätig, träge, faul, passiv, inaktiv.
vegetative endocarditis → verrucous endocarditis.
vegetative growth vegetatives Wachstum *nt*.
vegetative mycelium *micro.* Vegetationskörper *m*.
vegetative nervous system autonomes/vegetatives Nervensystem *nt abbr.* ANS, Pars autonomica systematis nervosi, Systema nervosum autonomicum.
vegetative period Vegetationsperiode *f*, -zeit *f*.
vegetative stage *embryo.* Ruhestadium *nt*.
vegetative tract vegetative Bahnen *pl*.
ve·hi·cle ['vi:ɪkl] *n* 1. *biochem.* Vehikel *nt*, Vehiculum *nt*, Träger *m*; Transportprotein *nt*. 2. *pharm.* Konstituens *nt*, Vehikel *nt*, Vehikulum *nt*. 3. *micro.* Übertrager *m*, Vehikel *nt*, Vehikulum *nt* Vektor *m*. 4. (Hilfs-)Mittel *nt*, Vehikel *nt*, Vermittler *m*.
ve·hic·u·lar accident [vɪ'hɪkjələr] Autounfall *m*, Verkehrsunfall *m*.
veil [veɪl] I *n* Schleier *m*; Schutz *m*. II *vt* verschleiern, verhüllen. III *vi* s. verschleiern, s. verhüllen.
veil cells *immun.* Schleierzellen *pl*.
veiled cells [veɪld] → veil cells.
Veil·lon·el·la [ˌveɪjə'nelə] *n micro.* Veillonella *f*.
Veil·lon·el·la·ce·ae [ˌveɪjəne'leɪsɪː] *pl micro.* Veilonellaceae *pl*.
vein [veɪn] *n* (Blut-)Ader *f*, Blutgefäß *nt*, Vene *f*, Vena *f*.
v. of aqueduct of cochlea V. aqu(a)eductus cochleae.
v. of aqueduct of vestibule → v. of cochlear canaliculus.
v. of bulb of penis Bulbusvene *f*, V. bulbi penis.
v. of bulb of vestibule Bulbusvene *f*, V. bulbi vestibuli.
v. of canaliculus of cochlea → v. cochlear canaliculus.

v.s of caudate nucleus Kaudatusvenen *pl*, Vv. nuclei caudati.
v.s of cerebellum Kleinhirnvenen *pl*, Vv. cerebelli.
v. of cochlear canaliculus Vene im Canaliculus cochleae, V. aqu(a)eductus vestibuli.
v.s of encephalic trunk → v.s of midbrain.
v.s of hypophyseoportal circulation Vv. portales hypophysiales.
v.s of inferior limbs Vv. membri inferioris.
v.s of kidney Nierenvenen *pl*, Vv. renalis/renis.
v.s of labyrinth 1. Labyrinthvenen *pl*, Vv. labyrinthi. 2. Vv. labyrinthinae.
v. of lateral recess of fourth ventricle V. rec. lateralis ventriculi quarti.
v. of Marshall Marshall'-Vene, V. obliqua atrii sinistri.
v.s of medulla oblongata Medulla (oblongata)-Venen *pl*, Vv. medullae oblongatae.
v.s of midbrain Mittelhirn-, Hirnstammvenen *pl*, Vv. mesencephalicae, Vv. trunci encephalici.
v. of olfactory gyrus Vene aus dem Gyrus olfactorius, V. gyri olfactorii.
v.s of pons Brückenvenen *pl*, Vv. pontis.
v. of pterygoid canal Begleitvene *f* der A. canalis pterygoidei, V. pterygoidea.
v.s of Sappey Sappey'-Venen *pl*, Vv. paraumbilicales.
v.s of spinal cord Rückenmarksvenen *pl*, Vv. medullae spinalis.
v.s of superior limbs Vv. membri superioris.
v.s of sylvian fossa Vv. mediae superficiales cerebri.
v.s of Thebesius kleinste Herzvenen *pl*, Thebesi'-Venen *pl*, Vv. cardiacae/cordis minimae.
v. of uncus V. uncialis.
v.s of vertebral column Vv. columnae vertebralis.
v.s of Vieussens vordere Herzvenen *pl*, Vv. cardiacae/cordis anteriores.
vein anesthesia intravenöse Regionalanästhesie *f abbr.* IVRA.
veined [veɪnd] *adj* → veinous 1.
vein graft Venentransplantat *nt*.
vein grafting *HTG* Venenverpflanzung *f*, -transplantation *f*.
interpositional v. Veneninterposition *f*.
vein·let ['veɪnlɪt] *n* Äderchen *nt*, kleine Vene *f*, Venole *f*, Venule *f*, Venula *f*.
vein·ous ['veɪnəs] *adj* 1. ad(e)rig, geädert. 2. → venous.
vein patch *HTG* Venenpatch *m*, -flicken *m*.
vein stone Venenstein *m*, Phlebolith *m*.
vein stripper *HTG* Venenstripper *m*.
vein stripping *HTG* Venenstripping *nt*.
vein·ule ['veɪnjuːl] *n* → veinlet.
vein·u·let ['veɪnjəlɪt] *n* → veinlet.
vein·y ['veɪnɪ] *adj* → veinous 1.
ve·la·men [və'leɪmən] *n*, *pl* **-lam·i·na** [-'læmɪnə] Membran *f*, Haut *f*, Velamen *nt*.
vel·a·men·tous [ˌvelə'mentəs] *adj* schleierartig umhüllend.
velamentous insertion *gyn.* Insertio velamentosa.
velamentous placenta *gyn.* Placenta velamentosa.
vel·a·men·tum [ˌ-'mentəm] *n*, *pl* **-ta** [-tə] Hülle *f*, Velamentum *nt*.
ve·lar ['viːlər] *adj* Velum betr., Velum-.
ve·li·form ['viːləfɔːrm] *adj* → velamentous.
vel·lus ['veləs] *n* Vellushaar *nt*.
ve·lo·cim·e·try [ˌviːləʊ'sɪmətrɪ] *n* Geschwindigkeitsmessung *f*.

ve·loc·i·ty [və'lɒsətɪ] *n*, *pl* **-ties** *phys.*, *techn.* Geschwindigkeit *f*.
v. of fall Fallgeschwindigkeit.
v. of flow Strömungsgeschwindigkeit.
velocity gradient Geschwindigkeitsgefälle *nt*, -gradient *m*.
velocity sensor Geschwindigkeitssensor *m*.
ve·lo·no·ski·as·co·py [ˌviːlənəʊskaɪ'æskəpɪ] *n ophthal.* Belonoskiaskopie *f*.
vel·o·pha·ryn·ge·al [ˌveləʊfə'rɪndʒɪəl] *adj* weichen Gaumen u. Pharynx betr., velopharyngeal.
Velpeau [vɛl'pəʊ]: **V.'s canal** Leistenkanal *m*, Canalis inguinalis.
V.'s deformity *ortho.* Bajonett-, Fourchette-, Gabelrückenstellung *f*.
V.'s fossa Fossa ischio-analis.
V.'s hernia Velpeau-Hernie *f*.
ve·lum ['viːləm] *n*, *pl* **-la** [-lə] *anat.* Segel *nt*, segelähnliche Struktur *f*, Velum *nt*.
ven- *pref.* → veno-.
ve·na ['viːnə] *n*, *pl* **-nae** [-niː] → vein.
vena ca·va ['keɪvə, 'kævə] Hohlvene *f*, *inf.* Kava *f*, Cava *f*, V. cava.
inferior v. untere Hohlvene, *inf.* Kava/Cava inferior, V. cava inferior.
superior v. obere Hohlvene, *inf.* Kava/Cava superior, V. cava superior.
vena caval anastomosis Kavaanastomose *f*, Vena-cava-Anastomose *f*.
vena caval foramen For. venae cavae.
ve·na·ca·vo·gram [ˌviːnə'keɪvəgræm] *n radiol.* Kavogramm *nt*.
ve·na·ca·vog·ra·phy [ˌ-'kɑːvəgrəfɪ] *n radiol.* Kontrastdarstellung *f* der V. cava, Kavographie *f*.
ve·nec·ta·sia [ˌvɪnek'teɪʒ(ɪ)ə] *n* Venenerweiterung *f*, Venektasie *f*, Phlebektasie *f*, Phlebectasia *f*.
ve·nec·to·my [vɪ'nektəmɪ] *n chir.* Venenresektion *f*, Phlebektomie *f*, Venektomie *f*.
ven·e·na·tion [ˌvenə'neɪʃn] *n* Vergiftung *f*, Venenatio(n) *f*.
ven·e·nif·er·ous [ˌ-'nɪfərəs] *adj* Gift-übertragend.
ven·e·nif·ic [ˌ-'nɪfɪk] *adj* giftbildend, -produzierend.
ven·e·no·sal·i·var·y [ˌvenənəʊ'sælɪˌverɪː, -vərɪ] *adj* Gift mit dem Speichel ausscheidend.
ven·e·nos·i·ty [ˌvenə'nɒsətɪ] *n* Giftigkeit *f*.
ven·e·nous ['venənəs] *adj* giftig, venenös.
ve·ne·num [və'niːnəm] *n* Gift *nt*, Venenum *nt*.
ven·e·punc·ture [ˌvenə'pʌŋktʃər] *n* → venipuncture.
ve·ne·re·al [və'nɪərɪəl] *adj* 1. geschlechtlich, sexuell, Geschlechts-, Sexual. 2. Geschlechtskrankheit betr., venerisch, Geschlechts-; geschlechtskrank.
venereal arthritis Reiter'-Krankheit *f*, -Syndrom *nt*, Fiessinger-Leroy-Reiter-Syndrom *nt*, Okulourethrosynovitis *f*, venerische Arthritis *f*.
venereal collar syphilitisches Leukoderm *nt*, Halsband *nt* der Venus.
venereal disease *abbr.* **VD** Geschlechtskrankheit *f*, venerische Erkrankung/Krankheit *f*.
fifth v. → fourth v.
fourth v. Morbus Durand-Nicolas-Favre *m*, klimatischer Bubo *m*, vierte Geschlechtskrankheit *f*, Lymphogranuloma inguinale/venereum *abbr.* LGV, Lymphopathia venerea, Poradenitis inguinalis.
sixth v. → fourth v.
venereal sore weicher Schanker *m*, Chankroid *nt*, Ulcus molle.
venereal ulcer → venereal sore.
venereal wart Feig-, Feuchtwarze *f*, spit-

venereologist

zes Kondylom *nt*, Condyloma acuminatum, Papilloma acuminatum/venereum.
ve·ne·re·ol·o·gist [vəˌnɪərɪ'ɑlədʒɪst] *n* Venerologe *m*, -login *f.*
ve·ne·re·ol·o·gy [ˌ-'ɑlədʒɪ] *n* Venerologie *f.*
ven·er·y ['venərɪ] *n* Geschlechtsverkehr *m*, Koitus *m*, Coitus *m.*
ven·e·sec·tion [ˌvenə'sekʃn] *n* **1.** Venenschnitt *m*, Phlebotomie *f*, Venaesectio *f.* **2.** Venenpunktion *f.* **3.** Veneneröffnung *f*, Venaesectio *f.*
ven·e·su·ture [ˌ-'suːtʃər] *n chir.* Venennaht *f*, Phleborrhaphie *f.*
Ven·e·zue·lan [venə'zweɪlən]: **V. equine encephalitis** *abbr.* **VEE** venezuelanische Pferdeenzephalitis *f*, Venezuelan equine encephalitis/encephalomyelitis *abbr.* VEE.
V. equine encephalitis virus *micro.* Venezuelan-Equine-Encephalitis-Virus *nt*, VEE-Virus *nt.*
V. equine encephalomyelitis → V. equine encephalitis.
V. equine encephalomyelitis virus → V. equine encephalitis virus.
veni- *pref.* veno-.
ven·i·plex ['venɪpleks] *n* venöser Plexus *m.*
ven·i·punc·ture [ˌvenɪ'pʌŋktʃər] *n* Venenpunktion *f.*
ven·i·su·ture [ˌ-'suːtʃər] *n chir.* Venennaht *f*, Phleborrhaphie *f.*
veno- *pref.* Venen-, Ven(o)-, Phleb(o)-.
ve·no·a·tri·al [ˌviːnə'eɪtrɪəl] *adj* Vena cava u. rechten Vorhof betr.
ve·no·au·ric·u·lar [ˌ-ɔː'rɪkjələr] *adj* → venoatrial.
ve·noc·ly·sis [vɪ'nɑkləsɪs] *n* intravenöse Infusion/Injektion *f.*
ve·no·gram ['viːnəɡræm] *n radiol.* Veno-, Phlebogramm *nt.*
ve·nog·ra·phy [vɪ'nɑɡrəfɪ] *n radiol.* Kontrastdarstellung *f* von Venen, Veno-, Phlebographie *f.*
ven·om ['venəm] *n* (tierisches) Gift *nt.*
ven·o·mo·sal·i·var·y [ˌvenəmoʊ'sæləˌveri:, -vərɪ] *adj* → venenosalivary.
ve·no·mo·tor [ˌviːnə'moʊtər] *adj* venomotorisch.
ven·o·mous ['venəməs] *adj* Gift sezernierend; giftig.
ve·no·per·i·to·ne·os·to·my [ˌviːnəˌperɪˌtoʊnɪ'ɑstəmɪ] *n chir.* Venoperitoneostomie *f.*
ve·no·scle·ro·sis [ˌ-sklɪ'roʊsɪs] *n* Phlebosklerose *f.*
ve·nose ['viːnoʊs] *adj* venenreich, Venen-.
ve·no·si·nal [ˌviːnə'saɪnl] *adj* → venoatrial.
ve·nos·ta·sis [vɪ'nɑstəsɪs] *n* venöse Stauung *f*, Venostase *f.*
ve·not·o·my [vɪ'nɑtəmɪ] *n* → venesection.
ve·nous ['viːnəs] *adj* Venen *od.* venöses System betr., venös, Adern-, Venen-, Veno-.
venous access *chir.* venöser Zugang *m.*
venous aneurysm venöses Aneurysma *nt*, Venenaneurysma *nt.*
venous angle Venenwinkel *m*, Angulus venosus.
venous arch Venenbogen *m*, Arcus venosus.
  dorsal v. of foot Venenbogen des Fußrückens, Arcus venosus dorsalis pedis.
  jugular v. Arcus venosus jugularis.
  v.s of kidney Bogenvenen *pl*, Venae arcuatae renis.
  palmar v., deep tiefer Venenbogen der Hohlhand, Arcus venosus palmaris profundus.
  palmar v., superficial oberflächlicher Venenbogen der Hohlhand, Arcus venosus palmaris superficialis.
  plantar v. Venenbogen der Fußsohle, Arcus venosus plantaris.
  volar v., deep → palmar v., deep.
  volar v., superficial → palmar v., superficial.
venous bleeding venöse Blutung *f.*
venous blood venöses/sauerstoffarmes Blut *nt.*
venous blood gases *abbr.* **VBG** venöse Blutgase *pl.*
venous capacitance system venöses Kapazitätssystem *nt.*
venous capillaries venöser Kapillarabschnitt/-schenkel *m*, venöse Kapillaren *pl.*
venous catheter Venenkatheter *m.*
venous congestion → venous hyperemia.
venous drainage venöser Abfluß *m.*
venous embolism venöse Embolie *f.*
venous foramen 1. For. venosum. **2.** → vena caval foramen.
venous gangrene Stauungsgangrän *f*, venöse Gangrän *f.*
venous gases → venous blood gases.
venous graft Venentransplantat *nt.*
venous grooves → venous sulci.
venous hematocrit *abbr.* **VH** venöser Hämatokrit *m.*
venous hemorrhage → venous bleeding.
venous hum *card.* Nonnensausen *nt*, -geräusch *nt*, Kreiselgeräusch *nt*, Bruit de diable.
venous hyperemia venöse/passive (Blut-)Stauung/Hyperämie *f.*
venous hypertension venöse Hypertonie *f.*
venous hypoxia venöse Hypoxie *f.*
venous impressions → venous sulci.
venous injury Venenverletzung *f.*
venous insufficiency Venen(klappen)insuffizienz *f.*
venous ligament of liver Lig. venosum (Arantii).
venous line → venous catheter.
venous mesocardium *embryo.* venöses Mesokard.
venous murmur Venengeräusch *nt.*
venous network → venous rete.
venous occlusion Venenverschluß *m.*
venous occlusion plethysmography Venenverschlußplethysmographie *f.*
venous patch *HTG* Venenpatch *m*, -flicken *m.*
venous plexus venöser Plexus *m*, Plexus venosus.
  areolar v. Venenplexus der Brustwarze, Plexus venosus areolaris.
  Batson's v. Venenplexus *pl* der Wirbelsäule, Plexus venosi vertebrales externi et interni.
  carotid v., internal Venenplexus im Karotiskanal, Plexus venosus caroticus internus.
  dorsal v. of foot Venenplexus des Fußrückens, Rete venosum dorsale pedis.
  dorsal v. of hand Venenplexus des Handrückens, Rete venosum dorsale manus.
  v. of foramen ovale Venengeflecht *nt* im For. ovale, Plexus venosus foraminis ovalis.
  hemorrhoidal v. → rectal v.
  v. of hypoglossal canal Venengeflecht *nt* im Hypoglossuskanal, Plexus venosus canalis hypoglossi.
  prostatic v. venöser Prostataplexus, Plexus venosus prostaticus.
  rectal v. rektaler Venenplexus, Hämorrhoidalplexus, Plexus h(a)emorrhoidalis, Plexus venosus rectalis.
  sacral v. sakraler Venenplexus, Plexus venosus sacralis.
  suboccipital v. subokzipitales Venengeflecht *nt*, Plexus venosus suboccipitalis.
  uterine v. venöser Uterusplexus, Plexus venosus uterinus.
  vertebral v., anterior external vorderes äußeres Venengeflecht *nt* der Wirbelsäule, Plexus venosus vertebralis externus anterior.
  vertebral v., anterior internal vorderes inneres Venengeflecht *nt* der Wirbelsäule, Plexus venosus vertebralis internus anterior.
  vertebral v., posterior external hinteres äußeres Venengeflecht *nt* der Wirbelsäule, Plexus venosus vertebralis externus posterior.
  vertebral v., posterior internal hinteres inneres Venengeflecht *nt* der Wirbelsäule, Plexus venosus vertebralis internus posterior.
  vesical v. Venengeflecht *nt* am Blasengrund, Plexus venosus vesicalis.
venous pooling venöses Pooling *nt.*
venous pressure Venendruck *m*, venöser Blutdruck *m.*
venous pulse Venenpuls *m*, Pulsus venosus.
venous rete Venengeflecht *nt*, Rete venosum.
  dorsal v. of foot Venengeflecht des Fußrückens, Rete venosum dorsale pedis.
  dorsal v. of hand Venengeflecht des Handrückens, Rete venosum dorsale manus.
venous return venöser Rückstrom *m.*
venous sinus venöser Sinus *m*, Sinus venosus.
v.es of dura mater Dura-Hirn-Sinus *pl*, Sinus der Dura mater encephali, Sinus venosi durales, Sinus durae matris.
v. of sclera Schlemm'-Kanal *m*, Sinus venosus sclerae.
venous stasis venöse Stauung *f*, Venostase *f.*
venous sulci Sulci venosi.
venous thrombosis Venenthrombose *f*; Phlebothrombose *f.*
venous tone Venentonus *m.*
venous valve Venenklappe *f*, Valvula venosa.
  left v. *embryo.* linke Venenklappe.
  right v. *embryo.* rechte Venenklappe.
ve·no·ve·nos·to·my [ˌviːnəvɪ'nɑstəmɪ] *n HTG* Venovenostomie *f*, Phlebophlebostomie *f.*
ve·no·ve·nous [ˌ-'viːnəs] *adj* venovenös.
venovenous bypass venovenöser Bypass *m.*
vent [vent] *n* **1.** (Abzugs-)Öffnung *f*, (Luft-)Loch *nt*, Schlitz *m*, Entlüftungsloch *nt*. **2.** After *m*, Kloake *f.*
ven·ti·late ['ventleɪt] *vt* **1.** (be-, ent-, durch-)lüften, ventilieren. **2.** *physiol.* Sauerstoff zuführen. **3.** (künstlich) beatmen. **4.** *chem.* mit Sauerstoff anreichern.
ven·ti·lat·ed patient ['ventleɪtɪd] Beatmungspatient(in *f*) *m*, beatmeter Patient *m.*
ven·ti·la·tion [ˌventə'leɪʃn] *n* **1.** Be-, Ent-, Durchlüften *nt*, Ventilation *f*. **2.** *physiol.* Ventilation *f*. **3.** Beatmung *f.*
ventilation disorder (*Lunge*) Ventilationsstörung *f.*
  obstructive v. obstruktive Ventilationsstörung.
  restrictive v. restriktive Ventilationsstörung.
ven·ti·la·tor ['ventleɪtər] *n* Beatmungsgerät *nt*, Ventilator *m.*
ven·ti·la·to·ry stenosis ['ventləˌtɔːrɪ, -tɔː-] respiratorische Ventilstenose *f.*
ventilatory support Atemhilfe *f.*
ventr- *pref.* → ventro-.
ven·tral ['ventrəl] *adj* Bauch *od.* Vorder-

seite betr., bauchwärts (liegend od. gerichtet), ventral; anterior.
ventral aorta embryo. ventrale Aorta f.
ventral border: v. of radius Radiusvorderkante f, Margo anterior radii.
   v. of ulna Ulnavorderrand m, Margo anterior ulnae.
ventral branch vorderer/ventraler Ast m, Bauchast m, Ramus ventralis.
   v.es of cervical nerves vordere/ventrale Halsnervenäste pl, Rami anteriores/ventrales nn. cervicalium.
   v. of coccygeal nerve vorderer/ventraler Ast m des N. coccygeus, Ramus anterior/ventralis n. coccygei.
   v.es of lumbar nerves vordere/ventrale Äste pl der Lumbalnerven, Rami anteriores/ventrales nn. lumbalium.
   v.es of sacral nerves ventrale Äste pl der Sakralnerven, Rami anteriores nn. sacralium.
   v. of spinal nerves vorderer Ast od. Bauchast m der Spinalnerven, Ramus anterior/ventralis nn. spinalium.
   v.es of thoracic nerves Interkostalnerven pl, Rami anteriores/ventrales nn. thoracicorum, Nn. intercostales.
ventral column of spinal cord Vordersäule f (der grauen Substanz), Columna anterior/ventralis medullae spinalis.
ventral decubitus Bauchlage f.
ventral divisions of trunks of brachial plexus vordere Äste pl der Trunci plexus brachialis, Divisiones anteriores/ventrales truncorum plexus brachialis.
ventral funiculus of spinal cord Vorderstrang m, Funiculus anterior/ventralis medullae spinalis.
ventral hernia Bauch(wand)hernie f, Laparozele f, Hernia abdominalis/ventralis.
ventral horn of spinal cord Vorderhorn nt des Rückenmarks, Cornu anterius/ventrale medullae spinalis.
ventral margin: v. of radius → ventral border of radius.
   v. of ulna → ventral border of ulna.
ventral mesentery embryo. ventrales Mesenterium nt.
ventral mesocardium embryo. ventrales Mesokard nt.
ventral mesogastrium embryo. ventrales Mesogastrium nt.
ventral nucleus: anterior v. of thalamus Nc. ventralis anterior (thalami).
   intermediate v. of thalamus Nc. ventralis intermedius.
   lateral v. of thalamus Ncc. ventrales laterales (thalami).
   medial v. of thalamus Nc. ventralis medialis thalami.
   posterior v.i of thalamus Ncc. ventrales posteriores (thalami).
   posterolateral v. of thalamus Nc. ventralis posterolateralis (thalami).
   posteromedial v. of thalamus Nc. ventralis posteromedialis (thalami).
   v.i of thalamus ventrale Thalamuskerne pl, Ncc. ventrales (thalami).
   v. of trapezoid body ventraler Trapezkern m, Nc. ventralis corporis trapezoidei.
ventral pancreas embryo. ventrales Pankreas nt.
ventral part: v. of cerebral peduncle Hirnschenkel m, Basis pedunculi cerebri, Crus cerebri, Pars anterior/ventralis pedunculi cerebri.
   v. of pons ventraler Brückenteil m, Pars basilaris/ventralis pontis.
   v. of substantia nigra Pars reticularis.
ventral plate embryo. Bodenplatte f.
ventral root (of spinal nerves) vordere/motorische (Spinal-)Nervenwurzel f,

Vorderwurzel f, Radix anterior/motoria/ventralis nn. spinalium.
ventral thalamus Subthalamus m, ventraler Thalamusabschnitt m, Thalamus ventralis.
ventri- pref. → ventro-.
ven·tri·cle ['vɛntrɪkl] n anat. 1. Kammer f, Ventrikel m, Ventriculus m. 2. (kleiner od. schmaler) Magen m, Ventriculus m, Gaster m. 3. (Hirn-)Kammer f, Ventrikel m, Ventriculus cerebri. 4. (Herz-)Kammer f, Ventrikel m, Ventriculus cordis.
   v. of Arantius 1. Cavum septi pellucidi. **2.** Rautengrube f, Fossa rhomboidea.
   v. of brain Hirnventrikel, Ventriculus cerebri.
   v. of cerebrum → v. of brain.
   v. of Galen Kehlkopfventrikel, Galen-Ventrikel, Morgagni'-Ventrikel, Kehlkopftasche f, Ventriculus laryngis.
   v. of Sylvius Cavum septi pellucidi.
ven·tri·cor·nu [ˌvɛntrɪˈkɔːrn(j)uː] n (Rückenmark) Vorderhorn nt, Cornu anterius (medullae spinalis).
ven·tri·cor·nu·al [ˌ-ˈkɔːrn(j)əwəl] adj Vorderhorn betr., Vorderhorn-.
ventriculo- pref. → ventriculo-.
ven·tric·u·lar [vɛnˈtrɪkjələr] adj Kammer/Ventrikel betr., ventrikulär, ventrikular, Kammer-, Ventrikel-, Ventrikulo-.
ventricular aneurysm Herzwand-, Kammerwand-, Ventrikelaneurysma nt, Aneurysma cordis.
ventricular aqueduct Aquädukt m, Aqu(a)eductus cerebri/mesencephalici.
ventricular arrhythmia ventrikuläre Arrhythmie f.
ventricular beat card. Kammersystole f.
   premature v. → ventricular extrasystole.
ventricular bigeminy card. Kammerbigeminie f.
ventricular block (ZNS) Ventrikelblockade f.
ventricular bradychardia card. Ventrikel-, Kammerbradykardie f, ventrikuläre Bradykardie f.
ventricular branch of left coronary artery, posterior linker Ast m zur Rückseite des linken Ventrikels, Ramus posterior ventriculi sinistri.
ventricular canal Magenstraße f, Canalis gastricus/ventriculi.
ventricular capture card. Capture beat (m).
ventricular complex card. EKG Kammerkomplex m.
ventricular conduction card. intraventrikuläre Erregungsleitung/Erregungsausbreitung f.
   aberrant v. aberrierende intraventrikuläre Erregungsleitung.
ventricular contraction card. Kammersystole f.
   premature v. abbr. **PVC** → ventricular extrasystole.
ventricular diastole card. Kammer-, Ventrikeldiastole f.
ventricular dilatation card. Kammer-, Ventrikeldilatation f.
ventricular excitation card. Kammer-, Ventrikelerregung f.
ventricular extrasystole card. ventrikuläre Extrasystole f, Kammerextrasystole f.
ventricular fibrillation card. Kammerflimmern nt.
ventricular flutter card. Kammerflattern nt.
ventricular fold Taschenfalte f, Plica ventricularis/vestibularis.
ventricular hypertrophy (Herz) Ventrikelhypertrophie f.

ventricular laryngocele HNO Laryngocele ventricularis.
ventricular ligament (of larynx) Taschenband nt, Lig. vestibulare.
ventricular mitosis histol. ventrikuläre Mitose f.
ventricular musculature (Herz) Kammer-, Ventrikelmuskulatur f.
ventricular myocardium (Herz) Kammer-, Ventrikelmyokard nt.
ventricular pacemaker (Herz) ventrikulärer Schrittmacher m.
ventricular preexcitation WPW-Syndrom nt, Wolff-Parkinson-White-Syndrom nt.
ventricular puncture Ventrikelpunktion f.
ventricular receptors (Herz) Kammer-, Ventrikelrezeptoren pl.
ventricular rhythm card. Kammerrhythmus m.
ventricular septal defect abbr. **VSD** card. Ventrikelseptumdefekt m abbr. VSD, Kammerseptumdefekt m abbr. KSD.
ventricular septum Kammer-, Interventrikular-, Ventrikelseptum nt, Septum interventriculare (cordis).
ventricular standstill card. Kammerstillstand m, -arrest m.
ventricular system Kammersystem nt.
ventricular systole card. Kammer-, Ventrikelsystole f.
   premature v. → ventricular extrasystole.
ventricular tachycardia card. ventrikuläre Tachykardie f.
ventricular tamponade card. Ventrikeltamponade f.
ventricular ulcer Magengeschwür nt, -ulkus nt, Ulcus ventriculi.
ventricular vein: v.s pl Venenäste pl aus der Ventrikelwand, Ventrikelvenen pl, Vv. ventriculares (cordis).
   inferior v. Ventricularis f inferior, V. ventricularis inferior.
ven·tric·u·li·tis [vɛnˌtrɪkjəˈlaɪtɪs] n neuro. (Gehirn) Ventrikelentzündung f, Ventrikulitis f.
ventriculo- pref. Ventrikel-, Kammer-, Ventrikul(o)-.
ven·tric·u·lo·a·tri·al [vɛnˌtrɪkjələʊˈeɪtrɪəl] adj abbr. **V-A** Kammer/Ventrikel u. Vorhof/Atrium betr., ventrikuloatrial, ventrikuloaurikulär; atrioventrikular.
ventriculoatrial conduction card. retrograde Erregungsleitung f.
ventriculoatrial shunt → ventriculoatriostomy.
ven·tric·u·lo·a·tri·os·to·my [ˌ-eɪtrɪˈɑstəmɪ] n neurochir. Ventrikel-Vorhof-Shunt m, Ventrikuloaurikulostomie f.
ven·tric·u·lo·cis·ter·nos·to·my [ˌ-sɪstərˈnɑstəmɪ] n neurochir. Torkildsen-Operation f, Ventrikulozisternostomie f.
ven·tric·u·lo·gram [vɛnˈtrɪkjələʊgræm] n radiol. Ventrikulogramm nt.
ven·tric·u·log·ra·phy [vɛnˌtrɪkjəˈlɑgrəfɪ] n radiol. **1.** (Gehirn) Ventrikeldarstellung f, Ventrikulographie f. **2.** card. (Herz-)Kammerdarstellung f, Ventrikulographie f.
ven·tric·u·lo·mas·toid·os·to·my [vɛnˌtrɪkjəlɑʊˌmæstɔɪˈdɑstəmɪ] n neurochir. Ventrikulomastoid(e)ostomie f.
ven·tric·u·lom·e·try [vɛnˌtrɪkjəˈlɑmətrɪ] n Ventrikulometrie f.
ven·tric·u·lo·my·ot·o·my [vɛnˌtrɪkjələʊmaɪˈɑtəmɪ] n HTG Ventrikulomyotomie f.
ven·tric·u·lo·nec·tor [ˌ-ˈnɛktər] n His'-Bündel nt, Fasciculus atrioventricularis.
ven·tric·u·lo·per·i·to·ne·al shunt [ˌ-ˌpɛrɪtəʊˈniːəl] ventrikuloperitonealer Shunt m.

ven·tric·u·lo·punc·ture [ˌ-'pʌŋktʃər] *n* neuro. Hirnkammer-, Ventrikelpunktion *f*.
ven·tric·u·lo·scope ['-skəʊp] *n* Ventrikuloskop *nt*.
ven·tric·u·los·co·py [venˌtrɪkjə'lɒskəpɪ] *n* Ventrikuloskopie *f*.
ven·tric·u·los·to·my [ˌ-'lɒstəmɪ] *n* neurochir. Ventrikulostomie *f*.
ven·tric·u·lot·o·my [ˌ-'lɒtəmɪ] *n* neurochir. Ventrikulotomie *f*.
ven·tric·u·lo·ve·nos·to·my [venˌtrɪkjələʊvɪ'nɒstəmɪ] *n* neurochir. Ventrikulovenostomie *f*, ventrikulovenöser Shunt *m*.
ven·tric·u·lo·ve·nous [ˌ-'viːnəs] *adj* ventrikulovenös.
ventriculovenous shunt → ventriculovenostomy.
ven·tric·u·lus [ven'trɪkjələs] *n, pl* **-li** [-laɪ] 1. *anat.* (kleiner *od.* schmaler) Magen *m*, Ventriculus *m*, Gaster *m*. 2. *anat.* Kammer *f*, Ventrikel *m*, Ventriculus *m*. 3. *bio.* Rumpfdarm *nt*.
ven·tri·cum·bent [ˌventrɪ'kʌmbənt] *adj* auf dem Bauch liegend, in Bauchlage.
ventro- *pref.* Ventri-, Ventr(o)-, Vorder-.
ven·tro·cys·tor·rha·phy [ˌventrəʊsɪs'tɒrəfɪ] *n chir.* Ventrozystorrhaphie *f*.
ven·tro·dor·sal [ˌ-'dɔːrsl] *adj anat.* ventral u. dorsal, ventrodorsal.
ven·tro·fix·a·tion [ˌ-fɪk'seɪʃn] *n gyn.* Ventrifixatio *f*, Ventrifixation *f*.
ven·tro·hys·ter·o·pex·y [ˌ-'hɪstərəʊpeksɪ] *n* → ventrofixation.
ven·tro·in·gui·nal [ˌ-'ɪŋgwɪnl] *adj* Abdomen u. Leistenregion betr., abdominoinguinal.
ven·tro·lat·er·al [ˌ-'lætərəl] *adj anat.* ventral u. lateral, ventrolateral.
ventrolateral groove: v. of medulla oblongata Vorderseitenfurche *f* der Medulla oblongata, Sulcus anterolateralis/ventrolateralis medullae oblongatae.
v. of spinal cord Vorderseitenfurche *f* des Rückenmarks, Sulcus anterolateralis/ventrolateralis medullae spinalis.
ventrolateral nucleus: v.i of thalamus ventrolaterale Kerngruppe *f* des Thalamus, Ncc. ventrolaterales thalami.
v. of ventral column of spinal cord Nc. anterolateralis.
ventrolateral sulcus: v. of medullae oblongata → ventrolateral groove of medulla oblongata.
v. of spinal cord → ventrolateral groove of spinal cord.
ven·tro·me·di·al [ˌ-'miːdɪəl] *adj anat.* ventral u. medial, ventromedial.
ventromedial nucleus Nc. ventromedialis.
v. of ventral column of spinal cord Nc. anteromedialis.
ven·tro·me·di·an [ˌ-'miːdɪən] *adj anat.* ventral u. median, ventromedian.
ven·tro·pos·te·ri·or [ˌ-pə'stɪərɪər, -pəʊ-] *adj anat.* ventral u. posterior, ventroposterior.
ven·trop·to·sia [ˌventrɒp'təʊsɪə] *n* → ventroptosis.
ven·trop·to·sis [ˌ-'təʊsɪs] *n* Magensenkung *f*, -tiefstand *m*, Gastroptose *f*.
ven·tro·sus·pen·sion [ˌventrəʊsə'spenʃn] *n* → ventrofixation.
ven·trot·o·my [ven'trɒtəmɪ] *n* 1. operative Eröffnung *f* der Bauchhöhle, Zölio-, Laparotomie *f*. 2. Bauch(decken)schnitt *m*.
Venturi [ven'tʊərɪ]: **V. effect** *phys.* Venturi-Effekt *m*.
ven·tu·rim·e·ter [ˌventʊ'rɪmɪtər] *n phys.* Venturimeter *nt*.
ven·u·la ['venjələ] *n, pl* **-lae** [-liː] → venule.

ven·u·lar ['venjələr] *adj* Venule betr., Venulen-.
ven·ule ['venjuːl] *n* kleine *od.* kleinste Vene *f*, Venole *f*, Venule *f*, Venula *f*.
ven·u·lous ['venjələs] *adj* → venular.
VEP *abbr.* → visual evoked potential.
ver·ap·a·mil [ver'æpəmɪl] *n pharm.* Verapamil *nt*.
ver·bal ['vɜrbl] *adj* mit Worten, wörtlich, Wort-; mündlich, verbal.
verbal agraphia verbale Agraphie *f*.
verbal amnesia verbale Amnesie *f*.
verbal aphasia motorische Aphasie *f*, Broca-Aphasie *f*.
verbal consent mündliche Einverständniserklärung *f*, mündliche Einwilligung *f*.
ver·big·er·a·tion [vərˌbɪdʒə'reɪʃn] *n psychia.* Verbigeration *f*.
ver·bo·ma·nia [ˌvɜrbəʊ'meɪnɪə, -jə] *n psychia.* krankhafte Geschwätzigkeit *f*, Verbomanie *f*.
ver·di·he·mo·glo·bin [ˌvɜrdɪ'hiːməgləʊbɪn, -'hemə-] *n* Verdiglobin *nt*.
ver·dine ['vɜrdɪn] *n* Biliverdin *nt*.
ver·do·glo·bin [ˌvɜrdəʊ'gləʊbɪn] *n* Verdoglobin *nt*.
ver·do·he·mo·glo·bin [ˌ-'hiːməgləʊbɪn, -'hemə-] *n* Choleglobin *nt*, Verdohämoglobin *nt*.
ver·do·per·ox·i·dase [ˌ-pə'rɒksɪdeɪz] *n* Myeloperoxidase *f abbr.* MPO.
verge [vɜrdʒ] **I** *n* (*a. fig.*) Rand *m*, Saum *m*, Grenze *f*. **II** *vi* 1. (*a. fig.*) grenzen (*on* an). 2. *s.* (hin-)neigen, *s.* erstrecken (*to, towards* nach).
ver·gence ['vɜrdʒəns] *n ophthal.* Vergenz *f*.
ver·gen·cy ['vɜrdʒənsɪ] *n* → vergence.
ver·i·fi·a·ble ['verəfaɪəbl] *adj* beweis-, nachweis-, nachprüf-, verifizierbar.
ver·i·fi·ca·tion [ˌverəfɪ'keɪʃn] *n* 1. (Nach-, Über-)Prüfung *f*, Verifizierung *f*. 2. Beglaubigung *f*, Beurkundung *f*; Echtheitsnachweis *m*, Verifizierung *f*. 3. (eidliche) Beglaubigung *f*.
ver·i·fy ['verəfaɪ] *vt* 1. (nach-, über-)prüfen, verifizieren. 2. die Richtigkeit *od.* Echtheit nachweisen, verifizieren; beglaubigen, beurkunden, belegen, beweisen. 3. (eidlich) beglaubigen *od.* bestätigen.
vermi- *pref.* Wurm-, Vermi-.
ver·mi·ci·dal [ˌvɜrmɪ'saɪdl] *adj* wurm(ab)tötend, vermizid.
ver·mi·cide ['vɜrmɪsaɪd] *n* Vermizid *nt*, Vermicidum *nt*.
ver·mic·u·lar [vɜr'mɪkjələr] *adj* → vermitoid.
vermicular colic Kolik *f od.* kolikartiger Schmerz *m* bei Appendizitis.
vermicular movement Peristaltik *f*.
ver·mic·u·la·tion [vərˌmɪkjə'leɪʃn] *n physiol.* Vermikulation *f*.
ver·mi·cule ['vɜrmɪkjuːl] *n* 1. wurmartige Struktur *f*. 2. *micro.* Ookinet *m*. 3. *micro.* Merozoit *m*.
ver·mic·u·lose [vɜr'mɪkjəʊs] *adj* → vermiculous.
ver·mic·u·lous [vɜr'mɪkjələs] *adj* 1. wurmartig, wurmähnlich, -förmig, vermiform. 2. von Würmern befallen, Wurm-.
ver·mi·form ['vɜrmɪfɔːrm] *adj anat.* wurmähnlich, -förmig, vermiform.
vermiform appendage → vermiform appendix.
vermiform appendix Wurmfortsatz *m* des Blinddarms, *inf.* Wurm *m*, *inf.* Blinddarm *m*, Appendix *f* (vermiformis).
vermiform artery Appendixarterie *f*, Appendikularis *f*, A. appendicularis.
vermiform granules Birbeck-Granula *pl*.
vermiform process → vermiform appendix.

ver·mif·u·gal [vɜr'mɪfjəgəl] *adj pharm.* wurmabtreibend, vermifug.
ver·mi·fuge ['vɜrmɪfjuːdʒ] *n* wurmabtreibendes Mittel *nt*, Vermifugum *nt*.
ver·min ['vɜrmɪn] *n micro.* tierischer Ektoparasit *m*.
ver·mi·nal ['vɜrmɪnl] *adj* → verminous.
ver·mi·na·tion [ˌvɜrmɪ'neɪʃn] *n* 1. Wurmbefall *m*. 2. Ektoparasitenbefall *m*.
ver·mi·no·sis [ˌ-'nəʊsɪs] *n* → vermination.
ver·mi·not·ic [ˌ-'nɒtɪk] *adj* 1. Wurminfektion betr., Wurm-. 2. Ektoparasitenbefall betr.
ver·mi·nous ['vɜrmɪnəs] *adj* Würmer betr., durch Würmer hervorgerufen, Wurm-.
verminous abscess Abszeß *m* bei Wurmbefall.
verminous appendicitis Appendizitis *f* durch Wurmbefall, Appendicitis helminthica/vermicularis.
verminous colic Darmkolik *f* bei Wurmbefall.
ver·mis ['vɜrmɪs] *n, pl* **-mes** [-miːz] 1. *bio.* Wurm *m*, Vermis *m*. 2. *anat.* → vermis cerebelli.
vermis cerebelli (Kleinhirn-)Wurm *m*, Vermis cerebelli.
ver·mi·toid ['vɜrmɪtɔɪd] *adj* wurmartig, -ähnlich, vermiform.
ver·mix ['vɜrmɪks] *n* → vermiform appendix.
ver·nal ['vɜrnl] *adj* im Frühling auftretend, Frühlings-, Frühjahr(s)-.
vernal catarrh Frühjahrskonjunktivitis *f*, -katarrh *m*, Conjunctivitis vernalis.
vernal conjunctivitis → vernal catarrh.
vernal encephalitis russische Früh(jahr)-Sommer-Enzephalitis *f abbr.* RSSE, russische Zeckenenzephalitis *f*.
Verner-Morrison ['vɜrnər 'mɒrəsən]: **V.-M. syndrome** Verner-Morrison-Syndrom *nt*, pankreatische Cholera *f*.
Vernet [vɛr'ne]: **V.'s syndrome** Vernet-Syndrom *nt*.
ver·nix caseosa ['vɜrnɪks] *gyn.*, *ped.* Frucht-, Käseschmiere *f*, Vernix caseosa.
ver·nos·ti·val ['vɜrnəʊ'estɪvəl] → vernal encephalitis.
ver·o·nal buffer ['verɒnəl, -næl, -nl] Veronalpuffer *m*.
ve·ro·tox·in [verə'tɒksɪn] *n* Verotoxin *nt*.
ver·ru·ca [və'ruːkə] *n, pl* **-cae** [-siː] 1. (virusbedingte) Warze *f*, Verruca *f*. 2. warzenähnliche Hautveränderung *f*.
verruca peruana Peruwarze *f*, Verruca peruana.
verruca peruviana → verruca peruana.
ver·ru·ci·form [və'ruːsəfɔːrm] *adj* warzenähnlich, -förmig.
ver·ru·cose ['verəkəʊs, və'ruːkəʊs] *adj* → verrucous.
ver·ru·co·sis [ˌverə'kəʊsɪs] *n* Verrucosis *f*.
ver·ru·cous ['verəkəs, və'ruː-] *adj* warzenartig, warzig, verrukös.
verrucous carditis → verrucous endocarditis.
verrucous endocarditis verruköse Endokarditis *f*, Endocarditis verrucosa.
atypical v. atypische verruköse Endokarditis, Libman-Sacks-Syndrom *nt*, Endokarditis-Libman-Sacks, Endocarditis thrombotica.
nonbacterial v. → atypical v.
simple v. Endocarditis verrucosa simplex.
verrucous nevus hyperkeratotischer Nävus *m*, harter Nävus *m*, harter epidermaler Nävus *m*, Naevus verrucosus.
ver·ru·ga [və'ruːgə] *n* → verruca.
verruga peruana → verruca peruana.
ver·sa·tile ['vɜrsətl; *Brit.* -taɪl] *adj* 1. vielseitig (verwendbar), versatil. 2. *bio.* frei

beweglich. **3.** wendig, beweglich, gewandt, vielseitig, flexibel.
ver·sa·til·i·ty [ˌvɜrsə'tɪlətɪ] *n* **1.** Vielseitigkeit *f*, vielseitige Anwendbarkeit *f*. **2.** *bio.* freie Beweglichkeit *f*. **3.** Wendigkeit *f*, Gewandtheit *f*, (geistige) Beweglichkeit *f*.
Verse ['vɜrs]: **V.'s disease** Calcinosis intervertebralis.
ver·sion ['vɜrʒn] *n* **1.** *gyn.* Gebärmutterneigung *f*, Versio uteri. **2.** *gyn.* Wendung *f*, Drehung *f*, Versio *f*. **3.** *ophthal.* Version *f*.
vertebr- *pref.* → vertebro-.
ver·te·bra ['vɜrtəbrə] *n, pl* **-bras, -brae** [-briː] *anat.* Wirbel *m*, Vertebra *f*.
vertebra fusion *ortho.* operative Wirbelsäulenversteifung *f*, Spondylodese *f*.
ver·te·bral ['vɜrtəbrəl] *adj* Wirbel(säule) betr., vertebral, Wirbel-, Wirbelsäulen-, Vertebral-, Vertebro-.
vertebral angiography Vertebralisangiographie *f*.
vertebral ankylosis Wirbelsäulenversteifung *f*, Spondylose *f*, Spondylosis *f*.
vertebral anomaly *ortho.* Wirbelkörperanomalie *f*, -fehlbildung *f*.
vertebral aponeurosis Fascia thoracolumbalis.
vertebral arch Wirbelbogen *m*, Arcus vertebrae/vertebralis.
vertebral artery Wirbelarterie *f*, Vertebralis *f*, A. vertebralis.
vertebral body Wirbelkörper *m*, Corpus vertebrae/vertebrale.
vertebral border of scapula medialer Skapularand *m*, Margo medialis scapulae.
vertebral canal Wirbel(säulen)-, Vertebralkanal *m*, Canalis vertebralis.
vertebral column Wirbelsäule *f*, Rückgrat *nt*, Columna vertebralis.
vertebral epiphysitis Morbus Scheuermann *m*, Scheuermann'-Krankheit *f*, Adoleszentenkyphose *f*, Osteochondritis/Osteochondrosis deformans juvenilis.
vertebral foramen Wirbelloch *nt*, For. vertebrale.
vertebral ganglion Ggl. vertebrale.
vertebral incisure: greater/inferior v. Inc. vertebralis inferior.
lesser/superior v. Inc. vertebralis superior.
vertebral line Linea vertebralis.
vertebral margin of scapula → vertebral border of scapula.
vertebral nerve N. vertebralis.
vertebral notch: greater/inferior v. Inc. vertebralis inferior.
lesser/superior v. Inc. vertebralis superior.
vertebral plexus vegetatives Geflecht *nt* der A. vertebralis, Plexus vertebralis.
vertebral region *anat.* Wirbelsäulengegend *f*, -region *f*, Vertebralregion *f*, Regio vertebralis.
vertebral ribs Costae fluitantes.
vertebral vein Begleitvene *f* der A. vertebralis, V. vertebralis.
accessory v. V. vertebralis accessoria.
anterior v. Begleitvene der A. cervicalis ascendens, V. vertebralis anterior.
ver·te·brar·i·um [ˌvɜrtə'brɛərɪəm] *n* → vertebral column.
ver·te·brar·te·ri·al [ˌ-brɑːr'tɪərɪəl] *adj* A. vertebralis betr., Vertebralis-.
Ver·te·bra·ta [ˌ-'breɪtə, -'brɑː-] *pl bio.* Wirbeltiere *pl*, Vertebraten *pl*, Vertebrata *pl*.
ver·te·brate [-'brɪt, -breɪt] **I** *n bio.* Wirbeltier *nt*, Vertebrat *m*. **II** *adj* **1.** mit einer Wirbelsäule/mit Wirbel(n) versehen, Wirbel-. **2.** zu den Vertebraten gehörig.
ver·te·brec·to·my [ˌ-'brɛktəmɪ] *n ortho., neurochir.* Wirbelentfernung *f*, -exzision *f*.

vertebro- *pref.* Wirbel-, Wirbelsäulen-, Vertebral-, Vertebro-.
ver·te·bro·ar·te·ri·al [ˌvɜrtəbroʊɑːr'tɪərɪəl] *adj* → vertebrarterial.
vertebroarterial foramen For. proc. transversi, For. vertebroarteriale, For. transversarium.
ver·te·bro·bas·i·lar insufficiency [ˌ-'bæsɪlər] vertebrobasiläre Insuffizienz *f*, A.-vertebralis-Insuffizienz *f*.
ver·te·bro·chon·dral [ˌ-'kɑndrəl] *adj* Wirbel u. Rippenknorpel betr., vertebrochondral.
ver·te·bro·cos·tal [ˌ-'kɑstl] *adj* Wirbel u. Rippe(n) betr., vertebrokostal, kostovertebral.
ver·te·bro·did·y·mus [ˌ-'dɪdəməs] *n embryo.* Vertebro(di)dymus *m*.
ver·te·brod·y·mus [ˌvɜrtə'brɑdɪməs] *n* → vertebrodidymus.
ver·te·bro·fem·o·ral [ˌvɜrtəbroʊ'fɛmərəl] *adj* vertebrofemoral.
ver·te·bro·il·i·ac [ˌ-'ɪlɪæk] *adj* Wirbel u. Os ilium betr., vertebroiliakal.
ver·te·bro·sa·cral [ˌ-'seɪkrəl, -'sæk-] *adj* Wirbel u. Kreuzbein/Sacrum betr., vertebrosakral, sakrovertebral.
ver·te·bro·ster·nal [ˌ-'stɜrnl] *adj* Wirbel u. Brustbein/Sternum betr., vertebrosternal, sternovertebral.
vertebrosternal ribs echte Rippen *pl*, Costae verae.
ver·tex ['vɜrtɛks] *n, pl* **-tex·es, -ti·ces** [-tɪsiːz] **1.** *anat.* Scheitel *m*, Vertex *m*. **2.** *mathe., fig.* Scheitel(punkt *m*) *m*, Spitze *f*, Vertex *m*.
v. of urinary bladder (Harn-)Blasenspitze *f*, Apex vesicae/vesicalis (urinariae).
vertex presentation *gyn.* Hinterhauptslage *f*.
ver·ti·cal ['vɜrtɪkl] **I** *n* Senkrechte *f*. **II** *adj* **1.** senkrecht, vertikal. **2.** Scheitel/Vertex betr., Scheitel-.
vertical heart *physiol.* Steiltyp *m*.
ver·ti·ca·lis linguae (muscle) [ˌvɜrtɪ'keɪlɪs] Vertikalis *m* linguae, M. verticalis linguae.
ver·ti·cal·i·ty [ˌvɜrtɪ'kælətɪ] *n* senkrechte Lage/Haltung/Stellung *f*, Vertikalität *f*.
vertical movement Vertikalbewegung *f*.
vertical muscle of tongue → verticalis linguae (muscle).
vertical nystagmus vertikaler Nystagmus *m*.
vertical plane Vertikalebene *f*.
vertical talus *ortho.* Plattfuß *m*, Pes planus.
vertical transmission vertikale Infektionsübertragung/Transmission *f*.
vertical vertigo vertikaler Schwindel *m*.
ver·ti·co·men·tal [ˌvɜrtɪkoʊ'mɛntl] *anat.* Scheitelkinnlinie *f*.
ver·tig·i·nous [vər'tɪdʒənəs] *adj* schwind(e)lig, vertiginös, Schwindel-.
ver·ti·go ['vɜrtɪgoʊ] *n* Schwindel *m*, Vertigo *f*.
ver·u·mon·ta·ni·tis [ˌvɛrjuˌmɑntə'naɪtɪs] *n urol.* Samenhügelentzündung *f*, Kolliculitis *f*, Colliculitis *f*.
ver·u·mon·ta·num [ˌvɛrjuːmɑn'teɪnəm] *n* Samenhügel *m*, Colliculus seminalis.
ver·y low-density lipoprotein ['vɛrɪ] *abbr.* VLDL Lipoprotein *nt* mit sehr geringer Dichte, very low-density lipoprotein *abbr.* VLDL, prä-β-Lipoprotein *nt*.
Vesalius [vɪ'seɪljəs, -lɪəs]: **V.' foramen** For. venosum.
ligament of V. Leistenband *nt*, Lig. inguinale, Arcus inguinale.
vesic- *pref.* → vesico-.
ve·si·ca [və'saɪkə, -'siː-, 'vɛsɪkə] *n, pl* **-cae**

[-siː, -kiː] *anat.* **1.** Blase *f*, Vesica *f*. **2.** Blase *f*, Sack *m*, Bulla *f*.
ves·i·cal ['vɛsɪkl] *adj* **1.** Blase/Vesica betr., vesikal, Vesiko-, Blasen-. **2.** Bläschen/Vesicula betr., mit Bläschenbildung einhergehend, vesikulär, bläschenartig, Vesikular-, Vesikulo-. **3.** Hautbläschen betr.
vesical artery: inferior v. untere (Harn-)Blasenarterie *f*, Vesicalis *f* inferior, A. vesicalis inferior.
superior v.s obere (Harn-)Blasenarterien *pl*, Aa. vesicales superiores.
vesical calculus Blasenstein *m*, Zystolith *m*, Calculus vesicae.
vesical center Blasenzentrum *nt*.
vesical crisis *neuro.* Blasenkrise *f*.
vesical diverticulum (Harn-)Blasendivertikel *nt*.
vesical fistula (Harn-)Blasenfistel *f*, Fistula vesicalis.
vesical fold, transverse quere (Harn-)Blasenfalte *f*, Plica vesicalis transversa.
vesical hernia Blasenhernie *f*, -bruch *m*, -vorfall *m*, Zystozele *f*, Cystocele *f*.
vesical lithotomy *urol.* Blasensteinschnitt *m*, Lithozystotomie *f*.
vesical plexus 1. Harnblasengeflecht *nt*, Plexus vesicalis. **2.** Plexus venosus vesicalis.
vesical reflex Blasenentleerungsreflex *m*.
vesical schistosomiasis Blasen-, Harnblasen-, Urogenitalbilharziose *f*, Schistosomiasis urogenitalis.
vesical sphincter, involuntary unwillkürlicher Blasenschließmuskel *m*.
vesical surface of uterus Blasenfläche *f* des Uterus, Facies vesicalis (uteri).
vesical tenesmus schmerzhafter Harndrang *m*, Tenesmus vesicae.
vesical triangle (Harn-)Blasendreieck *nt*, Lieutaud'-Dreieck *nt*, Trigonum vesicae.
vesical trigone → vesical triangle.
vesical veins Blasenvenen *pl*, Vv. vesicales.
ves·i·cant ['vɛsɪkənt] **I** *n* blasenziehendes/blasentreibendes Mittel *nt*, Vesikans *nt*, Vesikatorium *nt*. **II** *adj* blasenziehend, -treibend.
ves·i·cate ['vɛsɪkeɪt] *vt, vi* Blasen ziehen.
ves·i·ca·tion [ˌvɛsɪ'keɪʃn] *n* **1.** Blasenbildung *f*, Vesikation *f*. **2.** Blase *f*.
ves·i·ca·to·ry ['vɛsɪkətɔːriː, -təʊ-] *n, adj* → vesicant.
ves·i·cle ['vɛsɪkl] *n* **1.** *anat.* kleine Blase *f*, Bläschen *nt*, Vesikel *nt*, Vesicula *f*. **2.** *patho.* kleines Hautbläschen *nt*, Vesicula cutanea.
vesico- *pref.* Blasen-, Vesik(o)-.
ves·i·co·ab·dom·i·nal [ˌvɛsɪkoʊæb'dɑmɪnl] *adj* Harnblase u. Abdomen betr. *od.* verbindend, vesikoabdominal.
ves·i·co·cav·ern·ous [ˌ-'kævərnəs] *adj* vesikokavernös.
ves·i·co·cele ['-siːl] *n* Blasenbruch *m*, -vorfall *m*, -hernie *f*, Zystozele *f*, Cystocele *f*.
ves·i·co·cer·vi·cal [ˌ-'sɜrvɪkl] *adj* Harnblase u. Cervix uteri betr. *od.* verbindend, vesikozervikal.
ves·i·coc·ly·sis [vɛsɪ'kɑklɪsɪs] *n* Blasenspülung *f*.
ves·i·co·col·ic [ˌvɛsɪkoʊ'kɑlɪk] *adj* Harnblase u. Kolon betr. *od.* verbindend, vesikokolisch.
vesicocolic fistula (Harn-)Blasen-Kolon-Fistel *f*, Fistula vesicocolica.
ves·i·co·co·lon·ic [ˌ-koʊ'lɑnɪk, -kə-] *adj* → vesicocolic.
ves·i·co·cu·ta·ne·ous fistula [ˌ-kjuː'teɪnɪəs] adj *patho.* (Harn-)Blasenfistel *f*, vesikokutane Fistel *f*, Fistula vesicocutanea.
ves·i·co·en·ter·ic [ˌ-en'tɛrɪk] *adj* → vesicointestinal.

vesicofixation 816

ves·i·co·fix·a·tion [ˌ-fɪk'seɪʃn] *n urol.* (Harn-)Blasenanheftung *f*, Zystopexie *f*.
ves·i·co·in·tes·ti·nal [ˌ-ɪn'testənl] *adj* Harnblase u. Intestinum betr. *od.* verbindend, vesikointestinal.
vesicointestinal fistula (Harn-)Blasen-Darm-Fistel *f*, vesikointestinale Fistel *f*.
ves·i·co·li·thi·a·sis [ˌ-lɪ'θaɪəsɪs] *n urol.* Blasensteinleiden *nt*, Zystolithiasis *f*.
ves·i·co·per·i·neal [ˌ-perɪ'niːəl] *adj* (Harn-)Blase u. Damm/Perineum betr. *od.* verbindend, vesikoperineal.
vesicoperineal fistula *patho.* (Harn-)-Blasen-Damm-Fistel *f*, vesikoperineale Fistel *f*, Fistula vesicoperinealis.
ves·i·co·pros·tat·ic [ˌ-prɒs'tætɪk] *adj* Harnblase u. Prostata betr. *od.* verbindend, vesikoprostatisch.
ves·i·co·pu·bic [ˌ-'pjuːbɪk] *adj* Harnblase u. Scham(gegend)/Pubes betr., vesikopubisch.
vesicopubic ligament Lig. pubovesicale.
ves·i·co·rec·tal [ˌ-'rektl] *adj* Harnblase u. Rektum betr. *od.* verbindend, vesikorektal.
vesicorectal fistula *patho.* (Harn-)Blasen-Rektum-Fistel *f*, vesikorektale Fistel *f*, Fistula vesicorectalis.
ves·i·co·rec·tos·to·my [ˌ-rek'tɒstəmɪ] *n chir., urol.* (Harn-)Blasen-Rektum-Fistel *f*, Vesikorektostomie *f*.
ves·i·co·re·nal [ˌ-'riːnl] *adj* Harnblase u. Niere/Ren betr., vesikorenal.
ves·i·co·sig·moid [ˌ-'sɪgmɔɪd] *adj* Harnblase u. Sigma betr., vesikosigmoid.
ves·i·co·sig·moid·os·to·my [ˌ-sɪgmɔɪ'dɒstəmɪ] *n urol., chir.* (Harn-)Blasen-Sigma-Fistel *f*, Vesikosigmoid(e)ostomie *f*.
ves·i·co·spi·nal [ˌ-'spaɪnl] *adj* Harnblase u. Wirbelsäule *od.* Rückenmark betr., vesikospinal.
vesicospinal center vesikospinales Zentrum *nt*, Centrum vesicospinale.
ves·i·cos·to·my [vesɪ'kɒstəmɪ] *n urol.* äußere Blasenfistel *f*, Vesikostomie *f*.
ves·i·cot·o·my [vesɪ'kɒtəmɪ] *n urol.* (Harn-)Blasenschnitt *m*, Zystotomie *f*.
ves·i·co·um·bil·i·cal [ˌvesɪkəʊʌm'bɪlɪkl] *adj* Harnblase u. Nabel betr. *od.* verbindend, vesikoumbilikal.
vesicoumbilical fistula (Harn-)Blasen-Nabel-Fistel *f*, vesikoumbilikale Fistel *f*, Fistula vesicoumbilicalis.
vesicoumbilical ligament Lig. umbilicale mediale.
ves·i·co·u·re·ter·al [ˌ-jʊə'riːtərəl] *adj* → vesicoureteric.
vesicoureteral reflux vesiko-ureteraler Reflux *m*.
vesicoureteral regurgitation → vesicoureteral reflux.
ves·i·co·u·re·ter·ic [ˌ-jʊərɪ'terɪk] *adj* Harnblase u. Harnleiter/Ureter betr. *od.* verbindend, vesikoureterisch.
vesicoureteric reflux → vesicoureteral reflux.
ves·i·co·u·re·thral [ˌ-jʊə'riːθrəl] *adj* Harnblase u. Harnröhre/Urethra betr. *od.* verbindend, vesikourethral.
vesicourethral angle Blasen-Harnröhren-Winkel *m*.
anterior v. vorderer Blasen-Harnröhren-Winkel.
posterior v. hinterer Blasen-Harnröhren-Winkel.
vesicourethral opening innere Harnröhrenöffnung *f*, Harnröhrenanfang *m*, Ostium urethrae internum.
vesicourethral orifice → vesicourethral opening.
ves·i·co·u·ter·ine [ˌ-'juːtərɪn, -raɪn] *adj*

Harnblase u. Uterus betr. *od.* verbindend, vesikouterin.
vesicouterine excavation vorderer Douglas'-Raum *m*, Excavatio vesicouterina.
vesicouterine fistula *patho.* (Harn-)Blasen-Gebärmutter-Fistel, vesikouterine Fistel *f*, Fistula vesicouterina.
vesicouterine ligament äußerer Schenkel *m* des Blasenpfeilers, Lig. vesicouterinum.
vesicouterine pouch → vesicouterine excavation.
ves·i·co·u·ter·o·vag·i·nal [ˌ-juːtərəʊ-'vædʒɪnl] *adj* vesikouterovaginal.
ves·i·co·vag·i·nal [ˌ-'vædʒənl] *adj* Harnblase u. Scheide/Vagina betr. *od.* verbindend, vesikovaginal.
vesicovaginal fistula (Harn-)Blasen-Scheiden-Fistel *f*, Vesikovaginalfistel *f*, vesikovaginale Fistel *f*, Fistula vesicovaginalis.
ves·i·co·vag·i·no·rec·tal [ˌ-ˌvædʒɪnəʊ-'rektl] *adj* vesikovaginorektal.
ve·sic·u·la [və'sɪkjələ] *n, pl* **-lae** [-liː, -laɪ] → vesicle 1.
ve·sic·u·lar [və'sɪkjələr] *adj* (Haut-)Bläschen/Vesicula betr., aus Bläschen bestehend, blasig, bläschenförmig, -artig, vesikulär, Vesikulär-, Vesikulo-.
vesicular appendages (of epoophoron) Morgagni-Hydatiden *pl*, Appendices vesiculosae (epoophorontis).
vesicular blood fluke *micro.* Blasenpärchenegel *m*, Schistosoma haematobium.
vesicular brain *patho.* Blasenhirn *nt*, Hydranzephalie *f*.
vesicular breathing Vesikulär-, Bläschenatmen *nt*, vesikuläres Atemgeräusch *nt*.
vesicular bronchiolitis Bronchopneumonie *f*, lobuläre Pneumonie *f*.
vesicular bursa, iliopubic Bursa iliopectinea.
vesicular cartilage *histol.* Blasenknorpel *m*.
vesicular cartilage zone *histol.* Zone *f* des Blasenknorpels.
vesicular gland Bläschendrüse *f*, Samenblase *f*, -bläschen *nt*, Gonozystis *f*, Spermatozystis *f*, Vesicula seminalis.
vesicular keratitis Keratitis vesicularis.
vesicular mole *gyn.* Blasenmole *f*, Mola hydatidosa.
vesicular murmur Vesikulär-, Bläschenatmen *nt*, vesikuläres Atemgeräusch *nt*.
vesicular ovarian follicles Tertiärfollikel *pl*, Folliculi ovarici vesiculosi.
vesicular rales (Lunge) feinblasiges Knisterrasseln *nt*.
vesicular respiration Vesikuläratmen *nt*, Bläschenatmen *nt*, vesikuläres Atmen *nt*.
vesicular rickettsiosis Pockenfleckfieber *nt*, Rickettsienpocken *pl*.
vesicular stomatitis aphthöse Stomatitis *f*, Gingivostomatitis/Stomatitis herpetica.
ve·sic·u·late [və'sɪkjəlɪt, -lɪt] *adj* blasig, bläschenartig; mit Bläschen bedeckt.
ve·sic·u·lat·ed [və'sɪkjəlɪtɪd] *adj* → vesiculate.
ve·sic·u·la·tion [vəˌsɪkjə'leɪʃn] *n* Bläschenbildung *f*, Vesikulation *f*.
ve·sic·u·lec·to·my [vəˌsɪkjə'lektəmɪ] *n urol.* Samenblasenresektion *f*, -exzision *f*, Vesikulektomie *f*.
ve·sic·u·li·form [və'sɪkjəlɪfɔːrm] *adj* bläschenförmig.
ve·sic·u·li·tis [vəˌsɪkjə'laɪtɪs] *n urol.* Samenblasenentzündung *f*, Vesikulitis *f*, Vesiculitis *f*, Spermatozystitis *f*.
ve·sic·u·lo·bron·chi·al [vəˌsɪkjəlɒʊ'brɒŋkɪəl] *adj* vesikulobronchial, bronchovesikulär.

ve·sic·u·lo·cav·ern·ous [ˌ-'kævərnəs] *adj* vesikulokavernös, vesikulär-kavernös.
ve·sic·u·lo·gram ['-græm] *n radiol., urol.* Vesikulogramm *nt*.
ve·sic·u·log·ra·phy [vəˌsɪkjə'lɒgrəfɪ] *n urol., radiol.* Kontrastdarstellung *f* der Samenbläschen, Vesikulographie *f*.
ve·sic·u·lo·pap·u·lar [vəˌsɪkjələʊ'pæpjələr] *adj* vesikulopapulär, vesikulär-papulär.
ve·sic·u·lo·pus·tu·lar [ˌ-'pʌstʃələr] *adj* vesikulopustulär.
ve·sic·u·lot·o·my [vəˌsɪkjə'lɒtəmɪ] *n urol.* Vesikulotomie *f*.
ve·sic·u·lo·tu·bu·lar [vəˌsɪkjələʊ't(j)uːbjələr] *adj* vesikulotubulär.
ve·sic·u·lo·tym·pan·ic [ˌ-tɪm'pænɪk] *adj* vesikulotympanisch.
vesiculotympanic resonance hypersonorer Klopfschall *m*.
ve·sic·u·lo·tym·pa·nit·ic resonance [ˌ-ˌtɪmpə'nɪtɪk] → vesiculotympanic resonance.
ves·sel ['vesl] *n anat.* Gefäß *nt*; Ader *f*.
v.s of internal ear Innenohrgefäße *pl*, Vasa auris interna.
v.s of vessels Vasa vasorum.
vessel clamp *chir.* Gefäßklemme *f*, -klammer *f*.
vessel injury Gefäßverletzung *f*, -trauma *nt*.
ves·tib·u·lar [və'stɪbjələr] *adj anat.* Vorhof/Vestibulum betr., vestibulär, Vestibular-, Vestibulo-.
vestibular apparatus Vestibularapparat *m*, Gleichgewichtsorgan *nt*.
vestibular aqueduct Felsenbeinkanal *m*, Aqu(a)eductus vestibuli.
vestibular area Area vestibularis.
inferior v. of internal acoustic meatus Area vestibularis inferior.
superior v. of internal acoustic meatus Area vestibularis superior.
vestibular arteries Rami vestibulares a. labyrinthi.
vestibular ataxia vestibuläre/labyrinthäre Ataxie *f*.
vestibular branches of labyrinthine artery → vestibular arteries.
vestibular caecum of cochlear duct blindes Vestibulumende *nt* des Ductus cochlearis, Caecum vestibulare ductus cochlearis.
vestibular canal → vestibular scala.
vestibular crest Crista vestibuli.
vestibular disorder Vestibularisstörung *f*.
central v. zentrale Vestibularisstörung.
functional v. funktionelle Vestibularisstörung, vestibuläre Funktionsstörung.
peripheral v. periphere Vestibularisstörung.
vestibular fibers vestibuläre Fasern *pl*.
vestibular fold Taschenfalte *f*, Plica ventricularis/vestibularis.
vestibular fossa Fossa vestibuli vaginae.
vestibular ganglion Scarpa'-Ganglion *nt*, Rosenthal-Ferré'-Ganglion *nt*, Ggl. vestibulare.
vestibular glands Scheidenvorhofdrüsen *pl*, Gll. vestibulares.
greater v. Bartholin'-Drüsen *pl*, Gll. vestibulares majores.
lesser v. Gll. vestibulares minores.
vestibular haircells vestibuläre Haarzellen *pl*.
vestibular-induced nystagmus → vestibular nystagmus.
vestibular labyrinth Vorhoflabyrinth *nt*, Labyrinthus vestibularis.
vestibular ligament Taschenband *nt*, Lig. vestibulare.
vestibular lip of limb of spiral lamina Labium limbi vestibulare.

vestibular membrane of cochlear duct Reissner'-Membran *f*, Membrana vestibularis, Paries vestibularis ductus cochlearis.
vestibular nerve Gleichgewichtsnerv *m*, Vestibularis *m*, N. vestibularis, Pars vestibularis n. vestibulocochlearis.
vestibular neuronitis akuter unilateraler Vestibularisausfall *m*, Vestibularisneuronitis *f*, Neuronitis vestibularis.
vestibular nucleus: v.i *pl* Vestibulariskerne *pl*, Ncc. vestibulares.
 caudal/inferior v. Roller'-Kern *m*, Nc. vestibularis caudalis/inferior.
 lateral v. Deiters'-Kern *m*, Nc. vestibularis lateralis.
 medial v. Schwalbe'-Kern *m*, Nc. vestibularis medialis.
 rostral/superior v. Bechterew'-Kern *m*, Nc. vestibularis superior.
vestibular nystagmus vestibulärer Nystagmus *m*.
vestibular part of medial longitudinal fasciculus vestibulärer Anteil *m* des Fasciculus longitudinalis medialis.
vestibular reflex Vestibularisreflex *m*.
vestibular root of vestibulocochlear nerve oberer vestibulärer Anteil *m* des N. vestibulocochlearis, Radix superior/vestibularis n. vestibulocochlearis.
vestibular scala Scala vestibuli.
vestibular-semicircular canal system (*Ohr*) Vorhof-Bogengangssystem *nt*.
vestibular tracts vestibuläre Bahnen *pl*.
vestibular veins Bogengangsvenen *pl*, Vv. vestibulares.
vestibular vertigo Vestibularisschwindel *m*, Vertigo vestibularis.
vestibular wall of cochlear duct → vestibular membrane of cochlear duct.
vestibular window ovales Fenster *nt*, Vorhoffenster *nt*, Fenestra ovalis/vestibuli.
ves·ti·bule ['vestɪbju:l] *n anat.* Vorhof *m*, Eingang *m*, Vestibulum *nt*.
 v. of ear Innenohrvorhof, Vestibulum auris.
 v. of nose Nasenvorhof, -eingang, Vestibulum nasale/nasi.
 v. of omental bursa Vorhof des Netzbeutels, Vestibulum bursae omentalis.
 v. of vagina Scheidenvorhof, Vestibulum vaginae.
ves·tib·u·lo·cer·e·bel·lar ataxia [və‚stɪbjələʊ‚serə'belər] vestibulozerebelläre Ataxie *f*.
vestibulocerebellar fibers vestibulozerebelläre Fasern *pl*.
vestibulocerebellar tract Tractus vestibulocerebellaris.
ves·tib·u·lo·cer·e·bel·lum [‚-‚serə'beləm] *n* Arch(a)eocerebellum *nt*, Archicerebellum *nt*.
ves·tib·u·lo·coch·le·ar nerve [‚-'kɒklər, -'koʊ-] Akustikus *m*, Vestibulokochlearis *m*, VIII. Hirnnerv *m*, N. acusticus/vestibulocochlearis.
vestibulocochlear nuclei Vestibulokochleariskerne *pl*, Ncc. n. vestibulocochlearis.
vestibulocochlear organ Gehör- u. Gleichgewichtsorgan *nt*, Organon auditus, Organum vestibulocochleare/statoacusticum/vestibulocochlearis.
ves·tib·u·lo·cor·ti·cal [‚-'kɔ:rtɪkl] *adj* vestibulokortikal.
ves·tib·u·lo·oc·u·lar reflex [‚-'ɒkjələr] vestibulookulärer Reflex *m abbr.* VOR.
ves·tib·u·lo·plas·ty ['-‚plæstɪ] *n HNO* Vestibuloplastik *f*.
ves·tib·u·lo·spi·nal tract [‚-'spaɪnl] Held'-Bündel *nt*, Tractus vestibulospinalis.
ves·tib·u·lot·o·my [və‚stɪbjə'lɒtəmɪ] *n HNO* Vestibulotomie *f*.
ves·tib·u·lo·tox·ic [və‚stɪbjələʊ'tɒksɪk] *adj* vestibulotoxisch.
ves·tib·u·lo·u·re·thral [‚-jʊə'ri:θrəl] *adj* vestibulourethral.
ves·tib·u·lo·vag·i·nal bulb [‚-'vædʒɪnl] Schwellkörper *m* des Scheidenvorhofes, Bulbus vestibuli (vaginae).
ves·tib·u·lum [və'stɪbjələm] *n, pl* **-la** [-lə] → vestibule.
 v. of larynx Kehlkopfvorhof *m*, oberer Kehlkopfinnenraum *m*, Vestibulum laryngis.
 v. of mouth Mundvorhof *m*, Vestibulum oris.
 v. of omental bursa Vorhof *m* des Netzbeutels, Vestibulum bursae omentalis.
 v. of vulva Scheidenvorhof *m*, Vestibulum vaginae.
ves·tige ['vestɪdʒ] *n* Überbleibsel *nt*, -rest *m*, Spur *f*; Rudiment *nt*.
 v. of vaginal process Cloquet-Band *nt*, Vestigium proc. vaginalis.
ves·tig·i·al [ve'stɪdʒ(ɪ)əl] *adj* verkümmert, rudimentär.
vestigial deferent duct Ductus deferens vestigialis.
vestigial fold of Marshall Marshall-Falte *f*, Plica venae cavae sinistrae.
ves·tig·i·um [ve'stɪdʒɪəm] *n, pl* **-tig·ia** [-dʒɪə] *anat.* Vestigium *nt*.
vet [vet] *inf.* **I** *n* → veterinary **I. II** *vt* (*Tiere*) untersuchen *od.* behandeln.
vet·er·i·nar·i·an [‚vetərɪ'neərɪən] *n* → veterinary **I**.
vet·er·i·nar·y ['vetərɪnerɪ, 'vetrə-] **I** *n, pl* **-nar·ies** Tierarzt *m*, -ärztin *f*, Veterinär *m*. **II** *adj* Tiermedizin betr., veterinär, veterinärmedizinisch, Veterinär-, Tier-.
veterinary medicine Tier-, Veterinärmedizin *f*, Tierheilkunde *f*.
ve·to cells ['vi:təʊ] *immun.* Veto-Zellen *pl*.
v.G. *abbr.* → van Gieson's stain.
VH *abbr.* → venous hematocrit.
via ['vaɪə, 'vi:ə] **I** *n, pl* **vi·ae** ['vaɪi:] Weg *m*, Passage *f*, Zugang *m*, Via *f*. **II** *prep* **1.** durch, mit Hilfe, mittels, über, via. **2.** über, via.
vi·a·bil·i·ty [vaɪə'bɪlətɪ] *n* Lebensfähigkeit *f*.
vi·a·ble ['vaɪəbl] *adj* lebensfähig.
Vi agglutination Vi-Agglutination *f*.
vi·al ['vaɪəl] *n* (Glas-)Fläschchen *nt*, Phiole *f*.
Vi antigen Vi-Antigen *nt*.
vi·bex ['vaɪbeks] *n, pl* **vi·bi·ces** ['vaɪbəsi:z] streifenförmiger Bluterguß *m*, Striemen *m*, Strieme *f*, Vibex *f*.
vi·brate ['vaɪbreɪt] **I** *vt* zum Vibrieren/Schwingen bringen, vibrieren *od.* schwingen lassen. **II** *vi* (*a. fig.*) zittern, beben (*with* vor); vibrieren, schwingen, oszillieren, pulsieren (*with* von).
vi·bra·tile ['vaɪbrətɪl, -taɪl] *adj* schwingungsfähig, schwingend, oszillierend, vibrierend, Schwingungs-.
vi·bra·tion [vaɪ'breɪʃn] *n* **1.** Schwingen *nt*, Vibrieren *nt*, Beben *nt*, Zittern *nt*. **2.** *phys.* Vibration *f*, Schwingung *f*, Oszillation *f*. **3.** Vibration(smassage *f*) *f*.
vi·bra·tion·al [vaɪ'breɪʃnl] *adj* Schwingungs-, Vibrations-.
vibrational load Vibrationsbelastung *f*.
vibration-damping *adj* schwingungsdämpfend.
vibration receptor Vibrationsrezeptor *m*.
vibration sensation Vibrationsempfindung *f*.
vibration sensor Vibrationssensor *m*.
vi·bra·tor ['vaɪbreɪtər] *n* Vibrationsapparat *m*, Vibrator *m*.
vi·bra·to·ry ['vaɪbrətɔ:rɪ, -təʊ-] *adj* schwingend, schwingungsfähig, vibrierend, Schwing(ungs)-, Vibrations-.
vibratory nystagmus Pendelnystagmus *m*.
vibratory sensibility *neuro.* Vibrationsempfindung *f*, Pallästhesie *f*.
Vib·ri·o ['vɪbrɪəʊ] *n micro.* Vibrio *m*.
 V. cholerae Komma-Bazillus *m*, Vibrio cholerae/comma.
 V. cholerae biotype eltor Vibrio El-tor, Vibrio cholerae biovar eltor.
 V. cholerae (serogroup) non-01 nicht--agglutinable Vibrionen *pl*, NAG--Vibrionen *pl*, Vibrio cholerae non-01.
 V. cholerae (subgroup) 01 Vibrio cholerae 0:1.
 V. comma → V. cholerae.
 V. eltor → V. cholerae biotype eltor.
 V. septicus Pararauschbrandbazillus *m*, Clostridium septicum.
vib·rio ['vɪbrɪəʊ] *n, pl* **-ri·os** *micro.* Vibrio *m*.
Vibrio cholerae enterotoxin Choleraenterotoxin *nt*, Choleragen *nt*.
vib·ri·o·ci·dal [‚vɪbrɪəʊ'saɪdl] *adj* vibrio(ab)tötend, vibrionen(ab)tötend, vibriozid.
Vib·ri·o·na·ce·ae [‚vɪbrɪə'neɪsɪi:] *pl micro.* Vibrionaceae *pl*.
vib·ri·on sep·tique [vibri'ɔ̃ sɛp'tik] *French micro.* Pararauschbrandbazillus *m*, Clostridium septicum.
vib·ri·o·sis [vɪbrɪ'əʊsɪs] *n* Vibrioinfektion *f*.
vi·bris·sae [vaɪ'brɪsi:] *pl* Nasenhaare *pl*, Vibrissae *pl*.
vi·car·i·ous [vaɪ'keərɪəs] *adj* stellvertretend, ersatzweise, vikariierend.
vicarious hypertrophy vikariierende Hypertrophie *f*.
vicarious menstruation vikariierende Menstruation *f*.
vic·i·nal ['vɪsɪnl] *adj* umliegend, nah, benachbart.
vi·cin·i·ty [vɪ'sɪnətɪ] *n* Nähe *f*, Nachbarschaft *f*, (nähere) Umgebung *f*. **in the ~** in der Nähe (*of* von).
vi·cious ['vɪʃəs] *adj* **1.** fehler-, mangelhaft. **2.** bösartig, boshaft, tückisch, gemein, vitiosus.
vicious circle Teufelskreis *m*, Circulus vitiosus.
Vickers ['vɪkərz]: **V. hardness number** Vickers-Pyramidendruckhärte *f*.
Vicq d'Azyr [vik da'zi:r]: **V.'s band** → fasciculus of V.
 body of V. *old* schwarzer Kern *m*, Substantia nigra.
 bundle of V. → fasciculus of V.
 fasciculus of V. Vicq d'Azyr'-Bündel *nt*, Fasciculus mamillothalamicus.
 tract of V. → fasciculus of V.
 V.'s foramen For. caecum.
Vidal [vi'dal]: **V.'s disease** Vidal'-Krankheit *f*, Lichen Vidal *m*, Lichen simplex chronicus (Vidal), Neurodermitis circumscriptus.
vi·dar·a·bine [vaɪ'dærəbi:n] *n pharm.* Vidarabin *nt*, Adenin-Arabinosid *nt*, Ara-A *nt*.
vid·e·o ['vɪdɪəʊ] **I** *n* **1.** Videotechnik *f*. **2.** Videogerät *nt*. **3.** Bildschirm-, Bildsicht-, Datensichtgerät *nt*. **II** *adj* Video-.
video-tape I *n* Videoband *nt*. **II** *vt* auf Videoband aufnehmen.
vid·i·an artery ['vɪdɪən] A. canalis pterygoidei.
vidian canal Canalis pterygoideus/Vidii.
vidian nerve Radix facialis, N. Vidianus/Vidii, N. canalis pterygoidei.
 deep v. N. petrosus profundus.
vidian vein Begleitvene *f* der A. canalis pterygoidei, V. pterygoidea.
Vi·en·na encephalitis [vɪ'enə] (von)

Vieth-Müller

Economo-Krankheit f, -Enzephalitis f, europäische Schlafkrankheit f, Encephalitis epidemica/lethargica.
Vieth-Müller [viːt 'mjuːlə(r), 'mıl-; 'mylər]: **V.-M. circle/horopter** ophthal. Vieth-Müller-Kreis m.
Vieussens [vjøˈsã]: **ansa of V.** Ansa subclavia.
V.'s foramina Forr. venarum minimarum.
V.'s ganglion Plexus coeliacus.
V.'s isthmus Limbus fossae ovalis.
loop of V. → ansa of V.
V.'s ring Limbus fossae ovalis.
V.'s valve Velum medulare superius.
veins of V. vordere Herzvenen pl, Vv. cordis/cardiacae anteriores.
V.'s ventricle Cavum septi pellucidi.
view [vjuː] I n 1. (An-, Hin-, Zu-)Sehen nt, Betrachtung f. 2. Sicht f, Ansicht f. **in ~** sichtbar. **out of ~** außer Sicht. **to come in ~** sichtbar werden. **to keep in ~** beobachten, etw. im Auge behalten. 3. photo., radiol. Aufnahme f, Bild nt, Projektion f. 4. Prüfung f, Untersuchung f; (kritischer) Überblick m. 5. fig. Ansicht f, Anschauung f, Auffassung f, Meinung f, Urteil nt (of, on über). **to form a ~** s. ein Urteil bilden (on über). **to have/hold/keep/take a (strong) ~ of** eine (feste) Meinung haben über. 6. Absicht f, Intention f. **to have sth. in ~** etw. beabsichtigen. II vt 7. (s.) ansehen, betrachten, besichtigen, in Augenschein nehmen, prüfen. 8. beurteilen, auffassen, meinen.
vig·il·am·bu·lism [ˌvıdʒıl'æmbjəlızəm] n Vigilambulismus m.
vig·i·lance ['vıdʒələns] n 1. Aufmerksamkeit f, Reaktionsbereitschaft f, Vigilanz f, Vigilität f. 2. Schlaflosigkeit f, Wachheit f, Insomnie f.
vig·i·lant ['vıdʒələnt] adj aufmerksam, wachsam, vigilant.
vig·or ['vıgər] n (Körper-, Geistes-)Kraft f, Vitalität f; Aktivität f, Energie f; Lebenskraft f.
vig·or·ous ['vıgərəs] adj kräftig, kraftvoll, vital; lebhaft, aktiv, tatkräftig; energisch; nachhaltig.
vig·our n Brit. → vigor.
Villaret [vilaˈre]: **V.'s syndrome** Villaret-Syndrom nt.
vil·li·form ['vılıfɔːrm] adj bio. zottenförmig, villös.
vil·li·ki·nin [vıləˈkaının] n Villikinin nt.
vil·lo·ma [vıˈləʊmə] n Papillom(a) nt.
vil·lo·nod·u·lar [ˌvıləˈnɒdʒələr] adj villonodulär.
villonodular synovitis → villous synovitis.
vil·lose ['vıləʊs] adj → villous.
vil·los·ec·to·my [vıləˈsɛktəmı] n ortho. Synovialisentfernung f, -exzision f, -resektion f, Synovektomie f, Synovialektomie f.
vil·lo·si·tis [vıləʊˈsaıtıs] n gyn. Villositis f.
vil·lous ['vıləs] adj anat. mit Zotten/Villi besetzt, zottig, villös, Zotten-.
villous adenoma villöses Adenom nt.
villous arthritis, chronic Arthritis villosa chronica.
villous blood vessel Zottengefäß nt.
villous cancer → villous carcinoma.
villous capillary Zottenkapillare f.
villous carcinoma Zottenkrebs m, Ca. villosum f.
villous folds of stomach Plicae villosae.
villous papillae fadenförmige Papillen pl, Papillae filiformis.
villous papilloma Papillom(a) nt.
villous placenta Placenta villosa.
villous stem histol. Zottenstamm m.

villous synovitis villöse/villonoduläre Synovitis f, Synovitis villosa.
villous tumor Papillom nt.
villous vessel → villous blood vessel.
vil·lus ['vıləs] n, pl **-li** [-laı] anat. Zotte f, zottenartiges Gebilde nt, Villus m.
v.i of small intestine Darmzotten pl, Villi intestinales.
vi·lox·a·zine [vıˈlɒksəziːn] n pharm. Viloxazin nt.
Vim-Silverman [vım ˈsılvərmən]: **V.-S. needle** Vim-Silverman-Nadel f.
vin·blas·tine [vınˈblæstiːn] n pharm. Vinblastin nt, Vincaleukoblastin nt.
Vin·ca ['vıŋkə] n bio., pharm. Vinca f.
vin·ca alkaloids ['vıŋkə] Vinca-rosea-Alkaloide pl.
vin·ca·leu·ko·blas·tine [ˌvıŋkəˌluːkəˈblæstiːn] n → vinblastine.
vin·ca·mine ['vıŋkəmiːn] n pharm. Vincamin nt.
Vincent ['vınsent] : **V.'s angina** Vincent-Angina f, -Krankheit f, Plaut-Vincent-Angina f, Angina Plaut-Vincenti, Angina ulcerosa/ulceromembranacea, Fusospirochätose f, Fusospirillose f.
V.'s disease → V.'s angina.
V.'s infection → V.'s angina.
spirillum of V. Treponema/Borrelia/Spirochaeta vincentii.
V.'s stomatitis → V.'s angina.
vin·co·fos ['vıŋkəʊfəs] n pharm. Vincofos nt.
vin·cris·tine [vınˈkrıstiːn] n pharm. Vincristin nt.
vin·cu·lum ['vıŋkjələm] n, pl **-la** [-lə] 1. anat. Band nt, Fessel f, Vinculum f. 2. fig. Band nt.
v.la of tendons Fesselband, Vincula tendinum.
v.la of tendons of fingers Vincula tendinum digitorum manus.
v.la of tendons of toes Vincula tendinum digitorum pedis.
vinculum breve Vinculum breve.
vinculum longum Vinculum longum.
vin·de·sine ['vındəsiːn] n pharm. Vindesin nt, VP-16 nt.
Vineberg ['vaınbərg]: **V.'s operation** Vineberg-Operation f.
vin·e·gar ['vınəgər] n 1. Essig m, Acetum nt. 2. Essig(säure)lösung f.
vinegar bacteria micro. Essig(säure)bakterien pl, Acetobacter m.
Vinson ['vınsən]: **V.'s syndrome** Plummer-Vinson-Syndrom nt, Paterson-Brown-Syndrom nt, Kelly-Paterson-Syndrom nt, sideropenische Dysphagie f.
vi·nyl ['vaınl] n Vinyl-(Radikal nt).
vinyl acetate Vinylacetat nt.
vinyl chloride Vinylchlorid nt abbr. VC.
vi·o·cid ['vaıəsıd] n Gentianaviolett nt.
vi·o·late ['vaıəleıt] vt schänden, vergewaltigen, notzüchten.
vi·o·la·tion [vaıəˈleıʃn] n 1. Verletzung f, Übertretung f, Bruch m, Zuwiderhandlung f. 2. Notzucht f, Vergewaltigung f, Schändung f.
vi·o·lence ['vaıələns] n 1. Gewalt f, Gewalttätigkeit f. 2. Gewalttat f, -anwendung f, Gewalt f. 3. Verletzung f, Unrecht nt, Schändung f. 4. Heftigkeit f, Ungestüm nt.
vi·o·lent ['vaıələnt] adj 1. gewaltig, stark, heftig. 2. gewaltsam, gewalttätig, Gewalt-. 3. heftig, ungestüm, leidenschaftlich. 4. grell, laut.
vi·o·let ['vaıəlıt] I n Violett nt, violette Farbe f. II adj violett.
violet G Gentianaviolett nt.
vi·o·my·cin ['vaıəmaısın] n pharm. Viomycin nt.

vi·os·ter·ol [vaıˈɒstərɒl, -rɒl] n → vitamin D_2.
VIP abbr. → vasoactive intestinal peptide.
vi·per ['vaıpər] n bio. 1. Viper f, Otter f, Natter f. 2. Giftschlange f.
Vi·pera ['vaıpərə] f bio. Vipera f.
vi·per·id ['vaıpərıd] adj → viperine II.
Vi·per·i·dae [vaıˈpɛrədiː] pl bio. Viperidae pl.
vi·per·ine ['vaıpərın, -raın] bio. I n echte Otter f. II adj vipernartig, Vipern-.
vi·per·ish ['vaıpərıʃ] adj → viperine II.
vi·per·ous ['vaıpərəs] adj → viperine II.
VIPoma n → vipoma.
vi·po·ma [vıˈpəʊmə] n Vipom nt, VIPom nt, VIP-produzierendes Inselzelladenom nt, D_1-Tumor m.
vir·a·gin·i·ty [ˌvaırəˈdʒınətı, ˌvıərə-] n Viragenität f.
vi·ral ['vaırəl] adj Virus betr., durch Viren verursacht, viral, Virus-.
viral antigen Virusantigen nt.
viral antiserum Virusantiserum nt.
viral chromosome Viruschromosom nt.
viral deoxyribonuclease virale Desoxyribonuklease f, virale DNase f.
viral disease Viruserkrankung f, -krankheit f.
viral DNA Virus-DNA f, virale DNA f, Virus-DNS f, virale DNS f.
viral dysentery Virusdysenterie f.
viral encephalomyelitis Virusenzephalomyelitis f.
viral exanthema Virusexanthem nt.
viral genetics Virusgenetik f.
viral genome Virusgenom nt.
viral hemorrhagic fever 1. hämorrhagisches Fieber nt abbr. HF. 2. Ebola-Fieber nt, Ebola hämorrhagisches Fieber nt.
viral hepatitis Virushepatitis f.
acute v. akute Virushepatitis.
chronic v. chronische Virushepatitis.
type A v. (Virus-)Hepatitis A f abbr. HA, epidemische Hepatitis f, Hepatitis epidemica.
type B v. (Virus-)Hepatitis B f abbr. HB, Serumhepatitis f.
viral infection Virusinfektion f.
viral keratoconjunctivitis epidemische Keratokonjunktivitis f, Keratoconjunctivitis epidemica.
viral lysozyme virales Lysozym nt.
viral meningitis Virusmeningitis f, virale Meningitis f.
viral morphogenesis Virusmorphogenese f.
viral myocarditis Virusmyokarditis f.
viral oncogene virales Onkogen nt.
viral oncogenesis virale/virusinduzierte Tumorbildung f/Onkogenese f.
viral particle → virion.
viral pneumonia Viruspneumonie f.
viral protein Virusprotein nt.
viral recombination virale Rekombination f.
viral RNA Virus-RNA f, virale RNA f, Virus-RNS f, virale RNS f.
viral spread Virusausbreitung f, -verbreitung f.
viral structure Virusstruktur f.
viral titer Virustiter m.
viral vaccine Virusimpfstoff m, -vakzine f.
vi·ra·zole ['vaırəzəʊl] n Virazol nt, Ribavirin nt.
Virchow ['vıərçəʊ]: **V.'s cells** 1. (Virchow'-)Leprazellen pl. 2. Hornhautkörperchen pl.
V.'s corpuscles → V.'s cells 2.
V.'s crystals Virchow'-Kristalle pl.
V.'s degeneration → V.'s disease.
V.'s disease amyloide Degeneration f; Amyloidose f.

V.'s gland Klavikulardrüse f, Virchow'-Knötchen nt, -Knoten m, -Drüse f.
V.'s granulations Virchow-Granula pl.
V.'s hydatid alveoläre Echinokokkose f.
V.'s law Virchow-Regel f, -Gesetz nt.
V.'s node → V.'s gland.
V.'s psammoma Sandgeschwulst f, Psammom nt.
Virchow-Hassall ['hæsəl]: **V.-H. bodies** Hassall'-Körperchen pl.
Virchow-Robin [rɔ'bɛ̃]: **V.-R.'s space** Virchow-Robin'-Raum m, -Spalt m.
vi·re·mia [vaɪ'riːmɪə] n Virämie f.
vir·gin ['vɜrdʒɪn] I n Jungfrau f. II adj 1. → virginal. 2. techn. rein, unvermischt.
vir·gin·al ['vɜrdʒɪnl] adj 1. jungfräulich, Jungfern-. 2. bio. unbefruchtet.
virginal membrane Jungfernhäutchen nt, Hymen nt/m.
virgin-born adj bio. parthenogenetisch.
vir·gin·i·ty [vər'dʒɪnətɪ] n Unschuld f; Jungfräulichkeit, Jungfernschaft f, Virginität f.
vi·ri·ci·dal [vaɪrɪ'saɪdl, vɪr-] adj → virucidal.
vi·ri·cide ['vaɪrɪsaɪd, vɪr-] n → virucide.
vir·i·dans endocarditis ['vɪrɪdænz] Viridans-Endokarditis f, Endokarditis f durch Streptococcus viridans.
viridans streptococci micro. vergrünende Streptokokken pl, Viridans-Streptokokken pl, Streptococcus viridans.
vir·ile ['vɪraɪl; Brit. -raɪl] adj 1. männlich, maskulin, viril. 2. männlich, viril, zeugungskräftig, potent.
virile member (männliches) Glied nt, Penis m, Phallus m, Membrum virile.
vir·i·les·cence [vɪrə'lesəns] n → virilization.
vi·ril·ia [vaɪ'rɪlɪə] pl männliche Geschlechtsorgane pl, Organa genitalia masculina.
vir·i·lism ['vɪrəlɪzəm] n Virilismus m.
vi·ril·i·ty [və'rɪlətɪ] n 1. Männlichkeit f. 2. Mannes-, Zeugungskraft f, Potenz f, Virilität f.
vir·il·i·za·tion [ˌvɪrəlaɪ'zeɪʃn] n Vermännlichung f, Virilisierung f, Maskulinisierung f.
vi·ri·on ['vaɪrɪˌɑn, 'vɪrɪ-] n Viruspartikel m, Virion nt.
vi·rip·o·tent [vaɪ'rɪpətənt] adj geschlechtsreif.
vi·ro·ge·net·ic [ˌvaɪrədʒɪ'netɪk] adj durch Viren verursacht, von Viren abstammend, virogen.
vi·roid ['vaɪrɔɪd] n micro. nacktes Minivirus nt, Viroid nt.
vi·ro·lac·tia [ˌvaɪrə'læktɪə] n gyn. Virolaktie f.
vi·rol·o·gist [vaɪ'rɑlədʒɪst] n Virologe m, -login f.
vi·rol·o·gy [vaɪ'rɑlədʒɪ] n Virologie f.
vi·ro·pex·is [ˌvaɪrə'peksɪs] n immun. Viropexis f.
vi·ro·sis [vaɪ'rəʊsɪs] n Viruserkrankung f, Virose f.
vi·ro·stat·ic [ˌvaɪrə'stætɪk] I n Virostatikum nt, Virustatikum nt. II adj virostatisch.
vir·tu·al ['vɜrtʃəwəl] adj 1. tatsächlich, praktisch, faktisch, eigentlich. 2. phys. virtuell, virtual.
virtual image virtuelles/scheinbares Bild nt.
vi·ru·ci·dal [ˌvaɪrə'saɪdl] adj viruzid.
vi·ru·cide ['vaɪrəsaɪd] n Viruzid nt.
vi·ru·co·pria [ˌvaɪrə'kəʊprɪə] n Virusausscheidung f im Stuhl, Virukoprie f.
vir·u·lence ['vɪr(j)ələns] n immun. Virulenz f.
virulence-associated protein → virulence-associated surface protein.
virulence-associated surface protein virulenz-assoziiertes (Oberflächen-)Protein nt.
virulence factor Virulenzfaktor m.
vir·u·lent ['vɪr(j)ələnt] adj Virulenz betr., infektionsfähig, virulent; giftig; ansteckend.
virulent bacteriophage nichttemperenter/lytischer/virulenter Bakteriophage m.
virulent bubo schankröser/virulenter Bubo m.
virulent phage → virulent bacteriophage.
vir·u·lif·er·ous [vɪrə'lɪfərəs] adj virenübertragend.
vir·u·ria [vaɪ'r(j)ʊərɪə] n Virusausscheidung f im Harn, Virurie f.
vi·rus ['vaɪrəs] n, pl **-rus·es** 1. Virus nt. 2. → viral disease.
virus architecture Virusarchitektur f.
virus blockade Virusinterferenz f.
virus capsid antigen abbr. **VCA** virales Capsid-Antigen nt abbr. VCA, virus capsid antigen.
virus-coded adj viruscodiert.
virus diarrhea Virusdiarrhö f.
vi·rus·e·mia [ˌvaɪrə'siːmɪə] n → viremia.
virus encephalomyelitis → viral encephalomyelitis.
virus-encoded adj viruscodiert.
virus-encoded growth factor viruscodierter Wachstumsfaktor m.
virus expression Virusexpression f.
virus hepatitis Virushepatitis f.
anicteric v. anikterische Virushepatitis.
virus-host relationship Virus-Wirtbeziehung f.
virus-induced adj virusinduziert.
virus-infected adj virusinfiziert.
virus interference Virusinterferenz f.
virus maturation Virusreifung f.
virus particle → virion.
virus persistence Viruspersistenz f.
virus progeny Virusnachkommen(schaft f) pl.
virus replication Virusvermehrung f, -replikation f.
virus-specific adj virusspezifisch.
vir·u·stat·ic [ˌvɪrə'stætɪk] adj virostatisch.
vis [vɪs; wiːs] n, pl **vi·res** ['vaɪriːz; 'wiːraɪs] Kraft f, Energie f, Vis f.
viscer- pref. → viscero-.
vis·cer·a ['vɪsərə] pl, sing **vis·cus** ['vɪskəs] anat. Eingeweide pl, innere Organe der Körperhöhlen, Viszera pl, Viscera pl.
vis·cer·al ['vɪsərəl] adj Eingeweide/Viscera betr., viszeral, Eingeweide-, Viszeral-, Viszero-.
visceral abscess Eingeweideabszeß m.
visceral afferents physiol. Eingeweideafferenzen pl, viszerale Afferenzen pl.
visceral anesthesia Verlust m der Eingeweidesensibilität.
visceral angiography radiol. Eingeweideangiographie f.
visceral arteritis, localized Immunkomplexvaskulitis f, leukozytoklastische Vaskulitis f, Vasculitis allergica, Vasculitis hyperergica cutis, Arteriitis allergica cutis.
visceral brain limbisches System nt.
visceral cranium → viscerocranium.
visceral crisis neuro. Eingeweidekrise f, viszerale Krise f.
visceral disease virus micro. Zyto-, Cytomegalievirus nt abbr. CMV.
visceral ganglia vegetative/autonome Grenzstrangganglien pl, Ggll. autonomica/visceralia.
vis·cer·al·gia [vɪsə'rældʒ(ɪ)ə] n Eingeweideschmerz m, Viszeralgie f; Viszeralneuralgie f.

visceral herniation Eingeweidevorfall m.
visceral inversion Situs inversus.
visceral layer: v. of pelvic fascia Fascia pelvis visceralis.
v. of pericardium → visceral pericardium.
v. of tunica vaginalis testis Lamina visceralis tunicae vaginalis testis.
visceral leishmaniasis viszerale Leishmaniose/Leishmaniase f, Kala-Azar f, Splenomegalia tropica.
visceral mesoderm viszerales Mesoderm nt.
visceral metastasis Eingeweidemetastase f.
visceral muscle Eingeweide-, Viszeralmuskel m.
visceral nervous system autonomes/vegetatives Nervensystem nt abbr. ANS, Pars autonomica systematis nervosi, Systema nervosum autonomicum.
visceral neurofibers viszerale Nervenfasern pl, Neurofibrae viscerales.
visceral pain Viszeral-, Eingeweideschmerz m, viszeraler Schmerz m.
visceral pericardium Epikard nt, viszerales Perikard nt, Lamina visceralis pericardii, Epicardium f.
visceral perforation chir. Eingeweideperforation f.
visceral peritoneum Peritoneum nt der Baucheingeweide, viszerales Peritoneum nt, Peritoneum viscerale.
visceral pleura Lungenfell nt, Viszeralpleura f der Lunge, Pleura visceralis/pulmonis.
visceral pleurisy Lungenfellentzündung f.
visceral plexus autonomes/vegetatives Nervengeflecht nt, autonomer/vegetativer (Nerven-)Plexus m, Plexus autonomicus/visceralis.
visceral reflex Eingeweidereflex m, viszeraler Reflex m.
visceral schistosomiasis viszerale Schistosomiasis f, Schistosomiasis visceralis.
visceral sense Eingeweidesinn m.
visceral sensibility viszerale Sensibilität f, Eingeweidesensibilität f.
visceral skeleton Viszeralskelett nt.
visceral substance, second Substantia visceralis secundaria.
vis·cer·i·mo·tor [ˌvɪsərɪ'məʊtər] adj → visceromotor.
viscero- pref. Eingeweide-, Viszer(o)-, Viszeral-.
vis·cer·o·car·di·ac reflex [ˌvɪsərəʊ'kɑːrdɪæk] viszerokardialer Reflex m.
vis·cer·o·cep·tion [ˌ-'septʃn] n Viszero-, Interozeption f.
vis·cer·o·cra·ni·um [ˌ-'kreɪnɪəm] n Eingeweideschädel m, Viszerokranium nt, -cranium nt, Splanchnokranium nt, -cranium nt, Cranium viscerale.
vis·cer·o·gen·ic [ˌ-'dʒenɪk] adj von den Eingeweiden abstammend, viszerogen.
viscerogenic reflex viszerogener Reflex m.
vis·cer·o·in·hib·i·to·ry [ˌ-ɪn'hɪbətɔːriː, -təʊ-] adj viszeroinhibitorisch.
vis·cer·o·meg·a·ly [ˌ-'megəlɪ] n Eingeweidevergrößerung f, Splanchno-, Viszeromegalie f.
vis·cer·o·mo·tor [ˌ-'məʊtər] adj viszeromotorisch.
visceromotor fiber viszeromotorische Faser f.
visceromotor nuclei viszeromotorische Kerne pl.
visceromotor reflex viszeromotorischer Reflex m.
visceromotor system Viszeromotorik f, viszeromotorisches System nt.

visceroparietal

vis·cer·o·pa·ri·e·tal [ˌ-pəˈraɪɪtl] *adj* viszeroparietal.
vis·cer·o·per·i·to·ne·al [ˌ-perɪtəʊˈniːəl] *adj* Eingeweide u. Peritoneum betr., visceroperitoneal.
vis·cer·o·pleur·al [ˌ-ˈplʊərəl] *adj* Eingeweide u. Pleura betr., visceropleural.
vis·cer·op·to·sia [ˌvɪsərɒpˈtəʊsɪə] *n* → visceroptosis.
vis·cer·op·to·sis [ˌvɪsərɒpˈtəʊsɪs] *n* Eingeweidesenkung *f*, Splanchno-, Entero-, Viszeroptose *f*.
vis·cer·o·re·cep·tor [ˌvɪsərəʊrɪˈseptər] *n* Viszerorezeptor *m*.
vis·cer·o·sen·so·ry [ˌ-ˈsensərɪ] *adj* viszerosensorisch.
viscerosensory fiber viszerosensorische Faser *f*.
viscerosensory reflex viszerosensorischer Reflex *m*.
vis·cer·o·skel·e·tal [ˌ-ˈskelɪtl] *adj* viszeroskelettal.
vis·cer·o·ske·le·ton [ˌ-ˈskelɪtn] *n* Viszeralskelett *nt*.
vis·cer·o·so·mat·ic [ˌ-səʊˈmætɪk] *adj* splanchno-, viszerosomatisch.
vis·cer·o·tome [ˈ-təʊm] *n* 1. *patho., chir.* Viszerotom *nt*. 2. *anat.* Viszerotom *nt*.
vis·ce·rot·o·my [vɪsəˈrɒtəmɪ] *n chir.* Viszerotomie *f*.
vis·cer·o·troph·ic [ˌvɪsərəʊˈtrɒfɪk] *adj* viszerotroph.
vis·cer·o·trop·ic [ˌ-ˈtrɒpɪk] *adj* mit besonderer Affinität zu den Eingeweiden, splanchno-, viszerotrop.
viscero-visceral reflex viszero-viszeraler Reflex *m*.
vis·cid [ˈvɪsɪd] *adj* → viscous.
vis·cid·i·ty [vɪˈsɪdətɪ] *n* Zähflüssigkeit *f*, Zähigkeit *f*, Klebrigkeit *f*.
vis·cid·ness [ˈvɪsɪdnɪs] *n* → viscidity.
vis·ci·do·sis [vɪsəˈdəʊsɪs] *n* zystische (Pankreas-)Fibrose *f*, Mukoviszidose *f*, Fibrosis pancreatica cystica.
vis·co·e·las·tic [ˌvɪskəʊɪˈlæstɪk] *adj* viskoelastisch, viskös-elastisch.
vis·co·gel [ˈvɪskəʊdʒel] *n* Viskogel *nt*.
vis·com·e·ter [vɪsˈkɒmɪtər] *n* → viscosimeter.
vis·com·e·try [vɪsˈkɒmətrɪ] *n* → viscosimetry.
vis·cose [ˈvɪskəʊs] I *n* Viskose *f*; Viskose-, Zellstoffseide *f*. II *adj* → viscous.
vis·co·sim·e·ter [ˌvɪskəʊˈsɪmɪtər] *n* Viskosimeter *nt*.
vis·co·si·met·ric [ˌvɪskəʊsɪˈmetrɪk] *adj* viskosimetrisch.
vis·co·sim·e·try [ˌvɪskəʊˈsɪmətrɪ] *n* Viskositätsmessung *f*, Viskosimetrie *f*.
vis·cos·i·ty [vɪsˈkɒsətɪ] *n* Zähigkeit *f*, innere Reibung *f*, Viskosität *f*.
vis·cous [ˈvɪskəs] *adj* 1. zäh, zähflüssig, -fließend, viskös, viskos. 2. klebrig, leimartig.
viscous metamorphosis *patho.* viskose Metamorphose *f*.
viscous resistance viskoser/nichtelastischer Widerstand *m*.
vis·cus *sing* → viscera.
vis·i·bil·i·ty [ˌvɪzəˈbɪlɪtɪ] *n* Sichtbarkeit *f*.
vis·i·ble [ˈvɪzəbl] *adj* 1. sichtbar; *ophthal.* Sicht-. 2. *fig.* offensichtlich, deutlich, merklich.
visible angle *ophthal.* Gesichtsfeld-, Sehwinkel *m*.
minimum v. kleinster Sehwinkel, Grenzwinkel, Minimum separabile.
visible spectrum (*Licht*) sichtbares Spektrum *nt*, Spektrum *nt* des sichtbaren Lichtes.
vis·ile [ˈvɪzaɪl] *adj* 1. *neuro.* (*Typ*) visuell. 2. → visual.

vi·sion [ˈvɪʒn] *n* 1. Sehen *nt*, Vision *f*; Sehvermögen *nt*, Sehkraft *f*. 2. Erscheinung *f*, Vision *f*; Halluzination *f*. 3. *ophthal.* Sehschwäche *f*, Visus *m*.
vision-testing chart Sehproben-, Sehprüftafel *f*.
vis·it [ˈvɪzɪt] I *n* Besuch *m*; Arztbesuch *m*, Visite *f*. to make/pay a ~ einen Besuch machen. II *vt* 1. be-, aufsuchen. 2. (*Krankheit*) befallen, heimsuchen.
vis·na viruses [ˈvɪznə] *micro.* Visna-Viren *pl*.
vis·u·al [ˈvɪʒəwəl, -ʒəl] *adj* Sehen betr., visuell, Seh-, Gesichts-; sichtbar, Sicht-.
visual acuity *abbr.* VA Sehschärfe *f*, Visus *m*.
visual agnosia Seelenblindheit *f*, optische/visuelle Agnosie *f*.
visual allesthesia visuelle Allästhesie *f*.
visual amnesia Leseunfähigkeit *f*, -unvermögen *nt*, Alexie *f*.
visual angle → visible angle.
visual aphasia 1. optische Aphasie *f*. 2. → visual amnesia.
visual area → visual cortex.
visual aura *neuro.* visuelle/optische Aura *f*.
visual axis 1. Gesichtslinie *f*, Axis visualis. 2. (optische) Augen-/Sehachse *f*, Axis opticus (bulbi oculi).
visual blackout Amaurosis fugax der Flieger.
visual cell Photorezeptor-, Sehzelle *f*.
visual center *physiol.* Sehzentrum *nt*.
visual cone Sehkegel *m*.
visual cortex Sehrinde *f*, visueller Kortex *m*.
primary v. primäre Sehrinde, Area striata.
secondary v. sekundäre Sehrinde.
visual cycle *physiol.* Sehzyklus *m*, -vorgang *m*.
visual disturbance Sehstörung *f*, Störung *f* des Sehvermögens.
visual ectoderm *embryo.* Gesichtsektoderm *nt*.
visual evoked potential *abbr.* VEP visuell evoziertes Potential *nt abbr.* VEP.
pattern-reversal v. Musterwechsel-VEP *nt*.
visual display (*Computer*) (Sicht-)Anzeige *f*.
visual field Augenfeld *nt*; Blick-, Gesichtsfeld *nt*.
visual-field boundaries Gesichtsfeldgrenzen *pl*.
visual-field defect *ophthal.* Gesichtsfeldausfall *m*, -defekt *m*.
visual hallucination visuelle Halluzination *f*.
visual hearing Lippenlesen *nt*.
vis·u·al·i·za·tion [ˌvɪʒələˈzeɪʃn, ˌvɪʒwələ-] *n radiol.* Sichtbarmachung *f*, Visualisieren *nt*.
vis·u·al·ize [ˈvɪʒəlaɪz, ˈvɪʒwəlaɪz] I *vt* 1. s. vorstellen, s. vergegenwärtigen, s. ein Bild machen von. 2. *radiol.* sichtbar machen, darstellen (*by, with*). 3. erwarten, rechnen mit. II *vi radiol.* sichtbar werden.
vis·u·al·iz·er [ˈvɪʒəlaɪzər, ˈvɪʒwə-] *n neuro., psycho.* visueller Typ *m*.
visual light sichtbares Licht *nt*.
visual line *ophthal.* optische Augenachse *f*, Sehachse *f*, Axis opticus.
visual memory visuelles Gedächtnis *nt*.
visual organ Sehorgan *nt*, Organum visus *nt*.
visual pathway Sehbahn *f*.
visual perseveration *ophthal.* Palinopsie *f*.
visual physiology Sehphysiologie *f*, Physiologie *f* des Sehens.

visual pigment Sehfarbstoff *m*, -pigment *nt*.
visual plane Sehebene *f*.
visual purple Sehpurpur *m*, Rhodopsin *nt*.
visual radiation Gratiolet'-Sehstrahlung *f*, Radiatio optica.
visual-spatial agnosia visuell-räumliche Agnosie *f*.
visual test Augen-, Sehtest *m*.
visual violet Jodopsin *nt*.
visual white Sehweiß *nt*, Leukopsin *nt*.
visual yellow Sehgelb *nt*, Xanthopsin *nt*, all-trans Retinal *nt*.
vis·u·o·au·di·to·ry [ˌvɪʒwəʊˈɔːdɪt(ə)rɪ, -təʊ-] *adj* Hören u. Sehen betr., audiovisuell.
vi·tag·o·nist [vaɪˈtægənɪst] *n* Vitaminantagonist *m*.
vi·tal [ˈvaɪtl] I ~s *pl* 1. lebenswichtige Organe *pl*; Vitalfunktionen *pl*. 2. *fig.* das Wesentliche. II *adj* 3. vital, (lebens-)wichtig (*to* für); wesentlich, grundlegend, Lebens-, Vital-. 4. voller Leben, lebendig; vital, kraftvoll, leistungsfähig; lebensbejahend. 5. lebensgefährlich, -bedrohend, tödlich.
vital capacity *abbr.* VC (*Lunge*) Vitalkapazität *abbr.* VK.
vital dye Vitalfarbstoff *m*.
vital energy Lebenskraft *f*.
vital function lebenswichtige Organfunktion *f*, Vitalfunktion *f*.
Vitali [vɪˈtæliː]: V.'s test Vitali-Probe *f*.
vi·tal·ism [ˈvaɪtlɪzəm] *n bio.* Vitalismus *m*.
vi·tal·i·ty [vaɪˈtælətɪ] *n* 1. Lebenskraft *f*, Vitalität *f*. 2. Lebensfähigkeit *f*, -dauer *f*.
vi·tal·i·za·tion [ˌvaɪtləˈzeɪʃn] *n* Belebung *f*, Kräftigung *f*, Anregung *f*, Aktivierung *f*.
vi·tal·ize [ˈvaɪtəlaɪz] *vt* beleben, kräftigen, anregen, vitalisieren.
vital phenomena *histol.* Lebenserscheinungen *pl*.
vital power → vital energy.
vital red *histol.* Brillantrot *nt*.
vital stain Intravital-, Vitalfärbung *f*.
vital staining → vital stain.
vi·ta·min [ˈvaɪtəmɪn; *Brit.* ˈvɪtə-] *n* Vitamin *nt*.
vitamin A 1. Vitamin A *nt*. 2. → vitamin A$_1$.
vitamin A$_1$ Retinol *nt*, Vitamin A$_1$ *nt*, Vitamin A-Alkohol *m*.
vitamin A$_2$ (3-)Dehydroretinol *nt*, Vitamin A$_2$ *nt*.
vitamin A acid Retinsäure *f*, Vitamin A$_1$-Säure *f*, Tretinoin *nt*.
vitamin A deficiency Vitamin A-Mangel *m*.
vitamin B$_1$ Thiamin *nt*, Vitamin B$_1$ *nt*.
vitamin B$_2$ Ribo-, Lactoflavin *nt*, Vitamin B$_2$ *nt*.
vitamin B$_6$ Vitamin B$_6$ *nt*.
vitamin B$_{12}$ Zyano-, Cyanocobalamin *nt*, Vitamin B$_{12}$ *nt*.
Vitamin B$_{12b}$ Hydroxocobalamin *nt*, Aquocobalamin *nt*, Vitamin B$_{12b}$ *nt*.
vitamin B$_{12}$-binding globulin Transcobalamin *nt abbr.* TC, Vitamin-B$_{12}$-bindendes Globulin *nt*.
vitamin B complex Vitamin B-Komplex *m*.
vitamin B$_6$ deficiency anemia Vitamin B$_6$-Mangelanämie *f*.
vitamin B$_{12}$ deficiency anemia Vitamin-B$_{12}$-Mangelanämie *f*.
vitamin B$_{12}$-neuropathy Lichtheim-Syndrom *nt*, Dana-Lichtheim-Krankheit *f*, Dana-Syndrom *nt* Dana-Lichtheim-Putnam-Syndrom *nt*, funikuläre Spinalerkrankung/Myelose *f*.
vitamin B$_c$ *old* → folic acid.

vitamin C Askorbin-, Ascorbinsäure *f*, Vitamin C *nt*.
vitamin C deficiency anemia Vitamin C-Mangelanämie *f*.
vitamin concentrate Vitaminkonzentrat *nt*.
vitamin D Calciferol *nt*, Vitamin D *nt*.
vitamin D₂ Ergocalciferol *nt*, Vitamin D₂ *nt*.
vitamin D₃ Cholecalciferol *nt*, Vitamin D₃ *nt*.
vitamin D₄ Dihydrocalciferol *nt*, Vitamin D₄ *nt*.
vitamin D deficiency Vitamin D-Mangel *m*.
vitamin deficiency Vitaminmangel(krankheit *f*) *m*.
vitamin-deficiency disease Vitaminmangelkrankheit *f*, Hypovitaminose *f*; Avitaminose *f*.
vitamin D refractory rickets → vitamin D resistant rickets.
vitamin D-resistant osteomalacia Vitamin D-resistente Osteomalazie *f*.
vitamin D resistant rickets familiäre Hypophosphatämie *f*, Vitamin D-resistente Rachitis *f*, refraktäre Rachitis *f*, Vitamin D-refraktäre Rachitis *f*.
vitamin E α-Tocopherol *nt*, Vitamin E *nt*.
vi·ta·mine *n* → vitamin.
vitamin G → vitamin B₂.
vitamin H Biotin *nt*, Vitamin H *nt*.
vi·ta·min·ize ['vaɪtəmɪnaɪz] *vt* (*Lebensmittel*) mit Vitaminen anreichern, vitaminisieren, vitaminieren.
vitamin K Phyllochinone *pl*, Vitamin K *nt*.
vitamin K₁ Phytomenadion *nt*, Vitamin K₁ *nt*.
vitamin K₂ Menachinon *nt*, Vitamin K₂ *nt*.
vitamin K₃ Menadion *nt*, Vitamin K₃ *nt*.
vitamin K antagonist Vitamin K-Antagonist.
vitamin K deficiency Vitamin K-Mangel *m*.
vitamin K-dependent Vitamin K-abhängig.
vitamin M old → folic acid.
vi·tam·i·no·gen·ic [vaɪˌtæmənəʊ'dʒenɪk] *adj* durch ein Vitamin hervorgerufen, durch Vitamine verursacht, vitaminogen.
vi·tel·lar·i·um [vaɪtə'leərɪəm] *n* micro. Vitellarium *nt*, Dotterdrüse *f*, -stock *m*.
vi·tel·lary ['vaɪtəleriː, vaɪ'telərɪ] *adj* → vitelline.
vi·tel·line [vaɪ'telɪn, vɪ-, -liːn, -laɪn] *adj* vitellin, Dotter-, Eidotter-, Eigelb-.
vitelline circulation embryo. Dottersackkreislauf *m*.
vitelline cyst Dottergangszyste *f*, Enterozyste *f*, Enterokystom *nt*.
vitelline duct Darmstiel *m*, Dotter(sack)gang *m*, Ductus omphalo(mes)entericus.
vitelline fistula Dottergangsfistel *f*, Fistula omphaloenterica.
vitelline gland → vitellarium.
vitelline membrane Dotterhaut *f*.
vitelline reservoir → vitellarium.
vitelline sac Nabelbläschen *nt*, Dottersack *m*.
vitelline vessels Dottergefäße *pl*, Vasa omphalomesentericae.
vi·tel·lo·gen·e·sis [vɪˌtelǝʊ'dʒenǝsɪs] *n* embryo. Dotterbildung *f*.
vi·tel·lo·in·tes·ti·nal cyst [ˌ-ɪn'testǝnl] Nabelzyste *f*.
vitellointestinal duct → vitelline duct.
vi·tel·lus [vaɪ'telǝs, vɪ-] *n, pl* **-lus·es** (Ei-)Dotter *m*, Vitellus *m*.
vi·ti·ate ['vɪʃɪeɪt] *vt* (*Leistung*) beeinträchtigen, reduzieren; (*Luft*) verunreinigen, verpesten.

vi·ti·a·tion [vɪʃɪ'eɪʃn] *n* (*Leistung*) Beeinträchtigung *f*, Reduktion *f*; (*Luft*) Verunreinigung *f*, Verpestung *f*.
vit·i·lig·i·nous [vɪtǝ'lɪdʒǝnǝs] *adj* derm. Vitiligo betr., in Art einer Vitiligo, vitiliginös.
vit·i·li·go [vɪtǝ'laɪgǝʊ] *n* derm. Weißfleckenkrankheit *f*, Scheckhaut *f*, Vitiligo *f*.
vit·i·li·goi·dea [ˌvɪtǝlaɪ'gɔɪdɪǝ] *n* Xanthom(a) *nt*.
vi·ti·um ['vɪʃɪǝm] *n, pl* **-tia** [-ʃɪǝ] 1. Fehler *m*, Vitium *nt*. 2. Herzfehler *m*, (Herz-)Vitium *nt*, Vitium cordis.
vitre- *pref*. → vitreo-.
vi·trec·to·my [vɪ'trektǝmɪ] *n* ophthal. Glaskörperresektion *f*, Vitrektomie *f*.
vitreo- *pref*. Glaskörper-, Vitre(o)-.
vit·re·o·cap·su·li·tis [ˌvɪtrɪǝʊˌkæpsǝ'laɪtɪs] *n* Entzündung *f* der Glaskörperkapsel, Vitreokapsulitis *f*.
vit·re·o·ret·i·nal [ˌ-'retɪnl] *adj* vitreoretinal.
vitreoretinal dystrophy ophthal. Wagner'-Krankheit *f*.
vit·re·ous ['vɪtrɪǝs] I *n* → vitreous body. II *adj* gläsern, glasig, glasartig, hyalin, Glas-.
vitreous abscess ophthal. Glaskörperabszeß *m*.
vitreous body Glaskörper *m*, Corpus vitreum.
vitreous chamber Glaskörperraum *m*, Camera vitrea (bulbi).
vitreous degeneration old → hyalinosis.
vitreous floaters ophthal. Mückensehen *nt*, Mouches volantes.
vitreous humor → vitreous body.
vitreous lamina Bruch'-Membran *f*, Complexus/Lamina basalis (choroideae).
vitreous membrane Glaskörpermembran *f*, Membrana vitrea/hyaloidea.
vitreous stroma Glaskörperfaserwerk *nt*, -stroma *nt*, Stroma vitreum.
vitreous table Lamina interna.
vit·re·um ['vɪtrɪǝm] *n* → vitreous body.
vit·ri·ol ['vɪtrɪǝl] *n* Schwefelsäure *f*, Vitriol *nt*.
vi·vax fever ['vaɪvæks] → vivax malaria.
vivax malaria 1. Vivax-Malaria *f*. **2.** Tertiana *f*, Dreitagefieber *nt*, Malaria tertiana.
viv·i·di·al·y·sis [ˌvɪvǝdaɪ'ælǝsɪs] *n* Vividialyse *f*.
viv·i·par·i·ty [ˌ-'pærǝtɪ] *n* bio. Lebendgebären *nt*, Viviparie *f*.
vi·vip·a·rous [vaɪ'vɪpǝrǝs, vɪ-] *adj* bio. lebendgebärend, vivipar.
viv·i·sect ['vɪvǝsekt] *vt, vi* vivsezieren.
viv·i·sec·tion [ˌ-'sekʃn] *n* Vivisektion *f*.
viv·i·sec·tion·al [ˌ-'sekʃnl] *adj* Vivisektion betr., vivisektionell, Vivisektions-.
viv·i·sec·tion·ist [ˌ-'sekʃǝnɪst] *n* → vivisector.
viv·i·sec·tor [ˌ-'sektǝr] *n* Vivisektor *m*.
Vladimiroff-Mikulicz [ˌvlædɪ'mɪǝrǝf 'mɪkjǝlɪtʃ]: **V.-M. amputation/operation** ortho. Fußamputation *f* nach Vladimiroff-Mikulicz.
VLDL *abbr*. → very low-density lipoprotein.
VMA *abbr*. → vanillylmandelic acid.
vo·cal ['vǝʊkl] I *n* Vokal-, Stimmlaut *m*. II *adj* **1.** Stimme betr., stimmlich, mündlich, vokal, Stimm-, Sprech, Vokal-. **2.** klingend, wiederhallend. **3.** stimmhaft, vokalisch.
vocal cord → vocal fold.
false v. → vocal fold, false.
vocal cord paralysis Stimmbandlähmung *f*.
vocal cord paresis → vocal cord paralysis.

vocal cord polyp Stimmbandpolyp *m*.
vocal fold Stimmlippe *f*, -falte *f*, Plica vocalis; clin. Stimmband *nt*.
false v. Taschenfalte, Plica vestibularis.
vocal fremitus Stimmfremitus *m*, Fremitus pectoralis.
vo·ca·lis [vǝʊ'keɪlɪz] *n* → vocalis muscle.
vo·cal·i·sa·tion [ˌvǝʊkǝlaɪ'zeɪʃn] *n* Stimmbildung *f*, Vokalisation *f*.
vocalis muscle Stimmbandmuskel *m*, Vokalis *m*, M. vocalis.
vocal ligament Stimmband *nt*, Lig. vocale.
vocal muscle → vocalis muscle.
vocal nodule Sängerknötchen *nt*, Nodulus vocalis.
vocal process of arytenoid cartilage Stimmbandfortsatz *m* des Aryknorpels, Proc. vocalis (cartilaginis arytaenoideae).
Voelcker ['fœlkǝr]: **V.'s test** urol. Voelcker-Probe *f*, Blauprobe *f*.
Voges-Proskauer ['fǝʊgǝs 'prɔskaʊǝr, 'foːgǝs]: **V.-P. reaction/test** Voges-Proskauer-Reaktion *f*.
Vogt [fǝʊgt; foːkt]: **V.'s cephalodactyly** Apert-Crouzon-Syndrom *nt*, Akrozephalosyndaktylie *f* Typ IIa.
V.'s disease Vogt-Syndrom *nt*, -Erkrankung *f*, Status marmoratus.
V.'s syndrome → V.'s disease.
Vogt-Koyanagi [kɔɪǝ'nɑːgɪ]: **V.-K. syndrome** Vogt-Koyanagi(-Harada)-Syndrom *nt*, okulokutanes Syndrom *nt*.
Vogt-Spielmeyer ['spiːlmaɪǝr]: **V.-S. disease** Stock-Vogt-Spielmeyer-Syndrom *nt*, Batten-Spielmeyer-Vogt-Syndrom *nt*, neuronale/juvenile Zeroidlipofuszinose *f*, Ceroidlipofuscinose *f*, juvenile Form *f* der amaurotischen Idiotie.
Vohwinkel [fǝʊ'vɪŋkl, 'foːvɪŋkǝl]: **V.'s syndrome** Vohwinkel-Syndrom *nt*, Pseudoainhum-artige Dermatose *f*, Keratoma hereditarium mutilans, Keratosis palmoplantaris mutilans.
voice [vɔɪs] I *n* **1.** Stimme *f*; stimmhafter Laut *m*; Stimmton *m*, Stimmhaftigkeit *f*. **2.** Stimme *f*, Stimmrecht *nt*; Stimme *f*, Sprachrohr *nt*. II *vt* **3.** stimmhaft aussprechen. **4.** äußern, Ausdruck geben.
voice box Kehlkopf *m*; anat. Larynx *m*.
voice disorder Stimmstörung *f*.
voice·less ['vɔɪslɪs] *adj* **1.** sprachlos. **2.** stumm, ohne Stimme, stimmlos.
voice production Stimm-, Lautbildung *f*, Phonation *f*.
void [vɔɪd] I *n* (*a. fig.*) Leere *f*. II *adj* **1.** leer. **2. ~ of** ohne, frei von, arm an. III *vt* entleeren, ausscheiden.
void·ing cystography ['vɔɪdɪŋ] urol. Ausscheidungs-, Miktionszystographie *f*.
voiding cystourethrography urol. Ausscheidungs-, Miktionszystourethrographie *f* abbr. MZU.
voiding reflex Entleerungsreflex *m*.
vo·lar ['vǝʊlǝr] *adj* anat. zur Hohlhand gehörend, auf der Hohlhandseite (liegend), volar; palmar.
volar branch of ulnar nerve Hohlhand-/Palmarast *m* des N. ulnaris, Ramus palmaris n. ulnaris.
vo·lar·dor·sal [ˌvǝʊlǝr'dɔːrsl] *adj* volardorsal.
volar fascia Palmaraponeurose *f*, Aponeurosis palmaris.
volar flexion Palmar-, Volarflexion *f*.
volar margin of radius Margo anterior radii.
volar psoriasis derm. **1.** Psoriasis inversa. **2.** Psoriasis palmarum.
vol·a·tile ['vɒlǝtl, -tɪl; Brit. -taɪl] *adj* chem. (leicht) flüchtig, verdunstend, verdamp-

volatile alkali

fend, ätherisch, volatil. **to make ~** verflüchtigen.
volatile alkali 1. Ammoniak *nt.* **2.** Ammoniumkarbonat *nt.*
volatile anesthetic volatiles Anästhetikum *nt.*
volatile oil *chem.* ätherisches Öl *nt.*
volatile salt Riechsalz *nt.*
vol·a·til·i·ty [ˌvaləˈtılətı] *n* (leichte) Flüchtigkeit *f*, Verdunstbarkeit *f*, Verdampfbarkeit *f*.
vol·a·til·iz·a·ble [ˈvalətəˌlaızəbl] *adj* (leicht) verdampfbar.
vol·a·til·i·za·tion [ˌvalətlıˈzeıʃn] *n* Verflüchtigung *f*, Verdampfung *f*; Verdampfen *nt*, Verdunsten *nt.*
vol·a·til·ize [ˈvalətlaız] **I** *vt* verflüchtigen, verdampfen. **II** *vi s.* verflüchtigen, verdampfen, verdunsten.
vol·a·til·iz·er [ˈvalətlaızər] *n* Verdampfer *m.*
vol·can·ic mud [valˈkænık] Fango *m.*
vo·li·tion [vəʊˈlıʃn, və-] *n* Wille *m*, Willenskraft *f*, Wollen *nt.*
vo·li·tion·al [vəʊˈlıʃnəl] *adj* willensmäßig, willensstark, Willens-.
Volkmann [ˈfɔlkmən; ˈfɔlkman]: **V.'s canals** Volkmann'-Kanäle *pl*, -Kanälchen *pl.*
V.'s cheilitis Volkmann'-Cheilitis *f*, -Krankheit *f*, Cheilitis glandularis apostematosa.
V.'s contracture Volkmann ischämische Kontraktur *f*, Volkmann-Kontraktur *f*, -Lähmung *f.*
V.'s deformity → V.'s disease.
V.'s disease Volkmann-Deformität *f.*
V.'s ischemic contracture → V.'s contracture.
V.'s ischemic paralysis → V.'s contracture.
V.'s perforating vessels (perforierende) Volkmann'-Gefäße *pl.*
V.'s subluxation → V.'s disease.
V.'s syndrome → V.'s contracture.
V.'s vessels → V.'s perforating vessels.
vol·ley [ˈvalı] *n* Salve *f*, Gruppe *f*; Strom *m*, Flut *f.*
volt [vəʊlt] *n abbr.* **V** Volt *nt abbr.* V.
volt·age [ˈvəʊltıdʒ] *n* elektrische Spannung *f* (*in* Volt).
voltage clamp *physiol.* Spannungsklemme *f*, Voltage-Clamp (*f*).
voltage-dependence *n* Spannungsabhängigkeit *f.*
voltage difference Spannungsdifferenz *f*, elektrische Spannung *f.*
voltage gradient Spannungsgefälle *nt*, -gradient *m.*
voltage pulse *phys.* Spannungsimpuls *m.*
volt·a·ic [valˈteık] *adj* galvanisch.
volt·a·ism [ˈvəʊltaızəm, ˈval-] *n* **1.** Berührungselektrizität *f*, Galvanismus *m.* **2.** Behandlung *f* mit galvanischem Strom, Galvanotherapie *f.*
volt·am·me·ter [ˈvəʊltˌæmıtər] *n* Voltamperemeter *m.*
volt·am·pere [vəʊltˈæmpıər, -æmˈpıər] *n abbr.* **VA** Voltampere *nt abbr.* VA.
volt·me·ter [ˈvəʊltmiːtər] *n* Spannungsmesser *m*, Voltmeter *nt.*
Voltolini [ˌvaltəʊˈliːnı]: **V.'s sign** Burger-Zeichen *nt*, Heryng-Zeichen *nt.*
vol·u·ble speech [ˈvaljəbl] *neuro.*, *psychia.* Tachylalie *f.*
vol·ume [ˈvaljuːm, -jəm] *n* **1.** *phys.*, *mathe.* (Raum-)Inhalt *m*, Gesamtmenge *f*, Volumen *nt.* **2.** Umfang *m*, Ausmaß *nt*, Volumen *nt.* **3.** *phys.* Lautstärke *f.*
v. of packed red cells *abbr.* **VPRC** (venöser) Hämatokrit *m.*

volume-control system Volumenkontrollsystem *nt.*
volume dose *radiol.* Integraldosis *f.*
volume elasticity coefficient *abbr.* **E'** *phys.* Volumenelastizitätskoeffizient *m abbr.* E'.
volume flow *physiol.* Stromzeitvolumen *nt.*
volume load Volumenbelastung *f.*
vol·u·me·nom·e·ter [ˌvaljəmıˈnamıtər] *n* → volumometer.
volume pulse Querschnitts-, Volumenpuls *m.*
volume receptor Volumenrezeptor *m.*
volume replacement Volumenersatz *m.*
volume sensor Volumensensor *m.*
vol·u·met·ric [ˌvaljəˈmetrık] *adj* Volumetrie betr., volumetrisch.
vol·u·met·ri·cal [ˌ-ˈmetrıkl] *adj* → volumetric.
volumetric analysis Volumetrie *f*, Maßanalyse *f*, Titrimetrie *f.*
volumetric density Raumdichte *f.*
volumetric flask Meßkolben *m.*
vol·u·mi·nal [vəˈluːmınl] *adj* Volumen-, Umfangs-.
vol·u·mom·e·ter [ˌvaljəˈmamıtər] *n* Volumenometer *nt.*
vol·un·tar·y [ˈvalənˌterıː, -trı] *adj* **1.** freiwillig, aus eigenem Antrieb, frei, spontan. **2.** *physiol.* willkürlich, willentlich.
voluntary abortion Schwangerschaftsunterbrechung *f*, -abbruch *m*, Abtreibung *f.*
voluntary death Freitod *m*, Selbstmord *m*, Suizid *m.*
voluntary movement(s) Willkürbewegung *f*, -motorik *f.*
voluntary muscles willkürliche quergestreifte Muskulatur *f.*
voluntary mutism *psychia.* elektiver Mutismus *m.*
vol·un·teer [ˌvalənˈtıər] **I** *n* Freiwillige(r *m*) *f.* **II** *adj* freiwillig, Freiwilligen-. **III** *vt* (*Arbeit*) freiwillig anbieten *od.* leisten. **IV** *vi s.* freiwillig melden *od.* anbieten (*for* für, zu).
vo·lup·tu·a·ry [vəˈlʌptʃəweriː] **I** *n*, *pl* **-ries** Lüstling *m*, sinnlicher Mensch *m.* **II** *adj* → voluptuous.
vo·lup·tu·ous [vəˈlʌptʃəwəs] *adj* wollüstig, sinnlich; lüstern; *inf.* geil.
vo·lup·tu·ous·ness [vəˈlʌptʃəwəsnıs] *n* Wollust *f*, Sinnlichkeit *f*; Lüsternheit *f*; *inf.* Geilheit *f.*
vo·lute [vəˈluːt] **I** *n* Spirale *f.* **II** *adj* gewunden, spiral-, schneckenförmig, spiralig.
vo·lut·ed [vəˈluːtıd] *adj* → volute II.
vol·u·tin [vəˈluːtın] *n* Volutin *nt.*
volutin granules Volutinkörnchen *pl*, metachromatische Granula *pl*, Babès-Ernst-Körperchen *pl.*
vo·lu·tion [vəˈluːʃn] *n* Drehung *f*, Windung *f.*
vol·vu·lo·sis [ˌvalvjəˈləʊsıs] *n* Knotenfiliariose *f*, Onchocerca-volvulus-Infektion *f*, Onchozerkose *f*, -cercose *f*, -cerciasis *f.*
vol·vu·lus [ˈvalvjələs] *n*, *pl* **-lus·es 1.** Stiel-, Achsendrehung *f*, Verschlingung *f*, Volvulus *m.* **2.** Darmverschlingung *f*, Volvulus *m.* intestini.
vo·mer [ˈvəʊmər] *n anat.* Flugscharbein *nt*, Vomer *m.*
vomeral groove Sulcus vomeris.
vomeral sulcus → vomeral groove.
vomer bone Pflugscharbein *nt*, Vomer *m.*
vo·mer·ine [ˈvəʊmərain, -rın, ˈvam-] *adj* Vomer betr., Vomer-, Vomero-.
vomerine canal → vomerovaginal canal.
vom·er·o·na·sal cartilage [ˌvamərəʊˈneızl, ˌvəʊm-] Jacobson'-Knorpel *m*, Cartilago vomeronasalis.

vomeronasal organ Jacobson'-Organ *nt*, Vomeronasalorgan *nt*, Organum vomeronasale.
vom·er·o·ros·tral canal [ˌ-ˈrastrəl] Canalis vomerorostralis.
vom·er·o·vag·i·nal canal [ˌ-ˈvædʒınl] Canalis vomerovaginalis.
vomerovaginal groove → vomerovaginal sulcus.
vomerovaginal sulcus Sulcus vomerovaginalis.
vom·i·ca [ˈvamıkə] *n*, *pl* **-cae** [-siː] diffuse Eiterung *f.*
vom·i·cose [ˈvamıkəʊs] *adj* diffus eiternd.
vom·it [ˈvamıt] **I** *n* **1.** Erbrechen *nt*, Emesis *f*, Vomitus *m*, Vomitio *f.* **2.** Erbrochene(s) *nt.* **II** *vt* (er-, aus-)brechen. **III** *vi s.* erbrechen, brechen, *s.* übergeben.
vom·it·ing [ˈvamıtıŋ] *n* (Er-)Brechen *nt*, Vomitus *m*, Emesis *f*, Vomitio *f.*
v. of pregnancy Schwangerschaftserbrechen *nt*, Erbrechen *nt* in der Schwangerschaft.
vomiting center Brechzentrum *nt.*
vomiting reflex Brechreflex *m.*
vo·mi·tion [vəˈmıʃn] *n* → vomit I.
vom·i·tive [ˈvamıtıv] **I** *n* Brechmittel *nt*, Vomitivum *nt*, Emetikum *nt.* **II** *adj* Erbrechen verursachend, emetisch, Brech-.
vom·i·to·ri·um [ˌvaməˈtɔːrıəm, -ˈtəʊ-] *n* → vomitive I.
vom·i·to·ry [ˈvamətəːrı, -təʊ-] *n*, *adj* → vomitive.
vom·i·tous [ˈvamıtəs] *adj* → vomitive II.
vom·i·tu·ri·tion [ˌvamıtjʊəˈrıʃn] *n* Brechreiz *m*, Würgen *m.*
vom·i·tus [ˈvamıtəs] *n* → vomit I.
von Economo [van eıˈkanəməʊ; fɒn]: **v.E.'s disease/encephalitis** europäische Schlafkrankheit *f*, (von) Economo-Krankheit *f*, -Enzephalitis *f*, Encephalitis epidemica/lethargica.
von Gierke [ˈɡıərkə]: **v.G.'s disease** (von) Gierke-Krankheit *f*, van Creveld-von Gierke-Krankheit *f*, hepatorenale Glykogenose *f*, Glykogenose *f* Typ I.
von Graefe [ˈɡreıfı; ˈɡrɛːfə]: **v.G.'s sign** von Graefe-Zeichen *nt.*
von Hippel [ˈhıpl]: **v.H.'s disease** → von Hippel-Lindau disease.
von Hippel-Lindau [ˈlındaʊ]: **v.H.-L. disease** (von) Hippel-Lindau-Syndrom *nt*, Netzhautangiomatose *f*, Angiomatosis retinae cystica, Angiomatosis cerebelli et retinae.
von Jaksch [jakʃ]: **v.J.'s anemia/disease** von Jaksch-Hayem-Anämie *f*, -Syndrom *nt*, Anaemia pseudoleucaemica infantum.
von Kossa [ˈkasə]: **v.K.'s silver stain** (von) Kossa-Versilberung *f.*
von Kupffer [ˈkʊpfər]: **v.K.'s cells** (von) Kupffer'-(Stern-)Zellen *pl.*
von Meyenburg [ˈmeıənbɜːrɡ; ˈmaıənbʊrk]: **v.M.'s disease** (von) Meyenburg-Altherr-Uehlinger-Syndrom *nt*, rezidivierende Polychondritis *f*, systematisierte Chondromalazie *f.*
von Monakow [manˈækəf]: **v.M.'s fibers** Ansa lenticularis.
von Pirquet [parˈkeı; pırˈkɛ]: **v.P.'s reaction/test** Pirquet-Reaktion *f*, -Tuberkulinprobe *f.*
von Recklinghausen [ˈrɛklıŋhaʊzn]:
v.R.'s disease (von) Recklinghausen-Krankheit *f*, Neurofibromatosis generalisata.
v.R.'s disease of bone Engel-(von) Recklinghausen-Syndrom *nt*, (von) Recklinghausen-Krankheit *f*, Osteodystrophia fibrosa cystica generalisata, Ostitis fibrosa cystica (generalisata).

von Recklinghausen-Applebaum ['æplbaʊm]: **v.R.-A. disease** (von) Recklinghausen-Applebaum-Krankheit f, idiopathische Hämochromatose f.
von Rosen ['raʊzn]: **v.R. splint** ortho. von Rosen-Schiene f.
von Saar [sɑːr]: **v.S.'s epithelium** von Saar'-Epithel nt.
von Willebrand ['vɪləbrant]: **v.W.'s disease** (von) Willebrand-Jürgens-Syndrom nt, konstitutionelle Thrombopathie f, hereditäre/vaskuläre Pseudohämophilie f, Angiohämophilie f.
v.W. factor abbr. vWF von Willebrand--Faktor m abbr. vWF, Faktor VIII assoziiertes-Antigen nt.
v.W.'s syndrome → v.W.'s disease.
von Zumbusch ['tsʊmbʊʃ]: **v.Z.'s psoriasis** derm. Psoriasis pustulosa vom Typ Zumbusch, Psoriasis pustulosa generalisata, Psoriasis pustulosa gravis Zumbusch.
Voorhoeve [fəʊr'həʊv]: **V.'s disease** Voorhoeve-Syndrom nt, -Erkrankung f, Osteopathia striata.
vor·tex ['vɔːrteks] n, pl **-tex·es, -ti·ces** [-tɪsiːz] 1. anat. Wirbel m, Vortex m. 2. (a. fig.) Wirbel m, Strudel m.
v. of heart Herzwirbel, Vortex (cordis).
v. of urinary bladder 1. (Harn-)Blasengrund m, Fundus vesicae (urinariae). 2. (Harn-)Blasenspitze f, Apex vesicae/vesicalis (urinariae).
vortex motion Wirbelbewegung f.
vor·ti·cal ['vɔːrtɪkl] adj → vorticose.
vor·ti·cose ['vɔːrtɪkəʊs] adj wirbel-, strudelartig, wirbelig, wirbelbildend, Wirbel-.
vorticose veins hintere Ziliarvenen pl, Vv. vorticosae, Vv. choroideae oculi.
vow·el ['vaʊəl] **I** n Selbstlaut m, Vokal m. **II** adj vokalisch, Vokal-.
vox [vɒks] n Stimme f, Vox f.
vo·yeur [vwɑːˈjɜr, vɔɪ-] n psycho., psychia. Voyeur m; inf. Spanner m.
vo·yeur·ism [vwɑːˈjɜrɪzəm] n psychia.,

psycho. Voyeurismus m, Voyeurtum nt.
VP abbr. → vasopressin.
VP-16 n → vindesine.
VPRC abbr. → volume of packed red cells.
V region → variable region.
Vrolik ['vrɒlɪk]: **V.'s disease** Vrolik-Krankheit f, Vrolik-Typ m der Osteogenesis imperfecta, Osteogenesis imperfecta congenita, Osteogenesis imperfecta Typ Vrolik.
VSD abbr. → ventricular septal defect.
V-shaped fracture V-förmige Fraktur f.
V-shaped line of tongue Terminalsulkus m, V-Linguae nt, Sulcus terminalis linguae.
V_T abbr. → tidal volume.
vul·can·i·za·tion [ˌvʌlkənɪˈzeɪʃn] n chem. Vulkanisierung f, Vulkanisation f.
vul·can·ize ['vʌlkənaɪz] vt chem. vulkanisieren.
vul·gar ['vʌlɡər] adj gewöhnlich, allgemein, gemein, vulgär.
vulgar ichthyosis Fischschuppenkrankheit f, Ichthyosis simplex/vulgaris.
vul·ner·a·bil·i·ty [ˌvʌlnərəˈbɪlətɪ] n Verwundbarkeit f, Verletzbarkeit f, Vulnerabilität f.
vul·ner·a·ble ['vʌlnərəbl] adj verwundbar, verletzbar, verletzlich, vulnerabel, anfällig (to für).
vul·ner·a·ble·ness ['vʌlnərəblnɪs] n → vulnerability.
vul·ner·ant ['vʌlnərənt] adj verletzend, schädigend.
vul·ner·ar·y ['vʌlnərerɪ] **I** n Wundheilmittel nt. **II** adj Wunde betr., heilend, heilungsfördernd, Wund-, Heil(ungs)-.
vul·nus ['vʌlnəs] n, pl **-ner·a** [-nərə] Wunde f, Vulnus nt.
Vulpian ['vʌlpɪən; vylˈpjɑ̃]: **V.'s atrophy** Vulpian-Atrophie f, -Syndrom nt, Vulpian-Bernhard-Atrophie f, -Syndrom nt, adult-proximale/skapulohumerale

Form f der spinalen Muskelatrophie.
V.'s disease → V.'s atrophy.
vul·va ['vʌlvə] n, pl **-vas, -vae** [-viː] anat. (weibliche) Scham f, Schamgegend f, äußere (weibliche) Geschlechtsorgane/Genitalien pl, Vulva f.
vul·val ['vʌlvəl] adj Vulva betr., Scham(lippen)-, Vulvo-, Vulva-.
vulval cleft Schamspalte f, Rima pudendi.
vul·var ['vʌlvər] adj → vulval.
vulvar slit → vulval cleft.
vul·vec·to·my [vʌlˈvektəmɪ] n gyn. Vulvaexzision f, Vulvektomie f.
vul·vis·mus [vʌlˈvɪzməs] n → vaginismus.
vul·vi·tis [vʌlˈvaɪtɪs] n gyn. Vulvaentzündung f, Vulvitis f.
vulvo- pref. Scham-, Schamlippen-, Vulvo-, Vulva-.
vul·vo·cru·ral [ˌvʌlvəˈkrʊərəl] adj vulvokrural.
vul·vop·a·thy [vʌlˈvɒpəθɪ] n Vulvaerkrankung f, Vulvopathie f.
vul·vo·rec·tal [ˌvʌlvəˈrektl] adj Scham/Vulva u. Rektum betr. od. verbindend, vulvorektal.
vulvorectal fistula patho. Vulva-Rektum--Fistel f, vulvorektale Fistel f.
vul·vo·u·ter·ine [ˌ-ˈjuːtərɪn, -raɪn] adj Scham/Vulva u. Gebärmutter/Uterus betr., vulvouterin.
vulvouterine canal → vaginal canal.
vul·vo·vag·i·nal [ˌ-ˈvædʒɪnl] adj Scham/Vulva u. Scheide/Vagina betr., vulvovaginal.
vul·vo·vag·i·ni·tis [ˌ-ˌvædʒəˈnaɪtɪs] n gyn. Entzündung f von Vulva u. Scheide, Vulvovaginitis f.
v wave card. v-Welle f.
vWF abbr. → von Willebrand factor.
V-Y flap chir. V-Y-Lappen m.
V-Y plasty chir. V-Y-Plastik f.
V-Y procedure → V-Y plasty.
VZIG abbr. → varicella-zoster immune globulin.
VZV abbr. → varicella-zoster virus.

W

W *abbr.* **1.** → watt. **2.** → wolfram.
W₁₇₀ *abbr.* → physical work capacity.
Waaler-Rose ['vɑːlər rəʊz]: **W.-R. test** Rose-Waaler-Test *m*, Waaler-Rose-Test *m*.
Waardenburg ['vɑːrdnbɜrg]: **W.'s syndrome 1.** (Vogt-)Waardenburg-Syndrom *nt*, Dyszephalosyndaktylie *f*. **2.** (Klein-)Waardenburg-Syndrom *nt*.
Wachendorf ['vaxəndɔrf]: **W.'s membrane** *embryo*. Membrana pupillaris.
wad·ding ['wɑdɪŋ] **I** *n* **1.** Einlage *f*, Füllmaterial *nt*. **2.** Watte *f*. **3.** Polsterung *f*, Wattierung *f*. **II** *adj* Wattier-.
wad·dle ['wɑdl] **I** *n* → waddle gait. **II** *vi* watscheln.
waddle gait watschelnder Gang *m*, Watschelgang *m*, Watscheln *nt*.
wad·dling gait ['wɑdlɪŋ] → waddle gait.
wage [weɪdʒ] *n* (Arbeits-)Lohn *m*.
Wagner ['wægnər; 'vɑːg-]: **W.'s corpuscles** Meissner'-(Tast-)Körperchen *pl*, Corpuscula tactus.
W.'s disease/dystrophy *ophthal*. Wagner'-Krankheit *f*, hereditäre vitreoretinale Degeneration *f*.
WAIS *abbr.* → Wechsler Adult Intelligence Scale.
waist [weɪst] *n* **1.** Taille *f*. **2.** Mittelstück *nt*, Mitte *f*, schmalste Stelle *f*.
waist triangle Taillendreieck *nt*.
wait·ing list ['weɪtɪŋ] Warteliste *f*.
wake [weɪk] (*v* woke; woken) **I** *n* **1.** Totenwache *f*. **II** *vt* → wake up I. **III** *vi* **1.** → wake up II. **2.** wachen, wach sein *od*. bleiben.
wake up I *vt* (auf-)wecken, wachrütteln. **II** *vi* (auf-, er-)wachen, wach werden.
wake·ful ['weɪkfəl] *adj* **1.** wachend. **2.** ruhelos, schlaflos. **3.** *fig*. wachsam.
wake·ful coma Agrypnocoma *nt*.
wake·ful·ness ['weɪkfəlnɪs] *n* **1.** Wachen *nt* **2.** Schlaf-, Ruhelosigkeit *f*. **3.** *fig*. Wachsamkeit *f*.
wak·ing ['weɪkɪŋ] **I** *n* (Er-)Wachen *nt*. **on ~** beim Erwachen. **II** *adj* wachsam, wach, Wach-.
waking dream Wach-, Tagtraum *m*.
Walcher ['wɔːlʃər; 'valçər]: **W.'s position** *gyn*. Walcher-Hängelage *f*.
Walden ['wɔldən; 'valdən]: **W.'s inversion** Walden-Umkehr *f*, -Inversion *f*.
Waldenström ['valdənstrem]: **W.'s disease** Perthes-Krankheit *f*, Morbus Perthes *m*, Perthes-Legg-Calvé-Krankheit *f*, Legg-Calvé-Perthes-Krankheit *f*, Legg-Calvé-Perthes-Waldenström-Krankheit *f*, Osteochondropathia deformans coxae juvenilis, Coxa plana (idiopathica).
W.'s macroglobulinemia Waldenström-Krankheit *f*, Morbus Waldenström *m*, Makroglobulinämie (Waldenström) *f*.
W.'s purpura 1. Purpura hyperglobinaemica (Waldenström). **2.** → W.'s macroglobulinemia.
W.'s syndrome → W.'s macroglobulinemia.

Waldeyer ['valdaɪər]: **preurethral ligament of W.** Lig. transversum perinei.
W.'s ring lymphatischer Rachenring *m*, Waldeyer'-Rachenring *m*.
W.'s sheath → W.'s space.
W.'s space *urol*. Waldeyer-Scheide *f*.
W.'s tonsillar ring → W.'s ring.
W.'s tract Lissauer'-Randbündel *nt*, Tractus dorsolateralis.
W.'s zonal layer → W.'s tract.
walk [wɔːk] **I** *n* **1.** Gehen *nt*; Gang(art *f*) *m*, Schritt *m*. **2.** Spaziergang *m*; (Spazier-)Weg *m*, Strecke *f*. **II** *vi* gehen, laufen; spazierengehen; wandern.
walk·ing ['wɔːkɪŋ] **I** *n* (Zufuß-)Gehen *nt*; Spazierengehen *nt*; Wandern *nt*. **II** *adj* gehend, Geh-, Wander-.
w. on straight line *neuro*. Strichgang *m*.
walking aid Gehhilfe *f*.
walking cast *ortho*. Gehgips *m*.
walking typhoid Typhus ambulatorius/levissimus.
wall [wɔːl] **I** *n* Wand *f*, Innenwand *f*, Wall *m*; *anat*. Paries *m*. **II** *vt* mit einer Mauer/Wand umgeben, ein-, ummauern; befestigen.
Wallace ['wɑlɪs, 'wɔ-]: **W.'s rule of nine** Wallace'-Neunerregel *f*.
wall-defective microbial form *abbr*.
WDMF *micro*. L-Form *f*, L-Phase *f*, L-Organismus *m*.
walled-of perforation *n chir*. gedeckte Perforation *f*.
Wallenberg ['valənbɜrg; -bɛrk]: **W.'s syndrome** Wallenberg-Syndrom *nt*, dorsolaterales Oblongata-Syndrom *nt*.
Waller ['wɑlər, 'wɔl-]: **W.'s law** Waller'-Gesetz *nt*.
wal·le·ri·an [wɑ'lɪərɪən]: **w. degeneration** *neuro*. Waller'-Degeneration *f*, sekundäre/orthograde Degeneration *f*.
w. law →wallerian degeneration.
wall·eye ['wɔːlaɪ] *n ophthal*. **1.** weißer Hornhautfleck *m*, Albugo *f*, Leukoma corneae. **2.** Auswärtsschielen *nt*, Exotropie *f*, Strabismus divergens.
wall tension Wandspannung *f*.
Walther ['wɔːltər; 'valtər]: **W.'s canals** → W.'s ducts.
W.'s ducts Ausführungsgänge *pl* der kleinen Unterzungendrüsen, Ductus sublinguales minores.
W.'s ganglion Ggl. impar.
W.'s oblique ligament Lig. talofibulare posterius.
Walton ['wɔːltn]: **W.'s law** Gesetz *nt* der multiplen Proportionen.
wan·der·ing abscess ['wɑndərɪŋ] Senkungsabszeß *m*.
wandering cell 1. Wanderzelle *f*. **2.** amöboid-bewegliche Zelle *f*.
resting w. ruhende Wanderzelle; Histiozyt *m*.
wandering erysipelas Erysipelas migrans.
wandering gallbladder flottierende Gallenblase *f*.

wandering goiter Tauchkropf *m*.
wandering kidney *patho*. Wanderniere *f*, Ren mobilis/migrans.
wandering liver Lebersenkung *f*, -tiefstand *m*, Wanderleber *f*, Hepatoptose *f*, Hepar migrans/mobile.
wandering pacemaker wandernder Schrittmacher *m*.
wandering pneumonia wandernde Pneumonie *f*, Pneumonia migrans.
wandering rash Landkartenzunge *f*, Wanderplaques *pl*, Lingua geographica, Exfoliatio areata linguae/dolorosa, Glossitis exfoliativa marginata, Glossitis areata exsudativa.
wandering spleen *patho*. Wandermilz *f*, Lien migrans/mobilis.
wane [weɪn] **I** *n* Abnahme *f*, Nachlassen *nt*, Abnehmen *nt*, Schwinden *nt*. **II** *vi* abnehmen, nachlassen, schwinden, schwächer werden.
Wangensteen ['wæŋənstiːn]: **W.'s apparatus/tube** *chir*. Wangensteen-Drainage *f*.
Wangensteen-Rice ['raɪs]: **W.-R. roentgenogram** *radiol*. Röntgenaufnahme *f* nach Wangensteen.
W antigen W-Antigen *nt*.
war·ble botfly ['wɔːrbl] *micro*. Dasselfliege *f*, Dermatobia hominis.
Warburg ['wɔːrbɜrg; 'varbʊrk]: **W. apparatus** Warburg'-Apparat *m*.
W.'s coenzyme Nicotinamid-adenin-dinucleotid-phosphat *nt abbr.* NADP, Triphosphopyridinnucleotid *abbr.* TPN, Cohydrase II *f*, Coenzym II *nt*.
W.'s hypothesis *biochem*. Warburg'-Hypothese *f*.
Warburg-Barcroft ['bɑːrkrɒft]: **W.-B. apparatus** Warburg'-Apparat *m*.
Warburg-Lipmann-Dickens ['lɪpmən 'dɪkəns]: **W.-L.-D. shunt** Pentosephosphatzyklus *m*, Phosphogluconatweg *m*.
ward [wɔːrd] *n* **1.** (Krankenhaus-)Station *f*, Abteilung *f*; (Kranken-)Saal *m*, (-)Zimmer *nt*. **in/on the ~** auf Station. **2.** (Stadt-)Bezirk *m*.
ward·en ['wɔːrdn] *n* Aufseher(in *f*) *m*; Portier *m*, Pförtner *m*.
Ward-Romano [wɔːrd rəʊmɑːnəʊ]: **W.-R. syndrome** Romano-Ward-Syndrom *nt*.
war dropsy [wɔːr] → war edema.
ward round Visite *f*.
war edema Hungerödem *nt*.
war·fa·rin ['wɔːrfərɪn] *n pharm*. Warfarin *nt*.
war fever epidemisches/klassisches Fleckfieber *nt*, Läusefleckfieber *nt*, Fleck-, Hunger-, Kriegstyphus *m*, Typhus exanthematicus.
warm [wɔːrm] **I** *n* (An-, Auf-)Wärmen *nt*. **to give sth. a ~** etw. (an-, auf-)wärmen. **II** *adj* warm; heiß, erhitzt. **I am/feel ~** mir ist warm. **III** *vt* **1.** (an-, er-)wärmen, warm machen. **IV** *vi* warm *od*. wärmer werden, s. erwärmen; (*Sport*) s. aufwärmen.

warm up I *vt* → warm III. II *vi* → warm IV.
warm agglutinin Wärmeagglutinin *nt*.
warm antibody Wärmeantikörper *m*.
warm-blooded *adj bio*. warmblütig.
warm-cold hemolysin Kalt-Warm-Hämolysin *nt*.
warm·er ['wɔːrmər] *n* Wärmer *m*.
warm fiber *physiol*. Warmfaser *f*.
warm hemagglutinin Wärmehämagglutinin *nt*.
warm·ing ['wɔːrmɪŋ] *n* (An-, Auf-)Wärmen *nt*, Erwärmung *f*.
warming pad Heizkissen *nt*.
warming pan Wärmflasche *f*.
warm ischemia warme Ischämie *f*.
warm·ish ['wɔːrmɪʃ] *adj* lauwarm.
warm point *physiol*. Warmpunkt *m*.
warm-reactive antibody Wärmeantikörper *m*.
warm receptor *physiol*. Warmrezeptor *m*.
warm sensation *physiol*. Warmempfindung *f*.
warm-sensitive cells *physiol*. warmsensitive Zellen *pl*.
warm sensor *physiol*. Warmsensor *m*.
warm shock warmer/roter Schock *m*.
warm spots Warmpunkte *pl*.
warmth [wɔːrmθ] *n* (*a. fig.*) Wärme *f*.
war·rant ['wɔrənt, 'war-] I *n* 1. Vollmacht *f*. 2. Rechtfertigung *f*, Berechtigung *f*. II *vt* 3. bevollmächtigen. 4. rechtfertigen, berechtigen.
wart [wɔːrt] *n* 1. (virusbedingte) Warze *f*, Verruca *f*. 2. warzenähnliche Hautveränderung *f*.
Wartenberg ['wɔːrtənbɑrg]: **W.'s disease** 1. Ch(e)iralgia paraesthetica. 2. idiopathische Akroparästhesie *f*, Wartenberg-Syndrom *nt*, Brachialgia statica paraesthetica.
W.'s symptom 1. Wartenberg-Reflex *m*, Daumenzeichen. 2. → W.'s disease 2.
Warthin-Finkeldey ['wɔːrθɪn 'fɪŋkldi]: **W.-F. cells** Warthin-Finkeldey-Riesenzellen *pl*.
Warthin-Starry ['stɑːri]: **W.-S. silver stain** Silberimprägnierung *f* nach Warthin-Starry.
wart·y ['wɔːrtɪ] *adj* Warzen betr., von Warzen bedeckt, warzig, Warzen-.
warty dyskeratoma warziges Dyskeratom *nt*, Dyskeratoma segregans/verrucosum/lymphadenoides, Dyskeratosis segregans, Dyskeratosis follicularis isolata.
warty horn *derm*. Hauthorn *nt*, Cornu cutaneum, Keratoma giganteum.
warty tuberculosis Wilk'-Krankheit *f*, warzige Tuberkulose *f* der Haut, Leichentuberkel *m*, Schlachttuberkulose *f*, Tuberculosis cutis verrucosa, Verruca necrogenica, Tuberculum anatomicum.
warty ulcer Marjolin-Ulkus *nt*.
wash [wɑʃ] I *n* 1. Waschen *nt*, Waschung *f*, Wäsche *f*. **to give sth. a ~** etw. (ab-)waschen. **to have a ~** s. waschen. 2. (*Magen*) Spülung *f*; Aus-, Umspülen *nt*. 3. Wäsche *f*. 4. Waschwasser *nt*, -lauge *f*; Spülwasser *nt*. 5. (Haar-)Wasser *nt*; Spülflüssigkeit *f*. 6. *pharm*. Waschung *f*. 7. *techn*. Bad *nt*. II *adj* waschbar, Wasch-. III *vt* 8. waschen. **to ~ o.s.** s. waschen. **to ~ one's hands** s. die Hände waschen. 9. (ab-, um-, weg-, aus-)spülen, reinigen, (aus-)waschen.
wash away *vt* abwaschen, wegspülen.
wash down *vt* (*Tablette*) hinunterspülen.
wash off *vt* abwaschen, wegspülen.
wash out *vt* auswaschen, (aus-)spülen.
wash·ba·sin ['wɑʃbeɪsən] *n* Waschbecken *nt*.
wash bottle *chem*. 1. Spritzflasche *f*. 2. (*Gas*) Waschflasche *f*.

wash·cloth ['wɑʃklɔθ] *n* Waschlappen *nt*.
washed clot [wɑʃt] *patho*. Abscheidungsthrombus *m*, weißer/grauer Thrombus *m*.
wash·er ['wɑʃər] *n* 1. *lab*. Spülapparat *m*, -maschine *f*. 2. Dichtung(sring *m*, -scheibe *f*) *f*, Unterlegscheibe *f*.
wash·ing ['wɑʃɪŋ] *n* 1. Waschen *nt*, Waschung *f*, Wäsche *f*. 2. Wäsche *f*. 3. *techn*. Bad *nt*.
washing soda Soda *f*, Natriumkarbonat *nt*.
wash·out ['wɑʃaʊt] *n* Ausspülung *f*, -waschung *f*.
washout method *physiol*. Auswaschmethode *f*.
washout pyelography *urol.*, *radiol*. Auswaschpyelographie *f*.
wash-rag ['wɑʃræg] *n* → washcloth.
wash·room ['wɑʃrʊm, -ruːm] *n* Waschraum *m*.
wash·tub ['wɑʃtʌb] *n* Waschwanne *f*.
Wasmann ['wɑsmən; 'vɑːsman]: **W.'s glands** Magendrüsen *f*, Fundus- u. Korpusdrüsen *pl*, Gll. gastricae propriae.
wasp [wɑsp] *n* Wespe *f*.
was·ser·hel·le cells ['wɑsərhelɪ; 'vɑsərhelə] wasserhelle Zellen *pl*.
Wassermann ['wɑsərmən; 'vɑsərman]: **W. antibody** Wassermann-Antikörper *m*.
W. reaction *abbr*. **W.r.** Wassermann-Test *m*, -Reaktion *f abbr*. WaR, Komplementbindungsreaktion *f* nach Wassermann.
W. test → W. reaction.
waste [weɪst] I *n* 1. Verschwendung *f*, -geudung *f*. 2. Abfall(stoffe *pl*) *m*, Müll *m*. 3. Verfall *m*, Verschleiß *m*, Schwund *m*, Verlust *m*. II *adj* 4. ungenutzt, überschüssig, überflüssig. 5. Abfall-, Abfluß-, Ablauf-; *bio*. Ausscheidungs-. III *vt* 6. verschwenden, vergeuden. 7. aus-, aufzehren, schwächen. IV *vi* 8. verschwendet werden. 9. verfallen, verkümmern, schwächer werden, schwinden.
waste away *vi* dahinsiechen, -schwinden.
waste drain Abzugskanal *m*.
waste gas *techn*. Abgas *nt*.
waste materials Abfall *m*, Abfallmaterial *nt*, -stoffe *pl*.
waste product 1. *techn*. Abfallprodukt *nt*. 2. *physiol*. Ausscheidungsstoff *m*.
waste·wa·ter ['weɪst͵wɔːtər] *n* Abwasser *nt*.
wast·ing ['weɪstɪŋ] I *n* 1. → waste 1. u. 3. 2. *patho*. Auszehrung *f*, Kräftezerfall *m*; Schwund *m*. II *adj* 3. (aus-, ab-)zehrend, schwächend. 4. abnehmend, schwindend.
wasting paralysis spinale Muskelatrophie *f*.
watch [wɑtʃ] I *n* 1. Wache *f*; Wachen *nt*. **to be on the ~** aufpassen. **to keep (a) ~** wachen (*on, over* über); aufpassen (*on, over* auf); jdn. im Auge behalten. 2. Wachsamkeit *f*. II *vt* überwachen, aufpassen auf, beobachten. III *vi* 3. wachen (*with* bei). 4. zusehen, zuschauen; Ausschau halten (*for* nach).
watch over *vi* bewachen, aufpassen, wachen über.
watch·ful ['wɑtʃfəl] *adj* wachsam, aufmerksam (*of* auf).
watch·ful·ness ['wɑtʃfəlnɪs] *n* Wachsamkeit *f*.
wat·er ['wɔːtər] I *n* 1. Wasser *nt*; (*a. ~s pl*) Mineralquelle *f*, -wasser *nt*, Heilquelle *f*, -wasser *nt*. **to drink/take the ~s** eine (Trink-)Kur machen. 2. *chem*. Wasserlösung *f*. 3. *physiol*. Wasser *nt*, Sekret *nt*; **the ~s** *pl* Fruchtwasser *nt*. II *vt* 4. mit Wasser versorgen. 5. wässern, einweichen, befeuchten. 6. verwässern, verdün-

nen. III *vi* (*Mund*) wäßrig werden (*for nach*); (*Augen*) tränen.
water down *vt* verwässern, (mit Wasser) verdünnen, abschwächen.
w. on the brain Wasserkopf *m*, Hydrozephalus *m*, Hydrocephalus *m*.
w. of combustion Verbrennungswasser.
w. of crystallization Kristallwasser.
w. on the knee Kniegelenk(s)erguß *m*.
w. of metabolism *biochem*. Oxidations-, Verbrennungswasser.
w. of oxidation *biochem*. Oxidations-, Verbrennungswasser.
water balance Wasserhaushalt *m*, -bilanz *f*.
water bath *chem*. Wasserbad *nt*.
wa·ter·bed ['wɔːtərbed] *n* Wasserbett *nt*.
Christine's w. Christine'-Wasserbett.
water blister Wasserblase *f*.
water-borne *adj* (*Krankheit*) durch (Trink-)Wasser übertragen.
water brash Sodbrennen *nt*, Pyrosis *f*.
water canker Noma *f*, Wangenbrand *m*, Wasserkrebs *m*, infektiöse Gangrän *f* des Mundes, Cancer aquaticus, Chancrum oris, Stomatitis gangraenosa.
water-clear cells wasserhelle Zellen *pl*.
water closet (Wasser-)Klosett *nt*.
water content Wassergehalt *m*.
water cure Wasserkur *f*; Wasserheilkunde *f*, -verfahren *nt*, Hydriatrie *f*, Hydrotherapie *f*.
water deficiency Wassermangel *m*.
water dermatitis creeping disease (*nt*), Hautmaulwurf *m*, Larva migrans, Myiasis linearis migrans.
water diuresis Wasserdiurese *f*.
water drinker 1. Wassertrinker(in *f*) *m*. 2. Antialkoholiker(in *f*) *m*.
wa·ter·drop ['wɔːtər͵drɑp] *n* Wassertropfen *m*; Träne *f*.
water excretion Wasserausscheidung *f*.
water·fall stomach ['wɔːtərfɔːl] Kaskadenmagen *m*.
water gas *chem*. Wassergas *nt*.
water glass 1. *chem*. Wasserglas *nt*, wasserlösliche Alkalisilikate *pl*. 2. Wasserglas *nt*.
water-hammer pulse Wasserhammerpuls *m*.
Waterhouse-Friderichsen ['wɔːtərhaʊs ͵frɪdə'rɪksən]: **W.-F. syndrome** Waterhouse-Friderichsen-Syndrom *nt*.
wa·ter·i·ness ['wɔːtərɪnɪs] *n* Wässerigkeit *f*, Wäßrigkeit *f*.
wa·ter·ing ['wɔːtərɪŋ] *adj* wasserspendend, -produzierend, Kur-, Bade-.
water-insoluble *adj* wasserunlöslich, unlöslich in Wasser.
water intoxication Wasserintoxikation *f*.
water lens *opt*. Flüssigkeitslinse *f*.
wa·ter·less ['wɔːtərlɪs] *adj* wasserlos; trocken.
water loss Wasserabgabe *f*, -verlust *m*.
evaporative Wasserverlust durch Verdampfen, evaporativer Wasserverlust.
extraglandular w. extraglanduläre Wasserabgabe, Perspiratio insensibilis.
glandular w. glanduläre Wasserabgabe, Schwitzen *nt*, Transpiration *f*, Perspiratio sensibilis.
insensible w. → extraglandular w.
sensible w. → glandular w.
water-miscible *adj* mit Wasser mischbar.
water permeability Wasserdurchlässigkeit *f*.
water pill *inf*. Wassertablette *f*; *pharm*. harntreibendes Mittel *nt*, Diuretikum *nt*.
water pollution Wasserverschmutzung *f*, -unreinigung *f*.
water-repellent *adj* wasserabstoßend.

water-soluble *adj* wasserlöslich, löslich in Wasser.
water-soluble vitamin wasserlösliches Vitamin *nt*.
Waterstone ['wɔːtərstəʊn]: **W. operation** Waterstone-Anastomose *f*.
water store Wasserspeicher *m*.
water-stroke *n* ödem-bedingte Apoplexie *f*.
water thesaurismosis Ödem *nt*, Oedema *nt*.
water vapor Wasserdampf *m*.
water-vapor partial pressure Wasserdampfpartialdruck *m*.
water-vapor saturation Wasserdampfsättigung *f*.
water-wheel sound *card.* Mühlradgeräusch *nt*, Bruit de moulin.
wa·ter·works ['wɔːtərwɜːrks] *pl sl.* **1.** Tränen *pl.* **2.** Nieren *pl*; ableitende Harnwege *pl*.
wa·ter·y ['wɔːtərɪ] *adj* Wasser enthaltend, wäßrig, wässerig, wasserähnlich; (*Augen*) tränend; feucht, naß, voller Wasser; verwässert.
watery diarrhea seröser/wäßriger Durchfall *m*, Diarrhoea serosa.
watery eyes Tränenträufeln *nt*, Epiphora *f*, Dakryorrhoe *f*.
watery secretion wäßriges Sekret *nt*.
Watson-Crick ['wɑtsən krɪk]: **W.-C. helix/model** Watson-Crick-Modell *n*, Doppelhelix *f*.
Wat·so·ni·us wat·so·ni [wɑt'səʊnɪəs wɑt-'səʊnaɪ] *micro.* Watsonius watsoni.
Watson-Schwartz [ʃwɔːrts]: **W.-S. test** Watson-Schwartz-Test *m*.
watt [wɑt] *n abbr.* **W** Watt *nt abbr.* W.
watt·age ['wɑtɪdʒ] *n* Wattleistung *f*.
watt-hour *n abbr.* **Wh** Wattstunde *f abbr.* Wh.
watt·me·ter ['wɑtmiːtər] *n phys.* Leistungsmesser *m*, Wattmeter *nt*.
watt-second *n abbr.* **Ws** Wattsekunde *f abbr.* Ws.
wave [weɪv] **I** *n* **1.** (*a. fig.*) Welle *f*, Woge *f*. **in ~s** schubweise, in Wellen. **2.** *phys.* Welle *f*. **3.** *physiol., anat.* Welle *f*, wellenförmige Struktur *f*. **4.** (Haar-)Welle *f*. **II** *vt* wellenförmig bewegen. **III** *vi* **5.** wogen, s. wellenartig bewegen. **6.** (*Haar*) s. wellen.
wave equation *phys.* Wellengleichung *f*.
wave·length ['weɪv‚leŋ(k)θ] *n phys.* Wellenlänge *f*.
wave·like ['weɪvlaɪk] *adj* wellenförmig, -artig, -ähnlich.
wave·me·ter ['weɪvmiːtər] *n phys.* Wellenmesser *m*.
wave number *phys.* Wellenzahl *f*.
wave-resistance *n* Wellenwiderstand *m*.
wave theory *phys.* Wellentheorie *f*.
wav·y ['weɪvɪ] *adj* wellig, gewellt, Wellen-.
wax [wæks] **I** *n* **1.** (Bienen-, Pflanzen-)Wachs *nt*, Cera *f*. **2.** Ohr(en)schmalz *nt*, Zerumen *nt*, Cerumen *nt*. **3.** *chem.* Wachs *nt*. **II** *adj* wächsern, Wachs-. **III** *vt* (ein-)wachsen.
wax bath Paraffinbad *nt*.
wax·en ['wæksən] *adj* **1.** wachshaltig. **2.** wie Wachs, wachsartig, wächsern, Wachs-; (*Gesicht*) bleich, wächsern.
wax·y ['wæksɪ] *adj* ~ waxen.
waxy cast (*Harn*) Wachszylinder *m*.
waxy degeneration amyloide Degeneration *f*, Amyloidose *f*.
waxy flexibility *psychia.* wachsartige Biegsamkeit *f*, Flexibilitas cerea.
waxy kidney Amyloid(schrumpf)niere *f*, Wachs-, Speckniere *f*.
waxy liver Amyloidleber *f*.
waxy spleen Wachsmilz *f*.
way [weɪ] *n* **1.** Weg *m*, Bahn *f*; Richtung *f*.

2. Durchgang *m*, Öffnung *f*. **3.** *fig.* Lauf *m*, Gang *m*. **4.** Methode *f*, Verfahren *nt*, Art u. Weise. **5.** (Gesundheits-)Zustand *m*, Lage *f*. **in a bad ~** in schlimmer Verfassung.
w. of living Lebensweise.
Wayson ['weɪsən]: **W.'s stain** Wayson-Färbung *f*.
WBC *abbr.* **1.** → white blood cell. **2.** [white blood count] → white cell count.
WCC *abbr.* → white cell count.
W chromosome W-Chromosom *nt*.
WDHA syndrome [watery diarrhea, hypocalemia, achlorhydria] pankreatische Cholera *f*, Verner-Morrison-Syndrom *nt*.
WDL *abbr.* → well-differentiated lymphocytic lymphoma.
WDLL *abbr.* → well-differentiated lymphocytic lymphoma.
WDMF *abbr.* → wall-defective microbial form.
weak [wiːk] *adj* **1.** schwach. **2.** empfindlich, kränklich, gebrechlich, schwach. **to feel/go ~ at the knees** wacklig auf den Beinen sein. **3.** labil, haltlos, (charakter-)schwach. **4.** (*Lösung, Getränk*) schwach, dünn.
weak·en ['wiːkən] **I** *vt* etw. (ab-)schwächen; verdünnen. **II** *vi* schwach/schwächer werden, nachlassen; (*Kraft*) erlahmen.
weak·en·ing ['wiːkənɪŋ] *n* (Ab-)Schwächung *f*, Schwächen *nt*, Schwachwerden *nt*.
weak interaction *phys.* schwache Wechselwirkung *f*.
weak·ly ['wiːklɪ] **I** *adj* kränklich, schwächlich. **II** *adv* schwach.
weak-minded *adj* **1.** schwachsinnig. **2.** willens-, charakterschwach.
weak·ness ['wiːknɪs] *n* **1.** Schwäche *f*. **2.** Kränklichkeit *f*, Schwächlichkeit *f*. **3.** (Charakter-)Schwäche *f*.
weak pulse kleiner Puls *m*, Pulsus parvus.
weak-sighted *adj* schwachsichtig.
weak-willed *adj* willensschwach.
wean [wiːn] *vt* **1.** *ped.* entwöhnen (*off, from*); abstillen. **2.** abbringen (*away from von*); abgewöhnen, entwöhnen.
wean·er ['wiːnər] *n, adj* → weanling.
wean·ing ['wiːnɪŋ] *n* Entwöhnung *f*.
wean·ling ['wiːnlɪŋ] **I** *n* vor Kurzem entwöhntes Kind. **II** *adj* frisch entwöhnt.
wear [weər] (*v* **wore; worn**) **I** *n* **1.** Tragen *nt*. **2.** Abnutzung *f*, Verschleiß *m*. **3.** Haltbarkeit *f*, Strapazierfähigkeit *f*. **II** *vt* **4.** tragen. **5.** abtragen, abnutzen. **III** *vi* **6.** s. tragen; s. erhalten, halten, haltbar sein. **7.** s. abnutzen *od.* verbrauchen.
wear away I *vt* **1.** abnutzen, abtragen. **2.** auswaschen, aushöhlen. **II** *vi* s. abnutzen, s. abtragen, vermindern, verwischen, verrinnen, langsam vergehen.
wear down I *vt* **1.** abnutzen; verbrauchen. **2.** *fig.* zermürben, mürbe *od.* weichmachen, fix u. fertig machen. **II** *vi* s. abnutzen, s. verbrauchen.
wear off *vi* nachlassen, s. verlieren; abgehen, s. abnutzen; (*Wirkung*) s. verlieren, nachlassen, abklingen.
wear on *vi* s. hinziehen, s. (da-)hinschleppen.
wear out I *vt* abnutzen, abtragen; ermüden, erschöpfen. **II** *vi* s. abnutzen, s. abnutzen, verschleißen; *fig.* s. erschöpfen.
wear and tear Abnutzung *f*, Verschleiß (erscheinungen *pl*) *m*.
wear and tear pigment 1. Abnutzungspigment *nt*, Lipofuszin *nt*. **2. ~s** *pl* Lipochrome *pl*.
wea·ri·ness ['wɪərɪnɪs] *n* Müdigkeit *f*, Mattigkeit *f*, Lustlosigkeit *f*.

wea·ry ['wɪərɪ] *adj* **1.** müde, matt, lustlos (*with von, vor*). **2.** ermüdend.
web [web] *n* Gewebe *nt*, Netz *nt*, Gespinst *nt*; Schwimmhaut *f*; HNO Web *nt*.
webbed neck [webd] Pterygium colli.
webbed penis Penis palmatus.
web·bing ['webɪŋ] *n patho.* Schwimmhautbildung *f*.
Weber ['webər; 'veɪbər]: **W.'s corpuscle** Utriculus prostaticus.
W.'s disease Sturge-Weber(-Krabbe)-Krankheit *f*, -Syndrom *nt*, enzephalofaziale Angiomatose *f*, Neuroangiomatosis encephalofacialis, Angiomatosis encephalo-oculo-cutanea, Angiomatosis encephalotrigeminalis.
W.'s fraction Weber-Quotient *m*.
W.'s law Weber'-Gesetz *nt*.
W.'s organ Utriculus prostaticus.
W.'s paralysis → W.'s syndrome.
W.'s sign → W.'s syndrome.
W.'s symptom → W.'s syndrome.
W.'s syndrome Weber-Syndrom *nt*, Hemiplegia alternans oculomotorica.
W.'s test Weber-Versuch *m*.
W.'s zone Zona orbicularis.
Weber-Christian ['krɪstʃən]: **W.-C. disease/panniculitis** → W.-C. syndrome.
W.-C. syndrome Weber-Christian-Syndrom *nt*, Pfeiffer-Weber-Christian-Syndrom *nt*, rezidivierende fieberhafte nicht-eitrige Pannikulitis *f*, Panniculitis nodularis nonsuppurativa febrilis et recidivans.
Weber-Cockayne [kɑ'keɪn]: **W.-C. syndrome** Weber-Cockayne-Syndrom *nt*, Epidermolysis bullosa simplex Weber-Cockayne, Epidermolysis bullosa manuum et pedum aestivalis.
Weber-Dubler ['djuːblər]: **W.-D. syndrome** → Weber's syndrome.
Weber-Fechner ['feknər; 'fɛç-]: **W.-F. law** Weber-Fechner-Gesetz *nt*.
Weber-Ramstedt ['rɑːmstet; 'ramʃtɛt]: **W.-R. operation** *chir.* Weber-Ramstedt-Operation *f*, Ramstedt-Operation *f*, Pyloro(myo)tomie *f*.
web eye [web] *ophthal.* Flügelfell *nt*, Pterygium *nt*.
web space Interdigitalraum *m*.
web space infection Infektion *f* des Interdigitalraums.
Webster ['webstər]: **W.'s operation** Baldy-Webster-Operation *f*.
Wechsler ['wekslər]: **W. Adult Intelligence Scale** *abbr.* **WAIS** Hamburg-Wechsler-Intelligenztest *m* für Erwachsene *abbr.* HAWIE.
W. Intelligence Scale for Children *abbr.* **WISC** Hamburg-Wechsler-Intelligenztest *m* für Kinder *abbr.* HAWIK.
wed·dell·ite calculus [wə'delaɪt, 'wedlaɪt] *urol.* Calciumoxalatdihydrat-Stein *m*.
Wedensky [wə'denskɪ]: **W. inhibition** Wedensky-Hemmung *f*.
wedge [wedʒ] **I** *n* Keil *m*, keilförmige Struktur *f*. **II** *vt* (ver-)keilen, mit einem Keil festklemmen; (ein-)keilen. **III** *vi* s. festklemmen, s. verkeilen.
wedge biopsy Keilbiopsie *f*, -exzision *f*.
wedge compression fracture (*Wirbelkörper*) Stauchungsbruch *m* mit Keilbildung.
wedge osteotomy *ortho.* Keilosteotomie *f*.
wedge resection *chir., ortho.* Keilresektion *f*.
wedge resection osteotomy → wedge osteotomy.
wedge-shaped fasciculus Burdach'-Strang *m*, Fasciculus cuneatus medullae spinalis.
wedge-shaped vertebra Keilwirbel *m*.

WEE abbr. → Western equine encephalitis.
Weeks [wiːks]: **W.' bacillus** micro. Koch-Weeks-Bazillus m, Haemophilus aegypti(c)us/conjunctivitidis.
weep [wiːp] (v wept; wept) **I** n Weinen nt. **II** vt weinen. **III** vi 1. weinen. 2. triefen, tropfen, tröpfeln. 3. (Wunde) nässen, Serum ausscheiden.
WEE virus → Western equine encephalitis virus.
Wegener ['vegənər]: **W.'s granulomatosis/syndrome** Wegener-Granulomatose f, Wegener-Klinger-Granulomatose f.
Wegner ['vegnər]: **W.'s disease** Wegner'-Krankheit f, (kongenitale) Knochensyphilis f, Osteochondritis syphilitica.
Weichselbaum ['vaɪksəlbaʊm]: **W.'s coccus/diplococcus** Meningokokkus m, Neisseria meningitidis.
Weidel [vaɪdl]: **W.'s test** (for uric acid) Murexidprobe f.
Weigert ['vaɪgərt]: **W.'s fibrin stain** Weigert'-Fibrinfärbung f.
W.'s resorcin-fuchsin stain Weigert'-Elastikafärbung f, Weigert'-Resorcin-Fuchsin-Färbung f.
weigh [weɪ] **I** vt 1. wiegen. 2. fig. erwägen, abwägen (with, against gegen). **II** vi wiegen.
weigh up vt → weigh 2.
weight [weɪt] n 1. Gewicht nt, Last f; Gewichtseinheit f. 2. (Körper-)Gewicht nt. **to put on/gain** ~ zunehmen. **to lose** ~ abnehmen. 3. phys. Schwere f, (Massen-)Anziehungskraft f. 4. fig. Last f, Belastung f. 5. Wucht f, Heftigkeit f; Druck m.
weight density spezifisches Gewicht nt.
weight gain Gewichtszunahme f.
weight-i-ness ['weɪtɪnɪs] n Gewicht nt, Schwere f.
weight-less ['weɪtlɪs] adj schwerelos.
weight-less-ness ['weɪtlɪsnɪs] n Schwerelosigkeit f.
weight loss Gewichtsverlust m.
weight per volume abbr. **w./v.** Gewicht nt pro Volumeneinheit, spezifisches Gewicht nt.
weight problem Gewichtsprobleme pl.
weight reduction Gewichtsabnahme f, -reduktion f.
Weil [waɪl; vaɪl]: **W.'s basal layer** Weil'-Basalschicht f.
W.'s basal zone → **W.'s basal layer**.
W.'s disease 1. Weil'-Krankheit f, Leptospirosis icterohaemorrhagica. **2.** Weilähnliche-Erkrankung f.
W.'s syndrome → **W.'s disease**.
Weil-Felix ['fiːlɪks; 'feː-]: **W.-F. reaction/test** Weil-Felix-Reaktion f, -Test m.
Weill-Marchesani ['weɪ mɑrtʃə'sɑːnɪ]: **W.-M. syndrome** Marchesani-Syndrom nt, Weill-Marchesani-Syndrom nt.
Weinberg ['waɪnbɑrɡ]: **W.'s rule** genet. Weinberg-Methode f.
Weingrow ['waɪnɡroʊ] : **W.'s reflex** Weingrow-Reflex m.
Weir-Mitchell [wɪər 'mɪtʃl]: **W.-M.'s disease** Gerhardt-Syndrom nt, Weir-Mitchell-Gerhardt-Syndrom nt, Weir-Mitchell-Krankheit f, Erythromelalgie f, Erythralgie f, Erythermalgie f, Akromelalgie f.
Weiss [vaɪs]: **W.'s sign** neuro. Chvostek-Zeichen nt.
Weitbrecht ['vaɪtbrɛkt, -brɛçt]: **W.'s cartilage** Weitbrecht'-Knorpel m, Discus articularis artic. acromioclavicularis.
W.'s cord Chorda obliqua.
W.'s ligament Chorda obliqua.
prismatic ligament of W. Lig. capitis femoris.

Welch [weltʃ]: **W.'s abscess** Gasabszeß m.
W.'s bacillus Welch-Fränkel-(Gasbrand-)Bazillus m, Clostridium perfringens.
Welcker ['velkər]: **W.'s angle** Angulus sphenoidalis (ossis parietalis).
weld-er's conjunctivitis ['weldər] ophthal. Conjunctivitis actinica/photoelectrica, Keratoconjunctivitis/Ophthalmia photoelectrica.
wel-fare ['welfɛər] n 1. Wohl nt, Wohlergehen nt. 2. Sozialhilfe f; Fürsorge f, Wohlfahrt f. **to be on** ~ Sozialhilfe beziehen.
welfare case Sozialfall m.
welfare recipient Sozialhilfeempfänger(in f) m.
welfare state Wohlfahrtsstaat m.
welfare work Sozial-, Fürsorgearbeit f.
welfare worker Sozialarbeiter(in f) m, Fürsorger(in f) m.
well¹ [wel] adj 1. wohl, gesund. **to be/feel** ~ s. wohl fühlen. **to look** ~ gesund od. gut aussehen. 2. in Ordnung, richtig, gut.
well² [wel] **I** n Brunnen m; (Heil-)Quelle f, Mineralbrunnen m. **II** vi quellen (from aus).
well out vi hervorquellen.
well over vi überfließen.
well up vi (Tränen) aufsteigen; hervorbrechen, -schießen.
well-advised adj wohlüberlegt, klug.
well-balanced adj im Gleichgewicht befindlich; (Person) ausgeglichen, (Diät) ausgewogen.
well-being n Wohlbefinden nt, Gesundheit f, Wohl nt.
well-defined adj klar abgegrenzt, gut umrissen, gut zu unterscheiden; eindeutig definiert.
well-differentiated carcinoma hochdifferenziertes Karzinom nt.
well-differentiated lymphocytic lymphoma abbr. **WDLL, WDL** well-differentiated lymphocytic lymphoma abbr. WDLL, WDL.
well-fed adj wohlernährt.
well-fitting adj (richtig/gut) passend, sitzend.
well-kept adj gepflegt.
well-preserved adj guterhalten.
well-regulated adj geregelt, geordnet.
well-tried adj erprobt, bewährt.
welt [welt] n → **wheal**.
wen [wen] n 1. piläre Hautzyste f. 2. Epidermoid nt, Epidermal-, Epidermis-, Epidermoidzyste f, (echtes) Atherom nt, Talgretentionszyste f.
Wenckebach ['weŋkəbæk; -bax]: **W. block** Wenckebach-Periode f, AV-Block m II. Grades Typ I.
W.'s disease Herzsenkung f, -tiefstand m, Wanderherz m, Kardioptose f.
W. heart block → **W. block**.
W. period → **W. block**.
W. phenomenon Wenckebach-Phänomen nt.
Wepfer ['wepfər]: **W.'s glands** Brunner'-Drüsen pl, Duodenaldrüsen pl, Gll. duodenales.
Werdnig-Hoffmann ['verdnɪɡ 'hɑfmən]: **W.-H. atrophy** → **W.-H. disease**.
W.-H. disease Werdnig-Hoffmann-Krankheit f, -Syndrom nt, infantile spinale Muskelatrophie f (Werdnig-Hoffmann).
W.-H. paralysis → **W.-H. disease**.
W.-H. spinal muscular atrophy → **W.-H. disease**.
W.-H. type → **W.-H. disease**.
Werlhof ['verlhɔf]: **W.'s disease** idiopathische thrombozytopenische Purpura f abbr. ITP, Morbus Werlhof m, essentielle/idiopathische Thrombozytopenie f.
Wermer ['wɜrmər]: **W.'s syndrome** Wermer-Syndrom nt, MEN-Typ I m, MEA-Typ I m.
Werner ['wɜrnər; 'vɛrnər]: **W. syndrome** Werner-Syndrom nt, Progeria adultorum, Pangerie f.
Werner-His [hɪz]: **W.-H. disease** Wolhyn'-Fieber nt, Fünftagefieber nt, Wolhynienfieber nt, Febris quintana.
Werner-Schultz [ʃʊlts]: **W.-S. disease** Agranulozytose f, maligne/perniziöse Neutropenie f.
Wernicke ['vɛrnɪkə]: **W.'s aphasia** sensorische Aphasie f, Wernicke-Aphasie f.
W.'s area 1. → **W.'s speech center**. **2.** → **W.'s temporal speech area**.
W.'s center → **W.'s speech center**.
W.'s dementia Presbyophrenie f.
W.'s disease Wernicke-Enzephalopathie f, -Syndrom nt, Polioencephalitis haemorrhagica superior (Wernicke).
W.'s encephalopathy → **W.'s disease**.
W.'s reaction → **W.'s sign**.
W.'s sign Wernicke-Phänomen nt.
W.'s speech area → **W.'s temporal speech area**.
W.'s speech center Wernicke'-Sprachzentrum nt, akustisches/sensorisches Sprachzentrum nt.
W.'s speech field/region/zone → **W.'s temporal speech area**.
W.'s symptom Wernicke-Phänomen nt.
W.'s syndrome → **W.'s disease**.
W.'s temporal speech area Wernicke'-Sprachregion f, temporale Sprachregion f.
W.'s temporal speech field/region/zone → **W.'s temporal speech area**.
W.'s test Wernicke-Phänomen nt.
W.'s zone 1. → **W.'s speech center**. **2.** → **W.'s temporal speech area**.
Wernicke-Korsakoff ['kɔːrsəkɔf]: **W.-K. syndrome** Wernicke-Korsakoff-Syndrom nt.
Wernicke-Mann [mæn; man]: **W.-M. hemiplegia/type** Hemiplegie f Typ Wernicke-Mann, Wernicke-Prädilektionsparese f.
Wertheim ['verthaɪm]: **W. clamp** Wertheim-Klemme f.
W.'s operation gyn. Wertheim-Operation f.
Wes-sels-bron virus ['weslzbrɔn] Wesselsbron-Virus nt.
West [west]: **W.'s syndrome** West-Syndrom nt.
West Af·ri·can [west 'æfrɪkən]: **W. A. fever** Schwarzwasserfieber nt, Febris biliosa et haemoglobinurica.
W. A. sleeping sickness → **W. A. trypanosomiasis**.
W. A. trypanosomiasis westafrikanische Schlafkrankheit/Trypano(so)miasis f.
Westergren ['westərgren]: **W. method** Westergren-Methode f.
W. tube Westergren-Röhrchen nt.
West-ern ['westərn]: **W. blot technique** immun. Western-Blot-Technik f.
W. equine encephalitis abbr. **WEE** westliche Pferdeenzephalitis f, Western equine encephalitis/encephalomyelitis abbr. WEE.
W. equine encephalitis virus micro. Western-Equine-Enzephalitis-Virus nt, WEE-Virus nt.
W. equine encephalomyelitis → **W. equine encephalitis**.
W. equine encephalomyelitis virus → **W. equine encephalitis virus**.
West Nile [west naɪl]: **W. N. encephalitis** West-Nile-Fieber nt, -Enzephalitis f.

Westphal

W. N. fever → W. N. encephalitis.
W. N. nile fever virus *micro.* West-Nile-Fieber-Virus *nt.*
Westphal ['vɛstfɑːl]: W.'s disease → Westphal-Strümpell disease.
W.'s phenomenon 1. *neuro.* Westphal-Zeichen *nt,* -Reflex *m.* 2. Westphal-Piltz-Phänomen *nt,* Orbikularisphänomen *nt,* Lid-Pupillen-Reflex *m.*
W.'s pseudosclerosis → Westphal-Strümpell disease.
W.'s pupillary reflex → W.'s phenomenon 2.
W.'s sign Westphal-Zeichen *nt,* -Reflex *m,* Erb-Westphal-Zeichen *nt.*
W.'s symptom → W.'s sign.
Westphal-Erb [ɜrb]: W.-E. sign Westphal-Zeichen *nt,* -Reflex *m,* Erb-Westphal-Zeichen *nt.*
Westphal-Piltz [pɪlts]: W.-P. phenomenon/pupil/reflex → W.-P. sign.
W.-P. sign Westphal-Piltz-Phänomen *nt,* Orbikularisphänomen *nt,* Lid-Pupillen-Reflex *m.*
Westphal-Strümpell ['strɪmpəl; 'ʃtrʏmpəl]: W.-S. disease Westphal-Strümpell-Syndrom *nt.*
W.-S. pseudosclerosis/syndrome → W.-S. disease.
wet [wet] (*v* wet; wetted) I *n* Nässe *f,* Feuchtigkeit *f.* II *adj* naß, feucht, durchnäßt (*with* von); Naß-. III *vt* anfeuchten, naßmachen, benetzen. to ~ o.s. in die Hose machen. to ~ the bed bettnässen. to ~ through durchnässen. IV *vi* nässen, naß werden.
wet beriberi feuchte Form *f* der Beriberi.
wet-bulb thermometer Verdunstungsthermometer *nt.*
wet cell *phys.* Naßelement *nt,* nasse Zelle *f.*
wet colostomy *chir.* feuchte Kolostomie *f.*
wet cough Husten *m* mit Auswurf.
wet gangrene feuchte Gangrän *f.*
wet lung 1. Schocklunge *f,* adult respiratory distress syndrome *abbr.* ARDS. 2. Lungenödem *nt.*
wet·ness ['wetnɪs] *n* Nässe *f,* Feuchtigkeit *f.*
wet nurse Amme *f.*
wet-nurse *vt* (als Amme) säugen.
wet pack feuchter Umschlag *m,* feuchte Packung *f,* Wickel *m.*
wet pleurisy exsudative Brustfellentzündung/Pleuritis *f,* Pleuritis exsudativa.
wet sheet pack → wet pack.
wet shock Insulinschock *m.*
wet·ta·ble ['wetəbl] *adj phys.* benetzbar.
wettable surface *phys.* benetzbare Oberfläche *f.*
wet·ting ['wetɪŋ] *n* 1. Durchnässung *f.* 2. Befeuchtung *f.*
wetting agent *chem.* Netzmittel *nt.*
wet·tish ['wetɪʃ] *adj* etw. feucht.
Wever-Bray ['wiːvər breɪ]: W.-B. phenomenon (kochleäres) Mikropotential *nt.*
Weyers-Thier ['weɪɚs θɪər; 'vaɪərs tɪər]: W.-T. syndrome Weyers-Thier-Syndrom *nt,* okulovertebrales Syndrom *nt.*
Wh *abbr.* → watt-hour.
Whartin ['(h)wɔrtɪn]: W.'s tumor Whartin-Tumor *m,* Whartin-Albrecht-Arzt-Tumor *m,* Adenolymphom *nt,* Cystadenoma lymphomatosum, Cystadenolymphoma papilliferum.
Wharton ['(h)wɔrtn]: W.'s duct Wharton'-Gang *m,* Ductus submandibularis.
W.'s gelatine Wharton'-Sulze *f.*
W.'s jelly → W.'s gelatine.
wheal [(h)wiːl] *n derm.* Quaddel *f.*
wheat [(h)wiːt] *n* Weizen *m.*

Wheatstone ['(h)wiːtstəʊn]: W. bridge *phys.* Wheatstone'-Brücke *f.*
wheel [(h)wiːl] *n* 1. Rad *nt.* 2. (Steuer-, Lenk-)Rad *nt.* 3. Drehung *f,* Kreisbewegung *f.*
Wheeler ['(h)wiːlɚ]: W. method *ophthal.* Wheeler-Operation *f.*
wheeze [(h)wiːz] I *n* Keuchen *nt,* pfeifendes Atmen/Atemgeräusch *nt.* II *vi* keuchen, pfeifend atmen, pfeifen, schnaufen.
W hernia retrograde Hernie *f,* Hernie en W.
whet-stone crystals ['(h)wetstəʊn] *urol.* (*Harn*) Wetzsteinformen *pl.*
whew-ell-ite calculus ['hjuːəlaɪt] *urol.* Calciumoxalatmonohydrat-Stein *m.*
whey [(h)weɪ] *n* Molke *f.*
whey·ey ['(h)weɪɪ] *adj* molkig.
whey-faced ['(h)weɪfeɪst] *adj* käsig, käseweiß, käsebleich.
whip-lash ['(h)wɪplæʃ] *n* Schleudertrauma *nt* (der Halswirbelsäule), whiplash injury.
whiplash injury → whiplash.
Whipple ['(h)wɪpl]: W.'s disease Whipple'-Krankheit *f,* Morbus Whipple *m,* intestinale Lipodystrophie *f,* lipophage Intestinalgranulomatose *f,* Lipodystrophia intestinalis.
W.'s operation Whipple-Operation *f,* Pankreatikoduodenektomie *f.*
W. procedure 1. distale Pankreasresektion *f,* Linksresektion *f.* 2. → W.'s operation.
W.'s resection → W.'s operation.
W.'s triad Whipple-Trias *f.*
whip-worm ['(h)wɪpwɜrm] *n micro.* Peitschenwurm *m,* Trichuris trichiura, Trichocephalus dispar.
whis·per ['(h)wɪspɚ] I *n* Flüstern *nt,* Wispern *nt,* Geflüster *nt,* Gewisper *nt.* II *vt, vi* wispern, flüstern, leise sprechen.
whis-pered speech ['(h)wɪspərd] Flüstersprache *f.*
whis·tling face syndrome ['(h)wɪslɪŋ] Freeman-Sheldon-Syndrom *nt,* kranio-karpo-tarsales Dysplasie-Syndrom *nt,* Dysplasia cranio-carpo-tarsalis.
whistling rales pfeifende Rasselgeräusche *pl.*
white [(h)waɪt] I *n* (*Farbe*) Weiß *nt;* (*Rasse*) Weiße(r *m*) *f;* (etw.) Weißes, weißer Teil *m.* II *adj* weiß, Weiß-; hell(farbig); licht; blaß, bleich.
w. of egg Eiweiß *nt.*
white asphyxia weiße Apnoe/Asphyxie *f,* Asphyxia pallida.
white atrophy Atrophie blanche (Milian); Capillaritis alba.
white bile weiße Galle *f.*
white blood cell *abbr.* **WBC** weiße Blutzelle *f,* weißes Blutkörperchen *nt,* Leukozyt *m.*
white blood count *abbr.* **WBC** → white cell count.
white body of ovary Weißkörper *m,* Corpus albicans.
white bread Weiß-, Weizenbrot *nt.*
white cell → white blood cell.
white cell count *abbr.* **WCC** 1. Leukozytenzahl *f.* 2. Leukozytenzählung *f.*
differential w. Differentialblutbild *nt,* weißes Blutbild *m.*
white clot → white thrombus.
white coat Tunica albuginea testis/ovarii.
white commissure of spinal cord Commissura alba medullae spinalis.
lateral w. Seitenstrang *m* (des Rückenmarks), Funiculus lateralis (medullae spinalis).
white dermatographism weißer Dermographismus *m,* Dermographismus albus.
white-faced *adj* bleich, blaß.

white fat weißes Fett(gewebe *nt*) *nt.*
white fiber Kollagenfaser *f.*
white-haired *adj* weißhaarig; hellhaarig.
Whitehead ['(h)waɪthed]: W.'s operation *chir.* Whitehead-Operation *f.*
white-head ['(h)waɪthed] *n derm.* Hautgrieß *m,* Milium *nt,* Milie *f.*
white-headed *adj* → white-haired.
white infarct ischämischer/anämischer/weißer/blasser Infarkt *m.*
white laminae of cerebellum → white layers of cerebellum.
white layer: w.s of cerebellum Laminae albae (cerebelli).
w.s of cranial colliculus → w.s of rostral colliculus.
w.s of rostral colliculus Strata (grisea et alba) colliculi superioris.
w.s of superior colliculus → w.s of rostral colliculus.
white-leg ['(h)waɪtleg] *n* Milchbein *nt,* Leukophlegmasie *f,* Phlegmasia alba dolens.
white light *phys.* weißes *od.* farbloses Licht *nt.*
white line Linea alba (abdominis).
w. of abdomen → white line.
w. of Hilton Hilton'-Linie *f.*
w. of ischiococcygeal muscle Lig. anococcygeum
white lung Pneumocystis-Pneumonie *f,* interstitielle plasmazelluläre Pneumonie *f,* Pneumonia alba.
white matter → white substance.
central w. of cerebellum Kleinhirnmark *nt,* Corpus medullare cerebelli.
w. of spinal cord → white substance of spinal cord.
white muscle weißes Muskelgewebe *nt,* weiße Muskelfaser *f.*
whit·en ['(h)waɪtn] I *vt* weiß machen, weißen; bleichen. II *vi* (*Haar*) weiß werden.
white·ness ['(h)waɪtnɪs] *n* 1. Weiße *f.* 2. Blässe *f.*
white night schlaflose Nacht *f.*
whit·en·ing ['(h)waɪtnɪŋ] *n* 1. Weißen *nt.* 2. Bleichen *nt.* 3. Tünchen *nt.* 4. Weißwerden *nt.*
white noise weißes Rauschen *nt,* white noise.
white phosphorus weißer/gelber/gewöhnlicher Phosphor *m.*
white piedra Beigel'-Krankheit *f,* (weiße) Piedra *f,* Piedra alba, Trichomycosis nodosa.
white plague Tuberkulose *f abbr.* Tb, Tbc, Tbk, Tuberculosis *f.*
white pneumonia Pneumonia alba.
white-pox ['(h)waɪtpɑks] *n* weiße Pocken *pl,* Alastrim *nt,* Variola minor.
white pulp (*Milz*) weiße Pulpa *f,* Folliculi lymphatici splenici.
white ramus, communicans Ramus communicans albus.
white sponge nevus *derm.* weißer Schleimhautnävus *m,* Naevus spongiosus albus mucosae.
white-spot disease 1. Weißfleckenkrankheit *f,* White-Spot-Disease (*nt*), Lichen sclerosus et atrophicus, Lichen albus. 2. Morphaea guttata.
white substance weiße Hirn- u. Rückenmarkssubstanz *f,* Substantia alba.
arboreous w. of cerebellum (*Kleinhirn*) Markkörper *m,* Arbor vitae (cerebelli).
central w. of cerebellum Kleinhirnmark *nt,* Corpus medullare cerebelli.
w. of spinal cord weiße Rückenmarkssubstanz *f,* Substantia alba medullae spinalis.
white thrombus Abscheidungs-, Konglutinationsthrombus *m,* weißer/grauer Thrombus *m.*

whit·low ['(h)wɪtləʊ] *n* eitrige Fingerspitzenerkrankung *f*; tiefes Fingerpanaritium *nt*.
Whitmore ['(h)wɪtmɔʊr]: **W.'s bacillus** *micro*. Pseudomonas/Malleomyces/Actinobacillus pseudomallei.
W.'s disease Whitmore'-Krankheit *f*, Pseudomalleus *m*, Pseudorotz *m*, Melioidose *f*, Malleoidose *f*, Melioidosis *f*.
W.'s fever → W.'s disease.
whole [həʊl] **I** *n* das Ganze, die Gesamtheit; Einheit *f*, Ganze(s) *nt*. **II** *adj* **1.** ganz, gesamt, vollständig, völlig. **2.** ganz, unzerteilt. **3.** heil, unverletzt, unversehrt, unbeschädigt, ganz.
whole blood → whole human blood.
whole-body counter *radiol*. Ganzkörperzähler *m*.
whole-body irradiation → whole-body radiation.
whole-body radiation *radiol*. Ganzkörperbestrahlung *f*.
whole-brain irradiation → whole-brain radiation.
whole-brain radiation *radiol*. Ganzhirnbestrahlung *f*.
whole human blood Vollblut *nt*.
whole-virus vaccine Ganzvirusimpfstoff *m*.
whoop [(h)wuːp, (h)wʊp] *vi* keuchen, keuchend atmen.
whoop·ing cough ['(h)wuːpɪŋ, '(h)wʊp-] Keuchhusten *m*, Pertussis *f*, Tussis convulsiva.
whooping cough toxin *old* Pertussistoxin *nt abbr*. PT.
whooping-cough vaccine Pertussisvakzine *f*, -impfstoff *m*, Keuchhustenvakzine *f*, -impfstoff *m*.
whorl [(h)wɜrl, (h)wɔːrl] *n* **1.** *anat.*, *bio.* Windung *f*, Wirtel *m*, Quirl *m*. **2.** Windung *f*, Wirtel *m*.
Whytt [(h)wɪt]: **W.'s disease** Hydrocephalus internus.
Wichmann ['wɪkmən; 'vɪçman]: **W.'s asthma** Stimmritzenkrampf *m*, Laryngismus stridulus.
wick [wɪk] *n* **1.** Gazetampon *m*. **2.** Docht *m*.
Widal [viˈdal]: **W.'s reaction** Widal'-Reaktion *f*, -Test *m*, Gruber-Widal'-Reaktion *f*, -Test *m*.
W.'s serum test → W.'s reaction.
W.'s syndrome Widal-Abrami-Anämie *f*, -Ikterus *m*, Widal-Anämie *f*, -Ikterus *m*.
W.'s test → W.'s reaction.
wide [waɪd] *adj* **1.** breit; weit; groß; ausgedehnt. **2.** (*Augen*) aufgerissen. **3.** groß, beträchtlich. **4.** *fig*. umfangreich, umfassend, weitreichend; vielfältig.
wide-angle glaucoma Simplex-, Weitwinkelglaukom *nt*, Glaucoma simplex.
wide-awake *adj* **1.** hellwach. **2.** *fig*. aufmerksam, wachsam; aufgeweckt.
wide-eyed *adj* mit großen Augen.
wid·en [waɪdn] **I** *vt* erweitern, verbreitern, breiter machen; dehnen; dilatieren. **II** *vi* s. ausweiten, s. verbreitern, breiter werden.
widen out *vi* s. erweitern (*into* zu); s. ausweiten.
wide-necked *adj lab*. (*Flasche*) weithalsig.
wide·ness ['waɪdnɪs] *n* Breite *f*; Weite *f*; Ausgedehntheit *f*, Ausdehnung *f*.
wid·en·ing ['waɪdnɪŋ] *n* Dehnung *f*, Erweiterung *f*.
wide-open *adj* weit offen, weit geöffnet; weit aufgerissen.
wide-spread *adj* **1.** ausgedehnt, weit ausgebreitet. **2.** weitverbreitet.
Widmark ['wɪdmɑːrk]: **W.'s test** Widmark-Probe *f*, -Bestimmung *f*.
wid·ow ['wɪdəʊ] *n* Witwe *f*.

wid·owed ['wɪdəʊd] *adj* verwitwet.
wid·ow·er ['wɪdəʊər] *n* Witwer *m*.
width [wɪdθ, wɪtθ] *n* Weite *f*, Breite *f*.
Wigand ['viːgænt; -gant]: **W.'s maneuver/version** *gyn*. Wigand-Handgriff *m*.
Wilcoxon [wɪlˈkɑksən]: **W.'s (rank sum) test** *stat*. Wilcoxon-Test *m*, Rangsummentest *m*.
Wilde [waɪld]: **W.'s triangle** Trommelfell-, Lichtreflex *m*.
Wildervanck ['wɪldərvæŋk]: **W. syndrome** Wildervanck-Syndrom *nt*.
wild·fire pemphigus ['waɪldfaɪər] brasilianischer Pemphigus *m*, brasilianischer Pemphigus foliaceus *m*, Pemphigus brasiliensis, Fogo Salvagem.
wildfire rash *derm*. Roter Hund *m*, tropische Flechte *f*, Miliaria rubra.
wild type [waɪld] *bio.*, *genet*. Wildtyp *m*, -form *f*.
wild-type gene *genet*. Wildtypgen *nt*.
wild-type virus *micro*. Wildtypvirus *nt*.
Willebrand ['vɪləbrant]: **W.'s syndrome** (von) Willebrand-Jürgens-Syndrom *nt*, konstitutionelle Thrombopathie *f*, hereditäre/vaskuläre Pseudohämophilie *f*, Angiohämophilie *f*.
Williams ['wɪljəmz]: **W.'** **syndrome** Williams-Syndrom *nt*.
Williams-Campbell ['kæmbəl]: **W.-C. syndrome** Williams-Campbell-Syndrom *nt*.
Willis ['wɪlɪz]: **arterial circle of W.** Willis'-Anastomosenkranz *m*, Circulus arteriosus cerebri.
nerve of W. Akzessorius *m*, XI. Hirnerv *m*, N. accessorius.
W.'s pancreas Proc. uncinatus pancreatis.
paracusis of W. Paracusis Willisii.
W.' pouch kleines Netz *nt*, Omentum minus.
W.' valve Velum medulare superius.
wil·low fracture ['wɪləʊ] Grünholzbruch *m*, -fraktur *f*.
Wills [wɪlz]: **W.' factor** Fol(in)säure *f*, Folacin *nt*, Pteroylglutaminsäure *f*, Vitamin B$_c$ *nt*.
Wilms [wɪlmz]: **W.' tumor** Wilms-Tumor *m*, embryonales Adeno(myo)sarkom *nt*, Nephroblastom *nt*, Adenomyorhabdosarkom *nt* der Niere.
Wilson ['wɪlsən]: **W.'s block** *card*. Wilson-Block *m*.
W.'s degeneration → W.'s disease 1.
W.'s disease 1. Wilson-Krankheit *f*, -Syndrom *m*, Morbus Wilson *m*, hepatolentikuläre/hepatozerebrale Degeneration *f*. **2.** Wilson-Krankheit *f*, Dermatitis exfoliativa.
W.'s muscle M. sphincter urethrae.
W.'s precordial leads (*EKG*) (Brustwand-)Ableitungen *pl* nach Wilson.
W.'s syndrome → W.'s disease 1.
Wilson-Blair [blɛər]: **W.-B. agar** Wilson-Blair-Agar *m/nt*, Wismutsulfitagar *m/nt* nach Wilson u. Blair.
W.-B. culture medium → W.-B. agar.
Wilson-Mikity ['mɪkətɪ]: **W.-M. syndrome** Wilson-Mikity-Syndrom *nt*, bronchopulmonale Dysplasie *f*.
wind [wɪnd] *n* **1.** Wind *m*. **2.** Blähung(en *pl*) *f*, Wind *m*. **to break ~** einen Wind abgehen lassen. **to suffer from ~** Blähungen haben. **3.** Atem *m*, Atmen *nt*. **to be short of ~** außer Atem sein. **to catch one's ~/to get one's ~ back** wieder zu Atem kommen. **to have a good ~** eine gute Lunge haben.
wind-burn ['wɪndbɜrn] *n* Hauterythem *nt* durch scharfen Wind.
wind·chill ['wɪn(d)tʃɪl] *n phys*. Windabkühlung *f*, Abkühlung *f* durch Luftzug.

windchill factor *phys*. Windabkühlungsfaktor *m*.
wind·ed ['wɪndɪd] *adj* außer Atem, atemlos.
wind·kes·sel function ['wɪndkɛsl; 'vɪntkɛsəl] *physiol*. Windkesselfunktion *f*.
wind·lass ['wɪndləs] **I** *n techn*. Winde *f*. **II** *vi* hochwinden.
win·dow ['wɪndəʊ] *n* **1.** Fenster(öffnung *f*) *nt*; *anat*. Fenestra *f*. **2.** *pharm*. therapeutische Breite *f*.
win·dowed ['wɪndəʊd] *adj* mit Fenster(n) (versehen), gefenstert.
wind·pipe ['wɪndpaɪp] *n* Luftröhre *f*; *anat*. Trachea *f*.
wind velocity Windgeschwindigkeit *f*.
wind·y ['wɪndɪ] *adj* **1.** windig, stürmisch. **2.** blähend.
wing [wɪŋ] *n allg*. Flügel *m*, flügelähnliche Struktur *f*, *anat*. Ala *f*.
w. of crista galli Ala cristae galli.
w. of ilium Becken-, Darmschaufel *f*, Ala ossis ilii.
w. of nose Nasenflügel, Ala nasi.
w. of sacrum Ala sacralis.
w. of vomer Ala vomeris.
wing cells Flügelzellen *pl*.
winged scapula [wɪŋd] flügelförmig abstehende Skapula *f*, Scapula alata.
winged tick flies *micro*. Hippobosca *f*.
wing plate *embryo*. Flügelplatte *f*, Lamina alaris.
Winiwarter-Buerger ['wɪnɪwɑːrtər 'bɜrgər]: **W.-B. disease** Winiwarter-Buerger-Krankheit *f*, Morbus Winiwarter-Buerger *m*, Endangiitis/Thrombangiitis/Thrombendangiitis obliterans.
wink [wɪŋk] **I** *n* Blinzeln *nt*; Zwinkern *nt*. **II** *vt*, *vi* blinzeln, zwinkern.
wink·ing ['wɪŋkɪŋ] *n* Blinzeln *nt*; Zwinkern *nt*.
winking spasm Blinzelkrampf *m*, Spasmus nictitans.
Winkler ['wɪŋklər; 'vɪŋk-]: **W.'s disease** schmerzhaftes Ohrknötchen *nt*, Chondrodermatitis nodularis circumscripta helicis.
wink reflex Blinzelreflex *m*.
Winslow ['wɪnsləʊ]: **W.'s foramen** Winslow'-Loch *nt*, -Foramen *nt*, For. epiploicum/omentale (Winslow).
hiatus of W. → W.'s foramen.
W.'s ligament Lig. popliteum obliquum.
W.'s pancreas Proc. uncinatus pancreatis.
Winter ['wɪntər]: **W.'s syndrome** Winter-Syndrom *nt*, Winter-Kohn-Mellmann-Wagner-Syndrom *nt*.
win·ter eczema ['wɪntər] Exsikkationsekzem *nt*, -dermatitis *f*, asteatotisches/xerotisches Ekzem *nt*, Austrocknungsekzem *nt*, Exsikkationsekzematid *nt*, Asteatosis cutis, Xerosis *f*.
winter itch 1. Winterjucken *nt*, Pruritus hiemalis. **2.** → winter eczema.
Wintersteiner ['wɪntərstaɪnər; 'vɪntərʃtaɪnər]: **W.'s F compound** Kortison *nt*, Cortison *nt*.
winter tick *micro*. Dermacentor albipictus.
Wintrich ['wɪntrɪk; 'vɪntrɪç]: **W.'s sign** Wintrich-Schallwechsel *m*.
Wintrobe ['wɪntrəʊb]: **W. hematocrit** Wintrobe-Hämatokritbestimmung *f*.
W. method Wintrobe-Methode *f*.
wire [waɪər] **I** *n* **1.** Draht *m*. **2.** Leitung(sdraht *m*) *f*. **II** *adj* Draht-. **III** *vt* **3.** mit Draht anbinden *od*. zusammenbinden *od*. befestigen. **4.** *phys*. verdrahten, Leitungen verlegen.
wire brush Drahtbürste *f*.
wire cutter Drahtschneider *m*.
wired [waɪərd] *adj* **1.** mit Draht verstärkt.

wire fixation

2. *phys.* verdrahtet, mit Leitungen versehen.
wire fixation *ortho.* Verdrahtung *f*, Verdrahten *nt*, Drahtosteosynthese *f*.
wire loop Drahtschlinge *f*, -öse *f*.
wire snare Drahtschlinge *f*, -schleife *f*.
wire-worm ['waɪərwɜrm] *n micro.* Haemonchus contortus.
wir·ing ['waɪrɪŋ] *n* 1. Befestigen *nt* mit Draht. 2. *phys.* Verdrahtung *f*.
Wirsung ['vɪrzʊŋ]: **W.'s canal/duct** Wirsung'-Gang *m*, Pankreasgang *m*, Ductus pancreaticus.
WISC *abbr.* → Wechsler Intelligence Scale for Children.
wis·dom tooth ['wɪzdəm] Weisheitszahn *m*, dritter Molar *m*, Dens serotinus.
Wiskott-Aldrich ['vɪskɔt 'ɔːldrɪtʃ]: **W.-A. syndrome** Wiskott-Aldrich-Syndrom *nt*.
witch's milk [wɪtʃ] *gyn.* Hexenmilch *f*, Lac neonatorum.
with·draw [wɪð'drɔː, wɪθ-] I *vt* 1. zurückziehen, -nehmen herausziehen, entfernen (*from* von, aus). 2. (*Flüssigkeit*) entziehen; ab-, heraussaugen; (*Blut*) ab-, entnehmen. 3. jdn. entziehen. II *vi* 4. s. zurückziehen (*from* von, aus); s. entfernen. 5. eine Entziehungskur machen, s. einer Entziehungskur unterziehen.
w. of a specimen Probenentnahme.
with·draw·al [wɪð'drɔːəl, wɪθ-] *n* 1. Zurückziehen *nt*, -nehmen *nt*; Zurückziehung *f*, -nahme *f* (*from*); (Blut-)Entnahme *f*. 2. Koitus/Coitus interruptus. 3. (*Drogen*) Entzug *m*, Entziehung *f* (*from*).
withdrawal cure Entziehungskur *f*, Entwöhnung *f*.
withdrawal reflex 1. Wegziehreflex *m*, Fluchtreflex *m*. 2. Beuge-, Flexorreflex *m*.
withdrawal symptoms Entzugserscheinungen *pl*, -syndrom *nt*, Entziehungserscheinungen *pl*, -syndrom *nt*, Abstinenzerscheinungen *pl*, -syndrom *nt*.
withdrawal syndrome → withdrawal symptoms.
with·hold [wɪð'hoʊld, wɪθ-] *vt* 1. verweigern, vorenthalten (*sth. from sth.* jdm etw.). **to ~ one's consent** seine Zustimmung verweigern. 2. zurück-, abhalten (*s.o. from sth.* jdn. von etw.).
with·stand [wɪð'stænd, wɪθ-] I *vt* s. widersetzen, widerstehen, standhalten. II *vi* Widerstand leisten.
Witkop ['wɪtkɔp]: **W.'s disease** hereditäre benigne intraepitheliale Dyskeratose *f*.
Witkop-von Sallmann [van 'sælmən]: **W.-v.-S. disease** → Witkop's disease.
Witzel ['wɪtsəl]: **W.'s gastrostomy/operation** Witzel-Fistel *f*, -Gastrostomie *f*.
wit·zel·sucht ['vɪtsəlzuːkt; 'vɪtsəlzɔxt] *n psychia.* Witzelsucht *f*, Moria *f*.
Wladimiroff-Mikulicz [vlædə'mɪərɔf 'mɪkjəlɪtʃ]: **W.-M. amputation/operation** *ortho.* Fußamputation *f* nach Vladimiroff-Mikulicz.
W-neuron W-Neuron *nt*, Neuron *nt* der Latenzklasse III.
wob·ble ['wɑbl] I *n* Wackeln *nt*, Wanken *nt*, Schwanken *nt*, Schlottern *nt*. II *vi* wackeln, wanken, schwanken; (*Knie*) schlottern.
wobble base *biochem.* Wackel-, Wobble-Base *f*.
wobble hypothesis Wackel-, Wobble-Hypothese *f*.
wob·bly ['wɑblɪ] *adj* wack(e)lig; unsicher.
Wohl·fahr·tia [vəʊl'fɑrtɪə] *n bio., micro.* Wohlfahrtia *f*.
W. magnifica Schmeißfliege *f*, Wohlfahrtia magnifica.
Wohlfahrt-Kugelberg-Welander ['vəʊlfɑːrt 'kuːɡəlbɜrɡ 'welændər]: **W.-K.-W. disease** Kugelberg-Welander-Krankheit *f*, -Syndrom *nt*, juvenile Form *f* der spinalen Muskelatrophie, Atrophia musculorum spinalis pseudomyopathica (Kugelberg-Welander).
Wolbach ['wɑlbæk]: **sclerosing hemangioma of W.** Histiozytom *nt*, Histiocytoma *nt*.
Wolfe [wʊlf]: **W.'s graft** Wolfe-Krause-Lappen *m*, Krause-Wolfe-Lappen *m*.
Wolfe-Krause [wʊlf kraʊs; 'vɔlfə 'kraʊzə]: **W.-K. graft** → Wolfe's graft.
Wolff ['wʊlf, 'vɔlf]: **duct of W.** → wolffian duct.
wolff·i·an ['wʊlfɪən, 'vɔːl-]: **w. body** *embryo.* Urniere *f*, Wolff'-Körper *m*, Mesonephron *nt*, Mesonephros *m*.
w. duct Wolff'-Gang *m*, Urnierengang *m*, Ductus mesonephricus.
w. ridge *embryo.* Urnierenleiste *f*.
Wolff-Parkinson-White ['pɑːrkɪnsən (h)waɪt]: **W.-P.-W. syndrome** *abbr.* **WPW** Wolff-Parkinson-White-Syndrom *nt*, WPW-Syndrom *nt*.
Wolf-Hirschhorn ['wʊlf 'hɪrʃhɔːrn]: **W.-H. syndrome** Wolf-Syndrom *nt*, 4-Deletions-Syndrom *nt*.
Wölfler ['welflər; 'vœlf-]: **W.'s glands** akzessorische Schilddrüsen *pl*, Gll. thyroideae accessoriae.
W.'s operation *chir.* Wölfler-Operation *f*.
wolf·ram ['wʊlfrəm] *n abbr.* **W** Wolfram *nt abbr.* W.
wolfs·bane ['wʊlfsbeɪn] *n pharm.* Bergwohlverleih *m*, Arnika *f*, Arnica montana.
Wol·hyn·ia fever [wɑl'hɪnɪə] Wolhyn'-Fieber *nt*, Fünftagefieber *nt*, Wolhynienfieber *nt*, Febris quintana.
Wolman ['wɑlmən]: **W.'s disease/xanthomatosis** Wolman'-Krankheit *f*.
wom·an ['wʊmən] I *n, pl* **wom·en** ['wɪmɪn] Frau *f*. II *adj* womanish. III *vt* Frauen einstellen in.
woman doctor Ärztin *f*.
wom·an·hood ['wʊmənhʊd] *n* 1. Fraulichkeit *f*, Weiblichkeit *f*. 2. Frauen *pl*.
wom·an·ish ['wʊmənɪʃ] *adj* 1. weibisch. 2. fraulich, weiblich, Frauen-.
wom·an·ish·ness ['wʊmənɪʃnɪs] *n* 1. weibisches Wesen *nt*. 2. Weiblichkeit *f*, Fraulichkeit *f*.
wom·an·kind ['wʊmənkaɪnd] *n* Frauen *pl*, Weiblichkeit *f*.
woman-like *adj* → womanish.
wom·an·li·ness ['wʊmənlɪnɪs] *n* Weiblichkeit *f*, Fraulichkeit *f*.
wom·an·ly ['wʊmənlɪ] *adj* → womanish.
womb [wuːm] *n* Gebärmutter *f*, Uterus *m*, Metra *f*.
womb stone *gyn.* Gebärmutter-, Uterusstein *m*, Uterolith *m*, Hysterolith *m*.
Wood ['wʊd]: **W.'s glass** Wood-Glas *nt*.
W.'s lamp Wood'-Lampe *f*.
W.'s light Wood-Licht *nt*.
W.'s metal Wood'-Metall *nt*.
W.'s sign Wood-Zeichen *nt*.
wood-cut·ter's encephalitis ['wʊdkʌtər] russische Früh(jahr)-Sommer-Enzephalitis *f abbr.* RSSE, russische Zeckenenzephalitis *f*.
wood·en belly ['wʊdn] bretthartes Abdomen *nt*.
wooden resonance hypersonorer Klopfschall *m*.
wooden-shoe heart *card.* Holzschuhform *f*, Coeur en sabot.
wood sugar Holzzucker *m*, Xylose *f*.
wood tick 1. Holzzecke *f*, Dermacentor andersoni. 2. Dermacentor occidentalis.
wood·y thyroiditis ['wʊdɪ] eisenharte Struma Riedel *f*, Riedel-Struma *f*, chronische hypertrophische Thyreoiditis *f*.
wool [wʊl] I *n* 1. Wolle *f*. 2. Baumwolle *f*; Glaswolle *f*; Pflanzenwolle *f*. 3. *bio.* Haare *pl*, Pelz *m*. II *adj* wollen, Woll-.**wool fat**
wool fat Wollwachs *nt*, Lanolin *nt*.
wool grease → wool fat.
wool·ly ['wʊlɪ] *adj* wollig, weich, flaumig.
woolly-hair nevus Kräuselhaarnävus *m*, Wollhaarnävus *m*.
wool·sort·er's disease ['wʊlsɔːrtər] → woolsorter's pneumonia.
woolsorter's pneumonia Lungenmilzbrand *m*, Wollsortierer-, Lumpensortierer-, Hadernkrankheit *f*.
word blindness [wɜrd] Leseunfähigkeit *f*, -unvermögen *nt*, Alexie *f*.
word comprehension *neuro.* Wortverständnis *nt*, -verstehen *nt*. **total w.** Gesamtwortverstehen.
word deafness Worttaubheit *f*, akustische Aphasie *f*.
word salad *psychia.* Wortsalat *m*.
Woringer-Kolopp ['wɔrɪndʒər kə'lɔp, 'vɔrɪŋ'ɡe]: **W.-K. disease/syndrome** Morbus Woringer-Kolopp *m*, pagetoide/epidermotrope Retikulose *f*.
work [wɜrk] I *n* Arbeit *f*, Beschäftigung *f*, Tätigkeit *f*; Aufgabe *f*; Leistung *f*; *phys.* Arbeit *f*. **to do ~** arbeiten. II *vt* 1. arbeiten an; ver-, durch-, bearbeiten; (ver-)formen, gestalten (*into* zu). 2. jdn. bearbeiten. 3. (*Maschine*) bedienen, betätigen. 4. hervorbringen, herbeiführen, bewirken, verursachen, führen zu. III *vi* 5. arbeiten (*at, on* an); s. beschäftigen (*at, on* mit). 6. funktionieren, gehen, in Gang sein, arbeiten. 7. wirken, s. auswirken (*on, upon, with* auf). 8. (*Mund*) zucken; (*Zähne*) mahlen.
work in *vt* (*Salbe*) einreiben, einmassieren.
work off *vi* s. lockern, s. allmählich lösen, abgehen.
work on *vi* jdn. bearbeiten.
work out *vi* (*Sport*) trainieren.
work up 1. verarbeiten (*onto* zu). 2. (*Patient*) gründlich untersuchen.
work·a·hol·ic [ˌwɜrkə'hɔlɪk] *n* Arbeitssüchtige(r *m*) *f*.
work·a·hol·ism ['wɜrkəhɔlɪzəm] *n* Arbeitssucht *f*, -besessenheit *f*.
work diagram Arbeitsdiagramm *nt*.
work·er ['wɜrkər] *n* Arbeiter(in *f*) *m*; Forscher(in *f*) *m*.
work hypertrophy *physiol.* Arbeits-, Aktivitätshypertrophie *f*.
work·ing ['wɜrkɪŋ] I *n* (*a. physiol.*) Tätigkeit *f*, Funktion *f*, Arbeit *f*; Wirken *nt*, Tun *nt*, Arbeiten *nt*; *techn.* Funktionieren *nt*. II *adj* arbeitend, funktionierend, Arbeits-; berufstätig.
working cell Interphasenzelle *f*.
working conditions Arbeitsbedingungen *pl*.
working metabolic rate *physiol.* Arbeitsumsatz *m*.
working method Arbeitsverfahren *nt*, -technik *f*.
working myocardium (*Herz*) Arbeitsmuskulatur *f*, -myokard *nt*.
working power *phys.* Arbeitskraft *f*.
work leukocytosis Arbeitsleukozytose *f*.
work load Arbeitsbelastung *f*, Arbeit(slast *f*) *f*; Arbeitspensum *nt*.
work physiologist Arbeitsphysiologe *m*, -login *f*.
work physiology Arbeitsphysiologie *f*.
work·out ['wɜrkaʊt] *n* (*Sport*) Training *nt*. **to have a ~** trainieren.
work-up *n* (gründliche) medizinische Untersuchung *f*.

worm [wɜrm] *n* **1.** *bio., micro.* Wurm *m*; Made *f*; Raupe *f.* **2.** *patho.* ~s *pl* Wurmkrankheit *f*, Würmer *pl*, Helminthiase *f.* **3.** *anat.* wurmartige Struktur *f* Wurm *m*, Vermis *m.*
w. of cerebellum Kleinhirnwurm, Vermis cerebelli.
worm abscess Abszeß *m* bei Wurmbefall.
worm colic Darmkolik *f* bei Wurmbefall.
wor·mer ['wɜrmər] *n* Wurmmittel *nt.*
wor·mi·an bones ['wɔːrmɪən] Schalt-, Nahtknochen *pl*, Ossa suturalia.
worm·like ['wɜrmlaɪk] *adj* wurmähnlich, vermiform, helminthoid.
worm-seed oil ['wɜrmsiːd] *pharm.* Wurmsamenöl *nt.*
worm·y ['wɜrmɪ] *adj* voller Würmer, wurmig; wurmartig.
wors·en ['wɜrsn] **I** *vt* verschlechtern, schlechtern machen; etw. verschlimmern. **II** *vi* s. verschlechtern, s. verschlimmern.
wors·en·ing ['wɜrsnɪŋ] *n* Verschlechterung *f*, Verschlimmerung *f.*
wound [wuːnd] **I** *n* **1. the ~ed** die Verwundeten. **2.** *patho.* Wunde *f*, Vulnus *nt*; Verletzung *f.* **3.** *chir.* (Operations-)Wunde *f.* **II** *vt* verwunden, verletzen.
w. of entry (*Gewehr*) Einschuß.
w. of exit (*Gewehr*) Ausschuß.
wound abscess Wundabszeß *m.*
wound care Wundversorgung *f*, -behandlung *f.*
wound closure Wundverschluß *m*, -naht *f.*
delayed primary w. aufgeschobene Primärversorgung *f abbr.* APV, primär verzögerter Wundverschluß.
wound contraction Wundzusammenziehung *f*, -kontraktion *f.*
wound coverage Wundabdeckung *f.*
wound dehiscence Wunddehiszenz *f.*
wound drainage Wunddrainage *f.*
wound dystrophy Wunddystrophie *f.*
wound edge Wundrand *m.*
wound fever Wundfieber *nt*, Febris traumatica.
wound healing Wundheilung *f.*
wound hematoma Wundhämatom *nt.*
wound infection Wundinfektion *f.*
wound management Wundversorgung *f.*
wound sepsis Wundsepsis *f.*
wound suture *chir.* Wundverschluß *m*, -naht *f.*
wound toilet Wundtoilette *f*, Debridement *nt.*
wo·ven bone ['wəʊvən] Geflechtknochen *m.*
W-plasty *n chir.* W-Plastik *f.*
WPW *abbr.* → Wolff-Parkinson-White syndrome.
W.r. *abbr.* → Wassermann reaction.
wrin·kle ['rɪŋkl] **I** *n* (*Haut*) Fältchen *nt*, Runzel *f*, Falte *f.* **II** *vt* runzelig od. faltig machen; (*Stirn, Augenbrauen*) runzeln; (*Nase*) rümpfen; (*Augen*) zusammenkneifen. **III** *vi* **1.** runz(e)lig werden, Runzeln bekommen. **2.** s. falten, Falten werfen, (ver-)knittern, faltig werden.
wrin·kled ['rɪŋkld] *adj* gerunzelt; runz(e)lig, faltig.
wrinkled tongue Faltenzunge *f*, Lingua plicata/scrotalis.
wrin·kly ['rɪŋklɪ] *adj* → wrinkled.
Wrisberg ['rɪzbɜrɡ; 'vrɪsbɛrk]: **W.'s cartilage** Wrisberg-Knorpel *m*, Cartilago cuneiformis.
W.'s ganglia Wrisberg'-Ganglien *pl*, Ggll. cardiaca.
W.'s ligament Lig. meniscofemorale posterius.
W.'s nerve 1. Intermedius *m*, N. intermedius. **2.** medialer Hautnerv *m* des Oberarms, N. cutaneus brachii medialis.
W.'s tubercle Wrisberg'-Höckerchen *nt*, -Knötchen *nt*, Tuberculum cuneiforme.
wrist [rɪst] *n* **1.** Handwurzel *f*, Karpus *m*, Carpus *m.* **2.** (proximales) Handgelenk *nt*, Artic. radiocarpalis/radiocarpea.
wrist clonus Handklonus *m.*
wrist disarticulation *ortho.* Handgelenk(s)exartikulation *f*, Absetzung/Amputation *f* im Handgelenk.
wrist-drop ['rɪstdrɒp] *n neuro.* Fall-, Kußhand *f.*
wrist fracture Handgelenksbruch *m*, -fraktur *f.*
wrist injury 1. Handgelenksverletzung *f.* **2.** Handwurzelverletzung *f.*
wrist joint → wrist 2.
writ·er's cramp ['raɪtər] Schreibkrampf *m*, Graphospasmus *m*, Mogigraphie *f.*
writer's paralysis/spasm → writer's cramp.
writ·ten consent ['rɪtn] schriftliche Einverständniserklärung *f*, schriftliche Einwilligung *f.*
wry neck [raɪ] Schiefhals *m*, Torticollis *m*, Caput obstipum.
wry·neck ['raɪnek] *n* → wry neck.
Ws *abbr.* → watt-second.
Wuch·e·re·ria [ˌvʊkəˈriːrɪə] *n micro.* Wuchereria *f.*
W. bancrofti Bancroft-Filarie *f*, Wuchereria bancrofti.
W. brugi → W. malayi.
W. malayi Malayenfilarie *f*, Brugia/Wuchereria malayi.
wuch·e·ri·a·sis [ˌvʊkəriˈraɪəsɪs] *n* Wuchereria-Infektion *f*, Wuchereriose *f*, Wuchereriasis *f.*
w./v. *abbr.* → weight per volume.
WV vaccine → whole-virus vaccine.

X

X *abbr.* → xanthosine.
xan·chro·mat·ic [ˌzænkrəʊ'mætɪk] *adj* → xanthochromic.
xanth- *pref.* → xantho-.
xan·the·las·ma [ˌzænθe'læzmə] *n* 1. Lidxanthelasma *nt*, Xanthelasma palpebrarum. 2. → xanthoma.
xan·the·las·ma·to·sis [-ˌlæzmə'təʊsɪs] *n* → xanthomatosis.
xan·the·mia [zæn'θiːmɪə] *n* Karotinämie *f*, Carotinämie *f*.
xan·thene ['zænθiːn] *n* Xanthen *nt*.
xan·thic ['zænθɪk] *adj* 1. gelb. 2. Xanthin betr., Xanthin-.
xanthic calculus/stone Xanthinstein *m*.
xan·thine ['zænθiːn, -θɪn] *n* 2,6-Dihydroxypurin *nt*, Xanthin *nt*.
xanthine base Purinbase *f*.
xanthine body → xanthine base.
xanthine calculus → xanthic calculus.
xanthine oxidase Xanthinoxidase *f abbr.* XO, Schardinger'-Enzym *nt*.
xanthine oxidase inhibitor Xanthinoxidasehemmer *m*.
xanthine stone → xanthic calculus.
xan·thin·u·ria [ˌzænθɪ'n(j)ʊərɪə] *n* Xanthinausscheidung *f* im Harn, Xanthinurie *f*.
xan·thin·u·ric [-'n(j)ʊərɪk] *adj* Xanthinurie betr., xanthinurisch.
xan·thi·u·ria [ˌ-'(j)ʊərɪə] *n* → xanthinuria.
xantho- *pref.* Gelb-, Xanth(o)-.
xan·tho·chro·mat·ic [ˌzænθəʊkrəʊ'mætɪk] *adj* → xanthochromic.
xan·tho·chro·mia [ˌ-'krəʊmɪə] *n* 1. Gelbfärbung *f*, Xanthochromie *f*. 2. *neuro.* Liquorxanthochromie *f*. 3. *derm.* Xanthosis *f*, Xanthodermie *f*.
xan·tho·chro·mic [ˌ-'krəʊmɪk] *adj* gelb, xanthochrom.
xan·tho·der·ma [ˌ-'dɜrmə] *n* Gelbfärbung *f* der Haut, Xanthodermie *f*, Xanthosis *f*.
xan·tho·e·ryth·ro·der·mia [-ˌɪˌrɪθrə'dɜrmɪə] *n* Xanthoerythrodermie *f*.
xan·tho·fi·bro·ma [-ˌfaɪ'brəʊmə] *n* Xanthofibrom(a) *nt*.
xan·tho·gran·u·lo·ma [ˌ-ˌgrænjə'ləʊmə] *n* Xanthogranulom(a) *nt*.
x. of bone nicht-osteogenes/nicht-ossifizierendes (Knochen-)Fibrom *nt*, xanthomatöser/fibröser Riesenzelltumor *m* des Knochens, Xanthogranuloma *nt* des Knochens.
xan·tho·gran·u·lom·a·tous pyelonephritis [ˌ-ˌgrænjə'ləʊmətəs] xantho(granulo)matöse Pyelonephritis *f*.
xan·tho·ma [zæn'θəʊmə] *n* Xanthom(a) *nt*.
xanthoma cell Schaum-, Xanthomzelle *f*.
xan·tho·ma·to·sis [ˌzænθəmə'təʊsɪs] *n* Xanthomatose *f*.
x. of bone Chester-Erkrankung *f*, -Syndrom *nt*, Chester-Erdheim-Erkrankung *f*, -Syndrom *nt*, Knochenxanthomatose *f*.
xan·thom·a·tous [zæn'θəmətəs] *adj* Xanthom betr., xanthomatös.
xanthomatous inflammation verfettete Entzündung *f*.

xanthomatous pneumonia xanthomatöse Pneumonie *f*.
xanthomatous pyelonephritis → xanthogranulomatous pyelonephritis.
Xan·thom·o·nas [zæn'θəmənəs] *n micro.* Xanthomonas *f*.
xan·thop·a·thy [zæn'θəpəθɪ] *n* → xanthochromia.
xan·tho·phyll ['zænθəfɪl] *n* Xanthophyll *nt*.
xan·tho·pia [zæn'θəʊpɪə] *n* → xanthopsia.
xan·tho·pro·te·ic reaction [ˌ-'prəʊ'tiːɪk] Xanthoprotein-Reaktion *f*.
xan·tho·pro·te·in [ˌ-'prəʊtiːn, -tiːɪn] *n* Xanthoprotein *nt*.
xan·thop·sia [zæn'θəpsɪə] *n* Gelbsehen *nt*, Xanthop(s)ie *f*.
xan·thop·sin [zæn'θəpsɪn] *n* Sehgelb *nt*, Xanthopsin *nt*, all-trans Retinal *nt*.
xan·thop·ter·in [zæn'θəptərɪn] *n* Xanthopterin *nt*.
xan·tho·sar·co·ma [ˌzænθəʊsɑːr'kəʊmə] *n* Riesenzelltumor *m* der Sehnenscheide, pigmentierte villonoduläre Synovitis *f abbr.* PVNS, benignes Synovialom *nt*, Tendosynovitis nodosa.
xan·tho·sine ['zænθəsiːn, -sɪn] *n abbr.* X Xanthosin *nt abbr.* X.
xanthosine monophosphate *abbr.* XMP Xanthosinmonophosphat *nt abbr.* XMP, Xanthylsäure *f*.
xan·tho·sis [zæn'θəʊsɪs] *n* Gelbfärbung *f*, Xanthose *f*, Xanthosis *f*.
xan·thous ['zænθəs] *adj* gelb, gelblich.
xanthous albinism Yellow-Typ *m* des okulokutanen Albinismus.
xanth·u·ren·ic acid [ˌzænθ(j)ə'renɪk] Xanthurensäure *f*.
xan·thu·ria [zæn'θ(j)ʊərɪə] *n* → xanthinuria.
xan·thyl ['zænθɪl] *n* Xanthyl-(Radikal *nt*).
xan·thyl·ic [zæn'θɪlɪk] *adj* Xanthin betr., Xanthin-.
xanthylic acid → xanthosine monophosphate.
X chromosome X-Chromosom *nt*.
Xe *abbr.* → xenon.
xen(o)- *pref.* Fremd-, Xen(o)-.
xen·o·an·ti·gen [ˌzenə'æntɪdʒən] *n immun.* Xenoantigen *nt*.
xen·o·bi·ot·ic [ˌ-baɪ'ətɪk] *n* Xenobiotikum *nt*.
xen·o·di·ag·no·sis [ˌ-daɪəg'nəʊsɪs] *n* Xenodiagnose *f*, -diagnostik *f*.
xen·o·di·ag·nos·tic [ˌ-daɪəg'nəstɪk] *adj* Xenodiagnose betr., xenodiagnostisch.
xen·o·gen·ic [ˌ-'dʒenɪk] *adj* 1. → xenogeneic. 2. → xenogenous.
xen·o·ge·ne·ic [ˌ-dʒə'niːɪk] *adj embryo.* xenogen, xenogenetisch; heterogen.
xenogeneic antigen xenogenes/heterogenes Antigen *nt*, Heteroantigen *nt*.
xenogeneic graft → xenograft.
xenogeneic transplantation → xenotransplantation.
xen·o·gen·e·sis [ˌ-'dʒenəsɪs] *n* Xenogenese *f*; Heterogenese *f*.
xe·nog·e·nous [zə'nədʒənəs] *adj* durch

einen Fremdkörper hervorgerufen, von außen stammend, xenogen; exogen.
xen·o·graft ['zenəgræft] *n* heterogenes/ heterologes/xenogenes/xenogenetisches Transplantat *nt*, Xeno-, Heterotransplantat *nt*.
xe·nol·o·gy [zə'nɑlədʒɪ] *n* Xenologie *f*.
xen·o·me·nia [ˌzenə'miːnɪə] *n gyn.* vikariierende Menstruation *f*.
xe·non ['ziːnɑn, 'ze-] *n abbr.* **Xe** Xenon *nt abbr.* Xe.
xen·o·par·a·site [ˌzenə'pærəsaɪt] *n micro.* Xenoparasit *m*.
xen·o·pho·bia [ˌ-'fəʊbɪə] *n* krankhafte Angst *f* vor Fremden *od.* Fremdem, Xenophobie *f*.
xen·o·pho·nia [ˌ-'fəʊnɪə] *n neuro.*, *HNO* Xenophonie *f*.
xen·oph·thal·mia [ˌzenəf'θælmɪə] *n ophthal.* Xenophthalmie *f*.
Xen·op·syl·la [ˌzenəp'sɪlə, ˌzenəʊ'sɪlə] *n micro.* Xenopsylla *f*.
X. cheopis Pestfloh *m*, Xenopsylla cheopis.
xen·o·rex·ia [ˌzenə'reksɪə] *n psychia.* Xenorexie *f*.
xen·o·trans·plan·ta·tion [ˌ-ˌtrænsplæn'teɪʃn] *n* heterogene/heterologe/xenogene/ xenogenetische Transplantation *f*, Xeno-, Heterotransplantation *f*, Xeno-, Heteroplastik *f*.
xen·o·trop·ic virus [ˌ-'trɑpɪk, -'trəʊ-] *micro.* xenotropes Virus *nt*.
xen·yl ['zenl, 'ziːnl] *n* Xenyl-(Radikal *nt*).
xer- *pref.* → xero-.
xe·ran·sis [zɪ'rænsɪs] *n* Austrocknung *f*.
xe·ran·tic [zɪ'ræntɪk] *adj* (aus-)trocknend.
xero- *pref.* Trocken-, Xer(o)-.
xe·ro·chi·lia [ˌzɪərə'kaɪlɪə] *n* Trockenheit *f* der Lippen, Xeroch(e)ilie *f*.
xe·ro·der·ma [ˌ-'dɜrmə] *n* trockene Haut *f*, Xerodermie *f*, -dermia *f*, Xeroderma *nt*.
xe·ro·der·mat·ic [ˌ-dɜr'mætɪk] *adj* Xerodermie betr.
xe·ro·der·mia [ˌ-'dɜrmɪə] *n* → xeroderma.
xe·ro·der·mic idiocy [ˌ-'dɜrmɪk] De Sanctis-Cacchione-Syndrom *nt*.
xe·rog·ra·phy [zɪ'rɑgrəfɪ] *n* → xeroradiography.
xe·ro·ma [zɪ'rəʊmə] *n* → xerophthalmia.
xe·ro·mam·mog·ra·phy [ˌzɪərəmə'mɑgrəfɪ] *n abbr.* **XMM** *radiol.* Xeromammographie *f*, Xeroradiographie *f* der Mamma/ Brust.
xe·ro·me·nia [ˌ-'miːnɪə] *n gyn.* Xeromenie *f*.
xe·ro·myc·te·ria [ˌ-mɪk'tɪərɪə] *n* extreme Trockenheit *f* der Nasenschleimhaut.
xe·roph·thal·mia [ˌzɪərɑf'θælmɪə] *n ophthal.* Xerophthalmie *f*.
xe·roph·thal·mus [ˌzɪərɑf'θælməs] *n* → xerophthalmia.
xe·ro·ra·di·og·ra·phy [ˌzɪərəˌreɪdɪ'ɑgrəfɪ] *n radiol.* Xero(radio)graphie *f*, Röntgenphotographie *f*.
xe·ro·sis [zɪ'rəʊsɪs] *n*, *pl* **-ses** [-siːz] *patho.* pathologische Trockenheit *f* der Haut *od.* Schleimhaut, Xerosis *f*, Xerose *f*.

xe·ro·sto·mia [ˌzɪərə'stəʊmɪə] *n* pathologische Trockenheit *f* der Mundhöhle, Xerostomie *f*.
xe·ro·tes [zɪ'rəʊtiːz] *n* Trockenheit *f* (*des Körpers*).
xe·rot·ic [zɪ'rɒtɪk] *adj* Xerose betr., trocken, xerotisch.
xerotic eczema Exsikkationsekzem *nt*, -dermatitis *f*, asteatotisches/xerotisches Ekzem *nt*, Austrocknungsekzem *nt*, Exsikkationsekzematid *nt*, Asteatosis cutis, Xerosis *f*.
xerotic keratitis 1. Keratitis sicca. 2. Keratomalazie *f*, -malacia *f*.
xe·ro·trip·sis [ˌzɪərə'trɪpsɪs] *n* trockene Reibung *f*.
xip·a·mide ['zɪpəmaɪd] *n pharm.* Xipamid *nt*.
xiph·i·ster·nal [ˌzɪfɪ'stɜrnl] *adj* → xiphosternal.
xiph·i·ster·num [ˌ-'stɜrnəm] *n*, *pl* **-na** [-nə] → xiphoid process.
xiph·o·cos·tal [ˌzɪfəʊ'kɒstl] *adj* xiphokostal.
xiphocostal ligaments of Macalister Ligg. costoxiphoidea.
xiph·o·did·y·mus [ˌ-'dɪdəməs] *n* → xiphopagus.
xi·phod·y·mus [zɪ'fɑdɪməs] *n* → xiphopagus.
xiph·o·dyn·ia [ˌzɪfə'diːnɪə] *n* Xiphalgie *f*, Xiphoidalgie *f*.
xiph·oid ['zɪfɔɪd, 'zaɪ-] **I** *n* → xiphoid process. **II** *adj* schwertförmig, Schwertfortsatz-.
xiph·oid·al·gia [ˌzɪfɔɪ'dældʒ(ɪ)ə] *n* → xiphodynia.
xiphoid appendix → xiphoid process.
xiphoid bone Brustbein *nt*, Sternum *nt*.
xiphoid cartilage → xiphoid process.
xiph·oid·i·tis [ˌzɪfɔɪ'daɪtɪs] *n* Entzündung *f* des Proc. xiphoideus, Xiphoiditis *f*.
xiphoid ligaments → xiphocostal ligaments of Macalister.
xiphoid process Schwertfortsatz *m*, Proc. xiphoideus.
xi·phop·a·gus [zɪ'fɑpəgəs, zaɪ-] *n embryo.* Xiphopagus *m*.
xiph·o·ster·nal [ˌzɪfə'stɜrnl, ˌzaɪ-] *adj* Corpus sterni u. Proc. xiphoideus betr., xiphosternal

xiphosternal joint Synchondrosis xiphosternalis.
xiphosternal synchondrosis → xiphosternal joint.
X-linked *adj* X-gebunden.
X-linked agammaglobulinemia Bruton-Typ *m* der Agammaglobulinämie, infantile X-chromosomale Agammaglobulinämie *f*, kongenitale (geschlechtsgebundene) Agammaglobulinämie *f*.
X-linked gene X-gebundenes Gen *nt*.
X-linked heredity geschlechtsgebundene Vererbung *f*.
X-linked hypogammaglobulinemia → X-linked agammaglobulinemia.
X-linked ichthyosis X-chromosomal rezessive Ichthyosis *f*, geschlechtsgebundene/rezessive Ichthyosis vulgaris.
X-linked infantile agammaglobulinemia → X-linked agammaglobulinemia.
X-linked inheritance X-chromosomale Vererbung *f*.
X-linked lymphoproliferative syndrome Duncan-Syndrom *nt*.
XMM *abbr.* → xeromammography.
XMP *abbr.* → xanthosine monophosphate.
X-neuron *n* X-Neuron *nt*, Neuron *nt* der Latenzklasse II.
XO syndrome Ullrich-Turner-Syndrom *nt*.
x-radiation *n* Röntgenstrahlen *pl*, -strahlung *f*.
x-ray ['eksraɪ] **I** *n* 1. Röntgenstrahl *m*. 2. Röntgenaufnahme *f*, -bild *nt*. **to take an ~** ein Röntgenbild machen (*of* von). **II** *adj* Röntgen-. **III** *vt* 3. röntgen, ein Röntgenbild machen (*of* von); durchleuchten. **4.** mit Röntgenstrahlen behandeln, bestrahlen.
x-ray analysis *phys.* Röntgenanalyse *f*.
x-ray anatomy radiologische Anatomie *f*.
x-ray beam Röntgenstrahl *m*.
x-ray dermatitis → radiation dermatitis.
x-ray diffraction analysis *phys.* Röntgenstrukturanalyse *f*, Röntgenstreuungsanalyse *f*.
x-ray examination Röntgenuntersuchung *f*.
x-ray film 1. Röntgenfilm *m*. 2. Röntgenaufnahme *f*, -bild *nt*.
x-ray fluoroscopy (Röntgen-)Durchleuchtung *f*, Fluoroskopie *f*.
x-ray photograph → x-ray picture.
x-ray picture Röntgenbild *nt*, -aufnahme *f*.
x-ray sickness Strahlenkrankheit *f*.
x-ray spectrum Röntgenspektrum *nt*.
x-ray therapy Röntgentherapie *f*, -behandlung *f*.
x-ray tube Röntgenröhre *f*.
x-ray unit Röntgenanlage *f*.
X^2 test *stat.* Chi-Quadrat-Test *m*, χ^2-Test *m*.
x wave *card.* x-Welle *f*.
XXY syndrome Klinefelter Syndrom *nt*.
xyl- *pref.* → xylo-.
xy·lan ['zaɪlæn] *n* Holzgummi *nt/m*, Xylan *nt*.
xy·lene ['zaɪliːn] *n* 1. Xylol *nt*, Dimethylbenzol *nt*. 2. **~s** *pl* Xylole *pl*.
xy·li·tol ['zaɪlɪtɒl, -tɑl] *n* Xylit *nt*, Xylitol *nt*.
xylitol dehydrogenase → xylulose reductase.
xylo- *pref.* Holz-, Xyl(o)-.
xy·lo·gen ['zaɪlədʒən] *n* Lignin *nt*.
xy·lo·ke·tose [ˌzaɪlə'kiːtəʊs] *n* → xylulose.
xy·lol ['zaɪlɒl, -lɑl] *n* → xylene.
xy·lo·met·a·zo·line [ˌzaɪləˌmetə'zəʊliːn] *n pharm.* Xylometazolin *nt*.
xy·lo·py·ra·nose [ˌ-'paɪrənəʊz] *n* Xylopyranose *f*.
xy·lose ['zaɪləʊs] *n* Holzzucker *m*, Xylose *f*.
D-xylose absorption test D-Xyloseabsorptionstest *m*, D-Xylosetoleranztest *m*.
D-xylose tolerance test → D-xylose absorption test.
xy·lo·su·ria [ˌzaɪlə's(j)ʊərɪə] *n* Xyloseausscheidung *f* im Harn, Xylosurie *f*.
xy·lu·lose ['zaɪl(j)ələʊz] *n* Xylulose *f*.
xylulose-5-phosphate *n* Xylulose-5-Phosphat *nt*.
xylulose reductase Xylulosereduktase *f*.
L-xy·lu·lo·su·ria [ˌzaɪl(j)ələʊ's(j)ʊərɪə] *n* benigne essentielle Pentosurie *f*, Xylulosurie *f*.
xy·phoid ['zaɪfɔɪd] **I** *n* → xiphoid process. **II** *adj* → xiphoid II.
xys·ter ['zɪstər] *n chir.* Knochenschaber *m*, Raspatorium *nt*.
XYY syndrome XYY-Syndrom *nt*, YY-Syndrom *nt*.

Y

Y *abbr.* → yttrium.
Yang·tze Valley fever ['jæŋ(t)siː] japanische Schistosomiasis/Bilharziose *f*, Schistosomiasis japonica.
yard [jɑːrd] *n* Yard *nt*.
yaw [jɔː] *n* Yaws-Papel *f*, Pianom *nt*.
yawn [jɔːn] **I** *n* Gähnen *nt*; Gähner *m*. **II** *vi* **1.** gähnen. **2.** gähnen, klaffen, s. weit auftun.
yawn·ing ['jɔːnɪŋ] *n* Gähnen *nt*.
yaws [jɔːz] *n* Frambösie *f*, Pian *f*, Parangi *f*, Yaws *f*, Framboesia tropica.
Yb *abbr.* → ytterbium.
Y cartilage Y-Knorpel *m*, Y-Fuge *f*.
Y chromosome Y-Chromosom *nt*.
yeast [jiːst] *n micro.* Hefe *f*, Sproßpilz *m*.
yeast eluate factor Pyridoxin *nt*, Vitamin B₆ *nt*.
yeast extract agar Hefeextraktagar *m/nt*.
yeast filtrate factor Pantothensäure *f*, Vitamin B₃ *nt*.
yeast fungus *micro.* Hefe-, Sproßpilz *m*, Blastomyzet *m*.
yeast-like fungus → yeast fungus.
yel·low ['jeləʊ] **I** *n* **1.** (*Farbe*) Gelb *nt*. **2.** Eigelb *nt*. **II** *adj* gelb; (*Rasse*) gelb(häutig). **III** *vt* gelb färben. **IV** *vi* gelb werden, s. gelb färben; vergilben.
yellow atrophy akute gelbe Leberatrophie *f*.
yellow-blue-system neuron Neuron *nt* des Gelb-Blau-Systems.
yellow body Gelbkörper *m*, Corpus luteum.
 y. of menstruation Corpus luteum menstruationis.
 y. of ovary Gelbkörper, Corpus luteum.
 y. of pregnancy Gelbkörper der Schwangerschaft, Corpus luteum graviditatis.
yellow cartilage → yellow fiber.
yellow cross Gelbkreuz *nt*, Senfgas *nt*, Lost *nt*, Dichlordiäthylsulfid *nt*.
yellow fever *abbr.* **Y.F.** Gelbfieber *nt*.
 classic y. → urban y.
 jungle y. Buschgelbfieber, Dschungel-(gelb)fieber, sylvatisches Gelbfieber.
 rural y. → jungle y.
 sylvan y. → jungle y.
 urban y. klassisches/urbanes Gelbfieber, Stadtgelbfieber.

yellow-fever mosquito *micro.* Aedes aegypti.
yellow fever vaccine Gelbfieberimpfstoff *m*, -vakzine *f*.
yellow fever virus *micro.* Gelbfiebervirus *nt*.
yellow fiber elastische Faser *f*.
yellow hepatization *patho.* gelbe Hepatisation *f*.
yel·low·ish ['jeləʊɪʃ] *adj* gelblich.
yellow jack → yellow fever.
yellow ligaments gelbe Bänder *pl*, Ligg. flava.
yellow marrow gelbes fetthaltiges Knochenmark *nt*, Fettmark *nt*, Medulla ossium flava.
yellow mutant oculocutaneous albinism Yellow-Typ *m* des okulokutanen Albinismus.
yellow nail syndrome Syndrom *nt* der gelben Fingernägel, Yellow-nail-Syndrom *nt*.
yellow phosphorus weißer/gelber/gewöhnlicher Phosphor *m*.
yellow spot gelber Fleck *m*, Makula *f*, Macula (lutea/retinae).
yellow tubercle *patho.* verkäsender Tuberkel *m*.
yellow vernix syndrome Plazentainsuffizienzsyndrom *nt*.
yellow vision Gelbsehen *nt*, Xanthop(s)ie *f*.
yel·low·y ['jeləʊɪ] *adj* gelblich.
Yer·sin·ia [jerˈsɪnɪə] *n micro.* Yersinia *f*.
 Y. pestis Pestbakterium *nt*, Yersinia/Pasteurella pestis.
yer·sin·i·o·sis [jersɪnɪˈəʊsɪs] *n* Yersinia-Infektion *f*, Yersiniose *f*.
Y.F. *abbr.* → yellow fever.
yield [jiːld] **I** *n chem., techn., phys.* Ausbeute *f*, Ertrag *m*, Gewinn *m*; Ergebnis *nt*. **II** *vt* (hervor-, ein-)bringen, tragen, abwerfen; (*Resultat*) liefern, ergeben.
 y. of radiation Strahlungsausbeute, -ertrag.
yin-yang hypothesis [jɪn jæŋ] *biochem.* Yin-yang-Hypothese *f*.
Y ligament Lig. iliofemorale.
Y-linked gene Y-gebundenes Gen *nt*, holandrisches Gen *nt*.

Y-linked inheritance Y-gebundene/holandrische Vererbung *f*.
Y-neuron *n* Y-Neuron *nt*, Neuron *nt* der Latenzklasse I.
yo·ghurt ['jɔʊgərt] *n* Joghurt *m/nt*, Yoghurt *m/nt*.
yo-gurt *n* → yoghurt.
yo·him·bine [jəʊˈhɪmbiːn] *n pharm.* Yohimbin *nt*.
yoke [jəʊk] *n anat.* Jugum *nt*.
yolk [jəʊk] *n* (Ei-)Dotter *m*, Eigelb *nt*, Vitellus *m*.
yolk gland *micro.* Vitellarium *nt*, Dotterdrüse *f*, -stock *m*.
yolk granules Dottergranula *pl*.
yolk sac Nabelbläschen *nt*, Dottersack *m*.
 definitive y. sekundärer Dottersack.
 primitive y. primärer Dottersack.
 secondary y. → definitive y.
yolk sac placenta Placenta choriovitellina.
yolk sac stalk → yolk stalk.
yolk stalk Darmstiel *m*, Dotter(sack)gang *m*, Ductus omphalo(mes)entericus.
young [jʌŋ] *adj* jung, Jung-; klein; neu; jugendlich; unreif, unerfahren.
young child Kleinkind *nt*.
young form jugendlicher Granulozyt *m*, Metamyelozyt *m*; *inf.* Jugendlicher *m*.
Young [jʌŋ]: **Y.'s syndrome** Young-Syndrom *nt*.
Young-Helmholtz [ˈhelmhəʊlts]: **Y.-H. theory** *physiol.* Dreifarbentheorie *f*, Young-Helmholtz-Theorie *f*.
y·per·ite [ˈiːpəraɪt] *n* → yellow cross.
y-plate *n ortho.* Y-Platte *f*.
yp·sil·i·form [ɪpˈsɪləfɔːrm] *adj* → ypsiloid.
yp·si·loid [ˈɪpsələɪd] *adj* Y-förmig.
Y-shaped cartilage Y-Fuge *f*, Y-Knorpel *m*.
Y-shaped fracture Y-förmige Fraktur *f*.
Y-shaped ligament Lig. iliofemorale.
yt·ter·bi·um [ɪˈtɜːrbɪəm] *n abbr.* **Yb** Ytterbium *nt abbr.* Yb.
yt·tri·um [ˈɪtrɪəm] *n abbr.* **Y** Yttrium *nt abbr.* Y.
Y-V flap Y-V-Plastik *f*.
y wave *card.* y-Welle *f*.

Z

Z *abbr.* 1. → atomic number. 2. → impedance 1.
Zahn [tsaːn]: **Z.'s infarct** Zahn'-Infarkt *m*.
 Z.'s lines Zahn'-Linien *pl*.
 Z.'s striae → Z.'s lines.
 striae of Z. → Z.'s lines.
Zahorsky [zə'hɔːrskɪ]: **Z.'s disease** Dreitagefieber *nt*, sechste Krankheit *f*, Exanthema subitum, Roseola infantum.
Zander ['zændər]: **Z.'s cells** *embryo.* Zander-Zellen *pl*.
Zang [zæŋ; tsaŋ]: **Z.'s space** Fossa supraclavicularis minor.
Zappert ['tsæpərt, 'tsap-]: **Z.'s counting chamber** Zappert'-Zählkammer *f*.
Z band Z-Linie *f*, Z-Streifen *m*, Zwischenscheibe *f*, Telophragma *nt*.
Z chromosome Z-Chromosom *nt*.
Z disk → Z band.
ze·a·tin ['zɪətɪn] *n bio.* Zeatin *nt*.
ze·a·xan·thin [ˌziːə'zænθɪːn, -θɪn] *n* Zeaxanthin *nt*.
ze·bra bodies ['ziːbrə; *Brit.* 'zeb-] Zebra-Bodies *pl*, -Körper *pl*.
Zeeman ['tsiːmən]: **Z. effect** *phys.* Zeeman-Effekt *m*.
ze·in ['ziːɪn] *n* Zein *nt*.
Zeis [zaɪs; tsaɪs]: **glands of Z.** Zeis'-Drüsen *pl*, Gll. sebaceae conjunctivales.
Zellweger ['zɛlwegər]: **Z. syndrome** Zellweger-Syndrom *nt*, zerebrohepatorenales Syndrom *nt*, ZHR-Syndrom *nt*.
Zenker ['zɛŋkər; 'tsɛŋ-]: **Z.'s degeneration** Zenker-Degeneration *f*, wachsartige Degeneration *f* der Skelettmuskulatur.
 Z.'s diverticulum Zenker'-Divertikel *nt*, pharyngoösophageales Divertikel *nt*.
 Z.'s necrosis → Z.'s degeneration.
 Z.'s pouch → Z.'s diverticulum.
ze·ro ['zɪərəʊ] I *n*, *pl* **-ros, -roes** 1. Null *f*. 2. *phys.* Null(punkt *m*) *f*; (*Skala*) Ausgangspunkt *m*; (*Temperatur*) Gefrierpunkt *m*; *mathe.* Nullpunkt *m*, -stelle *f*. 3. *fig.* Tiefpunkt *m*. **at a ~** auf dem Nullpunkt (angelangt). II *adj* Null-. III *vt* auf Null einstellen, nullen.
zero adjustment 1. Nullpunkteinstellung *f*. 2. *electr.* Nullabgleich *m*.
zero axis Nullachse *f*.
zero conductor *electr.* Nulleiter *m*.
zero-order reaction *chem.* Reaktion *f* nullter Ordnung.
zero pressure breathing *abbr.* **ZPB** Atmung *f* unter Umgebungsdruck.
ze·roth law of thermodynamics ['zɪərəʊθ] nullter Hauptsatz *m* der Thermodynamik.
Z.-E. syndrome → Zollinger-Ellison syndrome.
ze·ta potential ['zeɪtə, ziː-] Zeta-Potential *nt*.
Z-E tumor → Zollinger-Ellison tumor.
Z-flap *n chir.* Z-Plastik *f*.
Zickel ['zɪkl]: **Z. nail** *ortho.* Zickel-Nagel *m*.
zi·do·vu·dine [zaɪ'dəʊvjuːdiːn] *n pharm.* Azidothymidin *nt abbr.* AZT.

Ziehen-Oppenheim ['ziːhən 'ɑpənhaɪm; 'tsiːən]: **Z.-O. disease** Torsionsneurose *f*, Ziehen-Oppenheim-Syndrom *nt*, -Krankheit *f*, Torsionsdystonie *f*, Dysbasia lordotica.
Ziehl-Neelsen [ziːl 'niːlsn; tsiːl]: **Z.-N. stain** Ziehl-Neelsen-Färbung *f*.
Zieve ['ziːv]: **Z. syndrome** Zieve-Syndrom *nt*.
zig·zag·plas·ty ['zɪgzægplæstɪ] *n chir.* Zickzackschnitt *m*, -plastik *f*.
Zika ['zɪkə]: **Z. virus** *micro* Zika-Virus *nt*.
Zimmerlin ['zɪmərlɪn; 'tsɪmər-]: **Z.'s atrophy/type** *ortho.*, *neuro.* Zimmerlin--Typ *m*.
Zimmermann ['zɪmərmən; 'tsɪmərman]: **Z.'s elementary particle** → Z.'s granule.
 Z.'s granule (Blut-)Plättchen *nt*, Thrombozyt *m*.
zinc [zɪŋk] *n abbr.* **Zn** Zink *nt*, *chem.* Zincum *nt abbr.* Zn.
zinc acetate Zinkazetat *nt*.
zinc·a·lism ['zɪŋkəlɪzəm] *n* Zinkvergiftung *f*.
zinc chill → zinc fume fever.
zinc chloride Zinkchlorid *nt*.
zinc colic Zinkkolik *f*, Darmkolik *f* bei Zinkvergiftung.
zinc fume chill → zinc fume fever.
zinc fume fever Gieß(er)fieber *nt*, Zinkfieber *nt*.
zinc·if·er·ous [zɪŋ'kɪfərəs] *adj* zinkhaltig, Zink-.
zinc oxide Zinkoxid *nt*.
zinc poisoning Zinkvergiftung *f*.
Zinn [zɪn; tsɪn]: **aponeurosis of Z.** Aufhängefasern *pl* der Linse, Zonularfasern *pl*, Fibrae zonulares.
 Z.'s artery zentrale Netzhautschlagader/ -arterie *f*, A. centralis retinae.
 circle of Z. Haller'-Gefäßkranz *m*, Zinn'-Gefäßkranz *m*, Circulus vasculosus n. optici.
 Z.'s corona → circle of Z.
 Z.'s ligament → Z.'s ring.
 Z.'s membrane → zonule of Z.
 Z.'s ring Zinn'-Sehnenring *m*, An(n)ulus tendineus communis.
 Z.'s tendon → zonule of Z.
 zonule of Z. Zinn'-(Strahlen-)Zone *f*, Zonula ciliaris.
Zinsser-Cole-Engman ['zɪnsər kəʊl 'eŋmən; 'tsɪn-]: **Z.-C.-E. syndrome** Zinsser--Cole-Engman-Syndrom *nt*, kongenitale Dyskeratose *f*, Dyskeratosis congenita, Polydysplasia ectodermica Typ Cole--Rauschkolb-Toomey.
zir·co·ni·um [zɜr'kəʊnɪəm] *n abbr.* **Zr** Zirkonium *nt abbr.* Zn.
zirconium granuloma Zirkonium-, Deodorant-, Desodorantiengranulom *nt*.
Z line → Z band.
Zn *abbr.* → zinc.
zo- *pref.* → zoo-.
zo·e·scope ['zəʊɪskəʊp] *n* Stroboskop *nt*.
zo·et·ic [zəʊ'etɪk] *adj* Lebens-.
Zollinger-Ellison ['zɑlɪndʒər 'elɪsən]: **Z.-E.**

syndrome Zollinger-Ellison-Syndrom *nt*.
 Z.-E. tumor Zollinger-Ellison-Tumor *m*.
zo·na ['zəʊnə] *n*, *pl* **-nae** [-niː, -naɪ] 1. → zone 1. 2. Gürtelrose *f*, Zoster *m*, Zona *f*, Herpes zoster.
zon·al ['zəʊnl] *adj* → zonary.
zonal centrifugation Dichtegradienten-, Zonenzentrifugation *f*.
zonal layer of cerebral cortex Molekularschicht *f*, Lamina molecularis/plexiformis corticis cerebri.
zo·na (pellucida) reaction ['zəʊnə] *embryo.* Zona-pellucida-Reaktion *f*.
zo·na·ry ['zəʊnərɪ] *adj* zonen-, gürtelförmig, Zonen-, Zonular-.
zonary placenta 1. Placenta zonaria. 2. Ring-, Gürtelplazenta *f*, Placenta anularis.
Zondek-Aschheim ['zɑndɪk 'æʃhaɪm]: **Z.-A. test** *gyn.* Aschheim-Zondek-Reaktion *f abbr.* AZR.
zone [zəʊn] *n* 1. *anat.* (Körper-)Gegend *f*, Bereich *m*, Zona *f*. 2. Zone *f*, Bereich *m*, Bezirk *m*, Gürtel *m*.
 z. of antibody excess *immun.* Präzone, Zone des Antikörperüberschusses.
 z. of antigen excess *immun.* Postzone, Zone des Antigenüberschusses.
 z. of coagulation *patho.* Koagulationszone.
 z. of complete compensation *physiol.* Zone der vollständigen Kompensation.
 z. of condensation Verdichtungszone.
 z.s of hyperalgesia Head'-Zonen *pl*.
 z. of hyperemia *patho.* hyperämische Zone.
 z. of incomplete compensation *physiol.* Zone der unvollständigen Kompensation, Gefahrenzone.
 z.s of Schreger *dent.* Schreger-Hunter'--Linien *pl*.
 z. of Zinn Zinn'-(Strahlen-)Zone, Zonula ciliaris.
zone electrophoresis Zonenelektrophorese *f*.
zo·nes·the·sia [ˌzəʊnes'θiːʒ(ɪ)ə] *n neuro.* Gürtelgefühl *nt*, Zonästhesie *f*.
zo·nif·u·gal [zəʊ'nɪfjəgəl] *adj* von einer Zone/Region weg, zonifugal.
zon·ing ['zəʊnɪŋ] *n immun.* Zoning *nt*, Zonenreaktion *f*.
zo·nip·e·tal [zəʊ'nɪpətəl] *adj* auf eine Zone/ Region zu, zonipetal.
zon·u·la ['zəʊnjələ, -zɑn-] *n*, *pl* **-las, -lae** [-liː, -laɪ] *anat.* kleiner Gürtel *od.* Bezirk *m*, kleine Zone *f*, Zonula *f*.
zonula adherens Haftzone *f*, Zonula adherens.
zonula occludens Verschlußkontakt *m*, Zonula occludens.
zo·nu·lar ['zəʊnjʊlər] *adj* → zonary.
zonular band Zona orbicularis.
zonular cataract Schichtstar *m*, Cataracta zonularis.
zonular fibers Aufhängefasern *pl* der Linse, Zonularfasern *pl*, Fibrae zonulares.
zonular keratitis bandförmige Keratitis *f*.

zonular placenta

zonular placenta → zonary placenta.
zonular spaces Petit'-Kanal *m*, Spatia zonularia.
zo·nule ['zəʊnjuːl, 'zɑn-] *n* → zonula.
z. of Zinn Zinn'-(Strahlen-)Zone *f*, Zonula ciliaris.
zo·nu·li·tis [ˌzəʊnjə'laɪtɪs, ˌzɑn-] *n ophthal.* Entzündung *f* der Zonula ciliaris, Zonulitis *f*.
zon·u·lol·y·sis [ˌ-'lɑləsɪs] *n* → zonulysis.
zon·u·lot·o·my [ˌ-'lɑtəmɪ] *n ophthal.* Zonulotomie *f*.
zon·u·ly·sis [ˌ-'laɪsɪs] *n ophthal.* Zonulolyse *f*.
zoo- *pref.* Tier-, Zo(o)-.
zoo-agglutinin *n embryo.* Zooagglutinin *nt*.
zo·o·an·thro·po·no·sis [ˌzəʊəˌænθrəpə'nəʊsɪs] *n* Anthropozoonose *f*, Zooanthroponose *f*.
zo·o·bi·ol·o·gy [ˌ-baɪ'ɑlədʒɪ] *n* Zoobiologie *f*.
zo·o·blast ['-blæst] *n* tierische Zelle *f*, Zooblast *m*.
zo·o·chem·is·try [ˌ-'kemɪstrɪ] *n* Zoochemie *f*.
zo·o·e·ras·tia [ˌ-ɪ'ræstɪə] *n psychia.* Zooerastie *f*, Sodomie *f*.
zo·o·flag·el·late [ˌ-'flædʒəlɪt, -leɪt] *n micro.* Zooflagellat *m*.
zo·og·e·nous [zəʊ'ɑdʒənəs] *adj bio.* lebendgebärend, vivipar.
zo·og·o·ny [zəʊ'ɑgənɪ] *n bio.* Lebendgebären *nt*, Viviparie *f*.
zo·o·lag·nia [ˌzəʊə'lægnɪə] *n psychia.* Zoolagnie *f*.
zo·ol·o·gy [zəʊ'ɑlədʒɪ] *n* Zoologie *f*.
zo·o·ma·nia [ˌzəʊə'meɪnɪə, -jə] *n psychia.* krankhafte Tierliebe *f*, Zoomanie *f*.
Zo·o·mas·ti·gi·na [ˌ-mæstɪ'dʒaɪnə] *pl* → Zoomastigophorea.
Zo·o·mas·ti·goph·o·ra [ˌ-mæstɪ'gɑfərə] *pl* → Zoomastigophorea.
Zo·o·mas·ti·go·pho·ras·i·da [ˌ-ˌmæstɪgəʊfə'ræsədeɪ] *pl* → Zoomastigophorea.
Zo·o·mas·ti·go·pho·rea [ˌ-ˌmæstɪgəʊ'fɔːrɪə] *pl micro.* Zoomastigophorea *pl*.
Zoon [zəʊn]: **balanitis of Z.** → **Z.'s erythroplasia**.
Z.'s erythroplasia Balanitis chronica circumscripta benigna plasmacellularis Zoon, Balanoposthitis (chronica) circumscripta plasmacellularis.
zo·on·o·my [zəʊ'ɑnəmɪ] *n* → zoobiology.
zo·o·no·sis [ˌzəʊə'nəʊsɪs] *n, pl* **-ses** [-siːz] Zoonose *f*.
zo·o·not·ic [ˌ-'nɑtɪk] *adj* Zoonose betr.
zo·o·par·a·site [ˌ-'pærəsaɪt] *n* tierischer Parasit *m*, Zooparasit *m*.
zo·o·par·a·sit·ic [ˌ-ˌpærə'sɪtɪk] *adj* Zooparasit(en) betr.
zo·oph·a·gous [zəʊ'ɑfəgəs] *adj* zoophag, fleischfressend, karnivor.
zo·o·phil·ia [ˌzəʊə'fɪlɪə] *n psychia.* 1. krankhaft übertriebene Tierliebe *f*, Zoophilie *f*. 2. Zoophilia erotica; Zoophilie *f*; Sodomie *f*.
zo·o·phil·ic [ˌ-'fɪlɪk] *adj* 1. tierliebend. 2. *psychia.* zoophil.
zo·oph·i·lism [zəʊ'ɑfəlɪzəm] *n* → zoophilia.
zo·oph·i·lous [zəʊ'ɑfɪləs] *adj* → zoophilic.
zo·o·pho·bia [ˌzəʊə'fəʊbɪə] *n psychia.* krankhafte Angst *f* vor Tieren, Zoophobie *f*.
zo·o·phyte ['-faɪt] *n bio.* Pflanzentier *nt*, Zoophyt *m*.
zo·o·plank·ton [ˌ-'plæŋktən] *n* Zooplankton *nt*.
zo·o·pre·cip·i·tin [ˌ-prɪ'sɪpətɪn] *n immun.* Zoopräziptin *nt*.
zo·op·sia [zəʊ'ɑpsɪə] *n psychia.* Zoopsie *f*.

zo·o·sperm ['zəʊəspɜrm] *n* männliche Keimzelle *f*, Spermium *nt*, Spermie *f*, Samenfaden *m*, Spermatozoon *nt*.
zo·o·sper·mia [ˌ-'spɜrmɪə] *n* Zoospermie *f*.
zo·o·spo·ran·gi·um [ˌ-spə'rændʒɪəm] *n, pl* **-gia** [-dʒɪə] Zoosporangium *nt*.
zo·o·spore ['-spəʊər, -spɔːr] *n* Schwärmspore *f*, -zelle *f*, Schwärmer *m*, Plano-, Zoospore *f*.
zo·os·te·rol [zəʊ'ɑstərɔl, -əʊl] *n* Zoosterin *nt*.
zo·o·tox·in [ˌzəʊə'tɑksɪn] *n* Tiergift *nt*, Zootoxin *nt*.
zos·ter ['zɑstər] *n* Gürtelrose *f*, Zoster *m*, Zona *f*, Herpes zoster.
zoster encephalitis Zoster-Enzephalitis *f*.
zoster encephalomyelitis Zoster-Enzephalomyelitis *f*.
zos·ter·i·form [zɑs'terɪfɔːrm] *adj* zosterartig, -ähnlich.
zoster meningitis Zoster-Meningitis *f*.
zos·ter·oid ['zɑstərɔɪd] *adj* → zosteriform.
zoster vesicles Zosterbläschen *pl*.
ZPB *abbr.* → zero pressure breathing.
Z-plasty *n chir.* Z-Plastik *f*.
Zr *abbr.* → zirconium.
Zsigmondy [sɪg'mɑndɪː]: **Z.'s movement** *phys.* Brown'-Molekularbewegung *f*.
Z-type incision Z-förmige Schnittführung *f*.
zucker·guss·le·ber ['tsʊkərgʊsleːbər] *n patho.* Zuckergußleber *f*, Perihepatitis chronica hyperplastica.
Zuckerkandl ['tsʊkərkændl]: **Z.'s body** Zuckerkandl'-Organ *nt*, Paraganglion aorticum abdominale.
Z.'s convolution Gyrus paraterminalis.
Z.'s gland → Z.'s body.
Zuelzer ['zʊlzər; 'tsyltsər]: **Z. plate** *ortho.* Zuelzer-Klammer *f*.
Zumbusch ['tsʊmbʊʃ]: **generalized pustular psoriasis of Z.** *derm.* Psoriasis pustulosa vom Typ Zumbusch, Psoriasis pustulosa generalisata, Psoriasis pustulosa gravis Zumbusch.
zwi·schen·fer·ment ['tsvɪʃnfɛr'mɛnt] *n* Glukose-6-phosphatdehydrogenase *f* *abbr.* G-6-PDH, GPP.
zwit·ter·i·on ['tsvɪtə'raɪən] *n* dipolares Ion *nt*, Zwitterion *nt*.
zyg- *pref.* → zygo-.
zyg·a·po·phys·e·al [ˌzaɪgəpəʊ'fɪzɪəl, ˌzɪg-] *adj* Zygapophysis betr.
zyg·a·po·phys·i·al *adj* → zygapophyseal.
zygapophysial joints Articc. zygapophysiales.
zyg·a·poph·y·sis [ˌzaɪgə'pɑfəsɪs, ˌzɪg-] *n, pl* **-ses** [-siːz] Zygapophysis *f*, Proc. articularis vertebrarum.
zyg·i·on ['zɪgɪən, 'zɪdʒ-] *n, pl* **-gia** [-gɪə, -dʒɪə] *anat.* Zygion *nt*.
zygo- *pref.* Zyg(o)-.
zy·go·dac·ty·ly [ˌzaɪgəʊ'dæktəlɪ] *n* Verwachsung *f* von Fingern *od.* Zehen, Syndaktylie *f*.
zy·go·ma [zaɪ'gəʊmə, zɪ-] *n, pl* **-mas, -mata** [-mətə] 1. → zygomatic arch. 2. → zygomatic bone. 3. → zygomatic process of temporal bone.
zy·go·mat·ic [zaɪgəʊ'mætɪk] *adj* Jochbogen/Arcus zygomaticus betr., zum Jochbogen gehörend, zygomatisch.
zygomatic arch Jochbogen *m*, Arcus zygomaticus.
zygomatic bone Jochbein *nt*, Os zygomaticum.
zygomatic branches of facial nerve Rami zygomatici n. facialis.
zygomatic foramen: anterior/external/facial z. → zygomaticofacial foramen.
inferior/internal/orbital z. → zygomaticoorbital foramen.

posterior/temporal z. → zygomaticotemporal foramen.
zygomatic fossa Unterschläfengrube *f*, Fossa infratemporalis.
zygomatic margin of great wing of sphenoid bone Margo zygomaticus (alae majoris).
zygomatic muscle: greater z. → zygomaticus major (muscle).
lesser z. → zygomaticus minor (muscle).
zygomatic nerve N. zygomaticus.
zy·go·mat·i·co·fa·cial [zaɪgəˌmætɪkəʊ'feɪʃl] *adj* Jochbein u. Gesicht betr., zygomatikofazial.
zygomaticofacial branch of zygomatic nerve Ramus zygomaticofacialis n. zygomatici.
zygomaticofacial canal → zygomaticofacial foramen.
zygomaticofacial foramen For. zygomaticofaciale.
zygomaticofacial nerve Ramus zygomaticofacialis n. zygomatici.
zy·go·mat·i·co·fron·tal [ˌ-'frʌntl] *adj* Jochbein u. Stirnbein betr., zygomatikofrontal.
zy·go·mat·i·co·max·il·lary [ˌ-'mæksɪlerɪː] *adj* Jochbein u. Oberkiefer/Maxilla betr., zygomatikomaxillar.
zygomaticomaxillary suture Sutura zygomaticomaxillaris.
zy·go·mat·i·co·or·bi·tal [ˌ-'ɔːrbɪtl] *adj* Jochbein u. Orbita betr., zygomatikoorbital.
zygomaticoorbital artery A. zygomatico-orbitalis.
zygomaticoorbital foramen For. zygomatico-orbitale.
zy·go·mat·i·co·sphe·noid [ˌ-'sfiːnɔɪd] *adj* Jochbein u. Keilbein betr., zygomatikosphenoidal.
zy·go·mat·i·co·tem·por·al [ˌ-'temp(ə)rəl] *adj* Jochbein u. Schläfenbein betr., zygomatikotemporal.
zygomaticotemporal branch of zygomatic nerve Ramus zygomaticotemporalis n. zygomatici.
zygomaticotemporal canal → zygomaticotemporal foramen.
zygomaticotemporal foramen For. zygomaticotemporale.
zygomaticotemporal nerve Ramus zygomaticotemporalis n. zygomatici.
zygomatic process Jochfortsatz *m*, Proc. zygomaticus.
z. of frontal bone Jochfortsatz des Stirnbeins, Proc. zygomaticus ossis frontalis.
z. of maxilla Jochfortsatz des Oberkiefers, Proc. zygomaticus maxillae.
z. of temporal bone Jochfortsatz des Schläfenbeins, Proc. zygomaticus ossis temporalis.
zygomatic region *anat.* Jochbeingegend *f*, -region *f*, Regio zygomatica.
zygomatic tubercle Tuberculum articulare (ossis zygomatici).
zy·go·mat·i·cus major (muscle) [ˌzaɪgə'mætɪkəs] großer Jochbeinmuskel *m*, Zygomatikus *m* major, M. zygomaticus major.
zygomaticus minor (muscle) kleiner Jochbeinmuskel *m*, Zygomatikus *m* minor, M. zygomaticus minor.
zy·go·max·il·lar·y [ˌ-'mæksəˌlerɪː] *adj* → zygomaticomaxillary.
Zy·go·my·ce·tes [zaɪ'maɪsiːtiːz] *pl micro.* Zygomyceten *pl*, -mycetes *pl*, -mycetales *pl*.
zy·go·my·co·sis [ˌ-maɪ'kəʊsɪs] *n* Zygomyzeteninfektion *f*, Zygomykose *f*.
zy·go·sis [zaɪ'gəʊsɪs, zɪ-] *n bio., micro.* Zygose *f*, Zygosis *f*.

zy·go·sperm ['zaɪgəspɜrm] *n* → zygospore.
zy·go·sphere ['-sfɪər] *n* Zygosphäre *f*.
zy·go·spore ['-spəʊər, -spɔːr] *n* Zygospore *f*.
zy·gote ['zaɪgəʊt] *n* befruchtete Eizelle *f*, Zygote *f*.
zy·go·tene ['zaɪgətiːn] *n* Zygotän *nt*, Synaptän *nt*.
zy·got·ic [zaɪ'gɑtɪk] *adj* Zygote betr., zygotisch, Zygoten-.
zy·go·to·blast [zaɪ'gəʊtəblæst] *n micro.* Sporozoit *m*.
zy·go·to·mere [zaɪ'gəʊtəmɪər] *n* Sporoblast *m*.
zym- *pref.* → zymo-.
zy·mase ['zaɪmeɪz] *n* Zymase *f*.

zyme [zaɪm] *n* Enzym *nt*.
zy·min ['zaɪmɪn] *n* Enzym *nt*.
zymo- *pref.* Enzym-, Zym(o)-.
zy·mo·chem·is·try [ˌzaɪməʊ'kemətrɪ] *n* Chemie *f* der Gärung, Zymochemie *f*.
zy·mo·gen ['zaɪmədʒən] *n* Enzymvorstufe *f*, Zymogen *nt*, Enzymogen *nt*, Proenzym *nt*.
zymogen granules Zymogengranula *pl*, -körnchen *pl*.
zy·mo·gen·ic [ˌ-'dʒenɪk] *adj* Gärung betr. *od.* auslösend, zymogen, Gärungs-.
zymogenic cells (*Magen*) Hauptzellen *pl*.
zy·mog·e·nous [zaɪ'mɑdʒənəs] *adj* → zymogenic.

zy·mog·ic [zaɪ'mɑdʒɪk] *adj* → zymogenic.
zy·mo·gram ['zaɪməgræm] *n lab.* Zymogramm *nt*.
zy·moid ['zaɪmɔɪd] **I** *n* Zymoid *nt*. **II** *adj* enzymartig, zymoid.
Zy·mo·mo·nas [ˌzaɪmə'məʊnəs] *n micro.* Zymomonas *f*.
Zy·mo·ne·ma [ˌ-'niːmə] *n micro.* Zymonema *f*.
zy·mo·san ['-sæn] *n* Zymosan *nt*.
zy·mos·ter·ol [zaɪ'mɑstərɔl, -rɑl] *n* Zymosterin *nt*.
zy·mot·ic papilloma [zaɪ'mɑtɪk] Frambösie *f*, Pian *f*, Parangi *f*, Yaws *f*, Framboesia tropica.

Appendix / Anhang

Appendix	page/Seite	Anhang
Contents Appendix	A1	**Inhaltsverzeichnis Anhang**
Weights and Measures	A2	**Maße und Gewichte**
I. Linear Measures	A2	I. Längenmaße
II. Square Measures	A3	II. Flächenmaße
III. Cubic Measures	A3	III. Raummaße
IV. Measures of Capacity	A4	IV. Hohlmaße
V. Weights	A5	V. Gewichte
Conversion Tables for Temperatures	A7	**Umrechnungstabellen für Temperaturen**
Anatomical Plates	A8 - A65	**Anatomische Tafeln**
Plate I: regions of the body	A8	Tafel I: Regionen des Körpers
Plate II: skeleton	A10	Tafel II: Knochenskelett
Plate III: bones	A12	Tafel III: Knochen
Plate IV: skull	A14	Tafel IV: Schädel
Plate V: thoracic cavity	A16	Tafel V: Brustraum
Plate VI: heart I	A18	Tafel VI: Herz I
Plate VII: heart II	A20	Tafel VII: Herz II
Plate VIII: upper abdominal organs	A22	Tafel VIII: Oberbauchorgane
Plate IX: lower abdominal organs/ retroperitoneum	A24	Tafel IX: Unterbauchorgane/ Retroperitoneum
Plate X: pelvic organs	A26	Tafel X: Beckenorgane
Plate XI: vessels I	A28	Tafel XI: Gefäße I
Plate XII: vessels II	A30	Tafel XII: Gefäße II
Plate XIII: vessels III	A32	Tafel XIII: Gefäße III
Plate XIV: vessels IV	A34	Tafel XIV: Gefäße IV
Plate XV: vessels V	A36	Tafel XV: Gefäße V
Plate XVI: vessels VI	A38	Tafel XVI: Gefäße VI
Plate XVII: lymphatic vessels	A40	Tafel XVII: Lymphbahnen
Plate XVIII: nervous system I	A42	Tafel XVIII: Nervensystem I
Plate XIX: nervous system II	A44	Tafel XIX: Nervensystem II
Plate XX: nervous system III	A46	Tafel XX: Nervensystem III
Plate XXI: nervous system IV	A48	Tafel XXI: Nervensystem IV
Plate XXII: nervous system V	A50	Tafel XXII: Nervensystem V
Plate XXIII: nervous system VI	A52	Tafel XXIII: Nervensystem VI
Plate XXIV: muscles I	A54	Tafel XXIV: Muskeln I
Plate XXV: muscles II	A56	Tafel XXV: Muskeln II
Plate XXVI: muscles III	A58	Tafel XXVI: Muskeln III
Plate XXVII: muscles IV	A60	Tafel XXVII: Muskeln IV
Plate XXVIII: muscles V	A62	Tafel XXVIII: Muskeln V
Plate XXIX: muscles VI	A64	Tafel XXIX: Muskeln VI

Weights and Measures — Maße und Gewichte

I. Linear Measures — Längenmaße

1. American Linear Measure — Amerikanische Längenmaße

1 (statute) mile = 8 furlongs = 320 rods = 1760 yards = 5280 feet = 1, 6093 km

1 furlong = 40 rods = 220 yards = 660 feet = 201,168 m

1 rod = 5½ yards = 16½ feet = 5, 029 m

1 yard = 3 feet = 36 inches = 0,9144 m = 91,44 cm

1 foot = 12 inches = 0,3048 m = 30,48 cm

1 inch = 2,54 cm = 25,4 mm

2. German Linear Measure — Deutsche Längenmaße

1 km = 1000 m = 0.6214 mile

1 m = 10 dm = 100 cm = 1000 mm = 1.0936 yards = 3.2808 feet

1 dm = 10 cm = 100 mm = 0.3281 foot = 3.9370 inches

1 cm = 10 mm = 0.3937 inch

1 mm = 0.0394 inch

3. Conversion Table — Umrechnungstabelle
Inches into Centimters — Inches in Zentimeter

inches	0	1	2	3	4	5	6	7	8	9
0		2,540	5,080	7,620	10,160	12,700	15,240	17,780	20,320	22,860
10	25,400	27,940	30,480	33,020	35,560	38,100	40,640	43,180	45,720	48,260
20	50,800	53,340	55,880	58,420	60,960	63,500	66,040	68,580	71,120	73,660
30	76,200	78,740	81,280	83,820	86,360	88,900	91,440	93,980	96,520	99,060

4. Conversion Table — Umrechnungstabelle
Feet and Inches into Centimeters — Feet und Inches in Zentimeter

feet ↓ \ inches →	0	1	2	3	4	5	6	7	8	9	10	11
3	91,44	93,98	96,52	99,06	101,60	104,14	106,68	109,22	111,76	114,30	116,84	119,38
4	121,92	124,46	127,00	129,54	132,08	134,62	137,16	139,70	142,24	144,78	147,32	149,86
5	152,40	154,94	157,48	160,02	162,56	165,50	167,64	170,18	172,72	175,26	177,80	180,34
6	182,88	185,42	187,96	190,50	193,04	195,58	198,12	200,66	203,20	205,74	208,28	210,82

II. Square Measures —— Flächenmaße

1. American Square Measure —— Amerikanische Flächenmaße

1 square mile = 640 acres = 2,59 km²

1 acre = 160 square rods = 4840 square yards = 4046,8 m²

1 square rod = 30¼ square yards = 25,29 m²

1 square yard = 9 square feet = 0,8361 m² = 8361,26 cm²

1 square foot = 144 square inches = 0,0929 m² = 929,03 cm²

1 square inch = 6,45 cm² = 645,16 mm²

2. German Square Measure —— Deutsche Flächenmaße

1 km² = 100 ha = 247.11 acres = 0.3861 square mile

1 ha = 100 a = 2.47 acres

1 a = 100 m² = 119.6 square yards

1 m² = 100 dm² = 1.196 square yards = 10.7639 square feet

1 dm² = 100 cm² = 0.1076 square foot = 15.499 square inches

1 cm² = 100 mm² = 0.155 square inch

III. Cubic Measures —— Raummaße

1. American Cubic Measure —— Amerikanische Raummaße

1 cubic yard = 27 cubic feet = 0,7646 m³

1 cubic foot = 1728 cubic inches = 0,0283 m³

1 cubic inch = 16,387 cm³

2. German Cubic Measure —— Deutsche Raummaße

1 m³ = 1000 dm³ = 1.31 cubic yards = 35.315 cubic feet

1 dm³ = 1000 cm³ = 61.024 cubic inches

1 cm³ = 1000 mm³ = 0.061 cubic inch

IV. Measures of Capacity — Hohlmaße

1. American Measure of Capacity — Amerikanische Hohlmaße

A. Liquid Measure — Flüssigkeitsmaße

1 hogshead = 2 barrels = 63 gallons = 238,456 l

1 barrel = 31.5 gallons = 119,228 l

1 gallon = 4 quarts = 8 pints = 3,7853 l

1 quart = 2 pints = 0,9464 l = 946,4 ml

1 pint = 4 gills = 0,4732 l = 473,2 ml

1 gill = 0,1183 l = 118,3 ml

B. Dry Measure — Trockenmaße

1 bushel = 4 pecks = 35,2383 l

1 peck = 2 gallons = 8,8096 l

1 gallon = 4 quarts = 8 pints = 4,405 l

1 quart = 2 pints = 1,1012 l = 1101,2 ml

1 pint = 0,5506 l = 550,6 ml

2. British Measure of Capacity — Britische Hohlmaße

A. Liquid Measure — Flüssigkeitsmaße

1 barrel = 36 (imperial) gallons = 163,656 l

1 (imperial) gallon = 4 quarts = 8 pints = 4,5459 l

1 quart = 2 pints = 1,136 l = 1136 ml

1 pint = 4 gills = 0,568 l = 568 ml

1 gill = 5 fluid ounces = 0,142 l = 142 ml

1 fluid ounce = 28,4 ml

B. Dry Measure — Trockenmaße

1 quarter = 8 bushels = 290,935 l

1 bushel = 4 pecks = 36,368 l

1 peck = 2 gallons = 9,092 l

1 gallon = 4 quarts = 8 pints = 4,5459 l

1 quart = 2 pints = 1,136 l = 1136 ml

1 pint = 4 gills = 0,568 l = 568 ml

1 gill = 5 fluid ounces = 0,142 l = 142 ml

1 fluid ounce = 28,4 ml

3. German Measure of Capacity — Deutsche Hohlmaße

1 hl = 10 dkl = 100 l = 26.418 gallons = 21.998 (imperial) gallons

1 dkl = 10 l = 2.64 gallons = 2.1998 (imperial) gallons

1 l = 10 dl = 2.113 pints (US) = 1.76 pints (British)

1 dl = 10 cl = 100 ml = 3.38 fluid ounces (US) = 3.52 fluid ounces (British)

1 cl = 10 ml = 0.338 fluid ounce (US) = 0.352 fluid ounce (British)

V. Weights — Gewichte

1. American Avoirdupois Weight — Amerikanische Handelsgewichte

1 stone = 14 pounds = 6,35 kg

1 pound = 16 ounces = 453,59 g

1 ounce = 16 drams = 28,35 g

1 dram = 1,772 g

2. German Weight — Deutsche Handelsgewichte

1 kg = 1000 g = 2.205 pounds

(1 Pfd = ½ kg = 500 g = 1.1023 pounds)

100 g = 3.5273 ounces

1 g = 0.564 dram

3. Conversion Table
Pounds and Ounces into Grams

Umrechnungstabelle
Pfund und Unzen in Gramm

pounds ↓ \ ounces →	0	4	8	12
1	453,59	566,99	680,39	793,79
2	907,18	1020,58	1133,98	1247,38
3	1360,78	1474,18	1587,59	1700,97
4	1814,36	1927,76	2041,16	2154,56
5	2267,96	2381,36	2494,75	2608,15
6	2721,54	2834,94	2948,34	3061,74
7	3175,13	3288,53	3401,93	3515,33
8	3628,72	3742,12	3855,52	3968,92
9	4082,31	4195,71	4309,11	4422,51

4. Conversion Table
Pounds into Kilograms

Umrechnungstabelle
Pfund in Kilogramm

pounds	0	1	2	3	4	5	6	7	8	9
0		0,45	0,91	1,36	1,81	2,27	2,72	3,18	3,63	4,08
10	4,54	4,99	5,44	5,90	6,35	6,80	7,26	7,71	8,16	8,62
20	9,07	9,53	9,98	10,43	10,89	11,34	11,79	12,25	12,70	13,15
30	13,61	14,06	14,51	14,97	15,42	15,88	16,33	16,78	17,24	17,69
40	18,14	18,60	19,05	19,50	19,96	20,41	20,87	21,32	21,77	22,23
50	22,68	23,13	23,59	24,04	24,49	24,95	25,40	25,85	26,31	26,76
60	27,22	27,67	28,12	28,58	29,03	29,48	29,94	30,39	30,84	31,30
70	31,75	32,21	32,66	33,11	33,57	34,02	34,47	34,93	35,38	35,83
80	36,29	36,74	37,19	37,65	38,10	38,56	39,01	39,46	39,92	40,37
90	40,82	41,28	41,73	42,18	42,64	43,09	43,54	44,00	44,45	44,91
100	45,36	45,81	46,27	46,72	47,17	47,63	48,08	48,53	48,99	49,44
110	49,90	50,35	50,80	51,26	51,71	52,16	52,62	53,07	53,52	53,98
120	54,43	54,88	55,34	55,79	56,25	56,70	57,15	57,61	58,06	58,51
130	58,97	59,42	59,87	60,33	60,78	61,23	61,69	62,14	62,60	63,05
140	63,50	63,96	64,41	64,86	65,32	65,77	66,22	66,68	67,13	67,59
150	68,04	68,49	68,95	69,40	69,85	70,31	70,76	71,21	71,67	72,12
160	72,57	73,03	73,48	73,94	74,39	74,84	75,30	75,75	76,20	76,66
170	77,11	77,56	78,02	78,47	78,93	79,38	79,83	80,29	80,74	81,19
180	81,65	82,10	82,55	83,01	83,46	83,91	84,37	84,82	85,28	85,37
190	86,18	86,64	87,09	87,54	88,00	88,45	88,90	89,36	89,81	90,26
200	90,72	91,17	91,63	92,08	92,53	92,99	93,44	93,89	94,35	94,80
210	95,25	95,71	96,16	96,62	97,07	97,52	97,98	98,43	98,88	99,34
220	99,79	100,24	100,70	101,15	101,60	102,06	102,51	102,97	103,42	103,87
230	104,33	104,78	105,23	105,69	106,14	106,59	107,05	107,50	107,96	108,41
240	108,86	109,32	109,77	110,22	110,68	111,13	111,58	112,04	112,49	112,94
250	113,40	113,85	114,31	114,76	115,21	115,67	116,12	116,57	117,03	117,48
260	117,93	118,39	118,84	119,29	119,75	120,20	120,66	121,66	121,56	122,02
270	122,47	122,92	123,38	123,83	124,28	124,74	125,19	125,65	126,10	126,55
280	127,01	127,46	127,91	128,37	128,82	129,27	129,73	130,18	130,63	131,09
290	131,54	132,00	132,45	132,90	133,36	133,81	134,26	134,72	135,17	135,62
300	136,08	136,53	136,98	137,44	137,89	138,35	138,80	139,25	139,71	140,16

Conversion Tables for Temperatures

A. Degress Fahrenheit into Degrees Celsius

Umrechnungstabelle für Temperaturen

B. Degrees Celsius into Degress Fahrenheit

A. Grad Fahrenheit in Grad Celsius

B. Grad Celsius in Grad Fahrenheit

Fahrenheit	Celsius
400	204
350	177
300	149
250	121
200	93
150	66
130	54
110	43,3
109	42,8
108	42,2
107	41,7
106	41,1
105	40,6
104	40,0
103	39,4
102	38,9
101	38,3
100	37,8
99	37,2
98	36,7
97	36,1
96	35,6
95	35,0
94	34,4
93	33,9
92	33,3
91	32,8
90	33,2
85	29,4
80	26,7
70	21,1
60	15,6
50	10,0
40	4,4
32	0
30	- 1,1
25	- 3,9
20	- 6,7
15	- 9,4
10	- 12,2
5	- 15,0
0	- 17,8
- 10	- 23,3
- 20	- 28,9
- 30	- 34,4
- 40	- 40,0
- 50	- 45,6
- 100	- 73,3

Celsius	Fahrenheit
400	752
350	662
300	572
250	482
200	392
150	302
100	212
90	194
80	176
70	158
60	140
50	122
49	120.2
48	118.4
47	116.6
46	114.8
45	113.0
44	111.2
43	109.4
42	107.6
41	105.8
40	104.0
39	102.2
38	100.4
37	98.6
36	96.8
35	95.0
34	93.2
33	91.4
32	89.6
31	87.8
30	86.0
29	84.2
28	82.4
27	80.6
26	78.8
25	77
20	68
15	59
10	50
5	41
0	32
- 5	23
- 10	14
- 15	5
- 20	- 4
- 25	- 13
- 30	- 22
- 40	- 40
- 50	- 58
- 100	- 148

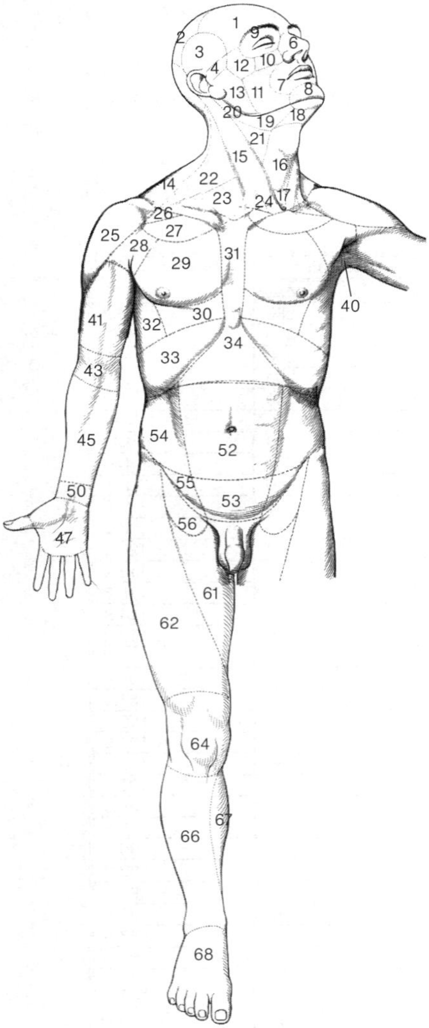

Plate I Tafel I A8

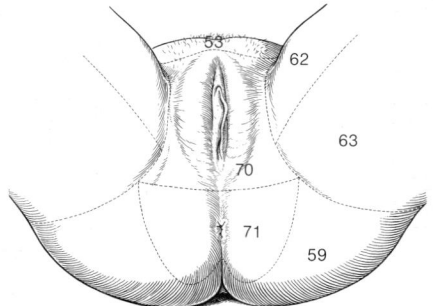

regions of the body, anterior view
Körperregionen, von vorne

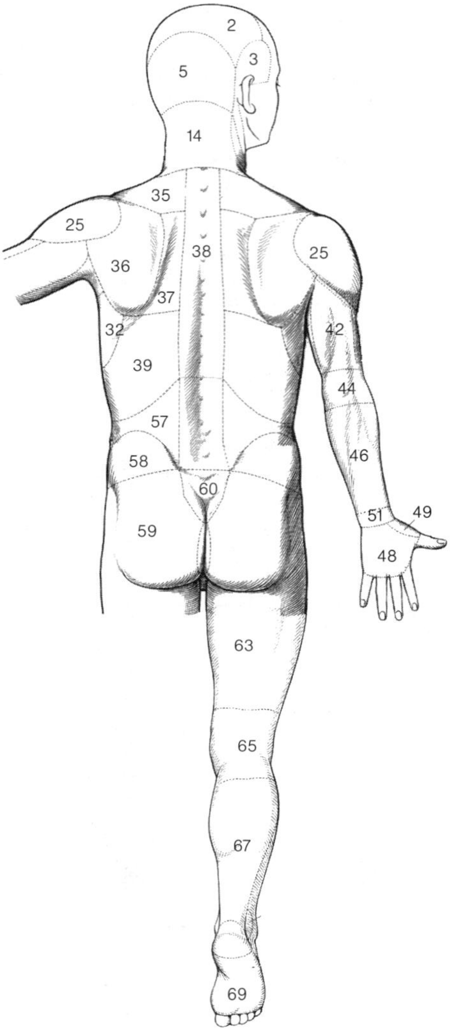

regions of the body, posterior view
Körperregionen, von hinten

genital and perineal regions
Regionen im Genital- und Dammbereich

Plate I

regions of the body, anterior view

regions of the body, posterior view

genital and perineal regions

1 frontal region
2 parietal region
3 temporal region
4 infratemporal fossa/region, zygomatic fossa
5 occipital region
6 nasal region, region of the nose
7 oral region
8 mental region, region of the chin
9 orbital region, ocular region
10 infraorbital region
11 buccal region, region of the cheek
12 zygomatic region
13 parotideomasseteric region
14 posterior cervical region, posterior region of the neck, nuchal region, back of the neck
15 sternocleidomastoid region
16 median cervical region
17 jugular fossa, suprasternal space
18 suprahyoid region
19 submandibular trigone
20 retromandibular fossa
21 carotid trigone/triangle
22 lateral cervical region, lateral region of the neck, posterior triangle of the neck
23 omoclavicular triangle, subclavian triangle
24 Zang's space, lesser supraclavicular fossa
25 deltoid region
26 clavipectoral trigone/triangle
27 Mohrenheim's fossa/triangle, infraclavicular fossa
28 axillary region
29 mammary region
30 inframammary region
31 presternal region
32 lateral thoracic region
33 hypochondriac region, hypochondrium
34 epigastric region, epigastrium
35 suprascapular region
36 scapular region
37 interscapular region
38 vertebral region
39 infrascapular region
40 armpit, axilla, axillary space/fossa
41 anterior region of the arm, anterior brachial region/facies
42 posterior region of the arm, posterior brachial region/facies
43 anterior cubital region/facies
44 posterior cubital region/facies
45 anterior region of the forearm, anterior antebrachial region/facies
46 posterior region of the forearm, posterior antebrachial region/facies
47 palm (of the hand)
48 back of the hand
49 anatomical snuff-box
50 anterior carpal region
51 posterior carpal region
52 umbilical region
53 pubic region, hypogastric region, hypogastrium
54 lateral region
55 inguinal region, iliac region
56 subinguinal region
57 lumbar region
58 region of the hip
59 gluteal region, region of the buttocks
60 sacral region
61 Scarpa's triangle, femoral trigone/triangle
62 anterior region of the thigh
63 posterior region of the thigh
64 anterior region of the knee
65 posterior region of the knee
66 anterior region of the leg, anterior crural region
67 posterior region of the leg, posterior crural region
68 back of the foot
69 sole (of the foot)
70 urogenital region/triangle
71 anal region/triangle

Tafel I

Körperregionen, von vorne

Körperregionen, von hinten

Regionen im Genital- und Dammbereich

1 Stirnregion, Regio frontalis
2 Scheitelregion, Regio parietalis
3 Schläfenregion, Regio temporalis
4 Infratemporalregion, Unterschläfengrube, Fossa infratemporalis
5 Hinterhauptsregion, Regio occipitalis
6 Nasenregion, Regio nasalis
7 Mundregion, Regio oralis
8 Kinnregion, Regio mentalis
9 Augenregion, Regio orbitalis
10 Infraorbitalregion, Regio infraorbitalis
11 Wangenregion, Regio buccalis
12 Jochbeinregion, Regio zygomatica
13 Regio parotideomasseterica
14 Nacken(region), Regio cervicalis posterior, Regio nuchalis
15 Regio sternocleidomastoidea
16 mittlere Halsregion, Regio mediana cervicalis
17 Drosselgrube, Fossa jugularis
18 Regio suprahyoidea
19 Trigonum submandibulare
20 Fossa retromandibularis
21 Karotisdreieck, Trigonum caroticum
22 hinteres Halsdreieck, Trigonum cervicale posterius, Regio cervicalis lateralis
23 Trigonum omoclaviculare
24 Fossa supraclavicularis minor
25 Regio deltoidea
26 Trigonum clavipectorale
27 Mohrenheim'-Grube, Fossa infraclavicularis
28 Achselregion, Regio axillaris
29 Brustregion, Regio mammaria
30 Regio inframammaria
31 Prästernalregion, Regio pr(a)esternalis
32 seitliche Brustregion, Regio thoracica lateralis
33 Hypochondrium, Regio hypochondriaca
34 Oberbauch, Epigastrium, Regio epigastrica
35 Supraskapularregion, Regio suprascapularis
36 Schulterblattregion, Regio scapularis
37 Interskapularregion, Regio interscapularis
38 Wirbelsäulenregion, Regio vertebralis
39 Infraskapularregion, Regio infrascapularis
40 Achselhöhle, Fossa axillaris
41 vordere Oberarmregion, Regio/Facies brachialis anterior
42 hintere Oberarmregion, Regio/Facies brachialis posterior
43 vordere Ellenbogenregion, Regio/Facies cubitalis anterior
44 hintere Ellenbogenregion, Regio/Facies cubitalis posterior
45 vordere Unterarmregion, Regio/Facies antebrachialis anterior
46 hintere Unterarmregion, Regio/Facies antebrachialis posterior
47 Handteller, Palma manus
48 Handrücken, Dorsum manus
49 Tabatière, Foveola radialis
50 vordere Handwurzelregion, Regio carpalis anterior
51 hintere Handwurzelregion, Regio carpalis posterior
52 Nabelregion, Regio umbilicalis
53 Unterbauch, Hypogastrium, Regio pubica
54 Seitenregion der Bauchwand, Regio lateralis
55 Leistenregion, Regio inguinalis
56 Subinguinalregion, Regio subinguinalis
57 Lendenregion, Regio lumbaris/lumbalis
58 Hüftbeinregion, Regio coxae
59 Gesäßregion, Regio glut(a)ealis
60 Kreuzbeinregion, Regio sacralis
61 Oberschenkeldreieck, Trigonum femorale
62 vordere Oberschenkelregion, Regio/Facies femoralis anterior
63 hintere Oberschenkelregion, Regio/Facies femoralis posterior
64 vordere Knieregion, Regio genus anterior
65 hintere Knieregion, Regio genus posterior
66 vordere Unterschenkelregion, Regio/Facies cruralis anterior
67 hintere Unterschenkelregion, Regio/Facies cruralis posterior
68 Fußrücken, Dorsum pedis, Regio dorsalis pedis
69 Fußsohle, Planta pedis, Regio plantaris pedis
70 Urogenitalregion, Regio urogenitalis
71 Analregion, Regio analis

Plate II   Tafel II   A10

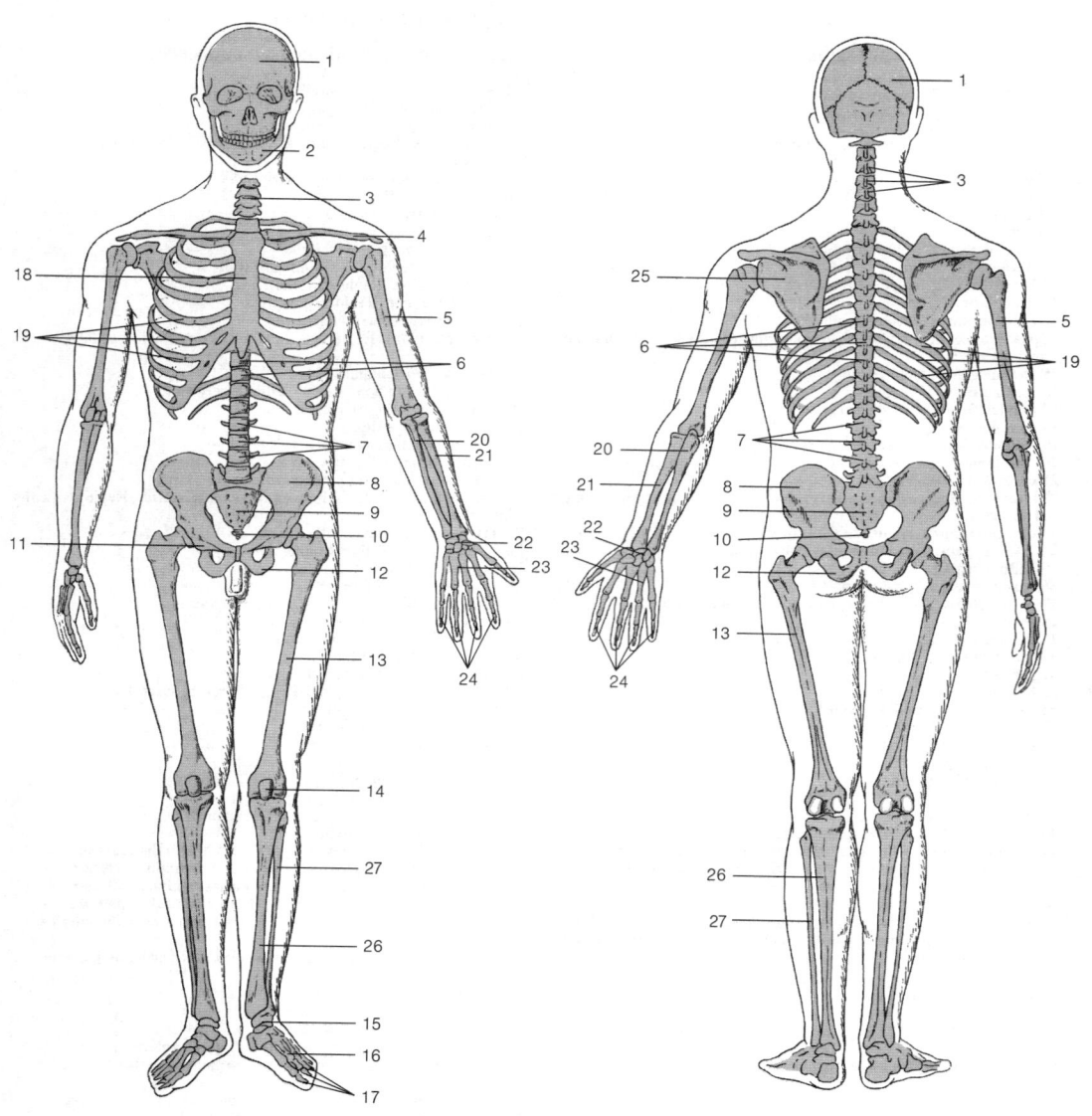

skeleton, anterior view
Knochenskelett, von vorne

skeleton, posterior view
Knochenskelett, von hinten

Plate II

skeleton, anterior view

skeleton, posterior view

1 cranium, skull
2 lower jaw, jaw bone, mandible
3 cervical vertebrae
4 collar bone, clavicle, cavicula
5 bone of the upper arm, humerus
6 thoracic vertebrae, dorsal vertebrae
7 lumbar vertebrae
8 iliac bone, flank, ilium
9 sacrum
10 coccygeal bone, tail bone, coccyx
11 pubic bone, pubis
12 ischial bone, ischium
13 thigh bone, femur
14 knee cap
15 root of the foot, tarsus
16 metatarsus
17 toes
18 breast bone, sternum
19 ribs
20 elbow bone, ulna
21 radial bone, radius
22 wrist, carpus
23 metacarpus
24 fingers
25 shoulder blade, scapula
26 shin bone, tibia
27 calf bone, fibula

Tafel II

Knochenskelett, von vorne

Knochenskelett, von hinten

1 (knöcherner) Schädel, Cranium
2 Unterkiefer(knochen), Mandibula
3 Halswirbel, Vertebrae cervicales
4 Schlüsselbein, Klavikula, Clavicula
5 Oberarmknochen, Humerus
6 Brustwirbel, Vertebrae thoracicae
7 Lendenwirbel, Vertebrae lumbales/lumbares
8 Darmbein, Ilium, Os ilii/iliacum
9 Kreuzbein, Sakrum, Os sacrum/sacrale, Vertebrae sacrales
10 Steißbein, Coccyx, Os coccygis, Vertebrae coccygeae
11 Schambein, Pubis, Os pubis
12 Sitzbein, Ischium, Os ischii
13 Oberschenkelknochen, Femur, Os femoris
14 Kniescheibe, Patella
15 Fußwurzel, Tarsus
16 Mittelfuß, Metatarsus
17 Zehen, Digiti pedis
18 Brustbein, Sternum
19 Rippen, Costae
20 Elle, Ulna
21 Speiche, Radius
22 Handwurzel, Carpus
23 Mittelhand, Metacarpus
24 Finger, Digiti manus
25 Schulterblatt, Skapula, Scapula
26 Schienbein, Tibia
27 Wadenbein, Fibula

Plate III Tafel III A12

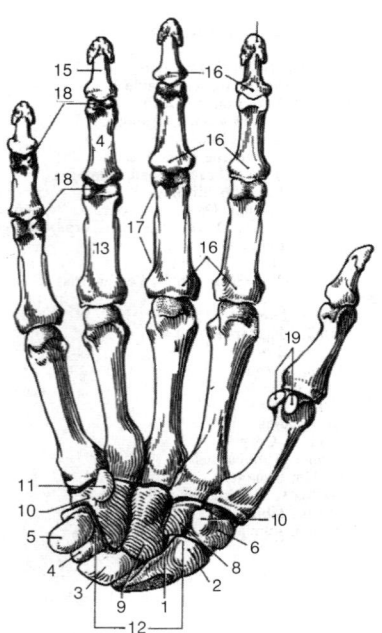

skeleton of right hand, palmar view
rechtes Handskelett, von palmar

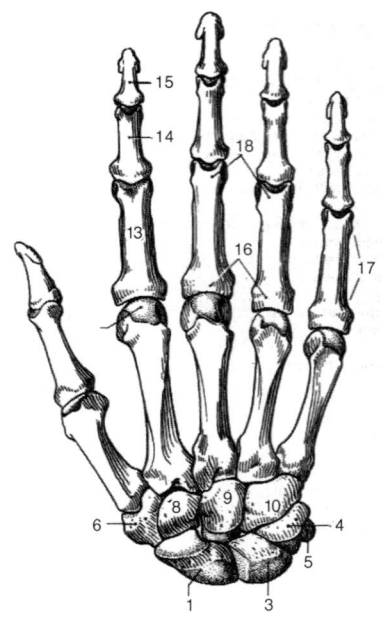

skeleton of right hand, dorsal view
rechtes Handskelett, von dorsal

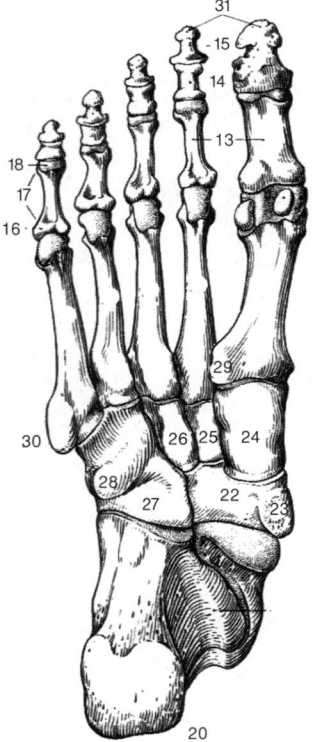

skeleton of right foot, inferior view
rechtes Fußskelett, von unten

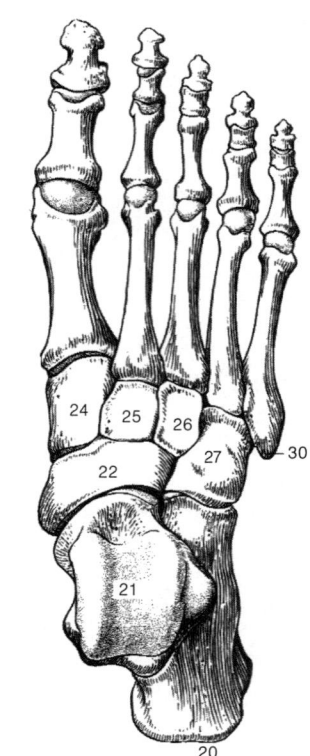

skeleton of right foot, superior view
rechtes Fußskelett, von oben

Plate III

skeleton of right hand, palmar view
skeleton of right hand, dorsal view
skeleton of right foot, inferior view
skeleton of right foor, superior view

1 scaphoid bone
2 scaphoid tubercle
3 lunate bone, semilunar bone, lunare
4 triangular/triquetral bone
5 pisiform bone, lentiform bone
6 trapezium bone, greater multangular bone
7 tubercle of trapezium
8 trapezoid bone, lesser multangular bone
9 capitate bone, capitate
10 hamate bone, hooked bone, unciform bone
11 hamulus of hamate bone
12 carpal sulcus
13 proximal phalanx
14 middle phalanx
15 distal phalanx
16 base of phalanx
17 body/shaft of phalanx
18 head of phalanx
19 sesamoid bones
20 heel bone, calcaneal bone, calcaneus
21 ankle bone, talus
22 navicular bone
23 tuberosity of navicular bone
24 medial/first cuneiform bone
25 intermediate/second cuneiform bone
26 lateral/third cuneiform bone
27 cuboid bone
28 tuberosity of cuboid bone
29 tuberosity of first metatarsal bone
30 tuberosity of fifth metatarsal bone
31 tuberosity of distal phalanx

Tafel III

rechtes Handskelett, von palmar
rechtes Handskelett, von dorsal
rechtes Fußskelett, von unten
rechtes Fußskelett, von oben

1 Kahnbein, Os scaphoideum
2 Tuberculum ossis scaphoidei
3 Mondbein, Os lunatum
4 Dreiecksbein, Os triquetrum
5 Erbsenbein, Os pisiforme
6 großes Vieleckbein, Os trapezium
7 Tuberculum ossis trapezii
8 kleines Vieleckbein, Os trapezoideum
9 Kopfbein, Os capitatum
10 Hakenbein, Os hamatum
11 Hamulus ossis hamati
12 Sulcus carpi
13 Grundphalanx, Phalanx proximalis
14 Mittelphalanx, Phalanx media
15 Endphalanx, Phalanx distalis
16 Fingerknochenbasis, Basis phalangis
17 Fingerknochenschaft, Corpus phalangis
18 Fingerknochenkopf, Caput phalangis
19 Sesamknochen, -beine, Ossa sesamoidea
20 Fersenbein, Kalkaneus, Calcaneus
21 Sprungbein, Talus
22 Kahnbein, Os naviculare
23 Tuberositas ossis navicularis
24 inneres Keilbein, Os cuneiforme mediale
25 mittleres Keilbein, Os cuneiforme intermedium
26 äußeres Keilbein, Os cuneiforme laterale
27 Würfelbein, Os cuboideum
28 Tuberositas ossis cuboidei
29 Tuberositas ossis metatarsalis primi
30 Tuberositas ossis metatarsalis quinti
31 Tuberositas phalangis distalis

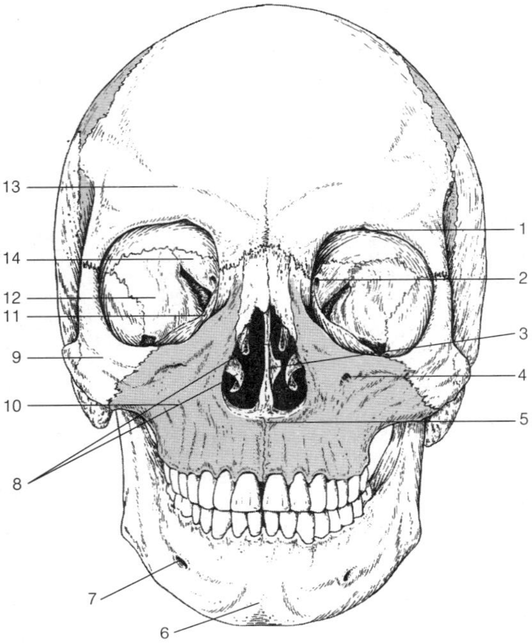

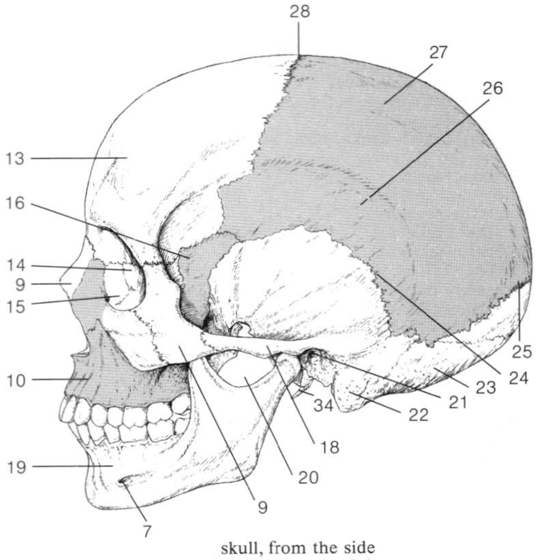

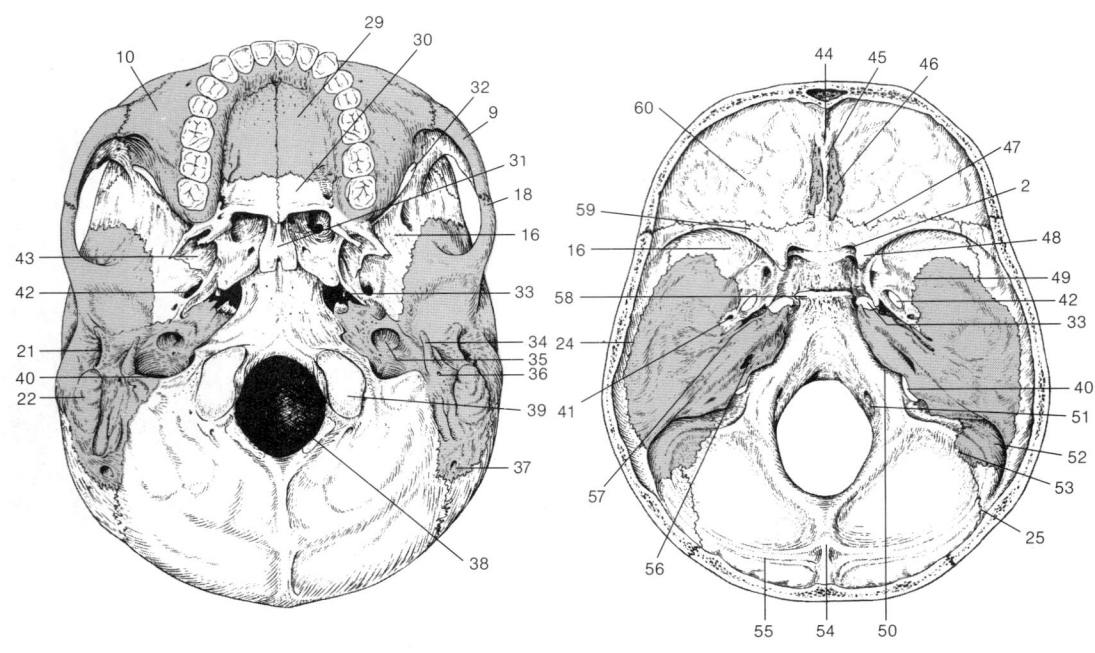

Plate IV

skull, frontal view

skull, from the side

base of skull, from below

base of skull, superior view

1 supraorbital incisure/notch/foramen
2 optic canal, optic foramen of sphenoid bone
3 bony/osseous septum of nose, bony/osseous nasal septum
4 infraorbital foramen
5 anterior nasal spine
6 mental protuberance
7 mental foramen
8 inferior and middle nasal concha

9 zygomatic bone
10 upper jaw bone, maxilla
11 palatine bone
12 sphenoid bone
13 frontal bone
14 ethmoid bone
15 lacrimal bone
16 great(er) wing of sphenoid bone, ali sphenoid bone
17 nasal bone
18 zygomatic arch, malar arch
19 lower jaw bone, jaw bone, mandible
20 mandibular notch, incisure of mandible
21 external acoustic meatus, external auditory meatus
22 mastoid process (of temporal bone)
23 occipital bone
24 squamous suture
25 lambdoid suture
26 temporal bone
27 parietal bone
28 coronal suture
29 palatine process (of maxilla)
30 horizontal plate of palatine bone
31 vomer
32 inferior orbital fissure, inferior sphenoidal fissure, sphenomaxillary fissure
33 lacerate foramen
34 styloid process of temporal bone

35 carotid canal
36 stylomastoid foramen
37 mastoid foramen
38 great (occipital) foramen
39 occipital condyle
40 jugular foramen
41 spinous foramen
42 oval foramen (of sphenoid bone)
43 pterygoid fossa (of sphenoid bone)
44 cecal foramen, foramen cecum of frontal bone
45 crista galli
46 cribriform lamina of ethmoid bone
47 sphenofrontal suture
48 anterior clinoid process
49 sphenosquamous suture
50 petro-occipital fissure, petrobasilar fissure
51 hypoglossal canal, anterior condyloid canal/foramen
52 sulcus of sigmoid sinus
53 occipitomastoid suture
54 internal occipital protuberance
55 sulcus of transverse sinus
56 internal acoustic meatus
57 sulcus of greater petrosal nerve
58 posterior clinoid process
59 small(er) wing of sphenoid bone
60 frontoethmoidal suture

Tafel IV

Schädel, von vorne

Schädel, von der Seite

Schädelbasis, von unten

Schädelbasis, von innen

1 Inc. supraorbitalis, For. supraorbitale
2 Sehnervenkanal, Optikuskanal, Canalis opticus
3 knöchernes Nasenseptum, Septum nasi osseum
4 For. infraorbitale
5 Spina nasalis anterior
6 Kinnvorsprung, Protuberantia mentalis
7 For. mentale
8 mittlere und untere Nasenmuschel, Concha nasalis media und Concha nasalis inferior
9 Jochbein, Os zygomaticum
10 Oberkiefer(knochen), Maxilla
11 Gaumenbein, Os palatinum
12 Keil-, Flügelbein, Os sphenoidale
13 Stirnbein, Os frontale
14 Siebbein, Os ethmoidale
15 Tränenbein, Os lacrimale
16 großer Keilbeinflügel, Ala major
17 Nasenbein, Os nasale
18 Jochbogen, Arcus zygomaticus
19 Unterkiefer(knochen), Mandibula
20 Inc. mandibulae
21 äußerer Gehörgang, Meatus acusticus externus
22 Warzenfortsatz, Proc. mastoideus
23 Hinterhauptsbein, Os occipitale
24 Schuppennaht, Sutura squamosa
25 Lambdanaht, Sutura lambdoidea
26 Schläfenbein, Os temporale
27 Scheitelbein, Os parietale
28 Kranznaht, Sutura coronalis
29 Gaumenfortsatz des Oberkiefers, Proc. palatinus
30 Lamina horizontalis (ossis palatini)
31 Flugscharbein, Vomer
32 Fissura orbitalis inferior

33 For. lacerum
34 Griffelfortsatz des Schläfenbeins, Proc. styloideus ossis temporalis
35 Karotiskanal, Canalis caroticus
36 For. stylomastoideum
37 For. mastoideum
38 großes Hinterhauptsloch, For. magnum
39 Hinterhauptskondyle, Condylus occipitalis
40 For. jugulare
41 For. spinosum
42 For. ovale
43 Fossa pterygoidea
44 For. caecum
45 Hahnenkamm, Crista galli
46 Siebbeinplatte, Lamina cribrosa
47 Sutura sphenofrontalis
48 Proc. clinoideus anterior
49 Sutura sphenosquamosa
50 Fissura petro-occipitalis
51 Hypoglossuskanal, Canalis hypoglossi
52 Sulcus sinus sigmoidei
53 Sutura occipitomastoidea
54 Protuberantia occipitalis interna
55 Sulcus sinus transversi
56 innerer Gehörgang, Meatus acusticus internus
57 Sulcus n. petrosi majoris
58 Proc. clinoideus posterior
59 kleiner Keilbeinflügel, Ala minor
60 Sutura fronto-ethmoidalis

Plate V   Tafel V   A16

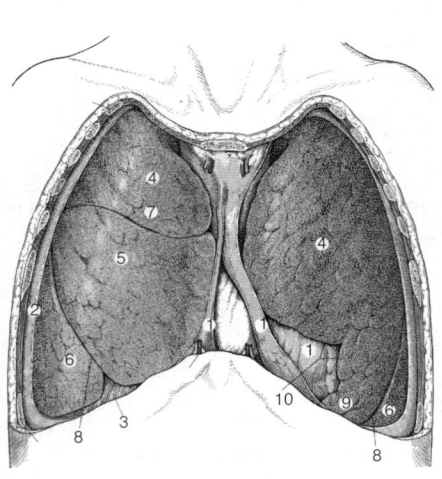

thoracic cavity, frontal view
Brusthöhle, von vorne

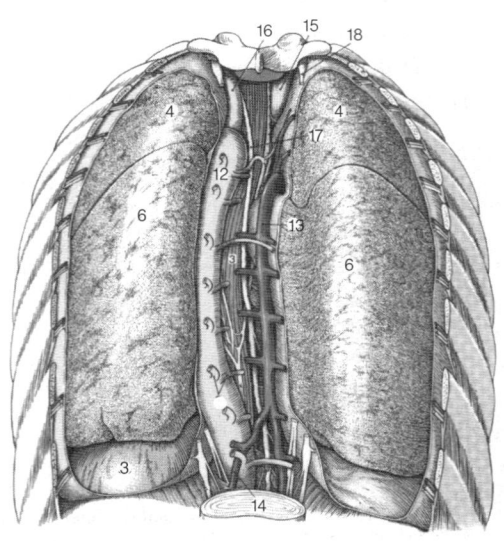

mediastinum, dorsal view
Mediastinum, von dorsal

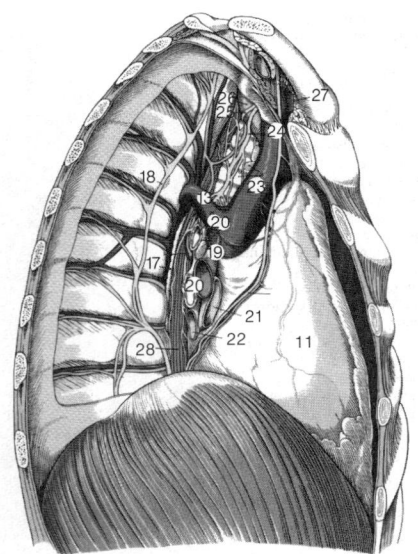

mediastinum, from the right
Mediastinum, von rechts

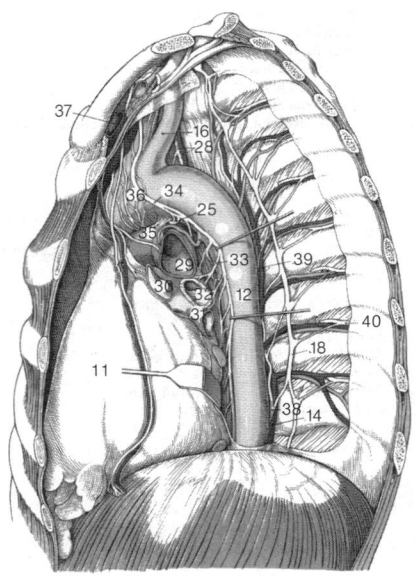

mediastinum, from the left
Mediastinum, von links

Plate V

thoracic cavity, frontal view
mediastinum, dorsal view
mediastinum, from the right
mediastinum, from the left

1 mediastinal pleura
2 costal pleura
3 diaphragmatic pleura
4 superior lobe
5 middle lobe
6 inferior lobe
7 horizontal fissure
8 oblique fissure
9 lingula of left lung
10 cardiac notch of left lung
11 pericardium
12 thoracic aorta
13 azygos vein
14 hemiazygos vein
15 brachiocephalic trunk
16 left subclavian artery
17 thoracic duct
18 sympathetic trunk
19 right pulmonary artery
20 right main bronchus

21 right superior pulmonary vein
22 right inferior pulmonary vein
23 superior vena cava
24 right vagus (nerve)
25 recurrent laryngeal nerve
26 right subclavian artery
27 right subclavian vein
28 esophagus, gullet
29 left pulmonary artery
30 left superior pulmonary vein
31 left inferior pulmonary vein
32 left main bronchus

33 bronchial branches of vagus (nerve)
34 left vagus (nerve)
35 ligament of Botallo
36 arch of aorta
37 left subclavian vein
38 greater splanchnic nerve
39 accessory hemiazygos vein
40 intercostal nerve

Tafel V

Brusthöhle, von vorne
Mediastinum, von dorsal
Mediastinum, von rechts
Mediastinum, von links

1 Pleura mediastinalis, Pars mediastinalis
2 Rippenfell, Pleura costalis, Pars costalis
3 Pleura diaphragmatica, Pars diaphragmatica
4 Oberlappen, Lobus superior
5 Mittellappen, Lobus medius (pulmonis dextri)
6 Unterlappen, Lobus inferior
7 Fissura horizontalis (pulmonis dextri)
8 Fissura obliqua
9 Lingula pulmonis sinistri
10 Inc. cardiaca (pulmonis dextri)
11 Herzbeutel, Perikard, Pericardium
12 Brustaorta, Aorta thoracica, Pars thoracica aortae
13 Azygos, V. azygos
14 Hemiazygos, V. hemiazygos
15 Truncus brachiocephalicus
16 linke Subklavia, A. subclavia sinistra
17 Brustmilchgang, Ductus thoracicus
18 Grenzstrang, Truncus sympatheticus
19 rechte Pulmonalis/Pulmonalarterie, A. pulmonalis dextra
20 rechter Hauptbronchus/Stammbronchus, Bronchus principalis dexter

21 rechte obere Lungenvene, V. pulmonalis dextra superior
22 rechte untere Lungenvene, V. pulmonalis dextra inferior
23 obere Hohlvene/Kava, Kava superior, Vena cava superior
24 rechter Vagus, N. vagus dexter
25 Rekurrens, N. laryngealis recurrens
26 rechte Subklavia, A. subclavia dextra
27 V. subclavia dextra
28 Speiseröhre, Ösophagus, Oesophagus
29 linke Pulmonalis/Pulmonalarterie, A. pulmonalis sinistra
30 linke obere Lungenvene, V. pulmonalis sinistra superior
31 linke untere Lungenvene, V. pulmonalis sinistra inferior
32 linker Hauptbronchus/Stammbronchus, Bronchus principalis sinister

33 Bronchialäste des N. vagus, Rami bronchiales n. vagi
34 linker Vagus, N. vagus sinister
35 Botalli'-Ligament, Lig. arteriosum
36 Aortenbogen, Arcus aortae
37 V. subclavia sinistra
38 Splanchnikus major, N. splanchnicus major
39 Hemiazygos accessoria, V. hemiazygos accessoria
40 Interkostalnerv, N. intercostalis, Ramus intercostalis

Plate VI   Tafel VI   A18

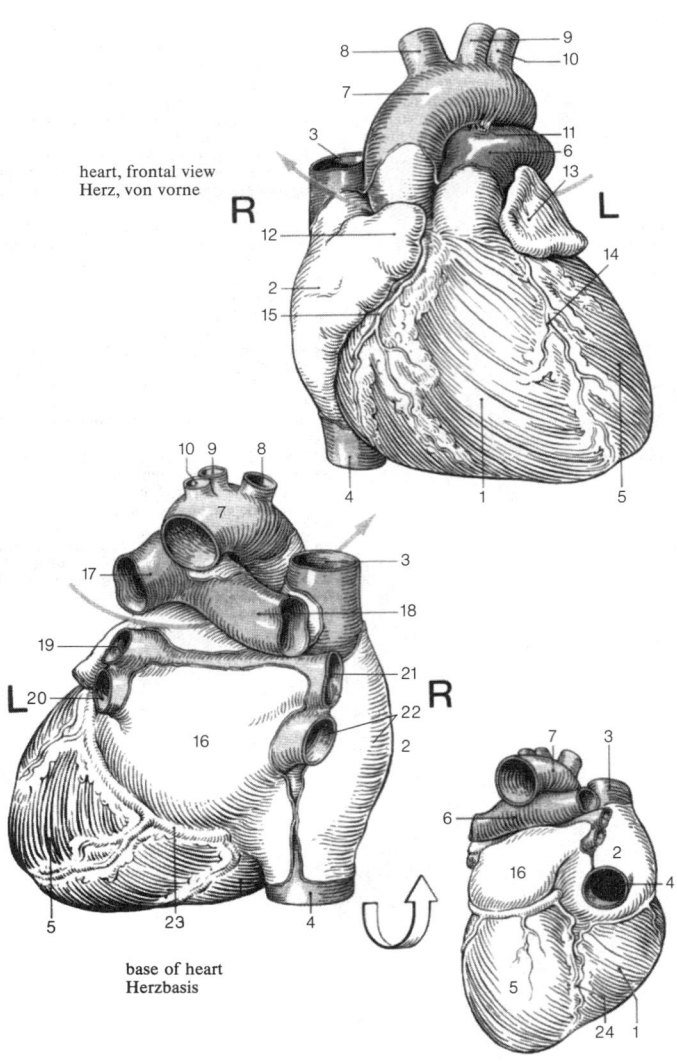

heart, frontal view
Herz, von vorne

base of heart
Herzbasis

heart, from below
Herz, von unten

Tafel VI

Herz, von vorne

Herzbasis

Herz, von unten

 1 rechte (Herz-)Kammer, rechter Ventrikel, Ventriculus dexter
 2 rechter Vorhof, rechtes Atrium, Atrium dextrum
 3 obere Hohlvene/Kava, Kava superior, V. cava superior
 4 untere Hohlvene/Kava, Kava inferior, V. cava inferior
 5 linke (Herz-)Kammer, linker Ventrikel, Ventriculus sinister
 6 Truncus pulmonalis
 7 Aortenbogen, Arcus aortae
 8 Truncus brachiocephalicus
 9 linke Karotis communis, A. carotis communis sinistra
10 linke Subklavia, A. subclavia sinistra
11 Botalli'-Ligament, Lig. arteriosum
12 rechtes Herzohr, Auricula dextra
13 linkes Herzohr, Auricula sinistra
14 Sulcus interventricularis anterior
15 Kranzfurche, Sulcus coronarius
16 linker Vorhof, linkes Atrium, Atrium sinistrum
17 linke Pulmonalarterie/Pulmonalis, A. pulmonalis sinistra
18 rechte Pulmonalarterie/Pulmonalis, A. pulmonalis dextra
19 linke obere Lungenvene, V. pulmonalis sinistra superior
20 linke untere Lungenvene, V. pulmonalis sinistra inferior
21 rechte obere Lungenvene, V. pulmonalis dextra superior
22 rechte untere Lungenvene, V. pulmonalis dextra inferior
23 Sinus coronarius
24 Sulcus interventricularis posterior

Plate VI

heart, frontal view

base of heart

heart, from below

 1 right ventricle
 2 right atrium
 3 superior vena cava
 4 inferior vena cava
 5 left ventricle
 6 pulmonary artery/trunk
 7 arch of aorta
 8 brachiocephalic trunk, innominate artery
 9 left common carotid (artery)
10 left subclavian artery
11 ligament of Botallo
12 right auricle
13 left auricle
14 anterior interventricular sulcus
15 coronary sulcus
16 left atrium
17 left pulmonary artery
18 right pulmonary artery
19 left superior pulmonary vein
20 left inferior pulmonary vein
21 right superior pulmonary vein
22 right inferior pulmonary vein
23 coronary sinus
24 posterior interventricular sulcus

Plate VII Tafel VII A20

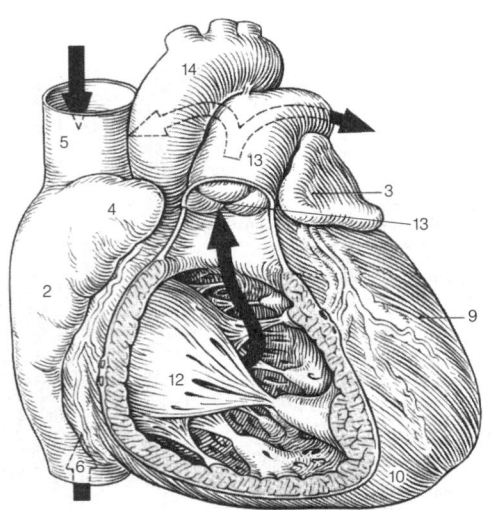

heart, right ventricle
Herz, rechte Kammer

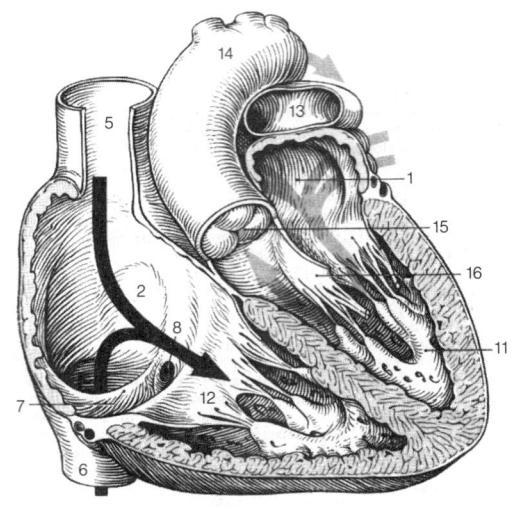

heart, ventricles and atria
Herz, Kammern und Vorhöfe

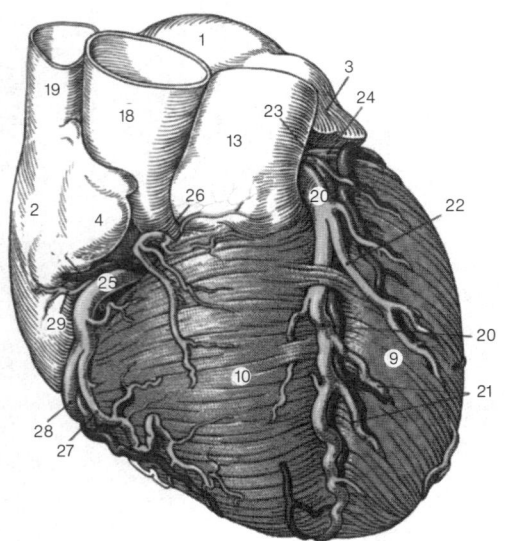

coronary vessels, sternocostal surface
Herzkranzgefäße, Facies sternocostalis

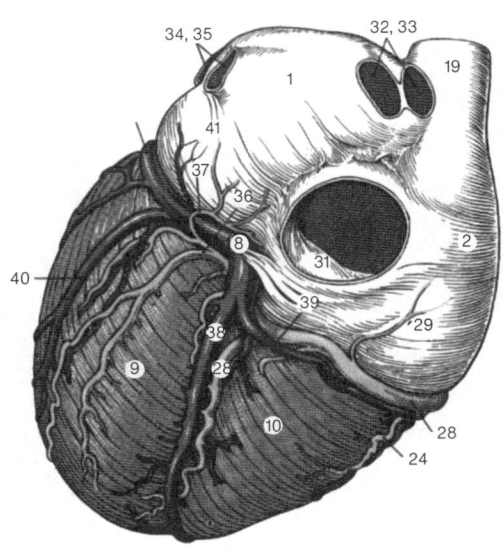

coronary vessels, diaphragmatic surface
Herzkranzgefäße, Facies diaphragmatica

Plate VII

heart, right ventricle

heart, ventricles and atria

coronary vessels, sternocostal surface

coronary vessels, diaphragmatic surface

1 left atrium
2 right atrium
3 left auricle
4 right auricle
5 opening of superior vena cava
6 opening of inferior vena cava
7 eustachian valve, valve of inferior vena cava

8 coronary sinus
9 left ventricle
10 right ventricle
11 trabeculae carneae
12 tricuspid valve, right atrioventricular valve
13 pulmonary artery/trunk
14 aorta
15 aortic valve
16 mitral valve, bicuspid valve, left atrioventricular valve

17 pulmonary valve, valve of pulmonary trunk
18 ascending (part of) aorta
19 superior vena cava
20 anterior interventricular branch
21 septal interventricular branches
22 lateral branch
23 left marginal branch
24 circumflex banch
25 right coronary artery
26 conal artery, conus artery
27 right marginal branch
28 posterior interventricular branch
29 intermediate atrial artery
30 anterior interventricular vein
31 inferior vena cava
32 left superior pulmonary vein
33 left inferior pulmonary vein
34 right superior pulmonary vein
35 right inferior pulmonary vein
36 right posterolateral branch
37 atrioventricular nodal artery
38 coronary sinus
39 posterior interventricular vein
40 small cardiac vein
41 posterior vein of left ventricle
42 oblique vein of left atrium

Tafel VII

Herz, rechte Kammer

Herz, Kammern und Vorhöfe

Herzkranzgefäße, Facies sternocostalis

Herzkranzgefäße, Facies diaphragmatica

1 linker Vorhof, linkes Atrium, Atrium sinistrum
2 rechter Vorhof, rechtes Atrium, Atrium dextrum
3 linkes Herzohr, Auricula sinistra
4 rechtes Herzohr, Auricula dextra
5 Ostium venae cavae superioris
6 Ostium venae cavae inferioris
7 Eustachio'-Klappe, Sylvius'-Klappe, Valvula v. cavae inferioris
8 Sinus coronarius
9 linke (Herz-)Kammer, linker Ventrikel, Ventriculus sinister
10 rechte (Herz-)Kammer, rechter Ventrikel, Ventriculus dexter
11 Trabeculae carneae
12 Trikuspidalklappe, Trikuspidalis, Valva tricuspidalis, Valva atrioventricularis dextra
13 Truncus pulmonalis
14 Aorta
15 Aortenklappe, Valva aortae
16 Mitralklappe, Mitralis, Bikuspidalklappe, Valva mitralis, Valva atrioventricularis sinistra
17 Pulmonalklappe, Valva trunci pulmonalis
18 aufsteigende Aorta, Aorta ascendens, Pars ascendens aortae
19 obere Hohlvene/Kava, Kava superior, V. cava superior
20 Ramus interventricularis anterior *abbr.* RIVA
21 Rami interventriculares septales
22 Ramus lateralis
23 Ramus marginalis sinister
24 Ramus circumflexus
25 rechte Kranzschlagader/Koronararterie, A. coronaria dextra
26 Ramus coni arteriosi
27 Ramus marginalis dexter
28 Ramus interventricularis posterior
29 Ramus atrialis intermedius
30 V. interventricularis anterior
31 untere Hohlvene/Kava, Kava inferior, V. cava inferior
32 linke obere Lungenvene, V. pulmonalis sinistra superior
33 linke untere Lungenvene, V. pulmonalis sinistra inferior
34 rechte obere Lungenvene, V. pulmonalis dextra superior
35 rechte untere Lungenvene, V. pulmonalis dextra inferior
36 Ramus posterolateralis dexter
37 Ramus nodi atrioventricularis
38 V. interventricularis posterior
39 V. cardiaca parva
40 V. ventriculi sinistri posterior
41 V. obliqua atrii sinistri

Plate VIII   Tafel VIII   A22

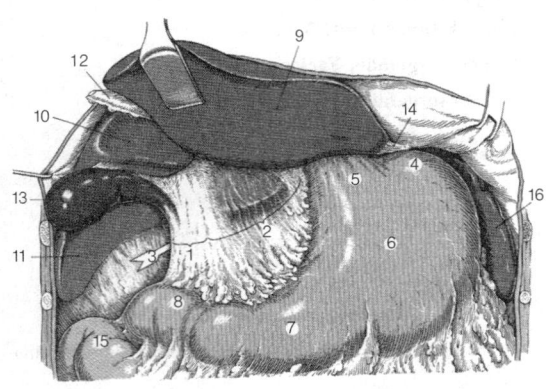

upper abdominal organs I
Oberbauchorgane I

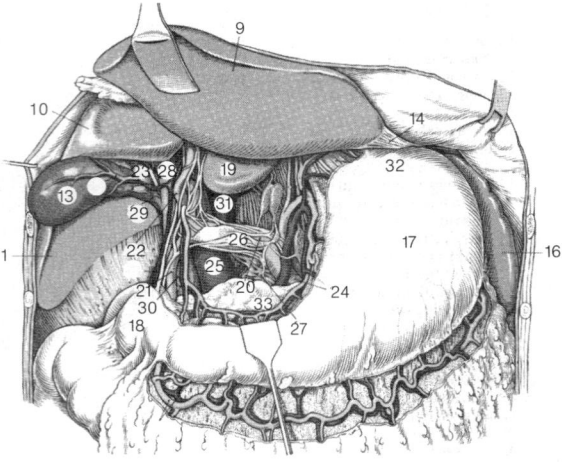

upper abdominal organs II
Oberbauchorgane II

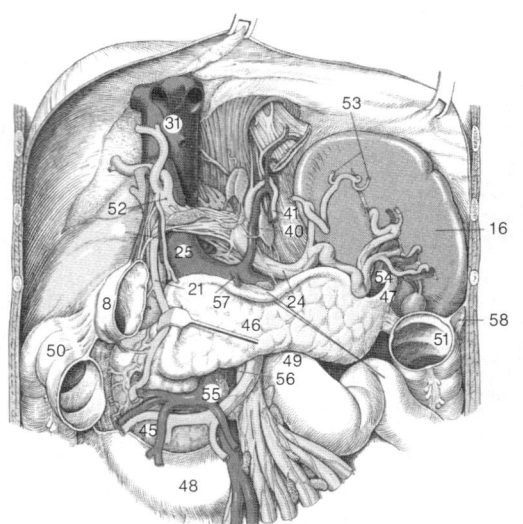

upper abdominal organs III
Oberbauchorgane III

upper abdominal organs IV
Oberbauchorgane IV

Plate VIII

upper abdominal organs I

upper abdominal organs II

upper abdominal organs III

upper abdominal organs IV

1 hepatoduodenal ligament
2 hepatogastric ligament
3 epiploic foramen, omental foramen
4 gastric fundus, fundus of stomach
5 cardia, cardiac part of stomach
6 gastric body, body of stomach
7 pyloric part of stomach
8 superior part of duodenum
9 left lobe of liver
10 quadrate lobe of liver
11 right lobe of liver
12 round ligament of liver
13 gallbladder
14 fibrous appendix of liver
15 right colic flexure, hepatic flexure of colon
16 spleen
17 stomach
18 duodenal ampulla/cap, ampulla of duodenum
19 caudate lobe of liver, spigelian lobe, Spigelius' lobe
20 common hepatic artery
21 gastroduodenal artery
22 left branch of proper hepatic artery
23 right branch of proper hepatic artery
24 splenic artery
25 portal vein
26 gastric plexus
27 celiac plexus, solar plexus
28 common hepatic duct
29 cystic duct, duct of gallbladder
30 choledochal duct, biliary duct, common bile duct *abbr.* CBD
31 inferior vena cava
32 abdominal part of esophagus
33 pancreas
34 right hepatic duct
35 left hepatic duct
36 left branch of portal vein (transverse part)
37 left branch of portal vein (umbilical part)
38 cystic vein
39 esophageal hiatus
40 left gastric vein
41 left gastric artery
42 anterior vagal trunk
43 posterior vagal trunk
44 hepatic plexus
45 head of pancreas
46 body of pancreas
47 tail of pancreas
48 inferior part of duodenum
49 duodenojejunal flexure, duodenal flexure
50 transverse colon
51 descending colon
52 proper hepatic artery
53 short gastric arteries
54 splenic vein
55 superior mesenteric vein
56 superior mesenteric artery

57 accessory pancreatic vein
58 phrenicocolic ligament

Tafel VIII

Oberbauchorgane I

Oberbauchorgane II

Oberbauchorgane III

Oberbauchorgane IV

1 Lig. hepatoduodenale
2 Lig. hepatogastricum
3 For. omentale/epiploicum
4 Magengrund, Fundus, Fundus gastricus/ventricularis
5 Kardia, Pars cardiaca
6 Magenkörper, Korpus, Corpus gastricum/ventriculare
7 Pars pylorica
8 Pars superior duodeni
9 linker Leberlappen, Lobus hepatis sinister
10 viereckiger Leberlappen, Lobus quadratus
11 rechter Leberlappen, Lobus hepatis dexter
12 rundes Leberband, Lig. teres hepatis
13 Gallenblase, Vesica biliaris/fellea
14 Appendix fibrosa hepatis
15 rechte Kolonflexur, Flexura coli dextra
16 Milz, Lien, Splen
17 Magen, Gaster, Ventriculus
18 Ampulla duodeni
19 Spieghel'-Leberlappen, Lobus caudatus
20 Hepatika/Hepatica communis, A. hepatica communis
21 Gastroduodenalis, A. gastroduodenalis
22 Ramus sinister a. hepaticae propriae
23 Ramus dexter a. hepaticae propriae
24 Milzschlagader, Lienalis, A. lienalis/splenica
25 Pfortader, V. portae hepatis
26 Plexus gastrici
27 Sonnengeflecht, Plexus solaris, Plexus coeliacus
28 Hauptgallengang, Ductus hepaticus communis
29 Gallenblasengang, Zystikus, Ductus cysticus
30 Choledochus, Ductus choledochus/biliaris
31 untere Hohlvene/Kava, Kava inferior, V. cava inferior
32 Bauchabschnitt der Speiseröhre, Pars abdominalis oesophagi
33 Bauchspeicheldrüse, Pankreas, Pancreas
34 Ductus hepaticus dexter
35 Ductus hepaticus sinister
36 Ramus sinister v. portae (Pars transversa)
37 Ramus sinister v. portae (Pars umbilicalis)
38 Gallenblasenvene, V. cystica
39 Hiatus oesophageus
40 V. gastrica sinistra
41 linke Magenschlagader, Gastrika sinistra, A. gastrica sinistra
42 vorderer/linker Vagusstamm, Truncus vagalis anterior
43 hinterer/rechter Vagusstamm, Truncus vagalis posterior
44 Plexus hepaticus
45 Pankreaskopf, Caput pancreatis
46 Pankreaskörper, Corpus pancreatis
47 Pankreasschwanz, Cauda pancreatis
48 Pars horizontalis/inferior duodeni
49 Flexura duodenojejunalis
50 Querkolon, Transversum, Colon transversum
51 absteigendes Kolon, Colon descendens
52 Hepatika/Hepatica propria, A. hepatica propria
53 kurze Magenschlagadern, Aa. gastrici breves
54 Milzvene, V. splenica
55 obere Mesenterialvene, V. mesenterica superior
56 obere Mesenterialarterie, Mesenterika superior, A. mesenterica superior
57 V. pancreatica accessoria
58 Lig. phrenicocolicum

Plate IX   Tafel IX   A24

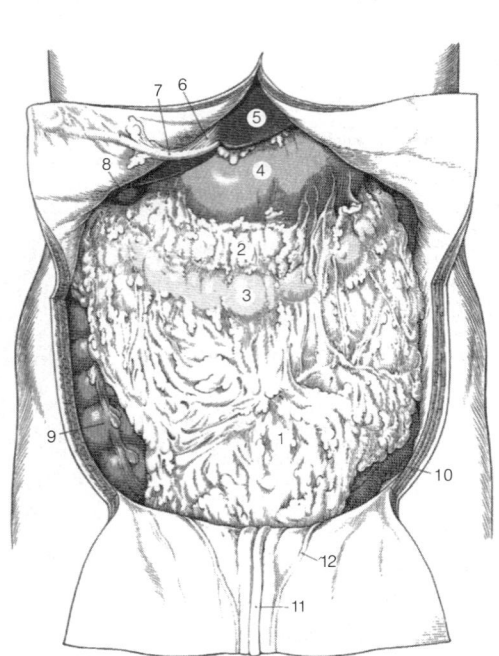

lower abdominal organs I
Unterbauchorgane I

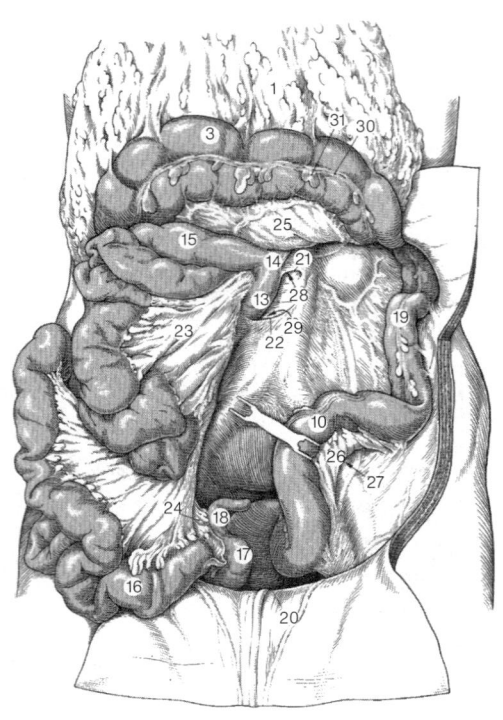

lower abdominal organs II
Unterbauchorgane II

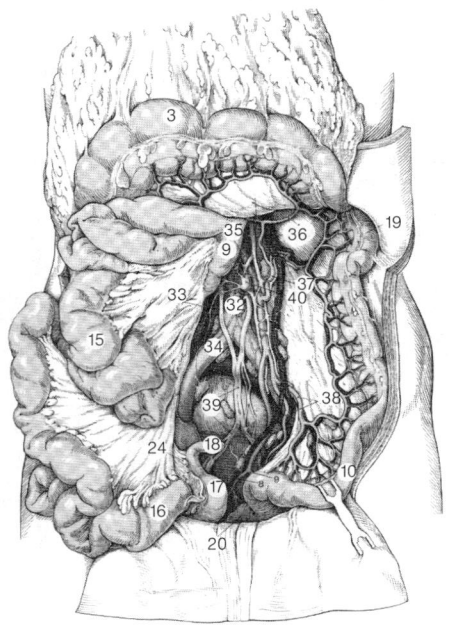

lower abdominal organs III
Unterbauchorgane III

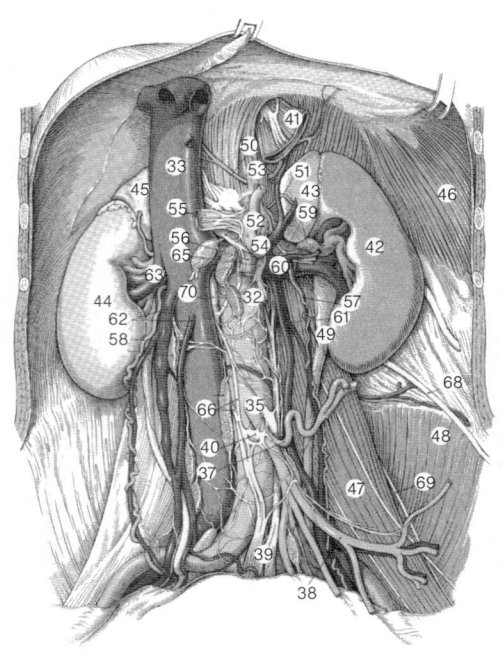

retroperitoneum
Retroperitoneum

Plate IX

lower abdominal organs I

lower abdominal organs II

lower abdominal organs III

retroperitoneum

1 greater omentum, gastrocolic omentum
2 gastrocolic ligament
3 transverse colon
4 stomach
5 left lobe of liver
6 falciform ligament (of liver), broad ligament of liver
7 round ligament of liver
8 gallbladder
9 ascending colon
10 sigmoid colon
11 median umbilical fold, middle umbilical fold, urachal fold
12 medial umbilical fold
13 ascending part of duodenum
14 duodenojejunal flexure
15 jejunum
16 ileum
17 cecum, blind gut
18 vermiform appendix/appendage/process, vermix, *inf.* appendix
19 descending colon
20 rectum
21 superior duodenal fold
22 inferior duodenal fold
23 mesentery
24 mesoappendix, mesentery of the appendix
25 transverse mesocolon
26 sigmoid mesocolon, pelvic mesocolon
27 intersigmoid recess
28 superior duodenal recess/fossa, duodenojejunal recess/fossa, Jonnesco's fossa
29 inferior duodenal recess/fossa, Gruber-Landzert fossa
30 free band of colon
31 epiploic appendices/appendages, omental appendices/appendages
32 abdominal aorta
33 inferior vena cava
34 right common iliac artery
35 inferior mesenteric artery

36 inferior mesenteric vein
37 left colic artery
38 sigmoid arteries
39 superior hypogastric plexus, presacral nerve, Latarjet's nerve

40 inferior mesenteric plexus
41 esophagus, gullet
42 left kidney
43 left suprarenal gland/body, left adrenal gland/body
44 right kidney
45 right suprarenal gland/body, right adrenal gland/body
46 diaphragm
47 greater psoas muscle, psoas major (muscle)
48 iliac muscle, iliacus (muscle)
49 ureter
50 inferior phrenic artery
51 middle suprarenal artery

52 celiac trunk/artery, Haller's tripod
53 left gastric artery
54 splenic artery, lienal artery
55 common hepatic artery
56 superior mesenteric artery
57 left ovarian artery
58 right ovarian artery
59 left renal artery
60 left renal vein
61 left ovarian vein
62 right ovarian vein
63 right renal vein
64 celiac plexus, solar plexus
65 superior mesenteric plexus
66 lumbar splanchnic nerves

67 subcostal nerve
68 iliohypogastric nerve
69 ilioinguinal nerve
70 chyle cistern, cistern of Pecquet, chylocyst

Tafel IX

Unterbauchorgane I

Unterbauchorgane II

Unterbauchorgane III

Retroperitoneum

1 großes Netz, Darmnetz, Omentum majus
2 Lig. gastrocolicum
3 Querkolon, Transversum, Colon transversum
4 Magen, Gaster, Ventriculus
5 linker Leberlappen, Lobus hepatis sinister
6 sichelförmiges Leberband, Lig. falciforme (hepatis)
7 rundes Leberband, Lig. teres hepatis
8 Gallenblase, Vesica biliaris/fellea
9 aufsteigendes Kolon, Colon ascendens
10 Sigma, Sigmoid, Colon sigmoideum
11 Plica umbilicalis mediana
12 Plica umbilicalis medialis
13 Pars ascendens duodeni
14 Flexura duodenojejunalis
15 Leerdarm, Intestinum tenue, Jejunum
16 Krummdarm, Intestinum ileum, Ileum
17 Blinddarm, Zäkum, Zökum, Intestinum caecum, Caecum
18 Wurmfortsatz, *inf.* Wurm, *inf.* Blinddarm, Appendix vermiformis
19 absteigendes Kolon, Colon descendens
20 Mastdarm, Enddarm, Rektum, Rectum
21 Plica duodenalis superior, Plica duodenojejunalis
22 Plica duodenalis inferior, Plica duodenomesocolica
23 Dünndarmgekröse, Mesostenium, Mesenterium
24 Meso-appendix
25 Meso(kolon) des Querkolons, Mesocolon transversum
26 Meso(kolon) des Sigmas, Mesosigma, Mesocolon sigmoideum
27 Rec. intersigmoideus
28 Rec. duodenalis superior

29 Rec. duodenalis inferior
30 freie Kolontänie, Taenia libera
31 Appendices epiploicae/omentales

32 Bauchaorta, Aorta abdominalis, Pars abdominalis aortae
33 untere Hohlvene/Kava, Kava inferior, V. cava inferior
34 rechte Iliaka communis, A. iliaca communis dextra
35 untere Mesenterialarterie, Mesenterika inferior, A. mesenterica inferior
36 untere Mesenterialvene, V. mesenterica inferior
37 linke Kolonschlagader, A. colica sinistra
38 Sigmaarterien, Aa. sigmoideae
39 Präsakralnerv, Plexus hypogastricus superior, N. pr(a)esacralis
40 Plexus mesentericus inferior
41 Speiseröhre, Ösophagus, Oesophagus
42 linke Niere
43 linke Nebenniere
44 rechte Niere
45 rechte Nebenniere
46 Zwerchfell, Diaphragma (thoraco-abdominale)
47 Psoas major, M. psoas major
48 Darmbeinmuskel, Iliakus, M. iliacus
49 Harnleiter, Ureter
50 untere Zwerchfellarterie, A. phrenica inferior
51 Suprarenalis/Adrenalis media, A. suprarenalis/adrenalis media
52 Truncus coeliacus
53 linke Magenschlagader, Gastrika sinistra, A. gastrica sinistra
54 Milzschlagader, Lienalis, A. lienalis/splenica
55 Hepatika/Hepatica communis, A. hepatica communis
56 obere Mesenterialarterie, Mesenterika superior, A. mesenterica superior
57 linke Eierstockschlagader, A. ovarica sinistra
58 rechte Eierstockschlagader, A. ovarica dextra
59 linke Nierenschlagader, A. renalis sinistra
60 linke Nierenvene, V. renalis sinistra
61 linke Eierstockvene, V. ovarica sinistra
62 rechte Eierstockvene, V. ovarica dextra
63 rechte Nierenvene, V. renalis dextra
64 Sonnengeflecht, Plexus solaris, Plexus coeliacus
65 Plexus mesentericus superior
66 lumbale Eingeweidenerven, Nn. splanchnici lumbales/lumbares
67 Subkostalis, N. subcostalis
68 Iliohypogastrikus, N. iliohypogastricus
69 Ilioinguinalis, N. ilio-inguinalis
70 Cisterna chyli

Plate X / Tafel X — A26

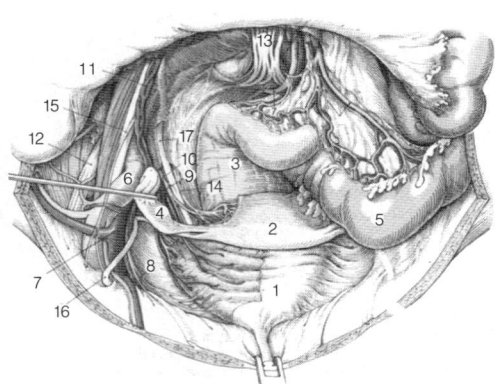

female pelvic organs, from above
weibliche Beckenorgane, von oben

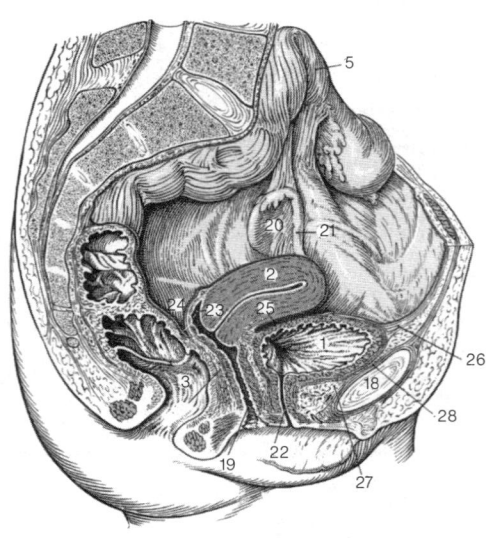

female pelvic organs, median section
weibliches Becken, Medianschnitt

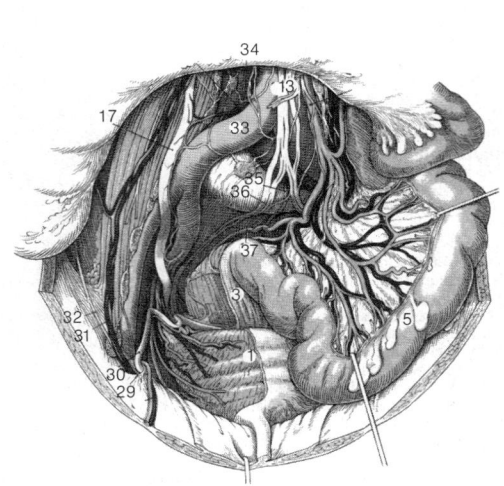

male pelvic organs, from above
männliche Beckenorgane, von oben

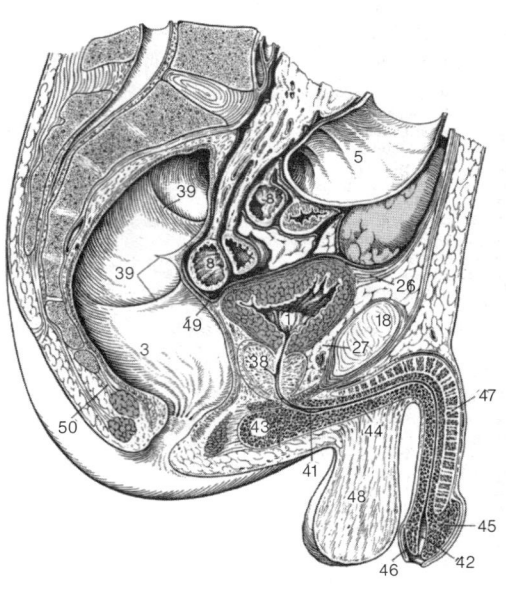

male pelvic organs, median section
männliches Becken, Medianschnitt

Plate X

female pelvic organs, from above

female pelvic organs, median section

male pelvic organs, from above

male pelvic organs, median section

1 urinary bladder, bladder
2 womb, metra, uterus
3 rectum
4 ovary
5 sigmoid colon
6 right external iliac artery
7 right external iliac vein
8 superior vesical arteries
9 inferior vesical artery
10 uterine artery
11 ovarian artery and vein
12 femoral nerve
13 superior hypogastric plexus, presacral nerve, Latarjet's nerve
14 uterovaginal plexus
15 genitofemoral nerve, genitocrural nerve
16 round ligament of uterus, Hunter's ligament
17 ureter
18 interpubic disk
19 vagina
20 left ovary
21 left uterine tube, left fallopian tube, left salpinx
22 urethra
23 fornix of vagina, fundus of vagina
24 Douglas' space/pouch/cul-de-sac, rectouterine pouch/excavation, rectovaginal pouch, rectovaginouterine pouch
25 vesicouterine pouch, uterovesical pouch
26 urachus
27 Retzius' cavity/space, retropubic space
28 pubovesical ligament
29 deep/internal inguinal ring
30 deferent duct/canal, spermatic duct, testicular duct
31 testicular artery with pampiniform plexus
32 ilioinguinal nerve
33 right common iliac artery
34 inferior vena cava
35 median/middle sacral artery
36 right hypogastric nerve
37 superior rectal artery, superior hemorrhoidal artery
38 prostate (gland)
39 transverse rectal folds, rectal valves, Houston's folds/valves, Kohlrausch's valves
40 anal canal
41 spongy/penile urethra, spongy part of male urethra
42 Morgagni's fossa/fovea, navicular fossa of urethra
43 bulb of penis, bulb of urethra
44 spongy body of penis, spongy body of (male) urethra
45 balanus, glans penis
46 foreskin, prepuce (of penis)
47 cavernous body of penis
48 scrotal septum
49 Proust's space, rectovesical pouch/excavation
50 anococcygeal ligament/body, Symington's (anococcygeal) body

Tafel X

weibliche Beckenorgane, von oben

weibliches Becken, Medianschnitt

männliche Beckenorgane, von oben

männliches Becken, Medianschnitt

1 Harnblase, Blase, Vesica urinaria
2 Gebärmutter, Metra, Uterus
3 Mastdarm, Enddarm, Rektum, Rectum
4 Eierstock, Ovarium
5 Sigma, Sigmoid, Colon sigmoideum
6 rechte Iliaka externa, A. iliaca externa dextra
7 V. iliaca externa dextra
8 obere Blasenschlagadern, Aa. vesicales superiores
9 untere Blasenschlagader, A. vesicalis inferior
10 Gebärmutterschlagader, Uterina, A. uterina
11 Eierstockschlagader und -vene
12 N. femoralis
13 Präsakralnerv, Plexus hypogastricus superior, N. pr(a)esacralis
14 Plexus uterovaginalis
15 Genitofemoralis, N. genitofemoralis
16 Hunter'-Band, rundes Mutterband, Lig. teres uteri
17 Harnleiter, Ureter
18 Discus interpubicus
19 Scheide, Vagina
20 linker Eierstock, Ovarium sinistrum
21 linker Eileiter, linke Tube, Tuba uterina sinistra
22 Harnröhre, Urethra
23 Scheidengewölbe, Fornix vaginae
24 Douglas'-Raum, Excavatio recto-uterina

25 vorderer Douglas'-Raum, Excavatio vesico-uterina
26 Harngang, Urachus
27 Retzius'-Raum, Spatium retropubicum
28 Lig. pubovesicale
29 innerer Leistenring, Anulus inguinalis profundus
30 Samenleiter, Ductus deferens
31 A. testicularis mit Plexus pampiniformis
32 Ilioinguinalis, N. ilioinguinalis
33 rechte Iliaka communis, A. iliaca communis dextra
34 untere Hohlvene/Kava, Kava inferior, V. cava inferior
35 mittlere Kreuzbeinschlagader, A. sacralis mediana
36 N. hypogastricus dexter
37 obere Rektumschlagader, A. rectalis superior
38 Vorsteherdrüse, Prostata
39 Plicae transversae recti

40 Analkanal, Canalis analis
41 Penisabschnitt der Harnröhre, Pars spongiosa
42 Fossa navicularis urethrae
43 Bulbus penis
44 Harnröhrenschwellkörper, Corpus spongiosum penis
45 Eichel, Glans penis
46 Vorhaut, Präputium, Pr(a)eputium penis
47 Penisschwellkörper, Corpus cavernosum penis
48 Septum scroti/scrotale
49 Proust'-Raum, Excavatio rectovesicalis
50 Lig. anococcygeum

Plate XI Tafel XI A28

aorta, main branches
Aorta, direkte Äste

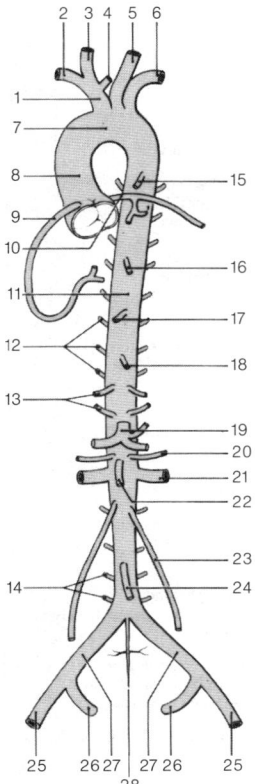

caval and azygos veins
Venae cavae und Azygossystem

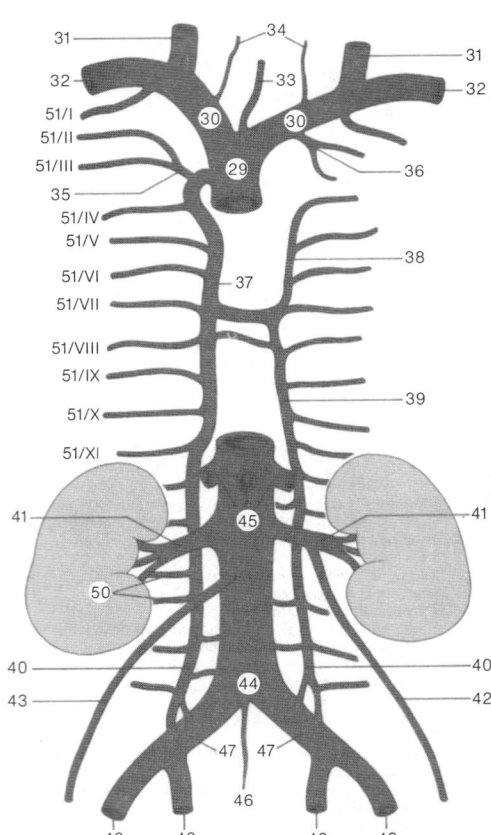

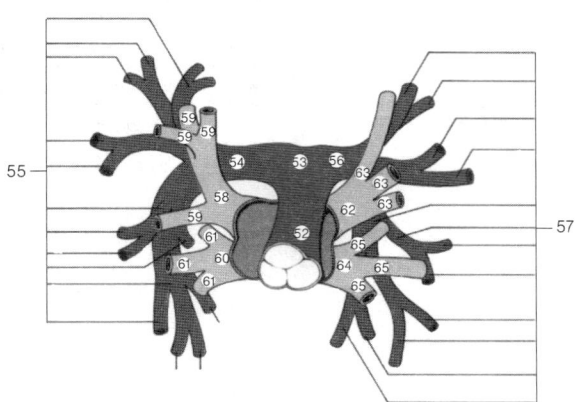

pulmonary trunk and pulmonary veins
Truncus pulmonalis und Venae pulmonales

Plate XI

aorta, main branches

caval and azygos veins

pulmonary trunk and pulmonary veins

1 brachiocephalic trunk, innominate artery
2 right subclavian artery
3 right common carotid (artery)
4 lowest thyroid artery
5 left common carotid (artery)
6 left subclavian artery
7 arch of aorta
8 ascending (part of) aorta
9 right coronary artery

10 left coronary artery

11 descending (part of) aorta
12 posterior intercostal arteries
13 superior phrenic arteries, superior diaphragmatic arteries
14 lumbal arteries
15 bronchial arteries, bronchial branches of thoracic aorta
16 esophageal branches of thoracic aorta
17 pericardiac branches of thoracic aorta
18 mediastinal branches of thoracic aorta
19 celiac trunk, celiac artery/axis
20 middle suprarenal artery, aortic suprarenal artery

21 renal artery, emulgent artery
22 superior mesenteric artery

23 testicular/funicular/ovarian/tubo-ovarian artery
24 inferior mesenteric artery

25 external iliac artery, anterior iliac artery
26 internal iliac artery, hypogastric artery
27 common iliac artery
28 median/middle sacral artery, coccygeal/sacrococcygeal artery
29 superior vena cava
30 (right/left) brachiocephalic vein, (right/left) innominate vein
31 internal jugular (vein)
32 subclavian vein
33 inferior thyroid veins
34 thymic veins
35 right superior intercostal vein
36 left superior intercostal vein
37 azygos (vein)
38 accessory hemiazygos (vein)
39 hemiazygos (vein)
40 ascending lumbar vein
41 renal vein
42 left testicular/ovarian vein

43 right testicular/ovarian vein

44 inferior vena cava
45 hepatic veins
46 median/middle sacral vein
47 common iliac vein
48 internal iliac vein, hypogastric vein
49 external iliac vein
50 lumbar veins
51/I - XI posterior intercostal veins I - XI
52 pulmonary trunk, pulmonary/venous artery
53 bifurcation of (the) pulmonary trunk
54 right pulmonary artery
55 pulmonary branches of right pulmonary artery
56 left pulmonary artery
57 pulmonary branches of left pulmonary artery
58 right superior pulmonary vein
59 pulmonary branches of right superior pulmonary vein
60 right inferior pulmonary vein
61 pulmonary branches of right inferior pulmonary vein
62 left superior pulmonary vein
63 pulmonary branches of left superior pulmonary vein
64 left inferior pulmonary vein
65 pulmonary branches of left inferior pulmonary vein

Tafel XI

Aorta, direkte Äste

Venae cavae und Azygossystem

Truncus pulmonalis und Venae pulmonales

1 Truncus brachiocephalicus
2 rechte Subklavia, A. subclavia dextra
3 rechte Karotis/Carotis communis, A. carotis communis dextra
4 unterste Schilddrüsenschlagader, A. thyroidea ima
5 linke Karotis/Carotis communis, A. carotis communis sinistra
6 linke Subklavia, A. subclavia sinistra
7 Aortenbogen, Arcus aortae
8 aufsteigende Aorta, Aorta ascendens, Pars ascendens aortae
9 rechte Herzkranzschlagader/Koronararterie, A. coronaria dextra
10 linke Herzkranzschlagader/Koronararterie, A. coronaria sinistra
11 absteigende Aorta, Aorta descendens, Pars descendens aortae
12 hintere Interkostalarterien, Aa. intercostales posteriores
13 obere Zwerchfellschlagadern, Aa. phrenicae superiores
14 Lendenschlagadern, Lumbalarterien, Aa. lumbales
15 Bronchialäste, Bronchialarterien, Rami bronchiales
16 Speiseröhrenäste, Rami oesophageales
17 Perikardäste, Rami pericardiaci
18 Mediastinumäste, Rami mediastinales
19 Truncus coeliacus
20 mittlere Nebennierenschlagader, A. suprarenalis/adrenalis media
21 Nierenschlagader, A. renalis
22 obere Mesenterialarterie, Mesenterika superior, A. mesenterica superior
23 Hodenschlagader/Eierstockschlagader, A. testicularis/ovarica
24 untere Mesenterialarterie, Mesenterika inferior, A. mesenterica inferior
25 Iliaka/Iliaca externa, A. iliaca externa
26 Iliaka/Iliaca interna, A. iliaca interna
27 Iliaka/Iliaca communis, A. iliaca communis
28 mittlere Kreuzbeinschlagader, A. sacralis mediana
29 obere Hohlvene/Kava, Kava superior, V. cava superior
30 V. brachiocephalica (dextra/sinistra)
31 Jugularis interna, V. jugularis interna
32 V. subclavia
33 unteren Schilddrüsenvenen, Vv. thyroideae inferiores
34 Thymusvenen, Vv. thymicales
35 V. intercostalis superior dextra
36 V. intercostalis superior sinistra
37 Azygos, V. azygos
38 Hemiazygos accessoria, V. hemiazygos accessoria
39 Hemiazygos, V. hemiazygos
40 V. lumbalis ascendens
41 Nierenvene, V. renalis
42 linke Hodenvene/Eierstockvene, V. testicularis/ovarica sinistra
43 rechte Hodenvene/Eierstockvene, V. testicularis/adrenalis/ovarica dextra
44 untere Hohlvene/Kava, Kava inferior, V. cava inferior
45 Lebervenen, Vv. hepaticae
46 V. sacralis mediana
47 V. iliaca communis
48 V. iliaca interna
49 V. iliaca externa
50 Lenden-, Lumbalvenen, Vv. lumbales
51/I - XI Vv. intercostales posteriores I - XI
52 Truncus pulmonalis
53 Bifurcatio trunci pulmonalis
54 rechte Pulmonalis/Pulmonalarterie, A. pulmonalis dextra
55 Lungenäste der A. pulmonalis dextra
56 linke Pulmonalis/Pulmonalarterie, A. pulmonalis sinistra
57 Lungenäste der A. pulmonalis sinistra
58 rechte obere Lungenvene, V. pulmonalis dextra superior
59 Lungenäste der V. pulmonalis dextra superior
60 rechte untere Lungenvene, V. pulmonalis dextra inferior
61 Lungenäste der V. pulmonalis dextra inferior
62 linke obere Lungenvene, V. pulmonalis sinistra superior
63 Lungenäste der V. pulmonalis sinistra superior
64 linke untere Lungenvene, V. pulmonalis sinistra inferior
65 Lungenäste der V. pulmonalis sinistra inferior

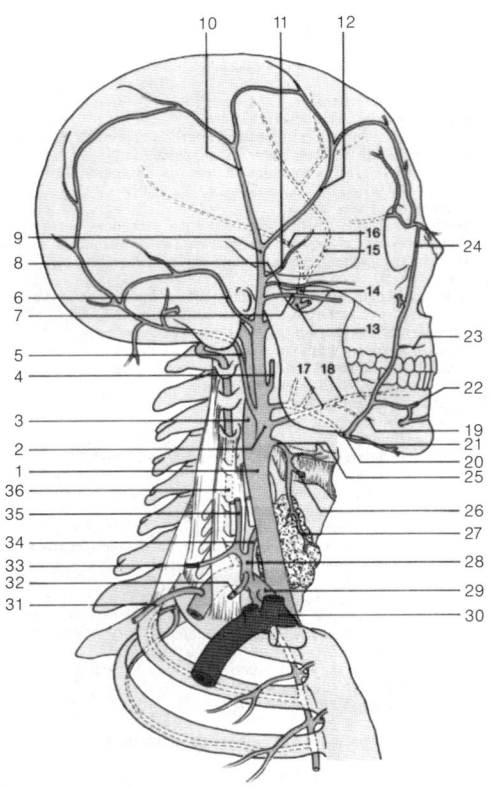

external carotid artery, subclavian artery
A. carotis externa, A. subclavia

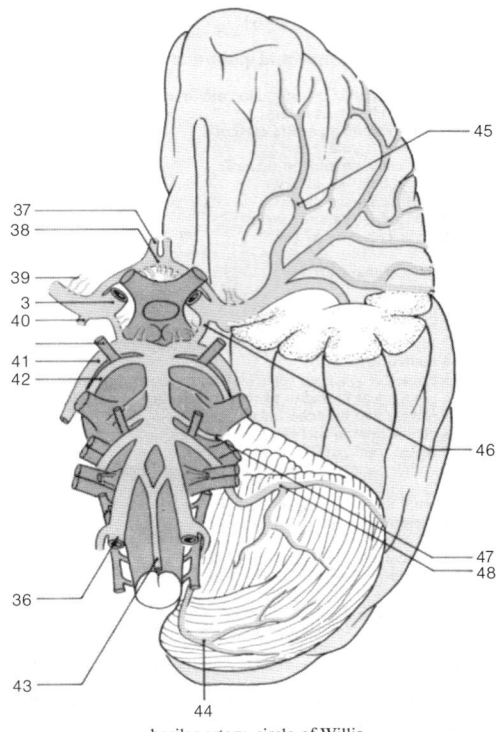

basilar artery, circle of Willis
A. basilaris, Circulus arteriosus cerebri

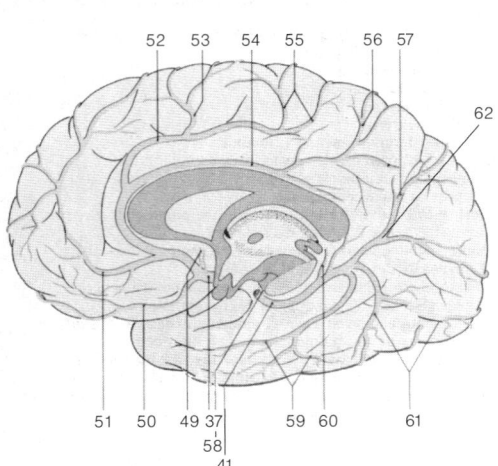

anterior and posterior cerebral artery
A. cerebri anterior, A. cerebri posterior

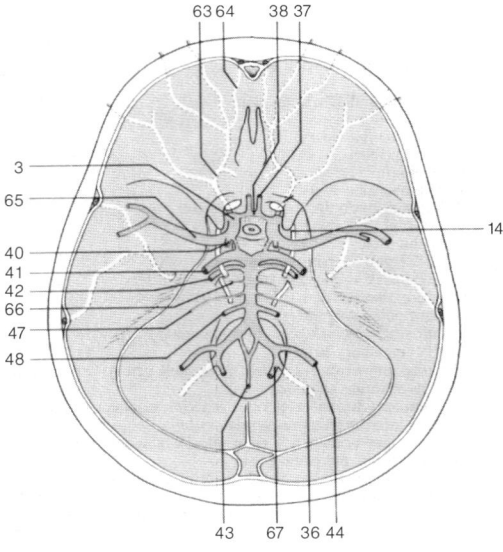

basilar artery, middle cerebral artery
A. basilaris, A. cerebri media

Plate XII

external carotid artery, subclavian artery

basilar artery, middle cerebral artery

anterior and posterior cerebral artery

basilar artery, circle of Willis

 1 common carotid (artery), cephalic artery
 2 external carotid (artery)

 3 internal carotid (artery)

 4 ascending pharyngeal artery
 5 occipital artery
 6 posterior auricular artery
 7 transverse facial artery
 8 zygomatico-orbital artery
 9 superficial temporal artery
10 parietal branch of superficial temporal artery
11 middle temporal artery
12 frontal branch of superficial temporal artery
13 maxillary artery, internal maxillary artery
14 middle meningeal artery

15 frontal branch of middle meningeal artery
16 parietal branch of middle meningeal artery
17 lingual artery
18 deep lingual artery, ranine artery
19 sublingual artery
20 facial artery, external maxillary artery
21 submental artery
22 inferior labial artery
23 superior labial artery
24 angular artery
25 superior thyroid artery

26 superior laryngeal artery

27 anterior (glandular) branch of superior thyroid artery

28 thyrocervical trunk, thyroid axis
29 subclavian artery
30 subclavian vein
31 transverse cervical artery, transverse artery of the neck
32 suprascapular artery, transverse scapular artery
33 descending cervical artery
34 inferior thyroid artery

35 ascending cervical artery
36 vertebral artery
37 anterior cerebral artery
38 anterior communicating artery (of cerebrum)
39 anterolateral central/thalamostriate arteries
40 anterior choroidal artery
41 posterior cerebral artery
42 superior cerebellar artery
43 anterior spinal artery

44 posterior inferior cerebellar artery
45 lateral frontobasal artery, lateral orbitofrontal branch
46 posterior communicating artery (of cerebrum)
47 labyrinthine artery, artery of the labyrinth
48 anterior inferior cerebellar artery
49 anteromedial central/thalamostriate arteries
50 medial frontobasal artery, medial orbitofrontal branch
51 anteromedial frontal branch of callosomarginal artery
52 callosomarginal artery
53 mediomedial frontal branch and posteromedial frontal branch of callosomarginal artery
54 pericallosal artery, postcommunical part
55 paracentral artery
56 precuneal artery, inferior internal parietal artery
57 parieto-occipital artery
58 posterolateral central arteries
59 temporal branches of posterior temporal artery
60 medial posterior choroid branches of posterior cerebral artery
61 occipitotemporal branch of posterior cerebral artery
62 parieto-occipital branch and calcarine branch of posterior cerebral artery
63 ophthalmic artery
64 supratrochlear artery, frontal artery
65 middle cerebral artery, sylvian artery
66 pontine arteries, arteries of the pons
67 posterior spinal artery

Tafel XII

A. carotis externa, A. subclavia

A. basilaris, A. cerebri media

A. cerebri anterior, A. cerebri posterior

A. basilaris, Circulus arteriosus cerebri

 1 Karotis/Carotis communis, A. carotis communis
 2 äußere Kopfschlagader, Karotis/Carotis externa, A. carotis externa
 3 innere Kopfschlagader, Karotis/Carotis interna, A. carotis interna
 4 Pharyngea ascendens, A. pharyngea ascendens
 5 Hinterhaupt(s)schlagader, Okzipitalis, A. occipitalis
 6 Aurikularis posterior, A. auricularis posterior
 7 Transversa faciais, A. transversa faciei/facialis
 8 Zygomaticoorbitalis, A. zygomatico-orbitalis
 9 Temporalis superficialis, A. temporalis superficialis
10 Ramus parietalis der Temporalis superficialis
11 Temporalis media, A. temporalis media
12 Ramus frontalis der Temporalis superficialis
13 Oberkieferschlagader, Maxillaris, A. maxillaris
14 mittlere Hirnhautschlagader, Meningea media, *inf.* Media, A. meningea media
15 Ramus frontalis der Meningea media
16 Ramus parietalis der Meningea media
17 Zungenschlagader, Lingualis, A. lingualis
18 tiefe Zungenschlagader, Profunda linguae, A. profunda linguae
19 Unterzungenschlagader, Sublingualis, A. sublingualis
20 Gesichtsschlagader, Fazialis, A. facialis
21 Unterkinnschlagader, Submentalis, A. submentalis
22 Unterlippenschlagader, Labialis inferior, A. labialis inferior
23 Oberlippenschlagader, Labialis superior, A. labialis superior
24 Angularis, A. angularis
25 obere Schilddrüsenschlagader, Thyroidea superior, A. thyroidea superior
26 obere Kehlkopfschlagader, Laryngea superior, A. laryngea superior
27 vorderer Drüsenast der Thyroidea superior, Ramus glandularis anterior
28 Truncus thyrocervicalis *abbr.* TTC
29 Unterschlüsselbeinschlagader, Subklavia, A. subclavia
30 V. subclavia
31 Transversa colli, A. transversa (colli)
32 Supraskapularis, A. suprascapularis
33 Cervicalis descendens, A. cervicalis descendens
34 untere Schilddrüsenschlagader, Thyroidea inferior, A. thyroidea inferior
35 Cervicalis ascendens, A. cervicalis ascendens
36 Wirbelschlagader, Vertebralis, A. vertebralis
37 Cerebri anterior, A. cerebri anterior
38 Communicans anterior, A. communicans anterior
39 Aa. centrales/thalamostriatae anterolaterales
40 Choroidea anterior, A. choroidea anterior
41 Cerebri posterior, A. cerebri posterior
42 Cerebelli superior, A. superior cerebelli
43 vordere Rückenmark(s)arterie, Spinalis anterior, A. spinalis anterior
44 A. inferior posterior cerebelli
45 A. frontobasalis lateralis, Ramus orbitofrontalis lateralis
46 Communicans posterior, A. communicans posterior
47 Labyrinthschlagader, A. labyrinthi
48 A. inferior anterior cerebelli
49 aa. centrales/thalamostriatae anteromediales
50 A. frontobasalis medialis, Ramus orbitofrontalis medialis
51 Ramus frontalis anteromedialis
52 Callosomarginalis, A. callosomarginalis
53 Ramus frontalis mediomedalis und Ramus frontalis posteromedialis
54 Pericallosa, A. pericallosa, Pars postcommunicalis
55 Paracentralis, A. paracentralis
56 Präcunealis, A. pr(a)ecunealis
57 Parietookzipitalis, A. parieto-occipitalis
58 Aa. centrales posterolaterales
59 Rami temporales der A. cerebri posterior
60 Rami choroidei posteriores mediales der A. cerebri posterior
61 Ramus occipitotemporalis der A. cerebri posterior
62 Ramus parieto-occipitalis und Ramus calcarinus der A. cerebri posterior
63 Augenschlagader, Ophthalmika, A. ophthalmica
64 Supratrochlearis, A. supratrochlearis
65 Cerebri media, *inf.* Media, A. cerebri media
66 Brückenarterien, Aa. pontis
67 hintere Rückenmark(s)arterie, Spinalis posterior, A. spinalis posterior

Plate XIII — Tafel XIII — A32

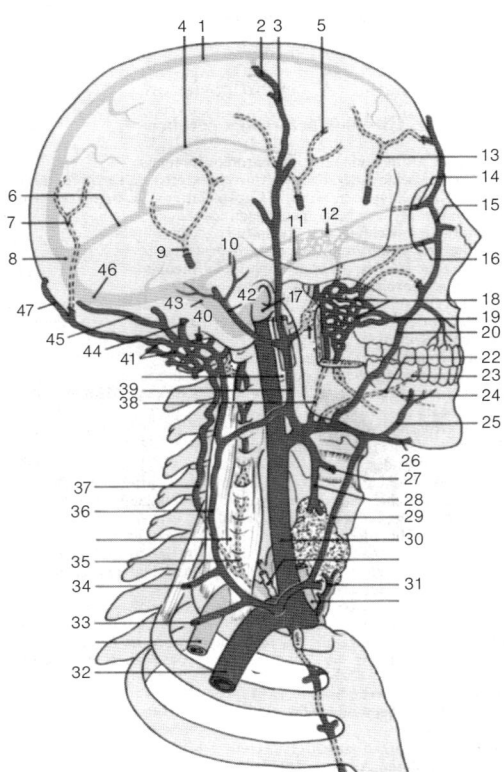

veins of head and neck, sinuses of dura mater
Kopf-, Halsvenen, Sinus durae matris

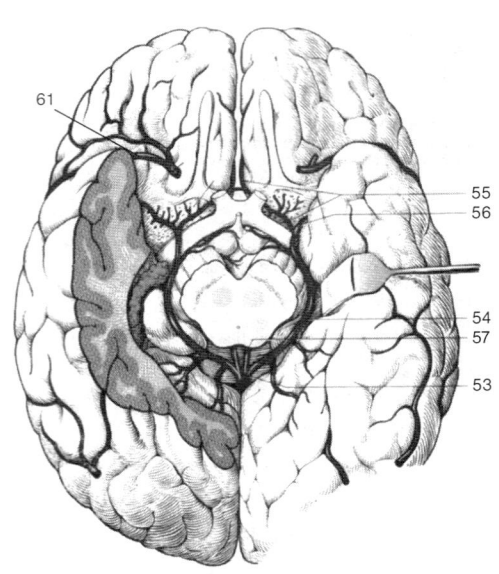

basal veins of the brain
basale Hirnvenen

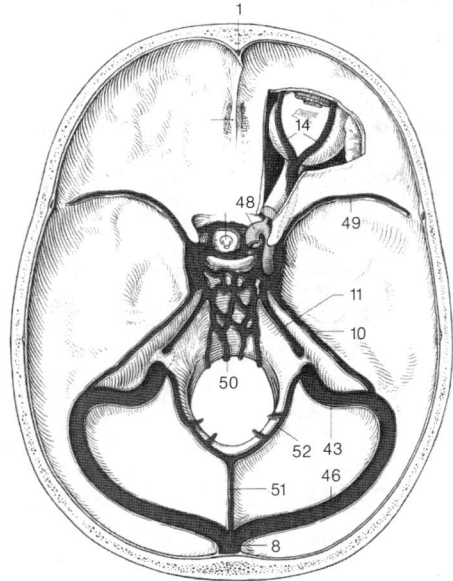

venous sinuses at the base of the cranium
Blutleiter der Schädelbasis

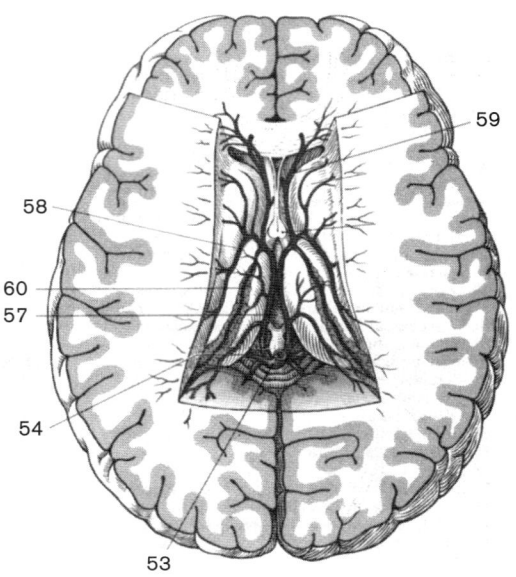

deep veins of the brain, from above
tiefe Hirnvenen, von oben

Plate XIII

veins of head and neck, sinuses of dura mater

venous sinuses at the base of the cranium

basal veins of the brain

deep veins of the brain, from above

1 superior sagittal sinus, superior longitudinal sinus
2 parietal emissary vein, Santorini's vein
3 superficial temporal veins
4 inferior sagittal sinus, inferior longitudinal sinus
5 anterior temporal diploic vein
6 straight sinus, tentorial sinus
7 occipital diploic vein
8 confluence of sinuses
9 posterior temporal diploic vein
10 superior petrosal sinus
11 inferior petrosal sinus, Englisch's sinus
12 cavernous sinus
13 frontal diploic vein
14 superior ophthalmic vein
15 angular vein
16 inferior ophthalmic vein
17 superior bulb of jugular vein, Heister's diverticulum

18 pterygoid plexus
19 deep facial vein
20 facial vein
21 maxillary veins
22 lingual vein
23 deep lingual vein
24 sublingual vein
25 inferior labial veins
26 submental vein
27 superior laryngeal vein
28 superior thyroid vein
29 anterior jugular (vein)

30 internal jugular (vein)

31 inferior thyroid veins
32 subclavian vein
33 suprascapular vein, transverse scapular vein
34 transverse cervical veins, transverse veins of the neck
35 vertebral vein
36 external jugular (vein)

37 deep cervical vein
38 external palatine vein
39 retromandibular vein, posterior facial vein, temporomaxillary vein
40 condylar emissary vein
41 suboccipital venous plexus
42 posterior auricular vein
43 sigmoid sinus
44 mastoid emissary vein
45 occipital vein
46 transverse sinus, lateral sinus
47 occipital emissary vein
48 internal carotid (artery)

49 sphenoparietal sinus, Breschet's sinus
50 basilar plexus
51 occipital sinus
52 marginal sinus
53 great cerebral vein, great vein of Galen
54 basal vein, Rosenthal's vein, basal vein of Rosenthal
55 anterior cerebral veins
56 deep middle cerebral vein
57 internal cerebral veins
58 terminal vein, superior thalamostriate vein
59 anterior vein of septum pellucidum
60 superior choroid artery
61 superficial middle cerebral veins

Tafel XIII

Kopf-, Halsvenen, Sinus durae matris

Blutleiter der Schädelbasis

basale Hirnvenen

tiefe Hirnvenen, von oben

1 oberer Sichelsinus, Sinus sagittalis superior *abbr.* SSS
2 V. emissaria parietalis
3 Vv. temporales superficiales
4 unterer Sichelsinus, Sinus sagittalis inferior
5 V. diploica temporalis anterior
6 Sinus rectus
7 V. diploica occipitalis
8 Confluens sinuum
9 V. diploica temporalis posterior
10 Sinus petrosus superior
11 Sinus petrosus inferior
12 Sinus cavernosus
13 V. diploica frontalis
14 obere Augenvene, V. ophthalmica superior
15 V. angularis
16 untere Augenvene, V. ophthalmica inferior
17 oberer Bulbus der V. jugularis interna, Bulbus superior v. jugularis
18 Plexus pterygoideus
19 tiefe Gesichtsvene, V. profunda faciei/facialis
20 Gesichtsvene, V. facialis
21 Vv. maxillares
22 Zungenvene, V. lingualis
23 tiefe Zungenvene, V. profunda linguae
24 Unterzungenvene, V. sublingualis
25 Unterlippenvenen, Vv. labiales inferiores
26 Unterkinnvene, V. submentalis
27 obere Kehlkopfvene, V. laryngealis superior
28 obere Schilddrüsenvene, V. thyroidea superior
29 vordere Drosselvene/Jugularvene, Jugularis anterior, V. jugularis anterior
30 innere Drosselvene/Jugularvene, Jugularis interna, V. jugularis interna
31 untere Schilddrüsenvenen, Vv. thyroideae inferiores
32 V. subclavia
33 V. suprascapularis
34 Vv. transversae cervicis
35 Wirbelvene, V. vertebralis
36 äußere Drosselvene/Jugularvene, Jugularis externa, V. jugularis externa
37 V. cervicalis profunda
38 V. palatina externa
39 V. retromandibularis
40 V. emissaria condylaris
41 Plexus venosus suboccipitalis
42 V. auricularis posterior
43 Sinus sigmoideus
44 V. emissaria mastoidea
45 Hinterhauptsvene, V. occipitalis
46 Sinus transversus
47 V. emissaria occipitalis
48 innere Kopfschlagader, Karotis/Carotis interna, A. carotis interna
49 Sinus sphenoparietalis
50 Plexus basilaris
51 Sinus occipitalis
52 Sinus marginalis
53 große Hirnvene, Galen'-Vene, V. magna cerebri
54 Rosenthal'-Vene, V. basalis
55 vordere Hirnvenen, Vv. anteriores cerebri
56 V. media profunda cerebri
57 innere Hirnvenen, Vv. internae cerebri
58 Terminalis, V. thalamostriata superior, V. terminalis
59 V. anterior septi pellucidi
60 V. choroidea superior
61 Vv. mediae superficiales cerebri

Plate XIV **Tafel XIV** A34

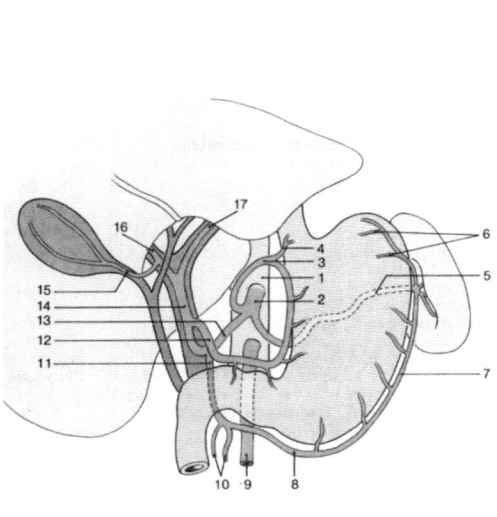

celiac trunk
Truncus coeliacus

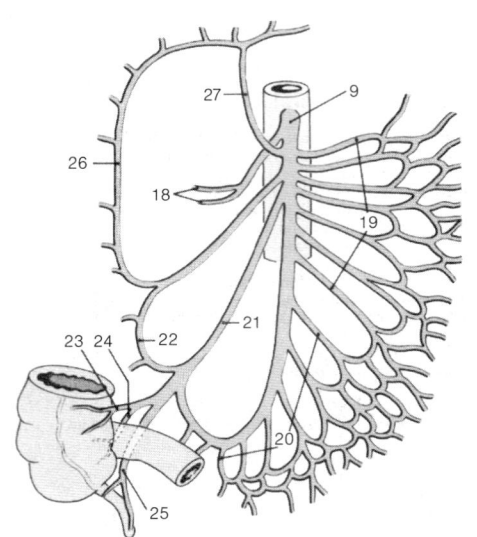

superior mesenteric artery
A. mesenterica superior

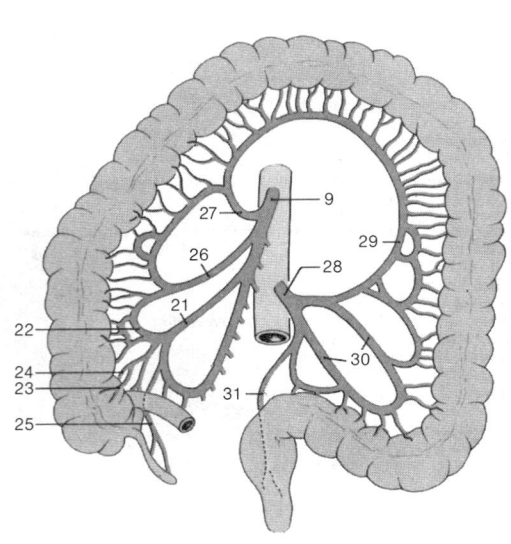

arteries of the large intestine
Dickdarmarterien

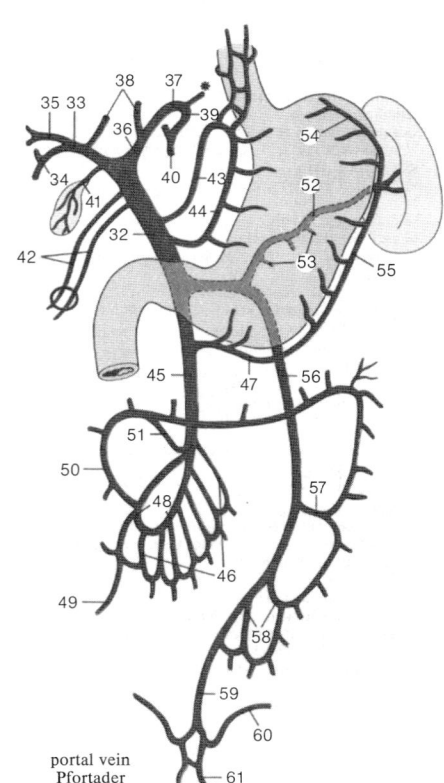

portal vein
Pfortader

Plate XIV

celiac trunk

superior mesenteric artery

arteries of the large intestine

portal vein

1 abdominal (part of) aorta
2 celiac trunk, celiac artery/axis
3 left gastric artery, left coronary artery of stomach

4 esophageal branches of left gastric artery
5 splenic artery, lienal artery
6 short gastric arteries
7 left gastro-omental artery, left gastro-epiploic artery, left inferior gastric artery
8 right gastro-omental artery, right gastro-epiploic artery, right inferior gastric artery
9 superior mesenteric artery

10 anterior/posterior pancreaticoduodenal artery
11 gastroduodenal artery
12 right gastric artery, right coronary artery of stomach, pyloric artery
13 common hepatic artery
14 proper hepatic artery
15 cystic artery
16 right branch of proper hepatic artery
17 left branch of proper hepatic artery
18 inferior pancreaticoduodenal artery
19 jejunal arteries
20 ileal arteries
21 ileocolic artery, inferior right colic artery
22 colic branch of ileocolic artery, ascending ileocolic artery
23 anterior cecal artery
24 posterior cecal artery
25 appendicular artery, vermiform artery
26 right colic artery

27 middle colic artery, accessory superior colic artery

28 inferior mesenteric artery

29 left colic artery

30 sigmoid arteries
31 superior rectal artery, superior hemorrhoidal artery

32 portal vein (of liver)
33 right branch of portal vein
34 anterior branch of right branch of portal vein
35 posterior branch of right branch of portal vein
36 left branch of portal vein
37 transverse part of left branch of portal vein
38 caudate branches (of left branch of portal vein)
39 umbilical part (of left branch of portal vein) and lateral branches
40 medial branch of left branch of portal vein
41 cystic vein
42 paraumbilical veins, Sappey's veins
43 left gastric vein
44 right gastric vein
45 superior mesenteric vein
46 jejunal and ileal veins
47 right gastro-omental vein, right gastro-epiploic vein
48 ileocolic vein
49 appendicular vein
50 right colic vein
51 middle/intermediate colic vein
52 splenic vein
53 pancreatic veins
54 short gastric veins
55 left gastro-omental vein, left gastro-epiploic vein
56 inferior mesenteric vein
57 left colic vein
58 sigmoid veins
59 superior rectal vein, superior hemorrhoidal vein
60 middle rectal veins, middle hemorrhoidal veins

61 inferior rectal veins, inferior hemorrhoidal veins

Tafel XIV

Truncus coeliacus

A. mesenterica superior

Dickdarmarterien

Pfortader

1 Bauchaorta, Aorta abdominalis, Pars abdominalis aortae
2 Truncus coeliacus
3 linke Magenschlagader/Magenkranzarterie, Gastrika sinistra, A. gastrica sinistra
4 Speiseröhrenäste der Gastrika sinistra, Rami oesophageales
5 Milzschlagader, Lienalis, A. lienalis/splenica
6 kurze Magenschlagadern, Aa. gastrici breves
7 linke Gastroomentalis/Gastroepiploika, A. gastro-omentalis/gastro-epiploica sinistra
8 rechte Gastroomentalis, A. gastro-omentalis dextra
9 obere Mesenterialarterie, Mesenterika superior, A. mesenterica superior
10 A. pancreaticoduodenalis superior anterior/posterior
11 Gastroduodenalis, A. gastroduodenalis
12 rechte Magenschlagader/Magenkranzarterie, Gastrika dextra, A. gastrica dextra
13 Hepatika/Hepatica communis, A. hepatica communis
14 Hepatika/Hepatica propria, A. hepatica propria
15 Gallenblasenschlagader, Zystika, Cystica, A. cystica
16 rechter Ast der A. hepatica propria, Ramus dexter
17 linker Ast der A. hepatica propria, Ramus sinister
18 A. pancreaticoduodenalis inferior
19 Jejunumschlagadern, -arterien, Aa. jejunales
20 Ileumschlagadern, -arterien, Aa. ileales
21 Ileokolika, A. ileocolica
22 Kolonast der A. ileocolica, Ramus colicus
23 vordere Zäkalarterie/Zökalarterie, A. caecalis anterior
24 hintere Zäkalarterie/Zökalarterie, A. caecalis posterior
25 Appendixschlagader, Appendikularis, A. appendicularis
26 rechte Kolonschlagader, Kolika/Colica dextra, A. colica dextra
27 mittlere Kolonschlagader, Kolika/Colica media, A. colica media
28 untere Mesenterialarterie, Mesenterika inferior, A. mesenterica inferior
29 linke Kolonschlagader, Kolika/Colica sinistra, A. colica sinistra
30 Sigmaschlagadern, Aa. sigmoideae
31 obere Rektumschlagader, Rektalis superior, A. rectalis superior
32 Pfortader, V. portae hepatis
33 rechter Ast der Pfortader, Ramus dexter
34 vorderer Ast des rechten Pfortaderastes, Ramus anterior
35 hinterer Ast des rechten Pfortaderastes, Ramus posterior
36 linker Ast der Pfortader, Ramus sinister
37 Pars transversa (des linken Pfortaderastes)
38 Pfortaderäste zum Lobus caudatus, Rami caudati
39 Pars umbilicalis (des linken Pfortaderastes) und Rami laterales
40 Rami mediales (des linken Pfortaderastes)
41 Gallenblasenvene, V. cystica
42 Paraumbilikalvenen, Vv. para-umbilicales
43 linke Magenvene, V. gastrica sinistra
44 rechte Magenvene, V. gastrica dextra
45 obere Mesenterialvene, V. mesenterica superior
46 Jejunum- und Ileumvenen, Vv. jejunales et ileales
47 V. gastro-omentalis/gastro-epiploica dextra
48 V. ileocolica
49 Appendixvene, V. appendicularis
50 rechte Kolonvene, V. colica dextra
51 mittlere Kolonvene, V. colica media/intermedia
52 Milzvene, V. splenica
53 Pankreasvenen, Vv. pancreaticae
54 kurze Magenvenen, Vv. gastricae breves
55 V. gastro-omentalis/gastro-epiploica sinistra
56 untere Mesenterialvene, V. mesenterica inferior
57 linke Kolonvene, V. colica sinistra
58 Sigmavenen, Vv. sigmoideae
59 obere Rektumvene/Hämorrhoidalvene, V. rectalis superior
60 mittlere Rektumvenen/Hämorrhoidalvenen, Vv. rectales mediae
61 untere Rektumvenen/Hämorrhoidalvenen, Vv. rectales inferiores

Plate XV   Tafel XV   A36

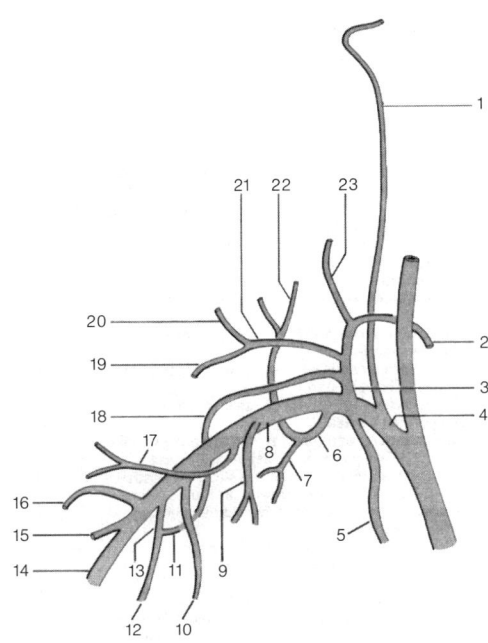

subclavian and axillary artery
A. sublavia und A. axillaris

axillary artery
A. axillaris

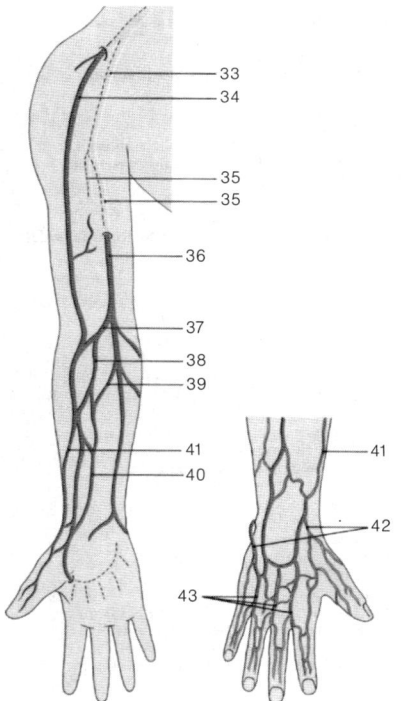

superficial veins of arm and hand
oberflächliche Venen von Arm und Hand

Plate XV

subclavian and axillary artery

axillary artery

superficial veins of arm and hand

1 vertebral artery
2 inferior thyroid artery

3 thyrocervical trunk, thyroid axis
4 subclavian artery
5 internal thoracic artery, internal mammary artery

6 costocervical trunk, costocervical artery
7 highest/supreme/anterior intercostal artery

8 axillary artery
9 superior/highest thoracic artery

10 lateral/long thoracic artery, external mammary artery

11 circumflex artery of scapula, circumflex scapular artery

12 thoracodorsal artery, dorsal thoracic artery

13 subscapular artery
14 brachial artery, humeral artery
15 anterior circumflex humeral artery

16 posterior circumflex humeral artery

17 thoracoacromial artery, thoracic axis, acromiothoracic artery
18 suprascapular artery, transverse scapular artery

19 deep branch of transverse cervical artery, dorsal/descending scapular artery
20 superficial branch of transverse cervical artery, superficial cervical artery
21 transverse cervical artery, transverse artery of the neck
22 deep cervical artery

23 ascending cervical artery

24 ulnar artery
25 common interosseous artery
26 proper palmar digital arteries, collateral digital arteries
27 common palmar digital arteries, ulnar metacarpal arteries
28 superficial palmar arterial arch
29 deep palmar arterial arch
30 radial artery
31 superior ulnar collateral artery
32 radial collateral artery
33 axillary vein
34 cephalic vein
35 brachial veins
36 basilic vein
37 intermediate/median cubital vein, intermediate/median vein of the elbow
38 intermediate/median cephalic vein
39 intermediate/median basilic vein
40 intermediate/median antebrachial vein, intermediate/median vein of the forearm
41 accessory cephalic vein
42 dorsal venous rete/network of the hand
43 dorsal metacarpal veins

Tafel XV

A. sublavia und A. axillaris

A. axillaris

oberflächliche Venen von Arm und Hand

1 Wirbelschlagader, Vertebralis, A. vertebralis
2 untere Schilddrüsenschlagader, Thyroidea inferior, A. thyroidea inferior
3 Truncus thyrocervicalis *abbr.* TTC
4 Unterschlüsselbeinschlagader, Subklavia, A. subclavia
5 innere Brustkorbschlagader, Thoracica/Mammaria interna, A. thoracica interna
6 Truncus costocervicalis
7 oberste Interkostalarterie, Interkostalis suprema, A. intercostalis suprema
8 Achselschlagader, Axillaris, A. axillaris
9 obere Brustkorbschlagader, Thoracica superior, A. thoracica superior
10 seitliche Brustkorbschlagader, Thoracica lateralis, A. thoracica lateralis
11 Kranzarterie des Schulterblattes, Circumflexa scapulae, A. circumflexa scapulae
12 hintere Brustwandschlagader, Thorakodorsalis, A. thoracodorsalis
13 Subskapularis, A. subscapularis
14 Armschlagader, Brachialis, A. brachialis
15 vordere Kranzarterie des Humerus, A. circumflexa anterior humeri
16 hintere Kranzarterie des Humerus, A. circumflexa posterior humeri
17 Thorakoakromialis, A. thoraco-acromialis
18 obere Schulterblattarterie, Supraskapularis, A. suprascapularis
19 Ramus profundus (der A. transversa colli), A. scapularis dorsalis
20 Ramus superficialis (der A. transversa colli), A. cervicalis superficialis
21 quere Halsschlagader, Transversa colli, A. transversa (colli)
22 tiefe Halsschlagader, Zervikalis/Cervicalis profunda, A. cervicalis profunda
23 aufsteigende Halsschlagader, Zervikalis/Cervicalis ascendens, A. cervicalis ascendens
24 Ulnaris, A. ulnaris
25 Interossea communis, A. interossea communis
26 Aa. digitales palmares propriae
27 Aa. digitales palmares communes
28 oberflächlicher Hohlhandbogen, Arcus palmaris superficialis
29 tiefer Hohlhandbogen, Arcus palmaris profundus
30 Radialis, A. radialis
31 A. collateralis ulnaris superior
32 A. collateralis radialis
33 Achselvene, V. axillaris
34 Cephalica, V. cephalica
35 Vv. brachiales
36 Basilika, V. basilica
37 Mediana cubiti, V. mediana cubiti

38 Mediana cephalica, V. mediana cephalica
39 Mediana basilica, V. mediana basilica
40 Mediana antebrachii, V. mediana antebrachii

41 Cephalica accessoria, V. cephalica accessoria
42 Venennetz des Handrückens, Rete venosum dorsale manus
43 dorsale Mittelhandvenen, Vv. metacarpales dorsales

Plate XVI Tafel XVI A38

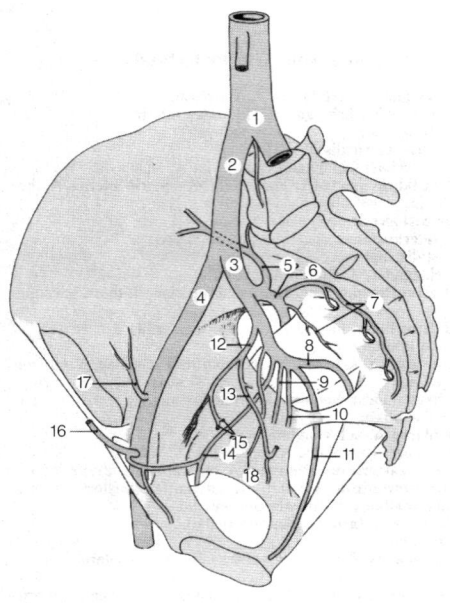

external and internal iliac artery
A. iliaca externa, A. iliaca interna

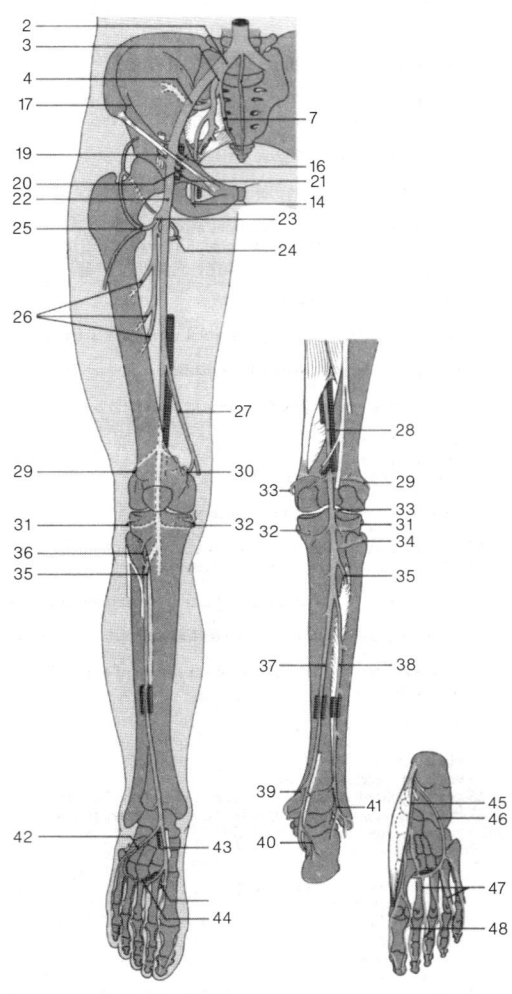

femoral artery
A. femoralis

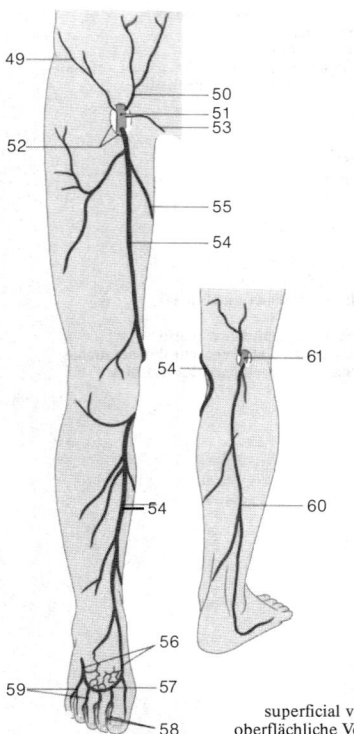

superficial veins of leg and foot
oberflächliche Venen von Bein und Fuß

Plate XVI

external and internal iliac artery

femoral artery

superficial veins of leg and foot

1 bifurcation of (the) aorta
2 common iliac artery
3 internal iliac artery, hypogastric artery
4 external iliac artery
5 iliolumbar artery, small iliac artery
6 superior gluteal artery
7 lateral sacral arteries
8 inferior gluteal artery
9 vaginal artery
10 middle rectal artery, middle hemorrhoidal artery
11 internal pudendal artery
12 umbilical artery
13 uterine artery, fallopian artery
14 obturator artery
15 superior vesical arteries
16 inferior epigastric vein, deep epigastric vein
17 deep circumflex iliac artery, external epigastric artery
18 inferior vesical artery
19 superficial circumflex iliac artery

20 superficial epigastric artery
21 external pudendal artery
22 femoral artery, crural artery
23 deep femoral artery, deep artery of the thigh
24 medial circumflex femoral artery, medial circumflex artery of the thigh
25 lateral circumflex femoral artery, lateral circumflex artery of the thigh
26 perforating arteries
27 descending genicular artery, descending artery of the knee
28 popliteal artery
29 lateral superior genicular artery, lateral superior artery of the knee
30 medial superior genicular artery, medial superior artery of the knee
31 lateral inferior genicular artery, lateral inferior artery of the knee
32 medial inferior genicular artery, medial inferior artery of the knee
33 middle genicular artery, middle artery of the knee
34 fibular circumflex branch/artery
35 anterior tibial artery
36 anterior tibial recurrent artery
37 posterior tibial artery
38 fibular artery, peroneal artery
39 medial malleolar branches of posterior tibial artery

40 calcaneal branches of posterior tibial artery
41 lateral malleolar branches of fibular artery
42 lateral tarsal artery
43 dorsal artery of the foot
44 arcuate artery (of the foot), metatarsal artery
45 medial plantar artery
46 lateral/external plantar artery
47 plantar metatarsal arteries
48 proper plantar digital arteries
49 superficial circumflex iliac vein
50 superficial epigatric vein
51 femoral vein
52 saphenous hiatus, oval fossa of the thigh
53 external pudendal veins
54 great saphenous vein, large/long saphenous vein
55 accessory saphenous vein
56 dorsal venous rete/network of the foot
57 dorsal venous arch of the foot
58 dorsal digital veins of the foot/of the toes
59 dorsal metatarsal veins
60 small saphenous vein, short saphenous vein
61 popliteal vein

Tafel XVI

A. iliaca externa, A. iliaca interna

A. femoralis

oberflächliche Venen von Bein und Fuß

1 Aortenbifurkation, Bifurcatio aortae
2 Iliaka/Iliaca communis, A. iliaca communis
3 Iliaka/Iliaca interna, A. iliaca interna
4 Iliaka/Iliaca externa, A. iliaca externa
5 Iliolumbalis, A. iliolumbalis
6 Glutaea superior, A. glut(a)ealis superior
7 Aa. sacrales laterales
8 Glutaea inferior, A. glut(a)ealis inferior
9 Scheidenschlagader, Vaginalis, A. vaginalis
10 mittlere Rektumschlagader, Rektalis media, A. rectalis media
11 Pudenda interna, A. pudenda interna
12 Nabelschlagader, Umbilikalis, A.umbilicalis
13 Gebärmutterschlagader, Uterina, A. uterina
14 Obturatoria, A. obturatoria
15 obere Blasenarterien, Aa. vesicales superiores
16 Epigastrika inferior, A. epigastrica inferior
17 tiefe Kranzarterie der Hüfte, A. circumflexa iliaca profunda
18 untere Blasenarterien, Vesikalis inferior, A. vesicalis inferior
19 oberflächliche Kranzarterie der Hüfte, A. circumflexa iliaca superficialis
20 Epigastrika superficialis, A. epigastrica superficialis
21 Pudenda externa, A. pudenda externa
22 Oberschenkelschlagader, Femoralis, A. femoralis
23 Profunda femoris, A. profunda femoris
24 mediale Femurkranzarterie, A. circumflexa femoris medialis

25 laterale Femurkranzarterie, A. circumflexa femoris lateralis

26 Perforansarterien, Aa. perforantes
27 A. descendens genicularis
28 Kniekehlenschlagader, Poplitea, A. poplitea
29 A. superior lateralis genus

30 A. superior medialis genus

31 A. inferior lateralis genus

32 A. inferior medialis genus

33 A. media genus
34 Ramus circumflexus fibularis (der A. tibialis posterior)
35 Tibialis anterior, A. tibialis anterior
36 A. recurrens tibialis anterior
37 Tibialis posterior, A. tibialis posterior
38 Wadenbeinschlagader, Fibularis, A. fibularis
39 Innenknöcheläste der A. tibialis posterior, Rami malleolares mediales
40 Kalkaneusäste der A. tibialis posterior, Rami calcanei
41 Außenknöcheläste der A. fibularis, Rami malleolares laterales
42 Tarsalis lateralis, A. tarsalis lateralis
43 Fußrückenschlagader, Dorsalis pedis, A. dorsalis pedis
44 Bogenschlagader, A. arcuata
45 Plantaris medialis, A. plantaris medialis
46 Plantaris lateralis, A. plantaris lateralis
47 plantare Mittelfußarterien, Aa. metatarales plantares
48 Aa. digitales plantares propriae
49 V. circumflexa iliaca superficialis
50 V. epigastrica superficialis
51 Oberschenkelvene, V. femoralis
52 Hiatus saphenus
53 Vv. pudendae externae
54 Saphena magna, V. saphena magna
55 Saphena accessoria, V. saphena accessoria
56 Venennetz des Fußrückens, Rete venosum dorsale pedis
57 Venenbogen des Fußrückens, Arcus venosus dorsalis pedis
58 Vv. digitales dorsales pedis
59 dorsale Mittelfußvenen, Vv. metatarsales dorsales
60 Saphena parva, V. saphena parva
61 Kniekehlenvene, V. poplitea

Plate XVII — Tafel XVII

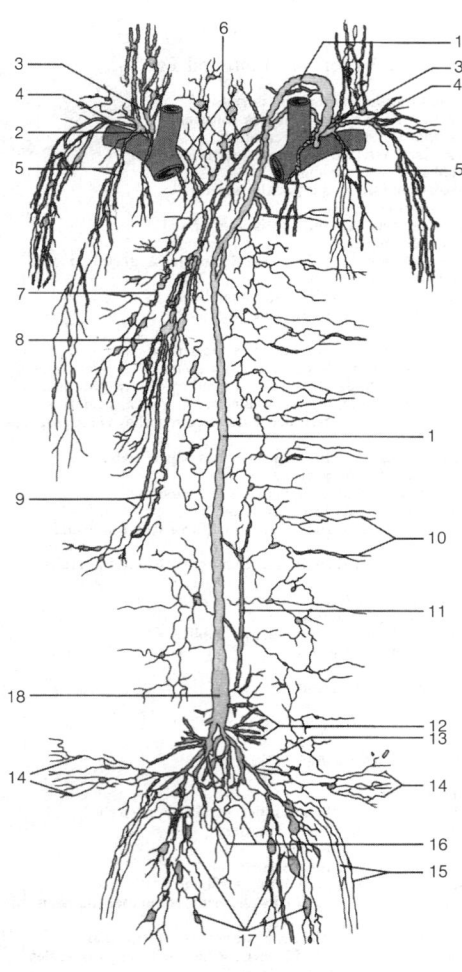

central lymphatic trunks
zentrale Lymphstämme

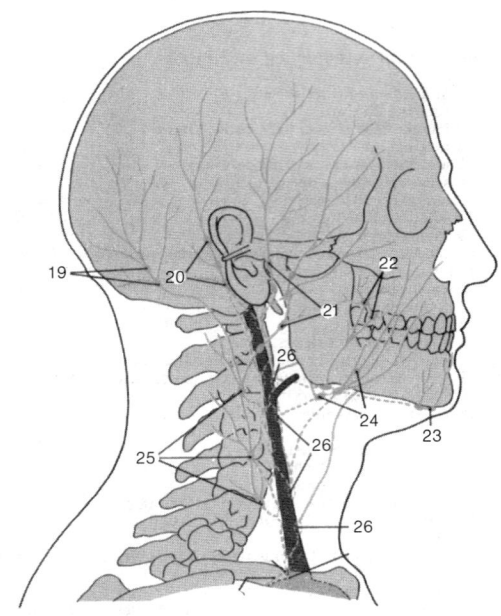

lymph nodes of head and neck
Lymphknoten von Kopf und Hals

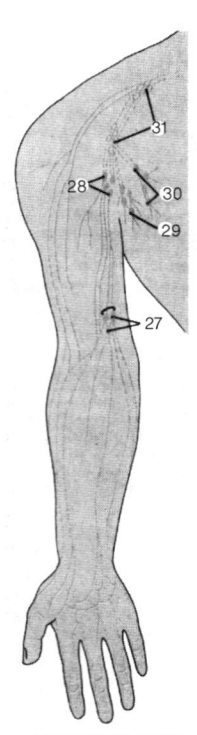

axillary lymph nodes
axilläre Lymphknoten

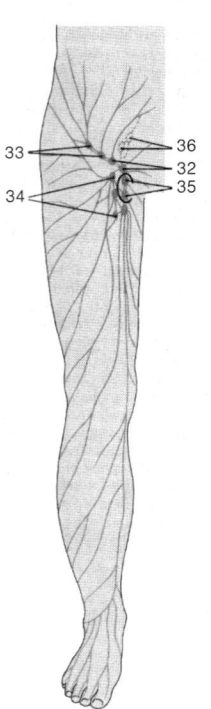

inguinal lymph nodes
Leistenlymphknoten

Plate XVII

central lymphatic trunks

lymph nodes of head and neck

axillary lymph nodes

inguinal lymph nodes

1 thoracic duct
2 right lymphatic duct, right thoracic duct

3 right/left jugular trunk
4 right/left subclavian trunk
5 right/left bronchomediastinal trunk
6 lymphatic vessels of the posterior mediastinum
7 lymphatic vessels of the lung
8 lymphatic vessels of the esophagus
9 posterior lymphatic vessels of the diaphragm
10 lymphatic vessels of the intercostal space
11 descending intercostal lymphatic trunk
12 anterior and lateral lymphatic vessels of diaphragm
13 intestinal trunks
14 lymphatic vessels of the kidney
15 lymphatic vessels of the testicle/of the ovary
16 celiac (lymphatic) plexus
17 right/left lumbar trunk
18 cistern of Pecquet, chylocyst, chyle cistern
19 occipital lymph nodes
20 mastoid lymph nodes, retroauricular lymph nodes
21 deep and superficial parotid lymph nodes
22 facial lymph nodes (buccal lymph nodes)
23 submental lymph nodes
24 mandibular lymph node and submandibular lymph nodes
25 superficial lateral cervical lymph nodes

26 deep lateral cervical lymph nodes

27 cubital lymph nodes, supratrochlear lymph nodes
28 brachial lymph nodes, lateral axillary lymph nodes
29 subscapular axillary lymph nodes

30 pectoral axillary lymph nodes

31 deep axillary lymph nodes
32 superomedial inguinal lymph nodes
33 superolateral inguinal lymph nodes
34 inferior superficial inguinal lymph nodes
35 deep inguinal lymph nodes
36 external iliac lymph nodes

Tafel XVII

zentrale Lymphstämme

Lymphknoten von Kopf und Hals

axilläre Lymphknoten

Leistenlymphknoten

1 Brustmilchgang, Ductus thoracicus
2 rechter Brustmilchgang, Ductus thoracicus dexter, Ductus lymphaticus dexter
3 Truncus jugularis dexter/sinister
4 Truncus subclavius dexter/sinister
5 Truncus bronchomediastinalis dexter/sinister
6 Lymphgefäße des hinteren Mediastinums
7 Lymphgefäße aus der Lunge
8 Lymphgefäße der Speiseröhre
9 hintere Lymphgefäße des Zwerchfells
10 Lymphgefäße des Interkostalraums
11 Truncus lymphaticus intercostalis descendens
12 vordere und seitliche Lymphgefäße des Zwerchfells
13 Trunci intestinales
14 Lymphgefäße aus der Niere
15 Lymphgefäße aus dem Hoden/Ovar
16 Plexus lymphaticus coeliacus
17 Truncus lumbalis dexter/sinister
18 Cisterna chyli
19 Okzipitallymphknoten, Nodi lymphatici occipitales
20 retroaurikuläre Lymphknoten, Nodi lymphatici mastoidei
21 oberflächliche und tiefe Parotislymphknoten, Nodi lymphatici parotidei superficiales et profundi
22 Nodi lymphatici faciales (buccinatorii)
23 Nodi lymphatici submentales
24 Nodus mandibularis und Nodi lymphatici submandibulares
25 oberflächliche seitliche Halslymphknoten, Nodi lymphatici cervicales laterales superficiales
26 tiefe seitliche Halslymphknoten, Nodi lymphatici cervicales laterales profundi
27 Lymphknoten der Ellenbeuge, Nodi lymphatici cubitales
28 Oberarmlymphknoten, Nodi lymphatici brachiales
29 subskapuläre Lymphknoten, Nodi lymphatici axillares subscapulares
30 pektorale Achsellymphknoten, Nodi lymphatici axillares pectorales
31 tiefe Achsellymphknoten, Nodi lymphatici (axillares) profundi
32 Nodi lymphatici inguinales superficiales superomediales
33 Nodi lymphatici inguinales superficiales superolaterales
34 Nodi lymphatici inguinales superficiales inferiores
35 tiefe Leistenlymphknoten, Nodi lymphatici inguinales profundi
36 Nodi lymphatici iliaci externi

Plate XVIII   Tafel XVIII   A42

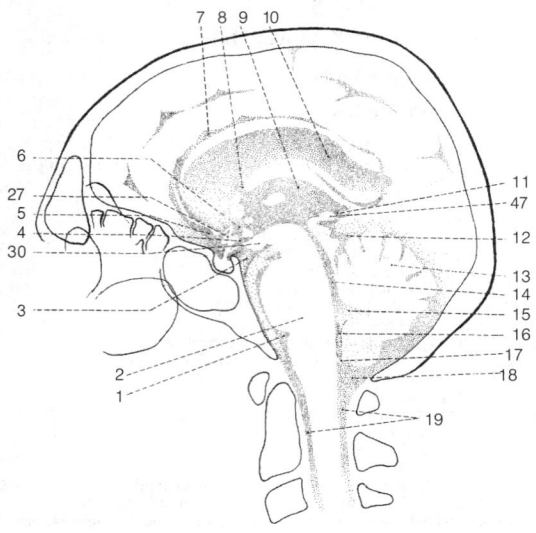

external and internal cerebrospinal fluid spaces
äußere und innere Liquorräume

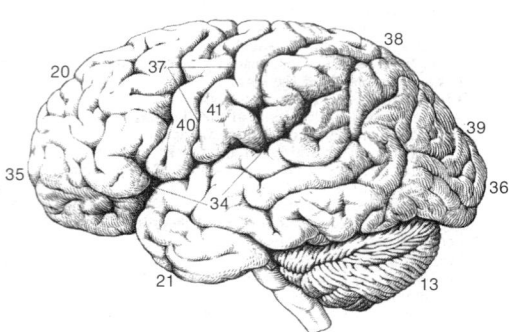

brain, lateral view
Gehirn, Seitenansicht

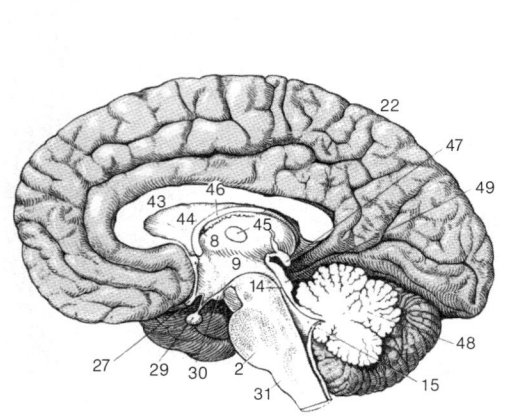

brain, median section
Gehirn, Medianschnitt

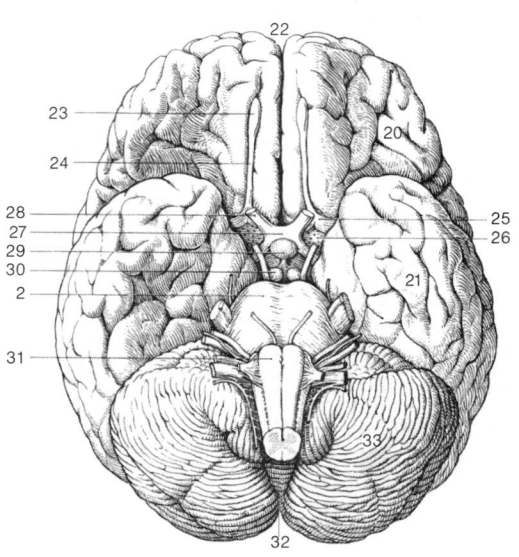

brain, from below
Gehirn, von basal

Plate XVIII

external and internal cerebrospinal fluid spaces

brain, lateral view

brain, median section

brain, from below

1 pontocerebellar cistern
2 bridge of Varolius, pons
3 interpeduncular cistern, basal cistern
4 recess of infundibulum
5 chiasmatic cistern, cistern of chiasma
6 optic recess
7 pericallosal cistern
8 foramen of Monro, interventricular foramen
9 third ventricle
10 lateral ventricle
11 suprapineal recess
12 ambient cistern, Bichat's canal/foramen, cistern of the great vein of cerebrum
13 cerebellum
14 aqueduct of Sylvius, aqueduct of mesencephalon, cerebral aqueduct
15 fourth ventricle
16 tela choroidea of fourth ventricle
17 median aperture of fourth ventricle, foramen of Magendie
18 great/posterior/cerebellomedullary cistern
19 subarachnoid cavity/space
20 frontal lobe
21 temporal lobe
22 longitudinal fissure of cerebrum
23 Morgagni's tubercle, olfactory bulb
24 olfactory tract
25 olfactory trigone/triangle
26 anterior perforated substance, olfactory area
27 optic chiasm/decussation, decussation of optic nerve
28 optic nerve, 2nd cranial nerve
29 pituitary, pituitary gland/body
30 mamillary body
31 medulla oblongata, myelencephalon, bulb
32 vermis
33 cerebellar hemisphere
34 lateral cerebral sulcus, fissure/fossa of Sylvius, sylvian fissure/fossa
35 frontal pole
36 occipital pole
37 central sulcus of cerebrum
38 parietal lobe
39 occipital lobe
40 precentral gyrus, anterior central gyrus
41 postcentral gyrus, posterior central gyrus
42 betweenbrain, interbrain, 'tween brain, diencephalon
43 corpus callosum
44 pellucid septum
45 interthalamic adhesion, intermediate mass
46 fornix of cerebrum
47 pineal body/gland
48 medullary body of vermis, arborescent white substance of cerebellum
49 quadrigeminal plate, tectal lamina of mesencephalon

Tafel XVIII

äußere und innere Liquorräume

Gehirn, Seitenansicht

Gehirn, Medianschnitt

Gehirn, von basal

1 Cisterna pontocerebellaris
2 Brücke, Pons
3 Cisterna interpeduncularis
4 Rec. infundibuli/infundibularis
5 Cisterna chiasmatica
6 Rec. opticus
7 Cisterna pericallosa
8 For. interventriculare
9 III. Ventrikel, Ventriculus tertius
10 Seitenventrikel, Ventriculus lateralis
11 Rec. suprapinealis
12 Cisterna ambiens
13 Kleinhirn, Cerebellum
14 Aqu(a)eductus cerebri/mesencephalici
15 IV. Ventrikel, Ventriculus quartus
16 Tela choroidea ventriculi quarti
17 Apertura mediana
18 Cisterna cerebellomedullaris/magna
19 Subarachnoidalraum, Spatium subarachnoideum
20 Stirn-, Frontallappen, Lobus frontalis
21 Schläfen-, Temporallappen, Lobus temporalis
22 Fissura longitudinalis cerebralis
23 Riechkolben, Bulbus olfactorius
24 Tractus olfactorius
25 Trigonum olfactorium
26 Substantia perforata anterior
27 Sehnervenkreuzung, Chiasma opticum
28 Sehnerv, Optikus, II. Hirnnerv, N. opticus
29 Hirnanhangsdrüse, Hypophyse, Gl. pituitaria, Hypophysis
30 Corpus mamillare
31 verlängertes Mark, Medulla oblongata, Bulbus
32 Kleinhirnwurm, Vermis cerebelli
33 Kleinhirnhemisphäre, Hemisph(a)erium cerebelli
34 Sylvius'-Furche, Sulcus lateralis
35 Frontalpol, Polus frontalis
36 Okzipitalpol, Polus occipitalis
37 Rolando'-Fissur, Zentralfurche, Sulcus centralis
38 Scheitel-, Parietallappen, Lobus parietalis
39 Hinterhaupts-, Okzipitallappen, Lobus occipitalis
40 vordere Zentralwindung, Gyrus pr(a)ecentralis
41 hintere Zentralwindung, Gyrus postcentralis
42 Zwischenhirn, Dienzephalon, Diencephalon
43 Balken, Corpus callosum
44 Septum pellucidum
45 Adh(a)esio interthalamica
46 Hirngewölbe, Fornix
47 Zirbeldrüse, Epiphyse, Epiphysis, Corpus pineale
48 Arbor vitae (cerebelli)
49 Vierhügelplatte, Lamina tectalis

Plate XIX
Tafel XIX
A44

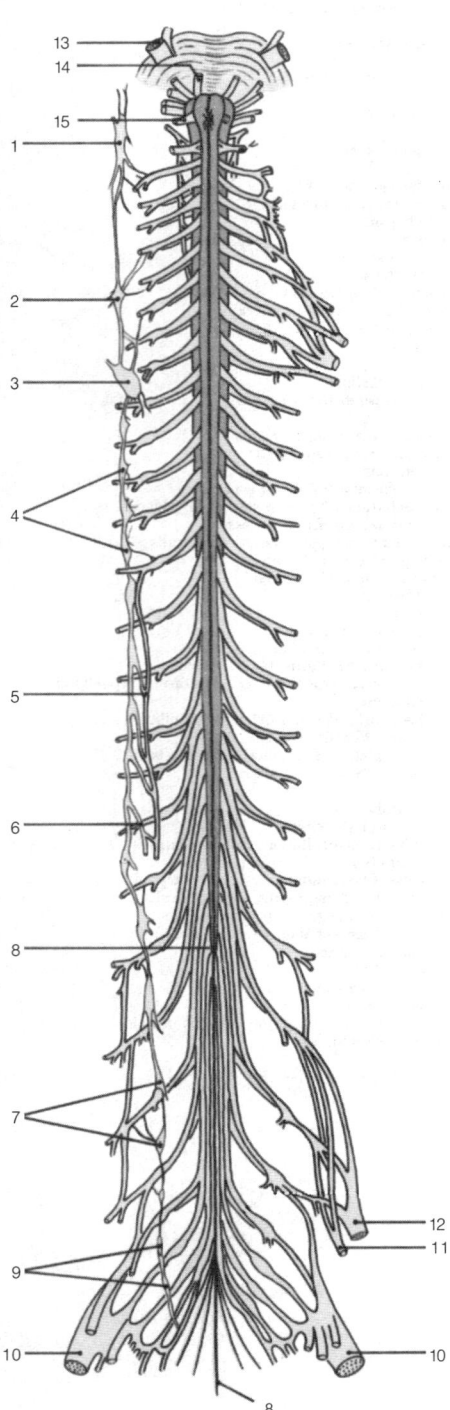

spinal chord, spinal nerves and sympathetic trunk
Rückenmark, Spinalnerven und Grenzstrang

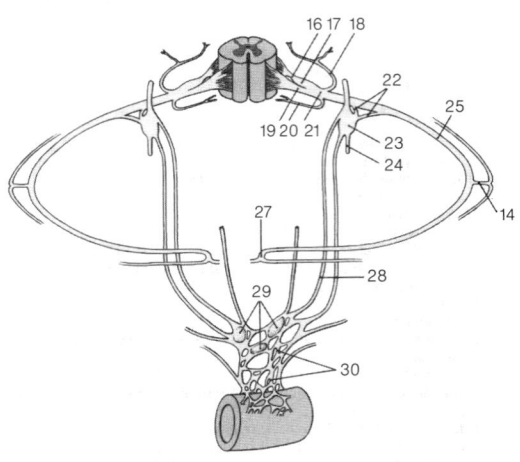

roots and branches of spinal nerves
Wurzeln und Äste der Spinalnerven

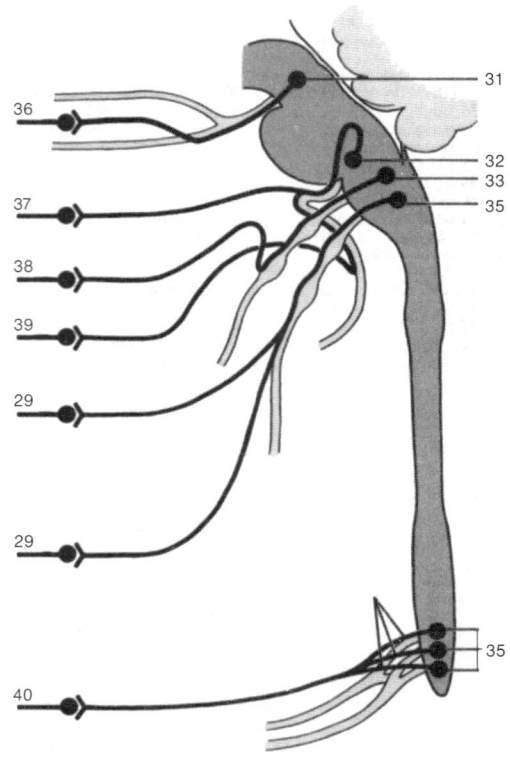

parasympathetic nervous system
parasympathisches Nervensystem

Plate XIX

spinal chord, spinal nerves and sympathetic trunk

roots and branches of spinal nerves

parasympathetic nervous system

   1 superior cervical ganglion
   2 middle cervical ganglion
   3 cervicothoracic/stellate ganglion
   4 thoracic ganglia
   5 greater (thoracic) splanchnic nerve

   6 lesser (thoracic) splanchnic nerve

   7 lumbar ganglia
   8 terminal/spinal/meningeal filament, filament of meningeum
   9 sacral ganglia
10 sciatic nerve
11 obturator nerve
12 femoral nerve
13 trigeminal nerve, 5th cranial nerve
14 abducens nerve, 6th cranial nerve
15 hypoglossal nerve, 12th cranial nerve
16 posterior/dorsal/sensory root of spinal nerves
17 spinal/sensory ganglia
18 dorsal/posterior branch of spinal nerves
19 anterior/motor/ventral root of spinal nerves
20 meningeal branch of spinal nerves
21 trunk of spinal nerve
22 communicating branches of spinal nerves
23 ganglion of sympathetic trunk
24 interganglionic branch
25 anterior/ventral branch of spinal nerves
26 (pectoral/abdominal) lateral cutaneous branch

27 (pectoral/abdominal) anterior cutaneous branch

28 splanchnic nerves of sympathetic trunk

29 ganglia of autonomic plexuses, ganglia of sympathetic plexuses, ganglia of visceral plexuses
30 autonomic/visceral plexuses

31 Edinger-Westphal nucleus, Edinger's nucleus, accessory oculomotor nucleus
32 superior/rostral salivatory nucleus
33 inferior/caudal salivatory nucleus
34 dorsal nucleus of vagus nerve, dorsal vagal nucleus
35 parasympathetic sacral nuclei
36 Schacher's ganglion, ciliary ganglion
37 Meckel's ganglion, pterygopalatine ganglion, sphenopalatine ganglion
38 Arnold's ganglion, otic ganglion
39 submandibular ganglion, submaxillary ganglion, Blandin's ganglion
40 pelvic ganglia

Tafel XIX

Rückenmark, Spinalnerven und Grenzstrang

Wurzeln und Äste der Spinalnerven

parasymphatisches Nervensystem

   1 oberes Halsganglion, Ggl. cervicale superius
   2 mittleres Halsganglion, Ggl. cervicale medium
   3 Ggl. cervicothoracicum/stellatum
   4 thorakale Grenzstrangganglien, Ggll. thoracica
   5 großer Eingeweidenerv, Splanchnikus major, N. splanchnicus major
   6 kleiner Eingeweidenerv, Splanchnikus minor, N. splanchnicus minor
   7 lumbale Grenzstrangganglien, Ggll. lumbalia/lumbaria
   8 Filum terminale/spinale
   9 sakrale Grenzstrangganglien, Ggll. sacralia
10 Ischiasnerv, N. ischiadicus/sciaticus
11 N. obturatorius
12 N. femoralis
13 Trigeminus, V. Hirnnerv, N. trigeminus
14 Abduzens, VI. Hirnnerv, N. abducens
15 Hypoglossus, XII. Hirnnerv, N. hypoglossus
16 hintere Spinalnervenwurzel, Radix posterior/sensoria
17 Spinalganglion, Ggl. spinale/sensorium
18 hinterer Spinalnervenast, Ramus posterior
19 vordere Spinalnervenwurzel, Radix anterior/motoria
20 Meningealast, Ramus meningeus
21 Spinalnervenstamm, Truncus n. spinalis
22 Rami communicantes
23 Grenzstrangganglion, Ggl. trunci sympathici
24 Ramus interganglionaris
25 Vorderast, Ramus anterior
26 seitlicher Hautast, Ramus cutaneus lateralis (pectoralis/abdominalis)
27 vorderer Hautast, Ramus cutaneus anterior (pectoralis/abdominalis)
28 Eingeweidenerven des Grenzstranges, Nn. splanchnici trunci sympathici
29 Ganglien der vegetativen Plexus, Ggll. plexuum autonomicorum/visceralium
30 vegetative/automome Nervengeflechte, Plexus autonomici/viscerales
31 Edinger-Westphal-Kern, akzessorischer Okulomotoriuskern, Nc. oculomotorius accessorius/autonomicus
32 Nc. salivarius superior
33 Nc. salivarius inferior
34 hinterer Vaguskern, Nc. dorsalis n. vagi, Nc. vagalis dorsalis
35 sakrale Parasympathikuskerne, Ncc. parasympathici sacrales
36 Schacher-Ganglion, Ziliarganglion, Ggl. ciliare
37 Meckel'-Ganglion, Ggl. pterygopalatinum

38 Arnold'-Ganglion, Ggl. oticum
39 Faesebeck'-Ganglion, Blandin'-Ganglion, Ggl. submandibulare
40 Beckenganglien des Parasympathikus, Ggll. pelvica

Plate XX — Tafel XX — A46

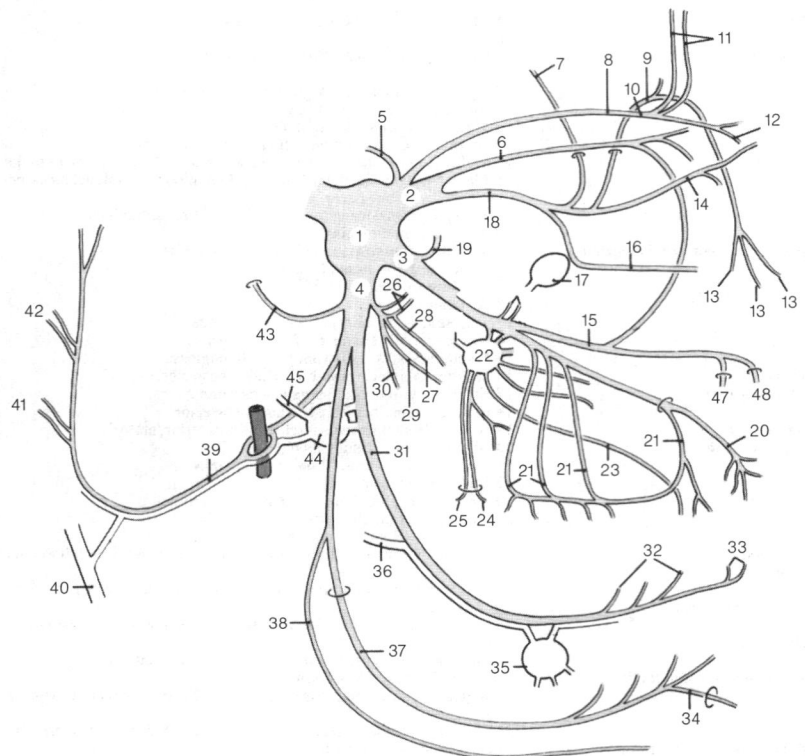

trigeminal nerve
N. trigeminus

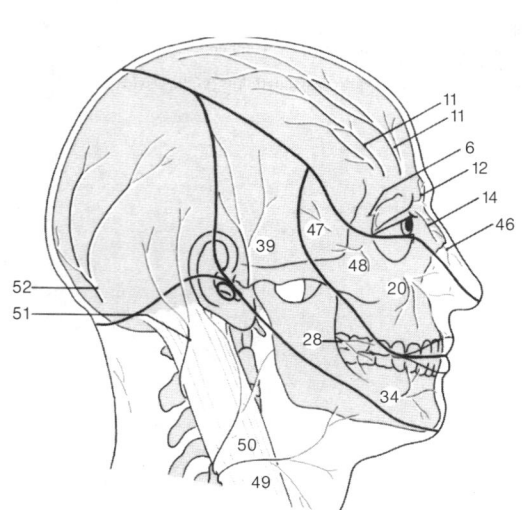

cutaneous nerves of head and neck
Hautnerven von Kopf und Hals

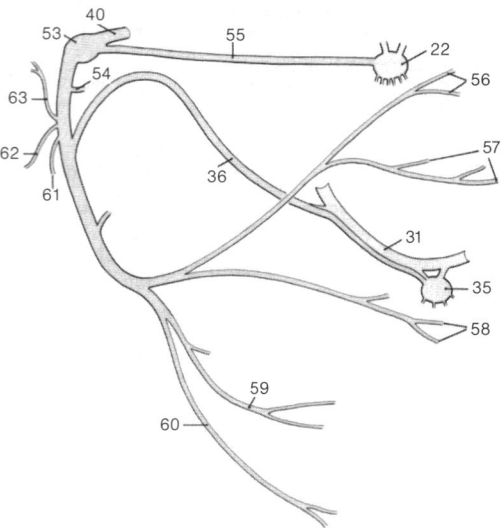

facial nerve
N. facialis

Plate XX

trigeminal nerve

cutaneous nerves of head and neck

facial nerve

1 Gasser's ganglion, gasserian ganglion, semilunar ganglion, trigeminal ganglion, ganglion of trigeminal nerve
2 ophthalmic nerve
3 maxillary nerve
4 mandibular nerve
5 tentorial/meningeal branch of ophthalmic nerve
6 lacrimal nerve
7 posterior ethmoidal nerve
8 frontal nerve
9 anterior ethmoidal nerve
10 supraorbital nerve
11 medial and lateral branch of supraorbital nerve
12 supratrochlear nerve
13 nasal branches of anterior ethmoidal nerve
14 infratrochlear nerve
15 zygomatic nerve
16 long ciliary nerves
17 Schacher's ganglion, ciliary ganglion
18 nasociliary nerve
19 middle meningeal branch of maxillary nerve, meningeal nerve
20 infraorbital nerve
21 superior alveolar nerves, superior dental nerves
22 Meckel's ganglion, pterygopalatine ganglion, sphenopalatine ganglion
23 nasopalatine nerve
24 greater palatine nerve
25 lesser palatine nerves
26 deep temporal nerves
27 masseteric nerve
28 buccal nerve
29 lateral/external pterygoid nerve
30 medial/internal pterygoid nerve
31 lingual nerve
32 lingual branches of lingual nerve
33 sublingual nerve
34 mental nerve
35 Blandin's ganglion, submandibular ganglion, submaxillary ganglion
36 chorda tympani
37 inferior alveolar nerve, inferior dental nerve
38 mylohyoid nerve
39 auriculotemporal nerve
40 facial nerve, 7th cranial nerve
41 nerve of the external acoustic meatus
42 anterior auricular nerves
43 meningeal branch of mandibular nerve
44 Arnold's ganglion, otic ganglion
45 lesser petrosal nerve
46 external nasal branch of anterior ethmoidal nerve
47 zygomaticotemporal branch of zygomatic nerve
48 zygomaticofacial branch of zygomatic nerve
49 transverse nerve of the neck, superficial cervical nerve, cutaneous cervical nerve
50 great auricular nerve
51 lesser occipital nerve
52 greater occipital nerve
53 knee/geniculum of facial canal and geniculate ganglion

54 nerve to stapedius muscle
55 greater petrosal nerve
56 temporal branches of facial nerve
57 zygomatic branches of facial nerve
58 buccal branches of facial nerve
59 marginal mandibular branch of facial nerve
60 cervical branch of facial nerve
61 stylohyoid branch of facial nerve
62 digastric branch of facial nerve
63 posterior auricular nerve

Tafel XX

N. trigeminus

Hautnerven von Kopf und Hals

N. facialis

1 Gasser'-Ganglion, Trigeminusganglion, Ggl. trigeminale
2 Ophthalmikus, N. ophthalmicus
3 Maxillaris, N. maxillaris
4 Mandibularis, N. mandibularis
5 Tentoriumast des N. ophthalmicus, Ramus tentorii/meningeus
6 N. lacrimalis
7 N. ethmoidalis posterior
8 N. frontalis
9 N. ethmoidalis anterior
10 N. supraorbitalis
11 Ramus medialis und Ramus lateralis des N. supraorbitalis
12 N. supratrochlearis
13 Nasenäste des N. ethmoidalis anterior
14 N. infratrochlearis
15 N. zygomaticus
16 lange Ziliarnerven, Nn. ciliares longi
17 Schacher-Ganglion, Ziliarganglion, Ganglon ciliare
18 N. nasociliaris
19 Hirnhautast des N. maxillaris, Ramus meningeus (medius)
20 N. infraorbitalis
21 Nn. alveolares superiores
22 Ggl. pterygopalatinum
23 N. nasopalatinus
24 N. palatinus major
25 Nn. palatini minores
26 Nn. temporales profundi
27 N. massetericus
28 N. buccalis
29 N. pterygoideus lateralis
30 N. pterygoideus medialis
31 N. lingualis
32 Zungenäste des N. lingualis, Rami linguales
33 N. sublingualis
34 N. mentalis
35 Ggl. submandibulare
36 Chorda tympani
37 N. alveolaris inferior
38 N. mylohyoideus
39 N. auriculotemporalis
40 Fazialis, VII. Hirnnerv, N. facialis
41 N. meatus acustici externi
42 Nn. auriculares anteriores
43 Hirnhautast des N. mandibularis
44 Arnold'-Ganglion, Ggl. oticum
45 N. petrosus minor
46 Ramus nasalis externus des N. ethmoidalis anterior
47 Ramus zygomaticotemporalis des N. zygomaticus
48 Ramus zygomaticofacialis des N. zygomaticus
49 N. transversus colli
50 N. auricularis magnus
51 N. occipitalis minor
52 N. occipitalis major
53 Fazialisknie/Geniculum n. facialis und Ggl. geniculi/geniculatum
54 N. stapedius
55 N. petrosus major
56 Rami temporales des N. facialis
57 Rami zygomatici des N. facialis
58 Rami buccales des N. facialis
59 Ramus marginalis mandibularis des N. facialis
60 Ramus colli/cervicalis des N. facialis
61 Ramus stylohyoideus des N. facialis
62 Ramus digastricus des N. facialis
63 N. auricularis posterior

Plate XXI Tafel XXI A48

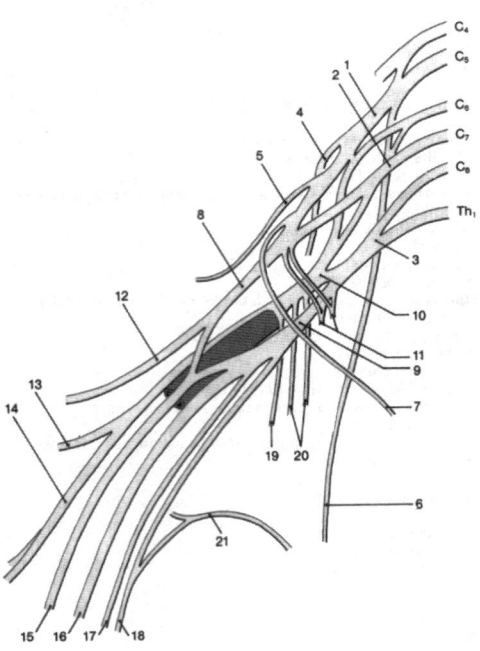

brachial plexus
Plexus brachialis

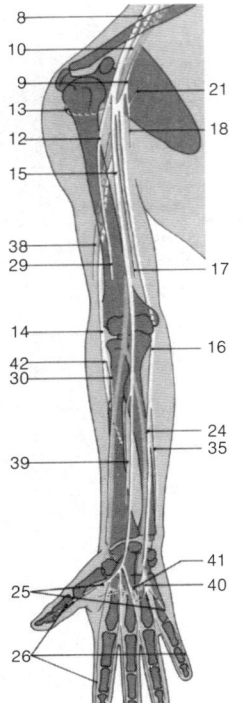

brachial plexus, nerves of the infraclavicular part
Plexus brachialis, Nerven der Pars infraclavicularis

cutaneous nerves of brachial plexus
Hautnerven des Plexus brachialis

Plate XXI

brachial plexus

cutaneous nerves of brachial plexus

brachial plexus, nerves of the infraclavicular part

1 superior trunk
2 middle trunk
3 inferior trunk
4 dorsal nerve of the scapula, posterior/dorsal scapular nerve
5 suprascapular nerve
6 long thoracic nerve, posterior thoracic nerve, Bell's respiratory nerve
7 subclavian nerve
8 lateral chord of brachial plexus
9 medial chord of brachial plexus
10 posterior chord of brachial plexus
11 medial and lateral pectoral nerve
12 musculocutaneous nerve
13 axillary nerve
14 radial nerve, musculospiral nerve
15 median nerve
16 ulnar nerve, cubital nerve
17 medial cutaneous nerve of the forearm
18 medial cutaneous nerve of the arm, Wrisberg's nerve, lesser internal cutaneous nerve
19 thoracodorsal nerve, long subscapular nerve
20 subscapular nerves
21 intercostobrachial nerve, intercostohumeral nerve
22 anterior branch of the medial cutaneous nerve of the forearm
23 posterior branch of the medial cutaneous nerve of the forearm
24 palmar/volar branch of ulnar nerve
25 ulnar nerve, superficial branch: common palmar digital nerves
26 ulnar nerve, superficial branch: proper palmar digital nerves
27 upper lateral cutaneous nerve of the arm
28 lower lateral cutaneous nerve of the arm
29 lateral cutaneous nerve of the forearm
30 superficial branch of radial nerve
31 palmar/volar branch of median nerve
32 median nerve: common palmar digital nerves
33 median nerve: proper palmar digital nerves
34 posterior cutaneous nerve of the arm
35 dorsal branch of ulnar nerve
36 ulnar nerve, dorsal branch: dorsal digital nerves
37 radial nerve, superficial branch: dorsal digital nerves
38 dorsal/posterior cutaneous nerve of the forearm
39 anterior interosseous nerve, anterior antebrachial nerve
40 superficial branch of ulnar nerve
41 deep branch of ulnar nerve
42 deep branch of radial nerve

Tafel XXI

Plexus brachialis

Hautnerven des Plexus brachialis

Plexus brachialis, Nerven der Pars infraclavicularis

1 oberer Primärstrang, Truncus superior
2 mittlerer Primärstrang, Truncus medius
3 unterer Primärstrang, Truncus inferior
4 N. dorsalis scapulae
5 N. suprascapularis
6 N. thoracicus longus
7 N. subclavius
8 seitlicher/lateraler Faszikel, Fasciculus lateralis
9 medialer Faszikel, Fasciculus medialis
10 hinterer Faszikel, Fasciculus posterior
11 N. pectoralis medialis und N. pectoralis lateralis
12 Musculocutaneus, N. musculocutaneus
13 Axillaris, N. axillaris
14 Radialis, N. radialis
15 Medianus, N. medianus
16 Ulnaris, N. ulnaris
17 N. cutaneus antebrachii medialis
18 N. cutaneus brachii medialis
19 N. thoracodorsalis
20 Nn. subscapulares
21 N. intercostobrachialis
22 Ramus anterior des N. cutaneus antebrachii medialis
23 Ramus posterior des N. cutaneus antebrachii medialis
24 Palmarast des N. ulnaris, Ramus palmaris n. ulnaris
25 N. ulnaris, Ramus superficialis: Nn. digitales palmares communes
26 N. ulnaris, Ramus superficialis: Nn. digitales palmares proprii
27 N. cutaneus brachii lateralis superior
28 N. cutaneus brachii lateralis inferior
29 N. cutaneus antebrachii lateralis
30 oberflächlicher Radialisast, Ramus superficialis
31 Palmarast des N. medianus, Ramus palmaris n. mediani
32 N. medianus: Nn. digitales palmares communes
33 N. medianus: Nn. digitales palmares proprii
34 N. cutaneus brachii posterior
35 Ramus dorsalis des N. ulnaris, Ramus dorsalis n. ulnaris
36 N. ulnaris, Ramus dorsalis: Nn. digitales dorsales
37 N. radialis, Ramus superficialis: Nn. digitales dorsales
38 N. cutaneus antebrachii dorsalis
39 N. interosseus/antebrachii anterior
40 oberflächlicher Ulnarisast, Ramus superficialis n. ulnaris
41 tiefer Ulnarisast, Ramus profundus n. ulnaris
42 tiefer Radialisast, Ramus profundus

Plate XXII   Tafel XXII   A50

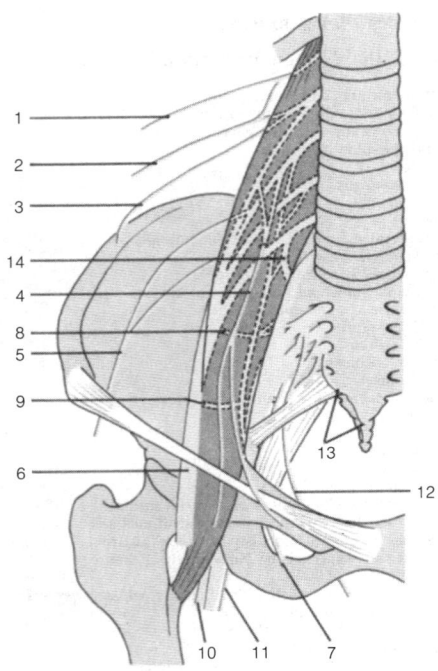

lumbosacral plexus
Plexus lumbosacralis

cutaneous nerves of lumbosacral plexus
Hautnerven des Plexus lumbosacralis

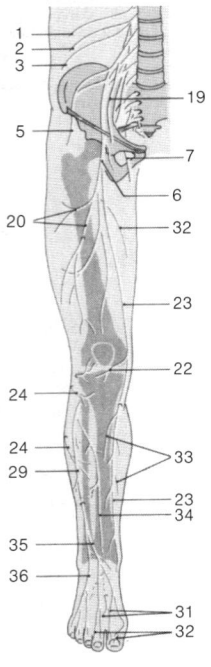

sacral plexus
Plexus sacralis

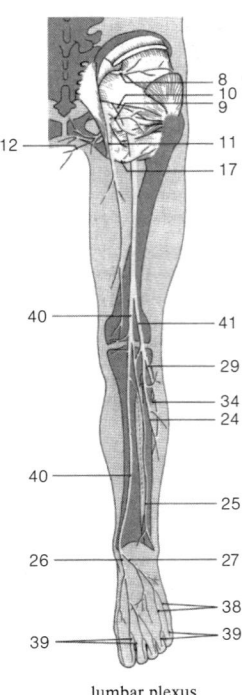

lumbar plexus
Plexus lumbalis

Plate XXII

lumbosacral plexus

cutaneous nerves of lumbosacral plexus

lumbar plexus

sacral plexus

1 subcostal nerve
2 iliohypogastric nerve
3 ilioinguinal nerve
4 genitofemoral nerve, genitocrural nerve
5 lateral cutaneous nerve of the thigh
6 femoral nerve, anterior crural nerve
7 obturator nerve
8 superior gluteal nerve
9 inferior gluteal nerve
10 sciatic nerve
11 posterior cutaneous nerve of the thigh
12 pudendal nerve, pudic nerve
13 coccygeal plexus
14 lumbosacral trunk
15 superior cluneal nerves, superior cluneal branches
16 middle cluneal nerves, middle cluneal branches
17 inferior cluneal nerves, inferior cluneal branches
18 lateral cutaneous branch of iliohypogastric nerve
19 genital branch of genitofemoral nerve, external spermatic nerve
20 anterior cutaneous branches of femoral nerve
21 cutaneous branch of obturator nerve
22 infrapatellar branch of saphenous nerve
23 saphenous nerve
24 lateral cutaneous nerve of the calf
25 sural nerve, short/external saphenous nerve
26 medial plantar nerve
27 lateral plantar nerve
28 femoral branch of genitofemoral nerve
29 superficial peroneal/fibular nerve, musculocutaneous nerve of the leg
30 dorsal lateral cutaneous nerve
31 cutaneous nerve of the skin of the great toe and medial surface of the second toe
32 muscular branches of femoral nerve
33 medial crural cutaneous branches of femoral nerve
34 deep peroneal/fibular nerve, anterior tibial nerve
35 dorsal medial cutaneous nerve
36 intermediate dorsal cutaneous nerve
37 dorsal digital nerves of the foot, dorsal nerves of the toes
38 common plantar digital nerves
39 proper plantar digital nerves
40 tibial nerve, middle popliteal nerve
41 common peroneal nerve, common fibular nerve, lateral popliteal nerve

Tafel XXII

Plexus lumbosacralis

Hautnerven des Plexus lumbosacralis

Plexus lumbalis

Plexus sacralis

1 Subkostalis, N. subcostalis
2 Iliohypogastrikus, N. iliohypogastricus
3 Ilioinguinalis, N. ilioinguinalis
4 Genitofemoralis, N. genitofemoralis
5 N. cutaneus femoris lateralis
6 N. femoralis
7 N. obturatorius
8 N. glut(a)eus superior
9 N. glut(a)eus inferior
10 Ischiasnerv, N. ischiadicus/sciaticus
11 N. cutaneus femoris posterior
12 Pudendus, N. pudendus
13 Plexus coccygeus
14 Truncus lumbosacralis
15 Rami clunium/glut(a)eales superiores
16 Rami clunium/glut(a)eales medii
17 Rami clunium/glut(a)eales inferiores
18 seitlicher Hautast des N. iliohypogastricus, Ramus cutaneus lateralis
19 Genitalast des N. genitofemoralis, Ramus genitalis
20 vordere Hautäste des N. femoralis, Rami cutanei anteriores
21 Hautast des N. obturatorius, Ramus cutaneus
22 Infrapatellarast des N. saphenus, Ramus infrapatellaris
23 Saphenus, N. saphenus
24 N. cutaneus surae lateralis
25 Suralis, N. suralis
26 N. plantaris medialis
27 N. plantaris lateralis
28 Oberschenkelast des N. genitofemoralis, Ramus femoralis
29 N. fibularis superficialis
30 N. cutaneus dorsalis lateralis
31 Nn. digitales dorsales pedis (hallucis lateralis et digiti secundi medialis)
32 Muskeläste des N. femoralis, Rami musculares
33 Rami cutanei cruris mediales (des N. femoralis)
34 N. fibularis profundus
35 N. cutaneus dorsalis medialis
36 N. cutaneus dorsalis intermedius
37 Nn. digitales dorsales pedis
38 Nn. digitales plantares communes
39 Nn. digitales plantares proprii
40 N. tibialis
41 N. fibularis communis

Plate XXIII   Tafel XXIII   A52

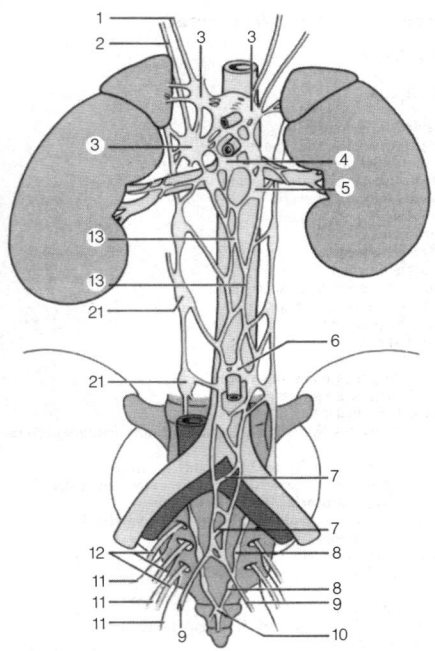

autonomic nervous system, autonomic plexuses
autonomes Nervensystem, vegetative Plexus

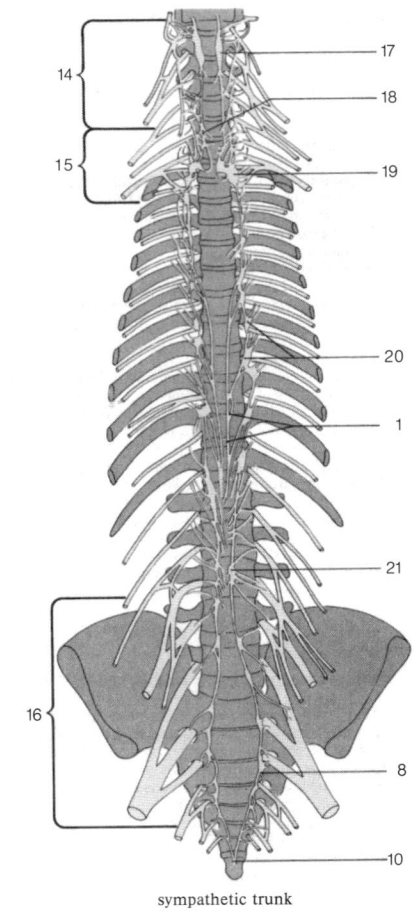

sympathetic trunk
Grenzstrang

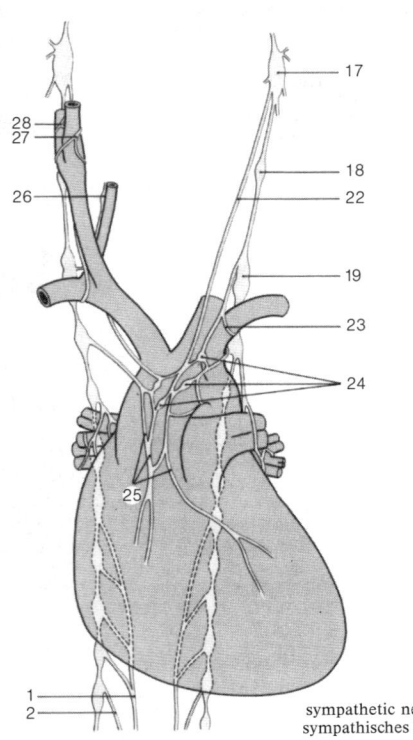

sympathetic nervous system
sympathisches Nervensystem

parasympathetic nervous system, innervation of the stomach
parasympathisches Nervensystem, Innervation des Magens

Plate XXIII

autonomic nervous system, autonomic plexuses

sympathetic trunk

sympathetic nervous system

parasympathetic nervous system, innervation of the stomach

 1 greater (thoracic) splanchnic nerve
 2 lesser (thoracic) splanchnic nerve
 3 celiac ganglia, solar ganglia
 4 superior mesenteric ganglion
 5 aorticorenal ganglia
 6 inferior mesenteric ganglion
 7 presacral nerve, Latarjet's nerve, superior hypogastric plexus
 8 sacral ganglia
 9 hypogastric nerve
10 Walther's ganglion, coccygeal ganglion
11 pelvic splanchnic nerves
12 sacral nerves
13 intermesenteric plexus and renal plexus
14 cervical plexus
15 brachial plexus
16 lumbosacral plexus
17 superior cervical ganglion
18 middle cervical ganglion
19 cervicothoracic ganglion, stellate ganglion
20 Lobstein's ganglion, splanchnic (thoracic) ganglion
21 lumbar ganglia
22 superior cervical cardiac nerve
23 Vieussens' loop/ansa, subclavian loop
24 Wrisberg's ganglia, cardiac ganglia
25 cardiac plexus
26 vertebral ganglia
27 external carotid nerves
28 internal carotid nerve
29 anterior/left vagal trunk
30 posterior/right vagal trunk
31 anterior gastric branches of the vagus nerve
32 posterior gastric branches of the vagus nerve
33 hepatic branches of the vagus nerve

Tafel XXIII

autonomes Nervensystem, vegetative Plexus

Grenzstrang

sympathisches Nervensystem

parasympathisches Nervensystem, Innervation des Magens

 1 großer Eingeweidenerv, Splanchnikus major, N. splanchnicus major
 2 kleiner Eingeweidenerv, Splanchnikus minor, N. splanchnicus minor
 3 Ggll. coeliaca
 4 Ggl. mesentericum superius
 5 Ggll. aorticorenalia
 6 Ggl. mesentericum inferius
 7 Präsakralnerv, Plexus hypogastricus superior, N. pr(a)esacralis
 8 sakrale Grenzstrangganglien, Ggll. sacralia
 9 Hypogastrikus, N. hypogastricus
10 Ggl. impar
11 Nn. pelvici splanchnici, Nn. erigentes
12 Nn. sacrales
13 Plexus intermesentericus und Plexus renalis
14 Halsgeflecht, -plexus, Plexus cervicalis
15 Armgeflecht, -plexus, Plexus brachialis
16 Plexus lumbosacralis
17 oberes Halsganglion, Ggl. cervicale superius
18 mittleres Halsganglion, Ggl. cervicale medium
19 Ggl. cervicothoracicum/stellatum
20 Ggl. thoracicum splanchnicum
21 lumbale Grenzstrangganglien, Ggll. lumbalia/lumbaria
22 N. cardiacus cervicalis superior
23 Subklaviaschlinge, Ansa subclavia
24 Ggll. cardiaca
25 Plexus cardiacus
26 Ggl. vertebrale
27 Nn. carotici externi
28 N. caroticus internus
29 vorderer/linker Vagusstamm, Truncus vagalis anterior
30 hinterer/rechter Vagusstamm, Truncus vagalis posterior
31 vordere Magenäste des Vagus, Rami gastrici anteriores
32 hintere Magenäste des Vagus, Rami gastrici posteriores
33 Leberäste des Vagus, Rami hepatici

Plate XXIV   Tafel XXIV   A54

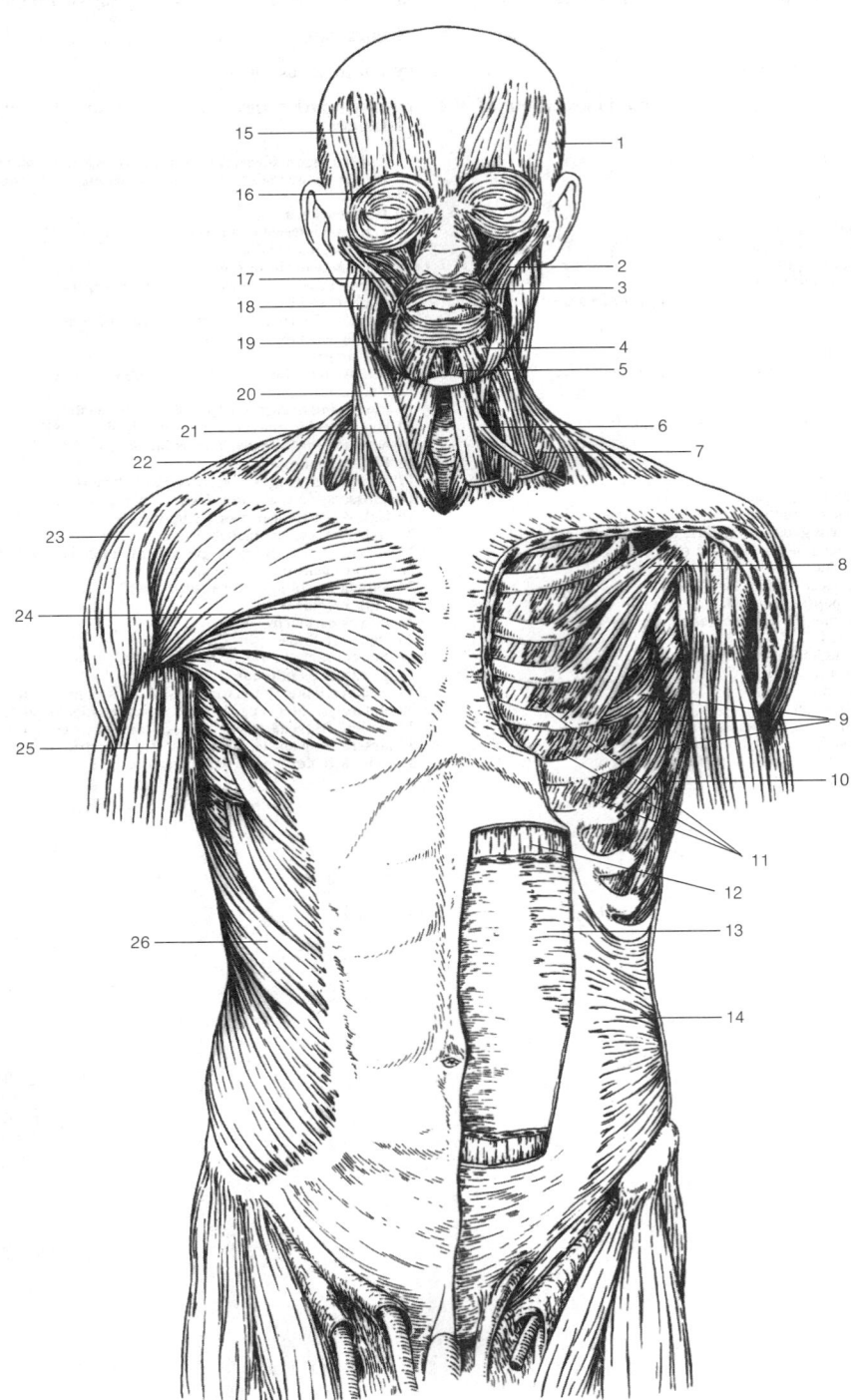

muscles of head, neck and trunk, anterior view
Muskeln von Kopf, Hals und Rumpf, von vorne

Plate XXIV

muscles of head, neck and trunk, anterior view

1 superior auricular muscle, auricularis superior (muscle)
2 greater zygomatic muscle, zygomaticus major (muscle)
3 orbicular muscle of the mouth, orbicularis oris (muscle)
4 depressor muscle of the lower lip, depressor labii inferioris (muscle)
5 mental muscle, mentalis (muscle)
6 omohyoid muscle, omohyoideus (muscle)
7 levator muscle of scapula, levator scapulae (muscle)
8 smaller pectoral muscle, pectoralis minor (muscle)
9 anterior serratus muscle, serratus anterior (muscle)
10 latissimus dorsi (muscle)
11 external intercostal muscles
12 straight muscle of abdomen, rectus abdominis (muscle)
13 transverse muscle of abdomen, transversus abdominis (muscle)
14 internal oblique muscle of abdomen, obliquus internus abdominis (muscle)
15 frontal muscle, frontal belly of occipitofrontal muscle
16 orbicular muscle of the eye, orbicularis oculi (muscle)
17 levator muscle of the upper lip, levator labii superioris (muscle)
18 masseter (muscle)
19 depressor muscle of the angle of the mouth, depressor anguli oris (muscle)
20 sternohyoid muscle, sternohyoideus (muscle)
21 sternocleidomastoid muscle, sternocleidomastoideus (muscle)
22 trapezius (muscle)
23 deltoid muscle, deltoideus (muscle)
24 greater pectoral muscle, pectoralis major (muscle)
25 biceps muscle of arm, biceps brachii (muscle)
26 external oblique muscle of abdomen, obliquus externus abdominis (muscle)

Tafel XXIV

Muskeln von Kopf, Hals und Rumpf, von vorne

1 Aurikularis superior, M. auricularis superior
2 Zygomatikus major, M. zygomaticus major
3 Orbikularis oris, M. orbicularis oris
4 Depressor labii inferioris, M. depressor labii inferioris
5 Kinnmuskel, Mentalis, M. mentalis
6 Omohyoideus, M. omohyoideus
7 Levator scapulae, M. levator scapulae
8 kleiner Brustmuskel, Pektoralis minor, M. pectoralis minor
9 Serratus anterior, M. serratus anterior
10 Latissimus dorsi, M. latissimus dorsi
11 äußere Interkostalmuskulatur/Interkostalmuskeln, Mm. intercostales externi
12 Rektus abdominis, M. rectus abdominis
13 Transversus abdominis, M. transversus abdominis
14 Obliquus internus, M. obliquus internus abdominis
15 Stirnmuskel, M. frontalis, Venter frontalis m. occipitofrontalis
16 Orbikularis oculi, M. orbicularis oculi
17 Levator labii superioris, M. levator labii superioris
18 Masseter, M. masseter
19 Depressor anguli oris, M. depressor anguli oris
20 Sternohyoideus, M. sternohyoideus
21 Sternkleidomastoideus, M. sternocleidomastoideus
22 Trapezius, M. trapezius
23 Deltamuskel, M. deltoideus
24 großer Brustmuskel, Pektoralis major, M. pectoralis major
25 Bizeps, Biceps brachii, M. biceps brachii
26 Obliquus externus, M. obliquus externus abdominis

Plate XXV **Tafel XXV** A56

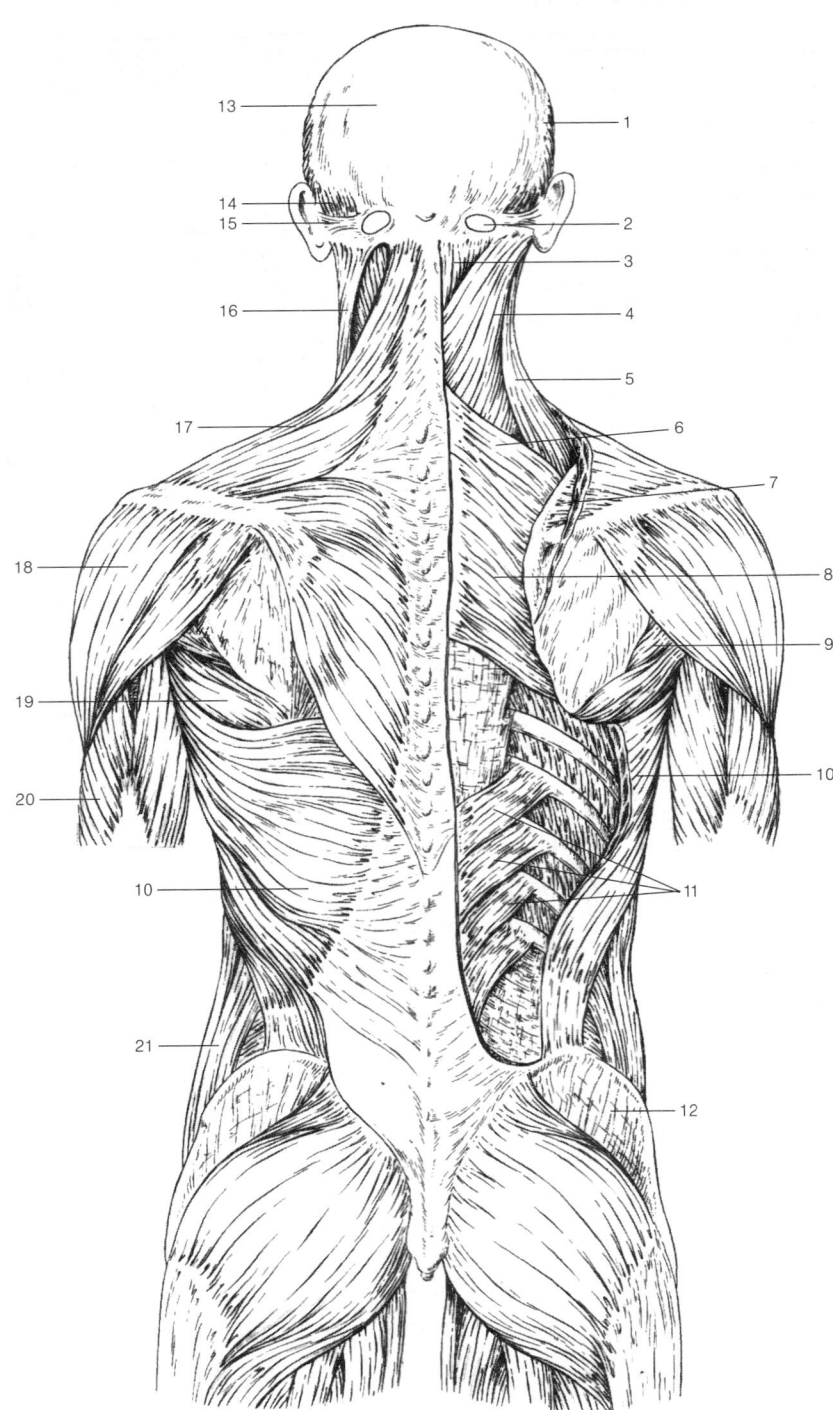

muscles of head, neck and trunk, posterior view
Muskeln von Kopf, Hals und Rumpf, von hinten

Plate XXV

muscles of head, neck and trunk, posterior view

1 superior auricular muscle, auricularis superior (muscle)
2 transverse muscle of nape, transversus nuchae (muscle)
3 semispinalis capitis (muscle)
4 splenius capitis (muscle) and splenius cervicis (muscle)

5 levator muscle of scapula, levator scapulae (muscle)
6 lesser rhomboid muscle, rhomboideus minor (muscle)

7 supraspinous muscle, supraspinatus (muscle)
8 greater rhomboid muscle, rhomboideus major (muscle)

9 teres minor (muscle)
10 latissimus dorsi (muscle)
11 serratus posterior inferior (muscle)
12 middle gluteal muscle, gluteus medius (muscle)
13 galea aponeurotica
14 occipital muscle, occipital belly of occipitofrontal muscle

15 posterior auricular muscle, auricularis posterior (muscle)
16 sternocleidomastoid muscle, sternocleidomastoideus (muscle)
17 trapezius (muscle)
18 deltoid muscle, deltoideus (muscle)
19 teres major (muscle)
20 triceps muscle of arm, triceps brachii (muscle)
21 external oblique muscle of abdomen, obliquus externus abdominis (muscle)

Tafel XXV

Muskeln von Kopf, Hals und Rumpf, von hinten

1 Aurikularis superior, M. auricularis superior
2 Transversus nuchae, M. transversus nuchae
3 Semispinalis capitis, M. semispinalis capitis
4 Splenius capitis und Splenius cervicis, M. splenius capitis und M. splenius cervicis
5 Levator scapulae, M. levator scapulae
6 kleiner Rautenmuskel, Rhomboideus minor, M. rhomboideus minor
7 Supraspinatus, M. supraspinatus
8 großer Rautenmuskel, Rhomboideus major, M. rhomboideus major
9 Teres minor, M. teres minor
10 Latissimus dorsi, M. latissimus dorsi
11 Serratus posterior inferior, M. serratus posterior inferior
12 Glutaeus medius, M. glut(a)eus medius
13 Galea aponeurotica
14 Okzipitalis, M. occipitalis, Venter occipitalis m. occipitofrontalis
15 Aurikularis posterior, M. auricularis posterior
16 Sternokleidomastoideus, M. sternocleidomastoideus
17 Trapezius, M. trapezius
18 Deltamuskel, M. deltoideus
19 Teres major, M. teres major
20 Trizeps, Triceps brachii, M. triceps brachii
21 Obliquus externus, M. obliquus externus abdominis

Plate XXVI Tafel XXVI A58

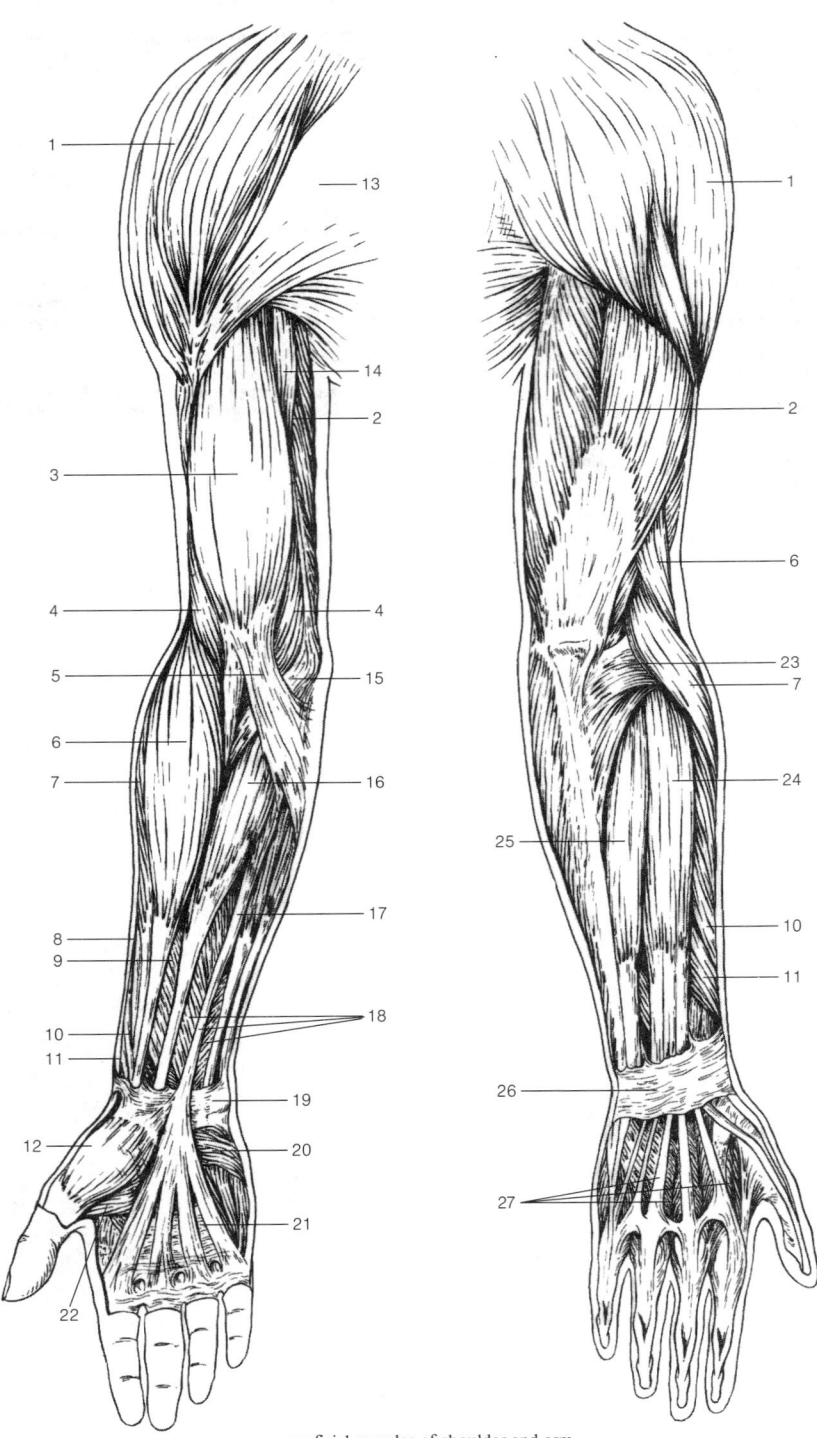

superficial muscles of shoulder and arm
oberflächliche Muskeln von Schulter und Arm

Plate XXVI
superficial muscles of shoulder and arm

1 deltoid muscle, deltoideus (muscle)
2 triceps muscle of arm, triceps brachii (muscle)
3 biceps muscle of arm, biceps brachii (muscle)
4 brachial muscle, brachialis (muscle)
5 bicipital aponeurosis, bicipital/semilunar fascia
6 brachioradial muscle, brachioradialis (muscle)
7 long radial extensor muscle of wrist, extensor carpi radialis longus (muscle)
8 short radial extensor muscle of wrist, extensor carpi radialis brevis (muscle)
9 long flexor muscle of thumb, flexor pollicis longus (muscle)
10 long abductor muscle of thumb, abductor pollicis longus (muscle)
11 short extensor muscle of thumb, extensor pollicis brevis (muscle)
12 short abductor muscle of thumb, abductor pollicis brevis (muscle)
13 greater pectoral muscle, pectoralis major (muscle)
14 coracobrachial muscle, coracobrachialis (muscle)
15 pronator teres (muscle)
16 radial flexor muscle of wrist, flexor carpi radialis (muscle)
17 long palmar muscle, palmaris longus (muscle)
18 superficial flexor muscle of fingers, flexor digitorum superficialis (muscle)
19 flexor retinaculum of hand
20 short palmar muscle, palmaris brevis (muscle)
21 Dupuytren's fascia, palmar aponeurosis/fascia
22 adductor muscle of thumb, adductor pollicis (muscle)
23 anconeus (muscle)
24 extensor muscle of fingers, extensor digitorum (muscle)
25 ulnar extensor muscle of wrist, extensor carpi ulnaris (muscle)
26 extensor retinaculum of hand
27 dorsal interosseous muscles of hand

Tafel XXVI
oberflächliche Muskeln von Schulter und Arm

1 Deltamuskel, M. deltoideus
2 Trizeps, Triceps brachii, M. triceps brachii
3 Bizeps, Biceps brachii, M. biceps brachii
4 Brachialis, M. brachialis
5 Bizepsaponeurose, Aponeurosis m. bicipitis brachii
6 Brachioradialis, M. brachioradialis
7 Extensor carpi radialis longus, M. extensor carpi radialis longus
8 Extensor carpi radialis brevis, M. extensor carpi radialis brevis
9 langer Daumenbeuger, Flexor pollicis longus, M. flexor pollicis longus
10 Abduktor pollicis longus, M. abductor pollicis longus
11 Extensor pollicis brevis, M. extensor pollicis brevis
12 Abduktor pollicis brevis, M. abductor pollicis brevis
13 großer Brustmuskel, Pektoralis major, M. pectoralis major
14 Korakobrachialis, M. coracobrachialis
15 Pronator teres, M. pronator teres
16 Flexor carpi radialis, M. flexor carpi radialis
17 Palmaris longus, M. palmaris longus
18 oberflächlicher Fingerbeuger, Flexor digitorum superficialis, M. flexor digitorum superficialis
19 Retinaculum flexorum
20 Palmaris brevis, M. palmaris brevis
21 Palmaraponeurose, Aponeurosis palmaris
22 Adduktor pollicis, M. adductor pollicis
23 Anconeus, M. anconeus
24 Fingerstrecker, M. extensor digitorum
25 Extensor carpi ulnaris, M. extensor carpi ulnaris
26 Retinaculum extensorum
27 Mm. interossei dorsales manus

Plate XXVII   Tafel XXVII   A60

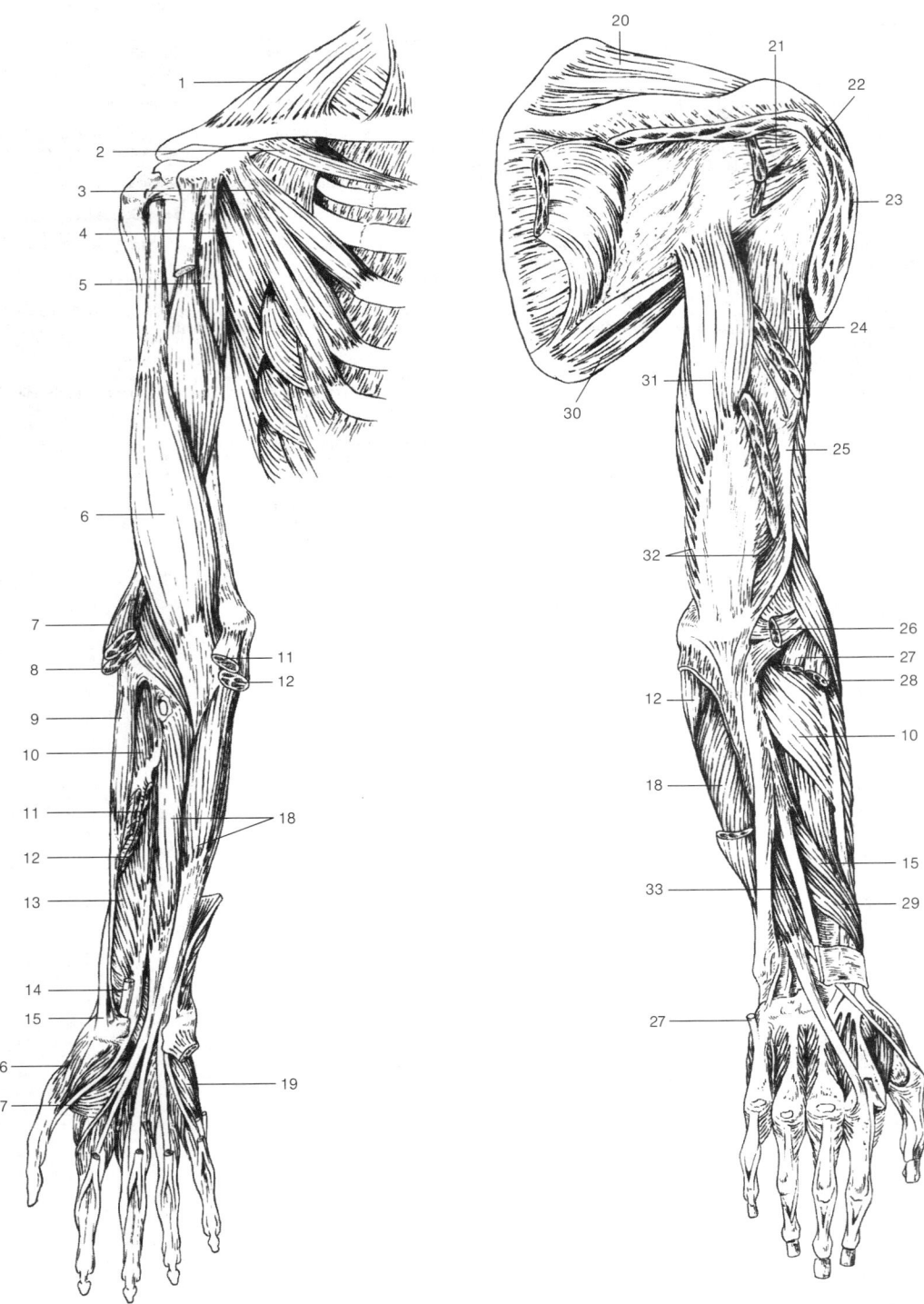

deep muscles of shoulder and arm
tiefe Muskeln von Schulter und Arm

Plate XXVII

deep muscles of shoulder and arm

1 trapezius (muscle)
2 subclavius (muscle)
3 smaller pectoral muscle, pectoralis minor (muscle)
4 subscapular muscle, subscapularis (muscle)
5 coracobrachial muscle, coracobrachialis (muscle)
6 brachial muscle, brachialis (muscle)
7 brachioradial muscle, brachioradialis (muscle)
8 long radial extensor muscle of wrist, extensor carpi radialis longus (muscle)
9 short radial extensor muscle of wrist, extensor carpi radialis brevis (muscle)
10 supinator (muscle)
11 pronator teres (muscle)
12 superficial flexor muscle of fingers, flexor digitorum superficialis (muscle)
13 long flexor muscle of thumb, flexor pollicis longus (muscle)
14 radial flexor muscle of wrist, flexor carpi radialis (muscle)
15 long abductor muscle of thumb, abductor pollicis longus (muscle)
16 opposing muscle of thumb, opponens pollicis (muscle)
17 short flexor muscle of thumb, flexor pollicis brevis (muscle)
18 deep flexor muscle of fingers, flexor digitorum profundus (muscle)
19 opposing muscle of little finger, opponens digiti minimi (muscle)
20 supraspinous muscle, supraspinatus (muscle)
21 infraspinous muscle, infraspinatus (muscle)
22 teres minor (muscle)
23 deltoid muscle, deltoideus (muscle)
24 triceps muscle of arm: lateral head
25 lateral intermuscular septum of arm
26 annular ligament of radius
27 ulnar extensor muscle of wrist, extensor carpi ulnaris (muscle)
28 extensor muscle of fingers, extensor digitorum (muscle)
29 short extensor muscle of thumb, extensor pollicis brevis (muscle)
30 teres major (muscle)
31 triceps muscle of arm: long head
32 triceps muscle of arm: medial head
33 long extensor muscle of thumb/extensor pollicis longus (muscle) and extensor muscle of index/extensor indicis (muscle)

Tafel XXVII

tiefe Muskeln von Schulter und Arm

1 Trapezius, M. trapezius
2 Subklavius, M. subclavius
3 kleiner Brustmuskel, Pektoralis minor, M. pectoralis minor
4 Subskapularis, M. subscapularis
5 Korakobrachialis, M. coracobrachialis
6 Brachialis, M. brachialis
7 Brachioradialis, M. brachioradialis
8 Extensor carpi radialis longus, M. extensor carpi radialis longus
9 Extensor carpi radialis brevis, M. extensor carpi radialis brevis
10 Supinator, M. supinator
11 Pronator teres, M. pronator teres
12 oberflächlicher Fingerbeuger, Flexor digitorum superficialis, M. flexor digitorum superficialis
13 langer Daumenbeuger, Flexor pollicis longus, M. flexor pollicis longus
14 Flexor carpi radialis, M. flexor carpi radialis
15 Abduktor pollicis longus, M. abductor pollicis longus
16 Opponens pollicis, M. opponens pollicis
17 kurzer Daumenbeuger, Flexor pollicis brevis, M. flexor pollicis brevis
18 tiefer Fingerbeuger, Flexor digitorum profundus, M. flexor digitorum profundus
19 Opponens digiti minimi, M. opponens digiti minimi
20 Supraspinatus, M. supraspinatus
21 Infraspinatus, M. infraspinatus
22 Teres minor, M. teres minor
23 Deltamuskel, M. deltoideus
24 M. triceps: Caput laterale
25 Septum intermusculare brachii laterale
26 Lig. anulare radii
27 Extensor carpi ulnaris, M. extensor carpi ulnaris
28 Extensor digitorum, M. extensor digitorum
29 Extensor pollicis brevis, M. extensor pollicis brevis
30 Teres major, M. teres major
31 M. triceps: Caput longum
32 M. triceps: Caput mediale
33 Extensor pollicis longus/M. extensor pollicis longus und Extensor indicis/M. extensor indicis

Plate XXVIII Tafel XXVIII A62

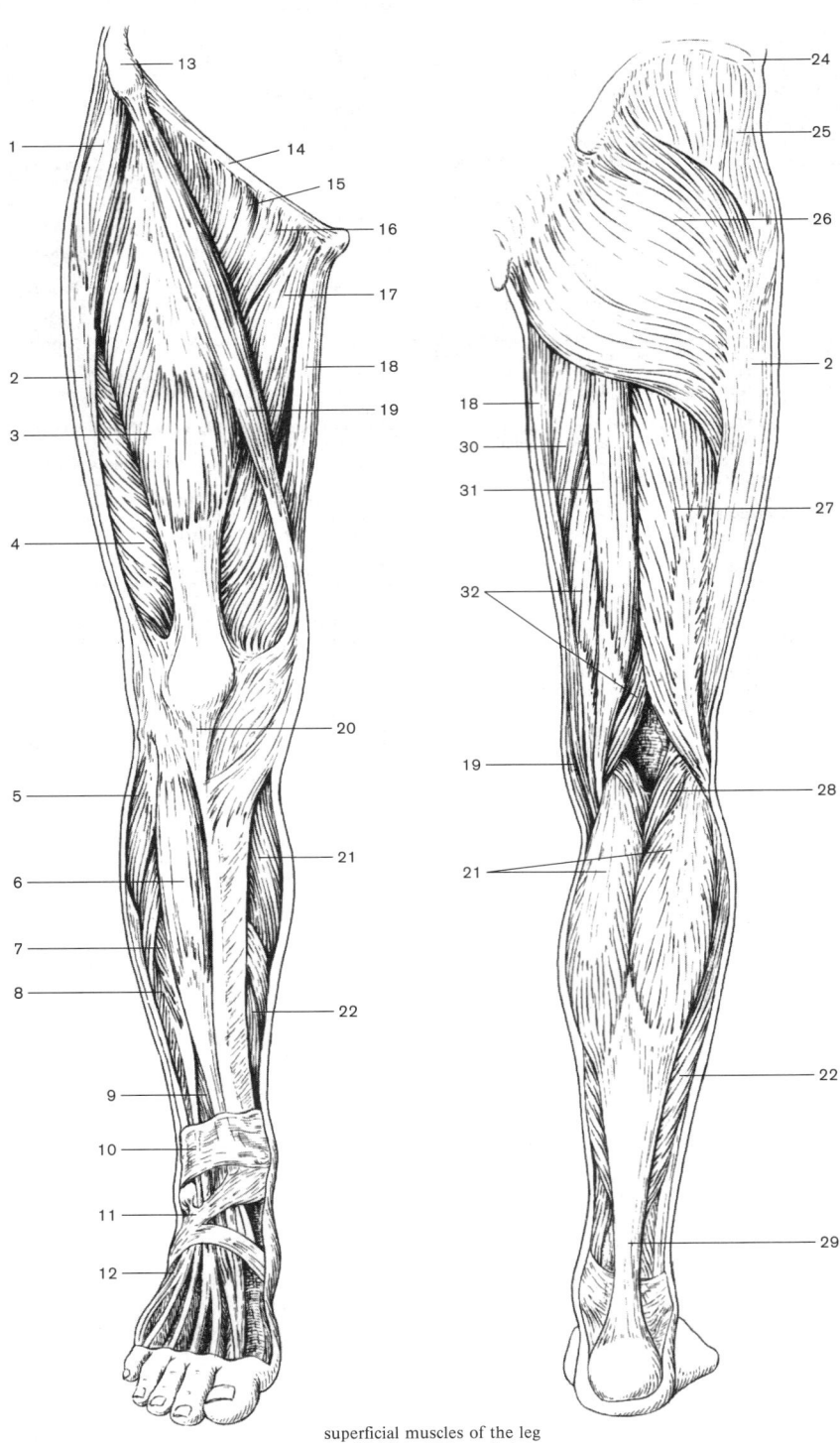

superficial muscles of the leg
oberflächliche Beinmuskulatur

Plate XXVIII

superficial muscles of the leg

1 tensor muscle of fascia lata, tensor fasciae latae (muscle)
2 Maissiat's band, iliotibial band/tract
3 straight muscle of thigh, rectus femoris (muscle)
4 vastus lateralis (muscle)
5 long peroneal muscle, long fibular muscle, peroneus longus (muscle), fibularis longus (muscle)
6 anterior tibial muscle, tibialis anterior (muscle)
7 long extensor muscle of toes, extensor digitorum longus (muscle)
8 short peroneal muscle, short fibular muscle, peroneus brevis (muscle), fibularis brevis (muscle)
9 long extensor muscle of great toe, extensor hallucis longus (muscle)
10 superior extensor retinaculum of foot
11 inferior extensor retinaculum of foot
12 short extensor muscle of toes, extensor digitorum brevis (muscle)
13 anterior superior iliac spine
14 Poupart's ligament, inguinal ligament, crural/femoral/fallopian arch
15 iliopsoas (muscle)
16 pectineal muscle, pectineus (muscle)
17 long adductor muscle, adductor longus (muscle)
18 gracilis (muscle)
19 tailor's muscle, sartorius (muscle)
20 patellar ligament
21 gastrocnemius (muscle)
22 soleus (muscle)
23 dorsal interosseus muscles of foot
24 iliac crest
25 middle gluteal muscle, gluteus medius (muscle)
26 greatest gluteal muscle, gluteus maximus (muscle)
27 biceps muscle of thigh, biceps femoris (muscle)
28 plantar muscle, plantaris (muscle)
29 Achilles tendon, calcanean/heel tendon
30 great adductor muscle, adductor magnus (muscle)
31 semitendinous muscle, semitendinosus (muscle)
32 semimembranous muscle, semimembranosus (muscle)

Tafel XXVIII

oberflächliche Beinmuskulatur

1 Tensor fasciae latae, M. tensor fasciae latae
2 Maissiat'-Band, Tractus iliotibialis
3 Rektus femoris, M. rectus femoris
4 Vastus lateralis, M. vastus lateralis
5 Peronäus/Fibularis longus, M. peron(a)eus/fibularis longus
6 Tibialis anterior, M. tibialis anterior
7 langer Zehenstrecker, Extensor digitorum longus, M. extensor digitorum longus
8 Peronäus/Fibularis brevis, M. peron(a)eus/fibularis brevis
9 Extensor hallucis longus, M. extensor hallucis longus
10 Retinaculum mm. extensorum superius
11 Retinaculum mm. extensorum inferius
12 kurzer Zehenstrecker, Extensor digitorum brevis, M. extensor digitorum brevis
13 Spina iliaca anterior superior
14 Leistenband, Lig. inguinale, Arcus inguinalis
15 Iliopsoas, M. iliopsoas
16 Pectineus, M. pectineus
17 Adduktor longus, M. adductor longus
18 Gracilis, M. gracilis
19 Schneidermuskel, Sartorius, M. sartorius
20 Lig. patellae
21 Gastrocnemius, M. gastrocnemius
22 Soleus, M. soleus
23 Mm. interossei dorsales pedis
24 Beckenkamm, Crista iliaca
25 Glutaeus medius, M. glut(a)eus medius
26 Glutaeus maximus, M. glut(a)eus maximus
27 Biceps femoris, M. biceps femoris
28 Plantaris, M. plantaris
29 Achilles-Sehne, Tendo calcaneus
30 Adduktor magnus, M. adductor magnus
31 Semitendinosus, M. semitendinosus
32 Semimembranosus, M. semimembranosus

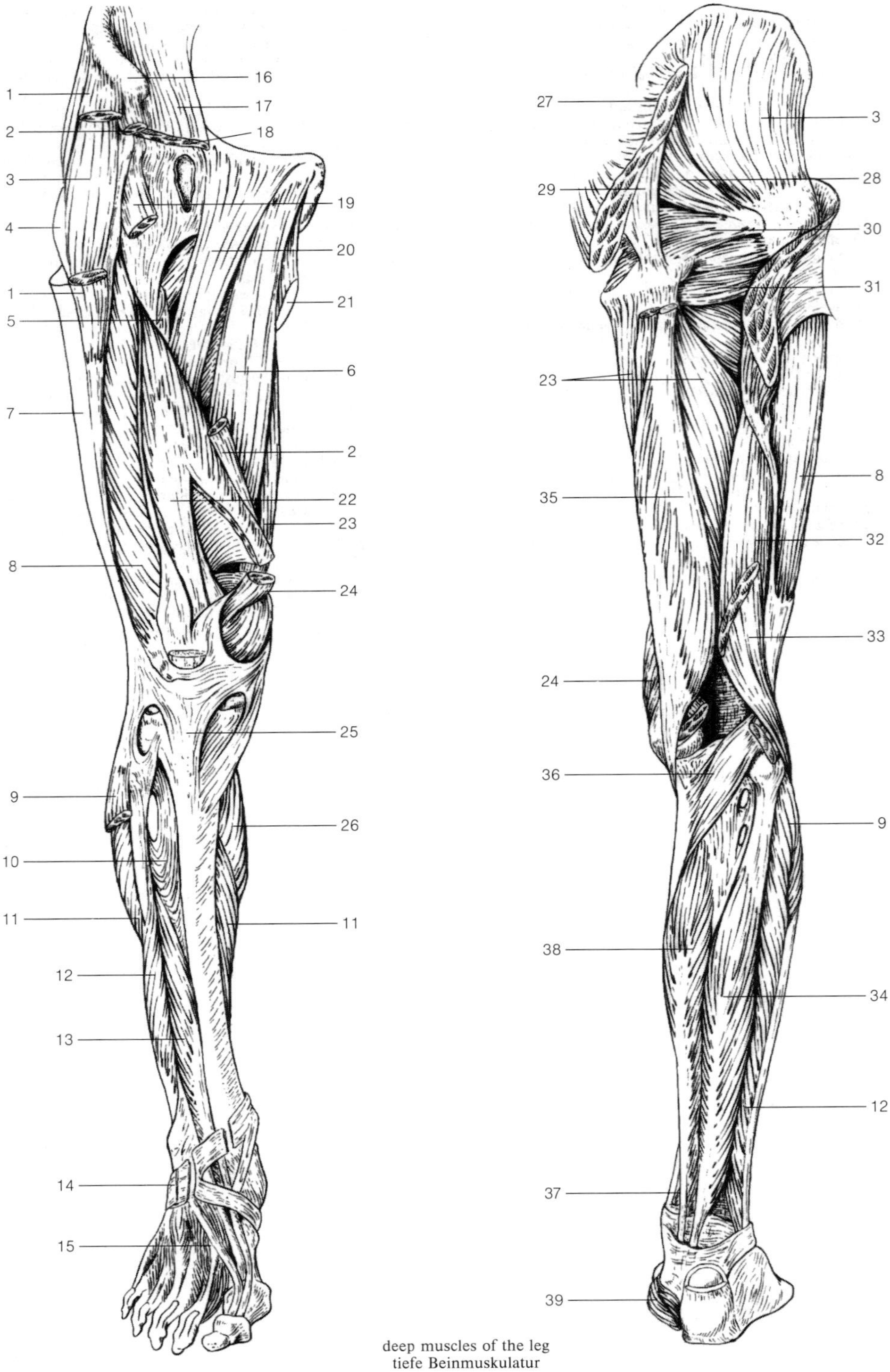

Plate XXIX   Tafel XXIX   A64

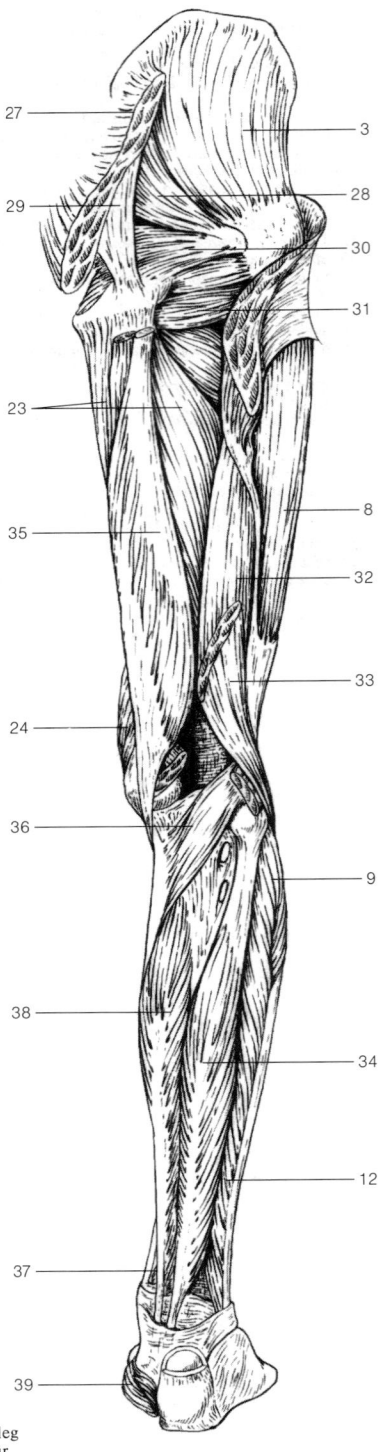

deep muscles of the leg
tiefe Beinmuskulatur

Plate XXIX

deep muscles of the leg

1 tensor fascia lata, tensor fasciae latae (muscle)
2 tailor... ...torius (muscle)
3 ...cle, gluteus medius (muscle)
4 ...(muscle)
... muscle, adductor longus (muscle)
... iliotibial band/tract
...(muscle)
...uscle, long fibular muscle, peroneus longus (muscle),
...(muscle)
...membrana of the leg
...)
...l muscle, short fibular muscle, peroneus brevis (muscle)
...brevis (muscle)
...r muscle of great toe, extensor hallucis longus (muscle)
...ensor retinaculum of the foot
...sor muscle of toes, extensor digitorum brevis (muscle)
...perior iliac spine
...scle, iliacus (muscle)
...er psoas muscle, psoas major (muscle)
...raight muscle of thigh, rectus femoris (muscle)
20 pectineal muscle, pectineus (muscle)
21 gracilis (muscle)
22 vastus intermedius (muscle)
23 great adductor muscle, adductor magnus (muscle)
24 vastus medialis (muscle)
25 patellar ligament
26 gastrocnemius (muscle)
27 greatest gluteal muscle, gluteus maximus (muscle)
28 piriform muscle, piriformis (muscle)
29 sacrotuberous ligament, posterior sacrosciatic ligament
30 internal obturator muscle, obturator internus (muscle)
31 quadrate muscle of thigh, quadratus femoris (muscle)
32 biceps muscle of thigh: short head
33 biceps muscle of thigh: long head
34 long flexor muscle of great toe, flexor hallucis longus (muscle)
35 semimembranous muscle, semimembranosus (muscle)
36 popliteal muscle, popliteus (muscle)
37 posterior tibial muscle, tibialis posterior (muscle)
38 long flexor muscle of toes, flexor digitorum longus (muscle)

39 adductor muscle of great toe, adductor hallucis (muscle)

Tafel XXIX

tiefe Beinmuskulatur

1 Tensor fasciae latae, M. tensor fasciae latae
2 Schneidermuskel, Sartorius, M. sartorius
3 Glutaeus medius, M. glut(a)eus medius
4 Trochanter major
5 Iliopsoas, M. iliopsoas
6 Adduktor longus, M. adductor longus
7 Maissiat'-Band, Tractus iliotibialis
8 Vastus lateralis, M. vastus lateralis
9 Peronäus/Fibularis longus, M. peron(a)eus/fibularis longus
10 Membrana interossea cruris
11 Soleus, M. soleus
12 Peronäus/Fibularis brevis, M. peron(a)eus/fibularis brevis
13 Extensor hallucis longus, M. extensor hallucis longus
14 Retinaculum mm. extensorum inferius
15 kurzer Zehenstrecker, Extensor digitorum brevis, M. extensor digitorum brevis
16 Spina iliaca anterior superior
17 Iliakus, M. iliacus
18 Psoas major, M. psoas major
19 Rektus femoris, M. rectus femoris
20 Pectineus, M. pectineus
21 Gracilis, M. gracilis
22 Vastus intermedius, M. vastus intermedius
23 Adduktor magnus, M. adductor magnus
24 Vastus medialis, M. vastus medialis
25 Lig. patellae
26 Gastrocnemius, M. gastrocnemius
27 Glutaeus maximus, M. glut(a)eus maximus
28 Piriformis, M. piriformis
29 Lig. sacrotuberale
30 Obturator internus, M. obturator internus
31 Quadratus femoris, M. quadratus femoris
32 M. biceps: Caput breve
33 M. biceps: Caput longum
34 Flexor hallucis longus, M. flexor hallucis longus
35 Semimembranosus, M. semimembranosus
36 Popliteus, M. popliteus
37 Tibialis posterior, M. tibialis posterior
38 langer Zehenbeuger, Flexor digitorum longus, M. flexor digitorum longus
39 Adduktor hallucis, M. adductor hallucis